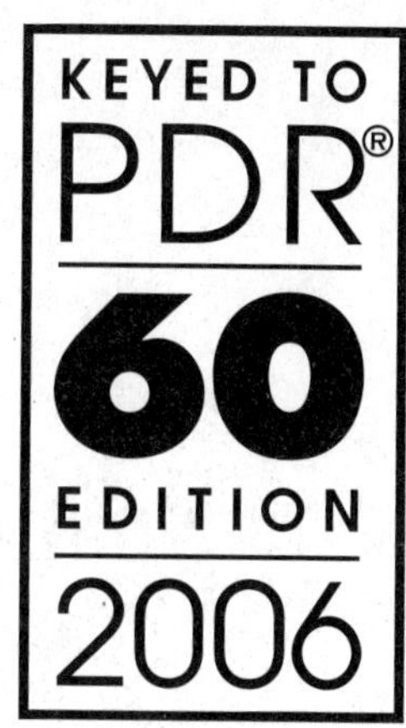

PDR®

Guide to Drug Interactions, Side Effects, and Indications

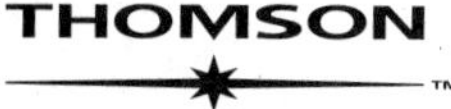

ISBN: 1-56363-529-1

CONTENTS

Section 1
Interactions Index 1

Section 2
Food Interactions Cross-Reference 1405

Section 3
Side Effects Index 1415

Section 4
Indications Index 1693

Section 5
Contraindications Index 1757

Section 6
International Drug Name Index 1773

Section 7
Generic Availability Guide 1913

Section 8
Imprint Identification Guide 1925

Key to Controlled Substances Categories 2137
Gives the definition of each category and the prescribing limitations that apply.

Key to FDA Use-In-Pregnancy Ratings 2137
Provides at-a-glance description of each risk/benefit rating.

U.S. Food and Drug Administration Telephone Directory 2139
Gives numbers of key reporting programs and information services.

Poison Control Centers 2141
A national directory arranged alphabetically by state and city.

Drug Information Centers 2147
A national directory arranged alphabetically by state and city.

MedWatch Adverse Event Report Form 2153
Includes master copy and instructions for completion.

SECTION 1

INTERACTIONS INDEX

Cataloged in this section are all interactions found during a review of the labeling published in *PDR®*, *PDR For Nonprescription Drugs and Dietary Supplements™*, and *PDR For Ophthalmic Medicines™*. The list is arranged alphabetically by brand or, when applicable, generic name.

Whenever appropriate, each brand-name heading is followed by a summary of the major pharmaceutical categories with which the product is said to interact. Beneath this summary is an alphabetical list of the compounds in these categories, each followed by a brief notation regarding the results of concurrent administration with the brand in question. After each notation is an alphabetical list of the brands of the compound found in *PDR®* and its companion volumes. Page numbers refer to the 2006 editions of *PDR®* and *PDR for Ophthalmic Medicines™* and the 2005 edition of *PDR for Nonprescription Drugs and Dietary Supplements™*, which is published later each year. A key to the symbols denoting the companion volumes appears in the bottom margin of every other page.

Following the list of interactive drugs is a similar list of foods. Note that interactions with alcohol are listed here as well.

This index lists only interactions cited in official prescribing information as published by *PDR®*. Because product labeling varies in the scope of its interaction reporting, the most prudent course is to check each product in the patient's regimen. Note also that cross-sensitivity reactions and effects on laboratory results are not included in the listings.

ABELCET INJECTION
(Amphotericin B Lipid Complex) 1119
May interact with aminoglycosides, antineoplastics, corticosteroids, curariform skeletal muscle relaxants, cardiac glycosides, imidazoles, and certain other agents. Compounds in these categories include:

ACTH (Concurrent use may potentiate hypokalemia which could predispose the patient to cardiac dysfunction).
No products indexed under this heading.

Altretamine (Concurrent use may enhance the potential for renal toxicity, bronchospasm and hypotension). Products include:
Hexalen Capsules 2101

Amikacin Sulfate (Concurrent use may enhance the potential for drug-induced renal toxicity).
No products indexed under this heading.

Anastrozole (Concurrent use may enhance the potential for renal toxicity, bronchospasm and hypotension). Products include:
Arimidex Tablets 665

Asparaginase (Concurrent use may enhance the potential for renal toxicity, bronchospasm and hypotension). Products include:
Elspar for Injection 1943

Atracurium Besylate (Amphotericin B-induced hypokalemia may enhance the curariform effect of skeletal relaxants).
No products indexed under this heading.

Betamethasone Acetate (Concurrent use may potentiate hypokalemia which could predispose the patient to cardiac dysfunction).
No products indexed under this heading.

Betamethasone Sodium Phosphate (Concurrent use may potentiate hypokalemia which could predispose the patient to cardiac dysfunction).
No products indexed under this heading.

Bicalutamide (Concurrent use may enhance the potential for renal toxicity, bronchospasm and hypotension). Products include:
Casodex Tablets 670

Bleomycin Sulfate (Concurrent use may enhance the potential for renal toxicity, bronchospasm and hypotension).
No products indexed under this heading.

Busulfan (Concurrent use may enhance the potential for renal toxicity, bronchospasm and hypotension). Products include:
I.V. Busulfex 1125
Myleran Tablets 1492

Carboplatin (Concurrent use may enhance the potential for renal toxicity, bronchospasm and hypotension).
No products indexed under this heading.

Carmustine (BCNU) (Concurrent use may enhance the potential for renal toxicity, bronchospasm and hypotension).
No products indexed under this heading.

Chlorambucil (Concurrent use may enhance the potential for renal toxicity, bronchospasm and hypotension). Products include:
Leukeran Tablets 1472

Cisatracurium Besylate (Amphotericin B-induced hypokalemia may enhance the curariform effect of skeletal relaxants). Products include:
Nimbex Injection 494

Cisplatin (Concurrent use may enhance the potential for renal toxicity, bronchospasm and hypotension).
No products indexed under this heading.

Clotrimazole (Antagonism between amphotericin B and imidazole derivatives, which inhibit ergosterol synthesis, has been reported; clinical significance of this finding has not been determined). Products include:
Lotrimin 3053
Lotrisone 3054

Cortisone Acetate (Concurrent use may potentiate hypokalemia which could predispose the patient to cardiac dysfunction).
No products indexed under this heading.

Cyclophosphamide (Concurrent use may enhance the potential for renal toxicity, bronchospasm and hypotension).
No products indexed under this heading.

Cyclosporine (Concurrent initiation of cyclosporine and Abelcet within several days of bone marrow ablation may be associated with increased nephrotoxicity). Products include:
Gengraf Capsules 458
Neoral Soft Gelatin Capsules 2247
Neoral Oral Solution 2247
Restasis Ophthalmic Emulsion 570
Sandimmune 2259

Dacarbazine (Concurrent use may enhance the potential for renal toxicity, bronchospasm and hypotension).
No products indexed under this heading.

Daunorubicin Citrate (Concurrent use may enhance the potential for renal toxicity, bronchospasm and hypotension).
No products indexed under this heading.

Daunorubicin Hydrochloride (Concurrent use may enhance the potential for renal toxicity, bronchospasm and hypotension). Products include:

Cerubidine for Injection 788

Denileukin Diftitox (Concurrent use may enhance the potential for renal toxicity, bronchospasm and hypotension). Products include:
Ontak Vials 1717

Deslanoside (Concurrent use may induce hypokalemia and may potentiate digitalis toxicity).
No products indexed under this heading.

Dexamethasone (Concurrent use may potentiate hypokalemia which could predispose the patient to cardiac dysfunction). Products include:
Ciprodex Otic Suspension 555
Decadron Tablets 1929
TobraDex Ophthalmic Ointment 558
TobraDex Ophthalmic Suspension ... 558

Dexamethasone Acetate (Concurrent use may potentiate hypokalemia which could predispose the patient to cardiac dysfunction).
No products indexed under this heading.

Dexamethasone Sodium Phosphate (Concurrent use may potentiate hypokalemia which could predispose the patient to cardiac dysfunction). Products include:
Decadron Phosphate Injection 1931

Digitalis Glycoside Preparations (Concurrent use may induce hypokalemia and may potentiate digitalis toxicity).
No products indexed under this heading.

Digitoxin (Concurrent use may induce hypokalemia and may potentiate digitalis toxicity).
No products indexed under this heading.

Digoxin (Concurrent use may induce hypokalemia and may potentiate digitalis toxicity). Products include:
Digitek Tablets 2146
Lanoxicaps Capsules 1458
Lanoxin Injection 1462
Lanoxin Tablets 1468
Lanoxin Injection Pediatric 1465

Docetaxel (Concurrent use may enhance the potential for renal toxicity, bronchospasm and hypotension). Products include:
Taxotere Injection Concentrate 2947

Doxacurium Chloride (Amphotericin B-induced hypokalemia may enhance the curariform effect of skeletal relaxants).
No products indexed under this heading.

Doxorubicin Hydrochloride (Concurrent use may enhance the potential for renal toxicity, bronchospasm and hypotension). Products include:
Adriamycin for Injection, USP 786
Adriamycin Injection, USP 786

Epirubicin Hydrochloride (Concurrent use may enhance the potential for renal toxicity, bronchospasm and hypotension). Products include:
Ellence Injection 2632

Estramustine Phosphate Sodium (Concurrent use may enhance the potential for renal toxicity, bronchospasm and hypotension). Products include:
Emcyt Capsules 3137

Etoposide (Concurrent use may enhance the potential for renal toxicity, bronchospasm and hypotension).
No products indexed under this heading.

Exemestane (Concurrent use may enhance the potential for renal toxicity, bronchospasm and hypotension). Products include:
Aromasin Tablets 2600

Floxuridine (Concurrent use may enhance the potential for renal toxicity, bronchospasm and hypotension).
No products indexed under this heading.

Fluconazole (Antagonism between amphotericin B and imidazole derivatives, which inhibit ergosterol synthesis, has been reported; clinical significance of this finding has not been determined).
No products indexed under this heading.

Flucytosine (Concurrent use may increase the toxicity of flucytosine by possibly increasing its cellular uptake and/or impairing its renal excretion).
No products indexed under this heading.

Fludrocortisone Acetate (Concurrent use may potentiate hypokalemia which could predispose the patient to cardiac dysfunction).
No products indexed under this heading.

Fluorouracil (Concurrent use may enhance the potential for renal toxicity, bronchospasm and hypotension). Products include:
Carac Cream, 0.5% 1048
Efudex 3348

Flutamide (Concurrent use may enhance the potential for renal toxicity, bronchospasm and hypotension). Products include:
Eulexin Capsules 3023

Gemcitabine Hydrochloride (Concurrent use may enhance the potential for renal toxicity, bronchospasm and hypotension). Products include:
Gemzar for Injection 1743

Gentamicin Sulfate (Concurrent use may enhance the potential for drug-induced renal toxicity). Products include:
Garamycin Injectable 3028
Genoptic Sterile Ophthalmic Solution.. ⊙ 227
Pred-G Ophthalmic Suspension ...... ⊙ 234
Pred-G Sterile Ophthalmic Ointment...................................... ⊙ 235

Hydrocortisone (Concurrent use may potentiate hypokalemia which could predispose the patient to cardiac dysfunction). Products include:
Cortizone•5 Ointment .... ▣ 699
Cortizone•10 Creme .... ▣ 699
Cortizone•10 Ointment .... ▣ 699
Cortizone•10 Plus Creme .... ▣ 700
Cortizone•10 Maximum Strength Quick Shot Spray........................ ▣ 700
Hydrocortone Tablets 1963
Preparation H Hydrocortisone Cream .... ▣ 748

Hydrocortisone Acetate (Concurrent use may potentiate hypokalemia which could predispose the patient to cardiac dysfunction). Products include:
Analpram-HC 1136
Pramosone 1139
ProctoFoam-HC 3113
Tucks Anti-Itch Ointment .... ▣ 712
U-cort 1% Cream 3289

Hydrocortisone Sodium Phosphate (Concurrent use may potentiate hypokalemia which could predispose the patient to cardiac dysfunction).
No products indexed under this heading.

Hydrocortisone Sodium Succinate (Concurrent use may potentiate hypokalemia which could predispose the patient to cardiac dysfunction).
No products indexed under this heading.

Hydroxyurea (Concurrent use may enhance the potential for renal toxicity, bronchospasm and hypotension).
No products indexed under this heading.

Idarubicin Hydrochloride (Concurrent use may enhance the potential for renal toxicity, bronchospasm and hypotension). Products include:
Idamycin PFS Injection 2645

Ifosfamide (Concurrent use may enhance the potential for renal toxicity, bronchospasm and hypotension).
No products indexed under this heading.

Interferon alfa-2a, Recombinant (Concurrent use may enhance the potential for renal toxicity, bronchospasm and hypotension). Products include:
Roferon-A Injection 2805

Interferon alfa-2b, Recombinant (Concurrent use may enhance the potential for renal toxicity, bronchospasm and hypotension). Products include:
Intron A for Injection 3038
Rebetron Combination Therapy 3078

Irinotecan Hydrochloride (Concurrent use may enhance the potential for renal toxicity, bronchospasm and hypotension). Products include:
Camptosar Injection 2602

Kanamycin Sulfate (Concurrent use may enhance the potential for drug-induced renal toxicity).
No products indexed under this heading.

Ketoconazole (Antagonism between amphotericin B and imidazole derivatives, which inhibit ergosterol synthesis, has been reported; clinical significance of this finding has not been determined). Products include:
Nizoral A-D Shampoo, 1% 1839
Nizoral 2% Shampoo 1838

Leukocyte Transfusions (Concurrent use has resulted in acute pulmonary toxicity; concurrent use should be avoided).
No products indexed under this heading.

Levamisole Hydrochloride (Concurrent use may enhance the potential for renal toxicity, bronchospasm and hypotension).
No products indexed under this heading.

Lomustine (CCNU) (Concurrent use may enhance the potential for renal toxicity, bronchospasm and hypotension).
No products indexed under this heading.

Mechlorethamine Hydrochloride (Concurrent use may enhance the potential for renal toxicity, bronchospasm and hypotension). Products include:
Mustargen for Injection 2007

Megestrol Acetate (Concurrent use may enhance the potential for renal toxicity, bronchospasm and hypotension). Products include:
Megace ES Oral Suspension 2492

Melphalan (Concurrent use may enhance the potential for renal toxicity, bronchospasm and hypotension). Products include:
Alkeran Tablets 977

Mercaptopurine (Concurrent use may enhance the potential for renal toxicity, bronchospasm and hypotension). Products include:
Purinethol Tablets 1222

Methotrexate Sodium (Concurrent use may enhance the potential for renal toxicity, bronchospasm and hypotension).
No products indexed under this heading.

Methylprednisolone Acetate (Concurrent use may potentiate hypokalemia which could predispose the patient to cardiac dysfunction). Products include:
Depo-Medrol Injectable Suspension 2615
Depo-Medrol Single-Dose Vial 2617

Methylprednisolone Sodium Succinate (Concurrent use may potentiate hypokalemia which could predispose the patient to cardiac dysfunction).
No products indexed under this heading.

Metocurine Iodide (Amphotericin B-induced hypokalemia may enhance the curariform effect of skeletal relaxants).
No products indexed under this heading.

Miconazole (Antagonism between amphotericin B and imidazole derivatives, which inhibit ergosterol synthesis, has been reported; clinical significance of this finding has not been determined).
No products indexed under this heading.

Miconazole Nitrate (Antagonism between amphotericin B and imidazole derivatives, which inhibit ergosterol synthesis, has been reported; clinical significance of this finding has not been determined). Products include:
Desenex .... ▣ 674
Desenex Jock Itch Spray Powder ... ▣ 674

Mitomycin (Mitomycin-C) (Concurrent use may enhance the potential for renal toxicity, bronchospasm and hypotension).
No products indexed under this heading.

Mitotane (Concurrent use may enhance the potential for renal toxicity, bronchospasm and hypotension).
No products indexed under this heading.

Mitoxantrone Hydrochloride (Concurrent use may enhance the potential for renal toxicity, bronchospasm and hypotension). Products include:
Novantrone for Injection Concentrate 3158

Mivacurium Chloride (Amphotericin B-induced hypokalemia may enhance the curariform effect of skeletal relaxants). Products include:
Mivacron Injection 489

Oxaliplatin (Concurrent use may enhance the potential for renal toxicity, bronchospasm and hypotension). Products include:
Eloxatin for Injection 2908

Paclitaxel (Concurrent use may enhance the potential for renal toxicity, bronchospasm and hypotension).
No products indexed under this heading.

Pancuronium Bromide (Amphotericin B-induced hypokalemia may enhance the curariform effect of skeletal relaxants).
No products indexed under this heading.

Pentamidine Isethionate (Concurrent use may enhance the potential for drug-induced renal toxicity).
No products indexed under this heading.

Pipecuronium Bromide (Amphotericin B-induced hypokalemia may enhance the curariform effect of skeletal relaxants).
No products indexed under this heading.

Prednisolone Acetate (Concurrent use may potentiate hypokalemia which could predispose the patient to cardiac dysfunction). Products include:
- Blephamide Ophthalmic Ointment 563
- Blephamide Ophthalmic Suspension 564
- Poly-Pred Liquifilm Ophthalmic Suspension .... ⊙231
- Pred Forte Ophthalmic Suspension .... ⊙233
- Pred Mild Sterile Ophthalmic Suspension .... ⊙236
- Pred-G Ophthalmic Suspension .... ⊙234
- Pred-G Sterile Ophthalmic Ointment .... ⊙235

Prednisolone Sodium Phosphate (Concurrent use may potentiate hypokalemia which could predispose the patient to cardiac dysfunction). Products include:
- Pediapred Oral Solution 3319

Prednisolone Tebutate (Concurrent use may potentiate hypokalemia which could predispose the patient to cardiac dysfunction).
No products indexed under this heading.

Prednisone (Concurrent use may potentiate hypokalemia which could predispose the patient to cardiac dysfunction).
No products indexed under this heading.

Procarbazine Hydrochloride (Concurrent use may enhance the potential for renal toxicity, bronchospasm and hypotension). Products include:
- Matulane Capsules 3188

Rapacuronium Bromide (Amphotericin B-induced hypokalemia may enhance the curariform effect of skeletal relaxants).
No products indexed under this heading.

Rocuronium Bromide (Amphotericin B-induced hypokalemia may enhance the curariform effect of skeletal relaxants). Products include:
- Zemuron Injection 2363

Streptomycin Sulfate (Concurrent use may enhance the potential for drug-induced renal toxicity).
No products indexed under this heading.

Streptozocin (Concurrent use may enhance the potential for renal toxicity, bronchospasm and hypotension).
No products indexed under this heading.

Tamoxifen Citrate (Concurrent use may enhance the potential for renal toxicity, bronchospasm and hypotension).
No products indexed under this heading.

Teniposide (Concurrent use may enhance the potential for renal toxicity, bronchospasm and hypotension).
No products indexed under this heading.

Thioguanine (Concurrent use may enhance the potential for renal toxicity, bronchospasm and hypotension). Products include:
- Tabloid Tablets 1545

Thiotepa (Concurrent use may enhance the potential for renal toxicity, bronchospasm and hypotension).
No products indexed under this heading.

Tobramycin (Concurrent use may enhance the potential for drug-induced renal toxicity). Products include:
- TOBI Solution for Inhalation 1015
- TobraDex Ophthalmic Ointment 558
- TobraDex Ophthalmic Suspension 558
- Zylet Ophthalmic Suspension 3508

Tobramycin Sulfate (Concurrent use may enhance the potential for drug-induced renal toxicity).
No products indexed under this heading.

Topotecan Hydrochloride (Concurrent use may enhance the potential for renal toxicity, bronchospasm and hypotension). Products include:
- Hycamtin for Injection 1427

Toremifene Citrate (Concurrent use may enhance the potential for renal toxicity, bronchospasm and hypotension).
No products indexed under this heading.

Triamcinolone (Concurrent use may potentiate hypokalemia which could predispose the patient to cardiac dysfunction).
No products indexed under this heading.

Triamcinolone Acetonide (Concurrent use may potentiate hypokalemia which could predispose the patient to cardiac dysfunction). Products include:
- Azmacort Inhalation Aerosol 1701
- Nasacort HFA Inhalation Aerosol 2939
- Nasacort AQ Nasal Spray 2937

Triamcinolone Diacetate (Concurrent use may potentiate hypokalemia which could predispose the patient to cardiac dysfunction).
No products indexed under this heading.

Triamcinolone Hexacetonide (Concurrent use may potentiate hypokalemia which could predispose the patient to cardiac dysfunction).
No products indexed under this heading.

Tubocurarine Chloride (Amphotericin B-induced hypokalemia may enhance the curariform effect of skeletal muscle relaxants).
No products indexed under this heading.

Valrubicin (Concurrent use may enhance the potential for renal toxicity, bronchospasm and hypotension).
No products indexed under this heading.

Vecuronium Bromide (Amphotericin B-induced hypokalemia may enhance the curariform effect of skeletal relaxants).
No products indexed under this heading.

Vincristine Sulfate (Concurrent use may enhance the potential for renal toxicity, bronchospasm and hypotension).
No products indexed under this heading.

Vinorelbine Tartrate (Concurrent use may enhance the potential for renal toxicity, bronchospasm and hypotension). Products include:
- Navelbine Injection 1494

Zidovudine (Potential for increased myelotoxicity and nephrotoxicity). Products include:
- Combivir Tablets 1373
- Retrovir 1533
- Retrovir IV Infusion 1537
- Trizivir Tablets 1565

ABILIFY TABLETS

(Aripiprazole) 916

May interact with cytochrome p450 2d6 inhibitors (selected), cytochrome p450 3a4 inducers (selected), cytochrome p450 3a4 inhibitors (selected), and certain other agents. Compounds in these categories include:

Acetazolamide (Inhibitors of CYP3A4 or CYP2D6 can inhibit aripiprazole elimination and cause increased blood levels).
No products indexed under this heading.

Allium sativum (Agents that induce CYP3A4 could cause an increase in aripiprazole clearance and lower blood levels).
No products indexed under this heading.

Amiodarone Hydrochloride (Inhibitors of CYP3A4 or CYP2D6 can inhibit aripiprazole elimination and cause increased blood levels). Products include:
- Pacerone Tablets 3337

Amitriptyline Hydrochloride (Inhibitors of CYP3A4 or CYP2D6 can inhibit aripiprazole elimination and cause increased blood levels).
No products indexed under this heading.

Amoxapine (Inhibitors of CYP3A4 or CYP2D6 can inhibit aripiprazole elimination and cause increased blood levels).
No products indexed under this heading.

Amprenavir (Inhibitors of CYP3A4 or CYP2D6 can inhibit aripiprazole elimination and cause increased blood levels). Products include:
- Agenerase Capsules 1299
- Agenerase Oral Solution 1304

Anastrozole (Inhibitors of CYP3A4 or CYP2D6 can inhibit aripiprazole elimination and cause increased blood levels). Products include:
- Arimidex Tablets 665

Aprepitant (Inhibitors of CYP3A4 or CYP2D6 can inhibit aripiprazole elimination and cause increased blood levels). Products include:
- Emend Capsules 1944

Betamethasone Acetate (Agents that induce CYP3A4 could cause an increase in aripiprazole clearance and lower blood levels).
No products indexed under this heading.

Betamethasone Sodium Phosphate (Agents that induce CYP3A4 could cause an increase in aripiprazole clearance and lower blood levels).
No products indexed under this heading.

Bupropion Hydrochloride (Inhibitors of CYP3A4 or CYP2D6 can inhibit aripiprazole elimination and cause increased blood levels). Products include:
- Wellbutrin Tablets 1579
- Wellbutrin SR Sustained-Release Tablets 1583
- Wellbutrin XL Extended-Release Tablets 1588
- Zyban Sustained-Release Tablets 1620

Carbamazepine (Agents that induce CYP3A4 could cause an increase in aripiprazole clearance and lower blood levels). Products include:
- Carbatrol Capsules 3174
- Equetro Extended-Release Capsules 3178
- Tegretol/Tegretol-XR 2278

Celecoxib (Inhibitors of CYP3A4 or CYP2D6 can inhibit aripiprazole elimination and cause increased blood levels). Products include:
- Celebrex Capsules 3130

Chloroquine Hydrochloride (Inhibitors of CYP3A4 or CYP2D6 can inhibit aripiprazole elimination and cause increased blood levels).
No products indexed under this heading.

Chloroquine Phosphate (Inhibitors of CYP3A4 or CYP2D6 can inhibit aripiprazole elimination and cause increased blood levels).
No products indexed under this heading.

Chlorpheniramine (Inhibitors of CYP3A4 or CYP2D6 can inhibit aripiprazole elimination and cause increased blood levels).
No products indexed under this heading.

Chlorpheniramine Maleate (Inhibitors of CYP3A4 or CYP2D6 can inhibit aripiprazole elimination and cause increased blood levels). Products include:
- Advil Allergy Sinus Caplets 737
- Advil Multi-Symptom Cold Caplets 738
- BC Allergy Sinus Cold Powder 612
- Contac Severe Cold and Flu Caplets Maximum Strength 615
- Hycomine Compound Tablets 1105
- PediaCare Multi-Symptom Cold Liquid 704
- PediaCare NightRest Cough & Cold Liquid 704
- Robitussin Flu Liquid 752
- Robitussin PM Cough & Cold Liquid 752
- Singlet Caplets 636
- Sudafed Sinus & Allergy Tablets 710
- TheraFlu Cold & Cough Hot Liquid 680
- TheraFlu Cold & Sore Throat Hot Liquid 680
- TheraFlu Flu & Sore Throat Hot Liquid 681
- TheraFlu Severe Cold & Cough Hot Liquid 683
- TheraFlu Severe Cold Caplets 679
- TheraFlu Severe Cold Hot Liquid 682
- Triaminic Cold & Allergy Liquid 685
- Triaminic Cold & Cough Liquid 685
- Triaminic Flu, Cough & Fever Liquid 685
- Triaminic Night Time Cough & Cold Liquid 685
- Triaminic Allergy Runny Nose & Congestion Softchews 688
- Triaminic Cold & Cough Softchews 688
- Children's Tylenol Plus Cold NightTime Suspension Liquid 1851
- Children's Tylenol Plus Cold & Cough Suspension Liquid and Chewable Tablets 1851
- Children's Tylenol Plus Cold Chewable Tablets 1851

Children's Tylenol Plus Flu Suspension Liquid **1853**
Tylenol Allergy Complete Multi-Symptom Caplets and Gelcaps with Cool Burst **1844**
Multi-Symptom Tylenol Cold Night Time Caplets **1845**
Vicks 44M Cough, Cold & Flu Relief **2676**
Pediatric Vicks 44m Cough & Cold Relief **2673**
Children's Vicks NyQuil Cold/Cough Relief **2671**

Chlorpheniramine Polistirex (Inhibitors of CYP3A4 or CYP2D6 can inhibit aripiprazole elimination and cause increased blood levels). Products include:
Tussionex Pennkinetic Extended-Release Suspension **3322**

Chlorpheniramine Tannate (Inhibitors of CYP3A4 or CYP2D6 can inhibit aripiprazole elimination and cause increased blood levels).
No products indexed under this heading.

Cimetidine (Inhibitors of CYP3A4 or CYP2D6 can inhibit aripiprazole elimination and cause increased blood levels). Products include:
Tagamet HB 200 Tablets .... ▣**637**
Tagamet Tablets **1547**

Cimetidine Hydrochloride (Inhibitors of CYP3A4 or CYP2D6 can inhibit aripiprazole elimination and cause increased blood levels).
No products indexed under this heading.

Ciprofloxacin (Inhibitors of CYP3A4 or CYP2D6 can inhibit aripiprazole elimination and cause increased blood levels). Products include:
Cipro I.V. **2998**
Cipro I.V. Pharmacy Bulk Package **3509**
Cipro Oral Suspension **2991**
Cipro XR Tablets **3004**
Ciprodex Otic Suspension **555**

Ciprofloxacin Hydrochloride (Agents that induce CYP3A4 could cause an increase in aripiprazole clearance and lower blood levels). Products include:
Ciloxan Ophthalmic Ointment **554**
Cipro Tablets **2991**

Cisplatin (Agents that induce CYP3A4 could cause an increase in aripiprazole clearance and lower blood levels).
No products indexed under this heading.

Citalopram Hydrobromide (Inhibitors of CYP3A4 or CYP2D6 can inhibit aripiprazole elimination and cause increased blood levels). Products include:
Celexa **1177**

Clarithromycin (Inhibitors of CYP3A4 or CYP2D6 can inhibit aripiprazole elimination and cause increased blood levels). Products include:
Biaxin/Biaxin XL **402**
PREVPAC **3281**

Clomipramine Hydrochloride (Inhibitors of CYP3A4 or CYP2D6 can inhibit aripiprazole elimination and cause increased blood levels).
No products indexed under this heading.

Clotrimazole (Inhibitors of CYP3A4 or CYP2D6 can inhibit aripiprazole elimination and cause increased blood levels). Products include:
Lotrimin **3053**
Lotrisone **3054**

Cocaine Hydrochloride (Inhibitors of CYP3A4 or CYP2D6 can inhibit aripiprazole elimination and cause increased blood levels).
No products indexed under this heading.

Cortisone Acetate (Agents that induce CYP3A4 could cause an increase in aripiprazole clearance and lower blood levels).
No products indexed under this heading.

Cyclosporine (Inhibitors of CYP3A4 or CYP2D6 can inhibit aripiprazole elimination and cause increased blood levels). Products include:
Gengraf Capsules **458**
Neoral Soft Gelatin Capsules **2247**
Neoral Oral Solution **2247**
Restasis Ophthalmic Emulsion **570**
Sandimmune **2259**

Dalfopristin (Inhibitors of CYP3A4 or CYP2D6 can inhibit aripiprazole elimination and cause increased blood levels). Products include:
Synercid I.V. **1690**

Danazol (Inhibitors of CYP3A4 or CYP2D6 can inhibit aripiprazole elimination and cause increased blood levels).
No products indexed under this heading.

Delavirdine Mesylate (Inhibitors of CYP3A4 or CYP2D6 can inhibit aripiprazole elimination and cause increased blood levels). Products include:
Rescriptor Tablets **2535**

Desipramine Hydrochloride (Inhibitors of CYP3A4 or CYP2D6 can inhibit aripiprazole elimination and cause increased blood levels).
No products indexed under this heading.

Dexamethasone (Agents that induce CYP3A4 could cause an increase in aripiprazole clearance and lower blood levels). Products include:
Ciprodex Otic Suspension **555**
Decadron Tablets **1929**
TobraDex Ophthalmic Ointment **558**
TobraDex Ophthalmic Suspension **558**

Dexamethasone Acetate (Agents that induce CYP3A4 could cause an increase in aripiprazole clearance and lower blood levels).
No products indexed under this heading.

Dexamethasone Sodium Phosphate (Agents that induce CYP3A4 could cause an increase in aripiprazole clearance and lower blood levels). Products include:
Decadron Phosphate Injection **1931**

Diltiazem Hydrochloride (Inhibitors of CYP3A4 or CYP2D6 can inhibit aripiprazole elimination and cause increased blood levels). Products include:
Cardizem LA Extended Release Tablets **1699**
Tiazac Capsules **1204**

Diltiazem Maleate (Inhibitors of CYP3A4 or CYP2D6 can inhibit aripiprazole elimination and cause increased blood levels).
No products indexed under this heading.

Diphenhydramine (Inhibitors of CYP3A4 or CYP2D6 can inhibit aripiprazole elimination and cause increased blood levels). Products include:
Tylenol Sore Throat NightTime Liquid with Cool Burst **1849**

Diphenhydramine Hydrochloride (Inhibitors of CYP3A4 or CYP2D6 can inhibit aripiprazole elimination and cause increased blood levels). Products include:
Benadryl Allergy & Cold Tablets .... ▣**692**
Benadryl Allergy .... ▣**691**
Benadryl Allergy & Sinus Headache Caplets & Gelcaps .... ▣**693**
Children's Benadryl Allergy Liquid .... ▣**695**
Children's Benadryl Dye-Free Allergy Liquid .... ▣**695**
Benadryl Dye-Free Allergy Liqui-Gels Softgels .... ▣**692**
Benadryl Itch Relief Stick Extra Strength .... ▣**696**
Benadryl Itch Stopping Cream Extra Strength .... ▣**697**
Benadryl Itch Stopping Gel Extra Strength .... ▣**697**
Benadryl Itch Stopping Spray Extra Strength .... ▣**697**
Benadryl Maximum Strength Severe Allergy & Sinus Headache Caplets .... ▣**694**
Children's Benadryl D Liquid Medication .... ▣**693**
Benadryl D Tablets .... ▣**694**
Nytol QuickCaps Caplets .... ▣**635**
Maximum Strength Nytol QuickGels Softgels .... ▣**635**
Simply Sleep Caplets **1841**
Sominex Original Formula Tablets .... ▣**637**
TheraFlu Thin Strips Multi Symptom .... ▣**684**
Triaminic Thin Strips Cough & Runny Nose .... ▣**690**
Children's Tylenol Plus Cold & Allergy Suspension Liquid **1850**
Tylenol Allergy Complete Night Time Caplets **1844**
Tylenol Severe Allergy Caplets **1844**
Tylenol Flu NightTime Gelcaps **1846**
Extra Strength Tylenol PM Caplets, Geltabs, Gelcaps and Liquid **1847**
Unisom Maximum Strength SleepGels .... ▣**712**

Doxepin Hydrochloride (Inhibitors of CYP3A4 or CYP2D6 can inhibit aripiprazole elimination and cause increased blood levels).
No products indexed under this heading.

Doxorubicin Hydrochloride (Agents that induce CYP3A4 could cause an increase in aripiprazole clearance and lower blood levels). Products include:
Adriamycin for Injection, USP **786**
Adriamycin Injection, USP **786**

Efavirenz (Inhibitors of CYP3A4 or CYP2D6 can inhibit aripiprazole elimination and cause increased blood levels). Products include:
Sustiva Capsules **957**

Erythromycin (Inhibitors of CYP3A4 or CYP2D6 can inhibit aripiprazole elimination and cause increased blood levels). Products include:
Erygel Topical Gel **2096**
Ery-Tab Tablets **447**
Erythromycin Base Filmtab Tablets **454**
Erythromycin Delayed-Release Capsules, USP **456**
PCE Dispertab Tablets **510**

Erythromycin Estolate (Inhibitors of CYP3A4 or CYP2D6 can inhibit aripiprazole elimination and cause increased blood levels).
No products indexed under this heading.

Erythromycin Ethylsuccinate (Inhibitors of CYP3A4 or CYP2D6 can inhibit aripiprazole elimination and cause increased blood levels). Products include:
E.E.S. **449**
EryPed **445**

Erythromycin Gluceptate (Inhibitors of CYP3A4 or CYP2D6 can inhibit aripiprazole elimination and cause increased blood levels).
No products indexed under this heading.

Erythromycin Lactobionate (Inhibitors of CYP3A4 or CYP2D6 can inhibit aripiprazole elimination and cause increased blood levels).
No products indexed under this heading.

Erythromycin Stearate (Inhibitors of CYP3A4 or CYP2D6 can inhibit aripiprazole elimination and cause increased blood levels). Products include:
Erythrocin Stearate Filmtab Tablets **452**

Escitalopram Oxalate (Inhibitors of CYP3A4 or CYP2D6 can inhibit aripiprazole elimination and cause increased blood levels). Products include:
Lexapro Oral Solution **1193**
Lexapro Tablets **1193**

Esomeprazole Magnesium (Inhibitors of CYP3A4 or CYP2D6 can inhibit aripiprazole elimination and cause increased blood levels). Products include:
Nexium Delayed-Release Capsules **645**

Ethosuximide (Agents that induce CYP3A4 could cause an increase in aripiprazole clearance and lower blood levels).
No products indexed under this heading.

Felbamate (Agents that induce CYP3A4 could cause an increase in aripiprazole clearance and lower blood levels).
No products indexed under this heading.

Fluconazole (Inhibitors of CYP3A4 or CYP2D6 can inhibit aripiprazole elimination and cause increased blood levels).
No products indexed under this heading.

Fludrocortisone Acetate (Agents that induce CYP3A4 could cause an increase in aripiprazole clearance and lower blood levels).
No products indexed under this heading.

Fluoxetine (Inhibitors of CYP3A4 or CYP2D6 can inhibit aripiprazole elimination and cause increased blood levels).
No products indexed under this heading.

Fluoxetine Hydrochloride (Inhibitors of CYP3A4 or CYP2D6 can inhibit aripiprazole elimination and cause increased blood levels). Products include:
Prozac Pulvules and Liquid **1771**
Symbyax Capsules **1788**

Fluphenazine Decanoate (Inhibitors of CYP3A4 or CYP2D6 can inhibit aripiprazole elimination and cause increased blood levels).
No products indexed under this heading.

Fluphenazine Enanthate (Inhibitors of CYP3A4 or CYP2D6 can inhibit aripiprazole elimination and cause increased blood levels).
No products indexed under this heading.

Fluphenazine Hydrochloride (Inhibitors of CYP3A4 or CYP2D6 can inhibit aripiprazole elimination and cause increased blood levels).
No products indexed under this heading.

Fluvoxamine Maleate (Inhibitors of CYP3A4 or CYP2D6 can inhibit aripiprazole elimination and cause increased blood levels).
No products indexed under this heading.

Fosamprenavir Calcium (Inhibitors of CYP3A4 or CYP2D6 can inhibit aripiprazole elimination and cause increased blood levels). Products include:
Lexiva Tablets 1473

Fosphenytoin Sodium (Agents that induce CYP3A4 could cause an increase in aripiprazole clearance and lower blood levels).
No products indexed under this heading.

Garlic Extract (Agents that induce CYP3A4 could cause an increase in aripiprazole clearance and lower blood levels).
No products indexed under this heading.

Garlic Oil (Agents that induce CYP3A4 could cause an increase in aripiprazole clearance and lower blood levels).
No products indexed under this heading.

Halofantrine Hydrochloride (Inhibitors of CYP3A4 or CYP2D6 can inhibit aripiprazole elimination and cause increased blood levels).
No products indexed under this heading.

Haloperidol (Inhibitors of CYP3A4 or CYP2D6 can inhibit aripiprazole elimination and cause increased blood levels).
No products indexed under this heading.

Haloperidol Decanoate (Inhibitors of CYP3A4 or CYP2D6 can inhibit aripiprazole elimination and cause increased blood levels).
No products indexed under this heading.

Hydrocortisone (Agents that induce CYP3A4 could cause an increase in aripiprazole clearance and lower blood levels). Products include:
Cortizone•5 Ointment 699
Cortizone•10 Creme 699
Cortizone•10 Ointment 699
Cortizone•10 Plus Creme 700
Cortizone•10 Maximum Strength Quick Shot Spray 700
Hydrocortone Tablets 1963
Preparation H Hydrocortisone Cream 748

Hydrocortisone Acetate (Agents that induce CYP3A4 could cause an increase in aripiprazole clearance and lower blood levels). Products include:
Analpram-HC 1136
Pramosone 1139
ProctoFoam-HC 3113
Tucks Anti-Itch Ointment 712
U-cort 1% Cream 3289

Hydrocortisone Butyrate (Agents that induce CYP3A4 could cause an increase in aripiprazole clearance and lower blood levels). Products include:
Locoid 1138
Locoid Lipocream Cream 1138

Hydrocortisone Cypionate (Agents that induce CYP3A4 could cause an increase in aripiprazole clearance and lower blood levels).
No products indexed under this heading.

Hydrocortisone Hemisuccinate (Agents that induce CYP3A4 could cause an increase in aripiprazole clearance and lower blood levels).
No products indexed under this heading.

Hydrocortisone Probutate (Agents that induce CYP3A4 could cause an increase in aripiprazole clearance and lower blood levels). Products include:
Pandel Cream, 0.1% 1017

Hydrocortisone Sodium Phosphate (Agents that induce CYP3A4 could cause an increase in aripiprazole clearance and lower blood levels).
No products indexed under this heading.

Hydrocortisone Sodium Succinate (Agents that induce CYP3A4 could cause an increase in aripiprazole clearance and lower blood levels).
No products indexed under this heading.

Hydrocortisone Valerate (Agents that induce CYP3A4 could cause an increase in aripiprazole clearance and lower blood levels).
No products indexed under this heading.

Hydroxychloroquine Sulfate (Inhibitors of CYP3A4 or CYP2D6 can inhibit aripiprazole elimination and cause increased blood levels).
No products indexed under this heading.

Hypericum (Agents that induce CYP3A4 could cause an increase in aripiprazole clearance and lower blood levels).
No products indexed under this heading.

Hypericum Perforatum (Agents that induce CYP3A4 could cause an increase in aripiprazole clearance and lower blood levels).
No products indexed under this heading.

Imatinib Mesylate (Inhibitors of CYP3A4 or CYP2D6 can inhibit aripiprazole elimination and cause increased blood levels). Products include:
Gleevec Tablets 2221

Imipramine Hydrochloride (Inhibitors of CYP3A4 or CYP2D6 can inhibit aripiprazole elimination and cause increased blood levels).
No products indexed under this heading.

Imipramine Pamoate (Inhibitors of CYP3A4 or CYP2D6 can inhibit aripiprazole elimination and cause increased blood levels).
No products indexed under this heading.

Indinavir Sulfate (Inhibitors of CYP3A4 or CYP2D6 can inhibit aripiprazole elimination and cause increased blood levels). Products include:
Crixivan Capsules 1918

Isoniazid (Inhibitors of CYP3A4 or CYP2D6 can inhibit aripiprazole elimination and cause increased blood levels).
No products indexed under this heading.

Itraconazole (Inhibitors of CYP3A4 or CYP2D6 can inhibit aripiprazole elimination and cause increased blood levels).
No products indexed under this heading.

Ketoconazole (Inhibitors of CYP3A4 or CYP2D6 can inhibit aripiprazole elimination and cause increased blood levels). Products include:
Nizoral A-D Shampoo, 1% 1839
Nizoral 2% Shampoo 1838

Lopinavir (Inhibitors of CYP3A4 or CYP2D6 can inhibit aripiprazole elimination and cause increased blood levels). Products include:
Kaletra 474

Loratadine (Inhibitors of CYP3A4 or CYP2D6 can inhibit aripiprazole elimination and cause increased blood levels). Products include:
Alavert Allergy & Sinus D-12 Hour Tablets 743
Alavert 743
Children's Claritin 24 Hour Non-Drowsy Allergy Syrup 732
Claritin Non-Drowsy 24 Hour Tablets 731
Non-Drowsy Claritin Hives Relief Tablets 733
Claritin Reditabs 24 Hour Non-Drowsy Tablets 732
Claritin-D Non-Drowsy 12 Hour Tablets 731
Claritin-D Non-Drowsy 24 Hour Tablets 731
Children's Dimetapp ND Non-Drowsy Allergy Syrup 746
Triaminic Allerchews 684

Maprotiline Hydrochloride (Inhibitors of CYP3A4 or CYP2D6 can inhibit aripiprazole elimination and cause increased blood levels).
No products indexed under this heading.

Mephenytoin (Agents that induce CYP3A4 could cause an increase in aripiprazole clearance and lower blood levels).
No products indexed under this heading.

Methadone Hydrochloride (Inhibitors of CYP3A4 or CYP2D6 can inhibit aripiprazole elimination and cause increased blood levels).
No products indexed under this heading.

Methsuximide (Agents that induce CYP3A4 could cause an increase in aripiprazole clearance and lower blood levels).
No products indexed under this heading.

Methylprednisolone (Agents that induce CYP3A4 could cause an increase in aripiprazole clearance and lower blood levels).
No products indexed under this heading.

Methylprednisolone Acetate (Agents that induce CYP3A4 could cause an increase in aripiprazole clearance and lower blood levels). Products include:
Depo-Medrol Injectable Suspension 2615
Depo-Medrol Single-Dose Vial 2617

Methylprednisolone Sodium Succinate (Agents that induce CYP3A4 could cause an increase in aripiprazole clearance and lower blood levels).
No products indexed under this heading.

Metronidazole (Inhibitors of CYP3A4 or CYP2D6 can inhibit aripiprazole elimination and cause increased blood levels). Products include:
Metrogel 1% 1212
MetroGel-Vaginal Gel 1822
Noritate Cream, 1% 1051

Metronidazole Benzoate (Inhibitors of CYP3A4 or CYP2D6 can inhibit aripiprazole elimination and cause increased blood levels).
No products indexed under this heading.

Metronidazole Hydrochloride (Inhibitors of CYP3A4 or CYP2D6 can inhibit aripiprazole elimination and cause increased blood levels).
No products indexed under this heading.

Mibefradil Dihydrochloride (Inhibitors of CYP3A4 or CYP2D6 can inhibit aripiprazole elimination and cause increased blood levels).
No products indexed under this heading.

Miconazole (Inhibitors of CYP3A4 or CYP2D6 can inhibit aripiprazole elimination and cause increased blood levels).
No products indexed under this heading.

Miconazole Nitrate (Inhibitors of CYP3A4 or CYP2D6 can inhibit aripiprazole elimination and cause increased blood levels). Products include:
Desenex 674
Desenex Jock Itch Spray Powder 674

Moclobemide (Inhibitors of CYP3A4 or CYP2D6 can inhibit aripiprazole elimination and cause increased blood levels).
No products indexed under this heading.

Modafinil (Agents that induce CYP3A4 could cause an increase in aripiprazole clearance and lower blood levels). Products include:
Provigil Tablets 1002

Nefazodone Hydrochloride (Inhibitors of CYP3A4 or CYP2D6 can inhibit aripiprazole elimination and cause increased blood levels).
No products indexed under this heading.

Nelfinavir Mesylate (Inhibitors of CYP3A4 or CYP2D6 can inhibit aripiprazole elimination and cause increased blood levels). Products include:
Viracept 2556

Nevirapine (Inhibitors of CYP3A4 or CYP2D6 can inhibit aripiprazole elimination and cause increased blood levels). Products include:
Viramune Oral Suspension 903
Viramune Tablets 903

Niacinamide (Inhibitors of CYP3A4 or CYP2D6 can inhibit aripiprazole elimination and cause increased blood levels).
No products indexed under this heading.

Nicotinamide (Inhibitors of CYP3A4 or CYP2D6 can inhibit aripiprazole elimination and cause increased blood levels). Products include:
Nicomide Tablets 3190

Nifedipine (Inhibitors of CYP3A4 or CYP2D6 can inhibit aripiprazole elimination and cause increased blood levels). Products include:
Adalat CC Tablets 2978

Norfloxacin (Inhibitors of CYP3A4 or CYP2D6 can inhibit aripiprazole elimination and cause increased blood levels). Products include:

Noroxin Tablets 2009

Nortriptyline Hydrochloride (Inhibitors of CYP3A4 or CYP2D6 can inhibit aripiprazole elimination and cause increased blood levels).
No products indexed under this heading.

Omeprazole (Inhibitors of CYP3A4 or CYP2D6 can inhibit aripiprazole elimination and cause increased blood levels). Products include:
Zegerid Powder for Oral Solution 2972

Oxcarbazepine (Agents that induce CYP3A4 could cause an increase in aripiprazole clearance and lower blood levels). Products include:
Trileptal Oral Suspension 2281
Trileptal Tablets 2281

Paroxetine Hydrochloride (Inhibitors of CYP3A4 or CYP2D6 can inhibit aripiprazole elimination and cause increased blood levels). Products include:
Paxil CR Controlled-Release Tablets 1509
Paxil 1501

Perphenazine (Inhibitors of CYP3A4 or CYP2D6 can inhibit aripiprazole elimination and cause increased blood levels).
No products indexed under this heading.

Phenobarbital (Agents that induce CYP3A4 could cause an increase in aripiprazole clearance and lower blood levels).
No products indexed under this heading.

Phenobarbital Sodium (Agents that induce CYP3A4 could cause an increase in aripiprazole clearance and lower blood levels).
No products indexed under this heading.

Phenytoin (Agents that induce CYP3A4 could cause an increase in aripiprazole clearance and lower blood levels).
No products indexed under this heading.

Phenytoin Sodium (Agents that induce CYP3A4 could cause an increase in aripiprazole clearance and lower blood levels). Products include:
Phenytek Capsules 2153

Prednisolone Acetate (Agents that induce CYP3A4 could cause an increase in aripiprazole clearance and lower blood levels). Products include:
Blephamide Ophthalmic Ointment 563
Blephamide Ophthalmic Suspension.................................. 564
Poly-Pred Liquifilm Ophthalmic Suspension .... ⊙231
Pred Forte Ophthalmic Suspension .... ⊙233
Pred Mild Sterile Ophthalmic Suspension .... ⊙236
Pred-G Ophthalmic Suspension ...... ⊙234
Pred-G Sterile Ophthalmic Ointment .... ⊙235

Prednisolone Sodium Phosphate (Agents that induce CYP3A4 could cause an increase in aripiprazole clearance and lower blood levels). Products include:
Pediapred Oral Solution 3319

Prednisolone Tebutate (Agents that induce CYP3A4 could cause an increase in aripiprazole clearance and lower blood levels).
No products indexed under this heading.

Prednisone (Agents that induce CYP3A4 could cause an increase in aripiprazole clearance and lower blood levels).
No products indexed under this heading.

Primidone (Agents that induce CYP3A4 could cause an increase in aripiprazole clearance and lower blood levels).
No products indexed under this heading.

Propafenone Hydrochloride (Inhibitors of CYP3A4 or CYP2D6 can inhibit aripiprazole elimination and cause increased blood levels). Products include:
Rythmol SR Capsules 2736

Propoxyphene Hydrochloride (Inhibitors of CYP3A4 or CYP2D6 can inhibit aripiprazole elimination and cause increased blood levels).
No products indexed under this heading.

Propoxyphene Napsylate (Inhibitors of CYP3A4 or CYP2D6 can inhibit aripiprazole elimination and cause increased blood levels). Products include:
Darvocet A 500 Tablets 3497

Protriptyline Hydrochloride (Inhibitors of CYP3A4 or CYP2D6 can inhibit aripiprazole elimination and cause increased blood levels). Products include:
Vivactil Tablets 2350

Quinacrine Hydrochloride (Inhibitors of CYP3A4 or CYP2D6 can inhibit aripiprazole elimination and cause increased blood levels).
No products indexed under this heading.

Quinidine (Inhibitors of CYP3A4 or CYP2D6 can inhibit aripiprazole elimination and cause increased blood levels).
No products indexed under this heading.

Quinidine Gluconate (Inhibitors of CYP3A4 or CYP2D6 can inhibit aripiprazole elimination and cause increased blood levels).
No products indexed under this heading.

Quinidine Hydrochloride (Inhibitors of CYP3A4 or CYP2D6 can inhibit aripiprazole elimination and cause increased blood levels).
No products indexed under this heading.

Quinidine Polygalacturonate (Inhibitors of CYP3A4 or CYP2D6 can inhibit aripiprazole elimination and cause increased blood levels).
No products indexed under this heading.

Quinidine Sulfate (Inhibitors of CYP3A4 or CYP2D6 can inhibit aripiprazole elimination and cause increased blood levels).
No products indexed under this heading.

Quinine (Inhibitors of CYP3A4 or CYP2D6 can inhibit aripiprazole elimination and cause increased blood levels).
No products indexed under this heading.

Quinine Sulfate (Inhibitors of CYP3A4 or CYP2D6 can inhibit aripiprazole elimination and cause increased blood levels).
No products indexed under this heading.

Quinupristin (Inhibitors of CYP3A4 or CYP2D6 can inhibit aripiprazole elimination and cause increased blood levels). Products include:
Synercid I.V. 1690

Ranitidine Bismuth Citrate (Inhibitors of CYP3A4 or CYP2D6 can inhibit aripiprazole elimination and cause increased blood levels).
No products indexed under this heading.

Ranitidine Hydrochloride (Inhibitors of CYP3A4 or CYP2D6 can inhibit aripiprazole elimination and cause increased blood levels). Products include:
Zantac 1597
Zantac Injection 1593
Zantac 75 Tablets .... ▣715
Zantac 150 Maximum Strength Tablets.. ▣715
Zantac Injection Pharmacy Bulk Package... 1595

Rifabutin (Agents that induce CYP3A4 could cause an increase in aripiprazole clearance and lower blood levels).
No products indexed under this heading.

Rifampicin (Agents that induce CYP3A4 could cause an increase in aripiprazole clearance and lower blood levels).
No products indexed under this heading.

Rifampin (Agents that induce CYP3A4 could cause an increase in aripiprazole clearance and lower blood levels).
No products indexed under this heading.

Rifapentine (Agents that induce CYP3A4 could cause an increase in aripiprazole clearance and lower blood levels).
No products indexed under this heading.

Ritonavir (Inhibitors of CYP3A4 or CYP2D6 can inhibit aripiprazole elimination and cause increased blood levels). Products include:
Kaletra 474
Norvir 499

Saquinavir (Inhibitors of CYP3A4 or CYP2D6 can inhibit aripiprazole elimination and cause increased blood levels).
No products indexed under this heading.

Saquinavir Mesylate (Inhibitors of CYP3A4 or CYP2D6 can inhibit aripiprazole elimination and cause increased blood levels). Products include:
Invirase 2776

Sertraline Hydrochloride (Inhibitors of CYP3A4 or CYP2D6 can inhibit aripiprazole elimination and cause increased blood levels). Products include:
Zoloft 2581

Sulfinpyrazone (Agents that induce CYP3A4 could cause an increase in aripiprazole clearance and lower blood levels).
No products indexed under this heading.

Telithromycin (Inhibitors of CYP3A4 or CYP2D6 can inhibit aripiprazole elimination and cause increased blood levels). Products include:
Ketek Tablets 2920

Terbinafine Hydrochloride (Inhibitors of CYP3A4 or CYP2D6 can inhibit aripiprazole elimination and cause increased blood levels). Products include:
Lamisil AT Creams (Athlete's Foot & Jock Itch)................................ ▣676
Lamisil Tablets 2226

Theophylline (Agents that induce CYP3A4 could cause an increase in aripiprazole clearance and lower blood levels).
No products indexed under this heading.

Thioridazine Hydrochloride (Inhibitors of CYP3A4 or CYP2D6 can inhibit aripiprazole elimination and cause increased blood levels). Products include:
Thioridazine Hydrochloride Tablets 2122

Triamcinolone (Agents that induce CYP3A4 could cause an increase in aripiprazole clearance and lower blood levels).
No products indexed under this heading.

Triamcinolone Acetonide (Agents that induce CYP3A4 could cause an increase in aripiprazole clearance and lower blood levels). Products include:
Azmacort Inhalation Aerosol 1701
Nasacort HFA Inhalation Aerosol 2939
Nasacort AQ Nasal Spray 2937

Triamcinolone Diacetate (Agents that induce CYP3A4 could cause an increase in aripiprazole clearance and lower blood levels).
No products indexed under this heading.

Triamcinolone Hexacetonide (Agents that induce CYP3A4 could cause an increase in aripiprazole clearance and lower blood levels).
No products indexed under this heading.

Trimipramine Maleate (Inhibitors of CYP3A4 or CYP2D6 can inhibit aripiprazole elimination and cause increased blood levels). Products include:
Surmontil Capsules 2347

Troglitazone (Agents that induce CYP3A4 could cause an increase in aripiprazole clearance and lower blood levels).
No products indexed under this heading.

Troleandomycin (Inhibitors of CYP3A4 or CYP2D6 can inhibit aripiprazole elimination and cause increased blood levels).
No products indexed under this heading.

Valproate Sodium (Inhibitors of CYP3A4 or CYP2D6 can inhibit aripiprazole elimination and cause increased blood levels). Products include:
Depacon Injection 412

Verapamil Hydrochloride (Inhibitors of CYP3A4 or CYP2D6 can inhibit aripiprazole elimination and cause increased blood levels). Products include:
Covera-HS Tablets 3135
Tarka Tablets 519
Verelan PM Capsules 3120

Voriconazole (Inhibitors of CYP3A4 or CYP2D6 can inhibit aripiprazole elimination and cause increased blood levels). Products include:
VFEND I.V. 2543
VFEND Oral Suspension 2543
VFEND Tablets 2543

Zafirlukast (Inhibitors of CYP3A4 or CYP2D6 can inhibit aripiprazole elimination and cause increased blood levels). Products include:
- Accolate Tablets ... 663

Zileuton (Inhibitors of CYP3A4 or CYP2D6 can inhibit aripiprazole elimination and cause increased blood levels).
- No products indexed under this heading.

Food Interactions

Grapefruit (Inhibitors of CYP3A4 or CYP2D6 can inhibit aripiprazole elimination and cause increased blood levels).

Grapefruit Juice (Inhibitors of CYP3A4 or CYP2D6 can inhibit aripiprazole elimination and cause increased blood levels).

ABILIFY TABLETS

(Aripiprazole) ... 2472
May interact with cytochrome p450 2d6 inhibitors (selected), cytochrome p450 3a4 inducers (selected), cytochrome p450 3a4 inhibitors (selected), and certain other agents. Compounds in these categories include:

Acetazolamide (Inhibitors of CYP3A4 or CYP2D6 can inhibit aripiprazole elimination and cause increased blood levels).
- No products indexed under this heading.

Allium sativum (Agents that induce CYP3A4 could cause an increase in aripiprazole clearance and lower blood levels).
- No products indexed under this heading.

Amiodarone Hydrochloride (Inhibitors of CYP3A4 or CYP2D6 can inhibit aripiprazole elimination and cause increased blood levels). Products include:
- Pacerone Tablets ... 3337

Amitriptyline Hydrochloride (Inhibitors of CYP3A4 or CYP2D6 can inhibit aripiprazole elimination and cause increased blood levels).
- No products indexed under this heading.

Amoxapine (Inhibitors of CYP3A4 or CYP2D6 can inhibit aripiprazole elimination and cause increased blood levels).
- No products indexed under this heading.

Amprenavir (Inhibitors of CYP3A4 or CYP2D6 can inhibit aripiprazole elimination and cause increased blood levels). Products include:
- Agenerase Capsules ... 1299
- Agenerase Oral Solution ... 1304

Anastrozole (Inhibitors of CYP3A4 or CYP2D6 can inhibit aripiprazole elimination and cause increased blood levels). Products include:
- Arimidex Tablets ... 665

Aprepitant (Inhibitors of CYP3A4 or CYP2D6 can inhibit aripiprazole elimination and cause increased blood levels). Products include:
- Emend Capsules ... 1944

Betamethasone Acetate (Agents that induce CYP3A4 could cause an increase in aripiprazole clearance and lower blood levels).
- No products indexed under this heading.

Betamethasone Sodium Phosphate (Agents that induce CYP3A4 could cause an increase in aripiprazole clearance and lower blood levels).
- No products indexed under this heading.

Bupropion Hydrochloride (Inhibitors of CYP3A4 or CYP2D6 can inhibit aripiprazole elimination and cause increased blood levels). Products include:
- Wellbutrin Tablets ... 1579
- Wellbutrin SR Sustained-Release Tablets ... 1583
- Wellbutrin XL Extended-Release Tablets ... 1588
- Zyban Sustained-Release Tablets ... 1620

Carbamazepine (Agents that induce CYP3A4 could cause an increase in aripiprazole clearance and lower blood levels). Products include:
- Carbatrol Capsules ... 3174
- Equetro Extended-Release Capsules ... 3178
- Tegretol/Tegretol-XR ... 2278

Celecoxib (Inhibitors of CYP3A4 or CYP2D6 can inhibit aripiprazole elimination and cause increased blood levels). Products include:
- Celebrex Capsules ... 3130

Chloroquine Hydrochloride (Inhibitors of CYP3A4 or CYP2D6 can inhibit aripiprazole elimination and cause increased blood levels).
- No products indexed under this heading.

Chloroquine Phosphate (Inhibitors of CYP3A4 or CYP2D6 can inhibit aripiprazole elimination and cause increased blood levels).
- No products indexed under this heading.

Chlorpheniramine (Inhibitors of CYP3A4 or CYP2D6 can inhibit aripiprazole elimination and cause increased blood levels).
- No products indexed under this heading.

Chlorpheniramine Maleate (Inhibitors of CYP3A4 or CYP2D6 can inhibit aripiprazole elimination and cause increased blood levels). Products include:
- Advil Allergy Sinus Caplets ... ■737
- Advil Multi-Symptom Cold Caplets ... ■738
- BC Allergy Sinus Cold Powder ... ■612
- Contac Severe Cold and Flu Caplets Maximum Strength ... ■615
- Hycomine Compound Tablets ... 1105
- PediaCare Multi-Symptom Cold Liquid ... ■704
- PediaCare NightRest Cough & Cold Liquid ... ■704
- Robitussin Flu Liquid ... ■752
- Robitussin PM Cough & Cold Liquid ... ■752
- Singlet Caplets ... ■636
- Sudafed Sinus & Allergy Tablets ... ■710
- TheraFlu Cold & Cough Hot Liquid ... ■680
- TheraFlu Cold & Sore Throat Hot Liquid ... ■680
- TheraFlu Flu & Sore Throat Hot Liquid ... ■681
- TheraFlu Severe Cold & Cough Hot Liquid ... ■683
- TheraFlu Severe Cold Caplets ... ■679
- TheraFlu Severe Cold Hot Liquid ... ■682
- Triaminic Cold & Allergy Liquid ... ■685
- Triaminic Cold & Cough Liquid ... ■685
- Triaminic Flu, Cough & Fever Liquid ... ■685
- Triaminic Night Time Cough & Cold Liquid ... ■685
- Triaminic Allergy Runny Nose & Congestion Softchews ... ■688
- Triaminic Cold & Cough Softchews ... ■688
- Children's Tylenol Plus Cold NightTime Suspension Liquid ... 1851
- Children's Tylenol Plus Cold & Cough Suspension Liquid and Chewable Tablets ... 1851
- Children's Tylenol Plus Cold Chewable Tablets ... 1851
- Children's Tylenol Plus Flu Suspension Liquid ... 1853
- Tylenol Allergy Complete Multi-Symptom Caplets and Gelcaps with Cool Burst ... 1844
- Multi-Symptom Tylenol Cold Night Time Caplets ... 1845
- Vicks 44M Cough, Cold & Flu Relief ... 2676
- Pediatric Vicks 44m Cough & Cold Relief ... 2673
- Children's Vicks NyQuil Cold/Cough Relief ... 2671

Chlorpheniramine Polistirex (Inhibitors of CYP3A4 or CYP2D6 can inhibit aripiprazole elimination and cause increased blood levels). Products include:
- Tussionex Pennkinetic Extended-Release Suspension ... 3322

Chlorpheniramine Tannate (Inhibitors of CYP3A4 or CYP2D6 can inhibit aripiprazole elimination and cause increased blood levels).
- No products indexed under this heading.

Cimetidine (Inhibitors of CYP3A4 or CYP2D6 can inhibit aripiprazole elimination and cause increased blood levels). Products include:
- Tagamet HB 200 Tablets ... ■637
- Tagamet Tablets ... 1547

Cimetidine Hydrochloride (Inhibitors of CYP3A4 or CYP2D6 can inhibit aripiprazole elimination and cause increased blood levels).
- No products indexed under this heading.

Ciprofloxacin (Inhibitors of CYP3A4 or CYP2D6 can inhibit aripiprazole elimination and cause increased blood levels). Products include:
- Cipro I.V. ... 2998
- Cipro I.V. Pharmacy Bulk Package ... 3509
- Cipro Oral Suspension ... 2991
- Cipro XR Tablets ... 3004
- Ciprodex Otic Suspension ... 555

Ciprofloxacin Hydrochloride (Agents that induce CYP3A4 could cause an increase in aripiprazole clearance and lower blood levels). Products include:
- Ciloxan Ophthalmic Ointment ... 554
- Cipro Tablets ... 2991

Cisplatin (Agents that induce CYP3A4 could cause an increase in aripiprazole clearance and lower blood levels).
- No products indexed under this heading.

Citalopram Hydrobromide (Inhibitors of CYP3A4 or CYP2D6 can inhibit aripiprazole elimination and cause increased blood levels). Products include:
- Celexa ... 1177

Clarithromycin (Inhibitors of CYP3A4 or CYP2D6 can inhibit aripiprazole elimination and cause increased blood levels). Products include:
- Biaxin/Biaxin XL ... 402
- PREVPAC ... 3281

Clomipramine Hydrochloride (Inhibitors of CYP3A4 or CYP2D6 can inhibit aripiprazole elimination and cause increased blood levels).
- No products indexed under this heading.

Clotrimazole (Inhibitors of CYP3A4 or CYP2D6 can inhibit aripiprazole elimination and cause increased blood levels). Products include:
- Lotrimin ... 3053
- Lotrisone ... 3054

Cocaine Hydrochloride (Inhibitors of CYP3A4 or CYP2D6 can inhibit aripiprazole elimination and cause increased blood levels).
- No products indexed under this heading.

Cortisone Acetate (Agents that induce CYP3A4 could cause an increase in aripiprazole clearance and lower blood levels).
- No products indexed under this heading.

Cyclosporine (Inhibitors of CYP3A4 or CYP2D6 can inhibit aripiprazole elimination and cause increased blood levels). Products include:
- Gengraf Capsules ... 458
- Neoral Soft Gelatin Capsules ... 2247
- Neoral Oral Solution ... 2247
- Restasis Ophthalmic Emulsion ... 570
- Sandimmune ... 2259

Dalfopristin (Inhibitors of CYP3A4 or CYP2D6 can inhibit aripiprazole elimination and cause increased blood levels). Products include:
- Synercid I.V. ... 1690

Danazol (Inhibitors of CYP3A4 or CYP2D6 can inhibit aripiprazole elimination and cause increased blood levels).
- No products indexed under this heading.

Delavirdine Mesylate (Inhibitors of CYP3A4 or CYP2D6 can inhibit aripiprazole elimination and cause increased blood levels). Products include:
- Rescriptor Tablets ... 2535

Desipramine Hydrochloride (Inhibitors of CYP3A4 or CYP2D6 can inhibit aripiprazole elimination and cause increased blood levels).
- No products indexed under this heading.

Dexamethasone (Agents that induce CYP3A4 could cause an increase in aripiprazole clearance and lower blood levels). Products include:
- Ciprodex Otic Suspension ... 555
- Decadron Tablets ... 1929
- TobraDex Ophthalmic Ointment ... 558
- TobraDex Ophthalmic Suspension ... 558

Dexamethasone Acetate (Agents that induce CYP3A4 could cause an increase in aripiprazole clearance and lower blood levels).
- No products indexed under this heading.

Dexamethasone Sodium Phosphate (Agents that induce CYP3A4 could cause an increase in aripiprazole clearance and lower blood levels). Products include:
- Decadron Phosphate Injection ... 1931

Diltiazem Hydrochloride (Inhibitors of CYP3A4 or CYP2D6 can inhibit aripiprazole elimination and cause increased blood levels). Products include:
- Cardizem LA Extended Release Tablets ... 1699
- Tiazac Capsules ... 1204

Diltiazem Maleate (Inhibitors of CYP3A4 or CYP2D6 can inhibit aripiprazole elimination and cause increased blood levels).
- No products indexed under this heading.

Diphenhydramine (Inhibitors of CYP3A4 or CYP2D6 can inhibit arip-

iprazole elimination and cause increased blood levels). Products include:
- Tylenol Sore Throat NightTime Liquid with Cool Burst 1849

Diphenhydramine Hydrochloride (Inhibitors of CYP3A4 or CYP2D6 can inhibit aripiprazole elimination and cause increased blood levels). Products include:
- Benadryl Allergy & Cold Tablets ..... ▣692
- Benadryl Allergy .... ▣691
- Benadryl Allergy & Sinus Headache Caplets & Gelcaps .... ▣693
- Children's Benadryl Allergy Liquid ... ▣695
- Children's Benadryl Dye-Free Allergy Liquid .... ▣695
- Benadryl Dye-Free Allergy Liqui-Gels Softgels .... ▣692
- Benadryl Itch Relief Stick Extra Strength .... ▣696
- Benadryl Itch Stopping Cream Extra Strength .... ▣697
- Benadryl Itch Stopping Gel Extra Strength .... ▣697
- Benadryl Itch Stopping Spray Extra Strength .... ▣697
- Benadryl Maximum Strength Severe Allergy & Sinus Headache Caplets .... ▣694
- Children's Benadryl D Liquid Medication .... ▣693
- Benadryl D Tablets .... ▣694
- Nytol QuickCaps Caplets .... ▣635
- Maximum Strength Nytol QuickGels Softgels .... ▣635
- Simply Sleep Caplets 1841
- Sominex Original Formula Tablets .. ▣637
- TheraFlu Thin Strips Multi Symptom .... ▣684
- Triaminic Thin Strips Cough & Runny Nose .... ▣690
- Children's Tylenol Plus Cold & Allergy Suspension Liquid 1850
- Tylenol Allergy Complete Night Time Caplets 1844
- Tylenol Severe Allergy Caplets 1844
- Tylenol Flu NightTime Gelcaps 1846
- Extra Strength Tylenol PM Caplets, Geltabs, Gelcaps and Liquid 1847
- Unisom Maximum Strength SleepGels .... ▣712

Doxepin Hydrochloride (Inhibitors of CYP3A4 or CYP2D6 can inhibit aripiprazole elimination and cause increased blood levels).
No products indexed under this heading.

Doxorubicin Hydrochloride (Agents that induce CYP3A4 could cause an increase in aripiprazole clearance and lower blood levels). Products include:
- Adriamycin for Injection, USP 786
- Adriamycin Injection, USP 786

Efavirenz (Inhibitors of CYP3A4 or CYP2D6 can inhibit aripiprazole elimination and cause increased blood levels). Products include:
- Sustiva Capsules 957

Erythromycin (Inhibitors of CYP3A4 or CYP2D6 can inhibit aripiprazole elimination and cause increased blood levels). Products include:
- Erygel Topical Gel 2096
- Ery-Tab Tablets 447
- Erythromycin Base Filmtab Tablets 454
- Erythromycin Delayed-Release Capsules, USP 456
- PCE Dispertab Tablets 510

Erythromycin Estolate (Inhibitors of CYP3A4 or CYP2D6 can inhibit aripiprazole elimination and cause increased blood levels).
No products indexed under this heading.

Erythromycin Ethylsuccinate (Inhibitors of CYP3A4 or CYP2D6 can inhibit aripiprazole elimination and cause increased blood levels). Products include:
- E.E.S. 449
- EryPed 445

Erythromycin Gluceptate (Inhibitors of CYP3A4 or CYP2D6 can inhibit aripiprazole elimination and cause increased blood levels).
No products indexed under this heading.

Erythromycin Lactobionate (Inhibitors of CYP3A4 or CYP2D6 can inhibit aripiprazole elimination and cause increased blood levels).
No products indexed under this heading.

Erythromycin Stearate (Inhibitors of CYP3A4 or CYP2D6 can inhibit aripiprazole elimination and cause increased blood levels). Products include:
- Erythrocin Stearate Filmtab Tablets 452

Escitalopram Oxalate (Inhibitors of CYP3A4 or CYP2D6 can inhibit aripiprazole elimination and cause increased blood levels). Products include:
- Lexapro Oral Solution 1193
- Lexapro Tablets 1193

Esomeprazole Magnesium (Inhibitors of CYP3A4 or CYP2D6 can inhibit aripiprazole elimination and cause increased blood levels). Products include:
- Nexium Delayed-Release Capsules 645

Ethosuximide (Agents that induce CYP3A4 could cause an increase in aripiprazole clearance and lower blood levels).
No products indexed under this heading.

Felbamate (Agents that induce CYP3A4 could cause an increase in aripiprazole clearance and lower blood levels).
No products indexed under this heading.

Fluconazole (Inhibitors of CYP3A4 or CYP2D6 can inhibit aripiprazole elimination and cause increased blood levels).
No products indexed under this heading.

Fludrocortisone Acetate (Agents that induce CYP3A4 could cause an increase in aripiprazole clearance and lower blood levels).
No products indexed under this heading.

Fluoxetine (Inhibitors of CYP3A4 or CYP2D6 can inhibit aripiprazole elimination and cause increased blood levels).
No products indexed under this heading.

Fluoxetine Hydrochloride (Inhibitors of CYP3A4 or CYP2D6 can inhibit aripiprazole elimination and cause increased blood levels). Products include:
- Prozac Pulvules and Liquid 1771
- Symbyax Capsules 1788

Fluphenazine Decanoate (Inhibitors of CYP3A4 or CYP2D6 can inhibit aripiprazole elimination and cause increased blood levels).
No products indexed under this heading.

Fluphenazine Enanthate (Inhibitors of CYP3A4 or CYP2D6 can inhibit aripiprazole elimination and cause increased blood levels).
No products indexed under this heading.

Fluphenazine Hydrochloride (Inhibitors of CYP3A4 or CYP2D6 can inhibit aripiprazole elimination and cause increased blood levels).
No products indexed under this heading.

Fluvoxamine Maleate (Inhibitors of CYP3A4 or CYP2D6 can inhibit aripiprazole elimination and cause increased blood levels).
No products indexed under this heading.

Fosamprenavir Calcium (Inhibitors of CYP3A4 or CYP2D6 can inhibit aripiprazole elimination and cause increased blood levels). Products include:
- Lexiva Tablets 1473

Fosphenytoin Sodium (Agents that induce CYP3A4 could cause an increase in aripiprazole clearance and lower blood levels).
No products indexed under this heading.

Garlic Extract (Agents that induce CYP3A4 could cause an increase in aripiprazole clearance and lower blood levels).
No products indexed under this heading.

Garlic Oil (Agents that induce CYP3A4 could cause an increase in aripiprazole clearance and lower blood levels).
No products indexed under this heading.

Halofantrine Hydrochloride (Inhibitors of CYP3A4 or CYP2D6 can inhibit aripiprazole elimination and cause increased blood levels).
No products indexed under this heading.

Haloperidol (Inhibitors of CYP3A4 or CYP2D6 can inhibit aripiprazole elimination and cause increased blood levels).
No products indexed under this heading.

Haloperidol Decanoate (Inhibitors of CYP3A4 or CYP2D6 can inhibit aripiprazole elimination and cause increased blood levels).
No products indexed under this heading.

Hydrocortisone (Agents that induce CYP3A4 could cause an increase in aripiprazole clearance and lower blood levels). Products include:
- Cortizone•5 Ointment .... ▣699
- Cortizone•10 Creme .... ▣699
- Cortizone•10 Ointment .... ▣699
- Cortizone•10 Plus Creme .... ▣700
- Cortizone•10 Maximum Strength Quick Shot Spray .... ▣700
- Hydrocortone Tablets 1963
- Preparation H Hydrocortisone Cream .... ▣748

Hydrocortisone Acetate (Agents that induce CYP3A4 could cause an increase in aripiprazole clearance and lower blood levels). Products include:
- Analpram-HC 1136
- Pramosone 1139
- ProctoFoam-HC 3113
- Tucks Anti-Itch Ointment .... ▣712
- U-cort 1% Cream 3289

Hydrocortisone Butyrate (Agents that induce CYP3A4 could cause an increase in aripiprazole clearance and lower blood levels). Products include:
- Locoid 1138
- Locoid Lipocream Cream 1138

Hydrocortisone Cypionate (Agents that induce CYP3A4 could cause an increase in aripiprazole clearance and lower blood levels).
No products indexed under this heading.

Hydrocortisone Hemisuccinate (Agents that induce CYP3A4 could cause an increase in aripiprazole clearance and lower blood levels).
No products indexed under this heading.

Hydrocortisone Probutate (Agents that induce CYP3A4 could cause an increase in aripiprazole clearance and lower blood levels). Products include:
- Pandel Cream, 0.1% 1017

Hydrocortisone Sodium Phosphate (Agents that induce CYP3A4 could cause an increase in aripiprazole clearance and lower blood levels).
No products indexed under this heading.

Hydrocortisone Sodium Succinate (Agents that induce CYP3A4 could cause an increase in aripiprazole clearance and lower blood levels).
No products indexed under this heading.

Hydrocortisone Valerate (Agents that induce CYP3A4 could cause an increase in aripiprazole clearance and lower blood levels).
No products indexed under this heading.

Hydroxychloroquine Sulfate (Inhibitors of CYP3A4 or CYP2D6 can inhibit aripiprazole elimination and cause increased blood levels).
No products indexed under this heading.

Hypericum (Agents that induce CYP3A4 could cause an increase in aripiprazole clearance and lower blood levels).
No products indexed under this heading.

Hypericum Perforatum (Agents that induce CYP3A4 could cause an increase in aripiprazole clearance and lower blood levels).
No products indexed under this heading.

Imatinib Mesylate (Inhibitors of CYP3A4 or CYP2D6 can inhibit aripiprazole elimination and cause increased blood levels). Products include:
- Gleevec Tablets 2221

Imipramine Hydrochloride (Inhibitors of CYP3A4 or CYP2D6 can inhibit aripiprazole elimination and cause increased blood levels).
No products indexed under this heading.

Imipramine Pamoate (Inhibitors of CYP3A4 or CYP2D6 can inhibit aripiprazole elimination and cause increased blood levels).
No products indexed under this heading.

Indinavir Sulfate (Inhibitors of CYP3A4 or CYP2D6 can inhibit aripiprazole elimination and cause increased blood levels). Products include:
- Crixivan Capsules 1918

Isoniazid (Inhibitors of CYP3A4 or CYP2D6 can inhibit aripiprazole elimination and cause increased blood levels).
No products indexed under this heading.

Itraconazole (Inhibitors of CYP3A4 or CYP2D6 can inhibit aripiprazole elimination and cause increased blood levels).
No products indexed under this heading.

Ketoconazole (Inhibitors of CYP3A4 or CYP2D6 can inhibit aripiprazole elimination and cause increased blood levels). Products include:
Nizoral A-D Shampoo, 1% 1839
Nizoral 2% Shampoo 1838

Lopinavir (Inhibitors of CYP3A4 or CYP2D6 can inhibit aripiprazole elimination and cause increased blood levels). Products include:
Kaletra 474

Loratadine (Inhibitors of CYP3A4 or CYP2D6 can inhibit aripiprazole elimination and cause increased blood levels). Products include:
Alavert Allergy & Sinus D-12 Hour Tablets.. ▣ 743
Alavert .... ▣ 743
Children's Claritin 24 Hour Non-Drowsy Allergy Syrup........... ▣ 732
Claritin Non-Drowsy 24 Hour Tablets.. ▣ 731
Non-Drowsy Claritin Hives Relief Tablets.. ▣ 733
Claritin Reditabs 24 Hour Non-Drowsy Tablets.................... ▣ 732
Claritin-D Non-Drowsy 12 Hour Tablets.. ▣ 731
Claritin-D Non-Drowsy 24 Hour Tablets.. ▣ 731
Children's Dimetapp ND Non-Drowsy Allergy Syrup........... ▣ 746
Triaminic Allerchews .... ▣ 684

Maprotiline Hydrochloride (Inhibitors of CYP3A4 or CYP2D6 can inhibit aripiprazole elimination and cause increased blood levels).
No products indexed under this heading.

Mephenytoin (Agents that induce CYP3A4 could cause an increase in aripiprazole clearance and lower blood levels).
No products indexed under this heading.

Methadone Hydrochloride (Inhibitors of CYP3A4 or CYP2D6 can inhibit aripiprazole elimination and cause increased blood levels).
No products indexed under this heading.

Methsuximide (Agents that induce CYP3A4 could cause an increase in aripiprazole clearance and lower blood levels).
No products indexed under this heading.

Methylprednisolone (Agents that induce CYP3A4 could cause an increase in aripiprazole clearance and lower blood levels).
No products indexed under this heading.

Methylprednisolone Acetate (Agents that induce CYP3A4 could cause an increase in aripiprazole clearance and lower blood levels). Products include:
Depo-Medrol Injectable Suspension 2615
Depo-Medrol Single-Dose Vial 2617

Methylprednisolone Sodium Succinate (Agents that induce CYP3A4 could cause an increase in aripiprazole clearance and lower blood levels).
No products indexed under this heading.

Metronidazole (Inhibitors of CYP3A4 or CYP2D6 can inhibit aripiprazole elimination and cause increased blood levels). Products include:
Metrogel 1% 1212
MetroGel-Vaginal Gel 1822
Noritate Cream, 1% 1051

Metronidazole Benzoate (Inhibitors of CYP3A4 or CYP2D6 can inhibit aripiprazole elimination and cause increased blood levels).
No products indexed under this heading.

Metronidazole Hydrochloride (Inhibitors of CYP3A4 or CYP2D6 can inhibit aripiprazole elimination and cause increased blood levels).
No products indexed under this heading.

Mibefradil Dihydrochloride (Inhibitors of CYP3A4 or CYP2D6 can inhibit aripiprazole elimination and cause increased blood levels).
No products indexed under this heading.

Miconazole (Inhibitors of CYP3A4 or CYP2D6 can inhibit aripiprazole elimination and cause increased blood levels).
No products indexed under this heading.

Miconazole Nitrate (Inhibitors of CYP3A4 or CYP2D6 can inhibit aripiprazole elimination and cause increased blood levels). Products include:
Desenex .... ▣ 674
Desenex Jock Itch Spray Powder ... ▣ 674

Moclobemide (Inhibitors of CYP3A4 or CYP2D6 can inhibit aripiprazole elimination and cause increased blood levels).
No products indexed under this heading.

Modafinil (Agents that induce CYP3A4 could cause an increase in aripiprazole clearance and lower blood levels). Products include:
Provigil Tablets 1002

Nefazodone Hydrochloride (Inhibitors of CYP3A4 or CYP2D6 can inhibit aripiprazole elimination and cause increased blood levels).
No products indexed under this heading.

Nelfinavir Mesylate (Inhibitors of CYP3A4 or CYP2D6 can inhibit aripiprazole elimination and cause increased blood levels). Products include:
Viracept 2556

Nevirapine (Inhibitors of CYP3A4 or CYP2D6 can inhibit aripiprazole elimination and cause increased blood levels). Products include:
Viramune Oral Suspension 903
Viramune Tablets 903

Niacinamide (Inhibitors of CYP3A4 or CYP2D6 can inhibit aripiprazole elimination and cause increased blood levels).
No products indexed under this heading.

Nicotinamide (Inhibitors of CYP3A4 or CYP2D6 can inhibit aripiprazole elimination and cause increased blood levels). Products include:
Nicomide Tablets 3190

Nifedipine (Inhibitors of CYP3A4 or CYP2D6 can inhibit aripiprazole elimination and cause increased blood levels). Products include:
Adalat CC Tablets 2978

Norfloxacin (Inhibitors of CYP3A4 or CYP2D6 can inhibit aripiprazole elimination and cause increased blood levels). Products include:
Noroxin Tablets 2009

Nortriptyline Hydrochloride (Inhibitors of CYP3A4 or CYP2D6 can inhibit aripiprazole elimination and cause increased blood levels).
No products indexed under this heading.

Omeprazole (Inhibitors of CYP3A4 or CYP2D6 can inhibit aripiprazole elimination and cause increased blood levels). Products include:
Zegerid Powder for Oral Solution 2972

Oxcarbazepine (Agents that induce CYP3A4 could cause an increase in aripiprazole clearance and lower blood levels). Products include:
Trileptal Oral Suspension 2281
Trileptal Tablets 2281

Paroxetine Hydrochloride (Inhibitors of CYP3A4 or CYP2D6 can inhibit aripiprazole elimination and cause increased blood levels). Products include:
Paxil CR Controlled-Release Tablets 1509
Paxil 1501

Perphenazine (Inhibitors of CYP3A4 or CYP2D6 can inhibit aripiprazole elimination and cause increased blood levels).
No products indexed under this heading.

Phenobarbital (Agents that induce CYP3A4 could cause an increase in aripiprazole clearance and lower blood levels).
No products indexed under this heading.

Phenobarbital Sodium (Agents that induce CYP3A4 could cause an increase in aripiprazole clearance and lower blood levels).
No products indexed under this heading.

Phenytoin (Agents that induce CYP3A4 could cause an increase in aripiprazole clearance and lower blood levels).
No products indexed under this heading.

Phenytoin Sodium (Agents that induce CYP3A4 could cause an increase in aripiprazole clearance and lower blood levels). Products include:
Phenytek Capsules 2153

Prednisolone Acetate (Agents that induce CYP3A4 could cause an increase in aripiprazole clearance and lower blood levels). Products include:
Blephamide Ophthalmic Ointment 563
Blephamide Ophthalmic Suspension.................................. 564
Poly-Pred Liquifilm Ophthalmic Suspension .... ⊙ 231
Pred Forte Ophthalmic Suspension .... ⊙ 233
Pred Mild Sterile Ophthalmic Suspension .... ⊙ 236
Pred-G Ophthalmic Suspension ...... ⊙ 234
Pred-G Sterile Ophthalmic Ointment.................................... ⊙ 235

Prednisolone Sodium Phosphate (Agents that induce CYP3A4 could cause an increase in aripiprazole clearance and lower blood levels). Products include:
Pediapred Oral Solution 3319

Prednisolone Tebutate (Agents that induce CYP3A4 could cause an increase in aripiprazole clearance and lower blood levels).
No products indexed under this heading.

Prednisone (Agents that induce CYP3A4 could cause an increase in aripiprazole clearance and lower blood levels).
No products indexed under this heading.

Primidone (Agents that induce CYP3A4 could cause an increase in aripiprazole clearance and lower blood levels).
No products indexed under this heading.

Propafenone Hydrochloride (Inhibitors of CYP3A4 or CYP2D6 can inhibit aripiprazole elimination and cause increased blood levels). Products include:
Rythmol SR Capsules 2736

Propoxyphene Hydrochloride (Inhibitors of CYP3A4 or CYP2D6 can inhibit aripiprazole elimination and cause increased blood levels).
No products indexed under this heading.

Propoxyphene Napsylate (Inhibitors of CYP3A4 or CYP2D6 can inhibit aripiprazole elimination and cause increased blood levels). Products include:
Darvocet A 500 Tablets 3497

Protriptyline Hydrochloride (Inhibitors of CYP3A4 or CYP2D6 can inhibit aripiprazole elimination and cause increased blood levels). Products include:
Vivactil Tablets 2350

Quinacrine Hydrochloride (Inhibitors of CYP3A4 or CYP2D6 can inhibit aripiprazole elimination and cause increased blood levels).
No products indexed under this heading.

Quinidine (Inhibitors of CYP3A4 or CYP2D6 can inhibit aripiprazole elimination and cause increased blood levels).
No products indexed under this heading.

Quinidine Gluconate (Inhibitors of CYP3A4 or CYP2D6 can inhibit aripiprazole elimination and cause increased blood levels).
No products indexed under this heading.

Quinidine Hydrochloride (Inhibitors of CYP3A4 or CYP2D6 can inhibit aripiprazole elimination and cause increased blood levels).
No products indexed under this heading.

Quinidine Polygalacturonate (Inhibitors of CYP3A4 or CYP2D6 can inhibit aripiprazole elimination and cause increased blood levels).
No products indexed under this heading.

Quinidine Sulfate (Inhibitors of CYP3A4 or CYP2D6 can inhibit aripiprazole elimination and cause increased blood levels).
No products indexed under this heading.

Quinine (Inhibitors of CYP3A4 or CYP2D6 can inhibit aripiprazole elimination and cause increased blood levels).
No products indexed under this heading.

Quinine Sulfate (Inhibitors of CYP3A4 or CYP2D6 can inhibit aripiprazole elimination and cause increased blood levels).
No products indexed under this heading.

Quinupristin (Inhibitors of CYP3A4 or CYP2D6 can inhibit aripiprazole elimination and cause increased blood levels). Products include:
- Synercid I.V. **1690**

Ranitidine Bismuth Citrate (Inhibitors of CYP3A4 or CYP2D6 can inhibit aripiprazole elimination and cause increased blood levels).
- No products indexed under this heading.

Ranitidine Hydrochloride (Inhibitors of CYP3A4 or CYP2D6 can inhibit aripiprazole elimination and cause increased blood levels). Products include:
- Zantac **1597**
- Zantac Injection **1593**
- Zantac 75 Tablets .... ▣**715**
- Zantac 150 Maximum Strength Tablets .... ▣**715**
- Zantac Injection Pharmacy Bulk Package **1595**

Rifabutin (Agents that induce CYP3A4 could cause an increase in aripiprazole clearance and lower blood levels).
- No products indexed under this heading.

Rifampicin (Agents that induce CYP3A4 could cause an increase in aripiprazole clearance and lower blood levels).
- No products indexed under this heading.

Rifampin (Agents that induce CYP3A4 could cause an increase in aripiprazole clearance and lower blood levels).
- No products indexed under this heading.

Rifapentine (Agents that induce CYP3A4 could cause an increase in aripiprazole clearance and lower blood levels).
- No products indexed under this heading.

Ritonavir (Inhibitors of CYP3A4 or CYP2D6 can inhibit aripiprazole elimination and cause increased blood levels). Products include:
- Kaletra **474**
- Norvir **499**

Saquinavir (Inhibitors of CYP3A4 or CYP2D6 can inhibit aripiprazole elimination and cause increased blood levels).
- No products indexed under this heading.

Saquinavir Mesylate (Inhibitors of CYP3A4 or CYP2D6 can inhibit aripiprazole elimination and cause increased blood levels). Products include:
- Invirase **2776**

Sertraline Hydrochloride (Inhibitors of CYP3A4 or CYP2D6 can inhibit aripiprazole elimination and cause increased blood levels). Products include:
- Zoloft **2581**

Sulfinpyrazone (Agents that induce CYP3A4 could cause an increase in aripiprazole clearance and lower blood levels).
- No products indexed under this heading.

Telithromycin (Inhibitors of CYP3A4 or CYP2D6 can inhibit aripiprazole elimination and cause increased blood levels). Products include:
- Ketek Tablets **2920**

Terbinafine Hydrochloride (Inhibitors of CYP3A4 or CYP2D6 can inhibit aripiprazole elimination and cause increased blood levels). Products include:
- Lamisil [AT] Creams (Athlete's Foot & Jock Itch) .... ▣**676**
- Lamisil Tablets **2226**

Theophylline (Agents that induce CYP3A4 could cause an increase in aripiprazole clearance and lower blood levels).
- No products indexed under this heading.

Thioridazine Hydrochloride (Inhibitors of CYP3A4 or CYP2D6 can inhibit aripiprazole elimination and cause increased blood levels). Products include:
- Thioridazine Hydrochloride Tablets **2122**

Triamcinolone (Agents that induce CYP3A4 could cause an increase in aripiprazole clearance and lower blood levels).
- No products indexed under this heading.

Triamcinolone Acetonide (Agents that induce CYP3A4 could cause an increase in aripiprazole clearance and lower blood levels). Products include:
- Azmacort Inhalation Aerosol **1701**
- Nasacort HFA Inhalation Aerosol **2939**
- Nasacort AQ Nasal Spray **2937**

Triamcinolone Diacetate (Agents that induce CYP3A4 could cause an increase in aripiprazole clearance and lower blood levels).
- No products indexed under this heading.

Triamcinolone Hexacetonide (Agents that induce CYP3A4 could cause an increase in aripiprazole clearance and lower blood levels).
- No products indexed under this heading.

Trimipramine Maleate (Inhibitors of CYP3A4 or CYP2D6 can inhibit aripiprazole elimination and cause increased blood levels). Products include:
- Surmontil Capsules **2347**

Troglitazone (Agents that induce CYP3A4 could cause an increase in aripiprazole clearance and lower blood levels).
- No products indexed under this heading.

Troleandomycin (Inhibitors of CYP3A4 or CYP2D6 can inhibit aripiprazole elimination and cause increased blood levels).
- No products indexed under this heading.

Valproate Sodium (Inhibitors of CYP3A4 or CYP2D6 can inhibit aripiprazole elimination and cause increased blood levels). Products include:
- Depacon Injection **412**

Verapamil Hydrochloride (Inhibitors of CYP3A4 or CYP2D6 can inhibit aripiprazole elimination and cause increased blood levels). Products include:
- Covera-HS Tablets **3135**
- Tarka Tablets **519**
- Verelan PM Capsules **3120**

Voriconazole (Inhibitors of CYP3A4 or CYP2D6 can inhibit aripiprazole elimination and cause increased blood levels). Products include:
- VFEND I.V. **2543**
- VFEND Oral Suspension **2543**
- VFEND Tablets **2543**

Zafirlukast (Inhibitors of CYP3A4 or CYP2D6 can inhibit aripiprazole elimination and cause increased blood levels). Products include:
- Accolate Tablets **663**

Zileuton (Inhibitors of CYP3A4 or CYP2D6 can inhibit aripiprazole elimination and cause increased blood levels).
- No products indexed under this heading.

Food Interactions

Grapefruit (Inhibitors of CYP3A4 or CYP2D6 can inhibit aripiprazole elimination and cause increased blood levels).

Grapefruit Juice (Inhibitors of CYP3A4 or CYP2D6 can inhibit aripiprazole elimination and cause increased blood levels).

ABREVA CREAM

(Docosanol) .... ▣**612**

None cited in PDR database.

ACCOLATE TABLETS

(Zafirlukast) **663**

May interact with dihydropyridine calcium channel blockers, erythromycin, phenytoin, xanthines, and certain other agents. Compounds in these categories include:

Aminophylline (Rare cases of patients experiencing increased theophylline levels with or without clinical signs or symptoms of theophylline toxicity after addition of zafirlukast to an existing theophylline regimen have been reported; co-administration with liquid theophylline products has resulted in a decrease in the mean plasma levels of zafirlukast by approximately 30%).
- No products indexed under this heading.

Amlodipine Besylate (Zafirlukast is a known inhibitor of CYP3A4 in vitro; co-administration with other drugs known to be metabolized by this isoenzyme, such as dihydropyridine calcium channel blockers, should be undertaken with reasonable clinical monitoring; no formal interaction studies have been conducted). Products include:
- Caduet Tablets **2507**
- Lotrel Capsules **2238**
- Norvasc Tablets **2529**

Aspirin (Co-administration has resulted in mean increased plasma levels of zafirlukast by approximately 45%). Products include:
- Aggrenox Capsules **855**
- Bayer, Aspirin Regimen .... ▣**606**
- Bayer Aspirin Tablets **3515**
- BC Powder .... ▣**612**
- BC Allergy Sinus Cold Powder .... ▣**612**
- Arthritis Strength BC Powder .... ▣**612**
- BC Sinus Cold Powder .... ▣**612**
- Ecotrin Enteric Coated Aspirin Low, Regular and Maximum Strength Tablets **1627**
- Goody's Body Pain Formula Powder .... ▣**621**
- Goody's Extra Strength Headache Powder .... ▣**621**
- Goody's Extra Strength Pain Relief Tablets .... ▣**621**
- Percodan Tablets **1115**
- St. Joseph 81 mg Aspirin Chewable and Enteric Coated Tablets **1841**

Astemizole (Zafirlukast is a known inhibitor of CYP3A4 in vitro; co-administration with other drugs known to be metabolized by this isoenzyme, such as astemizole, should be undertaken with reasonable clinical monitoring; no formal interaction studies have been conducted).
- No products indexed under this heading.

Carbamazepine (Zafirlukast is a known inhibitor of the cytochrome P4502C9 isoenzyme; co-administration with other drugs known to be metabolized by this isoenzyme, such as carbamazepine, should be undertaken with caution; no formal interaction studies have been conducted). Products include:
- Carbatrol Capsules **3174**
- Equetro Extended-Release Capsules **3178**
- Tegretol/Tegretol-XR **2278**

Cisapride (Zafirlukast is a known inhibitor of CYP3A4 in vitro; co-administration with other drugs known to be metabolized by this isoenzyme, such as cisapride, should be undertaken with reasonable clinical monitoring; no formal interaction studies have been conducted).
- No products indexed under this heading.

Cyclosporine (Zafirlukast is a known inhibitor of CYP3A4 in vitro; co-administration with other drugs known to be metabolized by this isoenzyme, such as cyclosporine, should be undertaken with reasonable clinical monitoring; no formal interaction studies have been conducted). Products include:
- Gengraf Capsules **458**
- Neoral Soft Gelatin Capsules **2247**
- Neoral Oral Solution **2247**
- Restasis Ophthalmic Emulsion **570**
- Sandimmune **2259**

Dyphylline (Rare cases of patients experiencing increased theophylline levels with or without clinical signs or symptoms of theophylline toxicity after addition of zafirlukast to an existing theophylline regimen have been reported; co-administration with liquid theophylline products has resulted in a decrease in the mean plasma levels of zafirlukast by approximately 30%).
- No products indexed under this heading.

Erythromycin (Co-administration results in a decrease in the mean plasma levels of zafirlukast by approximately 40% due to decrease in zafirlukast bioavailability). Products include:
- Erygel Topical Gel **2096**
- Ery-Tab Tablets **447**
- Erythromycin Base Filmtab Tablets **454**
- Erythromycin Delayed-Release Capsules, USP **456**
- PCE Dispertab Tablets **510**

Erythromycin Estolate (Co-administration results in a decrease in the mean plasma levels of zafirlukast by approximately 40% due to decrease in zafirlukast bioavailability).
- No products indexed under this heading.

Erythromycin Ethylsuccinate (Co-administration results in a decrease in the mean plasma levels of zafirlukast by approximately 40% due to decrease in zafirlukast bioavailability). Products include:
- E.E.S. **449**

EryPed **445**

Erythromycin Gluceptate (Co-administration results in a decrease in the mean plasma levels of zafirlukast by approximately 40% due to decrease in zafirlukast bioavailability).
No products indexed under this heading.

Erythromycin Lactobionate (Co-administration results in a decrease in the mean plasma levels of zafirlukast by approximately 40% due to decrease in zafirlukast bioavailability).
No products indexed under this heading.

Erythromycin Stearate (Co-administration results in a decrease in the mean plasma levels of zafirlukast by approximately 40% due to decrease in zafirlukast bio-availability). Products include:
Erythrocin Stearate Filmtab Tablets **452**

Felodipine (Zafirlukast is a known inhibitor of CYP3A4 in vitro; co-administration with other drugs known to be metabolized by this iso-enzyme, such as dihydropyridine calcium channel blockers, should be undertaken with reasonable clinical monitoring; no formal interaction studies have been conducted). Products include:
Plendil Extended-Release Tablets **651**

Fosphenytoin Sodium (Zafirlukast is a known inhibitor of the cyto-chrome P4502C9 isoenzyme; co-administration with other drugs known to be metabolized by this iso-enzyme, such as phenytoin, should be undertaken with caution; no for-mal interaction studies have been conducted).
No products indexed under this heading.

Isradipine (Zafirlukast is a known inhibitor of CYP3A4 in vitro; co-administration with other drugs known to be metabolized by this iso-enzyme, such as dihydropyridine calcium channel blockers, should be undertaken with reasonable clinical monitoring; no formal interaction studies have been conducted). Products include:
DynaCirc CR Tablets **2726**

Nicardipine Hydrochloride (Zafirlukast is a known inhibitor of CYP3A4 in vitro; co-administration with other drugs known to be metab-olized by this isoenzyme, such as dihydropyridine calcium channel blockers, should be undertaken with reasonable clinical monitoring; no formal interaction studies have been conducted). Products include:
Cardene I.V. **1129**

Nifedipine (Zafirlukast is a known inhibitor of CYP3A4 in vitro; co-administration with other drugs known to be metabolized by this iso-enzyme, such as dihydropyridine calcium channel blockers, should be undertaken with reasonable clinical monitoring; no formal interaction studies have been conducted). Products include:
Adalat CC Tablets **2978**

Nimodipine (Zafirlukast is a known inhibitor of CYP3A4 in vitro; co-administration with other drugs known to be metabolized by this iso-enzyme, such as dihydropyridine calcium channel blockers, should be undertaken with reasonable clinical monitoring; no formal interaction studies have been conducted). Products include:
Nimotop Capsules **774**

Phenytoin (Zafirlukast is a known inhibitor of the cytochrome P4502C9 isoenzyme; co-administration with other drugs known to be metabolized by this iso-enzyme, such as phenytoin, should be undertaken with caution; no for-mal interaction studies have been conducted).
No products indexed under this heading.

Phenytoin Sodium (Zafirlukast is a known inhibitor of the cytochrome P4502C9 isoenzyme; co-administration with other drugs known to be metabolized by this iso-enzyme, such as phenytoin, should be undertaken with caution; no for-mal interaction studies have been conducted). Products include:
Phenytek Capsules **2153**

Terfenadine (Co-administration results in a decrease in the mean Cmax (66%) and AUC (54%) of zafirlukast; no effect of zafirlukast on terfenadine plasma concentrations or ECG parameters).
No products indexed under this heading.

Theophylline (Rare cases of patients experiencing increased the-ophylline levels with or without clini-cal signs or symptoms of theophyl-line toxicity after addition of zafirlukast to an existing theophylline regimen have been reported; co-administration with liquid theophylline products has resulted in a decrease in the mean plasma levels of zafirlukast by approximately 30%).
No products indexed under this heading.

Theophylline Anhydrous (Rare cases of patients experiencing increased theophylline levels with or without clinical signs or symptoms of theophylline toxicity after addition of zafirlukast to an existing theophylline regimen have been reported; co-administration with liquid theophylline products has resulted in a decrease in the mean plasma levels of zafirlukast by approximately 30%). Products include:
Uniphyl Tablets **2708**

Theophylline Calcium Salicylate (Rare cases of patients experiencing increased theophylline levels with or without clinical signs or symptoms of theophylline toxicity after addition of zafirlukast to an existing theophylline regimen have been reported; co-administration with liquid theophylline products has resulted in a decrease in the mean plasma levels of zafirlukast by approximately 30%).
No products indexed under this heading.

Theophylline Dihydroxypropyl (Glyceryl) (Rare cases of patients experiencing increased theophylline levels with or without clinical signs or symptoms of theophylline toxicity after addition of zafirlukast to an existing theophylline regimen have been reported; co-administration with liquid theophylline products has resulted in a decrease in the mean plasma levels of zafirlukast by approximately 30%).
No products indexed under this heading.

Theophylline Ethylenediamine (Rare cases of patients experiencing increased theophylline levels with or without clinical signs or symptoms of theophylline toxicity after addition of zafirlukast to an existing theophylline regimen have been reported; co-administration with liquid theophylline products has resulted in a decrease in the mean plasma levels of zafirlukast by approximately 30%).
No products indexed under this heading.

Theophylline Sodium Glycinate (Rare cases of patients experiencing increased theophylline levels with or without clinical signs or symptoms of theophylline toxicity after addition of zafirlukast to an existing theophylline regimen have been reported; co-administration with liquid theophylline products has resulted in a decrease in the mean plasma levels of zafirlukast by approximately 30%).
No products indexed under this heading.

Tolbutamide (Zafirlukast is a known inhibitor of the cytochrome P4502C9 isoenzyme; co-administration with other drugs known to be metabolized by this iso-enzyme, such as tolbutamide, should be undertaken with caution; no formal interaction studies have been conducted).
No products indexed under this heading.

Warfarin Sodium (Co-administration results in a significant increase in the mean AUC and half-life of S-warfarin producing a clinical-ly significant increase in prothrombin time). Products include:
Coumadin for Injection **932**
Coumadin Tablets **932**

Food Interactions

Food, unspecified (Co-administration with food reduces mean bioavailability by approximately 40%; patients should be instructed to take Accolate at least 1 hour before or 2 hours after meals).

ACCUNEB INHALATION SOLUTION

(Albuterol Sulfate) **1055**

May interact with beta blockers, monoamine oxidase inhibitors, po-tassium-depleting diuretics, sym-pathomimetics, tricyclic antidepres-sants, and certain other agents. Compounds in these categories in-clude:

Acebutolol Hydrochloride (Co-administration with beta blockers inhibits the effects of each other).
No products indexed under this heading.

Albuterol (Co-administration with other sympathomimetic agents increases the risk of adverse cardio-vascular effects). Products include:
Proventil Inhalation Aerosol **3067**

Amitriptyline Hydrochloride (Co-administration with tricyclic antide-pressants can potentiate the action of albuterol on the cardiovascular system).
No products indexed under this heading.

Amoxapine (Co-administration with tricyclic antidepressants can potenti-ate the action of albuterol on the cardiovascular system).
No products indexed under this heading.

Atenolol (Co-administration with beta blockers inhibits the effects of each other). Products include:
Tenormin I.V. Injection **698**
Tenormin Tablets **695**

Bendroflumethiazide (Co-administration with non-potassium sparing diuretics can result in acute worsening of ECG changes and/or hypokalemia, especially when recom-mended dose of the beta agonist is exceeded; clinical significance of this interaction is unknown).
No products indexed under this heading.

Betaxolol Hydrochloride (Co-administration with beta blockers inhibits the effects of each other). Products include:
Betoptic S Ophthalmic Suspension.................................. **554**

Bisoprolol Fumarate (Co-administration with beta blockers inhibits the effects of each other).
No products indexed under this heading.

Bumetanide (Co-administration with non-potassium sparing diuretics can result in acute worsening of ECG changes and/or hypokalemia, espe-cially when recommended dose of the beta agonist is exceeded; clinical significance of this interaction is unknown).
No products indexed under this heading.

Carteolol Hydrochloride (Co-administration with beta blockers inhibits the effects of each other). Products include:
Carteolol Hydrochloride Ophthalmic Solution USP, 1%....... ⊙**246**

Chlorothiazide (Co-administration with non-potassium sparing diuretics can result in acute worsening of ECG changes and/or hypokalemia, espe-cially when recommended dose of the beta agonist is exceeded; clinical significance of this interaction is unknown). Products include:
Aldoclor Tablets **1881**
Diuril Oral **1936**

Chlorothiazide Sodium (Co-administration with non-potassium sparing diuretics can result in acute worsening of ECG changes and/or hypokalemia, especially when recom-mended dose of the beta agonist is exceeded; clinical significance of this interaction is unknown). Products include:
Diuril Sodium Intravenous **1934**

Clomipramine Hydrochloride (Co-administration with tricyclic anti-depressants can potentiate the action of albuterol on the cardiovas-cular system).
No products indexed under this heading.

Desipramine Hydrochloride (Co-administration with tricyclic antide-pressants can potentiate the action of albuterol on the cardiovascular system).
No products indexed under this heading.

Digoxin (Mean decreases of 16% to 22% in serum digoxin levels were demonstrated after single dose IV and oral albuterol, respectively; the clinical significance of this interac-tion is unknown). Products include:
Digitek Tablets **2146**
Lanoxicaps Capsules **1458**
Lanoxin Injection **1462**
Lanoxin Tablets **1468**
Lanoxin Injection Pediatric **1465**

Dobutamine Hydrochloride (Co-administration with other sympathomimetic agents increases the risk of adverse cardiovascular effects).
No products indexed under this heading.

Dopamine Hydrochloride (Co-administration with other sympathomimetic agents increases the risk of adverse cardiovascular effects).
No products indexed under this heading.

Doxepin Hydrochloride (Co-administration with tricyclic antidepressants can potentiate the action of albuterol on the cardiovascular system).
No products indexed under this heading.

Ephedrine Hydrochloride (Co-administration with other sympathomimetic agents increases the risk of adverse cardiovascular effects).
Products include:
Primatene Tablets .... ▣749

Ephedrine Sulfate (Co-administration with other sympathomimetic agents increases the risk of adverse cardiovascular effects).
No products indexed under this heading.

Ephedrine Tannate (Co-administration with other sympathomimetic agents increases the risk of adverse cardiovascular effects).
No products indexed under this heading.

Epinephrine (Co-administration with other sympathomimetic agents increases the risk of adverse cardiovascular effects). Products include:
EpiPen 1061
Primatene Mist .... ▣749

Epinephrine Bitartrate (Co-administration with other sympathomimetic agents increases the risk of adverse cardiovascular effects).
No products indexed under this heading.

Epinephrine Hydrochloride (Co-administration with other sympathomimetic agents increases the risk of adverse cardiovascular effects).
No products indexed under this heading.

Esmolol Hydrochloride (Co-administration with beta blockers inhibits the effects of each other).
Products include:
Brevibloc Concentrate 766
Brevibloc Injection 766
Brevibloc Double Strength Injection.................................... 766
Brevibloc Premixed Injection 766
Brevibloc Double Strength Premixed Injection 766

Ethacrynic Acid (Co-administration with non-potassium sparing diuretics can result in acute worsening of ECG changes and/or hypokalemia, especially when recommended dose of the beta agonist is exceeded; clinical significance of this interaction is unknown). Products include:
Edecrin Tablets 1941

Furosemide (Co-administration with non-potassium sparing diuretics can result in acute worsening of ECG changes and/or hypokalemia, especially when recommended dose of the beta agonist is exceeded; clinical significance of this interaction is unknown). Products include:
Furosemide Tablets 2117

Hydrochlorothiazide (Co-administration with non-potassium sparing diuretics can result in acute worsening of ECG changes and/or hypokalemia, especially when recommended dose of the beta agonist is exceeded; clinical significance of this interaction is unknown).
Products include:
Aldoril Tablets 1884
Atacand HCT 637
Avalide Tablets 2889
Avalide Tablets 922
Benicar HCT Tablets 2852
Diovan HCT Tablets 2195
Dyazide Capsules 1389
Hyzaar 1964
Lotensin HCT Tablets 2235
Maxzide 2150
Micardis HCT Tablets 886
Moduretic Tablets 2003
Prinzide Tablets 2033
Teveten HCT Tablets 1710
Timolide Tablets 2056
Uniretic Tablets 3114
Vaseretic Tablets 2073
Zestoretic Tablets 701

Hydroflumethiazide (Co-administration with non-potassium sparing diuretics can result in acute worsening of ECG changes and/or hypokalemia, especially when recommended dose of the beta agonist is exceeded; clinical significance of this interaction is unknown).
No products indexed under this heading.

Imipramine Hydrochloride (Co-administration with tricyclic antidepressants can potentiate the action of albuterol on the cardiovascular system).
No products indexed under this heading.

Imipramine Pamoate (Co-administration with tricyclic antidepressants can potentiate the action of albuterol on the cardiovascular system).
No products indexed under this heading.

Isocarboxazid (Co-administration with MAO inhibitors can potentiate the action of albuterol on the cardiovascular system).
No products indexed under this heading.

Isoproterenol Hydrochloride (Co-administration with other sympathomimetic agents increases the risk of adverse cardiovascular effects).
No products indexed under this heading.

Isoproterenol Sulfate (Co-administration with other sympathomimetic agents increases the risk of adverse cardiovascular effects).
No products indexed under this heading.

Labetalol Hydrochloride (Co-administration with beta blockers inhibits the effects of each other).
No products indexed under this heading.

Levalbuterol Hydrochloride (Co-administration with other sympathomimetic agents increases the risk of adverse cardiovascular effects).
Products include:
Xopenex Inhalation Solution 3143
Xopenex Inhalation Solution Concentrate 3147

Levobunolol Hydrochloride (Co-administration with beta blockers inhibits the effects of each other).
Products include:
Betagan Ophthalmic Solution, USP.. ⊙217

Maprotiline Hydrochloride (Co-administration with tricyclic antidepressants can potentiate the action of albuterol on the cardiovascular system).
No products indexed under this heading.

Metaproterenol Sulfate (Co-administration with other sympathomimetic agents increases the risk of adverse cardiovascular effects).
Products include:
Alupent Inhalation Aerosol 858

Metaraminol Bitartrate (Co-administration with other sympathomimetic agents increases the risk of adverse cardiovascular effects).
Products include:
Aramine Injection 1889

Methoxamine Hydrochloride (Co-administration with other sympathomimetic agents increases the risk of adverse cardiovascular effects).
No products indexed under this heading.

Methyclothiazide (Co-administration with non-potassium sparing diuretics can result in acute worsening of ECG changes and/or hypokalemia, especially when recommended dose of the beta agonist is exceeded; clinical significance of this interaction is unknown).
No products indexed under this heading.

Metipranolol Hydrochloride (Co-administration with beta blockers inhibits the effects of each other).
No products indexed under this heading.

Metoprolol Succinate (Co-administration with beta blockers inhibits the effects of each other).
Products include:
Toprol-XL Tablets 660

Metoprolol Tartrate (Co-administration with beta blockers inhibits the effects of each other).
No products indexed under this heading.

Moclobemide (Co-administration with MAO inhibitors can potentiate the action of albuterol on the cardiovascular system).
No products indexed under this heading.

Nadolol (Co-administration with beta blockers inhibits the effects of each other). Products include:
Nadolol Tablets 2121

Norepinephrine Bitartrate (Co-administration with other sympathomimetic agents increases the risk of adverse cardiovascular effects).
No products indexed under this heading.

Nortriptyline Hydrochloride (Co-administration with tricyclic antidepressants can potentiate the action of albuterol on the cardiovascular system).
No products indexed under this heading.

Pargyline Hydrochloride (Co-administration with MAO inhibitors can potentiate the action of albuterol on the cardiovascular system).
No products indexed under this heading.

Penbutolol Sulfate (Co-administration with beta blockers inhibits the effects of each other).
No products indexed under this heading.

Phenelzine Sulfate (Co-administration with MAO inhibitors can potentiate the action of albuterol on the cardiovascular system).
No products indexed under this heading.

Phenylephrine Bitartrate (Co-administration with other sympathomimetic agents increases the risk of adverse cardiovascular effects).
No products indexed under this heading.

Phenylephrine Hydrochloride (Co-administration with other sympathomimetic agents increases the risk of adverse cardiovascular effects).
Products include:
Alacol DM Syrup 739
Hycomine Compound Tablets 1105
Preparation H Maximum Strength Cream .... ▣747
Preparation H Cooling Gel .... ▣747
Preparation H .... ▣747
Sudafed PE Tablets .... ▣711
Vicks Sinex Nasal Spray and Ultra Fine Mist for Sinus Relief.............. 2677
Zicam Concentrated Cough Mist for Kids Plus D Cool Cherry......... ▣643
Zicam Concentrated Cough Mist Plus D Cool Cherry..................... ▣642

Phenylephrine Tannate (Co-administration with other sympathomimetic agents increases the risk of adverse cardiovascular effects).
No products indexed under this heading.

Phenylpropanolamine Hydrochloride (Co-administration with other sympathomimetic agents increases the risk of adverse cardiovascular effects).
No products indexed under this heading.

Pindolol (Co-administration with beta blockers inhibits the effects of each other).
No products indexed under this heading.

Pirbuterol Acetate (Co-administration with other sympathomimetic agents increases the risk of adverse cardiovascular effects).
Products include:
Maxair Autohaler 1820

Polythiazide (Co-administration with non-potassium sparing diuretics can result in acute worsening of ECG changes and/or hypokalemia, especially when recommended dose of the beta agonist is exceeded; clinical significance of this interaction is unknown).
No products indexed under this heading.

Procarbazine Hydrochloride (Co-administration with MAO inhibitors can potentiate the action of albuterol on the cardiovascular system).
Products include:
Matulane Capsules 3188

Propranolol Hydrochloride (Co-administration with beta blockers inhibits the effects of each other).
Products include:
Inderal LA Long-Acting Capsules 3421
InnoPran XL Capsules 2728

Protriptyline Hydrochloride (Co-administration with tricyclic antidepressants can potentiate the action of albuterol on the cardiovascular system). Products include:
Vivactil Tablets 2350

Pseudoephedrine Hydrochloride (Co-administration with other sympathomimetic agents increases the risk of adverse cardiovascular effects).
Products include:

Advil Allergy Sinus Caplets 737
Advil Cold & Sinus 739
Advil Flu & Body Ache Caplets 739
Children's Advil Cold Suspension ... 741
Advil Multi-Symptom Cold Caplets 738
Allegra-D 12 Hour Extended-Release Tablets 2860
Allegra-D 24 Hour Extended-Release Tablets 2862
Balamine DM 739
BC Cold Powder 612
Benadryl Allergy & Cold Tablets 692
Benadryl Allergy & Sinus Headache Caplets & Gelcaps 693
Children's Benadryl Allergy & Cold Fastmelt Tablets 695
Benadryl Maximum Strength Severe Allergy & Sinus Headache Caplets 694
Children's Benadryl D Allergy & Sinus Fastmelt Tablets 694
Children's Benadryl D Liquid Medication 693
Benadryl D Tablets 694
Contac Non-Drowsy 12 Hour Cold Caplets 614
Contac Non-Drowsy Timed Release 12 Hour Cold Caplets 615
Contac Severe Cold and Flu Caplets Maximum Strength 615
Contac Severe Cold and Flu Caplets Non-Drowsy 615
Children's Dimetapp Cold & Allergy Elixir 745
Children's Dimetapp DM Cold & Cough Elixir 745
Children's Dimetapp Long Acting Cough Plus Cold Syrup 746
Dimetapp Infant Drops Decongestant Plus Cough 746
Children's Motrin Cold Non-Staining Dye-Free Oral Suspension 1838
Children's Motrin Cold Oral Suspension 1838
Motrin Cold & Sinus Caplets 1836
PediaCare Decongestant & Cough Infant Drops 705
PediaCare Decongestant Infants' Drops 705
PediaCare Long-Acting Cough Plus Cold Liquid 704
PediaCare Multi-Symptom Cold Liquid 704
PediaCare NightRest Cough & Cold Liquid 704
Robitussin Allergy & Cough Syrup .. 750
Robitussin CF Liquid 755
Robitussin Cough & Cold Liquid-filled Capsules 750
Robitussin Cough, Cold & Flu Liquid-filled Capsules 750
Robitussin Cough & Cold Infant Drops 755
Robitussin Flu Liquid 752
Robitussin Maximum Strength Cough & Cold Liquid 754
Robitussin PE Syrup 753
Robitussin Pediatric Cough & Cold Liquid 754
Robitussin PM Cough & Cold Liquid 752
Robitussin Severe Congestion Liquid-filled Capsules 751
Simply Stuffy Liquid 1841
Singlet Caplets 636
Sudafed 12 Hour Caplets 708
Sudafed 24 Hour Tablets 709
Sudafed Nasal Decongestant Tablets 709
Sudafed Severe Cold 710
Sudafed Non-Drying Sinus Liquid Caps 709
Sudafed Sinus & Allergy Tablets 710
Sudafed Sinus Headache 711
TheraFlu Cold & Cough Hot Liquid 680
TheraFlu Cold & Sore Throat Hot Liquid 680
TheraFlu Flu & Chest Congestion Non-Drowsy Hot Liquid 681
TheraFlu Flu & Sore Throat Hot Liquid 681
TheraFlu Severe Cold Non-Drowsy Hot Liquid 683
TheraFlu Severe Cold & Cough Hot Liquid 683
TheraFlu Severe Cold Caplets 679
TheraFlu Severe Cold Hot Liquid 682
TheraFlu Severe Cold Non-Drowsy Caplets 679
Triaminic Chest & Nasal Congestion Liquid 685
Triaminic Cold & Allergy Liquid 685
Triaminic Cold & Cough Liquid 685
Triaminic Cough Liquid 687
Triaminic Cough & Nasal Congestion Liquid 687
Triaminic Cough & Sore Throat Liquid 687
Triaminic Flu, Cough & Fever Liquid 685
Triaminic Night Time Cough & Cold Liquid 685
Triaminic Allergy Runny Nose & Congestion Softchews 688
Triaminic Cold & Cough Softchews 688
Triaminic Cough & Sore Throat Softchews 689
Tylenol Sinus NightTime Caplets 663
Children's Tylenol Plus Cold & Allergy Suspension Liquid 1850
Children's Tylenol Plus Cold NightTime Suspension Liquid 1851
Children's Tylenol Plus Cold & Cough Suspension Liquid and Chewable Tablets 1851
Children's Tylenol Plus Cold Chewable Tablets 1851
Children's Tylenol Plus Cold Daytime Non-Drowsy Suspension Liquid 1851
Children's Tylenol Plus Flu Suspension Liquid 1853
Concentrated Tylenol Infants' Drops Plus Cold 1851
Concentrated Tylenol Infants' Drops Plus Cold and Cough 1851
Tylenol Cold & Flu Severe Daytime Liquid with Cool Bust 1846
Tylenol Cold & Flu Severe NightTime Liquid with Cool Burst 1846
Tylenol Cold Severe Congestion Non-Drowsy Caplets with Cool Burst 1846
Tylenol Allergy Complete Night Time Caplets 1844
Tylenol Allergy Complete Multi-Symptom Caplets and Gelcaps with Cool Burst 1844
Tylenol Flu NightTime Gelcaps 1846
Tylenol Flu Day Non-Drowsy Gelcaps 1846
Concentrated Tylenol Infants' Drops Plus Cold Nasal Congestant, Fever Reducer & Pain Reliever 668
Concentrated Tylenol Infants' Drops Plus Cold & Cough Nasal Decongestant, Fever Reducer & Pain Reliever 668
Multi-Symptom Tylenol Cold Night Time Caplets 1845
Multi-Symptom Tylenol Cold Day Non-Drowsy Caplets and Gelcaps 1845
Tylenol Sinus Day Non-Drowsy 1848
Tylenol Sinus Night Time Caplets 1848
Tylenol Sinus Severe Congestion Caplets with Cool Burst 1848
Vicks 44D Cough & Head Congestion Relief 2676
Vicks 44D Cough & Head Congestion Relief Liquid 721
Vicks 44M Cough, Cold & Flu Relief 2676
Pediatric Vicks 44m Cough & Cold Relief 2673
Vicks DayQuil LiquiCaps/Liquid Multi-Symptom Cold/Flu Relief..... 723
Vicks DayQuil Multi-Symptom Cold/Flu Relief LiquiCaps 2675
Vicks DayQuil Multi-Symptom Cold/Flu Relief Liquid 2675
Children's Vicks NyQuil Cold/Cough Relief 2671
Vicks NyQuil LiquiCaps 2677
Vicks NyQuil LiquiCaps/Liquid Multi-Symptom Cold/Flu Relief..... 725
Vicks NyQuil Liquid 2677
Zyrtec-D 12 Hour Extended Release Tablets 2591

Pseudoephedrine Sulfate (Co-administration with other sympathomimetic agents increases the risk of adverse cardiovascular effects). Products include:

Alavert Allergy & Sinus D-12 Hour Tablets 743
Clarinex-D 24-Hour Extended-Release Tablets 3012
Claritin-D Non-Drowsy 12 Hour Tablets 731
Claritin-D Non-Drowsy 24 Hour Tablets 731

Salmeterol Xinafoate (Co-administration with other sympathomimetic agents increases the risk of adverse cardiovascular effects). Products include:

Advair Diskus 100/50 1291
Advair Diskus 250/50 1291
Advair Diskus 500/50 1291
Serevent Diskus 1540

Selegiline Hydrochloride (Co-administration with MAO inhibitors can potentiate the action of albuterol on the cardiovascular system). Products include:

Eldepryl Capsules 3209

Sotalol Hydrochloride (Co-administration with beta blockers inhibits the effects of each other).

No products indexed under this heading.

Terbutaline Sulfate (Co-administration with other sympathomimetic agents increases the risk of adverse cardiovascular effects).

No products indexed under this heading.

Timolol Hemihydrate (Co-administration with beta blockers inhibits the effects of each other). Products include:

Betimol Ophthalmic Solution 3371
Betimol Ophthalmic Solution .... ⊙283

Timolol Maleate (Co-administration with beta blockers inhibits the effects of each other). Products include:

Blocadren Tablets 1891
Cosopt Sterile Ophthalmic Solution 1910
Timolide Tablets 2056
Timoptic in Ocudose 2061
Timoptic Sterile Ophthalmic Solution 2058
Timoptic-XE Sterile Ophthalmic Gel Forming Solution 2062

Torsemide (Co-administration with non-potassium sparing diuretics can result in acute worsening of ECG changes and/or hypokalemia, especially when recommended dose of the beta agonist is exceeded; clinical significance of this interaction is unknown).

No products indexed under this heading.

Tranylcypromine Sulfate (Co-administration with MAO inhibitors can potentiate the action of albuterol on the cardiovascular system). Products include:

Parnate Tablets 1499

Trimipramine Maleate (Co-administration with tricyclic antidepressants can potentiate the action of albuterol on the cardiovascular system). Products include:

Surmontil Capsules 2347

ACCUTANE CAPSULES

(Isotretinoin) 2740

May interact with corticosteroids, phenytoin, tetracyclines, and certain other agents. Compounds in these categories include:

Betamethasone Acetate (Systemic corticosteroids are known to cause osteoporosis; caution is advised if used concurrently because of potential interactive effect on bone loss between systemic corticosteroids and Accutane).

No products indexed under this heading.

Betamethasone Sodium Phosphate (Systemic corticosteroids are known to cause osteoporosis; caution is advised if used concurrently because of potential interactive effect on bone loss between systemic corticosteroids and Accutane).

No products indexed under this heading.

Cortisone Acetate (Systemic corticosteroids are known to cause osteoporosis; caution is advised if used concurrently because of potential interactive effect on bone loss between systemic corticosteroids and Accutane).

No products indexed under this heading.

Demeclocycline Hydrochloride (Concomitant treatment with Accutane and tetracyclines should be avoided because Accutane is associated with a number of cases of pseudotumor cerebri, some of which involved concomitant use of tetracyclines).

No products indexed under this heading.

Dexamethasone (Systemic corticosteroids are known to cause osteoporosis; caution is advised if used concurrently because of potential interactive effect on bone loss between systemic corticosteroids and Accutane). Products include:

Ciprodex Otic Suspension 555
Decadron Tablets 1929
TobraDex Ophthalmic Ointment 558
TobraDex Ophthalmic Suspension ... 558

Dexamethasone Acetate (Systemic corticosteroids are known to cause osteoporosis; caution is advised if used concurrently because of potential interactive effect on bone loss between systemic corticosteroids and Accutane).

No products indexed under this heading.

Dexamethasone Sodium Phosphate (Systemic corticosteroids are known to cause osteoporosis; caution is advised if used concurrently because of potential interactive effect on bone loss between systemic corticosteroids and Accutane). Products include:

Decadron Phosphate Injection 1931

Doxycycline Calcium (Concomitant treatment with Accutane and tetracyclines should be avoided because Accutane is associated with a number of cases of pseudotumor cerebri, some of which involved concomitant use of tetracyclines).

No products indexed under this heading.

Doxycycline Hyclate (Concomitant treatment with Accutane and tetracyclines should be avoided because Accutane is associated with a number of cases of pseudotumor cerebri, some of which involved concomitant use of tetracyclines).

No products indexed under this heading.

Doxycycline Monohydrate (Concomitant treatment with Accutane and tetracyclines should be avoided because Accutane is associated with a number of cases of pseudotumor cerebri, some of which involved concomitant use of tetracyclines).

No products indexed under this heading.

Fludrocortisone Acetate (Systemic corticosteroids are known to cause osteoporosis; caution is advised if used concurrently because of potential interactive effect on bone loss between systemic corticosteroids and Accutane).

No products indexed under this heading.

Fosphenytoin Sodium (Phenytoin is known to cause osteomalacia; caution is advised if used concurrently because of potential interactive effect on bone loss between phenytoin and Accutane).

No products indexed under this heading.

Hydrocortisone (Systemic corticosteroids are known to cause osteoporosis; caution is advised if used concurrently because of potential interactive effect on bone loss between systemic corticosteroids and Accutane). Products include:

Cortizone•5 Ointment .... ■699
Cortizone•10 Creme .... ■699
Cortizone•10 Ointment .... ■699
Cortizone•10 Plus Creme .... ■700
Cortizone•10 Maximum Strength Quick Shot Spray........................ ■700
Hydrocortone Tablets 1963
Preparation H Hydrocortisone Cream .... ■748

Hydrocortisone Acetate (Systemic corticosteroids are known to cause osteoporosis; caution is advised if used concurrently because of potential interactive effect on bone loss between systemic corticosteroids and Accutane). Products include:

Analpram-HC 1136
Pramosone 1139
ProctoFoam-HC 3113
Tucks Anti-Itch Ointment .... ■712
U-cort 1% Cream 3289

Hydrocortisone Sodium Phosphate (Systemic corticosteroids are known to cause osteoporosis; caution is advised if used concurrently because of potential interactive effect on bone loss between systemic corticosteroids and Accutane).

No products indexed under this heading.

Hydrocortisone Sodium Succinate (Systemic corticosteroids are known to cause osteoporosis; caution is advised if used concurrently because of potential interactive effect on bone loss between systemic corticosteroids and Accutane).

No products indexed under this heading.

Hypericum (Avoid St. John's Wort due to a possible interaction based on reports of breakthrough bleeding being reported on oral contraceptives shortly after starting St. John's Wort. Pregnancies have been reported by users of combined hormonal contraceptives who also used some form of St. John's Wort).

No products indexed under this heading.

Methacycline Hydrochloride (Concomitant treatment with Accutane and tetracyclines should be avoided because Accutane is associated with a number of cases of pseudotumor cerebri, some of which involved concomitant use of tetracyclines).

No products indexed under this heading.

Methylprednisolone Acetate (Systemic corticosteroids are known to cause osteoporosis; caution is advised if used concurrently because of potential interactive effect on bone loss between systemic corticosteroids and Accutane). Products include:

Depo-Medrol Injectable Suspension 2615
Depo-Medrol Single-Dose Vial 2617

Methylprednisolone Sodium Succinate (Systemic corticosteroids are known to cause osteoporosis; caution is advised if used concurrently because of potential interactive effect on bone loss between systemic corticosteroids and Accutane).

No products indexed under this heading.

Minocycline Hydrochloride (Concomitant treatment with Accutane and tetracyclines should be avoided because Accutane is associated with a number of cases of pseudotumor cerebri, some of which involved concomitant use of tetracyclines). Products include:

Dynacin Tablets 1859

Norethindrone (Microdosed progesterone preparations (minipills) may be an inadequate method of contraception during Accutane therapy). Products include:

Ortho Micronor Tablets 2411

Oxytetracycline Hydrochloride (Concomitant treatment with Accutane and tetracyclines should be avoided because Accutane is associated with a number of cases of pseudotumor cerebri, some of which involved concomitant use of tetracyclines).

No products indexed under this heading.

Phenytoin (Phenytoin is known to cause osteomalacia; caution is advised if used concurrently because of potential interactive effect on bone loss between phenytoin and Accutane).

No products indexed under this heading.

Phenytoin Sodium (Phenytoin is known to cause osteomalacia; caution is advised if used concurrently because of potential interactive effect on bone loss between phenytoin and Accutane). Products include:

Phenytek Capsules 2153

Prednisolone Acetate (Systemic corticosteroids are known to cause osteoporosis; caution is advised if used concurrently because of potential interactive effect on bone loss between systemic corticosteroids and Accutane). Products include:

Blephamide Ophthalmic Ointment 563
Blephamide Ophthalmic Suspension.................................. 564
Poly-Pred Liquifilm Ophthalmic Suspension .... ⊙231
Pred Forte Ophthalmic Suspension .... ⊙233
Pred Mild Sterile Ophthalmic Suspension .... ⊙236
Pred-G Ophthalmic Suspension ...... ⊙234
Pred-G Sterile Ophthalmic Ointment .... ⊙235

Prednisolone Sodium Phosphate (Systemic corticosteroids are known to cause osteoporosis; caution is advised if used concurrently because of potential interactive effect on bone loss between systemic corticosteroids and Accutane). Products include:

Pediapred Oral Solution 3319

Prednisolone Tebutate (Systemic corticosteroids are known to cause osteoporosis; caution is advised if used concurrently because of potential interactive effect on bone loss between systemic corticosteroids and Accutane).

No products indexed under this heading.

Prednisone (Systemic corticosteroids are known to cause osteoporosis; caution is advised if used concurrently because of potential interactive effect on bone loss between systemic corticosteroids and Accutane).

No products indexed under this heading.

Tetracycline Hydrochloride (Concomitant treatment with Accutane and tetracyclines should be avoided because Accutane is associated with a number of cases of pseudotumor cerebri, some of which involved concomitant use of tetracyclines).

No products indexed under this heading.

Triamcinolone (Systemic corticosteroids are known to cause osteoporosis; caution is advised if used concurrently because of potential interactive effect on bone loss between systemic corticosteroids and Accutane).

No products indexed under this heading.

Triamcinolone Acetonide (Systemic corticosteroids are known to cause osteoporosis; caution is advised if used concurrently because of potential interactive effect on bone loss between systemic corticosteroids and Accutane). Products include:

Azmacort Inhalation Aerosol 1701
Nasacort HFA Inhalation Aerosol 2939
Nasacort AQ Nasal Spray 2937

Triamcinolone Diacetate (Systemic corticosteroids are known to cause osteoporosis; caution is advised if used concurrently because of potential interactive effect on bone loss between systemic corticosteroids and Accutane).

No products indexed under this heading.

Triamcinolone Hexacetonide (Systemic corticosteroids are known to cause osteoporosis; caution is advised if used concurrently because of potential interactive effect on bone loss between systemic corticosteroids and Accutane).

No products indexed under this heading.

Vitamin A (Additive Vitamin A toxicity). Products include:

Visutein Capsules 3328

ACCUZYME DEBRIDING OINTMENT

(Papain, Urea) 1636
None cited in PDR database.

ACCUZYME SPRAY

(Papain, Urea) 1637
May interact with:

Heavy metal salts, unspecified (Papain may be inactivated by the salts of heavy metals).

No products indexed under this heading.

Hydrogen Peroxide (May inactivate papain).

No products indexed under this heading.

ACEON TABLETS (2 MG, 4 MG, 8 MG)

(Perindopril Erbumine) 3191
May interact with diuretics, lithium preparations, potassium preparations, potassium sparing diuretics, and certain other agents. Compounds in these categories include:

Amiloride Hydrochloride (Coadministration of perindopril with potassium-sparing diuretics may increase the risk of hyperkalemia). Products include:

Midamor Tablets 2000
Moduretic Tablets 2003

Bendroflumethiazide (Patients on diuretics, and especially those started recently, may occasionally experience an excessive reduction in blood pressure after initiation of perindopril therapy; co-administration has resulted in reduced bioavailability of perindopril).

No products indexed under this heading.

Bumetanide (Patients on diuretics, and especially those started recently, may occasionally experience an excessive reduction in blood pressure after initiation of perindopril therapy; co-administration has resulted in reduced bioavailability of perindopril).

No products indexed under this heading.

Chlorothiazide (Patients on diuretics, and especially those started recently, may occasionally experience an excessive reduction in blood pressure after initiation of perindopril therapy; co-administration has resulted in reduced bioavailability of perindopril). Products include:

Aldoclor Tablets 1881
Diuril Oral 1936

Chlorothiazide Sodium (Patients on diuretics, and especially those started recently, may occasionally experience an excessive reduction in blood pressure after initiation of perindopril therapy; co-administration has resulted in reduced bioavailability of perindopril). Products include:

Diuril Sodium Intravenous 1934

Chlorthalidone (Patients on diuretics, and especially those started recently, may occasionally experience an excessive reduction in blood pressure after initiation of perindopril therapy; co-administration has resulted in reduced bioavailability of perindopril). Products include:

Clorpres Tablets 2139

Cyclosporine (Co-administration of perindopril with other drugs capable of increasing serum potassium, such as cyclosporine, may increase the risk of hyperkalemia). Products include:

Gengraf Capsules ... 458
Neoral Soft Gelatin Capsules ... 2247
Neoral Oral Solution ... 2247
Restasis Ophthalmic Emulsion ... 570
Sandimmune ... 2259

Ethacrynic Acid (Patients on diuretics, and especially those started recently, may occasionally experience an excessive reduction in blood pressure after initiation of perindopril therapy; co-administration has resulted in reduced bioavailability of perindopril). Products include:

Edecrin Tablets ... 1941

Furosemide (Patients on diuretics, and especially those started recently, may occasionally experience an excessive reduction in blood pressure after initiation of perindopril therapy; co-administration has resulted in reduced bioavailability of perindopril). Products include:

Furosemide Tablets ... 2117

Gentamicin Sulfate (Animal data have suggested the possibility of interaction between gentamicin and perindopril; co-administration should proceed with caution). Products include:

Garamycin Injectable ... 3028
Genoptic Sterile Ophthalmic Solution ... ⊙227
Pred-G Ophthalmic Suspension ... ⊙234
Pred-G Sterile Ophthalmic Ointment ... ⊙235

Heparin Sodium (Co-administration of perindopril with other drugs capable of increasing serum potassium, such as heparin, may increase the risk of hyperkalemia).

No products indexed under this heading.

Hydrochlorothiazide (Patients on diuretics, and especially those started recently, may occasionally experience an excessive reduction in blood pressure after initiation of perindopril therapy; co-administration has resulted in reduced bioavailability of perindopril). Products include:

Aldoril Tablets ... 1884
Atacand HCT ... 637
Avalide Tablets ... 2889
Avalide Tablets ... 922
Benicar HCT Tablets ... 2852
Diovan HCT Tablets ... 2195
Dyazide Capsules ... 1389
Hyzaar ... 1964
Lotensin HCT Tablets ... 2235
Maxzide ... 2150
Micardis HCT Tablets ... 886
Moduretic Tablets ... 2003
Prinzide Tablets ... 2033
Teveten HCT Tablets ... 1710
Timolide Tablets ... 2056
Uniretic Tablets ... 3114
Vaseretic Tablets ... 2073
Zestoretic Tablets ... 701

Hydroflumethiazide (Patients on diuretics, and especially those started recently, may occasionally experience an excessive reduction in blood pressure after initiation of perindopril therapy; co-administration has resulted in reduced bioavailability of perindopril).

No products indexed under this heading.

Indapamide (Patients on diuretics, and especially those started recently, may occasionally experience an excessive reduction in blood pressure after initiation of perindopril therapy; co-administration has resulted in reduced bioavailability of perindopril). Products include:

Indapamide Tablets ... 2119

Indomethacin (Co-administration of perindopril with other drugs capable of increasing serum potassium, such as indomethacin, may increase the risk of hyperkalemia). Products include:

Indocin ... 1968

Lithium (Co-administration of ACE inhibitors and lithium has resulted in increased serum lithium levels and symptoms of lithium toxicity).

No products indexed under this heading.

Lithium Carbonate (Co-administration of ACE inhibitors and lithium has resulted in increased serum lithium levels and symptoms of lithium toxicity). Products include:

Eskalith ... 1406
Lithobid Tablets ... 1670

Lithium Citrate (Co-administration of ACE inhibitors and lithium has resulted in increased serum lithium levels and symptoms of lithium toxicity).

No products indexed under this heading.

Methyclothiazide (Patients on diuretics, and especially those started recently, may occasionally experience an excessive reduction in blood pressure after initiation of perindopril therapy; co-administration has resulted in reduced bioavailability of perindopril).

No products indexed under this heading.

Metolazone (Patients on diuretics, and especially those started recently, may occasionally experience an excessive reduction in blood pressure after initiation of perindopril therapy; co-administration has resulted in reduced bioavailability of perindopril).

No products indexed under this heading.

Polythiazide (Patients on diuretics, and especially those started recently, may occasionally experience an excessive reduction in blood pressure after initiation of perindopril therapy; co-administration has resulted in reduced bioavailability of perindopril).

No products indexed under this heading.

Potassium Acid Phosphate (Co-administration of perindopril with potassium supplements may increase the risk of hyperkalemia). Products include:

K-Phos Original (Sodium Free) Tablets ... 785

Potassium Bicarbonate (Co-administration of perindopril with potassium supplements may increase the risk of hyperkalemia).

No products indexed under this heading.

Potassium Chloride (Co-administration of perindopril with potassium supplements may increase the risk of hyperkalemia). Products include:

Colyte with Flavor Packs for Oral Solution ... 3102
HalfLytely and Bisacodyl Tablets Bowel Prep Kit with Flavors Packs ... 915
K-Dur Extended-Relase Tablets ... 3047
K-Lor Powder Packets ... 472
K-Tab Filmtab Tablets ... 473
TriLyte with Flavor Packs for Oral Solution ... 3114

Potassium Citrate (Co-administration of perindopril with potassium supplements may increase the risk of hyperkalemia). Products include:

Urocit-K Tablets ... 2109

Potassium Gluconate (Co-administration of perindopril with potassium supplements may increase the risk of hyperkalemia).

No products indexed under this heading.

Potassium Phosphate (Co-administration of perindopril with potassium supplements may increase the risk of hyperkalemia). Products include:

K-Phos Neutral Tablets ... 785

Spironolactone (Co-administration of perindopril with potassium-sparing diuretics may increase the risk of hyperkalemia).

No products indexed under this heading.

Torsemide (Patients on diuretics, and especially those started recently, may occasionally experience an excessive reduction in blood pressure after initiation of perindopril therapy; co-administration has resulted in reduced bioavailability of perindopril).

No products indexed under this heading.

Triamterene (Co-administration of perindopril with potassium-sparing diuretics may increase the risk of hyperkalemia). Products include:

Dyazide Capsules ... 1389
Dyrenium Capsules ... 3390
Maxzide ... 2150

Food Interactions

Food, unspecified (The presence of food in the GI tract does not affect the rate or extent of absorption of perindopril but reduces bioavailability of perindoprilat by about 35%; in clinical trials, perindopril was generally administered in a non-fasting state).

ACIPHEX TABLETS

(Rabeprazole Sodium) ... 1081

May interact with iron containing oral preparations and certain other agents. Compounds in these categories include:

Bacampicillin Hydrochloride (Rabeprazole produces sustained inhibition of gastric acid secretion; rabeprazole may interfere with the absorption of certain drugs, such as bacampicillin, where gastric pH is an important determinant of the bioavailability).

No products indexed under this heading.

Digoxin (Co-administration has resulted in an increase in the AUC and Cmax for digoxin of 19% and 29%, respectively). Products include:

Digitek Tablets ... 2146
Lanoxicaps Capsules ... 1458
Lanoxin Injection ... 1462
Lanoxin Tablets ... 1468
Lanoxin Injection Pediatric ... 1465

Ferrous Fumarate (Rabeprazole produces sustained inhibition of gastric acid secretion; rabeprazole may interfere with the absorption of certain drugs, such as iron salts, where gastric pH is an important determinant of the bioavailability). Products include:

Chromagen Forte Soft Gelatin Capsules ... 3296
Ferretts Tablets ... ▣773
Repliva 21/7 Tablets ... 3301

Ferrous Gluconate (Rabeprazole produces sustained inhibition of gastric acid secretion; rabeprazole may interfere with the absorption of certain drugs, such as iron salts, where gastric pH is an important determinant of the bioavailability).

No products indexed under this heading.

Ferrous Sulfate (Rabeprazole produces sustained inhibition of gastric acid secretion; rabeprazole may interfere with the absorption of certain drugs, such as iron salts, where gastric pH is an important determinant of the bioavailability). Products include:

Feosol Tablets ... 1629
Slow Fe Iron Tablets ... ▣772
Slow Fe with Folic Acid Tablets ... ▣773

Iron (Rabeprazole produces sustained inhibition of gastric acid secretion; rabeprazole may interfere with the absorption of certain drugs, such as iron salts, where gastric pH is an important determinant of the bioavailability). Products include:

Chromagen Forte Soft Gelatin Capsules ... 3296
Ferretts IPS Liquid ... ▣773
OptiNate ... 1162
Repliva 21/7 Tablets ... 3301

Ketoconazole (Co-administration has resulted in an approximately 30% decrease in the bioavailability of ketoconazole and an increase in the AUC). Products include:

Nizoral A-D Shampoo, 1% ... 1839
Nizoral 2% Shampoo ... 1838

Polysaccharide Iron Complex (Rabeprazole produces sustained inhibition of gastric acid secretion; rabeprazole may interfere with the absorption of certain drugs, such as iron salts, where gastric pH is an important determinant of the bioavailability). Products include:

Niferex-150 Forte Capsules ... 3299
Nu-Iron 150 Capsules ... 2098

Warfarin Sodium (Co-administration has resulted in increased INR and prothrombin time, which may lead to abnormal bleeding and even death). Products include:

Coumadin for Injection ... 932
Coumadin Tablets ... 932

ACLOVATE CREAM

(Alclometasone Dipropionate) ... 1290

None cited in PDR database.

ACLOVATE OINTMENT

(Alclometasone Dipropionate) ... 1290

None cited in PDR database.

ACTHREL FOR INJECTION

(Corticorelin Ovine Triflutate) ... 3528

May interact with dexamethasone and certain other agents. Compounds in these categories include:

Dexamethasone (The plasma ACTH response to corticorelin injection is inhibited or blunted in normal subjects pretreated with dexamethasone). Products include:

Ciprodex Otic Suspension ... 555
Decadron Tablets ... 1929
TobraDex Ophthalmic Ointment ... 558
TobraDex Ophthalmic Suspension ... 558

IMPORTANT NOTE: Always consult each drug listing in the patient's regimen for possible interactions.

Dexamethasone Acetate (The plasma ACTH response to corticorelin injection is inhibited or blunted in normal subjects pretreated with dexamethasone).
No products indexed under this heading.

Dexamethasone Sodium Phosphate (The plasma ACTH response to corticorelin injection is inhibited or blunted in normal subjects pretreated with dexamethasone).
Products include:
Decadron Phosphate Injection **1931**

Heparin Sodium (A possible interaction between corticorelin and heparin may be associated with a major hypotensive reaction; use of heparin to maintain i.v. canula patency during corticorelin test is not recommended).
No products indexed under this heading.

ACTICIN CREAM

(Permethrin) **2125**
None cited in PDR database.

ACTIMMUNE

(Interferon Gamma-1B) **1646**
May interact with:

Bone Marrow Depressants, unspecified (Caution should be exercised when administering with other potentially myelosuppressive agents).
No products indexed under this heading.

ACTIQ

(Fentanyl Citrate) **993**
May interact with antihistamines, central nervous system depressants, erythromycin, general anesthetics, hypnotics and sedatives, monoamine oxidase inhibitors, narcotic analgesics, phenothiazines, tranquilizers, and certain other agents. Compounds in these categories include:

Acrivastine (Co-administration may result in increased depressant effects).
No products indexed under this heading.

Alfentanil Hydrochloride (Co-administration may result in increased depressant effects; hypoventilation, hypotension, and profound sedation may occur).
No products indexed under this heading.

Alprazolam (Co-administration may result in increased depressant effects; hypoventilation, hypotension, and profound sedation may occur). Products include:
Niravam Orally Disintegrating Tablets.. **3106**
Xanax XR Tablets **2655**

Aprobarbital (Co-administration may result in increased depressant effects; hypoventilation, hypotension, and profound sedation may occur).
No products indexed under this heading.

Astemizole (Co-administration may result in increased depressant effects).
No products indexed under this heading.

Azatadine Maleate (Co-administration may result in increased depressant effects).
No products indexed under this heading.

Bromodiphenhydramine Hydrochloride (Co-administration may result in increased depressant effects).
No products indexed under this heading.

Brompheniramine Maleate (Co-administration may result in increased depressant effects).
Products include:
Alacol DM Syrup **739**
Children's Dimetapp Cold & Allergy Elixir.......................... ▣**745**
Children's Dimetapp DM Cold & Cough Elixir .... ▣**745**
Robitussin Allergy & Cough Syrup .. ▣**750**

Buprenorphine Hydrochloride (Co-administration may result in increased depressant effects; hypoventilation, hypotension, and profound sedation may occur). Products include:
Buprenex Injectable **2718**
Suboxone Tablets **2719**
Subutex Tablets **2719**

Buspirone Hydrochloride (Co-administration may result in increased depressant effects; hypoventilation, hypotension, and profound sedation may occur).
No products indexed under this heading.

Butabarbital (Co-administration may result in increased depressant effects; hypoventilation, hypotension, and profound sedation may occur).
No products indexed under this heading.

Butalbital (Co-administration may result in increased depressant effects; hypoventilation, hypotension, and profound sedation may occur). Products include:
Sedapap Tablets 50 mg/650 mg **2098**

Cetirizine Hydrochloride (Co-administration may result in increased depressant effects).
Products include:
Zyrtec Chewable Tablets **2589**
Zyrtec **2589**
Zyrtec-D 12 Hour Extended Release Tablets........................... **2591**

Chlordiazepoxide (Co-administration may result in increased depressant effects; hypoventilation, hypotension, and profound sedation may occur).
No products indexed under this heading.

Chlordiazepoxide Hydrochloride (Co-administration may result in increased depressant effects; hypoventilation, hypotension, and profound sedation may occur). Products include:
Librium Capsules **3349**

Chlorpheniramine Maleate (Co-administration may result in increased depressant effects).
Products include:
Advil Allergy Sinus Caplets .... ▣**737**
Advil Multi-Symptom Cold Caplets.. ▣**738**
BC Allergy Sinus Cold Powder .... ▣**612**
Contac Severe Cold and Flu Caplets Maximum Strength......... ▣**615**
Hycomine Compound Tablets **1105**
PediaCare Multi-Symptom Cold Liquid .... ▣**704**
PediaCare NightRest Cough & Cold Liquid.................................. ▣**704**
Robitussin Flu Liquid .... ▣**752**
Robitussin PM Cough & Cold Liquid .... ▣**752**
Singlet Caplets .... ▣**636**
Sudafed Sinus & Allergy Tablets ..... ▣**710**
TheraFlu Cold & Cough Hot Liquid .... ▣**680**
TheraFlu Cold & Sore Throat Hot Liquid .... ▣**680**
TheraFlu Flu & Sore Throat Hot Liquid .... ▣**681**
TheraFlu Severe Cold & Cough Hot Liquid.................................... ▣**683**
TheraFlu Severe Cold Caplets .... ▣**679**
TheraFlu Severe Cold Hot Liquid .... ▣**682**
Triaminic Cold & Allergy Liquid .... ▣**685**
Triaminic Cold & Cough Liquid .... ▣**685**
Triaminic Flu, Cough & Fever Liquid .... ▣**685**
Triaminic Night Time Cough & Cold Liquid.................................... ▣**685**
Triaminic Allergy Runny Nose & Congestion Softchews............... ▣**688**
Triaminic Cold & Cough Softchews.. ▣**688**
Children's Tylenol Plus Cold NightTime Suspension Liquid........ **1851**
Children's Tylenol Plus Cold & Cough Suspension Liquid and Chewable Tablets **1851**
Children's Tylenol Plus Cold Chewable Tablets **1851**
Children's Tylenol Plus Flu Suspension Liquid **1853**
Tylenol Allergy Complete Multi-Symptom Caplets and Gelcaps with Cool Burst............... **1844**
Multi-Symptom Tylenol Cold Night Time Caplets **1845**
Vicks 44M Cough, Cold & Flu Relief.. **2676**
Pediatric Vicks 44m Cough & Cold Relief.................................... **2673**
Children's Vicks NyQuil Cold/Cough Relief **2671**

Chlorpheniramine Polistirex (Co-administration may result in increased depressant effects).
Products include:
Tussionex Pennkinetic Extended-Release Suspension...... **3322**

Chlorpheniramine Tannate (Co-administration may result in increased depressant effects).
No products indexed under this heading.

Chlorpromazine (Co-administration may result in increased depressant effects; hypoventilation, hypotension, and profound sedation may occur).
No products indexed under this heading.

Chlorpromazine Hydrochloride (Co-administration may result in increased depressant effects; hypoventilation, hypotension, and profound sedation may occur).
No products indexed under this heading.

Chlorprothixene (Co-administration may result in increased depressant effects; hypoventilation, hypotension, and profound sedation may occur).
No products indexed under this heading.

Chlorprothixene Hydrochloride (Co-administration may result in increased depressant effects; hypoventilation, hypotension, and profound sedation may occur).
No products indexed under this heading.

Chlorprothixene Lactate (Co-administration may result in increased depressant effects; hypoventilation, hypotension, and profound sedation may occur).
No products indexed under this heading.

Clemastine Fumarate (Co-administration may result in increased depressant effects).
No products indexed under this heading.

Clorazepate Dipotassium (Co-administration may result in increased depressant effects; hypoventilation, hypotension, and profound sedation may occur). Products include:
Tranxene **2488**

Clozapine (Co-administration may result in increased depressant effects; hypoventilation, hypotension, and profound sedation may occur). Products include:
Clozapine Tablets **2141**
Clozaril Tablets **2174**
FazaClo Orally Disintegrating Tablets **547**

Codeine Phosphate (Co-administration may result in increased depressant effects; hypoventilation, hypotension, and profound sedation may occur). Products include:
Tylenol with Codeine **2461**

Cyproheptadine Hydrochloride (Co-administration may result in increased depressant effects).
No products indexed under this heading.

Desflurane (Co-administration may result in increased depressant effects; hypoventilation, hypotension, and profound sedation may occur). Products include:
Suprane Liquid for Inhalation **770**

Dexchlorpheniramine Maleate (Co-administration may result in increased depressant effects).
No products indexed under this heading.

Dezocine (Co-administration may result in increased depressant effects; hypoventilation, hypotension, and profound sedation may occur).
No products indexed under this heading.

Diazepam (Co-administration may result in increased depressant effects; hypoventilation, hypotension, and profound sedation may occur). Products include:
Diastat Rectal Delivery System **3344**
Valium Tablets **2822**

Diphenhydramine Citrate (Co-administration may result in increased depressant effects).
Products include:
Children's Benadryl Allergy & Cold Fastmelt Tablets.................. ▣**695**
Children's Benadryl D Allergy & Sinus Fastmelt Tablets .... ▣**694**
Children's Benadryl Allergy Fastmelt Tablets .... ▣**696**
Goody's PM Powder .... ▣**622**

Diphenhydramine Hydrochloride (Co-administration may result in increased depressant effects).
Products include:
Benadryl Allergy & Cold Tablets ..... ▣**692**
Benadryl Allergy .... ▣**691**
Benadryl Allergy & Sinus Headache Caplets & Gelcaps...... ▣**693**
Children's Benadryl Allergy Liquid ... ▣**695**
Children's Benadryl Dye-Free Allergy Liquid............................ ▣**695**
Benadryl Dye-Free Allergy Liqui-Gels Softgels...................... ▣**692**
Benadryl Itch Relief Stick Extra Strength .... ▣**696**
Benadryl Itch Stopping Cream Extra Strength .... ▣**697**
Benadryl Itch Stopping Gel Extra Strength .... ▣**697**
Benadryl Itch Stopping Spray Extra Strength .... ▣**697**
Benadryl Maximum Strength Severe Allergy & Sinus Headache Caplets...................... ▣**694**
Children's Benadryl D Liquid Medication..................................... ▣**693**
Benadryl D Tablets .... ▣**694**
Nytol QuickCaps Caplets .... ▣**635**

Maximum Strength Nytol QuickGels Softgels ▣ **635**
Simply Sleep Caplets **1841**
Sominex Original Formula Tablets ▣ **637**
TheraFlu Thin Strips Multi Symptom ▣ **684**
Triaminic Thin Strips Cough & Runny Nose ▣ **690**
Children's Tylenol Plus Cold & Allergy Suspension Liquid **1850**
Tylenol Allergy Complete Night Time Caplets **1844**
Tylenol Severe Allergy Caplets **1844**
Tylenol Flu NightTime Gelcaps **1846**
Extra Strength Tylenol PM Caplets, Geltabs, Gelcaps and Liquid **1847**
Unisom Maximum Strength SleepGels ▣ **712**

Diphenylpyraline Hydrochloride (Co-administration may result in increased depressant effects).
No products indexed under this heading.

Droperidol (Co-administration may result in increased depressant effects; hypoventilation, hypotension, and profound sedation may occur).
No products indexed under this heading.

Enflurane (Co-administration may result in increased depressant effects; hypoventilation, hypotension, and profound sedation may occur).
No products indexed under this heading.

Erythromycin (Co-administration with potent inhibitors of CYP4503A4 isoform, such as erythromycin, may increase the bioavailability of swallowed fentanyl by decreasing intestinal and hepatic first pass metabolism and may decrease the systemic clearance resulting in increased or prolonged opioid effects). Products include:
Erygel Topical Gel **2096**
Ery-Tab Tablets **447**
Erythromycin Base Filmtab Tablets **454**
Erythromycin Delayed-Release Capsules, USP **456**
PCE Dispertab Tablets **510**

Erythromycin Estolate (Co-administration with potent inhibitors of CYP4503A4 isoform, such as erythromycin, may increase the bioavailability of swallowed fentanyl by decreasing intestinal and hepatic first pass metabolism and may decrease the systemic clearance resulting in increased or prolonged opioid effects).
No products indexed under this heading.

Erythromycin Ethylsuccinate (Co-administration with potent inhibitors of CYP4503A4 isoform, such as erythromycin, may increase the bioavailability of swallowed fentanyl by decreasing intestinal and hepatic first pass metabolism and may decrease the systemic clearance resulting in increased or prolonged opioid effects). Products include:
E.E.S. **449**
EryPed **445**

Erythromycin Gluceptate (Co-administration with potent inhibitors of CYP4503A4 isoform, such as erythromycin, may increase the bioavailability of swallowed fentanyl by decreasing intestinal and hepatic first pass metabolism and may decrease the systemic clearance resulting in increased or prolonged opioid effects).
No products indexed under this heading.

Erythromycin Lactobionate (Co-administration with potent inhibitors of CYP4503A4 isoform, such as erythromycin, may increase the bioavailability of swallowed fentanyl by decreasing intestinal and hepatic first pass metabolism and may decrease the systemic clearance resulting in increased or prolonged opioid effects).
No products indexed under this heading.

Erythromycin Stearate (Co-administration with potent inhibitors of CYP4503A4 isoform, such as erythromycin, may increase the bioavailability of swallowed fentanyl by decreasing intestinal and hepatic first pass metabolism and may decrease the systemic clearance resulting in increased or prolonged opioid effects). Products include:
Erythrocin Stearate Filmtab Tablets **452**

Estazolam (Co-administration may result in increased depressant effects; hypoventilation, hypotension, and profound sedation may occur). Products include:
ProSom Tablets **512**

Ethanol (Co-administration may result in increased depressant effects; hypoventilation, hypotension, and profound sedation may occur).
No products indexed under this heading.

Ethchlorvynol (Co-administration may result in increased depressant effects; hypoventilation, hypotension, and profound sedation may occur).
No products indexed under this heading.

Ethinamate (Co-administration may result in increased depressant effects; hypoventilation, hypotension, and profound sedation may occur).
No products indexed under this heading.

Ethyl Alcohol (Co-administration may result in increased depressant effects; hypoventilation, hypotension, and profound sedation may occur).
No products indexed under this heading.

Fentanyl (Co-administration may result in increased depressant effects; hypoventilation, hypotension, and profound sedation may occur). Products include:
Duragesic Transdermal System **2448**

Fexofenadine Hydrochloride (Co-administration may result in increased depressant effects). Products include:
Allegra **2857**
Allegra-D 12 Hour Extended-Release Tablets **2860**
Allegra-D 24 Hour Extended-Release Tablets **2862**

Fluphenazine Decanoate (Co-administration may result in increased depressant effects; hypoventilation, hypotension, and profound sedation may occur).
No products indexed under this heading.

Fluphenazine Enanthate (Co-administration may result in increased depressant effects; hypoventilation, hypotension, and profound sedation may occur).
No products indexed under this heading.

Fluphenazine Hydrochloride (Co-administration may result in increased depressant effects; hypoventilation, hypotension, and profound sedation may occur).
No products indexed under this heading.

Flurazepam Hydrochloride (Co-administration may result in increased depressant effects; hypoventilation, hypotension, and profound sedation may occur). Products include:
Dalmane Capsules **3343**

Glutethimide (Co-administration may result in increased depressant effects; hypoventilation, hypotension, and profound sedation may occur).
No products indexed under this heading.

Haloperidol (Co-administration may result in increased depressant effects; hypoventilation, hypotension, and profound sedation may occur).
No products indexed under this heading.

Haloperidol Decanoate (Co-administration may result in increased depressant effects; hypoventilation, hypotension, and profound sedation may occur).
No products indexed under this heading.

Hydrocodone Bitartrate (Co-administration may result in increased depressant effects; hypoventilation, hypotension, and profound sedation may occur). Products include:
Hycodan **1104**
Hycomine Compound Tablets **1105**
Hycotuss Expectorant Syrup **1106**
Lortab **3315**
Lortab Elixir **3312**
Vicodin Tablets **530**
Vicodin ES Tablets **531**
Vicodin HP Tablets **532**
Vicoprofen Tablets **533**
Zydone Tablets **1118**

Hydrocodone Polistirex (Co-administration may result in increased depressant effects; hypoventilation, hypotension, and profound sedation may occur). Products include:
Tussionex Pennkinetic Extended-Release Suspension **3322**

Hydromorphone Hydrochloride (Co-administration may result in increased depressant effects; hypoventilation, hypotension, and profound sedation may occur). Products include:
Dilaudid **439**
Dilaudid Oral Liquid **443**
Dilaudid Non-Sterile Powder **439**
Dilaudid Rectal Suppositories **439**
Dilaudid Tablets **439**
Dilaudid Tablets - 8 mg **443**
Dilaudid-HP **441**

Hydroxyzine Hydrochloride (Co-administration may result in increased depressant effects; hypoventilation, hypotension, and profound sedation may occur).
No products indexed under this heading.

Isocarboxazid (Concurrent and/or sequential use with MAO inhibitors is not recommended; potential for severe and unpredictable potentiation of MAO inhibitors has been reported with opioid analgesics).
No products indexed under this heading.

Isoflurane (Co-administration may result in increased depressant effects; hypoventilation, hypotension, and profound sedation may occur).
No products indexed under this heading.

Itraconazole (Co-administration with potent inhibitors of CYP4503A4 isoform, such as azole antifungal itraconazole, may increase the bioavailability of swallowed fentanyl by decreasing intestinal and hepatic first pass metabolism and may decrease the systemic clearance resulting in increased or prolonged opioid effects).
No products indexed under this heading.

Ketamine Hydrochloride (Co-administration may result in increased depressant effects; hypoventilation, hypotension, and profound sedation may occur).
No products indexed under this heading.

Ketoconazole (Co-administration with potent inhibitors of CYP4503A4 isoform, such as azole antifungal ketoconazole, may increase the bioavailability of swallowed fentanyl by decreasing intestinal and hepatic first pass metabolism and may decrease the systemic clearance resulting in increased or prolonged opioid effects). Products include:
Nizoral A-D Shampoo, 1% **1839**
Nizoral 2% Shampoo **1838**

Levomethadyl Acetate Hydrochloride (Co-administration may result in increased depressant effects; hypoventilation, hypotension, and profound sedation may occur).
No products indexed under this heading.

Levorphanol Tartrate (Co-administration may result in increased depressant effects; hypoventilation, hypotension, and profound sedation may occur).
No products indexed under this heading.

Loratadine (Co-administration may result in increased depressant effects). Products include:
Alavert Allergy & Sinus D-12 Hour Tablets ▣ **743**
Alavert ▣ **743**
Children's Claritin 24 Hour Non-Drowsy Allergy Syrup ▣ **732**
Claritin Non-Drowsy 24 Hour Tablets ▣ **731**
Non-Drowsy Claritin Hives Relief Tablets ▣ **733**
Claritin Reditabs 24 Hour Non-Drowsy Tablets ▣ **732**
Claritin-D Non-Drowsy 12 Hour Tablets ▣ **731**
Claritin-D Non-Drowsy 24 Hour Tablets ▣ **731**
Children's Dimetapp ND Non-Drowsy Allergy Syrup ▣ **746**
Triaminic Allerchews ▣ **684**

Lorazepam (Co-administration may result in increased depressant effects; hypoventilation, hypotension, and profound sedation may occur).
No products indexed under this heading.

Loxapine Hydrochloride (Co-administration may result in increased depressant effects; hypoventilation, hypotension, and profound sedation may occur).
No products indexed under this heading.

Loxapine Succinate (Co-administration may result in increased depressant effects; hypoventilation, hypotension, and profound sedation may occur).
No products indexed under this heading.

Meperidine Hydrochloride (Co-administration may result in increased depressant effects; hypoventilation, hypotension, and profound sedation may occur).
No products indexed under this heading.

Mephobarbital (Co-administration may result in increased depressant effects; hypoventilation, hypotension, and profound sedation may occur). Products include:
Mebaral Tablets, USP 2483

Meprobamate (Co-administration may result in increased depressant effects; hypoventilation, hypotension, and profound sedation may occur).
No products indexed under this heading.

Mesoridazine Besylate (Co-administration may result in increased depressant effects; hypoventilation, hypotension, and profound sedation may occur).
No products indexed under this heading.

Methadone Hydrochloride (Co-administration may result in increased depressant effects; hypoventilation, hypotension, and profound sedation may occur).
No products indexed under this heading.

Methdilazine Hydrochloride (Co-administration may result in increased depressant effects).
No products indexed under this heading.

Methohexital Sodium (Co-administration may result in increased depressant effects; hypoventilation, hypotension, and profound sedation may occur).
No products indexed under this heading.

Methotrimeprazine (Co-administration may result in increased depressant effects; hypoventilation, hypotension, and profound sedation may occur).
No products indexed under this heading.

Methoxyflurane (Co-administration may result in increased depressant effects; hypoventilation, hypotension, and profound sedation may occur).
No products indexed under this heading.

Midazolam Hydrochloride (Co-administration may result in increased depressant effects; hypoventilation, hypotension, and profound sedation may occur).
No products indexed under this heading.

Moclobemide (Concurrent and/or sequential use with MAO inhibitors is not recommended; potential for severe and unpredictable potentiation of MAO inhibitors has been reported with opioid analgesics).
No products indexed under this heading.

Molindone Hydrochloride (Co-administration may result in increased depressant effects; hypoventilation, hypotension, and profound sedation may occur). Products include:
Moban Tablets 1108

Morphine Sulfate (Co-administration may result in increased depressant effects; hypoventilation, hypotension, and profound sedation may occur). Products include:
Avinza Capsules 1714
Kadian Capsules 572
MS Contin Tablets 2703

Olanzapine (Co-administration may result in increased depressant effects; hypoventilation, hypotension, and profound sedation may occur). Products include:
Symbyax Capsules 1788
Zyprexa Tablets 1798
Zyprexa IntraMuscular 1798
Zyprexa ZYDIS Orally Disintegrating Tablets 1798

Oxazepam (Co-administration may result in increased depressant effects; hypoventilation, hypotension, and profound sedation may occur).
No products indexed under this heading.

Oxycodone Hydrochloride (Co-administration may result in increased depressant effects; hypoventilation, hypotension, and profound sedation may occur). Products include:
Combunox Tablets 1183
OxyContin Tablets 2699
OxyFast Oral Concentrate Solution 2704
OxyIR Capsules 2704
Percocet Tablets 1114
Percodan Tablets 1115

Pargyline Hydrochloride (Concurrent and/or sequential use with MAO inhibitors is not recommended; potential for severe and unpredictable potentiation of MAO inhibitors has been reported with opioid analgesics).
No products indexed under this heading.

Pentobarbital Sodium (Co-administration may result in increased depressant effects; hypoventilation, hypotension, and profound sedation may occur). Products include:
Nembutal Sodium Solution, USP 2484

Perphenazine (Co-administration may result in increased depressant effects; hypoventilation, hypotension, and profound sedation may occur).
No products indexed under this heading.

Phenelzine Sulfate (Concurrent and/or sequential use with MAO inhibitors is not recommended; potential for severe and unpredictable potentiation of MAO inhibitors has been reported with opioid analgesics).
No products indexed under this heading.

Phenobarbital (Co-administration may result in increased depressant effects; hypoventilation, hypotension, and profound sedation may occur).
No products indexed under this heading.

Prazepam (Co-administration may result in increased depressant effects; hypoventilation, hypotension, and profound sedation may occur).
No products indexed under this heading.

Procarbazine Hydrochloride (Concurrent and/or sequential use with MAO inhibitors is not recommended; potential for severe and unpredictable potentiation of MAO inhibitors has been reported with opioid analgesics). Products include:
Matulane Capsules 3188

Prochlorperazine (Co-administration may result in increased depressant effects; hypoventilation, hypotension, and profound sedation may occur).
No products indexed under this heading.

Promethazine Hydrochloride (Co-administration may result in increased depressant effects). Products include:
Phenergan 3438

Propofol (Co-administration may result in increased depressant effects; hypoventilation, hypotension, and profound sedation may occur). Products include:
Diprivan Injectable Emulsion 676

Propoxyphene Hydrochloride (Co-administration may result in increased depressant effects; hypoventilation, hypotension, and profound sedation may occur).
No products indexed under this heading.

Propoxyphene Napsylate (Co-administration may result in increased depressant effects; hypoventilation, hypotension, and profound sedation may occur). Products include:
Darvocet A 500 Tablets 3497

Pyrilamine Maleate (Co-administration may result in increased depressant effects).
No products indexed under this heading.

Pyrilamine Tannate (Co-administration may result in increased depressant effects).
No products indexed under this heading.

Quazepam (Co-administration may result in increased depressant effects; hypoventilation, hypotension, and profound sedation may occur).
No products indexed under this heading.

Quetiapine Fumarate (Co-administration may result in increased depressant effects; hypoventilation, hypotension, and profound sedation may occur). Products include:
Seroquel Tablets 691

Remifentanil Hydrochloride (Co-administration may result in increased depressant effects; hypoventilation, hypotension, and profound sedation may occur).
No products indexed under this heading.

Risperidone (Co-administration may result in increased depressant effects; hypoventilation, hypotension, and profound sedation may occur). Products include:
Risperdal Consta Long-Acting Injection 1664
Risperdal M-Tab Orally Disintegrating Tablets 1658
Risperdal 1658

Ritonavir (Co-administration with potent inhibitors of CYP4503A4 isoform, such as protease inhibitor ritonavir, may increase the bioavailability of swallowed fentanyl by decreasing intestinal and hepatic first pass metabolism and may decrease the systemic clearance resulting in increased or prolonged opioid effects). Products include:
Kaletra 474
Norvir 499

Secobarbital Sodium (Co-administration may result in increased depressant effects; hypoventilation, hypotension, and profound sedation may occur).
No products indexed under this heading.

Selegiline Hydrochloride (Concurrent and/or sequential use with MAO inhibitors is not recommended; potential for severe and unpredictable potentiation of MAO inhibitors has been reported with opioid analgesics). Products include:
Eldepryl Capsules 3209

Sevoflurane (Co-administration may result in increased depressant effects; hypoventilation, hypotension, and profound sedation may occur). Products include:
Ultane Liquid for Inhalation 526

Sufentanil Citrate (Co-administration may result in increased depressant effects; hypoventilation, hypotension, and profound sedation may occur).
No products indexed under this heading.

Temazepam (Co-administration may result in increased depressant effects; hypoventilation, hypotension, and profound sedation may occur).
No products indexed under this heading.

Terfenadine (Co-administration may result in increased depressant effects).
No products indexed under this heading.

Thiamylal Sodium (Co-administration may result in increased depressant effects; hypoventilation, hypotension, and profound sedation may occur).
No products indexed under this heading.

Thioridazine Hydrochloride (Co-administration may result in increased depressant effects; hypoventilation, hypotension, and profound sedation may occur). Products include:
Thioridazine Hydrochloride Tablets 2122

Thiothixene (Co-administration may result in increased depressant effects; hypoventilation, hypotension, and profound sedation may occur). Products include:
Thiothixene Capsules 2124

Tranylcypromine Sulfate (Concurrent and/or sequential use with MAO inhibitors is not recommended; potential for severe and unpredictable potentiation of MAO inhibitors has been reported with opioid analgesics). Products include:
Parnate Tablets 1499

Triazolam (Co-administration may result in increased depressant effects; hypoventilation, hypotension, and profound sedation may occur).
No products indexed under this heading.

Trifluoperazine Hydrochloride (Co-administration may result in increased depressant effects; hypoventilation, hypotension, and profound sedation may occur).
No products indexed under this heading.

Trimeprazine Tartrate (Co-administration may result in increased depressant effects).
No products indexed under this heading.

Tripelennamine Hydrochloride (Co-administration may result in increased depressant effects).
No products indexed under this heading.

Triprolidine Hydrochloride (Co-administration may result in increased depressant effects).
No products indexed under this heading.

Zaleplon (Co-administration may result in increased depressant effects; hypoventilation, hypotension, and profound sedation may occur). Products include:
Sonata Capsules 1686

Ziprasidone Hydrochloride (Co-administration may result in increased depressant effects; hypoventilation, hypotension, and profound sedation may occur). Products include:
Geodon Capsules 2514

Zolpidem Tartrate (Co-administration may result in increased depressant effects; hypoventilation, hypotension, and profound sedation may occur). Products include:
Ambien Tablets 2867

Food Interactions

Alcohol (Concurrent use with alcoholic beverages may result in increased depressant effects; hypoventilation, hypotension, and profound sedation may occur).

ACTIVASE I.V.

(Alteplase) 1225
May interact with ACE inhibitors, vitamin K antagonists, and certain other agents. Compounds in these categories include:

Abciximab (Drugs that alter platelet function, such as abciximab, may increase the risk of bleeding if administered prior to or after alteplase therapy). Products include:
ReoPro Vials 1779

Aspirin (Drugs that alter platelet function, such as aspirin, may increase the risk of bleeding if administered prior to or after alteplase therapy). Products include:
Aggrenox Capsules 855
Bayer, Aspirin Regimen .... ◼◻606
Bayer Aspirin Tablets 3515
BC Powder .... ◼◻612
BC Allergy Sinus Cold Powder .... ◼◻612
Arthritis Strength BC Powder .... ◼◻612
BC Sinus Cold Powder .... ◼◻612
Ecotrin Enteric Coated Aspirin Low, Regular and Maximum Strength Tablets 1627
Goody's Body Pain Formula Powder .... ◼◻621
Goody's Extra Strength Headache Powder .... ◼◻621
Goody's Extra Strength Pain Relief Tablets .... ◼◻621
Percodan Tablets 1115
St. Joseph 81 mg Aspirin Chewable and Enteric Coated Tablets 1841

Benazepril Hydrochloride (Post-marketing reports of orolingual angioedema associated with alteplase have primarily been in acute ischemic stroke patients receiving concomitant ACE inhibitors). Products include:
Lotensin Tablets 2232
Lotensin HCT Tablets 2235
Lotrel Capsules 2238

Captopril (Post-marketing reports of orolingual angioedema associated with alteplase have primarily been in acute ischemic stroke patients receiving concomitant ACE inhibitors). Products include:
Captopril Tablets 2114

Clopidogrel Bisulfate (Drugs that alter platelet function, such as clopidogrel, may increase the risk of bleeding if administered prior to or after alteplase therapy). Products include:
Plavix Tablets 940
Plavix Tablets 2942

Dicumarol (Co-administration increases the risk of bleeding).
No products indexed under this heading.

Dipyridamole (Drugs that alter platelet function, such as dipyridamole, may increase the risk of bleeding if administered prior to or after alteplase therapy). Products include:
Aggrenox Capsules 855
Persantine Tablets 898

Enalapril Maleate (Post-marketing reports of orolingual angioedema associated with alteplase have primarily been in acute ischemic stroke patients receiving concomitant ACE inhibitors). Products include:
Vaseretic Tablets 2073
Vasotec I.V. Injection 2076

Enalaprilat (Post-marketing reports of orolingual angioedema associated with alteplase have primarily been in acute ischemic stroke patients receiving concomitant ACE inhibitors).
No products indexed under this heading.

Eptifibatide (Drugs that alter platelet function, such as eptifibatide, may increase the risk of bleeding if administered prior to or after alteplase therapy). Products include:
Integrilin Injection 3034

Fosinopril Sodium (Post-marketing reports of orolingual angioedema associated with alteplase have primarily been in acute ischemic stroke patients receiving concomitant ACE inhibitors).
No products indexed under this heading.

Heparin Sodium (Co-administration increases the risk of bleeding).
No products indexed under this heading.

Lisinopril (Post-marketing reports of orolingual angioedema associated with alteplase have primarily been in acute ischemic stroke patients receiving concomitant ACE inhibitors). Products include:
Prinivil Tablets 2029
Prinzide Tablets 2033
Zestoretic Tablets 701
Zestril Tablets 704

Moexipril Hydrochloride (Post-marketing reports of orolingual angioedema associated with alteplase have primarily been in acute ischemic stroke patients receiving concomitant ACE inhibitors). Products include:
Uniretic Tablets 3114
Univasc Tablets 3118

Perindopril Erbumine (Post-marketing reports of orolingual angioedema associated with alteplase have primarily been in acute ischemic stroke patients receiving concomitant ACE inhibitors). Products include:
Aceon Tablets (2 mg, 4 mg, 8 mg) 3191

Quinapril Hydrochloride (Post-marketing reports of orolingual angioedema associated with alteplase have primarily been in acute ischemic stroke patients receiving concomitant ACE inhibitors).
No products indexed under this heading.

Ramipril (Post-marketing reports of orolingual angioedema associated with alteplase have primarily been in acute ischemic stroke patients receiving concomitant ACE inhibitors). Products include:
Altace Capsules 1673

Spirapril Hydrochloride (Post-marketing reports of orolingual angioedema associated with alteplase have primarily been in acute ischemic stroke patients receiving concomitant ACE inhibitors).
No products indexed under this heading.

Ticlopidine Hydrochloride (Drugs that alter platelet function, such as ticlopidine, may increase the risk of bleeding if administered prior to or after alteplase therapy). Products include:
Ticlid Tablets 2813

Tirofiban Hydrochloride (Drugs that alter platelet function, such as tirofiban, may increase the risk of bleeding if administered prior to or after alteplase therapy). Products include:
Aggrastat 1878

Trandolapril (Post-marketing reports of orolingual angioedema associated with alteplase have primarily been in acute ischemic stroke patients receiving concomitant ACE inhibitors). Products include:
Mavik Tablets 482
Tarka Tablets 519

Warfarin Sodium (Co-administration increases the risk of bleeding). Products include:
Coumadin for Injection 932
Coumadin Tablets 932

ACTIVE CALCIUM TABLETS

(Calcium Citrate, Vitamin D) 3342
None cited in PDR database.

ACTIVELLA TABLETS

(Estradiol, Norethindrone Acetate) 2311
None cited in PDR database.

ACTONEL TABLETS

(Risedronate Sodium) 2679
May interact with antacids containing aluminum, calcium and magnesium, calcium preparations, and certain other agents. Compounds in these categories include:

Aluminum Carbonate (Antacids may interfere with the absorption of risedronate sodium; antacids should be taken at a different time of the day).
No products indexed under this heading.

Aluminum Hydroxide (Antacids may interfere with the absorption of risedronate sodium; antacids should be taken at a different time of the day). Products include:
Gaviscon Regular Strength Liquid .. ◼◻620
Gaviscon Regular Strength Tablets .... ◼◻619
Gaviscon Extra Strength Liquid .... ◼◻620
Gaviscon Extra Strength Tablets .... ◼◻619
Maalox Max Maximum Strength Antacid/Anti-Gas Liquid 2165
Maalox Regular Strength Antacid/Antigas Liquid 2164

Aspirin (The incidence of gastrointestinal adverse events is, in general, higher with co-administration; caution should be used). Products include:
Aggrenox Capsules 855
Bayer, Aspirin Regimen .... ◼◻606
Bayer Aspirin Tablets 3515
BC Powder .... ◼◻612
BC Allergy Sinus Cold Powder .... ◼◻612
Arthritis Strength BC Powder .... ◼◻612
BC Sinus Cold Powder .... ◼◻612
Ecotrin Enteric Coated Aspirin Low, Regular and Maximum Strength Tablets 1627
Goody's Body Pain Formula Powder .... ◼◻621
Goody's Extra Strength Headache Powder .... ◼◻621
Goody's Extra Strength Pain Relief Tablets .... ◼◻621
Percodan Tablets 1115
St. Joseph 81 mg Aspirin Chewable and Enteric Coated Tablets 1841

Calcium Carbonate (Calcium-containing preparations may interfere with the absorption of risedronate sodium; calcium preparations should be taken at a different time of the day). Products include:
Actonel with Calcium Tablets 2684
Caltrate 600 PLUS Chewables .... ◼◻779
Caltrate 600 PLUS Tablets .... ◼◻779
Caltrate 600 + D Tablets .... ◼◻779
Encora Capsules 3298
Encora AM Tablets 3298
Encora PM Tablets 3298
Gas-X with Maalox .... ◼◻675
Maalox Regular Strength Antacid Tablets 2166
Quick Dissolve Maalox Max Maximum Strength Antacid/Antigas Tablets 2165
Maalox Max Quick Dissolve Maximum Strength Chewable Tablets .... ◼◻678
Os-Cal Chewable Tablets .... ◼◻765
Pepcid Complete Chewable Tablets 1672
PremCal Light, Regular, and Extra Strength Tablets .... ◼◻762
Rolaids Tablets .... ◼◻707
Extra Strength Rolaids Softchews .... ◼◻708
Extra Strength Rolaids Tablets .... ◼◻707
Rolaids Multi-Symptom Antacid & Antigas Tablets .... ◼◻708
Tums .... ◼◻639

IMPORTANT NOTE: Always consult each drug listing in the patient's regimen for possible interactions.

Calcium Chloride (Calcium-containing preparations may interfere with the absorption of risedronate sodium; calcium preparations should be taken at a different time of the day).
No products indexed under this heading.

Calcium Citrate (Calcium-containing preparations may interfere with the absorption of risedronate sodium; calcium preparations should be taken at a different time of the day). Products include:
Active Calcium Tablets 3342
Citracal Tablets 2108

Calcium Glubionate (Calcium-containing preparations may interfere with the absorption of risedronate sodium; calcium preparations should be taken at a different time of the day).
No products indexed under this heading.

Magaldrate (Antacids may interfere with the absorption of risedronate sodium; antacids should be taken at a different time of the day).
No products indexed under this heading.

Magnesium Hydroxide (Antacids may interfere with the absorption of risedronate sodium; antacids should be taken at a different time of the day). Products include:
Maalox Max Maximum Strength Antacid/Anti-Gas Liquid 2165
Maalox Regular Strength Antacid/Antigas Liquid 2164
Pepcid Complete Chewable Tablets 1672
Rolaids Tablets .... ▣707
Extra Strength Rolaids Tablets .... ▣707
Rolaids Multi-Symptom Antacid & Antigas Tablets .... ▣708

Magnesium Oxide (Antacids may interfere with the absorption of risedronate sodium; antacids should be taken at a different time of the day). Products include:
Beelith Tablets 784
PremCal Light, Regular, and Extra Strength Tablets .... ▣762

Food Interactions

Food, unspecified (Mean oral bioavailability is decreased when risedronate is administered with food; risedronate sodium is effective when administered at least 30 minutes before breakfast).

ACTONEL WITH CALCIUM TABLETS

(Calcium Carbonate, Risedronate Sodium) 2684

May interact with antacids, antacids containing aluminum, calcium and magnesium, bisphosphonates, calcium preparations, cations, fluoroquinolone antibiotics, glucocorticoids, iron containing oral preparations, tetracyclines, thiazides, and certain other agents. Compounds in these categories include:

Alatrofloxacin Mesylate (Concomitant administration of a fluoroquinolone and calcium carbonate may decrease the absorption of the flouroquinolone).
No products indexed under this heading.

Alendronate Sodium (Co-administration with calcium may lead to a decrease in biphosphonate absorption). Products include:
Fosamax 1949
Fosamax Plus D Tablets 1956

Aluminum Carbonate (Antacids may interfere with the absorption of risedronate sodium; antacids should be taken at a different time of the day).
No products indexed under this heading.

Aluminum-containing Compounds, unspecified (Co-administration of risedronate sodium and calcium, antacids, or oral medications containing divalent cations will interfere with the absorption of risedronate sodium).
No products indexed under this heading.

Aluminum Hydroxide (Antacids may interfere with the absorption of risedronate sodium; antacids should be taken at a different time of the day). Products include:
Gaviscon Regular Strength Liquid .... ▣620
Gaviscon Regular Strength Tablets .... ▣619
Gaviscon Extra Strength Liquid .... ▣620
Gaviscon Extra Strength Tablets .... ▣619
Maalox Max Maximum Strength Antacid/Anti-Gas Liquid 2165
Maalox Regular Strength Antacid/Antigas Liquid 2164

Aspirin (The incidence of gastrointestinal adverse events is, in general, higher with co-administration; caution should be used). Products include:
Aggrenox Capsules 855
Bayer, Aspirin Regimen .... ▣606
Bayer Aspirin Tablets 3515
BC Powder .... ▣612
BC Allergy Sinus Cold Powder .... ▣612
Arthritis Strength BC Powder .... ▣612
BC Sinus Cold Powder .... ▣612
Ecotrin Enteric Coated Aspirin Low, Regular and Maximum Strength Tablets 1627
Goody's Body Pain Formula Powder .... ▣621
Goody's Extra Strength Headache Powder .... ▣621
Goody's Extra Strength Pain Relief Tablets .... ▣621
Percodan Tablets 1115
St. Joseph 81 mg Aspirin Chewable and Enteric Coated Tablets 1841

Bendroflumethiazide (Reduced urinary excretion of calcium has been reported during concomitant use of calcium carbonate and thiazide diuretics).
No products indexed under this heading.

Betamethasone Acetate (Calcium absorption is reduced when calcium carbonate is taken concomitantly with systemic glucocorticoids).
No products indexed under this heading.

Betamethasone Sodium Phosphate (Calcium absorption is reduced when calcium carbonate is taken concomitantly with systemic glucocorticoids).
No products indexed under this heading.

Calcitriol (Absorption of calcium may be increased when calcium carbonate is given concomitantly with vitamin D analogues). Products include:
Calcijex Injection 411

Calcium (Co-administration of risedronate sodium and calcium, antacids, or oral medications containing divalent cations will interfere with the absorption of risedronate sodium). Products include:
Os-Cal 250 + D Tablets .... ▣765
Os-Cal 500 Tablets .... ▣765
Os-Cal 500 + D Tablets .... ▣766
Perdiem Overnight Relief Pills 2166
Slow-Mag Tablets 2717

Calcium Chloride (Co-administration of risedronate sodium and calcium, antacids, or oral medications containing divalent cations will interfere with the absorption of risedronate sodium).
No products indexed under this heading.

Calcium Citrate (Co-administration of risedronate sodium and calcium, antacids, or oral medications containing divalent cations will interfere with the absorption of risedronate sodium). Products include:
Active Calcium Tablets 3342
Citracal Tablets 2108

Calcium Glubionate (Co-administration of risedronate sodium and calcium, antacids, or oral medications containing divalent cations will interfere with the absorption of risedronate sodium).
No products indexed under this heading.

Chlorothiazide (Reduced urinary excretion of calcium has been reported during concomitant use of calcium carbonate and thiazide diuretics). Products include:
Aldoclor Tablets 1881
Diuril Oral 1936

Chlorothiazide Sodium (Reduced urinary excretion of calcium has been reported during concomitant use of calcium carbonate and thiazide diuretics). Products include:
Diuril Sodium Intravenous 1934

Ciprofloxacin (Concomitant administration of a fluoroquinolone and calcium carbonate may decrease the absorption of the flouroquinolone). Products include:
Cipro I.V. 2998
Cipro I.V. Pharmacy Bulk Package 3509
Cipro Oral Suspension 2991
Cipro XR Tablets 3004
Ciprodex Otic Suspension 555

Ciprofloxacin Hydrochloride (Concomitant administration of a fluoroquinolone and calcium carbonate may decrease the absorption of the flouroquinolone). Products include:
Ciloxan Ophthalmic Ointment 554
Cipro Tablets 2991

Cortisone Acetate (Calcium absorption is reduced when calcium carbonate is taken concomitantly with systemic glucocorticoids).
No products indexed under this heading.

Demeclocycline Hydrochloride (Concomitant administration of a tetracycline and a calcium carbonate may decrease the absorption of the tetracycline).
No products indexed under this heading.

Dexamethasone (Calcium absorption is reduced when calcium carbonate is taken concomitantly with systemic glucocorticoids). Products include:
Ciprodex Otic Suspension 555
Decadron Tablets 1929
TobraDex Ophthalmic Ointment 558
TobraDex Ophthalmic Suspension 558

Dexamethasone Acetate (Calcium absorption is reduced when calcium carbonate is taken concomitantly with systemic glucocorticoids).
No products indexed under this heading.

Dexamethasone Sodium Phosphate (Calcium absorption is reduced when calcium carbonate is taken concomitantly with systemic glucocorticoids). Products include:
Decadron Phosphate Injection 1931

Doxercalciferol (Absorption of calcium may be increased when calcium carbonate is given concomitantly with vitamin D analogues). Products include:
Hectorol Capsules 909
Hectorol Injection 911

Doxycycline Calcium (Concomitant administration of a tetracycline and a calcium carbonate may decrease the absorption of the tetracycline).
No products indexed under this heading.

Doxycycline Hyclate (Concomitant administration of a tetracycline and a calcium carbonate may decrease the absorption of the tetracycline).
No products indexed under this heading.

Doxycycline Monohydrate (Concomitant administration of a tetracycline and a calcium carbonate may decrease the absorption of the tetracycline).
No products indexed under this heading.

Enoxacin (Concomitant administration of a fluoroquinolone and calcium carbonate may decrease the absorption of the flouroquinolone).
No products indexed under this heading.

Etidronate Disodium (Co-administration with calcium may lead to a decrease in biphosphonate absorption). Products include:
Didronel Tablets 2693

Ferrous Fumarate (Calcium may interfere with the absorption of iron. Patients being treated for iron-deficiency should take iron and calcium at different times of the day). Products include:
Chromagen Forte Soft Gelatin Capsules 3296
Ferretts Tablets .... ▣773
Repliva 21/7 Tablets 3301

Ferrous Gluconate (Calcium may interfere with the absorption of iron. Patients being treated for iron-deficiency should take iron and calcium at different times of the day).
No products indexed under this heading.

Ferrous Sulfate (Calcium may interfere with the absorption of iron. Patients being treated for iron-deficiency should take iron and calcium at different times of the day). Products include:
Feosol Tablets 1629
Slow Fe Iron Tablets .... ▣772
Slow Fe with Folic Acid Tablets .... ▣773

Fludrocortisone Acetate (Calcium absorption is reduced when calcium carbonate is taken concomitantly with systemic glucocorticoids).
No products indexed under this heading.

Grepafloxacin Hydrochloride (Concomitant administration of a fluoroquinolone and calcium carbonate may decrease the absorption of the flouroquinolone).
No products indexed under this heading.

Hydrochlorothiazide (Reduced urinary excretion of calcium has

been reported during concomitant use of calcium carbonate and thiazide diuretics). Products include:

- Aldoril Tablets ... 1884
- Atacand HCT ... 637
- Avalide Tablets ... 2889
- Avalide Tablets ... 922
- Benicar HCT Tablets ... 2852
- Diovan HCT Tablets ... 2195
- Dyazide Capsules ... 1389
- Hyzaar ... 1964
- Lotensin HCT Tablets ... 2235
- Maxzide ... 2150
- Micardis HCT Tablets ... 886
- Moduretic Tablets ... 2003
- Prinzide Tablets ... 2033
- Teveten HCT Tablets ... 1710
- Timolide Tablets ... 2056
- Uniretic Tablets ... 3114
- Vaseretic Tablets ... 2073
- Zestoretic Tablets ... 701

Hydrocortisone (Calcium absorption is reduced when calcium carbonate is taken concomitantly with systemic glucocorticoids). Products include:

- Cortizone•5 Ointment ... ▣699
- Cortizone•10 Creme ... ▣699
- Cortizone•10 Ointment ... ▣699
- Cortizone•10 Plus Creme ... ▣700
- Cortizone•10 Maximum Strength Quick Shot Spray ... ▣700
- Hydrocortone Tablets ... 1963
- Preparation H Hydrocortisone Cream ... ▣748

Hydrocortisone Acetate (Calcium absorption is reduced when calcium carbonate is taken concomitantly with systemic glucocorticoids). Products include:

- Analpram-HC ... 1136
- Pramosone ... 1139
- ProctoFoam-HC ... 3113
- Tucks Anti-Itch Ointment ... ▣712
- U-cort 1% Cream ... 3289

Hydrocortisone Sodium Phosphate (Calcium absorption is reduced when calcium carbonate is taken concomitantly with systemic glucocorticoids).
No products indexed under this heading.

Hydrocortisone Sodium Succinate (Calcium absorption is reduced when calcium carbonate is taken concomitantly with systemic glucocorticoids).
No products indexed under this heading.

Hydroflumethiazide (Reduced urinary excretion of calcium has been reported during concomitant use of calcium carbonate and thiazide diuretics).
No products indexed under this heading.

Iron (Calcium may interfere with the absorption of iron. Patients being treated for iron-deficiency should take iron and calcium at different times of the day). Products include:

- Chromagen Forte Soft Gelatin Capsules ... 3296
- Ferretts IPS Liquid ... ▣773
- OptiNate ... 1162
- Repliva 21/7 Tablets ... 3301

Levothyroxine Sodium (Concomitant intake of levothyroxine and calcium carbonate was found to reduce levothyroxine absorption and increase serum thyrotropin levels). Products include:

- Levothroid Tablets ... 1189
- Levoxyl Tablets ... 1680
- Synthroid Tablets ... 515
- Unithroid Tablets ... 3521

Lomefloxacin Hydrochloride (Concomitant administration of a fluoroquinolone and calcium carbonate may decrease the absorption of the flouroquinolone).
No products indexed under this heading.

Magaldrate (Antacids may interfere with the absorption of risedronate sodium; antacids should be taken at a different time of the day).
No products indexed under this heading.

Magnesium (Co-administration of risedronate sodium and calcium, antacids, or oral medications containing divalent cations will interfere with the absorption of risedronate sodium).
No products indexed under this heading.

Magnesium Hydroxide (Antacids may interfere with the absorption of risedronate sodium; antacids should be taken at a different time of the day). Products include:

- Maalox Max Maximum Strength Antacid/Anti-Gas Liquid ... 2165
- Maalox Regular Strength Antacid/Antigas Liquid ... 2164
- Pepcid Complete Chewable Tablets ... 1672
- Rolaids Tablets ... ▣707
- Extra Strength Rolaids Tablets ... ▣707
- Rolaids Multi-Symptom Antacid & Antigas Tablets ... ▣708

Magnesium Oxide (Antacids may interfere with the absorption of risedronate sodium; antacids should be taken at a different time of the day). Products include:

- Beelith Tablets ... 784
- PremCal Light, Regular, and Extra Strength Tablets ... ▣762

Methacycline Hydrochloride (Concomitant administration of a tetracycline and a calcium carbonate may decrease the absorption of the tetracycline).
No products indexed under this heading.

Methyclothiazide (Reduced urinary excretion of calcium has been reported during concomitant use of calcium carbonate and thiazide diuretics).
No products indexed under this heading.

Methylprednisolone Acetate (Calcium absorption is reduced when calcium carbonate is taken concomitantly with systemic glucocorticoids). Products include:

- Depo-Medrol Injectable Suspension ... 2615
- Depo-Medrol Single-Dose Vial ... 2617

Methylprednisolone Sodium Succinate (Calcium absorption is reduced when calcium carbonate is taken concomitantly with systemic glucocorticoids).
No products indexed under this heading.

Minocycline Hydrochloride (Concomitant administration of a tetracycline and a calcium carbonate may decrease the absorption of the tetracycline). Products include:

- Dynacin Tablets ... 1859

Moxifloxacin Hydrochloride (Concomitant administration of a fluoroquinolone and calcium carbonate may decrease the absorption of the flouroquinolone). Products include:

- Avelox ... 2984
- Vigamox Ophthalmic Solution ... 560

Norfloxacin (Concomitant administration of a fluoroquinolone and calcium carbonate may decrease the absorption of the flouroquinolone). Products include:

- Noroxin Tablets ... 2009

Ofloxacin (Concomitant administration of a fluoroquinolone and calcium carbonate may decrease the absorption of the flouroquinolone). Products include:

- Floxin Otic Singles ... 1045
- Floxin Otic Solution ... 1043

Oxytetracycline Hydrochloride (Concomitant administration of a tetracycline and a calcium carbonate may decrease the absorption of the tetracycline).
No products indexed under this heading.

Paricalcitol (Absorption of calcium may be increased when calcium carbonate is given concomitantly with vitamin D analogues). Products include:

- Zemplar Capsules ... 535
- Zemplar Injection ... 538

Polysaccharide Iron Complex (Calcium may interfere with the absorption of iron. Patients being treated for iron-deficiency should take iron and calcium at different times of the day). Products include:

- Niferex-150 Forte Capsules ... 3299
- Nu-Iron 150 Capsules ... 2098

Polythiazide (Reduced urinary excretion of calcium has been reported during concomitant use of calcium carbonate and thiazide diuretics).
No products indexed under this heading.

Prednisolone Acetate (Calcium absorption is reduced when calcium carbonate is taken concomitantly with systemic glucocorticoids). Products include:

- Blephamide Ophthalmic Ointment ... 563
- Blephamide Ophthalmic Suspension ... 564
- Poly-Pred Liquifilm Ophthalmic Suspension ... ⊙231
- Pred Forte Ophthalmic Suspension ... ⊙233
- Pred Mild Sterile Ophthalmic Suspension ... ⊙236
- Pred-G Ophthalmic Suspension ... ⊙234
- Pred-G Sterile Ophthalmic Ointment ... ⊙235

Prednisolone Sodium Phosphate (Calcium absorption is reduced when calcium carbonate is taken concomitantly with systemic glucocorticoids). Products include:

- Pediapred Oral Solution ... 3319

Prednisolone Tebutate (Calcium absorption is reduced when calcium carbonate is taken concomitantly with systemic glucocorticoids).
No products indexed under this heading.

Prednisone (Calcium absorption is reduced when calcium carbonate is taken concomitantly with systemic glucocorticoids).
No products indexed under this heading.

Sodium Bicarbonate (Co-administration of risedronate sodium and calcium, antacids, or oral medications containing divalent cations will interfere with the absorption of risedronate sodium). Products include:

- Ceo-Two Evacuant Suppository ... ▣607
- Colyte with Flavor Packs for Oral Solution ... 3102
- HalfLytely and Bisacodyl Tablets Bowel Prep Kit with Flavors Packs ... 915
- TriLyte with Flavor Packs for Oral Solution ... 3114

Tetracycline Hydrochloride (Concomitant administration of a tetracycline and a calcium carbonate may decrease the absorption of the tetracycline).
No products indexed under this heading.

Tiludronate Disodium (Co-administration with calcium may lead to a decrease in biphosphonate absorption).
No products indexed under this heading.

Triamcinolone (Calcium absorption is reduced when calcium carbonate is taken concomitantly with systemic glucocorticoids).
No products indexed under this heading.

Triamcinolone Acetonide (Calcium absorption is reduced when calcium carbonate is taken concomitantly with systemic glucocorticoids). Products include:

- Azmacort Inhalation Aerosol ... 1701
- Nasacort HFA Inhalation Aerosol ... 2939
- Nasacort AQ Nasal Spray ... 2937

Triamcinolone Diacetate (Calcium absorption is reduced when calcium carbonate is taken concomitantly with systemic glucocorticoids).
No products indexed under this heading.

Triamcinolone Hexacetonide (Calcium absorption is reduced when calcium carbonate is taken concomitantly with systemic glucocorticoids).
No products indexed under this heading.

Trovafloxacin Mesylate (Concomitant administration of a fluoroquinolone and calcium carbonate may decrease the absorption of the flouroquinolone).
No products indexed under this heading.

Vitamin D (Absorption of calcium may be increased when calcium carbonate is given concomitantly with vitamin D analogues). Products include:

- Active Calcium Tablets ... 3342
- Caltrate 600 PLUS Chewables ... ▣779
- Caltrate 600 PLUS Tablets ... ▣779
- Caltrate 600 + D Tablets ... ▣779
- Os-Cal 250 + D Tablets ... ▣765
- Os-Cal 500 + D Tablets ... ▣766

Zinc (Co-administration of risedronate sodium and calcium, antacids, or oral medications containing divalent cations will interfere with the absorption of risedronate sodium). Products include:

- Visutein Capsules ... 3328

Food Interactions

Food, unspecified (Mean oral bioavailability is decreased when risedronate is administered with food; risedronate sodium is effective when administered at least 30 minutes before breakfast).

ACTOPLUS MET TABLETS

(Metformin Hydrochloride, Pioglitazone Hydrochloride) ... 3219

May interact with cationic drugs that are eliminated by renal tubular, calcium channel blockers, corticosteroids, cytochrome p450 3a4 substrates (selected), diuretics, estrogens, oral hypoglycemic agents, insulin, oral contraceptives, phenothiazines, phenytoin, sympathomimetics, thiazides, thyroid preparations, and certain other agents. Compounds in these categories include:

Acarbose (Pioglitazone, like other thiazolidinediones, can cause fluid

retention when used alone or in combination with other antihyperglycemic agents, including insulin). Products include:
Precose Tablets 776

Albuterol (Certain drugs, including sympathomimetics, tend to produce hyperglycemia and may lead to loss of glycemic control. When such drugs are administered to a patient receiving Actoplus Met, the patient should be closely observed to maintain adequate glycemic control). Products include:
Proventil Inhalation Aerosol 3067

Albuterol Sulfate (Certain drugs, including sympathomimetics, tend to produce hyperglycemia and may lead to loss of glycemic control. When such drugs are administered to a patient receiving Actoplus Met, the patient should be closely observed to maintain adequate glycemic control). Products include:
AccuNeb Inhalation Solution 1055
Combivent Inhalation Aerosol 878
DuoNeb Inhalation Solution 1058
Proventil Inhalation Solution 0.083% 3069
Proventil HFA Inhalation Aerosol 3071
Ventolin HFA Inhalation Aerosol 1576
VoSpire Extended-Release Tablets 2352

Alfentanil Hydrochloride (Studies have suggested that pioglitazone may be a weak inducer of CYP450 isoform 3A4 substrate).
No products indexed under this heading.

Alprazolam (Studies have suggested that pioglitazone may be a weak inducer of CYP450 isoform 3A4 substrate). Products include:
Niravam Orally Disintegrating Tablets 3106
Xanax XR Tablets 2655

Amiloride Hydrochloride (Cationic drugs that are eliminated by renal tubular secretion theoretically have the potential for interaction with metformin by competing for common renal tubular transport systems. Although such interactions remain theoretical, careful patient monitoring and dose adjustment of Actoplus Met and/or the interfering drug is recommended in patients who are taking cationic medications that are excreted via the proximal renal tubular secretory system). Products include:
Midamor Tablets 2000
Moduretic Tablets 2003

Amitriptyline Hydrochloride (Studies have suggested that pioglitazone may be a weak inducer of CYP450 isoform 3A4 substrate).
No products indexed under this heading.

Amlodipine Besylate (Certain drugs, including calcium channel blockers, tend to produce hyperglycemia and may lead to loss of glycemic control. When such drugs are administered to a patient receiving Actoplus Met, the patient should be closely observed to maintain adequate glycemic control). Products include:
Caduet Tablets 2507
Lotrel Capsules 2238
Norvasc Tablets 2529

Aprepitant (Studies have suggested that pioglitazone may be a weak inducer of CYP450 isoform 3A4 substrate). Products include:
Emend Capsules 1944

Astemizole (Studies have suggested that pioglitazone may be a weak inducer of CYP450 isoform 3A4 substrate).
No products indexed under this heading.

Atorvastatin Calcium (Studies have suggested that pioglitazone may be a weak inducer of CYP450 isoform 3A4 substrate). Products include:
Caduet Tablets 2507
Lipitor Tablets 2495

Belladonna Ergotamine (Studies have suggested that pioglitazone may be a weak inducer of CYP450 isoform 3A4 substrate).
No products indexed under this heading.

Bendroflumethiazide (Certain drugs, including thiazide diuretics, tend to produce hyperglycemia and may lead to loss of glycemic control. When such drugs are administered to a patient receiving Actoplus Met, the patient should be closely observed to maintain adequate glycemic control).
No products indexed under this heading.

Bepridil Hydrochloride (Certain drugs, including calcium channel blockers, tend to produce hyperglycemia and may lead to loss of glycemic control. When such drugs are administered to a patient receiving Actoplus Met, the patient should be closely observed to maintain adequate glycemic control).
No products indexed under this heading.

Betamethasone Acetate (Certain drugs, including corticosteroids, tend to produce hyperglycemia and may lead to loss of glycemic control. When such drugs are administered to a patient receiving Actoplus Met, the patient should be closely observed to maintain adequate glycemic control).
No products indexed under this heading.

Betamethasone Sodium Phosphate (Certain drugs, including corticosteroids, tend to produce hyperglycemia and may lead to loss of glycemic control. When such drugs are administered to a patient receiving Actoplus Met, the patient should be closely observed to maintain adequate glycemic control).
No products indexed under this heading.

Bumetanide (Certain drugs, including diuretics, tend to produce hyperglycemia and may lead to loss of glycemic control. When such drugs are administered to a patient receiving Actoplus Met, the patient should be closely observed to maintain adequate glycemic control).
No products indexed under this heading.

Buspirone Hydrochloride (Studies have suggested that pioglitazone may be a weak inducer of CYP450 isoform 3A4 substrate).
No products indexed under this heading.

Busulfan (Studies have suggested that pioglitazone may be a weak inducer of CYP450 isoform 3A4 substrate). Products include:
I.V. Busulfex 1125
Myleran Tablets 1492

Carbamazepine (Studies have suggested that pioglitazone may be a weak inducer of CYP450 isoform 3A4 substrate). Products include:
Carbatrol Capsules 3174
Equetro Extended-Release Capsules 3178
Tegretol/Tegretol-XR 2278

Cerivastatin Sodium (Studies have suggested that pioglitazone may be a weak inducer of CYP450 isoform 3A4 substrate).
No products indexed under this heading.

Chlorothiazide (Certain drugs, including thiazide diuretics, tend to produce hyperglycemia and may lead to loss of glycemic control. When such drugs are administered to a patient receiving Actoplus Met, the patient should be closely observed to maintain adequate glycemic control). Products include:
Aldoclor Tablets 1881
Diuril Oral 1936

Chlorothiazide Sodium (Certain drugs, including thiazide diuretics, tend to produce hyperglycemia and may lead to loss of glycemic control. When such drugs are administered to a patient receiving Actoplus Met, the patient should be closely observed to maintain adequate glycemic control). Products include:
Diuril Sodium Intravenous 1934

Chlorotrianisene (Certain drugs, including estrogens, tend to produce hyperglycemia and may lead to loss of glycemic control. When such drugs are administered to a patient receiving Actoplus Met, the patient should be closely observed to maintain adequate glycemic control).
No products indexed under this heading.

Chlorpheniramine (Studies have suggested that pioglitazone may be a weak inducer of CYP450 isoform 3A4 substrate).
No products indexed under this heading.

Chlorpheniramine Maleate (Studies have suggested that pioglitazone may be a weak inducer of CYP450 isoform 3A4 substrate). Products include:
Advil Allergy Sinus Caplets .... ▣ 737
Advil Multi-Symptom Cold Caplets .... ▣ 738
BC Allergy Sinus Cold Powder .... ▣ 612
Contac Severe Cold and Flu Caplets Maximum Strength .... ▣ 615
Hycomine Compound Tablets 1105
PediaCare Multi-Symptom Cold Liquid .... ▣ 704
PediaCare NightRest Cough & Cold Liquid .... ▣ 704
Robitussin Flu Liquid .... ▣ 752
Robitussin PM Cough & Cold Liquid .... ▣ 752
Singlet Caplets .... ▣ 636
Sudafed Sinus & Allergy Tablets .... ▣ 710
TheraFlu Cold & Cough Hot Liquid .... ▣ 680
TheraFlu Cold & Sore Throat Hot Liquid .... ▣ 680
TheraFlu Flu & Sore Throat Hot Liquid .... ▣ 681
TheraFlu Severe Cold & Cough Hot Liquid .... ▣ 683
TheraFlu Severe Cold Caplets .... ▣ 679
TheraFlu Severe Cold Hot Liquid .... ▣ 682
Triaminic Cold & Allergy Liquid .... ▣ 685
Triaminic Cold & Cough Liquid .... ▣ 685
Triaminic Flu, Cough & Fever Liquid .... ▣ 685
Triaminic Night Time Cough & Cold Liquid .... ▣ 685
Triaminic Allergy Runny Nose & Congestion Softchews .... ▣ 688
Triaminic Cold & Cough Softchews .... ▣ 688
Children's Tylenol Plus Cold NightTime Suspension Liquid 1851
Children's Tylenol Plus Cold & Cough Suspension Liquid and Chewable Tablets 1851
Children's Tylenol Plus Cold Chewable Tablets 1851
Children's Tylenol Plus Flu Suspension Liquid 1853
Tylenol Allergy Complete Multi-Symptom Caplets and Gelcaps with Cool Burst 1844
Multi-Symptom Tylenol Cold Night Time Caplets 1845
Vicks 44M Cough, Cold & Flu Relief 2676
Pediatric Vicks 44m Cough & Cold Relief 2673
Children's Vicks NyQuil Cold/Cough Relief 2671

Chlorpheniramine Polistirex (Studies have suggested that pioglitazone may be a weak inducer of CYP450 isoform 3A4 substrate). Products include:
Tussionex Pennkinetic Extended-Release Suspension 3322

Chlorpheniramine Tannate (Studies have suggested that pioglitazone may be a weak inducer of CYP450 isoform 3A4 substrate).
No products indexed under this heading.

Chlorpromazine (Certain drugs, including phenothiazines, tend to produce hyperglycemia and may lead to loss of glycemic control. When such drugs are administered to a patient receiving Actoplus Met, the patient should be closely observed to maintain adequate glycemic control).
No products indexed under this heading.

Chlorpromazine Hydrochloride (Certain drugs, including phenothiazines, tend to produce hyperglycemia and may lead to loss of glycemic control. When such drugs are administered to a patient receiving Actoplus Met, the patient should be closely observed to maintain adequate glycemic control).
No products indexed under this heading.

Chlorpropamide (Pioglitazone, like other thiazolidinediones, can cause fluid retention when used alone or in combination with other antihyperglycemic agents, including insulin).
No products indexed under this heading.

Chlorthalidone (Certain drugs, including diuretics, tend to produce hyperglycemia and may lead to loss of glycemic control. When such drugs are administered to a patient receiving Actoplus Met, the patient should be closely observed to maintain adequate glycemic control). Products include:
Clorpres Tablets 2139

Cimetidine (Cationic drugs that are eliminated by renal tubulare secretion and theoretically have the potential for interaction with metformin by competing for common renal tubular transport systems. Althought such interactions remain theoretical (except for cimetidine), careful patient monitoring and dose adjustment of Actolus Met and/or the interfering drug is recommended in patients who are taking cationic medications that are excreted via the proximal renal tubular secretory system). Products include:

Tagamet HB 200 Tablets 637
Tagamet Tablets 1547

Cimetidine Hydrochloride (Cationic drugs that are eliminated by renal tubulare secreation and theoretically have the potential for interaction with metformin by competing for common renal tubular transport systems. Althought such interactions remain theoretical (except for cimetidine), careful patient monitoring and dose adjustment of Actolus Met and/or the interfering drug is recommended in patients who are taking cationic medications that are excreted via the proximal renal tubular secretory system).
No products indexed under this heading.

Cisapride (Studies have suggested that pioglitazone may be a weak inducer of CYP450 isoform 3A4 substrate).
No products indexed under this heading.

Clarithromycin (Studies have suggested that pioglitazone may be a weak inducer of CYP450 isoform 3A4 substrate). Products include:
Biaxin/Biaxin XL 402
PREVPAC 3281

Cortisone Acetate (Certain drugs, including corticosteroids, tend to produce hyperglycemia and may lead to loss of glycemic control. When such drugs are administered to a patient receiving Actoplus Met, the patient should be closely observed to maintain adequate glycemic control).
No products indexed under this heading.

Cyclosporine (Studies have suggested that pioglitazone may be a weak inducer of CYP450 isoform 3A4 substrate). Products include:
Gengraf Capsules 458
Neoral Soft Gelatin Capsules 2247
Neoral Oral Solution 2247
Restasis Ophthalmic Emulsion 570
Sandimmune 2259

Desogestrel (Certain drugs, including oral contraceptives, tend to produce hyperglycemia and may lead to loss of glycemic control. When such drugs are administered to a patient receiving Actoplus Met, the patient should be closely observed to maintain adequate glycemic control). Products include:
Ortho-Cept Tablets 2395

Dexamethasone (Certain drugs, including corticosteroids, tend to produce hyperglycemia and may lead to loss of glycemic control. When such drugs are administered to a patient receiving Actoplus Met, the patient should be closely observed to maintain adequate glycemic control). Products include:
Ciprodex Otic Suspension 555
Decadron Tablets 1929
TobraDex Ophthalmic Ointment 558
TobraDex Ophthalmic Suspension ... 558

Dexamethasone Acetate (Certain drugs, including corticosteroids, tend to produce hyperglycemia and may lead to loss of glycemic control. When such drugs are administered to a patient receiving Actoplus Met, the patient should be closely observed to maintain adequate glycemic control).
No products indexed under this heading.

Dexamethasone Sodium Phosphate (Certain drugs, including corticosteroids, tend to produce hyperglycemia and may lead to loss of glycemic control. When such drugs are administered to a patient receiving Actoplus Met, the patient should be closely observed to maintain adequate glycemic control). Products include:
Decadron Phosphate Injection 1931

Diazepam (Studies have suggested that pioglitazone may be a weak inducer of CYP450 isoform 3A4 substrate). Products include:
Diastat Rectal Delivery System 3344
Valium Tablets 2822

Dienestrol (Certain drugs, including estrogens, tend to produce hyperglycemia and may lead to loss of glycemic control. When such drugs are administered to a patient receiving Actoplus Met, the patient should be closely observed to maintain adequate glycemic control).
No products indexed under this heading.

Diethylstilbestrol (Certain drugs, including estrogens, tend to produce hyperglycemia and may lead to loss of glycemic control. When such drugs are administered to a patient receiving Actoplus Met, the patient should be closely observed to maintain adequate glycemic control).
No products indexed under this heading.

Digoxin (Cationic drugs that are eliminated by renal tubular secretion theoretically have the potential for interaction with metformin by competing for common renal tubular transport systems. Although such interactions remain theoretical, careful patient monitoring and dose adjustment of Actoplus Met and/or the interfering drug is recommended in patients who are taking cationic medications that are excreted via the proximal renal tubular secretory system). Products include:
Digitek Tablets 2146
Lanoxicaps Capsules 1458
Lanoxin Injection 1462
Lanoxin Tablets 1468
Lanoxin Injection Pediatric 1465

Dihydroergotamine Mesylate (Studies have suggested that pioglitazone may be a weak inducer of CYP450 isoform 3A4 substrate). Products include:
Migranal Nasal Spray 3350

Diltiazem Hydrochloride (Certain drugs, including calcium channel blockers, tend to produce hyperglycemia and may lead to loss of glycemic control. When such drugs are administered to a patient receiving Actoplus Met, the patient should be closely observed to maintain adequate glycemic control). Products include:
Cardizem LA Extended Release Tablets 1699
Tiazac Capsules 1204

Diltiazem Maleate (Studies have suggested that pioglitazone may be a weak inducer of CYP450 isoform 3A4 substrate).
No products indexed under this heading.

Disopyramide (Studies have suggested that pioglitazone may be a weak inducer of CYP450 isoform 3A4 substrate).
No products indexed under this heading.

Disopyramide Phosphate (Studies have suggested that pioglitazone may be a weak inducer of CYP450 isoform 3A4 substrate).
No products indexed under this heading.

Disulfiram (Studies have suggested that pioglitazone may be a weak inducer of CYP450 isoform 3A4 substrate). Products include:
Antabuse Tablets 2343

Dobutamine Hydrochloride (Certain drugs, including sympathomimetics, tend to produce hyperglycemia and may lead to loss of glycemic control. When such drugs are administered to a patient receiving Actoplus Met, the patient should be closely observed to maintain adequate glycemic control).
No products indexed under this heading.

Dopamine Hydrochloride (Certain drugs, including sympathomimetics, tend to produce hyperglycemia and may lead to loss of glycemic control. When such drugs are administered to a patient receiving Actoplus Met, the patient should be closely observed to maintain adequate glycemic control).
No products indexed under this heading.

Doxorubicin Hydrochloride (Studies have suggested that pioglitazone may be a weak inducer of CYP450 isoform 3A4 substrate). Products include:
Adriamycin for Injection, USP 786
Adriamycin Injection, USP 786

Dronabinol (Studies have suggested that pioglitazone may be a weak inducer of CYP450 isoform 3A4 substrate). Products include:
Marinol Capsules 3334

Ephedrine Hydrochloride (Certain drugs, including sympathomimetics, tend to produce hyperglycemia and may lead to loss of glycemic control. When such drugs are administered to a patient receiving Actoplus Met, the patient should be closely observed to maintain adequate glycemic control). Products include:
Primatene Tablets 749

Ephedrine Sulfate (Certain drugs, including sympathomimetics, tend to produce hyperglycemia and may lead to loss of glycemic control. When such drugs are administered to a patient receiving Actoplus Met, the patient should be closely observed to maintain adequate glycemic control).
No products indexed under this heading.

Ephedrine Tannate (Certain drugs, including sympathomimetics, tend to produce hyperglycemia and may lead to loss of glycemic control. When such drugs are administered to a patient receiving Actoplus Met, the patient should be closely observed to maintain adequate glycemic control).
No products indexed under this heading.

Epinephrine (Certain drugs, including sympathomimetics, tend to produce hyperglycemia and may lead to loss of glycemic control. When such drugs are administered to a patient receiving Actoplus Met, the patient should be closely observed to maintain adequate glycemic control). Products include:
EpiPen 1061
Primatene Mist 749

Epinephrine Bitartrate (Certain drugs, including sympathomimetics, tend to produce hyperglycemia and may lead to loss of glycemic control. When such drugs are administered to a patient receiving Actoplus Met, the patient should be closely observed to maintain adequate glycemic control).
No products indexed under this heading.

Epinephrine Hydrochloride (Certain drugs, including sympathomimetics, tend to produce hyperglycemia and may lead to loss of glycemic control. When such drugs are administered to a patient receiving Actoplus Met, the patient should be closely observed to maintain adequate glycemic control).
No products indexed under this heading.

Ergotamine Tartrate (Studies have suggested that pioglitazone may be a weak inducer of CYP450 isoform 3A4 substrate).
No products indexed under this heading.

Erythromycin (Studies have suggested that pioglitazone may be a weak inducer of CYP450 isoform 3A4 substrate). Products include:
Erygel Topical Gel 2096
Ery-Tab Tablets 447
Erythromycin Base Filmtab Tablets 454
Erythromycin Delayed-Release Capsules, USP 456
PCE Dispertab Tablets 510

Erythromycin Estolate (Studies have suggested that pioglitazone may be a weak inducer of CYP450 isoform 3A4 substrate).
No products indexed under this heading.

Erythromycin Ethylsuccinate (Studies have suggested that pioglitazone may be a weak inducer of CYP450 isoform 3A4 substrate). Products include:
E.E.S. 449
EryPed 445

Erythromycin Gluceptate (Studies have suggested that pioglitazone may be a weak inducer of CYP450 isoform 3A4 substrate).
No products indexed under this heading.

Erythromycin Lactobionate (Studies have suggested that pioglitazone may be a weak inducer of CYP450 isoform 3A4 substrate).
No products indexed under this heading.

Erythromycin Stearate (Studies have suggested that pioglitazone may be a weak inducer of CYP450 isoform 3A4 substrate). Products include:
Erythrocin Stearate Filmtab Tablets 452

Estradiol (Certain drugs, including estrogens, tend to produce hyperglycemia and may lead to loss of glycemic control. When such drugs are administered to a patient receiving Actoplus Met, the patient should be closely observed to maintain adequate glycemic control). Products include:
Activella Tablets 2311
Climara Transdermal System 795
Climara Pro Transdermal System 800
CombiPatch Transdermal System 2180
Estrogel 0.06% 3200
Menostar Transdermal System 805

Prefest Tablets **1069**
Vagifem Tablets **2340**
Vivelle Transdermal System **2288**
Vivelle-Dot Transdermal System **2293**

Estradiol Benzoate (Studies have suggested that pioglitazone may be a weak inducer of CYP450 isoform 3A4 substrate).
No products indexed under this heading.

Estradiol Cypionate (Studies have suggested that pioglitazone may be a weak inducer of CYP450 isoform 3A4 substrate).
No products indexed under this heading.

Estradiol Valerate (Studies have suggested that pioglitazone may be a weak inducer of CYP450 isoform 3A4 substrate).
No products indexed under this heading.

Estrogens, Conjugated (Certain drugs, including estrogens, tend to produce hyperglycemia and may lead to loss of glycemic control. When such drugs are administered to a patient receiving Actoplus Met, the patient should be closely observed to maintain adequate glycemic control). Products include:
Premarin Intravenous **3440**
Premarin Tablets **3443**
Premarin Vaginal Cream **3449**
Premphase Tablets **3452**
Prempro Tablets **3452**

Estrogens, Esterified (Certain drugs, including estrogens, tend to produce hyperglycemia and may lead to loss of glycemic control. When such drugs are administered to a patient receiving Actoplus Met, the patient should be closely observed to maintain adequate glycemic control). Products include:
Estratest Tablets **3196**
Estratest H.S. Tablets **3196**

Estropipate (Certain drugs, including estrogens, tend to produce hyperglycemia and may lead to loss of glycemic control. When such drugs are administered to a patient receiving Actoplus Met, the patient should be closely observed to maintain adequate glycemic control).
No products indexed under this heading.

Ethacrynic Acid (Certain drugs, including diuretics, tend to produce hyperglycemia and may lead to loss of glycemic control. When such drugs are administered to a patient receiving Actoplus Met, the patient should be closely observed to maintain adequate glycemic control). Products include:
Edecrin Tablets **1941**

Ethinyl Estradiol (Certain drugs, including oral contraceptives, tend to produce hyperglycemia and may lead to loss of glycemic control. When such drugs are administered to a patient receiving Actoplus Met, the patient should be closely observed to maintain adequate glycemic control). Products include:
Alesse-28 Tablets **3392**
Lo/Ovral-28 Tablets **3423**
NuvaRing **2357**
Ortho-Cept Tablets **2395**
Ortho-Cyclen/Ortho Tri-Cyclen **2414**
Ortho Evra Transdermal System **2402**
Ortho Tri-Cyclen Lo Tablets **2421**
Seasonale Tablets **1073**
Triphasil-28 Tablets **3483**
Yasmin 28 Tablets **818**

Ethosuximide (Studies have suggested that pioglitazone may be a weak inducer of CYP450 isoform 3A4 substrate).
No products indexed under this heading.

Ethyl Alcohol (Alcohol is known to potentiate the effect of metformin on lactate metabolism. Patients, therefore, should be warned against excessive alcohol intake, acute or chronic, while receiving Actoplus Met).
No products indexed under this heading.

Ethynodiol Diacetate (Certain drugs, including oral contraceptives, tend to produce hyperglycemia and may lead to loss of glycemic control. When such drugs are administered to a patient receiving Actoplus Met, the patient should be closely observed to maintain adequate glycemic control).
No products indexed under this heading.

Etoposide (Studies have suggested that pioglitazone may be a weak inducer of CYP450 isoform 3A4 substrate).
No products indexed under this heading.

Etoposide Phosphate (Studies have suggested that pioglitazone may be a weak inducer of CYP450 isoform 3A4 substrate).
No products indexed under this heading.

Felodipine (Certain drugs, including calcium channel blockers, tend to produce hyperglycemia and may lead to loss of glycemic control. When such drugs are administered to a patient receiving Actoplus Met, the patient should be closely observed to maintain adequate glycemic control). Products include:
Plendil Extended-Release Tablets **651**

Fentanyl (Studies have suggested that pioglitazone may be a weak inducer of CYP450 isoform 3A4 substrate). Products include:
Duragesic Transdermal System **2448**

Fentanyl Citrate (Studies have suggested that pioglitazone may be a weak inducer of CYP450 isoform 3A4 substrate). Products include:
Actiq **993**

Fludrocortisone Acetate (Certain drugs, including corticosteroids, tend to produce hyperglycemia and may lead to loss of glycemic control. When such drugs are administered to a patient receiving Actoplus Met, the patient should be closely observed to maintain adequate glycemic control).
No products indexed under this heading.

Fluphenazine Decanoate (Certain drugs, including phenothiazines, tend to produce hyperglycemia and may lead to loss of glycemic control. When such drugs are administered to a patient receiving Actoplus Met, the patient should be closely observed to maintain adequate glycemic control).
No products indexed under this heading.

Fluphenazine Enanthate (Certain drugs, including phenothiazines, tend to produce hyperglycemia and may lead to loss of glycemic control. When such drugs are administered to a patient receiving Actoplus Met, the patient should be closely observed to maintain adequate glycemic control).
No products indexed under this heading.

Fluphenazine Hydrochloride (Certain drugs, including phenothiazines, tend to produce hyperglycemia and may lead to loss of glycemic control. When such drugs are administered to a patient receiving Actoplus Met, the patient should be closely observed to maintain adequate glycemic control).
No products indexed under this heading.

Fosphenytoin Sodium (Certain drugs, including phenytoin, tend to produce hyperglycemia and may lead to loss of glycemic control. When such drugs are administered to a patient receiving Actoplus Met, the patient should be closely observed to maintain adequate glycemic control).
No products indexed under this heading.

Furosemide (A single-dose, metformin-furosemide drug interaction study in healthy subjects demonstrated that pharmacokinetic parameters of both compounds were affected by co-administration. Furosemide increased the metformin plasma and blood Cmax by 22% and blood AUC by 15%, without any significant change in metformin renal clearance. When administered with metformin, the Cmax and AUC of furosemide were 31% and 12% smaller, respectively, than when administered alone and the terminal half-life was decreased by 31%,without any significant change in furosemide renal clearance. No information is available about the interaction of metformin and furosemide when coadministerd chronically). Products include:
Furosemide Tablets **2117**

Glimepiride (Pioglitazone, like other thiazolidinediones, can cause fluid retention when used alone or in combination with other antihyperglycemic agents, including insulin). Products include:
Amaryl Tablets **2864**

Glipizide (Pioglitazone, like other thiazolidinediones, can cause fluid retention when used alone or in combination with other antihyperglycemic agents, including insulin).
No products indexed under this heading.

Glyburide (Pioglitazone, like other thiazolidinediones, can cause fluid retention when used alone or in combination with other antihyperglycemic agents, including insulin).
No products indexed under this heading.

Haloperidol (Studies have suggested that pioglitazone may be a weak inducer of CYP450 isoform 3A4 substrate).
No products indexed under this heading.

Haloperidol Decanoate (Studies have suggested that pioglitazone may be a weak inducer of CYP450 isoform 3A4 substrate).
No products indexed under this heading.

Haloperidol Lactate (Studies have suggested that pioglitazone may be a weak inducer of CYP450 isoform 3A4 substrate).
No products indexed under this heading.

Hydrochlorothiazide (Certain drugs, including thiazide diuretics, tend to produce hyperglycemia and may lead to loss of glycemic control. When such drugs are administered to a patient receiving Actoplus Met, the patient should be closely observed to maintain adequate glycemic control). Products include:
Aldoril Tablets **1884**
Atacand HCT **637**
Avalide Tablets **2889**
Avalide Tablets **922**
Benicar HCT Tablets **2852**
Diovan HCT Tablets **2195**
Dyazide Capsules **1389**
Hyzaar **1964**
Lotensin HCT Tablets **2235**
Maxzide **2150**
Micardis HCT Tablets **886**
Moduretic Tablets **2003**
Prinzide Tablets **2033**
Teveten HCT Tablets **1710**
Timolide Tablets **2056**
Uniretic Tablets **3114**
Vaseretic Tablets **2073**
Zestoretic Tablets **701**

Hydrocortisone (Certain drugs, including corticosteroids, tend to produce hyperglycemia and may lead to loss of glycemic control. When such drugs are administered to a patient receiving Actoplus Met, the patient should be closely observed to maintain adequate glycemic control). Products include:
Cortizone•5 Ointment .... ▣**699**
Cortizone•10 Creme .... ▣**699**
Cortizone•10 Ointment .... ▣**699**
Cortizone•10 Plus Creme .... ▣**700**
Cortizone•10 Maximum Strength Quick Shot Spray .... ▣**700**
Hydrocortone Tablets **1963**
Preparation H Hydrocortisone Cream .... ▣**748**

Hydrocortisone Acetate (Certain drugs, including corticosteroids, tend to produce hyperglycemia and may lead to loss of glycemic control. When such drugs are administered to a patient receiving Actoplus Met, the patient should be closely observed to maintain adequate glycemic control). Products include:
Analpram-HC **1136**
Pramosone **1139**
ProctoFoam-HC **3113**
Tucks Anti-Itch Ointment .... ▣**712**
U-cort 1% Cream **3289**

Hydrocortisone Sodium Phosphate (Certain drugs, including corticosteroids, tend to produce hyperglycemia and may lead to loss of glycemic control. When such drugs are administered to a patient receiving Actoplus Met, the patient should be closely observed to maintain adequate glycemic control).
No products indexed under this heading.

Hydrocortisone Sodium Succinate (Certain drugs, including corticosteroids, tend to produce hyperglycemia and may lead to loss of glycemic control. When such drugs are administered to a patient receiving Actoplus Met, the patient should be closely observed to maintain adequate glycemic control).
No products indexed under this heading.

Hydroflumethiazide (Certain drugs, including thiazide diuretics, tend to produce hyperglycemia and may lead to loss of glycemic control. When such drugs are administered to a patient receiving Actoplus Met, the patient should be closely observed to maintain adequate glycemic control).
No products indexed under this heading.

Indapamide (Certain drugs, including diuretics, tend to produce hyperglycemia and may lead to loss of glycemic control. When such drugs are administered to a patient receiving Actoplus Met, the patient should be closely observed to maintain adequate glycemic control). Products include:
Indapamide Tablets ... 2119

Indinavir Sulfate (Studies have suggested that pioglitazone may be a weak inducer of CYP450 isoform 3A4 substrate). Products include:
Crixivan Capsules ... 1918

Insulin, Human, Zinc Suspension (Pioglitazone, like other thiazolidinediones, can cause fluid retention when used alone or in combination with other antihyperglycemic agents, including insulin). Products include:
Humulin L, 100 Units ... 1763
Humulin U, 100 Units ... 1770

Insulin, Human NPH (Pioglitazone, like other thiazolidinediones, can cause fluid retention when used alone or in combination with other antihyperglycemic agents, including insulin). Products include:
Humulin N, 100 Units ... 1764
Humulin N Pen ... 1765
Novolin N Human Insulin 10 ml Vials ... 2322
Novolin N InnoLet ... 2322
Novolin N PenFill 3 ml Cartridges ... 2325
Novolin R InnoLet ... 2322

Insulin, Human Regular (Pioglitazone, like other thiazolidinediones, can cause fluid retention when used alone or in combination with other antihyperglycemic agents, including insulin). Products include:
Humulin R (U-500) ... 1768
Humulin R, 100 Units ... 1767
Novolin R Human Insulin 10 ml Vials ... 2322
Novolin R PenFill ... 2325

Insulin, Human Regular and Human NPH Mixture (Pioglitazone, like other thiazolidinediones, can cause fluid retention when used alone or in combination with other antihyperglycemic agents, including insulin). Products include:
Humulin 50/50, 100 Units ... 1760
Humulin 70/30 Pen ... 1761
Novolin 70/30 Human Insulin 10 ml Vials ... 2321
Novolin 70/30 InnoLet ... 2322
Novolin 70/30 PenFill 3 ml Cartridges ... 2325

Insulin, NPH (Pioglitazone, like other thiazolidinediones, can cause fluid retention when used alone or in combination with other antihyperglycemic agents, including insulin).
No products indexed under this heading.

Insulin, Regular (Pioglitazone, like other thiazolidinediones, can cause fluid retention when used alone or in combination with other antihyperglycemic agents, including insulin).
No products indexed under this heading.

Insulin, Zinc Crystals (Pioglitazone, like other thiazolidinediones, can cause fluid retention when used alone or in combination with other antihyperglycemic agents, including insulin).
No products indexed under this heading.

Insulin, Zinc Suspension (Pioglitazone, like other thiazolidinediones, can cause fluid retention when used alone or in combination with other antihyperglycemic agents, including insulin).
No products indexed under this heading.

Insulin Aspart, Human Regular (Pioglitazone, like other thiazolidinediones, can cause fluid retention when used alone or in combination with other antihyperglycemic agents, including insulin). Products include:
NovoLog Injection ... 2326

Insulin glargine (Pioglitazone, like other thiazolidinediones, can cause fluid retention when used alone or in combination with other antihyperglycemic agents, including insulin). Products include:
Lantus Injection ... 2925

Insulin Lispro, Human (Pioglitazone, like other thiazolidinediones, can cause fluid retention when used alone or in combination with other antihyperglycemic agents, including insulin). Products include:
Humalog-Pen ... 1751
Humalog Mix 75/25-Pen ... 1754

Insulin Lispro Protamine, Human (Pioglitazone, like other thiazolidinediones, can cause fluid retention when used alone or in combination with other antihyperglycemic agents, including insulin). Products include:
Humalog Mix 75/25-Pen ... 1754

Isoniazid (Certain drugs, including isoniazid, tend to produce hyperglycemia and may lead to loss of glycemic control. When such drugs are administered to a patient receiving Actoplus Met, the patient should be closely observed to maintain adequate glycemic control).
No products indexed under this heading.

Isoproterenol Hydrochloride (Certain drugs, including sympathomimetics, tend to produce hyperglycemia and may lead to loss of glycemic control. When such drugs are administered to a patient receiving Actoplus Met, the patient should be closely observed to maintain adequate glycemic control).
No products indexed under this heading.

Isoproterenol Sulfate (Certain drugs, including sympathomimetics, tend to produce hyperglycemia and may lead to loss of glycemic control. When such drugs are administered to a patient receiving Actoplus Met, the patient should be closely observed to maintain adequate glycemic control).
No products indexed under this heading.

Isradipine (Certain drugs, including calcium channel blockers, tend to produce hyperglycemia and may lead to loss of glycemic control. When such drugs are administered to a patient receiving Actoplus Met, the patient should be closely observed to maintain adequate glycemic control). Products include:
DynaCirc CR Tablets ... 2726

Itraconazole (Studies have suggested that pioglitazone may be a weak inducer of CYP450 isoform 3A4 substrate).
No products indexed under this heading.

Ketoconazole (Studies have suggested that pioglitazone may be a weak inducer of CYP450 isoform 3A4 substrate). Products include:
Nizoral A-D Shampoo, 1% ... 1839
Nizoral 2% Shampoo ... 1838

Levalbuterol Hydrochloride (Certain drugs, including sympathomimetics, tend to produce hyperglycemia and may lead to loss of glycemic control. When such drugs are administered to a patient receiving Actoplus Met, the patient should be closely observed to maintain adequate glycemic control). Products include:
Xopenex Inhalation Solution ... 3143
Xopenex Inhalation Solution Concentrate ... 3147

Levonorgestrel (Certain drugs, including oral contraceptives, tend to produce hyperglycemia and may lead to loss of glycemic control. When such drugs are administered to a patient receiving Actoplus Met, the patient should be closely observed to maintain adequate glycemic control). Products include:
Alesse-28 Tablets ... 3392
Climara Pro Transdermal System ... 800
Mirena Intrauterine System ... 810
Plan B Tablets ... 1068
Seasonale Tablets ... 1073
Triphasil-28 Tablets ... 3483

Levothyroxine Sodium (Certain drugs, including thyroid products, tend to produce hyperglycemia and may lead to loss of glycemic control. When such drugs are administered to a patient receiving Actoplus Met, the patient should be closely observed to maintain adequate glycemic control). Products include:
Levothroid Tablets ... 1189
Levoxyl Tablets ... 1680
Synthroid Tablets ... 515
Unithroid Tablets ... 3521

Lidocaine (Studies have suggested that pioglitazone may be a weak inducer of CYP450 isoform 3A4 substrate). Products include:
Lidoderm Patch ... 1107

Lidocaine Hydrochloride (Studies have suggested that pioglitazone may be a weak inducer of CYP450 isoform 3A4 substrate).
No products indexed under this heading.

Liothyronine Sodium (Certain drugs, including thyroid products, tend to produce hyperglycemia and may lead to loss of glycemic control. When such drugs are administered to a patient receiving Actoplus Met, the patient should be closely observed to maintain adequate glycemic control). Products include:
Cytomel Tablets ... 1678

Liotrix (Certain drugs, including thyroid products, tend to produce hyperglycemia and may lead to loss of glycemic control. When such drugs are administered to a patient receiving Actoplus Met, the patient should be closely observed to maintain adequate glycemic control). Products include:
Thyrolar ... 1203

Lovastatin (Studies have suggested that pioglitazone may be a weak inducer of CYP450 isoform 3A4 substrate). Products include:
Advicor Tablets ... 1694
Altoprev Extended-Release Tablets ... 1151
Mevacor Tablets ... 1996

Mesoridazine Besylate (Certain drugs, including phenothiazines, tend to produce hyperglycemia and may lead to loss of glycemic control. When such drugs are administered to a patient receiving Actoplus Met, the patient should be closely observed to maintain adequate glycemic control).
No products indexed under this heading.

Mestranol (Certain drugs, including oral contraceptives, tend to produce hyperglycemia and may lead to loss of glycemic control. When such drugs are administered to a patient receiving Actoplus Met, the patient should be closely observed to maintain adequate glycemic control).
No products indexed under this heading.

Metaproterenol Sulfate (Certain drugs, including sympathomimetics, tend to produce hyperglycemia and may lead to loss of glycemic control. When such drugs are administered to a patient receiving Actoplus Met, the patient should be closely observed to maintain adequate glycemic control). Products include:
Alupent Inhalation Aerosol ... 858

Metaraminol Bitartrate (Certain drugs, including sympathomimetics, tend to produce hyperglycemia and may lead to loss of glycemic control. When such drugs are administered to a patient receiving Actoplus Met, the patient should be closely observed to maintain adequate glycemic control). Products include:
Aramine Injection ... 1889

Methadone Hydrochloride (Studies have suggested that pioglitazone may be a weak inducer of CYP450 isoform 3A4 substrate).
No products indexed under this heading.

Methotrimeprazine (Certain drugs, including phenothiazines, tend to produce hyperglycemia and may lead to loss of glycemic control. When such drugs are administered to a patient receiving Actoplus Met, the patient should be closely observed to maintain adequate glycemic control).
No products indexed under this heading.

Methoxamine Hydrochloride (Certain drugs, including sympathomimetics, tend to produce hyperglycemia and may lead to loss of glycemic control. When such drugs are administered to a patient receiving Actoplus Met, the patient should be closely observed to maintain adequate glycemic control).
No products indexed under this heading.

Methyclothiazide (Certain drugs, including thiazide diuretics, tend to produce hyperglycemia and may lead to loss of glycemic control. When such drugs are administered to a patient receiving Actoplus Met, the patient should be closely observed to maintain adequate glycemic control).
No products indexed under this heading.

Methylprednisolone Acetate (Certain drugs, including corticosteroids, tend to produce hyperglycemia and may lead to loss of glycemic control. When such drugs are administered to a patient receiving Actoplus Met, the patient should be closely observed to maintain adequate glycemic control). Products include:
- Depo-Medrol Injectable Suspension 2615
- Depo-Medrol Single-Dose Vial 2617

Methylprednisolone Sodium Succinate (Certain drugs, including corticosteroids, tend to produce hyperglycemia and may lead to loss of glycemic control. When such drugs are administered to a patient receiving Actoplus Met, the patient should be closely observed to maintain adequate glycemic control).
No products indexed under this heading.

Metolazone (Certain drugs, including diuretics, tend to produce hyperglycemia and may lead to loss of glycemic control. When such drugs are administered to a patient receiving Actoplus Met, the patient should be closely observed to maintain adequate glycemic control).
No products indexed under this heading.

Mibefradil Dihydrochloride (Certain drugs, including calcium channel blockers, tend to produce hyperglycemia and may lead to loss of glycemic control. When such drugs are administered to a patient receiving Actoplus Met, the patient should be closely observed to maintain adequate glycemic control).
No products indexed under this heading.

Midazolam Hydrochloride (Studies have suggested that pioglitazone may be a weak inducer of CYP450 isoform 3A4 substrate).
No products indexed under this heading.

Miglitol (Pioglitazone, like other thiazolidinediones, can cause fluid retention when used alone or in combination with other antihyperglycemic agents, including insulin).
No products indexed under this heading.

Morphine Sulfate (Cationic drugs that are eliminated by renal tubular secretion theoretically have the potential for interaction with metformin by competing for common renal tubular transport systems. Although such interactions remain theoretical, careful patient monitoring and dose adjustment of Actoplus Met and/or the interfering drug is recommended in patients who are taking cationic medications that are excreted via the proximal renal tubular secretory system). Products include:
- Avinza Capsules 1714
- Kadian Capsules 572
- MS Contin Tablets 2703

Nefazodone Hydrochloride (Studies have suggested that pioglitazone may be a weak inducer of CYP450 isoform 3A4 substrate).
No products indexed under this heading.

Nelfinavir Mesylate (Studies have suggested that pioglitazone may be a weak inducer of CYP450 isoform 3A4 substrate). Products include:
- Viracept 2556

Nicardipine Hydrochloride (Certain drugs, including calcium channel blockers, tend to produce hyperglycemia and may lead to loss of glycemic control. When such drugs are administered to a patient receiving Actoplus Met, the patient should be closely observed to maintain adequate glycemic control). Products include:
- Cardene I.V. 1129

Nicotinic Acid (Certain drugs, including nicotinic acid, tend to produce hyperglycemia and may lead to loss of glycemic control. When such drugs are administered to a patient receiving Actoplus Met, the patient should be closely observed to maintain adequate glycemic control).
No products indexed under this heading.

Nifedipine (A single-dose, metformin-nifedipine drug interaction study in normal healthy volunteers demonstrated that co-administration of nifedipine increased plasma metformin Cmax and AUC by 20% and 9%, respectively, and increased the amount excreted in the urine.Tmax and half-life were unaffected. Nifedipine appears to enhance the absorption of metformin. Metformin had minimal effects on nifedipine). Products include:
- Adalat CC Tablets 2978

Nimodipine (Certain drugs, including calcium channel blockers, tend to produce hyperglycemia and may lead to loss of glycemic control. When such drugs are administered to a patient receiving Actoplus Met, the patient should be closely observed to maintain adequate glycemic control). Products include:
- Nimotop Capsules 774

Nisoldipine (Certain drugs, including calcium channel blockers, tend to produce hyperglycemia and may lead to loss of glycemic control. When such drugs are administered to a patient receiving Actoplus Met, the patient should be closely observed to maintain adequate glycemic control). Products include:
- Sular Tablets 1163

Nitrendipine (Studies have suggested that pioglitazone may be a weak inducer of CYP450 isoform 3A4 substrate).
No products indexed under this heading.

Norepinephrine Bitartrate (Certain drugs, including sympathomimetics, tend to produce hyperglycemia and may lead to loss of glycemic control. When such drugs are administered to a patient receiving Actoplus Met, the patient should be closely observed to maintain adequate glycemic control).
No products indexed under this heading.

Norethindrone (Certain drugs, including oral contraceptives, tend to produce hyperglycemia and may lead to loss of glycemic control. When such drugs are administered to a patient receiving Actoplus Met, the patient should be closely observed to maintain adequate glycemic control). Products include:
- Ortho Micronor Tablets 2411

Norethindrone Acetate (Studies have suggested that pioglitazone may be a weak inducer of CYP450 isoform 3A4 substrate). Products include:
- Activella Tablets 2311
- Aygestin Tablets 1062
- CombiPatch Transdermal System 2180

Norethynodrel (Certain drugs, including oral contraceptives, tend to produce hyperglycemia and may lead to loss of glycemic control. When such drugs are administered to a patient receiving Actoplus Met, the patient should be closely observed to maintain adequate glycemic control).
No products indexed under this heading.

Norgestimate (Certain drugs, including oral contraceptives, tend to produce hyperglycemia and may lead to loss of glycemic control. When such drugs are administered to a patient receiving Actoplus Met, the patient should be closely observed to maintain adequate glycemic control). Products include:
- Ortho-Cyclen/Ortho Tri-Cyclen 2414
- Ortho Tri-Cyclen Lo Tablets 2421
- Prefest Tablets 1069

Norgestrel (Certain drugs, including oral contraceptives, tend to produce hyperglycemia and may lead to loss of glycemic control. When such drugs are administered to a patient receiving Actoplus Met, the patient should be closely observed to maintain adequate glycemic control). Products include:
- Lo/Ovral-28 Tablets 3423

Ondansetron (Studies have suggested that pioglitazone may be a weak inducer of CYP450 isoform 3A4 substrate). Products include:
- Zofran ODT Orally Disintegrating Tablets 1613

Ondansetron Hydrochloride (Studies have suggested that pioglitazone may be a weak inducer of CYP450 isoform 3A4 substrate). Products include:
- Zofran Injection 1607
- Zofran 1613

Paclitaxel (Studies have suggested that pioglitazone may be a weak inducer of CYP450 isoform 3A4 substrate).
No products indexed under this heading.

Perphenazine (Certain drugs, including phenothiazines, tend to produce hyperglycemia and may lead to loss of glycemic control. When such drugs are administered to a patient receiving Actoplus Met, the patient should be closely observed to maintain adequate glycemic control).
No products indexed under this heading.

Phenylephrine Bitartrate (Certain drugs, including sympathomimetics, tend to produce hyperglycemia and may lead to loss of glycemic control. When such drugs are administered to a patient receiving Actoplus Met, the patient should be closely observed to maintain adequate glycemic control).
No products indexed under this heading.

Phenylephrine Hydrochloride (Certain drugs, including sympathomimetics, tend to produce hyperglycemia and may lead to loss of glycemic control. When such drugs are administered to a patient receiving Actoplus Met, the patient should be closely observed to maintain adequate glycemic control). Products include:
- Alacol DM Syrup 739
- Hycomine Compound Tablets 1105
- Preparation H Maximum Strength Cream .... ▣747
- Preparation H Cooling Gel .... ▣747
- Preparation H .... ▣747
- Sudafed PE Tablets .... ▣711
- Vicks Sinex Nasal Spray and Ultra Fine Mist for Sinus Relief 2677
- Zicam Concentrated Cough Mist for Kids Plus D Cool Cherry .... ▣643
- Zicam Concentrated Cough Mist Plus D Cool Cherry .... ▣642

Phenylephrine Tannate (Certain drugs, including sympathomimetics, tend to produce hyperglycemia and may lead to loss of glycemic control. When such drugs are administered to a patient receiving Actoplus Met, the patient should be closely observed to maintain adequate glycemic control).
No products indexed under this heading.

Phenylpropanolamine Hydrochloride (Certain drugs, including sympathomimetics, tend to produce hyperglycemia and may lead to loss of glycemic control. When such drugs are administered to a patient receiving Actoplus Met, the patient should be closely observed to maintain adequate glycemic control).
No products indexed under this heading.

Phenytoin (Certain drugs, including phenytoin, tend to produce hyperglycemia and may lead to loss of glycemic control. When such drugs are administered to a patient receiving Actoplus Met, the patient should be closely observed to maintain adequate glycemic control).
No products indexed under this heading.

Phenytoin Sodium (Certain drugs, including phenytoin, tend to produce hyperglycemia and may lead to loss of glycemic control. When such drugs are administered to a patient receiving Actoplus Met, the patient should be closely observed to maintain adequate glycemic control). Products include:
- Phenytek Capsules 2153

Pimozide (Studies have suggested that pioglitazone may be a weak inducer of CYP450 isoform 3A4 substrate). Products include:
- Orap Tablets ... 1220

Pirbuterol Acetate (Certain drugs, including sympathomimetics, tend to produce hyperglycemia and may lead to loss of glycemic control. When such drugs are administered to a patient receiving Actoplus Met, the patient should be closely observed to maintain adequate glycemic control). Products include:
- Maxair Autohaler ... 1820

Polyestradiol Phosphate (Certain drugs, including estrogens, tend to produce hyperglycemia and may lead to loss of glycemic control. When such drugs are administered to a patient receiving Actoplus Met, the patient should be closely observed to maintain adequate glycemic control).
- No products indexed under this heading.

Polythiazide (Certain drugs, including thiazide diuretics, tend to produce hyperglycemia and may lead to loss of glycemic control. When such drugs are administered to a patient receiving Actoplus Met, the patient should be closely observed to maintain adequate glycemic control).
- No products indexed under this heading.

Prednisolone Acetate (Certain drugs, including corticosteroids, tend to produce hyperglycemia and may lead to loss of glycemic control. When such drugs are administered to a patient receiving Actoplus Met, the patient should be closely observed to maintain adequate glycemic control). Products include:
- Blephamide Ophthalmic Ointment ... 563
- Blephamide Ophthalmic Suspension ... 564
- Poly-Pred Liquifilm Ophthalmic Suspension ... ⊙231
- Pred Forte Ophthalmic Suspension ... ⊙233
- Pred Mild Sterile Ophthalmic Suspension ... ⊙236
- Pred-G Ophthalmic Suspension ... ⊙234
- Pred-G Sterile Ophthalmic Ointment ... ⊙235

Prednisolone Sodium Phosphate (Certain drugs, including corticosteroids, tend to produce hyperglycemia and may lead to loss of glycemic control. When such drugs are administered to a patient receiving Actoplus Met, the patient should be closely observed to maintain adequate glycemic control). Products include:
- Pediapred Oral Solution ... 3319

Prednisolone Tebutate (Certain drugs, including corticosteroids, tend to produce hyperglycemia and may lead to loss of glycemic control. When such drugs are administered to a patient receiving Actoplus Met, the patient should be closely observed to maintain adequate glycemic control).
- No products indexed under this heading.

Prednisone (Certain drugs, including corticosteroids, tend to produce hyperglycemia and may lead to loss of glycemic control. When such drugs are administered to a patient receiving Actoplus Met, the patient should be closely observed to maintain adequate glycemic control).
- No products indexed under this heading.

Procainamide Hydrochloride (Cationic drugs that are eliminated by renal tubular secretion theoretically have the potential for interaction with metformin by competing for common renal tubular transport systems. Although such interactions remain theoretical, careful patient monitoring and dose adjustment of Actoplus Met and/or the interfering drug is recommended in patients who are taking cationic medications that are excreted via the proximal renal tubular secretory system).
- No products indexed under this heading.

Prochlorperazine (Certain drugs, including phenothiazines, tend to produce hyperglycemia and may lead to loss of glycemic control. When such drugs are administered to a patient receiving Actoplus Met, the patient should be closely observed to maintain adequate glycemic control).
- No products indexed under this heading.

Promethazine Hydrochloride (Certain drugs, including phenothiazines, tend to produce hyperglycemia and may lead to loss of glycemic control. When such drugs are administered to a patient receiving Actoplus Met, the patient should be closely observed to maintain adequate glycemic control). Products include:
- Phenergan ... 3438

Pseudoephedrine Hydrochloride (Certain drugs, including sympathomimetics, tend to produce hyperglycemia and may lead to loss of glycemic control. When such drugs are administered to a patient receiving Actoplus Met, the patient should be closely observed to maintain adequate glycemic control). Products include:
- Advil Allergy Sinus Caplets ... ▣737
- Advil Cold & Sinus ... ▣739
- Advil Flu & Body Ache Caplets ... ▣739
- Children's Advil Cold Suspension ... ▣741
- Advil Multi-Symptom Cold Caplets ... ▣738
- Allegra-D 12 Hour Extended-Release Tablets ... 2860
- Allegra-D 24 Hour Extended-Release Tablets ... 2862
- Balamine DM ... 739
- BC Cold Powder ... ▣612
- Benadryl Allergy & Cold Tablets ... ▣692
- Benadryl Allergy & Sinus Headache Caplets & Gelcaps ... ▣693
- Children's Benadryl Allergy & Cold Fastmelt Tablets ... ▣695
- Benadryl Maximum Strength Severe Allergy & Sinus Headache Caplets ... ▣694
- Children's Benadryl D Allergy & Sinus Fastmelt Tablets ... ▣694
- Children's Benadryl D Liquid Medication ... ▣693
- Benadryl D Tablets ... ▣694
- Contac Non-Drowsy 12 Hour Cold Caplets ... ▣614
- Contac Non-Drowsy Timed Release 12 Hour Cold Caplets ... ▣615
- Contac Severe Cold and Flu Caplets Maximum Strength ... ▣615
- Contac Severe Cold and Flu Caplets Non-Drowsy ... ▣615
- Children's Dimetapp Cold & Allergy Elixir ... ▣745
- Children's Dimetapp DM Cold & Cough Elixir ... ▣745
- Children's Dimetapp Long Acting Cough Plus Cold Syrup ... ▣746
- Dimetapp Infant Drops Decongestant Plus Cough ... ▣746
- Children's Motrin Cold Non-Staining Dye-Free Oral Suspension ... 1838
- Children's Motrin Cold Oral Suspension ... 1838
- Motrin Cold & Sinus Caplets ... 1836
- PediaCare Decongestant & Cough Infant Drops ... ▣705
- PediaCare Decongestant Infants' Drops ... ▣705
- PediaCare Long-Acting Cough Plus Cold Liquid ... ▣704
- PediaCare Multi-Symptom Cold Liquid ... ▣704
- PediaCare NightRest Cough & Cold Liquid ... ▣704
- Robitussin Allergy & Cough Syrup ... ▣750
- Robitussin CF Liquid ... ▣755
- Robitussin Cough & Cold Liquid-filled Capsules ... ▣750
- Robitussin Cough, Cold & Flu Liquid-filled Capsules ... ▣750
- Robitussin Cough & Cold Infant Drops ... ▣755
- Robitussin Flu Liquid ... ▣752
- Robitussin Maximum Strength Cough & Cold Liquid ... ▣754
- Robitussin PE Syrup ... ▣753
- Robitussin Pediatric Cough & Cold Liquid ... ▣754
- Robitussin PM Cough & Cold Liquid ... ▣752
- Robitussin Severe Congestion Liquid-filled Capsules ... ▣751
- Simply Stuffy Liquid ... 1841
- Singlet Caplets ... ▣636
- Sudafed 12 Hour Caplets ... ▣708
- Sudafed 24 Hour Tablets ... ▣709
- Sudafed Nasal Decongestant Tablets ... ▣709
- Sudafed Severe Cold ... ▣710
- Sudafed Non-Drying Sinus Liquid Caps ... ▣709
- Sudafed Sinus & Allergy Tablets ... ▣710
- Sudafed Sinus Headache ... ▣711
- TheraFlu Cold & Cough Hot Liquid ... ▣680
- TheraFlu Cold & Sore Throat Hot Liquid ... ▣680
- TheraFlu Flu & Chest Congestion Non-Drowsy Hot Liquid ... ▣681
- TheraFlu Flu & Sore Throat Hot Liquid ... ▣681
- TheraFlu Severe Cold Non-Drowsy Hot Liquid ... ▣683
- TheraFlu Severe Cold & Cough Hot Liquid ... ▣683
- TheraFlu Severe Cold Caplets ... ▣679
- TheraFlu Severe Cold Hot Liquid ... ▣682
- TheraFlu Severe Cold Non-Drowsy Caplets ... ▣679
- Triaminic Chest & Nasal Congestion Liquid ... ▣685
- Triaminic Cold & Allergy Liquid ... ▣685
- Triaminic Cold & Cough Liquid ... ▣685
- Triaminic Cough Liquid ... ▣687
- Triaminic Cough & Nasal Congestion Liquid ... ▣687
- Triaminic Cough & Sore Throat Liquid ... ▣687
- Triaminic Flu, Cough & Fever Liquid ... ▣685
- Triaminic Night Time Cough & Cold Liquid ... ▣685
- Triaminic Allergy Runny Nose & Congestion Softchews ... ▣688
- Triaminic Cold & Cough Softchews ... ▣688
- Triaminic Cough & Sore Throat Softchews ... ▣689
- Tylenol Sinus NightTime Caplets ... ▣663
- Children's Tylenol Plus Cold & Allergy Suspension Liquid ... 1850
- Children's Tylenol Plus Cold NightTime Suspension Liquid ... 1851
- Children's Tylenol Plus Cold & Cough Suspension Liquid and Chewable Tablets ... 1851
- Children's Tylenol Plus Cold Chewable Tablets ... 1851
- Children's Tylenol Plus Cold Daytime Non-Drowsy Suspension Liquid ... 1851
- Children's Tylenol Plus Flu Suspension Liquid ... 1853
- Concentrated Tylenol Infants' Drops Plus Cold ... 1851
- Concentrated Tylenol Infants' Drops Plus Cold and Cough ... 1851
- Tylenol Cold & Flu Severe Daytime Liquid with Cool Bust ... 1846
- Tylenol Cold & Flu Severe NightTime Liquid with Cool Burst ... 1846
- Tylenol Cold Severe Congestion Non-Drowsy Caplets with Cool Burst ... 1846
- Tylenol Allergy Complete Night Time Caplets ... 1844
- Tylenol Allergy Complete Multi-Symptom Caplets and Gelcaps with Cool Burst ... 1844
- Tylenol Flu NightTime Gelcaps ... 1846
- Tylenol Flu Day Non-Drowsy Gelcaps ... 1846
- Concentrated Tylenol Infants' Drops Plus Cold Nasal Congestant, Fever Reducer & Pain Reliever ... ▣668
- Concentrated Tylenol Infants' Drops Plus Cold & Cough Nasal Decongestant, Fever Reducer & Pain Reliever ... ▣668
- Multi-Symptom Tylenol Cold Night Time Caplets ... 1845
- Multi-Symptom Tylenol Cold Day Non-Drowsy Caplets and Gelcaps ... 1845
- Tylenol Sinus Day Non-Drowsy ... 1848
- Tylenol Sinus Night Time Caplets ... 1848
- Tylenol Sinus Severe Congestion Caplets with Cool Burst ... 1848
- Vicks 44D Cough & Head Congestion Relief ... 2676
- Vicks 44D Cough & Head Congestion Relief Liquid ... ▣721
- Vicks 44M Cough, Cold & Flu Relief ... 2676
- Pediatric Vicks 44m Cough & Cold Relief ... 2673
- Vicks DayQuil LiquiCaps/Liquid Multi-Symptom Cold/Flu Relief ... ▣723
- Vicks DayQuil Multi-Symptom Cold/Flu Relief LiquiCaps ... 2675
- Vicks DayQuil Multi-Symptom Cold/Flu Relief Liquid ... 2675
- Children's Vicks NyQuil Cold/Cough Relief ... 2671
- Vicks NyQuil LiquiCaps ... 2677
- Vicks NyQuil LiquiCaps/Liquid Multi-Symptom Cold/Flu Relief ... ▣725
- Vicks NyQuil Liquid ... 2677
- Zyrtec-D 12 Hour Extended Release Tablets ... 2591

Pseudoephedrine Sulfate (Certain drugs, including sympathomimetics, tend to produce hyperglycemia and may lead to loss of glycemic control. When such drugs are administered to a patient receiving Actoplus Met, the patient should be closely observed to maintain adequate glycemic control). Products include:
- Alavert Allergy & Sinus D-12 Hour Tablets ... ▣743
- Clarinex-D 24-Hour Extended-Release Tablets ... 3012
- Claritin-D Non-Drowsy 12 Hour Tablets ... ▣731
- Claritin-D Non-Drowsy 24 Hour Tablets ... ▣731

Quinestrol (Certain drugs, including estrogens, tend to produce hyperglycemia and may lead to loss of glycemic control. When such drugs are administered to a patient receiving Actoplus Met, the patient should be closely observed to maintain adequate glycemic control).
- No products indexed under this heading.

Quinidine Gluconate (Cationic drugs that are eliminated by renal tubular secretion theoretically have the potential for interaction with metformin by competing for common renal tubular transport systems. Although such interactions remain theoretical, careful patient monitoring and dose adjustment of Actoplus Met and/or the interfering drug is recommended in patients who are

IMPORTANT NOTE: Always consult each drug listing in the patient's regimen for possible interactions.

taking cationic medications that are excreted via the proximal renal tubular secretory system).
No products indexed under this heading.

Quinidine Polygalacturonate (Cationic drugs that are eliminated by renal tubular secretion theoretically have the potential for interaction with metformin by competing for common renal tubular transport systems. Although such interactions remain theoretical, careful patient monitoring and dose adjustment of Actoplus Met and/or the interfering drug is recommended in patients who are taking cationic medications that are excreted via the proximal renal tubular secretory system).
No products indexed under this heading.

Quinidine Sulfate (Cationic drugs that are eliminated by renal tubular secretion theoretically have the potential for interaction with metformin by competing for common renal tubular transport systems. Although such interactions remain theoretical, careful patient monitoring and dose adjustment of Actoplus Met and/or the interfering drug is recommended in patients who are taking cationic medications that are excreted via the proximal renal tubular secretory system).
No products indexed under this heading.

Quinine Sulfate (Cationic drugs that are eliminated by renal tubular secretion theoretically have the potential for interaction with metformin by competing for common renal tubular transport systems. Although such interactions remain theoretical, careful patient monitoring and dose adjustment of Actoplus Met and/or the interfering drug is recommended in patients who are taking cationic medications that are excreted via the proximal renal tubular secretory system).
No products indexed under this heading.

Ranitidine Hydrochloride (Cationic drugs that are eliminated by renal tubular secretion theoretically have the potential for interaction with metformin by competing for common renal tubular transport systems. Although such interactions remain theoretical, careful patient monitoring and dose adjustment of Actoplus Met and/or the interfering drug is recommended in patients who are taking cationic medications that are excreted via the proximal renal tubular secretory system). Products include:
Zantac **1597**
Zantac Injection **1593**
Zantac 75 Tablets .... **▣715**
Zantac 150 Maximum Strength Tablets .... **▣715**
Zantac Injection Pharmacy Bulk Package **1595**

Repaglinide (Pioglitazone, like other thiazolidinediones, can cause fluid retention when used alone or in combination with other antihyperglycemic agents, including insulin). Products include:
Prandin Tablets (0.5, 1, and 2 mg) **2337**

Rifabutin (Studies have suggested that pioglitazone may be a weak inducer of CYP450 isoform 3A4 substrate).
No products indexed under this heading.

Ritonavir (Studies have suggested that pioglitazone may be a weak inducer of CYP450 isoform 3A4 substrate). Products include:
Kaletra **474**
Norvir **499**

Rosiglitazone Maleate (Pioglitazone, like other thiazolidinediones, can cause fluid retention when used alone or in combination with other antihyperglycemic agents, including insulin). Products include:
Avandamet Tablets **1343**
Avandia Tablets **1348**

Salmeterol Xinafoate (Certain drugs, including sympathomimetics, tend to produce hyperglycemia and may lead to loss of glycemic control. When such drugs are administered to a patient receiving Actoplus Met, the patient should be closely observed to maintain adequate glycemic control). Products include:
Advair Diskus 100/50 .... **1291**
Advair Diskus 250/50 .... **1291**
Advair Diskus 500/50 .... **1291**
Serevent Diskus **1540**

Saquinavir (Studies have suggested that pioglitazone may be a weak inducer of CYP450 isoform 3A4 substrate).
No products indexed under this heading.

Saquinavir Mesylate (Studies have suggested that pioglitazone may be a weak inducer of CYP450 isoform 3A4 substrate). Products include:
Invirase **2776**

Sertraline Hydrochloride (Studies have suggested that pioglitazone may be a weak inducer of CYP450 isoform 3A4 substrate). Products include:
Zoloft **2581**

Sildenafil Citrate (Studies have suggested that pioglitazone may be a weak inducer of CYP450 isoform 3A4 substrate). Products include:
Revatio Tablets **2541**
Viagra Tablets **2552**

Simvastatin (Studies have suggested that pioglitazone may be a weak inducer of CYP450 isoform 3A4 substrate). Products include:
Vytorin 10/10 Tablets **2084**
Vytorin 10/10 Tablets **3092**
Vytorin 10/20 Tablets **2084**
Vytorin 10/20 Tablets **3092**
Vytorin 10/40 Tablets **3092**
Vytorin 10/40 Tablets **2084**
Vytorin 10/80 Tablets **2084**
Vytorin 10/80 Tablets **3092**
Zocor Tablets **2078**

Sirolimus (Studies have suggested that pioglitazone may be a weak inducer of CYP450 isoform 3A4 substrate). Products include:
Rapamune Oral Solution and Tablets **3472**

Spironolactone (Certain drugs, including diuretics, tend to produce hyperglycemia and may lead to loss of glycemic control. When such drugs are administered to a patient receiving Actoplus Met, the patient should be closely observed to maintain adequate glycemic control).
No products indexed under this heading.

Tacrolimus (Studies have suggested that pioglitazone may be a weak inducer of CYP450 isoform 3A4 substrate). Products include:
Prograf Capsules and Injection **624**
Protopic Ointment **629**

Tamoxifen Citrate (Studies have suggested that pioglitazone may be a weak inducer of CYP450 isoform 3A4 substrate).
No products indexed under this heading.

Terbutaline Sulfate (Certain drugs, including sympathomimetics, tend to produce hyperglycemia and may lead to loss of glycemic control. When such drugs are administered to a patient receiving Actoplus Met, the patient should be closely observed to maintain adequate glycemic control).
No products indexed under this heading.

Thioridazine Hydrochloride (Certain drugs, including phenothiazines, tend to produce hyperglycemia and may lead to loss of glycemic control. When such drugs are administered to a patient receiving Actoplus Met, the patient should be closely observed to maintain adequate glycemic control). Products include:
Thioridazine Hydrochloride Tablets **2122**

Thyroglobulin (Certain drugs, including thyroid products, tend to produce hyperglycemia and may lead to loss of glycemic control. When such drugs are administered to a patient receiving Actoplus Met, the patient should be closely observed to maintain adequate glycemic control).
No products indexed under this heading.

Thyroid (Certain drugs, including thyroid products, tend to produce hyperglycemia and may lead to loss of glycemic control. When such drugs are administered to a patient receiving Actoplus Met, the patient should be closely observed to maintain adequate glycemic control).
No products indexed under this heading.

Thyroxine (Certain drugs, including thyroid products, tend to produce hyperglycemia and may lead to loss of glycemic control. When such drugs are administered to a patient receiving Actoplus Met, the patient should be closely observed to maintain adequate glycemic control).
No products indexed under this heading.

Thyroxine Sodium (Certain drugs, including thyroid products, tend to produce hyperglycemia and may lead to loss of glycemic control. When such drugs are administered to a patient receiving Actoplus Met, the patient should be closely observed to maintain adequate glycemic control).
No products indexed under this heading.

Tiagabine Hydrochloride (Studies have suggested that pioglitazone may be a weak inducer of CYP450 isoform 3A4 substrate). Products include:
Gabitril Tablets **998**

Tolazamide (Pioglitazone, like other thiazolidinediones, can cause fluid retention when used alone or in combination with other antihyperglycemic agents, including insulin).
No products indexed under this heading.

Tolbutamide (Pioglitazone, like other thiazolidinediones, can cause fluid retention when used alone or in combination with other antihyperglycemic agents, including insulin).
No products indexed under this heading.

Tolterodine Tartrate (Studies have suggested that pioglitazone may be a weak inducer of CYP450 isoform 3A4 substrate). Products include:
Detrol Tablets **2626**
Detrol LA Capsules **2629**

Torsemide (Certain drugs, including diuretics, tend to produce hyperglycemia and may lead to loss of glycemic control. When such drugs are administered to a patient receiving Actoplus Met, the patient should be closely observed to maintain adequate glycemic control).
No products indexed under this heading.

Trazodone Hydrochloride (Studies have suggested that pioglitazone may be a weak inducer of CYP450 isoform 3A4 substrate).
No products indexed under this heading.

Triamcinolone (Certain drugs, including corticosteroids, tend to produce hyperglycemia and may lead to loss of glycemic control. When such drugs are administered to a patient receiving Actoplus Met, the patient should be closely observed to maintain adequate glycemic control).
No products indexed under this heading.

Triamcinolone Acetonide (Certain drugs, including corticosteroids, tend to produce hyperglycemia and may lead to loss of glycemic control. When such drugs are administered to a patient receiving Actoplus Met, the patient should be closely observed to maintain adequate glycemic control). Products include:
Azmacort Inhalation Aerosol **1701**
Nasacort HFA Inhalation Aerosol **2939**
Nasacort AQ Nasal Spray **2937**

Triamcinolone Diacetate (Certain drugs, including corticosteroids, tend to produce hyperglycemia and may lead to loss of glycemic control. When such drugs are administered to a patient receiving Actoplus Met, the patient should be closely observed to maintain adequate glycemic control).
No products indexed under this heading.

Triamcinolone Hexacetonide (Certain drugs, including corticosteroids, tend to produce hyperglycemia and may lead to loss of glycemic control. When such drugs are administered to a patient receiving Actoplus Met, the patient should be closely observed to maintain adequate glycemic control).
No products indexed under this heading.

Triamterene (Cationic drugs that are eliminated by renal tubular secretion theoretically have the potential for interaction with metformin by competing for common renal tubular transport systems. Although such

interactions remain theoretical, careful patient monitoring and dose adjustment of Actoplus Met and/or the interfering drug is recommended in patients who are taking cationic medications that are excreted via the proximal renal tubular secretory system). Products include:

Dyazide Capsules ... **1389**
Dyrenium Capsules ... **3390**
Maxzide ... **2150**

Triazolam (Studies have suggested that pioglitazone may be a weak inducer of CYP450 isoform 3A4 substrate).
No products indexed under this heading.

Trifluoperazine Hydrochloride (Certain drugs, including phenothiazines, tend to produce hyperglycemia and may lead to loss of glycemic control. When such drugs are administered to a patient receiving Actoplus Met, the patient should be closely observed to maintain adequate glycemic control).
No products indexed under this heading.

Trimethoprim (Cationic drugs that are eliminated by renal tubular secretion theoretically have the potential for interaction with metformin by competing for common renal tubular transport systems. Although such interactions remain theoretical, careful patient monitoring and dose adjustment of Actoplus Met and/or the interfering drug is recommended in patients who are taking cationic medications that are excreted via the proximal renal tubular secretory system).
No products indexed under this heading.

Trimethoprim Sulfate (Cationic drugs that are eliminated by renal tubular secretion theoretically have the potential for interaction with metformin by competing for common renal tubular transport systems. Although such interactions remain theoretical, careful patient monitoring and dose adjustment of Actoplus Met and/or the interfering drug is recommended in patients who are taking cationic medications that are excreted via the proximal renal tubular secretory system). Products include:

Polytrim Ophthalmic Solution ... **570**

Troglitazone (Pioglitazone, like other thiazolidinediones, can cause fluid retention when used alone or in combination with other antihyperglycemic agents, including insulin).
No products indexed under this heading.

Vancomycin Hydrochloride (Cationic drugs that are eliminated by renal tubular secretion theoretically have the potential for interaction with metformin by competing for common renal tubular transport systems. Although such interactions remain theoretical, careful patient monitoring and dose adjustment of Actoplus Met and/or the interfering drug is recommended in patients who are taking cationic medications that are excreted via the proximal renal tubular secretory system). Products include:

Vancocin HCl Capsules, USP ... **3370**

Verapamil Hydrochloride (Certain drugs, including calcium channel blockers, tend to produce hyperglycemia and may lead to loss of glycemic control. When such drugs are administered to a patient receiving Actoplus Met, the patient should be closely observed to maintain adequate glycemic control). Products include:

Covera-HS Tablets ... **3135**
Tarka Tablets ... **519**
Verelan PM Capsules ... **3120**

Vinblastine Sulfate (Studies have suggested that pioglitazone may be a weak inducer of CYP450 isoform 3A4 substrate).
No products indexed under this heading.

Vincristine Sulfate (Studies have suggested that pioglitazone may be a weak inducer of CYP450 isoform 3A4 substrate).
No products indexed under this heading.

Warfarin Sodium (Studies have suggested that pioglitazone may be a weak inducer of CYP450 isoform 3A4 substrate). Products include:

Coumadin for Injection ... **932**
Coumadin Tablets ... **932**

Food Interactions

Alcohol (Alcohol is known to potentiate the effect of metformin on lactate metabolism. Patients, therefore, should be warned against excessive alcohol intake, acute or chronic, while receiving Actoplus Met).

ACTOS TABLETS

(Pioglitazone Hydrochloride) ... **3224**

May interact with oral contraceptives and certain other agents. Compounds in these categories include:

Atorvastatin Calcium (Atorvastatin appears to induce the metabolism of pioglitazone; pioglitazone appears to induce the metabolism of atorvastatin). Products include:

Caduet Tablets ... **2507**
Lipitor Tablets ... **2495**

Desogestrel (Co-administration of pioglitazone hydrochloride (45mg once daily) and an oral contraceptive (1mg norethindrone plus 0.035mg ethinyl estradiol once daily) for 21 days, resulted in an 11% decrease in ethinyl estradiol AUC (0-24h) and an 11% to 14% decrease in Cmax. There were no significant changes in norethindrone AUC (0-24h) and Cmax). Products include:

Ortho-Cept Tablets ... **2395**

Ethinyl Estradiol (Co-administration of pioglitazone hydrochloride (45mg once daily) and an oral contraceptive (1mg norethindrone plus 0.035mg ethinyl estradiol once daily) for 21 days, resulted in an 11% decrease in ethinyl estradiol AUC (0-24h) and an 11% to 14% decrease in Cmax. There were no significant changes in norethindrone AUC (0-24h) and Cmax). Products include:

Alesse-28 Tablets ... **3392**
Lo/Ovral-28 Tablets ... **3423**
NuvaRing ... **2357**
Ortho-Cept Tablets ... **2395**
Ortho-Cyclen/Ortho Tri-Cyclen ... **2414**
Ortho Evra Transdermal System ... **2402**
Ortho Tri-Cyclen Lo Tablets ... **2421**
Seasonale Tablets ... **1073**
Triphasil-28 Tablets ... **3483**
Yasmin 28 Tablets ... **818**

Ethynodiol Diacetate (Co-administration of pioglitazone hydrochloride (45mg once daily) and an oral contraceptive (1mg norethindrone plus 0.035mg ethinyl estradiol once daily) for 21 days, resulted in an 11% decrease in ethinyl estradiol AUC (0-24h) and an 11% to 14% decrease in Cmax. There were no significant changes in norethindrone AUC (0-24h) and Cmax).
No products indexed under this heading.

Ketoconazole (In vitro, ketoconazole appears to significantly inhibit metabolism of pioglitazone). Products include:

Nizoral A-D Shampoo, 1% ... **1839**
Nizoral 2% Shampoo ... **1838**

Levonorgestrel (Co-administration of pioglitazone hydrochloride (45mg once daily) and an oral contraceptive (1mg norethindrone plus 0.035mg ethinyl estradiol once daily) for 21 days, resulted in an 11% decrease in ethinyl estradiol AUC (0-24h) and an 11% to 14% decrease in Cmax. There were no significant changes in norethindrone AUC (0-24h) and Cmax). Products include:

Alesse-28 Tablets ... **3392**
Climara Pro Transdermal System ... **800**
Mirena Intrauterine System ... **810**
Plan B Tablets ... **1068**
Seasonale Tablets ... **1073**
Triphasil-28 Tablets ... **3483**

Mestranol (Co-administration of pioglitazone hydrochloride (45mg once daily) and an oral contraceptive (1mg norethindrone plus 0.035mg ethinyl estradiol once daily) for 21 days, resulted in an 11% decrease in ethinyl estradiol AUC (0-24h) and an 11% to 14% decrease in Cmax. There were no significant changes in norethindrone AUC (0-24h) and Cmax).
No products indexed under this heading.

Midazolam Hydrochloride (Pioglitazone appears to induce the metabolism of midazolam with a 26% reduction of midazolam Cmax and AUC).
No products indexed under this heading.

Nifedipine (Co-administration of pioglitazone and nifedipine ER has resulted in increased metabolism of nifedipine; in view of the high variability of nifedipine pharmacokinetics, the clinical significance of the finding is unknown). Products include:

Adalat CC Tablets ... **2978**

Norethindrone (Co-administration of pioglitazone hydrochloride (45mg once daily) and an oral contraceptive (1mg norethindrone plus 0.035mg ethinyl estradiol once daily) for 21 days, resulted in an 11% decrease in ethinyl estradiol AUC (0-24h) and an 11% to 14% decrease in Cmax. There were no significant changes in norethindrone AUC (0-24h) and Cmax). Products include:

Ortho Micronor Tablets ... **2411**

Norethynodrel (Co-administration of pioglitazone hydrochloride (45mg once daily) and an oral contraceptive (1mg norethindrone plus 0.035mg ethinyl estradiol once daily) for 21 days, resulted in an 11% decrease in ethinyl estradiol AUC (0-24h) and an 11% to 14% decrease in Cmax. There were no significant changes in norethindrone AUC (0-24h) and Cmax).
No products indexed under this heading.

Norgestimate (Co-administration of pioglitazone hydrochloride (45mg once daily) and an oral contraceptive (1mg norethindrone plus 0.035mg ethinyl estradiol once daily) for 21 days, resulted in an 11% decrease in ethinyl estradiol AUC (0-24h) and an 11% to 14% decrease in Cmax. There were no significant changes in norethindrone AUC (0-24h) and Cmax). Products include:

Ortho-Cyclen/Ortho Tri-Cyclen ... **2414**
Ortho Tri-Cyclen Lo Tablets ... **2421**
Prefest Tablets ... **1069**

Norgestrel (Co-administration of pioglitazone hydrochloride (45mg once daily) and an oral contraceptive (1mg norethindrone plus 0.035mg ethinyl estradiol once daily) for 21 days, resulted in an 11% decrease in ethinyl estradiol AUC (0-24h) and an 11% to 14% decrease in Cmax. There were no significant changes in norethindrone AUC (0-24h) and Cmax). Products include:

Lo/Ovral-28 Tablets ... **3423**

ACULAR OPHTHALMIC SOLUTION

(Ketorolac Tromethamine) ... **561**

May interact with:

Warfarin Sodium (Potential for increased bleeding time; concurrent use with other agents which prolong bleeding time requires caution). Products include:

Coumadin for Injection ... **932**
Coumadin Tablets ... **932**

ACULAR LS OPHTHALMIC SOLUTION

(Ketorolac Tromethamine) ... **562**

None cited in PDR database.

ADACEL VACCINE

(Diphtheria & Tetanus Toxoids and Acellular Pertussis Vaccine Adsorbed) ... **2959**

May interact with alkylating agents, antimetabolites, corticosteroids, cytotoxic drugs, and immunosuppressive agents. Compounds in these categories include:

Azathioprine (Concurrent immunosuppressive therapy may reduce the immune response to vaccine). Products include:

Azasan Tablets ... **2844**

Basiliximab (Concurrent immunosuppressive therapy may reduce the immune response to vaccine). Products include:

Simulect for Injection ... **2268**

Betamethasone Acetate (Concurrent immunosuppressive therapy with greater than physiologic doses of corticosteroids may reduce the immune response to vaccine).
No products indexed under this heading.

Betamethasone Sodium Phosphate (Concurrent immunosuppressive therapy with greater than physiologic doses of corticosteroids may reduce the immune response to vaccine).
No products indexed under this heading.

Bleomycin Sulfate (Cytotoxic drugs may reduce the immune response to vaccine).
No products indexed under this heading.

Busulfan (Alkylating drugs may reduce the immune response to vaccine). Products include:

I.V. Busulfex 1125
Myleran Tablets 1492

Capecitabine (Immunosuppressive therapies may reduce the immune response to vaccines). Products include:
Xeloda Tablets 2825

Carmustine (BCNU) (Alkylating drugs may reduce the immune response to vaccine).
No products indexed under this heading.

Chlorambucil (Alkylating drugs may reduce the immune response to vaccine). Products include:
Leukeran Tablets 1472

Cladribine (Immunosuppressive therapies may reduce the immune response to vaccines). Products include:
Leustatin Injection 2368

Cortisone Acetate (Concurrent immunosuppressive therapy with greater than physiologic doses of corticosteroids may reduce the immune response to vaccine).
No products indexed under this heading.

Cyclophosphamide (Alkylating drugs may reduce the immune response to vaccine).
No products indexed under this heading.

Cyclosporine (Concurrent immunosuppressive therapy may reduce the immune response to vaccine). Products include:
Gengraf Capsules 458
Neoral Soft Gelatin Capsules 2247
Neoral Oral Solution 2247
Restasis Ophthalmic Emulsion 570
Sandimmune 2259

Cytarabine (Immunosuppressive therapies may reduce the immune response to vaccines).
No products indexed under this heading.

Dacarbazine (Alkylating drugs may reduce the immune response to vaccine).
No products indexed under this heading.

Daunorubicin Hydrochloride (Cytotoxic drugs may reduce the immune response to vaccine). Products include:
Cerubidine for Injection 788

Dexamethasone (Concurrent immunosuppressive therapy with greater than physiologic doses of corticosteroids may reduce the immune response to vaccine). Products include:
Ciprodex Otic Suspension 555
Decadron Tablets 1929
TobraDex Ophthalmic Ointment 558
TobraDex Ophthalmic Suspension 558

Dexamethasone Acetate (Concurrent immunosuppressive therapy with greater than physiologic doses of corticosteroids may reduce the immune response to vaccine).
No products indexed under this heading.

Dexamethasone Sodium Phosphate (Concurrent immunosuppressive therapy with greater than physiologic doses of corticosteroids may reduce the immune response to vaccine). Products include:
Decadron Phosphate Injection 1931

Doxorubicin Hydrochloride (Cytotoxic drugs may reduce the immune response to vaccine). Products include:
Adriamycin for Injection, USP 786
Adriamycin Injection, USP 786

Epirubicin Hydrochloride (Cytotoxic drugs may reduce the immune response to vaccine). Products include:
Ellence Injection 2632

Floxuridine (Immunosuppressive therapies may reduce the immune response to vaccines).
No products indexed under this heading.

Fludarabine Phosphate (Immunosuppressive therapies may reduce the immune response to vaccines).
No products indexed under this heading.

Fludrocortisone Acetate (Concurrent immunosuppressive therapy with greater than physiologic doses of corticosteroids may reduce the immune response to vaccine).
No products indexed under this heading.

Fluorouracil (Immunosuppressive therapies may reduce the immune response to vaccines). Products include:
Carac Cream, 0.5% 1048
Efudex 3348

Gemcitabine Hydrochloride (Immunosuppressive therapies may reduce the immune response to vaccines). Products include:
Gemzar for Injection 1743

Hydrocortisone (Concurrent immunosuppressive therapy with greater than physiologic doses of corticosteroids may reduce the immune response to vaccine). Products include:
Cortizone•5 Ointment .... ▣699
Cortizone•10 Creme .... ▣699
Cortizone•10 Ointment .... ▣699
Cortizone•10 Plus Creme .... ▣700
Cortizone•10 Maximum Strength Quick Shot Spray .... ▣700
Hydrocortone Tablets 1963
Preparation H Hydrocortisone Cream .... ▣748

Hydrocortisone Acetate (Concurrent immunosuppressive therapy with greater than physiologic doses of corticosteroids may reduce the immune response to vaccine). Products include:
Analpram-HC 1136
Pramosone 1139
ProctoFoam-HC 3113
Tucks Anti-Itch Ointment .... ▣712
U-cort 1% Cream 3289

Hydrocortisone Sodium Phosphate (Concurrent immunosuppressive therapy with greater than physiologic doses of corticosteroids may reduce the immune response to vaccine).
No products indexed under this heading.

Hydrocortisone Sodium Succinate (Concurrent immunosuppressive therapy with greater than physiologic doses of corticosteroids may reduce the immune response to vaccine).
No products indexed under this heading.

Hydroxyurea (Cytotoxic drugs may reduce the immune response to vaccine).
No products indexed under this heading.

Lomustine (CCNU) (Alkylating drugs may reduce the immune response to vaccine).
No products indexed under this heading.

Mechlorethamine Hydrochloride (Alkylating drugs may reduce the immune response to vaccine). Products include:
Mustargen for Injection 2007

Melphalan (Alkylating drugs may reduce the immune response to vaccine). Products include:
Alkeran Tablets 977

Mercaptopurine (Immunosuppressive therapies may reduce the immune response to vaccines). Products include:
Purinethol Tablets 1222

Methotrexate (Immunosuppressive therapies may reduce the immune response to vaccines).
No products indexed under this heading.

Methotrexate Sodium (Cytotoxic drugs may reduce the immune response to vaccine).
No products indexed under this heading.

Methylprednisolone Acetate (Concurrent immunosuppressive therapy with greater than physiologic doses of corticosteroids may reduce the immune response to vaccine). Products include:
Depo-Medrol Injectable Suspension 2615
Depo-Medrol Single-Dose Vial 2617

Methylprednisolone Sodium Succinate (Concurrent immunosuppressive therapy with greater than physiologic doses of corticosteroids may reduce the immune response to vaccine).
No products indexed under this heading.

Mitotane (Cytotoxic drugs may reduce the immune response to vaccine).
No products indexed under this heading.

Mitoxantrone Hydrochloride (Cytotoxic drugs may reduce the immune response to vaccine). Products include:
Novantrone for Injection Concentrate 3158

Muromonab-CD3 (Concurrent immunosuppressive therapy may reduce the immune response to vaccine). Products include:
Orthoclone OKT3 Sterile Solution 2370

Mycophenolate Mofetil (Concurrent immunosuppressive therapy may reduce the immune response to vaccine). Products include:
CellCept Capsules 2751
CellCept Oral Suspension 2751
CellCept Tablets 2751

Pentostatin (Immunosuppressive therapies may reduce the immune response to vaccines). Products include:
Nipent for Injection 3216

Prednisolone Acetate (Concurrent immunosuppressive therapy with greater than physiologic doses of corticosteroids may reduce the immune response to vaccine). Products include:
Blephamide Ophthalmic Ointment 563
Blephamide Ophthalmic Suspension 564
Poly-Pred Liquifilm Ophthalmic Suspension .... ⊙231
Pred Forte Ophthalmic Suspension .... ⊙233
Pred Mild Sterile Ophthalmic Suspension .... ⊙236
Pred-G Ophthalmic Suspension ...... ⊙234
Pred-G Sterile Ophthalmic Ointment .... ⊙235

Prednisolone Sodium Phosphate (Concurrent immunosuppressive therapy with greater than physiologic doses of corticosteroids may reduce the immune response to vaccine). Products include:
Pediapred Oral Solution 3319

Prednisolone Tebutate (Concurrent immunosuppressive therapy with greater than physiologic doses of corticosteroids may reduce the immune response to vaccine).
No products indexed under this heading.

Prednisone (Concurrent immunosuppressive therapy with greater than physiologic doses of corticosteroids may reduce the immune response to vaccine).
No products indexed under this heading.

Procarbazine Hydrochloride (Cytotoxic drugs may reduce the immune response to vaccine). Products include:
Matulane Capsules 3188

Sirolimus (Concurrent immunosuppressive therapy may reduce the immune response to vaccine). Products include:
Rapamune Oral Solution and Tablets 3472

Tacrolimus (Concurrent immunosuppressive therapy may reduce the immune response to vaccine). Products include:
Prograf Capsules and Injection 624
Protopic Ointment 629

Tamoxifen Citrate (Cytotoxic drugs may reduce the immune response to vaccine).
No products indexed under this heading.

Thioguanine (Immunosuppressive therapies may reduce the immune response to vaccines). Products include:
Tabloid Tablets 1545

Thiotepa (Alkylating drugs may reduce the immune response to vaccine).
No products indexed under this heading.

Triamcinolone (Concurrent immunosuppressive therapy with greater than physiologic doses of corticosteroids may reduce the immune response to vaccine).
No products indexed under this heading.

Triamcinolone Acetonide (Concurrent immunosuppressive therapy with greater than physiologic doses of corticosteroids may reduce the immune response to vaccine). Products include:
Azmacort Inhalation Aerosol 1701
Nasacort HFA Inhalation Aerosol 2939
Nasacort AQ Nasal Spray 2937

Triamcinolone Diacetate (Concurrent immunosuppressive therapy with greater than physiologic doses of corticosteroids may reduce the immune response to vaccine).
No products indexed under this heading.

Triamcinolone Hexacetonide (Concurrent immunosuppressive therapy with greater than physiologic doses of corticosteroids may reduce the immune response to vaccine).
No products indexed under this heading.

(▣ Described in PDR For Nonprescription Drugs) (⊙ Described in PDR For Ophthalmic Medicines™)

Vincristine Sulfate (Cytotoxic drugs may reduce the immune response to vaccine).
No products indexed under this heading.

ADALAT CC TABLETS

(Nifedipine) 2978

May interact with antihypertensives, beta blockers, oral anticoagulants, cytochrome p450 3a4 inducers (selected), cytochrome p450 3a4 inhibitors (selected), cytochrome p450 3a substrates (selected), erythromycin, cardiac glycosides, narcotic analgesics, phenytoin, and certain other agents. Compounds in these categories include:

Acarbose (Nifedipine tends to produce hyperglycemia and may lead to loss of glucose control. Blood glucose levels should be monitored when used in combination with nifedipine). Products include:
Precose Tablets 776

Acebutolol Hydrochloride (Combination of nifedipine and beta-blockers may increase the likelihood of congestive heart failure, severe hypotension, or exacerbation of angina).
No products indexed under this heading.

Acetazolamide (Nifedipine is mainly eliminated by metabolism and is a substrate of CYP3A4. Inhibitors of CYP3A4 can impact the exposure to nifedipine and consequently its desirable and undesirable effects).
No products indexed under this heading.

Alfentanil Hydrochloride (Potential for severe hypotension and/or increased fluid volume requirements cannot be ruled out when nifedipine is co-administered with a beta-blocker and a narcotic analgesic).
No products indexed under this heading.

Allium sativum (Nifedipine is mainly eliminated by metabolism and is a substrate of CYP3A4. Inducers of CYP3A4 can impact the exposure to nifedipine and consequently its desirable and undesirable effects).
No products indexed under this heading.

Alprazolam (Data indicates that nifedipine can inhibit the metabolism of drugs that are substrates of CYP3A, thereby increasing the exposure to other drugs). Products include:
Niravam Orally Disintegrating Tablets 3106
Xanax XR Tablets 2655

Aminophylline (Data indicates that nifedipine can inhibit the metabolism of drugs that are substrates of CYP3A, thereby increasing the exposure to other drugs).
No products indexed under this heading.

Amiodarone Hydrochloride (Nifedipine is mainly eliminated by metabolism and is a substrate of CYP3A4. Inhibitors of CYP3A4 can impact the exposure to nifedipine and consequently its desirable and undesirable effects). Products include:
Pacerone Tablets 3337

Amitriptyline Hydrochloride (Data indicates that nifedipine can inhibit the metabolism of drugs that are substrates of CYP3A, thereby increasing the exposure to other drugs).
No products indexed under this heading.

Amlodipine Besylate (Data indicates that nifedipine can inhibit the metabolism of drugs that are substrates of CYP3A, thereby increasing the exposure to other drugs). Products include:
Caduet Tablets 2507
Lotrel Capsules 2238
Norvasc Tablets 2529

Amprenavir (Co-administration of nifedipine with CYP3A4 inhibitors, such as amprenavir, may cause an increase in nifedipine plasma concentrations; a reduction in nifedipine dosage may be considered). Products include:
Agenerase Capsules 1299
Agenerase Oral Solution 1304

Anastrozole (Nifedipine is mainly eliminated by metabolism and is a substrate of CYP3A4. Inhibitors of CYP3A4 can impact the exposure to nifedipine and consequently its desirable and undesirable effects). Products include:
Arimidex Tablets 665

Anisindione (There have been rare reports of increased prothrombin time in patients taking coumarin anticoagulants to whom nifedipine was administered). Products include:
Miradon Tablets 3056

Aprepitant (Nifedipine is mainly eliminated by metabolism and is a substrate of CYP3A4. Inhibitors of CYP3A4 can impact the exposure to nifedipine and consequently its desirable and undesirable effects). Products include:
Emend Capsules 1944

Astemizole (Data indicates that nifedipine can inhibit the metabolism of drugs that are substrates of CYP3A, thereby increasing the exposure to other drugs).
No products indexed under this heading.

Atanazavir (Co-administration of nifedipine with CYP3A4 inhibitors, such as atanazavir, may cause an increase in nifedipine plasma concentrations; a reduction in nifedipine dosage may be considered).
No products indexed under this heading.

Atenolol (Combination of nifedipine and beta-blockers may increase the likelihood of congestive heart failure, severe hypotension, or exacerbation of angina). Products include:
Tenormin I.V. Injection 698
Tenormin Tablets 695

Atorvastatin Calcium (Data indicates that nifedipine can inhibit the metabolism of drugs that are substrates of CYP3A, thereby increasing the exposure to other drugs). Products include:
Caduet Tablets 2507
Lipitor Tablets 2495

Benazepril Hydrochloride (Co-administration with nifedipine can cause a hypotensive effect and attenuate the tachycardic effect of nifedipine). Products include:
Lotensin Tablets 2232
Lotensin HCT Tablets 2235
Lotrel Capsules 2238

Bendroflumethiazide (Nifedipine is a vasodilator, and co-administration of other drugs affecting blood pressure may result in pharmacodynamic interactions).
No products indexed under this heading.

Betamethasone Acetate (Nifedipine is mainly eliminated by metabolism and is a substrate of CYP3A4. Inducers of CYP3A4 can impact the exposure to nifedipine and consequently its desirable and undesirable effects).
No products indexed under this heading.

Betamethasone Sodium Phosphate (Nifedipine is mainly eliminated by metabolism and is a substrate of CYP3A4. Inducers of CYP3A4 can impact the exposure to nifedipine and consequently its desirable and undesirable effects).
No products indexed under this heading.

Betaxolol Hydrochloride (Combination of nifedipine and beta-blockers may increase the likelihood of congestive heart failure, severe hypotension, or exacerbation of angina). Products include:
Betoptic S Ophthalmic Suspension 554

Bisoprolol Fumarate (Combination of nifedipine and beta-blockers may increase the likelihood of congestive heart failure, severe hypotension, or exacerbation of angina).
No products indexed under this heading.

Buprenorphine Hydrochloride (Potential for severe hypotension and/or increased fluid volume requirements cannot be ruled out when nifedipine is co-administered with a beta-blocker and a narcotic analgesic). Products include:
Buprenex Injectable 2718
Suboxone Tablets 2719
Subutex Tablets 2719

Buspirone Hydrochloride (Data indicates that nifedipine can inhibit the metabolism of drugs that are substrates of CYP3A, thereby increasing the exposure to other drugs).
No products indexed under this heading.

Busulfan (Data indicates that nifedipine can inhibit the metabolism of drugs that are substrates of CYP3A, thereby increasing the exposure to other drugs). Products include:
I.V. Busulfex 1125
Myleran Tablets 1492

Candesartan Cilexetil (Nifedipine is a vasodilator, and co-administration of other drugs affecting blood pressure may result in pharmacodynamic interactions). Products include:
Atacand Tablets 634
Atacand HCT 637

Captopril (Nifedipine is a vasodilator, and co-administration of other drugs affecting blood pressure may result in pharmacodynamic interactions). Products include:
Captopril Tablets 2114

Carbamazepine (Carbamazepine has been shown to reduce plasma concentrations of other calcium channel blockers due to enzyme induction; a similar interaction with nifedipine leading to a decrease in nifedipine plasma concentrations and a decrease in efficacy cannot be excluded; a dosage adjustment of nifedipine may be needed). Products include:
Carbatrol Capsules 3174
Equetro Extended-Release Capsules 3178
Tegretol/Tegretol-XR 2278

Carteolol Hydrochloride (Combination of nifedipine and beta-blockers may increase the likelihood of congestive heart failure, severe hypotension, or exacerbation of angina). Products include:
Carteolol Hydrochloride Ophthalmic Solution USP, 1% .... ⊙246

Cerivastatin Sodium (Data indicates that nifedipine can inhibit the metabolism of drugs that are substrates of CYP3A, thereby increasing the exposure to other drugs).
No products indexed under this heading.

Chlorothiazide (Nifedipine is a vasodilator, and co-administration of other drugs affecting blood pressure may result in pharmacodynamic interactions). Products include:
Aldoclor Tablets 1881
Diuril Oral 1936

Chlorothiazide Sodium (Nifedipine is a vasodilator, and co-administration of other drugs affecting blood pressure may result in pharmacodynamic interactions). Products include:
Diuril Sodium Intravenous 1934

Chlorpheniramine (Data indicates that nifedipine can inhibit the metabolism of drugs that are substrates of CYP3A, thereby increasing the exposure to other drugs).
No products indexed under this heading.

Chlorpheniramine Maleate (Data indicates that nifedipine can inhibit the metabolism of drugs that are substrates of CYP3A, thereby increasing the exposure to other drugs). Products include:
Advil Allergy Sinus Caplets 737
Advil Multi-Symptom Cold Caplets 738
BC Allergy Sinus Cold Powder 612
Contac Severe Cold and Flu Caplets Maximum Strength 615
Hycomine Compound Tablets 1105
PediaCare Multi-Symptom Cold Liquid 704
PediaCare NightRest Cough & Cold Liquid 704
Robitussin Flu Liquid 752
Robitussin PM Cough & Cold Liquid 752
Singlet Caplets 636
Sudafed Sinus & Allergy Tablets 710
TheraFlu Cold & Cough Hot Liquid 680
TheraFlu Cold & Sore Throat Hot Liquid 680
TheraFlu Flu & Sore Throat Hot Liquid 681
TheraFlu Severe Cold & Cough Hot Liquid 683
TheraFlu Severe Cold Caplets 679
TheraFlu Severe Cold Hot Liquid 682
Triaminic Cold & Allergy Liquid 685
Triaminic Cold & Cough Liquid 685
Triaminic Flu, Cough & Fever Liquid 685
Triaminic Night Time Cough & Cold Liquid 685
Triaminic Allergy Runny Nose & Congestion Softchews 688
Triaminic Cold & Cough Softchews 688
Children's Tylenol Plus Cold NightTime Suspension Liquid 1851
Children's Tylenol Plus Cold & Cough Suspension Liquid and Chewable Tablets 1851

IMPORTANT NOTE: Always consult each drug listing in the patient's regimen for possible interactions.

Children's Tylenol Plus Cold Chewable Tablets **1851**
Children's Tylenol Plus Flu Suspension Liquid **1853**
Tylenol Allergy Complete Multi-Symptom Caplets and Gelcaps with Cool Burst **1844**
Multi-Symptom Tylenol Cold Night Time Caplets **1845**
Vicks 44M Cough, Cold & Flu Relief **2676**
Pediatric Vicks 44m Cough & Cold Relief **2673**
Children's Vicks NyQuil Cold/Cough Relief **2671**

Chlorpheniramine Polistirex (Data indicates that nifedipine can inhibit the metabolism of drugs that are substrates of CYP3A, thereby increasing the exposure to other drugs). Products include:
Tussionex Pennkinetic Extended-Release Suspension **3322**

Chlorpheniramine Tannate (Data indicates that nifedipine can inhibit the metabolism of drugs that are substrates of CYP3A, thereby increasing the exposure to other drugs).
No products indexed under this heading.

Chlorthalidone (Nifedipine is a vasodilator, and co-administration of other drugs affecting blood pressure may result in pharmacodynamic interactions). Products include:
Clorpres Tablets **2139**

Cimetidine (Both the peak plasma level of nifedipine and AUC may increase in the presence of cimetidine. Cautious titration of nifedipine is advised; relevant changes in blood pressure was experienced; a reduction in nifedipine dosage may be considered). Products include:
Tagamet HB 200 Tablets .... ▣**637**
Tagamet Tablets **1547**

Cimetidine Hydrochloride (Both the peak plasma level of nifedipine and AUC may increase in the presence of cimetidine. Cautious titration of nifedipine is advised; relevant changes in blood pressure was experienced; a reduction in nifedipine dosage may be considered).
No products indexed under this heading.

Ciprofloxacin (Nifedipine is mainly eliminated by metabolism and is a substrate of CYP3A4. Inhibitors of CYP3A4 can impact the exposure to nifedipine and consequently its desirable and undesirable effects). Products include:
Cipro I.V. **2998**
Cipro I.V. Pharmacy Bulk Package ... **3509**
Cipro Oral Suspension **2991**
Cipro XR Tablets **3004**
Ciprodex Otic Suspension **555**

Ciprofloxacin Hydrochloride (Nifedipine is mainly eliminated by metabolism and is a substrate of CYP3A4. Inducers of CYP3A4 can impact the exposure to nifedipine and consequently its desirable and undesirable effects). Products include:
Ciloxan Ophthalmic Ointment **554**
Cipro Tablets **2991**

Cisapride (Concomitant administration may lead to increased plasma concentrations of nifedipine).
No products indexed under this heading.

Cisplatin (Nifedipine is mainly eliminated by metabolism and is a substrate of CYP3A4. Inducers of CYP3A4 can impact the exposure to nifedipine and consequently its desirable and undesirable effects).
No products indexed under this heading.

Clarithromycin (Nifedipine is mainly eliminated by metabolism and is a substrate of CYP3A4. Inhibitors of CYP3A4 can impact the exposure to nifedipine and consequently its desirable and undesirable effects). Products include:
Biaxin/Biaxin XL **402**
PREVPAC **3281**

Clonidine (Nifedipine is a vasodilator, and co-administration of other drugs affecting blood pressure may result in pharmacodynamic interactions). Products include:
Catapres-TTS **875**

Clonidine Hydrochloride (Nifedipine is a vasodilator, and co-administration of other drugs affecting blood pressure may result in pharmacodynamic interactions). Products include:
Catapres Tablets **874**
Clorpres Tablets **2139**

Clotrimazole (Nifedipine is mainly eliminated by metabolism and is a substrate of CYP3A4. Inhibitors of CYP3A4 can impact the exposure to nifedipine and consequently its desirable and undesirable effects). Products include:
Lotrimin **3053**
Lotrisone **3054**

Codeine Phosphate (Potential for severe hypotension and/or increased fluid volume requirements cannot be ruled out when nifedipine is co-administered with a beta-blocker and a narcotic analgesic). Products include:
Tylenol with Codeine **2461**

Cortisone Acetate (Nifedipine is mainly eliminated by metabolism and is a substrate of CYP3A4. Inducers of CYP3A4 can impact the exposure to nifedipine and consequently its desirable and undesirable effects).
No products indexed under this heading.

Cyclosporine (Nifedipine is mainly eliminated by metabolism and is a substrate of CYP3A4. Inhibitors of CYP3A4 can impact the exposure to nifedipine and consequently its desirable and undesirable effects). Products include:
Gengraf Capsules **458**
Neoral Soft Gelatin Capsules **2247**
Neoral Oral Solution **2247**
Restasis Ophthalmic Emulsion **570**
Sandimmune **2259**

Dalfopristin (Concomitant administration may lead to increased plasma concentrations of nifedipine; a reduction in nifedipine dosage may be considered). Products include:
Synercid I.V. **1690**

Danazol (Nifedipine is mainly eliminated by metabolism and is a substrate of CYP3A4. Inhibitors of CYP3A4 can impact the exposure to nifedipine and consequently its desirable and undesirable effects).
No products indexed under this heading.

Delavirdine Mesylate (Nifedipine is mainly eliminated by metabolism and is a substrate of CYP3A4. Inhibitors of CYP3A4 can impact the exposure to nifedipine and consequently its desirable and undesirable effects). Products include:
Rescriptor Tablets **2535**

Delavirine (Co-administration of nifedipine with CYP3A4 inhibitors, such as delavirine, may cause an increase in nifedipine plasma concentrations; a reduction in nifedipine dosage may be considered).
No products indexed under this heading.

Deserpidine (Nifedipine is a vasodilator, and co-administration of other drugs affecting blood pressure may result in pharmacodynamic interactions).
No products indexed under this heading.

Deslanoside (Potential of elevated digoxin levels).
No products indexed under this heading.

Desogestrel (Data indicates that nifedipine can inhibit the metabolism of drugs that are substrates of CYP3A, thereby increasing the exposure to other drugs). Products include:
Ortho-Cept Tablets **2395**

Dexamethasone (Nifedipine is mainly eliminated by metabolism and is a substrate of CYP3A4. Inducers of CYP3A4 can impact the exposure to nifedipine and consequently its desirable and undesirable effects). Products include:
Ciprodex Otic Suspension **555**
Decadron Tablets **1929**
TobraDex Ophthalmic Ointment **558**
TobraDex Ophthalmic Suspension ... **558**

Dexamethasone Acetate (Nifedipine is mainly eliminated by metabolism and is a substrate of CYP3A4. Inducers of CYP3A4 can impact the exposure to nifedipine and consequently its desirable and undesirable effects).
No products indexed under this heading.

Dexamethasone Phosphate (Data indicates that nifedipine can inhibit the metabolism of drugs that are substrates of CYP3A, thereby increasing the exposure to other drugs).
No products indexed under this heading.

Dexamethasone Sodium (Data indicates that nifedipine can inhibit the metabolism of drugs that are substrates of CYP3A, thereby increasing the exposure to other drugs).
No products indexed under this heading.

Dexamethasone Sodium Phosphate (Nifedipine is mainly eliminated by metabolism and is a substrate of CYP3A4. Inducers of CYP3A4 can impact the exposure to nifedipine and consequently its desirable and undesirable effects). Products include:
Decadron Phosphate Injection **1931**

Dezocine (Potential for severe hypotension and/or increased fluid volume requirements cannot be ruled out when nifedipine is co-administered with a beta-blocker and a narcotic analgesic).
No products indexed under this heading.

Diazepam (Data indicates that nifedipine can inhibit the metabolism of drugs that are substrates of CYP3A, thereby increasing the exposure to other drugs). Products include:
Diastat Rectal Delivery System **3344**
Valium Tablets **2822**

Diazoxide (Nifedipine is a vasodilator, and co-administration of other drugs affecting blood pressure may result in pharmacodynamic interactions). Products include:
Hyperstat I.V. Injection **3031**

Dicumarol (There have been rare reports of increased prothrombin time in patients taking coumarin anticoagulants to whom nifedipine was administered).
No products indexed under this heading.

Digitalis Glycoside Preparations (Potential of elevated digoxin levels).
No products indexed under this heading.

Digitoxin (Potential of elevated digoxin levels).
No products indexed under this heading.

Digoxin (Potential of elevated digoxin levels). Products include:
Digitek Tablets **2146**
Lanoxicaps Capsules **1458**
Lanoxin Injection **1462**
Lanoxin Tablets **1468**
Lanoxin Injection Pediatric **1465**

Dihydroergotamine Mesylate (Data indicates that nifedipine can inhibit the metabolism of drugs that are substrates of CYP3A, thereby increasing the exposure to other drugs). Products include:
Migranal Nasal Spray **3350**

Diltiazem Hydrochloride (Co-administration can increase nifedipine Cmax and AUC by 2.0 and 2.2 respectively; use with caution and consider dose reducation of nifedipine). Products include:
Cardizem LA Extended Release Tablets **1699**
Tiazac Capsules **1204**

Diltiazem Maleate (Nifedipine is mainly eliminated by metabolism and is a substrate of CYP3A4. Inhibitors of CYP3A4 can impact the exposure to nifedipine and consequently its desirable and undesirable effects).
No products indexed under this heading.

Disopyramide Phosphate (Data indicates that nifedipine can inhibit the metabolism of drugs that are substrates of CYP3A, thereby increasing the exposure to other drugs).
No products indexed under this heading.

Doxazosin Mesylate (Co-administration of nifedipine with CYP3A4 inhibitors, such as doxazosin, may cause an increase in nifedipine plasma concentrations; a reduction in nifedipine dosage may be considered).
No products indexed under this heading.

Doxorubicin Hydrochloride (Nifedipine is mainly eliminated by metabolism and is a substrate of CYP3A4. Inducers of CYP3A4 can impact the exposure to nifedipine and consequently its desirable and undesirable effects). Products include:
Adriamycin for Injection, USP **786**
Adriamycin Injection, USP **786**

Dronabinol (Data indicates that nifedipine can inhibit the metabolism of drugs that are substrates of

CYP3A, thereby increasing the exposure to other drugs). Products include:

Marinol Capsules ... 3334

Dyphylline (Data indicates that nifedipine can inhibit the metabolism of drugs that are substrates of CYP3A, thereby increasing the exposure to other drugs).

No products indexed under this heading.

Efavirenz (Nifedipine is mainly eliminated by metabolism and is a substrate of CYP3A4. Inhibitors of CYP3A4 can impact the exposure to nifedipine and consequently its desirable and undesirable effects). Products include:

Sustiva Capsules ... 957

Enalapril Maleate (Nifedipine is a vasodilator, and co-administration of other drugs affecting blood pressure may result in pharmacodynamic interactions). Products include:

Vaseretic Tablets ... 2073
Vasotec I.V. Injection ... 2076

Enalaprilat (Nifedipine is a vasodilator, and co-administration of other drugs affecting blood pressure may result in pharmacodynamic interactions).

No products indexed under this heading.

Eprosartan Mesylate (Nifedipine is a vasodilator, and co-administration of other drugs affecting blood pressure may result in pharmacodynamic interactions). Products include:

Teveten Tablets ... 1707
Teveten HCT Tablets ... 1710

Ergotamine Tartrate (Data indicates that nifedipine can inhibit the metabolism of drugs that are substrates of CYP3A, thereby increasing the exposure to other drugs).

No products indexed under this heading.

Erythromycin (Co-administration of nifedipine with CYP3A4 inhibitors, such as erythromycin, may cause an increase in nifedipine plasma concentrations; a reduction in nifedipine dosage may be considered). Products include:

Erygel Topical Gel ... 2096
Ery-Tab Tablets ... 447
Erythromycin Base Filmtab Tablets ... 454
Erythromycin Delayed-Release Capsules, USP ... 456
PCE Dispertab Tablets ... 510

Erythromycin Estolate (Co-administration of nifedipine with CYP3A4 inhibitors, such as erythromycin, may cause an increase in nifedipine plasma concentrations; a reduction in nifedipine dosage may be considered).

No products indexed under this heading.

Erythromycin Ethylsuccinate (Co-administration of nifedipine with CYP3A4 inhibitors, such as erythromycin, may cause an increase in nifedipine plasma concentrations; a reduction in nifedipine dosage may be considered). Products include:

E.E.S. ... 449
EryPed ... 445

Erythromycin Gluceptate (Co-administration of nifedipine with CYP3A4 inhibitors, such as erythromycin, may cause an increase in nifedipine plasma concentrations; a reduction in nifedipine dosage may be considered).

No products indexed under this heading.

Erythromycin Lactobionate (Co-administration of nifedipine with CYP3A4 inhibitors, such as erythromycin, may cause an increase in nifedipine plasma concentrations; a reduction in nifedipine dosage may be considered).

No products indexed under this heading.

Erythromycin Stearate (Co-administration of nifedipine with CYP3A4 inhibitors, such as erythromycin, may cause an increase in nifedipine plasma concentrations; a reduction in nifedipine dosage may be considered). Products include:

Erythrocin Stearate Filmtab Tablets ... 452

Esmolol Hydrochloride (Combination of nifedipine and beta-blockers may increase the likelihood of congestive heart failure, severe hypotension, or exacerbation of angina). Products include:

Brevibloc Concentrate ... 766
Brevibloc Injection ... 766
Brevibloc Double Strength Injection ... 766
Brevibloc Premixed Injection ... 766
Brevibloc Double Strength Premixed Injection ... 766

Esomeprazole Magnesium (Nifedipine is mainly eliminated by metabolism and is a substrate of CYP3A4. Inhibitors of CYP3A4 can impact the exposure to nifedipine and consequently its desirable and undesirable effects). Products include:

Nexium Delayed-Release Capsules ... 645

Estrogen (Data indicates that nifedipine can inhibit the metabolism of drugs that are substrates of CYP3A, thereby increasing the exposure to other drugs).

No products indexed under this heading.

Estrogens, Conjugated (Data indicates that nifedipine can inhibit the metabolism of drugs that are substrates of CYP3A, thereby increasing the exposure to other drugs). Products include:

Premarin Intravenous ... 3440
Premarin Tablets ... 3443
Premarin Vaginal Cream ... 3449
Premphase Tablets ... 3452
Prempro Tablets ... 3452

Estrogens, Conjugated, Synthetic A (Data indicates that nifedipine can inhibit the metabolism of drugs that are substrates of CYP3A, thereby increasing the exposure to other drugs). Products include:

Cenestin Tablets, 0.45mg, 0.625mg, 0.9mg, 1.25mg ... 1063
Cenestin Tablets, 0.3mg ... 1063

Estrogens, Esterified (Data indicates that nifedipine can inhibit the metabolism of drugs that are substrates of CYP3A, thereby increasing the exposure to other drugs). Products include:

Estratest Tablets ... 3196
Estratest H.S. Tablets ... 3196

Ethinyl Estradiol (Data indicates that nifedipine can inhibit the metabolism of drugs that are substrates of CYP3A, thereby increasing the exposure to other drugs). Products include:

Alesse-28 Tablets ... 3392
Lo/Ovral-28 Tablets ... 3423
NuvaRing ... 2357
Ortho-Cept Tablets ... 2395
Ortho-Cyclen/Ortho Tri-Cyclen ... 2414
Ortho Evra Transdermal System ... 2402
Ortho Tri-Cyclen Lo Tablets ... 2421
Seasonale Tablets ... 1073
Triphasil-28 Tablets ... 3483
Yasmin 28 Tablets ... 818

Ethosuximide (Nifedipine is mainly eliminated by metabolism and is a substrate of CYP3A4. Inducers of CYP3A4 can impact the exposure to nifedipine and consequently its desirable and undesirable effects).

No products indexed under this heading.

Ethynodiol Diacetate (Data indicates that nifedipine can inhibit the metabolism of drugs that are substrates of CYP3A, thereby increasing the exposure to other drugs).

No products indexed under this heading.

Etoposide (Data indicates that nifedipine can inhibit the metabolism of drugs that are substrates of CYP3A, thereby increasing the exposure to other drugs).

No products indexed under this heading.

Etoposide Phosphate (Data indicates that nifedipine can inhibit the metabolism of drugs that are substrates of CYP3A, thereby increasing the exposure to other drugs).

No products indexed under this heading.

Felbamate (Nifedipine is mainly eliminated by metabolism and is a substrate of CYP3A4. Inducers of CYP3A4 can impact the exposure to nifedipine and consequently its desirable and undesirable effects).

No products indexed under this heading.

Felodipine (Data indicates that nifedipine can inhibit the metabolism of drugs that are substrates of CYP3A, thereby increasing the exposure to other drugs). Products include:

Plendil Extended-Release Tablets ... 651

Fentanyl (Severe hypotension and/or increased fluid volume requirements have been reported when nifedipine was co-administered with a beta-blocker and high-dose fentanyl anesthesia. If permitted, sufficient time (at least 36 hours) should be allowed for nifedipine to be washed out of the body prior to surgery). Products include:

Duragesic Transdermal System ... 2448

Fentanyl Citrate (Severe hypotension and/or increased fluid volume requirements have been reported when nifedipine was co-administered with a beta-blocker and high-dose fentanyl anesthesia. If permitted, sufficient time (at least 36 hours) should be allowed for nifedipine to be washed out of the body prior to surgery). Products include:

Actiq ... 993

Fluconazole (Co-administration of nifedipine with CYP3A4 inhibitors, such as fluconazole, may cause an increase in nifedipine plasma concentrations; a reduction in nifedipine dosage may be considered).

No products indexed under this heading.

Fludrocortisone Acetate (Nifedipine is mainly eliminated by metabolism and is a substrate of CYP3A4. Inducers of CYP3A4 can impact the exposure to nifedipine and consequently its desirable and undesirable effects).

No products indexed under this heading.

Fluoxetine (Co-administration of nifedipine with CYP3A4 inhibitors, such as fluoxetine, may cause an increase in nifedipine plasma concentrations; a reduction in nifedipine dosage may be considered).

No products indexed under this heading.

Fluoxetine Hydrochloride (Co-administration of nifedipine with CYP3A4 inhibitors, such as fluoxetine, may cause an increase in nifedipine plasma concentrations; a reduction in nifedipine dosage may be considered). Products include:

Prozac Pulvules and Liquid ... 1771
Symbyax Capsules ... 1788

Fluvoxamine Maleate (Nifedipine is mainly eliminated by metabolism and is a substrate of CYP3A4. Inhibitors of CYP3A4 can impact the exposure to nifedipine and consequently its desirable and undesirable effects).

No products indexed under this heading.

Fosamprenavir Calcium (Nifedipine is mainly eliminated by metabolism and is a substrate of CYP3A4. Inhibitors of CYP3A4 can impact the exposure to nifedipine and consequently its desirable and undesirable effects). Products include:

Lexiva Tablets ... 1473

Fosinopril Sodium (Nifedipine is a vasodilator, and co-administration of other drugs affecting blood pressure may result in pharmacodynamic interactions).

No products indexed under this heading.

Fosphenytoin Sodium (Co-administration of nifedipine and phenytoin, an inducer of CYP3A4, lowered AUC and Cmax of nifedipine by approximately 70%).

No products indexed under this heading.

Furosemide (Nifedipine is a vasodilator, and co-administration of other drugs affecting blood pressure may result in pharmacodynamic interactions). Products include:

Furosemide Tablets ... 2117

Garlic Extract (Nifedipine is mainly eliminated by metabolism and is a substrate of CYP3A4. Inducers of CYP3A4 can impact the exposure to nifedipine and consequently its desirable and undesirable effects).

No products indexed under this heading.

Garlic Oil (Nifedipine is mainly eliminated by metabolism and is a substrate of CYP3A4. Inducers of CYP3A4 can impact the exposure to nifedipine and consequently its desirable and undesirable effects).

No products indexed under this heading.

Glyburide (Data indicates that nifedipine can inhibit the metabolism of drugs that are substrates of CYP3A, thereby increasing the exposure to other drugs).

No products indexed under this heading.

IMPORTANT NOTE: Always consult each drug listing in the patient's regimen for possible interactions.

Guanabenz Acetate (Nifedipine is a vasodilator, and co-administration of other drugs affecting blood pressure may result in pharmacodynamic interactions).
No products indexed under this heading.

Guanethidine Monosulfate (Nifedipine is a vasodilator, and co-administration of other drugs affecting blood pressure may result in pharmacodynamic interactions).
No products indexed under this heading.

Haloperidol (Data indicates that nifedipine can inhibit the metabolism of drugs that are substrates of CYP3A, thereby increasing the exposure to other drugs).
No products indexed under this heading.

Haloperidol Decanoate (Data indicates that nifedipine can inhibit the metabolism of drugs that are substrates of CYP3A, thereby increasing the exposure to other drugs).
No products indexed under this heading.

Hydralazine Hydrochloride (Nifedipine is a vasodilator, and co-administration of other drugs affecting blood pressure may result in pharmacodynamic interactions).
Products include:
BiDil Tablets 2161

Hydrochlorothiazide (Nifedipine is a vasodilator, and co-administration of other drugs affecting blood pressure may result in pharmacodynamic interactions). Products include:
Aldoril Tablets 1884
Atacand HCT 637
Avalide Tablets 2889
Avalide Tablets 922
Benicar HCT Tablets 2852
Diovan HCT Tablets 2195
Dyazide Capsules 1389
Hyzaar 1964
Lotensin HCT Tablets 2235
Maxzide 2150
Micardis HCT Tablets 886
Moduretic Tablets 2003
Prinzide Tablets 2033
Teveten HCT Tablets 1710
Timolide Tablets 2056
Uniretic Tablets 3114
Vaseretic Tablets 2073
Zestoretic Tablets 701

Hydrocodone Bitartrate (Potential for severe hypotension and/or increased fluid volume requirements cannot be ruled out when nifedipine is co-administered with a beta-blocker and a narcotic analgesic).
Products include:
Hycodan 1104
Hycomine Compound Tablets 1105
Hycotuss Expectorant Syrup 1106
Lortab 3315
Lortab Elixir 3312
Vicodin Tablets 530
Vicodin ES Tablets 531
Vicodin HP Tablets 532
Vicoprofen Tablets 533
Zydone Tablets 1118

Hydrocodone Polistirex (Potential for severe hypotension and/or increased fluid volume requirements cannot be ruled out when nifedipine is co-administered with a beta-blocker and a narcotic analgesic).
Products include:
Tussionex Pennkinetic Extended-Release Suspension...... 3322

Hydrocortisone (Nifedipine is mainly eliminated by metabolism and is a substrate of CYP3A4. Inducers of CYP3A4 can impact the exposure to nifedipine and consequently its desirable and undesirable effects).
Products include:
Cortizone•5 Ointment .... ▣ 699
Cortizone•10 Creme .... ▣ 699
Cortizone•10 Ointment .... ▣ 699
Cortizone•10 Plus Creme .... ▣ 700
Cortizone•10 Maximum Strength Quick Shot Spray .... ▣ 700
Hydrocortone Tablets 1963
Preparation H Hydrocortisone Cream .... ▣ 748

Hydrocortisone Acetate (Nifedipine is mainly eliminated by metabolism and is a substrate of CYP3A4. Inducers of CYP3A4 can impact the exposure to nifedipine and consequently its desirable and undesirable effects). Products include:
Analpram-HC 1136
Pramosone 1139
ProctoFoam-HC 3113
Tucks Anti-Itch Ointment .... ▣ 712
U-cort 1% Cream 3289

Hydrocortisone Butyrate (Nifedipine is mainly eliminated by metabolism and is a substrate of CYP3A4. Inducers of CYP3A4 can impact the exposure to nifedipine and consequently its desirable and undesirable effects). Products include:
Locoid 1138
Locoid Lipocream Cream 1138

Hydrocortisone Cypionate (Nifedipine is mainly eliminated by metabolism and is a substrate of CYP3A4. Inducers of CYP3A4 can impact the exposure to nifedipine and consequently its desirable and undesirable effects).
No products indexed under this heading.

Hydrocortisone Hemisuccinate (Nifedipine is mainly eliminated by metabolism and is a substrate of CYP3A4. Inducers of CYP3A4 can impact the exposure to nifedipine and consequently its desirable and undesirable effects).
No products indexed under this heading.

Hydrocortisone Probutate (Nifedipine is mainly eliminated by metabolism and is a substrate of CYP3A4. Inducers of CYP3A4 can impact the exposure to nifedipine and consequently its desirable and undesirable effects). Products include:
Pandel Cream, 0.1% 1017

Hydrocortisone Sodium Phosphate (Nifedipine is mainly eliminated by metabolism and is a substrate of CYP3A4. Inducers of CYP3A4 can impact the exposure to nifedipine and consequently its desirable and undesirable effects).
No products indexed under this heading.

Hydrocortisone Sodium Succinate (Nifedipine is mainly eliminated by metabolism and is a substrate of CYP3A4. Inducers of CYP3A4 can impact the exposure to nifedipine and consequently its desirable and undesirable effects).
No products indexed under this heading.

Hydrocortisone Valerate (Nifedipine is mainly eliminated by metabolism and is a substrate of CYP3A4. Inducers of CYP3A4 can impact the exposure to nifedipine and consequently its desirable and undesirable effects).
No products indexed under this heading.

Hydroflumethiazide (Nifedipine is a vasodilator, and co-administration of other drugs affecting blood pressure may result in pharmacodynamic interactions).
No products indexed under this heading.

Hydromorphone Hydrochloride (Potential for severe hypotension and/or increased fluid volume requirements cannot be ruled out when nifedipine is co-administered with a beta-blocker and a narcotic analgesic). Products include:
Dilaudid 439
Dilaudid Oral Liquid 443
Dilaudid Non-Sterile Powder 439
Dilaudid Rectal Suppositories 439
Dilaudid Tablets 439
Dilaudid Tablets - 8 mg 443
Dilaudid-HP 441

Hypericum (Co-administration of nifedipine with CYP3A4 inducers, such as St. John's Wort, may cause a decrease in nifedipine plasma concentrations; a dosage adjustment may be needed).
No products indexed under this heading.

Hypericum Perforatum (Nifedipine is mainly eliminated by metabolism and is a substrate of CYP3A4. Inducers of CYP3A4 can impact the exposure to nifedipine and consequently its desirable and undesirable effects).
No products indexed under this heading.

Imipramine Hydrochloride (Data indicates that nifedipine can inhibit the metabolism of drugs that are substrates of CYP3A, thereby increasing the exposure to other drugs).
No products indexed under this heading.

Imipramine Pamoate (Data indicates that nifedipine can inhibit the metabolism of drugs that are substrates of CYP3A, thereby increasing the exposure to other drugs).
No products indexed under this heading.

Indapamide (Nifedipine is a vasodilator, and co-administration of other drugs affecting blood pressure may result in pharmacodynamic interactions). Products include:
Indapamide Tablets 2119

Indinavir Sulfate (Co-administration of nifedipine with CYP3A4 inhibitors, such as indinavir, may cause an increase in nifedipine plasma concentrations; a reduction in nifedipine dosage may be considered). Products include:
Crixivan Capsules 1918

Irbesartan (Nifedipine is a vasodilator, and co-administration of other drugs affecting blood pressure may result in pharmacodynamic interactions). Products include:
Avalide Tablets 922
Avalide Tablets 2889
Avapro Tablets 925
Avapro Tablets 2886

Isoniazid (Nifedipine is mainly eliminated by metabolism and is a substrate of CYP3A4. Inhibitors of CYP3A4 can impact the exposure to nifedipine and consequently its desirable and undesirable effects).
No products indexed under this heading.

Isradipine (Data indicates that nifedipine can inhibit the metabolism of drugs that are substrates of CYP3A, thereby increasing the exposure to other drugs). Products include:
DynaCirc CR Tablets 2726

Itraconazole (Co-administration of nifedipine with CYP3A4 inhibitors, such as itraconazole, may cause an increase in nifedipine plasma concentrations; a reduction in nifedipine dosage may be considered).
No products indexed under this heading.

Ketoconazole (Co-administration of nifedipine with CYP3A4 inhibitors, such as ketoconazol, may cause an increase in nifedipine plasma concentrations; a reduction in nifedipine dosage may be considered).
Products include:
Nizoral A-D Shampoo, 1% 1839
Nizoral 2% Shampoo 1838

Labetalol Hydrochloride (Combination of nifedipine and beta-blockers may increase the likelihood of congestive heart failure, severe hypotension, or exacerbation of angina).
No products indexed under this heading.

Levobunolol Hydrochloride (Combination of nifedipine and beta-blockers may increase the likelihood of congestive heart failure, severe hypotension, or exacerbation of angina). Products include:
Betagan Ophthalmic Solution, USP .... ⊙ 217

Levonorgestrel (Data indicates that nifedipine can inhibit the metabolism of drugs that are substrates of CYP3A, thereby increasing the exposure to other drugs). Products include:
Alesse-28 Tablets 3392
Climara Pro Transdermal System 800
Mirena Intrauterine System 810
Plan B Tablets 1068
Seasonale Tablets 1073
Triphasil-28 Tablets 3483

Levorphanol Tartrate (Potential for severe hypotension and/or increased fluid volume requirements cannot be ruled out when nifedipine is co-administered with a beta-blocker and a narcotic analgesic).
No products indexed under this heading.

Lidocaine (Data indicates that nifedipine can inhibit the metabolism of drugs that are substrates of CYP3A, thereby increasing the exposure to other drugs). Products include:
Lidoderm Patch 1107

Lidocaine Hydrochloride (Data indicates that nifedipine can inhibit the metabolism of drugs that are substrates of CYP3A, thereby increasing the exposure to other drugs).
No products indexed under this heading.

Lisinopril (Nifedipine is a vasodilator, and co-administration of other drugs affecting blood pressure may result in pharmacodynamic interactions). Products include:
Prinivil Tablets 2029
Prinzide Tablets 2033
Zestoretic Tablets 701
Zestril Tablets 704

Lopinavir (Nifedipine is mainly eliminated by metabolism and is a substrate of CYP3A4. Inhibitors of CYP3A4 can impact the exposure to nifedipine and consequently its desirable and undesirable effects).
Products include:

Kaletra **474**

Loratadine (Nifedipine is mainly eliminated by metabolism and is a substrate of CYP3A4. Inhibitors of CYP3A4 can impact the exposure to nifedipine and consequently its desirable and undesirable effects). Products include:

Alavert Allergy & Sinus D-12 Hour Tablets.. **743**
Alavert **743**
Children's Claritin 24 Hour Non-Drowsy Allergy Syrup........... **732**
Claritin Non-Drowsy 24 Hour Tablets.. **731**
Non-Drowsy Claritin Hives Relief Tablets.. **733**
Claritin Reditabs 24 Hour Non-Drowsy Tablets.................... **732**
Claritin-D Non-Drowsy 12 Hour Tablets.. **731**
Claritin-D Non-Drowsy 24 Hour Tablets.. **731**
Children's Dimetapp ND Non-Drowsy Allergy Syrup........... **746**
Triaminic Allerchews **684**

Losartan Potassium (Nifedipine is a vasodilator, and co-administration of other drugs affecting blood pressure may result in pharmacodynamic interactions). Products include:

Cozaar Tablets **1913**
Hyzaar **1964**

Lovastatin (Data indicates that nifedipine can inhibit the metabolism of drugs that are substrates of CYP3A, thereby increasing the exposure to other drugs). Products include:

Advicor Tablets **1694**
Altoprev Extended-Release Tablets **1151**
Mevacor Tablets **1996**

Mecamylamine Hydrochloride (Nifedipine is a vasodilator, and co-administration of other drugs affecting blood pressure may result in pharmacodynamic interactions). Products include:

Inversine Tablets **3286**

Meperidine Hydrochloride (Potential for severe hypotension and/or increased fluid volume requirements cannot be ruled out when nifedipine is co-administered with a beta-blocker and a narcotic analgesic).

No products indexed under this heading.

Mephenytoin (Nifedipine is mainly eliminated by metabolism and is a substrate of CYP3A4. Inducers of CYP3A4 can impact the exposure to nifedipine and consequently its desirable and undesirable effects).

No products indexed under this heading.

Mestranol (Data indicates that nifedipine can inhibit the metabolism of drugs that are substrates of CYP3A, thereby increasing the exposure to other drugs).

No products indexed under this heading.

Metformin Hydrochloride (Co-administration with nifedipine can increase Cmax of metformin hydrochloride, AUC of metformin hydrochloride and amount of metformin hydrochloride excreted in urine). Products include:

ActoPlus Met Tablets **3219**
Avandamet Tablets **1343**
Fortamet Extended-Release Tablets **1156**

Methadone Hydrochloride (Potential for severe hypotension and/or increased fluid volume requirements cannot be ruled out when nifedipine is co-administered with a beta-blocker and a narcotic analgesic).

No products indexed under this heading.

Methsuximide (Nifedipine is mainly eliminated by metabolism and is a substrate of CYP3A4. Inducers of CYP3A4 can impact the exposure to nifedipine and consequently its desirable and undesirable effects).

No products indexed under this heading.

Methyclothiazide (Nifedipine is a vasodilator, and co-administration of other drugs affecting blood pressure may result in pharmacodynamic interactions).

No products indexed under this heading.

Methyldopa (Nifedipine is a vasodilator, and co-administration of other drugs affecting blood pressure may result in pharmacodynamic interactions). Products include:

Aldoclor Tablets **1881**
Aldoril Tablets **1884**

Methyldopate Hydrochloride (Nifedipine is a vasodilator, and co-administration of other drugs affecting blood pressure may result in pharmacodynamic interactions).

No products indexed under this heading.

Methylprednisolone (Nifedipine is mainly eliminated by metabolism and is a substrate of CYP3A4. Inducers of CYP3A4 can impact the exposure to nifedipine and consequently its desirable and undesirable effects).

No products indexed under this heading.

Methylprednisolone Acetate (Nifedipine is mainly eliminated by metabolism and is a substrate of CYP3A4. Inducers of CYP3A4 can impact the exposure to nifedipine and consequently its desirable and undesirable effects). Products include:

Depo-Medrol Injectable Suspension **2615**
Depo-Medrol Single-Dose Vial **2617**

Methylprednisolone Sodium Succinate (Nifedipine is mainly eliminated by metabolism and is a substrate of CYP3A4. Inducers of CYP3A4 can impact the exposure to nifedipine and consequently its desirable and undesirable effects).

No products indexed under this heading.

Metipranolol Hydrochloride (Combination of nifedipine and beta-blockers may increase the likelihood of congestive heart failure, severe hypotension, or exacerbation of angina).

No products indexed under this heading.

Metolazone (Nifedipine is a vasodilator, and co-administration of other drugs affecting blood pressure may result in pharmacodynamic interactions).

No products indexed under this heading.

Metoprolol Succinate (Combination of nifedipine and beta-blockers may increase the likelihood of congestive heart failure, severe hypotension, or exacerbation of angina). Products include:

Toprol-XL Tablets **660**

Metoprolol Tartrate (Combination of nifedipine and beta-blockers may increase the likelihood of congestive heart failure, severe hypotension, or exacerbation of angina).

No products indexed under this heading.

Metronidazole (Nifedipine is mainly eliminated by metabolism and is a substrate of CYP3A4. Inhibitors of CYP3A4 can impact the exposure to nifedipine and consequently its desirable and undesirable effects). Products include:

Metrogel 1% **1212**
MetroGel-Vaginal Gel **1822**
Noritate Cream, 1% **1051**

Metronidazole Benzoate (Nifedipine is mainly eliminated by metabolism and is a substrate of CYP3A4. Inhibitors of CYP3A4 can impact the exposure to nifedipine and consequently its desirable and undesirable effects).

No products indexed under this heading.

Metronidazole Hydrochloride (Nifedipine is mainly eliminated by metabolism and is a substrate of CYP3A4. Inhibitors of CYP3A4 can impact the exposure to nifedipine and consequently its desirable and undesirable effects).

No products indexed under this heading.

Metyrosine (Nifedipine is a vasodilator, and co-administration of other drugs affecting blood pressure may result in pharmacodynamic interactions). Products include:

Demser Capsules **1933**

Mibefradil Dihydrochloride (Nifedipine is a vasodilator, and co-administration of other drugs affecting blood pressure may result in pharmacodynamic interactions).

No products indexed under this heading.

Miconazole (Nifedipine is mainly eliminated by metabolism and is a substrate of CYP3A4. Inhibitors of CYP3A4 can impact the exposure to nifedipine and consequently its desirable and undesirable effects).

No products indexed under this heading.

Miconazole Nitrate (Nifedipine is mainly eliminated by metabolism and is a substrate of CYP3A4. Inhibitors of CYP3A4 can impact the exposure to nifedipine and consequently its desirable and undesirable effects). Products include:

Desenex **674**
Desenex Jock Itch Spray Powder ... **674**

Midazolam Hydrochloride (Data indicates that nifedipine can inhibit the metabolism of drugs that are substrates of CYP3A, thereby increasing the exposure to other drugs).

No products indexed under this heading.

Minoxidil (Nifedipine is a vasodilator, and co-administration of other drugs affecting blood pressure may result in pharmacodynamic interactions). Products include:

Men's Rogaine Extra Strength Topical Solution, Ocean Rush Scent and Original Unscented..... **706**
Women's Rogaine Topical Solution, Spring Bloom Scent and Original Unscented.............. **707**

Modafinil (Nifedipine is mainly eliminated by metabolism and is a substrate of CYP3A4. Inducers of CYP3A4 can impact the exposure to nifedipine and consequently its desirable and undesirable effects). Products include:

Provigil Tablets **1002**

Moexipril Hydrochloride (Nifedipine is a vasodilator, and co-administration of other drugs affecting blood pressure may result in pharmacodynamic interactions). Products include:

Uniretic Tablets **3114**
Univasc Tablets **3118**

Morphine Sulfate (Potential for severe hypotension and/or increased fluid volume requirements cannot be ruled out when nifedipine is co-administered with a beta-blocker and a narcotic analgesic). Products include:

Avinza Capsules .... **17**[illegible]
Kadian Capsules .... **5**[illegible]
MS Contin Tablets .... [illegible]

Nadolol (Combination of nifedipine and beta-blockers may increase the likelihood of congestive heart failure, severe hypotension, or exacerbation of angina). Products include:

Nadolol Tablets **2121**

Nefazodone Hydrochloride (Co-administration of nifedipine with CYP3A4 inhibitors, such as nefazodone, may cause an increase in nifedipine plasma concentrations; a reduction in nifedipine dosage may be considered).

No products indexed under this heading.

Nelfinavir Mesylate (Co-administration of nifedipine with CYP3A4 inhibitors, such as nelfinavir, may cause an increase in nifedipine plasma concentrations; a reduction in nifedipine dosage may be considered). Products include:

Viracept **2556**

Nevirapine (Nifedipine is mainly eliminated by metabolism and is a substrate of CYP3A4. Inhibitors of CYP3A4 can impact the exposure to nifedipine and consequently its desirable and undesirable effects). Products include:

Viramune Oral Suspension **903**
Viramune Tablets **903**

Niacinamide (Nifedipine is mainly eliminated by metabolism and is a substrate of CYP3A4. Inhibitors of CYP3A4 can impact the exposure to nifedipine and consequently its desirable and undesirable effects).

No products indexed under this heading.

Nicardipine (Data indicates that nifedipine can inhibit the metabolism of drugs that are substrates of CYP3A, thereby increasing the exposure to other drugs).

No products indexed under this heading.

Nicardipine Hydrochloride (Data indicates that nifedipine can inhibit the metabolism of drugs that are substrates of CYP3A, thereby increasing the exposure to other drugs). Products include:

Cardene I.V. **1129**

Nicotinamide (Nifedipine is mainly eliminated by metabolism and is a substrate of CYP3A4. Inhibitors of CYP3A4 can impact the exposure to nifedipine and consequently its desirable and undesirable effects). Products include:

Nicomide Tablets **3190**

Nimodipine (Data indicates that nifedipine can inhibit the metabolism of drugs that are substrates of CYP3A, thereby increasing the exposure to other drugs). Products include:
- Nimotop Capsules 774

Nisoldipine (Data indicates that nifedipine can inhibit the metabolism of drugs that are substrates of CYP3A, thereby increasing the exposure to other drugs). Products include:
- Sular Tablets 1163

Nitroglycerin (Nifedipine is a vasodilator, and co-administration of other drugs affecting blood pressure may result in pharmacodynamic interactions). Products include:
- Nitro-Dur Transdermal Infusion System.. 3060
- Nitrolingual Pumpspray 1161

Norethindrone (Data indicates that nifedipine can inhibit the metabolism of drugs that are substrates of CYP3A, thereby increasing the exposure to other drugs). Products include:
- Ortho Micronor Tablets 2411

Norfloxacin (Nifedipine is mainly eliminated by metabolism and is a substrate of CYP3A4. Inhibitors of CYP3A4 can impact the exposure to nifedipine and consequently its desirable and undesirable effects). Products include:
- Noroxin Tablets 2009

Norgestrel (Data indicates that nifedipine can inhibit the metabolism of drugs that are substrates of CYP3A, thereby increasing the exposure to other drugs). Products include:
- Lo/Ovral-28 Tablets 3423

Omeprazole (Nifedipine is mainly eliminated by metabolism and is a substrate of CYP3A4. Inhibitors of CYP3A4 can impact the exposure to nifedipine and consequently its desirable and undesirable effects). Products include:
- Zegerid Powder for Oral Solution 2972

Ondansetron Hydrochloride (Data indicates that nifedipine can inhibit the metabolism of drugs that are substrates of CYP3A, thereby increasing the exposure to other drugs). Products include:
- Zofran Injection 1607
- Zofran 1613

Oxcarbazepine (Nifedipine is mainly eliminated by metabolism and is a substrate of CYP3A4. Inducers of CYP3A4 can impact the exposure to nifedipine and consequently its desirable and undesirable effects). Products include:
- Trileptal Oral Suspension 2281
- Trileptal Tablets 2281

Oxycodone Hydrochloride (Potential for severe hypotension and/or increased fluid volume requirements cannot be ruled out when nifedipine is co-administered with a beta-blocker and a narcotic analgesic). Products include:
- Combunox Tablets 1183
- OxyContin Tablets 2699
- OxyFast Oral Concentrate Solution...................................... 2704
- OxyIR Capsules 2704
- Percocet Tablets 1114
- Percodan Tablets 1115

Paclitaxel (Data indicates that nifedipine can inhibit the metabolism of drugs that are substrates of CYP3A, thereby increasing the exposure to other drugs).
No products indexed under this heading.

Paroxetine Hydrochloride (Nifedipine is mainly eliminated by metabolism and is a substrate of CYP3A4. Inhibitors of CYP3A4 can impact the exposure to nifedipine and consequently its desirable and undesirable effects). Products include:
- Paxil CR Controlled-Release Tablets 1509
- Paxil 1501

Penbutolol Sulfate (Combination of nifedipine and beta-blockers may increase the likelihood of congestive heart failure, severe hypotension, or exacerbation of angina).
No products indexed under this heading.

Perindopril Erbumine (Nifedipine is a vasodilator, and co-administration of other drugs affecting blood pressure may result in pharmacodynamic interactions). Products include:
- Aceon Tablets (2 mg, 4 mg, 8 mg)... 3191

Phenobarbital (Phenobarbital has been shown to reduce plasma concentrations of other calcium channel blockers due to enzyme induction; a similar interaction with nifedipine leading to a decrease in nifedipine plasma concentrations and a decrease in efficacy cannot be excluded; a dosage adjustment of nifedipine may be needed).
No products indexed under this heading.

Phenobarbital Sodium (Phenobarbital has been shown to reduce plasma concentrations of other calcium channel blockers due to enzyme induction; a similar interaction with nifedipine leading to a decrease in nifedipine plasma concentrations and a decrease in efficacy cannot be excluded, a dosage adjustment of nifedipine may be needed).
No products indexed under this heading.

Phenoxybenzamine Hydrochloride (Nifedipine is a vasodilator, and co-administration of other drugs affecting blood pressure may result in pharmacodynamic interactions). Products include:
- Dibenzyline Capsules 3390

Phentolamine Mesylate (Nifedipine is a vasodilator, and co-administration of other drugs affecting blood pressure may result in pharmacodynamic interactions).
No products indexed under this heading.

Phenytoin (Co-administration of nifedipine and phenytoin, an inducer of CYP3A4, lowered AUC and Cmax of nifedipine by approximately 70%; a dosage adjustment of nifedipine may be needed).
No products indexed under this heading.

Phenytoin Sodium (Co-administration of nifedipine and phenytoin, an inducer of CYP3A4, lowered AUC and Cmax of nifedipine by approximately 70%; a dosage adjustment of nifedipine may be needed). Products include:
- Phenytek Capsules 2153

Pimozide (Data indicates that nifedipine can inhibit the metabolism of drugs that are substrates of CYP3A, thereby increasing the exposure to other drugs). Products include:
- Orap Tablets 1220

Pindolol (Combination of nifedipine and beta-blockers may increase the likelihood of congestive heart failure, severe hypotension, or exacerbation of angina).
No products indexed under this heading.

Polythiazide (Nifedipine is a vasodilator, and co-administration of other drugs affecting blood pressure may result in pharmacodynamic interactions).
No products indexed under this heading.

Prazosin Hydrochloride (Nifedipine is a vasodilator, and co-administration of other drugs affecting blood pressure may result in pharmacodynamic interactions).
No products indexed under this heading.

Prednisolone Acetate (Nifedipine is mainly eliminated by metabolism and is a substrate of CYP3A4. Inducers of CYP3A4 can impact the exposure to nifedipine and consequently its desirable and undesirable effects). Products include:
- Blephamide Ophthalmic Ointment 563
- Blephamide Ophthalmic Suspension................................. 564
- Poly-Pred Liquifilm Ophthalmic Suspension .... ⊙ 231
- Pred Forte Ophthalmic Suspension .... ⊙ 233
- Pred Mild Sterile Ophthalmic Suspension .... ⊙ 236
- Pred-G Ophthalmic Suspension ...... ⊙ 234
- Pred-G Sterile Ophthalmic Ointment .... ⊙ 235

Prednisolone Sodium Phosphate (Nifedipine is mainly eliminated by metabolism and is a substrate of CYP3A4. Inducers of CYP3A4 can impact the exposure to nifedipine and consequently its desirable and undesirable effects). Products include:
- Pediapred Oral Solution 3319

Prednisolone Tebutate (Nifedipine is mainly eliminated by metabolism and is a substrate of CYP3A4. Inducers of CYP3A4 can impact the exposure to nifedipine and consequently its desirable and undesirable effects).
No products indexed under this heading.

Prednisone (Nifedipine is mainly eliminated by metabolism and is a substrate of CYP3A4. Inducers of CYP3A4 can impact the exposure to nifedipine and consequently its desirable and undesirable effects).
No products indexed under this heading.

Primidone (Nifedipine is mainly eliminated by metabolism and is a substrate of CYP3A4. Inducers of CYP3A4 can impact the exposure to nifedipine and consequently its desirable and undesirable effects).
No products indexed under this heading.

Propoxyphene Hydrochloride (Potential for severe hypotension and/or increased fluid volume requirements cannot be ruled out when nifedipine is co-administered with a beta-blocker and a narcotic analgesic).
No products indexed under this heading.

Propoxyphene Napsylate (Potential for severe hypotension and/or increased fluid volume requirements cannot be ruled out when nifedipine is co-administered with a beta-blocker and a narcotic analgesic). Products include:
- Darvocet A 500 Tablets 3497

Propranolol Hydrochloride (Combination of nifedipine and beta-blockers may increase the likelihood of congestive heart failure, severe hypotension, or exacerbation of angina). Products include:
- Inderal LA Long-Acting Capsules 3421
- InnoPran XL Capsules 2728

Quinapril Hydrochloride (Nifedipine is a vasodilator, and co-administration of other drugs affecting blood pressure may result in pharmacodynamic interactions).
No products indexed under this heading.

Quinidine (Nifedipine is mainly eliminated by metabolism and is a substrate of CYP3A4. Inhibitors of CYP3A4 can impact the exposure to nifedipine and consequently its desirable and undesirable effects).
No products indexed under this heading.

Quinidine Gluconate (Co-administration with nifedipine can increase nifedipine Cmax and AUC by 2.30 and 1.37 respectively. Heart rate will increase by 17.9 beats/minute).
No products indexed under this heading.

Quinidine Hydrochloride (Nifedipine is mainly eliminated by metabolism and is a substrate of CYP3A4. Inhibitors of CYP3A4 can impact the exposure to nifedipine and consequently its desirable and undesirable effects).
No products indexed under this heading.

Quinidine Polygalacturonate (Co-administration with nifedipine can increase nifedipine Cmax and AUC by 2.30 and 1.37 respectively. Heart rate will increase by 17.9 beats/minute).
No products indexed under this heading.

Quinidine Sulfate (Co-administration with nifedipine can increase nifedipine Cmax and AUC by 2.30 and 1.37 respectively. Heart rate will increase by 17.9 beats/minute).
No products indexed under this heading.

Quinine (Nifedipine is mainly eliminated by metabolism and is a substrate of CYP3A4. Inhibitors of CYP3A4 can impact the exposure to nifedipine and consequently its desirable and undesirable effects).
No products indexed under this heading.

Quinine Sulfate (Nifedipine is mainly eliminated by metabolism and is a substrate of CYP3A4. Inhibitors of CYP3A4 can impact the exposure to nifedipine and consequently its desirable and undesirable effects).
No products indexed under this heading.

Quinupristin (Concomitant administration may lead to increased plasma concentrations of nifedipine; a reduction in nifedipine dosage may be considered). Products include:
Synercid I.V. 1690

Ramipril (Nifedipine is a vasodilator, and co-administration of other drugs affecting blood pressure may result in pharmacodynamic interactions). Products include:
Altace Capsules 1673

Ranitidine Bismuth Citrate (Nifedipine is mainly eliminated by metabolism and is a substrate of CYP3A4. Inhibitors of CYP3A4 can impact the exposure to nifedipine and consequently its desirable and undesirable effects).
No products indexed under this heading.

Ranitidine Hydrochloride (Produces smaller, non-significant increases in peak nifedipine plasma levels and AUC). Products include:
Zantac 1597
Zantac Injection 1593
Zantac 75 Tablets 715
Zantac 150 Maximum Strength Tablets... 715
Zantac Injection Pharmacy Bulk Package....................................... 1595

Rauwolfia Serpentina (Nifedipine is a vasodilator, and co-administration of other drugs affecting blood pressure may result in pharmacodynamic interactions).
No products indexed under this heading.

Remifentanil Hydrochloride (Potential for severe hypotension and/or increased fluid volume requirements cannot be ruled out when nifedipine is co-administered with a beta-blocker and a narcotic analgesic).
No products indexed under this heading.

Rescinnamine (Nifedipine is a vasodilator, and co-administration of other drugs affecting blood pressure may result in pharmacodynamic interactions).
No products indexed under this heading.

Reserpine (Nifedipine is a vasodilator, and co-administration of other drugs affecting blood pressure may result in pharmacodynamic interactions).
No products indexed under this heading.

Rifabutin (Nifedipine is mainly eliminated by metabolism and is a substrate of CYP3A4. Inducers of CYP3A4 can impact the exposure to nifedipine and consequently its desirable and undesirable effects).
No products indexed under this heading.

Rifampicin (Rifampicin strongly induces CYP3A4, and upon co-administration with rifampicin, the bioavailability of nifedipine is distinctly reduced and its efficacy weakened. Rifampicin should be avoided in patients receiving nifedipine).
No products indexed under this heading.

Rifampin (Co-administration with nifedipine can decrease the exposure of oral nifedipine; a dosage adjustment of nifedipine may be needed).
No products indexed under this heading.

Rifapentine (Co-administration with a CYP3A4 inducer, such as rifapentine, will decrease the exposure to nifedipine; a dosage adjustment of nifedipine may be needed).
No products indexed under this heading.

Ritonavir (Co-administration of nifedipine with CYP3A4 inhibitors, such as ritonavir, may cause an increase in nifedipine plasma concentrations; a reduction in nifedipine dosage may be considered). Products include:
Kaletra 474
Norvir 499

Saquinavir (Co-administration of nifedipine with CYP3A4 inhibitors, such as saquinavir, may cause an increase in nifedipine plasma concentrations; a reduction in nifedipine dosage may be considered).
No products indexed under this heading.

Saquinavir Mesylate (Co-administration of nifedipine with CYP3A4 inhibitors, such as saquinavir, may cause an increase in nifedipine plasma concentrations; a reduction in nifedipine dosage may be considered). Products include:
Invirase 2776

Sertraline Hydrochloride (Nifedipine is mainly eliminated by metabolism and is a substrate of CYP3A4. Inhibitors of CYP3A4 can impact the exposure to nifedipine and consequently its desirable and undesirable effects). Products include:
Zoloft 2581

Sildenafil Citrate (Data indicates that nifedipine can inhibit the metabolism of drugs that are substrates of CYP3A, thereby increasing the exposure to other drugs). Products include:
Revatio Tablets 2541
Viagra Tablets 2552

Simvastatin (Data indicates that nifedipine can inhibit the metabolism of drugs that are substrates of CYP3A, thereby increasing the exposure to other drugs). Products include:
Vytorin 10/10 Tablets 2084
Vytorin 10/10 Tablets 3092
Vytorin 10/20 Tablets 2084
Vytorin 10/20 Tablets 3092
Vytorin 10/40 Tablets 3092
Vytorin 10/40 Tablets 2084
Vytorin 10/80 Tablets 2084
Vytorin 10/80 Tablets 3092
Zocor Tablets 2078

Sirolimus (Data indicates that nifedipine can inhibit the metabolism of drugs that are substrates of CYP3A, thereby increasing the exposure to other drugs). Products include:
Rapamune Oral Solution and Tablets 3472

Sodium Nitroprusside (Nifedipine is a vasodilator, and co-administration of other drugs affecting blood pressure may result in pharmacodynamic interactions).
No products indexed under this heading.

Sotalol Hydrochloride (Combination of nifedipine and beta-blockers may increase the likelihood of congestive heart failure, severe hypotension, or exacerbation of angina).
No products indexed under this heading.

Spirapril Hydrochloride (Nifedipine is a vasodilator, and co-administration of other drugs affecting blood pressure may result in pharmacodynamic interactions).
No products indexed under this heading.

Sufentanil Citrate (Potential for severe hypotension and/or increased fluid volume requirements cannot be ruled out when nifedipine is co-administered with a beta-blocker and a narcotic analgesic).
No products indexed under this heading.

Sulfinpyrazone (Nifedipine is mainly eliminated by metabolism and is a substrate of CYP3A4. Inducers of CYP3A4 can impact the exposure to nifedipine and consequently its desirable and undesirable effects).
No products indexed under this heading.

Tacrolimus (If co-administered with nifedipine, tacrolimus plasma concentrations should be monitored and a reduction in tacrolimus dosage may be considered). Products include:
Prograf Capsules and Injection 624
Protopic Ointment 629

Tamoxifen Citrate (Data indicates that nifedipine can inhibit the metabolism of drugs that are substrates of CYP3A, thereby increasing the exposure to other drugs).
No products indexed under this heading.

Telithromycin (Nifedipine is mainly eliminated by metabolism and is a substrate of CYP3A4. Inhibitors of CYP3A4 can impact the exposure to nifedipine and consequently its desirable and undesirable effects). Products include:
Ketek Tablets 2920

Telmisartan (Nifedipine is a vasodilator, and co-administration of other drugs affecting blood pressure may result in pharmacodynamic interactions). Products include:
Micardis Tablets 884
Micardis HCT Tablets 886

Terazosin Hydrochloride (Nifedipine is a vasodilator, and co-administration of other drugs affecting blood pressure may result in pharmacodynamic interactions). Products include:
Hytrin Capsules 469

Terfenadine (Data indicates that nifedipine can inhibit the metabolism of drugs that are substrates of CYP3A, thereby increasing the exposure to other drugs).
No products indexed under this heading.

Testosterone (Data indicates that nifedipine can inhibit the metabolism of drugs that are substrates of CYP3A, thereby increasing the exposure to other drugs). Products include:
AndroGel 3330
Striant Mucoadhesive 1022
Testim 1% Gel 722

Testosterone Cypionate (Data indicates that nifedipine can inhibit the metabolism of drugs that are substrates of CYP3A, thereby increasing the exposure to other drugs).
No products indexed under this heading.

Testosterone Enanthate (Data indicates that nifedipine can inhibit the metabolism of drugs that are substrates of CYP3A, thereby increasing the exposure to other drugs). Products include:
Delatestryl Injection 2976

Testosterone Propionate (Data indicates that nifedipine can inhibit the metabolism of drugs that are substrates of CYP3A, thereby increasing the exposure to other drugs).
No products indexed under this heading.

Theophylline (Nifedipine is mainly eliminated by metabolism and is a substrate of CYP3A4. Inducers of CYP3A4 can impact the exposure to nifedipine and consequently its desirable and undesirable effects).
No products indexed under this heading.

Theophylline Anhydrous (Data indicates that nifedipine can inhibit the metabolism of drugs that are substrates of CYP3A, thereby increasing the exposure to other drugs). Products include:
Uniphyl Tablets 2708

Theophylline Calcium Salicylate (Data indicates that nifedipine can inhibit the metabolism of drugs that are substrates of CYP3A, thereby increasing the exposure to other drugs).
No products indexed under this heading.

Theophylline Sodium Glycinate (Data indicates that nifedipine can inhibit the metabolism of drugs that are substrates of CYP3A, thereby increasing the exposure to other drugs).
No products indexed under this heading.

Tiagabine Hydrochloride (Data indicates that nifedipine can inhibit the metabolism of drugs that are substrates of CYP3A, thereby increasing the exposure to other drugs). Products include:
Gabitril Tablets 998

Timolol Hemihydrate (Combination of nifedipine and beta-blockers may increase the likelihood of congestive heart failure, severe hypotension, or exacerbation of angina). Products include:
Betimol Ophthalmic Solution 3371
Betimol Ophthalmic Solution .... ⊙283

Timolol Maleate (Combination of nifedipine and beta-blockers may increase the likelihood of congestive heart failure, severe hypotension, or exacerbation of angina). Products include:
Blocadren Tablets 1891
Cosopt Sterile Ophthalmic Solution... 1910
Timolide Tablets 2056
Timoptic in Ocudose 2061
Timoptic Sterile Ophthalmic Solution.. 2058
Timoptic-XE Sterile Ophthalmic Gel Forming Solution 2062

Tolterodine Tartrate (Data indicates that nifedipine can inhibit the metabolism of drugs that are sub-

strates of CYP3A, thereby increasing the exposure to other drugs). Products include:

Detrol Tablets 2626
Detrol LA Capsules 2629

Torsemide (Nifedipine is a vasodilator, and co-administration of other drugs affecting blood pressure may result in pharmacodynamic interactions).
No products indexed under this heading.

Trandolapril (Nifedipine is a vasodilator, and co-administration of other drugs affecting blood pressure may result in pharmacodynamic interactions). Products include:

Mavik Tablets 482
Tarka Tablets 519

Trazodone Hydrochloride (Data indicates that nifedipine can inhibit the metabolism of drugs that are substrates of CYP3A, thereby increasing the exposure to other drugs).
No products indexed under this heading.

Triamcinolone (Nifedipine is mainly eliminated by metabolism and is a substrate of CYP3A4. Inducers of CYP3A4 can impact the exposure to nifedipine and consequently its desirable and undesirable effects).
No products indexed under this heading.

Triamcinolone Acetonide (Nifedipine is mainly eliminated by metabolism and is a substrate of CYP3A4. Inducers of CYP3A4 can impact the exposure to nifedipine and consequently its desirable and undesirable effects). Products include:

Azmacort Inhalation Aerosol 1701
Nasacort HFA Inhalation Aerosol 2939
Nasacort AQ Nasal Spray 2937

Triamcinolone Diacetate (Nifedipine is mainly eliminated by metabolism and is a substrate of CYP3A4. Inducers of CYP3A4 can impact the exposure to nifedipine and consequently its desirable and undesirable effects).
No products indexed under this heading.

Triamcinolone Hexacetonide (Nifedipine is mainly eliminated by metabolism and is a substrate of CYP3A4. Inducers of CYP3A4 can impact the exposure to nifedipine and consequently its desirable and undesirable effects).
No products indexed under this heading.

Triazolam (Data indicates that nifedipine can inhibit the metabolism of drugs that are substrates of CYP3A, thereby increasing the exposure to other drugs).
No products indexed under this heading.

Trimethaphan Camsylate (Nifedipine is a vasodilator, and co-administration of other drugs affecting blood pressure may result in pharmacodynamic interactions).
No products indexed under this heading.

Troglitazone (Nifedipine is mainly eliminated by metabolism and is a substrate of CYP3A4. Inhibitors of CYP3A4 can impact the exposure to nifedipine and consequently its desirable and undesirable effects).
No products indexed under this heading.

Troleandomycin (Nifedipine is mainly eliminated by metabolism and is a substrate of CYP3A4. Inhibitors of CYP3A4 can impact the exposure to nifedipine and consequently its desirable and undesirable effects).
No products indexed under this heading.

Valproate Sodium (Nifedipine is mainly eliminated by metabolism and is a substrate of CYP3A4. Inhibitors of CYP3A4 can impact the exposure to nifedipine and consequently its desirable and undesirable effects). Products include:

Depacon Injection 412

Valproic Acid (Valproic acid has been shown to elevate plasma concentrations of other calcium channel blockers due to enzyme inhibition; a similar interaction with nifedipine leading to an increase in nifedipine plasma concentrations and an increase in efficacy cannot be excluded). Products include:

Depakene 417

Valsartan (Nifedipine is a vasodilator, and co-administration of other drugs affecting blood pressure may result in pharmacodynamic interactions). Products include:

Diovan HCT Tablets 2195
Diovan Tablets 2191

Venlafaxine Hydrochloride (Data indicates that nifedipine can inhibit the metabolism of drugs that are substrates of CYP3A, thereby increasing the exposure to other drugs). Products include:

Effexor Tablets 3405
Effexor XR Capsules 3411

Verapamil Hydrochloride (Co-administration of nifedipine with CYP3A4 inhibitors, such as verapamil hydrochloride, may cause an increase in nifedipine plasma concentration; a reduction in nifedipine dosage may be considered). Products include:

Covera-HS Tablets 3135
Tarka Tablets 519
Verelan PM Capsules 3120

Vinblastine Sulfate (Data indicates that nifedipine can inhibit the metabolism of drugs that are substrates of CYP3A, thereby increasing the exposure to other drugs).
No products indexed under this heading.

Vincristine Sulfate (Data indicates that nifedipine can inhibit the metabolism of drugs that are substrates of CYP3A, thereby increasing the exposure to other drugs).
No products indexed under this heading.

Voriconazole (Nifedipine is mainly eliminated by metabolism and is a substrate of CYP3A4. Inhibitors of CYP3A4 can impact the exposure to nifedipine and consequently its desirable and undesirable effects). Products include:

VFEND I.V. 2543
VFEND Oral Suspension 2543
VFEND Tablets 2543

Warfarin Sodium (There have been rare reports of increased prothrombin time in patients taking coumarin anticoagulants to whom nifedipine was administered). Products include:

Coumadin for Injection 932
Coumadin Tablets 932

Zafirlukast (Nifedipine is mainly eliminated by metabolism and is a substrate of CYP3A4. Inhibitors of CYP3A4 can impact the exposure to nifedipine and consequently its desirable and undesirable effects). Products include:

Accolate Tablets 663

Zileuton (Nifedipine is mainly eliminated by metabolism and is a substrate of CYP3A4. Inhibitors of CYP3A4 can impact the exposure to nifedipine and consequently its desirable and undesirable effects).
No products indexed under this heading.

Food Interactions

Diet, high-lipid (High-fat meal increases peak plasma nifedipine concentrations by 60%, a prolongation in the time to peak concentration, but no significant change in the AUC; administer on an empty stomach).

Grapefruit (Nifedipine is mainly eliminated by metabolism and is a substrate of CYP3A4. Inhibitors of CYP3A4 can impact the exposure to nifedipine and consequently its desirable and undesirable effects).

Grapefruit Juice (Co-administration of nifedipine with grapefruit juice results in up to a 2-fold increase in AUC and Cmax, due to inhibition of CYP3A4-related first-pass metabolism. This effect of grapefruit juice may last for at least 3 days; co-administration should beavoided).

ADDERALL TABLETS

(Amphetamine Aspartate, Amphetamine Sulfate, Dextroamphetamine Saccharate, Dextroamphetamine Sulfate) 3168
See Adderall XR Capsules

ADDERALL XR CAPSULES

(Amphetamine Aspartate, Amphetamine Sulfate, Dextroamphetamine Saccharate, Dextroamphetamine Sulfate) 3169
May interact with antacids, antihistamines, antihypertensives, beta blockers, monoamine oxidase inhibitors, methenamine, phenytoin, thiazides, tricyclic antidepressants, urinary alkalinizing agents, veratrum alkaloids, and certain other agents. Compounds in these categories include:

Acebutolol Hydrochloride (Adrenergic blockers are inhibited by amphetamines; amphetamines may antagonize the hypotensive effects of antihypertensives).
No products indexed under this heading.

Acetazolamide (Co-administration with urinary alkalinizing agents, such as acetazolamide, increase the concentration of the non-ionized species of the amphetamine molecule, thereby decreasing urinary excretion resulting in increased blood levels and potentiate the actions of amphetamines).
No products indexed under this heading.

Acetazolamide Sodium (Co-administration with urinary alkalinizing agents, such as acetazolamide, increase the concentration of the non-ionized species of the amphetamine molecule, thereby decreasing urinary excretion resulting in increased blood levels and potentiate the actions of amphetamines).
No products indexed under this heading.

Acrivastine (Amphetamines may counteract the sedative effect of antihistamines).
No products indexed under this heading.

Aluminum Carbonate (Co-administration with gastrointestinal alkalinizing agents, such as antacids, may increase the absorption of amphetamines; concurrent use should be avoided).
No products indexed under this heading.

Aluminum Hydroxide (Co-administration with gastrointestinal alkalinizing agents, such as antacids, may increase the absorption of amphetamines; concurrent use should be avoided). Products include:

Gaviscon Regular Strength Liquid .. ▣620
Gaviscon Regular Strength Tablets .... ▣619
Gaviscon Extra Strength Liquid .... ▣620
Gaviscon Extra Strength Tablets .... ▣619
Maalox Max Maximum Strength Antacid/Anti-Gas Liquid 2165
Maalox Regular Strength Antacid/Antigas Liquid 2164

Amitriptyline Hydrochloride (Enhanced activity of tricyclic antidepressants or sympathomimetics; possible increases in d-amphetamine resulting in potentiation of cardiovascular effects).
No products indexed under this heading.

Amlodipine Besylate (Amphetamines may antagonize the hypotensive effects of antihypertensives). Products include:

Caduet Tablets 2507
Lotrel Capsules 2238
Norvasc Tablets 2529

Ammonium Chloride (Co-administration with urinary acidifying agents increases the concentration of the ionized species of the amphetamine molecule, thereby increasing urinary excretion resulting in reduced blood levels and efficacy of amphetamines).
No products indexed under this heading.

Amoxapine (Enhanced activity of tricyclic antidepressants or sympathomimetics; possible increases in d-amphetamine resulting in potentiation of cardiovascular effects).
No products indexed under this heading.

Astemizole (Amphetamines may counteract the sedative effect of antihistamines).
No products indexed under this heading.

Atenolol (Adrenergic blockers are inhibited by amphetamines; amphetamines may antagonize the hypotensive effects of antihypertensives). Products include:

Tenormin I.V. Injection 698
Tenormin Tablets 695

Azatadine Maleate (Amphetamines may counteract the sedative effect of antihistamines).
No products indexed under this heading.

Benazepril Hydrochloride (Amphetamines may antagonize the hypotensive effects of antihypertensives). Products include:

Lotensin Tablets 2232
Lotensin HCT Tablets 2235
Lotrel Capsules 2238

Bendroflumethiazide (Co-administration with urinary alkalinizing agents, such as certain thiazides, increase the concentration of the non-ionized species of the amphetamine molecule, thereby decreasing urinary excretion resulting in increased blood levels and potentiation of actions of amphetamines; amphetamines may antagonize the hypotensive effects of antihypertensives).
No products indexed under this heading.

Betaxolol Hydrochloride (Adrenergic blockers are inhibited by amphetamines; amphetamines may antagonize the hypotensive effects of antihypertensives). Products include:
Betoptic S Ophthalmic Suspension.................................... 554

Bisoprolol Fumarate (Adrenergic blockers are inhibited by amphetamines; amphetamines may antagonize the hypotensive effects of antihypertensives).
No products indexed under this heading.

Bromodiphenhydramine Hydrochloride (Amphetamines may counteract the sedative effect of antihistamines).
No products indexed under this heading.

Brompheniramine Maleate (Amphetamines may counteract the sedative effect of antihistamines). Products include:
Alacol DM Syrup.............................. 739
Children's Dimetapp Cold & Allergy Elixir................................ 745
Children's Dimetapp DM Cold & Cough Elixir................................ 745
Robitussin Allergy & Cough Syrup .. 750

Candesartan Cilexetil (Amphetamines may antagonize the hypotensive effects of antihypertensives). Products include:
Atacand Tablets 634
Atacand HCT 637

Captopril (Amphetamines may antagonize the hypotensive effects of antihypertensives). Products include:
Captopril Tablets 2114

Carteolol Hydrochloride (Adrenergic blockers are inhibited by amphetamines; amphetamines may antagonize the hypotensive effects of antihypertensives). Products include:
Carteolol Hydrochloride Ophthalmic Solution USP, 1%....... ⊙246

Cetirizine Hydrochloride (Amphetamines may counteract the sedative effect of antihistamines). Products include:
Zyrtec Chewable Tablets 2589
Zyrtec 2589
Zyrtec-D 12 Hour Extended Release Tablets............................ 2591

Chlorothiazide (Co-administration with urinary alkalinizing agents, such as certain thiazides, increase the concentration of the non-ionized species of the amphetamine molecule, thereby decreasing urinary excretion resulting in increased blood levels and potentiation of actions of amphetamines; amphetamines may antagonize the hypotensive effects of antihypertensives). Products include:
Aldoclor Tablets 1881
Diuril Oral 1936

Chlorothiazide Sodium (Co-administration with urinary alkalinizing agents, such as certain thiazides, increase the concentration of the non-ionized species of the amphetamine molecule, thereby decreasing urinary excretion resulting in increased blood levels and potentiation of actions of amphetamines; amphetamines may antagonize the hypotensive effects of antihypertensives). Products include:
Diuril Sodium Intravenous 1934

Chlorpheniramine Maleate (Amphetamines may counteract the sedative effect of antihistamines). Products include:
Advil Allergy Sinus Caplets 737
Advil Multi-Symptom Cold Caplets....................................... 738
BC Allergy Sinus Cold Powder 612
Contac Severe Cold and Flu Caplets Maximum Strength......... 615
Hycomine Compound Tablets 1105
PediaCare Multi-Symptom Cold Liquid 704
PediaCare NightRest Cough & Cold Liquid.................................. 704
Robitussin Flu Liquid 752
Robitussin PM Cough & Cold Liquid 752
Singlet Caplets 636
Sudafed Sinus & Allergy Tablets 710
TheraFlu Cold & Cough Hot Liquid 680
TheraFlu Cold & Sore Throat Hot Liquid 680
TheraFlu Flu & Sore Throat Hot Liquid 681
TheraFlu Severe Cold & Cough Hot Liquid.................................... 683
TheraFlu Severe Cold Caplets 679
TheraFlu Severe Cold Hot Liquid 682
Triaminic Cold & Allergy Liquid 685
Triaminic Cold & Cough Liquid 685
Triaminic Flu, Cough & Fever Liquid 685
Triaminic Night Time Cough & Cold Liquid.................................. 685
Triaminic Allergy Runny Nose & Congestion Softchews................ 688
Triaminic Cold & Cough Softchews..................................... 688
Children's Tylenol Plus Cold NightTime Suspension Liquid........ 1851
Children's Tylenol Plus Cold & Cough Suspension Liquid and Chewable Tablets 1851
Children's Tylenol Plus Cold Chewable Tablets 1851
Children's Tylenol Plus Flu Suspension Liquid 1853
Tylenol Allergy Complete Multi-Symptom Caplets and Gelcaps with Cool Burst................ 1844
Multi-Symptom Tylenol Cold Night Time Caplets............................... 1845
Vicks 44M Cough, Cold & Flu Relief... 2676
Pediatric Vicks 44m Cough & Cold Relief.................................... 2673
Children's Vicks NyQuil Cold/Cough Relief........................ 2671

Chlorpheniramine Polistirex (Amphetamines may counteract the sedative effect of antihistamines). Products include:
Tussionex Pennkinetic Extended-Release Suspension...... 3322

Chlorpheniramine Tannate (Amphetamines may counteract the sedative effect of antihistamines).
No products indexed under this heading.

Chlorpromazine (Blocks the dopamine and norepinephrine receptors, thus inhibiting the central stimulant effects of amphetamines).
No products indexed under this heading.

Chlorpromazine Hydrochloride (Blocks the dopamine and norepinephrine receptors, thus inhibiting the central stimulant effects of amphetamines).
No products indexed under this heading.

Chlorthalidone (Amphetamines may antagonize the hypotensive effects of antihypertensives). Products include:
Clorpres Tablets 2139

Clemastine Fumarate (Amphetamines may counteract the sedative effect of antihistamines).
No products indexed under this heading.

Clomipramine Hydrochloride (Enhanced activity of tricyclic antidepressants or sympathomimetics; possible increases in d-amphetamine resulting in potentiation of cardiovascular effects).
No products indexed under this heading.

Clonidine (Amphetamines may antagonize the hypotensive effects of antihypertensives). Products include:
Catapres-TTS 875

Clonidine Hydrochloride (Amphetamines may antagonize the hypotensive effects of antihypertensives). Products include:
Catapres Tablets 874
Clorpres Tablets 2139

Cryptenamine Preparations (Amphetamines inhibit the hypotensive effect of veratrum alkaloids).
No products indexed under this heading.

Cyproheptadine Hydrochloride (Amphetamines may counteract the sedative effect of antihistamines).
No products indexed under this heading.

Deserpidine (Amphetamines may antagonize the hypotensive effects of antihypertensives).
No products indexed under this heading.

Desipramine Hydrochloride (Enhanced activity of tricyclic antidepressants or sympathomimetics; possible increases in d-amphetamine resulting in potentiation of cardiovascular effects).
No products indexed under this heading.

Dexchlorpheniramine Maleate (Amphetamines may counteract the sedative effect of antihistamines).
No products indexed under this heading.

Diazoxide (Amphetamines may antagonize the hypotensive effects of antihypertensives). Products include:
Hyperstat I.V. Injection 3031

Diltiazem Hydrochloride (Amphetamines may antagonize the hypotensive effects of antihypertensives). Products include:
Cardizem LA Extended Release Tablets.. 1699
Tiazac Capsules 1204

Diphenhydramine Citrate (Amphetamines may counteract the sedative effect of antihistamines). Products include:
Children's Benadryl Allergy & Cold Fastmelt Tablets.................. 695
Children's Benadryl D Allergy & Sinus Fastmelt Tablets................ 694
Children's Benadryl Allergy Fastmelt Tablets 696
Goody's PM Powder 622

Diphenhydramine Hydrochloride (Amphetamines may counteract the sedative effect of antihistamines). Products include:
Benadryl Allergy & Cold Tablets 692
Benadryl Allergy 691
Benadryl Allergy & Sinus Headache Caplets & Gelcaps...... 693
Children's Benadryl Allergy Liquid ... 695
Children's Benadryl Dye-Free Allergy Liquid 695
Benadryl Dye-Free Allergy Liqui-Gels Softgels........................ 692
Benadryl Itch Relief Stick Extra Strength 696
Benadryl Itch Stopping Cream Extra Strength 697
Benadryl Itch Stopping Gel Extra Strength 697
Benadryl Itch Stopping Spray Extra Strength 697
Benadryl Maximum Strength Severe Allergy & Sinus Headache Caplets......................... 694
Children's Benadryl D Liquid Medication................................. 693
Benadryl D Tablets 694
Nytol QuickCaps Caplets 635
Maximum Strength Nytol QuickGels Softgels..................... 635
Simply Sleep Caplets 1841
Sominex Original Formula Tablets .. 637
TheraFlu Thin Strips Multi Symptom.................................... 684
Triaminic Thin Strips Cough & Runny Nose 690
Children's Tylenol Plus Cold & Allergy Suspension Liquid............ 1850
Tylenol Allergy Complete Night Time Caplets............................... 1844
Tylenol Severe Allergy Caplets 1844
Tylenol Flu NightTime Gelcaps 1846
Extra Strength Tylenol PM Caplets, Geltabs, Gelcaps and Liquid 1847
Unisom Maximum Strength SleepGels................................... 712

Diphenylpyraline Hydrochloride (Amphetamines may counteract the sedative effect of antihistamines).
No products indexed under this heading.

Doxazosin Mesylate (Amphetamines may antagonize the hypotensive effects of antihypertensives).
No products indexed under this heading.

Doxepin Hydrochloride (Enhanced activity of tricyclic antidepressants or sympathomimetics; possible increases in d-amphetamine resulting in potentiation of cardiovascular effects).
No products indexed under this heading.

Enalapril Maleate (Amphetamines may antagonize the hypotensive effects of antihypertensives). Products include:
Vaseretic Tablets 2073
Vasotec I.V. Injection 2076

Enalaprilat (Amphetamines may antagonize the hypotensive effects of antihypertensives).
No products indexed under this heading.

Eprosartan Mesylate (Amphetamines may antagonize the hypotensive effects of antihypertensives). Products include:
Teveten Tablets 1707
Teveten HCT Tablets 1710

Esmolol Hydrochloride (Adrenergic blockers are inhibited by amphetamines; amphetamines may antagonize the hypotensive effects of antihypertensives). Products include:
Brevibloc Concentrate 766
Brevibloc Injection 766

IMPORTANT NOTE: Always consult each drug listing in the patient's regimen for possible interactions.

Brevibloc Double Strength Injection.. 766
Brevibloc Premixed Injection 766
Brevibloc Double Strength Premixed Injection 766

Ethosuximide (Amphetamines may delay intestinal absorption of ethosuximide).
No products indexed under this heading.

Felodipine (Amphetamines may antagonize the hypotensive effects of antihypertensives). Products include:
Plendil Extended-Release Tablets 651

Fexofenadine Hydrochloride (Amphetamines may counteract the sedative effect of antihistamines). Products include:
Allegra 2857
Allegra-D 12 Hour Extended-Release Tablets............ 2860
Allegra-D 24 Hour Extended-Release Tablets............ 2862

Fosinopril Sodium (Amphetamines may antagonize the hypotensive effects of antihypertensives).
No products indexed under this heading.

Fosphenytoin Sodium (Amphetamines may delay intestinal absorption of phenytoin; co-administration may produce a synergistic anticonvulsant action).
No products indexed under this heading.

Furazolidone (Concurrent use with metabolite of furazolidone may result in hypertensive crises; may slow the metabolism of amphetamines with resultant increase in their effect on release of norepinephrine and other monoamines from adrenergic nerve ending; this can cause headaches and other signs of hypertensice crises).
No products indexed under this heading.

Furosemide (Amphetamines may antagonize the hypotensive effects of antihypertensives). Products include:
Furosemide Tablets 2117

Glutamic Acid Hydrochloride (Co-administration with gastrointestinal acidifying agents, such as glutamic acid, lowers absorption of amphetamines resulting in reduced blood levels and efficacy of amphetamines).
No products indexed under this heading.

Guanabenz Acetate (Amphetamines may antagonize the hypotensive effects of antihypertensives).
No products indexed under this heading.

Guanethidine Monosulfate (Co-administration with gastrointestinal acidifying agents, such as guanethidine, lowers absorption of amphetamines resulting in reduced blood levels and efficacy of amphetamines; amphetamines may antagonize the hypotensive effects of antihypertensives).
No products indexed under this heading.

Haloperidol (Blocks the dopamine receptors, thus inhibiting the central stimulant effects of amphetamines).
No products indexed under this heading.

Haloperidol Decanoate (Blocks the dopamine receptors, thus inhibiting the central stimulant effects of amphetamines).
No products indexed under this heading.

Hydralazine Hydrochloride (Amphetamines may antagonize the hypotensive effects of antihypertensives). Products include:
BiDil Tablets 2161

Hydrochlorothiazide (Co-administration with urinary alkalinizing agents, such as certain thiazides, increase the concentration of the non-ionized species of the amphetamine molecule, thereby decreasing urinary excretion resulting in increased blood levels and potentiation of actions of amphetamines; amphetamines may antagonize the hypotensive effects of antihypertensives). Products include:
Aldoril Tablets 1884
Atacand HCT 637
Avalide Tablets 2889
Avalide Tablets 922
Benicar HCT Tablets 2852
Diovan HCT Tablets 2195
Dyazide Capsules 1389
Hyzaar 1964
Lotensin HCT Tablets 2235
Maxzide 2150
Micardis HCT Tablets 886
Moduretic Tablets 2003
Prinzide Tablets 2033
Teveten HCT Tablets 1710
Timolide Tablets 2056
Uniretic Tablets 3114
Vaseretic Tablets 2073
Zestoretic Tablets 701

Hydroflumethiazide (Co-administration with urinary alkalinizing agents, such as certain thiazides, increase the concentration of the non-ionized species of the amphetamine molecule, thereby decreasing urinary excretion resulting in increased blood levels and potentiation of actions of amphetamines; amphetamines may antagonize the hypotensive effects of antihypertensives).
No products indexed under this heading.

Imipramine Hydrochloride (Enhanced activity of tricyclic antidepressants or sympathomimetics; possible increases in d-amphetamine resulting in potentiation of cardiovascular effects).
No products indexed under this heading.

Imipramine Pamoate (Enhanced activity of tricyclic antidepressants or sympathomimetics; possible increases in d-amphetamine resulting in potentiation of cardiovascular effects).
No products indexed under this heading.

Indapamide (Amphetamines may antagonize the hypotensive effects of antihypertensives). Products include:
Indapamide Tablets 2119

Irbesartan (Amphetamines may antagonize the hypotensive effects of antihypertensives). Products include:
Avalide Tablets 922
Avalide Tablets 2889
Avapro Tablets 925
Avapro Tablets 2886

Isocarboxazid (Concurrent and/or sequential use may result in hypertensive crises; MAOI may slow the metabolism of amphetamines with resultant increase in their effect on release of norepinephrine and other monoamines from adrenergic nerve ending; this can cause headaches and other signs of hypertensive crises; concurrent and/or sequential use is contraindicated).
No products indexed under this heading.

Isradipine (Amphetamines may antagonize the hypotensive effects of antihypertensives). Products include:
DynaCirc CR Tablets 2726

Labetalol Hydrochloride (Adrenergic blockers are inhibited by amphetamines; amphetamines may antagonize the hypotensive effects of antihypertensives).
No products indexed under this heading.

Levobunolol Hydrochloride (Adrenergic blockers are inhibited by amphetamines; amphetamines may antagonize the hypotensive effects of antihypertensives). Products include:
Betagan Ophthalmic Solution, USP.. ⊙217

Lisinopril (Amphetamines may antagonize the hypotensive effects of antihypertensives). Products include:
Prinivil Tablets 2029
Prinzide Tablets 2033
Zestoretic Tablets 701
Zestril Tablets 704

Lithium Carbonate (Anorectic and stimulatory effects of amphetamines may be inhibited by lithium carbonate). Products include:
Eskalith 1406
Lithobid Tablets 1670

Loratadine (Amphetamines may counteract the sedative effect of antihistamines). Products include:
Alavert Allergy & Sinus D-12 Hour Tablets.. ▣743
Alavert .... ▣743
Children's Claritin 24 Hour Non-Drowsy Allergy Syrup........... ▣732
Claritin Non-Drowsy 24 Hour Tablets.. ▣731
Non-Drowsy Claritin Hives Relief Tablets.. ▣733
Claritin Reditabs 24 Hour Non-Drowsy Tablets.................... ▣732
Claritin-D Non-Drowsy 12 Hour Tablets.. ▣731
Claritin-D Non-Drowsy 24 Hour Tablets.. ▣731
Children's Dimetapp ND Non-Drowsy Allergy Syrup........... ▣746
Triaminic Allerchews .... ▣684

Losartan Potassium (Amphetamines may antagonize the hypotensive effects of antihypertensives). Products include:
Cozaar Tablets 1913
Hyzaar 1964

Magaldrate (Co-administration with gastrointestinal alkalinizing agents, such as antacids, may increase the absorption of amphetamines; concurrent use should be avoided).
No products indexed under this heading.

Magnesium Hydroxide (Co-administration with gastrointestinal alkalinizing agents, such as antacids, may increase the absorption of amphetamines; concurrent use should be avoided). Products include:
Maalox Max Maximum Strength Antacid/Anti-Gas Liquid................ 2165
Maalox Regular Strength Antacid/Antigas Liquid................. 2164
Pepcid Complete Chewable Tablets 1672
Rolaids Tablets .... ▣707
Extra Strength Rolaids Tablets ...... ▣707
Rolaids Multi-Symptom Antacid & Antigas Tablets .... ▣708

Magnesium Oxide (Co-administration with gastrointestinal alkalinizing agents, such as antacids, may increase the absorption of amphetamines; concurrent use should be avoided). Products include:
Beelith Tablets 784
PremCal Light, Regular, and Extra Strength Tablets................ ▣762

Maprotiline Hydrochloride (Enhanced activity of tricyclic antidepressants or sympathomimetics; possible increases in d-amphetamine resulting in potentiation of cardiovascular effects).
No products indexed under this heading.

Mecamylamine Hydrochloride (Amphetamines may antagonize the hypotensive effects of antihypertensives). Products include:
Inversine Tablets 3286

Meperidine Hydrochloride (Amphetamines potentiate the analgesic effect of meperidine).
No products indexed under this heading.

Methdilazine Hydrochloride (Amphetamines may counteract the sedative effect of antihistamines).
No products indexed under this heading.

Methenamine (Urinary excretion of amphetamines is increased, and efficacy is reduced by acidifying agents used in methenamine therapy).
No products indexed under this heading.

Methenamine Hippurate (Urinary excretion of amphetamines is increased, and efficacy is reduced by acidifying agents used in methenamine therapy).
No products indexed under this heading.

Methenamine Mandelate (Urinary excretion of amphetamines is increased, and efficacy is reduced by acidifying agents used in methenamine therapy). Products include:
Uroqid-Acid No. 2 Tablets 785

Methyclothiazide (Co-administration with urinary alkalinizing agents, such as certain thiazides, increase the concentration of the non-ionized species of the amphetamine molecule, thereby decreasing urinary excretion resulting in increased blood levels and potentiation of actions of amphetamines; amphetamines may antagonize the hypotensive effects of antihypertensives).
No products indexed under this heading.

Methyldopa (Amphetamines may antagonize the hypotensive effects of antihypertensives). Products include:
Aldoclor Tablets 1881
Aldoril Tablets 1884

Methyldopate Hydrochloride (Amphetamines may antagonize the hypotensive effects of antihypertensives).
No products indexed under this heading.

Metipranolol Hydrochloride (Adrenergic blockers are inhibited by amphetamines; amphetamines may antagonize the hypotensive effects of antihypertensives).
No products indexed under this heading.

Metolazone (Amphetamines may antagonize the hypotensive effects of antihypertensives).
No products indexed under this heading.

Metoprolol Succinate (Adrenergic blockers are inhibited by amphetamines; amphetamines may antagonize the hypotensive effects of antihypertensives). Products include:
Toprol-XL Tablets 660

Metoprolol Tartrate (Adrenergic blockers are inhibited by amphetamines; amphetamines may antagonize the hypotensive effects of antihypertensives).
No products indexed under this heading.

Metyrosine (Amphetamines may antagonize the hypotensive effects of antihypertensives). Products include:
Demser Capsules 1933

Mibefradil Dihydrochloride (Amphetamines may antagonize the hypotensive effects of antihypertensives).
No products indexed under this heading.

Minoxidil (Amphetamines may antagonize the hypotensive effects of antihypertensives). Products include:
Men's Rogaine Extra Strength Topical Solution, Ocean Rush Scent and Original Unscented 706
Women's Rogaine Topical Solution, Spring Bloom Scent and Original Unscented 707

Moclobemide (Concurrent and/or sequential use may result in hypertensive crises; MAOI may slow the metabolism of amphetamines with resultant increase in their effect on release of norepinephrine and other monoamines from adrenergic nerve ending; this can cause headaches and other signs of hypertensive crises; concurrent and/or sequential use is contraindicated).
No products indexed under this heading.

Moexipril Hydrochloride (Amphetamines may antagonize the hypotensive effects of antihypertensives). Products include:
Uniretic Tablets 3114
Univasc Tablets 3118

Nadolol (Adrenergic blockers are inhibited by amphetamines; amphetamines may antagonize the hypotensive effects of antihypertensives). Products include:
Nadolol Tablets 2121

Nicardipine Hydrochloride (Amphetamines may antagonize the hypotensive effects of antihypertensives). Products include:
Cardene I.V. 1129

Nifedipine (Amphetamines may antagonize the hypotensive effects of antihypertensives). Products include:
Adalat CC Tablets 2978

Nisoldipine (Amphetamines may antagonize the hypotensive effects of antihypertensives). Products include:
Sular Tablets 1163

Nitroglycerin (Amphetamines may antagonize the hypotensive effects of antihypertensives). Products include:
Nitro-Dur Transdermal Infusion System 3060
Nitrolingual Pumpspray 1161

Norepinephrine Bitartrate (Amphetamines enhance the adrenergic effect of norepinephrine).
No products indexed under this heading.

Nortriptyline Hydrochloride (Enhanced activity of tricyclic antidepressants or sympathomimetics; possible increases in d-amphetamine resulting in potentiation of cardiovascular effects).
No products indexed under this heading.

Pargyline Hydrochloride (Concurrent and/or sequential use may result in hypertensive crises; MAOI may slow the metabolism of amphetamines with resultant increase in their effect on release of norepinephrine and other monoamines from adrenergic nerve ending; this can cause headaches and other signs of hypertensive crises; concurrent and/or sequential use is contraindicated).
No products indexed under this heading.

Penbutolol Sulfate (Adrenergic blockers are inhibited by amphetamines; amphetamines may antagonize the hypotensive effects of antihypertensives).
No products indexed under this heading.

Perindopril Erbumine (Amphetamines may antagonize the hypotensive effects of antihypertensives). Products include:
Aceon Tablets (2 mg, 4 mg, 8 mg) 3191

Phenelzine Sulfate (Concurrent and/or sequential use may result in hypertensive crises; MAOI may slow the metabolism of amphetamines with resultant increase in their effect on release of norepinephrine and other monoamines from adrenergic nerve ending; this can cause headaches and other signs of hypertensive crises; concurrent and/or sequential use is contraindicated).
No products indexed under this heading.

Phenobarbital (Amphetamines may delay intestinal absorption of phenobarbital; co-administration may produce a synergistic anticonvulsant action).
No products indexed under this heading.

Phenoxybenzamine Hydrochloride (Amphetamines may antagonize the hypotensive effects of antihypertensives). Products include:
Dibenzyline Capsules 3390

Phentolamine Mesylate (Amphetamines may antagonize the hypotensive effects of antihypertensives).
No products indexed under this heading.

Phenytoin (Amphetamines may delay intestinal absorption of phenytoin; co-administration may produce a synergistic anticonvulsant action).
No products indexed under this heading.

Phenytoin Sodium (Amphetamines may delay intestinal absorption of phenytoin; co-administration may produce a synergistic anticonvulsant action). Products include:
Phenytek Capsules 2153

Pindolol (Adrenergic blockers are inhibited by amphetamines; amphetamines may antagonize the hypotensive effects of antihypertensives).
No products indexed under this heading.

Polythiazide (Co-administration with urinary alkalinizing agents, such as certain thiazides, increase the concentration of the non-ionized species of the amphetamine molecule, thereby decreasing urinary excretion resulting in increased blood levels and potentiation of actions of amphetamines; amphetamines may antagonize the hypotensive effects of antihypertensives).
No products indexed under this heading.

Potassium Citrate (Co-administration with urinary acidifying agents increases the concentration of the ionized species of the amphetamine molecule, thereby increasing urinary excretion resulting in reduced blood levels and efficacy of amphetamines). Products include:
Urocit-K Tablets 2109

Prazosin Hydrochloride (Amphetamines may antagonize the hypotensive effects of antihypertensives).
No products indexed under this heading.

Procarbazine Hydrochloride (Concurrent and/or sequential use may result in hypertensive crises; MAOI may slow the metabolism of amphetamines with resultant increase in their effect on release of norepinephrine and other monoamines from adrenergic nerve ending; this can cause headaches and other signs of hypertensive crises; concurrent and/or sequential use is contraindicated). Products include:
Matulane Capsules 3188

Promethazine Hydrochloride (Amphetamines may counteract the sedative effect of antihistamines). Products include:
Phenergan 3438

Propoxyphene Hydrochloride (In cases of propoxyphene overdosage, amphetamine CNS stimulation is potentiated and fatal convulstions can occur).
No products indexed under this heading.

Propoxyphene Napsylate (In cases of propoxyphene overdosage, amphetamine CNS stimulation is potentiated and fatal convulstions can occur). Products include:
Darvocet A 500 Tablets 3497

Propranolol Hydrochloride (Adrenergic blockers are inhibited by amphetamines; amphetamines may antagonize the hypotensive effects of antihypertensives). Products include:
Inderal LA Long-Acting Capsules 3421
InnoPran XL Capsules 2728

Protriptyline Hydrochloride (Enhanced activity of tricyclic antidepressants or sympathomimetics; possible increases in d-amphetamine resulting in potentiation of cardiovascular effects). Products include:
Vivactil Tablets 2350

Pyrilamine Maleate (Amphetamines may counteract the sedative effect of antihistamines).
No products indexed under this heading.

Pyrilamine Tannate (Amphetamines may counteract the sedative effect of antihistamines).
No products indexed under this heading.

Quinapril Hydrochloride (Amphetamines may antagonize the hypotensive effects of antihypertensives).
No products indexed under this heading.

Ramipril (Amphetamines may antagonize the hypotensive effects of antihypertensives). Products include:
Altace Capsules 1673

Rauwolfia Serpentina (Amphetamines may antagonize the hypotensive effects of antihypertensives).
No products indexed under this heading.

Rescinnamine (Amphetamines may antagonize the hypotensive effects of antihypertensives).
No products indexed under this heading.

Reserpine (Co-administration with gastrointestinal acidifying agents, such as reserpine, lowers absorption of amphetamines resulting in reduced blood levels and efficacy of amphetamines; amphetamines may antagonize the hypotensive effects of antihypertensives).
No products indexed under this heading.

Selegiline Hydrochloride (Concurrent and/or sequential use may result in hypertensive crises; MAOI may slow the metabolism of amphetamines with resultant increase in their effect on release of norepinephrine and other monoamines from adrenergic nerve ending; this can cause headaches and other signs of hypertensive crises; concurrent and/or sequential use is contraindicated). Products include:
Eldepryl Capsules 3209

Sodium Bicarbonate (Co-administration with gastrointestinal alkalinizing agents, such as systemic disodium bicarbonate, increases the absorption of amphetamines). Products include:
Ceo-Two Evacuant Suppository 607
Colyte with Flavor Packs for Oral Solution 3102
HalfLytely and Bisacodyl Tablets Bowel Prep Kit with Flavors Packs 915
TriLyte with Flavor Packs for Oral Solution 3114

Sodium Citrate (Co-administration with urinary acidifying agents increases the concentration of the ionized species of the amphetamine molecule, thereby increasing urinary excretion resulting in reduced blood levels and efficacy of amphetamines).
No products indexed under this heading.

Sodium Nitroprusside (Amphetamines may antagonize the hypotensive effects of antihypertensives).
No products indexed under this heading.

Sotalol Hydrochloride (Adrenergic blockers are inhibited by amphetamines; amphetamines may antagonize the hypotensive effects of antihypertensives).
No products indexed under this heading.

Spirapril Hydrochloride (Amphetamines may antagonize the hypotensive effects of antihypertensives).
No products indexed under this heading.

Telmisartan (Amphetamines may antagonize the hypotensive effects of antihypertensives). Products include:
Micardis Tablets 884
Micardis HCT Tablets 886

Terazosin Hydrochloride (Amphetamines may antagonize the hypotensive effects of antihypertensives). Products include:
Hytrin Capsules 469

Terfenadine (Amphetamines may counteract the sedative effect of antihistamines).
No products indexed under this heading.

Timolol Hemihydrate (Adrenergic blockers are inhibited by amphetamines; amphetamines may antagonize the hypotensive effects of antihypertensives). Products include:
Betimol Ophthalmic Solution 3371
Betimol Ophthalmic Solution .... ⊙283

Timolol Maleate (Adrenergic blockers are inhibited by amphetamines; amphetamines may antagonize the hypotensive effects of antihypertensives). Products include:
Blocadren Tablets 1891
Cosopt Sterile Ophthalmic Solution 1910
Timolide Tablets 2056
Timoptic in Ocudose 2061
Timoptic Sterile Ophthalmic Solution 2058
Timoptic-XE Sterile Ophthalmic Gel Forming Solution 2062

Torsemide (Amphetamines may antagonize the hypotensive effects of antihypertensives).
No products indexed under this heading.

Trandolapril (Amphetamines may antagonize the hypotensive effects of antihypertensives). Products include:
Mavik Tablets 482
Tarka Tablets 519

Tranylcypromine Sulfate (Concurrent and/or sequential use may result in hypertensive crises; MAOI may slow the metabolism of amphetamines with resultant increase in their effect on release of norepinephrine and other monoamines from adrenergic nerve ending; this can cause headaches and other signs of hypertensive crises; concurrent and/or sequential use is contraindicated). Products include:
Parnate Tablets 1499

Trimeprazine Tartrate (Amphetamines may counteract the sedative effect of antihistamines).
No products indexed under this heading.

Trimethaphan Camsylate (Amphetamines may antagonize the hypotensive effects of antihypertensives).
No products indexed under this heading.

Trimipramine Maleate (Enhanced activity of tricyclic antidepressants or sympathomimetics; possible increases in d-amphetamine resulting in potentiation of cardiovascular effects). Products include:
Surmontil Capsules 2347

Tripelennamine Hydrochloride (Amphetamines may counteract the sedative effect of antihistamines).
No products indexed under this heading.

Triprolidine Hydrochloride (Amphetamines may counteract the sedative effect of antihistamines).
No products indexed under this heading.

Valsartan (Amphetamines may antagonize the hypotensive effects of antihypertensives). Products include:
Diovan HCT Tablets 2195
Diovan Tablets 2191

Verapamil Hydrochloride (Amphetamines may antagonize the hypotensive effects of antihypertensives). Products include:
Covera-HS Tablets 3135
Tarka Tablets 519
Verelan PM Capsules 3120

Vitamin C (Co-administration with gastrointestinal acidifying agents, such as vitamin C, lowers absorption of amphetamines resulting in reduced blood levels and efficacy of amphetamines). Products include:
Chromagen Forte Soft Gelatin Capsules 3296
Halls Defense Sugarfree Vitamin C Drops .... ▣611
Niferex-150 Forte Capsules 3299
Peridin-C Tablets .... ▣761
Repliva 21/7 Tablets 3301

Food Interactions

Food, unspecified (Concurrent use with food prolongs T_{max} by 2.5 hours, however, food does not affect the extent of absorption).

ADENOCARD INJECTION

(Adenosine) 612

May interact with cardiac glycosides, xanthines, and certain other agents. Compounds in these categories include:

Aminophylline (The effects of adenosine are antagonized by co-administration with methylxanthines, such as theophylline; larger doses of adenosine may be required or adenosine may not be effective).
No products indexed under this heading.

Caffeine (The effects of adenosine are antagonized by co-administration with methylxanthines, such as caffeine; larger doses of adenosine may be required or adenosine may not be effective). Products include:
Athena Hair System Shampoo .... ▣767
BC Powder .... ▣612
Arthritis Strength BC Powder .... ▣612
Goody's Extra Strength Headache Powder .... ▣621
Goody's Extra Strength Pain Relief Tablets .... ▣621
Hycomine Compound Tablets 1105
Spartan Hair System Shampoo .... ▣767
Vivarin .... ▣639

Carbamazepine (Adenosine decreases the conduction through AV node, higher degrees of heart block may be produced in the presence of carbamazepine). Products include:
Carbatrol Capsules 3174
Equetro Extended-Release Capsules 3178
Tegretol/Tegretol-XR 2278

Deslanoside (The use of adenosine in patients receiving digitalis may be rarely associated with ventricular fibrillation).
No products indexed under this heading.

Digitalis Glycoside Preparations (The use of adenosine in patients receiving digitalis may be rarely associated with ventricular fibrillation).
No products indexed under this heading.

Digitoxin (The use of adenosine in patients receiving digitalis may be rarely associated with ventricular fibrillation).
No products indexed under this heading.

Digoxin (The use of adenosine in patients receiving digitalis may be rarely associated with ventricular fibrillation). Products include:
Digitek Tablets 2146
Lanoxicaps Capsules 1458
Lanoxin Injection 1462
Lanoxin Tablets 1468
Lanoxin Injection Pediatric 1465

Dipyridamole (Adenosine effects are potentiated by dipyridamole; smaller doses of adenosine may be effective with concurrent use). Products include:
Aggrenox Capsules 855
Persantine Tablets 898

Dyphylline (The effects of adenosine are antagonized by co-administration with methylxanthines, such as theophylline; larger doses of adenosine may be required or adenosine may not be effective).
No products indexed under this heading.

Theophylline (The effects of adenosine are antagonized by co-administration with methylxanthines, such as theophylline; larger doses of adenosine may be required or adenosine may not be effective).
No products indexed under this heading.

Theophylline Anhydrous (The effects of adenosine are antagonized by co-administration with methylxanthines, such as theophylline; larger doses of adenosine may be required or adenosine may not be effective). Products include:
Uniphyl Tablets 2708

Theophylline Calcium Salicylate (The effects of adenosine are antagonized by co-administration with methylxanthines, such as theophylline; larger doses of adenosine may be required or adenosine may not be effective).
No products indexed under this heading.

Theophylline Dihydroxypropyl (Glyceryl) (The effects of adenosine are antagonized by co-administration with methylxanthines, such as theophylline; larger doses of adenosine may be required or adenosine may not be effective).
No products indexed under this heading.

Theophylline Ethylenediamine (The effects of adenosine are antagonized by co-administration with methylxanthines, such as theophylline; larger doses of adenosine may be required or adenosine may not be effective).
No products indexed under this heading.

Theophylline Sodium Glycinate (The effects of adenosine are antagonized by co-administration with methylxanthines, such as theophylline; larger doses of adenosine may be required or adenosine may not be effective).
No products indexed under this heading.

Verapamil Hydrochloride (Digoxin and verapamil use may be rarely associated with ventricular fibrillation when combined with adenosine; potential for additive or synergistic depressant effects on the SA and AV nodes). Products include:
Covera-HS Tablets 3135
Tarka Tablets 519
Verelan PM Capsules 3120

ADENOSCAN

(Adenosine) 613

May interact with adenosine receptor antagonists, beta blockers, calcium channel blockers, cardiac glycosides, and nucleoside transport inhibitors. Compounds in these categories include:

Acebutolol Hydrochloride (Potential for additive or synergistic depressant effects on the SA or AV nodes; adenosine should be used with caution in the presence of these agents; no adverse interactions have been reported when co-administered).
No products indexed under this heading.

Aminophylline (The vasoactive effects of adenosine are inhibited by adenosine receptor antagonists such as alkylxanthines).
No products indexed under this heading.

Amlodipine Besylate (Potential for additive or synergistic depressant effects on the SA or AV nodes; adenosine should be used with caution in the presence of these agents; no adverse interactions have been reported when co-administered). Products include:
Caduet Tablets 2507
Lotrel Capsules 2238
Norvasc Tablets 2529

Atenolol (Potential for additive or synergistic depressant effects on the SA or AV nodes; adenosine should be used with caution in the presence of these agents; no adverse interactions have been reported when co-administered). Products include:
Tenormin I.V. Injection 698
Tenormin Tablets 695

Bepridil Hydrochloride (Potential for additive or synergistic depressant effects on the SA or AV nodes; adenosine should be used with caution in the presence of these agents; no adverse interactions have been reported when co-administered).
No products indexed under this heading.

Betaxolol Hydrochloride (Potential for additive or synergistic depressant effects on the SA or AV nodes; adenosine should be used with caution in the presence of these agents; no adverse interactions have been reported when co-administered). Products include:
Betoptic S Ophthalmic Suspension 554

Bisoprolol Fumarate (Potential for additive or synergistic depressant effects on the SA or AV nodes; adenosine should be used with caution in the presence of these agents; no adverse interactions have been reported when co-administered).
No products indexed under this heading.

Caffeine (The vasoactive effects of adenosine are inhibited by adenosine receptor antagonists such as alkylxanthines). Products include:
Athena Hair System Shampoo .... ▣767
BC Powder .... ▣612
Arthritis Strength BC Powder .... ▣612
Goody's Extra Strength Headache Powder....................... ▣621
Goody's Extra Strength Pain Relief Tablets............................. ▣621
Hycomine Compound Tablets 1105
Spartan Hair System Shampoo ...... ▣767
Vivarin .... ▣639

Carteolol Hydrochloride (Potential for additive or synergistic depressant effects on the SA or AV nodes; adenosine should be used with caution in the presence of these agents; no adverse interactions have been reported when co-administered). Products include:
Carteolol Hydrochloride Ophthalmic Solution USP, 1%....... ⊙246

Deslanoside (Potential for additive or synergistic depressant effects on the SA or AV nodes; adenosine should be used with caution in the presence of these agents; no adverse interactions have been reported when co-administered).
No products indexed under this heading.

Digitalis Glycoside Preparations (Potential for additive or synergistic depressant effects on the SA or AV nodes; adenosine should be used with caution in the presence of these agents; no adverse interactions have been reported when co-administered).
No products indexed under this heading.

Digitoxin (Potential for additive or synergistic depressant effects on the SA or AV nodes; adenosine should be used with caution in the presence of these agents; no adverse interactions have been reported when co-administered).
No products indexed under this heading.

Digoxin (Potential for additive or synergistic depressant effects on the SA or AV nodes; adenosine should be used with caution in the presence of these agents; no adverse interactions have been reported when co-administered). Products include:
Digitek Tablets 2146
Lanoxicaps Capsules 1458
Lanoxin Injection 1462
Lanoxin Tablets 1468
Lanoxin Injection Pediatric 1465

Diltiazem Hydrochloride (Potential for additive or synergistic depressant effects on the SA or AV nodes; adenosine should be used with caution in the presence of these agents; no adverse interactions have been reported when co-administered). Products include:
Cardizem LA Extended Release Tablets.. 1699
Tiazac Capsules 1204

Dipyridamole (Vasoactive effects of adenosine are potentiated by nucleoside transport inhibitors). Products include:
Aggrenox Capsules 855
Persantine Tablets 898

Dyphylline (The vasoactive effects of adenosine are inhibited by adenosine receptor antagonists such as alkylxanthines).
No products indexed under this heading.

Esmolol Hydrochloride (Potential for additive or synergistic depressant effects on the SA or AV nodes; adenosine should be used with caution in the presence of these agents; no adverse interactions have been reported when co-administered). Products include:
Brevibloc Concentrate 766
Brevibloc Injection 766
Brevibloc Double Strength Injection.. 766
Brevibloc Premixed Injection 766
Brevibloc Double Strength Premixed Injection........................ 766

Felodipine (Potential for additive or synergistic depressant effects on the SA or AV nodes; adenosine should be used with caution in the presence of these agents; no adverse interactions have been reported when co-administered). Products include:
Plendil Extended-Release Tablets 651

Isradipine (Potential for additive or synergistic depressant effects on the SA or AV nodes; adenosine should be used with caution in the presence of these agents; no adverse interactions have been reported when co-administered). Products include:
DynaCirc CR Tablets 2726

Labetalol Hydrochloride (Potential for additive or synergistic depressant effects on the SA or AV nodes; adenosine should be used with caution in the presence of these agents; no adverse interactions have been reported when co-administered).
No products indexed under this heading.

Levobunolol Hydrochloride (Potential for additive or synergistic depressant effects on the SA or AV nodes; adenosine should be used with caution in the presence of these agents; no adverse interactions have been reported when co-administered). Products include:
Betagan Ophthalmic Solution, USP.. ⊙217

Metipranolol Hydrochloride (Potential for additive or synergistic depressant effects on the SA or AV nodes; adenosine should be used with caution in the presence of these agents; no adverse interactions have been reported when co-administered).
No products indexed under this heading.

Metoprolol Succinate (Potential for additive or synergistic depressant effects on the SA or AV nodes; adenosine should be used with caution in the presence of these agents; no adverse interactions have been reported when co-administered). Products include:
Toprol-XL Tablets 660

Metoprolol Tartrate (Potential for additive or synergistic depressant effects on the SA or AV nodes; adenosine should be used with caution in the presence of these agents; no adverse interactions have been reported when co-administered).
No products indexed under this heading.

Mibefradil Dihydrochloride (Potential for additive or synergistic depressant effects on the SA or AV nodes; adenosine should be used with caution in the presence of these agents; no adverse interactions have been reported when co-administered).
No products indexed under this heading.

Nadolol (Potential for additive or synergistic depressant effects on the SA or AV nodes; adenosine should be used with caution in the presence of these agents; no adverse interactions have been reported when co-administered). Products include:
Nadolol Tablets 2121

Nicardipine Hydrochloride (Potential for additive or synergistic depressant effects on the SA or AV nodes; adenosine should be used with caution in the presence of these agents; no adverse interactions have been reported when co-administered). Products include:
Cardene I.V. 1129

Nifedipine (Potential for additive or synergistic depressant effects on the SA or AV nodes; adenosine should be used with caution in the presence of these agents; no adverse interactions have been reported when co-administered). Products include:
Adalat CC Tablets 2978

Nimodipine (Potential for additive or synergistic depressant effects on the SA or AV nodes; adenosine should be used with caution in the presence of these agents; no adverse interactions have been reported when co-administered). Products include:
Nimotop Capsules 774

Nisoldipine (Potential for additive or synergistic depressant effects on the SA or AV nodes; adenosine should be used with caution in the presence of these agents; no adverse interactions have been reported when co-administered). Products include:
Sular Tablets 1163

Penbutolol Sulfate (Potential for additive or synergistic depressant effects on the SA or AV nodes; adenosine should be used with caution in the presence of these agents; no adverse interactions have been reported when co-administered).
No products indexed under this heading.

Pindolol (Potential for additive or synergistic depressant effects on the SA or AV nodes; adenosine should be used with caution in the presence of these agents; no adverse interactions have been reported when co-administered).
No products indexed under this heading.

Propranolol Hydrochloride (Potential for additive or synergistic depressant effects on the SA or AV nodes; adenosine should be used with caution in the presence of these agents; no adverse interactions have been reported when co-administered). Products include:
Inderal LA Long-Acting Capsules 3421
InnoPran XL Capsules 2728

Sotalol Hydrochloride (Potential for additive or synergistic depressant effects on the SA or AV nodes; adenosine should be used with caution in the presence of these agents; no adverse interactions have been reported when co-administered).
No products indexed under this heading.

Theophylline (The vasoactive effects of adenosine are inhibited by adenosine receptor antagonists such as alkylxanthines).
No products indexed under this heading.

Theophylline Calcium Salicylate (The vasoactive effects of adenosine are inhibited by adenosine receptor antagonists such as alkylxanthines).
No products indexed under this heading.

Theophylline Sodium Glycinate (The vasoactive effects of adenosine are inhibited by adenosine receptor antagonists such as alkylxanthines).
No products indexed under this heading.

Timolol Hemihydrate (Potential for additive or synergistic depressant effects on the SA or AV nodes; adenosine should be used with caution in the presence of these agents; no adverse interactions have been reported when co-administered). Products include:
Betimol Ophthalmic Solution 3371
Betimol Ophthalmic Solution .... ⊙283

Timolol Maleate (Potential for additive or synergistic depressant effects on the SA or AV nodes; adenosine should be used with caution in the presence of these agents; no adverse interactions have been reported when co-administered). Products include:
Blocadren Tablets 1891
Cosopt Sterile Ophthalmic Solution.. 1910
Timolide Tablets 2056
Timoptic in Ocudose 2061
Timoptic Sterile Ophthalmic Solution.. 2058
Timoptic-XE Sterile Ophthalmic Gel Forming Solution.................... 2062

Verapamil Hydrochloride (Potential for additive or synergistic depressant effects on the SA or AV nodes; adenosine should be used with caution in the presence of these agents; no adverse interactions have been reported when co-administered). Products include:
Covera-HS Tablets 3135
Tarka Tablets 519
Verelan PM Capsules 3120

ADIPEX-P CAPSULES

(Phentermine Hydrochloride) 1216
See Adipex-P Tablets

ADIPEX-P TABLETS

(Phentermine Hydrochloride) 1216
May interact with insulin, monoamine oxidase inhibitors, selective serotonin reuptake inhibitors, and certain other agents. Compounds in these categories include:

Citalopram Hydrobromide (The safety and efficacy of combination therapy with phentermine and any other drug products for weight loss, including selective serotonin reuptake inhibitors, have not been

established; co-administration of these products for weight loss is not recommended). Products include:
Celexa 1177

Dexfenfluramine Hydrochloride (Co-administration has resulted in primary pulmonary hypertension, a rare, frequently fatal disease of the lungs and serious regurgitant cardiac valvular disease).
No products indexed under this heading.

Escitalopram Oxalate (The safety and efficacy of combination therapy with phentermine and any other drug products for weight loss, including selective serotonin reuptake inhibitors, have not been established; co-administration of these products for weight loss is not recommended).
Products include:
Lexapro Oral Solution 1193
Lexapro Tablets 1193

Fenfluramine Hydrochloride (Co-administration has resulted in primary pulmonary hypertension, a rare, frequently fatal disease of the lungs and serious regurgitant cardiac valvular disease).
No products indexed under this heading.

Fluoxetine Hydrochloride (The safety and efficacy of combination therapy with phentermine and any other drug products for weight loss, including selective serotonin reuptake inhibitors, have not been established; co-administration of these products for weight loss is not recommended). Products include:
Prozac Pulvules and Liquid 1771
Symbyax Capsules 1788

Fluvoxamine Maleate (The safety and efficacy of combination therapy with phentermine and any other drug products for weight loss, including selective serotonin reuptake inhibitors, have not been established; co-administration of these products for weight loss is not recommended).
No products indexed under this heading.

Guanethidine Monosulfate (Decreased hypotensive effect of guanethidine).
No products indexed under this heading.

Insulin, Human, Zinc Suspension (Insulin requirement may be altered).
Products include:
Humulin L, 100 Units 1763
Humulin U, 100 Units 1770

Insulin, Human NPH (Insulin requirement may be altered).
Products include:
Humulin N, 100 Units 1764
Humulin N Pen 1765
Novolin N Human Insulin 10 ml Vials 2322
Novolin N InnoLet 2322
Novolin N PenFill 3 ml Cartridges 2325
Novolin R InnoLet 2322

Insulin, Human Regular (Insulin requirement may be altered).
Products include:
Humulin R (U-500) 1768
Humulin R, 100 Units 1767
Novolin R Human Insulin 10 ml Vials 2322
Novolin R PenFill 2325

Insulin, Human Regular and Human NPH Mixture (Insulin requirement may be altered).
Products include:
Humulin 50/50, 100 Units 1760
Humulin 70/30 Pen 1761
Novolin 70/30 Human Insulin 10 ml Vials 2321
Novolin 70/30 InnoLet 2322
Novolin 70/30 PenFill 3 ml Cartridges 2325

Insulin, NPH (Insulin requirement may be altered).
No products indexed under this heading.

Insulin, Regular (Insulin requirement may be altered).
No products indexed under this heading.

Insulin, Zinc Crystals (Insulin requirement may be altered).
No products indexed under this heading.

Insulin, Zinc Suspension (Insulin requirement may be altered).
No products indexed under this heading.

Insulin Aspart, Human Regular (Insulin requirement may be altered).
Products include:
NovoLog Injection 2326

Insulin glargine (Insulin requirement may be altered). Products include:
Lantus Injection 2925

Insulin Lispro, Human (Insulin requirement may be altered).
Products include:
Humalog-Pen 1751
Humalog Mix 75/25-Pen 1754

Insulin Lispro Protamine, Human (Insulin requirement may be altered).
Products include:
Humalog Mix 75/25-Pen 1754

Isocarboxazid (Concurrent and/or sequential administration with MAO inhibitors may result in hypertensive crises; co-administration is contraindicated).
No products indexed under this heading.

Moclobemide (Concurrent and/or sequential administration with MAO inhibitors may result in hypertensive crises; co-administration is contraindicated).
No products indexed under this heading.

Pargyline Hydrochloride (Concurrent and/or sequential administration with MAO inhibitors may result in hypertensive crises; co-administration is contraindicated).
No products indexed under this heading.

Paroxetine Hydrochloride (The safety and efficacy of combination therapy with phentermine and any other drug products for weight loss, including selective serotonin reuptake inhibitors, have not been established; co-administration of these products for weight loss is not recommended). Products include:
Paxil CR Controlled-Release Tablets 1509
Paxil 1501

Phenelzine Sulfate (Concurrent and/or sequential administration with MAO inhibitors may result in hypertensive crises; co-administration is contraindicated).
No products indexed under this heading.

Procarbazine Hydrochloride (Concurrent and/or sequential administration with MAO inhibitors may result in hypertensive crises; co-administration is contraindicated).
Products include:
Matulane Capsules 3188

Selegiline Hydrochloride (Concurrent and/or sequential administration with MAO inhibitors may result in hypertensive crises; co-administration is contraindicated).
Products include:
Eldepryl Capsules 3209

Sertraline Hydrochloride (The safety and efficacy of combination therapy with phentermine and any other drug products for weight loss, including selective serotonin reuptake inhibitors, have not been established; co-administration of these products for weight loss is not recommended). Products include:
Zoloft 2581

Tranylcypromine Sulfate (Concurrent and/or sequential administration with MAO inhibitors may result in hypertensive crises; co-administration is contraindicated).
Products include:
Parnate Tablets 1499

Food Interactions

Alcohol (May result in adverse drug interaction).

ADRIAMYCIN FOR INJECTION, USP

(Doxorubicin Hydrochloride) 786
See Adriamycin Injection, USP

ADRIAMYCIN INJECTION, USP

(Doxorubicin Hydrochloride) 786
May interact with calcium channel blockers, antineoplastics, phenytoin, and certain other agents. Compounds in these categories include:

Altretamine (Doxorubicin may potentiate the toxicity of other anticancer therapies). Products include:
Hexalen Capsules 2101

Amlodipine Besylate (Co-administration of doxorubicin and calcium channel entry blockers may increase the risk of doxorubicin cardiotoxicity). Products include:
Caduet Tablets 2507
Lotrel Capsules 2238
Norvasc Tablets 2529

Anastrozole (Doxorubicin may potentiate the toxicity of other anticancer therapies). Products include:
Arimidex Tablets 665

Asparaginase (Doxorubicin may potentiate the toxicity of other anticancer therapies). Products include:
Elspar for Injection 1943

Bepridil Hydrochloride (Co-administration of doxorubicin and calcium channel entry blockers may increase the risk of doxorubicin cardiotoxicity).
No products indexed under this heading.

Bicalutamide (Doxorubicin may potentiate the toxicity of other anticancer therapies). Products include:
Casodex Tablets 670

Bleomycin Sulfate (Doxorubicin may potentiate the toxicity of other anticancer therapies).
No products indexed under this heading.

Busulfan (Doxorubicin may potentiate the toxicity of other anticancer therapies). Products include:
I.V. Busulfex 1125
Myleran Tablets 1492

Carboplatin (Doxorubicin may potentiate the toxicity of other anticancer therapies).
No products indexed under this heading.

Carmustine (BCNU) (Doxorubicin may potentiate the toxicity of other anticancer therapies).
No products indexed under this heading.

Chlorambucil (Doxorubicin may potentiate the toxicity of other anticancer therapies). Products include:
Leukeran Tablets 1472

Cisplatin (Doxorubicin may potentiate the toxicity of other anticancer therapies).
No products indexed under this heading.

Cyclophosphamide (Co-administration of doxorubicin with cyclophosphamide has resulted in exacerbation of cyclophosphamide-induced hemorrhagic cystitis; cardiac toxicity may occur at lower cumulative doses in patients who are receiving cyclophosphamide).
No products indexed under this heading.

Cyclosporine (Co-administration of doxorubicin may result in increases in AUC for both doxorubicin and doxorubicinol possibly due to a decrease in clearance of parent drug and a decrease in metabolism of doxorubicin; potential for more profound and prolonged hematologic toxicity is associated with combined use; coma and seizures have also been reported). Products include:
Gengraf Capsules 458
Neoral Soft Gelatin Capsules 2247
Neoral Oral Solution 2247
Restasis Ophthalmic Emulsion 570
Sandimmune 2259

Cytarabine (Combination therapy results in necrotizing colitis, typhilitis, bloody stools and severe infections).
No products indexed under this heading.

Dacarbazine (Doxorubicin may potentiate the toxicity of other anticancer therapies).
No products indexed under this heading.

Daunorubicin Citrate (Doxorubicin may potentiate the toxicity of other anticancer therapies).
No products indexed under this heading.

Daunorubicin Hydrochloride (Doxorubicin may potentiate the toxicity of other anticancer therapies).
Products include:
Cerubidine for Injection 788

Denileukin Diftitox (Doxorubicin may potentiate the toxicity of other anticancer therapies). Products include:
Ontak Vials 1717

Diltiazem Hydrochloride (Co-administration of doxorubicin and calcium channel entry blockers may increase the risk of doxorubicin cardiotoxicity). Products include:
Cardizem LA Extended Release Tablets 1699
Tiazac Capsules 1204

Docetaxel (Doxorubicin may potentiate the toxicity of other anticancer therapies). Products include:
Taxotere Injection Concentrate 2947

Epirubicin Hydrochloride (Doxorubicin may potentiate the toxicity of other anticancer therapies).
Products include:
Ellence Injection 2632

Estramustine Phosphate Sodium (Doxorubicin may potentiate the toxicity of other anticancer therapies). Products include:
Emcyt Capsules 3137
Etoposide (Doxorubicin may potentiate the toxicity of other anticancer therapies).
No products indexed under this heading.
Exemestane (Doxorubicin may potentiate the toxicity of other anticancer therapies). Products include:
Aromasin Tablets 2600
Felodipine (Co-administration of doxorubicin and calcium channel entry blockers may increase the risk of doxorubicin cardiotoxicity). Products include:
Plendil Extended-Release Tablets 651
Floxuridine (Doxorubicin may potentiate the toxicity of other anticancer therapies).
No products indexed under this heading.
Fluorouracil (Doxorubicin may potentiate the toxicity of other anticancer therapies). Products include:
Carac Cream, 0.5% 1048
Efudex 3348
Flutamide (Doxorubicin may potentiate the toxicity of other anticancer therapies). Products include:
Eulexin Capsules 3023
Fosphenytoin Sodium (Co-administration may result in decreased phenytoin levels).
No products indexed under this heading.
Gemcitabine Hydrochloride (Doxorubicin may potentiate the toxicity of other anticancer therapies). Products include:
Gemzar for Injection 1743
Hydroxyurea (Doxorubicin may potentiate the toxicity of other anticancer therapies).
No products indexed under this heading.
Idarubicin Hydrochloride (Doxorubicin may potentiate the toxicity of other anticancer therapies; concurrent use is contraindicated in patients who have received previous treatment with complete cumulative doses of idarubicin). Products include:
Idamycin PFS Injection 2645
Ifosfamide (Doxorubicin may potentiate the toxicity of other anticancer therapies).
No products indexed under this heading.
Interferon alfa-2a, Recombinant (Doxorubicin may potentiate the toxicity of other anticancer therapies). Products include:
Roferon-A Injection 2805
Interferon alfa-2b, Recombinant (Doxorubicin may potentiate the toxicity of other anticancer therapies). Products include:
Intron A for Injection 3038
Rebetron Combination Therapy 3078
Irinotecan Hydrochloride (Doxorubicin may potentiate the toxicity of other anticancer therapies). Products include:
Camptosar Injection 2602
Isradipine (Co-administration of doxorubicin and calcium channel entry blockers may increase the risk of doxorubicin cardiotoxicity). Products include:
DynaCirc CR Tablets 2726
Levamisole Hydrochloride (Doxorubicin may potentiate the toxicity of other anticancer therapies).
No products indexed under this heading.
Live Virus Vaccines (Administration of live vaccine to immunocompromised patients, including those undergoing cytotoxic chemotherapy, may be hazardous).
No products indexed under this heading.
Lomustine (CCNU) (Doxorubicin may potentiate the toxicity of other anticancer therapies).
No products indexed under this heading.
Mechlorethamine Hydrochloride (Doxorubicin may potentiate the toxicity of other anticancer therapies). Products include:
Mustargen for Injection 2007
Medroxyprogesterone Acetate (Co-administration of intravenous progesterone to patients with advanced malignancies at high doses with conventional formulation of fixed doxorubicin dose via bolus enhances doxorubicin-induced neutropenia and thrombocytopenia). Products include:
Depo-Provera Contraceptive Injection 2619
depo-subQ provera 104 Injectable Suspension................... 2622
Premphase Tablets 3452
Prempro Tablets 3452
Megestrol Acetate (Doxorubicin may potentiate the toxicity of other anticancer therapies). Products include:
Megace ES Oral Suspension 2492
Melphalan (Doxorubicin may potentiate the toxicity of other anticancer therapies). Products include:
Alkeran Tablets 977
Mercaptopurine (Co-administration of doxorubicin with 6-mercaptopurine has resulted in enhancement of hepatotoxicity of 6-mercaptopurine). Products include:
Purinethol Tablets 1222
Methotrexate Sodium (Doxorubicin may potentiate the toxicity of other anticancer therapies).
No products indexed under this heading.
Mibefradil Dihydrochloride (Co-administration of doxorubicin and calcium channel entry blockers may increase the risk of doxorubicin cardiotoxicity).
No products indexed under this heading.
Mitomycin (Mitomycin-C) (Doxorubicin may potentiate the toxicity of other anticancer therapies).
No products indexed under this heading.
Mitotane (Doxorubicin may potentiate the toxicity of other anticancer therapies).
No products indexed under this heading.
Mitoxantrone Hydrochloride (Doxorubicin may potentiate the toxicity of other anticancer therapies). Products include:
Novantrone for Injection Concentrate................................. 3158
Nicardipine Hydrochloride (Co-administration of doxorubicin and calcium channel entry blockers may increase the risk of doxorubicin cardiotoxicity). Products include:
Cardene I.V. 1129
Nifedipine (Co-administration of doxorubicin and calcium channel entry blockers may increase the risk of doxorubicin cardiotoxicity). Products include:
Adalat CC Tablets 2978
Nimodipine (Co-administration of doxorubicin and calcium channel entry blockers may increase the risk of doxorubicin cardiotoxicity). Products include:
Nimotop Capsules 774
Nisoldipine (Co-administration of doxorubicin and calcium channel entry blockers may increase the risk of doxorubicin cardiotoxicity). Products include:
Sular Tablets 1163
Oxaliplatin (Doxorubicin may potentiate the toxicity of other anticancer therapies). Products include:
Eloxatin for Injection 2908
Paclitaxel (Admisistration of paclitaxel infused over 24 hours followed by conventional formulation of doxorubicin administered over 48 hours resulted in a significant decrease in doxorubicin clearance with more profound neutropenic and stomatitis episodes than the reverse sequence of administration).
No products indexed under this heading.
Phenobarbital (Increases the elimination of doxorubicin).
No products indexed under this heading.
Phenytoin (Co-administration may result in decreased phenytoin levels).
No products indexed under this heading.
Phenytoin Sodium (Co-administration may result in decreased phenytoin levels). Products include:
Phenytek Capsules 2153
Procarbazine Hydrochloride (Doxorubicin may potentiate the toxicity of other anticancer therapies). Products include:
Matulane Capsules 3188
Progesterone (Co-administration of intravenous progesterone to patients with advanced malignancies at high doses with conventional formulation of fixed doxorubicin dose via bolus enhances doxorubicin-induced neutropenia and thrombocytopenia). Products include:
Prochieve 4% Gel 1018
Prochieve 8% Gel 1018
Prometrium Capsules (100 mg, 200 mg).. 3205
Streptozocin (May inhibit the hepatic metabolism; doxorubicin may potentiate the toxicity of other anticancer therapies).
No products indexed under this heading.
Tamoxifen Citrate (Doxorubicin may potentiate the toxicity of other anticancer therapies).
No products indexed under this heading.
Teniposide (Doxorubicin may potentiate the toxicity of other anticancer therapies).
No products indexed under this heading.
Thioguanine (Doxorubicin may potentiate the toxicity of other anticancer therapies). Products include:
Tabloid Tablets 1545
Thiotepa (Doxorubicin may potentiate the toxicity of other anticancer therapies).
No products indexed under this heading.
Topotecan Hydrochloride (Doxorubicin may potentiate the toxicity of other anticancer therapies). Products include:
Hycamtin for Injection 1427
Toremifene Citrate (Doxorubicin may potentiate the toxicity of other anticancer therapies).
No products indexed under this heading.
Valrubicin (Doxorubicin may potentiate the toxicity of other anticancer therapies).
No products indexed under this heading.
Verapamil Hydrochloride (Co-administration of doxorubicin in animal studies has resulted in higher initial peak concentrations of doxorubicin in the heart with a higher incidence and severity of degenerative changes in cardiac tissue resulting in a shorter survival). Products include:
Covera-HS Tablets 3135
Tarka Tablets 519
Verelan PM Capsules 3120
Vincristine Sulfate (Doxorubicin may potentiate the toxicity of other anticancer therapies).
No products indexed under this heading.
Vinorelbine Tartrate (Doxorubicin may potentiate the toxicity of other anticancer therapies). Products include:
Navelbine Injection 1494

ADVAIR DISKUS 100/50
(Fluticasone Propionate, Salmeterol Xinafoate)......................... 1291
May interact with beta blockers, monoamine oxidase inhibitors, potassium-depleting diuretics, tricyclic antidepressants, and certain other agents. Compounds in these categories include:

Acebutolol Hydrochloride (Co-administration with beta-blockers not only blocks the pulmonary effect of beta-agonists, such as salmeterol, but may produce severe bronchospasm in patients with asthma).
No products indexed under this heading.
Amitriptyline Hydrochloride (Concurrent and/or sequential administration with tricyclic antidepressants may potentiate the action of salmeterol on the vascular system).
No products indexed under this heading.
Amoxapine (Concurrent and/or sequential administration with tricyclic antidepressants may potentiate the action of salmeterol on the vascular system).
No products indexed under this heading.
Atenolol (Co-administration with beta-blockers not only blocks the pulmonary effect of beta-agonists, such as salmeterol, but may produce severe bronchospasm in patients with asthma). Products include:
Tenormin I.V. Injection 698
Tenormin Tablets 695

Bendroflumethiazide (The ECG changes and/or hypokalemia that may result from the administration of non-potassium sparing diuretics can be acutely worsened by beta-agonists, especially when the recommended dose of beta-agonist is exceeded).
No products indexed under this heading.

Betaxolol Hydrochloride (Co-administration with beta-blockers not only blocks the pulmonary effect of beta-agonists, such as salmeterol, but may produce severe bronchospasm in patients with asthma).
Products include:
Betoptic S Ophthalmic Suspension.................................. 554

Bisoprolol Fumarate (Co-administration with beta-blockers not only blocks the pulmonary effect of beta-agonists, such as salmeterol, but may produce severe bronchospasm in patients with asthma).
No products indexed under this heading.

Bumetanide (The ECG changes and/or hypokalemia that may result from the administration of non-potassium sparing diuretics can be acutely worsened by beta-agonists, especially when the recommended dose of beta-agonist is exceeded).
No products indexed under this heading.

Carteolol Hydrochloride (Co-administration with beta-blockers not only blocks the pulmonary effect of beta-agonists, such as salmeterol, but may produce severe bronchospasm in patients with asthma).
Products include:
Carteolol Hydrochloride Ophthalmic Solution USP, 1%....... ⊙246

Chlorothiazide (The ECG changes and/or hypokalemia that may result from the administration of non-potassium sparing diuretics can be acutely worsened by beta-agonists, especially when the recommended dose of beta-agonist is exceeded).
Products include:
Aldoclor Tablets 1881
Diuril Oral 1936

Chlorothiazide Sodium (The ECG changes and/or hypokalemia that may result from the administration of non-potassium sparing diuretics can be acutely worsened by beta-agonists, especially when the recommended dose of beta-agonist is exceeded). Products include:
Diuril Sodium Intravenous 1934

Clomipramine Hydrochloride (Concurrent and/or sequential administration with tricyclic antidepressants may potentiate the action of salmeterol on the vascular system).
No products indexed under this heading.

Desipramine Hydrochloride (Concurrent and/or sequential administration with tricyclic antidepressants may potentiate the action of salmeterol on the vascular system).
No products indexed under this heading.

Doxepin Hydrochloride (Concurrent and/or sequential administration with tricyclic antidepressants may potentiate the action of salmeterol on the vascular system).
No products indexed under this heading.

Esmolol Hydrochloride (Co-administration with beta-blockers not only blocks the pulmonary effect of beta-agonists, such as salmeterol, but may produce severe bronchospasm in patients with asthma).
Products include:
Brevibloc Concentrate 766
Brevibloc Injection 766
Brevibloc Double Strength Injection... 766
Brevibloc Premixed Injection 766
Brevibloc Double Strength Premixed Injection....................... 766

Ethacrynic Acid (The ECG changes and/or hypokalemia that may result from the administration of non-potassium sparing diuretics can be acutely worsened by beta-agonists, especially when the recommended dose of beta-agonist is exceeded).
Products include:
Edecrin Tablets 1941

Furosemide (The ECG changes and/or hypokalemia that may result from the administration of non-potassium sparing diuretics can be acutely worsened by beta-agonists, especially when the recommended dose of beta-agonist is exceeded).
Products include:
Furosemide Tablets 2117

Hydrochlorothiazide (The ECG changes and/or hypokalemia that may result from the administration of non-potassium sparing diuretics can be acutely worsened by beta-agonists, especially when the recommended dose of beta-agonist is exceeded). Products include:
Aldoril Tablets 1884
Atacand HCT 637
Avalide Tablets 2889
Avalide Tablets 922
Benicar HCT Tablets 2852
Diovan HCT Tablets 2195
Dyazide Capsules 1389
Hyzaar 1964
Lotensin HCT Tablets 2235
Maxzide 2150
Micardis HCT Tablets 886
Moduretic Tablets 2003
Prinzide Tablets 2033
Teveten HCT Tablets 1710
Timolide Tablets 2056
Uniretic Tablets 3114
Vaseretic Tablets 2073
Zestoretic Tablets 701

Hydroflumethiazide (The ECG changes and/or hypokalemia that may result from the administration of non-potassium sparing diuretics can be acutely worsened by beta-agonists, especially when the recommended dose of beta-agonist is exceeded).
No products indexed under this heading.

Imipramine Hydrochloride (Concurrent and/or sequential administration with tricyclic antidepressants may potentiate the action of salmeterol on the vascular system).
No products indexed under this heading.

Imipramine Pamoate (Concurrent and/or sequential administration with tricyclic antidepressants may potentiate the action of salmeterol on the vascular system).
No products indexed under this heading.

Isocarboxazid (Concurrent and/or sequential administration with MAO inhibitors may potentiate the action of salmeterol on the vascular system).
No products indexed under this heading.

Ketoconazole (Co-administration of a single dose of fluticasone with multiple doses of ketoconazole, a potent CYP3A4 inhibitor, to steady state has resulted in increased fluticasone exposure, a reduction in plasma cortisol AUC and no effect on urinary excretion of cortisol).
Products include:
Nizoral A-D Shampoo, 1%................ 1839
Nizoral 2% Shampoo 1838

Labetalol Hydrochloride (Co-administration with beta-blockers not only blocks the pulmonary effect of beta-agonists, such as salmeterol, but may produce severe bronchospasm in patients with asthma).
No products indexed under this heading.

Levobunolol Hydrochloride (Co-administration with beta-blockers not only blocks the pulmonary effect of beta-agonists, such as salmeterol, but may produce severe bronchospasm in patients with asthma).
Products include:
Betagan Ophthalmic Solution, USP.. ⊙217

Maprotiline Hydrochloride (Concurrent and/or sequential administration with tricyclic antidepressants may potentiate the action of salmeterol on the vascular system).
No products indexed under this heading.

Methyclothiazide (The ECG changes and/or hypokalemia that may result from the administration of non-potassium sparing diuretics can be acutely worsened by beta-agonists, especially when the recommended dose of beta-agonist is exceeded).
No products indexed under this heading.

Metipranolol Hydrochloride (Co-administration with beta-blockers not only blocks the pulmonary effect of beta-agonists, such as salmeterol, but may produce severe bronchospasm in patients with asthma).
No products indexed under this heading.

Metoprolol Succinate (Co-administration with beta-blockers not only blocks the pulmonary effect of beta-agonists, such as salmeterol, but may produce severe bronchospasm in patients with asthma).
Products include:
Toprol-XL Tablets 660

Metoprolol Tartrate (Co-administration with beta-blockers not only blocks the pulmonary effect of beta-agonists, such as salmeterol, but may produce severe bronchospasm in patients with asthma).
No products indexed under this heading.

Moclobemide (Concurrent and/or sequential administration with MAO inhibitors may potentiate the action of salmeterol on the vascular system).
No products indexed under this heading.

Nadolol (Co-administration with beta-blockers not only blocks the pulmonary effect of beta-agonists, such as salmeterol, but may produce severe bronchospasm in patients with asthma). Products include:
Nadolol Tablets 2121

Nortriptyline Hydrochloride (Concurrent and/or sequential administration with tricyclic antidepressants may potentiate the action of salmeterol on the vascular system).
No products indexed under this heading.

Pargyline Hydrochloride (Concurrent and/or sequential administration with MAO inhibitors may potentiate the action of salmeterol on the vascular system).
No products indexed under this heading.

Penbutolol Sulfate (Co-administration with beta-blockers not only blocks the pulmonary effect of beta-agonists, such as salmeterol, but may produce severe bronchospasm in patients with asthma).
No products indexed under this heading.

Phenelzine Sulfate (Concurrent and/or sequential administration with MAO inhibitors may potentiate the action of salmeterol on the vascular system).
No products indexed under this heading.

Pindolol (Co-administration with beta-blockers not only blocks the pulmonary effect of beta-agonists, such as salmeterol, but may produce severe bronchospasm in patients with asthma).
No products indexed under this heading.

Polythiazide (The ECG changes and/or hypokalemia that may result from the administration of non-potassium sparing diuretics can be acutely worsened by beta-agonists, especially when the recommended dose of beta-agonist is exceeded).
No products indexed under this heading.

Procarbazine Hydrochloride (Concurrent and/or sequential administration with MAO inhibitors may potentiate the action of salmeterol on the vascular system).
Products include:
Matulane Capsules 3188

Propranolol Hydrochloride (Co-administration with beta-blockers not only blocks the pulmonary effect of beta-agonists, such as salmeterol, but may produce severe bronchospasm in patients with asthma).
Products include:
Inderal LA Long-Acting Capsules 3421
InnoPran XL Capsules 2728

Protriptyline Hydrochloride (Concurrent and/or sequential administration with tricyclic antidepressants may potentiate the action of salmeterol on the vascular system).
Products include:
Vivactil Tablets 2350

Ritonavir (Ritonavir, a potent CYP3A4 inhibitor, can significantly increase plasma fluticasone exposure, resulting in reduced serum cortisol concentrations. Cushing syndrome and adrenal suppression have been reported; therefore, co-administration is not recommended unless the potential benefit outweighs the risks). Products include:
Kaletra 474
Norvir 499

Selegiline Hydrochloride (Concurrent and/or sequential administration with MAO inhibitors may potentiate the action of salmeterol on the vascular system). Products include:

Eldepryl Capsules 3209

Sotalol Hydrochloride (Co-administration with beta-blockers not only blocks the pulmonary effect of beta-agonists, such as salmeterol, but may produce severe broncho-spasm in patients with asthma).
No products indexed under this heading.

Timolol Hemihydrate (Co-administration with beta-blockers not only blocks the pulmonary effect of beta-agonists, such as salmeterol, but may produce severe broncho-spasm in patients with asthma). Products include:
Betimol Ophthalmic Solution 3371
Betimol Ophthalmic Solution .... ⊙ 283

Timolol Maleate (Co-administration with beta-blockers not only blocks the pulmonary effect of beta-agonists, such as salmeterol, but may produce severe bronchospasm in patients with asthma). Products include:
Blocadren Tablets 1891
Cosopt Sterile Ophthalmic Solution....................................... 1910
Timolide Tablets 2056
Timoptic in Ocudose 2061
Timoptic Sterile Ophthalmic Solution....................................... 2058
Timoptic-XE Sterile Ophthalmic Gel Forming Solution 2062

Torsemide (The ECG changes and/or hypokalemia that may result from the administration of non-potassium sparing diuretics can be acutely worsened by beta-agonists, especially when the recommended dose of beta-agonist is exceeded).
No products indexed under this heading.

Tranylcypromine Sulfate (Concurrent and/or sequential administration with MAO inhibitors may potentiate the action of salmeterol on the vascular system). Products include:
Parnate Tablets 1499

Trimipramine Maleate (Concurrent and/or sequential administration with tricyclic antidepressants may potentiate the action of salmeterol on the vascular system). Products include:
Surmontil Capsules 2347

ADVAIR DISKUS 250/50

(Fluticasone Propionate, Salmeterol Xinafoate)......................... 1291
See Advair Diskus 100/50

ADVAIR DISKUS 500/50

(Fluticasone Propionate, Salmeterol Xinafoate)......................... 1291
See Advair Diskus 100/50

ADVATE INJECTION

(Antihemophilic Factor (Recombinant)).................................. 742
None cited in PDR database.

ADVICOR TABLETS

(Lovastatin, Niacin) 1694
May interact with azole antifungals, beta blockers, calcium channel blockers, oral anticoagulants, erythromycin, fibrates, nitrates and nitrites, protease inhibitors, and certain other agents. Compounds in these categories include:

Acebutolol Hydrochloride (Co-administration of niacin with vasoactive drugs, such as adrenergic blocking agents, may result in postural hypotension, particularly in patients with unstable angina or acute phase of myocardial infarction).
No products indexed under this heading.

Amlodipine Besylate (Co-administration of niacin with vasoactive drugs, such as calcium channel blockers, may result in postural hypotension, particularly in patients with unstable angina or acute phase of myocardial infarction). Products include:
Caduet Tablets 2507
Lotrel Capsules 2238
Norvasc Tablets 2529

Amprenavir (Co-administration results in serious skeletal muscle disorders, such as rhabdomyolysis and myopathy). Products include:
Agenerase Capsules 1299
Agenerase Oral Solution 1304

Amyl Nitrite (Co-administration of niacin with vasoactive drugs, such as nitrates, may result in postural hypotension, particularly in patients with unstable angina or acute phase of myocardial infarction).
No products indexed under this heading.

Anisindione (Co-administration has resulted in increased bleeding and/or prothrombin time). Products include:
Miradon Tablets 3056

Aspirin (May decrease the metabolic clearance of niacin; the clinical relevance of this finding is unclear). Products include:
Aggrenox Capsules 855
Bayer, Aspirin Regimen .... ▣ 606
Bayer Aspirin Tablets 3515
BC Powder .... ▣ 612
BC Allergy Sinus Cold Powder .... ▣ 612
Arthritis Strength BC Powder .... ▣ 612
BC Sinus Cold Powder .... ▣ 612
Ecotrin Enteric Coated Aspirin Low, Regular and Maximum Strength Tablets.......................... 1627
Goody's Body Pain Formula Powder...................................... ▣ 621
Goody's Extra Strength Headache Powder........................ ▣ 621
Goody's Extra Strength Pain Relief Tablets............................. ▣ 621
Percodan Tablets 1115
St. Joseph 81 mg Aspirin Chewable and Enteric Coated Tablets.. 1841

Atenolol (Co-administration of niacin with vasoactive drugs, such as adrenergic blocking agents, may result in postural hypotension, particularly in patients with unstable angina or acute phase of myocardial infarction). Products include:
Tenormin I.V. Injection 698
Tenormin Tablets 695

Bepridil Hydrochloride (Co-administration of niacin with vasoactive drugs, such as calcium channel blockers, may result in postural hypotension, particularly in patients with unstable angina or acute phase of myocardial infarction).
No products indexed under this heading.

Betaxolol Hydrochloride (Co-administration of niacin with vasoactive drugs, such as adrenergic blocking agents, may result in postural hypotension, particularly in patients with unstable angina or acute phase of myocardial infarction). Products include:
Betoptic S Ophthalmic Suspension.................................. 554

Bisoprolol Fumarate (Co-administration of niacin with vasoactive drugs, such as adrenergic blocking agents, may result in postural hypotension, particularly in patients with unstable angina or acute phase of myocardial infarction).
No products indexed under this heading.

Carteolol Hydrochloride (Co-administration of niacin with vasoactive drugs, such as adrenergic blocking agents, may result in postural hypotension, particularly in patients with unstable angina or acute phase of myocardial infarction). Products include:
Carteolol Hydrochloride Ophthalmic Solution USP, 1%....... ⊙ 246

Cholestyramine (In-vitro study resulted in approximately 10% to 30% of available niacin bound to cholestyramine; 4 to 6 hours should elapse between ingestion of bile acid-binding resins and the administration of Advicor).
No products indexed under this heading.

Clarithromycin (Co-administration results in serious skeletal muscle disorders, such as rhabdomyolysis and myopathy). Products include:
Biaxin/Biaxin XL 402
PREVPAC 3281

Clofibrate (The incidence and severity of myopathy are increased by co-administration of Advicor with drugs that cause myopathy when given alone, such as fibrates; combined use should be avoided).
No products indexed under this heading.

Clotrimazole (Co-administration results in serious skeletal muscle disorders, such as rhabdomyolysis and myopathy). Products include:
Lotrimin 3053
Lotrisone 3054

Colestipol Hydrochloride (In-vitro study resulted in approximately 90% of available niacin bound to colestipol; 4 to 6 hours should elapse between ingestion of bile acid-binding resins and the administration of Advicor).
No products indexed under this heading.

Cyclosporine (Co-administration results in serious skeletal muscle disorders, such as rhabdomyolysis and myopathy). Products include:
Gengraf Capsules 458
Neoral Soft Gelatin Capsules 2247
Neoral Oral Solution 2247
Restasis Ophthalmic Emulsion 570
Sandimmune 2259

Dicumarol (Co-administration has resulted in increased bleeding and/or prothrombin time).
No products indexed under this heading.

Diltiazem Hydrochloride (Co-administration of niacin with vasoactive drugs, such as calcium channel blockers, may result in postural hypotension, particularly in patients with unstable angina or acute phase of myocardial infarction). Products include:
Cardizem LA Extended Release Tablets.. 1699
Tiazac Capsules 1204

Erythrityl Tetranitrate (Co-administration of niacin with vasoactive drugs, such as nitrates, may result in postural hypotension, particularly in patients with unstable angina or acute phase of myocardial infarction).
No products indexed under this heading.

Erythromycin (Co-administration results in serious skeletal muscle disorders, such as rhabdomyolysis and myopathy). Products include:
Erygel Topical Gel 2096
Ery-Tab Tablets 447
Erythromycin Base Filmtab Tablets 454
Erythromycin Delayed-Release Capsules, USP............................. 456
PCE Dispertab Tablets 510

Erythromycin Estolate (Co-administration results in serious skeletal muscle disorders, such as rhabdomyolysis and myopathy).
No products indexed under this heading.

Erythromycin Ethylsuccinate (Co-administration results in serious skeletal muscle disorders, such as rhabdomyolysis and myopathy). Products include:
E.E.S. 449
EryPed 445

Erythromycin Gluceptate (Co-administration results in serious skeletal muscle disorders, such as rhabdomyolysis and myopathy).
No products indexed under this heading.

Erythromycin Lactobionate (Co-administration results in serious skeletal muscle disorders, such as rhabdomyolysis and myopathy).
No products indexed under this heading.

Erythromycin Stearate (Co-administration results in serious skeletal muscle disorders, such as rhabdomyolysis and myopathy). Products include:
Erythrocin Stearate Filmtab Tablets 452

Esmolol Hydrochloride (Co-administration of niacin with vasoactive drugs, such as adrenergic blocking agents, may result in postural hypotension, particularly in patients with unstable angina or acute phase of myocardial infarction). Products include:
Brevibloc Concentrate 766
Brevibloc Injection 766
Brevibloc Double Strength Injection.. 766
Brevibloc Premixed Injection 766
Brevibloc Double Strength Premixed Injection........................ 766

Felodipine (Co-administration of niacin with vasoactive drugs, such as calcium channel blockers, may result in postural hypotension, particularly in patients with unstable angina or acute phase of myocardial infarction). Products include:
Plendil Extended-Release Tablets 651

Fenofibrate (The incidence and severity of myopathy are increased by co-administration of Advicor with drugs that cause myopathy when given alone, such as fibrates; combined use should be avoided). Products include:
Antara Capsules 2723
Lofibra Capsules 1217
Tricor Tablets 523
Triglide Tablets 1165

Fluconazole (Co-administration results in serious skeletal muscle disorders, such as rhabdomyolysis and myopathy).
No products indexed under this heading.

Gemfibrozil (The incidence and severity of myopathy are increased by co-administration of Advicor with drugs that cause myopathy when given alone, such as fibrates; combined use should be avoided).
No products indexed under this heading.

Indinavir Sulfate (Co-administration results in serious skeletal muscle disorders, such as rhabdomyolysis and myopathy). Products include:
Crixivan Capsules 1918

Isosorbide Dinitrate (Co-administration of niacin with vasoactive drugs, such as nitrates, may result in postural hypotension, particularly in patients with unstable angina or acute phase of myocardial infarction). Products include:
BiDil Tablets 2161

Isosorbide Mononitrate (Co-administration of niacin with vasoactive drugs, such as nitrates, may result in postural hypotension, particularly in patients with unstable angina or acute phase of myocardial infarction). Products include:
Imdur Tablets 3032

Isradipine (Co-administration of niacin with vasoactive drugs, such as calcium channel blockers, may result in postural hypotension, particularly in patients with unstable angina or acute phase of myocardial infarction). Products include:
DynaCirc CR Tablets 2726

Itraconazole (Co-administration results in serious skeletal muscle disorders, such as rhabdomyolysis and myopathy).
No products indexed under this heading.

Ketoconazole (Co-administration results in serious skeletal muscle disorders, such as rhabdomyolysis and myopathy). Products include:
Nizoral A-D Shampoo, 1% 1839
Nizoral 2% Shampoo 1838

Labetalol Hydrochloride (Co-administration of niacin with vasoactive drugs, such as adrenergic blocking agents, may result in postural hypotension, particularly in patients with unstable angina or acute phase of myocardial infarction).
No products indexed under this heading.

Levobunolol Hydrochloride (Co-administration of niacin with vasoactive drugs, such as adrenergic blocking agents, may result in postural hypotension, particularly in patients with unstable angina or acute phase of myocardial infarction). Products include:
Betagan Ophthalmic Solution, USP .... ⊙217

Lopinavir (Co-administration results in serious skeletal muscle disorders, such as rhabdomyolysis and myopathy). Products include:
Kaletra 474

Metipranolol Hydrochloride (Co-administration of niacin with vasoactive drugs, such as adrenergic blocking agents, may result in postural hypotension, particularly in patients with unstable angina or acute phase of myocardial infarction).
No products indexed under this heading.

Metoprolol Succinate (Co-administration of niacin with vasoactive drugs, such as adrenergic blocking agents, may result in postural hypotension, particularly in patients with unstable angina or acute phase of myocardial infarction). Products include:
Toprol-XL Tablets 660

Metoprolol Tartrate (Co-administration of niacin with vasoactive drugs, such as adrenergic blocking agents, may result in postural hypotension, particularly in patients with unstable angina or acute phase of myocardial infarction).
No products indexed under this heading.

Mibefradil Dihydrochloride (Co-administration of niacin with vasoactive drugs, such as calcium channel blockers, may result in postural hypotension, particularly in patients with unstable angina or acute phase of myocardial infarction).
No products indexed under this heading.

Miconazole (Co-administration results in serious skeletal muscle disorders, such as rhabdomyolysis and myopathy).
No products indexed under this heading.

Nadolol (Co-administration of niacin with vasoactive drugs, such as adrenergic blocking agents, may result in postural hypotension, particularly in patients with unstable angina or acute phase of myocardial infarction). Products include:
Nadolol Tablets 2121

Nefazodone Hydrochloride (Co-administration results in serious skeletal muscle disorders, such as rhabdomyolysis and myopathy).
No products indexed under this heading.

Nelfinavir Mesylate (Co-administration results in serious skeletal muscle disorders, such as rhabdomyolysis and myopathy). Products include:
Viracept 2556

Nicardipine Hydrochloride (Co-administration of niacin with vasoactive drugs, such as calcium channel blockers, may result in postural hypotension, particularly in patients with unstable angina or acute phase of myocardial infarction). Products include:
Cardene I.V. 1129

Nicotinamide (May potentiate the adverse effects of Advicor). Products include:
Nicomide Tablets 3190

Nifedipine (Co-administration of niacin with vasoactive drugs, such as calcium channel blockers, may result in postural hypotension, particularly in patients with unstable angina or acute phase of myocardial infarction). Products include:
Adalat CC Tablets 2978

Nimodipine (Co-administration of niacin with vasoactive drugs, such as calcium channel blockers, may result in postural hypotension, particularly in patients with unstable angina or acute phase of myocardial infarction). Products include:
Nimotop Capsules 774

Nisoldipine (Co-administration of niacin with vasoactive drugs, such as calcium channel blockers, may result in postural hypotension, particularly in patients with unstable angina or acute phase of myocardial infarction). Products include:
Sular Tablets 1163

Nitroglycerin (Co-administration of niacin with vasoactive drugs, such as nitrates, may result in postural hypotension, particularly in patients with unstable angina or acute phase of myocardial infarction). Products include:
Nitro-Dur Transdermal Infusion System 3060
Nitrolingual Pumpspray 1161

Oxiconazole Nitrate (Co-administration results in serious skeletal muscle disorders, such as rhabdomyolysis and myopathy). Products include:
Oxistat 1498

Penbutolol Sulfate (Co-administration of niacin with vasoactive drugs, such as adrenergic blocking agents, may result in postural hypotension, particularly in patients with unstable angina or acute phase of myocardial infarction).
No products indexed under this heading.

Pentaerythritol Tetranitrate (Co-administration of niacin with vasoactive drugs, such as nitrates, may result in postural hypotension, particularly in patients with unstable angina or acute phase of myocardial infarction).
No products indexed under this heading.

Pindolol (Co-administration of niacin with vasoactive drugs, such as adrenergic blocking agents, may result in postural hypotension, particularly in patients with unstable angina or acute phase of myocardial infarction).
No products indexed under this heading.

Propranolol Hydrochloride (Co-administration of niacin with vasoactive drugs, such as adrenergic blocking agents, may result in postural hypotension, particularly in patients with unstable angina or acute phase of myocardial infarction). Products include:
Inderal LA Long-Acting Capsules 3421
InnoPran XL Capsules 2728

Ritonavir (Co-administration results in serious skeletal muscle disorders, such as rhabdomyolysis and myopathy). Products include:
Kaletra 474
Norvir 499

Saquinavir (Co-administration results in serious skeletal muscle disorders, such as rhabdomyolysis and myopathy).
No products indexed under this heading.

Saquinavir Mesylate (Co-administration results in serious skeletal muscle disorders, such as rhabdomyolysis and myopathy). Products include:
Invirase 2776

Sotalol Hydrochloride (Co-administration of niacin with vasoactive drugs, such as adrenergic blocking agents, may result in postural hypotension, particularly in patients with unstable angina or acute phase of myocardial infarction).
No products indexed under this heading.

Terconazole (Co-administration results in serious skeletal muscle disorders, such as rhabdomyolysis and myopathy).
No products indexed under this heading.

Timolol Hemihydrate (Co-administration of niacin with vasoactive drugs, such as adrenergic blocking agents, may result in postural hypotension, particularly in patients with unstable angina or acute phase of myocardial infarction). Products include:
Betimol Ophthalmic Solution 3371
Betimol Ophthalmic Solution .... ⊙283

Timolol Maleate (Co-administration of niacin with vasoactive drugs, such as adrenergic blocking agents, may result in postural hypotension, particularly in patients with unstable angina or acute phase of myocardial infarction). Products include:
Blocadren Tablets 1891
Cosopt Sterile Ophthalmic Solution 1910
Timolide Tablets 2056
Timoptic in Ocudose 2061
Timoptic Sterile Ophthalmic Solution 2058
Timoptic-XE Sterile Ophthalmic Gel Forming Solution 2062

Verapamil Hydrochloride (Co-administration of niacin with vasoactive drugs, such as calcium channel blockers, may result in postural hypotension, particularly in patients with unstable angina or acute phase of myocardial infarction). Products include:
Covera-HS Tablets 3135
Tarka Tablets 519
Verelan PM Capsules 3120

Warfarin Sodium (Co-administration has resulted in increased bleeding and/or prothrombin time). Products include:
Coumadin for Injection 932
Coumadin Tablets 932

Food Interactions

Alcohol (Concomitant alcohol may increase the flushing and its use should be avoided around the time of Advicor administration).

Drinks, hot, unspecified (Concomitant hot drinks may increase the flushing and its use should be avoided around the time of Advicor administration).

Grapefruit Juice (Inhibits CYP3A4 and can increase the plasma concentration of lovastatin; concurrent use should be avoided).

ADVIL ALLERGY SINUS CAPLETS

(Chlorpheniramine Maleate, Ibuprofen, Pseudoephedrine Hydrochloride) .... ▣737
May interact with hypnotics and sedatives, monoamine oxidase inhibitors, tranquilizers, and certain other agents. Compounds in these categories include:

Alprazolam (Concurrent use with sedatives or tranquilizers may increase drowsiness). Products include:

Niravam Orally Disintegrating Tablets 3106
Xanax XR Tablets 2655

Buspirone Hydrochloride (Concurrent use with sedatives or tranquilizers may increase drowsiness).
No products indexed under this heading.

Chlordiazepoxide (Concurrent use with sedatives or tranquilizers may increase drowsiness).
No products indexed under this heading.

Chlordiazepoxide Hydrochloride (Concurrent use with sedatives or tranquilizers may increase drowsiness). Products include:
Librium Capsules 3349

Chlorpromazine (Concurrent use with sedatives or tranquilizers may increase drowsiness).
No products indexed under this heading.

Chlorpromazine Hydrochloride (Concurrent use with sedatives or tranquilizers may increase drowsiness).
No products indexed under this heading.

Chlorprothixene (Concurrent use with sedatives or tranquilizers may increase drowsiness).
No products indexed under this heading.

Chlorprothixene Hydrochloride (Concurrent use with sedatives or tranquilizers may increase drowsiness).
No products indexed under this heading.

Clorazepate Dipotassium (Concurrent use with sedatives or tranquilizers may increase drowsiness). Products include:
Tranxene 2488

Diazepam (Concurrent use with sedatives or tranquilizers may increase drowsiness). Products include:
Diastat Rectal Delivery System 3344
Valium Tablets 2822

Droperidol (Concurrent use with sedatives or tranquilizers may increase drowsiness).
No products indexed under this heading.

Estazolam (Concurrent use with sedatives or tranquilizers may increase drowsiness). Products include:
ProSom Tablets 512

Ethchlorvynol (Concurrent use with sedatives or tranquilizers may increase drowsiness).
No products indexed under this heading.

Ethinamate (Concurrent use with sedatives or tranquilizers may increase drowsiness).
No products indexed under this heading.

Fluphenazine Decanoate (Concurrent use with sedatives or tranquilizers may increase drowsiness).
No products indexed under this heading.

Fluphenazine Enanthate (Concurrent use with sedatives or tranquilizers may increase drowsiness).
No products indexed under this heading.

Fluphenazine Hydrochloride (Concurrent use with sedatives or tranquilizers may increase drowsiness).
No products indexed under this heading.

Flurazepam Hydrochloride (Concurrent use with sedatives or tranquilizers may increase drowsiness). Products include:
Dalmane Capsules 3343

Glutethimide (Concurrent use with sedatives or tranquilizers may increase drowsiness).
No products indexed under this heading.

Haloperidol (Concurrent use with sedatives or tranquilizers may increase drowsiness).
No products indexed under this heading.

Haloperidol Decanoate (Concurrent use with sedatives or tranquilizers may increase drowsiness).
No products indexed under this heading.

Hydroxyzine Hydrochloride (Concurrent use with sedatives or tranquilizers may increase drowsiness).
No products indexed under this heading.

Isocarboxazid (Do not use while taking, or for up to two weeks after stopping, MAO inhibitors).
No products indexed under this heading.

Lorazepam (Concurrent use with sedatives or tranquilizers may increase drowsiness).
No products indexed under this heading.

Loxapine Hydrochloride (Concurrent use with sedatives or tranquilizers may increase drowsiness).
No products indexed under this heading.

Loxapine Succinate (Concurrent use with sedatives or tranquilizers may increase drowsiness).
No products indexed under this heading.

Meprobamate (Concurrent use with sedatives or tranquilizers may increase drowsiness).
No products indexed under this heading.

Mesoridazine Besylate (Concurrent use with sedatives or tranquilizers may increase drowsiness).
No products indexed under this heading.

Midazolam Hydrochloride (Concurrent use with sedatives or tranquilizers may increase drowsiness).
No products indexed under this heading.

Moclobemide (Do not use while taking, or for up to two weeks after stopping, MAO inhibitors).
No products indexed under this heading.

Molindone Hydrochloride (Concurrent use with sedatives or tranquilizers may increase drowsiness). Products include:
Moban Tablets 1108

Oxazepam (Concurrent use with sedatives or tranquilizers may increase drowsiness).
No products indexed under this heading.

Pargyline Hydrochloride (Do not use while taking, or for up to two weeks after stopping, MAO inhibitors).
No products indexed under this heading.

Perphenazine (Concurrent use with sedatives or tranquilizers may increase drowsiness).
No products indexed under this heading.

Phenelzine Sulfate (Do not use while taking, or for up to two weeks after stopping, MAO inhibitors).
No products indexed under this heading.

Prazepam (Concurrent use with sedatives or tranquilizers may increase drowsiness).
No products indexed under this heading.

Procarbazine Hydrochloride (Do not use while taking, or for up to two weeks after stopping, MAO inhibitors). Products include:
Matulane Capsules 3188

Prochlorperazine (Concurrent use with sedatives or tranquilizers may increase drowsiness).
No products indexed under this heading.

Promethazine Hydrochloride (Concurrent use with sedatives or tranquilizers may increase drowsiness). Products include:
Phenergan 3438

Propofol (Concurrent use with sedatives or tranquilizers may increase drowsiness). Products include:
Diprivan Injectable Emulsion 676

Quazepam (Concurrent use with sedatives or tranquilizers may increase drowsiness).
No products indexed under this heading.

Secobarbital Sodium (Concurrent use with sedatives or tranquilizers may increase drowsiness).
No products indexed under this heading.

Selegiline Hydrochloride (Do not use while taking, or for up to two weeks after stopping, MAO inhibitors). Products include:
Eldepryl Capsules 3209

Temazepam (Concurrent use with sedatives or tranquilizers may increase drowsiness).
No products indexed under this heading.

Thioridazine Hydrochloride (Concurrent use with sedatives or tranquilizers may increase drowsiness). Products include:
Thioridazine Hydrochloride Tablets 2122

Thiothixene (Concurrent use with sedatives or tranquilizers may increase drowsiness). Products include:
Thiothixene Capsules 2124

Tranylcypromine Sulfate (Do not use while taking, or for up to two weeks after stopping, MAO inhibitors). Products include:
Parnate Tablets 1499

Triazolam (Concurrent use with sedatives or tranquilizers may increase drowsiness).
No products indexed under this heading.

Trifluoperazine Hydrochloride (Concurrent use with sedatives or tranquilizers may increase drowsiness).
No products indexed under this heading.

Zaleplon (Concurrent use with sedatives or tranquilizers may increase drowsiness). Products include:
Sonata Capsules 1686

Zolpidem Tartrate (Concurrent use with sedatives or tranquilizers may increase drowsiness). Products include:
Ambien Tablets 2867

Food Interactions

Alcohol (Avoid alcohol; concurrent use may increase drowsiness. Heavy alcohol users, three or more drinks per day, should consult their physician for advice on when and how they should take pain relievers/fever reducers, including ibuprofen).

ADVIL CAPLETS
(Ibuprofen) .... ▣737
See Advil Tablets

ADVIL GEL CAPLETS
(Ibuprofen) .... ▣737
See Advil Tablets

ADVIL LIQUI-GELS
(Ibuprofen) .... ▣737
See Advil Tablets

ADVIL TABLETS
(Ibuprofen) .... ▣737
None cited in PDR database.

CHILDREN'S ADVIL SUSPENSION
(Ibuprofen) .... ▣742
None cited in PDR database.

CHILDREN'S ADVIL CHEWABLE TABLETS
(Ibuprofen) .... ▣741
None cited in PDR database.

ADVIL COLD & SINUS CAPLETS
(Ibuprofen, Pseudoephedrine Hydrochloride) .... ▣739
See Advil Cold & Sinus Tablets

ADVIL COLD & SINUS LIQUI-GELS
(Ibuprofen, Pseudoephedrine Hydrochloride) .... ▣739
See Advil Cold & Sinus Tablets

ADVIL COLD & SINUS TABLETS
(Ibuprofen, Pseudoephedrine Hydrochloride) .... ▣739
May interact with monoamine oxidase inhibitors. Compounds in these categories include:

Isocarboxazid (Concurrent and/or sequential use with MAO inhibitors is not recommended).
No products indexed under this heading.

Moclobemide (Concurrent and/or sequential use with MAO inhibitors is not recommended).
No products indexed under this heading.

Pargyline Hydrochloride (Concurrent and/or sequential use with MAO inhibitors is not recommended).
No products indexed under this heading.

Phenelzine Sulfate (Concurrent and/or sequential use with MAO inhibitors is not recommended).
No products indexed under this heading.

Procarbazine Hydrochloride (Concurrent and/or sequential use with MAO inhibitors is not recommended). Products include:
Matulane Capsules 3188

Selegiline Hydrochloride (Concurrent and/or sequential use with MAO inhibitors is not recommended). Products include:
Eldepryl Capsules 3209

Tranylcypromine Sulfate (Concurrent and/or sequential use with MAO inhibitors is not recommended). Products include:
Parnate Tablets 1499

ADVIL FLU & BODY ACHE CAPLETS

(Ibuprofen, Pseudoephedrine Hydrochloride).................................. ■□739
May interact with monoamine oxidase inhibitors. Compounds in these categories include:

Isocarboxazid (Concurrent and/or sequential use with MAO inhibitors is not recommended).
No products indexed under this heading.

Moclobemide (Concurrent and/or sequential use with MAO inhibitors is not recommended).
No products indexed under this heading.

Pargyline Hydrochloride (Concurrent and/or sequential use with MAO inhibitors is not recommended).
No products indexed under this heading.

Phenelzine Sulfate (Concurrent and/or sequential use with MAO inhibitors is not recommended).
No products indexed under this heading.

Procarbazine Hydrochloride (Concurrent and/or sequential use with MAO inhibitors is not recommended). Products include:
Matulane Capsules 3188

Selegiline Hydrochloride (Concurrent and/or sequential use with MAO inhibitors is not recommended). Products include:
Eldepryl Capsules 3209

Tranylcypromine Sulfate (Concurrent and/or sequential use with MAO inhibitors is not recommended). Products include:
Parnate Tablets 1499

CHILDREN'S ADVIL COLD SUSPENSION

(Ibuprofen, Pseudoephedrine Hydrochloride).................................. ■□741
May interact with monoamine oxidase inhibitors. Compounds in these categories include:

Isocarboxazid (Concurrent and/or sequential use up to 14 days with MAO inhibitors is not recommended).
No products indexed under this heading.

Moclobemide (Concurrent and/or sequential use up to 14 days with MAO inhibitors is not recommended).
No products indexed under this heading.

Pargyline Hydrochloride (Concurrent and/or sequential use up to 14 days with MAO inhibitors is not recommended).
No products indexed under this heading.

Phenelzine Sulfate (Concurrent and/or sequential use up to 14 days with MAO inhibitors is not recommended).
No products indexed under this heading.

Procarbazine Hydrochloride (Concurrent and/or sequential use up to 14 days with MAO inhibitors is not recommended). Products include:
Matulane Capsules 3188

Selegiline Hydrochloride (Concurrent and/or sequential use up to 14 days with MAO inhibitors is not recommended). Products include:
Eldepryl Capsules 3209

Tranylcypromine Sulfate (Concurrent and/or sequential use up to 14 days with MAO inhibitors is not recommended). Products include:
Parnate Tablets 1499

INFANTS' ADVIL CONCENTRATED DROPS

(Ibuprofen) .... ■□743
None cited in PDR database.

JUNIOR STRENGTH ADVIL SWALLOW TABLETS

(Ibuprofen) .... ■□740
None cited in PDR database.

ADVIL MIGRAINE LIQUIGELS

(Ibuprofen) .... ■□740
None cited in PDR database.

ADVIL MULTI-SYMPTOM COLD CAPLETS

(Chlorpheniramine Maleate, Ibuprofen, Pseudoephedrine Hydrochloride)................................ ■□738
May interact with hypnotics and sedatives, monoamine oxidase inhibitors, tranquilizers, and certain other agents. Compounds in these categories include:

Alprazolam (Concurrent use with sedatives or tranquilizers may increase drowsiness). Products include:
Niravam Orally Disintegrating Tablets 3106
Xanax XR Tablets 2655

Buspirone Hydrochloride (Concurrent use with sedatives or tranquilizers may increase drowsiness).
No products indexed under this heading.

Chlordiazepoxide (Concurrent use with sedatives or tranquilizers may increase drowsiness).
No products indexed under this heading.

Chlordiazepoxide Hydrochloride (Concurrent use with sedatives or tranquilizers may increase drowsiness). Products include:
Librium Capsules 3349

Chlorpromazine (Concurrent use with sedatives or tranquilizers may increase drowsiness).
No products indexed under this heading.

Chlorpromazine Hydrochloride (Concurrent use with sedatives or tranquilizers may increase drowsiness).
No products indexed under this heading.

Chlorprothixene (Concurrent use with sedatives or tranquilizers may increase drowsiness).
No products indexed under this heading.

Chlorprothixene Hydrochloride (Concurrent use with sedatives or tranquilizers may increase drowsiness).
No products indexed under this heading.

Clorazepate Dipotassium (Concurrent use with sedatives or tranquilizers may increase drowsiness). Products include:
Tranxene 2488

Diazepam (Concurrent use with sedatives or tranquilizers may increase drowsiness). Products include:
Diastat Rectal Delivery System 3344
Valium Tablets 2822

Droperidol (Concurrent use with sedatives or tranquilizers may increase drowsiness).
No products indexed under this heading.

Estazolam (Concurrent use with sedatives or tranquilizers may increase drowsiness). Products include:
ProSom Tablets 512

Ethchlorvynol (Concurrent use with sedatives or tranquilizers may increase drowsiness).
No products indexed under this heading.

Ethinamate (Concurrent use with sedatives or tranquilizers may increase drowsiness).
No products indexed under this heading.

Fluphenazine Decanoate (Concurrent use with sedatives or tranquilizers may increase drowsiness).
No products indexed under this heading.

Fluphenazine Enanthate (Concurrent use with sedatives or tranquilizers may increase drowsiness).
No products indexed under this heading.

Fluphenazine Hydrochloride (Concurrent use with sedatives or tranquilizers may increase drowsiness).
No products indexed under this heading.

Flurazepam Hydrochloride (Concurrent use with sedatives or tranquilizers may increase drowsiness). Products include:
Dalmane Capsules 3343

Glutethimide (Concurrent use with sedatives or tranquilizers may increase drowsiness).
No products indexed under this heading.

Haloperidol (Concurrent use with sedatives or tranquilizers may increase drowsiness).
No products indexed under this heading.

Haloperidol Decanoate (Concurrent use with sedatives or tranquilizers may increase drowsiness).
No products indexed under this heading.

Hydroxyzine Hydrochloride (Concurrent use with sedatives or tranquilizers may increase drowsiness).
No products indexed under this heading.

Isocarboxazid (Do not use while taking, or for up to two weeks after stopping, MAO inhibitors).
No products indexed under this heading.

Lorazepam (Concurrent use with sedatives or tranquilizers may increase drowsiness).
No products indexed under this heading.

Loxapine Hydrochloride (Concurrent use with sedatives or tranquilizers may increase drowsiness).
No products indexed under this heading.

Loxapine Succinate (Concurrent use with sedatives or tranquilizers may increase drowsiness).
No products indexed under this heading.

Meprobamate (Concurrent use with sedatives or tranquilizers may increase drowsiness).
No products indexed under this heading.

Mesoridazine Besylate (Concurrent use with sedatives or tranquilizers may increase drowsiness).
No products indexed under this heading.

Midazolam Hydrochloride (Concurrent use with sedatives or tranquilizers may increase drowsiness).
No products indexed under this heading.

Moclobemide (Do not use while taking, or for up to two weeks after stopping, MAO inhibitors).
No products indexed under this heading.

Molindone Hydrochloride (Concurrent use with sedatives or tranquilizers may increase drowsiness). Products include:
Moban Tablets 1108

Oxazepam (Concurrent use with sedatives or tranquilizers may increase drowsiness).
No products indexed under this heading.

Pargyline Hydrochloride (Do not use while taking, or for up to two weeks after stopping, MAO inhibitors).
No products indexed under this heading.

Perphenazine (Concurrent use with sedatives or tranquilizers may increase drowsiness).
No products indexed under this heading.

Phenelzine Sulfate (Do not use while taking, or for up to two weeks after stopping, MAO inhibitors).
No products indexed under this heading.

Prazepam (Concurrent use with sedatives or tranquilizers may increase drowsiness).
No products indexed under this heading.

Procarbazine Hydrochloride (Do not use while taking, or for up to two weeks after stopping, MAO inhibitors). Products include:
Matulane Capsules 3188

Prochlorperazine (Concurrent use with sedatives or tranquilizers may increase drowsiness).
No products indexed under this heading.

Promethazine Hydrochloride (Concurrent use with sedatives or tranquilizers may increase drowsiness). Products include:

Phenergan 3438

Propofol (Concurrent use with sedatives or tranquilizers may increase drowsiness). Products include:

Diprivan Injectable Emulsion 676

Quazepam (Concurrent use with sedatives or tranquilizers may increase drowsiness).

No products indexed under this heading.

Secobarbital Sodium (Concurrent use with sedatives or tranquilizers may increase drowsiness).

No products indexed under this heading.

Selegiline Hydrochloride (Do not use while taking, or for up to two weeks after stopping, MAO inhibitors). Products include:

Eldepryl Capsules 3209

Temazepam (Concurrent use with sedatives or tranquilizers may increase drowsiness).

No products indexed under this heading.

Thioridazine Hydrochloride (Concurrent use with sedatives or tranquilizers may increase drowsiness). Products include:

Thioridazine Hydrochloride Tablets 2122

Thiothixene (Concurrent use with sedatives or tranquilizers may increase drowsiness). Products include:

Thiothixene Capsules 2124

Tranylcypromine Sulfate (Do not use while taking, or for up to two weeks after stopping, MAO inhibitors). Products include:

Parnate Tablets 1499

Triazolam (Concurrent use with sedatives or tranquilizers may increase drowsiness).

No products indexed under this heading.

Trifluoperazine Hydrochloride (Concurrent use with sedatives or tranquilizers may increase drowsiness).

No products indexed under this heading.

Zaleplon (Concurrent use with sedatives or tranquilizers may increase drowsiness). Products include:

Sonata Capsules 1686

Zolpidem Tartrate (Concurrent use with sedatives or tranquilizers may increase drowsiness). Products include:

Ambien Tablets 2867

Food Interactions

Alcohol (Avoid alcohol; concurrent use may increase drowsiness. Heavy alcohol users, three or more drinks per day, should consult their physician for advice on when and how they should take pain relievers/fever reducers, including ibuprofen).

AEROBID INHALER SYSTEM

(Flunisolide) 1172

None cited in PDR database.

AEROBID-M INHALER SYSTEM

(Flunisolide) 1172

None cited in PDR database.

AEROCHAMBER PLUS AND AEROCHAMBER PLUS WITH MASK

(Spacer, Inhalation) 1174

None cited in PDR database.

AGENERASE CAPSULES

(Amprenavir) 1299

See Agenerase Oral Solution

AGENERASE ORAL SOLUTION

(Amprenavir) 1304

May interact with antacids containing aluminum, calcium and magnesium, calcium channel blockers, dexamethasone, ergot-containing drugs, oral hypoglycemic agents, insulin, oral contraceptives, phenytoin, protease inhibitors, quinidine, and certain other agents. Compounds in these categories include:

Acarbose (New onset diabetes mellitus, exacerbation of pre-existing diabetes mellitus, and hyperglycemia have been reported in HIV-infected patients receiving protease inhibitors; some patients may require dose adjustments). Products include:

Precose Tablets 776

Alprazolam (Increased benzodiazepine plasma concentrations; clinical significance is unknown; however, a decrease in benzodiazepine dose may be needed). Products include:

Niravam Orally Disintegrating Tablets 3106

Xanax XR Tablets 2655

Aluminum Carbonate (Antacids decrease amprenavir plasma concentrations; Agenerase should be taken at least one hour before or after antacids).

No products indexed under this heading.

Aluminum Hydroxide (Antacids decrease amprenavir plasma concentrations; Agenerase should be taken at least one hour before or after antacids). Products include:

Gaviscon Regular Strength Liquid 620

Gaviscon Regular Strength Tablets 619

Gaviscon Extra Strength Liquid 620

Gaviscon Extra Strength Tablets 619

Maalox Max Maximum Strength Antacid/Anti-Gas Liquid 2165

Maalox Regular Strength Antacid/Antigas Liquid 2164

Amiodarone Hydrochloride (Increases antiarrhythmics plasma concentrations). Products include:

Pacerone Tablets 3337

Amitriptyline Hydrochloride (Increase in tricyclic antidepressant plasma concentrations).

No products indexed under this heading.

Amlodipine Besylate (Increased calcium channel blockers plasma concentrations). Products include:

Caduet Tablets 2507

Lotrel Capsules 2238

Norvasc Tablets 2529

Amoxapine (Co-administration could result in serious and/or life-threatening drug interactions).

No products indexed under this heading.

Atorvastatin Calcium (Increased atorvastatin plasma concentrations). Products include:

Caduet Tablets 2507

Lipitor Tablets 2495

Bepridil Hydrochloride (Increases bepridil plasma concentrations; increased bepridil exposure may be associated with life-threatening reactions, such as cardiac arrhythmias).

No products indexed under this heading.

Carbamazepine (Decreases amprenavir plasma concentrations potentially reducing effectiveness of amprenavir). Products include:

Carbatrol Capsules 3174

Equetro Extended-Release Capsules 3178

Tegretol/Tegretol-XR 2278

Chlorpropamide (New onset diabetes mellitus, exacerbation of pre-existing diabetes mellitus, and hyperglycemia have been reported in HIV-infected patients receiving protease inhibitors; some patients may require dose adjustments).

No products indexed under this heading.

Cisapride (Co-administration of amprenavir is contraindicated with drugs that are highly dependant of CYP3A4 for clearance and for which elevated plasma concentrations are associated with serious and/or life-threatening events).

No products indexed under this heading.

Clarithromycin (Co-administration has resulted in 15% increase in Cmax, 18% increase in AUC, and 39% increase in Cmin of amprenavir; 10% decrease in clarithromycin Cmax was reported). Products include:

Biaxin/Biaxin XL 402

PREVPAC 3281

Clomipramine Hydrochloride (Co-administration could result in serious and/or life-threatening drug interactions).

No products indexed under this heading.

Clorazepate Dipotassium (Increased benzodiazepine plasma concentrations; clinical significance is unknown; however, a decrease in benzodiazepine dose may be needed). Products include:

Tranxene 2488

Clozapine (May result in increased plasma concentrations of clozapine). Products include:

Clozapine Tablets 2141

Clozaril Tablets 2174

FazaClo Orally Disintegrating Tablets 547

Cyclosporine (Increased immunosuppressant plasma concentrations). Products include:

Gengraf Capsules 458

Neoral Soft Gelatin Capsules 2247

Neoral Oral Solution 2247

Restasis Ophthalmic Emulsion 570

Sandimmune 2259

Dapsone (Co-administration with dapsone may result in increased plasma concentrations of dapsone). Products include:

Dapsone Tablets USP 1656

Delavirdine Mesylate (Co-administration may lead to loss of virologic response and possible resistance to delavirdine. Co-administration has resulted in a 40% increase in Cmax, 130% increase in AUC, and 125% increase in Cmin of amprenavir. A 47% decrease in delavirdine Cmax, 61% decrease in delavirdine AUC, and 88% decrease in delavirdine Cmin). Products include:

Rescriptor Tablets 2535

Desogestrel (May lead to loss of virologic response and possible resistance to amprenavir; alternative methods of non-hormonal contraception are recommended). Products include:

Ortho-Cept Tablets 2395

Dexamethasone (Decreases amprenavir plasma concentrations potentially reducing effectiveness of amprenavir). Products include:

Ciprodex Otic Suspension 555

Decadron Tablets 1929

TobraDex Ophthalmic Ointment 558

TobraDex Ophthalmic Suspension 558

Dexamethasone Acetate (Decreases amprenavir plasma concentrations potentially reducing effectiveness of amprenavir).

No products indexed under this heading.

Dexamethasone Sodium Phosphate (Decreases amprenavir plasma concentrations potentially reducing effectiveness of amprenavir). Products include:

Decadron Phosphate Injection 1931

Diazepam (Increased benzodiazepine plasma concentrations; clinical significance is unknown; however, a decrease in benzodiazepine dose may be needed). Products include:

Diastat Rectal Delivery System 3344

Valium Tablets 2822

Didanosine (Didanosine secondary to the antacid content has not been specifically studied; however, based upon data with other protease inhibitors, it is advisable that antacids not be taken at the same time as amprenavir because of potential interference with absorption; it is recommended that their administration be separated by at least an hour).

No products indexed under this heading.

Dihydroergotamine Mesylate (Co-administration of amprenavir is contraindicated with drugs that are highly dependant of CYP3A4, such as ergot derivatives, for clearance and for which elevated plasma concentrations are associated with serious and/or life-threatening events, such as acute ergot toxicity characterized by peripheral vasospasm and ischemia of the extremities and other tissues). Products include:

Migranal Nasal Spray 3350

Diltiazem Hydrochloride (Increased calcium channel blockers plasma concentrations). Products include:

Cardizem LA Extended Release Tablets 1699

Tiazac Capsules 1204

Disulfiram (Agenerase Oral Solution contains a large amount of propylene glycol and because of the potential risk of toxicity from the large amount of this excipient; co-administration with disulfiram is contraindicated). Products include:

Antabuse Tablets 2343

Ergonovine Maleate (Co-administration of amprenavir is contraindicated with drugs that are highly dependant of CYP3A4, such as ergot derivatives, for clearance and for which elevated plasma concentrations are associated with serious and/or life-threatening events, such as acute ergot toxicity characterized by peripheral vasospasm and ischemia of the extremities and other tissues).

No products indexed under this heading.

Ergotamine Tartrate (Co-administration of amprenavir is contraindicated with drugs that are highly dependant of CYP3A4, such as ergot derivatives, for clearance and for which elevated plasma concentrations are associated with serious and/or life-threatening events, such as acute ergot toxicity characterized by peripheral vasospasm and ischemia of the extremities and other tissues).
No products indexed under this heading.

Ethinyl Estradiol (Co-administration has resulted in a 22% decrease in AUC and 20% decrease in Cmin of amprenavir. Ethinyl estradiol Cmin also increased 32%). Products include:
- Alesse-28 Tablets 3392
- Lo/Ovral-28 Tablets 3423
- NuvaRing 2357
- Ortho-Cept Tablets 2395
- Ortho-Cyclen/Ortho Tri-Cyclen 2414
- Ortho Evra Transdermal System 2402
- Ortho Tri-Cyclen Lo Tablets 2421
- Seasonale Tablets 1073
- Triphasil-28 Tablets 3483
- Yasmin 28 Tablets 818

Ethynodiol Diacetate (May lead to loss of virologic response and possible resistance to amprenavir; alternative methods of non-hormonal contraception are recommended).
No products indexed under this heading.

Felodipine (Increased calcium channel blockers plasma concentrations). Products include:
- Plendil Extended-Release Tablets 651

Flecainide Acetate (If amprenavir is co-administered with ritonavir capsules, concurrent use of flecainide is contraindicated). Products include:
- Tambocor Tablets 1824

Flurazepam Hydrochloride (Increased benzodiazepine plasma concentrations; clinical significance is unknown; however, a decrease in benzodiazepine dose may be needed). Products include:
- Dalmane Capsules 3343

Fluticasone Propionate (Concurrent use will result in significantly decreased serum cortisol concentrations). Products include:
- Advair Diskus 100/50 1291
- Advair Diskus 250/50 1291
- Advair Diskus 500/50 1291
- Cutivate Cream 1381
- Cutivate Lotion 0.05% 1383
- Cutivate Ointment 1384
- Flonase Nasal Spray 1412
- Flovent Diskus 100 mcg 1418
- Flovent Diskus 50 mcg 1415

Fosphenytoin Sodium (Decreases amprenavir plasma concentrations potentially reducing effectiveness of amprenavir).
No products indexed under this heading.

Glimepiride (New onset diabetes mellitus, exacerbation of pre-existing diabetes mellitus, and hyperglycemia have been reported in HIV-infected patients receiving protease inhibitors; some patients may require dose adjustments). Products include:
- Amaryl Tablets 2864

Glipizide (New onset diabetes mellitus, exacerbation of pre-existing diabetes mellitus, and hyperglycemia have been reported in HIV-infected patients receiving protease inhibitors; some patients may require dose adjustments).
No products indexed under this heading.

Glyburide (New onset diabetes mellitus, exacerbation of pre-existing diabetes mellitus, and hyperglycemia have been reported in HIV-infected patients receiving protease inhibitors; some patients may require dose adjustments).
No products indexed under this heading.

Hypericum (Co-administration of amprenavir and St. John's Wort or products containing St. John's Wort is expected to substantially decrease protease inhibitor concentrations and may result in suboptimal levels of amprenavir and lead to loss of virologic response and possible resistance to amprenavir; concurrent use is not recommended).
No products indexed under this heading.

Imipramine Hydrochloride (Increase in tricyclic antidepressant plasma concentrations).
No products indexed under this heading.

Imipramine Pamoate (Increase in tricyclic antidepressant plasma concentrations).
No products indexed under this heading.

Indinavir Sulfate (Increases amprenavir plasma concentrations). Products include:
- Crixivan Capsules 1918

Insulin, Human, Zinc Suspension (New onset diabetes mellitus, exacerbation of pre-existing diabetes mellitus, and hyperglycemia have been reported in HIV-infected patients receiving protease inhibitors; some patients may require dose adjustments). Products include:
- Humulin L, 100 Units 1763
- Humulin U, 100 Units 1770

Insulin, Human NPH (New onset diabetes mellitus, exacerbation of pre-existing diabetes mellitus, and hyperglycemia have been reported in HIV-infected patients receiving protease inhibitors; some patients may require dose adjustments). Products include:
- Humulin N, 100 Units 1764
- Humulin N Pen 1765
- Novolin N Human Insulin 10 ml Vials 2322
- Novolin N InnoLet 2322
- Novolin N PenFill 3 ml Cartridges 2325
- Novolin R InnoLet 2322

Insulin, Human Regular (New onset diabetes mellitus, exacerbation of pre-existing diabetes mellitus, and hyperglycemia have been reported in HIV-infected patients receiving protease inhibitors; some patients may require dose adjustments). Products include:
- Humulin R (U-500) 1768
- Humulin R, 100 Units 1767
- Novolin R Human Insulin 10 ml Vials 2322
- Novolin R PenFill 2325

Insulin, Human Regular and Human NPH Mixture (New onset diabetes mellitus, exacerbation of pre-existing diabetes mellitus, and hyperglycemia have been reported in HIV-infected patients receiving protease inhibitors; some patients may require dose adjustments). Products include:
- Humulin 50/50, 100 Units 1760
- Humulin 70/30 Pen 1761
- Novolin 70/30 Human Insulin 10 ml Vials 2321
- Novolin 70/30 InnoLet 2322
- Novolin 70/30 PenFill 3 ml Cartridges 2325

Insulin, NPH (New onset diabetes mellitus, exacerbation of pre-existing diabetes mellitus, and hyperglycemia have been reported in HIV-infected patients receiving protease inhibitors; some patients may require dose adjustments).
No products indexed under this heading.

Insulin, Regular (New onset diabetes mellitus, exacerbation of pre-existing diabetes mellitus, and hyperglycemia have been reported in HIV-infected patients receiving protease inhibitors; some patients may require dose adjustments).
No products indexed under this heading.

Insulin, Zinc Crystals (New onset diabetes mellitus, exacerbation of pre-existing diabetes mellitus, and hyperglycemia have been reported in HIV-infected patients receiving protease inhibitors; some patients may require dose adjustments).
No products indexed under this heading.

Insulin, Zinc Suspension (New onset diabetes mellitus, exacerbation of pre-existing diabetes mellitus, and hyperglycemia have been reported in HIV-infected patients receiving protease inhibitors; some patients may require dose adjustments).
No products indexed under this heading.

Insulin Aspart, Human Regular (New onset diabetes mellitus, exacerbation of pre-existing diabetes mellitus, and hyperglycemia have been reported in HIV-infected patients receiving protease inhibitors; some patients may require dose adjustments). Products include:
- NovoLog Injection 2326

Insulin glargine (New onset diabetes mellitus, exacerbation of pre-existing diabetes mellitus, and hyperglycemia have been reported in HIV-infected patients receiving protease inhibitors; some patients may require dose adjustments). Products include:
- Lantus Injection 2925

Insulin Lispro, Human (New onset diabetes mellitus, exacerbation of pre-existing diabetes mellitus, and hyperglycemia have been reported in HIV-infected patients receiving protease inhibitors; some patients may require dose adjustments). Products include:
- Humalog-Pen 1751
- Humalog Mix 75/25-Pen 1754

Insulin Lispro Protamine, Human (New onset diabetes mellitus, exacerbation of pre-existing diabetes mellitus, and hyperglycemia have been reported in HIV-infected patients receiving protease inhibitors; some patients may require dose adjustments). Products include:
- Humalog Mix 75/25-Pen 1754

Isradipine (Increased calcium channel blockers plasma concentrations). Products include:
- DynaCirc CR Tablets 2726

Itraconazole (Increased itraconazole plasma concentrations; dose reduction of itraconazole may be needed for patients receiving more than 400 mg itraconazole per day).
No products indexed under this heading.

Ketoconazole (Increased ketoconazole plasma concentrations; dose reduction of ketoconazole may be needed for patients receiving more than 400 mg ketoconazole per day). Products include:
- Nizoral A-D Shampoo, 1% 1839
- Nizoral 2% Shampoo 1838

Levonorgestrel (May lead to loss of virologic response and possible resistance to amprenavir; alternative methods of non-hormonal contraception are recommended). Products include:
- Alesse-28 Tablets 3392
- Climara Pro Transdermal System 800
- Mirena Intrauterine System 810
- Plan B Tablets 1068
- Seasonale Tablets 1073
- Triphasil-28 Tablets 3483

Lidocaine Hydrochloride (Increases antiarrhythmics plasma concentrations).
No products indexed under this heading.

Lopinavir (Increases amprenavir plasma concentrations). Products include:
- Kaletra 474

Loratadine (May result in increased plasma concentrations of loratadine). Products include:
- Alavert Allergy & Sinus D-12 Hour Tablets .... ▣743
- Alavert .... ▣743
- Children's Claritin 24 Hour Non-Drowsy Allergy Syrup .... ▣732
- Claritin Non-Drowsy 24 Hour Tablets .... ▣731
- Non-Drowsy Claritin Hives Relief Tablets .... ▣733
- Claritin Reditabs 24 Hour Non-Drowsy Tablets .... ▣732
- Claritin-D Non-Drowsy 12 Hour Tablets .... ▣731
- Claritin-D Non-Drowsy 24 Hour Tablets .... ▣731
- Children's Dimetapp ND Non-Drowsy Allergy Syrup .... ▣746
- Triaminic Allerchews .... ▣684

Lovastatin (Co-administration increases the serum concentrations of lovastatin resulting in increased activity as well as toxicity, such as myopathy and rhabdomyolysis; concurrent use is not recommended). Products include:
- Advicor Tablets 1694
- Altoprev Extended-Release Tablets 1151
- Mevacor Tablets 1996

Magaldrate (Antacids decrease amprenavir plasma concentrations; Agenerase should be taken at least one hour before or after antacids).
No products indexed under this heading.

Magnesium Hydroxide (Antacids decrease amprenavir plasma concentrations; Agenerase should be taken at least one hour before or after antacids). Products include:
- Maalox Max Maximum Strength Antacid/Anti-Gas Liquid 2165
- Maalox Regular Strength Antacid/Antigas Liquid 2164
- Pepcid Complete Chewable Tablets 1672
- Rolaids Tablets .... ▣707
- Extra Strength Rolaids Tablets .... ▣707
- Rolaids Multi-Symptom Antacid & Antigas Tablets .... ▣708

Magnesium Oxide (Antacids decrease amprenavir plasma concentrations; Agenerase should be taken at least one hour before or after antacids). Products include:
Beelith Tablets 784
PremCal Light, Regular, and Extra Strength Tablets 762

Mestranol (May lead to loss of virologic response and possible resistance to amprenavir; alternative methods of non-hormonal contraception are recommended).
No products indexed under this heading.

Metformin Hydrochloride (New onset diabetes mellitus, exacerbation of pre-existing diabetes mellitus, and hyperglycemia have been reported in HIV-infected patients receiving protease inhibitors; some patients may require dose adjustments). Products include:
ActoPlus Met Tablets 3219
Avandamet Tablets 1343
Fortamet Extended-Release Tablets 1156

Methadone Hydrochloride (Co-administration of amprenavir and methadone can decrease plasma levels of methadone. Co-administration of amprenavir and methadone as compared to a non-matched historical control group resulted in a 30%, 27% and 25% decrease in serum amprenavir AUC, Cmax and Cmin, respectively. Alternative antiretroviral therapy should be considered).
No products indexed under this heading.

Methylergonovine Maleate (Co-administration of amprenavir is contraindicated with drugs that are highly dependant of CYP3A4, such as ergot derivatives, for clearance and for which elevated plasma concentrations are associated with serious and/or life-threatening events, such as acute ergot toxicity characterized by peripheral vasospasm and ischemia of the extremities and other tissues).
No products indexed under this heading.

Methysergide Maleate (Co-administration of amprenavir is contraindicated with drugs that are highly dependant of CYP3A4, such as ergot derivatives, for clearance and for which elevated plasma concentrations are associated with serious and/or life-threatening events, such as acute ergot toxicity characterized by peripheral vasospasm and ischemia of the extremities and other tissues).
No products indexed under this heading.

Metronidazole (Agenerase Oral Solution contains a large amount of propylene glycol and because of the potential risk of toxicity from the large amount of this excipient; co-administration with metronidazole is contraindicated). Products include:
Metrogel 1% 1212
MetroGel-Vaginal Gel 1822
Noritate Cream, 1% 1051

Metronidazole Hydrochloride (Agenerase Oral Solution contains a large amount of propylene glycol and because of the potential risk of toxicity from the large amount of this excipient; co-administration with metronidazole is contraindicated).
No products indexed under this heading.

Mibefradil Dihydrochloride (Increased calcium channel blockers plasma concentrations).
No products indexed under this heading.

Midazolam Hydrochloride (Co-administration of amprenavir is contraindicated with drugs that are highly dependant of CYP3A4 for clearance and for which elevated plasma concentrations are associated with serious and/or life-threatening events, such as prolonged or increased sedation or respiratory depression).
No products indexed under this heading.

Miglitol (New onset diabetes mellitus, exacerbation of pre-existing diabetes mellitus, and hyperglycemia have been reported in HIV-infected patients receiving protease inhibitors; some patients may require dose adjustments).
No products indexed under this heading.

Nelfinavir Mesylate (Increases amprenavir plasma concentrations). Products include:
Viracept 2556

Nicardipine Hydrochloride (Increased calcium channel blockers plasma concentrations). Products include:
Cardene I.V. 1129

Nifedipine (Increased calcium channel blockers plasma concentrations). Products include:
Adalat CC Tablets 2978

Nimodipine (Increased calcium channel blockers plasma concentrations). Products include:
Nimotop Capsules 774

Nisoldipine (Increased calcium channel blockers plasma concentrations). Products include:
Sular Tablets 1163

Norethindrone (Co-administration has resulted in a 22% decrease in AUC and 20% decrease in Cmin of amprenavir. Norethindrone AUC and Cmin increased 18% and 45%, respectively). Products include:
Ortho Micronor Tablets 2411

Norethynodrel (May lead to loss of virologic response and possible resistance to amprenavir; alternative methods of non-hormonal contraception are recommended).
No products indexed under this heading.

Norgestimate (May lead to loss of virologic response and possible resistance to amprenavir; alternative methods of non-hormonal contraception are recommended). Products include:
Ortho-Cyclen/Ortho Tri-Cyclen 2414
Ortho Tri-Cyclen Lo Tablets 2421
Prefest Tablets 1069

Norgestrel (May lead to loss of virologic response and possible resistance to amprenavir; alternative methods of non-hormonal contraception are recommended). Products include:
Lo/Ovral-28 Tablets 3423

Phenobarbital (Decreases amprenavir plasma concentrations potentially reducing effectiveness of amprenavir).
No products indexed under this heading.

Phenytoin (Decreases amprenavir plasma concentrations potentially reducing effectiveness of amprenavir).
No products indexed under this heading.

Phenytoin Sodium (Decreases amprenavir plasma concentrations potentially reducing effectiveness of amprenavir). Products include:
Phenytek Capsules 2153

Pimozide (Co-administration of amprenavir is contraindicated with drugs that are highly dependant of CYP3A4 for clearance and for which elevated plasma concentrations are associated with serious and/or life-threatening events, such as cardiac arrhythmias). Products include:
Orap Tablets 1220

Pioglitazone Hydrochloride (New onset diabetes mellitus, exacerbation of pre-existing diabetes mellitus, and hyperglycemia have been reported in HIV-infected patients receiving protease inhibitors; some patients may require dose adjustments). Products include:
ActoPlus Met Tablets 3219
Actos Tablets 3224

Pravastatin Sodium (Co-administration increases the serum concentrations of pravastatin resulting in increased activity as well as toxicity, such as myopathy and rhabdomyolysis; caution should be exercised if used concurrently). Products include:
Pravachol Tablets 943

Propafenone Hydrochloride (If amprenavir is co-administered with ritonavir capsules; concurrent use of propafenone is contraindicated). Products include:
Rythmol SR Capsules 2736

Protriptyline Hydrochloride (Co-administration could result in serious and/or life-threatening drug interactions). Products include:
Vivactil Tablets 2350

Quinidine (Increases quinidine plasma concentrations; caution is warranted and therapeutic monitoring is recommended).
No products indexed under this heading.

Quinidine Gluconate (Increases quinidine plasma concentrations; caution is warranted and therapeutic monitoring is recommended).
No products indexed under this heading.

Quinidine Hydrochloride (Increases quinidine plasma concentrations; caution is warranted and therapeutic monitoring is recommended).
No products indexed under this heading.

Quinidine Polygalacturonate (Increases quinidine plasma concentrations; caution is warranted and therapeutic monitoring is recommended).
No products indexed under this heading.

Quinidine Sulfate (Increases quinidine plasma concentrations; caution is warranted and therapeutic monitoring is recommended).
No products indexed under this heading.

Rapamycin (Increased immunosuppressant plasma concentrations).
No products indexed under this heading.

Repaglinide (New onset diabetes mellitus, exacerbation of pre-existing diabetes mellitus, and hyperglycemia have been reported in HIV-infected patients receiving protease inhibitors; some patients may require dose adjustments). Products include:
Prandin Tablets (0.5, 1, and 2 mg) 2337

Rifabutin (Increased rifabutin and rifabutin metabolite plasma concentrations; dosage reduction of rifabutin to at least half the recommended dose is required when used concurrently).
No products indexed under this heading.

Rifampin (Co-administration may lead to loss of virologic response and possible resistance to amprenavir or the class of protease inhibitors).
No products indexed under this heading.

Ritonavir (Concurrent use of Agenerase Oral Solution and Norvir Oral Solution is not recommended because the large amount of propylene glycol in Agenerase Oral Solution and ethanol in Norvir Oral Solution may compete for the same metabolic pathway for elimination; concurrent use has been associated with elevation of ALT and AST as well as cholesterol and triglycerides). Products include:
Kaletra 474
Norvir 499

Rosiglitazone Maleate (New onset diabetes mellitus, exacerbation of pre-existing diabetes mellitus, and hyperglycemia have been reported in HIV-infected patients receiving protease inhibitors; some patients may require dose adjustments). Products include:
Avandamet Tablets 1343
Avandia Tablets 1348

Saquinavir (Decreases amprenavir plasma concentrations).
No products indexed under this heading.

Saquinavir Mesylate (Decreases amprenavir plasma concentrations). Products include:
Invirase 2776

Sildenafil Citrate (Increase in sildenafil plasma concentrations; use with caution at reduced doses of 25 mg every 48 hours with increased monitoring for adverse events). Products include:
Revatio Tablets 2541
Viagra Tablets 2552

Simvastatin (Co-administration increases the serum concentrations of simvastatin resulting in increased activity as well as toxicity, such as myopathy and rhabdomyolysis; concurrent use is not recommended). Products include:
Vytorin 10/10 Tablets 2084
Vytorin 10/10 Tablets 3092
Vytorin 10/20 Tablets 2084
Vytorin 10/20 Tablets 3092
Vytorin 10/40 Tablets 3092
Vytorin 10/40 Tablets 2084
Vytorin 10/80 Tablets 2084
Vytorin 10/80 Tablets 3092
Zocor Tablets 2078

Tacrolimus (Increased immunosuppressant plasma concentrations). Products include:
Prograf Capsules and Injection 624
Protopic Ointment 629

IMPORTANT NOTE: Always consult each drug listing in the patient's regimen for possible interactions.

Tolazamide (New onset diabetes mellitus, exacerbation of pre-existing diabetes mellitus, and hyperglycemia have been reported in HIV-infected patients receiving protease inhibitors; some patients may require dose adjustments).
No products indexed under this heading.

Tolbutamide (New onset diabetes mellitus, exacerbation of pre-existing diabetes mellitus, and hyperglycemia have been reported in HIV-infected patients receiving protease inhibitors; some patients may require dose adjustments).
No products indexed under this heading.

Trazodone Hydrochloride (Concomitant use may increase plasma concentrations of trazodone).
No products indexed under this heading.

Triazolam (Co-administration of amprenavir is contraindicated with drugs that are highly dependant of CYP3A4 for clearance and for which elevated plasma concentrations are associated with serious and/or life-threatening events, such as prolonged or increased sedation or respiratory depression).
No products indexed under this heading.

Trimipramine Maleate (Co-administration could result in serious and/or life-threatening drug interactions). Products include:
Surmontil Capsules 2347

Troglitazone (New onset diabetes mellitus, exacerbation of pre-existing diabetes mellitus, and hyperglycemia have been reported in HIV-infected patients receiving protease inhibitors; some patients may require dose adjustments).
No products indexed under this heading.

Verapamil Hydrochloride (Increased calcium channel blockers plasma concentrations). Products include:
Covera-HS Tablets 3135
Tarka Tablets 519
Verelan PM Capsules 3120

Vitamin E (Amprenavir formulations contain large amounts of vitamin E; high vitamin E doses may exacerbate the blood coagulation defect of vitamin K deficiency caused by anticoagulant therapy; concurrent use with additional vitamin E should be avoided). Products include:
MarineOmega Softgel Capsules 2669
Unique E Vitamin E Concentrate Capsules .... ▣602

Warfarin Sodium (Concentrations of warfarin may be affected with concurrent use; monitor INR). Products include:
Coumadin for Injection 932
Coumadin Tablets 932

Zidovudine (Co-administration has resulted in 13% increase in AUC of amprenavir; 40% increase in Cmax and 31% increase in AUC for zidovudine have been reported). Products include:
Combivir Tablets 1373
Retrovir 1533
Retrovir IV Infusion 1537
Trizivir Tablets 1565

Food Interactions

Alcohol (Concurrent use of Agenerase Oral Solution with alcoholic beverages is not recommended).

Food, unspecified (High-fat meals may decrease the absorption of Agenerase and should be avoided; Agenerase may be taken with meals of normal fat content).

AGGRASTAT INJECTION

(Tirofiban Hydrochloride) 1878
May interact with glycoprotein (GP) IIb/IIIa inhibitors and certain other agents. Compounds in these categories include:

Abciximab (Concomitant use with another parenteral GP IIb/IIIa inhibitor is contraindicated). Products include:
ReoPro Vials 1779

Aspirin (The use of tirofiban in combination with aspirin has been associated with an increase in bleeding compared to aspirin alone). Products include:
Aggrenox Capsules 855
Bayer, Aspirin Regimen .... ▣606
Bayer Aspirin Tablets 3515
BC Powder .... ▣612
BC Allergy Sinus Cold Powder .... ▣612
Arthritis Strength BC Powder .... ▣612
BC Sinus Cold Powder .... ▣612
Ecotrin Enteric Coated Aspirin Low, Regular and Maximum Strength Tablets 1627
Goody's Body Pain Formula Powder .... ▣621
Goody's Extra Strength Headache Powder .... ▣621
Goody's Extra Strength Pain Relief Tablets .... ▣621
Percodan Tablets 1115
St. Joseph 81 mg Aspirin Chewable and Enteric Coated Tablets 1841

Eptifibatide (Concomitant use with another parenteral GP IIb/IIIa inhibitor is contraindicated). Products include:
Integrilin Injection 3034

Heparin Sodium (The use of tirofiban in combination with heparin has been associated with an increase in bleeding compared to heparin alone).
No products indexed under this heading.

Levothyroxine Sodium (Co-administration has resulted in a higher rate of clearance of tirofiban; the clinical significance of this is unknown). Products include:
Levothroid Tablets 1189
Levoxyl Tablets 1680
Synthroid Tablets 515
Unithroid Tablets 3521

Omeprazole (Co-administration has resulted in a higher rate of clearance of tirofiban; the clinical significance of this is unknown). Products include:
Zegerid Powder for Oral Solution 2972

AGGRASTAT INJECTION PREMIXED

(Tirofiban Hydrochloride) 1878
See Aggrastat Injection

AGGRENOX CAPSULES

(Aspirin, Dipyridamole) 855
May interact with ACE inhibitors, anticholinesterase drugs, beta blockers, anticoagulants, diuretics, oral hypoglycemic agents, non-steroidal anti-inflammatory agents, phenytoin, valproate, and certain other agents. Compounds in these categories include:

Acarbose (Moderate doses of aspirin may increase the effectiveness of renal hypoglycemic drugs, leading to hypoglycemia). Products include:
Precose Tablets 776

Acebutolol Hydrochloride (The hypertensive effects of beta-blockers may be diminished by the concomitant administration of aspirin due to inhibition of renal prostaglandins, leading to decreased renal blood flow and salt and fluid retention).
No products indexed under this heading.

Acetazolamide (Co-administration can lead to high serum concentrations of acetazolamide (and toxicity) due to competition at the renal tube for secretion).
No products indexed under this heading.

Acetazolamide Sodium (Co-administration can lead to high serum concentrations of acetazolamide (and toxicity) due to competition at the renal tube for secretion).
No products indexed under this heading.

Adenosine (Dipyridamole has been reported to increase the plasma levels and cardiovascular effects of adenosine). Products include:
Adenocard Injection 612
Adenoscan 613

Amiloride Hydrochloride (The effectiveness of diuretics in patients with underlying renal or cardiovascular disease may be diminished by co-administration of aspirin due to inhibition of renal prostaglandins, leading to decreased renal blood flow and salt and fluid retention). Products include:
Midamor Tablets 2000
Moduretic Tablets 2003

Anisindione (Patients on anticoagulation therapy are at risk for bleeding). Products include:
Miradon Tablets 3056

Ardeparin Sodium (Patients on anticoagulation therapy are at risk for bleeding).
No products indexed under this heading.

Atenolol (The hypertensive effects of beta-blockers may be diminished by the concomitant administration of aspirin due to inhibition of renal prostaglandins, leading to decreased renal blood flow and salt and fluid retention). Products include:
Tenormin I.V. Injection 698
Tenormin Tablets 695

Benazepril Hydrochloride (Co-administration can result in diminished hypotensive and hyponatremic effects of ACE inhibitors due to the effect of aspirin on the renin-angiotensin conversion pathway). Products include:
Lotensin Tablets 2232
Lotensin HCT Tablets 2235
Lotrel Capsules 2238

Bendroflumethiazide (The effectiveness of diuretics in patients with underlying renal or cardiovascular disease may be diminished by co-administration of aspirin due to inhibition of renal prostaglandins, leading to decreased renal blood flow and salt and fluid retention).
No products indexed under this heading.

Betaxolol Hydrochloride (The hypertensive effects of beta-blockers may be diminished by the concomitant administration of aspirin due to inhibition of renal prostaglandins, leading to decreased renal blood flow and salt and fluid retention). Products include:
Betoptic S Ophthalmic Suspension 554

Bisoprolol Fumarate (The hypertensive effects of beta-blockers may be diminished by the concomitant administration of aspirin due to inhibition of renal prostaglandins, leading to decreased renal blood flow and salt and fluid retention).
No products indexed under this heading.

Bumetanide (The effectiveness of diuretics in patients with underlying renal or cardiovascular disease may be diminished by co-administration of aspirin due to inhibition of renal prostaglandins, leading to decreased renal blood flow and salt and fluid retention).
No products indexed under this heading.

Captopril (Co-administration can result in diminished hypotensive and hyponatremic effects of ACE inhibitors due to the effect of aspirin on the renin-angiotensin conversion pathway). Products include:
Captopril Tablets 2114

Carteolol Hydrochloride (The hypertensive effects of beta-blockers may be diminished by the concomitant administration of aspirin due to inhibition of renal prostaglandins, leading to decreased renal blood flow and salt and fluid retention). Products include:
Carteolol Hydrochloride Ophthalmic Solution USP, 1% .... ⊙246

Celecoxib (Co-administration of non-steroidal anti-inflammatory drugs with aspirin may increase bleeding or lead to decreased renal function). Products include:
Celebrex Capsules 3130

Chlorothiazide (The effectiveness of diuretics in patients with underlying renal or cardiovascular disease may be diminished by co-administration of aspirin due to inhibition of renal prostaglandins, leading to decreased renal blood flow and salt and fluid retention). Products include:
Aldoclor Tablets 1881
Diuril Oral 1936

Chlorothiazide Sodium (The effectiveness of diuretics in patients with underlying renal or cardiovascular disease may be diminished by co-administration of aspirin due to inhibition of renal prostaglandins, leading to decreased renal blood flow and salt and fluid retention). Products include:
Diuril Sodium Intravenous 1934

Chlorpropamide (Moderate doses of aspirin may increase the effectiveness of renal hypoglycemic drugs, leading to hypoglycemia).
No products indexed under this heading.

Chlorthalidone (The effectiveness of diuretics in patients with underlying renal or cardiovascular disease may be diminished by co-administration of aspirin due to inhibition of renal prostaglandins, leading to decreased renal blood flow and salt and fluid retention). Products include:
Clorpres Tablets 2139

Dalteparin Sodium (Patients on anticoagulation therapy are at risk for bleeding). Products include:

Fragmin Injection 2638

Danaparoid Sodium (Patients on anticoagulation therapy are at risk for bleeding).
No products indexed under this heading.

Diclofenac Potassium (Co-administration of non-steroidal anti-inflammatory drugs with aspirin may increase bleeding or lead to decreased renal function). Products include:
Cataflam Tablets 2173

Diclofenac Sodium (Co-administration of non-steroidal anti-inflammatory drugs with aspirin may increase bleeding or lead to decreased renal function). Products include:
Arthrotec Tablets 3126
Voltaren Ophthalmic Solution 2300
Voltaren Tablets 2298
Voltaren-XR Tablets 2301

Dicumarol (Patients on anticoagulation therapy are at risk for bleeding).
No products indexed under this heading.

Divalproex Sodium (Salicylic acid can displace protein-bound valproic acid leading to an increase in serum valproic acid levels). Products include:
Depakote Sprinkle Capsules 422
Depakote Tablets 427
Depakote ER Tablets 433

Donepezil Hydrochloride (Dipyridamole may counteract the anticholinesterase effect of cholinesterase inhibitors, thereby potentially aggravating myasthenia gravis). Products include:
Aricept Tablets 1086
Aricept ODT Tablets 1086

Enalapril Maleate (Co-administration can result in diminished hypotensive and hyponatremic effects of ACE inhibitors due to the effect of aspirin on the renin angiotensin conversion pathway). Products include:
Vaseretic Tablets 2073
Vasotec I.V. Injection 2076

Enalaprilat (Co-administration can result in diminished hypotensive and hyponatremic effects of ACE inhibitors due to the effect of aspirin on the renin-angiotensin conversion pathway).
No products indexed under this heading.

Enoxaparin Sodium (Patients on anticoagulation therapy are at risk for bleeding). Products include:
Lovenox Injection 2931

Esmolol Hydrochloride (The hypertensive effects of beta-blockers may be diminished by the concomitant administration of aspirin due to inhibition of renal prostaglandins, leading to decreased renal blood flow and salt and fluid retention). Products include:
Brevibloc Concentrate 766
Brevibloc Injection 766
Brevibloc Double Strength Injection............................ 766
Brevibloc Premixed Injection 766
Brevibloc Double Strength Premixed Injection 766

Ethacrynic Acid (The effectiveness of diuretics in patients with underlying renal or cardiovascular disease may be diminished by co-administration of aspirin due to inhibition of renal prostaglandins, leading to decreased renal blood flow and salt and fluid retention). Products include:
Edecrin Tablets 1941

Etodolac (Co-administration of non-steroidal anti-inflammatory drugs with aspirin may increase bleeding or lead to decreased renal function).
No products indexed under this heading.

Fenoprofen Calcium (Co-administration of non-steroidal anti-inflammatory drugs with aspirin may increase bleeding or lead to decreased renal function). Products include:
Nalfon Capsules 2504

Flurbiprofen (Co-administration of non-steroidal anti-inflammatory drugs with aspirin may increase bleeding or lead to decreased renal function).
No products indexed under this heading.

Fondaparinux Sodium (Patients on anticoagulation therapy are at risk for bleeding). Products include:
Arixtra Injection 1325

Fosinopril Sodium (Co-administration can result in diminished hypotensive and hyponatremic effects of ACE inhibitors due to the effect of aspirin on the renin-angiotensin conversion pathway).
No products indexed under this heading.

Fosphenytoin Sodium (Salicylic acid can displace protein-bound phenytoin leading to a decrease in the total concentration of phenytoin).
No products indexed under this heading.

Furosemide (The effectiveness of diuretics in patients with underlying renal or cardiovascular disease may be diminished by co-administration of aspirin due to inhibition of renal prostaglandins, leading to decreased renal blood flow and salt and fluid retention). Products include:
Furosemide Tablets 2117

Galantamine Hydrobromide (Dipyridamole may counteract the anticholinesterase effect of cholinesterase inhibitors, thereby potentially aggravating myasthenia gravis). Products include:
Razadyne ER Extended-Release Capsules 2434
Razadyne 2434

Glimepiride (Moderate doses of aspirin may increase the effectiveness of renal hypoglycemic drugs, leading to hypoglycemia). Products include:
Amaryl Tablets 2864

Glipizide (Moderate doses of aspirin may increase the effectiveness of renal hypoglycemic drugs, leading to hypoglycemia).
No products indexed under this heading.

Glyburide (Moderate doses of aspirin may increase the effectiveness of renal hypoglycemic drugs, leading to hypoglycemia).
No products indexed under this heading.

Heparin Calcium (Patients on anticoagulation therapy are at risk for bleeding).
No products indexed under this heading.

Heparin Sodium (Aspirin can increase the anticoagulant activity of heparin, increasing bleeding risk).
No products indexed under this heading.

Hydrochlorothiazide (The effectiveness of diuretics in patients with underlying renal or cardiovascular disease may be diminished by co-administration of aspirin due to inhibition of renal prostaglandins, leading to decreased renal blood flow and salt and fluid retention). Products include:
Aldoril Tablets 1884
Atacand HCT 637
Avalide Tablets 2889
Avalide Tablets 922
Benicar HCT Tablets 2852
Diovan HCT Tablets 2195
Dyazide Capsules 1389
Hyzaar 1964
Lotensin HCT Tablets 2235
Maxzide 2150
Micardis HCT Tablets 886
Moduretic Tablets 2003
Prinzide Tablets 2033
Teveten HCT Tablets 1710
Timolide Tablets 2056
Uniretic Tablets 3114
Vaseretic Tablets 2073
Zestoretic Tablets 701

Hydroflumethiazide (The effectiveness of diuretics in patients with underlying renal or cardiovascular disease may be diminished by co-administration of aspirin due to inhibition of renal prostaglandins, leading to decreased renal blood flow and salt and fluid retention).
No products indexed under this heading.

Ibuprofen (Co-administration of non-steroidal anti-inflammatory drugs with aspirin may increase bleeding or lead to decreased renal function). Products include:
Advil Allergy Sinus Caplets .... ▣737
Advil .... ▣737
Children's Advil Suspension .... ▣742
Children's Advil Chewable Tablets .. ▣741
Advil Cold & Sinus .... ▣739
Advil Flu & Body Ache Caplets .... ▣739
Children's Advil Cold Suspension ... ▣741
Infants' Advil Concentrated Drops .. ▣743
Junior Strength Advil Swallow Tablets............................ ▣740
Advil Migraine Liquigels .... ▣740
Advil Multi-Symptom Cold Caplets............................ ▣738
Combunox Tablets 1183
Children's Motrin Oral Suspension and Chewable Tablets............................ 1837
Children's Motrin Cold Non-Staining Dye-Free Oral Suspension 1838
Children's Motrin Cold Oral Suspension 1838
Children's Motrin Non-Staining Dye-Free Oral Suspension............ 1837
Motrin Cold & Sinus Caplets 1836
Motrin IB Tablets and Caplets 1836
Infants' Motrin Concentrated Drops............................ 1837
Infants' Motrin Non-Staining Dye-Free Drops............................ 1837
Junior Strength Motrin Caplets and Chewable Tablets............................ 1837
Vicoprofen Tablets 533

Indapamide (The effectiveness of diuretics in patients with underlying renal or cardiovascular disease may be diminished by co-administration of aspirin due to inhibition of renal prostaglandins, leading to decreased renal blood flow and salt and fluid retention). Products include:
Indapamide Tablets 2119

Indomethacin (Co-administration of non-steroidal anti-inflammatory drugs with aspirin may increase bleeding or lead to decreased renal function). Products include:
Indocin 1968

Indomethacin Sodium Trihydrate (Co-administration of non-steroidal anti-inflammatory drugs with aspirin may increase bleeding or lead to decreased renal function). Products include:
Indocin I.V. 1973

Ketoprofen (Co-administration of non-steroidal anti-inflammatory drugs with aspirin may increase bleeding or lead to decreased renal function).
No products indexed under this heading.

Ketorolac Tromethamine (Co-administration of non-steroidal anti-inflammatory drugs with aspirin may increase bleeding or lead to decreased renal function). Products include:
Acular Ophthalmic Solution 561
Acular LS Ophthalmic Solution 562

Labetalol Hydrochloride (The hypertensive effects of beta-blockers may be diminished by the concomitant administration of aspirin due to inhibition of renal prostaglandins, leading to decreased renal blood flow and salt and fluid retention).
No products indexed under this heading.

Levobunolol Hydrochloride (The hypertensive effects of beta-blockers may be diminished by the concomitant administration of aspirin due to inhibition of renal prostaglandins, leading to decreased renal blood flow and salt and fluid retention). Products include:
Betagan Ophthalmic Solution, USP............................ ⊙217

Lisinopril (Co-administration can result in diminished hypotensive and hyponatremic effects of ACE inhibitors due to the effect of aspirin on the renin-angiotensin conversion pathway). Products include:
Prinivil Tablets 2029
Prinzide Tablets 2033
Zestoretic Tablets 701
Zestril Tablets 704

Low Molecular Weight Heparins (Patients on anticoagulation therapy are at risk for bleeding).
No products indexed under this heading.

Meclofenamate Sodium (Co-administration of non-steroidal anti-inflammatory drugs with aspirin may increase bleeding or lead to decreased renal function).
No products indexed under this heading.

Mefenamic Acid (Co-administration of non-steroidal anti-inflammatory drugs with aspirin may increase bleeding or lead to decreased renal function).
No products indexed under this heading.

Meloxicam (Co-administration of non-steroidal anti-inflammatory drugs with aspirin may increase bleeding or lead to decreased renal function). Products include:
Mobic Oral Suspension 893
Mobic Tablets 893

Metformin Hydrochloride (Moderate doses of aspirin may increase the effectiveness of renal hypoglycemic drugs, leading to hypoglycemia). Products include:
ActoPlus Met Tablets 3219

Avandamet Tablets 1343
Fortamet Extended-Release Tablets 1156

Methotrexate Sodium (Salicylic acid can inhibit renal clearance of methotrexate, leading to bone marrow toxicity, especially in the elderly or renal impaired).
No products indexed under this heading.

Methyclothiazide (The effectiveness of diuretics in patients with underlying renal or cardiovascular disease may be diminished by co-administration of aspirin due to inhibition of renal prostaglandins, leading to decreased renal blood flow and salt and fluid retention).
No products indexed under this heading.

Metipranolol Hydrochloride (The hypertensive effects of beta-blockers may be diminished by the concomitant administration of aspirin due to inhibition of renal prostaglandins, leading to decreased renal blood flow and salt and fluid retention).
No products indexed under this heading.

Metolazone (The effectiveness of diuretics in patients with underlying renal or cardiovascular disease may be diminished by co-administration of aspirin due to inhibition of renal prostaglandins, leading to decreased renal blood flow and salt and fluid retention).
No products indexed under this heading.

Metoprolol Succinate (The hypertensive effects of beta-blockers may be diminished by the concomitant administration of aspirin due to inhibition of renal prostaglandins, leading to decreased renal blood flow and salt and fluid retention).
Products include:
Toprol-XL Tablets 660

Metoprolol Tartrate (The hypertensive effects of beta-blockers may be diminished by the concomitant administration of aspirin due to inhibition of renal prostaglandins, leading to decreased renal blood flow and salt and fluid retention).
No products indexed under this heading.

Miglitol (Moderate doses of aspirin may increase the effectiveness of renal hypoglycemic drugs, leading to hypoglycemia).
No products indexed under this heading.

Moexipril Hydrochloride (Co-administration can result in diminished hypotensive and hyponatremic effects of ACE inhibitors due to the effect of aspirin on the renin-angiotensin conversion pathway).
Products include:
Uniretic Tablets 3114
Univasc Tablets 3118

Nabumetone (Co-administration of non-steroidal anti-inflammatory drugs with aspirin may increase bleeding or lead to decreased renal function).
Products include:
Relafen Tablets 1523

Nadolol (The hypertensive effects of beta-blockers may be diminished by the concomitant administration of aspirin due to inhibition of renal prostaglandins, leading to decreased renal blood flow and salt and fluid retention). Products include:
Nadolol Tablets 2121

Naproxen (Co-administration of non-steroidal anti-inflammatory drugs with aspirin may increase bleeding or lead to decreased renal function).
Products include:
EC-Naprosyn Delayed-Release Tablets 2769
Naprosyn Suspension 2769
Naprosyn Tablets 2769
Prevacid NapraPAC 3277

Naproxen Sodium (Co-administration of non-steroidal anti-inflammatory drugs with aspirin may increase bleeding or lead to decreased renal function). Products include:
Aleve Tablets, Caplets and Gelcaps .... ■605
Anaprox Tablets 2769
Anaprox DS Tablets 2769

Neostigmine Bromide (Dipyridamole may counteract the anticholinesterase effect of cholinesterase inhibitors, thereby potentially aggravating myasthenia gravis).
No products indexed under this heading.

Neostigmine Methylsulfate (Dipyridamole may counteract the anticholinesterase effect of cholinesterase inhibitors, thereby potentially aggravating myasthenia gravis).
No products indexed under this heading.

Oxaprozin (Co-administration of non-steroidal anti-inflammatory drugs with aspirin may increase bleeding or lead to decreased renal function).
No products indexed under this heading.

Penbutolol Sulfate (The hypertensive effects of beta-blockers may be diminished by the concomitant administration of aspirin due to inhibition of renal prostaglandins, leading to decreased renal blood flow and salt and fluid retention).
No products indexed under this heading.

Perindopril Erbumine (Co-administration can result in diminished hypotensive and hyponatremic effects of ACE inhibitors due to the effect of aspirin on the renin-angiotensin conversion pathway).
Products include:
Aceon Tablets (2 mg, 4 mg, 8 mg) 3191

Phenylbutazone (Co-administration of non-steroidal anti-inflammatory drugs with aspirin may increase bleeding or lead to decreased renal function).
No products indexed under this heading.

Phenytoin (Salicylic acid can displace protein-bound phenytoin leading to a decrease in the total concentration of phenytoin).
No products indexed under this heading.

Phenytoin Sodium (Salicylic acid can displace protein-bound phenytoin leading to a decrease in the total concentration of phenytoin).
Products include:
Phenytek Capsules 2153

Pindolol (The hypertensive effects of beta-blockers may be diminished by the concomitant administration of aspirin due to inhibition of renal prostaglandins, leading to decreased renal blood flow and salt and fluid retention).
No products indexed under this heading.

Pioglitazone Hydrochloride (Moderate doses of aspirin may increase the effectiveness of renal hypoglycemic drugs, leading to hypoglycemia).
Products include:
ActoPlus Met Tablets 3219
Actos Tablets 3224

Piroxicam (Co-administration of non-steroidal anti-inflammatory drugs with aspirin may increase bleeding or lead to decreased renal function).
No products indexed under this heading.

Polythiazide (The effectiveness of diuretics in patients with underlying renal or cardiovascular disease may be diminished by co-administration of aspirin due to inhibition of renal prostaglandins, leading to decreased renal blood flow and salt and fluid retention).
No products indexed under this heading.

Probenecid (Salicylates antagonize the uricosuric action of uricosuric agents, such as probenecid).
No products indexed under this heading.

Propranolol Hydrochloride (The hypertensive effects of beta-blockers may be diminished by the concomitant administration of aspirin due to inhibition of renal prostaglandins, leading to decreased renal blood flow and salt and fluid retention). Products include:
Inderal LA Long-Acting Capsules 3421
InnoPran XL Capsules 2728

Pyridostigmine Bromide (Dipyridamole may counteract the anticholinesterase effect of cholinesterase inhibitors, thereby potentially aggravating myasthenia gravis).
No products indexed under this heading.

Quinapril Hydrochloride (Co-administration can result in diminished hypotensive and hyponatremic effects of ACE inhibitors due to the effect of aspirin on the renin-angiotensin conversion pathway).
No products indexed under this heading.

Ramipril (Co-administration can result in diminished hypotensive and hyponatremic effects of ACE inhibitors due to the effect of aspirin on the renin-angiotensin conversion pathway). Products include:
Altace Capsules 1673

Repaglinide (Moderate doses of aspirin may increase the effectiveness of renal hypoglycemic drugs, leading to hypoglycemia). Products include:
Prandin Tablets (0.5, 1, and 2 mg) 2337

Rivastigmine Tartrate (Dipyridamole may counteract the anticholinesterase effect of cholinesterase inhibitors, thereby potentially aggravating myasthenia gravis). Products include:
Exelon Capsules 2204

Rofecoxib (Co-administration of non-steroidal anti-inflammatory drugs with aspirin may increase bleeding or lead to decreased renal function).
No products indexed under this heading.

Rosiglitazone Maleate (Moderate doses of aspirin may increase the effectiveness of renal hypoglycemic drugs, leading to hypoglycemia).
Products include:
Avandamet Tablets 1343
Avandia Tablets 1348

Sotalol Hydrochloride (The hypertensive effects of beta-blockers may be diminished by the concomitant administration of aspirin due to inhibition of renal prostaglandins, leading to decreased renal blood flow and salt and fluid retention).
No products indexed under this heading.

Spirapril Hydrochloride (Co-administration can result in diminished hypotensive and hyponatremic effects of ACE inhibitors due to the effect of aspirin on the renin-angiotensin conversion pathway).
No products indexed under this heading.

Spironolactone (The effectiveness of diuretics in patients with underlying renal or cardiovascular disease may be diminished by co-administration of aspirin due to inhibition of renal prostaglandins, leading to decreased renal blood flow and salt and fluid retention).
No products indexed under this heading.

Sulfinpyrazone (Salicylates antagonize the uricosuric action of uricosuric agents, such as sulfinpyrazone).
No products indexed under this heading.

Sulindac (Co-administration of non-steroidal anti-inflammatory drugs with aspirin may increase bleeding or lead to decreased renal function).
Products include:
Clinoril Tablets 1899

Tacrine Hydrochloride (Dipyridamole may counteract the anticholinesterase effect of cholinesterase inhibitors, thereby potentially aggravating myasthenia gravis).
No products indexed under this heading.

Timolol Hemihydrate (The hypertensive effects of beta-blockers may be diminished by the concomitant administration of aspirin due to inhibition of renal prostaglandins, leading to decreased renal blood flow and salt and fluid retention).
Products include:
Betimol Ophthalmic Solution 3371
Betimol Ophthalmic Solution .... ⊙283

Timolol Maleate (The hypertensive effects of beta-blockers may be diminished by the concomitant administration of aspirin due to inhibition of renal prostaglandins, leading to decreased renal blood flow and salt and fluid retention).
Products include:
Blocadren Tablets 1891
Cosopt Sterile Ophthalmic Solution 1910
Timolide Tablets 2056
Timoptic in Ocudose 2061
Timoptic Sterile Ophthalmic Solution 2058
Timoptic-XE Sterile Ophthalmic Gel Forming Solution 2062

Tinzaparin Sodium (Patients on anticoagulation therapy are at risk for bleeding).
No products indexed under this heading.

Tolazamide (Moderate doses of aspirin may increase the effectiveness of renal hypoglycemic drugs, leading to hypoglycemia).
No products indexed under this heading.

Tolbutamide (Moderate doses of aspirin may increase the effectiveness of renal hypoglycemic drugs, leading to hypoglycemia).
No products indexed under this heading.

Tolmetin Sodium (Co-administration of non-steroidal anti-inflammatory drugs with aspirin may increase bleeding or lead to decreased renal function).
No products indexed under this heading.

Torsemide (The effectiveness of diuretics in patients with underlying renal or cardiovascular disease may be diminished by co-administration of aspirin due to inhibition of renal prostaglandins, leading to decreased renal blood flow and salt and fluid retention).
No products indexed under this heading.

Trandolapril (Co-administration can result in diminished hypotensive and hyponatremic effects of ACE inhibitors due to the effect of aspirin on the renin-angiotensin conversion pathway). Products include:
Mavik Tablets 482
Tarka Tablets 519

Triamterene (The effectiveness of diuretics in patients with underlying renal or cardiovascular disease may be diminished by co-administration of aspirin due to inhibition of renal prostaglandins, leading to decreased renal blood flow and salt and fluid retention). Products include:
Dyazide Capsules 1389
Dyrenium Capsules 3390
Maxzide 2150

Troglitazone (Moderate doses of aspirin may increase the effectiveness of renal hypoglycemic drugs, leading to hypoglycemia).
No products indexed under this heading.

Valdecoxib (Co-administration of non-steroidal anti-inflammatory drugs with aspirin may increase bleeding or lead to decreased renal function).
No products indexed under this heading.

Valproate Sodium (Salicylic acid can displace protein-bound valproic acid leading to an increase in serum valproic acid levels). Products include:
Depacon Injection 412

Valproic Acid (Salicylic acid can displace protein-bound valproic acid leading to an increase in serum valproic acid levels). Products include:
Depakene 417

Warfarin Sodium (Aspirin can displace warfarin from protein binding sites, leading to a prolongation of both the prothrombin time and the bleeding time). Products include:
Coumadin for Injection 932
Coumadin Tablets 932

Food Interactions

Alcohol (Patients who consume three or more alcoholic drinks every day should be counseled about the bleeding risks involved with chronic, heavy alcohol use while taking aspirin).

AGRYLIN CAPSULES

(Anagrelide Hydrochloride) 3172
May interact with aspirin-acetylsalicylic acid, cytochrome p450 1a2 inhibitors (selected), cytochrome p450 1a2 substrates (selected), and certain other agents. Compounds in these categories include:

Acetaminophen (Anagrelide demonstrates some limited inhibitory activity towards CYP1A2 which may present a theoretical potential for interaction with other co-administered medicinal products sharing that clearance mechanism). Products include:
Benadryl Allergy & Cold Tablets 692
Benadryl Allergy & Sinus Headache Caplets & Gelcaps 693
Benadryl Maximum Strength Severe Allergy & Sinus Headache Caplets 694
Contac Severe Cold and Flu Caplets Maximum Strength 615
Contac Severe Cold and Flu Caplets Non-Drowsy 615
Darvocet A 500 Tablets 3497
Goody's Body Pain Formula Powder 621
Goody's Extra Strength Headache Powder 621
Goody's Extra Strength Pain Relief Tablets 621
Goody's PM Powder 622
Hycomine Compound Tablets 1105
Lortab 3315
Lortab Elixir 3312
Percocet Tablets 1114
Robitussin Cough, Cold & Flu Liquid-filled Capsules 750
Robitussin Flu Liquid 752
Sedapap Tablets 50 mg/650 mg 2098
Singlet Caplets 636
Sudafed Severe Cold 710
Sudafed Sinus Headache 711
TheraFlu Cold & Cough Hot Liquid 680
TheraFlu Cold & Sore Throat Hot Liquid 680
TheraFlu Flu & Chest Congestion Non-Drowsy Hot Liquid 681
TheraFlu Flu & Sore Throat Hot Liquid 681
TheraFlu Severe Cold Non-Drowsy Hot Liquid 683
TheraFlu Severe Cold & Cough Hot Liquid 683
TheraFlu Severe Cold Caplets 679
TheraFlu Severe Cold Hot Liquid 682
TheraFlu Severe Cold Non-Drowsy Caplets 679
Triaminic Cough & Sore Throat Liquid 687
Triaminic Flu, Cough & Fever Liquid 685
Triaminic Cough & Sore Throat Softchews 689
Tylenol 8 Hour Extended Release Geltabs and Caplets 1843
Tylenol Sinus NightTime Caplets 663
Children's Tylenol Suspension Liquid and Meltaways 1850
Children's Tylenol Plus Cold & Allergy Suspension Liquid 1850
Children's Tylenol Plus Cold NightTime Suspension Liquid 1851
Children's Tylenol Plus Cold & Cough Suspension Liquid and Chewable Tablets 1851
Children's Tylenol Plus Cold Chewable Tablets 1851
Children's Tylenol Plus Cold Daytime Non-Drowsy Suspension Liquid 1851
Children's Tylenol Plus Flu Suspension Liquid 1853
Concentrated Tylenol Infants' Drops Plus Cold 1851
Concentrated Tylenol Infants' Drops Plus Cold and Cough 1851
Concentrated Tylenol Infants' Drops 1850
Junior Tylenol Meltaways 1850
Tylenol Cold & Flu Severe Daytime Liquid with Cool Bust 1846
Tylenol Cold & Flu Severe NightTime Liquid with Cool Burst 1846
Tylenol Cold Severe Congestion Non-Drowsy Caplets with Cool Burst 1846
Tylenol Cough & Sore Throat Daytime Liquid with Cool Burst 1849
Tylenol Cough & Sore Throat NightTime Liquid with Cool Burst 1849
Tylenol 1843
Extra Strength Tylenol Rapid Release Gels 1843
Tylenol 1843
Tylenol Allergy Complete Night Time Caplets 1844
Tylenol Allergy Complete Multi-Symptom Caplets and Gelcaps with Cool Burst 1844
Tylenol Severe Allergy Caplets 1844
Tylenol Flu NightTime Gelcaps 1846
Tylenol Flu Day Non-Drowsy Gelcaps 1846
Concentrated Tylenol Infants' Drops Plus Cold Nasal Congestant, Fever Reducer & Pain Reliever 668
Concentrated Tylenol Infants' Drops Plus Cold & Cough Nasal Decongestant, Fever Reducer & Pain Reliever 668
Multi-Symptom Tylenol Cold Night Time Caplets 1845
Multi-Symptom Tylenol Cold Day Non-Drowsy Caplets and Gelcaps 1845
Extra Strength Tylenol PM Caplets, Geltabs, Gelcaps and Liquid 1847
Tylenol Sinus Day Non-Drowsy 1848
Tylenol Sinus Night Time Caplets 1848
Tylenol Sinus Severe Congestion Caplets with Cool Burst 1848
Tylenol Sore Throat Daytime Liquid with Cool Burst 1849
Tylenol Sore Throat NightTime Liquid with Cool Burst 1849
Tylenol with Codeine 2461
Women's Tylenol Menstrual Relief Caplets 1849
Ultracet Tablets 2462
Vicks 44M Cough, Cold & Flu Relief 2676
Vicks DayQuil LiquiCaps/Liquid Multi-Symptom Cold/Flu Relief 723
Vicks DayQuil Multi-Symptom Cold/Flu Relief LiquiCaps 2675
Vicks DayQuil Multi-Symptom Cold/Flu Relief Liquid 2675
Vicks NyQuil LiquiCaps 2677
Vicks NyQuil LiquiCaps/Liquid Multi-Symptom Cold/Flu Relief 725
Vicks NyQuil Liquid 2677
Vicodin Tablets 530
Vicodin ES Tablets 531
Vicodin HP Tablets 532
Zydone Tablets 1118

Alatrofloxacin Mesylate (Anagrelide is metabolized at least in part by CYP1A2. Therefore, CYP1A2 inhibitors could theoretically adversely influence the clearance of anagrelide).
No products indexed under this heading.

Amiodarone Hydrochloride (Anagrelide is metabolized at least in part by CYP1A2. Therefore, CYP1A2 inhibitors could theoretically adversely influence the clearance of anagrelide). Products include:
Pacerone Tablets 3337

Amitriptyline Hydrochloride (Anagrelide demonstrates some limited inhibitory activity towards CYP1A2 which may present a theoretical potential for interaction with other co-administered medicinal products sharing that clearance mechanism).
No products indexed under this heading.

Amoxapine (Anagrelide demonstrates some limited inhibitory activity towards CYP1A2 which may present a theoretical potential for interaction with other co-administered medicinal products sharing that clearance mechanism).
No products indexed under this heading.

Amrinone Lactate (Anagrelide is an inhibitor of AMP PDE III. The effects of medicinal products with similar properties, such as amrinone, may be exacerbated by anagrelide).
No products indexed under this heading.

Anastrozole (Anagrelide is metabolized at least in part by CYP1A2. Therefore, CYP1A2 inhibitors could theoretically adversely influence the clearance of anagrelide). Products include:
Arimidex Tablets 665

Aspirin (Anagrelide may slightly enhance the inhibition of platelet aggregation by aspirin). Products include:
Aggrenox Capsules 855
Bayer, Aspirin Regimen 606
Bayer Aspirin Tablets 3515
BC Powder 612
BC Allergy Sinus Cold Powder 612
Arthritis Strength BC Powder 612
BC Sinus Cold Powder 612
Ecotrin Enteric Coated Aspirin Low, Regular and Maximum Strength Tablets 1627
Goody's Body Pain Formula Powder 621
Goody's Extra Strength Headache Powder 621
Goody's Extra Strength Pain Relief Tablets 621
Percodan Tablets 1115
St. Joseph 81 mg Aspirin Chewable and Enteric Coated Tablets 1841

Aspirin, Enteric Coated (Anagrelide may slightly enhance the inhibition of platelet aggregation by aspirin).
No products indexed under this heading.

Aspirin Buffered (Anagrelide may slightly enhance the inhibition of platelet aggregation by aspirin).
No products indexed under this heading.

Caffeine (Anagrelide demonstrates some limited inhibitory activity towards CYP1A2 which may present a theoretical potential for interaction with other co-administered medicinal products sharing that clearance mechanism). Products include:
Athena Hair System Shampoo 767
BC Powder 612
Arthritis Strength BC Powder 612
Goody's Extra Strength Headache Powder 621
Goody's Extra Strength Pain Relief Tablets 621
Hycomine Compound Tablets 1105
Spartan Hair System Shampoo 767
Vivarin 639

Caffeine Anhydrous (Anagrelide demonstrates some limited inhibitory activity towards CYP1A2 which may present a theoretical potential for interaction with other co-administered medicinal products sharing that clearance mechanism).
No products indexed under this heading.

Chlordiazepoxide (Anagrelide demonstrates some limited inhibitory activity towards CYP1A2 which may present a theoretical potential for interaction with other co-administered medicinal products sharing that clearance mechanism).
No products indexed under this heading.

Chlordiazepoxide Hydrochloride (Anagrelide demonstrates some limited inhibitory activity towards CYP1A2 which may present a theoretical potential for interaction with other co-administered medicinal products sharing that clearance mechanism). Products include:
Librium Capsules ... **3349**

Cilostazol (Anagrelide is an inhibitor of AMP PDE III. The effects of medicinal products with similar properties, such as cilostazol, may be exacerbated by anagrelide). Products include:
Pletal Tablets ... **2478**

Cimetidine (Anagrelide is metabolized at least in part by CYP1A2. Therefore, CYP1A2 inhibitors could theoretically adversely influence the clearance of anagrelide). Products include:
Tagamet HB 200 Tablets ... ▣**637**
Tagamet Tablets ... **1547**

Cimetidine Hydrochloride (Anagrelide is metabolized at least in part by CYP1A2. Therefore, CYP1A2 inhibitors could theoretically adversely influence the clearance of anagrelide).
No products indexed under this heading.

Ciprofloxacin (Anagrelide is metabolized at least in part by CYP1A2. Therefore, CYP1A2 inhibitors could theoretically adversely influence the clearance of anagrelide). Products include:
Cipro I.V. ... **2998**
Cipro I.V. Pharmacy Bulk Package ... **3509**
Cipro Oral Suspension ... **2991**
Cipro XR Tablets ... **3004**
Ciprodex Otic Suspension ... **555**

Ciprofloxacin Hydrochloride (Anagrelide is metabolized at least in part by CYP1A2. Therefore, CYP1A2 inhibitors could theoretically adversely influence the clearance of anagrelide). Products include:
Ciloxan Ophthalmic Ointment ... **554**
Cipro Tablets ... **2991**

Clarithromycin (Anagrelide is metabolized at least in part by CYP1A2. Therefore, CYP1A2 inhibitors could theoretically adversely influence the clearance of anagrelide). Products include:
Biaxin/Biaxin XL ... **402**
PREVPAC ... **3281**

Clomipramine Hydrochloride (Anagrelide demonstrates some limited inhibitory activity towards CYP1A2 which may present a theoretical potential for interaction with other co-administered medicinal products sharing that clearance mechanism).
No products indexed under this heading.

Clopidogrel Bisulfate (Anagrelide demonstrates some limited inhibitory activity towards CYP1A2 which may present a theoretical potential for interaction with other co-administered medicinal products sharing that clearance mechanism). Products include:
Plavix Tablets ... **940**
Plavix Tablets ... **2942**

Clozapine (Anagrelide demonstrates some limited inhibitory activity towards CYP1A2 which may present a theoretical potential for interaction with other co-administered medicinal products sharing that clearance mechanism). Products include:
Clozapine Tablets ... **2141**
Clozaril Tablets ... **2174**
FazaClo Orally Disintegrating Tablets ... **547**

Cyclobenzaprine (Anagrelide demonstrates some limited inhibitory activity towards CYP1A2 which may present a theoretical potential for interaction with other co-administered medicinal products sharing that clearance mechanism).
No products indexed under this heading.

Cyclobenzaprine Hydrochloride (Anagrelide demonstrates some limited inhibitory activity towards CYP1A2 which may present a theoretical potential for interaction with other co-administered medicinal products sharing that clearance mechanism). Products include:
Flexeril Tablets ... **1832**

Desipramine Hydrochloride (Anagrelide demonstrates some limited inhibitory activity towards CYP1A2 which may present a theoretical potential for interaction with other co-administered medicinal products sharing that clearance mechanism).
No products indexed under this heading.

Desogestrel (Anagrelide is metabolized at least in part by CYP1A2. Therefore, CYP1A2 inhibitors could theoretically adversely influence the clearance of anagrelide). Products include:
Ortho-Cept Tablets ... **2395**

Diazepam (Anagrelide demonstrates some limited inhibitory activity towards CYP1A2 which may present a theoretical potential for interaction with other co-administered medicinal products sharing that clearance mechanism). Products include:
Diastat Rectal Delivery System ... **3344**
Valium Tablets ... **2822**

Diltiazem Hydrochloride (Anagrelide demonstrates some limited inhibitory activity towards CYP1A2 which may present a theoretical potential for interaction with other co-administered medicinal products sharing that clearance mechanism). Products include:
Cardizem LA Extended Release Tablets ... **1699**
Tiazac Capsules ... **1204**

Diltiazem Maleate (Anagrelide demonstrates some limited inhibitory activity towards CYP1A2 which may present a theoretical potential for interaction with other co-administered medicinal products sharing that clearance mechanism).
No products indexed under this heading.

Doxepin Hydrochloride (Anagrelide demonstrates some limited inhibitory activity towards CYP1A2 which may present a theoretical potential for interaction with other co-administered medicinal products sharing that clearance mechanism).
No products indexed under this heading.

Enoxacin (Anagrelide is metabolized at least in part by CYP1A2. Therefore, CYP1A2 inhibitors could theoretically adversely influence the clearance of anagrelide).
No products indexed under this heading.

Enoximone (Anagrelide is an inhibitor of AMP PDE III. The effects of medicinal products with similar properties, such as enoximone, may be exacerbated by anagrelide).
No products indexed under this heading.

Erythromycin (Anagrelide demonstrates some limited inhibitory activity towards CYP1A2 which may present a theoretical potential for interaction with other co-administered medicinal products sharing that clearance mechanism). Products include:
Erygel Topical Gel ... **2096**
Ery-Tab Tablets ... **447**
Erythromycin Base Filmtab Tablets ... **454**
Erythromycin Delayed-Release Capsules, USP ... **456**
PCE Dispertab Tablets ... **510**

Erythromycin Estolate (Anagrelide demonstrates some limited inhibitory activity towards CYP1A2 which may present a theoretical potential for interaction with other co-administered medicinal products sharing that clearance mechanism).
No products indexed under this heading.

Erythromycin Ethylsuccinate (Anagrelide demonstrates some limited inhibitory activity towards CYP1A2 which may present a theoretical potential for interaction with other co-administered medicinal products sharing that clearance mechanism). Products include:
E.E.S. ... **449**
EryPed ... **445**

Erythromycin Gluceptate (Anagrelide demonstrates some limited inhibitory activity towards CYP1A2 which may present a theoretical potential for interaction with other co-administered medicinal products sharing that clearance mechanism).
No products indexed under this heading.

Erythromycin Lactobionate (Anagrelide demonstrates some limited inhibitory activity towards CYP1A2 which may present a theoretical potential for interaction with other co-administered medicinal products sharing that clearance mechanism).
No products indexed under this heading.

Erythromycin Stearate (Anagrelide demonstrates some limited inhibitory activity towards CYP1A2 which may present a theoretical potential for interaction with other co-administered medicinal products sharing that clearance mechanism). Products include:
Erythrocin Stearate Filmtab Tablets ... **452**

Estradiol (Anagrelide demonstrates some limited inhibitory activity towards CYP1A2 which may present a theoretical potential for interaction with other co-administered medicinal products sharing that clearance mechanism). Products include:
Activella Tablets ... **2311**
Climara Transdermal System ... **795**
Climara Pro Transdermal System ... **800**
CombiPatch Transdermal System ... **2180**
Estrogel 0.06% ... **3200**
Menostar Transdermal System ... **805**
Prefest Tablets ... **1069**
Vagifem Tablets ... **2340**
Vivelle Transdermal System ... **2288**
Vivelle-Dot Transdermal System ... **2293**

Estradiol Benzoate (Anagrelide demonstrates some limited inhibitory activity towards CYP1A2 which may present a theoretical potential for interaction with other co-administered medicinal products sharing that clearance mechanism).
No products indexed under this heading.

Estradiol Cypionate (Anagrelide demonstrates some limited inhibitory activity towards CYP1A2 which may present a theoretical potential for interaction with other co-administered medicinal products sharing that clearance mechanism).
No products indexed under this heading.

Ethinyl Estradiol (Anagrelide is metabolized at least in part by CYP1A2. Therefore, CYP1A2 inhibitors could theoretically adversely influence the clearance of anagrelide). Products include:
Alesse-28 Tablets ... **3392**
Lo/Ovral-28 Tablets ... **3423**
NuvaRing ... **2357**
Ortho-Cept Tablets ... **2395**
Ortho-Cyclen/Ortho Tri-Cyclen ... **2414**
Ortho Evra Transdermal System ... **2402**
Ortho Tri-Cyclen Lo Tablets ... **2421**
Seasonale Tablets ... **1073**
Triphasil-28 Tablets ... **3483**
Yasmin 28 Tablets ... **818**

Flutamide (Anagrelide demonstrates some limited inhibitory activity towards CYP1A2 which may present a theoretical potential for interaction with other co-administered medicinal products sharing that clearance mechanism). Products include:
Eulexin Capsules ... **3023**

Fluticasone Propionate (Anagrelide demonstrates some limited inhibitory activity towards CYP1A2 which may present a theoretical potential for interaction with other co-administered medicinal products sharing that clearance mechanism). Products include:
Advair Diskus 100/50 ... **1291**
Advair Diskus 250/50 ... **1291**
Advair Diskus 500/50 ... **1291**
Cutivate Cream ... **1381**
Cutivate Lotion 0.05% ... **1383**
Cutivate Ointment ... **1384**
Flonase Nasal Spray ... **1412**
Flovent Diskus 100 mcg ... **1418**
Flovent Diskus 50 mcg ... **1415**

Fluvoxamine (Anagrelide is metabolized at least in part by CYP1A2. Therefore, CYP1A2 inhibitors could theoretically adversely influence the clearance of anagrelide).
No products indexed under this heading.

Fluvoxamine Maleate (Anagrelide is metabolized at least in part by CYP1A2. Therefore, CYP1A2 inhibitors could theoretically adversely influence the clearance of anagrelide).
No products indexed under this heading.

Gatifloxacin (Anagrelide is metabolized at least in part by CYP1A2. Therefore, CYP1A2 inhibitors could theoretically adversely influence the clearance of anagrelide). Products include:

Tequin Injection 964
Tequin Tablets 964
Zymar Ophthalmic Solution 571

Gemifloxacin Mesylate
(Anagrelide is metabolized at least in part by CYP1A2. Therefore, CYP1A2 inhibitors could theoretically adversely influence the clearance of anagrelide). Products include:
Factive Tablets 2464

Grepafloxacin Hydrochloride
(Anagrelide is metabolized at least in part by CYP1A2. Therefore, CYP1A2 inhibitors could theoretically adversely influence the clearance of anagrelide).
No products indexed under this heading.

Haloperidol (Anagrelide demonstrates some limited inhibitory activity towards CYP1A2 which may present a theoretical potential for interaction with other co-administered medicinal products sharing that clearance mechanism).
No products indexed under this heading.

Haloperidol Decanoate
(Anagrelide demonstrates some limited inhibitory activity towards CYP1A2 which may present a theoretical potential for interaction with other co-administered medicinal products sharing that clearance mechanism).
No products indexed under this heading.

Haloperidol Lactate (Anagrelide demonstrates some limited inhibitory activity towards CYP1A2 which may present a theoretical potential for interaction with other co-administered medicinal products sharing that clearance mechanism).
No products indexed under this heading.

Imipramine Hydrochloride
(Anagrelide demonstrates some limited inhibitory activity towards CYP1A2 which may present a theoretical potential for interaction with other co-administered medicinal products sharing that clearance mechanism).
No products indexed under this heading.

Imipramine Pamoate (Anagrelide demonstrates some limited inhibitory activity towards CYP1A2 which may present a theoretical potential for interaction with other co-administered medicinal products sharing that clearance mechanism).
No products indexed under this heading.

Isoniazid (Anagrelide is metabolized at least in part by CYP1A2. Therefore, CYP1A2 inhibitors could theoretically adversely influence the clearance of anagrelide).
No products indexed under this heading.

Ketoconazole (Anagrelide is metabolized at least in part by CYP1A2. Therefore, CYP1A2 inhibitors could theoretically adversely influence the clearance of anagrelide). Products include:
Nizoral A-D Shampoo, 1% 1839
Nizoral 2% Shampoo 1838

Levobupivacaine Hydrochloride
(Anagrelide demonstrates some limited inhibitory activity towards CYP1A2 which may present a theoretical potential for interaction with other co-administered medicinal products sharing that clearance mechanism).
No products indexed under this heading.

Levofloxacin (Anagrelide is metabolized at least in part by CYP1A2. Therefore, CYP1A2 inhibitors could theoretically adversely influence the clearance of anagrelide). Products include:
Levaquin in 5% Dextrose Injection 2453
Levaquin 2453
Quixin Ophthalmic Solution 3373

Levonorgestrel (Anagrelide is metabolized at least in part by CYP1A2. Therefore, CYP1A2 inhibitors could theoretically adversely influence the clearance of anagrelide). Products include:
Alesse-28 Tablets 3392
Climara Pro Transdermal System 800
Mirena Intrauterine System 810
Plan B Tablets 1068
Seasonale Tablets 1073
Triphasil-28 Tablets 3483

Lomefloxacin Hydrochloride
(Anagrelide is metabolized at least in part by CYP1A2. Therefore, CYP1A2 inhibitors could theoretically adversely influence the clearance of anagrelide).
No products indexed under this heading.

Maprotiline Hydrochloride
(Anagrelide demonstrates some limited inhibitory activity towards CYP1A2 which may present a theoretical potential for interaction with other co-administered medicinal products sharing that clearance mechanism).
No products indexed under this heading.

Mestranol (Anagrelide is metabolized at least in part by CYP1A2. Therefore, CYP1A2 inhibitors could theoretically adversely influence the clearance of anagrelide).
No products indexed under this heading.

Methadone Hydrochloride
(Anagrelide demonstrates some limited inhibitory activity towards CYP1A2 which may present a theoretical potential for interaction with other co-administered medicinal products sharing that clearance mechanism).
No products indexed under this heading.

Methoxsalen (Anagrelide is metabolized at least in part by CYP1A2. Therefore, CYP1A2 inhibitors could theoretically adversely influence the clearance of anagrelide). Products include:
Oxsoralen Lotion 1% 3354
Oxsoralen-Ultra Capsules 3354

Mexiletine Hydrochloride
(Anagrelide is metabolized at least in part by CYP1A2. Therefore, CYP1A2 inhibitors could theoretically adversely influence the clearance of anagrelide).
No products indexed under this heading.

Mibefradil Dihydrochloride
(Anagrelide is metabolized at least in part by CYP1A2. Therefore, CYP1A2 inhibitors could theoretically adversely influence the clearance of anagrelide).
No products indexed under this heading.

Milrinone Lactate (Anagrelide is an inhibitor of cyclic AMP PDE III. The effects of medicinal products with similar properties, such as milrinone, may be exacerbated by anagrelide).
No products indexed under this heading.

Mirtazapine (Anagrelide demonstrates some limited inhibitory activity towards CYP1A2 which may present a theoretical potential for interaction with other co-administered medicinal products sharing that clearance mechanism).
No products indexed under this heading.

Moxifloxacin Hydrochloride
(Anagrelide is metabolized at least in part by CYP1A2. Therefore, CYP1A2 inhibitors could theoretically adversely influence the clearance of anagrelide). Products include:
Avelox 2984
Vigamox Ophthalmic Solution 560

Nafcillin Sodium (Anagrelide demonstrates some limited inhibitory activity towards CYP1A2 which may present a theoretical potential for interaction with other co-administered medicinal products sharing that clearance mechanism).
No products indexed under this heading.

Nalidixic Acid (Anagrelide is metabolized at least in part by CYP1A2. Therefore, CYP1A2 inhibitors could theoretically adversely influence the clearance of anagrelide).
No products indexed under this heading.

Naproxen (Anagrelide demonstrates some limited inhibitory activity towards CYP1A2 which may present a theoretical potential for interaction with other co-administered medicinal products sharing that clearance mechanism). Products include:
EC-Naprosyn Delayed-Release Tablets 2769
Naprosyn Suspension 2769
Naprosyn Tablets 2769
Prevacid NapraPAC 3277

Naproxen Sodium (Anagrelide demonstrates some limited inhibitory activity towards CYP1A2 which may present a theoretical potential for interaction with other co-administered medicinal products sharing that clearance mechanism). Products include:
Aleve Tablets, Caplets and Gelcaps 605
Anaprox Tablets 2769
Anaprox DS Tablets 2769

Nicotine Polacrilex (Anagrelide demonstrates some limited inhibitory activity towards CYP1A2 which may present a theoretical potential for interaction with other co-administered medicinal products sharing that clearance mechanism). Products include:
Commit Lozenges 1625
Nicorette Gum 1632

Nicotine Salicylate (Anagrelide demonstrates some limited inhibitory activity towards CYP1A2 which may present a theoretical potential for interaction with other co-administered medicinal products sharing that clearance mechanism).
No products indexed under this heading.

Nicotine Sulfate (Anagrelide demonstrates some limited inhibitory activity towards CYP1A2 which may present a theoretical potential for interaction with other co-administered medicinal products sharing that clearance mechanism).
No products indexed under this heading.

Norethindrone (Anagrelide is metabolized at least in part by CYP1A2. Therefore, CYP1A2 inhibitors could theoretically adversely influence the clearance of anagrelide). Products include:
Ortho Micronor Tablets 2411

Norethindrone Acetate
(Anagrelide demonstrates some limited inhibitory activity towards CYP1A2 which may present a theoretical potential for interaction with other co-administered medicinal products sharing that clearance mechanism). Products include:
Activella Tablets 2311
Aygestin Tablets 1062
CombiPatch Transdermal System 2180

Norfloxacin (Anagrelide is metabolized at least in part by CYP1A2. Therefore, CYP1A2 inhibitors could theoretically adversely influence the clearance of anagrelide). Products include:
Noroxin Tablets 2009

Norgestrel (Anagrelide is metabolized at least in part by CYP1A2. Therefore, CYP1A2 inhibitors could theoretically adversely influence the clearance of anagrelide). Products include:
Lo/Ovral-28 Tablets 3423

Nortriptyline Hydrochloride
(Anagrelide demonstrates some limited inhibitory activity towards CYP1A2 which may present a theoretical potential for interaction with other co-administered medicinal products sharing that clearance mechanism).
No products indexed under this heading.

Ofloxacin (Anagrelide is metabolized at least in part by CYP1A2. Therefore, CYP1A2 inhibitors could theoretically adversely influence the clearance of anagrelide). Products include:
Floxin Otic Singles 1045
Floxin Otic Solution 1043

Olanzapine (Anagrelide demonstrates some limited inhibitory activity towards CYP1A2 which may present a theoretical potential for interaction with other co-administered medicinal products sharing that clearance mechanism). Products include:
Symbyax Capsules 1788
Zyprexa Tablets 1798
Zyprexa IntraMuscular 1798
Zyprexa ZYDIS Orally Disintegrating Tablets.................. 1798

Olprinone (Anagrelide is an inhibitor of AMP PDE III. The effects of medicinal products with similar properties, such as olprinone, may be exacerbated by anagrelide).
No products indexed under this heading.

Omeprazole (Anagrelide is metabolized at least in part by CYP1A2. Therefore, CYP1A2 inhibitors could theoretically adversely influence the clearance of anagrelide). Products include:
Zegerid Powder for Oral Solution 2972

Ondansetron (Anagrelide demonstrates some limited inhibitory activity towards CYP1A2 which may present a theoretical potential for interaction with other co-administered medicinal products sharing that clearance mechanism). Products include:
Zofran ODT Orally Disintegrating Tablets 1613

Ondansetron Hydrochloride (Anagrelide demonstrates some limited inhibitory activity towards CYP1A2 which may present a theoretical potential for interaction with other co-administered medicinal products sharing that clearance mechanism). Products include:
Zofran Injection 1607
Zofran 1613

Paroxetine Hydrochloride (Anagrelide is metabolized at least in part by CYP1A2. Therefore, CYP1A2 inhibitors could theoretically adversely influence the clearance of anagrelide). Products include:
Paxil CR Controlled-Release Tablets 1509
Paxil 1501

Phenobarbital Sodium (Anagrelide demonstrates some limited inhibitory activity towards CYP1A2 which may present a theoretical potential for interaction with other co-administered medicinal products sharing that clearance mechanism).
No products indexed under this heading.

Phenytoin Sodium (Anagrelide demonstrates some limited inhibitory activity towards CYP1A2 which may present a theoretical potential for interaction with other co-administered medicinal products sharing that clearance mechanism). Products include:
Phenytek Capsules 2153

Propafenone Hydrochloride (Anagrelide demonstrates some limited inhibitory activity towards CYP1A2 which may present a theoretical potential for interaction with other co-administered medicinal products sharing that clearance mechanism). Products include:
Rythmol SR Capsules 2736

Propranolol Hydrochloride (Anagrelide demonstrates some limited inhibitory activity towards CYP1A2 which may present a theoretical potential for interaction with other co-administered medicinal products sharing that clearance mechanism). Products include:
Inderal LA Long-Acting Capsules 3421
InnoPran XL Capsules 2728

Protriptyline Hydrochloride (Anagrelide demonstrates some limited inhibitory activity towards CYP1A2 which may present a theoretical potential for interaction with other co-administered medicinal products sharing that clearance mechanism). Products include:
Vivactil Tablets 2350

Ranitidine Hydrochloride (Anagrelide is metabolized at least in part by CYP1A2. Therefore, CYP1A2 inhibitors could theoretically adversely influence the clearance of anagrelide). Products include:
Zantac 1597
Zantac Injection 1593
Zantac 75 Tablets ..... ▣715
Zantac 150 Maximum Strength Tablets ..... ▣715
Zantac Injection Pharmacy Bulk Package 1595

Riluzole (Anagrelide demonstrates some limited inhibitory activity towards CYP1A2 which may present a theoretical potential for interaction with other co-administered medicinal products sharing that clearance mechanism). Products include:
Rilutek Tablets 2945

Ritonavir (Anagrelide is metabolized at least in part by CYP1A2. Therefore, CYP1A2 inhibitors could theoretically adversely influence the clearance of anagrelide). Products include:
Kaletra 474
Norvir 499

Ropinirole Hydrochloride (Anagrelide demonstrates some limited inhibitory activity towards CYP1A2 which may present a theoretical potential for interaction with other co-administered medicinal products sharing that clearance mechanism). Products include:
Requip Tablets 1528

Ropivacaine Hydrochloride (Anagrelide demonstrates some limited inhibitory activity towards CYP1A2 which may present a theoretical potential for interaction with other co-administered medicinal products sharing that clearance mechanism). Products include:
Naropin Injection 640

Sparfloxacin (Anagrelide is metabolized at least in part by CYP1A2. Therefore, CYP1A2 inhibitors could theoretically adversely influence the clearance of anagrelide).
No products indexed under this heading.

Sucralfate (There is a single case report which suggests that sucralfate may interfere with anagrelide absorption). Products include:
Carafate Suspension 727
Carafate Tablets 728

Tacrine Hydrochloride (Anagrelide is metabolized at least in part by CYP1A2. Therefore, CYP1A2 inhibitors could theoretically adversely influence the clearance of anagrelide).
No products indexed under this heading.

Tamoxifen Citrate (Anagrelide demonstrates some limited inhibitory activity towards CYP1A2 which may present a theoretical potential for interaction with other co-administered medicinal products sharing that clearance mechanism).
No products indexed under this heading.

Theophylline (Anagrelide demonstrates some limited inhibitory activity towards CYP1A2 which may present a theoretical potential for interaction with other co-administered medicinal products sharing that clearance mechanism).
No products indexed under this heading.

Theophylline Anhydrous (Anagrelide demonstrates some limited inhibitory activity towards CYP1A2 which may present a theoretical potential for interaction with other co-administered medicinal products sharing that clearance mechanism). Products include:
Uniphyl Tablets 2708

Ticlopidine Hydrochloride (Anagrelide is metabolized at least in part by CYP1A2. Therefore, CYP1A2 inhibitors could theoretically adversely influence the clearance of anagrelide). Products include:
Ticlid Tablets 2813

Trimethaphan Camsylate (Anagrelide demonstrates some limited inhibitory activity towards CYP1A2 which may present a theoretical potential for interaction with other co-administered medicinal products sharing that clearance mechanism).
No products indexed under this heading.

Trimipramine Maleate (Anagrelide demonstrates some limited inhibitory activity towards CYP1A2 which may present a theoretical potential for interaction with other co-administered medicinal products sharing that clearance mechanism). Products include:
Surmontil Capsules 2347

Troleandomycin (Anagrelide is metabolized at least in part by CYP1A2. Therefore, CYP1A2 inhibitors could theoretically adversely influence the clearance of anagrelide).
No products indexed under this heading.

Trovafloxacin Mesylate (Anagrelide is metabolized at least in part by CYP1A2. Therefore, CYP1A2 inhibitors could theoretically adversely influence the clearance of anagrelide).
No products indexed under this heading.

Verapamil Hydrochloride (Anagrelide demonstrates some limited inhibitory activity towards CYP1A2 which may present a theoretical potential for interaction with other co-administered medicinal products sharing that clearance mechanism). Products include:
Covera-HS Tablets 3135
Tarka Tablets 519
Verelan PM Capsules 3120

Warfarin Sodium (Anagrelide demonstrates some limited inhibitory activity towards CYP1A2 which may present a theoretical potential for interaction with other co-administered medicinal products sharing that clearance mechanism). Products include:
Coumadin for Injection 932
Coumadin Tablets 932

Zileuton (Anagrelide is metabolized at least in part by CYP1A2. Therefore, CYP1A2 inhibitors could theoretically adversely influence the clearance of anagrelide).
No products indexed under this heading.

Zolmitriptan (Anagrelide demonstrates some limited inhibitory activity towards CYP1A2 which may present a theoretical potential for interaction with other co-administered medicinal products sharing that clearance mechanism). Products include:
Zomig Nasal Spray 718
Zomig Tablets 714
Zomig-ZMT Tablets 714

Food Interactions

Grapefruit Juice (Anagrelide is metabolized at least in part by CYP1A2. Therefore, CYP1A2 inhibitors could theoretically adversely influence the clearance of anagrelide).

ALACOL DM SYRUP

(Brompheniramine Maleate, Dextromethorphan Hydrobromide, Phenylephrine Hydrochloride)..... 739
May interact with antihypertensives, central nervous system depressants, monoamine oxidase inhibitors, and certain other agents. Compounds in these categories include:

Acebutolol Hydrochloride (Sympathomimetics may reduce the effects of antihypertensives).
No products indexed under this heading.

Alfentanil Hydrochloride (Potential for additive effects).
No products indexed under this heading.

Alprazolam (Potential for additive effects). Products include:
Niravam Orally Disintegrating Tablets 3106
Xanax XR Tablets 2655

Amlodipine Besylate (Sympathomimetics may reduce the effects of antihypertensives). Products include:
Caduet Tablets 2507
Lotrel Capsules 2238
Norvasc Tablets 2529

Aprobarbital (Potential for additive effects).
No products indexed under this heading.

Atenolol (Sympathomimetics may reduce the effects of antihypertensives). Products include:
Tenormin I.V. Injection 698
Tenormin Tablets 695

Benazepril Hydrochloride (Sympathomimetics may reduce the effects of antihypertensives). Products include:
Lotensin Tablets 2232
Lotensin HCT Tablets 2235
Lotrel Capsules 2238

Bendroflumethiazide (Sympathomimetics may reduce the effects of antihypertensives).
No products indexed under this heading.

Betaxolol Hydrochloride (Sympathomimetics may reduce the effects of antihypertensives). Products include:
Betoptic S Ophthalmic Suspension 554

Bisoprolol Fumarate (Sympathomimetics may reduce the effects of antihypertensives).
No products indexed under this heading.

Buprenorphine Hydrochloride (Potential for additive effects). Products include:
Buprenex Injectable ... 2718
Suboxone Tablets ... 2719
Subutex Tablets ... 2719

Buspirone Hydrochloride (Potential for additive effects).
No products indexed under this heading.

Butabarbital (Potential for additive effects).
No products indexed under this heading.

Butalbital (Potential for additive effects). Products include:
Sedapap Tablets 50 mg/650 mg ... 2098

Candesartan Cilexetil (Sympathomimetics may reduce the effects of antihypertensives). Products include:
Atacand Tablets ... 634
Atacand HCT ... 637

Captopril (Sympathomimetics may reduce the effects of antihypertensives). Products include:
Captopril Tablets ... 2114

Carteolol Hydrochloride (Sympathomimetics may reduce the effects of antihypertensives). Products include:
Carteolol Hydrochloride Ophthalmic Solution USP, 1% ... ⊙246

Chlordiazepoxide (Potential for additive effects).
No products indexed under this heading.

Chlordiazepoxide Hydrochloride (Potential for additive effects). Products include:
Librium Capsules ... 3349

Chlorothiazide (Sympathomimetics may reduce the effects of antihypertensives). Products include:
Aldoclor Tablets ... 1881
Diuril Oral ... 1936

Chlorothiazide Sodium (Sympathomimetics may reduce the effects of antihypertensives). Products include:
Diuril Sodium Intravenous ... 1934

Chlorpromazine (Potential for additive effects).
No products indexed under this heading.

Chlorpromazine Hydrochloride (Potential for additive effects).
No products indexed under this heading.

Chlorprothixene (Potential for additive effects).
No products indexed under this heading.

Chlorprothixene Hydrochloride (Potential for additive effects).
No products indexed under this heading.

Chlorprothixene Lactate (Potential for additive effects).
No products indexed under this heading.

Chlorthalidone (Sympathomimetics may reduce the effects of antihypertensives). Products include:
Clorpres Tablets ... 2139

Clonidine (Sympathomimetics may reduce the effects of antihypertensives). Products include:
Catapres-TTS ... 875

Clonidine Hydrochloride (Sympathomimetics may reduce the effects of antihypertensives). Products include:
Catapres Tablets ... 874
Clorpres Tablets ... 2139

Clorazepate Dipotassium (Potential for additive effects). Products include:
Tranxene ... 2488

Clozapine (Potential for additive effects). Products include:
Clozapine Tablets ... 2141
Clozaril Tablets ... 2174
FazaClo Orally Disintegrating Tablets ... 547

Codeine Phosphate (Potential for additive effects). Products include:
Tylenol with Codeine ... 2461

Deserpidine (Sympathomimetics may reduce the effects of antihypertensives).
No products indexed under this heading.

Desflurane (Potential for additive effects). Products include:
Suprane Liquid for Inhalation ... 770

Dezocine (Potential for additive effects).
No products indexed under this heading.

Diazepam (Potential for additive effects). Products include:
Diastat Rectal Delivery System ... 3344
Valium Tablets ... 2822

Diazoxide (Sympathomimetics may reduce the effects of antihypertensives). Products include:
Hyperstat I.V. Injection ... 3031

Diltiazem Hydrochloride (Sympathomimetics may reduce the effects of antihypertensives). Products include:
Cardizem LA Extended Release Tablets ... 1699
Tiazac Capsules ... 1204

Doxazosin Mesylate (Sympathomimetics may reduce the effects of antihypertensives).
No products indexed under this heading.

Droperidol (Potential for additive effects).
No products indexed under this heading.

Enalapril Maleate (Sympathomimetics may reduce the effects of antihypertensives). Products include:
Vaseretic Tablets ... 2073
Vasotec I.V. Injection ... 2076

Enalaprilat (Sympathomimetics may reduce the effects of antihypertensives).
No products indexed under this heading.

Enflurane (Potential for additive effects).
No products indexed under this heading.

Eprosartan Mesylate (Sympathomimetics may reduce the effects of antihypertensives). Products include:
Teveten Tablets ... 1707
Teveten HCT Tablets ... 1710

Esmolol Hydrochloride (Sympathomimetics may reduce the effects of antihypertensives). Products include:
Brevibloc Concentrate ... 766
Brevibloc Injection ... 766
Brevibloc Double Strength Injection ... 766
Brevibloc Premixed Injection ... 766
Brevibloc Double Strength Premixed Injection ... 766

Estazolam (Potential for additive effects). Products include:
ProSom Tablets ... 512

Ethanol (Potential for additive effects).
No products indexed under this heading.

Ethchlorvynol (Potential for additive effects).
No products indexed under this heading.

Ethinamate (Potential for additive effects).
No products indexed under this heading.

Ethyl Alcohol (Potential for additive effects).
No products indexed under this heading.

Felodipine (Sympathomimetics may reduce the effects of antihypertensives). Products include:
Plendil Extended-Release Tablets ... 651

Fentanyl (Potential for additive effects). Products include:
Duragesic Transdermal System ... 2448

Fentanyl Citrate (Potential for additive effects). Products include:
Actiq ... 993

Fluphenazine Decanoate (Potential for additive effects).
No products indexed under this heading.

Fluphenazine Enanthate (Potential for additive effects).
No products indexed under this heading.

Fluphenazine Hydrochloride (Potential for additive effects).
No products indexed under this heading.

Flurazepam Hydrochloride (Potential for additive effects). Products include:
Dalmane Capsules ... 3343

Fosinopril Sodium (Sympathomimetics may reduce the effects of antihypertensives).
No products indexed under this heading.

Furosemide (Sympathomimetics may reduce the effects of antihypertensives). Products include:
Furosemide Tablets ... 2117

Glutethimide (Potential for additive effects).
No products indexed under this heading.

Guanabenz Acetate (Sympathomimetics may reduce the effects of antihypertensives).
No products indexed under this heading.

Guanethidine Monosulfate (Sympathomimetics may reduce the effects of antihypertensives).
No products indexed under this heading.

Haloperidol (Potential for additive effects).
No products indexed under this heading.

Haloperidol Decanoate (Potential for additive effects).
No products indexed under this heading.

Hydralazine Hydrochloride (Sympathomimetics may reduce the effects of antihypertensives). Products include:
BiDil Tablets ... 2161

Hydrochlorothiazide (Sympathomimetics may reduce the effects of antihypertensives). Products include:
Aldoril Tablets ... 1884
Atacand HCT ... 637
Avalide Tablets ... 2889
Avalide Tablets ... 922
Benicar HCT Tablets ... 2852
Diovan HCT Tablets ... 2195
Dyazide Capsules ... 1389
Hyzaar ... 1964
Lotensin HCT Tablets ... 2235
Maxzide ... 2150
Micardis HCT Tablets ... 886
Moduretic Tablets ... 2003
Prinzide Tablets ... 2033
Teveten HCT Tablets ... 1710
Timolide Tablets ... 2056
Uniretic Tablets ... 3114
Vaseretic Tablets ... 2073
Zestoretic Tablets ... 701

Hydrocodone Bitartrate (Potential for additive effects). Products include:
Hycodan ... 1104
Hycomine Compound Tablets ... 1105
Hycotuss Expectorant Syrup ... 1106
Lortab ... 3315
Lortab Elixir ... 3312
Vicodin Tablets ... 530
Vicodin ES Tablets ... 531
Vicodin HP Tablets ... 532
Vicoprofen Tablets ... 533
Zydone Tablets ... 1118

Hydrocodone Polistirex (Potential for additive effects). Products include:
Tussionex Pennkinetic Extended-Release Suspension ... 3322

Hydroflumethiazide (Sympathomimetics may reduce the effects of antihypertensives).
No products indexed under this heading.

Hydromorphone Hydrochloride (Potential for additive effects). Products include:
Dilaudid ... 439
Dilaudid Oral Liquid ... 443
Dilaudid Non-Sterile Powder ... 439
Dilaudid Rectal Suppositories ... 439
Dilaudid Tablets ... 439
Dilaudid Tablets - 8 mg ... 443
Dilaudid-HP ... 441

Hydroxyzine Hydrochloride (Potential for additive effects).
No products indexed under this heading.

Indapamide (Sympathomimetics may reduce the effects of antihypertensives). Products include:
Indapamide Tablets ... 2119

Irbesartan (Sympathomimetics may reduce the effects of antihypertensives). Products include:
Avalide Tablets ... 922
Avalide Tablets ... 2889
Avapro Tablets ... 925
Avapro Tablets ... 2886

Isocarboxazid (MAO inhibitors may enhance the effects of phenylephrine; concurrent and/or sequential use is contraindicated; MAO inhibitors prolong and intensify the anticholinergic effects of antihistamines).
No products indexed under this heading.

Isoflurane (Potential for additive effects).
No products indexed under this heading.

Isradipine (Sympathomimetics may reduce the effects of antihypertensives). Products include:
DynaCirc CR Tablets ... 2726

Ketamine Hydrochloride (Potential for additive effects).
No products indexed under this heading.

Labetalol Hydrochloride (Sympathomimetics may reduce the effects of antihypertensives).
No products indexed under this heading.

IMPORTANT NOTE: Always consult each drug listing in the patient's regimen for possible interactions.

Levomethadyl Acetate Hydrochloride (Potential for additive effects).
No products indexed under this heading.

Levorphanol Tartrate (Potential for additive effects).
No products indexed under this heading.

Lisinopril (Sympathomimetics may reduce the effects of antihypertensives). Products include:
Prinivil Tablets 2029
Prinzide Tablets 2033
Zestoretic Tablets 701
Zestril Tablets 704

Lorazepam (Potential for additive effects).
No products indexed under this heading.

Losartan Potassium (Sympathomimetics may reduce the effects of antihypertensives). Products include:
Cozaar Tablets 1913
Hyzaar 1964

Loxapine Hydrochloride (Potential for additive effects).
No products indexed under this heading.

Loxapine Succinate (Potential for additive effects).
No products indexed under this heading.

Mecamylamine Hydrochloride (Sympathomimetics may reduce the effects of antihypertensives). Products include:
Inversine Tablets 3286

Meperidine Hydrochloride (Potential for additive effects).
No products indexed under this heading.

Mephobarbital (Potential for additive effects). Products include:
Mebaral Tablets, USP 2483

Meprobamate (Potential for additive effects).
No products indexed under this heading.

Mesoridazine Besylate (Potential for additive effects).
No products indexed under this heading.

Methadone Hydrochloride (Potential for additive effects).
No products indexed under this heading.

Methohexital Sodium (Potential for additive effects).
No products indexed under this heading.

Methotrimeprazine (Potential for additive effects).
No products indexed under this heading.

Methoxyflurane (Potential for additive effects).
No products indexed under this heading.

Methyclothiazide (Sympathomimetics may reduce the effects of antihypertensives).
No products indexed under this heading.

Methyldopa (Sympathomimetics may reduce the effects of antihypertensives). Products include:
Aldoclor Tablets 1881
Aldoril Tablets 1884

Methyldopate Hydrochloride (Sympathomimetics may reduce the effects of antihypertensives).
No products indexed under this heading.

Metolazone (Sympathomimetics may reduce the effects of antihypertensives).
No products indexed under this heading.

Metoprolol Succinate (Sympathomimetics may reduce the effects of antihypertensives). Products include:
Toprol-XL Tablets 660

Metoprolol Tartrate (Sympathomimetics may reduce the effects of antihypertensives).
No products indexed under this heading.

Metyrosine (Sympathomimetics may reduce the effects of antihypertensives). Products include:
Demser Capsules 1933

Mibefradil Dihydrochloride (Sympathomimetics may reduce the effects of antihypertensives).
No products indexed under this heading.

Midazolam Hydrochloride (Potential for additive effects).
No products indexed under this heading.

Minoxidil (Sympathomimetics may reduce the effects of antihypertensives). Products include:
Men's Rogaine Extra Strength Topical Solution, Ocean Rush Scent and Original Unscented .... ▣706
Women's Rogaine Topical Solution, Spring Bloom Scent and Original Unscented .... ▣707

Moclobemide (MAO inhibitors may enhance the effects of phenylephrine; concurrent and/or sequential use is contraindicated; MAO inhibitors prolong and intensify the anticholinergic effects of antihistamines).
No products indexed under this heading.

Moexipril Hydrochloride (Sympathomimetics may reduce the effects of antihypertensives). Products include:
Uniretic Tablets 3114
Univasc Tablets 3118

Molindone Hydrochloride (Potential for additive effects). Products include:
Moban Tablets 1108

Morphine Sulfate (Potential for additive effects). Products include:
Avinza Capsules 1714
Kadian Capsules 572
MS Contin Tablets 2703

Nadolol (Sympathomimetics may reduce the effects of antihypertensives). Products include:
Nadolol Tablets 2121

Nicardipine Hydrochloride (Sympathomimetics may reduce the effects of antihypertensives). Products include:
Cardene I.V. 1129

Nifedipine (Sympathomimetics may reduce the effects of antihypertensives). Products include:
Adalat CC Tablets 2978

Nisoldipine (Sympathomimetics may reduce the effects of antihypertensives). Products include:
Sular Tablets 1163

Nitroglycerin (Sympathomimetics may reduce the effects of antihypertensives). Products include:
Nitro-Dur Transdermal Infusion System 3060
Nitrolingual Pumpspray 1161

Olanzapine (Potential for additive effects). Products include:
Symbyax Capsules 1788
Zyprexa Tablets 1798
Zyprexa IntraMuscular 1798
Zyprexa ZYDIS Orally Disintegrating Tablets 1798

Oxazepam (Potential for additive effects).
No products indexed under this heading.

Oxycodone Hydrochloride (Potential for additive effects). Products include:
Combunox Tablets 1183
OxyContin Tablets 2699
OxyFast Oral Concentrate Solution 2704
OxyIR Capsules 2704
Percocet Tablets 1114
Percodan Tablets 1115

Pargyline Hydrochloride (MAO inhibitors may enhance the effects of phenylephrine; concurrent and/or sequential use is contraindicated; MAO inhibitors prolong and intensify the anticholinergic effects of antihistamines).
No products indexed under this heading.

Penbutolol Sulfate (Sympathomimetics may reduce the effects of antihypertensives).
No products indexed under this heading.

Pentobarbital Sodium (Potential for additive effects). Products include:
Nembutal Sodium Solution, USP 2484

Perindopril Erbumine (Sympathomimetics may reduce the effects of antihypertensives). Products include:
Aceon Tablets (2 mg, 4 mg, 8 mg) 3191

Perphenazine (Potential for additive effects).
No products indexed under this heading.

Phenelzine Sulfate (MAO inhibitors may enhance the effects of phenylephrine; concurrent and/or sequential use is contraindicated; MAO inhibitors prolong and intensify the anticholinergic effects of antihistamines).
No products indexed under this heading.

Phenobarbital (Potential for additive effects).
No products indexed under this heading.

Phenoxybenzamine Hydrochloride (Sympathomimetics may reduce the effects of antihypertensives). Products include:
Dibenzyline Capsules 3390

Phentolamine Mesylate (Sympathomimetics may reduce the effects of antihypertensives).
No products indexed under this heading.

Pindolol (Sympathomimetics may reduce the effects of antihypertensives).
No products indexed under this heading.

Polythiazide (Sympathomimetics may reduce the effects of antihypertensives).
No products indexed under this heading.

Prazepam (Potential for additive effects).
No products indexed under this heading.

Prazosin Hydrochloride (Sympathomimetics may reduce the effects of antihypertensives).
No products indexed under this heading.

Procarbazine Hydrochloride (MAO inhibitors may enhance the effects of phenylephrine; concurrent and/or sequential use is contraindicated; MAO inhibitors prolong and intensify the anticholinergic effects of antihistamines). Products include:
Matulane Capsules 3188

Prochlorperazine (Potential for additive effects).
No products indexed under this heading.

Promethazine Hydrochloride (Potential for additive effects). Products include:
Phenergan 3438

Propofol (Potential for additive effects). Products include:
Diprivan Injectable Emulsion 676

Propoxyphene Hydrochloride (Potential for additive effects).
No products indexed under this heading.

Propoxyphene Napsylate (Potential for additive effects). Products include:
Darvocet A 500 Tablets 3497

Propranolol Hydrochloride (Sympathomimetics may reduce the effects of antihypertensives). Products include:
Inderal LA Long-Acting Capsules 3421
InnoPran XL Capsules 2728

Quazepam (Potential for additive effects).
No products indexed under this heading.

Quetiapine Fumarate (Potential for additive effects). Products include:
Seroquel Tablets 691

Quinapril Hydrochloride (Sympathomimetics may reduce the effects of antihypertensives).
No products indexed under this heading.

Ramipril (Sympathomimetics may reduce the effects of antihypertensives). Products include:
Altace Capsules 1673

Rauwolfia Serpentina (Sympathomimetics may reduce the effects of antihypertensives).
No products indexed under this heading.

Remifentanil Hydrochloride (Potential for additive effects).
No products indexed under this heading.

Rescinnamine (Sympathomimetics may reduce the effects of antihypertensives).
No products indexed under this heading.

Reserpine (Sympathomimetics may reduce the effects of antihypertensives).
No products indexed under this heading.

Risperidone (Potential for additive effects). Products include:
Risperdal Consta Long-Acting Injection 1664
Risperdal M-Tab Orally Disintegrating Tablets 1658
Risperdal 1658

Secobarbital Sodium (Potential for additive effects).
No products indexed under this heading.

Selegiline Hydrochloride (MAO inhibitors may enhance the effects of phenylephrine; concurrent and/or sequential use is contraindicated;

MAO inhibitors prolong and intensify the anticholinergic effects of antihistamines). Products include:
Eldepryl Capsules 3209

Sevoflurane (Potential for additive effects). Products include:
Ultane Liquid for Inhalation 526

Sodium Nitroprusside (Sympathomimetics may reduce the effects of antihypertensives).
No products indexed under this heading.

Sodium Oxybate (Potential for additive effects).
No products indexed under this heading.

Sotalol Hydrochloride (Sympathomimetics may reduce the effects of antihypertensives).
No products indexed under this heading.

Spirapril Hydrochloride (Sympathomimetics may reduce the effects of antihypertensives).
No products indexed under this heading.

Sufentanil Citrate (Potential for additive effects).
No products indexed under this heading.

Telmisartan (Sympathomimetics may reduce the effects of antihypertensives). Products include:
Micardis Tablets 884
Micardis HCT Tablets 886

Temazepam (Potential for additive effects).
No products indexed under this heading.

Terazosin Hydrochloride (Sympathomimetics may reduce the effects of antihypertensives). Products include:
Hytrin Capsules 469

Thiamylal Sodium (Potential for additive effects).
No products indexed under this heading.

Thioridazine Hydrochloride (Potential for additive effects). Products include:
Thioridazine Hydrochloride Tablets 2122

Thiothixene (Potential for additive effects). Products include:
Thiothixene Capsules 2124

Timolol Maleate (Sympathomimetics may reduce the effects of antihypertensives). Products include:
Blocadren Tablets 1891
Cosopt Sterile Ophthalmic Solution 1910
Timolide Tablets 2056
Timoptic in Ocudose 2061
Timoptic Sterile Ophthalmic Solution 2058
Timoptic-XE Sterile Ophthalmic Gel Forming Solution 2062

Torsemide (Sympathomimetics may reduce the effects of antihypertensives).
No products indexed under this heading.

Trandolapril (Sympathomimetics may reduce the effects of antihypertensives). Products include:
Mavik Tablets 482
Tarka Tablets 519

Tranylcypromine Sulfate (MAO inhibitors may enhance the effects of phenylephrine; concurrent and/or sequential use is contraindicated; MAO inhibitors prolong and intensify the anticholinergic effects of antihistamines). Products include:
Parnate Tablets 1499

Triazolam (Potential for additive effects).
No products indexed under this heading.

Trifluoperazine Hydrochloride (Potential for additive effects).
No products indexed under this heading.

Trimethaphan Camsylate (Sympathomimetics may reduce the effects of antihypertensives).
No products indexed under this heading.

Valsartan (Sympathomimetics may reduce the effects of antihypertensives). Products include:
Diovan HCT Tablets 2195
Diovan Tablets 2191

Verapamil Hydrochloride (Sympathomimetics may reduce the effects of antihypertensives). Products include:
Covera-HS Tablets 3135
Tarka Tablets 519
Verelan PM Capsules 3120

Zaleplon (Potential for additive effects). Products include:
Sonata Capsules 1686

Ziprasidone Hydrochloride (Potential for additive effects). Products include:
Geodon Capsules 2514

Zolpidem Tartrate (Potential for additive effects). Products include:
Ambien Tablets 2867

Food Interactions

Alcohol (Antihistamines have additive effects with alcohol).

ALAMAST OPHTHALMIC SOLUTION

(Pemirolast Potassium) 3371
None cited in PDR database.

ALAVERT ALLERGY & SINUS D-12 HOUR TABLETS

(Loratadine, Pseudoephedrine Sulfate) 743
May interact with monoamine oxidase inhibitors. Compounds in these categories include:

Isocarboxazid (Do not use while taking, or for two weeks after stopping, MAO inhibitors).
No products indexed under this heading.

Moclobemide (Do not use while taking, or for two weeks after stopping, MAO inhibitors).
No products indexed under this heading.

Pargyline Hydrochloride (Do not use while taking, or for two weeks after stopping, MAO inhibitors).
No products indexed under this heading.

Phenelzine Sulfate (Do not use while taking, or for two weeks after stopping, MAO inhibitors).
No products indexed under this heading.

Procarbazine Hydrochloride (Do not use while taking, or for two weeks after stopping, MAO inhibitors). Products include:
Matulane Capsules 3188

Selegiline Hydrochloride (Do not use while taking, or for two weeks after stopping, MAO inhibitors). Products include:
Eldepryl Capsules 3209

Tranylcypromine Sulfate (Do not use while taking, or for two weeks after stopping, MAO inhibitors). Products include:
Parnate Tablets 1499

ALAVERT ORALLY DISINTEGRATING TABLETS

(Loratadine) 743
None cited in PDR database.

ALAVERT SWALLOW TABLETS

(Loratadine) 743
None cited in PDR database.

ALBALON OPHTHALMIC SOLUTION

(Naphazoline Hydrochloride) .... ⊙216
May interact with monoamine oxidase inhibitors, tricyclic antidepressants, and certain other agents. Compounds in these categories include:

Amitriptyline Hydrochloride (May potentiate the pressor effect of naphazoline).
No products indexed under this heading.

Amoxapine (May potentiate the pressor effect of naphazoline).
No products indexed under this heading.

Clomipramine Hydrochloride (May potentiate the pressor effect of naphazoline).
No products indexed under this heading.

Desipramine Hydrochloride (May potentiate the pressor effect of naphazoline).
No products indexed under this heading.

Doxepin Hydrochloride (May potentiate the pressor effect of naphazoline).
No products indexed under this heading.

Imipramine Hydrochloride (May potentiate the pressor effect of naphazoline).
No products indexed under this heading.

Imipramine Pamoate (May potentiate the pressor effect of naphazoline).
No products indexed under this heading.

Isocarboxazid (Severe hypertensive crisis).
No products indexed under this heading.

Maprotiline Hydrochloride (May potentiate the pressor effect of naphazoline).
No products indexed under this heading.

Moclobemide (Severe hypertensive crisis).
No products indexed under this heading.

Nortriptyline Hydrochloride (May potentiate the pressor effect of naphazoline).
No products indexed under this heading.

Pargyline Hydrochloride (Severe hypertensive crisis).
No products indexed under this heading.

Phenelzine Sulfate (Severe hypertensive crisis).
No products indexed under this heading.

Procarbazine Hydrochloride (Severe hypertensive crisis). Products include:
Matulane Capsules 3188

Protriptyline Hydrochloride (May potentiate the pressor effect of naphazoline). Products include:
Vivactil Tablets 2350

Selegiline Hydrochloride (Severe hypertensive crisis). Products include:
Eldepryl Capsules 3209

Tranylcypromine Sulfate (Severe hypertensive crisis). Products include:
Parnate Tablets 1499

Trimipramine Maleate (May potentiate the pressor effect of naphazoline). Products include:
Surmontil Capsules 2347

ALBENZA TABLETS

(Albendazole) 1310
May interact with:

Cimetidine (Co-administration has resulted in increased albendazole sulfoxide concentrations in bile and cystic fluid in hydatid cyst). Products include:
Tagamet HB 200 Tablets 637
Tagamet Tablets 1547

Cimetidine Hydrochloride (Co-administration has resulted in increased albendazole sulfoxide concentrations in bile and cystic fluid in hydatid cyst).
No products indexed under this heading.

Dexamethasone (Co-administration has resulted in higher steady-state trough concentrations of albendazole sulfoxide). Products include:
Ciprodex Otic Suspension 555
Decadron Tablets 1929
TobraDex Ophthalmic Ointment 558
TobraDex Ophthalmic Suspension 558

Dexamethasone Acetate (Co-administration has resulted in higher steady-state trough concentrations of albendazole sulfoxide).
No products indexed under this heading.

Dexamethasone Sodium Phosphate (Co-administration has resulted in higher steady-state trough concentrations of albendazole sulfoxide). Products include:
Decadron Phosphate Injection 1931

Praziquantel (Co-administration has resulted in increased mean maximum plasma concentration and area under the curve of albendazole sulfoxide). Products include:
Biltricide Tablets 2990

Food Interactions

Diet, high-lipid (Oral bioavailability appears to be enhanced when albendazole is co-administered with a fatty meal).

ALDARA CREAM, 5%

(Imiquimod) 1814
None cited in PDR database.

ALDOCLOR TABLETS
(Chlorothiazide, Methyldopa) 1881
May interact with antihypertensives, barbiturates, corticosteroids, general anesthetics, cardiac glycosides, oral hypoglycemic agents, insulin, lithium preparations, monoamine oxidase inhibitors, narcotic analgesics, non-steroidal anti-inflammatory agents, and certain other agents. Compounds in these categories include:

Acarbose (Dosage adjustment of the antidiabetic drug may be required). Products include:
Precose Tablets 776

Acebutolol Hydrochloride (Potentiation of antihypertensive effect).
No products indexed under this heading.

ACTH (Hypokalemia may result).
No products indexed under this heading.

Alfentanil Hydrochloride (Aggravates orthostatic hypotension).
No products indexed under this heading.

Amlodipine Besylate (Potentiation of antihypertensive effect). Products include:
Caduet Tablets 2507
Lotrel Capsules 2238
Norvasc Tablets 2529

Aprobarbital (Aggravates orthostatic hypotension).
No products indexed under this heading.

Atenolol (Potentiation of antihypertensive effect). Products include:
Tenormin I.V. Injection 698
Tenormin Tablets 695

Benazepril Hydrochloride (Potentiation of antihypertensive effect). Products include:
Lotensin Tablets 2232
Lotensin HCT Tablets 2235
Lotrel Capsules 2238

Bendroflumethiazide (Potentiation of antihypertensive effect).
No products indexed under this heading.

Betamethasone Acetate (Hypokalemia may result).
No products indexed under this heading.

Betamethasone Sodium Phosphate (Hypokalemia may result).
No products indexed under this heading.

Betaxolol Hydrochloride (Potentiation of antihypertensive effect). Products include:
Betoptic S Ophthalmic Suspension.................................. 554

Bisoprolol Fumarate (Potentiation of antihypertensive effect).
No products indexed under this heading.

Buprenorphine Hydrochloride (Aggravates orthostatic hypotension). Products include:
Buprenex Injectable 2718
Suboxone Tablets 2719
Subutex Tablets 2719

Butabarbital (Aggravates orthostatic hypotension).
No products indexed under this heading.

Butalbital (Aggravates orthostatic hypotension). Products include:
Sedapap Tablets 50 mg/650 mg 2098

Candesartan Cilexetil (Potentiation of antihypertensive effect). Products include:
Atacand Tablets 634
Atacand HCT 637

Captopril (Potentiation of antihypertensive effect). Products include:
Captopril Tablets 2114

Carteolol Hydrochloride (Potentiation of antihypertensive effect). Products include:
Carteolol Hydrochloride Ophthalmic Solution USP, 1%....... ⊙246

Celecoxib (May result in reduced diuretic effect). Products include:
Celebrex Capsules 3130

Chlorothiazide Sodium (Potentiation of antihypertensive effect). Products include:
Diuril Sodium Intravenous 1934

Chlorpropamide (Dosage adjustment of the antidiabetic drug may be required).
No products indexed under this heading.

Chlorthalidone (Potentiation of antihypertensive effect). Products include:
Clorpres Tablets 2139

Cholestyramine (Cholestyramine resin has the potential of binding thiazide diuretics and reducing absorption from the gastrointestinal tract).
No products indexed under this heading.

Clonidine (Potentiation of antihypertensive effect). Products include:
Catapres-TTS 875

Clonidine Hydrochloride (Potentiation of antihypertensive effect). Products include:
Catapres Tablets 874
Clorpres Tablets 2139

Codeine Phosphate (Aggravates orthostatic hypotension). Products include:
Tylenol with Codeine 2461

Colestipol Hydrochloride (Colestipole resin has the potential of binding thiazide diuretics and reducing absorption from the gastrointestinal tract).
No products indexed under this heading.

Cortisone Acetate (Hypokalemia may result).
No products indexed under this heading.

Deserpidine (Potentiation of antihypertensive effect).
No products indexed under this heading.

Deslanoside (Thiazide-induced hypokalemia may cause cardiac arrhythmia and may also sensitize or exaggerate the response of the heart to the toxic effects of digitalis).
No products indexed under this heading.

Dexamethasone (Hypokalemia may result). Products include:
Ciprodex Otic Suspension 555
Decadron Tablets 1929
TobraDex Ophthalmic Ointment 558
TobraDex Ophthalmic Suspension ... 558

Dexamethasone Acetate (Hypokalemia may result).
No products indexed under this heading.

Dexamethasone Sodium Phosphate (Hypokalemia may result). Products include:
Decadron Phosphate Injection 1931

Dezocine (Aggravates orthostatic hypotension).
No products indexed under this heading.

Diazoxide (Potentiation of antihypertensive effect). Products include:
Hyperstat I.V. Injection 3031

Diclofenac Potassium (May result in reduced diuretic effect). Products include:
Cataflam Tablets 2173

Diclofenac Sodium (May result in reduced diuretic effect). Products include:
Arthrotec Tablets 3126
Voltaren Ophthalmic Solution 2300
Voltaren Tablets 2298
Voltaren-XR Tablets 2301

Digitalis Glycoside Preparations (Thiazide-induced hypokalemia may cause cardiac arrhythmia and may also sensitize or exaggerate the response of the heart to the toxic effects of digitalis).
No products indexed under this heading.

Digitoxin (Thiazide-induced hypokalemia may cause cardiac arrhythmia and may also sensitize or exaggerate the response of the heart to the toxic effects of digitalis).
No products indexed under this heading.

Digoxin (Thiazide-induced hypokalemia may cause cardiac arrhythmia and may also sensitize or exaggerate the response of the heart to the toxic effects of digitalis). Products include:
Digitek Tablets 2146
Lanoxicaps Capsules 1458
Lanoxin Injection 1462
Lanoxin Tablets 1468
Lanoxin Injection Pediatric 1465

Diltiazem Hydrochloride (Potentiation of antihypertensive effect). Products include:
Cardizem LA Extended Release Tablets....................................... 1699
Tiazac Capsules 1204

Doxazosin Mesylate (Potentiation of antihypertensive effect).
No products indexed under this heading.

Enalapril Maleate (Potentiation of antihypertensive effect). Products include:
Vaseretic Tablets 2073
Vasotec I.V. Injection 2076

Enalaprilat (Potentiation of antihypertensive effect).
No products indexed under this heading.

Enflurane (May require reduced dose of anesthetics).
No products indexed under this heading.

Eprosartan Mesylate (Potentiation of antihypertensive effect). Products include:
Teveten Tablets 1707
Teveten HCT Tablets 1710

Esmolol Hydrochloride (Potentiation of antihypertensive effect). Products include:
Brevibloc Concentrate 766
Brevibloc Injection 766
Brevibloc Double Strength Injection.. 766
Brevibloc Premixed Injection 766
Brevibloc Double Strength Premixed Injection........................ 766

Etodolac (May result in reduced diuretic effect).
No products indexed under this heading.

Felodipine (Potentiation of antihypertensive effect). Products include:
Plendil Extended-Release Tablets 651

Fenoprofen Calcium (May result in reduced diuretic effect). Products include:
Nalfon Capsules 2504

Fentanyl (Aggravates orthostatic hypotension). Products include:
Duragesic Transdermal System 2448

Fentanyl Citrate (Aggravates orthostatic hypotension). Products include:
Actiq 993

Ferrous Gluconate (Co-administration results in a decrease in the bioavailability of methyldopa; this may adversely affect blood pressure control in patients treated with methlydopa; concurrent use is not recommended).
No products indexed under this heading.

Ferrous Sulfate (Co-administration results in a decrease in the bioavailability of methyldopa; this may adversely affect blood pressure control in patients treated with methyldopa; concurrent use is not recommended). Products include:
Feosol Tablets 1629
Slow Fe Iron Tablets .... ▣772
Slow Fe with Folic Acid Tablets .... ▣773

Fludrocortisone Acetate (Hypokalemia may result).
No products indexed under this heading.

Flurbiprofen (May result in reduced diuretic effect).
No products indexed under this heading.

Fosinopril Sodium (Potentiation of antihypertensive effect).
No products indexed under this heading.

Furosemide (Potentiation of antihypertensive effect). Products include:
Furosemide Tablets 2117

Glimepiride (Dosage adjustment of the antidiabetic drug may be required). Products include:
Amaryl Tablets 2864

Glipizide (Dosage adjustment of the antidiabetic drug may be required).
No products indexed under this heading.

Glyburide (Dosage adjustment of the antidiabetic drug may be required).
No products indexed under this heading.

Guanabenz Acetate (Potentiation of antihypertensive effect).
No products indexed under this heading.

Guanethidine Monosulfate (Potentiation of antihypertensive effect).
No products indexed under this heading.

Hydralazine Hydrochloride (Potentiation of antihypertensive effect). Products include:
BiDil Tablets 2161

Hydrochlorothiazide (Potentiation of antihypertensive effect). Products include:
Aldoril Tablets 1884
Atacand HCT 637
Avalide Tablets 2889
Avalide Tablets 922
Benicar HCT Tablets 2852
Diovan HCT Tablets 2195
Dyazide Capsules 1389
Hyzaar 1964
Lotensin HCT Tablets 2235
Maxzide 2150
Micardis HCT Tablets 886
Moduretic Tablets 2003
Prinzide Tablets 2033
Teveten HCT Tablets 1710
Timolide Tablets 2056
Uniretic Tablets 3114
Vaseretic Tablets 2073

Zestoretic Tablets 701

Hydrocodone Bitartrate (Aggravates orthostatic hypotension). Products include:
Hycodan 1104
Hycomine Compound Tablets 1105
Hycotuss Expectorant Syrup 1106
Lortab 3315
Lortab Elixir 3312
Vicodin Tablets 530
Vicodin ES Tablets 531
Vicodin HP Tablets 532
Vicoprofen Tablets 533
Zydone Tablets 1118

Hydrocodone Polistirex (Aggravates orthostatic hypotension). Products include:
Tussionex Pennkinetic Extended-Release Suspension 3322

Hydrocortisone (Hypokalemia may result). Products include:
Cortizone•5 Ointment ▣699
Cortizone•10 Creme ▣699
Cortizone•10 Ointment ▣699
Cortizone•10 Plus Creme ▣700
Cortizone•10 Maximum Strength Quick Shot Spray ▣700
Hydrocortone Tablets 1963
Preparation H Hydrocortisone Cream ▣748

Hydrocortisone Acetate (Hypokalemia may result). Products include:
Analpram-HC 1136
Pramosone 1139
ProctoFoam-HC 3113
Tucks Anti-Itch Ointment ▣712
U-cort 1% Cream 3289

Hydrocortisone Sodium Phosphate (Hypokalemia may result).
No products indexed under this heading.

Hydrocortisone Sodium Succinate (Hypokalemia may result).
No products indexed under this heading.

Hydroflumethiazide (Potentiation of antihypertensive effect).
No products indexed under this heading.

Hydromorphone Hydrochloride (Aggravates orthostatic hypotension). Products include:
Dilaudid 439
Dilaudid Oral Liquid 443
Dilaudid Non-Sterile Powder 439
Dilaudid Rectal Suppositories 439
Dilaudid Tablets 439
Dilaudid Tablets - 8 mg 443
Dilaudid-HP 441

Ibuprofen (May result in reduced diuretic effect). Products include:
Advil Allergy Sinus Caplets ▣737
Advil ▣737
Children's Advil Suspension ▣742
Children's Advil Chewable Tablets ▣741
Advil Cold & Sinus ▣739
Advil Flu & Body Ache Caplets ▣739
Children's Advil Cold Suspension ▣741
Infants' Advil Concentrated Drops ▣743
Junior Strength Advil Swallow Tablets ▣740
Advil Migraine Liquigels ▣740
Advil Multi-Symptom Cold Caplets ▣738
Combunox Tablets 1183
Children's Motrin Oral Suspension and Chewable Tablets 1837
Children's Motrin Cold Non-Staining Dye-Free Oral Suspension 1838
Children's Motrin Cold Oral Suspension 1838
Children's Motrin Non-Staining Dye-Free Oral Suspension 1837
Motrin Cold & Sinus Caplets 1836
Motrin IB Tablets and Caplets 1836
Infants' Motrin Concentrated Drops 1837
Infants' Motrin Non-Staining Dye-Free Drops 1837
Junior Strength Motrin Caplets and Chewable Tablets 1837
Vicoprofen Tablets 533

Indapamide (Potentiation of antihypertensive effect). Products include:
Indapamide Tablets 2119

Indomethacin (May result in reduced diuretic effect). Products include:
Indocin 1968

Indomethacin Sodium Trihydrate (May result in reduced diuretic effect). Products include:
Indocin I.V. 1973

Insulin, Human, Zinc Suspension (May alter insulin requirements). Products include:
Humulin L, 100 Units 1763
Humulin U, 100 Units 1770

Insulin, Human NPH (May alter insulin requirements). Products include:
Humulin N, 100 Units 1764
Humulin N Pen 1765
Novolin N Human Insulin 10 ml Vials 2322
Novolin N InnoLet 2322
Novolin N PenFill 3 ml Cartridges 2325
Novolin R InnoLet 2322

Insulin, Human Regular (May alter insulin requirements). Products include:
Humulin R (U-500) 1768
Humulin R, 100 Units 1767
Novolin R Human Insulin 10 ml Vials 2322
Novolin R PenFill 2325

Insulin, Human Regular and Human NPH Mixture (May alter insulin requirements). Products include:
Humulin 50/50, 100 Units 1760
Humulin 70/30 Pen 1761
Novolin 70/30 Human Insulin 10 ml Vials 2321
Novolin 70/30 InnoLet 2322
Novolin 70/30 PenFill 3 ml Cartridges 2325

Insulin, NPH (May alter insulin requirements).
No products indexed under this heading.

Insulin, Regular (May alter insulin requirements).
No products indexed under this heading.

Insulin, Zinc Crystals (May alter insulin requirements).
No products indexed under this heading.

Insulin, Zinc Suspension (May alter insulin requirements).
No products indexed under this heading.

Insulin Aspart, Human Regular (May alter insulin requirements). Products include:
NovoLog Injection 2326

Insulin glargine (May alter insulin requirements). Products include:
Lantus Injection 2925

Insulin Lispro, Human (May alter insulin requirements). Products include:
Humalog-Pen 1751
Humalog Mix 75/25-Pen 1754

Insulin Lispro Protamine, Human (May alter insulin requirements). Products include:
Humalog Mix 75/25-Pen 1754

Irbesartan (Potentiation of antihypertensive effect). Products include:
Avalide Tablets 922
Avalide Tablets 2889
Avapro Tablets 925
Avapro Tablets 2886

Isocarboxazid (Concurrent use is contraindicated).
No products indexed under this heading.

Isoflurane (May require reduced dose of anesthetics).
No products indexed under this heading.

Isradipine (Potentiation of antihypertensive effect). Products include:
DynaCirc CR Tablets 2726

Ketamine Hydrochloride (May require reduced dose of anesthetics).
No products indexed under this heading.

Ketoprofen (May result in reduced diuretic effect).
No products indexed under this heading.

Ketorolac Tromethamine (May result in reduced diuretic effect). Products include:
Acular Ophthalmic Solution 561
Acular LS Ophthalmic Solution 562

Labetalol Hydrochloride (Potentiation of antihypertensive effect).
No products indexed under this heading.

Levorphanol Tartrate (Aggravates orthostatic hypotension).
No products indexed under this heading.

Lisinopril (Potentiation of antihypertensive effect). Products include:
Prinivil Tablets 2029
Prinzide Tablets 2033
Zestoretic Tablets 701
Zestril Tablets 704

Lithium (High risk of lithium toxicity).
No products indexed under this heading.

Lithium Carbonate (High risk of lithium toxicity). Products include:
Eskalith 1406
Lithobid Tablets 1670

Lithium Citrate (High risk of lithium toxicity).
No products indexed under this heading.

Losartan Potassium (Potentiation of antihypertensive effect). Products include:
Cozaar Tablets 1913
Hyzaar 1964

Mecamylamine Hydrochloride (Potentiation of antihypertensive effect). Products include:
Inversine Tablets 3286

Meclofenamate Sodium (May result in reduced diuretic effect).
No products indexed under this heading.

Mefenamic Acid (May result in reduced diuretic effect).
No products indexed under this heading.

Meloxicam (May result in reduced diuretic effect). Products include:
Mobic Oral Suspension 893
Mobic Tablets 893

Meperidine Hydrochloride (Aggravates orthostatic hypotension).
No products indexed under this heading.

Mephobarbital (Aggravates orthostatic hypotension). Products include:
Mebaral Tablets, USP 2483

Metformin Hydrochloride (Dosage adjustment of the antidiabetic drug may be required). Products include:
ActoPlus Met Tablets 3219
Avandamet Tablets 1343
Fortamet Extended-Release Tablets 1156

Methadone Hydrochloride (Aggravates orthostatic hypotension).
No products indexed under this heading.

Methohexital Sodium (May require reduced dose of anesthetics).
No products indexed under this heading.

Methoxyflurane (May require reduced dose of anesthetics).
No products indexed under this heading.

Methyclothiazide (Potentiation of antihypertensive effect).
No products indexed under this heading.

Methyldopate Hydrochloride (Potentiation of antihypertensive effect).
No products indexed under this heading.

Methylprednisolone Acetate (Hypokalemia may result). Products include:
Depo-Medrol Injectable Suspension 2615
Depo-Medrol Single-Dose Vial 2617

Methylprednisolone Sodium Succinate (Hypokalemia may result).
No products indexed under this heading.

Metolazone (Potentiation of antihypertensive effect).
No products indexed under this heading.

Metoprolol Succinate (Potentiation of antihypertensive effect). Products include:
Toprol-XL Tablets 660

Metoprolol Tartrate (Potentiation of antihypertensive effect).
No products indexed under this heading.

Metyrosine (Potentiation of antihypertensive effect). Products include:
Demser Capsules 1933

Mibefradil Dihydrochloride (Potentiation of antihypertensive effect).
No products indexed under this heading.

Miglitol (Dosage adjustment of the antidiabetic drug may be required).
No products indexed under this heading.

Minoxidil (Potentiation of antihypertensive effect). Products include:
Men's Rogaine Extra Strength Topical Solution, Ocean Rush Scent and Original Unscented ▣706
Women's Rogaine Topical Solution, Spring Bloom Scent and Original Unscented ▣707

Moclobemide (Concurrent use is contraindicated).
No products indexed under this heading.

Moexipril Hydrochloride (Potentiation of antihypertensive effect). Products include:
Uniretic Tablets 3114
Univasc Tablets 3118

Morphine Sulfate (Aggravates orthostatic hypotension). Products include:
Avinza Capsules 1714
Kadian Capsules 572
MS Contin Tablets 2703

Nabumetone (May result in reduced diuretic effect). Products include:
- Relafen Tablets ... 1523

Nadolol (Potentiation of antihypertensive effect). Products include:
- Nadolol Tablets ... 2121

Naproxen (May result in reduced diuretic effect). Products include:
- EC-Naprosyn Delayed-Release Tablets ... 2769
- Naprosyn Suspension ... 2769
- Naprosyn Tablets ... 2769
- Prevacid NapraPAC ... 3277

Naproxen Sodium (May result in reduced diuretic effect). Products include:
- Aleve Tablets, Caplets and Gelcaps ... ◼◻605
- Anaprox Tablets ... 2769
- Anaprox DS Tablets ... 2769

Nicardipine Hydrochloride (Potentiation of antihypertensive effect). Products include:
- Cardene I.V. ... 1129

Nifedipine (Potentiation of antihypertensive effect). Products include:
- Adalat CC Tablets ... 2978

Nisoldipine (Potentiation of antihypertensive effect). Products include:
- Sular Tablets ... 1163

Nitroglycerin (Potentiation of antihypertensive effect). Products include:
- Nitro-Dur Transdermal Infusion System ... 3060
- Nitrolingual Pumpspray ... 1161

Norepinephrine Bitartrate (May decrease arterial responsiveness to norepinephrine).
No products indexed under this heading.

Oxaprozin (May result in reduced diuretic effect).
No products indexed under this heading.

Oxycodone Hydrochloride (Aggravates orthostatic hypotension). Products include:
- Combunox Tablets ... 1183
- OxyContin Tablets ... 2699
- OxyFast Oral Concentrate Solution ... 2704
- OxyIR Capsules ... 2704
- Percocet Tablets ... 1114
- Percodan Tablets ... 1115

Pargyline Hydrochloride (Concurrent use is contraindicated).
No products indexed under this heading.

Penbutolol Sulfate (Potentiation of antihypertensive effect).
No products indexed under this heading.

Pentobarbital Sodium (Aggravates orthostatic hypotension). Products include:
- Nembutal Sodium Solution, USP ... 2484

Perindopril Erbumine (Potentiation of antihypertensive effect). Products include:
- Aceon Tablets (2 mg, 4 mg, 8 mg) ... 3191

Phenelzine Sulfate (Concurrent use is contraindicated).
No products indexed under this heading.

Phenobarbital (Aggravates orthostatic hypotension).
No products indexed under this heading.

Phenoxybenzamine Hydrochloride (Potentiation of antihypertensive effect). Products include:
- Dibenzyline Capsules ... 3390

Phentolamine Mesylate (Potentiation of antihypertensive effect).
No products indexed under this heading.

Phenylbutazone (May result in reduced diuretic effect).
No products indexed under this heading.

Pindolol (Potentiation of antihypertensive effect).
No products indexed under this heading.

Pioglitazone Hydrochloride (Dosage adjustment of the antidiabetic drug may be required). Products include:
- ActoPlus Met Tablets ... 3219
- Actos Tablets ... 3224

Piroxicam (May result in reduced diuretic effect).
No products indexed under this heading.

Polythiazide (Potentiation of antihypertensive effect).
No products indexed under this heading.

Prazosin Hydrochloride (Potentiation of antihypertensive effect).
No products indexed under this heading.

Prednisolone Acetate (Hypokalemia may result). Products include:
- Blephamide Ophthalmic Ointment ... 563
- Blephamide Ophthalmic Suspension ... 564
- Poly-Pred Liquifilm Ophthalmic Suspension ... ⊙231
- Pred Forte Ophthalmic Suspension ... ⊙233
- Pred Mild Sterile Ophthalmic Suspension ... ⊙236
- Pred-G Ophthalmic Suspension ... ⊙234
- Pred-G Sterile Ophthalmic Ointment ... ⊙235

Prednisolone Sodium Phosphate (Hypokalemia may result). Products include:
- Pediapred Oral Solution ... 3319

Prednisolone Tebutate (Hypokalemia may result).
No products indexed under this heading.

Prednisone (Hypokalemia may result).
No products indexed under this heading.

Procarbazine Hydrochloride (Concurrent use is contraindicated). Products include:
- Matulane Capsules ... 3188

Propofol (May require reduced dose of anesthetics). Products include:
- Diprivan Injectable Emulsion ... 676

Propoxyphene Hydrochloride (Aggravates orthostatic hypotension).
No products indexed under this heading.

Propoxyphene Napsylate (Aggravates orthostatic hypotension). Products include:
- Darvocet A 500 Tablets ... 3497

Propranolol Hydrochloride (Potentiation of antihypertensive effect). Products include:
- Inderal LA Long-Acting Capsules ... 3421
- InnoPran XL Capsules ... 2728

Quinapril Hydrochloride (Potentiation of antihypertensive effect).
No products indexed under this heading.

Ramipril (Potentiation of antihypertensive effect). Products include:
- Altace Capsules ... 1673

Rauwolfia Serpentina (Potentiation of antihypertensive effect).
No products indexed under this heading.

Remifentanil Hydrochloride (Aggravates orthostatic hypotension).
No products indexed under this heading.

Repaglinide (Dosage adjustment of the antidiabetic drug may be required). Products include:
- Prandin Tablets (0.5, 1, and 2 mg) ... 2337

Rescinnamine (Potentiation of antihypertensive effect).
No products indexed under this heading.

Reserpine (Potentiation of antihypertensive effect).
No products indexed under this heading.

Rofecoxib (May result in reduced diuretic effect).
No products indexed under this heading.

Rosiglitazone Maleate (Dosage adjustment of the antidiabetic drug may be required). Products include:
- Avandamet Tablets ... 1343
- Avandia Tablets ... 1348

Secobarbital Sodium (Aggravates orthostatic hypotension).
No products indexed under this heading.

Selegiline Hydrochloride (Concurrent use is contraindicated). Products include:
- Eldepryl Capsules ... 3209

Sevoflurane (May require reduced dose of anesthetics). Products include:
- Ultane Liquid for Inhalation ... 526

Sodium Nitroprusside (Potentiation of antihypertensive effect).
No products indexed under this heading.

Sotalol Hydrochloride (Potentiation of antihypertensive effect).
No products indexed under this heading.

Spirapril Hydrochloride (Potentiation of antihypertensive effect).
No products indexed under this heading.

Sufentanil Citrate (Aggravates orthostatic hypotension).
No products indexed under this heading.

Sulindac (May result in reduced diuretic effect). Products include:
- Clinoril Tablets ... 1899

Telmisartan (Potentiation of antihypertensive effect). Products include:
- Micardis Tablets ... 884
- Micardis HCT Tablets ... 886

Terazosin Hydrochloride (Potentiation of antihypertensive effect). Products include:
- Hytrin Capsules ... 469

Thiamylal Sodium (Aggravates orthostatic hypotension).
No products indexed under this heading.

Timolol Maleate (Potentiation of antihypertensive effect). Products include:
- Blocadren Tablets ... 1891
- Cosopt Sterile Ophthalmic Solution ... 1910
- Timolide Tablets ... 2056
- Timoptic in Ocudose ... 2061
- Timoptic Sterile Ophthalmic Solution ... 2058
- Timoptic-XE Sterile Ophthalmic Gel Forming Solution ... 2062

Tolazamide (Dosage adjustment of the antidiabetic drug may be required).
No products indexed under this heading.

Tolbutamide (Dosage adjustment of the antidiabetic drug may be required).
No products indexed under this heading.

Tolmetin Sodium (May result in reduced diuretic effect).
No products indexed under this heading.

Torsemide (Potentiation of antihypertensive effect).
No products indexed under this heading.

Trandolapril (Potentiation of antihypertensive effect). Products include:
- Mavik Tablets ... 482
- Tarka Tablets ... 519

Tranylcypromine Sulfate (Concurrent use is contraindicated). Products include:
- Parnate Tablets ... 1499

Triamcinolone (Hypokalemia may result).
No products indexed under this heading.

Triamcinolone Acetonide (Hypokalemia may result). Products include:
- Azmacort Inhalation Aerosol ... 1701
- Nasacort HFA Inhalation Aerosol ... 2939
- Nasacort AQ Nasal Spray ... 2937

Triamcinolone Diacetate (Hypokalemia may result).
No products indexed under this heading.

Triamcinolone Hexacetonide (Hypokalemia may result).
No products indexed under this heading.

Trimethaphan Camsylate (Potentiation of antihypertensive effect).
No products indexed under this heading.

Troglitazone (Dosage adjustment of the antidiabetic drug may be required).
No products indexed under this heading.

Tubocurarine Chloride (Increased responsiveness to tubocurarine).
No products indexed under this heading.

Valdecoxib (May result in reduced diuretic effect).
No products indexed under this heading.

Valsartan (Potentiation of antihypertensive effect). Products include:
- Diovan HCT Tablets ... 2195
- Diovan Tablets ... 2191

Verapamil Hydrochloride (Potentiation of antihypertensive effect). Products include:
- Covera-HS Tablets ... 3135
- Tarka Tablets ... 519
- Verelan PM Capsules ... 3120

Food Interactions

Alcohol (Aggravates orthostatic hypotension).

ALDORIL TABLETS

(Hydrochlorothiazide, Methyldopa) **1884**

May interact with antihypertensives, barbiturates, corticosteroids, general anesthetics, cardiac glycosides, oral hypoglycemic agents, insulin, lithium preparations, monoamine oxidase inhibitors, narcotic analgesics, non-steroidal anti-inflammatory agents, and certain other agents. Compounds in these categories include:

Acarbose (Dosage adjustment of the antidiabetic drug may be required). Products include:
- Precose Tablets 776

Acebutolol Hydrochloride (Potentiation of antihypertensive effect).
- No products indexed under this heading.

ACTH (Hypokalemia may result).
- No products indexed under this heading.

Alfentanil Hydrochloride (Aggravates orthostatic hypotension).
- No products indexed under this heading.

Amlodipine Besylate (Potentiation of antihypertensive effect). Products include:
- Caduet Tablets 2507
- Lotrel Capsules 2238
- Norvasc Tablets 2529

Aprobarbital (Aggravates orthostatic hypotension).
- No products indexed under this heading.

Atenolol (Potentiation of antihypertensive effect). Products include:
- Tenormin I.V. Injection 698
- Tenormin Tablets 695

Benazepril Hydrochloride (Potentiation of antihypertensive effect). Products include:
- Lotensin Tablets 2232
- Lotensin HCT Tablets 2235
- Lotrel Capsules 2238

Bendroflumethiazide (Potentiation of antihypertensive effect).
- No products indexed under this heading.

Betamethasone Acetate (Hypokalemia may result).
- No products indexed under this heading.

Betamethasone Sodium Phosphate (Hypokalemia may result).
- No products indexed under this heading.

Betaxolol Hydrochloride (Potentiation of antihypertensive effect). Products include:
- Betoptic S Ophthalmic Suspension 554

Bisoprolol Fumarate (Potentiation of antihypertensive effect).
- No products indexed under this heading.

Buprenorphine Hydrochloride (Aggravates orthostatic hypotension). Products include:
- Buprenex Injectable 2718
- Suboxone Tablets 2719
- Subutex Tablets 2719

Butabarbital (Aggravates orthostatic hypotension).
- No products indexed under this heading.

Butalbital (Aggravates orthostatic hypotension). Products include:
- Sedapap Tablets 50 mg/650 mg 2098

Candesartan Cilexetil (Potentiation of antihypertensive effect). Products include:
- Atacand Tablets 634
- Atacand HCT 637

Captopril (Potentiation of antihypertensive effect). Products include:
- Captopril Tablets 2114

Carteolol Hydrochloride (Potentiation of antihypertensive effect). Products include:
- Carteolol Hydrochloride Ophthalmic Solution USP, 1%....... ⊙246

Celecoxib (May result in reduced diuretic effect). Products include:
- Celebrex Capsules 3130

Chlorothiazide (Potentiation of antihypertensive effect). Products include:
- Aldoclor Tablets 1881
- Diuril Oral 1936

Chlorothiazide Sodium (Potentiation of antihypertensive effect). Products include:
- Diuril Sodium Intravenous 1934

Chlorpropamide (Dosage adjustment of the antidiabetic drug may be required).
- No products indexed under this heading.

Chlorthalidone (Potentiation of antihypertensive effect). Products include:
- Clorpres Tablets 2139

Cholestyramine (Binds the hydrochlorothiazide and reduces its absorption from gastrointestinal tract by up to 85%).
- No products indexed under this heading.

Clonidine (Potentiation of antihypertensive effect). Products include:
- Catapres-TTS 875

Clonidine Hydrochloride (Potentiation of antihypertensive effect). Products include:
- Catapres Tablets 874
- Clorpres Tablets 2139

Codeine Phosphate (Aggravates orthostatic hypotension). Products include:
- Tylenol with Codeine 2461

Colestipol Hydrochloride (Binds the hydrochlorothiazide and reduces its absorption from gastrointestinal tract by up to 43%).
- No products indexed under this heading.

Cortisone Acetate (Hypokalemia may result).
- No products indexed under this heading.

Deserpidine (Potentiation of antihypertensive effect).
- No products indexed under this heading.

Deslanoside (Hypokalemia may exaggerate cardiac toxicity of digitalis).
- No products indexed under this heading.

Dexamethasone (Hypokalemia may result). Products include:
- Ciprodex Otic Suspension 555
- Decadron Tablets 1929
- TobraDex Ophthalmic Ointment 558
- TobraDex Ophthalmic Suspension ... 558

Dexamethasone Acetate (Hypokalemia may result).
- No products indexed under this heading.

Dexamethasone Sodium Phosphate (Hypokalemia may result). Products include:
- Decadron Phosphate Injection 1931

Dezocine (Aggravates orthostatic hypotension).
- No products indexed under this heading.

Diazoxide (Potentiation of antihypertensive effect). Products include:
- Hyperstat I.V. Injection 3031

Diclofenac Potassium (May result in reduced diuretic effect). Products include:
- Cataflam Tablets 2173

Diclofenac Sodium (May result in reduced diuretic effect). Products include:
- Arthrotec Tablets 3126
- Voltaren Ophthalmic Solution 2300
- Voltaren Tablets 2298
- Voltaren-XR Tablets 2301

Digitalis Glycoside Preparations (Hypokalemia may exaggerate cardiac toxicity of digitalis).
- No products indexed under this heading.

Digitoxin (Hypokalemia may exaggerate cardiac toxicity of digitalis).
- No products indexed under this heading.

Digoxin (Hypokalemia may exaggerate cardiac toxicity of digitalis). Products include:
- Digitek Tablets 2146
- Lanoxicaps Capsules 1458
- Lanoxin Injection 1462
- Lanoxin Tablets 1468
- Lanoxin Injection Pediatric 1465

Diltiazem Hydrochloride (Potentiation of antihypertensive effect). Products include:
- Cardizem LA Extended Release Tablets 1699
- Tiazac Capsules 1204

Doxazosin Mesylate (Potentiation of antihypertensive effect).
- No products indexed under this heading.

Enalapril Maleate (Potentiation of antihypertensive effect). Products include:
- Vaseretic Tablets 2073
- Vasotec I.V. Injection 2076

Enalaprilat (Potentiation of antihypertensive effect).
- No products indexed under this heading.

Enflurane (May require reduced dose of anesthetics).
- No products indexed under this heading.

Eprosartan Mesylate (Potentiation of antihypertensive effect). Products include:
- Teveten Tablets 1707
- Teveten HCT Tablets 1710

Esmolol Hydrochloride (Potentiation of antihypertensive effect). Products include:
- Brevibloc Concentrate 766
- Brevibloc Injection 766
- Brevibloc Double Strength Injection 766
- Brevibloc Premixed Injection 766
- Brevibloc Double Strength Premixed Injection 766

Etodolac (May result in reduced diuretic effect).
- No products indexed under this heading.

Felodipine (Potentiation of antihypertensive effect). Products include:
- Plendil Extended-Release Tablets 651

Fenoprofen Calcium (May result in reduced diuretic effect). Products include:
- Nalfon Capsules 2504

Fentanyl (Aggravates orthostatic hypotension). Products include:
- Duragesic Transdermal System 2448

Fentanyl Citrate (Aggravates orthostatic hypotension). Products include:
- Actiq 993

Ferrous Gluconate (Co-administration results in a decrease in the bioavailability of methyldopa; this may adversely affect blood pressure control in patients treated with methlydopa; concurrent use is not recommended).
- No products indexed under this heading.

Ferrous Sulfate (Co-administration results in a decrease in the bioavailability of methyldopa; this may adversely affect blood pressure control in patients treated with methyldopa; concurrent use is not recommended). Products include:
- Feosol Tablets 1629
- Slow Fe Iron Tablets .... ▣772
- Slow Fe with Folic Acid Tablets .... ▣773

Fludrocortisone Acetate (Hypokalemia may result).
- No products indexed under this heading.

Flurbiprofen (May result in reduced diuretic effect).
- No products indexed under this heading.

Fosinopril Sodium (Potentiation of antihypertensive effect).
- No products indexed under this heading.

Furosemide (Potentiation of antihypertensive effect). Products include:
- Furosemide Tablets 2117

Glimepiride (Dosage adjustment of the antidiabetic drug may be required). Products include:
- Amaryl Tablets 2864

Glipizide (Dosage adjustment of the antidiabetic drug may be required).
- No products indexed under this heading.

Glyburide (Dosage adjustment of the antidiabetic drug may be required).
- No products indexed under this heading.

Guanabenz Acetate (Potentiation of antihypertensive effect).
- No products indexed under this heading.

Guanethidine Monosulfate (Potentiation of antihypertensive effect).
- No products indexed under this heading.

Hydralazine Hydrochloride (Potentiation of antihypertensive effect). Products include:
- BiDil Tablets 2161

Hydrocodone Bitartrate (Aggravates orthostatic hypotension). Products include:
- Hycodan 1104
- Hycomine Compound Tablets 1105
- Hycotuss Expectorant Syrup 1106
- Lortab 3315
- Lortab Elixir 3312
- Vicodin Tablets 530
- Vicodin ES Tablets 531
- Vicodin HP Tablets 532
- Vicoprofen Tablets 533
- Zydone Tablets 1118

Hydrocodone Polistirex (Aggravates orthostatic hypotension). Products include:
- Tussionex Pennkinetic Extended-Release Suspension 3322

Hydrocortisone (Hypokalemia may result). Products include:
- Cortizone•5 Ointment .... ▣699
- Cortizone•10 Creme .... ▣699
- Cortizone•10 Ointment .... ▣699
- Cortizone•10 Plus Creme .... ▣700
- Cortizone•10 Maximum Strength Quick Shot Spray .... ▣700
- Hydrocortone Tablets 1963

Preparation H Hydrocortisone Cream .... ▣ 748

Hydrocortisone Acetate (Hypokalemia may result). Products include:
Analpram-HC 1136
Pramosone 1139
ProctoFoam-HC 3113
Tucks Anti-Itch Ointment .... ▣ 712
U-cort 1% Cream 3289

Hydrocortisone Sodium Phosphate (Hypokalemia may result).
No products indexed under this heading.

Hydrocortisone Sodium Succinate (Hypokalemia may result).
No products indexed under this heading.

Hydroflumethiazide (Potentiation of antihypertensive effect).
No products indexed under this heading.

Hydromorphone Hydrochloride (Aggravates orthostatic hypotension). Products include:
Dilaudid 439
Dilaudid Oral Liquid 443
Dilaudid Non-Sterile Powder 439
Dilaudid Rectal Suppositories 439
Dilaudid Tablets 439
Dilaudid Tablets - 8 mg 443
Dilaudid-HP 441

Ibuprofen (May result in reduced diuretic effect). Products include:
Advil Allergy Sinus Caplets .... ▣ 737
Advil .... ▣ 737
Children's Advil Suspension .... ▣ 742
Children's Advil Chewable Tablets .. ▣ 741
Advil Cold & Sinus .... ▣ 739
Advil Flu & Body Ache Caplets .... ▣ 739
Children's Advil Cold Suspension ... ▣ 741
Infants' Advil Concentrated Drops .. ▣ 743
Junior Strength Advil Swallow Tablets .... ▣ 740
Advil Migraine Liquigels .... ▣ 740
Advil Multi-Symptom Cold Caplets .... ▣ 738
Combunox Tablets 1183
Children's Motrin Oral Suspension and Chewable Tablets 1837
Children's Motrin Cold Non-Staining Dye-Free Oral Suspension 1838
Children's Motrin Cold Oral Suspension 1838
Children's Motrin Non-Staining Dye-Free Oral Suspension 1837
Motrin Cold & Sinus Caplets 1836
Motrin IB Tablets and Caplets 1836
Infants' Motrin Concentrated Drops 1837
Infants' Motrin Non-Staining Dye-Free Drops 1837
Junior Strength Motrin Caplets and Chewable Tablets 1837
Vicoprofen Tablets 533

Indapamide (Potentiation of antihypertensive effect). Products include:
Indapamide Tablets 2119

Indomethacin (May result in reduced diuretic effect). Products include:
Indocin 1968

Indomethacin Sodium Trihydrate (May result in reduced diuretic effect). Products include:
Indocin I.V. 1973

Insulin, Human, Zinc Suspension (Insulin requirement may be altered). Products include:
Humulin L, 100 Units 1763
Humulin U, 100 Units 1770

Insulin, Human NPH (Insulin requirement may be altered). Products include:
Humulin N, 100 Units 1764
Humulin N Pen 1765
Novolin N Human Insulin 10 ml Vials 2322
Novolin N InnoLet 2322
Novolin N PenFill 3 ml Cartridges 2325
Novolin R InnoLet 2322

Insulin, Human Regular (Insulin requirement may be altered). Products include:
Humulin R (U-500) 1768
Humulin R, 100 Units 1767
Novolin R Human Insulin 10 ml Vials 2322
Novolin R PenFill 2325

Insulin, Human Regular and Human NPH Mixture (Insulin requirement may be altered). Products include:
Humulin 50/50, 100 Units 1760
Humulin 70/30 Pen 1761
Novolin 70/30 Human Insulin 10 ml Vials 2321
Novolin 70/30 InnoLet 2322
Novolin 70/30 PenFill 3 ml Cartridges 2325

Insulin, NPH (Insulin requirement may be altered).
No products indexed under this heading.

Insulin, Regular (Insulin requirement may be altered).
No products indexed under this heading.

Insulin, Zinc Crystals (Insulin requirement may be altered).
No products indexed under this heading.

Insulin, Zinc Suspension (Insulin requirement may be altered).
No products indexed under this heading.

Insulin Aspart, Human Regular (Insulin requirement may be altered). Products include:
NovoLog Injection 2326

Insulin glargine (Insulin requirement may be altered). Products include:
Lantus Injection 2925

Insulin Lispro, Human (Insulin requirement may be altered). Products include:
Humalog-Pen 1751
Humalog Mix 75/25-Pen 1754

Insulin Lispro Protamine, Human (Insulin requirement may be altered). Products include:
Humalog Mix 75/25-Pen 1754

Irbesartan (Potentiation of antihypertensive effect). Products include:
Avalide Tablets 922
Avalide Tablets 2889
Avapro Tablets 925
Avapro Tablets 2886

Isocarboxazid (Concurrent use is contraindicated).
No products indexed under this heading.

Isoflurane (May require reduced dose of anesthetics).
No products indexed under this heading.

Isradipine (Potentiation of antihypertensive effect). Products include:
DynaCirc CR Tablets 2726

Ketamine Hydrochloride (May require reduced dose of anesthetics).
No products indexed under this heading.

Ketoprofen (May result in reduced diuretic effect).
No products indexed under this heading.

Ketorolac Tromethamine (May result in reduced diuretic effect). Products include:
Acular Ophthalmic Solution 561
Acular LS Ophthalmic Solution 562

Labetalol Hydrochloride (Potentiation of antihypertensive effect).
No products indexed under this heading.

Levorphanol Tartrate (Aggravates orthostatic hypotension).
No products indexed under this heading.

Lisinopril (Potentiation of antihypertensive effect). Products include:
Prinivil Tablets 2029
Prinzide Tablets 2033
Zestoretic Tablets 701
Zestril Tablets 704

Lithium (High risk of lithium toxicity).
No products indexed under this heading.

Lithium Carbonate (High risk of lithium toxicity). Products include:
Eskalith 1406
Lithobid Tablets 1670

Lithium Citrate (High risk of lithium toxicity).
No products indexed under this heading.

Losartan Potassium (Potentiation of antihypertensive effect). Products include:
Cozaar Tablets 1913
Hyzaar 1964

Mecamylamine Hydrochloride (Potentiation of antihypertensive effect). Products include:
Inversine Tablets 3286

Meclofenamate Sodium (May result in reduced diuretic effect).
No products indexed under this heading.

Mefenamic Acid (May result in reduced diuretic effect).
No products indexed under this heading.

Meloxicam (May result in reduced diuretic effect). Products include:
Mobic Oral Suspension 893
Mobic Tablets 893

Meperidine Hydrochloride (Aggravates orthostatic hypotension).
No products indexed under this heading.

Mephobarbital (Aggravates orthostatic hypotension). Products include:
Mebaral Tablets, USP 2483

Metformin Hydrochloride (Dosage adjustment of the antidiabetic drug may be required). Products include:
ActoPlus Met Tablets 3219
Avandamet Tablets 1343
Fortamet Extended-Release Tablets 1156

Methadone Hydrochloride (Aggravates orthostatic hypotension).
No products indexed under this heading.

Methohexital Sodium (May require reduced dose of anesthetics).
No products indexed under this heading.

Methoxyflurane (May require reduced dose of anesthetics).
No products indexed under this heading.

Methyclothiazide (Potentiation of antihypertensive effect).
No products indexed under this heading.

Methyldopate Hydrochloride (Potentiation of antihypertensive effect).
No products indexed under this heading.

Methylprednisolone Acetate (Hypokalemia may result). Products include:
Depo-Medrol Injectable Suspension 2615
Depo-Medrol Single-Dose Vial 2617

Methylprednisolone Sodium Succinate (Hypokalemia may result).
No products indexed under this heading.

Metolazone (Potentiation of antihypertensive effect).
No products indexed under this heading.

Metoprolol Succinate (Potentiation of antihypertensive effect). Products include:
Toprol-XL Tablets 660

Metoprolol Tartrate (Potentiation of antihypertensive effect).
No products indexed under this heading.

Metyrosine (Potentiation of antihypertensive effect). Products include:
Demser Capsules 1933

Mibefradil Dihydrochloride (Potentiation of antihypertensive effect).
No products indexed under this heading.

Miglitol (Dosage adjustment of the antidiabetic drug may be required).
No products indexed under this heading.

Minoxidil (Potentiation of antihypertensive effect). Products include:
Men's Rogaine Extra Strength Topical Solution, Ocean Rush Scent and Original Unscented ..... ▣ 706
Women's Rogaine Topical Solution, Spring Bloom Scent and Original Unscented .... ▣ 707

Moclobemide (Concurrent use is contraindicated).
No products indexed under this heading.

Moexipril Hydrochloride (Potentiation of antihypertensive effect). Products include:
Uniretic Tablets 3114
Univasc Tablets 3118

Morphine Sulfate (Aggravates orthostatic hypotension). Products include:
Avinza Capsules 1714
Kadian Capsules 572
MS Contin Tablets 2703

Nabumetone (May result in reduced diuretic effect). Products include:
Relafen Tablets 1523

Nadolol (Potentiation of antihypertensive effect). Products include:
Nadolol Tablets 2121

Naproxen (May result in reduced diuretic effect). Products include:
EC-Naprosyn Delayed-Release Tablets 2769
Naprosyn Suspension 2769
Naprosyn Tablets 2769
Prevacid NapraPAC 3277

Naproxen Sodium (May result in reduced diuretic effect). Products include:
Aleve Tablets, Caplets and Gelcaps .... ▣ 605
Anaprox Tablets 2769
Anaprox DS Tablets 2769

Nicardipine Hydrochloride (Potentiation of antihypertensive effect). Products include:
Cardene I.V. 1129

Nifedipine (Potentiation of antihypertensive effect). Products include:
Adalat CC Tablets 2978

Nisoldipine (Potentiation of antihypertensive effect). Products include:
Sular Tablets ... 1163

Nitroglycerin (Potentiation of antihypertensive effect). Products include:
Nitro-Dur Transdermal Infusion System ... 3060
Nitrolingual Pumpspray ... 1161

Norepinephrine Bitartrate (Decreased arterial responsiveness to norepinephrine).
No products indexed under this heading.

Oxaprozin (May result in reduced diuretic effect).
No products indexed under this heading.

Oxycodone Hydrochloride (Aggravates orthostatic hypotension). Products include:
Combunox Tablets ... 1183
OxyContin Tablets ... 2699
OxyFast Oral Concentrate Solution ... 2704
OxyIR Capsules ... 2704
Percocet Tablets ... 1114
Percodan Tablets ... 1115

Pargyline Hydrochloride (Concurrent use is contraindicated).
No products indexed under this heading.

Penbutolol Sulfate (Potentiation of antihypertensive effect).
No products indexed under this heading.

Pentobarbital Sodium (Aggravates orthostatic hypotension). Products include:
Nembutal Sodium Solution, USP ... 2484

Perindopril Erbumine (Potentiation of antihypertensive effect). Products include:
Aceon Tablets (2 mg, 4 mg, 8 mg) ... 3191

Phenelzine Sulfate (Concurrent use is contraindicated).
No products indexed under this heading.

Phenobarbital (Aggravates orthostatic hypotension).
No products indexed under this heading.

Phenoxybenzamine Hydrochloride (Potentiation of antihypertensive effect). Products include:
Dibenzyline Capsules ... 3390

Phentolamine Mesylate (Potentiation of antihypertensive effect).
No products indexed under this heading.

Phenylbutazone (May result in reduced diuretic effect).
No products indexed under this heading.

Pindolol (Potentiation of antihypertensive effect).
No products indexed under this heading.

Pioglitazone Hydrochloride (Dosage adjustment of the antidiabetic drug may be required). Products include:
ActoPlus Met Tablets ... 3219
Actos Tablets ... 3224

Piroxicam (May result in reduced diuretic effect).
No products indexed under this heading.

Polythiazide (Potentiation of antihypertensive effect).
No products indexed under this heading.

Prazosin Hydrochloride (Potentiation of antihypertensive effect).
No products indexed under this heading.

Prednisolone Acetate (Hypokalemia may result). Products include:
Blephamide Ophthalmic Ointment ... 563
Blephamide Ophthalmic Suspension ... 564
Poly-Pred Liquifilm Ophthalmic Suspension ... ⊙231
Pred Forte Ophthalmic Suspension ... ⊙233
Pred Mild Sterile Ophthalmic Suspension ... ⊙236
Pred-G Ophthalmic Suspension ... ⊙234
Pred-G Sterile Ophthalmic Ointment ... ⊙235

Prednisolone Sodium Phosphate (Hypokalemia may result). Products include:
Pediapred Oral Solution ... 3319

Prednisolone Tebutate (Hypokalemia may result).
No products indexed under this heading.

Prednisone (Hypokalemia may result).
No products indexed under this heading.

Procarbazine Hydrochloride (Concurrent use is contraindicated). Products include:
Matulane Capsules ... 3188

Propofol (May require reduced dose of anesthetics). Products include:
Diprivan Injectable Emulsion ... 676

Propoxyphene Hydrochloride (Aggravates orthostatic hypotension).
No products indexed under this heading.

Propoxyphene Napsylate (Aggravates orthostatic hypotension). Products include:
Darvocet A 500 Tablets ... 3497

Propranolol Hydrochloride (Potentiation of antihypertensive effect). Products include:
Inderal LA Long-Acting Capsules ... 3421
InnoPran XL Capsules ... 2728

Quinapril Hydrochloride (Potentiation of antihypertensive effect).
No products indexed under this heading.

Ramipril (Potentiation of antihypertensive effect). Products include:
Altace Capsules ... 1673

Rauwolfia Serpentina (Potentiation of antihypertensive effect).
No products indexed under this heading.

Remifentanil Hydrochloride (Aggravates orthostatic hypotension).
No products indexed under this heading.

Repaglinide (Dosage adjustment of the antidiabetic drug may be required). Products include:
Prandin Tablets (0.5, 1, and 2 mg) ... 2337

Rescinnamine (Potentiation of antihypertensive effect).
No products indexed under this heading.

Reserpine (Potentiation of antihypertensive effect).
No products indexed under this heading.

Rofecoxib (May result in reduced diuretic effect).
No products indexed under this heading.

Rosiglitazone Maleate (Dosage adjustment of the antidiabetic drug may be required). Products include:
Avandamet Tablets ... 1343
Avandia Tablets ... 1348

Secobarbital Sodium (Aggravates orthostatic hypotension).
No products indexed under this heading.

Selegiline Hydrochloride (Concurrent use is contraindicated). Products include:
Eldepryl Capsules ... 3209

Sevoflurane (May require reduced dose of anesthetics). Products include:
Ultane Liquid for Inhalation ... 526

Sodium Nitroprusside (Potentiation of antihypertensive effect).
No products indexed under this heading.

Sotalol Hydrochloride (Potentiation of antihypertensive effect).
No products indexed under this heading.

Spirapril Hydrochloride (Potentiation of antihypertensive effect).
No products indexed under this heading.

Sufentanil Citrate (Aggravates orthostatic hypotension).
No products indexed under this heading.

Sulindac (May result in reduced diuretic effect). Products include:
Clinoril Tablets ... 1899

Telmisartan (Potentiation of antihypertensive effect). Products include:
Micardis Tablets ... 884
Micardis HCT Tablets ... 886

Terazosin Hydrochloride (Potentiation of antihypertensive effect). Products include:
Hytrin Capsules ... 469

Thiamylal Sodium (Aggravates orthostatic hypotension).
No products indexed under this heading.

Timolol Maleate (Potentiation of antihypertensive effect). Products include:
Blocadren Tablets ... 1891
Cosopt Sterile Ophthalmic Solution ... 1910
Timolide Tablets ... 2056
Timoptic in Ocudose ... 2061
Timoptic Sterile Ophthalmic Solution ... 2058
Timoptic-XE Sterile Ophthalmic Gel Forming Solution ... 2062

Tolazamide (Dosage adjustment of the antidiabetic drug may be required).
No products indexed under this heading.

Tolbutamide (Dosage adjustment of the antidiabetic drug may be required).
No products indexed under this heading.

Tolmetin Sodium (May result in reduced diuretic effect).
No products indexed under this heading.

Torsemide (Potentiation of antihypertensive effect).
No products indexed under this heading.

Trandolapril (Potentiation of antihypertensive effect). Products include:
Mavik Tablets ... 482
Tarka Tablets ... 519

Tranylcypromine Sulfate (Concurrent use is contraindicated). Products include:
Parnate Tablets ... 1499

Triamcinolone (Hypokalemia may result).
No products indexed under this heading.

Triamcinolone Acetonide (Hypokalemia may result). Products include:
Azmacort Inhalation Aerosol ... 1701
Nasacort HFA Inhalation Aerosol ... 2939
Nasacort AQ Nasal Spray ... 2937

Triamcinolone Diacetate (Hypokalemia may result).
No products indexed under this heading.

Triamcinolone Hexacetonide (Hypokalemia may result).
No products indexed under this heading.

Trimethaphan Camsylate (Potentiation of antihypertensive effect).
No products indexed under this heading.

Troglitazone (Dosage adjustment of the antidiabetic drug may be required).
No products indexed under this heading.

Tubocurarine Chloride (Increased responsiveness to tubocurarine).
No products indexed under this heading.

Valdecoxib (May result in reduced diuretic effect).
No products indexed under this heading.

Valsartan (Potentiation of antihypertensive effect). Products include:
Diovan HCT Tablets ... 2195
Diovan Tablets ... 2191

Verapamil Hydrochloride (Potentiation of antihypertensive effect). Products include:
Covera-HS Tablets ... 3135
Tarka Tablets ... 519
Verelan PM Capsules ... 3120

Food Interactions

Alcohol (Aggravates orthostatic hypotension).

ALDURAZYME FOR INTRAVENOUS INFUSION

(Laronidase) ... 1261
None cited in PDR database.

ALESSE-28 TABLETS

(Ethinyl Estradiol, Levonorgestrel) ... 3392
May interact with barbiturates, corticosteroids, cytochrome p450 3a4 inhibitors (selected), anticonvulsants, penicillins, phenytoin, protease inhibitors, tetracyclines, xanthines, and certain other agents. Compounds in these categories include:

Acetaminophen (May increase plasma ethinyl estradiol concentrations by competitive inhibition of sulfation of ethinyl estradiol; may also decrease plasma levels of acetaminophen due to induction of conjugation). Products include:
Benadryl Allergy & Cold Tablets ... ■692
Benadryl Allergy & Sinus Headache Caplets & Gelcaps ... ■693
Benadryl Maximum Strength Severe Allergy & Sinus Headache Caplets ... ■694
Contac Severe Cold and Flu Caplets Maximum Strength ... ■615
Contac Severe Cold and Flu Caplets Non-Drowsy ... ■615
Darvocet A 500 Tablets ... 3497
Goody's Body Pain Formula Powder ... ■621
Goody's Extra Strength Headache Powder ... ■621
Goody's Extra Strength Pain Relief Tablets ... ■621
Goody's PM Powder ... ■622
Hycomine Compound Tablets ... 1105
Lortab ... 3315

IMPORTANT NOTE: Always consult each drug listing in the patient's regimen for possible interactions.

Lortab Elixir 3312
Percocet Tablets 1114
Robitussin Cough, Cold & Flu Liquid-filled Capsules........ ▣750
Robitussin Flu Liquid .... ▣752
Sedapap Tablets 50 mg/650 mg 2098
Singlet Caplets .... ▣636
Sudafed Severe Cold .... ▣710
Sudafed Sinus Headache .... ▣711
TheraFlu Cold & Cough Hot Liquid .... ▣680
TheraFlu Cold & Sore Throat Hot Liquid .... ▣680
TheraFlu Flu & Chest Congestion Non-Drowsy Hot Liquid........ ▣681
TheraFlu Flu & Sore Throat Hot Liquid .... ▣681
TheraFlu Severe Cold Non-Drowsy Hot Liquid .... ▣683
TheraFlu Severe Cold & Cough Hot Liquid .... ▣683
TheraFlu Severe Cold Caplets .... ▣679
TheraFlu Severe Cold Hot Liquid .... ▣682
TheraFlu Severe Cold Non-Drowsy Caplets........ ▣679
Triaminic Cough & Sore Throat Liquid .... ▣687
Triaminic Flu, Cough & Fever Liquid .... ▣685
Triaminic Cough & Sore Throat Softchews .... ▣689
Tylenol 8 Hour Extended Release Geltabs and Caplets 1843
Tylenol Sinus NightTime Caplets .... ▣663
Children's Tylenol Suspension Liquid and Meltaways........ 1850
Children's Tylenol Plus Cold & Allergy Suspension Liquid........ 1850
Children's Tylenol Plus Cold NightTime Suspension Liquid........ 1851
Children's Tylenol Plus Cold & Cough Suspension Liquid and Chewable Tablets 1851
Children's Tylenol Plus Cold Chewable Tablets 1851
Children's Tylenol Plus Cold Daytime Non-Drowsy Suspension Liquid 1851
Children's Tylenol Plus Flu Suspension Liquid 1853
Concentrated Tylenol Infants' Drops Plus Cold........ 1851
Concentrated Tylenol Infants' Drops Plus Cold and Cough 1851
Concentrated Tylenol Infants' Drops........ 1850
Junior Tylenol Meltaways 1850
Tylenol Cold & Flu Severe Daytime Liquid with Cool Bust....... 1846
Tylenol Cold & Flu Severe NightTime Liquid with Cool Burst........ 1846
Tylenol Cold Severe Congestion Non-Drowsy Caplets with Cool Burst........ 1846
Tylenol Cough & Sore Throat Daytime Liquid with Cool Burst...... 1849
Tylenol Cough & Sore Throat NightTime Liquid with Cool Burst........ 1849
Tylenol 1843
Extra Strength Tylenol Rapid Release Gels........ 1843
Tylenol 1843
Tylenol Allergy Complete Night Time Caplets........ 1844
Tylenol Allergy Complete Multi-Symptom Caplets and Gelcaps with Cool Burst........ 1844
Tylenol Severe Allergy Caplets 1844
Tylenol Flu NightTime Gelcaps 1846
Tylenol Flu Day Non-Drowsy Gelcaps........ 1846
Concentrated Tylenol Infants' Drops Plus Cold Nasal Congestant, Fever Reducer & Pain Reliever........ ▣668
Concentrated Tylenol Infants' Drops Plus Cold & Cough Nasal Decongestant, Fever Reducer & Pain Reliever........ ▣668
Multi-Symptom Tylenol Cold Night Time Caplets........ 1845
Multi-Symptom Tylenol Cold Day Non-Drowsy Caplets and Gelcaps........ 1845
Extra Strength Tylenol PM Caplets, Geltabs, Gelcaps and Liquid........ 1847
Tylenol Sinus Day Non-Drowsy........ 1848
Tylenol Sinus Night Time Caplets..... 1848
Tylenol Sinus Severe Congestion Caplets with Cool Burst........ 1848
Tylenol Sore Throat Daytime Liquid with Cool Burst........ 1849
Tylenol Sore Throat NightTime Liquid with Cool Burst........ 1849
Tylenol with Codeine 2461
Women's Tylenol Menstrual Relief Caplets........ 1849
Ultracet Tablets 2462
Vicks 44M Cough, Cold & Flu Relief........ 2676
Vicks DayQuil LiquiCaps/Liquid Multi-Symptom Cold/Flu Relief..... ▣723
Vicks DayQuil Multi-Symptom Cold/Flu Relief LiquiCaps........ 2675
Vicks DayQuil Multi-Symptom Cold/Flu Relief Liquid........ 2675
Vicks NyQuil LiquiCaps 2677
Vicks NyQuil LiquiCaps/Liquid Multi-Symptom Cold/Flu Relief..... ▣725
Vicks NyQuil Liquid 2677
Vicodin Tablets 530
Vicodin ES Tablets 531
Vicodin HP Tablets 532
Zydone Tablets 1118

Acetazolamide (Co-administration may increase plasma hormone levels).
No products indexed under this heading.

Aminophylline (Ethinyl estradiol may interfere with the mechanism of other drugs by inhibiting hepatic microsomal enzymes, or by inducing hepatic drug conjugation; tissue concentrations of theophylline may be increased).
No products indexed under this heading.

Amiodarone Hydrochloride (Co-administration may increase plasma hormone levels). Products include:
Pacerone Tablets 3337

Amoxicillin (May decrease plasma ethinyl estradiol concentrations by reducing gut transit time and a decrease of enterohepatic circulation of estrogens; may cause contraceptive failure and breakthrough bleeding). Products include:
Amoxil Capsules 1315
Amoxil Chewable Tablets 1315
Amoxil Pediatric Drops for Oral Suspension........ 1315
Amoxil Powder for Oral Suspension........ 1315
Amoxil Tablets 1315
Augmentin 1331
Augmentin Tablets 1334
Augmentin XR Extended-Release Tablets........ 1340
Augmentin ES-600 Powder for Oral Suspension........ 1337
PREVPAC 3281

Amoxicillin Trihydrate (May decrease plasma ethinyl estradiol concentrations by reducing gut transit time and a decrease of enterohepatic circulation of estrogens; may cause contraceptive failure and breakthrough bleeding).
No products indexed under this heading.

Ampicillin (May decrease plasma ethinyl estradiol concentrations by reducing gut transit time and a decrease of enterohepatic circulation of estrogens; may cause contraceptive failure and breakthrough bleeding).
No products indexed under this heading.

Ampicillin Sodium (May decrease plasma ethinyl estradiol concentrations by reducing gut transit time and a decrease of enterohepatic circulation of estrogens; may cause contraceptive failure and breakthrough bleeding).
No products indexed under this heading.

Ampicillin Trihydrate (May decrease plasma ethinyl estradiol concentrations by reducing gut transit time and a decrease of enterohepatic circulation of estrogens; may cause contraceptive failure and breakthrough bleeding).
No products indexed under this heading.

Amprenavir (Significant changes (increase and decrease) in plasma levels of the estrogen and progestin have been noted; safety and efficacy of oral contraceptive products may be altered with co-administration of anti-HIV protease inhibitors). Products include:
Agenerase Capsules 1299
Agenerase Oral Solution 1304

Anastrozole (Co-administration may increase plasma hormone levels). Products include:
Arimidex Tablets 665

Aprepitant (Co-administration may increase plasma hormone levels). Products include:
Emend Capsules 1944

Aprobarbital (Co-administration with barbiturates results in decreased plasma concentrations of ethinyl estradiol; a reduction in contraceptive effectiveness and increased incidence of breakthrough bleeding and menstrual irregularities have been associated with concomitant use of barbiturates).
No products indexed under this heading.

Atorvastatin Calcium (May increase plasma ethinyl estradiol concentrations). Products include:
Caduet Tablets 2507
Lipitor Tablets 2495

Azlocillin Sodium (May decrease plasma ethinyl estradiol concentrations by reducing gut transit time and a decrease of enterohepatic circulation of estrogens; may cause contraceptive failure and breakthrough bleeding).
No products indexed under this heading.

Bacampicillin Hydrochloride (May decrease plasma ethinyl estradiol concentrations by reducing gut transit time and a decrease of enterohepatic circulation of estrogens; may cause contraceptive failure and breakthrough bleeding).
No products indexed under this heading.

Betamethasone Acetate (Ethinyl estradiol may interfere with the mechanism of other drugs by inhibiting hepatic microsomal enzymes, or by inducing hepatic drug conjugation; tissue concentrations of corticosteroids may be increased).
No products indexed under this heading.

Betamethasone Sodium Phosphate (Ethinyl estradiol may interfere with the mechanism of other drugs by inhibiting hepatic microsomal enzymes, or by inducing hepatic drug conjugation; tissue concentrations of corticosteroids may be increased).
No products indexed under this heading.

Butabarbital (Co-administration with barbiturates results in decreased plasma concentrations of ethinyl estradiol; a reduction in contraceptive effectiveness and increased incidence of breakthrough bleeding and menstrual irregularities have been associated with concomitant use of barbiturates).
No products indexed under this heading.

Butalbital (Co-administration with barbiturates results in decreased plasma concentrations of ethinyl estradiol; a reduction in contraceptive effectiveness and increased incidence of breakthrough bleeding and menstrual irregularities have been associated with concomitant use of barbiturates). Products include:
Sedapap Tablets 50 mg/650 mg 2098

Carbamazepine (Contraceptive effectiveness may be reduced when hormonal contraceptives are co-administered with anticonvulsants and other drugs that increase the metabolism of contraceptive steroids. This could result in unintended pregnancy or breakthrough bleeding). Products include:
Carbatrol Capsules 3174
Equetro Extended-Release Capsules........ 3178
Tegretol/Tegretol-XR 2278

Carbenicillin Disodium (May decrease plasma ethinyl estradiol concentrations by reducing gut transit time and a decrease of enterohepatic circulation of estrogens; may cause contraceptive failure and breakthrough bleeding).
No products indexed under this heading.

Carbenicillin Indanyl Sodium (May decrease plasma ethinyl estradiol concentrations by reducing gut transit time and a decrease of enterohepatic circulation of estrogens; may cause contraceptive failure and breakthrough bleeding).
No products indexed under this heading.

Cimetidine (Co-administration may increase plasma hormone levels). Products include:
Tagamet HB 200 Tablets .... ▣637
Tagamet Tablets 1547

Cimetidine Hydrochloride (Co-administration may increase plasma hormone levels).
No products indexed under this heading.

Ciprofloxacin (Co-administration may increase plasma hormone levels). Products include:
Cipro I.V. 2998
Cipro I.V. Pharmacy Bulk Package ... 3509
Cipro Oral Suspension 2991
Cipro XR Tablets 3004
Ciprodex Otic Suspension 555

Clarithromycin (Co-administration may increase plasma hormone levels). Products include:
Biaxin/Biaxin XL 402
PREVPAC 3281

Clotrimazole (Co-administration may increase plasma hormone levels). Products include:
- Lotrimin 3053
- Lotrisone 3054

Cortisone Acetate (Ethinyl estradiol may interfere with the mechanism of other drugs by inhibiting hepatic microsomal enzymes, or by inducing hepatic drug conjugation; tissue concentrations of corticosteroids may be increased).
No products indexed under this heading.

Cyclosporine (Ethinyl estradiol may interfere with the mechanism of other drugs by inhibiting hepatic microsomal enzymes, or by inducing hepatic drug conjugation; tissue concentrations of cyclosporine may be increased). Products include:
- Gengraf Capsules 458
- Neoral Soft Gelatin Capsules 2247
- Neoral Oral Solution 2247
- Restasis Ophthalmic Emulsion 570
- Sandimmune 2259

Dalfopristin (Co-administration may increase plasma hormone levels). Products include:
- Synercid I.V. 1690

Danazol (Co-administration may increase plasma hormone levels).
No products indexed under this heading.

Delavirdine Mesylate (Co-administration may increase plasma hormone levels). Products include:
- Rescriptor Tablets 2535

Demeclocycline Hydrochloride (May decrease plasma ethinyl estradiol concentrations by reducing gut transit time and a decrease of enterohepatic circulation of estrogens; may cause contraceptive failure and breakthrough bleeding).
No products indexed under this heading.

Dexamethasone (Ethinyl estradiol may interfere with the mechanism of other drugs by inhibiting hepatic microsomal enzymes, or by inducing hepatic drug conjugation; tissue concentrations of corticosteroids may be increased). Products include:
- Ciprodex Otic Suspension 555
- Decadron Tablets 1929
- TobraDex Ophthalmic Ointment 558
- TobraDex Ophthalmic Suspension ... 558

Dexamethasone Acetate (Ethinyl estradiol may interfere with the mechanism of other drugs by inhibiting hepatic microsomal enzymes, or by inducing hepatic drug conjugation; tissue concentrations of corticosteroids may be increased).
No products indexed under this heading.

Dexamethasone Sodium Phosphate (Ethinyl estradiol may interfere with the mechanism of other drugs by inhibiting hepatic microsomal enzymes, or by inducing hepatic drug conjugation; tissue concentrations of corticosteroids may be increased). Products include:
- Decadron Phosphate Injection 1931

Dicloxacillin Sodium (May decrease plasma ethinyl estradiol concentrations by reducing gut transit time and a decrease of enterohepatic circulation of estrogens; may cause contraceptive failure and breakthrough bleeding).
No products indexed under this heading.

Diltiazem Hydrochloride (Co-administration may increase plasma hormone levels). Products include:
- Cardizem LA Extended Release Tablets 1699
- Tiazac Capsules 1204

Diltiazem Maleate (Co-administration may increase plasma hormone levels).
No products indexed under this heading.

Divalproex Sodium (Contraceptive effectiveness may be reduced when hormonal contraceptives are co-administered with anticonvulsants and other drugs that increase the metabolism of contraceptive steroids. This could result in unintended pregnancy or breakthrough bleeding). Products include:
- Depakote Sprinkle Capsules 422
- Depakote Tablets 427
- Depakote ER Tablets 433

Doxycycline Calcium (May decrease plasma ethinyl estradiol concentrations by reducing gut transit time and a decrease of enterohepatic circulation of estrogens; may cause contraceptive failure and breakthrough bleeding).
No products indexed under this heading.

Doxycycline Hyclate (May decrease plasma ethinyl estradiol concentrations by reducing gut transit time and a decrease of enterohepatic circulation of estrogens; may cause contraceptive failure and breakthrough bleeding).
No products indexed under this heading.

Doxycycline Monohydrate (May decrease plasma ethinyl estradiol concentrations by reducing gut transit time and a decrease of enterohepatic circulation of estrogens; may cause contraceptive failure and breakthrough bleeding).
No products indexed under this heading.

Dyphylline (Ethinyl estradiol may interfere with the mechanism of other drugs by inhibiting hepatic microsomal enzymes, or by inducing hepatic drug conjugation; tissue concentrations of theophylline may be increased).
No products indexed under this heading.

Efavirenz (Co-administration may increase plasma hormone levels). Products include:
- Sustiva Capsules 957

Erythromycin (Co-administration may increase plasma hormone levels). Products include:
- Erygel Topical Gel 2096
- Ery-Tab Tablets 447
- Erythromycin Base Filmtab Tablets 454
- Erythromycin Delayed-Release Capsules, USP 456
- PCE Dispertab Tablets 510

Erythromycin Estolate (Co-administration may increase plasma hormone levels).
No products indexed under this heading.

Erythromycin Ethylsuccinate (Co-administration may increase plasma hormone levels). Products include:
- E.E.S. 449
- EryPed 445

Erythromycin Gluceptate (Co-administration may increase plasma hormone levels).
No products indexed under this heading.

Erythromycin Lactobionate (Co-administration may increase plasma hormone levels).
No products indexed under this heading.

Erythromycin Stearate (Co-administration may increase plasma hormone levels). Products include:
- Erythrocin Stearate Filmtab Tablets 452

Esomeprazole Magnesium (Co-administration may increase plasma hormone levels). Products include:
- Nexium Delayed-Release Capsules 645

Ethosuximide (Contraceptive effectiveness may be reduced when hormonal contraceptives are co-administered with anticonvulsants and other drugs that increase the metabolism of contraceptive steroids. This could result in unintended pregnancy or breakthrough bleeding).
No products indexed under this heading.

Ethotoin (Contraceptive effectiveness may be reduced when hormonal contraceptives are co-administered with anticonvulsants and other drugs that increase the metabolism of contraceptive steroids. This could result in unintended pregnancy or breakthrough bleeding). Products include:
- Peganone Tablets, USP 2487

Felbamate (Contraceptive effectiveness may be reduced when hormonal contraceptives are co-administered with anticonvulsants and other drugs that increase the metabolism of contraceptive steroids. This could result in unintended pregnancy or breakthrough bleeding).
No products indexed under this heading.

Fluconazole (May increase plasma ethinyl estradiol concentrations by inhibition of CYP450 3A4 isoenzymes).
No products indexed under this heading.

Fludrocortisone Acetate (Ethinyl estradiol may interfere with the mechanism of other drugs by inhibiting hepatic microsomal enzymes, or by inducing hepatic drug conjugation; tissue concentrations of corticosteroids may be increased).
No products indexed under this heading.

Fluoxetine Hydrochloride (Co-administration may increase plasma hormone levels). Products include:
- Prozac Pulvules and Liquid 1771
- Symbyax Capsules 1788

Fluvoxamine Maleate (Co-administration may increase plasma hormone levels).
No products indexed under this heading.

Fosamprenavir Calcium (Co-administration may increase plasma hormone levels). Products include:
- Lexiva Tablets 1473

Fosphenytoin (Contraceptive effectiveness may be reduced when hormonal contraceptives are co-administered with anticonvulsants and other drugs that increase the metabolism of contraceptive steroids. This could result in unintended pregnancy or breakthrough bleeding).
No products indexed under this heading.

Fosphenytoin Sodium (Co-administration with phenytoin results in decreased plasma concentrations of ethinyl estradiol; a reduction in contraceptive effectiveness and increased incidence of breakthrough bleeding and menstrual irregularities have been associated with concomitant use of phenytoin).
No products indexed under this heading.

Gabapentin (Contraceptive effectiveness may be reduced when hormonal contraceptives are co-administered with anticonvulsants and other drugs that increase the metabolism of contraceptive steroids. This could result in unintended pregnancy or breakthrough bleeding). Products include:
- Neurontin Capsules 2498
- Neurontin Oral Solution 2498
- Neurontin Tablets 2498

Griseofulvin (Co-administration with griseofulvin results in decreased plasma concentrations of ethinyl estradiol; a reduction in contraceptive effectiveness and increased incidence of breakthrough bleeding and menstrual irregularities have been associated with concomitant use of griseofulvin). Products include:
- Grifulvin V Tablets Microsize and Oral Suspension Microsize 2384
- Gris-PEG Tablets 2504

Hydrocortisone (Ethinyl estradiol may interfere with the mechanism of other drugs by inhibiting hepatic microsomal enzymes, or by inducing hepatic drug conjugation; tissue concentrations of corticosteroids may be increased). Products include:
- Cortizone•5 Ointment .... ▣699
- Cortizone•10 Creme .... ▣699
- Cortizone•10 Ointment .... ▣699
- Cortizone•10 Plus Creme .... ▣700
- Cortizone•10 Maximum Strength Quick Shot Spray .... ▣700
- Hydrocortone Tablets 1963
- Preparation H Hydrocortisone Cream .... ▣748

Hydrocortisone Acetate (Ethinyl estradiol may interfere with the mechanism of other drugs by inhibiting hepatic microsomal enzymes, or by inducing hepatic drug conjugation; tissue concentrations of corticosteroids may be increased). Products include:
- Analpram-HC 1136
- Pramosone 1139
- ProctoFoam-HC 3113
- Tucks Anti-Itch Ointment .... ▣712
- U-cort 1% Cream 3289

Hydrocortisone Sodium Phosphate (Ethinyl estradiol may interfere with the mechanism of other drugs by inhibiting hepatic microsomal enzymes, or by inducing hepatic drug conjugation; tissue concentrations of corticosteroids may be increased).
No products indexed under this heading.

Hydrocortisone Sodium Succinate (Ethinyl estradiol may interfere with the mechanism of other drugs by inhibiting hepatic microsomal enzymes, or by inducing hepatic drug conjugation; tissue concentrations of corticosteroids may be increased).
No products indexed under this heading.

Hypericum (May induce hepatic enzymes (cytochrome P450) and p-glycoprotein transporter; may reduce the effectiveness of contraceptive steroid and result in breakthrough bleeding).
No products indexed under this heading.

Indinavir Sulfate (May increase plasma ethinyl estradiol concentrations by inhibition of CYP450 3A4). Products include:
Crixivan Capsules **1918**

Isoniazid (Co-administration may increase plasma hormone levels).
No products indexed under this heading.

Itraconazole (Co-administration may increase plasma hormone levels).
No products indexed under this heading.

Ketoconazole (Co-administration may increase plasma hormone levels). Products include:
Nizoral A-D Shampoo, 1% **1839**
Nizoral 2% Shampoo **1838**

Lamotrigine (Contraceptive effectiveness may be reduced when hormonal contraceptives are co-administered with anticonvulsants and other drugs that increase the metabolism of contraceptive steroids. This could result in unintended pregnancy or breakthrough bleeding). Products include:
Lamictal **1449**

Levetiracetam (Contraceptive effectiveness may be reduced when hormonal contraceptives are co-administered with anticonvulsants and other drugs that increase the metabolism of contraceptive steroids. This could result in unintended pregnancy or breakthrough bleeding). Products include:
Keppra Oral Solution **3307**
Keppra Tablets **3307**

Lopinavir (Significant changes (increase and decrease) in plasma levels of the estrogen and progestin have been noted; safety and efficacy of oral contraceptive products may be altered with co-administration of anti-HIV protease inhibitors). Products include:
Kaletra **474**

Loratadine (Co-administration may increase plasma hormone levels). Products include:
Alavert Allergy & Sinus D-12 Hour Tablets .... ▣ **743**
Alavert .... ▣ **743**
Children's Claritin 24 Hour Non-Drowsy Allergy Syrup .... ▣ **732**
Claritin Non-Drowsy 24 Hour Tablets .... ▣ **731**
Non-Drowsy Claritin Hives Relief Tablets .... ▣ **733**
Claritin Reditabs 24 Hour Non-Drowsy Tablets .... ▣ **732**
Claritin-D Non-Drowsy 12 Hour Tablets .... ▣ **731**
Claritin-D Non-Drowsy 24 Hour Tablets .... ▣ **731**
Children's Dimetapp ND Non-Drowsy Allergy Syrup .... ▣ **746**
Triaminic Allerchews .... ▣ **684**

Mephenytoin (Contraceptive effectiveness may be reduced when hormonal contraceptives are co-administered with anticonvulsants and other drugs that increase the metabolism of contraceptive steroids. This could result in unintended pregnancy or breakthrough bleeding).
No products indexed under this heading.

Mephobarbital (Co-administration with barbiturates results in decreased plasma concentrations of ethinyl estradiol; a reduction in contraceptive effectiveness and increased incidence of breakthrough bleeding and menstrual irregularities have been associated with concomitant use of barbiturates). Products include:
Mebaral Tablets, USP **2483**

Methacycline Hydrochloride (May decrease plasma ethinyl estradiol concentrations by reducing gut transit time and a decrease of enterohepatic circulation of estrogens; may cause contraceptive failure and breakthrough bleeding).
No products indexed under this heading.

Methsuximide (Contraceptive effectiveness may be reduced when hormonal contraceptives are co-administered with anticonvulsants and other drugs that increase the metabolism of contraceptive steroids. This could result in unintended pregnancy or breakthrough bleeding).
No products indexed under this heading.

Methylprednisolone Acetate (Ethinyl estradiol may interfere with the mechanism of other drugs by inhibiting hepatic microsomal enzymes, or by inducing hepatic drug conjugation; tissue concentrations of corticosteroids may be increased). Products include:
Depo-Medrol Injectable Suspension **2615**
Depo-Medrol Single-Dose Vial **2617**

Methylprednisolone Sodium Succinate (Ethinyl estradiol may interfere with the mechanism of other drugs by inhibiting hepatic microsomal enzymes, or by inducing hepatic drug conjugation; tissue concentrations of corticosteroids may be increased).
No products indexed under this heading.

Metronidazole (Co-administration may increase plasma hormone levels). Products include:
Metrogel 1% **1212**
MetroGel-Vaginal Gel **1822**
Noritate Cream, 1% **1051**

Metronidazole Benzoate (Co-administration may increase plasma hormone levels).
No products indexed under this heading.

Metronidazole Hydrochloride (Co-administration may increase plasma hormone levels).
No products indexed under this heading.

Mezlocillin Sodium (May decrease plasma ethinyl estradiol concentrations by reducing gut transit time and a decrease of enterohepatic circulation of estrogens; may cause contraceptive failure and breakthrough bleeding).
No products indexed under this heading.

Miconazole (Co-administration may increase plasma hormone levels).
No products indexed under this heading.

Miconazole Nitrate (Co-administration may increase plasma hormone levels). Products include:
Desenex .... ▣ **674**
Desenex Jock Itch Spray Powder .... ▣ **674**

Minocycline Hydrochloride (May decrease plasma ethinyl estradiol concentrations by reducing gut transit time and a decrease of enterohepatic circulation of estrogens; may cause contraceptive failure and breakthrough bleeding). Products include:
Dynacin Tablets **1859**

Modafinil (Co-administration with modafinil results in decreased plasma concentrations of ethinyl estradiol; a reduction in contraceptive effectiveness and increased incidence of breakthrough bleeding and menstrual irregularities have been associated with concomitant use of modafinil). Products include:
Provigil Tablets **1002**

Nafcillin Sodium (May decrease plasma ethinyl estradiol concentrations by reducing gut transit time and a decrease of enterohepatic circulation of estrogens; may cause contraceptive failure and breakthrough bleeding).
No products indexed under this heading.

Nefazodone Hydrochloride (Co-administration may increase plasma hormone levels).
No products indexed under this heading.

Nelfinavir Mesylate (Significant changes (increase and decrease) in plasma levels of the estrogen and progestin have been noted; safety and efficacy of oral contraceptive products may be altered with co-administration of anti-HIV protease inhibitors). Products include:
Viracept **2556**

Nevirapine (Co-administration may increase plasma hormone levels). Products include:
Viramune Oral Suspension **903**
Viramune Tablets **903**

Niacinamide (Co-administration may increase plasma hormone levels).
No products indexed under this heading.

Nicotinamide (Co-administration may increase plasma hormone levels). Products include:
Nicomide Tablets **3190**

Nifedipine (Co-administration may increase plasma hormone levels). Products include:
Adalat CC Tablets **2978**

Norfloxacin (Co-administration may increase plasma hormone levels). Products include:
Noroxin Tablets **2009**

Omeprazole (Co-administration may increase plasma hormone levels). Products include:
Zegerid Powder for Oral Solution **2972**

Oxcarbazepine (Contraceptive effectiveness may be reduced when hormonal contraceptives are co-administered with anticonvulsants and other drugs that increase the metabolism of contraceptive steroids. This could result in unintended pregnancy or breakthrough bleeding). Products include:
Trileptal Oral Suspension **2281**
Trileptal Tablets **2281**

Oxytetracycline Hydrochloride (May decrease plasma ethinyl estradiol concentrations by reducing gut transit time and a decrease of enterohepatic circulation of estrogens; may cause contraceptive failure and breakthrough bleeding).
No products indexed under this heading.

Paramethadione (Contraceptive effectiveness may be reduced when hormonal contraceptives are co-administered with anticonvulsants and other drugs that increase the metabolism of contraceptive steroids. This could result in unintended pregnancy or breakthrough bleeding).
No products indexed under this heading.

Paroxetine Hydrochloride (Co-administration may increase plasma hormone levels). Products include:
Paxil CR Controlled-Release Tablets **1509**
Paxil **1501**

Penicillin G Benzathine (May decrease plasma ethinyl estradiol concentrations by reducing gut transit time and a decrease of enterohepatic circulation of estrogens; may cause contraceptive failure and breakthrough bleeding).
No products indexed under this heading.

Penicillin G Potassium (May decrease plasma ethinyl estradiol concentrations by reducing gut transit time and a decrease of enterohepatic circulation of estrogens; may cause contraceptive failure and breakthrough bleeding).
No products indexed under this heading.

Penicillin G Procaine (May decrease plasma ethinyl estradiol concentrations by reducing gut transit time and a decrease of enterohepatic circulation of estrogens; may cause contraceptive failure and breakthrough bleeding).
No products indexed under this heading.

Penicillin G Sodium (May decrease plasma ethinyl estradiol concentrations by reducing gut transit time and a decrease of enterohepatic circulation of estrogens; may cause contraceptive failure and breakthrough bleeding).
No products indexed under this heading.

Penicillin V Potassium (May decrease plasma ethinyl estradiol concentrations by reducing gut transit time and a decrease of enterohepatic circulation of estrogens; may cause contraceptive failure and breakthrough bleeding).
No products indexed under this heading.

Pentobarbital Sodium (Co-administration with barbiturates results in decreased plasma concentrations of ethinyl estradiol; a reduction in contraceptive effectiveness and increased incidence of breakthrough bleeding and menstrual irregularities have been associated with concomitant use of barbiturates). Products include:
Nembutal Sodium Solution, USP **2484**

Phenacemide (Contraceptive effectiveness may be reduced when hormonal contraceptives are co-administered with anticonvulsants and other drugs that increase the metabolism of contraceptive steroids. This could result in unintended pregnancy or breakthrough bleeding).
No products indexed under this heading.

Phenobarbital (Contraceptive effectiveness may be reduced when hormonal contraceptives are co-administered with anticonvulsants and other drugs that increase the metabolism of contraceptive steroids. This could result in unintended pregnancy or breakthrough bleeding).
No products indexed under this heading.

Phensuximide (Contraceptive effectiveness may be reduced when hormonal contraceptives are co-administered with anticonvulsants and other drugs that increase the metabolism of contraceptive steroids. This could result in unintended pregnancy or breakthrough bleeding).
No products indexed under this heading.

Phenylbutazone (Co-administration with phenylbutazone results in decreased plasma concentrations of ethinyl estradiol; a reduction in contraceptive effectiveness and increased incidence of breakthrough bleeding and menstrual irregularities have been associated with concomitant use of phenylbutazone).
No products indexed under this heading.

Phenytoin (Co-administration with phenytoin results in decreased plasma concentrations of ethinyl estradiol; a reduction in contraceptive effectiveness and increased incidence of breakthrough bleeding and menstrual irregularities have been associated with concomitant use of phenytoin).
No products indexed under this heading.

Phenytoin Sodium (Co-administration with phenytoin results in decreased plasma concentrations of ethinyl estradiol; a reduction in contraceptive effectiveness and increased incidence of breakthrough bleeding and menstrual irregularities have been associated with concomitant use of phenytoin). Products include:
Phenytek Capsules 2153

Prednisolone Acetate (Ethinyl estradiol may interfere with the mechanism of other drugs by inhibiting hepatic microsomal enzymes, or by inducing hepatic drug conjugation; tissue concentrations of corticosteroids may be increased).
Products include:
Blephamide Ophthalmic Ointment 563
Blephamide Ophthalmic Suspension 564
Poly-Pred Liquifilm Ophthalmic Suspension .... ⊙231
Pred Forte Ophthalmic Suspension .... ⊙233
Pred Mild Sterile Ophthalmic Suspension .... ⊙236
Pred-G Ophthalmic Suspension ...... ⊙234
Pred-G Sterile Ophthalmic Ointment .... ⊙235

Prednisolone Sodium Phosphate (Ethinyl estradiol may interfere with the mechanism of other drugs by inhibiting hepatic microsomal enzymes, or by inducing hepatic drug conjugation; tissue concentrations of corticosteroids may be increased). Products include:
Pediapred Oral Solution 3319

Prednisolone Tebutate (Ethinyl estradiol may interfere with the mechanism of other drugs by inhibiting hepatic microsomal enzymes, or by inducing hepatic drug conjugation; tissue concentrations of corticosteroids may be increased).
No products indexed under this heading.

Prednisone (Ethinyl estradiol may interfere with the mechanism of other drugs by inhibiting hepatic microsomal enzymes, or by inducing hepatic drug conjugation; tissue concentrations of corticosteroids may be increased).
No products indexed under this heading.

Primidone (Contraceptive effectiveness may be reduced when hormonal contraceptives are co-administered with anticonvulsants and other drugs that increase the metabolism of contraceptive steroids. This could result in unintended pregnancy or breakthrough bleeding).
No products indexed under this heading.

Propoxyphene Hydrochloride (Co-administration may increase plasma hormone levels).
No products indexed under this heading.

Propoxyphene Napsylate (Co-administration may increase plasma hormone levels). Products include:
Darvocet A 500 Tablets 3497

Quinidine (Co-administration may increase plasma hormone levels).
No products indexed under this heading.

Quinidine Hydrochloride (Co-administration may increase plasma hormone levels).
No products indexed under this heading.

Quinidine Polygalacturonate (Co-administration may increase plasma hormone levels).
No products indexed under this heading.

Quinidine Sulfate (Co-administration may increase plasma hormone levels).
No products indexed under this heading.

Quinine (Co-administration may increase plasma hormone levels).
No products indexed under this heading.

Quinine Sulfate (Co-administration may increase plasma hormone levels).
No products indexed under this heading.

Quinupristin (Co-administration may increase plasma hormone levels). Products include:
Synercid I.V. 1690

Ranitidine Bismuth Citrate (Co-administration may increase plasma hormone levels).
No products indexed under this heading.

Ranitidine Hydrochloride (Co-administration may increase plasma hormone levels). Products include:
Zantac 1597
Zantac Injection 1593
Zantac 75 Tablets .... ▣715
Zantac 150 Maximum Strength Tablets .... ▣715
Zantac Injection Pharmacy Bulk Package 1595

Rifabutin (Co-administration with rifabutin results in decreased plasma concentrations of ethinyl estradiol; a reduction in contraceptive effectiveness and increased incidence of breakthrough bleeding and menstrual irregularities have been associated with concomitant use of rifabutin).
No products indexed under this heading.

Rifampin (Co-administration with rifampin results in decreased plasma concentrations of ethinyl estradiol; a reduction in contraceptive effectiveness and increased incidence of breakthrough bleeding and menstrual irregularities have been associated with concomitant use of rifampin).
No products indexed under this heading.

Ritonavir (Significant changes (increase and decrease) in plasma levels of the estrogen and progestin have been noted; safety and efficacy of oral contraceptive products may be altered with co-administration of anti-HIV protease inhibitors).
Products include:
Kaletra 474
Norvir 499

Saquinavir (Significant changes (increase and decrease) in plasma levels of the estrogen and progestin have been noted; safety and efficacy of oral contraceptive products may be altered with co-administration of anti-HIV protease inhibitors).
No products indexed under this heading.

Saquinavir Mesylate (Significant changes (increase and decrease) in plasma levels of the estrogen and progestin have been noted; safety and efficacy of oral contraceptive products may be altered with co-administration of anti-HIV protease inhibitors). Products include:
Invirase 2776

Secobarbital Sodium (Co-administration with barbiturates results in decreased plasma concentrations of ethinyl estradiol; a reduction in contraceptive effectiveness and increased incidence of breakthrough bleeding and menstrual irregularities have been associated with concomitant use of barbiturates).
No products indexed under this heading.

Sertraline Hydrochloride (Co-administration may increase plasma hormone levels). Products include:
Zoloft 2581

Telithromycin (Co-administration may increase plasma hormone levels). Products include:
Ketek Tablets 2920

Tetracycline Hydrochloride (May decrease plasma ethinyl estradiol concentrations by reducing gut transit time and a decrease of enterohepatic circulation of estrogens; may cause contraceptive failure and breakthrough bleeding).
No products indexed under this heading.

Theophylline (Ethinyl estradiol may interfere with the mechanism of other drugs by inhibiting hepatic microsomal enzymes, or by inducing hepatic drug conjugation; tissue concentrations of theophylline may be increased).
No products indexed under this heading.

Theophylline Anhydrous (Ethinyl estradiol may interfere with the mechanism of other drugs by inhibiting hepatic microsomal enzymes, or by inducing hepatic drug conjugation; tissue concentrations of theophylline may be increased). Products include:
Uniphyl Tablets 2708

Theophylline Calcium Salicylate (Ethinyl estradiol may interfere with the mechanism of other drugs by inhibiting hepatic microsomal enzymes, or by inducing hepatic drug conjugation; tissue concentrations of theophylline may be increased).
No products indexed under this heading.

Theophylline Dihydroxypropyl (Glyceryl) (Ethinyl estradiol may interfere with the mechanism of other drugs by inhibiting hepatic microsomal enzymes, or by inducing hepatic drug conjugation; tissue concentrations of theophylline may be increased).
No products indexed under this heading.

Theophylline Ethylenediamine (Ethinyl estradiol may interfere with the mechanism of other drugs by inhibiting hepatic microsomal enzymes, or by inducing hepatic drug conjugation; tissue concentrations of theophylline may be increased).
No products indexed under this heading.

Theophylline Sodium Glycinate (Ethinyl estradiol may interfere with the mechanism of other drugs by inhibiting hepatic microsomal enzymes, or by inducing hepatic drug conjugation; tissue concentrations of theophylline may be increased).
No products indexed under this heading.

Thiamylal Sodium (Co-administration with barbiturates results in decreased plasma concentrations of ethinyl estradiol; a reduction in contraceptive effectiveness and increased incidence of breakthrough bleeding and menstrual irregularities have been associated with concomitant use of barbiturates).
No products indexed under this heading.

Tiagabine Hydrochloride (Contraceptive effectiveness may be reduced when hormonal contraceptives are co-administered with anticonvulsants and other drugs that increase the metabolism of contraceptive steroids. This could result in unintended pregnancy or breakthrough bleeding). Products include:
Gabitril Tablets 998

Ticarcillin Disodium (May decrease plasma ethinyl estradiol concentrations by reducing gut transit time and a decrease of enterohepatic circulation of estrogens; may

cause contraceptive failure and breakthrough bleeding). Products include:

Timentin ADD-Vantage 1556
Timentin Injection Galaxy Container 1559
Timentin IV Infusion 1553
Timentin Pharmacy Bulk Package 1562

Topiramate (Co-administration with topiramate results in decreased plasma concentrations of ethinyl estradiol; a reduction in contraceptive effectiveness and increased incidence of breakthrough bleeding and menstrual irregularities have been associated with concomitant use of topiramate). Products include:

Topamax Sprinkle Capsules 2438
Topamax Tablets 2438

Triamcinolone (Ethinyl estradiol may interfere with the mechanism of other drugs by inhibiting hepatic microsomal enzymes, or by inducing hepatic drug conjugation; tissue concentrations of corticosteroids may be increased).

No products indexed under this heading.

Triamcinolone Acetonide (Ethinyl estradiol may interfere with the mechanism of other drugs by inhibiting hepatic microsomal enzymes, or by inducing hepatic drug conjugation; tissue concentrations of corticosteroids may be increased). Products include:

Azmacort Inhalation Aerosol 1701
Nasacort HFA Inhalation Aerosol 2939
Nasacort AQ Nasal Spray 2937

Triamcinolone Diacetate (Ethinyl estradiol may interfere with the mechanism of other drugs by inhibiting hepatic microsomal enzymes, or by inducing hepatic drug conjugation; tissue concentrations of corticosteroids may be increased).

No products indexed under this heading.

Triamcinolone Hexacetonide (Ethinyl estradiol may interfere with the mechanism of other drugs by inhibiting hepatic microsomal enzymes, or by inducing hepatic drug conjugation; tissue concentrations of corticosteroids may be increased).

No products indexed under this heading.

Trimethadione (Contraceptive effectiveness may be reduced when hormonal contraceptives are co-administered with anticonvulsants and other drugs that increase the metabolism of contraceptive steroids. This could result in unintended pregnancy or breakthrough bleeding).

No products indexed under this heading.

Troglitazone (Co-administration may increase plasma hormone levels).

No products indexed under this heading.

Troleandomycin (May increase plasma ethinyl estradiol concentrations by inhibition of CYP450 3A4 isoenzymes; may increase the risk of intrahepatic cholestasis during co-administration with combination oral contraceptives).

No products indexed under this heading.

Valproate Sodium (Contraceptive effectiveness may be reduced when hormonal contraceptives are co-administered with anticonvulsants and other drugs that increase the metabolism of contraceptive steroids. This could result in unintended pregnancy or breakthrough bleeding). Products include:

Depacon Injection 412

Valproic Acid (Contraceptive effectiveness may be reduced when hormonal contraceptives are co-administered with anticonvulsants and other drugs that increase the metabolism of contraceptive steroids. This could result in unintended pregnancy or breakthrough bleeding). Products include:

Depakene 417

Verapamil Hydrochloride (Co-administration may increase plasma hormone levels). Products include:

Covera-HS Tablets 3135
Tarka Tablets 519
Verelan PM Capsules 3120

Vitamin C (May increase plasma ethinyl estradiol concentrations by competitive inhibition of sulfation of ethinyl estradiol). Products include:

Chromagen Forte Soft Gelatin Capsules 3296
Halls Defense Sugarfree Vitamin C Drops .... ▣611
Niferex-150 Forte Capsules 3299
Peridin-C Tablets .... ▣761
Repliva 21/7 Tablets 3301

Voriconazole (Co-administration may increase plasma hormone levels). Products include:

VFEND I.V. 2543
VFEND Oral Suspension 2543
VFEND Tablets 2543

Zafirlukast (Co-administration may increase plasma hormone levels). Products include:

Accolate Tablets 663

Zileuton (Co-administration may increase plasma hormone levels).

No products indexed under this heading.

Zonisamide (Contraceptive effectiveness may be reduced when hormonal contraceptives are co-administered with anticonvulsants and other drugs that increase the metabolism of contraceptive steroids. This could result in unintended pregnancy or breakthrough bleeding). Products include:

Zonegran Capsules 1089

Food Interactions

Grapefruit (Co-administration may increase plasma hormone levels).

Grapefruit Juice (Co-administration may increase plasma hormone levels).

ALEVE TABLETS, CAPLETS AND GELCAPS

(Naproxen Sodium) .... ▣605

Food Interactions

Alcohol (Individuals consuming 3 or more alcohol-containing drinks per day should consult their physicians for advice on when and how they should take this product).

ALFERON N INJECTION

(Interferon alfa-N3 (Human Leukocyte Derived)) 1640

None cited in PDR database.

ALIMTA FOR INJECTION

(Pemetrexed) 1722

May interact with nephrotoxic agents, non-steroidal anti-inflammatory agents, and certain other agents. Compounds in these categories include:

Abacavir Sulfate (Concomitant administration of nephrotoxic drugs could result in delayed clearance of pemetrexed). Products include:

Epzicom Tablets 1402
Trizivir Tablets 1565
Ziagen 1600

Acyclovir (Concomitant administration of nephrotoxic drugs could result in delayed clearance of pemetrexed). Products include:

Zovirax 1616
Zovirax Cream 853
Zovirax Ointment 854

Acyclovir Sodium (Concomitant administration of nephrotoxic drugs could result in delayed clearance of pemetrexed). Products include:

Zovirax for Injection 1618

Alatrofloxacin Mesylate (Concomitant administration of nephrotoxic drugs could result in delayed clearance of pemetrexed).

No products indexed under this heading.

Aldesleukin (Concomitant administration of nephrotoxic drugs could result in delayed clearance of pemetrexed). Products include:

Proleukin for Injection 1007

Amikacin Sulfate (Concomitant administration of nephrotoxic drugs could result in delayed clearance of pemetrexed).

No products indexed under this heading.

Amoxicillin (Concomitant administration of nephrotoxic drugs could result in delayed clearance of pemetrexed). Products include:

Amoxil Capsules 1315
Amoxil Chewable Tablets 1315
Amoxil Pediatric Drops for Oral Suspension 1315
Amoxil Powder for Oral Suspension 1315
Amoxil Tablets 1315
Augmentin 1331
Augmentin Tablets 1334
Augmentin XR Extended-Release Tablets 1340
Augmentin ES-600 Powder for Oral Suspension 1337
PREVPAC 3281

Amoxicillin Trihydrate (Concomitant administration of nephrotoxic drugs could result in delayed clearance of pemetrexed).

No products indexed under this heading.

Amphotericin B (Concomitant administration of nephrotoxic drugs could result in delayed clearance of pemetrexed).

No products indexed under this heading.

Amphotericin B, liposomal (Concomitant administration of nephrotoxic drugs could result in delayed clearance of pemetrexed). Products include:

AmBisome for Injection 615

Amphotericin B Cholesteryl Sulfate (Concomitant administration of nephrotoxic drugs could result in delayed clearance of pemetrexed).

No products indexed under this heading.

Amphotericin B Lipid Complex (Concomitant administration of nephrotoxic drugs could result in delayed clearance of pemetrexed). Products include:

Abelcet Injection 1119

Ampicillin (Concomitant administration of nephrotoxic drugs could result in delayed clearance of pemetrexed).

No products indexed under this heading.

Ampicillin Sodium (Concomitant administration of nephrotoxic drugs could result in delayed clearance of pemetrexed).

No products indexed under this heading.

Ampicillin Trihydrate (Concomitant administration of nephrotoxic drugs could result in delayed clearance of pemetrexed).

No products indexed under this heading.

Amprenavir (Concomitant administration of nephrotoxic drugs could result in delayed clearance of pemetrexed). Products include:

Agenerase Capsules 1299
Agenerase Oral Solution 1304

Aspirin (Concomitant administration of nephrotoxic drugs could result in delayed clearance of pemetrexed). Products include:

Aggrenox Capsules 855
Bayer, Aspirin Regimen .... ▣606
Bayer Aspirin Tablets 3515
BC Powder .... ▣612
BC Allergy Sinus Cold Powder .... ▣612
Arthritis Strength BC Powder .... ▣612
BC Sinus Cold Powder .... ▣612
Ecotrin Enteric Coated Aspirin Low, Regular and Maximum Strength Tablets 1627
Goody's Body Pain Formula Powder .... ▣621
Goody's Extra Strength Headache Powder .... ▣621
Goody's Extra Strength Pain Relief Tablets .... ▣621
Percodan Tablets 1115
St. Joseph 81 mg Aspirin Chewable and Enteric Coated Tablets 1841

Atazanavir (Concomitant administration of nephrotoxic drugs could result in delayed clearance of pemetrexed).

No products indexed under this heading.

Atorvastatin Calcium (Concomitant administration of nephrotoxic drugs could result in delayed clearance of pemetrexed). Products include:

Caduet Tablets 2507
Lipitor Tablets 2495

Azithromycin Dihydrate (Concomitant administration of nephrotoxic drugs could result in delayed clearance of pemetrexed). Products include:

Zithromax 2568
Zithromax for IV Infusion 2573
Zithromax for Oral Suspension, 300 mg, 600 mg, 900 mg, 1200 mg 2561
Zithromax Tablets, 250 mg, 500 mg 2561
Zithromax Tri-Pak 2561
Zithromax Z-Pak 2568

Azlocillin Sodium (Concomitant administration of nephrotoxic drugs could result in delayed clearance of pemetrexed).

No products indexed under this heading.

Aztreonam (Concomitant administration of nephrotoxic drugs could result in delayed clearance of pemetrexed).

No products indexed under this heading.

Bacampicillin Hydrochloride (Concomitant administration of nephrotoxic drugs could result in delayed clearance of pemetrexed).

No products indexed under this heading.

Balsalazide Disodium (Concomitant administration of nephrotoxic

drugs could result in delayed clearance of pemetrexed). Products include:
- Colazal Capsules 2845

Benazepril Hydrochloride (Concomitant administration of nephrotoxic drugs could result in delayed clearance of pemetrexed). Products include:
- Lotensin Tablets 2232
- Lotensin HCT Tablets 2235
- Lotrel Capsules 2238

Bendroflumethiazide (Concomitant administration of nephrotoxic drugs could result in delayed clearance of pemetrexed).
- No products indexed under this heading.

Caffeine (Concomitant administration of nephrotoxic drugs could result in delayed clearance of pemetrexed). Products include:
- Athena Hair System Shampoo 767
- BC Powder 612
- Arthritis Strength BC Powder 612
- Goody's Extra Strength Headache Powder 621
- Goody's Extra Strength Pain Relief Tablets 621
- Hycomine Compound Tablets 1105
- Spartan Hair System Shampoo 767
- Vivarin 639

Captopril (Concomitant administration of nephrotoxic drugs could result in delayed clearance of pemetrexed). Products include:
- Captopril Tablets 2114

Carbenicillin Disodium (Concomitant administration of nephrotoxic drugs could result in delayed clearance of pemetrexed).
- No products indexed under this heading.

Carbenicillin Indanyl Sodium (Concomitant administration of nephrotoxic drugs could result in delayed clearance of pemetrexed).
- No products indexed under this heading.

Carboplatin (Concomitant administration of nephrotoxic drugs could result in delayed clearance of pemetrexed).
- No products indexed under this heading.

Carmustine (BCNU) (Concomitant administration of nephrotoxic drugs could result in delayed clearance of pemetrexed).
- No products indexed under this heading.

Cefaclor (Concomitant administration of nephrotoxic drugs could result in delayed clearance of pemetrexed).
- No products indexed under this heading.

Cefadroxil (Concomitant administration of nephrotoxic drugs could result in delayed clearance of pemetrexed).
- No products indexed under this heading.

Cefamandole Nafate (Concomitant administration of nephrotoxic drugs could result in delayed clearance of pemetrexed).
- No products indexed under this heading.

Cefazolin Sodium (Concomitant administration of nephrotoxic drugs could result in delayed clearance of pemetrexed). Products include:
- Ancef for Injection 1318

Cefdinir (Concomitant administration of nephrotoxic drugs could result in delayed clearance of pemetrexed). Products include:
- Omnicef Capsules 506
- Omnicef for Oral Suspension 506

Cefepime Hydrochloride (Concomitant administration of nephrotoxic drugs could result in delayed clearance of pemetrexed). Products include:
- Maxipime for Injection 1093

Cefixime (Concomitant administration of nephrotoxic drugs could result in delayed clearance of pemetrexed). Products include:
- Suprax 1811

Cefmetazole Sodium (Concomitant administration of nephrotoxic drugs could result in delayed clearance of pemetrexed).
- No products indexed under this heading.

Cefonicid Sodium (Concomitant administration of nephrotoxic drugs could result in delayed clearance of pemetrexed).
- No products indexed under this heading.

Cefoperazone Sodium (Concomitant administration of nephrotoxic drugs could result in delayed clearance of pemetrexed).
- No products indexed under this heading.

Ceforanide (Concomitant administration of nephrotoxic drugs could result in delayed clearance of pemetrexed).
- No products indexed under this heading.

Cefotaxime Sodium (Concomitant administration of nephrotoxic drugs could result in delayed clearance of pemetrexed).
- No products indexed under this heading.

Cefotetan (Concomitant administration of nephrotoxic drugs could result in delayed clearance of pemetrexed).
- No products indexed under this heading.

Cefoxitin Sodium (Concomitant administration of nephrotoxic drugs could result in delayed clearance of pemetrexed). Products include:
- Mefoxin for Injection 1987
- Mefoxin Premixed Intravenous Solution 1990

Cefpodoxime Proxetil (Concomitant administration of nephrotoxic drugs could result in delayed clearance of pemetrexed). Products include:
- Vantin Tablets and Oral Suspension 2650

Cefprozil (Concomitant administration of nephrotoxic drugs could result in delayed clearance of pemetrexed).
- No products indexed under this heading.

Ceftazidime (Concomitant administration of nephrotoxic drugs could result in delayed clearance of pemetrexed). Products include:
- Fortaz for Injection 1422

Ceftizoxime Sodium (Concomitant administration of nephrotoxic drugs could result in delayed clearance of pemetrexed).
- No products indexed under this heading.

Ceftriaxone Sodium (Concomitant administration of nephrotoxic drugs could result in delayed clearance of pemetrexed). Products include:
- Rocephin Injectable Vials, ADD-Vantage, Galaxy, Bulk 2801

Cefuroxime Axetil (Concomitant administration of nephrotoxic drugs could result in delayed clearance of pemetrexed). Products include:
- Ceftin 1369

Cefuroxime Sodium (Concomitant administration of nephrotoxic drugs could result in delayed clearance of pemetrexed).
- No products indexed under this heading.

Celecoxib (Patients with mild to moderate renal insufficiency should avoid NSAIDs with short elimination half-lives two days before, the day of, and two days following administration of pemetrexed. All patients should avoid NSAIDs with longer half-lives at least five days before, the day of, and two days following pemetrexed administration. If concomitant administration of an NSAID is necessary, patients should be monitored closely for toxicity, especially myelosuppression, renal and gastrointestinal toxicity). Products include:
- Celebrex Capsules 3130

Cephalexin (Concomitant administration of nephrotoxic drugs could result in delayed clearance of pemetrexed).
- No products indexed under this heading.

Cephalothin Sodium (Concomitant administration of nephrotoxic drugs could result in delayed clearance of pemetrexed).
- No products indexed under this heading.

Cephapirin Sodium (Concomitant administration of nephrotoxic drugs could result in delayed clearance of pemetrexed).
- No products indexed under this heading.

Cephradine (Concomitant administration of nephrotoxic drugs could result in delayed clearance of pemetrexed).
- No products indexed under this heading.

Cerivastatin Sodium (Concomitant administration of nephrotoxic drugs could result in delayed clearance of pemetrexed).
- No products indexed under this heading.

Chlorothiazide (Concomitant administration of nephrotoxic drugs could result in delayed clearance of pemetrexed). Products include:
- Aldoclor Tablets 1881
- Diuril Oral 1936

Chlorothiazide Sodium (Concomitant administration of nephrotoxic drugs could result in delayed clearance of pemetrexed). Products include:
- Diuril Sodium Intravenous 1934

Chlorpropamide (Concomitant administration of nephrotoxic drugs could result in delayed clearance of pemetrexed).
- No products indexed under this heading.

Cidofovir (Concomitant administration of nephrotoxic drugs could result in delayed clearance of pemetrexed).
- No products indexed under this heading.

Cilastatin Sodium (Concomitant administration of nephrotoxic drugs could result in delayed clearance of pemetrexed). Products include:
- Primaxin I.M. 2022
- Primaxin I.V. 2024

Cimetidine (Concomitant administration of nephrotoxic drugs could result in delayed clearance of pemetrexed). Products include:
- Tagamet HB 200 Tablets 637
- Tagamet Tablets 1547

Cimetidine Hydrochloride (Concomitant administration of nephrotoxic drugs could result in delayed clearance of pemetrexed).
- No products indexed under this heading.

Cisplatin (Concomitant administration of nephrotoxic drugs could result in delayed clearance of pemetrexed).
- No products indexed under this heading.

Cladribine (Concomitant administration of nephrotoxic drugs could result in delayed clearance of pemetrexed). Products include:
- Leustatin Injection 2368

Clozapine (Concomitant administration of nephrotoxic drugs could result in delayed clearance of pemetrexed). Products include:
- Clozapine Tablets 2141
- Clozaril Tablets 2174
- FazaClo Orally Disintegrating Tablets 547

Colistimethate Sodium (Concomitant administration of nephrotoxic drugs could result in delayed clearance of pemetrexed).
- No products indexed under this heading.

Colistin Sulfate (Concomitant administration of nephrotoxic drugs could result in delayed clearance of pemetrexed).
- No products indexed under this heading.

Cyclophosphamide (Concomitant administration of nephrotoxic drugs could result in delayed clearance of pemetrexed).
- No products indexed under this heading.

Cyclosporine (Concomitant administration of nephrotoxic drugs could result in delayed clearance of pemetrexed). Products include:
- Gengraf Capsules 458
- Neoral Soft Gelatin Capsules 2247
- Neoral Oral Solution 2247
- Restasis Ophthalmic Emulsion 570
- Sandimmune 2259

Cytarabine (Concomitant administration of nephrotoxic drugs could result in delayed clearance of pemetrexed).
- No products indexed under this heading.

Cytarabine Liposome (Concomitant administration of nephrotoxic drugs could result in delayed clearance of pemetrexed). Products include:
- DepoCyt Injection 1121

Delavirdine Mesylate (Concomitant administration of nephrotoxic drugs could result in delayed clearance of pemetrexed). Products include:

Rescriptor Tablets 2535

Diatrizoate Meglumine (Concomitant administration of nephrotoxic drugs could result in delayed clearance of pemetrexed).
No products indexed under this heading.

Diatrizoate Sodium (Concomitant administration of nephrotoxic drugs could result in delayed clearance of pemetrexed).
No products indexed under this heading.

Diclofenac Potassium (Patients with mild to moderate renal insufficiency should avoid NSAIDs with short elimination half-lives two days before, the day of, and two days following administration of pemetrexed. All patients should avoid NSAIDs with longer half-lives at least five days before, the day of, and two days following pemetrexed administration. If concomitant administration of an NSAID is necessary, patients should be monitored closely for toxicity, especially myelosuppression, renal and gastrointestinal toxicity). Products include:
Cataflam Tablets 2173

Diclofenac Sodium (Patients with mild to moderate renal insufficiency should avoid NSAIDs with short elimination half-lives two days before, the day of, and two days following administration of pemetrexed. All patients should avoid NSAIDs with longer half-lives at least five days before, the day of, and two days following pemetrexed administration. If concomitant administration of an NSAID is necessary, patients should be monitored closely for toxicity, especially myelosuppression, renal and gastrointestinal toxicity). Products include:
Arthrotec Tablets 3126
Voltaren Ophthalmic Solution 2300
Voltaren Tablets 2298
Voltaren-XR Tablets 2301

Dicloxacillin Sodium (Concomitant administration of nephrotoxic drugs could result in delayed clearance of pemetrexed).
No products indexed under this heading.

Didanosine (Concomitant administration of nephrotoxic drugs could result in delayed clearance of pemetrexed).
No products indexed under this heading.

Efavirenz (Concomitant administration of nephrotoxic drugs could result in delayed clearance of pemetrexed). Products include:
Sustiva Capsules 957

Emtricitabine (Concomitant administration of nephrotoxic drugs could result in delayed clearance of pemetrexed). Products include:
Emtriva Capsules 1272
Truvada Tablets 1279

Enalapril Maleate (Concomitant administration of nephrotoxic drugs could result in delayed clearance of pemetrexed). Products include:
Vaseretic Tablets 2073
Vasotec I.V. Injection 2076

Enalaprilat (Concomitant administration of nephrotoxic drugs could result in delayed clearance of pemetrexed).
No products indexed under this heading.

Enfuvirtide (Concomitant administration of nephrotoxic drugs could result in delayed clearance of pemetrexed). Products include:
Fuzeon Injection 2772

Ethiodized Oil (Concomitant administration of nephrotoxic drugs could result in delayed clearance of pemetrexed).
No products indexed under this heading.

Etodolac (Patients with mild to moderate renal insufficiency should avoid NSAIDs with short elimination half-lives two days before, the day of, and two days following administration of pemetrexed. All patients should avoid NSAIDs with longer half-lives at least five days before, the day of, and two days following pemetrexed administration. If concomitant administration of an NSAID is necessary, patients should be monitored closely for toxicity, especially myelosuppression, renal and gastrointestinal toxicity).
No products indexed under this heading.

Fenoprofen Calcium (Patients with mild to moderate renal insufficiency should avoid NSAIDs with short elimination half-lives two days before, the day of, and two days following administration of pemetrexed. All patients should avoid NSAIDs with longer half-lives at least five days before, the day of, and two days following pemetrexed administration. If concomitant administration of an NSAID is necessary, patients should be monitored closely for toxicity, especially myelosuppression, renal and gastrointestinal toxicity). Products include:
Nalfon Capsules 2504

Filgrastim (Concomitant administration of nephrotoxic drugs could result in delayed clearance of pemetrexed). Products include:
Neupogen for Injection 598

Fluorouracil (Concomitant administration of nephrotoxic drugs could result in delayed clearance of pemetrexed). Products include:
Carac Cream, 0.5% 1048
Efudex 3348

Flurbiprofen (Patients with mild to moderate renal insufficiency should avoid NSAIDs with short elimination half-lives two days before, the day of, and two days following administration of pemetrexed. All patients should avoid NSAIDs with longer half-lives at least five days before, the day of, and two days following pemetrexed administration. If concomitant administration of an NSAID is necessary, patients should be monitored closely for toxicity, especially myelosuppression, renal and gastrointestinal toxicity).
No products indexed under this heading.

Fluvastatin Sodium (Concomitant administration of nephrotoxic drugs could result in delayed clearance of pemetrexed). Products include:
Lescol Capsules 2227
Lescol 2730
Lescol XL Tablets 2227

Foscarnet Sodium (Concomitant administration of nephrotoxic drugs could result in delayed clearance of pemetrexed).
No products indexed under this heading.

Fosinopril Sodium (Concomitant administration of nephrotoxic drugs could result in delayed clearance of pemetrexed).
No products indexed under this heading.

Furosemide (Concomitant administration of nephrotoxic drugs could result in delayed clearance of pemetrexed). Products include:
Furosemide Tablets 2117

Gadopentetate Dimeglumine (Concomitant administration of nephrotoxic drugs could result in delayed clearance of pemetrexed).
No products indexed under this heading.

Gentamicin (Concomitant administration of nephrotoxic drugs could result in delayed clearance of pemetrexed).
No products indexed under this heading.

Gentamicin Sulfate (Concomitant administration of nephrotoxic drugs could result in delayed clearance of pemetrexed). Products include:
Garamycin Injectable 3028
Genoptic Sterile Ophthalmic Solution .... ⊙227
Pred-G Ophthalmic Suspension ...... ⊙234
Pred-G Sterile Ophthalmic Ointment .... ⊙235

Glipizide (Concomitant administration of nephrotoxic drugs could result in delayed clearance of pemetrexed).
No products indexed under this heading.

Globulin, Immune (Human) (Concomitant administration of nephrotoxic drugs could result in delayed clearance of pemetrexed). Products include:
GamaSTAN 3231

Glyburide (Concomitant administration of nephrotoxic drugs could result in delayed clearance of pemetrexed).
No products indexed under this heading.

Gold Therapy (Concomitant administration of nephrotoxic drugs could result in delayed clearance of pemetrexed).
No products indexed under this heading.

HMG-CoA Reductase Inhibitors (Concomitant administration of nephrotoxic drugs could result in delayed clearance of pemetrexed).
No products indexed under this heading.

Hydrochlorothiazide (Concomitant administration of nephrotoxic drugs could result in delayed clearance of pemetrexed). Products include:
Aldoril Tablets 1884
Atacand HCT 637
Avalide Tablets 2889
Avalide Tablets 922
Benicar HCT Tablets 2852
Diovan HCT Tablets 2195
Dyazide Capsules 1389
Hyzaar 1964
Lotensin HCT Tablets 2235
Maxzide 2150
Micardis HCT Tablets 886
Moduretic Tablets 2003
Prinzide Tablets 2033
Teveten HCT Tablets 1710
Timolide Tablets 2056
Uniretic Tablets 3114
Vaseretic Tablets 2073
Zestoretic Tablets 701

Hydroflumethiazide (Concomitant administration of nephrotoxic drugs could result in delayed clearance of pemetrexed).
No products indexed under this heading.

Ibuprofen (Caution should be used when administering ibuprofen concurrently with pemetrexed to patients with mild to moderate renal insufficiency (CrCl 45-79 mL/min)). Products include:
Advil Allergy Sinus Caplets .... ■737
Advil .... ■737
Children's Advil Suspension .... ■742
Children's Advil Chewable Tablets .. ■741
Advil Cold & Sinus .... ■739
Advil Flu & Body Ache Caplets .... ■739
Children's Advil Cold Suspension ... ■741
Infants' Advil Concentrated Drops .. ■743
Junior Strength Advil Swallow Tablets .... ■740
Advil Migraine Liquigels .... ■740
Advil Multi-Symptom Cold Caplets .... ■738
Combunox Tablets 1183
Children's Motrin Oral Suspension and Chewable Tablets 1837
Children's Motrin Cold Non-Staining Dye-Free Oral Suspension 1838
Children's Motrin Cold Oral Suspension 1838
Children's Motrin Non-Staining Dye-Free Oral Suspension 1837
Motrin Cold & Sinus Caplets 1836
Motrin IB Tablets and Caplets 1836
Infants' Motrin Concentrated Drops 1837
Infants' Motrin Non-Staining Dye-Free Drops 1837
Junior Strength Motrin Caplets and Chewable Tablets 1837
Vicoprofen Tablets 533

Idarubicin Hydrochloride (Concomitant administration of nephrotoxic drugs could result in delayed clearance of pemetrexed). Products include:
Idamycin PFS Injection 2645

Ifosfamide (Concomitant administration of nephrotoxic drugs could result in delayed clearance of pemetrexed).
No products indexed under this heading.

Imipenem (Concomitant administration of nephrotoxic drugs could result in delayed clearance of pemetrexed). Products include:
Primaxin I.M. 2022
Primaxin I.V. 2024

Immune Globulin Intravenous (Human) (Concomitant administration of nephrotoxic drugs could result in delayed clearance of pemetrexed). Products include:
Carimune NF 3501
Gammagard Liquid 751
Gammagard S/D 754
Gamunex Immune Globulin I.V., 10% 3232
Iveegam EN 759

Indinavir Sulfate (Concomitant administration of nephrotoxic drugs could result in delayed clearance of pemetrexed). Products include:
Crixivan Capsules 1918

Indomethacin (Patients with mild to moderate renal insufficiency should avoid NSAIDs with short elimination half-lives two days before, the day of, and two days following administration of pemetrexed. All patients should avoid NSAIDs with longer half-lives at least five days before, the day of, and two days following pemetrexed administration. If concomitant administration of an NSAID is necessary, patients should be

monitored closely for toxicity, especially myelosuppression, renal and gastrointestinal toxicity). Products include:
Indocin 1968

Indomethacin Sodium Trihydrate (Patients with mild to moderate renal insufficiency should avoid NSAIDs with short elimination half-lives two days before, the day of, and two days following administration of pemetrexed. All patients should avoid NSAIDs with longer half-lives at least five days before, the day of, and two days following pemetrexed administration. If concomitant administration of an NSAID is necessary, patients should be monitored closely for toxicity, especially myelosuppression, renal and gastrointestinal toxicity). Products include:
Indocin I.V. 1973

Interferon Beta-1b (Concomitant administration of nephrotoxic drugs could result in delayed clearance of pemetrexed). Products include:
Betaseron for SC Injection 791

Interleuken-2 (Concomitant administration of nephrotoxic drugs could result in delayed clearance of pemetrexed).
No products indexed under this heading.

Iodamide Meglumine (Concomitant administration of nephrotoxic drugs could result in delayed clearance of pemetrexed).
No products indexed under this heading.

Iohexol (Concomitant administration of nephrotoxic drugs could result in delayed clearance of pemetrexed).
No products indexed under this heading.

Iopamidol (Concomitant administration of nephrotoxic drugs could result in delayed clearance of pemetrexed).
No products indexed under this heading.

Iopanoic Acid (Concomitant administration of nephrotoxic drugs could result in delayed clearance of pemetrexed).
No products indexed under this heading.

Iothalamate Meglumine (Concomitant administration of nephrotoxic drugs could result in delayed clearance of pemetrexed).
No products indexed under this heading.

Ioxaglate Meglumine (Concomitant administration of nephrotoxic drugs could result in delayed clearance of pemetrexed).
No products indexed under this heading.

Ioxaglate Sodium (Concomitant administration of nephrotoxic drugs could result in delayed clearance of pemetrexed).
No products indexed under this heading.

Kanamycin Sulfate (Concomitant administration of nephrotoxic drugs could result in delayed clearance of pemetrexed).
No products indexed under this heading.

Ketoprofen (Patients with mild to moderate renal insufficiency should avoid NSAIDs with short elimination half-lives two days before, the day of, and two days following administration of pemetrexed. All patients should avoid NSAIDs with longer half-lives at least five days before, the day of, and two days following pemetrexed administration. If concomitant administration of an NSAID is necessary, patients should be monitored closely for toxicity, especially myelosuppression, renal and gastrointestinal toxicity).
No products indexed under this heading.

Ketorolac Tromethamine (Patients with mild to moderate renal insufficiency should avoid NSAIDs with short elimination half-lives two days before, the day of, and two days following administration of pemetrexed. All patients should avoid NSAIDs with longer half-lives at least five days before, the day of, and two days following pemetrexed administration. If concomitant administration of an NSAID is necessary, patients should be monitored closely for toxicity, especially myelosuppression, renal and gastrointestinal toxicity). Products include:
Acular Ophthalmic Solution 561
Acular LS Ophthalmic Solution 562

Lamium album (Concomitant administration of nephrotoxic drugs could result in delayed clearance of pemetrexed).
No products indexed under this heading.

Lisinopril (Concomitant administration of nephrotoxic drugs could result in delayed clearance of pemetrexed). Products include:
Prinivil Tablets 2029
Prinzide Tablets 2033
Zestoretic Tablets 701
Zestril Tablets 704

Lithium (Concomitant administration of nephrotoxic drugs could result in delayed clearance of pemetrexed).
No products indexed under this heading.

Lithium Carbonate (Concomitant administration of nephrotoxic drugs could result in delayed clearance of pemetrexed). Products include:
Eskalith 1406
Lithobid Tablets 1670

Lithium Citrate (Concomitant administration of nephrotoxic drugs could result in delayed clearance of pemetrexed).
No products indexed under this heading.

Lopinavir (Concomitant administration of nephrotoxic drugs could result in delayed clearance of pemetrexed). Products include:
Kaletra 474

Loracarbef (Concomitant administration of nephrotoxic drugs could result in delayed clearance of pemetrexed).
No products indexed under this heading.

Lovastatin (Concomitant administration of nephrotoxic drugs could result in delayed clearance of pemetrexed). Products include:
Advicor Tablets 1694
Altoprev Extended-Release Tablets 1151
Mevacor Tablets 1996

Meclofenamate Sodium (Patients with mild to moderate renal insufficiency should avoid NSAIDs with short elimination half-lives two days before, the day of, and two days following administration of pemetrexed. All patients should avoid NSAIDs with longer half-lives at least five days before, the day of, and two days following pemetrexed administration. If concomitant administration of an NSAID is necessary, patients should be monitored closely for toxicity, especially myelosuppression, renal and gastrointestinal toxicity).
No products indexed under this heading.

Mefenamic Acid (Patients with mild to moderate renal insufficiency should avoid NSAIDs with short elimination half-lives two days before, the day of, and two days following administration of pemetrexed. All patients should avoid NSAIDs with longer half-lives at least five days before, the day of, and two days following pemetrexed administration. If concomitant administration of an NSAID is necessary, patients should be monitored closely for toxicity, especially myelosuppression, renal and gastrointestinal toxicity).
No products indexed under this heading.

Meloxicam (Patients with mild to moderate renal insufficiency should avoid NSAIDs with short elimination half-lives two days before, the day of, and two days following administration of pemetrexed. All patients should avoid NSAIDs with longer half-lives at least five days before, the day of, and two days following pemetrexed administration. If concomitant administration of an NSAID is necessary, patients should be monitored closely for toxicity, especially myelosuppression, renal and gastrointestinal toxicity). Products include:
Mobic Oral Suspension 893
Mobic Tablets 893

Melphalan Hydrochloride (Concomitant administration of nephrotoxic drugs could result in delayed clearance of pemetrexed). Products include:
Alkeran for Injection 976

Mesalamine (Concomitant administration of nephrotoxic drugs could result in delayed clearance of pemetrexed). Products include:
Asacol Delayed-Release Tablets 2688
Canasa Rectal Suppositories 726
Pentasa Capsules 3182

Methimazole (Concomitant administration of nephrotoxic drugs could result in delayed clearance of pemetrexed).
No products indexed under this heading.

Methotrexate (Concomitant administration of nephrotoxic drugs could result in delayed clearance of pemetrexed).
No products indexed under this heading.

Methotrexate Sodium (Concomitant administration of nephrotoxic drugs could result in delayed clearance of pemetrexed).
No products indexed under this heading.

Methyclothiazide (Concomitant administration of nephrotoxic drugs could result in delayed clearance of pemetrexed).
No products indexed under this heading.

Mezlocillin Sodium (Concomitant administration of nephrotoxic drugs could result in delayed clearance of pemetrexed).
No products indexed under this heading.

Minocycline Hydrochloride (Concomitant administration of nephrotoxic drugs could result in delayed clearance of pemetrexed). Products include:
Dynacin Tablets 1859

Mitomycin (Mitomycin-C) (Concomitant administration of nephrotoxic drugs could result in delayed clearance of pemetrexed).
No products indexed under this heading.

Moexipril Hydrochloride (Concomitant administration of nephrotoxic drugs could result in delayed clearance of pemetrexed). Products include:
Uniretic Tablets 3114
Univasc Tablets 3118

Muromonab-CD3 (Concomitant administration of nephrotoxic drugs could result in delayed clearance of pemetrexed). Products include:
Orthoclone OKT3 Sterile Solution 2370

Nabumetone (Patients with mild to moderate renal insufficiency should avoid NSAIDs with short elimination half-lives two days before, the day of, and two days following administration of pemetrexed. All patients should avoid NSAIDs with longer half-lives at least five days before, the day of, and two days following pemetrexed administration. If concomitant administration of an NSAID is necessary, patients should be monitored closely for toxicity, especially myelosuppression, renal and gastrointestinal toxicity). Products include:
Relafen Tablets 1523

Nafcillin Sodium (Concomitant administration of nephrotoxic drugs could result in delayed clearance of pemetrexed).
No products indexed under this heading.

Naproxen (Patients with mild to moderate renal insufficiency should avoid NSAIDs with short elimination half-lives two days before, the day of, and two days following administration of pemetrexed. All patients should avoid NSAIDs with longer half-lives at least five days before, the day of, and two days following pemetrexed administration. If concomitant administration of an NSAID is necessary, patients should be monitored closely for toxicity, especially myelosuppression, renal and gastrointestinal toxicity). Products include:
EC-Naprosyn Delayed-Release Tablets 2769
Naprosyn Suspension 2769
Naprosyn Tablets 2769
Prevacid NapraPAC 3277

Naproxen Sodium (Patients with mild to moderate renal insufficiency should avoid NSAIDs with short elimination half-lives two days before, the day of, and two days following administration of pemetrexed. All patients should avoid NSAIDs with longer half-lives at least five days before, the day of, and two days following pemetrexed administration. If concomitant administration of an NSAID is necessary, patients should be monitored closely for toxicity,

especially myelosuppression, renal and gastrointestinal toxicity). Products include:
Aleve Tablets, Caplets and Gelcaps .... ▣605
Anaprox Tablets 2769
Anaprox DS Tablets 2769

Nelfinavir Mesylate (Concomitant administration of nephrotoxic drugs could result in delayed clearance of pemetrexed). Products include:
Viracept 2556

Neomycin (Concomitant administration of nephrotoxic drugs could result in delayed clearance of pemetrexed). Products include:
Neosporin Ointment .... ▣702
Neosporin + Pain Relief Maximum Strength Cream........ ▣703
Neosporin + Pain Relief Maximum Strength Ointment........ ▣703

Neomycin, oral (Concomitant administration of nephrotoxic drugs could result in delayed clearance of pemetrexed).
No products indexed under this heading.

Neomycin Sulfate (Concomitant administration of nephrotoxic drugs could result in delayed clearance of pemetrexed). Products include:
Poly-Pred Liquifilm Ophthalmic Suspension........ ⊙231

Nevirapine (Concomitant administration of nephrotoxic drugs could result in delayed clearance of pemetrexed). Products include:
Viramune Oral Suspension........ 903
Viramune Tablets........ 903

Norfloxacin (Concomitant administration of nephrotoxic drugs could result in delayed clearance of pemetrexed). Products include:
Noroxin Tablets........ 2009

Olsalazine Sodium (Concomitant administration of nephrotoxic drugs could result in delayed clearance of pemetrexed).
No products indexed under this heading.

Omeprazole (Concomitant administration of nephrotoxic drugs could result in delayed clearance of pemetrexed). Products include:
Zegerid Powder for Oral Solution........ 2972

Oxaprozin (Patients with mild to moderate renal insufficiency should avoid NSAIDs with short elimination half-lives two days before, the day of, and two days following administration of pemetrexed. All patients should avoid NSAIDs with longer half-lives at least five days before, the day of, and two days following pemetrexed administration. If concomitant administration of an NSAID is necessary, patients should be monitored closely for toxicity, especially myelosuppression, renal and gastrointestinal toxicity).
No products indexed under this heading.

Pamidronate Disodium (Concomitant administration of nephrotoxic drugs could result in delayed clearance of pemetrexed). Products include:
Aredia for Injection........ 2168

Paroxetine Hydrochloride (Concomitant administration of nephrotoxic drugs could result in delayed clearance of pemetrexed). Products include:
Paxil CR Controlled-Release Tablets........ 1509
Paxil........ 1501

Penicillamine (Concomitant administration of nephrotoxic drugs could result in delayed clearance of pemetrexed). Products include:
Cuprimine Capsules........ 1925

Penicillin G Benzathine (Concomitant administration of nephrotoxic drugs could result in delayed clearance of pemetrexed).
No products indexed under this heading.

Penicillin G Potassium (Concomitant administration of nephrotoxic drugs could result in delayed clearance of pemetrexed).
No products indexed under this heading.

Penicillin G Procaine (Concomitant administration of nephrotoxic drugs could result in delayed clearance of pemetrexed).
No products indexed under this heading.

Penicillin G Sodium (Concomitant administration of nephrotoxic drugs could result in delayed clearance of pemetrexed).
No products indexed under this heading.

Penicillin V Potassium (Concomitant administration of nephrotoxic drugs could result in delayed clearance of pemetrexed).
No products indexed under this heading.

Pentamidine Isethionate (Concomitant administration of nephrotoxic drugs could result in delayed clearance of pemetrexed).
No products indexed under this heading.

Perindopril Erbumine (Concomitant administration of nephrotoxic drugs could result in delayed clearance of pemetrexed). Products include:
Aceon Tablets (2 mg, 4 mg, 8 mg)........ 3191

Phenylbutazone (Patients with mild to moderate renal insufficiency should avoid NSAIDs with short elimination half-lives two days before, the day of, and two days following administration of pemetrexed. All patients should avoid NSAIDs with longer half-lives at least five days before, the day of, and two days following pemetrexed administration. If concomitant administration of an NSAID is necessary, patients should be monitored closely for toxicity, especially myelosuppression, renal and gastrointestinal toxicity).
No products indexed under this heading.

Piroxicam (Patients with mild to moderate renal insufficiency should avoid NSAIDs with short elimination half-lives two days before, the day of, and two days following administration of pemetrexed. All patients should avoid NSAIDs with longer half-lives at least five days before, the day of, and two days following pemetrexed administration. If concomitant administration of an NSAID is necessary, patients should be monitored closely for toxicity, especially myelosuppression, renal and gastrointestinal toxicity).
No products indexed under this heading.

Plicamycin (Concomitant administration of nephrotoxic drugs could result in delayed clearance of pemetrexed).
No products indexed under this heading.

Polymyxin (Concomitant administration of nephrotoxic drugs could result in delayed clearance of pemetrexed).
No products indexed under this heading.

Polymyxin B Sulfate (Concomitant administration of nephrotoxic drugs could result in delayed clearance of pemetrexed). Products include:
Neosporin Ointment........ ▣702
Neosporin + Pain Relief Maximum Strength Cream........ ▣703
Neosporin + Pain Relief Maximum Strength Ointment........ ▣703
Poly-Pred Liquifilm Ophthalmic Suspension........ ⊙231
Polysporin Ointment........ ▣706
Polytrim Ophthalmic Solution........ 570

Polythiazide (Concomitant administration of nephrotoxic drugs could result in delayed clearance of pemetrexed).
No products indexed under this heading.

Pravastatin Sodium (Concomitant administration of nephrotoxic drugs could result in delayed clearance of pemetrexed). Products include:
Pravachol Tablets........ 943

Probenecid (Concomitant administration of substances that are also tubularly secreted (e.g., probenecid) could potentially result in delayed clearance of pemetrexed).
No products indexed under this heading.

Quinapril Hydrochloride (Concomitant administration of nephrotoxic drugs could result in delayed clearance of pemetrexed).
No products indexed under this heading.

Rabeprazole Sodium (Concomitant administration of nephrotoxic drugs could result in delayed clearance of pemetrexed). Products include:
Aciphex Tablets........ 1081

Ramipril (Concomitant administration of nephrotoxic drugs could result in delayed clearance of pemetrexed). Products include:
Altace Capsules........ 1673

Rifampin (Concomitant administration of nephrotoxic drugs could result in delayed clearance of pemetrexed).
No products indexed under this heading.

Riluzole (Concomitant administration of nephrotoxic drugs could result in delayed clearance of pemetrexed). Products include:
Rilutek Tablets........ 2945

Ritonavir (Concomitant administration of nephrotoxic drugs could result in delayed clearance of pemetrexed). Products include:
Kaletra........ 474
Norvir........ 499

Rofecoxib (Patients with mild to moderate renal insufficiency should avoid NSAIDs with short elimination half-lives two days before, the day of, and two days following administration of pemetrexed. All patients should avoid NSAIDs with longer half-lives at least five days before, the day of, and two days following pemetrexed administration. If concomitant administration of an NSAID is necessary, patients should be monitored closely for toxicity, especially myelosuppression, renal and gastrointestinal toxicity).
No products indexed under this heading.

Saquinavir (Concomitant administration of nephrotoxic drugs could result in delayed clearance of pemetrexed).
No products indexed under this heading.

Sibutramine Hydrochloride Monohydrate (Concomitant administration of nephrotoxic drugs could result in delayed clearance of pemetrexed). Products include:
Meridia Capsules........ 485

Simvastatin (Concomitant administration of nephrotoxic drugs could result in delayed clearance of pemetrexed). Products include:
Vytorin 10/10 Tablets........ 2084
Vytorin 10/10 Tablets........ 3092
Vytorin 10/20 Tablets........ 2084
Vytorin 10/20 Tablets........ 3092
Vytorin 10/40 Tablets........ 3092
Vytorin 10/40 Tablets........ 2084
Vytorin 10/80 Tablets........ 2084
Vytorin 10/80 Tablets........ 3092
Zocor Tablets........ 2078

Spirapril Hydrochloride (Concomitant administration of nephrotoxic drugs could result in delayed clearance of pemetrexed).
No products indexed under this heading.

Stavudine (Concomitant administration of nephrotoxic drugs could result in delayed clearance of pemetrexed). Products include:
Zerit........ 971

Streptomycin Sulfate (Concomitant administration of nephrotoxic drugs could result in delayed clearance of pemetrexed).
No products indexed under this heading.

Streptozocin (Concomitant administration of nephrotoxic drugs could result in delayed clearance of pemetrexed).
No products indexed under this heading.

Sulfacytine (Concomitant administration of nephrotoxic drugs could result in delayed clearance of pemetrexed).
No products indexed under this heading.

Sulfamethizole (Concomitant administration of nephrotoxic drugs could result in delayed clearance of pemetrexed).
No products indexed under this heading.

Sulfamethoxazole (Concomitant administration of nephrotoxic drugs could result in delayed clearance of pemetrexed).
No products indexed under this heading.

Sulfasalazine (Concomitant administration of nephrotoxic drugs could result in delayed clearance of pemetrexed).
No products indexed under this heading.

Sulfinpyrazone (Concomitant administration of nephrotoxic drugs could result in delayed clearance of pemetrexed).
No products indexed under this heading.

Sulfisoxazole (Concomitant administration of nephrotoxic drugs could result in delayed clearance of pemetrexed).
No products indexed under this heading.

Sulfisoxazole Acetyl (Concomitant administration of nephrotoxic drugs could result in delayed clearance of pemetrexed).
No products indexed under this heading.

Sulfisoxazole Diolamine (Concomitant administration of nephrotoxic drugs could result in delayed clearance of pemetrexed).
No products indexed under this heading.

Sulindac (Patients with mild to moderate renal insufficiency should avoid NSAIDs with short elimination half-lives two days before, the day of, and two days following administration of pemetrexed. All patients should avoid NSAIDs with longer half-lives at least five days before, the day of, and two days following pemetrexed administration. If concomitant administration of an NSAID is necessary, patients should be monitored closely for toxicity, especially myelosuppression, renal and gastrointestinal toxicity). Products include:
Clinoril Tablets 1899

Tacrolimus (Concomitant administration of nephrotoxic drugs could result in delayed clearance of pemetrexed). Products include:
Prograf Capsules and Injection 624
Protopic Ointment 629

Tenofovir Disoproxil Fumarate (Concomitant administration of nephrotoxic drugs could result in delayed clearance of pemetrexed). Products include:
Truvada Tablets 1279
Viread Tablets 1284

Thioguanine (Concomitant administration of nephrotoxic drugs could result in delayed clearance of pemetrexed). Products include:
Tabloid Tablets 1545

Ticarcillin Disodium (Concomitant administration of nephrotoxic drugs could result in delayed clearance of pemetrexed). Products include:
Timentin ADD-Vantage 1556
Timentin Injection Galaxy Container 1559
Timentin IV Infusion 1553
Timentin Pharmacy Bulk Package 1562

Tobramycin (Concomitant administration of nephrotoxic drugs could result in delayed clearance of pemetrexed). Products include:
TOBI Solution for Inhalation 1015
TobraDex Ophthalmic Ointment 558
TobraDex Ophthalmic Suspension 558
Zylet Ophthalmic Suspension 3508

Tobramycin Sulfate (Concomitant administration of nephrotoxic drugs could result in delayed clearance of pemetrexed).
No products indexed under this heading.

Tolazamide (Concomitant administration of nephrotoxic drugs could result in delayed clearance of pemetrexed).
No products indexed under this heading.

Tolbutamide (Concomitant administration of nephrotoxic drugs could result in delayed clearance of pemetrexed).
No products indexed under this heading.

Tolmetin Sodium (Patients with mild to moderate renal insufficiency should avoid NSAIDs with short elimination half-lives two days before, the day of, and two days following administration of pemetrexed. All patients should avoid NSAIDs with longer half-lives at least five days before, the day of, and two days following pemetrexed administration. If concomitant administration of an NSAID is necessary, patients should be monitored closely for toxicity, especially myelosuppression, renal and gastrointestinal toxicity).
No products indexed under this heading.

Trandolapril (Concomitant administration of nephrotoxic drugs could result in delayed clearance of pemetrexed). Products include:
Mavik Tablets 482
Tarka Tablets 519

Triamterene (Concomitant administration of nephrotoxic drugs could result in delayed clearance of pemetrexed). Products include:
Dyazide Capsules 1389
Dyrenium Capsules 3390
Maxzide 2150

Trimethadione (Concomitant administration of nephrotoxic drugs could result in delayed clearance of pemetrexed).
No products indexed under this heading.

Trovafloxacin Mesylate (Concomitant administration of nephrotoxic drugs could result in delayed clearance of pemetrexed).
No products indexed under this heading.

Tyropanoate Sodium (Concomitant administration of nephrotoxic drugs could result in delayed clearance of pemetrexed).
No products indexed under this heading.

Valacyclovir Hydrochloride (Concomitant administration of nephrotoxic drugs could result in delayed clearance of pemetrexed). Products include:
Valtrex Caplets 1573

Valdecoxib (Patients with mild to moderate renal insufficiency should avoid NSAIDs with short elimination half-lives two days before, the day of, and two days following administration of pemetrexed. All patients should avoid NSAIDs with longer half-lives at least five days before, the day of, and two days following pemetrexed administration. If concomitant administration of an NSAID is necessary, patients should be monitored closely for toxicity, especially myelosuppression, renal and gastrointestinal toxicity).
No products indexed under this heading.

Vancomycin Hydrochloride (Concomitant administration of nephrotoxic drugs could result in delayed clearance of pemetrexed). Products include:
Vancocin HCl Capsules, USP 3370

Voriconazole (Concomitant administration of nephrotoxic drugs could result in delayed clearance of pemetrexed). Products include:
VFEND I.V. 2543
VFEND Oral Suspension 2543
VFEND Tablets 2543

Zalcitabine (Concomitant administration of nephrotoxic drugs could result in delayed clearance of pemetrexed).
No products indexed under this heading.

Zidovudine (Concomitant administration of nephrotoxic drugs could result in delayed clearance of pemetrexed). Products include:
Combivir Tablets 1373
Retrovir 1533
Retrovir IV Infusion 1537
Trizivir Tablets 1565

Zoledronic acid (Concomitant administration of nephrotoxic drugs could result in delayed clearance of pemetrexed). Products include:
Zometa for Intravenous Infusion 2306

ALINIA FOR ORAL SUSPENSION

(Nitazoxanide) 2840
May interact with highly protein bound drugs (selected). Compounds in these categories include:

Amiodarone Hydrochloride (Metabolite is highly bound to plasma protein. Use caution when administering nitazoxanide concurrently with other highly plasma protein-bound drugs with narrow therapeutic indices). Products include:
Pacerone Tablets 3337

Amitriptyline Hydrochloride (Metabolite is highly bound to plasma protein. Use caution when administering nitazoxanide concurrently with other highly plasma protein-bound drugs with narrow therapeutic indices).
No products indexed under this heading.

Atovaquone (Metabolite is highly bound to plasma protein. Use caution when administering nitazoxanide concurrently with other highly plasma protein-bound drugs with narrow therapeutic indices). Products include:
Malarone Tablets 1484
Malarone Pediatric Tablets 1484
Mepron Suspension 1487

Cefonicid Sodium (Metabolite is highly bound to plasma protein. Use caution when administering nitazoxanide concurrently with other highly plasma protein-bound drugs with narrow therapeutic indices).
No products indexed under this heading.

Celecoxib (Metabolite is highly bound to plasma protein. Use caution when administering nitazoxanide concurrently with other highly plasma protein-bound drugs with narrow therapeutic indices). Products include:
Celebrex Capsules 3130

Chlordiazepoxide (Metabolite is highly bound to plasma protein. Use caution when administering nitazoxanide concurrently with other highly plasma protein-bound drugs with narrow therapeutic indices).
No products indexed under this heading.

Chlordiazepoxide Hydrochloride (Metabolite is highly bound to plasma protein. Use caution when administering nitazoxanide concurrently with other highly plasma protein-bound drugs with narrow therapeutic indices). Products include:
Librium Capsules 3349

Chlorpromazine (Metabolite is highly bound to plasma protein. Use caution when administering nitazoxanide concurrently with other highly plasma protein-bound drugs with narrow therapeutic indices).
No products indexed under this heading.

Chlorpromazine Hydrochloride (Metabolite is highly bound to plasma protein. Use caution when administering nitazoxanide concurrently with other highly plasma protein-bound drugs with narrow therapeutic indices).
No products indexed under this heading.

Clomipramine Hydrochloride (Metabolite is highly bound to plasma protein. Use caution when administering nitazoxanide concurrently with other highly plasma protein-bound drugs with narrow therapeutic indices).
No products indexed under this heading.

Clozapine (Metabolite is highly bound to plasma protein. Use caution when administering nitazoxanide concurrently with other highly plasma protein-bound drugs with narrow therapeutic indices). Products include:
Clozapine Tablets 2141
Clozaril Tablets 2174
FazaClo Orally Disintegrating Tablets 547

Cyclosporine (Metabolite is highly bound to plasma protein. Use caution when administering nitazoxanide concurrently with other highly plasma protein-bound drugs with narrow therapeutic indices). Products include:
Gengraf Capsules 458
Neoral Soft Gelatin Capsules 2247
Neoral Oral Solution 2247
Restasis Ophthalmic Emulsion 570
Sandimmune 2259

Diazepam (Metabolite is highly bound to plasma protein. Use caution when administering nitazoxanide concurrently with other highly plasma protein-bound drugs with narrow therapeutic indices). Products include:
Diastat Rectal Delivery System 3344
Valium Tablets 2822

Diclofenac Potassium (Metabolite is highly bound to plasma protein. Use caution when administering nitazoxanide concurrently with other highly plasma protein-bound drugs with narrow therapeutic indices). Products include:
Cataflam Tablets 2173

Diclofenac Sodium (Metabolite is highly bound to plasma protein. Use caution when administering nitazoxanide concurrently with other highly plasma protein-bound drugs with narrow therapeutic indices). Products include:
Arthrotec Tablets 3126
Voltaren Ophthalmic Solution 2300
Voltaren Tablets 2298
Voltaren-XR Tablets 2301

Dipyridamole (Metabolite is highly bound to plasma protein. Use caution when administering nitazoxanide concurrently with other highly plasma protein-bound drugs with narrow therapeutic indices). Products include:
Aggrenox Capsules 855
Persantine Tablets 898

Fenoprofen Calcium (Metabolite is highly bound to plasma protein. Use caution when administering nitazoxanide concurrently with other highly plasma protein-bound drugs with narrow therapeutic indices). Products include:

Nalfon Capsules 2504

Flurazepam Hydrochloride (Metabolite is highly bound to plasma protein. Use caution when administering nitazoxanide concurrently with other highly plasma protein-bound drugs with narrow therapeutic indices). Products include:

Dalmane Capsules 3343

Flurbiprofen (Metabolite is highly bound to plasma protein. Use caution when administering nitazoxanide concurrently with other highly plasma protein-bound drugs with narrow therapeutic indices).

No products indexed under this heading.

Glipizide (Metabolite is highly bound to plasma protein. Use caution when administering nitazoxanide concurrently with other highly plasma protein-bound drugs with narrow therapeutic indices).

No products indexed under this heading.

Ibuprofen (Metabolite is highly bound to plasma protein. Use caution when administering nitazoxanide concurrently with other highly plasma protein-bound drugs with narrow therapeutic indices). Products include:

Advil Allergy Sinus Caplets .... ▣737
Advil .... ▣737
Children's Advil Suspension .... ▣742
Children's Advil Chewable Tablets .. ▣741
Advil Cold & Sinus .... ▣739
Advil Flu & Body Ache Caplets .... ▣739
Children's Advil Cold Suspension ... ▣741
Infants' Advil Concentrated Drops .. ▣743
Junior Strength Advil Swallow Tablets .... ▣740
Advil Migraine Liquigels .... ▣740
Advil Multi-Symptom Cold Caplets .... ▣738
Combunox Tablets 1183
Children's Motrin Oral Suspension and Chewable Tablets 1837
Children's Motrin Cold Non-Staining Dye-Free Oral Suspension 1838
Children's Motrin Cold Oral Suspension 1838
Children's Motrin Non-Staining Dye-Free Oral Suspension 1837
Motrin Cold & Sinus Caplets 1836
Motrin IB Tablets and Caplets 1836
Infants' Motrin Concentrated Drops 1837
Infants' Motrin Non-Staining Dye-Free Drops 1837
Junior Strength Motrin Caplets and Chewable Tablets 1837
Vicoprofen Tablets 533

Imipramine Hydrochloride (Metabolite is highly bound to plasma protein. Use caution when administering nitazoxanide concurrently with other highly plasma protein-bound drugs with narrow therapeutic indices).

No products indexed under this heading.

Imipramine Pamoate (Metabolite is highly bound to plasma protein. Use caution when administering nitazoxanide concurrently with other highly plasma protein-bound drugs with narrow therapeutic indices).

No products indexed under this heading.

Indomethacin (Metabolite is highly bound to plasma protein. Use caution when administering nitazoxanide concurrently with other highly plasma protein-bound drugs with narrow therapeutic indices). Products include:

Indocin 1968

Indomethacin Sodium Trihydrate (Metabolite is highly bound to plasma protein. Use caution when administering nitazoxanide concurrently with other highly plasma protein-bound drugs with narrow therapeutic indices). Products include:

Indocin I.V. 1973

Ketoprofen (Metabolite is highly bound to plasma protein. Use caution when administering nitazoxanide concurrently with other highly plasma protein-bound drugs with narrow therapeutic indices).

No products indexed under this heading.

Ketorolac Tromethamine (Metabolite is highly bound to plasma protein. Use caution when administering nitazoxanide concurrently with other highly plasma protein-bound drugs with narrow therapeutic indices). Products include:

Acular Ophthalmic Solution 561
Acular LS Ophthalmic Solution 562

Meclofenamate Sodium (Metabolite is highly bound to plasma protein. Use caution when administering nitazoxanide concurrently with other highly plasma protein-bound drugs with narrow therapeutic indices).

No products indexed under this heading.

Mefenamic Acid (Metabolite is highly bound to plasma protein. Use caution when administering nitazoxanide concurrently with other highly plasma protein-bound drugs with narrow therapeutic indices).

No products indexed under this heading.

Midazolam Hydrochloride (Metabolite is highly bound to plasma protein. Use caution when administering nitazoxanide concurrently with other highly plasma protein-bound drugs with narrow therapeutic indices).

No products indexed under this heading.

Naproxen (Metabolite is highly bound to plasma protein. Use caution when administering nitazoxanide concurrently with other highly plasma protein-bound drugs with narrow therapeutic indices). Products include:

EC-Naprosyn Delayed-Release Tablets 2769
Naprosyn Suspension 2769
Naprosyn Tablets 2769
Prevacid NapraPAC 3277

Naproxen Sodium (Metabolite is highly bound to plasma protein. Use caution when administering nitazoxanide concurrently with other highly plasma protein-bound drugs with narrow therapeutic indices). Products include:

Aleve Tablets, Caplets and Gelcaps .... ▣605
Anaprox Tablets 2769
Anaprox DS Tablets 2769

Nortriptyline Hydrochloride (Metabolite is highly bound to plasma protein. Use caution when administering nitazoxanide concurrently with other highly plasma protein-bound drugs with narrow therapeutic indices).

No products indexed under this heading.

Oxaprozin (Metabolite is highly bound to plasma protein. Use caution when administering nitazoxanide concurrently with other highly plasma protein-bound drugs with narrow therapeutic indices).

No products indexed under this heading.

Oxazepam (Metabolite is highly bound to plasma protein. Use caution when administering nitazoxanide concurrently with other highly plasma protein-bound drugs with narrow therapeutic indices).

No products indexed under this heading.

Phenylbutazone (Metabolite is highly bound to plasma protein. Use caution when administering nitazoxanide concurrently with other highly plasma protein-bound drugs with narrow therapeutic indices).

No products indexed under this heading.

Piroxicam (Metabolite is highly bound to plasma protein. Use caution when administering nitazoxanide concurrently with other highly plasma protein-bound drugs with narrow therapeutic indices).

No products indexed under this heading.

Propranolol Hydrochloride (Metabolite is highly bound to plasma protein. Use caution when administering nitazoxanide concurrently with other highly plasma protein-bound drugs with narrow therapeutic indices). Products include:

Inderal LA Long-Acting Capsules 3421
InnoPran XL Capsules 2728

Sulindac (Metabolite is highly bound to plasma protein. Use caution when administering nitazoxanide concurrently with other highly plasma protein-bound drugs with narrow therapeutic indices). Products include:

Clinoril Tablets 1899

Temazepam (Metabolite is highly bound to plasma protein. Use caution when administering nitazoxanide concurrently with other highly plasma protein-bound drugs with narrow therapeutic indices).

No products indexed under this heading.

Tolbutamide (Metabolite is highly bound to plasma protein. Use caution when administering nitazoxanide concurrently with other highly plasma protein-bound drugs with narrow therapeutic indices).

No products indexed under this heading.

Tolmetin Sodium (Metabolite is highly bound to plasma protein. Use caution when administering nitazoxanide concurrently with other highly plasma protein-bound drugs with narrow therapeutic indices).

No products indexed under this heading.

Trimipramine Maleate (Metabolite is highly bound to plasma protein. Use caution when administering nitazoxanide concurrently with other highly plasma protein-bound drugs with narrow therapeutic indices). Products include:

Surmontil Capsules 2347

Warfarin Sodium (Metabolite is highly bound to plasma protein. Use caution when administering nitazoxanide concurrently with other highly plasma protein-bound drugs with narrow therapeutic indices). Products include:

Coumadin for Injection 932
Coumadin Tablets 932

ALINIA TABLETS

(Nitazoxanide) 2840
See Alinia for Oral Suspension

ALKERAN FOR INJECTION

(Melphalan Hydrochloride) 976
May interact with:

Carmustine (BCNU) (Reduced threshold for BCNU lung toxicity).

No products indexed under this heading.

Cisplatin (Affects melphalan kinetics by inducing renal dysfunction and subsequently altering melphalan clearance).

No products indexed under this heading.

Cyclosporine (Potential for severe renal failure). Products include:

Gengraf Capsules 458
Neoral Soft Gelatin Capsules 2247
Neoral Oral Solution 2247
Restasis Ophthalmic Emulsion 570
Sandimmune 2259

Nalidixic Acid (Increased incidence of severe hemorrhagic necrotic enterocolitis).

No products indexed under this heading.

ALKERAN TABLETS

(Melphalan) 977
None cited in PDR database.

ALL-BASIC CAPSULES

(Amino Acid Preparations) 2110
None cited in PDR database.

ALLEGRA CAPSULES

(Fexofenadine Hydrochloride) 2857
May interact with erythromycin and certain other agents. Compounds in these categories include:

Aluminum Hydroxide (Administration of fexofenadine within 15 minutes of an aluminum and magnesium containing antacid decreased fexofenadine AUC by 41% and Cmax by 43%; Allegra should not be taken closely in time with aluminum and magnesium containing antacids). Products include:

Gaviscon Regular Strength Liquid .. ▣620
Gaviscon Regular Strength Tablets .... ▣619
Gaviscon Extra Strength Liquid .... ▣620
Gaviscon Extra Strength Tablets .... ▣619
Maalox Max Maximum Strength Antacid/Anti-Gas Liquid 2165
Maalox Regular Strength Antacid/Antigas Liquid 2164

Erythromycin (Co-administration with erythromycin enhances fexofenadine gastrointestinal absorption thereby increasing plasma levels of fexofenadine; in vivo animal studies suggest that erythromycin may also decrease biliary excretion). Products include:

Erygel Topical Gel 2096
Ery-Tab Tablets 447

Erythromycin Base Filmtab Tablets 454
Erythromycin Delayed-Release Capsules, USP 456
PCE Dispertab Tablets 510

Erythromycin Estolate (Co-administration with erythromycin enhances fexofenadine gastrointestinal absorption thereby increasing plasma levels of fexofenadine; in vivo animal studies suggest that erythromycin may also decrease biliary excretion).
No products indexed under this heading.

Erythromycin Ethylsuccinate (Co-administration with erythromycin enhances fexofenadine gastrointestinal absorption thereby increasing plasma levels of fexofenadine; in vivo animal studies suggest that erythromycin may also decrease biliary excretion). Products include:
E.E.S. 449
EryPed 445

Erythromycin Gluceptate (Co-administration with erythromycin enhances fexofenadine gastrointestinal absorption thereby increasing plasma levels of fexofenadine; in vivo animal studies suggest that erythromycin may also decrease biliary excretion).
No products indexed under this heading.

Erythromycin Lactobionate (Co-administration with erythromycin enhances fexofenadine gastrointestinal absorption thereby increasing plasma levels of fexofenadine; in vivo animal studies suggest that erythromycin may also decrease biliary excretion).
No products indexed under this heading.

Erythromycin Stearate (Co-administration with erythromycin enhances fexofenadine gastrointestinal absorption thereby increasing plasma levels of fexofenadine; in vivo animal studies suggest that erythromycin may also decrease biliary excretion). Products include:
Erythrocin Stearate Filmtab Tablets 452

Ketoconazole (Co-administration with ketoconazole enhances fexofenadine gastrointestinal absorption thereby increasing plasma levels of fexofenadine; in vivo animal studies suggest that ketoconazole may also decrease fexofenadine gastrointestinal secretion). Products include:
Nizoral A-D Shampoo, 1% 1839
Nizoral 2% Shampoo 1838

Magnesium Hydroxide (Administration of fexofenadine within 15 minutes of an aluminum and magnesium containing antacid decreased fexofenadine AUC by 41% and Cmax by 43%; Allegra should not be taken closely in time with aluminum and magnesium containing antacids). Products include:
Maalox Max Maximum Strength Antacid/Anti-Gas Liquid 2165
Maalox Regular Strength Antacid/Antigas Liquid 2164
Pepcid Complete Chewable Tablets 1672
Rolaids Tablets 707
Extra Strength Rolaids Tablets 707
Rolaids Multi-Symptom Antacid & Antigas Tablets 708

ALLEGRA TABLETS

(Fexofenadine Hydrochloride) 2857
See Allegra Capsules

ALLEGRA-D 12 HOUR EXTENDED-RELEASE TABLETS

(Fexofenadine Hydrochloride, Pseudoephedrine Hydrochloride) 2860
May interact with antacids, erythromycin, cardiac glycosides, monoamine oxidase inhibitors, sympathomimetics, and certain other agents. Compounds in these categories include:

Albuterol (Combined effects of pseudoephedrine with other sympathomimetics on cardiovascular system may be harmful to the patient). Products include:
Proventil Inhalation Aerosol 3067

Albuterol Sulfate (Combined effects of pseudoephedrine with other sympathomimetics on cardiovascular system may be harmful to the patient). Products include:
AccuNeb Inhalation Solution 1055
Combivent Inhalation Aerosol 878
DuoNeb Inhalation Solution 1058
Proventil Inhalation Solution 0.083% 3069
Proventil HFA Inhalation Aerosol 3071
Ventolin HFA Inhalation Aerosol 1576
VoSpire Extended-Release Tablets 2352

Aluminum Carbonate (Co-administration with fexofenadine HCL may decrease fexofenadine AUC by 41% and Cmax by 43%).
No products indexed under this heading.

Aluminum Hydroxide (Co-administration with fexofenadine HCL may decrease fexofenadine AUC by 41% and Cmax by 43%). Products include:
Gaviscon Regular Strength Liquid 620
Gaviscon Regular Strength Tablets 619
Gaviscon Extra Strength Liquid 620
Gaviscon Extra Strength Tablets 619
Maalox Max Maximum Strength Antacid/Anti-Gas Liquid 2165
Maalox Regular Strength Antacid/Antigas Liquid 2164

Apple Juice (Co-administration with grapefruit, orange or apple juice will reduce the bioavailability and exposure or fexofenadine).
No products indexed under this heading.

Deslanoside (Increased ectopic pacemaker activity can occur when pseudoephedrine is used concomitantly with digitalis).
No products indexed under this heading.

Digitalis Glycoside Preparations (Increased ectopic pacemaker activity can occur when pseudoephedrine is used concomitantly with digitalis).
No products indexed under this heading.

Digitoxin (Increased ectopic pacemaker activity can occur when pseudoephedrine is used concomitantly with digitalis).
No products indexed under this heading.

Digoxin (Increased ectopic pacemaker activity can occur when pseudoephedrine is used concomitantly with digitalis). Products include:
Digitek Tablets 2146
Lanoxicaps Capsules 1458
Lanoxin Injection 1462
Lanoxin Tablets 1468
Lanoxin Injection Pediatric 1465

Dobutamine Hydrochloride (Combined effects of pseudoephedrine with other sympathomimetics on cardiovascular system may be harmful to the patient).
No products indexed under this heading.

Dopamine Hydrochloride (Combined effects of pseudoephedrine with other sympathomimetics on cardiovascular system may be harmful to the patient).
No products indexed under this heading.

Ephedrine Hydrochloride (Combined effects of pseudoephedrine with other sympathomimetics on cardiovascular system may be harmful to the patient). Products include:
Primatene Tablets 749

Ephedrine Sulfate (Combined effects of pseudoephedrine with other sympathomimetics on cardiovascular system may be harmful to the patient).
No products indexed under this heading.

Ephedrine Tannate (Combined effects of pseudoephedrine with other sympathomimetics on cardiovascular system may be harmful to the patient).
No products indexed under this heading.

Epinephrine (Combined effects of pseudoephedrine with other sympathomimetics on cardiovascular system may be harmful to the patient). Products include:
EpiPen 1061
Primatene Mist 749

Epinephrine Bitartrate (Combined effects of pseudoephedrine with other sympathomimetics on cardiovascular system may be harmful to the patient).
No products indexed under this heading.

Epinephrine Hydrochloride (Combined effects of pseudoephedrine with other sympathomimetics on cardiovascular system may be harmful to the patient).
No products indexed under this heading.

Erythromycin (Co-administration with erythromycin enhances fexofenadine gastrointestinal absorption thereby increasing plasma levels of fexofenadine; in vivo animal studies suggest that erythromycin may also decrease biliary excretion). Products include:
Erygel Topical Gel 2096
Ery-Tab Tablets 447
Erythromycin Base Filmtab Tablets 454
Erythromycin Delayed-Release Capsules, USP 456
PCE Dispertab Tablets 510

Erythromycin Estolate (Co-administration with erythromycin enhances fexofenadine gastrointestinal absorption thereby increasing plasma levels of fexofenadine; in vivo animal studies suggest that erythromycin may also decrease biliary excretion).
No products indexed under this heading.

Erythromycin Ethylsuccinate (Co-administration with erythromycin enhances fexofenadine gastrointestinal absorption thereby increasing plasma levels of fexofenadine; in vivo animal studies suggest that erythromycin may also decrease biliary excretion). Products include:
E.E.S. 449
EryPed 445

Erythromycin Gluceptate (Co-administration with erythromycin enhances fexofenadine gastrointestinal absorption thereby increasing plasma levels of fexofenadine; in vivo animal studies suggest that erythromycin may also decrease biliary excretion).
No products indexed under this heading.

Erythromycin Lactobionate (Co-administration with erythromycin enhances fexofenadine gastrointestinal absorption thereby increasing plasma levels of fexofenadine; in vivo animal studies suggest that erythromycin may also decrease biliary excretion).
No products indexed under this heading.

Erythromycin Stearate (Co-administration with erythromycin enhances fexofenadine gastrointestinal absorption thereby increasing plasma levels of fexofenadine; in vivo animal studies suggest that erythromycin may also decrease biliary excretion). Products include:
Erythrocin Stearate Filmtab Tablets 452

Isocarboxazid (Concurrent and/or sequential use with MAO inhibitors is contraindicated).
No products indexed under this heading.

Isoproterenol Hydrochloride (Combined effects of pseudoephedrine with other sympathomimetics on cardiovascular system may be harmful to the patient).
No products indexed under this heading.

Isoproterenol Sulfate (Combined effects of pseudoephedrine with other sympathomimetics on cardiovascular system may be harmful to the patient).
No products indexed under this heading.

Ketoconazole (Co-administration with ketoconazole enhances fexofenadine gastrointestinal absorption thereby increasing plasma levels of fexofenadine; in vivo animal studies suggest that ketoconazole may also decrease fexofenadine gastrointestinal secretion). Products include:
Nizoral A-D Shampoo, 1% 1839
Nizoral 2% Shampoo 1838

Levalbuterol Hydrochloride (Combined effects of pseudoephedrine with other sympathomimetics on cardiovascular system may be harmful to the patient). Products include:
Xopenex Inhalation Solution 3143
Xopenex Inhalation Solution Concentrate 3147

Magaldrate (Co-administration with fexofenadine HCL may decrease fexofenadine AUC by 41% and Cmax by 43%).
No products indexed under this heading.

Magnesium Hydroxide (Co-administration with fexofenadine HCL may decrease fexofenadine AUC by 41% and Cmax by 43%). Products include:
Maalox Max Maximum Strength Antacid/Anti-Gas Liquid 2165
Maalox Regular Strength Antacid/Antigas Liquid 2164
Pepcid Complete Chewable Tablets 1672
Rolaids Tablets 707

Extra Strength Rolaids Tablets .... ■707
Rolaids Multi-Symptom Antacid & Antigas Tablets .... ■708

Magnesium Oxide (Co-administration with fexofenadine HCL may decrease fexofenadine AUC by 41% and Cmax by 43%). Products include:
Beelith Tablets 784
PremCal Light, Regular, and Extra Strength Tablets................ ■762

Mecamylamine Hydrochloride (Reduced antihypertensive effects). Products include:
Inversine Tablets 3286

Metaproterenol Sulfate (Combined effects of pseudoephedrine with other sympathomimetics on cardiovascular system may be harmful to the patient). Products include:
Alupent Inhalation Aerosol 858

Metaraminol Bitartrate (Combined effects of pseudoephedrine with other sympathomimetics on cardiovascular system may be harmful to the patient). Products include:
Aramine Injection 1889

Methoxamine Hydrochloride (Combined effects of pseudoephedrine with other sympathomimetics on cardiovascular system may be harmful to the patient).
No products indexed under this heading.

Methyldopa (Reduced antihypertensive effects). Products include:
Aldoclor Tablets 1881
Aldoril Tablets 1884

Methyldopate Hydrochloride (Reduced antihypertensive effects).
No products indexed under this heading.

Moclobemide (Concurrent and/or sequential use with MAO inhibitors is contraindicated).
No products indexed under this heading.

Norepinephrine Bitartrate (Combined effects of pseudoephedrine with other sympathomimetics on cardiovascular system may be harmful to the patient).
No products indexed under this heading.

Pargyline Hydrochloride (Concurrent and/or sequential use with MAO inhibitors is contraindicated).
No products indexed under this heading.

Phenelzine Sulfate (Concurrent and/or sequential use with MAO inhibitors is contraindicated).
No products indexed under this heading.

Phenylephrine Bitartrate (Combined effects of pseudoephedrine with other sympathomimetics on cardiovascular system may be harmful to the patient).
No products indexed under this heading.

Phenylephrine Hydrochloride (Combined effects of pseudoephedrine with other sympathomimetics on cardiovascular system may be harmful to the patient). Products include:
Alacol DM Syrup 739
Hycomine Compound Tablets 1105
Preparation H Maximum Strength Cream.. ■747
Preparation H Cooling Gel............. ■747
Preparation H .... ■747
Sudafed PE Tablets .... ■711
Vicks Sinex Nasal Spray and Ultra Fine Mist for Sinus Relief............... 2677
Zicam Concentrated Cough Mist for Kids Plus D Cool Cherry......... ■643
Zicam Concentrated Cough Mist Plus D Cool Cherry...................... ■642

Phenylephrine Tannate (Combined effects of pseudoephedrine with other sympathomimetics on cardiovascular system may be harmful to the patient).
No products indexed under this heading.

Phenylpropanolamine Hydrochloride (Combined effects of pseudoephedrine with other sympathomimetics on cardiovascular system may be harmful to the patient).
No products indexed under this heading.

Pirbuterol Acetate (Combined effects of pseudoephedrine with other sympathomimetics on cardiovascular system may be harmful to the patient). Products include:
Maxair Autohaler 1820

Procarbazine Hydrochloride (Concurrent and/or sequential use with MAO inhibitors is contraindicated). Products include:
Matulane Capsules 3188

Pseudoephedrine Sulfate (Combined effects of pseudoephedrine with other sympathomimetics on cardiovascular system may be harmful to the patient). Products include:
Alavert Allergy & Sinus D-12 Hour Tablets.. ■743
Clarinex-D 24-Hour Extended-Release Tablets............ 3012
Claritin-D Non-Drowsy 12 Hour Tablets.. ■731
Claritin-D Non-Drowsy 24 Hour Tablets.. ■731

Reserpine (Reduced antihypertensive effects).
No products indexed under this heading.

Salmeterol Xinafoate (Combined effects of pseudoephedrine with other sympathomimetics on cardiovascular system may be harmful to the patient). Products include:
Advair Diskus 100/50 1291
Advair Diskus 250/50 1291
Advair Diskus 500/50 1291
Serevent Diskus 1540

Selegiline Hydrochloride (Concurrent and/or sequential use with MAO inhibitors is contraindicated). Products include:
Eldepryl Capsules 3209

Sodium Bicarbonate (Co-administration with fexofenadine HCL may decrease fexofenadine AUC by 41% and Cmax by 43%). Products include:
Ceo-Two Evacuant Suppository ...... ■607
Colyte with Flavor Packs for Oral Solution.. 3102
HalfLytely and Bisacodyl Tablets Bowel Prep Kit with Flavors Packs.. 915
TriLyte with Flavor Packs for Oral Solution.. 3114

Terbutaline Sulfate (Combined effects of pseudoephedrine with other sympathomimetics on cardiovascular system may be harmful to the patient).
No products indexed under this heading.

Tranylcypromine Sulfate (Concurrent and/or sequential use with MAO inhibitors is contraindicated). Products include:
Parnate Tablets 1499

Food Interactions

Diet, high-lipid (Co-administration with a high-fat meal decreased fexofenadine plasma concentrations Cmax and AUC, and Tmax was delayed by 50%; the rate of extent of pseudoephedrine absorption was not affected by food; administration of Allegra-D with food should be avoided).

Grapefruit Juice (Co-administration with grapefruit, orange or apple juice will reduce the bioavailability and exposure or fexofenadine).

Orange Juice (Co-administration with grapefruit, orange or apple juice will reduce the bioavailability and exposure or fexofenadine).

ALLEGRA-D 24 HOUR EXTENDED-RELEASE TABLETS
(Fexofenadine Hydrochloride, Pseudoephedrine Hydrochloride)........ 2862
See Allegra-D 12 Hour Extended-Release Tablets

ALLUNA SLEEP TABLETS
(Valeriana officinalis) .... ■763
None cited in PDR database.

ALOPRIM FOR INJECTION
(Allopurinol Sodium) 2156
May interact with cytotoxic drugs, thiazides, and certain other agents. Compounds in these categories include:

Amoxicillin Trihydrate (Co-administration of amoxicillin with allopurinol increases the frequency of rash).
No products indexed under this heading.

Ampicillin (Co-administration of ampicillin with allopurinol increases the frequency of rash).
No products indexed under this heading.

Ampicillin Sodium (Co-administration of ampicillin with allopurinol increases the frequency of rash).
No products indexed under this heading.

Azathioprine (Allopurinol inhibits the enzymatic oxidation of azathioprine to 6-thiouric acid; this interaction has been observed with oral allopurinol, usually with longer term therapy, reduction in oral dose of allopurinol has been suggested). Products include:
Azasan Tablets 2844

Bendroflumethiazide (Co-administration of allopurinol and thiazide diuretics contribute to increased allopurinol toxicity).
No products indexed under this heading.

Bleomycin Sulfate (Co-administration of allopurinol with cytotoxic agents including cyclophosphamide in patients with neoplastic disease, except leukemia, enhances the bone marrow suppression).
No products indexed under this heading.

Chlorothiazide (Co-administration of allopurinol and thiazide diuretics contribute to increased allopurinol toxicity). Products include:
Aldoclor Tablets 1881
Diuril Oral 1936

Chlorothiazide Sodium (Co-administration of allopurinol and thiazide diuretics contribute to increased allopurinol toxicity). Products include:
Diuril Sodium Intravenous 1934

Chlorpropamide (The half-life of chlorpropamide in the plasma may be prolonged by allopurinol, since allopurinol and chlorpropamide may compete for excretion in the renal tubule; the risk of hypoglycemia secondary to this interaction may be increased if used concurrently).
No products indexed under this heading.

Cyclophosphamide (Co-administration of allopurinol with cyclophosphamide in patients with neoplastic disease, except leukemia, enhances the bone marrow suppression).
No products indexed under this heading.

Cyclosporine (Co-administration may result in increased cyclosporine levels). Products include:
Gengraf Capsules 458
Neoral Soft Gelatin Capsules 2247
Neoral Oral Solution 2247
Restasis Ophthalmic Emulsion 570
Sandimmune 2259

Daunorubicin Hydrochloride (Co-administration of allopurinol with cytotoxic agents including cyclophosphamide in patients with neoplastic disease, except leukemia, enhances the bone marrow suppression). Products include:
Cerubidine for Injection 788

Dicumarol (Allopurinol prolongs the half-life of dicumarol).
No products indexed under this heading.

Doxorubicin Hydrochloride (Co-administration of allopurinol with cytotoxic agents including cyclophosphamide in patients with neoplastic disease, except leukemia, enhances the bone marrow suppression). Products include:
Adriamycin for Injection, USP 786
Adriamycin Injection, USP 786

Epirubicin Hydrochloride (Co-administration of allopurinol with cytotoxic agents including cyclophosphamide in patients with neoplastic disease, except leukemia, enhances the bone marrow suppression). Products include:
Ellence Injection 2632

Fluorouracil (Co-administration of allopurinol with cytotoxic agents including cyclophosphamide in patients with neoplastic disease, except leukemia, enhances the bone marrow suppression). Products include:
Carac Cream, 0.5% 1048
Efudex 3348

Hydrochlorothiazide (Co-administration of allopurinol and thiazide diuretics contribute to increased allopurinol toxicity). Products include:
Aldoril Tablets 1884
Atacand HCT 637
Avalide Tablets 2889
Avalide Tablets 922
Benicar HCT Tablets 2852
Diovan HCT Tablets 2195
Dyazide Capsules 1389
Hyzaar 1964
Lotensin HCT Tablets 2235
Maxzide 2150
Micardis HCT Tablets 886
Moduretic Tablets 2003
Prinzide Tablets 2033
Teveten HCT Tablets 1710
Timolide Tablets 2056
Uniretic Tablets 3114
Vaseretic Tablets 2073
Zestoretic Tablets 701

Hydroflumethiazide (Co-administration of allopurinol and thiazide diuretics contribute to increased allopurinol toxicity).
No products indexed under this heading.

Hydroxyurea (Co-administration of allopurinol with cytotoxic agents including cyclophosphamide in patients with neoplastic disease, except leukemia, enhances the bone marrow suppression).
No products indexed under this heading.

Mercaptopurine (Allopurinol inhibits the enzymatic oxidation of mercaptopurine to 6-thiouric acid; this interaction has been observed with oral allopurinol, usually with longer term therapy, reduction in oral dose of allopurinol has been suggested). Products include:
Purinethol Tablets 1222

Methotrexate Sodium (Co-administration of allopurinol with cytotoxic agents including cyclophosphamide in patients with neoplastic disease, except leukemia, enhances the bone marrow suppression).
No products indexed under this heading.

Methyclothiazide (Co-administration of allopurinol and thiazide diuretics contribute to increased allopurinol toxicity).
No products indexed under this heading.

Mitotane (Co-administration of allopurinol with cytotoxic agents including cyclophosphamide in patients with neoplastic disease, except leukemia, enhances the bone marrow suppression).
No products indexed under this heading.

Mitoxantrone Hydrochloride (Co-administration of allopurinol with cytotoxic agents including cyclophosphamide in patients with neoplastic disease, except leukemia, enhances the bone marrow suppression). Products include:
Novantrone for Injection Concentrate 3158

Polythiazide (Co-administration of allopurinol and thiazide diuretics contribute to increased allopurinol toxicity).
No products indexed under this heading.

Probenecid (Co-administration of uricosuric agents decreases the inhibition of xanthine by oxypurinol and increases the urinary excretion of uric acid).
No products indexed under this heading.

Procarbazine Hydrochloride (Co-administration of allopurinol with cytotoxic agents including cyclophosphamide in patients with neoplastic disease, except leukemia, enhances the bone marrow suppression). Products include:
Matulane Capsules 3188

Sulfinpyrazone (Co-administration of uricosuric agents decreases the inhibition of xanthine by oxypurinol and increases the urinary excretion of uric acid).
No products indexed under this heading.

Tamoxifen Citrate (Co-administration of allopurinol with cytotoxic agents including cyclophosphamide in patients with neoplastic disease, except leukemia, enhances the bone marrow suppression).
No products indexed under this heading.

Vincristine Sulfate (Co-administration of allopurinol with cytotoxic agents including cyclophosphamide in patients with neoplastic disease, except leukemia, enhances the bone marrow suppression).
No products indexed under this heading.

ALOXI INJECTION

(Palonosetron Hydrochloride) 2099
None cited in PDR database.

ALPHAGAN P OPHTHALMIC SOLUTION

(Brimonidine Tartrate) 563
May interact with anesthetics, antihypertensives, barbiturates, beta blockers, central nervous system depressants, cardiac glycosides, hypnotics and sedatives, monoamine oxidase inhibitors, narcotic analgesics, tricyclic antidepressants, and certain other agents. Compounds in these categories include:

Acebutolol Hydrochloride (Concurrent use of brimonidine, an alpha adrenergic agonist, with beta blockers (ophthalmic and systemic) may reduce pulse and blood pressure, however, in clinical trials brimonidine did not have any significant effects on pulse and blood pressure).
No products indexed under this heading.

Alfentanil Hydrochloride (Possible additive or potentiating effect with CNS depressants).
No products indexed under this heading.

Alprazolam (Possible additive or potentiating effect with CNS depressants). Products include:
Niravam Orally Disintegrating Tablets 3106
Xanax XR Tablets 2655

Amitriptyline Hydrochloride (Tricyclic antidepressants have been reported to blunt the hypotensive effect of systemic clonidine, an alpha adrenergic agonist; it is not known whether the concurrent use of these agents with brimonidine can lead to interference in IOP-lowering effect; caution is advised).
No products indexed under this heading.

Amlodipine Besylate (Concurrent use of brimonidine, an alpha adrenergic agonist, with antihypertensives may reduce pulse and blood pressure, however, in clinical trials brimonidine did not have any significant effects on pulse and blood pressure). Products include:
Caduet Tablets 2507
Lotrel Capsules 2238
Norvasc Tablets 2529

Amoxapine (Tricyclic antidepressants have been reported to blunt the hypotensive effect of systemic clonidine, an alpha adrenergic agonist; it is not known whether the concurrent use of these agents with brimonidine can lead to interference in IOP-lowering effect; caution is advised).
No products indexed under this heading.

Aprobarbital (Possible additive or potentiating effect with CNS depressants).
No products indexed under this heading.

Atenolol (Concurrent use of brimonidine, an alpha adrenergic agonist, with beta blockers (ophthalmic and systemic) may reduce pulse and blood pressure, however, in clinical trials brimonidine did not have any significant effects on pulse and blood pressure). Products include:
Tenormin I.V. Injection 698
Tenormin Tablets 695

Benazepril Hydrochloride (Concurrent use of brimonidine, an alpha adrenergic agonist, with antihypertensives may reduce pulse and blood pressure, however, in clinical trials brimonidine did not have any significant effects on pulse and blood pressure). Products include:
Lotensin Tablets 2232
Lotensin HCT Tablets 2235
Lotrel Capsules 2238

Bendroflumethiazide (Concurrent use of brimonidine, an alpha adrenergic agonist, with antihypertensives may reduce pulse and blood pressure, however, in clinical trials brimonidine did not have any significant effects on pulse and blood pressure).
No products indexed under this heading.

Betaxolol Hydrochloride (Concurrent use of brimonidine, an alpha adrenergic agonist, with beta blockers (ophthalmic and systemic) may reduce pulse and blood pressure, however, in clinical trials brimonidine did not have any significant effects on pulse and blood pressure). Products include:
Betoptic S Ophthalmic Suspension................................. 554

Bisoprolol Fumarate (Concurrent use of brimonidine, an alpha adrenergic agonist, with beta blockers (ophthalmic and systemic) may reduce pulse and blood pressure, however, in clinical trials brimonidine did not have any significant effects on pulse and blood pressure).
No products indexed under this heading.

Buprenorphine Hydrochloride (Possible additive or potentiating effect with CNS depressants). Products include:
Buprenex Injectable 2718
Suboxone Tablets 2719
Subutex Tablets 2719

Buspirone Hydrochloride (Possible additive or potentiating effect with CNS depressants).
No products indexed under this heading.

Butabarbital (Possible additive or potentiating effect with CNS depressants).
No products indexed under this heading.

Butalbital (Possible additive or potentiating effect with CNS depressants). Products include:
Sedapap Tablets 50 mg/650 mg 2098

Candesartan Cilexetil (Concurrent use of brimonidine, an alpha adrenergic agonist, with antihypertensives may reduce pulse and blood pressure, however, in clinical trials brimonidine did not have any significant effects on pulse and blood pressure). Products include:
Atacand Tablets 634
Atacand HCT 637

Captopril (Concurrent use of brimonidine, an alpha adrenergic agonist, with antihypertensives may reduce pulse and blood pressure, however, in clinical trials brimonidine did not have any significant effects on pulse and blood pressure). Products include:
Captopril Tablets 2114

Carteolol Hydrochloride (Concurrent use of brimonidine, an alpha adrenergic agonist, with beta blockers (ophthalmic and systemic) may reduce pulse and blood pressure, however, in clinical trials brimonidine did not have any significant effects on pulse and blood pressure). Products include:
Carteolol Hydrochloride Ophthalmic Solution USP, 1%....... ⊙246

Chlordiazepoxide (Possible additive or potentiating effect with CNS depressants).
No products indexed under this heading.

Chlordiazepoxide Hydrochloride (Possible additive or potentiating effect with CNS depressants). Products include:
Librium Capsules 3349

Chlorothiazide (Concurrent use of brimonidine, an alpha adrenergic agonist, with antihypertensives may reduce pulse and blood pressure, however, in clinical trials brimonidine did not have any significant effects on pulse and blood pressure). Products include:
Aldoclor Tablets 1881
Diuril Oral 1936

Chlorothiazide Sodium (Concurrent use of brimonidine, an alpha adrenergic agonist, with antihypertensives may reduce pulse and blood pressure, however, in clinical trials brimonidine did not have any significant effects on pulse and blood pressure). Products include:
Diuril Sodium Intravenous 1934

Chlorpromazine (Possible additive or potentiating effect with CNS depressants).
No products indexed under this heading.

Chlorpromazine Hydrochloride (Possible additive or potentiating effect with CNS depressants).
No products indexed under this heading.

Chlorprothixene (Possible additive or potentiating effect with CNS depressants).
No products indexed under this heading.

Chlorprothixene Hydrochloride (Possible additive or potentiating effect with CNS depressants).
No products indexed under this heading.

Chlorprothixene Lactate (Possible additive or potentiating effect with CNS depressants).
No products indexed under this heading.

Chlorthalidone (Concurrent use of brimonidine, an alpha adrenergic

agonist, with antihypertensives may reduce pulse and blood pressure, however, in clinical trials brimonidine did not have any significant effects on pulse and blood pressure). Products include:
Clorpres Tablets ... 2139

Clomipramine Hydrochloride (Tricyclic antidepressants have been reported to blunt the hypotensive effect of systemic clonidine, an alpha adrenergic agonist; it is not known whether the concurrent use of these agents with brimonidine can lead to interference in IOP-lowering effect; caution is advised).
No products indexed under this heading.

Clonidine (Concurrent use of brimonidine, an alpha adrenergic agonist, with antihypertensives may reduce pulse and blood pressure, however, in clinical trials brimonidine did not have any significant effects on pulse and blood pressure). Products include:
Catapres-TTS ... 875

Clonidine Hydrochloride (Concurrent use of brimonidine, an alpha adrenergic agonist, with antihypertensives may reduce pulse and blood pressure, however, in clinical trials brimonidine did not have any significant effects on pulse and blood pressure). Products include:
Catapres Tablets ... 874
Clorpres Tablets ... 2139

Clorazepate Dipotassium (Possible additive or potentiating effect with CNS depressants). Products include:
Tranxene ... 2488

Clozapine (Possible additive or potentiating effect with CNS depressants). Products include:
Clozapine Tablets ... 2141
Clozaril Tablets ... 2174
FazaClo Orally Disintegrating Tablets ... 547

Codeine Phosphate (Possible additive or potentiating effect with CNS depressants). Products include:
Tylenol with Codeine ... 2461

Deserpidine (Concurrent use of brimonidine, an alpha adrenergic agonist, with antihypertensives may reduce pulse and blood pressure, however, in clinical trials brimonidine did not have any significant effects on pulse and blood pressure).
No products indexed under this heading.

Desflurane (Possible additive or potentiating effect with CNS depressants). Products include:
Suprane Liquid for Inhalation ... 770

Desipramine Hydrochloride (Tricyclic antidepressants have been reported to blunt the hypotensive effect of systemic clonidine, an alpha adrenergic agonist; it is not known whether the concurrent use of these agents with brimonidine can lead to interference in IOP-lowering effect; caution is advised).
No products indexed under this heading.

Deslanoside (Concurrent use of brimonidine, an alpha adrenergic agonist, with cardiac glycosides may reduce pulse and blood pressure, however, in clinical trials brimonidine did not have any significant effects on pulse and blood pressure).
No products indexed under this heading.

Dezocine (Possible additive or potentiating effect with CNS depressants).
No products indexed under this heading.

Diazepam (Possible additive or potentiating effect with CNS depressants). Products include:
Diastat Rectal Delivery System ... 3344
Valium Tablets ... 2822

Diazoxide (Concurrent use of brimonidine, an alpha adrenergic agonist, with antihypertensives may reduce pulse and blood pressure, however, in clinical trials brimonidine did not have any significant effects on pulse and blood pressure). Products include:
Hyperstat I.V. Injection ... 3031

Digitalis Glycoside Preparations (Concurrent use of brimonidine, an alpha adrenergic agonist, with cardiac glycosides may reduce pulse and blood pressure, however, in clinical trials brimonidine did not have any significant effects on pulse and blood pressure).
No products indexed under this heading.

Digitoxin (Concurrent use of brimonidine, an alpha adrenergic agonist, with cardiac glycosides may reduce pulse and blood pressure, however, in clinical trials brimonidine did not have any significant effects on pulse and blood pressure).
No products indexed under this heading.

Digoxin (Concurrent use of brimonidine, an alpha adrenergic agonist, with cardiac glycosides may reduce pulse and blood pressure, however, in clinical trials brimonidine did not have any significant effects on pulse and blood pressure). Products include:
Digitek Tablets ... 2146
Lanoxicaps Capsules ... 1458
Lanoxin Injection ... 1462
Lanoxin Tablets ... 1468
Lanoxin Injection Pediatric ... 1465

Diltiazem Hydrochloride (Concurrent use of brimonidine, an alpha adrenergic agonist, with antihypertensives may reduce pulse and blood pressure, however, in clinical trials brimonidine did not have any significant effects on pulse and blood pressure). Products include:
Cardizem LA Extended Release Tablets ... 1699
Tiazac Capsules ... 1204

Doxazosin Mesylate (Concurrent use of brimonidine, an alpha adrenergic agonist, with antihypertensives may reduce pulse and blood pressure, however, in clinical trials brimonidine did not have any significant effects on pulse and blood pressure).
No products indexed under this heading.

Doxepin Hydrochloride (Tricyclic antidepressants have been reported to blunt the hypotensive effect of systemic clonidine, an alpha adrenergic agonist; it is not known whether the concurrent use of these agents with brimonidine can lead to interference in IOP-lowering effect; caution is advised).
No products indexed under this heading.

Droperidol (Possible additive or potentiating effect with CNS depressants).
No products indexed under this heading.

Enalapril Maleate (Concurrent use of brimonidine, an alpha adrenergic agonist, with antihypertensives may reduce pulse and blood pressure, however, in clinical trials brimonidine did not have any significant effects on pulse and blood pressure). Products include:
Vaseretic Tablets ... 2073
Vasotec I.V. Injection ... 2076

Enalaprilat (Concurrent use of brimonidine, an alpha adrenergic agonist, with antihypertensives may reduce pulse and blood pressure, however, in clinical trials brimonidine did not have any significant effects on pulse and blood pressure).
No products indexed under this heading.

Enflurane (Possible additive or potentiating effect with CNS depressants).
No products indexed under this heading.

Eprosartan Mesylate (Concurrent use of brimonidine, an alpha adrenergic agonist, with antihypertensives may reduce pulse and blood pressure, however, in clinical trials brimonidine did not have any significant effects on pulse and blood pressure). Products include:
Teveten Tablets ... 1707
Teveten HCT Tablets ... 1710

Esmolol Hydrochloride (Concurrent use of brimonidine, an alpha adrenergic agonist, with beta blockers (ophthalmic and systemic) may reduce pulse and blood pressure, however, in clinical trials brimonidine did not have any significant effects on pulse and blood pressure). Products include:
Brevibloc Concentrate ... 766
Brevibloc Injection ... 766
Brevibloc Double Strength Injection ... 766
Brevibloc Premixed Injection ... 766
Brevibloc Double Strength Premixed Injection ... 766

Estazolam (Possible additive or potentiating effect with CNS depressants). Products include:
ProSom Tablets ... 512

Ethanol (Possible additive or potentiating effect with CNS depressants).
No products indexed under this heading.

Ethchlorvynol (Possible additive or potentiating effect with CNS depressants).
No products indexed under this heading.

Ethinamate (Possible additive or potentiating effect with CNS depressants).
No products indexed under this heading.

Ethyl Alcohol (Possible additive or potentiating effect with CNS depressants).
No products indexed under this heading.

Felodipine (Concurrent use of brimonidine, an alpha adrenergic agonist, with antihypertensives may reduce pulse and blood pressure, however, in clinical trials brimonidine did not have any significant effects on pulse and blood pressure). Products include:
Plendil Extended-Release Tablets ... 651

Fentanyl (Possible additive or potentiating effect with CNS depressants). Products include:
Duragesic Transdermal System ... 2448

Fentanyl Citrate (Possible additive or potentiating effect with CNS depressants). Products include:
Actiq ... 993

Fluphenazine Decanoate (Possible additive or potentiating effect with CNS depressants).
No products indexed under this heading.

Fluphenazine Enanthate (Possible additive or potentiating effect with CNS depressants).
No products indexed under this heading.

Fluphenazine Hydrochloride (Possible additive or potentiating effect with CNS depressants).
No products indexed under this heading.

Flurazepam Hydrochloride (Possible additive or potentiating effect with CNS depressants). Products include:
Dalmane Capsules ... 3343

Fosinopril Sodium (Concurrent use of brimonidine, an alpha adrenergic agonist, with antihypertensives may reduce pulse and blood pressure, however, in clinical trials brimonidine did not have any significant effects on pulse and blood pressure).
No products indexed under this heading.

Furosemide (Concurrent use of brimonidine, an alpha adrenergic agonist, with antihypertensives may reduce pulse and blood pressure, however, in clinical trials brimonidine did not have any significant effects on pulse and blood pressure). Products include:
Furosemide Tablets ... 2117

Glutethimide (Possible additive or potentiating effect with CNS depressants).
No products indexed under this heading.

Guanabenz Acetate (Concurrent use of brimonidine, an alpha adrenergic agonist, with antihypertensives may reduce pulse and blood pressure, however, in clinical trials brimonidine did not have any significant effects on pulse and blood pressure).
No products indexed under this heading.

Guanethidine Monosulfate (Concurrent use of brimonidine, an alpha adrenergic agonist, with antihypertensives may reduce pulse and blood pressure, however, in clinical trials brimonidine did not have any significant effects on pulse and blood pressure).
No products indexed under this heading.

Haloperidol (Possible additive or potentiating effect with CNS depressants).
No products indexed under this heading.

Haloperidol Decanoate (Possible additive or potentiating effect with CNS depressants).
No products indexed under this heading.

Halothane (Possible additive or potentiating effect with CNS depressants).
No products indexed under this heading.

Hydralazine Hydrochloride (Concurrent use of brimonidine, an alpha adrenergic agonist, with antihypertensives may reduce pulse and

blood pressure, however, in clinical trials brimonidine did not have any significant effects on pulse and blood pressure). Products include:
BiDil Tablets 2161

Hydrochlorothiazide (Concurrent use of brimonidine, an alpha adrenergic agonist, with antihypertensives may reduce pulse and blood pressure, however, in clinical trials brimonidine did not have any significant effects on pulse and blood pressure). Products include:
Aldoril Tablets 1884
Atacand HCT 637
Avalide Tablets 2889
Avalide Tablets 922
Benicar HCT Tablets 2852
Diovan HCT Tablets 2195
Dyazide Capsules 1389
Hyzaar 1964
Lotensin HCT Tablets 2235
Maxzide 2150
Micardis HCT Tablets 886
Moduretic Tablets 2003
Prinzide Tablets 2033
Teveten HCT Tablets 1710
Timolide Tablets 2056
Uniretic Tablets 3114
Vaseretic Tablets 2073
Zestoretic Tablets 701

Hydrocodone Bitartrate (Possible additive or potentiating effect with CNS depressants). Products include:
Hycodan 1104
Hycomine Compound Tablets 1105
Hycotuss Expectorant Syrup 1106
Lortab 3315
Lortab Elixir 3312
Vicodin Tablets 530
Vicodin ES Tablets 531
Vicodin HP Tablets 532
Vicoprofen Tablets 533
Zydone Tablets 1118

Hydrocodone Polistirex (Possible additive or potentiating effect with CNS depressants). Products include:
Tussionex Pennkinetic Extended-Release Suspension 3322

Hydroflumethiazide (Concurrent use of brimonidine, an alpha adrenergic agonist, with antihypertensives may reduce pulse and blood pressure, however, in clinical trials brimonidine did not have any significant effects on pulse and blood pressure).
No products indexed under this heading.

Hydromorphone Hydrochloride (Possible additive or potentiating effect with CNS depressants). Products include:
Dilaudid 439
Dilaudid Oral Liquid 443
Dilaudid Non-Sterile Powder 439
Dilaudid Rectal Suppositories 439
Dilaudid Tablets 439
Dilaudid Tablets - 8 mg 443
Dilaudid-HP 441

Hydroxyzine Hydrochloride (Possible additive or potentiating effect with CNS depressants).
No products indexed under this heading.

Imipramine Hydrochloride (Tricyclic antidepressants have been reported to blunt the hypotensive effect of systemic clonidine, an alpha adrenergic agonist; it is not known whether the concurrent use of these agents with brimonidine can lead to interference in IOP-lowering effect; caution is advised).
No products indexed under this heading.

Imipramine Pamoate (Tricyclic antidepressants have been reported to blunt the hypotensive effect of systemic clonidine, an alpha adrenergic agonist; it is not known whether the concurrent use of these agents with brimonidine can lead to interference in IOP-lowering effect; caution is advised).
No products indexed under this heading.

Indapamide (Concurrent use of brimonidine, an alpha adrenergic agonist, with antihypertensives may reduce pulse and blood pressure, however, in clinical trials brimonidine did not have any significant effects on pulse and blood pressure). Products include:
Indapamide Tablets 2119

Irbesartan (Concurrent use of brimonidine, an alpha adrenergic agonist, with antihypertensives may reduce pulse and blood pressure, however, in clinical trials brimonidine did not have any significant effects on pulse and blood pressure). Products include:
Avalide Tablets 922
Avalide Tablets 2889
Avapro Tablets 925
Avapro Tablets 2886

Isocarboxazid (Concurrent use of brimonidine, an alpha adrenergic agonist, and MAO inhibitor is contraindicated).
No products indexed under this heading.

Isoflurane (Possible additive or potentiating effect with CNS depressants).
No products indexed under this heading.

Isradipine (Concurrent use of brimonidine, an alpha adrenergic agonist, with antihypertensives may reduce pulse and blood pressure, however, in clinical trials brimonidine did not have any significant effects on pulse and blood pressure). Products include:
DynaCirc CR Tablets 2726

Ketamine Hydrochloride (Possible additive or potentiating effect with CNS depressants).
No products indexed under this heading.

Labetalol Hydrochloride (Concurrent use of brimonidine, an alpha adrenergic agonist, with beta blockers (ophthalmic and systemic) may reduce pulse and blood pressure, however, in clinical trials brimonidine did not have any significant effects on pulse and blood pressure).
No products indexed under this heading.

Levobunolol Hydrochloride (Concurrent use of brimonidine, an alpha adrenergic agonist, with beta blockers (ophthalmic and systemic) may reduce pulse and blood pressure, however, in clinical trials brimonidine did not have any significant effects on pulse and blood pressure). Products include:
Betagan Ophthalmic Solution, USP .... ⊙217

Levomethadyl Acetate Hydrochloride (Possible additive or potentiating effect with CNS depressants).
No products indexed under this heading.

Levorphanol Tartrate (Possible additive or potentiating effect with CNS depressants).
No products indexed under this heading.

Lisinopril (Concurrent use of brimonidine, an alpha adrenergic agonist, with antihypertensives may reduce pulse and blood pressure, however, in clinical trials brimonidine did not have any significant effects on pulse and blood pressure). Products include:
Prinivil Tablets 2029
Prinzide Tablets 2033
Zestoretic Tablets 701
Zestril Tablets 704

Lorazepam (Possible additive or potentiating effect with CNS depressants).
No products indexed under this heading.

Losartan Potassium (Concurrent use of brimonidine, an alpha adrenergic agonist, with antihypertensives may reduce pulse and blood pressure, however, in clinical trials brimonidine did not have any significant effects on pulse and blood pressure). Products include:
Cozaar Tablets 1913
Hyzaar 1964

Loxapine Hydrochloride (Possible additive or potentiating effect with CNS depressants).
No products indexed under this heading.

Loxapine Succinate (Possible additive or potentiating effect with CNS depressants).
No products indexed under this heading.

Maprotiline Hydrochloride (Tricyclic antidepressants have been reported to blunt the hypotensive effect of systemic clonidine, an alpha adrenergic agonist; it is not known whether the concurrent use of these agents with brimonidine can lead to interference in IOP-lowering effect; caution is advised).
No products indexed under this heading.

Mecamylamine Hydrochloride (Concurrent use of brimonidine, an alpha adrenergic agonist, with antihypertensives may reduce pulse and blood pressure, however, in clinical trials brimonidine did not have any significant effects on pulse and blood pressure). Products include:
Inversine Tablets 3286

Meperidine Hydrochloride (Possible additive or potentiating effect with CNS depressants).
No products indexed under this heading.

Mephobarbital (Possible additive or potentiating effect with CNS depressants). Products include:
Mebaral Tablets, USP 2483

Meprobamate (Possible additive or potentiating effect with CNS depressants).
No products indexed under this heading.

Mesoridazine Besylate (Possible additive or potentiating effect with CNS depressants).
No products indexed under this heading.

Methadone Hydrochloride (Possible additive or potentiating effect with CNS depressants).
No products indexed under this heading.

Methohexital Sodium (Possible additive or potentiating effect with CNS depressants).
No products indexed under this heading.

Methotrimeprazine (Possible additive or potentiating effect with CNS depressants).
No products indexed under this heading.

Methoxyflurane (Possible additive or potentiating effect with CNS depressants).
No products indexed under this heading.

Methyclothiazide (Concurrent use of brimonidine, an alpha adrenergic agonist, with antihypertensives may reduce pulse and blood pressure, however, in clinical trials brimonidine did not have any significant effects on pulse and blood pressure).
No products indexed under this heading.

Methyldopa (Concurrent use of brimonidine, an alpha adrenergic agonist, with antihypertensives may reduce pulse and blood pressure, however, in clinical trials brimonidine did not have any significant effects on pulse and blood pressure). Products include:
Aldoclor Tablets 1881
Aldoril Tablets 1884

Methyldopate Hydrochloride (Concurrent use of brimonidine, an alpha adrenergic agonist, with antihypertensives may reduce pulse and blood pressure, however, in clinical trials brimonidine did not have any significant effects on pulse and blood pressure).
No products indexed under this heading.

Metipranolol Hydrochloride (Concurrent use of brimonidine, an alpha adrenergic agonist, with beta blockers (ophthalmic and systemic) may reduce pulse and blood pressure, however, in clinical trials brimonidine did not have any significant effects on pulse and blood pressure).
No products indexed under this heading.

Metolazone (Concurrent use of brimonidine, an alpha adrenergic agonist, with antihypertensives may reduce pulse and blood pressure, however, in clinical trials brimonidine did not have any significant effects on pulse and blood pressure).
No products indexed under this heading.

Metoprolol Succinate (Concurrent use of brimonidine, an alpha adrenergic agonist, with beta blockers (ophthalmic and systemic) may reduce pulse and blood pressure, however, in clinical trials brimonidine did not have any significant effects on pulse and blood pressure). Products include:
Toprol-XL Tablets 660

Metoprolol Tartrate (Concurrent use of brimonidine, an alpha adrenergic agonist, with beta blockers (ophthalmic and systemic) may reduce pulse and blood pressure, however, in clinical trials brimonidine did not have any significant effects on pulse and blood pressure).
No products indexed under this heading.

Metyrosine (Concurrent use of brimonidine, an alpha adrenergic agonist, with antihypertensives may reduce pulse and blood pressure,

however, in clinical trials brimonidine did not have any significant effects on pulse and blood pressure). Products include:
Demser Capsules 1933

Mibefradil Dihydrochloride (Concurrent use of brimonidine, an alpha adrenergic agonist, with antihypertensives may reduce pulse and blood pressure, however, in clinical trials brimonidine did not have any significant effects on pulse and blood pressure).
No products indexed under this heading.

Midazolam Hydrochloride (Possible additive or potentiating effect with CNS depressants).
No products indexed under this heading.

Minoxidil (Concurrent use of brimonidine, an alpha adrenergic agonist, with antihypertensives may reduce pulse and blood pressure, however, in clinical trials brimonidine did not have any significant effects on pulse and blood pressure). Products include:
Men's Rogaine Extra Strength Topical Solution, Ocean Rush Scent and Original Unscented ..... ■706
Women's Rogaine Topical Solution, Spring Bloom Scent and Original Unscented .... ■707

Moclobemide (Concurrent use of brimonidine, an alpha adrenergic agonist, and MAO inhibitor is contraindicated).
No products indexed under this heading.

Moexipril Hydrochloride (Concurrent use of brimonidine, an alpha adrenergic agonist, with antihypertensives may reduce pulse and blood pressure, however, in clinical trials brimonidine did not have any significant effects on pulse and blood pressure). Products include:
Uniretic Tablets 3114
Univasc Tablets 3118

Molindone Hydrochloride (Possible additive or potentiating effect with CNS depressants). Products include:
Moban Tablets 1108

Morphine Sulfate (Possible additive or potentiating effect with CNS depressants). Products include:
Avinza Capsules 1714
Kadian Capsules 572
MS Contin Tablets 2703

Nadolol (Concurrent use of brimonidine, an alpha adrenergic agonist, with beta blockers (ophthalmic and systemic) may reduce pulse and blood pressure, however, in clinical trials brimonidine did not have any significant effects on pulse and blood pressure). Products include:
Nadolol Tablets 2121

Nicardipine Hydrochloride (Concurrent use of brimonidine, an alpha adrenergic agonist, with antihypertensives may reduce pulse and blood pressure, however, in clinical trials brimonidine did not have any significant effects on pulse and blood pressure). Products include:
Cardene I.V. 1129

Nifedipine (Concurrent use of brimonidine, an alpha adrenergic agonist, with antihypertensives may reduce pulse and blood pressure, however, in clinical trials brimonidine did not have any significant effects on pulse and blood pressure). Products include:
Adalat CC Tablets 2978

Nisoldipine (Concurrent use of brimonidine, an alpha adrenergic agonist, with antihypertensives may reduce pulse and blood pressure, however, in clinical trials brimonidine did not have any significant effects on pulse and blood pressure). Products include:
Sular Tablets 1163

Nitroglycerin (Concurrent use of brimonidine, an alpha adrenergic agonist, with antihypertensives may reduce pulse and blood pressure, however, in clinical trials brimonidine did not have any significant effects on pulse and blood pressure). Products include:
Nitro-Dur Transdermal Infusion System....................................... 3060
Nitrolingual Pumpspray 1161

Nortriptyline Hydrochloride (Tricyclic antidepressants have been reported to blunt the hypotensive effect of systemic clonidine, an alpha adrenergic agonist; it is not known whether the concurrent use of these agents with brimonidine can lead to interference in IOP-lowering effect; caution is advised).
No products indexed under this heading.

Olanzapine (Possible additive or potentiating effect with CNS depressants). Products include:
Symbyax Capsules 1788
Zyprexa Tablets 1798
Zyprexa IntraMuscular 1798
Zyprexa ZYDIS Orally Disintegrating Tablets.................. 1798

Oxazepam (Possible additive or potentiating effect with CNS depressants).
No products indexed under this heading.

Oxycodone Hydrochloride (Possible additive or potentiating effect with CNS depressants). Products include:
Combunox Tablets 1183
OxyContin Tablets 2699
OxyFast Oral Concentrate Solution....................................... 2704
OxyIR Capsules 2704
Percocet Tablets 1114
Percodan Tablets 1115

Pargyline Hydrochloride (Concurrent use of brimonidine, an alpha adrenergic agonist, and MAO inhibitor is contraindicated).
No products indexed under this heading.

Penbutolol Sulfate (Concurrent use of brimonidine, an alpha adrenergic agonist, with beta blockers (ophthalmic and systemic) may reduce pulse and blood pressure, however, in clinical trials brimonidine did not have any significant effects on pulse and blood pressure).
No products indexed under this heading.

Pentobarbital Sodium (Possible additive or potentiating effect with CNS depressants). Products include:
Nembutal Sodium Solution, USP 2484

Perindopril Erbumine (Concurrent use of brimonidine, an alpha adrenergic agonist, with antihypertensives may reduce pulse and blood pressure, however, in clinical trials brimonidine did not have any significant effects on pulse and blood pressure). Products include:
Aceon Tablets (2 mg, 4 mg, 8 mg).. 3191

Perphenazine (Possible additive or potentiating effect with CNS depressants).
No products indexed under this heading.

Phenelzine Sulfate (Concurrent use of brimonidine, an alpha adrenergic agonist, and MAO inhibitor is contraindicated).
No products indexed under this heading.

Phenobarbital (Possible additive or potentiating effect with CNS depressants).
No products indexed under this heading.

Phenoxybenzamine Hydrochloride (Concurrent use of brimonidine, an alpha adrenergic agonist, with antihypertensives may reduce pulse and blood pressure, however, in clinical trials brimonidine did not have any significant effects on pulse and blood pressure). Products include:
Dibenzyline Capsules 3390

Phentolamine Mesylate (Concurrent use of brimonidine, an alpha adrenergic agonist, with antihypertensives may reduce pulse and blood pressure, however, in clinical trials brimonidine did not have any significant effects on pulse and blood pressure).
No products indexed under this heading.

Pindolol (Concurrent use of brimonidine, an alpha adrenergic agonist, with beta blockers (ophthalmic and systemic) may reduce pulse and blood pressure, however, in clinical trials brimonidine did not have any significant effects on pulse and blood pressure).
No products indexed under this heading.

Polythiazide (Concurrent use of brimonidine, an alpha adrenergic agonist, with antihypertensives may reduce pulse and blood pressure, however, in clinical trials brimonidine did not have any significant effects on pulse and blood pressure).
No products indexed under this heading.

Prazepam (Possible additive or potentiating effect with CNS depressants).
No products indexed under this heading.

Prazosin Hydrochloride (Concurrent use of brimonidine, an alpha adrenergic agonist, with antihypertensives may reduce pulse and blood pressure, however, in clinical trials brimonidine did not have any significant effects on pulse and blood pressure).
No products indexed under this heading.

Procarbazine Hydrochloride (Concurrent use of brimonidine, an alpha adrenergic agonist, and MAO inhibitor is contraindicated). Products include:
Matulane Capsules 3188

Prochlorperazine (Possible additive or potentiating effect with CNS depressants).
No products indexed under this heading.

Promethazine Hydrochloride (Possible additive or potentiating effect with CNS depressants). Products include:
Phenergan 3438

Propofol (Possible additive or potentiating effect with CNS depressants). Products include:
Diprivan Injectable Emulsion 676

Propoxyphene Hydrochloride (Possible additive or potentiating effect with CNS depressants).
No products indexed under this heading.

Propoxyphene Napsylate (Possible additive or potentiating effect with CNS depressants). Products include:
Darvocet A 500 Tablets 3497

Propranolol Hydrochloride (Concurrent use of brimonidine, an alpha adrenergic agonist, with beta blockers (ophthalmic and systemic) may reduce pulse and blood pressure, however, in clinical trials brimonidine did not have any significant effects on pulse and blood pressure). Products include:
Inderal LA Long-Acting Capsules 3421
InnoPran XL Capsules 2728

Protriptyline Hydrochloride (Tricyclic antidepressants have been reported to blunt the hypotensive effect of systemic clonidine, an alpha adrenergic agonist; it is not known whether the concurrent use of these agents with brimonidine can lead to interference in IOP-lowering effect; caution is advised). Products include:
Vivactil Tablets 2350

Quazepam (Possible additive or potentiating effect with CNS depressants).
No products indexed under this heading.

Quetiapine Fumarate (Possible additive or potentiating effect with CNS depressants). Products include:
Seroquel Tablets 691

Quinapril Hydrochloride (Concurrent use of brimonidine, an alpha adrenergic agonist, with antihypertensives may reduce pulse and blood pressure, however, in clinical trials brimonidine did not have any significant effects on pulse and blood pressure).
No products indexed under this heading.

Ramipril (Concurrent use of brimonidine, an alpha adrenergic agonist, with antihypertensives may reduce pulse and blood pressure, however, in clinical trials brimonidine did not have any significant effects on pulse and blood pressure). Products include:
Altace Capsules 1673

Rauwolfia Serpentina (Concurrent use of brimonidine, an alpha adrenergic agonist, with antihypertensives may reduce pulse and blood pressure, however, in clinical trials brimonidine did not have any significant effects on pulse and blood pressure).
No products indexed under this heading.

Remifentanil Hydrochloride (Possible additive or potentiating effect with CNS depressants).
No products indexed under this heading.

Rescinnamine (Concurrent use of brimonidine, an alpha adrenergic agonist, with antihypertensives may reduce pulse and blood pressure, however, in clinical trials brimonidine did not have any significant effects on pulse and blood pressure).
No products indexed under this heading.

Reserpine (Concurrent use of brimonidine, an alpha adrenergic agonist, with antihypertensives may reduce pulse and blood pressure, however, in clinical trials brimonidine did not have any significant effects on pulse and blood pressure).
No products indexed under this heading.

Risperidone (Possible additive or potentiating effect with CNS depressants). Products include:
Risperdal Consta Long-Acting Injection 1664
Risperdal M-Tab Orally Disintegrating Tablets 1658
Risperdal 1658

Secobarbital Sodium (Possible additive or potentiating effect with CNS depressants).
No products indexed under this heading.

Selegiline Hydrochloride (Concurrent use of brimonidine, an alpha adrenergic agonist, and MAO inhibitor is contraindicated). Products include:
Eldepryl Capsules 3209

Sevoflurane (Possible additive or potentiating effect with CNS depressants). Products include:
Ultane Liquid for Inhalation 526

Sodium Nitroprusside (Concurrent use of brimonidine, an alpha adrenergic agonist, with antihypertensives may reduce pulse and blood pressure, however, in clinical trials brimonidine did not have any significant effects on pulse and blood pressure).
No products indexed under this heading.

Sodium Oxybate (Possible additive or potentiating effect with CNS depressants).
No products indexed under this heading.

Sotalol Hydrochloride (Concurrent use of brimonidine, an alpha adrenergic agonist, with beta blockers (ophthalmic and systemic) may reduce pulse and blood pressure, however, in clinical trials brimonidine did not have any significant effects on pulse and blood pressure).
No products indexed under this heading.

Spirapril Hydrochloride (Concurrent use of brimonidine, an alpha adrenergic agonist, with antihypertensives may reduce pulse and blood pressure, however, in clinical trials brimonidine did not have any significant effects on pulse and blood pressure).
No products indexed under this heading.

Sufentanil Citrate (Possible additive or potentiating effect with CNS depressants).
No products indexed under this heading.

Telmisartan (Concurrent use of brimonidine, an alpha adrenergic agonist, with antihypertensives may reduce pulse and blood pressure, however, in clinical trials brimonidine did not have any significant effects on pulse and blood pressure). Products include:
Micardis Tablets 884
Micardis HCT Tablets 886

Temazepam (Possible additive or potentiating effect with CNS depressants).
No products indexed under this heading.

Terazosin Hydrochloride (Concurrent use of brimonidine, an alpha adrenergic agonist, with antihypertensives may reduce pulse and blood pressure, however, in clinical trials brimonidine did not have any significant effects on pulse and blood pressure). Products include:
Hytrin Capsules 469

Thiamylal Sodium (Possible additive or potentiating effect with CNS depressants).
No products indexed under this heading.

Thioridazine Hydrochloride (Possible additive or potentiating effect with CNS depressants). Products include:
Thioridazine Hydrochloride Tablets 2122

Thiothixene (Possible additive or potentiating effect with CNS depressants). Products include:
Thiothixene Capsules 2124

Timolol Hemihydrate (Concurrent use of brimonidine, an alpha adrenergic agonist, with beta blockers (ophthalmic and systemic) may reduce pulse and blood pressure, however, in clinical trials brimonidine did not have any significant effects on pulse and blood pressure). Products include:
Betimol Ophthalmic Solution 3371
Betimol Ophthalmic Solution .... ⊙283

Timolol Maleate (Concurrent use of brimonidine, an alpha adrenergic agonist, with beta blockers (ophthalmic and systemic) may reduce pulse and blood pressure, however, in clinical trials brimonidine did not have any significant effects on pulse and blood pressure). Products include:
Blocadren Tablets 1891
Cosopt Sterile Ophthalmic Solution 1910
Timolide Tablets 2056
Timoptic in Ocudose 2061
Timoptic Sterile Ophthalmic Solution 2058
Timoptic-XE Sterile Ophthalmic Gel Forming Solution 2062

Torsemide (Concurrent use of brimonidine, an alpha adrenergic agonist, with antihypertensives may reduce pulse and blood pressure, however, in clinical trials brimonidine did not have any significant effects on pulse and blood pressure).
No products indexed under this heading.

Trandolapril (Concurrent use of brimonidine, an alpha adrenergic agonist, with antihypertensives may reduce pulse and blood pressure, however, in clinical trials brimonidine did not have any significant effects on pulse and blood pressure). Products include:
Mavik Tablets 482
Tarka Tablets 519

Tranylcypromine Sulfate (Concurrent use of brimonidine, an alpha adrenergic agonist, and MAO inhibitor is contraindicated). Products include:
Parnate Tablets 1499

Triazolam (Possible additive or potentiating effect with CNS depressants).
No products indexed under this heading.

Trifluoperazine Hydrochloride (Possible additive or potentiating effect with CNS depressants).
No products indexed under this heading.

Trimethaphan Camsylate (Concurrent use of brimonidine, an alpha adrenergic agonist, with antihypertensives may reduce pulse and blood pressure, however, in clinical trials brimonidine did not have any significant effects on pulse and blood pressure).
No products indexed under this heading.

Trimipramine Maleate (Tricyclic antidepressants have been reported to blunt the hypotensive effect of systemic clonidine, an alpha adrenergic agonist; it is not known whether the concurrent use of these agents with brimonidine can lead to interference in IOP-lowering effect; caution is advised). Products include:
Surmontil Capsules 2347

Valsartan (Concurrent use of brimonidine, an alpha adrenergic agonist, with antihypertensives may reduce pulse and blood pressure, however, in clinical trials brimonidine did not have any significant effects on pulse and blood pressure). Products include:
Diovan HCT Tablets 2195
Diovan Tablets 2191

Verapamil Hydrochloride (Concurrent use of brimonidine, an alpha adrenergic agonist, with antihypertensives may reduce pulse and blood pressure, however, in clinical trials brimonidine did not have any significant effects on pulse and blood pressure). Products include:
Covera-HS Tablets 3135
Tarka Tablets 519
Verelan PM Capsules 3120

Zaleplon (Possible additive or potentiating effect with CNS depressants). Products include:
Sonata Capsules 1686

Ziprasidone Hydrochloride (Possible additive or potentiating effect with CNS depressants). Products include:
Geodon Capsules 2514

Zolpidem Tartrate (Possible additive or potentiating effect with CNS depressants). Products include:
Ambien Tablets 2867

Food Interactions

Alcohol (Possible additive or potentiating effect with CNS depressants).

ALREX OPHTHALMIC SUSPENSION 0.2%

(Loteprednol Etabonate) .... ⊙243
None cited in PDR database.

ALTACE CAPSULES

(Ramipril) 1673
May interact with diuretics, oral hypoglycemic agents, insulin, lithium preparations, non-steroidal anti-inflammatory agents, potassium preparations, potassium sparing diuretics, and certain other agents. Compounds in these categories include:

Acarbose (There have been rare reports of hypoglycemia reported during ramipril therapy when given to patients concomitantly taking oral hypoglycemic agents or insulin). Products include:
Precose Tablets 776

Amiloride Hydrochloride (May result in excessive reduction of blood pressure after initiation of therapy; increased risk of hyperkalemia). Products include:
Midamor Tablets 2000
Moduretic Tablets 2003

Bendroflumethiazide (May result in excessive reduction of blood pressure after initiation of therapy).
No products indexed under this heading.

Bumetanide (May result in excessive reduction of blood pressure after initiation of therapy).
No products indexed under this heading.

Celecoxib (Co-administration of ACE inhibitors with NSAIDs have been associated with worsening of renal failure and hyperkalemia). Products include:
Celebrex Capsules 3130

Chlorothiazide (May result in excessive reduction of blood pressure after initiation of therapy). Products include:
Aldoclor Tablets 1881
Diuril Oral 1936

Chlorothiazide Sodium (May result in excessive reduction of blood pressure after initiation of therapy). Products include:
Diuril Sodium Intravenous 1934

Chlorpropamide (There have been rare reports of hypoglycemia reported during ramipril therapy when given to patients concomitantly taking oral hypoglycemic agents or insulin).
No products indexed under this heading.

Chlorthalidone (May result in excessive reduction of blood pressure after initiation of therapy). Products include:
Clorpres Tablets 2139

Diclofenac Potassium (Co-administration of ACE inhibitors with NSAIDs have been associated with worsening of renal failure and hyperkalemia). Products include:
Cataflam Tablets 2173

Diclofenac Sodium (Co-administration of ACE inhibitors with NSAIDs have been associated with worsening of renal failure and hyperkalemia). Products include:
Arthrotec Tablets 3126
Voltaren Ophthalmic Solution 2300
Voltaren Tablets 2298
Voltaren-XR Tablets 2301

Ethacrynic Acid (May result in excessive reduction of blood pressure after initiation of therapy). Products include:
Edecrin Tablets 1941

Etodolac (Co-administration of ACE inhibitors with NSAIDs have been associated with worsening of renal failure and hyperkalemia).
No products indexed under this heading.

Fenoprofen Calcium (Co-administration of ACE inhibitors with NSAIDs have been associated with worsening of renal failure and hyperkalemia). Products include:
Nalfon Capsules 2504

Flurbiprofen (Co-administration of ACE inhibitors with NSAIDs have been associated with worsening of renal failure and hyperkalemia).
No products indexed under this heading.

Furosemide (May result in excessive reduction of blood pressure after initiation of therapy). Products include:
Furosemide Tablets 2117

Glimepiride (There have been rare reports of hypoglycemia reported during ramipril therapy when given to patients concomitantly taking oral hypoglycemic agents or insulin). Products include:
Amaryl Tablets 2864

Glipizide (There have been rare reports of hypoglycemia reported during ramipril therapy when given to patients concomitantly taking oral hypoglycemic agents or insulin).
No products indexed under this heading.

Glyburide (There have been rare reports of hypoglycemia reported during ramipril therapy when given to patients concomitantly taking oral hypoglycemic agents or insulin).
No products indexed under this heading.

Hydrochlorothiazide (May result in excessive reduction of blood pressure after initiation of therapy). Products include:
Aldoril Tablets 1884
Atacand HCT 637
Avalide Tablets 2889
Avalide Tablets 922
Benicar HCT Tablets 2852
Diovan HCT Tablets 2195
Dyazide Capsules 1389
Hyzaar 1964
Lotensin HCT Tablets 2235
Maxzide 2150
Micardis HCT Tablets 886
Moduretic Tablets 2003
Prinzide Tablets 2033
Teveten HCT Tablets 1710
Timolide Tablets 2056
Uniretic Tablets 3114
Vaseretic Tablets 2073
Zestoretic Tablets 701

Hydroflumethiazide (May result in excessive reduction of blood pressure after initiation of therapy).
No products indexed under this heading.

Ibuprofen (Co-administration of ACE inhibitors with NSAIDs have been associated with worsening of renal failure and hyperkalemia). Products include:
Advil Allergy Sinus Caplets .... ▣737
Advil .... ▣737
Children's Advil Suspension .... ▣742
Children's Advil Chewable Tablets .... ▣741
Advil Cold & Sinus .... ▣739
Advil Flu & Body Ache Caplets .... ▣739
Children's Advil Cold Suspension .... ▣741
Infants' Advil Concentrated Drops .... ▣743
Junior Strength Advil Swallow Tablets .... ▣740
Advil Migraine Liquigels .... ▣740
Advil Multi-Symptom Cold Caplets .... ▣738
Combunox Tablets 1183
Children's Motrin Oral Suspension and Chewable Tablets 1837
Children's Motrin Cold Non-Staining Dye-Free Oral Suspension 1838
Children's Motrin Cold Oral Suspension 1838
Children's Motrin Non-Staining Dye-Free Oral Suspension 1837
Motrin Cold & Sinus Caplets 1836
Motrin IB Tablets and Caplets 1836
Infants' Motrin Concentrated Drops 1837
Infants' Motrin Non-Staining Dye-Free Drops 1837
Junior Strength Motrin Caplets and Chewable Tablets 1837
Vicoprofen Tablets 533

Indapamide (May result in excessive reduction of blood pressure after initiation of therapy). Products include:
Indapamide Tablets 2119

Indomethacin (Co-administration of ACE inhibitors with NSAIDs have been associated with worsening of renal failure and hyperkalemia). Products include:
Indocin 1968

Indomethacin Sodium Trihydrate (Co-administration of ACE inhibitors with NSAIDs have been associated with worsening of renal failure and hyperkalemia). Products include:
Indocin I.V. 1973

Insulin, Human, Zinc Suspension (There have been rare reports of hypoglycemia reported during ramipril therapy when given to patients concomitantly taking oral hypoglycemic agents or insulin). Products include:
Humulin L, 100 Units 1763
Humulin U, 100 Units 1770

Insulin, Human NPH (There have been rare reports of hypoglycemia reported during ramipril therapy when given to patients concomitantly taking oral hypoglycemic agents or insulin). Products include:
Humulin N, 100 Units 1764
Humulin N Pen 1765
Novolin N Human Insulin 10 ml Vials 2322
Novolin N InnoLet 2322
Novolin N PenFill 3 ml Cartridges 2325
Novolin R InnoLet 2322

Insulin, Human Regular (There have been rare reports of hypoglycemia reported during ramipril therapy when given to patients concomitantly taking oral hypoglycemic agents or insulin). Products include:
Humulin R (U-500) 1768
Humulin R, 100 Units 1767
Novolin R Human Insulin 10 ml Vials 2322
Novolin R PenFill 2325

Insulin, Human Regular and Human NPH Mixture (There have been rare reports of hypoglycemia reported during ramipril therapy when given to patients concomitantly taking oral hypoglycemic agents or insulin). Products include:
Humulin 50/50, 100 Units 1760
Humulin 70/30 Pen 1761
Novolin 70/30 Human Insulin 10 ml Vials 2321
Novolin 70/30 InnoLet 2322
Novolin 70/30 PenFill 3 ml Cartridges 2325

Insulin, NPH (There have been rare reports of hypoglycemia reported during ramipril therapy when given to patients concomitantly taking oral hypoglycemic agents or insulin).
No products indexed under this heading.

Insulin, Regular (There have been rare reports of hypoglycemia reported during ramipril therapy when given to patients concomitantly taking oral hypoglycemic agents or insulin).
No products indexed under this heading.

Insulin, Zinc Crystals (There have been rare reports of hypoglycemia reported during ramipril therapy when given to patients concomitantly taking oral hypoglycemic agents or insulin).
No products indexed under this heading.

Insulin, Zinc Suspension (There have been rare reports of hypoglycemia reported during ramipril therapy when given to patients concomitantly taking oral hypoglycemic agents or insulin).
No products indexed under this heading.

Insulin Aspart, Human Regular (There have been rare reports of hypoglycemia reported during ramipril therapy when given to patients concomitantly taking oral hypoglycemic agents or insulin). Products include:
NovoLog Injection 2326

Insulin glargine (There have been rare reports of hypoglycemia reported during ramipril therapy when given to patients concomitantly taking oral hypoglycemic agents or insulin). Products include:
Lantus Injection 2925

Insulin Lispro, Human (There have been rare reports of hypoglycemia reported during ramipril therapy when given to patients concomitantly taking oral hypoglycemic agents or insulin). Products include:
Humalog-Pen 1751
Humalog Mix 75/25-Pen 1754

Insulin Lispro Protamine, Human (There have been rare reports of hypoglycemia reported during ramipril therapy when given to patients concomitantly taking oral hypoglycemic agents or insulin). Products include:
Humalog Mix 75/25-Pen 1754

Ketoprofen (Co-administration of ACE inhibitors with NSAIDs have been associated with worsening of renal failure and hyperkalemia).
No products indexed under this heading.

Ketorolac Tromethamine (Co-administration of ACE inhibitors with NSAIDs have been associated with worsening of renal failure and hyperkalemia). Products include:
Acular Ophthalmic Solution 561
Acular LS Ophthalmic Solution 562

Lithium (Increased serum lithium levels and symptoms of lithium toxicity).
No products indexed under this heading.

Lithium Carbonate (Increased serum lithium levels and symptoms of lithium toxicity). Products include:
Eskalith 1406
Lithobid Tablets 1670

Lithium Citrate (Increased serum lithium levels and symptoms of lithium toxicity).
No products indexed under this heading.

Meclofenamate Sodium (Co-administration of ACE inhibitors with NSAIDs have been associated with worsening of renal failure and hyperkalemia).
No products indexed under this heading.

Mefenamic Acid (Co-administration of ACE inhibitors with NSAIDs have been associated with worsening of renal failure and hyperkalemia).
No products indexed under this heading.

Meloxicam (Co-administration of ACE inhibitors with NSAIDs have been associated with worsening of renal failure and hyperkalemia). Products include:
Mobic Oral Suspension 893
Mobic Tablets 893

Metformin Hydrochloride (There have been rare reports of hypoglycemia reported during ramipril therapy when given to patients concomitantly taking oral hypoglycemic agents or insulin). Products include:
ActoPlus Met Tablets 3219
Avandamet Tablets 1343
Fortamet Extended-Release Tablets 1156

Methyclothiazide (May result in excessive reduction of blood pressure after initiation of therapy).
No products indexed under this heading.

Metolazone (May result in excessive reduction of blood pressure after initiation of therapy).
No products indexed under this heading.

Miglitol (There have been rare reports of hypoglycemia reported during ramipril therapy when given to patients concomitantly taking oral hypoglycemic agents or insulin).
No products indexed under this heading.

Nabumetone (Co-administration of ACE inhibitors with NSAIDs have been associated with worsening of renal failure and hyperkalemia). Products include:
Relafen Tablets 1523

Naproxen (Co-administration of ACE inhibitors with NSAIDs have been associated with worsening of renal failure and hyperkalemia). Products include:
EC-Naprosyn Delayed-Release Tablets 2769
Naprosyn Suspension 2769
Naprosyn Tablets 2769
Prevacid NapraPAC 3277

Naproxen Sodium (Co-administration of ACE inhibitors with NSAIDs have been associated with worsening of renal failure and hyperkalemia). Products include:
Aleve Tablets, Caplets and Gelcaps .... ▣605
Anaprox Tablets 2769
Anaprox DS Tablets 2769

Oxaprozin (Co-administration of ACE inhibitors with NSAIDs have been associated with worsening of renal failure and hyperkalemia).
No products indexed under this heading.

Phenylbutazone (Co-administration of ACE inhibitors with NSAIDs have been associated with worsening of renal failure and hyperkalemia).
No products indexed under this heading.

Pioglitazone Hydrochloride (There have been rare reports of hypoglycemia reported during ramipril therapy when given to patients concomitantly taking oral hypoglycemic agents or insulin). Products include:
ActoPlus Met Tablets 3219
Actos Tablets 3224

Piroxicam (Co-administration of ACE inhibitors with NSAIDs have been associated with worsening of renal failure and hyperkalemia).
No products indexed under this heading.

Polythiazide (May result in excessive reduction of blood pressure after initiation of therapy).
No products indexed under this heading.

Potassium Acid Phosphate (Increased risk of hyperkalemia). Products include:
K-Phos Original (Sodium Free) Tablets 785

Potassium Bicarbonate (Increased risk of hyperkalemia).
No products indexed under this heading.

Potassium Chloride (Increased risk of hyperkalemia). Products include:
Colyte with Flavor Packs for Oral Solution 3102
HalfLytely and Bisacodyl Tablets Bowel Prep Kit with Flavors Packs 915
K-Dur Extended-Relase Tablets 3047
K-Lor Powder Packets 472
K-Tab Filmtab Tablets 473
TriLyte with Flavor Packs for Oral Solution 3114

Potassium Citrate (Increased risk of hyperkalemia). Products include:
Urocit-K Tablets 2109

Potassium Gluconate (Increased risk of hyperkalemia).
No products indexed under this heading.

Potassium Phosphate (Increased risk of hyperkalemia). Products include:
K-Phos Neutral Tablets 785

Repaglinide (There have been rare reports of hypoglycemia reported during ramipril therapy when given to patients concomitantly taking oral hypoglycemic agents or insulin). Products include:
Prandin Tablets (0.5, 1, and 2 mg) 2337

Rofecoxib (Co-administration of ACE inhibitors with NSAIDs have been associated with worsening of renal failure and hyperkalemia).
No products indexed under this heading.

Rosiglitazone Maleate (There have been rare reports of hypoglycemia reported during ramipril therapy when given to patients concomitantly taking oral hypoglycemic agents or insulin). Products include:
Avandamet Tablets 1343
Avandia Tablets 1348

Spironolactone (May result in excessive reduction of blood pressure after initiation of therapy; increased risk of hyperkalemia).
No products indexed under this heading.

Sulindac (Co-administration of ACE inhibitors with NSAIDs have been associated with worsening of renal failure and hyperkalemia). Products include:
Clinoril Tablets 1899

Tolazamide (There have been rare reports of hypoglycemia reported during ramipril therapy when given to patients concomitantly taking oral hypoglycemic agents or insulin).
No products indexed under this heading.

Tolbutamide (There have been rare reports of hypoglycemia reported during ramipril therapy when given to patients concomitantly taking oral hypoglycemic agents or insulin).
No products indexed under this heading.

Tolmetin Sodium (Co-administration of ACE inhibitors with NSAIDs have been associated with worsening of renal failure and hyperkalemia).
No products indexed under this heading.

Torsemide (May result in excessive reduction of blood pressure after initiation of therapy).
No products indexed under this heading.

Triamterene (May result in excessive reduction of blood pressure after initiation of therapy; increased risk of hyperkalemia). Products include:
Dyazide Capsules 1389
Dyrenium Capsules 3390
Maxzide 2150

Troglitazone (There have been rare reports of hypoglycemia reported during ramipril therapy when given to patients concomitantly taking oral hypoglycemic agents or insulin).
No products indexed under this heading.

Valdecoxib (Co-administration of ACE inhibitors with NSAIDs have been associated with worsening of renal failure and hyperkalemia).
No products indexed under this heading.

Food Interactions

Food, unspecified (The rate of absorption is reduced, not the extent of absorption).

Salt Substitutes, Potassium-Containing (Increases risk of hyperkalemia).

ALTOPREV EXTENDED-RELEASE TABLETS

(Lovastatin) 1151
May interact with oral anticoagulants, erythromycin, fibrates, protease inhibitors, and certain other agents. Compounds in these categories include:

Amiodarone Hydrochloride (Co-administration with potent CYP3A4 inhibitors, such as cyclosporine, increases the risk of myopathy/rhabdomyolysis; the dose of lovastatin should not exceed 40 mg/day). Products include:
Pacerone Tablets 3337

Amprenavir (Co-administration with potent CYP3A4 inhibitors, such as HIV protease inhibitors, increases the risk of myopathy/rhabdomyolysis; concurrent use should be avoided). Products include:
Agenerase Capsules 1299
Agenerase Oral Solution 1304

Anisindione (Co-administration has resulted in increased bleeding and/or prothrombin time in a few patients). Products include:
Miradon Tablets 3056

Cimetidine (May blunt adrenal and/or gonadal steroid production. Co-administration with drugs that may decrease the levels or activity of endogenous steroid hormones, like cimetidine, should be done with caution). Products include:
Tagamet HB 200 Tablets 637
Tagamet Tablets 1547

Cimetidine Hydrochloride (May blunt adrenal and/or gonadal steroid production. Co-administration with drugs that may decrease the levels or activity of endogenous steroid hormones, like cimetidine, should be done with caution).
No products indexed under this heading.

Clarithromycin (Co-administration with potent CYP3A4 inhibitors, such as cyclosporine, increases the risk of myopathy/rhabdomyolysis; the dose of lovastatin should not exceed 20 mg/day). Products include:
Biaxin/Biaxin XL 402
PREVPAC 3281

Clofibrate (Co-administration with other lipid lowering drugs that can cause myopathy when given alone, such as fibrates, increases the risk of myopathy/rhabdomyolysis; concurrent use should be avoided unless the benefit outweights the risk. The dose of lovastatin should not exceed 20 mg/day if given concurrently).
No products indexed under this heading.

Cyclosporine (Co-administration with potent CYP3A4 inhibitors, such as cyclosporine, increases the risk of myopathy/rhabdomyolysis; the dose of lovastatin should not exceed 20 mg/day). Products include:
Gengraf Capsules 458
Neoral Soft Gelatin Capsules 2247
Neoral Oral Solution 2247
Restasis Ophthalmic Emulsion 570
Sandimmune 2259

Dicumarol (Co-administration has resulted in increased bleeding and/or prothrombin time in a few patients).
No products indexed under this heading.

Erythromycin (Co-administration with potent CYP3A4 inhibitors, such as erythromycin, increases the risk of myopathy/rhabdomyolysis; concurrent use should be avoided). Products include:
Erygel Topical Gel 2096
Ery-Tab Tablets 447
Erythromycin Base Filmtab Tablets 454
Erythromycin Delayed-Release Capsules, USP 456
PCE Dispertab Tablets 510

Erythromycin Estolate (Co-administration with potent CYP3A4 inhibitors, such as erythromycin, increases the risk of myopathy/rhabdomyolysis; concurrent use should be avoided).
No products indexed under this heading.

Erythromycin Ethylsuccinate (Co-administration with potent CYP3A4 inhibitors, such as erythromycin, increases the risk of myopathy/rhabdomyolysis; concurrent use should be avoided). Products include:
E.E.S. 449
EryPed 445

Erythromycin Gluceptate (Co-administration with potent CYP3A4 inhibitors, such as erythromycin, increases the risk of myopathy/rhabdomyolysis; concurrent use should be avoided).
No products indexed under this heading.

Erythromycin Lactobionate (Co-administration with potent CYP3A4 inhibitors, such as erythromycin, increases the risk of myopathy/rhabdomyolysis; concurrent use should be avoided).
No products indexed under this heading.

Erythromycin Stearate (Co-administration with potent CYP3A4 inhibitors, such as erythromycin, increases the risk of myopathy/rhabdomyolysis; concurrent use should be avoided). Products include:
Erythrocin Stearate Filmtab Tablets 452

Fenofibrate (Co-administration with other lipid lowering drugs that can cause myopathy when given alone, such as fibrates, increases the risk of myopathy/rhabdomyolysis; concurrent use should be avoided unless the benefit outweights the risk. The dose of lovastatin should not exceed 20 mg/day if given concurrently). Products include:
Antara Capsules 2723
Lofibra Capsules 1217
Tricor Tablets 523
Triglide Tablets 1165

Gemfibrozil (Co-administration with other lipid lowering drugs that can cause myopathy when given alone, such as fibrates, increases the risk of myopathy/rhabdomyolysis; concurrent use should be avoided unless the benefit outweights the risk. The dose of lovastatin should not exceed 20 mg/day if given concurrently).
No products indexed under this heading.

Indinavir Sulfate (Co-administration with potent CYP3A4 inhibitors, such as HIV protease inhibitors, increases the risk of myopathy/rhabdomyolysis; concurrent use should be avoided). Products include:
Crixivan Capsules 1918

Itraconazole (Co-administration with potent CYP3A4 inhibitors, such as itraconazole, increases the risk of myopathy/rhabdomyolysis; concurrent use should be avoided).
No products indexed under this heading.

Ketoconazole (Co-administration with potent CYP3A4 inhibitors, such as ketoconazole, increases the risk of myopathy/rhabdomyolysis; concurrent use should be avoided). Products include:
Nizoral A-D Shampoo, 1% 1839
Nizoral 2% Shampoo 1838

Lopinavir (Co-administration with potent CYP3A4 inhibitors, such as HIV protease inhibitors, increases the risk of myopathy/rhabdomyolysis; concurrent use should be avoided). Products include:
Kaletra 474

Nefazodone Hydrochloride (Co-administration with the potent CYP3A4 inhibitors, such as nefazodone, increases the risk of myopathy/rhabdomyolysis; concurrent use should be avoided).
No products indexed under this heading.

Nelfinavir Mesylate (Co-administration with potent CYP3A4 inhibitors, such as HIV protease inhibitors, increases the risk of

myopathy/rhabdomyolysis; concurrent use should be avoided). Products include:

Viracept 2556

Niacin (Co-administration with niacin (greater than or equal to 1 g/day) increases the risk of myopathy/ rhabdomyolysis; concurrent use should be avoided unless the benefit outweighs the risk. The dose of lovastatin should not exceed 20 mg/ day if given concurrently). Products include:

Advicor Tablets 1694
Niaspan Extended-Release Tablets 1703

Ritonavir (Co-administration with potent CYP3A4 inhibitors, such as HIV protease inhibitors, increases the risk of myopathy/ rhabdomyolysis; concurrent use should be avoided). Products include:

Kaletra 474
Norvir 499

Saquinavir (Co-administration with potent CYP3A4 inhibitors, such as HIV protease inhibitors, increases the risk of myopathy/ rhabdomyolysis; concurrent use should be avoided).

No products indexed under this heading.

Saquinavir Mesylate (Co-administration with potent CYP3A4 inhibitors, such as HIV protease inhibitors, increases the risk of myopathy/rhabdomyolysis; concurrent use should be avoided). Products include:

Invirase 2776

Spironolactone (May blunt adrenal and/or gonadal steroid production. Co-administration with drugs that may decrease the levels or activity of endogenous steroid hormones, like spironolactone, should be done with caution).

No products indexed under this heading.

Verapamil Hydrochloride (Co-administration with potent CYP3A4 inhibitors, such as verapamil, increases the risk of myopathy/ rhabdomyolysis; the dose of lovastatin should not exceed 40 mg/day). Products include:

Covera-HS Tablets 3135
Tarka Tablets 519
Verelan PM Capsules 3120

Warfarin Sodium (Co-administration has resulted in increased bleeding and/or prothrombin time in a few patients). Products include:

Coumadin for Injection 932
Coumadin Tablets 932

Food Interactions

Food, unspecified (Decreases the bioavailability of Altoprev).

Grapefruit Juice (Co-administration with potent CYP3A4 inhibitors, such as large quantities of grapefruit juice (greater than 1 quart daily), increases the risk of myopathy/rhabdomyolysis; concurrent use should be avoided).

ALUPENT INHALATION AEROSOL

(Metaproterenol Sulfate) 858

May interact with monoamine oxidase inhibitors, sympathomimetic aerosol bronchodilators, and tricyclic antidepressants. Compounds in these categories include:

Albuterol (Possible potentiation of adrenergic effects with beta adrenergic aerosol bronchodilators). Products include:

Proventil Inhalation Aerosol 3067

Amitriptyline Hydrochloride (The action of beta adrenergic agonists on the vascular system may be potentiated).

No products indexed under this heading.

Amoxapine (The action of beta adrenergic agonists on the vascular system may be potentiated).

No products indexed under this heading.

Bitolterol Mesylate (Possible potentiation of adrenergic effects with beta adrenergic aerosol bronchodilators).

No products indexed under this heading.

Clomipramine Hydrochloride (The action of beta adrenergic agonists on the vascular system may be potentiated).

No products indexed under this heading.

Desipramine Hydrochloride (The action of beta adrenergic agonists on the vascular system may be potentiated).

No products indexed under this heading.

Doxepin Hydrochloride (The action of beta adrenergic agonists on the vascular system may be potentiated).

No products indexed under this heading.

Imipramine Hydrochloride (The action of beta adrenergic agonists on the vascular system may be potentiated).

No products indexed under this heading.

Imipramine Pamoate (The action of beta adrenergic agonists on the vascular system may be potentiated).

No products indexed under this heading.

Isocarboxazid (The action of beta adrenergic agonists on the vascular system may be potentiated).

No products indexed under this heading.

Isoetharine (Possible potentiation of adrenergic effects with beta adrenergic aerosol bronchodilators).

No products indexed under this heading.

Isoproterenol Hydrochloride (Possible potentiation of adrenergic effects with beta adrenergic aerosol bronchodilators).

No products indexed under this heading.

Levalbuterol Hydrochloride (Possible potentiation of adrenergic effects with beta adrenergic aerosol bronchodilators). Products include:

Xopenex Inhalation Solution 3143
Xopenex Inhalation Solution Concentrate 3147

Maprotiline Hydrochloride (The action of beta adrenergic agonists on the vascular system may be potentiated).

No products indexed under this heading.

Moclobemide (The action of beta adrenergic agonists on the vascular system may be potentiated).

No products indexed under this heading.

Nortriptyline Hydrochloride (The action of beta adrenergic agonists on the vascular system may be potentiated).

No products indexed under this heading.

Pargyline Hydrochloride (The action of beta adrenergic agonists on the vascular system may be potentiated).

No products indexed under this heading.

Phenelzine Sulfate (The action of beta adrenergic agonists on the vascular system may be potentiated).

No products indexed under this heading.

Pirbuterol Acetate (Possible potentiation of adrenergic effects with beta adrenergic aerosol bronchodilators). Products include:

Maxair Autohaler 1820

Procarbazine Hydrochloride (The action of beta adrenergic agonists on the vascular system may be potentiated). Products include:

Matulane Capsules 3188

Protriptyline Hydrochloride (The action of beta adrenergic agonists on the vascular system may be potentiated). Products include:

Vivactil Tablets 2350

Salmeterol Xinafoate (Possible potentiation of adrenergic effects with beta adrenergic aerosol bronchodilators). Products include:

Advair Diskus 100/50 1291
Advair Diskus 250/50 1291
Advair Diskus 500/50 1291
Serevent Diskus 1540

Selegiline Hydrochloride (The action of beta adrenergic agonists on the vascular system may be potentiated). Products include:

Eldepryl Capsules 3209

Terbutaline Sulfate (Possible potentiation of adrenergic effects with beta adrenergic aerosol bronchodilators).

No products indexed under this heading.

Tranylcypromine Sulfate (The action of beta adrenergic agonists on the vascular system may be potentiated). Products include:

Parnate Tablets 1499

Trimipramine Maleate (The action of beta adrenergic agonists on the vascular system may be potentiated). Products include:

Surmontil Capsules 2347

AMARYL TABLETS

(Glimepiride) 2864

May interact with beta blockers, corticosteroids, oral anticoagulants, diuretics, estrogens, insulin, monoamine oxidase inhibitors, non-steroidal anti-inflammatory agents, oral contraceptives, phenothiazines, salicylates, sulfonamides, sympathomimetics, thiazides, thyroid preparations, and certain other agents. Compounds in these categories include:

Acebutolol Hydrochloride (May potentiate hypoglycemic action).

No products indexed under this heading.

Albuterol (Sympathomimetics tend to produce hyperglycemia and concurrent use may lead to loss of control). Products include:

Proventil Inhalation Aerosol 3067

Albuterol Sulfate (Sympathomimetics tend to produce hyperglycemia and concurrent use may lead to loss of control). Products include:

AccuNeb Inhalation Solution 1055
Combivent Inhalation Aerosol 878
DuoNeb Inhalation Solution 1058
Proventil Inhalation Solution 0.083% 3069
Proventil HFA Inhalation Aerosol 3071
Ventolin HFA Inhalation Aerosol 1576
VoSpire Extended-Release Tablets 2352

Amiloride Hydrochloride (Diuretics tend to produce hyperglycemia and concurrent use may lead to loss of control). Products include:

Midamor Tablets 2000
Moduretic Tablets 2003

Anisindione (May potentiate hypoglycemic action). Products include:

Miradon Tablets 3056

Aspirin (Co-administration of aspirin (1 g tid) led to a 34% decrease in the mean glimepiride AUC and, therefore, a 34% increase in the mean CL/f; no hypoglycemic symptoms were reported). Products include:

Aggrenox Capsules 855
Bayer, Aspirin Regimen .... ■ 606
Bayer Aspirin Tablets 3515
BC Powder .... ■ 612
BC Allergy Sinus Cold Powder .... ■ 612
Arthritis Strength BC Powder .... ■ 612
BC Sinus Cold Powder .... ■ 612
Ecotrin Enteric Coated Aspirin Low, Regular and Maximum Strength Tablets 1627
Goody's Body Pain Formula Powder .... ■ 621
Goody's Extra Strength Headache Powder .... ■ 621
Goody's Extra Strength Pain Relief Tablets .... ■ 621
Percodan Tablets 1115
St. Joseph 81 mg Aspirin Chewable and Enteric Coated Tablets 1841

Aspirin, Enteric Coated (May potentiate hypoglycemic action; clinical trials data indicate no evidence of significant adverse interaction with concurrent use).

No products indexed under this heading.

Aspirin Buffered (May potentiate hypoglycemic action; clinical trials data indicate no evidence of significant adverse interaction with concurrent use).

No products indexed under this heading.

Atenolol (May potentiate hypoglycemic action). Products include:

Tenormin I.V. Injection 698
Tenormin Tablets 695

Bendroflumethiazide (Diuretics tend to produce hyperglycemia and concurrent use may lead to loss of control).
No products indexed under this heading.

Betamethasone Acetate (Corticosteroids tend to produce hyperglycemia and concurrent use may lead to loss of control).
No products indexed under this heading.

Betamethasone Sodium Phosphate (Corticosteroids tend to produce hyperglycemia and concurrent use may lead to loss of control).
No products indexed under this heading.

Betaxolol Hydrochloride (May potentiate hypoglycemic action). Products include:
- Betoptic S Ophthalmic Suspension 554

Bisoprolol Fumarate (May potentiate hypoglycemic action).
No products indexed under this heading.

Bumetanide (Diuretics tend to produce hyperglycemia and concurrent use may lead to loss of control).
No products indexed under this heading.

Carteolol Hydrochloride (May potentiate hypoglycemic action). Products include:
- Carteolol Hydrochloride Ophthalmic Solution USP, 1% .... ⊙246

Celecoxib (May potentiate hypoglycemic action). Products include:
- Celebrex Capsules 3130

Chloramphenicol (May potentiate hypoglycemic action).
No products indexed under this heading.

Chloramphenicol Palmitate (May potentiate hypoglycemic action).
No products indexed under this heading.

Chloramphenicol Sodium Succinate (May potentiate hypoglycemic action).
No products indexed under this heading.

Chlorothiazide (Diuretics tend to produce hyperglycemia and concurrent use may lead to loss of control). Products include:
- Aldoclor Tablets 1881
- Diuril Oral 1936

Chlorothiazide Sodium (Diuretics tend to produce hyperglycemia and concurrent use may lead to loss of control). Products include:
- Diuril Sodium Intravenous 1934

Chlorotrianisene (Estrogens tend to produce hyperglycemia and concurrent use may lead to loss of control).
No products indexed under this heading.

Chlorpromazine (Phenothiazines tend to produce hyperglycemia and concurrent use may lead to loss of control).
No products indexed under this heading.

Chlorpromazine Hydrochloride (Phenothiazines tend to produce hyperglycemia and concurrent use may lead to loss of control).
No products indexed under this heading.

Chlorpropamide (May potentiate hypoglycemic action).
No products indexed under this heading.

Chlorthalidone (Diuretics tend to produce hyperglycemia and concurrent use may lead to loss of control). Products include:
- Clorpres Tablets 2139

Choline Magnesium Trisalicylate (May potentiate hypoglycemic action; clinical trials data indicate no evidence of significant adverse interaction with concurrent use).
No products indexed under this heading.

Cortisone Acetate (Corticosteroids tend to produce hyperglycemia and concurrent use may lead to loss of control).
No products indexed under this heading.

Desogestrel (Oral contraceptives tend to produce hyperglycemia and concurrent use may lead to loss of control). Products include:
- Ortho-Cept Tablets 2395

Dexamethasone (Corticosteroids tend to produce hyperglycemia and concurrent use may lead to loss of control). Products include:
- Ciprodex Otic Suspension 555
- Decadron Tablets 1929
- TobraDex Ophthalmic Ointment 558
- TobraDex Ophthalmic Suspension 558

Dexamethasone Acetate (Corticosteroids tend to produce hyperglycemia and concurrent use may lead to loss of control).
No products indexed under this heading.

Dexamethasone Sodium Phosphate (Corticosteroids tend to produce hyperglycemia and concurrent use may lead to loss of control). Products include:
- Decadron Phosphate Injection 1931

Diclofenac Potassium (May potentiate hypoglycemic action). Products include:
- Cataflam Tablets 2173

Diclofenac Sodium (May potentiate hypoglycemic action). Products include:
- Arthrotec Tablets 3126
- Voltaren Ophthalmic Solution 2300
- Voltaren Tablets 2298
- Voltaren-XR Tablets 2301

Dicumarol (May potentiate hypoglycemic action).
No products indexed under this heading.

Dienestrol (Estrogens tend to produce hyperglycemia and concurrent use may lead to loss of control).
No products indexed under this heading.

Diethylstilbestrol (Estrogens tend to produce hyperglycemia and concurrent use may lead to loss of control).
No products indexed under this heading.

Diflunisal (May potentiate hypoglycemic action; clinical trials data indicate no evidence of significant adverse interaction with concurrent use). Products include:
- Dolobid Tablets 1937

Dobutamine Hydrochloride (Sympathomimetics tend to produce hyperglycemia and concurrent use may lead to loss of control).
No products indexed under this heading.

Dopamine Hydrochloride (Sympathomimetics tend to produce hyperglycemia and concurrent use may lead to loss of control).
No products indexed under this heading.

Ephedrine Hydrochloride (Sympathomimetics tend to produce hyperglycemia and concurrent use may lead to loss of control). Products include:
- Primatene Tablets .... ▣749

Ephedrine Sulfate (Sympathomimetics tend to produce hyperglycemia and concurrent use may lead to loss of control).
No products indexed under this heading.

Ephedrine Tannate (Sympathomimetics tend to produce hyperglycemia and concurrent use may lead to loss of control).
No products indexed under this heading.

Epinephrine (Sympathomimetics tend to produce hyperglycemia and concurrent use may lead to loss of control). Products include:
- EpiPen 1061
- Primatene Mist .... ▣749

Epinephrine Bitartrate (Sympathomimetics tend to produce hyperglycemia and concurrent use may lead to loss of control).
No products indexed under this heading.

Epinephrine Hydrochloride (Sympathomimetics tend to produce hyperglycemia and concurrent use may lead to loss of control).
No products indexed under this heading.

Esmolol Hydrochloride (May potentiate hypoglycemic action). Products include:
- Brevibloc Concentrate 766
- Brevibloc Injection 766
- Brevibloc Double Strength Injection 766
- Brevibloc Premixed Injection 766
- Brevibloc Double Strength Premixed Injection 766

Estradiol (Estrogens tend to produce hyperglycemia and concurrent use may lead to loss of control). Products include:
- Activella Tablets 2311
- Climara Transdermal System 795
- Climara Pro Transdermal System 800
- CombiPatch Transdermal System 2180
- Estrogel 0.06% 3200
- Menostar Transdermal System 805
- Prefest Tablets 1069
- Vagifem Tablets 2340
- Vivelle Transdermal System 2288
- Vivelle-Dot Transdermal System 2293

Estrogens, Conjugated (Estrogens tend to produce hyperglycemia and concurrent use may lead to loss of control). Products include:
- Premarin Intravenous 3440
- Premarin Tablets 3443
- Premarin Vaginal Cream 3449
- Premphase Tablets 3452
- Prempro Tablets 3452

Estrogens, Esterified (Estrogens tend to produce hyperglycemia and concurrent use may lead to loss of control). Products include:
- Estratest Tablets 3196
- Estratest H.S. Tablets 3196

Estropipate (Estrogens tend to produce hyperglycemia and concurrent use may lead to loss of control).
No products indexed under this heading.

Ethacrynic Acid (Diuretics tend to produce hyperglycemia and concurrent use may lead to loss of control). Products include:
- Edecrin Tablets 1941

Ethinyl Estradiol (Estrogens tend to produce hyperglycemia and concurrent use may lead to loss of control). Products include:
- Alesse-28 Tablets 3392
- Lo/Ovral-28 Tablets 3423
- NuvaRing 2357
- Ortho-Cept Tablets 2395
- Ortho-Cyclen/Ortho Tri-Cyclen 2414
- Ortho Evra Transdermal System 2402
- Ortho Tri-Cyclen Lo Tablets 2421
- Seasonale Tablets 1073
- Triphasil-28 Tablets 3483
- Yasmin 28 Tablets 818

Ethynodiol Diacetate (Oral contraceptives tend to produce hyperglycemia and concurrent use may lead to loss of control).
No products indexed under this heading.

Etodolac (May potentiate hypoglycemic action).
No products indexed under this heading.

Fenoprofen Calcium (May potentiate hypoglycemic action). Products include:
- Nalfon Capsules 2504

Fludrocortisone Acetate (Corticosteroids tend to produce hyperglycemia and concurrent use may lead to loss of control).
No products indexed under this heading.

Fluphenazine Decanoate (Phenothiazines tend to produce hyperglycemia and concurrent use may lead to loss of control).
No products indexed under this heading.

Fluphenazine Enanthate (Phenothiazines tend to produce hyperglycemia and concurrent use may lead to loss of control).
No products indexed under this heading.

Fluphenazine Hydrochloride (Phenothiazines tend to produce hyperglycemia and concurrent use may lead to loss of control).
No products indexed under this heading.

Flurbiprofen (May potentiate hypoglycemic action).
No products indexed under this heading.

Furosemide (Diuretics tend to produce hyperglycemia and concurrent use may lead to loss of control). Products include:
- Furosemide Tablets 2117

Glipizide (May potentiate hypoglycemic action).
No products indexed under this heading.

Glyburide (May potentiate hypoglycemic action).
No products indexed under this heading.

Hydrochlorothiazide (Diuretics tend to produce hyperglycemia and concurrent use may lead to loss of control). Products include:
- Aldoril Tablets 1884
- Atacand HCT 637
- Avalide Tablets 2889
- Avalide Tablets 922
- Benicar HCT Tablets 2852
- Diovan HCT Tablets 2195
- Dyazide Capsules 1389
- Hyzaar 1964
- Lotensin HCT Tablets 2235
- Maxzide 2150
- Micardis HCT Tablets 886
- Moduretic Tablets 2003
- Prinzide Tablets 2033
- Teveten HCT Tablets 1710

IMPORTANT NOTE: Always consult each drug listing in the patient's regimen for possible interactions.

Timolide Tablets 2056
Uniretic Tablets 3114
Vaseretic Tablets 2073
Zestoretic Tablets 701

Hydrocortisone (Corticosteroids tend to produce hyperglycemia and concurrent use may lead to loss of control). Products include:
Cortizone•5 Ointment .... ▣699
Cortizone•10 Creme .... ▣699
Cortizone•10 Ointment .... ▣699
Cortizone•10 Plus Creme .... ▣700
Cortizone•10 Maximum Strength Quick Shot Spray .... ▣700
Hydrocortone Tablets 1963
Preparation H Hydrocortisone Cream .... ▣748

Hydrocortisone Acetate (Corticosteroids tend to produce hyperglycemia and concurrent use may lead to loss of control). Products include:
Analpram-HC 1136
Pramosone 1139
ProctoFoam-HC 3113
Tucks Anti-Itch Ointment .... ▣712
U-cort 1% Cream 3289

Hydrocortisone Sodium Phosphate (Corticosteroids tend to produce hyperglycemia and concurrent use may lead to loss of control).
No products indexed under this heading.

Hydrocortisone Sodium Succinate (Corticosteroids tend to produce hyperglycemia and concurrent use may lead to loss of control).
No products indexed under this heading.

Hydroflumethiazide (Diuretics tend to produce hyperglycemia and concurrent use may lead to loss of control).
No products indexed under this heading.

Ibuprofen (May potentiate hypoglycemic action). Products include:
Advil Allergy Sinus Caplets .... ▣737
Advil .... ▣737
Children's Advil Suspension .... ▣742
Children's Advil Chewable Tablets .... ▣741
Advil Cold & Sinus .... ▣739
Advil Flu & Body Ache Caplets .... ▣739
Children's Advil Cold Suspension .... ▣741
Infants' Advil Concentrated Drops .... ▣743
Junior Strength Advil Swallow Tablets .... ▣740
Advil Migraine Liquigels .... ▣740
Advil Multi-Symptom Cold Caplets .... ▣738
Combunox Tablets 1183
Children's Motrin Oral Suspension and Chewable Tablets 1837
Children's Motrin Cold Non-Staining Dye-Free Oral Suspension 1838
Children's Motrin Cold Oral Suspension 1838
Children's Motrin Non-Staining Dye-Free Oral Suspension 1837
Motrin Cold & Sinus Caplets 1836
Motrin IB Tablets and Caplets 1836
Infants' Motrin Concentrated Drops 1837
Infants' Motrin Non-Staining Dye-Free Drops 1837
Junior Strength Motrin Caplets and Chewable Tablets 1837
Vicoprofen Tablets 533

Indapamide (Diuretics tend to produce hyperglycemia and concurrent use may lead to loss of control). Products include:
Indapamide Tablets 2119

Indomethacin (May potentiate hypoglycemic action). Products include:
Indocin 1968

Indomethacin Sodium Trihydrate (May potentiate hypoglycemic action). Products include:
Indocin I.V. 1973

Insulin, Human, Zinc Suspension (Co-administration of glimepiride with insulin may increase the potential for hypoglycemia). Products include:
Humulin L, 100 Units 1763
Humulin U, 100 Units 1770

Insulin, Human NPH (Co-administration of glimepiride with insulin may increase the potential for hypoglycemia). Products include:
Humulin N, 100 Units 1764
Humulin N Pen 1765
Novolin N Human Insulin 10 ml Vials 2322
Novolin N InnoLet 2322
Novolin N PenFill 3 ml Cartridges 2325
Novolin R InnoLet 2322

Insulin, Human Regular (Co-administration of glimepiride with insulin may increase the potential for hypoglycemia). Products include:
Humulin R (U-500) 1768
Humulin R, 100 Units 1767
Novolin R Human Insulin 10 ml Vials 2322
Novolin R PenFill 2325

Insulin, Human Regular and Human NPH Mixture (Co-administration of glimepiride with insulin may increase the potential for hypoglycemia). Products include:
Humulin 50/50, 100 Units 1760
Humulin 70/30 Pen 1761
Novolin 70/30 Human Insulin 10 ml Vials 2321
Novolin 70/30 InnoLet 2322
Novolin 70/30 PenFill 3 ml Cartridges 2325

Insulin, NPH (Co-administration of glimepiride with insulin may increase the potential for hypoglycemia).
No products indexed under this heading.

Insulin, Regular (Co-administration of glimepiride with insulin may increase the potential for hypoglycemia).
No products indexed under this heading.

Insulin, Zinc Crystals (Co-administration of glimepiride with insulin may increase the potential for hypoglycemia).
No products indexed under this heading.

Insulin, Zinc Suspension (Co-administration of glimepiride with insulin may increase the potential for hypoglycemia).
No products indexed under this heading.

Insulin Aspart, Human Regular (Co-administration of glimepiride with insulin may increase the potential for hypoglycemia). Products include:
NovoLog Injection 2326

Insulin glargine (Co-administration of glimepiride with insulin may increase the potential for hypoglycemia). Products include:
Lantus Injection 2925

Insulin Lispro, Human (Co-administration of glimepiride with insulin may increase the potential for hypoglycemia). Products include:
Humalog-Pen 1751
Humalog Mix 75/25-Pen 1754

Insulin Lispro Protamine, Human (Co-administration of glimepiride with insulin may increase the potential for hypoglycemia). Products include:
Humalog Mix 75/25-Pen 1754

Isocarboxazid (May potentiate hypoglycemic action).
No products indexed under this heading.

Isoniazid (Isoniazid tends to produce hyperglycemia and concurrent use may lead to loss of control).
No products indexed under this heading.

Isoproterenol Hydrochloride (Sympathomimetics tend to produce hyperglycemia and concurrent use may lead to loss of control).
No products indexed under this heading.

Isoproterenol Sulfate (Sympathomimetics tend to produce hyperglycemia and concurrent use may lead to loss of control).
No products indexed under this heading.

Ketoprofen (May potentiate hypoglycemic action).
No products indexed under this heading.

Ketorolac Tromethamine (May potentiate hypoglycemic action). Products include:
Acular Ophthalmic Solution 561
Acular LS Ophthalmic Solution 562

Labetalol Hydrochloride (May potentiate hypoglycemic action).
No products indexed under this heading.

Levalbuterol Hydrochloride (Sympathomimetics tend to produce hyperglycemia and concurrent use may lead to loss of control). Products include:
Xopenex Inhalation Solution 3143
Xopenex Inhalation Solution Concentrate 3147

Levobunolol Hydrochloride (May potentiate hypoglycemic action). Products include:
Betagan Ophthalmic Solution, USP .... ⊙217

Levonorgestrel (Oral contraceptives tend to produce hyperglycemia and concurrent use may lead to loss of control). Products include:
Alesse-28 Tablets 3392
Climara Pro Transdermal System 800
Mirena Intrauterine System 810
Plan B Tablets 1068
Seasonale Tablets 1073
Triphasil-28 Tablets 3483

Levothyroxine Sodium (Thyroid products tend to produce hyperglycemia and concurrent use may lead to loss of control). Products include:
Levothroid Tablets 1189
Levoxyl Tablets 1680
Synthroid Tablets 515
Unithroid Tablets 3521

Liothyronine Sodium (Thyroid products tend to produce hyperglycemia and concurrent use may lead to loss of control). Products include:
Cytomel Tablets 1678

Liotrix (Thyroid products tend to produce hyperglycemia and concurrent use may lead to loss of control). Products include:
Thyrolar 1203

Magnesium Salicylate (May potentiate hypoglycemic action; clinical trials data indicate no evidence of significant adverse interaction with concurrent use).
No products indexed under this heading.

Meclofenamate Sodium (May potentiate hypoglycemic action).
No products indexed under this heading.

Mefenamic Acid (May potentiate hypoglycemic action).
No products indexed under this heading.

Meloxicam (May potentiate hypoglycemic action). Products include:
Mobic Oral Suspension 893
Mobic Tablets 893

Mesoridazine Besylate (Phenothiazines tend to produce hyperglycemia and concurrent use may lead to loss of control).
No products indexed under this heading.

Mestranol (Oral contraceptives tend to produce hyperglycemia and concurrent use may lead to loss of control).
No products indexed under this heading.

Metaproterenol Sulfate (Sympathomimetics tend to produce hyperglycemia and concurrent use may lead to loss of control). Products include:
Alupent Inhalation Aerosol 858

Metaraminol Bitartrate (Sympathomimetics tend to produce hyperglycemia and concurrent use may lead to loss of control). Products include:
Aramine Injection 1889

Metformin Hydrochloride (Co-administration of glimepiride with metformin may increase the potential for hypoglycemia). Products include:
ActoPlus Met Tablets 3219
Avandamet Tablets 1343
Fortamet Extended-Release Tablets 1156

Methotrimeprazine (Phenothiazines tend to produce hyperglycemia and concurrent use may lead to loss of control).
No products indexed under this heading.

Methoxamine Hydrochloride (Sympathomimetics tend to produce hyperglycemia and concurrent use may lead to loss of control).
No products indexed under this heading.

Methyclothiazide (Diuretics tend to produce hyperglycemia and concurrent use may lead to loss of control).
No products indexed under this heading.

Methylprednisolone Acetate (Corticosteroids tend to produce hyperglycemia and concurrent use may lead to loss of control). Products include:
Depo-Medrol Injectable Suspension 2615
Depo-Medrol Single-Dose Vial 2617

Methylprednisolone Sodium Succinate (Corticosteroids tend to produce hyperglycemia and concurrent use may lead to loss of control).
No products indexed under this heading.

Metipranolol Hydrochloride (May potentiate hypoglycemic action).
No products indexed under this heading.

Metolazone (Diuretics tend to produce hyperglycemia and concurrent use may lead to loss of control).
No products indexed under this heading.

Metoprolol Succinate (May potentiate hypoglycemic action). Products include:
Toprol-XL Tablets 660

Metoprolol Tartrate (May potentiate hypoglycemic action).
No products indexed under this heading.

Miconazole (A potential interaction between oral miconazole and oral hypoglycemic agents leading to severe hypoglycemia has been reported).
No products indexed under this heading.

Moclobemide (May potentiate hypoglycemic action).
No products indexed under this heading.

Nabumetone (May potentiate hypoglycemic action). Products include:
Relafen Tablets 1523

Nadolol (May potentiate hypoglycemic action). Products include:
Nadolol Tablets 2121

Naproxen (May potentiate hypoglycemic action). Products include:
EC-Naprosyn Delayed-Release Tablets 2769
Naprosyn Suspension 2769
Naprosyn Tablets 2769
Prevacid NapraPAC 3277

Naproxen Sodium (May potentiate hypoglycemic action). Products include:
Aleve Tablets, Caplets and Gelcaps 605
Anaprox Tablets 2769
Anaprox DS Tablets 2769

Nicotinic Acid (Nicotinic acid tends to produce hyperglycemia and concurrent use may lead to loss of control).
No products indexed under this heading.

Norepinephrine Bitartrate (Sympathomimetics tend to produce hyperglycemia and concurrent use may lead to loss of control).
No products indexed under this heading.

Norethindrone (Oral contraceptives tend to produce hyperglycemia and concurrent use may lead to loss of control). Products include:
Ortho Micronor Tablets 2411

Norethynodrel (Oral contraceptives tend to produce hyperglycemia and concurrent use may lead to loss of control).
No products indexed under this heading.

Norgestimate (Oral contraceptives tend to produce hyperglycemia and concurrent use may lead to loss of control). Products include:
Ortho-Cyclen/Ortho Tri-Cyclen 2414
Ortho Tri-Cyclen Lo Tablets 2421
Prefest Tablets 1069

Norgestrel (Oral contraceptives tend to produce hyperglycemia and concurrent use may lead to loss of control). Products include:
Lo/Ovral-28 Tablets 3423

Oxaprozin (May potentiate hypoglycemic action).
No products indexed under this heading.

Pargyline Hydrochloride (May potentiate hypoglycemic action).
No products indexed under this heading.

Penbutolol Sulfate (May potentiate hypoglycemic action).
No products indexed under this heading.

Perphenazine (Phenothiazines tend to produce hyperglycemia and concurrent use may lead to loss of control).
No products indexed under this heading.

Phenelzine Sulfate (May potentiate hypoglycemic action).
No products indexed under this heading.

Phenylbutazone (May potentiate hypoglycemic action).
No products indexed under this heading.

Phenylephrine Bitartrate (Sympathomimetics tend to produce hyperglycemia and concurrent use may lead to loss of control).
No products indexed under this heading.

Phenylephrine Hydrochloride (Sympathomimetics tend to produce hyperglycemia and concurrent use may lead to loss of control). Products include:
Alacol DM Syrup 739
Hycomine Compound Tablets 1105
Preparation H Maximum Strength Cream 747
Preparation H Cooling Gel 747
Preparation H 747
Sudafed PE Tablets 711
Vicks Sinex Nasal Spray and Ultra Fine Mist for Sinus Relief 2677
Zicam Concentrated Cough Mist for Kids Plus D Cool Cherry 643
Zicam Concentrated Cough Mist Plus D Cool Cherry 642

Phenylephrine Tannate (Sympathomimetics tend to produce hyperglycemia and concurrent use may lead to loss of control).
No products indexed under this heading.

Phenylpropanolamine Hydrochloride (Sympathomimetics tend to produce hyperglycemia and concurrent use may lead to loss of control).
No products indexed under this heading.

Phenytoin (Phenytoin tends to produce hyperglycemia and concurrent use may lead to loss of control).
No products indexed under this heading.

Phenytoin Sodium (Phenytoin tends to produce hyperglycemia and concurrent use may lead to loss of control). Products include:
Phenytek Capsules 2153

Pindolol (May potentiate hypoglycemic action).
No products indexed under this heading.

Pirbuterol Acetate (Sympathomimetics tend to produce hyperglycemia and concurrent use may lead to loss of control). Products include:
Maxair Autohaler 1820

Piroxicam (May potentiate hypoglycemic action).
No products indexed under this heading.

Polyestradiol Phosphate (Estrogens tend to produce hyperglycemia and concurrent use may lead to loss of control).
No products indexed under this heading.

Polythiazide (Diuretics tend to produce hyperglycemia and concurrent use may lead to loss of control).
No products indexed under this heading.

Prednisolone Acetate (Corticosteroids tend to produce hyperglycemia and concurrent use may lead to loss of control). Products include:
Blephamide Ophthalmic Ointment 563
Blephamide Ophthalmic Suspension 564
Poly-Pred Liquifilm Ophthalmic Suspension ⊙231
Pred Forte Ophthalmic Suspension ⊙233
Pred Mild Sterile Ophthalmic Suspension ⊙236
Pred-G Ophthalmic Suspension ⊙234
Pred-G Sterile Ophthalmic Ointment ⊙235

Prednisolone Sodium Phosphate (Corticosteroids tend to produce hyperglycemia and concurrent use may lead to loss of control). Products include:
Pediapred Oral Solution 3319

Prednisolone Tebutate (Corticosteroids tend to produce hyperglycemia and concurrent use may lead to loss of control).
No products indexed under this heading.

Prednisone (Corticosteroids tend to produce hyperglycemia and concurrent use may lead to loss of control).
No products indexed under this heading.

Probenecid (May potentiate hypoglycemic action).
No products indexed under this heading.

Procarbazine Hydrochloride (May potentiate hypoglycemic action). Products include:
Matulane Capsules 3188

Prochlorperazine (Phenothiazines tend to produce hyperglycemia and concurrent use may lead to loss of control).
No products indexed under this heading.

Promethazine Hydrochloride (Phenothiazines tend to produce hyperglycemia and concurrent use may lead to loss of control). Products include:
Phenergan 3438

Propranolol Hydrochloride (Co-administration increases Cmax AUC, and T1/2 of glimepiride by 23%, 22% and 15% respectively and it decreased CL/f by 18%; no evidence of clinically significant adverse interactions). Products include:
Inderal LA Long-Acting Capsules 3421
InnoPran XL Capsules 2728

Pseudoephedrine Hydrochloride (Sympathomimetics tend to produce hyperglycemia and concurrent use may lead to loss of control). Products include:
Advil Allergy Sinus Caplets 737
Advil Cold & Sinus 739
Advil Flu & Body Ache Caplets 739
Children's Advil Cold Suspension 741
Advil Multi-Symptom Cold Caplets 738
Allegra-D 12 Hour Extended-Release Tablets 2860
Allegra-D 24 Hour Extended-Release Tablets 2862
Balamine DM 739
BC Cold Powder 612
Benadryl Allergy & Cold Tablets 692
Benadryl Allergy & Sinus Headache Caplets & Gelcaps 693
Children's Benadryl Allergy & Cold Fastmelt Tablets 695
Benadryl Maximum Strength Severe Allergy & Sinus Headache Caplets 694
Children's Benadryl D Allergy & Sinus Fastmelt Tablets 694
Children's Benadryl D Liquid Medication 693
Benadryl D Tablets 694
Contac Non-Drowsy 12 Hour Cold Caplets 614
Contac Non-Drowsy Timed Release 12 Hour Cold Caplets 615
Contac Severe Cold and Flu Caplets Maximum Strength 615
Contac Severe Cold and Flu Caplets Non-Drowsy 615
Children's Dimetapp Cold & Allergy Elixir 745
Children's Dimetapp DM Cold & Cough Elixir 745
Children's Dimetapp Long Acting Cough Plus Cold Syrup 746
Dimetapp Infant Drops Decongestant Plus Cough 746
Children's Motrin Cold Non-Staining Dye-Free Oral Suspension 1838
Children's Motrin Cold Oral Suspension 1838
Motrin Cold & Sinus Caplets 1836
PediaCare Decongestant & Cough Infant Drops 705
PediaCare Decongestant Infants' Drops 705
PediaCare Long-Acting Cough Plus Cold Liquid 704
PediaCare Multi-Symptom Cold Liquid 704
PediaCare NightRest Cough & Cold Liquid 704
Robitussin Allergy & Cough Syrup 750
Robitussin CF Liquid 755
Robitussin Cough & Cold Liquid-filled Capsules 750
Robitussin Cough, Cold & Flu Liquid-filled Capsules 750
Robitussin Cough & Cold Infant Drops 755
Robitussin Flu Liquid 752
Robitussin Maximum Strength Cough & Cold Liquid 754
Robitussin PE Syrup 753
Robitussin Pediatric Cough & Cold Liquid 754
Robitussin PM Cough & Cold Liquid 752
Robitussin Severe Congestion Liquid-filled Capsules 751
Simply Stuffy Liquid 1841
Singlet Caplets 636
Sudafed 12 Hour Caplets 708
Sudafed 24 Hour Tablets 709
Sudafed Nasal Decongestant Tablets 709
Sudafed Severe Cold 710
Sudafed Non-Drying Sinus Liquid Caps 709
Sudafed Sinus & Allergy Tablets 710
Sudafed Sinus Headache 711
TheraFlu Cold & Cough Hot Liquid 680
TheraFlu Cold & Sore Throat Hot Liquid 680
TheraFlu Flu & Chest Congestion Non-Drowsy Hot Liquid 681
TheraFlu Flu & Sore Throat Hot Liquid 681
TheraFlu Severe Cold Non-Drowsy Hot Liquid 683
TheraFlu Severe Cold & Cough Hot Liquid 683
TheraFlu Severe Cold Caplets 679
TheraFlu Severe Cold Hot Liquid 682
TheraFlu Severe Cold Non-Drowsy Caplets 679
Triaminic Chest & Nasal Congestion Liquid 685
Triaminic Cold & Allergy Liquid 685
Triaminic Cold & Cough Liquid 685
Triaminic Cough Liquid 687
Triaminic Cough & Nasal Congestion Liquid 687
Triaminic Cough & Sore Throat Liquid 687
Triaminic Flu, Cough & Fever Liquid 685
Triaminic Night Time Cough & Cold Liquid 685
Triaminic Allergy Runny Nose & Congestion Softchews 688
Triaminic Cold & Cough Softchews 688
Triaminic Cough & Sore Throat Softchews 689
Tylenol Sinus NightTime Caplets 663
Children's Tylenol Plus Cold & Allergy Suspension Liquid 1850

IMPORTANT NOTE: Always consult each drug listing in the patient's regimen for possible interactions.

Children's Tylenol Plus Cold NightTime Suspension Liquid........ 1851
Children's Tylenol Plus Cold & Cough Suspension Liquid and Chewable Tablets........................ 1851
Children's Tylenol Plus Cold Chewable Tablets........................ 1851
Children's Tylenol Plus Cold Daytime Non-Drowsy Suspension Liquid........................ 1851
Children's Tylenol Plus Flu Suspension Liquid........................ 1853
Concentrated Tylenol Infants' Drops Plus Cold........................ 1851
Concentrated Tylenol Infants' Drops Plus Cold and Cough.......... 1851
Tylenol Cold & Flu Severe Daytime Liquid with Cool Bust....... 1846
Tylenol Cold & Flu Severe NightTime Liquid with Cool Burst.. 1846
Tylenol Cold Severe Congestion Non-Drowsy Caplets with Cool Burst.. 1846
Tylenol Allergy Complete Night Time Caplets.............................. 1844
Tylenol Allergy Complete Multi-Symptom Caplets and Gelcaps with Cool Burst............... 1844
Tylenol Flu NightTime Gelcaps.......... 1846
Tylenol Flu Day Non-Drowsy Gelcaps.. 1846
Concentrated Tylenol Infants' Drops Plus Cold Nasal Congestant, Fever Reducer & Pain Reliever............................ ■□668
Concentrated Tylenol Infants' Drops Plus Cold & Cough Nasal Decongestant, Fever Reducer & Pain Reliever............. ■□668
Multi-Symptom Tylenol Cold Night Time Caplets.............................. 1845
Multi-Symptom Tylenol Cold Day Non-Drowsy Caplets and Gelcaps.. 1845
Tylenol Sinus Day Non-Drowsy.......... 1848
Tylenol Sinus Night Time Caplets..... 1848
Tylenol Sinus Severe Congestion Caplets with Cool Burst............... 1848
Vicks 44D Cough & Head Congestion Relief........................ 2676
Vicks 44D Cough & Head Congestion Relief Liquid............ ■□721
Vicks 44M Cough, Cold & Flu Relief.. 2676
Pediatric Vicks 44m Cough & Cold Relief.. 2673
Vicks DayQuil LiquiCaps/Liquid Multi-Symptom Cold/Flu Relief...... ■□723
Vicks DayQuil Multi-Symptom Cold/Flu Relief LiquiCaps.............. 2675
Vicks DayQuil Multi-Symptom Cold/Flu Relief Liquid.................... 2675
Children's Vicks NyQuil Cold/Cough Relief........................ 2671
Vicks NyQuil LiquiCaps.................... 2677
Vicks NyQuil LiquiCaps/Liquid Multi-Symptom Cold/Flu Relief..... ■□725
Vicks NyQuil Liquid.......................... 2677
Zyrtec-D 12 Hour Extended Release Tablets........................ 2591

Pseudoephedrine Sulfate (Sympathomimetics tend to produce hyperglycemia and concurrent use may lead to loss of control). Products include:
Alavert Allergy & Sinus D-12 Hour Tablets.. ■□743
Clarinex-D 24-Hour Extended-Release Tablets.............. 3012
Claritin-D Non-Drowsy 12 Hour Tablets.. ■□731
Claritin-D Non-Drowsy 24 Hour Tablets.. ■□731

Quinestrol (Estrogens tend to produce hyperglycemia and concurrent use may lead to loss of control).
No products indexed under this heading.

Rofecoxib (May potentiate hypoglycemic action).
No products indexed under this heading.

Salmeterol Xinafoate (Sympathomimetics tend to produce hyperglycemia and concurrent use may lead to loss of control). Products include:
Advair Diskus 100/50.................... 1291
Advair Diskus 250/50.................... 1291
Advair Diskus 500/50.................... 1291
Serevent Diskus............................ 1540

Salsalate (May potentiate hypoglycemic action; clinical trials data indicate no evidence of significant adverse interaction with concurrent use).
No products indexed under this heading.

Selegiline Hydrochloride (May potentiate hypoglycemic action). Products include:
Eldepryl Capsules............................ 3209

Sotalol Hydrochloride (May potentiate hypoglycemic action).
No products indexed under this heading.

Spironolactone (Diuretics tend to produce hyperglycemia and concurrent use may lead to loss of control).
No products indexed under this heading.

Sulfacytine (May potentiate hypoglycemic action).
No products indexed under this heading.

Sulfamethizole (May potentiate hypoglycemic action).
No products indexed under this heading.

Sulfamethoxazole (May potentiate hypoglycemic action).
No products indexed under this heading.

Sulfasalazine (May potentiate hypoglycemic action).
No products indexed under this heading.

Sulfinpyrazone (May potentiate hypoglycemic action).
No products indexed under this heading.

Sulfisoxazole (May potentiate hypoglycemic action).
No products indexed under this heading.

Sulfisoxazole Acetyl (May potentiate hypoglycemic action).
No products indexed under this heading.

Sulfisoxazole Diolamine (May potentiate hypoglycemic action).
No products indexed under this heading.

Sulindac (May potentiate hypoglycemic action). Products include:
Clinoril Tablets.............................. 1899

Terbutaline Sulfate (Sympathomimetics tend to produce hyperglycemia and concurrent use may lead to loss of control).
No products indexed under this heading.

Thioridazine Hydrochloride (Phenothiazines tend to produce hyperglycemia and concurrent use may lead to loss of control). Products include:
Thioridazine Hydrochloride Tablets.. 2122

Thyroglobulin (Thyroid products tend to produce hyperglycemia and concurrent use may lead to loss of control).
No products indexed under this heading.

Thyroid (Thyroid products tend to produce hyperglycemia and concurrent use may lead to loss of control).
No products indexed under this heading.

Thyroxine (Thyroid products tend to produce hyperglycemia and concurrent use may lead to loss of control).
No products indexed under this heading.

Thyroxine Sodium (Thyroid products tend to produce hyperglycemia and concurrent use may lead to loss of control).
No products indexed under this heading.

Timolol Hemihydrate (May potentiate hypoglycemic action). Products include:
Betimol Ophthalmic Solution........... 3371
Betimol Ophthalmic Solution......... ⊙283

Timolol Maleate (May potentiate hypoglycemic action). Products include:
Blocadren Tablets............................ 1891
Cosopt Sterile Ophthalmic Solution.. 1910
Timolide Tablets.............................. 2056
Timoptic in Ocudose........................ 2061
Timoptic Sterile Ophthalmic Solution.. 2058
Timoptic-XE Sterile Ophthalmic Gel Forming Solution.................... 2062

Tolazamide (May potentiate hypoglycemic action).
No products indexed under this heading.

Tolbutamide (May potentiate hypoglycemic action).
No products indexed under this heading.

Tolmetin Sodium (May potentiate hypoglycemic action).
No products indexed under this heading.

Torsemide (Diuretics tend to produce hyperglycemia and concurrent use may lead to loss of control).
No products indexed under this heading.

Tranylcypromine Sulfate (May potentiate hypoglycemic action). Products include:
Parnate Tablets.............................. 1499

Triamcinolone (Corticosteroids tend to produce hyperglycemia and concurrent use may lead to loss of control).
No products indexed under this heading.

Triamcinolone Acetonide (Corticosteroids tend to produce hyperglycemia and concurrent use may lead to loss of control). Products include:
Azmacort Inhalation Aerosol........... 1701
Nasacort HFA Inhalation Aerosol...... 2939
Nasacort AQ Nasal Spray............... 2937

Triamcinolone Diacetate (Corticosteroids tend to produce hyperglycemia and concurrent use may lead to loss of control).
No products indexed under this heading.

Triamcinolone Hexacetonide (Corticosteroids tend to produce hyperglycemia and concurrent use may lead to loss of control).
No products indexed under this heading.

Triamterene (Diuretics tend to produce hyperglycemia and concurrent use may lead to loss of control). Products include:
Dyazide Capsules............................ 1389
Dyrenium Capsules.......................... 3390
Maxzide.. 2150

Trifluoperazine Hydrochloride (Phenothiazines tend to produce hyperglycemia and concurrent use may lead to loss of control).
No products indexed under this heading.

Valdecoxib (May potentiate hypoglycemic action).
No products indexed under this heading.

Warfarin Sodium (May potentiate hypoglycemic action). Products include:
Coumadin for Injection.................... 932
Coumadin Tablets............................ 932

Food Interactions

Meal, unspecified (When glimepiride is given with meals the mean Tmax is slightly increased (12%) and mean Cmax and AUC are slightly decreased).

AMBIEN TABLETS

(Zolpidem Tartrate)........................... 2867
May interact with central nervous system depressants and certain other agents. Compounds in these categories include:

Alfentanil Hydrochloride (Potential for enhanced CNS depressant effects of zolpidem).
No products indexed under this heading.

Alprazolam (Potential for enhanced CNS depressant effects of zolpidem). Products include:
Niravam Orally Disintegrating Tablets.. 3106
Xanax XR Tablets............................ 2655

Aprobarbital (Potential for enhanced CNS depressant effects of zolpidem).
No products indexed under this heading.

Buprenorphine Hydrochloride (Potential for enhanced CNS depressant effects of zolpidem). Products include:
Buprenex Injectable......................... 2718
Suboxone Tablets............................ 2719
Subutex Tablets.............................. 2719

Buspirone Hydrochloride (Potential for enhanced CNS depressant effects of zolpidem).
No products indexed under this heading.

Butabarbital (Potential for enhanced CNS depressant effects of zolpidem).
No products indexed under this heading.

Butalbital (Potential for enhanced CNS depressant effects of zolpidem). Products include:
Sedapap Tablets 50 mg/650 mg.... 2098

Chlordiazepoxide (Potential for enhanced CNS depressant effects of zolpidem).
No products indexed under this heading.

Chlordiazepoxide Hydrochloride (Potential for enhanced CNS depressant effects of zolpidem). Products include:
Librium Capsules............................ 3349

Chlorpromazine (Additive effect of decreased alertness and psychomotor performance; potential for enhanced CNS depressant effects of zolpidem).
No products indexed under this heading.

Chlorpromazine Hydrochloride (Additive effect of decreased alertness and psychomotor performance; potential for enhanced CNS depressant effects of zolpidem).
No products indexed under this heading.

Chlorprothixene (Potential for enhanced CNS depressant effects of zolpidem).
No products indexed under this heading.

Chlorprothixene Hydrochloride (Potential for enhanced CNS depressant effects of zolpidem).
No products indexed under this heading.

Chlorprothixene Lactate (Potential for enhanced CNS depressant effects of zolpidem).
No products indexed under this heading.

Clorazepate Dipotassium (Potential for enhanced CNS depressant effects of zolpidem). Products include:
Tranxene **2488**

Clozapine (Potential for enhanced CNS depressant effects of zolpidem). Products include:
Clozapine Tablets **2141**
Clozaril Tablets **2174**
FazaClo Orally Disintegrating Tablets **547**

Codeine Phosphate (Potential for enhanced CNS depressant effects of zolpidem). Products include:
Tylenol with Codeine **2461**

Desflurane (Potential for enhanced CNS depressant effects of zolpidem). Products include:
Suprane Liquid for Inhalation **770**

Dezocine (Potential for enhanced CNS depressant effects of zolpidem).
No products indexed under this heading.

Diazepam (Potential for enhanced CNS depressant effects of zolpidem). Products include:
Diastat Rectal Delivery System **3344**
Valium Tablets **2822**

Droperidol (Potential for enhanced CNS depressant effects of zolpidem).
No products indexed under this heading.

Enflurane (Potential for enhanced CNS depressant effects of zolpidem).
No products indexed under this heading.

Estazolam (Potential for enhanced CNS depressant effects of zolpidem). Products include:
ProSom Tablets **512**

Ethanol (Potential for enhanced CNS depressant effects of zolpidem).
No products indexed under this heading.

Ethchlorvynol (Potential for enhanced CNS depressant effects of zolpidem).
No products indexed under this heading.

Ethinamate (Potential for enhanced CNS depressant effects of zolpidem).
No products indexed under this heading.

Ethyl Alcohol (Potential for enhanced CNS depressant effects of zolpidem).
No products indexed under this heading.

Fentanyl (Potential for enhanced CNS depressant effects of zolpidem). Products include:
Duragesic Transdermal System **2448**

Fentanyl Citrate (Potential for enhanced CNS depressant effects of zolpidem). Products include:
Actiq **993**

Flumazenil (Zolpidem's sedative/hypnotic effect was reversed by flumazenil; however, no significant alterations in zolpidem pharmacokinetics was found).
No products indexed under this heading.

Fluoxetine Hydrochloride (Co-administration during multiple doses of both drugs at steady-state concentrations has resulted in a 17% increase in the zolpidem half-life; there was no evidence of an additive effect in psychomotor performance). Products include:
Prozac Pulvules and Liquid **1771**
Symbyax Capsules **1788**

Fluphenazine Decanoate (Potential for enhanced CNS depressant effects of zolpidem).
No products indexed under this heading.

Fluphenazine Enanthate (Potential for enhanced CNS depressant effects of zolpidem).
No products indexed under this heading.

Fluphenazine Hydrochloride (Potential for enhanced CNS depressant effects of zolpidem).
No products indexed under this heading.

Flurazepam Hydrochloride (Potential for enhanced CNS depressant effects of zolpidem). Products include:
Dalmane Capsules **3343**

Glutethimide (Potential for enhanced CNS depressant effects of zolpidem).
No products indexed under this heading.

Haloperidol (Co-administration in a single study revealed no effect on the pharmacokinetics or pharmacodynamics of zolpidem; however, there is a potential for enhanced CNS depressant effect of zolpidem).
No products indexed under this heading.

Haloperidol Decanoate (Co-administration in a single study revealed no effect on the pharmacokinetics or pharmacodynamics of zolpidem; however, there is a potential for enhanced CNS depressant effect of zolpidem).
No products indexed under this heading.

Hydrocodone Bitartrate (Potential for enhanced CNS depressant effects of zolpidem). Products include:
Hycodan **1104**
Hycomine Compound Tablets **1105**
Hycotuss Expectorant Syrup **1106**
Lortab **3315**
Lortab Elixir **3312**
Vicodin Tablets **530**
Vicodin ES Tablets **531**
Vicodin HP Tablets **532**
Vicoprofen Tablets **533**
Zydone Tablets **1118**

Hydrocodone Polistirex (Potential for enhanced CNS depressant effects of zolpidem). Products include:
Tussionex Pennkinetic Extended-Release Suspension **3322**

Hydromorphone Hydrochloride (Potential for enhanced CNS depressant effects of zolpidem). Products include:
Dilaudid **439**
Dilaudid Oral Liquid **443**
Dilaudid Non-Sterile Powder **439**
Dilaudid Rectal Suppositories **439**
Dilaudid Tablets **439**
Dilaudid Tablets - 8 mg **443**
Dilaudid-HP **441**

Hydroxyzine Hydrochloride (Potential for enhanced CNS depressant effects of zolpidem).
No products indexed under this heading.

Imipramine Hydrochloride (Co-administration produces 20% decrease in peak levels of imipramine with an additive effect of decreased alertness).
No products indexed under this heading.

Imipramine Pamoate (Co-administration produces 20% decrease in peak levels of imipramine with an additive effect of decreased alertness).
No products indexed under this heading.

Isoflurane (Potential for enhanced CNS depressant effects of zolpidem).
No products indexed under this heading.

Itraconazole (Co-administration has resulted in a 34% increse in AUC0-infinity of zolpidem; there were no significant pharmacodynamic effects of zolpidem on subjective drowsiness, postural sway, or pychomotor performance).
No products indexed under this heading.

Ketamine Hydrochloride (Potential for enhanced CNS depressant effects of zolpidem).
No products indexed under this heading.

Levomethadyl Acetate Hydrochloride (Potential for enhanced CNS depressant effects of zolpidem).
No products indexed under this heading.

Levorphanol Tartrate (Potential for enhanced CNS depressant effects of zolpidem).
No products indexed under this heading.

Lorazepam (Potential for enhanced CNS depressant effects of zolpidem).
No products indexed under this heading.

Loxapine Hydrochloride (Potential for enhanced CNS depressant effects of zolpidem).
No products indexed under this heading.

Loxapine Succinate (Potential for enhanced CNS depressant effects of zolpidem).
No products indexed under this heading.

Meperidine Hydrochloride (Potential for enhanced CNS depressant effects of zolpidem).
No products indexed under this heading.

Mephobarbital (Potential for enhanced CNS depressant effects of zolpidem). Products include:
Mebaral Tablets, USP **2483**

Meprobamate (Potential for enhanced CNS depressant effects of zolpidem).
No products indexed under this heading.

Mesoridazine Besylate (Potential for enhanced CNS depressant effects of zolpidem).
No products indexed under this heading.

Methadone Hydrochloride (Potential for enhanced CNS depressant effects of zolpidem).
No products indexed under this heading.

Methohexital Sodium (Potential for enhanced CNS depressant effects of zolpidem).
No products indexed under this heading.

Methotrimeprazine (Potential for enhanced CNS depressant effects of zolpidem).
No products indexed under this heading.

Methoxyflurane (Potential for enhanced CNS depressant effects of zolpidem).
No products indexed under this heading.

Midazolam Hydrochloride (Potential for enhanced CNS depressant effects of zolpidem).
No products indexed under this heading.

Molindone Hydrochloride (Potential for enhanced CNS depressant effects of zolpidem). Products include:
Moban Tablets **1108**

Morphine Sulfate (Potential for enhanced CNS depressant effects of zolpidem). Products include:
Avinza Capsules **1714**
Kadian Capsules **572**
MS Contin Tablets **2703**

Olanzapine (Potential for enhanced CNS depressant effects of zolpidem). Products include:
Symbyax Capsules **1788**
Zyprexa Tablets **1798**
Zyprexa IntraMuscular **1798**
Zyprexa ZYDIS Orally Disintegrating Tablets **1798**

Oxazepam (Potential for enhanced CNS depressant effects of zolpidem).
No products indexed under this heading.

Oxycodone Hydrochloride (Potential for enhanced CNS depressant effects of zolpidem). Products include:
Combunox Tablets **1183**
OxyContin Tablets **2699**
OxyFast Oral Concentrate Solution **2704**
OxyIR Capsules **2704**
Percocet Tablets **1114**
Percodan Tablets **1115**

Pentobarbital Sodium (Potential for enhanced CNS depressant effects of zolpidem). Products include:
Nembutal Sodium Solution, USP **2484**

Perphenazine (Potential for enhanced CNS depressant effects of zolpidem).
No products indexed under this heading.

Phenobarbital (Potential for enhanced CNS depressant effects of zolpidem).
No products indexed under this heading.

Prazepam (Potential for enhanced CNS depressant effects of zolpidem).
No products indexed under this heading.

Prochlorperazine (Potential for enhanced CNS depressant effects of zolpidem).
No products indexed under this heading.

Promethazine Hydrochloride (Potential for enhanced CNS depressant effects of zolpidem). Products include:
Phenergan 3438

Propofol (Potential for enhanced CNS depressant effects of zolpidem). Products include:
Diprivan Injectable Emulsion 676

Propoxyphene Hydrochloride (Potential for enhanced CNS depressant effects of zolpidem).
No products indexed under this heading.

Propoxyphene Napsylate (Potential for enhanced CNS depressant effects of zolpidem). Products include:
Darvocet A 500 Tablets 3497

Quazepam (Potential for enhanced CNS depressant effects of zolpidem).
No products indexed under this heading.

Quetiapine Fumarate (Potential for enhanced CNS depressant effects of zolpidem). Products include:
Seroquel Tablets 691

Remifentanil Hydrochloride (Potential for enhanced CNS depressant effects of zolpidem).
No products indexed under this heading.

Rifampin (Co-administration has resulted in significant reductions of the AUC, Cmax, and $T_{1/2}$ of zolpidem together with significant reductions in the pharmacodynamic effects of zolpidem).
No products indexed under this heading.

Risperidone (Potential for enhanced CNS depressant effects of zolpidem). Products include:
Risperdal Consta Long-Acting Injection 1664
Risperdal M-Tab Orally Disintegrating Tablets 1658
Risperdal 1658

Secobarbital Sodium (Potential for enhanced CNS depressant effects of zolpidem).
No products indexed under this heading.

Sertraline Hydrochloride (Co-administration following consecutive nightly doses has resulted in significantly higher (43%) Cmax and significantly lower Tmax (53%) of zolpidem). Products include:
Zoloft 2581

Sevoflurane (Potential for enhanced CNS depressant effects of zolpidem). Products include:
Ultane Liquid for Inhalation 526

Sufentanil Citrate (Potential for enhanced CNS depressant effects of zolpidem).
No products indexed under this heading.

Temazepam (Potential for enhanced CNS depressant effects of zolpidem).
No products indexed under this heading.

Thiamylal Sodium (Potential for enhanced CNS depressant effects of zolpidem).
No products indexed under this heading.

Thioridazine Hydrochloride (Potential for enhanced CNS depressant effects of zolpidem). Products include:
Thioridazine Hydrochloride Tablets 2122

Thiothixene (Potential for enhanced CNS depressant effects of zolpidem). Products include:
Thiothixene Capsules 2124

Triazolam (Potential for enhanced CNS depressant effects of zolpidem).
No products indexed under this heading.

Trifluoperazine Hydrochloride (Potential for enhanced CNS depressant effects of zolpidem).
No products indexed under this heading.

Zaleplon (Potential for enhanced CNS depressant effects of zolpidem). Products include:
Sonata Capsules 1686

Ziprasidone Hydrochloride (Potential for enhanced CNS depressant effects of zolpidem). Products include:
Geodon Capsules 2514

Food Interactions

Alcohol (Co-administration produces additive effects on psychomotor performance).

Meal, unspecified (Mean AUC and Cmax decreased by 15% and 25% respectively, while Tmax was prolonged by 60%; for faster sleep onset, Ambien should not be administered with or immediately after meal).

AMBISOME FOR INJECTION

(Amphotericin B, liposomal) 615
May interact with aminoglycosides, antineoplastics, corticosteroids, curariform skeletal muscle relaxants, cardiac glycosides, imidazoles, and certain other agents. Compounds in these categories include:

ACTH (Concurrent use of ACTH and amphotericin B may potentiate hypokalemia which could predispose the patient to cardiac dysfunction).
No products indexed under this heading.

Altretamine (Concurrent use of antineoplastic agents and amphotericin B may enhance the potential for renal toxicity, bronchospasm, and hypotension). Products include:
Hexalen Capsules 2101

Amikacin Sulfate (Concurrent use of amphotericin B and other nephrotoxic agents, such as aminoglycosides, may enhance the potential for drug-induced renal toxicity).
No products indexed under this heading.

Anastrozole (Concurrent use of antineoplastic agents and amphotericin B may enhance the potential for renal toxicity, bronchospasm, and hypotension). Products include:
Arimidex Tablets 665

Asparaginase (Concurrent use of antineoplastic agents and amphotericin B may enhance the potential for renal toxicity, bronchospasm, and hypotension). Products include:
Elspar for Injection 1943

Atracurium Besylate (Amphotericin B-induced hypokalemia may enhance the curariform effect of skeletal relaxants).
No products indexed under this heading.

Betamethasone Acetate (Concurrent use of corticosteroids and amphotericin B may potentiate hypokalemia which could predispose the patient to cardiac dysfunction).
No products indexed under this heading.

Betamethasone Sodium Phosphate (Concurrent use of corticosteroids and amphotericin B may potentiate hypokalemia which could predispose the patient to cardiac dysfunction).
No products indexed under this heading.

Bicalutamide (Concurrent use of antineoplastic agents and amphotericin B may enhance the potential for renal toxicity, bronchospasm, and hypotension). Products include:
Casodex Tablets 670

Bleomycin Sulfate (Concurrent use of antineoplastic agents and amphotericin B may enhance the potential for renal toxicity, bronchospasm, and hypotension).
No products indexed under this heading.

Busulfan (Concurrent use of antineoplastic agents and amphotericin B may enhance the potential for renal toxicity, bronchospasm, and hypotension). Products include:
I.V. Busulfex 1125
Myleran Tablets 1492

Carboplatin (Concurrent use of antineoplastic agents and amphotericin B may enhance the potential for renal toxicity, bronchospasm, and hypotension).
No products indexed under this heading.

Carmustine (BCNU) (Concurrent use of antineoplastic agents and amphotericin B may enhance the potential for renal toxicity, bronchospasm, and hypotension).
No products indexed under this heading.

Chlorambucil (Concurrent use of antineoplastic agents and amphotericin B may enhance the potential for renal toxicity, bronchospasm, and hypotension). Products include:
Leukeran Tablets 1472

Cisatracurium Besylate (Amphotericin B-induced hypokalemia may enhance the curariform effect of skeletal relaxants). Products include:
Nimbex Injection 494

Cisplatin (Concurrent use of antineoplastic agents and amphotericin B may enhance the potential for renal toxicity, bronchospasm, and hypotension).
No products indexed under this heading.

Clotrimazole (Imidazoles may induce fungal resistance to amphotericin B; combination therapy should be administered with caution, especially in immunocompromised patients). Products include:
Lotrimin 3053
Lotrisone 3054

Cortisone Acetate (Concurrent use of corticosteroids and amphotericin B may potentiate hypokalemia which could predispose the patient to cardiac dysfunction).
No products indexed under this heading.

Cyclophosphamide (Concurrent use of antineoplastic agents and amphotericin B may enhance the potential for renal toxicity, bronchospasm, and hypotension).
No products indexed under this heading.

Cyclosporine (Concurrent use of amphotericin B and other nephrotoxic agents, such as cyclosporine, may enhance the potential for drug-induced renal toxicity). Products include:
Gengraf Capsules 458
Neoral Soft Gelatin Capsules 2247
Neoral Oral Solution 2247
Restasis Ophthalmic Emulsion 570
Sandimmune 2259

Dacarbazine (Concurrent use of antineoplastic agents and amphotericin B may enhance the potential for renal toxicity, bronchospasm, and hypotension).
No products indexed under this heading.

Daunorubicin Citrate (Concurrent use of antineoplastic agents and amphotericin B may enhance the potential for renal toxicity, bronchospasm, and hypotension).
No products indexed under this heading.

Daunorubicin Hydrochloride (Concurrent use of antineoplastic agents and amphotericin B may enhance the potential for renal toxicity, bronchospasm, and hypotension). Products include:
Cerubidine for Injection 788

Denileukin Diftitox (Concurrent use of antineoplastic agents and amphotericin B may enhance the potential for renal toxicity, bronchospasm, and hypotension). Products include:
Ontak Vials 1717

Deslanoside (Concurrent use of digitalis and amphotericin B may induce hypokalemia and may potentiate digitalis toxicity).
No products indexed under this heading.

Dexamethasone (Concurrent use of corticosteroids and amphotericin B may potentiate hypokalemia which could predispose the patient to cardiac dysfunction). Products include:
Ciprodex Otic Suspension 555
Decadron Tablets 1929
TobraDex Ophthalmic Ointment 558
TobraDex Ophthalmic Suspension 558

Dexamethasone Acetate (Concurrent use of corticosteroids and amphotericin B may potentiate hypokalemia which could predispose the patient to cardiac dysfunction).
No products indexed under this heading.

Dexamethasone Sodium Phosphate (Concurrent use of corticosteroids and amphotericin B may potentiate hypokalemia which could predispose the patient to cardiac dysfunction). Products include:
Decadron Phosphate Injection 1931

Digitalis Glycoside Preparations (Concurrent use of digitalis and amphotericin B may induce hypokalemia and may potentiate digitalis toxicity).
No products indexed under this heading.

Digitoxin (Concurrent use of digitalis and amphotericin B may induce hypokalemia and may potentiate digitalis toxicity).
No products indexed under this heading.

Digoxin (Concurrent use of digitalis and amphotericin B may induce hypokalemia and may potentiate digitalis toxicity). Products include:
Digitek Tablets 2146
Lanoxicaps Capsules 1458
Lanoxin Injection 1462
Lanoxin Tablets 1468
Lanoxin Injection Pediatric 1465

Docetaxel (Concurrent use of antineoplastic agents and amphotericin B may enhance the potential for renal toxicity, bronchospasm, and hypotension). Products include:
Taxotere Injection Concentrate 2947

Doxacurium Chloride (Amphotericin B-induced hypokalemia may enhance the curariform effect of skeletal relaxants).
No products indexed under this heading.

Doxorubicin Hydrochloride (Concurrent use of antineoplastic agents and amphotericin B may enhance the potential for renal toxicity, bronchospasm, and hypotension). Products include:
Adriamycin for Injection, USP 786
Adriamycin Injection, USP 786

Epirubicin Hydrochloride (Concurrent use of antineoplastic agents and amphotericin B may enhance the potential for renal toxicity, bronchospasm, and hypotension). Products include:
Ellence Injection 2632

Estramustine Phosphate Sodium (Concurrent use of antineoplastic agents and amphotericin B may enhance the potential for renal toxicity, bronchospasm, and hypotension). Products include:
Emcyt Capsules 3137

Etoposide (Concurrent use of antineoplastic agents and amphotericin B may enhance the potential for renal toxicity, bronchospasm, and hypotension).
No products indexed under this heading.

Exemestane (Concurrent use of antineoplastic agents and amphotericin B may enhance the potential for renal toxicity, bronchospasm, and hypotension). Products include:
Aromasin Tablets 2600

Floxuridine (Concurrent use of antineoplastic agents and amphotericin B may enhance the potential for renal toxicity, bronchospasm, and hypotension).
No products indexed under this heading.

Fluconazole (Imidazoles may induce fungal resistance to amphotericin B; combination therapy should be administered with caution, especially in immunocompromised patients).
No products indexed under this heading.

Flucytosine (Concurrent use may increase the toxicity of flucytosine by possibly increasing its cellular uptake and/or impairing its renal excretion).
No products indexed under this heading.

Fludrocortisone Acetate (Concurrent use of corticosteroids and amphotericin B may potentiate hypokalemia which could predispose the patient to cardiac dysfunction).
No products indexed under this heading.

Fluorouracil (Concurrent use of antineoplastic agents and amphotericin B may enhance the potential for renal toxicity, bronchospasm, and hypotension). Products include:
Carac Cream, 0.5% 1048
Efudex 3348

Flutamide (Concurrent use of antineoplastic agents and amphotericin B may enhance the potential for renal toxicity, bronchospasm, and hypotension). Products include:
Eulexin Capsules 3023

Gemcitabine Hydrochloride (Concurrent use of antineoplastic agents and amphotericin B may enhance the potential for renal toxicity, bronchospasm, and hypotension). Products include:
Gemzar for Injection 1743

Gentamicin Sulfate (Concurrent use of amphotericin B and other nephrotoxic agents, such as aminoglycosides, may enhance the potential for drug-induced renal toxicity). Products include:
Garamycin Injectable 3028
Genoptic Sterile Ophthalmic Solution .... ⊙ 227
Pred-G Ophthalmic Suspension .... ⊙ 234
Pred-G Sterile Ophthalmic Ointment .... ⊙ 235

Hydrocortisone (Concurrent use of corticosteroids and amphotericin B may potentiate hypokalemia which could predispose the patient to cardiac dysfunction). Products include:
Cortizone•5 Ointment .... ▣ 699
Cortizone•10 Creme .... ▣ 699
Cortizone•10 Ointment .... ▣ 699
Cortizone•10 Plus Creme .... ▣ 700
Cortizone•10 Maximum Strength Quick Shot Spray .... ▣ 700
Hydrocortone Tablets 1963
Preparation H Hydrocortisone Cream .... ▣ 748

Hydrocortisone Acetate (Concurrent use of corticosteroids and amphotericin B may potentiate hypokalemia which could predispose the patient to cardiac dysfunction). Products include:
Analpram-HC 1136
Pramosone 1139
ProctoFoam-HC 3113
Tucks Anti-Itch Ointment .... ▣ 712
U-cort 1% Cream 3289

Hydrocortisone Sodium Phosphate (Concurrent use of corticosteroids and amphotericin B may potentiate hypokalemia which could predispose the patient to cardiac dysfunction).
No products indexed under this heading.

Hydrocortisone Sodium Succinate (Concurrent use of corticosteroids and amphotericin B may potentiate hypokalemia which could predispose the patient to cardiac dysfunction).
No products indexed under this heading.

Hydroxyurea (Concurrent use of antineoplastic agents and amphotericin B may enhance the potential for renal toxicity, bronchospasm, and hypotension).
No products indexed under this heading.

Idarubicin Hydrochloride (Concurrent use of antineoplastic agents and amphotericin B may enhance the potential for renal toxicity, bronchospasm, and hypotension). Products include:
Idamycin PFS Injection 2645

Ifosfamide (Concurrent use of antineoplastic agents and amphotericin B may enhance the potential for renal toxicity, bronchospasm, and hypotension).
No products indexed under this heading.

Interferon alfa-2a, Recombinant (Concurrent use of antineoplastic agents and amphotericin B may enhance the potential for renal toxicity, bronchospasm, and hypotension). Products include:
Roferon-A Injection 2805

Interferon alfa-2b, Recombinant (Concurrent use of antineoplastic agents and amphotericin B may enhance the potential for renal toxicity, bronchospasm, and hypotension). Products include:
Intron A for Injection 3038
Rebetron Combination Therapy 3078

Irinotecan Hydrochloride (Concurrent use of antineoplastic agents and amphotericin B may enhance the potential for renal toxicity, bronchospasm, and hypotension). Products include:
Camptosar Injection 2602

Kanamycin Sulfate (Concurrent use of amphotericin B and other nephrotoxic agents, such as aminoglycosides, may enhance the potential for drug-induced renal toxicity).
No products indexed under this heading.

Ketoconazole (Imidazoles may induce fungal resistance to amphotericin B; combination therapy should be administered with caution, especially in immunocompromised patients). Products include:
Nizoral A-D Shampoo, 1% 1839
Nizoral 2% Shampoo 1838

Levamisole Hydrochloride (Concurrent use of antineoplastic agents and amphotericin B may enhance the potential for renal toxicity, bronchospasm, and hypotension).
No products indexed under this heading.

Lomustine (CCNU) (Concurrent use of antineoplastic agents and amphotericin B may enhance the potential for renal toxicity, bronchospasm, and hypotension).
No products indexed under this heading.

Mechlorethamine Hydrochloride (Concurrent use of antineoplastic agents and amphotericin B may enhance the potential for renal toxicity, bronchospasm, and hypotension). Products include:
Mustargen for Injection 2007

Megestrol Acetate (Concurrent use of antineoplastic agents and amphotericin B may enhance the potential for renal toxicity, bronchospasm, and hypotension). Products include:
Megace ES Oral Suspension 2492

Melphalan (Concurrent use of antineoplastic agents and amphotericin B may enhance the potential for renal toxicity, bronchospasm, and hypotension). Products include:
Alkeran Tablets 977

Mercaptopurine (Concurrent use of antineoplastic agents and amphotericin B may enhance the potential for renal toxicity, bronchospasm, and hypotension). Products include:
Purinethol Tablets 1222

Methotrexate Sodium (Concurrent use of antineoplastic agents and amphotericin B may enhance the potential for renal toxicity, bronchospasm, and hypotension).
No products indexed under this heading.

Methylprednisolone Acetate (Concurrent use of corticosteroids and amphotericin B may potentiate hypokalemia which could predispose the patient to cardiac dysfunction). Products include:
Depo-Medrol Injectable Suspension 2615
Depo-Medrol Single-Dose Vial 2617

Methylprednisolone Sodium Succinate (Concurrent use of corticosteroids and amphotericin B may potentiate hypokalemia which could predispose the patient to cardiac dysfunction).
No products indexed under this heading.

Metocurine Iodide (Amphotericin B-induced hypokalemia may enhance the curariform effect of skeletal relaxants).
No products indexed under this heading.

Miconazole (Imidazoles may induce fungal resistance to amphotericin B; combination therapy should be administered with caution, especially in immunocompromised patients).
No products indexed under this heading.

Miconazole Nitrate (Imidazoles may induce fungal resistance to amphotericin B; combination therapy should be administered with caution, especially in immunocompromised patients). Products include:
Desenex .... ▣ 674
Desenex Jock Itch Spray Powder .... ▣ 674

Mitomycin (Mitomycin-C) (Concurrent use of antineoplastic agents and amphotericin B may enhance the potential for renal toxicity, bronchospasm, and hypotension).
No products indexed under this heading.

Mitotane (Concurrent use of antineoplastic agents and amphotericin B may enhance the potential for renal toxicity, bronchospasm, and hypotension).
No products indexed under this heading.

Mitoxantrone Hydrochloride (Concurrent use of antineoplastic agents and amphotericin B may enhance the potential for renal toxicity, bronchospasm, and hypotension). Products include:
Novantrone for Injection Concentrate 3158

Mivacurium Chloride (Amphotericin B-induced hypokalemia may enhance the curariform effect of skeletal relaxants). Products include:
Mivacron Injection 489

Oxaliplatin (Concurrent use of antineoplastic agents and amphotericin

B may enhance the potential for renal toxicity, bronchospasm, and hypotension). Products include:

Eloxatin for Injection 2908

Paclitaxel (Concurrent use of antineoplastic agents and amphotericin B may enhance the potential for renal toxicity, bronchospasm, and hypotension).

No products indexed under this heading.

Pancuronium Bromide (Amphotericin B-induced hypokalemia may enhance the curariform effect of skeletal relaxants).

No products indexed under this heading.

Pentamidine Isethionate (Concurrent use of amphotericin B and other nephrotoxic agents, such as pentamidine, may enhance the potential for drug-induced renal toxicity).

No products indexed under this heading.

Pipecuronium Bromide (Amphotericin B-induced hypokalemia may enhance the curariform effect of skeletal relaxants).

No products indexed under this heading.

Prednisolone Acetate (Concurrent use of corticosteroids and amphotericin B may potentiate hypokalemia which could predispose the patient to cardiac dysfunction). Products include:

Blephamide Ophthalmic Ointment 563
Blephamide Ophthalmic Suspension.................................. 564
Poly-Pred Liquifilm Ophthalmic Suspension .... ⊙231
Pred Forte Ophthalmic Suspension .... ⊙233
Pred Mild Sterile Ophthalmic Suspension .... ⊙236
Pred-G Ophthalmic Suspension ...... ⊙234
Pred-G Sterile Ophthalmic Ointment.................................... ⊙235

Prednisolone Sodium Phosphate (Concurrent use of corticosteroids and amphotericin B may potentiate hypokalemia which could predispose the patient to cardiac dysfunction). Products include:

Pediapred Oral Solution 3319

Prednisolone Tebutate (Concurrent use of corticosteroids and amphotericin B may potentiate hypokalemia which could predispose the patient to cardiac dysfunction).

No products indexed under this heading.

Prednisone (Concurrent use of corticosteroids and amphotericin B may potentiate hypokalemia which could predispose the patient to cardiac dysfunction).

No products indexed under this heading.

Procarbazine Hydrochloride (Concurrent use of antineoplastic agents and amphotericin B may enhance the potential for renal toxicity, bronchospasm, and hypotension). Products include:

Matulane Capsules 3188

Rapacuronium Bromide (Amphotericin B-induced hypokalemia may enhance the curariform effect of skeletal relaxants).

No products indexed under this heading.

Rocuronium Bromide (Amphotericin B-induced hypokalemia may enhance the curariform effect of skeletal relaxants). Products include:

Zemuron Injection 2363

Streptomycin Sulfate (Concurrent use of amphotericin B and other nephrotoxic agents, such as aminoglycosides, may enhance the potential for drug-induced renal toxicity).

No products indexed under this heading.

Streptozocin (Concurrent use of antineoplastic agents and amphotericin B may enhance the potential for renal toxicity, bronchospasm, and hypotension).

No products indexed under this heading.

Tamoxifen Citrate (Concurrent use of antineoplastic agents and amphotericin B may enhance the potential for renal toxicity, bronchospasm, and hypotension).

No products indexed under this heading.

Teniposide (Concurrent use of antineoplastic agents and amphotericin B may enhance the potential for renal toxicity, bronchospasm, and hypotension).

No products indexed under this heading.

Thioguanine (Concurrent use of antineoplastic agents and amphotericin B may enhance the potential for renal toxicity, bronchospasm, and hypotension). Products include:

Tabloid Tablets 1545

Thiotepa (Concurrent use of antineoplastic agents and amphotericin B may enhance the potential for renal toxicity, bronchospasm, and hypotension).

No products indexed under this heading.

Tobramycin (Concurrent use of amphotericin B and other nephrotoxic agents, such as aminoglycosides, may enhance the potential for drug-induced renal toxicity). Products include:

TOBI Solution for Inhalation 1015
TobraDex Ophthalmic Ointment 558
TobraDex Ophthalmic Suspension ... 558
Zylet Ophthalmic Suspension 3508

Tobramycin Sulfate (Concurrent use of amphotericin B and other nephrotoxic agents, such as aminoglycosides, may enhance the potential for drug-induced renal toxicity).

No products indexed under this heading.

Topotecan Hydrochloride (Concurrent use of antineoplastic agents and amphotericin B may enhance the potential for renal toxicity, bronchospasm, and hypotension). Products include:

Hycamtin for Injection 1427

Toremifene Citrate (Concurrent use of antineoplastic agents and amphotericin B may enhance the potential for renal toxicity, bronchospasm, and hypotension).

No products indexed under this heading.

Triamcinolone (Concurrent use of corticosteroids and amphotericin B may potentiate hypokalemia which could predispose the patient to cardiac dysfunction).

No products indexed under this heading.

Triamcinolone Acetonide (Concurrent use of corticosteroids and amphotericin B may potentiate hypokalemia which could predispose the patient to cardiac dysfunction). Products include:

Azmacort Inhalation Aerosol 1701
Nasacort HFA Inhalation Aerosol 2939
Nasacort AQ Nasal Spray 2937

Triamcinolone Diacetate (Concurrent use of corticosteroids and amphotericin B may potentiate hypokalemia which could predispose the patient to cardiac dysfunction).

No products indexed under this heading.

Triamcinolone Hexacetonide (Concurrent use of corticosteroids and amphotericin B may potentiate hypokalemia which could predispose the patient to cardiac dysfunction).

No products indexed under this heading.

Tubocurarine Chloride (Amphotericin B-induced hypokalemia may enhance the curariform effect of skeletal relaxants).

No products indexed under this heading.

Valrubicin (Concurrent use of antineoplastic agents and amphotericin B may enhance the potential for renal toxicity, bronchospasm, and hypotension).

No products indexed under this heading.

Vecuronium Bromide (Amphotericin B-induced hypokalemia may enhance the curariform effect of skeletal relaxants).

No products indexed under this heading.

Vincristine Sulfate (Concurrent use of antineoplastic agents and amphotericin B may enhance the potential for renal toxicity, bronchospasm, and hypotension).

No products indexed under this heading.

Vinorelbine Tartrate (Concurrent use of antineoplastic agents and amphotericin B may enhance the potential for renal toxicity, bronchospasm, and hypotension). Products include:

Navelbine Injection 1494

AMBROTOSE AO CAPSULES

(Herbals with Vitamins) .... ▣769
None cited in PDR database.

AMBROTOSE CAPSULES

(Herbals, Multiple) .... ▣768
None cited in PDR database.

AMBROTOSE POWDER

(Glucosamine Hydrochloride, Herbals, Multiple)............................. ▣768
None cited in PDR database.

AMBROTOSE WITH LECITHIN CAPSULES

(Herbals, Multiple, Lecithin) .... ▣768
None cited in PDR database.

AMERGE TABLETS

(Naratriptan Hydrochloride) 1312

May interact with 5HT1-receptor agonists, ergot-containing drugs, oral contraceptives, and selective serotonin reuptake inhibitors. Compounds in these categories include:

Citalopram Hydrobromide (Co-administration of 5-HT$_1$ agonists with selective serotonin reuptake inhibitors (SSRIs) has resulted, rarely, in hyperreflexia, weakness, and incoordination). Products include:

Celexa 1177

Desogestrel (Co-administration with oral contraceptives has resulted in reduced clearance by 32% and volume of distribution by 22%, producing slightly higher concentrations of naratriptan). Products include:

Ortho-Cept Tablets 2395

Dihydroergotamine Mesylate (Ergot-containing drugs have been reported to cause prolonged vasospastic reactions; because there is a theoretical basis that these effects may be additive, use of ergot-type agents and naratriptan within 24 hours is contraindicated). Products include:

Migranal Nasal Spray 3350

Ergonovine Maleate (Ergot-containing drugs have been reported to cause prolonged vasospastic reactions; because there is a theoretical basis that these effects may be additive, use of ergot-type agents and naratriptan within 24 hours is contraindicated).

No products indexed under this heading.

Ergotamine Tartrate (Ergot-containing drugs have been reported to cause prolonged vasospastic reactions; because there is a theoretical basis that these effects may be additive, use of ergot-type agents and naratriptan within 24 hours is contraindicated).

No products indexed under this heading.

Ethinyl Estradiol (Co-administration with oral contraceptives has resulted in reduced clearance by 32% and volume of distribution by 22%, producing slightly higher concentrations of naratriptan). Products include:

Alesse-28 Tablets 3392
Lo/Ovral-28 Tablets 3423
NuvaRing 2357
Ortho-Cept Tablets 2395
Ortho-Cyclen/Ortho Tri-Cyclen 2414
Ortho Evra Transdermal System 2402
Ortho Tri-Cyclen Lo Tablets 2421
Seasonale Tablets 1073
Triphasil-28 Tablets 3483
Yasmin 28 Tablets 818

Ethynodiol Diacetate (Co-administration with oral contraceptives has resulted in reduced clearance by 32% and volume of distribution by 22%, producing slightly higher concentrations of naratriptan).

No products indexed under this heading.

Fluoxetine Hydrochloride (Co-administration of 5-HT$_1$ agonists with selective serotonin reuptake inhibitors (SSRIs) has resulted, rarely, in hyperreflexia, weakness, and incoordination). Products include:

Prozac Pulvules and Liquid 1771
Symbyax Capsules 1788

Fluvoxamine Maleate (Co-administration of 5-HT$_1$ agonists with selective serotonin reuptake inhibitors (SSRIs) has resulted, rarely, in hyperreflexia, weakness, and incoordination).

No products indexed under this heading.

Levonorgestrel (Co-administration with oral contraceptives has resulted in reduced clearance by 32% and volume of distribution by 22%, producing slightly higher concentrations of naratriptan). Products include:

Alesse-28 Tablets 3392
Climara Pro Transdermal System 800
Mirena Intrauterine System 810
Plan B Tablets 1068
Seasonale Tablets 1073

Triphasil-28 Tablets 3483

Mestranol (Co-administration with oral contraceptives has resulted in reduced clearance by 32% and volume of distribution by 22%, producing slightly higher concentrations of naratriptan).
No products indexed under this heading.

Methylergonovine Maleate (Ergot-containing drugs have been reported to cause prolonged vasospastic reactions; because there is a theoretical basis that these effects may be additive, use of ergot-type agents and naratriptan within 24 hours is contraindicated).
No products indexed under this heading.

Methysergide Maleate (Ergot-containing drugs have been reported to cause prolonged vasospastic reactions; because there is a theoretical basis that these effects may be additive, use of ergot-type agents and naratriptan within 24 hours is contraindicated).
No products indexed under this heading.

Norethindrone (Co-administration with oral contraceptives has resulted in reduced clearance by 32% and volume of distribution by 22%, producing slightly higher concentrations of naratriptan). Products include:
Ortho Micronor Tablets 2411

Norethynodrel (Co-administration with oral contraceptives has resulted in reduced clearance by 32% and volume of distribution by 22%, producing slightly higher concentrations of naratriptan).
No products indexed under this heading.

Norgestimate (Co-administration with oral contraceptives has resulted in reduced clearance by 32% and volume of distribution by 22%, producing slightly higher concentrations of naratriptan). Products include:
Ortho-Cyclen/Ortho Tri-Cyclen 2414
Ortho Tri-Cyclen Lo Tablets 2421
Prefest Tablets 1069

Norgestrel (Co-administration with oral contraceptives has resulted in reduced clearance by 32% and volume of distribution by 22%, producing slightly higher concentrations of naratriptan). Products include:
Lo/Ovral-28 Tablets 3423

Paroxetine Hydrochloride (Co-administration of 5-HT_1 agonists with selective serotonin reuptake inhibitors (SSRIs) has resulted, rarely, in hyperreflexia, weakness, and incoordination). Products include:
Paxil CR Controlled-Release Tablets 1509
Paxil 1501

Rizatriptan Benzoate (Co-administration with other 5-HT_1 agonists within 24 hours of each other is contraindicated because of the vasospastic effects may be additive). Products include:
Maxalt Tablets 1983
Maxalt-MLT Orally Disintegrating Tablets 1983

Sertraline Hydrochloride (Co-administration of 5-HT_1 agonists with selective serotonin reuptake inhibitors (SSRIs) has resulted, rarely, in hyperreflexia, weakness, and incoordination). Products include:
Zoloft 2581

Sumatriptan (Co-administration with other 5-HT_1 agonists within 24 hours of each other is contraindicated because of the vasospastic effects may be additive). Products include:
Imitrex Nasal Spray 1435

Sumatriptan Succinate (Co-administration with other 5-HT_1 agonists within 24 hours of each other is contraindicated because of the vasospastic effects may be additive). Products include:
Imitrex Injection 1431
Imitrex Tablets 1440

Zolmitriptan (Co-administration with other 5-HT_1 agonists within 24 hours of each other is contraindicated because of the vasospastic effects may be additive). Products include:
Zomig Nasal Spray 718
Zomig Tablets 714
Zomig-ZMT Tablets 714

AMEVIVE

(Alefacept) 836
None cited in PDR database.

AMINOHIPPURATE SODIUM "PAH" INJECTION

(Aminohippurate Sodium) 1886
May interact with sulfonamides and certain other agents. Compounds in these categories include:

Bendroflumethiazide (Co-administration with sulfonamides interfere with chemical color development essential to the analytical procedures).
No products indexed under this heading.

Chlorothiazide (Co-administration with sulfonamides interfere with chemical color development essential to the analytical procedures). Products include:
Aldoclor Tablets 1881
Diuril Oral 1936

Chlorothiazide Sodium (Co-administration with sulfonamides interfere with chemical color development essential to the analytical procedures). Products include:
Diuril Sodium Intravenous 1934

Chlorpropamide (Co-administration with sulfonamides interfere with chemical color development essential to the analytical procedures).
No products indexed under this heading.

Glipizide (Co-administration with sulfonamides interfere with chemical color development essential to the analytical procedures).
No products indexed under this heading.

Glyburide (Co-administration with sulfonamides interfere with chemical color development essential to the analytical procedures).
No products indexed under this heading.

Hydrochlorothiazide (Co-administration with sulfonamides interfere with chemical color development essential to the analytical procedures). Products include:
Aldoril Tablets 1884
Atacand HCT 637
Avalide Tablets 2889
Avalide Tablets 922
Benicar HCT Tablets 2852
Diovan HCT Tablets 2195
Dyazide Capsules 1389
Hyzaar 1964
Lotensin HCT Tablets 2235
Maxzide 2150
Micardis HCT Tablets 886
Moduretic Tablets 2003
Prinzide Tablets 2033
Teveten HCT Tablets 1710
Timolide Tablets 2056
Uniretic Tablets 3114
Vaseretic Tablets 2073
Zestoretic Tablets 701

Hydroflumethiazide (Co-administration with sulfonamides interfere with chemical color development essential to the analytical procedures).
No products indexed under this heading.

Methyclothiazide (Co-administration with sulfonamides interfere with chemical color development essential to the analytical procedures).
No products indexed under this heading.

Polythiazide (Co-administration with sulfonamides interfere with chemical color development essential to the analytical procedures).
No products indexed under this heading.

Probenecid (Tubular secretion of PAH depressed).
No products indexed under this heading.

Procaine Hydrochloride (Renal clearance measurements impaired).
No products indexed under this heading.

Sulfacytine (Co-administration with sulfonamides interfere with chemical color development essential to the analytical procedures).
No products indexed under this heading.

Sulfamethizole (Co-administration with sulfonamides interfere with chemical color development essential to the analytical procedures).
No products indexed under this heading.

Sulfamethoxazole (Co-administration with sulfonamides interfere with chemical color development essential to the analytical procedures).
No products indexed under this heading.

Sulfasalazine (Co-administration with sulfonamides interfere with chemical color development essential to the analytical procedures).
No products indexed under this heading.

Sulfinpyrazone (Co-administration with sulfonamides interfere with chemical color development essential to the analytical procedures).
No products indexed under this heading.

Sulfisoxazole (Co-administration with sulfonamides interfere with chemical color development essential to the analytical procedures).
No products indexed under this heading.

Sulfisoxazole Acetyl (Co-administration with sulfonamides interfere with chemical color development essential to the analytical procedures).
No products indexed under this heading.

Sulfisoxazole Diolamine (Co-administration with sulfonamides interfere with chemical color development essential to the analytical procedures).
No products indexed under this heading.

Tolazamide (Co-administration with sulfonamides interfere with chemical color development essential to the analytical procedures).
No products indexed under this heading.

Tolbutamide (Co-administration with sulfonamides interfere with chemical color development essential to the analytical procedures).
No products indexed under this heading.

AMMONUL INJECTION

(Sodium Benzoate, Sodium Phenylacelate) 3323
May interact with penicillins and certain other agents. Compounds in these categories include:

5-Amino-Salicylic Acid (Some antibiotics, such as penicillin, may compete with phenylacetylglutamine and hippurate for active secretion by renal tubules, which may affect the overall disposition of the infused drug).
No products indexed under this heading.

Amoxicillin (Some antibiotics, such as penicillin, may compete with phenylacetylglutamine and hippurate for active secretion by renal tubules, which may affect the overall disposition of the infused drug). Products include:
Amoxil Capsules 1315
Amoxil Chewable Tablets 1315
Amoxil Pediatric Drops for Oral Suspension 1315
Amoxil Powder for Oral Suspension 1315
Amoxil Tablets 1315
Augmentin 1331
Augmentin Tablets 1334
Augmentin XR Extended-Release Tablets 1340
Augmentin ES-600 Powder for Oral Suspension 1337
PREVPAC 3281

Amoxicillin Trihydrate (Some antibiotics, such as penicillin, may compete with phenylacetylglutamine and hippurate for active secretion by renal tubules, which may affect the overall disposition of the infused drug).
No products indexed under this heading.

Ampicillin (Some antibiotics, such as penicillin, may compete with phenylacetylglutamine and hippurate for active secretion by renal tubules, which may affect the overall disposition of the infused drug).
No products indexed under this heading.

Ampicillin Sodium (Some antibiotics, such as penicillin, may compete with phenylacetylglutamine and hippurate for active secretion by renal tubules, which may affect the overall disposition of the infused drug).
No products indexed under this heading.

Ampicillin Trihydrate (Some antibiotics, such as penicillin, may compete with phenylacetylglutamine and hippurate for active secretion by renal tubules, which may affect the overall disposition of the infused drug).
No products indexed under this heading.

Azlocillin Sodium (Some antibiotics, such as penicillin, may compete with phenylacetylglutamine and hippurate for active secretion by renal tubules, which may affect the overall disposition of the infused drug).
No products indexed under this heading.

Bacampicillin Hydrochloride (Some antibiotics, such as penicillin, may compete with phenylacetylglutamine and hippurate for active secretion by renal tubules, which may affect the overall disposition of the infused drug).
No products indexed under this heading.

Carbenicillin Disodium (Some antibiotics, such as penicillin, may compete with phenylacetylglutamine and hippurate for active secretion by renal tubules, which may affect the overall disposition of the infused drug).
No products indexed under this heading.

Carbenicillin Indanyl Sodium (Some antibiotics, such as penicillin, may compete with phenylacetylglutamine and hippurate for active secretion by renal tubules, which may affect the overall disposition of the infused drug).
No products indexed under this heading.

Dicloxacillin Sodium (Some antibiotics, such as penicillin, may compete with phenylacetylglutamine and hippurate for active secretion by renal tubules, which may affect the overall disposition of the infused drug).
No products indexed under this heading.

Mezlocillin Sodium (Some antibiotics, such as penicillin, may compete with phenylacetylglutamine and hippurate for active secretion by renal tubules, which may affect the overall disposition of the infused drug).
No products indexed under this heading.

Nafcillin Sodium (Some antibiotics, such as penicillin, may compete with phenylacetylglutamine and hippurate for active secretion by renal tubules, which may affect the overall disposition of the infused drug).
No products indexed under this heading.

Penicillin G Benzathine (Some antibiotics, such as penicillin, may compete with phenylacetylglutamine and hippurate for active secretion by renal tubules, which may affect the overall disposition of the infused drug).
No products indexed under this heading.

Penicillin G Potassium (Some antibiotics, such as penicillin, may compete with phenylacetylglutamine and hippurate for active secretion by renal tubules, which may affect the overall disposition of the infused drug).
No products indexed under this heading.

Penicillin G Procaine (Some antibiotics, such as penicillin, may compete with phenylacetylglutamine and hippurate for active secretion by renal tubules, which may affect the overall disposition of the infused drug).
No products indexed under this heading.

Penicillin G Sodium (Some antibiotics, such as penicillin, may compete with phenylacetylglutamine and hippurate for active secretion by renal tubules, which may affect the overall disposition of the infused drug).
No products indexed under this heading.

Penicillin V Potassium (Some antibiotics, such as penicillin, may compete with phenylacetylglutamine and hippurate for active secretion by renal tubules, which may affect the overall disposition of the infused drug).
No products indexed under this heading.

Probenecid (Probenecid is known to inhibit the renal transport of many organic compounds including aminohippuric acid, and may affect renal excretion of phenylacetylglutamine and hippurate).
No products indexed under this heading.

Ticarcillin Disodium (Some antibiotics, such as penicillin, may compete with phenylacetylglutamine and hippurate for active secretion by renal tubules, which may affect the overall disposition of the infused drug). Products include:
Timentin ADD-Vantage 1556
Timentin Injection Galaxy Container 1559
Timentin IV Infusion 1553
Timentin Pharmacy Bulk Package 1562

Valproic Acid (There have been reports that valproic acid can induce hyperammonemia through inhibition of the synthesis of N-acetylglutamate, a co-factor for carbamyl phosphate synthetase. Therefore, administration of valproic acid to patients with urea cycle disorders may exercerbate their condition and antagonize the efficacy of Ammonul). Products include:
Depakene 417

AMNESTEEM CAPSULES

(Isotretinoin) 2126
May interact with tetracyclines and certain other agents. Compounds in these categories include:

Demeclocycline Hydrochloride (Concomitant treatment with isotretinoin and tetracyclines should be avoided because isotretinoin use has been associated with a number of cases of pseudotumor cerebri, some of which involved concomitant use of tetracyclines).
No products indexed under this heading.

Doxycycline Calcium (Concomitant treatment with isotretinoin and tetracyclines should be avoided because isotretinoin use has been associated with a number of cases of pseudotumor cerebri, some of which involved concomitant use of tetracyclines).
No products indexed under this heading.

Doxycycline Hyclate (Concomitant treatment with isotretinoin and tetracyclines should be avoided because isotretinoin use has been associated with a number of cases of pseudotumor cerebri, some of which involved concomitant use of tetracyclines).
No products indexed under this heading.

Doxycycline Monohydrate (Concomitant treatment with isotretinoin and tetracyclines should be avoided because isotretinoin use has been associated with a number of cases of pseudotumor cerebri, some of which involved concomitant use of tetracyclines).
No products indexed under this heading.

Methacycline Hydrochloride (Concomitant treatment with isotretinoin and tetracyclines should be avoided because isotretinoin use has been associated with a number of cases of pseudotumor cerebri, some of which involved concomitant use of tetracyclines).
No products indexed under this heading.

Minocycline Hydrochloride (Concomitant treatment with isotretinoin and tetracyclines should be avoided because isotretinoin use has been associated with a number of cases of pseudotumor cerebri, some of which involved concomitant use of tetracyclines). Products include:
Dynacin Tablets 1859

Norethindrone (Micro-dosed progesterone preparations may be an inadequate method of contraception during isotretinoin capsules therapy). Products include:
Ortho Micronor Tablets 2411

Norgestrel (Micro-dosed progesterone preparations may be an inadequate method of contraception during isotretinoin capsules therapy). Products include:
Lo/Ovral-28 Tablets 3423

Oxytetracycline Hydrochloride (Concomitant treatment with isotretinoin and tetracyclines should be avoided because isotretinoin use has been associated with a number of cases of pseudotumor cerebri, some of which involved concomitant use of tetracyclines).
No products indexed under this heading.

Phenytoin (If acitretin is given concurrently with phenytoin, the protein binding of phenytoin may be reduced).
No products indexed under this heading.

Tetracycline Hydrochloride (Concomitant treatment with isotretinoin and tetracyclines should be avoided because isotretinoin use has been associated with a number of cases of pseudotumor cerebri, some of which involved concomitant use of tetracyclines).
No products indexed under this heading.

Vitamin A (Concomitant administration of vitamin A and/or other oral retinoids with acitretin must be avoided because of the risk of hypervitaminosis A). Products include:
Visutein Capsules 3328

AMOXIL CAPSULES

(Amoxicillin) 1315
See Amoxil Tablets

AMOXIL CHEWABLE TABLETS

(Amoxicillin) 1315
See Amoxil Tablets

AMOXIL PEDIATRIC DROPS FOR ORAL SUSPENSION

(Amoxicillin) 1315
May interact with:

See (Amoxil Tablets).

AMOXIL POWDER FOR ORAL SUSPENSION

(Amoxicillin) 1315
See Amoxil Tablets

AMOXIL TABLETS

(Amoxicillin) 1315
May interact with macrolide antibiotics, tetracyclines, and certain other agents. Compounds in these categories include:

Azithromycin Dihydrate (May interfere with bactericidal effects of penicillin. This has been demonstrated in vitro; however, the clinical significance of the interaction is not well documented). Products include:
Zithromax 2568
Zithromax for IV Infusion 2573
Zithromax for Oral Suspension, 300 mg, 600 mg, 900 mg, 1200 mg 2561
Zithromax Tablets, 250 mg, 500 mg 2561
Zithromax Tri-Pak 2561
Zithromax Z-Pak 2568

Chloramphenicol Sodium Succinate (May interfere with bactericidal effects of penicillin. This has been demonstrated in vitro; however, the clinical significance of the interaction is not well documented).
No products indexed under this heading.

Clarithromycin (May interfere with bactericidal effects of penicillin. This has been demonstrated in vitro; however, the clinical significance of the interaction is not well documented). Products include:
Biaxin/Biaxin XL 402
PREVPAC 3281

Demeclocycline Hydrochloride (May interfere with bactericidal effects of penicillin. This has been demonstrated in vitro; however, the clinical significance of the interaction is not well documented).
No products indexed under this heading.

Dirithromycin (May interfere with bactericidal effects of penicillin. This has been demonstrated in vitro; however, the clinical significance of the interaction is not well documented).
No products indexed under this heading.

Doxycycline Calcium (May interfere with bactericidal effects of penicillin. This has been demonstrated in vitro; however, the clinical significance of the interaction is not well documented).
No products indexed under this heading.

Doxycycline Hyclate (May interfere with bactericidal effects of penicillin. This has been demonstrated in vitro; however, the clinical significance of the interaction is not well documented).
No products indexed under this heading.

Doxycycline Monohydrate (May interfere with bactericidal effects of penicillin. This has been demonstrated in vitro; however, the clinical significance of the interaction is not well documented).
No products indexed under this heading.

Erythromycin (May interfere with bactericidal effects of penicillin. This has been demonstrated in vitro; however, the clinical significance of the interaction is not well documented).
Products include:
Erygel Topical Gel **2096**
Ery-Tab Tablets **447**
Erythromycin Base Filmtab Tablets **454**
Erythromycin Delayed-Release Capsules, USP **456**
PCE Dispertab Tablets **510**

Erythromycin Estolate (May interfere with bactericidal effects of penicillin. This has been demonstrated in vitro; however, the clinical significance of the interaction is not well documented).
No products indexed under this heading.

Erythromycin Ethylsuccinate (May interfere with bactericidal effects of penicillin. This has been demonstrated in vitro; however, the clinical significance of the interaction is not well documented). Products include:
E.E.S. **449**
EryPed **445**

Erythromycin Gluceptate (May interfere with bactericidal effects of penicillin. This has been demonstrated in vitro; however, the clinical significance of the interaction is not well documented).
No products indexed under this heading.

Erythromycin Stearate (May interfere with bactericidal effects of penicillin. This has been demonstrated in vitro; however, the clinical significance of the interaction is not well documented). Products include:
Erythrocin Stearate Filmtab Tablets **452**

Methacycline Hydrochloride (May interfere with bactericidal effects of penicillin. This has been demonstrated in vitro; however, the clinical significance of the interaction is not well documented).
No products indexed under this heading.

Minocycline Hydrochloride (May interfere with bactericidal effects of penicillin. This has been demonstrated in vitro; however, the clinical significance of the interaction is not well documented). Products include:
Dynacin Tablets **1859**

Oxytetracycline Hydrochloride (May interfere with bactericidal effects of penicillin. This has been demonstrated in vitro; however, the clinical significance of the interaction is not well documented).
No products indexed under this heading.

Probenecid (Decreases the renal tubular secretion of amoxicillin; concurrent use may result in increased and prolonged blood levels).
No products indexed under this heading.

Sulfamethoxazole (May interfere with bactericidal effects of penicillin. This has been demonstrated in vitro; however, the clinical significance of the interaction is not well documented).
No products indexed under this heading.

Sulfisoxazole Acetyl (May interfere with bactericidal effects of penicillin. This has been demonstrated in vitro; however, the clinical significance of the interaction is not well documented).
No products indexed under this heading.

Tetracycline Hydrochloride (May interfere with bactericidal effects of penicillin. This has been demonstrated in vitro; however, the clinical significance of the interaction is not well documented).
No products indexed under this heading.

Troleandomycin (May interfere with bactericidal effects of penicillin. This has been demonstrated in vitro; however, the clinical significance of the interaction is not well documented).
No products indexed under this heading.

AMVISC PLUS

(Sodium Hyaluronate) .... ⊙289
None cited in PDR database.

ANADROL-50 TABLETS

(Oxymetholone) **3329**
May interact with oral anticoagulants, oral hypoglycemic agents, and insulin. Compounds in these categories include:

Acarbose (Anabolic steroids tend to decrease glucose tolerance; oral hypoglycemic dosage may need to be adjusted in diabetic patients).
Products include:
Precose Tablets **776**

Anisindione (Anabolic steroids may increase sensitivity to oral anticoagulants. Dosage of the anticoagulant may have to be decreased in order to maintain the desired prothrombin time. Patients receiving oral anticoagulant therapy require close monitoring, especially when anabolic steroids are started or stopped).
Products include:
Miradon Tablets **3056**

Chlorpropamide (Anabolic steroids tend to decrease glucose tolerance; oral hypoglycemic dosage may need to be adjusted in diabetic patients).
No products indexed under this heading.

Dicumarol (Anabolic steroids may increase sensitivity to oral anticoagulants. Dosage of the anticoagulant may have to be decreased in order to maintain the desired prothrombin time. Patients receiving oral anticoagulant therapy require close monitoring, especially when anabolic steroids are started or stopped).
No products indexed under this heading.

Glimepiride (Anabolic steroids tend to decrease glucose tolerance; oral hypoglycemic dosage may need to be adjusted in diabetic patients).
Products include:
Amaryl Tablets **2864**

Glipizide (Anabolic steroids tend to decrease glucose tolerance; oral hypoglycemic dosage may need to be adjusted in diabetic patients).
No products indexed under this heading.

Glyburide (Anabolic steroids tend to decrease glucose tolerance; oral hypoglycemic dosage may need to be adjusted in diabetic patients).
No products indexed under this heading.

Insulin, Human, Zinc Suspension (Anabolic steroids tend to decrease glucose tolerance; insulin dosage may need to be adjusted in diabetic patients). Products include:
Humulin L, 100 Units **1763**
Humulin U, 100 Units **1770**

Insulin, Human NPH (Anabolic steroids tend to decrease glucose tolerance; insulin dosage may need to be adjusted in diabetic patients).
Products include:
Humulin N, 100 Units **1764**
Humulin N Pen **1765**
Novolin N Human Insulin 10 ml Vials **2322**
Novolin N InnoLet **2322**
Novolin N PenFill 3 ml Cartridges **2325**
Novolin R InnoLet **2322**

Insulin, Human Regular (Anabolic steroids tend to decrease glucose tolerance; insulin dosage may need to be adjusted in diabetic patients).
Products include:
Humulin R (U-500) **1768**
Humulin R, 100 Units **1767**
Novolin R Human Insulin 10 ml Vials **2322**
Novolin R PenFill **2325**

Insulin, Human Regular and Human NPH Mixture (Anabolic steroids tend to decrease glucose tolerance; insulin dosage may need to be adjusted in diabetic patients).
Products include:
Humulin 50/50, 100 Units **1760**
Humulin 70/30 Pen **1761**
Novolin 70/30 Human Insulin 10 ml Vials **2321**
Novolin 70/30 InnoLet **2322**
Novolin 70/30 PenFill 3 ml Cartridges **2325**

Insulin, NPH (Anabolic steroids tend to decrease glucose tolerance; insulin dosage may need to be adjusted in diabetic patients).
No products indexed under this heading.

Insulin, Regular (Anabolic steroids tend to decrease glucose tolerance; insulin dosage may need to be adjusted in diabetic patients).
No products indexed under this heading.

Insulin, Zinc Crystals (Anabolic steroids tend to decrease glucose tolerance; insulin dosage may need to be adjusted in diabetic patients).
No products indexed under this heading.

Insulin, Zinc Suspension (Anabolic steroids tend to decrease glucose tolerance; insulin dosage may need to be adjusted in diabetic patients).
No products indexed under this heading.

Insulin Aspart, Human Regular (Anabolic steroids tend to decrease glucose tolerance; insulin dosage may need to be adjusted in diabetic patients). Products include:
NovoLog Injection **2326**

Insulin glargine (Anabolic steroids tend to decrease glucose tolerance; insulin dosage may need to be adjusted in diabetic patients).
Products include:
Lantus Injection **2925**

Insulin Lispro, Human (Anabolic steroids tend to decrease glucose tolerance; insulin dosage may need to be adjusted in diabetic patients).
Products include:
Humalog-Pen **1751**
Humalog Mix 75/25-Pen **1754**

Insulin Lispro Protamine, Human (Anabolic steroids tend to decrease glucose tolerance; insulin dosage may need to be adjusted in diabetic patients). Products include:
Humalog Mix 75/25-Pen **1754**

Metformin Hydrochloride (Anabolic steroids tend to decrease glucose tolerance; oral hypoglycemic dosage may need to be adjusted in diabetic patients). Products include:
ActoPlus Met Tablets **3219**
Avandamet Tablets **1343**
Fortamet Extended-Release Tablets **1156**

Miglitol (Anabolic steroids tend to decrease glucose tolerance; oral hypoglycemic dosage may need to be adjusted in diabetic patients).
No products indexed under this heading.

Pioglitazone Hydrochloride (Anabolic steroids tend to decrease glucose tolerance; oral hypoglycemic dosage may need to be adjusted in diabetic patients). Products include:
ActoPlus Met Tablets **3219**
Actos Tablets **3224**

Repaglinide (Anabolic steroids tend to decrease glucose tolerance; oral hypoglycemic dosage may need to be adjusted in diabetic patients).
Products include:
Prandin Tablets (0.5, 1, and 2 mg) **2337**

Rosiglitazone Maleate (Anabolic steroids tend to decrease glucose tolerance; oral hypoglycemic dosage may need to be adjusted in diabetic patients). Products include:
Avandamet Tablets **1343**
Avandia Tablets **1348**

Tolazamide (Anabolic steroids tend to decrease glucose tolerance; oral hypoglycemic dosage may need to be adjusted in diabetic patients).
No products indexed under this heading.

Tolbutamide (Anabolic steroids tend to decrease glucose tolerance; oral hypoglycemic dosage may need to be adjusted in diabetic patients).
No products indexed under this heading.

Troglitazone (Anabolic steroids tend to decrease glucose tolerance; oral hypoglycemic dosage may need to be adjusted in diabetic patients).
No products indexed under this heading.

Warfarin Sodium (Anabolic steroids may increase sensitivity to oral anticoagulants. Dosage of the anticoagulant may have to be decreased in order to maintain the desired prothrombin time. Patients receiving oral anticoagulant therapy require close monitoring, especially when anabolic steroids are started or stopped). Products include:
Coumadin for Injection **932**
Coumadin Tablets **932**

ANALPRAM HC CREAM, 1% AND 2.5%
(Hydrocortisone Acetate, Pramoxine Hydrochloride)................... 1136
None cited in PDR database.

ANALPRAM HC LOTION, 2.5%
(Hydrocortisone Acetate, Pramoxine Hydrochloride)................... 1136
None cited in PDR database.

ANAPROX TABLETS
(Naproxen Sodium) 2769
See EC-Naprosyn Delayed-Release Tablets

ANAPROX DS TABLETS
(Naproxen Sodium) 2769
See EC-Naprosyn Delayed-Release Tablets

ANBESOL COLD SORE THERAPY OINTMENT
(Allantoin, Benzocaine, Camphor, Petrolatum, White)............................ ▣745
None cited in PDR database.

BABY ANBESOL GEL
(Benzocaine) .... ▣744
None cited in PDR database.

JUNIOR ANBESOL GEL
(Benzocaine) .... ▣744
None cited in PDR database.

MAXIMUM STRENGTH ANBESOL GEL
(Benzocaine) .... ▣744
None cited in PDR database.

MAXIMUM STRENGTH ANBESOL LIQUID
(Benzocaine) .... ▣744
None cited in PDR database.

ANCEF FOR INJECTION
(Cefazolin Sodium) 1318
May interact with:

Probenecid (Increased and prolonged cephalosporin blood levels).
No products indexed under this heading.

ANDROGEL
(Testosterone) 3330
May interact with corticosteroids, insulin, and certain other agents. Compounds in these categories include:

ACTH (Co-administration of testosterone with ACTH may enhance edema formation).
No products indexed under this heading.

Betamethasone Acetate (Co-administration of testosterone with corticosteroids may enhance edema formation).
No products indexed under this heading.

Betamethasone Sodium Phosphate (Co-administration of testosterone with corticosteroids may enhance edema formation).
No products indexed under this heading.

Cortisone Acetate (Co-administration of testosterone with corticosteroids may enhance edema formation).
No products indexed under this heading.

Dexamethasone (Co-administration of testosterone with corticosteroids may enhance edema formation). Products include:
Ciprodex Otic Suspension 555
Decadron Tablets 1929
TobraDex Ophthalmic Ointment 558
TobraDex Ophthalmic Suspension ... 558

Dexamethasone Acetate (Co-administration of testosterone with corticosteroids may enhance edema formation).
No products indexed under this heading.

Dexamethasone Sodium Phosphate (Co-administration of testosterone with corticosteroids may enhance edema formation). Products include:
Decadron Phosphate Injection 1931

Fludrocortisone Acetate (Co-administration of testosterone with corticosteroids may enhance edema formation).
No products indexed under this heading.

Hydrocortisone (Co-administration of testosterone with corticosteroids may enhance edema formation). Products include:
Cortizone•5 Ointment .... ▣699
Cortizone•10 Creme .... ▣699
Cortizone•10 Ointment .... ▣699
Cortizone•10 Plus Creme .... ▣700
Cortizone•10 Maximum Strength Quick Shot Spray........................ ▣700
Hydrocortone Tablets 1963
Preparation H Hydrocortisone Cream .... ▣748

Hydrocortisone Acetate (Co-administration of testosterone with corticosteroids may enhance edema formation). Products include:
Analpram-HC 1136
Pramosone 1139
ProctoFoam-HC 3113
Tucks Anti-Itch Ointment .... ▣712
U-cort 1% Cream 3289

Hydrocortisone Sodium Phosphate (Co-administration of testosterone with corticosteroids may enhance edema formation).
No products indexed under this heading.

Hydrocortisone Sodium Succinate (Co-administration of testosterone with corticosteroids may enhance edema formation).
No products indexed under this heading.

Insulin, Human, Zinc Suspension (In diabetic patients, the metabolic effects of androgens may decrease blood glucose and, therefore, insulin requirements). Products include:
Humulin L, 100 Units 1763
Humulin U, 100 Units 1770

Insulin, Human NPH (In diabetic patients, the metabolic effects of androgens may decrease blood glucose and, therefore, insulin requirements). Products include:
Humulin N, 100 Units 1764
Humulin N Pen 1765
Novolin N Human Insulin 10 ml Vials 2322
Novolin N InnoLet 2322
Novolin N PenFill 3 ml Cartridges 2325
Novolin R InnoLet 2322

Insulin, Human Regular (In diabetic patients, the metabolic effects of androgens may decrease blood glucose and, therefore, insulin requirements). Products include:
Humulin R (U-500) 1768
Humulin R, 100 Units 1767
Novolin R Human Insulin 10 ml Vials 2322
Novolin R PenFill 2325

Insulin, Human Regular and Human NPH Mixture (In diabetic patients, the metabolic effects of androgens may decrease blood glucose and, therefore, insulin requirements). Products include:
Humulin 50/50, 100 Units 1760
Humulin 70/30 Pen 1761
Novolin 70/30 Human Insulin 10 ml Vials 2321
Novolin 70/30 InnoLet 2322
Novolin 70/30 PenFill 3 ml Cartridges 2325

Insulin, NPH (In diabetic patients, the metabolic effects of androgens may decrease blood glucose and, therefore, insulin requirements).
No products indexed under this heading.

Insulin, Regular (In diabetic patients, the metabolic effects of androgens may decrease blood glucose and, therefore, insulin requirements).
No products indexed under this heading.

Insulin, Zinc Crystals (In diabetic patients, the metabolic effects of androgens may decrease blood glucose and, therefore, insulin requirements).
No products indexed under this heading.

Insulin, Zinc Suspension (In diabetic patients, the metabolic effects of androgens may decrease blood glucose and, therefore, insulin requirements).
No products indexed under this heading.

Insulin Aspart, Human Regular (In diabetic patients, the metabolic effects of androgens may decrease blood glucose and, therefore, insulin requirements). Products include:
NovoLog Injection 2326

Insulin glargine (In diabetic patients, the metabolic effects of androgens may decrease blood glucose and, therefore, insulin requirements). Products include:
Lantus Injection 2925

Insulin Lispro, Human (In diabetic patients, the metabolic effects of androgens may decrease blood glucose and, therefore, insulin requirements). Products include:
Humalog-Pen 1751
Humalog Mix 75/25-Pen 1754

Insulin Lispro Protamine, Human (In diabetic patients, the metabolic effects of androgens may decrease blood glucose and, therefore, insulin requirements). Products include:
Humalog Mix 75/25-Pen 1754

Methylprednisolone Acetate (Co-administration of testosterone with corticosteroids may enhance edema formation). Products include:
Depo-Medrol Injectable Suspension 2615
Depo-Medrol Single-Dose Vial 2617

Methylprednisolone Sodium Succinate (Co-administration of testosterone with corticosteroids may enhance edema formation).
No products indexed under this heading.

Oxyphenbutazone (Co-administration of androgens and oxyphenbutazone may result in elevated serum levels of oxyphenbutazone).
No products indexed under this heading.

Prednisolone Acetate (Co-administration of testosterone with corticosteroids may enhance edema formation). Products include:
Blephamide Ophthalmic Ointment 563
Blephamide Ophthalmic Suspension.................................. 564
Poly-Pred Liquifilm Ophthalmic Suspension .... ⊙231
Pred Forte Ophthalmic Suspension .... ⊙233
Pred Mild Sterile Ophthalmic Suspension .... ⊙236
Pred-G Ophthalmic Suspension ...... ⊙234
Pred-G Sterile Ophthalmic Ointment.................................... ⊙235

Prednisolone Sodium Phosphate (Co-administration of testosterone with corticosteroids may enhance edema formation). Products include:
Pediapred Oral Solution 3319

Prednisolone Tebutate (Co-administration of testosterone with corticosteroids may enhance edema formation).
No products indexed under this heading.

Prednisone (Co-administration of testosterone with corticosteroids may enhance edema formation).
No products indexed under this heading.

Propranolol Hydrochloride (Co-administration of injectable testosterone cypionate has resulted in an increased clearance of propranolol). Products include:
Inderal LA Long-Acting Capsules 3421
InnoPran XL Capsules 2728

Triamcinolone (Co-administration of testosterone with corticosteroids may enhance edema formation).
No products indexed under this heading.

Triamcinolone Acetonide (Co-administration of testosterone with corticosteroids may enhance edema formation). Products include:
Azmacort Inhalation Aerosol 1701
Nasacort HFA Inhalation Aerosol 2939
Nasacort AQ Nasal Spray 2937

Triamcinolone Diacetate (Co-administration of testosterone with corticosteroids may enhance edema formation).
No products indexed under this heading.

Triamcinolone Hexacetonide (Co-administration of testosterone with corticosteroids may enhance edema formation).
No products indexed under this heading.

ANGIOMAX FOR INJECTION
(Bivalirudin) 1856
May interact with thrombolytics and certain other agents. Compounds in these categories include:

Alteplase (Co-administration was associated with increased risks of major bleeding events). Products include:
Activase I.V. 1225
Cathflo Activase 1232

Anistreplase (Co-administration was associated with increased risks of major bleeding events).
No products indexed under this heading.

Heparin Sodium (Co-administration was associated with increased risks of major bleeding events).
No products indexed under this heading.

Reteplase (Co-administration was associated with increased risks of major bleeding events). Products include:
Retavase 1131

Streptokinase (Co-administration was associated with increased risks of major bleeding events).
No products indexed under this heading.

Urokinase (Co-administration was associated with increased risks of major bleeding events).
No products indexed under this heading.

Warfarin Sodium (Co-administration was associated with increased risks of major bleeding events). Products include:
Coumadin for Injection 932
Coumadin Tablets 932

ANTABUSE TABLETS
(Disulfiram) 2343
May interact with oral anticoagulants and phenytoin. Compounds in these categories include:

Anisindione (Disulfiram may prolong prothrombin time). Products include:
Miradon Tablets 3056

Dicumarol (Disulfiram may prolong prothrombin time).
No products indexed under this heading.

Fosphenytoin Sodium (Co-administration can result in an increase in phenytoin levels leading to phenytoin intoxication).
No products indexed under this heading.

Isoniazid (Co-administration may lead to unsteady gait or mixed changes in mental status).
No products indexed under this heading.

Metronidazole (Co-administration has resulted in psychotic reactions; concurrent use is contraindicated). Products include:
Metrogel 1% 1212
MetroGel-Vaginal Gel 1822
Noritate Cream, 1% 1051

Metronidazole Hydrochloride (Co-administration has resulted in psychotic reactions; concurrent use is contraindicated).
No products indexed under this heading.

Paraldehyde (Concurrent use is contraindicated due to possibility of disulfiram-alcohol reactions).
No products indexed under this heading.

Phenytoin (Co-administration can result in an increase in phenytoin levels leading to phenytoin intoxication).
No products indexed under this heading.

Phenytoin Sodium (Co-administration can result in an increase in phenytoin levels leading to phenytoin intoxication). Products include:
Phenytek Capsules 2153

Warfarin Sodium (Disulfiram may prolong prothrombin time). Products include:
Coumadin for Injection 932
Coumadin Tablets 932

Food Interactions

Alcohol (Disulfiram plus alcohol, even small amounts, produce flushing, throbbing in head and neck, throbbing headache, respiratory difficulty, nausea, vomiting, and confusion; concurrent use with alcohol-containing preparations, such as cough syrups, tonics, sauces, vinegars, and even aftershave lotion and back rubs should be avoided).

ANTARA CAPSULES
(Fenofibrate) 2723
May interact with bile acid sequestering agents, oral anticoagulants, HMG-CoA reductase inhibitors, and certain other agents. Compounds in these categories include:

Anisindione (Caution should be exercised when coumarin anticoagulants are given in conjunction with fenofibrate. The dosage of the anticoagulants should be reduced to maintain the prothrombin time/INR at the desired level to prevent bleeding complications. Frequent prothrombin time/INR determinations are advisable until it has been definitely determined that the prothrombin time/INR has stabilized). Products include:
Miradon Tablets 3056

Atorvastatin Calcium (The combined use of fenofibrate and HMG-CoA reductase inhibitors should be avoided unless the benefit of further alterations in lipid levels is likely to outweigh the increased risk of this drug combination). Products include:
Caduet Tablets 2507
Lipitor Tablets 2495

Cerivastatin Sodium (The combined use of fenofibrate and HMG-CoA reductase inhibitors should be avoided unless the benefit of further alterations in lipid levels is likely to outweigh the increased risk of this drug combination).
No products indexed under this heading.

Cholestyramine (Since bile acid sequestrants may bind other drugs given concurrently, patients should take Antara at least one hour before, or 4-6 hours after, a bile acid binding resin to avoid impeding its absorption).
No products indexed under this heading.

Colesevelam Hydrochloride (Since bile acid sequestrants may bind other drugs given concurrently, patients should take Antara at least one hour before, or 4-6 hours after, a bile acid binding resin to avoid impeding its absorption). Products include:
WelChol Tablets 2855

Colestipol Hydrochloride (Since bile acid sequestrants may bind other drugs given concurrently, patients should take Antara at least one hour before, or 4-6 hours after, a bile acid binding resin to avoid impeding its absorption).
No products indexed under this heading.

Cyclosporine (Because cyclosporine can produce nephrotoxicity with decreases in creatinine clearance and rises in serum creatinine and because renal excretion is the primary elimination route of fibrate drugs including fenofibrate, there is a risk that an interaction will lead to deterioration. The benefits and risks of using Antara with immunosuppressants and other potentially nephrotoxic agents should be carefully considered, and the lowest effective dose employed). Products include:
Gengraf Capsules 458
Neoral Soft Gelatin Capsules 2247
Neoral Oral Solution 2247
Restasis Ophthalmic Emulsion 570
Sandimmune 2259

Dicumarol (Caution should be exercised when coumarin anticoagulants are given in conjunction with fenofibrate. The dosage of the anticoagulants should be reduced to maintain the prothrombin time/INR at the desired level to prevent bleeding complications. Frequent prothrombin time/INR determinations are advisable until it has been definitely determined that the prothrombin time/INR has stabilized).
No products indexed under this heading.

Fluvastatin Sodium (The combined use of fenofibrate and HMG-CoA reductase inhibitors should be avoided unless the benefit of further alterations in lipid levels is likely to outweigh the increased risk of this drug combination). Products include:
Lescol Capsules 2227
Lescol 2730
Lescol XL Tablets 2227

Lovastatin (The combined use of fenofibrate and HMG-CoA reductase inhibitors should be avoided unless the benefit of further alterations in lipid levels is likely to outweigh the increased risk of this drug combination). Products include:
Advicor Tablets 1694
Altoprev Extended-Release Tablets 1151
Mevacor Tablets 1996

Pravastatin Sodium (The combined use of fenofibrate and HMG-CoA reductase inhibitors should be avoided unless the benefit of further alterations in lipid levels is likely to outweigh the increased risk of this drug combination). Products include:
Pravachol Tablets 943

Simvastatin (The combined use of fenofibrate and HMG-CoA reductase inhibitors should be avoided unless the benefit of further alterations in lipid levels is likely to outweigh the increased risk of this drug combination). Products include:
Vytorin 10/10 Tablets 2084
Vytorin 10/10 Tablets 3092
Vytorin 10/20 Tablets 2084
Vytorin 10/20 Tablets 3092
Vytorin 10/40 Tablets 3092
Vytorin 10/40 Tablets 2084
Vytorin 10/80 Tablets 2084
Vytorin 10/80 Tablets 3092
Zocor Tablets 2078

Warfarin Sodium (Caution should be exercised when coumarin anticoagulants are given in conjunction with fenofibrate. The dosage of the anticoagulants should be reduced to maintain the prothrombin time/INR at the desired level to prevent bleeding complications. Frequent prothrombin time/INR determinations are advisable until it has been definitely determined that the prothrombin time/INR has stabilized). Products include:
Coumadin for Injection 932
Coumadin Tablets 932

ANTIVENIN (BLACK WIDOW SPIDER ANTIVENIN)
(Black Widow Spider Antivenin (Equine)) 1887
None cited in PDR database.

ANTIVENIN (MICRURUS FULVIUS)
(Antivenin (Micrurus Fulvius)) 3401
May interact with beta blockers and narcotic analgesics. Compounds in these categories include:

Acebutolol Hydrochloride (Co-administration with beta-adrenergic blockers has been associated with an increased severity of acute anaphylaxis; anaphylaxis may be resistant and prolonged; altered or larger than usual doses of epinephrine may be required to treat anaphylaxis).
No products indexed under this heading.

Alfentanil Hydrochloride (Co-administration with drugs that depress respiration, such as narcotic analgesics, are contraindicated).
No products indexed under this heading.

Atenolol (Co-administration with beta-adrenergic blockers has been associated with an increased severity of acute anaphylaxis; anaphylaxis may be resistant and prolonged; altered or larger than usual doses of epinephrine may be required to treat anaphylaxis). Products include:
Tenormin I.V. Injection 698
Tenormin Tablets 695

Betaxolol Hydrochloride (Co-administration with beta-adrenergic blockers has been associated with an increased severity of acute anaphylaxis; anaphylaxis may be resistant and prolonged; altered or larger than usual doses of epinephrine may be required to treat anaphylaxis). Products include:
Betoptic S Ophthalmic Suspension.................................. 554

Bisoprolol Fumarate (Co-administration with beta-adrenergic blockers has been associated with an increased severity of acute anaphylaxis; anaphylaxis may be resistant and prolonged; altered or larger than usual doses of epinephrine may be required to treat anaphylaxis).
No products indexed under this heading.

Buprenorphine Hydrochloride (Co-administration with drugs that depress respiration, such as narcotic analgesics, are contraindicated). Products include:
Buprenex Injectable 2718
Suboxone Tablets 2719
Subutex Tablets 2719

Carteolol Hydrochloride (Co-administration with beta-adrenergic blockers has been associated with an increased severity of acute anaphylaxis; anaphylaxis may be resistant and prolonged; altered or larger than usual doses of epinephrine may be required to treat anaphylaxis). Products include:
Carteolol Hydrochloride Ophthalmic Solution USP, 1%....... ⊙246

Codeine Phosphate (Co-administration with drugs that depress respiration, such as narcotic analgesics, are contraindicated). Products include:
Tylenol with Codeine 2461

Dezocine (Co-administration with drugs that depress respiration, such as narcotic analgesics, are contraindicated).
No products indexed under this heading.

Esmolol Hydrochloride (Co-administration with beta-adrenergic

blockers has been associated with an increased severity of acute anaphylaxis; anaphylaxis may be resistant and prolonged; altered or larger than usual doses of epinephrine may be required to treat anaphylaxis). Products include:

- Brevibloc Concentrate 766
- Brevibloc Injection 766
- Brevibloc Double Strength Injection.. 766
- Brevibloc Premixed Injection 766
- Brevibloc Double Strength Premixed Injection........................ 766

Fentanyl (Co-administration with drugs that depress respiration, such as narcotic analgesics, are contraindicated). Products include:

- Duragesic Transdermal System 2448

Fentanyl Citrate (Co-administration with drugs that depress respiration, such as narcotic analgesics, are contraindicated). Products include:

- Actiq 993

Hydrocodone Bitartrate (Co-administration with drugs that depress respiration, such as narcotic analgesics, are contraindicated). Products include:

- Hycodan 1104
- Hycomine Compound Tablets 1105
- Hycotuss Expectorant Syrup 1106
- Lortab 3315
- Lortab Elixir 3312
- Vicodin Tablets 530
- Vicodin ES Tablets 531
- Vicodin HP Tablets 532
- Vicoprofen Tablets 533
- Zydone Tablets 1118

Hydrocodone Polistirex (Co-administration with drugs that depress respiration, such as narcotic analgesics, are contraindicated). Products include:

- Tussionex Pennkinetic Extended-Release Suspension...... 3322

Hydromorphone Hydrochloride (Co-administration with drugs that depress respiration, such as narcotic analgesics, are contraindicated). Products include:

- Dilaudid 439
- Dilaudid Oral Liquid 443
- Dilaudid Non-Sterile Powder 439
- Dilaudid Rectal Suppositories 439
- Dilaudid Tablets 439
- Dilaudid Tablets - 8 mg 443
- Dilaudid-HP 441

Labetalol Hydrochloride (Co-administration with beta-adrenergic blockers has been associated with an increased severity of acute anaphylaxis; anaphylaxis may be resistant and prolonged; altered or larger than usual doses of epinephrine may be required to treat anaphylaxis).
No products indexed under this heading.

Levobunolol Hydrochloride (Co-administration with beta-adrenergic blockers has been associated with an increased severity of acute anaphylaxis; anaphylaxis may be resistant and prolonged; altered or larger than usual doses of epinephrine may be required to treat anaphylaxis). Products include:

- Betagan Ophthalmic Solution, USP.. ⊙ 217

Levorphanol Tartrate (Co-administration with drugs that depress respiration, such as narcotic analgesics, are contraindicated).
No products indexed under this heading.

Meperidine Hydrochloride (Co-administration with drugs that depress respiration, such as narcotic analgesics, are contraindicated).
No products indexed under this heading.

Methadone Hydrochloride (Co-administration with drugs that depress respiration, such as narcotic analgesics, are contraindicated).
No products indexed under this heading.

Metipranolol Hydrochloride (Co-administration with beta-adrenergic blockers has been associated with an increased severity of acute anaphylaxis; anaphylaxis may be resistant and prolonged; altered or larger than usual doses of epinephrine may be required to treat anaphylaxis).
No products indexed under this heading.

Metoprolol Succinate (Co-administration with beta-adrenergic blockers has been associated with an increased severity of acute anaphylaxis; anaphylaxis may be resistant and prolonged; altered or larger than usual doses of epinephrine may be required to treat anaphylaxis). Products include:

- Toprol-XL Tablets 660

Metoprolol Tartrate (Co-administration with beta-adrenergic blockers has been associated with an increased severity of acute anaphylaxis; anaphylaxis may be resistant and prolonged; altered or larger than usual doses of epinephrine may be required to treat anaphylaxis).
No products indexed under this heading.

Morphine Sulfate (Co-administration with drugs that depress respiration, such as narcotic analgesics, are contraindicated). Products include:

- Avinza Capsules 1714
- Kadian Capsules 572
- MS Contin Tablets 2703

Nadolol (Co-administration with beta-adrenergic blockers has been associated with an increased severity of acute anaphylaxis; anaphylaxis may be resistant and prolonged; altered or larger than usual doses of epinephrine may be required to treat anaphylaxis). Products include:

- Nadolol Tablets 2121

Oxycodone Hydrochloride (Co-administration with drugs that depress respiration, such as narcotic analgesics, are contraindicated). Products include:

- Combunox Tablets 1183
- OxyContin Tablets 2699
- OxyFast Oral Concentrate Solution.. 2704
- OxyIR Capsules 2704
- Percocet Tablets 1114
- Percodan Tablets 1115

Penbutolol Sulfate (Co-administration with beta-adrenergic blockers has been associated with an increased severity of acute anaphylaxis; anaphylaxis may be resistant and prolonged; altered or larger than usual doses of epinephrine may be required to treat anaphylaxis).
No products indexed under this heading.

Pindolol (Co-administration with beta-adrenergic blockers has been associated with an increased severity of acute anaphylaxis; anaphylaxis may be resistant and prolonged; altered or larger than usual doses of epinephrine may be required to treat anaphylaxis).
No products indexed under this heading.

Propoxyphene Hydrochloride (Co-administration with drugs that depress respiration, such as narcotic analgesics, are contraindicated).
No products indexed under this heading.

Propoxyphene Napsylate (Co-administration with drugs that depress respiration, such as narcotic analgesics, are contraindicated). Products include:

- Darvocet A 500 Tablets 3497

Propranolol Hydrochloride (Co-administration with beta-adrenergic blockers has been associated with an increased severity of acute anaphylaxis; anaphylaxis may be resistant and prolonged; altered or larger than usual doses of epinephrine may be required to treat anaphylaxis). Products include:

- Inderal LA Long-Acting Capsules 3421
- InnoPran XL Capsules 2728

Remifentanil Hydrochloride (Co-administration with drugs that depress respiration, such as narcotic analgesics, are contraindicated).
No products indexed under this heading.

Sotalol Hydrochloride (Co-administration with beta-adrenergic blockers has been associated with an increased severity of acute anaphylaxis; anaphylaxis may be resistant and prolonged; altered or larger than usual doses of epinephrine may be required to treat anaphylaxis).
No products indexed under this heading.

Sufentanil Citrate (Co-administration with drugs that depress respiration, such as narcotic analgesics, are contraindicated).
No products indexed under this heading.

Timolol Hemihydrate (Co-administration with beta-adrenergic blockers has been associated with an increased severity of acute anaphylaxis; anaphylaxis may be resistant and prolonged; altered or larger than usual doses of epinephrine may be required to treat anaphylaxis). Products include:

- Betimol Ophthalmic Solution 3371
- Betimol Ophthalmic Solution .... ⊙ 283

Timolol Maleate (Co-administration with beta-adrenergic blockers has been associated with an increased severity of acute anaphylaxis; anaphylaxis may be resistant and prolonged; altered or larger than usual doses of epinephrine may be required to treat anaphylaxis). Products include:

- Blocadren Tablets 1891
- Cosopt Sterile Ophthalmic Solution.. 1910
- Timolide Tablets 2056
- Timoptic in Ocudose 2061
- Timoptic Sterile Ophthalmic Solution.. 2058
- Timoptic-XE Sterile Ophthalmic Gel Forming Solution 2062

ANTIVENIN POLYVALENT

(Antivenin (Crotalidae) Polyvalent) 3399
May interact with beta blockers. Compounds in these categories include:

Acebutolol Hydrochloride (Co-administration with beta-adrenergic blockers has been associated with an increased severity of acute anaphylaxis; anaphylaxis may be resistant and prolonged; altered or larger than usual doses of epinephrine may be required to treat anaphylaxis).
No products indexed under this heading.

Atenolol (Co-administration with beta-adrenergic blockers has been associated with an increased severity of acute anaphylaxis; anaphylaxis may be resistant and prolonged; altered or larger than usual doses of epinephrine may be required to treat anaphylaxis). Products include:

- Tenormin I.V. Injection 698
- Tenormin Tablets 695

Betaxolol Hydrochloride (Co-administration with beta-adrenergic blockers has been associated with an increased severity of acute anaphylaxis; anaphylaxis may be resistant and prolonged; altered or larger than usual doses of epinephrine may be required to treat anaphylaxis). Products include:

- Betoptic S Ophthalmic Suspension.. 554

Bisoprolol Fumarate (Co-administration with beta-adrenergic blockers has been associated with an increased severity of acute anaphylaxis; anaphylaxis may be resistant and prolonged; altered or larger than usual doses of epinephrine may be required to treat anaphylaxis).
No products indexed under this heading.

Carteolol Hydrochloride (Co-administration with beta-adrenergic blockers has been associated with an increased severity of acute anaphylaxis; anaphylaxis may be resistant and prolonged; altered or larger than usual doses of epinephrine may be required to treat anaphylaxis). Products include:

- Carteolol Hydrochloride Ophthalmic Solution USP, 1%....... ⊙ 246

Esmolol Hydrochloride (Co-administration with beta-adrenergic blockers has been associated with an increased severity of acute anaphylaxis; anaphylaxis may be resistant and prolonged; altered or larger than usual doses of epinephrine may be required to treat anaphylaxis). Products include:

- Brevibloc Concentrate 766
- Brevibloc Injection 766
- Brevibloc Double Strength Injection.. 766
- Brevibloc Premixed Injection 766
- Brevibloc Double Strength Premixed Injection........................ 766

Labetalol Hydrochloride (Co-administration with beta-adrenergic blockers has been associated with an increased severity of acute anaphylaxis; anaphylaxis may be resistant and prolonged; altered or larger than usual doses of epinephrine may be required to treat anaphylaxis).
No products indexed under this heading.

Levobunolol Hydrochloride (Co-administration with beta-adrenergic blockers has been associated with an increased severity of acute anaphylaxis; anaphylaxis may be resis-

tant and prolonged; altered or larger than usual doses of epinephrine may be required to treat anaphylaxis). Products include:
Betagan Ophthalmic Solution, USP .... ⊙217

Metipranolol Hydrochloride (Co-administration with beta-adrenergic blockers has been associated with an increased severity of acute anaphylaxis; anaphylaxis may be resistant and prolonged; altered or larger than usual doses of epinephrine may be required to treat anaphylaxis).
No products indexed under this heading.

Metoprolol Succinate (Co-administration with beta-adrenergic blockers has been associated with an increased severity of acute anaphylaxis; anaphylaxis may be resistant and prolonged; altered or larger than usual doses of epinephrine may be required to treat anaphylaxis). Products include:
Toprol-XL Tablets 660

Metoprolol Tartrate (Co-administration with beta-adrenergic blockers has been associated with an increased severity of acute anaphylaxis; anaphylaxis may be resistant and prolonged; altered or larger than usual doses of epinephrine may be required to treat anaphylaxis).
No products indexed under this heading.

Nadolol (Co-administration with beta-adrenergic blockers has been associated with an increased severity of acute anaphylaxis; anaphylaxis may be resistant and prolonged; altered or larger than usual doses of epinephrine may be required to treat anaphylaxis). Products include:
Nadolol Tablets 2121

Penbutolol Sulfate (Co-administration with beta-adrenergic blockers has been associated with an increased severity of acute anaphylaxis; anaphylaxis may be resistant and prolonged; altered or larger than usual doses of epinephrine may be required to treat anaphylaxis).
No products indexed under this heading.

Pindolol (Co-administration with beta-adrenergic blockers has been associated with an increased severity of acute anaphylaxis; anaphylaxis may be resistant and prolonged; altered or larger than usual doses of epinephrine may be required to treat anaphylaxis).
No products indexed under this heading.

Propranolol Hydrochloride (Co-administration with beta-adrenergic blockers has been associated with an increased severity of acute anaphylaxis; anaphylaxis may be resistant and prolonged; altered or larger than usual doses of epinephrine may be required to treat anaphylaxis). Products include:
Inderal LA Long-Acting Capsules 3421
InnoPran XL Capsules 2728

Sotalol Hydrochloride (Co-administration with beta-adrenergic blockers has been associated with an increased severity of acute anaphylaxis; anaphylaxis may be resistant and prolonged; altered or larger than usual doses of epinephrine may be required to treat anaphylaxis).
No products indexed under this heading.

Timolol Hemihydrate (Co-administration with beta-adrenergic blockers has been associated with an increased severity of acute anaphylaxis; anaphylaxis may be resistant and prolonged; altered or larger than usual doses of epinephrine may be required to treat anaphylaxis). Products include:
Betimol Ophthalmic Solution 3371
Betimol Ophthalmic Solution .... ⊙283

Timolol Maleate (Co-administration with beta-adrenergic blockers has been associated with an increased severity of acute anaphylaxis; anaphylaxis may be resistant and prolonged; altered or larger than usual doses of epinephrine may be required to treat anaphylaxis). Products include:
Blocadren Tablets 1891
Cosopt Sterile Ophthalmic Solution 1910
Timolide Tablets 2056
Timoptic in Ocudose 2061
Timoptic Sterile Ophthalmic Solution 2058
Timoptic-XE Sterile Ophthalmic Gel Forming Solution 2062

ANZEMET INJECTION

(Dolasetron Mesylate) 2871
See Anzemet Tablets

ANZEMET TABLETS

(Dolasetron Mesylate) 2874
May interact with:

Atenolol (Decreases hydrodolasetron clearance by 27%). Products include:
Tenormin I.V. Injection 698
Tenormin Tablets 695

Cimetidine (Co-administration of dolasetron with cimetidine, a nonselective inhibitor of CYP450, has resulted in increased blood levels of dolasetron by 24%). Products include:
Tagamet HB 200 Tablets .... ▣637
Tagamet Tablets 1547

Cimetidine Hydrochloride (Co-administration of dolasetron with cimetidine, a nonselective inhibitor of CYP450, has resulted in increased blood levels of dolasetron by 24%).
No products indexed under this heading.

Rifampin (Co-administration of dolasetron with rifampin, a potent inducer of CYP450, has resulted in decreased blood levels of dolasetron by 28%).
No products indexed under this heading.

APIDRA INJECTION

(Insulin Glulisine) 2876
May interact with ACE inhibitors, atypical antipsychotics, beta blockers, corticosteroids, diuretics, estrogens, fibrates, oral hypoglycemic agents, lithium preparations, monoamine oxidase inhibitors, phenothiazines, progestins, protease inhibitors, salicylates, sulfonamides, sympathomimetics, thyroid preparations, and certain other agents. Compounds in these categories include:

Acarbose (Oral antidiabetic products may increase the blood glucose-lowering effect and susceptibility to hypoglycemia of insulin). Products include:
Precose Tablets 776

Acebutolol Hydrochloride (Beta-blockers may either potentiate or weaken the blood glucose-lowering effect of insulin and reduce or hide the signs of hypoglycemia).
No products indexed under this heading.

Albuterol (Sympathomimetic agents may reduce the blood glucose-lowering effect of insulin). Products include:
Proventil Inhalation Aerosol 3067

Albuterol Sulfate (Sympathomimetic agents may reduce the blood glucose-lowering effect of insulin). Products include:
AccuNeb Inhalation Solution 1055
Combivent Inhalation Aerosol 878
DuoNeb Inhalation Solution 1058
Proventil Inhalation Solution 0.083% 3069
Proventil HFA Inhalation Aerosol 3071
Ventolin HFA Inhalation Aerosol 1576
VoSpire Extended-Release Tablets 2352

Amiloride Hydrochloride (Diuretics may reduce the blood glucose-lowering effect of insulin). Products include:
Midamor Tablets 2000
Moduretic Tablets 2003

Amprenavir (Protease inhibitors may reduce the blood glucose-lowering effect of insulin). Products include:
Agenerase Capsules 1299
Agenerase Oral Solution 1304

Aripiprazole (Atypical antipsychotics may reduce the blood glucose-lowering effect of insulin). Products include:
Abilify Tablets 2472
Abilify Tablets 916

Aspirin (Salicylates may increase the blood glucose-lowering effect and susceptibility to hypoglycemia of insulin). Products include:
Aggrenox Capsules 855
Bayer, Aspirin Regimen .... ▣606
Bayer Aspirin Tablets 3515
BC Powder .... ▣612
BC Allergy Sinus Cold Powder .... ▣612
Arthritis Strength BC Powder .... ▣612
BC Sinus Cold Powder .... ▣612
Ecotrin Enteric Coated Aspirin Low, Regular and Maximum Strength Tablets 1627
Goody's Body Pain Formula Powder .... ▣621
Goody's Extra Strength Headache Powder .... ▣621
Goody's Extra Strength Pain Relief Tablets .... ▣621
Percodan Tablets 1115
St. Joseph 81 mg Aspirin Chewable and Enteric Coated Tablets 1841

Aspirin, Enteric Coated (Salicylates may increase the blood glucose-lowering effect and susceptibility to hypoglycemia of insulin).
No products indexed under this heading.

Aspirin Buffered (Salicylates may increase the blood glucose-lowering effect and susceptibility to hypoglycemia of insulin).
No products indexed under this heading.

Atenolol (Beta-blockers may either potentiate or weaken the blood glucose-lowering effect of insulin and reduce or hide the signs of hypoglycemia). Products include:
Tenormin I.V. Injection 698
Tenormin Tablets 695

Benazepril Hydrochloride (ACE inhibitors may increase the blood glucose-lowering effect and susceptibility to hypoglycemia of insulin). Products include:
Lotensin Tablets 2232
Lotensin HCT Tablets 2235
Lotrel Capsules 2238

Bendroflumethiazide (Diuretics may reduce the blood glucose-lowering effect of insulin).
No products indexed under this heading.

Betamethasone Acetate (Corticosteroids may reduce the blood glucose-lowering effect of insulin).
No products indexed under this heading.

Betamethasone Sodium Phosphate (Corticosteroids may reduce the blood glucose-lowering effect of insulin).
No products indexed under this heading.

Betaxolol Hydrochloride (Beta-blockers may either potentiate or weaken the blood glucose-lowering effect of insulin and reduce or hide the signs of hypoglycemia). Products include:
Betoptic S Ophthalmic Suspension 554

Bisoprolol Fumarate (Beta-blockers may either potentiate or weaken the blood glucose-lowering effect of insulin and reduce or hide the signs of hypoglycemia).
No products indexed under this heading.

Bumetanide (Diuretics may reduce the blood glucose-lowering effect of insulin).
No products indexed under this heading.

Captopril (ACE inhibitors may increase the blood glucose-lowering effect and susceptibility to hypoglycemia of insulin). Products include:
Captopril Tablets 2114

Carteolol Hydrochloride (Beta-blockers may either potentiate or weaken the blood glucose-lowering effect of insulin and reduce or hide the signs of hypoglycemia). Products include:
Carteolol Hydrochloride Ophthalmic Solution USP, 1% .... ⊙246

Chlorothiazide (Diuretics may reduce the blood glucose-lowering effect of insulin). Products include:
Aldoclor Tablets 1881
Diuril Oral 1936

Chlorothiazide Sodium (Diuretics may reduce the blood glucose-lowering effect of insulin). Products include:
Diuril Sodium Intravenous 1934

Chlorotrianisene (Estrogens may reduce the blood glucose-lowering effect of insulin).
No products indexed under this heading.

Chlorpromazine (Phenothiazine derivatives may reduce the blood glucose-lowering effect of insulin).
No products indexed under this heading.

Chlorpromazine Hydrochloride (Phenothiazine derivatives may reduce the blood glucose-lowering effect of insulin).
No products indexed under this heading.

Chlorpropamide (Oral antidiabetic products may increase the blood glucose-lowering effect and susceptibility to hypoglycemia of insulin).
No products indexed under this heading.

IMPORTANT NOTE: Always consult each drug listing in the patient's regimen for possible interactions.

Chlorthalidone (Diuretics may reduce the blood glucose-lowering effect of insulin). Products include:
Clorpres Tablets 2139

Choline Magnesium Trisalicylate (Salicylates may increase the blood glucose-lowering effect and susceptibility to hypoglycemia of insulin).
No products indexed under this heading.

Clofibrate (Fibrates may increase the blood glucose-lowering effect and susceptibility to hypoglycemia of insulin).
No products indexed under this heading.

Clonidine (Clonidine may either potentiate or weaken the blood glucose-lowering effect of insulin and reduce or hide the signs of hypoglycemia). Products include:
Catapres-TTS 875

Clonidine Hydrochloride (Clonidine may either potentiate or weaken the blood glucose-lowering effect of insulin and reduce or hide the signs of hypoglycemia). Products include:
Catapres Tablets 874
Clorpres Tablets 2139

Clozapine (Atypical antipsychotics may reduce the blood glucose-lowering effect of insulin). Products include:
Clozapine Tablets 2141
Clozaril Tablets 2174
FazaClo Orally Disintegrating Tablets 547

Cortisone Acetate (Corticosteroids may reduce the blood glucose-lowering effect of insulin).
No products indexed under this heading.

Danazol (Danazol may reduce the blood glucose-lowering effect of insulin).
No products indexed under this heading.

Desogestrel (Progestogens may reduce the blood glucose-lowering effect of insulin). Products include:
Ortho-Cept Tablets 2395

Dexamethasone (Corticosteroids may reduce the blood glucose-lowering effect of insulin). Products include:
Ciprodex Otic Suspension 555
Decadron Tablets 1929
TobraDex Ophthalmic Ointment 558
TobraDex Ophthalmic Suspension ... 558

Dexamethasone Acetate (Corticosteroids may reduce the blood glucose-lowering effect of insulin).
No products indexed under this heading.

Dexamethasone Sodium Phosphate (Corticosteroids may reduce the blood glucose-lowering effect of insulin). Products include:
Decadron Phosphate Injection 1931

Diazoxide (Diazoxide may reduce the blood glucose-lowering effect of insulin). Products include:
Hyperstat I.V. Injection 3031

Dienestrol (Estrogens may reduce the blood glucose-lowering effect of insulin).
No products indexed under this heading.

Diethylstilbestrol (Estrogens may reduce the blood glucose-lowering effect of insulin).
No products indexed under this heading.

Diflunisal (Salicylates may increase the blood glucose-lowering effect and susceptibility to hypoglycemia of insulin). Products include:
Dolobid Tablets 1937

Disopyramide (Disopyramide may increase the blood glucose-lowering effect and susceptibility to hypoglycemia of insulin).
No products indexed under this heading.

Disopyramide Phosphate (Disopyramide may increase the blood glucose-lowering effect and susceptibility to hypoglycemia of insulin).
No products indexed under this heading.

Dobutamine Hydrochloride (Sympathomimetic agents may reduce the blood glucose-lowering effect of insulin).
No products indexed under this heading.

Dopamine Hydrochloride (Sympathomimetic agents may reduce the blood glucose-lowering effect of insulin).
No products indexed under this heading.

Enalapril Maleate (ACE inhibitors may increase the blood glucose-lowering effect and susceptibility to hypoglycemia of insulin). Products include:
Vaseretic Tablets 2073
Vasotec I.V. Injection 2076

Enalaprilat (ACE inhibitors may increase the blood glucose-lowering effect and susceptibility to hypoglycemia of insulin).
No products indexed under this heading.

Ephedrine Hydrochloride (Sympathomimetic agents may reduce the blood glucose-lowering effect of insulin). Products include:
Primatene Tablets .... ▣ 749

Ephedrine Sulfate (Sympathomimetic agents may reduce the blood glucose-lowering effect of insulin).
No products indexed under this heading.

Ephedrine Tannate (Sympathomimetic agents may reduce the blood glucose-lowering effect of insulin).
No products indexed under this heading.

Epinephrine (Sympathomimetic agents may reduce the blood glucose-lowering effect of insulin). Products include:
EpiPen 1061
Primatene Mist .... ▣ 749

Epinephrine Bitartrate (Sympathomimetic agents may reduce the blood glucose-lowering effect of insulin).
No products indexed under this heading.

Epinephrine Hydrochloride (Sympathomimetic agents may reduce the blood glucose-lowering effect of insulin).
No products indexed under this heading.

Esmolol Hydrochloride (Beta-blockers may either potentiate or weaken the blood glucose-lowering effect of insulin and reduce or hide the signs of hypoglycemia). Products include:
Brevibloc Concentrate 766
Brevibloc Injection 766
Brevibloc Double Strength Injection 766
Brevibloc Premixed Injection 766
Brevibloc Double Strength Premixed Injection 766

Estradiol (Estrogens may reduce the blood glucose-lowering effect of insulin). Products include:
Activella Tablets 2311
Climara Transdermal System 795
Climara Pro Transdermal System 800
CombiPatch Transdermal System 2180
Estrogel 0.06% 3200
Menostar Transdermal System 805
Prefest Tablets 1069
Vagifem Tablets 2340
Vivelle Transdermal System 2288
Vivelle-Dot Transdermal System 2293

Estrogens, Conjugated (Estrogens may reduce the blood glucose-lowering effect of insulin). Products include:
Premarin Intravenous 3440
Premarin Tablets 3443
Premarin Vaginal Cream 3449
Premphase Tablets 3452
Prempro Tablets 3452

Estrogens, Esterified (Estrogens may reduce the blood glucose-lowering effect of insulin). Products include:
Estratest Tablets 3196
Estratest H.S. Tablets 3196

Estropipate (Estrogens may reduce the blood glucose-lowering effect of insulin).
No products indexed under this heading.

Ethacrynic Acid (Diuretics may reduce the blood glucose-lowering effect of insulin). Products include:
Edecrin Tablets 1941

Ethinyl Estradiol (Estrogens may reduce the blood glucose-lowering effect of insulin). Products include:
Alesse-28 Tablets 3392
Lo/Ovral-28 Tablets 3423
NuvaRing 2357
Ortho-Cept Tablets 2395
Ortho-Cyclen/Ortho Tri-Cyclen 2414
Ortho Evra Transdermal System 2402
Ortho Tri-Cyclen Lo Tablets 2421
Seasonale Tablets 1073
Triphasil-28 Tablets 3483
Yasmin 28 Tablets 818

Fenofibrate (Fibrates may increase the blood glucose-lowering effect and susceptibility to hypoglycemia of insulin). Products include:
Antara Capsules 2723
Lofibra Capsules 1217
Tricor Tablets 523
Triglide Tablets 1165

Fludrocortisone Acetate (Corticosteroids may reduce the blood glucose-lowering effect of insulin).
No products indexed under this heading.

Fluoxetine (Fluoxetine may increase the blood glucose-lowering effect and susceptibility to hypoglycemia of insulin).
No products indexed under this heading.

Fluoxetine Hydrochloride (Fluoxetine may increase the blood glucose-lowering effect and susceptibility to hypoglycemia of insulin). Products include:
Prozac Pulvules and Liquid 1771
Symbyax Capsules 1788

Fluphenazine Decanoate (Phenothiazine derivatives may reduce the blood glucose-lowering effect of insulin).
No products indexed under this heading.

Fluphenazine Enanthate (Phenothiazine derivatives may reduce the blood glucose-lowering effect of insulin).
No products indexed under this heading.

Fluphenazine Hydrochloride (Phenothiazine derivatives may reduce the blood glucose-lowering effect of insulin).
No products indexed under this heading.

Fosinopril Sodium (ACE inhibitors may increase the blood glucose-lowering effect and susceptibility to hypoglycemia of insulin).
No products indexed under this heading.

Furosemide (Diuretics may reduce the blood glucose-lowering effect of insulin). Products include:
Furosemide Tablets 2117

Gemfibrozil (Fibrates may increase the blood glucose-lowering effect and susceptibility to hypoglycemia of insulin).
No products indexed under this heading.

Glimepiride (Oral antidiabetic products may increase the blood glucose-lowering effect and susceptibility to hypoglycemia of insulin). Products include:
Amaryl Tablets 2864

Glipizide (Oral antidiabetic products may increase the blood glucose-lowering effect and susceptibility to hypoglycemia of insulin).
No products indexed under this heading.

Glucagon (Glucagon may reduce the blood glucose-lowering effect of insulin). Products include:
GlucaGen for Injection 790
Glucagon for Injection Vials and Emergency Kit 1749

Glyburide (Oral antidiabetic products may increase the blood glucose-lowering effect and susceptibility to hypoglycemia of insulin).
No products indexed under this heading.

Guanethidine (Under the influence of sympatholytic medicinal products, such as guanethidine, the signs of hypoglycemia may be reduced or absent).
No products indexed under this heading.

Guanethidine Monosulfate (Under the influence of sympatholytic medicinal products, such as guanethidine, the signs of hypoglycemia may be reduced or absent).
No products indexed under this heading.

Guanethidine Sulfate (Under the influence of sympatholytic medicinal products, such as guanethidine, the signs of hypoglycemia may be reduced or absent).
No products indexed under this heading.

Hydrochlorothiazide (Diuretics may reduce the blood glucose-lowering effect of insulin). Products include:
Aldoril Tablets 1884
Atacand HCT 637
Avalide Tablets 2889
Avalide Tablets 922
Benicar HCT Tablets 2852
Diovan HCT Tablets 2195
Dyazide Capsules 1389
Hyzaar 1964
Lotensin HCT Tablets 2235
Maxzide 2150
Micardis HCT Tablets 886
Moduretic Tablets 2003
Prinzide Tablets 2033
Teveten HCT Tablets 1710
Timolide Tablets 2056
Uniretic Tablets 3114

Vaseretic Tablets 2073
Zestoretic Tablets 701

Hydrocortisone (Corticosteroids may reduce the blood glucose-lowering effect of insulin). Products include:
Cortizone•5 Ointment 699
Cortizone•10 Creme 699
Cortizone•10 Ointment 699
Cortizone•10 Plus Creme 700
Cortizone•10 Maximum Strength Quick Shot Spray 700
Hydrocortone Tablets 1963
Preparation H Hydrocortisone Cream 748

Hydrocortisone Acetate (Corticosteroids may reduce the blood glucose-lowering effect of insulin). Products include:
Analpram-HC 1136
Pramosone 1139
ProctoFoam-HC 3113
Tucks Anti-Itch Ointment 712
U-cort 1% Cream 3289

Hydrocortisone Sodium Phosphate (Corticosteroids may reduce the blood glucose-lowering effect of insulin).
No products indexed under this heading.

Hydrocortisone Sodium Succinate (Corticosteroids may reduce the blood glucose-lowering effect of insulin).
No products indexed under this heading.

Hydroflumethiazide (Diuretics may reduce the blood glucose-lowering effect of insulin).
No products indexed under this heading.

Indapamide (Diuretics may reduce the blood glucose-lowering effect of insulin). Products include:
Indapamide Tablets 2119

Indinavir Sulfate (Protease inhibitors may reduce the blood glucose-lowering effect of insulin). Products include:
Crixivan Capsules 1918

Isocarboxazid (MAO inhibitors may increase the blood glucose-lowering effect and susceptibility to hypoglycemia of insulin).
No products indexed under this heading.

Isoniazid (Isoniazid may reduce the blood glucose-lowering effect of insulin).
No products indexed under this heading.

Isoproterenol Hydrochloride (Sympathomimetic agents may reduce the blood glucose-lowering effect of insulin).
No products indexed under this heading.

Isoproterenol Sulfate (Sympathomimetic agents may reduce the blood glucose-lowering effect of insulin).
No products indexed under this heading.

Labetalol Hydrochloride (Beta-blockers may either potentiate or weaken the blood glucose-lowering effect of insulin and reduce or hide the signs of hypoglycemia).
No products indexed under this heading.

Levalbuterol Hydrochloride (Sympathomimetic agents may reduce the blood glucose-lowering effect of insulin). Products include:
Xopenex Inhalation Solution 3143
Xopenex Inhalation Solution Concentrate 3147

Levobunolol Hydrochloride (Beta-blockers may either potentiate or weaken the blood glucose-lowering effect of insulin and reduce or hide the signs of hypoglycemia). Products include:
Betagan Ophthalmic Solution, USP .... ⊙217

Levothyroxine Sodium (Thyroid hormones may reduce the blood glucose-lowering effect of insulin). Products include:
Levothroid Tablets 1189
Levoxyl Tablets 1680
Synthroid Tablets 515
Unithroid Tablets 3521

Liothyronine Sodium (Thyroid hormones may reduce the blood glucose-lowering effect of insulin). Products include:
Cytomel Tablets 1678

Liotrix (Thyroid hormones may reduce the blood glucose-lowering effect of insulin). Products include:
Thyrolar 1203

Lisinopril (ACE inhibitors may increase the blood glucose-lowering effect and susceptibility to hypoglycemia of insulin). Products include:
Prinivil Tablets 2029
Prinzide Tablets 2033
Zestoretic Tablets 701
Zestril Tablets 704

Lithium (Lithium salts may either potentiate or weaken the blood-glucose-lowering effect of insulin).
No products indexed under this heading.

Lithium Carbonate (Lithium salts may either potentiate or weaken the blood-glucose-lowering effect of insulin). Products include:
Eskalith 1406
Lithobid Tablets 1670

Lithium Citrate (Lithium salts may either potentiate or weaken the blood-glucose-lowering effect of insulin).
No products indexed under this heading.

Lopinavir (Protease inhibitors may reduce the blood glucose-lowering effect of insulin). Products include:
Kaletra 474

Magnesium Salicylate (Salicylates may increase the blood glucose-lowering effect and susceptibility to hypoglycemia of insulin).
No products indexed under this heading.

Medroxyprogesterone Acetate (Progestogens may reduce the blood glucose-lowering effect of insulin). Products include:
Depo-Provera Contraceptive Injection 2619
depo-subQ provera 104 Injectable Suspension 2622
Premphase Tablets 3452
Prempro Tablets 3452

Megestrol Acetate (Progestogens may reduce the blood glucose-lowering effect of insulin). Products include:
Megace ES Oral Suspension 2492

Mesoridazine Besylate (Phenothiazine derivatives may reduce the blood glucose-lowering effect of insulin).
No products indexed under this heading.

Metaproterenol Sulfate (Sympathomimetic agents may reduce the blood glucose-lowering effect of insulin). Products include:
Alupent Inhalation Aerosol 858

Metaraminol Bitartrate (Sympathomimetic agents may reduce the blood glucose-lowering effect of insulin). Products include:
Aramine Injection 1889

Metformin Hydrochloride (Oral antidiabetic products may increase the blood glucose-lowering effect and susceptibility to hypoglycemia of insulin). Products include:
ActoPlus Met Tablets 3219
Avandamet Tablets 1343
Fortamet Extended-Release Tablets 1156

Methotrimeprazine (Phenothiazine derivatives may reduce the blood glucose-lowering effect of insulin).
No products indexed under this heading.

Methoxamine Hydrochloride (Sympathomimetic agents may reduce the blood glucose-lowering effect of insulin).
No products indexed under this heading.

Methyclothiazide (Diuretics may reduce the blood glucose-lowering effect of insulin).
No products indexed under this heading.

Methylprednisolone Acetate (Corticosteroids may reduce the blood glucose-lowering effect of insulin). Products include:
Depo-Medrol Injectable Suspension 2615
Depo-Medrol Single-Dose Vial 2617

Methylprednisolone Sodium Succinate (Corticosteroids may reduce the blood glucose-lowering effect of insulin).
No products indexed under this heading.

Metipranolol Hydrochloride (Beta-blockers may either potentiate or weaken the blood glucose-lowering effect of insulin and reduce or hide the signs of hypoglycemia).
No products indexed under this heading.

Metolazone (Diuretics may reduce the blood glucose-lowering effect of insulin).
No products indexed under this heading.

Metoprolol Succinate (Beta-blockers may either potentiate or weaken the blood glucose-lowering effect of insulin and reduce or hide the signs of hypoglycemia). Products include:
Toprol-XL Tablets 660

Metoprolol Tartrate (Beta-blockers may either potentiate or weaken the blood glucose-lowering effect of insulin and reduce or hide the signs of hypoglycemia).
No products indexed under this heading.

Miglitol (Oral antidiabetic products may increase the blood glucose-lowering effect and susceptibility to hypoglycemia of insulin).
No products indexed under this heading.

Moclobemide (MAO inhibitors may increase the blood glucose-lowering effect and susceptibility to hypoglycemia of insulin).
No products indexed under this heading.

Moexipril Hydrochloride (ACE inhibitors may increase the blood glucose-lowering effect and susceptibility to hypoglycemia of insulin). Products include:
Uniretic Tablets 3114
Univasc Tablets 3118

Nadolol (Beta-blockers may either potentiate or weaken the blood glucose-lowering effect of insulin and reduce or hide the signs of hypoglycemia). Products include:
Nadolol Tablets 2121

Nelfinavir Mesylate (Protease inhibitors may reduce the blood glucose-lowering effect of insulin). Products include:
Viracept 2556

Norepinephrine Bitartrate (Sympathomimetic agents may reduce the blood glucose-lowering effect of insulin).
No products indexed under this heading.

Norgestimate (Progestogens may reduce the blood glucose-lowering effect of insulin). Products include:
Ortho-Cyclen/Ortho Tri-Cyclen 2414
Ortho Tri-Cyclen Lo Tablets 2421
Prefest Tablets 1069

Olanzapine (Atypical antipsychotics may reduce the blood glucose-lowering effect of insulin). Products include:
Symbyax Capsules 1788
Zyprexa Tablets 1798
Zyprexa IntraMuscular 1798
Zyprexa ZYDIS Orally Disintegrating Tablets 1798

Pargyline Hydrochloride (MAO inhibitors may increase the blood glucose-lowering effect and susceptibility to hypoglycemia of insulin).
No products indexed under this heading.

Penbutolol Sulfate (Beta-blockers may either potentiate or weaken the blood glucose-lowering effect of insulin and reduce or hide the signs of hypoglycemia).
No products indexed under this heading.

Pentamidine Isethionate (Pentamidine may cause hypoglycemia, which may sometimes be followed by hyperglycemia).
No products indexed under this heading.

Pentoxifylline (Pentoxifylline may increase the blood glucose-lowering effect and susceptibility to hypoglycemia of insulin).
No products indexed under this heading.

Perindopril Erbumine (ACE inhibitors may increase the blood glucose-lowering effect and susceptibility to hypoglycemia of insulin). Products include:
Aceon Tablets (2 mg, 4 mg, 8 mg) 3191

Perphenazine (Phenothiazine derivatives may reduce the blood glucose-lowering effect of insulin).
No products indexed under this heading.

Phenelzine Sulfate (MAO inhibitors may increase the blood glucose-lowering effect and susceptibility to hypoglycemia of insulin).
No products indexed under this heading.

Phenylephrine Bitartrate (Sympathomimetic agents may reduce the blood glucose-lowering effect of insulin).
No products indexed under this heading.

Phenylephrine Hydrochloride (Sympathomimetic agents may reduce the blood glucose-lowering effect of insulin). Products include:

Alacol DM Syrup 739
Hycomine Compound Tablets 1105
Preparation H Maximum Strength Cream .... ▣747
Preparation H Cooling Gel .... ▣747
Preparation H .... ▣747
Sudafed PE Tablets .... ▣711
Vicks Sinex Nasal Spray and Ultra Fine Mist for Sinus Relief 2677
Zicam Concentrated Cough Mist for Kids Plus D Cool Cherry .... ▣643
Zicam Concentrated Cough Mist Plus D Cool Cherry .... ▣642

Phenylephrine Tannate (Sympathomimetic agents may reduce the blood glucose-lowering effect of insulin).
No products indexed under this heading.

Phenylpropanolamine Hydrochloride (Sympathomimetic agents may reduce the blood glucose-lowering effect of insulin).
No products indexed under this heading.

Pindolol (Beta-blockers may either potentiate or weaken the blood glucose-lowering effect of insulin and reduce or hide the signs of hypoglycemia).
No products indexed under this heading.

Pioglitazone Hydrochloride (Oral antidiabetic products may increase the blood glucose-lowering effect and susceptibility to hypoglycemia of insulin). Products include:
ActoPlus Met Tablets 3219
Actos Tablets 3224

Pirbuterol Acetate (Sympathomimetic agents may reduce the blood glucose-lowering effect of insulin). Products include:
Maxair Autohaler 1820

Polyestradiol Phosphate (Estrogens may reduce the blood glucose-lowering effect of insulin).
No products indexed under this heading.

Polythiazide (Diuretics may reduce the blood glucose-lowering effect of insulin).
No products indexed under this heading.

Prednisolone Acetate (Corticosteroids may reduce the blood glucose-lowering effect of insulin). Products include:
Blephamide Ophthalmic Ointment 563
Blephamide Ophthalmic Suspension 564
Poly-Pred Liquifilm Ophthalmic Suspension .... ⊙231
Pred Forte Ophthalmic Suspension .... ⊙233
Pred Mild Sterile Ophthalmic Suspension .... ⊙236
Pred-G Ophthalmic Suspension .... ⊙234
Pred-G Sterile Ophthalmic Ointment .... ⊙235

Prednisolone Sodium Phosphate (Corticosteroids may reduce the blood glucose-lowering effect of insulin). Products include:
Pediapred Oral Solution 3319

Prednisolone Tebutate (Corticosteroids may reduce the blood glucose-lowering effect of insulin).
No products indexed under this heading.

Prednisone (Corticosteroids may reduce the blood glucose-lowering effect of insulin).
No products indexed under this heading.

Procarbazine Hydrochloride (MAO inhibitors may increase the blood glucose-lowering effect and susceptibility to hypoglycemia of insulin). Products include:
Matulane Capsules 3188

Prochlorperazine (Phenothiazine derivatives may reduce the blood glucose-lowering effect of insulin).
No products indexed under this heading.

Promethazine Hydrochloride (Phenothiazine derivatives may reduce the blood glucose-lowering effect of insulin). Products include:
Phenergan 3438

Propoxyphene Hydrochloride (Propoxyphene may increase the blood glucose-lowering effect and susceptibility to hypoglycemia of insulin).
No products indexed under this heading.

Propoxyphene Napsylate (Propoxyphene may increase the blood glucose-lowering effect and susceptibility to hypoglycemia of insulin). Products include:
Darvocet A 500 Tablets 3497

Propranolol Hydrochloride (Beta-blockers may either potentiate or weaken the blood glucose-lowering effect of insulin and reduce or hide the signs of hypoglycemia). Products include:
Inderal LA Long-Acting Capsules 3421
InnoPran XL Capsules 2728

Pseudoephedrine Hydrochloride (Sympathomimetic agents may reduce the blood glucose-lowering effect of insulin). Products include:
Advil Allergy Sinus Caplets .... ▣737
Advil Cold & Sinus .... ▣739
Advil Flu & Body Ache Caplets .... ▣739
Children's Advil Cold Suspension .... ▣741
Advil Multi-Symptom Cold Caplets .... ▣738
Allegra-D 12 Hour Extended-Release Tablets 2860
Allegra-D 24 Hour Extended-Release Tablets 2862
Balamine DM 739
BC Cold Powder .... ▣612
Benadryl Allergy & Cold Tablets .... ▣692
Benadryl Allergy & Sinus Headache Caplets & Gelcaps .... ▣693
Children's Benadryl Allergy & Cold Fastmelt Tablets .... ▣695
Benadryl Maximum Strength Severe Allergy & Sinus Headache Caplets .... ▣694
Children's Benadryl D Allergy & Sinus Fastmelt Tablets .... ▣694
Children's Benadryl D Liquid Medication .... ▣693
Benadryl D Tablets .... ▣694
Contac Non-Drowsy 12 Hour Cold Caplets .... ▣614
Contac Non-Drowsy Timed Release 12 Hour Cold Caplets .... ▣615
Contac Severe Cold and Flu Caplets Maximum Strength .... ▣615
Contac Severe Cold and Flu Caplets Non-Drowsy .... ▣615
Children's Dimetapp Cold & Allergy Elixir .... ▣745
Children's Dimetapp DM Cold & Cough Elixir .... ▣745
Children's Dimetapp Long Acting Cough Plus Cold Syrup .... ▣746
Dimetapp Infant Drops Decongestant Plus Cough .... ▣746
Children's Motrin Cold Non-Staining Dye-Free Oral Suspension 1838
Children's Motrin Cold Oral Suspension 1838
Motrin Cold & Sinus Caplets 1836
PediaCare Decongestant & Cough Infant Drops .... ▣705
PediaCare Decongestant Infants' Drops .... ▣705
PediaCare Long-Acting Cough Plus Cold Liquid .... ▣704
PediaCare Multi-Symptom Cold Liquid .... ▣704
PediaCare NightRest Cough & Cold Liquid .... ▣704
Robitussin Allergy & Cough Syrup .... ▣750
Robitussin CF Liquid .... ▣755
Robitussin Cough & Cold Liquid-filled Capsules .... ▣750
Robitussin Cough, Cold & Flu Liquid-filled Capsules .... ▣750
Robitussin Cough & Cold Infant Drops .... ▣755
Robitussin Flu Liquid .... ▣752
Robitussin Maximum Strength Cough & Cold Liquid .... ▣754
Robitussin PE Syrup .... ▣753
Robitussin Pediatric Cough & Cold Liquid .... ▣754
Robitussin PM Cough & Cold Liquid .... ▣752
Robitussin Severe Congestion Liquid-filled Capsules .... ▣751
Simply Stuffy Liquid 1841
Singlet Caplets .... ▣636
Sudafed 12 Hour Caplets .... ▣708
Sudafed 24 Hour Tablets .... ▣709
Sudafed Nasal Decongestant Tablets .... ▣709
Sudafed Severe Cold .... ▣710
Sudafed Non-Drying Sinus Liquid Caps .... ▣709
Sudafed Sinus & Allergy Tablets .... ▣710
Sudafed Sinus Headache .... ▣711
TheraFlu Cold & Cough Hot Liquid .... ▣680
TheraFlu Cold & Sore Throat Hot Liquid .... ▣680
TheraFlu Flu & Chest Congestion Non-Drowsy Hot Liquid .... ▣681
TheraFlu Flu & Sore Throat Hot Liquid .... ▣681
TheraFlu Severe Cold Non-Drowsy Hot Liquid .... ▣683
TheraFlu Severe Cold & Cough Hot Liquid .... ▣683
TheraFlu Severe Cold Caplets .... ▣679
TheraFlu Severe Cold Hot Liquid .... ▣682
TheraFlu Severe Cold Non-Drowsy Caplets .... ▣679
Triaminic Chest & Nasal Congestion Liquid .... ▣685
Triaminic Cold & Allergy Liquid .... ▣685
Triaminic Cold & Cough Liquid .... ▣685
Triaminic Cough Liquid .... ▣687
Triaminic Cough & Nasal Congestion Liquid .... ▣687
Triaminic Cough & Sore Throat Liquid .... ▣687
Triaminic Flu, Cough & Fever Liquid .... ▣685
Triaminic Night Time Cough & Cold Liquid .... ▣685
Triaminic Allergy Runny Nose & Congestion Softchews .... ▣688
Triaminic Cold & Cough Softchews .... ▣688
Triaminic Cough & Sore Throat Softchews .... ▣689
Tylenol Sinus NightTime Caplets .... ▣663
Children's Tylenol Plus Cold & Allergy Suspension Liquid 1850
Children's Tylenol Plus Cold NightTime Suspension Liquid 1851
Children's Tylenol Plus Cold & Cough Suspension Liquid and Chewable Tablets 1851
Children's Tylenol Plus Cold Chewable Tablets 1851
Children's Tylenol Plus Cold Daytime Non-Drowsy Suspension Liquid 1851
Children's Tylenol Plus Flu Suspension Liquid 1853
Concentrated Tylenol Infants' Drops Plus Cold 1851
Concentrated Tylenol Infants' Drops Plus Cold and Cough 1851
Tylenol Cold & Flu Severe Daytime Liquid with Cool Bust 1846
Tylenol Cold & Flu Severe NightTime Liquid with Cool Burst 1846
Tylenol Cold Severe Congestion Non-Drowsy Caplets with Cool Burst 1846
Tylenol Allergy Complete Night Time Caplets 1844
Tylenol Allergy Complete Multi-Symptom Caplets and Gelcaps with Cool Burst 1844
Tylenol Flu NightTime Gelcaps 1846
Tylenol Flu Day Non-Drowsy Gelcaps 1846
Concentrated Tylenol Infants' Drops Plus Cold Nasal Congestant, Fever Reducer & Pain Reliever .... ▣668
Concentrated Tylenol Infants' Drops Plus Cold & Cough Nasal Decongestant, Fever Reducer & Pain Reliever .... ▣668
Multi-Symptom Tylenol Cold Night Time Caplets 1845
Multi-Symptom Tylenol Cold Day Non-Drowsy Caplets and Gelcaps 1845
Tylenol Sinus Day Non-Drowsy 1848
Tylenol Sinus Night Time Caplets 1848
Tylenol Sinus Severe Congestion Caplets with Cool Burst 1848
Vicks 44D Cough & Head Congestion Relief 2676
Vicks 44D Cough & Head Congestion Relief Liquid .... ▣721
Vicks 44M Cough, Cold & Flu Relief 2676
Pediatric Vicks 44m Cough & Cold Relief 2673
Vicks DayQuil LiquiCaps/Liquid Multi-Symptom Cold/Flu Relief .... ▣723
Vicks DayQuil Multi-Symptom Cold/Flu Relief LiquiCaps 2675
Vicks DayQuil Multi-Symptom Cold/Flu Relief Liquid 2675
Children's Vicks NyQuil Cold/Cough Relief 2671
Vicks NyQuil LiquiCaps 2677
Vicks NyQuil LiquiCaps/Liquid Multi-Symptom Cold/Flu Relief .... ▣725
Vicks NyQuil Liquid 2677
Zyrtec-D 12 Hour Extended Release Tablets 2591

Pseudoephedrine Sulfate (Sympathomimetic agents may reduce the blood glucose-lowering effect of insulin). Products include:
Alavert Allergy & Sinus D-12 Hour Tablets .... ▣743
Clarinex-D 24-Hour Extended-Release Tablets 3012
Claritin-D Non-Drowsy 12 Hour Tablets .... ▣731
Claritin-D Non-Drowsy 24 Hour Tablets .... ▣731

Quetiapine Fumarate (Atypical antipsychotics may reduce the blood glucose-lowering effect of insulin). Products include:
Seroquel Tablets 691

Quinapril Hydrochloride (ACE inhibitors may increase the blood glucose-lowering effect and susceptibility to hypoglycemia of insulin).
No products indexed under this heading.

Quinestrol (Estrogens may reduce the blood glucose-lowering effect of insulin).
No products indexed under this heading.

Ramipril (ACE inhibitors may increase the blood glucose-lowering effect and susceptibility to hypoglycemia of insulin). Products include:
Altace Capsules 1673

Repaglinide (Oral antidiabetic products may increase the blood glucose-lowering effect and susceptibility to hypoglycemia of insulin). Products include:
Prandin Tablets (0.5, 1, and 2 mg) 2337

Reserpine (Under the influence of sympatholytic medicinal products, such as reserpine, the signs of hypoglycemia may be reduced or absent).
No products indexed under this heading.

Risperidone (Atypical antipsychotics may reduce the blood glucose-lowering effect of insulin). Products include:
Risperdal Consta Long-Acting Injection 1664
Risperdal M-Tab Orally Disintegrating Tablets 1658
Risperdal 1658

Ritonavir (Protease inhibitors may reduce the blood glucose-lowering effect of insulin). Products include:
Kaletra 474
Norvir 499

Rosiglitazone Maleate (Oral antidiabetic products may increase the blood glucose-lowering effect and susceptibility to hypoglycemia of insulin). Products include:
Avandamet Tablets 1343
Avandia Tablets 1348

Salmeterol Xinafoate (Sympathomimetic agents may reduce the blood glucose-lowering effect of insulin). Products include:
Advair Diskus 100/50 1291
Advair Diskus 250/50 1291
Advair Diskus 500/50 1291
Serevent Diskus 1540

Salsalate (Salicylates may increase the blood glucose-lowering effect and susceptibility to hypoglycemia of insulin).
No products indexed under this heading.

Saquinavir (Protease inhibitors may reduce the blood glucose-lowering effect of insulin).
No products indexed under this heading.

Saquinavir Mesylate (Protease inhibitors may reduce the blood glucose-lowering effect of insulin). Products include:
Invirase 2776

Selegiline Hydrochloride (MAO inhibitors may increase the blood glucose-lowering effect and susceptibility to hypoglycemia of insulin). Products include:
Eldepryl Capsules 3209

Somatropin (Somatropin may reduce the blood glucose-lowering effect of insulin). Products include:
Genotropin Lyophilized Powder 2642
Humatrope Vials and Cartridges 1756
Norditropin Cartridges 2318
Nutropin for Injection 1238
Nutropin AQ Injection 1241
Nutropin AQ Pen 1241
Nutropin AQ Pen Cartridge 1241

Sotalol Hydrochloride (Beta-blockers may either potentiate or weaken the blood glucose-lowering effect of insulin and reduce or hide the signs of hypoglycemia).
No products indexed under this heading.

Spirapril Hydrochloride (ACE inhibitors may increase the blood glucose-lowering effect and susceptibility to hypoglycemia of insulin).
No products indexed under this heading.

Spironolactone (Diuretics may reduce the blood glucose-lowering effect of insulin).
No products indexed under this heading.

Sulfacytine (Sulfonamide antibiotics may increase the blood glucose-lowering effect and susceptibility to hypoglycemia of insulin).
No products indexed under this heading.

Sulfamethizole (Sulfonamide antibiotics may increase the blood glucose-lowering effect and susceptibility to hypoglycemia of insulin).
No products indexed under this heading.

Sulfamethoxazole (Sulfonamide antibiotics may increase the blood glucose-lowering effect and susceptibility to hypoglycemia of insulin).
No products indexed under this heading.

Sulfasalazine (Sulfonamide antibiotics may increase the blood glucose-lowering effect and susceptibility to hypoglycemia of insulin).
No products indexed under this heading.

Sulfinpyrazone (Sulfonamide antibiotics may increase the blood glucose-lowering effect and susceptibility to hypoglycemia of insulin).
No products indexed under this heading.

Sulfisoxazole (Sulfonamide antibiotics may increase the blood glucose-lowering effect and susceptibility to hypoglycemia of insulin).
No products indexed under this heading.

Sulfisoxazole Acetyl (Sulfonamide antibiotics may increase the blood glucose-lowering effect and susceptibility to hypoglycemia of insulin).
No products indexed under this heading.

Sulfisoxazole Diolamine (Sulfonamide antibiotics may increase the blood glucose-lowering effect and susceptibility to hypoglycemia of insulin).
No products indexed under this heading.

Terbutaline Sulfate (Sympathomimetic agents may reduce the blood glucose-lowering effect of insulin).
No products indexed under this heading.

Thioridazine Hydrochloride (Phenothiazine derivatives may reduce the blood glucose-lowering effect of insulin). Products include:
Thioridazine Hydrochloride Tablets 2122

Thyroglobulin (Thyroid hormones may reduce the blood glucose-lowering effect of insulin).
No products indexed under this heading.

Thyroid (Thyroid hormones may reduce the blood glucose-lowering effect of insulin).
No products indexed under this heading.

Thyroxine (Thyroid hormones may reduce the blood glucose-lowering effect of insulin).
No products indexed under this heading.

Thyroxine Sodium (Thyroid hormones may reduce the blood glucose-lowering effect of insulin).
No products indexed under this heading.

Timolol Hemihydrate (Beta-blockers may either potentiate or weaken the blood glucose-lowering effect of insulin and reduce or hide the signs of hypoglycemia). Products include:
Betimol Ophthalmic Solution 3371
Betimol Ophthalmic Solution .... ⊙ 283

Timolol Maleate (Beta-blockers may either potentiate or weaken the blood glucose-lowering effect of insulin and reduce or hide the signs of hypoglycemia). Products include:
Blocadren Tablets 1891
Cosopt Sterile Ophthalmic Solution 1910
Timolide Tablets 2056
Timoptic in Ocudose 2061
Timoptic Sterile Ophthalmic Solution 2058
Timoptic-XE Sterile Ophthalmic Gel Forming Solution 2062

Tolazamide (Oral antidiabetic products may increase the blood glucose-lowering effect and susceptibility to hypoglycemia of insulin).
No products indexed under this heading.

Tolbutamide (Oral antidiabetic products may increase the blood glucose-lowering effect and susceptibility to hypoglycemia of insulin).
No products indexed under this heading.

Torsemide (Diuretics may reduce the blood glucose-lowering effect of insulin).
No products indexed under this heading.

Trandolapril (ACE inhibitors may increase the blood glucose-lowering effect and susceptibility to hypoglycemia of insulin). Products include:
Mavik Tablets 482
Tarka Tablets 519

Tranylcypromine Sulfate (MAO inhibitors may increase the blood glucose-lowering effect and susceptibility to hypoglycemia of insulin). Products include:
Parnate Tablets 1499

Triamcinolone (Corticosteroids may reduce the blood glucose-lowering effect of insulin).
No products indexed under this heading.

Triamcinolone Acetonide (Corticosteroids may reduce the blood glucose-lowering effect of insulin). Products include:
Azmacort Inhalation Aerosol 1701
Nasacort HFA Inhalation Aerosol 2939
Nasacort AQ Nasal Spray 2937

Triamcinolone Diacetate (Corticosteroids may reduce the blood glucose-lowering effect of insulin).
No products indexed under this heading.

Triamcinolone Hexacetonide (Corticosteroids may reduce the blood glucose-lowering effect of insulin).
No products indexed under this heading.

Triamterene (Diuretics may reduce the blood glucose-lowering effect of insulin). Products include:
Dyazide Capsules 1389
Dyrenium Capsules 3390
Maxzide 2150

Trifluoperazine Hydrochloride (Phenothiazine derivatives may reduce the blood glucose-lowering effect of insulin).
No products indexed under this heading.

Troglitazone (Oral antidiabetic products may increase the blood glucose-lowering effect and susceptibility to hypoglycemia of insulin).
No products indexed under this heading.

Ziprasidone Hydrochloride (Atypical antipsychotics may reduce the blood glucose-lowering effect of insulin). Products include:
Geodon Capsules 2514

Ziprasidone Mesylate (Atypical antipsychotics may reduce the blood glucose-lowering effect of insulin). Products include:
Geodon for Injection 2514

Food Interactions

Alcohol (Alcohol may either potentiate or weaken the blood glucose-lowering effect of insulin).

APOKYN INJECTION

(Apomorphine Hydrochloride) 2132
May interact with dopamine antagonists, antihypertensives, butyrophenones, phenothiazines, drugs that prolong the QT interval, vasodilators, and certain other agents. Compounds in these categories include:

Acebutolol Hydrochloride (The following adverse events were experienced more commonly in patients receiving concomitant antihypertensive medications: hypotension, myocardial infarction, serious pneumonia, serious falls, and bone and joint injuries. The mechanism underlying many of these events is unknown, but may represent increased hypotension).
No products indexed under this heading.

Alosetron Hydrochloride (Based on reports of profound hypotension and loss of consciousness, the concomitant use of apomorphine with drugs of the 5HT3 antagonist class is contraindicated). Products include:
Lotronex Tablets 1479

Amiodarone Hydrochloride (Caution should be exercised when prescribing apomorphine concomitantly with drugs that prolong the QT/QTc interval). Products include:
Pacerone Tablets 3337

Amitriptyline Hydrochloride (Caution should be exercised when prescribing apomorphine concomitantly with drugs that prolong the QT/QTc interval).
No products indexed under this heading.

Amlodipine Besylate (The following adverse events were experienced more commonly in patients receiving concomitant antihypertensive medications: hypotension, myocardial infarction, serious pneumonia, serious falls, and bone and joint injuries. The mechanism underlying many of these events is unknown, but may represent increased hypotension). Products include:
Caduet Tablets 2507
Lotrel Capsules 2238
Norvasc Tablets 2529

Amoxapine (Caution should be exercised when prescribing apomorphine concomitantly with drugs that prolong the QT/QTc interval).
No products indexed under this heading.

Amyl Nitrite (The following adverse events were experienced more commonly in patients receiving concomitant vasodilators: hypotension, myocardial infarction, serious pneumonia, serious falls, and bone and joint injuries. The mechanism underlying many of these events is unknown, but may represent increased hypotension).
No products indexed under this heading.

Astemizole (Caution should be exercised when prescribing apomorphine concomitantly with drugs that prolong the QT/QTc interval).
No products indexed under this heading.

Atenolol (The following adverse events were experienced more commonly in patients receiving concomitant antihypertensive medications: hypotension, myocardial infarction, serious pneumonia, serious falls, and bone and joint injuries. The mechanism underlying many of these events is unknown, but may represent increased hypotension). Products include:
Tenormin I.V. Injection 698
Tenormin Tablets 695

Benazepril Hydrochloride (The following adverse events were experienced more commonly in patients receiving concomitant antihypertensive medications: hypotension, myocardial infarction, serious pneumonia, serious falls, and bone and joint injuries. The mechanism underlying many of these events is unknown, but may represent increased hypotension). Products include:
Lotensin Tablets 2232
Lotensin HCT Tablets 2235
Lotrel Capsules 2238

Bendroflumethiazide (The following adverse events were experienced more commonly in patients receiving concomitant antihypertensive medications: hypotension, myocardial infarction, serious pneumonia, serious falls, and bone and joint injuries. The mechanism underlying many of these events is unknown, but may represent increased hypotension).
No products indexed under this heading.

Betaxolol Hydrochloride (The following adverse events were experienced more commonly in patients receiving concomitant antihypertensive medications: hypotension, myocardial infarction, serious pneumonia, serious falls, and bone and joint injuries. The mechanism underlying many of these events is unknown, but may represent increased hypotension). Products include:
Betoptic S Ophthalmic Suspension................................ 554

Bisoprolol Fumarate (The following adverse events were experienced more commonly in patients receiving concomitant antihypertensive medications: hypotension, myocardial infarction, serious pneumonia, serious falls, and bone and joint injuries. The mechanism underlying many of these events is unknown, but may represent increased hypotension).
No products indexed under this heading.

Bretylium Tosylate (Caution should be exercised when prescribing apomorphine concomitantly with drugs that prolong the QT/QTc interval).
No products indexed under this heading.

Candesartan Cilexetil (The following adverse events were experienced more commonly in patients receiving concomitant antihypertensive medications: hypotension, myocardial infarction, serious pneumonia, serious falls, and bone and joint injuries. The mechanism underlying many of these events is unknown, but may represent increased hypotension). Products include:
Atacand Tablets 634
Atacand HCT 637

Captopril (The following adverse events were experienced more commonly in patients receiving concomitant antihypertensive medications: hypotension, myocardial infarction, serious pneumonia, serious falls, and bone and joint injuries. The mechanism underlying many of these events is unknown, but may represent increased hypotension). Products include:
Captopril Tablets 2114

Carteolol Hydrochloride (The following adverse events were experienced more commonly in patients receiving concomitant antihypertensive medications: hypotension, myocardial infarction, serious pneumonia, serious falls, and bone and joint injuries. The mechanism underlying many of these events is unknown, but may represent increased hypotension). Products include:
Carteolol Hydrochloride Ophthalmic Solution USP, 1%....... ⊙246

Chlorothiazide (The following adverse events were experienced more commonly in patients receiving concomitant antihypertensive medications: hypotension, myocardial infarction, serious pneumonia, serious falls, and bone and joint injuries. The mechanism underlying many of these events is unknown, but may represent increased hypotension). Products include:
Aldoclor Tablets 1881
Diuril Oral 1936

Chlorothiazide Sodium (The following adverse events were experienced more commonly in patients receiving concomitant antihypertensive medications: hypotension, myocardial infarction, serious pneumonia, serious falls, and bone and joint injuries. The mechanism underlying many of these events is unknown, but may represent increased hypotension). Products include:
Diuril Sodium Intravenous 1934

Chlorpromazine (Dopamine antagonists may diminish the effectiveness of apomorphine. Patients with major psychotic disorders, treated with neuroleptics, should be treated with dopamine agonists only if the potential benefits outweigh the risks).
No products indexed under this heading.

Chlorpromazine Hydrochloride (Dopamine antagonists may diminish the effectiveness of apomorphine. Patients with major psychotic disorders, treated with neuroleptics, should be treated with dopamine agonists only if the potential benefits outweigh the risks).
No products indexed under this heading.

Chlorthalidone (The following adverse events were experienced more commonly in patients receiving concomitant antihypertensive medications: hypotension, myocardial infarction, serious pneumonia, serious falls, and bone and joint injuries. The mechanism underlying many of these events is unknown, but may represent increased hypotension). Products include:
Clorpres Tablets 2139

Clomipramine Hydrochloride (Caution should be exercised when prescribing apomorphine concomitantly with drugs that prolong the QT/QTc interval).
No products indexed under this heading.

Clonidine (The following adverse events were experienced more commonly in patients receiving concomitant antihypertensive medications: hypotension, myocardial infarction, serious pneumonia, serious falls, and bone and joint injuries. The mechanism underlying many of these events is unknown, but may represent increased hypotension). Products include:
Catapres-TTS 875

Clonidine Hydrochloride (The following adverse events were experienced more commonly in patients receiving concomitant antihypertensive medications: hypotension, myocardial infarction, serious pneumonia, serious falls, and bone and joint injuries. The mechanism underlying many of these events is unknown, but may represent increased hypotension). Products include:
Catapres Tablets 874
Clorpres Tablets 2139

Clozapine (Dopamine antagonists may diminish the effectiveness of apomorphine. Patients with major psychotic disorders, treated with neuroleptics, should be treated with dopamine agonists only if the potential benefits outweigh the risks). Products include:
Clozapine Tablets 2141
Clozaril Tablets 2174
FazaClo Orally Disintegrating Tablets 547

Deserpidine (The following adverse events were experienced more commonly in patients receiving concomitant antihypertensive medications: hypotension, myocardial infarction, serious pneumonia, serious falls, and bone and joint injuries. The mechanism underlying many of these events is unknown, but may represent increased hypotension).
No products indexed under this heading.

Desipramine Hydrochloride (Caution should be exercised when prescribing apomorphine concomitantly with drugs that prolong the QT/QTc interval).
No products indexed under this heading.

Diazoxide (The following adverse events were experienced more commonly in patients receiving concomitant antihypertensive medications: hypotension, myocardial infarction, serious pneumonia, serious falls, and bone and joint injuries. The mechanism underlying many of these events is unknown, but may represent increased hypotension). Products include:
Hyperstat I.V. Injection 3031

Diltiazem Hydrochloride (The following adverse events were experienced more commonly in patients receiving concomitant antihypertensive medications: hypotension, myocardial infarction, serious pneumonia, serious falls, and bone and joint injuries. The mechanism underlying many of these events is unknown, but may represent increased hypotension). Products include:
Cardizem LA Extended Release Tablets 1699
Tiazac Capsules 1204

Disopyramide Phosphate (Caution should be exercised when prescribing apomorphine concomitantly with drugs that prolong the QT/QTc interval).
No products indexed under this heading.

Dofetilide (Caution should be exercised when prescribing apomorphine concomitantly with drugs that prolong the QT/QTc interval).
No products indexed under this heading.

Dolasetron Mesylate (Based on reports of profound hypotension and loss of consciousness, the concomitant use of apomorphine with drugs of the 5HT3 antagonist class is contraindicated). Products include:
Anzemet Injection 2871
Anzemet Tablets 2874

Doxazosin Mesylate (The following adverse events were experienced more commonly in patients receiving concomitant antihypertensive medications: hypotension, myocardial infarction, serious pneumonia, serious falls, and bone and joint injuries. The mechanism underlying many of these events is unknown, but may represent increased hypotension).
No products indexed under this heading.

Doxepin Hydrochloride (Caution should be exercised when prescribing apomorphine concomitantly with drugs that prolong the QT/QTc interval).
No products indexed under this heading.

Enalapril Maleate (The following adverse events were experienced more commonly in patients receiving concomitant antihypertensive medications: hypotension, myocardial infarction, serious pneumonia, serious falls, and bone and joint injuries. The mechanism underlying many of these events is unknown, but may represent increased hypotension). Products include:
Vaseretic Tablets 2073
Vasotec I.V. Injection 2076

Enalaprilat (The following adverse events were experienced more commonly in patients receiving concomitant antihypertensive medications: hypotension, myocardial infarction, serious pneumonia, serious falls, and bone and joint injuries. The mechanism underlying many of these events is unknown, but may represent increased hypotension).
No products indexed under this heading.

Epoprostenol Sodium (The following adverse events were experienced more commonly in patients receiving concomitant vasodilators: hypotension, myocardial infarction, serious pneumonia, serious falls, and bone and joint injuries. The mechanism underlying many of these events is unknown, but may represent increased hypotension). Products include:
Flolan for Injection 1408

Eprosartan Mesylate (The following adverse events were experienced more commonly in patients receiving concomitant antihypertensive medications: hypotension, myocardial infarction, serious pneumonia, serious falls, and bone and joint injuries. The mechanism underlying

many of these events is unknown, but may represent increased hypotension). Products include:

- Teveten Tablets 1707
- Teveten HCT Tablets 1710

Esmolol Hydrochloride (The following adverse events were experienced more commonly in patients receiving concomitant antihypertensive medications: hypotension, myocardial infarction, serious pneumonia, serious falls, and bone and joint injuries. The mechanism underlying many of these events is unknown, but may represent increased hypotension). Products include:

- Brevibloc Concentrate 766
- Brevibloc Injection 766
- Brevibloc Double Strength Injection 766
- Brevibloc Premixed Injection 766
- Brevibloc Double Strength Premixed Injection 766

Ethaverine Hydrochloride (The following adverse events were experienced more commonly in patients receiving concomitant vasodilators: hypotension, myocardial infarction, serious pneumonia, serious falls, and bone and joint injuries. The mechanism underlying many of these events is unknown, but may represent increased hypotension).

No products indexed under this heading.

Felodipine (The following adverse events were experienced more commonly in patients receiving concomitant antihypertensive medications: hypotension, myocardial infarction, serious pneumonia, serious falls, and bone and joint injuries. The mechanism underlying many of these events is unknown, but may represent increased hypotension). Products include:

- Plendil Extended-Release Tablets 651

Flecainide Acetate (Caution should be exercised when prescribing apomorphine concomitantly with drugs that prolong the QT/QTc interval). Products include:

- Tambocor Tablets 1824

Fluphenazine Decanoate (Dopamine antagonists may diminish the effectiveness of apomorphine. Patients with major psychotic disorders, treated with neuroleptics, should be treated with dopamine agonists only if the potential benefits outweigh the risks).

No products indexed under this heading.

Fluphenazine Enanthate (Dopamine antagonists may diminish the effectiveness of apomorphine. Patients with major psychotic disorders, treated with neuroleptics, should be treated with dopamine agonists only if the potential benefits outweigh the risks).

No products indexed under this heading.

Fluphenazine Hydrochloride (Dopamine antagonists may diminish the effectiveness of apomorphine. Patients with major psychotic disorders, treated with neuroleptics, should be treated with dopamine agonists only if the potential benefits outweigh the risks).

No products indexed under this heading.

Fosinopril Sodium (The following adverse events were experienced more commonly in patients receiving concomitant antihypertensive medications: hypotension, myocardial infarction, serious pneumonia, serious falls, and bone and joint injuries. The mechanism underlying many of these events is unknown, but may represent increased hypotension).

No products indexed under this heading.

Furosemide (The following adverse events were experienced more commonly in patients receiving concomitant antihypertensive medications: hypotension, myocardial infarction, serious pneumonia, serious falls, and bone and joint injuries. The mechanism underlying many of these events is unknown, but may represent increased hypotension). Products include:

- Furosemide Tablets 2117

Granisetron Hydrochloride (Based on reports of profound hypotension and loss of consciousness, the concomitant use of apomorphine with drugs of the 5HT3 antagonist class is contraindicated). Products include:

- Kytril Injection 2785
- Kytril 2788

Guanabenz Acetate (The following adverse events were experienced more commonly in patients receiving concomitant antihypertensive medications: hypotension, myocardial infarction, serious pneumonia, serious falls, and bone and joint injuries. The mechanism underlying many of these events is unknown, but may represent increased hypotension).

No products indexed under this heading.

Guanethidine Monosulfate (The following adverse events were experienced more commonly in patients receiving concomitant antihypertensive medications: hypotension, myocardial infarction, serious pneumonia, serious falls, and bone and joint injuries. The mechanism underlying many of these events is unknown, but may represent increased hypotension).

No products indexed under this heading.

Haloperidol (Dopamine antagonists may diminish the effectiveness of apomorphine. Patients with major psychotic disorders, treated with neuroleptics, should be treated with dopamine agonists only if the potential benefits outweigh the risks).

No products indexed under this heading.

Haloperidol Decanoate (Dopamine antagonists may diminish the effectiveness of apomorphine. Patients with major psychotic disorders, treated with neuroleptics, should be treated with dopamine agonists only if the potential benefits outweigh the risks).

No products indexed under this heading.

Hydralazine Hydrochloride (The following adverse events were experienced more commonly in patients receiving concomitant antihypertensive medications: hypotension, myocardial infarction, serious pneumonia, serious falls, and bone and joint injuries. The mechanism underlying many of these events is unknown, but may represent increased hypotension). Products include:

- BiDil Tablets 2161

Hydrochlorothiazide (The following adverse events were experienced more commonly in patients receiving concomitant antihypertensive medications: hypotension, myocardial infarction, serious pneumonia, serious falls, and bone and joint injuries. The mechanism underlying many of these events is unknown, but may represent increased hypotension). Products include:

- Aldoril Tablets 1884
- Atacand HCT 637
- Avalide Tablets 2889
- Avalide Tablets 922
- Benicar HCT Tablets 2852
- Diovan HCT Tablets 2195
- Dyazide Capsules 1389
- Hyzaar 1964
- Lotensin HCT Tablets 2235
- Maxzide 2150
- Micardis HCT Tablets 886
- Moduretic Tablets 2003
- Prinzide Tablets 2033
- Teveten HCT Tablets 1710
- Timolide Tablets 2056
- Uniretic Tablets 3114
- Vaseretic Tablets 2073
- Zestoretic Tablets 701

Hydroflumethiazide (The following adverse events were experienced more commonly in patients receiving concomitant antihypertensive medications: hypotension, myocardial infarction, serious pneumonia, serious falls, and bone and joint injuries. The mechanism underlying many of these events is unknown, but may represent increased hypotension).

No products indexed under this heading.

Imipramine Hydrochloride (Caution should be exercised when prescribing apomorphine concomitantly with drugs that prolong the QT/QTc interval).

No products indexed under this heading.

Imipramine Pamoate (Caution should be exercised when prescribing apomorphine concomitantly with drugs that prolong the QT/QTc interval).

No products indexed under this heading.

Indapamide (The following adverse events were experienced more commonly in patients receiving concomitant antihypertensive medications: hypotension, myocardial infarction, serious pneumonia, serious falls, and bone and joint injuries. The mechanism underlying many of these events is unknown, but may represent increased hypotension). Products include:

- Indapamide Tablets 2119

Irbesartan (The following adverse events were experienced more commonly in patients receiving concomitant antihypertensive medications: hypotension, myocardial infarction, serious pneumonia, serious falls, and bone and joint injuries. The mechanism underlying many of these events is unknown, but may represent increased hypotension). Products include:

- Avalide Tablets 922
- Avalide Tablets 2889
- Avapro Tablets 925
- Avapro Tablets 2886

Isosorbide Dinitrate (The following adverse events were experienced more commonly in patients receiving concomitant vasodilators: hypotension, myocardial infarction, serious pneumonia, serious falls, and bone and joint injuries. The mechanism underlying many of these events is unknown, but may represent increased hypotension). Products include:

- BiDil Tablets 2161

Isosorbide Mononitrate (The following adverse events were experienced more commonly in patients receiving concomitant vasodilators: hypotension, myocardial infarction, serious pneumonia, serious falls, and bone and joint injuries. The mechanism underlying many of these events is unknown, but may represent increased hypotension). Products include:

- Imdur Tablets 3032

Isoxsuprine Hydrochloride (The following adverse events were experienced more commonly in patients receiving concomitant vasodilators: hypotension, myocardial infarction, serious pneumonia, serious falls, and bone and joint injuries. The mechanism underlying many of these events is unknown, but may represent increased hypotension).

No products indexed under this heading.

Isradipine (The following adverse events were experienced more commonly in patients receiving concomitant antihypertensive medications: hypotension, myocardial infarction, serious pneumonia, serious falls, and bone and joint injuries. The mechanism underlying many of these events is unknown, but may represent increased hypotension). Products include:

- DynaCirc CR Tablets 2726

Labetalol Hydrochloride (The following adverse events were experienced more commonly in patients receiving concomitant antihypertensive medications: hypotension, myocardial infarction, serious pneumonia, serious falls, and bone and joint injuries. The mechanism underlying many of these events is unknown, but may represent increased hypotension).

No products indexed under this heading.

Levodopa (The threshold levodopa concentration necessary for an improved motor response was reduced significantly, leading to an increased duration of effect, without a change in the maximal response to levodopa therapy). Products include:

- Parcopa Orally Disintegrating Tablets 3111
- Stalevo Tablets 2270

Lidocaine Hydrochloride (Caution should be exercised when prescribing apomorphine concomitantly with drugs that prolong the QT/QTc interval).

No products indexed under this heading.

Lisinopril (The following adverse events were experienced more commonly in patients receiving concomitant antihypertensive medications: hypotension, myocardial infarction, serious pneumonia, serious falls, and bone and joint injuries. The mechanism underlying many of these events is unknown, but may represent increased hypotension). Products include:

- Prinivil Tablets 2029
- Prinzide Tablets 2033
- Zestoretic Tablets 701
- Zestril Tablets 704

Losartan Potassium (The following adverse events were experienced more commonly in patients receiving concomitant antihypertensive medications: hypotension, myocardial infarction, serious pneumonia, serious falls, and bone and joint injuries. The mechanism underlying many of these events is unknown, but may represent increased hypotension). Products include:

Cozaar Tablets **1913**
Hyzaar **1964**

Maprotiline Hydrochloride (Caution should be exercised when prescribing apomorphine concomitantly with drugs that prolong the QT/QTc interval).

No products indexed under this heading.

Mecamylamine Hydrochloride (The following adverse events were experienced more commonly in patients receiving concomitant antihypertensive medications: hypotension, myocardial infarction, serious pneumonia, serious falls, and bone and joint injuries. The mechanism underlying many of these events is unknown, but may represent increased hypotension). Products include:

Inversine Tablets **3286**

Mesoridazine Besylate (Dopamine antagonists may diminish the effectiveness of apomorphine. Patients with major psychotic disorders, treated with neuroleptics, should be treated with dopamine agonists only if the potential benefits outweigh the risks).

No products indexed under this heading.

Methotrimeprazine (Dopamine antagonists may diminish the effectiveness of apomorphine. Patients with major psychotic disorders, treated with neuroleptics, should be treated with dopamine agonists only if the potential benefits outweigh the risks).

No products indexed under this heading.

Methyclothiazide (The following adverse events were experienced more commonly in patients receiving concomitant antihypertensive medications: hypotension, myocardial infarction, serious pneumonia, serious falls, and bone and joint injuries. The mechanism underlying many of these events is unknown, but may represent increased hypotension).

No products indexed under this heading.

Methyldopa (The following adverse events were experienced more commonly in patients receiving concomitant antihypertensive medications: hypotension, myocardial infarction, serious pneumonia, serious falls, and bone and joint injuries. The mechanism underlying many of these events is unknown, but may represent increased hypotension). Products include:

Aldoclor Tablets **1881**
Aldoril Tablets **1884**

Methyldopate Hydrochloride (The following adverse events were experienced more commonly in patients receiving concomitant antihypertensive medications: hypotension, myocardial infarction, serious pneumonia, serious falls, and bone and joint injuries. The mechanism underlying many of these events is unknown, but may represent increased hypotension).

No products indexed under this heading.

Metoclopramide Hydrochloride (Dopamine antagonists, such as metoclopramide, may diminish the effectiveness of apomorphine).

No products indexed under this heading.

Metolazone (The following adverse events were experienced more commonly in patients receiving concomitant antihypertensive medications: hypotension, myocardial infarction, serious pneumonia, serious falls, and bone and joint injuries. The mechanism underlying many of these events is unknown, but may represent increased hypotension).

No products indexed under this heading.

Metoprolol Succinate (The following adverse events were experienced more commonly in patients receiving concomitant antihypertensive medications: hypotension, myocardial infarction, serious pneumonia, serious falls, and bone and joint injuries. The mechanism underlying many of these events is unknown, but may represent increased hypotension). Products include:

Toprol-XL Tablets **660**

Metoprolol Tartrate (The following adverse events were experienced more commonly in patients receiving concomitant antihypertensive medications: hypotension, myocardial infarction, serious pneumonia, serious falls, and bone and joint injuries. The mechanism underlying many of these events is unknown, but may represent increased hypotension).

No products indexed under this heading.

Metyrosine (The following adverse events were experienced more commonly in patients receiving concomitant antihypertensive medications: hypotension, myocardial infarction, serious pneumonia, serious falls, and bone and joint injuries. The mechanism underlying many of these events is unknown, but may represent increased hypotension). Products include:

Demser Capsules **1933**

Mexiletine Hydrochloride (Caution should be exercised when prescribing apomorphine concomitantly with drugs that prolong the QT/QTc interval).

No products indexed under this heading.

Mibefradil Dihydrochloride (The following adverse events were experienced more commonly in patients receiving concomitant antihypertensive medications: hypotension, myocardial infarction, serious pneumonia, serious falls, and bone and joint injuries. The mechanism underlying many of these events is unknown, but may represent increased hypotension).

No products indexed under this heading.

Minoxidil (The following adverse events were experienced more commonly in patients receiving concomitant antihypertensive medications: hypotension, myocardial infarction, serious pneumonia, serious falls, and bone and joint injuries. The mechanism underlying many of these events is unknown, but may represent increased hypotension). Products include:

Men's Rogaine Extra Strength Topical Solution, Ocean Rush Scent and Original Unscented .... ⊡ **706**
Women's Rogaine Topical Solution, Spring Bloom Scent and Original Unscented .... ⊡ **707**

Moexipril Hydrochloride (The following adverse events were experienced more commonly in patients receiving concomitant antihypertensive medications: hypotension, myocardial infarction, serious pneumonia, serious falls, and bone and joint injuries. The mechanism underlying many of these events is unknown, but may represent increased hypotension). Products include:

Uniretic Tablets **3114**
Univasc Tablets **3118**

Nadolol (The following adverse events were experienced more commonly in patients receiving concomitant antihypertensive medications: hypotension, myocardial infarction, serious pneumonia, serious falls, and bone and joint injuries. The mechanism underlying many of these events is unknown, but may represent increased hypotension). Products include:

Nadolol Tablets **2121**

Nicardipine Hydrochloride (The following adverse events were experienced more commonly in patients receiving concomitant antihypertensive medications: hypotension, myocardial infarction, serious pneumonia, serious falls, and bone and joint injuries. The mechanism underlying many of these events is unknown, but may represent increased hypotension). Products include:

Cardene I.V. **1129**

Nifedipine (The following adverse events were experienced more commonly in patients receiving concomitant antihypertensive medications: hypotension, myocardial infarction, serious pneumonia, serious falls, and bone and joint injuries. The mechanism underlying many of these events is unknown, but may represent increased hypotension). Products include:

Adalat CC Tablets **2978**

Nisoldipine (The following adverse events were experienced more commonly in patients receiving concomitant antihypertensive medications: hypotension, myocardial infarction, serious pneumonia, serious falls, and bone and joint injuries. The mechanism underlying many of these events is unknown, but may represent increased hypotension). Products include:

Sular Tablets **1163**

Nitroglycerin (The following adverse events were experienced more commonly in patients receiving concomitant antihypertensive medications: hypotension, myocardial infarction, serious pneumonia, serious falls, and bone and joint injuries. The mechanism underlying many of these events is unknown, but may represent increased hypotension). Products include:

Nitro-Dur Transdermal Infusion System **3060**
Nitrolingual Pumpspray **1161**

Nitroglycerin, long-acting formulations (The following adverse events were experienced more commonly in patients receiving concomitant vasodilators: hypotension, myocardial infarction, serious pneumonia, serious falls, and bone and joint injuries. The mechanism underlying many of these events is unknown, but may represent increased hypotension).

No products indexed under this heading.

Nitroglycerin Intravenous (The following adverse events were experienced more commonly in patients receiving concomitant vasodilators: hypotension, myocardial infarction, serious pneumonia, serious falls, and bone and joint injuries. The mechanism underlying many of these events is unknown, but may represent increased hypotension).

No products indexed under this heading.

Nortriptyline Hydrochloride (Caution should be exercised when prescribing apomorphine concomitantly with drugs that prolong the QT/QTc interval).

No products indexed under this heading.

Olanzapine (Dopamine antagonists may diminish the effectiveness of apomorphine. Patients with major psychotic disorders, treated with neuroleptics, should be treated with dopamine agonists only if the potential benefits outweigh the risks). Products include:

Symbyax Capsules **1788**
Zyprexa Tablets **1798**
Zyprexa IntraMuscular **1798**
Zyprexa ZYDIS Orally Disintegrating Tablets **1798**

Ondansetron (Based on reports of profound hypotension and loss of consciousness, the concomitant use of apomorphine with drugs of the 5HT3 antagonist class is contraindicated). Products include:

Zofran ODT Orally Disintegrating Tablets **1613**

Ondansetron Hydrochloride (Based on reports of profound hypotension and loss of consciousness, the concomitant use of apomorphine with drugs of the 5HT3 antagonist class is contraindicated). Products include:

Zofran Injection **1607**
Zofran **1613**

Palonosetron Hydrochloride (Based on reports of profound hypotension and loss of consciousness, the concomitant use of apomorphine with drugs of the 5HT3 antagonist class is contraindicated). Products include:

Aloxi Injection **2099**

Papaverine (The following adverse events were experienced more commonly in patients receiving concomitant vasodilators: hypotension, myocardial infarction, serious pneumonia, serious falls, and bone and joint injuries. The mechanism underlying many of these events is unknown, but may represent increased hypotension).

No products indexed under this heading.

Papaverine Hydrochloride (The following adverse events were experienced more commonly in patients receiving concomitant vasodilators: hypotension, myocardial infarction, serious pneumonia, serious falls, and bone and joint injuries. The mechanism underlying many of these events is unknown, but may represent increased hypotension).
No products indexed under this heading.

Penbutolol Sulfate (The following adverse events were experienced more commonly in patients receiving concomitant antihypertensive medications: hypotension, myocardial infarction, serious pneumonia, serious falls, and bone and joint injuries. The mechanism underlying many of these events is unknown, but may represent increased hypotension).
No products indexed under this heading.

Perindopril Erbumine (The following adverse events were experienced more commonly in patients receiving concomitant antihypertensive medications: hypotension, myocardial infarction, serious pneumonia, serious falls, and bone and joint injuries. The mechanism underlying many of these events is unknown, but may represent increased hypotension). Products include:
Aceon Tablets (2 mg, 4 mg, 8 mg) **3191**

Perphenazine (Dopamine antagonists may diminish the effectiveness of apomorphine. Patients with major psychotic disorders, treated with neuroleptics, should be treated with dopamine agonists only if the potential benefits outweigh the risks).
No products indexed under this heading.

Phenoxybenzamine Hydrochloride (The following adverse events were experienced more commonly in patients receiving concomitant antihypertensive medications: hypotension, myocardial infarction, serious pneumonia, serious falls, and bone and joint injuries. The mechanism underlying many of these events is unknown, but may represent increased hypotension). Products include:
Dibenzyline Capsules **3390**

Phentolamine Mesylate (The following adverse events were experienced more commonly in patients receiving concomitant antihypertensive medications: hypotension, myocardial infarction, serious pneumonia, serious falls, and bone and joint injuries. The mechanism underlying many of these events is unknown, but may represent increased hypotension).
No products indexed under this heading.

Pimozide (Dopamine antagonists may diminish the effectiveness of apomorphine. Patients with major psychotic disorders, treated with neuroleptics, should be treated with dopamine agonists only if the potential benefits outweigh the risks). Products include:
Orap Tablets **1220**

Pindolol (The following adverse events were experienced more commonly in patients receiving concomitant antihypertensive medications: hypotension, myocardial infarction, serious pneumonia, serious falls, and bone and joint injuries. The mechanism underlying many of these events is unknown, but may represent increased hypotension).
No products indexed under this heading.

Polythiazide (The following adverse events were experienced more commonly in patients receiving concomitant antihypertensive medications: hypotension, myocardial infarction, serious pneumonia, serious falls, and bone and joint injuries. The mechanism underlying many of these events is unknown, but may represent increased hypotension).
No products indexed under this heading.

Prazosin Hydrochloride (The following adverse events were experienced more commonly in patients receiving concomitant antihypertensive medications: hypotension, myocardial infarction, serious pneumonia, serious falls, and bone and joint injuries. The mechanism underlying many of these events is unknown, but may represent increased hypotension).
No products indexed under this heading.

Procainamide Hydrochloride (Caution should be exercised when prescribing apomorphine concomitantly with drugs that prolong the QT/QTc interval).
No products indexed under this heading.

Prochlorperazine (Dopamine antagonists may diminish the effectiveness of apomorphine. Patients with major psychotic disorders, treated with neuroleptics, should be treated with dopamine agonists only if the potential benefits outweigh the risks).
No products indexed under this heading.

Promethazine Hydrochloride (Dopamine antagonists may diminish the effectiveness of apomorphine. Patients with major psychotic disorders, treated with neuroleptics, should be treated with dopamine agonists only if the potential benefits outweigh the risks). Products include:
Phenergan **3438**

Propafenone Hydrochloride (Caution should be exercised when prescribing apomorphine concomitantly with drugs that prolong the QT/QTc interval). Products include:
Rythmol SR Capsules **2736**

Propranolol Hydrochloride (The following adverse events were experienced more commonly in patients receiving concomitant antihypertensive medications: hypotension, myocardial infarction, serious pneumonia, serious falls, and bone and joint injuries. The mechanism underlying many of these events is unknown, but may represent increased hypotension). Products include:
Inderal LA Long-Acting Capsules **3421**
InnoPran XL Capsules **2728**

Protriptyline Hydrochloride (Caution should be exercised when prescribing apomorphine concomitantly with drugs that prolong the QT/QTc interval). Products include:
Vivactil Tablets **2350**

Quetiapine Fumarate (Dopamine antagonists may diminish the effectiveness of apomorphine. Patients with major psychotic disorders, treated with neuroleptics, should be treated with dopamine agonists only if the potential benefits outweigh the risks). Products include:
Seroquel Tablets **691**

Quinapril Hydrochloride (The following adverse events were experienced more commonly in patients receiving concomitant antihypertensive medications: hypotension, myocardial infarction, serious pneumonia, serious falls, and bone and joint injuries. The mechanism underlying many of these events is unknown, but may represent increased hypotension).
No products indexed under this heading.

Quinidine Gluconate (Caution should be exercised when prescribing apomorphine concomitantly with drugs that prolong the QT/QTc interval).
No products indexed under this heading.

Quinidine Polygalacturonate (Caution should be exercised when prescribing apomorphine concomitantly with drugs that prolong the QT/QTc interval).
No products indexed under this heading.

Quinidine Sulfate (Caution should be exercised when prescribing apomorphine concomitantly with drugs that prolong the QT/QTc interval).
No products indexed under this heading.

Ramipril (The following adverse events were experienced more commonly in patients receiving concomitant antihypertensive medications: hypotension, myocardial infarction, serious pneumonia, serious falls, and bone and joint injuries. The mechanism underlying many of these events is unknown, but may represent increased hypotension). Products include:
Altace Capsules **1673**

Rauwolfia Serpentina (The following adverse events were experienced more commonly in patients receiving concomitant antihypertensive medications: hypotension, myocardial infarction, serious pneumonia, serious falls, and bone and joint injuries. The mechanism underlying many of these events is unknown, but may represent increased hypotension).
No products indexed under this heading.

Rescinnamine (The following adverse events were experienced more commonly in patients receiving concomitant antihypertensive medications: hypotension, myocardial infarction, serious pneumonia, serious falls, and bone and joint injuries. The mechanism underlying many of these events is unknown, but may represent increased hypotension).
No products indexed under this heading.

Reserpine (The following adverse events were experienced more commonly in patients receiving concomitant antihypertensive medications: hypotension, myocardial infarction, serious pneumonia, serious falls, and bone and joint injuries. The mechanism underlying many of these events is unknown, but may represent increased hypotension).
No products indexed under this heading.

Sodium Nitroprusside (The following adverse events were experienced more commonly in patients receiving concomitant antihypertensive medications: hypotension, myocardial infarction, serious pneumonia, serious falls, and bone and joint injuries. The mechanism underlying many of these events is unknown, but may represent increased hypotension).
No products indexed under this heading.

Sotalol Hydrochloride (The following adverse events were experienced more commonly in patients receiving concomitant antihypertensive medications: hypotension, myocardial infarction, serious pneumonia, serious falls, and bone and joint injuries. The mechanism underlying many of these events is unknown, but may represent increased hypotension).
No products indexed under this heading.

Spirapril Hydrochloride (The following adverse events were experienced more commonly in patients receiving concomitant antihypertensive medications: hypotension, myocardial infarction, serious pneumonia, serious falls, and bone and joint injuries. The mechanism underlying many of these events is unknown, but may represent increased hypotension).
No products indexed under this heading.

Telmisartan (The following adverse events were experienced more commonly in patients receiving concomitant antihypertensive medications: hypotension, myocardial infarction, serious pneumonia, serious falls, and bone and joint injuries. The mechanism underlying many of these events is unknown, but may represent increased hypotension). Products include:
Micardis Tablets **884**
Micardis HCT Tablets **886**

Terazosin Hydrochloride (The following adverse events were experienced more commonly in patients receiving concomitant antihypertensive medications: hypotension, myocardial infarction, serious pneumonia, serious falls, and bone and joint injuries. The mechanism underlying many of these events is unknown, but may represent increased hypotension). Products include:
Hytrin Capsules **469**

Thioridazine Hydrochloride (Dopamine antagonists may diminish the effectiveness of apomorphine. Patients with major psychotic disorders, treated with neuroleptics, should be treated with dopamine agonists only if the potential benefits outweigh the risks). Products include:
Thioridazine Hydrochloride Tablets **2122**

IMPORTANT NOTE: Always consult each drug listing in the patient's regimen for possible interactions.

Timolol Maleate (The following adverse events were experienced more commonly in patients receiving concomitant antihypertensive medications: hypotension, myocardial infarction, serious pneumonia, serious falls, and bone and joint injuries. The mechanism underlying many of these events is unknown, but may represent increased hypotension). Products include:

Blocadren Tablets ... 1891
Cosopt Sterile Ophthalmic Solution ... 1910
Timolide Tablets ... 2056
Timoptic in Ocudose ... 2061
Timoptic Sterile Ophthalmic Solution ... 2058
Timoptic-XE Sterile Ophthalmic Gel Forming Solution ... 2062

Tocainide Hydrochloride (Caution should be exercised when prescribing apomorphine concomitantly with drugs that prolong the QT/QTc interval).

No products indexed under this heading.

Tolazoline Hydrochloride (The following adverse events were experienced more commonly in patients receiving concomitant vasodilators: hypotension, myocardial infarction, serious pneumonia, serious falls, and bone and joint injuries. The mechanism underlying many of these events is unknown, but may represent increased hypotension).

No products indexed under this heading.

Torsemide (The following adverse events were experienced more commonly in patients receiving concomitant antihypertensive medications: hypotension, myocardial infarction, serious pneumonia, serious falls, and bone and joint injuries. The mechanism underlying many of these events is unknown, but may represent increased hypotension).

No products indexed under this heading.

Trandolapril (The following adverse events were experienced more commonly in patients receiving concomitant antihypertensive medications: hypotension, myocardial infarction, serious pneumonia, serious falls, and bone and joint injuries. The mechanism underlying many of these events is unknown, but may represent increased hypotension). Products include:

Mavik Tablets ... 482
Tarka Tablets ... 519

Trifluoperazine Hydrochloride (Dopamine antagonists may diminish the effectiveness of apomorphine. Patients with major psychotic disorders, treated with neuroleptics, should be treated with dopamine agonists only if the potential benefits outweigh the risks).

No products indexed under this heading.

Trimethaphan Camsylate (The following adverse events were experienced more commonly in patients receiving concomitant antihypertensive medications: hypotension, myocardial infarction, serious pneumonia, serious falls, and bone and joint injuries. The mechanism underlying many of these events is unknown, but may represent increased hypotension).

No products indexed under this heading.

Trimipramine Maleate (Caution should be exercised when prescribing apomorphine concomitantly with drugs that prolong the QT/QTc interval). Products include:

Surmontil Capsules ... 2347

Valsartan (The following adverse events were experienced more commonly in patients receiving concomitant antihypertensive medications: hypotension, myocardial infarction, serious pneumonia, serious falls, and bone and joint injuries. The mechanism underlying many of these events is unknown, but may represent increased hypotension). Products include:

Diovan HCT Tablets ... 2195
Diovan Tablets ... 2191

Verapamil Hydrochloride (The following adverse events were experienced more commonly in patients receiving concomitant antihypertensive medications: hypotension, myocardial infarction, serious pneumonia, serious falls, and bone and joint injuries. The mechanism underlying many of these events is unknown, but may represent increased hypotension). Products include:

Covera-HS Tablets ... 3135
Tarka Tablets ... 519
Verelan PM Capsules ... 3120

Ziprasidone Hydrochloride (Caution should be exercised when prescribing apomorphine concomitantly with drugs that prolong the QT/QTc interval). Products include:

Geodon Capsules ... 2514

Food Interactions

Alcohol (The effects of apomorphine on blood pressure may be increased by the concomitant use of alcohol; concurrent use should be avoided).

APPEAREX TABLETS

(Biotin) ... 2095

May interact with phenytoin and certain other agents. Compounds in these categories include:

Antibiotics, unspecified (The use of antibiotics may reduce the contribution of biotin made by bacteria within the large intestine).

No products indexed under this heading.

Carbamazepine (May accelerate biotin metabolism, leading to a reduction in available biotin). Products include:

Carbatrol Capsules ... 3174
Equetro Extended-Release Capsules ... 3178
Tegretol/Tegretol-XR ... 2278

Fosphenytoin Sodium (May accelerate biotin metabolism, leading to a reduction in available biotin).

No products indexed under this heading.

Phenobarbital (May accelerate biotin metabolism, leading to a reduction in available biotin).

No products indexed under this heading.

Phenytoin (May accelerate biotin metabolism, leading to a reduction in available biotin).

No products indexed under this heading.

Phenytoin Sodium (May accelerate biotin metabolism, leading to a reduction in available biotin). Products include:

Phenytek Capsules ... 2153

Primidone (May accelerate biotin metabolism, leading to a reduction in available biotin).

No products indexed under this heading.

APTIVUS CAPSULES

(Tipranavir) ... 859

May interact with ergot-containing drugs, estrogens, oral contraceptives, quinidine, and certain other agents. Compounds in these categories include:

Abacavir Sulfate (Co-administration may decrease abacavir AUC by approximately 40%. Clinical relevance of reduction in abacavir levels has not been established. Dose adjustment of abacavir cannot be recommended at this time). Products include:

Epzicom Tablets ... 1402
Trizivir Tablets ... 1565
Ziagen ... 1600

Amiodarone Hydrochloride (Co-administration is contraindicated due to potential for serious and/or life-threatening reactions, such as cardiac arrhythmias secondary to increases in plasma concentrations of antiarrhythmics). Products include:

Pacerone Tablets ... 3337

Amprenavir (Co-administration may decrease amprenavir levels. Combining amprenavir, lopinavir or saquinavir with tipranavir/ritonavir is not recommended). Products include:

Agenerase Capsules ... 1299
Agenerase Oral Solution ... 1304

Astemizole (Co-administration is contraindicated due to potential for serious and/or life-threatening reactions, such as cardiac arrhythmias).

No products indexed under this heading.

Atorvastatin Calcium (Co-administration may increase tipranavir and/or atorvastatin levels and decrease hydroxy-atorvastatin levels. Start with the lowest possible dose of atorvastatin with careful monitoring or consider other HMG-CoA reductase inhibitors). Products include:

Caduet Tablets ... 2507
Lipitor Tablets ... 2495

Bepridil Hydrochloride (Co-administration is contraindicated due to potential for serious and/or life-threatening reactions, such as cardiac arrhythmias secondary to increases in plasma concentrations of antiarrhythmics).

No products indexed under this heading.

Chlorotrianisene (Co-administration may decrease ethinyl estradiol concentrations by 50%. Alternative methods of non-hormonal contraception should be used when estrogen-based oral contraceptives are co-administered with tipranavir and 200 mg of ritonavir. Patients using estrogens as hormone replacement therapy should be clinically monitored for signs of estrogen deficiency. Women using estrogens may have an increased risk of non serious rash).

No products indexed under this heading.

Cisapride (Co-administration is contraindicated due to potential for serious and/or life-threatening reactions, such as cardiac arrhythmias).

No products indexed under this heading.

Clarithromycin (Co-administration may increase tipranavir and/or clarithromycin levels and decrease 14-hydroxy-clarithromycin metabolite levels. No dose adjustment of tipranavir or clarithromycin for patients with normal renal function is necessary. For patients with renal impairment the following dosage adjustments should be considered: for patients with CrCl 30 - 60 mL/min the dose of clarithromycin should be reduced by 50%; for patients with CrCl < 30 mL/min the dose of clarithromycin should be decreased by 75%). Products include:

Biaxin/Biaxin XL ... 402
PREVPAC ... 3281

Cyclosporine (Co-administration may increase or decrease cyclosporine levels. More frequent concentration monitoring is recommended until blood levels have been stabilized). Products include:

Gengraf Capsules ... 458
Neoral Soft Gelatin Capsules ... 2247
Neoral Oral Solution ... 2247
Restasis Ophthalmic Emulsion ... 570
Sandimmune ... 2259

Desipramine Hydrochloride (Co-administration may lead to increased desipramine levels. Dosage reduction and concentration monitoring of desipramine is recommended).

No products indexed under this heading.

Desogestrel (Alternative methods of non-hormonal contraception should be used when estrogen-based oral contraceptives are co-administered with tipranavir and 200 mg of ritonavir). Products include:

Ortho-Cept Tablets ... 2395

Didanosine (Co-administration may decrease didanosine levels. Clinical relevance of reduction in didanosine levels has not been established. For optimal absorption, didanosine should be separated from tipranavir/ritonavir dosing by at least 2 hours).

No products indexed under this heading.

Dienestrol (Co-administration may decrease ethinyl estradiol concentrations by 50%. Alternative methods of non-hormonal contraception should be used when estrogen-based oral contraceptives are co-administered with tipranavir and 200 mg of ritonavir. Patients using estrogens as hormone replacement therapy should be clinically monitored for signs of estrogen deficiency. Women using estrogens may have an increased risk of non serious rash).

No products indexed under this heading.

Diethylstilbestrol (Co-administration may decrease ethinyl estradiol concentrations by 50%. Alternative methods of non-hormonal contraception should be used when estrogen-based oral contraceptives are co-administered with tipranavir and 200 mg of ritonavir. Patients using estrogens as hormone replacement therapy should be clinically monitored for signs of estrogen deficiency. Women using estrogens may have an increased risk of non

serious rash).
No products indexed under this heading.

Dihydroergotamine Mesylate (Co-administration is contraindicated due to potential for serious and/or life-threatening reactions, such as acute ergot toxicity characterized by peripheral vasospasm and ischemia of the extremities and other tissues). Products include:
Migranal Nasal Spray 3350

Diltiazem Hydrochloride (Co-administration may increase or decrease diltiazem levels. Caution is warranted and monitoring of patients is recommended). Products include:
Cardizem LA Extended Release Tablets 1699
Tiazac Capsules 1204

Diltiazem Maleate (Co-administration may increase or decrease diltiazem levels. Caution is warranted and monitoring of patients is recommended).
No products indexed under this heading.

Disulfiram (Aptivus capsules contain alcohol that can produce disulfiram-like reactions when co-administered with disulfiram or other drugs which produce this reaction). Products include:
Antabuse Tablets 2343

Ergonovine Maleate (Co-administration is contraindicated due to potential for serious and/or life-threatening reactions, such as acute ergot toxicity characterized by peripheral vasospasm and ischemia of the extremities and other tissues).
No products indexed under this heading.

Ergotamine Tartrate (Co-administration is contraindicated due to potential for serious and/or life-threatening reactions, such as acute ergot toxicity characterized by peripheral vasospasm and ischemia of the extremities and other tissues).
No products indexed under this heading.

Estradiol (Co-administration may decrease ethinyl estradiol concentrations by 50%. Alternative methods of non-hormonal contraception should be used when estrogen-based oral contraceptives are co-administered with tipranavir and 200 mg of ritonavir. Patients using estrogens as hormone replacement therapy should be clinically monitored for signs of estrogen deficiency. Women using estrogens may have an increased risk of non serious rash). Products include:
Activella Tablets 2311
Climara Transdermal System 795
Climara Pro Transdermal System 800
CombiPatch Transdermal System 2180
Estrogel 0.06% 3200
Menostar Transdermal System 805
Prefest Tablets 1069
Vagifem Tablets 2340
Vivelle Transdermal System 2288
Vivelle-Dot Transdermal System 2293

Estrogens, Conjugated (Co-administration may decrease ethinyl estradiol concentrations by 50%. Alternative methods of non-hormonal contraception should be used when estrogen-based oral contraceptives are co-administered with tipranavir and 200 mg of ritonavir. Patients using estrogens as hormone replacement therapy should be clinically monitored for signs of estrogen deficiency. Women using estrogens may have an increased risk of non serious rash). Products include:
Premarin Intravenous 3440
Premarin Tablets 3443
Premarin Vaginal Cream 3449
Premphase Tablets 3452
Prempro Tablets 3452

Estrogens, Esterified (Co-administration may decrease ethinyl estradiol concentrations by 50%. Alternative methods of non-hormonal contraception should be used when estrogen-based oral contraceptives are co-administered with tipranavir and 200 mg of ritonavir. Patients using estrogens as hormone replacement therapy should be clinically monitored for signs of estrogen deficiency. Women using estrogens may have an increased risk of non serious rash). Products include:
Estratest Tablets 3196
Estratest H.S. Tablets 3196

Estropipate (Co-administration may decrease ethinyl estradiol concentrations by 50%. Alternative methods of non-hormonal contraception should be used when estrogen-based oral contraceptives are co-administered with tipranavir and 200 mg of ritonavir. Patients using estrogens as hormone replacement therapy should be clinically monitored for signs of estrogen deficiency. Women using estrogens may have an increased risk of non serious rash).
No products indexed under this heading.

Ethinyl Estradiol (Co-administration may decrease ethinyl estradiol concentrations by 50%. Alternative methods of non-hormonal contraception should be used when estrogen-based oral contraceptives are co-administered with tipranavir and 200 mg of ritonavir. Patients using estrogens as hormone replacement therapy should be clinically monitored for signs of estrogen deficiency. Women using estrogens may have an increased risk of non-serious rash). Products include:
Alesse-28 Tablets 3392
Lo/Ovral-28 Tablets 3423
NuvaRing 2357
Ortho-Cept Tablets 2395
Ortho-Cyclen/Ortho Tri-Cyclen 2414
Ortho Evra Transdermal System 2402
Ortho Tri-Cyclen Lo Tablets 2421
Seasonale Tablets 1073
Triphasil-28 Tablets 3483
Yasmin 28 Tablets 818

Ethynodiol Diacetate (Alternative methods of non-hormonal contraception should be used when estrogen-based oral contraceptives are co-administered with tipranavir and 200 mg of ritonavir).
No products indexed under this heading.

Felodipine (Co-administration may increase felodipine levels. Caution is warranted and monitoring of patients is recommended). Products include:
Plendil Extended-Release Tablets 651

Flecainide Acetate (Co-administration is contraindicated due to potential for serious and/or life-threatening reactions, such as cardiac arrhythmias secondary to increases in plasma concentrations of antiarrhythmics). Products include:
Tambocor Tablets 1824

Fluconazole (Co-administration may increase tipranavir levels. Fluconazole increases tipranavir concentrations but dose adjustments are not needed. Fluconazole doses greater than 200 mg/day are not recommended).
No products indexed under this heading.

Fluoxetine (Co-administration may increase fluoxetine levels. Fluoxetine doses may need to be adjusted upon initiation of tipranavir/ritonavir therapy).
No products indexed under this heading.

Fluoxetine Hydrochloride (Co-administration may increase fluoxetine levels. Fluoxetine doses may need to be adjusted upon initiation of tipranavir/ritonavir therapy). Products include:
Prozac Pulvules and Liquid 1771
Symbyax Capsules 1788

Fosamprenavir Calcium (Co-administration may decrease amprenavir levels. Combining amprenavir with tipranavir/ritonavir is not recommended). Products include:
Lexiva Tablets 1473

Glimepiride (Co-administration may increase or decrease glimepiride levels. Careful glucose monitoring is warranted). Products include:
Amaryl Tablets 2864

Glipizide (Co-administration may increase or decrease glipizide levels. Careful glucose monitoring is warranted).
No products indexed under this heading.

Glyburide (Co-administration may increase or decrease glyburide levels. Careful glucose monitoring is warranted).
No products indexed under this heading.

Hypericum (Co-administration may lead to loss of virologic response and possible resistance to tipranavir or to the class of protease inhibitors).
No products indexed under this heading.

Itraconazole (Co-administration may increase itraconazole levels. Based on theoretical considerations itraconazole should be used with caution. High doses (200 mg/day) are not recommended).
No products indexed under this heading.

Ketoconazole (Co-administration may increase ketoconazole levels. Based on theoretical considerations ketoconazole should be used with caution. High doses (200 mg/day) are not recommended). Products include:
Nizoral A-D Shampoo, 1% 1839
Nizoral 2% Shampoo 1838

Levonorgestrel (Alternative methods of non-hormonal contraception should be used when estrogen-based oral contraceptives are co-administered with tipranavir and 200 mg of ritonavir). Products include:
Alesse-28 Tablets 3392
Climara Pro Transdermal System 800
Mirena Intrauterine System 810
Plan B Tablets 1068
Seasonale Tablets 1073
Triphasil-28 Tablets 3483

Lopinavir (Co-administration may decrease lopinavir levels. Combining lopinavir with tipranavir/ritonavir is not recommended). Products include:
Kaletra 474

Lovastatin (Co-administration may lead to potential for serious reactions, such as risk of myopathy including rhabdomyolysis. Concomitant use of tipranavir, coadministered with 200 mg of ritonavir, with lovastatin is not recommended). Products include:
Advicor Tablets 1694
Altoprev Extended-Release Tablets 1151
Mevacor Tablets 1996

Meperidine Hydrochloride (Co-administration may decrease meperidine levels and increase normeperidine levels. Dosage increase and long-term use of meperidine are not recommended due to increased concentrations of the metabolite normeperidine which has both analgesic activity and CNS stimulant activity (eg, seizures)).
No products indexed under this heading.

Mestranol (Alternative methods of non-hormonal contraception should be used when estrogen-based oral contraceptives are co-administered with tipranavir and 200 mg of ritonavir).
No products indexed under this heading.

Methadone Hydrochloride (Co-administration may decrease methadone levels by 50%. Dosage of methadone may need to be increased when co-administered with tipranavir and 200 mg of ritonavir).
No products indexed under this heading.

Methylergonovine Maleate (Co-administration is contraindicated due to potential for serious and/or life-threatening reactions, such as acute ergot toxicity characterized by peripheral vasospasm and ischemia of the extremities and other tissues).
No products indexed under this heading.

Methysergide Maleate (Co-administration is contraindicated due to potential for serious and/or life-threatening reactions, such as acute ergot toxicity characterized by peripheral vasospasm and ischemia of the extremities and other tissues).
No products indexed under this heading.

Metronidazole (Aptivus capsules contain alcohol that can produce disulfiram-like reactions when co-administered with metronidazole or other drugs which produce this reaction). Products include:
Metrogel 1% 1212
MetroGel-Vaginal Gel 1822
Noritate Cream, 1% 1051

Metronidazole Benzoate (Aptivus capsules contain alcohol that can produce disulfiram-like reactions when co-administered with metronidazole or other drugs which produce this reaction).
No products indexed under this heading.

Metronidazole Hydrochloride (Aptivus capsules contain alcohol that can produce disulfiram-like reactions when co-administered with metronidazole or other drugs which produce this reaction).
No products indexed under this heading.

IMPORTANT NOTE: Always consult each drug listing in the patient's regimen for possible interactions.

Metronidazole Sodium (Aptivus capsules contain alcohol that can produce disulfiram-like reactions when co-administered with metronidazole or other drugs which produce this reaction).
No products indexed under this heading.

Midazolam Hydrochloride (Co-administration is contraindicated due to potential for serious and/or life-threatening reactions, such as prolonged or increased sedation or respiratory depression).
No products indexed under this heading.

Nicardipine (Co-administration may increase or decrease nicardipine levels. Caution is warranted and monitoring of patients is recommended).
No products indexed under this heading.

Nicardipine Hydrochloride (Co-administration may increase or decrease nicardipine levels. Caution is warranted and monitoring of patients is recommended). Products include:
Cardene I.V. 1129

Nisoldipine (Co-administration may increase or decrease nisoldipine levels. Caution is warranted and monitoring of patients is recommended). Products include:
Sular Tablets 1163

Norethindrone (Alternative methods of non-hormonal contraception should be used when estrogen-based oral contraceptives are co-administered with tipranavir and 200 mg of ritonavir). Products include:
Ortho Micronor Tablets 2411

Norethynodrel (Alternative methods of non-hormonal contraception should be used when estrogen-based oral contraceptives are co-administered with tipranavir and 200 mg of ritonavir).
No products indexed under this heading.

Norgestimate (Alternative methods of non-hormonal contraception should be used when estrogen-based oral contraceptives are co-administered with tipranavir and 200 mg of ritonavir). Products include:
Ortho-Cyclen/Ortho Tri-Cyclen 2414
Ortho Tri-Cyclen Lo Tablets 2421
Prefest Tablets 1069

Norgestrel (Alternative methods of non-hormonal contraception should be used when estrogen-based oral contraceptives are co-administered with tipranavir and 200 mg of ritonavir). Products include:
Lo/Ovral-28 Tablets 3423

Paroxetine Hydrochloride (Co-administration may increase paroxetine levels. Paroxetine doses may need to be adjusted upon initiation of tipranavir/ritonavir therapy). Products include:
Paxil CR Controlled-Release Tablets 1509
Paxil 1501

Paroxetine Mesylate (Co-administration may increase paroxetine levels. Paroxetine doses may need to be adjusted upon initiation of tipranavir/ritonavir therapy).
No products indexed under this heading.

Pimozide (Co-administration is contraindicated due to potential for serious and/or life-threatening reactions, such as cardiac arrhythmias). Products include:
Orap Tablets 1220

Pioglitazone Hydrochloride (Co-administration may increase or decrease pioglitazone levels. Careful glucose monitoring is warranted). Products include:
ActoPlus Met Tablets 3219
Actos Tablets 3224

Polyestradiol Phosphate (Co-administration may decrease ethinyl estradiol concentrations by 50%. Alternative methods of non-hormonal contraception should be used when estrogen-based oral contraceptives are co-administered with tipranavir and 200 mg of ritonavir. Patients using estrogens as hormone replacement therapy should be clinically monitored for signs of estrogen deficiency. Women using estrogens may have an increased risk of non serious rash).
No products indexed under this heading.

Propafenone Hydrochloride (Co-administration is contraindicated due to potential for serious and/or life-threatening reactions, such as cardiac arrhythmias secondary to increases in plasma concentrations of antiarrhythmics). Products include:
Rythmol SR Capsules 2736

Quinestrol (Co-administration may decrease ethinyl estradiol concentrations by 50%. Alternative methods of non-hormonal contraception should be used when estrogen-based oral contraceptives are co-administered with tipranavir and 200 mg of ritonavir. Patients using estrogens as hormone replacement therapy should be clinically monitored for signs of estrogen deficiency. Women using estrogens may have an increased risk of non serious rash).
No products indexed under this heading.

Quinidine (Co-administration is contraindicated due to potential for serious and/or life-threatening reactions, such as cardiac arrhythmias secondary to increases in plasma concentrations of antiarrhythmics).
No products indexed under this heading.

Quinidine Gluconate (Co-administration is contraindicated due to potential for serious and/or life-threatening reactions, such as cardiac arrhythmias secondary to increases in plasma concentrations of antiarrhythmics).
No products indexed under this heading.

Quinidine Hydrochloride (Co-administration is contraindicated due to potential for serious and/or life-threatening reactions, such as cardiac arrhythmias secondary to increases in plasma concentrations of antiarrhythmics).
No products indexed under this heading.

Quinidine Polygalacturonate (Co-administration is contraindicated due to potential for serious and/or life-threatening reactions, such as cardiac arrhythmias secondary to increases in plasma concentrations of antiarrhythmics).
No products indexed under this heading.

Quinidine Sulfate (Co-administration is contraindicated due to potential for serious and/or life-threatening reactions, such as cardiac arrhythmias secondary to increases in plasma concentrations of antiarrhythmics).
No products indexed under this heading.

Repaglinide (Co-administration may increase or decrease repaglinide levels. Careful glucose monitoring is warranted). Products include:
Prandin Tablets (0.5, 1, and 2 mg) 2337

Rifabutin (Co-administration may increase levels of rifabutin and desacetyl-rifabutin. Dosage reductions of rifabutin by 75% are recommended (eg. 150 mg every other day). Increased monitoring for adverse events in patients receiving the combination is warranted. Further dosage reduction may be necessary).
No products indexed under this heading.

Rifampin (Co-administration may lead to loss of virologic response and possible resistance to tipranavir or to the class of protease inhibitors).
No products indexed under this heading.

Saquinavir (Co-administration may decrease saquinavir levels. Combining saquinavir with tipranavir/ritonavir is not recommended).
No products indexed under this heading.

Saquinavir Mesylate (Co-administration may decrease saquinavir levels. Combining saquinavir with tipranavir/ritonavir is not recommended). Products include:
Invirase 2776

Sertraline Hydrochloride (Co-administration may increase sertraline levels. Sertraline doses may need to be adjusted upon initiation of tipranavir/ritonavir therapy). Products include:
Zoloft 2581

Sildenafil Citrate (Co-administration may increase sildenafil levels. Concomitant use of PDE5 inhibitors with tipranavir and ritonavir should be used with caution and in no case should the starting dose of sildenafil exceed 25 mg within 48 hours). Products include:
Revatio Tablets 2541
Viagra Tablets 2552

Simvastatin (Co-administration may lead to potential for serious reactions, such as risk of myopathy including rhabdomyolysis. Concomitant use of tipranavir, co-administered with 200 mg of ritonavir, with simvastatin is not recommended). Products include:
Vytorin 10/10 Tablets 2084
Vytorin 10/10 Tablets 3092
Vytorin 10/20 Tablets 2084
Vytorin 10/20 Tablets 3092
Vytorin 10/40 Tablets 3092
Vytorin 10/40 Tablets 2084
Vytorin 10/80 Tablets 2084
Vytorin 10/80 Tablets 3092
Zocor Tablets 2078

Sirolimus (Co-administration may increase or decrease cyclosporine levels. More frequent concentration monitoring is recommended until blood levels have been stabilized). Products include:
Rapamune Oral Solution and Tablets 3472

Tacrolimus (Co-administration may increase or decrease cyclosporine levels. More frequent concentration monitoring is recommended until blood levels have been stabilized). Products include:
Prograf Capsules and Injection 624
Protopic Ointment 629

Tadalafil (Co-administration may increase tadalafil levels. Concomitant use of PDE5 inhibitors with tipranavir and ritonavir should be used with caution and in no case should the starting dose of tadalafil exceed 10 mg every 72 hours). Products include:
Cialis Tablets 1806

Terfenadine (Co-administration is contraindicated due to potential for serious and/or life-threatening reactions, such as cardiac arrhythmias).
No products indexed under this heading.

Tolbutamide (Co-administration may increase or decrease tolbutamide levels. Careful glucose monitoring is warranted).
No products indexed under this heading.

Tolbutamide Sodium (Co-administration may increase or decrease tolbutamide levels. Careful glucose monitoring is warranted).
No products indexed under this heading.

Triazolam (Co-administration is contraindicated due to potential for serious and/or life-threatening reactions, such as prolonged or increased sedation or respiratory depression).
No products indexed under this heading.

Vardenafil Hydrochloride (Co-administration may increase vardenafil levels. Concomitant use of PDE5 inhibitors with tipranavir and ritonavir should be used with caution and in no case should the starting dose of vardenafil exceed 2.5 mg every 72 hours). Products include:
Levitra Tablets 3048

Verapamil Hydrochloride (Co-administration may increase or decrease verapamil levels. Caution is warranted and monitoring of patients is recommended). Products include:
Covera-HS Tablets 3135
Tarka Tablets 519
Verelan PM Capsules 3120

Voriconazole (Co-administration may increase or decrease voriconazole levels. Due to multiple enzymes involved with voriconazole metabolism, it is difficult to predict the interaction). Products include:
VFEND I.V. 2543
VFEND Oral Suspension 2543
VFEND Tablets 2543

Warfarin Sodium (Frequent INR monitoring upon initiation of tipranavir/ritonavir therapy is recommended). Products include:
Coumadin for Injection 932
Coumadin Tablets 932

Zidovudine (Co-administration may decrease zidovudine AUC by approximately 35%. Clinical relevance of reduction in zidovudine levels has not been established. Dose adjustment of zidovudine cannot be recommended at this time). Products include:
Combivir Tablets 1373
Retrovir 1533

Retrovir IV Infusion 1537
Trizivir Tablets 1565

AQUACEL AG WITH HYDROFIBER

(Silver impregnated antimicrobial dressing).. 1035
None cited in PDR database.

AQUAMEPHYTON INJECTION

(Vitamin K_1) 1887
May interact with oral anticoagulants. Compounds in these categories include:

Anisindione (Temporary resistance to anticoagulants). Products include:
Miradon Tablets 3056

Dicumarol (Temporary resistance to anticoagulants).
No products indexed under this heading.

Warfarin Sodium (Temporary resistance to anticoagulants). Products include:
Coumadin for Injection 932
Coumadin Tablets 932

ARALAST

(Alpha$_1$-Proteinase Inhibitor (Human)).. 745
None cited in PDR database.

ARAMINE INJECTION

(Metaraminol Bitartrate) 1889
May interact with cardiac glycosides, monoamine oxidase inhibitors, tricyclic antidepressants, and certain other agents. Compounds in these categories include:

Amitriptyline Hydrochloride (Potentiates pressor effect).
No products indexed under this heading.

Amoxapine (Potentiates pressor effect).
No products indexed under this heading.

Clomipramine Hydrochloride (Potentiates pressor effect).
No products indexed under this heading.

Desipramine Hydrochloride (Potentiates pressor effect).
No products indexed under this heading.

Deslanoside (May cause ectopic arrhythmic reaction).
No products indexed under this heading.

Digitalis Glycoside Preparations (May cause ectopic arrhythmic reaction).
No products indexed under this heading.

Digitoxin (May cause ectopic arrhythmic reaction).
No products indexed under this heading.

Digoxin (May cause ectopic arrhythmic reaction). Products include:
Digitek Tablets 2146
Lanoxicaps Capsules 1458
Lanoxin Injection 1462
Lanoxin Tablets 1468
Lanoxin Injection Pediatric 1465

Doxepin Hydrochloride (Potentiates pressor effect).
No products indexed under this heading.

Halothane (Concurrent use should be avoided).
No products indexed under this heading.

Imipramine Hydrochloride (Potentiates pressor effect).
No products indexed under this heading.

Imipramine Pamoate (Potentiates pressor effect).
No products indexed under this heading.

Isocarboxazid (Potentiates pressor effect).
No products indexed under this heading.

Maprotiline Hydrochloride (Potentiates pressor effect).
No products indexed under this heading.

Moclobemide (Potentiates pressor effect).
No products indexed under this heading.

Nortriptyline Hydrochloride (Potentiates pressor effect).
No products indexed under this heading.

Pargyline Hydrochloride (Potentiates pressor effect).
No products indexed under this heading.

Phenelzine Sulfate (Potentiates pressor effect).
No products indexed under this heading.

Procarbazine Hydrochloride (Potentiates pressor effect). Products include:
Matulane Capsules 3188

Protriptyline Hydrochloride (Potentiates pressor effect). Products include:
Vivactil Tablets 2350

Selegiline Hydrochloride (Potentiates pressor effect). Products include:
Eldepryl Capsules 3209

Tranylcypromine Sulfate (Potentiates pressor effect). Products include:
Parnate Tablets 1499

Trimipramine Maleate (Potentiates pressor effect). Products include:
Surmontil Capsules 2347

ARANESP FOR INJECTION

(Darbepoetin alfa) 576
None cited in PDR database.

ARAVA TABLETS

(Leflunomide) 2881
May interact with:

Charcoal, Activated (Co-administration has resulted in a rapid and significant decrease in plasma M1 (the active metabolite of leflunomide) concentration).
No products indexed under this heading.

Cholestyramine (Co-administration has resulted in a rapid and significant decrease in plasma M1 (the active metabolite of leflunomide) concentration).
No products indexed under this heading.

Diclofenac Potassium (In vitro co-administration has resulted in an increase in free fraction of diclofenac; the clinical significance is unknown). Products include:
Cataflam Tablets 2173

Diclofenac Sodium (In vitro co-administration has resulted in an increase in free fraction of diclofenac; the clinical significance is unknown). Products include:
Arthrotec Tablets 3126
Voltaren Ophthalmic Solution 2300
Voltaren Tablets 2298
Voltaren-XR Tablets 2301

Hepatotoxic Drugs, unspecified (Leflunomide treatment is associated with elevations of liver enzymes; co-adminstration may increase the risk of hepatotoxicity).
No products indexed under this heading.

Ibuprofen (In vitro co-administration has resulted in an increase in free fraction of ibuprofen; the clinical significance is unknown). Products include:
Advil Allergy Sinus Caplets 737
Advil 737
Children's Advil Suspension 742
Children's Advil Chewable Tablets .. 741
Advil Cold & Sinus 739
Advil Flu & Body Ache Caplets 739
Children's Advil Cold Suspension ... 741
Infants' Advil Concentrated Drops .. 743
Junior Strength Advil Swallow Tablets.. 740
Advil Migraine Liquigels 740
Advil Multi-Symptom Cold Caplets...................................... 738
Combunox Tablets 1183
Children's Motrin Oral Suspension and Chewable Tablets.................. 1837
Children's Motrin Cold Non-Staining Dye-Free Oral Suspension 1838
Children's Motrin Cold Oral Suspension 1838
Children's Motrin Non-Staining Dye-Free Oral Suspension............ 1837
Motrin Cold & Sinus Caplets 1836
Motrin IB Tablets and Caplets 1836
Infants' Motrin Concentrated Drops.. 1837
Infants' Motrin Non-Staining Dye-Free Drops........................... 1837
Junior Strength Motrin Caplets and Chewable Tablets.................. 1837
Vicoprofen Tablets 533

Methotrexate Sodium (Co-administration increases the risk of hepatotoxicity; concurrent use has not demonstrated any pharmacokinetic interaction).
No products indexed under this heading.

Rifampin (Co-administration has resulted in increased M1 peak levels).
No products indexed under this heading.

Tolbutamide (In vitro co-administration has resulted in an increase in free fraction of tolbutamide).
No products indexed under this heading.

Warfarin Sodium (Increased INR when leflunomide and warfarin were co-administered has been rarely reported). Products include:
Coumadin for Injection 932
Coumadin Tablets 932

AREDIA FOR INJECTION

(Pamidronate Disodium) 2168
May interact with:

Nephrotoxic Drugs (Co-administration with nephrotoxic drugs requires caution due to the risk of clinically significant deterioration in renal function with the use of Aredia).
No products indexed under this heading.

ARGATROBAN INJECTION

(Argatroban) 1321
May interact with anticoagulants, thrombolytics, and certain other agents. Compounds in these categories include:

Alteplase (Co-administration with thrombolytic agents may increase the risk of bleeding). Products include:
Activase I.V. 1225
Cathflo Activase 1232

Anisindione (Co-administration with other anticoagulants may increase the risk of bleeding). Products include:
Miradon Tablets 3056

Anistreplase (Co-administration with thrombolytic agents may increase the risk of bleeding).
No products indexed under this heading.

Ardeparin Sodium (Co-administration with other anticoagulants may increase the risk of bleeding).
No products indexed under this heading.

Aspirin (Co-administration with antiplatelet agents, such as aspirin, may increase the risk of bleeding). Products include:
Aggrenox Capsules 855
Bayer, Aspirin Regimen 606
Bayer Aspirin Tablets 3515
BC Powder 612
BC Allergy Sinus Cold Powder 612
Arthritis Strength BC Powder 612
BC Sinus Cold Powder 612
Ecotrin Enteric Coated Aspirin Low, Regular and Maximum Strength Tablets.......................... 1627
Goody's Body Pain Formula Powder.. 621
Goody's Extra Strength Headache Powder........................ 621
Goody's Extra Strength Pain Relief Tablets 621
Percodan Tablets 1115
St. Joseph 81 mg Aspirin Chewable and Enteric Coated Tablets 1841

Clopidogrel Bisulfate (Co-administration with antiplatelet agents may increase the risk of bleeding). Products include:
Plavix Tablets 940
Plavix Tablets 2942

Dalteparin Sodium (Co-administration with other anticoagulants may increase the risk of bleeding). Products include:
Fragmin Injection 2638

Danaparoid Sodium (Co-administration with other anticoagulants may increase the risk of bleeding).
No products indexed under this heading.

Dicumarol (Co-administration with other anticoagulants may increase the risk of bleeding).
No products indexed under this heading.

Dipyridamole (Co-administration with antiplatelet agents may increase the risk of bleeding). Products include:
Aggrenox Capsules 855
Persantine Tablets 898

Enoxaparin Sodium (Co-administration with other anticoagulants may increase the risk of bleeding). Products include:
Lovenox Injection 2931

Fondaparinux Sodium (Co-administration with other anticoagulants may increase the risk of bleeding). Products include:
Arixtra Injection 1325

Heparin Calcium (Co-administration with other anticoagulants may increase the risk of bleeding).
No products indexed under this heading.

Heparin Sodium (Co-administration with other anticoagulants may increase the risk of bleeding).
No products indexed under this heading.

Low Molecular Weight Heparins (Co-administration with other anticoagulants may increase the risk of bleeding).
No products indexed under this heading.

Reteplase (Co-administration with thrombolytic agents may increase the risk of bleeding). Products include:
Retavase 1131

Streptokinase (Co-administration with thrombolytic agents may increase the risk of bleeding).
No products indexed under this heading.

Tinzaparin Sodium (Co-administration with other anticoagulants may increase the risk of bleeding).
No products indexed under this heading.

Urokinase (Co-administration with thrombolytic agents may increase the risk of bleeding).
No products indexed under this heading.

Warfarin Sodium (Co-administration with other anticoagulants may increase the risk of bleeding). Products include:
Coumadin for Injection 932
Coumadin Tablets 932

ARICEPT TABLETS

(Donepezil Hydrochloride) 1086
May interact with anticholinergics, cytochrome p450 2d6 inducers (selected), cytochrome p450 3a4 inducers (selected), dexamethasone, non-steroidal anti-inflammatory agents, phenytoin, quinidine, and certain other agents. Compounds in these categories include:

Allium sativum (Inducers of CYP3A4 could increase the rate of elimination of donepezil).
No products indexed under this heading.

Aprepitant (Inducers of CYP3A4 could increase the rate of elimination of donepezil). Products include:
Emend Capsules 1944

Atropine Sulfate (Donepezil, a cholinesterase inhibitor, has the potential to interfere with the activity of anticholinergic medications).
No products indexed under this heading.

Belladonna Alkaloids (Donepezil, a cholinesterase inhibitor, has the potential to interfere with the activity of anticholinergic medications). Products include:
Hyland's Teething Tablets .... ■736

Benztropine Mesylate (Donepezil, a cholinesterase inhibitor, has the potential to interfere with the activity of anticholinergic medications). Products include:
Cogentin Injection 1903

Betamethasone Acetate (Inducers of CYP3A4 could increase the rate of elimination of donepezil).
No products indexed under this heading.

Betamethasone Sodium Phosphate (Inducers of CYP3A4 could increase the rate of elimination of donepezil).
No products indexed under this heading.

Bethanechol Chloride (Potential for synergistic effect). Products include:
Urecholine Tablets 2349

Biperiden Hydrochloride (Donepezil, a cholinesterase inhibitor, has the potential to interfere with the activity of anticholinergic medications).
No products indexed under this heading.

Carbamazepine (Inducers of CYP2D6 and CYP3A4, such as carbamazepine, could increase the rate of elimination of donepezil). Products include:
Carbatrol Capsules 3174
Equetro Extended-Release Capsules 3178
Tegretol/Tegretol-XR 2278

Celecoxib (Cholinesterase inhibitors, such as donepezil, may be expected to increase gastric acid secretion due to increased cholinergic activity, therefore, patients on concurrent NSAID therapy should be monitored closely for increased risk of developing ulcers or symptoms of active or occult gastrointestinal bleeding). Products include:
Celebrex Capsules 3130

Ciprofloxacin Hydrochloride (Inducers of CYP3A4 could increase the rate of elimination of donepezil). Products include:
Ciloxan Ophthalmic Ointment 554
Cipro Tablets 2991

Cisplatin (Inducers of CYP3A4 could increase the rate of elimination of donepezil).
No products indexed under this heading.

Clidinium Bromide (Donepezil, a cholinesterase inhibitor, has the potential to interfere with the activity of anticholinergic medications).
No products indexed under this heading.

Cortisone Acetate (Inducers of CYP3A4 could increase the rate of elimination of donepezil).
No products indexed under this heading.

Dexamethasone (Inducers of CYP2D6 and CYP3A4, such as dexamethasone, could increase the rate of elimination of donepezil). Products include:
Ciprodex Otic Suspension 555
Decadron Tablets 1929
TobraDex Ophthalmic Ointment 558
TobraDex Ophthalmic Suspension 558

Dexamethasone Acetate (Inducers of CYP2D6 and CYP3A4, such as dexamethasone, could increase the rate of elimination of donepezil).
No products indexed under this heading.

Dexamethasone Sodium Phosphate (Inducers of CYP2D6 and CYP3A4, such as dexamethasone, could increase the rate of elimination of donepezil). Products include:
Decadron Phosphate Injection 1931

Diclofenac Potassium (Cholinesterase inhibitors, such as donepezil, may be expected to increase gastric acid secretion due to increased cholinergic activity, therefore, patients on concurrent NSAID therapy should be monitored closely for increased risk of developing ulcers or symptoms of active or occult gastrointestinal bleeding). Products include:
Cataflam Tablets 2173

Diclofenac Sodium (Cholinesterase inhibitors, such as donepezil, may be expected to increase gastric acid secretion due to increased cholinergic activity, therefore, patients on concurrent NSAID therapy should be monitored closely for increased risk of developing ulcers or symptoms of active or occult gastrointestinal bleeding). Products include:
Arthrotec Tablets 3126
Voltaren Ophthalmic Solution 2300
Voltaren Tablets 2298
Voltaren-XR Tablets 2301

Dicyclomine Hydrochloride (Donepezil, a cholinesterase inhibitor, has the potential to interfere with the activity of anticholinergic medications). Products include:
Bentyl Capsules 724
Bentyl Injection 724
Bentyl Syrup 724
Bentyl Tablets 724

Doxorubicin Hydrochloride (Inducers of CYP3A4 could increase the rate of elimination of donepezil). Products include:
Adriamycin for Injection, USP 786
Adriamycin Injection, USP 786

Efavirenz (Inducers of CYP3A4 could increase the rate of elimination of donepezil). Products include:
Sustiva Capsules 957

Ethanol (Inducers of CYP2D6 could increase the rate of elimination of donepezil).
No products indexed under this heading.

Ethosuximide (Inducers of CYP3A4 could increase the rate of elimination of donepezil).
No products indexed under this heading.

Etodolac (Cholinesterase inhibitors, such as donepezil, may be expected to increase gastric acid secretion due to increased cholinergic activity, therefore, patients on concurrent NSAID therapy should be monitored closely for increased risk of developing ulcers or symptoms of active or occult gastrointestinal bleeding).
No products indexed under this heading.

Felbamate (Inducers of CYP3A4 could increase the rate of elimination of donepezil).
No products indexed under this heading.

Fenoprofen Calcium (Cholinesterase inhibitors, such as donepezil, may be expected to increase gastric acid secretion due to increased cholinergic activity, therefore, patients on concurrent NSAID therapy should be monitored closely for increased risk of developing ulcers or symptoms of active or occult gastrointestinal bleeding). Products include:
Nalfon Capsules 2504

Fludrocortisone Acetate (Inducers of CYP3A4 could increase the rate of elimination of donepezil).
No products indexed under this heading.

Flurbiprofen (Cholinesterase inhibitors, such as donepezil, may be expected to increase gastric acid secretion due to increased cholinergic activity, therefore, patients on concurrent NSAID therapy should be monitored closely for increased risk of developing ulcers or symptoms of active or occult gastrointestinal bleeding).
No products indexed under this heading.

Fosphenytoin Sodium (Inducers of CYP2D6 and CYP3A4, such as phenytoin, could increase the rate of elimination of donepezil).
No products indexed under this heading.

Garlic Extract (Inducers of CYP3A4 could increase the rate of elimination of donepezil).
No products indexed under this heading.

Garlic Oil (Inducers of CYP3A4 could increase the rate of elimination of donepezil).
No products indexed under this heading.

Glycopyrrolate (Donepezil, a cholinesterase inhibitor, has the potential to interfere with the activity of anticholinergic medications).
No products indexed under this heading.

Hydrocortisone (Inducers of CYP3A4 could increase the rate of elimination of donepezil). Products include:
Cortizone•5 Ointment .... ■699
Cortizone•10 Creme .... ■699
Cortizone•10 Ointment .... ■699
Cortizone•10 Plus Creme .... ■700
Cortizone•10 Maximum Strength Quick Shot Spray .... ■700
Hydrocortone Tablets 1963
Preparation H Hydrocortisone Cream .... ■748

Hydrocortisone Acetate (Inducers of CYP3A4 could increase the rate of elimination of donepezil). Products include:
Analpram-HC 1136
Pramosone 1139
ProctoFoam-HC 3113
Tucks Anti-Itch Ointment .... ■712
U-cort 1% Cream 3289

Hydrocortisone Butyrate (Inducers of CYP3A4 could increase the rate of elimination of donepezil). Products include:
Locoid 1138
Locoid Lipocream Cream 1138

Hydrocortisone Cypionate (Inducers of CYP3A4 could increase the rate of elimination of donepezil).
No products indexed under this heading.

Hydrocortisone Hemisuccinate (Inducers of CYP3A4 could increase the rate of elimination of donepezil).
No products indexed under this heading.

Hydrocortisone Probutate (Inducers of CYP3A4 could increase the rate of elimination of donepezil). Products include:
Pandel Cream, 0.1% 1017

Hydrocortisone Sodium Phosphate (Inducers of CYP3A4 could increase the rate of elimination of donepezil).
No products indexed under this heading.

Hydrocortisone Sodium Succinate (Inducers of CYP3A4 could increase the rate of elimination of donepezil).
No products indexed under this heading.

Hydrocortisone Valerate (Inducers of CYP3A4 could increase the rate of elimination of donepezil).
No products indexed under this heading.

Hyoscyamine (Donepezil, a cholinesterase inhibitor, has the potential to interfere with the activity of anticholinergic medications).
No products indexed under this heading.

Hyoscyamine Sulfate (Donepezil, a cholinesterase inhibitor, has the potential to interfere with the activity of anticholinergic medications).
No products indexed under this heading.

Hypericum (Inducers of CYP3A4 could increase the rate of elimination of donepezil).
No products indexed under this heading.

Hypericum Perforatum (Inducers of CYP3A4 could increase the rate of elimination of donepezil).
No products indexed under this heading.

Ibuprofen (Cholinesterase inhibitors, such as donepezil, may be expected to increase gastric acid secretion due to increased cholinergic activity, therefore, patients on concurrent NSAID therapy should be monitored closely for increased risk of developing ulcers or symptoms of active or occult gastrointestinal bleeding). Products include:
- Advil Allergy Sinus Caplets .... ▣ **737**
- Advil .... ▣ **737**
- Children's Advil Suspension .... ▣ **742**
- Children's Advil Chewable Tablets .. ▣ **741**
- Advil Cold & Sinus .... ▣ **739**
- Advil Flu & Body Ache Caplets .... ▣ **739**
- Children's Advil Cold Suspension ... ▣ **741**
- Infants' Advil Concentrated Drops .. ▣ **743**
- Junior Strength Advil Swallow Tablets .... ▣ **740**
- Advil Migraine Liquigels .... ▣ **740**
- Advil Multi-Symptom Cold Caplets .... ▣ **738**
- Combunox Tablets **1183**
- Children's Motrin Oral Suspension and Chewable Tablets **1837**
- Children's Motrin Cold Non-Staining Dye-Free Oral Suspension **1838**
- Children's Motrin Cold Oral Suspension **1838**
- Children's Motrin Non-Staining Dye-Free Oral Suspension **1837**
- Motrin Cold & Sinus Caplets **1836**
- Motrin IB Tablets and Caplets **1836**
- Infants' Motrin Concentrated Drops **1837**
- Infants' Motrin Non-Staining Dye-Free Drops **1837**
- Junior Strength Motrin Caplets and Chewable Tablets **1837**
- Vicoprofen Tablets **533**

Indomethacin (Cholinesterase inhibitors, such as donepezil, may be expected to increase gastric acid secretion due to increased cholinergic activity, therefore, patients on concurrent NSAID therapy should be monitored closely for increased risk of developing ulcers or symptoms of active or occult gastrointestinal bleeding). Products include:
- Indocin **1968**

Indomethacin Sodium Trihydrate (Cholinesterase inhibitors, such as donepezil, may be expected to increase gastric acid secretion due to increased cholinergic activity, therefore, patients on concurrent NSAID therapy should be monitored closely for increased risk of developing ulcers or symptoms of active or occult gastrointestinal bleeding). Products include:
- Indocin I.V. **1973**

Ipratropium Bromide (Donepezil, a cholinesterase inhibitor, has the potential to interfere with the activity of anticholinergic medications). Products include:
- Atrovent HFA Inhalation Aerosol **872**
- Atrovent Inhalation Solution **868**
- Atrovent Nasal Spray 0.03% **869**
- Atrovent Nasal Spray 0.06% **870**
- Combivent Inhalation Aerosol **878**
- DuoNeb Inhalation Solution **1058**

Ketoconazole (Inhibitors of CYP450, 2D6 and 3A4, such as ketoconazole, inhibit donepezil metabolism in vitro. In a crossover study, ketoconazole increased mean donepezil concentrations by 36%; the clinical relevance is unknown). Products include:
- Nizoral A-D Shampoo, 1% **1839**
- Nizoral 2% Shampoo **1838**

Ketoprofen (Cholinesterase inhibitors, such as donepezil, may be expected to increase gastric acid secretion due to increased cholinergic activity, therefore, patients on concurrent NSAID therapy should be monitored closely for increased risk of developing ulcers or symptoms of active or occult gastrointestinal bleeding).
No products indexed under this heading.

Ketorolac Tromethamine (Cholinesterase inhibitors, such as donepezil, may be expected to increase gastric acid secretion due to increased cholinergic activity, therefore, patients on concurrent NSAID therapy should be monitored closely for increased risk of developing ulcers or symptoms of active or occult gastrointestinal bleeding). Products include:
- Acular Ophthalmic Solution **561**
- Acular LS Ophthalmic Solution **562**

Meclofenamate Sodium (Cholinesterase inhibitors, such as donepezil, may be expected to increase gastric acid secretion due to increased cholinergic activity, therefore, patients on concurrent NSAID therapy should be monitored closely for increased risk of developing ulcers or symptoms of active or occult gastrointestinal bleeding).
No products indexed under this heading.

Mefenamic Acid (Cholinesterase inhibitors, such as donepezil, may be expected to increase gastric acid secretion due to increased cholinergic activity, therefore, patients on concurrent NSAID therapy should be monitored closely for increased risk of developing ulcers or symptoms of active or occult gastrointestinal bleeding).
No products indexed under this heading.

Meloxicam (Cholinesterase inhibitors, such as donepezil, may be expected to increase gastric acid secretion due to increased cholinergic activity, therefore, patients on concurrent NSAID therapy should be monitored closely for increased risk of developing ulcers or symptoms of active or occult gastrointestinal bleeding). Products include:
- Mobic Oral Suspension **893**
- Mobic Tablets **893**

Mepenzolate Bromide (Donepezil, a cholinesterase inhibitor, has the potential to interfere with the activity of anticholinergic medications).
No products indexed under this heading.

Mephenytoin (Inducers of CYP3A4 could increase the rate of elimination of donepezil).
No products indexed under this heading.

Methsuximide (Inducers of CYP3A4 could increase the rate of elimination of donepezil).
No products indexed under this heading.

Methylprednisolone (Inducers of CYP3A4 could increase the rate of elimination of donepezil).
No products indexed under this heading.

Methylprednisolone Acetate (Inducers of CYP3A4 could increase the rate of elimination of donepezil). Products include:
- Depo-Medrol Injectable Suspension **2615**
- Depo-Medrol Single-Dose Vial **2617**

Methylprednisolone Sodium Succinate (Inducers of CYP3A4 could increase the rate of elimination of donepezil).
No products indexed under this heading.

Modafinil (Inducers of CYP3A4 could increase the rate of elimination of donepezil). Products include:
- Provigil Tablets **1002**

Nabumetone (Cholinesterase inhibitors, such as donepezil, may be expected to increase gastric acid secretion due to increased cholinergic activity, therefore, patients on concurrent NSAID therapy should be monitored closely for increased risk of developing ulcers or symptoms of active or occult gastrointestinal bleeding). Products include:
- Relafen Tablets **1523**

Naproxen (Cholinesterase inhibitors, such as donepezil, may be expected to increase gastric acid secretion due to increased cholinergic activity, therefore, patients on concurrent NSAID therapy should be monitored closely for increased risk of developing ulcers or symptoms of active or occult gastrointestinal bleeding). Products include:
- EC-Naprosyn Delayed-Release Tablets **2769**
- Naprosyn Suspension **2769**
- Naprosyn Tablets **2769**
- Prevacid NapraPAC **3277**

Naproxen Sodium (Cholinesterase inhibitors, such as donepezil, may be expected to increase gastric acid secretion due to increased cholinergic activity, therefore, patients on concurrent NSAID therapy should be monitored closely for increased risk of developing ulcers or symptoms of active or occult gastrointestinal bleeding). Products include:
- Aleve Tablets, Caplets and Gelcaps .... ▣ **605**
- Anaprox Tablets **2769**
- Anaprox DS Tablets **2769**

Nevirapine (Inducers of CYP3A4 could increase the rate of elimination of donepezil). Products include:
- Viramune Oral Suspension **903**
- Viramune Tablets **903**

Oxaprozin (Cholinesterase inhibitors, such as donepezil, may be expected to increase gastric acid secretion due to increased cholinergic activity, therefore, patients on concurrent NSAID therapy should be monitored closely for increased risk of developing ulcers or symptoms of active or occult gastrointestinal bleeding).
No products indexed under this heading.

Oxcarbazepine (Inducers of CYP3A4 could increase the rate of elimination of donepezil). Products include:
- Trileptal Oral Suspension **2281**
- Trileptal Tablets **2281**

Oxybutynin Chloride (Donepezil, a cholinesterase inhibitor, has the potential to interfere with the activity of anticholinergic medications). Products include:
- Ditropan XL Extended Release Tablets **2391**

Phenobarbital (Inducers of CYP2D6 and CYP3A4, such as phenobarbital, could increase the rate of elimination of donepezil).
No products indexed under this heading.

Phenobarbital Sodium (Inducers of CYP3A4 could increase the rate of elimination of donepezil).
No products indexed under this heading.

Phenylbutazone (Cholinesterase inhibitors, such as donepezil, may be expected to increase gastric acid secretion due to increased cholinergic activity, therefore, patients on concurrent NSAID therapy should be monitored closely for increased risk of developing ulcers or symptoms of active or occult gastrointestinal bleeding).
No products indexed under this heading.

Phenytoin (Inducers of CYP2D6 and CYP3A4, such as phenytoin, could increase the rate of elimination of donepezil).
No products indexed under this heading.

Phenytoin Sodium (Inducers of CYP2D6 and CYP3A4, such as phenytoin, could increase the rate of elimination of donepezil). Products include:
- Phenytek Capsules **2153**

Piroxicam (Cholinesterase inhibitors, such as donepezil, may be expected to increase gastric acid secretion due to increased cholinergic activity, therefore, patients on concurrent NSAID therapy should be monitored closely for increased risk of developing ulcers or symptoms of active or occult gastrointestinal bleeding).
No products indexed under this heading.

Prednisolone Acetate (Inducers of CYP3A4 could increase the rate of elimination of donepezil). Products include:
- Blephamide Ophthalmic Ointment **563**
- Blephamide Ophthalmic Suspension **564**
- Poly-Pred Liquifilm Ophthalmic Suspension .... ⊙ **231**
- Pred Forte Ophthalmic Suspension .... ⊙ **233**
- Pred Mild Sterile Ophthalmic Suspension .... ⊙ **236**
- Pred-G Ophthalmic Suspension .... ⊙ **234**

IMPORTANT NOTE: Always consult each drug listing in the patient's regimen for possible interactions.

Pred-G Sterile Ophthalmic Ointment ⊙235

Prednisolone Sodium Phosphate (Inducers of CYP3A4 could increase the rate of elimination of donepezil). Products include:

Pediapred Oral Solution 3319

Prednisolone Tebutate (Inducers of CYP3A4 could increase the rate of elimination of donepezil).

No products indexed under this heading.

Prednisone (Inducers of CYP3A4 could increase the rate of elimination of donepezil).

No products indexed under this heading.

Primidone (Inducers of CYP3A4 could increase the rate of elimination of donepezil).

No products indexed under this heading.

Procyclidine Hydrochloride (Donepezil, a cholinesterase inhibitor, has the potential to interfere with the activity of anticholinergic medications).

No products indexed under this heading.

Propantheline Bromide (Donepezil, a cholinesterase inhibitor, has the potential to interfere with the activity of anticholinergic medications).

No products indexed under this heading.

Quinidine (Inhibitors of CYP450, 2D6 and 3A4, such as quinidine, inhibit donepezil metabolism in vitro).

No products indexed under this heading.

Quinidine Gluconate (Inhibitors of CYP450, 2D6 and 3A4, such as quinidine, inhibit donepezil metabolism in vitro).

No products indexed under this heading.

Quinidine Hydrochloride (Inhibitors of CYP450, 2D6 and 3A4, such as quinidine, inhibit donepezil metabolism in vitro).

No products indexed under this heading.

Quinidine Polygalacturonate (Inhibitors of CYP450, 2D6 and 3A4, such as quinidine, inhibit donepezil metabolism in vitro).

No products indexed under this heading.

Quinidine Sulfate (Inhibitors of CYP450, 2D6 and 3A4, such as quinidine, inhibit donepezil metabolism in vitro).

No products indexed under this heading.

Rifabutin (Inducers of CYP3A4 could increase the rate of elimination of donepezil).

No products indexed under this heading.

Rifampicin (Inducers of CYP3A4 could increase the rate of elimination of donepezil).

No products indexed under this heading.

Rifampin (Inducers of CYP2D6 and CYP3A4, such as rifampin, could increase the rate of elimination of donepezil).

No products indexed under this heading.

Rifapentine (Inducers of CYP3A4 could increase the rate of elimination of donepezil).

No products indexed under this heading.

Ritonavir (Inducers of CYP2D6 could increase the rate of elimination of donepezil). Products include:

Kaletra 474
Norvir 499

Rofecoxib (Cholinesterase inhibitors, such as donepezil, may be expected to increase gastric acid secretion due to increased cholinergic activity, therefore, patients on concurrent NSAID therapy should be monitored closely for increased risk of developing ulcers or symptoms of active or occult gastrointestinal bleeding).

No products indexed under this heading.

Scopolamine (Donepezil, a cholinesterase inhibitor, has the potential to interfere with the activity of anticholinergic medications). Products include:

Transderm Scōp Transdermal Therapeutic System 2166

Scopolamine Hydrobromide (Donepezil, a cholinesterase inhibitor, has the potential to interfere with the activity of anticholinergic medications).

No products indexed under this heading.

Succinylcholine Chloride (Potential for synergistic effect).

No products indexed under this heading.

Sulfinpyrazone (Inducers of CYP3A4 could increase the rate of elimination of donepezil).

No products indexed under this heading.

Sulindac (Cholinesterase inhibitors, such as donepezil, may be expected to increase gastric acid secretion due to increased cholinergic activity, therefore, patients on concurrent NSAID therapy should be monitored closely for increased risk of developing ulcers or symptoms of active or occult gastrointestinal bleeding). Products include:

Clinoril Tablets 1899

Theophylline (Inducers of CYP3A4 could increase the rate of elimination of donepezil).

No products indexed under this heading.

Tolmetin Sodium (Cholinesterase inhibitors, such as donepezil, may be expected to increase gastric acid secretion due to increased cholinergic activity, therefore, patients on concurrent NSAID therapy should be monitored closely for increased risk of developing ulcers or symptoms of active or occult gastrointestinal bleeding).

No products indexed under this heading.

Tolterodine Tartrate (Donepezil, a cholinesterase inhibitor, has the potential to interfere with the activity of anticholinergic medications). Products include:

Detrol Tablets 2626
Detrol LA Capsules 2629

Triamcinolone (Inducers of CYP3A4 could increase the rate of elimination of donepezil).

No products indexed under this heading.

Triamcinolone Acetonide (Inducers of CYP3A4 could increase the rate of elimination of donepezil). Products include:

Azmacort Inhalation Aerosol 1701
Nasacort HFA Inhalation Aerosol 2939
Nasacort AQ Nasal Spray 2937

Triamcinolone Diacetate (Inducers of CYP3A4 could increase the rate of elimination of donepezil).

No products indexed under this heading.

Triamcinolone Hexacetonide (Inducers of CYP3A4 could increase the rate of elimination of donepezil).

No products indexed under this heading.

Tridihexethyl Chloride (Donepezil, a cholinesterase inhibitor, has the potential to interfere with the activity of anticholinergic medications).

No products indexed under this heading.

Trihexyphenidyl Hydrochloride (Donepezil, a cholinesterase inhibitor, has the potential to interfere with the activity of anticholinergic medications).

No products indexed under this heading.

Troglitazone (Inducers of CYP3A4 could increase the rate of elimination of donepezil).

No products indexed under this heading.

Valdecoxib (Cholinesterase inhibitors, such as donepezil, may be expected to increase gastric acid secretion due to increased cholinergic activity, therefore, patients on concurrent NSAID therapy should be monitored closely for increased risk of developing ulcers or symptoms of active or occult gastrointestinal bleeding).

No products indexed under this heading.

ARICEPT ODT TABLETS

(Donepezil Hydrochloride) 1086

See Aricept Tablets

ARIMIDEX TABLETS

(Anastrozole) 665

May interact with estrogens and certain other agents. Compounds in these categories include:

Chlorotrianisene (Estrogen-containing therapies should not be used with anastrozole as they may diminish its pharmacologic action).

No products indexed under this heading.

Dienestrol (Estrogen-containing therapies should not be used with anastrozole as they may diminish its pharmacologic action).

No products indexed under this heading.

Diethylstilbestrol (Estrogen-containing therapies should not be used with anastrozole as they may diminish its pharmacologic action).

No products indexed under this heading.

Estradiol (Estrogen-containing therapies should not be used with anastrozole as they may diminish its pharmacologic action). Products include:

Activella Tablets 2311
Climara Transdermal System 795
Climara Pro Transdermal System 800
CombiPatch Transdermal System 2180
Estrogel 0.06% 3200
Menostar Transdermal System 805
Prefest Tablets 1069
Vagifem Tablets 2340
Vivelle Transdermal System 2288
Vivelle-Dot Transdermal System 2293

Estrogens, Conjugated (Estrogen-containing therapies should not be used with anastrozole as they may diminish its pharmacologic action). Products include:

Premarin Intravenous 3440
Premarin Tablets 3443
Premarin Vaginal Cream 3449
Premphase Tablets 3452
Prempro Tablets 3452

Estrogens, Esterified (Estrogen-containing therapies should not be used with anastrozole as they may diminish its pharmacologic action). Products include:

Estratest Tablets 3196
Estratest H.S. Tablets 3196

Estropipate (Estrogen-containing therapies should not be used with anastrozole as they may diminish its pharmacologic action).

No products indexed under this heading.

Ethinyl Estradiol (Estrogen-containing therapies should not be used with anastrozole as they may diminish its pharmacologic action). Products include:

Alesse-28 Tablets 3392
Lo/Ovral-28 Tablets 3423
NuvaRing 2357
Ortho-Cept Tablets 2395
Ortho-Cyclen/Ortho Tri-Cyclen 2414
Ortho Evra Transdermal System 2402
Ortho Tri-Cyclen Lo Tablets 2421
Seasonale Tablets 1073
Triphasil-28 Tablets 3483
Yasmin 28 Tablets 818

Polyestradiol Phosphate (Estrogen-containing therapies should not be used with anastrozole as they may diminish its pharmacologic action).

No products indexed under this heading.

Quinestrol (Estrogen-containing therapies should not be used with anastrozole as they may diminish its pharmacologic action).

No products indexed under this heading.

Tamoxifen Citrate (Co-administration of tamoxifen and anastrozole may reduce anastrozole plasma concentration; avoid co-administration).

No products indexed under this heading.

ARIXTRA INJECTION

(Fondaparinux Sodium) 1325

May interact with anticoagulants, non-steroidal anti-inflammatory agents, and certain other agents. Compounds in these categories include:

Abciximab (Agents that may enhance the risk of hemorrhage, such as abciximab, should be discontinued prior to initiation of fondaparinux sodium therapy. If co-administration is essential, close monitoring may be appropriate). Products include:

ReoPro Vials 1779

Anisindione (Agents that may enhance the risk of hemorrhage, such as anticoagulants, should be discontinued prior to initiation of fondaparinux sodium therapy. If co-administration is essential, close monitoring may be appropriate). Products include:

Miradon Tablets 3056

Ardeparin Sodium (Agents that may enhance the risk of hemorrhage, such as anticoagulants, should be discontinued prior to initiation of fondaparinux sodium therapy. If co-administration is essential, close monitoring may be appropriate).
No products indexed under this heading.

Aspirin (Agents that may enhance the risk of hemorrhage, such as aspirin, should be discontinued prior to initiation of fondaparinux sodium therapy. If co-administration is essential, close monitoring may be appropriate). Products include:
Aggrenox Capsules 855
Bayer, Aspirin Regimen .... ▣606
Bayer Aspirin Tablets 3515
BC Powder .... ▣612
BC Allergy Sinus Cold Powder .... ▣612
Arthritis Strength BC Powder .... ▣612
BC Sinus Cold Powder .... ▣612
Ecotrin Enteric Coated Aspirin Low, Regular and Maximum Strength Tablets 1627
Goody's Body Pain Formula Powder .... ▣621
Goody's Extra Strength Headache Powder .... ▣621
Goody's Extra Strength Pain Relief Tablets .... ▣621
Percodan Tablets 1115
St. Joseph 81 mg Aspirin Chewable and Enteric Coated Tablets 1841

Celecoxib (Agents that may enhance the risk of hemorrhage, such as non-steroidal anti-inflammatory agents, should be discontinued prior to initiation of fondaparinux sodium therapy. If co-administration is essential, close monitoring may be appropriate). Products include:
Celebrex Capsules 3130

Clopidogrel Bisulfate (Agents that may enhance the risk of hemorrhage, such as clopidogrel bisulfate, should be discontinued prior to initiation of fondaparinux sodium therapy. If co-administration is essential, close monitoring may be appropriate). Products include:
Plavix Tablets 940
Plavix Tablets 2942

Dalteparin Sodium (Agents that may enhance the risk of hemorrhage, such as anticoagulants, should be discontinued prior to initiation of fondaparinux sodium therapy. If co-administration is essential, close monitoring may be appropriate). Products include:
Fragmin Injection 2638

Danaparoid Sodium (Agents that may enhance the risk of hemorrhage, such as anticoagulants, should be discontinued prior to initiation of fondaparinux sodium therapy. If co-administration is essential, close monitoring may be appropriate).
No products indexed under this heading.

Diclofenac Potassium (Agents that may enhance the risk of hemorrhage, such as non-steroidal anti-inflammatory agents, should be discontinued prior to initiation of fondaparinux sodium therapy. If co-administration is essential, close monitoring may be appropriate). Products include:
Cataflam Tablets 2173

Diclofenac Sodium (Agents that may enhance the risk of hemorrhage, such as non-steroidal anti-inflammatory agents, should be discontinued prior to initiation of fondaparinux sodium therapy. If co-administration is essential, close monitoring may be appropriate). Products include:
Arthrotec Tablets 3126
Voltaren Ophthalmic Solution 2300
Voltaren Tablets 2298
Voltaren-XR Tablets 2301

Dicumarol (Agents that may enhance the risk of hemorrhage, such as anticoagulants, should be discontinued prior to initiation of fondaparinux sodium therapy. If co-administration is essential, close monitoring may be appropriate).
No products indexed under this heading.

Dipyridamole (Agents that may enhance the risk of hemorrhage, such as dipyridamole, should be discontinued prior to initiation of fondaparinux sodium therapy. If co-administration is essential, close monitoring may be appropriate). Products include:
Aggrenox Capsules 855
Persantine Tablets 898

Enoxaparin Sodium (Agents that may enhance the risk of hemorrhage, such as anticoagulants, should be discontinued prior to initiation of fondaparinux sodium therapy. If co-administration is essential, close monitoring may be appropriate). Products include:
Lovenox Injection 2931

Eptifibatide (Agents that may enhance the risk of hemorrhage, such as eptifibatide, should be discontinued prior to initiation of fondaparinux sodium therapy. If co-administration is essential, close monitoring may be appropriate). Products include:
Integrilin Injection 3034

Etodolac (Agents that may enhance the risk of hemorrhage, such as non-steroidal anti-inflammatory agents, should be discontinued prior to initiation of fondaparinux sodium therapy. If co-administration is essential, close monitoring may be appropriate).
No products indexed under this heading.

Fenoprofen Calcium (Agents that may enhance the risk of hemorrhage, such as non-steroidal anti-inflammatory agents, should be discontinued prior to initiation of fondaparinux sodium therapy. If co-administration is essential, close monitoring may be appropriate). Products include:
Nalfon Capsules 2504

Flurbiprofen (Agents that may enhance the risk of hemorrhage, such as non-steroidal anti-inflammatory agents, should be discontinued prior to initiation of fondaparinux sodium therapy. If co-administration is essential, close monitoring may be appropriate).
No products indexed under this heading.

Heparin Calcium (Agents that may enhance the risk of hemorrhage, such as anticoagulants, should be discontinued prior to initiation of fondaparinux sodium therapy. If co-administration is essential, close monitoring may be appropriate).
No products indexed under this heading.

Heparin Sodium (Agents that may enhance the risk of hemorrhage, such as anticoagulants, should be discontinued prior to initiation of fondaparinux sodium therapy. If co-administration is essential, close monitoring may be appropriate).
No products indexed under this heading.

Ibuprofen (Agents that may enhance the risk of hemorrhage, such as non-steroidal anti-inflammatory agents, should be discontinued prior to initiation of fondaparinux sodium therapy. If co-administration is essential, close monitoring may be appropriate). Products include:
Advil Allergy Sinus Caplets .... ▣737
Advil .... ▣737
Children's Advil Suspension .... ▣742
Children's Advil Chewable Tablets .... ▣741
Advil Cold & Sinus .... ▣739
Advil Flu & Body Ache Caplets .... ▣739
Children's Advil Cold Suspension .... ▣741
Infants' Advil Concentrated Drops .... ▣743
Junior Strength Advil Swallow Tablets .... ▣740
Advil Migraine Liquigels .... ▣740
Advil Multi-Symptom Cold Caplets .... ▣738
Combunox Tablets 1183
Children's Motrin Oral Suspension and Chewable Tablets 1837
Children's Motrin Cold Non-Staining Dye-Free Oral Suspension 1838
Children's Motrin Cold Oral Suspension 1838
Children's Motrin Non-Staining Dye-Free Oral Suspension 1837
Motrin Cold & Sinus Caplets 1836
Motrin IB Tablets and Caplets 1836
Infants' Motrin Concentrated Drops 1837
Infants' Motrin Non-Staining Dye-Free Drops 1837
Junior Strength Motrin Caplets and Chewable Tablets 1837
Vicoprofen Tablets 533

Indomethacin (Agents that may enhance the risk of hemorrhage, such as non-steroidal anti-inflammatory agents, should be discontinued prior to initiation of fondaparinux sodium therapy. If co-administration is essential, close monitoring may be appropriate). Products include:
Indocin 1968

Indomethacin Sodium Trihydrate (Agents that may enhance the risk of hemorrhage, such as non-steroidal anti-inflammatory agents, should be discontinued prior to initiation of fondaparinux sodium therapy. If co-administration is essential, close monitoring may be appropriate). Products include:
Indocin I.V. 1973

Ketoprofen (Agents that may enhance the risk of hemorrhage, such as non-steroidal anti-inflammatory agents, should be discontinued prior to initiation of fondaparinux sodium therapy. If co-administration is essential, close monitoring may be appropriate).
No products indexed under this heading.

Ketorolac Tromethamine (Agents that may enhance the risk of hemorrhage, such as non-steroidal anti-inflammatory agents, should be discontinued prior to initiation of fondaparinux sodium therapy. If co-administration is essential, close monitoring may be appropriate). Products include:
Acular Ophthalmic Solution 561
Acular LS Ophthalmic Solution 562

Low Molecular Weight Heparins (Agents that may enhance the risk of hemorrhage, such as anticoagulants, should be discontinued prior to initiation of fondaparinux sodium therapy. If co-administration is essential, close monitoring may be appropriate).
No products indexed under this heading.

Meclofenamate Sodium (Agents that may enhance the risk of hemorrhage, such as non-steroidal anti-inflammatory agents, should be discontinued prior to initiation of fondaparinux sodium therapy. If co-administration is essential, close monitoring may be appropriate).
No products indexed under this heading.

Mefenamic Acid (Agents that may enhance the risk of hemorrhage, such as non-steroidal anti-inflammatory agents, should be discontinued prior to initiation of fondaparinux sodium therapy. If co-administration is essential, close monitoring may be appropriate).
No products indexed under this heading.

Meloxicam (Agents that may enhance the risk of hemorrhage, such as non-steroidal anti-inflammatory agents, should be discontinued prior to initiation of fondaparinux sodium therapy. If co-administration is essential, close monitoring may be appropriate). Products include:
Mobic Oral Suspension 893
Mobic Tablets 893

Nabumetone (Agents that may enhance the risk of hemorrhage, such as non-steroidal anti-inflammatory agents, should be discontinued prior to initiation of fondaparinux sodium therapy. If co-administration is essential, close monitoring may be appropriate). Products include:
Relafen Tablets 1523

Naproxen (Agents that may enhance the risk of hemorrhage, such as non-steroidal anti-inflammatory agents, should be discontinued prior to initiation of fondaparinux sodium therapy. If co-administration is essential, close monitoring may be appropriate). Products include:
EC-Naprosyn Delayed-Release Tablets 2769
Naprosyn Suspension 2769
Naprosyn Tablets 2769
Prevacid NapraPAC 3277

Naproxen Sodium (Agents that may enhance the risk of hemorrhage, such as non-steroidal anti-inflammatory agents, should be discontinued prior to initiation of fondaparinux sodium therapy. If co-administration is essential, close monitoring may be appropriate). Products include:
Aleve Tablets, Caplets and Gelcaps .... ▣605
Anaprox Tablets 2769
Anaprox DS Tablets 2769

Oxaprozin (Agents that may enhance the risk of hemorrhage, such as non-steroidal anti-inflammatory agents, should be discontinued prior to initiation of fondaparinux sodium therapy. If co-administration is essential, close monitoring may be appropriate).
No products indexed under this heading.

Phenylbutazone (Agents that may enhance the risk of hemorrhage, such as non-steroidal anti-inflammatory agents, should be discontinued prior to initiation of fondaparinux sodium therapy. If co-administration is essential, close monitoring may be appropriate).
No products indexed under this heading.

Piroxicam (Agents that may enhance the risk of hemorrhage, such as non-steroidal anti-inflammatory agents, should be discontinued prior to initiation of fondaparinux sodium therapy. If co-administration is essential, close monitoring may be appropriate).
No products indexed under this heading.

Rofecoxib (Agents that may enhance the risk of hemorrhage, such as non-steroidal anti-inflammatory agents, should be discontinued prior to initiation of fondaparinux sodium therapy. If co-administration is essential, close monitoring may be appropriate).
No products indexed under this heading.

Sulindac (Agents that may enhance the risk of hemorrhage, such as non-steroidal anti-inflammatory agents, should be discontinued prior to initiation of fondaparinux sodium therapy. If co-administration is essential, close monitoring may be appropriate). Products include:
Clinoril Tablets 1899

Tinzaparin Sodium (Agents that may enhance the risk of hemorrhage, such as anticoagulants, should be discontinued prior to initiation of fondaparinux sodium therapy. If co-administration is essential, close monitoring may be appropriate).
No products indexed under this heading.

Tirofiban Hydrochloride (Agents that may enhance the risk of hemorrhage, such as tirofiban hydrochloride, should be discontinued prior to initiation of fondaparinux sodium therapy. If co-administration is essential, close monitoring may be appropriate). Products include:
Aggrastat 1878

Tolmetin Sodium (Agents that may enhance the risk of hemorrhage, such as non-steroidal anti-inflammatory agents, should be discontinued prior to initiation of fondaparinux sodium therapy. If co-administration is essential, close monitoring may be appropriate).
No products indexed under this heading.

Valdecoxib (Agents that may enhance the risk of hemorrhage, such as non-steroidal anti-inflammatory agents, should be discontinued prior to initiation of fondaparinux sodium therapy. If co-administration is essential, close monitoring may be appropriate).
No products indexed under this heading.

Warfarin Sodium (Agents that may enhance the risk of hemorrhage, such as anticoagulants, should be discontinued prior to initiation of fondaparinux sodium therapy. If co-administration is essential, close monitoring may be appropriate). Products include:
Coumadin for Injection 932
Coumadin Tablets 932

AROMASIN TABLETS

(Exemestane) 2600
May interact with cytochrome p450 3a4 inducers (selected) and certain other agents. Compounds in these categories include:

Allium sativum (Co-medications that induce CYP3A4 may significantly decrease exposure to exemestane. Dose modification is recommended for patients receiving a potent CYP3A4 inducer).
No products indexed under this heading.

Aprepitant (Co-medications that induce CYP3A4 may significantly decrease exposure to exemestane. Dose modification is recommended for patients receiving a potent CYP3A4 inducer). Products include:
Emend Capsules 1944

Betamethasone Acetate (Co-medications that induce CYP3A4 may significantly decrease exposure to exemestane. Dose modification is recommended for patients receiving a potent CYP3A4 inducer).
No products indexed under this heading.

Betamethasone Sodium Phosphate (Co-medications that induce CYP3A4 may significantly decrease exposure to exemestane. Dose modification is recommended for patients receiving a potent CYP3A4 inducer).
No products indexed under this heading.

Carbamazepine (Co-medications that induce CYP3A4 may significantly decrease exposure to exemestane. Dose modification is recommended for patients receiving a potent CYP3A4 inducer). Products include:
Carbatrol Capsules 3174
Equetro Extended-Release Capsules 3178
Tegretol/Tegretol-XR 2278

Ciprofloxacin Hydrochloride (Co-medications that induce CYP3A4 may significantly decrease exposure to exemestane. Dose modification is recommended for patients receiving a potent CYP3A4 inducer). Products include:
Ciloxan Ophthalmic Ointment 554
Cipro Tablets 2991

Cisplatin (Co-medications that induce CYP3A4 may significantly decrease exposure to exemestane. Dose modification is recommended for patients receiving a potent CYP3A4 inducer).
No products indexed under this heading.

Cortisone Acetate (Co-medications that induce CYP3A4 may significantly decrease exposure to exemestane. Dose modification is recommended for patients receiving a potent CYP3A4 inducer).
No products indexed under this heading.

Dexamethasone (Co-medications that induce CYP3A4 may significantly decrease exposure to exemestane. Dose modification is recommended for patients receiving a potent CYP3A4 inducer). Products include:
Ciprodex Otic Suspension 555
Decadron Tablets 1929
TobraDex Ophthalmic Ointment 558
TobraDex Ophthalmic Suspension 558

Dexamethasone Acetate (Co-medications that induce CYP3A4 may significantly decrease exposure to exemestane. Dose modification is recommended for patients receiving a potent CYP3A4 inducer).
No products indexed under this heading.

Dexamethasone Sodium Phosphate (Co-medications that induce CYP3A4 may significantly decrease exposure to exemestane. Dose modification is recommended for patients receiving a potent CYP3A4 inducer). Products include:
Decadron Phosphate Injection 1931

Doxorubicin Hydrochloride (Co-medications that induce CYP3A4 may significantly decrease exposure to exemestane. Dose modification is recommended for patients receiving a potent CYP3A4 inducer). Products include:
Adriamycin for Injection, USP 786
Adriamycin Injection, USP 786

Efavirenz (Co-medications that induce CYP3A4 may significantly decrease exposure to exemestane. Dose modification is recommended for patients receiving a potent CYP3A4 inducer). Products include:
Sustiva Capsules 957

Ethosuximide (Co-medications that induce CYP3A4 may significantly decrease exposure to exemestane. Dose modification is recommended for patients receiving a potent CYP3A4 inducer).
No products indexed under this heading.

Felbamate (Co-medications that induce CYP3A4 may significantly decrease exposure to exemestane. Dose modification is recommended for patients receiving a potent CYP3A4 inducer).
No products indexed under this heading.

Fludrocortisone Acetate (Co-medications that induce CYP3A4 may significantly decrease exposure to exemestane. Dose modification is recommended for patients receiving a potent CYP3A4 inducer).
No products indexed under this heading.

Fosphenytoin Sodium (Co-medications that induce CYP3A4 may significantly decrease exposure to exemestane. Dose modification is recommended for patients receiving a potent CYP3A4 inducer).
No products indexed under this heading.

Garlic Extract (Co-medications that induce CYP3A4 may significantly decrease exposure to exemestane. Dose modification is recommended for patients receiving a potent CYP3A4 inducer).
No products indexed under this heading.

Garlic Oil (Co-medications that induce CYP3A4 may significantly decrease exposure to exemestane. Dose modification is recommended for patients receiving a potent CYP3A4 inducer).
No products indexed under this heading.

Hydrocortisone (Co-medications that induce CYP3A4 may significantly decrease exposure to exemestane. Dose modification is recommended for patients receiving a potent CYP3A4 inducer). Products include:
Cortizone•5 Ointment .... ▣699
Cortizone•10 Creme .... ▣699
Cortizone•10 Ointment .... ▣699
Cortizone•10 Plus Creme .... ▣700
Cortizone•10 Maximum Strength Quick Shot Spray .... ▣700
Hydrocortone Tablets 1963
Preparation H Hydrocortisone Cream .... ▣748

Hydrocortisone Acetate (Co-medications that induce CYP3A4 may significantly decrease exposure to exemestane. Dose modification is recommended for patients receiving a potent CYP3A4 inducer). Products include:
Analpram-HC 1136
Pramosone 1139
ProctoFoam-HC 3113
Tucks Anti-Itch Ointment .... ▣712
U-cort 1% Cream 3289

Hydrocortisone Butyrate (Co-medications that induce CYP3A4 may significantly decrease exposure to exemestane. Dose modification is recommended for patients receiving a potent CYP3A4 inducer). Products include:
Locoid 1138
Locoid Lipocream Cream 1138

Hydrocortisone Cypionate (Co-medications that induce CYP3A4 may significantly decrease exposure to exemestane. Dose modification is recommended for patients receiving a potent CYP3A4 inducer).
No products indexed under this heading.

Hydrocortisone Hemisuccinate (Co-medications that induce CYP3A4 may significantly decrease exposure to exemestane. Dose modification is recommended for patients receiving a potent CYP3A4 inducer).
No products indexed under this heading.

Hydrocortisone Probutate (Co-medications that induce CYP3A4 may significantly decrease exposure to exemestane. Dose modification is recommended for patients receiving a potent CYP3A4 inducer). Products include:
Pandel Cream, 0.1% 1017

Hydrocortisone Sodium Phosphate (Co-medications that induce CYP3A4 may significantly decrease exposure to exemestane. Dose modification is recommended for patients receiving a potent CYP3A4 inducer).
No products indexed under this heading.

Hydrocortisone Sodium Succinate (Co-medications that induce CYP3A4 may significantly decrease exposure to exemestane. Dose modification is recommended for patients receiving a potent CYP3A4 inducer).
No products indexed under this heading.

Hydrocortisone Valerate (Co-medications that induce CYP3A4 may significantly decrease exposure to exemestane. Dose modification is recommended for patients receiving a potent CYP3A4 inducer).
No products indexed under this heading.

Hypericum (Co-medications that induce CYP3A4 may significantly decrease exposure to exemestane. Dose modification is recommended for patients receiving a potent CYP3A4 inducer).
No products indexed under this heading.

Hypericum Perforatum (Co-medications that induce CYP3A4 may significantly decrease exposure to exemestane. Dose modification is recommended for patients receiving a potent CYP3A4 inducer).
No products indexed under this heading.

Mephenytoin (Co-medications that induce CYP3A4 may significantly decrease exposure to exemestane. Dose modification is recommended for patients receiving a potent CYP3A4 inducer).
No products indexed under this heading.

Methsuximide (Co-medications that induce CYP3A4 may significantly decrease exposure to exemestane. Dose modification is recommended for patients receiving a potent CYP3A4 inducer).
No products indexed under this heading.

Methylprednisolone (Co-medications that induce CYP3A4 may significantly decrease exposure to exemestane. Dose modification is recommended for patients receiving a potent CYP3A4 inducer).
No products indexed under this heading.

Methylprednisolone Acetate (Co-medications that induce CYP3A4 may significantly decrease exposure to exemestane. Dose modification is recommended for patients receiving a potent CYP3A4 inducer). Products include:
Depo-Medrol Injectable Suspension 2615
Depo-Medrol Single-Dose Vial 2617

Methylprednisolone Sodium Succinate (Co-medications that induce CYP3A4 may significantly decrease exposure to exemestane. Dose modification is recommended for patients receiving a potent CYP3A4 inducer).
No products indexed under this heading.

Modafinil (Co-medications that induce CYP3A4 may significantly decrease exposure to exemestane. Dose modification is recommended for patients receiving a potent CYP3A4 inducer). Products include:
Provigil Tablets 1002

Nevirapine (Co-medications that induce CYP3A4 may significantly decrease exposure to exemestane. Dose modification is recommended for patients receiving a potent CYP3A4 inducer). Products include:
Viramune Oral Suspension 903
Viramune Tablets 903

Oxcarbazepine (Co-medications that induce CYP3A4 may significantly decrease exposure to exemestane. Dose modification is recommended for patients receiving a potent CYP3A4 inducer). Products include:
Trileptal Oral Suspension 2281
Trileptal Tablets 2281

Phenobarbital (Co-medications that induce CYP3A4 may significantly decrease exposure to exemestane. Dose modification is recommended for patients receiving a potent CYP3A4 inducer).
No products indexed under this heading.

Phenobarbital Sodium (Co-medications that induce CYP3A4 may significantly decrease exposure to exemestane. Dose modification is recommended for patients receiving a potent CYP3A4 inducer).
No products indexed under this heading.

Phenytoin (Co-medications that induce CYP3A4 may significantly decrease exposure to exemestane. Dose modification is recommended for patients receiving a potent CYP3A4 inducer).
No products indexed under this heading.

Phenytoin Sodium (Co-medications that induce CYP3A4 may significantly decrease exposure to exemestane. Dose modification is recommended for patients receiving a potent CYP3A4 inducer). Products include:
Phenytek Capsules 2153

Prednisolone Acetate (Co-medications that induce CYP3A4 may significantly decrease exposure to exemestane. Dose modification is recommended for patients receiving a potent CYP3A4 inducer). Products include:
Blephamide Ophthalmic Ointment 563
Blephamide Ophthalmic Suspension 564
Poly-Pred Liquifilm Ophthalmic Suspension .... ⊙231
Pred Forte Ophthalmic Suspension .... ⊙233
Pred Mild Sterile Ophthalmic Suspension .... ⊙236
Pred-G Ophthalmic Suspension .... ⊙234
Pred-G Sterile Ophthalmic Ointment .... ⊙235

Prednisolone Sodium Phosphate (Co-medications that induce CYP3A4 may significantly decrease exposure to exemestane. Dose modification is recommended for patients receiving a potent CYP3A4 inducer). Products include:
Pediapred Oral Solution 3319

Prednisolone Tebutate (Co-medications that induce CYP3A4 may significantly decrease exposure to exemestane. Dose modification is recommended for patients receiving a potent CYP3A4 inducer).
No products indexed under this heading.

Prednisone (Co-medications that induce CYP3A4 may significantly decrease exposure to exemestane. Dose modification is recommended for patients receiving a potent CYP3A4 inducer).
No products indexed under this heading.

Primidone (Co-medications that induce CYP3A4 may significantly decrease exposure to exemestane. Dose modification is recommended for patients receiving a potent CYP3A4 inducer).
No products indexed under this heading.

Rifabutin (Co-medications that induce CYP3A4 may significantly decrease exposure to exemestane. Dose modification is recommended for patients receiving a potent CYP3A4 inducer).
No products indexed under this heading.

Rifampicin (When patients were pretreated with rifampicin, a potent CYP3A4 inducer, followed by a single dose of exemestane, the mean plasma Cmax and AUC of exemestane were decreased. Dose modification is recommended).
No products indexed under this heading.

Rifampin (Co-medications that induce CYP3A4 may significantly decrease exposure to exemestane. Dose modification is recommended for patients receiving a potent CYP3A4 inducer).
No products indexed under this heading.

Rifapentine (Co-medications that induce CYP3A4 may significantly decrease exposure to exemestane. Dose modification is recommended for patients receiving a potent CYP3A4 inducer).
No products indexed under this heading.

Sulfinpyrazone (Co-medications that induce CYP3A4 may significantly decrease exposure to exemestane. Dose modification is recommended for patients receiving a potent CYP3A4 inducer).
No products indexed under this heading.

Theophylline (Co-medications that induce CYP3A4 may significantly decrease exposure to exemestane. Dose modification is recommended for patients receiving a potent CYP3A4 inducer).
No products indexed under this heading.

Triamcinolone (Co-medications that induce CYP3A4 may significantly decrease exposure to exemestane. Dose modification is recommended for patients receiving a potent CYP3A4 inducer).
No products indexed under this heading.

Triamcinolone Acetonide (Co-medications that induce CYP3A4 may significantly decrease exposure to exemestane. Dose modification is recommended for patients receiving a potent CYP3A4 inducer). Products include:
Azmacort Inhalation Aerosol 1701
Nasacort HFA Inhalation Aerosol 2939
Nasacort AQ Nasal Spray 2937

Triamcinolone Diacetate (Co-medications that induce CYP3A4 may significantly decrease exposure to exemestane. Dose modification is recommended for patients receiving a potent CYP3A4 inducer).
No products indexed under this heading.

Triamcinolone Hexacetonide (Co-medications that induce CYP3A4 may significantly decrease exposure to exemestane. Dose modification is recommended for patients receiving a potent CYP3A4 inducer).
No products indexed under this heading.

Troglitazone (Co-medications that induce CYP3A4 may significantly decrease exposure to exemestane. Dose modification is recommended for patients receiving a potent CYP3A4 inducer).
No products indexed under this heading.

Food Interactions

Food, unspecified (Exemestane plasma levels increased approximately 40% after high-fat breakfast).

ARTHROTEC TABLETS

(Diclofenac Sodium, Misoprostol) 3126
May interact with antacids, antihypertensives, diuretics, oral hypoglycemic agents, insulin, lithium preparations, potassium sparing diuretics, and certain other agents. Compounds in these categories include:

Acarbose (Diclofenac may alter a diabetic patient's response to oral hypoglycemic agents; both hypo- and hyperglycemic effects have been reported). Products include:
Precose Tablets 776

Acebutolol Hydrochloride (NSAIDs can inhibit the activity of antihypertensives).
No products indexed under this heading.

Aluminum Carbonate (Antacids reduce the bioavailability of misoprostol acid and may delay absorption of diclofenac).
No products indexed under this heading.

Aluminum Hydroxide (Antacids reduce the bioavailability of misoprostol acid and may delay absorption of diclofenac). Products include:
Gaviscon Regular Strength Liquid .... ▣620
Gaviscon Regular Strength Tablets .... ▣619
Gaviscon Extra Strength Liquid .... ▣620
Gaviscon Extra Strength Tablets .... ▣619
Maalox Max Maximum Strength Antacid/Anti-Gas Liquid 2165
Maalox Regular Strength Antacid/Antigas Liquid 2164

Amiloride Hydrochloride (Co-administration with potassium-sparing diuretics may be associated with increased serum potassium levels). Products include:
Midamor Tablets 2000
Moduretic Tablets 2003

Amlodipine Besylate (NSAIDs can inhibit the activity of antihypertensives). Products include:
Caduet Tablets 2507
Lotrel Capsules 2238
Norvasc Tablets 2529

Aspirin (Co-administration is not recommended because diclofenac sodium is displaced from its binding sites by aspirin resulting in lower plasma concentrations, peak plasma levels and AUC values). Products include:
Aggrenox Capsules 855
Bayer, Aspirin Regimen .... ▣606
Bayer Aspirin Tablets 3515
BC Powder .... ▣612
BC Allergy Sinus Cold Powder .... ▣612
Arthritis Strength BC Powder .... ▣612
BC Sinus Cold Powder .... ▣612
Ecotrin Enteric Coated Aspirin Low, Regular and Maximum Strength Tablets 1627
Goody's Body Pain Formula Powder .... ▣621
Goody's Extra Strength Headache Powder .... ▣621
Goody's Extra Strength Pain Relief Tablets .... ▣621
Percodan Tablets 1115
St. Joseph 81 mg Aspirin Chewable and Enteric Coated Tablets 1841

Atenolol (NSAIDs can inhibit the activity of antihypertensives). Products include:
Tenormin I.V. Injection 698
Tenormin Tablets 695

Benazepril Hydrochloride (NSAIDs can inhibit the activity of antihypertensives). Products include:
Lotensin Tablets 2232
Lotensin HCT Tablets 2235
Lotrel Capsules 2238

Bendroflumethiazide (NSAIDs can inhibit the activity of diuretics).
No products indexed under this heading.

Betaxolol Hydrochloride (NSAIDs can inhibit the activity of antihypertensives). Products include:
Betoptic S Ophthalmic Suspension 554

Bisoprolol Fumarate (NSAIDs can inhibit the activity of antihypertensives).
No products indexed under this heading.

Bumetanide (NSAIDs can inhibit the activity of diuretics).
No products indexed under this heading.

Candesartan Cilexetil (NSAIDs can inhibit the activity of antihypertensives). Products include:
Atacand Tablets 634
Atacand HCT 637

Captopril (NSAIDs can inhibit the activity of antihypertensives). Products include:
Captopril Tablets 2114

Carteolol Hydrochloride (NSAIDs can inhibit the activity of antihypertensives). Products include:
Carteolol Hydrochloride Ophthalmic Solution USP, 1% .... ⊙246

Chlorothiazide (NSAIDs can inhibit the activity of diuretics). Products include:
Aldoclor Tablets 1881
Diuril Oral 1936

Chlorothiazide Sodium (NSAIDs can inhibit the activity of diuretics). Products include:
Diuril Sodium Intravenous 1934

Chlorpropamide (Diclofenac may alter a diabetic patient's response to oral hypoglycemic agents; both hypo- and hyperglycemic effects have been reported).
No products indexed under this heading.

Chlorthalidone (NSAIDs can inhibit the activity of diuretics). Products include:
Clorpres Tablets 2139

Clonidine (NSAIDs can inhibit the activity of antihypertensives). Products include:
Catapres-TTS 875

Clonidine Hydrochloride (NSAIDs can inhibit the activity of antihypertensives). Products include:
Catapres Tablets 874
Clorpres Tablets 2139

Cyclosporine (NSAIDs may affect renal prostaglandins and increase the toxicity of certain drugs, including cyclosporine; potential for increased cyclosporine-induced nephrotoxicity). Products include:
Gengraf Capsules 458
Neoral Soft Gelatin Capsules 2247
Neoral Oral Solution 2247
Restasis Ophthalmic Emulsion 570
Sandimmune 2259

Deserpidine (NSAIDs can inhibit the activity of antihypertensives).
No products indexed under this heading.

Diazoxide (NSAIDs can inhibit the activity of antihypertensives). Products include:
Hyperstat I.V. Injection 3031

Digoxin (Co-administration of digoxin with diclofenac has resulted in elevated digoxin levels). Products include:
Digitek Tablets 2146
Lanoxicaps Capsules 1458
Lanoxin Injection 1462
Lanoxin Tablets 1468
Lanoxin Injection Pediatric 1465

Diltiazem Hydrochloride (NSAIDs can inhibit the activity of antihypertensives). Products include:
Cardizem LA Extended Release Tablets 1699
Tiazac Capsules 1204

Doxazosin Mesylate (NSAIDs can inhibit the activity of antihypertensives).
No products indexed under this heading.

Enalapril Maleate (NSAIDs can inhibit the activity of antihypertensives). Products include:
Vaseretic Tablets 2073
Vasotec I.V. Injection 2076

Enalaprilat (NSAIDs can inhibit the activity of antihypertensives).
No products indexed under this heading.

Eprosartan Mesylate (NSAIDs can inhibit the activity of antihypertensives). Products include:
Teveten Tablets 1707
Teveten HCT Tablets 1710

Esmolol Hydrochloride (NSAIDs can inhibit the activity of antihypertensives). Products include:
Brevibloc Concentrate 766
Brevibloc Injection 766
Brevibloc Double Strength Injection 766
Brevibloc Premixed Injection 766
Brevibloc Double Strength Premixed Injection 766

Ethacrynic Acid (NSAIDs can inhibit the activity of diuretics). Products include:
Edecrin Tablets 1941

Felodipine (NSAIDs can inhibit the activity of antihypertensives). Products include:
Plendil Extended-Release Tablets 651

Fosinopril Sodium (NSAIDs can inhibit the activity of antihypertensives).
No products indexed under this heading.

Furosemide (NSAIDs can inhibit the activity of diuretics). Products include:
Furosemide Tablets 2117

Glimepiride (Diclofenac may alter a diabetic patient's response to oral hypoglycemic agents; both hypo- and hyperglycemic effects have been reported). Products include:
Amaryl Tablets 2864

Glipizide (Diclofenac may alter a diabetic patient's response to oral hypoglycemic agents; both hypo- and hyperglycemic effects have been reported).
No products indexed under this heading.

Glyburide (Diclofenac may alter a diabetic patient's response to oral hypoglycemic agents; both hypo- and hyperglycemic effects have been reported).
No products indexed under this heading.

Guanabenz Acetate (NSAIDs can inhibit the activity of antihypertensives).
No products indexed under this heading.

Guanethidine Monosulfate (NSAIDs can inhibit the activity of antihypertensives).
No products indexed under this heading.

Hydralazine Hydrochloride (NSAIDs can inhibit the activity of antihypertensives). Products include:
BiDil Tablets 2161

Hydrochlorothiazide (NSAIDs can inhibit the activity of diuretics). Products include:
Aldoril Tablets 1884
Atacand HCT 637
Avalide Tablets 2889
Avalide Tablets 922
Benicar HCT Tablets 2852
Diovan HCT Tablets 2195
Dyazide Capsules 1389
Hyzaar 1964
Lotensin HCT Tablets 2235
Maxzide 2150
Micardis HCT Tablets 886
Moduretic Tablets 2003
Prinzide Tablets 2033
Teveten HCT Tablets 1710
Timolide Tablets 2056
Uniretic Tablets 3114
Vaseretic Tablets 2073
Zestoretic Tablets 701

Hydroflumethiazide (NSAIDs can inhibit the activity of diuretics).
No products indexed under this heading.

Indapamide (NSAIDs can inhibit the activity of diuretics). Products include:
Indapamide Tablets 2119

Insulin, Human, Zinc Suspension (Diclofenac may alter a diabetic patient's response to insulin; both hypo- and hyperglycemic effects have been reported). Products include:
Humulin L, 100 Units 1763
Humulin U, 100 Units 1770

Insulin, Human NPH (Diclofenac may alter a diabetic patient's response to insulin; both hypo- and hyperglycemic effects have been reported). Products include:
Humulin N, 100 Units 1764
Humulin N Pen 1765
Novolin N Human Insulin 10 ml Vials 2322
Novolin N InnoLet 2322
Novolin N PenFill 3 ml Cartridges 2325
Novolin R InnoLet 2322

Insulin, Human Regular (Diclofenac may alter a diabetic patient's response to insulin; both hypo- and hyperglycemic effects have been reported). Products include:
Humulin R (U-500) 1768
Humulin R, 100 Units 1767
Novolin R Human Insulin 10 ml Vials 2322
Novolin R PenFill 2325

Insulin, Human Regular and Human NPH Mixture (Diclofenac may alter a diabetic patient's response to insulin; both hypo- and hyperglycemic effects have been reported). Products include:
Humulin 50/50, 100 Units 1760
Humulin 70/30 Pen 1761
Novolin 70/30 Human Insulin 10 ml Vials 2321
Novolin 70/30 InnoLet 2322
Novolin 70/30 PenFill 3 ml Cartridges 2325

Insulin, NPH (Diclofenac may alter a diabetic patient's response to insulin; both hypo- and hyperglycemic effects have been reported).
No products indexed under this heading.

Insulin, Regular (Diclofenac may alter a diabetic patient's response to insulin; both hypo- and hyperglycemic effects have been reported).
No products indexed under this heading.

Insulin, Zinc Crystals (Diclofenac may alter a diabetic patient's response to insulin; both hypo- and hyperglycemic effects have been reported).
No products indexed under this heading.

Insulin, Zinc Suspension (Diclofenac may alter a diabetic patient's response to insulin; both hypo- and hyperglycemic effects have been reported).
No products indexed under this heading.

Insulin Aspart, Human Regular (Diclofenac may alter a diabetic patient's response to insulin; both hypo- and hyperglycemic effects have been reported). Products include:
NovoLog Injection 2326

Insulin glargine (Diclofenac may alter a diabetic patient's response to insulin; both hypo- and hyperglycemic effects have been reported). Products include:
Lantus Injection 2925

Insulin Lispro, Human (Diclofenac may alter a diabetic patient's response to insulin; both hypo- and hyperglycemic effects have been reported). Products include:
Humalog-Pen 1751
Humalog Mix 75/25-Pen 1754

Insulin Lispro Protamine, Human (Diclofenac may alter a diabetic patient's response to insulin; both hypo- and hyperglycemic effects have been reported). Products include:
Humalog Mix 75/25-Pen 1754

Irbesartan (NSAIDs can inhibit the activity of antihypertensives). Products include:
Avalide Tablets 922
Avalide Tablets 2889
Avapro Tablets 925
Avapro Tablets 2886

Isradipine (NSAIDs can inhibit the activity of antihypertensives). Products include:
DynaCirc CR Tablets 2726

Labetalol Hydrochloride (NSAIDs can inhibit the activity of antihypertensives).
No products indexed under this heading.

Lisinopril (NSAIDs can inhibit the activity of antihypertensives). Products include:
Prinivil Tablets 2029
Prinzide Tablets 2033
Zestoretic Tablets 701
Zestril Tablets 704

Lithium (NSAIDs have produced an elevation of plasma lithium levels and a reduction in renal lithium clearance).
No products indexed under this heading.

Lithium Carbonate (NSAIDs have produced an elevation of plasma lithium levels and a reduction in renal lithium clearance). Products include:
Eskalith 1406
Lithobid Tablets 1670

Lithium Citrate (NSAIDs have produced an elevation of plasma lithium levels and a reduction in renal lithium clearance).
No products indexed under this heading.

Losartan Potassium (NSAIDs can inhibit the activity of antihypertensives). Products include:
Cozaar Tablets 1913

Hyzaar 1964

Magaldrate (Antacids reduce the bioavailability of misoprostol acid and may delay absorption of diclofenac).
No products indexed under this heading.

Magnesium Hydroxide (Antacids reduce the bioavailability of misoprostol acid and may delay absorption of diclofenac; magnesium-containing antacids exacerbate misoprostol-associated diarrhea). Products include:
Maalox Max Maximum Strength Antacid/Anti-Gas Liquid 2165
Maalox Regular Strength Antacid/Antigas Liquid 2164
Pepcid Complete Chewable Tablets 1672
Rolaids Tablets 707
Extra Strength Rolaids Tablets 707
Rolaids Multi-Symptom Antacid & Antigas Tablets 708

Magnesium Oxide (Antacids reduce the bioavailability of misoprostol acid and may delay absorption of diclofenac; magnesium-containing antacids exacerbate misoprostol-associated diarrhea). Products include:
Beelith Tablets 784
PremCal Light, Regular, and Extra Strength Tablets 762

Mecamylamine Hydrochloride (NSAIDs can inhibit the activity of antihypertensives). Products include:
Inversine Tablets 3286

Metformin Hydrochloride (Diclofenac may alter a diabetic patient's response to oral hypoglycemic agents; both hypo- and hyperglycemic effects have been reported). Products include:
ActoPlus Met Tablets 3219
Avandamet Tablets 1343
Fortamet Extended-Release Tablets 1156

Methotrexate Sodium (NSAIDs may affect renal prostaglandins and increase the toxicity of certain drugs, including methotrexate; potential for increased serum methotrexate concentrations).
No products indexed under this heading.

Methyclothiazide (NSAIDs can inhibit the activity of diuretics).
No products indexed under this heading.

Methyldopa (NSAIDs can inhibit the activity of antihypertensives). Products include:
Aldoclor Tablets 1881
Aldoril Tablets 1884

Methyldopate Hydrochloride (NSAIDs can inhibit the activity of antihypertensives).
No products indexed under this heading.

Metolazone (NSAIDs can inhibit the activity of diuretics).
No products indexed under this heading.

Metoprolol Succinate (NSAIDs can inhibit the activity of antihypertensives). Products include:
Toprol-XL Tablets 660

Metoprolol Tartrate (NSAIDs can inhibit the activity of antihypertensives).
No products indexed under this heading.

Metyrosine (NSAIDs can inhibit the activity of antihypertensives). Products include:
Demser Capsules 1933

Mibefradil Dihydrochloride (NSAIDs can inhibit the activity of antihypertensives).
No products indexed under this heading.

Miglitol (Diclofenac may alter a diabetic patient's response to oral hypoglycemic agents; both hypo- and hyperglycemic effects have been reported).
No products indexed under this heading.

Minoxidil (NSAIDs can inhibit the activity of antihypertensives). Products include:
Men's Rogaine Extra Strength Topical Solution, Ocean Rush Scent and Original Unscented 706
Women's Rogaine Topical Solution, Spring Bloom Scent and Original Unscented 707

Moexipril Hydrochloride (NSAIDs can inhibit the activity of antihypertensives). Products include:
Uniretic Tablets 3114
Univasc Tablets 3118

Nadolol (NSAIDs can inhibit the activity of antihypertensives). Products include:
Nadolol Tablets 2121

Nicardipine Hydrochloride (NSAIDs can inhibit the activity of antihypertensives). Products include:
Cardene I.V. 1129

Nifedipine (NSAIDs can inhibit the activity of antihypertensives). Products include:
Adalat CC Tablets 2978

Nisoldipine (NSAIDs can inhibit the activity of antihypertensives). Products include:
Sular Tablets 1163

Nitroglycerin (NSAIDs can inhibit the activity of antihypertensives). Products include:
Nitro-Dur Transdermal Infusion System 3060
Nitrolingual Pumpspray 1161

Penbutolol Sulfate (NSAIDs can inhibit the activity of antihypertensives).
No products indexed under this heading.

Perindopril Erbumine (NSAIDs can inhibit the activity of antihypertensives). Products include:
Aceon Tablets (2 mg, 4 mg, 8 mg) 3191

Phenobarbital (Co-administration in patients on chronic phenobarbital therapy has resulted in phenobarbital toxicity).
No products indexed under this heading.

Phenoxybenzamine Hydrochloride (NSAIDs can inhibit the activity of antihypertensives). Products include:
Dibenzyline Capsules 3390

Phentolamine Mesylate (NSAIDs can inhibit the activity of antihypertensives).
No products indexed under this heading.

Pindolol (NSAIDs can inhibit the activity of antihypertensives).
No products indexed under this heading.

Pioglitazone Hydrochloride (Diclofenac may alter a diabetic patient's response to oral hypoglycemic agents; both hypo- and hyperglycemic effects have been reported). Products include:
ActoPlus Met Tablets 3219
Actos Tablets 3224

Polythiazide (NSAIDs can inhibit the activity of diuretics).
No products indexed under this heading.

Prazosin Hydrochloride (NSAIDs can inhibit the activity of antihypertensives).
No products indexed under this heading.

Propranolol Hydrochloride (NSAIDs can inhibit the activity of antihypertensives). Products include:
Inderal LA Long-Acting Capsules 3421
InnoPran XL Capsules 2728

Quinapril Hydrochloride (NSAIDs can inhibit the activity of antihypertensives).
No products indexed under this heading.

Ramipril (NSAIDs can inhibit the activity of antihypertensives). Products include:
Altace Capsules 1673

Rauwolfia Serpentina (NSAIDs can inhibit the activity of antihypertensives).
No products indexed under this heading.

Repaglinide (Diclofenac may alter a diabetic patient's response to oral hypoglycemic agents; both hypo- and hyperglycemic effects have been reported). Products include:
Prandin Tablets (0.5, 1, and 2 mg) 2337

Rescinnamine (NSAIDs can inhibit the activity of antihypertensives).
No products indexed under this heading.

Reserpine (NSAIDs can inhibit the activity of antihypertensives).
No products indexed under this heading.

Rosiglitazone Maleate (Diclofenac may alter a diabetic patient's response to oral hypoglycemic agents; both hypo- and hyperglycemic effects have been reported). Products include:
Avandamet Tablets 1343
Avandia Tablets 1348

Sodium Bicarbonate (Antacids reduce the bioavailability of misoprostol acid and may delay absorption of diclofenac). Products include:
Ceo-Two Evacuant Suppository 607
Colyte with Flavor Packs for Oral Solution 3102
HalfLytely and Bisacodyl Tablets Bowel Prep Kit with Flavors Packs 915
TriLyte with Flavor Packs for Oral Solution 3114

Sodium Nitroprusside (NSAIDs can inhibit the activity of antihypertensives).
No products indexed under this heading.

Sotalol Hydrochloride (NSAIDs can inhibit the activity of antihypertensives).
No products indexed under this heading.

Spirapril Hydrochloride (NSAIDs can inhibit the activity of antihypertensives).
No products indexed under this heading.

Spironolactone (Co-administration with potassium-sparing diuretics may be associated with increased serum potassium levels).
No products indexed under this heading.

Telmisartan (NSAIDs can inhibit the activity of antihypertensives). Products include:
Micardis Tablets 884
Micardis HCT Tablets 886

Terazosin Hydrochloride (NSAIDs can inhibit the activity of antihypertensives). Products include:
Hytrin Capsules 469

Timolol Maleate (NSAIDs can inhibit the activity of antihypertensives). Products include:
Blocadren Tablets 1891
Cosopt Sterile Ophthalmic Solution 1910
Timolide Tablets 2056
Timoptic in Ocudose 2061
Timoptic Sterile Ophthalmic Solution 2058
Timoptic-XE Sterile Ophthalmic Gel Forming Solution 2062

Tolazamide (Diclofenac may alter a diabetic patient's response to oral hypoglycemic agents; both hypo- and hyperglycemic effects have been reported).
No products indexed under this heading.

Tolbutamide (Diclofenac may alter a diabetic patient's response to oral hypoglycemic agents; both hypo- and hyperglycemic effects have been reported).
No products indexed under this heading.

Torsemide (NSAIDs can inhibit the activity of diuretics).
No products indexed under this heading.

Trandolapril (NSAIDs can inhibit the activity of antihypertensives). Products include:
Mavik Tablets 482
Tarka Tablets 519

Triamterene (Co-administration with potassium-sparing diuretics may be associated with increased serum potassium levels). Products include:
Dyazide Capsules 1389
Dyrenium Capsules 3390
Maxzide 2150

Trimethaphan Camsylate (NSAIDs can inhibit the activity of antihypertensives).
No products indexed under this heading.

Troglitazone (Diclofenac may alter a diabetic patient's response to oral hypoglycemic agents; both hypo- and hyperglycemic effects have been reported).
No products indexed under this heading.

Valsartan (NSAIDs can inhibit the activity of antihypertensives). Products include:
Diovan HCT Tablets 2195
Diovan Tablets 2191

Verapamil Hydrochloride (NSAIDs can inhibit the activity of antihypertensives). Products include:
Covera-HS Tablets 3135
Tarka Tablets 519
Verelan PM Capsules 3120

Warfarin Sodium (The effects of warfarin and NSAIDs on GI bleeding are synergistic, such that users of both drugs together have a risk of serious bleeding greater than users of either drug alone). Products include:
Coumadin for Injection 932
Coumadin Tablets 932

ASACOL DELAYED-RELEASE TABLETS

(Mesalamine) 2688
None cited in PDR database.

ASMANEX TWISTHALER
(Mometasone Furoate) 2981
May interact with:

Ketoconazole (Ketoconazole may increase plasma levels of mometasone furoate during concomitant dosing. Since mometasone furoate plasma levels appear to increase plasma and cortisol levels appear to decrease upon concomitant administration of ketoconazole, caution should be exercised in the co-administration of these drugs). Products include:
- Nizoral A-D Shampoo, 1% 1839
- Nizoral 2% Shampoo 1838

ASTELIN NASAL SPRAY
(Azelastine Hydrochloride) 1876
May interact with antihistamines, central nervous system depressants, and certain other agents. Compounds in these categories include:

Acrivastine (Co-administration may result in additional reduction in alertness and impairment of CNS performance; concurrent use with other antihistamines should be avoided).
No products indexed under this heading.

Alfentanil Hydrochloride (Co-administration may result in additional reduction in alertness and impairment of CNS performance).
No products indexed under this heading.

Alprazolam (Co-administration may result in additional reduction in alertness and impairment of CNS performance). Products include:
- Niravam Orally Disintegrating Tablets 3106
- Xanax XR Tablets 2655

Aprobarbital (Co-administration may result in additional reduction in alertness and impairment of CNS performance).
No products indexed under this heading.

Astemizole (Co-administration may result in additional reduction in alertness and impairment of CNS performance; concurrent use with other antihistamines should be avoided).
No products indexed under this heading.

Azatadine Maleate (Co-administration may result in additional reduction in alertness and impairment of CNS performance; concurrent use with other antihistamines should be avoided).
No products indexed under this heading.

Bromodiphenhydramine Hydrochloride (Co-administration may result in additional reduction in alertness and impairment of CNS performance; concurrent use with other antihistamines should be avoided).
No products indexed under this heading.

Brompheniramine Maleate (Co-administration may result in additional reduction in alertness and impairment of CNS performance; concurrent use with other antihistamines should be avoided). Products include:
- Alacol DM Syrup 739
- Children's Dimetapp Cold & Allergy Elixir .... ▣ 745
- Children's Dimetapp DM Cold & Cough Elixir .... ▣ 745
- Robitussin Allergy & Cough Syrup .. ▣ 750

Buprenorphine Hydrochloride (Co-administration may result in additional reduction in alertness and impairment of CNS performance). Products include:
- Buprenex Injectable 2718
- Suboxone Tablets 2719
- Subutex Tablets 2719

Buspirone Hydrochloride (Co-administration may result in additional reduction in alertness and impairment of CNS performance).
No products indexed under this heading.

Butabarbital (Co-administration may result in additional reduction in alertness and impairment of CNS performance).
No products indexed under this heading.

Butalbital (Co-administration may result in additional reduction in alertness and impairment of CNS performance). Products include:
- Sedapap Tablets 50 mg/650 mg 2098

Cetirizine Hydrochloride (Co-administration may result in additional reduction in alertness and impairment of CNS performance; concurrent use with other antihistamines should be avoided). Products include:
- Zyrtec Chewable Tablets 2589
- Zyrtec 2589
- Zyrtec-D 12 Hour Extended Release Tablets 2591

Chlordiazepoxide (Co-administration may result in additional reduction in alertness and impairment of CNS performance).
No products indexed under this heading.

Chlordiazepoxide Hydrochloride (Co-administration may result in additional reduction in alertness and impairment of CNS performance). Products include:
- Librium Capsules 3349

Chlorpheniramine Maleate (Co-administration may result in additional reduction in alertness and impairment of CNS performance; concurrent use with other antihistamines should be avoided). Products include:
- Advil Allergy Sinus Caplets .... ▣ 737
- Advil Multi-Symptom Cold Caplets .... ▣ 738
- BC Allergy Sinus Cold Powder .... ▣ 612
- Contac Severe Cold and Flu Caplets Maximum Strength .... ▣ 615
- Hycomine Compound Tablets 1105
- PediaCare Multi-Symptom Cold Liquid .... ▣ 704
- PediaCare NightRest Cough & Cold Liquid .... ▣ 704
- Robitussin Flu Liquid .... ▣ 752
- Robitussin PM Cough & Cold Liquid .... ▣ 752
- Singlet Caplets .... ▣ 636
- Sudafed Sinus & Allergy Tablets ..... ▣ 710
- TheraFlu Cold & Cough Hot Liquid .... ▣ 680
- TheraFlu Cold & Sore Throat Hot Liquid .... ▣ 680
- TheraFlu Flu & Sore Throat Hot Liquid .... ▣ 681
- TheraFlu Severe Cold & Cough Hot Liquid .... ▣ 683
- TheraFlu Severe Cold Caplets .... ▣ 679
- TheraFlu Severe Cold Hot Liquid ..... ▣ 682
- Triaminic Cold & Allergy Liquid ...... ▣ 685
- Triaminic Cold & Cough Liquid .... ▣ 685
- Triaminic Flu, Cough & Fever Liquid .... ▣ 685
- Triaminic Night Time Cough & Cold Liquid .... ▣ 685
- Triaminic Allergy Runny Nose & Congestion Softchews .... ▣ 688
- Triaminic Cold & Cough Softchews .... ▣ 688
- Children's Tylenol Plus Cold NightTime Suspension Liquid 1851
- Children's Tylenol Plus Cold & Cough Suspension Liquid and Chewable Tablets 1851
- Children's Tylenol Plus Cold Chewable Tablets 1851
- Children's Tylenol Plus Flu Suspension Liquid 1853
- Tylenol Allergy Complete Multi-Symptom Caplets and Gelcaps with Cool Burst 1844
- Multi-Symptom Tylenol Cold Night Time Caplets 1845
- Vicks 44M Cough, Cold & Flu Relief 2676
- Pediatric Vicks 44m Cough & Cold Relief 2673
- Children's Vicks NyQuil Cold/Cough Relief 2671

Chlorpheniramine Polistirex (Co-administration may result in additional reduction in alertness and impairment of CNS performance; concurrent use with other antihistamines should be avoided). Products include:
- Tussionex Pennkinetic Extended-Release Suspension 3322

Chlorpheniramine Tannate (Co-administration may result in additional reduction in alertness and impairment of CNS performance; concurrent use with other antihistamines should be avoided).
No products indexed under this heading.

Chlorpromazine (Co-administration may result in additional reduction in alertness and impairment of CNS performance).
No products indexed under this heading.

Chlorpromazine Hydrochloride (Co-administration may result in additional reduction in alertness and impairment of CNS performance).
No products indexed under this heading.

Chlorprothixene (Co-administration may result in additional reduction in alertness and impairment of CNS performance).
No products indexed under this heading.

Chlorprothixene Hydrochloride (Co-administration may result in additional reduction in alertness and impairment of CNS performance).
No products indexed under this heading.

Chlorprothixene Lactate (Co-administration may result in additional reduction in alertness and impairment of CNS performance).
No products indexed under this heading.

Cimetidine (Increases the mean Cmax and AUC of orally administered azelastine by approximately 65%). Products include:
- Tagamet HB 200 Tablets .... ▣ 637
- Tagamet Tablets 1547

Cimetidine Hydrochloride (Co-administration of oral azelastine and cimetidine has resulted in increased mean Cmax and AUC of azelastine).
No products indexed under this heading.

Clemastine Fumarate (Co-administration may result in additional reduction in alertness and impairment of CNS performance; concurrent use with other antihistamines should be avoided).
No products indexed under this heading.

Clorazepate Dipotassium (Co-administration may result in additional reduction in alertness and impairment of CNS performance). Products include:
- Tranxene 2488

Clozapine (Co-administration may result in additional reduction in alertness and impairment of CNS performance). Products include:
- Clozapine Tablets 2141
- Clozaril Tablets 2174
- FazaClo Orally Disintegrating Tablets 547

Codeine Phosphate (Co-administration may result in additional reduction in alertness and impairment of CNS performance). Products include:
- Tylenol with Codeine 2461

Cyproheptadine Hydrochloride (Co-administration may result in additional reduction in alertness and impairment of CNS performance; concurrent use with other antihistamines should be avoided).
No products indexed under this heading.

Desflurane (Co-administration may result in additional reduction in alertness and impairment of CNS performance). Products include:
- Suprane Liquid for Inhalation 770

Dexchlorpheniramine Maleate (Co-administration may result in additional reduction in alertness and impairment of CNS performance; concurrent use with other antihistamines should be avoided).
No products indexed under this heading.

Dezocine (Co-administration may result in additional reduction in alertness and impairment of CNS performance).
No products indexed under this heading.

Diazepam (Co-administration may result in additional reduction in alertness and impairment of CNS performance). Products include:
- Diastat Rectal Delivery System 3344
- Valium Tablets 2822

Diphenhydramine Citrate (Co-administration may result in additional reduction in alertness and impairment of CNS performance; concurrent use with other antihistamines should be avoided). Products include:
- Children's Benadryl Allergy & Cold Fastmelt Tablets .... ▣ 695
- Children's Benadryl D Allergy & Sinus Fastmelt Tablets .... ▣ 694
- Children's Benadryl Allergy Fastmelt Tablets .... ▣ 696
- Goody's PM Powder .... ▣ 622

Diphenhydramine Hydrochloride (Co-administration may result in additional reduction in alertness and impairment of CNS performance; concurrent use with other antihistamines should be avoided). Products include:
- Benadryl Allergy & Cold Tablets ..... ▣ 692
- Benadryl Allergy .... ▣ 691
- Benadryl Allergy & Sinus Headache Caplets & Gelcaps ...... ▣ 693
- Children's Benadryl Allergy Liquid ... ▣ 695
- Children's Benadryl Dye-Free Allergy Liquid .... ▣ 695
- Benadryl Dye-Free Allergy Liqui-Gels Softgels .... ▣ 692
- Benadryl Itch Relief Stick Extra Strength .... ▣ 696
- Benadryl Itch Stopping Cream Extra Strength .... ▣ 697
- Benadryl Itch Stopping Gel Extra Strength .... ▣ 697

Benadryl Itch Stopping Spray Extra Strength 697
Benadryl Maximum Strength Severe Allergy & Sinus Headache Caplets 694
Children's Benadryl D Liquid Medication 693
Benadryl D Tablets 694
Nytol QuickCaps Caplets 635
Maximum Strength Nytol QuickGels Softgels 635
Simply Sleep Caplets 1841
Sominex Original Formula Tablets .. 637
TheraFlu Thin Strips Multi Symptom 684
Triaminic Thin Strips Cough & Runny Nose 690
Children's Tylenol Plus Cold & Allergy Suspension Liquid 1850
Tylenol Allergy Complete Night Time Caplets 1844
Tylenol Severe Allergy Caplets 1844
Tylenol Flu NightTime Gelcaps 1846
Extra Strength Tylenol PM Caplets, Geltabs, Gelcaps and Liquid 1847
Unisom Maximum Strength SleepGels 712

Diphenylpyraline Hydrochloride (Co-administration may result in additional reduction in alertness and impairment of CNS performance; concurrent use with other antihistamines should be avoided).
No products indexed under this heading.

Droperidol (Co-administration may result in additional reduction in alertness and impairment of CNS performance).
No products indexed under this heading.

Enflurane (Co-administration may result in additional reduction in alertness and impairment of CNS performance).
No products indexed under this heading.

Estazolam (Co-administration may result in additional reduction in alertness and impairment of CNS performance). Products include:
ProSom Tablets 512

Ethanol (Co-administration may result in additional reduction in alertness and impairment of CNS performance).
No products indexed under this heading.

Ethchlorvynol (Co-administration may result in additional reduction in alertness and impairment of CNS performance).
No products indexed under this heading.

Ethinamate (Co-administration may result in additional reduction in alertness and impairment of CNS performance).
No products indexed under this heading.

Ethyl Alcohol (Co-administration may result in additional reduction in alertness and impairment of CNS performance).
No products indexed under this heading.

Fentanyl (Co-administration may result in additional reduction in alertness and impairment of CNS performance). Products include:
Duragesic Transdermal System 2448

Fentanyl Citrate (Co-administration may result in additional reduction in alertness and impairment of CNS performance). Products include:
Actiq 993

Fexofenadine Hydrochloride (Co-administration may result in additional reduction in alertness and impairment of CNS performance; concurrent use with other antihistamines should be avoided). Products include:
Allegra 2857
Allegra-D 12 Hour Extended-Release Tablets 2860
Allegra-D 24 Hour Extended-Release Tablets 2862

Fluphenazine Decanoate (Co-administration may result in additional reduction in alertness and impairment of CNS performance).
No products indexed under this heading.

Fluphenazine Enanthate (Co-administration may result in additional reduction in alertness and impairment of CNS performance).
No products indexed under this heading.

Fluphenazine Hydrochloride (Co-administration may result in additional reduction in alertness and impairment of CNS performance).
No products indexed under this heading.

Flurazepam Hydrochloride (Co-administration may result in additional reduction in alertness and impairment of CNS performance).
Products include:
Dalmane Capsules 3343

Glutethimide (Co-administration may result in additional reduction in alertness and impairment of CNS performance).
No products indexed under this heading.

Haloperidol (Co-administration may result in additional reduction in alertness and impairment of CNS performance).
No products indexed under this heading.

Haloperidol Decanoate (Co-administration may result in additional reduction in alertness and impairment of CNS performance).
No products indexed under this heading.

Hydrocodone Bitartrate (Co-administration may result in additional reduction in alertness and impairment of CNS performance).
Products include:
Hycodan 1104
Hycomine Compound Tablets 1105
Hycotuss Expectorant Syrup 1106
Lortab 3315
Lortab Elixir 3312
Vicodin Tablets 530
Vicodin ES Tablets 531
Vicodin HP Tablets 532
Vicoprofen Tablets 533
Zydone Tablets 1118

Hydrocodone Polistirex (Co-administration may result in additional reduction in alertness and impairment of CNS performance).
Products include:
Tussionex Pennkinetic Extended-Release Suspension 3322

Hydromorphone Hydrochloride (Co-administration may result in additional reduction in alertness and impairment of CNS performance).
Products include:
Dilaudid 439
Dilaudid Oral Liquid 443
Dilaudid Non-Sterile Powder 439
Dilaudid Rectal Suppositories 439
Dilaudid Tablets 439
Dilaudid Tablets - 8 mg 443
Dilaudid-HP 441

Hydroxyzine Hydrochloride (Co-administration may result in additional reduction in alertness and impairment of CNS performance).
No products indexed under this heading.

Isoflurane (Co-administration may result in additional reduction in alertness and impairment of CNS performance).
No products indexed under this heading.

Ketamine Hydrochloride (Co-administration may result in additional reduction in alertness and impairment of CNS performance).
No products indexed under this heading.

Ketoconazole (Co-administration of oral azelastine and ketoconazole interfere with the measurement of azelastine plasma concentrations, however, no effects on QTc have been observed). Products include:
Nizoral A-D Shampoo, 1% 1839
Nizoral 2% Shampoo 1838

Levomethadyl Acetate Hydrochloride (Co-administration may result in additional reduction in alertness and impairment of CNS performance).
No products indexed under this heading.

Levorphanol Tartrate (Co-administration may result in additional reduction in alertness and impairment of CNS performance).
No products indexed under this heading.

Loratadine (Co-administration may result in additional reduction in alertness and impairment of CNS performance; concurrent use with other antihistamines should be avoided).
Products include:
Alavert Allergy & Sinus D-12 Hour Tablets 743
Alavert 743
Children's Claritin 24 Hour Non-Drowsy Allergy Syrup 732
Claritin Non-Drowsy 24 Hour Tablets 731
Non-Drowsy Claritin Hives Relief Tablets 733
Claritin Reditabs 24 Hour Non-Drowsy Tablets 732
Claritin-D Non-Drowsy 12 Hour Tablets 731
Claritin-D Non-Drowsy 24 Hour Tablets 731
Children's Dimetapp ND Non-Drowsy Allergy Syrup 746
Triaminic Allerchews 684

Lorazepam (Co-administration may result in additional reduction in alertness and impairment of CNS performance).
No products indexed under this heading.

Loxapine Hydrochloride (Co-administration may result in additional reduction in alertness and impairment of CNS performance).
No products indexed under this heading.

Loxapine Succinate (Co-administration may result in additional reduction in alertness and impairment of CNS performance).
No products indexed under this heading.

Meperidine Hydrochloride (Co-administration may result in additional reduction in alertness and impairment of CNS performance).
No products indexed under this heading.

Mephobarbital (Co-administration may result in additional reduction in alertness and impairment of CNS performance). Products include:
Mebaral Tablets, USP 2483

Meprobamate (Co-administration may result in additional reduction in alertness and impairment of CNS performance).
No products indexed under this heading.

Mesoridazine Besylate (Co-administration may result in additional reduction in alertness and impairment of CNS performance).
No products indexed under this heading.

Methadone Hydrochloride (Co-administration may result in additional reduction in alertness and impairment of CNS performance).
No products indexed under this heading.

Methdilazine Hydrochloride (Co-administration may result in additional reduction in alertness and impairment of CNS performance; concurrent use with other antihistamines should be avoided).
No products indexed under this heading.

Methohexital Sodium (Co-administration may result in additional reduction in alertness and impairment of CNS performance).
No products indexed under this heading.

Methotrimeprazine (Co-administration may result in additional reduction in alertness and impairment of CNS performance).
No products indexed under this heading.

Methoxyflurane (Co-administration may result in additional reduction in alertness and impairment of CNS performance).
No products indexed under this heading.

Midazolam Hydrochloride (Co-administration may result in additional reduction in alertness and impairment of CNS performance).
No products indexed under this heading.

Molindone Hydrochloride (Co-administration may result in additional reduction in alertness and impairment of CNS performance).
Products include:
Moban Tablets 1108

Morphine Sulfate (Co-administration may result in additional reduction in alertness and impairment of CNS performance).
Products include:
Avinza Capsules 1714
Kadian Capsules 572
MS Contin Tablets 2703

Olanzapine (Co-administration may result in additional reduction in alertness and impairment of CNS performance). Products include:
Symbyax Capsules 1788
Zyprexa Tablets 1798
Zyprexa IntraMuscular 1798
Zyprexa ZYDIS Orally Disintegrating Tablets 1798

Oxazepam (Co-administration may result in additional reduction in alertness and impairment of CNS performance).
No products indexed under this heading.

Oxycodone Hydrochloride (Co-administration may result in addition-

al reduction in alertness and impairment of CNS performance).
Products include:
Combunox Tablets 1183
OxyContin Tablets 2699
OxyFast Oral Concentrate Solution 2704
OxyIR Capsules 2704
Percocet Tablets 1114
Percodan Tablets 1115

Pentobarbital Sodium (Co-administration may result in additional reduction in alertness and impairment of CNS performance).
Products include:
Nembutal Sodium Solution, USP 2484

Perphenazine (Co-administration may result in additional reduction in alertness and impairment of CNS performance).
No products indexed under this heading.

Phenobarbital (Co-administration may result in additional reduction in alertness and impairment of CNS performance).
No products indexed under this heading.

Prazepam (Co-administration may result in additional reduction in alertness and impairment of CNS performance).
No products indexed under this heading.

Prochlorperazine (Co-administration may result in additional reduction in alertness and impairment of CNS performance).
No products indexed under this heading.

Promethazine Hydrochloride (Co-administration may result in additional reduction in alertness and impairment of CNS performance; concurrent use with other antihistamines should be avoided). Products include:
Phenergan 3438

Propofol (Co-administration may result in additional reduction in alertness and impairment of CNS performance). Products include:
Diprivan Injectable Emulsion 676

Propoxyphene Hydrochloride (Co-administration may result in additional reduction in alertness and impairment of CNS performance).
No products indexed under this heading.

Propoxyphene Napsylate (Co-administration may result in additional reduction in alertness and impairment of CNS performance).
Products include:
Darvocet A 500 Tablets 3497

Pyrilamine Maleate (Co-administration may result in additional reduction in alertness and impairment of CNS performance; concurrent use with other antihistamines should be avoided).
No products indexed under this heading.

Pyrilamine Tannate (Co-administration may result in additional reduction in alertness and impairment of CNS performance; concurrent use with other antihistamines should be avoided).
No products indexed under this heading.

Quazepam (Co-administration may result in additional reduction in alertness and impairment of CNS performance).
No products indexed under this heading.

Quetiapine Fumarate (Co-administration may result in additional reduction in alertness and impairment of CNS performance).
Products include:
Seroquel Tablets 691

Remifentanil Hydrochloride (Co-administration may result in additional reduction in alertness and impairment of CNS performance).
No products indexed under this heading.

Risperidone (Co-administration may result in additional reduction in alertness and impairment of CNS performance). Products include:
Risperdal Consta Long-Acting Injection 1664
Risperdal M-Tab Orally Disintegrating Tablets 1658
Risperdal 1658

Secobarbital Sodium (Co-administration may result in additional reduction in alertness and impairment of CNS performance).
No products indexed under this heading.

Sevoflurane (Co-administration may result in additional reduction in alertness and impairment of CNS performance). Products include:
Ultane Liquid for Inhalation 526

Sufentanil Citrate (Co-administration may result in additional reduction in alertness and impairment of CNS performance).
No products indexed under this heading.

Temazepam (Co-administration may result in additional reduction in alertness and impairment of CNS performance).
No products indexed under this heading.

Terfenadine (Co-administration may result in additional reduction in alertness and impairment of CNS performance; concurrent use with other antihistamines should be avoided).
No products indexed under this heading.

Thiamylal Sodium (Co-administration may result in additional reduction in alertness and impairment of CNS performance).
No products indexed under this heading.

Thioridazine Hydrochloride (Co-administration may result in additional reduction in alertness and impairment of CNS performance).
Products include:
Thioridazine Hydrochloride Tablets 2122

Thiothixene (Co-administration may result in additional reduction in alertness and impairment of CNS performance). Products include:
Thiothixene Capsules 2124

Triazolam (Co-administration may result in additional reduction in alertness and impairment of CNS performance).
No products indexed under this heading.

Trifluoperazine Hydrochloride (Co-administration may result in additional reduction in alertness and impairment of CNS performance).
No products indexed under this heading.

Trimeprazine Tartrate (Co-administration may result in additional reduction in alertness and impairment of CNS performance; concurrent use with other antihistamines should be avoided).
No products indexed under this heading.

Tripelennamine Hydrochloride (Co-administration may result in additional reduction in alertness and impairment of CNS performance; concurrent use with other antihistamines should be avoided).
No products indexed under this heading.

Triprolidine Hydrochloride (Co-administration may result in additional reduction in alertness and impairment of CNS performance; concurrent use with other antihistamines should be avoided).
No products indexed under this heading.

Zaleplon (Co-administration may result in additional reduction in alertness and impairment of CNS performance). Products include:
Sonata Capsules 1686

Ziprasidone Hydrochloride (Co-administration may result in additional reduction in alertness and impairment of CNS performance).
Products include:
Geodon Capsules 2514

Zolpidem Tartrate (Co-administration may result in additional reduction in alertness and impairment of CNS performance).
Products include:
Ambien Tablets 2867

Food Interactions

Alcohol (Concurrent use may result in additional reduction in alertness and impairment of CNS performance; alcohol intake should be avoided).

ATACAND TABLETS

(Candesartan Cilexetil) 634
May interact with lithium preparations. Compounds in these categories include:

Lithium (An increase in serum lithium concentration has been reported during concomitant administration of lithium with candesartan cilexetil, so careful monitoring of serum lithium levels is recommended during concomitant use).
No products indexed under this heading.

Lithium Carbonate (An increase in serum lithium concentration has been reported during concomitant administration of lithium with candesartan cilexetil, so careful monitoring of serum lithium levels is recommended during concomitant use).
Products include:
Eskalith 1406
Lithobid Tablets 1670

Lithium Citrate (An increase in serum lithium concentration has been reported during concomitant administration of lithium with candesartan cilexetil, so careful monitoring of serum lithium levels is recommended during concomitant use).
No products indexed under this heading.

ATACAND HCT 16-12.5 TABLETS

(Candesartan Cilexetil, Hydrochlorothiazide) 637
May interact with antihypertensives, barbiturates, corticosteroids, oral hypoglycemic agents, insulin, lithium preparations, narcotic analgesics, nondepolarizing neuromuscular blocking agents, non-steroidal anti-inflammatory agents, and certain other agents. Compounds in these categories include:

Acarbose (Hyperglycemia may occur with thiazide diuretics; dosage adjustment of the antidiabetic drugs may be required). Products include:
Precose Tablets 776

Acebutolol Hydrochloride (Co-administration with other antihypertensive drugs may result in additive effect or potentiation of the antihypertensive effects with a potential for aggravation of orthostatic hypotension).
No products indexed under this heading.

ACTH (Co-administration with ACTH intensifies the electrolyte depletion, particularly hypokalemia).
No products indexed under this heading.

Alfentanil Hydrochloride (Narcotics may aggravate orthostatic hypotension produced by hydrochlorothiazide).
No products indexed under this heading.

Amlodipine Besylate (Co-administration with other antihypertensive drugs may result in additive effect or potentiation of the antihypertensive effects with a potential for aggravation of orthostatic hypotension). Products include:
Caduet Tablets 2507
Lotrel Capsules 2238
Norvasc Tablets 2529

Aprobarbital (Barbiturates may aggravate orthostatic hypotension produced by hydrochlorothiazide).
No products indexed under this heading.

Atenolol (Co-administration with other antihypertensive drugs may result in additive effect or potentiation of the antihypertensive effects with a potential for aggravation of orthostatic hypotension). Products include:
Tenormin I.V. Injection 698
Tenormin Tablets 695

Atracurium Besylate (Possible increased responsiveness to the muscle relaxant).
No products indexed under this heading.

Benazepril Hydrochloride (Co-administration with other antihypertensive drugs may result in additive effect or potentiation of the antihypertensive effects with a potential for aggravation of orthostatic hypotension). Products include:
Lotensin Tablets 2232
Lotensin HCT Tablets 2235
Lotrel Capsules 2238

Bendroflumethiazide (Co-administration with other antihypertensive drugs may result in additive effect or potentiation of the antihypertensive effects with a potential for aggravation of orthostatic hypotension).
No products indexed under this heading.

Betamethasone Acetate (Co-administration with corticosteroids intensifies the electrolyte depletion, particularly hypokalemia).
No products indexed under this heading.

Betamethasone Sodium Phosphate (Co-administration with corticosteroids intensifies the electrolyte depletion, particularly hypokalemia).
No products indexed under this heading.

Betaxolol Hydrochloride (Co-administration with other antihypertensive drugs may result in additive effect or potentiation of the antihypertensive effects with a potential for aggravation of orthostatic hypotension). Products include:
Betoptic S Ophthalmic Suspension 554

Bisoprolol Fumarate (Co-administration with other antihypertensive drugs may result in additive effect or potentiation of the antihypertensive effects with a potential for aggravation of orthostatic hypotension).
No products indexed under this heading.

Buprenorphine Hydrochloride (Narcotics may aggravate orthostatic hypotension produced by hydrochlorothiazide). Products include:
Buprenex Injectable 2718
Suboxone Tablets 2719
Subutex Tablets 2719

Butabarbital (Barbiturates may aggravate orthostatic hypotension produced by hydrochlorothiazide).
No products indexed under this heading.

Butalbital (Barbiturates may aggravate orthostatic hypotension produced by hydrochlorothiazide). Products include:
Sedapap Tablets 50 mg/650 mg 2098

Captopril (Co-administration with other antihypertensive drugs may result in additive effect or potentiation of the antihypertensive effects with a potential for aggravation of orthostatic hypotension). Products include:
Captopril Tablets 2114

Carteolol Hydrochloride (Co-administration with other antihypertensive drugs may result in additive effect or potentiation of the antihypertensive effects with a potential for aggravation of orthostatic hypotension). Products include:
Carteolol Hydrochloride Ophthalmic Solution USP, 1% .... ⊙ 246

Celecoxib (Co-administration of non-steroidal anti-inflammatory agents can reduce the diuretic, natriuretic, and antihypertensive effects of thiazide diuretics). Products include:
Celebrex Capsules 3130

Chlorothiazide (Co-administration with other antihypertensive drugs may result in additive effect or potentiation of the antihypertensive effects with a potential for aggravation of orthostatic hypotension). Products include:
Aldoclor Tablets 1881
Diuril Oral 1936

Chlorothiazide Sodium (Co-administration with other antihypertensive drugs may result in additive effect or potentiation of the antihypertensive effects with a potential for aggravation of orthostatic hypotension). Products include:
Diuril Sodium Intravenous 1934

Chlorpropamide (Hyperglycemia may occur with thiazide diuretics; dosage adjustment of the antidiabetic drugs may be required).
No products indexed under this heading.

Chlorthalidone (Co-administration with other antihypertensive drugs may result in additive effect or potentiation of the antihypertensive effects with a potential for aggravation of orthostatic hypotension). Products include:
Clorpres Tablets 2139

Cholestyramine (Co-administration with anionic exchange resins, such as cholestyramine, binds the hydrochlorothiazide and reduces its absorption by up to 85 percent).
No products indexed under this heading.

Cisatracurium Besylate (Possible increased responsiveness to the muscle relaxant). Products include:
Nimbex Injection 494

Clonidine (Co-administration with other antihypertensive drugs may result in additive effect or potentiation of the antihypertensive effects with a potential for aggravation of orthostatic hypotension). Products include:
Catapres-TTS 875

Clonidine Hydrochloride (Co-administration with other antihypertensive drugs may result in additive effect or potentiation of the antihypertensive effects with a potential for aggravation of orthostatic hypotension). Products include:
Catapres Tablets 874
Clorpres Tablets 2139

Codeine Phosphate (Narcotics may aggravate orthostatic hypotension produced by hydrochlorothiazide). Products include:
Tylenol with Codeine 2461

Colestipol Hydrochloride (Co-administration with anionic exchange resins, such as colestipol, binds the hydrochlorothiazide and reduces its absorption by up to 43 percent).
No products indexed under this heading.

Cortisone Acetate (Co-administration with corticosteroids intensifies the electrolyte depletion, particularly hypokalemia).
No products indexed under this heading.

Deserpidine (Co-administration with other antihypertensive drugs may result in additive effect or potentiation of the antihypertensive effects with a potential for aggravation of orthostatic hypotension).
No products indexed under this heading.

Dexamethasone (Co-administration with corticosteroids intensifies the electrolyte depletion, particularly hypokalemia). Products include:
Ciprodex Otic Suspension 555
Decadron Tablets 1929
TobraDex Ophthalmic Ointment 558
TobraDex Ophthalmic Suspension 558

Dexamethasone Acetate (Co-administration with corticosteroids intensifies the electrolyte depletion, particularly hypokalemia).
No products indexed under this heading.

Dexamethasone Sodium Phosphate (Co-administration with corticosteroids intensifies the electrolyte depletion, particularly hypokalemia). Products include:
Decadron Phosphate Injection 1931

Dezocine (Narcotics may aggravate orthostatic hypotension produced by hydrochlorothiazide).
No products indexed under this heading.

Diazoxide (Co-administration with other antihypertensive drugs may result in additive effect or potentiation of the antihypertensive effects with a potential for aggravation of orthostatic hypotension). Products include:
Hyperstat I.V. Injection 3031

Diclofenac Potassium (Co-administration of non-steroidal anti-inflammatory agents can reduce the diuretic, natriuretic, and antihypertensive effects of thiazide diuretics). Products include:
Cataflam Tablets 2173

Diclofenac Sodium (Co-administration of non-steroidal anti-inflammatory agents can reduce the diuretic, natriuretic, and antihypertensive effects of thiazide diuretics). Products include:
Arthrotec Tablets 3126
Voltaren Ophthalmic Solution 2300
Voltaren Tablets 2298
Voltaren-XR Tablets 2301

Diltiazem Hydrochloride (Co-administration with other antihypertensive drugs may result in additive effect or potentiation of the antihypertensive effects with a potential for aggravation of orthostatic hypotension). Products include:
Cardizem LA Extended Release Tablets 1699
Tiazac Capsules 1204

Doxazosin Mesylate (Co-administration with other antihypertensive drugs may result in additive effect or potentiation of the antihypertensive effects with a potential for aggravation of orthostatic hypotension).
No products indexed under this heading.

Enalapril Maleate (Co-administration with other antihypertensive drugs may result in additive effect or potentiation of the antihypertensive effects with a potential for aggravation of orthostatic hypotension). Products include:
Vaseretic Tablets 2073
Vasotec I.V. Injection 2076

Enalaprilat (Co-administration with other antihypertensive drugs may result in additive effect or potentiation of the antihypertensive effects with a potential for aggravation of orthostatic hypotension).
No products indexed under this heading.

Eprosartan Mesylate (Co-administration with other antihypertensive drugs may result in additive effect or potentiation of the antihypertensive effects with a potential for aggravation of orthostatic hypotension). Products include:
Teveten Tablets 1707
Teveten HCT Tablets 1710

Esmolol Hydrochloride (Co-administration with other antihypertensive drugs may result in additive effect or potentiation of the antihypertensive effects with a potential for aggravation of orthostatic hypotension). Products include:
Brevibloc Concentrate 766
Brevibloc Injection 766
Brevibloc Double Strength Injection 766
Brevibloc Premixed Injection 766
Brevibloc Double Strength Premixed Injection 766

Etodolac (Co-administration of non-steroidal anti-inflammatory agents can reduce the diuretic, natriuretic, and antihypertensive effects of thiazide diuretics).
No products indexed under this heading.

Felodipine (Co-administration with other antihypertensive drugs may result in additive effect or potentiation of the antihypertensive effects with a potential for aggravation of orthostatic hypotension). Products include:
Plendil Extended-Release Tablets 651

Fenoprofen Calcium (Co-administration of non-steroidal anti-inflammatory agents can reduce the diuretic, natriuretic, and antihypertensive effects of thiazide diuretics). Products include:
Nalfon Capsules 2504

Fentanyl (Narcotics may aggravate orthostatic hypotension produced by hydrochlorothiazide). Products include:
Duragesic Transdermal System 2448

Fentanyl Citrate (Narcotics may aggravate orthostatic hypotension produced by hydrochlorothiazide). Products include:
Actiq 993

Fludrocortisone Acetate (Co-administration with corticosteroids intensifies the electrolyte depletion, particularly hypokalemia).
No products indexed under this heading.

Flurbiprofen (Co-administration of non-steroidal anti-inflammatory agents can reduce the diuretic, natriuretic, and antihypertensive effects of thiazide diuretics).
No products indexed under this heading.

Fosinopril Sodium (Co-administration with other antihypertensive drugs may result in additive effect or potentiation of the antihypertensive effects with a potential for aggravation of orthostatic hypotension).
No products indexed under this heading.

Furosemide (Co-administration with other antihypertensive drugs may result in additive effect or potentiation of the antihypertensive effects with a potential for aggravation of orthostatic hypotension). Products include:
Furosemide Tablets 2117

Glimepiride (Hyperglycemia may occur with thiazide diuretics; dosage adjustment of the antidiabetic drugs may be required). Products include:
Amaryl Tablets 2864

Glipizide (Hyperglycemia may occur with thiazide diuretics; dosage adjustment of the antidiabetic drugs may be required).
No products indexed under this heading.

Glyburide (Hyperglycemia may occur with thiazide diuretics; dosage adjustment of the antidiabetic drugs may be required).
No products indexed under this heading.

Guanabenz Acetate (Co-administration with other antihypertensive drugs may result in additive effect or potentiation of the antihypertensive effects with a potential for aggravation of orthostatic hypotension).
No products indexed under this heading.

Guanethidine Monosulfate (Co-administration with other antihypertensive drugs may result in additive effect or potentiation of the antihypertensive effects with a potential for aggravation of orthostatic hypotension).
No products indexed under this heading.

Hydralazine Hydrochloride (Co-administration with other antihypertensive drugs may result in additive effect or potentiation of the antihypertensive effects with a potential for aggravation of orthostatic hypotension). Products include:
- BiDil Tablets ... 2161

Hydrocodone Bitartrate (Narcotics may aggravate orthostatic hypotension produced by hydrochlorothiazide). Products include:
- Hycodan ... 1104
- Hycomine Compound Tablets ... 1105
- Hycotuss Expectorant Syrup ... 1106
- Lortab ... 3315
- Lortab Elixir ... 3312
- Vicodin Tablets ... 530
- Vicodin ES Tablets ... 531
- Vicodin HP Tablets ... 532
- Vicoprofen Tablets ... 533
- Zydone Tablets ... 1118

Hydrocodone Polistirex (Narcotics may aggravate orthostatic hypotension produced by hydrochlorothiazide). Products include:
- Tussionex Pennkinetic Extended-Release Suspension ... 3322

Hydrocortisone (Co-administration with corticosteroids intensifies the electrolyte depletion, particularly hypokalemia). Products include:
- Cortizone•5 Ointment ... ■ 699
- Cortizone•10 Creme ... ■ 699
- Cortizone•10 Ointment ... ■ 699
- Cortizone•10 Plus Creme ... ■ 700
- Cortizone•10 Maximum Strength Quick Shot Spray ... ■ 700
- Hydrocortone Tablets ... 1963
- Preparation H Hydrocortisone Cream ... ■ 748

Hydrocortisone Acetate (Co-administration with corticosteroids intensifies the electrolyte depletion, particularly hypokalemia). Products include:
- Analpram-HC ... 1136
- Pramosone ... 1139
- ProctoFoam-HC ... 3113
- Tucks Anti-Itch Ointment ... ■ 712
- U-cort 1% Cream ... 3289

Hydrocortisone Sodium Phosphate (Co-administration with corticosteroids intensifies the electrolyte depletion, particularly hypokalemia).
No products indexed under this heading.

Hydrocortisone Sodium Succinate (Co-administration with corticosteroids intensifies the electrolyte depletion, particularly hypokalemia).
No products indexed under this heading.

Hydroflumethiazide (Co-administration with other antihypertensive drugs may result in additive effect or potentiation of the antihypertensive effects with a potential for aggravation of orthostatic hypotension).
No products indexed under this heading.

Hydromorphone Hydrochloride (Narcotics may aggravate orthostatic hypotension produced by hydrochlorothiazide). Products include:
- Dilaudid ... 439
- Dilaudid Oral Liquid ... 443
- Dilaudid Non-Sterile Powder ... 439
- Dilaudid Rectal Suppositories ... 439
- Dilaudid Tablets ... 439
- Dilaudid Tablets - 8 mg ... 443
- Dilaudid-HP ... 441

Ibuprofen (Co-administration of non-steroidal anti-inflammatory agents can reduce the diuretic, natriuretic, and antihypertensive effects of thiazide diuretics). Products include:
- Advil Allergy Sinus Caplets ... ■ 737
- Advil ... ■ 737
- Children's Advil Suspension ... ■ 742
- Children's Advil Chewable Tablets ... ■ 741
- Advil Cold & Sinus ... ■ 739
- Advil Flu & Body Ache Caplets ... ■ 739
- Children's Advil Cold Suspension ... ■ 741
- Infants' Advil Concentrated Drops ... ■ 743
- Junior Strength Advil Swallow Tablets ... ■ 740
- Advil Migraine Liquigels ... ■ 740
- Advil Multi-Symptom Cold Caplets ... ■ 738
- Combunox Tablets ... 1183
- Children's Motrin Oral Suspension and Chewable Tablets ... 1837
- Children's Motrin Cold Non-Staining Dye-Free Oral Suspension ... 1838
- Children's Motrin Cold Oral Suspension ... 1838
- Children's Motrin Non-Staining Dye-Free Oral Suspension ... 1837
- Motrin Cold & Sinus Caplets ... 1836
- Motrin IB Tablets and Caplets ... 1836
- Infants' Motrin Concentrated Drops ... 1837
- Infants' Motrin Non-Staining Dye-Free Drops ... 1837
- Junior Strength Motrin Caplets and Chewable Tablets ... 1837
- Vicoprofen Tablets ... 533

Indapamide (Co-administration with other antihypertensive drugs may result in additive effect or potentiation of the antihypertensive effects with a potential for aggravation of orthostatic hypotension). Products include:
- Indapamide Tablets ... 2119

Indomethacin (Co-administration of non-steroidal anti-inflammatory agents can reduce the diuretic, natriuretic, and antihypertensive effects of thiazide diuretics). Products include:
- Indocin ... 1968

Indomethacin Sodium Trihydrate (Co-administration of non-steroidal anti-inflammatory agents can reduce the diuretic, natriuretic, and antihypertensive effects of thiazide diuretics). Products include:
- Indocin I.V. ... 1973

Insulin, Human, Zinc Suspension (Hyperglycemia may occur with thiazide diuretics; dosage adjustment of the insulin may be required). Products include:
- Humulin L, 100 Units ... 1763
- Humulin U, 100 Units ... 1770

Insulin, Human NPH (Hyperglycemia may occur with thiazide diuretics; dosage adjustment of the insulin may be required). Products include:
- Humulin N, 100 Units ... 1764
- Humulin N Pen ... 1765
- Novolin N Human Insulin 10 ml Vials ... 2322
- Novolin N InnoLet ... 2322
- Novolin N PenFill 3 ml Cartridges ... 2325
- Novolin R InnoLet ... 2322

Insulin, Human Regular (Hyperglycemia may occur with thiazide diuretics; dosage adjustment of the insulin may be required). Products include:
- Humulin R (U-500) ... 1768
- Humulin R, 100 Units ... 1767
- Novolin R Human Insulin 10 ml Vials ... 2322
- Novolin R PenFill ... 2325

Insulin, Human Regular and Human NPH Mixture (Hyperglycemia may occur with thiazide diuretics; dosage adjustment of the insulin may be required). Products include:
- Humulin 50/50, 100 Units ... 1760
- Humulin 70/30 Pen ... 1761
- Novolin 70/30 Human Insulin 10 ml Vials ... 2321
- Novolin 70/30 InnoLet ... 2322
- Novolin 70/30 PenFill 3 ml Cartridges ... 2325

Insulin, NPH (Hyperglycemia may occur with thiazide diuretics; dosage adjustment of the insulin may be required).
No products indexed under this heading.

Insulin, Regular (Hyperglycemia may occur with thiazide diuretics; dosage adjustment of the insulin may be required).
No products indexed under this heading.

Insulin, Zinc Crystals (Hyperglycemia may occur with thiazide diuretics; dosage adjustment of the insulin may be required).
No products indexed under this heading.

Insulin, Zinc Suspension (Hyperglycemia may occur with thiazide diuretics; dosage adjustment of the insulin may be required).
No products indexed under this heading.

Insulin Aspart, Human Regular (Hyperglycemia may occur with thiazide diuretics; dosage adjustment of the insulin may be required). Products include:
- NovoLog Injection ... 2326

Insulin glargine (Hyperglycemia may occur with thiazide diuretics; dosage adjustment of the insulin may be required). Products include:
- Lantus Injection ... 2925

Insulin Lispro, Human (Hyperglycemia may occur with thiazide diuretics; dosage adjustment of the insulin may be required). Products include:
- Humalog-Pen ... 1751
- Humalog Mix 75/25-Pen ... 1754

Insulin Lispro Protamine, Human (Hyperglycemia may occur with thiazide diuretics; dosage adjustment of the insulin may be required). Products include:
- Humalog Mix 75/25-Pen ... 1754

Irbesartan (Co-administration with other antihypertensive drugs may result in additive effect or potentiation of the antihypertensive effects with a potential for aggravation of orthostatic hypotension). Products include:
- Avalide Tablets ... 922
- Avalide Tablets ... 2889
- Avapro Tablets ... 925
- Avapro Tablets ... 2886

Isradipine (Co-administration with other antihypertensive drugs may result in additive effect or potentiation of the antihypertensive effects with a potential for aggravation of orthostatic hypotension). Products include:
- DynaCirc CR Tablets ... 2726

Ketoprofen (Co-administration of non-steroidal anti-inflammatory agents can reduce the diuretic, natriuretic, and antihypertensive effects of thiazide diuretics).
No products indexed under this heading.

Ketorolac Tromethamine (Co-administration of non-steroidal anti-inflammatory agents can reduce the diuretic, natriuretic, and antihypertensive effects of thiazide diuretics). Products include:
- Acular Ophthalmic Solution ... 561
- Acular LS Ophthalmic Solution ... 562

Labetalol Hydrochloride (Co-administration with other antihypertensive drugs may result in additive effect or potentiation of the antihypertensive effects with a potential for aggravation of orthostatic hypotension).
No products indexed under this heading.

Levorphanol Tartrate (Narcotics may aggravate orthostatic hypotension produced by hydrochlorothiazide).
No products indexed under this heading.

Lisinopril (Co-administration with other antihypertensive drugs may result in additive effect or potentiation of the antihypertensive effects with a potential for aggravation of orthostatic hypotension). Products include:
- Prinivil Tablets ... 2029
- Prinzide Tablets ... 2033
- Zestoretic Tablets ... 701
- Zestril Tablets ... 704

Lithium (Hydrochlorothiazide reduces the renal clearance of lithium and can cause a high risk of lithium toxicity; in general, lithium should not be given with diuretics. An increase in serum lithium concentration has been reported during concomitant administration of lithium with candesartan cilexetil; careful monitoring of serum lithium levels is recommended during concomitant use).
No products indexed under this heading.

Lithium Carbonate (Hydrochlorothiazide reduces the renal clearance of lithium and can cause a high risk of lithium toxicity; in general, lithium should not be given with diuretics. An increase in serum lithium concentration has been reported during concomitant administration of lithium with candesartan cilexetil; careful monitoring of serum lithium levels is recommended during concomitant use). Products include:
- Eskalith ... 1406
- Lithobid Tablets ... 1670

Lithium Citrate (Hydrochlorothiazide reduces the renal clearance of lithium and can cause a high risk of lithium toxicity; in general, lithium should not be given with diuretics. An increase in serum lithium concentration has been reported during concomitant administration of lithium with candesartan cilexetil; careful monitoring of serum lithium levels is

recommended during concomitant use).
No products indexed under this heading.

Losartan Potassium (Co-administration with other antihypertensive drugs may result in additive effect or potentiation of the antihypertensive effects with a potential for aggravation of orthostatic hypotension). Products include:
Cozaar Tablets 1913
Hyzaar 1964

Mecamylamine Hydrochloride (Co-administration with other antihypertensive drugs may result in additive effect or potentiation of the antihypertensive effects with a potential for aggravation of orthostatic hypotension). Products include:
Inversine Tablets 3286

Meclofenamate Sodium (Co-administration of non-steroidal anti-inflammatory agents can reduce the diuretic, natriuretic, and antihypertensive effects of thiazide diuretics).
No products indexed under this heading.

Mefenamic Acid (Co-administration of non-steroidal anti-inflammatory agents can reduce the diuretic, natriuretic, and antihypertensive effects of thiazide diuretics).
No products indexed under this heading.

Meloxicam (Co-administration of non-steroidal anti-inflammatory agents can reduce the diuretic, natriuretic, and antihypertensive effects of thiazide diuretics). Products include:
Mobic Oral Suspension 893
Mobic Tablets 893

Meperidine Hydrochloride (Narcotics may aggravate orthostatic hypotension produced by hydrochlorothiazide).
No products indexed under this heading.

Mephobarbital (Barbiturates may aggravate orthostatic hypotension produced by hydrochlorothiazide). Products include:
Mebaral Tablets, USP 2483

Metformin Hydrochloride (Hyperglycemia may occur with thiazide diuretics; dosage adjustment of the antidiabetic drugs may be required). Products include:
ActoPlus Met Tablets 3219
Avandamet Tablets 1343
Fortamet Extended-Release Tablets 1156

Methadone Hydrochloride (Narcotics may aggravate orthostatic hypotension produced by hydrochlorothiazide).
No products indexed under this heading.

Methyclothiazide (Co-administration with other antihypertensive drugs may result in additive effect or potentiation of the antihypertensive effects with a potential for aggravation of orthostatic hypotension).
No products indexed under this heading.

Methyldopa (Co-administration with other antihypertensive drugs may result in additive effect or potentiation of the antihypertensive effects with a potential for aggravation of orthostatic hypotension). Products include:
Aldoclor Tablets 1881
Aldoril Tablets 1884

Methyldopate Hydrochloride (Co-administration with other antihypertensive drugs may result in additive effect or potentiation of the antihypertensive effects with a potential for aggravation of orthostatic hypotension).
No products indexed under this heading.

Methylprednisolone Acetate (Co-administration with corticosteroids intensifies the electrolyte depletion, particularly hypokalemia). Products include:
Depo-Medrol Injectable Suspension 2615
Depo-Medrol Single-Dose Vial 2617

Methylprednisolone Sodium Succinate (Co-administration with corticosteroids intensifies the electrolyte depletion, particularly hypokalemia).
No products indexed under this heading.

Metocurine Iodide (Possible increased responsiveness to the muscle relaxant).
No products indexed under this heading.

Metolazone (Co-administration with other antihypertensive drugs may result in additive effect or potentiation of the antihypertensive effects with a potential for aggravation of orthostatic hypotension).
No products indexed under this heading.

Metoprolol Succinate (Co-administration with other antihypertensive drugs may result in additive effect or potentiation of the antihypertensive effects with a potential for aggravation of orthostatic hypotension). Products include:
Toprol-XL Tablets 660

Metoprolol Tartrate (Co-administration with other antihypertensive drugs may result in additive effect or potentiation of the antihypertensive effects with a potential for aggravation of orthostatic hypotension).
No products indexed under this heading.

Metyrosine (Co-administration with other antihypertensive drugs may result in additive effect or potentiation of the antihypertensive effects with a potential for aggravation of orthostatic hypotension). Products include:
Demser Capsules 1933

Mibefradil Dihydrochloride (Co-administration with other antihypertensive drugs may result in additive effect or potentiation of the antihypertensive effects with a potential for aggravation of orthostatic hypotension).
No products indexed under this heading.

Miglitol (Hyperglycemia may occur with thiazide diuretics; dosage adjustment of the antidiabetic drugs may be required).
No products indexed under this heading.

Minoxidil (Co-administration with other antihypertensive drugs may result in additive effect or potentiation of the antihypertensive effects with a potential for aggravation of orthostatic hypotension). Products include:
Men's Rogaine Extra Strength Topical Solution, Ocean Rush Scent and Original Unscented .... ◘ 706
Women's Rogaine Topical Solution, Spring Bloom Scent and Original Unscented .... ◘ 707

Mivacurium Chloride (Possible increased responsiveness to the muscle relaxant). Products include:
Mivacron Injection 489

Moexipril Hydrochloride (Co-administration with other antihypertensive drugs may result in additive effect or potentiation of the antihypertensive effects with a potential for aggravation of orthostatic hypotension). Products include:
Uniretic Tablets 3114
Univasc Tablets 3118

Morphine Sulfate (Narcotics may aggravate orthostatic hypotension produced by hydrochlorothiazide). Products include:
Avinza Capsules 1714
Kadian Capsules 572
MS Contin Tablets 2703

Nabumetone (Co-administration of non-steroidal anti-inflammatory agents can reduce the diuretic, natriuretic, and antihypertensive effects of thiazide diuretics). Products include:
Relafen Tablets 1523

Nadolol (Co-administration with other antihypertensive drugs may result in additive effect or potentiation of the antihypertensive effects with a potential for aggravation of orthostatic hypotension). Products include:
Nadolol Tablets 2121

Naproxen (Co-administration of non-steroidal anti-inflammatory agents can reduce the diuretic, natriuretic, and antihypertensive effects of thiazide diuretics). Products include:
EC-Naprosyn Delayed-Release Tablets 2769
Naprosyn Suspension 2769
Naprosyn Tablets 2769
Prevacid NapraPAC 3277

Naproxen Sodium (Co-administration of non-steroidal anti-inflammatory agents can reduce the diuretic, natriuretic, and antihypertensive effects of thiazide diuretics). Products include:
Aleve Tablets, Caplets and Gelcaps .... ◘ 605
Anaprox Tablets 2769
Anaprox DS Tablets 2769

Nicardipine Hydrochloride (Co-administration with other antihypertensive drugs may result in additive effect or potentiation of the antihypertensive effects with a potential for aggravation of orthostatic hypotension). Products include:
Cardene I.V. 1129

Nifedipine (Co-administration with other antihypertensive drugs may result in additive effect or potentiation of the antihypertensive effects with a potential for aggravation of orthostatic hypotension). Products include:
Adalat CC Tablets 2978

Nisoldipine (Co-administration with other antihypertensive drugs may result in additive effect or potentiation of the antihypertensive effects with a potential for aggravation of orthostatic hypotension). Products include:
Sular Tablets 1163

Nitroglycerin (Co-administration with other antihypertensive drugs may result in additive effect or potentiation of the antihypertensive effects with a potential for aggravation of orthostatic hypotension). Products include:
Nitro-Dur Transdermal Infusion System 3066
Nitrolingual Pumpspray 1161

Norepinephrine Bitartrate (Possible decreased response to pressor amines).
No products indexed under this heading.

Oxaprozin (Co-administration of non-steroidal anti-inflammatory agents can reduce the diuretic, natriuretic, and antihypertensive effects of thiazide diuretics).
No products indexed under this heading.

Oxycodone Hydrochloride (Narcotics may aggravate orthostatic hypotension produced by hydrochlorothiazide). Products include:
Combunox Tablets 1183
OxyContin Tablets 2699
OxyFast Oral Concentrate Solution 2704
OxyIR Capsules 2704
Percocet Tablets 1114
Percodan Tablets 1115

Pancuronium Bromide (Possible increased responsiveness to the muscle relaxant).
No products indexed under this heading.

Penbutolol Sulfate (Co-administration with other antihypertensive drugs may result in additive effect or potentiation of the antihypertensive effects with a potential for aggravation of orthostatic hypotension).
No products indexed under this heading.

Pentobarbital Sodium (Barbiturates may aggravate orthostatic hypotension produced by hydrochlorothiazide). Products include:
Nembutal Sodium Solution, USP 2484

Perindopril Erbumine (Co-administration with other antihypertensive drugs may result in additive effect or potentiation of the antihypertensive effects with a potential for aggravation of orthostatic hypotension). Products include:
Aceon Tablets (2 mg, 4 mg, 8 mg) 3191

Phenobarbital (Barbiturates may aggravate orthostatic hypotension produced by hydrochlorothiazide).
No products indexed under this heading.

Phenoxybenzamine Hydrochloride (Co-administration with other antihypertensive drugs may result in additive effect or potentiation of the antihypertensive effects with a potential for aggravation of orthostatic hypotension). Products include:
Dibenzyline Capsules 3390

Phentolamine Mesylate (Co-administration with other antihypertensive drugs may result in additive effect or potentiation of the antihypertensive effects with a potential for aggravation of orthostatic hypotension).
No products indexed under this heading.

Phenylbutazone (Co-administration of non-steroidal anti-inflammatory agents can reduce the diuretic, natriuretic, and antihypertensive effects of thiazide diuretics).
No products indexed under this heading.

Pindolol (Co-administration with other antihypertensive drugs may result in additive effect or potentiation of the antihypertensive effects with a potential for aggravation of orthostatic hypotension).
No products indexed under this heading.

Pioglitazone Hydrochloride (Hyperglycemia may occur with thiazide diuretics; dosage adjustment of the antidiabetic drugs may be required). Products include:
ActoPlus Met Tablets **3219**
Actos Tablets **3224**

Piroxicam (Co-administration of non-steroidal anti-inflammatory agents can reduce the diuretic, natriuretic, and antihypertensive effects of thiazide diuretics).
No products indexed under this heading.

Polythiazide (Co-administration with other antihypertensive drugs may result in additive effect or potentiation of the antihypertensive effects with a potential for aggravation of orthostatic hypotension).
No products indexed under this heading.

Prazosin Hydrochloride (Co-administration with other antihypertensive drugs may result in additive effect or potentiation of the antihypertensive effects with a potential for aggravation of orthostatic hypotension).
No products indexed under this heading.

Prednisolone Acetate (Co-administration with corticosteroids intensifies the electrolyte depletion, particularly hypokalemia). Products include:
Blephamide Ophthalmic Ointment **563**
Blephamide Ophthalmic Suspension.................... **564**
Poly-Pred Liquifilm Ophthalmic Suspension .... ⊙ **231**
Pred Forte Ophthalmic Suspension .... ⊙ **233**
Pred Mild Sterile Ophthalmic Suspension .... ⊙ **236**
Pred-G Ophthalmic Suspension ...... ⊙ **234**
Pred-G Sterile Ophthalmic Ointment .... ⊙ **235**

Prednisolone Sodium Phosphate (Co-administration with corticosteroids intensifies the electrolyte depletion, particularly hypokalemia). Products include:
Pediapred Oral Solution **3319**

Prednisolone Tebutate (Co-administration with corticosteroids intensifies the electrolyte depletion, particularly hypokalemia).
No products indexed under this heading.

Prednisone (Co-administration with corticosteroids intensifies the electrolyte depletion, particularly hypokalemia).
No products indexed under this heading.

Propoxyphene Hydrochloride (Narcotics may aggravate orthostatic hypotension produced by hydrochlorothiazide).
No products indexed under this heading.

Propoxyphene Napsylate (Narcotics may aggravate orthostatic hypotension produced by hydrochlorothiazide). Products include:
Darvocet A 500 Tablets **3497**

Propranolol Hydrochloride (Co-administration with other antihypertensive drugs may result in additive effect or potentiation of the antihypertensive effects with a potential for aggravation of orthostatic hypotension). Products include:
Inderal LA Long-Acting Capsules **3421**
InnoPran XL Capsules **2728**

Quinapril Hydrochloride (Co-administration with other antihypertensive drugs may result in additive effect or potentiation of the antihypertensive effects with a potential for aggravation of orthostatic hypotension).
No products indexed under this heading.

Ramipril (Co-administration with other antihypertensive drugs may result in additive effect or potentiation of the antihypertensive effects with a potential for aggravation of orthostatic hypotension). Products include:
Altace Capsules **1673**

Rapacuronium Bromide (Possible increased responsiveness to the muscle relaxant).
No products indexed under this heading.

Rauwolfia Serpentina (Co-administration with other antihypertensive drugs may result in additive effect or potentiation of the antihypertensive effects with a potential for aggravation of orthostatic hypotension).
No products indexed under this heading.

Remifentanil Hydrochloride (Narcotics may aggravate orthostatic hypotension produced by hydrochlorothiazide).
No products indexed under this heading.

Repaglinide (Hyperglycemia may occur with thiazide diuretics; dosage adjustment of the antidiabetic drugs may be required). Products include:
Prandin Tablets (0.5, 1, and 2 mg) **2337**

Rescinnamine (Co-administration with other antihypertensive drugs may result in additive effect or potentiation of the antihypertensive effects with a potential for aggravation of orthostatic hypotension).
No products indexed under this heading.

Reserpine (Co-administration with other antihypertensive drugs may result in additive effect or potentiation of the antihypertensive effects with a potential for aggravation of orthostatic hypotension).
No products indexed under this heading.

Rocuronium Bromide (Possible increased responsiveness to the muscle relaxant). Products include:
Zemuron Injection **2363**

Rofecoxib (Co-administration of non-steroidal anti-inflammatory agents can reduce the diuretic, natriuretic, and antihypertensive effects of thiazide diuretics).
No products indexed under this heading.

Rosiglitazone Maleate (Hyperglycemia may occur with thiazide diuretics; dosage adjustment of the antidiabetic drugs may be required). Products include:
Avandamet Tablets **1343**
Avandia Tablets **1348**

Secobarbital Sodium (Barbiturates may aggravate orthostatic hypotension produced by hydrochlorothiazide).
No products indexed under this heading.

Sodium Nitroprusside (Co-administration with other antihypertensive drugs may result in additive effect or potentiation of the antihypertensive effects with a potential for aggravation of orthostatic hypotension).
No products indexed under this heading.

Sotalol Hydrochloride (Co-administration with other antihypertensive drugs may result in additive effect or potentiation of the antihypertensive effects with a potential for aggravation of orthostatic hypotension).
No products indexed under this heading.

Spirapril Hydrochloride (Co-administration with other antihypertensive drugs may result in additive effect or potentiation of the antihypertensive effects with a potential for aggravation of orthostatic hypotension).
No products indexed under this heading.

Sufentanil Citrate (Narcotics may aggravate orthostatic hypotension produced by hydrochlorothiazide).
No products indexed under this heading.

Sulindac (Co-administration of non-steroidal anti-inflammatory agents can reduce the diuretic, natriuretic, and antihypertensive effects of thiazide diuretics). Products include:
Clinoril Tablets **1899**

Telmisartan (Co-administration with other antihypertensive drugs may result in additive effect or potentiation of the antihypertensive effects with a potential for aggravation of orthostatic hypotension). Products include:
Micardis Tablets **884**
Micardis HCT Tablets **886**

Terazosin Hydrochloride (Co-administration with other antihypertensive drugs may result in additive effect or potentiation of the antihypertensive effects with a potential for aggravation of orthostatic hypotension). Products include:
Hytrin Capsules **469**

Thiamylal Sodium (Barbiturates may aggravate orthostatic hypotension produced by hydrochlorothiazide).
No products indexed under this heading.

Timolol Maleate (Co-administration with other antihypertensive drugs may result in additive effect or potentiation of the antihypertensive effects with a potential for aggravation of orthostatic hypotension). Products include:
Blocadren Tablets **1891**
Cosopt Sterile Ophthalmic Solution.................... **1910**
Timolide Tablets **2056**
Timoptic in Ocudose **2061**
Timoptic Sterile Ophthalmic Solution **2058**
Timoptic-XE Sterile Ophthalmic Gel Forming Solution **2062**

Tolazamide (Hyperglycemia may occur with thiazide diuretics; dosage adjustment of the antidiabetic drugs may be required).
No products indexed under this heading.

Tolbutamide (Hyperglycemia may occur with thiazide diuretics; dosage adjustment of the antidiabetic drugs may be required).
No products indexed under this heading.

Tolmetin Sodium (Co-administration of non-steroidal anti-inflammatory agents can reduce the diuretic, natriuretic, and antihypertensive effects of thiazide diuretics).
No products indexed under this heading.

Torsemide (Co-administration with other antihypertensive drugs may result in additive effect or potentiation of the antihypertensive effects with a potential for aggravation of orthostatic hypotension).
No products indexed under this heading.

Trandolapril (Co-administration with other antihypertensive drugs may result in additive effect or potentiation of the antihypertensive effects with a potential for aggravation of orthostatic hypotension). Products include:
Mavik Tablets **482**
Tarka Tablets **519**

Triamcinolone (Co-administration with corticosteroids intensifies the electrolyte depletion, particularly hypokalemia).
No products indexed under this heading.

Triamcinolone Acetonide (Co-administration with corticosteroids intensifies the electrolyte depletion, particularly hypokalemia). Products include:
Azmacort Inhalation Aerosol **1701**
Nasacort HFA Inhalation Aerosol **2939**
Nasacort AQ Nasal Spray **2937**

Triamcinolone Diacetate (Co-administration with corticosteroids intensifies the electrolyte depletion, particularly hypokalemia).
No products indexed under this heading.

Triamcinolone Hexacetonide (Co-administration with corticosteroids intensifies the electrolyte depletion, particularly hypokalemia).
No products indexed under this heading.

Trimethaphan Camsylate (Co-administration with other antihypertensive drugs may result in additive effect or potentiation of the antihypertensive effects with a potential for aggravation of orthostatic hypotension).
No products indexed under this heading.

Troglitazone (Hyperglycemia may occur with thiazide diuretics; dosage adjustment of the antidiabetic drugs may be required).
No products indexed under this heading.

Tubocurarine Chloride (Possible increased responsiveness to the muscle relaxant).
No products indexed under this heading.

Valdecoxib (Co-administration of non-steroidal anti-inflammatory agents can reduce the diuretic, natriuretic, and antihypertensive effects of thiazide diuretics).
No products indexed under this heading.

Valsartan (Co-administration with other antihypertensive drugs may result in additive effect or potentiation of the antihypertensive effects with a potential for aggravation of orthostatic hypotension). Products include:
Diovan HCT Tablets 2195
Diovan Tablets 2191

Vecuronium Bromide (Possible increased responsiveness to the muscle relaxant).
No products indexed under this heading.

Verapamil Hydrochloride (Co-administration with other antihypertensive drugs may result in additive effect or potentiation of the antihypertensive effects with a potential for aggravation of orthostatic hypotension). Products include:
Covera-HS Tablets 3135
Tarka Tablets 519
Verelan PM Capsules 3120

Food Interactions

Alcohol (May aggravate orthostatic hypotension produced by hydrochlorothiazide).

ATACAND HCT 32-12.5 TABLETS

(Candesartan Cilexetil, Hydrochlorothiazide)........................ 637
See Atacand HCT 16-12.5 Tablets

ATHENA HAIR SYSTEM SUPPLEMENT

(Herbals with Vitamins) 767
None cited in PDR database.

ATHENA HAIR SYSTEM SHAMPOO

(Azelaic Acid, Biotin, Caffeine, Lecithin, Panthenol, Phytosterols, Serenoa repens, Tocopherol Acetate, Zinc Sulfate)........................ 767
None cited in PDR database.

ATROVENT HFA INHALATION AEROSOL

(Ipratropium Bromide) 872
May interact with anticholinergics. Compounds in these categories include:

Atropine Sulfate (Although ipratropium bromide is minimally absorbed into the systemic circulation, there is some potential for an additive interaction with concomitantly used anticholinergic medications. Caution is therefore advised in the co-administration of ipratropium bromide HFA Inhalation Aerosol with other anticholinergic-containing drugs).
No products indexed under this heading.

Belladonna Alkaloids (Although ipratropium bromide is minimally absorbed into the systemic circulation, there is some potential for an additive interaction with concomitantly used anticholinergic medications. Caution is therefore advised in the co-administration of ipratropium bromide HFA Inhalation Aerosol with other anticholinergic-containing drugs). Products include:
Hyland's Teething Tablets 736

Benztropine Mesylate (Although ipratropium bromide is minimally absorbed into the systemic circulation, there is some potential for an additive interaction with concomitantly used anticholinergic medications. Caution is therefore advised in the co-administration of ipratropium bromide HFA Inhalation Aerosol with other anticholinergic-containing drugs). Products include:
Cogentin Injection 1903

Biperiden Hydrochloride (Although ipratropium bromide is minimally absorbed into the systemic circulation, there is some potential for an additive interaction with concomitantly used anticholinergic medications. Caution is therefore advised in the co-administration of ipratropium bromide HFA Inhalation Aerosol with other anticholinergic-containing drugs).
No products indexed under this heading.

Clidinium Bromide (Although ipratropium bromide is minimally absorbed into the systemic circulation, there is some potential for an additive interaction with concomitantly used anticholinergic medications. Caution is therefore advised in the co-administration of ipratropium bromide HFA Inhalation Aerosol with other anticholinergic-containing drugs).
No products indexed under this heading.

Dicyclomine Hydrochloride (Although ipratropium bromide is minimally absorbed into the systemic circulation, there is some potential for an additive interaction with concomitantly used anticholinergic medications. Caution is therefore advised in the co-administration of ipratropium bromide HFA Inhalation Aerosol with other anticholinergic-containing drugs). Products include:
Bentyl Capsules 724
Bentyl Injection 724
Bentyl Syrup 724
Bentyl Tablets 724

Glycopyrrolate (Although ipratropium bromide is minimally absorbed into the systemic circulation, there is some potential for an additive interaction with concomitantly used anticholinergic medications. Caution is therefore advised in the co-administration of ipratropium bromide HFA Inhalation Aerosol with other anticholinergic-containing drugs).
No products indexed under this heading.

Hyoscyamine (Although ipratropium bromide is minimally absorbed into the systemic circulation, there is some potential for an additive interaction with concomitantly used anticholinergic medications. Caution is therefore advised in the co-administration of ipratropium bromide HFA Inhalation Aerosol with other anticholinergic-containing drugs).
No products indexed under this heading.

Hyoscyamine Sulfate (Although ipratropium bromide is minimally absorbed into the systemic circulation, there is some potential for an additive interaction with concomitantly used anticholinergic medications. Caution is therefore advised in the co-administration of ipratropium bromide HFA Inhalation Aerosol with other anticholinergic-containing drugs).
No products indexed under this heading.

Mepenzolate Bromide (Although ipratropium bromide is minimally absorbed into the systemic circulation, there is some potential for an additive interaction with concomitantly used anticholinergic medications. Caution is therefore advised in the co-administration of ipratropium bromide HFA Inhalation Aerosol with other anticholinergic-containing drugs).
No products indexed under this heading.

Oxybutynin Chloride (Although ipratropium bromide is minimally absorbed into the systemic circulation, there is some potential for an additive interaction with concomitantly used anticholinergic medications. Caution is therefore advised in the co-administration of ipratropium bromide HFA Inhalation Aerosol with other anticholinergic-containing drugs). Products include:
Ditropan XL Extended Release Tablets 2391

Procyclidine Hydrochloride (Although ipratropium bromide is minimally absorbed into the systemic circulation, there is some potential for an additive interaction with concomitantly used anticholinergic medications. Caution is therefore advised in the co-administration of ipratropium bromide HFA Inhalation Aerosol with other anticholinergic-containing drugs).
No products indexed under this heading.

Propantheline Bromide (Although ipratropium bromide is minimally absorbed into the systemic circulation, there is some potential for an additive interaction with concomitantly used anticholinergic medications. Caution is therefore advised in the co-administration of ipratropium bromide HFA Inhalation Aerosol with other anticholinergic-containing drugs).
No products indexed under this heading.

Scopolamine (Although ipratropium bromide is minimally absorbed into the systemic circulation, there is some potential for an additive interaction with concomitantly used anticholinergic medications. Caution is therefore advised in the co-administration of ipratropium bromide HFA Inhalation Aerosol with other anticholinergic-containing drugs). Products include:
Transderm Scōp Transdermal Therapeutic System 2166

Scopolamine Hydrobromide (Although ipratropium bromide is minimally absorbed into the systemic circulation, there is some potential for an additive interaction with concomitantly used anticholinergic medications. Caution is therefore advised in the co-administration of ipratropium bromide HFA Inhalation Aerosol with other anticholinergic-containing drugs).
No products indexed under this heading.

Tolterodine Tartrate (Although ipratropium bromide is minimally absorbed into the systemic circulation, there is some potential for an additive interaction with concomitantly used anticholinergic medications. Caution is therefore advised in the co-administration of ipratropium bromide HFA Inhalation Aerosol with other anticholinergic-containing drugs). Products include:
Detrol Tablets 2626
Detrol LA Capsules 2629

Tridihexethyl Chloride (Although ipratropium bromide is minimally absorbed into the systemic circulation, there is some potential for an additive interaction with concomitantly used anticholinergic medications. Caution is therefore advised in the co-administration of ipratropium bromide HFA Inhalation Aerosol with other anticholinergic-containing drugs).
No products indexed under this heading.

Trihexyphenidyl Hydrochloride (Although ipratropium bromide is minimally absorbed into the systemic circulation, there is some potential for an additive interaction with concomitantly used anticholinergic medications. Caution is therefore advised in the co-administration of ipratropium bromide HFA Inhalation Aerosol with other anticholinergic-containing drugs).
No products indexed under this heading.

ATROVENT INHALATION SOLUTION

(Ipratropium Bromide) 868
None cited in PDR database.

ATROVENT NASAL SPRAY 0.03%

(Ipratropium Bromide) 869
May interact with anticholinergics. Compounds in these categories include:

Atropine Sulfate (Some potential for an additive interaction with other concomitantly administered anticholinergic drugs).
No products indexed under this heading.

Belladonna Alkaloids (Some potential for an additive interaction with other concomitantly administered anticholinergic drugs). Products include:
Hyland's Teething Tablets 736

Benztropine Mesylate (Some potential for an additive interaction with other concomitantly administered anticholinergic drugs). Products include:
Cogentin Injection 1903

Biperiden Hydrochloride (Some potential for an additive interaction with other concomitantly administered anticholinergic drugs).
No products indexed under this heading.

Clidinium Bromide (Some potential for an additive interaction with other concomitantly administered anticholinergic drugs).
No products indexed under this heading.

Dicyclomine Hydrochloride (Some potential for an additive interaction with other concomitantly administered anticholinergic drugs). Products include:
Bentyl Capsules 724
Bentyl Injection 724
Bentyl Syrup 724
Bentyl Tablets 724

Glycopyrrolate (Some potential for an additive interaction with other concomitantly administered anticholinergic drugs).
No products indexed under this heading.

Hyoscyamine (Some potential for an additive interaction with other concomitantly administered anticholinergic drugs).
No products indexed under this heading.

Hyoscyamine Sulfate (Some potential for an additive interaction with other concomitantly administered anticholinergic drugs).
No products indexed under this heading.

Mepenzolate Bromide (Some potential for an additive interaction with other concomitantly administered anticholinergic drugs).
No products indexed under this heading.

Oxybutynin Chloride (Some potential for an additive interaction with other concomitantly administered anticholinergic drugs). Products include:
Ditropan XL Extended Release Tablets 2391

Procyclidine Hydrochloride (Some potential for an additive interaction with other concomitantly administered anticholinergic drugs).
No products indexed under this heading.

Propantheline Bromide (Some potential for an additive interaction with other concomitantly administered anticholinergic drugs).
No products indexed under this heading.

Scopolamine (Some potential for an additive interaction with other concomitantly administered anticholinergic drugs). Products include:
Transderm Scōp Transdermal Therapeutic System 2166

Scopolamine Hydrobromide (Some potential for an additive interaction with other concomitantly administered anticholinergic drugs).
No products indexed under this heading.

Tolterodine Tartrate (Some potential for an additive interaction with other concomitantly administered anticholinergic drugs). Products include:
Detrol Tablets 2626
Detrol LA Capsules 2629

Tridihexethyl Chloride (Some potential for an additive interaction with other concomitantly administered anticholinergic drugs).
No products indexed under this heading.

Trihexyphenidyl Hydrochloride (Some potential for an additive interaction with other concomitantly administered anticholinergic drugs).
No products indexed under this heading.

ATROVENT NASAL SPRAY 0.06%

(Ipratropium Bromide) 870
May interact with anticholinergics. Compounds in these categories include:

Atropine Sulfate (Some potential for an additive interaction with other concomitantly administered anticholinergic drugs).
No products indexed under this heading.

Belladonna Alkaloids (Some potential for an additive interaction with other concomitantly administered anticholinergic drugs). Products include:
Hyland's Teething Tablets .... ▣736

Benztropine Mesylate (Some potential for an additive interaction with other concomitantly administered anticholinergic drugs). Products include:
Cogentin Injection 1903

Biperiden Hydrochloride (Some potential for an additive interaction with other concomitantly administered anticholinergic drugs).
No products indexed under this heading.

Clidinium Bromide (Some potential for an additive interaction with other concomitantly administered anticholinergic drugs).
No products indexed under this heading.

Dicyclomine Hydrochloride (Some potential for an additive interaction with other concomitantly administered anticholinergic drugs). Products include:
Bentyl Capsules 724
Bentyl Injection 724
Bentyl Syrup 724
Bentyl Tablets 724

Glycopyrrolate (Some potential for an additive interaction with other concomitantly administered anticholinergic drugs).
No products indexed under this heading.

Hyoscyamine (Some potential for an additive interaction with other concomitantly administered anticholinergic drugs).
No products indexed under this heading.

Hyoscyamine Sulfate (Some potential for an additive interaction with other concomitantly administered anticholinergic drugs).
No products indexed under this heading.

Mepenzolate Bromide (Some potential for an additive interaction with other concomitantly administered anticholinergic drugs).
No products indexed under this heading.

Oxybutynin Chloride (Some potential for an additive interaction with other concomitantly administered anticholinergic drugs). Products include:
Ditropan XL Extended Release Tablets 2391

Procyclidine Hydrochloride (Some potential for an additive interaction with other concomitantly administered anticholinergic drugs).
No products indexed under this heading.

Propantheline Bromide (Some potential for an additive interaction with other concomitantly administered anticholinergic drugs).
No products indexed under this heading.

Scopolamine (Some potential for an additive interaction with other concomitantly administered anticholinergic drugs). Products include:
Transderm Scōp Transdermal Therapeutic System 2166

Scopolamine Hydrobromide (Some potential for an additive interaction with other concomitantly administered anticholinergic drugs).
No products indexed under this heading.

Tolterodine Tartrate (Some potential for an additive interaction with other concomitantly administered anticholinergic drugs). Products include:
Detrol Tablets 2626
Detrol LA Capsules 2629

Tridihexethyl Chloride (Some potential for an additive interaction with other concomitantly administered anticholinergic drugs).
No products indexed under this heading.

Trihexyphenidyl Hydrochloride (Some potential for an additive interaction with other concomitantly administered anticholinergic drugs).
No products indexed under this heading.

ATTENUVAX

(Measles Virus Vaccine Live) 1889
May interact with immunosuppressive agents. Compounds in these categories include:

Azathioprine (Concurrent use in individuals on immunosuppressive therapy is contraindicated). Products include:
Azasan Tablets 2844

Basiliximab (Concurrent use in individuals on immunosuppressive therapy is contraindicated). Products include:
Simulect for Injection 2268

Cyclosporine (Concurrent use in individuals on immunosuppressive therapy is contraindicated). Products include:
Gengraf Capsules 458
Neoral Soft Gelatin Capsules 2247
Neoral Oral Solution 2247
Restasis Ophthalmic Emulsion 570
Sandimmune 2259

Muromonab-CD3 (Concurrent use in individuals on immunosuppressive therapy is contraindicated). Products include:
Orthoclone OKT3 Sterile Solution 2370

Mycophenolate Mofetil (Concurrent use in individuals on immunosuppressive therapy is contraindicated). Products include:
CellCept Capsules 2751
CellCept Oral Suspension 2751
CellCept Tablets 2751

Sirolimus (Concurrent use in individuals on immunosuppressive therapy is contraindicated). Products include:
Rapamune Oral Solution and Tablets 3472

Tacrolimus (Concurrent use in individuals on immunosuppressive therapy is contraindicated). Products include:
Prograf Capsules and Injection 624
Protopic Ointment 629

AUGMENTIN CHEWABLE TABLETS

(Amoxicillin, Clavulanate Potassium) 1331
See Augmentin ES-600 Powder for Oral Suspension

AUGMENTIN POWDER FOR ORAL SUSPENSION

(Amoxicillin, Clavulanate Potassium) 1331
See Augmentin ES-600 Powder for Oral Suspension

AUGMENTIN TABLETS

(Amoxicillin, Clavulanate Potassium) 1334
See Augmentin ES-600 Powder for Oral Suspension

AUGMENTIN XR EXTENDED-RELEASE TABLETS

(Amoxicillin, Clavulanate Potassium) 1340
See Augmentin ES-600 Powder for Oral Suspension

AUGMENTIN ES-600 POWDER FOR ORAL SUSPENSION

(Amoxicillin, Clavulanate Potassium) 1337
May interact with oral contraceptives and certain other agents. Compounds in these categories include:

Allopurinol (Co-administration of ampicillin with allopurinol substantially increases the incidence of rashes; there are no data with Augmentin and allopurinol administered concurrently).
No products indexed under this heading.

Desogestrel (Potential for reduced efficacy of oral contraceptives). Products include:
Ortho-Cept Tablets 2395

Ethinyl Estradiol (Potential for reduced efficacy of oral contraceptives). Products include:
Alesse-28 Tablets 3392
Lo/Ovral-28 Tablets 3423
NuvaRing 2357
Ortho-Cept Tablets 2395
Ortho-Cyclen/Ortho Tri-Cyclen 2414
Ortho Evra Transdermal System 2402
Ortho Tri-Cyclen Lo Tablets 2421
Seasonale Tablets 1073
Triphasil-28 Tablets 3483
Yasmin 28 Tablets 818

Ethynodiol Diacetate (Potential for reduced efficacy of oral contraceptives).
No products indexed under this heading.

Levonorgestrel (Potential for reduced efficacy of oral contraceptives). Products include:
Alesse-28 Tablets 3392
Climara Pro Transdermal System 800
Mirena Intrauterine System 810
Plan B Tablets 1068
Seasonale Tablets 1073
Triphasil-28 Tablets 3483

Mestranol (Potential for reduced efficacy of oral contraceptives).
No products indexed under this heading.

Norethindrone (Potential for reduced efficacy of oral contraceptives). Products include:
Ortho Micronor Tablets 2411

Norethynodrel (Potential for reduced efficacy of oral contraceptives).
No products indexed under this heading.

Norgestimate (Potential for reduced efficacy of oral contraceptives). Products include:
Ortho-Cyclen/Ortho Tri-Cyclen 2414
Ortho Tri-Cyclen Lo Tablets 2421
Prefest Tablets 1069

Norgestrel (Potential for reduced efficacy of oral contraceptives). Products include:
Lo/Ovral-28 Tablets 3423

Probenecid (Decreases the renal tubular secretion of amoxicillin; concurrent use may result in increased and prolonged blood levels of amoxicillin; therefore, concomitant use is not recommended).
No products indexed under this heading.

AVALIDE TABLETS
(Hydrochlorothiazide, Irbesartan) 2889
May interact with antihypertensives, barbiturates, corticosteroids, cardiac glycosides, oral hypoglycemic agents, insulin, lithium preparations, narcotic analgesics, nondepolarizing neuromuscular blocking agents, nonsteroidal anti-inflammatory agents, and certain other agents. Compounds in these categories include:

Acarbose (Hydrochlorothiazide may cause hyperglycemia, therefore, dosage adjustment of oral hypoglycemic agent may be required). Products include:
Precose Tablets 776

Acebutolol Hydrochloride (Hydrochlorothiazide may add to or potentiate the therapeutic effect of other antihypertensive drugs).
No products indexed under this heading.

ACTH (Co-administration with ACTH intensifies electrolyte depletion particularly hypokalemia).
No products indexed under this heading.

Alfentanil Hydrochloride (Potentiation of orthostatic hypotension).
No products indexed under this heading.

Amlodipine Besylate (Hydrochlorothiazide may add to or potentiate the therapeutic effect of other antihypertensive drugs). Products include:
Caduet Tablets 2507
Lotrel Capsules 2238
Norvasc Tablets 2529

Aprobarbital (Potentiation of orthostatic hypotension).
No products indexed under this heading.

Atenolol (Hydrochlorothiazide may add to or potentiate the therapeutic effect of other antihypertensive drugs). Products include:
Tenormin I.V. Injection 698
Tenormin Tablets 695

Atracurium Besylate (Possible increased responsiveness to the muscle relaxants).
No products indexed under this heading.

Benazepril Hydrochloride (Hydrochlorothiazide may add to or potentiate the therapeutic effect of other antihypertensive drugs). Products include:
Lotensin Tablets 2232
Lotensin HCT Tablets 2235
Lotrel Capsules 2238

Bendroflumethiazide (Hydrochlorothiazide may add to or potentiate the therapeutic effect of other antihypertensive drugs).
No products indexed under this heading.

Betamethasone Acetate (Co-administration with corticosteroids intensifies electrolyte depletion particularly hypokalemia).
No products indexed under this heading.

Betamethasone Sodium Phosphate (Co-administration with corticosteroids intensifies electrolyte depletion particularly hypokalemia).
No products indexed under this heading.

Betaxolol Hydrochloride (Hydrochlorothiazide may add to or potentiate the therapeutic effect of other antihypertensive drugs). Products include:
Betoptic S Ophthalmic Suspension.................................. 554

Bisoprolol Fumarate (Hydrochlorothiazide may add to or potentiate the therapeutic effect of other antihypertensive drugs).
No products indexed under this heading.

Buprenorphine Hydrochloride (Potentiation of orthostatic hypotension). Products include:
Buprenex Injectable 2718
Suboxone Tablets 2719
Subutex Tablets 2719

Butabarbital (Potentiation of orthostatic hypotension).
No products indexed under this heading.

Butalbital (Potentiation of orthostatic hypotension). Products include:
Sedapap Tablets 50 mg/650 mg 2098

Candesartan Cilexetil (Hydrochlorothiazide may add to or potentiate the therapeutic effect of other antihypertensive drugs). Products include:
Atacand Tablets 634
Atacand HCT 637

Captopril (Hydrochlorothiazide may add to or potentiate the therapeutic effect of other antihypertensive drugs). Products include:
Captopril Tablets 2114

Carteolol Hydrochloride (Hydrochlorothiazide may add to or potentiate the therapeutic effect of other antihypertensive drugs). Products include:
Carteolol Hydrochloride Ophthalmic Solution USP, 1%....... ⊙246

Celecoxib (Co-administration with non-steroidal anti-inflammatory agents may reduce the natriuretic and antihypertensive effects of thiazides). Products include:
Celebrex Capsules 3130

Chlorothiazide (Hydrochlorothiazide may add to or potentiate the therapeutic effect of other antihypertensive drugs). Products include:
Aldoclor Tablets 1881
Diuril Oral 1936

Chlorothiazide Sodium (Hydrochlorothiazide may add to or potentiate the therapeutic effect of other antihypertensive drugs). Products include:
Diuril Sodium Intravenous 1934

Chlorpropamide (Hydrochlorothiazide may cause hyperglycemia, therefore, dosage adjustment of oral hypoglycemic agent may be required).
No products indexed under this heading.

Chlorthalidone (Hydrochlorothiazide may add to or potentiate the therapeutic effect of other antihypertensive drugs). Products include:
Clorpres Tablets 2139

Cholestyramine (Absorption of hydrochlorothiazide is impaired in the presence of anionic exchange resins; single dose of cholestyramine binds the hydrochlorothiazide and reduces its absorption from GI tract by 85%).
No products indexed under this heading.

Cisatracurium Besylate (Possible increased responsiveness to the muscle relaxants). Products include:
Nimbex Injection 494

Clonidine (Hydrochlorothiazide may add to or potentiate the therapeutic effect of other antihypertensive drugs). Products include:
Catapres-TTS 875

Clonidine Hydrochloride (Hydrochlorothiazide may add to or potentiate the therapeutic effect of other antihypertensive drugs). Products include:
Catapres Tablets 874
Clorpres Tablets 2139

Codeine Phosphate (Potentiation of orthostatic hypotension). Products include:
Tylenol with Codeine 2461

Colestipol Hydrochloride (Absorption of hydrochlorothiazide is impaired in the presence of anionic exchange resins; single dose of colestipol binds the hydrochlorothiazide and reduces its absorption from GI tract by 43%).
No products indexed under this heading.

Cortisone Acetate (Co-administration with corticosteroids intensifies electrolyte depletion particularly hypokalemia).
No products indexed under this heading.

Deserpidine (Hydrochlorothiazide may add to or potentiate the therapeutic effect of other antihypertensive drugs).
No products indexed under this heading.

Deslanoside (Concurrent digitalis therapy may exaggerate metabolic effects of hypokalemia, especially myocardial effects, e.g., increased ventricular irritability).
No products indexed under this heading.

Dexamethasone (Co-administration with corticosteroids intensifies electrolyte depletion particularly hypokalemia). Products include:
Ciprodex Otic Suspension 555
Decadron Tablets 1929
TobraDex Ophthalmic Ointment 558
TobraDex Ophthalmic Suspension ... 558

Dexamethasone Acetate (Co-administration with corticosteroids intensifies electrolyte depletion particularly hypokalemia).
No products indexed under this heading.

Dexamethasone Sodium Phosphate (Co-administration with corticosteroids intensifies electrolyte depletion particularly hypokalemia). Products include:
Decadron Phosphate Injection 1931

Dezocine (Potentiation of orthostatic hypotension).
No products indexed under this heading.

Diazoxide (Hydrochlorothiazide may add to or potentiate the therapeutic effect of other antihypertensive drugs). Products include:
Hyperstat I.V. Injection 3031

Diclofenac Potassium (Co-administration with non-steroidal anti-inflammatory agents may reduce the natriuretic and antihypertensive effects of thiazides). Products include:
Cataflam Tablets 2173

Diclofenac Sodium (Co-administration with non-steroidal anti-inflammatory agents may reduce the natriuretic and antihypertensive effects of thiazides). Products include:
Arthrotec Tablets 3126
Voltaren Ophthalmic Solution 2300
Voltaren Tablets 2298
Voltaren-XR Tablets 2301

Digitalis Glycoside Preparations (Concurrent digitalis therapy may exaggerate metabolic effects of hypokalemia, especially myocardial effects, e.g., increased ventricular irritability).
No products indexed under this heading.

Digitoxin (Concurrent digitalis therapy may exaggerate metabolic effects of hypokalemia, especially myocardial effects, e.g., increased ventricular irritability).
No products indexed under this heading.

Digoxin (Concurrent digitalis therapy may exaggerate metabolic effects of hypokalemia, especially myocardial effects, e.g., increased ventricular irritability). Products include:
Digitek Tablets 2146
Lanoxicaps Capsules 1458
Lanoxin Injection 1462
Lanoxin Tablets 1468
Lanoxin Injection Pediatric 1465

Diltiazem Hydrochloride (Hydrochlorothiazide may add to or potentiate the therapeutic effect of other antihypertensive drugs). Products include:
Cardizem LA Extended Release Tablets.. 1699
Tiazac Capsules 1204

Doxazosin Mesylate (Hydrochlorothiazide may add to or potentiate the therapeutic effect of other antihypertensive drugs).
No products indexed under this heading.

Enalapril Maleate (Hydrochlorothiazide may add to or potentiate the therapeutic effect of other antihypertensive drugs). Products include:
Vaseretic Tablets 2073
Vasotec I.V. Injection 2076

IMPORTANT NOTE: Always consult each drug listing in the patient's regimen for possible interactions.

Enalaprilat (Hydrochlorothiazide may add to or potentiate the therapeutic effect of other antihypertensive drugs).
No products indexed under this heading.

Eprosartan Mesylate (Hydrochlorothiazide may add to or potentiate the therapeutic effect of other antihypertensive drugs). Products include:
Teveten Tablets 1707
Teveten HCT Tablets 1710

Esmolol Hydrochloride (Hydrochlorothiazide may add to or potentiate the therapeutic effect of other antihypertensive drugs). Products include:
Brevibloc Concentrate 766
Brevibloc Injection 766
Brevibloc Double Strength Injection 766
Brevibloc Premixed Injection 766
Brevibloc Double Strength Premixed Injection 766

Etodolac (Co-administration with non-steroidal anti-inflammatory agents may reduce the natriuretic and antihypertensive effects of thiazides).
No products indexed under this heading.

Felodipine (Hydrochlorothiazide may add to or potentiate the therapeutic effect of other antihypertensive drugs). Products include:
Plendil Extended-Release Tablets 651

Fenoprofen Calcium (Co-administration with non-steroidal anti-inflammatory agents may reduce the natriuretic and antihypertensive effects of thiazides). Products include:
Nalfon Capsules 2504

Fentanyl (Potentiation of orthostatic hypotension). Products include:
Duragesic Transdermal System 2448

Fentanyl Citrate (Potentiation of orthostatic hypotension). Products include:
Actiq 993

Fludrocortisone Acetate (Co-administration with corticosteroids intensifies electrolyte depletion particularly hypokalemia).
No products indexed under this heading.

Flurbiprofen (Co-administration with non-steroidal anti-inflammatory agents may reduce the natriuretic and antihypertensive effects of thiazides).
No products indexed under this heading.

Fosinopril Sodium (Hydrochlorothiazide may add to or potentiate the therapeutic effect of other antihypertensive drugs).
No products indexed under this heading.

Furosemide (Hydrochlorothiazide may add to or potentiate the therapeutic effect of other antihypertensive drugs). Products include:
Furosemide Tablets 2117

Glimepiride (Hydrochlorothiazide may cause hyperglycemia, therefore, dosage adjustment of oral hypoglycemic agent may be required). Products include:
Amaryl Tablets 2864

Glipizide (Hydrochlorothiazide may cause hyperglycemia, therefore, dosage adjustment of oral hypoglycemic agent may be required).
No products indexed under this heading.

Glyburide (Hydrochlorothiazide may cause hyperglycemia, therefore, dosage adjustment of oral hypoglycemic agent may be required).
No products indexed under this heading.

Guanabenz Acetate (Hydrochlorothiazide may add to or potentiate the therapeutic effect of other antihypertensive drugs).
No products indexed under this heading.

Guanethidine Monosulfate (Hydrochlorothiazide may add to or potentiate the therapeutic effect of other antihypertensive drugs).
No products indexed under this heading.

Hydralazine Hydrochloride (Hydrochlorothiazide may add to or potentiate the therapeutic effect of other antihypertensive drugs). Products include:
BiDil Tablets 2161

Hydrocodone Bitartrate (Potentiation of orthostatic hypotension). Products include:
Hycodan 1104
Hycomine Compound Tablets 1105
Hycotuss Expectorant Syrup 1106
Lortab 3315
Lortab Elixir 3312
Vicodin Tablets 530
Vicodin ES Tablets 531
Vicodin HP Tablets 532
Vicoprofen Tablets 533
Zydone Tablets 1118

Hydrocodone Polistirex (Potentiation of orthostatic hypotension). Products include:
Tussionex Pennkinetic Extended-Release Suspension 3322

Hydrocortisone (Co-administration with corticosteroids intensifies electrolyte depletion particularly hypokalemia). Products include:
Cortizone•5 Ointment ▣699
Cortizone•10 Creme ▣699
Cortizone•10 Ointment ▣699
Cortizone•10 Plus Creme ▣700
Cortizone•10 Maximum Strength Quick Shot Spray ▣700
Hydrocortone Tablets 1963
Preparation H Hydrocortisone Cream ▣748

Hydrocortisone Acetate (Co-administration with corticosteroids intensifies electrolyte depletion particularly hypokalemia). Products include:
Analpram-HC 1136
Pramosone 1139
ProctoFoam-HC 3113
Tucks Anti-Itch Ointment ▣712
U-cort 1% Cream 3289

Hydrocortisone Sodium Phosphate (Co-administration with corticosteroids intensifies electrolyte depletion particularly hypokalemia).
No products indexed under this heading.

Hydrocortisone Sodium Succinate (Co-administration with corticosteroids intensifies electrolyte depletion particularly hypokalemia).
No products indexed under this heading.

Hydroflumethiazide (Hydrochlorothiazide may add to or potentiate the therapeutic effect of other antihypertensive drugs).
No products indexed under this heading.

Hydromorphone Hydrochloride (Potentiation of orthostatic hypotension). Products include:
Dilaudid 439
Dilaudid Oral Liquid 443
Dilaudid Non-Sterile Powder 439
Dilaudid Rectal Suppositories 439
Dilaudid Tablets 439
Dilaudid Tablets - 8 mg 443
Dilaudid-HP 441

Ibuprofen (Co-administration with non-steroidal anti-inflammatory agents may reduce the natriuretic and antihypertensive effects of thiazides). Products include:
Advil Allergy Sinus Caplets ▣737
Advil ▣737
Children's Advil Suspension ▣742
Children's Advil Chewable Tablets ▣741
Advil Cold & Sinus ▣739
Advil Flu & Body Ache Caplets ▣739
Children's Advil Cold Suspension ▣741
Infants' Advil Concentrated Drops ▣743
Junior Strength Advil Swallow Tablets ▣740
Advil Migraine Liquigels ▣740
Advil Multi-Symptom Cold Caplets ▣738
Combunox Tablets 1183
Children's Motrin Oral Suspension and Chewable Tablets 1837
Children's Motrin Cold Non-Staining Dye-Free Oral Suspension 1838
Children's Motrin Cold Oral Suspension 1838
Children's Motrin Non-Staining Dye-Free Oral Suspension 1837
Motrin Cold & Sinus Caplets 1836
Motrin IB Tablets and Caplets 1836
Infants' Motrin Concentrated Drops 1837
Infants' Motrin Non-Staining Dye-Free Drops 1837
Junior Strength Motrin Caplets and Chewable Tablets 1837
Vicoprofen Tablets 533

Indapamide (Hydrochlorothiazide may add to or potentiate the therapeutic effect of other antihypertensive drugs). Products include:
Indapamide Tablets 2119

Indomethacin (Co-administration with non-steroidal anti-inflammatory agents may reduce the natriuretic and antihypertensive effects of thiazides). Products include:
Indocin 1968

Indomethacin Sodium Trihydrate (Co-administration with non-steroidal anti-inflammatory agents may reduce the natriuretic and antihypertensive effects of thiazides). Products include:
Indocin I.V. 1973

Insulin, Human, Zinc Suspension (Hydrochlorothiazide may cause hyperglycemia, therefore, dosage adjustment of insulin may be required). Products include:
Humulin L, 100 Units 1763
Humulin U, 100 Units 1770

Insulin, Human NPH (Hydrochlorothiazide may cause hyperglycemia, therefore, dosage adjustment of insulin may be required). Products include:
Humulin N, 100 Units 1764
Humulin N Pen 1765
Novolin N Human Insulin 10 ml Vials 2322
Novolin N InnoLet 2322
Novolin N PenFill 3 ml Cartridges 2325
Novolin R InnoLet 2322

Insulin, Human Regular (Hydrochlorothiazide may cause hyperglycemia, therefore, dosage adjustment of insulin may be required). Products include:
Humulin R (U-500) 1768
Humulin R, 100 Units 1767
Novolin R Human Insulin 10 ml Vials 2322
Novolin R PenFill 2325

Insulin, Human Regular and Human NPH Mixture (Hydrochlorothiazide may cause hyperglycemia, therefore, dosage adjustment of insulin may be required). Products include:
Humulin 50/50, 100 Units 1760
Humulin 70/30 Pen 1761
Novolin 70/30 Human Insulin 10 ml Vials 2321
Novolin 70/30 InnoLet 2322
Novolin 70/30 PenFill 3 ml Cartridges 2325

Insulin, NPH (Hydrochlorothiazide may cause hyperglycemia, therefore, dosage adjustment of insulin may be required).
No products indexed under this heading.

Insulin, Regular (Hydrochlorothiazide may cause hyperglycemia, therefore, dosage adjustment of insulin may be required).
No products indexed under this heading.

Insulin, Zinc Crystals (Hydrochlorothiazide may cause hyperglycemia, therefore, dosage adjustment of insulin may be required).
No products indexed under this heading.

Insulin, Zinc Suspension (Hydrochlorothiazide may cause hyperglycemia, therefore, dosage adjustment of insulin may be required).
No products indexed under this heading.

Insulin Aspart, Human Regular (Hydrochlorothiazide may cause hyperglycemia, therefore, dosage adjustment of insulin may be required). Products include:
NovoLog Injection 2326

Insulin glargine (Hydrochlorothiazide may cause hyperglycemia, therefore, dosage adjustment of insulin may be required). Products include:
Lantus Injection 2925

Insulin Lispro, Human (Hydrochlorothiazide may cause hyperglycemia, therefore, dosage adjustment of insulin may be required). Products include:
Humalog-Pen 1751
Humalog Mix 75/25-Pen 1754

Insulin Lispro Protamine, Human (Hydrochlorothiazide may cause hyperglycemia, therefore, dosage adjustment of insulin may be required). Products include:
Humalog Mix 75/25-Pen 1754

Isradipine (Hydrochlorothiazide may add to or potentiate the therapeutic effect of other antihypertensive drugs). Products include:
DynaCirc CR Tablets 2726

Ketoprofen (Co-administration with non-steroidal anti-inflammatory agents may reduce the natriuretic and antihypertensive effects of thiazides).
No products indexed under this heading.

Ketorolac Tromethamine (Co-administration with non-steroidal anti-inflammatory agents may reduce the natriuretic and antihypertensive effects of thiazides). Products include:
Acular Ophthalmic Solution ⊙561
Acular LS Ophthalmic Solution ⊙562

Labetalol Hydrochloride (Hydrochlorothiazide may add to or potentiate the therapeutic effect of other antihypertensive drugs).
No products indexed under this heading.

Levorphanol Tartrate (Potentiation of orthostatic hypotension).
No products indexed under this heading.

Lisinopril (Hydrochlorothiazide may add to or potentiate the therapeutic effect of other antihypertensive drugs). Products include:
Prinivil Tablets ... 2029
Prinzide Tablets ... 2033
Zestoretic Tablets ... 701
Zestril Tablets ... 704

Lithium (Diuretics reduce lithium's renal clearance and add a high risk of lithium toxicity).
No products indexed under this heading.

Lithium Carbonate (Diuretics reduce lithium's renal clearance and add a high risk of lithium toxicity). Products include:
Eskalith ... 1406
Lithobid Tablets ... 1670

Lithium Citrate (Diuretics reduce lithium's renal clearance and add a high risk of lithium toxicity).
No products indexed under this heading.

Losartan Potassium (Hydrochlorothiazide may add to or potentiate the therapeutic effect of other antihypertensive drugs). Products include:
Cozaar Tablets ... 1913
Hyzaar ... 1964

Mecamylamine Hydrochloride (Hydrochlorothiazide may add to or potentiate the therapeutic effect of other antihypertensive drugs). Products include:
Inversine Tablets ... 3286

Meclofenamate Sodium (Co-administration with non-steroidal anti-inflammatory agents may reduce the natriuretic and antihypertensive effects of thiazides).
No products indexed under this heading.

Mefenamic Acid (Co-administration with non-steroidal anti-inflammatory agents may reduce the natriuretic and antihypertensive effects of thiazides).
No products indexed under this heading.

Meloxicam (Co-administration with non-steroidal anti-inflammatory agents may reduce the natriuretic and antihypertensive effects of thiazides). Products include:
Mobic Oral Suspension ... 893
Mobic Tablets ... 893

Meperidine Hydrochloride (Potentiation of orthostatic hypotension).
No products indexed under this heading.

Mephobarbital (Potentiation of orthostatic hypotension). Products include:
Mebaral Tablets, USP ... 2483

Metformin Hydrochloride (Hydrochlorothiazide may cause hyperglycemia, therefore, dosage adjustment of oral hypoglycemic agent may be required). Products include:
ActoPlus Met Tablets ... 3219
Avandamet Tablets ... 1343
Fortamet Extended-Release Tablets ... 1156

Methadone Hydrochloride (Potentiation of orthostatic hypotension).
No products indexed under this heading.

Methyclothiazide (Hydrochlorothiazide may add to or potentiate the therapeutic effect of other antihypertensive drugs).
No products indexed under this heading.

Methyldopa (Hydrochlorothiazide may add to or potentiate the therapeutic effect of other antihypertensive drugs). Products include:
Aldoclor Tablets ... 1881
Aldoril Tablets ... 1884

Methyldopate Hydrochloride (Hydrochlorothiazide may add to or potentiate the therapeutic effect of other antihypertensive drugs).
No products indexed under this heading.

Methylprednisolone Acetate (Co-administration with corticosteroids intensifies electrolyte depletion particularly hypokalemia). Products include:
Depo-Medrol Injectable Suspension ... 2615
Depo-Medrol Single-Dose Vial ... 2617

Methylprednisolone Sodium Succinate (Co-administration with corticosteroids intensifies electrolyte depletion particularly hypokalemia).
No products indexed under this heading.

Metocurine Iodide (Possible increased responsiveness to the muscle relaxants).
No products indexed under this heading.

Metolazone (Hydrochlorothiazide may add to or potentiate the therapeutic effect of other antihypertensive drugs).
No products indexed under this heading.

Metoprolol Succinate (Hydrochlorothiazide may add to or potentiate the therapeutic effect of other antihypertensive drugs). Products include:
Toprol-XL Tablets ... 660

Metoprolol Tartrate (Hydrochlorothiazide may add to or potentiate the therapeutic effect of other antihypertensive drugs).
No products indexed under this heading.

Metyrosine (Hydrochlorothiazide may add to or potentiate the therapeutic effect of other antihypertensive drugs). Products include:
Demser Capsules ... 1933

Mibefradil Dihydrochloride (Hydrochlorothiazide may add to or potentiate the therapeutic effect of other antihypertensive drugs).
No products indexed under this heading.

Miglitol (Hydrochlorothiazide may cause hyperglycemia, therefore, dosage adjustment of oral hypoglycemic agent may be required).
No products indexed under this heading.

Minoxidil (Hydrochlorothiazide may add to or potentiate the therapeutic effect of other antihypertensive drugs). Products include:
Men's Rogaine Extra Strength Topical Solution, Ocean Rush Scent and Original Unscented ... 706
Women's Rogaine Topical Solution, Spring Bloom Scent and Original Unscented ... 707

Mivacurium Chloride (Possible increased responsiveness to the muscle relaxants). Products include:
Mivacron Injection ... 489

Moexipril Hydrochloride (Hydrochlorothiazide may add to or potentiate the therapeutic effect of other antihypertensive drugs). Products include:
Uniretic Tablets ... 3114
Univasc Tablets ... 3118

Morphine Sulfate (Potentiation of orthostatic hypotension). Products include:
Avinza Capsules ... 1714
Kadian Capsules ... 572
MS Contin Tablets ... 2703

Nabumetone (Co-administration with non-steroidal anti-inflammatory agents may reduce the natriuretic and antihypertensive effects of thiazides). Products include:
Relafen Tablets ... 1523

Nadolol (Hydrochlorothiazide may add to or potentiate the therapeutic effect of other antihypertensive drugs). Products include:
Nadolol Tablets ... 2121

Naproxen (Co-administration with non-steroidal anti-inflammatory agents may reduce the natriuretic and antihypertensive effects of thiazides). Products include:
EC-Naprosyn Delayed-Release Tablets ... 2769
Naprosyn Suspension ... 2769
Naprosyn Tablets ... 2769
Prevacid NapraPAC ... 3277

Naproxen Sodium (Co-administration with non-steroidal anti-inflammatory agents may reduce the natriuretic and antihypertensive effects of thiazides). Products include:
Aleve Tablets, Caplets and Gelcaps ... 605
Anaprox Tablets ... 2769
Anaprox DS Tablets ... 2769

Nicardipine Hydrochloride (Hydrochlorothiazide may add to or potentiate the therapeutic effect of other antihypertensive drugs). Products include:
Cardene I.V. ... 1129

Nifedipine (In vitro studies show significant inhibition of the formation of oxidized irbesartan metabolites with the known cytochrome CYP 2C9 substrate/inhibitor, nifedipine; the pharmacokinetics of irbesartan were not affected by co-administration of nifedipine; hydrochlorothiazide may add to or potentiate the therapeutic effect of other antihypertensive drugs). Products include:
Adalat CC Tablets ... 2978

Nisoldipine (Hydrochlorothiazide may add to or potentiate the therapeutic effect of other antihypertensive drugs). Products include:
Sular Tablets ... 1163

Nitroglycerin (Hydrochlorothiazide may add to or potentiate the therapeutic effect of other antihypertensive drugs). Products include:
Nitro-Dur Transdermal Infusion System ... 3060
Nitrolingual Pumpspray ... 1161

Norepinephrine Bitartrate (Thiazides may decrease arterial responsiveness to norepinephrine).
No products indexed under this heading.

Oxaprozin (Co-administration with non-steroidal anti-inflammatory agents may reduce the natriuretic and antihypertensive effects of thiazides).
No products indexed under this heading.

Oxycodone Hydrochloride (Potentiation of orthostatic hypotension). Products include:
Combunox Tablets ... 1183
OxyContin Tablets ... 2699
OxyFast Oral Concentrate Solution ... 2704
OxyIR Capsules ... 2704
Percocet Tablets ... 1114
Percodan Tablets ... 1115

Pancuronium Bromide (Possible increased responsiveness to the muscle relaxants).
No products indexed under this heading.

Penbutolol Sulfate (Hydrochlorothiazide may add to or potentiate the therapeutic effect of other antihypertensive drugs).
No products indexed under this heading.

Pentobarbital Sodium (Potentiation of orthostatic hypotension). Products include:
Nembutal Sodium Solution, USP ... 2484

Perindopril Erbumine (Hydrochlorothiazide may add to or potentiate the therapeutic effect of other antihypertensive drugs). Products include:
Aceon Tablets (2 mg, 4 mg, 8 mg) ... 3191

Phenobarbital (Potentiation of orthostatic hypotension).
No products indexed under this heading.

Phenoxybenzamine Hydrochloride (Hydrochlorothiazide may add to or potentiate the therapeutic effect of other antihypertensive drugs). Products include:
Dibenzyline Capsules ... 3390

Phentolamine Mesylate (Hydrochlorothiazide may add to or potentiate the therapeutic effect of other antihypertensive drugs).
No products indexed under this heading.

Phenylbutazone (Co-administration with non-steroidal anti-inflammatory agents may reduce the natriuretic and antihypertensive effects of thiazides).
No products indexed under this heading.

Pindolol (Hydrochlorothiazide may add to or potentiate the therapeutic effect of other antihypertensive drugs).
No products indexed under this heading.

Pioglitazone Hydrochloride (Hydrochlorothiazide may cause hyperglycemia, therefore, dosage adjustment of oral hypoglycemic agent may be required). Products include:
ActoPlus Met Tablets ... 3219
Actos Tablets ... 3224

Piroxicam (Co-administration with non-steroidal anti-inflammatory agents may reduce the natriuretic and antihypertensive effects of thiazides).
No products indexed under this heading.

Polythiazide (Hydrochlorothiazide may add to or potentiate the therapeutic effect of other antihypertensive drugs).
No products indexed under this heading.

Prazosin Hydrochloride (Hydrochlorothiazide may add to or potentiate the therapeutic effect of other antihypertensive drugs).
No products indexed under this heading.

Prednisolone Acetate (Co-administration with corticosteroids

IMPORTANT NOTE: Always consult each drug listing in the patient's regimen for possible interactions.

intensifies electrolyte depletion particularly hypokalemia). Products include:
- Blephamide Ophthalmic Ointment 563
- Blephamide Ophthalmic Suspension 564
- Poly-Pred Liquifilm Ophthalmic Suspension .... ⊙231
- Pred Forte Ophthalmic Suspension .... ⊙233
- Pred Mild Sterile Ophthalmic Suspension .... ⊙236
- Pred-G Ophthalmic Suspension .... ⊙234
- Pred-G Sterile Ophthalmic Ointment .... ⊙235

Prednisolone Sodium Phosphate (Co-administration with corticosteroids intensifies electrolyte depletion particularly hypokalemia). Products include:
- Pediapred Oral Solution 3319

Prednisolone Tebutate (Co-administration with corticosteroids intensifies electrolyte depletion particularly hypokalemia).
No products indexed under this heading.

Prednisone (Co-administration with corticosteroids intensifies electrolyte depletion particularly hypokalemia).
No products indexed under this heading.

Propoxyphene Hydrochloride (Potentiation of orthostatic hypotension).
No products indexed under this heading.

Propoxyphene Napsylate (Potentiation of orthostatic hypotension). Products include:
- Darvocet A 500 Tablets 3497

Propranolol Hydrochloride (Hydrochlorothiazide may add to or potentiate the therapeutic effect of other antihypertensive drugs). Products include:
- Inderal LA Long-Acting Capsules 3421
- InnoPran XL Capsules 2728

Quinapril Hydrochloride (Hydrochlorothiazide may add to or potentiate the therapeutic effect of other antihypertensive drugs).
No products indexed under this heading.

Ramipril (Hydrochlorothiazide may add to or potentiate the therapeutic effect of other antihypertensive drugs). Products include:
- Altace Capsules 1673

Rapacuronium Bromide (Possible increased responsiveness to the muscle relaxants).
No products indexed under this heading.

Rauwolfia Serpentina (Hydrochlorothiazide may add to or potentiate the therapeutic effect of other antihypertensive drugs).
No products indexed under this heading.

Remifentanil Hydrochloride (Potentiation of orthostatic hypotension).
No products indexed under this heading.

Repaglinide (Hydrochlorothiazide may cause hyperglycemia, therefore, dosage adjustment of oral hypoglycemic agent may be required). Products include:
- Prandin Tablets (0.5, 1, and 2 mg) 2337

Rescinnamine (Hydrochlorothiazide may add to or potentiate the therapeutic effect of other antihypertensive drugs).
No products indexed under this heading.

Reserpine (Hydrochlorothiazide may add to or potentiate the therapeutic effect of other antihypertensive drugs).
No products indexed under this heading.

Rocuronium Bromide (Possible increased responsiveness to the muscle relaxants). Products include:
- Zemuron Injection 2363

Rofecoxib (Co-administration with non-steroidal anti-inflammatory agents may reduce the natriuretic and antihypertensive effects of thiazides).
No products indexed under this heading.

Rosiglitazone Maleate (Hydrochlorothiazide may cause hyperglycemia, therefore, dosage adjustment of oral hypoglycemic agent may be required). Products include:
- Avandamet Tablets 1343
- Avandia Tablets 1348

Secobarbital Sodium (Potentiation of orthostatic hypotension).
No products indexed under this heading.

Sodium Nitroprusside (Hydrochlorothiazide may add to or potentiate the therapeutic effect of other antihypertensive drugs).
No products indexed under this heading.

Sotalol Hydrochloride (Hydrochlorothiazide may add to or potentiate the therapeutic effect of other antihypertensive drugs).
No products indexed under this heading.

Spirapril Hydrochloride (Hydrochlorothiazide may add to or potentiate the therapeutic effect of other antihypertensive drugs).
No products indexed under this heading.

Sufentanil Citrate (Potentiation of orthostatic hypotension).
No products indexed under this heading.

Sulindac (Co-administration with non-steroidal anti-inflammatory agents may reduce the natriuretic and antihypertensive effects of thiazides). Products include:
- Clinoril Tablets 1899

Telmisartan (Hydrochlorothiazide may add to or potentiate the therapeutic effect of other antihypertensive drugs). Products include:
- Micardis Tablets 884
- Micardis HCT Tablets 886

Terazosin Hydrochloride (Hydrochlorothiazide may add to or potentiate the therapeutic effect of other antihypertensive drugs). Products include:
- Hytrin Capsules 469

Thiamylal Sodium (Potentiation of orthostatic hypotension).
No products indexed under this heading.

Timolol Maleate (Hydrochlorothiazide may add to or potentiate the therapeutic effect of other antihypertensive drugs). Products include:
- Blocadren Tablets 1891
- Cosopt Sterile Ophthalmic Solution 1910
- Timolide Tablets 2056
- Timoptic in Ocudose 2061
- Timoptic Sterile Ophthalmic Solution 2058
- Timoptic-XE Sterile Ophthalmic Gel Forming Solution 2062

Tolazamide (Hydrochlorothiazide may cause hyperglycemia, therefore, dosage adjustment of oral hypoglycemic agent may be required).
No products indexed under this heading.

Tolbutamide (In vitro studies show significant inhibition of the formation of oxidized irbesartan metabolites with the known cytochrome CYP 2C9 substrate/inhibitor, tolbutamide; hydrochlorothiazide may cause hyperglycemia, therefore dosage adjustment of oral hypoglycemic agent may be required).
No products indexed under this heading.

Tolmetin Sodium (Co-administration with non-steroidal anti-inflammatory agents may reduce the natriuretic and antihypertensive effects of thiazides).
No products indexed under this heading.

Torsemide (Hydrochlorothiazide may add to or potentiate the therapeutic effect of other antihypertensive drugs).
No products indexed under this heading.

Trandolapril (Hydrochlorothiazide may add to or potentiate the therapeutic effect of other antihypertensive drugs). Products include:
- Mavik Tablets 482
- Tarka Tablets 519

Triamcinolone (Co-administration with corticosteroids intensifies electrolyte depletion particularly hypokalemia).
No products indexed under this heading.

Triamcinolone Acetonide (Co-administration with corticosteroids intensifies electrolyte depletion particularly hypokalemia). Products include:
- Azmacort Inhalation Aerosol 1701
- Nasacort HFA Inhalation Aerosol 2939
- Nasacort AQ Nasal Spray 2937

Triamcinolone Diacetate (Co-administration with corticosteroids intensifies electrolyte depletion particularly hypokalemia).
No products indexed under this heading.

Triamcinolone Hexacetonide (Co-administration with corticosteroids intensifies electrolyte depletion particularly hypokalemia).
No products indexed under this heading.

Trimethaphan Camsylate (Hydrochlorothiazide may add to or potentiate the therapeutic effect of other antihypertensive drugs).
No products indexed under this heading.

Troglitazone (Hydrochlorothiazide may cause hyperglycemia, therefore, dosage adjustment of oral hypoglycemic agent may be required).
No products indexed under this heading.

Tubocurarine Chloride (Possible increased responsiveness to the muscle relaxants).
No products indexed under this heading.

Valdecoxib (Co-administration with non-steroidal anti-inflammatory agents may reduce the natriuretic and antihypertensive effects of thiazides).
No products indexed under this heading.

Valsartan (Hydrochlorothiazide may add to or potentiate the therapeutic effect of other antihypertensive drugs). Products include:
- Diovan HCT Tablets 2195
- Diovan Tablets 2191

Vecuronium Bromide (Possible increased responsiveness to the muscle relaxants).
No products indexed under this heading.

Verapamil Hydrochloride (Hydrochlorothiazide may add to or potentiate the therapeutic effect of other antihypertensive drugs). Products include:
- Covera-HS Tablets 3135
- Tarka Tablets 519
- Verelan PM Capsules 3120

Food Interactions

Alcohol (Potentiation of orthostatic hypotension).

AVALIDE TABLETS

(Hydrochlorothiazide, Irbesartan) 922
May interact with antihypertensives, barbiturates, corticosteroids, cardiac glycosides, oral hypoglycemic agents, insulin, lithium preparations, narcotic analgesics, nondepolarizing neuromuscular blocking agents, nonsteroidal anti-inflammatory agents, and certain other agents. Compounds in these categories include:

Acarbose (Hydrochlorothiazide may cause hyperglycemia, therefore, dosage adjustment of oral hypoglycemic agent may be required). Products include:
- Precose Tablets 776

Acebutolol Hydrochloride (Hydrochlorothiazide may add to or potentiate the therapeutic effect of other antihypertensive drugs).
No products indexed under this heading.

ACTH (Co-administration with ACTH intensifies electrolyte depletion particularly hypokalemia).
No products indexed under this heading.

Alfentanil Hydrochloride (Potentiation of orthostatic hypotension).
No products indexed under this heading.

Amlodipine Besylate (Hydrochlorothiazide may add to or potentiate the therapeutic effect of other antihypertensive drugs). Products include:
- Caduet Tablets 2507
- Lotrel Capsules 2238
- Norvasc Tablets 2529

Aprobarbital (Potentiation of orthostatic hypotension).
No products indexed under this heading.

Atenolol (Hydrochlorothiazide may add to or potentiate the therapeutic effect of other antihypertensive drugs). Products include:
- Tenormin I.V. Injection 698
- Tenormin Tablets 695

Atracurium Besylate (Possible increased responsiveness to the muscle relaxants).
No products indexed under this heading.

Benazepril Hydrochloride (Hydrochlorothiazide may add to or potenti-

ate the therapeutic effect of other antihypertensive drugs). Products include:
Lotensin Tablets 2232
Lotensin HCT Tablets 2235
Lotrel Capsules 2238

Bendroflumethiazide (Hydrochlorothiazide may add to or potentiate the therapeutic effect of other antihypertensive drugs).
No products indexed under this heading.

Betamethasone Acetate (Co-administration with corticosteroids intensifies electrolyte depletion particularly hypokalemia).
No products indexed under this heading.

Betamethasone Sodium Phosphate (Co-administration with corticosteroids intensifies electrolyte depletion particularly hypokalemia).
No products indexed under this heading.

Betaxolol Hydrochloride (Hydrochlorothiazide may add to or potentiate the therapeutic effect of other antihypertensive drugs). Products include:
Betoptic S Ophthalmic Suspension 554

Bisoprolol Fumarate (Hydrochlorothiazide may add to or potentiate the therapeutic effect of other antihypertensive drugs).
No products indexed under this heading.

Buprenorphine Hydrochloride (Potentiation of orthostatic hypotension). Products include:
Buprenex Injectable 2718
Suboxone Tablets 2719
Subutex Tablets 2719

Butabarbital (Potentiation of orthostatic hypotension).
No products indexed under this heading.

Butalbital (Potentiation of orthostatic hypotension). Products include:
Sedapap Tablets 50 mg/650 mg 2098

Candesartan Cilexetil (Hydrochlorothiazide may add to or potentiate the therapeutic effect of other antihypertensive drugs). Products include:
Atacand Tablets 634
Atacand HCT 637

Captopril (Hydrochlorothiazide may add to or potentiate the therapeutic effect of other antihypertensive drugs). Products include:
Captopril Tablets 2114

Carteolol Hydrochloride (Hydrochlorothiazide may add to or potentiate the therapeutic effect of other antihypertensive drugs). Products include:
Carteolol Hydrochloride Ophthalmic Solution USP, 1% .... ⊙246

Celecoxib (Co-administration with non-steroidal anti-inflammatory agents may reduce the natriuretic and antihypertensive effects of thiazides). Products include:
Celebrex Capsules 3130

Chlorothiazide (Hydrochlorothiazide may add to or potentiate the therapeutic effect of other antihypertensive drugs). Products include:
Aldoclor Tablets 1881
Diuril Oral 1936

Chlorothiazide Sodium (Hydrochlorothiazide may add to or potentiate the therapeutic effect of other antihypertensive drugs). Products include:
Diuril Sodium Intravenous 1934

Chlorpropamide (Hydrochlorothiazide may cause hyperglycemia, therefore, dosage adjustment of oral hypoglycemic agent may be required).
No products indexed under this heading.

Chlorthalidone (Hydrochlorothiazide may add to or potentiate the therapeutic effect of other antihypertensive drugs). Products include:
Clorpres Tablets 2139

Cholestyramine (Absorption of hydrochlorothiazide is impaired in the presence of anionic exchange resins; single dose of cholestyramine binds the hydrochlorothiazide and reduces its absorption from GI tract by 85%).
No products indexed under this heading.

Cisatracurium Besylate (Possible increased responsiveness to the muscle relaxants). Products include:
Nimbex Injection 494

Clonidine (Hydrochlorothiazide may add to or potentiate the therapeutic effect of other antihypertensive drugs). Products include:
Catapres-TTS 875

Clonidine Hydrochloride (Hydrochlorothiazide may add to or potentiate the therapeutic effect of other antihypertensive drugs). Products include:
Catapres Tablets 874
Clorpres Tablets 2139

Codeine Phosphate (Potentiation of orthostatic hypotension). Products include:
Tylenol with Codeine 2461

Colestipol Hydrochloride (Absorption of hydrochlorothiazide is impaired in the presence of anionic exchange resins; single dose of colestipol binds the hydrochlorothiazide and reduces its absorption from GI tract by 43%).
No products indexed under this heading.

Cortisone Acetate (Co-administration with corticosteroids intensifies electrolyte depletion particularly hypokalemia).
No products indexed under this heading.

Deserpidine (Hydrochlorothiazide may add to or potentiate the therapeutic effect of other antihypertensive drugs).
No products indexed under this heading.

Deslanoside (Concurrent digitalis therapy may exaggerate metabolic effects of hypokalemia, especially myocardial effects, e.g., increased ventricular irritability).
No products indexed under this heading.

Dexamethasone (Co-administration with corticosteroids intensifies electrolyte depletion particularly hypokalemia). Products include:
Ciprodex Otic Suspension 555
Decadron Tablets 1929
TobraDex Ophthalmic Ointment 558
TobraDex Ophthalmic Suspension ... 558

Dexamethasone Acetate (Co-administration with corticosteroids intensifies electrolyte depletion particularly hypokalemia).
No products indexed under this heading.

Dexamethasone Sodium Phosphate (Co-administration with corticosteroids intensifies electrolyte depletion particularly hypokalemia). Products include:
Decadron Phosphate Injection 1931

Dezocine (Potentiation of orthostatic hypotension).
No products indexed under this heading.

Diazoxide (Hydrochlorothiazide may add to or potentiate the therapeutic effect of other antihypertensive drugs). Products include:
Hyperstat I.V. Injection 3031

Diclofenac Potassium (Co-administration with non-steroidal anti-inflammatory agents may reduce the natriuretic and antihypertensive effects of thiazides). Products include:
Cataflam Tablets 2173

Diclofenac Sodium (Co-administration with non-steroidal anti-inflammatory agents may reduce the natriuretic and antihypertensive effects of thiazides). Products include:
Arthrotec Tablets 3126
Voltaren Ophthalmic Solution 2300
Voltaren Tablets 2298
Voltaren-XR Tablets 2301

Digitalis Glycoside Preparations (Concurrent digitalis therapy may exaggerate metabolic effects of hypokalemia, especially myocardial effects, e.g., increased ventricular irritability).
No products indexed under this heading.

Digitoxin (Concurrent digitalis therapy may exaggerate metabolic effects of hypokalemia, especially myocardial effects, e.g., increased ventricular irritability).
No products indexed under this heading.

Digoxin (Concurrent digitalis therapy may exaggerate metabolic effects of hypokalemia, especially myocardial effects, e.g., increased ventricular irritability). Products include:
Digitek Tablets 2146
Lanoxicaps Capsules 1458
Lanoxin Injection 1462
Lanoxin Tablets 1468
Lanoxin Injection Pediatric 1465

Diltiazem Hydrochloride (Hydrochlorothiazide may add to or potentiate the therapeutic effect of other antihypertensive drugs). Products include:
Cardizem LA Extended Release Tablets 1699
Tiazac Capsules 1204

Doxazosin Mesylate (Hydrochlorothiazide may add to or potentiate the therapeutic effect of other antihypertensive drugs).
No products indexed under this heading.

Enalapril Maleate (Hydrochlorothiazide may add to or potentiate the therapeutic effect of other antihypertensive drugs). Products include:
Vaseretic Tablets 2073
Vasotec I.V. Injection 2076

Enalaprilat (Hydrochlorothiazide may add to or potentiate the therapeutic effect of other antihypertensive drugs).
No products indexed under this heading.

Eprosartan Mesylate (Hydrochlorothiazide may add to or potentiate the therapeutic effect of other antihypertensive drugs). Products include:
Teveten Tablets 1707
Teveten HCT Tablets 1710

Esmolol Hydrochloride (Hydrochlorothiazide may add to or potentiate the therapeutic effect of other antihypertensive drugs). Products include:
Brevibloc Concentrate 766
Brevibloc Injection 766
Brevibloc Double Strength Injection 766
Brevibloc Premixed Injection 766
Brevibloc Double Strength Premixed Injection 766

Etodolac (Co-administration with non-steroidal anti-inflammatory agents may reduce the natriuretic and antihypertensive effects of thiazides).
No products indexed under this heading.

Felodipine (Hydrochlorothiazide may add to or potentiate the therapeutic effect of other antihypertensive drugs). Products include:
Plendil Extended-Release Tablets 651

Fenoprofen Calcium (Co-administration with non-steroidal anti-inflammatory agents may reduce the natriuretic and antihypertensive effects of thiazides). Products include:
Nalfon Capsules 2504

Fentanyl (Potentiation of orthostatic hypotension). Products include:
Duragesic Transdermal System 2448

Fentanyl Citrate (Potentiation of orthostatic hypotension). Products include:
Actiq 993

Fludrocortisone Acetate (Co-administration with corticosteroids intensifies electrolyte depletion particularly hypokalemia).
No products indexed under this heading.

Flurbiprofen (Co-administration with non-steroidal anti-inflammatory agents may reduce the natriuretic and antihypertensive effects of thiazides).
No products indexed under this heading.

Fosinopril Sodium (Hydrochlorothiazide may add to or potentiate the therapeutic effect of other antihypertensive drugs).
No products indexed under this heading.

Furosemide (Hydrochlorothiazide may add to or potentiate the therapeutic effect of other antihypertensive drugs). Products include:
Furosemide Tablets 2117

Glimepiride (Hydrochlorothiazide may cause hyperglycemia, therefore, dosage adjustment of oral hypoglycemic agent may be required). Products include:
Amaryl Tablets 2864

Glipizide (Hydrochlorothiazide may cause hyperglycemia, therefore, dosage adjustment of oral hypoglycemic agent may be required).
No products indexed under this heading.

Glyburide (Hydrochlorothiazide may cause hyperglycemia, therefore, dosage adjustment of oral hypoglycemic agent may be required).
No products indexed under this heading.

Guanabenz Acetate (Hydrochlorothiazide may add to or potentiate the therapeutic effect of other antihypertensive drugs).
No products indexed under this heading.

Guanethidine Monosulfate (Hydrochlorothiazide may add to or potentiate the therapeutic effect of other antihypertensive drugs).
No products indexed under this heading.

Hydralazine Hydrochloride (Hydrochlorothiazide may add to or potentiate the therapeutic effect of other antihypertensive drugs).
Products include:
BiDil Tablets 2161

Hydrocodone Bitartrate (Potentiation of orthostatic hypotension).
Products include:
Hycodan 1104
Hycomine Compound Tablets 1105
Hycotuss Expectorant Syrup 1106
Lortab 3315
Lortab Elixir 3312
Vicodin Tablets 530
Vicodin ES Tablets 531
Vicodin HP Tablets 532
Vicoprofen Tablets 533
Zydone Tablets 1118

Hydrocodone Polistirex (Potentiation of orthostatic hypotension).
Products include:
Tussionex Pennkinetic Extended-Release Suspension 3322

Hydrocortisone (Co-administration with corticosteroids intensifies electrolyte depletion particularly hypokalemia). Products include:
Cortizone•5 Ointment .... ▣699
Cortizone•10 Creme .... ▣699
Cortizone•10 Ointment .... ▣699
Cortizone•10 Plus Creme .... ▣700
Cortizone•10 Maximum Strength Quick Shot Spray .... ▣700
Hydrocortone Tablets 1963
Preparation H Hydrocortisone Cream .... ▣748

Hydrocortisone Acetate (Co-administration with corticosteroids intensifies electrolyte depletion particularly hypokalemia). Products include:
Analpram-HC 1136
Pramosone 1139
ProctoFoam-HC 3113
Tucks Anti-Itch Ointment .... ▣712
U-cort 1% Cream 3289

Hydrocortisone Sodium Phosphate (Co-administration with corticosteroids intensifies electrolyte depletion particularly hypokalemia).
No products indexed under this heading.

Hydrocortisone Sodium Succinate (Co-administration with corticosteroids intensifies electrolyte depletion particularly hypokalemia).
No products indexed under this heading.

Hydroflumethiazide (Hydrochlorothiazide may add to or potentiate the therapeutic effect of other antihypertensive drugs).
No products indexed under this heading.

Hydromorphone Hydrochloride (Potentiation of orthostatic hypotension). Products include:
Dilaudid 439
Dilaudid Oral Liquid 443
Dilaudid Non-Sterile Powder 439
Dilaudid Rectal Suppositories 439
Dilaudid Tablets 439
Dilaudid Tablets - 8 mg 443
Dilaudid-HP 441

Ibuprofen (Co-administration with non-steroidal anti-inflammatory agents may reduce the natriuretic and antihypertensive effects of thiazides). Products include:
Advil Allergy Sinus Caplets .... ▣737
Advil .... ▣737
Children's Advil Suspension .... ▣742
Children's Advil Chewable Tablets .. ▣741
Advil Cold & Sinus .... ▣739
Advil Flu & Body Ache Caplets .... ▣739
Children's Advil Cold Suspension ... ▣741
Infants' Advil Concentrated Drops .. ▣743
Junior Strength Advil Swallow Tablets .... ▣740
Advil Migraine Liquigels .... ▣740
Advil Multi-Symptom Cold Caplets .... ▣738
Combunox Tablets 1183
Children's Motrin Oral Suspension and Chewable Tablets 1837
Children's Motrin Cold Non-Staining Dye-Free Oral Suspension 1838
Children's Motrin Cold Oral Suspension 1838
Children's Motrin Non-Staining Dye-Free Oral Suspension 1837
Motrin Cold & Sinus Caplets 1836
Motrin IB Tablets and Caplets 1836
Infants' Motrin Concentrated Drops 1837
Infants' Motrin Non-Staining Dye-Free Drops 1837
Junior Strength Motrin Caplets and Chewable Tablets 1837
Vicoprofen Tablets 533

Indapamide (Hydrochlorothiazide may add to or potentiate the therapeutic effect of other antihypertensive drugs). Products include:
Indapamide Tablets 2119

Indomethacin (Co-administration with non-steroidal anti-inflammatory agents may reduce the natriuretic and antihypertensive effects of thiazides). Products include:
Indocin 1968

Indomethacin Sodium Trihydrate (Co-administration with non-steroidal anti-inflammatory agents may reduce the natriuretic and antihypertensive effects of thiazides).
Products include:
Indocin I.V. 1973

Insulin, Human, Zinc Suspension (Hydrochlorothiazide may cause hyperglycemia, therefore, dosage adjustment of insulin may be required). Products include:
Humulin L, 100 Units 1763
Humulin U, 100 Units 1770

Insulin, Human NPH (Hydrochlorothiazide may cause hyperglycemia, therefore, dosage adjustment of insulin may be required). Products include:
Humulin N, 100 Units 1764
Humulin N Pen 1765
Novolin N Human Insulin 10 ml Vials 2322
Novolin N InnoLet 2322
Novolin N PenFill 3 ml Cartridges 2325
Novolin R InnoLet 2322

Insulin, Human Regular (Hydrochlorothiazide may cause hyperglycemia, therefore, dosage adjustment of insulin may be required). Products include:
Humulin R (U-500) 1768
Humulin R, 100 Units 1767
Novolin R Human Insulin 10 ml Vials 2322
Novolin R PenFill 2325

Insulin, Human Regular and Human NPH Mixture (Hydrochlorothiazide may cause hyperglycemia, therefore, dosage adjustment of insulin may be required). Products include:
Humulin 50/50, 100 Units 1760
Humulin 70/30 Pen 1761
Novolin 70/30 Human Insulin 10 ml Vials 2321
Novolin 70/30 InnoLet 2322
Novolin 70/30 PenFill 3 ml Cartridges 2325

Insulin, NPH (Hydrochlorothiazide may cause hyperglycemia, therefore, dosage adjustment of insulin may be required).
No products indexed under this heading.

Insulin, Regular (Hydrochlorothiazide may cause hyperglycemia, therefore, dosage adjustment of insulin may be required).
No products indexed under this heading.

Insulin, Zinc Crystals (Hydrochlorothiazide may cause hyperglycemia, therefore, dosage adjustment of insulin may be required).
No products indexed under this heading.

Insulin, Zinc Suspension (Hydrochlorothiazide may cause hyperglycemia, therefore, dosage adjustment of insulin may be required).
No products indexed under this heading.

Insulin Aspart, Human Regular (Hydrochlorothiazide may cause hyperglycemia, therefore, dosage adjustment of insulin may be required). Products include:
NovoLog Injection 2326

Insulin glargine (Hydrochlorothiazide may cause hyperglycemia, therefore, dosage adjustment of insulin may be required). Products include:
Lantus Injection 2925

Insulin Lispro, Human (Hydrochlorothiazide may cause hyperglycemia, therefore, dosage adjustment of insulin may be required). Products include:
Humalog-Pen 1751
Humalog Mix 75/25-Pen 1754

Insulin Lispro Protamine, Human (Hydrochlorothiazide may cause hyperglycemia, therefore, dosage adjustment of insulin may be required). Products include:
Humalog Mix 75/25-Pen 1754

Isradipine (Hydrochlorothiazide may add to or potentiate the therapeutic effect of other antihypertensive drugs). Products include:
DynaCirc CR Tablets 2726

Ketoprofen (Co-administration with non-steroidal anti-inflammatory agents may reduce the natriuretic and antihypertensive effects of thiazides).
No products indexed under this heading.

Ketorolac Tromethamine (Co-administration with non-steroidal anti-inflammatory agents may reduce the natriuretic and antihypertensive effects of thiazides). Products include:
Acular Ophthalmic Solution 561
Acular LS Ophthalmic Solution 562

Labetalol Hydrochloride (Hydrochlorothiazide may add to or potentiate the therapeutic effect of other antihypertensive drugs).
No products indexed under this heading.

Levorphanol Tartrate (Potentiation of orthostatic hypotension).
No products indexed under this heading.

Lisinopril (Hydrochlorothiazide may add to or potentiate the therapeutic effect of other antihypertensive drugs). Products include:
Prinivil Tablets 2029
Prinzide Tablets 2033
Zestoretic Tablets 701
Zestril Tablets 704

Lithium (Diuretics reduce lithium's renal clearance and add a high risk of lithium toxicity).
No products indexed under this heading.

Lithium Carbonate (Diuretics reduce lithium's renal clearance and add a high risk of lithium toxicity).
Products include:
Eskalith 1406
Lithobid Tablets 1670

Lithium Citrate (Diuretics reduce lithium's renal clearance and add a high risk of lithium toxicity).
No products indexed under this heading.

Losartan Potassium (Hydrochlorothiazide may add to or potentiate the therapeutic effect of other antihypertensive drugs). Products include:
Cozaar Tablets 1913
Hyzaar 1964

Mecamylamine Hydrochloride (Hydrochlorothiazide may add to or potentiate the therapeutic effect of other antihypertensive drugs).
Products include:
Inversine Tablets 3286

Meclofenamate Sodium (Co-administration with non-steroidal anti-inflammatory agents may reduce the natriuretic and antihypertensive effects of thiazides).
No products indexed under this heading.

Mefenamic Acid (Co-administration with non-steroidal anti-inflammatory agents may reduce the natriuretic and antihypertensive effects of thiazides).
No products indexed under this heading.

Meloxicam (Co-administration with non-steroidal anti-inflammatory agents may reduce the natriuretic and antihypertensive effects of thiazides). Products include:
Mobic Oral Suspension 893
Mobic Tablets 893

Meperidine Hydrochloride (Potentiation of orthostatic hypotension).
No products indexed under this heading.

Mephobarbital (Potentiation of orthostatic hypotension). Products include:
Mebaral Tablets, USP 2483

Metformin Hydrochloride (Hydrochlorothiazide may cause hyperglycemia, therefore, dosage adjustment of oral hypoglycemic agent may be required). Products include:
ActoPlus Met Tablets 3219
Avandamet Tablets 1343
Fortamet Extended-Release Tablets 1156

Methadone Hydrochloride (Potentiation of orthostatic hypotension).
No products indexed under this heading.

Methyclothiazide (Hydrochlorothiazide may add to or potentiate the therapeutic effect of other antihypertensive drugs).
No products indexed under this heading.

Methyldopa (Hydrochlorothiazide may add to or potentiate the therapeutic effect of other antihypertensive drugs). Products include:
Aldoclor Tablets 1881
Aldoril Tablets 1884

Methyldopate Hydrochloride (Hydrochlorothiazide may add to or potentiate the therapeutic effect of other antihypertensive drugs).
No products indexed under this heading.

Methylprednisolone Acetate (Co-administration with corticosteroids intensifies electrolyte depletion particularly hypokalemia). Products include:
Depo-Medrol Injectable Suspension 2615
Depo-Medrol Single-Dose Vial 2617

Methylprednisolone Sodium Succinate (Co-administration with corticosteroids intensifies electrolyte depletion particularly hypokalemia).
No products indexed under this heading.

Metocurine Iodide (Possible increased responsiveness to the muscle relaxants).
No products indexed under this heading.

Metolazone (Hydrochlorothiazide may add to or potentiate the therapeutic effect of other antihypertensive drugs).
No products indexed under this heading.

Metoprolol Succinate (Hydrochlorothiazide may add to or potentiate the therapeutic effect of other antihypertensive drugs). Products include:
Toprol-XL Tablets 660

Metoprolol Tartrate (Hydrochlorothiazide may add to or potentiate the therapeutic effect of other antihypertensive drugs).
No products indexed under this heading.

Metyrosine (Hydrochlorothiazide may add to or potentiate the therapeutic effect of other antihypertensive drugs). Products include:
Demser Capsules 1933

Mibefradil Dihydrochloride (Hydrochlorothiazide may add to or potentiate the therapeutic effect of other antihypertensive drugs).
No products indexed under this heading.

Miglitol (Hydrochlorothiazide may cause hyperglycemia, therefore, dosage adjustment of oral hypoglycemic agent may be required).
No products indexed under this heading.

Minoxidil (Hydrochlorothiazide may add to or potentiate the therapeutic effect of other antihypertensive drugs). Products include:
Men's Rogaine Extra Strength Topical Solution, Ocean Rush Scent and Original Unscented 706
Women's Rogaine Topical Solution, Spring Bloom Scent and Original Unscented 707

Mivacurium Chloride (Possible increased responsiveness to the muscle relaxants). Products include:
Mivacron Injection 489

Moexipril Hydrochloride (Hydrochlorothiazide may add to or potentiate the therapeutic effect of other antihypertensive drugs). Products include:
Uniretic Tablets 3114
Univasc Tablets 3118

Morphine Sulfate (Potentiation of orthostatic hypotension). Products include:
Avinza Capsules 1714
Kadian Capsules 572
MS Contin Tablets 2703

Nabumetone (Co-administration with non-steroidal anti-inflammatory agents may reduce the natriuretic and antihypertensive effects of thiazides). Products include:
Relafen Tablets 1523

Nadolol (Hydrochlorothiazide may add to or potentiate the therapeutic effect of other antihypertensive drugs). Products include:
Nadolol Tablets 2121

Naproxen (Co-administration with non-steroidal anti-inflammatory agents may reduce the natriuretic and antihypertensive effects of thiazides). Products include:
EC-Naprosyn Delayed-Release Tablets 2769
Naprosyn Suspension 2769
Naprosyn Tablets 2769
Prevacid NapraPAC 3277

Naproxen Sodium (Co-administration with non-steroidal anti-inflammatory agents may reduce the natriuretic and antihypertensive effects of thiazides). Products include:
Aleve Tablets, Caplets and Gelcaps 605
Anaprox Tablets 2769
Anaprox DS Tablets 2769

Nicardipine Hydrochloride (Hydrochlorothiazide may add to or potentiate the therapeutic effect of other antihypertensive drugs). Products include:
Cardene I.V. 1129

Nifedipine (In vitro studies show significant inhibition of the formation of oxidized irbesartan metabolites with the known cytochrome CYP 2C9 substrate/inhibitor, nifedipine; the pharmacokinetics of irbesartan were not affected by co-administration of nifedipine; hydrochlorothiazide may add to or potentiate the therapeutic effect of other antihypertensive drugs). Products include:
Adalat CC Tablets 2978

Nisoldipine (Hydrochlorothiazide may add to or potentiate the therapeutic effect of other antihypertensive drugs). Products include:
Sular Tablets 1163

Nitroglycerin (Hydrochlorothiazide may add to or potentiate the therapeutic effect of other antihypertensive drugs). Products include:
Nitro-Dur Transdermal Infusion System 3060
Nitrolingual Pumpspray 1161

Norepinephrine Bitartrate (Thiazides may decrease arterial responsiveness to norepinephrine).
No products indexed under this heading.

Oxaprozin (Co-administration with non-steroidal anti-inflammatory agents may reduce the natriuretic and antihypertensive effects of thiazides).
No products indexed under this heading.

Oxycodone Hydrochloride (Potentiation of orthostatic hypotension). Products include:
Combunox Tablets 1183
OxyContin Tablets 2699
OxyFast Oral Concentrate Solution 2704
OxyIR Capsules 2704
Percocet Tablets 1114
Percodan Tablets 1115

Pancuronium Bromide (Possible increased responsiveness to the muscle relaxants).
No products indexed under this heading.

Penbutolol Sulfate (Hydrochlorothiazide may add to or potentiate the therapeutic effect of other antihypertensive drugs).
No products indexed under this heading.

Pentobarbital Sodium (Potentiation of orthostatic hypotension). Products include:
Nembutal Sodium Solution, USP 2484

Perindopril Erbumine (Hydrochlorothiazide may add to or potentiate the therapeutic effect of other antihypertensive drugs). Products include:
Aceon Tablets (2 mg, 4 mg, 8 mg) 3191

Phenobarbital (Potentiation of orthostatic hypotension).
No products indexed under this heading.

Phenoxybenzamine Hydrochloride (Hydrochlorothiazide may add to or potentiate the therapeutic effect of other antihypertensive drugs). Products include:
Dibenzyline Capsules 3390

Phentolamine Mesylate (Hydrochlorothiazide may add to or potentiate the therapeutic effect of other antihypertensive drugs).
No products indexed under this heading.

Phenylbutazone (Co-administration with non-steroidal anti-inflammatory agents may reduce the natriuretic and antihypertensive effects of thiazides).
No products indexed under this heading.

Pindolol (Hydrochlorothiazide may add to or potentiate the therapeutic effect of other antihypertensive drugs).
No products indexed under this heading.

Pioglitazone Hydrochloride (Hydrochlorothiazide may cause hyperglycemia, therefore, dosage adjustment of oral hypoglycemic agent may be required). Products include:
ActoPlus Met Tablets 3219
Actos Tablets 3224

Piroxicam (Co-administration with non-steroidal anti-inflammatory agents may reduce the natriuretic and antihypertensive effects of thiazides).
No products indexed under this heading.

Polythiazide (Hydrochlorothiazide may add to or potentiate the therapeutic effect of other antihypertensive drugs).
No products indexed under this heading.

Prazosin Hydrochloride (Hydrochlorothiazide may add to or potentiate the therapeutic effect of other antihypertensive drugs).
No products indexed under this heading.

Prednisolone Acetate (Co-administration with corticosteroids intensifies electrolyte depletion particularly hypokalemia). Products include:
Blephamide Ophthalmic Ointment 563
Blephamide Ophthalmic Suspension 564
Poly-Pred Liquifilm Ophthalmic Suspension .... ⊙231
Pred Forte Ophthalmic Suspension .... ⊙233
Pred Mild Sterile Ophthalmic Suspension .... ⊙236
Pred-G Ophthalmic Suspension ...... ⊙234
Pred-G Sterile Ophthalmic Ointment .... ⊙235

Prednisolone Sodium Phosphate (Co-administration with corticosteroids intensifies electrolyte depletion particularly hypokalemia). Products include:
Pediapred Oral Solution 3319

Prednisolone Tebutate (Co-administration with corticosteroids intensifies electrolyte depletion particularly hypokalemia).
No products indexed under this heading.

Prednisone (Co-administration with corticosteroids intensifies electrolyte depletion particularly hypokalemia).
No products indexed under this heading.

Propoxyphene Hydrochloride (Potentiation of orthostatic hypotension).
No products indexed under this heading.

Propoxyphene Napsylate (Potentiation of orthostatic hypotension). Products include:
Darvocet A 500 Tablets 3497

Propranolol Hydrochloride (Hydrochlorothiazide may add to or potentiate the therapeutic effect of other antihypertensive drugs). Products include:
Inderal LA Long-Acting Capsules 3421
InnoPran XL Capsules 2728

Quinapril Hydrochloride (Hydrochlorothiazide may add to or potentiate the therapeutic effect of other antihypertensive drugs).
No products indexed under this heading.

Ramipril (Hydrochlorothiazide may add to or potentiate the therapeutic effect of other antihypertensive drugs). Products include:
Altace Capsules 1673

Rapacuronium Bromide (Possible increased responsiveness to the muscle relaxants).
No products indexed under this heading.

Rauwolfia Serpentina (Hydrochlorothiazide may add to or potentiate the therapeutic effect of other antihypertensive drugs).
No products indexed under this heading.

Remifentanil Hydrochloride (Potentiation of orthostatic hypotension).
No products indexed under this heading.

Repaglinide (Hydrochlorothiazide may cause hyperglycemia, therefore, dosage adjustment of oral hypoglycemic agent may be required). Products include:
Prandin Tablets (0.5, 1, and 2 mg) 2337

Rescinnamine (Hydrochlorothiazide may add to or potentiate the therapeutic effect of other antihypertensive drugs).
No products indexed under this heading.

Reserpine (Hydrochlorothiazide may add to or potentiate the therapeutic effect of other antihypertensive drugs).
No products indexed under this heading.

Rocuronium Bromide (Possible increased responsiveness to the muscle relaxants). Products include:
Zemuron Injection 2363

IMPORTANT NOTE: Always consult each drug listing in the patient's regimen for possible interactions.

Rofecoxib (Co-administration with non-steroidal anti-inflammatory agents may reduce the natriuretic and antihypertensive effects of thiazides).
No products indexed under this heading.

Rosiglitazone Maleate (Hydrochlorothiazide may cause hyperglycemia, therefore, dosage adjustment of oral hypoglycemic agent may be required). Products include:
Avandamet Tablets 1343
Avandia Tablets 1348

Secobarbital Sodium (Potentiation of orthostatic hypotension).
No products indexed under this heading.

Sodium Nitroprusside (Hydrochlorothiazide may add to or potentiate the therapeutic effect of other antihypertensive drugs).
No products indexed under this heading.

Sotalol Hydrochloride (Hydrochlorothiazide may add to or potentiate the therapeutic effect of other antihypertensive drugs).
No products indexed under this heading.

Spirapril Hydrochloride (Hydrochlorothiazide may add to or potentiate the therapeutic effect of other antihypertensive drugs).
No products indexed under this heading.

Sufentanil Citrate (Potentiation of orthostatic hypotension).
No products indexed under this heading.

Sulindac (Co-administration with non-steroidal anti-inflammatory agents may reduce the natriuretic and antihypertensive effects of thiazides). Products include:
Clinoril Tablets 1899

Telmisartan (Hydrochlorothiazide may add to or potentiate the therapeutic effect of other antihypertensive drugs). Products include:
Micardis Tablets 884
Micardis HCT Tablets 886

Terazosin Hydrochloride (Hydrochlorothiazide may add to or potentiate the therapeutic effect of other antihypertensive drugs). Products include:
Hytrin Capsules 469

Thiamylal Sodium (Potentiation of orthostatic hypotension).
No products indexed under this heading.

Timolol Maleate (Hydrochlorothiazide may add to or potentiate the therapeutic effect of other antihypertensive drugs). Products include:
Blocadren Tablets 1891
Cosopt Sterile Ophthalmic Solution 1910
Timolide Tablets 2056
Timoptic in Ocudose 2061
Timoptic Sterile Ophthalmic Solution 2058
Timoptic-XE Sterile Ophthalmic Gel Forming Solution 2062

Tolazamide (Hydrochlorothiazide may cause hyperglycemia, therefore, dosage adjustment of oral hypoglycemic agent may be required).
No products indexed under this heading.

Tolbutamide (In vitro studies show significant inhibition of the formation of oxidized irbesartan metabolites with the known cytochrome CYP 2C9 substrate/inhibitor, tolbutamide; hydrochlorothiazide may cause hyperglycemia, therefore dosage adjustment of oral hypoglycemic agent may be required).
No products indexed under this heading.

Tolmetin Sodium (Co-administration with non-steroidal anti-inflammatory agents may reduce the natriuretic and antihypertensive effects of thiazides).
No products indexed under this heading.

Torsemide (Hydrochlorothiazide may add to or potentiate the therapeutic effect of other antihypertensive drugs).
No products indexed under this heading.

Trandolapril (Hydrochlorothiazide may add to or potentiate the therapeutic effect of other antihypertensive drugs). Products include:
Mavik Tablets 482
Tarka Tablets 519

Triamcinolone (Co-administration with corticosteroids intensifies electrolyte depletion particularly hypokalemia).
No products indexed under this heading.

Triamcinolone Acetonide (Co-administration with corticosteroids intensifies electrolyte depletion particularly hypokalemia). Products include:
Azmacort Inhalation Aerosol 1701
Nasacort HFA Inhalation Aerosol 2939
Nasacort AQ Nasal Spray 2937

Triamcinolone Diacetate (Co-administration with corticosteroids intensifies electrolyte depletion particularly hypokalemia).
No products indexed under this heading.

Triamcinolone Hexacetonide (Co-administration with corticosteroids intensifies electrolyte depletion particularly hypokalemia).
No products indexed under this heading.

Trimethaphan Camsylate (Hydrochlorothiazide may add to or potentiate the therapeutic effect of other antihypertensive drugs).
No products indexed under this heading.

Troglitazone (Hydrochlorothiazide may cause hyperglycemia, therefore, dosage adjustment of oral hypoglycemic agent may be required).
No products indexed under this heading.

Tubocurarine Chloride (Possible increased responsiveness to the muscle relaxants).
No products indexed under this heading.

Valdecoxib (Co-administration with non-steroidal anti-inflammatory agents may reduce the natriuretic and antihypertensive effects of thiazides).
No products indexed under this heading.

Valsartan (Hydrochlorothiazide may add to or potentiate the therapeutic effect of other antihypertensive drugs). Products include:
Diovan HCT Tablets 2195
Diovan Tablets 2191

Vecuronium Bromide (Possible increased responsiveness to the muscle relaxants).
No products indexed under this heading.

Verapamil Hydrochloride (Hydrochlorothiazide may add to or potentiate the therapeutic effect of other antihypertensive drugs). Products include:
Covera-HS Tablets 3135
Tarka Tablets 519
Verelan PM Capsules 3120

Food Interactions

Alcohol (Potentiation of orthostatic hypotension).

AVANDAMET TABLETS

(Metformin Hydrochloride, Rosiglitazone Maleate) 1343

May interact with cationic drugs that are eliminated by renal tubular, calcium channel blockers, corticosteroids, cytochrome p450 2c8 inducers (selected), cytochrome p450 2c8 inhibitors (selected), diuretics, estrogens, insulin, oral contraceptives, phenothiazines, phenytoin, quinidine, radiographic iodinated contrast media, sympathomimetics, thiazides, thyroid preparations, and certain other agents. Compounds in these categories include:

Albuterol (Certain drugs, such as sympathomimetics, tend to produce hyperglycemia and may lead to loss of glycemic control). Products include:
Proventil Inhalation Aerosol 3067

Albuterol Sulfate (Certain drugs, such as sympathomimetics, tend to produce hyperglycemia and may lead to loss of glycemic control). Products include:
AccuNeb Inhalation Solution 1055
Combivent Inhalation Aerosol 878
DuoNeb Inhalation Solution 1058
Proventil Inhalation Solution 0.083% 3069
Proventil HFA Inhalation Aerosol 3071
Ventolin HFA Inhalation Aerosol 1576
VoSpire Extended-Release Tablets 2352

Amiloride Hydrochloride (Potential for loss of glycemic control; theoretical potential for interaction with metformin by competing for common renal tubular transport system). Products include:
Midamor Tablets 2000
Moduretic Tablets 2003

Amlodipine Besylate (Certain drugs, such as calcium channel blockers, tend to produce hyperglycemia and may lead to loss of glycemic control). Products include:
Caduet Tablets 2507
Lotrel Capsules 2238
Norvasc Tablets 2529

Anastrozole (An inhibitor of CYP2C8 may increase the AUC of rosiglitazone). Products include:
Arimidex Tablets 665

Bendroflumethiazide (Certain drugs, such as thiazides and other diuretics, tend to produce hyperglycemia and may lead to loss of glycemic control).
No products indexed under this heading.

Bepridil Hydrochloride (Certain drugs, such as calcium channel blockers, tend to produce hyperglycemia and may lead to loss of glycemic control).
No products indexed under this heading.

Betamethasone Acetate (Certain drugs, such as corticosteroids, tend to produce hyperglycemia and may lead to loss of glycemic control).
No products indexed under this heading.

Betamethasone Sodium Phosphate (Certain drugs, such as corticosteroids, tend to produce hyperglycemia and may lead to loss of glycemic control).
No products indexed under this heading.

Bumetanide (Certain drugs, such as diuretics, tend to produce hyperglycemia and may lead to loss of glycemic control).
No products indexed under this heading.

Carbamazepine (An inducer of CYP2C8 may decrease the AUC of rosiglitazone). Products include:
Carbatrol Capsules 3174
Equetro Extended-Release Capsules 3178
Tegretol/Tegretol-XR 2278

Chlorothiazide (Certain drugs, such as thiazides and other diuretics, tend to produce hyperglycemia and may lead to loss of glycemic control). Products include:
Aldoclor Tablets 1881
Diuril Oral 1936

Chlorothiazide Sodium (Certain drugs, such as thiazides and other diuretics, tend to produce hyperglycemia and may lead to loss of glycemic control). Products include:
Diuril Sodium Intravenous 1934

Chlorotrianisene (Certain drugs, such as estrogens, tend to produce hyperglycemia and may lead to loss of glycemic control).
No products indexed under this heading.

Chlorpromazine (Certain drugs, such as phenothiazines, tend to produce hyperglycemia and may lead to loss of glycemic control).
No products indexed under this heading.

Chlorpromazine Hydrochloride (Certain drugs, such as phenothiazines, tend to produce hyperglycemia and may lead to loss of glycemic control).
No products indexed under this heading.

Chlorthalidone (Certain drugs, such as diuretics, tend to produce hyperglycemia and may lead to loss of glycemic control). Products include:
Clorpres Tablets 2139

Cimetidine (Co-administered with oral cimetidine may increase peak metformin plasma and whole blood concentrations by 60% and a 40% increase in plasma and whole blood metformin AUC). Products include:
Tagamet HB 200 Tablets .... ▣ 637
Tagamet Tablets 1547

Cimetidine Hydrochloride (An inhibitor of CYP2C8 may increase the AUC of rosiglitazone).
No products indexed under this heading.

Cortisone Acetate (Certain drugs, such as corticosteroids, tend to produce hyperglycemia and may lead to loss of glycemic control).
No products indexed under this heading.

Desogestrel (Certain drugs, such as oral contraceptives, tend to pro-

duce hyperglycemia and may lead to loss of glycemic control). Products include:

Ortho-Cept Tablets 2395

Dexamethasone (Certain drugs, such as corticosteroids, tend to produce hyperglycemia and may lead to loss of glycemic control). Products include:

Ciprodex Otic Suspension 555
Decadron Tablets 1929
TobraDex Ophthalmic Ointment 558
TobraDex Ophthalmic Suspension ... 558

Dexamethasone Acetate (Certain drugs, such as corticosteroids, tend to produce hyperglycemia and may lead to loss of glycemic control).

No products indexed under this heading.

Dexamethasone Sodium Phosphate (Certain drugs, such as corticosteroids, tend to produce hyperglycemia and may lead to loss of glycemic control). Products include:

Decadron Phosphate Injection 1931

Diatrizoate Meglumine (Potential for acute alteration of renal function; metformin should be temporarily withheld in patients undergoing radiologic studies involving parenteral iodinated contrast material).

No products indexed under this heading.

Diatrizoate Sodium (Potential for acute alteration of renal function; metformin should be temporarily withheld in patients undergoing radiologic studies involving parenteral iodinated contrast material).

No products indexed under this heading.

Dienestrol (Certain drugs, such as estrogens, tend to produce hyperglycemia and may lead to loss of glycemic control).

No products indexed under this heading.

Diethylstilbestrol (Certain drugs, such as estrogens, tend to produce hyperglycemia and may lead to loss of glycemic control).

No products indexed under this heading.

Digoxin (Theoretical potential for interaction with metformin by competing for common renal tubular transport system). Products include:

Digitek Tablets 2146
Lanoxicaps Capsules 1458
Lanoxin Injection 1462
Lanoxin Tablets 1468
Lanoxin Injection Pediatric 1465

Diltiazem Hydrochloride (Certain drugs, such as calcium channel blockers, tend to produce hyperglycemia and may lead to loss of glycemic control). Products include:

Cardizem LA Extended Release Tablets 1699
Tiazac Capsules 1204

Dobutamine Hydrochloride (Certain drugs, such as sympathomimetics, tend to produce hyperglycemia and may lead to loss of glycemic control).

No products indexed under this heading.

Dopamine Hydrochloride (Certain drugs, such as sympathomimetics, tend to produce hyperglycemia and may lead to loss of glycemic control).

No products indexed under this heading.

Ephedrine Hydrochloride (Certain drugs, such as sympathomimetics, tend to produce hyperglycemia and may lead to loss of glycemic control). Products include:

Primatene Tablets 749

Ephedrine Sulfate (Certain drugs, such as sympathomimetics, tend to produce hyperglycemia and may lead to loss of glycemic control).

No products indexed under this heading.

Ephedrine Tannate (Certain drugs, such as sympathomimetics, tend to produce hyperglycemia and may lead to loss of glycemic control).

No products indexed under this heading.

Epinephrine (Certain drugs, such as sympathomimetics, tend to produce hyperglycemia and may lead to loss of glycemic control). Products include:

EpiPen 1061
Primatene Mist 749

Epinephrine Bitartrate (Certain drugs, such as sympathomimetics, tend to produce hyperglycemia and may lead to loss of glycemic control).

No products indexed under this heading.

Epinephrine Hydrochloride (Certain drugs, such as sympathomimetics, tend to produce hyperglycemia and may lead to loss of glycemic control).

No products indexed under this heading.

Estradiol (Certain drugs, such as estrogens, tend to produce hyperglycemia and may lead to loss of glycemic control). Products include:

Activella Tablets 2311
Climara Transdermal System 795
Climara Pro Transdermal System 800
CombiPatch Transdermal System 2180
Estrogel 0.06% 3200
Menostar Transdermal System 805
Prefest Tablets 1069
Vagifem Tablets 2340
Vivelle Transdermal System 2288
Vivelle-Dot Transdermal System 2293

Estrogens, Conjugated (Certain drugs, such as estrogens, tend to produce hyperglycemia and may lead to loss of glycemic control). Products include:

Premarin Intravenous 3440
Premarin Tablets 3443
Premarin Vaginal Cream 3449
Premphase Tablets 3452
Prempro Tablets 3452

Estrogens, Esterified (Certain drugs, such as estrogens, tend to produce hyperglycemia and may lead to loss of glycemic control). Products include:

Estratest Tablets 3196
Estratest H.S. Tablets 3196

Estropipate (Certain drugs, such as estrogens, tend to produce hyperglycemia and may lead to loss of glycemic control).

No products indexed under this heading.

Ethacrynic Acid (Certain drugs, such as diuretics, tend to produce hyperglycemia and may lead to loss of glycemic control). Products include:

Edecrin Tablets 1941

Ethinyl Estradiol (Certain drugs, such as estrogens, tend to produce hyperglycemia and may lead to loss of glycemic control). Products include:

Alesse-28 Tablets 3392
Lo/Ovral-28 Tablets 3423
NuvaRing 2357
Ortho-Cept Tablets 2395
Ortho-Cyclen/Ortho Tri-Cyclen 2414
Ortho Evra Transdermal System 2402
Ortho Tri-Cyclen Lo Tablets 2421
Seasonale Tablets 1073
Triphasil-28 Tablets 3483
Yasmin 28 Tablets 818

Ethiodized Oil (Potential for acute alteration of renal function; metformin should be temporarily withheld in patients undergoing radiologic studies involving parenteral iodinated contrast material).

No products indexed under this heading.

Ethynodiol Diacetate (Certain drugs, such as oral contraceptives, tend to produce hyperglycemia and may lead to loss of glycemic control).

No products indexed under this heading.

Felodipine (Certain drugs, such as calcium channel blockers, tend to produce hyperglycemia and may lead to loss of glycemic control). Products include:

Plendil Extended-Release Tablets 651

Fludrocortisone Acetate (Certain drugs, such as corticosteroids, tend to produce hyperglycemia and may lead to loss of glycemic control).

No products indexed under this heading.

Fluphenazine Decanoate (Certain drugs, such as phenothiazines, tend to produce hyperglycemia and may lead to loss of glycemic control).

No products indexed under this heading.

Fluphenazine Enanthate (Certain drugs, such as phenothiazines, tend to produce hyperglycemia and may lead to loss of glycemic control).

No products indexed under this heading.

Fluphenazine Hydrochloride (Certain drugs, such as phenothiazines, tend to produce hyperglycemia and may lead to loss of glycemic control).

No products indexed under this heading.

Fosphenytoin Sodium (Certain drugs, such as phenytoin, tend to produce hyperglycemia and may lead to loss of glycemic control).

No products indexed under this heading.

Furosemide (Increases metformin plasma and blood Cmax by 22% and blood AUC by 15%; the Cmax and AUC of furosemide were 31% and 12% smaller when co-administered; potential for loss of glycemic control). Products include:

Furosemide Tablets 2117

Gadopentetate Dimeglumine (Potential for acute alteration of renal function; metformin should be temporarily withheld in patients undergoing radiologic studies involving parenteral iodinated contrast material).

No products indexed under this heading.

Gemfibrozil (Concomitant administration of gemfibrozil (600 mg bid), an inhibitor of CYP2C8, and rosiglitazone (4 mg qd) for 7 days increased rosiglitazone AUC by 127%, compared to administration of rosiglitazone (4 mg qd) alone).

No products indexed under this heading.

Glyburide (Decrease in glyburide AUC and Cmax have been observed, but were highly variable).

No products indexed under this heading.

Hydrochlorothiazide (Certain drugs, such as thiazides and other diuretics, tend to produce hyperglycemia and may lead to loss of glycemic control). Products include:

Aldoril Tablets 1884
Atacand HCT 637
Avalide Tablets 2889
Avalide Tablets 922
Benicar HCT Tablets 2852
Diovan HCT Tablets 2195
Dyazide Capsules 1389
Hyzaar 1964
Lotensin HCT Tablets 2235
Maxzide 2150
Micardis HCT Tablets 886
Moduretic Tablets 2003
Prinzide Tablets 2033
Teveten HCT Tablets 1710
Timolide Tablets 2056
Uniretic Tablets 3114
Vaseretic Tablets 2073
Zestoretic Tablets 701

Hydrocortisone (Certain drugs, such as corticosteroids, tend to produce hyperglycemia and may lead to loss of glycemic control). Products include:

Cortizone•5 Ointment 699
Cortizone•10 Creme 699
Cortizone•10 Ointment 699
Cortizone•10 Plus Creme 700
Cortizone•10 Maximum Strength Quick Shot Spray 700
Hydrocortone Tablets 1963
Preparation H Hydrocortisone Cream 748

Hydrocortisone Acetate (Certain drugs, such as corticosteroids, tend to produce hyperglycemia and may lead to loss of glycemic control). Products include:

Analpram-HC 1136
Pramosone 1139
ProctoFoam-HC 3113
Tucks Anti-Itch Ointment 712
U-cort 1% Cream 3289

Hydrocortisone Sodium Phosphate (Certain drugs, such as corticosteroids, tend to produce hyperglycemia and may lead to loss of glycemic control).

No products indexed under this heading.

Hydrocortisone Sodium Succinate (Certain drugs, such as corticosteroids, tend to produce hyperglycemia and may lead to loss of glycemic control).

No products indexed under this heading.

Hydroflumethiazide (Certain drugs, such as thiazides and other diuretics, tend to produce hyperglycemia and may lead to loss of glycemic control).

No products indexed under this heading.

Indapamide (Certain drugs, such as diuretics, tend to produce hyperglycemia and may lead to loss of glycemic control). Products include:

Indapamide Tablets 2119

Insulin, Human, Zinc Suspension (Co-administration of rosiglitazone with insulin has resulted in increased incidence of cardiac failure and other cardiovascular adverse events). Products include:

Humulin L, 100 Units 1763
Humulin U, 100 Units 1770

Insulin, Human NPH (Co-administration of rosiglitazone with insulin has resulted in increased inci-

dence of cardiac failure and other cardiovascular adverse events).
Products include:
Humulin N, 100 Units 1764
Humulin N Pen 1765
Novolin N Human Insulin 10 ml Vials 2322
Novolin N InnoLet 2322
Novolin N PenFill 3 ml Cartridges 2325
Novolin R InnoLet 2322

Insulin, Human Regular (Co-administration of rosiglitazone with insulin has resulted in increased incidence of cardiac failure and other cardiovascular adverse events).
Products include:
Humulin R (U-500) 1768
Humulin R, 100 Units 1767
Novolin R Human Insulin 10 ml Vials 2322
Novolin R PenFill 2325

Insulin, Human Regular and Human NPH Mixture (Co-administration of rosiglitazone with insulin has resulted in increased incidence of cardiac failure and other cardiovascular adverse events).
Products include:
Humulin 50/50, 100 Units 1760
Humulin 70/30 Pen 1761
Novolin 70/30 Human Insulin 10 ml Vials 2321
Novolin 70/30 InnoLet 2322
Novolin 70/30 PenFill 3 ml Cartridges 2325

Insulin, NPH (Co-administration of rosiglitazone with insulin has resulted in increased incidence of cardiac failure and other cardiovascular adverse events).
No products indexed under this heading.

Insulin, Regular (Co-administration of rosiglitazone with insulin has resulted in increased incidence of cardiac failure and other cardiovascular adverse events).
No products indexed under this heading.

Insulin, Zinc Crystals (Co-administration of rosiglitazone with insulin has resulted in increased incidence of cardiac failure and other cardiovascular adverse events).
No products indexed under this heading.

Insulin, Zinc Suspension (Co-administration of rosiglitazone with insulin has resulted in increased incidence of cardiac failure and other cardiovascular adverse events).
No products indexed under this heading.

Insulin Aspart, Human Regular (Co-administration of rosiglitazone with insulin has resulted in increased incidence of cardiac failure and other cardiovascular adverse events).
Products include:
NovoLog Injection 2326

Insulin glargine (Co-administration of rosiglitazone with insulin has resulted in increased incidence of cardiac failure and other cardiovascular adverse events). Products include:
Lantus Injection 2925

Insulin Lispro, Human (Co-administration of rosiglitazone with insulin has resulted in increased incidence of cardiac failure and other cardiovascular adverse events).
Products include:
Humalog-Pen 1751
Humalog Mix 75/25-Pen 1754

Insulin Lispro Protamine, Human (Co-administration of rosiglitazone with insulin has resulted in increased incidence of cardiac failure and other cardiovascular adverse events).
Products include:
Humalog Mix 75/25-Pen 1754

Iodamide Meglumine (Potential for acute alteration of renal function; metformin should be temporarily withheld in patients undergoing radiologic studies involving parenteral iodinated contrast material).
No products indexed under this heading.

Iohexol (Potential for acute alteration of renal function; metformin should be temporarily withheld in patients undergoing radiologic studies involving parenteral iodinated contrast material).
No products indexed under this heading.

Iopamidol (Potential for acute alteration of renal function; metformin should be temporarily withheld in patients undergoing radiologic studies involving parenteral iodinated contrast material).
No products indexed under this heading.

Iopanoic Acid (Potential for acute alteration of renal function; metformin should be temporarily withheld in patients undergoing radiologic studies involving parenteral iodinated contrast material).
No products indexed under this heading.

Iothalamate Meglumine (Potential for acute alteration of renal function; metformin should be temporarily withheld in patients undergoing radiologic studies involving parenteral iodinated contrast material).
No products indexed under this heading.

Ioxaglate Meglumine (Potential for acute alteration of renal function; metformin should be temporarily withheld in patients undergoing radiologic studies involving parenteral iodinated contrast material).
No products indexed under this heading.

Ioxaglate Sodium (Potential for acute alteration of renal function; metformin should be temporarily withheld in patients undergoing radiologic studies involving parenteral iodinated contrast material).
No products indexed under this heading.

Isoniazid (Certain drugs, such as isoniazid, tend to produce hyperglycemia and may lead to loss of glycemic control).
No products indexed under this heading.

Isoproterenol Hydrochloride (Certain drugs, such as sympathomimetics, tend to produce hyperglycemia and may lead to loss of glycemic control).
No products indexed under this heading.

Isoproterenol Sulfate (Certain drugs, such as sympathomimetics, tend to produce hyperglycemia and may lead to loss of glycemic control).
No products indexed under this heading.

Isradipine (Certain drugs, such as calcium channel blockers, tend to produce hyperglycemia and may lead to loss of glycemic control).
Products include:
DynaCirc CR Tablets 2726

Levalbuterol Hydrochloride (Certain drugs, such as sympathomimetics, tend to produce hyperglycemia and may lead to loss of glycemic control). Products include:
Xopenex Inhalation Solution 3143
Xopenex Inhalation Solution Concentrate 3147

Levonorgestrel (Certain drugs, such as oral contraceptives, tend to produce hyperglycemia and may lead to loss of glycemic control).
Products include:
Alesse-28 Tablets 3392
Climara Pro Transdermal System 800
Mirena Intrauterine System 810
Plan B Tablets 1068
Seasonale Tablets 1073
Triphasil-28 Tablets 3483

Levothyroxine Sodium (Certain drugs, such as thyroid products, tend to produce hyperglycemia and may lead to loss of glycemic control). Products include:
Levothroid Tablets 1189
Levoxyl Tablets 1680
Synthroid Tablets 515
Unithroid Tablets 3521

Liothyronine Sodium (Certain drugs, such as thyroid products, tend to produce hyperglycemia and may lead to loss of glycemic control). Products include:
Cytomel Tablets 1678

Liotrix (Certain drugs, such as thyroid products, tend to produce hyperglycemia and may lead to loss of glycemic control). Products include:
Thyrolar 1203

Mesoridazine Besylate (Certain drugs, such as phenothiazines, tend to produce hyperglycemia and may lead to loss of glycemic control).
No products indexed under this heading.

Mestranol (Certain drugs, such as oral contraceptives, tend to produce hyperglycemia and may lead to loss of glycemic control).
No products indexed under this heading.

Metaproterenol Sulfate (Certain drugs, such as sympathomimetics, tend to produce hyperglycemia and may lead to loss of glycemic control). Products include:
Alupent Inhalation Aerosol 858

Metaraminol Bitartrate (Certain drugs, such as sympathomimetics, tend to produce hyperglycemia and may lead to loss of glycemic control). Products include:
Aramine Injection 1889

Methotrimeprazine (Certain drugs, such as phenothiazines, tend to produce hyperglycemia and may lead to loss of glycemic control).
No products indexed under this heading.

Methoxamine Hydrochloride (Certain drugs, such as sympathomimetics, tend to produce hyperglycemia and may lead to loss of glycemic control).
No products indexed under this heading.

Methyclothiazide (Certain drugs, such as thiazides and other diuretics, tend to produce hyperglycemia and may lead to loss of glycemic control).
No products indexed under this heading.

Methylprednisolone Acetate (Certain drugs, such as corticosteroids, tend to produce hyperglycemia and may lead to loss of glycemic control). Products include:
Depo-Medrol Injectable Suspension 2615
Depo-Medrol Single-Dose Vial 2617

Methylprednisolone Sodium Succinate (Certain drugs, such as corticosteroids, tend to produce hyperglycemia and may lead to loss of glycemic control).
No products indexed under this heading.

Metolazone (Certain drugs, such as diuretics, tend to produce hyperglycemia and may lead to loss of glycemic control).
No products indexed under this heading.

Mibefradil Dihydrochloride (Certain drugs, such as calcium channel blockers, tend to produce hyperglycemia and may lead to loss of glycemic control).
No products indexed under this heading.

Morphine Sulfate (Theoretical potential for interaction with metformin by competing for common renal tubular transport system).
Products include:
Avinza Capsules 1714
Kadian Capsules 572
MS Contin Tablets 2703

Niacin (Certain drugs, such as niacin, tend to produce hyperglycemia and may lead to loss of glycemic control). Products include:
Advicor Tablets 1694
Niaspan Extended-Release Tablets 1703

Nicardipine Hydrochloride (Certain drugs, such as calcium channel blockers, tend to produce hyperglycemia and may lead to loss of glycemic control). Products include:
Cardene I.V. 1129

Nicotinic Acid (Potential for loss of glycemic control).
No products indexed under this heading.

Nifedipine (Enhances the absorption of metformin by increasing plasma metformin Cmax and AUC; potential for loss of glycemic control). Products include:
Adalat CC Tablets 2978

Nimodipine (Certain drugs, such as calcium channel blockers, tend to produce hyperglycemia and may lead to loss of glycemic control).
Products include:
Nimotop Capsules 774

Nisoldipine (Certain drugs, such as calcium channel blockers, tend to produce hyperglycemia and may lead to loss of glycemic control).
Products include:
Sular Tablets 1163

Norepinephrine Bitartrate (Certain drugs, such as sympathomimetics, tend to produce hyperglycemia and may lead to loss of glycemic control).
No products indexed under this heading.

Norethindrone (Certain drugs, such as oral contraceptives, tend to produce hyperglycemia and may lead to loss of glycemic control).
Products include:
Ortho Micronor Tablets 2411

Norethynodrel (Certain drugs, such as oral contraceptives, tend to produce hyperglycemia and may lead to loss of glycemic control).
No products indexed under this heading.

Norgestimate (Certain drugs, such as oral contraceptives, tend to produce hyperglycemia and may lead to loss of glycemic control). Products include:
Ortho-Cyclen/Ortho Tri-Cyclen 2414
Ortho Tri-Cyclen Lo Tablets 2421
Prefest Tablets 1069

Norgestrel (Certain drugs, such as oral contraceptives, tend to produce hyperglycemia and may lead to loss of glycemic control). Products include:
Lo/Ovral-28 Tablets 3423

Omeprazole (An inhibitor of CYP2C8 may increase the AUC of rosiglitazone). Products include:
Zegerid Powder for Oral Solution 2972

Perphenazine (Certain drugs, such as phenothiazines, tend to produce hyperglycemia and may lead to loss of glycemic control).
No products indexed under this heading.

Phenobarbital (An inducer of CYP2C8 may decrease the AUC of rosiglitazone).
No products indexed under this heading.

Phenylephrine Bitartrate (Certain drugs, such as sympathomimetics, tend to produce hyperglycemia and may lead to loss of glycemic control).
No products indexed under this heading.

Phenylephrine Hydrochloride (Certain drugs, such as sympathomimetics, tend to produce hyperglycemia and may lead to loss of glycemic control). Products include:
Alacol DM Syrup 739
Hycomine Compound Tablets 1105
Preparation H Maximum Strength Cream ▣747
Preparation H Cooling Gel ▣747
Preparation H ▣747
Sudafed PE Tablets ▣711
Vicks Sinex Nasal Spray and Ultra Fine Mist for Sinus Relief 2677
Zicam Concentrated Cough Mist for Kids Plus D Cool Cherry ▣643
Zicam Concentrated Cough Mist Plus D Cool Cherry ▣642

Phenylephrine Tannate (Certain drugs, such as sympathomimetics, tend to produce hyperglycemia and may lead to loss of glycemic control).
No products indexed under this heading.

Phenylpropanolamine Hydrochloride (Certain drugs, such as sympathomimetics, tend to produce hyperglycemia and may lead to loss of glycemic control).
No products indexed under this heading.

Phenytoin (Certain drugs, such as phenytoin, tend to produce hyperglycemia and may lead to loss of glycemic control).
No products indexed under this heading.

Phenytoin Sodium (Certain drugs, such as phenytoin, tend to produce hyperglycemia and may lead to loss of glycemic control). Products include:
Phenytek Capsules 2153

Pirbuterol Acetate (Certain drugs, such as sympathomimetics, tend to produce hyperglycemia and may lead to loss of glycemic control). Products include:
Maxair Autohaler 1820

Polyestradiol Phosphate (Certain drugs, such as estrogens, tend to produce hyperglycemia and may lead to loss of glycemic control).
No products indexed under this heading.

Polythiazide (Certain drugs, such as thiazides and other diuretics, tend to produce hyperglycemia and may lead to loss of glycemic control).
No products indexed under this heading.

Prednisolone Acetate (Certain drugs, such as corticosteroids, tend to produce hyperglycemia and may lead to loss of glycemic control). Products include:
Blephamide Ophthalmic Ointment 563
Blephamide Ophthalmic Suspension 564
Poly-Pred Liquifilm Ophthalmic Suspension ⊙231
Pred Forte Ophthalmic Suspension ⊙233
Pred Mild Sterile Ophthalmic Suspension ⊙236
Pred-G Ophthalmic Suspension ⊙234
Pred-G Sterile Ophthalmic Ointment ⊙235

Prednisolone Sodium Phosphate (Certain drugs, such as corticosteroids, tend to produce hyperglycemia and may lead to loss of glycemic control). Products include:
Pediapred Oral Solution 3319

Prednisolone Tebutate (Certain drugs, such as corticosteroids, tend to produce hyperglycemia and may lead to loss of glycemic control).
No products indexed under this heading.

Prednisone (Certain drugs, such as corticosteroids, tend to produce hyperglycemia and may lead to loss of glycemic control).
No products indexed under this heading.

Primidone (An inducer of CYP2C8 may decrease the AUC of rosiglitazone).
No products indexed under this heading.

Procainamide Hydrochloride (Theoretical potential for interaction with metformin by competing for common renal tubular transport system).
No products indexed under this heading.

Prochlorperazine (Certain drugs, such as phenothiazines, tend to produce hyperglycemia and may lead to loss of glycemic control).
No products indexed under this heading.

Promethazine Hydrochloride (Certain drugs, such as phenothiazines, tend to produce hyperglycemia and may lead to loss of glycemic control). Products include:
Phenergan 3438

Pseudoephedrine Hydrochloride (Certain drugs, such as sympathomimetics, tend to produce hyperglycemia and may lead to loss of glycemic control). Products include:
Advil Allergy Sinus Caplets ▣737
Advil Cold & Sinus ▣739
Advil Flu & Body Ache Caplets ▣739
Children's Advil Cold Suspension ▣741
Advil Multi-Symptom Cold Caplets ▣738
Allegra-D 12 Hour Extended-Release Tablets 2860
Allegra-D 24 Hour Extended-Release Tablets 2862
Balamine DM 739
BC Cold Powder ▣612
Benadryl Allergy & Cold Tablets ▣692
Benadryl Allergy & Sinus Headache Caplets & Gelcaps ▣693
Children's Benadryl Allergy & Cold Fastmelt Tablets ▣695
Benadryl Maximum Strength Severe Allergy & Sinus Headache Caplets ▣694
Children's Benadryl D Allergy & Sinus Fastmelt Tablets ▣694
Children's Benadryl D Liquid Medication ▣693
Benadryl D Tablets ▣694
Contac Non-Drowsy 12 Hour Cold Caplets ▣614
Contac Non-Drowsy Timed Release 12 Hour Cold Caplets ▣615
Contac Severe Cold and Flu Caplets Maximum Strength ▣615
Contac Severe Cold and Flu Caplets Non-Drowsy ▣615
Children's Dimetapp Cold & Allergy Elixir ▣745
Children's Dimetapp DM Cold & Cough Elixir ▣745
Children's Dimetapp Long Acting Cough Plus Cold Syrup ▣746
Dimetapp Infant Drops Decongestant Plus Cough ▣746
Children's Motrin Cold Non-Staining Dye-Free Oral Suspension 1838
Children's Motrin Cold Oral Suspension 1838
Motrin Cold & Sinus Caplets 1836
PediaCare Decongestant & Cough Infant Drops ▣705
PediaCare Decongestant Infants' Drops ▣705
PediaCare Long-Acting Cough Plus Cold Liquid ▣704
PediaCare Multi-Symptom Cold Liquid ▣704
PediaCare NightRest Cough & Cold Liquid ▣704
Robitussin Allergy & Cough Syrup ▣750
Robitussin CF Liquid ▣755
Robitussin Cough & Cold Liquid-filled Capsules ▣750
Robitussin Cough, Cold & Flu Liquid-filled Capsules ▣750
Robitussin Cough & Cold Infant Drops ▣755
Robitussin Flu Liquid ▣752
Robitussin Maximum Strength Cough & Cold Liquid ▣754
Robitussin PE Syrup ▣753
Robitussin Pediatric Cough & Cold Liquid ▣754
Robitussin PM Cough & Cold Liquid ▣752
Robitussin Severe Congestion Liquid-filled Capsules ▣751
Simply Stuffy Liquid 1841
Singlet Caplets ▣636
Sudafed 12 Hour Caplets ▣708
Sudafed 24 Hour Tablets ▣709
Sudafed Nasal Decongestant Tablets ▣709
Sudafed Severe Cold ▣710
Sudafed Non-Drying Sinus Liquid Caps ▣709
Sudafed Sinus & Allergy Tablets ▣710
Sudafed Sinus Headache ▣711
TheraFlu Cold & Cough Hot Liquid ▣680
TheraFlu Cold & Sore Throat Hot Liquid ▣680
TheraFlu Flu & Chest Congestion Non-Drowsy Hot Liquid ▣681
TheraFlu Flu & Sore Throat Hot Liquid ▣681
TheraFlu Severe Cold Non-Drowsy Hot Liquid ▣683
TheraFlu Severe Cold & Cough Hot Liquid ▣683
TheraFlu Severe Cold Caplets ▣679
TheraFlu Severe Cold Hot Liquid ▣682
TheraFlu Severe Cold Non-Drowsy Caplets ▣679
Triaminic Chest & Nasal Congestion Liquid ▣685
Triaminic Cold & Allergy Liquid ▣685
Triaminic Cold & Cough Liquid ▣685
Triaminic Cough Liquid ▣687
Triaminic Cough & Nasal Congestion Liquid ▣687
Triaminic Cough & Sore Throat Liquid ▣687
Triaminic Flu, Cough & Fever Liquid ▣685
Triaminic Night Time Cough & Cold Liquid ▣685
Triaminic Allergy Runny Nose & Congestion Softchews ▣688
Triaminic Cold & Cough Softchews ▣688
Triaminic Cough & Sore Throat Softchews ▣689
Tylenol Sinus NightTime Caplets ▣663
Children's Tylenol Plus Cold & Allergy Suspension Liquid 1850
Children's Tylenol Plus Cold NightTime Suspension Liquid 1851
Children's Tylenol Plus Cold & Cough Suspension Liquid and Chewable Tablets 1851
Children's Tylenol Plus Cold Chewable Tablets 1851
Children's Tylenol Plus Cold Daytime Non-Drowsy Suspension Liquid 1851
Children's Tylenol Plus Flu Suspension Liquid 1853
Concentrated Tylenol Infants' Drops Plus Cold 1851
Concentrated Tylenol Infants' Drops Plus Cold and Cough 1851
Tylenol Cold & Flu Severe Daytime Liquid with Cool Burst 1846
Tylenol Cold & Flu Severe NightTime Liquid with Cool Burst 1846
Tylenol Cold Severe Congestion Non-Drowsy Caplets with Cool Burst 1846
Tylenol Allergy Complete Night Time Caplets 1844
Tylenol Allergy Complete Multi-Symptom Caplets and Gelcaps with Cool Burst 1844
Tylenol Flu NightTime Gelcaps 1846
Tylenol Flu Day Non-Drowsy Gelcaps 1846
Concentrated Tylenol Infants' Drops Plus Cold Nasal Congestant, Fever Reducer & Pain Reliever ▣668
Concentrated Tylenol Infants' Drops Plus Cold & Cough Nasal Decongestant, Fever Reducer & Pain Reliever ▣668
Multi-Symptom Tylenol Cold Night Time Caplets 1845
Multi-Symptom Tylenol Cold Day Non-Drowsy Caplets and Gelcaps 1845
Tylenol Sinus Day Non-Drowsy 1848
Tylenol Sinus Night Time Caplets 1848
Tylenol Sinus Severe Congestion Caplets with Cool Burst 1848
Vicks 44D Cough & Head Congestion Relief 2676
Vicks 44D Cough & Head Congestion Relief Liquid ▣721
Vicks 44M Cough, Cold & Flu Relief 2676
Pediatric Vicks 44m Cough & Cold Relief 2673
Vicks DayQuil LiquiCaps/Liquid Multi-Symptom Cold/Flu Relief ▣723
Vicks DayQuil Multi-Symptom Cold/Flu Relief LiquiCaps 2675
Vicks DayQuil Multi-Symptom Cold/Flu Relief Liquid 2675
Children's Vicks NyQuil Cold/Cough Relief 2671
Vicks NyQuil LiquiCaps 2677
Vicks NyQuil LiquiCaps/Liquid Multi-Symptom Cold/Flu Relief ▣725
Vicks NyQuil Liquid 2677
Zyrtec-D 12 Hour Extended Release Tablets 2591

Pseudoephedrine Sulfate (Certain drugs, such as sympathomimet-

ics, tend to produce hyperglycemia and may lead to loss of glycemic control). Products include:
- Alavert Allergy & Sinus D-12 Hour Tablets .... ▣ **743**
- Clarinex-D 24-Hour Extended-Release Tablets **3012**
- Claritin-D Non-Drowsy 12 Hour Tablets .... ▣ **731**
- Claritin-D Non-Drowsy 24 Hour Tablets .... ▣ **731**

Quercetin (An inhibitor of CYP2C8 may increase the AUC of rosiglitazone).
No products indexed under this heading.

Quinestrol (Certain drugs, such as estrogens, tend to produce hyperglycemia and may lead to loss of glycemic control).
No products indexed under this heading.

Quinidine (Theoretical potential for interaction with metformin by competing for common renal tubular transport system).
No products indexed under this heading.

Quinidine Gluconate (Theoretical potential for interaction with metformin by competing for common renal tubular transport system).
No products indexed under this heading.

Quinidine Hydrochloride (Theoretical potential for interaction with metformin by competing for common renal tubular transport system).
No products indexed under this heading.

Quinidine Polygalacturonate (Theoretical potential for interaction with metformin by competing for common renal tubular transport system).
No products indexed under this heading.

Quinidine Sulfate (Theoretical potential for interaction with metformin by competing for common renal tubular transport system).
No products indexed under this heading.

Quinine Sulfate (Theoretical potential for interaction with metformin by competing for common renal tubular transport system).
No products indexed under this heading.

Ranitidine Hydrochloride (Theoretical potential for interaction with metformin by competing for common renal tubular transport system). Products include:
- Zantac **1597**
- Zantac Injection **1593**
- Zantac 75 Tablets .... ▣ **715**
- Zantac 150 Maximum Strength Tablets .... ▣ **715**
- Zantac Injection Pharmacy Bulk Package **1595**

Rifabutin (An inducer of CYP2C8 may decrease the AUC of rosiglitazone).
No products indexed under this heading.

Rifampin (Rifampin administration (600 mg qd) an inducer of CYP2C8, for 6 days is reported to decrease rosiglitazone AUC by 66%, compared to administration of rosiglitazone (8 mg) alone).
No products indexed under this heading.

Salmeterol Xinafoate (Certain drugs, such as sympathomimetics, tend to produce hyperglycemia and may lead to loss of glycemic control). Products include:
- Advair Diskus 100/50 .... **1291**
- Advair Diskus 250/50 .... **1291**
- Advair Diskus 500/50 .... **1291**
- Serevent Diskus **1540**

Spironolactone (Certain drugs, such as diuretics, tend to produce hyperglycemia and may lead to loss of glycemic control).
No products indexed under this heading.

Sulfaphenazole (An inhibitor of CYP2C8 may increase the AUC of rosiglitazone).
No products indexed under this heading.

Sulfinpyrazone (An inhibitor of CYP2C8 may increase the AUC of rosiglitazone).
No products indexed under this heading.

Terbutaline Sulfate (Certain drugs, such as sympathomimetics, tend to produce hyperglycemia and may lead to loss of glycemic control).
No products indexed under this heading.

Thioridazine Hydrochloride (Certain drugs, such as phenothiazines, tend to produce hyperglycemia and may lead to loss of glycemic control). Products include:
- Thioridazine Hydrochloride Tablets **2122**

Thyroglobulin (Certain drugs, such as thyroid products, tend to produce hyperglycemia and may lead to loss of glycemic control).
No products indexed under this heading.

Thyroid (Certain drugs, such as thyroid products, tend to produce hyperglycemia and may lead to loss of glycemic control).
No products indexed under this heading.

Thyroxine (Certain drugs, such as thyroid products, tend to produce hyperglycemia and may lead to loss of glycemic control).
No products indexed under this heading.

Thyroxine Sodium (Certain drugs, such as thyroid products, tend to produce hyperglycemia and may lead to loss of glycemic control).
No products indexed under this heading.

Torsemide (Certain drugs, such as diuretics, tend to produce hyperglycemia and may lead to loss of glycemic control).
No products indexed under this heading.

Triamcinolone (Certain drugs, such as corticosteroids, tend to produce hyperglycemia and may lead to loss of glycemic control).
No products indexed under this heading.

Triamcinolone Acetonide (Certain drugs, such as corticosteroids, tend to produce hyperglycemia and may lead to loss of glycemic control). Products include:
- Azmacort Inhalation Aerosol **1701**
- Nasacort HFA Inhalation Aerosol **2939**
- Nasacort AQ Nasal Spray **2937**

Triamcinolone Diacetate (Certain drugs, such as corticosteroids, tend to produce hyperglycemia and may lead to loss of glycemic control).
No products indexed under this heading.

Triamcinolone Hexacetonide (Certain drugs, such as corticosteroids, tend to produce hyperglycemia and may lead to loss of glycemic control).
No products indexed under this heading.

Triamterene (Potential for loss of glycemic control; theoretical potential for interaction with metformin by competing for common renal tubular transport system). Products include:
- Dyazide Capsules **1389**
- Dyrenium Capsules **3390**
- Maxzide **2150**

Trifluoperazine Hydrochloride (Certain drugs, such as phenothiazines, tend to produce hyperglycemia and may lead to loss of glycemic control).
No products indexed under this heading.

Trimethoprim (An inhibitor of CYP2C8 may increase the AUC of rosiglitazone).
No products indexed under this heading.

Trimethoprim Hydrochloride (An inhibitor of CYP2C8 may increase the AUC of rosiglitazone).
No products indexed under this heading.

Trimethoprim Sulfate (Theoretical potential for interaction with metformin by competing for common renal tubular transport system). Products include:
- Polytrim Ophthalmic Solution .... ⊙ **570**

Tyropanoate Sodium (Potential for acute alteration of renal function; metformin should be temporarily withheld in patients undergoing radiologic studies involving parenteral iodinated contrast material).
No products indexed under this heading.

Vancomycin Hydrochloride (Theoretical potential for interaction with metformin by competing for common renal tubular transport system). Products include:
- Vancocin HCl Capsules, USP **3370**

Verapamil Hydrochloride (Certain drugs, such as calcium channel blockers, tend to produce hyperglycemia and may lead to loss of glycemic control). Products include:
- Covera-HS Tablets **3135**
- Tarka Tablets **519**
- Verelan PM Capsules **3120**

Food Interactions

Alcohol (Alcohol potentiates the effect of metformin on lactate metabolism; patients should be warned against excessive alcohol intake, acute or chronic).

Food, unspecified (Food decreases the extent and slightly delays the absorption of metformin).

AVANDIA TABLETS

(Rosiglitazone Maleate) **1348**

May interact with cytochrome p450 2c8 inducers (selected), cytochrome p450 2c8 inhibitors (selected), insulin, and certain other agents. Compounds in these categories include:

Anastrozole (An inhibitor of CYP2C8 may decrease the AUC of rosiglitazone. Therefore, if an inducer of CYP2C8 is started or stopped during treatment with rosiglitazone, changes in diabetes treatment may be needed upon clinical response). Products include:
- Arimidex Tablets **665**

Carbamazepine (An inhibitor of CYP2C8 may decrease the AUC of rosiglitazone. Therefore, if an inducer of CYP2C8 is started or stopped during treatment with rosiglitazone, changes in diabetes treatment may be needed upon clinical response). Products include:
- Carbatrol Capsules **3174**
- Equetro Extended-Release Capsules **3178**
- Tegretol/Tegretol-XR **2278**

Cimetidine (An inhibitor of CYP2C8 may decrease the AUC of rosiglitazone. Therefore, if an inducer of CYP2C8 is started or stopped during treatment with rosiglitazone, changes in diabetes treatment may be needed upon clinical response). Products include:
- Tagamet HB 200 Tablets .... ▣ **637**
- Tagamet Tablets **1547**

Cimetidine Hydrochloride (An inhibitor of CYP2C8 may decrease the AUC of rosiglitazone. Therefore, if an inducer of CYP2C8 is started or stopped during treatment with rosiglitazone, changes in diabetes treatment may be needed upon clinical response).
No products indexed under this heading.

Gemfibrozil (Concomitant administration of gemfibrozil (600 mg twice daily), an inhibitor of CYP2C8, and rosiglitazone (4 mg once daily) for 7 days increased rosiglitazone AUC by 127% compared to the administration of rosiglitazone (4 mg once daily) alone. Given the potential for dose-related adverse events with rosiglitazone, a decrease in the dose of rosiglitazone may be needed when gemfibrozil is introduced).
No products indexed under this heading.

Glyburide (Rosiglitazone (2 mg twice daily) taken concomitantly with glyburide (3.75 to 10 mg/day) for 7 days did not alter the mean steady-state 24-hour plasma glucose concentrations in diabetic patients stabilized on glyburide therapy. Repeat doses of rosiglitazone (8 mg once daily) for 8 days in healthy adult Caucasian subjects caused a decrease in glyburide AUC (32%) and Cmax (35%). In Japanese subjects, glyburide AUC (14%) and Cmax (31%) slightly increased following co-administration of rosiglitazone).
No products indexed under this heading.

Insulin, Human, Zinc Suspension (Co-administration of rosiglitazone with insulin has resulted in increased incidence of cardiac failure and other cardiovascular adverse events). Products include:
- Humulin L, 100 Units **1763**
- Humulin U, 100 Units **1770**

Insulin, Human NPH (Co-administration of rosiglitazone with insulin has resulted in increased incidence of cardiac failure and other cardiovascular adverse events). Products include:
- Humulin N, 100 Units **1764**
- Humulin N Pen **1765**
- Novolin N Human Insulin 10 ml Vials **2322**
- Novolin N InnoLet **2322**
- Novolin N PenFill 3 ml Cartridges **2325**
- Novolin R InnoLet **2322**

Insulin, Human Regular (Co-administration of rosiglitazone with insulin has resulted in increased inci-

dence of cardiac failure and other cardiovascular adverse events).
Products include:
- Humulin R (U-500) **1768**
- Humulin R, 100 Units **1767**
- Novolin R Human Insulin 10 ml Vials **2322**
- Novolin R PenFill **2325**

Insulin, Human Regular and Human NPH Mixture (Co-administration of rosiglitazone with insulin has resulted in increased incidence of cardiac failure and other cardiovascular adverse events).
Products include:
- Humulin 50/50, 100 Units **1760**
- Humulin 70/30 Pen **1761**
- Novolin 70/30 Human Insulin 10 ml Vials **2321**
- Novolin 70/30 InnoLet **2322**
- Novolin 70/30 PenFill 3 ml Cartridges **2325**

Insulin, NPH (Co-administration of rosiglitazone with insulin has resulted in increased incidence of cardiac failure and other cardiovascular adverse events).
No products indexed under this heading.

Insulin, Regular (Co-administration of rosiglitazone with insulin has resulted in increased incidence of cardiac failure and other cardiovascular adverse events).
No products indexed under this heading.

Insulin, Zinc Crystals (Co-administration of rosiglitazone with insulin has resulted in increased incidence of cardiac failure and other cardiovascular adverse events).
No products indexed under this heading.

Insulin, Zinc Suspension (Co-administration of rosiglitazone with insulin has resulted in increased incidence of cardiac failure and other cardiovascular adverse events).
No products indexed under this heading.

Insulin Aspart, Human Regular (Co-administration of rosiglitazone with insulin has resulted in increased incidence of cardiac failure and other cardiovascular adverse events).
Products include:
- NovoLog Injection **2326**

Insulin glargine (Co-administration of rosiglitazone with insulin has resulted in increased incidence of cardiac failure and other cardiovascular adverse events). Products include:
- Lantus Injection **2925**

Insulin Lispro, Human (Co-administration of rosiglitazone with insulin has resulted in increased incidence of cardiac failure and other cardiovascular adverse events).
Products include:
- Humalog-Pen **1751**
- Humalog Mix 75/25-Pen **1754**

Insulin Lispro Protamine, Human (Co-administration of rosiglitazone with insulin has resulted in increased incidence of cardiac failure and other cardiovascular adverse events).
Products include:
- Humalog Mix 75/25-Pen **1754**

Nicardipine Hydrochloride (An inhibitor of CYP2C8 may decrease the AUC of rosiglitazone. Therefore, if an inducer of CYP2C8 is started or stopped during treatment with rosiglitazone, changes in diabetes treatment may be needed upon clinical response). Products include:
- Cardene I.V. **1129**

Omeprazole (An inhibitor of CYP2C8 may decrease the AUC of rosiglitazone. Therefore, if an inducer of CYP2C8 is started or stopped during treatment with rosiglitazone, changes in diabetes treatment may be needed upon clinical response).
Products include:
- Zegerid Powder for Oral Solution **2972**

Phenobarbital (An inhibitor of CYP2C8 may decrease the AUC of rosiglitazone. Therefore, if an inducer of CYP2C8 is started or stopped during treatment with rosiglitazone, changes in diabetes treatment may be needed upon clinical response).
No products indexed under this heading.

Primidone (An inhibitor of CYP2C8 may decrease the AUC of rosiglitazone. Therefore, if an inducer of CYP2C8 is started or stopped during treatment with rosiglitazone, changes in diabetes treatment may be needed upon clinical response).
No products indexed under this heading.

Quercetin (An inhibitor of CYP2C8 may decrease the AUC of rosiglitazone. Therefore, if an inducer of CYP2C8 is started or stopped during treatment with rosiglitazone, changes in diabetes treatment may be needed upon clinical response).
No products indexed under this heading.

Rifabutin (An inhibitor of CYP2C8 may decrease the AUC of rosiglitazone. Therefore, if an inducer of CYP2C8 is started or stopped during treatment with rosiglitazone, changes in diabetes treatment may be needed upon clinical response).
No products indexed under this heading.

Rifampin (Rifampin administration (600 mg twice daily), an inducer of CYP2C8, for 6 days is reported to decrease rosiglitazone AUC by 66%, compared to the administration of rosiglitazone (8 mg) alone).
No products indexed under this heading.

Sulfaphenazole (An inhibitor of CYP2C8 may decrease the AUC of rosiglitazone. Therefore, if an inducer of CYP2C8 is started or stopped during treatment with rosiglitazone, changes in diabetes treatment may be needed upon clinical response).
No products indexed under this heading.

Sulfinpyrazone (An inhibitor of CYP2C8 may decrease the AUC of rosiglitazone. Therefore, if an inducer of CYP2C8 is started or stopped during treatment with rosiglitazone, changes in diabetes treatment may be needed upon clinical response).
No products indexed under this heading.

Trimethoprim (An inhibitor of CYP2C8 may decrease the AUC of rosiglitazone. Therefore, if an inducer of CYP2C8 is started or stopped during treatment with rosiglitazone, changes in diabetes treatment may be needed upon clinical response).
No products indexed under this heading.

Trimethoprim Hydrochloride (An inhibitor of CYP2C8 may decrease the AUC of rosiglitazone. Therefore, if an inducer of CYP2C8 is started or stopped during treatment with rosiglitazone, changes in diabetes treatment may be needed upon clinical response).
No products indexed under this heading.

AVAPRO TABLETS
(Irbesartan) **2886**
None cited in PDR database.

AVAPRO TABLETS
(Irbesartan) **925**
None cited in PDR database.

AVAR CLEANSER
(Sodium Sulfacetamide, Sulfur) **3189**
None cited in PDR database.

AVAR GEL
(Sodium Sulfacetamide, Sulfur) **3189**
None cited in PDR database.

AVAR GREEN
(Sodium Sulfacetamide, Sulfur) **3189**
None cited in PDR database.

AVAR-E EMOLLIENT CREAM
(Sodium Sulfacetamide, Sulfur) **3189**
None cited in PDR database.

AVAR-E GREEN CREAM
(Sodium Sulfacetamide, Sulfur) **3189**
None cited in PDR database.

AVASTIN IV
(Bevacizumab) **1229**
None cited in PDR database.

AVELOX I.V.
(Moxifloxacin Hydrochloride) **2984**
See Avelox Tablets

AVELOX TABLETS
(Moxifloxacin Hydrochloride) **2984**
May interact with antacids containing aluminum, calcium and magnesium, corticosteroids, oral anticoagulants, erythromycin, iron containing oral preparations, non-steroidal anti-inflammatory agents, phenothiazines, quinidine, tricyclic antidepressants, and certain other agents. Compounds in these categories include:

Aluminum Carbonate (Co-administration of quinolones, such as moxifloxacin, with antacids containing magnesium, calcium, or aluminum may substantially interfere with the absorption of quinolones; moxifloxacin should be taken at least 4 hours before or 8 hours after ingestion of antacids).
No products indexed under this heading.

Aluminum Hydroxide (Co-administration of quinolones, such as moxifloxacin, with antacids containing magnesium, calcium, or aluminum may substantially interfere with the absorption of quinolones; moxifloxacin should be taken at least 4 hours before or 8 hours after ingestion of antacids). Products include:
- Gaviscon Regular Strength Liquid **620**
- Gaviscon Regular Strength Tablets **619**
- Gaviscon Extra Strength Liquid **620**
- Gaviscon Extra Strength Tablets **619**
- Maalox Max Maximum Strength Antacid/Anti-Gas Liquid **2165**
- Maalox Regular Strength Antacid/Antigas Liquid **2164**

Amiodarone Hydrochloride (Moxifloxacin has been shown to prolong the QT interval; concurrent use with class 1A antiarrhythmic agents, such as amiodarone, should be avoided).
Products include:
- Pacerone Tablets **3337**

Amitriptyline Hydrochloride (Moxifloxacin has been shown to prolong the QT interval; an additive effect with co-administration cannot be excluded).
No products indexed under this heading.

Amoxapine (Moxifloxacin has been shown to prolong the QT interval; an additive effect with co-administration cannot be excluded).
No products indexed under this heading.

Anisindione (Quinolones, including moxifloxacin, have been reported to enhance the anticoagulant effects of warfarin or its derivatives). Products include:
- Miradon Tablets **3056**

Atenolol (The mean Cmax of single dose atenolol decreased by about 10% following co-administration with a single dose of moxifloxacin).
Products include:
- Tenormin I.V. Injection **698**
- Tenormin Tablets **695**

Betamethasone Acetate (Achilles and other tendon rupture have been reported with quinolones; although not reported in clinical trials with moxifloxacin, post market surveillance reports indicate that the risk may be increased in patients on concomitant corticosteroids).
No products indexed under this heading.

Betamethasone Sodium Phosphate (Achilles and other tendon rupture have been reported with quinolones; although not reported in clinical trials with moxifloxacin, post market surveillance reports indicate that the risk may be increased in patients on concomitant corticosteroids).
No products indexed under this heading.

Calcium Carbonate (Co-administration of quinolones, such as moxifloxacin, with antacids containing magnesium, calcium or aluminum may substantially interfere with the absorption of quinolones; moxifloxacin should be taken at least 4 hours before or 8 hours after ingestion of antacids). Products include:
- Actonel with Calcium Tablets **2684**
- Caltrate 600 PLUS Chewables **779**
- Caltrate 600 PLUS Tablets **779**
- Caltrate 600 + D Tablets **779**
- Encora Capsules **3298**
- Encora AM Tablets **3298**
- Encora PM Tablets **3298**
- Gas-X with Maalox **675**
- Maalox Regular Strength Antacid Tablets **2166**
- Quick Dissolve Maalox Max Maximum Strength Antacid/Antigas Tablets **2165**
- Maalox Max Quick Dissolve Maximum Strength Chewable Tablets **678**
- Os-Cal Chewable Tablets **765**
- Pepcid Complete Chewable Tablets **1672**
- PremCal Light, Regular, and Extra Strength Tablets **762**
- Rolaids Tablets **707**

Extra Strength Rolaids Softchews ... ▣708
Extra Strength Rolaids Tablets ... ▣707
Rolaids Multi-Symptom Antacid & Antigas Tablets ... ▣708
Tums ... ▣639

Celecoxib (Co-administration of a non-steroidal anti-inflammatory agent with a quinolone may increase the risks of CNS stimulation and convulsions; this interaction has not been observed in moxifloxacin clinical and preclinical trials). Products include:
Celebrex Capsules ... 3130

Chlorpromazine (Moxifloxacin has been shown to prolong the QT interval; co-administration with antipsychotic phenothiazines cannot be excluded).
No products indexed under this heading.

Chlorpromazine Hydrochloride (Moxifloxacin has been shown to prolong the QT interval; co-administration with antipsychotic phenothiazines cannot be excluded).
No products indexed under this heading.

Cisapride (Moxifloxacin has been shown to prolong the QT interval; an additive effect with co-administration cannot be excluded).
No products indexed under this heading.

Clomipramine Hydrochloride (Moxifloxacin has been shown to prolong the QT interval; an additive effect with co-administration cannot be excluded).
No products indexed under this heading.

Cortisone Acetate (Achilles and other tendon rupture have been reported with quinolones; although not reported in clinical trials with moxifloxacin, post market surveillance reports indicate that the risk may be increased in patients on concomitant corticosteroids).
No products indexed under this heading.

Desipramine Hydrochloride (Moxifloxacin has been shown to prolong the QT interval; an additive effect with co-administration cannot be excluded).
No products indexed under this heading.

Dexamethasone (Achilles and other tendon rupture have been reported with quinolones; although not reported in clinical trials with moxifloxacin, post market surveillance reports indicate that the risk may be increased in patients on concomitant corticosteroids). Products include:
Ciprodex Otic Suspension ... 555
Decadron Tablets ... 1929
TobraDex Ophthalmic Ointment ... 558
TobraDex Ophthalmic Suspension ... 558

Dexamethasone Acetate (Achilles and other tendon rupture have been reported with quinolones; although not reported in clinical trials with moxifloxacin, post market surveillance reports indicate that the risk may be increased in patients on concomitant corticosteroids).
No products indexed under this heading.

Dexamethasone Sodium Phosphate (Achilles and other tendon rupture have been reported with quinolones; although not reported in clinical trials with moxifloxacin, post market surveillance reports indicate that the risk may be increased in patients on concomitant corticosteroids). Products include:
Decadron Phosphate Injection ... 1931

Diclofenac Potassium (Co-administration of a non-steroidal anti-inflammatory agent with a quinolone may increase the risks of CNS stimulation and convulsions; this interaction has not been observed in moxifloxacin clinical and preclinical trials). Products include:
Cataflam Tablets ... 2173

Diclofenac Sodium (Co-administration of a non-steroidal anti-inflammatory agent with a quinolone may increase the risks of CNS stimulation and convulsions; this interaction has not been observed in moxifloxacin clinical and preclinical trials). Products include:
Arthrotec Tablets ... 3126
Voltaren Ophthalmic Solution ... 2300
Voltaren Tablets ... 2298
Voltaren-XR Tablets ... 2301

Dicumarol (Quinolones, including moxifloxacin, have been reported to enhance the anticoagulant effects of warfarin or its derivatives).
No products indexed under this heading.

Didanosine (Co-administration of quinolones, such as moxifloxacin, with antacids contained in Videx chewable/buffered tablets or the pediatric powder for oral solution may substantially interfere with the absorption of quinolones; moxifloxacin should be taken at least 4 hours before or 8 hours after ingestion of Videx).
No products indexed under this heading.

Digoxin (Co-administration in healthy individuals has resulted in the increase in mean digoxin Cmax by about 50% during the distribution phase of digoxin; this transient increase in digoxin Cmax is not viewed to be clinically significant). Products include:
Digitek Tablets ... 2146
Lanoxicaps Capsules ... 1458
Lanoxin Injection ... 1462
Lanoxin Tablets ... 1468
Lanoxin Injection Pediatric ... 1465

Doxepin Hydrochloride (Moxifloxacin has been shown to prolong the QT interval; an additive effect with co-administration cannot be excluded).
No products indexed under this heading.

Erythromycin (Moxifloxacin has been shown to prolong the QT interval; an additive effect with co-administration cannot be excluded). Products include:
Erygel Topical Gel ... 2096
Ery-Tab Tablets ... 447
Erythromycin Base Filmtab Tablets ... 454
Erythromycin Delayed-Release Capsules, USP ... 456
PCE Dispertab Tablets ... 510

Erythromycin Estolate (Moxifloxacin has been shown to prolong the QT interval; an additive effect with co-administration cannot be excluded).
No products indexed under this heading.

Erythromycin Ethylsuccinate (Moxifloxacin has been shown to prolong the QT interval; an additive effect with co-administration cannot be excluded). Products include:
E.E.S. ... 449
EryPed ... 445

Erythromycin Gluceptate (Moxifloxacin has been shown to prolong the QT interval; an additive effect with co-administration cannot be excluded).
No products indexed under this heading.

Erythromycin Lactobionate (Moxifloxacin has been shown to prolong the QT interval; an additive effect with co-administration cannot be excluded).
No products indexed under this heading.

Erythromycin Stearate (Moxifloxacin has been shown to prolong the QT interval; an additive effect with co-administration cannot be excluded). Products include:
Erythrocin Stearate Filmtab Tablets ... 452

Etodolac (Co-administration of a non-steroidal anti-inflammatory agent with a quinolone may increase the risks of CNS stimulation and convulsions; this interaction has not been observed in moxifloxacin clinical and preclinical trials).
No products indexed under this heading.

Fenoprofen Calcium (Co-administration of a non-steroidal anti-inflammatory agent with a quinolone may increase the risks of CNS stimulation and convulsions; this interaction has not been observed in moxifloxacin clinical and preclinical trials). Products include:
Nalfon Capsules ... 2504

Ferrous Fumarate (Co-administration of quinolones, such as moxifloxacin, with iron-containing products may substantially interfere with the absorption of quinolones; moxifloxacin should be taken at least 4 hours before or 8 hours after ingestion of iron-containing products). Products include:
Chromagen Forte Soft Gelatin Capsules ... 3296
Ferretts Tablets ... ▣773
Repliva 21/7 Tablets ... 3301

Ferrous Gluconate (Co-administration of quinolones, such as moxifloxacin, with iron-containing products may substantially interfere with the absorption of quinolones; moxifloxacin should be taken at least 4 hours before or 8 hours after ingestion of iron-containing products).
No products indexed under this heading.

Ferrous Sulfate (Co-administration of moxifloxacin with ferrous sulfate has resulted in reduced mean AUC (39%) and Cmax (59%) of moxifloxacin; moxifloxacin should be taken at least 4 hours before or 8 hours after ingestion of ferrous sulfate). Products include:
Feosol Tablets ... 1629
Slow Fe Iron Tablets ... ▣772
Slow Fe with Folic Acid Tablets ... ▣773

Fludrocortisone Acetate (Achilles and other tendon rupture have been reported with quinolones; although not reported in clinical trials with moxifloxacin, post market surveillance reports indicate that the risk may be increased in patients on concomitant corticosteroids).
No products indexed under this heading.

Fluphenazine Decanoate (Moxifloxacin has been shown to prolong the QT interval; co-administration with antipsychotic phenothiazines cannot be excluded).
No products indexed under this heading.

Fluphenazine Enanthate (Moxifloxacin has been shown to prolong the QT interval; co-administration with antipsychotic phenothiazines cannot be excluded).
No products indexed under this heading.

Fluphenazine Hydrochloride (Moxifloxacin has been shown to prolong the QT interval; co-administration with antipsychotic phenothiazines cannot be excluded).
No products indexed under this heading.

Flurbiprofen (Co-administration of a non-steroidal anti-inflammatory agent with a quinolone may increase the risks of CNS stimulation and convulsions; this interaction has not been observed in moxifloxacin clinical and preclinical trials).
No products indexed under this heading.

Glyburide (Co-administration has resulted in reduced mean AUC and Cmax by 12% and 21%, respectively; blood glucose levels were decreased slightly in patients on concurrent therapy; these interaction results are not viewed as clinically significant).
No products indexed under this heading.

Hydrocortisone (Achilles and other tendon rupture have been reported with quinolones; although not reported in clinical trials with moxifloxacin, post market surveillance reports indicate that the risk may be increased in patients on concomitant corticosteroids). Products include:
Cortizone•5 Ointment ... ▣699
Cortizone•10 Creme ... ▣699
Cortizone•10 Ointment ... ▣699
Cortizone•10 Plus Creme ... ▣700
Cortizone•10 Maximum Strength Quick Shot Spray ... ▣700
Hydrocortone Tablets ... 1963
Preparation H Hydrocortisone Cream ... ▣748

Hydrocortisone Acetate (Achilles and other tendon rupture have been reported with quinolones; although not reported in clinical trials with moxifloxacin, post market surveillance reports indicate that the risk may be increased in patients on concomitant corticosteroids). Products include:
Analpram-HC ... 1136
Pramosone ... 1139
ProctoFoam-HC ... 3113
Tucks Anti-Itch Ointment ... ▣712
U-cort 1% Cream ... 3289

Hydrocortisone Sodium Phosphate (Achilles and other tendon rupture have been reported with quinolones; although not reported in clinical trials with moxifloxacin, post market surveillance reports indicate that the risk may be increased in patients on concomitant corticosteroids).
No products indexed under this heading.

Hydrocortisone Sodium Succinate (Achilles and other tendon rupture have been reported with quinolones; although not reported in clinical trials with moxifloxacin, post market surveillance reports indicate that the risk may be increased in patients on concomitant corticosteroids).
No products indexed under this heading.

Ibuprofen (Co-administration of a non-steroidal anti-inflammatory agent with a quinolone may increase the risks of CNS stimulation and convulsions; this interaction has not been observed in moxifloxacin clinical and preclinical trials). Products include:
Advil Allergy Sinus Caplets .... ■ **737**
Advil .... ■ **737**
Children's Advil Suspension .... ■ **742**
Children's Advil Chewable Tablets .. ■ **741**
Advil Cold & Sinus .... ■ **739**
Advil Flu & Body Ache Caplets .... ■ **739**
Children's Advil Cold Suspension ... ■ **741**
Infants' Advil Concentrated Drops .. ■ **743**
Junior Strength Advil Swallow Tablets .... ■ **740**
Advil Migraine Liquigels .... ■ **740**
Advil Multi-Symptom Cold Caplets .... ■ **738**
Combunox Tablets **1183**
Children's Motrin Oral Suspension and Chewable Tablets **1837**
Children's Motrin Cold Non-Staining Dye-Free Oral Suspension **1838**
Children's Motrin Cold Oral Suspension **1838**
Children's Motrin Non-Staining Dye-Free Oral Suspension **1837**
Motrin Cold & Sinus Caplets **1836**
Motrin IB Tablets and Caplets **1836**
Infants' Motrin Concentrated Drops **1837**
Infants' Motrin Non-Staining Dye-Free Drops **1837**
Junior Strength Motrin Caplets and Chewable Tablets **1837**
Vicoprofen Tablets **533**

Imipramine Hydrochloride (Moxifloxacin has been shown to prolong the QT interval; an additive effect with co-administration cannot be excluded).
No products indexed under this heading.

Imipramine Pamoate (Moxifloxacin has been shown to prolong the QT interval; an additive effect with co-administration cannot be excluded).
No products indexed under this heading.

Indomethacin (Co-administration of a non-steroidal anti-inflammatory agent with a quinolone may increase the risks of CNS stimulation and convulsions; this interaction has not been observed in moxifloxacin clinical and preclinical trials). Products include:
Indocin **1968**

Indomethacin Sodium Trihydrate (Co-administration of a non-steroidal anti-inflammatory agent with a quinolone may increase the risks of CNS stimulation and convulsions; this interaction has not been observed in moxifloxacin clinical and preclinical trials). Products include:
Indocin I.V. **1973**

Iron (Co-administration of quinolones, such as moxifloxacin, with iron-containing products may substantially interfere with the absorption of quinolones; moxifloxacin should be taken at least 4 hours before or 8 hours after ingestion of iron-containing products). Products include:
Chromagen Forte Soft Gelatin Capsules **3296**
Ferretts IPS Liquid .... ■ **773**
OptiNate **1162**
Repliva 21/7 Tablets **3301**

Ketoprofen (Co-administration of a non-steroidal anti-inflammatory agent with a quinolone may increase the risks of CNS stimulation and convulsions; this interaction has not been observed in moxifloxacin clinical and preclinical trials).
No products indexed under this heading.

Ketorolac Tromethamine (Co-administration of a non-steroidal anti-inflammatory agent with a quinolone may increase the risks of CNS stimulation and convulsions; this interaction has not been observed in moxifloxacin clinical and preclinical trials). Products include:
Acular Ophthalmic Solution **561**
Acular LS Ophthalmic Solution **562**

Magaldrate (Co-administration of quinolones, such as moxifloxacin, with antacids containing magnesium, calcium, or aluminum may substantially interfere with the absorption of quinolones; moxifloxacin should be taken at least 4 hours before or 8 hours after ingestion of antacids).
No products indexed under this heading.

Magnesium Hydroxide (Co-administration of quinolones, such as moxifloxacin, with antacids containing magnesium, calcium, or aluminum may substantially interfere with the absorption of quinolones; moxifloxacin should be taken at least 4 hours before or 8 hours after ingestion of antacids). Products include:
Maalox Max Maximum Strength Antacid/Anti-Gas Liquid **2165**
Maalox Regular Strength Antacid/Antigas Liquid **2164**
Pepcid Complete Chewable Tablets **1672**
Rolaids Tablets .... ■ **707**
Extra Strength Rolaids Tablets .... ■ **707**
Rolaids Multi-Symptom Antacid & Antigas Tablets .... ■ **708**

Magnesium Oxide (Co-administration of quinolones, such as moxifloxacin, with antacids containing magnesium, calcium, or aluminum may substantially interfere with the absorption of quinolones; moxifloxacin should be taken at least 4 hours before or 8 hours after ingestion of antacids). Products include:
Beelith Tablets **784**
PremCal Light, Regular, and Extra Strength Tablets .... ■ **762**

Maprotiline Hydrochloride (Moxifloxacin has been shown to prolong the QT interval; an additive effect with co-administration cannot be excluded).
No products indexed under this heading.

Meclofenamate Sodium (Co-administration of a non-steroidal anti-inflammatory agent with a quinolone may increase the risks of CNS stimulation and convulsions; this interaction has not been observed in moxifloxacin clinical and preclinical trials).
No products indexed under this heading.

Mefenamic Acid (Co-administration of a non-steroidal anti-inflammatory agent with a quinolone may increase the risks of CNS stimulation and convulsions; this interaction has not been observed in moxifloxacin clinical and preclinical trials).
No products indexed under this heading.

Meloxicam (Co-administration of a non-steroidal anti-inflammatory agent with a quinolone may increase the risks of CNS stimulation and convulsions; this interaction has not been observed in moxifloxacin clinical and preclinical trials). Products include:
Mobic Oral Suspension **893**
Mobic Tablets **893**

Mesoridazine Besylate (Moxifloxacin has been shown to prolong the QT interval; co-administration with antipsychotic phenothiazines cannot be excluded).
No products indexed under this heading.

Methotrimeprazine (Moxifloxacin has been shown to prolong the QT interval; co-administration with antipsychotic phenothiazines cannot be excluded).
No products indexed under this heading.

Methylprednisolone Acetate (Achilles and other tendon rupture have been reported with quinolones; although not reported in clinical trials with moxifloxacin, post market surveillance reports indicate that the risk may be increased in patients on concomitant corticosteroids). Products include:
Depo-Medrol Injectable Suspension **2615**
Depo-Medrol Single-Dose Vial **2617**

Methylprednisolone Sodium Succinate (Achilles and other tendon rupture have been reported with quinolones; although not reported in clinical trials with moxifloxacin, post market surveillance reports indicate that the risk may be increased in patients on concomitant corticosteroids).
No products indexed under this heading.

Nabumetone (Co-administration of a non-steroidal anti-inflammatory agent with a quinolone may increase the risks of CNS stimulation and convulsions; this interaction has not been observed in moxifloxacin clinical and preclinical trials). Products include:
Relafen Tablets **1523**

Naproxen (Co-administration of a non-steroidal anti-inflammatory agent with a quinolone may increase the risks of CNS stimulation and convulsions; this interaction has not been observed in moxifloxacin clinical and preclinical trials). Products include:
EC-Naprosyn Delayed-Release Tablets **2769**
Naprosyn Suspension **2769**
Naprosyn Tablets **2769**
Prevacid NapraPAC **3277**

Naproxen Sodium (Co-administration of a non-steroidal anti-inflammatory agent with a quinolone may increase the risks of CNS stimulation and convulsions; this interaction has not been observed in moxifloxacin clinical and preclinical trials). Products include:
Aleve Tablets, Caplets and Gelcaps .... ■ **605**
Anaprox Tablets **2769**
Anaprox DS Tablets **2769**

Nortriptyline Hydrochloride (Moxifloxacin has been shown to prolong the QT interval; an additive effect with co-administration cannot be excluded).
No products indexed under this heading.

Oxaprozin (Co-administration of a non-steroidal anti-inflammatory agent with a quinolone may increase the risks of CNS stimulation and convulsions; this interaction has not been observed in moxifloxacin clinical and preclinical trials).
No products indexed under this heading.

Perphenazine (Moxifloxacin has been shown to prolong the QT interval; co-administration with antipsychotic phenothiazines cannot be excluded).
No products indexed under this heading.

Phenylbutazone (Co-administration of a non-steroidal anti-inflammatory agent with a quinolone may increase the risks of CNS stimulation and convulsions; this interaction has not been observed in moxifloxacin clinical and preclinical trials).
No products indexed under this heading.

Piroxicam (Co-administration of a non-steroidal anti-inflammatory agent with a quinolone may increase the risks of CNS stimulation and convulsions; this interaction has not been observed in moxifloxacin clinical and preclinical trials).
No products indexed under this heading.

Polysaccharide Iron Complex (Co-administration of quinolones, such as moxifloxacin, with iron-containing products may substantially interfere with the absorption of quinolones; moxifloxacin should be taken at least 4 hours before or 8 hours after ingestion of iron-containing products). Products include:
Niferex-150 Forte Capsules **3299**
Nu-Iron 150 Capsules **2098**

Prednisolone Acetate (Achilles and other tendon rupture have been reported with quinolones; although not reported in clinical trials with moxifloxacin, post market surveillance reports indicate that the risk may be increased in patients on concomitant corticosteroids). Products include:
Blephamide Ophthalmic Ointment **563**
Blephamide Ophthalmic Suspension **564**
Poly-Pred Liquifilm Ophthalmic Suspension .... ⊙ **231**
Pred Forte Ophthalmic Suspension .... ⊙ **233**
Pred Mild Sterile Ophthalmic Suspension .... ⊙ **236**
Pred-G Ophthalmic Suspension .... ⊙ **234**
Pred-G Sterile Ophthalmic Ointment .... ⊙ **235**

Prednisolone Sodium Phosphate (Achilles and other tendon rupture have been reported with quinolones; although not reported in clinical trials with moxifloxacin, post market surveillance reports indicate that the risk may be increased in patients on concomitant corticosteroids). Products include:
Pediapred Oral Solution **3319**

Prednisolone Tebutate (Achilles and other tendon rupture have been reported with quinolones; although not reported in clinical trials with moxifloxacin, post market surveillance reports indicate that the risk may be increased in patients on concomitant corticosteroids).
No products indexed under this heading.

Prednisone (Achilles and other tendon rupture have been reported with quinolones; although not reported in clinical trials with moxifloxacin, post market surveillance reports indicate that the risk may be increased in patients on concomitant corticosteroids).
No products indexed under this heading.

Procainamide Hydrochloride (Moxifloxacin has been shown to prolong the QT interval; concurrent use with class 1A antiarrhythmic agents, such as procainamide, should be avoided).
No products indexed under this heading.

Prochlorperazine (Moxifloxacin has been shown to prolong the QT interval; co-administration with antipsychotic phenothiazines cannot be excluded).
No products indexed under this heading.

Promethazine Hydrochloride (Moxifloxacin has been shown to prolong the QT interval; co-administration with antipsychotic phenothiazines cannot be excluded). Products include:
Phenergan **3438**

Protriptyline Hydrochloride (Moxifloxacin has been shown to prolong the QT interval; an additive effect with co-administration cannot be excluded). Products include:
Vivactil Tablets **2350**

Quinidine (Moxifloxacin has been shown to prolong the QT interval; concurrent use with class 1A antiarrhythmic agents, such as quinidine, should be avoided).
No products indexed under this heading.

Quinidine Gluconate (Moxifloxacin has been shown to prolong the QT interval; concurrent use with class 1A antiarrhythmic agents, such as quinidine, should be avoided).
No products indexed under this heading.

Quinidine Hydrochloride (Moxifloxacin has been shown to prolong the QT interval; concurrent use with class 1A antiarrhythmic agents, such as quinidine, should be avoided).
No products indexed under this heading.

Quinidine Polygalacturonate (Moxifloxacin has been shown to prolong the QT interval; concurrent use with class 1A antiarrhythmic agents, such as quinidine, should be avoided).
No products indexed under this heading.

Quinidine Sulfate (Moxifloxacin has been shown to prolong the QT interval; concurrent use with class 1A antiarrhythmic agents, such as quinidine, should be avoided).
No products indexed under this heading.

Rofecoxib (Co-administration of a non-steroidal anti-inflammatory agent with a quinolone may increase the risks of CNS stimulation and convulsions; this interaction has not been observed in moxifloxacin clinical and preclinical trials).
No products indexed under this heading.

Sotalol Hydrochloride (Moxifloxacin has been shown to prolong the QT interval; concurrent use with class III antiarrhythmic agents, such as sotalol, should be avoided).
No products indexed under this heading.

Sucralfate (Co-administration of quinolones, such as moxifloxacin, with sucralfate may substantially interfere with the absorption of quinolones; moxifloxacin should be taken at least 4 hours before or 8 hours after ingestion of sucralfate). Products include:
Carafate Suspension **727**
Carafate Tablets **728**

Sulindac (Co-administration of a non-steroidal anti-inflammatory agent with a quinolone may increase the risks of CNS stimulation and convulsions; this interaction has not been observed in moxifloxacin clinical and preclinical trials). Products include:
Clinoril Tablets **1899**

Thioridazine Hydrochloride (Moxifloxacin has been shown to prolong the QT interval; co-administration with antipsychotic phenothiazines cannot be excluded). Products include:
Thioridazine Hydrochloride Tablets **2122**

Tolmetin Sodium (Co-administration of a non-steroidal anti-inflammatory agent with a quinolone may increase the risks of CNS stimulation and convulsions; this interaction has not been observed in moxifloxacin clinical and preclinical trials).
No products indexed under this heading.

Triamcinolone (Achilles and other tendon rupture have been reported with quinolones; although not reported in clinical trials with moxifloxacin, post market surveillance reports indicate that the risk may be increased in patients on concomitant corticosteroids).
No products indexed under this heading.

Triamcinolone Acetonide (Achilles and other tendon rupture have been reported with quinolones; although not reported in clinical trials with moxifloxacin, post market surveillance reports indicate that the risk may be increased in patients on concomitant corticosteroids). Products include:
Azmacort Inhalation Aerosol **1701**
Nasacort HFA Inhalation Aerosol **2939**
Nasacort AQ Nasal Spray **2937**

Triamcinolone Diacetate (Achilles and other tendon rupture have been reported with quinolones; although not reported in clinical trials with moxifloxacin, post market surveillance reports indicate that the risk may be increased in patients on concomitant corticosteroids).
No products indexed under this heading.

Triamcinolone Hexacetonide (Achilles and other tendon rupture have been reported with quinolones; although not reported in clinical trials with moxifloxacin, post market surveillance reports indicate that the risk may be increased in patients on concomitant corticosteroids).
No products indexed under this heading.

Trifluoperazine Hydrochloride (Moxifloxacin has been shown to prolong the QT interval; co-administration with antipsychotic phenothiazines cannot be excluded).
No products indexed under this heading.

Trimipramine Maleate (Moxifloxacin has been shown to prolong the QT interval; an additive effect with co-administration cannot be excluded). Products include:
Surmontil Capsules **2347**

Valdecoxib (Co-administration of a non-steroidal anti-inflammatory agent with a quinolone may increase the risks of CNS stimulation and convulsions; this interaction has not been observed in moxifloxacin clinical and preclinical trials).
No products indexed under this heading.

Warfarin Sodium (Quinolones, including moxifloxacin, have been reported to enhance the anticoagulant effects of warfarin or its derivatives). Products include:
Coumadin for Injection **932**
Coumadin Tablets **932**

Zinc Sulfate (Co-administration of quinolones, such as moxifloxacin, with zinc-containing products may substantially interfere with the absorption of quinolones; moxifloxacin should be taken at least 4 hours before or 8 hours after ingestion of zinc-containing products). Products include:
Athena Hair System Shampoo .... ▣ **767**
Spartan Hair System Shampoo ...... ▣ **767**
Visine A.C. Seasonal Itching and Redness Relief Drops .... ⊙ **278**
Zinc-220 Capsules **576**

AVINZA CAPSULES

(Morphine Sulfate) **1714**

May interact with central nervous system depressants, monoamine oxidase inhibitors, mixed agonist/antagonist opioid analgesics, muscle relaxants, and certain other agents. Compounds in these categories include:

Alfentanil Hydrochloride (Co-administration increases the risk of respiratory depression, hypotension, profound sedation, or coma).
No products indexed under this heading.

Alprazolam (Co-administration increases the risk of respiratory depression, hypotension, profound sedation, or coma). Products include:
Niravam Orally Disintegrating Tablets **3106**
Xanax XR Tablets **2655**

Aprobarbital (Co-administration increases the risk of respiratory depression, hypotension, profound sedation, or coma).
No products indexed under this heading.

Atracurium Besylate (Morphine may enhance the neuromuscular blocking action of skeletal muscle relaxants and produce an increased degree of respiratory depression).
No products indexed under this heading.

Baclofen (Morphine may enhance the neuromuscular blocking action of skeletal muscle relaxants and produce an increased degree of respiratory depression).
No products indexed under this heading.

Buprenorphine Hydrochloride (Mixed agonist/antagonist analgesics may reduce the analgesic effect and/or may precipitate withdrawal symptoms; mixed agonist/antagonist analgesics should NOT be administered to patients who have received or are receiving a course of therapy with pure opioid agonist analgesic). Products include:
Buprenex Injectable **2718**
Suboxone Tablets **2719**
Subutex Tablets **2719**

Buspirone Hydrochloride (Co-administration increases the risk of respiratory depression, hypotension, profound sedation, or coma).
No products indexed under this heading.

Butabarbital (Co-administration increases the risk of respiratory depression, hypotension, profound sedation, or coma).
No products indexed under this heading.

Butalbital (Co-administration increases the risk of respiratory depression, hypotension, profound sedation, or coma). Products include:
Sedapap Tablets 50 mg/650 mg **2098**

Butorphanol Tartrate (Mixed agonist/antagonist analgesics may reduce the analgesic effect and/or may precipitate withdrawal symptoms; mixed agonist/antagonist analgesics should NOT be administered to patients who have received or are receiving a course of therapy with pure opioid agonist analgesic).
No products indexed under this heading.

Carisoprodol (Morphine may enhance the neuromuscular blocking action of skeletal muscle relaxants and produce an increased degree of respiratory depression).
No products indexed under this heading.

Chlordiazepoxide (Co-administration increases the risk of respiratory depression, hypotension, profound sedation, or coma).
No products indexed under this heading.

Chlordiazepoxide Hydrochloride (Co-administration increases the risk of respiratory depression, hypotension, profound sedation, or coma). Products include:
Librium Capsules **3349**

Chlorpromazine (Co-administration increases the risk of respiratory depression, hypotension, profound sedation, or coma).
No products indexed under this heading.

Chlorpromazine Hydrochloride (Co-administration increases the risk of respiratory depression, hypotension, profound sedation, or coma).
No products indexed under this heading.

Chlorprothixene (Co-administration increases the risk of respiratory depression, hypotension, profound sedation, or coma).
No products indexed under this heading.

Chlorprothixene Hydrochloride (Co-administration increases the risk of respiratory depression, hypotension, profound sedation, or coma).
No products indexed under this heading.

Chlorprothixene Lactate (Co-administration increases the risk of respiratory depression, hypotension, profound sedation, or coma).
No products indexed under this heading.

Chlorzoxazone (Morphine may enhance the neuromuscular blocking action of skeletal muscle relaxants and produce an increased degree of respiratory depression).
No products indexed under this heading.

Cimetidine (Co-administration has been reported to precipitate apnea, confusion and muscle twitching in an isolated report). Products include:
Tagamet HB 200 Tablets 637
Tagamet Tablets 1547

Cisatracurium Besylate (Morphine may enhance the neuromuscular blocking action of skeletal muscle relaxants and produce an increased degree of respiratory depression). Products include:
Nimbex Injection 494

Clorazepate Dipotassium (Co-administration increases the risk of respiratory depression, hypotension, profound sedation, or coma). Products include:
Tranxene 2488

Clozapine (Co-administration increases the risk of respiratory depression, hypotension, profound sedation, or coma). Products include:
Clozapine Tablets 2141
Clozaril Tablets 2174
FazaClo Orally Disintegrating Tablets 547

Codeine Phosphate (Co-administration increases the risk of respiratory depression, hypotension, profound sedation, or coma). Products include:
Tylenol with Codeine 2461

Cyclobenzaprine Hydrochloride (Morphine may enhance the neuromuscular blocking action of skeletal muscle relaxants and produce an increased degree of respiratory depression). Products include:
Flexeril Tablets 1832

Dantrolene Sodium (Morphine may enhance the neuromuscular blocking action of skeletal muscle relaxants and produce an increased degree of respiratory depression). Products include:
Dantrium Capsules 2690
Dantrium Intravenous 2691

Desflurane (Co-administration increases the risk of respiratory depression, hypotension, profound sedation, or coma). Products include:
Suprane Liquid for Inhalation 770

Dezocine (Co-administration increases the risk of respiratory depression, hypotension, profound sedation, or coma).
No products indexed under this heading.

Diazepam (Co-administration increases the risk of respiratory depression, hypotension, profound sedation, or coma). Products include:
Diastat Rectal Delivery System 3344
Valium Tablets 2822

Doxacurium Chloride (Morphine may enhance the neuromuscular blocking action of skeletal muscle relaxants and produce an increased degree of respiratory depression).
No products indexed under this heading.

Droperidol (Co-administration increases the risk of respiratory depression, hypotension, profound sedation, or coma).
No products indexed under this heading.

Enflurane (Co-administration increases the risk of respiratory depression, hypotension, profound sedation, or coma).
No products indexed under this heading.

Estazolam (Co-administration increases the risk of respiratory depression, hypotension, profound sedation, or coma). Products include:
ProSom Tablets 512

Ethanol (Co-administration increases the risk of respiratory depression, hypotension, profound sedation, or coma).
No products indexed under this heading.

Ethchlorvynol (Co-administration increases the risk of respiratory depression, hypotension, profound sedation, or coma).
No products indexed under this heading.

Ethinamate (Co-administration increases the risk of respiratory depression, hypotension, profound sedation, or coma).
No products indexed under this heading.

Ethyl Alcohol (Co-administration increases the risk of respiratory depression, hypotension, profound sedation, or coma).
No products indexed under this heading.

Fentanyl (Co-administration increases the risk of respiratory depression, hypotension, profound sedation, or coma). Products include:
Duragesic Transdermal System 2448

Fentanyl Citrate (Co-administration increases the risk of respiratory depression, hypotension, profound sedation, or coma). Products include:
Actiq 993

Fluphenazine Decanoate (Co-administration increases the risk of respiratory depression, hypotension, profound sedation, or coma).
No products indexed under this heading.

Fluphenazine Enanthate (Co-administration increases the risk of respiratory depression, hypotension, profound sedation, or coma).
No products indexed under this heading.

Fluphenazine Hydrochloride (Co-administration increases the risk of respiratory depression, hypotension, profound sedation, or coma).
No products indexed under this heading.

Flurazepam Hydrochloride (Co-administration increases the risk of respiratory depression, hypotension, profound sedation, or coma). Products include:
Dalmane Capsules 3343

Glutethimide (Co-administration increases the risk of respiratory depression, hypotension, profound sedation, or coma).
No products indexed under this heading.

Haloperidol (Co-administration increases the risk of respiratory depression, hypotension, profound sedation, or coma).
No products indexed under this heading.

Haloperidol Decanoate (Co-administration increases the risk of respiratory depression, hypotension, profound sedation, or coma).
No products indexed under this heading.

Hydrocodone Bitartrate (Co-administration increases the risk of respiratory depression, hypotension, profound sedation, or coma). Products include:
Hycodan 1104
Hycomine Compound Tablets 1105
Hycotuss Expectorant Syrup 1106
Lortab 3315
Lortab Elixir 3312
Vicodin Tablets 530
Vicodin ES Tablets 531
Vicodin HP Tablets 532
Vicoprofen Tablets 533
Zydone Tablets 1118

Hydrocodone Polistirex (Co-administration increases the risk of respiratory depression, hypotension, profound sedation, or coma). Products include:
Tussionex Pennkinetic Extended-Release Suspension 3322

Hydromorphone Hydrochloride (Co-administration increases the risk of respiratory depression, hypotension, profound sedation, or coma). Products include:
Dilaudid 439
Dilaudid Oral Liquid 443
Dilaudid Non-Sterile Powder 439
Dilaudid Rectal Suppositories 439
Dilaudid Tablets 439
Dilaudid Tablets - 8 mg 443
Dilaudid-HP 441

Hydroxyzine Hydrochloride (Co-administration increases the risk of respiratory depression, hypotension, profound sedation, or coma).
No products indexed under this heading.

Isocarboxazid (MAO inhibitors markedly potentiate the action of morphine; concurrent and/or sequential use should be avoided).
No products indexed under this heading.

Isoflurane (Co-administration increases the risk of respiratory depression, hypotension, profound sedation, or coma).
No products indexed under this heading.

Ketamine Hydrochloride (Co-administration increases the risk of respiratory depression, hypotension, profound sedation, or coma).
No products indexed under this heading.

Levomethadyl Acetate Hydrochloride (Co-administration increases the risk of respiratory depression, hypotension, profound sedation, or coma).
No products indexed under this heading.

Levorphanol Tartrate (Co-administration increases the risk of respiratory depression, hypotension, profound sedation, or coma).
No products indexed under this heading.

Lorazepam (Co-administration increases the risk of respiratory depression, hypotension, profound sedation, or coma).
No products indexed under this heading.

Loxapine Hydrochloride (Co-administration increases the risk of respiratory depression, hypotension, profound sedation, or coma).
No products indexed under this heading.

Loxapine Succinate (Co-administration increases the risk of respiratory depression, hypotension, profound sedation, or coma).
No products indexed under this heading.

Meperidine Hydrochloride (Co-administration increases the risk of respiratory depression, hypotension, profound sedation, or coma).
No products indexed under this heading.

Mephobarbital (Co-administration increases the risk of respiratory depression, hypotension, profound sedation, or coma). Products include:
Mebaral Tablets, USP 2483

Meprobamate (Co-administration increases the risk of respiratory depression, hypotension, profound sedation, or coma).
No products indexed under this heading.

Mesoridazine Besylate (Co-administration increases the risk of respiratory depression, hypotension, profound sedation, or coma).
No products indexed under this heading.

Metaxalone (Morphine may enhance the neuromuscular blocking action of skeletal muscle relaxants and produce an increased degree of respiratory depression). Products include:
Skelaxin Tablets 1685

Methadone Hydrochloride (Co-administration increases the risk of respiratory depression, hypotension, profound sedation, or coma).
No products indexed under this heading.

Methocarbamol (Morphine may enhance the neuromuscular blocking action of skeletal muscle relaxants and produce an increased degree of respiratory depression).
No products indexed under this heading.

Methohexital Sodium (Co-administration increases the risk of respiratory depression, hypotension, profound sedation, or coma).
No products indexed under this heading.

Methotrimeprazine (Co-administration increases the risk of respiratory depression, hypotension, profound sedation, or coma).
No products indexed under this heading.

Methoxyflurane (Co-administration increases the risk of respiratory depression, hypotension, profound sedation, or coma).
No products indexed under this heading.

Metocurine Iodide (Morphine may enhance the neuromuscular blocking action of skeletal muscle relaxants and produce an increased degree of respiratory depression).
No products indexed under this heading.

Midazolam Hydrochloride (Co-administration increases the risk of respiratory depression, hypotension, profound sedation, or coma).
No products indexed under this heading.

Mivacurium Chloride (Morphine may enhance the neuromuscular blocking action of skeletal muscle relaxants and produce an increased degree of respiratory depression). Products include:
Mivacron Injection 489

Moclobemide (MAO inhibitors markedly potentiate the action of morphine; concurrent and/or sequential use should be avoided).
No products indexed under this heading.

Molindone Hydrochloride (Co-administration increases the risk of respiratory depression, hypotension, profound sedation, or coma). Products include:
Moban Tablets 1108

Nalbuphine Hydrochloride (Mixed agonist/antagonist analgesics may reduce the analgesic effect and/or may precipitate withdrawal symptoms; mixed agonist/antagonist analgesics should NOT be administered to patients who have received or are receiving a course of therapy with pure opioid agonist analgesic). Products include:
Nubain Injection 1111

Olanzapine (Co-administration increases the risk of respiratory depression, hypotension, profound sedation, or coma). Products include:
Symbyax Capsules 1788
Zyprexa Tablets 1798
Zyprexa IntraMuscular 1798
Zyprexa ZYDIS Orally Disintegrating Tablets 1798

Orphenadrine Citrate (Morphine may enhance the neuromuscular blocking action of skeletal muscle relaxants and produce an increased degree of respiratory depression). Products include:
Norflex Injection 1824

Oxazepam (Co-administration increases the risk of respiratory depression, hypotension, profound sedation, or coma).
No products indexed under this heading.

Oxycodone Hydrochloride (Co-administration increases the risk of respiratory depression, hypotension, profound sedation, or coma). Products include:
Combunox Tablets 1183
OxyContin Tablets 2699
OxyFast Oral Concentrate Solution 2704
OxyIR Capsules 2704
Percocet Tablets 1114
Percodan Tablets 1115

Pancuronium Bromide (Morphine may enhance the neuromuscular blocking action of skeletal muscle relaxants and produce an increased degree of respiratory depression).
No products indexed under this heading.

Pargyline Hydrochloride (MAO inhibitors markedly potentiate the action of morphine; concurrent and/or sequential use should be avoided).
No products indexed under this heading.

Pentazocine Hydrochloride (Mixed agonist/antagonist analgesics may reduce the analgesic effect and/or may precipitate withdrawal symptoms; mixed agonist/antagonist analgesics should NOT be administered to patients who have received or are receiving a course of therapy with pure opioid agonist analgesic).
No products indexed under this heading.

Pentazocine Lactate (Mixed agonist/antagonist analgesics may reduce the analgesic effect and/or may precipitate withdrawal symptoms; mixed agonist/antagonist analgesics should NOT be administered to patients who have received or are receiving a course of therapy with pure opioid agonist analgesic).
No products indexed under this heading.

Pentobarbital Sodium (Co-administration increases the risk of respiratory depression, hypotension, profound sedation, or coma). Products include:
Nembutal Sodium Solution, USP 2484

Perphenazine (Co-administration increases the risk of respiratory depression, hypotension, profound sedation, or coma).
No products indexed under this heading.

Phenelzine Sulfate (MAO inhibitors markedly potentiate the action of morphine; concurrent and/or sequential use should be avoided).
No products indexed under this heading.

Phenobarbital (Co-administration increases the risk of respiratory depression, hypotension, profound sedation, or coma).
No products indexed under this heading.

Prazepam (Co-administration increases the risk of respiratory depression, hypotension, profound sedation, or coma).
No products indexed under this heading.

Procarbazine Hydrochloride (MAO inhibitors markedly potentiate the action of morphine; concurrent and/or sequential use should be avoided). Products include:
Matulane Capsules 3188

Prochlorperazine (Co-administration increases the risk of respiratory depression, hypotension, profound sedation, or coma).
No products indexed under this heading.

Promethazine Hydrochloride (Co-administration increases the risk of respiratory depression, hypotension, profound sedation, or coma). Products include:
Phenergan 3438

Propofol (Co-administration increases the risk of respiratory depression, hypotension, profound sedation, or coma). Products include:
Diprivan Injectable Emulsion 676

Propoxyphene Hydrochloride (Co-administration increases the risk of respiratory depression, hypotension, profound sedation, or coma).
No products indexed under this heading.

Propoxyphene Napsylate (Co-administration increases the risk of respiratory depression, hypotension, profound sedation, or coma). Products include:
Darvocet A 500 Tablets 3497

Quazepam (Co-administration increases the risk of respiratory depression, hypotension, profound sedation, or coma).
No products indexed under this heading.

Quetiapine Fumarate (Co-administration increases the risk of respiratory depression, hypotension, profound sedation, or coma). Products include:
Seroquel Tablets 691

Rapacuronium Bromide (Morphine may enhance the neuromuscular blocking action of skeletal muscle relaxants and produce an increased degree of respiratory depression).
No products indexed under this heading.

Remifentanil Hydrochloride (Co-administration increases the risk of respiratory depression, hypotension, profound sedation, or coma).
No products indexed under this heading.

Risperidone (Co-administration increases the risk of respiratory depression, hypotension, profound sedation, or coma). Products include:
Risperdal Consta Long-Acting Injection 1664
Risperdal M-Tab Orally Disintegrating Tablets 1658
Risperdal 1658

Rocuronium Bromide (Morphine may enhance the neuromuscular blocking action of skeletal muscle relaxants and produce an increased degree of respiratory depression). Products include:
Zemuron Injection 2363

Secobarbital Sodium (Co-administration increases the risk of respiratory depression, hypotension, profound sedation, or coma).
No products indexed under this heading.

Selegiline Hydrochloride (MAO inhibitors markedly potentiate the action of morphine; concurrent and/or sequential use should be avoided). Products include:
Eldepryl Capsules 3209

Sevoflurane (Co-administration increases the risk of respiratory depression, hypotension, profound sedation, or coma). Products include:
Ultane Liquid for Inhalation 526

Sodium Oxybate (Co-administration increases the risk of respiratory depression, hypotension, profound sedation, or coma).
No products indexed under this heading.

Succinylcholine Chloride (Morphine may enhance the neuromuscular blocking action of skeletal muscle relaxants and produce an increased degree of respiratory depression).
No products indexed under this heading.

Sufentanil Citrate (Co-administration increases the risk of respiratory depression, hypotension, profound sedation, or coma).
No products indexed under this heading.

Temazepam (Co-administration increases the risk of respiratory depression, hypotension, profound sedation, or coma).
No products indexed under this heading.

Thiamylal Sodium (Co-administration increases the risk of respiratory depression, hypotension, profound sedation, or coma).
No products indexed under this heading.

Thioridazine Hydrochloride (Co-administration increases the risk of respiratory depression, hypotension, profound sedation, or coma). Products include:
Thioridazine Hydrochloride Tablets 2122

Thiothixene (Co-administration increases the risk of respiratory depression, hypotension, profound sedation, or coma). Products include:
Thiothixene Capsules 2124

Tranylcypromine Sulfate (MAO inhibitors markedly potentiate the action of morphine; concurrent and/or sequential use should be avoided). Products include:
Parnate Tablets 1499

Triazolam (Co-administration increases the risk of respiratory depression, hypotension, profound sedation, or coma).
No products indexed under this heading.

Trifluoperazine Hydrochloride (Co-administration increases the risk of respiratory depression, hypotension, profound sedation, or coma).
No products indexed under this heading.

Vecuronium Bromide (Morphine may enhance the neuromuscular blocking action of skeletal muscle relaxants and produce an increased degree of respiratory depression).
No products indexed under this heading.

Zaleplon (Co-administration increases the risk of respiratory depression, hypotension, profound sedation, or coma). Products include:
Sonata Capsules 1686

Ziprasidone Hydrochloride (Co-administration increases the risk of respiratory depression, hypotension, profound sedation, or coma). Products include:
Geodon Capsules 2514

Zolpidem Tartrate (Co-administration increases the risk of respiratory depression, hypotension, profound sedation, or coma). Products include:
Ambien Tablets 2867

Food Interactions

Alcohol (Concurrent use increases the risk of respiratory depression, hypotension, profound sedation, or coma).

AVITA CREAM

(Tretinoin) 2136

May interact with:

Concomitant Topical Acne Therapy (Effect not specified).
No products indexed under this heading.

Resorcinol (Caution should be exercised).
No products indexed under this heading.

Salicylic Acid (Caution should be exercised).
No products indexed under this heading.

Sulfur (Caution should be exercised). Products include:
Avar Cleanser 3189
Avar Gel 3189
Avar Green 3189
Avar-e Emollient Cream 3189
Avar-e Green Cream 3189
Plexion 1863
Rosac Cream with Sunscreens 3216
Zeel Solution 1639
Zicam Allergy Relief Nasal Pump ....

Topical Medications (Effect not specified).

AVITA GEL

(Tretinoin) 2138
See Avita Cream

AVODART SOFT GELATIN CAPSULES

(Dutasteride) 1353

May interact with cytochrome p450 3a4 inhibitors (selected) and certain other agents. Compounds in these categories include:

Acetazolamide (Blood concentrations of dutasteride may increase in the presence of CYP3A4 inhibitors).
No products indexed under this heading.

Amiodarone Hydrochloride (Blood concentrations of dutasteride may increase in the presence of CYP3A4 inhibitors). Products include:
Pacerone Tablets 3337

Amprenavir (Blood concentrations of dutasteride may increase in the presence of CYP3A4 inhibitors). Products include:
Agenerase Capsules 1299
Agenerase Oral Solution 1304

Anastrozole (Blood concentrations of dutasteride may increase in the presence of CYP3A4 inhibitors). Products include:
Arimidex Tablets 665

Aprepitant (Blood concentrations of dutasteride may increase in the presence of CYP3A4 inhibitors). Products include:
Emend Capsules 1944

Cimetidine (Blood concentrations of dutasteride may increase in the presence of CYP3A4 inhibitors). Products include:
Tagamet HB 200 Tablets 637
Tagamet Tablets 1547

Cimetidine Hydrochloride (Blood concentrations of dutasteride may increase in the presence of CYP3A4 inhibitors).
No products indexed under this heading.

Ciprofloxacin (Blood concentrations of dutasteride may increase in the presence of CYP3A4 inhibitors). Products include:
Cipro I.V. 2998
Cipro I.V. Pharmacy Bulk Package 3509
Cipro Oral Suspension 2991
Cipro XR Tablets 3004
Ciprodex Otic Suspension 555

Clarithromycin (Blood concentrations of dutasteride may increase in the presence of CYP3A4 inhibitors). Products include:
Biaxin/Biaxin XL 402
PREVPAC 3281

Clotrimazole (Blood concentrations of dutasteride may increase in the presence of CYP3A4 inhibitors). Products include:
Lotrimin 3053
Lotrisone 3054

Cyclosporine (Blood concentrations of dutasteride may increase in the presence of CYP3A4 inhibitors). Products include:
Gengraf Capsules 458
Neoral Soft Gelatin Capsules 2247
Neoral Oral Solution 2247
Restasis Ophthalmic Emulsion 570
Sandimmune 2259

Dalfopristin (Blood concentrations of dutasteride may increase in the presence of CYP3A4 inhibitors). Products include:
Synercid I.V. 1690

Danazol (Blood concentrations of dutasteride may increase in the presence of CYP3A4 inhibitors).
No products indexed under this heading.

Delavirdine Mesylate (Blood concentrations of dutasteride may increase in the presence of CYP3A4 inhibitors). Products include:
Rescriptor Tablets 2535

Diltiazem Hydrochloride (Blood concentrations of dutasteride may increase in the presence of CYP3A4 inhibitors). Products include:
Cardizem LA Extended Release Tablets 1699
Tiazac Capsules 1204

Diltiazem Maleate (Blood concentrations of dutasteride may increase in the presence of CYP3A4 inhibitors).
No products indexed under this heading.

Efavirenz (Blood concentrations of dutasteride may increase in the presence of CYP3A4 inhibitors). Products include:
Sustiva Capsules 957

Erythromycin (Blood concentrations of dutasteride may increase in the presence of CYP3A4 inhibitors). Products include:
Erygel Topical Gel 2096
Ery-Tab Tablets 447
Erythromycin Base Filmtab Tablets 454
Erythromycin Delayed-Release Capsules, USP 456
PCE Dispertab Tablets 510

Erythromycin Estolate (Blood concentrations of dutasteride may increase in the presence of CYP3A4 inhibitors).
No products indexed under this heading.

Erythromycin Ethylsuccinate (Blood concentrations of dutasteride may increase in the presence of CYP3A4 inhibitors). Products include:
E.E.S. 449
EryPed 445

Erythromycin Gluceptate (Blood concentrations of dutasteride may increase in the presence of CYP3A4 inhibitors).
No products indexed under this heading.

Erythromycin Lactobionate (Blood concentrations of dutasteride may increase in the presence of CYP3A4 inhibitors).
No products indexed under this heading.

Erythromycin Stearate (Blood concentrations of dutasteride may increase in the presence of CYP3A4 inhibitors). Products include:
Erythrocin Stearate Filmtab Tablets 452

Esomeprazole Magnesium (Blood concentrations of dutasteride may increase in the presence of CYP3A4 inhibitors). Products include:
Nexium Delayed-Release Capsules 645

Fluconazole (Blood concentrations of dutasteride may increase in the presence of CYP3A4 inhibitors).
No products indexed under this heading.

Fluoxetine Hydrochloride (Blood concentrations of dutasteride may increase in the presence of CYP3A4 inhibitors). Products include:
Prozac Pulvules and Liquid 1771
Symbyax Capsules 1788

Fluvoxamine Maleate (Blood concentrations of dutasteride may increase in the presence of CYP3A4 inhibitors).
No products indexed under this heading.

Fosamprenavir Calcium (Blood concentrations of dutasteride may increase in the presence of CYP3A4 inhibitors). Products include:
Lexiva Tablets 1473

Indinavir Sulfate (Blood concentrations of dutasteride may increase in the presence of CYP3A4 inhibitors). Products include:
Crixivan Capsules 1918

Isoniazid (Blood concentrations of dutasteride may increase in the presence of CYP3A4 inhibitors).
No products indexed under this heading.

Itraconazole (Blood concentrations of dutasteride may increase in the presence of CYP3A4 inhibitors).
No products indexed under this heading.

Ketoconazole (Blood concentrations of dutasteride may increase in the presence of CYP3A4 inhibitors). Products include:
Nizoral A-D Shampoo, 1% 1839
Nizoral 2% Shampoo 1838

Lopinavir (Blood concentrations of dutasteride may increase in the presence of CYP3A4 inhibitors). Products include:
Kaletra 474

Loratadine (Blood concentrations of dutasteride may increase in the presence of CYP3A4 inhibitors). Products include:
Alavert Allergy & Sinus D-12 Hour Tablets 743
Alavert 743
Children's Claritin 24 Hour Non-Drowsy Allergy Syrup 732
Claritin Non-Drowsy 24 Hour Tablets 731
Non-Drowsy Claritin Hives Relief Tablets 733
Claritin Reditabs 24 Hour Non-Drowsy Tablets 732
Claritin-D Non-Drowsy 12 Hour Tablets 731
Claritin-D Non-Drowsy 24 Hour Tablets 731
Children's Dimetapp ND Non-Drowsy Allergy Syrup 746
Triaminic Allerchews 684

Metronidazole (Blood concentrations of dutasteride may increase in the presence of CYP3A4 inhibitors). Products include:
Metrogel 1% 1212
MetroGel-Vaginal Gel 1822
Noritate Cream, 1% 1051

Metronidazole Benzoate (Blood concentrations of dutasteride may increase in the presence of CYP3A4 inhibitors).
No products indexed under this heading.

Metronidazole Hydrochloride (Blood concentrations of dutasteride may increase in the presence of CYP3A4 inhibitors).
No products indexed under this heading.

Miconazole (Blood concentrations of dutasteride may increase in the presence of CYP3A4 inhibitors).
No products indexed under this heading.

Miconazole Nitrate (Blood concentrations of dutasteride may increase in the presence of CYP3A4 inhibitors). Products include:
Desenex 674
Desenex Jock Itch Spray Powder 674

Nefazodone Hydrochloride (Blood concentrations of dutasteride may increase in the presence of CYP3A4 inhibitors).
No products indexed under this heading.

Nelfinavir Mesylate (Blood concentrations of dutasteride may increase in the presence of CYP3A4 inhibitors). Products include:
Viracept 2556

Nevirapine (Blood concentrations of dutasteride may increase in the presence of CYP3A4 inhibitors). Products include:
Viramune Oral Suspension 903
Viramune Tablets 903

Niacinamide (Blood concentrations of dutasteride may increase in the presence of CYP3A4 inhibitors).
No products indexed under this heading.

Nicotinamide (Blood concentrations of dutasteride may increase in the presence of CYP3A4 inhibitors). Products include:
Nicomide Tablets 3190

Nifedipine (Blood concentrations of dutasteride may increase in the presence of CYP3A4 inhibitors). Products include:
Adalat CC Tablets 2978

Norfloxacin (Blood concentrations of dutasteride may increase in the presence of CYP3A4 inhibitors). Products include:
Noroxin Tablets 2009

Omeprazole (Blood concentrations of dutasteride may increase in the presence of CYP3A4 inhibitors). Products include:
Zegerid Powder for Oral Solution 2972

Paroxetine Hydrochloride (Blood concentrations of dutasteride may increase in the presence of CYP3A4 inhibitors). Products include:
Paxil CR Controlled-Release Tablets 1509
Paxil 1501

Propoxyphene Hydrochloride (Blood concentrations of dutasteride may increase in the presence of CYP3A4 inhibitors).
No products indexed under this heading.

IMPORTANT NOTE: Always consult each drug listing in the patient's regimen for possible interactions.

Propoxyphene Napsylate (Blood concentrations of dutasteride may increase in the presence of CYP3A4 inhibitors). Products include:
Darvocet A 500 Tablets 3497

Quinidine (Blood concentrations of dutasteride may increase in the presence of CYP3A4 inhibitors).
No products indexed under this heading.

Quinidine Hydrochloride (Blood concentrations of dutasteride may increase in the presence of CYP3A4 inhibitors).
No products indexed under this heading.

Quinidine Polygalacturonate (Blood concentrations of dutasteride may increase in the presence of CYP3A4 inhibitors).
No products indexed under this heading.

Quinidine Sulfate (Blood concentrations of dutasteride may increase in the presence of CYP3A4 inhibitors).
No products indexed under this heading.

Quinine (Blood concentrations of dutasteride may increase in the presence of CYP3A4 inhibitors).
No products indexed under this heading.

Quinine Sulfate (Blood concentrations of dutasteride may increase in the presence of CYP3A4 inhibitors).
No products indexed under this heading.

Quinupristin (Blood concentrations of dutasteride may increase in the presence of CYP3A4 inhibitors). Products include:
Synercid I.V. 1690

Ranitidine Bismuth Citrate (Blood concentrations of dutasteride may increase in the presence of CYP3A4 inhibitors).
No products indexed under this heading.

Ranitidine Hydrochloride (Blood concentrations of dutasteride may increase in the presence of CYP3A4 inhibitors). Products include:
Zantac 1597
Zantac Injection 1593
Zantac 75 Tablets .... ▣715
Zantac 150 Maximum Strength Tablets .... ▣715
Zantac Injection Pharmacy Bulk Package 1595

Ritonavir (Blood concentrations of dutasteride may increase in the presence of CYP3A4 inhibitors). Products include:
Kaletra 474
Norvir 499

Saquinavir (Blood concentrations of dutasteride may increase in the presence of CYP3A4 inhibitors).
No products indexed under this heading.

Saquinavir Mesylate (Blood concentrations of dutasteride may increase in the presence of CYP3A4 inhibitors). Products include:
Invirase 2776

Sertraline Hydrochloride (Blood concentrations of dutasteride may increase in the presence of CYP3A4 inhibitors). Products include:
Zoloft 2581

Telithromycin (Blood concentrations of dutasteride may increase in the presence of CYP3A4 inhibitors). Products include:
Ketek Tablets 2920

Troglitazone (Blood concentrations of dutasteride may increase in the presence of CYP3A4 inhibitors).
No products indexed under this heading.

Troleandomycin (Blood concentrations of dutasteride may increase in the presence of CYP3A4 inhibitors).
No products indexed under this heading.

Valproate Sodium (Blood concentrations of dutasteride may increase in the presence of CYP3A4 inhibitors). Products include:
Depacon Injection 412

Verapamil Hydrochloride (Blood concentrations of dutasteride may increase in the presence of CYP3A4 inhibitors). Products include:
Covera-HS Tablets 3135
Tarka Tablets 519
Verelan PM Capsules 3120

Voriconazole (Blood concentrations of dutasteride may increase in the presence of CYP3A4 inhibitors). Products include:
VFEND I.V. 2543
VFEND Oral Suspension 2543
VFEND Tablets 2543

Zafirlukast (Blood concentrations of dutasteride may increase in the presence of CYP3A4 inhibitors). Products include:
Accolate Tablets 663

Zileuton (Blood concentrations of dutasteride may increase in the presence of CYP3A4 inhibitors).
No products indexed under this heading.

Food Interactions

Grapefruit (Blood concentrations of dutasteride may increase in the presence of CYP3A4 inhibitors).

Grapefruit Juice (Blood concentrations of dutasteride may increase in the presence of CYP3A4 inhibitors).

AVONEX

(Interferon Beta-1a) 839
None cited in PDR database.

AWARENESS CLEAR CAPSULES

(Herbals, Multiple) .... ▣759
None cited in PDR database.

AXERT TABLETS

(Almotriptan Malate) 2430
May interact with 5HT1-receptor agonists, ergot-containing drugs, erythromycin, selective serotonin reuptake inhibitors, and certain other agents. Compounds in these categories include:

Citalopram Hydrobromide (Co-administration of SSRI and 5HT1 agonist have been rarely reported to cause weakness, hyperreflexia, and incoordination). Products include:
Celexa 1177

Dihydroergotamine Mesylate (Ergot-containing drugs have been reported to cause prolonged vasospastic reactions; because there is a theoretical basis that these effects may be additive, use of ergot-type agents and almotriptan within 24 hours is contraindicated). Products include:
Migranal Nasal Spray 3350

Ergonovine Maleate (Ergot-containing drugs have been reported to cause prolonged vasospastic reactions; because there is a theoretical basis that these effects may be additive, use of ergot-type agents and almotriptan within 24 hours is contraindicated).
No products indexed under this heading.

Ergotamine Tartrate (Ergot-containing drugs have been reported to cause prolonged vasospastic reactions; because there is a theoretical basis that these effects may be additive, use of ergot-type agents and almotriptan within 24 hours is contraindicated).
No products indexed under this heading.

Erythromycin (Co-administration with other potent inhibitors of CYP3A4 inhibitors, such as erythromycin, may result in increased exposures to almotriptan). Products include:
Erygel Topical Gel 2096
Ery-Tab Tablets 447
Erythromycin Base Filmtab Tablets 454
Erythromycin Delayed-Release Capsules, USP 456
PCE Dispertab Tablets 510

Erythromycin Estolate (Co-administration with other potent inhibitors of CYP3A4 inhibitors, such as erythromycin, may result in increased exposures to almotriptan).
No products indexed under this heading.

Erythromycin Ethylsuccinate (Co-administration with other potent inhibitors of CYP3A4 inhibitors, such as erythromycin, may result in increased exposures to almotriptan). Products include:
E.E.S. 449
EryPed 445

Erythromycin Gluceptate (Co-administration with other potent inhibitors of CYP3A4 inhibitors, such as erythromycin, may result in increased exposures to almotriptan).
No products indexed under this heading.

Erythromycin Stearate (Co-administration with other potent inhibitors of CYP3A4 inhibitors, such as erythromycin, may result in increased exposures to almotriptan). Products include:
Erythrocin Stearate Filmtab Tablets 452

Fluoxetine Hydrochloride (Co-administration has resulted in an increase in maximal concentrations of almotriptan by 18%; this difference is not clinically significant; co-administration of SSRI and 5HT1 agonist have been rarely reported to cause weakness, hyperreflexia, and incoordination). Products include:
Prozac Pulvules and Liquid 1771
Symbyax Capsules 1788

Fluvoxamine Maleate (Co-administration of SSRI and 5HT1 agonist have been rarely reported to cause weakness, hyperreflexia, and incoordination).
No products indexed under this heading.

Itraconazole (Co-administration with other potent inhibitors of CYP3A4 inhibitors, such as itraconazole, may result in increased exposures to almotriptan).
No products indexed under this heading.

Ketoconazole (Co-administration has resulted in an approximately 60% increase in the AUC and maximal plasma concentrations of almotriptan). Products include:
Nizoral A-D Shampoo, 1% 1839
Nizoral 2% Shampoo 1838

Methylergonovine Maleate (Ergot-containing drugs have been reported to cause prolonged vasospastic reactions; because there is a theoretical basis that these effects may be additive, use of ergot-type agents and almotriptan within 24 hours is contraindicated).
No products indexed under this heading.

Methysergide Maleate (Ergot-containing drugs have been reported to cause prolonged vasospastic reactions; because there is a theoretical basis that these effects may be additive, use of ergot-type agents and almotriptan within 24 hours is contraindicated).
No products indexed under this heading.

Moclobemide (Co-administration has resulted in a 27% decrease in almotriptan clearance).
No products indexed under this heading.

Naratriptan Hydrochloride (Co-administration with other 5HT1 agonists within 24 hours of treatment with almotriptan is contraindicated). Products include:
Amerge Tablets 1312

Paroxetine Hydrochloride (Co-administration of SSRI and 5HT1 agonist have been rarely reported to cause weakness, hyperreflexia, and incoordination). Products include:
Paxil CR Controlled-Release Tablets 1509
Paxil 1501

Ritonavir (Co-administration with other potent inhibitors of CYP3A4 inhibitors, such as ritonavir, may result in increased exposures to almotriptan). Products include:
Kaletra 474
Norvir 499

Rizatriptan Benzoate (Co-administration with other 5HT1 agonists within 24 hours of treatment with almotriptan is contraindicated). Products include:
Maxalt Tablets 1983
Maxalt-MLT Orally Disintegrating Tablets 1983

Sertraline Hydrochloride (Co-administration of SSRI and 5HT1 agonist have been rarely reported to cause weakness, hyperreflexia, and incoordination). Products include:
Zoloft 2581

Sumatriptan (Co-administration with other 5HT1 agonists within 24 hours of treatment with almotriptan is contraindicated). Products include:
Imitrex Nasal Spray 1435

Sumatriptan Succinate (Co-administration with other 5HT1 agonists within 24 hours of treatment with almotriptan is contraindicated). Products include:
Imitrex Injection 1431
Imitrex Tablets 1440

Verapamil Hydrochloride (Co-administration has resulted in a 20% increase in AUC and a 24% increase in maximal plasma concentrations of almotriptan; neither of these changes is clinically significant). Products include:

Covera-HS Tablets 3135
Tarka Tablets 519
Verelan PM Capsules 3120

Zolmitriptan (Co-administration with other 5HT1 agonists within 24 hours of treatment with almotriptan is contraindicated). Products include:

Zomig Nasal Spray 718
Zomig Tablets 714
Zomig-ZMT Tablets 714

AXID ORAL SOLUTION

(Nizatidine) 913
May interact with:

Aspirin (Increased serum salicylate levels when nizatidine is given concurrently with very high doses (3,900 mg) of aspirin). Products include:

Aggrenox Capsules 855
Bayer, Aspirin Regimen 606
Bayer Aspirin Tablets 3515
BC Powder 612
BC Allergy Sinus Cold Powder 612
Arthritis Strength BC Powder 612
BC Sinus Cold Powder 612
Ecotrin Enteric Coated Aspirin Low, Regular and Maximum Strength Tablets 1627
Goody's Body Pain Formula Powder 621
Goody's Extra Strength Headache Powder 621
Goody's Extra Strength Pain Relief Tablets 621
Percodan Tablets 1115
St. Joseph 81 mg Aspirin Chewable and Enteric Coated Tablets 1841

AYGESTIN TABLETS

(Norethindrone Acetate) 1062
None cited in PDR database.

AZASAN TABLETS

(Azathioprine) 2844
May interact with ACE inhibitors, alkylating agents, drugs with myeloproliferative effects, and certain other agents. Compounds in these categories include:

Allopurinol (The principal pathway for detoxification of azathioprine is inhibited by allopurinol; patients on concurrent therapy should have a dose reduction of azathioprine by one-third to one-fourth the usual dose).

No products indexed under this heading.

Benazepril Hydrochloride (Co-administration has been reported to induce severe leukopenia). Products include:

Lotensin Tablets 2232
Lotensin HCT Tablets 2235
Lotrel Capsules 2238

Betamethasone Acetate (Drugs which may affect leukocyte production may lead to exaggerated leukopenia, especially in renal transplant recipients).

No products indexed under this heading.

Betamethasone Sodium Phosphate (Drugs which may affect leukocyte production may lead to exaggerated leukopenia, especially in renal transplant recipients).

No products indexed under this heading.

Busulfan (Patients with rheumatoid arthritis previously treated with alkylating agents may have a prohibitive risk of neoplasia if treated with azathioprine). Products include:

I.V. Busulfex 1125
Myleran Tablets 1492

Captopril (Co-administration has been reported to induce severe leukopenia). Products include:

Captopril Tablets 2114

Carmustine (BCNU) (Patients with rheumatoid arthritis previously treated with alkylating agents may have a prohibitive risk of neoplasia if treated with azathioprine).

No products indexed under this heading.

Chlorambucil (Patients with rheumatoid arthritis previously treated with alkylating agents may have a prohibitive risk of neoplasia if treated with azathioprine). Products include:

Leukeran Tablets 1472

Cortisone Acetate (Drugs which may affect leukocyte production may lead to exaggerated leukopenia, especially in renal transplant recipients).

No products indexed under this heading.

Cyclophosphamide (Patients with rheumatoid arthritis previously treated with alkylating agents may have a prohibitive risk of neoplasia if treated with azathioprine).

No products indexed under this heading.

Dacarbazine (Patients with rheumatoid arthritis previously treated with alkylating agents may have a prohibitive risk of neoplasia if treated with azathioprine).

No products indexed under this heading.

Dexamethasone (Drugs which may affect leukocyte production may lead to exaggerated leukopenia, especially in renal transplant recipients). Products include:

Ciprodex Otic Suspension 555
Decadron Tablets 1929
TobraDex Ophthalmic Ointment 558
TobraDex Ophthalmic Suspension ... 558

Dexamethasone Acetate (Drugs which may affect leukocyte production may lead to exaggerated leukopenia, especially in renal transplant recipients).

No products indexed under this heading.

Dexamethasone Sodium Phosphate (Drugs which may affect leukocyte production may lead to exaggerated leukopenia, especially in renal transplant recipients). Products include:

Decadron Phosphate Injection 1931

Enalapril Maleate (Co-administration has been reported to induce severe leukopenia). Products include:

Vaseretic Tablets 2073
Vasotec I.V. Injection 2076

Enalaprilat (Co-administration has been reported to induce severe leukopenia).

No products indexed under this heading.

Fosinopril Sodium (Co-administration has been reported to induce severe leukopenia).

No products indexed under this heading.

Hydrocortisone (Drugs which may affect leukocyte production may lead to exaggerated leukopenia, especially in renal transplant recipients). Products include:

Cortizone•5 Ointment 699
Cortizone•10 Creme 699
Cortizone•10 Ointment 699
Cortizone•10 Plus Creme 700
Cortizone•10 Maximum Strength Quick Shot Spray 700
Hydrocortone Tablets 1963
Preparation H Hydrocortisone Cream 748

Hydrocortisone Acetate (Drugs which may affect leukocyte production may lead to exaggerated leukopenia, especially in renal transplant recipients). Products include:

Analpram-HC 1136
Pramosone 1139
ProctoFoam-HC 3113
Tucks Anti-Itch Ointment 712
U-cort 1% Cream 3289

Hydrocortisone Sodium Phosphate (Drugs which may affect leukocyte production may lead to exaggerated leukopenia, especially in renal transplant recipients).

No products indexed under this heading.

Hydrocortisone Sodium Succinate (Drugs which may affect leukocyte production may lead to exaggerated leukopenia, especially in renal transplant recipients).

No products indexed under this heading.

Lisinopril (Co-administration has been reported to induce severe leukopenia). Products include:

Prinivil Tablets 2029
Prinzide Tablets 2033
Zestoretic Tablets 701
Zestril Tablets 704

Lithium Carbonate (Drugs which may affect leukocyte production may lead to exaggerated leukopenia, especially in renal transplant recipients). Products include:

Eskalith 1406
Lithobid Tablets 1670

Lithium Citrate (Drugs which may affect leukocyte production may lead to exaggerated leukopenia, especially in renal transplant recipients).

No products indexed under this heading.

Lomustine (CCNU) (Patients with rheumatoid arthritis previously treated with alkylating agents may have a prohibitive risk of neoplasia if treated with azathioprine).

No products indexed under this heading.

Mechlorethamine Hydrochloride (Patients with rheumatoid arthritis previously treated with alkylating agents may have a prohibitive risk of neoplasia if treated with azathioprine). Products include:

Mustargen for Injection 2007

Melphalan (Patients with rheumatoid arthritis previously treated with alkylating agents may have a prohibitive risk of neoplasia if treated with azathioprine). Products include:

Alkeran Tablets 977

Methylprednisolone Acetate (Drugs which may affect leukocyte production may lead to exaggerated leukopenia, especially in renal transplant recipients). Products include:

Depo-Medrol Injectable Suspension 2615
Depo-Medrol Single-Dose Vial 2617

Methylprednisolone Sodium Succinate (Drugs which may affect leukocyte production may lead to exaggerated leukopenia, especially in renal transplant recipients).

No products indexed under this heading.

Moexipril Hydrochloride (Co-administration has been reported to induce severe leukopenia). Products include:

Uniretic Tablets 3114
Univasc Tablets 3118

Perindopril Erbumine (Co-administration has been reported to induce severe leukopenia). Products include:

Aceon Tablets (2 mg, 4 mg, 8 mg) 3191

Prednisolone Sodium Phosphate (Drugs which may affect leukocyte production may lead to exaggerated leukopenia, especially in renal transplant recipients). Products include:

Pediapred Oral Solution 3319

Prednisolone Tebutate (Drugs which may affect leukocyte production may lead to exaggerated leukopenia, especially in renal transplant recipients).

No products indexed under this heading.

Prednisone (Drugs which may affect leukocyte production may lead to exaggerated leukopenia, especially in renal transplant recipients).

No products indexed under this heading.

Quinapril Hydrochloride (Co-administration has been reported to induce severe leukopenia).

No products indexed under this heading.

Ramipril (Co-administration has been reported to induce severe leukopenia). Products include:

Altace Capsules 1673

Spirapril Hydrochloride (Co-administration has been reported to induce severe leukopenia).

No products indexed under this heading.

Sulfamethoxazole (Drugs which may affect leukocyte production, including co-trimoxazole, may lead to exaggerated leukopenia, especially in renal transplant recipients).

No products indexed under this heading.

Thiotepa (Patients with rheumatoid arthritis previously treated with alkylating agents may have a prohibitive risk of neoplasia if treated with azathioprine).

No products indexed under this heading.

Trandolapril (Co-administration has been reported to induce severe leukopenia). Products include:

Mavik Tablets 482
Tarka Tablets 519

Triamcinolone (Drugs which may affect leukocyte production may lead to exaggerated leukopenia, especially in renal transplant recipients).

No products indexed under this heading.

Triamcinolone Acetonide (Drugs which may affect leukocyte production may lead to exaggerated leukopenia, especially in renal transplant recipients). Products include:

Azmacort Inhalation Aerosol 1701
Nasacort HFA Inhalation Aerosol 2939
Nasacort AQ Nasal Spray 2937

Triamcinolone Diacetate (Drugs which may affect leukocyte production may lead to exaggerated leukopenia, especially in renal transplant recipients).

No products indexed under this heading.

Triamcinolone Hexacetonide (Drugs which may affect leukocyte production may lead to exaggerated leukopenia, especially in renal transplant recipients).
No products indexed under this heading.

Trimethoprim (Drugs which may affect leukocyte production, including co-trimoxazole, may lead to exaggerated leukopenia, especially in renal transplant recipients).
No products indexed under this heading.

Trimethoprim Hydrochloride (Drugs which may affect leukocyte production, including co-trimoxazole, may lead to exaggerated leukopenia, especially in renal transplant recipients).
No products indexed under this heading.

Trimethoprim Sulfate (Drugs which may affect leukocyte production, including co-trimoxazole, may lead to exaggerated leukopenia, especially in renal transplant recipients). Products include:
Polytrim Ophthalmic Solution **570**

AZMACORT INHALATION AEROSOL

(Triamcinolone Acetonide) **1701**
May interact with:

Prednisone (Potential for increased likelihood of HPA suppression).
No products indexed under this heading.

AZOPT OPHTHALMIC SUSPENSION

(Brinzolamide) **553**
May interact with carbonic anhydrase inhibitors and salicylates. Compounds in these categories include:

Acetazolamide (There is a potential for an additive effect on the known systemic effects of carbonic anhydrase inhibition in patients receiving an oral carbonic anhydrase inhibitor and brinzolamide; co-administration is not recommended).
No products indexed under this heading.

Aspirin (Co-administration with high dose salicylate and oral carbonic anhydrase inhibitor has resulted in rare instances of drug interactions). Products include:
Aggrenox Capsules **855**
Bayer, Aspirin Regimen .... ■ **606**
Bayer Aspirin Tablets **3515**
BC Powder .... ■ **612**
BC Allergy Sinus Cold Powder .... ■ **612**
Arthritis Strength BC Powder .... ■ **612**
BC Sinus Cold Powder .... ■ **612**
Ecotrin Enteric Coated Aspirin Low, Regular and Maximum Strength Tablets **1627**
Goody's Body Pain Formula Powder .... ■ **621**
Goody's Extra Strength Headache Powder .... ■ **621**
Goody's Extra Strength Pain Relief Tablets .... ■ **621**
Percodan Tablets **1115**
St. Joseph 81 mg Aspirin Chewable and Enteric Coated Tablets **1841**

Aspirin, Enteric Coated (Co-administration with high dose salicylate and oral carbonic anhydrase inhibitor has resulted in rare instances of drug interactions).
No products indexed under this heading.

Aspirin Buffered (Co-administration with high dose salicylate and oral carbonic anhydrase inhibitor has resulted in rare instances of drug interactions).
No products indexed under this heading.

Choline Magnesium Trisalicylate (Co-administration with high dose salicylate and oral carbonic anhydrase inhibitor has resulted in rare instances of drug interactions).
No products indexed under this heading.

Dichlorphenamide (There is a potential for an additive effect on the known systemic effects of carbonic anhydrase inhibition in patients receiving an oral carbonic anhydrase inhibitor and brinzolamide; co-administration is not recommended). Products include:
Daranide Tablets **1928**

Diflunisal (Co-administration with high dose salicylate and oral carbonic anhydrase inhibitor has resulted in rare instances of drug interactions). Products include:
Dolobid Tablets **1937**

Dorzolamide Hydrochloride (There is a potential for an additive effect on the known systemic effects of carbonic anhydrase inhibition in patients receiving an oral carbonic anhydrase inhibitor and brinzolamide; co-administration is not recommended). Products include:
Cosopt Sterile Ophthalmic Solution **1910**
Trusopt Sterile Ophthalmic Solution **2065**

Magnesium Salicylate (Co-administration with high dose salicylate and oral carbonic anhydrase inhibitor has resulted in rare instances of drug interactions).
No products indexed under this heading.

Methazolamide (There is a potential for an additive effect on the known systemic effects of carbonic anhydrase inhibition in patients receiving an oral carbonic anhydrase inhibitor and brinzolamide; co-administration is not recommended).
No products indexed under this heading.

Salsalate (Co-administration with high dose salicylate and oral carbonic anhydrase inhibitor has resulted in rare instances of drug interactions).
No products indexed under this heading.

BACTROBAN CREAM

(Mupirocin Calcium) **1356**
None cited in PDR database.

BACTROBAN NASAL

(Mupirocin Calcium) **1357**
None cited in PDR database.

BACTROBAN OINTMENT

(Mupirocin) **1358**
None cited in PDR database.

BALAMINE DM ORAL DROPS

(Carbinoxamine Maleate, Dextromethorphan Hydrobromide, Pseudoephedrine Hydrochloride) **739**
May interact with beta blockers, central nervous system depressants, monoamine oxidase inhibitors, veratrum alkaloids, and certain other agents. Compounds in these categories include:

Acebutolol Hydrochloride (Effects of sympathomimetics are increased with beta-blockers).
No products indexed under this heading.

Alfentanil Hydrochloride (Potential for additive CNS depression effects).
No products indexed under this heading.

Alprazolam (Potential for additive CNS depression effects). Products include:
Niravam Orally Disintegrating Tablets **3106**
Xanax XR Tablets **2655**

Aprobarbital (Potential for additive CNS depression effects).
No products indexed under this heading.

Atenolol (Effects of sympathomimetics are increased with beta-blockers). Products include:
Tenormin I.V. Injection **698**
Tenormin Tablets **695**

Betaxolol Hydrochloride (Effects of sympathomimetics are increased with beta-blockers). Products include:
Betoptic S Ophthalmic Suspension **554**

Bisoprolol Fumarate (Effects of sympathomimetics are increased with beta-blockers).
No products indexed under this heading.

Buprenorphine Hydrochloride (Potential for additive CNS depression effects). Products include:
Buprenex Injectable **2718**
Suboxone Tablets **2719**
Subutex Tablets **2719**

Buspirone Hydrochloride (Potential for additive CNS depression effects).
No products indexed under this heading.

Butabarbital (Potential for additive CNS depression effects).
No products indexed under this heading.

Butalbital (Potential for additive CNS depression effects). Products include:
Sedapap Tablets 50 mg/650 mg **2098**

Carteolol Hydrochloride (Effects of sympathomimetics are increased with beta-blockers). Products include:
Carteolol Hydrochloride Ophthalmic Solution USP, 1%....... ⊙ **246**

Chlordiazepoxide (Potential for additive CNS depression effects).
No products indexed under this heading.

Chlordiazepoxide Hydrochloride (Potential for additive CNS depression effects). Products include:
Librium Capsules **3349**

Chlorpromazine (Potential for additive CNS depression effects).
No products indexed under this heading.

Chlorpromazine Hydrochloride (Potential for additive CNS depression effects).
No products indexed under this heading.

Chlorprothixene (Potential for additive CNS depression effects).
No products indexed under this heading.

Chlorprothixene Hydrochloride (Potential for additive CNS depression effects).
No products indexed under this heading.

Chlorprothixene Lactate (Potential for additive CNS depression effects).
No products indexed under this heading.

Clorazepate Dipotassium (Potential for additive CNS depression effects). Products include:
Tranxene **2488**

Clozapine (Potential for additive CNS depression effects). Products include:
Clozapine Tablets **2141**
Clozaril Tablets **2174**
FazaClo Orally Disintegrating Tablets **547**

Codeine Phosphate (Potential for additive CNS depression effects). Products include:
Tylenol with Codeine **2461**

Codeine Sulfate (Cough suppressant action of dextromethorphan and narcotic antitussives are additive; potential for additive CNS depression effects).
No products indexed under this heading.

Cryptenamine Preparations (Sympathomimetics may reduce the effects of veratrum alkaloids).
No products indexed under this heading.

Desflurane (Potential for additive CNS depression effects). Products include:
Suprane Liquid for Inhalation **770**

Dezocine (Potential for additive CNS depression effects).
No products indexed under this heading.

Diazepam (Potential for additive CNS depression effects). Products include:
Diastat Rectal Delivery System **3344**
Valium Tablets **2822**

Droperidol (Potential for additive CNS depression effects).
No products indexed under this heading.

Enflurane (Potential for additive CNS depression effects).
No products indexed under this heading.

Esmolol Hydrochloride (Effects of sympathomimetics are increased with beta-blockers). Products include:
Brevibloc Concentrate **766**
Brevibloc Injection **766**
Brevibloc Double Strength Injection.. **766**
Brevibloc Premixed Injection **766**
Brevibloc Double Strength Premixed Injection **766**

Estazolam (Potential for additive CNS depression effects). Products include:
ProSom Tablets **512**

Ethanol (Potential for additive CNS depression effects).
No products indexed under this heading.

Ethchlorvynol (Potential for additive CNS depression effects).
No products indexed under this heading.

Ethinamate (Potential for additive CNS depression effects).
No products indexed under this heading.

Ethyl Alcohol (Potential for additive CNS depression effects).
No products indexed under this heading.

Fentanyl (Potential for additive CNS depression effects). Products include:
Duragesic Transdermal System 2448

Fentanyl Citrate (Potential for additive CNS depression effects). Products include:
Actiq 993

Fluphenazine Decanoate (Potential for additive CNS depression effects).
No products indexed under this heading.

Fluphenazine Enanthate (Potential for additive CNS depression effects).
No products indexed under this heading.

Fluphenazine Hydrochloride (Potential for additive CNS depression effects).
No products indexed under this heading.

Flurazepam Hydrochloride (Potential for additive CNS depression effects). Products include:
Dalmane Capsules 3343

Glutethimide (Potential for additive CNS depression effects).
No products indexed under this heading.

Haloperidol (Potential for additive CNS depression effects).
No products indexed under this heading.

Haloperidol Decanoate (Potential for additive CNS depression effects).
No products indexed under this heading.

Hydrocodone Bitartrate (Cough suppressant action of dextromethorphan and narcotic antitussives are additive; potential for additive CNS depression effects). Products include:
Hycodan 1104
Hycomine Compound Tablets 1105
Hycotuss Expectorant Syrup 1106
Lortab 3315
Lortab Elixir 3312
Vicodin Tablets 530
Vicodin ES Tablets 531
Vicodin HP Tablets 532
Vicoprofen Tablets 533
Zydone Tablets 1118

Hydrocodone Polistirex (Cough suppressant action of dextromethorphan and narcotic antitussives are additive; potential for additive CNS depression effects). Products include:
Tussionex Pennkinetic Extended-Release Suspension...... 3322

Hydromorphone Hydrochloride (Potential for additive CNS depression effects). Products include:
Dilaudid 439
Dilaudid Oral Liquid 443
Dilaudid Non-Sterile Powder 439
Dilaudid Rectal Suppositories 439
Dilaudid Tablets 439
Dilaudid Tablets - 8 mg 443
Dilaudid-HP 441

Hydroxyzine Hydrochloride (Potential for additive CNS depression effects).
No products indexed under this heading.

Isocarboxazid (MAO inhibitors increase the effects of sympathomimetic amines; concurrent and/or sequential use with MAO inhibitors is contraindicated; MAO inhibitors prolong and intensify the anticholinergic effects of antihistamines).
No products indexed under this heading.

Isoflurane (Potential for additive CNS depression effects).
No products indexed under this heading.

Ketamine Hydrochloride (Potential for additive CNS depression effects).
No products indexed under this heading.

Labetalol Hydrochloride (Effects of sympathomimetics are increased with beta-blockers).
No products indexed under this heading.

Levobunolol Hydrochloride (Effects of sympathomimetics are increased with beta-blockers). Products include:
Betagan Ophthalmic Solution, USP............ ⊙217

Levomethadyl Acetate Hydrochloride (Potential for additive CNS depression effects).
No products indexed under this heading.

Levorphanol Tartrate (Potential for additive CNS depression effects).
No products indexed under this heading.

Lorazepam (Potential for additive CNS depression effects).
No products indexed under this heading.

Loxapine Hydrochloride (Potential for additive CNS depression effects).
No products indexed under this heading.

Loxapine Succinate (Potential for additive CNS depression effects).
No products indexed under this heading.

Mecamylamine Hydrochloride (Sympathomimetics may reduce the effects of mecamylamine). Products include:
Inversine Tablets 3286

Meperidine Hydrochloride (Potential for additive CNS depression effects).
No products indexed under this heading.

Mephobarbital (Potential for additive CNS depression effects). Products include:
Mebaral Tablets, USP 2483

Meprobamate (Potential for additive CNS depression effects).
No products indexed under this heading.

Mesoridazine Besylate (Potential for additive CNS depression effects).
No products indexed under this heading.

Methadone Hydrochloride (Potential for additive CNS depression effects).
No products indexed under this heading.

Methohexital Sodium (Potential for additive CNS depression effects).
No products indexed under this heading.

Methotrimeprazine (Potential for additive CNS depression effects).
No products indexed under this heading.

Methoxyflurane (Potential for additive CNS depression effects).
No products indexed under this heading.

Methyldopa (Sympathomimetics may reduce the effects of methyldopa). Products include:
Aldoclor Tablets 1881
Aldoril Tablets 1884

Metipranolol Hydrochloride (Effects of sympathomimetics are increased with beta-blockers).
No products indexed under this heading.

Metoprolol Succinate (Effects of sympathomimetics are increased with beta-blockers). Products include:
Toprol-XL Tablets 660

Metoprolol Tartrate (Effects of sympathomimetics are increased with beta-blockers).
No products indexed under this heading.

Midazolam Hydrochloride (Potential for additive CNS depression effects).
No products indexed under this heading.

Moclobemide (MAO inhibitors increase the effects of sympathomimetic amines; concurrent and/or sequential use with MAO inhibitors is contraindicated; MAO inhibitors prolong and intensify the anticholinergic effects of antihistamines).
No products indexed under this heading.

Molindone Hydrochloride (Potential for additive CNS depression effects). Products include:
Moban Tablets 1108

Morphine Sulfate (Potential for additive CNS depression effects). Products include:
Avinza Capsules 1714
Kadian Capsules 572
MS Contin Tablets 2703

Nadolol (Effects of sympathomimetics are increased with beta-blockers). Products include:
Nadolol Tablets 2121

Olanzapine (Potential for additive CNS depression effects). Products include:
Symbyax Capsules 1788
Zyprexa Tablets 1798
Zyprexa IntraMuscular 1798
Zyprexa ZYDIS Orally Disintegrating Tablets............ 1798

Oxazepam (Potential for additive CNS depression effects).
No products indexed under this heading.

Oxycodone Hydrochloride (Potential for additive CNS depression effects). Products include:
Combunox Tablets 1183
OxyContin Tablets 2699
OxyFast Oral Concentrate Solution............ 2704
OxyIR Capsules 2704
Percocet Tablets 1114
Percodan Tablets 1115

Pargyline Hydrochloride (MAO inhibitors increase the effects of sympathomimetic amines; concurrent and/or sequential use with MAO inhibitors is contraindicated; MAO inhibitors prolong and intensify the anticholinergic effects of antihistamines).
No products indexed under this heading.

Penbutolol Sulfate (Effects of sympathomimetics are increased with beta-blockers).
No products indexed under this heading.

Pentobarbital Sodium (Potential for additive CNS depression effects). Products include:
Nembutal Sodium Solution, USP...... 2484

Perphenazine (Potential for additive CNS depression effects).
No products indexed under this heading.

Phenelzine Sulfate (MAO inhibitors increase the effects of sympathomimetic amines; concurrent and/or sequential use with MAO inhibitors is contraindicated; MAO inhibitors prolong and intensify the anticholinergic effects of antihistamines).
No products indexed under this heading.

Phenobarbital (Potential for additive CNS depression effects).
No products indexed under this heading.

Pindolol (Effects of sympathomimetics are increased with beta-blockers).
No products indexed under this heading.

Prazepam (Potential for additive CNS depression effects).
No products indexed under this heading.

Procarbazine Hydrochloride (MAO inhibitors increase the effects of sympathomimetic amines; concurrent and/or sequential use with MAO inhibitors is contraindicated; MAO inhibitors prolong and intensify the anticholinergic effects of antihistamines). Products include:
Matulane Capsules 3188

Prochlorperazine (Potential for additive CNS depression effects).
No products indexed under this heading.

Promethazine Hydrochloride (Potential for additive CNS depression effects). Products include:
Phenergan 3438

Propofol (Potential for additive CNS depression effects). Products include:
Diprivan Injectable Emulsion 676

Propoxyphene Hydrochloride (Potential for additive CNS depression effects).
No products indexed under this heading.

Propoxyphene Napsylate (Potential for additive CNS depression effects). Products include:
Darvocet A 500 Tablets 3497

Propranolol Hydrochloride (Effects of sympathomimetics are increased with beta-blockers). Products include:
Inderal LA Long-Acting Capsules 3421
InnoPran XL Capsules 2728

Quazepam (Potential for additive CNS depression effects).
No products indexed under this heading.

Quetiapine Fumarate (Potential for additive CNS depression effects). Products include:
Seroquel Tablets 691

Remifentanil Hydrochloride (Potential for additive CNS depression effects).
No products indexed under this heading.

Reserpine (Sympathomimetics may reduce the effects of reserpine).
No products indexed under this heading.

Risperidone (Potential for additive CNS depression effects). Products include:
Risperdal Consta Long-Acting Injection 1664
Risperdal M-Tab Orally Disintegrating Tablets 1658
Risperdal 1658

Secobarbital Sodium (Potential for additive CNS depression effects).
No products indexed under this heading.

Selegiline Hydrochloride (MAO inhibitors increase the effects of sympathomimetic amines; concurrent and/or sequential use with MAO inhibitors is contraindicated; MAO inhibitors prolong and intensify the anticholinergic effects of antihistamines). Products include:
Eldepryl Capsules 3209

Sevoflurane (Potential for additive CNS depression effects). Products include:
Ultane Liquid for Inhalation 526

Sodium Oxybate (Potential for additive CNS depression effects).
No products indexed under this heading.

Sotalol Hydrochloride (Effects of sympathomimetics are increased with beta-blockers).
No products indexed under this heading.

Sufentanil Citrate (Potential for additive CNS depression effects).
No products indexed under this heading.

Temazepam (Potential for additive CNS depression effects).
No products indexed under this heading.

Thiamylal Sodium (Potential for additive CNS depression effects).
No products indexed under this heading.

Thioridazine Hydrochloride (Potential for additive CNS depression effects). Products include:
Thioridazine Hydrochloride Tablets 2122

Thiothixene (Potential for additive CNS depression effects). Products include:
Thiothixene Capsules 2124

Timolol Hemihydrate (Effects of sympathomimetics are increased with beta-blockers). Products include:
Betimol Ophthalmic Solution 3371
Betimol Ophthalmic Solution .... ⊙283

Timolol Maleate (Effects of sympathomimetics are increased with beta-blockers). Products include:
Blocadren Tablets 1891
Cosopt Sterile Ophthalmic Solution 1910
Timolide Tablets 2056
Timoptic in Ocudose 2061
Timoptic Sterile Ophthalmic Solution 2058
Timoptic-XE Sterile Ophthalmic Gel Forming Solution 2062

Tranylcypromine Sulfate (MAO inhibitors increase the effects of sympathomimetic amines; concurrent and/or sequential use with MAO inhibitors is contraindicated; MAO inhibitors prolong and intensify the anticholinergic effects of antihistamines). Products include:
Parnate Tablets 1499

Triazolam (Potential for additive CNS depression effects).
No products indexed under this heading.

Trifluoperazine Hydrochloride (Potential for additive CNS depression effects).
No products indexed under this heading.

Zaleplon (Potential for additive CNS depression effects). Products include:
Sonata Capsules 1686

Ziprasidone Hydrochloride (Potential for additive CNS depression effects). Products include:
Geodon Capsules 2514

Zolpidem Tartrate (Potential for additive CNS depression effects). Products include:
Ambien Tablets 2867

Food Interactions

Alcohol (Antihistamines have additive effects with alcohol).

BALAMINE DM SYRUP

(Carbinoxamine Maleate, Dextromethorphan Hydrobromide, Pseudoephedrine Hydrochloride) 739
See Balamine DM Oral Drops

BARACLUDE ORAL SOLUTION

(Entecavir) 928
See Baraclude Tablets

BARACLUDE TABLETS

(Entecavir) 928

May interact with nephrotoxic agents. Compounds in these categories include:

Abacavir Sulfate (Since entecavir is primarily eliminated by the kidneys co-administration of entecavir with drugs that reduce renal function or compete for active tubular secretion may increase serum concentrations of either entecavir or the co-administered drug). Products include:
Epzicom Tablets 1402
Trizivir Tablets 1565
Ziagen 1600

Acyclovir (Since entecavir is primarily eliminated by the kidneys co-administration of entecavir with drugs that reduce renal function or compete for active tubular secretion may increase serum concentrations of either entecavir or the co-administered drug). Products include:
Zovirax 1616
Zovirax Cream 853
Zovirax Ointment 854

Acyclovir Sodium (Since entecavir is primarily eliminated by the kidneys co-administration of entecavir with drugs that reduce renal function or compete for active tubular secretion may increase serum concentrations of either entecavir or the co-administered drug). Products include:
Zovirax for Injection 1618

Alatrofloxacin Mesylate (Since entecavir is primarily eliminated by the kidneys co-administration of entecavir with drugs that reduce renal function or compete for active tubular secretion may increase serum concentrations of either entecavir or the co-administered drug).
No products indexed under this heading.

Aldesleukin (Since entecavir is primarily eliminated by the kidneys co-administration of entecavir with drugs that reduce renal function or compete for active tubular secretion may increase serum concentrations of either entecavir or the co-administered drug). Products include:
Proleukin for Injection 1007

Amikacin Sulfate (Since entecavir is primarily eliminated by the kidneys co-administration of entecavir with drugs that reduce renal function or compete for active tubular secretion may increase serum concentrations of either entecavir or the co-administered drug).
No products indexed under this heading.

Amoxicillin (Since entecavir is primarily eliminated by the kidneys co-administration of entecavir with drugs that reduce renal function or compete for active tubular secretion may increase serum concentrations of either entecavir or the co-administered drug). Products include:
Amoxil Capsules 1315
Amoxil Chewable Tablets 1315
Amoxil Pediatric Drops for Oral Suspension 1315
Amoxil Powder for Oral Suspension 1315
Amoxil Tablets 1315
Augmentin 1331
Augmentin Tablets 1334
Augmentin XR Extended-Release Tablets 1340
Augmentin ES-600 Powder for Oral Suspension 1337
PREVPAC 3281

Amoxicillin Trihydrate (Since entecavir is primarily eliminated by the kidneys co-administration of entecavir with drugs that reduce renal function or compete for active tubular secretion may increase serum concentrations of either entecavir or the co-administered drug).
No products indexed under this heading.

Amphotericin B (Since entecavir is primarily eliminated by the kidneys co-administration of entecavir with drugs that reduce renal function or compete for active tubular secretion may increase serum concentrations of either entecavir or the co-administered drug).
No products indexed under this heading.

Amphotericin B, liposomal (Since entecavir is primarily eliminated by the kidneys co-administration of entecavir with drugs that reduce renal function or compete for active tubular secretion may increase serum concentrations of either entecavir or the co-administered drug). Products include:
AmBisome for Injection 615

Amphotericin B Cholesteryl Sulfate (Since entecavir is primarily eliminated by the kidneys co-administration of entecavir with drugs that reduce renal function or compete for active tubular secretion may increase serum concentrations of either entecavir or the co-administered drug).
No products indexed under this heading.

Amphotericin B Lipid Complex (Since entecavir is primarily eliminated by the kidneys co-administration of entecavir with drugs that reduce renal function or compete for active tubular secretion may increase serum concentrations of either entecavir or the co-administered drug). Products include:
Abelcet Injection 1119

Ampicillin (Since entecavir is primarily eliminated by the kidneys co-administration of entecavir with drugs that reduce renal function or compete for active tubular secretion may increase serum concentrations of either entecavir or the co-administered drug).
No products indexed under this heading.

Ampicillin Sodium (Since entecavir is primarily eliminated by the kidneys co-administration of entecavir with drugs that reduce renal function or compete for active tubular secretion may increase serum concentrations of either entecavir or the co-administered drug).
No products indexed under this heading.

Ampicillin Trihydrate (Since entecavir is primarily eliminated by the kidneys co-administration of entecavir with drugs that reduce renal function or compete for active tubular secretion may increase serum concentrations of either entecavir or the co-administered drug).
No products indexed under this heading.

Amprenavir (Since entecavir is primarily eliminated by the kidneys co-administration of entecavir with drugs that reduce renal function or compete for active tubular secretion may increase serum concentrations of either entecavir or the co-administered drug). Products include:
Agenerase Capsules 1299
Agenerase Oral Solution 1304

Aspirin (Since entecavir is primarily eliminated by the kidneys co-administration of entecavir with drugs that reduce renal function or compete for active tubular secretion may increase serum concentrations of either entecavir or the co-administered drug). Products include:
Aggrenox Capsules 855
Bayer, Aspirin Regimen .... ■606
Bayer Aspirin Tablets 3515
BC Powder .... ■612
BC Allergy Sinus Cold Powder .... ■612
Arthritis Strength BC Powder .... ■612
BC Sinus Cold Powder .... ■612
Ecotrin Enteric Coated Aspirin Low, Regular and Maximum Strength Tablets 1627
Goody's Body Pain Formula Powder .... ■621
Goody's Extra Strength Headache Powder .... ■621
Goody's Extra Strength Pain Relief Tablets .... ■621
Percodan Tablets 1115

St. Joseph 81 mg Aspirin Chewable and Enteric Coated Tablets 1841

Atazanavir (Since entecavir is primarily eliminated by the kidneys co-administration of entecavir with drugs that reduce renal function or compete for active tubular secretion may increase serum concentrations of either entecavir or the co-administered drug).
No products indexed under this heading.

Atorvastatin Calcium (Since entecavir is primarily eliminated by the kidneys co-administration of entecavir with drugs that reduce renal function or compete for active tubular secretion may increase serum concentrations of either entecavir or the co-administered drug). Products include:
Caduet Tablets 2507
Lipitor Tablets 2495

Azithromycin Dihydrate (Since entecavir is primarily eliminated by the kidneys co-administration of entecavir with drugs that reduce renal function or compete for active tubular secretion may increase serum concentrations of either entecavir or the co-administered drug). Products include:
Zithromax 2568
Zithromax for IV Infusion 2573
Zithromax for Oral Suspension, 300 mg, 600 mg, 900 mg, 1200 mg 2561
Zithromax Tablets, 250 mg, 500 mg 2561
Zithromax Tri-Pak 2561
Zithromax Z-Pak 2568

Azlocillin Sodium (Since entecavir is primarily eliminated by the kidneys co-administration of entecavir with drugs that reduce renal function or compete for active tubular secretion may increase serum concentrations of either entecavir or the co-administered drug).
No products indexed under this heading.

Aztreonam (Since entecavir is primarily eliminated by the kidneys co-administration of entecavir with drugs that reduce renal function or compete for active tubular secretion may increase serum concentrations of either entecavir or the co-administered drug).
No products indexed under this heading.

Bacampicillin Hydrochloride (Since entecavir is primarily eliminated by the kidneys co-administration of entecavir with drugs that reduce renal function or compete for active tubular secretion may increase serum concentrations of either entecavir or the co-administered drug).
No products indexed under this heading.

Balsalazide Disodium (Since entecavir is primarily eliminated by the kidneys co-administration of entecavir with drugs that reduce renal function or compete for active tubular secretion may increase serum concentrations of either entecavir or the co-administered drug). Products include:
Colazal Capsules 2845

Benazepril Hydrochloride (Since entecavir is primarily eliminated by the kidneys co-administration of entecavir with drugs that reduce renal function or compete for active tubular secretion may increase serum concentrations of either entecavir or the co-administered drug). Products include:
Lotensin Tablets 2232
Lotensin HCT Tablets 2235
Lotrel Capsules 2238

Bendroflumethiazide (Since entecavir is primarily eliminated by the kidneys co-administration of entecavir with drugs that reduce renal function or compete for active tubular secretion may increase serum concentrations of either entecavir or the co-administered drug).
No products indexed under this heading.

Caffeine (Since entecavir is primarily eliminated by the kidneys co-administration of entecavir with drugs that reduce renal function or compete for active tubular secretion may increase serum concentrations of either entecavir or the co-administered drug). Products include:
Athena Hair System Shampoo 767
BC Powder 612
Arthritis Strength BC Powder 612
Goody's Extra Strength Headache Powder 621
Goody's Extra Strength Pain Relief Tablets 621
Hycomine Compound Tablets 1105
Spartan Hair System Shampoo 767
Vivarin 639

Captopril (Since entecavir is primarily eliminated by the kidneys co-administration of entecavir with drugs that reduce renal function or compete for active tubular secretion may increase serum concentrations of either entecavir or the co-administered drug). Products include:
Captopril Tablets 2114

Carbenicillin Disodium (Since entecavir is primarily eliminated by the kidneys co-administration of entecavir with drugs that reduce renal function or compete for active tubular secretion may increase serum concentrations of either entecavir or the co-administered drug).
No products indexed under this heading.

Carbenicillin Indanyl Sodium (Since entecavir is primarily eliminated by the kidneys co-administration of entecavir with drugs that reduce renal function or compete for active tubular secretion may increase serum concentrations of either entecavir or the co-administered drug).
No products indexed under this heading.

Carboplatin (Since entecavir is primarily eliminated by the kidneys co-administration of entecavir with drugs that reduce renal function or compete for active tubular secretion may increase serum concentrations of either entecavir or the co-administered drug).
No products indexed under this heading.

Carmustine (BCNU) (Since entecavir is primarily eliminated by the kidneys co-administration of entecavir with drugs that reduce renal function or compete for active tubular secretion may increase serum concentrations of either entecavir or the co-administered drug).
No products indexed under this heading.

Cefaclor (Since entecavir is primarily eliminated by the kidneys co-administration of entecavir with drugs that reduce renal function or compete for active tubular secretion may increase serum concentrations of either entecavir or the co-administered drug).
No products indexed under this heading.

Cefadroxil (Since entecavir is primarily eliminated by the kidneys co-administration of entecavir with drugs that reduce renal function or compete for active tubular secretion may increase serum concentrations of either entecavir or the co-administered drug).
No products indexed under this heading.

Cefamandole Nafate (Since entecavir is primarily eliminated by the kidneys co-administration of entecavir with drugs that reduce renal function or compete for active tubular secretion may increase serum concentrations of either entecavir or the co-administered drug).
No products indexed under this heading.

Cefazolin Sodium (Since entecavir is primarily eliminated by the kidneys co-administration of entecavir with drugs that reduce renal function or compete for active tubular secretion may increase serum concentrations of either entecavir or the co-administered drug). Products include:
Ancef for Injection 1318

Cefdinir (Since entecavir is primarily eliminated by the kidneys co-administration of entecavir with drugs that reduce renal function or compete for active tubular secretion may increase serum concentrations of either entecavir or the co-administered drug). Products include:
Omnicef Capsules 506
Omnicef for Oral Suspension 506

Cefepime Hydrochloride (Since entecavir is primarily eliminated by the kidneys co-administration of entecavir with drugs that reduce renal function or compete for active tubular secretion may increase serum concentrations of either entecavir or the co-administered drug). Products include:
Maxipime for Injection 1093

Cefixime (Since entecavir is primarily eliminated by the kidneys co-administration of entecavir with drugs that reduce renal function or compete for active tubular secretion may increase serum concentrations of either entecavir or the co-administered drug). Products include:
Suprax 1811

Cefmetazole Sodium (Since entecavir is primarily eliminated by the kidneys co-administration of entecavir with drugs that reduce renal function or compete for active tubular secretion may increase serum concentrations of either entecavir or the co-administered drug).
No products indexed under this heading.

Cefonicid Sodium (Since entecavir is primarily eliminated by the kidneys co-administration of entecavir with drugs that reduce renal function or compete for active tubular secretion may increase serum concentrations of either entecavir or the co-administered drug).
No products indexed under this heading.

Cefoperazone Sodium (Since entecavir is primarily eliminated by the kidneys co-administration of entecavir with drugs that reduce renal function or compete for active tubular secretion may increase serum concentrations of either entecavir or the co-administered drug).
No products indexed under this heading.

Ceforanide (Since entecavir is primarily eliminated by the kidneys co-administration of entecavir with drugs that reduce renal function or compete for active tubular secretion may increase serum concentrations of either entecavir or the co-administered drug).
No products indexed under this heading.

Cefotaxime Sodium (Since entecavir is primarily eliminated by the kidneys co-administration of entecavir with drugs that reduce renal function or compete for active tubular secretion may increase serum concentrations of either entecavir or the co-administered drug).
No products indexed under this heading.

Cefotetan (Since entecavir is primarily eliminated by the kidneys co-administration of entecavir with drugs that reduce renal function or compete for active tubular secretion may increase serum concentrations of either entecavir or the co-administered drug).
No products indexed under this heading.

Cefoxitin Sodium (Since entecavir is primarily eliminated by the kidneys co-administration of entecavir with drugs that reduce renal function or compete for active tubular secretion may increase serum concentrations of either entecavir or the co-administered drug). Products include:
Mefoxin for Injection 1987
Mefoxin Premixed Intravenous Solution 1990

Cefpodoxime Proxetil (Since entecavir is primarily eliminated by the kidneys co-administration of entecavir with drugs that reduce renal function or compete for active tubular secretion may increase serum concentrations of either entecavir or the co-administered drug). Products include:
Vantin Tablets and Oral Suspension 2650

Cefprozil (Since entecavir is primarily eliminated by the kidneys co-administration of entecavir with drugs that reduce renal function or compete for active tubular secretion may increase serum concentrations of either entecavir or the co-administered drug).
No products indexed under this heading.

Ceftazidime (Since entecavir is primarily eliminated by the kidneys co-administration of entecavir with drugs that reduce renal function or compete for active tubular secretion

ay increase serum concentrations f either entecavir or the co-dministered drug). Products iclude:

Fortaz for Injection 1422

eftizoxime Sodium (Since ente-avir is primarily eliminated by the idneys co-administration of ente-avir with drugs that reduce renal unction or compete for active tubu-ar secretion may increase serum concentrations of either entecavir or he co-administered drug).

No products indexed under this heading.

Ceftriaxone Sodium (Since ente-cavir is primarily eliminated by the kidneys co-administration of ente-cavir with drugs that reduce renal function or compete for active tubu-ar secretion may increase serum concentrations of either entecavir or the co-administered drug). Products include:

Rocephin Injectable Vials, ADD-Vantage, Galaxy, Bulk........... 2801

Cefuroxime Axetil (Since entecavir is primarily eliminated by the kidneys co-administration of entecavir with drugs that reduce renal function or compete for active tubular secretion may increase serum concentrations of either entecavir or the co-administered drug). Products include:

Ceftin 1369

Cefuroxime Sodium (Since ente-cavir is primarily eliminated by the kidneys co-administration of ente-cavir with drugs that reduce renal function or compete for active tubu-lar secretion may increase serum concentrations of either entecavir or the co-administered drug).

No products indexed under this heading.

Celecoxib (Since entecavir is pri-marily eliminated by the kidneys co-administration of entecavir with drugs that reduce renal function or compete for active tubular secretion may increase serum concentrations of either entecavir or the co-administered drug). Products include:

Celebrex Capsules 3130

Cephalexin (Since entecavir is pri-marily eliminated by the kidneys co-administration of entecavir with drugs that reduce renal function or compete for active tubular secretion may increase serum concentrations of either entecavir or the co-administered drug).

No products indexed under this heading.

Cephalothin Sodium (Since ente-cavir is primarily eliminated by the kidneys co-administration of ente-cavir with drugs that reduce renal function or compete for active tubu-lar secretion may increase serum concentrations of either entecavir or the co-administered drug).

No products indexed under this heading.

Cephapirin Sodium (Since ente-cavir is primarily eliminated by the kidneys co-administration of ente-cavir with drugs that reduce renal function or compete for active tubu-lar secretion may increase serum concentrations of either entecavir or the co-administered drug).

No products indexed under this heading.

Cephradine (Since entecavir is pri-marily eliminated by the kidneys co-administration of entecavir with drugs that reduce renal function or compete for active tubular secretion may increase serum concentrations of either entecavir or the co-administered drug).

No products indexed under this heading.

Cerivastatin Sodium (Since ente-cavir is primarily eliminated by the kidneys co-administration of ente-cavir with drugs that reduce renal function or compete for active tubu-lar secretion may increase serum concentrations of either entecavir or the co-administered drug).

No products indexed under this heading.

Chlorothiazide (Since entecavir is primarily eliminated by the kidneys co-administration of entecavir with drugs that reduce renal function or compete for active tubular secretion may increase serum concentrations of either entecavir or the co-administered drug). Products include:

Aldoclor Tablets 1881
Diuril Oral 1936

Chlorothiazide Sodium (Since entecavir is primarily eliminated by the kidneys co-administration of entecavir with drugs that reduce renal function or compete for active tubular secretion may increase ser-um concentrations of either ente-cavir or the co-administered drug). Products include:

Diuril Sodium Intravenous 1934

Chlorpropamide (Since entecavir is primarily eliminated by the kidneys co-administration of entecavir with drugs that reduce renal function or compete for active tubular secretion may increase serum concentrations of either entecavir or the co-administered drug).

No products indexed under this heading.

Cidofovir (Since entecavir is primar-ily eliminated by the kidneys co-administration of entecavir with drugs that reduce renal function or compete for active tubular secretion may increase serum concentrations of either entecavir or the co-administered drug).

No products indexed under this heading.

Cilastatin Sodium (Since entecavir is primarily eliminated by the kidneys co-administration of entecavir with drugs that reduce renal function or compete for active tubular secretion may increase serum concentrations of either entecavir or the co-administered drug). Products include:

Primaxin I.M. 2022
Primaxin I.V. 2024

Cimetidine (Since entecavir is pri-marily eliminated by the kidneys co-administration of entecavir with drugs that reduce renal function or compete for active tubular secretion may increase serum concentrations of either entecavir or the co-administered drug). Products include:

Tagamet HB 200 Tablets .... ▣ 637
Tagamet Tablets 1547

Cimetidine Hydrochloride (Since entecavir is primarily eliminated by the kidneys co-administration of entecavir with drugs that reduce renal function or compete for active tubular secretion may increase ser-um concentrations of either ente-cavir or the co-administered drug).

No products indexed under this heading.

Cisplatin (Since entecavir is primari-ly eliminated by the kidneys co-administration of entecavir with drugs that reduce renal function or compete for active tubular secretion may increase serum concentrations of either entecavir or the co-administered drug).

No products indexed under this heading.

Cladribine (Since entecavir is pri-marily eliminated by the kidneys co-administration of entecavir with drugs that reduce renal function or compete for active tubular secretion may increase serum concentrations of either entecavir or the co-administered drug). Products include:

Leustatin Injection 2368

Clozapine (Since entecavir is pri-marily eliminated by the kidneys co-administration of entecavir with drugs that reduce renal function or compete for active tubular secretion may increase serum concentrations of either entecavir or the co-administered drug). Products include:

Clozapine Tablets 2141
Clozaril Tablets 2174
FazaClo Orally Disintegrating Tablets 547

Colistimethate Sodium (Since entecavir is primarily eliminated by the kidneys co-administration of entecavir with drugs that reduce renal function or compete for active tubular secretion may increase ser-um concentrations of either ente-cavir or the co-administered drug).

No products indexed under this heading.

Colistin Sulfate (Since entecavir is primarily eliminated by the kidneys co-administration of entecavir with drugs that reduce renal function or compete for active tubular secretion may increase serum concentrations of either entecavir or the co-administered drug).

No products indexed under this heading.

Cyclophosphamide (Since ente-cavir is primarily eliminated by the kidneys co-administration of ente-cavir with drugs that reduce renal function or compete for active tubu-lar secretion may increase serum concentrations of either entecavir or the co-administered drug).

No products indexed under this heading.

Cyclosporine (Since entecavir is primarily eliminated by the kidneys co-administration of entecavir with drugs that reduce renal function or compete for active tubular secretion may increase serum concentrations of either entecavir or the co-administered drug). Products include:

Gengraf Capsules 458
Neoral Soft Gelatin Capsules 2247
Neoral Oral Solution 2247
Restasis Ophthalmic Emulsion 570
Sandimmune 2259

Cytarabine (Since entecavir is pri-marily eliminated by the kidneys co-administration of entecavir with drugs that reduce renal function or compete for active tubular secretion may increase serum concentrations of either entecavir or the co-administered drug).

No products indexed under this heading.

Cytarabine Liposome (Since ente-cavir is primarily eliminated by the kidneys co-administration of ente-cavir with drugs that reduce renal function or compete for active tubu-lar secretion may increase serum concentrations of either entecavir or the co-administered drug). Products include:

DepoCyt Injection 1121

Delavirdine Mesylate (Since ente-cavir is primarily eliminated by the kidneys co-administration of ente-cavir with drugs that reduce renal function or compete for active tubu-lar secretion may increase serum concentrations of either entecavir or the co-administered drug). Products include:

Rescriptor Tablets 2535

Diatrizoate Meglumine (Since entecavir is primarily eliminated by the kidneys co-administration of entecavir with drugs that reduce renal function or compete for active tubular secretion may increase ser-um concentrations of either ente-cavir or the co-administered drug).

No products indexed under this heading.

Diatrizoate Sodium (Since ente-cavir is primarily eliminated by the kidneys co-administration of ente-cavir with drugs that reduce renal function or compete for active tubu-lar secretion may increase serum concentrations of either entecavir or the co-administered drug).

No products indexed under this heading.

Diclofenac Potassium (Since ente-cavir is primarily eliminated by the kidneys co-administration of ente-cavir with drugs that reduce renal function or compete for active tubu-lar secretion may increase serum concentrations of either entecavir or the co-administered drug). Products include:

Cataflam Tablets 2173

Diclofenac Sodium (Since ente-cavir is primarily eliminated by the kidneys co-administration of ente-cavir with drugs that reduce renal function or compete for active tubu-lar secretion may increase serum concentrations of either entecavir or the co-administered drug). Products include:

Arthrotec Tablets 3126
Voltaren Ophthalmic Solution 2300
Voltaren Tablets 2298
Voltaren-XR Tablets 2301

Dicloxacillin Sodium (Since ente-cavir is primarily eliminated by the kidneys co-administration of ente-cavir with drugs that reduce renal function or compete for active tubu-lar secretion may increase serum concentrations of either entecavir or the co-administered drug).

No products indexed under this heading.

Didanosine (Since entecavir is primarily eliminated by the kidneys co-administration of entecavir with drugs that reduce renal function or compete for active tubular secretion may increase serum concentrations of either entecavir or the co-administered drug).
No products indexed under this heading.

Efavirenz (Since entecavir is primarily eliminated by the kidneys co-administration of entecavir with drugs that reduce renal function or compete for active tubular secretion may increase serum concentrations of either entecavir or the co-administered drug). Products include:
Sustiva Capsules 957

Emtricitabine (Since entecavir is primarily eliminated by the kidneys co-administration of entecavir with drugs that reduce renal function or compete for active tubular secretion may increase serum concentrations of either entecavir or the co-administered drug). Products include:
Emtriva Capsules 1272
Truvada Tablets 1279

Enalapril Maleate (Since entecavir is primarily eliminated by the kidneys co-administration of entecavir with drugs that reduce renal function or compete for active tubular secretion may increase serum concentrations of either entecavir or the co-administered drug). Products include:
Vaseretic Tablets 2073
Vasotec I.V. Injection 2076

Enalaprilat (Since entecavir is primarily eliminated by the kidneys co-administration of entecavir with drugs that reduce renal function or compete for active tubular secretion may increase serum concentrations of either entecavir or the co-administered drug).
No products indexed under this heading.

Enfuvirtide (Since entecavir is primarily eliminated by the kidneys co-administration of entecavir with drugs that reduce renal function or compete for active tubular secretion may increase serum concentrations of either entecavir or the co-administered drug). Products include:
Fuzeon Injection 2772

Ethiodized Oil (Since entecavir is primarily eliminated by the kidneys co-administration of entecavir with drugs that reduce renal function or compete for active tubular secretion may increase serum concentrations of either entecavir or the co-administered drug).
No products indexed under this heading.

Etodolac (Since entecavir is primarily eliminated by the kidneys co-administration of entecavir with drugs that reduce renal function or compete for active tubular secretion may increase serum concentrations of either entecavir or the co-administered drug).
No products indexed under this heading.

Fenoprofen Calcium (Since entecavir is primarily eliminated by the kidneys co-administration of entecavir with drugs that reduce renal function or compete for active tubular secretion may increase serum concentrations of either entecavir or the co-administered drug). Products include:
Nalfon Capsules 2504

Filgrastim (Since entecavir is primarily eliminated by the kidneys co-administration of entecavir with drugs that reduce renal function or compete for active tubular secretion may increase serum concentrations of either entecavir or the co-administered drug). Products include:
Neupogen for Injection 598

Fluorouracil (Since entecavir is primarily eliminated by the kidneys co-administration of entecavir with drugs that reduce renal function or compete for active tubular secretion may increase serum concentrations of either entecavir or the co-administered drug). Products include:
Carac Cream, 0.5% 1048
Efudex 3348

Flurbiprofen (Since entecavir is primarily eliminated by the kidneys co-administration of entecavir with drugs that reduce renal function or compete for active tubular secretion may increase serum concentrations of either entecavir or the co-administered drug).
No products indexed under this heading.

Fluvastatin Sodium (Since entecavir is primarily eliminated by the kidneys co-administration of entecavir with drugs that reduce renal function or compete for active tubular secretion may increase serum concentrations of either entecavir or the co-administered drug). Products include:
Lescol Capsules 2227
Lescol 2730
Lescol XL Tablets 2227

Foscarnet Sodium (Since entecavir is primarily eliminated by the kidneys co-administration of entecavir with drugs that reduce renal function or compete for active tubular secretion may increase serum concentrations of either entecavir or the co-administered drug).
No products indexed under this heading.

Fosinopril Sodium (Since entecavir is primarily eliminated by the kidneys co-administration of entecavir with drugs that reduce renal function or compete for active tubular secretion may increase serum concentrations of either entecavir or the co-administered drug).
No products indexed under this heading.

Furosemide (Since entecavir is primarily eliminated by the kidneys co-administration of entecavir with drugs that reduce renal function or compete for active tubular secretion may increase serum concentrations of either entecavir or the co-administered drug). Products include:
Furosemide Tablets 2117

Gadopentetate Dimeglumine (Since entecavir is primarily eliminated by the kidneys co-administration of entecavir with drugs that reduce renal function or compete for active tubular secretion may increase serum concentrations of either entecavir or the co-administered drug).
No products indexed under this heading.

Gentamicin (Since entecavir is primarily eliminated by the kidneys co-administration of entecavir with drugs that reduce renal function or compete for active tubular secretion may increase serum concentrations of either entecavir or the co-administered drug).
No products indexed under this heading.

Gentamicin Sulfate (Since entecavir is primarily eliminated by the kidneys co-administration of entecavir with drugs that reduce renal function or compete for active tubular secretion may increase serum concentrations of either entecavir or the co-administered drug). Products include:
Garamycin Injectable 3028
Genoptic Sterile Ophthalmic Solution .... ⊙227
Pred-G Ophthalmic Suspension ...... ⊙234
Pred-G Sterile Ophthalmic Ointment .... ⊙235

Glipizide (Since entecavir is primarily eliminated by the kidneys co-administration of entecavir with drugs that reduce renal function or compete for active tubular secretion may increase serum concentrations of either entecavir or the co-administered drug).
No products indexed under this heading.

Globulin, Immune (Human) (Since entecavir is primarily eliminated by the kidneys co-administration of entecavir with drugs that reduce renal function or compete for active tubular secretion may increase serum concentrations of either entecavir or the co-administered drug). Products include:
GamaSTAN 3231

Glyburide (Since entecavir is primarily eliminated by the kidneys co-administration of entecavir with drugs that reduce renal function or compete for active tubular secretion may increase serum concentrations of either entecavir or the co-administered drug).
No products indexed under this heading.

Gold Therapy (Since entecavir is primarily eliminated by the kidneys co-administration of entecavir with drugs that reduce renal function or compete for active tubular secretion may increase serum concentrations of either entecavir or the co-administered drug).
No products indexed under this heading.

HMG-CoA Reductase Inhibitors (Since entecavir is primarily eliminated by the kidneys co-administration of entecavir with drugs that reduce renal function or compete for active tubular secretion may increase serum concentrations of either entecavir or the co-administered drug).
No products indexed under this heading.

Hydrochlorothiazide (Since entecavir is primarily eliminated by the kidneys co-administration of entecavir with drugs that reduce renal function or compete for active tubular secretion may increase serum concentrations of either entecavir or the co-administered drug). Products include:
Aldoril Tablets 1884
Atacand HCT 637
Avalide Tablets 2889
Avalide Tablets 922
Benicar HCT Tablets 2852
Diovan HCT Tablets 2195
Dyazide Capsules 1389
Hyzaar 1964
Lotensin HCT Tablets 2235
Maxzide 2150
Micardis HCT Tablets 886
Moduretic Tablets 2003
Prinzide Tablets 2033
Teveten HCT Tablets 1710
Timolide Tablets 2056
Uniretic Tablets 3114
Vaseretic Tablets 2073
Zestoretic Tablets 701

Hydroflumethiazide (Since entecavir is primarily eliminated by the kidneys co-administration of entecavir with drugs that reduce renal function or compete for active tubular secretion may increase serum concentrations of either entecavir or the co-administered drug).
No products indexed under this heading.

Ibuprofen (Since entecavir is primarily eliminated by the kidneys co-administration of entecavir with drugs that reduce renal function or compete for active tubular secretion may increase serum concentrations of either entecavir or the co-administered drug). Products include:
Advil Allergy Sinus Caplets .... ▣737
Advil .... ▣737
Children's Advil Suspension .... ▣742
Children's Advil Chewable Tablets .. ▣741
Advil Cold & Sinus .... ▣739
Advil Flu & Body Ache Caplets .... ▣739
Children's Advil Cold Suspension ... ▣741
Infants' Advil Concentrated Drops .. ▣743
Junior Strength Advil Swallow Tablets .... ▣740
Advil Migraine Liquigels .... ▣740
Advil Multi-Symptom Cold Caplets .... ▣738
Combunox Tablets 1183
Children's Motrin Oral Suspension and Chewable Tablets 1837
Children's Motrin Cold Non-Staining Dye-Free Oral Suspension 1838
Children's Motrin Cold Oral Suspension 1838
Children's Motrin Non-Staining Dye-Free Oral Suspension 1837
Motrin Cold & Sinus Caplets 1836
Motrin IB Tablets and Caplets 1836
Infants' Motrin Concentrated Drops 1837
Infants' Motrin Non-Staining Dye-Free Drops 1837
Junior Strength Motrin Caplets and Chewable Tablets 1837
Vicoprofen Tablets 533

Idarubicin Hydrochloride (Since entecavir is primarily eliminated by the kidneys co-administration of entecavir with drugs that reduce renal function or compete for active tubular secretion may increase serum concentrations of either entecavir or the co-administered drug). Products include:
Idamycin PFS Injection 2645

Ifosfamide (Since entecavir is primarily eliminated by the kidneys co-administration of entecavir with drugs that reduce renal function or compete for active tubular secretion may increase serum concentrations of either entecavir or the co-administered drug).
No products indexed under this heading.

Imipenem (Since entecavir is primarily eliminated by the kidneys co-administration of entecavir with drugs that reduce renal function or compete for active tubular secretion may increase serum concentrations

of either entecavir or the co-administered drug). Products include:

Primaxin I.M. 2022
Primaxin I.V. 2024

Immune Globulin Intravenous (Human) (Since entecavir is primarily eliminated by the kidneys co-administration of entecavir with drugs that reduce renal function or compete for active tubular secretion may increase serum concentrations of either entecavir or the co-administered drug). Products include:

Carimune NF 3501
Gammagard Liquid 751
Gammagard S/D 754
Gamunex Immune Globulin I.V., 10% 3232
Iveegam EN 759

Indinavir Sulfate (Since entecavir is primarily eliminated by the kidneys co-administration of entecavir with drugs that reduce renal function or compete for active tubular secretion may increase serum concentrations of either entecavir or the co-administered drug). Products include:

Crixivan Capsules 1918

Indomethacin (Since entecavir is primarily eliminated by the kidneys co-administration of entecavir with drugs that reduce renal function or compete for active tubular secretion may increase serum concentrations of either entecavir or the co-administered drug). Products include:

Indocin 1968

Indomethacin Sodium Trihydrate (Since entecavir is primarily eliminated by the kidneys co-administration of entecavir with drugs that reduce renal function or compete for active tubular secretion may increase serum concentrations of either entecavir or the co-administered drug). Products include:

Indocin I.V. 1973

Interferon Beta-1b (Since entecavir is primarily eliminated by the kidneys co-administration of entecavir with drugs that reduce renal function or compete for active tubular secretion may increase serum concentrations of either entecavir or the co-administered drug). Products include:

Betaseron for SC Injection 791

Interleuken-2 (Since entecavir is primarily eliminated by the kidneys co-administration of entecavir with drugs that reduce renal function or compete for active tubular secretion may increase serum concentrations of either entecavir or the co-administered drug).

No products indexed under this heading.

Iodamide Meglumine (Since entecavir is primarily eliminated by the kidneys co-administration of entecavir with drugs that reduce renal function or compete for active tubular secretion may increase serum concentrations of either entecavir or the co-administered drug).

No products indexed under this heading.

Iohexol (Since entecavir is primarily eliminated by the kidneys co-administration of entecavir with drugs that reduce renal function or compete for active tubular secretion may increase serum concentrations of either entecavir or the co-administered drug).

No products indexed under this heading.

Iopamidol (Since entecavir is primarily eliminated by the kidneys co-administration of entecavir with drugs that reduce renal function or compete for active tubular secretion may increase serum concentrations of either entecavir or the co-administered drug).

No products indexed under this heading.

Iopanoic Acid (Since entecavir is primarily eliminated by the kidneys co-administration of entecavir with drugs that reduce renal function or compete for active tubular secretion may increase serum concentrations of either entecavir or the co-administered drug).

No products indexed under this heading.

Iothalamate Meglumine (Since entecavir is primarily eliminated by the kidneys co-administration of entecavir with drugs that reduce renal function or compete for active tubular secretion may increase serum concentrations of either entecavir or the co-administered drug).

No products indexed under this heading.

Ioxaglate Meglumine (Since entecavir is primarily eliminated by the kidneys co-administration of entecavir with drugs that reduce renal function or compete for active tubular secretion may increase serum concentrations of either entecavir or the co-administered drug).

No products indexed under this heading.

Ioxaglate Sodium (Since entecavir is primarily eliminated by the kidneys co-administration of entecavir with drugs that reduce renal function or compete for active tubular secretion may increase serum concentrations of either entecavir or the co-administered drug).

No products indexed under this heading.

Kanamycin Sulfate (Since entecavir is primarily eliminated by the kidneys co-administration of entecavir with drugs that reduce renal function or compete for active tubular secretion may increase serum concentrations of either entecavir or the co-administered drug).

No products indexed under this heading.

Ketoprofen (Since entecavir is primarily eliminated by the kidneys co-administration of entecavir with drugs that reduce renal function or compete for active tubular secretion may increase serum concentrations of either entecavir or the co-administered drug).

No products indexed under this heading.

Ketorolac Tromethamine (Since entecavir is primarily eliminated by the kidneys co-administration of entecavir with drugs that reduce renal function or compete for active tubular secretion may increase serum concentrations of either entecavir or the co-administered drug). Products include:

Acular Ophthalmic Solution .... ⊙ 561
Acular LS Ophthalmic Solution .... ⊙ 562

Lamium album (Since entecavir is primarily eliminated by the kidneys co-administration of entecavir with drugs that reduce renal function or compete for active tubular secretion may increase serum concentrations of either entecavir or the co-administered drug).

No products indexed under this heading.

Lisinopril (Since entecavir is primarily eliminated by the kidneys co-administration of entecavir with drugs that reduce renal function or compete for active tubular secretion may increase serum concentrations of either entecavir or the co-administered drug). Products include:

Prinivil Tablets 2029
Prinzide Tablets 2033
Zestoretic Tablets 701
Zestril Tablets 704

Lithium (Since entecavir is primarily eliminated by the kidneys co-administration of entecavir with drugs that reduce renal function or compete for active tubular secretion may increase serum concentrations of either entecavir or the co-administered drug).

No products indexed under this heading.

Lithium Carbonate (Since entecavir is primarily eliminated by the kidneys co-administration of entecavir with drugs that reduce renal function or compete for active tubular secretion may increase serum concentrations of either entecavir or the co-administered drug). Products include:

Eskalith 1406
Lithobid Tablets 1670

Lithium Citrate (Since entecavir is primarily eliminated by the kidneys co-administration of entecavir with drugs that reduce renal function or compete for active tubular secretion may increase serum concentrations of either entecavir or the co-administered drug).

No products indexed under this heading.

Lopinavir (Since entecavir is primarily eliminated by the kidneys co-administration of entecavir with drugs that reduce renal function or compete for active tubular secretion may increase serum concentrations of either entecavir or the co-administered drug). Products include:

Kaletra 474

Loracarbef (Since entecavir is primarily eliminated by the kidneys co-administration of entecavir with drugs that reduce renal function or compete for active tubular secretion may increase serum concentrations of either entecavir or the co-administered drug).

No products indexed under this heading.

Lovastatin (Since entecavir is primarily eliminated by the kidneys co-administration of entecavir with drugs that reduce renal function or compete for active tubular secretion may increase serum concentrations of either entecavir or the co-administered drug). Products include:

Advicor Tablets 1694
Altoprev Extended-Release Tablets 1151
Mevacor Tablets 1996

Meclofenamate Sodium (Since entecavir is primarily eliminated by the kidneys co-administration of entecavir with drugs that reduce renal function or compete for active tubular secretion may increase serum concentrations of either entecavir or the co-administered drug).

No products indexed under this heading.

Mefenamic Acid (Since entecavir is primarily eliminated by the kidneys co-administration of entecavir with drugs that reduce renal function or compete for active tubular secretion may increase serum concentrations of either entecavir or the co-administered drug).

No products indexed under this heading.

Meloxicam (Since entecavir is primarily eliminated by the kidneys co-administration of entecavir with drugs that reduce renal function or compete for active tubular secretion may increase serum concentrations of either entecavir or the co-administered drug). Products include:

Mobic Oral Suspension 893
Mobic Tablets 893

Melphalan Hydrochloride (Since entecavir is primarily eliminated by the kidneys co-administration of entecavir with drugs that reduce renal function or compete for active tubular secretion may increase serum concentrations of either entecavir or the co-administered drug). Products include:

Alkeran for Injection 976

Mesalamine (Since entecavir is primarily eliminated by the kidneys co-administration of entecavir with drugs that reduce renal function or compete for active tubular secretion may increase serum concentrations of either entecavir or the co-administered drug). Products include:

Asacol Delayed-Release Tablets 2688
Canasa Rectal Suppositories 726
Pentasa Capsules 3182

Methimazole (Since entecavir is primarily eliminated by the kidneys co-administration of entecavir with drugs that reduce renal function or compete for active tubular secretion may increase serum concentrations of either entecavir or the co-administered drug).

No products indexed under this heading.

Methotrexate (Since entecavir is primarily eliminated by the kidneys co-administration of entecavir with drugs that reduce renal function or compete for active tubular secretion may increase serum concentrations of either entecavir or the co-administered drug).

No products indexed under this heading.

Methotrexate Sodium (Since entecavir is primarily eliminated by the kidneys co-administration of entecavir with drugs that reduce renal function or compete for active tubular secretion may increase serum concentrations of either entecavir or the co-administered drug).

No products indexed under this heading.

Methyclothiazide (Since entecavir is primarily eliminated by the kidneys co-administration of entecavir with drugs that reduce renal function or compete for active tubular secretion may increase serum concentrations of either entecavir or the co-administered drug).
No products indexed under this heading.

Mezlocillin Sodium (Since entecavir is primarily eliminated by the kidneys co-administration of entecavir with drugs that reduce renal function or compete for active tubular secretion may increase serum concentrations of either entecavir or the co-administered drug).
No products indexed under this heading.

Minocycline Hydrochloride (Since entecavir is primarily eliminated by the kidneys co-administration of entecavir with drugs that reduce renal function or compete for active tubular secretion may increase serum concentrations of either entecavir or the co-administered drug). Products include:
Dynacin Tablets **1859**

Mitomycin (Mitomycin-C) (Since entecavir is primarily eliminated by the kidneys co-administration of entecavir with drugs that reduce renal function or compete for active tubular secretion may increase serum concentrations of either entecavir or the co-administered drug).
No products indexed under this heading.

Moexipril Hydrochloride (Since entecavir is primarily eliminated by the kidneys co-administration of entecavir with drugs that reduce renal function or compete for active tubular secretion may increase serum concentrations of either entecavir or the co-administered drug). Products include:
Uniretic Tablets **3114**
Univasc Tablets **3118**

Muromonab-CD3 (Since entecavir is primarily eliminated by the kidneys co-administration of entecavir with drugs that reduce renal function or compete for active tubular secretion may increase serum concentrations of either entecavir or the co-administered drug). Products include:
Orthoclone OKT3 Sterile Solution **2370**

Nabumetone (Since entecavir is primarily eliminated by the kidneys co-administration of entecavir with drugs that reduce renal function or compete for active tubular secretion may increase serum concentrations of either entecavir or the co-administered drug). Products include:
Relafen Tablets **1523**

Nafcillin Sodium (Since entecavir is primarily eliminated by the kidneys co-administration of entecavir with drugs that reduce renal function or compete for active tubular secretion may increase serum concentrations of either entecavir or the co-administered drug).
No products indexed under this heading.

Naproxen (Since entecavir is primarily eliminated by the kidneys co-administration of entecavir with drugs that reduce renal function or compete for active tubular secretion may increase serum concentrations of either entecavir or the co-administered drug). Products include:
EC-Naprosyn Delayed-Release Tablets **2769**
Naprosyn Suspension **2769**
Naprosyn Tablets **2769**
Prevacid NapraPAC **3277**

Naproxen Sodium (Since entecavir is primarily eliminated by the kidneys co-administration of entecavir with drugs that reduce renal function or compete for active tubular secretion may increase serum concentrations of either entecavir or the co-administered drug). Products include:
Aleve Tablets, Caplets and Gelcaps **605**
Anaprox Tablets **2769**
Anaprox DS Tablets **2769**

Nelfinavir Mesylate (Since entecavir is primarily eliminated by the kidneys co-administration of entecavir with drugs that reduce renal function or compete for active tubular secretion may increase serum concentrations of either entecavir or the co-administered drug). Products include:
Viracept **2556**

Neomycin (Since entecavir is primarily eliminated by the kidneys co-administration of entecavir with drugs that reduce renal function or compete for active tubular secretion may increase serum concentrations of either entecavir or the co-administered drug). Products include:
Neosporin Ointment **702**
Neosporin + Pain Relief Maximum Strength Cream........... **703**
Neosporin + Pain Relief Maximum Strength Ointment....... **703**

Neomycin, oral (Since entecavir is primarily eliminated by the kidneys co-administration of entecavir with drugs that reduce renal function or compete for active tubular secretion may increase serum concentrations of either entecavir or the co-administered drug).
No products indexed under this heading.

Neomycin Sulfate (Since entecavir is primarily eliminated by the kidneys co-administration of entecavir with drugs that reduce renal function or compete for active tubular secretion may increase serum concentrations of either entecavir or the co-administered drug). Products include:
Poly-Pred Liquifilm Ophthalmic Suspension .... ⊙ **231**

Nevirapine (Since entecavir is primarily eliminated by the kidneys co-administration of entecavir with drugs that reduce renal function or compete for active tubular secretion may increase serum concentrations of either entecavir or the co-administered drug). Products include:
Viramune Oral Suspension **903**
Viramune Tablets **903**

Norfloxacin (Since entecavir is primarily eliminated by the kidneys co-administration of entecavir with drugs that reduce renal function or compete for active tubular secretion may increase serum concentrations of either entecavir or the co-administered drug). Products include:
Noroxin Tablets **2009**

Olsalazine Sodium (Since entecavir is primarily eliminated by the kidneys co-administration of entecavir with drugs that reduce renal function or compete for active tubular secretion may increase serum concentrations of either entecavir or the co-administered drug).
No products indexed under this heading.

Omeprazole (Since entecavir is primarily eliminated by the kidneys co-administration of entecavir with drugs that reduce renal function or compete for active tubular secretion may increase serum concentrations of either entecavir or the co-administered drug). Products include:
Zegerid Powder for Oral Solution **2972**

Oxaprozin (Since entecavir is primarily eliminated by the kidneys co-administration of entecavir with drugs that reduce renal function or compete for active tubular secretion may increase serum concentrations of either entecavir or the co-administered drug).
No products indexed under this heading.

Pamidronate Disodium (Since entecavir is primarily eliminated by the kidneys co-administration of entecavir with drugs that reduce renal function or compete for active tubular secretion may increase serum concentrations of either entecavir or the co-administered drug). Products include:
Aredia for Injection **2168**

Paroxetine Hydrochloride (Since entecavir is primarily eliminated by the kidneys co-administration of entecavir with drugs that reduce renal function or compete for active tubular secretion may increase serum concentrations of either entecavir or the co-administered drug). Products include:
Paxil CR Controlled-Release Tablets **1509**
Paxil **1501**

Penicillamine (Since entecavir is primarily eliminated by the kidneys co-administration of entecavir with drugs that reduce renal function or compete for active tubular secretion may increase serum concentrations of either entecavir or the co-administered drug). Products include:
Cuprimine Capsules **1925**

Penicillin G Benzathine (Since entecavir is primarily eliminated by the kidneys co-administration of entecavir with drugs that reduce renal function or compete for active tubular secretion may increase serum concentrations of either entecavir or the co-administered drug).
No products indexed under this heading.

Penicillin G Potassium (Since entecavir is primarily eliminated by the kidneys co-administration of entecavir with drugs that reduce renal function or compete for active tubular secretion may increase serum concentrations of either entecavir or the co-administered drug).
No products indexed under this heading.

Penicillin G Procaine (Since entecavir is primarily eliminated by the kidneys co-administration of entecavir with drugs that reduce renal function or compete for active tubular secretion may increase serum concentrations of either entecavir or the co-administered drug).
No products indexed under this heading.

Penicillin G Sodium (Since entecavir is primarily eliminated by the kidneys co-administration of entecavir with drugs that reduce renal function or compete for active tubular secretion may increase serum concentrations of either entecavir or the co-administered drug).
No products indexed under this heading.

Penicillin V Potassium (Since entecavir is primarily eliminated by the kidneys co-administration of entecavir with drugs that reduce renal function or compete for active tubular secretion may increase serum concentrations of either entecavir or the co-administered drug).
No products indexed under this heading.

Pentamidine Isethionate (Since entecavir is primarily eliminated by the kidneys co-administration of entecavir with drugs that reduce renal function or compete for active tubular secretion may increase serum concentrations of either entecavir or the co-administered drug).
No products indexed under this heading.

Perindopril Erbumine (Since entecavir is primarily eliminated by the kidneys co-administration of entecavir with drugs that reduce renal function or compete for active tubular secretion may increase serum concentrations of either entecavir or the co-administered drug). Products include:
Aceon Tablets (2 mg, 4 mg, 8 mg) **3191**

Phenylbutazone (Since entecavir is primarily eliminated by the kidneys co-administration of entecavir with drugs that reduce renal function or compete for active tubular secretion may increase serum concentrations of either entecavir or the co-administered drug).
No products indexed under this heading.

Piroxicam (Since entecavir is primarily eliminated by the kidneys co-administration of entecavir with drugs that reduce renal function or compete for active tubular secretion may increase serum concentrations of either entecavir or the co-administered drug).
No products indexed under this heading.

Plicamycin (Since entecavir is primarily eliminated by the kidneys co-administration of entecavir with drugs that reduce renal function or compete for active tubular secretion may increase serum concentrations of either entecavir or the co-administered drug).
No products indexed under this heading.

Polymyxin (Since entecavir is primarily eliminated by the kidneys co-administration of entecavir with drugs that reduce renal function or compete for active tubular secretion may increase serum concentrations of either entecavir or the co-administered drug).
No products indexed under this heading.

Polymyxin B Sulfate (Since entecavir is primarily eliminated by the kidneys co-administration of entecavir with drugs that reduce renal function or compete for active tubular secretion may increase serum concentrations of either entecavir or the co-administered drug). Products include:
Neosporin Ointment .... ▣ 702
Neosporin + Pain Relief Maximum Strength Cream........... ▣ 703
Neosporin + Pain Relief Maximum Strength Ointment....... ▣ 703
Poly-Pred Liquifilm Ophthalmic Suspension................................. ⊙ 231
Polysporin Ointment .... ▣ 706
Polytrim Ophthalmic Solution 570

Polythiazide (Since entecavir is primarily eliminated by the kidneys co-administration of entecavir with drugs that reduce renal function or compete for active tubular secretion may increase serum concentrations of either entecavir or the co-administered drug).
No products indexed under this heading.

Pravastatin Sodium (Since entecavir is primarily eliminated by the kidneys co-administration of entecavir with drugs that reduce renal function or compete for active tubular secretion may increase serum concentrations of either entecavir or the co-administered drug). Products include:
Pravachol Tablets 943

Probenecid (Since entecavir is primarily eliminated by the kidneys co-administration of entecavir with drugs that reduce renal function or compete for active tubular secretion may increase serum concentrations of either entecavir or the co-administered drug).
No products indexed under this heading.

Quinapril Hydrochloride (Since entecavir is primarily eliminated by the kidneys co-administration of entecavir with drugs that reduce renal function or compete for active tubular secretion may increase serum concentrations of either entecavir or the co-administered drug).
No products indexed under this heading.

Rabeprazole Sodium (Since entecavir is primarily eliminated by the kidneys co-administration of entecavir with drugs that reduce renal function or compete for active tubular secretion may increase serum concentrations of either entecavir or the co-administered drug). Products include:
Aciphex Tablets 1081

Ramipril (Since entecavir is primarily eliminated by the kidneys co-administration of entecavir with drugs that reduce renal function or compete for active tubular secretion may increase serum concentrations of either entecavir or the co-administered drug). Products include:
Altace Capsules 1673

Rifampin (Since entecavir is primarily eliminated by the kidneys co-administration of entecavir with drugs that reduce renal function or compete for active tubular secretion may increase serum concentrations of either entecavir or the co-administered drug).
No products indexed under this heading.

Riluzole (Since entecavir is primarily eliminated by the kidneys co-administration of entecavir with drugs that reduce renal function or compete for active tubular secretion may increase serum concentrations of either entecavir or the co-administered drug). Products include:
Rilutek Tablets 2945

Ritonavir (Since entecavir is primarily eliminated by the kidneys co-administration of entecavir with drugs that reduce renal function or compete for active tubular secretion may increase serum concentrations of either entecavir or the co-administered drug). Products include:
Kaletra 474
Norvir 499

Rofecoxib (Since entecavir is primarily eliminated by the kidneys co-administration of entecavir with drugs that reduce renal function or compete for active tubular secretion may increase serum concentrations of either entecavir or the co-administered drug).
No products indexed under this heading.

Saquinavir (Since entecavir is primarily eliminated by the kidneys co-administration of entecavir with drugs that reduce renal function or compete for active tubular secretion may increase serum concentrations of either entecavir or the co-administered drug).
No products indexed under this heading.

Sibutramine Hydrochloride Monohydrate (Since entecavir is primarily eliminated by the kidneys co-administration of entecavir with drugs that reduce renal function or compete for active tubular secretion may increase serum concentrations of either entecavir or the co-administered drug). Products include:
Meridia Capsules 485

Simvastatin (Since entecavir is primarily eliminated by the kidneys co-administration of entecavir with drugs that reduce renal function or compete for active tubular secretion may increase serum concentrations of either entecavir or the co-administered drug). Products include:
Vytorin 10/10 Tablets 2084
Vytorin 10/10 Tablets 3092
Vytorin 10/20 Tablets 2084
Vytorin 10/20 Tablets 3092
Vytorin 10/40 Tablets 3092
Vytorin 10/40 Tablets 2084
Vytorin 10/80 Tablets 2084
Vytorin 10/80 Tablets 3092
Zocor Tablets 2078

Spirapril Hydrochloride (Since entecavir is primarily eliminated by the kidneys co-administration of entecavir with drugs that reduce renal function or compete for active tubular secretion may increase serum concentrations of either entecavir or the co-administered drug).
No products indexed under this heading.

Stavudine (Since entecavir is primarily eliminated by the kidneys co-administration of entecavir with drugs that reduce renal function or compete for active tubular secretion may increase serum concentrations of either entecavir or the co-administered drug). Products include:
Zerit 971

Streptomycin Sulfate (Since entecavir is primarily eliminated by the kidneys co-administration of entecavir with drugs that reduce renal function or compete for active tubular secretion may increase serum concentrations of either entecavir or the co-administered drug).
No products indexed under this heading.

Streptozocin (Since entecavir is primarily eliminated by the kidneys co-administration of entecavir with drugs that reduce renal function or compete for active tubular secretion may increase serum concentrations of either entecavir or the co-administered drug).
No products indexed under this heading.

Sulfacytine (Since entecavir is primarily eliminated by the kidneys co-administration of entecavir with drugs that reduce renal function or compete for active tubular secretion may increase serum concentrations of either entecavir or the co-administered drug).
No products indexed under this heading.

Sulfamethizole (Since entecavir is primarily eliminated by the kidneys co-administration of entecavir with drugs that reduce renal function or compete for active tubular secretion may increase serum concentrations of either entecavir or the co-administered drug).
No products indexed under this heading.

Sulfamethoxazole (Since entecavir is primarily eliminated by the kidneys co-administration of entecavir with drugs that reduce renal function or compete for active tubular secretion may increase serum concentrations of either entecavir or the co-administered drug).
No products indexed under this heading.

Sulfasalazine (Since entecavir is primarily eliminated by the kidneys co-administration of entecavir with drugs that reduce renal function or compete for active tubular secretion may increase serum concentrations of either entecavir or the co-administered drug).
No products indexed under this heading.

Sulfinpyrazone (Since entecavir is primarily eliminated by the kidneys co-administration of entecavir with drugs that reduce renal function or compete for active tubular secretion may increase serum concentrations of either entecavir or the co-administered drug).
No products indexed under this heading.

Sulfisoxazole (Since entecavir is primarily eliminated by the kidneys co-administration of entecavir with drugs that reduce renal function or compete for active tubular secretion may increase serum concentrations of either entecavir or the co-administered drug).
No products indexed under this heading.

Sulfisoxazole Acetyl (Since entecavir is primarily eliminated by the kidneys co-administration of entecavir with drugs that reduce renal function or compete for active tubular secretion may increase serum concentrations of either entecavir or the co-administered drug).
No products indexed under this heading.

Sulfisoxazole Diolamine (Since entecavir is primarily eliminated by the kidneys co-administration of entecavir with drugs that reduce renal function or compete for active tubular secretion may increase serum concentrations of either entecavir or the co-administered drug).
No products indexed under this heading.

Sulindac (Since entecavir is primarily eliminated by the kidneys co-administration of entecavir with drugs that reduce renal function or compete for active tubular secretion may increase serum concentrations of either entecavir or the co-administered drug). Products include:
Clinoril Tablets 1899

Tacrolimus (Since entecavir is primarily eliminated by the kidneys co-administration of entecavir with drugs that reduce renal function or compete for active tubular secretion may increase serum concentrations of either entecavir or the co-administered drug). Products include:
Prograf Capsules and Injection 624
Protopic Ointment 629

Tenofovir Disoproxil Fumarate (Since entecavir is primarily eliminated by the kidneys co-administration of entecavir with drugs that reduce renal function or compete for active tubular secretion may increase serum concentrations of either entecavir or the co-administered drug). Products include:
Truvada Tablets 1279
Viread Tablets 1284

Thioguanine (Since entecavir is primarily eliminated by the kidneys co-administration of entecavir with drugs that reduce renal function or compete for active tubular secretion may increase serum concentrations of either entecavir or the co-administered drug). Products include:
Tabloid Tablets 1545

Ticarcillin Disodium (Since entecavir is primarily eliminated by the kidneys co-administration of entecavir with drugs that reduce renal function or compete for active tubular secretion may increase serum concentrations of either entecavir or the co-administered drug). Products include:
Timentin ADD-Vantage 1556
Timentin Injection Galaxy Container 1559
Timentin IV Infusion 1553
Timentin Pharmacy Bulk Package 1562

Tobramycin (Since entecavir is primarily eliminated by the kidneys co-administration of entecavir with drugs that reduce renal function or compete for active tubular secretion may increase serum concentrations of either entecavir or the co-administered drug). Products include:
- TOBI Solution for Inhalation **1015**
- TobraDex Ophthalmic Ointment **558**
- TobraDex Ophthalmic Suspension ... **558**
- Zylet Ophthalmic Suspension **3508**

Tobramycin Sulfate (Since entecavir is primarily eliminated by the kidneys co-administration of entecavir with drugs that reduce renal function or compete for active tubular secretion may increase serum concentrations of either entecavir or the co-administered drug).
No products indexed under this heading.

Tolazamide (Since entecavir is primarily eliminated by the kidneys co-administration of entecavir with drugs that reduce renal function or compete for active tubular secretion may increase serum concentrations of either entecavir or the co-administered drug).
No products indexed under this heading.

Tolbutamide (Since entecavir is primarily eliminated by the kidneys co-administration of entecavir with drugs that reduce renal function or compete for active tubular secretion may increase serum concentrations of either entecavir or the co-administered drug).
No products indexed under this heading.

Tolmetin Sodium (Since entecavir is primarily eliminated by the kidneys co-administration of entecavir with drugs that reduce renal function or compete for active tubular secretion may increase serum concentrations of either entecavir or the co-administered drug).
No products indexed under this heading.

Trandolapril (Since entecavir is primarily eliminated by the kidneys co-administration of entecavir with drugs that reduce renal function or compete for active tubular secretion may increase serum concentrations of either entecavir or the co-administered drug). Products include:
- Mavik Tablets **482**
- Tarka Tablets **519**

Triamterene (Since entecavir is primarily eliminated by the kidneys co-administration of entecavir with drugs that reduce renal function or compete for active tubular secretion may increase serum concentrations of either entecavir or the co-administered drug). Products include:
- Dyazide Capsules **1389**
- Dyrenium Capsules **3390**
- Maxzide **2150**

Trimethadione (Since entecavir is primarily eliminated by the kidneys co-administration of entecavir with drugs that reduce renal function or compete for active tubular secretion may increase serum concentrations of either entecavir or the co-administered drug).
No products indexed under this heading.

Trovafloxacin Mesylate (Since entecavir is primarily eliminated by the kidneys co-administration of entecavir with drugs that reduce renal function or compete for active tubular secretion may increase serum concentrations of either entecavir or the co-administered drug).
No products indexed under this heading.

Tyropanoate Sodium (Since entecavir is primarily eliminated by the kidneys co-administration of entecavir with drugs that reduce renal function or compete for active tubular secretion may increase serum concentrations of either entecavir or the co-administered drug).
No products indexed under this heading.

Valacyclovir Hydrochloride (Since entecavir is primarily eliminated by the kidneys co-administration of entecavir with drugs that reduce renal function or compete for active tubular secretion may increase serum concentrations of either entecavir or the co-administered drug). Products include:
- Valtrex Caplets **1573**

Valdecoxib (Since entecavir is primarily eliminated by the kidneys co-administration of entecavir with drugs that reduce renal function or compete for active tubular secretion may increase serum concentrations of either entecavir or the co-administered drug).
No products indexed under this heading.

Vancomycin Hydrochloride (Since entecavir is primarily eliminated by the kidneys co-administration of entecavir with drugs that reduce renal function or compete for active tubular secretion may increase serum concentrations of either entecavir or the co-administered drug). Products include:
- Vancocin HCl Capsules, USP **3370**

Voriconazole (Since entecavir is primarily eliminated by the kidneys co-administration of entecavir with drugs that reduce renal function or compete for active tubular secretion may increase serum concentrations of either entecavir or the co-administered drug). Products include:
- VFEND I.V. **2543**
- VFEND Oral Suspension **2543**
- VFEND Tablets **2543**

Zalcitabine (Since entecavir is primarily eliminated by the kidneys co-administration of entecavir with drugs that reduce renal function or compete for active tubular secretion may increase serum concentrations of either entecavir or the co-administered drug).
No products indexed under this heading.

Zidovudine (Since entecavir is primarily eliminated by the kidneys co-administration of entecavir with drugs that reduce renal function or compete for active tubular secretion may increase serum concentrations of either entecavir or the co-administered drug). Products include:
- Combivir Tablets **1373**
- Retrovir **1533**
- Retrovir IV Infusion **1537**
- Trizivir Tablets **1565**

Zoledronic acid (Since entecavir is primarily eliminated by the kidneys co-administration of entecavir with drugs that reduce renal function or compete for active tubular secretion may increase serum concentrations of either entecavir or the co-administered drug). Products include:
- Zometa for Intravenous Infusion **2306**

BAUSCH & LOMB PRESERVISION AREDS SOFTGELS

(Vitamins with Minerals) .... ⊙**244**
None cited in PDR database.

BAUSCH & LOMB PRESERVISION AREDS TABLETS

(Vitamins with Minerals) .... ⊙**252**
None cited in PDR database.

BAUSCH & LOMB PRESERVISION LUTEIN SOFTGELS

(Lutein, Vitamins with Minerals) .... ⊙**245**
None cited in PDR database.

BAUSCH & LOMB PRESERVISION AREDS EYE VITAMIN AND MINERAL SUPPLEMENT SOFTGELS

(Vitamins with Minerals) **760**
None cited in PDR database.

BAUSCH & LOMB PRESERVISION LUTEIN EYE VITAMIN AND MINERAL SUPPLEMENT SOFTGELS

(Lutein, Vitamins with Minerals) **760**
None cited in PDR database.

ASPIRIN REGIMEN BAYER ADULT LOW STRENGTH 81 MG TABLETS

(Aspirin) **606**
May interact with oral anticoagulants, oral hypoglycemic agents, and certain other agents. Compounds in these categories include:

Acarbose (Concurrent use should be avoided unless directed by a doctor). Products include:
- Precose Tablets **776**

Anisindione (Concurrent use should be avoided unless directed by a doctor). Products include:
- Miradon Tablets **3056**

Antiarthritic Drugs, unspecified (Concurrent use should be avoided unless directed by a doctor).
No products indexed under this heading.

Chlorpropamide (Concurrent use should be avoided unless directed by a doctor).
No products indexed under this heading.

Dicumarol (Concurrent use should be avoided unless directed by a doctor).
No products indexed under this heading.

Glimepiride (Concurrent use should be avoided unless directed by a doctor). Products include:
- Amaryl Tablets **2864**

Glipizide (Concurrent use should be avoided unless directed by a doctor).
No products indexed under this heading.

Glyburide (Concurrent use should be avoided unless directed by a doctor).
No products indexed under this heading.

Metformin Hydrochloride (Concurrent use should be avoided unless directed by a doctor). Products include:
- ActoPlus Met Tablets **3219**
- Avandamet Tablets **1343**
- Fortamet Extended-Release Tablets **1156**

Miglitol (Concurrent use should be avoided unless directed by a doctor).
No products indexed under this heading.

Pioglitazone Hydrochloride (Concurrent use should be avoided unless directed by a doctor). Products include:
- ActoPlus Met Tablets **3219**
- Actos Tablets **3224**

Probenecid (Concurrent use with gout medications should be avoided unless directed by a doctor).
No products indexed under this heading.

Repaglinide (Concurrent use should be avoided unless directed by a doctor). Products include:
- Prandin Tablets (0.5, 1, and 2 mg).. **2337**

Rosiglitazone Maleate (Concurrent use should be avoided unless directed by a doctor). Products include:
- Avandamet Tablets **1343**
- Avandia Tablets **1348**

Sulfinpyrazone (Concurrent use with gout medications should be avoided unless directed by a doctor).
No products indexed under this heading.

Tolazamide (Concurrent use should be avoided unless directed by a doctor).
No products indexed under this heading.

Tolbutamide (Concurrent use should be avoided unless directed by a doctor).
No products indexed under this heading.

Troglitazone (Concurrent use should be avoided unless directed by a doctor).
No products indexed under this heading.

Warfarin Sodium (Concurrent use should be avoided unless directed by a doctor). Products include:
- Coumadin for Injection **932**
- Coumadin Tablets **932**

Food Interactions

Alcohol (Chronic heavy alcohol users, 3 or more drinks per day, should consult their physicians for advice on when and how they should take pain relievers/fever reducers including aspirin).

ASPIRIN REGIMEN BAYER REGULAR STRENGTH 325 MG CAPLETS

(Aspirin) **606**
See Aspirin Regimen Bayer Adult Low Strength 81 mg Tablets

BAYER ASPIRIN TABLETS

(Aspirin) 3515
May interact with ACE inhibitors, beta blockers, anticoagulants, diuretics, oral hypoglycemic agents, non-steroidal anti-inflammatory agents, phenytoin, valproate, and certain other agents. Compounds in these categories include:

Acarbose (Moderate doses of aspirin may increase the effectiveness of oral hypoglycemic drugs, leading to hypoglycemia). Products include:
Precose Tablets 776

Acebutolol Hydrochloride (The hypotensive effects of beta blockers may be diminished by the concomitant administration of aspirin due to inhibition of renal prostaglandins, leading to decreased renal blood flow, and salt and fluid retention).
No products indexed under this heading.

Acetazolamide (Concurrent use of aspirin and acetazolamide can lead to high serum concentrations of acetazolamide (and toxicity) due to competition at the renal tubule for secretion).
No products indexed under this heading.

Acetazolamide Sodium (Concurrent use of aspirin and acetazolamide can lead to high serum concentrations of acetazolamide (and toxicity) due to competition at the renal tubule for secretion).
No products indexed under this heading.

Amiloride Hydrochloride (The effectiveness of diuretics in patients with underlying renal or cardiovascular disease may be diminished by the concomitant administration of aspirin due to inhibition of renal prostaglandins, leading to decreased renal blood flow, and salt and fluidretention). Products include:
Midamor Tablets 2000
Moduretic Tablets 2003

Anisindione (Patients on anticoagulation therapy are at increased risk for bleeding because of drug-drug interactions and the effect on platelets. Aspirin can displace warfarin from protein binding sites, leading to prolongation of both the prothrombin time and bleeding time. Aspirin can increase the anticoagulant activity of heparin, increasing bleeding risk). Products include:
Miradon Tablets 3056

Ardeparin Sodium (Patients on anticoagulation therapy are at increased risk for bleeding because of drug-drug interactions and the effect on platelets. Aspirin can displace warfarin from protein binding sites, leading to prolongation of both the prothrombin time and bleeding time. Aspirin can increase the anticoagulant activity of heparin, increasing bleeding risk).
No products indexed under this heading.

Atenolol (The hypotensive effects of beta blockers may be diminished by the concomitant administration of aspirin due to inhibition of renal prostaglandins, leading to decreased renal blood flow, and salt and fluid retention). Products include:
Tenormin I.V. Injection 698
Tenormin Tablets 695

Benazepril Hydrochloride (The hyponatremic and hypotensive effects of ACE inhibitors may be diminished by the concomitant administration of aspirin due to its indirect effect on the renin-angiotensin conversion pathway). Products include:
Lotensin Tablets 2232
Lotensin HCT Tablets 2235
Lotrel Capsules 2238

Bendroflumethiazide (The effectiveness of diuretics in patients with underlying renal or cardiovascular disease may be diminished by the concomitant administration of aspirin due to inhibition of renal prostaglandins, leading to decreased renal blood flow, and salt and fluidretention).
No products indexed under this heading.

Betaxolol Hydrochloride (The hypotensive effects of beta blockers may be diminished by the concomitant administration of aspirin due to inhibition of renal prostaglandins, leading to decreased renal blood flow, and salt and fluid retention). Products include:
Betoptic S Ophthalmic Suspension.. 554

Bisoprolol Fumarate (The hypotensive effects of beta blockers may be diminished by the concomitant administration of aspirin due to inhibition of renal prostaglandins, leading to decreased renal blood flow, and salt and fluid retention).
No products indexed under this heading.

Bumetanide (The effectiveness of diuretics in patients with underlying renal or cardiovascular disease may be diminished by the concomitant administration of aspirin due to inhibition of renal prostaglandins, leading to decreased renal blood flow, and salt and fluidretention).
No products indexed under this heading.

Captopril (The hyponatremic and hypotensive effects of ACE inhibitors may be diminished by the concomitant administration of aspirin due to its indirect effect on the renin-angiotensin conversion pathway). Products include:
Captopril Tablets 2114

Carteolol Hydrochloride (The hypotensive effects of beta blockers may be diminished by the concomitant administration of aspirin due to inhibition of renal prostaglandins, leading to decreased renal blood flow, and salt and fluid retention). Products include:
Carteolol Hydrochloride Ophthalmic Solution USP, 1%....... ⊙246

Celecoxib (The concurrent use of aspirin with other NSAIDs should be avoided because this may increase bleeding or lead to decreased renal function). Products include:
Celebrex Capsules 3130

Chlorothiazide (The effectiveness of diuretics in patients with underlying renal or cardiovascular disease may be diminished by the concomitant administration of aspirin due to inhibition of renal prostaglandins, leading to decreased renal blood flow, and salt and fluidretention). Products include:
Aldoclor Tablets 1881
Diuril Oral 1936

Chlorothiazide Sodium (The effectiveness of diuretics in patients with underlying renal or cardiovascular disease may be diminished by the concomitant administration of aspirin due to inhibition of renal prostaglandins, leading to decreased renal blood flow, and salt and fluidretention). Products include:
Diuril Sodium Intravenous 1934

Chlorpropamide (Moderate doses of aspirin may increase the effectiveness of oral hypoglycemic drugs, leading to hypoglycemia).
No products indexed under this heading.

Chlorthalidone (The effectiveness of diuretics in patients with underlying renal or cardiovascular disease may be diminished by the concomitant administration of aspirin due to inhibition of renal prostaglandins, leading to decreased renal blood flow, and salt and fluidretention). Products include:
Clorpres Tablets 2139

Dalteparin Sodium (Patients on anticoagulation therapy are at increased risk for bleeding because of drug-drug interactions and the effect on platelets. Aspirin can displace warfarin from protein binding sites, leading to prolongation of both the prothrombin time and bleeding time. Aspirin can increase the anticoagulant activity of heparin, increasing bleeding risk). Products include:
Fragmin Injection 2638

Danaparoid Sodium (Patients on anticoagulation therapy are at increased risk for bleeding because of drug-drug interactions and the effect on platelets. Aspirin can displace warfarin from protein binding sites, leading to prolongation of both the prothrombin time and bleeding time. Aspirin can increase the anticoagulant activity of heparin, increasing bleeding risk).
No products indexed under this heading.

Diclofenac Potassium (The concurrent use of aspirin with other NSAIDs should be avoided because this may increase bleeding or lead to decreased renal function). Products include:
Cataflam Tablets 2173

Diclofenac Sodium (The concurrent use of aspirin with other NSAIDs should be avoided because this may increase bleeding or lead to decreased renal function). Products include:
Arthrotec Tablets 3126
Voltaren Ophthalmic Solution 2300
Voltaren Tablets 2298
Voltaren-XR Tablets 2301

Dicumarol (Patients on anticoagulation therapy are at increased risk for bleeding because of drug-drug interactions and the effect on platelets. Aspirin can displace warfarin from protein binding sites, leading to prolongation of both the prothrombin time and bleeding time. Aspirin can increase the anticoagulant activity of heparin, increasing bleeding risk).
No products indexed under this heading.

Divalproex Sodium (Salicylate can displace protein-bound valproic acid, leading to an increase in serum valproic acid levels). Products include:
Depakote Sprinkle Capsules 422
Depakote Tablets 427
Depakote ER Tablets 433

Enalapril Maleate (The hyponatremic and hypotensive effects of ACE inhibitors may be diminished by the concomitant administration of aspirin due to its indirect effect on the renin-angiotensin conversion pathway). Products include:
Vaseretic Tablets 2073
Vasotec I.V. Injection 2076

Enalaprilat (The hyponatremic and hypotensive effects of ACE inhibitors may be diminished by the concomitant administration of aspirin due to its indirect effect on the renin-angiotensin conversion pathway).
No products indexed under this heading.

Enoxaparin Sodium (Patients on anticoagulation therapy are at increased risk for bleeding because of drug-drug interactions and the effect on platelets. Aspirin can displace warfarin from protein binding sites, leading to prolongation of both the prothrombin time and bleeding time. Aspirin can increase the anticoagulant activity of heparin, increasing bleeding risk). Products include:
Lovenox Injection 2931

Esmolol Hydrochloride (The hypotensive effects of beta blockers may be diminished by the concomitant administration of aspirin due to inhibition of renal prostaglandins, leading to decreased renal blood flow, and salt and fluid retention). Products include:
Brevibloc Concentrate 766
Brevibloc Injection 766
Brevibloc Double Strength Injection.. 766
Brevibloc Premixed Injection 766
Brevibloc Double Strength Premixed Injection 766

Ethacrynic Acid (The effectiveness of diuretics in patients with underlying renal or cardiovascular disease may be diminished by the concomitant administration of aspirin due to inhibition of renal prostaglandins, leading to decreased renal blood flow, and salt and fluidretention). Products include:
Edecrin Tablets 1941

Etodolac (The concurrent use of aspirin with other NSAIDs should be avoided because this may increase bleeding or lead to decreased renal function).
No products indexed under this heading.

Fenoprofen Calcium (The concurrent use of aspirin with other NSAIDs should be avoided because this may increase bleeding or lead to decreased renal function). Products include:
Nalfon Capsules 2504

Flurbiprofen (The concurrent use of aspirin with other NSAIDs should be avoided because this may increase bleeding or lead to decreased renal function).
No products indexed under this heading.

Fondaparinux Sodium (Patients on anticoagulation therapy are at increased risk for bleeding because of drug-drug interactions and the effect on platelets. Aspirin can displace warfarin from protein binding sites, leading to prolongation of both the prothrombin time and bleeding time. Aspirin can increase the anticoagulant activity of heparin, increasing bleeding risk). Products include:
Arixtra Injection 1325

Fosinopril Sodium (The hyponatremic and hypotensive effects of ACE inhibitors may be diminished by the concomitant administration of aspirin due to its indirect effect on the renin-angiotensin conversion pathway).
No products indexed under this heading.

Fosphenytoin Sodium (Salicylate can displace protein-bound phenytoin, leading to a decrease in the total concentration of phenytoin).
No products indexed under this heading.

Furosemide (The effectiveness of diuretics in patients with underlying renal or cardiovascular disease may be diminished by the concomitant administration of aspirin due to inhibition of renal prostaglandins, leading to decreased renal blood flow, and salt and fluidretention). Products include:
Furosemide Tablets 2117

Glimepiride (Moderate doses of aspirin may increase the effectiveness of oral hypoglycemic drugs, leading to hypoglycemia). Products include:
Amaryl Tablets 2864

Glipizide (Moderate doses of aspirin may increase the effectiveness of oral hypoglycemic drugs, leading to hypoglycemia).
No products indexed under this heading.

Glyburide (Moderate doses of aspirin may increase the effectiveness of oral hypoglycemic drugs, leading to hypoglycemia).
No products indexed under this heading.

Heparin Calcium (Patients on anticoagulation therapy are at increased risk for bleeding because of drug-drug interactions and the effect on platelets. Aspirin can displace warfarin from protein binding sites, leading to prolongation of both the prothrombin time and bleeding time. Aspirin can increase the anticoagulant activity of heparin, increasing bleeding risk).
No products indexed under this heading.

Heparin Sodium (Patients on anticoagulation therapy are at increased risk for bleeding because of drug-drug interactions and the effect on platelets. Aspirin can displace warfarin from protein binding sites, leading to prolongation of both the prothrombin time and bleeding time. Aspirin can increase the anticoagulant activity of heparin, increasing bleeding risk).
No products indexed under this heading.

Hydrochlorothiazide (The effectiveness of diuretics in patients with underlying renal or cardiovascular disease may be diminished by the concomitant administration of aspirin due to inhibition of renal prostaglandins, leading to decreased renal blood flow, and salt and fluidretention). Products include:
Aldoril Tablets 1884
Atacand HCT 637
Avalide Tablets 2889
Avalide Tablets 922
Benicar HCT Tablets 2852
Diovan HCT Tablets 2195
Dyazide Capsules 1389
Hyzaar 1964
Lotensin HCT Tablets 2235
Maxzide 2150
Micardis HCT Tablets 886
Moduretic Tablets 2003
Prinzide Tablets 2033
Teveten HCT Tablets 1710
Timolide Tablets 2056
Uniretic Tablets 3114
Vaseretic Tablets 2073
Zestoretic Tablets 701

Hydroflumethiazide (The effectiveness of diuretics in patients with underlying renal or cardiovascular disease may be diminished by the concomitant administration of aspirin due to inhibition of renal prostaglandins, leading to decreased renal blood flow, and salt and fluidretention).
No products indexed under this heading.

Ibuprofen (The concurrent use of aspirin with other NSAIDs should be avoided because this may increase bleeding or lead to decreased renal function). Products include:
Advil Allergy Sinus Caplets 737
Advil 737
Children's Advil Suspension 742
Children's Advil Chewable Tablets .. 741
Advil Cold & Sinus 739
Advil Flu & Body Ache Caplets 739
Children's Advil Cold Suspension ... 741
Infants' Advil Concentrated Drops .. 743
Junior Strength Advil Swallow Tablets 740
Advil Migraine Liquigels 740
Advil Multi-Symptom Cold Caplets 738
Combunox Tablets 1183
Children's Motrin Oral Suspension and Chewable Tablets 1837
Children's Motrin Cold Non-Staining Dye-Free Oral Suspension 1838
Children's Motrin Cold Oral Suspension 1838
Children's Motrin Non-Staining Dye-Free Oral Suspension 1837
Motrin Cold & Sinus Caplets 1836
Motrin IB Tablets and Caplets 1836
Infants' Motrin Concentrated Drops 1837
Infants' Motrin Non-Staining Dye-Free Drops 1837
Junior Strength Motrin Caplets and Chewable Tablets 1837
Vicoprofen Tablets 533

Indapamide (The effectiveness of diuretics in patients with underlying renal or cardiovascular disease may be diminished by the concomitant administration of aspirin due to inhibition of renal prostaglandins, leading to decreased renal blood flow, and salt and fluidretention). Products include:
Indapamide Tablets 2119

Indomethacin (The concurrent use of aspirin with other NSAIDs should be avoided because this may increase bleeding or lead to decreased renal function). Products include:
Indocin 1968

Indomethacin Sodium Trihydrate (The concurrent use of aspirin with other NSAIDs should be avoided because this may increase bleeding or lead to decreased renal function). Products include:
Indocin I.V. 1973

Ketoprofen (The concurrent use of aspirin with other NSAIDs should be avoided because this may increase bleeding or lead to decreased renal function).
No products indexed under this heading.

Ketorolac Tromethamine (The concurrent use of aspirin with other NSAIDs should be avoided because this may increase bleeding or lead to decreased renal function). Products include:
Acular Ophthalmic Solution 561
Acular LS Ophthalmic Solution 562

Labetalol Hydrochloride (The hypotensive effects of beta blockers may be diminished by the concomitant administration of aspirin due to inhibition of renal prostaglandins, leading to decreased renal blood flow, and salt and fluid retention).
No products indexed under this heading.

Levobunolol Hydrochloride (The hypotensive effects of beta blockers may be diminished by the concomitant administration of aspirin due to inhibition of renal prostaglandins, leading to decreased renal blood flow, and salt and fluid retention). Products include:
Betagan Ophthalmic Solution, USP .... ⊙ 217

Lisinopril (The hyponatremic and hypotensive effects of ACE inhibitors may be diminished by the concomitant administration of aspirin due to its indirect effect on the renin-angiotensin conversion pathway). Products include:
Prinivil Tablets 2029
Prinzide Tablets 2033
Zestoretic Tablets 701
Zestril Tablets 704

Low Molecular Weight Heparins (Patients on anticoagulation therapy are at increased risk for bleeding because of drug-drug interactions and the effect on platelets. Aspirin can displace warfarin from protein binding sites, leading to prolongation of both the prothrombin time and bleeding time. Aspirin can increase the anticoagulant activity of heparin, increasing bleeding risk).
No products indexed under this heading.

Meclofenamate Sodium (The concurrent use of aspirin with other NSAIDs should be avoided because this may increase bleeding or lead to decreased renal function).
No products indexed under this heading.

Mefenamic Acid (The concurrent use of aspirin with other NSAIDs should be avoided because this may increase bleeding or lead to decreased renal function).
No products indexed under this heading.

Meloxicam (The concurrent use of aspirin with other NSAIDs should be avoided because this may increase bleeding or lead to decreased renal function). Products include:
Mobic Oral Suspension 893
Mobic Tablets 893

Metformin Hydrochloride (Moderate doses of aspirin may increase the effectiveness of oral hypoglycemic drugs, leading to hypoglycemia). Products include:
ActoPlus Met Tablets 3219
Avandamet Tablets 1343
Fortamet Extended-Release Tablets 1156

Methotrexate (Salicylate can inhibit renal clearance of methotrexate, leading to bone marrow toxicity, especially in the elderly or renal-impaired).
No products indexed under this heading.

Methotrexate Sodium (Salicylate can inhibit renal clearance of methotrexate, leading to bone marrow toxicity, especially in the elderly or renal-impaired).
No products indexed under this heading.

Methyclothiazide (The effectiveness of diuretics in patients with underlying renal or cardiovascular disease may be diminished by the concomitant administration of aspirin due to inhibition of renal prostaglandins, leading to decreased renal blood flow, and salt and fluidretention).
No products indexed under this heading.

Metipranolol Hydrochloride (The hypotensive effects of beta blockers may be diminished by the concomitant administration of aspirin due to inhibition of renal prostaglandins, leading to decreased renal blood flow, and salt and fluid retention).
No products indexed under this heading.

Metolazone (The effectiveness of diuretics in patients with underlying renal or cardiovascular disease may be diminished by the concomitant administration of aspirin due to inhibition of renal prostaglandins, leading to decreased renal blood flow, and salt and fluidretention).
No products indexed under this heading.

Metoprolol Succinate (The hypotensive effects of beta blockers may be diminished by the concomitant administration of aspirin due to inhibition of renal prostaglandins, leading to decreased renal blood flow, and salt and fluid retention). Products include:
Toprol-XL Tablets 660

Metoprolol Tartrate (The hypotensive effects of beta blockers may be diminished by the concomitant administration of aspirin due to inhibition of renal prostaglandins, leading to decreased renal blood flow, and salt and fluid retention).
No products indexed under this heading.

Miglitol (Moderate doses of aspirin may increase the effectiveness of oral hypoglycemic drugs, leading to hypoglycemia).
No products indexed under this heading.

Moexipril Hydrochloride (The hyponatremic and hypotensive effects of ACE inhibitors may be diminished by the concomitant administration of aspirin due to its indirect effect on the renin-angiotensin conversion pathway). Products include:
Uniretic Tablets 3114
Univasc Tablets 3118

Nabumetone (The concurrent use of aspirin with other NSAIDs should be avoided because this may increase bleeding or lead to decreased renal function). Products include:
Relafen Tablets 1523

Nadolol (The hypotensive effects of beta blockers may be diminished by the concomitant administration of aspirin due to inhibition of renal prostaglandins, leading to decreased renal blood flow, and salt and fluid retention). Products include:
Nadolol Tablets 2121

Naproxen (The concurrent use of aspirin with other NSAIDs should be avoided because this may increase bleeding or lead to decreased renal function). Products include:
EC-Naprosyn Delayed-Release Tablets 2769
Naprosyn Suspension 2769
Naprosyn Tablets 2769
Prevacid NapraPAC 3277

Naproxen Sodium (The concurrent use of aspirin with other NSAIDs should be avoided because this may increase bleeding or lead to decreased renal function). Products include:
Aleve Tablets, Caplets and Gelcaps .... ▣605
Anaprox Tablets 2769
Anaprox DS Tablets 2769

Oxaprozin (The concurrent use of aspirin with other NSAIDs should be avoided because this may increase bleeding or lead to decreased renal function).
No products indexed under this heading.

Penbutolol Sulfate (The hypotensive effects of beta blockers may be diminished by the concomitant administration of aspirin due to inhibition of renal prostaglandins, leading to decreased renal blood flow, and salt and fluid retention).
No products indexed under this heading.

Perindopril Erbumine (The hyponatremic and hypotensive effects of ACE inhibitors may be diminished by the concomitant administration of aspirin due to its indirect effect on the renin-angiotensin conversion pathway). Products include:
Aceon Tablets (2 mg, 4 mg, 8 mg) 3191

Phenylbutazone (The concurrent use of aspirin with other NSAIDs should be avoided because this may increase bleeding or lead to decreased renal function).
No products indexed under this heading.

Phenytoin (Salicylate can displace protein-bound phenytoin, leading to a decrease in the total concentration of phenytoin).
No products indexed under this heading.

Phenytoin Sodium (Salicylate can displace protein-bound phenytoin, leading to a decrease in the total concentration of phenytoin). Products include:
Phenytek Capsules 2153

Pindolol (The hypotensive effects of beta blockers may be diminished by the concomitant administration of aspirin due to inhibition of renal prostaglandins, leading to decreased renal blood flow, and salt and fluid retention).
No products indexed under this heading.

Pioglitazone Hydrochloride (Moderate doses of aspirin may increase the effectiveness of oral hypoglycemic drugs, leading to hypoglycemia). Products include:
ActoPlus Met Tablets 3219
Actos Tablets 3224

Piroxicam (The concurrent use of aspirin with other NSAIDs should be avoided because this may increase bleeding or lead to decreased renal function).
No products indexed under this heading.

Polythiazide (The effectiveness of diuretics in patients with underlying renal or cardiovascular disease may be diminished by the concomitant administration of aspirin due to inhibition of renal prostaglandins, leading to decreased renal blood flow, and salt and fluidretention).
No products indexed under this heading.

Probenecid (Salicylates antagonize the uricosuric action of uricouric agents).
No products indexed under this heading.

Propranolol Hydrochloride (The hypotensive effects of beta blockers may be diminished by the concomitant administration of aspirin due to inhibition of renal prostaglandins, leading to decreased renal blood flow, and salt and fluid retention). Products include:
Inderal LA Long-Acting Capsules 3421
InnoPran XL Capsules 2728

Quinapril Hydrochloride (The hyponatremic and hypotensive effects of ACE inhibitors may be diminished by the concomitant administration of aspirin due to its indirect effect on the renin-angiotensin conversion pathway).
No products indexed under this heading.

Ramipril (The hyponatremic and hypotensive effects of ACE inhibitors may be diminished by the concomitant administration of aspirin due to its indirect effect on the renin-angiotensin conversion pathway). Products include:
Altace Capsules 1673

Repaglinide (Moderate doses of aspirin may increase the effectiveness of oral hypoglycemic drugs, leading to hypoglycemia). Products include:
Prandin Tablets (0.5, 1, and 2 mg) 2337

Rofecoxib (The concurrent use of aspirin with other NSAIDs should be avoided because this may increase bleeding or lead to decreased renal function).
No products indexed under this heading.

Rosiglitazone Maleate (Moderate doses of aspirin may increase the effectiveness of oral hypoglycemic drugs, leading to hypoglycemia). Products include:
Avandamet Tablets 1343
Avandia Tablets 1348

Sotalol Hydrochloride (The hypotensive effects of beta blockers may be diminished by the concomitant administration of aspirin due to inhibition of renal prostaglandins, leading to decreased renal blood flow, and salt and fluid retention).
No products indexed under this heading.

Spirapril Hydrochloride (The hyponatremic and hypotensive effects of ACE inhibitors may be diminished by the concomitant administration of aspirin due to its indirect effect on the renin-angiotensin conversion pathway).
No products indexed under this heading.

Spironolactone (The effectiveness of diuretics in patients with underlying renal or cardiovascular disease may be diminished by the concomitant administration of aspirin due to inhibition of renal prostaglandins, leading to decreased renal blood flow, and salt and fluidretention).
No products indexed under this heading.

Sulfinpyrazone (Salicylates antagonize the uricosuric action of uricouric agents).
No products indexed under this heading.

Sulindac (The concurrent use of aspirin with other NSAIDs should be avoided because this may increase bleeding or lead to decreased renal function). Products include:
Clinoril Tablets 1899

Timolol Hemihydrate (The hypotensive effects of beta blockers may be diminished by the concomitant administration of aspirin due to inhibition of renal prostaglandins, leading to decreased renal blood flow, and salt and fluid retention). Products include:
Betimol Ophthalmic Solution 3371
Betimol Ophthalmic Solution .... ⊙283

Timolol Maleate (The hypotensive effects of beta blockers may be diminished by the concomitant administration of aspirin due to inhibition of renal prostaglandins, leading to decreased renal blood flow, and salt and fluid retention). Products include:
Blocadren Tablets 1891
Cosopt Sterile Ophthalmic Solution 1910
Timolide Tablets 2056
Timoptic in Ocudose 2061
Timoptic Sterile Ophthalmic Solution 2058
Timoptic-XE Sterile Ophthalmic Gel Forming Solution 2062

Tinzaparin Sodium (Patients on anticoagulation therapy are at increased risk for bleeding because of drug-drug interactions and the effect on platelets. Aspirin can displace warfarin from protein binding sites, leading to prolongation of both the prothrombin time and bleeding time. Aspirin can increase the anticoagulant activity of heparin, increasing bleeding risk).
No products indexed under this heading.

Tolazamide (Moderate doses of aspirin may increase the effectiveness of oral hypoglycemic drugs, leading to hypoglycemia).
No products indexed under this heading.

Tolbutamide (Moderate doses of aspirin may increase the effectiveness of oral hypoglycemic drugs, leading to hypoglycemia).
No products indexed under this heading.

Tolmetin Sodium (The concurrent use of aspirin with other NSAIDs should be avoided because this may increase bleeding or lead to decreased renal function).
No products indexed under this heading.

Torsemide (The effectiveness of diuretics in patients with underlying renal or cardiovascular disease may be diminished by the concomitant administration of aspirin due to inhibition of renal prostaglandins, leading to decreased renal blood flow, and salt and fluidretention).
No products indexed under this heading.

Trandolapril (The hyponatremic and hypotensive effects of ACE inhibitors may be diminished by the concomitant administration of aspirin due to its indirect effect on the renin-angiotensin conversion pathway). Products include:
Mavik Tablets 482
Tarka Tablets 519

Triamterene (The effectiveness of diuretics in patients with underlying renal or cardiovascular disease may be diminished by the concomitant administration of aspirin due to inhibition of renal prostaglandins, leading to decreased renal blood flow, and salt and fluidretention). Products include:
Dyazide Capsules 1389
Dyrenium Capsules 3390
Maxzide 2150

Troglitazone (Moderate doses of aspirin may increase the effectiveness of oral hypoglycemic drugs, leading to hypoglycemia).
No products indexed under this heading.

Valdecoxib (The concurrent use of aspirin with other NSAIDs should be avoided because this may increase bleeding or lead to decreased renal function).
No products indexed under this heading.

Valproate Sodium (Salicylate can displace protein-bound valproic acid, leading to an increase in serum valproic acid levels). Products include:
Depacon Injection 412

Valproic Acid (Salicylate can displace protein-bound valproic acid, leading to an increase in serum valproic acid levels). Products include:
Depakene 417

Warfarin Sodium (Patients on anticoagulation therapy are at increased risk for bleeding because of drug-drug interactions and the effect on platelets. Aspirin can displace warfarin from protein binding sites, leading to prolongation of both the prothrombin time and bleeding time. Aspirin can increase the anticoagulant activity of heparin, increasing bleeding risk). Products include:
Coumadin for Injection 932
Coumadin Tablets 932

BC POWDER
(Aspirin, Caffeine, Salicylamide) .... ▣612
See BC Allergy Sinus Cold Powder

BC ALLERGY SINUS COLD POWDER
(Aspirin, Chlorpheniramine Maleate, Pseudoephedrine Hydrochloride) .... ▣612
May interact with oral anticoagulants, oral hypoglycemic agents, monoamine oxidase inhibitors, and certain other agents. Compounds in these categories include:

Acarbose (Concurrent use should be avoided unless directed by a physician). Products include:
Precose Tablets 776

Anisindione (Concurrent use should be avoided unless directed by a physician). Products include:
Miradon Tablets 3056

Chlorpropamide (Concurrent use should be avoided unless directed by a physician).
No products indexed under this heading.

Dicumarol (Concurrent use should be avoided unless directed by a physician).
No products indexed under this heading.

Glimepiride (Concurrent use should be avoided unless directed by a physician). Products include:
Amaryl Tablets 2864

Glipizide (Concurrent use should be avoided unless directed by a physician).
No products indexed under this heading.

Glyburide (Concurrent use should be avoided unless directed by a physician).
No products indexed under this heading.

Isocarboxazid (Concurrent use with MAO inhibitors is not recommended; consult your doctor).
No products indexed under this heading.

Metformin Hydrochloride (Concurrent use should be avoided unless directed by a physician). Products include:
ActoPlus Met Tablets 3219
Avandamet Tablets 1343
Fortamet Extended-Release Tablets 1156

Miglitol (Concurrent use should be avoided unless directed by a physician).
No products indexed under this heading.

Moclobemide (Concurrent use with MAO inhibitors is not recommended; consult your doctor).
No products indexed under this heading.

Pargyline Hydrochloride (Concurrent use with MAO inhibitors is not recommended; consult your doctor).
No products indexed under this heading.

Phenelzine Sulfate (Concurrent use with MAO inhibitors is not recommended; consult your doctor).
No products indexed under this heading.

Pioglitazone Hydrochloride (Concurrent use should be avoided unless directed by a physician). Products include:
ActoPlus Met Tablets 3219
Actos Tablets 3224

Procarbazine Hydrochloride (Concurrent use with MAO inhibitors is not recommended; consult your doctor). Products include:
Matulane Capsules 3188

Repaglinide (Concurrent use should be avoided unless directed by a physician). Products include:
Prandin Tablets (0.5, 1, and 2 mg) 2337

Rosiglitazone Maleate (Concurrent use should be avoided unless directed by a physician). Products include:
Avandamet Tablets 1343
Avandia Tablets 1348

Selegiline Hydrochloride (Concurrent use with MAO inhibitors is not recommended; consult your doctor). Products include:
Eldepryl Capsules 3209

Tolazamide (Concurrent use should be avoided unless directed by a physician).
No products indexed under this heading.

Tolbutamide (Concurrent use should be avoided unless directed by a physician).
No products indexed under this heading.

Tranylcypromine Sulfate (Concurrent use with MAO inhibitors is not recommended; consult your doctor). Products include:
Parnate Tablets 1499

Troglitazone (Concurrent use should be avoided unless directed by a physician).
No products indexed under this heading.

Warfarin Sodium (Concurrent use should be avoided unless directed by a physician). Products include:
Coumadin for Injection 932
Coumadin Tablets 932

Food Interactions

Alcohol (Individuals consuming 3 or more alcohol-containing drinks per day should consult their physician for advice on when and how they should take this product; increases drowsiness; avoid concurrent use).

ARTHRITIS STRENGTH BC POWDER

(Aspirin, Caffeine, Salicylamide) 612
See BC Allergy Sinus Cold Powder

BC SINUS COLD POWDER

(Aspirin, Pseudoephedrine Hydrochloride)................................ 612
See BC Allergy Sinus Cold Powder

BEANO LIQUID

(Alpha Galactosidase Enzyme) 764
None cited in PDR database.

BEANO TABLETS

(Alpha Galactosidase Enzyme) 764
None cited in PDR database.

BECONASE AQ NASAL SPRAY

(Beclomethasone Dipropionate Monohydrate)................................... 1359
None cited in PDR database.

BEELITH TABLETS

(Magnesium Oxide, Vitamin B_6) 784
May interact with:

Prescription Drugs, unspecified (Concurrent use should be avoided).

BENADRYL ALLERGY & COLD TABLETS

(Acetaminophen, Diphenhydramine Hydrochloride, Pseudoephedrine Hydrochloride)....... 692
May interact with hypnotics and sedatives, monoamine oxidase inhibitors, tranquilizers, and certain other agents. Compounds in these categories include:

Alprazolam (Concurrent use may increase drowsiness). Products include:
Niravam Orally Disintegrating Tablets 3106
Xanax XR Tablets 2655

Buspirone Hydrochloride (Concurrent use may increase drowsiness).
No products indexed under this heading.

Chlordiazepoxide (Concurrent use may increase drowsiness).
No products indexed under this heading.

Chlordiazepoxide Hydrochloride (Concurrent use may increase drowsiness). Products include:
Librium Capsules 3349

Chlorpromazine (Concurrent use may increase drowsiness).
No products indexed under this heading.

Chlorpromazine Hydrochloride (Concurrent use may increase drowsiness).
No products indexed under this heading.

Chlorprothixene (Concurrent use may increase drowsiness).
No products indexed under this heading.

Chlorprothixene Hydrochloride (Concurrent use may increase drowsiness).
No products indexed under this heading.

Clorazepate Dipotassium (Concurrent use may increase drowsiness). Products include:
Tranxene 2488

Diazepam (Concurrent use may increase drowsiness). Products include:
Diastat Rectal Delivery System 3344
Valium Tablets 2822

Droperidol (Concurrent use may increase drowsiness).
No products indexed under this heading.

Estazolam (Concurrent use may increase drowsiness). Products include:
ProSom Tablets 512

Ethchlorvynol (Concurrent use may increase drowsiness).
No products indexed under this heading.

Ethinamate (Concurrent use may increase drowsiness).
No products indexed under this heading.

Fluphenazine Decanoate (Concurrent use may increase drowsiness).
No products indexed under this heading.

Fluphenazine Enanthate (Concurrent use may increase drowsiness).
No products indexed under this heading.

Fluphenazine Hydrochloride (Concurrent use may increase drowsiness).
No products indexed under this heading.

Flurazepam Hydrochloride (Concurrent use may increase drowsiness). Products include:
Dalmane Capsules 3343

Glutethimide (Concurrent use may increase drowsiness).
No products indexed under this heading.

Haloperidol (Concurrent use may increase drowsiness).
No products indexed under this heading.

Haloperidol Decanoate (Concurrent use may increase drowsiness).
No products indexed under this heading.

Hydroxyzine Hydrochloride (Concurrent use may increase drowsiness).
No products indexed under this heading.

Isocarboxazid (Avoid use with, or for two weeks after stopping, MAOI drugs).
No products indexed under this heading.

Lorazepam (Concurrent use may increase drowsiness).
No products indexed under this heading.

Loxapine Hydrochloride (Concurrent use may increase drowsiness).
No products indexed under this heading.

Loxapine Succinate (Concurrent use may increase drowsiness).
No products indexed under this heading.

Meprobamate (Concurrent use may increase drowsiness).
No products indexed under this heading.

Mesoridazine Besylate (Concurrent use may increase drowsiness).
No products indexed under this heading.

Midazolam Hydrochloride (Concurrent use may increase drowsiness).
No products indexed under this heading.

Moclobemide (Avoid use with, or for two weeks after stopping, MAOI drugs).
No products indexed under this heading.

Molindone Hydrochloride (Concurrent use may increase drowsiness). Products include:
Moban Tablets 1108

Oxazepam (Concurrent use may increase drowsiness).
No products indexed under this heading.

Pargyline Hydrochloride (Avoid use with, or for two weeks after stopping, MAOI drugs).
No products indexed under this heading.

Perphenazine (Concurrent use may increase drowsiness).
No products indexed under this heading.

Phenelzine Sulfate (Avoid use with, or for two weeks after stopping, MAOI drugs).
No products indexed under this heading.

Prazepam (Concurrent use may increase drowsiness).
No products indexed under this heading.

Procarbazine Hydrochloride (Avoid use with, or for two weeks after stopping, MAOI drugs). Products include:
Matulane Capsules 3188

Prochlorperazine (Concurrent use may increase drowsiness).
No products indexed under this heading.

Promethazine Hydrochloride (Concurrent use may increase drowsiness). Products include:
Phenergan 3438

Propofol (Concurrent use may increase drowsiness). Products include:
Diprivan Injectable Emulsion 676

Quazepam (Concurrent use may increase drowsiness).
No products indexed under this heading.

Secobarbital Sodium (Concurrent use may increase drowsiness).
No products indexed under this heading.

Selegiline Hydrochloride (Avoid use with, or for two weeks after stopping, MAOI drugs). Products include:
Eldepryl Capsules 3209

Temazepam (Concurrent use may increase drowsiness).
No products indexed under this heading.

Thioridazine Hydrochloride (Concurrent use may increase drowsiness). Products include:
Thioridazine Hydrochloride Tablets.. 2122

Thiothixene (Concurrent use may increase drowsiness). Products include:
Thiothixene Capsules 2124

Tranylcypromine Sulfate (Avoid use with, or for two weeks after stopping, MAOI drugs). Products include:
Parnate Tablets 1499

Triazolam (Concurrent use may increase drowsiness).
No products indexed under this heading.

Trifluoperazine Hydrochloride (Concurrent use may increase drowsiness).
No products indexed under this heading.

Zaleplon (Concurrent use may increase drowsiness). Products include:
Sonata Capsules 1686

Zolpidem Tartrate (Concurrent use may increase drowsiness). Products include:
Ambien Tablets 2867

Food Interactions

Alcohol (Concurrent use may increase drowsiness).

BENADRYL ALLERGY KAPSEAL CAPSULES

(Diphenhydramine Hydrochloride) ..... ▣691

May interact with hypnotics and sedatives, tranquilizers, and certain other agents. Compounds in these categories include:

Alprazolam (May increase drowsiness effect). Products include:
Niravam Orally Disintegrating Tablets.. 3106
Xanax XR Tablets 2655

Buspirone Hydrochloride (May increase drowsiness effect).
No products indexed under this heading.

Chlordiazepoxide (May increase drowsiness effect).
No products indexed under this heading.

Chlordiazepoxide Hydrochloride (May increase drowsiness effect). Products include:
Librium Capsules 3349

Chlorpromazine (May increase drowsiness effect).
No products indexed under this heading.

Chlorpromazine Hydrochloride (May increase drowsiness effect).
No products indexed under this heading.

Chlorprothixene (May increase drowsiness effect).
No products indexed under this heading.

Chlorprothixene Hydrochloride (May increase drowsiness effect).
No products indexed under this heading.

Clorazepate Dipotassium (May increase drowsiness effect). Products include:
Tranxene 2488

Diazepam (May increase drowsiness effect). Products include:
Diastat Rectal Delivery System 3344
Valium Tablets 2822

Droperidol (May increase drowsiness effect).
No products indexed under this heading.

Estazolam (May increase drowsiness effect). Products include:
ProSom Tablets 512

Ethchlorvynol (May increase drowsiness effect).
No products indexed under this heading.

Ethinamate (May increase drowsiness effect).
No products indexed under this heading.

Fluphenazine Decanoate (May increase drowsiness effect).
No products indexed under this heading.

Fluphenazine Enanthate (May increase drowsiness effect).
No products indexed under this heading.

Fluphenazine Hydrochloride (May increase drowsiness effect).
No products indexed under this heading.

Flurazepam Hydrochloride (May increase drowsiness effect). Products include:
Dalmane Capsules 3343

Glutethimide (May increase drowsiness effect).
No products indexed under this heading.

Haloperidol (May increase drowsiness effect).
No products indexed under this heading.

Haloperidol Decanoate (May increase drowsiness effect).
No products indexed under this heading.

Hydroxyzine Hydrochloride (May increase drowsiness effect).
No products indexed under this heading.

Lorazepam (May increase drowsiness effect).
No products indexed under this heading.

Loxapine Hydrochloride (May increase drowsiness effect).
No products indexed under this heading.

Loxapine Succinate (May increase drowsiness effect).
No products indexed under this heading.

Meprobamate (May increase drowsiness effect).
No products indexed under this heading.

Mesoridazine Besylate (May increase drowsiness effect).
No products indexed under this heading.

Midazolam Hydrochloride (May increase drowsiness effect).
No products indexed under this heading.

Molindone Hydrochloride (May increase drowsiness effect). Products include:
Moban Tablets 1108

Oxazepam (May increase drowsiness effect).
No products indexed under this heading.

Perphenazine (May increase drowsiness effect).
No products indexed under this heading.

Prazepam (May increase drowsiness effect).
No products indexed under this heading.

Prochlorperazine (May increase drowsiness effect).
No products indexed under this heading.

Promethazine Hydrochloride (May increase drowsiness effect). Products include:
Phenergan 3438

Propofol (May increase drowsiness effect). Products include:
Diprivan Injectable Emulsion 676

Quazepam (May increase drowsiness effect).
No products indexed under this heading.

Secobarbital Sodium (May increase drowsiness effect).
No products indexed under this heading.

Temazepam (May increase drowsiness effect).
No products indexed under this heading.

Thioridazine Hydrochloride (May increase drowsiness effect). Products include:
Thioridazine Hydrochloride Tablets.. 2122

Thiothixene (May increase drowsiness effect). Products include:
Thiothixene Capsules 2124

Triazolam (May increase drowsiness effect).
No products indexed under this heading.

Trifluoperazine Hydrochloride (May increase drowsiness effect).
No products indexed under this heading.

Zaleplon (May increase drowsiness effect). Products include:
Sonata Capsules 1686

Zolpidem Tartrate (May increase drowsiness effect). Products include:
Ambien Tablets 2867

Food Interactions

Alcohol (May increase drowsiness effect).

BENADRYL ALLERGY ULTRATAB TABLETS

(Diphenhydramine Hydrochloride) ..... ▣691

See Benadryl Allergy Kapseal Capsules

BENADRYL ALLERGY & SINUS HEADACHE CAPLETS & GELCAPS

(Acetaminophen, Diphenhydramine Hydrochloride, Pseudoephedrine Hydrochloride)....... ▣693

See Benadryl D Tablets

CHILDREN'S BENADRYL ALLERGY LIQUID

(Diphenhydramine Hydrochloride) ..... ▣695

See Benadryl Allergy Kapseal Capsules

CHILDREN'S BENADRYL ALLERGY & COLD FASTMELT TABLETS

(Diphenhydramine Citrate, Pseudoephedrine Hydrochloride)....... ▣695

May interact with hypnotics and sedatives, monoamine oxidase inhibitors, tranquilizers, and certain other agents. Compounds in these categories include:

Alprazolam (May increase drowsiness effect; consult your physician). Products include:
Niravam Orally Disintegrating Tablets.. 3106
Xanax XR Tablets 2655

Buspirone Hydrochloride (May increase drowsiness effect; consult your physician).
No products indexed under this heading.

Chlordiazepoxide (May increase drowsiness effect; consult your physician).
No products indexed under this heading.

Chlordiazepoxide Hydrochloride (May increase drowsiness effect; consult your physician). Products include:
Librium Capsules 3349

Chlorpromazine (May increase drowsiness effect; consult your physician).
No products indexed under this heading.

Chlorpromazine Hydrochloride (May increase drowsiness effect; consult your physician).
No products indexed under this heading.

Chlorprothixene (May increase drowsiness effect; consult your physician).
No products indexed under this heading.

Chlorprothixene Hydrochloride (May increase drowsiness effect; consult your physician).
No products indexed under this heading.

Clorazepate Dipotassium (May increase drowsiness effect; consult your physician). Products include:
Tranxene 2488

Diazepam (May increase drowsiness effect; consult your physician). Products include:
Diastat Rectal Delivery System 3344
Valium Tablets 2822

Droperidol (May increase drowsiness effect; consult your physician).
No products indexed under this heading.

Estazolam (May increase drowsiness effect; consult your physician). Products include:
ProSom Tablets 512

Ethchlorvynol (May increase drowsiness effect; consult your physician).
No products indexed under this heading.

Ethinamate (May increase drowsiness effect; consult your physician).
No products indexed under this heading.

Fluphenazine Decanoate (May increase drowsiness effect; consult your physician).
No products indexed under this heading.

Fluphenazine Enanthate (May increase drowsiness effect; consult your physician).
No products indexed under this heading.

Fluphenazine Hydrochloride (May increase drowsiness effect; consult your physician).
No products indexed under this heading.

Flurazepam Hydrochloride (May increase drowsiness effect; consult your physician). Products include:
Dalmane Capsules **3343**

Glutethimide (May increase drowsiness effect; consult your physician).
No products indexed under this heading.

Haloperidol (May increase drowsiness effect; consult your physician).
No products indexed under this heading.

Haloperidol Decanoate (May increase drowsiness effect; consult your physician).
No products indexed under this heading.

Hydroxyzine Hydrochloride (May increase drowsiness effect; consult your physician).
No products indexed under this heading.

Isocarboxazid (Concurrent and/or sequential use with MAO inhibitors is not recommended).
No products indexed under this heading.

Lorazepam (May increase drowsiness effect; consult your physician).
No products indexed under this heading.

Loxapine Hydrochloride (May increase drowsiness effect; consult your physician).
No products indexed under this heading.

Loxapine Succinate (May increase drowsiness effect; consult your physician).
No products indexed under this heading.

Meprobamate (May increase drowsiness effect; consult your physician).
No products indexed under this heading.

Mesoridazine Besylate (May increase drowsiness effect; consult your physician).
No products indexed under this heading.

Midazolam Hydrochloride (May increase drowsiness effect; consult your physician).
No products indexed under this heading.

Moclobemide (Concurrent and/or sequential use with MAO inhibitors is not recommended).
No products indexed under this heading.

Molindone Hydrochloride (May increase drowsiness effect; consult your physician). Products include:
Moban Tablets **1108**

Oxazepam (May increase drowsiness effect; consult your physician).
No products indexed under this heading.

Pargyline Hydrochloride (Concurrent and/or sequential use with MAO inhibitors is not recommended).
No products indexed under this heading.

Perphenazine (May increase drowsiness effect; consult your physician).
No products indexed under this heading.

Phenelzine Sulfate (Concurrent and/or sequential use with MAO inhibitors is not recommended).
No products indexed under this heading.

Prazepam (May increase drowsiness effect; consult your physician).
No products indexed under this heading.

Procarbazine Hydrochloride (Concurrent and/or sequential use with MAO inhibitors is not recommended). Products include:
Matulane Capsules **3188**

Prochlorperazine (May increase drowsiness effect; consult your physician).
No products indexed under this heading.

Promethazine Hydrochloride (May increase drowsiness effect; consult your physician). Products include:
Phenergan **3438**

Propofol (May increase drowsiness effect; consult your physician). Products include:
Diprivan Injectable Emulsion **676**

Quazepam (May increase drowsiness effect; consult your physician).
No products indexed under this heading.

Secobarbital Sodium (May increase drowsiness effect; consult your physician).
No products indexed under this heading.

Selegiline Hydrochloride (Concurrent and/or sequential use with MAO inhibitors is not recommended). Products include:
Eldepryl Capsules **3209**

Temazepam (May increase drowsiness effect; consult your physician).
No products indexed under this heading.

Thioridazine Hydrochloride (May increase drowsiness effect; consult your physician). Products include:
Thioridazine Hydrochloride Tablets **2122**

Thiothixene (May increase drowsiness effect; consult your physician). Products include:
Thiothixene Capsules **2124**

Tranylcypromine Sulfate (Concurrent and/or sequential use with MAO inhibitors is not recommended). Products include:
Parnate Tablets **1499**

Triazolam (May increase drowsiness effect; consult your physician).
No products indexed under this heading.

Trifluoperazine Hydrochloride (May increase drowsiness effect; consult your physician).
No products indexed under this heading.

Zaleplon (May increase drowsiness effect; consult your physician). Products include:
Sonata Capsules **1686**

Zolpidem Tartrate (May increase drowsiness effect; consult your physician). Products include:
Ambien Tablets **2867**

Food Interactions

Alcohol (May increase drowsiness effect; avoid concurrent use).

CHILDREN'S BENADRYL DYE-FREE ALLERGY LIQUID

(Diphenhydramine Hydrochloride) **695**
May interact with hypnotics and sedatives, tranquilizers, and certain other agents. Compounds in these categories include:

Alprazolam (May increase the drowsiness effect). Products include:
Niravam Orally Disintegrating Tablets **3106**
Xanax XR Tablets **2655**

Buspirone Hydrochloride (May increase the drowsiness effect).
No products indexed under this heading.

Chlordiazepoxide (May increase the drowsiness effect).
No products indexed under this heading.

Chlordiazepoxide Hydrochloride (May increase the drowsiness effect). Products include:
Librium Capsules **3349**

Chlorpromazine (May increase the drowsiness effect).
No products indexed under this heading.

Chlorpromazine Hydrochloride (May increase the drowsiness effect).
No products indexed under this heading.

Chlorprothixene (May increase the drowsiness effect).
No products indexed under this heading.

Chlorprothixene Hydrochloride (May increase the drowsiness effect).
No products indexed under this heading.

Clorazepate Dipotassium (May increase the drowsiness effect). Products include:
Tranxene **2488**

Diazepam (May increase the drowsiness effect). Products include:
Diastat Rectal Delivery System **3344**
Valium Tablets **2822**

Droperidol (May increase the drowsiness effect).
No products indexed under this heading.

Estazolam (May increase the drowsiness effect). Products include:
ProSom Tablets **512**

Ethchlorvynol (May increase the drowsiness effect).
No products indexed under this heading.

Ethinamate (May increase the drowsiness effect).
No products indexed under this heading.

Fluphenazine Decanoate (May increase the drowsiness effect).
No products indexed under this heading.

Fluphenazine Enanthate (May increase the drowsiness effect).
No products indexed under this heading.

Fluphenazine Hydrochloride (May increase the drowsiness effect).
No products indexed under this heading.

Flurazepam Hydrochloride (May increase the drowsiness effect). Products include:
Dalmane Capsules **3343**

Glutethimide (May increase the drowsiness effect).
No products indexed under this heading.

Haloperidol (May increase the drowsiness effect).
No products indexed under this heading.

Haloperidol Decanoate (May increase the drowsiness effect).
No products indexed under this heading.

Hydroxyzine Hydrochloride (May increase the drowsiness effect).
No products indexed under this heading.

Lorazepam (May increase the drowsiness effect).
No products indexed under this heading.

Loxapine Hydrochloride (May increase the drowsiness effect).
No products indexed under this heading.

Loxapine Succinate (May increase the drowsiness effect).
No products indexed under this heading.

Meprobamate (May increase the drowsiness effect).
No products indexed under this heading.

Mesoridazine Besylate (May increase the drowsiness effect).
No products indexed under this heading.

Midazolam Hydrochloride (May increase the drowsiness effect).
No products indexed under this heading.

Molindone Hydrochloride (May increase the drowsiness effect). Products include:
Moban Tablets **1108**

Oxazepam (May increase the drowsiness effect).
No products indexed under this heading.

Perphenazine (May increase the drowsiness effect).
No products indexed under this heading.

Prazepam (May increase the drowsiness effect).
No products indexed under this heading.

Prochlorperazine (May increase the drowsiness effect).
No products indexed under this heading.

Promethazine Hydrochloride (May increase the drowsiness effect). Products include:
Phenergan **3438**

Propofol (May increase the drowsiness effect). Products include:
Diprivan Injectable Emulsion **676**

IMPORTANT NOTE: Always consult each drug listing in the patient's regimen for possible interactions.

Quazepam (May increase the drowsiness effect).
No products indexed under this heading.

Secobarbital Sodium (May increase the drowsiness effect).
No products indexed under this heading.

Temazepam (May increase the drowsiness effect).
No products indexed under this heading.

Thioridazine Hydrochloride (May increase the drowsiness effect). Products include:
Thioridazine Hydrochloride Tablets 2122

Thiothixene (May increase the drowsiness effect). Products include:
Thiothixene Capsules 2124

Triazolam (May increase the drowsiness effect).
No products indexed under this heading.

Trifluoperazine Hydrochloride (May increase the drowsiness effect).
No products indexed under this heading.

Zaleplon (May increase the drowsiness effect). Products include:
Sonata Capsules 1686

Zolpidem Tartrate (May increase the drowsiness effect). Products include:
Ambien Tablets 2867

Food Interactions

Alcohol (May increase the drowsiness effect).

BENADRYL DYE-FREE ALLERGY LIQUI-GELS SOFTGELS

(Diphenhydramine Hydrochloride) .... ▣692
See Benadryl Allergy Kapseal Capsules

BENADRYL ITCH RELIEF STICK EXTRA STRENGTH

(Diphenhydramine Hydrochloride, Zinc Acetate) .... ▣696
May interact with:

Diphenhydramine (Concurrent use with other diphenydramine-containing products is not recommended). Products include:
Tylenol Sore Throat NightTime Liquid with Cool Burst 1849

BENADRYL ITCH STOPPING CREAM EXTRA STRENGTH

(Diphenhydramine Hydrochloride, Zinc Acetate) .... ▣697
May interact with:

Diphenhydramine (Concurrent use with other diphenhydramine-containing products is not recommended). Products include:
Tylenol Sore Throat NightTime Liquid with Cool Burst 1849

BENADRYL ITCH STOPPING GEL EXTRA STRENGTH

(Diphenhydramine Hydrochloride) .... ▣697
May interact with:

Diphenhydramine (Concurrent use with other diphenhydramine-containing products is not recommended). Products include:
Tylenol Sore Throat NightTime Liquid with Cool Burst 1849

BENADRYL ITCH STOPPING SPRAY EXTRA STRENGTH

(Diphenhydramine Hydrochloride, Zinc Acetate) .... ▣697
May interact with:

Diphenhydramine (Concurrent use with other diphenhydramine-containing products is not recommended). Products include:
Tylenol Sore Throat NightTime Liquid with Cool Burst 1849

BENADRYL MAXIMUM STRENGTH SEVERE ALLERGY & SINUS HEADACHE CAPLETS

(Acetaminophen, Diphenhydramine Hydrochloride, Pseudoephedrine Hydrochloride) .... ▣694
See Benadryl D Tablets

CHILDREN'S BENADRYL D ALLERGY & SINUS FASTMELT TABLETS

(Diphenhydramine Citrate, Pseudoephedrine Hydrochloride) .... ▣694
See Benadryl D Tablets

CHILDREN'S BENADRYL D LIQUID MEDICATION

(Diphenhydramine Hydrochloride, Pseudoephedrine Hydrochloride) .... ▣693
See Benadryl D Tablets

BENADRYL D TABLETS

(Diphenhydramine Hydrochloride, Pseudoephedrine Hydrochloride) .... ▣694
May interact with hypnotics and sedatives, monoamine oxidase inhibitors, tranquilizers, and certain other agents. Compounds in these categories include:

Alprazolam (May increase drowsiness effect). Products include:
Niravam Orally Disintegrating Tablets 3106
Xanax XR Tablets 2655

Buspirone Hydrochloride (May increase drowsiness effect).
No products indexed under this heading.

Chlordiazepoxide (May increase drowsiness effect).
No products indexed under this heading.

Chlordiazepoxide Hydrochloride (May increase drowsiness effect). Products include:
Librium Capsules 3349

Chlorpromazine (May increase drowsiness effect).
No products indexed under this heading.

Chlorpromazine Hydrochloride (May increase drowsiness effect).
No products indexed under this heading.

Chlorprothixene (May increase drowsiness effect).
No products indexed under this heading.

Chlorprothixene Hydrochloride (May increase drowsiness effect).
No products indexed under this heading.

Clorazepate Dipotassium (May increase drowsiness effect). Products include:
Tranxene 2488

Diazepam (May increase drowsiness effect). Products include:
Diastat Rectal Delivery System 3344
Valium Tablets 2822

Diphenhydramine (Concurrent use with other diphenhydramine containing products is not recommended). Products include:
Tylenol Sore Throat NightTime Liquid with Cool Burst 1849

Droperidol (May increase drowsiness effect).
No products indexed under this heading.

Estazolam (May increase drowsiness effect). Products include:
ProSom Tablets 512

Ethchlorvynol (May increase drowsiness effect).
No products indexed under this heading.

Ethinamate (May increase drowsiness effect).
No products indexed under this heading.

Fluphenazine Decanoate (May increase drowsiness effect).
No products indexed under this heading.

Fluphenazine Enanthate (May increase drowsiness effect).
No products indexed under this heading.

Fluphenazine Hydrochloride (May increase drowsiness effect).
No products indexed under this heading.

Flurazepam Hydrochloride (May increase drowsiness effect). Products include:
Dalmane Capsules 3343

Glutethimide (May increase drowsiness effect).
No products indexed under this heading.

Haloperidol (May increase drowsiness effect).
No products indexed under this heading.

Haloperidol Decanoate (May increase drowsiness effect).
No products indexed under this heading.

Hydroxyzine Hydrochloride (May increase drowsiness effect).
No products indexed under this heading.

Isocarboxazid (Concurrent and/or sequential use with MAO inhibitors is not recommended).
No products indexed under this heading.

Lorazepam (May increase drowsiness effect).
No products indexed under this heading.

Loxapine Hydrochloride (May increase drowsiness effect).
No products indexed under this heading.

Loxapine Succinate (May increase drowsiness effect).
No products indexed under this heading.

Meprobamate (May increase drowsiness effect).
No products indexed under this heading.

Mesoridazine Besylate (May increase drowsiness effect).
No products indexed under this heading.

Midazolam Hydrochloride (May increase drowsiness effect).
No products indexed under this heading.

Moclobemide (Concurrent and/or sequential use with MAO inhibitors is not recommended).
No products indexed under this heading.

Molindone Hydrochloride (May increase drowsiness effect). Products include:
Moban Tablets 1108

Oxazepam (May increase drowsiness effect).
No products indexed under this heading.

Pargyline Hydrochloride (Concurrent and/or sequential use with MAO inhibitors is not recommended).
No products indexed under this heading.

Perphenazine (May increase drowsiness effect).
No products indexed under this heading.

Phenelzine Sulfate (Concurrent and/or sequential use with MAO inhibitors is not recommended).
No products indexed under this heading.

Prazepam (May increase drowsiness effect).
No products indexed under this heading.

Procarbazine Hydrochloride (Concurrent and/or sequential use with MAO inhibitors is not recommended). Products include:
Matulane Capsules 3188

Prochlorperazine (May increase drowsiness effect).
No products indexed under this heading.

Promethazine Hydrochloride (May increase drowsiness effect). Products include:
Phenergan 3438

Propofol (May increase drowsiness effect). Products include:
Diprivan Injectable Emulsion 676

Quazepam (May increase drowsiness effect).
No products indexed under this heading.

Secobarbital Sodium (May increase drowsiness effect).
No products indexed under this heading.

Selegiline Hydrochloride (Concurrent and/or sequential use with MAO inhibitors is not recommended). Products include:
Eldepryl Capsules 3209

Temazepam (May increase drowsiness effect).
No products indexed under this heading.

Thioridazine Hydrochloride (May increase drowsiness effect). Products include:
Thioridazine Hydrochloride Tablets 2122

Thiothixene (May increase drowsiness effect). Products include:
Thiothixene Capsules 2124

Tranylcypromine Sulfate (Concurrent and/or sequential use with MAO inhibitors is not recommended). Products include:
Parnate Tablets 1499

Triazolam (May increase drowsiness effect).
No products indexed under this heading.

Trifluoperazine Hydrochloride (May increase drowsiness effect).
No products indexed under this heading.

Zaleplon (May increase drowsiness effect). Products include:
Sonata Capsules 1686

Zolpidem Tartrate (May increase drowsiness effect). Products include:
Ambien Tablets 2867

Food Interactions

Alcohol (Increases drowsiness effect; avoid concomitant use).

BENEFIBER FIBER SUPPLEMENT CAPLETS

(Fiber, dietary) 772
None cited in PDR database.

BENEFIBER DIETARY FIBER SUPPLEMENT POWDER

(Fiber, dietary) 771
None cited in PDR database.

BENEFIBER DIETARY FIBER SUPPLEMENT CHEWABLE TABLETS

(Fiber, dietary) 772
None cited in PDR database.

BENEFIX FOR INJECTION

(Antihemophilic Factor (Recombinant)) 3402
None cited in PDR database.

BENGAY EXTERNAL ANALGESIC PRODUCTS

(Menthol, Methyl Salicylate) 698
None cited in PDR database.

BENGAY PAIN RELIEVING PATCH

(Menthol) 698
None cited in PDR database.

BENGAY ULTRA STRENGTH PAIN RELIEVING PATCH

(Menthol) 698
None cited in PDR database.

BENICAR TABLETS

(Olmesartan Medoxomil) 2850
None cited in PDR database.

BENICAR HCT TABLETS

(Hydrochlorothiazide, Olmesartan Medoxomil) 2852

May interact with angiotensin-II receptor antagonists, antihypertensives, barbiturates, corticosteroids, curariform skeletal muscle relaxants, oral hypoglycemic agents, insulin, lithium preparations, narcotic analgesics, non-steroidal anti-inflammatory agents, vasopressors, and certain other agents. Compounds in these categories include:

Acarbose (Co-administration may require a dosage adjustment of the antidiabetic drug). Products include:
Precose Tablets 776

Acebutolol Hydrochloride (Co-administration could have additive effect or potentiation).
No products indexed under this heading.

ACTH (Co-administration could cause intensified electrolyte depletion, particularly hypokalemia).
No products indexed under this heading.

Alfentanil Hydrochloride (Concurrent administration could cause potentiation of orthostatic hypotension).
No products indexed under this heading.

Amlodipine Besylate (Co-administration could have additive effect or potentiation). Products include:
Caduet Tablets 2507
Lotrel Capsules 2238
Norvasc Tablets 2529

Aprobarbital (Concurrent administration could cause potentiation of orthostatic hypotension).
No products indexed under this heading.

Atenolol (Co-administration could have additive effect or potentiation). Products include:
Tenormin I.V. Injection 698
Tenormin Tablets 695

Atracurium Besylate (Co-administration could cause possible increased responsiveness to the muscle relaxant).
No products indexed under this heading.

Benazepril Hydrochloride (Co-administration could have additive effect or potentiation). Products include:
Lotensin Tablets 2232
Lotensin HCT Tablets 2235
Lotrel Capsules 2238

Bendroflumethiazide (Co-administration could have additive effect or potentiation).
No products indexed under this heading.

Betamethasone Acetate (Co-administration could cause intensified electrolyte depletion, particularly hypokalemia).
No products indexed under this heading.

Betamethasone Sodium Phosphate (Co-administration could cause intensified electrolyte depletion, particularly hypokalemia).
No products indexed under this heading.

Betaxolol Hydrochloride (Co-administration could have additive effect or potentiation). Products include:
Betoptic S Ophthalmic Suspension 554

Bisoprolol Fumarate (Co-administration could have additive effect or potentiation).
No products indexed under this heading.

Buprenorphine Hydrochloride (Concurrent administration could cause potentiation of orthostatic hypotension). Products include:
Buprenex Injectable 2718
Suboxone Tablets 2719
Subutex Tablets 2719

Butabarbital (Concurrent administration could cause potentiation of orthostatic hypotension).
No products indexed under this heading.

Butalbital (Concurrent administration could cause potentiation of orthostatic hypotension). Products include:
Sedapap Tablets 50 mg/650 mg 2098

Candesartan Cilexetil (Co-administration could have additive effect or potentiation). Products include:
Atacand Tablets 634
Atacand HCT 637

Captopril (Co-administration could have additive effect or potentiation). Products include:
Captopril Tablets 2114

Carteolol Hydrochloride (Co-administration could have additive effect or potentiation). Products include:
Carteolol Hydrochloride Ophthalmic Solution USP, 1% .... ⊙246

Celecoxib (In some patients the administration of a non-steroidal anti-inflammatory agent can reduce the diuretic, natriuretic and antihypertensive effects of loop, potassium-sparing and thiazide diuretics). Products include:
Celebrex Capsules 3130

Chlorothiazide (Co-administration could have additive effect or potentiation). Products include:
Aldoclor Tablets 1881
Diuril Oral 1936

Chlorothiazide Sodium (Co-administration could have additive effect or potentiation). Products include:
Diuril Sodium Intravenous 1934

Chlorpropamide (Co-administration may require a dosage adjustment of the antidiabetic drug).
No products indexed under this heading.

Chlorthalidone (Co-administration could have additive effect or potentiation). Products include:
Clorpres Tablets 2139

Cholestyramine (Absorption of hydrochlorothiazide is impaired in the presence of anionic exchange resins; single doses of cholestyramine bind the hydrochlorothiazide and reduce its absorption from the gastrointestinal tract by 85%).
No products indexed under this heading.

Cisatracurium Besylate (Co-administration could cause possible increased responsiveness to the muscle relaxant). Products include:
Nimbex Injection 494

Clonidine (Co-administration could have additive effect or potentiation). Products include:
Catapres-TTS 875

Clonidine Hydrochloride (Co-administration could have additive effect or potentiation). Products include:
Catapres Tablets 874
Clorpres Tablets 2139

Codeine Phosphate (Concurrent administration could cause potentiation of orthostatic hypotension). Products include:
Tylenol with Codeine 2461

Colestipol (Absorption of hydrochlorothiazide is impaired in the presence of anionic exchange resins; single doses of colestipol bind the hydrochlorothiazide and reduce its absorption from the gastrointestinal tract by 43%).
No products indexed under this heading.

Colestipol Hydrochloride (Absorption of hydrochlorothiazide is impaired in the presence of anionic exchange resins; single doses of colestipol bind the hydrochlorothiazide and reduce its absorption from the gastrointestinal tract by 43%).
No products indexed under this heading.

Cortisone Acetate (Co-administration could cause intensified electrolyte depletion, particularly hypokalemia).
No products indexed under this heading.

Deserpidine (Co-administration could have additive effect or potentiation).
No products indexed under this heading.

Dexamethasone (Co-administration could cause intensified electrolyte depletion, particularly hypokalemia). Products include:
Ciprodex Otic Suspension 555
Decadron Tablets 1929
TobraDex Ophthalmic Ointment 558
TobraDex Ophthalmic Suspension ... 558

Dexamethasone Acetate (Co-administration could cause intensified electrolyte depletion, particularly hypokalemia).
No products indexed under this heading.

Dexamethasone Sodium Phosphate (Co-administration could cause intensified electrolyte depletion, particularly hypokalemia). Products include:
Decadron Phosphate Injection 1931

Dezocine (Concurrent administration could cause potentiation of orthostatic hypotension).
No products indexed under this heading.

Diazoxide (Co-administration could have additive effect or potentiation). Products include:
Hyperstat I.V. Injection 3031

Diclofenac Potassium (In some patients the administration of a non-steroidal anti-inflammatory agent can reduce the diuretic, natriuretic and antihypertensive effects of loop, potassium-sparing and thiazide diuretics). Products include:
Cataflam Tablets 2173

Diclofenac Sodium (In some patients the administration of a non-steroidal anti-inflammatory agent can reduce the diuretic, natriuretic and antihypertensive effects of loop, potassium-sparing and thiazide diuretics). Products include:
Arthrotec Tablets 3126
Voltaren Ophthalmic Solution 2300
Voltaren Tablets 2298
Voltaren-XR Tablets 2301

Diltiazem Hydrochloride (Co-administration could have additive effect or potentiation). Products include:
Cardizem LA Extended Release Tablets 1699
Tiazac Capsules 1204

Dobutamine (Co-administration could cause possible decreased response to pressor amines but not sufficient to preclude their use).
No products indexed under this heading.

Dobutamine Hydrochloride (Co-administration could cause possible decreased response to pressor amines but not sufficient to preclude their use).
No products indexed under this heading.

Dopamine Hydrochloride (Co-administration could cause possible decreased response to pressor amines but not sufficient to preclude their use).
No products indexed under this heading.

Doxacurium Chloride (Co-administration could cause possible increased responsiveness to the muscle relaxant).
No products indexed under this heading.

Doxazosin Mesylate (Co-administration could have additive effect or potentiation).
No products indexed under this heading.

Enalapril Maleate (Co-administration could have additive effect or potentiation). Products include:
Vaseretic Tablets 2073
Vasotec I.V. Injection 2076

Enalaprilat (Co-administration could have additive effect or potentiation).
No products indexed under this heading.

Ephedrine Sulfate (Co-administration could cause possible decreased response to pressor amines but not sufficient to preclude their use).
No products indexed under this heading.

Epinephrine Bitartrate (Co-administration could cause possible decreased response to pressor amines but not sufficient to preclude their use).
No products indexed under this heading.

Epinephrine Hydrochloride (Co-administration could cause possible decreased response to pressor amines but not sufficient to preclude their use).
No products indexed under this heading.

Eprosartan Mesylate (Co-administration could have additive effect or potentiation). Products include:
Teveten Tablets 1707
Teveten HCT Tablets 1710

Esmolol Hydrochloride (Co-administration could have additive effect or potentiation). Products include:
Brevibloc Concentrate 766
Brevibloc Injection 766
Brevibloc Double Strength Injection 766
Brevibloc Premixed Injection 766
Brevibloc Double Strength Premixed Injection 766

Etodolac (In some patients the administration of a non-steroidal anti-inflammatory agent can reduce the diuretic, natriuretic and antihypertensive effects of loop, potassium-sparing and thiazide diuretics).
No products indexed under this heading.

Felodipine (Co-administration could have additive effect or potentiation). Products include:
Plendil Extended-Release Tablets 651

Fenoprofen Calcium (In some patients the administration of a non-steroidal anti-inflammatory agent can reduce the diuretic, natriuretic and antihypertensive effects of loop, potassium-sparing and thiazide diuretics). Products include:
Nalfon Capsules 2504

Fentanyl (Concurrent administration could cause potentiation of orthostatic hypotension). Products include:
Duragesic Transdermal System 2448

Fentanyl Citrate (Concurrent administration could cause potentiation of orthostatic hypotension). Products include:
Actiq 993

Fludrocortisone Acetate (Co-administration could cause intensified electrolyte depletion, particularly hypokalemia).
No products indexed under this heading.

Flurbiprofen (In some patients the administration of a non-steroidal anti-inflammatory agent can reduce the diuretic, natriuretic and antihypertensive effects of loop, potassium-sparing and thiazide diuretics).
No products indexed under this heading.

Fosinopril Sodium (Co-administration could have additive effect or potentiation).
No products indexed under this heading.

Furosemide (Co-administration could have additive effect or potentiation). Products include:
Furosemide Tablets 2117

Glimepiride (Co-administration may require a dosage adjustment of the antidiabetic drug). Products include:
Amaryl Tablets 2864

Glipizide (Co-administration may require a dosage adjustment of the antidiabetic drug).
No products indexed under this heading.

Glyburide (Co-administration may require a dosage adjustment of the antidiabetic drug).
No products indexed under this heading.

Guanabenz Acetate (Co-administration could have additive effect or potentiation).
No products indexed under this heading.

Guanethidine Monosulfate (Co-administration could have additive effect or potentiation).
No products indexed under this heading.

Hydralazine Hydrochloride (Co-administration could have additive effect or potentiation). Products include:
BiDil Tablets 2161

Hydrocodone Bitartrate (Concurrent administration could cause potentiation of orthostatic hypotension). Products include:
Hycodan 1104
Hycomine Compound Tablets 1105
Hycotuss Expectorant Syrup 1106
Lortab 3315
Lortab Elixir 3312
Vicodin Tablets 530
Vicodin ES Tablets 531
Vicodin HP Tablets 532
Vicoprofen Tablets 533
Zydone Tablets 1118

Hydrocodone Polistirex (Concurrent administration could cause potentiation of orthostatic hypotension). Products include:
Tussionex Pennkinetic Extended-Release Suspension 3322

Hydrocortisone (Co-administration could cause intensified electrolyte depletion, particularly hypokalemia). Products include:
Cortizone•5 Ointment .... ▣ 699
Cortizone•10 Creme .... ▣ 699
Cortizone•10 Ointment .... ▣ 699
Cortizone•10 Plus Creme .... ▣ 700
Cortizone•10 Maximum Strength Quick Shot Spray .... ▣ 700
Hydrocortone Tablets 1963
Preparation H Hydrocortisone Cream .... ▣ 748

Hydrocortisone Acetate (Co-administration could cause intensified electrolyte depletion, particularly hypokalemia). Products include:
Analpram-HC 1136
Pramosone 1139
ProctoFoam-HC 3113
Tucks Anti-Itch Ointment .... ▣ 712
U-cort 1% Cream 3289

Hydrocortisone Sodium Phosphate (Co-administration could cause intensified electrolyte depletion, particularly hypokalemia).
No products indexed under this heading.

Hydrocortisone Sodium Succinate (Co-administration could cause intensified electrolyte depletion, particularly hypokalemia).
No products indexed under this heading.

Hydroflumethiazide (Co-administration could have additive effect or potentiation).
No products indexed under this heading.

Hydromorphone Hydrochloride (Concurrent administration could cause potentiation of orthostatic hypotension). Products include:
Dilaudid 439
Dilaudid Oral Liquid 443
Dilaudid Non-Sterile Powder 439
Dilaudid Rectal Suppositories 439
Dilaudid Tablets 439
Dilaudid Tablets - 8 mg 443
Dilaudid-HP 441

Ibuprofen (In some patients the administration of a non-steroidal anti-inflammatory agent can reduce the diuretic, natriuretic and antihypertensive effects of loop, potassium-sparing and thiazide diuretics). Products include:
Advil Allergy Sinus Caplets .... ▣ 737
Advil .... ▣ 737
Children's Advil Suspension .... ▣ 742
Children's Advil Chewable Tablets .... ▣ 741
Advil Cold & Sinus .... ▣ 739
Advil Flu & Body Ache Caplets .... ▣ 739
Children's Advil Cold Suspension .... ▣ 741
Infants' Advil Concentrated Drops .... ▣ 743
Junior Strength Advil Swallow Tablets .... ▣ 740
Advil Migraine Liquigels .... ▣ 740
Advil Multi-Symptom Cold Caplets .... ▣ 738
Combunox Tablets 1183
Children's Motrin Oral Suspension and Chewable Tablets 1837
Children's Motrin Cold Non-Staining Dye-Free Oral Suspension 1838
Children's Motrin Cold Oral Suspension 1838
Children's Motrin Non-Staining Dye-Free Oral Suspension 1837
Motrin Cold & Sinus Caplets 1836
Motrin IB Tablets and Caplets 1836
Infants' Motrin Concentrated Drops 1837
Infants' Motrin Non-Staining Dye-Free Drops 1837
Junior Strength Motrin Caplets and Chewable Tablets 1837
Vicoprofen Tablets 533

Indapamide (Co-administration could have additive effect or potentiation). Products include:
Indapamide Tablets 2119

Indomethacin (In some patients the administration of a non-steroidal anti-inflammatory agent can reduce the diuretic, natriuretic and antihypertensive effects of loop, potassium-sparing and thiazide diuretics). Products include:
Indocin 1968

Indomethacin Sodium Trihydrate (In some patients the administration of a non-steroidal anti-inflammatory agent can reduce the diuretic, natriuretic and antihypertensive effects of loop, potassium-sparing and thiazide diuretics). Products include:
Indocin I.V. 1973

Insulin, Human, Zinc Suspension (Co-administration may require a dosage adjustment of the antidiabetic drug). Products include:
Humulin L, 100 Units 1763
Humulin U, 100 Units 1770

Insulin, Human NPH (Co-administration may require a dosage adjustment of the antidiabetic drug). Products include:
Humulin N, 100 Units 1764
Humulin N Pen 1765
Novolin N Human Insulin 10 ml Vials 2322
Novolin N InnoLet 2322
Novolin N PenFill 3 ml Cartridges 2325
Novolin R InnoLet 2322

Insulin, Human Regular (Co-administration may require a dosage adjustment of the antidiabetic drug). Products include:
Humulin R (U-500) 1768
Humulin R, 100 Units 1767
Novolin R Human Insulin 10 ml Vials 2322
Novolin R PenFill 2325

Insulin, Human Regular and Human NPH Mixture (Co-administration may require a dosage adjustment of the antidiabetic drug). Products include:
Humulin 50/50, 100 Units 1760
Humulin 70/30 Pen 1761
Novolin 70/30 Human Insulin 10 ml Vials 2321
Novolin 70/30 InnoLet 2322
Novolin 70/30 PenFill 3 ml Cartridges 2325

Insulin, NPH (Co-administration may require a dosage adjustment of the antidiabetic drug).
No products indexed under this heading.

Insulin, Regular (Co-administration may require a dosage adjustment of the antidiabetic drug).
No products indexed under this heading.

Insulin, Zinc Crystals (Co-administration may require a dosage adjustment of the antidiabetic drug).
No products indexed under this heading.

Insulin, Zinc Suspension (Co-administration may require a dosage adjustment of the antidiabetic drug).
No products indexed under this heading.

Insulin Aspart, Human Regular (Co-administration may require a dosage adjustment of the antidiabetic drug). Products include:
NovoLog Injection 2326

Insulin glargine (Co-administration may require a dosage adjustment of the antidiabetic drug). Products include:
Lantus Injection 2925

Insulin Lispro, Human (Co-administration may require a dosage adjustment of the antidiabetic drug). Products include:
Humalog-Pen 1751
Humalog Mix 75/25-Pen 1754

Insulin Lispro Protamine, Human (Co-administration may require a dosage adjustment of the antidiabetic drug). Products include:
Humalog Mix 75/25-Pen 1754

Irbesartan (Co-administration could have additive effect or potentiation). Products include:
- Avalide Tablets ... 922
- Avalide Tablets ... 2889
- Avapro Tablets ... 925
- Avapro Tablets ... 2886

Isoproterenol Hydrochloride (Co-administration could cause possible decreased response to pressor amines but not sufficient to preclude their use).
- No products indexed under this heading.

Isoproterenol Sulfate (Co-administration could cause possible decreased response to pressor amines but not sufficient to preclude their use).
- No products indexed under this heading.

Isradipine (Co-administration could have additive effect or potentiation). Products include:
- DynaCirc CR Tablets ... 2726

Ketoprofen (In some patients the administration of a non-steroidal anti-inflammatory agent can reduce the diuretic, natriuretic and antihypertensive effects of loop, potassium-sparing and thiazide diuretics).
- No products indexed under this heading.

Ketorolac Tromethamine (In some patients the administration of a non-steroidal anti-inflammatory agent can reduce the diuretic, natriuretic and antihypertensive effects of loop, potassium-sparing and thiazide diuretics). Products include:
- Acular Ophthalmic Solution ... 561
- Acular LS Ophthalmic Solution ... 562

Labetalol Hydrochloride (Co-administration could have additive effect or potentiation).
- No products indexed under this heading.

Levorphanol Tartrate (Concurrent administration could cause potentiation of orthostatic hypotension).
- No products indexed under this heading.

Lisinopril (Co-administration could have additive effect or potentiation). Products include:
- Prinivil Tablets ... 2029
- Prinzide Tablets ... 2033
- Zestoretic Tablets ... 701
- Zestril Tablets ... 704

Lithium (Lithium should not generally be given with diuretics; diuretic agents reduce the renal clearance of lithium and add a high risk of lithium toxicity).
- No products indexed under this heading.

Lithium Carbonate (Lithium should not generally be given with diuretics; diuretic agents reduce the renal clearance of lithium and add a high risk of lithium toxicity). Products include:
- Eskalith ... 1406
- Lithobid Tablets ... 1670

Lithium Citrate (Lithium should not generally be given with diuretics; diuretic agents reduce the renal clearance of lithium and add a high risk of lithium toxicity).
- No products indexed under this heading.

Losartan Potassium (Co-administration could have additive effect or potentiation). Products include:
- Cozaar Tablets ... 1913
- Hyzaar ... 1964

Mecamylamine Hydrochloride (Co-administration could have additive effect or potentiation). Products include:
- Inversine Tablets ... 3286

Meclofenamate Sodium (In some patients the administration of a non-steroidal anti-inflammatory agent can reduce the diuretic, natriuretic and antihypertensive effects of loop, potassium-sparing and thiazide diuretics).
- No products indexed under this heading.

Mefenamic Acid (In some patients the administration of a non-steroidal anti-inflammatory agent can reduce the diuretic, natriuretic and antihypertensive effects of loop, potassium-sparing and thiazide diuretics).
- No products indexed under this heading.

Meloxicam (In some patients the administration of a non-steroidal anti-inflammatory agent can reduce the diuretic, natriuretic and antihypertensive effects of loop, potassium-sparing and thiazide diuretics). Products include:
- Mobic Oral Suspension ... 893
- Mobic Tablets ... 893

Meperidine Hydrochloride (Concurrent administration could cause potentiation of orthostatic hypotension).
- No products indexed under this heading.

Mephentermine Sulfate (Co-administration could cause possible decreased response to pressor amines but not sufficient to preclude their use).
- No products indexed under this heading.

Mephobarbital (Concurrent administration could cause potentiation of orthostatic hypotension). Products include:
- Mebaral Tablets, USP ... 2483

Metaraminol Bitartrate (Co-administration could cause possible decreased response to pressor amines but not sufficient to preclude their use). Products include:
- Aramine Injection ... 1889

Metformin Hydrochloride (Co-administration may require a dosage adjustment of the antidiabetic drug). Products include:
- ActoPlus Met Tablets ... 3219
- Avandamet Tablets ... 1343
- Fortamet Extended-Release Tablets ... 1156

Methadone Hydrochloride (Concurrent administration could cause potentiation of orthostatic hypotension).
- No products indexed under this heading.

Methoxamine Hydrochloride (Co-administration could cause possible decreased response to pressor amines but not sufficient to preclude their use).
- No products indexed under this heading.

Methyclothiazide (Co-administration could have additive effect or potentiation).
- No products indexed under this heading.

Methyldopa (Co-administration could have additive effect or potentiation). Products include:
- Aldoclor Tablets ... 1881
- Aldoril Tablets ... 1884

Methyldopate Hydrochloride (Co-administration could have additive effect or potentiation).
- No products indexed under this heading.

Methylprednisolone Acetate (Co-administration could cause intensified electrolyte depletion, particularly hypokalemia). Products include:
- Depo-Medrol Injectable Suspension ... 2615
- Depo-Medrol Single-Dose Vial ... 2617

Methylprednisolone Sodium Succinate (Co-administration could cause intensified electrolyte depletion, particularly hypokalemia).
- No products indexed under this heading.

Metocurine Iodide (Co-administration could cause possible increased responsiveness to the muscle relaxant).
- No products indexed under this heading.

Metolazone (Co-administration could have additive effect or potentiation).
- No products indexed under this heading.

Metoprolol Succinate (Co-administration could have additive effect or potentiation). Products include:
- Toprol-XL Tablets ... 660

Metoprolol Tartrate (Co-administration could have additive effect or potentiation).
- No products indexed under this heading.

Metyrosine (Co-administration could have additive effect or potentiation). Products include:
- Demser Capsules ... 1933

Mibefradil Dihydrochloride (Co-administration could have additive effect or potentiation).
- No products indexed under this heading.

Miglitol (Co-administration may require a dosage adjustment of the antidiabetic drug).
- No products indexed under this heading.

Minoxidil (Co-administration could have additive effect or potentiation). Products include:
- Men's Rogaine Extra Strength Topical Solution, Ocean Rush Scent and Original Unscented ... 706
- Women's Rogaine Topical Solution, Spring Bloom Scent and Original Unscented ... 707

Mivacurium Chloride (Co-administration could cause possible increased responsiveness to the muscle relaxant). Products include:
- Mivacron Injection ... 489

Moexipril Hydrochloride (Co-administration could have additive effect or potentiation). Products include:
- Uniretic Tablets ... 3114
- Univasc Tablets ... 3118

Morphine Sulfate (Concurrent administration could cause potentiation of orthostatic hypotension). Products include:
- Avinza Capsules ... 1714
- Kadian Capsules ... 572
- MS Contin Tablets ... 2703

Nabumetone (In some patients the administration of a non-steroidal anti-inflammatory agent can reduce the diuretic, natriuretic and antihypertensive effects of loop, potassium-sparing and thiazide diuretics). Products include:
- Relafen Tablets ... 1523

Nadolol (Co-administration could have additive effect or potentiation). Products include:
- Nadolol Tablets ... 2121

Naproxen (In some patients the administration of a non-steroidal anti-inflammatory agent can reduce the diuretic, natriuretic and antihypertensive effects of loop, potassium-sparing and thiazide diuretics). Products include:
- EC-Naprosyn Delayed-Release Tablets ... 2769
- Naprosyn Suspension ... 2769
- Naprosyn Tablets ... 2769
- Prevacid NapraPAC ... 3277

Naproxen Sodium (In some patients the administration of a non-steroidal anti-inflammatory agent can reduce the diuretic, natriuretic and antihypertensive effects of loop, potassium-sparing and thiazide diuretics). Products include:
- Aleve Tablets, Caplets and Gelcaps ... 605
- Anaprox Tablets ... 2769
- Anaprox DS Tablets ... 2769

Nicardipine Hydrochloride (Co-administration could have additive effect or potentiation). Products include:
- Cardene I.V. ... 1129

Nifedipine (Co-administration could have additive effect or potentiation). Products include:
- Adalat CC Tablets ... 2978

Nisoldipine (Co-administration could have additive effect or potentiation). Products include:
- Sular Tablets ... 1163

Nitroglycerin (Co-administration could have additive effect or potentiation). Products include:
- Nitro-Dur Transdermal Infusion System ... 3060
- Nitrolingual Pumpspray ... 1161

Norepinephrine Bitartrate (Co-administration could cause possible decreased response to pressor amines but not sufficient to preclude their use).
- No products indexed under this heading.

Oxaprozin (In some patients the administration of a non-steroidal anti-inflammatory agent can reduce the diuretic, natriuretic and antihypertensive effects of loop, potassium-sparing and thiazide diuretics).
- No products indexed under this heading.

Oxycodone Hydrochloride (Concurrent administration could cause potentiation of orthostatic hypotension). Products include:
- Combunox Tablets ... 1183
- OxyContin Tablets ... 2699
- OxyFast Oral Concentrate Solution ... 2704
- OxyIR Capsules ... 2704
- Percocet Tablets ... 1114
- Percodan Tablets ... 1115

Pancuronium Bromide (Co-administration could cause possible increased responsiveness to the muscle relaxant).
- No products indexed under this heading.

Penbutolol Sulfate (Co-administration could have additive effect or potentiation).
- No products indexed under this heading.

Pentobarbital Sodium (Concurrent administration could cause potentiation of orthostatic hypotension). Products include:
Nembutal Sodium Solution, USP 2484

Perindopril Erbumine (Co-administration could have additive effect or potentiation). Products include:
Aceon Tablets (2 mg, 4 mg, 8 mg) 3191

Phenobarbital (Concurrent administration could cause potentiation of orthostatic hypotension).
No products indexed under this heading.

Phenoxybenzamine Hydrochloride (Co-administration could have additive effect or potentiation). Products include:
Dibenzyline Capsules 3390

Phentolamine Mesylate (Co-administration could have additive effect or potentiation).
No products indexed under this heading.

Phenylbutazone (In some patients the administration of a non-steroidal anti-inflammatory agent can reduce the diuretic, natriuretic and antihypertensive effects of loop, potassium-sparing and thiazide diuretics).
No products indexed under this heading.

Phenylephrine Hydrochloride (Co-administration could cause possible decreased response to pressor amines but not sufficient to preclude their use). Products include:
Alacol DM Syrup 739
Hycomine Compound Tablets 1105
Preparation H Maximum Strength Cream ...... ■ 747
Preparation H Cooling Gel ...... ■ 747
Preparation H ...... ■ 747
Sudafed PE Tablets ...... ■ 711
Vicks Sinex Nasal Spray and Ultra Fine Mist for Sinus Relief 2677
Zicam Concentrated Cough Mist for Kids Plus D Cool Cherry ...... ■ 643
Zicam Concentrated Cough Mist Plus D Cool Cherry ...... ■ 642

Pindolol (Co-administration could have additive effect or potentiation).
No products indexed under this heading.

Pioglitazone Hydrochloride (Co-administration may require a dosage adjustment of the antidiabetic drug). Products include:
ActoPlus Met Tablets 3219
Actos Tablets 3224

Pipecuronium Bromide (Co-administration could cause possible increased responsiveness to the muscle relaxant).
No products indexed under this heading.

Piroxicam (In some patients the administration of a non-steroidal anti-inflammatory agent can reduce the diuretic, natriuretic and antihypertensive effects of loop, potassium-sparing and thiazide diuretics).
No products indexed under this heading.

Polythiazide (Co-administration could have additive effect or potentiation).
No products indexed under this heading.

Prazosin Hydrochloride (Co-administration could have additive effect or potentiation).
No products indexed under this heading.

Prednisolone Acetate (Co-administration could cause intensified electrolyte depletion, particularly hypokalemia). Products include:
Blephamide Ophthalmic Ointment 563
Blephamide Ophthalmic Suspension 564
Poly-Pred Liquifilm Ophthalmic Suspension ...... ⊙ 231
Pred Forte Ophthalmic Suspension ...... ⊙ 233
Pred Mild Sterile Ophthalmic Suspension ...... ⊙ 236
Pred-G Ophthalmic Suspension ...... ⊙ 234
Pred-G Sterile Ophthalmic Ointment ...... ⊙ 235

Prednisolone Sodium Phosphate (Co-administration could cause intensified electrolyte depletion, particularly hypokalemia). Products include:
Pediapred Oral Solution 3319

Prednisolone Tebutate (Co-administration could cause intensified electrolyte depletion, particularly hypokalemia).
No products indexed under this heading.

Prednisone (Co-administration could cause intensified electrolyte depletion, particularly hypokalemia).
No products indexed under this heading.

Propoxyphene Hydrochloride (Concurrent administration could cause potentiation of orthostatic hypotension).
No products indexed under this heading.

Propoxyphene Napsylate (Concurrent administration could cause potentiation of orthostatic hypotension). Products include:
Darvocet A 500 Tablets 3497

Propranolol Hydrochloride (Co-administration could have additive effect or potentiation). Products include:
Inderal LA Long-Acting Capsules 3421
InnoPran XL Capsules 2728

Quinapril Hydrochloride (Co-administration could have additive effect or potentiation).
No products indexed under this heading.

Ramipril (Co-administration could have additive effect or potentiation). Products include:
Altace Capsules 1673

Rapacuronium Bromide (Co-administration could cause possible increased responsiveness to the muscle relaxant).
No products indexed under this heading.

Rauwolfia Serpentina (Co-administration could have additive effect or potentiation).
No products indexed under this heading.

Remifentanil Hydrochloride (Concurrent administration could cause potentiation of orthostatic hypotension).
No products indexed under this heading.

Repaglinide (Co-administration may require a dosage adjustment of the antidiabetic drug). Products include:
Prandin Tablets (0.5, 1, and 2 mg) 2337

Rescinnamine (Co-administration could have additive effect or potentiation).
No products indexed under this heading.

Reserpine (Co-administration could have additive effect or potentiation).
No products indexed under this heading.

Rocuronium Bromide (Co-administration could cause possible increased responsiveness to the muscle relaxant). Products include:
Zemuron Injection 2363

Rofecoxib (In some patients the administration of a non-steroidal anti-inflammatory agent can reduce the diuretic, natriuretic and antihypertensive effects of loop, potassium-sparing and thiazide diuretics).
No products indexed under this heading.

Rosiglitazone Maleate (Co-administration may require a dosage adjustment of the antidiabetic drug). Products include:
Avandamet Tablets 1343
Avandia Tablets 1348

Secobarbital Sodium (Concurrent administration could cause potentiation of orthostatic hypotension).
No products indexed under this heading.

Sodium Nitroprusside (Co-administration could have additive effect or potentiation).
No products indexed under this heading.

Sotalol Hydrochloride (Co-administration could have additive effect or potentiation).
No products indexed under this heading.

Spirapril Hydrochloride (Co-administration could have additive effect or potentiation).
No products indexed under this heading.

Sufentanil Citrate (Concurrent administration could cause potentiation of orthostatic hypotension).
No products indexed under this heading.

Sulindac (In some patients the administration of a non-steroidal anti-inflammatory agent can reduce the diuretic, natriuretic and antihypertensive effects of loop, potassium-sparing and thiazide diuretics). Products include:
Clinoril Tablets 1899

Telmisartan (Co-administration could have additive effect or potentiation). Products include:
Micardis Tablets 884
Micardis HCT Tablets 886

Terazosin Hydrochloride (Co-administration could have additive effect or potentiation). Products include:
Hytrin Capsules 469

Thiamylal Sodium (Concurrent administration could cause potentiation of orthostatic hypotension).
No products indexed under this heading.

Timolol Maleate (Co-administration could have additive effect or potentiation). Products include:
Blocadren Tablets 1891
Cosopt Sterile Ophthalmic Solution 1910
Timolide Tablets 2056
Timoptic in Ocudose 2061
Timoptic Sterile Ophthalmic Solution 2058
Timoptic-XE Sterile Ophthalmic Gel Forming Solution 2062

Tolazamide (Co-administration may require a dosage adjustment of the antidiabetic drug).
No products indexed under this heading.

Tolbutamide (Co-administration may require a dosage adjustment of the antidiabetic drug).
No products indexed under this heading.

Tolmetin Sodium (In some patients the administration of a non-steroidal anti-inflammatory agent can reduce the diuretic, natriuretic and antihypertensive effects of loop, potassium-sparing and thiazide diuretics).
No products indexed under this heading.

Torsemide (Co-administration could have additive effect or potentiation).
No products indexed under this heading.

Trandolapril (Co-administration could have additive effect or potentiation). Products include:
Mavik Tablets 482
Tarka Tablets 519

Triamcinolone (Co-administration could cause intensified electrolyte depletion, particularly hypokalemia).
No products indexed under this heading.

Triamcinolone Acetonide (Co-administration could cause intensified electrolyte depletion, particularly hypokalemia). Products include:
Azmacort Inhalation Aerosol 1701
Nasacort HFA Inhalation Aerosol 2939
Nasacort AQ Nasal Spray 2937

Triamcinolone Diacetate (Co-administration could cause intensified electrolyte depletion, particularly hypokalemia).
No products indexed under this heading.

Triamcinolone Hexacetonide (Co-administration could cause intensified electrolyte depletion, particularly hypokalemia).
No products indexed under this heading.

Trimethaphan Camsylate (Co-administration could have additive effect or potentiation).
No products indexed under this heading.

Troglitazone (Co-administration may require a dosage adjustment of the antidiabetic drug).
No products indexed under this heading.

Tubocurarine Chloride (Co-administration could cause possible increased responsiveness to the muscle relaxant).
No products indexed under this heading.

Valdecoxib (In some patients the administration of a non-steroidal anti-inflammatory agent can reduce the diuretic, natriuretic and antihypertensive effects of loop, potassium-sparing and thiazide diuretics).
No products indexed under this heading.

Valsartan (Co-administration could have additive effect or potentiation). Products include:
Diovan HCT Tablets 2195
Diovan Tablets 2191

Vecuronium Bromide (Co-administration could cause possible increased responsiveness to the muscle relaxant).
No products indexed under this heading.

Verapamil Hydrochloride (Co-administration could have additive effect or potentiation). Products include:
Covera-HS Tablets 3135
Tarka Tablets 519
Verelan PM Capsules 3120

Food Interactions

Alcohol (Concurrent administration could cause potentiation of orthostatic hypotension).

BENTYL CAPSULES

(Dicyclomine Hydrochloride) 724
See Bentyl Tablets

BENTYL INJECTION

(Dicyclomine Hydrochloride) 724
See Bentyl Tablets

BENTYL SYRUP

(Dicyclomine Hydrochloride) 724
See Bentyl Tablets

BENTYL TABLETS

(Dicyclomine Hydrochloride) 724
May interact with agents used to treat achlorhydria and/or to test gastric secretion, antacids, antiglaucoma agents, antihistamines, corticosteroids, monoamine oxidase inhibitors, narcotic analgesics, antipsychotic agents, nitrates and nitrites, sympathomimetics, tricyclic antidepressants, type 1 antiarrhythmic drugs, and certain other agents. Compounds in these categories include:

Acetazolamide (Anticholinergics antagonize the effects of antiglaucoma agents).
No products indexed under this heading.

Acetylcholine Chloride (Anticholinergics antagonize the effects of antiglaucoma agents).
No products indexed under this heading.

Acrivastine (Antihistamines may increase certain actions or side effects of anticholinergic agents).
No products indexed under this heading.

Albuterol (Sympathomimetic agents may increase certain actions or side effects of anticholinergic agents). Products include:
Proventil Inhalation Aerosol 3067

Albuterol Sulfate (Sympathomimetic agents may increase certain actions or side effects of anticholinergic agents). Products include:
AccuNeb Inhalation Solution 1055
Combivent Inhalation Aerosol 878
DuoNeb Inhalation Solution 1058
Proventil Inhalation Solution 0.083% 3069
Proventil HFA Inhalation Aerosol 3071
Ventolin HFA Inhalation Aerosol 1576
VoSpire Extended-Release Tablets 2352

Alfentanil Hydrochloride (Narcotic analgesics may increase certain actions or side effects of anticholinergic agents).
No products indexed under this heading.

Aluminum Carbonate (Antacids may interfere with the absorption of anticholinergic agents; therefore, simultaneous use of these drugs should be avoided).
No products indexed under this heading.

Aluminum Hydroxide (Antacids may interfere with the absorption of anticholinergic agents; therefore, simultaneous use of these drugs should be avoided). Products include:
Gaviscon Regular Strength Liquid 620
Gaviscon Regular Strength Tablets 619
Gaviscon Extra Strength Liquid 620
Gaviscon Extra Strength Tablets 619
Maalox Max Maximum Strength Antacid/Anti-Gas Liquid 2165
Maalox Regular Strength Antacid/Antigas Liquid 2164

Amantadine Hydrochloride (Amantadine may increase certain actions or side effects of anticholinergic agents). Products include:
Symmetrel 1115

Amitriptyline Hydrochloride (Tricyclic antidepressants may increase certain actions or side effects of anticholinergic agents).
No products indexed under this heading.

Amoxapine (Tricyclic antidepressants may increase certain actions or side effects of anticholinergic agents).
No products indexed under this heading.

Amyl Nitrite (Nitrates and nitrites may increase certain actions or side effects of anticholinergic agents).
No products indexed under this heading.

Aripiprazole (Antipsychotic agents may increase certain actions or side effects of anticholinergic agents). Products include:
Abilify Tablets 2472
Abilify Tablets 916

Astemizole (Antihistamines may increase certain actions or side effects of anticholinergic agents).
No products indexed under this heading.

Azatadine Maleate (Antihistamines may increase certain actions or side effects of anticholinergic agents).
No products indexed under this heading.

Betamethasone Acetate (Anticholinergic drugs in the presence of increased intraocular pressure may be hazardous when taken concurrently with agents such as corticosteroids).
No products indexed under this heading.

Betamethasone Sodium Phosphate (Anticholinergic drugs in the presence of increased intraocular pressure may be hazardous when taken concurrently with agents such as corticosteroids).
No products indexed under this heading.

Betaxolol Hydrochloride (Anticholinergics antagonize the effects of antiglaucoma agents). Products include:
Betoptic S Ophthalmic Suspension 554

Bromodiphenhydramine Hydrochloride (Antihistamines may increase certain actions or side effects of anticholinergic agents).
No products indexed under this heading.

Brompheniramine Maleate (Antihistamines may increase certain actions or side effects of anticholinergic agents). Products include:
Alacol DM Syrup 739
Children's Dimetapp Cold & Allergy Elixir 745
Children's Dimetapp DM Cold & Cough Elixir 745
Robitussin Allergy & Cough Syrup 750

Buprenorphine Hydrochloride (Narcotic analgesics may increase certain actions or side effects of anticholinergic agents). Products include:
Buprenex Injectable 2718
Suboxone Tablets 2719
Subutex Tablets 2719

Carbachol (Anticholinergics antagonize the effects of antiglaucoma agents).
No products indexed under this heading.

Cetirizine Hydrochloride (Antihistamines may increase certain actions or side effects of anticholinergic agents). Products include:
Zyrtec Chewable Tablets 2589
Zyrtec 2589
Zyrtec-D 12 Hour Extended Release Tablets 2591

Chlorpheniramine Maleate (Antihistamines may increase certain actions or side effects of anticholinergic agents). Products include:
Advil Allergy Sinus Caplets 737
Advil Multi-Symptom Cold Caplets 738
BC Allergy Sinus Cold Powder 612
Contac Severe Cold and Flu Caplets Maximum Strength 615
Hycomine Compound Tablets 1105
PediaCare Multi-Symptom Cold Liquid 704
PediaCare NightRest Cough & Cold Liquid 704
Robitussin Flu Liquid 752
Robitussin PM Cough & Cold Liquid 752
Singlet Caplets 636
Sudafed Sinus & Allergy Tablets 710
TheraFlu Cold & Cough Hot Liquid 680
TheraFlu Cold & Sore Throat Hot Liquid 680
TheraFlu Flu & Sore Throat Hot Liquid 681
TheraFlu Severe Cold & Cough Hot Liquid 683
TheraFlu Severe Cold Caplets 679
TheraFlu Severe Cold Hot Liquid 682
Triaminic Cold & Allergy Liquid 685
Triaminic Cold & Cough Liquid 685
Triaminic Flu, Cough & Fever Liquid 685
Triaminic Night Time Cough & Cold Liquid 685
Triaminic Allergy Runny Nose & Congestion Softchews 688
Triaminic Cold & Cough Softchews 688
Children's Tylenol Plus Cold NightTime Suspension Liquid 1851
Children's Tylenol Plus Cold & Cough Suspension Liquid and Chewable Tablets 1851
Children's Tylenol Plus Cold Chewable Tablets 1851
Children's Tylenol Plus Flu Suspension Liquid 1853
Tylenol Allergy Complete Multi-Symptom Caplets and Gelcaps with Cool Burst 1844
Multi-Symptom Tylenol Cold Night Time Caplets 1845
Vicks 44M Cough, Cold & Flu Relief 2676
Pediatric Vicks 44m Cough & Cold Relief 2673
Children's Vicks NyQuil Cold/Cough Relief 2671

Chlorpheniramine Polistirex (Antihistamines may increase certain actions or side effects of anticholinergic agents). Products include:
Tussionex Pennkinetic Extended-Release Suspension 3322

Chlorpheniramine Tannate (Antihistamines may increase certain actions or side effects of anticholinergic agents).
No products indexed under this heading.

Chlorpromazine (Antipsychotic agents may increase certain actions or side effects of anticholinergic agents).
No products indexed under this heading.

Chlorpromazine Hydrochloride (Antipsychotic agents may increase certain actions or side effects of anticholinergic agents).
No products indexed under this heading.

Chlorprothixene (Antipsychotic agents may increase certain actions or side effects of anticholinergic agents).
No products indexed under this heading.

Chlorprothixene Hydrochloride (Antipsychotic agents may increase certain actions or side effects of anticholinergic agents).
No products indexed under this heading.

Cisapride (Anticholinergic drugs may antagonize the effects of drugs that alter gastrointestinal motility).
No products indexed under this heading.

Clemastine Fumarate (Antihistamines may increase certain actions or side effects of anticholinergic agents).
No products indexed under this heading.

Clomipramine Hydrochloride (Tricyclic antidepressants may increase certain actions or side effects of anticholinergic agents).
No products indexed under this heading.

Clozapine (Antipsychotic agents may increase certain actions or side effects of anticholinergic agents). Products include:
Clozapine Tablets 2141
Clozaril Tablets 2174
FazaClo Orally Disintegrating Tablets 547

Codeine Phosphate (Narcotic analgesics may increase certain actions or side effects of anticholinergic agents). Products include:
Tylenol with Codeine 2461

Cortisone Acetate (Anticholinergic drugs in the presence of increased intraocular pressure may be hazardous when taken concurrently with agents such as corticosteroids).
No products indexed under this heading.

Cyproheptadine Hydrochloride (Antihistamines may increase certain actions or side effects of anticholinergic agents).
No products indexed under this heading.

Demecarium Bromide (Anticholinergics antagonize the effects of antiglaucoma agents).
No products indexed under this heading.

Desipramine Hydrochloride (Tricyclic antidepressants may increase certain actions or side effects of anticholinergic agents).
No products indexed under this heading.

Dexamethasone (Anticholinergic drugs in the presence of increased intraocular pressure may be hazardous when taken concurrently with agents such as corticosteroids). Products include:
- Ciprodex Otic Suspension 555
- Decadron Tablets 1929
- TobraDex Ophthalmic Ointment 558
- TobraDex Ophthalmic Suspension 558

Dexamethasone Acetate (Anticholinergic drugs in the presence of increased intraocular pressure may be hazardous when taken concurrently with agents such as corticosteroids).
No products indexed under this heading.

Dexamethasone Sodium Phosphate (Anticholinergic drugs in the presence of increased intraocular pressure may be hazardous when taken concurrently with agents such as corticosteroids). Products include:
- Decadron Phosphate Injection 1931

Dexchlorpheniramine Maleate (Antihistamines may increase certain actions or side effects of anticholinergic agents).
No products indexed under this heading.

Dexpanthenol (Anticholinergic drugs may antagonize the effects of drugs that alter gastrointestinal motility).
No products indexed under this heading.

Dezocine (Narcotic analgesics may increase certain actions or side effects of anticholinergic agents).
No products indexed under this heading.

Dichlorphenamide (Anticholinergics antagonize the effects of antiglaucoma agents). Products include:
- Daranide Tablets 1928

Digoxin (Anticholinergic agents may affect gastrointestinal absorption of various drugs, such as slowly dissolving dosage forms of digoxin; increased serum digoxin concentrations may result). Products include:
- Digitek Tablets 2146
- Lanoxicaps Capsules 1458
- Lanoxin Injection 1462
- Lanoxin Tablets 1468
- Lanoxin Injection Pediatric 1465

Diphenhydramine Citrate (Antihistamines may increase certain actions or side effects of anticholinergic agents). Products include:
- Children's Benadryl Allergy & Cold Fastmelt Tablets .... ■ 695
- Children's Benadryl D Allergy & Sinus Fastmelt Tablets .... ■ 694
- Children's Benadryl Allergy Fastmelt Tablets .... ■ 696
- Goody's PM Powder .... ■ 622

Diphenhydramine Hydrochloride (Antihistamines may increase certain actions or side effects of anticholinergic agents). Products include:
- Benadryl Allergy & Cold Tablets .... ■ 692
- Benadryl Allergy .... ■ 691
- Benadryl Allergy & Sinus Headache Caplets & Gelcaps .... ■ 693
- Children's Benadryl Allergy Liquid .... ■ 695
- Children's Benadryl Dye-Free Allergy Liquid .... ■ 695
- Benadryl Dye-Free Allergy Liqui-Gels Softgels .... ■ 692
- Benadryl Itch Relief Stick Extra Strength .... ■ 696
- Benadryl Itch Stopping Cream Extra Strength .... ■ 697
- Benadryl Itch Stopping Gel Extra Strength .... ■ 697
- Benadryl Itch Stopping Spray Extra Strength .... ■ 697
- Benadryl Maximum Strength Severe Allergy & Sinus Headache Caplets .... ■ 694
- Children's Benadryl D Liquid Medication .... ■ 693
- Benadryl D Tablets .... ■ 694
- Nytol QuickCaps Caplets .... ■ 635
- Maximum Strength Nytol QuickGels Softgels .... ■ 635
- Simply Sleep Caplets 1841
- Sominex Original Formula Tablets .... ■ 637
- TheraFlu Thin Strips Multi Symptom .... ■ 684
- Triaminic Thin Strips Cough & Runny Nose .... ■ 690
- Children's Tylenol Plus Cold & Allergy Suspension Liquid 1850
- Tylenol Allergy Complete Night Time Caplets 1844
- Tylenol Severe Allergy Caplets 1844
- Tylenol Flu NightTime Gelcaps 1846
- Extra Strength Tylenol PM Caplets, Geltabs, Gelcaps and Liquid 1847
- Unisom Maximum Strength SleepGels .... ■ 712

Diphenylpyraline Hydrochloride (Antihistamines may increase certain actions or side effects of anticholinergic agents).
No products indexed under this heading.

Dipivefrin Hydrochloride (Anticholinergics antagonize the effects of antiglaucoma agents). Products include:
- Propine Ophthalmic Solution .... ⊙ 237

Disopyramide Phosphate (Class I antiarrhythmic agents may increase certain actions or side effects of anticholinergic agents).
No products indexed under this heading.

Dobutamine Hydrochloride (Sympathomimetic agents may increase certain actions or side effects of anticholinergic agents).
No products indexed under this heading.

Dopamine Hydrochloride (Sympathomimetic agents may increase certain actions or side effects of anticholinergic agents).
No products indexed under this heading.

Doxepin Hydrochloride (Tricyclic antidepressants may increase certain actions or side effects of anticholinergic agents).
No products indexed under this heading.

Echothiophate Iodide (Anticholinergics antagonize the effects of antiglaucoma agents).
No products indexed under this heading.

Ephedrine Hydrochloride (Sympathomimetic agents may increase certain actions or side effects of anticholinergic agents). Products include:
- Primatene Tablets .... ■ 749

Ephedrine Sulfate (Sympathomimetic agents may increase certain actions or side effects of anticholinergic agents).
No products indexed under this heading.

Ephedrine Tannate (Sympathomimetic agents may increase certain actions or side effects of anticholinergic agents).
No products indexed under this heading.

Epinephrine (Sympathomimetic agents may increase certain actions or side effects of anticholinergic agents). Products include:
- EpiPen 1061
- Primatene Mist .... ■ 749

Epinephrine Bitartrate (Sympathomimetic agents may increase certain actions or side effects of anticholinergic agents).
No products indexed under this heading.

Epinephrine Hydrochloride (Sympathomimetic agents may increase certain actions or side effects of anticholinergic agents).
No products indexed under this heading.

Epinephryl Borate (Anticholinergics antagonize the effects of antiglaucoma agents).
No products indexed under this heading.

Erythrityl Tetranitrate (Nitrates and nitrites may increase certain actions or side effects of anticholinergic agents).
No products indexed under this heading.

Fentanyl (Narcotic analgesics may increase certain actions or side effects of anticholinergic agents). Products include:
- Duragesic Transdermal System 2448

Fentanyl Citrate (Narcotic analgesics may increase certain actions or side effects of anticholinergic agents). Products include:
- Actiq 993

Fexofenadine Hydrochloride (Antihistamines may increase certain actions or side effects of anticholinergic agents). Products include:
- Allegra 2857
- Allegra-D 12 Hour Extended-Release Tablets 2860
- Allegra-D 24 Hour Extended-Release Tablets 2862

Fludrocortisone Acetate (Anticholinergic drugs in the presence of increased intraocular pressure may be hazardous when taken concurrently with agents such as corticosteroids).
No products indexed under this heading.

Fluphenazine Decanoate (Antipsychotic agents may increase certain actions or side effects of anticholinergic agents).
No products indexed under this heading.

Fluphenazine Enanthate (Antipsychotic agents may increase certain actions or side effects of anticholinergic agents).
No products indexed under this heading.

Fluphenazine Hydrochloride (Antipsychotic agents may increase certain actions or side effects of anticholinergic agents).
No products indexed under this heading.

Glutamic Acid Hydrochloride (The inhibiting effects of anticholinergic drugs on gastric hydrochloric acid secretion are antagonized by agents used to treat achlorhydria and those used to test gastric secretion).
No products indexed under this heading.

Haloperidol (Antipsychotic agents may increase certain actions or side effects of anticholinergic agents).
No products indexed under this heading.

Haloperidol Decanoate (Antipsychotic agents may increase certain actions or side effects of anticholinergic agents).
No products indexed under this heading.

Hydrocodone Bitartrate (Narcotic analgesics may increase certain actions or side effects of anticholinergic agents). Products include:
- Hycodan 1104
- Hycomine Compound Tablets 1105
- Hycotuss Expectorant Syrup 1106
- Lortab 3315
- Lortab Elixir 3312
- Vicodin Tablets 530
- Vicodin ES Tablets 531
- Vicodin HP Tablets 532
- Vicoprofen Tablets 533
- Zydone Tablets 1118

Hydrocodone Polistirex (Narcotic analgesics may increase certain actions or side effects of anticholinergic agents). Products include:
- Tussionex Pennkinetic Extended-Release Suspension 3322

Hydrocortisone (Anticholinergic drugs in the presence of increased intraocular pressure may be hazardous when taken concurrently with agents such as corticosteroids). Products include:
- Cortizone•5 Ointment .... ■ 699
- Cortizone•10 Creme .... ■ 699
- Cortizone•10 Ointment .... ■ 699
- Cortizone•10 Plus Creme .... ■ 700
- Cortizone•10 Maximum Strength Quick Shot Spray .... ■ 700
- Hydrocortone Tablets 1963
- Preparation H Hydrocortisone Cream .... ■ 748

Hydrocortisone Acetate (Anticholinergic drugs in the presence of increased intraocular pressure may be hazardous when taken concurrently with agents such as corticosteroids). Products include:
- Analpram-HC 1136
- Pramosone 1139
- ProctoFoam-HC 3113
- Tucks Anti-Itch Ointment .... ■ 712
- U-cort 1% Cream 3289

Hydrocortisone Sodium Phosphate (Anticholinergic drugs in the presence of increased intraocular pressure may be hazardous when taken concurrently with agents such as corticosteroids).
No products indexed under this heading.

Hydrocortisone Sodium Succinate (Anticholinergic drugs in the presence of increased intraocular pressure may be hazardous when taken concurrently with agents such as corticosteroids).
No products indexed under this heading.

Hydromorphone Hydrochloride (Narcotic analgesics may increase certain actions or side effects of anticholinergic agents). Products include:
- Dilaudid 439

Dilaudid Oral Liquid ... **443**
Dilaudid Non-Sterile Powder ... **439**
Dilaudid Rectal Suppositories ... **439**
Dilaudid Tablets ... **439**
Dilaudid Tablets - 8 mg ... **443**
Dilaudid-HP ... **441**

Imipramine Hydrochloride (Tricyclic antidepressants may increase certain actions or side effects of anticholinergic agents).
No products indexed under this heading.

Imipramine Pamoate (Tricyclic antidepressants may increase certain actions or side effects of anticholinergic agents).
No products indexed under this heading.

Isocarboxazid (MAO inhibitors may increase certain actions or side effects of anticholinergic agents).
No products indexed under this heading.

Isoflurophate (Anticholinergics antagonize the effects of antiglaucoma agents).
No products indexed under this heading.

Isoproterenol Hydrochloride (Sympathomimetic agents may increase certain actions or side effects of anticholinergic agents).
No products indexed under this heading.

Isoproterenol Sulfate (Sympathomimetic agents may increase certain actions or side effects of anticholinergic agents).
No products indexed under this heading.

Isosorbide Dinitrate (Nitrates and nitrites may increase certain actions or side effects of anticholinergic agents). Products include:
BiDil Tablets ... **2161**

Isosorbide Mononitrate (Nitrates and nitrites may increase certain actions or side effects of anticholinergic agents). Products include:
Imdur Tablets ... **3032**

Levalbuterol Hydrochloride (Sympathomimetic agents may increase certain actions or side effects of anticholinergic agents). Products include:
Xopenex Inhalation Solution ... **3143**
Xopenex Inhalation Solution Concentrate ... **3147**

Levobunolol Hydrochloride (Anticholinergics antagonize the effects of antiglaucoma agents). Products include:
Betagan Ophthalmic Solution, USP ... ⊙ **217**

Levorphanol Tartrate (Narcotic analgesics may increase certain actions or side effects of anticholinergic agents).
No products indexed under this heading.

Lithium Carbonate (Antipsychotic agents may increase certain actions or side effects of anticholinergic agents). Products include:
Eskalith ... **1406**
Lithobid Tablets ... **1670**

Lithium Citrate (Antipsychotic agents may increase certain actions or side effects of anticholinergic agents).
No products indexed under this heading.

Loratadine (Antihistamines may increase certain actions or side effects of anticholinergic agents). Products include:
Alavert Allergy & Sinus D-12 Hour Tablets ... **743**
Alavert ... **743**
Children's Claritin 24 Hour Non-Drowsy Allergy Syrup ... **732**
Claritin Non-Drowsy 24 Hour Tablets ... **731**
Non-Drowsy Claritin Hives Relief Tablets ... **733**
Claritin Reditabs 24 Hour Non-Drowsy Tablets ... **732**
Claritin-D Non-Drowsy 12 Hour Tablets ... **731**
Claritin-D Non-Drowsy 24 Hour Tablets ... **731**
Children's Dimetapp ND Non-Drowsy Allergy Syrup ... **746**
Triaminic Allerchews ... **684**

Loxapine Hydrochloride (Antipsychotic agents may increase certain actions or side effects of anticholinergic agents).
No products indexed under this heading.

Loxapine Succinate (Antipsychotic agents may increase certain actions or side effects of anticholinergic agents).
No products indexed under this heading.

Magaldrate (Antacids may interfere with the absorption of anticholinergic agents; therefore, simultaneous use of these drugs should be avoided).
No products indexed under this heading.

Magnesium Hydroxide (Antacids may interfere with the absorption of anticholinergic agents; therefore, simultaneous use of these drugs should be avoided). Products include:
Maalox Max Maximum Strength Antacid/Anti-Gas Liquid ... **2165**
Maalox Regular Strength Antacid/Antigas Liquid ... **2164**
Pepcid Complete Chewable Tablets ... **1672**
Rolaids Tablets ... **707**
Extra Strength Rolaids Tablets ... **707**
Rolaids Multi-Symptom Antacid & Antigas Tablets ... **708**

Magnesium Oxide (Antacids may interfere with the absorption of anticholinergic agents; therefore, simultaneous use of these drugs should be avoided). Products include:
Beelith Tablets ... **784**
PremCal Light, Regular, and Extra Strength Tablets ... **762**

Maprotiline Hydrochloride (Tricyclic antidepressants may increase certain actions or side effects of anticholinergic agents).
No products indexed under this heading.

Meperidine Hydrochloride (Narcotic analgesics may increase certain actions or side effects of anticholinergic agents).
No products indexed under this heading.

Mesoridazine Besylate (Antipsychotic agents may increase certain actions or side effects of anticholinergic agents).
No products indexed under this heading.

Metaproterenol Sulfate (Sympathomimetic agents may increase certain actions or side effects of anticholinergic agents). Products include:
Alupent Inhalation Aerosol ... **858**

Metaraminol Bitartrate (Sympathomimetic agents may increase certain actions or side effects of anticholinergic agents). Products include:
Aramine Injection ... **1889**

Methadone Hydrochloride (Narcotic analgesics may increase certain actions or side effects of anticholinergic agents).
No products indexed under this heading.

Methazolamide (Anticholinergics antagonize the effects of antiglaucoma agents).
No products indexed under this heading.

Methdilazine Hydrochloride (Antihistamines may increase certain actions or side effects of anticholinergic agents).
No products indexed under this heading.

Methotrimeprazine (Antipsychotic agents may increase certain actions or side effects of anticholinergic agents).
No products indexed under this heading.

Methoxamine Hydrochloride (Sympathomimetic agents may increase certain actions or side effects of anticholinergic agents).
No products indexed under this heading.

Methylprednisolone Acetate (Anticholinergic drugs in the presence of increased intraocular pressure may be hazardous when taken concurrently with agents such as corticosteroids). Products include:
Depo-Medrol Injectable Suspension ... **2615**
Depo-Medrol Single-Dose Vial ... **2617**

Methylprednisolone Sodium Succinate (Anticholinergic drugs in the presence of increased intraocular pressure may be hazardous when taken concurrently with agents such as corticosteroids).
No products indexed under this heading.

Metoclopramide Hydrochloride (Anticholinergic drugs may antagonize the effects of drugs that alter gastrointestinal motility).
No products indexed under this heading.

Moclobemide (MAO inhibitors may increase certain actions or side effects of anticholinergic agents).
No products indexed under this heading.

Molindone Hydrochloride (Antipsychotic agents may increase certain actions or side effects of anticholinergic agents). Products include:
Moban Tablets ... **1108**

Moricizine Hydrochloride (Class I antiarrhythmic agents may increase certain actions or side effects of anticholinergic agents).
No products indexed under this heading.

Morphine Sulfate (Narcotic analgesics may increase certain actions or side effects of anticholinergic agents). Products include:
Avinza Capsules ... **1714**
Kadian Capsules ... **572**
MS Contin Tablets ... **2703**

Nitroglycerin (Nitrates and nitrites may increase certain actions or side effects of anticholinergic agents). Products include:
Nitro-Dur Transdermal Infusion System ... **3060**
Nitrolingual Pumpspray ... **1161**

Norepinephrine Bitartrate (Sympathomimetic agents may increase certain actions or side effects of anticholinergic agents).
No products indexed under this heading.

Nortriptyline Hydrochloride (Tricyclic antidepressants may increase certain actions or side effects of anticholinergic agents).
No products indexed under this heading.

Olanzapine (Antipsychotic agents may increase certain actions or side effects of anticholinergic agents). Products include:
Symbyax Capsules ... **1788**
Zyprexa Tablets ... **1798**
Zyprexa IntraMuscular ... **1798**
Zyprexa ZYDIS Orally Disintegrating Tablets ... **1798**

Oxycodone Hydrochloride (Narcotic analgesics may increase certain actions or side effects of anticholinergic agents). Products include:
Combunox Tablets ... **1183**
OxyContin Tablets ... **2699**
OxyFast Oral Concentrate Solution ... **2704**
OxyIR Capsules ... **2704**
Percocet Tablets ... **1114**
Percodan Tablets ... **1115**

Pargyline Hydrochloride (MAO inhibitors may increase certain actions or side effects of anticholinergic agents).
No products indexed under this heading.

Pentaerythritol Tetranitrate (Nitrates and nitrites may increase certain actions or side effects of anticholinergic agents).
No products indexed under this heading.

Pentagastrin (The inhibiting effects of anticholinergic drugs on gastric hydrochloric acid secretion are antagonized by agents used to treat achlorhydria and those used to test gastric secretion).
No products indexed under this heading.

Perphenazine (Antipsychotic agents may increase certain actions or side effects of anticholinergic agents).
No products indexed under this heading.

Phenelzine Sulfate (MAO inhibitors may increase certain actions or side effects of anticholinergic agents).
No products indexed under this heading.

Phenylephrine Bitartrate (Sympathomimetic agents may increase certain actions or side effects of anticholinergic agents).
No products indexed under this heading.

Phenylephrine Hydrochloride (Sympathomimetic agents may increase certain actions or side effects of anticholinergic agents). Products include:
Alacol DM Syrup ... **739**
Hycomine Compound Tablets ... **1105**
Preparation H Maximum Strength Cream ... **747**
Preparation H Cooling Gel ... **747**
Preparation H ... **747**
Sudafed PE Tablets ... **711**
Vicks Sinex Nasal Spray and Ultra Fine Mist for Sinus Relief ... **2677**
Zicam Concentrated Cough Mist for Kids Plus D Cool Cherry ... **643**
Zicam Concentrated Cough Mist Plus D Cool Cherry ... **642**

Phenylephrine Tannate (Sympathomimetic agents may increase certain actions or side effects of anticholinergic agents).
No products indexed under this heading.

Phenylpropanolamine Hydrochloride (Sympathomimetic agents may increase certain actions or side effects of anticholinergic agents).
No products indexed under this heading.

Pilocarpine (Anticholinergics antagonize the effects of antiglaucoma agents).
No products indexed under this heading.

Pilocarpine Hydrochloride (Anticholinergics antagonize the effects of antiglaucoma agents).
No products indexed under this heading.

Pimozide (Antipsychotic agents may increase certain actions or side effects of anticholinergic agents). Products include:
Orap Tablets 1220

Pirbuterol Acetate (Sympathomimetic agents may increase certain actions or side effects of anticholinergic agents). Products include:
Maxair Autohaler 1820

Prednisolone Acetate (Anticholinergic drugs in the presence of increased intraocular pressure may be hazardous when taken concurrently with agents such as corticosteroids). Products include:
Blephamide Ophthalmic Ointment 563
Blephamide Ophthalmic Suspension 564
Poly-Pred Liquifilm Ophthalmic Suspension .... ⊙ 231
Pred Forte Ophthalmic Suspension .... ⊙ 233
Pred Mild Sterile Ophthalmic Suspension .... ⊙ 236
Pred-G Ophthalmic Suspension ...... ⊙ 234
Pred-G Sterile Ophthalmic Ointment .... ⊙ 235

Prednisolone Sodium Phosphate (Anticholinergic drugs in the presence of increased intraocular pressure may be hazardous when taken concurrently with agents such as corticosteroids). Products include:
Pediapred Oral Solution 3319

Prednisolone Tebutate (Anticholinergic drugs in the presence of increased intraocular pressure may be hazardous when taken concurrently with agents such as corticosteroids).
No products indexed under this heading.

Prednisone (Anticholinergic drugs in the presence of increased intraocular pressure may be hazardous when taken concurrently with agents such as corticosteroids).
No products indexed under this heading.

Procainamide Hydrochloride (Class I antiarrhythmic agents may increase certain actions or side effects of anticholinergic agents).
No products indexed under this heading.

Procarbazine Hydrochloride (MAO inhibitors may increase certain actions or side effects of anticholinergic agents). Products include:
Matulane Capsules 3188

Prochlorperazine (Antipsychotic agents may increase certain actions or side effects of anticholinergic agents).
No products indexed under this heading.

Promethazine Hydrochloride (Antihistamines may increase certain actions or side effects of anticholinergic agents). Products include:
Phenergan 3438

Propafenone Hydrochloride (Class I antiarrhythmic agents may increase certain actions or side effects of anticholinergic agents). Products include:
Rythmol SR Capsules 2736

Propoxyphene Hydrochloride (Narcotic analgesics may increase certain actions or side effects of anticholinergic agents).
No products indexed under this heading.

Propoxyphene Napsylate (Narcotic analgesics may increase certain actions or side effects of anticholinergic agents). Products include:
Darvocet A 500 Tablets 3497

Protriptyline Hydrochloride (Tricyclic antidepressants may increase certain actions or side effects of anticholinergic agents). Products include:
Vivactil Tablets 2350

Pseudoephedrine Hydrochloride (Sympathomimetic agents may increase certain actions or side effects of anticholinergic agents). Products include:
Advil Allergy Sinus Caplets .... ▣ 737
Advil Cold & Sinus .... ▣ 739
Advil Flu & Body Ache Caplets .... ▣ 739
Children's Advil Cold Suspension ... ▣ 741
Advil Multi-Symptom Cold Caplets .... ▣ 738
Allegra-D 12 Hour Extended-Release Tablets 2860
Allegra-D 24 Hour Extended-Release Tablets 2862
Balamine DM 739
BC Cold Powder .... ▣ 612
Benadryl Allergy & Cold Tablets ..... ▣ 692
Benadryl Allergy & Sinus Headache Caplets & Gelcaps ...... ▣ 693
Children's Benadryl Allergy & Cold Fastmelt Tablets .... ▣ 695
Benadryl Maximum Strength Severe Allergy & Sinus Headache Caplets .... ▣ 694
Children's Benadryl D Allergy & Sinus Fastmelt Tablets .... ▣ 694
Children's Benadryl D Liquid Medication .... ▣ 693
Benadryl D Tablets .... ▣ 694
Contac Non-Drowsy 12 Hour Cold Caplets .... ▣ 614
Contac Non-Drowsy Timed Release 12 Hour Cold Caplets .... ▣ 615
Contac Severe Cold and Flu Caplets Maximum Strength .... ▣ 615
Contac Severe Cold and Flu Caplets Non-Drowsy .... ▣ 615
Children's Dimetapp Cold & Allergy Elixir .... ▣ 745
Children's Dimetapp DM Cold & Cough Elixir .... ▣ 745
Children's Dimetapp Long Acting Cough Plus Cold Syrup .... ▣ 746
Dimetapp Infant Drops Decongestant Plus Cough .... ▣ 746
Children's Motrin Cold Non-Staining Dye-Free Oral Suspension 1838
Children's Motrin Cold Oral Suspension 1838
Motrin Cold & Sinus Caplets 1836
PediaCare Decongestant & Cough Infant Drops .... ▣ 705
PediaCare Decongestant Infants' Drops .... ▣ 705
PediaCare Long-Acting Cough Plus Cold Liquid .... ▣ 704
PediaCare Multi-Symptom Cold Liquid .... ▣ 704
PediaCare NightRest Cough & Cold Liquid .... ▣ 704
Robitussin Allergy & Cough Syrup .. ▣ 750
Robitussin CF Liquid .... ▣ 755
Robitussin Cough & Cold Liquid-filled Capsules .... ▣ 750
Robitussin Cough, Cold & Flu Liquid-filled Capsules .... ▣ 750
Robitussin Cough & Cold Infant Drops .... ▣ 755
Robitussin Flu Liquid .... ▣ 752
Robitussin Maximum Strength Cough & Cold Liquid .... ▣ 754
Robitussin PE Syrup .... ▣ 753
Robitussin Pediatric Cough & Cold Liquid .... ▣ 754
Robitussin PM Cough & Cold Liquid .... ▣ 752
Robitussin Severe Congestion Liquid-filled Capsules .... ▣ 751
Simply Stuffy Liquid 1841
Singlet Caplets .... ▣ 636
Sudafed 12 Hour Caplets .... ▣ 708
Sudafed 24 Hour Tablets .... ▣ 709
Sudafed Nasal Decongestant Tablets .... ▣ 709
Sudafed Severe Cold .... ▣ 710
Sudafed Non-Drying Sinus Liquid Caps .... ▣ 709
Sudafed Sinus & Allergy Tablets ..... ▣ 710
Sudafed Sinus Headache .... ▣ 711
TheraFlu Cold & Cough Hot Liquid .... ▣ 680
TheraFlu Cold & Sore Throat Hot Liquid .... ▣ 680
TheraFlu Flu & Chest Congestion Non-Drowsy Hot Liquid .... ▣ 681
TheraFlu Flu & Sore Throat Hot Liquid .... ▣ 681
TheraFlu Severe Cold Non-Drowsy Hot Liquid .... ▣ 683
TheraFlu Severe Cold & Cough Hot Liquid .... ▣ 683
TheraFlu Severe Cold Caplets .... ▣ 679
TheraFlu Severe Cold Hot Liquid .... ▣ 682
TheraFlu Severe Cold Non-Drowsy Caplets .... ▣ 679
Triaminic Chest & Nasal Congestion Liquid .... ▣ 685
Triaminic Cold & Allergy Liquid ...... ▣ 685
Triaminic Cold & Cough Liquid ...... ▣ 685
Triaminic Cough Liquid .... ▣ 687
Triaminic Cough & Nasal Congestion Liquid .... ▣ 687
Triaminic Cough & Sore Throat Liquid .... ▣ 687
Triaminic Flu, Cough & Fever Liquid .... ▣ 685
Triaminic Night Time Cough & Cold Liquid .... ▣ 685
Triaminic Allergy Runny Nose & Congestion Softchews .... ▣ 688
Triaminic Cold & Cough Softchews .... ▣ 688
Triaminic Cough & Sore Throat Softchews .... ▣ 689
Tylenol Sinus NightTime Caplets .... ▣ 663
Children's Tylenol Plus Cold & Allergy Suspension Liquid 1850
Children's Tylenol Plus Cold NightTime Suspension Liquid 1851
Children's Tylenol Plus Cold & Cough Suspension Liquid and Chewable Tablets 1851
Children's Tylenol Plus Cold Chewable Tablets 1851
Children's Tylenol Plus Cold Daytime Non-Drowsy Suspension Liquid 1851
Children's Tylenol Plus Flu Suspension Liquid 1853
Concentrated Tylenol Infants' Drops Plus Cold 1851
Concentrated Tylenol Infants' Drops Plus Cold and Cough 1851
Tylenol Cold & Flu Severe Daytime Liquid with Cool Bust 1846
Tylenol Cold & Flu Severe NightTime Liquid with Cool Burst 1846
Tylenol Cold Severe Congestion Non-Drowsy Caplets with Cool Burst 1846
Tylenol Allergy Complete Night Time Caplets 1844
Tylenol Allergy Complete Multi-Symptom Caplets and Gelcaps with Cool Burst 1844
Tylenol Flu NightTime Gelcaps 1846
Tylenol Flu Day Non-Drowsy Gelcaps 1846
Concentrated Tylenol Infants' Drops Plus Cold Nasal Congestant, Fever Reducer & Pain Reliever .... ▣ 668
Concentrated Tylenol Infants' Drops Plus Cold & Cough Nasal Decongestant, Fever Reducer & Pain Reliever .... ▣ 668
Multi-Symptom Tylenol Cold Night Time Caplets 1845
Multi-Symptom Tylenol Cold Day Non-Drowsy Caplets and Gelcaps 1845
Tylenol Sinus Day Non-Drowsy 1848
Tylenol Sinus Night Time Caplets 1848
Tylenol Sinus Severe Congestion Caplets with Cool Burst 1848
Vicks 44D Cough & Head Congestion Relief 2676
Vicks 44D Cough & Head Congestion Relief Liquid .... ▣ 721
Vicks 44M Cough, Cold & Flu Relief 2676
Pediatric Vicks 44m Cough & Cold Relief 2673
Vicks DayQuil LiquiCaps/Liquid Multi-Symptom Cold/Flu Relief ..... ▣ 723
Vicks DayQuil Multi-Symptom Cold/Flu Relief LiquiCaps 2675
Vicks DayQuil Multi-Symptom Cold/Flu Relief Liquid 2675
Children's Vicks NyQuil Cold/Cough Relief 2671
Vicks NyQuil LiquiCaps 2677
Vicks NyQuil LiquiCaps/Liquid Multi-Symptom Cold/Flu Relief ..... ▣ 725
Vicks NyQuil Liquid 2677
Zyrtec-D 12 Hour Extended Release Tablets 2591

Pseudoephedrine Sulfate (Sympathomimetic agents may increase certain actions or side effects of anticholinergic agents). Products include:
Alavert Allergy & Sinus D-12 Hour Tablets .... ▣ 743
Clarinex-D 24-Hour Extended-Release Tablets 3012
Claritin-D Non-Drowsy 12 Hour Tablets .... ▣ 731
Claritin-D Non-Drowsy 24 Hour Tablets .... ▣ 731

Pyrilamine Maleate (Antihistamines may increase certain actions or side effects of anticholinergic agents).
No products indexed under this heading.

Pyrilamine Tannate (Antihistamines may increase certain actions or side effects of anticholinergic agents).
No products indexed under this heading.

Quetiapine Fumarate (Antipsychotic agents may increase certain actions or side effects of anticholinergic agents). Products include:
Seroquel Tablets 691

Quinidine Gluconate (Class I antiarrhythmic agents may increase certain actions or side effects of anticholinergic agents).
No products indexed under this heading.

Quinidine Polygalacturonate (Class I antiarrhythmic agents may increase certain actions or side effects of anticholinergic agents).
No products indexed under this heading.

(▣ Described in PDR For Nonprescription Drugs) (⊙ Described in PDR For Ophthalmic Medicines™)

Quinidine Sulfate (Class I antiarrhythmic agents may increase certain actions or side effects of anticholinergic agents).
No products indexed under this heading.

Remifentanil Hydrochloride (Narcotic analgesics may increase certain actions or side effects of anticholinergic agents).
No products indexed under this heading.

Risperidone (Antipsychotic agents may increase certain actions or side effects of anticholinergic agents). Products include:
- Risperdal Consta Long-Acting Injection 1664
- Risperdal M-Tab Orally Disintegrating Tablets 1658
- Risperdal 1658

Salmeterol Xinafoate (Sympathomimetic agents may increase certain actions or side effects of anticholinergic agents). Products include:
- Advair Diskus 100/50 1291
- Advair Diskus 250/50 1291
- Advair Diskus 500/50 1291
- Serevent Diskus 1540

Selegiline Hydrochloride (MAO inhibitors may increase certain actions or side effects of anticholinergic agents). Products include:
- Eldepryl Capsules 3209

Sodium Bicarbonate (Antacids may interfere with the absorption of anticholinergic agents; therefore, simultaneous use of these drugs should be avoided). Products include:
- Ceo-Two Evacuant Suppository 607
- Colyte with Flavor Packs for Oral Solution 3102
- HalfLytely and Bisacodyl Tablets Bowel Prep Kit with Flavors Packs 915
- TriLyte with Flavor Packs for Oral Solution 3114

Sufentanil Citrate (Narcotic analgesics may increase certain actions or side effects of anticholinergic agents).
No products indexed under this heading.

Terbutaline Sulfate (Sympathomimetic agents may increase certain actions or side effects of anticholinergic agents).
No products indexed under this heading.

Terfenadine (Antihistamines may increase certain actions or side effects of anticholinergic agents).
No products indexed under this heading.

Thioridazine Hydrochloride (Antipsychotic agents may increase certain actions or side effects of anticholinergic agents). Products include:
- Thioridazine Hydrochloride Tablets 2122

Thiothixene (Antipsychotic agents may increase certain actions or side effects of anticholinergic agents). Products include:
- Thiothixene Capsules 2124

Timolol Maleate (Anticholinergics antagonize the effects of antiglaucoma agents). Products include:
- Blocadren Tablets 1891
- Cosopt Sterile Ophthalmic Solution 1910
- Timolide Tablets 2056
- Timoptic in Ocudose 2061
- Timoptic Sterile Ophthalmic Solution 2058
- Timoptic-XE Sterile Ophthalmic Gel Forming Solution 2062

Tranylcypromine Sulfate (MAO inhibitors may increase certain actions or side effects of anticholinergic agents). Products include:
- Parnate Tablets 1499

Triamcinolone (Anticholinergic drugs in the presence of increased intraocular pressure may be hazardous when taken concurrently with agents such as corticosteroids).
No products indexed under this heading.

Triamcinolone Acetonide (Anticholinergic drugs in the presence of increased intraocular pressure may be hazardous when taken concurrently with agents such as corticosteroids). Products include:
- Azmacort Inhalation Aerosol 1701
- Nasacort HFA Inhalation Aerosol 2939
- Nasacort AQ Nasal Spray 2937

Triamcinolone Diacetate (Anticholinergic drugs in the presence of increased intraocular pressure may be hazardous when taken concurrently with agents such as corticosteroids).
No products indexed under this heading.

Triamcinolone Hexacetonide (Anticholinergic drugs in the presence of increased intraocular pressure may be hazardous when taken concurrently with agents such as corticosteroids).
No products indexed under this heading.

Trifluoperazine Hydrochloride (Antipsychotic agents may increase certain actions or side effects of anticholinergic agents).
No products indexed under this heading.

Trimeprazine Tartrate (Antihistamines may increase certain actions or side effects of anticholinergic agents).
No products indexed under this heading.

Trimipramine Maleate (Tricyclic antidepressants may increase certain actions or side effects of anticholinergic agents). Products include:
- Surmontil Capsules 2347

Tripelennamine Hydrochloride (Antihistamines may increase certain actions or side effects of anticholinergic agents).
No products indexed under this heading.

Triprolidine Hydrochloride (Antihistamines may increase certain actions or side effects of anticholinergic agents).
No products indexed under this heading.

Ziprasidone Hydrochloride (Antipsychotic agents may increase certain actions or side effects of anticholinergic agents). Products include:
- Geodon Capsules 2514

BENZACLIN TOPICAL GEL

(Benzoyl Peroxide, Clindamycin Phosphate) 1046

May interact with peeling/desquamating agents and certain other agents. Compounds in these categories include:

Acitretin (Concomitant topical acne therapy should be used with caution because a possible cumulative irritancy may occur, especially with the use of peeling, desquamating or abrasive agents). Products include:
- Soriatane Capsules 1028

Adapalene (Concomitant topical acne therapy should be used with caution because a possible cumulative irritancy may occur, especially with the use of peeling, desquamating or abrasive agents). Products include:
- Differin Cream 1210
- Differin Gel 1211

Azelaic Acid (Concomitant topical acne therapy should be used with caution because a possible cumulative irritancy may occur, especially with the use of peeling, desquamating or abrasive agents). Products include:
- Athena Hair System Shampoo 767
- Finacea Gel 1644
- Spartan Hair System Shampoo 767

Calcipotriene (Concomitant topical acne therapy should be used with caution because a possible cumulative irritancy may occur, especially with the use of peeling, desquamating or abrasive agents). Products include:
- Dovonex Cream 0.005% 3374
- Dovonex Ointment 0.005% 3375
- Dovonex Scalp Solution 0.005% 3375

Clindamycin, Topical (Concomitant topical acne therapy should be used with caution because a possible cumulative irritancy may occur, especially with the use of peeling, desquamating or abrasive agents).
No products indexed under this heading.

Clotrimazole, Topical (Concomitant topical acne therapy should be used with caution because a possible cumulative irritancy may occur, especially with the use of peeling, desquamating or abrasive agents).
No products indexed under this heading.

Coal Tar (Concomitant topical acne therapy should be used with caution because a possible cumulative irritancy may occur, especially with the use of peeling, desquamating or abrasive agents). Products include:
- Tegrin Dandruff Shampoo - Extra Conditioning 637
- Tegrin Dandruff Shampoo - Fresh Herbal 638
- Tegrin Skin Cream 638

Concomitant Topical Acne Therapy (Possible cumulative irritancy effect may occur, especially with the use of peeling, desquamating, or abrasive agents).
No products indexed under this heading.

Erythromycin, Topical (Concomitant topical acne therapy should be used with caution because a possible cumulative irritancy may occur, especially with the use of peeling, desquamating or abrasive agents).
No products indexed under this heading.

Fluorouracil, Topical (Concomitant topical acne therapy should be used with caution because a possible cumulative irritancy may occur, especially with the use of peeling, desquamating or abrasive agents).
No products indexed under this heading.

Hydroquinone (Concomitant topical acne therapy should be used with caution because a possible cumulative irritancy may occur, especially with the use of peeling, desquamating or abrasive agents). Products include:
- Claripel Cream 3212
- Lustra Cream 3287
- Lustra-AF Cream 3287
- Lustra-Ultra Cream 3287
- Tri-Luma Cream 1213

Isotretinoin (Concomitant topical acne therapy should be used with caution because a possible cumulative irritancy may occur, especially with the use of peeling, desquamating or abrasive agents). Products include:
- Accutane Capsules 2740
- Amnesteem Capsules 2126

Mequinol (Concomitant topical acne therapy should be used with caution because a possible cumulative irritancy may occur, especially with the use of peeling, desquamating or abrasive agents). Products include:
- Solage Topical Solution 740

Podofilox (Concomitant topical acne therapy should be used with caution because a possible cumulative irritancy may occur, especially with the use of peeling, desquamating or abrasive agents).
No products indexed under this heading.

Salicylic Acid (Concomitant topical acne therapy should be used with caution because a possible cumulative irritancy may occur, especially with the use of peeling, desquamating or abrasive agents).
No products indexed under this heading.

Sulfur Preparations (Concomitant topical acne therapy should be used with caution because a possible cumulative irritancy may occur, especially with the use of peeling, desquamating or abrasive agents).
No products indexed under this heading.

Tazarotene (Concomitant topical acne therapy should be used with caution because a possible cumulative irritancy may occur, especially with the use of peeling, desquamating or abrasive agents).
No products indexed under this heading.

Tretinoin (Concomitant topical acne therapy should be used with caution because a possible cumulative irritancy may occur, especially with the use of peeling, desquamating or abrasive agents). Products include:
- Avita Cream 2136
- Avita Gel 2138
- Renova 0.02% Cream 2384
- Renova 0.05% Cream 2387
- Retin-A Micro 0.1%/0.04% 2388
- Solage Topical Solution 740
- Tri-Luma Cream 1213
- Vesanoid Capsules 2823

Zalcitabine (Concomitant topical acne therapy should be used with caution because a possible cumulative irritancy may occur, especially with the use of peeling, desquamating or abrasive agents).
No products indexed under this heading.

BETADINE 5% OPHTHALMIC SOLUTION

(Povidone Iodine) .... ⊙202
None cited in PDR database.

BETADINE SKIN CLEANSER

(Povidone Iodine) 2714
None cited in PDR database.

BETADINE SOLUTION

(Povidone Iodine) 2715
None cited in PDR database.

BETADINE SURGICAL SCRUB

(Povidone Iodine) 2715
None cited in PDR database.

BETAGAN OPHTHALMIC SOLUTION, USP

(Levobunolol Hydrochloride) .... ⊙217
May interact with beta blockers, cardiac glycosides, phenothiazines, and certain other agents. Compounds in these categories include:

Acebutolol Hydrochloride (Co-administration with oral beta blockers may result in additive effect either on intraocular pressure or on the known systemic effects of beta blockade).
No products indexed under this heading.

Atenolol (Co-administration with oral beta blockers may result in additive effect either on intraocular pressure or on the known systemic effects of beta blockade). Products include:
Tenormin I.V. Injection 698
Tenormin Tablets 695

Betaxolol Hydrochloride (Co-administration with oral beta blockers may result in additive effect either on intraocular pressure or on the known systemic effects of beta blockade). Products include:
Betoptic S Ophthalmic Suspension................................ 554

Bisoprolol Fumarate (Co-administration with oral beta blockers may result in additive effect either on intraocular pressure or on the known systemic effects of beta blockade).
No products indexed under this heading.

Carteolol Hydrochloride (Co-administration with oral beta blockers may result in additive effect either on intraocular pressure or on the known systemic effects of beta blockade). Products include:
Carteolol Hydrochloride Ophthalmic Solution USP, 1%..... ⊙246

Chlorpromazine (Co-administration with phenothiazine-related compounds may have an additive hypotensive effect due to inhibition of each other's metabolism).
No products indexed under this heading.

Chlorpromazine Hydrochloride (Co-administration with phenothiazine-related compounds may have an additive hypotensive effect due to inhibition of each other's metabolism).
No products indexed under this heading.

Deserpidine (Possible additive effects and production of hypotension and/or bradycardia when beta blocker is concurrently used with catecholamine-depleting drugs).
No products indexed under this heading.

Deslanoside (Co-administration with digitalis and calcium channel blockers may have an additive effect on prolonging atrioventricular conduction time).
No products indexed under this heading.

Digitalis Glycoside Preparations (Co-administration with digitalis and calcium channel blockers may have an additive effect on prolonging atrioventricular conduction time).
No products indexed under this heading.

Digitoxin (Co-administration with digitalis and calcium channel blockers may have an additive effect on prolonging atrioventricular conduction time).
No products indexed under this heading.

Digoxin (Co-administration with digitalis and calcium channel blockers may have an additive effect on prolonging atrioventricular conduction time). Products include:
Digitek Tablets 2146
Lanoxicaps Capsules 1458
Lanoxin Injection 1462
Lanoxin Tablets 1468
Lanoxin Injection Pediatric 1465

Epinephrine (Concurrent use in patients with history of atopy or severe anaphylactic reaction to allergens may be unresponsive to the usual doses of epinephrine used to treat anaphylactic reaction; mydriasis may result with concomitant epinephrine). Products include:
EpiPen 1061
Primatene Mist .... ▣749

Epinephrine Hydrochloride (Concurrent use in patients with history of atopy or severe anaphylactic reaction to allergens may be unresponsive to the usual doses of epinephrine used to treat anaphylactic reaction; mydriasis may result with concomitant epinephrine).
No products indexed under this heading.

Esmolol Hydrochloride (Co-administration with oral beta blockers may result in additive effect either on intraocular pressure or on the known systemic effects of beta blockade). Products include:
Brevibloc Concentrate 766
Brevibloc Injection 766
Brevibloc Double Strength Injection.. 766
Brevibloc Premixed Injection 766
Brevibloc Double Strength Premixed Injection 766

Fluphenazine Decanoate (Co-administration with phenothiazine-related compounds may have an additive hypotensive effect due to inhibition of each other's metabolism).
No products indexed under this heading.

Fluphenazine Enanthate (Co-administration with phenothiazine-related compounds may have an additive hypotensive effect due to inhibition of each other's metabolism).
No products indexed under this heading.

Fluphenazine Hydrochloride (Co-administration with phenothiazine-related compounds may have an additive hypotensive effect due to inhibition of each other's metabolism).
No products indexed under this heading.

Labetalol Hydrochloride (Co-administration with oral beta blockers may result in additive effect either on intraocular pressure or on the known systemic effects of beta blockade).
No products indexed under this heading.

Mesoridazine Besylate (Co-administration with phenothiazine-related compounds may have an additive hypotensive effect due to inhibition of each other's metabolism).
No products indexed under this heading.

Methotrimeprazine (Co-administration with phenothiazine-related compounds may have an additive hypotensive effect due to inhibition of each other's metabolism).
No products indexed under this heading.

Metipranolol Hydrochloride (Co-administration with oral beta blockers may result in additive effect either on intraocular pressure or on the known systemic effects of beta blockade).
No products indexed under this heading.

Metoprolol Succinate (Co-administration with oral beta blockers may result in additive effect either on intraocular pressure or on the known systemic effects of beta blockade). Products include:
Toprol-XL Tablets 660

Metoprolol Tartrate (Co-administration with oral beta blockers may result in additive effect either on intraocular pressure or on the known systemic effects of beta blockade).
No products indexed under this heading.

Nadolol (Co-administration with oral beta blockers may result in additive effect either on intraocular pressure or on the known systemic effects of beta blockade). Products include:
Nadolol Tablets 2121

Penbutolol Sulfate (Co-administration with oral beta blockers may result in additive effect either on intraocular pressure or on the known systemic effects of beta blockade).
No products indexed under this heading.

Perphenazine (Co-administration with phenothiazine-related compounds may have an additive hypotensive effect due to inhibition of each other's metabolism).
No products indexed under this heading.

Pindolol (Co-administration with oral beta blockers may result in additive effect either on intraocular pressure or on the known systemic effects of beta blockade).
No products indexed under this heading.

Prochlorperazine (Co-administration with phenothiazine-related compounds may have an additive hypotensive effect due to inhibition of each other's metabolism).
No products indexed under this heading.

Promethazine Hydrochloride (Co-administration with phenothiazine-related compounds may have an additive hypotensive effect due to inhibition of each other's metabolism). Products include:
Phenergan 3438

Propranolol Hydrochloride (Co-administration with oral beta blockers may result in additive effect either on intraocular pressure or on the known systemic effects of beta blockade). Products include:
Inderal LA Long-Acting Capsules 3421
InnoPran XL Capsules 2728

Rauwolfia Serpentina (Possible additive effects and production of hypotension and/or bradycardia when beta blocker is concurrently used with catecholamine-depleting drugs).
No products indexed under this heading.

Rescinnamine (Possible additive effects and production of hypotension and/or bradycardia when beta blocker is concurrently used with catecholamine-depleting drugs).
No products indexed under this heading.

Reserpine (Possible additive effects and production of hypotension and/or bradycardia when beta blocker is concurrently used with catecholamine-depleting drugs).
No products indexed under this heading.

Sotalol Hydrochloride (Co-administration with oral beta blockers may result in additive effect either on intraocular pressure or on the known systemic effects of beta blockade).
No products indexed under this heading.

Thioridazine Hydrochloride (Co-administration with phenothiazine-related compounds may have an additive hypotensive effect due to inhibition of each other's metabolism). Products include:
Thioridazine Hydrochloride Tablets 2122

Timolol Hemihydrate (Co-administration with oral beta blockers may result in additive effect either on intraocular pressure or on the known systemic effects of beta blockade). Products include:
Betimol Ophthalmic Solution 3371
Betimol Ophthalmic Solution .... ⊙283

Timolol Maleate (Co-administration with oral beta blockers may result in additive effect either on intraocular pressure or on the known systemic effects of beta blockade). Products include:
Blocadren Tablets 1891
Cosopt Sterile Ophthalmic Solution 1910
Timolide Tablets 2056
Timoptic in Ocudose 2061
Timoptic Sterile Ophthalmic Solution 2058
Timoptic-XE Sterile Ophthalmic Gel Forming Solution 2062

Trifluoperazine Hydrochloride (Co-administration with phenothiazine-related compounds may have an additive hypotensive effect due to inhibition of each other's metabolism).
No products indexed under this heading.

BETASEPT SURGICAL SCRUB

(Chlorhexidine Gluconate) 2715
None cited in PDR database.

BETASERON FOR SC INJECTION
(Interferon Beta-1b) 791
None cited in PDR database.

BETIMOL OPHTHALMIC SOLUTION
(Timolol Hemihydrate) 3371
May interact with beta blockers, calcium channel blockers, cardiac glycosides, and certain other agents. Compounds in these categories include:

Acebutolol Hydrochloride (Concurrent use with systemic beta blockers may result in additive effect either on the intraocular pressure or the known systemic effect of beta blockade).
No products indexed under this heading.

Amlodipine Besylate (Possible atrioventricular conduction disturbances, left ventricular failure, and hypotension). Products include:
Caduet Tablets 2507
Lotrel Capsules 2238
Norvasc Tablets 2529

Atenolol (Concurrent use with systemic beta blockers may result in additive effect either on the intraocular pressure or the known systemic effect of beta blockade). Products include:
Tenormin I.V. Injection 698
Tenormin Tablets 695

Bepridil Hydrochloride (Possible atrioventricular conduction disturbances, left ventricular failure, and hypotension).
No products indexed under this heading.

Betaxolol Hydrochloride (Concurrent use with systemic beta blockers may result in additive effect either on the intraocular pressure or the known systemic effect of beta blockade). Products include:
Betoptic S Ophthalmic Suspension.................................. 554

Bisoprolol Fumarate (Concurrent use with systemic beta blockers may result in additive effect either on the intraocular pressure or the known systemic effect of beta blockade).
No products indexed under this heading.

Carteolol Hydrochloride (Concurrent use with systemic beta blockers may result in additive effect either on the intraocular pressure or the known systemic effect of beta blockade). Products include:
Carteolol Hydrochloride Ophthalmic Solution USP, 1%....... ⊙246

Deslanoside (Concomitant use of beta blockers with digitalis and calcium antagonists may have additive effects in prolonging atrioventricular conduction time).
No products indexed under this heading.

Digitalis Glycoside Preparations (Concomitant use of beta blockers with digitalis and calcium antagonists may have additive effects in prolonging atrioventricular conduction time).
No products indexed under this heading.

Digitoxin (Concomitant use of beta blockers with digitalis and calcium antagonists may have additive effects in prolonging atrioventricular conduction time).
No products indexed under this heading.

Digoxin (Concomitant use of beta blockers with digitalis and calcium antagonists may have additive effects in prolonging atrioventricular conduction time). Products include:
Digitek Tablets 2146
Lanoxicaps Capsules 1458
Lanoxin Injection 1462
Lanoxin Tablets 1468
Lanoxin Injection Pediatric 1465

Diltiazem Hydrochloride (Possible atrioventricular conduction disturbances, left ventricular failure, and hypotension). Products include:
Cardizem LA Extended Release Tablets 1699
Tiazac Capsules 1204

Epinephrine (Patients with a history of atopy or anaphylactic reactions to a variety of allergens may be unresponsive to the usual dose of injectable epinephrine used to treat allergic reactions). Products include:
EpiPen 1061
Primatene Mist 749

Epinephrine Bitartrate (Patients with a history of atopy or anaphylactic reactions to a variety of allergens may be unresponsive to the usual dose of injectable epinephrine used to treat allergic reactions).
No products indexed under this heading.

Esmolol Hydrochloride (Concurrent use with systemic beta blockers may result in additive effect either on the intraocular pressure or the known systemic effect of beta blockade). Products include:
Brevibloc Concentrate 766
Brevibloc Injection 766
Brevibloc Double Strength Injection.. 766
Brevibloc Premixed Injection 766
Brevibloc Double Strength Premixed Injection.............................. 766

Felodipine (Possible atrioventricular conduction disturbances, left ventricular failure, and hypotension). Products include:
Plendil Extended-Release Tablets 651

Isradipine (Possible atrioventricular conduction disturbances, left ventricular failure, and hypotension). Products include:
DynaCirc CR Tablets 2726

Labetalol Hydrochloride (Concurrent use with systemic beta blockers may result in additive effect either on the intraocular pressure or the known systemic effect of beta blockade).
No products indexed under this heading.

Levobunolol Hydrochloride (Concurrent use with systemic beta blockers may result in additive effect either on the intraocular pressure or the known systemic effect of beta blockade). Products include:
Betagan Ophthalmic Solution, USP.. ⊙217

Metipranolol Hydrochloride (Concurrent use with systemic beta blockers may result in additive effect either on the intraocular pressure or the known systemic effect of beta blockade).
No products indexed under this heading.

Metoprolol Succinate (Concurrent use with systemic beta blockers may result in additive effect either on the intraocular pressure or the known systemic effect of beta blockade). Products include:
Toprol-XL Tablets 660

Metoprolol Tartrate (Concurrent use with systemic beta blockers may result in additive effect either on the intraocular pressure or the known systemic effect of beta blockade).
No products indexed under this heading.

Mibefradil Dihydrochloride (Possible atrioventricular conduction disturbances, left ventricular failure, and hypotension).
No products indexed under this heading.

Nadolol (Concurrent use with systemic beta blockers may result in additive effect either on the intraocular pressure or the known systemic effect of beta blockade). Products include:
Nadolol Tablets 2121

Nicardipine Hydrochloride (Possible atrioventricular conduction disturbances, left ventricular failure, and hypotension). Products include:
Cardene I.V. 1129

Nifedipine (Possible atrioventricular conduction disturbances, left ventricular failure, and hypotension). Products include:
Adalat CC Tablets 2978

Nimodipine (Possible atrioventricular conduction disturbances, left ventricular failure, and hypotension). Products include:
Nimotop Capsules 774

Nisoldipine (Possible atrioventricular conduction disturbances, left ventricular failure, and hypotension). Products include:
Sular Tablets 1163

Penbutolol Sulfate (Concurrent use with systemic beta blockers may result in additive effect either on the intraocular pressure or the known systemic effect of beta blockade).
No products indexed under this heading.

Pindolol (Concurrent use with systemic beta blockers may result in additive effect either on the intraocular pressure or the known systemic effect of beta blockade).
No products indexed under this heading.

Propranolol Hydrochloride (Concurrent use with systemic beta blockers may result in additive effect either on the intraocular pressure or the known systemic effect of beta blockade). Products include:
Inderal LA Long-Acting Capsules 3421
InnoPran XL Capsules 2728

Sotalol Hydrochloride (Concurrent use with systemic beta blockers may result in additive effect either on the intraocular pressure or the known systemic effect of beta blockade).
No products indexed under this heading.

Timolol Maleate (Concurrent use with systemic beta blockers may result in additive effect either on the intraocular pressure or the known systemic effect of beta blockade). Products include:
Blocadren Tablets 1891
Cosopt Sterile Ophthalmic Solution... 1910
Timolide Tablets 2056
Timoptic in Ocudose 2061
Timoptic Sterile Ophthalmic Solution... 2058
Timoptic-XE Sterile Ophthalmic Gel Forming Solution 2062

Verapamil Hydrochloride (Possible atrioventricular conduction disturbances, left ventricular failure, and hypotension). Products include:
Covera-HS Tablets 3135
Tarka Tablets 519
Verelan PM Capsules 3120

BETOPTIC S OPHTHALMIC SUSPENSION
(Betaxolol Hydrochloride) 554
May interact with adrenergic augmenting psychotropics, beta blockers, and certain other agents. Compounds in these categories include:

Acebutolol Hydrochloride (Co-administration with oral beta blockers may result in additive effects either on intraocular pressure or on the known systemic effects of beta blockade).
No products indexed under this heading.

Atenolol (Co-administration with oral beta blockers may result in additive effects either on intraocular pressure or on the known systemic effects of beta blockade). Products include:
Tenormin I.V. Injection 698
Tenormin Tablets 695

Bisoprolol Fumarate (Co-administration with oral beta blockers may result in additive effects either on intraocular pressure or on the known systemic effects of beta blockade).
No products indexed under this heading.

Carteolol Hydrochloride (Co-administration with oral beta blockers may result in additive effects either on intraocular pressure or on the known systemic effects of beta blockade). Products include:
Carteolol Hydrochloride Ophthalmic Solution USP, 1%....... ⊙246

Deserpidine (Possible additive effects and production of hypotension and/or bradycardia when beta blocker is concurrently used with catecholamine depleting drugs).
No products indexed under this heading.

Epinephrine (Concurrent use in patients with history of atopy or severe anaphylactic reaction to allergens may be unresponsive to the usual doses of epinephrine used to treat anaphylactic reaction). Products include:
EpiPen 1061
Primatene Mist 749

Epinephrine Hydrochloride (Concurrent use in patients with history of atopy or severe anaphylactic reaction to allergens may be unresponsive to the usual doses of epinephrine used to treat anaphylactic reaction).
No products indexed under this heading.

Esmolol Hydrochloride (Co-administration with oral beta blockers may result in additive effects either on intraocular pressure or on the known systemic effects of beta blockade). Products include:
Brevibloc Concentrate 766
Brevibloc Injection 766
Brevibloc Double Strength Injection.. 766
Brevibloc Premixed Injection 766
Brevibloc Double Strength Premixed Injection.............................. 766

Isocarboxazid (Exercise caution when used concurrently with adrenergic psychotropic drugs).
No products indexed under this heading.

Labetalol Hydrochloride (Co-administration with oral beta blockers may result in additive effects either on intraocular pressure or on the known systemic effects of beta blockade).
No products indexed under this heading.

Levobunolol Hydrochloride (Co-administration with oral beta blockers may result in additive effects either on intraocular pressure or on the known systemic effects of beta blockade). Products include:
Betagan Ophthalmic Solution, USP .... ⊙217

Metipranolol Hydrochloride (Co-administration with oral beta blockers may result in additive effects either on intraocular pressure or on the known systemic effects of beta blockade).
No products indexed under this heading.

Metoprolol Succinate (Co-administration with oral beta blockers may result in additive effects either on intraocular pressure or on the known systemic effects of beta blockade). Products include:
Toprol-XL Tablets 660

Metoprolol Tartrate (Co-administration with oral beta blockers may result in additive effects either on intraocular pressure or on the known systemic effects of beta blockade).
No products indexed under this heading.

Nadolol (Co-administration with oral beta blockers may result in additive effects either on intraocular pressure or on the known systemic effects of beta blockade). Products include:
Nadolol Tablets 2121

Pargyline Hydrochloride (Exercise caution when used concurrently with adrenergic psychotropic drugs).
No products indexed under this heading.

Penbutolol Sulfate (Co-administration with oral beta blockers may result in additive effects either on intraocular pressure or on the known systemic effects of beta blockade).
No products indexed under this heading.

Phenelzine Sulfate (Exercise caution when used concurrently with adrenergic psychotropic drugs).
No products indexed under this heading.

Pindolol (Co-administration with oral beta blockers may result in additive effects either on intraocular pressure or on the known systemic effects of beta blockade).
No products indexed under this heading.

Propranolol Hydrochloride (Co-administration with oral beta blockers may result in additive effects either on intraocular pressure or on the known systemic effects of beta blockade). Products include:
Inderal LA Long-Acting Capsules 3421
InnoPran XL Capsules 2728

Rauwolfia Serpentina (Possible additive effects and production of hypotension and/or bradycardia when beta blocker is concurrently used with catecholamine depleting drugs).
No products indexed under this heading.

Rescinnamine (Possible additive effects and production of hypotension and/or bradycardia when beta blocker is concurrently used with catecholamine depleting drugs).
No products indexed under this heading.

Reserpine (Possible additive effects and production of hypotension and/or bradycardia when beta blocker is concurrently used with catecholamine depleting drugs).
No products indexed under this heading.

Sotalol Hydrochloride (Co-administration with oral beta blockers may result in additive effects either on intraocular pressure or on the known systemic effects of beta blockade).
No products indexed under this heading.

Timolol Hemihydrate (Co-administration with oral beta blockers may result in additive effects either on intraocular pressure or on the known systemic effects of beta blockade). Products include:
Betimol Ophthalmic Solution 3371
Betimol Ophthalmic Solution .... ⊙283

Timolol Maleate (Co-administration with oral beta blockers may result in additive effects either on intraocular pressure or on the known systemic effects of beta blockade). Products include:
Blocadren Tablets 1891
Cosopt Sterile Ophthalmic Solution 1910
Timolide Tablets 2056
Timoptic in Ocudose 2061
Timoptic Sterile Ophthalmic Solution 2058
Timoptic-XE Sterile Ophthalmic Gel Forming Solution 2062

Tranylcypromine Sulfate (Exercise caution when used concurrently with adrenergic psychotropic drugs). Products include:
Parnate Tablets 1499

BEVITAMEL TABLETS

(Folic Acid, Melatonin, Vitamin B_{12}) 3392
None cited in PDR database.

BEXXAR

(Iodine I 131 Tositumomab, Tositumomab) 1360
May interact with anticoagulants, oral anticoagulants, and platelet inhibitors. Compounds in these categories include:

Anisindione (Due to the frequent occurrence of severe and prolonged thrombocytopenia, the potential benefits of medications that interfere with platelet function and/or anticoagulation should be weighed against the potential increased risk of bleeding and hemorrhage). Products include:
Miradon Tablets 3056

Ardeparin Sodium (Due to the frequent occurrence of severe and prolonged thrombocytopenia, the potential benefits of medications that interfere with platelet function and/or anticoagulation should be weighed against the potential increased risk of bleeding and hemorrhage).
No products indexed under this heading.

Aspirin (Due to the frequent occurrence of severe and prolonged thrombocytopenia, the potential benefits of medications that interfere with platelet function and/or anticoagulation should be weighed against the potential increased risk of bleeding and hemorrhage). Products include:
Aggrenox Capsules 855
Bayer, Aspirin Regimen .... ▣606
Bayer Aspirin Tablets 3515
BC Powder .... ▣612
BC Allergy Sinus Cold Powder .... ▣612
Arthritis Strength BC Powder .... ▣612
BC Sinus Cold Powder .... ▣612
Ecotrin Enteric Coated Aspirin Low, Regular and Maximum Strength Tablets 1627
Goody's Body Pain Formula Powder .... ▣621
Goody's Extra Strength Headache Powder .... ▣621
Goody's Extra Strength Pain Relief Tablets .... ▣621
Percodan Tablets 1115
St. Joseph 81 mg Aspirin Chewable and Enteric Coated Tablets 1841

Aspirin, Enteric Coated (Due to the frequent occurrence of severe and prolonged thrombocytopenia, the potential benefits of medications that interfere with platelet function and/or anticoagulation should be weighed against the potential increased risk of bleeding and hemorrhage).
No products indexed under this heading.

Aspirin Buffered (Due to the frequent occurrence of severe and prolonged thrombocytopenia, the potential benefits of medications that interfere with platelet function and/or anticoagulation should be weighed against the potential increased risk of bleeding and hemorrhage).
No products indexed under this heading.

Azlocillin Sodium (Due to the frequent occurrence of severe and prolonged thrombocytopenia, the potential benefits of medications that interfere with platelet function and/or anticoagulation should be weighed against the potential increased risk of bleeding and hemorrhage).
No products indexed under this heading.

Carbenicillin Indanyl Sodium (Due to the frequent occurrence of severe and prolonged thrombocytopenia, the potential benefits of medications that interfere with platelet function and/or anticoagulation should be weighed against the potential increased risk of bleeding and hemorrhage).
No products indexed under this heading.

Choline Magnesium Trisalicylate (Due to the frequent occurrence of severe and prolonged thrombocytopenia, the potential benefits of medications that interfere with platelet function and/or anticoagulation should be weighed against the potential increased risk of bleeding and hemorrhage).
No products indexed under this heading.

Clopidogrel Bisulfate (Due to the frequent occurrence of severe and prolonged thrombocytopenia, the potential benefits of medications that interfere with platelet function and/or anticoagulation should be weighed against the potential increased risk of bleeding and hemorrhage). Products include:
Plavix Tablets 940
Plavix Tablets 2942

Dalteparin Sodium (Due to the frequent occurrence of severe and prolonged thrombocytopenia, the potential benefits of medications that interfere with platelet function and/or anticoagulation should be weighed against the potential increased risk of bleeding and hemorrhage). Products include:
Fragmin Injection 2638

Danaparoid Sodium (Due to the frequent occurrence of severe and prolonged thrombocytopenia, the potential benefits of medications that interfere with platelet function and/or anticoagulation should be weighed against the potential increased risk of bleeding and hemorrhage).
No products indexed under this heading.

Diclofenac Potassium (Due to the frequent occurrence of severe and prolonged thrombocytopenia, the potential benefits of medications that interfere with platelet function and/or anticoagulation should be weighed against the potential increased risk of bleeding and hemorrhage). Products include:
Cataflam Tablets 2173

Diclofenac Sodium (Due to the frequent occurrence of severe and prolonged thrombocytopenia, the potential benefits of medications that interfere with platelet function and/or anticoagulation should be weighed against the potential increased risk of bleeding and hemorrhage). Products include:
Arthrotec Tablets 3126
Voltaren Ophthalmic Solution 2300
Voltaren Tablets 2298
Voltaren-XR Tablets 2301

Dicumarol (Due to the frequent occurrence of severe and prolonged thrombocytopenia, the potential benefits of medications that interfere with platelet function and/or anticoagulation should be weighed against the potential increased risk of bleeding and hemorrhage).
No products indexed under this heading.

Diflunisal (Due to the frequent occurrence of severe and prolonged thrombocytopenia, the potential benefits of medications that interfere with platelet function and/or anticoagulation should be weighed against the potential increased risk of bleeding and hemorrhage). Products include:
Dolobid Tablets 1937

Dipyridamole (Due to the frequent occurrence of severe and prolonged thrombocytopenia, the potential benefits of medications that interfere with platelet function and/or anticoagulation should be weighed against the potential increased risk of bleeding and hemorrhage). Products include:

Aggrenox Capsules 855
Persantine Tablets 898

Enoxaparin Sodium (Due to the frequent occurrence of severe and prolonged thrombocytopenia, the potential benefits of medications that interfere with platelet function and/ or anticoagulation should be weighed against the potential increased risk of bleeding and hemorrhage). Products include:

Lovenox Injection 2931

Fenoprofen Calcium (Due to the frequent occurrence of severe and prolonged thrombocytopenia, the potential benefits of medications that interfere with platelet function and/ or anticoagulation should be weighed against the potential increased risk of bleeding and hemorrhage). Products include:

Nalfon Capsules 2504

Flurbiprofen (Due to the frequent occurrence of severe and prolonged thrombocytopenia, the potential benefits of medications that interfere with platelet function and/or anticoagulation should be weighed against the potential increased risk of bleeding and hemorrhage).

No products indexed under this heading.

Fondaparinux Sodium (Due to the frequent occurrence of severe and prolonged thrombocytopenia, the potential benefits of medications that interfere with platelet function and/ or anticoagulation should be weighed against the potential increased risk of bleeding and hemorrhage). Products include:

Arixtra Injection 1325

Heparin Calcium (Due to the frequent occurrence of severe and prolonged thrombocytopenia, the potential benefits of medications that interfere with platelet function and/ or anticoagulation should be weighed against the potential increased risk of bleeding and hemorrhage).

No products indexed under this heading.

Heparin Sodium (Due to the frequent occurrence of severe and prolonged thrombocytopenia, the potential benefits of medications that interfere with platelet function and/ or anticoagulation should be weighed against the potential increased risk of bleeding and hemorrhage).

No products indexed under this heading.

Ibuprofen (Due to the frequent occurrence of severe and prolonged thrombocytopenia, the potential benefits of medications that interfere with platelet function and/or anticoagulation should be weighed against the potential increased risk of bleeding and hemorrhage). Products include:

Advil Allergy Sinus Caplets 737
Advil 737
Children's Advil Suspension 742
Children's Advil Chewable Tablets .. 741
Advil Cold & Sinus 739
Advil Flu & Body Ache Caplets 739
Children's Advil Cold Suspension ... 741
Infants' Advil Concentrated Drops .. 743
Junior Strength Advil Swallow Tablets 740
Advil Migraine Liquigels 740
Advil Multi-Symptom Cold Caplets 738
Combunox Tablets 1183
Children's Motrin Oral Suspension and Chewable Tablets 1837
Children's Motrin Cold Non-Staining Dye-Free Oral Suspension 1838
Children's Motrin Cold Oral Suspension 1838
Children's Motrin Non-Staining Dye-Free Oral Suspension............ 1837
Motrin Cold & Sinus Caplets 1836
Motrin IB Tablets and Caplets 1836
Infants' Motrin Concentrated Drops 1837
Infants' Motrin Non-Staining Dye-Free Drops........................... 1837
Junior Strength Motrin Caplets and Chewable Tablets.................. 1837
Vicoprofen Tablets 533

Indomethacin (Due to the frequent occurrence of severe and prolonged thrombocytopenia, the potential benefits of medications that interfere with platelet function and/or anticoagulation should be weighed against the potential increased risk of bleeding and hemorrhage). Products include:

Indocin 1968

Indomethacin Sodium Trihydrate (Due to the frequent occurrence of severe and prolonged thrombocytopenia, the potential benefits of medications that interfere with platelet function and/or anticoagulation should be weighed against the potential increased risk of bleeding and hemorrhage). Products include:

Indocin I.V. 1973

Ketoprofen (Due to the frequent occurrence of severe and prolonged thrombocytopenia, the potential benefits of medications that interfere with platelet function and/or anticoagulation should be weighed against the potential increased risk of bleeding and hemorrhage).

No products indexed under this heading.

Low Molecular Weight Heparins (Due to the frequent occurrence of severe and prolonged thrombocytopenia, the potential benefits of medications that interfere with platelet function and/or anticoagulation should be weighed against the potential increased risk of bleeding and hemorrhage).

No products indexed under this heading.

Magnesium Salicylate (Due to the frequent occurrence of severe and prolonged thrombocytopenia, the potential benefits of medications that interfere with platelet function and/ or anticoagulation should be weighed against the potential increased risk of bleeding and hemorrhage).

No products indexed under this heading.

Meclofenamate Sodium (Due to the frequent occurrence of severe and prolonged thrombocytopenia, the potential benefits of medications that interfere with platelet function and/or anticoagulation should be weighed against the potential increased risk of bleeding and hemorrhage).

No products indexed under this heading.

Mefenamic Acid (Due to the frequent occurrence of severe and prolonged thrombocytopenia, the potential benefits of medications that interfere with platelet function and/ or anticoagulation should be weighed against the potential increased risk of bleeding and hemorrhage).

No products indexed under this heading.

Mezlocillin Sodium (Due to the frequent occurrence of severe and prolonged thrombocytopenia, the potential benefits of medications that interfere with platelet function and/ or anticoagulation should be weighed against the potential increased risk of bleeding and hemorrhage).

No products indexed under this heading.

Nafcillin Sodium (Due to the frequent occurrence of severe and prolonged thrombocytopenia, the potential benefits of medications that interfere with platelet function and/ or anticoagulation should be weighed against the potential increased risk of bleeding and hemorrhage).

No products indexed under this heading.

Naproxen (Due to the frequent occurrence of severe and prolonged thrombocytopenia, the potential benefits of medications that interfere with platelet function and/or anticoagulation should be weighed against the potential increased risk of bleeding and hemorrhage). Products include:

EC-Naprosyn Delayed-Release Tablets 2769
Naprosyn Suspension 2769
Naprosyn Tablets 2769
Prevacid NapraPAC 3277

Naproxen Sodium (Due to the frequent occurrence of severe and prolonged thrombocytopenia, the potential benefits of medications that interfere with platelet function and/ or anticoagulation should be weighed against the potential increased risk of bleeding and hemorrhage). Products include:

Aleve Tablets, Caplets and Gelcaps 605
Anaprox Tablets 2769
Anaprox DS Tablets 2769

Penicillin G Benzathine (Due to the frequent occurrence of severe and prolonged thrombocytopenia, the potential benefits of medications that interfere with platelet function and/or anticoagulation should be weighed against the potential increased risk of bleeding and hemorrhage).

No products indexed under this heading.

Penicillin G Procaine (Due to the frequent occurrence of severe and prolonged thrombocytopenia, the potential benefits of medications that interfere with platelet function and/ or anticoagulation should be weighed against the potential increased risk of bleeding and hemorrhage).

No products indexed under this heading.

Phenylbutazone (Due to the frequent occurrence of severe and prolonged thrombocytopenia, the potential benefits of medications that interfere with platelet function and/ or anticoagulation should be weighed against the potential increased risk of bleeding and hemorrhage).

No products indexed under this heading.

Piroxicam (Due to the frequent occurrence of severe and prolonged thrombocytopenia, the potential benefits of medications that interfere with platelet function and/or anticoagulation should be weighed against the potential increased risk of bleeding and hemorrhage).

No products indexed under this heading.

Salsalate (Due to the frequent occurrence of severe and prolonged thrombocytopenia, the potential benefits of medications that interfere with platelet function and/or anticoagulation should be weighed against the potential increased risk of bleeding and hemorrhage).

No products indexed under this heading.

Sulindac (Due to the frequent occurrence of severe and prolonged thrombocytopenia, the potential benefits of medications that interfere with platelet function and/or anticoagulation should be weighed against the potential increased risk of bleeding and hemorrhage). Products include:

Clinoril Tablets 1899

Ticarcillin Disodium (Due to the frequent occurrence of severe and prolonged thrombocytopenia, the potential benefits of medications that interfere with platelet function and/ or anticoagulation should be weighed against the potential increased risk of bleeding and hemorrhage). Products include:

Timentin ADD-Vantage 1556
Timentin Injection Galaxy Container 1559
Timentin IV Infusion 1553
Timentin Pharmacy Bulk Package 1562

Ticlopidine Hydrochloride (Due to the frequent occurrence of severe and prolonged thrombocytopenia, the potential benefits of medications that interfere with platelet function and/or anticoagulation should be weighed against the potential increased risk of bleeding and hemorrhage). Products include:

Ticlid Tablets 2813

Tinzaparin Sodium (Due to the frequent occurrence of severe and prolonged thrombocytopenia, the potential benefits of medications that interfere with platelet function and/ or anticoagulation should be weighed against the potential increased risk of bleeding and hemorrhage).

No products indexed under this heading.

Tolmetin Sodium (Due to the frequent occurrence of severe and prolonged thrombocytopenia, the potential benefits of medications that interfere with platelet function and/ or anticoagulation should be weighed against the potential increased risk of bleeding and hemorrhage).

No products indexed under this heading.

IMPORTANT NOTE: Always consult each drug listing in the patient's regimen for possible interactions.

Warfarin Sodium (Due to the frequent occurrence of severe and prolonged thrombocytopenia, the potential benefits of medications that interfere with platelet function and/or anticoagulation should be weighed against the potential increased risk of bleeding and hemorrhage). Products include:
Coumadin for Injection ... 932
Coumadin Tablets ... 932

BIAFINE TOPICAL EMULSION
(Methylparaben, Propylene Glycol, Propylparaben, Stearic Acid, Triethanolamine) ... 2382
None cited in PDR database.

BIAXIN FILMTAB TABLETS
(Clarithromycin) ... 402
May interact with oral anticoagulants, oral hypoglycemic agents, insulin, phenytoin, valproate, xanthines, and certain other agents. Compounds in these categories include:

Acarbose (Clarithromycin, in rare cases, causes hypoglycemia, some of which have occurred in patients taking oral hypoglycemic agents). Products include:
Precose Tablets ... 776

Alfentanil Hydrochloride (Concurrent use of erythromycin and/or clarithromycin in patients receiving drugs metabolized by the cytochrome P450 system may be associated with elevation in serum levels of alfentanil).
No products indexed under this heading.

Aminophylline (Co-administration in patients who are receiving high doses of theophylline may be associated with an increase in serum theophylline levels and potential theophylline toxicity).
No products indexed under this heading.

Anisindione (Co-administration may result in the potentiation of oral anticoagulant effects). Products include:
Miradon Tablets ... 3056

Astemizole (Concurrent use of erythromycin in patients receiving astemizole has resulted in prolonged QT interval and torsade de pointes; because clarithromycin is metabolized by P450, co-administration is contraindicated).
No products indexed under this heading.

Bromocriptine Mesylate (Concurrent use of erythromycin and/or clarithromycin in patients receiving drugs metabolized by the cytochrome P450 system may be associated with elevation in serum levels of bromocriptine).
No products indexed under this heading.

Carbamazepine (Potential for increased serum concentration of carbamazepine). Products include:
Carbatrol Capsules ... 3174
Equetro Extended-Release Capsules ... 3178
Tegretol/Tegretol-XR ... 2278

Chlorpropamide (Clarithromycin, in rare cases, causes hypoglycemia, some of which have occurred in patients taking oral hypoglycemic agents).
No products indexed under this heading.

Cisapride (Concurrent use of erythromycin and/or clarithromycin in patients receiving cisapride has been reported to result in rare cases of cardiovascular adverse events including prolonged QT interval, ventricular tachycardia, ventricular fibrillation, and torsade de pointes, and death have been reported; co-administration is contraindicated).
No products indexed under this heading.

Colchicine (There have been post-marketing reports of colchicine toxicity with concomitant use of clarithromycin and colchicine, especially in the elderly, some of which occurred in patients with renal insufficiency).
No products indexed under this heading.

Cyclosporine (Concurrent use of erythromycin and/or clarithromycin in patients receiving drugs metabolized by the cytochrome P450 system may be associated with elevation in serum levels of cyclosporine). Products include:
Gengraf Capsules ... 458
Neoral Soft Gelatin Capsules ... 2247
Neoral Oral Solution ... 2247
Restasis Ophthalmic Emulsion ... 570
Sandimmune ... 2259

Dicumarol (Co-administration may result in the potentiation of oral anticoagulant effects).
No products indexed under this heading.

Digoxin (Concomitant use has resulted in elevated digoxin serum concentrations and some patients have shown signs of digoxin toxicity, including arrhythmias. Serum digoxin concentrations should be carefully monitored during co-administration). Products include:
Digitek Tablets ... 2146
Lanoxicaps Capsules ... 1458
Lanoxin Injection ... 1462
Lanoxin Tablets ... 1468
Lanoxin Injection Pediatric ... 1465

Dihydroergotamine Mesylate (Post-marketing reports indicate that co-administration of clarithromycin with dihydroergotamine has been associated with acute ergot toxicity characterized by vasospasm and ischemia of the extremities and other tissues including the central nervous system. Concomitant administration of clarithromycin with dihydroergotamine is contraindicated). Products include:
Migranal Nasal Spray ... 3350

Disopyramide Phosphate (Concurrent use of erythromycin and/or clarithromycin in patients receiving drugs metabolized by the cytochrome P450 system may be associated with elevation in serum levels of disopyramide).
No products indexed under this heading.

Divalproex Sodium (Concurrent use of erythromycin and/or clarithromycin in patients receiving drugs metabolized by the cytochrome P450 system may be associated with elevation in serum levels of valproate). Products include:
Depakote Sprinkle Capsules ... 422
Depakote Tablets ... 427
Depakote ER Tablets ... 433

Dyphylline (Co-administration in patients who are receiving high doses of theophylline may be associated with an increase in serum theophylline levels and potential theophylline toxicity).
No products indexed under this heading.

Ergotamine Tartrate (Post-marketing reports indicate that co-administration of clarithromycin with ergotamine has been associated with acute ergot toxicity characterized by vasospasm and ischemia of the extremities and other tissues including the central nervous system. Concomitant administration of clarithromycin with ergotamine is contraindicated).
No products indexed under this heading.

Fluconazole (Co-administration has resulted in increases in the mean steady-state clarithromycin Cmin and AUC).
No products indexed under this heading.

Fosphenytoin Sodium (Concurrent use of erythromycin and/or clarithromycin in patients receiving drugs metabolized by the cytochrome P450 system may be associated with elevation in serum levels of phenytoin).
No products indexed under this heading.

Glimepiride (Clarithromycin, in rare cases, causes hypoglycemia, some of which have occurred in patients taking oral hypoglycemic agents). Products include:
Amaryl Tablets ... 2864

Glipizide (Clarithromycin, in rare cases, causes hypoglycemia, some of which have occurred in patients taking oral hypoglycemic agents).
No products indexed under this heading.

Glyburide (Clarithromycin, in rare cases, causes hypoglycemia, some of which have occurred in patients taking oral hypoglycemic agents).
No products indexed under this heading.

Hexobarbital (Concurrent use of erythromycin and/or clarithromycin in patients receiving drugs metabolized by the cytochrome P450 system may be associated with elevation in serum levels of hexobarbital).
No products indexed under this heading.

Insulin, Human, Zinc Suspension (Clarithromycin, in rare cases, causes hypoglycemia, some of which have occurred in patients taking insulin). Products include:
Humulin L, 100 Units ... 1763
Humulin U, 100 Units ... 1770

Insulin, Human NPH (Clarithromycin, in rare cases, causes hypoglycemia, some of which have occurred in patients taking insulin). Products include:
Humulin N, 100 Units ... 1764
Humulin N Pen ... 1765
Novolin N Human Insulin 10 ml Vials ... 2322
Novolin N InnoLet ... 2322
Novolin N PenFill 3 ml Cartridges ... 2325
Novolin R InnoLet ... 2322

Insulin, Human Regular (Clarithromycin, in rare cases, causes hypoglycemia, some of which have occurred in patients taking insulin). Products include:
Humulin R (U-500) ... 1768
Humulin R, 100 Units ... 1767
Novolin R Human Insulin 10 ml Vials ... 2322
Novolin R PenFill ... 2325

Insulin, Human Regular and Human NPH Mixture (Clarithromycin, in rare cases, causes hypoglycemia, some of which have occurred in patients taking insulin). Products include:
Humulin 50/50, 100 Units ... 1760
Humulin 70/30 Pen ... 1761
Novolin 70/30 Human Insulin 10 ml Vials ... 2321
Novolin 70/30 InnoLet ... 2322
Novolin 70/30 PenFill 3 ml Cartridges ... 2325

Insulin, NPH (Clarithromycin, in rare cases, causes hypoglycemia, some of which have occurred in patients taking insulin).
No products indexed under this heading.

Insulin, Regular (Clarithromycin, in rare cases, causes hypoglycemia, some of which have occurred in patients taking insulin).
No products indexed under this heading.

Insulin, Zinc Crystals (Clarithromycin, in rare cases, causes hypoglycemia, some of which have occurred in patients taking insulin).
No products indexed under this heading.

Insulin, Zinc Suspension (Clarithromycin, in rare cases, causes hypoglycemia, some of which have occurred in patients taking insulin).
No products indexed under this heading.

Insulin Aspart, Human Regular (Clarithromycin, in rare cases, causes hypoglycemia, some of which have occurred in patients taking insulin). Products include:
NovoLog Injection ... 2326

Insulin glargine (Clarithromycin, in rare cases, causes hypoglycemia, some of which have occurred in patients taking insulin). Products include:
Lantus Injection ... 2925

Insulin Lispro, Human (Clarithromycin, in rare cases, causes hypoglycemia, some of which have occurred in patients taking insulin). Products include:
Humalog-Pen ... 1751
Humalog Mix 75/25-Pen ... 1754

Insulin Lispro Protamine, Human (Clarithromycin, in rare cases, causes hypoglycemia, some of which have occurred in patients taking insulin). Products include:
Humalog Mix 75/25-Pen ... 1754

Lovastatin (As with other macrolides, clarithromycin has been reported to increase concentrations of HMG-CoA reductase inhibitors, such as lovastatin, through inhibition of CYP450 metabolism of simvastatin; rare cases of rhabdomyolysis have been reported). Products include:
Advicor Tablets ... 1694
Altoprev Extended-Release Tablets ... 1151
Mevacor Tablets ... 1996

Metformin Hydrochloride (Clarithromycin, in rare cases, causes hypoglycemia, some of which have occurred in patients taking oral hypoglycemic agents). Products include:
ActoPlus Met Tablets ... 3219

Avandamet Tablets 1343
Fortamet Extended-Release Tablets 1156

iglitol (Clarithromycin, in rare ases, causes hypoglycemia, some f which have occurred in patients king oral hypoglycemic agents).
No products indexed under this heading.

meprazole (Co-administration creases the steady-state plasma oncentrations, Cmax, AUC 0-24, nd T 1/2 of omeprazole). Products clude:
Zegerid Powder for Oral Solution 2972

henytoin (Concurrent use of erythmycin and/or clarithromycin in atients receiving drugs metabolized y the cytochrome P450 system ay be associated with elevation in erum levels of phenytoin).
No products indexed under this heading.

henytoin Sodium (Concurrent se of erythromycin and/or clarithroycin in patients receiving drugs etabolized by the cytochrome 450 system may be associated ith elevation in serum levels of henytoin). Products include:
Phenytek Capsules 2153

imozide (Concurrent use of erythmycin and/or clarithromycin in atients receiving pimozide has been ported to result in rare cases of rdiovascular adverse events cluding prolonged QT interval, vencular tachycardia, ventricular fibriltion, and torsade de pointes, and eath; co-administration is contraincated). Products include:
Orap Tablets 1220

oglitazone Hydrochloride larithromycin, in rare cases, caus hypoglycemia, some of which ve occurred in patients taking oral poglycemic agents). Products clude:
ActoPlus Met Tablets 3219
Actos Tablets 3224

anitidine Bismuth Citrate (Coministration has resulted in creased plasma ranitidine concenations (57%), increased plasma smuth trough concentrations 8%), and increased 14-hydroxyarithromycin plasma concentrans (31%); these effects are clinilly insignificant).
No products indexed under this heading.

epaglinide (Clarithromycin, in rare ses, causes hypoglycemia, some which have occurred in patients king oral hypoglycemic agents). oducts include:
Prandin Tablets (0.5, 1, and 2 mg).. 2337

tonavir (Co-administration has sulted in a 77% increase in arithromycin AUC and a 100% crease in the AUC of 14-OH arithromycin; dosage adjustments ay be needed if clarithromycin is ministered to patients with renal pairment). Products include:
Kaletra 474
Norvir 499

osiglitazone Maleate (Clarithroycin, in rare cases, causes hypocemia, some of which have curred in patients taking oral poglycemic agents). Products clude:
Avandamet Tablets 1343
Avandia Tablets 1348

Simvastatin (As with other macrolides, clarithromycin has been reported to increase concentrations of HMG-CoA reductase inhibitors, such as simvastatin, through inhibition of CYP450 metabolism of simvastatin; rare cases of rhabdomyolysis have been reported). Products include:
Vytorin 10/10 Tablets 2084
Vytorin 10/10 Tablets 3092
Vytorin 10/20 Tablets 2084
Vytorin 10/20 Tablets 3092
Vytorin 10/40 Tablets 3092
Vytorin 10/40 Tablets 2084
Vytorin 10/80 Tablets 2084
Vytorin 10/80 Tablets 3092
Zocor Tablets 2078

Tacrolimus (Concurrent use of erythromycin and/or clarithromycin in patients receiving drugs metabolized by the cytochrome P450 system may be associated with elevation in serum levels of tacrolimus). Products include:
Prograf Capsules and Injection 624
Protopic Ointment 629

Terfenadine (Co-administration has resulted in increase in active metabolite of terfenadine by 3-fold; rare cases of cardiovascular adverse events including prolonged QT interval, ventricular tachycardia, ventricular fibrillation, and torsade de pointes, and death have been reported; co-administration is contraindicated).
No products indexed under this heading.

Theophylline (Co-administration in patients who are receiving high doses of theophylline may be associated with an increase in serum theophylline levels and potential theophylline toxicity).
No products indexed under this heading.

Theophylline Anhydrous (Co-administration in patients who are receiving high doses of theophylline may be associated with an increase in serum theophylline levels and potential theophylline toxicity). Products include:
Uniphyl Tablets 2708

Theophylline Calcium Salicylate (Co-administration in patients who are receiving high doses of theophylline may be associated with an increase in serum theophylline levels and potential theophylline toxicity).
No products indexed under this heading.

Theophylline Dihydroxypropyl (Glyceryl) (Co-administration in patients who are receiving high doses of theophylline may be associated with an increase in serum theophylline levels and potential theophylline toxicity).
No products indexed under this heading.

Theophylline Ethylenediamine (Co-administration in patients who are receiving high doses of theophylline may be associated with an increase in serum theophylline levels and potential theophylline toxicity).
No products indexed under this heading.

Theophylline Sodium Glycinate (Co-administration in patients who are receiving high doses of theophylline may be associated with an increase in serum theophylline levels and potential theophylline toxicity).
No products indexed under this heading.

Tolazamide (Clarithromycin, in rare cases, causes hypoglycemia, some of which have occurred in patients taking oral hypoglycemic agents).
No products indexed under this heading.

Tolbutamide (Clarithromycin, in rare cases, causes hypoglycemia, some of which have occurred in patients taking oral hypoglycemic agents).
No products indexed under this heading.

Triazolam (Erythromycin, another macrolide antibiotic, has been reported to decrease the clearance of triazolam and, thus, may increase the pharmacologic effect of the triazolam; concomitant use has resulted in somnolence and confusion).
No products indexed under this heading.

Troglitazone (Clarithromycin, in rare cases, causes hypoglycemia, some of which have occurred in patients taking oral hypoglycemic agents).
No products indexed under this heading.

Valproate Sodium (Concurrent use of erythromycin and/or clarithromycin in patients receiving drugs metabolized by the cytochrome P450 system may be associated with elevation in serum levels of valproate). Products include:
Depacon Injection 412

Valproic Acid (Concurrent use of erythromycin and/or clarithromycin in patients receiving drugs metabolized by the cytochrome P450 system may be associated with elevation in serum levels of valproate). Products include:
Depakene 417

Warfarin Sodium (Co-administration may result in the potentiation of oral anticoagulant effects). Products include:
Coumadin for Injection 932
Coumadin Tablets 932

Zidovudine (Potential for decreased steady-state zidovudine concentration). Products include:
Combivir Tablets 1373
Retrovir 1533
Retrovir IV Infusion 1537
Trizivir Tablets 1565

Food Interactions

Food, unspecified (Food slightly delays both the onset of absorption and the formation of the active metabolite, but does not affect the extent of bioavailability; Biaxin may be administered without regard to food).

BIAXIN GRANULES

(Clarithromycin) 402
See Biaxin Filmtab Tablets

BIAXIN XL FILMTAB TABLETS

(Clarithromycin) 402
See Biaxin Filmtab Tablets

BIDIL TABLETS

(Hydralazine Hydrochloride, Isosorbide Dinitrate)......................... 2161
May interact with antihypertensives, monoamine oxidase inhibitors, vasodilators, and certain other agents. Compounds in these categories include:

Acebutolol Hydrochloride (Increased risk of hypotension with concomitant antihypertensive drugs. Patients treated with BiDil who receive any potent parenteral antihypertensive agent should be continuously observed for several hours for excessive fall in blood pressure).
No products indexed under this heading.

Amlodipine Besylate (Increased risk of hypotension with concomitant antihypertensive drugs. Patients treated with BiDil who receive any potent parenteral antihypertensive agent should be continuously observed for several hours for excessive fall in blood pressure). Products include:
Caduet Tablets 2507
Lotrel Capsules 2238
Norvasc Tablets 2529

Amyl Nitrite (The effects of BiDil on vasodilators may be additive).
No products indexed under this heading.

Atenolol (Increased risk of hypotension with concomitant antihypertensive drugs. Patients treated with BiDil who receive any potent parenteral antihypertensive agent should be continuously observed for several hours for excessive fall in blood pressure). Products include:
Tenormin I.V. Injection 698
Tenormin Tablets 695

Benazepril Hydrochloride (Increased risk of hypotension with concomitant antihypertensive drugs. Patients treated with BiDil who receive any potent parenteral antihypertensive agent should be continuously observed for several hours for excessive fall in blood pressure). Products include:
Lotensin Tablets 2232
Lotensin HCT Tablets 2235
Lotrel Capsules 2238

Bendroflumethiazide (Increased risk of hypotension with concomitant antihypertensive drugs. Patients treated with BiDil who receive any potent parenteral antihypertensive agent should be continuously observed for several hours for excessive fall in blood pressure).
No products indexed under this heading.

Betaxolol Hydrochloride (Increased risk of hypotension with concomitant antihypertensive drugs. Patients treated with BiDil who receive any potent parenteral antihypertensive agent should be continuously observed for several hours for excessive fall in blood pressure). Products include:
Betoptic S Ophthalmic Suspension.................................. 554

Bisoprolol Fumarate (Increased risk of hypotension with concomitant antihypertensive drugs. Patients treated with BiDil who receive any potent parenteral antihypertensive agent should be continuously observed for several hours for excessive fall in blood pressure).
No products indexed under this heading.

Candesartan Cilexetil (Increased risk of hypotension with concomitant antihypertensive drugs. Patients treated with BiDil who receive any potent parenteral antihypertensive agent should be continuously observed for several hours for excessive fall in blood pressure). Products include:

Atacand Tablets 634
Atacand HCT 637

Captopril (Increased risk of hypotension with concomitant antihypertensive drugs. Patients treated with BiDil who receive any potent parenteral antihypertensive agent should be continuously observed for several hours for excessive fall in blood pressure). Products include:

Captopril Tablets 2114

Carteolol Hydrochloride (Increased risk of hypotension with concomitant antihypertensive drugs. Patients treated with BiDil who receive any potent parenteral antihypertensive agent should be continuously observed for several hours for excessive fall in blood pressure). Products include:

Carteolol Hydrochloride Ophthalmic Solution USP, 1% ⊙246

Chlorothiazide (Increased risk of hypotension with concomitant antihypertensive drugs. Patients treated with BiDil who receive any potent parenteral antihypertensive agent should be continuously observed for several hours for excessive fall in blood pressure). Products include:

Aldoclor Tablets 1881
Diuril Oral 1936

Chlorothiazide Sodium (Increased risk of hypotension with concomitant antihypertensive drugs. Patients treated with BiDil who receive any potent parenteral antihypertensive agent should be continuously observed for several hours for excessive fall in blood pressure). Products include:

Diuril Sodium Intravenous 1934

Chlorthalidone (Increased risk of hypotension with concomitant antihypertensive drugs. Patients treated with BiDil who receive any potent parenteral antihypertensive agent should be continuously observed for several hours for excessive fall in blood pressure). Products include:

Clorpres Tablets 2139

Clonidine (Increased risk of hypotension with concomitant antihypertensive drugs. Patients treated with BiDil who receive any potent parenteral antihypertensive agent should be continuously observed for several hours for excessive fall in blood pressure). Products include:

Catapres-TTS 875

Clonidine Hydrochloride (Increased risk of hypotension with concomitant antihypertensive drugs. Patients treated with BiDil who receive any potent parenteral antihypertensive agent should be continuously observed for several hours for excessive fall in blood pressure). Products include:

Catapres Tablets 874
Clorpres Tablets 2139

Deserpidine (Increased risk of hypotension with concomitant antihypertensive drugs. Patients treated with BiDil who receive any potent parenteral antihypertensive agent should be continuously observed for several hours for excessive fall in blood pressure).

No products indexed under this heading.

Diazoxide (Increased risk of hypotension with concomitant antihypertensive drugs. Patients treated with BiDil who receive any potent parenteral antihypertensive agent should be continuously observed for several hours for excessive fall in blood pressure). Products include:

Hyperstat I.V. Injection 3031

Diltiazem Hydrochloride (Increased risk of hypotension with concomitant antihypertensive drugs. Patients treated with BiDil who receive any potent parenteral antihypertensive agent should be continuously observed for several hours for excessive fall in blood pressure). Products include:

Cardizem LA Extended Release Tablets 1699
Tiazac Capsules 1204

Doxazosin Mesylate (Increased risk of hypotension with concomitant antihypertensive drugs. Patients treated with BiDil who receive any potent parenteral antihypertensive agent should be continuously observed for several hours for excessive fall in blood pressure).

No products indexed under this heading.

Enalapril Maleate (Increased risk of hypotension with concomitant antihypertensive drugs. Patients treated with BiDil who receive any potent parenteral antihypertensive agent should be continuously observed for several hours for excessive fall in blood pressure). Products include:

Vaseretic Tablets 2073
Vasotec I.V. Injection 2076

Enalaprilat (Increased risk of hypotension with concomitant antihypertensive drugs. Patients treated with BiDil who receive any potent parenteral antihypertensive agent should be continuously observed for several hours for excessive fall in blood pressure).

No products indexed under this heading.

Epoprostenol Sodium (The effects of BiDil on vasodilators may be additive). Products include:

Flolan for Injection 1408

Eprosartan Mesylate (Increased risk of hypotension with concomitant antihypertensive drugs. Patients treated with BiDil who receive any potent parenteral antihypertensive agent should be continuously observed for several hours for excessive fall in blood pressure). Products include:

Teveten Tablets 1707
Teveten HCT Tablets 1710

Esmolol Hydrochloride (Increased risk of hypotension with concomitant antihypertensive drugs. Patients treated with BiDil who receive any potent parenteral antihypertensive agent should be continuously observed for several hours for excessive fall in blood pressure). Products include:

Brevibloc Concentrate 766
Brevibloc Injection 766
Brevibloc Double Strength Injection 766
Brevibloc Premixed Injection 766
Brevibloc Double Strength Premixed Injection 766

Ethanol (The effects of BiDil on vasodilators, including alcohol, may be additive).

No products indexed under this heading.

Ethaverine Hydrochloride (The effects of BiDil on vasodilators may be additive).

No products indexed under this heading.

Felodipine (Increased risk of hypotension with concomitant antihypertensive drugs. Patients treated with BiDil who receive any potent parenteral antihypertensive agent should be continuously observed for several hours for excessive fall in blood pressure). Products include:

Plendil Extended-Release Tablets 651

Fosinopril Sodium (Increased risk of hypotension with concomitant antihypertensive drugs. Patients treated with BiDil who receive any potent parenteral antihypertensive agent should be continuously observed for several hours for excessive fall in blood pressure).

No products indexed under this heading.

Furosemide (Increased risk of hypotension with concomitant antihypertensive drugs. Patients treated with BiDil who receive any potent parenteral antihypertensive agent should be continuously observed for several hours for excessive fall in blood pressure). Products include:

Furosemide Tablets 2117

Guanabenz Acetate (Increased risk of hypotension with concomitant antihypertensive drugs. Patients treated with BiDil who receive any potent parenteral antihypertensive agent should be continuously observed for several hours for excessive fall in blood pressure).

No products indexed under this heading.

Guanethidine Monosulfate (Increased risk of hypotension with concomitant antihypertensive drugs. Patients treated with BiDil who receive any potent parenteral antihypertensive agent should be continuously observed for several hours for excessive fall in blood pressure).

No products indexed under this heading.

Hydrochlorothiazide (Increased risk of hypotension with concomitant antihypertensive drugs. Patients treated with BiDil who receive any potent parenteral antihypertensive agent should be continuously observed for several hours for excessive fall in blood pressure). Products include:

Aldoril Tablets 1884
Atacand HCT 637
Avalide Tablets 2889
Avalide Tablets 922
Benicar HCT Tablets 2852
Diovan HCT Tablets 2195
Dyazide Capsules 1389
Hyzaar 1964
Lotensin HCT Tablets 2235
Maxzide 2150
Micardis HCT Tablets 886
Moduretic Tablets 2003
Prinzide Tablets 2033
Teveten HCT Tablets 1710
Timolide Tablets 2056
Uniretic Tablets 3114
Vaseretic Tablets 2073
Zestoretic Tablets 701

Hydroflumethiazide (Increased risk of hypotension with concomitant antihypertensive drugs. Patients treated with BiDil who receive any potent parenteral antihypertensive agent should be continuously observed for several hours for excessive fall in blood pressure).

No products indexed under this heading.

Indapamide (Increased risk of hypotension with concomitant antihypertensive drugs. Patients treated with BiDil who receive any potent parenteral antihypertensive agent should be continuously observed for several hours for excessive fall in blood pressure). Products include:

Indapamide Tablets 2119

Irbesartan (Increased risk of hypotension with concomitant antihypertensive drugs. Patients treated with BiDil who receive any potent parenteral antihypertensive agent should be continuously observed for several hours for excessive fall in blood pressure). Products include:

Avalide Tablets 922
Avalide Tablets 2889
Avapro Tablets 925
Avapro Tablets 2886

Isocarboxazid (Due to the hydralazine component of BiDil, monoamine oxidase inhibitors should be used with caution in patients receiving BiDil).

No products indexed under this heading.

Isosorbide Mononitrate (The effects of BiDil on vasodilators may be additive). Products include:

Imdur Tablets 3032

Isoxsuprine Hydrochloride (The effects of BiDil on vasodilators may be additive).

No products indexed under this heading.

Isradipine (Increased risk of hypotension with concomitant antihypertensive drugs. Patients treated with BiDil who receive any potent parenteral antihypertensive agent should be continuously observed for several hours for excessive fall in blood pressure). Products include:

DynaCirc CR Tablets 2726

Labetalol Hydrochloride (Increased risk of hypotension with concomitant antihypertensive drugs. Patients treated with BiDil who receive any potent parenteral antihypertensive agent should be continuously observed for several hours for excessive fall in blood pressure).

No products indexed under this heading.

Lisinopril (Increased risk of hypotension with concomitant antihypertensive drugs. Patients treated with BiDil who receive any potent parenteral antihypertensive agent should be continuously observed for several hours for excessive fall in blood pressure). Products include:

Prinivil Tablets 2029
Prinzide Tablets 2033
Zestoretic Tablets 701
Zestril Tablets 704

Losartan Potassium (Increased risk of hypotension with concomitant antihypertensive drugs. Patients treated with BiDil who receive any potent parenteral antihypertensive agent should be continuously

›served for several hours for
‹cessive fall in blood pressure).
›oducts include:
Cozaar Tablets 1913
Hyzaar 1964

ecamylamine Hydrochloride
creased risk of hypotension with
›ncomitant antihypertensive drugs.
›tients treated with BiDil who
ceive any potent parenteral antihy-
›rtensive agent should be continu-
›sly observed for several hours for
cessive fall in blood pressure).
oducts include:
nversine Tablets 3286

ethyclothiazide (Increased risk
hypotension with concomitant
tihypertensive drugs. Patients
›ated with BiDil who receive any
›tent parenteral antihypertensive
ent should be continuously
served for several hours for
cessive fall in blood pressure).
No products indexed under this heading.

ethyldopa (Increased risk of
potension with concomitant antihy-
rtensive drugs. Patients treated
th BiDil who receive any potent
renteral antihypertensive agent
ould be continuously observed for
veral hours for excessive fall in
ood pressure). Products include:
Aldoclor Tablets 1881
Aldoril Tablets 1884

ethyldopate Hydrochloride
creased risk of hypotension with
ncomitant antihypertensive drugs.
tients treated with BiDil who
ceive any potent parenteral antihy-
rtensive agent should be continu-
sly observed for several hours for
cessive fall in blood pressure).
No products indexed under this heading.

etolazone (Increased risk of
potension with concomitant antihy-
rtensive drugs. Patients treated
h BiDil who receive any potent
renteral antihypertensive agent
ould be continuously observed for
veral hours for excessive fall in
od pressure).
No products indexed under this heading.

etoprolol Succinate (Increased
k of hypotension with concomitant
tihypertensive drugs. Patients
ated with BiDil who receive any
tent parenteral antihypertensive
ent should be continuously
served for several hours for
cessive fall in blood pressure).
oducts include:
oprol-XL Tablets 660

etoprolol Tartrate (Increased
k of hypotension with concomitant
tihypertensive drugs. Patients
ated with BiDil who receive any
tent parenteral antihypertensive
ent should be continuously
served for several hours for
cessive fall in blood pressure).
No products indexed under this heading.

etyrosine (Increased risk of hypo-
sion with concomitant antihyper-
sive drugs. Patients treated with
Dil who receive any potent paren-
al antihypertensive agent should
continuously observed for several
urs for excessive fall in blood
essure). Products include:
Demser Capsules 1933

Mibefradil Dihydrochloride (Increased risk of hypotension with concomitant antihypertensive drugs. Patients treated with BiDil who receive any potent parenteral antihypertensive agent should be continuously observed for several hours for excessive fall in blood pressure).
No products indexed under this heading.

Minoxidil (Increased risk of hypotension with concomitant antihypertensive drugs. Patients treated with BiDil who receive any potent parenteral antihypertensive agent should be continuously observed for several hours for excessive fall in blood pressure). Products include:
Men's Rogaine Extra Strength Topical Solution, Ocean Rush Scent and Original Unscented ..... ▣706
Women's Rogaine Topical Solution, Spring Bloom Scent and Original Unscented .... ▣707

Moclobemide (Due to the hydralazine component of BiDil, monoamine oxidase inhibitors should be used with caution in patients receiving BiDil).
No products indexed under this heading.

Moexipril Hydrochloride (Increased risk of hypotension with concomitant antihypertensive drugs. Patients treated with BiDil who receive any potent parenteral antihypertensive agent should be continuously observed for several hours for excessive fall in blood pressure). Products include:
Uniretic Tablets 3114
Univasc Tablets 3118

Nadolol (Increased risk of hypotension with concomitant antihypertensive drugs. Patients treated with BiDil who receive any potent parenteral antihypertensive agent should be continuously observed for several hours for excessive fall in blood pressure). Products include:
Nadolol Tablets 2121

Nicardipine Hydrochloride (Increased risk of hypotension with concomitant antihypertensive drugs. Patients treated with BiDil who receive any potent parenteral antihypertensive agent should be continuously observed for several hours for excessive fall in blood pressure). Products include:
Cardene I.V. 1129

Nifedipine (Increased risk of hypotension with concomitant antihypertensive drugs. Patients treated with BiDil who receive any potent parenteral antihypertensive agent should be continuously observed for several hours for excessive fall in blood pressure). Products include:
Adalat CC Tablets 2978

Nisoldipine (Increased risk of hypotension with concomitant antihypertensive drugs. Patients treated with BiDil who receive any potent parenteral antihypertensive agent should be continuously observed for several hours for excessive fall in blood pressure). Products include:
Sular Tablets 1163

Nitroglycerin (Increased risk of hypotension with concomitant antihypertensive drugs. Patients treated with BiDil who receive any potent parenteral antihypertensive agent should be continuously observed for several hours for excessive fall in blood pressure). Products include:
Nitro-Dur Transdermal Infusion System.. 3060
Nitrolingual Pumpspray 1161

Nitroglycerin, long-acting formulations (The effects of BiDil on vasodilators may be additive).
No products indexed under this heading.

Nitroglycerin Intravenous (The effects of BiDil on vasodilators may be additive).
No products indexed under this heading.

Papaverine (The effects of BiDil on vasodilators may be additive).
No products indexed under this heading.

Papaverine Hydrochloride (The effects of BiDil on vasodilators may be additive).
No products indexed under this heading.

Pargyline Hydrochloride (Due to the hydralazine component of BiDil, monoamine oxidase inhibitors should be used with caution in patients receiving BiDil).
No products indexed under this heading.

Penbutolol Sulfate (Increased risk of hypotension with concomitant antihypertensive drugs. Patients treated with BiDil who receive any potent parenteral antihypertensive agent should be continuously observed for several hours for excessive fall in blood pressure).
No products indexed under this heading.

Perindopril Erbumine (Increased risk of hypotension with concomitant antihypertensive drugs. Patients treated with BiDil who receive any potent parenteral antihypertensive agent should be continuously observed for several hours for excessive fall in blood pressure). Products include:
Aceon Tablets (2 mg, 4 mg, 8 mg)... 3191

Phenelzine Sulfate (Due to the hydralazine component of BiDil, monoamine oxidase inhibitors should be used with caution in patients receiving BiDil).
No products indexed under this heading.

Phenoxybenzamine Hydrochloride (Increased risk of hypotension with concomitant antihypertensive drugs. Patients treated with BiDil who receive any potent parenteral antihypertensive agent should be continuously observed for several hours for excessive fall in blood pressure). Products include:
Dibenzyline Capsules 3390

Phentolamine Mesylate (Increased risk of hypotension with concomitant antihypertensive drugs. Patients treated with BiDil who receive any potent parenteral antihypertensive agent should be continuously observed for several hours for excessive fall in blood pressure).
No products indexed under this heading.

Pindolol (Increased risk of hypotension with concomitant antihypertensive drugs. Patients treated with BiDil who receive any potent parenteral antihypertensive agent should be continuously observed for several hours for excessive fall in blood pressure).
No products indexed under this heading.

Polythiazide (Increased risk of hypotension with concomitant antihypertensive drugs. Patients treated with BiDil who receive any potent parenteral antihypertensive agent should be continuously observed for several hours for excessive fall in blood pressure).
No products indexed under this heading.

Prazosin Hydrochloride (Increased risk of hypotension with concomitant antihypertensive drugs. Patients treated with BiDil who receive any potent parenteral antihypertensive agent should be continuously observed for several hours for excessive fall in blood pressure).
No products indexed under this heading.

Procarbazine Hydrochloride (Due to the hydralazine component of BiDil, monoamine oxidase inhibitors should be used with caution in patients receiving BiDil). Products include:
Matulane Capsules 3188

Propranolol Hydrochloride (Increased risk of hypotension with concomitant antihypertensive drugs. Patients treated with BiDil who receive any potent parenteral antihypertensive agent should be continuously observed for several hours for excessive fall in blood pressure). Products include:
Inderal LA Long-Acting Capsules 3421
InnoPran XL Capsules 2728

Quinapril Hydrochloride (Increased risk of hypotension with concomitant antihypertensive drugs. Patients treated with BiDil who receive any potent parenteral antihypertensive agent should be continuously observed for several hours for excessive fall in blood pressure).
No products indexed under this heading.

Ramipril (Increased risk of hypotension with concomitant antihypertensive drugs. Patients treated with BiDil who receive any potent parenteral antihypertensive agent should be continuously observed for several hours for excessive fall in blood pressure). Products include:
Altace Capsules 1673

Rauwolfia Serpentina (Increased risk of hypotension with concomitant antihypertensive drugs. Patients treated with BiDil who receive any potent parenteral antihypertensive agent should be continuously observed for several hours for excessive fall in blood pressure).
No products indexed under this heading.

Rescinnamine (Increased risk of hypotension with concomitant antihypertensive drugs. Patients treated with BiDil who receive any potent parenteral antihypertensive agent should be continuously observed for several hours for excessive fall in blood pressure).
No products indexed under this heading.

Reserpine (Increased risk of hypotension with concomitant antihypertensive drugs. Patients treated with BiDil who receive any potent parenteral antihypertensive agent should be continuously observed for several hours for excessive fall in blood pressure).
No products indexed under this heading.

Selegiline Hydrochloride (Due to the hydralazine component of BiDil, monoamine oxidase inhibitors should be used with caution in patients receiving BiDil). Products include:

Eldepryl Capsules **3209**

Sildenafil Citrate (Augmentation of the vasodilatory effects of isosorbide dinitrate by phosphodiesterase inhibitors, such as sildenafil, could result in severe hypotension. The time course and dose dependence of this interaction have not been studied. Reasonable supportivecare should consist of those measures used to treat a nitrate overdose with elevation of the extremities and central volume expansion). Products include:

Revatio Tablets **2541**
Viagra Tablets **2552**

Sodium Nitroprusside (Increased risk of hypotension with concomitant antihypertensive drugs. Patients treated with BiDil who receive any potent parenteral antihypertensive agent should be continuously observed for several hours for excessive fall in blood pressure).

No products indexed under this heading.

Sotalol Hydrochloride (Increased risk of hypotension with concomitant antihypertensive drugs. Patients treated with BiDil who receive any potent parenteral antihypertensive agent should be continuously observed for several hours for excessive fall in blood pressure).

No products indexed under this heading.

Spirapril Hydrochloride (Increased risk of hypotension with concomitant antihypertensive drugs. Patients treated with BiDil who receive any potent parenteral antihypertensive agent should be continuously observed for several hours for excessive fall in blood pressure).

No products indexed under this heading.

Tadalafil (Augmentation of the vasodilatory effects of isosorbide dinitrate by phosphodiesterase inhibitors, such as tadalafil, could result in severe hypotension. The time course and dose dependence of this interaction have not been studied. Reasonable supportive care should consist of those measures used to treat a nitrate overdose with elevation of the extremities and central volume expansion). Products include:

Cialis Tablets **1806**

Telmisartan (Increased risk of hypotension with concomitant antihypertensive drugs. Patients treated with BiDil who receive any potent parenteral antihypertensive agent should be continuously observed for several hours for excessive fall in blood pressure). Products include:

Micardis Tablets **884**
Micardis HCT Tablets **886**

Terazosin Hydrochloride (Increased risk of hypotension with concomitant antihypertensive drugs. Patients treated with BiDil who receive any potent parenteral antihypertensive agent should be continuously observed for several hours for excessive fall in blood pressure). Products include:

Hytrin Capsules **469**

Timolol Maleate (Increased risk of hypotension with concomitant antihypertensive drugs. Patients treated with BiDil who receive any potent parenteral antihypertensive agent should be continuously observed for several hours for excessive fall in blood pressure). Products include:

Blocadren Tablets **1891**
Cosopt Sterile Ophthalmic Solution **1910**
Timolide Tablets **2056**
Timoptic in Ocudose **2061**
Timoptic Sterile Ophthalmic Solution **2058**
Timoptic-XE Sterile Ophthalmic Gel Forming Solution **2062**

Tolazoline Hydrochloride (The effects of BiDil on vasodilators may be additive).

No products indexed under this heading.

Torsemide (Increased risk of hypotension with concomitant antihypertensive drugs. Patients treated with BiDil who receive any potent parenteral antihypertensive agent should be continuously observed for several hours for excessive fall in blood pressure).

No products indexed under this heading.

Trandolapril (Increased risk of hypotension with concomitant antihypertensive drugs. Patients treated with BiDil who receive any potent parenteral antihypertensive agent should be continuously observed for several hours for excessive fall in blood pressure). Products include:

Mavik Tablets **482**
Tarka Tablets **519**

Tranylcypromine Sulfate (Due to the hydralazine component of BiDil, monoamine oxidase inhibitors should be used with caution in patients receiving BiDil). Products include:

Parnate Tablets **1499**

Trimethaphan Camsylate (Increased risk of hypotension with concomitant antihypertensive drugs. Patients treated with BiDil who receive any potent parenteral antihypertensive agent should be continuously observed for several hours for excessive fall in blood pressure).

No products indexed under this heading.

Valsartan (Increased risk of hypotension with concomitant antihypertensive drugs. Patients treated with BiDil who receive any potent parenteral antihypertensive agent should be continuously observed for several hours for excessive fall in blood pressure). Products include:

Diovan HCT Tablets **2195**
Diovan Tablets **2191**

Vardenafil Hydrochloride (Augmentation of the vasodilatory effects of isosorbide dinitrate by phosphodiesterase inhibitors, such as vardenafil, could result in severe hypotension. The time course and dose dependence of this interaction have not been studied. Reasonable supportivecare should consist of those measures used to treat a nitrate overdose with elevation of the extremities and central volume expansion). Products include:

Levitra Tablets **3048**

Verapamil Hydrochloride (Increased risk of hypotension with concomitant antihypertensive drugs. Patients treated with BiDil who receive any potent parenteral antihypertensive agent should be continuously observed for several hours for excessive fall in blood pressure). Products include:

Covera-HS Tablets **3135**
Tarka Tablets **519**
Verelan PM Capsules **3120**

Food Interactions

Alcohol (The effects of BiDil on vasodilators, including alcohol, may be additive).

BILTRICIDE TABLETS

(Praziquantel) **2990**

May interact with cytochrome p450 1a2 inducers (selected), cytochrome p450 1a2 inhibitors (selected), cytochrome p450 2c19 inducers (selected), cytochrome p450 2c19 inhibitors (selected), cytochrome p450 2c8 inducers (selected), cytochrome p450 2c8 inhibitors (selected), cytochrome p450 2c9 inducers (selected), cytochrome p450 2c9 inhibitors (selected), cytochrome p450 2d6 inducers (selected), cytochrome p450 2d6 inhibitors (selected), cytochrome p450 3a4 inducers (selected), cytochrome p450 3a4 inhibitors (selected), cytochrome p450 3a inducers (selected), cytochrome p450 3a inhibitors (selected), and certain other agents. Compounds in these categories include:

Acetazolamide (Concomitant administration of drugs that decrease the activity of drug metabolizing liver enzymes (Cytochrome P450) may increase plasma levels of praziquantel).

No products indexed under this heading.

Alatrofloxacin Mesylate (Concomitant administration of drugs that decrease the activity of drug metabolizing liver enzymes (Cytochrome P450) may increase plasma levels of praziqua).

No products indexed under this heading.

Allium sativum (Concomitant administration of drugs that increase the activity of drug metabolizing liver enzymes (Cytochrome P450) may reduce plasma levels of praziquantel).

No products indexed under this heading.

Amiodarone Hydrochloride (Concomitant administration of drugs that decrease the activity of drug metabolizing liver enzymes (Cytochrome P450) may increase plasma levels of praziqua). Products include:

Pacerone Tablets **3337**

Amitriptyline Hydrochloride (Concomitant administration of drugs that decrease the activity of drug metabolizing liver enzymes (Cytochrome P450) may increase plasma levels of praziquantel).

No products indexed under this heading.

Amoxapine (Concomitant administration of drugs that decrease the activity of drug metabolizing liver enzymes (Cytochrome P450) may increase plasma levels of praziquantel).

No products indexed under this heading.

Amprenavir (Concomitant administration of drugs that decrease the activity of drug metabolizing liver enzymes (Cytochrome P450) may increase plasma levels of praziquantel). Products include:

Agenerase Capsules **1299**
Agenerase Oral Solution **1304**

Anastrozole (Concomitant administration of drugs that decrease the activity of drug metabolizing liver enzymes (Cytochrome P450) may increase plasma levels of praziqua). Products include:

Arimidex Tablets **665**

Aprepitant (Concomitant administration of drugs that increase the activity of drug metabolizing liver enzymes (Cytochrome P450) may reduce plasma levels of praziquantel). Products include:

Emend Capsules **1944**

Bendroflumethiazide (Concomitant administration of drugs that decrease the activity of drug metabolizing liver enzymes (Cytochrome P450) may increase plasma levels of praziquantel).

No products indexed under this heading.

Betamethasone Acetate (Concomitant administration of drugs that increase the activity of drug metabolizing liver enzymes (Cytochrome P450) may reduce plasma levels of praziquantel).

No products indexed under this heading.

Betamethasone Sodium Phosphate (Concomitant administration of drugs that increase the activity of drug metabolizing liver enzymes (Cytochrome P450) may reduce plasma levels of praziquantel).

No products indexed under this heading.

Bupropion Hydrochloride (Concomitant administration of drugs that decrease the activity of drug metabolizing liver enzymes (Cytochrome P450) may increase plasma levels of praziquantel). Products include:

Wellbutrin Tablets **1579**
Wellbutrin SR Sustained-Release Tablets **1583**
Wellbutrin XL Extended-Release Tablets **1588**
Zyban Sustained-Release Tablets **1620**

Carbamazepine (Concomitant administration of drugs that increase the activity of drug metabolizing liver enzymes (Cytochrome P450) may reduce plasma levels of praziquantel). Products include:

Carbatrol Capsules **3174**
Equetro Extended-Release Capsules **3178**
Tegretol/Tegretol-XR **2278**

Celecoxib (Concomitant administration of drugs that decrease the activity of drug metabolizing liver enzymes (Cytochrome P450) may increase plasma levels of praziquantel). Products include:

Celebrex Capsules **3130**

Chloramphenicol (Concomitant administration of drugs that decrease the activity of drug metabolizing liver enzymes (Cytochrome P450) may increase plasma levels of praziquantel).

No products indexed under this heading.

Chloroquine (Co-administration may lead to lower concentrations of praziquantel).

No products indexed under this heading.

Chloroquine Hydrochloride (Co-administration may lead to lower concentrations of praziquantel).

No products indexed under this heading.

Chloroquine Phosphate (Coadministration may lead to lower concentrations of praziquantel).
No products indexed under this heading.

Chlorothiazide (Concomitant administration of drugs that decrease the activity of drug metabolizing liver enzymes (Cytochrome P450) may increase plasma levels of praziquantel). Products include:
- Aldoclor Tablets 1881
- Diuril Oral 1936

Chlorothiazide Sodium (Concomitant administration of drugs that decrease the activity of drug metabolizing liver enzymes (Cytochrome P450) may increase plasma levels of praziquantel). Products include:
- Diuril Sodium Intravenous 1934

Chlorpheniramine (Concomitant administration of drugs that decrease the activity of drug metabolizing liver enzymes (Cytochrome P450) may increase plasma levels of praziquantel).
No products indexed under this heading.

Chlorpheniramine Maleate (Concomitant administration of drugs that decrease the activity of drug metabolizing liver enzymes (Cytochrome P450) may increase plasma levels of praziquantel). Products include:
- Advil Allergy Sinus Caplets 737
- Advil Multi-Symptom Cold Caplets 738
- BC Allergy Sinus Cold Powder 612
- Contac Severe Cold and Flu Caplets Maximum Strength 615
- Hycomine Compound Tablets 1105
- PediaCare Multi-Symptom Cold Liquid 704
- PediaCare NightRest Cough & Cold Liquid 704
- Robitussin Flu Liquid 752
- Robitussin PM Cough & Cold Liquid 752
- Singlet Caplets 636
- Sudafed Sinus & Allergy Tablets 710
- TheraFlu Cold & Cough Hot Liquid 680
- TheraFlu Cold & Sore Throat Hot Liquid 680
- TheraFlu Flu & Sore Throat Hot Liquid 681
- TheraFlu Severe Cold & Cough Hot Liquid 683
- TheraFlu Severe Cold Caplets 679
- TheraFlu Severe Cold Hot Liquid 682
- Triaminic Cold & Allergy Liquid 685
- Triaminic Cold & Cough Liquid 685
- Triaminic Flu, Cough & Fever Liquid 685
- Triaminic Night Time Cough & Cold Liquid 685
- Triaminic Allergy Runny Nose & Congestion Softchews 688
- Triaminic Cold & Cough Softchews 688
- Children's Tylenol Plus Cold NightTime Suspension Liquid 1851
- Children's Tylenol Plus Cold & Cough Suspension Liquid and Chewable Tablets 1851
- Children's Tylenol Plus Cold Chewable Tablets 1851
- Children's Tylenol Plus Flu Suspension Liquid 1853
- Tylenol Allergy Complete Multi-Symptom Caplets and Gelcaps with Cool Burst 1844
- Multi-Symptom Tylenol Cold Night Time Caplets 1845
- Vicks 44M Cough, Cold & Flu Relief 2676
- Pediatric Vicks 44m Cough & Cold Relief 2673
- Children's Vicks NyQuil Cold/Cough Relief 2671

Chlorpheniramine Polistirex (Concomitant administration of drugs that decrease the activity of drug metabolizing liver enzymes (Cytochrome P450) may increase plasma levels of praziquantel). Products include:
- Tussionex Pennkinetic Extended-Release Suspension 3322

Chlorpheniramine Tannate (Concomitant administration of drugs that decrease the activity of drug metabolizing liver enzymes (Cytochrome P450) may increase plasma levels of praziquantel).
No products indexed under this heading.

Chlorpropamide (Concomitant administration of drugs that decrease the activity of drug metabolizing liver enzymes (Cytochrome P450) may increase plasma levels of praziquantel).
No products indexed under this heading.

Cimetidine (Concomitant administration of drugs that decrease the activity of drug metabolizing liver enzymes (Cytochrome P450) may increase plasma levels of praziqua). Products include:
- Tagamet HB 200 Tablets 637
- Tagamet Tablets 1547

Cimetidine Hydrochloride (Concomitant administration of drugs that decrease the activity of drug metabolizing liver enzymes (Cytochrome P450) may increase plasma levels of praziqua).
No products indexed under this heading.

Ciprofloxacin (Concomitant administration of drugs that decrease the activity of drug metabolizing liver enzymes (Cytochrome P450) may increase plasma levels of praziqua). Products include:
- Cipro I.V. 2998
- Cipro I.V. Pharmacy Bulk Package ... 3509
- Cipro Oral Suspension 2991
- Cipro XR Tablets 3004
- Ciprodex Otic Suspension 555

Ciprofloxacin Hydrochloride (Concomitant administration of drugs that increase the activity of drug metabolizing liver enzymes (Cytochrome P450) may reduce plasma levels of praziquantel). Products include:
- Ciloxan Ophthalmic Ointment 554
- Cipro Tablets 2991

Cisplatin (Concomitant administration of drugs that increase the activity of drug metabolizing liver enzymes (Cytochrome P450) may reduce plasma levels of praziquantel).
No products indexed under this heading.

Citalopram Hydrobromide (Concomitant administration of drugs that increase the activity of drug metabolizing liver enzymes (Cytochrome P450) may reduce plasma levels of praziquantel). Products include:
- Celexa 1177

Clarithromycin (Concomitant administration of drugs that decrease the activity of drug metabolizing liver enzymes (Cytochrome P450) may increase plasma levels of praziqua). Products include:
- Biaxin/Biaxin XL 402
- PREVPAC 3281

Clomipramine Hydrochloride (Concomitant administration of drugs that decrease the activity of drug metabolizing liver enzymes (Cytochrome P450) may increase plasma levels of praziquantel).
No products indexed under this heading.

Clopidogrel Hydrogen Sulfate (Concomitant administration of drugs that decrease the activity of drug metabolizing liver enzymes (Cytochrome P450) may increase plasma levels of praziquantel).
No products indexed under this heading.

Clotrimazole (Concomitant administration of drugs that decrease the activity of drug metabolizing liver enzymes (Cytochrome P450) may increase plasma levels of praziquantel). Products include:
- Lotrimin 3053
- Lotrisone 3054

Cocaine Hydrochloride (Concomitant administration of drugs that decrease the activity of drug metabolizing liver enzymes (Cytochrome P450) may increase plasma levels of praziquantel).
No products indexed under this heading.

Cortisone Acetate (Concomitant administration of drugs that increase the activity of drug metabolizing liver enzymes (Cytochrome P450) may reduce plasma levels of praziquantel).
No products indexed under this heading.

Cyclosporine (Concomitant administration of drugs that decrease the activity of drug metabolizing liver enzymes (Cytochrome P450) may increase plasma levels of praziquantel). Products include:
- Gengraf Capsules 458
- Neoral Soft Gelatin Capsules 2247
- Neoral Oral Solution 2247
- Restasis Ophthalmic Emulsion 570
- Sandimmune 2259

Dalfopristin (Concomitant administration of drugs that decrease the activity of drug metabolizing liver enzymes (Cytochrome P450) may increase plasma levels of praziquantel). Products include:
- Synercid I.V. 1690

Danazol (Concomitant administration of drugs that decrease the activity of drug metabolizing liver enzymes (Cytochrome P450) may increase plasma levels of praziquantel).
No products indexed under this heading.

Delavirdine Mesylate (Concomitant administration of drugs that decrease the activity of drug metabolizing liver enzymes (Cytochrome P450) may increase plasma levels of praziquantel). Products include:
- Rescriptor Tablets 2535

Desipramine Hydrochloride (Concomitant administration of drugs that decrease the activity of drug metabolizing liver enzymes (Cytochrome P450) may increase plasma levels of praziquantel).
No products indexed under this heading.

Desogestrel (Concomitant administration of drugs that decrease the activity of drug metabolizing liver enzymes (Cytochrome P450) may increase plasma levels of praziqua). Products include:
- Ortho-Cept Tablets 2395

Dexamethasone (Concomitant administration of drugs that increase the activity of drug metabolizing liver enzymes (Cytochrome P450) may reduce plasma levels of praziquantel). Products include:
- Ciprodex Otic Suspension 555
- Decadron Tablets 1929
- TobraDex Ophthalmic Ointment 558
- TobraDex Ophthalmic Suspension ... 558

Dexamethasone Acetate (Concomitant administration of drugs that increase the activity of drug metabolizing liver enzymes (Cytochrome P450) may reduce plasma levels of praziquantel).
No products indexed under this heading.

Dexamethasone Sodium Phosphate (Concomitant administration of drugs that increase the activity of drug metabolizing liver enzymes (Cytochrome P450) may reduce plasma levels of praziquantel). Products include:
- Decadron Phosphate Injection 1931

Diclofenac Potassium (Concomitant administration of drugs that decrease the activity of drug metabolizing liver enzymes (Cytochrome P450) may increase plasma levels of praziquantel). Products include:
- Cataflam Tablets 2173

Diclofenac Sodium (Concomitant administration of drugs that decrease the activity of drug metabolizing liver enzymes (Cytochrome P450) may increase plasma levels of praziquantel). Products include:
- Arthrotec Tablets 3126
- Voltaren Ophthalmic Solution 2300
- Voltaren Tablets 2298
- Voltaren-XR Tablets 2301

Diltiazem Hydrochloride (Concomitant administration of drugs that increase the activity of drug metabolizing liver enzymes (Cytochrome P450) may reduce plasma levels of praziquantel). Products include:
- Cardizem LA Extended Release Tablets 1699
- Tiazac Capsules 1204

Diltiazem Maleate (Concomitant administration of drugs that increase the activity of drug metabolizing liver enzymes (Cytochrome P450) may reduce plasma levels of praziquantel).
No products indexed under this heading.

Diphenhydramine (Concomitant administration of drugs that decrease the activity of drug metabolizing liver enzymes (Cytochrome P450) may increase plasma levels of praziquantel). Products include:
- Tylenol Sore Throat NightTime Liquid with Cool Burst 1849

Diphenhydramine Hydrochloride (Concomitant administration of drugs that decrease the activity of drug metabolizing liver enzymes (Cytochrome P450) may increase plasma levels of praziquantel). Products include:
- Benadryl Allergy & Cold Tablets 692
- Benadryl Allergy 691
- Benadryl Allergy & Sinus Headache Caplets & Gelcaps 693
- Children's Benadryl Allergy Liquid ... 695
- Children's Benadryl Dye-Free Allergy Liquid 695
- Benadryl Dye-Free Allergy Liqui-Gels Softgels 692
- Benadryl Itch Relief Stick Extra Strength 696
- Benadryl Itch Stopping Cream Extra Strength 697

Benadryl Itch Stopping Gel Extra Strength ▣ 697
Benadryl Itch Stopping Spray Extra Strength ▣ 697
Benadryl Maximum Strength Severe Allergy & Sinus Headache Caplets ▣ 694
Children's Benadryl D Liquid Medication ▣ 693
Benadryl D Tablets ▣ 694
Nytol QuickCaps Caplets ▣ 635
Maximum Strength Nytol QuickGels Softgels ▣ 635
Simply Sleep Caplets 1841
Sominex Original Formula Tablets ▣ 637
TheraFlu Thin Strips Multi Symptom ▣ 684
Triaminic Thin Strips Cough & Runny Nose ▣ 690
Children's Tylenol Plus Cold & Allergy Suspension Liquid 1850
Tylenol Allergy Complete Night Time Caplets 1844
Tylenol Severe Allergy Caplets 1844
Tylenol Flu NightTime Gelcaps 1846
Extra Strength Tylenol PM Caplets, Geltabs, Gelcaps and Liquid 1847
Unisom Maximum Strength SleepGels ▣ 712

Disulfiram (Concomitant administration of drugs that decrease the activity of drug metabolizing liver enzymes (Cytochrome P450) may increase plasma levels of praziquantel). Products include:
Antabuse Tablets 2343

Doxepin Hydrochloride (Concomitant administration of drugs that decrease the activity of drug metabolizing liver enzymes (Cytochrome P450) may increase plasma levels of praziquantel).
No products indexed under this heading.

Doxorubicin Hydrochloride (Concomitant administration of drugs that increase the activity of drug metabolizing liver enzymes (Cytochrome P450) may reduce plasma levels of praziquantel). Products include:
Adriamycin for Injection, USP 786
Adriamycin Injection, USP 786

Efavirenz (Concomitant administration of drugs that increase the activity of drug metabolizing liver enzymes (Cytochrome P450) may reduce plasma levels of praziquantel). Products include:
Sustiva Capsules 957

Enoxacin (Concomitant administration of drugs that decrease the activity of drug metabolizing liver enzymes (Cytochrome P450) may increase plasma levels of praziqua).
No products indexed under this heading.

Erythromycin (Concomitant administration of drugs that increase the activity of drug metabolizing liver enzymes (Cytochrome P450) may reduce plasma levels of praziquantel). Products include:
Erygel Topical Gel 2096
Ery-Tab Tablets 447
Erythromycin Base Filmtab Tablets 454
Erythromycin Delayed-Release Capsules, USP 456
PCE Dispertab Tablets 510

Erythromycin Estolate (Concomitant administration of drugs that increase the activity of drug metabolizing liver enzymes (Cytochrome P450) may reduce plasma levels of praziquantel).
No products indexed under this heading.

Erythromycin Ethylsuccinate (Concomitant administration of drugs that increase the activity of drug metabolizing liver enzymes (Cytochrome P450) may reduce plasma levels of praziquantel). Products include:
E.E.S. 449
EryPed 445

Erythromycin Gluceptate (Concomitant administration of drugs that increase the activity of drug metabolizing liver enzymes (Cytochrome P450) may reduce plasma levels of praziquantel).
No products indexed under this heading.

Erythromycin Lactobionate (Concomitant administration of drugs that increase the activity of drug metabolizing liver enzymes (Cytochrome P450) may reduce plasma levels of praziquantel).
No products indexed under this heading.

Erythromycin Stearate (Concomitant administration of drugs that increase the activity of drug metabolizing liver enzymes (Cytochrome P450) may reduce plasma levels of praziquantel). Products include:
Erythrocin Stearate Filmtab Tablets 452

Escitalopram Oxalate (Concomitant administration of drugs that decrease the activity of drug metabolizing liver enzymes (Cytochrome P450) may increase plasma levels of praziquantel). Products include:
Lexapro Oral Solution 1193
Lexapro Tablets 1193

Esomeprazole Magnesium (Concomitant administration of drugs that decrease the activity of drug metabolizing liver enzymes (Cytochrome P450) may increase plasma levels of praziquantel). Products include:
Nexium Delayed-Release Capsules 645

Ethanol (Concomitant administration of drugs that increase the activity of drug metabolizing liver enzymes (Cytochrome P450) may reduce plasma levels of praziquantel).
No products indexed under this heading.

Ethinyl Estradiol (Concomitant administration of drugs that decrease the activity of drug metabolizing liver enzymes (Cytochrome P450) may increase plasma levels of praziqua). Products include:
Alesse-28 Tablets 3392
Lo/Ovral-28 Tablets 3423
NuvaRing 2357
Ortho-Cept Tablets 2395
Ortho-Cyclen/Ortho Tri-Cyclen 2414
Ortho Evra Transdermal System 2402
Ortho Tri-Cyclen Lo Tablets 2421
Seasonale Tablets 1073
Triphasil-28 Tablets 3483
Yasmin 28 Tablets 818

Ethosuximide (Concomitant administration of drugs that increase the activity of drug metabolizing liver enzymes (Cytochrome P450) may reduce plasma levels of praziquantel).
No products indexed under this heading.

Ethynodiol Diacetate (Concomitant administration of drugs that decrease the activity of drug metabolizing liver enzymes (Cytochrome P450) may increase plasma levels of praziquantel).
No products indexed under this heading.

Felbamate (Concomitant administration of drugs that increase the activity of drug metabolizing liver enzymes (Cytochrome P450) may reduce plasma levels of praziquantel).
No products indexed under this heading.

Fenofibrate (Concomitant administration of drugs that decrease the activity of drug metabolizing liver enzymes (Cytochrome P450) may increase plasma levels of praziquantel). Products include:
Antara Capsules 2723
Lofibra Capsules 1217
Tricor Tablets 523
Triglide Tablets 1165

Fluconazole (Concomitant administration of drugs that decrease the activity of drug metabolizing liver enzymes (Cytochrome P450) may increase plasma levels of praziquantel).
No products indexed under this heading.

Fludrocortisone Acetate (Concomitant administration of drugs that increase the activity of drug metabolizing liver enzymes (Cytochrome P450) may reduce plasma levels of praziquantel).
No products indexed under this heading.

Fluorouracil (Concomitant administration of drugs that decrease the activity of drug metabolizing liver enzymes (Cytochrome P450) may increase plasma levels of praziquantel). Products include:
Carac Cream, 0.5% 1048
Efudex 3348

Fluoxetine (Concomitant administration of drugs that decrease the activity of drug metabolizing liver enzymes (Cytochrome P450) may increase plasma levels of praziquantel).
No products indexed under this heading.

Fluoxetine Hydrochloride (Concomitant administration of drugs that decrease the activity of drug metabolizing liver enzymes (Cytochrome P450) may increase plasma levels of praziquantel). Products include:
Prozac Pulvules and Liquid 1771
Symbyax Capsules 1788

Fluphenazine Decanoate (Concomitant administration of drugs that decrease the activity of drug metabolizing liver enzymes (Cytochrome P450) may increase plasma levels of praziquantel).
No products indexed under this heading.

Fluphenazine Enanthate (Concomitant administration of drugs that decrease the activity of drug metabolizing liver enzymes (Cytochrome P450) may increase plasma levels of praziquantel).
No products indexed under this heading.

Fluphenazine Hydrochloride (Concomitant administration of drugs that decrease the activity of drug metabolizing liver enzymes (Cytochrome P450) may increase plasma levels of praziquantel).
No products indexed under this heading.

Flurbiprofen (Concomitant administration of drugs that decrease the activity of drug metabolizing liver enzymes (Cytochrome P450) may increase plasma levels of praziquantel).
No products indexed under this heading.

Flurbiprofen Sodium (Concomitant administration of drugs that decrease the activity of drug metabolizing liver enzymes (Cytochrome P450) may increase plasma levels of praziquantel). Products include:
Ocufen Ophthalmic Solution ⊙ 230

Fluvastatin Sodium (Concomitant administration of drugs that decrease the activity of drug metabolizing liver enzymes (Cytochrome P450) may increase plasma levels of praziquantel). Products include:
Lescol Capsules 2227
Lescol 2730
Lescol XL Tablets 2227

Fluvoxamine (Concomitant administration of drugs that decrease the activity of drug metabolizing liver enzymes (Cytochrome P450) may increase plasma levels of praziqua).
No products indexed under this heading.

Fluvoxamine Maleate (Concomitant administration of drugs that increase the activity of drug metabolizing liver enzymes (Cytochrome P450) may reduce plasma levels of praziquantel).
No products indexed under this heading.

Fosamprenavir Calcium (Concomitant administration of drugs that decrease the activity of drug metabolizing liver enzymes (Cytochrome P450) may increase plasma levels of praziquantel). Products include:
Lexiva Tablets 1473

Fosphenytoin Sodium (Concomitant administration of drugs that increase the activity of drug metabolizing liver enzymes (Cytochrome P450) may reduce plasma levels of praziquantel).
No products indexed under this heading.

Garlic Extract (Concomitant administration of drugs that increase the activity of drug metabolizing liver enzymes (Cytochrome P450) may reduce plasma levels of praziquantel).
No products indexed under this heading.

Garlic Oil (Concomitant administration of drugs that increase the activity of drug metabolizing liver enzymes (Cytochrome P450) may reduce plasma levels of praziquantel).
No products indexed under this heading.

Gatifloxacin (Concomitant administration of drugs that decrease the activity of drug metabolizing liver enzymes (Cytochrome P450) may increase plasma levels of praziqua). Products include:
Tequin Injection 964
Tequin Tablets 964
Zymar Ophthalmic Solution 571

Gemfibrozil (Concomitant administration of drugs that decrease the activity of drug metabolizing liver enzymes (Cytochrome P450) may increase plasma levels of praziquantel).
No products indexed under this heading.

emifloxacin Mesylate (Concomi-
ınt administration of drugs that
ecrease the activity of drug metab-
lizing liver enzymes (Cytochrome
450) may increase plasma levels of
raziqua). Products include:
Factive Tablets 2464

lipizide (Concomitant administra-
on of drugs that decrease the activ-
y of drug metabolizing liver
nzymes (Cytochrome P450) may
crease plasma levels of
raziquantel).
No products indexed under this heading.

lyburide (Concomitant administra-
on of drugs that decrease the activ-
y of drug metabolizing liver
nzymes (Cytochrome P450) may
crease plasma levels of
raziquantel).
No products indexed under this heading.

repafloxacin Hydrochloride
oncomitant administration of
rugs that decrease the activity of
rug metabolizing liver enzymes
ytochrome P450) may increase
asma levels of praziqua).
No products indexed under this heading.

alofantrine Hydrochloride (Con-
omitant administration of drugs that
ecrease the activity of drug metab-
izing liver enzymes (Cytochrome
450) may increase plasma levels of
raziquantel).
No products indexed under this heading.

aloperidol (Concomitant adminis-
ation of drugs that decrease the
ctivity of drug metabolizing liver
nzymes (Cytochrome P450) may
crease plasma levels of
raziquantel).
No products indexed under this heading.

aloperidol Decanoate (Concomi-
nt administration of drugs that
ecrease the activity of drug metab-
izing liver enzymes (Cytochrome
450) may increase plasma levels of
raziquantel).
No products indexed under this heading.

ydrochlorothiazide (Concomitant
dministration of drugs that
ecrease the activity of drug metab-
izing liver enzymes (Cytochrome
450) may increase plasma levels of
raziquantel). Products include:
Aldoril Tablets 1884
Atacand HCT 637
Avalide Tablets 2889
Avalide Tablets 922
Benicar HCT Tablets 2852
Diovan HCT Tablets 2195
Dyazide Capsules 1389
Hyzaar 1964
Lotensin HCT Tablets 2235
Maxzide 2150
Micardis HCT Tablets 886
Moduretic Tablets 2003
Prinzide Tablets 2033
Teveten HCT Tablets 1710
Timolide Tablets 2056
Uniretic Tablets 3114
Vaseretic Tablets 2073
Zestoretic Tablets 701

ydrocortisone (Concomitant
dministration of drugs that increase
e activity of drug metabolizing liver
nzymes (Cytochrome P450) may
duce plasma levels of praziquan-
l). Products include:
Cortizone•5 Ointment 699
Cortizone•10 Creme 699
Cortizone•10 Ointment 699
Cortizone•10 Plus Creme 700
Cortizone•10 Maximum Strength Quick Shot Spray 700
Hydrocortone Tablets 1963
Preparation H Hydrocortisone Cream 748

Hydrocortisone Acetate (Concomitant administration of drugs that increase the activity of drug metabolizing liver enzymes (Cytochrome P450) may reduce plasma levels of praziquantel). Products include:
Analpram-HC 1136
Pramosone 1139
ProctoFoam-HC 3113
Tucks Anti-Itch Ointment 712
U-cort 1% Cream 3289

Hydrocortisone Butyrate (Concomitant administration of drugs that increase the activity of drug metabolizing liver enzymes (Cytochrome P450) may reduce plasma levels of praziquantel). Products include:
Locoid 1138
Locoid Lipocream Cream 1138

Hydrocortisone Cypionate (Concomitant administration of drugs that increase the activity of drug metabolizing liver enzymes (Cytochrome P450) may reduce plasma levels of praziquantel).
No products indexed under this heading.

Hydrocortisone Hemisuccinate (Concomitant administration of drugs that increase the activity of drug metabolizing liver enzymes (Cytochrome P450) may reduce plasma levels of praziquantel).
No products indexed under this heading.

Hydrocortisone Probutate (Concomitant administration of drugs that increase the activity of drug metabolizing liver enzymes (Cytochrome P450) may reduce plasma levels of praziquantel). Products include:
Pandel Cream, 0.1% 1017

Hydrocortisone Sodium Phosphate (Concomitant administration of drugs that increase the activity of drug metabolizing liver enzymes (Cytochrome P450) may reduce plasma levels of praziquantel).
No products indexed under this heading.

Hydrocortisone Sodium Succinate (Concomitant administration of drugs that increase the activity of drug metabolizing liver enzymes (Cytochrome P450) may reduce plasma levels of praziquantel).
No products indexed under this heading.

Hydrocortisone Valerate (Concomitant administration of drugs that increase the activity of drug metabolizing liver enzymes (Cytochrome P450) may reduce plasma levels of praziquantel).
No products indexed under this heading.

Hydroflumethiazide (Concomitant administration of drugs that decrease the activity of drug metabolizing liver enzymes (Cytochrome P450) may increase plasma levels of praziquantel).
No products indexed under this heading.

Hydroxychloroquine Sulfate (Concomitant administration of drugs that decrease the activity of drug metabolizing liver enzymes (Cytochrome P450) may increase plasma levels of praziquantel).
No products indexed under this heading.

Hypericum (Concomitant administration of drugs that increase the activity of drug metabolizing liver enzymes (Cytochrome P450) may reduce plasma levels of praziquantel).
No products indexed under this heading.

Hypericum Perforatum (Concomitant administration of drugs that increase the activity of drug metabolizing liver enzymes (Cytochrome P450) may reduce plasma levels of praziquantel).
No products indexed under this heading.

Imatinib Mesylate (Concomitant administration of drugs that decrease the activity of drug metabolizing liver enzymes (Cytochrome P450) may increase plasma levels of praziquantel). Products include:
Gleevec Tablets 2221

Imipramine Hydrochloride (Concomitant administration of drugs that decrease the activity of drug metabolizing liver enzymes (Cytochrome P450) may increase plasma levels of praziquantel).
No products indexed under this heading.

Imipramine Pamoate (Concomitant administration of drugs that decrease the activity of drug metabolizing liver enzymes (Cytochrome P450) may increase plasma levels of praziquantel).
No products indexed under this heading.

Indinavir Sulfate (Concomitant administration of drugs that decrease the activity of drug metabolizing liver enzymes (Cytochrome P450) may increase plasma levels of praziquantel). Products include:
Crixivan Capsules 1918

Indomethacin (Concomitant administration of drugs that decrease the activity of drug metabolizing liver enzymes (Cytochrome P450) may increase plasma levels of praziquantel). Products include:
Indocin 1968

Indomethacin Sodium Trihydrate (Concomitant administration of drugs that decrease the activity of drug metabolizing liver enzymes (Cytochrome P450) may increase plasma levels of praziquantel). Products include:
Indocin I.V. 1973

Insulin (Concomitant administration of drugs that increase the activity of drug metabolizing liver enzymes (Cytochrome P450) may reduce plasma levels of praziquantel).
No products indexed under this heading.

Isoniazid (Concomitant administration of drugs that decrease the activity of drug metabolizing liver enzymes (Cytochrome P450) may increase plasma levels of praziqua).
No products indexed under this heading.

Itraconazole (Concomitant administration of drugs that decrease the activity of drug metabolizing liver enzymes (Cytochrome P450) may increase plasma levels of praziquantel).
No products indexed under this heading.

Ketoconazole (Concomitant administration of drugs that decrease the activity of drug metabolizing liver enzymes (Cytochrome P450) may increase plasma levels of praziqua). Products include:
Nizoral A-D Shampoo, 1% 1839
Nizoral 2% Shampoo 1838

Ketoprofen (Concomitant administration of drugs that decrease the activity of drug metabolizing liver enzymes (Cytochrome P450) may increase plasma levels of praziquantel).
No products indexed under this heading.

Lansoprazole (Concomitant administration of drugs that increase the activity of drug metabolizing liver enzymes (Cytochrome P450) may reduce plasma levels of praziquantel). Products include:
Prevacid Delayed-Release Capsules 3268
Prevacid for Delayed-Release Oral Suspension 3268
Prevacid I.V. for Injection 3274
Prevacid NapraPAC 3277
Prevacid SoluTab Delayed-Release Orally Disintegrating Tablets 3268
PREVPAC 3281

Leflunomide (Concomitant administration of drugs that decrease the activity of drug metabolizing liver enzymes (Cytochrome P450) may increase plasma levels of praziquantel). Products include:
Arava Tablets 2881

Letrozole (Concomitant administration of drugs that decrease the activity of drug metabolizing liver enzymes (Cytochrome P450) may increase plasma levels of praziquantel). Products include:
Femara Tablets 2210

Levofloxacin (Concomitant administration of drugs that decrease the activity of drug metabolizing liver enzymes (Cytochrome P450) may increase plasma levels of praziqua). Products include:
Levaquin in 5% Dextrose Injection 2453
Levaquin 2453
Quixin Ophthalmic Solution 3373

Levonorgestrel (Concomitant administration of drugs that decrease the activity of drug metabolizing liver enzymes (Cytochrome P450) may increase plasma levels of praziqua). Products include:
Alesse-28 Tablets 3392
Climara Pro Transdermal System 800
Mirena Intrauterine System 810
Plan B Tablets 1068
Seasonale Tablets 1073
Triphasil-28 Tablets 3483

Lomefloxacin Hydrochloride (Concomitant administration of drugs that decrease the activity of drug metabolizing liver enzymes (Cytochrome P450) may increase plasma levels of praziqua).
No products indexed under this heading.

Lopinavir (Concomitant administration of drugs that decrease the activity of drug metabolizing liver enzymes (Cytochrome P450) may increase plasma levels of praziquantel). Products include:
Kaletra 474

Loratadine (Concomitant administration of drugs that decrease the activity of drug metabolizing liver enzymes (Cytochrome P450) may increase plasma levels of praziquantel). Products include:
Alavert Allergy & Sinus D-12 Hour Tablets 743
Alavert 743

IMPORTANT NOTE: Always consult each drug listing in the patient's regimen for possible interactions.

Children's Claritin 24 Hour Non-Drowsy Allergy Syrup .... ▣ **732**
Claritin Non-Drowsy 24 Hour Tablets .... ▣ **731**
Non-Drowsy Claritin Hives Relief Tablets .... ▣ **733**
Claritin Reditabs 24 Hour Non-Drowsy Tablets .... ▣ **732**
Claritin-D Non-Drowsy 12 Hour Tablets .... ▣ **731**
Claritin-D Non-Drowsy 24 Hour Tablets .... ▣ **731**
Children's Dimetapp ND Non-Drowsy Allergy Syrup .... ▣ **746**
Triaminic Allerchews .... ▣ **684**

Lovastatin (Concomitant administration of drugs that decrease the activity of drug metabolizing liver enzymes (Cytochrome P450) may increase plasma levels of praziquantel). Products include:
Advicor Tablets **1694**
Altoprev Extended-Release Tablets **1151**
Mevacor Tablets **1996**

Maprotiline Hydrochloride (Concomitant administration of drugs that decrease the activity of drug metabolizing liver enzymes (Cytochrome P450) may increase plasma levels of praziquantel).
No products indexed under this heading.

Mephenytoin (Concomitant administration of drugs that increase the activity of drug metabolizing liver enzymes (Cytochrome P450) may reduce plasma levels of praziquantel).
No products indexed under this heading.

Mestranol (Concomitant administration of drugs that decrease the activity of drug metabolizing liver enzymes (Cytochrome P450) may increase plasma levels of praziqua).
No products indexed under this heading.

Methadone Hydrochloride (Concomitant administration of drugs that decrease the activity of drug metabolizing liver enzymes (Cytochrome P450) may increase plasma levels of praziquantel).
No products indexed under this heading.

Methoxsalen (Concomitant administration of drugs that decrease the activity of drug metabolizing liver enzymes (Cytochrome P450) may increase plasma levels of praziqua). Products include:
Oxsoralen Lotion 1% **3354**
Oxsoralen-Ultra Capsules **3354**

Methsuximide (Concomitant administration of drugs that increase the activity of drug metabolizing liver enzymes (Cytochrome P450) may reduce plasma levels of praziquantel).
No products indexed under this heading.

Methyclothiazide (Concomitant administration of drugs that decrease the activity of drug metabolizing liver enzymes (Cytochrome P450) may increase plasma levels of praziquantel).
No products indexed under this heading.

Methylprednisolone (Concomitant administration of drugs that increase the activity of drug metabolizing liver enzymes (Cytochrome P450) may reduce plasma levels of praziquantel).
No products indexed under this heading.

Methylprednisolone Acetate (Concomitant administration of drugs that increase the activity of drug metabolizing liver enzymes (Cytochrome P450) may reduce plasma levels of praziquantel). Products include:
Depo-Medrol Injectable Suspension **2615**
Depo-Medrol Single-Dose Vial **2617**

Methylprednisolone Sodium Succinate (Concomitant administration of drugs that increase the activity of drug metabolizing liver enzymes (Cytochrome P450) may reduce plasma levels of praziquantel).
No products indexed under this heading.

Metronidazole (Concomitant administration of drugs that decrease the activity of drug metabolizing liver enzymes (Cytochrome P450) may increase plasma levels of praziquantel). Products include:
Metrogel 1% **1212**
MetroGel-Vaginal Gel **1822**
Noritate Cream, 1% **1051**

Metronidazole Benzoate (Concomitant administration of drugs that decrease the activity of drug metabolizing liver enzymes (Cytochrome P450) may increase plasma levels of praziquantel).
No products indexed under this heading.

Metronidazole Hydrochloride (Concomitant administration of drugs that decrease the activity of drug metabolizing liver enzymes (Cytochrome P450) may increase plasma levels of praziquantel).
No products indexed under this heading.

Mexiletine Hydrochloride (Concomitant administration of drugs that decrease the activity of drug metabolizing liver enzymes (Cytochrome P450) may increase plasma levels of praziqua).
No products indexed under this heading.

Mibefradil Dihydrochloride (Concomitant administration of drugs that decrease the activity of drug metabolizing liver enzymes (Cytochrome P450) may increase plasma levels of praziqua).
No products indexed under this heading.

Miconazole (Concomitant administration of drugs that decrease the activity of drug metabolizing liver enzymes (Cytochrome P450) may increase plasma levels of praziquantel).
No products indexed under this heading.

Miconazole Nitrate (Concomitant administration of drugs that decrease the activity of drug metabolizing liver enzymes (Cytochrome P450) may increase plasma levels of praziquantel). Products include:
Desenex .... ▣ **674**
Desenex Jock Itch Spray Powder .... ▣ **674**

Moclobemide (Concomitant administration of drugs that decrease the activity of drug metabolizing liver enzymes (Cytochrome P450) may increase plasma levels of praziquantel).
No products indexed under this heading.

Modafinil (Concomitant administration of drugs that increase the activity of drug metabolizing liver enzymes (Cytochrome P450) may reduce plasma levels of praziquantel). Products include:
Provigil Tablets **1002**

Moxifloxacin Hydrochloride (Concomitant administration of drugs that decrease the activity of drug metabolizing liver enzymes (Cytochrome P450) may increase plasma levels of praziqua). Products include:
Avelox **2984**
Vigamox Ophthalmic Solution **560**

Nafcillin Sodium (Concomitant administration of drugs that increase the activity of drug metabolizing liver enzymes (Cytochrome P450) may reduce plasma levels of praziquantel).
No products indexed under this heading.

Nalidixic Acid (Concomitant administration of drugs that decrease the activity of drug metabolizing liver enzymes (Cytochrome P450) may increase plasma levels of praziqua).
No products indexed under this heading.

Nefazodone Hydrochloride (Concomitant administration of drugs that decrease the activity of drug metabolizing liver enzymes (Cytochrome P450) may increase plasma levels of praziquantel).
No products indexed under this heading.

Nelfinavir Mesylate (Concomitant administration of drugs that decrease the activity of drug metabolizing liver enzymes (Cytochrome P450) may increase plasma levels of praziquantel). Products include:
Viracept **2556**

Nevirapine (Concomitant administration of drugs that increase the activity of drug metabolizing liver enzymes (Cytochrome P450) may reduce plasma levels of praziquantel). Products include:
Viramune Oral Suspension **903**
Viramune Tablets **903**

Niacinamide (Concomitant administration of drugs that decrease the activity of drug metabolizing liver enzymes (Cytochrome P450) may increase plasma levels of praziquantel).
No products indexed under this heading.

Nicardipine Hydrochloride (Concomitant administration of drugs that decrease the activity of drug metabolizing liver enzymes (Cytochrome P450) may increase plasma levels of praziquantel). Products include:
Cardene I.V. **1129**

Nicotinamide (Concomitant administration of drugs that decrease the activity of drug metabolizing liver enzymes (Cytochrome P450) may increase plasma levels of praziquantel). Products include:
Nicomide Tablets **3190**

Nicotine (Concomitant administration of drugs that increase the activity of drug metabolizing liver enzymes (Cytochrome P450) may reduce plasma levels of praziquantel). Products include:
Nicoderm CQ Patch **1629**
NicoDerm CQ Clear Patch .... ▣ **627**
Nicotrol Inhaler **2594**
Nicotrol NS **2596**

Nicotine Polacrilex (Concomitant administration of drugs that increase the activity of drug metabolizing liver enzymes (Cytochrome P450) may reduce plasma levels of praziquantel). Products include:
Commit Lozenges **1625**
Nicorette Gum **1632**

Nicotine Salicylate (Concomitant administration of drugs that increase the activity of drug metabolizing liver enzymes (Cytochrome P450) may reduce plasma levels of praziquantel).
No products indexed under this heading.

Nicotine Sulfate (Concomitant administration of drugs that increase the activity of drug metabolizing liver enzymes (Cytochrome P450) may reduce plasma levels of praziquantel).
No products indexed under this heading.

Nifedipine (Concomitant administration of drugs that decrease the activity of drug metabolizing liver enzymes (Cytochrome P450) may increase plasma levels of praziquantel). Products include:
Adalat CC Tablets **2978**

Norethindrone (Concomitant administration of drugs that increase the activity of drug metabolizing liver enzymes (Cytochrome P450) may reduce plasma levels of praziquantel). Products include:
Ortho Micronor Tablets **2411**

Norethindrone Acetate (Concomitant administration of drugs that increase the activity of drug metabolizing liver enzymes (Cytochrome P450) may reduce plasma levels of praziquantel). Products include:
Activella Tablets **2311**
Aygestin Tablets **1062**
CombiPatch Transdermal System **2180**

Norethynodrel (Concomitant administration of drugs that decrease the activity of drug metabolizing liver enzymes (Cytochrome P450) may increase plasma levels of praziquantel).
No products indexed under this heading.

Norfloxacin (Concomitant administration of drugs that decrease the activity of drug metabolizing liver enzymes (Cytochrome P450) may increase plasma levels of praziqua). Products include:
Noroxin Tablets **2009**

Norgestimate (Concomitant administration of drugs that decrease the activity of drug metabolizing liver enzymes (Cytochrome P450) may increase plasma levels of praziquantel). Products include:
Ortho-Cyclen/Ortho Tri-Cyclen **2414**
Ortho Tri-Cyclen Lo Tablets **2421**
Prefest Tablets **1069**

Norgestrel (Concomitant administration of drugs that decrease the activity of drug metabolizing liver enzymes (Cytochrome P450) may increase plasma levels of praziqua). Products include:
Lo/Ovral-28 Tablets **3423**

Nortriptyline Hydrochloride (Concomitant administration of drugs that decrease the activity of drug metabolizing liver enzymes (Cytochrome P450) may increase plasma levels of praziquantel).
No products indexed under this heading.

Ofloxacin (Concomitant administration of drugs that decrease the activity of drug metabolizing liver

enzymes (Cytochrome P450) may increase plasma levels of praziqua). Products include:

Floxin Otic Singles 1045
Floxin Otic Solution 1043

Omeprazole (Concomitant administration of drugs that increase the activity of drug metabolizing liver enzymes (Cytochrome P450) may reduce plasma levels of praziquantel). Products include:

Zegerid Powder for Oral Solution 2972

Oxcarbazepine (Concomitant administration of drugs that increase the activity of drug metabolizing liver enzymes (Cytochrome P450) may reduce plasma levels of praziquantel). Products include:

Trileptal Oral Suspension 2281
Trileptal Tablets 2281

Oxiconazole Nitrate (Concomitant administration of drugs that decrease the activity of drug metabolizing liver enzymes (Cytochrome P450) may increase plasma levels of praziquantel). Products include:

Oxistat 1498

Paroxetine Hydrochloride (Concomitant administration of drugs that decrease the activity of drug metabolizing liver enzymes (Cytochrome P450) may increase plasma levels of praziqua). Products include:

Paxil CR Controlled-Release Tablets 1509
Paxil 1501

Perphenazine (Concomitant administration of drugs that decrease the activity of drug metabolizing liver enzymes (Cytochrome P450) may increase plasma levels of praziquantel).

No products indexed under this heading.

Phenobarbital (Concomitant administration of drugs that increase the activity of drug metabolizing liver enzymes (Cytochrome P450) may reduce plasma levels of praziquantel).

No products indexed under this heading.

Phenobarbital Sodium (Concomitant administration of drugs that increase the activity of drug metabolizing liver enzymes (Cytochrome P450) may reduce plasma levels of praziquantel).

No products indexed under this heading.

Phenylbutazone (Concomitant administration of drugs that decrease the activity of drug metabolizing liver enzymes (Cytochrome P450) may increase plasma levels of praziquantel).

No products indexed under this heading.

Phenytoin (Concomitant administration of drugs that increase the activity of drug metabolizing liver enzymes (Cytochrome P450) may reduce plasma levels of praziquantel).

No products indexed under this heading.

Phenytoin Sodium (Concomitant administration of drugs that increase the activity of drug metabolizing liver enzymes (Cytochrome P450) may reduce plasma levels of praziquantel). Products include:

Phenytek Capsules 2153

Polythiazide (Concomitant administration of drugs that decrease the activity of drug metabolizing liver enzymes (Cytochrome P450) may increase plasma levels of praziquantel).

No products indexed under this heading.

Prednisolone Acetate (Concomitant administration of drugs that increase the activity of drug metabolizing liver enzymes (Cytochrome P450) may reduce plasma levels of praziquantel). Products include:

Blephamide Ophthalmic Ointment 563
Blephamide Ophthalmic Suspension 564
Poly-Pred Liquifilm Ophthalmic Suspension .... ⊙231
Pred Forte Ophthalmic Suspension .... ⊙233
Pred Mild Sterile Ophthalmic Suspension .... ⊙236
Pred-G Ophthalmic Suspension ...... ⊙234
Pred-G Sterile Ophthalmic Ointment .... ⊙235

Prednisolone Sodium Phosphate (Concomitant administration of drugs that increase the activity of drug metabolizing liver enzymes (Cytochrome P450) may reduce plasma levels of praziquantel). Products include:

Pediapred Oral Solution 3319

Prednisolone Tebutate (Concomitant administration of drugs that increase the activity of drug metabolizing liver enzymes (Cytochrome P450) may reduce plasma levels of praziquantel).

No products indexed under this heading.

Prednisone (Concomitant administration of drugs that increase the activity of drug metabolizing liver enzymes (Cytochrome P450) may reduce plasma levels of praziquantel).

No products indexed under this heading.

Primidone (Concomitant administration of drugs that increase the activity of drug metabolizing liver enzymes (Cytochrome P450) may reduce plasma levels of praziquantel).

No products indexed under this heading.

Propafenone Hydrochloride (Concomitant administration of drugs that decrease the activity of drug metabolizing liver enzymes (Cytochrome P450) may increase plasma levels of praziquantel). Products include:

Rythmol SR Capsules 2736

Propoxyphene Hydrochloride (Concomitant administration of drugs that decrease the activity of drug metabolizing liver enzymes (Cytochrome P450) may increase plasma levels of praziquantel).

No products indexed under this heading.

Propoxyphene Napsylate (Concomitant administration of drugs that decrease the activity of drug metabolizing liver enzymes (Cytochrome P450) may increase plasma levels of praziquantel). Products include:

Darvocet A 500 Tablets 3497

Protriptyline Hydrochloride (Concomitant administration of drugs that decrease the activity of drug metabolizing liver enzymes (Cytochrome P450) may increase plasma levels of praziquantel). Products include:

Vivactil Tablets 2350

Quercetin (Concomitant administration of drugs that decrease the activity of drug metabolizing liver enzymes (Cytochrome P450) may increase plasma levels of praziquantel).

No products indexed under this heading.

Quinacrine Hydrochloride (Concomitant administration of drugs that decrease the activity of drug metabolizing liver enzymes (Cytochrome P450) may increase plasma levels of praziquantel).

No products indexed under this heading.

Quinidine (Concomitant administration of drugs that decrease the activity of drug metabolizing liver enzymes (Cytochrome P450) may increase plasma levels of praziquantel).

No products indexed under this heading.

Quinidine Gluconate (Concomitant administration of drugs that decrease the activity of drug metabolizing liver enzymes (Cytochrome P450) may increase plasma levels of praziquantel).

No products indexed under this heading.

Quinidine Hydrochloride (Concomitant administration of drugs that decrease the activity of drug metabolizing liver enzymes (Cytochrome P450) may increase plasma levels of praziquantel).

No products indexed under this heading.

Quinidine Polygalacturonate (Concomitant administration of drugs that decrease the activity of drug metabolizing liver enzymes (Cytochrome P450) may increase plasma levels of praziquantel).

No products indexed under this heading.

Quinidine Sulfate (Concomitant administration of drugs that decrease the activity of drug metabolizing liver enzymes (Cytochrome P450) may increase plasma levels of praziquantel).

No products indexed under this heading.

Quinine (Concomitant administration of drugs that decrease the activity of drug metabolizing liver enzymes (Cytochrome P450) may increase plasma levels of praziquantel).

No products indexed under this heading.

Quinine Sulfate (Concomitant administration of drugs that decrease the activity of drug metabolizing liver enzymes (Cytochrome P450) may increase plasma levels of praziquantel).

No products indexed under this heading.

Quinupristin (Concomitant administration of drugs that decrease the activity of drug metabolizing liver enzymes (Cytochrome P450) may increase plasma levels of praziquantel). Products include:

Synercid I.V. 1690

Ranitidine Bismuth Citrate (Concomitant administration of drugs that decrease the activity of drug metabolizing liver enzymes (Cytochrome P450) may increase plasma levels of praziquantel).

No products indexed under this heading.

Ranitidine Hydrochloride (Concomitant administration of drugs that decrease the activity of drug metabolizing liver enzymes (Cytochrome P450) may increase plasma levels of praziqua). Products include:

Zantac 1597
Zantac Injection 1593
Zantac 75 Tablets .... ▣715
Zantac 150 Maximum Strength Tablets .... ▣715
Zantac Injection Pharmacy Bulk Package 1595

Rifabutin (Concomitant administration of drugs that increase the activity of drug metabolizing liver enzymes (Cytochrome P450) may reduce plasma levels of praziquantel).

No products indexed under this heading.

Rifampicin (Concomitant administration of drugs that increase the activity of drug metabolizing liver enzymes (Cytochrome P450) may reduce plasma levels of praziquantel).

No products indexed under this heading.

Rifampin (Concomitant administration of rifampin should be avoided).

No products indexed under this heading.

Rifapentine (Concomitant administration of drugs that increase the activity of drug metabolizing liver enzymes (Cytochrome P450) may reduce plasma levels of praziquantel).

No products indexed under this heading.

Ritonavir (Concomitant administration of drugs that increase the activity of drug metabolizing liver enzymes (Cytochrome P450) may reduce plasma levels of praziquantel). Products include:

Kaletra 474
Norvir 499

Saquinavir (Concomitant administration of drugs that decrease the activity of drug metabolizing liver enzymes (Cytochrome P450) may increase plasma levels of praziquantel).

No products indexed under this heading.

Saquinavir Mesylate (Concomitant administration of drugs that decrease the activity of drug metabolizing liver enzymes (Cytochrome P450) may increase plasma levels of praziquantel). Products include:

Invirase 2776

Secobarbital Sodium (Concomitant administration of drugs that increase the activity of drug metabolizing liver enzymes (Cytochrome P450) may reduce plasma levels of praziquantel).

No products indexed under this heading.

Sertraline Hydrochloride (Concomitant administration of drugs that decrease the activity of drug metabolizing liver enzymes (Cytochrome P450) may increase plasma levels of praziquantel). Products include:

Zoloft 2581

Sparfloxacin (Concomitant administration of drugs that decrease the activity of drug metabolizing liver enzymes (Cytochrome P450) may increase plasma levels of praziqua).

No products indexed under this heading.

Sulfacytine (Concomitant administration of drugs that decrease the activity of drug metabolizing liver enzymes (Cytochrome P450) may increase plasma levels of praziquantel).
No products indexed under this heading.

Sulfamethizole (Concomitant administration of drugs that decrease the activity of drug metabolizing liver enzymes (Cytochrome P450) may increase plasma levels of praziquantel).
No products indexed under this heading.

Sulfamethoxazole (Concomitant administration of drugs that decrease the activity of drug metabolizing liver enzymes (Cytochrome P450) may increase plasma levels of praziquantel).
No products indexed under this heading.

Sulfaphenazole (Concomitant administration of drugs that decrease the activity of drug metabolizing liver enzymes (Cytochrome P450) may increase plasma levels of praziquantel).
No products indexed under this heading.

Sulfasalazine (Concomitant administration of drugs that decrease the activity of drug metabolizing liver enzymes (Cytochrome P450) may increase plasma levels of praziquantel).
No products indexed under this heading.

Sulfinpyrazone (Concomitant administration of drugs that increase the activity of drug metabolizing liver enzymes (Cytochrome P450) may reduce plasma levels of praziquantel).
No products indexed under this heading.

Sulfisoxazole (Concomitant administration of drugs that decrease the activity of drug metabolizing liver enzymes (Cytochrome P450) may increase plasma levels of praziquantel).
No products indexed under this heading.

Sulfisoxazole Acetyl (Concomitant administration of drugs that decrease the activity of drug metabolizing liver enzymes (Cytochrome P450) may increase plasma levels of praziquantel).
No products indexed under this heading.

Sulfisoxazole Diolamine (Concomitant administration of drugs that decrease the activity of drug metabolizing liver enzymes (Cytochrome P450) may increase plasma levels of praziquantel).
No products indexed under this heading.

Tacrine Hydrochloride (Concomitant administration of drugs that decrease the activity of drug metabolizing liver enzymes (Cytochrome P450) may increase plasma levels of praziqua).
No products indexed under this heading.

Telithromycin (Concomitant administration of drugs that decrease the activity of drug metabolizing liver enzymes (Cytochrome P450) may increase plasma levels of praziquantel). Products include:
Ketek Tablets 2920

Telmisartan (Concomitant administration of drugs that decrease the activity of drug metabolizing liver enzymes (Cytochrome P450) may increase plasma levels of praziquantel). Products include:
Micardis Tablets 884
Micardis HCT Tablets 886

Terbinafine Hydrochloride (Concomitant administration of drugs that decrease the activity of drug metabolizing liver enzymes (Cytochrome P450) may increase plasma levels of praziquantel). Products include:
Lamisil AT Creams (Athlete's Foot & Jock Itch) .... ▣676
Lamisil Tablets 2226

Terconazole (Concomitant administration of drugs that decrease the activity of drug metabolizing liver enzymes (Cytochrome P450) may increase plasma levels of praziquantel).
No products indexed under this heading.

Theophylline (Concomitant administration of drugs that increase the activity of drug metabolizing liver enzymes (Cytochrome P450) may reduce plasma levels of praziquantel).
No products indexed under this heading.

Thioridazine Hydrochloride (Concomitant administration of drugs that decrease the activity of drug metabolizing liver enzymes (Cytochrome P450) may increase plasma levels of praziquantel). Products include:
Thioridazine Hydrochloride Tablets 2122

Ticlopidine Hydrochloride (Concomitant administration of drugs that decrease the activity of drug metabolizing liver enzymes (Cytochrome P450) may increase plasma levels of praziqua). Products include:
Ticlid Tablets 2813

Tobacco (Concomitant administration of drugs that increase the activity of drug metabolizing liver enzymes (Cytochrome P450) may reduce plasma levels of praziquantel).
No products indexed under this heading.

Tolazamide (Concomitant administration of drugs that decrease the activity of drug metabolizing liver enzymes (Cytochrome P450) may increase plasma levels of praziquantel).
No products indexed under this heading.

Tolbutamide (Concomitant administration of drugs that decrease the activity of drug metabolizing liver enzymes (Cytochrome P450) may increase plasma levels of praziquantel).
No products indexed under this heading.

Tolbutamide Sodium (Concomitant administration of drugs that decrease the activity of drug metabolizing liver enzymes (Cytochrome P450) may increase plasma levels of praziquantel).
No products indexed under this heading.

Topiramate (Concomitant administration of drugs that decrease the activity of drug metabolizing liver enzymes (Cytochrome P450) may increase plasma levels of praziquantel). Products include:
Topamax Sprinkle Capsules 2438
Topamax Tablets 2438

Triamcinolone (Concomitant administration of drugs that increase the activity of drug metabolizing liver enzymes (Cytochrome P450) may reduce plasma levels of praziquantel).
No products indexed under this heading.

Triamcinolone Acetonide (Concomitant administration of drugs that increase the activity of drug metabolizing liver enzymes (Cytochrome P450) may reduce plasma levels of praziquantel). Products include:
Azmacort Inhalation Aerosol 1701
Nasacort HFA Inhalation Aerosol 2939
Nasacort AQ Nasal Spray 2937

Triamcinolone Diacetate (Concomitant administration of drugs that increase the activity of drug metabolizing liver enzymes (Cytochrome P450) may reduce plasma levels of praziquantel).
No products indexed under this heading.

Triamcinolone Hexacetonide (Concomitant administration of drugs that increase the activity of drug metabolizing liver enzymes (Cytochrome P450) may reduce plasma levels of praziquantel).
No products indexed under this heading.

Trimethoprim (Concomitant administration of drugs that decrease the activity of drug metabolizing liver enzymes (Cytochrome P450) may increase plasma levels of praziquantel).
No products indexed under this heading.

Trimethoprim Hydrochloride (Concomitant administration of drugs that decrease the activity of drug metabolizing liver enzymes (Cytochrome P450) may increase plasma levels of praziquantel).
No products indexed under this heading.

Trimipramine Maleate (Concomitant administration of drugs that decrease the activity of drug metabolizing liver enzymes (Cytochrome P450) may increase plasma levels of praziquantel). Products include:
Surmontil Capsules 2347

Troglitazone (Concomitant administration of drugs that increase the activity of drug metabolizing liver enzymes (Cytochrome P450) may reduce plasma levels of praziquantel).
No products indexed under this heading.

Troleandomycin (Concomitant administration of drugs that decrease the activity of drug metabolizing liver enzymes (Cytochrome P450) may increase plasma levels of praziqua).
No products indexed under this heading.

Trovafloxacin Mesylate (Concomitant administration of drugs that decrease the activity of drug metabolizing liver enzymes (Cytochrome P450) may increase plasma levels of praziqua).
No products indexed under this heading.

Valproate Sodium (Concomitant administration of drugs that decrease the activity of drug metabolizing liver enzymes (Cytochrome P450) may increase plasma levels of praziquantel). Products include:
Depacon Injection 412

Venlafaxine Hydrochloride (Concomitant administration of drugs that decrease the activity of drug metabolizing liver enzymes (Cytochrome P450) may increase plasma levels of praziquantel). Products include:
Effexor Tablets 3405
Effexor XR Capsules 3411

Verapamil Hydrochloride (Concomitant administration of drugs that decrease the activity of drug metabolizing liver enzymes (Cytochrome P450) may increase plasma levels of praziquantel). Products include:
Covera-HS Tablets 3135
Tarka Tablets 519
Verelan PM Capsules 3120

Voriconazole (Concomitant administration of drugs that decrease the activity of drug metabolizing liver enzymes (Cytochrome P450) may increase plasma levels of praziquantel). Products include:
VFEND I.V. 2543
VFEND Oral Suspension 2543
VFEND Tablets 2543

Zafirlukast (Concomitant administration of drugs that decrease the activity of drug metabolizing liver enzymes (Cytochrome P450) may increase plasma levels of praziquantel). Products include:
Accolate Tablets 663

Zileuton (Concomitant administration of drugs that decrease the activity of drug metabolizing liver enzymes (Cytochrome P450) may increase plasma levels of praziqua).
No products indexed under this heading.

Food Interactions

Broccoli (Concomitant administration of drugs that increase the activity of drug metabolizing liver enzymes (Cytochrome P450) may reduce plasma levels of praziquantel).

Brussel Sprouts (Concomitant administration of drugs that increase the activity of drug metabolizing liver enzymes (Cytochrome P450) may reduce plasma levels of praziquantel).

Charbroiled Food (Concomitant administration of drugs that increase the activity of drug metabolizing liver enzymes (Cytochrome P450) may reduce plasma levels of praziquantel).

Grapefruit (Grapefruit juice was reported to produce a 1.6-fold increase in the Cmax and a 1.9-fold increase in the AUC of praziquantel).

Grapefruit Juice (Grapefruit juice was reported to produce a 1.6-fold increase in the Cmax and a 1.9-fold increase in the AUC of praziquantel).

BIOFREEZE PAIN RELIEVING GEL

(Camphor, Menthol) .... ▣691
May interact with:

Topical Medications (Do not use with other ointments, creams, sprays or liniments).
No products indexed under this heading.

BIOS LIFE 2 DRINK MIX

(Fiber, Vitamins with Minerals) 3328
None cited in PDR database.

BLEPH-10 OPHTHALMIC SOLUTION 10%
(Sulfacetamide Sodium) ⊙219
May interact with silver preparations. Compounds in these categories include:

Silver Acetate (Incompatible).
No products indexed under this heading.

Silver Nitrate (Incompatible).
No products indexed under this heading.

Silver Sulfadiazine (Incompatible).
No products indexed under this heading.

BLEPHAMIDE OPHTHALMIC OINTMENT
(Prednisolone Acetate, Sulfacetamide Sodium) 563
May interact with para-aminobenzoic acid based local anesthetics and silver preparations. Compounds in these categories include:

Procaine Hydrochloride (May antagonize the action of sulfonamide).
No products indexed under this heading.

Silver Acetate (Blephamide ointment is incompatible with silver preparations).
No products indexed under this heading.

Silver Nitrate (Blephamide ointment is incompatible with silver preparations).
No products indexed under this heading.

Silver Sulfadiazine (Blephamide ointment is incompatible with silver preparations).
No products indexed under this heading.

Tetracaine Hydrochloride (May antagonize the action of sulfonamide). Products include:
Cetacaine Topical Anesthetic 1007

BLEPHAMIDE OPHTHALMIC SUSPENSION
(Prednisolone Acetate, Sulfacetamide Sodium) 564
May interact with para-aminobenzoic acid based local anesthetics and certain other agents. Compounds in these categories include:

Procaine Hydrochloride (Local anesthetics related to p-amino benzoic acid may antagonize the action of the sulfonamides).
No products indexed under this heading.

Silver Nitrate (Blephamide ophthalmic suspension is incompatible with silver preparations).
No products indexed under this heading.

Tetracaine Hydrochloride (Local anesthetics related to p-amino benzoic acid may antagonize the action of the sulfonamides). Products include:
Cetacaine Topical Anesthetic 1007

BLOCADREN TABLETS
(Timolol Maleate) 1891
May interact with catecholamine depleting drugs, calcium channel blockers, cardiac glycosides, oral hypoglycemic agents, insulin, nonsteroidal anti-inflammatory agents, quinidine, and certain other agents. Compounds in these categories include:

Acarbose (Beta blockers may mask the signs and symptoms of acute hypoglycemia). Products include:
Precose Tablets 776

Amlodipine Besylate (Hypotension, AV conduction disturbances, and left ventricular failure have been reported in some patients receiving beta-adrenergic blocking agents when an oral calcium antagonist was added to the treatment regimen). Products include:
Caduet Tablets 2507
Lotrel Capsules 2238
Norvasc Tablets 2529

Bepridil Hydrochloride (Hypotension, AV conduction disturbances, and left ventricular failure have been reported in some patients receiving beta-adrenergic blocking agents when an oral calcium antagonist was added to the treatment regimen).
No products indexed under this heading.

Celecoxib (NSAIDs reduce the antihypertensive effects of Blocadren). Products include:
Celebrex Capsules 3130

Chlorpropamide (Beta blockers may mask the signs and symptoms of acute hypoglycemia).
No products indexed under this heading.

Clonidine (Beta adrenergic blocking agents may exacerbate the rebound hypertension). Products include:
Catapres-TTS 875

Clonidine Hydrochloride (Beta adrenergic blocking agents may exacerbate the rebound hypertension). Products include:
Catapres Tablets 874
Clorpres Tablets 2139

Deserpidine (Close observation of the patient is recommended when Blocadren is administered to patients receiving catecholamine-depleting drugs such as reserpine, because of possible additive effects and the production of hypotension and/or marked bradycardia, which may produce vertigo, syncope, or postural hypotension).
No products indexed under this heading.

Deslanoside (The concomitant use of beta-adrenergic blocking agents with digitalis and either diltiazem or verapamil may have additive effects in prolonging AV conduction time).
No products indexed under this heading.

Diclofenac Potassium (NSAIDs reduce the antihypertensive effects of Blocadren). Products include:
Cataflam Tablets 2173

Diclofenac Sodium (NSAIDs reduce the antihypertensive effects of Blocadren). Products include:
Arthrotec Tablets 3126
Voltaren Ophthalmic Solution 2300
Voltaren Tablets 2298
Voltaren-XR Tablets 2301

Digitalis Glycoside Preparations (The concomitant use of beta-adrenergic blocking agents with digitalis and either diltiazem or verapamil may have additive effects in prolonging AV conduction time).
No products indexed under this heading.

Digitoxin (The concomitant use of beta-adrenergic blocking agents with digitalis and either diltiazem or verapamil may have additive effects in prolonging AV conduction time).
No products indexed under this heading.

Digoxin (The concomitant use of beta-adrenergic blocking agents with digitalis and either diltiazem or verapamil may have additive effects in prolonging AV conduction time). Products include:
Digitek Tablets 2146
Lanoxicaps Capsules 1458
Lanoxin Injection 1462
Lanoxin Tablets 1468
Lanoxin Injection Pediatric 1465

Diltiazem Hydrochloride (Hypotension, AV conduction disturbances, and left ventricular failure have been reported in some patients receiving beta-adrenergic blocking agents when an oral calcium antagonist was added to the treatment regimen). Products include:
Cardizem LA Extended Release Tablets 1699
Tiazac Capsules 1204

Epinephrine (Patients with a history of atopy or severe anaphylactic reaction to a variety of allergens may be unresponsive to the usual dose of epinephrine to treat anaphylactic reactions). Products include:
EpiPen 1061
Primatene Mist ▣749

Epinephrine Hydrochloride (Patients with a history of atopy or severe anaphylactic reaction to a variety of allergens may be unresponsive to the usual dose of epinephrine to treat anaphylactic reactions).
No products indexed under this heading.

Etodolac (NSAIDs reduce the antihypertensive effects of Blocadren).
No products indexed under this heading.

Felodipine (Hypotension, AV conduction disturbances, and left ventricular failure have been reported in some patients receiving beta-adrenergic blocking agents when an oral calcium antagonist was added to the treatment regimen). Products include:
Plendil Extended-Release Tablets 651

Fenoprofen Calcium (NSAIDs reduce the antihypertensive effects of Blocadren). Products include:
Nalfon Capsules 2504

Flurbiprofen (NSAIDs reduce the antihypertensive effects of Blocadren).
No products indexed under this heading.

Glimepiride (Beta blockers may mask the signs and symptoms of acute hypoglycemia). Products include:
Amaryl Tablets 2864

Glipizide (Beta blockers may mask the signs and symptoms of acute hypoglycemia).
No products indexed under this heading.

Glyburide (Beta blockers may mask the signs and symptoms of acute hypoglycemia).
No products indexed under this heading.

Guanethidine Monosulfate (Close observation of the patient is recommended when Blocadren is administered to patients receiving catecholamine-depleting drugs such as reserpine, because of possible additive effects and the production of hypotension and/or marked bradycardia, which may produce vertigo, syncope, or postural hypotension).
No products indexed under this heading.

Ibuprofen (NSAIDs reduce the antihypertensive effects of Blocadren). Products include:
Advil Allergy Sinus Caplets ▣737
Advil ▣737
Children's Advil Suspension ▣742
Children's Advil Chewable Tablets ▣741
Advil Cold & Sinus ▣739
Advil Flu & Body Ache Caplets ▣739
Children's Advil Cold Suspension ▣741
Infants' Advil Concentrated Drops ▣743
Junior Strength Advil Swallow Tablets ▣740
Advil Migraine Liquigels ▣740
Advil Multi-Symptom Cold Caplets ▣738
Combunox Tablets 1183
Children's Motrin Oral Suspension and Chewable Tablets 1837
Children's Motrin Cold Non-Staining Dye-Free Oral Suspension 1838
Children's Motrin Cold Oral Suspension 1838
Children's Motrin Non-Staining Dye-Free Oral Suspension 1837
Motrin Cold & Sinus Caplets 1836
Motrin IB Tablets and Caplets 1836
Infants' Motrin Concentrated Drops 1837
Infants' Motrin Non-Staining Dye-Free Drops 1837
Junior Strength Motrin Caplets and Chewable Tablets 1837
Vicoprofen Tablets 533

Indomethacin (NSAIDs reduce the antihypertensive effects of Blocadren). Products include:
Indocin 1968

Indomethacin Sodium Trihydrate (NSAIDs reduce the antihypertensive effects of Blocadren). Products include:
Indocin I.V. 1973

Insulin, Human, Zinc Suspension (Beta blockers may mask the signs and symptoms of acute hypoglycemia; insulin requirements may be altered). Products include:
Humulin L, 100 Units 1763
Humulin U, 100 Units 1770

Insulin, Human NPH (Beta blockers may mask the signs and symptoms of acute hypoglycemia; insulin requirements may be altered). Products include:
Humulin N, 100 Units 1764
Humulin N Pen 1765
Novolin N Human Insulin 10 ml Vials 2322
Novolin N InnoLet 2322
Novolin N PenFill 3 ml Cartridges 2325
Novolin R InnoLet 2322

Insulin, Human Regular (Beta blockers may mask the signs and symptoms of acute hypoglycemia; insulin requirements may be altered). Products include:
Humulin R (U-500) 1768
Humulin R, 100 Units 1767
Novolin R Human Insulin 10 ml Vials 2322
Novolin R PenFill 2325

Insulin, Human Regular and Human NPH Mixture (Beta blockers may mask the signs and symptoms of acute hypoglycemia; insulin requirements may be altered). Products include:
Humulin 50/50, 100 Units 1760
Humulin 70/30 Pen 1761
Novolin 70/30 Human Insulin 10 ml Vials 2321
Novolin 70/30 InnoLet 2322
Novolin 70/30 PenFill 3 ml Cartridges 2325

Insulin, NPH (Beta blockers may mask the signs and symptoms of acute hypoglycemia; insulin requirements may be altered).
No products indexed under this heading.

Insulin, Regular (Beta blockers may mask the signs and symptoms of acute hypoglycemia; insulin requirements may be altered).
No products indexed under this heading.

Insulin, Zinc Crystals (Beta blockers may mask the signs and symptoms of acute hypoglycemia; insulin requirements may be altered).
No products indexed under this heading.

Insulin, Zinc Suspension (Beta blockers may mask the signs and symptoms of acute hypoglycemia; insulin requirements may be altered).
No products indexed under this heading.

Insulin Aspart, Human Regular (Beta blockers may mask the signs and symptoms of acute hypoglycemia; insulin requirements may be altered). Products include:
NovoLog Injection 2326

Insulin glargine (Beta blockers may mask the signs and symptoms of acute hypoglycemia; insulin requirements may be altered). Products include:
Lantus Injection 2925

Insulin Lispro, Human (Beta blockers may mask the signs and symptoms of acute hypoglycemia; insulin requirements may be altered). Products include:
Humalog-Pen 1751
Humalog Mix 75/25-Pen 1754

Insulin Lispro Protamine, Human (Beta blockers may mask the signs and symptoms of acute hypoglycemia; insulin requirements may be altered). Products include:
Humalog Mix 75/25-Pen 1754

Isradipine (Hypotension, AV conduction disturbances, and left ventricular failure have been reported in some patients receiving beta-adrenergic blocking agents when an oral calcium antagonist was added to the treatment regimen). Products include:
DynaCirc CR Tablets 2726

Ketoprofen (NSAIDs reduce the antihypertensive effects of Blocadren).
No products indexed under this heading.

Ketorolac Tromethamine (NSAIDs reduce the antihypertensive effects of Blocadren). Products include:
Acular Ophthalmic Solution 561
Acular LS Ophthalmic Solution 562

Meclofenamate Sodium (NSAIDs reduce the antihypertensive effects of Blocadren).
No products indexed under this heading.

Mefenamic Acid (NSAIDs reduce the antihypertensive effects of Blocadren).
No products indexed under this heading.

Meloxicam (NSAIDs reduce the antihypertensive effects of Blocadren). Products include:
Mobic Oral Suspension 893
Mobic Tablets 893

Metformin Hydrochloride (Beta blockers may mask the signs and symptoms of acute hypoglycemia). Products include:
ActoPlus Met Tablets 3219
Avandamet Tablets 1343
Fortamet Extended-Release Tablets 1156

Mibefradil Dihydrochloride (Hypotension, AV conduction disturbances, and left ventricular failure have been reported in some patients receiving beta-adrenergic blocking agents when an oral calcium antagonist was added to the treatment regimen).
No products indexed under this heading.

Miglitol (Beta blockers may mask the signs and symptoms of acute hypoglycemia).
No products indexed under this heading.

Nabumetone (NSAIDs reduce the antihypertensive effects of Blocadren). Products include:
Relafen Tablets 1523

Naproxen (NSAIDs reduce the antihypertensive effects of Blocadren). Products include:
EC-Naprosyn Delayed-Release Tablets 2769
Naprosyn Suspension 2769
Naprosyn Tablets 2769
Prevacid NapraPAC 3277

Naproxen Sodium (NSAIDs reduce the antihypertensive effects of Blocadren). Products include:
Aleve Tablets, Caplets and Gelcaps 605
Anaprox Tablets 2769
Anaprox DS Tablets 2769

Nicardipine Hydrochloride (Hypotension, AV conduction disturbances, and left ventricular failure have been reported in some patients receiving beta-adrenergic blocking agents when an oral calcium antagonist was added to the treatment regimen). Products include:
Cardene I.V. 1129

Nifedipine (Hypotension, AV conduction disturbances, and left ventricular failure have been reported in some patients receiving beta-adrenergic blocking agents when an oral calcium antagonist was added to the treatment regimen). Products include:
Adalat CC Tablets 2978

Nimodipine (Hypotension, AV conduction disturbances, and left ventricular failure have been reported in some patients receiving beta-adrenergic blocking agents when an oral calcium antagonist was added to the treatment regimen). Products include:
Nimotop Capsules 774

Nisoldipine (Hypotension, AV conduction disturbances, and left ventricular failure have been reported in some patients receiving beta-adrenergic blocking agents when an oral calcium antagonist was added to the treatment regimen). Products include:
Sular Tablets 1163

Oxaprozin (NSAIDs reduce the antihypertensive effects of Blocadren).
No products indexed under this heading.

Phenylbutazone (NSAIDs reduce the antihypertensive effects of Blocadren).
No products indexed under this heading.

Pioglitazone Hydrochloride (Beta blockers may mask the signs and symptoms of acute hypoglycemia). Products include:
ActoPlus Met Tablets 3219
Actos Tablets 3224

Piroxicam (NSAIDs reduce the antihypertensive effects of Blocadren).
No products indexed under this heading.

Quinidine (Co-administration has resulted in potentiated systemic beta-blockade, such as decreased heart rate).
No products indexed under this heading.

Quinidine Gluconate (Co-administration has resulted in potentiated systemic beta-blockade, such as decreased heart rate).
No products indexed under this heading.

Quinidine Hydrochloride (Co-administration has resulted in potentiated systemic beta-blockade, such as decreased heart rate).
No products indexed under this heading.

Quinidine Polygalacturonate (Co-administration has resulted in potentiated systemic beta-blockade, such as decreased heart rate).
No products indexed under this heading.

Quinidine Sulfate (Co-administration has resulted in potentiated systemic beta-blockade, such as decreased heart rate).
No products indexed under this heading.

Rauwolfia Serpentina (Close observation of the patient is recommended when Blocadren is administered to patients receiving catecholamine-depleting drugs such as reserpine, because of possible additive effects and the production of hypotension and/or marked bradycardia, which may produce vertigo, syncope, or postural hypotension).
No products indexed under this heading.

Repaglinide (Beta blockers may mask the signs and symptoms of acute hypoglycemia). Products include:
Prandin Tablets (0.5, 1, and 2 mg) 2337

Rescinnamine (Close observation of the patient is recommended when Blocadren is administered to patients receiving catecholamine-depleting drugs such as reserpine, because of possible additive effects and the production of hypotension and/or marked bradycardia, which may produce vertigo, syncope, or postural hypotension).
No products indexed under this heading.

Reserpine (Close observation of the patient is recommended when Blocadren is administered to patients receiving catecholamine-depleting drugs such as reserpine, because of possible additive effects and the production of hypotension and/or marked bradycardia, which may produce vertigo, syncope, or postural hypotension).
No products indexed under this heading.

Rofecoxib (NSAIDs reduce the antihypertensive effects of Blocadren).
No products indexed under this heading.

Rosiglitazone Maleate (Beta blockers may mask the signs and symptoms of acute hypoglycemia). Products include:
Avandamet Tablets 1343
Avandia Tablets 1348

Sulindac (NSAIDs reduce the antihypertensive effects of Blocadren). Products include:
Clinoril Tablets 1899

Tolazamide (Beta blockers may mask the signs and symptoms of acute hypoglycemia).
No products indexed under this heading.

Tolbutamide (Beta blockers may mask the signs and symptoms of acute hypoglycemia).
No products indexed under this heading.

Tolmetin Sodium (NSAIDs reduce the antihypertensive effects of Blocadren).
No products indexed under this heading.

Troglitazone (Beta blockers may mask the signs and symptoms of acute hypoglycemia).
No products indexed under this heading.

Valdecoxib (NSAIDs reduce the antihypertensive effects of Blocadren).
No products indexed under this heading.

Verapamil Hydrochloride (Hypotension, AV conduction disturbances, and left ventricular failure have been reported in some patients receiving beta-adrenergic blocking agents when an oral calcium antagonist was added to the treatment regimen). Products include:
Covera-HS Tablets 3135
Tarka Tablets 519
Verelan PM Capsules 3120

BONIVA TABLETS
(Ibandronate Sodium) 2747
May interact with antacids containing aluminum, calcium and magnesium, non-steroidal anti-inflammatory agents, and certain other agents. Compounds in these categories include:

Aluminum Carbonate (Products containing calcium and other multivalent cations (such as aluminum, magnesium, iron) are likely to interfere with absorption of ibandronate sodium. Ibandronate sodium should be taken at least 60 minutes before any oral medications containing multivalent cations (including antacids)).
No products indexed under this heading.

Aluminum Hydroxide (Products containing calcium and other multivalent cations (such as aluminum, magnesium, iron) are likely to interfere with absorption of ibandronate sodi-

um. Ibandronate sodium should be taken at least 60 minutes before any oral medications containing multivalent cations (including antacids)). Products include:

- Gaviscon Regular Strength Liquid .. 620
- Gaviscon Regular Strength Tablets 619
- Gaviscon Extra Strength Liquid 620
- Gaviscon Extra Strength Tablets 619
- Maalox Max Maximum Strength Antacid/Anti-Gas Liquid.......... 2165
- Maalox Regular Strength Antacid/Antigas Liquid.......... 2164

Aspirin (Since aspirin and bisphosphonates are associated with gastrointestinal irritation, caution should be exercised in the concomitant use of aspirin products with ibandronate sodium). Products include:

- Aggrenox Capsules 855
- Bayer, Aspirin Regimen 606
- Bayer Aspirin Tablets 3515
- BC Powder 612
- BC Allergy Sinus Cold Powder 612
- Arthritis Strength BC Powder 612
- BC Sinus Cold Powder 612
- Ecotrin Enteric Coated Aspirin Low, Regular and Maximum Strength Tablets 1627
- Goody's Body Pain Formula Powder 621
- Goody's Extra Strength Headache Powder 621
- Goody's Extra Strength Pain Relief Tablets 621
- Percodan Tablets 1115
- St. Joseph 81 mg Aspirin Chewable and Enteric Coated Tablets 1841

Aspirin, Enteric Coated (Since aspirin and bisphosphonates are associated with gastrointestinal irritation, caution should be exercised in the concomitant use of aspirin products with ibandronate sodium).

No products indexed under this heading.

Aspirin Buffered (Since aspirin and bisphosphonates are associated with gastrointestinal irritation, caution should be exercised in the concomitant use of aspirin products with ibandronate sodium).

No products indexed under this heading.

Calcium (Products containing calcium and other multivalent cations (such as aluminum, magnesium, iron) are likely to interfere with absorption of ibandronate sodium. Ibandronate sodium should be taken at least 60 minutes before any oral medications containing multivalent cations (including supplements and vitamins)). Products include:

- Os-Cal 250 + D Tablets 765
- Os-Cal 500 Tablets 765
- Os-Cal 500 + D Tablets 766
- Perdiem Overnight Relief Pills 2166
- Slow-Mag Tablets 2717

Calcium (Oyster Shell) (Products containing calcium and other multivalent cations (such as aluminum, magnesium, iron) are likely to interfere with absorption of ibandronate sodium. Ibandronate sodium should be taken at least 60 minutes before any oral medications containing multivalent cations (including supplements and vitamins)).

No products indexed under this heading.

Calcium Carbonate (Products containing calcium and other multivalent cations (such as aluminum, magnesium, iron) are likely to interfere with absorption of ibandronate sodium. Ibandronate sodium should be taken at least 60 minutes before any oral medications containing multivalent cations (including supplements and vitamins)). Products include:

- Actonel with Calcium Tablets 2684
- Caltrate 600 PLUS Chewables 779
- Caltrate 600 PLUS Tablets 779
- Caltrate 600 + D Tablets 779
- Encora Capsules 3298
- Encora AM Tablets 3298
- Encora PM Tablets 3298
- Gas-X with Maalox 675
- Maalox Regular Strength Antacid Tablets 2166
- Quick Dissolve Maalox Max Maximum Strength Antacid/Antigas Tablets 2165
- Maalox Max Quick Dissolve Maximum Strength Chewable Tablets 678
- Os-Cal Chewable Tablets 765
- Pepcid Complete Chewable Tablets 1672
- PremCal Light, Regular, and Extra Strength Tablets 762
- Rolaids Tablets 707
- Extra Strength Rolaids Softchews 708
- Extra Strength Rolaids Tablets 707
- Rolaids Multi-Symptom Antacid & Antigas Tablets 708
- Tums 639

Calcium Citrate (Products containing calcium and other multivalent cations (such as aluminum, magnesium, iron) are likely to interfere with absorption of ibandronate sodium. Ibandronate sodium should be taken at least 60 minutes before any oral medications containing multivalent cations (including supplements and vitamins)). Products include:

- Active Calcium Tablets 3342
- Citracal Tablets 2108

Celecoxib (Since NSAIDs and bisphosphonates are associated with gastrointestinal irritation, caution should be exercised in the concomitant use of NSAIDs with ibandronate sodium). Products include:

- Celebrex Capsules 3130

Diclofenac Potassium (Since NSAIDs and bisphosphonates are associated with gastrointestinal irritation, caution should be exercised in the concomitant use of NSAIDs with ibandronate sodium). Products include:

- Cataflam Tablets 2173

Diclofenac Sodium (Since NSAIDs and bisphosphonates are associated with gastrointestinal irritation, caution should be exercised in the concomitant use of NSAIDs with ibandronate sodium). Products include:

- Arthrotec Tablets 3126
- Voltaren Ophthalmic Solution 2300
- Voltaren Tablets 2298
- Voltaren-XR Tablets 2301

Etodolac (Since NSAIDs and bisphosphonates are associated with gastrointestinal irritation, caution should be exercised in the concomitant use of NSAIDs with ibandronate sodium).

No products indexed under this heading.

Fenoprofen Calcium (Since NSAIDs and bisphosphonates are associated with gastrointestinal irritation, caution should be exercised in the concomitant use of NSAIDs with ibandronate sodium). Products include:

- Nalfon Capsules 2504

Flurbiprofen (Since NSAIDs and bisphosphonates are associated with gastrointestinal irritation, caution should be exercised in the concomitant use of NSAIDs with ibandronate sodium).

No products indexed under this heading.

Ibuprofen (Since NSAIDs and bisphosphonates are associated with gastrointestinal irritation, caution should be exercised in the concomitant use of NSAIDs with ibandronate sodium). Products include:

- Advil Allergy Sinus Caplets 737
- Advil 737
- Children's Advil Suspension 742
- Children's Advil Chewable Tablets .. 741
- Advil Cold & Sinus 739
- Advil Flu & Body Ache Caplets 739
- Children's Advil Cold Suspension 741
- Infants' Advil Concentrated Drops .. 743
- Junior Strength Advil Swallow Tablets 740
- Advil Migraine Liquigels 740
- Advil Multi-Symptom Cold Caplets 738
- Combunox Tablets 1183
- Children's Motrin Oral Suspension and Chewable Tablets 1837
- Children's Motrin Cold Non-Staining Dye-Free Oral Suspension 1838
- Children's Motrin Cold Oral Suspension 1838
- Children's Motrin Non-Staining Dye-Free Oral Suspension 1837
- Motrin Cold & Sinus Caplets 1836
- Motrin IB Tablets and Caplets 1836
- Infants' Motrin Concentrated Drops 1837
- Infants' Motrin Non-Staining Dye-Free Drops 1837
- Junior Strength Motrin Caplets and Chewable Tablets 1837
- Vicoprofen Tablets 533

Indomethacin (Since NSAIDs and bisphosphonates are associated with gastrointestinal irritation, caution should be exercised in the concomitant use of NSAIDs with ibandronate sodium). Products include:

- Indocin 1968

Indomethacin Sodium Trihydrate (Since NSAIDs and bisphosphonates are associated with gastrointestinal irritation, caution should be exercised in the concomitant use of NSAIDs with ibandronate sodium). Products include:

- Indocin I.V. 1973

Iron (Products containing calcium and other multivalent cations (such as aluminum, magnesium, iron) are likely to interfere with absorption of ibandronate sodium. Ibandronate sodium should be taken at least 60 minutes before any oral medications containing multivalent cations (including supplements and vitamins)). Products include:

- Chromagen Forte Soft Gelatin Capsules 3296
- Ferretts IPS Liquid 773
- OptiNate 1162
- Repliva 21/7 Tablets 3301

Iron Supplements (Products containing calcium and other multivalent cations (such as aluminum, magnesium, iron) are likely to interfere with absorption of ibandronate sodium. Ibandronate sodium should be taken at least 60 minutes before any oral medications containing multivalent cations (including supplements and vitamins)).

No products indexed under this heading.

Ketoprofen (Since NSAIDs and bisphosphonates are associated with gastrointestinal irritation, caution should be exercised in the concomitant use of NSAIDs with ibandronate sodium).

No products indexed under this heading.

Ketorolac Tromethamine (Since NSAIDs and bisphosphonates are associated with gastrointestinal irritation, caution should be exercised in the concomitant use of NSAIDs with ibandronate sodium). Products include:

- Acular Ophthalmic Solution 561
- Acular LS Ophthalmic Solution 562

Magaldrate (Products containing calcium and other multivalent cations (such as aluminum, magnesium, iron) are likely to interfere with absorption of ibandronate sodium. Ibandronate sodium should be taken at least 60 minutes before any oral medications containing multivalent cations (including antacids)).

No products indexed under this heading.

Magnesium Hydroxide (Products containing calcium and other multivalent cations (such as aluminum, magnesium, iron) are likely to interfere with absorption of ibandronate sodium. Ibandronate sodium should be taken at least 60 minutes before any oral medications containing multivalent cations (including antacids)). Products include:

- Maalox Max Maximum Strength Antacid/Anti-Gas Liquid 2165
- Maalox Regular Strength Antacid/Antigas Liquid 2164
- Pepcid Complete Chewable Tablets 1672
- Rolaids Tablets 707
- Extra Strength Rolaids Tablets 707
- Rolaids Multi-Symptom Antacid & Antigas Tablets 708

Magnesium Oxide (Products containing calcium and other multivalent cations (such as aluminum, magnesium, iron) are likely to interfere with absorption of ibandronate sodium. Ibandronate sodium should be taken at least 60 minutes before any oral medications containing multivalent cations (including antacids)). Products include:

- Beelith Tablets 784
- PremCal Light, Regular, and Extra Strength Tablets 762

Meclofenamate Sodium (Since NSAIDs and bisphosphonates are associated with gastrointestinal irritation, caution should be exercised in the concomitant use of NSAIDs with ibandronate sodium).

No products indexed under this heading.

Mefenamic Acid (Since NSAIDs and bisphosphonates are associated with gastrointestinal irritation, caution should be exercised in the concomitant use of NSAIDs with ibandronate sodium).

No products indexed under this heading.

Meloxicam (Since NSAIDs and bisphosphonates are associated with gastrointestinal irritation, caution should be exercised in the concomitant use of NSAIDs with ibandronate sodium). Products include:

- Mobic Oral Suspension 893
- Mobic Tablets 893

Multivitamins (Products containing calcium and other multivalent cations (such as aluminum, magnesium, iron) are likely to interfere with absorption of ibandronate sodium. Ibandronate sodium should be taken at least 60 minutes before any oral medications containing multivalent cations (including vitamins)).
No products indexed under this heading.

Multivitamins with Minerals (Products containing calcium and other multivalent cations (such as aluminum, magnesium, iron) are likely to interfere with absorption of ibandronate sodium. Ibandronate sodium should be taken at least 60 minutes before any oral medications containing multivalent cations (including vitamins)). Products include:
Microdiet Dietary Supplement .... ▣775
Noni Plus Plus Liquid .... ▣759
OptiNate 1162

Nabumetone (Since NSAIDs and bisphosphonates are associated with gastrointestinal irritation, caution should be exercised in the concomitant use of NSAIDs with ibandronate sodium). Products include:
Relafen Tablets 1523

Naproxen (Since NSAIDs and bisphosphonates are associated with gastrointestinal irritation, caution should be exercised in the concomitant use of NSAIDs with ibandronate sodium). Products include:
EC-Naprosyn Delayed-Release Tablets 2769
Naprosyn Suspension 2769
Naprosyn Tablets 2769
Prevacid NapraPAC 3277

Naproxen Sodium (Since NSAIDs and bisphosphonates are associated with gastrointestinal irritation, caution should be exercised in the concomitant use of NSAIDs with ibandronate sodium). Products include:
Aleve Tablets, Caplets and Gelcaps .... ▣605
Anaprox Tablets 2769
Anaprox DS Tablets 2769

Oxaprozin (Since NSAIDs and bisphosphonates are associated with gastrointestinal irritation, caution should be exercised in the concomitant use of NSAIDs with ibandronate sodium).
No products indexed under this heading.

Phenylbutazone (Since NSAIDs and bisphosphonates are associated with gastrointestinal irritation, caution should be exercised in the concomitant use of NSAIDs with ibandronate sodium).
No products indexed under this heading.

Piroxicam (Since NSAIDs and bisphosphonates are associated with gastrointestinal irritation, caution should be exercised in the concomitant use of NSAIDs with ibandronate sodium).
No products indexed under this heading.

Rofecoxib (Since NSAIDs and bisphosphonates are associated with gastrointestinal irritation, caution should be exercised in the concomitant use of NSAIDs with ibandronate sodium).
No products indexed under this heading.

Sulindac (Since NSAIDs and bisphosphonates are associated with gastrointestinal irritation, caution should be exercised in the concomitant use of NSAIDs with ibandronate sodium). Products include:
Clinoril Tablets 1899

Tolmetin Sodium (Since NSAIDs and bisphosphonates are associated with gastrointestinal irritation, caution should be exercised in the concomitant use of NSAIDs with ibandronate sodium).
No products indexed under this heading.

Valdecoxib (Since NSAIDs and bisphosphonates are associated with gastrointestinal irritation, caution should be exercised in the concomitant use of NSAIDs with ibandronate sodium).
No products indexed under this heading.

Vitamins, Multiple (Products containing calcium and other multivalent cations (such as aluminum, magnesium, iron) are likely to interfere with absorption of ibandronate sodium. Ibandronate sodium should be taken at least 60 minutes before any oral medications containing multivalent cations (including vitamins)). Products include:
Encora Capsules 3298
Encora AM Tablets 3298
Encora PM Tablets 3298
Mega Antioxidant Tablets 3343

Vitamins with Iron (Products containing calcium and other multivalent cations (such as aluminum, magnesium, iron) are likely to interfere with absorption of ibandronate sodium. Ibandronate sodium should be taken at least 60 minutes before any oral medications containing multivalent cations (including vitamins)).
No products indexed under this heading.

BOOSTRIX

(Diphtheria & Tetanus Toxoids and Acellular Pertussis Vaccine Adsorbed) 1366

May interact with alkylating agents, antimetabolites, corticosteroids, cytotoxic drugs, immunosuppressive agents, and certain other agents. Compounds in these categories include:

Azathioprine (May reduce immune response to vaccines. When administered to patients who are receiving immunosuppressive therapy, who have an immunodeficiency disorder, or who have received a recent injection of immune globulin, an adequate immunologic response may not be obtained). Products include:
Azasan Tablets 2844

Basiliximab (May reduce immune response to vaccines. When administered to patients who are receiving immunosuppressive therapy, who have an immunodeficiency disorder, or who have received a recent injection of immune globulin, an adequate immunologic response may not be obtained). Products include:
Simulect for Injection 2268

Betamethasone Acetate (May reduce immune response to vaccines. When administered to patients who are receiving immunosuppressive therapy, who have an immunodeficiency disorder, or who have received a recent injection of immune globulin, an adequate immunologic response may not be obtained).
No products indexed under this heading.

Betamethasone Sodium Phosphate (May reduce immune response to vaccines. When administered to patients who are receiving immunosuppressive therapy, who have an immunodeficiency disorder, or who have received a recent injection of immune globulin, an adequate immunologic response may not be obtained).
No products indexed under this heading.

Bleomycin Sulfate (May reduce immune response to vaccines. When administered to patients who are receiving immunosuppressive therapy, who have an immunodeficiency disorder, or who have received a recent injection of immune globulin, an adequate immunologic response may not be obtained).
No products indexed under this heading.

Busulfan (May reduce immune response to vaccines. When administered to patients who are receiving immunosuppressive therapy, who have an immunodeficiency disorder, or who have received a recent injection of immune globulin, an adequate immunologic response may not be obtained). Products include:
I.V. Busulfex 1125
Myleran Tablets 1492

Capecitabine (May reduce immune response to vaccines. When administered to patients who are receiving immunosuppressive therapy, who have an immunodeficiency disorder, or who have received a recent injection of immune globulin, an adequate immunologic response may not be obtained). Products include:
Xeloda Tablets 2825

Carmustine (BCNU) (May reduce immune response to vaccines. When administered to patients who are receiving immunosuppressive therapy, who have an immunodeficiency disorder, or who have received a recent injection of immune globulin, an adequate immunologic response may not be obtained).
No products indexed under this heading.

Chlorambucil (May reduce immune response to vaccines. When administered to patients who are receiving immunosuppressive therapy, who have an immunodeficiency disorder, or who have received a recent injection of immune globulin, an adequate immunologic response may not be obtained). Products include:
Leukeran Tablets 1472

Cladribine (May reduce immune response to vaccines. When administered to patients who are receiving immunosuppressive therapy, who have an immunodeficiency disorder, or who have received a recent injection of immune globulin, an adequate immunologic response may not be obtained). Products include:
Leustatin Injection 2368

Cortisone Acetate (May reduce immune response to vaccines. When administered to patients who are receiving immunosuppressive therapy, who have an immunodeficiency disorder, or who have received a recent injection of immune globulin, an adequate immunologic response may not be obtained).
No products indexed under this heading.

Cyclophosphamide (May reduce immune response to vaccines. When administered to patients who are receiving immunosuppressive therapy, who have an immunodeficiency disorder, or who have received a recent injection of immune globulin, an adequate immunologic response may not be obtained).
No products indexed under this heading.

Cyclosporine (May reduce immune response to vaccines. When administered to patients who are receiving immunosuppressive therapy, who have an immunodeficiency disorder, or who have received a recent injection of immune globulin, an adequate immunologic response may not be obtained). Products include:
Gengraf Capsules 458
Neoral Soft Gelatin Capsules 2247
Neoral Oral Solution 2247
Restasis Ophthalmic Emulsion 570
Sandimmune 2259

Cytarabine (May reduce immune response to vaccines. When administered to patients who are receiving immunosuppressive therapy, who have an immunodeficiency disorder, or who have received a recent injection of immune globulin, an adequate immunologic response may not be obtained).
No products indexed under this heading.

Dacarbazine (May reduce immune response to vaccines. When administered to patients who are receiving immunosuppressive therapy, who have an immunodeficiency disorder, or who have received a recent injection of immune globulin, an adequate immunologic response may not be obtained).
No products indexed under this heading.

Daunorubicin Hydrochloride (May reduce immune response to vaccines. When administered to patients who are receiving immunosuppressive therapy, who have an immunodeficiency disorder, or who have received a recent injection of immune globulin, an adequate immunologic response may not be obtained). Products include:
Cerubidine for Injection 788

Dexamethasone (May reduce immune response to vaccines. When administered to patients who are receiving immunosuppressive therapy, who have an immunodeficiency disorder, or who have received a recent injection of immune globulin, an adequate immunologic response may not be obtained). Products include:
Ciprodex Otic Suspension 555
Decadron Tablets 1929
TobraDex Ophthalmic Ointment 558
TobraDex Ophthalmic Suspension 558

Dexamethasone Acetate (May reduce immune response to vaccines. When administered to patients who are receiving immunosuppressive therapy, who have an immunodeficiency disorder, or who have received a recent injection of immune globulin, an adequate immunologic response may not be obtained).
No products indexed under this heading.

Dexamethasone Sodium Phosphate (May reduce immune response to vaccines. When administered to patients who are receiving

immunosuppressive therapy, who have an immunodeficiency disorder, or who have received a recent injection of immune globulin, an adequate immunologic response may not be obtained). Products include:

- Decadron Phosphate Injection 1931

Doxorubicin Hydrochloride (May reduce immune response to vaccines. When administered to patients who are receiving immunosuppressive therapy, who have an immunodeficiency disorder, or who have received a recent injection of immune globulin, an adequate immunologic response may not be obtained). Products include:

- Adriamycin for Injection, USP 786
- Adriamycin Injection, USP 786

Epirubicin Hydrochloride (May reduce immune response to vaccines. When administered to patients who are receiving immunosuppressive therapy, who have an immunodeficiency disorder, or who have received a recent injection of immune globulin, an adequate immunologic response may not be obtained). Products include:

- Ellence Injection 2632

Floxuridine (May reduce immune response to vaccines. When administered to patients who are receiving immunosuppressive therapy, who have an immunodeficiency disorder, or who have received a recent injection of immune globulin, an adequate immunologic response may not be obtained).

No products indexed under this heading.

Fludarabine Phosphate (May reduce immune response to vaccines. When administered to patients who are receiving immunosuppressive therapy, who have an immunodeficiency disorder, or who have received a recent injection of immune globulin, an adequate immunologic response may not be obtained).

No products indexed under this heading.

Fludrocortisone Acetate (May reduce immune response to vaccines. When administered to patients who are receiving immunosuppressive therapy, who have an immunodeficiency disorder, or who have received a recent injection of immune globulin, an adequate immunologic response may not be obtained).

No products indexed under this heading.

Fluorouracil (May reduce immune response to vaccines. When administered to patients who are receiving immunosuppressive therapy, who have an immunodeficiency disorder, or who have received a recent injection of immune globulin, an adequate immunologic response may not be obtained). Products include:

- Carac Cream, 0.5% 1048
- Efudex 3348

Gemcitabine Hydrochloride (May reduce immune response to vaccines. When administered to patients who are receiving immunosuppressive therapy, who have an immunodeficiency disorder, or who have received a recent injection of immune globulin, an adequate immunologic response may not be obtained). Products include:

- Gemzar for Injection 1743

Hydrocortisone (May reduce immune response to vaccines. When administered to patients who are receiving immunosuppressive therapy, who have an immunodeficiency disorder, or who have received a recent injection of immune globulin, an adequate immunologic response may not be obtained). Products include:

- Cortizone•5 Ointment .... ▣699
- Cortizone•10 Creme .... ▣699
- Cortizone•10 Ointment .... ▣699
- Cortizone•10 Plus Creme .... ▣700
- Cortizone•10 Maximum Strength Quick Shot Spray .... ▣700
- Hydrocortone Tablets 1963
- Preparation H Hydrocortisone Cream .... ▣748

Hydrocortisone Acetate (May reduce immune response to vaccines. When administered to patients who are receiving immunosuppressive therapy, who have an immunodeficiency disorder, or who have received a recent injection of immune globulin, an adequate immunologic response may not be obtained). Products include:

- Analpram-HC 1136
- Pramosone 1139
- ProctoFoam-HC 3113
- Tucks Anti-Itch Ointment .... ▣712
- U-cort 1% Cream 3289

Hydrocortisone Sodium Phosphate (May reduce immune response to vaccines. When administered to patients who are receiving immunosuppressive therapy, who have an immunodeficiency disorder, or who have received a recent injection of immune globulin, an adequate immunologic response may not be obtained).

No products indexed under this heading.

Hydrocortisone Sodium Succinate (May reduce immune response to vaccines. When administered to patients who are receiving immunosuppressive therapy, who have an immunodeficiency disorder, or who have received a recent injection of immune globulin, an adequate immunologic response may not be obtained).

No products indexed under this heading.

Hydroxyurea (May reduce immune response to vaccines. When administered to patients who are receiving immunosuppressive therapy, who have an immunodeficiency disorder, or who have received a recent injection of immune globulin, an adequate immunologic response may not be obtained).

No products indexed under this heading.

Immune Globulin Intravenous (Human) (May reduce immune response to vaccines. When administered to patients who are receiving immunosuppressive therapy, who have an immunodeficiency disorder, or who have received a recent injection of immune globulin, an adequate immunologic response may not be obtained). Products include:

- Carimune NF 3501
- Gammagard Liquid 751
- Gammagard S/D 754
- Gamunex Immune Globulin I.V., 10% 3232
- Iveegam EN 759

Lomustine (CCNU) (May reduce immune response to vaccines. When administered to patients who are receiving immunosuppressive therapy, who have an immunodeficiency disorder, or who have received a recent injection of immune globulin, an adequate immunologic response may not be obtained).

No products indexed under this heading.

Mechlorethamine Hydrochloride (May reduce immune response to vaccines. When administered to patients who are receiving immunosuppressive therapy, who have an immunodeficiency disorder, or who have received a recent injection of immune globulin, an adequate immunologic response may not be obtained). Products include:

- Mustargen for Injection 2007

Melphalan (May reduce immune response to vaccines. When administered to patients who are receiving immunosuppressive therapy, who have an immunodeficiency disorder, or who have received a recent injection of immune globulin, an adequate immunologic response may not be obtained). Products include:

- Alkeran Tablets 977

Mercaptopurine (May reduce immune response to vaccines. When administered to patients who are receiving immunosuppressive therapy, who have an immunodeficiency disorder, or who have received a recent injection of immune globulin, an adequate immunologic response may not be obtained). Products include:

- Purinethol Tablets 1222

Methotrexate (May reduce immune response to vaccines. When administered to patients who are receiving immunosuppressive therapy, who have an immunodeficiency disorder, or who have received a recent injection of immune globulin, an adequate immunologic response may not be obtained).

No products indexed under this heading.

Methotrexate Sodium (May reduce immune response to vaccines. When administered to patients who are receiving immunosuppressive therapy, who have an immunodeficiency disorder, or who have received a recent injection of immune globulin, an adequate immunologic response may not be obtained).

No products indexed under this heading.

Methylprednisolone Acetate (May reduce immune response to vaccines. When administered to patients who are receiving immunosuppressive therapy, who have an immunodeficiency disorder, or who have received a recent injection of immune globulin, an adequate immunologic response may not be obtained). Products include:

- Depo-Medrol Injectable Suspension 2615
- Depo-Medrol Single-Dose Vial 2617

Methylprednisolone Sodium Succinate (May reduce immune response to vaccines. When administered to patients who are receiving immunosuppressive therapy, who have an immunodeficiency disorder, or who have received a recent injection of immune globulin, an adequate immunologic response may not be obtained).

No products indexed under this heading.

Mitotane (May reduce immune response to vaccines. When administered to patients who are receiving immunosuppressive therapy, who have an immunodeficiency disorder, or who have received a recent injection of immune globulin, an adequate immunologic response may not be obtained).

No products indexed under this heading.

Mitoxantrone Hydrochloride (May reduce immune response to vaccines. When administered to patients who are receiving immunosuppressive therapy, who have an immunodeficiency disorder, or who have received a recent injection of immune globulin, an adequate immunologic response may not be obtained). Products include:

- Novantrone for Injection Concentrate 3158

Muromonab-CD3 (May reduce immune response to vaccines. When administered to patients who are receiving immunosuppressive therapy, who have an immunodeficiency disorder, or who have received a recent injection of immune globulin, an adequate immunologic response may not be obtained). Products include:

- Orthoclone OKT3 Sterile Solution 2370

Mycophenolate Mofetil (May reduce immune response to vaccines. When administered to patients who are receiving immunosuppressive therapy, who have an immunodeficiency disorder, or who have received a recent injection of immune globulin, an adequate immunologic response may not be obtained). Products include:

- CellCept Capsules 2751
- CellCept Oral Suspension 2751
- CellCept Tablets 2751

Pentostatin (May reduce immune response to vaccines. When administered to patients who are receiving immunosuppressive therapy, who have an immunodeficiency disorder, or who have received a recent injection of immune globulin, an adequate immunologic response may not be obtained). Products include:

- Nipent for Injection 3216

Prednisolone Acetate (May reduce immune response to vaccines. When administered to patients who are receiving immunosuppressive therapy, who have an immunodeficiency disorder, or who have received a recent injection of immune globulin, an adequate immunologic response may not be obtained). Products include:

- Blephamide Ophthalmic Ointment 563
- Blephamide Ophthalmic Suspension.................................. 564
- Poly-Pred Liquifilm Ophthalmic Suspension .... ⊙231
- Pred Forte Ophthalmic Suspension .... ⊙233
- Pred Mild Sterile Ophthalmic Suspension .... ⊙236

Pred-G Ophthalmic Suspension ... ⊙ 234
Pred-G Sterile Ophthalmic Ointment ... ⊙ 235

Prednisolone Sodium Phosphate (May reduce immune response to vaccines. When administered to patients who are receiving immunosuppressive therapy, who have an immunodeficiency disorder, or who have received a recent injection of immune globulin, an adequate immunologic response may not be obtained). Products include:
Pediapred Oral Solution ... 3319

Prednisolone Tebutate (May reduce immune response to vaccines. When administered to patients who are receiving immunosuppressive therapy, who have an immunodeficiency disorder, or who have received a recent injection of immune globulin, an adequate immunologic response may not be obtained).
No products indexed under this heading.

Prednisone (May reduce immune response to vaccines. When administered to patients who are receiving immunosuppressive therapy, who have an immunodeficiency disorder, or who have received a recent injection of immune globulin, an adequate immunologic response may not be obtained).
No products indexed under this heading.

Procarbazine Hydrochloride (May reduce immune response to vaccines. When administered to patients who are receiving immunosuppressive therapy, who have an immunodeficiency disorder, or who have received a recent injection of immune globulin, an adequate immunologic response may not be obtained). Products include:
Matulane Capsules ... 3188

Sirolimus (May reduce immune response to vaccines. When administered to patients who are receiving immunosuppressive therapy, who have an immunodeficiency disorder, or who have received a recent injection of immune globulin, an adequate immunologic response may not be obtained). Products include:
Rapamune Oral Solution and Tablets ... 3472

Tacrolimus (May reduce immune response to vaccines. When administered to patients who are receiving immunosuppressive therapy, who have an immunodeficiency disorder, or who have received a recent injection of immune globulin, an adequate immunologic response may not be obtained). Products include:
Prograf Capsules and Injection ... 624
Protopic Ointment ... 629

Tamoxifen Citrate (May reduce immune response to vaccines. When administered to patients who are receiving immunosuppressive therapy, who have an immunodeficiency disorder, or who have received a recent injection of immune globulin, an adequate immunologic response may not be obtained).
No products indexed under this heading.

Thioguanine (May reduce immune response to vaccines. When administered to patients who are receiving immunosuppressive therapy, who have an immunodeficiency disorder, or who have received a recent injection of immune globulin, an adequate immunologic response may not be obtained). Products include:
Tabloid Tablets ... 1545

Thiotepa (May reduce immune response to vaccines. When administered to patients who are receiving immunosuppressive therapy, who have an immunodeficiency disorder, or who have received a recent injection of immune globulin, an adequate immunologic response may not be obtained).
No products indexed under this heading.

Triamcinolone (May reduce immune response to vaccines. When administered to patients who are receiving immunosuppressive therapy, who have an immunodeficiency disorder, or who have received a recent injection of immune globulin, an adequate immunologic response may not be obtained).
No products indexed under this heading.

Triamcinolone Acetonide (May reduce immune response to vaccines. When administered to patients who are receiving immunosuppressive therapy, who have an immunodeficiency disorder, or who have received a recent injection of immune globulin, an adequate immunologic response may not be obtained). Products include:
Azmacort Inhalation Aerosol ... 1701
Nasacort HFA Inhalation Aerosol ... 2939
Nasacort AQ Nasal Spray ... 2937

Triamcinolone Diacetate (May reduce immune response to vaccines. When administered to patients who are receiving immunosuppressive therapy, who have an immunodeficiency disorder, or who have received a recent injection of immune globulin, an adequate immunologic response may not be obtained).
No products indexed under this heading.

Triamcinolone Hexacetonide (May reduce immune response to vaccines. When administered to patients who are receiving immunosuppressive therapy, who have an immunodeficiency disorder, or who have received a recent injection of immune globulin, an adequate immunologic response may not be obtained).
No products indexed under this heading.

Vincristine Sulfate (May reduce immune response to vaccines. When administered to patients who are receiving immunosuppressive therapy, who have an immunodeficiency disorder, or who have received a recent injection of immune globulin, an adequate immunologic response may not be obtained).
No products indexed under this heading.

BOTOX PURIFIED NEUROTOXIN COMPLEX

(Botulinum Toxin Type A) ... 565
None cited in PDR database.

BRAVELLE FOR INTRAMUSCULAR OR SUBCUTANEOUS INJECTION

(Urofollitropin) ... 1140
None cited in PDR database.

BREVIBLOC CONCENTRATE

(Esmolol Hydrochloride) ... 766
See Brevibloc Injection

BREVIBLOC INJECTION

(Esmolol Hydrochloride) ... 766
May interact with oral hypoglycemic agents, insulin, and certain other agents. Compounds in these categories include:

Acarbose (Beta blockers may mask tachycardia occurring with hypoglycemia). Products include:
Precose Tablets ... 776

Chlorpropamide (Beta blockers may mask tachycardia occurring with hypoglycemia).
No products indexed under this heading.

Digoxin (Increased digoxin levels by 10-20% when concomitantly administered by intravenous route). Products include:
Digitek Tablets ... 2146
Lanoxicaps Capsules ... 1458
Lanoxin Injection ... 1462
Lanoxin Tablets ... 1468
Lanoxin Injection Pediatric ... 1465

Dopamine Hydrochloride (Concurrent use is not recommended to control supraventricular tachycardia because of the danger of blocking cardiac contractility when systemic vascular resistance is high).
No products indexed under this heading.

Epinephrine Hydrochloride (Concurrent use is not recommended to control supraventricular tachycardia because of the danger of blocking cardiac contractility when systemic vascular resistance is high; potential for unresponsiveness to the usual dose of epinephrine to treat allergic reaction).
No products indexed under this heading.

Glimepiride (Beta blockers may mask tachycardia occurring with hypoglycemia). Products include:
Amaryl Tablets ... 2864

Glipizide (Beta blockers may mask tachycardia occurring with hypoglycemia).
No products indexed under this heading.

Glyburide (Beta blockers may mask tachycardia occurring with hypoglycemia).
No products indexed under this heading.

Insulin, Human, Zinc Suspension (Beta blockers may mask tachycardia occurring with hypoglycemia). Products include:
Humulin L, 100 Units ... 1763
Humulin U, 100 Units ... 1770

Insulin, Human NPH (Beta blockers may mask tachycardia occurring with hypoglycemia). Products include:
Humulin N, 100 Units ... 1764
Humulin N Pen ... 1765
Novolin N Human Insulin 10 ml Vials ... 2322
Novolin N InnoLet ... 2322
Novolin N PenFill 3 ml Cartridges ... 2325
Novolin R InnoLet ... 2322

Insulin, Human Regular (Beta blockers may mask tachycardia occurring with hypoglycemia). Products include:
Humulin R (U-500) ... 1768
Humulin R, 100 Units ... 1767
Novolin R Human Insulin 10 ml Vials ... 2322
Novolin R PenFill ... 2325

Insulin, Human Regular and Human NPH Mixture (Beta blockers may mask tachycardia occurring with hypoglycemia). Products include:
Humulin 50/50, 100 Units ... 1760
Humulin 70/30 Pen ... 1761
Novolin 70/30 Human Insulin 10 ml Vials ... 2321
Novolin 70/30 InnoLet ... 2322
Novolin 70/30 PenFill 3 ml Cartridges ... 2325

Insulin, NPH (Beta blockers may mask tachycardia occurring with hypoglycemia).
No products indexed under this heading.

Insulin, Regular (Beta blockers may mask tachycardia occurring with hypoglycemia).
No products indexed under this heading.

Insulin, Zinc Crystals (Beta blockers may mask tachycardia occurring with hypoglycemia).
No products indexed under this heading.

Insulin, Zinc Suspension (Beta blockers may mask tachycardia occurring with hypoglycemia).
No products indexed under this heading.

Insulin Aspart, Human Regular (Beta blockers may mask tachycardia occurring with hypoglycemia). Products include:
NovoLog Injection ... 2326

Insulin glargine (Beta blockers may mask tachycardia occurring with hypoglycemia). Products include:
Lantus Injection ... 2925

Insulin Lispro, Human (Beta blockers may mask tachycardia occurring with hypoglycemia). Products include:
Humalog-Pen ... 1751
Humalog Mix 75/25-Pen ... 1754

Insulin Lispro Protamine, Human (Beta blockers may mask tachycardia occurring with hypoglycemia). Products include:
Humalog Mix 75/25-Pen ... 1754

Metformin Hydrochloride (Beta blockers may mask tachycardia occurring with hypoglycemia). Products include:
ActoPlus Met Tablets ... 3219
Avandamet Tablets ... 1343
Fortamet Extended-Release Tablets ... 1156

Miglitol (Beta blockers may mask tachycardia occurring with hypoglycemia).
No products indexed under this heading.

Morphine Sulfate (Intravenous morphine increases Brevibloc steady-state blood levels by 46%). Products include:
Avinza Capsules ... 1714
Kadian Capsules ... 572
MS Contin Tablets ... 2703

Norepinephrine Hydrochloride (Concurrent use is not recommended to control supraventricular tachycardia because of the danger of blocking cardiac contractility when systemic vascular resistance is high).
No products indexed under this heading.

Pioglitazone Hydrochloride (Beta blockers may mask tachycardia occurring with hypoglycemia). Products include:
ActoPlus Met Tablets 3219
Actos Tablets 3224

Repaglinide (Beta blockers may mask tachycardia occurring with hypoglycemia). Products include:
Prandin Tablets (0.5, 1, and 2 mg) 2337

Reserpine (Potential for additive effect; hypotension or marked bradycardia which may result in vertigo, syncope, or postural hypotension).
No products indexed under this heading.

Rosiglitazone Maleate (Beta blockers may mask tachycardia occurring with hypoglycemia). Products include:
Avandamet Tablets 1343
Avandia Tablets 1348

Succinylcholine Chloride (Prolonged neuromuscular blockade from five minutes to eight minutes).
No products indexed under this heading.

Tolazamide (Beta blockers may mask tachycardia occurring with hypoglycemia).
No products indexed under this heading.

Tolbutamide (Beta blockers may mask tachycardia occurring with hypoglycemia).
No products indexed under this heading.

Troglitazone (Beta blockers may mask tachycardia occurring with hypoglycemia).
No products indexed under this heading.

Verapamil Hydrochloride (Potential for fatal cardiac arrests in patients with depressed myocardial function). Products include:
Covera-HS Tablets 3135
Tarka Tablets 519
Verelan PM Capsules 3120

Warfarin Sodium (Brevibloc concentrations were equivocally higher when given with Warfarin). Products include:
Coumadin for Injection 932
Coumadin Tablets 932

BREVIBLOC DOUBLE STRENGTH INJECTION
(Esmolol Hydrochloride) 766
See Brevibloc Injection

BREVIBLOC PREMIXED INJECTION
(Esmolol Hydrochloride) 766
See Brevibloc Injection

BREVIBLOC DOUBLE STRENGTH PREMIXED INJECTION
(Esmolol Hydrochloride) 766
See Brevibloc Injection

BREVOXYL-4 CREAMY WASH
(Benzoyl Peroxide) 3212
None cited in PDR database.

BREVOXYL-4 GEL
(Benzoyl Peroxide) 3211
None cited in PDR database.

BREVOXYL-8 CREAMY WASH
(Benzoyl Peroxide) 3212
None cited in PDR database.

BREVOXYL-8 GEL
(Benzoyl Peroxide) 3211
None cited in PDR database.

BRIMONIDINE TARTRATE OPHTHALMIC SOLUTION 0.2%
(Brimonidine Tartrate) .... ⊙245
May interact with antihypertensives, beta blockers, central nervous system depressants, cardiac glycosides, monoamine oxidase inhibitors, and tricyclic antidepressants. Compounds in these categories include:

Acebutolol Hydrochloride (Caution is advised in concomitant use of beta-blockers and brimonidine).
No products indexed under this heading.

Alfentanil Hydrochloride (There may be an additive or potentiating effect with CNS depressants and brimonidine administered concomitantly).
No products indexed under this heading.

Alprazolam (There may be an additive or potentiating effect with CNS depressants and brimonidine administered concomitantly). Products include:
Niravam Orally Disintegrating Tablets 3106
Xanax XR Tablets 2655

Amitriptyline Hydrochloride (Caution is advised in concomitant use of tricyclic antidepressants and brimonidine).
No products indexed under this heading.

Amlodipine Besylate (Caution is advised in concomitant use of antihypertensives and brimonidine). Products include:
Caduet Tablets 2507
Lotrel Capsules 2238
Norvasc Tablets 2529

Amoxapine (Caution is advised in concomitant use of tricyclic antidepressants and brimonidine).
No products indexed under this heading.

Aprobarbital (There may be an additive or potentiating effect with CNS depressants and brimonidine administered concomitantly).
No products indexed under this heading.

Atenolol (Caution is advised in concomitant use of beta-blockers and brimonidine). Products include:
Tenormin I.V. Injection 698
Tenormin Tablets 695

Benazepril Hydrochloride (Caution is advised in concomitant use of antihypertensives and brimonidine). Products include:
Lotensin Tablets 2232
Lotensin HCT Tablets 2235
Lotrel Capsules 2238

Bendroflumethiazide (Caution is advised in concomitant use of antihypertensives and brimonidine).
No products indexed under this heading.

Betaxolol Hydrochloride (Caution is advised in concomitant use of beta-blockers and brimonidine). Products include:
Betoptic S Ophthalmic Suspension 554

Bisoprolol Fumarate (Caution is advised in concomitant use of beta-blockers and brimonidine).
No products indexed under this heading.

Buprenorphine Hydrochloride (There may be an additive or potentiating effect with CNS depressants and brimonidine administered concomitantly). Products include:
Buprenex Injectable 2718
Suboxone Tablets 2719
Subutex Tablets 2719

Buspirone Hydrochloride (There may be an additive or potentiating effect with CNS depressants and brimonidine administered concomitantly).
No products indexed under this heading.

Butabarbital (There may be an additive or potentiating effect with CNS depressants and brimonidine administered concomitantly).
No products indexed under this heading.

Butalbital (There may be an additive or potentiating effect with CNS depressants and brimonidine administered concomitantly). Products include:
Sedapap Tablets 50 mg/650 mg 2098

Candesartan Cilexetil (Caution is advised in concomitant use of antihypertensives and brimonidine). Products include:
Atacand Tablets 634
Atacand HCT 637

Captopril (Caution is advised in concomitant use of antihypertensives and brimonidine). Products include:
Captopril Tablets 2114

Carteolol Hydrochloride (Caution is advised in concomitant use of beta-blockers and brimonidine). Products include:
Carteolol Hydrochloride Ophthalmic Solution USP, 1% .... ⊙246

Chlordiazepoxide (There may be an additive or potentiating effect with CNS depressants and brimonidine administered concomitantly).
No products indexed under this heading.

Chlordiazepoxide Hydrochloride (There may be an additive or potentiating effect with CNS depressants and brimonidine administered concomitantly). Products include:
Librium Capsules 3349

Chlorothiazide (Caution is advised in concomitant use of antihypertensives and brimonidine). Products include:
Aldoclor Tablets 1881
Diuril Oral 1936

Chlorothiazide Sodium (Caution is advised in concomitant use of antihypertensives and brimonidine). Products include:
Diuril Sodium Intravenous 1934

Chlorpromazine (There may be an additive or potentiating effect with CNS depressants and brimonidine administered concomitantly).
No products indexed under this heading.

Chlorpromazine Hydrochloride (There may be an additive or potentiating effect with CNS depressants and brimonidine administered concomitantly).
No products indexed under this heading.

Chlorprothixene (There may be an additive or potentiating effect with CNS depressants and brimonidine administered concomitantly).
No products indexed under this heading.

Chlorprothixene Hydrochloride (There may be an additive or potentiating effect with CNS depressants and brimonidine administered concomitantly).
No products indexed under this heading.

Chlorprothixene Lactate (There may be an additive or potentiating effect with CNS depressants and brimonidine administered concomitantly).
No products indexed under this heading.

Chlorthalidone (Caution is advised in concomitant use of antihypertensives and brimonidine). Products include:
Clorpres Tablets 2139

Clomipramine Hydrochloride (Caution is advised in concomitant use of tricyclic antidepressants and brimonidine).
No products indexed under this heading.

Clonidine (Caution is advised in concomitant use of antihypertensives and brimonidine). Products include:
Catapres-TTS 875

Clonidine Hydrochloride (Caution is advised in concomitant use of antihypertensives and brimonidine). Products include:
Catapres Tablets 874
Clorpres Tablets 2139

Clorazepate Dipotassium (There may be an additive or potentiating effect with CNS depressants and brimonidine administered concomitantly). Products include:
Tranxene 2488

Clozapine (There may be an additive or potentiating effect with CNS depressants and brimonidine administered concomitantly). Products include:
Clozapine Tablets 2141
Clozaril Tablets 2174
FazaClo Orally Disintegrating Tablets 547

Codeine Phosphate (There may be an additive or potentiating effect with CNS depressants and brimonidine administered concomitantly). Products include:
Tylenol with Codeine 2461

Deserpidine (Caution is advised in concomitant use of antihypertensives and brimonidine).
No products indexed under this heading.

Desflurane (There may be an additive or potentiating effect with CNS depressants and brimonidine administered concomitantly). Products include:
Suprane Liquid for Inhalation 770

Desipramine Hydrochloride (Caution is advised in concomitant use of tricyclic antidepressants and brimonidine).
No products indexed under this heading.

Deslanoside (Caution is advised in concomitant use of cardiac glycosides and brimonidine).
No products indexed under this heading.

Dezocine (There may be an additive or potentiating effect with CNS depressants and brimonidine administered concomitantly).
No products indexed under this heading.

Diazepam (There may be an additive or potentiating effect with CNS depressants and brimonidine administered concomitantly). Products include:
Diastat Rectal Delivery System 3344
Valium Tablets 2822

Diazoxide (Caution is advised in concomitant use of antihypertensives and brimonidine). Products include:
Hyperstat I.V. Injection 3031

Digitalis Glycoside Preparations (Caution is advised in concomitant use of cardiac glycosides and brimonidine).
No products indexed under this heading.

Digitoxin (Caution is advised in concomitant use of cardiac glycosides and brimonidine).
No products indexed under this heading.

Digoxin (Caution is advised in concomitant use of cardiac glycosides and brimonidine). Products include:
Digitek Tablets 2146
Lanoxicaps Capsules 1458
Lanoxin Injection 1462
Lanoxin Tablets 1468
Lanoxin Injection Pediatric 1465

Diltiazem Hydrochloride (Caution is advised in concomitant use of antihypertensives and brimonidine). Products include:
Cardizem LA Extended Release Tablets 1699
Tiazac Capsules 1204

Doxazosin Mesylate (Caution is advised in concomitant use of antihypertensives and brimonidine).
No products indexed under this heading.

Doxepin Hydrochloride (Caution is advised in concomitant use of tricyclic antidepressants and brimonidine).
No products indexed under this heading.

Droperidol (There may be an additive or potentiating effect with CNS depressants and brimonidine administered concomitantly).
No products indexed under this heading.

Enalapril Maleate (Caution is advised in concomitant use of antihypertensives and brimonidine). Products include:
Vaseretic Tablets 2073
Vasotec I.V. Injection 2076

Enalaprilat (Caution is advised in concomitant use of antihypertensives and brimonidine).
No products indexed under this heading.

Enflurane (There may be an additive or potentiating effect with CNS depressants and brimonidine administered concomitantly).
No products indexed under this heading.

Eprosartan Mesylate (Caution is advised in concomitant use of antihypertensives and brimonidine). Products include:
Teveten Tablets 1707
Teveten HCT Tablets 1710

Esmolol Hydrochloride (Caution is advised in concomitant use of beta-blockers and brimonidine). Products include:
Brevibloc Concentrate 766
Brevibloc Injection 766
Brevibloc Double Strength Injection 766
Brevibloc Premixed Injection 766
Brevibloc Double Strength Premixed Injection 766

Estazolam (There may be an additive or potentiating effect with CNS depressants and brimonidine administered concomitantly). Products include:
ProSom Tablets 512

Ethanol (There may be an additive or potentiating effect with CNS depressants and brimonidine administered concomitantly).
No products indexed under this heading.

Ethchlorvynol (There may be an additive or potentiating effect with CNS depressants and brimonidine administered concomitantly).
No products indexed under this heading.

Ethinamate (There may be an additive or potentiating effect with CNS depressants and brimonidine administered concomitantly).
No products indexed under this heading.

Ethyl Alcohol (There may be an additive or potentiating effect with CNS depressants and brimonidine administered concomitantly).
No products indexed under this heading.

Felodipine (Caution is advised in concomitant use of antihypertensives and brimonidine). Products include:
Plendil Extended-Release Tablets 651

Fentanyl (There may be an additive or potentiating effect with CNS depressants and brimonidine administered concomitantly). Products include:
Duragesic Transdermal System 2448

Fentanyl Citrate (There may be an additive or potentiating effect with CNS depressants and brimonidine administered concomitantly). Products include:
Actiq 993

Fluphenazine Decanoate (There may be an additive or potentiating effect with CNS depressants and brimonidine administered concomitantly).
No products indexed under this heading.

Fluphenazine Enanthate (There may be an additive or potentiating effect with CNS depressants and brimonidine administered concomitantly).
No products indexed under this heading.

Fluphenazine Hydrochloride (There may be an additive or potentiating effect with CNS depressants and brimonidine administered concomitantly).
No products indexed under this heading.

Flurazepam Hydrochloride (There may be an additive or potentiating effect with CNS depressants and brimonidine administered concomitantly). Products include:
Dalmane Capsules 3343

Fosinopril Sodium (Caution is advised in concomitant use of antihypertensives and brimonidine).
No products indexed under this heading.

Furosemide (Caution is advised in concomitant use of antihypertensives and brimonidine). Products include:
Furosemide Tablets 2117

Glutethimide (There may be an additive or potentiating effect with CNS depressants and brimonidine administered concomitantly).
No products indexed under this heading.

Guanabenz Acetate (Caution is advised in concomitant use of antihypertensives and brimonidine).
No products indexed under this heading.

Guanethidine Monosulfate (Caution is advised in concomitant use of antihypertensives and brimonidine).
No products indexed under this heading.

Haloperidol (There may be an additive or potentiating effect with CNS depressants and brimonidine administered concomitantly).
No products indexed under this heading.

Haloperidol Decanoate (There may be an additive or potentiating effect with CNS depressants and brimonidine administered concomitantly).
No products indexed under this heading.

Hydralazine Hydrochloride (Caution is advised in concomitant use of antihypertensives and brimonidine). Products include:
BiDil Tablets 2161

Hydrochlorothiazide (Caution is advised in concomitant use of antihypertensives and brimonidine). Products include:
Aldoril Tablets 1884
Atacand HCT 637
Avalide Tablets 2889
Avalide Tablets 922
Benicar HCT Tablets 2852
Diovan HCT Tablets 2195
Dyazide Capsules 1389
Hyzaar 1964
Lotensin HCT Tablets 2235
Maxzide 2150
Micardis HCT Tablets 886
Moduretic Tablets 2003
Prinzide Tablets 2033
Teveten HCT Tablets 1710
Timolide Tablets 2056
Uniretic Tablets 3114
Vaseretic Tablets 2073
Zestoretic Tablets 701

Hydrocodone Bitartrate (There may be an additive or potentiating effect with CNS depressants and brimonidine administered concomitantly). Products include:
Hycodan 1104
Hycomine Compound Tablets 1105
Hycotuss Expectorant Syrup 1106
Lortab 3315
Lortab Elixir 3312
Vicodin Tablets 530
Vicodin ES Tablets 531
Vicodin HP Tablets 532
Vicoprofen Tablets 533
Zydone Tablets 1118

Hydrocodone Polistirex (There may be an additive or potentiating effect with CNS depressants and brimonidine administered concomitantly). Products include:
Tussionex Pennkinetic Extended-Release Suspension 3322

Hydroflumethiazide (Caution is advised in concomitant use of antihypertensives and brimonidine).
No products indexed under this heading.

Hydromorphone Hydrochloride (There may be an additive or potentiating effect with CNS depressants and brimonidine administered concomitantly). Products include:
Dilaudid 439
Dilaudid Oral Liquid 443
Dilaudid Non-Sterile Powder 439
Dilaudid Rectal Suppositories 439
Dilaudid Tablets 439
Dilaudid Tablets - 8 mg 443
Dilaudid-HP 441

Hydroxyzine Hydrochloride (There may be an additive or potentiating effect with CNS depressants and brimonidine administered concomitantly).
No products indexed under this heading.

Imipramine Hydrochloride (Caution is advised in concomitant use of tricyclic antidepressants and brimonidine).
No products indexed under this heading.

Imipramine Pamoate (Caution is advised in concomitant use of tricyclic antidepressants and brimonidine).
No products indexed under this heading.

Indapamide (Caution is advised in concomitant use of antihypertensives and brimonidine). Products include:
Indapamide Tablets 2119

Irbesartan (Caution is advised in concomitant use of antihypertensives and brimonidine). Products include:
Avalide Tablets 922
Avalide Tablets 2889
Avapro Tablets 925
Avapro Tablets 2886

Isocarboxazid (Concurrent administration of monoamine oxidase (MAO) inhibitors and brimonidine is contraindicated).
No products indexed under this heading.

Isoflurane (There may be an additive or potentiating effect with CNS depressants and brimonidine administered concomitantly).
No products indexed under this heading.

Isradipine (Caution is advised in concomitant use of antihypertensives and brimonidine). Products include:
DynaCirc CR Tablets 2726

Ketamine Hydrochloride (There may be an additive or potentiating effect with CNS depressants and brimonidine administered concomitantly).
No products indexed under this heading.

Labetalol Hydrochloride (Caution is advised in concomitant use of beta-blockers and brimonidine).
No products indexed under this heading.

Levobunolol Hydrochloride (Caution is advised in concomitant use of beta-blockers and brimonidine). Products include:
Betagan Ophthalmic Solution, USP .... ⊙217

Levomethadyl Acetate Hydrochloride (There may be an additive or potentiating effect with CNS depressants and brimonidine administered concomitantly).
No products indexed under this heading.

Levorphanol Tartrate (There may be an additive or potentiating effect with CNS depressants and brimonidine administered concomitantly).
No products indexed under this heading.

Lisinopril (Caution is advised in concomitant use of antihypertensives and brimonidine). Products include:
Prinivil Tablets 2029
Prinzide Tablets 2033
Zestoretic Tablets 701
Zestril Tablets 704

Lorazepam (There may be an additive or potentiating effect with CNS depressants and brimonidine administered concomitantly).
No products indexed under this heading.

Losartan Potassium (Caution is advised in concomitant use of antihypertensives and brimonidine). Products include:
Cozaar Tablets 1913
Hyzaar 1964

Loxapine Hydrochloride (There may be an additive or potentiating effect with CNS depressants and brimonidine administered concomitantly).
No products indexed under this heading.

Loxapine Succinate (There may be an additive or potentiating effect with CNS depressants and brimonidine administered concomitantly).
No products indexed under this heading.

Maprotiline Hydrochloride (Caution is advised in concomitant use of tricyclic antidepressants and brimonidine).
No products indexed under this heading.

Mecamylamine Hydrochloride (Caution is advised in concomitant use of antihypertensives and brimonidine). Products include:
Inversine Tablets 3286

Meperidine Hydrochloride (There may be an additive or potentiating effect with CNS depressants and brimonidine administered concomitantly).
No products indexed under this heading.

Mephobarbital (There may be an additive or potentiating effect with CNS depressants and brimonidine administered concomitantly). Products include:
Mebaral Tablets, USP 2483

Meprobamate (There may be an additive or potentiating effect with CNS depressants and brimonidine administered concomitantly).
No products indexed under this heading.

Mesoridazine Besylate (There may be an additive or potentiating effect with CNS depressants and brimonidine administered concomitantly).
No products indexed under this heading.

Methadone Hydrochloride (There may be an additive or potentiating effect with CNS depressants and brimonidine administered concomitantly).
No products indexed under this heading.

Methohexital Sodium (There may be an additive or potentiating effect with CNS depressants and brimonidine administered concomitantly).
No products indexed under this heading.

Methotrimeprazine (There may be an additive or potentiating effect with CNS depressants and brimonidine administered concomitantly).
No products indexed under this heading.

Methoxyflurane (There may be an additive or potentiating effect with CNS depressants and brimonidine administered concomitantly).
No products indexed under this heading.

Methyclothiazide (Caution is advised in concomitant use of antihypertensives and brimonidine).
No products indexed under this heading.

Methyldopa (Caution is advised in concomitant use of antihypertensives and brimonidine). Products include:
Aldoclor Tablets 1881
Aldoril Tablets 1884

Methyldopate Hydrochloride (Caution is advised in concomitant use of antihypertensives and brimonidine).
No products indexed under this heading.

Metipranolol Hydrochloride (Caution is advised in concomitant use of beta-blockers and brimonidine).
No products indexed under this heading.

Metolazone (Caution is advised in concomitant use of antihypertensives and brimonidine).
No products indexed under this heading.

Metoprolol Succinate (Caution is advised in concomitant use of beta-blockers and brimonidine). Products include:
Toprol-XL Tablets 660

Metoprolol Tartrate (Caution is advised in concomitant use of beta-blockers and brimonidine).
No products indexed under this heading.

Metyrosine (Caution is advised in concomitant use of antihypertensives and brimonidine). Products include:
Demser Capsules 1933

Mibefradil Dihydrochloride (Caution is advised in concomitant use of antihypertensives and brimonidine).
No products indexed under this heading.

Midazolam Hydrochloride (There may be an additive or potentiating effect with CNS depressants and brimonidine administered concomitantly).
No products indexed under this heading.

Minoxidil (Caution is advised in concomitant use of antihypertensives and brimonidine). Products include:
Men's Rogaine Extra Strength Topical Solution, Ocean Rush Scent and Original Unscented 706
Women's Rogaine Topical Solution, Spring Bloom Scent and Original Unscented 707

Moclobemide (Concurrent administration of monoamine oxidase (MAO) inhibitors and brimonidine is contraindicated).
No products indexed under this heading.

Moexipril Hydrochloride (Caution is advised in concomitant use of antihypertensives and brimonidine). Products include:
Uniretic Tablets 3114
Univasc Tablets 3118

Molindone Hydrochloride (There may be an additive or potentiating effect with CNS depressants and brimonidine administered concomitantly). Products include:
Moban Tablets 1108

Morphine Sulfate (There may be an additive or potentiating effect with CNS depressants and brimonidine administered concomitantly). Products include:
Avinza Capsules 1714
Kadian Capsules 572
MS Contin Tablets 2703

Nadolol (Caution is advised in concomitant use of beta-blockers and brimonidine). Products include:
Nadolol Tablets 2121

Nicardipine Hydrochloride (Caution is advised in concomitant use of antihypertensives and brimonidine). Products include:
Cardene I.V. 1129

Nifedipine (Caution is advised in concomitant use of antihypertensives and brimonidine). Products include:
Adalat CC Tablets 2978

Nisoldipine (Caution is advised in concomitant use of antihypertensives and brimonidine). Products include:
Sular Tablets 1163

Nitroglycerin (Caution is advised in concomitant use of antihypertensives and brimonidine). Products include:
Nitro-Dur Transdermal Infusion System 3060
Nitrolingual Pumpspray 1161

Nortriptyline Hydrochloride (Caution is advised in concomitant use of tricyclic antidepressants and brimonidine).
No products indexed under this heading.

Olanzapine (There may be an additive or potentiating effect with CNS depressants and brimonidine administered concomitantly). Products include:
Symbyax Capsules 1788
Zyprexa Tablets 1798
Zyprexa IntraMuscular 1798
Zyprexa ZYDIS Orally Disintegrating Tablets 1798

Oxazepam (There may be an additive or potentiating effect with CNS depressants and brimonidine administered concomitantly).
No products indexed under this heading.

Oxycodone Hydrochloride (There may be an additive or potentiating effect with CNS depressants and brimonidine administered concomitantly). Products include:
Combunox Tablets 1183
OxyContin Tablets 2699
OxyFast Oral Concentrate Solution 2704
OxyIR Capsules 2704
Percocet Tablets 1114
Percodan Tablets 1115

Pargyline Hydrochloride (Concurrent administration of monoamine oxidase (MAO) inhibitors and brimonidine is contraindicated).
No products indexed under this heading.

Penbutolol Sulfate (Caution is advised in concomitant use of beta-blockers and brimonidine).
No products indexed under this heading.

Pentobarbital Sodium (There may be an additive or potentiating effect with CNS depressants and brimonidine administered concomitantly). Products include:
Nembutal Sodium Solution, USP 2484

Perindopril Erbumine (Caution is advised in concomitant use of antihypertensives and brimonidine). Products include:
Aceon Tablets (2 mg, 4 mg, 8 mg) 3191

Perphenazine (There may be an additive or potentiating effect with CNS depressants and brimonidine administered concomitantly).
No products indexed under this heading.

Phenelzine Sulfate (Concurrent administration of monoamine oxidase (MAO) inhibitors and brimonidine is contraindicated).
No products indexed under this heading.

Phenobarbital (There may be an additive or potentiating effect with CNS depressants and brimonidine administered concomitantly).
No products indexed under this heading.

Phenoxybenzamine Hydrochloride (Caution is advised in concomitant use of antihypertensives and brimonidine). Products include:
Dibenzyline Capsules 3390

Phentolamine Mesylate (Caution is advised in concomitant use of antihypertensives and brimonidine).
No products indexed under this heading.

Pindolol (Caution is advised in concomitant use of beta-blockers and brimonidine).
No products indexed under this heading.

Polythiazide (Caution is advised in concomitant use of antihypertensives and brimonidine).
No products indexed under this heading.

Prazepam (There may be an additive or potentiating effect with CNS depressants and brimonidine administered concomitantly).
No products indexed under this heading.

Prazosin Hydrochloride (Caution is advised in concomitant use of antihypertensives and brimonidine).
No products indexed under this heading.

Procarbazine Hydrochloride (Concurrent administration of monoamine oxidase (MAO) inhibitors and brimonidine is contraindicated). Products include:
Matulane Capsules 3188

Prochlorperazine (There may be an additive or potentiating effect with CNS depressants and brimonidine administered concomitantly).
No products indexed under this heading.

Promethazine Hydrochloride (There may be an additive or potentiating effect with CNS depressants and brimonidine administered concomitantly). Products include:
Phenergan 3438

Propofol (There may be an additive or potentiating effect with CNS depressants and brimonidine administered concomitantly). Products include:
Diprivan Injectable Emulsion 676

Propoxyphene Hydrochloride (There may be an additive or potentiating effect with CNS depressants and brimonidine administered concomitantly).
No products indexed under this heading.

Propoxyphene Napsylate (There may be an additive or potentiating effect with CNS depressants and brimonidine administered concomitantly). Products include:
Darvocet A 500 Tablets 3497

Propranolol Hydrochloride (Caution is advised in concomitant use of beta-blockers and brimonidine). Products include:
Inderal LA Long-Acting Capsules 3421
InnoPran XL Capsules 2728

Protriptyline Hydrochloride (Caution is advised in concomitant use of tricyclic antidepressants and brimonidine). Products include:
Vivactil Tablets 2350

Quazepam (There may be an additive or potentiating effect with CNS depressants and brimonidine administered concomitantly).
No products indexed under this heading.

Quetiapine Fumarate (There may be an additive or potentiating effect with CNS depressants and brimonidine administered concomitantly). Products include:
Seroquel Tablets 691

Quinapril Hydrochloride (Caution is advised in concomitant use of antihypertensives and brimonidine).
No products indexed under this heading.

Ramipril (Caution is advised in concomitant use of antihypertensives and brimonidine). Products include:
Altace Capsules 1673

Rauwolfia Serpentina (Caution is advised in concomitant use of antihypertensives and brimonidine).
No products indexed under this heading.

Remifentanil Hydrochloride (There may be an additive or potentiating effect with CNS depressants and brimonidine administered concomitantly).
No products indexed under this heading.

Rescinnamine (Caution is advised in concomitant use of antihypertensives and brimonidine).
No products indexed under this heading.

Reserpine (Caution is advised in concomitant use of antihypertensives and brimonidine).
No products indexed under this heading.

Risperidone (There may be an additive or potentiating effect with CNS depressants and brimonidine administered concomitantly). Products include:
Risperdal Consta Long-Acting Injection 1664
Risperdal M-Tab Orally Disintegrating Tablets 1658
Risperdal 1658

Secobarbital Sodium (There may be an additive or potentiating effect with CNS depressants and brimonidine administered concomitantly).
No products indexed under this heading.

Selegiline Hydrochloride (Concurrent administration of monoamine oxidase (MAO) inhibitors and brimonidine is contraindicated). Products include:
Eldepryl Capsules 3209

Sevoflurane (There may be an additive or potentiating effect with CNS depressants and brimonidine administered concomitantly). Products include:
Ultane Liquid for Inhalation 526

Sodium Nitroprusside (Caution is advised in concomitant use of antihypertensives and brimonidine).
No products indexed under this heading.

Sodium Oxybate (There may be an additive or potentiating effect with CNS depressants and brimonidine administered concomitantly).
No products indexed under this heading.

Sotalol Hydrochloride (Caution is advised in concomitant use of beta-blockers and brimonidine).
No products indexed under this heading.

Spirapril Hydrochloride (Caution is advised in concomitant use of antihypertensives and brimonidine).
No products indexed under this heading.

Sufentanil Citrate (There may be an additive or potentiating effect with CNS depressants and brimonidine administered concomitantly).
No products indexed under this heading.

Telmisartan (Caution is advised in concomitant use of antihypertensives and brimonidine). Products include:
Micardis Tablets 884
Micardis HCT Tablets 886

Temazepam (There may be an additive or potentiating effect with CNS depressants and brimonidine administered concomitantly).
No products indexed under this heading.

Terazosin Hydrochloride (Caution is advised in concomitant use of antihypertensives and brimonidine). Products include:
Hytrin Capsules 469

Thiamylal Sodium (There may be an additive or potentiating effect with CNS depressants and brimonidine administered concomitantly).
No products indexed under this heading.

Thioridazine Hydrochloride (There may be an additive or potentiating effect with CNS depressants and brimonidine administered concomitantly). Products include:
Thioridazine Hydrochloride Tablets 2122

Thiothixene (There may be an additive or potentiating effect with CNS depressants and brimonidine administered concomitantly). Products include:
Thiothixene Capsules 2124

Timolol Hemihydrate (Caution is advised in concomitant use of beta-blockers and brimonidine). Products include:
Betimol Ophthalmic Solution 3371
Betimol Ophthalmic Solution .... ⊙283

Timolol Maleate (Caution is advised in concomitant use of beta-blockers and brimonidine). Products include:
Blocadren Tablets 1891
Cosopt Sterile Ophthalmic Solution 1910
Timolide Tablets 2056
Timoptic in Ocudose 2061
Timoptic Sterile Ophthalmic Solution 2058
Timoptic-XE Sterile Ophthalmic Gel Forming Solution 2062

Torsemide (Caution is advised in concomitant use of antihypertensives and brimonidine).
No products indexed under this heading.

Trandolapril (Caution is advised in concomitant use of antihypertensives and brimonidine). Products include:
Mavik Tablets 482
Tarka Tablets 519

Tranylcypromine Sulfate (Concurrent administration of monoamine oxidase (MAO) inhibitors and brimonidine is contraindicated). Products include:
Parnate Tablets 1499

Triazolam (There may be an additive or potentiating effect with CNS depressants and brimonidine administered concomitantly).
No products indexed under this heading.

Trifluoperazine Hydrochloride (There may be an additive or potentiating effect with CNS depressants and brimonidine administered concomitantly).
No products indexed under this heading.

Trimethaphan Camsylate (Caution is advised in concomitant use of antihypertensives and brimonidine).
No products indexed under this heading.

Trimipramine Maleate (Caution is advised in concomitant use of tricyclic antidepressants and brimonidine). Products include:
Surmontil Capsules 2347

Valsartan (Caution is advised in concomitant use of antihypertensives and brimonidine). Products include:
Diovan HCT Tablets 2195
Diovan Tablets 2191

Verapamil Hydrochloride (Caution is advised in concomitant use of antihypertensives and brimonidine). Products include:
Covera-HS Tablets 3135
Tarka Tablets 519
Verelan PM Capsules 3120

Zaleplon (There may be an additive or potentiating effect with CNS depressants and brimonidine administered concomitantly). Products include:
Sonata Capsules 1686

Ziprasidone Hydrochloride (There may be an additive or potentiating effect with CNS depressants and brimonidine administered concomitantly). Products include:
Geodon Capsules 2514

Zolpidem Tartrate (There may be an additive or potentiating effect with CNS depressants and brimonidine administered concomitantly). Products include:
Ambien Tablets 2867

BUMINATE 5% SOLUTION, USP

(Albumin (human)) 747
None cited in PDR database.

BUMINATE 25% SOLUTION, USP

(Albumin (human)) 748
None cited in PDR database.

BUPHENYL POWDER

(Sodium Phenylbutyrate) 3327
May interact with:

Probenecid (Probenecid is known to inhibit the renal transport of many organic compounds, including hippuric acid, and may affect renal excretion of the conjugated product of sodium phenylbutyrate as well as its metabolite).
No products indexed under this heading.

BUPHENYL TABLETS

(Sodium Phenylbutyrate) 3327
May interact with:

Probenecid (Probenecid is known to inhibit the renal transport of many organic compounds, including hippuric acid, and may affect renal excretion of the conjugated product of sodium phenylbutyrate as well as its metabolite).
No products indexed under this heading.

BUPRENEX INJECTABLE

(Buprenorphine Hydrochloride) 2718
May interact with antihistamines, benzodiazepines, central nervous system depressants, cytochrome p450 3a4 inducers (selected), cytochrome p450 3a4 inhibitors (selected), general anesthetics, hypnotics and sedatives, monoamine oxidase inhibitors, narcotic analgesics, phenothiazines, tranquilizers, and certain other agents. Compounds in these categories include:

Acetazolamide (Buprenorphine is metabolized by the CYP3A4 isoenzyme; co-administration with inhibitors of CYP3A4 may cause decrease in clearance of buprenorphine).
No products indexed under this heading.

Acrivastine (Increased CNS depression).
No products indexed under this heading.

Alfentanil Hydrochloride (Increased CNS depression).
No products indexed under this heading.

Allium sativum (Buprenorphine is metabolized by the CYP3A4 isoenzyme; co-administration with inducers of CYP3A4 may cause increase in clearance of buprenorphine).
No products indexed under this heading.

Alprazolam (Increased CNS depression). Products include:
Niravam Orally Disintegrating Tablets 3106
Xanax XR Tablets 2655

Amiodarone Hydrochloride (Buprenorphine is metabolized by the CYP3A4 isoenzyme; co-administration with inhibitors of

CYP3A4 may cause decrease in clearance of buprenorphine). Products include:
- Pacerone Tablets ... 3337

Amprenavir (Buprenorphine is metabolized by the CYP3A4 isoenzyme; co-administration with inhibitors of CYP3A4 may cause decrease in clearance of buprenorphine). Products include:
- Agenerase Capsules ... 1299
- Agenerase Oral Solution ... 1304

Anastrozole (Buprenorphine is metabolized by the CYP3A4 isoenzyme; co-administration with inhibitors of CYP3A4 may cause decrease in clearance of buprenorphine). Products include:
- Arimidex Tablets ... 665

Aprepitant (Buprenorphine is metabolized by the CYP3A4 isoenzyme; co-administration with inhibitors of CYP3A4 may cause decrease in clearance of buprenorphine). Products include:
- Emend Capsules ... 1944

Aprobarbital (Increased CNS depression).
No products indexed under this heading.

Astemizole (Increased CNS depression).
No products indexed under this heading.

Azatadine Maleate (Increased CNS depression).
No products indexed under this heading.

Betamethasone Acetate (Buprenorphine is metabolized by the CYP3A4 isoenzyme; co-administration with inducers of CYP3A4 may cause increase in clearance of buprenorphine).
No products indexed under this heading.

Betamethasone Sodium Phosphate (Buprenorphine is metabolized by the CYP3A4 isoenzyme; co-administration with inducers of CYP3A4 may cause increase in clearance of buprenorphine).
No products indexed under this heading.

Bromodiphenhydramine Hydrochloride (Increased CNS depression).
No products indexed under this heading.

Brompheniramine Maleate (Increased CNS depression). Products include:
- Alacol DM Syrup ... 739
- Children's Dimetapp Cold & Allergy Elixir ... 745
- Children's Dimetapp DM Cold & Cough Elixir ... 745
- Robitussin Allergy & Cough Syrup ... 750

Buspirone Hydrochloride (Increased CNS depression).
No products indexed under this heading.

Butabarbital (Increased CNS depression).
No products indexed under this heading.

Butalbital (Increased CNS depression). Products include:
- Sedapap Tablets 50 mg/650 mg ... 2098

Carbamazepine (Buprenorphine is metabolized by the CYP3A4 isoenzyme; co-administration with inducers of CYP3A4 may cause increase in clearance of buprenorphine). Products include:
- Carbatrol Capsules ... 3174
- Equetro Extended-Release Capsules ... 3178
- Tegretol/Tegretol-XR ... 2278

Cetirizine Hydrochloride (Increased CNS depression). Products include:
- Zyrtec Chewable Tablets ... 2589
- Zyrtec ... 2589
- Zyrtec-D 12 Hour Extended Release Tablets ... 2591

Chlordiazepoxide (Increased CNS depression).
No products indexed under this heading.

Chlordiazepoxide Hydrochloride (Increased CNS depression). Products include:
- Librium Capsules ... 3349

Chlorpheniramine Maleate (Increased CNS depression). Products include:
- Advil Allergy Sinus Caplets ... 737
- Advil Multi-Symptom Cold Caplets ... 738
- BC Allergy Sinus Cold Powder ... 612
- Contac Severe Cold and Flu Caplets Maximum Strength ... 615
- Hycomine Compound Tablets ... 1105
- PediaCare Multi-Symptom Cold Liquid ... 704
- PediaCare NightRest Cough & Cold Liquid ... 704
- Robitussin Flu Liquid ... 752
- Robitussin PM Cough & Cold Liquid ... 752
- Singlet Caplets ... 636
- Sudafed Sinus & Allergy Tablets ... 710
- TheraFlu Cold & Cough Hot Liquid ... 680
- TheraFlu Cold & Sore Throat Hot Liquid ... 680
- TheraFlu Flu & Sore Throat Hot Liquid ... 681
- TheraFlu Severe Cold & Cough Hot Liquid ... 683
- TheraFlu Severe Cold Caplets ... 679
- TheraFlu Severe Cold Hot Liquid ... 682
- Triaminic Cold & Allergy Liquid ... 685
- Triaminic Cold & Cough Liquid ... 685
- Triaminic Flu, Cough & Fever Liquid ... 685
- Triaminic Night Time Cough & Cold Liquid ... 685
- Triaminic Allergy Runny Nose & Congestion Softchews ... 688
- Triaminic Cold & Cough Softchews ... 688
- Children's Tylenol Plus Cold NightTime Suspension Liquid ... 1851
- Children's Tylenol Plus Cold & Cough Suspension Liquid and Chewable Tablets ... 1851
- Children's Tylenol Plus Cold Chewable Tablets ... 1851
- Children's Tylenol Plus Flu Suspension Liquid ... 1853
- Tylenol Allergy Complete Multi-Symptom Caplets and Gelcaps with Cool Burst ... 1844
- Multi-Symptom Tylenol Cold Night Time Caplets ... 1845
- Vicks 44M Cough, Cold & Flu Relief ... 2676
- Pediatric Vicks 44m Cough & Cold Relief ... 2673
- Children's Vicks NyQuil Cold/Cough Relief ... 2671

Chlorpheniramine Polistirex (Increased CNS depression). Products include:
- Tussionex Pennkinetic Extended-Release Suspension ... 3322

Chlorpheniramine Tannate (Increased CNS depression).
No products indexed under this heading.

Chlorpromazine (Increased CNS depression).
No products indexed under this heading.

Chlorpromazine Hydrochloride (Increased CNS depression).
No products indexed under this heading.

Chlorprothixene (Increased CNS depression).
No products indexed under this heading.

Chlorprothixene Hydrochloride (Increased CNS depression).
No products indexed under this heading.

Chlorprothixene Lactate (Increased CNS depression).
No products indexed under this heading.

Cimetidine (Buprenorphine is metabolized by the CYP3A4 isoenzyme; co-administration with inhibitors of CYP3A4 may cause decrease in clearance of buprenorphine). Products include:
- Tagamet HB 200 Tablets ... 637
- Tagamet Tablets ... 1547

Cimetidine Hydrochloride (Buprenorphine is metabolized by the CYP3A4 isoenzyme; co-administration with inhibitors of CYP3A4 may cause decrease in clearance of buprenorphine).
No products indexed under this heading.

Ciprofloxacin (Buprenorphine is metabolized by the CYP3A4 isoenzyme; co-administration with inhibitors of CYP3A4 may cause decrease in clearance of buprenorphine). Products include:
- Cipro I.V. ... 2998
- Cipro I.V. Pharmacy Bulk Package ... 3509
- Cipro Oral Suspension ... 2991
- Cipro XR Tablets ... 3004
- Ciprodex Otic Suspension ... 555

Ciprofloxacin Hydrochloride (Buprenorphine is metabolized by the CYP3A4 isoenzyme; co-administration with inducers of CYP3A4 may cause increase in clearance of buprenorphine). Products include:
- Ciloxan Ophthalmic Ointment ... 554
- Cipro Tablets ... 2991

Cisplatin (Buprenorphine is metabolized by the CYP3A4 isoenzyme; co-administration with inducers of CYP3A4 may cause increase in clearance of buprenorphine).
No products indexed under this heading.

Clarithromycin (Buprenorphine is metabolized by the CYP3A4 isoenzyme; co-administration with inhibitors of CYP3A4 may cause decrease in clearance of buprenorphine). Products include:
- Biaxin/Biaxin XL ... 402
- PREVPAC ... 3281

Clemastine Fumarate (Increased CNS depression).
No products indexed under this heading.

Clorazepate Dipotassium (Increased CNS depression). Products include:
- Tranxene ... 2488

Clotrimazole (Buprenorphine is metabolized by the CYP3A4 isoenzyme; co-administration with inhibitors of CYP3A4 may cause decrease in clearance of buprenorphine). Products include:
- Lotrimin ... 3053
- Lotrisone ... 3054

Clozapine (Increased CNS depression). Products include:
- Clozapine Tablets ... 2141
- Clozaril Tablets ... 2174
- FazaClo Orally Disintegrating Tablets ... 547

Codeine Phosphate (Increased CNS depression). Products include:
- Tylenol with Codeine ... 2461

Cortisone Acetate (Buprenorphine is metabolized by the CYP3A4 isoenzyme; co-administration with inducers of CYP3A4 may cause increase in clearance of buprenorphine).
No products indexed under this heading.

Cyclosporine (Buprenorphine is metabolized by the CYP3A4 isoenzyme; co-administration with inhibitors of CYP3A4 may cause decrease in clearance of buprenorphine). Products include:
- Gengraf Capsules ... 458
- Neoral Soft Gelatin Capsules ... 2247
- Neoral Oral Solution ... 2247
- Restasis Ophthalmic Emulsion ... 570
- Sandimmune ... 2259

Cyproheptadine Hydrochloride (Increased CNS depression).
No products indexed under this heading.

Dalfopristin (Buprenorphine is metabolized by the CYP3A4 isoenzyme; co-administration with inhibitors of CYP3A4 may cause decrease in clearance of buprenorphine). Products include:
- Synercid I.V. ... 1690

Danazol (Buprenorphine is metabolized by the CYP3A4 isoenzyme; co-administration with inhibitors of CYP3A4 may cause decrease in clearance of buprenorphine).
No products indexed under this heading.

Delavirdine Mesylate (Buprenorphine is metabolized by the CYP3A4 isoenzyme; co-administration with inhibitors of CYP3A4 may cause decrease in clearance of buprenorphine). Products include:
- Rescriptor Tablets ... 2535

Desflurane (Increased CNS depression). Products include:
- Suprane Liquid for Inhalation ... 770

Dexamethasone (Buprenorphine is metabolized by the CYP3A4 isoenzyme; co-administration with inducers of CYP3A4 may cause increase in clearance of buprenorphine). Products include:
- Ciprodex Otic Suspension ... 555
- Decadron Tablets ... 1929
- TobraDex Ophthalmic Ointment ... 558
- TobraDex Ophthalmic Suspension ... 558

Dexamethasone Acetate (Buprenorphine is metabolized by the CYP3A4 isoenzyme; co-administration with inducers of CYP3A4 may cause increase in clearance of buprenorphine).
No products indexed under this heading.

Dexamethasone Sodium Phosphate (Buprenorphine is metabolized by the CYP3A4 isoenzyme; co-administration with inducers of CYP3A4 may cause increase in clearance of buprenorphine). Products include:
- Decadron Phosphate Injection ... 1931

Dexchlorpheniramine Maleate (Increased CNS depression).
No products indexed under this heading.

Dezocine (Increased CNS depression).
No products indexed under this heading.

Diazepam (Concurrent use has resulted in respiratory and cardiovascular collapse; increased CNS depression). Products include:

Diastat Rectal Delivery System 3344
Valium Tablets 2822

Diltiazem Hydrochloride (Buprenorphine is metabolized by the CYP3A4 isoenzyme; co-administration with inhibitors of CYP3A4 may cause decrease in clearance of buprenorphine). Products include:

Cardizem LA Extended Release Tablets 1699
Tiazac Capsules 1204

Diltiazem Maleate (Buprenorphine is metabolized by the CYP3A4 isoenzyme; co-administration with inhibitors of CYP3A4 may cause decrease in clearance of buprenorphine).

No products indexed under this heading.

Diphenhydramine Citrate (Increased CNS depression). Products include:

Children's Benadryl Allergy & Cold Fastmelt Tablets .... ■ 695
Children's Benadryl D Allergy & Sinus Fastmelt Tablets .... ■ 694
Children's Benadryl Allergy Fastmelt Tablets .... ■ 696
Goody's PM Powder .... ■ 622

Diphenhydramine Hydrochloride (Increased CNS depression). Products include:

Benadryl Allergy & Cold Tablets .... ■ 692
Benadryl Allergy .... ■ 691
Benadryl Allergy & Sinus Headache Caplets & Gelcaps .... ■ 693
Children's Benadryl Allergy Liquid .... ■ 695
Children's Benadryl Dye-Free Allergy Liquid .... ■ 695
Benadryl Dye-Free Allergy Liqui-Gels Softgels .... ■ 692
Benadryl Itch Relief Stick Extra Strength .... ■ 696
Benadryl Itch Stopping Cream Extra Strength .... ■ 697
Benadryl Itch Stopping Gel Extra Strength .... ■ 697
Benadryl Itch Stopping Spray Extra Strength .... ■ 697
Benadryl Maximum Strength Severe Allergy & Sinus Headache Caplets .... ■ 694
Children's Benadryl D Liquid Medication .... ■ 693
Benadryl D Tablets .... ■ 694
Nytol QuickCaps Caplets .... ■ 635
Maximum Strength Nytol QuickGels Softgels .... ■ 635
Simply Sleep Caplets 1841
Sominex Original Formula Tablets .... ■ 637
TheraFlu Thin Strips Multi Symptom .... ■ 684
Triaminic Thin Strips Cough & Runny Nose .... ■ 690
Children's Tylenol Plus Cold & Allergy Suspension Liquid 1850
Tylenol Allergy Complete Night Time Caplets 1844
Tylenol Severe Allergy Caplets 1844
Tylenol Flu NightTime Gelcaps 1846
Extra Strength Tylenol PM Caplets, Geltabs, Gelcaps and Liquid 1847
Unisom Maximum Strength SleepGels .... ■ 712

Diphenylpyraline Hydrochloride (Increased CNS depression).

No products indexed under this heading.

Doxorubicin Hydrochloride (Buprenorphine is metabolized by the CYP3A4 isoenzyme; co-administration with inducers of CYP3A4 may cause increase in clearance of buprenorphine). Products include:

Adriamycin for Injection, USP 786
Adriamycin Injection, USP 786

Droperidol (Increased CNS depression).

No products indexed under this heading.

Efavirenz (Buprenorphine is metabolized by the CYP3A4 isoenzyme; co-administration with inhibitors of CYP3A4 may cause decrease in clearance of buprenorphine). Products include:

Sustiva Capsules 957

Enflurane (Increased CNS depression).

No products indexed under this heading.

Erythromycin (Buprenorphine is metabolized by the CYP3A4 isoenzyme; co-administration with inhibitors of CYP3A4 may cause decrease in clearance of buprenorphine). Products include:

Erygel Topical Gel 2096
Ery-Tab Tablets 447
Erythromycin Base Filmtab Tablets 454
Erythromycin Delayed-Release Capsules, USP 456
PCE Dispertab Tablets 510

Erythromycin Estolate (Buprenorphine is metabolized by the CYP3A4 isoenzyme; co-administration with inhibitors of CYP3A4 may cause decrease in clearance of buprenorphine).

No products indexed under this heading.

Erythromycin Ethylsuccinate (Buprenorphine is metabolized by the CYP3A4 isoenzyme; co-administration with inhibitors of CYP3A4 may cause decrease in clearance of buprenorphine). Products include:

E.E.S. 449
EryPed 445

Erythromycin Gluceptate (Buprenorphine is metabolized by the CYP3A4 isoenzyme; co-administration with inhibitors of CYP3A4 may cause decrease in clearance of buprenorphine).

No products indexed under this heading.

Erythromycin Lactobionate (Buprenorphine is metabolized by the CYP3A4 isoenzyme; co-administration with inhibitors of CYP3A4 may cause decrease in clearance of buprenorphine).

No products indexed under this heading.

Erythromycin Stearate (Buprenorphine is metabolized by the CYP3A4 isoenzyme; co-administration with inhibitors of CYP3A4 may cause decrease in clearance of buprenorphine). Products include:

Erythrocin Stearate Filmtab Tablets 452

Esomeprazole Magnesium (Buprenorphine is metabolized by the CYP3A4 isoenzyme; co-administration with inhibitors of CYP3A4 may cause decrease in clearance of buprenorphine). Products include:

Nexium Delayed-Release Capsules 645

Estazolam (Increased CNS depression). Products include:

ProSom Tablets 512

Ethanol (Increased CNS depression).

No products indexed under this heading.

Ethchlorvynol (Increased CNS depression).

No products indexed under this heading.

Ethinamate (Increased CNS depression).

No products indexed under this heading.

Ethosuximide (Buprenorphine is metabolized by the CYP3A4 isoenzyme; co-administration with inducers of CYP3A4 may cause increase in clearance of buprenorphine).

No products indexed under this heading.

Ethyl Alcohol (Increased CNS depression).

No products indexed under this heading.

Felbamate (Buprenorphine is metabolized by the CYP3A4 isoenzyme; co-administration with inducers of CYP3A4 may cause increase in clearance of buprenorphine).

No products indexed under this heading.

Fentanyl (Increased CNS depression). Products include:

Duragesic Transdermal System 2448

Fentanyl Citrate (Increased CNS depression). Products include:

Actiq 993

Fexofenadine Hydrochloride (Increased CNS depression). Products include:

Allegra 2857
Allegra-D 12 Hour Extended-Release Tablets 2860
Allegra-D 24 Hour Extended-Release Tablets 2862

Fluconazole (Buprenorphine is metabolized by the CYP3A4 isoenzyme; co-administration with inhibitors of CYP3A4 may cause decrease in clearance of buprenorphine).

No products indexed under this heading.

Fludrocortisone Acetate (Buprenorphine is metabolized by the CYP3A4 isoenzyme; co-administration with inducers of CYP3A4 may cause increase in clearance of buprenorphine).

No products indexed under this heading.

Fluoxetine Hydrochloride (Buprenorphine is metabolized by the CYP3A4 isoenzyme; co-administration with inhibitors of CYP3A4 may cause decrease in clearance of buprenorphine). Products include:

Prozac Pulvules and Liquid 1771
Symbyax Capsules 1788

Fluphenazine Decanoate (Increased CNS depression).

No products indexed under this heading.

Fluphenazine Enanthate (Increased CNS depression).

No products indexed under this heading.

Fluphenazine Hydrochloride (Increased CNS depression).

No products indexed under this heading.

Flurazepam Hydrochloride (Increased CNS depression). Products include:

Dalmane Capsules 3343

Fluvoxamine Maleate (Buprenorphine is metabolized by the CYP3A4 isoenzyme; co-administration with inhibitors of CYP3A4 may cause decrease in clearance of buprenorphine).

No products indexed under this heading.

Fosamprenavir Calcium (Buprenorphine is metabolized by the CYP3A4 isoenzyme; co-administration with inhibitors of CYP3A4 may cause decrease in clearance of buprenorphine). Products include:

Lexiva Tablets 1473

Fosphenytoin Sodium (Buprenorphine is metabolized by the CYP3A4 isoenzyme; co-administration with inducers of CYP3A4 may cause increase in clearance of buprenorphine).

No products indexed under this heading.

Garlic Extract (Buprenorphine is metabolized by the CYP3A4 isoenzyme; co-administration with inducers of CYP3A4 may cause increase in clearance of buprenorphine).

No products indexed under this heading.

Garlic Oil (Buprenorphine is metabolized by the CYP3A4 isoenzyme; co-administration with inducers of CYP3A4 may cause increase in clearance of buprenorphine).

No products indexed under this heading.

Glutethimide (Increased CNS depression).

No products indexed under this heading.

Halazepam (Increased CNS depression).

No products indexed under this heading.

Haloperidol (Increased CNS depression).

No products indexed under this heading.

Haloperidol Decanoate (Increased CNS depression).

No products indexed under this heading.

Hydrocodone Bitartrate (Increased CNS depression). Products include:

Hycodan 1104
Hycomine Compound Tablets 1105
Hycotuss Expectorant Syrup 1106
Lortab 3315
Lortab Elixir 3312
Vicodin Tablets 530
Vicodin ES Tablets 531
Vicodin HP Tablets 532
Vicoprofen Tablets 533
Zydone Tablets 1118

Hydrocodone Polistirex (Increased CNS depression). Products include:

Tussionex Pennkinetic Extended-Release Suspension 3322

Hydrocortisone (Buprenorphine is metabolized by the CYP3A4 isoenzyme; co-administration with inducers of CYP3A4 may cause increase in clearance of buprenorphine). Products include:

Cortizone•5 Ointment .... ■ 699
Cortizone•10 Creme .... ■ 699
Cortizone•10 Ointment .... ■ 699
Cortizone•10 Plus Creme .... ■ 700
Cortizone•10 Maximum Strength Quick Shot Spray .... ■ 700
Hydrocortone Tablets 1963
Preparation H Hydrocortisone Cream .... ■ 748

Hydrocortisone Acetate (Buprenorphine is metabolized by the CYP3A4 isoenzyme; co-administration with inducers of CYP3A4 may cause increase in clearance of buprenorphine). Products include:
Analpram-HC 1136
Pramosone 1139
ProctoFoam-HC 3113
Tucks Anti-Itch Ointment .... ▣712
U-cort 1% Cream 3289

Hydrocortisone Butyrate (Buprenorphine is metabolized by the CYP3A4 isoenzyme; co-administration with inducers of CYP3A4 may cause increase in clearance of buprenorphine). Products include:
Locoid 1138
Locoid Lipocream Cream 1138

Hydrocortisone Cypionate (Buprenorphine is metabolized by the CYP3A4 isoenzyme; co-administration with inducers of CYP3A4 may cause increase in clearance of buprenorphine).
No products indexed under this heading.

Hydrocortisone Hemisuccinate (Buprenorphine is metabolized by the CYP3A4 isoenzyme; co-administration with inducers of CYP3A4 may cause increase in clearance of buprenorphine).
No products indexed under this heading.

Hydrocortisone Probutate (Buprenorphine is metabolized by the CYP3A4 isoenzyme; co-administration with inducers of CYP3A4 may cause increase in clearance of buprenorphine). Products include:
Pandel Cream, 0.1% 1017

Hydrocortisone Sodium Phosphate (Buprenorphine is metabolized by the CYP3A4 isoenzyme; co-administration with inducers of CYP3A4 may cause increase in clearance of buprenorphine).
No products indexed under this heading.

Hydrocortisone Sodium Succinate (Buprenorphine is metabolized by the CYP3A4 isoenzyme; co-administration with inducers of CYP3A4 may cause increase in clearance of buprenorphine).
No products indexed under this heading.

Hydrocortisone Valerate (Buprenorphine is metabolized by the CYP3A4 isoenzyme; co-administration with inducers of CYP3A4 may cause increase in clearance of buprenorphine).
No products indexed under this heading.

Hydromorphone Hydrochloride (Increased CNS depression). Products include:
Dilaudid 439
Dilaudid Oral Liquid 443
Dilaudid Non-Sterile Powder 439
Dilaudid Rectal Suppositories 439
Dilaudid Tablets 439
Dilaudid Tablets - 8 mg 443
Dilaudid-HP 441

Hydroxyzine Hydrochloride (Increased CNS depression).
No products indexed under this heading.

Hypericum (Buprenorphine is metabolized by the CYP3A4 isoenzyme; co-administration with inducers of CYP3A4 may cause increase in clearance of buprenorphine).
No products indexed under this heading.

Hypericum Perforatum (Buprenorphine is metabolized by the CYP3A4 isoenzyme; co-administration with inducers of CYP3A4 may cause increase in clearance of buprenorphine).
No products indexed under this heading.

Indinavir Sulfate (Buprenorphine is metabolized by the CYP3A4 isoenzyme; co-administration with inhibitors of CYP3A4 may cause decrease in clearance of buprenorphine). Products include:
Crixivan Capsules 1918

Isocarboxazid (Effect unspecified; caution should be exercised).
No products indexed under this heading.

Isoflurane (Increased CNS depression).
No products indexed under this heading.

Isoniazid (Buprenorphine is metabolized by the CYP3A4 isoenzyme; co-administration with inhibitors of CYP3A4 may cause decrease in clearance of buprenorphine).
No products indexed under this heading.

Itraconazole (Buprenorphine is metabolized by the CYP3A4 isoenzyme; co-administration with inhibitors of CYP3A4 may cause decrease in clearance of buprenorphine).
No products indexed under this heading.

Ketamine Hydrochloride (Increased CNS depression).
No products indexed under this heading.

Ketoconazole (Buprenorphine is metabolized by the CYP3A4 isoenzyme; co-administration with inhibitors of CYP3A4 may cause decrease in clearance of buprenorphine). Products include:
Nizoral A-D Shampoo, 1% 1839
Nizoral 2% Shampoo 1838

Levomethadyl Acetate Hydrochloride (Increased CNS depression).
No products indexed under this heading.

Levorphanol Tartrate (Increased CNS depression).
No products indexed under this heading.

Lopinavir (Buprenorphine is metabolized by the CYP3A4 isoenzyme; co-administration with inhibitors of CYP3A4 may cause decrease in clearance of buprenorphine). Products include:
Kaletra 474

Loratadine (Increased CNS depression). Products include:
Alavert Allergy & Sinus D-12 Hour Tablets .... ▣743
Alavert .... ▣743
Children's Claritin 24 Hour Non-Drowsy Allergy Syrup .... ▣732
Claritin Non-Drowsy 24 Hour Tablets .... ▣731
Non-Drowsy Claritin Hives Relief Tablets .... ▣733
Claritin Reditabs 24 Hour Non-Drowsy Tablets .... ▣732
Claritin-D Non-Drowsy 12 Hour Tablets .... ▣731
Claritin-D Non-Drowsy 24 Hour Tablets .... ▣731
Children's Dimetapp ND Non-Drowsy Allergy Syrup .... ▣746
Triaminic Allerchews .... ▣684

Lorazepam (Increased CNS depression).
No products indexed under this heading.

Loxapine Hydrochloride (Increased CNS depression).
No products indexed under this heading.

Loxapine Succinate (Increased CNS depression).
No products indexed under this heading.

Meperidine Hydrochloride (Increased CNS depression).
No products indexed under this heading.

Mephenytoin (Buprenorphine is metabolized by the CYP3A4 isoenzyme; co-administration with inducers of CYP3A4 may cause increase in clearance of buprenorphine).
No products indexed under this heading.

Mephobarbital (Increased CNS depression). Products include:
Mebaral Tablets, USP 2483

Meprobamate (Increased CNS depression).
No products indexed under this heading.

Mesoridazine Besylate (Increased CNS depression).
No products indexed under this heading.

Methadone Hydrochloride (Increased CNS depression).
No products indexed under this heading.

Methdilazine Hydrochloride (Increased CNS depression).
No products indexed under this heading.

Methohexital Sodium (Increased CNS depression).
No products indexed under this heading.

Methotrimeprazine (Increased CNS depression).
No products indexed under this heading.

Methoxyflurane (Increased CNS depression).
No products indexed under this heading.

Methsuximide (Buprenorphine is metabolized by the CYP3A4 isoenzyme; co-administration with inducers of CYP3A4 may cause increase in clearance of buprenorphine).
No products indexed under this heading.

Methylprednisolone (Buprenorphine is metabolized by the CYP3A4 isoenzyme; co-administration with inducers of CYP3A4 may cause increase in clearance of buprenorphine).
No products indexed under this heading.

Methylprednisolone Acetate (Buprenorphine is metabolized by the CYP3A4 isoenzyme; co-administration with inducers of CYP3A4 may cause increase in clearance of buprenorphine). Products include:
Depo-Medrol Injectable Suspension 2615
Depo-Medrol Single-Dose Vial 2617

Methylprednisolone Sodium Succinate (Buprenorphine is metabolized by the CYP3A4 isoenzyme; co-administration with inducers of CYP3A4 may cause increase in clearance of buprenorphine).
No products indexed under this heading.

Metronidazole (Buprenorphine is metabolized by the CYP3A4 isoenzyme; co-administration with inhibitors of CYP3A4 may cause decrease in clearance of buprenorphine). Products include:
Metrogel 1% 1212
MetroGel-Vaginal Gel 1822
Noritate Cream, 1% 1051

Metronidazole Benzoate (Buprenorphine is metabolized by the CYP3A4 isoenzyme; co-administration with inhibitors of CYP3A4 may cause decrease in clearance of buprenorphine).
No products indexed under this heading.

Metronidazole Hydrochloride (Buprenorphine is metabolized by the CYP3A4 isoenzyme; co-administration with inhibitors of CYP3A4 may cause decrease in clearance of buprenorphine).
No products indexed under this heading.

Miconazole (Buprenorphine is metabolized by the CYP3A4 isoenzyme; co-administration with inhibitors of CYP3A4 may cause decrease in clearance of buprenorphine).
No products indexed under this heading.

Miconazole Nitrate (Buprenorphine is metabolized by the CYP3A4 isoenzyme; co-administration with inhibitors of CYP3A4 may cause decrease in clearance of buprenorphine). Products include:
Desenex .... ▣674
Desenex Jock Itch Spray Powder .... ▣674

Midazolam Hydrochloride (Increased CNS depression).
No products indexed under this heading.

Moclobemide (Effect unspecified; caution should be exercised).
No products indexed under this heading.

Modafinil (Buprenorphine is metabolized by the CYP3A4 isoenzyme; co-administration with inducers of CYP3A4 may cause increase in clearance of buprenorphine). Products include:
Provigil Tablets 1002

Molindone Hydrochloride (Increased CNS depression). Products include:
Moban Tablets 1108

Morphine Sulfate (Increased CNS depression). Products include:
Avinza Capsules 1714
Kadian Capsules 572
MS Contin Tablets 2703

Nefazodone Hydrochloride (Buprenorphine is metabolized by the CYP3A4 isoenzyme; co-administration with inhibitors of CYP3A4 may cause decrease in clearance of buprenorphine).
No products indexed under this heading.

Nelfinavir Mesylate (Buprenorphine is metabolized by the CYP3A4 isoenzyme; co-administration with inhibitors of CYP3A4 may cause decrease in clearance of buprenorphine). Products include:

Viracept 2556

Nevirapine (Buprenorphine is metabolized by the CYP3A4 isoenzyme; co-administration with inhibitors of CYP3A4 may cause decrease in clearance of buprenorphine). Products include:
- Viramune Oral Suspension 903
- Viramune Tablets 903

Niacinamide (Buprenorphine is metabolized by the CYP3A4 isoenzyme; co-administration with inhibitors of CYP3A4 may cause decrease in clearance of buprenorphine).
No products indexed under this heading.

Nicotinamide (Buprenorphine is metabolized by the CYP3A4 isoenzyme; co-administration with inhibitors of CYP3A4 may cause decrease in clearance of buprenorphine). Products include:
- Nicomide Tablets 3190

Nifedipine (Buprenorphine is metabolized by the CYP3A4 isoenzyme; co-administration with inhibitors of CYP3A4 may cause decrease in clearance of buprenorphine). Products include:
- Adalat CC Tablets 2978

Norfloxacin (Buprenorphine is metabolized by the CYP3A4 isoenzyme; co-administration with inhibitors of CYP3A4 may cause decrease in clearance of buprenorphine). Products include:
- Noroxin Tablets 2009

Olanzapine (Increased CNS depression). Products include:
- Symbyax Capsules 1788
- Zyprexa Tablets 1798
- Zyprexa IntraMuscular 1798
- Zyprexa ZYDIS Orally Disintegrating Tablets 1798

Omeprazole (Buprenorphine is metabolized by the CYP3A4 isoenzyme; co-administration with inhibitors of CYP3A4 may cause decrease in clearance of buprenorphine). Products include:
- Zegerid Powder for Oral Solution 2972

Oxazepam (Increased CNS depression).
No products indexed under this heading.

Oxcarbazepine (Buprenorphine is metabolized by the CYP3A4 isoenzyme; co-administration with inducers of CYP3A4 may cause increase in clearance of buprenorphine). Products include:
- Trileptal Oral Suspension 2281
- Trileptal Tablets 2281

Oxycodone Hydrochloride (Increased CNS depression). Products include:
- Combunox Tablets 1183
- OxyContin Tablets 2699
- OxyFast Oral Concentrate Solution 2704
- OxyIR Capsules 2704
- Percocet Tablets 1114
- Percodan Tablets 1115

Pargyline Hydrochloride (Effect unspecified; caution should be exercised).
No products indexed under this heading.

Paroxetine Hydrochloride (Buprenorphine is metabolized by the CYP3A4 isoenzyme; co-administration with inhibitors of CYP3A4 may cause decrease in clearance of buprenorphine). Products include:
- Paxil CR Controlled-Release Tablets 1509
- Paxil 1501

Pentobarbital Sodium (Increased CNS depression). Products include:
- Nembutal Sodium Solution, USP 2484

Perphenazine (Increased CNS depression).
No products indexed under this heading.

Phenelzine Sulfate (Effect unspecified; caution should be exercised).
No products indexed under this heading.

Phenobarbital (Increased CNS depression).
No products indexed under this heading.

Phenobarbital Sodium (Buprenorphine is metabolized by the CYP3A4 isoenzyme; co-administration with inducers of CYP3A4 may cause increase in clearance of buprenorphine).
No products indexed under this heading.

Phenprocoumon (Potential for purpura).
No products indexed under this heading.

Phenytoin (Buprenorphine is metabolized by the CYP3A4 isoenzyme; co-administration with inducers of CYP3A4 may cause increase in clearance of buprenorphine).
No products indexed under this heading.

Phenytoin Sodium (Buprenorphine is metabolized by the CYP3A4 isoenzyme; co-administration with inducers of CYP3A4 may cause increase in clearance of buprenorphine). Products include:
- Phenytek Capsules 2153

Prazepam (Increased CNS depression).
No products indexed under this heading.

Prednisolone Acetate (Buprenorphine is metabolized by the CYP3A4 isoenzyme; co-administration with inducers of CYP3A4 may cause increase in clearance of buprenorphine). Products include:
- Blephamide Ophthalmic Ointment 563
- Blephamide Ophthalmic Suspension 564
- Poly-Pred Liquifilm Ophthalmic Suspension .... ⊙231
- Pred Forte Ophthalmic Suspension .... ⊙233
- Pred Mild Sterile Ophthalmic Suspension .... ⊙236
- Pred-G Ophthalmic Suspension ...... ⊙234
- Pred-G Sterile Ophthalmic Ointment .... ⊙235

Prednisolone Sodium Phosphate (Buprenorphine is metabolized by the CYP3A4 isoenzyme; co-administration with inducers of CYP3A4 may cause increase in clearance of buprenorphine). Products include:
- Pediapred Oral Solution 3319

Prednisolone Tebutate (Buprenorphine is metabolized by the CYP3A4 isoenzyme; co-administration with inducers of CYP3A4 may cause increase in clearance of buprenorphine).
No products indexed under this heading.

Prednisone (Buprenorphine is metabolized by the CYP3A4 isoenzyme; co-administration with inducers of CYP3A4 may cause increase in clearance of buprenorphine).
No products indexed under this heading.

Primidone (Buprenorphine is metabolized by the CYP3A4 isoenzyme; co-administration with inducers of CYP3A4 may cause increase in clearance of buprenorphine).
No products indexed under this heading.

Procarbazine Hydrochloride (Effect unspecified; caution should be exercised). Products include:
- Matulane Capsules 3188

Prochlorperazine (Increased CNS depression).
No products indexed under this heading.

Promethazine Hydrochloride (Increased CNS depression). Products include:
- Phenergan 3438

Propofol (Increased CNS depression). Products include:
- Diprivan Injectable Emulsion 676

Propoxyphene Hydrochloride (Increased CNS depression).
No products indexed under this heading.

Propoxyphene Napsylate (Increased CNS depression). Products include:
- Darvocet A 500 Tablets 3497

Pyrilamine Maleate (Increased CNS depression).
No products indexed under this heading.

Pyrilamine Tannate (Increased CNS depression).
No products indexed under this heading.

Quazepam (Increased CNS depression).
No products indexed under this heading.

Quetiapine Fumarate (Increased CNS depression). Products include:
- Seroquel Tablets 691

Quinidine (Buprenorphine is metabolized by the CYP3A4 isoenzyme; co-administration with inhibitors of CYP3A4 may cause decrease in clearance of buprenorphine).
No products indexed under this heading.

Quinidine Hydrochloride (Buprenorphine is metabolized by the CYP3A4 isoenzyme; co-administration with inhibitors of CYP3A4 may cause decrease in clearance of buprenorphine).
No products indexed under this heading.

Quinidine Polygalacturonate (Buprenorphine is metabolized by the CYP3A4 isoenzyme; co-administration with inhibitors of CYP3A4 may cause decrease in clearance of buprenorphine).
No products indexed under this heading.

Quinidine Sulfate (Buprenorphine is metabolized by the CYP3A4 isoenzyme; co-administration with inhibitors of CYP3A4 may cause decrease in clearance of buprenorphine).
No products indexed under this heading.

Quinine (Buprenorphine is metabolized by the CYP3A4 isoenzyme; co-administration with inhibitors of CYP3A4 may cause decrease in clearance of buprenorphine).
No products indexed under this heading.

Quinine Sulfate (Buprenorphine is metabolized by the CYP3A4 isoenzyme; co-administration with inhibitors of CYP3A4 may cause decrease in clearance of buprenorphine).
No products indexed under this heading.

Quinupristin (Buprenorphine is metabolized by the CYP3A4 isoenzyme; co-administration with inhibitors of CYP3A4 may cause decrease in clearance of buprenorphine). Products include:
- Synercid I.V. 1690

Ranitidine Bismuth Citrate (Buprenorphine is metabolized by the CYP3A4 isoenzyme; co-administration with inhibitors of CYP3A4 may cause decrease in clearance of buprenorphine).
No products indexed under this heading.

Ranitidine Hydrochloride (Buprenorphine is metabolized by the CYP3A4 isoenzyme; co-administration with inhibitors of CYP3A4 may cause decrease in clearance of buprenorphine). Products include:
- Zantac 1597
- Zantac Injection 1593
- Zantac 75 Tablets .... ▣715
- Zantac 150 Maximum Strength Tablets .... ▣715
- Zantac Injection Pharmacy Bulk Package 1595

Remifentanil Hydrochloride (Increased CNS depression).
No products indexed under this heading.

Rifabutin (Buprenorphine is metabolized by the CYP3A4 isoenzyme; co-administration with inducers of CYP3A4 may cause increase in clearance of buprenorphine).
No products indexed under this heading.

Rifampicin (Buprenorphine is metabolized by the CYP3A4 isoenzyme; co-administration with inducers of CYP3A4 may cause increase in clearance of buprenorphine).
No products indexed under this heading.

Rifampin (Buprenorphine is metabolized by the CYP3A4 isoenzyme; co-administration with inducers of CYP3A4 may cause increase in clearance of buprenorphine).
No products indexed under this heading.

Rifapentine (Buprenorphine is metabolized by the CYP3A4 isoenzyme; co-administration with inducers of CYP3A4 may cause increase in clearance of buprenorphine).
No products indexed under this heading.

Risperidone (Increased CNS depression). Products include:
- Risperdal Consta Long-Acting Injection 1664
- Risperdal M-Tab Orally Disintegrating Tablets 1658
- Risperdal 1658

Ritonavir (Buprenorphine is metabolized by the CYP3A4 isoenzyme; co-administration with inhibitors of

CYP3A4 may cause decrease in clearance of buprenorphine). Products include:
- Kaletra 474
- Norvir 499

Saquinavir (Buprenorphine is metabolized by the CYP3A4 isoenzyme; co-administration with inhibitors of CYP3A4 may cause decrease in clearance of buprenorphine).
No products indexed under this heading.

Saquinavir Mesylate (Buprenorphine is metabolized by the CYP3A4 isoenzyme; co-administration with inhibitors of CYP3A4 may cause decrease in clearance of buprenorphine). Products include:
- Invirase 2776

Secobarbital Sodium (Increased CNS depression).
No products indexed under this heading.

Selegiline Hydrochloride (Effect unspecified; caution should be exercised). Products include:
- Eldepryl Capsules 3209

Sertraline Hydrochloride (Buprenorphine is metabolized by the CYP3A4 isoenzyme; co-administration with inhibitors of CYP3A4 may cause decrease in clearance of buprenorphine). Products include:
- Zoloft 2581

Sevoflurane (Increased CNS depression). Products include:
- Ultane Liquid for Inhalation 526

Sodium Oxybate (Increased CNS depression).
No products indexed under this heading.

Sufentanil Citrate (Increased CNS depression).
No products indexed under this heading.

Sulfinpyrazone (Buprenorphine is metabolized by the CYP3A4 isoenzyme; co-administration with inducers of CYP3A4 may cause increase in clearance of buprenorphine).
No products indexed under this heading.

Telithromycin (Buprenorphine is metabolized by the CYP3A4 isoenzyme; co-administration with inhibitors of CYP3A4 may cause decrease in clearance of buprenorphine). Products include:
- Ketek Tablets 2920

Temazepam (Increased CNS depression).
No products indexed under this heading.

Terfenadine (Increased CNS depression).
No products indexed under this heading.

Theophylline (Buprenorphine is metabolized by the CYP3A4 isoenzyme; co-administration with inducers of CYP3A4 may cause increase in clearance of buprenorphine).
No products indexed under this heading.

Thiamylal Sodium (Increased CNS depression).
No products indexed under this heading.

Thioridazine Hydrochloride (Increased CNS depression). Products include:
- Thioridazine Hydrochloride Tablets 2122

Thiothixene (Increased CNS depression). Products include:
- Thiothixene Capsules 2124

Tranylcypromine Sulfate (Effect unspecified; caution should be exercised). Products include:
- Parnate Tablets 1499

Triamcinolone (Buprenorphine is metabolized by the CYP3A4 isoenzyme; co-administration with inducers of CYP3A4 may cause increase in clearance of buprenorphine).
No products indexed under this heading.

Triamcinolone Acetonide (Buprenorphine is metabolized by the CYP3A4 isoenzyme; co-administration with inducers of CYP3A4 may cause increase in clearance of buprenorphine). Products include:
- Azmacort Inhalation Aerosol 1701
- Nasacort HFA Inhalation Aerosol 2939
- Nasacort AQ Nasal Spray 2937

Triamcinolone Diacetate (Buprenorphine is metabolized by the CYP3A4 isoenzyme; co-administration with inducers of CYP3A4 may cause increase in clearance of buprenorphine).
No products indexed under this heading.

Triamcinolone Hexacetonide (Buprenorphine is metabolized by the CYP3A4 isoenzyme; co-administration with inducers of CYP3A4 may cause increase in clearance of buprenorphine).
No products indexed under this heading.

Triazolam (Increased CNS depression).
No products indexed under this heading.

Trifluoperazine Hydrochloride (Increased CNS depression).
No products indexed under this heading.

Trimeprazine Tartrate (Increased CNS depression).
No products indexed under this heading.

Tripelennamine Hydrochloride (Increased CNS depression).
No products indexed under this heading.

Triprolidine Hydrochloride (Increased CNS depression).
No products indexed under this heading.

Troglitazone (Buprenorphine is metabolized by the CYP3A4 isoenzyme; co-administration with inhibitors of CYP3A4 may cause decrease in clearance of buprenorphine).
No products indexed under this heading.

Troleandomycin (Buprenorphine is metabolized by the CYP3A4 isoenzyme; co-administration with inhibitors of CYP3A4 may cause decrease in clearance of buprenorphine).
No products indexed under this heading.

Valproate Sodium (Buprenorphine is metabolized by the CYP3A4 isoenzyme; co-administration with inhibitors of CYP3A4 may cause decrease in clearance of buprenorphine). Products include:
- Depacon Injection 412

Verapamil Hydrochloride (Buprenorphine is metabolized by the CYP3A4 isoenzyme; co-administration with inhibitors of CYP3A4 may cause decrease in clearance of buprenorphine). Products include:
- Covera-HS Tablets 3135
- Tarka Tablets 519
- Verelan PM Capsules 3120

Voriconazole (Buprenorphine is metabolized by the CYP3A4 isoenzyme; co-administration with inhibitors of CYP3A4 may cause decrease in clearance of buprenorphine). Products include:
- VFEND I.V. 2543
- VFEND Oral Suspension 2543
- VFEND Tablets 2543

Zafirlukast (Buprenorphine is metabolized by the CYP3A4 isoenzyme; co-administration with inhibitors of CYP3A4 may cause decrease in clearance of buprenorphine). Products include:
- Accolate Tablets 663

Zaleplon (Increased CNS depression). Products include:
- Sonata Capsules 1686

Zileuton (Buprenorphine is metabolized by the CYP3A4 isoenzyme; co-administration with inhibitors of CYP3A4 may cause decrease in clearance of buprenorphine).
No products indexed under this heading.

Ziprasidone Hydrochloride (Increased CNS depression). Products include:
- Geodon Capsules 2514

Zolpidem Tartrate (Increased CNS depression). Products include:
- Ambien Tablets 2867

Food Interactions

Alcohol (Increased CNS depression).

Grapefruit (Buprenorphine is metabolized by the CYP3A4 isoenzyme; co-administration with inhibitors of CYP3A4 may cause decrease in clearance of buprenorphine).

Grapefruit Juice (Buprenorphine is metabolized by the CYP3A4 isoenzyme; co-administration with inhibitors of CYP3A4 may cause decrease in clearance of buprenorphine).

BYETTA INJECTION

(Exenatide) 605

May interact with bacteriostatic antibiotics, beta-lactams antibiotics, fluoroquinolone antibiotics, macrolide antibiotics, oral contraceptives, penicillins, tetracyclines, and certain other agents. Compounds in these categories include:

Alatrofloxacin Mesylate (The effect of exenatide to slow gastric emptying may reduce the extent and rate of absorption of orally administered drugs. Exenatide should be used with caution in patients receiving oral medications that require rapid gastrointestinal absorption. For oral medications that are dependent on threshold concentrations for efficacy, such as antibiotics, patients should be advised to take those drugs at least 1 hr before exenatide injection. If such drugs are to be administered with food, patients should be advised to take them with a meal or snack when exenatide is not administered).
No products indexed under this heading.

5-Amino-Salicylic Acid (The effect of exenatide to slow gastric emptying may reduce the extent and rate of absorption of orally administered drugs. Exenatide should be used with caution in patients receiving oral medications that require rapid gastrointestinal absorption. For oral medications that are dependent on threshold concentrations for efficacy, such as antibiotics, patients should be advised to take those drugs at least 1 hr before exenatide injection. If such drugs are to be administered with food, patients should be advised to take them with a meal or snack when exenatide is not administered).
No products indexed under this heading.

Amoxicillin (The effect of exenatide to slow gastric emptying may reduce the extent and rate of absorption of orally administered drugs. Exenatide should be used with caution in patients receiving oral medications that require rapid gastrointestinal absorption. For oral medications that are dependent on threshold concentrations for efficacy, such as antibiotics, patients should be advised to take those drugs at least 1 hr before exenatide injection. If such drugs are to be administered with food, patients should be advised to take them with a meal or snack when exenatide is not administered). Products include:
- Amoxil Capsules 1315
- Amoxil Chewable Tablets 1315
- Amoxil Pediatric Drops for Oral Suspension 1315
- Amoxil Powder for Oral Suspension 1315
- Amoxil Tablets 1315
- Augmentin 1331
- Augmentin Tablets 1334
- Augmentin XR Extended-Release Tablets 1340
- Augmentin ES-600 Powder for Oral Suspension 1337
- PREVPAC 3281

Amoxicillin Trihydrate (The effect of exenatide to slow gastric emptying may reduce the extent and rate of absorption of orally administered drugs. Exenatide should be used with caution in patients receiving oral medications that require rapid gastrointestinal absorption. For oral medications that are dependent on threshold concentrations for efficacy, such as antibiotics, patients should be advised to take those drugs at least 1 hr before exenatide injection. If such drugs are to be administered with food, patients should be advised to take them with a meal or snack when exenatide is not administered).
No products indexed under this heading.

Ampicillin (The effect of exenatide to slow gastric emptying may reduce the extent and rate of absorption of orally administered drugs. Exenatide should be used with caution in patients receiving oral medications that require rapid gastrointestinal absorption. For oral medications that are dependent on threshold concentrations for efficacy, such as antibiotics, patients should be advised to take those drugs at least 1 hr before exenatide injection. If such drugs are to be administered with food, patients should be advised to take them with a meal or snack when exenatide is not administered).
No products indexed under this heading.

Ampicillin Sodium (The effect of exenatide to slow gastric emptying may reduce the extent and rate of absorption of orally administered drugs. Exenatide should be used with caution in patients receiving oral

medications that require rapid gastrointestinal absorption. For oral medications that are dependent on threshold concentrations for efficacy, such as antibiotics, patients should be advised to take those drugs at least 1 hr before exenatide injection. If such drugs are to be administered with food, patients should be advised to take them with a meal or snack when exenatide is not administered).

No products indexed under this heading.

Ampicillin Trihydrate (The effect of exenatide to slow gastric emptying may reduce the extent and rate of absorption of orally administered drugs. Exenatide should be used with caution in patients receiving oral medications that require rapid gastrointestinal absorption. For oral medications that are dependent on threshold concentrations for efficacy, such as antibiotics, patients should be advised to take those drugs at least 1 hr before exenatide injection. If such drugs are to be administered with food, patients should be advised to take them with a meal or snack when exenatide is not administered).

No products indexed under this heading.

Azithromycin Dihydrate (The effect of exenatide to slow gastric emptying may reduce the extent and rate of absorption of orally administered drugs. Exenatide should be used with caution in patients receiving oral medications that require rapid gastrointestinal absorption. For oral medications that are dependent on threshold concentrations for efficacy, such as antibiotics, patients should be advised to take those drugs at least 1 hr before exenatide injection. If such drugs are to be administered with food, patients should be advised to take them with a meal or snack when exenatide is not administered). Products include:

Zithromax **2568**
Zithromax for IV Infusion **2573**
Zithromax for Oral Suspension, 300 mg, 600 mg, 900 mg, 1200 mg **2561**
Zithromax Tablets, 250 mg, 500 mg **2561**
Zithromax Tri-Pak **2561**
Zithromax Z-Pak **2568**

Azlocillin Sodium (The effect of exenatide to slow gastric emptying may reduce the extent and rate of absorption of orally administered drugs. Exenatide should be used with caution in patients receiving oral medications that require rapid gastrointestinal absorption. For oral medications that are dependent on threshold concentrations for efficacy, such as antibiotics, patients should be advised to take those drugs at least 1 hr before exenatide injection. If such drugs are to be administered with food, patients should be advised to take them with a meal or snack when exenatide is not administered).

No products indexed under this heading.

Aztreonam (The effect of exenatide to slow gastric emptying may reduce the extent and rate of absorption of orally administered drugs. Exenatide should be used with caution in patients receiving oral medications that require rapid gastrointestinal absorption. For oral medications that are dependent on threshold concentrations for efficacy, such as antibiotics, patients should be advised to take those drugs at least 1 hr before exenatide injection. If such drugs are to be administered with food, patients should be advised to take them with a meal or snack when exenatide is not administered).

No products indexed under this heading.

Bacampicillin Hydrochloride (The effect of exenatide to slow gastric emptying may reduce the extent and rate of absorption of orally administered drugs. Exenatide should be used with caution in patients receiving oral medications that require rapid gastrointestinal absorption. For oral medications that are dependent on threshold concentrations for efficacy, such as antibiotics, patients should be advised to take those drugs at least 1 hr before exenatide injection. If such drugs are to be administered with food, patients should be advised to take them with a meal or snack when exenatide is not administered).

No products indexed under this heading.

Carbenicillin Disodium (The effect of exenatide to slow gastric emptying may reduce the extent and rate of absorption of orally administered drugs. Exenatide should be used with caution in patients receiving oral medications that require rapid gastrointestinal absorption. For oral medications that are dependent on threshold concentrations for efficacy, such as antibiotics, patients should be advised to take those drugs at least 1 hr before exenatide injection. If such drugs are to be administered with food, patients should be advised to take them with a meal or snack when exenatide is not administered).

No products indexed under this heading.

Carbenicillin Indanyl Sodium (The effect of exenatide to slow gastric emptying may reduce the extent and rate of absorption of orally administered drugs. Exenatide should be used with caution in patients receiving oral medications that require rapid gastrointestinal absorption. For oral medications that are dependent on threshold concentrations for efficacy, such as antibiotics, patients should be advised to take those drugs at least 1 hr before exenatide injection. If such drugs are to be administered with food, patients should be advised to take them with a meal or snack when exenatide is not administered).

No products indexed under this heading.

Cefaclor (The effect of exenatide to slow gastric emptying may reduce the extent and rate of absorption of orally administered drugs. Exenatide should be used with caution in patients receiving oral medications that require rapid gastrointestinal absorption. For oral medications that are dependent on threshold concentrations for efficacy, such as antibiotics, patients should be advised to take those drugs at least 1 hr before exenatide injection. If such drugs are to be administered with food, patients should be advised to take them with a meal or snack when exenatide is not administered).

No products indexed under this heading.

Cefadroxil (The effect of exenatide to slow gastric emptying may reduce the extent and rate of absorption of orally administered drugs. Exenatide should be used with caution in patients receiving oral medications that require rapid gastrointestinal absorption. For oral medications that are dependent on threshold concentrations for efficacy, such as antibiotics, patients should be advised to take those drugs at least 1 hr before exenatide injection. If such drugs are to be administered with food, patients should be advised to take them with a meal or snack when exenatide is not administered).

No products indexed under this heading.

Cefamandole Nafate (The effect of exenatide to slow gastric emptying may reduce the extent and rate of absorption of orally administered drugs. Exenatide should be used with caution in patients receiving oral medications that require rapid gastrointestinal absorption. For oral medications that are dependent on threshold concentrations for efficacy, such as antibiotics, patients should be advised to take those drugs at least 1 hr before exenatide injection. If such drugs are to be administered with food, patients should be advised to take them with a meal or snack when exenatide is not administered).

No products indexed under this heading.

Cefazolin Sodium (The effect of exenatide to slow gastric emptying may reduce the extent and rate of absorption of orally administered drugs. Exenatide should be used with caution in patients receiving oral medications that require rapid gastrointestinal absorption. For oral medications that are dependent on threshold concentrations for efficacy, such as antibiotics, patients should be advised to take those drugs at least 1 hr before exenatide injection. If such drugs are to be administered with food, patients should be advised to take them with a meal or snack when exenatide is not administered). Products include:

Ancef for Injection **1318**

Cefixime (The effect of exenatide to slow gastric emptying may reduce the extent and rate of absorption of orally administered drugs. Exenatide should be used with caution in patients receiving oral medications that require rapid gastrointestinal absorption. For oral medications that are dependent on threshold concentrations for efficacy, such as antibiotics, patients should be advised to take those drugs at least 1 hr before exenatide injection. If such drugs are to be administered with food, patients should be advised to take them with a meal or snack when exenatide is not administered). Products include:

Suprax **1811**

Cefmetazole Sodium (The effect of exenatide to slow gastric emptying may reduce the extent and rate of absorption of orally administered drugs. Exenatide should be used with caution in patients receiving oral medications that require rapid gastrointestinal absorption. For oral medications that are dependent on threshold concentrations for efficacy, such as antibiotics, patients should be advised to take those drugs at least 1 hr before exenatide injection. If such drugs are to be administered with food, patients should be advised to take them with a meal or snack when exenatide is not administered).

No products indexed under this heading.

Cefonicid Sodium (The effect of exenatide to slow gastric emptying may reduce the extent and rate of absorption of orally administered drugs. Exenatide should be used with caution in patients receiving oral medications that require rapid gastrointestinal absorption. For oral medications that are dependent on threshold concentrations for efficacy, such as antibiotics, patients should be advised to take those drugs at least 1 hr before exenatide injection. If such drugs are to be administered with food, patients should be advised to take them with a meal or snack when exenatide is not administered).

No products indexed under this heading.

Cefoperazone Sodium (The effect of exenatide to slow gastric emptying may reduce the extent and rate of absorption of orally administered drugs. Exenatide should be used with caution in patients receiving oral medications that require rapid gastrointestinal absorption. For oral medications that are dependent on threshold concentrations for efficacy, such as antibiotics, patients should be advised to take those drugs at least 1 hr before exenatide injection. If such drugs are to be administered with food, patients should be advised to take them with a meal or snack when exenatide is not administered).

No products indexed under this heading.

Ceforanide (The effect of exenatide to slow gastric emptying may reduce the extent and rate of absorption of orally administered drugs. Exenatide should be used with caution in patients receiving oral medications that require rapid gastrointestinal absorption. For oral medications that are dependent on threshold concentrations for efficacy, such as antibiotics, patients should be advised to take those drugs at least 1 hr before exenatide injection. If such drugs are to be administered with food, patients should be advised to take them with a meal or snack when exenatide is not administered).

No products indexed under this heading.

Cefotaxime Sodium (The effect of exenatide to slow gastric emptying may reduce the extent and rate of absorption of orally administered drugs. Exenatide should be used with caution in patients receiving oral medications that require rapid gastrointestinal absorption. For oral medications that are dependent on threshold concentrations for efficacy, such as antibiotics, patients should be advised to take those drugs at least 1 hr before exenatide injection. If such drugs are to be administered with food, patients should be advised to take them with a meal or snack when exenatide is

not administered).
No products indexed under this heading.

Cefotetan (The effect of exenatide to slow gastric emptying may reduce the extent and rate of absorption of orally administered drugs. Exenatide should be used with caution in patients receiving oral medications that require rapid gastrointestinal absorption. For oral medications that are dependent on threshold concentrations for efficacy, such as antibiotics, patients should be advised to take those drugs at least 1 hr before exenatide injection. If such drugs are to be administered with food, patients should be advised to take them with a meal or snack when exenatide is not administered).
No products indexed under this heading.

Cefoxitin Sodium (The effect of exenatide to slow gastric emptying may reduce the extent and rate of absorption of orally administered drugs. Exenatide should be used with caution in patients receiving oral medications that require rapid gastrointestinal absorption. For oral medications that are dependent on threshold concentrations for efficacy, such as antibiotics, patients should be advised to take those drugs at least 1 hr before exenatide injection. If such drugs are to be administered with food, patients should be advised to take them with a meal or snack when exenatide is not administered). Products include:
Mefoxin for Injection **1987**
Mefoxin Premixed Intravenous Solution.. **1990**

Cefpodoxime Proxetil (The effect of exenatide to slow gastric emptying may reduce the extent and rate of absorption of orally administered drugs. Exenatide should be used with caution in patients receiving oral medications that require rapid gastrointestinal absorption. For oral medications that are dependent on threshold concentrations for efficacy, such as antibiotics, patients should be advised to take those drugs at least 1 hr before exenatide injection. If such drugs are to be administered with food, patients should be advised to take them with a meal or snack when exenatide is not administered). Products include:
Vantin Tablets and Oral Suspension **2650**

Cefprozil (The effect of exenatide to slow gastric emptying may reduce the extent and rate of absorption of orally administered drugs. Exenatide should be used with caution in patients receiving oral medications that require rapid gastrointestinal absorption. For oral medications that are dependent on threshold concentrations for efficacy, such as antibiotics, patients should be advised to take those drugs at least 1 hr before exenatide injection. If such drugs are to be administered with food, patients should be advised to take them with a meal or snack when exenatide is not administered).
No products indexed under this heading.

Ceftazidime (The effect of exenatide to slow gastric emptying may reduce the extent and rate of absorption of orally administered drugs. Exenatide should be used with caution in patients receiving oral medications that require rapid gastrointestinal absorption. For oral medications that are dependent on threshold concentrations for efficacy, such as antibiotics, patients should be advised to take those drugs at least 1 hr before exenatide injection. If such drugs are to be administered with food, patients should be advised to take them with a meal or snack when exenatide is not administered). Products include:
Fortaz for Injection **1422**

Ceftizoxime Sodium (The effect of exenatide to slow gastric emptying may reduce the extent and rate of absorption of orally administered drugs. Exenatide should be used with caution in patients receiving oral medications that require rapid gastrointestinal absorption. For oral medications that are dependent on threshold concentrations for efficacy, such as antibiotics, patients should be advised to take those drugs at least 1 hr before exenatide injection. If such drugs are to be administered with food, patients should be advised to take them with a meal or snack when exenatide is not administered).
No products indexed under this heading.

Ceftriaxone Sodium (The effect of exenatide to slow gastric emptying may reduce the extent and rate of absorption of orally administered drugs. Exenatide should be used with caution in patients receiving oral medications that require rapid gastrointestinal absorption. For oral medications that are dependent on threshold concentrations for efficacy, such as antibiotics, patients should be advised to take those drugs at least 1 hr before exenatide injection. If such drugs are to be administered with food, patients should be advised to take them with a meal or snack when exenatide is not administered). Products include:
Rocephin Injectable Vials, ADD-Vantage, Galaxy, Bulk........... **2801**

Cefuroxime Axetil (The effect of exenatide to slow gastric emptying may reduce the extent and rate of absorption of orally administered drugs. Exenatide should be used with caution in patients receiving oral medications that require rapid gastrointestinal absorption. For oral medications that are dependent on threshold concentrations for efficacy, such as antibiotics, patients should be advised to take those drugs at least 1 hr before exenatide injection. If such drugs are to be administered with food, patients should be advised to take them with a meal or snack when exenatide is not administered). Products include:
Ceftin **1369**

Cefuroxime Sodium (The effect of exenatide to slow gastric emptying may reduce the extent and rate of absorption of orally administered drugs. Exenatide should be used with caution in patients receiving oral medications that require rapid gastrointestinal absorption. For oral medications that are dependent on threshold concentrations for efficacy, such as antibiotics, patients should be advised to take those drugs at least 1 hr before exenatide injection. If such drugs are to be administered with food, patients should be advised to take them with a meal or snack when exenatide is not administered).
No products indexed under this heading.

Cephalexin (The effect of exenatide to slow gastric emptying may reduce the extent and rate of absorption of orally administered drugs. Exenatide should be used with caution in patients receiving oral medications that require rapid gastrointestinal absorption. For oral medications that are dependent on threshold concentrations for efficacy, such as antibiotics, patients should be advised to take those drugs at least 1 hr before exenatide injection. If such drugs are to be administered with food, patients should be advised to take them with a meal or snack when exenatide is not administered).
No products indexed under this heading.

Cephalothin Sodium (The effect of exenatide to slow gastric emptying may reduce the extent and rate of absorption of orally administered drugs. Exenatide should be used with caution in patients receiving oral medications that require rapid gastrointestinal absorption. For oral medications that are dependent on threshold concentrations for efficacy, such as antibiotics, patients should be advised to take those drugs at least 1 hr before exenatide injection. If such drugs are to be administered with food, patients should be advised to take them with a meal or snack when exenatide is not administered).
No products indexed under this heading.

Cephapirin Sodium (The effect of exenatide to slow gastric emptying may reduce the extent and rate of absorption of orally administered drugs. Exenatide should be used with caution in patients receiving oral medications that require rapid gastrointestinal absorption. For oral medications that are dependent on threshold concentrations for efficacy, such as antibiotics, patients should be advised to take those drugs at least 1 hr before exenatide injection. If such drugs are to be administered with food, patients should be advised to take them with a meal or snack when exenatide is not administered).
No products indexed under this heading.

Chloramphenicol (The effect of exenatide to slow gastric emptying may reduce the extent and rate of absorption of orally administered drugs. Exenatide should be used with caution in patients receiving oral medications that require rapid gastrointestinal absorption. For oral medications that are dependent on threshold concentrations for efficacy, such as antibiotics, patients should be advised to take those drugs at least 1 hr before exenatide injection. If such drugs are to be administered with food, patients should be advised to take them with a meal or snack when exenatide is not administered).
No products indexed under this heading.

Chloramphenicol Palmitate (The effect of exenatide to slow gastric emptying may reduce the extent and rate of absorption of orally administered drugs. Exenatide should be used with caution in patients receiving oral medications that require rapid gastrointestinal absorption. For oral medications that are dependent on threshold concentrations for efficacy, such as antibiotics, patients should be advised to take those drugs at least 1 hr before exenatide injection. If such drugs are to be administered with food, patients should be advised to take them with a meal or snack when exenatide is not administered).
No products indexed under this heading.

Chloramphenicol Sodium Succinate (The effect of exenatide to slow gastric emptying may reduce the extent and rate of absorption of orally administered drugs. Exenatide should be used with caution in patients receiving oral medications that require rapid gastrointestinal absorption. For oral medications that are dependent on threshold concentrations for efficacy, such as antibiotics, patients should be advised to take those drugs at least 1 hr before exenatide injection. If such drugs are to be administered with food, patients should be advised to take them with a meal or snack when exenatide is not administered).
No products indexed under this heading.

Cilastatin Sodium (The effect of exenatide to slow gastric emptying may reduce the extent and rate of absorption of orally administered drugs. Exenatide should be used with caution in patients receiving oral medications that require rapid gastrointestinal absorption. For oral medications that are dependent on threshold concentrations for efficacy, such as antibiotics, patients should be advised to take those drugs at least 1 hr before exenatide injection. If such drugs are to be administered with food, patients should be advised to take them with a meal or snack when exenatide is not administered). Products include:
Primaxin I.M. **2022**
Primaxin I.V. **2024**

Ciprofloxacin (The effect of exenatide to slow gastric emptying may reduce the extent and rate of absorption of orally administered drugs. Exenatide should be used with caution in patients receiving oral medications that require rapid gastrointestinal absorption. For oral medications that are dependent on threshold concentrations for efficacy, such as antibiotics, patients should be advised to take those drugs at least 1 hr before exenatide injection. If such drugs are to be administered with food, patients should be advised to take them with a meal or snack when exenatide is not administered). Products include:
Cipro I.V. **2998**
Cipro I.V. Pharmacy Bulk Package ... **3509**
Cipro Oral Suspension **2991**
Cipro XR Tablets **3004**
Ciprodex Otic Suspension **555**

Ciprofloxacin Hydrochloride (The effect of exenatide to slow gastric emptying may reduce the extent and rate of absorption of orally administered drugs. Exenatide should be used with caution in patients receiving oral medications that require rapid gastrointestinal absorption. For oral medications that are dependent

on threshold concentrations for efficacy, such as antibiotics, patients should be advised to take those drugs at least 1 hr before exenatide injection. If such drugs are to be administered with food, patients should be advised to take them with a meal or snack when exenatide is not administered). Products include:

Ciloxan Ophthalmic Ointment 554
Cipro Tablets 2991

Clarithromycin (The effect of exenatide to slow gastric emptying may reduce the extent and rate of absorption of orally administered drugs. Exenatide should be used with caution in patients receiving oral medications that require rapid gastrointestinal absorption. For oral medications that are dependent on threshold concentrations for efficacy, such as antibiotics, patients should be advised to take those drugs at least 1 hr before exenatide injection. If such drugs are to be administered with food, patients should be advised to take them with a meal or snack when exenatide is not administered). Products include:

Biaxin/Biaxin XL 402
PREVPAC 3281

Demeclocycline Hydrochloride (The effect of exenatide to slow gastric emptying may reduce the extent and rate of absorption of orally administered drugs. Exenatide should be used with caution in patients receiving oral medications that require rapid gastrointestinal absorption. For oral medications that are dependent on threshold concentrations for efficacy, such as antibiotics, patients should be advised to take those drugs at least 1 hr before exenatide injection. If such drugs are to be administered with food, patients should be advised to take them with a meal or snack when exenatide is not administered).

No products indexed under this heading.

Desogestrel (The effect of exenatide to slow gastric emptying may reduce the extent and rate of absorption of orally administered drugs. Exenatide should be used with caution in patients receiving oral medications that require rapid gastrointestinal absorption. For oral medications that are dependent on threshold concentrations for efficacy, such as contraceptives, patients should be advised to take those drugs at least 1 hr before exenatide injection. If such drugs are to be administered with food, patients should be advised to take them with a meal or snack when exenatide is not administered). Products include:

Ortho-Cept Tablets 2395

Dicloxacillin Sodium (The effect of exenatide to slow gastric emptying may reduce the extent and rate of absorption of orally administered drugs. Exenatide should be used with caution in patients receiving oral medications that require rapid gastrointestinal absorption. For oral medications that are dependent on threshold concentrations for efficacy, such as antibiotics, patients should be advised to take those drugs at least 1 hr before exenatide injection. If such drugs are to be administered with food, patients should be advised to take them with a meal or snack when exenatide is not administered).

No products indexed under this heading.

Dirithromycin (The effect of exenatide to slow gastric emptying may reduce the extent and rate of absorption of orally administered drugs. Exenatide should be used with caution in patients receiving oral medications that require rapid gastrointestinal absorption. For oral medications that are dependent on threshold concentrations for efficacy, such as antibiotics, patients should be advised to take those drugs at least 1 hr before exenatide injection. If such drugs are to be administered with food, patients should be advised to take them with a meal or snack when exenatide is not administered).

No products indexed under this heading.

Doxycycline Calcium (The effect of exenatide to slow gastric emptying may reduce the extent and rate of absorption of orally administered drugs. Exenatide should be used with caution in patients receiving oral medications that require rapid gastrointestinal absorption. For oral medications that are dependent on threshold concentrations for efficacy, such as antibiotics, patients should be advised to take those drugs at least 1 hr before exenatide injection. If such drugs are to be administered with food, patients should be advised to take them with a meal or snack when exenatide is not administered).

No products indexed under this heading.

Doxycycline Hyclate (The effect of exenatide to slow gastric emptying may reduce the extent and rate of absorption of orally administered drugs. Exenatide should be used with caution in patients receiving oral medications that require rapid gastrointestinal absorption. For oral medications that are dependent on threshold concentrations for efficacy, such as antibiotics, patients should be advised to take those drugs at least 1 hr before exenatide injection. If such drugs are to be administered with food, patients should be advised to take them with a meal or snack when exenatide is not administered).

No products indexed under this heading.

Doxycycline Monohydrate (The effect of exenatide to slow gastric emptying may reduce the extent and rate of absorption of orally administered drugs. Exenatide should be used with caution in patients receiving oral medications that require rapid gastrointestinal absorption. For oral medications that are dependent on threshold concentrations for efficacy, such as antibiotics, patients should be advised to take those drugs at least 1 hr before exenatide injection. If such drugs are to be administered with food, patients should be advised to take them with a meal or snack when exenatide is not administered).

No products indexed under this heading.

Enoxacin (The effect of exenatide to slow gastric emptying may reduce the extent and rate of absorption of orally administered drugs. Exenatide should be used with caution in patients receiving oral medications that require rapid gastrointestinal absorption. For oral medications that are dependent on threshold concentrations for efficacy, such as antibiotics, patients should be advised to take those drugs at least 1 hr before exenatide injection. If such drugs are to be administered with food, patients should be advised to take them with a meal or snack when exenatide is not administered).

No products indexed under this heading.

Erythromycin (The effect of exenatide to slow gastric emptying may reduce the extent and rate of absorption of orally administered drugs. Exenatide should be used with caution in patients receiving oral medications that require rapid gastrointestinal absorption. For oral medications that are dependent on threshold concentrations for efficacy, such as antibiotics, patients should be advised to take those drugs at least 1 hr before exenatide injection. If such drugs are to be administered with food, patients should be advised to take them with a meal or snack when exenatide is not administered). Products include:

Erygel Topical Gel 2096
Ery-Tab Tablets 447
Erythromycin Base Filmtab Tablets 454
Erythromycin Delayed-Release Capsules, USP 456
PCE Dispertab Tablets 510

Erythromycin Estolate (The effect of exenatide to slow gastric emptying may reduce the extent and rate of absorption of orally administered drugs. Exenatide should be used with caution in patients receiving oral medications that require rapid gastrointestinal absorption. For oral medications that are dependent on threshold concentrations for efficacy, such as antibiotics, patients should be advised to take those drugs at least 1 hr before exenatide injection. If such drugs are to be administered with food, patients should be advised to take them with a meal or snack when exenatide is not administered).

No products indexed under this heading.

Erythromycin Ethylsuccinate (The effect of exenatide to slow gastric emptying may reduce the extent and rate of absorption of orally administered drugs. Exenatide should be used with caution in patients receiving oral medications that require rapid gastrointestinal absorption. For oral medications that are dependent on threshold concentrations for efficacy, such as antibiotics, patients should be advised to take those drugs at least 1 hr before exenatide injection. If such drugs are to be administered with food, patients should be advised to take them with a meal or snack when exenatide is not administered). Products include:

E.E.S. 449
EryPed 445

Erythromycin Gluceptate (The effect of exenatide to slow gastric emptying may reduce the extent and rate of absorption of orally administered drugs. Exenatide should be used with caution in patients receiving oral medications that require rapid gastrointestinal absorption. For oral medications that are dependent on threshold concentrations for efficacy, such as antibiotics, patients should be advised to take those drugs at least 1 hr before exenatide injection. If such drugs are to be administered with food, patients should be advised to take them with a meal or snack when exenatide is not administered).

No products indexed under this heading.

Erythromycin Stearate (The effect of exenatide to slow gastric emptying may reduce the extent and rate of absorption of orally administered drugs. Exenatide should be used with caution in patients receiving oral medications that require rapid gastrointestinal absorption. For oral medications that are dependent on threshold concentrations for efficacy, such as antibiotics, patients should be advised to take those drugs at least 1 hr before exenatide injection. If such drugs are to be administered with food, patients should be advised to take them with a meal or snack when exenatide is not administered). Products include:

Erythrocin Stearate Filmtab Tablets 452

Ethinyl Estradiol (The effect of exenatide to slow gastric emptying may reduce the extent and rate of absorption of orally administered drugs. Exenatide should be used with caution in patients receiving oral medications that require rapid gastrointestinal absorption. For oral medications that are dependent on threshold concentrations for efficacy, such as contraceptives, patients should be advised to take those drugs at least 1 hr before exenatide injection. If such drugs are to be administered with food, patients should be advised to take them with a meal or snack when exenatide is not administered). Products include:

Alesse-28 Tablets 3392
Lo/Ovral-28 Tablets 3423
NuvaRing 2357
Ortho-Cept Tablets 2395
Ortho-Cyclen/Ortho Tri-Cyclen 2414
Ortho Evra Transdermal System 2402
Ortho Tri-Cyclen Lo Tablets 2421
Seasonale Tablets 1073
Triphasil-28 Tablets 3483
Yasmin 28 Tablets 818

Ethynodiol Diacetate (The effect of exenatide to slow gastric emptying may reduce the extent and rate of absorption of orally administered drugs. Exenatide should be used with caution in patients receiving oral medications that require rapid gastrointestinal absorption. For oral medications that are dependent on threshold concentrations for efficacy, such as contraceptives, patients should be advised to take those drugs at least 1 hr before exenatide injection. If such drugs are to be administered with food, patients should be advised to take them with a meal or snack when exenatide is not administered).

No products indexed under this heading.

Grepafloxacin Hydrochloride (The effect of exenatide to slow gastric emptying may reduce the extent and rate of absorption of orally administered drugs. Exenatide should be used with caution in patients receiving oral medications that require rapid gastrointestinal absorption. For oral medications that

are dependent on threshold concentrations for efficacy, such as antibiotics, patients should be advised to take those drugs at least 1 hr before exenatide injection. If such drugs are to be administered with food, patients should be advised to take them with a meal or snack when exenatide is not administered).

No products indexed under this heading.

Imipenem (The effect of exenatide to slow gastric emptying may reduce the extent and rate of absorption of orally administered drugs. Exenatide should be used with caution in patients receiving oral medications that require rapid gastrointestinal absorption. For oral medications that are dependent on threshold concentrations for efficacy, such as antibiotics, patients should be advised to take those drugs at least 1 hr before exenatide injection. If such drugs are to be administered with food, patients should be advised to take them with a meal or snack when exenatide is not administered). Products include:

Primaxin I.M. **2022**
Primaxin I.V. **2024**

Levonorgestrel (The effect of exenatide to slow gastric emptying may reduce the extent and rate of absorption of orally administered drugs. Exenatide should be used with caution in patients receiving oral medications that require rapid gastrointestinal absorption. For oral medications that are dependent on threshold concentrations for efficacy, such as contraceptives, patients should be advised to take those drugs at least 1 hr before exenatide injection. If such drugs are to be administered with food, patients should be advised to take them with a meal or snack when exenatide is not administered). Products include:

Alesse-28 Tablets **3392**
Climara Pro Transdermal System **800**
Mirena Intrauterine System **810**
Plan B Tablets **1068**
Seasonale Tablets **1073**
Triphasil-28 Tablets **3483**

Lomefloxacin Hydrochloride (The effect of exenatide to slow gastric emptying may reduce the extent and rate of absorption of orally administered drugs. Exenatide should be used with caution in patients receiving oral medications that require rapid gastrointestinal absorption. For oral medications that are dependent on threshold concentrations for efficacy, such as antibiotics, patients should be advised to take those drugs at least 1 hr before exenatide injection. If such drugs are to be administered with food, patients should be advised to take them with a meal or snack when exenatide is not administered).

No products indexed under this heading.

Loracarbef (The effect of exenatide to slow gastric emptying may reduce the extent and rate of absorption of orally administered drugs. Exenatide should be used with caution in patients receiving oral medications that require rapid gastrointestinal absorption. For oral medications that are dependent on threshold concentrations for efficacy, such as antibiotics, patients should be advised to take those drugs at least 1 hr before exenatide injection. If such drugs are to be administered with food, patients should be advised to take them with a meal or snack when exenatide is not administered).

No products indexed under this heading.

Mestranol (The effect of exenatide to slow gastric emptying may reduce the extent and rate of absorption of orally administered drugs. Exenatide should be used with caution in patients receiving oral medications that require rapid gastrointestinal absorption. For oral medications that are dependent on threshold concentrations for efficacy, such as contraceptives, patients should be advised to take those drugs at least 1 hr before exenatide injection. If such drugs are to be administered with food, patients should be advised to take them with a meal or snack when exenatide is not administered).

No products indexed under this heading.

Methacycline Hydrochloride (The effect of exenatide to slow gastric emptying may reduce the extent and rate of absorption of orally administered drugs. Exenatide should be used with caution in patients receiving oral medications that require rapid gastrointestinal absorption. For oral medications that are dependent on threshold concentrations for efficacy, such as antibiotics, patients should be advised to take those drugs at least 1 hr before exenatide injection. If such drugs are to be administered with food, patients should be advised to take them with a meal or snack when exenatide is not administered).

No products indexed under this heading.

Mezlocillin Sodium (The effect of exenatide to slow gastric emptying may reduce the extent and rate of absorption of orally administered drugs. Exenatide should be used with caution in patients receiving oral medications that require rapid gastrointestinal absorption. For oral medications that are dependent on threshold concentrations for efficacy, such as antibiotics, patients should be advised to take those drugs at least 1 hr before exenatide injection. If such drugs are to be administered with food, patients should be advised to take them with a meal or snack when exenatide is not administered).

No products indexed under this heading.

Minocycline Hydrochloride (The effect of exenatide to slow gastric emptying may reduce the extent and rate of absorption of orally administered drugs. Exenatide should be used with caution in patients receiving oral medications that require rapid gastrointestinal absorption. For oral medications that are dependent on threshold concentrations for efficacy, such as antibiotics, patients should be advised to take those drugs at least 1 hr before exenatide injection. If such drugs are to be administered with food, patients should be advised to take them with a meal or snack when exenatide is not administered). Products include:

Dynacin Tablets **1859**

Moxifloxacin Hydrochloride (The effect of exenatide to slow gastric emptying may reduce the extent and rate of absorption of orally administered drugs. Exenatide should be used with caution in patients receiving oral medications that require rapid gastrointestinal absorption. For oral medications that are dependent on threshold concentrations for efficacy, such as antibiotics, patients should be advised to take those drugs at least 1 hr before exenatide injection. If such drugs are to be administered with food, patients should be advised to take them with a meal or snack when exenatide is not administered). Products include:

Avelox **2984**
Vigamox Ophthalmic Solution **560**

Nafcillin Sodium (The effect of exenatide to slow gastric emptying may reduce the extent and rate of absorption of orally administered drugs. Exenatide should be used with caution in patients receiving oral medications that require rapid gastrointestinal absorption. For oral medications that are dependent on threshold concentrations for efficacy, such as antibiotics, patients should be advised to take those drugs at least 1 hr before exenatide injection. If such drugs are to be administered with food, patients should be advised to take them with a meal or snack when exenatide is not administered).

No products indexed under this heading.

Norethindrone (The effect of exenatide to slow gastric emptying may reduce the extent and rate of absorption of orally administered drugs. Exenatide should be used with caution in patients receiving oral medications that require rapid gastrointestinal absorption. For oral medications that are dependent on threshold concentrations for efficacy, such as contraceptives, patients should be advised to take those drugs at least 1 hr before exenatide injection. If such drugs are to be administered with food, patients should be advised to take them with a meal or snack when exenatide is not administered). Products include:

Ortho Micronor Tablets **2411**

Norethynodrel (The effect of exenatide to slow gastric emptying may reduce the extent and rate of absorption of orally administered drugs. Exenatide should be used with caution in patients receiving oral medications that require rapid gastrointestinal absorption. For oral medications that are dependent on threshold concentrations for efficacy, such as contraceptives, patients should be advised to take those drugs at least 1 hr before exenatide injection. If such drugs are to be administered with food, patients should be advised to take them with a meal or snack when exenatide is not administered).

No products indexed under this heading.

Norfloxacin (The effect of exenatide to slow gastric emptying may reduce the extent and rate of absorption of orally administered drugs. Exenatide should be used with caution in patients receiving oral medications that require rapid gastrointestinal absorption. For oral medications that are dependent on threshold concentrations for efficacy, such as antibiotics, patients should be advised to take those drugs at least 1 hr before exenatide injection. If such drugs are to be administered with food, patients should be advised to take them with a meal or snack when exenatide is not administered). Products include:

Noroxin Tablets **2009**

Norgestimate (The effect of exenatide to slow gastric emptying may reduce the extent and rate of absorption of orally administered drugs. Exenatide should be used with caution in patients receiving oral medications that require rapid gastrointestinal absorption. For oral medications that are dependent on threshold concentrations for efficacy, such as contraceptives, patients should be advised to take those drugs at least 1 hr before exenatide injection. If such drugs are to be administered with food, patients should be advised to take them with a meal or snack when exenatide is not administered). Products include:

Ortho-Cyclen/Ortho Tri-Cyclen **2414**
Ortho Tri-Cyclen Lo Tablets **2421**
Prefest Tablets **1069**

Norgestrel (The effect of exenatide to slow gastric emptying may reduce the extent and rate of absorption of orally administered drugs. Exenatide should be used with caution in patients receiving oral medications that require rapid gastrointestinal absorption. For oral medications that are dependent on threshold concentrations for efficacy, such as contraceptives, patients should be advised to take those drugs at least 1 hr before exenatide injection. If such drugs are to be administered with food, patients should be advised to take them with a meal or snack when exenatide is not administered). Products include:

Lo/Ovral-28 Tablets **3423**

Ofloxacin (The effect of exenatide to slow gastric emptying may reduce the extent and rate of absorption of orally administered drugs. Exenatide should be used with caution in patients receiving oral medications that require rapid gastrointestinal absorption. For oral medications that are dependent on threshold concentrations for efficacy, such as antibiotics, patients should be advised to take those drugs at least 1 hr before exenatide injection. If such drugs are to be administered with food, patients should be advised to take them with a meal or snack when exenatide is not administered). Products include:

Floxin Otic Singles **1045**
Floxin Otic Solution **1043**

Oral Medications, unspecified (The effect of exenatide to slow gastric emptying may reduce the extent and rate of absorption of orally administered drugs. Exenatide should be used with caution in patients receiving oral medications that require rapid gastrointestinal absorption).

No products indexed under this heading.

Oxytetracycline Hydrochloride (The effect of exenatide to slow gastric emptying may reduce the extent and rate of absorption of orally administered drugs. Exenatide should be used with caution in patients receiving oral medications that require rapid gastrointestinal absorption. For oral medications that are dependent on threshold concentrations for efficacy, such as antibiot-

ics, patients should be advised to take those drugs at least 1 hr before exenatide injection. If such drugs are to be administered with food, patients should be advised to take them with a meal or snack when exenatide is not administered).
No products indexed under this heading.

Penicillin G Benzathine (The effect of exenatide to slow gastric emptying may reduce the extent and rate of absorption of orally administered drugs. Exenatide should be used with caution in patients receiving oral medications that require rapid gastrointestinal absorption. For oral medications that are dependent on threshold concentrations for efficacy, such as antibiotics, patients should be advised to take those drugs at least 1 hr before exenatide injection. If such drugs are to be administered with food, patients should be advised to take them with a meal or snack when exenatide is not administered).
No products indexed under this heading.

Penicillin G Potassium (The effect of exenatide to slow gastric emptying may reduce the extent and rate of absorption of orally administered drugs. Exenatide should be used with caution in patients receiving oral medications that require rapid gastrointestinal absorption. For oral medications that are dependent on threshold concentrations for efficacy, such as antibiotics, patients should be advised to take those drugs at least 1 hr before exenatide injection. If such drugs are to be administered with food, patients should be advised to take them with a meal or snack when exenatide is not administered).
No products indexed under this heading.

Penicillin G Procaine (The effect of exenatide to slow gastric emptying may reduce the extent and rate of absorption of orally administered drugs. Exenatide should be used with caution in patients receiving oral medications that require rapid gastrointestinal absorption. For oral medications that are dependent on threshold concentrations for efficacy, such as antibiotics, patients should be advised to take those drugs at least 1 hr before exenatide injection. If such drugs are to be administered with food, patients should be advised to take them with a meal or snack when exenatide is not administered).
No products indexed under this heading.

Penicillin G Sodium (The effect of exenatide to slow gastric emptying may reduce the extent and rate of absorption of orally administered drugs. Exenatide should be used with caution in patients receiving oral medications that require rapid gastrointestinal absorption. For oral medications that are dependent on threshold concentrations for efficacy, such as antibiotics, patients should be advised to take those drugs at least 1 hr before exenatide injection. If such drugs are to be administered with food, patients should be advised to take them with a meal or snack when exenatide is not administered).
No products indexed under this heading.

Penicillin V Potassium (The effect of exenatide to slow gastric emptying may reduce the extent and rate of absorption of orally administered drugs. Exenatide should be used with caution in patients receiving oral medications that require rapid gastrointestinal absorption. For oral medications that are dependent on threshold concentrations for efficacy, such as antibiotics, patients should be advised to take those drugs at least 1 hr before exenatide injection. If such drugs are to be administered with food, patients should be advised to take them with a meal or snack when exenatide is not administered).
No products indexed under this heading.

Sulfamethizole (The effect of exenatide to slow gastric emptying may reduce the extent and rate of absorption of orally administered drugs. Exenatide should be used with caution in patients receiving oral medications that require rapid gastrointestinal absorption. For oral medications that are dependent on threshold concentrations for efficacy, such as antibiotics, patients should be advised to take those drugs at least 1 hr before exenatide injection. If such drugs are to be administered with food, patients should be advised to take them with a meal or snack when exenatide is not administered).
No products indexed under this heading.

Sulfamethoxazole (The effect of exenatide to slow gastric emptying may reduce the extent and rate of absorption of orally administered drugs. Exenatide should be used with caution in patients receiving oral medications that require rapid gastrointestinal absorption. For oral medications that are dependent on threshold concentrations for efficacy, such as antibiotics, patients should be advised to take those drugs at least 1 hr before exenatide injection. If such drugs are to be administered with food, patients should be advised to take them with a meal or snack when exenatide is not administered).
No products indexed under this heading.

Sulfisoxazole (The effect of exenatide to slow gastric emptying may reduce the extent and rate of absorption of orally administered drugs. Exenatide should be used with caution in patients receiving oral medications that require rapid gastrointestinal absorption. For oral medications that are dependent on threshold concentrations for efficacy, such as antibiotics, patients should be advised to take those drugs at least 1 hr before exenatide injection. If such drugs are to be administered with food, patients should be advised to take them with a meal or snack when exenatide is not administered).
No products indexed under this heading.

Sulfisoxazole Acetyl (The effect of exenatide to slow gastric emptying may reduce the extent and rate of absorption of orally administered drugs. Exenatide should be used with caution in patients receiving oral medications that require rapid gastrointestinal absorption. For oral medications that are dependent on threshold concentrations for efficacy, such as antibiotics, patients should be advised to take those drugs at least 1 hr before exenatide injection. If such drugs are to be administered with food, patients should be advised to take them with a meal or snack when exenatide is not administered).
No products indexed under this heading.

Tetracycline Hydrochloride (The effect of exenatide to slow gastric emptying may reduce the extent and rate of absorption of orally administered drugs. Exenatide should be used with caution in patients receiving oral medications that require rapid gastrointestinal absorption. For oral medications that are dependent on threshold concentrations for efficacy, such as antibiotics, patients should be advised to take those drugs at least 1 hr before exenatide injection. If such drugs are to be administered with food, patients should be advised to take them with a meal or snack when exenatide is not administered).
No products indexed under this heading.

Ticarcillin Disodium (The effect of exenatide to slow gastric emptying may reduce the extent and rate of absorption of orally administered drugs. Exenatide should be used with caution in patients receiving oral medications that require rapid gastrointestinal absorption. For oral medications that are dependent on threshold concentrations for efficacy, such as antibiotics, patients should be advised to take those drugs at least 1 hr before exenatide injection. If such drugs are to be administered with food, patients should be advised to take them with a meal or snack when exenatide is not administered). Products include:
Timentin ADD-Vantage **1556**
Timentin Injection Galaxy Container **1559**
Timentin IV Infusion **1553**
Timentin Pharmacy Bulk Package **1562**

Troleandomycin (The effect of exenatide to slow gastric emptying may reduce the extent and rate of absorption of orally administered drugs. Exenatide should be used with caution in patients receiving oral medications that require rapid gastrointestinal absorption. For oral medications that are dependent on threshold concentrations for efficacy, such as antibiotics, patients should be advised to take those drugs at least 1 hr before exenatide injection. If such drugs are to be administered with food, patients should be advised to take them with a meal or snack when exenatide is not administered).
No products indexed under this heading.

Trovafloxacin Mesylate (The effect of exenatide to slow gastric emptying may reduce the extent and rate of absorption of orally administered drugs. Exenatide should be used with caution in patients receiving oral medications that require rapid gastrointestinal absorption. For oral medications that are dependent on threshold concentrations for efficacy, such as antibiotics, patients should be advised to take those drugs at least 1 hr before exenatide injection. If such drugs are to be administered with food, patients should be advised to take them with a meal or snack when exenatide is not administered).
No products indexed under this heading.

CADUET TABLETS

(Amlodipine Besylate, Atorvastatin Calcium) **2507**
May interact with azole antifungals, erythromycin, fibrates, and certain other agents. Compounds in these categories include:

Aluminum Hydroxide (Co-administration with aluminum hydroxide/magnesium hydroxide antacid has resulted in decreased atorvastatin plasma concentrations by 35%; LDL-C reduction was unaltered). Products include:
Gaviscon Regular Strength Liquid .. ■**620**
Gaviscon Regular Strength Tablets .... ■**619**
Gaviscon Extra Strength Liquid .... ■**620**
Gaviscon Extra Strength Tablets .... ■**619**
Maalox Max Maximum Strength Antacid/Anti-Gas Liquid **2165**
Maalox Regular Strength Antacid/Antigas Liquid **2164**

Clofibrate (Co-administration with fibric acid derivatives increases the risk of myopathy).
No products indexed under this heading.

Clotrimazole (Co-administration with azole antifungals increases the risk of myopathy). Products include:
Lotrimin **3053**
Lotrisone **3054**

Colestipol Hydrochloride (Co-administration has resulted in decreased atorvastatin plasma concentrations by 25%, however; LDL-C reduction was greater when these drugs were given together than when either drug was given alone).
No products indexed under this heading.

Cyclosporine (Co-administration increases the risk of myopathy). Products include:
Gengraf Capsules **458**
Neoral Soft Gelatin Capsules **2247**
Neoral Oral Solution **2247**
Restasis Ophthalmic Emulsion **570**
Sandimmune **2259**

Digoxin (Co-administration has resulted in increased steady-state digoxin plasma concentrations by 20%). Products include:
Digitek Tablets **2146**
Lanoxicaps Capsules **1458**
Lanoxin Injection **1462**
Lanoxin Tablets **1468**
Lanoxin Injection Pediatric **1465**

Erythromycin (Co-administration increases the risk of myopathy; plasma concentrations of atorvastatin has increased by 40% when co-administered with erythromycin, a known inhibitor of cytochrome P4503A4). Products include:
Erygel Topical Gel **2096**
Ery-Tab Tablets **447**
Erythromycin Base Filmtab Tablets **454**
Erythromycin Delayed-Release Capsules, USP **456**
PCE Dispertab Tablets **510**

Erythromycin Estolate (Co-administration increases the risk of myopathy; plasma concentrations of atorvastatin has increased by 40% when co-administered with erythromycin, a known inhibitor of cytochrome P4503A4).
No products indexed under this heading.

Erythromycin Ethylsuccinate (Co-administration increases the risk of myopathy; plasma concentrations of atorvastatin has increased by 40% when co-administered with erythromycin, a known inhibitor of cytochrome P4503A4). Products include:
E.E.S. ... 449
EryPed ... 445

Erythromycin Gluceptate (Co-administration increases the risk of myopathy; plasma concentrations of atorvastatin has increased by 40% when co-administered with erythromycin, a known inhibitor of cytochrome P4503A4).
No products indexed under this heading.

Erythromycin Lactobionate (Co-administration increases the risk of myopathy; plasma concentrations of atorvastatin has increased by 40% when co-administered with erythromycin, a known inhibitor of cytochrome P4503A4).
No products indexed under this heading.

Erythromycin Stearate (Co-administration increases the risk of myopathy; plasma concentrations of atorvastatin has increased by 40% when co-administered with erythromycin, a known inhibitor of cytochrome P4503A4). Products include:
Erythrocin Stearate Filmtab Tablets ... 452

Ethinyl Estradiol (Co-administration with an oral contraceptive has increased AUC values for norethindrone and ethinyl estradiol by 30% and 20%, respectively). Products include:
Alesse-28 Tablets ... 3392
Lo/Ovral-28 Tablets ... 3423
NuvaRing ... 2357
Ortho-Cept Tablets ... 2395
Ortho-Cyclen/Ortho Tri-Cyclen ... 2414
Ortho Evra Transdermal System ... 2402
Ortho Tri-Cyclen Lo Tablets ... 2421
Seasonale Tablets ... 1073
Triphasil-28 Tablets ... 3483
Yasmin 28 Tablets ... 818

Fenofibrate (Co-administration with fibric acid derivatives increases the risk of myopathy). Products include:
Antara Capsules ... 2723
Lofibra Capsules ... 1217
Tricor Tablets ... 523
Triglide Tablets ... 1165

Fluconazole (Co-administration with azole antifungals increases the risk of myopathy).
No products indexed under this heading.

Gemfibrozil (Co-administration with fibric acid derivatives increases the risk of myopathy).
No products indexed under this heading.

Itraconazole (Co-administration with azole antifungals increases the risk of myopathy).
No products indexed under this heading.

Ketoconazole (Co-administration with azole antifungals increases the risk of myopathy). Products include:
Nizoral A-D Shampoo, 1% ... 1839
Nizoral 2% Shampoo ... 1838

Miconazole (Co-administration with azole antifungals increases the risk of myopathy).
No products indexed under this heading.

Niacin (Co-administration increases the risk of myopathy). Products include:
Advicor Tablets ... 1694
Niaspan Extended-Release Tablets ... 1703

Norethindrone (Co-administration with an oral contraceptive has increased AUC values for norethindrone and ethinyl estradiol by 30% and 20%; respectively). Products include:
Ortho Micronor Tablets ... 2411

Oxiconazole Nitrate (Co-administration with azole antifungals increases the risk of myopathy). Products include:
Oxistat ... 1498

Terconazole (Co-administration with azole antifungals increases the risk of myopathy).
No products indexed under this heading.

CAFCIT INJECTION

(Caffeine Citrate) ... 1854
May interact with cytochrome p450 1a2 inducers (selected), cytochrome p450 1a2 inhibitors (selected), cytochrome p450 1a2 substrates (selected), phenytoin, xanthines, and certain other agents. Compounds in these categories include:

Acetaminophen (Caffeine has the potential to interact with drugs that are substrates for CYP1A2). Products include:
Benadryl Allergy & Cold Tablets ... ■692
Benadryl Allergy & Sinus Headache Caplets & Gelcaps ... ■693
Benadryl Maximum Strength Severe Allergy & Sinus Headache Caplets ... ■694
Contac Severe Cold and Flu Caplets Maximum Strength ... ■615
Contac Severe Cold and Flu Caplets Non-Drowsy ... ■615
Darvocet A 500 Tablets ... 3497
Goody's Body Pain Formula Powder ... ■621
Goody's Extra Strength Headache Powder ... ■621
Goody's Extra Strength Pain Relief Tablets ... ■621
Goody's PM Powder ... ■622
Hycomine Compound Tablets ... 1105
Lortab ... 3315
Lortab Elixir ... 3312
Percocet Tablets ... 1114
Robitussin Cough, Cold & Flu Liquid-filled Capsules ... ■750
Robitussin Flu Liquid ... ■752
Sedapap Tablets 50 mg/650 mg ... 2098
Singlet Caplets ... ■636
Sudafed Severe Cold ... ■710
Sudafed Sinus Headache ... ■711
TheraFlu Cold & Cough Hot Liquid ... ■680
TheraFlu Cold & Sore Throat Hot Liquid ... ■680
TheraFlu Flu & Chest Congestion Non-Drowsy Hot Liquid ... ■681
TheraFlu Flu & Sore Throat Hot Liquid ... ■681
TheraFlu Severe Cold Non-Drowsy Hot Liquid ... ■683
TheraFlu Severe Cold & Cough Hot Liquid ... ■683
TheraFlu Severe Cold Caplets ... ■679
TheraFlu Severe Cold Hot Liquid ... ■682
TheraFlu Severe Cold Non-Drowsy Caplets ... ■679
Triaminic Cough & Sore Throat Liquid ... ■687
Triaminic Flu, Cough & Fever Liquid ... ■685
Triaminic Cough & Sore Throat Softchews ... ■689
Tylenol 8 Hour Extended Release Geltabs and Caplets ... 1843
Tylenol Sinus NightTime Caplets ... ■663
Children's Tylenol Suspension Liquid and Meltaways ... 1850
Children's Tylenol Plus Cold & Allergy Suspension Liquid ... 1850
Children's Tylenol Plus Cold NightTime Suspension Liquid ... 1851
Children's Tylenol Plus Cold & Cough Suspension Liquid and Chewable Tablets ... 1851
Children's Tylenol Plus Cold Chewable Tablets ... 1851
Children's Tylenol Plus Cold Daytime Non-Drowsy Suspension Liquid ... 1851
Children's Tylenol Plus Flu Suspension Liquid ... 1853
Concentrated Tylenol Infants' Drops Plus Cold ... 1851
Concentrated Tylenol Infants' Drops Plus Cold and Cough ... 1851
Concentrated Tylenol Infants' Drops ... 1850
Junior Tylenol Meltaways ... 1850
Tylenol Cold & Flu Severe Daytime Liquid with Cool Burst ... 1846
Tylenol Cold & Flu Severe NightTime Liquid with Cool Burst ... 1846
Tylenol Cold Severe Congestion Non-Drowsy Caplets with Cool Burst ... 1846
Tylenol Cough & Sore Throat Daytime Liquid with Cool Burst ... 1849
Tylenol Cough & Sore Throat NightTime Liquid with Cool Burst ... 1849
Tylenol ... 1843
Extra Strength Tylenol Rapid Release Gels ... 1843
Tylenol ... 1843
Tylenol Allergy Complete Night Time Caplets ... 1844
Tylenol Allergy Complete Multi-Symptom Caplets and Gelcaps with Cool Burst ... 1844
Tylenol Severe Allergy Caplets ... 1844
Tylenol Flu NightTime Gelcaps ... 1846
Tylenol Flu Day Non-Drowsy Gelcaps ... 1846
Concentrated Tylenol Infants' Drops Plus Cold Nasal Congestant, Fever Reducer & Pain Reliever ... ■668
Concentrated Tylenol Infants' Drops Plus Cold & Cough Nasal Decongestant, Fever Reducer & Pain Reliever ... ■668
Multi-Symptom Tylenol Cold Night Time Caplets ... 1845
Multi-Symptom Tylenol Cold Day Non-Drowsy Caplets and Gelcaps ... 1845
Extra Strength Tylenol PM Caplets, Geltabs, Gelcaps and Liquid ... 1847
Tylenol Sinus Day Non-Drowsy ... 1848
Tylenol Sinus Night Time Caplets ... 1848
Tylenol Sinus Severe Congestion Caplets with Cool Burst ... 1848
Tylenol Sore Throat Daytime Liquid with Cool Burst ... 1849
Tylenol Sore Throat NightTime Liquid with Cool Burst ... 1849
Tylenol with Codeine ... 2461
Women's Tylenol Menstrual Relief Caplets ... 1849
Ultracet Tablets ... 2462
Vicks 44M Cough, Cold & Flu Relief ... 2676
Vicks DayQuil LiquiCaps/Liquid Multi-Symptom Cold/Flu Relief ... ■723
Vicks DayQuil Multi-Symptom Cold/Flu Relief LiquiCaps ... 2675
Vicks DayQuil Multi-Symptom Cold/Flu Relief Liquid ... 2675
Vicks NyQuil LiquiCaps ... 2677
Vicks NyQuil LiquiCaps/Liquid Multi-Symptom Cold/Flu Relief ... ■725
Vicks NyQuil Liquid ... 2677
Vicodin Tablets ... 530
Vicodin ES Tablets ... 531
Vicodin HP Tablets ... 532
Zydone Tablets ... 1118

Alatrofloxacin Mesylate (Caffeine has the potential to interact with drugs that inhibit CYP1A2).
No products indexed under this heading.

Aminophylline (Interconversion between caffeine and theophylline has been reported in preterm neonates; the concurrent use of these drugs is not recommended).
No products indexed under this heading.

Amiodarone Hydrochloride (Caffeine has the potential to interact with drugs that inhibit CYP1A2). Products include:
Pacerone Tablets ... 3337

Amitriptyline Hydrochloride (Caffeine has the potential to interact with drugs that are substrates for CYP1A2).
No products indexed under this heading.

Amoxapine (Caffeine has the potential to interact with drugs that are substrates for CYP1A2).
No products indexed under this heading.

Anagrelide Hydrochloride (Caffeine has the potential to interact with drugs that are substrates for CYP1A2). Products include:
Agrylin Capsules ... 3172

Anastrozole (Caffeine has the potential to interact with drugs that inhibit CYP1A2). Products include:
Arimidex Tablets ... 665

Caffeine (Caffeine has the potential to interact with drugs that are substrates for CYP1A2). Products include:
Athena Hair System Shampoo ... ■767
BC Powder ... ■612
Arthritis Strength BC Powder ... ■612
Goody's Extra Strength Headache Powder ... ■621
Goody's Extra Strength Pain Relief Tablets ... ■621
Hycomine Compound Tablets ... 1105
Spartan Hair System Shampoo ... ■767
Vivarin ... ■639

Caffeine Anhydrous (Caffeine has the potential to interact with drugs that are substrates for CYP1A2).
No products indexed under this heading.

Carbamazepine (Caffeine has the potential to interact with drugs that induce CYP1A2). Products include:
Carbatrol Capsules ... 3174
Equetro Extended-Release Capsules ... 3178
Tegretol/Tegretol-XR ... 2278

Chlordiazepoxide (Caffeine has the potential to interact with drugs that are substrates for CYP1A2).
No products indexed under this heading.

Chlordiazepoxide Hydrochloride (Caffeine has the potential to interact with drugs that are substrates for CYP1A2). Products include:
Librium Capsules ... 3349

Cimetidine (Co-administration of caffeine with cimetidine may result in reduced caffeine elimination; lower doses of caffeine may be needed). Products include:
Tagamet HB 200 Tablets ... ■637
Tagamet Tablets ... 1547

Cimetidine Hydrochloride (Co-administration of caffeine with cimetidine may result in reduced caffeine elimination; lower doses of caffeine may be needed).
No products indexed under this heading.

Ciprofloxacin (Caffeine has the potential to interact with drugs that inhibit CYP1A2). Products include:
Cipro I.V. ... 2998
Cipro I.V. Pharmacy Bulk Package ... 3509
Cipro Oral Suspension ... 2991
Cipro XR Tablets ... 3004
Ciprodex Otic Suspension ... 555

Ciprofloxacin Hydrochloride (Caffeine has the potential to interact with drugs that inhibit CYP1A2). Products include:
Ciloxan Ophthalmic Ointment ... 554
Cipro Tablets ... 2991

Citalopram Hydrobromide (Caffeine has the potential to interact with drugs that induce CYP1A2). Products include:
Celexa ... 1177

Clarithromycin (Caffeine has the potential to interact with drugs that inhibit CYP1A2). Products include:
Biaxin/Biaxin XL ... 402
PREVPAC ... 3281

Clomipramine Hydrochloride (Caffeine has the potential to interact with drugs that are substrates for CYP1A2).
No products indexed under this heading.

Clopidogrel Bisulfate (Caffeine has the potential to interact with drugs that are substrates for CYP1A2). Products include:
Plavix Tablets ... 940
Plavix Tablets ... 2942

Clozapine (Caffeine has the potential to interact with drugs that are substrates for CYP1A2). Products include:
Clozapine Tablets ... 2141
Clozaril Tablets ... 2174
FazaClo Orally Disintegrating Tablets ... 547

Cyclobenzaprine (Caffeine has the potential to interact with drugs that are substrates for CYP1A2).
No products indexed under this heading.

Cyclobenzaprine Hydrochloride (Caffeine has the potential to interact with drugs that are substrates for CYP1A2). Products include:
Flexeril Tablets ... 1832

Desipramine Hydrochloride (Caffeine has the potential to interact with drugs that are substrates for CYP1A2).
No products indexed under this heading.

Desogestrel (Caffeine has the potential to interact with drugs that inhibit CYP1A2). Products include:
Ortho-Cept Tablets ... 2395

Diazepam (Caffeine has the potential to interact with drugs that are substrates for CYP1A2). Products include:
Diastat Rectal Delivery System ... 3344
Valium Tablets ... 2822

Diltiazem Hydrochloride (Caffeine has the potential to interact with drugs that induce CYP1A2). Products include:
Cardizem LA Extended Release Tablets ... 1699
Tiazac Capsules ... 1204

Diltiazem Maleate (Caffeine has the potential to interact with drugs that induce CYP1A2).
No products indexed under this heading.

Doxepin Hydrochloride (Caffeine has the potential to interact with drugs that are substrates for CYP1A2).
No products indexed under this heading.

Dyphylline (Interconversion between caffeine and theophylline has been reported in preterm neonates; the concurrent use of these drugs is not recommended).
No products indexed under this heading.

Enoxacin (Caffeine has the potential to interact with drugs that inhibit CYP1A2).
No products indexed under this heading.

Erythromycin (Caffeine has the potential to interact with drugs that induce CYP1A2). Products include:
Erygel Topical Gel ... 2096
Ery-Tab Tablets ... 447
Erythromycin Base Filmtab Tablets ... 454
Erythromycin Delayed-Release Capsules, USP ... 456
PCE Dispertab Tablets ... 510

Erythromycin Estolate (Caffeine has the potential to interact with drugs that induce CYP1A2).
No products indexed under this heading.

Erythromycin Ethylsuccinate (Caffeine has the potential to interact with drugs that induce CYP1A2). Products include:
E.E.S. ... 449
EryPed ... 445

Erythromycin Gluceptate (Caffeine has the potential to interact with drugs that induce CYP1A2).
No products indexed under this heading.

Erythromycin Lactobionate (Caffeine has the potential to interact with drugs that induce CYP1A2).
No products indexed under this heading.

Erythromycin Stearate (Caffeine has the potential to interact with drugs that induce CYP1A2). Products include:
Erythrocin Stearate Filmtab Tablets ... 452

Estradiol (Caffeine has the potential to interact with drugs that are substrates for CYP1A2). Products include:
Activella Tablets ... 2311
Climara Transdermal System ... 795
Climara Pro Transdermal System ... 800
CombiPatch Transdermal System ... 2180
Estrogel 0.06% ... 3200
Menostar Transdermal System ... 805
Prefest Tablets ... 1069
Vagifem Tablets ... 2340
Vivelle Transdermal System ... 2288
Vivelle-Dot Transdermal System ... 2293

Estradiol Benzoate (Caffeine has the potential to interact with drugs that are substrates for CYP1A2).
No products indexed under this heading.

Estradiol Cypionate (Caffeine has the potential to interact with drugs that are substrates for CYP1A2).
No products indexed under this heading.

Ethinyl Estradiol (Caffeine has the potential to interact with drugs that inhibit CYP1A2). Products include:
Alesse-28 Tablets ... 3392
Lo/Ovral-28 Tablets ... 3423
NuvaRing ... 2357
Ortho-Cept Tablets ... 2395
Ortho-Cyclen/Ortho Tri-Cyclen ... 2414
Ortho Evra Transdermal System ... 2402
Ortho Tri-Cyclen Lo Tablets ... 2421
Seasonale Tablets ... 1073
Triphasil-28 Tablets ... 3483
Yasmin 28 Tablets ... 818

Flutamide (Caffeine has the potential to interact with drugs that are substrates for CYP1A2). Products include:
Eulexin Capsules ... 3023

Fluticasone Propionate (Caffeine has the potential to interact with drugs that are substrates for CYP1A2). Products include:
Advair Diskus 100/50 ... 1291
Advair Diskus 250/50 ... 1291
Advair Diskus 500/50 ... 1291
Cutivate Cream ... 1381
Cutivate Lotion 0.05% ... 1383
Cutivate Ointment ... 1384
Flonase Nasal Spray ... 1412
Flovent Diskus 100 mcg ... 1418
Flovent Diskus 50 mcg ... 1415

Fluvoxamine (Caffeine has the potential to interact with drugs that inhibit CYP1A2).
No products indexed under this heading.

Fluvoxamine Maleate (Caffeine has the potential to interact with drugs that induce CYP1A2).
No products indexed under this heading.

Fosphenytoin Sodium (Co-administration of caffeine with phenytoin may result in increased caffeine elimination; higher doses of caffeine may be needed).
No products indexed under this heading.

Gatifloxacin (Caffeine has the potential to interact with drugs that inhibit CYP1A2). Products include:
Tequin Injection ... 964
Tequin Tablets ... 964
Zymar Ophthalmic Solution ... 571

Gemifloxacin Mesylate (Caffeine has the potential to interact with drugs that inhibit CYP1A2). Products include:
Factive Tablets ... 2464

Grepafloxacin Hydrochloride (Caffeine has the potential to interact with drugs that inhibit CYP1A2).
No products indexed under this heading.

Haloperidol (Caffeine has the potential to interact with drugs that are substrates for CYP1A2).
No products indexed under this heading.

Haloperidol Decanoate (Caffeine has the potential to interact with drugs that are substrates for CYP1A2).
No products indexed under this heading.

Haloperidol Lactate (Caffeine has the potential to interact with drugs that are substrates for CYP1A2).
No products indexed under this heading.

Hypericum (Caffeine has the potential to interact with drugs that induce CYP1A2).
No products indexed under this heading.

Imipramine Hydrochloride (Caffeine has the potential to interact with drugs that are substrates for CYP1A2).
No products indexed under this heading.

Imipramine Pamoate (Caffeine has the potential to interact with drugs that are substrates for CYP1A2).
No products indexed under this heading.

Insulin (Caffeine has the potential to interact with drugs that induce CYP1A2).
No products indexed under this heading.

Isoniazid (Caffeine has the potential to interact with drugs that inhibit CYP1A2).
No products indexed under this heading.

Ketoconazole (Co-administration of caffeine with ketoconazole may result in reduced caffeine elimination; lower doses of caffeine may be needed). Products include:
Nizoral A-D Shampoo, 1% ... 1839
Nizoral 2% Shampoo ... 1838

Ketoprofen (Co-administration results in reduced urine volume in healthy volunteers).
No products indexed under this heading.

Lansoprazole (Caffeine has the potential to interact with drugs that induce CYP1A2). Products include:
Prevacid Delayed-Release Capsules ... 3268
Prevacid for Delayed-Release Oral Suspension ... 3268
Prevacid I.V. for Injection ... 3274
Prevacid NapraPAC ... 3277
Prevacid SoluTab Delayed-Release Orally Disintegrating Tablets ... 3268
PREVPAC ... 3281

Levobupivacaine Hydrochloride (Caffeine has the potential to interact with drugs that are substrates for CYP1A2).
No products indexed under this heading.

Levofloxacin (Caffeine has the potential to interact with drugs that inhibit CYP1A2). Products include:
Levaquin in 5% Dextrose Injection ... 2453
Levaquin ... 2453
Quixin Ophthalmic Solution ... 3373

Levonorgestrel (Caffeine has the potential to interact with drugs that inhibit CYP1A2). Products include:
Alesse-28 Tablets ... 3392
Climara Pro Transdermal System ... 800
Mirena Intrauterine System ... 810
Plan B Tablets ... 1068
Seasonale Tablets ... 1073
Triphasil-28 Tablets ... 3483

Lomefloxacin Hydrochloride (Caffeine has the potential to interact with drugs that inhibit CYP1A2).
No products indexed under this heading.

Maprotiline Hydrochloride (Caffeine has the potential to interact with drugs that are substrates for CYP1A2).
No products indexed under this heading.

Mestranol (Caffeine has the potential to interact with drugs that inhibit CYP1A2).
No products indexed under this heading.

Methadone Hydrochloride (Caffeine has the potential to interact with drugs that are substrates for CYP1A2).
No products indexed under this heading.

Methoxsalen (Caffeine has the potential to interact with drugs that inhibit CYP1A2). Products include:

Oxsoralen Lotion 1% 3354
Oxsoralen-Ultra Capsules 3354

Mexiletine Hydrochloride (Caffeine has the potential to interact with drugs that inhibit CYP1A2).
No products indexed under this heading.

Mibefradil Dihydrochloride (Caffeine has the potential to interact with drugs that inhibit CYP1A2).
No products indexed under this heading.

Mirtazapine (Caffeine has the potential to interact with drugs that are substrates for CYP1A2).
No products indexed under this heading.

Moxifloxacin Hydrochloride (Caffeine has the potential to interact with drugs that inhibit CYP1A2). Products include:
Avelox 2984
Vigamox Ophthalmic Solution 560

Nafcillin Sodium (Caffeine has the potential to interact with drugs that induce CYP1A2).
No products indexed under this heading.

Nalidixic Acid (Caffeine has the potential to interact with drugs that inhibit CYP1A2).
No products indexed under this heading.

Naproxen (Caffeine has the potential to interact with drugs that are substrates for CYP1A2). Products include:
EC-Naprosyn Delayed-Release Tablets 2769
Naprosyn Suspension 2769
Naprosyn Tablets 2769
Prevacid NapraPAC 3277

Naproxen Sodium (Caffeine has the potential to interact with drugs that are substrates for CYP1A2). Products include:
Aleve Tablets, Caplets and Gelcaps 605
Anaprox Tablets 2769
Anaprox DS Tablets 2769

Nicotine (Caffeine has the potential to interact with drugs that induce CYP1A2). Products include:
Nicoderm CQ Patch 1629
NicoDerm CQ Clear Patch 627
Nicotrol Inhaler 2594
Nicotrol NS 2596

Nicotine Polacrilex (Caffeine has the potential to interact with drugs that induce CYP1A2). Products include:
Commit Lozenges 1625
Nicorette Gum 1632

Nicotine Salicylate (Caffeine has the potential to interact with drugs that induce CYP1A2).
No products indexed under this heading.

Nicotine Sulfate (Caffeine has the potential to interact with drugs that induce CYP1A2).
No products indexed under this heading.

Norethindrone (Caffeine has the potential to interact with drugs that inhibit CYP1A2). Products include:
Ortho Micronor Tablets 2411

Norethindrone Acetate (Caffeine has the potential to interact with drugs that are substrates for CYP1A2). Products include:
Activella Tablets 2311
Aygestin Tablets 1062
CombiPatch Transdermal System 2180

Norfloxacin (Caffeine has the potential to interact with drugs that inhibit CYP1A2). Products include:
Noroxin Tablets 2009

Norgestrel (Caffeine has the potential to interact with drugs that inhibit CYP1A2). Products include:
Lo/Ovral-28 Tablets 3423

Nortriptyline Hydrochloride (Caffeine has the potential to interact with drugs that are substrates for CYP1A2).
No products indexed under this heading.

Ofloxacin (Caffeine has the potential to interact with drugs that inhibit CYP1A2). Products include:
Floxin Otic Singles 1045
Floxin Otic Solution 1043

Olanzapine (Caffeine has the potential to interact with drugs that are substrates for CYP1A2). Products include:
Symbyax Capsules 1788
Zyprexa Tablets 1798
Zyprexa IntraMuscular 1798
Zyprexa ZYDIS Orally Disintegrating Tablets 1798

Omeprazole (Caffeine has the potential to interact with drugs that induce CYP1A2). Products include:
Zegerid Powder for Oral Solution 2972

Ondansetron (Caffeine has the potential to interact with drugs that are substrates for CYP1A2). Products include:
Zofran ODT Orally Disintegrating Tablets 1613

Ondansetron Hydrochloride (Caffeine has the potential to interact with drugs that are substrates for CYP1A2). Products include:
Zofran Injection 1607
Zofran 1613

Paroxetine Hydrochloride (Caffeine has the potential to interact with drugs that inhibit CYP1A2). Products include:
Paxil CR Controlled-Release Tablets 1509
Paxil 1501

Phenobarbital (Co-administration of caffeine with phenobarbital may result in increased caffeine elimination; higher doses of caffeine may be needed).
No products indexed under this heading.

Phenobarbital Sodium (Caffeine has the potential to interact with drugs that are substrates for CYP1A2).
No products indexed under this heading.

Phenytoin (Co-administration of caffeine with phenytoin may result in increased caffeine elimination; higher doses of caffeine may be needed).
No products indexed under this heading.

Phenytoin Sodium (Co-administration of caffeine with phenytoin may result in increased caffeine elimination; higher doses of caffeine may be needed). Products include:
Phenytek Capsules 2153

Primidone (Caffeine has the potential to interact with drugs that induce CYP1A2).
No products indexed under this heading.

Propafenone Hydrochloride (Caffeine has the potential to interact with drugs that are substrates for CYP1A2). Products include:
Rythmol SR Capsules 2736

Propranolol Hydrochloride (Caffeine has the potential to interact with drugs that are substrates for CYP1A2). Products include:
Inderal LA Long-Acting Capsules 3421
InnoPran XL Capsules 2728

Protriptyline Hydrochloride (Caffeine has the potential to interact with drugs that are substrates for CYP1A2). Products include:
Vivactil Tablets 2350

Ranitidine Hydrochloride (Caffeine has the potential to interact with drugs that inhibit CYP1A2). Products include:
Zantac 1597
Zantac Injection 1593
Zantac 75 Tablets 715
Zantac 150 Maximum Strength Tablets 715
Zantac Injection Pharmacy Bulk Package 1595

Rifampicin (Caffeine has the potential to interact with drugs that induce CYP1A2).
No products indexed under this heading.

Rifampin (Caffeine has the potential to interact with drugs that induce CYP1A2).
No products indexed under this heading.

Riluzole (Caffeine has the potential to interact with drugs that are substrates for CYP1A2). Products include:
Rilutek Tablets 2945

Ritonavir (Caffeine has the potential to interact with drugs that induce CYP1A2). Products include:
Kaletra 474
Norvir 499

Ropinirole Hydrochloride (Caffeine has the potential to interact with drugs that are substrates for CYP1A2). Products include:
Requip Tablets 1528

Ropivacaine Hydrochloride (Caffeine has the potential to interact with drugs that are substrates for CYP1A2). Products include:
Naropin Injection 640

Sparfloxacin (Caffeine has the potential to interact with drugs that inhibit CYP1A2).
No products indexed under this heading.

Tacrine Hydrochloride (Caffeine has the potential to interact with drugs that inhibit CYP1A2).
No products indexed under this heading.

Tamoxifen Citrate (Caffeine has the potential to interact with drugs that are substrates for CYP1A2).
No products indexed under this heading.

Theophylline (Interconversion between caffeine and theophylline has been reported in preterm neonates; the concurrent use of these drugs is not recommended).
No products indexed under this heading.

Theophylline Anhydrous (Interconversion between caffeine and theophylline has been reported in preterm neonates; the concurrent use of these drugs is not recommended). Products include:
Uniphyl Tablets 2708

Theophylline Calcium Salicylate (Interconversion between caffeine and theophylline has been reported in preterm neonates; the concurrent use of these drugs is not recommended).
No products indexed under this heading.

Theophylline Dihydroxypropyl (Glyceryl) (Interconversion between caffeine and theophylline has been reported in preterm neonates; the concurrent use of these drugs is not recommended).
No products indexed under this heading.

Theophylline Ethylenediamine (Interconversion between caffeine and theophylline has been reported in preterm neonates; the concurrent use of these drugs is not recommended).
No products indexed under this heading.

Theophylline Sodium Glycinate (Interconversion between caffeine and theophylline has been reported in preterm neonates; the concurrent use of these drugs is not recommended).
No products indexed under this heading.

Ticlopidine Hydrochloride (Caffeine has the potential to interact with drugs that inhibit CYP1A2). Products include:
Ticlid Tablets 2813

Tobacco (Caffeine has the potential to interact with drugs that induce CYP1A2).
No products indexed under this heading.

Trimethaphan Camsylate (Caffeine has the potential to interact with drugs that are substrates for CYP1A2).
No products indexed under this heading.

Trimipramine Maleate (Caffeine has the potential to interact with drugs that are substrates for CYP1A2). Products include:
Surmontil Capsules 2347

Troleandomycin (Caffeine has the potential to interact with drugs that inhibit CYP1A2).
No products indexed under this heading.

Trovafloxacin Mesylate (Caffeine has the potential to interact with drugs that inhibit CYP1A2).
No products indexed under this heading.

Verapamil Hydrochloride (Caffeine has the potential to interact with drugs that are substrates for CYP1A2). Products include:
Covera-HS Tablets 3135
Tarka Tablets 519
Verelan PM Capsules 3120

Warfarin Sodium (Caffeine has the potential to interact with drugs that are substrates for CYP1A2). Products include:
Coumadin for Injection 932
Coumadin Tablets 932

Zileuton (Caffeine has the potential to interact with drugs that inhibit CYP1A2).
No products indexed under this heading.

Zolmitriptan (Caffeine has the potential to interact with drugs that are substrates for CYP1A2). Products include:
Zomig Nasal Spray 718

Zomig Tablets 714
Zomig-ZMT Tablets 714

Food Interactions

Broccoli (Caffeine has the potential to interact with drugs that induce CYP1A2).

Brussel Sprouts (Caffeine has the potential to interact with drugs that induce CYP1A2).

Charbroiled Food (Caffeine has the potential to interact with drugs that induce CYP1A2).

Grapefruit Juice (Caffeine has the potential to interact with drugs that inhibit CYP1A2).

CAFCIT ORAL SOLUTION

(Caffeine Citrate) 1854
May interact with:

See (Cafcit Injection).

CALCIJEX INJECTION

(Calcitriol) 411
May interact with:

Magnesium Carbonate (Co-administration with magnesium-containing antacids may lead to the development of hypermagnesemia; concurrent use should be avoided). Products include:
Gaviscon Regular Strength Liquid .. ▣620
Gaviscon Extra Strength Liquid ...... ▣620
Gaviscon Extra Strength Tablets .... ▣619

Magnesium Hydroxide (Co-administration with magnesium-containing antacids may lead to the development of hypermagnesemia; concurrent use should be avoided). Products include:
Maalox Max Maximum Strength Antacid/Anti-Gas Liquid................ 2165
Maalox Regular Strength Antacid/Antigas Liquid.................. 2164
Pepcid Complete Chewable Tablets.. 1672
Rolaids Tablets .... ▣707
Extra Strength Rolaids Tablets .... ▣707
Rolaids Multi-Symptom Antacid & Antigas Tablets........................... ▣708

Vitamin D (Since calcitriol is the most potent metabolite of vitamin D available, vitamin D and its derivatives should be withheld during treatment). Products include:
Active Calcium Tablets 3342
Caltrate 600 PLUS Chewables .... ▣779
Caltrate 600 PLUS Tablets .... ▣779
Caltrate 600 + D Tablets .... ▣779
Os-Cal 250 + D Tablets .... ▣765
Os-Cal 500 + D Tablets .... ▣766

CALCIUM DISODIUM VERSENATE INJECTION

(Calcium Disodium Edetate) 1819
May interact with:

Insulin, Human, Zinc Suspension (Interference with the action of zinc insulin by chelating the zinc). Products include:
Humulin L, 100 Units 1763
Humulin U, 100 Units 1770

Insulin, Zinc Crystals (Interference with the action of zinc insulin by chelating the zinc).
No products indexed under this heading.

Insulin, Zinc Suspension (Interference with the action of zinc insulin by chelating the zinc).
No products indexed under this heading.

Steroids, unspecified (Enhances renal toxicity of edetate calcium disodium in animals).
No products indexed under this heading.

CALTRATE 600 PLUS CHEWABLES

(Calcium Carbonate, Minerals, Multiple, Vitamin D)......................... ▣779
None cited in PDR database.

CALTRATE 600 PLUS TABLETS

(Calcium Carbonate, Minerals, Multiple, Vitamin D)......................... ▣779
None cited in PDR database.

CALTRATE 600 + D TABLETS

(Calcium Carbonate, Vitamin D) .... ▣779
None cited in PDR database.

CAMPATH AMPULES

(Alemtuzumab) 826
May interact with:

Live Virus Vaccines (Patients who have recently received Campath, should not be immunized with live viral vaccines due to their immunosuppression).
No products indexed under this heading.

CAMPRAL TABLETS

(Acamprosate Calcium) 1175
May interact with antidepressant drugs and certain other agents. Compounds in these categories include:

Amitriptyline Hydrochloride (Patients taking acaprosate calcium concomitantly with antidepressants more commonly reported both weight gain and weight loss, compared with patients taking either medication alone).
No products indexed under this heading.

Amoxapine (Patients taking acaprosate calcium concomitantly with antidepressants more commonly reported both weight gain and weight loss, compared with patients taking either medication alone).
No products indexed under this heading.

Bupropion Hydrochloride (Patients taking acaprosate calcium concomitantly with antidepressants more commonly reported both weight gain and weight loss, compared with patients taking either medication alone). Products include:
Wellbutrin Tablets 1579
Wellbutrin SR Sustained-Release Tablets.. 1583
Wellbutrin XL Extended-Release Tablets.. 1588
Zyban Sustained-Release Tablets 1620

Citalopram Hydrobromide (Patients taking acaprosate calcium concomitantly with antidepressants more commonly reported both weight gain and weight loss, compared with patients taking either medication alone). Products include:
Celexa 1177

Desipramine Hydrochloride (Patients taking acaprosate calcium concomitantly with antidepressants more commonly reported both weight gain and weight loss, compared with patients taking either medication alone).
No products indexed under this heading.

Doxepin Hydrochloride (Patients taking acaprosate calcium concomitantly with antidepressants more commonly reported both weight gain and weight loss, compared with patients taking either medication alone).
No products indexed under this heading.

Escitalopram Oxalate (Patients taking acaprosate calcium concomitantly with antidepressants more commonly reported both weight gain and weight loss, compared with patients taking either medication alone). Products include:
Lexapro Oral Solution 1193
Lexapro Tablets 1193

Fluoxetine Hydrochloride (Patients taking acaprosate calcium concomitantly with antidepressants more commonly reported both weight gain and weight loss, compared with patients taking either medication alone). Products include:
Prozac Pulvules and Liquid 1771
Symbyax Capsules 1788

Imipramine Hydrochloride (Patients taking acaprosate calcium concomitantly with antidepressants more commonly reported both weight gain and weight loss, compared with patients taking either medication alone).
No products indexed under this heading.

Imipramine Pamoate (Patients taking acaprosate calcium concomitantly with antidepressants more commonly reported both weight gain and weight loss, compared with patients taking either medication alone).
No products indexed under this heading.

Isocarboxazid (Patients taking acaprosate calcium concomitantly with antidepressants more commonly reported both weight gain and weight loss, compared with patients taking either medication alone).
No products indexed under this heading.

Maprotiline Hydrochloride (Patients taking acaprosate calcium concomitantly with antidepressants more commonly reported both weight gain and weight loss, compared with patients taking either medication alone).
No products indexed under this heading.

Mirtazapine (Patients taking acaprosate calcium concomitantly with antidepressants more commonly reported both weight gain and weight loss, compared with patients taking either medication alone).
No products indexed under this heading.

Naltrexone Hydrochloride (Co-administration of naltrexone with acamprosate calcium produced a 25% increase in AUC and a 33% increase in the Cmax of acamprosate. No adjustment of dosage is recommended in such patients).
No products indexed under this heading.

Nefazodone Hydrochloride (Patients taking acaprosate calcium concomitantly with antidepressants more commonly reported both weight gain and weight loss, compared with patients taking either medication alone).
No products indexed under this heading.

Nortriptyline Hydrochloride (Patients taking acaprosate calcium concomitantly with antidepressants more commonly reported both weight gain and weight loss, compared with patients taking either medication alone).
No products indexed under this heading.

Paroxetine Hydrochloride (Patients taking acaprosate calcium concomitantly with antidepressants more commonly reported both weight gain and weight loss, compared with patients taking either medication alone). Products include:
Paxil CR Controlled-Release Tablets.. 1509
Paxil 1501

Phenelzine Sulfate (Patients taking acaprosate calcium concomitantly with antidepressants more commonly reported both weight gain and weight loss, compared with patients taking either medication alone).
No products indexed under this heading.

Protriptyline Hydrochloride (Patients taking acaprosate calcium concomitantly with antidepressants more commonly reported both weight gain and weight loss, compared with patients taking either medication alone). Products include:
Vivactil Tablets 2350

Sertraline Hydrochloride (Patients taking acaprosate calcium concomitantly with antidepressants more commonly reported both weight gain and weight loss, compared with patients taking either medication alone). Products include:
Zoloft 2581

Tranylcypromine Sulfate (Patients taking acaprosate calcium concomitantly with antidepressants more commonly reported both weight gain and weight loss, compared with patients taking either medication alone). Products include:
Parnate Tablets 1499

Trazodone Hydrochloride (Patients taking acaprosate calcium concomitantly with antidepressants more commonly reported both weight gain and weight loss, compared with patients taking either medication alone).
No products indexed under this heading.

Trimipramine Maleate (Patients taking acaprosate calcium concomitantly with antidepressants more commonly reported both weight gain and weight loss, compared with patients taking either medication alone). Products include:
Surmontil Capsules 2347

Venlafaxine Hydrochloride (Patients taking acaprosate calcium concomitantly with antidepressants more commonly reported both weight gain and weight loss, compared with patients taking either medication alone). Products include:
Effexor Tablets 3405
Effexor XR Capsules 3411

CAMPTOSAR INJECTION

(Irinotecan Hydrochloride) 2602
May interact with antineoplastics, dexamethasone, diuretics, oral hypoglycemic agents, insulin, laxatives, phenytoin, and certain other agents. Compounds in these categories include:

Acarbose (Hyperglycemia has been reported in patients receiving irinote-

can and it is probable that the administration of dexamethasone as antiemetic prophylaxis may have contributed to hyperglycemia in some patients). Products include:

Precose Tablets ... 776

Altretamine (Co-administration may exacerbate the adverse effects of irinotecan, such as myelosuppression and diarrhea). Products include:

Hexalen Capsules ... 2101

Amiloride Hydrochloride (Co-administration with diuretics may increase the potential risk of dehydration secondary to vomiting and/or diarrhea induced by irinotecan; the physician may wish to withhold diuretics during dosing with Camptosar and, certainly, during periods of active vomiting or diarrhea). Products include:

Midamor Tablets ... 2000
Moduretic Tablets ... 2003

Anastrozole (Co-administration may exacerbate the adverse effects of irinotecan, such as myelosuppression and diarrhea). Products include:

Arimidex Tablets ... 665

Asparaginase (Co-administration may exacerbate the adverse effects of irinotecan, such as myelosuppression and diarrhea). Products include:

Elspar for Injection ... 1943

Bendroflumethiazide (Co-administration with diuretics may increase the potential risk of dehydration secondary to vomiting and/or diarrhea induced by irinotecan; the physician may wish to withhold diuretics during dosing with Camptosar and, certainly, during periods of active vomiting or diarrhea).

No products indexed under this heading.

Bicalutamide (Co-administration may exacerbate the adverse effects of irinotecan, such as myelosuppression and diarrhea). Products include:

Casodex Tablets ... 670

Bisacodyl (Co-administration with laxatives may worsen the incidence or severity of diarrhea). Products include:

Dulcolax Suppositories ... 608
Dulcolax Tablets ... 607
Fleet Bisacodyl Laxatives ... 1169
Fleet Prep Kits ... 1172
HalfLytely and Bisacodyl Tablets Bowel Prep Kit with Flavors Packs ... 915

Bleomycin Sulfate (Co-administration may exacerbate the adverse effects of irinotecan, such as myelosuppression and diarrhea).

No products indexed under this heading.

Bumetanide (Co-administration with diuretics may increase the potential risk of dehydration secondary to vomiting and/or diarrhea induced by irinotecan; the physician may wish to withhold diuretics during dosing with Camptosar and, certainly, during periods of active vomiting or diarrhea).

No products indexed under this heading.

Busulfan (Co-administration may exacerbate the adverse effects of irinotecan, such as myelosuppression and diarrhea). Products include:

I.V. Busulfex ... 1125
Myleran Tablets ... 1492

Carbamazepine (Exposure to irinotecan and its active metabolite SN-38 is substantially reduced in adult and pediatric patients concomitantly receiving the CYP3A4 enzyme-inducing anticonvulsants phenytoin, phenobarbital, or carbamazepine. The appropriate starting dose for patients taking these anticonvulsants has not been formally defined. For patients requiring anticonvulsant treatment, consideration should be given to substituting non-enzyme inducing anticonvulsants at least 2 weeks prior to initiation of irinotecan-therapy). Products include:

Carbatrol Capsules ... 3174
Equetro Extended-Release Capsules ... 3178
Tegretol/Tegretol-XR ... 2278

Carboplatin (Co-administration may exacerbate the adverse effects of irinotecan, such as myelosuppression and diarrhea).

No products indexed under this heading.

Carmustine (BCNU) (Co-administration may exacerbate the adverse effects of irinotecan, such as myelosuppression and diarrhea).

No products indexed under this heading.

Cascara Sagrada (Co-administration with laxatives may worsen the incidence or severity of diarrhea).

No products indexed under this heading.

Castor Oil (Co-administration with laxatives may worsen the incidence or severity of diarrhea). Products include:

Xenaderm Ointment ... 1638

Chlorambucil (Co-administration may exacerbate the adverse effects of irinotecan, such as myelosuppression and diarrhea). Products include:

Leukeran Tablets ... 1472

Chlorothiazide (Co-administration with diuretics may increase the potential risk of dehydration secondary to vomiting and/or diarrhea induced by irinotecan; the physician may wish to withhold diuretics during dosing with Camptosar and, certainly, during periods of active vomiting or diarrhea). Products include:

Aldoclor Tablets ... 1881
Diuril Oral ... 1936

Chlorothiazide Sodium (Co-administration with diuretics may increase the potential risk of dehydration secondary to vomiting and/or diarrhea induced by irinotecan; the physician may wish to withhold diuretics during dosing with Camptosar and, certainly, during periods of active vomiting or diarrhea). Products include:

Diuril Sodium Intravenous ... 1934

Chlorpropamide (Hyperglycemia has been reported in patients receiving irinotecan and it is probable that the administration of dexamethasone as antiemetic prophylaxis may have contributed to hyperglycemia in some patients).

No products indexed under this heading.

Chlorthalidone (Co-administration with diuretics may increase the potential risk of dehydration secondary to vomiting and/or diarrhea induced by irinotecan; the physician may wish to withhold diuretics during dosing with Camptosar and, certainly, during periods of active vomiting or diarrhea). Products include:

Clorpres Tablets ... 2139

Cisplatin (Co-administration may exacerbate the adverse effects of irinotecan, such as myelosuppression and diarrhea).

No products indexed under this heading.

Cyclophosphamide (Co-administration may exacerbate the adverse effects of irinotecan, such as myelosuppression and diarrhea).

No products indexed under this heading.

Dacarbazine (Co-administration may exacerbate the adverse effects of irinotecan, such as myelosuppression and diarrhea).

No products indexed under this heading.

Daunorubicin Citrate (Co-administration may exacerbate the adverse effects of irinotecan, such as myelosuppression and diarrhea).

No products indexed under this heading.

Daunorubicin Hydrochloride (Co-administration may exacerbate the adverse effects of irinotecan, such as myelosuppression and diarrhea). Products include:

Cerubidine for Injection ... 788

Denileukin Diftitox (Co-administration may exacerbate the adverse effects of irinotecan, such as myelosuppression and diarrhea). Products include:

Ontak Vials ... 1717

Dexamethasone (Lymphocytopenia has been reported in patients receiving irinotecan and it is possible that the administration of dexamethasone as antiemetic prophylaxis may have enhanced the likelihood of this effect. Dexamethasone does not appear to alter the pharmacokinetics of irinotecan). Products include:

Ciprodex Otic Suspension ... 555
Decadron Tablets ... 1929
TobraDex Ophthalmic Ointment ... 558
TobraDex Ophthalmic Suspension ... 558

Dexamethasone Acetate (Lymphocytopenia has been reported in patients receiving irinotecan and it is possible that the administration of dexamethasone as antiemetic prophylaxis may have enhanced the likelihood of this effect. Dexamethasone does not appear to alter the pharmacokinetics of irinotecan).

No products indexed under this heading.

Dexamethasone Sodium Phosphate (Lymphocytopenia has been reported in patients receiving irinotecan and it is possible that the administration of dexamethasone as antiemetic prophylaxis may have enhanced the likelihood of this effect. Dexamethasone does not appear to alter the pharmacokinetics of irinotecan). Products include:

Decadron Phosphate Injection ... 1931

Docetaxel (Co-administration may exacerbate the adverse effects of irinotecan, such as myelosuppression and diarrhea). Products include:

Taxotere Injection Concentrate ... 2947

Docusate Sodium (Co-administration with laxatives may worsen the incidence or severity of diarrhea). Products include:

Colace Capsules ... 729
Colace Capsules 50 mg ... 2715
Colace Capsules 100 mg ... 2715
Colace Liquid 1% Solution ... 2716
Colace Syrup ... 2716
Dulcolax Stool Softener ... 608
Peri-Colace Tablets ... 2716
Senokot-S Tablets ... 2717

Doxorubicin Hydrochloride (Co-administration may exacerbate the adverse effects of irinotecan, such as myelosuppression and diarrhea). Products include:

Adriamycin for Injection, USP ... 786
Adriamycin Injection, USP ... 786

Epirubicin Hydrochloride (Co-administration may exacerbate the adverse effects of irinotecan, such as myelosuppression and diarrhea). Products include:

Ellence Injection ... 2632

Estramustine Phosphate Sodium (Co-administration may exacerbate the adverse effects of irinotecan, such as myelosuppression and diarrhea). Products include:

Emcyt Capsules ... 3137

Ethacrynic Acid (Co-administration with diuretics may increase the potential risk of dehydration secondary to vomiting and/or diarrhea induced by irinotecan; the physician may wish to withhold diuretics during dosing with Camptosar and, certainly, during periods of active vomiting or diarrhea). Products include:

Edecrin Tablets ... 1941

Etoposide (Co-administration may exacerbate the adverse effects of irinotecan, such as myelosuppression and diarrhea).

No products indexed under this heading.

Exemestane (Co-administration may exacerbate the adverse effects of irinotecan, such as myelosuppression and diarrhea). Products include:

Aromasin Tablets ... 2600

Floxuridine (Co-administration may exacerbate the adverse effects of irinotecan, such as myelosuppression and diarrhea).

No products indexed under this heading.

Fluorouracil (Co-administration may exacerbate the adverse effects of irinotecan, such as myelosuppression and diarrhea). Products include:

Carac Cream, 0.5% ... 1048
Efudex ... 3348

Flutamide (Co-administration may exacerbate the adverse effects of irinotecan, such as myelosuppression and diarrhea). Products include:

Eulexin Capsules ... 3023

Fosphenytoin Sodium (Exposure to irinotecan and its active metabolite SN-38 is substantially reduced in adult and pediatric patients concomitantly receiving the CYP3A4 enzyme-inducing anticonvulsants phenytoin, phenobarbital, or carbamazepine. The appropriate starting dose for patients taking these anticonvulsants has not been formally defined. For patients requiring anticonvulsant treatment, consideration should be given to substituting non-enzyme inducing anticonvulsants at least 2 weeks prior to initiation of irinotecantherapy).

No products indexed under this heading.

Furosemide (Co-administration with diuretics may increase the potential risk of dehydration secondary to vomiting and/or diarrhea induced by irinotecan; the physician may wish to withhold diuretics during dosing with Camptosar and, certainly, during periods of active vomiting or diarrhea). Products include:

Furosemide Tablets ... 2117

Gemcitabine Hydrochloride (Co-administration may exacerbate the adverse effects of irinotecan, such as myelosuppression and diarrhea). Products include:
Gemzar for Injection 1743

Glimepiride (Hyperglycemia has been reported in patients receiving irinotecan and it is probable that the administration of dexamethasone as antiemetic prophylaxis may have contributed to hyperglycemia in some patients). Products include:
Amaryl Tablets 2864

Glipizide (Hyperglycemia has been reported in patients receiving irinotecan and it is probable that the administration of dexamethasone as antiemetic prophylaxis may have contributed to hyperglycemia in some patients).
No products indexed under this heading.

Glyburide (Hyperglycemia has been reported in patients receiving irinotecan and it is probable that the administration of dexamethasone as antiemetic prophylaxis may have contributed to hyperglycemia in some patients).
No products indexed under this heading.

Hydrochlorothiazide (Co-administration with diuretics may increase the potential risk of dehydration secondary to vomiting and/or diarrhea induced by irinotecan; the physician may wish to withhold diuretics during dosing with Camptosar and, certainly, during periods of active vomiting or diarrhea). Products include:
Aldoril Tablets 1884
Atacand HCT 637
Avalide Tablets 2889
Avalide Tablets 922
Benicar HCT Tablets 2852
Diovan HCT Tablets 2195
Dyazide Capsules 1389
Hyzaar 1964
Lotensin HCT Tablets 2235
Maxzide 2150
Micardis HCT Tablets 886
Moduretic Tablets 2003
Prinzide Tablets 2033
Teveten HCT Tablets 1710
Timolide Tablets 2056
Uniretic Tablets 3114
Vaseretic Tablets 2073
Zestoretic Tablets 701

Hydroflumethiazide (Co-administration with diuretics may increase the potential risk of dehydration secondary to vomiting and/or diarrhea induced by irinotecan; the physician may wish to withhold diuretics during dosing with Camptosar and, certainly, during periods of active vomiting or diarrhea).
No products indexed under this heading.

Hydroxyurea (Co-administration may exacerbate the adverse effects of irinotecan, such as myelosuppression and diarrhea).
No products indexed under this heading.

Hypericum (St. John's Wort is an inducer of CYP2A4 enzymes. Exposure to the active metabolite SN-38 is reduced in patients receiving concomitant St. John's Wort. St. John's Wort should be discontinued at least 2 weeks prior to the first cycle of irinotecan and St. John's Wort is contraindicated during irinotecan therapy).
No products indexed under this heading.

Idarubicin Hydrochloride (Co-administration may exacerbate the adverse effects of irinotecan, such as myelosuppression and diarrhea). Products include:
Idamycin PFS Injection 2645

Ifosfamide (Co-administration may exacerbate the adverse effects of irinotecan, such as myelosuppression and diarrhea).
No products indexed under this heading.

Indapamide (Co-administration with diuretics may increase the potential risk of dehydration secondary to vomiting and/or diarrhea induced by irinotecan; the physician may wish to withhold diuretics during dosing with Camptosar and, certainly, during periods of active vomiting or diarrhea). Products include:
Indapamide Tablets 2119

Insulin, Human, Zinc Suspension (Hyperglycemia has been reported in patients receiving irinotecan and it is probable that the administration of dexamethasone as antiemetic prophylaxis may have contributed to hyperglycemia in some patients). Products include:
Humulin L, 100 Units 1763
Humulin U, 100 Units 1770

Insulin, Human NPH (Hyperglycemia has been reported in patients receiving irinotecan and it is probable that the administration of dexamethasone as antiemetic prophylaxis may have contributed to hyperglycemia in some patients). Products include:
Humulin N, 100 Units 1764
Humulin N Pen 1765
Novolin N Human Insulin 10 ml Vials 2322
Novolin N InnoLet 2322
Novolin N PenFill 3 ml Cartridges 2325
Novolin R InnoLet 2322

Insulin, Human Regular (Hyperglycemia has been reported in patients receiving irinotecan and it is probable that the administration of dexamethasone as antiemetic prophylaxis may have contributed to hyperglycemia in some patients). Products include:
Humulin R (U-500) 1768
Humulin R, 100 Units 1767
Novolin R Human Insulin 10 ml Vials 2322
Novolin R PenFill 2325

Insulin, Human Regular and Human NPH Mixture (Hyperglycemia has been reported in patients receiving irinotecan and it is probable that the administration of dexamethasone as antiemetic prophylaxis may have contributed to hyperglycemia in some patients). Products include:
Humulin 50/50, 100 Units 1760
Humulin 70/30 Pen 1761
Novolin 70/30 Human Insulin 10 ml Vials 2321
Novolin 70/30 InnoLet 2322
Novolin 70/30 PenFill 3 ml Cartridges 2325

Insulin, NPH (Hyperglycemia has been reported in patients receiving irinotecan and it is probable that the administration of dexamethasone as antiemetic prophylaxis may have contributed to hyperglycemia in some patients).
No products indexed under this heading.

Insulin, Regular (Hyperglycemia has been reported in patients receiving irinotecan and it is probable that the administration of dexamethasone as antiemetic prophylaxis may have contributed to hyperglycemia in some patients).
No products indexed under this heading.

Insulin, Zinc Crystals (Hyperglycemia has been reported in patients receiving irinotecan and it is probable that the administration of dexamethasone as antiemetic prophylaxis may have contributed to hyperglycemia in some patients).
No products indexed under this heading.

Insulin, Zinc Suspension (Hyperglycemia has been reported in patients receiving irinotecan and it is probable that the administration of dexamethasone as antiemetic prophylaxis may have contributed to hyperglycemia in some patients).
No products indexed under this heading.

Insulin Aspart, Human Regular (Hyperglycemia has been reported in patients receiving irinotecan and it is probable that the administration of dexamethasone as antiemetic prophylaxis may have contributed to hyperglycemia in some patients). Products include:
NovoLog Injection 2326

Insulin glargine (Hyperglycemia has been reported in patients receiving irinotecan and it is probable that the administration of dexamethasone as antiemetic prophylaxis may have contributed to hyperglycemia in some patients). Products include:
Lantus Injection 2925

Insulin Lispro, Human (Hyperglycemia has been reported in patients receiving irinotecan and it is probable that the administration of dexamethasone as antiemetic prophylaxis may have contributed to hyperglycemia in some patients). Products include:
Humalog-Pen 1751
Humalog Mix 75/25-Pen 1754

Insulin Lispro Protamine, Human (Hyperglycemia has been reported in patients receiving irinotecan and it is probable that the administration of dexamethasone as antiemetic prophylaxis may have contributed to hyperglycemia in some patients). Products include:
Humalog Mix 75/25-Pen 1754

Interferon alfa-2a, Recombinant (Co-administration may exacerbate the adverse effects of irinotecan, such as myelosuppression and diarrhea). Products include:
Roferon-A Injection 2805

Interferon alfa-2b, Recombinant (Co-administration may exacerbate the adverse effects of irinotecan, such as myelosuppression and diarrhea). Products include:
Intron A for Injection 3038
Rebetron Combination Therapy 3078

Ketoconazole (Ketoconazole is a strong inhibitor of CYP3A4 enzymes. Patients receiving concomitant ketoconazole have increased exposure to irinotecan and its active metabolite SN-38. Patients should discontinue ketoconazole at least 1 week prior to starting irinotecan therapy and ketoconazole is contraindicated during irinotecan therapy). Products include:
Nizoral A-D Shampoo, 1% 1839
Nizoral 2% Shampoo 1838

Lactulose (Co-administration with laxatives may worsen the incidence or severity of diarrhea). Products include:
Kristalose for Oral Solution 2149

Levamisole Hydrochloride (Co-administration may exacerbate the adverse effects of irinotecan, such as myelosuppression and diarrhea).
No products indexed under this heading.

Lomustine (CCNU) (Co-administration may exacerbate the adverse effects of irinotecan, such as myelosuppression and diarrhea).
No products indexed under this heading.

Mechlorethamine Hydrochloride (Co-administration may exacerbate the adverse effects of irinotecan, such as myelosuppression and diarrhea). Products include:
Mustargen for Injection 2007

Megestrol Acetate (Co-administration may exacerbate the adverse effects of irinotecan, such as myelosuppression and diarrhea). Products include:
Megace ES Oral Suspension 2492

Melphalan (Co-administration may exacerbate the adverse effects of irinotecan, such as myelosuppression and diarrhea). Products include:
Alkeran Tablets 977

Mercaptopurine (Co-administration may exacerbate the adverse effects of irinotecan, such as myelosuppression and diarrhea). Products include:
Purinethol Tablets 1222

Metformin Hydrochloride (Hyperglycemia has been reported in patients receiving irinotecan and it is probable that the administration of dexamethasone as antiemetic prophylaxis may have contributed to hyperglycemia in some patients). Products include:
ActoPlus Met Tablets 3219
Avandamet Tablets 1343
Fortamet Extended-Release Tablets 1156

Methotrexate Sodium (Co-administration may exacerbate the adverse effects of irinotecan, such as myelosuppression and diarrhea).
No products indexed under this heading.

Methyclothiazide (Co-administration with diuretics may increase the potential risk of dehydration secondary to vomiting and/or diarrhea induced by irinotecan; the physician may wish to withhold diuretics during dosing with Camptosar and, certainly, during periods of active vomiting or diarrhea).
No products indexed under this heading.

Methylcellulose (Co-administration with laxatives may worsen the incidence or severity of diarrhea). Products include:
Citrucel Caplets .... ■□614
Citrucel Orange Flavor Powder ...... ■□613
Citrucel Sugar Free Orange Flavor Powder .... ■□613

Metolazone (Co-administration with diuretics may increase the potential risk of dehydration secondary to vomiting and/or diarrhea induced by irinotecan; the physician may wish to withhold diuretics during dosing with Camptosar and, certainly, during periods of active vomiting or diarrhea).
No products indexed under this heading.

Miglitol (Hyperglycemia has been reported in patients receiving irinotecan and it is probable that the administration of dexamethasone as antiemetic prophylaxis may have contributed to hyperglycemia in some patients).
No products indexed under this heading.

Mitomycin (Mitomycin-C) (Co-administration may exacerbate the adverse effects of irinotecan, such as myelosuppression and diarrhea).
No products indexed under this heading.

Mitotane (Co-administration may exacerbate the adverse effects of irinotecan, such as myelosuppression and diarrhea).
No products indexed under this heading.

Mitoxantrone Hydrochloride (Co-administration may exacerbate the adverse effects of irinotecan, such as myelosuppression and diarrhea). Products include:
Novantrone for Injection Concentrate **3158**

Oxaliplatin (Co-administration may exacerbate the adverse effects of irinotecan, such as myelosuppression and diarrhea). Products include:
Eloxatin for Injection **2908**

Paclitaxel (Co-administration may exacerbate the adverse effects of irinotecan, such as myelosuppression and diarrhea).
No products indexed under this heading.

Phenobarbital (Exposure to irinotecan and its active metabolite SN-38 is substantially reduced in adult and pediatric patients concomitantly receiving the CYP3A4 enzyme-inducing anticonvulsants phenytoin, phenobarbital, or carbamazepine. The appropriate starting dose for patients taking these anticonvulsants has not been formally defined. For patients requiring anticonvulsant treatment, consideration should be given to substituting non-enzyme inducing anticonvulsants at least 2 weeks prior to initiation of irinotecantherapy).
No products indexed under this heading.

Phenobarbital Sodium (Exposure to irinotecan and its active metabolite SN-38 is substantially reduced in adult and pediatric patients concomitantly receiving the CYP3A4 enzyme-inducing anticonvulsants phenytoin, phenobarbital, or carbamazepine. The appropriate starting dose for patients taking these anticonvulsants has not been formally defined. For patients requiring anticonvulsant treatment, consideration should be given to substituting non-enzyme inducing anticonvulsants at least 2 weeks prior to initiation of irinotecantherapy).
No products indexed under this heading.

Phenolphthalein (Co-administration with laxatives may worsen the incidence or severity of diarrhea).
No products indexed under this heading.

Phenytoin (Exposure to irinotecan and its active metabolite SN-38 is substantially reduced in adult and pediatric patients concomitantly receiving the CYP3A4 enzyme-inducing anticonvulsants phenytoin, phenobarbital, or carbamazepine. The appropriate starting dose for patients taking these anticonvulsants has not been formally defined. For patients requiring anticonvulsant treatment, consideration should be given to substituting non-enzyme inducing anticonvulsants at least 2 weeks prior to initiation of irinotecantherapy).
No products indexed under this heading.

Phenytoin Sodium (Exposure to irinotecan and its active metabolite SN-38 is substantially reduced in adult and pediatric patients concomitantly receiving the CYP3A4 enzyme-inducing anticonvulsants phenytoin, phenobarbital, or carbamazepine. The appropriate starting dose for patients taking these anticonvulsants has not been formally defined. For patients requiring anticonvulsant treatment, consideration should be given to substituting non-enzyme inducing anticonvulsants at least 2 weeks prior to initiation of irinotecan-therapy). Products include:
Phenytek Capsules **2153**

Pioglitazone Hydrochloride (Hyperglycemia has been reported in patients receiving irinotecan and it is probable that the administration of dexamethasone as antiemetic prophylaxis may have contributed to hyperglycemia in some patients). Products include:
ActoPlus Met Tablets **3219**
Actos Tablets **3224**

Polythiazide (Co-administration with diuretics may increase the potential risk of dehydration secondary to vomiting and/or diarrhea induced by irinotecan; the physician may wish to withhold diuretics during dosing with Camptosar and, certainly, during periods of active vomiting or diarrhea).
No products indexed under this heading.

Procarbazine Hydrochloride (Co-administration may exacerbate the adverse effects of irinotecan, such as myelosuppression and diarrhea). Products include:
Matulane Capsules **3188**

Prochlorperazine (May increase the incidence of akathisia).
No products indexed under this heading.

Psyllium Preparations (Co-administration with laxatives may worsen the incidence or severity of diarrhea). Products include:
Experience Capsules **760**
Metamucil Capsules **2672**
Metamucil **2672**
Metamucil Dietary Fiber Supplement **774**

Repaglinide (Hyperglycemia has been reported in patients receiving irinotecan and it is probable that the administration of dexamethasone as antiemetic prophylaxis may have contributed to hyperglycemia in some patients). Products include:
Prandin Tablets (0.5, 1, and 2 mg) **2337**

Rosiglitazone Maleate (Hyperglycemia has been reported in patients receiving irinotecan and it is probable that the administration of dexamethasone as antiemetic prophylaxis may have contributed to hyperglycemia in some patients). Products include:
Avandamet Tablets **1343**
Avandia Tablets **1348**

Senna (Co-administration with laxatives may worsen the incidence or severity of diarrhea). Products include:
Peri-Colace Tablets **730**
Senokot Tablets **2717**
Senokot-S Tablets **2717**

Spironolactone (Co-administration with diuretics may increase the potential risk of dehydration secondary to vomiting and/or diarrhea induced by irinotecan; the physician may wish to withhold diuretics during dosing with Camptosar and, certainly, during periods of active vomiting or diarrhea).
No products indexed under this heading.

Streptozocin (Co-administration may exacerbate the adverse effects of irinotecan, such as myelosuppression and diarrhea).
No products indexed under this heading.

Tamoxifen Citrate (Co-administration may exacerbate the adverse effects of irinotecan, such as myelosuppression and diarrhea).
No products indexed under this heading.

Teniposide (Co-administration may exacerbate the adverse effects of irinotecan, such as myelosuppression and diarrhea).
No products indexed under this heading.

Thioguanine (Co-administration may exacerbate the adverse effects of irinotecan, such as myelosuppression and diarrhea). Products include:
Tabloid Tablets **1545**

Thiotepa (Co-administration may exacerbate the adverse effects of irinotecan, such as myelosuppression and diarrhea).
No products indexed under this heading.

Tolazamide (Hyperglycemia has been reported in patients receiving irinotecan and it is probable that the administration of dexamethasone as antiemetic prophylaxis may have contributed to hyperglycemia in some patients).
No products indexed under this heading.

Tolbutamide (Hyperglycemia has been reported in patients receiving irinotecan and it is probable that the administration of dexamethasone as antiemetic prophylaxis may have contributed to hyperglycemia in some patients).
No products indexed under this heading.

Topotecan Hydrochloride (Co-administration may exacerbate the adverse effects of irinotecan, such as myelosuppression and diarrhea). Products include:
Hycamtin for Injection **1427**

Toremifene Citrate (Co-administration may exacerbate the adverse effects of irinotecan, such as myelosuppression and diarrhea).
No products indexed under this heading.

Torsemide (Co-administration with diuretics may increase the potential risk of dehydration secondary to vomiting and/or diarrhea induced by irinotecan; the physician may wish to withhold diuretics during dosing with Camptosar and, certainly, during periods of active vomiting or diarrhea).
No products indexed under this heading.

Triamterene (Co-administration with diuretics may increase the potential risk of dehydration secondary to vomiting and/or diarrhea induced by irinotecan; the physician may wish to withhold diuretics during dosing with Camptosar and, certainly, during periods of active vomiting or diarrhea). Products include:
Dyazide Capsules **1389**
Dyrenium Capsules **3390**
Maxzide **2150**

Troglitazone (Hyperglycemia has been reported in patients receiving irinotecan and it is probable that the administration of dexamethasone as antiemetic prophylaxis may have contributed to hyperglycemia in some patients).
No products indexed under this heading.

Valrubicin (Co-administration may exacerbate the adverse effects of irinotecan, such as myelosuppression and diarrhea).
No products indexed under this heading.

Vincristine Sulfate (Co-administration may exacerbate the adverse effects of irinotecan, such as myelosuppression and diarrhea).
No products indexed under this heading.

Vinorelbine Tartrate (Co-administration may exacerbate the adverse effects of irinotecan, such as myelosuppression and diarrhea). Products include:
Navelbine Injection **1494**

CANASA RECTAL SUPPOSITORIES

(Mesalamine) **726**
May interact with:

Sulfasalazine (Patients on concurrent oral products that contain or release mesalamine should be carefully monitored with urinalysis, BUN and creatinine testing).
No products indexed under this heading.

CANCIDAS FOR INJECTION

(Caspofungin acetate) **1894**
May interact with dexamethasone, phenytoin, and certain other agents. Compounds in these categories include:

Carbamazepine (The results from regression analyses of patient pharmacokinetic data suggest that co-administration of inducers of drug clearance and/or mixed inducers/inhibitors with caspofungin may result in clinically meaningful reductions in caspofungin concentrations; an increase in the daily dose of caspofungin to 70 mg, following the

usual 70-mg loading dose, should be considered in patients who are not clinically responding during concomitant therapy). Products include:
Carbatrol Capsules 3174
Equetro Extended-Release Capsules 3178
Tegretol/Tegretol-XR 2278

Cyclosporine (Co-administration with cyclosporine results in increased AUC of caspofungin by approximately 35%; there were transient increases in liver ALT and AST during co-administration; concomitant use is not recommended unless the potential benefit outweighs the potential risk to the patient). Products include:
Gengraf Capsules 458
Neoral Soft Gelatin Capsules 2247
Neoral Oral Solution 2247
Restasis Ophthalmic Emulsion 570
Sandimmune 2259

Dexamethasone (The results from regression analyses of patient pharmacokinetic data suggest that co-administration of inducers of drug clearance and/or mixed inducers/inhibitors with caspofungin may result in clinically meaningful reductions in caspofungin concentrations; an increase in the daily dose of caspofungin to 70 mg, following the usual 70-mg loading dose, should be considered in patients who are not clinically responding during concomitant therapy). Products include:
Ciprodex Otic Suspension 555
Decadron Tablets 1929
TobraDex Ophthalmic Ointment 558
TobraDex Ophthalmic Suspension 558

Dexamethasone Acetate (The results from regression analyses of patient pharmacokinetic data suggest that co-administration of inducers of drug clearance and/or mixed inducers/inhibitors with caspofungin may result in clinically meaningful reductions in caspofungin concentrations; an increase in the daily dose of caspofungin to 70 mg, following the usual 70-mg loading dose, should be considered in patients who are not clinically responding during concomitant therapy).
No products indexed under this heading.

Dexamethasone Sodium Phosphate (The results from regression analyses of patient pharmacokinetic data suggest that co-administration of inducers of drug clearance and/or mixed inducers/inhibitors with caspofungin may result in clinically meaningful reductions in caspofungin concentrations; an increase in the daily dose of caspofungin to 70 mg, following the usual 70-mg loading dose, should be considered in patients who are not clinically responding during concomitant therapy). Products include:
Decadron Phosphate Injection 1931

Efavirenz (The results from regression analyses of patient pharmacokinetic data suggest that co-administration of inducers of drug clearance and/or mixed inducers/inhibitors with caspofungin may result in clinically meaningful reductions in caspofungin concentrations; an increase in the daily dose of caspofungin to 70 mg, following the usual 70-mg loading dose, should be considered in patients who are not clinically responding during concomitant therapy). Products include:
Sustiva Capsules 957

Fosphenytoin Sodium (The results from regression analyses of patient pharmacokinetic data suggest that co-administration of inducers of drug clearance and/or mixed inducers/inhibitors with caspofungin may result in clinically meaningful reductions in caspofungin concentrations; an increase in the daily dose of caspofungin to 70 mg, following the usual 70-mg loading dose, should be considered in patients who are not clinically responding during concomitant therapy).
No products indexed under this heading.

Nelfinavir Mesylate (The results from regression analyses of patient pharmacokinetic data suggest that co-administration of inducers of drug clearance and/or mixed inducers/inhibitors with caspofungin may result in clinically meaningful reductions in caspofungin concentrations; an increase in the daily dose of caspofungin to 70 mg, following the usual 70-mg loading dose, should be considered in patients who are not clinically responding during concomitant therapy). Products include:
Viracept 2556

Nevirapine (The results from regression analyses of patient pharmacokinetic data suggest that co-administration of inducers of drug clearance and/or mixed inducers/inhibitors with caspofungin may result in clinically meaningful reductions in caspofungin concentrations; an increase in the daily dose of caspofungin to 70 mg, following the usual 70-mg loading dose, should be considered in patients who are not clinically responding during concomitant therapy). Products include:
Viramune Oral Suspension 903
Viramune Tablets 903

Phenytoin (The results from regression analyses of patient pharmacokinetic data suggest that co-administration of inducers of drug clearance and/or mixed inducers/inhibitors with caspofungin may result in clinically meaningful reductions in caspofungin concentrations; an increase in the daily dose of caspofungin to 70 mg, following the usual 70-mg loading dose, should be considered in patients who are not clinically responding during concomitant therapy).
No products indexed under this heading.

Phenytoin Sodium (The results from regression analyses of patient pharmacokinetic data suggest that co-administration of inducers of drug clearance and/or mixed inducers/inhibitors with caspofungin may result in clinically meaningful reductions in caspofungin concentrations; an increase in the daily dose of caspofungin to 70 mg, following the usual 70-mg loading dose, should be considered in patients who are not clinically responding during concomitant therapy). Products include:
Phenytek Capsules 2153

Rifampin (The results from regression analyses of patient pharmacokinetic data suggest that co-administration of inducers of drug clearance and/or mixed inducers/inhibitors with caspofungin may result in clinically meaningful reductions in caspofungin concentrations; an increase in the daily dose of caspofungin to 70 mg, following the usual 70-mg loading dose, should be considered in patients who are not clinically responding during concomitant therapy).
No products indexed under this heading.

Tacrolimus (Co-administration with tacrolimus reduces the AUC of tacrolimus by approximately 20%, peak blood concentration by 16% and 12-hour blood concentration by 26%; standard monitoring of tacrolimus blood concentrations and appropriate tacrolimus dosage adjustments are recommended). Products include:
Prograf Capsules and Injection 624
Protopic Ointment 629

CAPASTAT SULFATE FOR INJECTION

(Capreomycin Sulfate) 1728
May interact with aminoglycosides, antituberculosis drugs, and certain other agents. Compounds in these categories include:

Amikacin Sulfate (Additive ototoxicity and/or nephrotoxicity).
No products indexed under this heading.

Aminosalicylic Acid (Potential for febrile reactions and abnormal liver function tests). Products include:
Paser Granules 1657

p-Aminosalicylic Acid (Potential for febrile reactions and abnormal liver function tests).
No products indexed under this heading.

Colistin Sulfate (Additive ototoxicity and/or nephrotoxicity).
No products indexed under this heading.

Cycloserine (Potential for febrile reactions and abnormal liver function tests). Products include:
Seromycin Capsules 1783

Ethambutol Hydrochloride (Potential for febrile reactions and abnormal liver function tests).
No products indexed under this heading.

Ether (May enhance the partial neuromuscular blockade caused by capreomycin).
No products indexed under this heading.

Gentamicin Sulfate (Additive ototoxicity and/or nephrotoxicity). Products include:
Garamycin Injectable 3028
Genoptic Sterile Ophthalmic Solution .... ⊙ 227
Pred-G Ophthalmic Suspension .... ⊙ 234
Pred-G Sterile Ophthalmic Ointment .... ⊙ 235

Isoniazid (Potential for febrile reactions and abnormal liver function tests).
No products indexed under this heading.

Kanamycin Sulfate (Additive ototoxicity and/or nephrotoxicity).
No products indexed under this heading.

Neomycin, oral (Additive ototoxicity and/or nephrotoxicity).
No products indexed under this heading.

Neostigmine Bromide (May antagonize the partial neuromuscular blockade caused by capreomycin).
No products indexed under this heading.

Neostigmine Methylsulfate (May antagonize the partial neuromuscular blockade caused by capreomycin).
No products indexed under this heading.

Paromomycin Sulfate (Additive ototoxicity and/or nephrotoxicity).
No products indexed under this heading.

Polymyxin B Sulfate (Additive ototoxicity and/or nephrotoxicity). Products include:
Neosporin Ointment .... ■ 702
Neosporin + Pain Relief Maximum Strength Cream .... ■ 703
Neosporin + Pain Relief Maximum Strength Ointment .... ■ 703
Poly-Pred Liquifilm Ophthalmic Suspension .... ⊙ 231
Polysporin Ointment .... ■ 706
Polytrim Ophthalmic Solution 570

Pyrazinamide (Potential for febrile reactions and abnormal liver function tests).
No products indexed under this heading.

Rifampin (Potential for febrile reactions and abnormal liver function tests).
No products indexed under this heading.

Rifapentine (Potential for febrile reactions and abnormal liver function tests).
No products indexed under this heading.

Streptomycin Sulfate (Additive ototoxicity and/or nephrotoxicity).
No products indexed under this heading.

Tobramycin (Additive ototoxicity and/or nephrotoxicity). Products include:
TOBI Solution for Inhalation 1015
TobraDex Ophthalmic Ointment 558
TobraDex Ophthalmic Suspension 558
Zylet Ophthalmic Suspension 3508

Tobramycin Sulfate (Additive ototoxicity and/or nephrotoxicity).
No products indexed under this heading.

Vancomycin Hydrochloride (Additive ototoxicity and/or nephrotoxicity). Products include:
Vancocin HCl Capsules, USP 3370

Viomycin (Additive ototoxicity and/or nephrotoxicity).

CAPTOPRIL TABLETS

(Captopril) 2114
May interact with beta blockers, diuretics, ganglionic blocking agents, lithium preparations, nitrates and nitrites, non-steroidal anti-inflammatory agents, peripheral adrenergic blockers, potassium preparations, inhibitors of endogenous prostaglandin synthesis, potassium sparing diuretics, agents causing renin release, thiazides, vasodilators, and certain other agents. Compounds in these categories include:

Acebutolol Hydrochloride (Less than additive antihypertensive effect).
No products indexed under this heading.

Amiloride Hydrochloride (Hypotension; increased serum potassium). Products include:
Midamor Tablets 2000
Moduretic Tablets 2003

Amyl Nitrite (Discontinue before starting captopril; if resumed administer at lower dosage).
No products indexed under this heading.

Aspirin (Antihypertensive effects of captopril reduced). Products include:
- Aggrenox Capsules 855
- Bayer, Aspirin Regimen .... ▣606
- Bayer Aspirin Tablets 3515
- BC Powder .... ▣612
- BC Allergy Sinus Cold Powder .... ▣612
- Arthritis Strength BC Powder .... ▣612
- BC Sinus Cold Powder .... ▣612
- Ecotrin Enteric Coated Aspirin Low, Regular and Maximum Strength Tablets 1627
- Goody's Body Pain Formula Powder .... ▣621
- Goody's Extra Strength Headache Powder .... ▣621
- Goody's Extra Strength Pain Relief Tablets .... ▣621
- Percodan Tablets 1115
- St. Joseph 81 mg Aspirin Chewable and Enteric Coated Tablets 1841

Atenolol (Less than additive antihypertensive effect). Products include:
- Tenormin I.V. Injection 698
- Tenormin Tablets 695

Bendroflumethiazide (Captopril's effect will be augmented).
No products indexed under this heading.

Betaxolol Hydrochloride (Less than additive antihypertensive effect). Products include:
- Betoptic S Ophthalmic Suspension 554

Bisoprolol Fumarate (Less than additive antihypertensive effect).
No products indexed under this heading.

Bumetanide (Captopril's effect will be augmented; hypotension).
No products indexed under this heading.

Carteolol Hydrochloride (Less than additive antihypertensive effect). Products include:
- Carteolol Hydrochloride Ophthalmic Solution USP, 1% .... ⊙246

Celecoxib (Antihypertensive effects of captopril reduced). Products include:
- Celebrex Capsules 3130

Chlorothiazide (Captopril's effect will be augmented). Products include:
- Aldoclor Tablets 1881
- Diuril Oral 1936

Chlorothiazide Sodium (Captopril's effect will be augmented). Products include:
- Diuril Sodium Intravenous 1934

Chlorthalidone (Captopril's effect will be augmented; hypotension; increased serum potassium). Products include:
- Clorpres Tablets 2139

Deserpidine (Use with caution).
No products indexed under this heading.

Diazoxide (Drugs having vasodilator activity should, if possible, be discontinued before starting captopril). Products include:
- Hyperstat I.V. Injection 3031

Diclofenac Potassium (Antihypertensive effects of captopril reduced). Products include:
- Cataflam Tablets 2173

Diclofenac Sodium (Antihypertensive effects of captopril reduced). Products include:
- Arthrotec Tablets 3126
- Voltaren Ophthalmic Solution 2300
- Voltaren Tablets 2298
- Voltaren-XR Tablets 2301

Epoprostenol Sodium (Drugs having vasodilator activity should, if possible, be discontinued before starting captopril). Products include:
- Flolan for Injection 1408

Erythrityl Tetranitrate (Discontinue before starting captopril; if resumed administer at lower dosage).
No products indexed under this heading.

Esmolol Hydrochloride (Less than additive antihypertensive effect). Products include:
- Brevibloc Concentrate 766
- Brevibloc Injection 766
- Brevibloc Double Strength Injection 766
- Brevibloc Premixed Injection 766
- Brevibloc Double Strength Premixed Injection 766

Ethacrynic Acid (Captopril's effect will be augmented; hypotension). Products include:
- Edecrin Tablets 1941

Ethaverine Hydrochloride (Drugs having vasodilator activity should, if possible, be discontinued before starting captopril).
No products indexed under this heading.

Etodolac (Antihypertensive effects of captopril reduced).
No products indexed under this heading.

Fenoprofen Calcium (Antihypertensive effects of captopril reduced). Products include:
- Nalfon Capsules 2504

Flurbiprofen (Antihypertensive effects of captopril reduced).
No products indexed under this heading.

Furosemide (Captopril's effect will be augmented; hypotension). Products include:
- Furosemide Tablets 2117

Guanethidine Monosulfate (Use with caution).
No products indexed under this heading.

Hydralazine Hydrochloride (Drugs having vasodilator activity should, if possible, be discontinued before starting captopril). Products include:
- BiDil Tablets 2161

Hydrochlorothiazide (Captopril's effect will be augmented). Products include:
- Aldoril Tablets 1884
- Atacand HCT 637
- Avalide Tablets 2889
- Avalide Tablets 922
- Benicar HCT Tablets 2852
- Diovan HCT Tablets 2195
- Dyazide Capsules 1389
- Hyzaar 1964
- Lotensin HCT Tablets 2235
- Maxzide 2150
- Micardis HCT Tablets 886
- Moduretic Tablets 2003
- Prinzide Tablets 2033
- Teveten HCT Tablets 1710
- Timolide Tablets 2056
- Uniretic Tablets 3114
- Vaseretic Tablets 2073
- Zestoretic Tablets 701

Hydroflumethiazide (Captopril's effect will be augmented).
No products indexed under this heading.

Ibuprofen (Antihypertensive effects of captopril reduced). Products include:
- Advil Allergy Sinus Caplets .... ▣737
- Advil .... ▣737
- Children's Advil Suspension .... ▣742
- Children's Advil Chewable Tablets .... ▣741
- Advil Cold & Sinus .... ▣739
- Advil Flu & Body Ache Caplets .... ▣739
- Children's Advil Cold Suspension .... ▣741
- Infants' Advil Concentrated Drops .... ▣743
- Junior Strength Advil Swallow Tablets .... ▣740
- Advil Migraine Liquigels .... ▣740
- Advil Multi-Symptom Cold Caplets .... ▣738
- Combunox Tablets 1183
- Children's Motrin Oral Suspension and Chewable Tablets 1837
- Children's Motrin Cold Non-Staining Dye-Free Oral Suspension 1838
- Children's Motrin Cold Oral Suspension 1838
- Children's Motrin Non-Staining Dye-Free Oral Suspension 1837
- Motrin Cold & Sinus Caplets 1836
- Motrin IB Tablets and Caplets 1836
- Infants' Motrin Concentrated Drops 1837
- Infants' Motrin Non-Staining Dye-Free Drops 1837
- Junior Strength Motrin Caplets and Chewable Tablets 1837
- Vicoprofen Tablets 533

Indapamide (Captopril's effect will be augmented; hypotension). Products include:
- Indapamide Tablets 2119

Indomethacin (Antihypertensive effects of captopril reduced). Products include:
- Indocin 1968

Indomethacin Sodium Trihydrate (Antihypertensive effects of captopril reduced). Products include:
- Indocin I.V. 1973

Isosorbide Dinitrate (Discontinue before starting captopril; if resumed administer at lower dosage). Products include:
- BiDil Tablets 2161

Isosorbide Mononitrate (Discontinue before starting captopril; if resumed administer at lower dosage). Products include:
- Imdur Tablets 3032

Isoxsuprine Hydrochloride (Drugs having vasodilator activity should, if possible, be discontinued before starting captopril).
No products indexed under this heading.

Ketoprofen (Antihypertensive effects of captopril reduced).
No products indexed under this heading.

Ketorolac Tromethamine (Antihypertensive effects of captopril reduced). Products include:
- Acular Ophthalmic Solution 561
- Acular LS Ophthalmic Solution 562

Labetalol Hydrochloride (Less than additive antihypertensive effect).
No products indexed under this heading.

Levobunolol Hydrochloride (Less than additive antihypertensive effect). Products include:
- Betagan Ophthalmic Solution, USP .... ⊙217

Lithium (Increased serum lithium levels and symptoms of lithium toxicity).
No products indexed under this heading.

Lithium Carbonate (Increased serum lithium levels and symptoms of lithium toxicity). Products include:
- Eskalith 1406
- Lithobid Tablets 1670

Lithium Citrate (Increased serum lithium levels and symptoms of lithium toxicity).
No products indexed under this heading.

Mecamylamine Hydrochloride (Use with caution). Products include:
- Inversine Tablets 3286

Meclofenamate Sodium (Antihypertensive effects of captopril reduced).
No products indexed under this heading.

Mefenamic Acid (Antihypertensive effects of captopril reduced).
No products indexed under this heading.

Meloxicam (Antihypertensive effects of captopril reduced). Products include:
- Mobic Oral Suspension 893
- Mobic Tablets 893

Methyclothiazide (Captopril's effect will be augmented).
No products indexed under this heading.

Metipranolol Hydrochloride (Less than additive antihypertensive effect).
No products indexed under this heading.

Metolazone (Captopril's effect will be augmented; hypotension).
No products indexed under this heading.

Metoprolol Succinate (Less than additive antihypertensive effect). Products include:
- Toprol-XL Tablets 660

Metoprolol Tartrate (Less than additive antihypertensive effect).
No products indexed under this heading.

Minoxidil (Drugs having vasodilator activity should, if possible, be discontinued before starting captopril). Products include:
- Men's Rogaine Extra Strength Topical Solution, Ocean Rush Scent and Original Unscented .... ▣706
- Women's Rogaine Topical Solution, Spring Bloom Scent and Original Unscented .... ▣707

Nabumetone (Antihypertensive effects of captopril reduced). Products include:
- Relafen Tablets 1523

Nadolol (Less than additive antihypertensive effect). Products include:
- Nadolol Tablets 2121

Naproxen (Antihypertensive effects of captopril reduced). Products include:
- EC-Naprosyn Delayed-Release Tablets 2769
- Naprosyn Suspension 2769
- Naprosyn Tablets 2769
- Prevacid NapraPAC 3277

Naproxen Sodium (Antihypertensive effects of captopril reduced). Products include:
- Aleve Tablets, Caplets and Gelcaps .... ▣605
- Anaprox Tablets 2769
- Anaprox DS Tablets 2769

Nitroglycerin (Discontinue before starting captopril; if resumed administer at lower dosage). Products include:
- Nitro-Dur Transdermal Infusion System 3060
- Nitrolingual Pumpspray 1161

Nitroglycerin, long-acting formulations (Drugs having vasodilator activity should, if possible, be discontinued before starting captopril).
No products indexed under this heading.

Nitroglycerin Intravenous (Drugs having vasodilator activity should, if possible, be discontinued before starting captopril).
No products indexed under this heading.

Oxaprozin (Antihypertensive effects of captopril reduced).
No products indexed under this heading.

Papaverine (Drugs having vasodilator activity should, if possible, be discontinued before starting captopril).
No products indexed under this heading.

Papaverine Hydrochloride (Drugs having vasodilator activity should, if possible, be discontinued before starting captopril).
No products indexed under this heading.

Penbutolol Sulfate (Less than additive antihypertensive effect).
No products indexed under this heading.

Pentaerythritol Tetranitrate (Discontinue before starting captopril; if resumed administer at lower dosage).
No products indexed under this heading.

Phenylbutazone (Antihypertensive effects of captopril reduced).
No products indexed under this heading.

Pindolol (Less than additive antihypertensive effect).
No products indexed under this heading.

Piroxicam (Antihypertensive effects of captopril reduced).
No products indexed under this heading.

Polythiazide (Captopril's effect will be augmented).
No products indexed under this heading.

Potassium Acid Phosphate (Potential for significant increase in serum potassium). Products include:
K-Phos Original (Sodium Free) Tablets 785

Potassium Bicarbonate (Potential for significant increase in serum potassium).
No products indexed under this heading.

Potassium Chloride (Potential for significant increase in serum potassium). Products include:
Colyte with Flavor Packs for Oral Solution 3102
HalfLytely and Bisacodyl Tablets Bowel Prep Kit with Flavors Packs 915
K-Dur Extended-Relase Tablets 3047
K-Lor Powder Packets 472
K-Tab Filmtab Tablets 473
TriLyte with Flavor Packs for Oral Solution 3114

Potassium Citrate (Potential for significant increase in serum potassium). Products include:
Urocit-K Tablets 2109

Potassium Gluconate (Potential for significant increase in serum potassium).
No products indexed under this heading.

Potassium Phosphate (Potential for significant increase in serum potassium). Products include:
K-Phos Neutral Tablets 785

Prazosin Hydrochloride (Use with caution).
No products indexed under this heading.

Propranolol Hydrochloride (Less than additive antihypertensive effect). Products include:
Inderal LA Long-Acting Capsules 3421
InnoPran XL Capsules 2728

Rauwolfia Serpentina (Use with caution).
No products indexed under this heading.

Rescinnamine (Use with caution).
No products indexed under this heading.

Reserpine (Use with caution).
No products indexed under this heading.

Rofecoxib (Antihypertensive effects of captopril reduced).
No products indexed under this heading.

Sotalol Hydrochloride (Less than additive antihypertensive effect).
No products indexed under this heading.

Spironolactone (Captopril's effect will be augmented; hypotension; increased serum potassium).
No products indexed under this heading.

Sulindac (Antihypertensive effects of captopril reduced). Products include:
Clinoril Tablets 1899

Terazosin Hydrochloride (Use with caution). Products include:
Hytrin Capsules 469

Timolol Hemihydrate (Less than additive antihypertensive effect). Products include:
Betimol Ophthalmic Solution 3371
Betimol Ophthalmic Solution .... ⊙283

Timolol Maleate (Less than additive antihypertensive effect). Products include:
Blocadren Tablets 1891
Cosopt Sterile Ophthalmic Solution 1910
Timolide Tablets 2056
Timoptic in Ocudose 2061
Timoptic Sterile Ophthalmic Solution 2058
Timoptic-XE Sterile Ophthalmic Gel Forming Solution 2062

Tolazoline Hydrochloride (Drugs having vasodilator activity should, if possible, be discontinued before starting captopril).
No products indexed under this heading.

Tolmetin Sodium (Antihypertensive effects of captopril reduced).
No products indexed under this heading.

Torsemide (Captopril's effect will be augmented; hypotension).
No products indexed under this heading.

Triamterene (Captopril's effect will be augmented; hypotension; increased serum potassium). Products include:
Dyazide Capsules 1389
Dyrenium Capsules 3390
Maxzide 2150

Trimethaphan Camsylate (Use with caution).
No products indexed under this heading.

Valdecoxib (Antihypertensive effects of captopril reduced).
No products indexed under this heading.

Food Interactions

Alcohol (Drugs having vasodilator activity should, if possible, be discontinued before starting captopril).

Food, unspecified (Reduces absorption by about 30% to 40%; should be given one hour before meals).

CARAC CREAM, 0.5%

(Fluorouracil) 1048
None cited in PDR database.

CARAFATE SUSPENSION

(Sucralfate) 727
May interact with fluoroquinolone antibiotics, quinidine, xanthines, and certain other agents. Compounds in these categories include:

Alatrofloxacin Mesylate (Potential for reduced extent of absorption (bioavailability) with concomitant oral administration; dosing the concomitant medication 2 hours before sucralfate eliminates the interaction).
No products indexed under this heading.

Aluminum Carbonate (Simultaneous administration within one-half hour before or after sucralfate should be avoided; may increase the total body burden of aluminum).
No products indexed under this heading.

Aluminum Hydroxide (Simultaneous administration within one-half hour before or after sucralfate should be avoided; may increase the total body burden of aluminum). Products include:
Gaviscon Regular Strength Liquid .... ▣620
Gaviscon Regular Strength Tablets .... ▣619
Gaviscon Extra Strength Liquid .... ▣620
Gaviscon Extra Strength Tablets .... ▣619
Maalox Max Maximum Strength Antacid/Anti-Gas Liquid 2165
Maalox Regular Strength Antacid/Antigas Liquid 2164

Aminophylline (Simultaneous administration results in reduced oral absorption of theophylline).
No products indexed under this heading.

Cimetidine (Simultaneous administration results in reduced oral absorption of oral cimetidine; dosing the concomitant medication 2 hours before sucralfate eliminates the interaction). Products include:
Tagamet HB 200 Tablets .... ▣637
Tagamet Tablets 1547

Cimetidine Hydrochloride (Simultaneous administration results in reduced oral absorption of oral cimetidine; dosing the concomitant medication 2 hours before sucralfate eliminates the interaction).
No products indexed under this heading.

Ciprofloxacin (Potential for reduced extent of absorption (bioavailability) with concomitant oral administration; dosing the concomitant medication 2 hours before sucralfate eliminates the interaction). Products include:
Cipro I.V. 2998
Cipro I.V. Pharmacy Bulk Package 3509
Cipro Oral Suspension 2991
Cipro XR Tablets 3004
Ciprodex Otic Suspension 555

Ciprofloxacin Hydrochloride (Potential for reduced extent of absorption (bioavailability) with concomitant oral administration; dosing the concomitant medication 2 hours before sucralfate eliminates the interaction). Products include:
Ciloxan Ophthalmic Ointment 554
Cipro Tablets 2991

Digoxin (Simultaneous administration results in reduced oral absorption of oral digoxin; dosing the concomitant medication 2 hours before sucralfate eliminates the interaction). Products include:
Digitek Tablets 2146
Lanoxicaps Capsules 1458
Lanoxin Injection 1462
Lanoxin Tablets 1468
Lanoxin Injection Pediatric 1465

Dyphylline (Simultaneous administration results in reduced oral absorption of theophylline).
No products indexed under this heading.

Enoxacin (Potential for reduced extent of absorption (bioavailability) with concomitant oral administration; dosing the concomitant medication 2 hours before sucralfate eliminates the interaction).
No products indexed under this heading.

Grepafloxacin Hydrochloride (Potential for reduced extent of absorption (bioavailability) with concomitant oral administration; dosing the concomitant medication 2 hours before sucralfate eliminates the interaction).
No products indexed under this heading.

Ketoconazole (Simultaneous administration results in reduced oral absorption of oral ketoconazole). Products include:
Nizoral A-D Shampoo, 1% 1839
Nizoral 2% Shampoo 1838

Levothyroxine Sodium (Potential for reduced extent of absorption (bioavailability) with concomitant oral administration). Products include:
Levothroid Tablets 1189
Levoxyl Tablets 1680
Synthroid Tablets 515
Unithroid Tablets 3521

Lomefloxacin Hydrochloride (Potential for reduced extent of absorption (bioavailability) with concomitant oral administration; dosing the concomitant medication 2 hours before sucralfate eliminates the interaction).
No products indexed under this heading.

Magnesium Hydroxide (Simultaneous administration within one-half hour before or after sucralfate should be avoided; may increase the total body burden of aluminum). Products include:
Maalox Max Maximum Strength Antacid/Anti-Gas Liquid 2165
Maalox Regular Strength Antacid/Antigas Liquid 2164
Pepcid Complete Chewable Tablets 1672
Rolaids Tablets .... ▣707
Extra Strength Rolaids Tablets .... ▣707
Rolaids Multi-Symptom Antacid & Antigas Tablets .... ▣708

Magnesium Oxide (Simultaneous administration within one-half hour before or after sucralfate should be

avoided; may increase the total body burden of aluminum). Products include:

- Beelith Tablets ... 784
- PremCal Light, Regular, and Extra Strength Tablets ... 762

Moxifloxacin Hydrochloride (Potential for reduced extent of absorption (bioavailability) with concomitant oral administration; dosing the concomitant medication 2 hours before sucralfate eliminates the interaction). Products include:

- Avelox ... 2984
- Vigamox Ophthalmic Solution ... 560

Norfloxacin (Potential for reduced extent of absorption (bioavailability) with concomitant oral administration; dosing the concomitant medication 2 hours before sucralfate eliminates the interaction). Products include:

- Noroxin Tablets ... 2009

Ofloxacin (Potential for reduced extent of absorption (bioavailability) with concomitant oral administration; dosing the concomitant medication 2 hours before sucralfate eliminates the interaction). Products include:

- Floxin Otic Singles ... 1045
- Floxin Otic Solution ... 1043

Phenytoin (Simultaneous administration results in reduced oral absorption of oral phenytoin).

No products indexed under this heading.

Phenytoin Sodium (Simultaneous administration results in reduced oral absorption of oral phenytoin). Products include:

- Phenytek Capsules ... 2153

Quinidine (Potential for reduced extent of absorption (bioavailability) with concomitant oral administration).

No products indexed under this heading.

Quinidine Gluconate (Potential for reduced extent of absorption (bioavailability) with concomitant oral administration).

No products indexed under this heading.

Quinidine Hydrochloride (Potential for reduced extent of absorption (bioavailability) with concomitant oral administration).

No products indexed under this heading.

Quinidine Polygalacturonate (Potential for reduced extent of absorption (bioavailability) with concomitant oral administration).

No products indexed under this heading.

Quinidine Sulfate (Potential for reduced extent of absorption (bioavailability) with concomitant oral administration).

No products indexed under this heading.

Ranitidine Hydrochloride (Simultaneous administration results in reduced oral absorption of oral ranitidine; dosing the concomitant medication 2 hours before sucralfate eliminates the interaction). Products include:

- Zantac ... 1597
- Zantac Injection ... 1593
- Zantac 75 Tablets ... 715
- Zantac 150 Maximum Strength Tablets ... 715
- Zantac Injection Pharmacy Bulk Package ... 1595

Tetracycline Hydrochloride (Simultaneous administration results in reduced oral absorption of oral tetracycline).

No products indexed under this heading.

Theophylline (Simultaneous administration results in reduced oral absorption of theophylline).

No products indexed under this heading.

Theophylline Anhydrous (Simultaneous administration results in reduced oral absorption of theophylline). Products include:

- Uniphyl Tablets ... 2708

Theophylline Calcium Salicylate (Simultaneous administration results in reduced oral absorption of theophylline).

No products indexed under this heading.

Theophylline Dihydroxypropyl (Glyceryl) (Simultaneous administration results in reduced oral absorption of theophylline).

No products indexed under this heading.

Theophylline Ethylenediamine (Simultaneous administration results in reduced oral absorption of theophylline).

No products indexed under this heading.

Theophylline Sodium Glycinate (Simultaneous administration results in reduced oral absorption of theophylline).

No products indexed under this heading.

Trovafloxacin Mesylate (Potential for reduced extent of absorption (bioavailability) with concomitant oral administration; dosing the concomitant medication 2 hours before sucralfate eliminates the interaction).

No products indexed under this heading.

Warfarin Sodium (Subtherapeutic prothrombin times with concomitant warfarin and sucralfate have been reported in spontaneous and published reports; clinical studies have demonstrated no changes in the prothrombin time with the addition of sucralfate to chronic warfarin therapy). Products include:

- Coumadin for Injection ... 932
- Coumadin Tablets ... 932

CARAFATE TABLETS

(Sucralfate) ... 728

May interact with fluoroquinolone antibiotics, quinidine, xanthines, and certain other agents. Compounds in these categories include:

Alatrofloxacin Mesylate (Potential for reduced extent of absorption (bioavailability) with concomitant oral administration; dosing the concomitant medication 2 hours before sucralfate eliminates the interaction).

No products indexed under this heading.

Aluminum Carbonate (Simultaneous administration within one-half hour before or after sucralfate should be avoided; may increase the total body burden of aluminum).

No products indexed under this heading.

Aluminum Hydroxide (Simultaneous administration within one-half hour before or after sucralfate should be avoided; may increase the total body burden of aluminum). Products include:

- Gaviscon Regular Strength Liquid ... 620
- Gaviscon Regular Strength Tablets ... 619
- Gaviscon Extra Strength Liquid ... 620
- Gaviscon Extra Strength Tablets ... 619
- Maalox Max Maximum Strength Antacid/Anti-Gas Liquid ... 2165
- Maalox Regular Strength Antacid/Antigas Liquid ... 2164

Aminophylline (Simultaneous administration results in reduced oral absorption of theophylline).

No products indexed under this heading.

Cimetidine (Simultaneous administration results in reduced oral absorption of oral cimetidine; dosing the concomitant medication 2 hours before sucralfate eliminates the interaction). Products include:

- Tagamet HB 200 Tablets ... 637
- Tagamet Tablets ... 1547

Cimetidine Hydrochloride (Simultaneous administration results in reduced oral absorption of oral cimetidine; dosing the concomitant medication 2 hours before sucralfate eliminates the interaction).

No products indexed under this heading.

Ciprofloxacin (Potential for reduced extent of absorption (bioavailability) with concomitant oral administration; dosing the concomitant medication 2 hours before sucralfate eliminates the interaction). Products include:

- Cipro I.V. ... 2998
- Cipro I.V. Pharmacy Bulk Package ... 3509
- Cipro Oral Suspension ... 2991
- Cipro XR Tablets ... 3004
- Ciprodex Otic Suspension ... 555

Ciprofloxacin Hydrochloride (Potential for reduced extent of absorption (bioavailability) with concomitant oral administration; dosing the concomitant medication 2 hours before sucralfate eliminates the interaction). Products include:

- Ciloxan Ophthalmic Ointment ... 554
- Cipro Tablets ... 2991

Digoxin (Simultaneous administration results in reduced oral absorption of oral digoxin; dosing the concomitant medication 2 hours before sucralfate eliminates the interaction). Products include:

- Digitek Tablets ... 2146
- Lanoxicaps Capsules ... 1458
- Lanoxin Injection ... 1462
- Lanoxin Tablets ... 1468
- Lanoxin Injection Pediatric ... 1465

Dyphylline (Simultaneous administration results in reduced oral absorption of theophylline).

No products indexed under this heading.

Enoxacin (Potential for reduced extent of absorption (bioavailability) with concomitant oral administration; dosing the concomitant medication 2 hours before sucralfate eliminates the interaction).

No products indexed under this heading.

Grepafloxacin Hydrochloride (Potential for reduced extent of absorption (bioavailability) with concomitant oral administration; dosing the concomitant medication 2 hours before sucralfate eliminates the interaction).

No products indexed under this heading.

Ketoconazole (Simultaneous administration results in reduced oral absorption of oral ketoconazole). Products include:

- Nizoral A-D Shampoo, 1% ... 1839
- Nizoral 2% Shampoo ... 1838

Levothyroxine Sodium (Potential for reduced extent of absorption (bioavailability) with concomitant oral administration). Products include:

- Levothroid Tablets ... 1189
- Levoxyl Tablets ... 1680
- Synthroid Tablets ... 515
- Unithroid Tablets ... 3521

Lomefloxacin Hydrochloride (Potential for reduced extent of absorption (bioavailability) with concomitant oral administration; dosing the concomitant medication 2 hours before sucralfate eliminates the interaction).

No products indexed under this heading.

Magnesium Hydroxide (Simultaneous administration within one-half hour before or after sucralfate should be avoided; may increase the total body burden of aluminum). Products include:

- Maalox Max Maximum Strength Antacid/Anti-Gas Liquid ... 2165
- Maalox Regular Strength Antacid/Antigas Liquid ... 2164
- Pepcid Complete Chewable Tablets ... 1672
- Rolaids Tablets ... 707
- Extra Strength Rolaids Tablets ... 707
- Rolaids Multi-Symptom Antacid & Antigas Tablets ... 708

Magnesium Oxide (Simultaneous administration within one-half hour before or after sucralfate should be avoided; may increase the total body burden of aluminum). Products include:

- Beelith Tablets ... 784
- PremCal Light, Regular, and Extra Strength Tablets ... 762

Moxifloxacin Hydrochloride (Potential for reduced extent of absorption (bioavailability) with concomitant oral administration; dosing the concomitant medication 2 hours before sucralfate eliminates the interaction). Products include:

- Avelox ... 2984
- Vigamox Ophthalmic Solution ... 560

Norfloxacin (Potential for reduced extent of absorption (bioavailability) with concomitant oral administration; dosing the concomitant medication 2 hours before sucralfate eliminates the interaction). Products include:

- Noroxin Tablets ... 2009

Ofloxacin (Potential for reduced extent of absorption (bioavailability) with concomitant oral administration; dosing the concomitant medication 2 hours before sucralfate eliminates the interaction). Products include:

- Floxin Otic Singles ... 1045
- Floxin Otic Solution ... 1043

Phenytoin (Simultaneous administration results in reduced oral absorption of oral phenytoin).

No products indexed under this heading.

Phenytoin Sodium (Simultaneous administration results in reduced oral absorption of oral phenytoin). Products include:

- Phenytek Capsules ... 2153

Quinidine (Potential for reduced extent of absorption (bioavailability) with concomitant oral administration).

No products indexed under this heading.

Quinidine Gluconate (Potential for reduced extent of absorption (bioavailability) with concomitant oral administration).
No products indexed under this heading.

Quinidine Hydrochloride (Potential for reduced extent of absorption (bioavailability) with concomitant oral administration).
No products indexed under this heading.

Quinidine Polygalacturonate (Potential for reduced extent of absorption (bioavailability) with concomitant oral administration).
No products indexed under this heading.

Quinidine Sulfate (Potential for reduced extent of absorption (bioavailability) with concomitant oral administration).
No products indexed under this heading.

Ranitidine Hydrochloride (Simultaneous administration results in reduced oral absorption of oral ranitidine; dosing the concomitant medication 2 hours before sucralfate eliminates the interaction). Products include:
Zantac 1597
Zantac Injection 1593
Zantac 75 Tablets .... ■715
Zantac 150 Maximum Strength Tablets .... ■715
Zantac Injection Pharmacy Bulk Package 1595

Tetracycline Hydrochloride (Simultaneous administration results in reduced oral absorption of oral tetracycline).
No products indexed under this heading.

Theophylline (Simultaneous administration results in reduced oral absorption of theophylline).
No products indexed under this heading.

Theophylline Anhydrous (Simultaneous administration results in reduced oral absorption of theophylline). Products include:
Uniphyl Tablets 2708

Theophylline Calcium Salicylate (Simultaneous administration results in reduced oral absorption of theophylline).
No products indexed under this heading.

Theophylline Dihydroxypropyl (Glyceryl) (Simultaneous administration results in reduced oral absorption of theophylline).
No products indexed under this heading.

Theophylline Ethylenediamine (Simultaneous administration results in reduced oral absorption of theophylline).
No products indexed under this heading.

Theophylline Sodium Glycinate (Simultaneous administration results in reduced oral absorption of theophylline).
No products indexed under this heading.

Trovafloxacin Mesylate (Potential for reduced extent of absorption (bioavailability) with concomitant oral administration; dosing the concomitant medication 2 hours before sucralfate eliminates the interaction).
No products indexed under this heading.

Warfarin Sodium (Subtherapeutic prothrombin times with concomitant warfarin and sucralfate have been reported in spontaneous and published reports; clinical studies have demonstrated no changes in the prothrombin time with the addition of sucralfate to chronic warfarin therapy). Products include:
Coumadin for Injection 932
Coumadin Tablets 932

CARBATROL CAPSULES

(Carbamazepine) 3174

May interact with antimalarials, cytochrome p450 1a2 substrates (selected), cytochrome p450 3a4 inducers (selected), cytochrome p450 3a4 inhibitors (selected), cytochrome p450 3a4 substrates (selected), doxycycline, anticonvulsants, erythromycin, lithium preparations, macrolide antibiotics, monoamine oxidase inhibitors, antipsychotic agents, oral contraceptives, phenytoin, valproate, xanthines, and certain other agents. Compounds in these categories include:

Acetaminophen (Carbamazepine induces hepatic CYP activity and causes or would be expected to decrease plasma levels of acetaminophen). Products include:
Benadryl Allergy & Cold Tablets .... ■692
Benadryl Allergy & Sinus Headache Caplets & Gelcaps .... ■693
Benadryl Maximum Strength Severe Allergy & Sinus Headache Caplets .... ■694
Contac Severe Cold and Flu Caplets Maximum Strength .... ■615
Contac Severe Cold and Flu Caplets Non-Drowsy .... ■615
Darvocet A 500 Tablets 3497
Goody's Body Pain Formula Powder .... ■621
Goody's Extra Strength Headache Powder .... ■621
Goody's Extra Strength Pain Relief Tablets .... ■621
Goody's PM Powder .... ■622
Hycomine Compound Tablets 1105
Lortab 3315
Lortab Elixir 3312
Percocet Tablets 1114
Robitussin Cough, Cold & Flu Liquid-filled Capsules .... ■750
Robitussin Flu Liquid .... ■752
Sedapap Tablets 50 mg/650 mg 2098
Singlet Caplets .... ■636
Sudafed Severe Cold .... ■710
Sudafed Sinus Headache .... ■711
TheraFlu Cold & Cough Hot Liquid .... ■680
TheraFlu Cold & Sore Throat Hot Liquid .... ■680
TheraFlu Flu & Chest Congestion Non-Drowsy Hot Liquid .... ■681
TheraFlu Flu & Sore Throat Hot Liquid .... ■681
TheraFlu Severe Cold Non-Drowsy Hot Liquid .... ■683
TheraFlu Severe Cold & Cough Hot Liquid .... ■683
TheraFlu Severe Cold Caplets .... ■679
TheraFlu Severe Cold Hot Liquid .... ■682
TheraFlu Severe Cold Non-Drowsy Caplets .... ■679
Triaminic Cough & Sore Throat Liquid .... ■687
Triaminic Flu, Cough & Fever Liquid .... ■685
Triaminic Cough & Sore Throat Softchews .... ■689
Tylenol 8 Hour Extended Release Geltabs and Caplets 1843
Tylenol Sinus NightTime Caplets .... ■663
Children's Tylenol Suspension Liquid and Meltaways 1850
Children's Tylenol Plus Cold & Allergy Suspension Liquid 1850
Children's Tylenol Plus Cold NightTime Suspension Liquid 1851
Children's Tylenol Plus Cold & Cough Suspension Liquid and Chewable Tablets 1851
Children's Tylenol Plus Cold Chewable Tablets 1851
Children's Tylenol Plus Cold Daytime Non-Drowsy Suspension Liquid 1851
Children's Tylenol Plus Flu Suspension Liquid 1853
Concentrated Tylenol Infants' Drops Plus Cold 1851
Concentrated Tylenol Infants' Drops Plus Cold and Cough 1851
Concentrated Tylenol Infants' Drops 1850
Junior Tylenol Meltaways 1850
Tylenol Cold & Flu Severe Daytime Liquid with Cool Bust 1846
Tylenol Cold & Flu Severe NightTime Liquid with Cool Burst 1846
Tylenol Cold Severe Congestion Non-Drowsy Caplets with Cool Burst 1846
Tylenol Cough & Sore Throat Daytime Liquid with Cool Burst 1849
Tylenol Cough & Sore Throat NightTime Liquid with Cool Burst 1849
Tylenol 1843
Extra Strength Tylenol Rapid Release Gels 1843
Tylenol 1843
Tylenol Allergy Complete Night Time Caplets 1844
Tylenol Allergy Complete Multi-Symptom Caplets and Gelcaps with Cool Burst 1844
Tylenol Severe Allergy Caplets 1844
Tylenol Flu NightTime Gelcaps 1846
Tylenol Flu Day Non-Drowsy Gelcaps 1846
Concentrated Tylenol Infants' Drops Plus Cold Nasal Congestant, Fever Reducer & Pain Reliever .... ■668
Concentrated Tylenol Infants' Drops Plus Cold & Cough Nasal Decongestant, Fever Reducer & Pain Reliever .... ■668
Multi-Symptom Tylenol Cold Night Time Caplets 1845
Multi-Symptom Tylenol Cold Day Non-Drowsy Caplets and Gelcaps 1845
Extra Strength Tylenol PM Caplets, Geltabs, Gelcaps and Liquid 1847
Tylenol Sinus Day Non-Drowsy 1848
Tylenol Sinus Night Time Caplets 1848
Tylenol Sinus Severe Congestion Caplets with Cool Burst 1848
Tylenol Sore Throat Daytime Liquid with Cool Burst 1849
Tylenol Sore Throat NightTime Liquid with Cool Burst 1849
Tylenol with Codeine 2461
Women's Tylenol Menstrual Relief Caplets 1849
Ultracet Tablets 2462
Vicks 44M Cough, Cold & Flu Relief 2676
Vicks DayQuil LiquiCaps/Liquid Multi-Symptom Cold/Flu Relief .... ■723
Vicks DayQuil Multi-Symptom Cold/Flu Relief LiquiCaps 2675
Vicks DayQuil Multi-Symptom Cold/Flu Relief Liquid 2675
Vicks NyQuil LiquiCaps 2677
Vicks NyQuil LiquiCaps/Liquid Multi-Symptom Cold/Flu Relief .... ■725
Vicks NyQuil Liquid 2677
Vicodin Tablets 530
Vicodin ES Tablets 531
Vicodin HP Tablets 532
Zydone Tablets 1118

Acetazolamide (Carbamazepine is metabolized mainly by cytochrome P450 (CYP) 3A4 to the active carbamazepine 10,11 -epoxide, which is further metabolized to the trans-diol by epoxide hydrolase. Therefore, the potential exists for interaction between carbamazepine and any agent that inhibits CYP3A4 and/or epoxide hydrolase).
No products indexed under this heading.

Alatrofloxacin Mesylate (Carbamazepine is known to induce CYP1A2 and CYP3A4. Therefore, the potential exists for interaction between carbamazepine and any agent metabolized by one (or more) of these enzymes).
No products indexed under this heading.

Alfentanil Hydrochloride (Carbamazepine is known to induce CYP1A2 and CYP3A4. Therefore, the potential exists for interaction between carbamazepine and any agent metabolized by one (or more) of these enzymes).
No products indexed under this heading.

Allium sativum (Carbamazepine is metabolized by CYP3A4. Therefore, the potential exists for interaction between caramazepine and any agent that induces CYP3A4).
No products indexed under this heading.

Alprazolam (Carbamazepine induces hepatic CYP activity and causes or would be expected to decrease plasma levels of alprazolam). Products include:
Niravam Orally Disintegrating Tablets 3106
Xanax XR Tablets 2655

Aminophylline (Inducers of CYP3A4, such as theophylline, can increase the rate of carbamazepine metabolism and can thus decrease plasma carbamazepine levels; carbamazepine induces hepatic CYP activity and causes or would be expected to decrease plasma levels of theophylline).
No products indexed under this heading.

Amiodarone Hydrochloride (Carbamazepine is metabolized mainly by cytochrome P450 (CYP) 3A4 to the active carbamazepine 10,11 -epoxide, which is further metabolized to the trans-diol by epoxide hydrolase. Therefore, the potential exists for interaction between carbamazepine and any agent that inhibits its CYP3A4 and/or epoxide hydrolase). Products include:
Pacerone Tablets 3337

Amitriptyline Hydrochloride (Carbamazepine is known to induce CYP1A2 and CYP3A4. Therefore, the potential exists for interaction between carbamazepine and any agent metabolized by one (or more) of these enzymes).
No products indexed under this heading.

Amlodipine Besylate (Carbamazepine is known to induce CYP1A2 and CYP3A4. Therefore, the potential exists for interaction between carbamazepine and any agent metabolized by one (or more) of these enzymes). Products include:
Caduet Tablets 2507

Lotrel Capsules 2238
Norvasc Tablets 2529

Amoxapine (Carbamazepine is known to induce CYP1A2 and CYP3A4. Therefore, the potential exists for interaction between carbamazepine and any agent metabolized by one (or more) of these enzymes).
No products indexed under this heading.

Amprenavir (Carbamazepine is metabolized mainly by cytochrome P450 (CYP) 3A4 to the active carbamazepine 10,11 -epoxide, which is further metabolized to the transdiol by epoxide hydrolase. Therefore, the potential exists for interaction between carbamazepine and any agent that inhibits CYP3A4 and/or epoxide hydrolase). Products include:
Agenerase Capsules 1299
Agenerase Oral Solution 1304

Anagrelide Hydrochloride (Carbamazepine is known to induce CYP1A2 and CYP3A4. Therefore, the potential exists for interaction between carbamazepine and any agent metabolized by one (or more) of these enzymes). Products include:
Agrylin Capsules 3172

Anastrozole (Carbamazepine is metabolized mainly by cytochrome P450 (CYP) 3A4 to the active carbamazepine 10,11 -epoxide, which is further metabolized to the transdiol by epoxide hydrolase. Therefore, the potential exists for interaction between carbamazepine and any agent that inhibits CYP3A4 and/or epoxide hydrolase). Products include:
Arimidex Tablets 665

Aprepitant (Carbamazepine is metabolized mainly by cytochrome P450 (CYP) 3A4 to the active carbamazepine 10,11 -epoxide, which is further metabolized to the transdiol by epoxide hydrolase. Therefore, the potential exists for interaction between carbamazepine and any agent that inhibits CYP3A4 and/or epoxide hydrolase). Products include:
Emend Capsules 1944

Aripiprazole (Co-administration with psychotropic agents has resulted in isolated cases of neuroleptic malignant syndrome). Products include:
Abilify Tablets 2472
Abilify Tablets 916

Astemizole (Carbamazepine is known to induce CYP1A2 and CYP3A4. Therefore, the potential exists for interaction between carbamazepine and any agent metabolized by one (or more) of these enzymes).
No products indexed under this heading.

Atorvastatin Calcium (Carbamazepine is known to induce CYP1A2 and CYP3A4. Therefore, the potential exists for interaction between carbamazepine and any agent metabolized by one (or more) of these enzymes). Products include:
Caduet Tablets 2507
Lipitor Tablets 2495

Azithromycin Dihydrate (Inhibitors of CYP3A4, such as macrolides, inhibit carbamazepine metabolism and thus increase plasma carbamazepine levels). Products include:
Zithromax 2568
Zithromax for IV Infusion 2573
Zithromax for Oral Suspension, 300 mg, 600 mg, 900 mg, 1200 mg 2561
Zithromax Tablets, 250 mg, 500 mg 2561
Zithromax Tri-Pak 2561
Zithromax Z-Pak 2568

Belladonna Ergotamine (Carbamazepine is known to induce CYP1A2 and CYP3A4. Therefore, the potential exists for interaction between carbamazepine and any agent metabolized by one (or more) of these enzymes).
No products indexed under this heading.

Betamethasone Acetate (Carbamazepine is metabolized by CYP3A4. Therefore, the potential exists for interaction between caramazepine and any agent that induces CYP3A4).
No products indexed under this heading.

Betamethasone Sodium Phosphate (Carbamazepine is metabolized by CYP3A4. Therefore, the potential exists for interaction between caramazepine and any agent that induces CYP3A4).
No products indexed under this heading.

Buspirone Hydrochloride (Carbamazepine is known to induce CYP1A2 and CYP3A4. Therefore, the potential exists for interaction between carbamazepine and any agent metabolized by one (or more) of these enzymes).
No products indexed under this heading.

Busulfan (Carbamazepine is known to induce CYP1A2 and CYP3A4. Therefore, the potential exists for interaction between carbamazepine and any agent metabolized by one (or more) of these enzymes). Products include:
I.V. Busulfex 1125
Myleran Tablets 1492

Caffeine (Carbamazepine is known to induce CYP1A2 and CYP3A4. Therefore, the potential exists for interaction between carbamazepine and any agent metabolized by one (or more) of these enzymes). Products include:
Athena Hair System Shampoo 767
BC Powder 612
Arthritis Strength BC Powder 612
Goody's Extra Strength Headache Powder 621
Goody's Extra Strength Pain Relief Tablets 621
Hycomine Compound Tablets 1105
Spartan Hair System Shampoo 767
Vivarin 639

Caffeine Anhydrous (Carbamazepine is known to induce CYP1A2 and CYP3A4. Therefore, the potential exists for interaction between carbamazepine and any agent metabolized by one (or more) of these enzymes).
No products indexed under this heading.

Cerivastatin Sodium (Carbamazepine is known to induce CYP1A2 and CYP3A4. Therefore, the potential exists for interaction between carbamazepine and any agent metabolized by one (or more) of these enzymes).
No products indexed under this heading.

Chlordiazepoxide (Carbamazepine is known to induce CYP1A2 and CYP3A4. Therefore, the potential exists for interaction between carbamazepine and any agent metabolized by one (or more) of these enzymes).
No products indexed under this heading.

Chlordiazepoxide Hydrochloride (Carbamazepine is known to induce CYP1A2 and CYP3A4. Therefore, the potential exists for interaction between carbamazepine and any agent metabolized by one (or more) of these enzymes). Products include:
Librium Capsules 3349

Chloroquine Hydrochloride (Antimalarial drugs, such as chloroquine and mefloquine, may antagonize the activity of carbamazepine).
No products indexed under this heading.

Chloroquine Phosphate (Antimalarial drugs, such as chloroquine and mefloquine, may antagonize the activity of carbamazepine).
No products indexed under this heading.

Chlorpheniramine (Carbamazepine is known to induce CYP1A2 and CYP3A4. Therefore, the potential exists for interaction between carbamazepine and any agent metabolized by one (or more) of these enzymes).
No products indexed under this heading.

Chlorpheniramine Maleate (Carbamazepine is known to induce CYP1A2 and CYP3A4. Therefore, the potential exists for interaction between carbamazepine and any agent metabolized by one (or more) of these enzymes). Products include:
Advil Allergy Sinus Caplets 737
Advil Multi-Symptom Cold Caplets 738
BC Allergy Sinus Cold Powder 612
Contac Severe Cold and Flu Caplets Maximum Strength 615
Hycomine Compound Tablets 1105
PediaCare Multi-Symptom Cold Liquid 704
PediaCare NightRest Cough & Cold Liquid 704
Robitussin Flu Liquid 752
Robitussin PM Cough & Cold Liquid 752
Singlet Caplets 636
Sudafed Sinus & Allergy Tablets 710
TheraFlu Cold & Cough Hot Liquid 680
TheraFlu Cold & Sore Throat Hot Liquid 680
TheraFlu Flu & Sore Throat Hot Liquid 681
TheraFlu Severe Cold & Cough Hot Liquid 683
TheraFlu Severe Cold Caplets 679
TheraFlu Severe Cold Hot Liquid 682
Triaminic Cold & Allergy Liquid 685
Triaminic Cold & Cough Liquid 685
Triaminic Flu, Cough & Fever Liquid 685
Triaminic Night Time Cough & Cold Liquid 685
Triaminic Allergy Runny Nose & Congestion Softchews 688
Triaminic Cold & Cough Softchews 688
Children's Tylenol Plus Cold NightTime Suspension Liquid 1851
Children's Tylenol Plus Cold & Cough Suspension Liquid and Chewable Tablets 1851
Children's Tylenol Plus Cold Chewable Tablets 1851
Children's Tylenol Plus Flu Suspension Liquid 1853
Tylenol Allergy Complete Multi-Symptom Caplets and Gelcaps with Cool Burst 1844
Multi-Symptom Tylenol Cold Night Time Caplets 1845
Vicks 44M Cough, Cold & Flu Relief 2676
Pediatric Vicks 44m Cough & Cold Relief 2673
Children's Vicks NyQuil Cold/Cough Relief 2671

Chlorpheniramine Polistirex (Carbamazepine is known to induce CYP1A2 and CYP3A4. Therefore, the potential exists for interaction between carbamazepine and any agent metabolized by one (or more) of these enzymes). Products include:
Tussionex Pennkinetic Extended-Release Suspension 3322

Chlorpheniramine Tannate (Carbamazepine is known to induce CYP1A2 and CYP3A4. Therefore, the potential exists for interaction between carbamazepine and any agent metabolized by one (or more) of these enzymes).
No products indexed under this heading.

Chlorpromazine (Co-administration with psychotropic agents has resulted in isolated cases of neuroleptic malignant syndrome).
No products indexed under this heading.

Chlorpromazine Hydrochloride (Co-administration with psychotropic agents has resulted in isolated cases of neuroleptic malignant syndrome).
No products indexed under this heading.

Chlorprothixene (Co-administration with psychotropic agents has resulted in isolated cases of neuroleptic malignant syndrome).
No products indexed under this heading.

Chlorprothixene Hydrochloride (Co-administration with psychotropic agents has resulted in isolated cases of neuroleptic malignant syndrome).
No products indexed under this heading.

Cimetidine (Inhibitors of CYP3A4, such as cimetidine, inhibit carbamazepine metabolism and thus increase plasma carbamazepine levels). Products include:
Tagamet HB 200 Tablets 637
Tagamet Tablets 1547

Cimetidine Hydrochloride (Inhibitors of CYP3A4, such as cimetidine, inhibit carbamazepine metabolism and thus increase plasma carbamazepine levels).
No products indexed under this heading.

Ciprofloxacin (Carbamazepine is metabolized mainly by cytochrome P450 (CYP) 3A4 to the active carbamazepine 10,11 -epoxide, which is further metabolized to the transdiol by epoxide hydrolase. Therefore, the potential exists for interaction between carbamazepine and any agent that inhibits CYP3A4 and/or epoxide hydrolase). Products include:
Cipro I.V. 2998
Cipro I.V. Pharmacy Bulk Package ... 3509
Cipro Oral Suspension 2991
Cipro XR Tablets 3004
Ciprodex Otic Suspension 555

Ciprofloxacin Hydrochloride (Carbamazepine is metabolized by

CYP3A4. Therefore, the potential exists for interaction between caramazepine and any agent that induces CYP3A4). Products include:
Ciloxan Ophthalmic Ointment 554
Cipro Tablets 2991

Cisapride (Carbamazepine is known to induce CYP1A2 and CYP3A4. Therefore, the potential exists for interaction between carbamazepine and any agent metabolized by one (or more) of these enzymes).
No products indexed under this heading.

Cisplatin (Inducers of CYP3A4, such as cisplatin, can increase the rate of carbamazepine metabolism and can thus decrease plasma carbamazepine levels).
No products indexed under this heading.

Clarithromycin (Inhibitors of CYP3A4, such as clarithromycin, inhibit carbamazepine metabolism and thus increase plasma carbamazepine levels). Products include:
Biaxin/Biaxin XL 402
PREVPAC 3281

Clomipramine Hydrochloride (Carbamazepine can increase plasma levels of clomipramine).
No products indexed under this heading.

Clonazepam (Carbamazepine induces hepatic CYP activity and causes or would be expected to decrease plasma levels of clonazepine; alterations of thyroid function have been reported in combination therapy with other anticonvulsants). Products include:
Klonopin 2782

Clopidogrel Bisulfate (Carbamazepine is known to induce CYP1A2 and CYP3A4. Therefore, the potential exists for interaction between carbamazepine and any agent metabolized by one (or more) of these enzymes). Products include:
Plavix Tablets 940
Plavix Tablets 2942

Clotrimazole (Carbamazepine is metabolized mainly by cytochrome P450 (CYP) 3A4 to the active carbamazepine 10,11 -epoxide, which is further metabolized to the trans-diol by epoxide hydrolase. Therefore, the potential exists for interaction between carbamazepine and any agent that inhibits CYP3A4 and/ or epoxide hydrolase). Products include:
Lotrimin 3053
Lotrisone 3054

Clozapine (Carbamazepine induces hepatic CYP activity and causes or would be expected to decrease plasma levels of clozapine). Products include:
Clozapine Tablets 2141
Clozaril Tablets 2174
FazaClo Orally Disintegrating Tablets 547

Cortisone Acetate (Carbamazepine is metabolized by CYP3A4. Therefore, the potential exists for interaction between caramazepine and any agent that induces CYP3A4).
No products indexed under this heading.

Cyclobenzaprine (Carbamazepine is known to induce CYP1A2 and CYP3A4. Therefore, the potential exists for interaction between carbamazepine and any agent metabolized by one (or more) of these enzymes).
No products indexed under this heading.

Cyclobenzaprine Hydrochloride (Carbamazepine is known to induce CYP1A2 and CYP3A4. Therefore, the potential exists for interaction between carbamazepine and any agent metabolized by one (or more) of these enzymes). Products include:
Flexeril Tablets 1832

Cyclosporine (Carbamazepine is metabolized mainly by cytochrome P450 (CYP) 3A4 to the active carbamazepine 10,11 -epoxide, which is further metabolized to the trans-diol by epoxide hydrolase. Therefore, the potential exists for interaction between carbamazepine and any agent that inhibits CYP3A4 and/ or epoxide hydrolase). Products include:
Gengraf Capsules 458
Neoral Soft Gelatin Capsules 2247
Neoral Oral Solution 2247
Restasis Ophthalmic Emulsion 570
Sandimmune 2259

Dalfopristin (Carbamazepine is metabolized mainly by cytochrome P450 (CYP) 3A4 to the active carbamazepine 10,11 -epoxide, which is further metabolized to the trans-diol by epoxide hydrolase. Therefore, the potential exists for interaction between carbamazepine and any agent that inhibits CYP3A4 and/ or epoxide hydrolase). Products include:
Synercid I.V. 1690

Danazol (Inhibitors of CYP3A4, such as danazol, inhibit carbamazepine metabolism and thus increase plasma carbamazepine levels).
No products indexed under this heading.

Delavirdine Mesylate (Carbamazepine is metabolized mainly by cytochrome P450 (CYP) 3A4 to the active carbamazepine 10,11 -epoxide, which is further metabolized to the trans-diol by epoxide hydrolase. Therefore, the potential exists for interaction between carbamazepine and any agent that inhibits CYP3A4 and/or epoxide hydrolase). Products include:
Rescriptor Tablets 2535

Desipramine Hydrochloride (Carbamazepine is known to induce CYP1A2 and CYP3A4. Therefore, the potential exists for interaction between carbamazepine and any agent metabolized by one (or more) of these enzymes).
No products indexed under this heading.

Desogestrel (Carbamazepine induces hepatic CYP activity and causes or would be expected to decrease plasma levels of oral contraceptives; breakthrough bleeding has been reported among patients receiving concomitant oral contraceptives and their reliability may be adversely affected). Products include:
Ortho-Cept Tablets 2395

Dexamethasone (Carbamazepine is metabolized by CYP3A4. Therefore, the potential exists for interaction between caramazepine and any agent that induces CYP3A4). Products include:
Ciprodex Otic Suspension 555
Decadron Tablets 1929
TobraDex Ophthalmic Ointment 558
TobraDex Ophthalmic Suspension ... 558

Dexamethasone Acetate (Carbamazepine is metabolized by CYP3A4. Therefore, the potential exists for interaction between caramazepine and any agent that induces CYP3A4).
No products indexed under this heading.

Dexamethasone Sodium Phosphate (Carbamazepine is metabolized by CYP3A4. Therefore, the potential exists for interaction between caramazepine and any agent that induces CYP3A4). Products include:
Decadron Phosphate Injection 1931

Diazepam (Carbamazepine is known to induce CYP1A2 and CYP3A4. Therefore, the potential exists for interaction between carbamazepine and any agent metabolized by one (or more) of these enzymes). Products include:
Diastat Rectal Delivery System 3344
Valium Tablets 2822

Dicumarol (Carbamazepine induces hepatic CYP activity and causes or would be expected to decrease plasma levels of dicumarol).
No products indexed under this heading.

Dihydroergotamine Mesylate (Carbamazepine is known to induce CYP1A2 and CYP3A4. Therefore, the potential exists for interaction between carbamazepine and any agent metabolized by one (or more) of these enzymes). Products include:
Migranal Nasal Spray 3350

Diltiazem Hydrochloride (Inhibitors of CYP3A4, such as diltiazem, inhibit carbamazepine metabolism and thus increase plasma carbamazepine levels). Products include:
Cardizem LA Extended Release Tablets 1699
Tiazac Capsules 1204

Diltiazem Maleate (Carbamazepine is metabolized mainly by cytochrome P450 (CYP) 3A4 to the active carbamazepine 10,11 -epoxide, which is further metabolized to the trans-diol by epoxide hydrolase. Therefore, the potential exists for interaction between carbamazepine and any agent that inhibits CYP3A4 and/or epoxide hydrolase).
No products indexed under this heading.

Dirithromycin (Inhibitors of CYP3A4, such as macrolides, inhibit carbamazepine metabolism and thus increase plasma carbamazepine levels).
No products indexed under this heading.

Disopyramide (Carbamazepine is known to induce CYP1A2 and CYP3A4. Therefore, the potential exists for interaction between carbamazepine and any agent metabolized by one (or more) of these enzymes).
No products indexed under this heading.

Disopyramide Phosphate (Carbamazepine is known to induce CYP1A2 and CYP3A4. Therefore, the potential exists for interaction between carbamazepine and any agent metabolized by one (or more) of these enzymes).
No products indexed under this heading.

Disulfiram (Carbamazepine is known to induce CYP1A2 and CYP3A4. Therefore, the potential exists for interaction between carbamazepine and any agent metabolized by one (or more) of these enzymes). Products include:
Antabuse Tablets 2343

Divalproex Sodium (Alterations of thyroid function have been reported in combination therapy with other anticonvulsants). Products include:
Depakote Sprinkle Capsules 422
Depakote Tablets 427
Depakote ER Tablets 433

Doxepin Hydrochloride (Carbamazepine is known to induce CYP1A2 and CYP3A4. Therefore, the potential exists for interaction between carbamazepine and any agent metabolized by one (or more) of these enzymes).
No products indexed under this heading.

Doxorubicin Hydrochloride (Inducers of CYP3A4, such as doxorubicin, can increase the rate of carbamazepine metabolism and can thus decrease plasma carbamazepine levels). Products include:
Adriamycin for Injection, USP 786
Adriamycin Injection, USP 786

Doxycycline Calcium (Carbamazepine induces hepatic CYP activity and causes or would be expected to decrease plasma levels of doxycycline).
No products indexed under this heading.

Doxycycline Hyclate (Carbamazepine induces hepatic CYP activity and causes or would be expected to decrease plasma levels of doxycycline).
No products indexed under this heading.

Doxycycline Monohydrate (Carbamazepine induces hepatic CYP activity and causes or would be expected to decrease plasma levels of doxycycline).
No products indexed under this heading.

Dronabinol (Carbamazepine is known to induce CYP1A2 and CYP3A4. Therefore, the potential exists for interaction between carbamazepine and any agent metabolized by one (or more) of these enzymes). Products include:
Marinol Capsules 3334

Dyphylline (Inducers of CYP3A4, such as theophylline, can increase the rate of carbamazepine metabolism and can thus decrease plasma carbamazepine levels; carbamazepine induces hepatic CYP activity and causes or would be expected to decrease plasma levels of theophylline).
No products indexed under this heading.

Efavirenz (Carbamazepine is metabolized mainly by cytochrome P450 (CYP) 3A4 to the active carbamazepine 10,11 -epoxide, which is further metabolized to the trans-diol by epoxide hydrolase. There-

fore, the potential exists for interaction between carbamazepine and any agent that inhibits CYP3A4 and/or epoxide hydrolase). Products include:

Sustiva Capsules 957

Enoxacin (Carbamazepine is known to induce CYP1A2 and CYP3A4. Therefore, the potential exists for interaction between carbamazepine and any agent metabolized by one (or more) of these enzymes).

No products indexed under this heading.

Ergotamine Tartrate (Carbamazepine is known to induce CYP1A2 and CYP3A4. Therefore, the potential exists for interaction between carbamazepine and any agent metabolized by one (or more) of these enzymes).

No products indexed under this heading.

Erythromycin (Inhibitors of CYP3A4, such as erythromycin, inhibit carbamazepine metabolism and thus increase plasma carbamazepine levels). Products include:

Erygel Topical Gel 2096
Ery-Tab Tablets 447
Erythromycin Base Filmtab Tablets 454
Erythromycin Delayed-Release Capsules, USP 456
PCE Dispertab Tablets 510

Erythromycin Estolate (Inhibitors of CYP3A4, such as erythromycin, inhibit carbamazepine metabolism and thus increase plasma carbamazepine levels).

No products indexed under this heading.

Erythromycin Ethylsuccinate (Inhibitors of CYP3A4, such as erythromycin, inhibit carbamazepine metabolism and thus increase plasma carbamazepine levels). Products include:

E.E.S. 449
EryPed 445

Erythromycin Gluceptate (Inhibitors of CYP3A4, such as erythromycin, inhibit carbamazepine metabolism and thus increase plasma carbamazepine levels).

No products indexed under this heading.

Erythromycin Lactobionate (Inhibitors of CYP3A4, such as erythromycin, inhibit carbamazepine metabolism and thus increase plasma carbamazepine levels).

No products indexed under this heading.

Erythromycin Stearate (Inhibitors of CYP3A4, such as erythromycin, inhibit carbamazepine metabolism and thus increase plasma carbamazepine levels). Products include:

Erythrocin Stearate Filmtab Tablets 452

Esomeprazole Magnesium (Carbamazepine is metabolized mainly by cytochrome P450 (CYP) 3A4 to the active carbamazepine 10,11 -epoxide, which is further metabolized to the trans-diol by epoxide hydrolase. Therefore, the potential exists for interaction between carbamazepine and any agent that inhibits CYP3A4 and/or epoxide hydrolase). Products include:

Nexium Delayed-Release Capsules 645

Estradiol (Carbamazepine is known to induce CYP1A2 and CYP3A4. Therefore, the potential exists for interaction between carbamazepine and any agent metabolized by one (or more) of these enzymes). Products include:

Activella Tablets 2311
Climara Transdermal System 795
Climara Pro Transdermal System 800
CombiPatch Transdermal System 2180
Estrogel 0.06% 3200
Menostar Transdermal System 805
Prefest Tablets 1069
Vagifem Tablets 2340
Vivelle Transdermal System 2288
Vivelle-Dot Transdermal System 2293

Estradiol Benzoate (Carbamazepine is known to induce CYP1A2 and CYP3A4. Therefore, the potential exists for interaction between carbamazepine and any agent metabolized by one (or more) of these enzymes).

No products indexed under this heading.

Estradiol Cypionate (Carbamazepine is known to induce CYP1A2 and CYP3A4. Therefore, the potential exists for interaction between carbamazepine and any agent metabolized by one (or more) of these enzymes).

No products indexed under this heading.

Estradiol Valerate (Carbamazepine is known to induce CYP1A2 and CYP3A4. Therefore, the potential exists for interaction between carbamazepine and any agent metabolized by one (or more) of these enzymes).

No products indexed under this heading.

Ethinyl Estradiol (Carbamazepine induces hepatic CYP activity and causes or would be expected to decrease plasma levels of oral contraceptives; breakthrough bleeding has been reported among patients receiving concomitant oral contraceptives and their reliability may be adversely affected). Products include:

Alesse-28 Tablets 3392
Lo/Ovral-28 Tablets 3423
NuvaRing 2357
Ortho-Cept Tablets 2395
Ortho-Cyclen/Ortho Tri-Cyclen 2414
Ortho Evra Transdermal System 2402
Ortho Tri-Cyclen Lo Tablets 2421
Seasonale Tablets 1073
Triphasil-28 Tablets 3483
Yasmin 28 Tablets 818

Ethosuximide (Carbamazepine induces hepatic CYP activity and causes or would be expected to decrease plasma levels of ethosuximide; alterations of thyroid function have been reported in combination therapy with other anticonvulsants).

No products indexed under this heading.

Ethotoin (Alterations of thyroid function have been reported in combination therapy with other anticonvulsants). Products include:

Peganone Tablets, USP 2487

Ethynodiol Diacetate (Carbamazepine induces hepatic CYP activity and causes or would be expected to decrease plasma levels of oral contraceptives; breakthrough bleeding has been reported among patients receiving concomitant oral contraceptives and their reliability may be adversely affected).

No products indexed under this heading.

Etoposide (Carbamazepine is known to induce CYP1A2 and CYP3A4. Therefore, the potential exists for interaction between carbamazepine and any agent metabolized by one (or more) of these enzymes).

No products indexed under this heading.

Etoposide Phosphate (Carbamazepine is known to induce CYP1A2 and CYP3A4. Therefore, the potential exists for interaction between carbamazepine and any agent metabolized by one (or more) of these enzymes).

No products indexed under this heading.

Felbamate (Inducers of CYP3A4, such as felbamate, can increase the rate of carbamazepine metabolism and can thus decrease plasma carbamazepine levels; alterations of thyroid function have been reported in combination therapy with other anticonvulsants).

No products indexed under this heading.

Felodipine (Carbamazepine is known to induce CYP1A2 and CYP3A4. Therefore, the potential exists for interaction between carbamazepine and any agent metabolized by one (or more) of these enzymes). Products include:

Plendil Extended-Release Tablets 651

Fentanyl (Carbamazepine is known to induce CYP1A2 and CYP3A4. Therefore, the potential exists for interaction between carbamazepine and any agent metabolized by one (or more) of these enzymes). Products include:

Duragesic Transdermal System 2448

Fentanyl Citrate (Carbamazepine is known to induce CYP1A2 and CYP3A4. Therefore, the potential exists for interaction between carbamazepine and any agent metabolized by one (or more) of these enzymes). Products include:

Actiq 993

Fluconazole (Carbamazepine is metabolized mainly by cytochrome P450 (CYP) 3A4 to the active carbamazepine 10,11 -epoxide, which is further metabolized to the trans-diol by epoxide hydrolase. Therefore, the potential exists for interaction between carbamazepine and any agent that inhibits CYP3A4 and/or epoxide hydrolase).

No products indexed under this heading.

Fludrocortisone Acetate (Carbamazepine is metabolized by CYP3A4. Therefore, the potential exists for interaction between caramazepine and any agent that induces CYP3A4).

No products indexed under this heading.

Fluoxetine Hydrochloride (Inhibitors of CYP3A4, such as fluoxetine, inhibit carbamazepine metabolism and thus increase plasma carbamazepine levels). Products include:

Prozac Pulvules and Liquid 1771
Symbyax Capsules 1788

Fluphenazine Decanoate (Co-administration with psychotropic agents has resulted in isolated cases of neuroleptic malignant syndrome).

No products indexed under this heading.

Fluphenazine Enanthate (Co-administration with psychotropic agents has resulted in isolated cases of neuroleptic malignant syndrome).

No products indexed under this heading.

Fluphenazine Hydrochloride (Co-administration with psychotropic agents has resulted in isolated cases of neuroleptic malignant syndrome).

No products indexed under this heading.

Flutamide (Carbamazepine is known to induce CYP1A2 and CYP3A4. Therefore, the potential exists for interaction between carbamazepine and any agent metabolized by one (or more) of these enzymes). Products include:

Eulexin Capsules 3023

Fluticasone Propionate (Carbamazepine is known to induce CYP1A2 and CYP3A4. Therefore, the potential exists for interaction between carbamazepine and any agent metabolized by one (or more) of these enzymes). Products include:

Advair Diskus 100/50 1291
Advair Diskus 250/50 1291
Advair Diskus 500/50 1291
Cutivate Cream 1381
Cutivate Lotion 0.05% 1383
Cutivate Ointment 1384
Flonase Nasal Spray 1412
Flovent Diskus 100 mcg 1418
Flovent Diskus 50 mcg 1415

Fluvoxamine Maleate (Carbamazepine is metabolized mainly by cytochrome P450 (CYP) 3A4 to the active carbamazepine 10,11 -epoxide, which is further metabolized to the trans-diol by epoxide hydrolase. Therefore, the potential exists for interaction between carbamazepine and any agent that inhibits its CYP3A4 and/or epoxide hydrolase).

No products indexed under this heading.

Fosamprenavir Calcium (Carbamazepine is metabolized mainly by cytochrome P450 (CYP) 3A4 to the active carbamazepine 10,11 -epoxide, which is further metabolized to the trans-diol by epoxide hydrolase. Therefore, the potential exists for interaction between carbamazepine and any agent that inhibits its CYP3A4 and/or epoxide hydrolase). Products include:

Lexiva Tablets 1473

Fosphenytoin (Alterations of thyroid function have been reported in combination therapy with other anticonvulsants).

No products indexed under this heading.

Fosphenytoin Sodium (Alterations of thyroid function have been reported in combination therapy with other anticonvulsants).

No products indexed under this heading.

Gabapentin (Alterations of thyroid function have been reported in combination therapy with other anticonvulsants). Products include:

Neurontin Capsules 2498
Neurontin Oral Solution 2498
Neurontin Tablets 2498

IMPORTANT NOTE: Always consult each drug listing in the patient's regimen for possible interactions.

Garlic Extract (Carbamazepine is metabolized by CYP3A4. Therefore, the potential exists for interaction between caramazepine and any agent that induces CYP3A4).
No products indexed under this heading.

Garlic Oil (Carbamazepine is metabolized by CYP3A4. Therefore, the potential exists for interaction between caramazepine and any agent that induces CYP3A4).
No products indexed under this heading.

Grepafloxacin Hydrochloride (Carbamazepine is known to induce CYP1A2 and CYP3A4. Therefore, the potential exists for interaction between carbamazepine and any agent metabolized by one (or more) of these enzymes).
No products indexed under this heading.

Haloperidol (Carbamazepine induces hepatic CYP activity and causes or would be expected to decrease plasma levels of haloperidol).
No products indexed under this heading.

Haloperidol Decanoate (Carbamazepine induces hepatic CYP activity and causes or would be expected to decrease plasma levels of haloperidol).
No products indexed under this heading.

Haloperidol Lactate (Carbamazepine is known to induce CYP1A2 and CYP3A4. Therefore, the potential exists for interaction between carbamazepine and any agent metabolized by one (or more) of these enzymes).
No products indexed under this heading.

Hydrocortisone (Carbamazepine is metabolized by CYP3A4. Therefore, the potential exists for interaction between caramazepine and any agent that induces CYP3A4).
Products include:
- Cortizone•5 Ointment ... ▣699
- Cortizone•10 Creme ... ▣699
- Cortizone•10 Ointment ... ▣699
- Cortizone•10 Plus Creme ... ▣700
- Cortizone•10 Maximum Strength Quick Shot Spray ... ▣700
- Hydrocortone Tablets ... 1963
- Preparation H Hydrocortisone Cream ... ▣748

Hydrocortisone Acetate (Carbamazepine is metabolized by CYP3A4. Therefore, the potential exists for interaction between caramazepine and any agent that induces CYP3A4). Products include:
- Analpram-HC ... 1136
- Pramosone ... 1139
- ProctoFoam-HC ... 3113
- Tucks Anti-Itch Ointment ... ▣712
- U-cort 1% Cream ... 3289

Hydrocortisone Butyrate (Carbamazepine is metabolized by CYP3A4. Therefore, the potential exists for interaction between caramazepine and any agent that induces CYP3A4). Products include:
- Locoid ... 1138
- Locoid Lipocream Cream ... 1138

Hydrocortisone Cypionate (Carbamazepine is metabolized by CYP3A4. Therefore, the potential exists for interaction between caramazepine and any agent that induces CYP3A4).
No products indexed under this heading.

Hydrocortisone Hemisuccinate (Carbamazepine is metabolized by CYP3A4. Therefore, the potential exists for interaction between caramazepine and any agent that induces CYP3A4).
No products indexed under this heading.

Hydrocortisone Probutate (Carbamazepine is metabolized by CYP3A4. Therefore, the potential exists for interaction between caramazepine and any agent that induces CYP3A4). Products include:
- Pandel Cream, 0.1% ... 1017

Hydrocortisone Sodium Phosphate (Carbamazepine is metabolized by CYP3A4. Therefore, the potential exists for interaction between caramazepine and any agent that induces CYP3A4).
No products indexed under this heading.

Hydrocortisone Sodium Succinate (Carbamazepine is metabolized by CYP3A4. Therefore, the potential exists for interaction between caramazepine and any agent that induces CYP3A4).
No products indexed under this heading.

Hydrocortisone Valerate (Carbamazepine is metabolized by CYP3A4. Therefore, the potential exists for interaction between caramazepine and any agent that induces CYP3A4).
No products indexed under this heading.

Hypericum (Carbamazepine is metabolized by CYP3A4. Therefore, the potential exists for interaction between caramazepine and any agent that induces CYP3A4).
No products indexed under this heading.

Hypericum Perforatum (Carbamazepine is metabolized by CYP3A4. Therefore, the potential exists for interaction between caramazepine and any agent that induces CYP3A4).
No products indexed under this heading.

Imipramine Hydrochloride (Carbamazepine is known to induce CYP1A2 and CYP3A4. Therefore, the potential exists for interaction between carbamazepine and any agent metabolized by one (or more) of these enzymes).
No products indexed under this heading.

Imipramine Pamoate (Carbamazepine is known to induce CYP1A2 and CYP3A4. Therefore, the potential exists for interaction between carbamazepine and any agent metabolized by one (or more) of these enzymes).
No products indexed under this heading.

Indinavir Sulfate (Carbamazepine is metabolized mainly by cytochrome P450 (CYP) 3A4 to the active carbamazepine 10,11 -epoxide, which is further metabolized to the trans-diol by epoxide hydrolase. Therefore, the potential exists for interaction between carbamazepine and any agent that inhibits CYP3A4 and/or epoxide hydrolase). Products include:
- Crixivan Capsules ... 1918

Isocarboxazid (Because of the relationship of carbamazepine to other tricyclic compounds, on theoretical grounds, co-administration with MAO inhibitors is contraindicated).
No products indexed under this heading.

Isoniazid (Inhibitors of CYP3A4, such as isoniazid, inhibit carbamazepine metabolism and thus increase plasma carbamazepine levels).
No products indexed under this heading.

Isradipine (Carbamazepine is known to induce CYP1A2 and CYP3A4. Therefore, the potential exists for interaction between carbamazepine and any agent metabolized by one (or more) of these enzymes). Products include:
- DynaCirc CR Tablets ... 2726

Itraconazole (Inhibitors of CYP3A4, such as itraconazole, inhibit carbamazepine metabolism and thus increase plasma carbamazepine levels).
No products indexed under this heading.

Ketoconazole (Inhibitors of CYP3A4, such as ketoconazole, inhibit carbamazepine metabolism and thus increase plasma carbamazepine levels). Products include:
- Nizoral A-D Shampoo, 1% ... 1839
- Nizoral 2% Shampoo ... 1838

Lamotrigine (Alterations of thyroid function have been reported in combination therapy with other anticonvulsants). Products include:
- Lamictal ... 1449

Levetiracetam (Alterations of thyroid function have been reported in combination therapy with other anticonvulsants). Products include:
- Keppra Oral Solution ... 3307
- Keppra Tablets ... 3307

Levobupivacaine Hydrochloride (Carbamazepine is known to induce CYP1A2 and CYP3A4. Therefore, the potential exists for interaction between carbamazepine and any agent metabolized by one (or more) of these enzymes).
No products indexed under this heading.

Levonorgestrel (Carbamazepine induces hepatic CYP activity and causes or would be expected to decrease plasma levels of oral contraceptives; breakthrough bleeding has been reported among patients receiving concomitant oral contraceptives and their reliability may be adversely affected). Products include:
- Alesse-28 Tablets ... 3392
- Climara Pro Transdermal System ... 800
- Mirena Intrauterine System ... 810
- Plan B Tablets ... 1068
- Seasonale Tablets ... 1073
- Triphasil-28 Tablets ... 3483

Lidocaine (Carbamazepine is known to induce CYP1A2 and CYP3A4. Therefore, the potential exists for interaction between carbamazepine and any agent metabolized by one (or more) of these enzymes). Products include:
- Lidoderm Patch ... 1107

Lidocaine Hydrochloride (Carbamazepine is known to induce CYP1A2 and CYP3A4. Therefore, the potential exists for interaction between carbamazepine and any agent metabolized by one (or more) of these enzymes).
No products indexed under this heading.

Lithium (Co-administration may increase the risk of neurotoxic side effects).
No products indexed under this heading.

Lithium Carbonate (Co-administration with psychotropic agents has resulted in isolated cases of neuroleptic malignant syndrome). Products include:
- Eskalith ... 1406
- Lithobid Tablets ... 1670

Lithium Citrate (Co-administration with psychotropic agents has resulted in isolated cases of neuroleptic malignant syndrome).
No products indexed under this heading.

Lomefloxacin Hydrochloride (Carbamazepine is known to induce CYP1A2 and CYP3A4. Therefore, the potential exists for interaction between carbamazepine and any agent metabolized by one (or more) of these enzymes).
No products indexed under this heading.

Lopinavir (Carbamazepine is metabolized mainly by cytochrome P450 (CYP) 3A4 to the active carbamazepine 10,11 -epoxide, which is further metabolized to the trans-diol by epoxide hydrolase. Therefore, the potential exists for interaction between carbamazepine and any agent that inhibits CYP3A4 and/or epoxide hydrolase). Products include:
- Kaletra ... 474

Loratadine (Inhibitors of CYP3A4, such as loratadine, inhibit carbamazepine metabolism and thus increase plasma carbamazepine levels).
Products include:
- Alavert Allergy & Sinus D-12 Hour Tablets ... ▣743
- Alavert ... ▣743
- Children's Claritin 24 Hour Non-Drowsy Allergy Syrup ... ▣732
- Claritin Non-Drowsy 24 Hour Tablets ... ▣731
- Non-Drowsy Claritin Hives Relief Tablets ... ▣733
- Claritin Reditabs 24 Hour Non-Drowsy Tablets ... ▣732
- Claritin-D Non-Drowsy 12 Hour Tablets ... ▣731
- Claritin-D Non-Drowsy 24 Hour Tablets ... ▣731
- Children's Dimetapp ND Non-Drowsy Allergy Syrup ... ▣746
- Triaminic Allerchews ... ▣684

Lovastatin (Carbamazepine is known to induce CYP1A2 and CYP3A4. Therefore, the potential exists for interaction between carbamazepine and any agent metabolized by one (or more) of these enzymes). Products include:
- Advicor Tablets ... 1694
- Altoprev Extended-Release Tablets ... 1151
- Mevacor Tablets ... 1996

Loxapine Hydrochloride (Co-administration with psychotropic agents has resulted in isolated cases of neuroleptic malignant syndrome).
No products indexed under this heading.

Loxapine Succinate (Co-administration with psychotropic agents has resulted in isolated cases of neuroleptic malignant syndrome).
No products indexed under this heading.

Maprotiline Hydrochloride (Carbamazepine is known to induce CYP1A2 and CYP3A4. Therefore, the potential exists for interaction between carbamazepine and any agent metabolized by one (or more) of these enzymes).
No products indexed under this heading.

Mefloquine Hydrochloride (Antimalarial drugs, such as chloroquine and mefloquine, may antagonize the activity of carbamazepine). Products include:
Lariam Tablets 2790

Mephenytoin (Alterations of thyroid function have been reported in combination therapy with other anticonvulsants).
No products indexed under this heading.

Mesoridazine Besylate (Co-administration with psychotropic agents has resulted in isolated cases of neuroleptic malignant syndrome).
No products indexed under this heading.

Mestranol (Carbamazepine induces hepatic CYP activity and causes or would be expected to decrease plasma levels of oral contraceptives; breakthrough bleeding has been reported among patients receiving concomitant oral contraceptives and their reliability may be adversely affected).
No products indexed under this heading.

Methadone Hydrochloride (Carbamazepine is known to induce CYP1A2 and CYP3A4. Therefore, the potential exists for interaction between carbamazepine and any agent metabolized by one (or more) of these enzymes).
No products indexed under this heading.

Methotrimeprazine (Co-administration with psychotropic agents has resulted in isolated cases of neuroleptic malignant syndrome).
No products indexed under this heading.

Methsuximide (Carbemezapine induces hepatic CYP activity and causes or would be expected to decrease plasma levels of methsuximide; alterations of thyroid function have been reported in combination therapy with other anticonvulsants).
No products indexed under this heading.

Methylprednisolone (Carbamazepine is metabolized by CYP3A4. Therefore, the potential exists for interaction between caramazepine and any agent that induces CYP3A4).
No products indexed under this heading.

Methylprednisolone Acetate (Carbamazepine is metabolized by CYP3A4. Therefore, the potential exists for interaction between caramazepine and any agent that induces CYP3A4). Products include:
Depo-Medrol Injectable Suspension 2615
Depo-Medrol Single-Dose Vial 2617

Methylprednisolone Sodium Succinate (Carbamazepine is metabolized by CYP3A4. Therefore, the potential exists for interaction between caramazepine and any agent that induces CYP3A4).
No products indexed under this heading.

Metronidazole (Carbamazepine is metabolized mainly by cytochrome P450 (CYP) 3A4 to the active carbamazepine 10,11 -epoxide, which is further metabolized to the trans-diol by epoxide hydrolase. Therefore, the potential exists for interaction between carbamazepine and any agent that inhibits CYP3A4 and/or epoxide hydrolase). Products include:
Metrogel 1% 1212
MetroGel-Vaginal Gel 1822
Noritate Cream, 1% 1051

Metronidazole Benzoate (Carbamazepine is metabolized mainly by cytochrome P450 (CYP) 3A4 to the active carbamazepine 10,11 -epoxide, which is further metabolized to the trans-diol by epoxide hydrolase. Therefore, the potential exists for interaction between carbamazepine and any agent that inhibits CYP3A4 and/or epoxide hydrolase).
No products indexed under this heading.

Metronidazole Hydrochloride (Carbamazepine is metabolized mainly by cytochrome P450 (CYP) 3A4 to the active carbamazepine 10,11 -epoxide, which is further metabolized to the trans-diol by epoxide hydrolase. Therefore, the potential exists for interaction between carbamazepine and any agent that inhibits CYP3A4 and/or epoxide hydrolase).
No products indexed under this heading.

Mexiletine Hydrochloride (Carbamazepine is known to induce CYP1A2 and CYP3A4. Therefore, the potential exists for interaction between carbamazepine and any agent metabolized by one (or more) of these enzymes).
No products indexed under this heading.

Miconazole (Carbamazepine is metabolized mainly by cytochrome P450 (CYP) 3A4 to the active carbamazepine 10,11 -epoxide, which is further metabolized to the trans-diol by epoxide hydrolase. Therefore, the potential exists for interaction between carbamazepine and any agent that inhibits CYP3A4 and/or epoxide hydrolase).
No products indexed under this heading.

Miconazole Nitrate (Carbamazepine is metabolized mainly by cytochrome P450 (CYP) 3A4 to the active carbamazepine 10,11 -epoxide, which is further metabolized to the trans-diol by epoxide hydrolase. Therefore, the potential exists for interaction between carbamazepine and any agent that inhibits CYP3A4 and/or epoxide hydrolase). Products include:
Desenex .... ▣ 674
Desenex Jock Itch Spray Powder ... ▣ 674

Midazolam Hydrochloride (Carbamazepine is known to induce CYP1A2 and CYP3A4. Therefore, the potential exists for interaction between carbamazepine and any agent metabolized by one (or more) of these enzymes).
No products indexed under this heading.

Mirtazapine (Carbamazepine is known to induce CYP1A2 and CYP3A4. Therefore, the potential exists for interaction between carbamazepine and any agent metabolized by one (or more) of these enzymes).
No products indexed under this heading.

Moclobemide (Because of the relationship of carbamazepine to other tricyclic compounds, on theoretical grounds, co-administration with MAO inhibitors is contraindicated).
No products indexed under this heading.

Modafinil (Carbamazepine is metabolized by CYP3A4. Therefore, the potential exists for interaction between caramazepine and any agent that induces CYP3A4). Products include:
Provigil Tablets 1002

Molindone Hydrochloride (Co-administration with psychotropic agents has resulted in isolated cases of neuroleptic malignant syndrome). Products include:
Moban Tablets 1108

Moxifloxacin Hydrochloride (Carbamazepine is known to induce CYP1A2 and CYP3A4. Therefore, the potential exists for interaction between carbamazepine and any agent metabolized by one (or more) of these enzymes). Products include:
Avelox 2984
Vigamox Ophthalmic Solution 560

Nafcillin Sodium (Carbamazepine is known to induce CYP1A2 and CYP3A4. Therefore, the potential exists for interaction between carbamazepine and any agent metabolized by one (or more) of these enzymes).
No products indexed under this heading.

Naproxen (Carbamazepine is known to induce CYP1A2 and CYP3A4. Therefore, the potential exists for interaction between carbamazepine and any agent metabolized by one (or more) of these enzymes). Products include:
EC-Naprosyn Delayed-Release Tablets 2769
Naprosyn Suspension 2769
Naprosyn Tablets 2769
Prevacid NapraPAC 3277

Naproxen Sodium (Carbamazepine is known to induce CYP1A2 and CYP3A4. Therefore, the potential exists for interaction between carbamazepine and any agent metabolized by one (or more) of these enzymes). Products include:
Aleve Tablets, Caplets and Gelcaps .... ▣ 605
Anaprox Tablets 2769
Anaprox DS Tablets 2769

Nefazodone Hydrochloride (Carbamazepine is metabolized mainly by cytochrome P450 (CYP) 3A4 to the active carbamazepine 10,11 -epoxide, which is further metabolized to the trans-diol by epoxide hydrolase. Therefore, the potential exists for interaction between carbamazepine and any agent that inhibits its CYP3A4 and/or epoxide hydrolase).
No products indexed under this heading.

Nelfinavir Mesylate (Carbamazepine is metabolized mainly by cytochrome P450 (CYP) 3A4 to the active carbamazepine 10,11 -epoxide, which is further metabolized to the trans-diol by epoxide hydrolase. Therefore, the potential exists for interaction between carbamazepine and any agent that inhibits its CYP3A4 and/or epoxide hydrolase). Products include:
Viracept 2556

Nevirapine (Carbamazepine is metabolized mainly by cytochrome P450 (CYP) 3A4 to the active carbamazepine 10,11 -epoxide, which is further metabolized to the trans-diol by epoxide hydrolase. Therefore, the potential exists for interaction between carbamazepine and any agent that inhibits CYP3A4 and/or epoxide hydrolase). Products include:
Viramune Oral Suspension 903
Viramune Tablets 903

Niacinamide (Inhibitors of CYP3A4, such as niacinamide, inhibit carbamazepine metabolism and thus increase plasma carbamazepine levels).
No products indexed under this heading.

Nicardipine Hydrochloride (Carbamazepine is known to induce CYP1A2 and CYP3A4. Therefore, the potential exists for interaction between carbamazepine and any agent metabolized by one (or more) of these enzymes). Products include:
Cardene I.V. 1129

Nicotinamide (Inhibitors of CYP3A4, such as nicotinamide, inhibit carbamazepine metabolism and thus increase plasma carbamazepine levels). Products include:
Nicomide Tablets 3190

Nicotine Polacrilex (Carbamazepine is known to induce CYP1A2 and CYP3A4. Therefore, the potential exists for interaction between carbamazepine and any agent metabolized by one (or more) of these enzymes). Products include:
Commit Lozenges 1625
Nicorette Gum 1632

Nicotine Salicylate (Carbamazepine is known to induce CYP1A2 and CYP3A4. Therefore, the potential exists for interaction between carbamazepine and any agent metabolized by one (or more) of these enzymes).
No products indexed under this heading.

Nicotine Sulfate (Carbamazepine is known to induce CYP1A2 and CYP3A4. Therefore, the potential exists for interaction between carbamazepine and any agent metabolized by one (or more) of these enzymes).
No products indexed under this heading.

Nifedipine (Carbamazepine is metabolized mainly by cytochrome P450 (CYP) 3A4 to the active carbamazepine 10,11 -epoxide, which is further metabolized to the trans-diol by epoxide hydrolase. Therefore, the potential exists for interaction between carbamazepine and any agent that inhibits CYP3A4 and/or epoxide hydrolase). Products include:

Adalat CC Tablets 2978

Nimodipine (Carbamazepine is known to induce CYP1A2 and CYP3A4. Therefore, the potential exists for interaction between carbamazepine and any agent metabolized by one (or more) of these enzymes). Products include:

Nimotop Capsules 774

Nisoldipine (Carbamazepine is known to induce CYP1A2 and CYP3A4. Therefore, the potential exists for interaction between carbamazepine and any agent metabolized by one (or more) of these enzymes). Products include:

Sular Tablets 1163

Nitrendipine (Carbamazepine is known to induce CYP1A2 and CYP3A4. Therefore, the potential exists for interaction between carbamazepine and any agent metabolized by one (or more) of these enzymes).

No products indexed under this heading.

Norethindrone (Carbamazepine induces hepatic CYP activity and causes or would be expected to decrease plasma levels of oral contraceptives; breakthrough bleeding has been reported among patients receiving concomitant oral contraceptives and their reliability may be adversely affected). Products include:

Ortho Micronor Tablets 2411

Norethindrone Acetate (Carbamazepine is known to induce CYP1A2 and CYP3A4. Therefore, the potential exists for interaction between carbamazepine and any agent metabolized by one (or more) of these enzymes). Products include:

Activella Tablets 2311
Aygestin Tablets 1062
CombiPatch Transdermal System 2180

Norethynodrel (Carbamazepine induces hepatic CYP activity and causes or would be expected to decrease plasma levels of oral contraceptives; breakthrough bleeding has been reported among patients receiving concomitant oral contraceptives and their reliability may be adversely affected).

No products indexed under this heading.

Norfloxacin (Carbamazepine is metabolized mainly by cytochrome P450 (CYP) 3A4 to the active carbamazepine 10,11 -epoxide, which is further metabolized to the trans-diol by epoxide hydrolase. Therefore, the potential exists for interaction between carbamazepine and any agent that inhibits CYP3A4 and/or epoxide hydrolase). Products include:

Noroxin Tablets 2009

Norgestimate (Carbamazepine induces hepatic CYP activity and causes or would be expected to decrease plasma levels of oral contraceptives; breakthrough bleeding has been reported among patients receiving concomitant oral contraceptives and their reliability may be adversely affected). Products include:

Ortho-Cyclen/Ortho Tri-Cyclen 2414
Ortho Tri-Cyclen Lo Tablets 2421
Prefest Tablets 1069

Norgestrel (Carbamazepine induces hepatic CYP activity and causes or would be expected to decrease plasma levels of oral contraceptives; breakthrough bleeding has been reported among patients receiving concomitant oral contraceptives and their reliability may be adversely affected). Products include:

Lo/Ovral-28 Tablets 3423

Nortriptyline Hydrochloride (Carbamazepine is known to induce CYP1A2 and CYP3A4. Therefore, the potential exists for interaction between carbamazepine and any agent metabolized by one (or more) of these enzymes).

No products indexed under this heading.

Ofloxacin (Carbamazepine is known to induce CYP1A2 and CYP3A4. Therefore, the potential exists for interaction between carbamazepine and any agent metabolized by one (or more) of these enzymes). Products include:

Floxin Otic Singles 1045
Floxin Otic Solution 1043

Olanzapine (Co-administration with psychotropic agents has resulted in isolated cases of neuroleptic malignant syndrome). Products include:

Symbyax Capsules 1788
Zyprexa Tablets 1798
Zyprexa IntraMuscular 1798
Zyprexa ZYDIS Orally Disintegrating Tablets 1798

Omeprazole (Carbamazepine is metabolized mainly by cytochrome P450 (CYP) 3A4 to the active carbamazepine 10,11 -epoxide, which is further metabolized to the trans-diol by epoxide hydrolase. Therefore, the potential exists for interaction between carbamazepine and any agent that inhibits CYP3A4 and/or epoxide hydrolase). Products include:

Zegerid Powder for Oral Solution 2972

Ondansetron (Carbamazepine is known to induce CYP1A2 and CYP3A4. Therefore, the potential exists for interaction between carbamazepine and any agent metabolized by one (or more) of these enzymes). Products include:

Zofran ODT Orally Disintegrating Tablets 1613

Ondansetron Hydrochloride (Carbamazepine is known to induce CYP1A2 and CYP3A4. Therefore, the potential exists for interaction between carbamazepine and any agent metabolized by one (or more) of these enzymes). Products include:

Zofran Injection 1607
Zofran 1613

Oxcarbazepine (Alterations of thyroid function have been reported in combination therapy with other anticonvulsants). Products include:

Trileptal Oral Suspension 2281
Trileptal Tablets 2281

Paclitaxel (Carbamazepine is known to induce CYP1A2 and CYP3A4. Therefore, the potential exists for interaction between carbamazepine and any agent metabolized by one (or more) of these enzymes).

No products indexed under this heading.

Paramethadione (Alterations of thyroid function have been reported in combination therapy with other anticonvulsants).

No products indexed under this heading.

Pargyline Hydrochloride (Because of the relationship of carbamazepine to other tricyclic compounds, on theoretical grounds, co-administration with MAO inhibitors is contraindicated).

No products indexed under this heading.

Paroxetine Hydrochloride (Carbamazepine is metabolized mainly by cytochrome P450 (CYP) 3A4 to the active carbamazepine 10,11 -epoxide, which is further metabolized to the trans-diol by epoxide hydrolase. Therefore, the potential exists for interaction between carbamazepine and any agent that inhibits CYP3A4 and/or epoxide hydrolase). Products include:

Paxil CR Controlled-Release Tablets 1509
Paxil 1501

Perphenazine (Co-administration with psychotropic agents has resulted in isolated cases of neuroleptic malignant syndrome).

No products indexed under this heading.

Phenacemide (Alterations of thyroid function have been reported in combination therapy with other anticonvulsants).

No products indexed under this heading.

Phenelzine Sulfate (Because of the relationship of carbamazepine to other tricyclic compounds, on theoretical grounds, co-administration with MAO inhibitors is contraindicated).

No products indexed under this heading.

Phenobarbital (Inducers of CYP3A4, such as phenobarbital, can increase the rate of carbamazepine metabolism and can thus decrease plasma carbamazepine levels; alterations of thyroid function have been reported in combination therapy with other anticonvulsants).

No products indexed under this heading.

Phenobarbital Sodium (Carbamazepine is metabolized by CYP3A4. Therefore, the potential exists for interaction between caramazepine and any agent that induces CYP3A4).

No products indexed under this heading.

Phensuximide (Carbamezapine induces hepatic CYP activity and causes or would be expected to decrease plasma levels of phensuximide; alterations of thyroid function have been reported in combination therapy with other anticonvulsants).

No products indexed under this heading.

Phenytoin (Alterations of thyroid function have been reported in combination therapy with other anticonvulsants).

No products indexed under this heading.

Phenytoin Sodium (Alterations of thyroid function have been reported in combination therapy with other anticonvulsants). Products include:

Phenytek Capsules 2153

Pimozide (Co-administration with psychotropic agents has resulted in isolated cases of neuroleptic malignant syndrome). Products include:

Orap Tablets 1220

Polyestradiol Phosphate (Carbamazepine is known to induce CYP1A2 and CYP3A4. Therefore, the potential exists for interaction between carbamazepine and any agent metabolized by one (or more) of these enzymes).

No products indexed under this heading.

Prednisolone Acetate (Carbamazepine is metabolized by CYP3A4. Therefore, the potential exists for interaction between caramazepine and any agent that induces CYP3A4). Products include:

Blephamide Ophthalmic Ointment 563
Blephamide Ophthalmic Suspension 564
Poly-Pred Liquifilm Ophthalmic Suspension .... ⊙ 231
Pred Forte Ophthalmic Suspension .... ⊙ 233
Pred Mild Sterile Ophthalmic Suspension .... ⊙ 236
Pred-G Ophthalmic Suspension .... ⊙ 234
Pred-G Sterile Ophthalmic Ointment .... ⊙ 235

Prednisolone Sodium Phosphate (Carbamazepine is metabolized by CYP3A4. Therefore, the potential exists for interaction between caramazepine and any agent that induces CYP3A4). Products include:

Pediapred Oral Solution 3319

Prednisolone Tebutate (Carbamazepine is metabolized by CYP3A4. Therefore, the potential exists for interaction between caramazepine and any agent that induces CYP3A4).

No products indexed under this heading.

Prednisone (Carbamazepine is metabolized by CYP3A4. Therefore, the potential exists for interaction between caramazepine and any agent that induces CYP3A4).

No products indexed under this heading.

Primidone (Inducers of CYP3A4, such as primidone, can increase the rate of carbamazepine metabolism and can thus decrease plasma carbamazepine levels; carbamazepine increases levels of primidone; alterations of thyroid function have been reported in combination therapy with other anticonvulsants).

No products indexed under this heading.

Procarbazine Hydrochloride (Because of the relationship of carbamazepine to other tricyclic compounds, on theoretical grounds, co-administration with MAO inhibitors is contraindicated). Products include:

Matulane Capsules 3188

Prochlorperazine (Co-administration with psychotropic agents has resulted in isolated cases of neuroleptic malignant syndrome).
No products indexed under this heading.

Promethazine Hydrochloride (Co-administration with psychotropic agents has resulted in isolated cases of neuroleptic malignant syndrome). Products include:
Phenergan 3438

Propafenone Hydrochloride (Carbamazepine is known to induce CYP1A2 and CYP3A4. Therefore, the potential exists for interaction between carbamazepine and any agent metabolized by one (or more) of these enzymes). Products include:
Rythmol SR Capsules 2736

Propoxyphene Hydrochloride (Inhibitors of CYP3A4, such as propoxyphene, inhibit carbamazepine metabolism and thus increase plasma carbamazepine levels).
No products indexed under this heading.

Propoxyphene Napsylate (Inhibitors of CYP3A4, such as propoxyphene, inhibit carbamazepine metabolism and thus increase plasma carbamazepine levels). Products include:
Darvocet A 500 Tablets 3497

Propranolol Hydrochloride (Carbamazepine is known to induce CYP1A2 and CYP3A4. Therefore, the potential exists for interaction between carbamazepine and any agent metabolized by one (or more) of these enzymes). Products include:
Inderal LA Long-Acting Capsules 3421
InnoPran XL Capsules 2728

Protriptyline Hydrochloride (Carbamazepine is known to induce CYP1A2 and CYP3A4. Therefore, the potential exists for interaction between carbamazepine and any agent metabolized by one (or more) of these enzymes). Products include:
Vivactil Tablets 2350

Pyrimethamine (Anti-malarial drugs, such as chloroquine and mefloquine, may antagonize the activity of carbamazepine). Products include:
Daraprim Tablets 1385

Quetiapine Fumarate (Co-administration with psychotropic agents has resulted in isolated cases of neuroleptic malignant syndrome). Products include:
Seroquel Tablets 691

Quinidine (Carbamazepine is metabolized mainly by cytochrome P450 (CYP) 3A4 to the active carbamazepine 10,11 -epoxide, which is further metabolized to the trans-diol by epoxide hydrolase. Therefore, the potential exists for interaction between carbamazepine and any agent that inhibits CYP3A4 and/or epoxide hydrolase).
No products indexed under this heading.

Quinidine Gluconate (Carbamazepine is known to induce CYP1A2 and CYP3A4. Therefore, the potential exists for interaction between carbamazepine and any agent metabolized by one (or more) of these enzymes).
No products indexed under this heading.

Quinidine Hydrochloride (Carbamazepine is metabolized mainly by cytochrome P450 (CYP) 3A4 to the active carbamazepine 10,11 -epoxide, which is further metabolized to the trans-diol by epoxide hydrolase. Therefore, the potential exists for interaction between carbamazepine and any agent that inhibits CYP3A4 and/or epoxide hydrolase).
No products indexed under this heading.

Quinidine Polygalacturonate (Carbamazepine is metabolized mainly by cytochrome P450 (CYP) 3A4 to the active carbamazepine 10,11 -epoxide, which is further metabolized to the trans-diol by epoxide hydrolase. Therefore, the potential exists for interaction between carbamazepine and any agent that inhibits CYP3A4 and/or epoxide hydrolase).
No products indexed under this heading.

Quinidine Sulfate (Carbamazepine is metabolized mainly by cytochrome P450 (CYP) 3A4 to the active carbamazepine 10,11 -epoxide, which is further metabolized to the trans-diol by epoxide hydrolase. Therefore, the potential exists for interaction between carbamazepine and any agent that inhibits CYP3A4 and/or epoxide hydrolase).
No products indexed under this heading.

Quinine (Carbamazepine is metabolized mainly by cytochrome P450 (CYP) 3A4 to the active carbamazepine 10,11 -epoxide, which is further metabolized to the trans-diol by epoxide hydrolase. Therefore, the potential exists for interaction between carbamazepine and any agent that inhibits CYP3A4 and/or epoxide hydrolase).
No products indexed under this heading.

Quinine Sulfate (Carbamazepine is metabolized mainly by cytochrome P450 (CYP) 3A4 to the active carbamazepine 10,11 -epoxide, which is further metabolized to the trans-diol by epoxide hydrolase. Therefore, the potential exists for interaction between carbamazepine and any agent that inhibits CYP3A4 and/or epoxide hydrolase).
No products indexed under this heading.

Quinupristin (Carbamazepine is metabolized mainly by cytochrome P450 (CYP) 3A4 to the active carbamazepine 10,11 -epoxide, which is further metabolized to the trans-diol by epoxide hydrolase. Therefore, the potential exists for interaction between carbamazepine and any agent that inhibits CYP3A4 and/or epoxide hydrolase). Products include:
Synercid I.V. 1690

Ranitidine Bismuth Citrate (Carbamazepine is metabolized mainly by cytochrome P450 (CYP) 3A4 to the active carbamazepine 10,11 -epoxide, which is further metabolized to the trans-diol by epoxide hydrolase. Therefore, the potential exists for interaction between carbamazepine and any agent that inhibits CYP3A4 and/or epoxide hydrolase).
No products indexed under this heading.

Ranitidine Hydrochloride (Carbamazepine is metabolized mainly by cytochrome P450 (CYP) 3A4 to the active carbamazepine 10,11 -epoxide, which is further metabolized to the trans-diol by epoxide hydrolase. Therefore, the potential exists for interaction between carbamazepine and any agent that inhibits CYP3A4 and/or epoxide hydrolase). Products include:
Zantac 1597
Zantac Injection 1593
Zantac 75 Tablets 715
Zantac 150 Maximum Strength Tablets 715
Zantac Injection Pharmacy Bulk Package 1595

Rifabutin (Carbamazepine is metabolized by CYP3A4. Therefore, the potential exists for interaction between caramazepine and any agent that induces CYP3A4).
No products indexed under this heading.

Rifampicin (Carbamazepine is metabolized by CYP3A4. Therefore, the potential exists for interaction between caramazepine and any agent that induces CYP3A4).
No products indexed under this heading.

Rifampin (Inducers of CYP3A4, such as rifampin, can increase the rate of carbamazepine metabolism and can thus decrease plasma carbamazepine levels).
No products indexed under this heading.

Rifapentine (Carbamazepine is metabolized by CYP3A4. Therefore, the potential exists for interaction between caramazepine and any agent that induces CYP3A4).
No products indexed under this heading.

Riluzole (Carbamazepine is known to induce CYP1A2 and CYP3A4. Therefore, the potential exists for interaction between carbamazepine and any agent metabolized by one (or more) of these enzymes). Products include:
Rilutek Tablets 2945

Risperidone (Co-administration with psychotropic agents has resulted in isolated cases of neuroleptic malignant syndrome). Products include:
Risperdal Consta Long-Acting Injection 1664
Risperdal M-Tab Orally Disintegrating Tablets 1658
Risperdal 1658

Ritonavir (Carbamazepine is metabolized mainly by cytochrome P450 (CYP) 3A4 to the active carbamazepine 10,11 -epoxide, which is further metabolized to the trans-diol by epoxide hydrolase. Therefore, the potential exists for interaction between carbamazepine and any agent that inhibits CYP3A4 and/or epoxide hydrolase). Products include:
Kaletra 474
Norvir 499

Ropinirole Hydrochloride (Carbamazepine is known to induce CYP1A2 and CYP3A4. Therefore, the potential exists for interaction between carbamazepine and any agent metabolized by one (or more) of these enzymes). Products include:
Requip Tablets 1528

Ropivacaine Hydrochloride (Carbamazepine is known to induce CYP1A2 and CYP3A4. Therefore, the potential exists for interaction between carbamazepine and any agent metabolized by one (or more) of these enzymes). Products include:
Naropin Injection 640

Saquinavir (Carbamazepine is metabolized mainly by cytochrome P450 (CYP) 3A4 to the active carbamazepine 10,11 -epoxide, which is further metabolized to the trans-diol by epoxide hydrolase. Therefore, the potential exists for interaction between carbamazepine and any agent that inhibits CYP3A4 and/or epoxide hydrolase).
No products indexed under this heading.

Saquinavir Mesylate (Carbamazepine is metabolized mainly by cytochrome P450 (CYP) 3A4 to the active carbamazepine 10,11 -epoxide, which is further metabolized to the trans-diol by epoxide hydrolase. Therefore, the potential exists for interaction between carbamazepine and any agent that inhibits CYP3A4 and/or epoxide hydrolase). Products include:
Invirase 2776

Selegiline Hydrochloride (Because of the relationship of carbamazepine to other tricyclic compounds, on theoretical grounds, co-administration with MAO inhibitors is contraindicated). Products include:
Eldepryl Capsules 3209

Sertraline Hydrochloride (Carbamazepine is metabolized mainly by cytochrome P450 (CYP) 3A4 to the active carbamazepine 10,11 -epoxide, which is further metabolized to the trans-diol by epoxide hydrolase. Therefore, the potential exists for interaction between carbamazepine and any agent that inhibits CYP3A4 and/or epoxide hydrolase). Products include:
Zoloft 2581

Sildenafil Citrate (Carbamazepine is known to induce CYP1A2 and CYP3A4. Therefore, the potential exists for interaction between carbamazepine and any agent metabolized by one (or more) of these enzymes). Products include:
Revatio Tablets 2541
Viagra Tablets 2552

Simvastatin (Carbamazepine is known to induce CYP1A2 and CYP3A4. Therefore, the potential exists for interaction between carbamazepine and any agent metabolized by one (or more) of these enzymes). Products include:
Vytorin 10/10 Tablets 2084
Vytorin 10/10 Tablets 3092
Vytorin 10/20 Tablets 2084
Vytorin 10/20 Tablets 3092
Vytorin 10/40 Tablets 3092
Vytorin 10/40 Tablets 2084
Vytorin 10/80 Tablets 2084
Vytorin 10/80 Tablets 3092
Zocor Tablets 2078

Sirolimus (Carbamazepine is known to induce CYP1A2 and CYP3A4. Therefore, the potential exists for interaction between carbamazepine and any agent metabolized by one (or more) of these enzymes). Products include:
Rapamune Oral Solution and Tablets 3472

Sulfinpyrazone (Carbamazepine is metabolized by CYP3A4. Therefore, the potential exists for interaction between caramazepine and any agent that induces CYP3A4).
No products indexed under this heading.

Tacrine Hydrochloride (Carbamazepine is known to induce CYP1A2 and CYP3A4. Therefore, the potential exists for interaction between carbamazepine and any agent metabolized by one (or more) of these enzymes).
No products indexed under this heading.

Tacrolimus (Carbamazepine is known to induce CYP1A2 and CYP3A4. Therefore, the potential exists for interaction between carbamazepine and any agent metabolized by one (or more) of these enzymes). Products include:
Prograf Capsules and Injection 624
Protopic Ointment 629

Tamoxifen Citrate (Carbamazepine is known to induce CYP1A2 and CYP3A4. Therefore, the potential exists for interaction between carbamazepine and any agent metabolized by one (or more) of these enzymes).
No products indexed under this heading.

Telithromycin (Carbamazepine is metabolized mainly by cytochrome P450 (CYP) 3A4 to the active carbamazepine 10,11 -epoxide, which is further metabolized to the transdiol by epoxide hydrolase. Therefore, the potential exists for interaction between carbamazepine and any agent that inhibits CYP3A4 and/or epoxide hydrolase). Products include:
Ketek Tablets 2920

Terfenadine (Inhibitors of CYP3A4, such as terfenadine, inhibit carbamazepine metabolism and thus increase plasma carbamazepine levels).
No products indexed under this heading.

Theophylline (Inducers of CYP3A4, such as theophylline, can increase the rate of carbamazepine metabolism and can thus decrease plasma carbamazepine levels; carbamazepine induces hepatic CYP activity and causes or would be expected to decrease plasma levels of theophylline).
No products indexed under this heading.

Theophylline Anhydrous (Inducers of CYP3A4, such as theophylline, can increase the rate of carbamazepine metabolism and can thus decrease plasma carbamazepine levels; carbamazepine induces hepatic CYP activity and causes or would be expected to decrease plasma levels of theophylline). Products include:
Uniphyl Tablets 2708

Theophylline Calcium Salicylate (Inducers of CYP3A4, such as theophylline, can increase the rate of carbamazepine metabolism and can thus decrease plasma carbamazepine levels; carbamazepine induces hepatic CYP activity and causes or would be expected to decrease plasma levels of theophylline).
No products indexed under this heading.

Theophylline Dihydroxypropyl (Glyceryl) (Inducers of CYP3A4, such as theophylline, can increase the rate of carbamazepine metabolism and can thus decrease plasma carbamazepine levels; carbamazepine induces hepatic CYP activity and causes or would be expected to decrease plasma levels of theophylline).
No products indexed under this heading.

Theophylline Ethylenediamine (Inducers of CYP3A4, such as theophylline, can increase the rate of carbamazepine metabolism and can thus decrease plasma carbamazepine levels; carbamazepine induces hepatic CYP activity and causes or would be expected to decrease plasma levels of theophylline).
No products indexed under this heading.

Theophylline Sodium Glycinate (Inducers of CYP3A4, such as theophylline, can increase the rate of carbamazepine metabolism and can thus decrease plasma carbamazepine levels; carbamazepine induces hepatic CYP activity and causes or would be expected to decrease plasma levels of theophylline).
No products indexed under this heading.

Thioridazine Hydrochloride (Co-administration with psychotropic agents has resulted in isolated cases of neuroleptic malignant syndrome). Products include:
Thioridazine Hydrochloride Tablets 2122

Thiothixene (Co-administration with psychotropic agents has resulted in isolated cases of neuroleptic malignant syndrome). Products include:
Thiothixene Capsules 2124

Tiagabine Hydrochloride (Alterations of thyroid function have been reported in combination therapy with other anticonvulsants). Products include:
Gabitril Tablets 998

Tolterodine Tartrate (Carbamazepine is known to induce CYP1A2 and CYP3A4. Therefore, the potential exists for interaction between carbamazepine and any agent metabolized by one (or more) of these enzymes). Products include:
Detrol Tablets 2626
Detrol LA Capsules 2629

Topiramate (Alterations of thyroid function have been reported in combination therapy with other anticonvulsants). Products include:
Topamax Sprinkle Capsules 2438
Topamax Tablets 2438

Tranylcypromine Sulfate (Because of the relationship of carbamazepine to other tricyclic compounds, on theoretical grounds, co-administration with MAO inhibitors is contraindicated). Products include:
Parnate Tablets 1499

Trazodone Hydrochloride (Carbamazepine is known to induce CYP1A2 and CYP3A4. Therefore, the potential exists for interaction between carbamazepine and any agent metabolized by one (or more) of these enzymes).
No products indexed under this heading.

Triamcinolone (Carbamazepine is metabolized by CYP3A4. Therefore, the potential exists for interaction between caramazepine and any agent that induces CYP3A4).
No products indexed under this heading.

Triamcinolone Acetonide (Carbamazepine is metabolized by CYP3A4. Therefore, the potential exists for interaction between carамazepine and any agent that induces CYP3A4). Products include:
Azmacort Inhalation Aerosol 1701
Nasacort HFA Inhalation Aerosol 2939
Nasacort AQ Nasal Spray 2937

Triamcinolone Diacetate (Carbamazepine is metabolized by CYP3A4. Therefore, the potential exists for interaction between caramazepine and any agent that induces CYP3A4).
No products indexed under this heading.

Triamcinolone Hexacetonide (Carbamazepine is metabolized by CYP3A4. Therefore, the potential exists for interaction between caramazepine and any agent that induces CYP3A4).
No products indexed under this heading.

Triazolam (Carbamazepine is known to induce CYP1A2 and CYP3A4. Therefore, the potential exists for interaction between carbamazepine and any agent metabolized by one (or more) of these enzymes).
No products indexed under this heading.

Trifluoperazine Hydrochloride (Co-administration with psychotropic agents has resulted in isolated cases of neuroleptic malignant syndrome).
No products indexed under this heading.

Trimethadione (Alterations of thyroid function have been reported in combination therapy with other anticonvulsants).
No products indexed under this heading.

Trimethaphan Camsylate (Carbamazepine is known to induce CYP1A2 and CYP3A4. Therefore, the potential exists for interaction between carbamazepine and any agent metabolized by one (or more) of these enzymes).
No products indexed under this heading.

Trimipramine Maleate (Carbamazepine is known to induce CYP1A2 and CYP3A4. Therefore, the potential exists for interaction between carbamazepine and any agent metabolized by one (or more) of these enzymes). Products include:
Surmontil Capsules 2347

Troglitazone (Carbamazepine is metabolized mainly by cytochrome P450 (CYP) 3A4 to the active carbamazepine 10,11 -epoxide, which is further metabolized to the transdiol by epoxide hydrolase. Therefore, the potential exists for interaction between carbamazepine and any agent that inhibits CYP3A4 and/or epoxide hydrolase).
No products indexed under this heading.

Troleandomycin (Inhibitors of CYP3A4, such as troleandomycin, inhibit carbamazepine metabolism and thus increase plasma carbamazepine levels).
No products indexed under this heading.

Trovafloxacin Mesylate (Carbamazepine is known to induce CYP1A2 and CYP3A4. Therefore, the potential exists for interaction between carbamazepine and any agent metabolized by one (or more) of these enzymes).
No products indexed under this heading.

Valproate Sodium (Alterations of thyroid function have been reported in combination therapy with other anticonvulsants). Products include:
Depacon Injection 412

Valproic Acid (Alterations of thyroid function have been reported in combination therapy with other anticonvulsants). Products include:
Depakene 417

Verapamil Hydrochloride (Inhibitors of CYP3A4, such as verapamil, inhibit carbamazepine metabolism and thus increase plasma carbamazepine levels). Products include:
Covera-HS Tablets 3135
Tarka Tablets 519
Verelan PM Capsules 3120

Vinblastine Sulfate (Carbamazepine is known to induce CYP1A2 and CYP3A4. Therefore, the potential exists for interaction between carbamazepine and any agent metabolized by one (or more) of these enzymes).
No products indexed under this heading.

Vincristine Sulfate (Carbamazepine is known to induce CYP1A2 and CYP3A4. Therefore, the potential exists for interaction between carbamazepine and any agent metabolized by one (or more) of these enzymes).
No products indexed under this heading.

Voriconazole (Carbamazepine is metabolized mainly by cytochrome P450 (CYP) 3A4 to the active carbamazepine 10,11 -epoxide, which is further metabolized to the transdiol by epoxide hydrolase. Therefore, the potential exists for interaction between carbamazepine and any agent that inhibits CYP3A4 and/or epoxide hydrolase). Products include:
VFEND I.V. 2543
VFEND Oral Suspension 2543
VFEND Tablets 2543

Warfarin Sodium (Carbamezapine induces hepatic CYP activity and causes or would be expected to decrease plasma levels of warfarin). Products include:
Coumadin for Injection 932
Coumadin Tablets 932

Zafirlukast (Carbamazepine is metabolized mainly by cytochrome P450 (CYP) 3A4 to the active carbamazepine 10,11 -epoxide, which is further metabolized to the transdiol by epoxide hydrolase. Therefore, the potential exists for interaction between carbamazepine and any agent that inhibits CYP3A4 and/or epoxide hydrolase). Products include:
Accolate Tablets 663

Zileuton (Carbamazepine is metabolized mainly by cytochrome P450 (CYP) 3A4 to the active carbamazepine 10,11 -epoxide, which is further metabolized to the trans-diol by epoxide hydrolase. Therefore, the potential exists for interaction between carbamazepine and any agent that inhibits CYP3A4 and/or epoxide hydrolase).
No products indexed under this heading.

Ziprasidone Hydrochloride (Co-administration with psychotropic agents has resulted in isolated cases of neuroleptic malignant syndrome). Products include:
Geodon Capsules 2514

Zolmitriptan (Carbamazepine is known to induce CYP1A2 and CYP3A4. Therefore, the potential exists for interaction between carbamazepine and any agent metabolized by one (or more) of these enzymes). Products include:
Zomig Nasal Spray 718
Zomig Tablets 714
Zomig-ZMT Tablets 714

Zonisamide (Alterations of thyroid function have been reported in combination therapy with other anticonvulsants). Products include:
Zonegran Capsules 1089

Food Interactions

Food, unspecified (A high fat meal increased the rat of absorption of a single 400 mg dose but not the AUC; elimination half-life remains unchanged between fasting and fed states).

Grapefruit (Carbamazepine is metabolized mainly by cytochrome P450 (CYP) 3A4 to the active carbamazepine 10,11 -epoxide, which is further metabolized to the trans-diol by epoxide hydrolase. Therefore, the potential exists for interaction between carbamazepine and any agent that inhibits CYP3A4 and/or epoxide hydrolase).

Grapefruit Juice (Carbamazepine is metabolized mainly by cytochrome P450 (CYP) 3A4 to the active carbamazepine 10,11 -epoxide, which is further metabolized to the trans-diol by epoxide hydrolase. Therefore, the potential exists for interaction between carbamazepine and any agent that inhibits CYP3A4 and/or epoxide hydrolase).

CARDENE I.V.

(Nicardipine Hydrochloride) 1129
May interact with beta blockers and certain other agents. Compounds in these categories include:

Acebutolol Hydrochloride (In vitro and in some patients a negative inotropic effect has been observed with Cardene I.V., therefore, caution should be exercised when co-administered with beta blockers in patients with CHF or significant left ventricular dysfunction).
No products indexed under this heading.

Atenolol (In vitro and in some patients a negative inotropic effect has been observed with Cardene I.V., therefore, caution should be exercised when co-administered with beta blockers in patients with CHF or significant left ventricular dysfunction). Products include:
Tenormin I.V. Injection 698
Tenormin Tablets 695

Beta Blockers (Cardene I.V. may be safely used concomitantly with beta-blockers. However, exercise caution when using Cardene I.V. in combination with a beta-blocker in CHF patients).
No products indexed under this heading.

Betaxolol Hydrochloride (In vitro and in some patients a negative inotropic effect has been observed with Cardene I.V., therefore, caution should be exercised when co-administered with beta blockers in patients with CHF or significant left ventricular dysfunction). Products include:
Betoptic S Ophthalmic Suspension.................................. 554

Bisoprolol Fumarate (In vitro and in some patients a negative inotropic effect has been observed with Cardene I.V., therefore, caution should be exercised when co-administered with beta blockers in patients with CHF or significant left ventricular dysfunction).
No products indexed under this heading.

Carteolol Hydrochloride (In vitro and in some patients a negative inotropic effect has been observed with Cardene I.V., therefore, caution should be exercised when co-administered with beta blockers in patients with CHF or significant left ventricular dysfunction). Products include:
Carteolol Hydrochloride Ophthalmic Solution USP, 1%....... ⊙246

Cimetidine (Co-administration of cimetidine with Cardene I.V. increases nicardipine plasma concentration. Carefully monitor). Products include:
Tagamet HB 200 Tablets 637
Tagamet Tablets 1547

Cimetidine Hydrochloride (Co-administration of cimetidine with Cardene I.V. increases nicardipine plasma concentration).
No products indexed under this heading.

Cyclosporine (Co-administration of Cardene I.V. and cyclosporine results in elevated plasma cyclosporine levels. Closely monitor plasma concentrations of cyclosporine and reduce dose accordingly). Products include:
Gengraf Capsules 458
Neoral Soft Gelatin Capsules 2247
Neoral Oral Solution 2247
Restasis Ophthalmic Emulsion 570
Sandimmune 2259

Digoxin (No alteration in digoxin plasma levels, however, as a precaution, digoxin levels should be evaluated when concomitant therapy is initiated). Products include:
Digitek Tablets 2146
Lanoxicaps Capsules 1458
Lanoxin Injection 1462
Lanoxin Tablets 1468
Lanoxin Injection Pediatric 1465

Esmolol Hydrochloride (In vitro and in some patients a negative inotropic effect has been observed with Cardene I.V., therefore, caution should be exercised when co-administered with beta blockers in patients with CHF or significant left ventricular dysfunction). Products include:
Brevibloc Concentrate 766
Brevibloc Injection 766
Brevibloc Double Strength Injection....................................... 766
Brevibloc Premixed Injection 766
Brevibloc Double Strength Premixed Injection 766

Fentanyl (Potential for hypotension with fentanyl anesthesia when used with calcium channel blockers and beta blockers; such reaction has not been observed with Cardene I.V. during clinical trials). Products include:
Duragesic Transdermal System 2448

Fentanyl Citrate (Potential for hypotension with fentanyl anesthesia when used with calcium channel blockers and beta blockers; such reaction has not been observed with Cardene I.V. during clinical trials). Products include:
Actiq 993

Labetalol Hydrochloride (In vitro and in some patients a negative inotropic effect has been observed with Cardene I.V., therefore, caution should be exercised when co-administered with beta blockers in patients with CHF or significant left ventricular dysfunction).
No products indexed under this heading.

Levobunolol Hydrochloride (In vitro and in some patients a negative inotropic effect has been observed with Cardene I.V., therefore, caution should be exercised when co-administered with beta blockers in patients with CHF or significant left ventricular dysfunction). Products include:
Betagan Ophthalmic Solution, USP.. ⊙217

Metipranolol Hydrochloride (In vitro and in some patients a negative inotropic effect has been observed with Cardene I.V., therefore, caution should be exercised when co-administered with beta blockers in patients with CHF or significant left ventricular dysfunction).
No products indexed under this heading.

Metoprolol Succinate (In vitro and in some patients a negative inotropic effect has been observed with Cardene I.V., therefore, caution should be exercised when co-administered with beta blockers in patients with CHF or significant left ventricular dysfunction). Products include:
Toprol-XL Tablets 660

Metoprolol Tartrate (In vitro and in some patients a negative inotropic effect has been observed with Cardene I.V., therefore, caution should be exercised when co-administered with beta blockers in patients with CHF or significant left ventricular dysfunction).
No products indexed under this heading.

Nadolol (In vitro and in some patients a negative inotropic effect has been observed with Cardene I.V., therefore, caution should be exercised when co-administered with beta blockers in patients with CHF or significant left ventricular dysfunction). Products include:
Nadolol Tablets 2121

Penbutolol Sulfate (In vitro and in some patients a negative inotropic effect has been observed with Cardene I.V., therefore, caution should be exercised when co-administered with beta blockers in patients with CHF or significant left ventricular dysfunction).
No products indexed under this heading.

Pindolol (In vitro and in some patients a negative inotropic effect has been observed with Cardene I.V., therefore, caution should be exercised when co-administered with beta blockers in patients with CHF or significant left ventricular dysfunction).
No products indexed under this heading.

Propranolol Hydrochloride (In vitro and in some patients a negative inotropic effect has been observed with Cardene I.V., therefore, caution should be exercised when co-administered with beta blockers in patients with CHF or significant left ventricular dysfunction). Products include:
Inderal LA Long-Acting Capsules 3421
InnoPran XL Capsules 2728

Sotalol Hydrochloride (In vitro and in some patients a negative inotropic effect has been observed with Cardene I.V., therefore, caution should be exercised when co-administered with beta blockers in patients with CHF or significant left ventricular dysfunction).
No products indexed under this heading.

Timolol Hemihydrate (In vitro and in some patients a negative inotropic effect has been observed with Cardene I.V., therefore, caution should be exercised when co-administered with beta blockers in patients with CHF or significant left ventricular dysfunction). Products include:
Betimol Ophthalmic Solution 3371
Betimol Ophthalmic Solution .... ⊙283

Timolol Maleate (In vitro and in some patients a negative inotropic effect has been observed with Cardene I.V., therefore, caution should be exercised when co-administered with beta blockers in patients with CHF or significant left ventricular dysfunction). Products include:
Blocadren Tablets 1891
Cosopt Sterile Ophthalmic Solution.. 1910
Timolide Tablets 2056
Timoptic in Ocudose 2061
Timoptic Sterile Ophthalmic Solution.. 2058
Timoptic-XE Sterile Ophthalmic Gel Forming Solution 2062

CARDIO ESSENTIALS CAPSULES

(Coenzyme Q-10) 3328
None cited in PDR database.

CARDIZEM LA EXTENDED RELEASE TABLETS

(Diltiazem Hydrochloride) 1699
May interact with anesthetics, benzodiazepines, beta blockers, cardiac glycosides, and certain other agents. Compounds in these categories include:

Acebutolol Hydrochloride (Pharmacologic studies indicate that there may be additive effects in prolonging A-V conduction when using beta-blockers or digitalis concomitantly with diltiazem).
No products indexed under this heading.

Alfentanil Hydrochloride (The depression of cardiac contractility, conductivity, and automaticity, as well as the vascular dilation associated with anesthetics, may be potentiated by calcium channel blockers).
No products indexed under this heading.

Alprazolam (Studies showed that diltiazem increased the AUC of midazolam and triazolam by 3- to 4-fold and the Cmax by 2-fold, compared to placebo. The elimination half-life of midazolam and triazolam also increased during co-administration with diltiazem). Products include:
Niravam Orally Disintegrating Tablets 3106
Xanax XR Tablets 2655

Atenolol (Pharmacologic studies indicate that there may be additive effects in prolonging A-V conduction when using beta-blockers or digitalis concomitantly with diltiazem). Products include:
Tenormin I.V. Injection 698
Tenormin Tablets 695

Betaxolol Hydrochloride (Pharmacologic studies indicate that there may be additive effects in prolonging A-V conduction when using beta-blockers or digitalis concomitantly with diltiazem). Products include:
Betoptic S Ophthalmic Suspension 554

Bisoprolol Fumarate (Pharmacologic studies indicate that there may be additive effects in prolonging A-V conduction when using beta-blockers or digitalis concomitantly with diltiazem).
No products indexed under this heading.

Carbamazepine (Concomitant administration of diltiazem with carbamazepine has been reported to result in elevated serum levels of carbamazepine (40% to 72% increase), resulting in toxicity in some cases). Products include:
Carbatrol Capsules 3174
Equetro Extended-Release Capsules 3178
Tegretol/Tegretol-XR 2278

Carteolol Hydrochloride (Pharmacologic studies indicate that there may be additive effects in prolonging A-V conduction when using beta-blockers or digitalis concomitantly with diltiazem). Products include:
Carteolol Hydrochloride Ophthalmic Solution USP, 1% .... ⊙246

Chlordiazepoxide (Studies showed that diltiazem increased the AUC of midazolam and triazolam by 3- to 4-fold and the Cmax by 2-fold, compared to placebo. The elimination half-life of midazolam and triazolam also increased during co-administration with diltiazem).
No products indexed under this heading.

Chlordiazepoxide Hydrochloride (Studies showed that diltiazem increased the AUC of midazolam and triazolam by 3- to 4-fold and the Cmax by 2-fold, compared to placebo. The elimination half-life of midazolam and triazolam also increased during co-administration with diltiazem). Products include:
Librium Capsules 3349

Cimetidine (A study in six healthy volunteers has shown a significant increase in peak diltiazem plasma levels (58%) and AUC (53%) after a 1-week course of cimetidine at 1200 mg per day and a single dose of diltiazem 60 mg). Products include:
Tagamet HB 200 Tablets .... ◙637
Tagamet Tablets 1547

Cimetidine Hydrochloride (A study in six healthy volunteers has shown a significant increase in peak diltiazem plasma levels (58%) and AUC (53%) after a 1-week course of cimetidine at 1200 mg per day and a single dose of diltiazem 60 mg).
No products indexed under this heading.

Clorazepate Dipotassium (Studies showed that diltiazem increased the AUC of midazolam and triazolam by 3- to 4-fold and the Cmax by 2-fold, compared to placebo. The elimination half-life of midazolam and triazolam also increased during co-administration with diltiazem). Products include:
Tranxene 2488

Cyclosporine (In renal and cardiac transplant recipients, a reduction of cyclosporine dose ranging from 15% to 48% was necessary to maintain cyclosporine trough concentrations similar to those seen prior to the addition of diltiazem. If these agents are to be administered concurrently, cyclosporine concentrations should be monitored, especially when diltiazem therapy is initiated, adjusted or discontinued). Products include:
Gengraf Capsules 458
Neoral Soft Gelatin Capsules 2247
Neoral Oral Solution 2247
Restasis Ophthalmic Emulsion 570
Sandimmune 2259

Deslanoside (Pharmacologic studies indicate that there may be additive effects in prolonging A-V conduction when using beta-blockers or digitalis concomitantly with diltiazem).
No products indexed under this heading.

Diazepam (Studies showed that diltiazem increased the AUC of midazolam and triazolam by 3- to 4-fold and the Cmax by 2-fold, compared to placebo. The elimination half-life of midazolam and triazolam also increased during co-administration with diltiazem). Products include:
Diastat Rectal Delivery System 3344
Valium Tablets 2822

Digitalis Glycoside Preparations (Pharmacologic studies indicate that there may be additive effects in prolonging A-V conduction when using beta-blockers or digitalis concomitantly with diltiazem).
No products indexed under this heading.

Digitoxin (Pharmacologic studies indicate that there may be additive effects in prolonging A-V conduction when using beta-blockers or digitalis concomitantly with diltiazem).
No products indexed under this heading.

Digoxin (Pharmacologic studies indicate that there may be additive effects in prolonging A-V conduction when using beta-blockers or digitalis concomitantly with diltiazem). Products include:
Digitek Tablets 2146
Lanoxicaps Capsules 1458
Lanoxin Injection 1462
Lanoxin Tablets 1468
Lanoxin Injection Pediatric 1465

Enflurane (The depression of cardiac contractility, conductivity, and automaticity, as well as the vascular dilation associated with anesthetics, may be potentiated by calcium channel blockers).
No products indexed under this heading.

Esmolol Hydrochloride (Pharmacologic studies indicate that there may be additive effects in prolonging A-V conduction when using beta-blockers or digitalis concomitantly with diltiazem). Products include:
Brevibloc Concentrate 766
Brevibloc Injection 766
Brevibloc Double Strength Injection 766
Brevibloc Premixed Injection 766
Brevibloc Double Strength Premixed Injection 766

Estazolam (Studies showed that diltiazem increased the AUC of midazolam and triazolam by 3- to 4-fold and the Cmax by 2-fold, compared to placebo. The elimination half-life of midazolam and triazolam also increased during co-administration with diltiazem). Products include:
ProSom Tablets 512

Fentanyl Citrate (The depression of cardiac contractility, conductivity, and automaticity, as well as the vascular dilation associated with anesthetics, may be potentiated by calcium channel blockers). Products include:
Actiq 993

Flurazepam Hydrochloride (Studies showed that diltiazem increased the AUC of midazolam and triazolam by 3- to 4-fold and the Cmax by 2-fold, compared to placebo. The elimination half-life of midazolam and triazolam also increased during co-administration with diltiazem). Products include:
Dalmane Capsules 3343

Halazepam (Studies showed that diltiazem increased the AUC of midazolam and triazolam by 3- to 4-fold and the Cmax by 2-fold, compared to placebo. The elimination half-life of midazolam and triazolam also increased during co-administration with diltiazem).
No products indexed under this heading.

Halothane (The depression of cardiac contractility, conductivity, and automaticity, as well as the vascular dilation associated with anesthetics, may be potentiated by calcium channel blockers).
No products indexed under this heading.

Isoflurane (The depression of cardiac contractility, conductivity, and automaticity, as well as the vascular dilation associated with anesthetics, may be potentiated by calcium channel blockers).
No products indexed under this heading.

Ketamine Hydrochloride (The depression of cardiac contractility, conductivity, and automaticity, as well as the vascular dilation associated with anesthetics, may be potentiated by calcium channel blockers).
No products indexed under this heading.

Labetalol Hydrochloride (Pharmacologic studies indicate that there may be additive effects in prolonging A-V conduction when using beta-blockers or digitalis concomitantly with diltiazem).
No products indexed under this heading.

Levobunolol Hydrochloride (Pharmacologic studies indicate that there may be additive effects in prolonging A-V conduction when using beta-blockers or digitalis concomitantly with diltiazem). Products include:
Betagan Ophthalmic Solution, USP .... ⊙217

Lorazepam (Studies showed that diltiazem increased the AUC of midazolam and triazolam by 3- to 4-fold and the Cmax by 2-fold, compared to placebo. The elimination half-life of midazolam and triazolam also increased during co-administration with diltiazem).
No products indexed under this heading.

Lovastatin (In a ten-subject study, co-administration of diltiazem (120 mg bid diltiazem SR) with lovastatin resulted in a 3-4 times increase in mean lovastatin AUC and Cmax versus lovastatin alone). Products include:
Advicor Tablets 1694
Altoprev Extended-Release Tablets 1151
Mevacor Tablets 1996

Methohexital Sodium (The depression of cardiac contractility, conductivity, and automaticity, as well as the vascular dilation associated with anesthetics, may be potentiated by calcium channel blockers).
No products indexed under this heading.

Metipranolol Hydrochloride (Pharmacologic studies indicate that there may be additive effects in prolonging A-V conduction when using beta-blockers or digitalis concomitantly with diltiazem).
No products indexed under this heading.

Metoprolol Succinate (Pharmacologic studies indicate that there may be additive effects in prolonging A-V conduction when using beta-blockers or digitalis concomitantly with diltiazem). Products include:
Toprol-XL Tablets 660

Metoprolol Tartrate (Pharmacologic studies indicate that there may be additive effects in prolonging A-V conduction when using beta-blockers or digitalis concomitantly with diltiazem).
No products indexed under this heading.

Midazolam Hydrochloride (The depression of cardiac contractility, conductivity, and automaticity, as well as the vascular dilation associated with anesthetics, may be potentiated by calcium channel blockers).
No products indexed under this heading.

Nadolol (Pharmacologic studies indicate that there may be additive effects in prolonging A-V conduction when using beta-blockers or digitalis concomitantly with diltiazem). Products include:
Nadolol Tablets 2121

Oxazepam (Studies showed that diltiazem increased the AUC of midazolam and triazolam by 3- to 4-fold and the Cmax by 2-fold, compared to placebo. The elimination half-life of midazolam and triazolam also increased during co-administration with diltiazem).
No products indexed under this heading.

Penbutolol Sulfate (Pharmacologic studies indicate that there may be additive effects in prolonging A-V conduction when using beta-blockers or digitalis concomitantly with diltiazem).
No products indexed under this heading.

Pindolol (Pharmacologic studies indicate that there may be additive effects in prolonging A-V conduction when using beta-blockers or digitalis concomitantly with diltiazem).
No products indexed under this heading.

Prazepam (Studies showed that diltiazem increased the AUC of midazolam and triazolam by 3- to 4-fold and the Cmax by 2-fold, compared to placebo. The elimination half-life of midazolam and triazolam also increased during co-administration with diltiazem).
No products indexed under this heading.

Propofol (The depression of cardiac contractility, conductivity, and automaticity, as well as the vascular dilation associated with anesthetics, may be potentiated by calcium channel blockers). Products include:
Diprivan Injectable Emulsion 676

Propranolol Hydrochloride (Pharmacologic studies indicate that there may be additive effects in prolonging A-V conduction when using beta-blockers or digitalis concomitantly with diltiazem). Products include:
Inderal LA Long-Acting Capsules 3421
InnoPran XL Capsules 2728

Quazepam (Studies showed that diltiazem increased the AUC of midazolam and triazolam by 3- to 4-fold and the Cmax by 2-fold, compared to placebo. The elimination half-life of midazolam and triazolam also increased during co-administration with diltiazem).
No products indexed under this heading.

Remifentanil Hydrochloride (The depression of cardiac contractility, conductivity, and automaticity, as well as the vascular dilation associated with anesthetics, may be potentiated by calcium channel blockers).
No products indexed under this heading.

Rifampin (Co-administration of rifampin with diltiazem lowered the diltiazem plasma concentrations to undetectable levels. Co-administration of diltiazem with rifampin or any known CYP3A4 inducer should be avoided when possible and alternative therapy considered).
No products indexed under this heading.

Sotalol Hydrochloride (Pharmacologic studies indicate that there may be additive effects in prolonging A-V conduction when using beta-blockers or digitalis concomitantly with diltiazem).
No products indexed under this heading.

Sufentanil Citrate (The depression of cardiac contractility, conductivity, and automaticity, as well as the vascular dilation associated with anesthetics, may be potentiated by calcium channel blockers).
No products indexed under this heading.

Temazepam (Studies showed that diltiazem increased the AUC of midazolam and triazolam by 3- to 4-fold and the Cmax by 2-fold, compared to placebo. The elimination half-life of midazolam and triazolam also increased during co-administration with diltiazem).
No products indexed under this heading.

Thiamylal Sodium (The depression of cardiac contractility, conductivity, and automaticity, as well as the vascular dilation associated with anesthetics, may be potentiated by calcium channel blockers).
No products indexed under this heading.

Timolol Hemihydrate (Pharmacologic studies indicate that there may be additive effects in prolonging A-V conduction when using beta-blockers or digitalis concomitantly with diltiazem). Products include:
Betimol Ophthalmic Solution 3371
Betimol Ophthalmic Solution .... ⊙283

Timolol Maleate (Pharmacologic studies indicate that there may be additive effects in prolonging A-V conduction when using beta-blockers or digitalis concomitantly with diltiazem). Products include:
Blocadren Tablets 1891
Cosopt Sterile Ophthalmic Solution....................................... 1910
Timolide Tablets 2056
Timoptic in Ocudose 2061
Timoptic Sterile Ophthalmic Solution....................................... 2058
Timoptic-XE Sterile Ophthalmic Gel Forming Solution 2062

Triazolam (Studies showed that diltiazem increased the AUC of midazolam and triazolam by 3- to 4-fold and the Cmax by 2-fold, compared to placebo. The elimination half-life of midazolam and triazolam also increased during co-administration with diltiazem).
No products indexed under this heading.

CARIMUNE NF

(Immune Globulin Intravenous (Human)).. 3501
May interact with:

Measles, Mumps & Rubella Virus Vaccine, Live (Antibodies in immune globulin intravenous (human) may impair the efficacy of live attenuated viral vaccines). Products include:
M-M-R II 1980

Measles & Rubella Virus Vaccine Live (Antibodies in immune globulin intravenous (human) may impair the efficacy of live attenuated viral vaccines).
No products indexed under this heading.

Measles Virus Vaccine Live (Antibodies in immune globulin intravenous (human) may impair the efficacy of live attenuated viral vaccines). Products include:
Attenuvax 1889

Mumps Virus Vaccine, Live (Antibodies in immune globulin intravenous (human) may impair the efficacy of live attenuated viral vaccines). Products include:
Mumpsvax 2005

Rubella & Mumps Virus Vaccine Live (Antibodies in immune globulin intravenous (human) may impair the efficacy of live attenuated viral vaccines).
No products indexed under this heading.

Rubella Virus Vaccine Live (Antibodies in immune globulin intravenous (human) may impair the efficacy of live attenuated viral vaccines). Products include:
Meruvax II 1994

CARNITOR INJECTION

(Levocarnitine) 3185
None cited in PDR database.

CARNITOR TABLETS AND ORAL SOLUTION

(Levocarnitine) 3187
None cited in PDR database.

CARTEOLOL HYDROCHLORIDE OPHTHALMIC SOLUTION USP, 1%

(Carteolol Hydrochloride) .... ⊙246
May interact with beta blockers and certain other agents. Compounds in these categories include:

Acebutolol Hydrochloride (Co-administration with oral beta-adrenergic blocking agents may result in potential additive effects on systemic beta-blockade).
No products indexed under this heading.

Atenolol (Co-administration with oral beta-adrenergic blocking agents may result in potential additive effects on systemic beta-blockade). Products include:
Tenormin I.V. Injection 698
Tenormin Tablets 695

Betaxolol Hydrochloride (Co-administration with oral beta-adrenergic blocking agents may result in potential additive effects on systemic beta-blockade). Products include:
Betoptic S Ophthalmic Suspension................................. 554

Bisoprolol Fumarate (Co-administration with oral beta-adrenergic blocking agents may result in potential additive effects on systemic beta-blockade).
No products indexed under this heading.

Esmolol Hydrochloride (Co-administration with oral beta-adrenergic blocking agents may result in potential additive effects on systemic beta-blockade). Products include:
Brevibloc Concentrate 766
Brevibloc Injection 766
Brevibloc Double Strength Injection....................................... 766
Brevibloc Premixed Injection 766
Brevibloc Double Strength Premixed Injection 766

Guanethidine Monosulfate (Co-administration with catecholamine-depleting drugs, such as guanethidine, may result in possible additive effects and production of hypotension and/or marked bradycardia, which may produce vertigo, syncope, or postural hypertension).
No products indexed under this heading.

Labetalol Hydrochloride (Co-administration with oral beta-adrenergic blocking agents may result in potential additive effects on systemic beta-blockade).
No products indexed under this heading.

Levobunolol Hydrochloride (Co-administration with oral beta-adrenergic blocking agents may result in potential additive effects on systemic beta-blockade). Products include:
Betagan Ophthalmic Solution, USP... ⊙217

Metipranolol Hydrochloride (Co-administration with oral beta-adrenergic blocking agents may result in potential additive effects on systemic beta-blockade).
No products indexed under this heading.

Metoprolol Succinate (Co-administration with oral beta-adrenergic blocking agents may result in potential additive effects on systemic beta-blockade). Products include:
Toprol-XL Tablets 660

Metoprolol Tartrate (Co-administration with oral beta-adrenergic blocking agents may result in potential additive effects on systemic beta-blockade).
No products indexed under this heading.

Nadolol (Co-administration with oral beta-adrenergic blocking agents may result in potential additive effects on systemic beta-blockade). Products include:
Nadolol Tablets 2121

Penbutolol Sulfate (Co-administration with oral beta-adrenergic blocking agents may result in potential additive effects on systemic beta-blockade).
No products indexed under this heading.

Pindolol (Co-administration with oral beta-adrenergic blocking agents may result in potential additive effects on systemic beta-blockade).
No products indexed under this heading.

Propranolol Hydrochloride (Co-administration with oral beta-adrenergic blocking agents may result in potential additive effects on systemic beta-blockade). Products include:
Inderal LA Long-Acting Capsules 3421
InnoPran XL Capsules 2728

Reserpine (Co-administration with catecholamine-depleting drugs, such as reserpine, may result in possible additive effects and production of hypotension and/or marked bradycardia, which may produce vertigo, syncope, or postural hypertension).
No products indexed under this heading.

Sotalol Hydrochloride (Co-administration with oral beta-adrenergic blocking agents may result in potential additive effects on systemic beta-blockade).
No products indexed under this heading.

Timolol Hemihydrate (Co-administration with oral beta-adrenergic blocking agents may result in potential additive effects on systemic beta-blockade). Products include:
Betimol Ophthalmic Solution 3371
Betimol Ophthalmic Solution .... ⊙283

Timolol Maleate (Co-administration with oral beta-adrenergic blocking

agents may result in potential additive effects on systemic beta-blockade). Products include:

Blocadren Tablets 1891
Cosopt Sterile Ophthalmic Solution 1910
Timolide Tablets 2056
Timoptic in Ocudose 2061
Timoptic Sterile Ophthalmic Solution 2058
Timoptic-XE Sterile Ophthalmic Gel Forming Solution 2062

CASODEX TABLETS

(Bicalutamide) 670

May interact with oral anticoagulants. Compounds in these categories include:

Anisindione (Bicalutamide can displace coumarin anticoagulant from their protein-binding sites as shown in *in vitro* studies; close monitoring of prothrombin time is advised). Products include:

Miradon Tablets 3056

Dicumarol (Bicalutamide can displace coumarin anticoagulant from their protein-binding sites as shown in *in vitro* studies; close monitoring of prothrombin time is advised).

No products indexed under this heading.

Warfarin Sodium (Bicalutamide can displace coumarin anticoagulant from their protein-binding sites as shown in *in vitro* studies; close monitoring of prothrombin time is advised). Products include:

Coumadin for Injection 932
Coumadin Tablets 932

CATAFLAM TABLETS

(Diclofenac Potassium) 2173

May interact with ACE inhibitors, lithium preparations, thiazides, and certain other agents. Compounds in these categories include:

Aspirin (When diclofenac is administered with aspirin, its protein binding is reduced; the clinical significance of this interaction is not known). Products include:

Aggrenox Capsules 855
Bayer, Aspirin Regimen .... ▣606
Bayer Aspirin Tablets 3515
BC Powder .... ▣612
BC Allergy Sinus Cold Powder .... ▣612
Arthritis Strength BC Powder .... ▣612
BC Sinus Cold Powder .... ▣612
Ecotrin Enteric Coated Aspirin Low, Regular and Maximum Strength Tablets 1627
Goody's Body Pain Formula Powder .... ▣621
Goody's Extra Strength Headache Powder .... ▣621
Goody's Extra Strength Pain Relief Tablets .... ▣621
Percodan Tablets 1115
St. Joseph 81 mg Aspirin Chewable and Enteric Coated Tablets 1841

Benazepril Hydrochloride (Reports suggest that NSAIDs may diminish the antihypertensive effect of ACE inhibitors; this interaction should be given consideration in patients taking NSAIDs concomitantly with ACE inhibitors). Products include:

Lotensin Tablets 2232
Lotensin HCT Tablets 2235
Lotrel Capsules 2238

Bendroflumethiazide (Studies have shown that diclofenac can reduce the natriuretic effect of furosemide and thiazides in some patients; during concomitant therapy with NSAIDs, the patient should be observed closely for signs of renal failure, as well as to assure diuretic efficacy).

No products indexed under this heading.

Captopril (Reports suggest that NSAIDs may diminish the antihypertensive effect of ACE inhibitors; this interaction should be given consideration in patients taking NSAIDs concomitantly with ACE inhibitors). Products include:

Captopril Tablets 2114

Chlorothiazide (Studies have shown that diclofenac can reduce the natriuretic effect of furosemide and thiazides in some patients; during concomitant therapy with NSAIDs, the patient should be observed closely for signs of renal failure, as well as to assure diuretic efficacy). Products include:

Aldoclor Tablets 1881
Diuril Oral 1936

Chlorothiazide Sodium (Studies have shown that diclofenac can reduce the natriuretic effect of furosemide and thiazides in some patients; during concomitant therapy with NSAIDs, the patient should be observed closely for signs of renal failure, as well as to assure diuretic efficacy). Products include:

Diuril Sodium Intravenous 1934

Cyclosporine (Diclofenac may affect renal prostaglandins and increase the toxicity of certain drugs; concomitant therapy with diclofenac may increase cyclosporine's nephrotoxicity; caution should be used when administered concomitantly with cyclosporine). Products include:

Gengraf Capsules 458
Neoral Soft Gelatin Capsules 2247
Neoral Oral Solution 2247
Restasis Ophthalmic Emulsion 570
Sandimmune 2259

Enalapril Maleate (Reports suggest that NSAIDs may diminish the antihypertensive effect of ACE inhibitors; this interaction should be given consideration in patients taking NSAIDs concomitantly with ACE inhibitors). Products include:

Vaseretic Tablets 2073
Vasotec I.V. Injection 2076

Enalaprilat (Reports suggest that NSAIDs may diminish the antihypertensive effect of ACE inhibitors; this interaction should be given consideration in patients taking NSAIDs concomitantly with ACE inhibitors).

No products indexed under this heading.

Fosinopril Sodium (Reports suggest that NSAIDs may diminish the antihypertensive effect of ACE inhibitors; this interaction should be given consideration in patients taking NSAIDs concomitantly with ACE inhibitors).

No products indexed under this heading.

Furosemide (Studies have shown that diclofenac can reduce the natriuretic effect of furosemide and thiazides in some patients; during concomitant therapy with NSAIDs, the patient should be observed closely for signs of renal failure, as well as to assure diuretic efficacy). Products include:

Furosemide Tablets 2117

Hydrochlorothiazide (Studies have shown that diclofenac can reduce the natriuretic effect of furosemide and thiazides in some patients; during concomitant therapy with NSAIDs, the patient should be observed closely for signs of renal failure, as well as to assure diuretic efficacy). Products include:

Aldoril Tablets 1884
Atacand HCT 637
Avalide Tablets 2889
Avalide Tablets 922
Benicar HCT Tablets 2852
Diovan HCT Tablets 2195
Dyazide Capsules 1389
Hyzaar 1964
Lotensin HCT Tablets 2235
Maxzide 2150
Micardis HCT Tablets 886
Moduretic Tablets 2003
Prinzide Tablets 2033
Teveten HCT Tablets 1710
Timolide Tablets 2056
Uniretic Tablets 3114
Vaseretic Tablets 2073
Zestoretic Tablets 701

Hydroflumethiazide (Studies have shown that diclofenac can reduce the natriuretic effect of furosemide and thiazides in some patients; during concomitant therapy with NSAIDs, the patient should be observed closely for signs of renal failure, as well as to assure diuretic efficacy).

No products indexed under this heading.

Lisinopril (Reports suggest that NSAIDs may diminish the antihypertensive effect of ACE inhibitors; this interaction should be given consideration in patients taking NSAIDs concomitantly with ACE inhibitors). Products include:

Prinivil Tablets 2029
Prinzide Tablets 2033
Zestoretic Tablets 701
Zestril Tablets 704

Lithium (NSAIDs have produced an elevation of plasma lithium levels and a reduction in renal lithium clearance; these effects have been attributed to inhibition of renal prostaglandin synthesis by the NSAID; monitor for signs of lithium toxicity).

No products indexed under this heading.

Lithium Carbonate (NSAIDs have produced an elevation of plasma lithium levels and a reduction in renal lithium clearance; these effects have been attributed to inhibition of renal prostaglandin synthesis by the NSAID; monitor for signs of lithium toxicity). Products include:

Eskalith 1406
Lithobid Tablets 1670

Lithium Citrate (NSAIDs have produced an elevation of plasma lithium levels and a reduction in renal lithium clearance; these effects have been attributed to inhibition of renal prostaglandin synthesis by the NSAID; monitor for signs of lithium toxicity).

No products indexed under this heading.

Methotrexate Sodium (NSAIDs have been reported to competitively inhibit methotrexate accumulation in animal studies; this may indicate that they could enhance the toxicity of methotrexate; caution should be given when NSAIDs are administered concomitantly with methotrexate).

No products indexed under this heading.

Methyclothiazide (Studies have shown that diclofenac can reduce the natriuretic effect of furosemide and thiazides in some patients; during concomitant therapy with NSAIDs, the patient should be observed closely for signs of renal failure, as well as to assure diuretic efficacy).

No products indexed under this heading.

Moexipril Hydrochloride (Reports suggest that NSAIDs may diminish the antihypertensive effect of ACE inhibitors; this interaction should be given consideration in patients taking NSAIDs concomitantly with ACE inhibitors). Products include:

Uniretic Tablets 3114
Univasc Tablets 3118

Perindopril Erbumine (Reports suggest that NSAIDs may diminish the antihypertensive effect of ACE inhibitors; this interaction should be given consideration in patients taking NSAIDs concomitantly with ACE inhibitors). Products include:

Aceon Tablets (2 mg, 4 mg, 8 mg) 3191

Polythiazide (Studies have shown that diclofenac can reduce the natriuretic effect of furosemide and thiazides in some patients; during concomitant therapy with NSAIDs, the patient should be observed closely for signs of renal failure, as well as to assure diuretic efficacy).

No products indexed under this heading.

Quinapril Hydrochloride (Reports suggest that NSAIDs may diminish the antihypertensive effect of ACE inhibitors; this interaction should be given consideration in patients taking NSAIDs concomitantly with ACE inhibitors).

No products indexed under this heading.

Ramipril (Reports suggest that NSAIDs may diminish the antihypertensive effect of ACE inhibitors; this interaction should be given consideration in patients taking NSAIDs concomitantly with ACE inhibitors). Products include:

Altace Capsules 1673

Spirapril Hydrochloride (Reports suggest that NSAIDs may diminish the antihypertensive effect of ACE inhibitors; this interaction should be given consideration in patients taking NSAIDs concomitantly with ACE inhibitors).

No products indexed under this heading.

Trandolapril (Reports suggest that NSAIDs may diminish the antihypertensive effect of ACE inhibitors; this interaction should be given consideration in patients taking NSAIDs concomitantly with ACE inhibitors). Products include:

Mavik Tablets 482
Tarka Tablets 519

Warfarin Sodium (The effects of warfarin and NSAIDs on GI bleeding are synergistic such that users of

both drugs together have a risk of serious GI bleeding higher than users of either drug alone). Products include:

Coumadin for Injection 932
Coumadin Tablets 932

CATAPRES TABLETS

(Clonidine Hydrochloride) 874

May interact with barbiturates, beta blockers, calcium channel blockers, cardiac glycosides, hypnotics and sedatives, tricyclic antidepressants, and certain other agents. Compounds in these categories include:

Acebutolol Hydrochloride (Co-administration with agents known to affect sinus node function or AV nodal conduction, such as beta blockers, may result in additive effects such as bradycardia and AV block).
No products indexed under this heading.

Amitriptyline Hydrochloride (Co-administration may reduce the hypotensive effects; dosage adjustment may be necessary; concurrent use has resulted in corneal lesions in rats within 5 days).
No products indexed under this heading.

Amlodipine Besylate (Co-administration with agents known to affect sinus node function or AV nodal conduction, such as calcium channel blockers, may result in additive effects such as bradycardia and AV block). Products include:

Caduet Tablets 2507
Lotrel Capsules 2238
Norvasc Tablets 2529

Amoxapine (Co-administration may reduce the hypotensive effects; dosage adjustment may be necessary).
No products indexed under this heading.

Aprobarbital (Clonidine may potentiate the CNS-depressive effects).
No products indexed under this heading.

Atenolol (Co-administration with agents known to affect sinus node function or AV nodal conduction, such as beta blockers, may result in additive effects such as bradycardia and AV block). Products include:

Tenormin I.V. Injection 698
Tenormin Tablets 695

Bepridil Hydrochloride (Co-administration with agents known to affect sinus node function or AV nodal conduction, such as calcium channel blockers, may result in additive effects such as bradycardia and AV block).
No products indexed under this heading.

Betaxolol Hydrochloride (Co-administration with agents known to affect sinus node function or AV nodal conduction, such as beta blockers, may result in additive effects such as bradycardia and AV block). Products include:

Betoptic S Ophthalmic Suspension................................... 554

Bisoprolol Fumarate (Co-administration with agents known to affect sinus node function or AV nodal conduction, such as beta blockers, may result in additive effects such as bradycardia and AV block).
No products indexed under this heading.

Butabarbital (Clonidine may potentiate the CNS-depressive effects).
No products indexed under this heading.

Butalbital (Clonidine may potentiate the CNS-depressive effects). Products include:

Sedapap Tablets 50 mg/650 mg 2098

Carteolol Hydrochloride (Co-administration with agents known to affect sinus node function or AV nodal conduction, such as beta blockers, may result in additive effects such as bradycardia and AV block). Products include:

Carteolol Hydrochloride Ophthalmic Solution USP, 1%....... ⊙246

Clomipramine Hydrochloride (Co-administration may reduce the hypotensive effects; dosage adjustment may be necessary).
No products indexed under this heading.

Desipramine Hydrochloride (Co-administration may reduce the hypotensive effects; dosage adjustment may be necessary).
No products indexed under this heading.

Deslanoside (Co-administration with agents known to affect sinus node function or AV nodal conduction, such as digitalis, may result in additive effects such as bradycardia and AV block).
No products indexed under this heading.

Digitalis Glycoside Preparations (Co-administration with agents known to affect sinus node function or AV nodal conduction, such as digitalis, may result in additive effects such as bradycardia and AV block).
No products indexed under this heading.

Digitoxin (Co-administration with agents known to affect sinus node function or AV nodal conduction, such as digitalis, may result in additive effects such as bradycardia and AV block).
No products indexed under this heading.

Digoxin (Co-administration with agents known to affect sinus node function or AV nodal conduction, such as digitalis, may result in additive effects such as bradycardia and AV block). Products include:

Digitek Tablets 2146
Lanoxicaps Capsules 1458
Lanoxin Injection 1462
Lanoxin Tablets 1468
Lanoxin Injection Pediatric 1465

Diltiazem Hydrochloride (Co-administration with agents known to affect sinus node function or AV nodal conduction, such as calcium channel blockers, may result in additive effects such as bradycardia and AV block). Products include:

Cardizem LA Extended Release Tablets.. 1699
Tiazac Capsules 1204

Doxepin Hydrochloride (Co-administration may reduce the hypotensive effects; dosage adjustment may be necessary).
No products indexed under this heading.

Esmolol Hydrochloride (Co-administration with agents known to affect sinus node function or AV nodal conduction, such as beta blockers, may result in additive effects such as bradycardia and AV block). Products include:

Brevibloc Concentrate 766
Brevibloc Injection 766
Brevibloc Double Strength Injection... 766
Brevibloc Premixed Injection 766
Brevibloc Double Strength Premixed Injection........................ 766

Estazolam (Clonidine may potentiate the CNS-depressive effects). Products include:

ProSom Tablets 512

Ethchlorvynol (Clonidine may potentiate the CNS-depressive effects).
No products indexed under this heading.

Ethinamate (Clonidine may potentiate the CNS-depressive effects).
No products indexed under this heading.

Felodipine (Co-administration with agents known to affect sinus node function or AV nodal conduction, such as calcium channel blockers, may result in additive effects such as bradycardia and AV block). Products include:

Plendil Extended-Release Tablets 651

Flurazepam Hydrochloride (Clonidine may potentiate the CNS-depressive effects). Products include:

Dalmane Capsules 3343

Glutethimide (Clonidine may potentiate the CNS-depressive effects).
No products indexed under this heading.

Imipramine Hydrochloride (Co-administration may reduce the hypotensive effects; dosage adjustment may be necessary).
No products indexed under this heading.

Imipramine Pamoate (Co-administration may reduce the hypotensive effects; dosage adjustment may be necessary).
No products indexed under this heading.

Isradipine (Co-administration with agents known to affect sinus node function or AV nodal conduction, such as calcium channel blockers, may result in additive effects such as bradycardia and AV block). Products include:

DynaCirc CR Tablets 2726

Labetalol Hydrochloride (Co-administration with agents known to affect sinus node function or AV nodal conduction, such as beta blockers, may result in additive effects such as bradycardia and AV block).
No products indexed under this heading.

Levobunolol Hydrochloride (Co-administration with agents known to affect sinus node function or AV nodal conduction, such as beta blockers, may result in additive effects such as bradycardia and AV block). Products include:

Betagan Ophthalmic Solution, USP.. ⊙217

Lorazepam (Clonidine may potentiate the CNS-depressive effects).
No products indexed under this heading.

Maprotiline Hydrochloride (Co-administration may reduce the hypotensive effects; dosage adjustment may be necessary).
No products indexed under this heading.

Mephobarbital (Clonidine may potentiate the CNS-depressive effects). Products include:

Mebaral Tablets, USP 2483

Metipranolol Hydrochloride (Co-administration with agents known to affect sinus node function or AV nodal conduction, such as beta blockers, may result in additive effects such as bradycardia and AV block).
No products indexed under this heading.

Metoprolol Succinate (Co-administration with agents known to affect sinus node function or AV nodal conduction, such as beta blockers, may result in additive effects such as bradycardia and AV block). Products include:

Toprol-XL Tablets 660

Metoprolol Tartrate (Co-administration with agents known to affect sinus node function or AV nodal conduction, such as beta blockers, may result in additive effects such as bradycardia and AV block).
No products indexed under this heading.

Mibefradil Dihydrochloride (Co-administration with agents known to affect sinus node function or AV nodal conduction, such as calcium channel blockers, may result in additive effects such as bradycardia and AV block).
No products indexed under this heading.

Midazolam Hydrochloride (Clonidine may potentiate the CNS-depressive effects).
No products indexed under this heading.

Nadolol (Co-administration with agents known to affect sinus node function or AV nodal conduction, such as beta blockers, may result in additive effects such as bradycardia and AV block). Products include:

Nadolol Tablets 2121

Nicardipine Hydrochloride (Co-administration with agents known to affect sinus node function or AV nodal conduction, such as calcium channel blockers, may result in additive effects such as bradycardia and AV block). Products include:

Cardene I.V. 1129

Nifedipine (Co-administration with agents known to affect sinus node function or AV nodal conduction, such as calcium channel blockers, may result in additive effects such as bradycardia and AV block). Products include:

Adalat CC Tablets 2978

Nimodipine (Co-administration with agents known to affect sinus node function or AV nodal conduction, such as calcium channel blockers, may result in additive effects such as bradycardia and AV block). Products include:

Nimotop Capsules 774

Nisoldipine (Co-administration with agents known to affect sinus node function or AV nodal conduction, such as calcium channel blockers, may result in additive effects such as bradycardia and AV block). Products include:

Sular Tablets 1163

Nortriptyline Hydrochloride (Co-administration may reduce the hypotensive effects; dosage adjustment may be necessary).
No products indexed under this heading.

Penbutolol Sulfate (Co-administration with agents known to affect sinus node function or AV nodal conduction, such as beta blockers, may result in additive effects such as bradycardia and AV block).
No products indexed under this heading.

Pentobarbital Sodium (Clonidine may potentiate the CNS-depressive effects). Products include:
Nembutal Sodium Solution, USP **2484**

Phenobarbital (Clonidine may potentiate the CNS-depressive effects).
No products indexed under this heading.

Pindolol (Co-administration with agents known to affect sinus node function or AV nodal conduction, such as beta blockers, may result in additive effects such as bradycardia and AV block).
No products indexed under this heading.

Propofol (Clonidine may potentiate the CNS-depressive effects). Products include:
Diprivan Injectable Emulsion **676**

Propranolol Hydrochloride (Co-administration with agents known to affect sinus node function or AV nodal conduction, such as beta blockers, may result in additive effects such as bradycardia and AV block). Products include:
Inderal LA Long-Acting Capsules **3421**
InnoPran XL Capsules **2728**

Protriptyline Hydrochloride (Co-administration may reduce the hypotensive effects; dosage adjustment may be necessary). Products include:
Vivactil Tablets **2350**

Quazepam (Clonidine may potentiate the CNS-depressive effects).
No products indexed under this heading.

Secobarbital Sodium (Clonidine may potentiate the CNS-depressive effects).
No products indexed under this heading.

Sotalol Hydrochloride (Co-administration with agents known to affect sinus node function or AV nodal conduction, such as beta blockers, may result in additive effects such as bradycardia and AV block).
No products indexed under this heading.

Temazepam (Clonidine may potentiate the CNS-depressive effects).
No products indexed under this heading.

Thiamylal Sodium (Clonidine may potentiate the CNS-depressive effects).
No products indexed under this heading.

Timolol Hemihydrate (Co-administration with agents known to affect sinus node function or AV nodal conduction, such as beta blockers, may result in additive effects such as bradycardia and AV block). Products include:
Betimol Ophthalmic Solution **3371**
Betimol Ophthalmic Solution .... ⊙**283**

Timolol Maleate (Co-administration with agents known to affect sinus node function or AV nodal conduction, such as beta blockers, may result in additive effects such as bradycardia and AV block). Products include:
Blocadren Tablets **1891**
Cosopt Sterile Ophthalmic Solution **1910**
Timolide Tablets **2056**
Timoptic in Ocudose **2061**
Timoptic Sterile Ophthalmic Solution **2058**
Timoptic-XE Sterile Ophthalmic Gel Forming Solution **2062**

Triazolam (Clonidine may potentiate the CNS-depressive effects).
No products indexed under this heading.

Trimipramine Maleate (Co-administration may reduce the hypotensive effects; dosage adjustment may be necessary). Products include:
Surmontil Capsules **2347**

Verapamil Hydrochloride (Co-administration with agents known to affect sinus node function or AV nodal conduction, such as calcium channel blockers, may result in additive effects such as bradycardia and AV block). Products include:
Covera-HS Tablets **3135**
Tarka Tablets **519**
Verelan PM Capsules **3120**

Zaleplon (Clonidine may potentiate the CNS-depressive effects). Products include:
Sonata Capsules **1686**

Zolpidem Tartrate (Clonidine may potentiate the CNS-depressive effects). Products include:
Ambien Tablets **2867**

Food Interactions

Alcohol (Clonidine may potentiate the CNS-depressive effects).

CATAPRES-TTS

(Clonidine) **875**

May interact with barbiturates, beta blockers, calcium channel blockers, cardiac glycosides, hypnotics and sedatives, tricyclic antidepressants, and certain other agents. Compounds in these categories include:

Acebutolol Hydrochloride (Co-administration with agents known to affect sinus node function or AV nodal conduction, such as beta blockers, may result in additive effects such as bradycardia and AV block).
No products indexed under this heading.

Amitriptyline Hydrochloride (Co-administration may reduce the hypotensive effects; dosage adjustment may be necessary; concurrent use has resulted in corneal lesions in rats within 5 days).
No products indexed under this heading.

Amlodipine Besylate (Co-administration with agents known to affect sinus node function or AV nodal conduction, such as calcium channel blockers, may result in additive effects such as bradycardia and AV block). Products include:
Caduet Tablets **2507**
Lotrel Capsules **2238**
Norvasc Tablets **2529**

Amoxapine (Co-administration may reduce the hypotensive effects; dosage adjustment may be necessary).
No products indexed under this heading.

Aprobarbital (Clonidine may potentiate the CNS-depressive effects).
No products indexed under this heading.

Atenolol (Co-administration with agents known to affect sinus node function or AV nodal conduction, such as beta blockers, may result in additive effects such as bradycardia and AV block). Products include:
Tenormin I.V. Injection **698**
Tenormin Tablets **695**

Bepridil Hydrochloride (Co-administration with agents known to affect sinus node function or AV nodal conduction, such as calcium channel blockers, may result in additive effects such as bradycardia and AV block).
No products indexed under this heading.

Betaxolol Hydrochloride (Co-administration with agents known to affect sinus node function or AV nodal conduction, such as beta blockers, may result in additive effects such as bradycardia and AV block). Products include:
Betoptic S Ophthalmic Suspension.................................. **554**

Bisoprolol Fumarate (Co-administration with agents known to affect sinus node function or AV nodal conduction, such as beta blockers, may result in additive effects such as bradycardia and AV block).
No products indexed under this heading.

Butabarbital (Clonidine may potentiate the CNS-depressive effects).
No products indexed under this heading.

Butalbital (Clonidine may potentiate the CNS-depressive effects). Products include:
Sedapap Tablets 50 mg/650 mg **2098**

Carteolol Hydrochloride (Co-administration with agents known to affect sinus node function or AV nodal conduction, such as beta blockers, may result in additive effects such as bradycardia and AV block). Products include:
Carteolol Hydrochloride Ophthalmic Solution USP, 1%....... ⊙**246**

Clomipramine Hydrochloride (Co-administration may reduce the hypotensive effects; dosage adjustment may be necessary).
No products indexed under this heading.

Desipramine Hydrochloride (Co-administration may reduce the hypotensive effects; dosage adjustment may be necessary).
No products indexed under this heading.

Deslanoside (Co-administration with agents known to affect sinus node function or AV nodal conduction, such as digitalis, may result in additive effects such as bradycardia and AV block).
No products indexed under this heading.

Digitalis Glycoside Preparations (Co-administration with agents known to affect sinus node function or AV nodal conduction, such as digitalis, may result in additive effects such as bradycardia and AV block).
No products indexed under this heading.

Digitoxin (Co-administration with agents known to affect sinus node function or AV nodal conduction, such as digitalis, may result in additive effects such as bradycardia and AV block).
No products indexed under this heading.

Digoxin (Co-administration with agents known to affect sinus node function or AV nodal conduction, such as digitalis, may result in additive effects such as bradycardia and AV block). Products include:
Digitek Tablets **2146**
Lanoxicaps Capsules **1458**
Lanoxin Injection **1462**
Lanoxin Tablets **1468**
Lanoxin Injection Pediatric **1465**

Diltiazem Hydrochloride (Co-administration with agents known to affect sinus node function or AV nodal conduction, such as calcium channel blockers, may result in additive effects such as bradycardia and AV block). Products include:
Cardizem LA Extended Release Tablets **1699**
Tiazac Capsules **1204**

Doxepin Hydrochloride (Co-administration may reduce the hypotensive effects; dosage adjustment may be necessary).
No products indexed under this heading.

Esmolol Hydrochloride (Co-administration with agents known to affect sinus node function or AV nodal conduction, such as beta blockers, may result in additive effects such as bradycardia and AV block). Products include:
Brevibloc Concentrate **766**
Brevibloc Injection **766**
Brevibloc Double Strength Injection.. **766**
Brevibloc Premixed Injection **766**
Brevibloc Double Strength Premixed Injection.............................. **766**

Estazolam (Clonidine may potentiate the CNS-depressive effects). Products include:
ProSom Tablets **512**

Ethchlorvynol (Clonidine may potentiate the CNS-depressive effects).
No products indexed under this heading.

Ethinamate (Clonidine may potentiate the CNS-depressive effects).
No products indexed under this heading.

Felodipine (Co-administration with agents known to affect sinus node function or AV nodal conduction, such as calcium channel blockers, may result in additive effects such as bradycardia and AV block). Products include:
Plendil Extended-Release Tablets **651**

Flurazepam Hydrochloride (Clonidine may potentiate the CNS-depressive effects). Products include:
Dalmane Capsules **3343**

Glutethimide (Clonidine may potentiate the CNS-depressive effects).
No products indexed under this heading.

Imipramine Hydrochloride (Co-administration may reduce the hypotensive effects; dosage adjustment may be necessary).
No products indexed under this heading.

Imipramine Pamoate (Co-administration may reduce the hypotensive effects; dosage adjustment may be necessary).
No products indexed under this heading.

Isradipine (Co-administration with agents known to affect sinus node function or AV nodal conduction, such as calcium channel blockers, may result in additive effects such as bradycardia and AV block). Products include:
DynaCirc CR Tablets 2726

Labetalol Hydrochloride (Co-administration with agents known to affect sinus node function or AV nodal conduction, such as beta blockers, may result in additive effects such as bradycardia and AV block).
No products indexed under this heading.

Levobunolol Hydrochloride (Co-administration with agents known to affect sinus node function or AV nodal conduction, such as beta blockers, may result in additive effects such as bradycardia and AV block). Products include:
Betagan Ophthalmic Solution, USP .... ⊙217

Lorazepam (Clonidine may potentiate the CNS-depressive effects).
No products indexed under this heading.

Maprotiline Hydrochloride (Co-administration may reduce the hypotensive effects; dosage adjustment may be necessary).
No products indexed under this heading.

Mephobarbital (Clonidine may potentiate the CNS-depressive effects). Products include:
Mebaral Tablets, USP 2483

Metipranolol Hydrochloride (Co-administration with agents known to affect sinus node function or AV nodal conduction, such as beta blockers, may result in additive effects such as bradycardia and AV block).
No products indexed under this heading.

Metoprolol Succinate (Co-administration with agents known to affect sinus node function or AV nodal conduction, such as beta blockers, may result in additive effects such as bradycardia and AV block). Products include:
Toprol-XL Tablets 660

Metoprolol Tartrate (Co-administration with agents known to affect sinus node function or AV nodal conduction, such as beta blockers, may result in additive effects such as bradycardia and AV block).
No products indexed under this heading.

Mibefradil Dihydrochloride (Co-administration with agents known to affect sinus node function or AV nodal conduction, such as calcium channel blockers, may result in additive effects such as bradycardia and AV block).
No products indexed under this heading.

Midazolam Hydrochloride (Clonidine may potentiate the CNS-depressive effects).
No products indexed under this heading.

Nadolol (Co-administration with agents known to affect sinus node function or AV nodal conduction, such as beta blockers, may result in additive effects such as bradycardia and AV block). Products include:
Nadolol Tablets 2121

Nicardipine Hydrochloride (Co-administration with agents known to affect sinus node function or AV nodal conduction, such as calcium channel blockers, may result in additive effects such as bradycardia and AV block). Products include:
Cardene I.V. 1129

Nifedipine (Co-administration with agents known to affect sinus node function or AV nodal conduction, such as calcium channel blockers, may result in additive effects such as bradycardia and AV block). Products include:
Adalat CC Tablets 2978

Nimodipine (Co-administration with agents known to affect sinus node function or AV nodal conduction, such as calcium channel blockers, may result in additive effects such as bradycardia and AV block). Products include:
Nimotop Capsules 774

Nisoldipine (Co-administration with agents known to affect sinus node function or AV nodal conduction, such as calcium channel blockers, may result in additive effects such as bradycardia and AV block). Products include:
Sular Tablets 1163

Nortriptyline Hydrochloride (Co-administration may reduce the hypotensive effects; dosage adjustment may be necessary).
No products indexed under this heading.

Penbutolol Sulfate (Co-administration with agents known to affect sinus node function or AV nodal conduction, such as beta blockers, may result in additive effects such as bradycardia and AV block).
No products indexed under this heading.

Pentobarbital Sodium (Clonidine may potentiate the CNS-depressive effects). Products include:
Nembutal Sodium Solution, USP 2484

Phenobarbital (Clonidine may potentiate the CNS-depressive effects).
No products indexed under this heading.

Pindolol (Co-administration with agents known to affect sinus node function or AV nodal conduction, such as beta blockers, may result in additive effects such as bradycardia and AV block).
No products indexed under this heading.

Propofol (Clonidine may potentiate the CNS-depressive effects). Products include:
Diprivan Injectable Emulsion 676

Propranolol Hydrochloride (Co-administration with agents known to affect sinus node function or AV nodal conduction, such as beta blockers, may result in additive effects such as bradycardia and AV block). Products include:
Inderal LA Long-Acting Capsules 3421
InnoPran XL Capsules 2728

Protriptyline Hydrochloride (Co-administration may reduce the hypotensive effects; dosage adjustment may be necessary). Products include:
Vivactil Tablets 2350

Quazepam (Clonidine may potentiate the CNS-depressive effects).
No products indexed under this heading.

Secobarbital Sodium (Clonidine may potentiate the CNS-depressive effects).
No products indexed under this heading.

Sotalol Hydrochloride (Co-administration with agents known to affect sinus node function or AV nodal conduction, such as beta blockers, may result in additive effects such as bradycardia and AV block).
No products indexed under this heading.

Temazepam (Clonidine may potentiate the CNS-depressive effects).
No products indexed under this heading.

Thiamylal Sodium (Clonidine may potentiate the CNS-depressive effects).
No products indexed under this heading.

Timolol Hemihydrate (Co-administration with agents known to affect sinus node function or AV nodal conduction, such as beta blockers, may result in additive effects such as bradycardia and AV block). Products include:
Betimol Ophthalmic Solution 3371
Betimol Ophthalmic Solution .... ⊙283

Timolol Maleate (Co-administration with agents known to affect sinus node function or AV nodal conduction, such as beta blockers, may result in additive effects such as bradycardia and AV block). Products include:
Blocadren Tablets 1891
Cosopt Sterile Ophthalmic Solution 1910
Timolide Tablets 2056
Timoptic in Ocudose 2061
Timoptic Sterile Ophthalmic Solution 2058
Timoptic-XE Sterile Ophthalmic Gel Forming Solution 2062

Triazolam (Clonidine may potentiate the CNS-depressive effects).
No products indexed under this heading.

Trimipramine Maleate (Co-administration may reduce the hypotensive effects; dosage adjustment may be necessary). Products include:
Surmontil Capsules 2347

Verapamil Hydrochloride (Co-administration with agents known to affect sinus node function or AV nodal conduction, such as calcium channel blockers, may result in additive effects such as bradycardia and AV block). Products include:
Covera-HS Tablets 3135
Tarka Tablets 519
Verelan PM Capsules 3120

Zaleplon (Clonidine may potentiate the CNS-depressive effects). Products include:
Sonata Capsules 1686

Zolpidem Tartrate (Clonidine may potentiate the CNS-depressive effects). Products include:
Ambien Tablets 2867

Food Interactions

Alcohol (Clonidine may potentiate the CNS-depressive effects).

CATHFLO ACTIVASE
(Alteplase) 1232
See Activase I.V.

CAVERJECT IMPULSE INJECTION
(Alprostadil) 2610
May interact with:

Heparin Sodium (Patients on anticoagulants, such as heparin, may have increased propensity for bleeding after intracavernosal injection).
No products indexed under this heading.

Sildenafil Citrate (The safety and efficacy of combination therapy with other vasoactive agents, such as sildenafil, have not been studied; therefore, such combinations are not recommended). Products include:
Revatio Tablets 2541
Viagra Tablets 2552

Warfarin Sodium (Patients on anticoagulants, such as warfarin, may have increased propensity for bleeding after intracavernosal injection). Products include:
Coumadin for Injection 932
Coumadin Tablets 932

CEFTIN FOR ORAL SUSPENSION
(Cefuroxime Axetil) 1369
See Ceftin Tablets

CEFTIN TABLETS
(Cefuroxime Axetil) 1369
May interact with oral anticoagulants, drugs that reduce gastric acidity, and certain other agents. Compounds in these categories include:

Aluminum Carbonate (Drugs that reduce gastric acidity may result in a lower bioavailability of Ceftin compared with that of fasting state and tend to cancel the effect of postprandial absorption).
No products indexed under this heading.

Aluminum Hydroxide (Drugs that reduce gastric acidity may result in a lower bioavailability of Ceftin compared with that of fasting state and tend to cancel the effect of postprandial absorption). Products include:
Gaviscon Regular Strength Liquid .... ▣620
Gaviscon Regular Strength Tablets .... ▣619
Gaviscon Extra Strength Liquid .... ▣620
Gaviscon Extra Strength Tablets .... ▣619
Maalox Max Maximum Strength Antacid/Anti-Gas Liquid 2165
Maalox Regular Strength Antacid/Antigas Liquid 2164

Anisindione (Cephalosporins may be associated with a fall in prothrombin activity; those at risk include patients previously stabilized on anticoagulant therapy). Products include:
Miradon Tablets 3056

Cimetidine (Drugs that reduce gastric acidity may result in a lower bioavailability of Ceftin compared with that of fasting state and tend to cancel the effect of postprandial absorption). Products include:
Tagamet HB 200 Tablets .... ▣637

Tagamet Tablets 1547

Cimetidine Hydrochloride (Drugs that reduce gastric acidity may result in a lower bioavailability of Ceftin compared with that of fasting state and tend to cancel the effect of postprandial absorption).
No products indexed under this heading.

Dicumarol (Cephalosporins may be associated with a fall in prothrombin activity; those at risk include patients previously stabilized on anticoagulant therapy).
No products indexed under this heading.

Esomeprazole Magnesium (Drugs that reduce gastric acidity may result in a lower bioavailability of Ceftin compared with that of fasting state and tend to cancel the effect of postprandial absorption). Products include:
Nexium Delayed-Release Capsules 645

Famotidine (Drugs that reduce gastric acidity may result in a lower bioavailability of Ceftin compared with that of fasting state and tend to cancel the effect of postprandial absorption). Products include:
Pepcid AC Chewable Tablets 1672
Pepcid AC Gelcaps 1672
Pepcid AC Tablets 1672
Maximum Strength Pepcid AC Tablets 1672
Pepcid Complete Chewable Tablets 1672
Pepcid Injection 2017
Pepcid 2014

Lansoprazole (Drugs that reduce gastric acidity may result in a lower bioavailability of Ceftin compared with that of fasting state and tend to cancel the effect of postprandial absorption). Products include:
Prevacid Delayed-Release Capsules 3268
Prevacid for Delayed-Release Oral Suspension 3268
Prevacid I.V. for Injection 3274
Prevacid NapraPAC 3277
Prevacid SoluTab Delayed-Release Orally Disintegrating Tablets 3268
PREVPAC 3281

Magnesium Hydroxide (Drugs that reduce gastric acidity may result in a lower bioavailability of Ceftin compared with that of fasting state and tend to cancel the effect of postprandial absorption). Products include:
Maalox Max Maximum Strength Antacid/Anti-Gas Liquid 2165
Maalox Regular Strength Antacid/Antigas Liquid 2164
Pepcid Complete Chewable Tablets 1672
Rolaids Tablets .... ▣707
Extra Strength Rolaids Tablets ...... ▣707
Rolaids Multi-Symptom Antacid & Antigas Tablets .... ▣708

Nizatidine (Drugs that reduce gastric acidity may result in a lower bioavailability of Ceftin compared with that of fasting state and tend to cancel the effect of postprandial absorption). Products include:
Axid Oral Solution 913

Omeprazole (Drugs that reduce gastric acidity may result in a lower bioavailability of Ceftin compared with that of fasting state and tend to cancel the effect of postprandial absorption). Products include:
Zegerid Powder for Oral Solution 2972

Probenecid (Increases serum concentration of cefuroxime).
No products indexed under this heading.

Rabeprazole Sodium (Drugs that reduce gastric acidity may result in a lower bioavailability of Ceftin compared with that of fasting state and tend to cancel the effect of postprandial absorption). Products include:
Aciphex Tablets 1081

Ranitidine Hydrochloride (Drugs that reduce gastric acidity may result in a lower bioavailability of Ceftin compared with that of fasting state and tend to cancel the effect of postprandial absorption). Products include:
Zantac 1597
Zantac Injection 1593
Zantac 75 Tablets .... ▣715
Zantac 150 Maximum Strength Tablets .... ▣715
Zantac Injection Pharmacy Bulk Package 1595

Warfarin Sodium (Cephalosporins may be associated with a fall in prothrombin activity; those at risk include patients previously stabilized on anticoagulant therapy). Products include:
Coumadin for Injection 932
Coumadin Tablets 932

Food Interactions

Food, unspecified (Absorption is greater when taken after food).

CELEBREX CAPSULES

(Celecoxib) 3130
May interact with ACE inhibitors, antacids containing aluminum, calcium and magnesium, oral anticoagulants, lithium preparations, thiazides, and certain other agents. Compounds in these categories include:

Aluminum Carbonate (Co-administration with an aluminum-and-magnesium-containing antacid resulted in a reduction in plasma celecoxib concentration with a decrease of 37% in Cmax and 10% in AUC).
No products indexed under this heading.

Aluminum Hydroxide (Co-administration with an aluminum-and-magnesium-containing antacid resulted in a reduction in plasma celecoxib concentration with a decrease of 37% in Cmax and 10% in AUC). Products include:
Gaviscon Regular Strength Liquid .. ▣620
Gaviscon Regular Strength Tablets .... ▣619
Gaviscon Extra Strength Liquid ...... ▣620
Gaviscon Extra Strength Tablets .... ▣619
Maalox Max Maximum Strength Antacid/Anti-Gas Liquid 2165
Maalox Regular Strength Antacid/Antigas Liquid 2164

Amiodarone Hydrochloride (Co-administration of celecoxib with drugs known to inhibit CYP4502C9, such as amiodarone, may result in increased plasma concentration; caution should be exercised if used concurrently). Products include:
Pacerone Tablets 3337

Anisindione (Serious bleeding events, some of which were fatal, have been reported, predominately in the elderly, in association with increases in prothrombin time in patients receiving celecoxib concurrently with warfarin. Anticoagulant activity should be monitored,particulary in the first few days, after initiating or changing celecoxib therapy in patients receiving warfarin or similar agents, since these patients are at an increased risk of bleeding complications). Products include:
Miradon Tablets 3056

Aspirin (Co-administration may result in an increased rate of GI ulceration or other complications; low dose of aspirin can be used with celecoxib). Products include:
Aggrenox Capsules 855
Bayer, Aspirin Regimen .... ▣606
Bayer Aspirin Tablets 3515
BC Powder .... ▣612
BC Allergy Sinus Cold Powder .... ▣612
Arthritis Strength BC Powder .... ▣612
BC Sinus Cold Powder .... ▣612
Ecotrin Enteric Coated Aspirin Low, Regular and Maximum Strength Tablets 1627
Goody's Body Pain Formula Powder .... ▣621
Goody's Extra Strength Headache Powder .... ▣621
Goody's Extra Strength Pain Relief Tablets .... ▣621
Percodan Tablets 1115
St. Joseph 81 mg Aspirin Chewable and Enteric Coated Tablets 1841

Benazepril Hydrochloride (Co-administration of NSAIDs with ACE inhibitors may result in diminished antihypertensive effect of ACE inhibitors). Products include:
Lotensin Tablets 2232
Lotensin HCT Tablets 2235
Lotrel Capsules 2238

Bendroflumethiazide (Co-administration of NSAIDs with thiazides may result in reduced natriuretic effect of thiazide diuretics).
No products indexed under this heading.

Captopril (Co-administration of NSAIDs with ACE inhibitors may result in diminished antihypertensive effect of ACE inhibitors). Products include:
Captopril Tablets 2114

Chlorothiazide (Co-administration of NSAIDs with thiazides may result in reduced natriuretic effect of thiazide diuretics). Products include:
Aldoclor Tablets 1881
Diuril Oral 1936

Chlorothiazide Sodium (Co-administration of NSAIDs with thiazides may result in reduced natriuretic effect of thiazide diuretics). Products include:
Diuril Sodium Intravenous 1934

Dicumarol (Serious bleeding events, some of which were fatal, have been reported, predominately in the elderly, in association with increases in prothrombin time in patients receiving celecoxib concurrently with warfarin. Anticoagulant activity should be monitored,particulary in the first few days, after initiating or changing celecoxib therapy in patients receiving warfarin or similar agents, since these patients are at an increased risk of bleeding complications).
No products indexed under this heading.

Enalapril Maleate (Co-administration of NSAIDs with ACE inhibitors may result in diminished antihypertensive effect of ACE inhibitors). Products include:
Vaseretic Tablets 2073
Vasotec I.V. Injection 2076

Enalaprilat (Co-administration of NSAIDs with ACE inhibitors may result in diminished antihypertensive effect of ACE inhibitors).
No products indexed under this heading.

Fluconazole (Co-administration has resulted in a two-fold increase in celecoxib plasma concentration due to inhibition of celecoxib metabolism via P4502C9).
No products indexed under this heading.

Fosinopril Sodium (Co-administration of NSAIDs with ACE inhibitors may result in diminished antihypertensive effect of ACE inhibitors).
No products indexed under this heading.

Furosemide (Co-administration of NSAIDs with thiazides may result in reduced natriuretic effect of furosemide). Products include:
Furosemide Tablets 2117

Hydrochlorothiazide (Co-administration of NSAIDs with thiazides may result in reduced natriuretic effect of thiazide diuretics). Products include:
Aldoril Tablets 1884
Atacand HCT 637
Avalide Tablets 2889
Avalide Tablets 922
Benicar HCT Tablets 2852
Diovan HCT Tablets 2195
Dyazide Capsules 1389
Hyzaar 1964
Lotensin HCT Tablets 2235
Maxzide 2150
Micardis HCT Tablets 886
Moduretic Tablets 2003
Prinzide Tablets 2033
Teveten HCT Tablets 1710
Timolide Tablets 2056
Uniretic Tablets 3114
Vaseretic Tablets 2073
Zestoretic Tablets 701

Hydroflumethiazide (Co-administration of NSAIDs with thiazides may result in reduced natriuretic effect of thiazide diuretics).
No products indexed under this heading.

Itraconazole (Co-administration of celecoxib with drugs known to inhibit CYP4502C9, such as itraconazole, may result in increased plasma concentration; caution should be exercised if used concurrently).
No products indexed under this heading.

Ketoconazole (Co-administration of celecoxib with drugs known to inhibit CYP4502C9, such as ketoconazole, may result in increased plasma concentration; caution should be exercised if used concurrently). Products include:
Nizoral A-D Shampoo, 1% 1839
Nizoral 2% Shampoo 1838

Lisinopril (Co-administration of NSAIDs with ACE inhibitors may result in diminished antihypertensive effect of ACE inhibitors). Products include:
Prinivil Tablets 2029
Prinzide Tablets 2033
Zestoretic Tablets 701
Zestril Tablets 704

Lithium (Co-administration has resulted in increased steady-state lithium plasma levels).
No products indexed under this heading.

Lithium Carbonate (Co-administration has resulted in increased steady-state lithium plasma levels). Products include:
- Eskalith 1406
- Lithobid Tablets 1670

Lithium Citrate (Co-administration has resulted in increased steady-state lithium plasma levels).
No products indexed under this heading.

Magaldrate (Co-administration with an aluminum-and-magnesium-containing antacid resulted in a reduction in plasma celecoxib concentration with a decrease of 37% in Cmax and 10% in AUC).
No products indexed under this heading.

Magnesium Hydroxide (Co-administration with an aluminum-and-magnesium-containing antacid resulted in a reduction in plasma celecoxib concentration with a decrease of 37% in Cmax and 10% in AUC). Products include:
- Maalox Max Maximum Strength Antacid/Anti-Gas Liquid 2165
- Maalox Regular Strength Antacid/Antigas Liquid 2164
- Pepcid Complete Chewable Tablets 1672
- Rolaids Tablets .... ▣707
- Extra Strength Rolaids Tablets .... ▣707
- Rolaids Multi-Symptom Antacid & Antigas Tablets .... ▣708

Magnesium Oxide (Co-administration with an aluminum-and-magnesium-containing antacid resulted in a reduction in plasma celecoxib concentration with a decrease of 37% in Cmax and 10% in AUC). Products include:
- Beelith Tablets 784
- PremCal Light, Regular, and Extra Strength Tablets .... ▣762

Methyclothiazide (Co-administration of NSAIDs with thiazides may result in reduced natriuretic effect of thiazide diuretics).
No products indexed under this heading.

Moexipril Hydrochloride (Co-administration of NSAIDs with ACE inhibitors may result in diminished antihypertensive effect of ACE inhibitors). Products include:
- Uniretic Tablets 3114
- Univasc Tablets 3118

Perindopril Erbumine (Co-administration of NSAIDs with ACE inhibitors may result in diminished antihypertensive effect of ACE inhibitors). Products include:
- Aceon Tablets (2 mg, 4 mg, 8 mg) 3191

Polythiazide (Co-administration of NSAIDs with thiazides may result in reduced natriuretic effect of thiazide diuretics).
No products indexed under this heading.

Quinapril Hydrochloride (Co-administration of NSAIDs with ACE inhibitors may result in diminished antihypertensive effect of ACE inhibitors).
No products indexed under this heading.

Ramipril (Co-administration of NSAIDs with ACE inhibitors may result in diminished antihypertensive effect of ACE inhibitors). Products include:
- Altace Capsules 1673

Spirapril Hydrochloride (Co-administration of NSAIDs with ACE inhibitors may result in diminished antihypertensive effect of ACE inhibitors).
No products indexed under this heading.

Trandolapril (Co-administration of NSAIDs with ACE inhibitors may result in diminished antihypertensive effect of ACE inhibitors). Products include:
- Mavik Tablets 482
- Tarka Tablets 519

Warfarin Sodium (Serious bleeding events, some of which were fatal, have been reported, predominately in the elderly, in association with increases in prothrombin time in patients receiving celecoxib concurrently with warfarin. Anticoagulant activity should be monitored,particulary in the first few days, after initiating or changing celecoxib therapy in patients receiving warfarin or similar agents, since these patients are at an increased risk of bleeding complications). Products include:
- Coumadin for Injection 932
- Coumadin Tablets 932

Food Interactions

Food, unspecified (Co-administration with a high-fat meal delayed peak plasma levels for about 1 to 2 hours with an increase in total absorption (AUC) of 10% to 20%; Celebrex can be administered without regard to the timing of meals).

CELEXA ORAL SOLUTION

(Citalopram Hydrobromide) 1177
See Celexa Tablets

CELEXA TABLETS

(Citalopram Hydrobromide) 1177
May interact with anticoagulants, erythromycin, lithium preparations, macrolide antibiotics, monoamine oxidase inhibitors, non-steroidal anti-inflammatory agents, tricyclic antidepressants, and certain other agents. Compounds in these categories include:

Amitriptyline Hydrochloride (Co-administration of imipramine with citalopram has resulted in a 50% increase in active metabolite, desipramine concentration; the clinical significance of these findings is unknown; caution is indicated if tricyclic antidepressants are co-administered with citalopram, a relatively weak inhibitor of CYP2D6).
No products indexed under this heading.

Amoxapine (Co-administration of imipramine with citalopram has resulted in a 50% increase in active metabolite, desipramine concentration; the clinical significance of these findings is unknown; caution is indicated if tricyclic antidepressants are co-administered with citalopram, a relatively weak inhibitor of CYP2D6).
No products indexed under this heading.

Anisindione (The combined use of psychotropic drugs that interfere with serotonin reuptake and drugs that affect coagulation has been associated with an increased risk of bleeding). Products include:
- Miradon Tablets 3056

Ardeparin Sodium (The combined use of psychotropic drugs that interfere with serotonin reuptake and drugs that affect coagulation has been associated with an increased risk of bleeding).
No products indexed under this heading.

Aspirin (The combined use of psychotropic drugs that interfere with serotonin reuptake and drugs that affect coagulation has been associated with an increased risk of bleeding; use caution when co-administering). Products include:
- Aggrenox Capsules 855
- Bayer, Aspirin Regimen .... ▣606
- Bayer Aspirin Tablets 3515
- BC Powder .... ▣612
- BC Allergy Sinus Cold Powder .... ▣612
- Arthritis Strength BC Powder .... ▣612
- BC Sinus Cold Powder .... ▣612
- Ecotrin Enteric Coated Aspirin Low, Regular and Maximum Strength Tablets 1627
- Goody's Body Pain Formula Powder .... ▣621
- Goody's Extra Strength Headache Powder .... ▣621
- Goody's Extra Strength Pain Relief Tablets .... ▣621
- Percodan Tablets 1115
- St. Joseph 81 mg Aspirin Chewable and Enteric Coated Tablets 1841

Aspirin, Enteric Coated (The combined use of psychotropic drugs that interfere with serotonin reuptake and drugs that affect coagulation has been associated with an increased risk of bleeding; use caution when co-administering).
No products indexed under this heading.

Aspirin Buffered (The combined use of psychotropic drugs that interfere with serotonin reuptake and drugs that affect coagulation has been associated with an increased risk of bleeding; use caution when co-administering).
No products indexed under this heading.

Azithromycin Dihydrate (Co-administration with potent inhibitors of CYP3A4, such as macrolide antibiotics, may decrease the clearance of citalopram). Products include:
- Zithromax 2568
- Zithromax for IV Infusion 2573
- Zithromax for Oral Suspension, 300 mg, 600 mg, 900 mg, 1200 mg 2561
- Zithromax Tablets, 250 mg, 500 mg 2561
- Zithromax Tri-Pak 2561
- Zithromax Z-Pak 2568

Carbamazepine (Given the enzyme inducing properties of carbamazepine, the possibility that carbamazepine might increase the clearance of citalopram should be considered if the two drugs are co-administered; during pharmacokinetic studies, the citalopram levels were unaffected with concurrent use). Products include:
- Carbatrol Capsules 3174
- Equetro Extended-Release Capsules 3178
- Tegretol/Tegretol-XR 2278

Celecoxib (The combined use of psychotropic drugs that interfere with serotonin reuptake and drugs that affect coagulation has been associated with an increased risk of bleeding; use caution when co-administering). Products include:
- Celebrex Capsules 3130

Cimetidine (Co-administration has resulted in an increase in citalopram AUC and Cmax by 43% and 39% respectively; the clinical significance of these findings is unknown). Products include:
- Tagamet HB 200 Tablets .... ▣637
- Tagamet Tablets 1547

Cimetidine Hydrochloride (Co-administration has resulted in an increase in citalopram AUC and Cmax by 43% and 39% respectively; the clinical significance of these findings is unknown).
No products indexed under this heading.

Clarithromycin (Co-administration with potent inhibitors of CYP3A4, such as macrolide antibiotics, may decrease the clearance of citalopram). Products include:
- Biaxin/Biaxin XL 402
- PREVPAC 3281

Clomipramine Hydrochloride (Co-administration of imipramine with citalopram has resulted in a 50% increase in active metabolite, desipramine concentration; the clinical significance of these findings is unknown; caution is indicated if tricyclic antidepressants are co-administered with citalopram, a relatively weak inhibitor of CYP2D6).
No products indexed under this heading.

Dalteparin Sodium (The combined use of psychotropic drugs that interfere with serotonin reuptake and drugs that affect coagulation has been associated with an increased risk of bleeding). Products include:
- Fragmin Injection 2638

Danaparoid Sodium (The combined use of psychotropic drugs that interfere with serotonin reuptake and drugs that affect coagulation has been associated with an increased risk of bleeding).
No products indexed under this heading.

Desipramine Hydrochloride (Co-administration of imipramine with citalopram has resulted in a 50% increase in active metabolite, desipramine concentration; the clinical significance of these findings is unknown; caution is indicated if tricyclic antidepressants are co-administered with citalopram, a relatively weak inhibitor of CYP2D6).
No products indexed under this heading.

Diclofenac Potassium (The combined use of psychotropic drugs that interfere with serotonin reuptake and drugs that affect coagulation has been associated with an increased risk of bleeding; use caution when co-administering). Products include:
- Cataflam Tablets 2173

Diclofenac Sodium (The combined use of psychotropic drugs that interfere with serotonin reuptake and drugs that affect coagulation has been associated with an increased risk of bleeding; use caution when co-administering). Products include:
- Arthrotec Tablets 3126
- Voltaren Ophthalmic Solution 2300
- Voltaren Tablets 2298
- Voltaren-XR Tablets 2301

Dicumarol (The combined use of psychotropic drugs that interfere with serotonin reuptake and drugs that affect coagulation has been associated with an increased risk of bleeding).
No products indexed under this heading.

Dirithromycin (Co-administration with potent inhibitors of CYP3A4, such as macrolide antibiotics, may decrease the clearance of citalopram).
No products indexed under this heading.

Doxepin Hydrochloride (Co-administration of imipramine with citalopram has resulted in a 50% increase in active metabolite, desipramine concentration; the clinical significance of these findings is unknown; caution is indicated if tricyclic antidepressants are co-administered with citalopram, a relatively weak inhibitor of CYP2D6).
No products indexed under this heading.

Enoxaparin Sodium (The combined use of psychotropic drugs that interfere with serotonin reuptake and drugs that affect coagulation has been associated with an increased risk of bleeding). Products include:
Lovenox Injection 2931

Erythromycin (Co-administration with potent inhibitors of CYP3A4, such as macrolide antibiotics, may decrease the clearance of citalopram). Products include:
Erygel Topical Gel 2096
Ery-Tab Tablets 447
Erythromycin Base Filmtab Tablets 454
Erythromycin Delayed-Release Capsules, USP 456
PCE Dispertab Tablets 510

Erythromycin Estolate (Co-administration with potent inhibitors of CYP3A4, such as macrolide antibiotics, may decrease the clearance of citalopram).
No products indexed under this heading.

Erythromycin Ethylsuccinate (Co-administration with potent inhibitors of CYP3A4, such as macrolide antibiotics, may decrease the clearance of citalopram). Products include:
E.E.S. 449
EryPed 445

Erythromycin Gluceptate (Co-administration with potent inhibitors of CYP3A4, such as macrolide antibiotics, may decrease the clearance of citalopram).
No products indexed under this heading.

Erythromycin Lactobionate (Co-administration with potent inhibitors of CYP3A4, such as erythromycin, may decrease the clearance of citalopram).
No products indexed under this heading.

Erythromycin Stearate (Co-administration with potent inhibitors of CYP3A4, such as macrolide antibiotics, may decrease the clearance of citalopram). Products include:
Erythrocin Stearate Filmtab Tablets 452

Etodolac (The combined use of psychotropic drugs that interfere with serotonin reuptake and drugs that affect coagulation has been associated with an increased risk of bleeding; use caution when co-administering).
No products indexed under this heading.

Fenoprofen Calcium (The combined use of psychotropic drugs that interfere with serotonin reuptake and drugs that affect coagulation has been associated with an increased risk of bleeding; use caution when co-administering). Products include:
Nalfon Capsules 2504

Fluconazole (Co-administration with potent inhibitors of CYP3A4, such as fluconazole, may decrease the clearance of citalopram).
No products indexed under this heading.

Flurbiprofen (The combined use of psychotropic drugs that interfere with serotonin reuptake and drugs that affect coagulation has been associated with an increased risk of bleeding; use caution when co-administering).
No products indexed under this heading.

Fondaparinux Sodium (The combined use of psychotropic drugs that interfere with serotonin reuptake and drugs that affect coagulation has been associated with an increased risk of bleeding). Products include:
Arixtra Injection 1325

Heparin Calcium (The combined use of psychotropic drugs that interfere with serotonin reuptake and drugs that affect coagulation has been associated with an increased risk of bleeding).
No products indexed under this heading.

Heparin Sodium (The combined use of psychotropic drugs that interfere with serotonin reuptake and drugs that affect coagulation has been associated with an increased risk of bleeding).
No products indexed under this heading.

Ibuprofen (The combined use of psychotropic drugs that interfere with serotonin reuptake and drugs that affect coagulation has been associated with an increased risk of bleeding; use caution when co-administering). Products include:
Advil Allergy Sinus Caplets .... ▣ 737
Advil .... ▣ 737
Children's Advil Suspension .... ▣ 742
Children's Advil Chewable Tablets .. ▣ 741
Advil Cold & Sinus .... ▣ 739
Advil Flu & Body Ache Caplets .... ▣ 739
Children's Advil Cold Suspension ... ▣ 741
Infants' Advil Concentrated Drops .. ▣ 743
Junior Strength Advil Swallow Tablets .... ▣ 740
Advil Migraine Liquigels .... ▣ 740
Advil Multi-Symptom Cold Caplets .... ▣ 738
Combunox Tablets 1183
Children's Motrin Oral Suspension and Chewable Tablets 1837
Children's Motrin Cold Non-Staining Dye-Free Oral Suspension 1838
Children's Motrin Cold Oral Suspension 1838
Children's Motrin Non-Staining Dye-Free Oral Suspension 1837
Motrin Cold & Sinus Caplets 1836
Motrin IB Tablets and Caplets 1836
Infants' Motrin Concentrated Drops 1837
Infants' Motrin Non-Staining Dye-Free Drops 1837
Junior Strength Motrin Caplets and Chewable Tablets 1837
Vicoprofen Tablets 533

Imipramine Hydrochloride (Co-administration of imipramine with citalopram has resulted in a 50% increase in active metabolite, desipramine concentration; the clinical significance of these findings is unknown; caution is indicated if tricyclic antidepressants are co-administered with citalopram, a relatively weak inhibitor of CYP2D6).
No products indexed under this heading.

Imipramine Pamoate (Co-administration of imipramine with citalopram has resulted in a 50% increase in active metabolite, desipramine concentration; the clinical significance of these findings is unknown; caution is indicated if tricyclic antidepressants are co-administered with citalopram, a relatively weak inhibitor of CYP2D6).
No products indexed under this heading.

Indomethacin (The combined use of psychotropic drugs that interfere with serotonin reuptake and drugs that affect coagulation has been associated with an increased risk of bleeding; use caution when co-administering). Products include:
Indocin 1968

Indomethacin Sodium Trihydrate (The combined use of psychotropic drugs that interfere with serotonin reuptake and drugs that affect coagulation has been associated with an increased risk of bleeding; use caution when co-administering). Products include:
Indocin I.V. 1973

Isocarboxazid (Co-administration of serotonin reuptake inhibitors and MAO inhibitors has resulted in serious, sometimes fatal, reactions including hyperthermia, rigidity, myoclonus, and other potentially serious adverse reactions; concurrent and/or sequential use is contraindicated).
No products indexed under this heading.

Itraconazole (Co-administration with potent inhibitors of CYP3A4, such as itraconazole, may decrease the clearance of citalopram).
No products indexed under this heading.

Ketoconazole (Co-administration resulted in decreased Cmax and AUC of ketoconazole by 21% and 10% respectively, and did not significantly affect the pharmacokinetics of citalopram). Products include:
Nizoral A-D Shampoo, 1% 1839
Nizoral 2% Shampoo 1838

Ketoprofen (The combined use of psychotropic drugs that interfere with serotonin reuptake and drugs that affect coagulation has been associated with an increased risk of bleeding; use caution when co-administering).
No products indexed under this heading.

Ketorolac Tromethamine (The combined use of psychotropic drugs that interfere with serotonin reuptake and drugs that affect coagulation has been associated with an increased risk of bleeding; use caution when co-administering). Products include:
Acular Ophthalmic Solution 561
Acular LS Ophthalmic Solution 562

Lithium (Plasma lithium levels should be monitored; if used concurrently, lithium may enhance the serotonergic effects of citalopram; co-administration during clinical trials had no significant effect on the pharmacokinetics of either drug).
No products indexed under this heading.

Lithium Carbonate (Plasma lithium levels should be monitored; if used concurrently, lithium may enhance the serotonergic effects of citalopram; co-administration during clinical trials had no significant effect on the pharmacokinetics of either drug). Products include:
Eskalith 1406
Lithobid Tablets 1670

Lithium Citrate (Plasma lithium levels should be monitored; if used concurrently, lithium may enhance the serotonergic effects of citalopram; co-administration during clinical trials had no significant effect on the pharmacokinetics of either drug).
No products indexed under this heading.

Low Molecular Weight Heparins (The combined use of psychotropic drugs that interfere with serotonin reuptake and drugs that affect coagulation has been associated with an increased risk of bleeding).
No products indexed under this heading.

Maprotiline Hydrochloride (Co-administration of imipramine with citalopram has resulted in a 50% increase in active metabolite, desipramine concentration; the clinical significance of these findings is unknown; caution is indicated if tricyclic antidepressants are co-administered with citalopram, a relatively weak inhibitor of CYP2D6).
No products indexed under this heading.

Meclofenamate Sodium (The combined use of psychotropic drugs that interfere with serotonin reuptake and drugs that affect coagulation has been associated with an increased risk of bleeding; use caution when co-administering).
No products indexed under this heading.

Mefenamic Acid (The combined use of psychotropic drugs that interfere with serotonin reuptake and drugs that affect coagulation has been associated with an increased risk of bleeding; use caution when co-administering).
No products indexed under this heading.

Meloxicam (The combined use of psychotropic drugs that interfere with serotonin reuptake and drugs that affect coagulation has been associated with an increased risk of bleeding; use caution when co-administering). Products include:
Mobic Oral Suspension 893
Mobic Tablets 893

Metoprolol Succinate (Co-administration has resulted in a two-fold increase in the plasma levels of metoprolol; increased plasma levels of metoprolol have been associated with decreased cardioselectivity; no clinically significant effects on the blood pressure or heart rate have been reported with concurrent use). Products include:

Toprol-XL Tablets 660

Metoprolol Tartrate (Co-administration has resulted in a two-fold increase in the plasma levels of metoprolol; increased plasma levels of metoprolol have been associated with decreased cardioselectivity; no clinically significant effects on the blood pressure or heart rate have been reported with concurrent use).
No products indexed under this heading.

Moclobemide (Co-administration of serotonin reuptake inhibitors and MAO inhibitors has resulted in serious, sometimes fatal, reactions including hyperthermia, rigidity, myoclonus, and other potentially serious adverse reactions; concurrent and/or sequential use is contraindicated).
No products indexed under this heading.

Nabumetone (The combined use of psychotropic drugs that interfere with serotonin reuptake and drugs that affect coagulation has been associated with an increased risk of bleeding; use caution when co-administering). Products include:
Relafen Tablets 1523

Naproxen (The combined use of psychotropic drugs that interfere with serotonin reuptake and drugs that affect coagulation has been associated with an increased risk of bleeding; use caution when co-administering). Products include:
EC-Naprosyn Delayed-Release Tablets 2769
Naprosyn Suspension 2769
Naprosyn Tablets 2769
Prevacid NapraPAC 3277

Naproxen Sodium (The combined use of psychotropic drugs that interfere with serotonin reuptake and drugs that affect coagulation has been associated with an increased risk of bleeding; use caution when co-administering). Products include:
Aleve Tablets, Caplets and Gelcaps 605
Anaprox Tablets 2769
Anaprox DS Tablets 2769

Nortriptyline Hydrochloride (Co-administration of imipramine with citalopram has resulted in a 50% increase in active metabolite, desipramine concentration; the clinical significance of these findings is unknown; caution is indicated if tricyclic antidepressants are co-administered with citalopram, a relatively weak inhibitor of CYP2D6).
No products indexed under this heading.

Omeprazole (Co-administration with potent inhibitors of CYP2C19, such as omeprazole, may decrease the clearance of citalopram). Products include:
Zegerid Powder for Oral Solution 2972

Oxaprozin (The combined use of psychotropic drugs that interfere with serotonin reuptake and drugs that affect coagulation has been associated with an increased risk of bleeding; use caution when co-administering).
No products indexed under this heading.

Pargyline Hydrochloride (Co-administration of serotonin reuptake inhibitors and MAO inhibitors has resulted in serious, sometimes fatal, reactions including hyperthermia, rigidity, myoclonus, and other potentially serious adverse reactions; concurrent and/or sequential use is contraindicated).
No products indexed under this heading.

Phenelzine Sulfate (Co-administration of serotonin reuptake inhibitors and MAO inhibitors has resulted in serious, sometimes fatal, reactions including hyperthermia, rigidity, myoclonus, and other potentially serious adverse reactions; concurrent and/or sequential use is contraindicated).
No products indexed under this heading.

Phenylbutazone (The combined use of psychotropic drugs that interfere with serotonin reuptake and drugs that affect coagulation has been associated with an increased risk of bleeding; use caution when co-administering).
No products indexed under this heading.

Pimozide (In a controlled study, a single dose of pimozide 2 mg co-administered with citalopram 40 mg given once daily for 11 days was associated with a mean increase in QTc values of approximately 10 msec. compared to pimozide given alone). Products include:
Orap Tablets 1220

Piroxicam (The combined use of psychotropic drugs that interfere with serotonin reuptake and drugs that affect coagulation has been associated with an increased risk of bleeding; use caution when co-administering).
No products indexed under this heading.

Procarbazine Hydrochloride (Co-administration of serotonin reuptake inhibitors and MAO inhibitors has resulted in serious, sometimes fatal, reactions including hyperthermia, rigidity, myoclonus, and other potentially serious adverse reactions; concurrent and/or sequential use is contraindicated). Products include:
Matulane Capsules 3188

Protriptyline Hydrochloride (Co-administration of imipramine with citalopram has resulted in a 50% increase in active metabolite, desipramine concentration; the clinical significance of these findings is unknown; caution is indicated if tricyclic antidepressants are co-administered with citalopram, a relatively weak inhibitor of CYP2D6). Products include:
Vivactil Tablets 2350

Rofecoxib (The combined use of psychotropic drugs that interfere with serotonin reuptake and drugs that affect coagulation has been associated with an increased risk of bleeding; use caution when co-administering).
No products indexed under this heading.

Selegiline Hydrochloride (Co-administration of serotonin reuptake inhibitors and MAO inhibitors has resulted in serious, sometimes fatal, reactions including hyperthermia, rigidity, myoclonus, and other potentially serious adverse reactions; concurrent and/or sequential use is contraindicated). Products include:
Eldepryl Capsules 3209

Sulindac (The combined use of psychotropic drugs that interfere with serotonin reuptake and drugs that affect coagulation has been associated with an increased risk of bleeding; use caution when co-administering). Products include:
Clinoril Tablets 1899

Sumatriptan (Co-administration of SSRIs and sumatriptan has resulted in weakness, hyperreflexia, and incoordination). Products include:
Imitrex Nasal Spray 1435

Sumatriptan Succinate (Co-administration of SSRIs and sumatriptan has resulted in weakness, hyperreflexia, and incoordination). Products include:
Imitrex Injection 1431
Imitrex Tablets 1440

Tinzaparin Sodium (The combined use of psychotropic drugs that interfere with serotonin reuptake and drugs that affect coagulation has been associated with an increased risk of bleeding).
No products indexed under this heading.

Tolmetin Sodium (The combined use of psychotropic drugs that interfere with serotonin reuptake and drugs that affect coagulation has been associated with an increased risk of bleeding; use caution when co-administering).
No products indexed under this heading.

Tranylcypromine Sulfate (Co-administration of serotonin reuptake inhibitors and MAO inhibitors has resulted in serious, sometimes fatal, reactions including hyperthermia, rigidity, myoclonus, and other potentially serious adverse reactions; concurrent and/or sequential use is contraindicated). Products include:
Parnate Tablets 1499

Trimipramine Maleate (Co-administration of imipramine with citalopram has resulted in a 50% increase in active metabolite, desipramine concentration; the clinical significance of these findings is unknown; caution is indicated if tricyclic antidepressants are co-administered with citalopram, a relatively weak inhibitor of CYP2D6). Products include:
Surmontil Capsules 2347

Troleandomycin (Co-administration with potent inhibitors of CYP3A4, such as macrolide antibiotics, may decrease the clearance of citalopram).
No products indexed under this heading.

Valdecoxib (The combined use of psychotropic drugs that interfere with serotonin reuptake and drugs that affect coagulation has been associated with an increased risk of bleeding; use caution when co-administering).
No products indexed under this heading.

Warfarin Sodium (The combined use of psychotropic drugs that interfere with serotonin reuptake and drugs that affect coagulation has been associated with an increased risk of bleeding). Products include:
Coumadin for Injection 932
Coumadin Tablets 932

Food Interactions

Alcohol (Although citalopram did not potentiate cognitive and motor effects of alcohol, concurrent use is not recommended).

CELLCEPT CAPSULES

(Mycophenolate Mofetil) 2751
May interact with:

Acyclovir (Potential for these two drugs to compete for tubular secretion further increasing the concentrations of both drugs; AUCs were increased 10.6% for phenolic glucuronide of mycophenolate mofetil and 21.9% for acyclovir). Products include:
Zovirax 1616
Zovirax Cream 853
Zovirax Ointment 854

Acyclovir Sodium (Potential for these two drugs to compete for tubular secretion further increasing the concentrations of both drugs; AUCs were increased 10.6% for phenolic glucuronide of mycophenolate mofetil and 21.9% for acyclovir). Products include:
Zovirax for Injection 1618

Aluminum Hydroxide (Potential for decreased absorption when CellCept is administered with the antacids containing aluminum and magnesium hydroxide; avoid simultaneous administration). Products include:
Gaviscon Regular Strength Liquid 620
Gaviscon Regular Strength Tablets 619
Gaviscon Extra Strength Liquid 620
Gaviscon Extra Strength Tablets 619
Maalox Max Maximum Strength Antacid/Anti-Gas Liquid 2165
Maalox Regular Strength Antacid/Antigas Liquid 2164

Antibiotics, unspecified (Drugs that alter gastrointestinal flora may interact with mycophenolate mofetil by disrupting enterohepatic recirculation).
No products indexed under this heading.

Azathioprine (Concomitant administration is not recommended because such co-administration has not been studied clinically). Products include:
Azasan Tablets 2844

Azathioprine Sodium (Concomitant administration is not recommended because such co-administration has not been studied clinically).
No products indexed under this heading.

Cholestyramine (Decreased AUC of mycophenolate mofetil by approximately 40%; concomitant use with agents that may interfere with enterohepatic circulation should be avoided).
No products indexed under this heading.

Ethinyl Estradiol (Possibility of changes in the pharmacokinetics of the oral contraceptives under long term dosing conditions with CellCept which might adversely affect the efficacy of the oral contraceptive). Products include:
Alesse-28 Tablets 3392
Lo/Ovral-28 Tablets 3423
NuvaRing 2357
Ortho-Cept Tablets 2395
Ortho-Cyclen/Ortho Tri-Cyclen 2414
Ortho Evra Transdermal System 2402
Ortho Tri-Cyclen Lo Tablets 2421

Seasonale Tablets 1073
Triphasil-28 Tablets 3483
Yasmin 28 Tablets 818

Ganciclovir Sodium (Potential for these two drugs to compete for tubular secretion further increasing the concentrations of both drugs). Products include:
Cytovene-IV 2763

Magnesium Hydroxide (Potential for decreased absorption when CellCept is administered with the antacids containing aluminum and magnesium hydroxide; avoid simultaneous administration). Products include:
Maalox Max Maximum Strength Antacid/Anti-Gas Liquid.......... 2165
Maalox Regular Strength Antacid/Antigas Liquid.......... 2164
Pepcid Complete Chewable Tablets.......... 1672
Rolaids Tablets .... ▣707
Extra Strength Rolaids Tablets .... ▣707
Rolaids Multi-Symptom Antacid & Antigas Tablets.......... ▣708

Norethindrone (Possibility of changes in the pharmacokinetics of the oral contraceptives under long term dosing conditions with CellCept which might adversely affect the efficacy of the oral contraceptive). Products include:
Ortho Micronor Tablets 2411

Probenecid (Potential for increased plasma concentration of MPA).
No products indexed under this heading.

Food Interactions

Food, unspecified (Food has no effect on MPA AUC, but has been shown to decrease MPA Cmax by 40%; it is recommended that CellCept be administered on an empty stomach).

CELLCEPT INTRAVENOUS

(Mycophenolate Mofetil Hydrochloride).......... 2751
See CellCept Capsules

CELLCEPT ORAL SUSPENSION

(Mycophenolate Mofetil) 2751
See CellCept Capsules

CELLCEPT TABLETS

(Mycophenolate Mofetil) 2751
See CellCept Capsules

CENESTIN TABLETS, 0.45MG, 0.625MG, 0.9MG, 1.25MG

(Estrogens, Conjugated, Synthetic A).......... 1063
May interact with cytochrome p450 3a4 inducers (selected), cytochrome p450 3a4 inhibitors (selected), and certain other agents. Compounds in these categories include:

Acetazolamide (Co-administration of estrogens with CYP3A4 inhibitors may increase plasma concentrations of estrogens and may result in side effects).
No products indexed under this heading.

Allium sativum (Co-administration of estrogens with CYP3A4 inducers may reduce plasma concentrations of estrogens, possibly resulting in decreased therapeutic effects and/or changes in uterine bleeding profile).
No products indexed under this heading.

Amiodarone Hydrochloride (Co-administration of estrogens with CYP3A4 inhibitors may increase plasma concentrations of estrogens and may result in side effects). Products include:
Pacerone Tablets 3337

Amprenavir (Co-administration of estrogens with CYP3A4 inhibitors may increase plasma concentrations of estrogens and may result in side effects). Products include:
Agenerase Capsules 1299
Agenerase Oral Solution 1304

Anastrozole (Co-administration of estrogens with CYP3A4 inhibitors may increase plasma concentrations of estrogens and may result in side effects). Products include:
Arimidex Tablets 665

Aprepitant (Co-administration of estrogens with CYP3A4 inhibitors may increase plasma concentrations of estrogens and may result in side effects). Products include:
Emend Capsules 1944

Betamethasone Acetate (Co-administration of estrogens with CYP3A4 inducers may reduce plasma concentrations of estrogens, possibly resulting in decreased therapeutic effects and/or changes in uterine bleeding profile).
No products indexed under this heading.

Betamethasone Sodium Phosphate (Co-administration of estrogens with CYP3A4 inducers may reduce plasma concentrations of estrogens, possibly resulting in decreased therapeutic effects and/or changes in uterine bleeding profile).
No products indexed under this heading.

Carbamazepine (Co-administration of estrogens with CYP3A4 inducers may reduce plasma concentrations of estrogens, possibly resulting in decreased therapeutic effects and/or changes in uterine bleeding profile). Products include:
Carbatrol Capsules 3174
Equetro Extended-Release Capsules.......... 3178
Tegretol/Tegretol-XR 2278

Cimetidine (Co-administration of estrogens with CYP3A4 inhibitors may increase plasma concentrations of estrogens and may result in side effects). Products include:
Tagamet HB 200 Tablets .... ▣637
Tagamet Tablets 1547

Cimetidine Hydrochloride (Co-administration of estrogens with CYP3A4 inhibitors may increase plasma concentrations of estrogens and may result in side effects).
No products indexed under this heading.

Ciprofloxacin (Co-administration of estrogens with CYP3A4 inhibitors may increase plasma concentrations of estrogens and may result in side effects). Products include:
Cipro I.V. 2998
Cipro I.V. Pharmacy Bulk Package ... 3509
Cipro Oral Suspension.......... 2991
Cipro XR Tablets 3004
Ciprodex Otic Suspension 555

Ciprofloxacin Hydrochloride (Co-administration of estrogens with CYP3A4 inducers may reduce plasma concentrations of estrogens, possibly resulting in decreased therapeutic effects and/or changes in uterine bleeding profile). Products include:
Ciloxan Ophthalmic Ointment 554
Cipro Tablets 2991

Cisplatin (Co-administration of estrogens with CYP3A4 inducers may reduce plasma concentrations of estrogens, possibly resulting in decreased therapeutic effects and/or changes in uterine bleeding profile).
No products indexed under this heading.

Clarithromycin (Co-administration of estrogens with CYP3A4 inhibitors may increase plasma concentrations of estrogens and may result in side effects). Products include:
Biaxin/Biaxin XL 402
PREVPAC 3281

Clotrimazole (Co-administration of estrogens with CYP3A4 inhibitors may increase plasma concentrations of estrogens and may result in side effects). Products include:
Lotrimin 3053
Lotrisone 3054

Cortisone Acetate (Co-administration of estrogens with CYP3A4 inducers may reduce plasma concentrations of estrogens, possibly resulting in decreased therapeutic effects and/or changes in uterine bleeding profile).
No products indexed under this heading.

Cyclosporine (Co-administration of estrogens with CYP3A4 inhibitors may increase plasma concentrations of estrogens and may result in side effects). Products include:
Gengraf Capsules 458
Neoral Soft Gelatin Capsules 2247
Neoral Oral Solution 2247
Restasis Ophthalmic Emulsion 570
Sandimmune 2259

Dalfopristin (Co-administration of estrogens with CYP3A4 inhibitors may increase plasma concentrations of estrogens and may result in side effects). Products include:
Synercid I.V. 1690

Danazol (Co-administration of estrogens with CYP3A4 inhibitors may increase plasma concentrations of estrogens and may result in side effects).
No products indexed under this heading.

Delavirdine Mesylate (Co-administration of estrogens with CYP3A4 inhibitors may increase plasma concentrations of estrogens and may result in side effects). Products include:
Rescriptor Tablets 2535

Dexamethasone (Co-administration of estrogens with CYP3A4 inducers may reduce plasma concentrations of estrogens, possibly resulting in decreased therapeutic effects and/or changes in uterine bleeding profile). Products include:
Ciprodex Otic Suspension 555
Decadron Tablets 1929
TobraDex Ophthalmic Ointment 558
TobraDex Ophthalmic Suspension ... 558

Dexamethasone Acetate (Co-administration of estrogens with CYP3A4 inducers may reduce plasma concentrations of estrogens, possibly resulting in decreased therapeutic effects and/or changes in uterine bleeding profile).
No products indexed under this heading.

Dexamethasone Sodium Phosphate (Co-administration of estrogens with CYP3A4 inducers may reduce plasma concentrations of estrogens, possibly resulting in decreased therapeutic effects and/or changes in uterine bleeding profile). Products include:
Decadron Phosphate Injection 1931

Diltiazem Hydrochloride (Co-administration of estrogens with CYP3A4 inhibitors may increase plasma concentrations of estrogens and may result in side effects). Products include:
Cardizem LA Extended Release Tablets 1699
Tiazac Capsules 1204

Diltiazem Maleate (Co-administration of estrogens with CYP3A4 inhibitors may increase plasma concentrations of estrogens and may result in side effects).
No products indexed under this heading.

Doxorubicin Hydrochloride (Co-administration of estrogens with CYP3A4 inducers may reduce plasma concentrations of estrogens, possibly resulting in decreased therapeutic effects and/or changes in uterine bleeding profile). Products include:
Adriamycin for Injection, USP 786
Adriamycin Injection, USP 786

Efavirenz (Co-administration of estrogens with CYP3A4 inhibitors may increase plasma concentrations of estrogens and may result in side effects). Products include:
Sustiva Capsules 957

Erythromycin (Co-administration of estrogens with CYP3A4 inhibitors may increase plasma concentrations of estrogens and may result in side effects). Products include:
Erygel Topical Gel 2096
Ery-Tab Tablets 447
Erythromycin Base Filmtab Tablets 454
Erythromycin Delayed-Release Capsules, USP.......... 456
PCE Dispertab Tablets 510

Erythromycin Estolate (Co-administration of estrogens with CYP3A4 inhibitors may increase plasma concentrations of estrogens and may result in side effects).
No products indexed under this heading.

Erythromycin Ethylsuccinate (Co-administration of estrogens with CYP3A4 inhibitors may increase plasma concentrations of estrogens and may result in side effects). Products include:
E.E.S. 449
EryPed 445

Erythromycin Gluceptate (Co-administration of estrogens with CYP3A4 inhibitors may increase plasma concentrations of estrogens and may result in side effects).
No products indexed under this heading.

Erythromycin Lactobionate (Co-administration of estrogens with CYP3A4 inhibitors may increase plasma concentrations of estrogens and may result in side effects).
No products indexed under this heading.

Erythromycin Stearate (Co-administration of estrogens with CYP3A4 inhibitors may increase plasma concentrations of estrogens and may result in side effects). Products include:
Erythrocin Stearate Filmtab Tablets 452

Esomeprazole Magnesium (Co-administration of estrogens with CYP3A4 inhibitors may increase plasma concentrations of estrogens and may result in side effects). Products include:
- Nexium Delayed-Release Capsules ... 645

Ethosuximide (Co-administration of estrogens with CYP3A4 inducers may reduce plasma concentrations of estrogens, possibly resulting in decreased therapeutic effects and/or changes in uterine bleeding profile).
No products indexed under this heading.

Felbamate (Co-administration of estrogens with CYP3A4 inducers may reduce plasma concentrations of estrogens, possibly resulting in decreased therapeutic effects and/or changes in uterine bleeding profile).
No products indexed under this heading.

Fluconazole (Co-administration of estrogens with CYP3A4 inhibitors may increase plasma concentrations of estrogens and may result in side effects).
No products indexed under this heading.

Fludrocortisone Acetate (Co-administration of estrogens with CYP3A4 inducers may reduce plasma concentrations of estrogens, possibly resulting in decreased therapeutic effects and/or changes in uterine bleeding profile).
No products indexed under this heading.

Fluoxetine Hydrochloride (Co-administration of estrogens with CYP3A4 inhibitors may increase plasma concentrations of estrogens and may result in side effects). Products include:
- Prozac Pulvules and Liquid ... 1771
- Symbyax Capsules ... 1788

Fluvoxamine Maleate (Co-administration of estrogens with CYP3A4 inhibitors may increase plasma concentrations of estrogens and may result in side effects).
No products indexed under this heading.

Fosamprenavir Calcium (Co-administration of estrogens with CYP3A4 inhibitors may increase plasma concentrations of estrogens and may result in side effects). Products include:
- Lexiva Tablets ... 1473

Fosphenytoin Sodium (Co-administration of estrogens with CYP3A4 inducers may reduce plasma concentrations of estrogens, possibly resulting in decreased therapeutic effects and/or changes in uterine bleeding profile).
No products indexed under this heading.

Garlic Extract (Co-administration of estrogens with CYP3A4 inducers may reduce plasma concentrations of estrogens, possibly resulting in decreased therapeutic effects and/or changes in uterine bleeding profile).
No products indexed under this heading.

Garlic Oil (Co-administration of estrogens with CYP3A4 inducers may reduce plasma concentrations of estrogens, possibly resulting in decreased therapeutic effects and/or changes in uterine bleeding profile).
No products indexed under this heading.

Hydrocortisone (Co-administration of estrogens with CYP3A4 inducers may reduce plasma concentrations of estrogens, possibly resulting in decreased therapeutic effects and/or changes in uterine bleeding profile). Products include:
- Cortizone•5 Ointment ... 699
- Cortizone•10 Creme ... 699
- Cortizone•10 Ointment ... 699
- Cortizone•10 Plus Creme ... 700
- Cortizone•10 Maximum Strength Quick Shot Spray ... 700
- Hydrocortone Tablets ... 1963
- Preparation H Hydrocortisone Cream ... 748

Hydrocortisone Acetate (Co-administration of estrogens with CYP3A4 inducers may reduce plasma concentrations of estrogens, possibly resulting in decreased therapeutic effects and/or changes in uterine bleeding profile). Products include:
- Analpram-HC ... 1136
- Pramosone ... 1139
- ProctoFoam-HC ... 3113
- Tucks Anti-Itch Ointment ... 712
- U-cort 1% Cream ... 3289

Hydrocortisone Butyrate (Co-administration of estrogens with CYP3A4 inducers may reduce plasma concentrations of estrogens, possibly resulting in decreased therapeutic effects and/or changes in uterine bleeding profile). Products include:
- Locoid ... 1138
- Locoid Lipocream Cream ... 1138

Hydrocortisone Cypionate (Co-administration of estrogens with CYP3A4 inducers may reduce plasma concentrations of estrogens, possibly resulting in decreased therapeutic effects and/or changes in uterine bleeding profile).
No products indexed under this heading.

Hydrocortisone Hemisuccinate (Co-administration of estrogens with CYP3A4 inducers may reduce plasma concentrations of estrogens, possibly resulting in decreased therapeutic effects and/or changes in uterine bleeding profile).
No products indexed under this heading.

Hydrocortisone Probutate (Co-administration of estrogens with CYP3A4 inducers may reduce plasma concentrations of estrogens, possibly resulting in decreased therapeutic effects and/or changes in uterine bleeding profile). Products include:
- Pandel Cream, 0.1% ... 1017

Hydrocortisone Sodium Phosphate (Co-administration of estrogens with CYP3A4 inducers may reduce plasma concentrations of estrogens, possibly resulting in decreased therapeutic effects and/or changes in uterine bleeding profile).
No products indexed under this heading.

Hydrocortisone Sodium Succinate (Co-administration of estrogens with CYP3A4 inducers may reduce plasma concentrations of estrogens, possibly resulting in decreased therapeutic effects and/or changes in uterine bleeding profile).
No products indexed under this heading.

Hydrocortisone Valerate (Co-administration of estrogens with CYP3A4 inducers may reduce plasma concentrations of estrogens, possibly resulting in decreased therapeutic effects and/or changes in uterine bleeding profile).
No products indexed under this heading.

Hypericum (Co-administration of estrogens with CYP3A4 inducers may reduce plasma concentrations of estrogens, possibly resulting in decreased therapeutic effects and/or changes in uterine bleeding profile).
No products indexed under this heading.

Hypericum Perforatum (Co-administration of estrogens with CYP3A4 inducers may reduce plasma concentrations of estrogens, possibly resulting in decreased therapeutic effects and/or changes in uterine bleeding profile).
No products indexed under this heading.

Indinavir Sulfate (Co-administration of estrogens with CYP3A4 inhibitors may increase plasma concentrations of estrogens and may result in side effects). Products include:
- Crixivan Capsules ... 1918

Isoniazid (Co-administration of estrogens with CYP3A4 inhibitors may increase plasma concentrations of estrogens and may result in side effects).
No products indexed under this heading.

Itraconazole (Co-administration of estrogens with CYP3A4 inhibitors may increase plasma concentrations of estrogens and may result in side effects).
No products indexed under this heading.

Ketoconazole (Co-administration of estrogens with CYP3A4 inhibitors may increase plasma concentrations of estrogens and may result in side effects). Products include:
- Nizoral A-D Shampoo, 1% ... 1839
- Nizoral 2% Shampoo ... 1838

Lopinavir (Co-administration of estrogens with CYP3A4 inhibitors may increase plasma concentrations of estrogens and may result in side effects). Products include:
- Kaletra ... 474

Loratadine (Co-administration of estrogens with CYP3A4 inhibitors may increase plasma concentrations of estrogens and may result in side effects). Products include:
- Alavert Allergy & Sinus D-12 Hour Tablets ... 743
- Alavert ... 743
- Children's Claritin 24 Hour Non-Drowsy Allergy Syrup ... 732
- Claritin Non-Drowsy 24 Hour Tablets ... 731
- Non-Drowsy Claritin Hives Relief Tablets ... 733
- Claritin Reditabs 24 Hour Non-Drowsy Tablets ... 732
- Claritin-D Non-Drowsy 12 Hour Tablets ... 731
- Claritin-D Non-Drowsy 24 Hour Tablets ... 731
- Children's Dimetapp ND Non-Drowsy Allergy Syrup ... 746
- Triaminic Allerchews ... 684

Mephenytoin (Co-administration of estrogens with CYP3A4 inducers may reduce plasma concentrations of estrogens, possibly resulting in decreased therapeutic effects and/or changes in uterine bleeding profile).
No products indexed under this heading.

Methsuximide (Co-administration of estrogens with CYP3A4 inducers may reduce plasma concentrations of estrogens, possibly resulting in decreased therapeutic effects and/or changes in uterine bleeding profile).
No products indexed under this heading.

Methylprednisolone (Co-administration of estrogens with CYP3A4 inducers may reduce plasma concentrations of estrogens, possibly resulting in decreased therapeutic effects and/or changes in uterine bleeding profile).
No products indexed under this heading.

Methylprednisolone Acetate (Co-administration of estrogens with CYP3A4 inducers may reduce plasma concentrations of estrogens, possibly resulting in decreased therapeutic effects and/or changes in uterine bleeding profile). Products include:
- Depo-Medrol Injectable Suspension ... 2615
- Depo-Medrol Single-Dose Vial ... 2617

Methylprednisolone Sodium Succinate (Co-administration of estrogens with CYP3A4 inducers may reduce plasma concentrations of estrogens, possibly resulting in decreased therapeutic effects and/or changes in uterine bleeding profile).
No products indexed under this heading.

Metronidazole (Co-administration of estrogens with CYP3A4 inhibitors may increase plasma concentrations of estrogens and may result in side effects). Products include:
- Metrogel 1% ... 1212
- MetroGel-Vaginal Gel ... 1822
- Noritate Cream, 1% ... 1051

Metronidazole Benzoate (Co-administration of estrogens with CYP3A4 inhibitors may increase plasma concentrations of estrogens and may result in side effects).
No products indexed under this heading.

Metronidazole Hydrochloride (Co-administration of estrogens with CYP3A4 inhibitors may increase plasma concentrations of estrogens and may result in side effects).
No products indexed under this heading.

Miconazole (Co-administration of estrogens with CYP3A4 inhibitors may increase plasma concentrations of estrogens and may result in side effects).
No products indexed under this heading.

Miconazole Nitrate (Co-administration of estrogens with CYP3A4 inhibitors may increase plasma concentrations of estrogens and may result in side effects). Products include:

Desenex .... ▣674
Desenex Jock Itch Spray Powder ... ▣674

Modafinil (Co-administration of estrogens with CYP3A4 inducers may reduce plasma concentrations of estrogens, possibly resulting in decreased therapeutic effects and/ or changes in uterine bleeding profile). Products include:
Provigil Tablets 1002

Nefazodone Hydrochloride (Co-administration of estrogens with CYP3A4 inhibitors may increase plasma concentrations of estrogens and may result in side effects).
No products indexed under this heading.

Nelfinavir Mesylate (Co-administration of estrogens with CYP3A4 inhibitors may increase plasma concentrations of estrogens and may result in side effects). Products include:
Viracept 2556

Nevirapine (Co-administration of estrogens with CYP3A4 inhibitors may increase plasma concentrations of estrogens and may result in side effects). Products include:
Viramune Oral Suspension 903
Viramune Tablets 903

Niacinamide (Co-administration of estrogens with CYP3A4 inhibitors may increase plasma concentrations of estrogens and may result in side effects).
No products indexed under this heading.

Nicotinamide (Co-administration of estrogens with CYP3A4 inhibitors may increase plasma concentrations of estrogens and may result in side effects). Products include:
Nicomide Tablets 3190

Nifedipine (Co-administration of estrogens with CYP3A4 inhibitors may increase plasma concentrations of estrogens and may result in side effects). Products include:
Adalat CC Tablets 2978

Norfloxacin (Co-administration of estrogens with CYP3A4 inhibitors may increase plasma concentrations of estrogens and may result in side effects). Products include:
Noroxin Tablets 2009

Omeprazole (Co-administration of estrogens with CYP3A4 inhibitors may increase plasma concentrations of estrogens and may result in side effects). Products include:
Zegerid Powder for Oral Solution 2972

Oxcarbazepine (Co-administration of estrogens with CYP3A4 inducers may reduce plasma concentrations of estrogens, possibly resulting in decreased therapeutic effects and/ or changes in uterine bleeding profile). Products include:
Trileptal Oral Suspension 2281
Trileptal Tablets 2281

Paroxetine Hydrochloride (Co-administration of estrogens with CYP3A4 inhibitors may increase plasma concentrations of estrogens and may result in side effects). Products include:
Paxil CR Controlled-Release Tablets 1509
Paxil 1501

Phenobarbital (Co-administration of estrogens with CYP3A4 inducers may reduce plasma concentrations of estrogens, possibly resulting in decreased therapeutic effects and/ or changes in uterine bleeding profile).
No products indexed under this heading.

Phenobarbital Sodium (Co-administration of estrogens with CYP3A4 inducers may reduce plasma concentrations of estrogens, possibly resulting in decreased therapeutic effects and/or changes in uterine bleeding profile).
No products indexed under this heading.

Phenytoin (Co-administration of estrogens with CYP3A4 inducers may reduce plasma concentrations of estrogens, possibly resulting in decreased therapeutic effects and/ or changes in uterine bleeding profile).
No products indexed under this heading.

Phenytoin Sodium (Co-administration of estrogens with CYP3A4 inducers may reduce plasma concentrations of estrogens, possibly resulting in decreased therapeutic effects and/or changes in uterine bleeding profile). Products include:
Phenytek Capsules 2153

Prednisolone Acetate (Co-administration of estrogens with CYP3A4 inducers may reduce plasma concentrations of estrogens, possibly resulting in decreased therapeutic effects and/or changes in uterine bleeding profile). Products include:
Blephamide Ophthalmic Ointment 563
Blephamide Ophthalmic Suspension 564
Poly-Pred Liquifilm Ophthalmic Suspension .... ⊙231
Pred Forte Ophthalmic Suspension .... ⊙233
Pred Mild Sterile Ophthalmic Suspension .... ⊙236
Pred-G Ophthalmic Suspension ...... ⊙234
Pred-G Sterile Ophthalmic Ointment .... ⊙235

Prednisolone Sodium Phosphate (Co-administration of estrogens with CYP3A4 inducers may reduce plasma concentrations of estrogens, possibly resulting in decreased therapeutic effects and/or changes in uterine bleeding profile). Products include:
Pediapred Oral Solution 3319

Prednisolone Tebutate (Co-administration of estrogens with CYP3A4 inducers may reduce plasma concentrations of estrogens, possibly resulting in decreased therapeutic effects and/or changes in uterine bleeding profile).
No products indexed under this heading.

Prednisone (Co-administration of estrogens with CYP3A4 inducers may reduce plasma concentrations of estrogens, possibly resulting in decreased therapeutic effects and/ or changes in uterine bleeding profile).
No products indexed under this heading.

Primidone (Co-administration of estrogens with CYP3A4 inducers may reduce plasma concentrations of estrogens, possibly resulting in decreased therapeutic effects and/ or changes in uterine bleeding profile).
No products indexed under this heading.

Propoxyphene Hydrochloride (Co-administration of estrogens with CYP3A4 inhibitors may increase plasma concentrations of estrogens and may result in side effects).
No products indexed under this heading.

Propoxyphene Napsylate (Co-administration of estrogens with CYP3A4 inhibitors may increase plasma concentrations of estrogens and may result in side effects). Products include:
Darvocet A 500 Tablets 3497

Quinidine (Co-administration of estrogens with CYP3A4 inhibitors may increase plasma concentrations of estrogens and may result in side effects).
No products indexed under this heading.

Quinidine Hydrochloride (Co-administration of estrogens with CYP3A4 inhibitors may increase plasma concentrations of estrogens and may result in side effects).
No products indexed under this heading.

Quinidine Polygalacturonate (Co-administration of estrogens with CYP3A4 inhibitors may increase plasma concentrations of estrogens and may result in side effects).
No products indexed under this heading.

Quinidine Sulfate (Co-administration of estrogens with CYP3A4 inhibitors may increase plasma concentrations of estrogens and may result in side effects).
No products indexed under this heading.

Quinine (Co-administration of estrogens with CYP3A4 inhibitors may increase plasma concentrations of estrogens and may result in side effects).
No products indexed under this heading.

Quinine Sulfate (Co-administration of estrogens with CYP3A4 inhibitors may increase plasma concentrations of estrogens and may result in side effects).
No products indexed under this heading.

Quinupristin (Co-administration of estrogens with CYP3A4 inhibitors may increase plasma concentrations of estrogens and may result in side effects). Products include:
Synercid I.V. 1690

Ranitidine Bismuth Citrate (Co-administration of estrogens with CYP3A4 inhibitors may increase plasma concentrations of estrogens and may result in side effects).
No products indexed under this heading.

Ranitidine Hydrochloride (Co-administration of estrogens with CYP3A4 inhibitors may increase plasma concentrations of estrogens and may result in side effects). Products include:
Zantac 1597
Zantac Injection 1593
Zantac 75 Tablets .... ▣715
Zantac 150 Maximum Strength Tablets .... ▣715
Zantac Injection Pharmacy Bulk Package 1595

Rifabutin (Co-administration of estrogens with CYP3A4 inducers may reduce plasma concentrations of estrogens, possibly resulting in decreased therapeutic effects and/ or changes in uterine bleeding profile).
No products indexed under this heading.

Rifampicin (Co-administration of estrogens with CYP3A4 inducers may reduce plasma concentrations of estrogens, possibly resulting in decreased therapeutic effects and/ or changes in uterine bleeding profile).
No products indexed under this heading.

Rifampin (Co-administration of estrogens with CYP3A4 inducers may reduce plasma concentrations of estrogens, possibly resulting in decreased therapeutic effects and/ or changes in uterine bleeding profile).
No products indexed under this heading.

Rifapentine (Co-administration of estrogens with CYP3A4 inducers may reduce plasma concentrations of estrogens, possibly resulting in decreased therapeutic effects and/ or changes in uterine bleeding profile).
No products indexed under this heading.

Ritonavir (Co-administration of estrogens with CYP3A4 inhibitors may increase plasma concentrations of estrogens and may result in side effects). Products include:
Kaletra 474
Norvir 499

Saquinavir (Co-administration of estrogens with CYP3A4 inhibitors may increase plasma concentrations of estrogens and may result in side effects).
No products indexed under this heading.

Saquinavir Mesylate (Co-administration of estrogens with CYP3A4 inhibitors may increase plasma concentrations of estrogens and may result in side effects). Products include:
Invirase 2776

Sertraline Hydrochloride (Co-administration of estrogens with CYP3A4 inhibitors may increase plasma concentrations of estrogens and may result in side effects). Products include:
Zoloft 2581

Sulfinpyrazone (Co-administration of estrogens with CYP3A4 inducers may reduce plasma concentrations of estrogens, possibly resulting in decreased therapeutic effects and/ or changes in uterine bleeding profile).
No products indexed under this heading.

Telithromycin (Co-administration of estrogens with CYP3A4 inhibitors may increase plasma concentrations of estrogens and may result in side effects). Products include:
Ketek Tablets 2920

Theophylline (Co-administration of estrogens with CYP3A4 inducers may reduce plasma concentrations of estrogens, possibly resulting in decreased therapeutic effects and/or changes in uterine bleeding profile).
No products indexed under this heading.

Triamcinolone (Co-administration of estrogens with CYP3A4 inducers may reduce plasma concentrations of estrogens, possibly resulting in decreased therapeutic effects and/or changes in uterine bleeding profile).
No products indexed under this heading.

Triamcinolone Acetonide (Co-administration of estrogens with CYP3A4 inducers may reduce plasma concentrations of estrogens, possibly resulting in decreased therapeutic effects and/or changes in uterine bleeding profile). Products include:
Azmacort Inhalation Aerosol 1701
Nasacort HFA Inhalation Aerosol 2939
Nasacort AQ Nasal Spray 2937

Triamcinolone Diacetate (Co-administration of estrogens with CYP3A4 inducers may reduce plasma concentrations of estrogens, possibly resulting in decreased therapeutic effects and/or changes in uterine bleeding profile).
No products indexed under this heading.

Triamcinolone Hexacetonide (Co-administration of estrogens with CYP3A4 inducers may reduce plasma concentrations of estrogens, possibly resulting in decreased therapeutic effects and/or changes in uterine bleeding profile).
No products indexed under this heading.

Troglitazone (Co-administration of estrogens with CYP3A4 inducers may reduce plasma concentrations of estrogens, possibly resulting in decreased therapeutic effects and/or changes in uterine bleeding profile).
No products indexed under this heading.

Troleandomycin (Co-administration of estrogens with CYP3A4 inhibitors may increase plasma concentrations of estrogens and may result in side effects).
No products indexed under this heading.

Valproate Sodium (Co-administration of estrogens with CYP3A4 inhibitors may increase plasma concentrations of estrogens and may result in side effects). Products include:
Depacon Injection 412

Verapamil Hydrochloride (Co-administration of estrogens with CYP3A4 inhibitors may increase plasma concentrations of estrogens and may result in side effects). Products include:
Covera-HS Tablets 3135
Tarka Tablets 519
Verelan PM Capsules 3120

Voriconazole (Co-administration of estrogens with CYP3A4 inhibitors may increase plasma concentrations of estrogens and may result in side effects). Products include:
VFEND I.V. 2543
VFEND Oral Suspension 2543
VFEND Tablets 2543

Zafirlukast (Co-administration of estrogens with CYP3A4 inhibitors may increase plasma concentrations of estrogens and may result in side effects). Products include:
Accolate Tablets 663

Zileuton (Co-administration of estrogens with CYP3A4 inhibitors may increase plasma concentrations of estrogens and may result in side effects).
No products indexed under this heading.

Food Interactions

Grapefruit (Co-administration of estrogens with CYP3A4 inhibitors may increase plasma concentrations of estrogens and may result in side effects).

Grapefruit Juice (Co-administration of estrogens with CYP3A4 inhibitors, such as grapefruit juice, may increase plasma concentrations of estrogens and may result in side effects).

CENESTIN TABLETS, 0.3MG

(Estrogens, Conjugated, Synthetic A) 1063
See Cenestin Tablets, 0.45mg, 0.625mg, 0.9mg, 1.25mg

CENTANY OINTMENT, 2%

(Mupirocin) 2382
None cited in PDR database.

CENTRUM TABLETS

(Vitamins with Minerals) .... ▣780
May interact with:

Vitamin A (Concurrent use with other Vitamin A supplements is not recommended). Products include:
Visutein Capsules 3328

CENTRUM KIDS RUGRATS COMPLETE CHILDREN'S CHEWABLES

(Vitamins with Minerals) .... ▣780
None cited in PDR database.

CENTRUM PERFORMANCE COMPLETE MULTIVITAMIN TABLETS

(Vitamins with Minerals) .... ▣781
May interact with:

Prescription Drugs, unspecified (Contact physician before using product).
No products indexed under this heading.

Vitamin A (Concurrent use with other Vitamin A supplements is not recommended). Products include:
Visutein Capsules 3328

CENTRUM SILVER TABLETS

(Vitamins with Minerals) .... ▣781
May interact with:

Vitamin A (Concurrent use with other Vitamin A supplements is not recommended). Products include:
Visutein Capsules 3328

CEO-TWO EVACUANT SUPPOSITORY

(Potassium Bitartrate, Sodium Bicarbonate) .... ▣607
None cited in PDR database.

CEREZYME FOR INJECTION

(Imiglucerase) 1263
None cited in PDR database.

CERUBIDINE FOR INJECTION

(Daunorubicin Hydrochloride) 788
May interact with:

Bone Marrow Depressants, unspecified (Therapy with Cerubidine should not be started in patients with pre-existing drug-induced myelosuppression).
No products indexed under this heading.

Cyclophosphamide (Co-administration increases the risk of cardiotoxicity).
No products indexed under this heading.

Doxorubicin Hydrochloride (Use of daunorubicin in a patient who has previously received doxorubicin increases the risk of cardiotoxicity; daunorubicin should not be used in patients who have previously received the recommended maximum cumulative doses of doxorubicin or daunorubicin). Products include:
Adriamycin for Injection, USP 786
Adriamycin Injection, USP 786

Methotrexate Sodium (Co-administration with hepatotoxic drugs, such as methotrexate, may impair liver function and increase the risk of toxicity).
No products indexed under this heading.

CERVIDIL VAGINAL INSERT

(Dinoprostone) 1182
May interact with oxytocic drugs. Compounds in these categories include:

Ergonovine Maleate (Dinoprostone may augment the activity of oxytocic agents and concomitant use is not recommended; a dosing interval of at least 30 minutes is recommended for sequential use).
No products indexed under this heading.

Methylergonovine Maleate (Dinoprostone may augment the activity of oxytocic agents and concomitant use is not recommended; a dosing interval of at least 30 minutes is recommended for sequential use).
No products indexed under this heading.

Oxytocin (Dinoprostone may augment the activity of oxytocic agents and concomitant use is not recommended; a dosing interval of at least 30 minutes is recommended for sequential use).
No products indexed under this heading.

CETACAINE TOPICAL ANESTHETIC

(Benzocaine, Butyl Aminobenzoate, Tetracaine Hydrochloride) 1007
None cited in PDR database.

CHELATED MINERAL TABLETS

(Minerals, Multiple) 3342
None cited in PDR database.

CHEMET CAPSULES

(Succimer) 2480
May interact with:

Calcium Disodium Edetate (Concomitant administration is not recommended). Products include:
Calcium Disodium Versenate Injection 1819

CHILDREN'S BENADRYL ALLERGY FASTMELT TABLETS

(Diphenhydramine Citrate) .... ▣696
May interact with hypnotics and sedatives, tranquilizers, and certain other agents. Compounds in these categories include:

Alprazolam (Tranquilizers may increase drowsiness). Products include:
Niravam Orally Disintegrating Tablets 3106
Xanax XR Tablets 2655

Buspirone Hydrochloride (Tranquilizers may increase drowsiness).
No products indexed under this heading.

Chlordiazepoxide (Tranquilizers may increase drowsiness).
No products indexed under this heading.

Chlordiazepoxide Hydrochloride (Tranquilizers may increase drowsiness). Products include:
Librium Capsules 3349

Chlorpromazine (Tranquilizers may increase drowsiness).
No products indexed under this heading.

Chlorpromazine Hydrochloride (Tranquilizers may increase drowsiness).
No products indexed under this heading.

Chlorprothixene (Tranquilizers may increase drowsiness).
No products indexed under this heading.

Chlorprothixene Hydrochloride (Tranquilizers may increase drowsiness).
No products indexed under this heading.

Clorazepate Dipotassium (Tranquilizers may increase drowsiness). Products include:
Tranxene 2488

Diazepam (Tranquilizers may increase drowsiness). Products include:
Diastat Rectal Delivery System 3344
Valium Tablets 2822

Droperidol (Tranquilizers may increase drowsiness).
No products indexed under this heading.

Estazolam (Sedatives may increase drowsiness). Products include:
ProSom Tablets 512

Ethchlorvynol (Sedatives may increase drowsiness).
No products indexed under this heading.

Ethinamate (Sedatives may increase drowsiness).
No products indexed under this heading.

Fluphenazine Decanoate (Tranquilizers may increase drowsiness).
No products indexed under this heading.

Fluphenazine Enanthate (Tranquilizers may increase drowsiness).
No products indexed under this heading.

Fluphenazine Hydrochloride (Tranquilizers may increase drowsiness).
No products indexed under this heading.

Flurazepam Hydrochloride (Sedatives may increase drowsiness). Products include:
Dalmane Capsules 3343

Glutethimide (Sedatives may increase drowsiness).
No products indexed under this heading.

Haloperidol (Tranquilizers may increase drowsiness).
No products indexed under this heading.

Haloperidol Decanoate (Tranquilizers may increase drowsiness).
No products indexed under this heading.

Hydroxyzine Hydrochloride (Tranquilizers may increase drowsiness).
No products indexed under this heading.

Lorazepam (Sedatives may increase drowsiness).
No products indexed under this heading.

Loxapine Hydrochloride (Tranquilizers may increase drowsiness).
No products indexed under this heading.

Loxapine Succinate (Tranquilizers may increase drowsiness).
No products indexed under this heading.

Meprobamate (Tranquilizers may increase drowsiness).
No products indexed under this heading.

Mesoridazine Besylate (Tranquilizers may increase drowsiness).
No products indexed under this heading.

Midazolam Hydrochloride (Sedatives may increase drowsiness).
No products indexed under this heading.

Molindone Hydrochloride (Tranquilizers may increase drowsiness). Products include:
Moban Tablets 1108

Oxazepam (Tranquilizers may increase drowsiness).
No products indexed under this heading.

Perphenazine (Tranquilizers may increase drowsiness).
No products indexed under this heading.

Prazepam (Tranquilizers may increase drowsiness).
No products indexed under this heading.

Prochlorperazine (Tranquilizers may increase drowsiness).
No products indexed under this heading.

Promethazine Hydrochloride (Tranquilizers may increase drowsiness). Products include:
Phenergan 3438

Propofol (Sedatives may increase drowsiness). Products include:
Diprivan Injectable Emulsion 676

Quazepam (Sedatives may increase drowsiness).
No products indexed under this heading.

Secobarbital Sodium (Sedatives may increase drowsiness).
No products indexed under this heading.

Temazepam (Sedatives may increase drowsiness).
No products indexed under this heading.

Thioridazine Hydrochloride (Tranquilizers may increase drowsiness). Products include:
Thioridazine Hydrochloride Tablets 2122

Thiothixene (Tranquilizers may increase drowsiness). Products include:
Thiothixene Capsules 2124

Triazolam (Sedatives may increase drowsiness).
No products indexed under this heading.

Trifluoperazine Hydrochloride (Tranquilizers may increase drowsiness).
No products indexed under this heading.

Zaleplon (Sedatives may increase drowsiness). Products include:
Sonata Capsules 1686

Zolpidem Tartrate (Sedatives may increase drowsiness). Products include:
Ambien Tablets 2867

Food Interactions

Alcohol (Alcohol may increase drowsiness. Avoid alcoholic drinks).

CHROMAGEN FORTE SOFT GELATIN CAPSULES

(Ferrous Fumarate, Folic Acid, Iron, Vitamin B_{12}, Vitamin C) 3296
None cited in PDR database.

CIALIS TABLETS

(Tadalafil) 1806
May interact with alpha adrenergic blockers, angiotensin-II receptor antagonists, antacids, cytochrome p450 3a4 inducers (selected), cytochrome p450 3a4 inhibitors (selected), erythromycin, nitrates and nitrites, phenytoin, protease inhibitors, and certain other agents. Compounds in these categories include:

Acetazolamide (Tadalafil is metabolized predominantly by CYP3A4 in the liver. The dose of tadalafil should be limited to 10 mg no more than once every 72 hours in patients taking potent inhibitors of CYP3A4).
No products indexed under this heading.

Allium sativum (Drugs that induce CYP3A4 can increase tadalafil exposure).
No products indexed under this heading.

Aluminum Carbonate (Simultaneous administration of an antacid (magnesium hydroxide/aluminum hydroxide) and tadalafil reduced the apparent rate of absorption of tadalafil without altering exposure (AUC) to tadalafil).
No products indexed under this heading.

Aluminum Hydroxide (Simultaneous administration of an antacid (magnesium hydroxide/aluminum hydroxide) and tadalafil reduced the apparent rate of absorption of tadalafil without altering exposure (AUC) to tadalafil). Products include:
Gaviscon Regular Strength Liquid .. ▣ 620
Gaviscon Regular Strength Tablets....................................... ▣ 619
Gaviscon Extra Strength Liquid ...... ▣ 620
Gaviscon Extra Strength Tablets .... ▣ 619
Maalox Max Maximum Strength Antacid/Anti-Gas Liquid.................. 2165
Maalox Regular Strength Antacid/Antigas Liquid.................. 2164

Amiodarone Hydrochloride (Tadalafil is metabolized predominantly by CYP3A4 in the liver. The dose of tadalafil should be limited to 10 mg no more than once every 72 hours in patients taking potent inhibitors of CYP3A4). Products include:
Pacerone Tablets 3337

Amlodipine Besylate (A study was conducted to assess the interaction of amlodipine (5mg daily) and tadalafil 10mg. There were no effects of tadalafil on amlodipine blood levels and no effect of amlodipine on tadalafil blood levels. The mean reduction in supine systolic/diastolic blood pressure due to tadalafil 10mg in subjects taking amlodipine was 3/2mm Hg, compare to placebo). Products include:
Caduet Tablets 2507
Lotrel Capsules 2238
Norvasc Tablets 2529

Amprenavir (Tadalafil is metabolized predominantly by CYP3A4 in the liver. The dose of tadalafil should be limited to 10 mg no more than once every 72 hours in patients taking potent inhibitors of CYP3A4). Products include:
Agenerase Capsules 1299
Agenerase Oral Solution 1304

Amyl Nitrite (Administration of tadalafil to patients using any form of organic nitrate, either regularly and/or intermittently, is contraindicated).
No products indexed under this heading.

Anastrozole (Tadalafil is metabolized predominantly by CYP3A4 in the liver. The dose of tadalafil should be limited to 10 mg no more than once every 72 hours in patients taking potent inhibitors of CYP3A4). Products include:
Arimidex Tablets 665

Aprepitant (Tadalafil is metabolized predominantly by CYP3A4 in the liver. The dose of tadalafil should be limited to 10 mg no more than once every 72 hours in patients taking potent inhibitors of CYP3A4). Products include:
Emend Capsules 1944

Bendrofluazide (A study was conducted to assess the interaction of bendrofluazide (2.5mg daily) and tadalafil 10mg. Following dosing, the mean reduction in supine systolic diastolic blood pressure due to tadalafil 10mg in subjects taking bendrofluazide was 6/4mm Hg, compared to placebo).
No products indexed under this heading.

Betamethasone Acetate (Drugs that induce CYP3A4 can increase tadalafil exposure).
No products indexed under this heading.

Betamethasone Sodium Phosphate (Drugs that induce CYP3A4 can increase tadalafil exposure).
No products indexed under this heading.

Candesartan Cilexetil (A study was conducted to assess the interaction of angiotensin II receptor blockers and tadalafil 20mg. Following dosing, ambulatory measurements of blood pressure revealed differences between tadalafil and placebo of 8/4mm Hg in systolic/diastolic blood pressure). Products include:
Atacand Tablets 634
Atacand HCT 637

Carbamazepine (CYP3A4 inducers, such as carbamazepine, may decrease tadalafil exposure. No dose adjustment is warranted). Products include:
Carbatrol Capsules 3174
Equetro Extended-Release Capsules.. 3178
Tegretol/Tegretol-XR 2278

Cimetidine (Tadalafil is metabolized predominantly by CYP3A4 in the liver. The dose of tadalafil should be limited to 10 mg no more than once every 72 hours in patients taking potent inhibitors of CYP3A4). Products include:
Tagamet HB 200 Tablets .... ▣ 637
Tagamet Tablets 1547

Cimetidine Hydrochloride (Tadalafil is metabolized predominantly by CYP3A4 in the liver. The dose of tadalafil should be limited to 10 mg no more than once every 72 hours in patients taking potent inhibitors of CYP3A4).
No products indexed under this heading.

Ciprofloxacin (Tadalafil is metabolized predominantly by CYP3A4 in the liver. The dose of tadalafil should be limited to 10 mg no more than once every 72 hours in patients taking potent inhibitors of CYP3A4). Products include:
Cipro I.V. 2998
Cipro I.V. Pharmacy Bulk Package ... 3509
Cipro Oral Suspension 2991
Cipro XR Tablets 3004
Ciprodex Otic Suspension 555

Ciprofloxacin Hydrochloride (Drugs that induce CYP3A4 can increase tadalafil exposure). Products include:
Ciloxan Ophthalmic Ointment 554
Cipro Tablets 2991

Cisplatin (Drugs that induce CYP3A4 can increase tadalafil exposure).
No products indexed under this heading.

Clarithromycin (Tadalafil is metabolized predominantly by CYP3A4 in the liver. The dose of tadalafil should be limited to 10 mg no more than once every 72 hours in patients taking potent inhibitors of CYP3A4). Products include:
Biaxin/Biaxin XL 402
PREVPAC 3281

Clotrimazole (Tadalafil is metabolized predominantly by CYP3A4 in the liver. The dose of tadalafil should be limited to 10 mg no more than once every 72 hours in patients taking potent inhibitors of CYP3A4). Products include:
Lotrimin 3053
Lotrisone 3054

Cortisone Acetate (Drugs that induce CYP3A4 can increase tadalafil exposure).
No products indexed under this heading.

Cyclosporine (Tadalafil is metabolized predominantly by CYP3A4 in the liver. The dose of tadalafil should be limited to 10 mg no more than once every 72 hours in patients taking potent inhibitors of CYP3A4). Products include:
Gengraf Capsules 458
Neoral Soft Gelatin Capsules 2247
Neoral Oral Solution 2247
Restasis Ophthalmic Emulsion 570
Sandimmune 2259

Dalfopristin (Tadalafil is metabolized predominantly by CYP3A4 in the liver. The dose of tadalafil should be limited to 10 mg no more than

once every 72 hours in patients taking potent inhibitors of CYP3A4). Products include:

Synercid I.V. 1690

Danazol (Tadalafil is metabolized predominantly by CYP3A4 in the liver. The dose of tadalafil should be limited to 10 mg no more than once every 72 hours in patients taking potent inhibitors of CYP3A4).

No products indexed under this heading.

Delavirdine Mesylate (Tadalafil is metabolized predominantly by CYP3A4 in the liver. The dose of tadalafil should be limited to 10 mg no more than once every 72 hours in patients taking potent inhibitors of CYP3A4). Products include:

Rescriptor Tablets 2535

Dexamethasone (Drugs that induce CYP3A4 can increase tadalafil exposure). Products include:

Ciprodex Otic Suspension 555
Decadron Tablets 1929
TobraDex Ophthalmic Ointment 558
TobraDex Ophthalmic Suspension 558

Dexamethasone Acetate (Drugs that induce CYP3A4 can increase tadalafil exposure).

No products indexed under this heading.

Dexamethasone Sodium Phosphate (Drugs that induce CYP3A4 can increase tadalafil exposure). Products include:

Decadron Phosphate Injection 1931

Diltiazem Hydrochloride (Tadalafil is metabolized predominantly by CYP3A4 in the liver. The dose of tadalafil should be limited to 10 mg no more than once every 72 hours in patients taking potent inhibitors of CYP3A4). Products include:

Cardizem LA Extended Release Tablets 1699
Tiazac Capsules 1204

Diltiazem Maleate (Tadalafil is metabolized predominantly by CYP3A4 in the liver. The dose of tadalafil should be limited to 10 mg no more than once every 72 hours in patients taking potent inhibitors of CYP3A4).

No products indexed under this heading.

Doxazosin Mesylate (Caution is advised when PDE5 inhibitors are co-administered with alpha-blockers. PDE5 inhibitors, including tadalafil, and alpha-adrenergic blocking agents are both vasodilators with blood-pressure lowering effects. When vasodilators are used in combination, an additive effect on blood pressure may be anticipated. In some patients, concomitant use of these two drug classes can lower blood presure significantly, which may lead to symptomatic hypotension (e.g., fainting)).

No products indexed under this heading.

Doxorubicin Hydrochloride (Drugs that induce CYP3A4 can increase tadalafil exposure). Products include:

Adriamycin for Injection, USP 786
Adriamycin Injection, USP 786

Efavirenz (Tadalafil is metabolized predominantly by CYP3A4 in the liver. The dose of tadalafil should be limited to 10 mg no more than once every 72 hours in patients taking potent inhibitors of CYP3A4). Products include:

Sustiva Capsules 957

Enalapril Maleate (Following dosing with enalapril (10-20mg daily) and tadalafil 10mg, the mean reduction in supine systolic/diastolic blood pressure due to tadalafil 10mg in subjects taking analapril was 4/1mm Hg, compared to placebo). Products include:

Vaseretic Tablets 2073
Vasotec I.V. Injection 2076

Enalaprilat (Following dosing with enalapril (10-20mg daily) and tadalafil 10mg, the mean reduction in supine systolic/diastolic blood pressure due to tadalafil 10mg in subjects taking analapril was 4/1mm Hg, compared to placebo).

No products indexed under this heading.

Eprosartan Mesylate (A study was conducted to assess the interaction of angiotensin II receptor blockers and tadalafil 20mg. Following dosing, ambulatory measurements of blood pressure revealed differences between tadalafil and placebo of 8/4mm Hg in systolic/diastolic blood pressure). Products include:

Teveten Tablets 1707
Teveten HCT Tablets 1710

Erythrityl Tetranitrate (Administration of tadalafil to patients using any form of organic nitrate, either regularly and/or intermittently, is contraindicated).

No products indexed under this heading.

Erythromycin (Tadalafil is metabolized predominantly by CYP3A4 in the liver. The dose of tadalafil should be limited to 10 mg no more than once every 72 hours in patients taking potent inhibitors of CYP3A4). Products include:

Erygel Topical Gel 2096
Ery-Tab Tablets 447
Erythromycin Base Filmtab Tablets 454
Erythromycin Delayed-Release Capsules, USP 456
PCE Dispertab Tablets 510

Erythromycin Estolate (Tadalafil is metabolized predominantly by CYP3A4 in the liver. The dose of tadalafil should be limited to 10 mg no more than once every 72 hours in patients taking potent inhibitors of CYP3A4).

No products indexed under this heading.

Erythromycin Ethylsuccinate (Tadalafil is metabolized predominantly by CYP3A4 in the liver. The dose of tadalafil should be limited to 10 mg no more than once every 72 hours in patients taking potent inhibitors of CYP3A4). Products include:

E.E.S. 449
EryPed 445

Erythromycin Gluceptate (Tadalafil is metabolized predominantly by CYP3A4 in the liver. The dose of tadalafil should be limited to 10 mg no more than once every 72 hours in patients taking potent inhibitors of CYP3A4).

No products indexed under this heading.

Erythromycin Lactobionate (Tadalafil is metabolized predominantly by CYP3A4 in the liver. The dose of tadalafil should be limited to 10 mg no more than once every 72 hours in patients taking potent inhibitors of CYP3A4).

No products indexed under this heading.

Erythromycin Stearate (Tadalafil is metabolized predominantly by CYP3A4 in the liver. The dose of tadalafil should be limited to 10 mg no more than once every 72 hours in patients taking potent inhibitors of CYP3A4). Products include:

Erythrocin Stearate Filmtab Tablets 452

Esomeprazole Magnesium (Tadalafil is metabolized predominantly by CYP3A4 in the liver. The dose of tadalafil should be limited to 10 mg no more than once every 72 hours in patients taking potent inhibitors of CYP3A4). Products include:

Nexium Delayed-Release Capsules 645

Ethosuximide (Drugs that induce CYP3A4 can increase tadalafil exposure).

No products indexed under this heading.

Felbamate (Drugs that induce CYP3A4 can increase tadalafil exposure).

No products indexed under this heading.

Fluconazole (Tadalafil is metabolized predominantly by CYP3A4 in the liver. The dose of tadalafil should be limited to 10 mg no more than once every 72 hours in patients taking potent inhibitors of CYP3A4).

No products indexed under this heading.

Fludrocortisone Acetate (Drugs that induce CYP3A4 can increase tadalafil exposure).

No products indexed under this heading.

Fluoxetine Hydrochloride (Tadalafil is metabolized predominantly by CYP3A4 in the liver. The dose of tadalafil should be limited to 10 mg no more than once every 72 hours in patients taking potent inhibitors of CYP3A4). Products include:

Prozac Pulvules and Liquid 1771
Symbyax Capsules 1788

Fluvoxamine Maleate (Tadalafil is metabolized predominantly by CYP3A4 in the liver. The dose of tadalafil should be limited to 10 mg no more than once every 72 hours in patients taking potent inhibitors of CYP3A4).

No products indexed under this heading.

Fosamprenavir Calcium (Tadalafil is metabolized predominantly by CYP3A4 in the liver. The dose of tadalafil should be limited to 10 mg no more than once every 72 hours in patients taking potent inhibitors of CYP3A4). Products include:

Lexiva Tablets 1473

Fosphenytoin Sodium (Drugs that induce CYP3A4 can increase tadalafil exposure).

No products indexed under this heading.

Garlic Extract (Drugs that induce CYP3A4 can increase tadalafil exposure).

No products indexed under this heading.

Garlic Oil (Drugs that induce CYP3A4 can increase tadalafil exposure).

No products indexed under this heading.

Hydrocortisone (Drugs that induce CYP3A4 can increase tadalafil exposure). Products include:

Cortizone•5 Ointment 699
Cortizone•10 Creme 699
Cortizone•10 Ointment 699
Cortizone•10 Plus Creme 700
Cortizone•10 Maximum Strength Quick Shot Spray 700
Hydrocortone Tablets 1963
Preparation H Hydrocortisone Cream 748

Hydrocortisone Acetate (Drugs that induce CYP3A4 can increase tadalafil exposure). Products include:

Analpram-HC 1136
Pramosone 1139
ProctoFoam-HC 3113
Tucks Anti-Itch Ointment 712
U-cort 1% Cream 3289

Hydrocortisone Butyrate (Drugs that induce CYP3A4 can increase tadalafil exposure). Products include:

Locoid 1138
Locoid Lipocream Cream 1138

Hydrocortisone Cypionate (Drugs that induce CYP3A4 can increase tadalafil exposure).

No products indexed under this heading.

Hydrocortisone Hemisuccinate (Drugs that induce CYP3A4 can increase tadalafil exposure).

No products indexed under this heading.

Hydrocortisone Probutate (Drugs that induce CYP3A4 can increase tadalafil exposure). Products include:

Pandel Cream, 0.1% 1017

Hydrocortisone Sodium Phosphate (Drugs that induce CYP3A4 can increase tadalafil exposure).

No products indexed under this heading.

Hydrocortisone Sodium Succinate (Drugs that induce CYP3A4 can increase tadalafil exposure).

No products indexed under this heading.

Hydrocortisone Valerate (Drugs that induce CYP3A4 can increase tadalafil exposure).

No products indexed under this heading.

Hypericum (Drugs that induce CYP3A4 can increase tadalafil exposure).

No products indexed under this heading.

Hypericum Perforatum (Drugs that induce CYP3A4 can increase tadalafil exposure).

No products indexed under this heading.

Indinavir Sulfate (Tadalafil is metabolized predominantly by CYP3A4 in the liver. The dose of tadalafil should be limited to 10 mg no more than once every 72 hours in patients taking potent inhibitors of CYP3A4). Products include:

Crixivan Capsules 1918

Irbesartan (A study was conducted to assess the interaction of angiotensin II receptor blockers and tadalafil 20mg. Following dosing, ambulatory measurements of blood pressure revealed differences between tadalafil and placebo of 8/4mm Hg in systolic/diastolic blood pressure). Products include:

Avalide Tablets 922
Avalide Tablets 2889
Avapro Tablets 925
Avapro Tablets 2886

IMPORTANT NOTE: Always consult each drug listing in the patient's regimen for possible interactions.

soniazid (Tadalafil is metabolized redominantly by CYP3A4 in the liv- er. The dose of tadalafil should be mited to 10 mg no more than once every 72 hours in patients taking potent inhibitors of CYP3A4).
No products indexed under this heading.

sosorbide Dinitrate (Administra- tion of tadalafil to patients using any form of organic nitrate, either regu- arly and/or intermittently, is contra- ndicated). Products include:
BiDil Tablets 2161

Isosorbide Mononitrate (Adminis- tration of tadalafil to patients using any form of organic nitrate, either regularly and/or intermittently, is contraindicated). Products include:
Imdur Tablets 3032

Itraconazole (CYP3A4 inhibitors such as itraconazole may likely increase tadalafil exposure).
No products indexed under this heading.

Ketoconazole (Ketoconazole increased tadalafil 20mg single dose exposure (AUC) by 312% and Cmax by 22%, relative to the values for tadalafil 20mg alone. Ketoconazole increased tadalafil 10mg single dose exposure (AUC) by 107% and Cmax by 15%, relative to the values for tadalafil 10mg alone. Based on these results, the dose of tadalafil should not exceed 10mg and tadala- fil should not be taken more fre- quently than once in 72 hours).
Products include:
Nizoral A-D Shampoo, 1% 1839
Nizoral 2% Shampoo 1838

Lopinavir (Tadalafil is metabolized predominantly by CYP3A4 in the liv- er. The dose of tadalafil should be limited to 10 mg no more than once every 72 hours in patients taking potent inhibitors of CYP3A4).
Products include:
Kaletra 474

Loratadine (Tadalafil is metabolized predominantly by CYP3A4 in the liv- er. The dose of tadalafil should be limited to 10 mg no more than once every 72 hours in patients taking potent inhibitors of CYP3A4).
Products include:
Alavert Allergy & Sinus D-12 Hour Tablets .... ▣743
Alavert .... ▣743
Children's Claritin 24 Hour Non-Drowsy Allergy Syrup .... ▣732
Claritin Non-Drowsy 24 Hour Tablets .... ▣731
Non-Drowsy Claritin Hives Relief Tablets .... ▣733
Claritin Reditabs 24 Hour Non-Drowsy Tablets .... ▣732
Claritin-D Non-Drowsy 12 Hour Tablets .... ▣731
Claritin-D Non-Drowsy 24 Hour Tablets .... ▣731
Children's Dimetapp ND Non-Drowsy Allergy Syrup .... ▣746
Triaminic Allerchews .... ▣684

Losartan Potassium (A study was conducted to assess the interaction of angiotensin II receptor blockers and tadalafil 20mg. Following dos- ing, ambulatory measurements of blood pressure revealed differences between tadalafil and placebo of 8/4mm Hg in systolic/diastolic blood pressure). Products include:
Cozaar Tablets 1913
Hyzaar 1964

Magaldrate (Simultaneous adminis- tration of an antacid (magnesium hydroxide/aluminum hydroxide) and tadalafil reduced the apparent rate of absorption of tadalafil without altering exposure (AUC) to tadalafil).
No products indexed under this heading.

Magnesium Hydroxide (Simulta- neous administration of an antacid (magnesium hydroxide/aluminum hydroxide) and tadalafil reduced the apparent rate of absorption of tad- alafil without altering exposure (AUC) to tadalafil). Products include:
Maalox Max Maximum Strength Antacid/Anti-Gas Liquid 2165
Maalox Regular Strength Antacid/Antigas Liquid 2164
Pepcid Complete Chewable Tablets 1672
Rolaids Tablets .... ▣707
Extra Strength Rolaids Tablets .... ▣707
Rolaids Multi-Symptom Antacid & Antigas Tablets .... ▣708

Magnesium Oxide (Simultaneous administration of an antacid (magne- sium hydroxide/aluminum hydroxide) and tadalafil reduced the apparent rate of absorption of tadalafil without altering exposure (AUC) to tadalafil).
Products include:
Beelith Tablets 784
PremCal Light, Regular, and Extra Strength Tablets .... ▣762

Mephenytoin (Drugs that induce CYP3A4 can increase tadalafil exposure).
No products indexed under this heading.

Methsuximide (Drugs that induce CYP3A4 can increase tadalafil exposure).
No products indexed under this heading.

Methylprednisolone (Drugs that induce CYP3A4 can increase tadala- fil exposure).
No products indexed under this heading.

Methylprednisolone Acetate (Drugs that induce CYP3A4 can increase tadalafil exposure).
Products include:
Depo-Medrol Injectable Suspension 2615
Depo-Medrol Single-Dose Vial 2617

Methylprednisolone Sodium Succinate (Drugs that induce CYP3A4 can increase tadalafil exposure).
No products indexed under this heading.

Metoprolol Succinate (Following dosing with sustained-release meto- prolol (25-200mg daily) and tadalafil 10mg, the mean reduction in supine systolic/diastolic blood pressure due to tadalafil 10mg in subjects taking metoprolol was 5/3mm Hg, com- pared to placebo). Products include:
Toprol-XL Tablets 660

Metoprolol Tartrate (Following dosing with sustained-release meto- prolol (25-200mg daily) and tadalafil 10mg, the mean reduction in supine systolic/diastolic blood pressure due to tadalafil 10mg in subjects taking metoprolol was 5/3mm Hg, com- pared to placebo).
No products indexed under this heading.

Metronidazole (Tadalafil is metabo- lized predominantly by CYP3A4 in the liver. The dose of tadalafil should be limited to 10 mg no more than once every 72 hours in patients tak- ing potent inhibitors of CYP3A4).
Products include:
Metrogel 1% 1212
MetroGel-Vaginal Gel 1822
Noritate Cream, 1% 1051

Metronidazole Benzoate (Tadalafil is metabolized predominantly by CYP3A4 in the liver. The dose of tad- alafil should be limited to 10 mg no more than once every 72 hours in patients taking potent inhibitors of CYP3A4).
No products indexed under this heading.

Metronidazole Hydrochloride (Tadalafil is metabolized predomi- nantly by CYP3A4 in the liver. The dose of tadalafil should be limited to 10 mg no more than once every 72 hours in patients taking potent inhibi- tors of CYP3A4).
No products indexed under this heading.

Miconazole (Tadalafil is metabo- lized predominantly by CYP3A4 in the liver. The dose of tadalafil should be limited to 10 mg no more than once every 72 hours in patients tak- ing potent inhibitors of CYP3A4).
No products indexed under this heading.

Miconazole Nitrate (Tadalafil is metabolized predominantly by CYP3A4 in the liver. The dose of tad- alafil should be limited to 10 mg no more than once every 72 hours in patients taking potent inhibitors of CYP3A4). Products include:
Desenex .... ▣674
Desenex Jock Itch Spray Powder ... ▣674

Modafinil (Drugs that induce CYP3A4 can increase tadalafil expo- sure). Products include:
Provigil Tablets 1002

Nefazodone Hydrochloride (Tad- alafil is metabolized predominantly by CYP3A4 in the liver. The dose of tadalafil should be limited to 10 mg no more than once every 72 hours in patients taking potent inhibitors of CYP3A4).
No products indexed under this heading.

Nelfinavir Mesylate (Tadalafil is metabolized predominantly by CYP3A4 in the liver. The dose of tad- alafil should be limited to 10 mg no more than once every 72 hours in patients taking potent inhibitors of CYP3A4). Products include:
Viracept 2556

Nevirapine (Tadalafil is metabolized predominantly by CYP3A4 in the liv- er. The dose of tadalafil should be limited to 10 mg no more than once every 72 hours in patients taking potent inhibitors of CYP3A4).
Products include:
Viramune Oral Suspension 903
Viramune Tablets 903

Niacinamide (Tadalafil is metabo- lized predominantly by CYP3A4 in the liver. The dose of tadalafil should be limited to 10 mg no more than once every 72 hours in patients tak- ing potent inhibitors of CYP3A4).
No products indexed under this heading.

Nicotinamide (Tadalafil is metabo- lized predominantly by CYP3A4 in the liver. The dose of tadalafil should be limited to 10 mg no more than once every 72 hours in patients tak- ing potent inhibitors of CYP3A4).
Products include:
Nicomide Tablets 3190

Nifedipine (Tadalafil is metabolized predominantly by CYP3A4 in the liv- er. The dose of tadalafil should be limited to 10 mg no more than once every 72 hours in patients taking potent inhibitors of CYP3A4).
Products include:
Adalat CC Tablets 2978

Nitroglycerin (Administration of tadalafil to patients using any form of organic nitrate, either regularly and/ or intermittently, is contraindicated).
Products include:
Nitro-Dur Transdermal Infusion System 3060
Nitrolingual Pumpspray 1161

Norfloxacin (Tadalafil is metabo- lized predominantly by CYP3A4 in the liver. The dose of tadalafil should be limited to 10 mg no more than once every 72 hours in patients tak- ing potent inhibitors of CYP3A4).
Products include:
Noroxin Tablets 2009

Omeprazole (Tadalafil is metabo- lized predominantly by CYP3A4 in the liver. The dose of tadalafil should be limited to 10 mg no more than once every 72 hours in patients tak- ing potent inhibitors of CYP3A4).
Products include:
Zegerid Powder for Oral Solution 2972

Oxcarbazepine (Drugs that induce CYP3A4 can increase tadalafil expo- sure). Products include:
Trileptal Oral Suspension 2281
Trileptal Tablets 2281

Paroxetine Hydrochloride (Tad- alafil is metabolized predominantly by CYP3A4 in the liver. The dose of tadalafil should be limited to 10 mg no more than once every 72 hours in patients taking potent inhibitors of CYP3A4). Products include:
Paxil CR Controlled-Release Tablets 1509
Paxil 1501

Pentaerythritol Tetranitrate (Administration of tadalafil to patients using any form of organic nitrate, either regularly and/or inter- mittently, is contraindicated).
No products indexed under this heading.

Phenobarbital (CYP3A4 inducers, such as phenobarbital, may decrease tadalafil exposure. No dose adjustment is warranted).
No products indexed under this heading.

Phenobarbital Sodium (CYP3A4 inducers, such as phenobarbital, may decrease tadalafil exposure. No dose adjustment is warranted).
No products indexed under this heading.

Phenytoin (Drugs that induce CYP3A4 can increase tadalafil exposure).
No products indexed under this heading.

Phenytoin Sodium (Drugs that induce CYP3A4 can increase tadala- fil exposure). Products include:
Phenytek Capsules 2153

Prazosin Hydrochloride (Caution is advised when PDE5 inhibitors are co-administered with alpha-blockers. PDE5 inhibitors, including tadalafil, and alpha-adrenergic blocking agents are both vasodilators with blood-pressure lowering effects. When vasodilators are used in com- bination, an additive effect on blood pressure may be anticipated. In some patients, concomitant use of these two drug classes can lower

blood presure significantly, which may lead to symptomatic hypotension (e.g., fainting)).
No products indexed under this heading.

Prednisolone Acetate (Drugs that induce CYP3A4 can increase tadalafil exposure). Products include:
Blephamide Ophthalmic Ointment 563
Blephamide Ophthalmic Suspension 564
Poly-Pred Liquifilm Ophthalmic Suspension .... ⊙231
Pred Forte Ophthalmic Suspension .... ⊙233
Pred Mild Sterile Ophthalmic Suspension .... ⊙236
Pred-G Ophthalmic Suspension .... ⊙234
Pred-G Sterile Ophthalmic Ointment .... ⊙235

Prednisolone Sodium Phosphate (Drugs that induce CYP3A4 can increase tadalafil exposure). Products include:
Pediapred Oral Solution 3319

Prednisolone Tebutate (Drugs that induce CYP3A4 can increase tadalafil exposure).
No products indexed under this heading.

Prednisone (Drugs that induce CYP3A4 can increase tadalafil exposure).
No products indexed under this heading.

Primidone (Drugs that induce CYP3A4 can increase tadalafil exposure).
No products indexed under this heading.

Propoxyphene Hydrochloride (Tadalafil is metabolized predominantly by CYP3A4 in the liver. The dose of tadalafil should be limited to 10 mg no more than once every 72 hours in patients taking potent inhibitors of CYP3A4).
No products indexed under this heading.

Propoxyphene Napsylate (Tadalafil is metabolized predominantly by CYP3A4 in the liver. The dose of tadalafil should be limited to 10 mg no more than once every 72 hours in patients taking potent inhibitors of CYP3A4). Products include:
Darvocet A 500 Tablets 3497

Quinidine (Tadalafil is metabolized predominantly by CYP3A4 in the liver. The dose of tadalafil should be limited to 10 mg no more than once every 72 hours in patients taking potent inhibitors of CYP3A4).
No products indexed under this heading.

Quinidine Hydrochloride (Tadalafil is metabolized predominantly by CYP3A4 in the liver. The dose of tadalafil should be limited to 10 mg no more than once every 72 hours in patients taking potent inhibitors of CYP3A4).
No products indexed under this heading.

Quinidine Polygalacturonate (Tadalafil is metabolized predominantly by CYP3A4 in the liver. The dose of tadalafil should be limited to 10 mg no more than once every 72 hours in patients taking potent inhibitors of CYP3A4).
No products indexed under this heading.

Quinidine Sulfate (Tadalafil is metabolized predominantly by CYP3A4 in the liver. The dose of tadalafil should be limited to 10 mg no more than once every 72 hours in patients taking potent inhibitors of CYP3A4).
No products indexed under this heading.

Quinine (Tadalafil is metabolized predominantly by CYP3A4 in the liver. The dose of tadalafil should be limited to 10 mg no more than once every 72 hours in patients taking potent inhibitors of CYP3A4).
No products indexed under this heading.

Quinine Sulfate (Tadalafil is metabolized predominantly by CYP3A4 in the liver. The dose of tadalafil should be limited to 10 mg no more than once every 72 hours in patients taking potent inhibitors of CYP3A4).
No products indexed under this heading.

Quinupristin (Tadalafil is metabolized predominantly by CYP3A4 in the liver. The dose of tadalafil should be limited to 10 mg no more than once every 72 hours in patients taking potent inhibitors of CYP3A4). Products include:
Synercid I.V. 1690

Ranitidine Bismuth Citrate (Tadalafil is metabolized predominantly by CYP3A4 in the liver. The dose of tadalafil should be limited to 10 mg no more than once every 72 hours in patients taking potent inhibitors of CYP3A4).
No products indexed under this heading.

Ranitidine Hydrochloride (Tadalafil is metabolized predominantly by CYP3A4 in the liver. The dose of tadalafil should be limited to 10 mg no more than once every 72 hours in patients taking potent inhibitors of CYP3A4). Products include:
Zantac 1597
Zantac Injection 1593
Zantac 75 Tablets 715
Zantac 150 Maximum Strength Tablets 715
Zantac Injection Pharmacy Bulk Package 1595

Rifabutin (Drugs that induce CYP3A4 can increase tadalafil exposure).
No products indexed under this heading.

Rifampicin (Drugs that induce CYP3A4 can increase tadalafil exposure).
No products indexed under this heading.

Rifampin (Rifampin reduced tadalafil 10mg single dose exposure (AUC) by 88% and Cmax by 46% relative to the values for tadalafil 10mg alone. No dose adjustment is warranted).
No products indexed under this heading.

Rifapentine (Drugs that induce CYP3A4 can increase tadalafil exposure).
No products indexed under this heading.

Ritonavir (Ritonavir increased tadalafil 20mg single dose exposure (AUC) by 124% with no change in Cmax, relative to the values for tadalafil 20mg alone. Based on these results, the dose of tadalafil should not exceed 10mg and tadalafil should not be taken more frequently than once in 72 hours). Products include:
Kaletra 474
Norvir 499

Saquinavir (Tadalafil is metabolized predominantly by CYP3A4 in the liver. The dose of tadalafil should be limited to 10 mg no more than once every 72 hours in patients taking potent inhibitors of CYP3A4).
No products indexed under this heading.

Saquinavir Mesylate (Tadalafil is metabolized predominantly by CYP3A4 in the liver. The dose of tadalafil should be limited to 10 mg no more than once every 72 hours in patients taking potent inhibitors of CYP3A4). Products include:
Invirase 2776

Sertraline Hydrochloride (Tadalafil is metabolized predominantly by CYP3A4 in the liver. The dose of tadalafil should be limited to 10 mg no more than once every 72 hours in patients taking potent inhibitors of CYP3A4). Products include:
Zoloft 2581

Sodium Bicarbonate (Simultaneous administration of an antacid (magnesium hydroxide/aluminum hydroxide) and tadalafil reduced the apparent rate of absorption of tadalafil without altering exposure (AUC) to tadalafil). Products include:
Ceo-Two Evacuant Suppository 607
Colyte with Flavor Packs for Oral Solution 3102
HalfLytely and Bisacodyl Tablets Bowel Prep Kit with Flavors Packs 915
TriLyte with Flavor Packs for Oral Solution 3114

Sulfinpyrazone (Drugs that induce CYP3A4 can increase tadalafil exposure).
No products indexed under this heading.

Tamsulosin Hydrochloride (Caution is advised when PDE5 inhibitors are co-administered with alpha-blockers. PDE5 inhibitors, including tadalafil, and alpha-adrenergic blocking agents are both vasodilators with blood-pressure lowering effects. When vasodilators are used in combination, an additive effect on blood pressure may be anticipated. In some patients, concomitant use of these two drug classes can lower blood presure significantly, which may lead to symptomatic hypotension (e.g., fainting)). Products include:
Flomax Capsules 881

Telithromycin (Tadalafil is metabolized predominantly by CYP3A4 in the liver. The dose of tadalafil should be limited to 10 mg no more than once every 72 hours in patients taking potent inhibitors of CYP3A4). Products include:
Ketek Tablets 2920

Telmisartan (A study was conducted to assess the interaction of angiotensin II receptor blockers and tadalafil 20mg. Following dosing, ambulatory measurements of blood pressure revealed differences between tadalafil and placebo of 8/4mm Hg in systolic/diastolic blood pressure). Products include:
Micardis Tablets 884
Micardis HCT Tablets 886

Terazosin Hydrochloride (Caution is advised when PDE5 inhibitors are co-administered with alpha-blockers. PDE5 inhibitors, including tadalafil, and alpha-adrenergic blocking agents are both vasodilators with blood-pressure lowering effects. When vasodilators are used in combination, an additive effect on blood pressure may be anticipated. In some patients, concomitant use of these two drug classes can lower blood presure significantly, which may lead to symptomatic hypotension (e.g., fainting)). Products include:
Hytrin Capsules 469

Theophylline (Drugs that induce CYP3A4 can increase tadalafil exposure).
No products indexed under this heading.

Triamcinolone (Drugs that induce CYP3A4 can increase tadalafil exposure).
No products indexed under this heading.

Triamcinolone Acetonide (Drugs that induce CYP3A4 can increase tadalafil exposure). Products include:
Azmacort Inhalation Aerosol 1701
Nasacort HFA Inhalation Aerosol 2939
Nasacort AQ Nasal Spray 2937

Triamcinolone Diacetate (Drugs that induce CYP3A4 can increase tadalafil exposure).
No products indexed under this heading.

Triamcinolone Hexacetonide (Drugs that induce CYP3A4 can increase tadalafil exposure).
No products indexed under this heading.

Troglitazone (Tadalafil is metabolized predominantly by CYP3A4 in the liver. The dose of tadalafil should be limited to 10 mg no more than once every 72 hours in patients taking potent inhibitors of CYP3A4).
No products indexed under this heading.

Troleandomycin (Tadalafil is metabolized predominantly by CYP3A4 in the liver. The dose of tadalafil should be limited to 10 mg no more than once every 72 hours in patients taking potent inhibitors of CYP3A4).
No products indexed under this heading.

Valproate Sodium (Tadalafil is metabolized predominantly by CYP3A4 in the liver. The dose of tadalafil should be limited to 10 mg no more than once every 72 hours in patients taking potent inhibitors of CYP3A4). Products include:
Depacon Injection 412

Valsartan (A study was conducted to assess the interaction of angiotensin II receptor blockers and tadalafil 20mg. Following dosing, ambulatory measurements of blood pressure revealed differences between tadalafil and placebo of 8/4mm Hg in systolic/diastolic blood pressure). Products include:
Diovan HCT Tablets 2195
Diovan Tablets 2191

Verapamil Hydrochloride (Tadalafil is metabolized predominantly by CYP3A4 in the liver. The dose of tadalafil should be limited to 10 mg no more than once every 72 hours in patients taking potent inhibitors of CYP3A4). Products include:
Covera-HS Tablets 3135
Tarka Tablets 519
Verelan PM Capsules 3120

Voriconazole (Tadalafil is metabolized predominantly by CYP3A4 in the liver. The dose of tadalafil should be limited to 10 mg no more than

once every 72 hours in patients taking potent inhibitors of CYP3A4). Products include:

- VFEND I.V. 2543
- VFEND Oral Suspension 2543
- VFEND Tablets 2543

Zafirlukast (Tadalafil is metabolized predominantly by CYP3A4 in the liver. The dose of tadalafil should be limited to 10 mg no more than once every 72 hours in patients taking potent inhibitors of CYP3A4). Products include:

- Accolate Tablets 663

Zileuton (Tadalafil is metabolized predominantly by CYP3A4 in the liver. The dose of tadalafil should be limited to 10 mg no more than once every 72 hours in patients taking potent inhibitors of CYP3A4).

No products indexed under this heading.

Food Interactions

Alcohol (Both tadalafil and alcohol act as mild vasodilators. When mild vasodilators are taken in combination, blood-pressure lowering effects of each individual compound may be increased. Substantial consumption of alcohol in combination with tadalafil may increase the potential for orthostatic signs and symptoms, including increase in heart rate, decrease in standing blood pressure, dizziness, and headache).

Grapefruit (Tadalafil is metabolized predominantly by CYP3A4 in the liver. The dose of tadalafil should be limited to 10 mg no more than once every 72 hours in patients taking potent inhibitors of CYP3A4).

Grapefruit Juice (YP3A4 inhibitors such as grapefruit juice may likely increase tadalafil exposure).

CILOXAN OPHTHALMIC OINTMENT

(Ciprofloxacin Hydrochloride) 554

May interact with oral anticoagulants, xanthines, and certain other agents. Compounds in these categories include:

Aminophylline (Systemic administration of quinolones elevates plasma concentrations of theophylline).

No products indexed under this heading.

Anisindione (Enhanced anticoagulant effect with systemic quinolones). Products include:

- Miradon Tablets 3056

Caffeine (Systemic administration of quinolones has shown to interfere with caffeine metabolism). Products include:

- Athena Hair System Shampoo .... ▣767
- BC Powder .... ▣612
- Arthritis Strength BC Powder .... ▣612
- Goody's Extra Strength Headache Powder .... ▣621
- Goody's Extra Strength Pain Relief Tablets .... ▣621
- Hycomine Compound Tablets 1105
- Spartan Hair System Shampoo .... ▣767
- Vivarin .... ▣639

Caffeine Citrate (Systemic administration of quinolones has shown to interfere with caffeine metabolism). Products include:

- Cafcit 1854

Cyclosporine (Concomitant administration with systemic quinolones may result in transient elevations in serum creatinine). Products include:

- Gengraf Capsules 458
- Neoral Soft Gelatin Capsules 2247
- Neoral Oral Solution 2247
- Restasis Ophthalmic Emulsion 570
- Sandimmune 2259

Dicumarol (Enhanced anticoagulant effect with systemic quinolones).

No products indexed under this heading.

Dyphylline (Systemic administration of quinolones elevates plasma concentrations of theophylline).

No products indexed under this heading.

Theophylline (Systemic administration of quinolones elevates plasma concentrations of theophylline).

No products indexed under this heading.

Theophylline Anhydrous (Systemic administration of quinolones elevates plasma concentrations of theophylline). Products include:

- Uniphyl Tablets 2708

Theophylline Calcium Salicylate (Systemic administration of quinolones elevates plasma concentrations of theophylline).

No products indexed under this heading.

Theophylline Dihydroxypropyl (Glyceryl) (Systemic administration of quinolones elevates plasma concentrations of theophylline).

No products indexed under this heading.

Theophylline Ethylenediamine (Systemic administration of quinolones elevates plasma concentrations of theophylline).

No products indexed under this heading.

Theophylline Sodium Glycinate (Systemic administration of quinolones elevates plasma concentrations of theophylline).

No products indexed under this heading.

Warfarin Sodium (Enhanced anticoagulant effect with systemic quinolones). Products include:

- Coumadin for Injection 932
- Coumadin Tablets 932

CIPRO I.V.

(Ciprofloxacin) 2998

May interact with antacids containing aluminum, calcium and magnesium, calcium preparations, corticosteroids, oral anticoagulants, cytochrome p450 1a2 substrates (selected), iron containing oral preparations, non-steroidal anti-inflammatory agents, phenytoin, xanthines, and certain other agents. Compounds in these categories include:

Acetaminophen (Ciprofloxacin is a moderate inhibitor of CYP450 1A2 isoenzymes. Co-administration of ciprofloxacin and other drugs primarily metabolized by the CYP450 1A2 enzyme pathway may result in increased plasma concentrations of the co-administered drug and couldlead to clinically significant pharmacodynamic side effects). Products include:

- Benadryl Allergy & Cold Tablets .... ▣692
- Benadryl Allergy & Sinus Headache Caplets & Gelcaps .... ▣693
- Benadryl Maximum Strength Severe Allergy & Sinus Headache Caplets .... ▣694
- Contac Severe Cold and Flu Caplets Maximum Strength .... ▣615
- Contac Severe Cold and Flu Caplets Non-Drowsy .... ▣615
- Darvocet A 500 Tablets 3497
- Goody's Body Pain Formula Powder .... ▣621
- Goody's Extra Strength Headache Powder .... ▣621
- Goody's Extra Strength Pain Relief Tablets .... ▣621
- Goody's PM Powder .... ▣622
- Hycomine Compound Tablets 1105
- Lortab 3315
- Lortab Elixir 3312
- Percocet Tablets 1114
- Robitussin Cough, Cold & Flu Liquid-filled Capsules .... ▣750
- Robitussin Flu Liquid .... ▣752
- Sedapap Tablets 50 mg/650 mg 2098
- Singlet Caplets .... ▣636
- Sudafed Severe Cold .... ▣710
- Sudafed Sinus Headache .... ▣711
- TheraFlu Cold & Cough Hot Liquid .... ▣680
- TheraFlu Cold & Sore Throat Hot Liquid .... ▣680
- TheraFlu Flu & Chest Congestion Non-Drowsy Hot Liquid .... ▣681
- TheraFlu Flu & Sore Throat Hot Liquid .... ▣681
- TheraFlu Severe Cold Non-Drowsy Hot Liquid .... ▣683
- TheraFlu Severe Cold & Cough Hot Liquid .... ▣683
- TheraFlu Severe Cold Caplets .... ▣679
- TheraFlu Severe Cold Hot Liquid .... ▣682
- TheraFlu Severe Cold Non-Drowsy Caplets .... ▣679
- Triaminic Cough & Sore Throat Liquid .... ▣687
- Triaminic Flu, Cough & Fever Liquid .... ▣685
- Triaminic Cough & Sore Throat Softchews .... ▣689
- Tylenol 8 Hour Extended Release Geltabs and Caplets 1843
- Tylenol Sinus NightTime Caplets .... ▣663
- Children's Tylenol Suspension Liquid and Meltaways 1850
- Children's Tylenol Plus Cold & Allergy Suspension Liquid 1850
- Children's Tylenol Plus Cold NightTime Suspension Liquid 1851
- Children's Tylenol Plus Cold & Cough Suspension Liquid and Chewable Tablets 1851
- Children's Tylenol Plus Cold Chewable Tablets 1851
- Children's Tylenol Plus Cold Daytime Non-Drowsy Suspension Liquid 1851
- Children's Tylenol Plus Flu Suspension Liquid 1853
- Concentrated Tylenol Infants' Drops Plus Cold 1851
- Concentrated Tylenol Infants' Drops Plus Cold and Cough 1851
- Concentrated Tylenol Infants' Drops 1850
- Junior Tylenol Meltaways 1850
- Tylenol Cold & Flu Severe Daytime Liquid with Cool Bust 1846
- Tylenol Cold & Flu Severe NightTime Liquid with Cool Burst 1846
- Tylenol Cold Severe Congestion Non-Drowsy Caplets with Cool Burst 1846
- Tylenol Cough & Sore Throat Daytime Liquid with Cool Burst 1849
- Tylenol Cough & Sore Throat NightTime Liquid with Cool Burst 1849
- Tylenol 1843
- Extra Strength Tylenol Rapid Release Gels 1843
- Tylenol 1843
- Tylenol Allergy Complete Night Time Caplets 1844
- Tylenol Allergy Complete Multi-Symptom Caplets and Gelcaps with Cool Burst 1844
- Tylenol Severe Allergy Caplets 1844
- Tylenol Flu NightTime Gelcaps 1846
- Tylenol Flu Day Non-Drowsy Gelcaps 1846
- Concentrated Tylenol Infants' Drops Plus Cold Nasal Congestant, Fever Reducer & Pain Reliever .... ▣668
- Concentrated Tylenol Infants' Drops Plus Cold & Cough Nasal Decongestant, Fever Reducer & Pain Reliever .... ▣668
- Multi-Symptom Tylenol Cold Night Time Caplets 1845
- Multi-Symptom Tylenol Cold Day Non-Drowsy Caplets and Gelcaps 1845
- Extra Strength Tylenol PM Caplets, Geltabs, Gelcaps and Liquid 1847
- Tylenol Sinus Day Non-Drowsy 1848
- Tylenol Sinus Night Time Caplets 1848
- Tylenol Sinus Severe Congestion Caplets with Cool Burst 1848
- Tylenol Sore Throat Daytime Liquid with Cool Burst 1849
- Tylenol Sore Throat NightTime Liquid with Cool Burst 1849
- Tylenol with Codeine 2461
- Women's Tylenol Menstrual Relief Caplets 1849
- Ultracet Tablets 2462
- Vicks 44M Cough, Cold & Flu Relief 2676
- Vicks DayQuil LiquiCaps/Liquid Multi-Symptom Cold/Flu Relief .... ▣723
- Vicks DayQuil Multi-Symptom Cold/Flu Relief LiquiCaps 2675
- Vicks DayQuil Multi-Symptom Cold/Flu Relief Liquid 2675
- Vicks NyQuil LiquiCaps 2677
- Vicks NyQuil LiquiCaps/Liquid Multi-Symptom Cold/Flu Relief .... ▣725
- Vicks NyQuil Liquid 2677
- Vicodin Tablets 530
- Vicodin ES Tablets 531
- Vicodin HP Tablets 532
- Zydone Tablets 1118

Alatrofloxacin Mesylate (Ciprofloxacin is a moderate inhibitor of CYP450 1A2 isoenzymes. Co-administration of ciprofloxacin and other drugs primarily metabolized by the CYP450 1A2 enzyme pathway may result in increased plasma concentrations of the co-administered drug and couldlead to clinically significant pharmacodynamic side effects).

No products indexed under this heading.

Aluminum Carbonate (Concurrent administration of these antacids may substantially interfere with the oral absorption of ciprofloxacin; antacids may be administered either two hours after or six hours before ciprofloxacin dosing without a significant decrease in bioavailability).

No products indexed under this heading.

Aluminum Hydroxide (Concurrent administration of these antacids may substantially interfere with the oral absorption of ciprofloxacin; antacids may be administered either two hours after or six hours before ciprofloxacin dosing without a significant decrease in bioavailability). Products include:

- Gaviscon Regular Strength Liquid .... ▣620
- Gaviscon Regular Strength Tablets .... ▣619
- Gaviscon Extra Strength Liquid .... ▣620
- Gaviscon Extra Strength Tablets .... ▣619
- Maalox Max Maximum Strength Antacid/Anti-Gas Liquid 2165
- Maalox Regular Strength Antacid/Antigas Liquid 2164

Aminophylline (Potential for severe and fatal reactions including cardiac arrest, seizures, respiratory failure and status epilepticus; concurrent use should be avoided or serum levels of theophylline should be monitored carefully).

No products indexed under this heading.

Amiodarone Hydrochloride (Ciprofloxacin is a moderate inhibitor of CYP450 1A2 isoenzymes. Co-administration of ciprofloxacin and other drugs primarily metabolized by the CYP450 1A2 enzyme pathway

may result in increased plasma concentrations of the co-administered drug and couldlead to clinically significant pharmacodynamic side effects). Products include:
- Pacerone Tablets 3337

Amitriptyline Hydrochloride (Ciprofloxacin is a moderate inhibitor of CYP450 1A2 isoenzymes. Co-administration of ciprofloxacin and other drugs primarily metabolized by the CYP450 1A2 enzyme pathway may result in increased plasma concentrations of the co-administered drug and couldlead to clinically significant pharmacodynamic side effects).
- No products indexed under this heading.

Amoxapine (Ciprofloxacin is a moderate inhibitor of CYP450 1A2 isoenzymes. Co-administration of ciprofloxacin and other drugs primarily metabolized by the CYP450 1A2 enzyme pathway may result in increased plasma concentrations of the co-administered drug and couldlead to clinically significant pharmacodynamic side effects).
- No products indexed under this heading.

Anagrelide Hydrochloride (Ciprofloxacin is a moderate inhibitor of CYP450 1A2 isoenzymes. Co-administration of ciprofloxacin and other drugs primarily metabolized by the CYP450 1A2 enzyme pathway may result in increased plasma concentrations of the co-administered drug and couldlead to clinically significant pharmacodynamic side effects). Products include:
- Agrylin Capsules 3172

Anisindione (Enhanced effects of anticoagulant). Products include:
- Miradon Tablets 3056

Betamethasone Acetate (Risk of ruptures of the shoulder, hand, Achilles tendon or other tendons may be increased in patients receiving concomitant corticosteroids, especially in the elderly).
- No products indexed under this heading.

Betamethasone Sodium Phosphate (Risk of ruptures of the shoulder, hand, Achilles tendon or other tendons may be increased in patients receiving concomitant corticosteroids, especially in the elderly).
- No products indexed under this heading.

Caffeine (Reduced clearance of caffeine and a prolongation of its serum half-life). Products include:
- Athena Hair System Shampoo 767
- BC Powder 612
- Arthritis Strength BC Powder 612
- Goody's Extra Strength Headache Powder 621
- Goody's Extra Strength Pain Relief Tablets 621
- Hycomine Compound Tablets 1105
- Spartan Hair System Shampoo 767
- Vivarin 639

Caffeine Anhydrous (Ciprofloxacin is a moderate inhibitor of CYP450 1A2 isoenzymes. Co-administration of ciprofloxacin and other drugs primarily metabolized by the CYP450 1A2 enzyme pathway may result in increased plasma concentrations of the co-administered drug and couldlead to clinically significant pharmacodynamic side effects).
- No products indexed under this heading.

Caffeine Citrate (Reduced clearance of caffeine and a prolongation of its serum half-life). Products include:
- Cafcit 1854

Calcium Carbonate (Co-administration with calcium-containing products may substantially interfere with the oral absorption of quinolones; these preparations may be taken six hours before or two hours after taking ciprofloxacin). Products include:
- Actonel with Calcium Tablets 2684
- Caltrate 600 PLUS Chewables 779
- Caltrate 600 PLUS Tablets 779
- Caltrate 600 + D Tablets 779
- Encora Capsules 3298
- Encora AM Tablets 3298
- Encora PM Tablets 3298
- Gas-X with Maalox 675
- Maalox Regular Strength Antacid Tablets 2166
- Quick Dissolve Maalox Max Maximum Strength Antacid/Antigas Tablets 2165
- Maalox Max Quick Dissolve Maximum Strength Chewable Tablets 678
- Os-Cal Chewable Tablets 765
- Pepcid Complete Chewable Tablets 1672
- PremCal Light, Regular, and Extra Strength Tablets 762
- Rolaids Tablets 707
- Extra Strength Rolaids Softchews 708
- Extra Strength Rolaids Tablets 707
- Rolaids Multi-Symptom Antacid & Antigas Tablets 708
- Tums 639

Calcium Chloride (Co-administration with calcium-containing products may substantially interfere with the oral absorption of quinolones; these preparations may be taken six hours before or two hours after taking ciprofloxacin).
- No products indexed under this heading.

Calcium Citrate (Co-administration with calcium-containing products may substantially interfere with the oral absorption of quinolones; these preparations may be taken six hours before or two hours after taking ciprofloxacin). Products include:
- Active Calcium Tablets 3342
- Citracal Tablets 2108

Calcium Glubionate (Co-administration with calcium-containing products may substantially interfere with the oral absorption of quinolones; these preparations may be taken six hours before or two hours after taking ciprofloxacin).
- No products indexed under this heading.

Celecoxib (NSAIDs in combination with very high doses of quinolones have been shown to provoke convulsions in pre-clinical trials). Products include:
- Celebrex Capsules 3130

Chlordiazepoxide (Ciprofloxacin is a moderate inhibitor of CYP450 1A2 isoenzymes. Co-administration of ciprofloxacin and other drugs primarily metabolized by the CYP450 1A2 enzyme pathway may result in increased plasma concentrations of the co-administered drug and couldlead to clinically significant pharmacodynamic side effects).
- No products indexed under this heading.

Chlordiazepoxide Hydrochloride (Ciprofloxacin is a moderate inhibitor of CYP450 1A2 isoenzymes. Co-administration of ciprofloxacin and other drugs primarily metabolized by the CYP450 1A2 enzyme pathway may result in increased plasma concentrations of the co-administered drug and couldlead to clinically significant pharmacodynamic side effects). Products include:
- Librium Capsules 3349

Cimetidine Hydrochloride (Ciprofloxacin is a moderate inhibitor of CYP450 1A2 isoenzymes. Co-administration of ciprofloxacin and other drugs primarily metabolized by the CYP450 1A2 enzyme pathway may result in increased plasma concentrations of the co-administered drug and couldlead to clinically significant pharmacodynamic side effects).
- No products indexed under this heading.

Ciprofloxacin Hydrochloride (Ciprofloxacin is a moderate inhibitor of CYP450 1A2 isoenzymes. Co-administration of ciprofloxacin and other drugs primarily metabolized by the CYP450 1A2 enzyme pathway may result in increased plasma concentrations of the co-administered drug and couldlead to clinically significant pharmacodynamic side effects). Products include:
- Ciloxan Ophthalmic Ointment 554
- Cipro Tablets 2991

Clomipramine Hydrochloride (Ciprofloxacin is a moderate inhibitor of CYP450 1A2 isoenzymes. Co-administration of ciprofloxacin and other drugs primarily metabolized by the CYP450 1A2 enzyme pathway may result in increased plasma concentrations of the co-administered drug and couldlead to clinically significant pharmacodynamic side effects).
- No products indexed under this heading.

Clopidogrel Bisulfate (Ciprofloxacin is a moderate inhibitor of CYP450 1A2 isoenzymes. Co-administration of ciprofloxacin and other drugs primarily metabolized by the CYP450 1A2 enzyme pathway may result in increased plasma concentrations of the co-administered drug and couldlead to clinically significant pharmacodynamic side effects). Products include:
- Plavix Tablets 940
- Plavix Tablets 2942

Clozapine (Ciprofloxacin is a moderate inhibitor of CYP450 1A2 isoenzymes. Co-administration of ciprofloxacin and other drugs primarily metabolized by the CYP450 1A2 enzyme pathway may result in increased plasma concentrations of the co-administered drug and couldlead to clinically significant pharmacodynamic side effects). Products include:
- Clozapine Tablets 2141
- Clozaril Tablets 2174
- FazaClo Orally Disintegrating Tablets 547

Cortisone Acetate (Risk of ruptures of the shoulder, hand, Achilles tendon or other tendons may be increased in patients receiving concomitant corticosteroids, especially in the elderly).
- No products indexed under this heading.

Cyclobenzaprine (Ciprofloxacin is a moderate inhibitor of CYP450 1A2 isoenzymes. Co-administration of ciprofloxacin and other drugs primarily metabolized by the CYP450 1A2 enzyme pathway may result in increased plasma concentrations of the co-administered drug and couldlead to clinically significant pharmacodynamic side effects).
- No products indexed under this heading.

Cyclobenzaprine Hydrochloride (Ciprofloxacin is a moderate inhibitor of CYP450 1A2 isoenzymes. Co-administration of ciprofloxacin and other drugs primarily metabolized by the CYP450 1A2 enzyme pathway may result in increased plasma concentrations of the co-administered drug and couldlead to clinically significant pharmacodynamic side effects). Products include:
- Flexeril Tablets 1832

Cyclosporine (Transient elevations in serum creatinine). Products include:
- Gengraf Capsules 458
- Neoral Soft Gelatin Capsules 2247
- Neoral Oral Solution 2247
- Restasis Ophthalmic Emulsion 570
- Sandimmune 2259

Desipramine Hydrochloride (Ciprofloxacin is a moderate inhibitor of CYP450 1A2 isoenzymes. Co-administration of ciprofloxacin and other drugs primarily metabolized by the CYP450 1A2 enzyme pathway may result in increased plasma concentrations of the co-administered drug and couldlead to clinically significant pharmacodynamic side effects).
- No products indexed under this heading.

Dexamethasone (Risk of ruptures of the shoulder, hand, Achilles tendon or other tendons may be increased in patients receiving concomitant corticosteroids, especially in the elderly). Products include:
- Ciprodex Otic Suspension 555
- Decadron Tablets 1929
- TobraDex Ophthalmic Ointment 558
- TobraDex Ophthalmic Suspension 558

Dexamethasone Acetate (Risk of ruptures of the shoulder, hand, Achilles tendon or other tendons may be increased in patients receiving concomitant corticosteroids, especially in the elderly).
- No products indexed under this heading.

Dexamethasone Sodium Phosphate (Risk of ruptures of the shoulder, hand, Achilles tendon or other tendons may be increased in patients receiving concomitant corticosteroids, especially in the elderly). Products include:
- Decadron Phosphate Injection 1931

Diazepam (Ciprofloxacin is a moderate inhibitor of CYP450 1A2 isoenzymes. Co-administration of ciprofloxacin and other drugs primarily metabolized by the CYP450 1A2 enzyme pathway may result in increased plasma concentrations of the co-administered drug and couldlead to clinically significant pharmacodynamic side effects). Products include:
- Diastat Rectal Delivery System 3344
- Valium Tablets 2822

Diclofenac Potassium (NSAIDs in combination with very high doses of

quinolones have been shown to provoke convulsions in pre-clinical trials). Products include:
Cataflam Tablets **2173**

Diclofenac Sodium (NSAIDs in combination with very high doses of quinolones have been shown to provoke convulsions in pre-clinical trials). Products include:
Arthrotec Tablets **3126**
Voltaren Ophthalmic Solution **2300**
Voltaren Tablets **2298**
Voltaren-XR Tablets **2301**

Dicumarol (Enhanced effects of anticoagulant).
No products indexed under this heading.

Didanosine (Didanosine (Videx) chewable tablets or pediatric powder for oral solution contains aluminum-magnesium-based antacid; co-administration may interfere with Cipro oral absorption; these preparations may be taken six hours before or two hours after taking ciprofloxacin).
No products indexed under this heading.

Diltiazem Hydrochloride (Ciprofloxacin is a moderate inhibitor of CYP450 1A2 isoenzymes. Co-administration of ciprofloxacin and other drugs primarily metabolized by the CYP450 1A2 enzyme pathway may result in increased plasma concentrations of the co-administered drug and couldlead to clinically significant pharmacodynamic side effects). Products include:
Cardizem LA Extended Release Tablets **1699**
Tiazac Capsules **1204**

Diltiazem Maleate (Ciprofloxacin is a moderate inhibitor of CYP450 1A2 isoenzymes. Co-administration of ciprofloxacin and other drugs primarily metabolized by the CYP450 1A2 enzyme pathway may result in increased plasma concentrations of the co-administered drug and could-lead to clinically significant pharmacodynamic side effects).
No products indexed under this heading.

Doxepin Hydrochloride (Ciprofloxacin is a moderate inhibitor of CYP450 1A2 isoenzymes. Co-administration of ciprofloxacin and other drugs primarily metabolized by the CYP450 1A2 enzyme pathway may result in increased plasma concentrations of the co-administered drug and couldlead to clinically significant pharmacodynamic side effects).
No products indexed under this heading.

Dyphylline (Potential for severe and fatal reactions including cardiac arrest, seizures, respiratory failure and status epilepticus; concurrent use should be avoided or serum levels of theophylline should be monitored carefully).
No products indexed under this heading.

Enoxacin (Ciprofloxacin is a moderate inhibitor of CYP450 1A2 isoenzymes. Co-administration of ciprofloxacin and other drugs primarily metabolized by the CYP450 1A2 enzyme pathway may result in increased plasma concentrations of the co-administered drug and could-lead to clinically significant pharmacodynamic side effects).
No products indexed under this heading.

Erythromycin (Ciprofloxacin is a moderate inhibitor of CYP450 1A2 isoenzymes. Co-administration of ciprofloxacin and other drugs primarily metabolized by the CYP450 1A2 enzyme pathway may result in increased plasma concentrations of the co-administered drug and could-lead to clinically significant pharmacodynamic side effects). Products include:
Erygel Topical Gel **2096**
Ery-Tab Tablets **447**
Erythromycin Base Filmtab Tablets **454**
Erythromycin Delayed-Release Capsules, USP **456**
PCE Dispertab Tablets **510**

Erythromycin Estolate (Ciprofloxacin is a moderate inhibitor of CYP450 1A2 isoenzymes. Co-administration of ciprofloxacin and other drugs primarily metabolized by the CYP450 1A2 enzyme pathway may result in increased plasma concentrations of the co-administered drug and couldlead to clinically significant pharmacodynamic side effects).
No products indexed under this heading.

Erythromycin Ethylsuccinate (Ciprofloxacin is a moderate inhibitor of CYP450 1A2 isoenzymes. Co-administration of ciprofloxacin and other drugs primarily metabolized by the CYP450 1A2 enzyme pathway may result in increased plasma concentrations of the co-administered drug and couldlead to clinically significant pharmacodynamic side effects). Products include:
E.E.S. **449**
EryPed **445**

Erythromycin Gluceptate (Ciprofloxacin is a moderate inhibitor of CYP450 1A2 isoenzymes. Co-administration of ciprofloxacin and other drugs primarily metabolized by the CYP450 1A2 enzyme pathway may result in increased plasma concentrations of the co-administered drug and couldlead to clinically significant pharmacodynamic side effects).
No products indexed under this heading.

Erythromycin Lactobionate (Ciprofloxacin is a moderate inhibitor of CYP450 1A2 isoenzymes. Co-administration of ciprofloxacin and other drugs primarily metabolized by the CYP450 1A2 enzyme pathway may result in increased plasma concentrations of the co-administered drug and couldlead to clinically significant pharmacodynamic side effects).
No products indexed under this heading.

Erythromycin Stearate (Ciprofloxacin is a moderate inhibitor of CYP450 1A2 isoenzymes. Co-administration of ciprofloxacin and other drugs primarily metabolized by the CYP450 1A2 enzyme pathway may result in increased plasma concentrations of the co-administered drug and couldlead to clinically significant pharmacodynamic side effects). Products include:
Erythrocin Stearate Filmtab Tablets **452**

Estradiol (Ciprofloxacin is a moderate inhibitor of CYP450 1A2 isoenzymes. Co-administration of ciprofloxacin and other drugs primarily metabolized by the CYP450 1A2 enzyme pathway may result in increased plasma concentrations of the co-administered drug and could-lead to clinically significant pharmacodynamic side effects). Products include:
Activella Tablets **2311**
Climara Transdermal System **795**
Climara Pro Transdermal System **800**
CombiPatch Transdermal System **2180**
Estrogel 0.06% **3200**
Menostar Transdermal System **805**
Prefest Tablets **1069**
Vagifem Tablets **2340**
Vivelle Transdermal System **2288**
Vivelle-Dot Transdermal System **2293**

Estradiol Benzoate (Ciprofloxacin is a moderate inhibitor of CYP450 1A2 isoenzymes. Co-administration of ciprofloxacin and other drugs primarily metabolized by the CYP450 1A2 enzyme pathway may result in increased plasma concentrations of the co-administered drug and could-lead to clinically significant pharmacodynamic side effects).
No products indexed under this heading.

Estradiol Cypionate (Ciprofloxacin is a moderate inhibitor of CYP450 1A2 isoenzymes. Co-administration of ciprofloxacin and other drugs primarily metabolized by the CYP450 1A2 enzyme pathway may result in increased plasma concentrations of the co-administered drug and could-lead to clinically significant pharmacodynamic side effects).
No products indexed under this heading.

Etodolac (NSAIDs in combination with very high doses of quinolones have been shown to provoke convulsions in pre-clinical trials).
No products indexed under this heading.

Fenoprofen Calcium (NSAIDs in combination with very high doses of quinolones have been shown to provoke convulsions in pre-clinical trials). Products include:
Nalfon Capsules **2504**

Ferrous Fumarate (Co-administration with iron-containing products may substantially interfere with the oral absorption of quinolones; these preparations may be taken six hours before or two hours after taking ciprofloxacin). Products include:
Chromagen Forte Soft Gelatin Capsules **3296**
Ferretts Tablets .... ▣**773**
Repliva 21/7 Tablets **3301**

Ferrous Gluconate (Co-administration with iron-containing products may substantially interfere with the oral absorption of quinolones; these preparations may be taken six hours before or two hours after taking ciprofloxacin).
No products indexed under this heading.

Ferrous Sulfate (Co-administration with iron-containing products may substantially interfere with the oral absorption of quinolones; these preparations may be taken six hours before or two hours after taking ciprofloxacin). Products include:
Feosol Tablets **1629**
Slow Fe Iron Tablets .... ▣**772**
Slow Fe with Folic Acid Tablets .... ▣**773**

Fludrocortisone Acetate (Risk of ruptures of the shoulder, hand, Achilles tendon or other tendons may be increased in patients receiving concomitant corticosteroids, especially in the elderly).
No products indexed under this heading.

Flurbiprofen (NSAIDs in combination with very high doses of quinolones have been shown to provoke convulsions in pre-clinical trials).
No products indexed under this heading.

Flutamide (Ciprofloxacin is a moderate inhibitor of CYP450 1A2 isoenzymes. Co-administration of ciprofloxacin and other drugs primarily metabolized by the CYP450 1A2 enzyme pathway may result in increased plasma concentrations of the co-administered drug and could-lead to clinically significant pharmacodynamic side effects). Products include:
Eulexin Capsules **3023**

Fluticasone Propionate (Ciprofloxacin is a moderate inhibitor of CYP450 1A2 isoenzymes. Co-administration of ciprofloxacin and other drugs primarily metabolized by the CYP450 1A2 enzyme pathway may result in increased plasma concentrations of the co-administered drug and couldlead to clinically significant pharmacodynamic side effects). Products include:
Advair Diskus 100/50 .... **1291**
Advair Diskus 250/50 .... **1291**
Advair Diskus 500/50 .... **1291**
Cutivate Cream **1381**
Cutivate Lotion 0.05% **1383**
Cutivate Ointment **1384**
Flonase Nasal Spray **1412**
Flovent Diskus 100 mcg **1418**
Flovent Diskus 50 mcg **1415**

Fluvoxamine Maleate (Ciprofloxacin is a moderate inhibitor of CYP450 1A2 isoenzymes. Co-administration of ciprofloxacin and other drugs primarily metabolized by the CYP450 1A2 enzyme pathway may result in increased plasma concentrations of the co-administered drug and couldlead to clinically significant pharmacodynamic side effects).
No products indexed under this heading.

Fosphenytoin Sodium (Potential for change in serum phenytoin levels).
No products indexed under this heading.

Glyburide (Co-administration, on rare occasions, has resulted in severe hypoglycemia).
No products indexed under this heading.

Grepafloxacin Hydrochloride (Ciprofloxacin is a moderate inhibitor of CYP450 1A2 isoenzymes. Co-administration of ciprofloxacin and other drugs primarily metabolized by the CYP450 1A2 enzyme pathway may result in increased plasma concentrations of the co-administered drug and couldlead to clinically significant pharmacodynamic side effects).
No products indexed under this heading.

Haloperidol (Ciprofloxacin is a moderate inhibitor of CYP450 1A2 isoenzymes. Co-administration of ciprofloxacin and other drugs primarily metabolized by the CYP450 1A2 enzyme pathway may result in increased plasma concentrations of the co-administered drug and couldlead to clinically significant pharmacodynamic side effects).
No products indexed under this heading.

Haloperidol Decanoate (Ciprofloxacin is a moderate inhibitor of CYP450 1A2 isoenzymes. Co-administration of ciprofloxacin and other drugs primarily metabolized by the CYP450 1A2 enzyme pathway may result in increased plasma concentrations of the co-administered drug and couldlead to clinically significant pharmacodynamic side effects).
No products indexed under this heading.

Haloperidol Lactate (Ciprofloxacin is a moderate inhibitor of CYP450 1A2 isoenzymes. Co-administration of ciprofloxacin and other drugs primarily metabolized by the CYP450 1A2 enzyme pathway may result in increased plasma concentrations of the co-administered drug and couldlead to clinically significant pharmacodynamic side effects).
No products indexed under this heading.

Hydrocortisone (Risk of ruptures of the shoulder, hand, Achilles tendon or other tendons may be increased in patients receiving concomitant corticosteroids, especially in the elderly). Products include:
Cortizone•5 Ointment 699
Cortizone•10 Creme 699
Cortizone•10 Ointment 699
Cortizone•10 Plus Creme 700
Cortizone•10 Maximum Strength Quick Shot Spray 700
Hydrocortone Tablets 1963
Preparation H Hydrocortisone Cream 748

Hydrocortisone Acetate (Risk of ruptures of the shoulder, hand, Achilles tendon or other tendons may be increased in patients receiving concomitant corticosteroids, especially in the elderly). Products include:
Analpram-HC 1136
Pramosone 1139
ProctoFoam-HC 3113
Tucks Anti-Itch Ointment 712
U-cort 1% Cream 3289

Hydrocortisone Sodium Phosphate (Risk of ruptures of the shoulder, hand, Achilles tendon or other tendons may be increased in patients receiving concomitant corticosteroids, especially in the elderly).
No products indexed under this heading.

Hydrocortisone Sodium Succinate (Risk of ruptures of the shoulder, hand, Achilles tendon or other tendons may be increased in patients receiving concomitant corticosteroids, especially in the elderly).
No products indexed under this heading.

Ibuprofen (NSAIDs in combination with very high doses of quinolones have been shown to provoke convulsions in pre-clinical trials). Products include:
Advil Allergy Sinus Caplets 737
Advil 737
Children's Advil Suspension 742
Children's Advil Chewable Tablets .. 741
Advil Cold & Sinus 739
Advil Flu & Body Ache Caplets 739
Children's Advil Cold Suspension ... 741
Infants' Advil Concentrated Drops .. 743
Junior Strength Advil Swallow Tablets 740
Advil Migraine Liquigels 740
Advil Multi-Symptom Cold Caplets 738
Combunox Tablets 1183
Children's Motrin Oral Suspension and Chewable Tablets 1837
Children's Motrin Cold Non-Staining Dye-Free Oral Suspension 1838
Children's Motrin Cold Oral Suspension 1838
Children's Motrin Non-Staining Dye-Free Oral Suspension............ 1837
Motrin Cold & Sinus Caplets 1836
Motrin IB Tablets and Caplets 1836
Infants' Motrin Concentrated Drops 1837
Infants' Motrin Non-Staining Dye-Free Drops............................ 1837
Junior Strength Motrin Caplets and Chewable Tablets.................. 1837
Vicoprofen Tablets 533

Imipramine Hydrochloride (Ciprofloxacin is a moderate inhibitor of CYP450 1A2 isoenzymes. Co-administration of ciprofloxacin and other drugs primarily metabolized by the CYP450 1A2 enzyme pathway may result in increased plasma concentrations of the co-administered drug and couldlead to clinically significant pharmacodynamic side effects).
No products indexed under this heading.

Imipramine Pamoate (Ciprofloxacin is a moderate inhibitor of CYP450 1A2 isoenzymes. Co-administration of ciprofloxacin and other drugs primarily metabolized by the CYP450 1A2 enzyme pathway may result in increased plasma concentrations of the co-administered drug and couldlead to clinically significant pharmacodynamic side effects).
No products indexed under this heading.

Indomethacin (NSAIDs in combination with very high doses of quinolones have been shown to provoke convulsions in pre-clinical trials). Products include:
Indocin 1968

Indomethacin Sodium Trihydrate (NSAIDs in combination with very high doses of quinolones have been shown to provoke convulsions in pre-clinical trials). Products include:
Indocin I.V. 1973

Iron (Co-administration with iron-containing products may substantially interfere with the oral absorption of quinolones; these preparations may be taken six hours before or two hours after taking ciprofloxacin). Products include:
Chromagen Forte Soft Gelatin Capsules 3296
Ferretts IPS Liquid 773
OptiNate 1162
Repliva 21/7 Tablets 3301

Ketoprofen (NSAIDs in combination with very high doses of quinolones have been shown to provoke convulsions in pre-clinical trials).
No products indexed under this heading.

Ketorolac Tromethamine (NSAIDs in combination with very high doses of quinolones have been shown to provoke convulsions in pre-clinical trials). Products include:
Acular Ophthalmic Solution 561
Acular LS Ophthalmic Solution 562

Levobupivacaine Hydrochloride (Ciprofloxacin is a moderate inhibitor of CYP450 1A2 isoenzymes. Co-administration of ciprofloxacin and other drugs primarily metabolized by the CYP450 1A2 enzyme pathway may result in increased plasma concentrations of the co-administered drug and couldlead to clinically significant pharmacodynamic side effects).
No products indexed under this heading.

Lomefloxacin Hydrochloride (Ciprofloxacin is a moderate inhibitor of CYP450 1A2 isoenzymes. Co-administration of ciprofloxacin and other drugs primarily metabolized by the CYP450 1A2 enzyme pathway may result in increased plasma concentrations of the co-administered drug and couldlead to clinically significant pharmacodynamic side effects).
No products indexed under this heading.

Magaldrate (Concurrent administration of these antacids may substantially interfere with the oral absorption of ciprofloxacin; antacids may be administered either two hours after or six hours before ciprofloxacin dosing without a significant decrease in bioavailability).
No products indexed under this heading.

Magnesium Hydroxide (Concurrent administration of these antacids may substantially interfere with the oral absorption of ciprofloxacin; antacids may be administered either two hours after or six hours before ciprofloxacin dosing without a significant decrease in bioavailability). Products include:
Maalox Max Maximum Strength Antacid/Anti-Gas Liquid................ 2165
Maalox Regular Strength Antacid/Antigas Liquid................. 2164
Pepcid Complete Chewable Tablets 1672
Rolaids Tablets 707
Extra Strength Rolaids Tablets 707
Rolaids Multi-Symptom Antacid & Antigas Tablets 708

Magnesium Oxide (Concurrent administration of these antacids may substantially interfere with the oral absorption of ciprofloxacin; antacids may be administered either two hours after or six hours before ciprofloxacin dosing without a significant decrease in bioavailability). Products include:
Beelith Tablets 784
PremCal Light, Regular, and Extra Strength Tablets................ 762

Maprotiline Hydrochloride (Ciprofloxacin is a moderate inhibitor of CYP450 1A2 isoenzymes. Co-administration of ciprofloxacin and other drugs primarily metabolized by the CYP450 1A2 enzyme pathway may result in increased plasma concentrations of the co-administered drug and couldlead to clinically significant pharmacodynamic side effects).
No products indexed under this heading.

Meclofenamate Sodium (NSAIDs in combination with very high doses of quinolones have been shown to provoke convulsions in pre-clinical trials).
No products indexed under this heading.

Mefenamic Acid (NSAIDs in combination with very high doses of quinolones have been shown to provoke convulsions in pre-clinical trials).
No products indexed under this heading.

Meloxicam (NSAIDs in combination with very high doses of quinolones have been shown to provoke convulsions in pre-clinical trials). Products include:
Mobic Oral Suspension 893
Mobic Tablets 893

Methadone Hydrochloride (Ciprofloxacin is a moderate inhibitor of CYP450 1A2 isoenzymes. Co-administration of ciprofloxacin and other drugs primarily metabolized by the CYP450 1A2 enzyme pathway may result in increased plasma concentrations of the co-administered drug and couldlead to clinically significant pharmacodynamic side effects).
No products indexed under this heading.

Methotrexate (Renal tubular transport of methotrexate may be inhibited by concomitant administration of ciprofloxacin potentially leading to increased plasma levels of methotrexate).
No products indexed under this heading.

Methotrexate Sodium (Renal tubular transport of methotrexate may be inhibited by concomitant administration of ciprofloxacin potentially leading to increased plasma levels of methotrexate).
No products indexed under this heading.

Methylprednisolone Acetate (Risk of ruptures of the shoulder, hand, Achilles tendon or other tendons may be increased in patients receiving concomitant corticosteroids, especially in the elderly). Products include:
Depo-Medrol Injectable Suspension 2615
Depo-Medrol Single-Dose Vial 2617

Methylprednisolone Sodium Succinate (Risk of ruptures of the shoulder, hand, Achilles tendon or other tendons may be increased in patients receiving concomitant corticosteroids, especially in the elderly).
No products indexed under this heading.

Metoclopramide Hydrochloride (Metoclopramide significantly accelerates the absorption of oral ciprofloxacin resulting in a shorter time to reach maximum plasma concentrations).
No products indexed under this heading.

Mexiletine Hydrochloride (Ciprofloxacin is a moderate inhibitor of CYP450 1A2 isoenzymes. Co-administration of ciprofloxacin and other drugs primarily metabolized by the CYP450 1A2 enzyme pathway may result in increased plasma concentrations of the co-administered drug and couldlead to clinically significant pharmacodynamic side effects).
No products indexed under this heading.

Mirtazapine (Ciprofloxacin is a moderate inhibitor of CYP450 1A2 isoenzymes. Co-administration of ciprofloxacin and other drugs primarily metabolized by the CYP450 1A2 enzyme pathway may result in increased plasma concentrations of the co-administered drug and couldlead to clinically significant pharmacodynamic side effects).
No products indexed under this heading.

Moxifloxacin Hydrochloride (Ciprofloxacin is a moderate inhibitor of CYP450 1A2 isoenzymes. Co-administration of ciprofloxacin and other drugs primarily metabolized by the CYP450 1A2 enzyme pathway may result in increased plasma concentrations of the co-administered drug and couldlead to clinically significant pharmacodynamic side effects). Products include:
Avelox 2984
Vigamox Ophthalmic Solution 560

Nabumetone (NSAIDs in combination with very high doses of quinolones have been shown to provoke convulsions in pre-clinical trials). Products include:
Relafen Tablets 1523

Nafcillin Sodium (Ciprofloxacin is a moderate inhibitor of CYP450 1A2 isoenzymes. Co-administration of ciprofloxacin and other drugs primarily metabolized by the CYP450 1A2 enzyme pathway may result in increased plasma concentrations of the co-administered drug and couldlead to clinically significant pharmacodynamic side effects).
No products indexed under this heading.

Naproxen (NSAIDs in combination with very high doses of quinolones have been shown to provoke convulsions in pre-clinical trials). Products include:
EC-Naprosyn Delayed-Release Tablets 2769
Naprosyn Suspension 2769
Naprosyn Tablets 2769
Prevacid NapraPAC 3277

Naproxen Sodium (NSAIDs in combination with very high doses of quinolones have been shown to provoke convulsions in pre-clinical trials). Products include:
Aleve Tablets, Caplets and Gelcaps .... ▣605
Anaprox Tablets 2769
Anaprox DS Tablets 2769

Nicotine Polacrilex (Ciprofloxacin is a moderate inhibitor of CYP450 1A2 isoenzymes. Co-administration of ciprofloxacin and other drugs primarily metabolized by the CYP450 1A2 enzyme pathway may result in increased plasma concentrations of the co-administered drug and couldlead to clinically significant pharmacodynamic side effects). Products include:
Commit Lozenges 1625
Nicorette Gum 1632

Nicotine Salicylate (Ciprofloxacin is a moderate inhibitor of CYP450 1A2 isoenzymes. Co-administration of ciprofloxacin and other drugs primarily metabolized by the CYP450 1A2 enzyme pathway may result in increased plasma concentrations of the co-administered drug and couldlead to clinically significant pharmacodynamic side effects).
No products indexed under this heading.

Nicotine Sulfate (Ciprofloxacin is a moderate inhibitor of CYP450 1A2 isoenzymes. Co-administration of ciprofloxacin and other drugs primarily metabolized by the CYP450 1A2 enzyme pathway may result in increased plasma concentrations of the co-administered drug and couldlead to clinically significant pharmacodynamic side effects).
No products indexed under this heading.

Norethindrone Acetate (Ciprofloxacin is a moderate inhibitor of CYP450 1A2 isoenzymes. Co-administration of ciprofloxacin and other drugs primarily metabolized by the CYP450 1A2 enzyme pathway may result in increased plasma concentrations of the co-administered drug and couldlead to clinically significant pharmacodynamic side effects). Products include:
Activella Tablets 2311
Aygestin Tablets 1062
CombiPatch Transdermal System 2180

Norfloxacin (Ciprofloxacin is a moderate inhibitor of CYP450 1A2 isoenzymes. Co-administration of ciprofloxacin and other drugs primarily metabolized by the CYP450 1A2 enzyme pathway may result in increased plasma concentrations of the co-administered drug and couldlead to clinically significant pharmacodynamic side effects). Products include:
Noroxin Tablets 2009

Nortriptyline Hydrochloride (Ciprofloxacin is a moderate inhibitor of CYP450 1A2 isoenzymes. Co-administration of ciprofloxacin and other drugs primarily metabolized by the CYP450 1A2 enzyme pathway may result in increased plasma concentrations of the co-administered drug and couldlead to clinically significant pharmacodynamic side effects).
No products indexed under this heading.

Ofloxacin (Ciprofloxacin is a moderate inhibitor of CYP450 1A2 isoenzymes. Co-administration of ciprofloxacin and other drugs primarily metabolized by the CYP450 1A2 enzyme pathway may result in increased plasma concentrations of the co-administered drug and couldlead to clinically significant pharmacodynamic side effects). Products include:
Floxin Otic Singles 1045
Floxin Otic Solution 1043

Olanzapine (Ciprofloxacin is a moderate inhibitor of CYP450 1A2 isoenzymes. Co-administration of ciprofloxacin and other drugs primarily metabolized by the CYP450 1A2 enzyme pathway may result in increased plasma concentrations of the co-administered drug and couldlead to clinically significant pharmacodynamic side effects). Products include:
Symbyax Capsules 1788
Zyprexa Tablets 1798
Zyprexa IntraMuscular 1798
Zyprexa ZYDIS Orally Disintegrating Tablets 1798

Ondansetron (Ciprofloxacin is a moderate inhibitor of CYP450 1A2 isoenzymes. Co-administration of ciprofloxacin and other drugs primarily metabolized by the CYP450 1A2 enzyme pathway may result in increased plasma concentrations of the co-administered drug and couldlead to clinically significant pharmacodynamic side effects). Products include:
Zofran ODT Orally Disintegrating Tablets 1613

Ondansetron Hydrochloride (Ciprofloxacin is a moderate inhibitor of CYP450 1A2 isoenzymes. Co-administration of ciprofloxacin and other drugs primarily metabolized by the CYP450 1A2 enzyme pathway may result in increased plasma concentrations of the co-administered drug and couldlead to clinically significant pharmacodynamic side effects). Products include:
Zofran Injection 1607
Zofran 1613

Oxaprozin (NSAIDs in combination with very high doses of quinolones have been shown to provoke convulsions in pre-clinical trials).
No products indexed under this heading.

Phenobarbital Sodium (Ciprofloxacin is a moderate inhibitor of CYP450 1A2 isoenzymes. Co-administration of ciprofloxacin and other drugs primarily metabolized by the CYP450 1A2 enzyme pathway may result in increased plasma concentrations of the co-administered drug and couldlead to clinically significant pharmacodynamic side effects).
No products indexed under this heading.

Phenylbutazone (NSAIDs in combination with very high doses of quinolones have been shown to provoke convulsions in pre-clinical trials).
No products indexed under this heading.

Phenytoin (Potential for change in serum phenytoin levels).
No products indexed under this heading.

Phenytoin Sodium (Potential for change in serum phenytoin levels). Products include:
Phenytek Capsules 2153

Piroxicam (NSAIDs in combination with very high doses of quinolones have been shown to provoke convulsions in pre-clinical trials).
No products indexed under this heading.

Polysaccharide Iron Complex (Co-administration with iron-containing products may substantially interfere with the oral absorption of quinolones; these preparations may be taken six hours before or two hours after taking ciprofloxacin). Products include:
Niferex-150 Forte Capsules 3299
Nu-Iron 150 Capsules 2098

Prednisolone Acetate (Risk of ruptures of the shoulder, hand, Achilles tendon or other tendons may be increased in patients receiving concomitant corticosteroids, especially in the elderly). Products include:
Blephamide Ophthalmic Ointment 563
Blephamide Ophthalmic Suspension 564
Poly-Pred Liquifilm Ophthalmic Suspension .... ⊙231
Pred Forte Ophthalmic Suspension .... ⊙233
Pred Mild Sterile Ophthalmic Suspension .... ⊙236
Pred-G Ophthalmic Suspension .... ⊙234
Pred-G Sterile Ophthalmic Ointment .... ⊙235

Prednisolone Sodium Phosphate (Risk of ruptures of the shoulder, hand, Achilles tendon or other tendons may be increased in patients receiving concomitant corticosteroids, especially in the elderly). Products include:
Pediapred Oral Solution 3319

Prednisolone Tebutate (Risk of ruptures of the shoulder, hand, Achilles tendon or other tendons may be increased in patients receiving concomitant corticosteroids, especially in the elderly).
No products indexed under this heading.

Prednisone (Risk of ruptures of the shoulder, hand, Achilles tendon or other tendons may be increased in patients receiving concomitant corticosteroids, especially in the elderly).
No products indexed under this heading.

Probenecid (Interferes with renal tubular secretion of ciprofloxacin).
No products indexed under this heading.

Propafenone Hydrochloride (Ciprofloxacin is a moderate inhibitor of CYP450 1A2 isoenzymes. Co-administration of ciprofloxacin and other drugs primarily metabolized by the CYP450 1A2 enzyme pathway may result in increased plasma concentrations of the co-administered drug and couldlead to clinically significant pharmacodynamic side effects). Products include:
Rythmol SR Capsules 2736

Propranolol Hydrochloride (Ciprofloxacin is a moderate inhibitor of CYP450 1A2 isoenzymes. Co-administration of ciprofloxacin and other drugs primarily metabolized by the CYP450 1A2 enzyme pathway may result in increased plasma concentrations of the co-administered drug and couldlead to clinically significant pharmacodynamic side effects). Products include:
Inderal LA Long-Acting Capsules 3421
InnoPran XL Capsules 2728

Protriptyline Hydrochloride (Ciprofloxacin is a moderate inhibitor of CYP450 1A2 isoenzymes. Co-administration of ciprofloxacin and other drugs primarily metabolized by the CYP450 1A2 enzyme pathway may result in increased plasma concentrations of the co-administered drug and couldlead to clinically significant pharmacodynamic side effects). Products include:
Vivactil Tablets 2350

Riluzole (Ciprofloxacin is a moderate inhibitor of CYP450 1A2 isoenzymes. Co-administration of ciprofloxacin and other drugs primarily metabolized by the CYP450 1A2 enzyme pathway may result in increased plasma concentrations of the co-administered drug and couldlead to clinically significant pharmacodynamic side effects). Products include:
Rilutek Tablets 2945

Ritonavir (Ciprofloxacin is a moderate inhibitor of CYP450 1A2 isoenzymes. Co-administration of ciprofloxacin and other drugs primarily metabolized by the CYP450 1A2 enzyme pathway may result in increased plasma concentrations of the co-administered drug and couldlead to clinically significant pharmacodynamic side effects). Products include:
Kaletra 474
Norvir 499

Rofecoxib (NSAIDs in combination with very high doses of quinolones have been shown to provoke convulsions in pre-clinical trials).
No products indexed under this heading.

Ropinirole Hydrochloride (Ciprofloxacin is a moderate inhibitor of CYP450 1A2 isoenzymes. Co-administration of ciprofloxacin and other drugs primarily metabolized by the CYP450 1A2 enzyme pathway may result in increased plasma concentrations of the co-administered drug and couldlead to clinically significant pharmacodynamic side effects). Products include:
Requip Tablets 1528

Ropivacaine Hydrochloride (Ciprofloxacin is a moderate inhibitor of CYP450 1A2 isoenzymes. Co-administration of ciprofloxacin and other drugs primarily metabolized by the CYP450 1A2 enzyme pathway may result in increased plasma concentrations of the co-administered drug and couldlead to clinically significant pharmacodynamic side effects). Products include:
Naropin Injection 640

Sucralfate (Co-administration with sucralfate may substantially interfere with the oral absorption of quinolones; these preparations may be taken six hours before or two hours after taking ciprofloxacin). Products include:
Carafate Suspension 727
Carafate Tablets 728

Sulindac (NSAIDs in combination with very high doses of quinolones have been shown to provoke convulsions in pre-clinical trials). Products include:
Clinoril Tablets 1899

Tacrine Hydrochloride (Ciprofloxacin is a moderate inhibitor of CYP450 1A2 isoenzymes. Co-administration of ciprofloxacin and other drugs primarily metabolized by the CYP450 1A2 enzyme pathway may result in increased plasma concentrations of the co-administered drug and couldlead to clinically significant pharmacodynamic side effects).
No products indexed under this heading.

Tamoxifen Citrate (Ciprofloxacin is a moderate inhibitor of CYP450 1A2 isoenzymes. Co-administration of ciprofloxacin and other drugs primarily metabolized by the CYP450 1A2 enzyme pathway may result in increased plasma concentrations of the co-administered drug and couldlead to clinically significant pharmacodynamic side effects).
No products indexed under this heading.

Theophylline (Potential for severe and fatal reactions including cardiac arrest, seizures, respiratory failure and status epilepticus; concurrent use should be avoided or serum levels of theophylline should be monitored carefully).
No products indexed under this heading.

Theophylline Anhydrous (Potential for severe and fatal reactions including cardiac arrest, seizures, respiratory failure and status epilepticus; concurrent use should be avoided or serum levels of theophylline should be monitored carefully). Products include:
Uniphyl Tablets 2708

Theophylline Calcium Salicylate (Potential for severe and fatal reactions including cardiac arrest, seizures, respiratory failure and status epilepticus; concurrent use should be avoided or serum levels of theophylline should be monitored carefully).
No products indexed under this heading.

Theophylline Dihydroxypropyl (Glyceryl) (Potential for severe and fatal reactions including cardiac arrest, seizures, respiratory failure and status epilepticus; concurrent use should be avoided or serum levels of theophylline should be monitored carefully).
No products indexed under this heading.

Theophylline Ethylenediamine (Potential for severe and fatal reactions including cardiac arrest, seizures, respiratory failure and status epilepticus; concurrent use should be avoided or serum levels of theophylline should be monitored carefully).
No products indexed under this heading.

Theophylline Sodium Glycinate (Potential for severe and fatal reactions including cardiac arrest, seizures, respiratory failure and status epilepticus; concurrent use should be avoided or serum levels of theophylline should be monitored carefully).
No products indexed under this heading.

Tizanidine Hydrochloride (Co-administration of ciprofloxacin with tizanidine can significantly increase tizanidine serum concentrations. Potentiated hypotensive and sedative effects have been observed. Co-administation of tizanidine and ciprofloxacin must be avoided).
No products indexed under this heading.

Tolmetin Sodium (NSAIDs in combination with very high doses of quinolones have been shown to provoke convulsions in pre-clinical trials).
No products indexed under this heading.

Triamcinolone (Risk of ruptures of the shoulder, hand, Achilles tendon or other tendons may be increased in patients receiving concomitant corticosteroids, especially in the elderly).
No products indexed under this heading.

Triamcinolone Acetonide (Risk of ruptures of the shoulder, hand, Achilles tendon or other tendons may be increased in patients receiving concomitant corticosteroids, especially in the elderly). Products include:
Azmacort Inhalation Aerosol 1701
Nasacort HFA Inhalation Aerosol 2939
Nasacort AQ Nasal Spray 2937

Triamcinolone Diacetate (Risk of ruptures of the shoulder, hand, Achilles tendon or other tendons may be increased in patients receiving concomitant corticosteroids, especially in the elderly).
No products indexed under this heading.

Triamcinolone Hexacetonide (Risk of ruptures of the shoulder, hand, Achilles tendon or other tendons may be increased in patients receiving concomitant corticosteroids, especially in the elderly).
No products indexed under this heading.

Trimethaphan Camsylate (Ciprofloxacin is a moderate inhibitor of CYP450 1A2 isoenzymes. Co-administration of ciprofloxacin and other drugs primarily metabolized by the CYP450 1A2 enzyme pathway may result in increased plasma concentrations of the co-administered drug and couldlead to clinically significant pharmacodynamic side effects).
No products indexed under this heading.

Trimipramine Maleate (Ciprofloxacin is a moderate inhibitor of CYP450 1A2 isoenzymes. Co-administration of ciprofloxacin and other drugs primarily metabolized by the CYP450 1A2 enzyme pathway may result in increased plasma concentrations of the co-administered drug and couldlead to clinically significant pharmacodynamic side effects). Products include:
Surmontil Capsules 2347

Trovafloxacin Mesylate (Ciprofloxacin is a moderate inhibitor of CYP450 1A2 isoenzymes. Co-administration of ciprofloxacin and other drugs primarily metabolized by the CYP450 1A2 enzyme pathway may result in increased plasma concentrations of the co-administered drug and couldlead to clinically significant pharmacodynamic side effects).
No products indexed under this heading.

Valdecoxib (NSAIDs in combination with very high doses of quinolones have been shown to provoke convulsions in pre-clinical trials).
No products indexed under this heading.

Verapamil Hydrochloride (Ciprofloxacin is a moderate inhibitor of CYP450 1A2 isoenzymes. Co-administration of ciprofloxacin and other drugs primarily metabolized by the CYP450 1A2 enzyme pathway may result in increased plasma concentrations of the co-administered drug and couldlead to clinically significant pharmacodynamic side effects). Products include:
Covera-HS Tablets 3135
Tarka Tablets 519
Verelan PM Capsules 3120

Warfarin Sodium (Enhanced effects of anticoagulant). Products include:
Coumadin for Injection 932
Coumadin Tablets 932

Zileuton (Ciprofloxacin is a moderate inhibitor of CYP450 1A2 isoenzymes. Co-administration of ciprofloxacin and other drugs primarily metabolized by the CYP450 1A2 enzyme pathway may result in increased plasma concentrations of the co-administered drug and couldlead to clinically significant pharmacodynamic side effects).
No products indexed under this heading.

Zinc Sulfate (Co-administration with zinc-containing products may substantially interfere with the oral absorption of quinolones; these preparations may be taken six hours before or two hours after taking ciprofloxacin). Products include:
Athena Hair System Shampoo 767
Spartan Hair System Shampoo 767
Visine A.C. Seasonal Itching and Redness Relief Drops .... ⊙ 278
Zinc-220 Capsules 576

Zolmitriptan (Ciprofloxacin is a moderate inhibitor of CYP450 1A2 isoenzymes. Co-administration of ciprofloxacin and other drugs primarily metabolized by the CYP450 1A2 enzyme pathway may result in increased plasma concentrations of the co-administered drug and couldlead to clinically significant pharmacodynamic side effects). Products include:
Zomig Nasal Spray 718
Zomig Tablets 714
Zomig-ZMT Tablets 714

Food Interactions

Dairy products (Oral ciprofloxacin should not be taken concurrently with milk or yogurt alone, since absorption of ciprofloxacin may be significantly reduced; dietary calcium as part of a meal; however, does not significantly affect ciprofloxacin absorption).

Food, unspecified (Delays the oral absorption of the drug resulting in peak concentrations that are closer to two hours after dosing).

CIPRO I.V. PHARMACY BULK PACKAGE

(Ciprofloxacin) 3509
May interact with:

See (Cipro I.V).

CIPRO ORAL SUSPENSION

(Ciprofloxacin) 2991
See Cipro Tablets

CIPRO TABLETS

(Ciprofloxacin Hydrochloride) 2991
May interact with antacids containing aluminum, calcium and magnesium, calcium preparations, corticosteroids, oral anticoagulants, iron containing oral preparations, nonsteroidal anti-inflammatory agents, phenytoin, xanthines, and certain other agents. Compounds in these categories include:

Aluminum Carbonate (Concurrent administration of these antacids may substantially interfere with the oral absorption of ciprofloxacin; antacids may be administered either two hours after or six hours before ciprofloxacin dosing without a significant decrease in bioavailability).
No products indexed under this heading.

Aluminum Hydroxide (Concurrent administration of these antacids may substantially interfere with the oral absorption of ciprofloxacin; antacids may be administered either two hours after or six hours before ciprofloxacin dosing without a significant decrease in bioavailability). Products include:
Gaviscon Regular Strength Liquid .. 620
Gaviscon Regular Strength Tablets 619
Gaviscon Extra Strength Liquid 620
Gaviscon Extra Strength Tablets 619
Maalox Max Maximum Strength Antacid/Anti-Gas Liquid 2165
Maalox Regular Strength Antacid/Antigas Liquid 2164

Aminophylline (Potential for severe and fatal reactions including cardiac arrest, seizures, respiratory failure and status epilepticus; concurrent use should be avoided or serum levels of theophylline should be monitored carefully).
No products indexed under this heading.

Anisindione (Enhanced effects of anticoagulant). Products include:
- Miradon Tablets ... 3056

Betamethasone Acetate (Risk of ruptures of the shoulder, hand, Achilles tendon or other tendons may be increased in patients receiving concomitant corticosteroids, especially in the elderly).
No products indexed under this heading.

Betamethasone Sodium Phosphate (Risk of ruptures of the shoulder, hand, Achilles tendon or other tendons may be increased in patients receiving concomitant corticosteroids, especially in the elderly).
No products indexed under this heading.

Caffeine (Reduced clearance of caffeine and a prolongation of its serum half-life). Products include:
- Athena Hair System Shampoo ... ■767
- BC Powder ... ■612
- Arthritis Strength BC Powder ... ■612
- Goody's Extra Strength Headache Powder ... ■621
- Goody's Extra Strength Pain Relief Tablets ... ■621
- Hycomine Compound Tablets ... 1105
- Spartan Hair System Shampoo ... ■767
- Vivarin ... ■639

Caffeine Citrate (Reduced clearance of caffeine and a prolongation of its serum half-like). Products include:
- Cafcit ... 1854

Calcium Carbonate (Co-administration with calcium-containing products may substantially interfere with the oral absorption of quinolones; these preparations may be taken six hours before or two hours after taking ciprofloxacin). Products include:
- Actonel with Calcium Tablets ... 2684
- Caltrate 600 PLUS Chewables ... ■779
- Caltrate 600 PLUS Tablets ... ■779
- Caltrate 600 + D Tablets ... ■779
- Encora Capsules ... 3298
- Encora AM Tablets ... 3298
- Encora PM Tablets ... 3298
- Gas-X with Maalox ... ■675
- Maalox Regular Strength Antacid Tablets ... 2166
- Quick Dissolve Maalox Max Maximum Strength Antacid/Antigas Tablets ... 2165
- Maalox Max Quick Dissolve Maximum Strength Chewable Tablets ... ■678
- Os-Cal Chewable Tablets ... ■765
- Pepcid Complete Chewable Tablets ... 1672
- PremCal Light, Regular, and Extra Strength Tablets ... ■762
- Rolaids Tablets ... ■707
- Extra Strength Rolaids Softchews ... ■708
- Extra Strength Rolaids Tablets ... ■707
- Rolaids Multi-Symptom Antacid & Antigas Tablets ... ■708
- Tums ... ■639

Calcium Chloride (Co-administration with calcium-containing products may substantially interfere with the oral absorption of quinolones; these preparations may be taken six hours before or two hours after taking ciprofloxacin).
No products indexed under this heading.

Calcium Citrate (Co-administration with calcium-containing products may substantially interfere with the oral absorption of quinolones; these preparations may be taken six hours before or two hours after taking ciprofloxacin). Products include:
- Active Calcium Tablets ... 3342
- Citracal Tablets ... 2108

Calcium Glubionate (Co-administration with calcium-containing products may substantially interfere with the oral absorption of quinolones; these preparations may be taken six hours before or two hours after taking ciprofloxacin).
No products indexed under this heading.

Celecoxib (NSAIDs in combination with very high doses of quinolones have been shown to provoke convulsions in pre-clinical trials). Products include:
- Celebrex Capsules ... 3130

Cortisone Acetate (Risk of ruptures of the shoulder, hand, Achilles tendon or other tendons may be increased in patients receiving concomitant corticosteroids, especially in the elderly).
No products indexed under this heading.

Cyclosporine (Transient elevations in serum creatinine). Products include:
- Gengraf Capsules ... 458
- Neoral Soft Gelatin Capsules ... 2247
- Neoral Oral Solution ... 2247
- Restasis Ophthalmic Emulsion ... 570
- Sandimmune ... 2259

Dexamethasone (Risk of ruptures of the shoulder, hand, Achilles tendon or other tendons may be increased in patients receiving concomitant corticosteroids, especially in the elderly). Products include:
- Ciprodex Otic Suspension ... 555
- Decadron Tablets ... 1929
- TobraDex Ophthalmic Ointment ... 558
- TobraDex Ophthalmic Suspension ... 558

Dexamethasone Acetate (Risk of ruptures of the shoulder, hand, Achilles tendon or other tendons may be increased in patients receiving concomitant corticosteroids, especially in the elderly).
No products indexed under this heading.

Dexamethasone Sodium Phosphate (Risk of ruptures of the shoulder, hand, Achilles tendon or other tendons may be increased in patients receiving concomitant corticosteroids, especially in the elderly). Products include:
- Decadron Phosphate Injection ... 1931

Diclofenac Potassium (NSAIDs in combination with very high doses of quinolones have been shown to provoke convulsions in pre-clinical trials). Products include:
- Cataflam Tablets ... 2173

Diclofenac Sodium (NSAIDs in combination with very high doses of quinolones have been shown to provoke convulsions in pre-clinical trials). Products include:
- Arthrotec Tablets ... 3126
- Voltaren Ophthalmic Solution ... 2300
- Voltaren Tablets ... 2298
- Voltaren-XR Tablets ... 2301

Dicumarol (Enhanced effects of anticoagulant).
No products indexed under this heading.

Didanosine (Didanosine (Videx) chewable tablets or pediatric powder for oral solution contains aluminum-magnesium-based antacid; co-administration may interfere with Cipro oral absorption; these preparations may be taken six hours before or two hours after taking ciprofloxacin).
No products indexed under this heading.

Dyphylline (Potential for severe and fatal reactions including cardiac arrest, seizures, respiratory failure and status epilepticus; concurrent use should be avoided or serum levels of theophylline should be monitored carefully).
No products indexed under this heading.

Etodolac (NSAIDs in combination with very high doses of quinolones have been shown to provoke convulsions in pre-clinical trials).
No products indexed under this heading.

Fenoprofen Calcium (NSAIDs in combination with very high doses of quinolones have been shown to provoke convulsions in pre-clinical trials). Products include:
- Nalfon Capsules ... 2504

Ferrous Fumarate (Co-administration with iron-containing products may substantially interfere with the oral absorption of quinolones; these preparations may be taken six hours before or two hours after taking ciprofloxacin). Products include:
- Chromagen Forte Soft Gelatin Capsules ... 3296
- Ferretts Tablets ... ■773
- Repliva 21/7 Tablets ... 3301

Ferrous Gluconate (Co-administration with iron-containing products may substantially interfere with the oral absorption of quinolones; these preparations may be taken six hours before or two hours after taking ciprofloxacin).
No products indexed under this heading.

Ferrous Sulfate (Co-administration with iron-containing products may substantially interfere with the oral absorption of quinolones; these preparations may be taken six hours before or two hours after taking ciprofloxacin). Products include:
- Feosol Tablets ... 1629
- Slow Fe Iron Tablets ... ■772
- Slow Fe with Folic Acid Tablets ... ■773

Fludrocortisone Acetate (Risk of ruptures of the shoulder, hand, Achilles tendon or other tendons may be increased in patients receiving concomitant corticosteroids, especially in the elderly).
No products indexed under this heading.

Flurbiprofen (NSAIDs in combination with very high doses of quinolones have been shown to provoke convulsions in pre-clinical trials).
No products indexed under this heading.

Fosphenytoin Sodium (Potential for change in serum phenytoin levels).
No products indexed under this heading.

Glyburide (Co-administration, on rare occasions, has resulted in severe hypoglycemia).
No products indexed under this heading.

Hydrocortisone (Risk of ruptures of the shoulder, hand, Achilles tendon or other tendons may be increased in patients receiving concomitant corticosteroids, especially in the elderly). Products include:
- Cortizone•5 Ointment ... ■699
- Cortizone•10 Creme ... ■699
- Cortizone•10 Ointment ... ■699
- Cortizone•10 Plus Creme ... ■700
- Cortizone•10 Maximum Strength Quick Shot Spray ... ■700
- Hydrocortone Tablets ... 1963
- Preparation H Hydrocortisone Cream ... ■748

Hydrocortisone Acetate (Risk of ruptures of the shoulder, hand, Achilles tendon or other tendons may be increased in patients receiving concomitant corticosteroids, especially in the elderly). Products include:
- Analpram-HC ... 1136
- Pramosone ... 1139
- ProctoFoam-HC ... 3113
- Tucks Anti-Itch Ointment ... ■712
- U-cort 1% Cream ... 3289

Hydrocortisone Sodium Phosphate (Risk of ruptures of the shoulder, hand, Achilles tendon or other tendons may be increased in patients receiving concomitant corticosteroids, especially in the elderly).
No products indexed under this heading.

Hydrocortisone Sodium Succinate (Risk of ruptures of the shoulder, hand, Achilles tendon or other tendons may be increased in patients receiving concomitant corticosteroids, especially in the elderly).
No products indexed under this heading.

Ibuprofen (NSAIDs in combination with very high doses of quinolones have been shown to provoke convulsions in pre-clinical trials). Products include:
- Advil Allergy Sinus Caplets ... ■737
- Advil ... ■737
- Children's Advil Suspension ... ■742
- Children's Advil Chewable Tablets ... ■741
- Advil Cold & Sinus ... ■739
- Advil Flu & Body Ache Caplets ... ■739
- Children's Advil Cold Suspension ... ■741
- Infants' Advil Concentrated Drops ... ■743
- Junior Strength Advil Swallow Tablets ... ■740
- Advil Migraine Liquigels ... ■740
- Advil Multi-Symptom Cold Caplets ... ■738
- Combunox Tablets ... 1183
- Children's Motrin Oral Suspension and Chewable Tablets ... 1837
- Children's Motrin Cold Non-Staining Dye-Free Oral Suspension ... 1838
- Children's Motrin Cold Oral Suspension ... 1838
- Children's Motrin Non-Staining Dye-Free Oral Suspension ... 1837
- Motrin Cold & Sinus Caplets ... 1836
- Motrin IB Tablets and Caplets ... 1836
- Infants' Motrin Concentrated Drops ... 1837
- Infants' Motrin Non-Staining Dye-Free Drops ... 1837
- Junior Strength Motrin Caplets and Chewable Tablets ... 1837
- Vicoprofen Tablets ... 533

Indomethacin (NSAIDs in combination with very high doses of quinolo-

nes have been shown to provoke convulsions in pre-clinical trials). Products include:

Indocin 1968

Indomethacin Sodium Trihydrate (NSAIDs in combination with very high doses of quinolones have been shown to provoke convulsions in pre-clinical trials). Products include:

Indocin I.V. 1973

Iron (Co-administration with iron-containing products may substantially interfere with the oral absorption of quinolones; these preparations may be taken six hours before or two hours after taking ciprofloxacin). Products include:

Chromagen Forte Soft Gelatin Capsules 3296
Ferretts IPS Liquid .... ◙ 773
OptiNate 1162
Repliva 21/7 Tablets 3301

Ketoprofen (NSAIDs in combination with very high doses of quinolones have been shown to provoke convulsions in pre-clinical trials).

No products indexed under this heading.

Ketorolac Tromethamine (NSAIDs in combination with very high doses of quinolones have been shown to provoke convulsions in pre-clinical trials). Products include:

Acular Ophthalmic Solution 561
Acular LS Ophthalmic Solution 562

Magaldrate (Concurrent administration of these antacids may substantially interfere with the oral absorption of ciprofloxacin; antacids may be administered either two hours after or six hours before ciprofloxacin dosing without a significant decrease in bioavailability).

No products indexed under this heading.

Magnesium Hydroxide (Concurrent administration of these antacids may substantially interfere with the oral absorption of ciprofloxacin; antacids may be administered either two hours after or six hours before ciprofloxacin dosing without a significant decrease in bioavailability). Products include:

Maalox Max Maximum Strength Antacid/Anti-Gas Liquid 2165
Maalox Regular Strength Antacid/Antigas Liquid 2164
Pepcid Complete Chewable Tablets 1672
Rolaids Tablets .... ◙ 707
Extra Strength Rolaids Tablets .... ◙ 707
Rolaids Multi-Symptom Antacid & Antigas Tablets .... ◙ 708

Magnesium Oxide (Concurrent administration of these antacids may substantially interfere with the oral absorption of ciprofloxacin; antacids may be administered either two hours after or six hours before ciprofloxacin dosing without a significant decrease in bioavailability). Products include:

Beelith Tablets 784
PremCal Light, Regular, and Extra Strength Tablets .... ◙ 762

Meclofenamate Sodium (NSAIDs in combination with very high doses of quinolones have been shown to provoke convulsions in pre-clinical trials).

No products indexed under this heading.

Mefenamic Acid (NSAIDs in combination with very high doses of quinolones have been shown to provoke convulsions in pre-clinical trials).

No products indexed under this heading.

Meloxicam (NSAIDs in combination with very high doses of quinolones have been shown to provoke convulsions in pre-clinical trials). Products include:

Mobic Oral Suspension 893
Mobic Tablets 893

Methotrexate (Renal tubular transport of methotrexate may be inhibited by concomitant administration of ciprofloxacin potentially leading to increased plasma levels of methotrexate).

No products indexed under this heading.

Methotrexate Sodium (Renal tubular transport of methotrexate may be inhibited by concomitant administration of ciprofloxacin potentially leading to increased plasma levels of methotrexate).

No products indexed under this heading.

Methylprednisolone Acetate (Risk of ruptures of the shoulder, hand, Achilles tendon or other tendons may be increased in patients receiving concomitant corticosteroids, especially in the elderly). Products include:

Depo-Medrol Injectable Suspension 2615
Depo-Medrol Single-Dose Vial 2617

Methylprednisolone Sodium Succinate (Risk of ruptures of the shoulder, hand, Achilles tendon or other tendons may be increased in patients receiving concomitant corticosteroids, especially in the elderly).

No products indexed under this heading.

Metoclopramide Hydrochloride (Metoclopramide significantly accelerates the absorption of oral ciprofloxacin resulting in a shorter time to reach maximum plasma concentrations).

No products indexed under this heading.

Nabumetone (NSAIDs in combination with very high doses of quinolones have been shown to provoke convulsions in pre-clinical trials). Products include:

Relafen Tablets 1523

Naproxen (NSAIDs in combination with very high doses of quinolones have been shown to provoke convulsions in pre-clinical trials). Products include:

EC-Naprosyn Delayed-Release Tablets 2769
Naprosyn Suspension 2769
Naprosyn Tablets 2769
Prevacid NapraPAC 3277

Naproxen Sodium (NSAIDs in combination with very high doses of quinolones have been shown to provoke convulsions in pre-clinical trials). Products include:

Aleve Tablets, Caplets and Gelcaps .... ◙ 605
Anaprox Tablets 2769
Anaprox DS Tablets 2769

Oxaprozin (NSAIDs in combination with very high doses of quinolones have been shown to provoke convulsions in pre-clinical trials).

No products indexed under this heading.

Phenylbutazone (NSAIDs in combination with very high doses of quinolones have been shown to provoke convulsions in pre-clinical trials).

No products indexed under this heading.

Phenytoin (Potential for change in serum phenytoin levels).

No products indexed under this heading.

Phenytoin Sodium (Potential for change in serum phenytoin levels). Products include:

Phenytek Capsules 2153

Piroxicam (NSAIDs in combination with very high doses of quinolones have been shown to provoke convulsions in pre-clinical trials).

No products indexed under this heading.

Polysaccharide Iron Complex (Co-administration with iron-containing products may substantially interfere with the oral absorption of quinolones; these preparations may be taken six hours before or two hours after taking ciprofloxacin). Products include:

Niferex-150 Forte Capsules 3299
Nu-Iron 150 Capsules 2098

Prednisolone Acetate (Risk of ruptures of the shoulder, hand, Achilles tendon or other tendons may be increased in patients receiving concomitant corticosteroids, especially in the elderly). Products include:

Blephamide Ophthalmic Ointment 563
Blephamide Ophthalmic Suspension................................. 564
Poly-Pred Liquifilm Ophthalmic Suspension .... ⊙ 231
Pred Forte Ophthalmic Suspension .... ⊙ 233
Pred Mild Sterile Ophthalmic Suspension .... ⊙ 236
Pred-G Ophthalmic Suspension ...... ⊙ 234
Pred-G Sterile Ophthalmic Ointment .... ⊙ 235

Prednisolone Sodium Phosphate (Risk of ruptures of the shoulder, hand, Achilles tendon or other tendons may be increased in patients receiving concomitant corticosteroids, especially in the elderly). Products include:

Pediapred Oral Solution 3319

Prednisolone Tebutate (Risk of ruptures of the shoulder, hand, Achilles tendon or other tendons may be increased in patients receiving concomitant corticosteroids, especially in the elderly).

No products indexed under this heading.

Prednisone (Risk of ruptures of the shoulder, hand, Achilles tendon or other tendons may be increased in patients receiving concomitant corticosteroids, especially in the elderly).

No products indexed under this heading.

Probenecid (Interferes with renal tubular secretion of ciprofloxacin).

No products indexed under this heading.

Rofecoxib (NSAIDs in combination with very high doses of quinolones have been shown to provoke convulsions in pre-clinical trials).

No products indexed under this heading.

Sucralfate (Co-administration with sucralfate may substantially interfere with the oral absorption of quinolones; these preparations may be taken six hours before or two hours after taking ciprofloxacin). Products include:

Carafate Suspension 727
Carafate Tablets 728

Sulindac (NSAIDs in combination with very high doses of quinolones have been shown to provoke convulsions in pre-clinical trials). Products include:

Clinoril Tablets 1899

Theophylline (Potential for severe and fatal reactions including cardiac arrest, seizures, respiratory failure and status epilepticus; concurrent use should be avoided or serum levels of theophylline should be monitored carefully).

No products indexed under this heading.

Theophylline Anhydrous (Potential for severe and fatal reactions including cardiac arrest, seizures, respiratory failure and status epilepticus; concurrent use should be avoided or serum levels of theophylline should be monitored carefully). Products include:

Uniphyl Tablets 2708

Theophylline Calcium Salicylate (Potential for severe and fatal reactions including cardiac arrest, seizures, respiratory failure and status epilepticus; concurrent use should be avoided or serum levels of theophylline should be monitored carefully).

No products indexed under this heading.

Theophylline Dihydroxypropyl (Glyceryl) (Potential for severe and fatal reactions including cardiac arrest, seizures, respiratory failure and status epilepticus; concurrent use should be avoided or serum levels of theophylline should be monitored carefully).

No products indexed under this heading.

Theophylline Ethylenediamine (Potential for severe and fatal reactions including cardiac arrest, seizures, respiratory failure and status epilepticus; concurrent use should be avoided or serum levels of theophylline should be monitored carefully).

No products indexed under this heading.

Theophylline Sodium Glycinate (Potential for severe and fatal reactions including cardiac arrest, seizures, respiratory failure and status epilepticus; concurrent use should be avoided or serum levels of theophylline should be monitored carefully).

No products indexed under this heading.

Tolmetin Sodium (NSAIDs in combination with very high doses of quinolones have been shown to provoke convulsions in pre-clinical trials).

No products indexed under this heading.

Triamcinolone (Risk of ruptures of the shoulder, hand, Achilles tendon or other tendons may be increased in patients receiving concomitant corticosteroids, especially in the elderly).

No products indexed under this heading.

Triamcinolone Acetonide (Risk of ruptures of the shoulder, hand, Achilles tendon or other tendons may be increased in patients receiving concomitant corticosteroids, especially in the elderly). Products include:

Azmacort Inhalation Aerosol 1701
Nasacort HFA Inhalation Aerosol 2939
Nasacort AQ Nasal Spray 2937

Triamcinolone Diacetate (Risk of ruptures of the shoulder, hand, Achilles tendon or other tendons may be increased in patients receiving concomitant corticosteroids, especially in the elderly).
No products indexed under this heading.

Triamcinolone Hexacetonide (Risk of ruptures of the shoulder, hand, Achilles tendon or other tendons may be increased in patients receiving concomitant corticosteroids, especially in the elderly).
No products indexed under this heading.

Valdecoxib (NSAIDs in combination with very high doses of quinolones have been shown to provoke convulsions in pre-clinical trials).
No products indexed under this heading.

Warfarin Sodium (Enhanced effects of anticoagulant). Products include:
Coumadin for Injection 932
Coumadin Tablets 932

Zinc Sulfate (Co-administration with zinc-containing products may substantially interfere with the oral absorption of quinolones; these preparations may be taken six hours before or two hours after taking ciprofloxacin). Products include:
Athena Hair System Shampoo .... ▣ 767
Spartan Hair System Shampoo ...... ▣ 767
Visine A.C. Seasonal Itching and Redness Relief Drops .... ⊙ 278
Zinc-220 Capsules 576

Food Interactions

Dairy products (Oral ciprofloxacin should not be taken concurrently with milk or yogurt alone, since absorption of ciprofloxacin may be significantly reduced; dietary calcium as part of a meal, however, does not significantly affect ciprofloxacin absorption).

Food, unspecified (Delays the oral absorption of the drug resulting in peak concentrations that are closer to two hours after dosing).

CIPRO XR TABLETS

(Ciprofloxacin) 3004

May interact with antacids containing aluminum, calcium and magnesium, nonabsorbable antacids, calcium preparations, cations, corticosteroids, oral anticoagulants, iron containing oral preparations, nonsteroidal anti-inflammatory agents, phenytoin, xanthines, and certain other agents. Compounds in these categories include:

Aluminum Carbonate (Concurrent administration may substantially interfere with the absorption of ciprofloxacin, resulting in serum and urine levels of ciprofloxacin considerably lower than desired. Ciprofloxacin extended-release tablets should be administered at least 2 hours before or 6 hours after antacids containing magnesium or aluminum).
No products indexed under this heading.

Aluminum-containing Compounds, unspecified (Concurrent administration may substantially interfere with the absorption of ciprofloxacin, resulting in serum and urine levels of ciprofloxacin considerably lower than desired. Ciprofloxacin extended-release tablets should be administered at least 2 hours before or 6 hours after metal cations).
No products indexed under this heading.

Aluminum Hydroxide (Concurrent administration may substantially interfere with the absorption of ciprofloxacin, resulting in serum and urine levels of ciprofloxacin considerably lower than desired. Ciprofloxacin extended-release tablets should be administered at least 2 hours before or 6 hours after antacids containing magnesium or aluminum). Products include:
Gaviscon Regular Strength Liquid .. ▣ 620
Gaviscon Regular Strength Tablets.. ▣ 619
Gaviscon Extra Strength Liquid ...... ▣ 620
Gaviscon Extra Strength Tablets .... ▣ 619
Maalox Max Maximum Strength Antacid/Anti-Gas Liquid................ 2165
Maalox Regular Strength Antacid/Antigas Liquid................. 2164

Aminophylline (Concurrent administration of ciprofloxacin and theophylline may lead to elevated serum concentrations of theophylline and prolongation of its elimination half-life. Serious and fatal reactions have been reported in patients receiving concurrent administration. These reactions have included cardiac arrest, seizure, status epilepticus, and respiratory failure).
No products indexed under this heading.

Anisindione (Quinolones have been reported to enhance the effects of the oral anticoagulant warfarin or its derivatives). Products include:
Miradon Tablets 3056

Betamethasone Acetate (Risk of ruptures of the shoulder, hand, Achilles tendon or other tendons may be increased in patients receiving concomitant corticosteroids, especially in the elderly).
No products indexed under this heading.

Betamethasone Sodium Phosphate (Risk of ruptures of the shoulder, hand, Achilles tendon or other tendons may be increased in patients receiving concomitant corticosteroids, especially in the elderly).
No products indexed under this heading.

Caffeine (Concurrent administration of ciprofloxacin and caffeine may lead to reduced clearance of caffeine and a prolongation of its serum half-life). Products include:
Athena Hair System Shampoo .... ▣ 767
BC Powder .... ▣ 612
Arthritis Strength BC Powder .... ▣ 612
Goody's Extra Strength Headache Powder....................... ▣ 621
Goody's Extra Strength Pain Relief Tablets .... ▣ 621
Hycomine Compound Tablets 1105
Spartan Hair System Shampoo ...... ▣ 767
Vivarin .... ▣ 639

Calcium (Concurrent administration may substantially interfere with the absorption of ciprofloxacin, resulting in serum and urine levels of ciprofloxacin considerably lower than desired. Ciprofloxacin extended-release tablets should be administered at least 2 hours before or 6 hours after metal cations). Products include:
Os-Cal 250 + D Tablets .... ▣ 765
Os-Cal 500 Tablets .... ▣ 765
Os-Cal 500 + D Tablets .... ▣ 766
Perdiem Overnight Relief Pills 2166
Slow-Mag Tablets 2717

Calcium Carbonate (Concurrent administration may substantially interfere with the absorption of ciprofloxacin, resulting in serum and urine levels of ciprofloxacin considerably lower than desired). Products include:
Actonel with Calcium Tablets 2684
Caltrate 600 PLUS Chewables .... ▣ 779
Caltrate 600 PLUS Tablets .... ▣ 779
Caltrate 600 + D Tablets .... ▣ 779
Encora Capsules 3298
Encora AM Tablets 3298
Encora PM Tablets 3298
Gas-X with Maalox .... ▣ 675
Maalox Regular Strength Antacid Tablets 2166
Quick Dissolve Maalox Max Maximum Strength Antacid/Antigas Tablets................ 2165
Maalox Max Quick Dissolve Maximum Strength Chewable Tablets.. ▣ 678
Os-Cal Chewable Tablets .... ▣ 765
Pepcid Complete Chewable Tablets 1672
PremCal Light, Regular, and Extra Strength Tablets................ ▣ 762
Rolaids Tablets .... ▣ 707
Extra Strength Rolaids Softchews .... ▣ 708
Extra Strength Rolaids Tablets .... ▣ 707
Rolaids Multi-Symptom Antacid & Antigas Tablets .... ▣ 708
Tums .... ▣ 639

Calcium Chloride (Concurrent administration may substantially interfere with the absorption of ciprofloxacin, resulting in serum and urine levels of ciprofloxacin considerably lower than desired).
No products indexed under this heading.

Calcium Citrate (Concurrent administration may substantially interfere with the absorption of ciprofloxacin, resulting in serum and urine levels of ciprofloxacin considerably lower than desired). Products include:
Active Calcium Tablets 3342
Citracal Tablets 2108

Calcium Glubionate (Concurrent administration may substantially interfere with the absorption of ciprofloxacin, resulting in serum and urine levels of ciprofloxacin considerably lower than desired).
No products indexed under this heading.

Celecoxib (NSAIDs in combination with very high doses of quinolones have been shown to provoke convulsions in pre-clinical trials). Products include:
Celebrex Capsules 3130

Cortisone Acetate (Risk of ruptures of the shoulder, hand, Achilles tendon or other tendons may be increased in patients receiving concomitant corticosteroids, especially in the elderly).
No products indexed under this heading.

Cyclosporine (Transient elevations in serum creatinine have been reported in patients receiving ciprofloxacin and cyclosporine concomitantly). Products include:
Gengraf Capsules 458
Neoral Soft Gelatin Capsules 2247
Neoral Oral Solution 2247
Restasis Ophthalmic Emulsion 570
Sandimmune 2259

Dexamethasone (Risk of ruptures of the shoulder, hand, Achilles tendon or other tendons may be increased in patients receiving concomitant corticosteroids, especially in the elderly). Products include:
Ciprodex Otic Suspension 555
Decadron Tablets 1929
TobraDex Ophthalmic Ointment 558
TobraDex Ophthalmic Suspension ... 558

Dexamethasone Acetate (Risk of ruptures of the shoulder, hand, Achilles tendon or other tendons may be increased in patients receiving concomitant corticosteroids, especially in the elderly).
No products indexed under this heading.

Dexamethasone Sodium Phosphate (Risk of ruptures of the shoulder, hand, Achilles tendon or other tendons may be increased in patients receiving concomitant corticosteroids, especially in the elderly). Products include:
Decadron Phosphate Injection 1931

Diclofenac Potassium (NSAIDs in combination with very high doses of quinolones have been shown to provoke convulsions in pre-clinical trials). Products include:
Cataflam Tablets 2173

Diclofenac Sodium (NSAIDs in combination with very high doses of quinolones have been shown to provoke convulsions in pre-clinical trials). Products include:
Arthrotec Tablets 3126
Voltaren Ophthalmic Solution 2300
Voltaren Tablets 2298
Voltaren-XR Tablets 2301

Dicumarol (Quinolones have been reported to enhance the effects of the oral anticoagulant warfarin or its derivatives).
No products indexed under this heading.

Didanosine (Concurrent administration may substantially interfere with the absorption of ciprofloxacin, resulting in serum and urine levels of ciprofloxacin considerably lower than desired. Ciprofloxacin extended-release tablets should be administered at least 2 hours before or 6 hours after didanosine chewable/buffered tablets or pediatric powder).
No products indexed under this heading.

Dyphylline (Concurrent administration of ciprofloxacin and theophylline may lead to elevated serum concentrations of theophylline and prolongation of its elimination half-life. Serious and fatal reactions have been reported in patients receiving concurrent administration. These reactions have included cardiac arrest, seizure, status epilepticus, and respiratory failure).
No products indexed under this heading.

Etodolac (NSAIDs in combination with very high doses of quinolones have been shown to provoke convulsions in pre-clinical trials).
No products indexed under this heading.

Fenoprofen Calcium (NSAIDs in combination with very high doses of quinolones have been shown to provoke convulsions in pre-clinical trials). Products include:
Nalfon Capsules 2504

Ferrous Fumarate (Concurrent administration may substantially interfere with the absorption of ciprofloxacin, resulting in serum and urine levels of ciprofloxacin considerably lower than desired. Ciprofloxacin extended-release tablets should be administered at least 2 hours before or 6 hours after metal cations, such as iron). Products include:

- Chromagen Forte Soft Gelatin Capsules ... 3296
- Ferretts Tablets ... 773
- Repliva 21/7 Tablets ... 3301

Ferrous Gluconate (Concurrent administration may substantially interfere with the absorption of ciprofloxacin, resulting in serum and urine levels of ciprofloxacin considerably lower than desired. Ciprofloxacin extended-release tablets should be administered at least 2 hours before or 6 hours after metal cations, such as iron).

No products indexed under this heading.

Ferrous Sulfate (Concurrent administration may substantially interfere with the absorption of ciprofloxacin, resulting in serum and urine levels of ciprofloxacin considerably lower than desired. Ciprofloxacin extended-release tablets should be administered at least 2 hours before or 6 hours after metal cations, such as iron). Products include:

- Feosol Tablets ... 1629
- Slow Fe Iron Tablets ... 772
- Slow Fe with Folic Acid Tablets ... 773

Fludrocortisone Acetate (Risk of ruptures of the shoulder, hand, Achilles tendon or other tendons may be increased in patients receiving concomitant corticosteroids, especially in the elderly).

No products indexed under this heading.

Flurbiprofen (NSAIDs in combination with very high doses of quinolones have been shown to provoke convulsions in pre-clinical trials).

No products indexed under this heading.

Fosphenytoin Sodium (Altered serum levels of phenytoin (increased and decreased) have been reported in patients receiving concomitant ciprofloxacin).

No products indexed under this heading.

Glyburide (The concomitant administration of ciprofloxacin with glyburide has, on rare occasions, resulted in severe hypoglycemia).

No products indexed under this heading.

Hydrocortisone (Risk of ruptures of the shoulder, hand, Achilles tendon or other tendons may be increased in patients receiving concomitant corticosteroids, especially in the elderly). Products include:

- Cortizone•5 Ointment ... 699
- Cortizone•10 Creme ... 699
- Cortizone•10 Ointment ... 699
- Cortizone•10 Plus Creme ... 700
- Cortizone•10 Maximum Strength Quick Shot Spray ... 700
- Hydrocortone Tablets ... 1963
- Preparation H Hydrocortisone Cream ... 748

Hydrocortisone Acetate (Risk of ruptures of the shoulder, hand, Achilles tendon or other tendons may be increased in patients receiving concomitant corticosteroids, especially in the elderly). Products include:

- Analpram-HC ... 1136
- Pramosone ... 1139
- ProctoFoam-HC ... 3113
- Tucks Anti-Itch Ointment ... 712
- U-cort 1% Cream ... 3289

Hydrocortisone Sodium Phosphate (Risk of ruptures of the shoulder, hand, Achilles tendon or other tendons may be increased in patients receiving concomitant corticosteroids, especially in the elderly).

No products indexed under this heading.

Hydrocortisone Sodium Succinate (Risk of ruptures of the shoulder, hand, Achilles tendon or other tendons may be increased in patients receiving concomitant corticosteroids, especially in the elderly).

No products indexed under this heading.

Ibuprofen (NSAIDs in combination with very high doses of quinolones have been shown to provoke convulsions in pre-clinical trials). Products include:

- Advil Allergy Sinus Caplets ... 737
- Advil ... 737
- Children's Advil Suspension ... 742
- Children's Advil Chewable Tablets ... 741
- Advil Cold & Sinus ... 739
- Advil Flu & Body Ache Caplets ... 739
- Children's Advil Cold Suspension ... 741
- Infants' Advil Concentrated Drops ... 743
- Junior Strength Advil Swallow Tablets ... 740
- Advil Migraine Liquigels ... 740
- Advil Multi-Symptom Cold Caplets ... 738
- Combunox Tablets ... 1183
- Children's Motrin Oral Suspension and Chewable Tablets ... 1837
- Children's Motrin Cold Non-Staining Dye-Free Oral Suspension ... 1838
- Children's Motrin Cold Oral Suspension ... 1838
- Children's Motrin Non-Staining Dye-Free Oral Suspension ... 1837
- Motrin Cold & Sinus Caplets ... 1836
- Motrin IB Tablets and Caplets ... 1836
- Infants' Motrin Concentrated Drops ... 1837
- Infants' Motrin Non-Staining Dye-Free Drops ... 1837
- Junior Strength Motrin Caplets and Chewable Tablets ... 1837
- Vicoprofen Tablets ... 533

Indomethacin (NSAIDs in combination with very high doses of quinolones have been shown to provoke convulsions in pre-clinical trials). Products include:

- Indocin ... 1968

Indomethacin Sodium Trihydrate (NSAIDs in combination with very high doses of quinolones have been shown to provoke convulsions in pre-clinical trials). Products include:

- Indocin I.V. ... 1973

Iron (Concurrent administration may substantially interfere with the absorption of ciprofloxacin, resulting in serum and urine levels of ciprofloxacin considerably lower than desired. Ciprofloxacin extended-release tablets should be administered at least 2 hours before or 6 hours after metal cations, such as iron). Products include:

- Chromagen Forte Soft Gelatin Capsules ... 3296
- Ferretts IPS Liquid ... 773
- OptiNate ... 1162
- Repliva 21/7 Tablets ... 3301

Ketoprofen (NSAIDs in combination with very high doses of quinolones have been shown to provoke convulsions in pre-clinical trials).

No products indexed under this heading.

Ketorolac Tromethamine (NSAIDs in combination with very high doses of quinolones have been shown to provoke convulsions in pre-clinical trials). Products include:

- Acular Ophthalmic Solution ... 561
- Acular LS Ophthalmic Solution ... 562

Magaldrate (Concurrent administration may substantially interfere with the absorption of ciprofloxacin, resulting in serum and urine levels of ciprofloxacin considerably lower than desired. Ciprofloxacin extended-release tablets should be administered at least 2 hours before or 6 hours after antacids containing magnesium or aluminum).

No products indexed under this heading.

Magnesium (Concurrent administration may substantially interfere with the absorption of ciprofloxacin, resulting in serum and urine levels of ciprofloxacin considerably lower than desired. Ciprofloxacin extended-release tablets should be administered at least 2 hours before or 6 hours after metal cations).

No products indexed under this heading.

Magnesium Carbonate (Concurrent administration may substantially interfere with the absorption of ciprofloxacin, resulting in serum and urine levels of ciprofloxacin considerably lower than desired). Products include:

- Gaviscon Regular Strength Liquid ... 620
- Gaviscon Extra Strength Liquid ... 620
- Gaviscon Extra Strength Tablets ... 619

Magnesium Hydroxide (Concurrent administration may substantially interfere with the absorption of ciprofloxacin, resulting in serum and urine levels of ciprofloxacin considerably lower than desired. Ciprofloxacin extended-release tablets should be administered at least 2 hours before or 6 hours after antacids containing magnesium or aluminum). Products include:

- Maalox Max Maximum Strength Antacid/Anti-Gas Liquid ... 2165
- Maalox Regular Strength Antacid/Antigas Liquid ... 2164
- Pepcid Complete Chewable Tablets ... 1672
- Rolaids Tablets ... 707
- Extra Strength Rolaids Tablets ... 707
- Rolaids Multi-Symptom Antacid & Antigas Tablets ... 708

Magnesium Oxide (Concurrent administration may substantially interfere with the absorption of ciprofloxacin, resulting in serum and urine levels of ciprofloxacin considerably lower than desired. Ciprofloxacin extended-release tablets should be administered at least 2 hours before or 6 hours after antacids containing magnesium or aluminum). Products include:

- Beelith Tablets ... 784
- PremCal Light, Regular, and Extra Strength Tablets ... 762

Meclofenamate Sodium (NSAIDs in combination with very high doses of quinolones have been shown to provoke convulsions in pre-clinical trials).

No products indexed under this heading.

Mefenamic Acid (NSAIDs in combination with very high doses of quinolones have been shown to provoke convulsions in pre-clinical trials).

No products indexed under this heading.

Meloxicam (NSAIDs in combination with very high doses of quinolones have been shown to provoke convulsions in pre-clinical trials). Products include:

- Mobic Oral Suspension ... 893
- Mobic Tablets ... 893

Methotrexate (Renal tubular transport of methotrexate may be inhibited by concomitant administration of ciprofloxacin potentially leading to increased plasma levels of methotrexate).

No products indexed under this heading.

Methotrexate Sodium (Renal tubular transport of methotrexate may be inhibited by concomitant administration of ciprofloxacin potentially leading to increased plasma levels of methotrexate).

No products indexed under this heading.

Methylprednisolone Acetate (Risk of ruptures of the shoulder, hand, Achilles tendon or other tendons may be increased in patients receiving concomitant corticosteroids, especially in the elderly). Products include:

- Depo-Medrol Injectable Suspension ... 2615
- Depo-Medrol Single-Dose Vial ... 2617

Methylprednisolone Sodium Succinate (Risk of ruptures of the shoulder, hand, Achilles tendon or other tendons may be increased in patients receiving concomitant corticosteroids, especially in the elderly).

No products indexed under this heading.

Metoclopramide Hydrochloride (Metoclopramide significantly accelerates the absorption of oral ciprofloxacin resulting in a shorter time to reach maximum plasma concentrations).

No products indexed under this heading.

Nabumetone (NSAIDs in combination with very high doses of quinolones have been shown to provoke convulsions in pre-clinical trials). Products include:

- Relafen Tablets ... 1523

Naproxen (NSAIDs in combination with very high doses of quinolones have been shown to provoke convulsions in pre-clinical trials). Products include:

- EC-Naprosyn Delayed-Release Tablets ... 2769
- Naprosyn Suspension ... 2769
- Naprosyn Tablets ... 2769
- Prevacid NapraPAC ... 3277

Naproxen Sodium (NSAIDs in combination with very high doses of quinolones have been shown to provoke convulsions in pre-clinical trials). Products include:

- Aleve Tablets, Caplets and Gelcaps ... 605
- Anaprox Tablets ... 2769
- Anaprox DS Tablets ... 2769

Omeprazole (Absorption of the Cipro XR tablet was slightly diminished (20%) when given concomitantly with omeprazole). Products include:

- Zegerid Powder for Oral Solution ... 2972

IMPORTANT NOTE: Always consult each drug listing in the patient's regimen for possible interactions.

Oxaprozin (NSAIDs in combination with very high doses of quinolones have been shown to provoke convulsions in pre-clinical trials).
No products indexed under this heading.

Phenylbutazone (NSAIDs in combination with very high doses of quinolones have been shown to provoke convulsions in pre-clinical trials).
No products indexed under this heading.

Phenytoin (Altered serum levels of phenytoin (increased and decreased) have been reported in patients receiving concomitant ciprofloxacin).
No products indexed under this heading.

Phenytoin Sodium (Altered serum levels of phenytoin (increased and decreased) have been reported in patients receiving concomitant ciprofloxacin). Products include:
Phenytek Capsules 2153

Piroxicam (NSAIDs in combination with very high doses of quinolones have been shown to provoke convulsions in pre-clinical trials).
No products indexed under this heading.

Polysaccharide Iron Complex (Concurrent administration may substantially interfere with the absorption of ciprofloxacin, resulting in serum and urine levels of ciprofloxacin considerably lower than desired. Ciprofloxacin extended-release tablets should be administered at least 2 hours before or 6 hours after metal cations, such as iron). Products include:
Niferex-150 Forte Capsules 3299
Nu-Iron 150 Capsules 2098

Prednisolone Acetate (Risk of ruptures of the shoulder, hand, Achilles tendon or other tendons may be increased in patients receiving concomitant corticosteroids, especially in the elderly). Products include:
Blephamide Ophthalmic Ointment 563
Blephamide Ophthalmic Suspension 564
Poly-Pred Liquifilm Ophthalmic Suspension .... ⊙231
Pred Forte Ophthalmic Suspension .... ⊙233
Pred Mild Sterile Ophthalmic Suspension .... ⊙236
Pred-G Ophthalmic Suspension .... ⊙234
Pred-G Sterile Ophthalmic Ointment .... ⊙235

Prednisolone Sodium Phosphate (Risk of ruptures of the shoulder, hand, Achilles tendon or other tendons may be increased in patients receiving concomitant corticosteroids, especially in the elderly). Products include:
Pediapred Oral Solution 3319

Prednisolone Tebutate (Risk of ruptures of the shoulder, hand, Achilles tendon or other tendons may be increased in patients receiving concomitant corticosteroids, especially in the elderly).
No products indexed under this heading.

Prednisone (Risk of ruptures of the shoulder, hand, Achilles tendon or other tendons may be increased in patients receiving concomitant corticosteroids, especially in the elderly).
No products indexed under this heading.

Probenecid (Probenecid interferes with renal tubular secretion of ciprofloxacin and produces an increase in the level of ciprofloxacin in the serum).
No products indexed under this heading.

Rofecoxib (NSAIDs in combination with very high doses of quinolones have been shown to provoke convulsions in pre-clinical trials).
No products indexed under this heading.

Sucralfate (Concurrent administration may substantially interfere with the absorption of ciprofloxacin, resulting in serum and urine levels of ciprofloxacin considerably lower than desired. Ciprofloxacin extended-release tablets should be administered at least 2 hours before or 6 hours after sucralfate). Products include:
Carafate Suspension 727
Carafate Tablets 728

Sulindac (NSAIDs in combination with very high doses of quinolones have been shown to provoke convulsions in pre-clinical trials). Products include:
Clinoril Tablets 1899

Theophylline (Concurrent administration of ciprofloxacin and theophylline may lead to elevated serum concentrations of theophylline and prolongation of its elimination half-life. Serious and fatal reactions have been reported in patients receiving concurrent administration. These reactions have included cardiac arrest, seizure, status epilepticus, and respiratory failure).
No products indexed under this heading.

Theophylline Anhydrous (Concurrent administration of ciprofloxacin and theophylline may lead to elevated serum concentrations of theophylline and prolongation of its elimination half-life. Serious and fatal reactions have been reported in patients receiving concurrent administration. These reactions have included cardiac arrest, seizure, status epilepticus, and respiratory failure). Products include:
Uniphyl Tablets 2708

Theophylline Calcium Salicylate (Concurrent administration of ciprofloxacin and theophylline may lead to elevated serum concentrations of theophylline and prolongation of its elimination half-life. Serious and fatal reactions have been reported in patients receiving concurrent administration. These reactions have included cardiac arrest, seizure, status epilepticus, and respiratory failure).
No products indexed under this heading.

Theophylline Dihydroxypropyl (Glyceryl) (Concurrent administration of ciprofloxacin and theophylline may lead to elevated serum concentrations of theophylline and prolongation of its elimination half-life. Serious and fatal reactions have been reported in patients receiving concurrent administration. These reactions have included cardiac arrest, seizure, status epilepticus, and respiratory failure).
No products indexed under this heading.

Theophylline Ethylenediamine (Concurrent administration of ciprofloxacin and theophylline may lead to elevated serum concentrations of theophylline and prolongation of its elimination half-life. Serious and fatal reactions have been reported in patients receiving concurrent administration. These reactions have included cardiac arrest, seizure, status epilepticus, and respiratory failure).
No products indexed under this heading.

Theophylline Sodium Glycinate (Concurrent administration of ciprofloxacin and theophylline may lead to elevated serum concentrations of theophylline and prolongation of its elimination half-life. Serious and fatal reactions have been reported in patients receiving concurrent administration. These reactions have included cardiac arrest, seizure, status epilepticus, and respiratory failure).
No products indexed under this heading.

Tolmetin Sodium (NSAIDs in combination with very high doses of quinolones have been shown to provoke convulsions in pre-clinical trials).
No products indexed under this heading.

Triamcinolone (Risk of ruptures of the shoulder, hand, Achilles tendon or other tendons may be increased in patients receiving concomitant corticosteroids, especially in the elderly).
No products indexed under this heading.

Triamcinolone Acetonide (Risk of ruptures of the shoulder, hand, Achilles tendon or other tendons may be increased in patients receiving concomitant corticosteroids, especially in the elderly). Products include:
Azmacort Inhalation Aerosol 1701
Nasacort HFA Inhalation Aerosol 2939
Nasacort AQ Nasal Spray 2937

Triamcinolone Diacetate (Risk of ruptures of the shoulder, hand, Achilles tendon or other tendons may be increased in patients receiving concomitant corticosteroids, especially in the elderly).
No products indexed under this heading.

Triamcinolone Hexacetonide (Risk of ruptures of the shoulder, hand, Achilles tendon or other tendons may be increased in patients receiving concomitant corticosteroids, especially in the elderly).
No products indexed under this heading.

Valdecoxib (NSAIDs in combination with very high doses of quinolones have been shown to provoke convulsions in pre-clinical trials).
No products indexed under this heading.

Warfarin Sodium (Quinolones have been reported to enhance the effects of the oral anticoagulant warfarin or its derivatives). Products include:
Coumadin for Injection 932
Coumadin Tablets 932

Zinc (Concurrent administration may substantially interfere with the absorption of ciprofloxacin, resulting in serum and urine levels of ciprofloxacin considerably lower than desired. Ciprofloxacin extended-release tablets should be administered at least 2 hours before or 6 hours after zinc-containing products). Products include:
Visutein Capsules 3328

Zinc Acetate (Concurrent administration may substantially interfere with the absorption of ciprofloxacin, resulting in serum and urine levels of ciprofloxacin considerably lower than desired. Ciprofloxacin extended-release tablets should be administered at least 2 hours before or 6 hours after zinc-containing products). Products include:
Benadryl Itch Relief Stick Extra Strength .... ▣696
Benadryl Itch Stopping Cream Extra Strength .... ▣697
Benadryl Itch Stopping Spray Extra Strength .... ▣697

Zinc Chloride (Concurrent administration may substantially interfere with the absorption of ciprofloxacin, resulting in serum and urine levels of ciprofloxacin considerably lower than desired. Ciprofloxacin extended-release tablets should be administered at least 2 hours before or 6 hours after zinc-containing products).
No products indexed under this heading.

Zinc Citrate (Concurrent administration may substantially interfere with the absorption of ciprofloxacin, resulting in serum and urine levels of ciprofloxacin considerably lower than desired. Ciprofloxacin extended-release tablets should be administered at least 2 hours before or 6 hours after zinc-containing products).
No products indexed under this heading.

Zinc-Containing Multivitamins (Concurrent administration may substantially interfere with the absorption of ciprofloxacin, resulting in serum and urine levels of ciprofloxacin considerably lower than desired. Ciprofloxacin extended-release tablets should be administered at least 2 hours before or 6 hours after multivitamin preparations with zinc).
No products indexed under this heading.

Zinc Gluconate (Concurrent administration may substantially interfere with the absorption of ciprofloxacin, resulting in serum and urine levels of ciprofloxacin considerably lower than desired. Ciprofloxacin extended-release tablets should be administered at least 2 hours before or 6 hours after zinc-containing products).
No products indexed under this heading.

Zinc Oxide (Concurrent administration may substantially interfere with the absorption of ciprofloxacin, resulting in serum and urine levels of ciprofloxacin considerably lower than desired. Ciprofloxacin extended-release tablets should be administered at least 2 hours before or 6 hours after zinc-containing products). Products include:
Desitin Creamy Ointment .... ▣700
Desitin Ointment .... ▣700
Nicomide Tablets 3190
Tucks Hemorrhoidal Ointment .... ▣711

Zinc Phenosulfonate (Concurrent administration may substantially interfere with the absorption of ciprofloxacin, resulting in serum and urine levels of ciprofloxacin considerably lower than desired. Ciprofloxacin extended-release tablets should be administered at least 2 hours before or 6 hours after zinc-containing products).
No products indexed under this heading.

Zinc Pyrithione (Concurrent administration may substantially interfere with the absorption of ciprofloxacin, resulting in serum and urine levels of ciprofloxacin considerably lower than desired. Ciprofloxacin extended-release tablets should be administered at least 2 hours before or 6 hours after zinc-containing products).
No products indexed under this heading.

Zinc Sulfate (Concurrent administration may substantially interfere with the absorption of ciprofloxacin, resulting in serum and urine levels of ciprofloxacin considerably lower than desired. Ciprofloxacin extended-release tablets should be administered at least 2 hours before or 6 hours after zinc-containing products). Products include:
Athena Hair System Shampoo .... ▣767
Spartan Hair System Shampoo ...... ▣767
Visine A.C. Seasonal Itching and Redness Relief Drops .... ⊙278
Zinc-220 Capsules 576

Zinc Undecylenate (Concurrent administration may substantially interfere with the absorption of ciprofloxacin, resulting in serum and urine levels of ciprofloxacin considerably lower than desired. Ciprofloxacin extended-release tablets should be administered at least 2 hours before or 6 hours after zinc-containing products).
No products indexed under this heading.

Food Interactions

Dairy products (Concurrent administration of ciprofloxacin with dairy products should be avoided since decreased absorption of ciprofloxacin is possible).

Food, calcium-rich (Concurrent administration of ciprofloxacin with calcium-fortified juices should be avoided since decreased absorption of ciprofloxacin is possible).

CIPRODEX OTIC SUSPENSION
(Ciprofloxacin, Dexamethasone) 555
None cited in PDR database.

CITRACAL PRENATAL RX TABLETS
(Vitamins, Prenatal) 2108
None cited in PDR database.

CITRACAL TABLETS
(Calcium Citrate) 2108
None cited in PDR database.

CITRUCEL CAPLETS
(Methylcellulose) .... ▣614
None cited in PDR database.

CITRUCEL ORANGE FLAVOR POWDER
(Methylcellulose) .... ▣613
None cited in PDR database.

CITRUCEL SUGAR FREE ORANGE FLAVOR POWDER
(Methylcellulose) .... ▣613
None cited in PDR database.

CLARINEX SYRUP
(Desloratadine) 3009
See Clarinex Tablets

CLARINEX TABLETS
(Desloratadine) 3009
May interact with erythromycin and certain other agents. Compounds in these categories include:

Azithromycin Dihydrate (Co-administration resulted in increased Cmax and AUC of desloratadine by 15% and 5% respectively; Cmax and AUC of 3-hydroxydesloratadine increased by 15% and 4% respectively; there were no clinically relevant changes in the safety profile of desloratadine). Products include:
Zithromax 2568
Zithromax for IV Infusion 2573
Zithromax for Oral Suspension, 300 mg, 600 mg, 900 mg, 1200 mg 2561
Zithromax Tablets, 250 mg, 500 mg 2561
Zithromax Tri-Pak 2561
Zithromax Z-Pak 2568

Cimetidine (Co-administration resulted in increased Cmax and AUC of desloratadine by 12% and 19% respectively; Cmax and AUC of 3-hydroxydesloratadine decreased by 11% and 3% respectively; there were no clinically relevant changes in the safety profile of desloratadine). Products include:
Tagamet HB 200 Tablets .... ▣637
Tagamet Tablets 1547

Cimetidine Hydrochloride (Co-administration resulted in increased Cmax and AUC of desloratadine by 12% and 19% respectively; Cmax and AUC of 3-hydroxydesloratadine decreased by 11% and 3% respectively; there were no clinically relevant changes in the safety profile of desloratadine).
No products indexed under this heading.

Erythromycin (Co-administration resulted in increased Cmax and AUC of desloratadine by 24% and 14% respectively; Cmax and AUC of 3-hydroxydesloratadine increased by 43% and 40% respectively; there were no clinically relevant changes in the safety profile of desloratadine). Products include:
Erygel Topical Gel 2096
Ery-Tab Tablets 447
Erythromycin Base Filmtab Tablets 454
Erythromycin Delayed-Release Capsules, USP 456
PCE Dispertab Tablets 510

Erythromycin Estolate (Co-administration resulted in increased Cmax and AUC of desloratadine by 24% and 14% respectively; Cmax and AUC of 3-hydroxydesloratadine increased by 43% and 40% respectively; there were no clinically relevant changes in the safety profile of desloratadine).
No products indexed under this heading.

Erythromycin Ethylsuccinate (Co-administration resulted in increased Cmax and AUC of desloratadine by 24% and 14% respectively; Cmax and AUC of 3-hydroxydesloratadine increased by 43% and 40% respectively; there were no clinically relevant changes in the safety profile of desloratadine). Products include:
E.E.S. 449
EryPed 445

Erythromycin Gluceptate (Co-administration resulted in increased Cmax and AUC of desloratadine by 24% and 14% respectively; Cmax and AUC of 3-hydroxydesloratadine increased by 43% and 40% respectively; there were no clinically relevant changes in the safety profile of desloratadine).
No products indexed under this heading.

Erythromycin Lactobionate (Co-administration resulted in increased Cmax and AUC of desloratadine by 24% and 14% respectively; Cmax and AUC of 3-hydroxydesloratadine increased by 43% and 40% respectively; there were no clinically relevant changes in the safety profile of desloratadine).
No products indexed under this heading.

Erythromycin Stearate (Co-administration resulted in increased Cmax and AUC of desloratadine by 24% and 14% respectively; Cmax and AUC of 3-hydroxydesloratadine increased by 43% and 40% respectively; there were no clinically relevant changes in the safety profile of desloratadine). Products include:
Erythrocin Stearate Filmtab Tablets 452

Fluoxetine Hydrochloride (Co-administration resulted in increased Cmax of desloratadine by 15%; Cmax and AUC of 3-hydroxydesloratadine increased by 17% and 13% respectively; there were no clinically relevant changes in the safety profile of desloratadine). Products include:
Prozac Pulvules and Liquid 1771
Symbyax Capsules 1788

Ketoconazole (Co-administration resulted in increased Cmax and AUC of desloratadine by 45% and 39% respectively; Cmax and AUC of 3-hydroxydesloratadine increased by 43% and 72% respectively; there were no clinically relevant changes in the safety profile of desloratadine). Products include:
Nizoral A-D Shampoo, 1% 1839
Nizoral 2% Shampoo 1838

CLARINEX REDITABS TABLETS
(Desloratadine) 3009
See Clarinex Tablets

CLARINEX-D 24-HOUR EXTENDED-RELEASE TABLETS
(Desloratadine, Pseudoephedrine Sulfate) 3012
May interact with beta blockers, cardiac glycosides, monoamine oxidase inhibitors, veratrum alkaloids, and certain other agents. Compounds in these categories include:

Acebutolol Hydrochloride (The antihypertensive effects of beta-adrenergic blocking agents may be reduced by sympathomimetics).
No products indexed under this heading.

Atenolol (The antihypertensive effects of beta-adrenergic blocking agents may be reduced by sympathomimetics). Products include:
Tenormin I.V. Injection 698
Tenormin Tablets 695

Betaxolol Hydrochloride (The antihypertensive effects of beta-adrenergic blocking agents may be reduced by sympathomimetics). Products include:
Betoptic S Ophthalmic Suspension 554

Bisoprolol Fumarate (The antihypertensive effects of beta-adrenergic blocking agents may be reduced by sympathomimetics).
No products indexed under this heading.

Carteolol Hydrochloride (The antihypertensive effects of beta-adrenergic blocking agents may be reduced by sympathomimetics). Products include:
Carteolol Hydrochloride Ophthalmic Solution USP, 1% .... ⊙246

Cryptenamine Preparations (The antihypertensive effects of veratrum alkaloids may be reduced by sympathomimetics).
No products indexed under this heading.

Deslanoside (Increased ectopic pacemaker activity can occur when pseudoephedrine is used concomitantly with digitalis).
No products indexed under this heading.

Digitalis Glycoside Preparations (Increased ectopic pacemaker activity can occur when pseudoephedrine is used concomitantly with digitalis).
No products indexed under this heading.

Digitoxin (Increased ectopic pacemaker activity can occur when pseudoephedrine is used concomitantly with digitalis).
No products indexed under this heading.

Digoxin (Increased ectopic pacemaker activity can occur when pseudoephedrine is used concomitantly with digitalis). Products include:
Digitek Tablets 2146
Lanoxicaps Capsules 1458
Lanoxin Injection 1462
Lanoxin Tablets 1468
Lanoxin Injection Pediatric 1465

Esmolol Hydrochloride (The antihypertensive effects of beta-adrenergic blocking agents may be reduced by sympathomimetics). Products include:
Brevibloc Concentrate 766
Brevibloc Injection 766
Brevibloc Double Strength Injection 766
Brevibloc Premixed Injection 766
Brevibloc Double Strength Premixed Injection 766

Isocarboxazid (Due to the pseudoephedrine component, Clarinex-D 24 Hour extended-release tablets should not be used by patients taking monoamine oxidase inhibitors or within 14 days after stopping such treatment).
No products indexed under this heading.

Labetalol Hydrochloride (The antihypertensive effects of beta-adrenergic blocking agents may be reduced by sympathomimetics).
No products indexed under this heading.

Levobunolol Hydrochloride (The antihypertensive effects of beta-adrenergic blocking agents may be reduced by sympathomimetics). Products include:

Betagan Ophthalmic Solution, USP ⊙217

Mecamylamine Hydrochloride (The antihypertensive effects of mecamylamine may be reduced by sympathomimetics). Products include:

Inversine Tablets 3286

Methyldopa (The antihypertensive effects of methyldopa may be reduced by sympathomimetics). Products include:

Aldoclor Tablets 1881
Aldoril Tablets 1884

Methyldopate Hydrochloride (The antihypertensive effects of methyldopa may be reduced by sympathomimetics).

No products indexed under this heading.

Metipranolol Hydrochloride (The antihypertensive effects of beta-adrenergic blocking agents may be reduced by sympathomimetics).

No products indexed under this heading.

Metoprolol Succinate (The antihypertensive effects of beta-adrenergic blocking agents may be reduced by sympathomimetics). Products include:

Toprol-XL Tablets 660

Metoprolol Tartrate (The antihypertensive effects of beta-adrenergic blocking agents may be reduced by sympathomimetics).

No products indexed under this heading.

Moclobemide (Due to the pseudoephedrine component, Clarinex-D 24 Hour extended-release tablets should not be used by patients taking monoamine oxidase inhibitors or within 14 days after stopping such treatment).

No products indexed under this heading.

Nadolol (The antihypertensive effects of beta-adrenergic blocking agents may be reduced by sympathomimetics). Products include:

Nadolol Tablets 2121

Pargyline Hydrochloride (Due to the pseudoephedrine component, Clarinex-D 24 Hour extended-release tablets should not be used by patients taking monoamine oxidase inhibitors or within 14 days after stopping such treatment).

No products indexed under this heading.

Penbutolol Sulfate (The antihypertensive effects of beta-adrenergic blocking agents may be reduced by sympathomimetics).

No products indexed under this heading.

Phenelzine Sulfate (Due to the pseudoephedrine component, Clarinex-D 24 Hour extended-release tablets should not be used by patients taking monoamine oxidase inhibitors or within 14 days after stopping such treatment).

No products indexed under this heading.

Pindolol (The antihypertensive effects of beta-adrenergic blocking agents may be reduced by sympathomimetics).

No products indexed under this heading.

Procarbazine Hydrochloride (Due to the pseudoephedrine component, Clarinex-D 24 Hour extended-release tablets should not be used by patients taking monoamine oxidase inhibitors or within 14 days after stopping such treatment). Products include:

Matulane Capsules 3188

Propranolol Hydrochloride (The antihypertensive effects of beta-adrenergic blocking agents may be reduced by sympathomimetics). Products include:

Inderal LA Long-Acting Capsules 3421
InnoPran XL Capsules 2728

Reserpine (The antihypertensive effects of reserpine may be reduced by sympathomimetics).

No products indexed under this heading.

Selegiline Hydrochloride (Due to the pseudoephedrine component, Clarinex-D 24 Hour extended-release tablets should not be used by patients taking monoamine oxidase inhibitors or within 14 days after stopping such treatment). Products include:

Eldepryl Capsules 3209

Sotalol Hydrochloride (The antihypertensive effects of beta-adrenergic blocking agents may be reduced by sympathomimetics).

No products indexed under this heading.

Timolol Hemihydrate (The antihypertensive effects of beta-adrenergic blocking agents may be reduced by sympathomimetics). Products include:

Betimol Ophthalmic Solution 3371
Betimol Ophthalmic Solution ⊙283

Timolol Maleate (The antihypertensive effects of beta-adrenergic blocking agents may be reduced by sympathomimetics). Products include:

Blocadren Tablets 1891
Cosopt Sterile Ophthalmic Solution 1910
Timolide Tablets 2056
Timoptic in Ocudose 2061
Timoptic Sterile Ophthalmic Solution 2058
Timoptic-XE Sterile Ophthalmic Gel Forming Solution 2062

Tranylcypromine Sulfate (Due to the pseudoephedrine component, Clarinex-D 24 Hour extended-release tablets should not be used by patients taking monoamine oxidase inhibitors or within 14 days after stopping such treatment). Products include:

Parnate Tablets 1499

CLARIPEL CREAM

(Hydroquinone) 3212
None cited in PDR database.

CHILDREN'S CLARITIN 24 HOUR NON-DROWSY ALLERGY SYRUP

(Loratadine) ▣732
None cited in PDR database.

CLARITIN NON-DROWSY 24 HOUR TABLETS

(Loratadine) ▣731
None cited in PDR database.

NON-DROWSY CLARITIN HIVES RELIEF TABLETS

(Loratadine) ▣733
None cited in PDR database.

CLARITIN REDITABS 24 HOUR NON-DROWSY TABLETS

(Loratadine) ▣732
None cited in PDR database.

CLARITIN-D NON-DROWSY 12 HOUR TABLETS

(Loratadine, Pseudoephedrine Sulfate) ▣731
May interact with monoamine oxidase inhibitors. Compounds in these categories include:

Isocarboxazid (Concurrent and/or sequential use with MAO inhibitors is not recommended).

No products indexed under this heading.

Moclobemide (Concurrent and/or sequential use with MAO inhibitors is not recommended).

No products indexed under this heading.

Pargyline Hydrochloride (Concurrent and/or sequential use with MAO inhibitors is not recommended).

No products indexed under this heading.

Phenelzine Sulfate (Concurrent and/or sequential use with MAO inhibitors is not recommended).

No products indexed under this heading.

Procarbazine Hydrochloride (Concurrent and/or sequential use with MAO inhibitors is not recommended). Products include:

Matulane Capsules 3188

Selegiline Hydrochloride (Concurrent and/or sequential use with MAO inhibitors is not recommended). Products include:

Eldepryl Capsules 3209

Tranylcypromine Sulfate (Concurrent and/or sequential use with MAO inhibitors is not recommended). Products include:

Parnate Tablets 1499

CLARITIN-D NON-DROWSY 24 HOUR TABLETS

(Loratadine, Pseudoephedrine Sulfate) ▣731
See Claritin-D Non-Drowsy 12 Hour Tablets

CLEOCIN VAGINAL OVULES

(Clindamycin Hydrochloride) 2613
May interact with erythromycin, neuromuscular blocking agents, and certain other agents. Compounds in these categories include:

Atracurium Besylate (Co-administration with clindamycin will enhance the action of other neuromuscular blocking agents).

No products indexed under this heading.

Cisatracurium Besylate (Co-administration with clindamycin will enhance the action of other neuromuscular blocking agents). Products include:

Nimbex Injection 494

Diphenoxylate Hydrochloride (May prolong and/or worsen colitis).

No products indexed under this heading.

Doxacurium Chloride (Co-administration with clindamycin will enhance the action of other neuromuscular blocking agents).

No products indexed under this heading.

Erythromycin (Antagonism has been demonstrated between clindamycin and erythromycin in vitro because of possible clinical significance; these two drugs should not be administered concurrently). Products include:

Erygel Topical Gel 2096
Ery-Tab Tablets 447
Erythromycin Base Filmtab Tablets 454
Erythromycin Delayed-Release Capsules, USP 456
PCE Dispertab Tablets 510

Erythromycin Estolate (Antagonism has been demonstrated between clindamycin and erythromycin in vitro because of possible clinical significance; these two drugs should not be administered concurrently).

No products indexed under this heading.

Erythromycin Ethylsuccinate (Antagonism has been demonstrated between clindamycin and erythromycin in vitro because of possible clinical significance; these two drugs should not be administered concurrently). Products include:

E.E.S. 449
EryPed 445

Erythromycin Gluceptate (Antagonism has been demonstrated between clindamycin and erythromycin in vitro because of possible clinical significance; these two drugs should not be administered concurrently).

No products indexed under this heading.

Erythromycin Lactobionate (Antagonism has been demonstrated between clindamycin and erythromycin in vitro because of possible clinical significance; these two drugs should not be administered concurrently).

No products indexed under this heading.

Erythromycin Stearate (Antagonism has been demonstrated between clindamycin and erythromycin in vitro because of possible clinical significance; these two drugs should not be administered concurrently). Products include:

Erythrocin Stearate Filmtab Tablets 452

Metocurine Iodide (Co-administration with clindamycin will enhance the action of other neuromuscular blocking agents).

No products indexed under this heading.

Mivacurium Chloride (Co-administration with clindamycin will enhance the action of other neuromuscular blocking agents). Products include:

Mivacron Injection 489

Pancuronium Bromide (Co-administration with clindamycin will enhance the action of other neuromuscular blocking agents).

No products indexed under this heading.

Rapacuronium Bromide (Co-administration with clindamycin will enhance the action of other neuromuscular blocking agents).

No products indexed under this heading.

Rocuronium Bromide (Co-administration with clindamycin will enhance the action of other neuromuscular blocking agents). Products include:

Zemuron Injection 2363

Succinylcholine Chloride (Co-administration with clindamycin will enhance the action of other neuromuscular blocking agents).
No products indexed under this heading.

Vecuronium Bromide (Co-administration with clindamycin will enhance the action of other neuromuscular blocking agents).
No products indexed under this heading.

CLIMARA TRANSDERMAL SYSTEM

(Estradiol) 795
May interact with erythromycin. Compounds in these categories include:

Carbamazepine (Inducers of CYP3A4, such as carbamazepine, may be reduce plasma concentrations of estrogens, possibly resulting in a decrease in therapuetic effects and/or changes in uterine bleeding profile). Products include:
Carbatrol Capsules 3174
Equetro Extended-Release Capsules 3178
Tegretol/Tegretol-XR 2278

Clarithromycin (Inducers of CYP3A4, such as clarithromycin, may increase plasma concentrations of estrogens and may result in side effects). Products include:
Biaxin/Biaxin XL 402
PREVPAC 3281

Erythromycin (Inducers of CYP3A4, such as erythromycin, may increase plasma concentrations of estrogens and may result in side effects). Products include:
Erygel Topical Gel 2096
Ery-Tab Tablets 447
Erythromycin Base Filmtab Tablets 454
Erythromycin Delayed-Release Capsules, USP............................. 456
PCE Dispertab Tablets 510

Erythromycin Estolate (Inducers of CYP3A4, such as erythromycin, may increase plasma concentrations of estrogens and may result in side effects).
No products indexed under this heading.

Erythromycin Ethylsuccinate (Inducers of CYP3A4, such as erythromycin, may increase plasma concentrations of estrogens and may result in side effects). Products include:
E.E.S. 449
EryPed 445

Erythromycin Gluceptate (Inducers of CYP3A4, such as erythromycin, may increase plasma concentrations of estrogens and may result in side effects).
No products indexed under this heading.

Erythromycin Lactobionate (Inducers of CYP3A4, such as erythromycin, may increase plasma concentrations of estrogens and may result in side effects).
No products indexed under this heading.

Erythromycin Stearate (Inducers of CYP3A4, such as erythromycin, may increase plasma concentrations of estrogens and may result in side effects). Products include:
Erythrocin Stearate Filmtab Tablets 452

Hypericum Perforatum (Inducers of CYP3A4, such as St. John's Wort preparations (Hypericum perforatum) may reduce plasma concentrations of estrogens, possibly resulting in a decrease in therapuetic effects and/or changes in uterine bleeding profile).
No products indexed under this heading.

Itraconazole (Inducers of CYP3A4, such as itraconazole, may increase plasma concentrations of estrogens and may result in side effects).
No products indexed under this heading.

Ketoconazole (Inducers of CYP3A4, such as ketoconazole, may increase plasma concentrations of estrogens and may result in side effects). Products include:
Nizoral A-D Shampoo, 1% 1839
Nizoral 2% Shampoo 1838

Phenobarbital (Inducers of CYP3A4, such as phenobarbital, may be reduce plasma concentrations of estrogens, possibly resulting in a decrease in therapuetic effects and/or changes in uterine bleeding profile).
No products indexed under this heading.

Rifampin (Inducers of CYP3A4, such as rifampin, may reduce plasma concentrations of estrogens, possibly resulting in a decrease in therapuetic effects and/or changes in uterine bleeding profile).
No products indexed under this heading.

Ritonavir (Inducers of CYP3A4, such as ritonavir, may increase plasma concentrations of estrogens and may result in side effects). Products include:
Kaletra 474
Norvir 499

Food Interactions

Grapefruit Juice (Inducers of CYP3A4, such as grapefruit juice, may increase plasma concentrations of estrogens and may result in side effects).

CLIMARA PRO TRANSDERMAL SYSTEM

(Estradiol, Levonorgestrel) 800
May interact with cytochrome p450 3a4 inducers (selected) and cytochrome p450 3a4 inhibitors (selected). Compounds in these categories include:

Acetazolamide (Inhibitors of CYP3A4 such as erythromycin, clarithromycin, ketoconazole, itraconazole, ritonavir and grapefruit juice may increase plasma concentrations of estrogens and may result in side effects).
No products indexed under this heading.

Allium sativum (Inducers of CYP3A4 may reduce plasma concentrations of estrogens, possibly resulting in a decrease in therapeutic effects and/or changes in the uterine bleeding profile).
No products indexed under this heading.

Amiodarone Hydrochloride (Inhibitors of CYP3A4 such as erythromycin, clarithromycin, ketoconazole, itraconazole, ritonavir and grapefruit juice may increase plasma concentrations of estrogens and may result in side effects). Products include:
Pacerone Tablets 3337

Amprenavir (Inhibitors of CYP3A4 such as erythromycin, clarithromycin, ketoconazole, itraconazole, ritonavir and grapefruit juice may increase plasma concentrations of estrogens and may result in side effects). Products include:
Agenerase Capsules 1299
Agenerase Oral Solution 1304

Anastrozole (Inhibitors of CYP3A4 such as erythromycin, clarithromycin, ketoconazole, itraconazole, ritonavir and grapefruit juice may increase plasma concentrations of estrogens and may result in side effects). Products include:
Arimidex Tablets 665

Aprepitant (Inducers of CYP3A4 may reduce plasma concentrations of estrogens, possibly resulting in a decrease in therapeutic effects and/or changes in the uterine bleeding profile). Products include:
Emend Capsules 1944

Betamethasone Acetate (Inducers of CYP3A4 may reduce plasma concentrations of estrogens, possibly resulting in a decrease in therapeutic effects and/or changes in the uterine bleeding profile).
No products indexed under this heading.

Betamethasone Sodium Phosphate (Inducers of CYP3A4 may reduce plasma concentrations of estrogens, possibly resulting in a decrease in therapeutic effects and/or changes in the uterine bleeding profile).
No products indexed under this heading.

Carbamazepine (Inducers of CYP3A4 may reduce plasma concentrations of estrogens, possibly resulting in a decrease in therapeutic effects and/or changes in the uterine bleeding profile). Products include:
Carbatrol Capsules 3174
Equetro Extended-Release Capsules 3178
Tegretol/Tegretol-XR 2278

Cimetidine (Inhibitors of CYP3A4 such as erythromycin, clarithromycin, ketoconazole, itraconazole, ritonavir and grapefruit juice may increase plasma concentrations of estrogens and may result in side effects). Products include:
Tagamet HB 200 Tablets 637
Tagamet Tablets 1547

Cimetidine Hydrochloride (Inhibitors of CYP3A4 such as erythromycin, clarithromycin, ketoconazole, itraconazole, ritonavir and grapefruit juice may increase plasma concentrations of estrogens and may result in side effects).
No products indexed under this heading.

Ciprofloxacin (Inhibitors of CYP3A4 such as erythromycin, clarithromycin, ketoconazole, itraconazole, ritonavir and grapefruit juice may increase plasma concentrations of estrogens and may result in side effects). Products include:
Cipro I.V. 2998
Cipro I.V. Pharmacy Bulk Package ... 3509
Cipro Oral Suspension 2991
Cipro XR Tablets 3004
Ciprodex Otic Suspension 555

Ciprofloxacin Hydrochloride (Inducers of CYP3A4 may reduce plasma concentrations of estrogens, possibly resulting in a decrease in therapeutic effects and/or changes in the uterine bleeding profile). Products include:
Ciloxan Ophthalmic Ointment 554
Cipro Tablets 2991

Cisplatin (Inducers of CYP3A4 may reduce plasma concentrations of estrogens, possibly resulting in a decrease in therapeutic effects and/or changes in the uterine bleeding profile).
No products indexed under this heading.

Clarithromycin (Inhibitors of CYP3A4 such as erythromycin, clarithromycin, ketoconazole, itraconazole, ritonavir and grapefruit juice may increase plasma concentrations of estrogens and may result in side effects). Products include:
Biaxin/Biaxin XL 402
PREVPAC 3281

Clotrimazole (Inhibitors of CYP3A4 such as erythromycin, clarithromycin, ketoconazole, itraconazole, ritonavir and grapefruit juice may increase plasma concentrations of estrogens and may result in side effects). Products include:
Lotrimin 3053
Lotrisone 3054

Cortisone Acetate (Inducers of CYP3A4 may reduce plasma concentrations of estrogens, possibly resulting in a decrease in therapeutic effects and/or changes in the uterine bleeding profile).
No products indexed under this heading.

Cyclosporine (Inhibitors of CYP3A4 such as erythromycin, clarithromycin, ketoconazole, itraconazole, ritonavir and grapefruit juice may increase plasma concentrations of estrogens and may result in side effects). Products include:
Gengraf Capsules 458
Neoral Soft Gelatin Capsules 2247
Neoral Oral Solution 2247
Restasis Ophthalmic Emulsion 570
Sandimmune 2259

Dalfopristin (Inhibitors of CYP3A4 such as erythromycin, clarithromycin, ketoconazole, itraconazole, ritonavir and grapefruit juice may increase plasma concentrations of estrogens and may result in side effects). Products include:
Synercid I.V. 1690

Danazol (Inhibitors of CYP3A4 such as erythromycin, clarithromycin, ketoconazole, itraconazole, ritonavir and grapefruit juice may increase plasma concentrations of estrogens and may result in side effects).
No products indexed under this heading.

Delavirdine Mesylate (Inhibitors of CYP3A4 such as erythromycin, clarithromycin, ketoconazole, itraconazole, ritonavir and grapefruit juice may increase plasma concentrations of estrogens and may result in side effects). Products include:
Rescriptor Tablets 2535

Dexamethasone (Inducers of CYP3A4 may reduce plasma concentrations of estrogens, possibly resulting in a decrease in therapeutic effects and/or changes in the uterine bleeding profile). Products include:
Ciprodex Otic Suspension 555
Decadron Tablets 1929
TobraDex Ophthalmic Ointment 558
TobraDex Ophthalmic Suspension ... 558

Dexamethasone Acetate (Inducers of CYP3A4 may reduce plasma concentrations of estrogens, possibly resulting in a decrease in therapeutic effects and/or changes in the uterine bleeding profile).
No products indexed under this heading.

Dexamethasone Sodium Phosphate (Inducers of CYP3A4 may reduce plasma concentrations of estrogens, possibly resulting in a decrease in therapeutic effects and/or changes in the uterine bleeding profile). Products include:
Decadron Phosphate Injection 1931

Diltiazem Hydrochloride (Inhibitors of CYP3A4 such as erythromycin, clarithromycin, ketoconazole, itraconazole, ritonavir and grapefruit juice may increase plasma concentrations of estrogens and may result in side effects). Products include:
Cardizem LA Extended Release Tablets 1699
Tiazac Capsules 1204

Diltiazem Maleate (Inhibitors of CYP3A4 such as erythromycin, clarithromycin, ketoconazole, itraconazole, ritonavir and grapefruit juice may increase plasma concentrations of estrogens and may result in side effects).
No products indexed under this heading.

Doxorubicin Hydrochloride (Inducers of CYP3A4 may reduce plasma concentrations of estrogens, possibly resulting in a decrease in therapeutic effects and/or changes in the uterine bleeding profile). Products include:
Adriamycin for Injection, USP 786
Adriamycin Injection, USP 786

Efavirenz (Inducers of CYP3A4 may reduce plasma concentrations of estrogens, possibly resulting in a decrease in therapeutic effects and/or changes in the uterine bleeding profile). Products include:
Sustiva Capsules 957

Erythromycin (Inhibitors of CYP3A4 such as erythromycin, clarithromycin, ketoconazole, itraconazole, ritonavir and grapefruit juice may increase plasma concentrations of estrogens and may result in side effects). Products include:
Erygel Topical Gel 2096
Ery-Tab Tablets 447
Erythromycin Base Filmtab Tablets 454
Erythromycin Delayed-Release Capsules, USP 456
PCE Dispertab Tablets 510

Erythromycin Estolate (Inhibitors of CYP3A4 such as erythromycin, clarithromycin, ketoconazole, itraconazole, ritonavir and grapefruit juice may increase plasma concentrations of estrogens and may result in side effects).
No products indexed under this heading.

Erythromycin Ethylsuccinate (Inhibitors of CYP3A4 such as erythromycin, clarithromycin, ketoconazole, itraconazole, ritonavir and grapefruit juice may increase plasma concentrations of estrogens and may result in side effects). Products include:
E.E.S. 449
EryPed 445

Erythromycin Gluceptate (Inhibitors of CYP3A4 such as erythromycin, clarithromycin, ketoconazole, itraconazole, ritonavir and grapefruit juice may increase plasma concentrations of estrogens and may result in side effects).
No products indexed under this heading.

Erythromycin Lactobionate (Inhibitors of CYP3A4 such as erythromycin, clarithromycin, ketoconazole, itraconazole, ritonavir and grapefruit juice may increase plasma concentrations of estrogens and may result in side effects).
No products indexed under this heading.

Erythromycin Stearate (Inhibitors of CYP3A4 such as erythromycin, clarithromycin, ketoconazole, itraconazole, ritonavir and grapefruit juice may increase plasma concentrations of estrogens and may result in side effects). Products include:
Erythrocin Stearate Filmtab Tablets 452

Esomeprazole Magnesium (Inhibitors of CYP3A4 such as erythromycin, clarithromycin, ketoconazole, itraconazole, ritonavir and grapefruit juice may increase plasma concentrations of estrogens and may result in side effects). Products include:
Nexium Delayed-Release Capsules 645

Ethosuximide (Inducers of CYP3A4 may reduce plasma concentrations of estrogens, possibly resulting in a decrease in therapeutic effects and/or changes in the uterine bleeding profile).
No products indexed under this heading.

Felbamate (Inducers of CYP3A4 may reduce plasma concentrations of estrogens, possibly resulting in a decrease in therapeutic effects and/or changes in the uterine bleeding profile).
No products indexed under this heading.

Fluconazole (Inhibitors of CYP3A4 such as erythromycin, clarithromycin, ketoconazole, itraconazole, ritonavir and grapefruit juice may increase plasma concentrations of estrogens and may result in side effects).
No products indexed under this heading.

Fludrocortisone Acetate (Inducers of CYP3A4 may reduce plasma concentrations of estrogens, possibly resulting in a decrease in therapeutic effects and/or changes in the uterine bleeding profile).
No products indexed under this heading.

Fluoxetine Hydrochloride (Inhibitors of CYP3A4 such as erythromycin, clarithromycin, ketoconazole, itraconazole, ritonavir and grapefruit juice may increase plasma concentrations of estrogens and may result in side effects). Products include:
Prozac Pulvules and Liquid 1771
Symbyax Capsules 1788

Fluvoxamine Maleate (Inhibitors of CYP3A4 such as erythromycin, clarithromycin, ketoconazole, itraconazole, ritonavir and grapefruit juice may increase plasma concentrations of estrogens and may result in side effects).
No products indexed under this heading.

Fosamprenavir Calcium (Inhibitors of CYP3A4 such as erythromycin, clarithromycin, ketoconazole, itraconazole, ritonavir and grapefruit juice may increase plasma concentrations of estrogens and may result in side effects). Products include:
Lexiva Tablets 1473

Fosphenytoin Sodium (Inducers of CYP3A4 may reduce plasma concentrations of estrogens, possibly resulting in a decrease in therapeutic effects and/or changes in the uterine bleeding profile).
No products indexed under this heading.

Garlic Extract (Inducers of CYP3A4 may reduce plasma concentrations of estrogens, possibly resulting in a decrease in therapeutic effects and/or changes in the uterine bleeding profile).
No products indexed under this heading.

Garlic Oil (Inducers of CYP3A4 may reduce plasma concentrations of estrogens, possibly resulting in a decrease in therapeutic effects and/or changes in the uterine bleeding profile).
No products indexed under this heading.

Hydrocortisone (Inducers of CYP3A4 may reduce plasma concentrations of estrogens, possibly resulting in a decrease in therapeutic effects and/or changes in the uterine bleeding profile). Products include:
Cortizone•5 Ointment .... ■699
Cortizone•10 Creme .... ■699
Cortizone•10 Ointment .... ■699
Cortizone•10 Plus Creme .... ■700
Cortizone•10 Maximum Strength Quick Shot Spray .... ■700
Hydrocortone Tablets 1963
Preparation H Hydrocortisone Cream .... ■748

Hydrocortisone Acetate (Inducers of CYP3A4 may reduce plasma concentrations of estrogens, possibly resulting in a decrease in therapeutic effects and/or changes in the uterine bleeding profile). Products include:
Analpram-HC 1136
Pramosone 1139
ProctoFoam-HC 3113
Tucks Anti-Itch Ointment .... ■712
U-cort 1% Cream 3289

Hydrocortisone Butyrate (Inducers of CYP3A4 may reduce plasma concentrations of estrogens, possibly resulting in a decrease in therapeutic effects and/or changes in the uterine bleeding profile). Products include:
Locoid 1138
Locoid Lipocream Cream 1138

Hydrocortisone Cypionate (Inducers of CYP3A4 may reduce plasma concentrations of estrogens, possibly resulting in a decrease in therapeutic effects and/or changes in the uterine bleeding profile).
No products indexed under this heading.

Hydrocortisone Hemisuccinate (Inducers of CYP3A4 may reduce plasma concentrations of estrogens, possibly resulting in a decrease in therapeutic effects and/or changes in the uterine bleeding profile).
No products indexed under this heading.

Hydrocortisone Probutate (Inducers of CYP3A4 may reduce plasma concentrations of estrogens, possibly resulting in a decrease in therapeutic effects and/or changes in the uterine bleeding profile). Products include:
Pandel Cream, 0.1% 1017

Hydrocortisone Sodium Phosphate (Inducers of CYP3A4 may reduce plasma concentrations of estrogens, possibly resulting in a decrease in therapeutic effects and/or changes in the uterine bleeding profile).
No products indexed under this heading.

Hydrocortisone Sodium Succinate (Inducers of CYP3A4 may reduce plasma concentrations of estrogens, possibly resulting in a decrease in therapeutic effects and/or changes in the uterine bleeding profile).
No products indexed under this heading.

Hydrocortisone Valerate (Inducers of CYP3A4 may reduce plasma concentrations of estrogens, possibly resulting in a decrease in therapeutic effects and/or changes in the uterine bleeding profile).
No products indexed under this heading.

Hypericum (Inducers of CYP3A4 may reduce plasma concentrations of estrogens, possibly resulting in a decrease in therapeutic effects and/or changes in the uterine bleeding profile).
No products indexed under this heading.

Hypericum Perforatum (Inducers of CYP3A4 may reduce plasma concentrations of estrogens, possibly resulting in a decrease in therapeutic effects and/or changes in the uterine bleeding profile).
No products indexed under this heading.

Indinavir Sulfate (Inhibitors of CYP3A4 such as erythromycin, clarithromycin, ketoconazole, itraconazole, ritonavir and grapefruit juice may increase plasma concentrations of estrogens and may result in side effects). Products include:
Crixivan Capsules 1918

Isoniazid (Inhibitors of CYP3A4 such as erythromycin, clarithromycin, ketoconazole, itraconazole, ritonavir and grapefruit juice may increase plasma concentrations of estrogens and may result in side effects).
No products indexed under this heading.

Itraconazole (Inhibitors of CYP3A4 such as erythromycin, clarithromycin, ketoconazole, itraconazole, ritonavir and grapefruit juice may increase plasma concentrations of estrogens and may result in side effects).
No products indexed under this heading.

Ketoconazole (Inhibitors of CYP3A4 such as erythromycin, clarithromycin, ketoconazole, itra-

conazole, ritonavir and grapefruit juice may increase plasma concentrations of estrogens and may result in side effects). Products include:

Nizoral A-D Shampoo, 1% ... 1839
Nizoral 2% Shampoo ... 1838

Lopinavir (Inhibitors of CYP3A4 such as erythromycin, clarithromycin, ketoconazole, itraconazole, ritonavir and grapefruit juice may increase plasma concentrations of estrogens and may result in side effects). Products include:

Kaletra ... 474

Loratadine (Inhibitors of CYP3A4 such as erythromycin, clarithromycin, ketoconazole, itraconazole, ritonavir and grapefruit juice may increase plasma concentrations of estrogens and may result in side effects). Products include:

Alavert Allergy & Sinus D-12 Hour Tablets ... 743
Alavert ... 743
Children's Claritin 24 Hour Non-Drowsy Allergy Syrup ... 732
Claritin Non-Drowsy 24 Hour Tablets ... 731
Non-Drowsy Claritin Hives Relief Tablets ... 733
Claritin Reditabs 24 Hour Non-Drowsy Tablets ... 732
Claritin-D Non-Drowsy 12 Hour Tablets ... 731
Claritin-D Non-Drowsy 24 Hour Tablets ... 731
Children's Dimetapp ND Non-Drowsy Allergy Syrup ... 746
Triaminic Allerchews ... 684

Mephenytoin (Inducers of CYP3A4 may reduce plasma concentrations of estrogens, possibly resulting in a decrease in therapeutic effects and/or changes in the uterine bleeding profile).

No products indexed under this heading.

Methsuximide (Inducers of CYP3A4 may reduce plasma concentrations of estrogens, possibly resulting in a decrease in therapeutic effects and/or changes in the uterine bleeding profile).

No products indexed under this heading.

Methylprednisolone (Inducers of CYP3A4 may reduce plasma concentrations of estrogens, possibly resulting in a decrease in therapeutic effects and/or changes in the uterine bleeding profile).

No products indexed under this heading.

Methylprednisolone Acetate (Inducers of CYP3A4 may reduce plasma concentrations of estrogens, possibly resulting in a decrease in therapeutic effects and/or changes in the uterine bleeding profile). Products include:

Depo-Medrol Injectable Suspension ... 2615
Depo-Medrol Single-Dose Vial ... 2617

Methylprednisolone Sodium Succinate (Inducers of CYP3A4 may reduce plasma concentrations of estrogens, possibly resulting in a decrease in therapeutic effects and/or changes in the uterine bleeding profile).

No products indexed under this heading.

Metronidazole (Inhibitors of CYP3A4 such as erythromycin, clarithromycin, ketoconazole, itraconazole, ritonavir and grapefruit juice may increase plasma concentrations of estrogens and may result in side effects). Products include:

Metrogel 1% ... 1212
MetroGel-Vaginal Gel ... 1822
Noritate Cream, 1% ... 1051

Metronidazole Benzoate (Inhibitors of CYP3A4 such as erythromycin, clarithromycin, ketoconazole, itraconazole, ritonavir and grapefruit juice may increase plasma concentrations of estrogens and may result in side effects).

No products indexed under this heading.

Metronidazole Hydrochloride (Inhibitors of CYP3A4 such as erythromycin, clarithromycin, ketoconazole, itraconazole, ritonavir and grapefruit juice may increase plasma concentrations of estrogens and may result in side effects).

No products indexed under this heading.

Miconazole (Inhibitors of CYP3A4 such as erythromycin, clarithromycin, ketoconazole, itraconazole, ritonavir and grapefruit juice may increase plasma concentrations of estrogens and may result in side effects).

No products indexed under this heading.

Miconazole Nitrate (Inhibitors of CYP3A4 such as erythromycin, clarithromycin, ketoconazole, itraconazole, ritonavir and grapefruit juice may increase plasma concentrations of estrogens and may result in side effects). Products include:

Desenex ... 674
Desenex Jock Itch Spray Powder ... 674

Modafinil (Inducers of CYP3A4 may reduce plasma concentrations of estrogens, possibly resulting in a decrease in therapeutic effects and/or changes in the uterine bleeding profile). Products include:

Provigil Tablets ... 1002

Nefazodone Hydrochloride (Inhibitors of CYP3A4 such as erythromycin, clarithromycin, ketoconazole, itraconazole, ritonavir and grapefruit juice may increase plasma concentrations of estrogens and may result in side effects).

No products indexed under this heading.

Nelfinavir Mesylate (Inhibitors of CYP3A4 such as erythromycin, clarithromycin, ketoconazole, itraconazole, ritonavir and grapefruit juice may increase plasma concentrations of estrogens and may result in side effects). Products include:

Viracept ... 2556

Nevirapine (Inducers of CYP3A4 may reduce plasma concentrations of estrogens, possibly resulting in a decrease in therapeutic effects and/or changes in the uterine bleeding profile). Products include:

Viramune Oral Suspension ... 903
Viramune Tablets ... 903

Niacinamide (Inhibitors of CYP3A4 such as erythromycin, clarithromycin, ketoconazole, itraconazole, ritonavir and grapefruit juice may increase plasma concentrations of estrogens and may result in side effects).

No products indexed under this heading.

Nicotinamide (Inhibitors of CYP3A4 such as erythromycin, clarithromycin, ketoconazole, itraconazole, ritonavir and grapefruit juice may increase plasma concentrations of estrogens and may result in side effects). Products include:

Nicomide Tablets ... 3190

Nifedipine (Inhibitors of CYP3A4 such as erythromycin, clarithromycin, ketoconazole, itraconazole, ritonavir and grapefruit juice may increase plasma concentrations of estrogens and may result in side effects). Products include:

Adalat CC Tablets ... 2978

Norfloxacin (Inhibitors of CYP3A4 such as erythromycin, clarithromycin, ketoconazole, itraconazole, ritonavir and grapefruit juice may increase plasma concentrations of estrogens and may result in side effects). Products include:

Noroxin Tablets ... 2009

Omeprazole (Inhibitors of CYP3A4 such as erythromycin, clarithromycin, ketoconazole, itraconazole, ritonavir and grapefruit juice may increase plasma concentrations of estrogens and may result in side effects). Products include:

Zegerid Powder for Oral Solution ... 2972

Oxcarbazepine (Inducers of CYP3A4 may reduce plasma concentrations of estrogens, possibly resulting in a decrease in therapeutic effects and/or changes in the uterine bleeding profile). Products include:

Trileptal Oral Suspension ... 2281
Trileptal Tablets ... 2281

Paroxetine Hydrochloride (Inhibitors of CYP3A4 such as erythromycin, clarithromycin, ketoconazole, itraconazole, ritonavir and grapefruit juice may increase plasma concentrations of estrogens and may result in side effects). Products include:

Paxil CR Controlled-Release Tablets ... 1509
Paxil ... 1501

Phenobarbital (Inducers of CYP3A4 may reduce plasma concentrations of estrogens, possibly resulting in a decrease in therapeutic effects and/or changes in the uterine bleeding profile).

No products indexed under this heading.

Phenobarbital Sodium (Inducers of CYP3A4 may reduce plasma concentrations of estrogens, possibly resulting in a decrease in therapeutic effects and/or changes in the uterine bleeding profile).

No products indexed under this heading.

Phenytoin (Inducers of CYP3A4 may reduce plasma concentrations of estrogens, possibly resulting in a decrease in therapeutic effects and/or changes in the uterine bleeding profile).

No products indexed under this heading.

Phenytoin Sodium (Inducers of CYP3A4 may reduce plasma concentrations of estrogens, possibly resulting in a decrease in therapeutic effects and/or changes in the uterine bleeding profile). Products include:

Phenytek Capsules ... 2153

Prednisolone Acetate (Inducers of CYP3A4 may reduce plasma concentrations of estrogens, possibly resulting in a decrease in therapeutic effects and/or changes in the uterine bleeding profile). Products include:

Blephamide Ophthalmic Ointment ... 563
Blephamide Ophthalmic Suspension ... 564
Poly-Pred Liquifilm Ophthalmic Suspension ... ⊙231
Pred Forte Ophthalmic Suspension ... ⊙233
Pred Mild Sterile Ophthalmic Suspension ... ⊙236
Pred-G Ophthalmic Suspension ... ⊙234
Pred-G Sterile Ophthalmic Ointment ... ⊙235

Prednisolone Sodium Phosphate (Inducers of CYP3A4 may reduce plasma concentrations of estrogens, possibly resulting in a decrease in therapeutic effects and/or changes in the uterine bleeding profile). Products include:

Pediapred Oral Solution ... 3319

Prednisolone Tebutate (Inducers of CYP3A4 may reduce plasma concentrations of estrogens, possibly resulting in a decrease in therapeutic effects and/or changes in the uterine bleeding profile).

No products indexed under this heading.

Prednisone (Inducers of CYP3A4 may reduce plasma concentrations of estrogens, possibly resulting in a decrease in therapeutic effects and/or changes in the uterine bleeding profile).

No products indexed under this heading.

Primidone (Inducers of CYP3A4 may reduce plasma concentrations of estrogens, possibly resulting in a decrease in therapeutic effects and/or changes in the uterine bleeding profile).

No products indexed under this heading.

Propoxyphene Hydrochloride (Inhibitors of CYP3A4 such as erythromycin, clarithromycin, ketoconazole, itraconazole, ritonavir and grapefruit juice may increase plasma concentrations of estrogens and may result in side effects).

No products indexed under this heading.

Propoxyphene Napsylate (Inhibitors of CYP3A4 such as erythromycin, clarithromycin, ketoconazole, itraconazole, ritonavir and grapefruit juice may increase plasma concentrations of estrogens and may result in side effects). Products include:

Darvocet A 500 Tablets ... 3497

Quinidine (Inhibitors of CYP3A4 such as erythromycin, clarithromycin, ketoconazole, itraconazole, ritonavir and grapefruit juice may increase plasma concentrations of estrogens and may result in side effects).

No products indexed under this heading.

Quinidine Hydrochloride (Inhibitors of CYP3A4 such as erythromycin, clarithromycin, ketoconazole, itraconazole, ritonavir and grapefruit juice may increase plasma concentrations of estrogens and may result in side effects).

No products indexed under this heading.

Quinidine Polygalacturonate (Inhibitors of CYP3A4 such as erythromycin, clarithromycin, ketoconazole, itraconazole, ritonavir and grapefruit juice may increase plasma concentrations of estrogens and may result in side effects).

No products indexed under this heading.

Quinidine Sulfate (Inhibitors of CYP3A4 such as erythromycin, clarithromycin, ketoconazole, itraconazole, ritonavir and grapefruit juice may increase plasma concentrations of estrogens and may result in side effects).
No products indexed under this heading.

Quinine (Inhibitors of CYP3A4 such as erythromycin, clarithromycin, ketoconazole, itraconazole, ritonavir and grapefruit juice may increase plasma concentrations of estrogens and may result in side effects).
No products indexed under this heading.

Quinine Sulfate (Inhibitors of CYP3A4 such as erythromycin, clarithromycin, ketoconazole, itraconazole, ritonavir and grapefruit juice may increase plasma concentrations of estrogens and may result in side effects).
No products indexed under this heading.

Quinupristin (Inhibitors of CYP3A4 such as erythromycin, clarithromycin, ketoconazole, itraconazole, ritonavir and grapefruit juice may increase plasma concentrations of estrogens and may result in side effects). Products include:
Synercid I.V. 1690

Ranitidine Bismuth Citrate (Inhibitors of CYP3A4 such as erythromycin, clarithromycin, ketoconazole, itraconazole, ritonavir and grapefruit juice may increase plasma concentrations of estrogens and may result in side effects).
No products indexed under this heading.

Ranitidine Hydrochloride (Inhibitors of CYP3A4 such as erythromycin, clarithromycin, ketoconazole, itraconazole, ritonavir and grapefruit juice may increase plasma concentrations of estrogens and may result in side effects). Products include:
Zantac 1597
Zantac Injection 1593
Zantac 75 Tablets .... ■715
Zantac 150 Maximum Strength Tablets.. ■715
Zantac Injection Pharmacy Bulk Package.. 1595

Rifabutin (Inducers of CYP3A4 may reduce plasma concentrations of estrogens, possibly resulting in a decrease in therapeutic effects and/or changes in the uterine bleeding profile).
No products indexed under this heading.

Rifampicin (Inducers of CYP3A4 may reduce plasma concentrations of estrogens, possibly resulting in a decrease in therapeutic effects and/or changes in the uterine bleeding profile).
No products indexed under this heading.

Rifampin (Inducers of CYP3A4 may reduce plasma concentrations of estrogens, possibly resulting in a decrease in therapeutic effects and/or changes in the uterine bleeding profile).
No products indexed under this heading.

Rifapentine (Inducers of CYP3A4 may reduce plasma concentrations of estrogens, possibly resulting in a decrease in therapeutic effects and/or changes in the uterine bleeding profile).
No products indexed under this heading.

Ritonavir (Inhibitors of CYP3A4 such as erythromycin, clarithromycin, ketoconazole, itraconazole, ritonavir and grapefruit juice may increase plasma concentrations of estrogens and may result in side effects). Products include:
Kaletra 474
Norvir 499

Saquinavir (Inhibitors of CYP3A4 such as erythromycin, clarithromycin, ketoconazole, itraconazole, ritonavir and grapefruit juice may increase plasma concentrations of estrogens and may result in side effects).
No products indexed under this heading.

Saquinavir Mesylate (Inhibitors of CYP3A4 such as erythromycin, clarithromycin, ketoconazole, itraconazole, ritonavir and grapefruit juice may increase plasma concentrations of estrogens and may result in side effects). Products include:
Invirase 2776

Sertraline Hydrochloride (Inhibitors of CYP3A4 such as erythromycin, clarithromycin, ketoconazole, itraconazole, ritonavir and grapefruit juice may increase plasma concentrations of estrogens and may result in side effects). Products include:
Zoloft 2581

Sulfinpyrazone (Inducers of CYP3A4 may reduce plasma concentrations of estrogens, possibly resulting in a decrease in therapeutic effects and/or changes in the uterine bleeding profile).
No products indexed under this heading.

Telithromycin (Inhibitors of CYP3A4 such as erythromycin, clarithromycin, ketoconazole, itraconazole, ritonavir and grapefruit juice may increase plasma concentrations of estrogens and may result in side effects). Products include:
Ketek Tablets 2920

Theophylline (Inducers of CYP3A4 may reduce plasma concentrations of estrogens, possibly resulting in a decrease in therapeutic effects and/or changes in the uterine bleeding profile).
No products indexed under this heading.

Triamcinolone (Inducers of CYP3A4 may reduce plasma concentrations of estrogens, possibly resulting in a decrease in therapeutic effects and/or changes in the uterine bleeding profile).
No products indexed under this heading.

Triamcinolone Acetonide (Inducers of CYP3A4 may reduce plasma concentrations of estrogens, possibly resulting in a decrease in therapeutic effects and/or changes in the uterine bleeding profile). Products include:
Azmacort Inhalation Aerosol 1701
Nasacort HFA Inhalation Aerosol 2939
Nasacort AQ Nasal Spray 2937

Triamcinolone Diacetate (Inducers of CYP3A4 may reduce plasma concentrations of estrogens, possibly resulting in a decrease in therapeutic effects and/or changes in the uterine bleeding profile).
No products indexed under this heading.

Triamcinolone Hexacetonide (Inducers of CYP3A4 may reduce plasma concentrations of estrogens, possibly resulting in a decrease in therapeutic effects and/or changes in the uterine bleeding profile).
No products indexed under this heading.

Troglitazone (Inducers of CYP3A4 may reduce plasma concentrations of estrogens, possibly resulting in a decrease in therapeutic effects and/or changes in the uterine bleeding profile).
No products indexed under this heading.

Troleandomycin (Inhibitors of CYP3A4 such as erythromycin, clarithromycin, ketoconazole, itraconazole, ritonavir and grapefruit juice may increase plasma concentrations of estrogens and may result in side effects).
No products indexed under this heading.

Valproate Sodium (Inhibitors of CYP3A4 such as erythromycin, clarithromycin, ketoconazole, itraconazole, ritonavir and grapefruit juice may increase plasma concentrations of estrogens and may result in side effects). Products include:
Depacon Injection 412

Verapamil Hydrochloride (Inhibitors of CYP3A4 such as erythromycin, clarithromycin, ketoconazole, itraconazole, ritonavir and grapefruit juice may increase plasma concentrations of estrogens and may result in side effects). Products include:
Covera-HS Tablets 3135
Tarka Tablets 519
Verelan PM Capsules 3120

Voriconazole (Inhibitors of CYP3A4 such as erythromycin, clarithromycin, ketoconazole, itraconazole, ritonavir and grapefruit juice may increase plasma concentrations of estrogens and may result in side effects). Products include:
VFEND I.V. 2543
VFEND Oral Suspension 2543
VFEND Tablets 2543

Zafirlukast (Inhibitors of CYP3A4 such as erythromycin, clarithromycin, ketoconazole, itraconazole, ritonavir and grapefruit juice may increase plasma concentrations of estrogens and may result in side effects). Products include:
Accolate Tablets 663

Zileuton (Inhibitors of CYP3A4 such as erythromycin, clarithromycin, ketoconazole, itraconazole, ritonavir and grapefruit juice may increase plasma concentrations of estrogens and may result in side effects).
No products indexed under this heading.

Food Interactions

Grapefruit (Inhibitors of CYP3A4 such as erythromycin, clarithromycin, ketoconazole, itraconazole, ritonavir and grapefruit juice may increase plasma concentrations of estrogens and may result in side effects).

Grapefruit Juice (Inhibitors of CYP3A4 such as erythromycin, clarithromycin, ketoconazole, itraconazole, ritonavir and grapefruit juice may increase plasma concentrations of estrogens and may result in side effects).

CLINAC BPO 7 GEL USP

(Benzoyl Peroxide) 1137
None cited in PDR database.

CLINDAGEL

(Clindamycin Phosphate) 1207
May interact with neuromuscular blocking agents. Compounds in these categories include:

Atracurium Besylate (Clindamycin has neuromuscular blocking properties that may enhance the action of other neuromuscular blocking agents).
No products indexed under this heading.

Cisatracurium Besylate (Clindamycin has neuromuscular blocking properties that may enhance the action of other neuromuscular blocking agents). Products include:
Nimbex Injection 494

Doxacurium Chloride (Clindamycin has neuromuscular blocking properties that may enhance the action of other neuromuscular blocking agents).
No products indexed under this heading.

Metocurine Iodide (Clindamycin has neuromuscular blocking properties that may enhance the action of other neuromuscular blocking agents).
No products indexed under this heading.

Mivacurium Chloride (Clindamycin has neuromuscular blocking properties that may enhance the action of other neuromuscular blocking agents). Products include:
Mivacron Injection 489

Pancuronium Bromide (Clindamycin has neuromuscular blocking properties that may enhance the action of other neuromuscular blocking agents).
No products indexed under this heading.

Rapacuronium Bromide (Clindamycin has neuromuscular blocking properties that may enhance the action of other neuromuscular blocking agents).
No products indexed under this heading.

Rocuronium Bromide (Clindamycin has neuromuscular blocking properties that may enhance the action of other neuromuscular blocking agents). Products include:
Zemuron Injection 2363

Succinylcholine Chloride (Clindamycin has neuromuscular blocking properties that may enhance the action of other neuromuscular blocking agents).
No products indexed under this heading.

Vecuronium Bromide (Clindamycin has neuromuscular blocking properties that may enhance the action of other neuromuscular blocking agents).
No products indexed under this heading.

CLINDESSE VAGINAL CREAM

(Clindamycin Phosphate) 3296

May interact with neuromuscular blocking agents. Compounds in these categories include:

Atracurium Besylate (Clindamycin has been shown to have neuromuscular blocking properties that may enhance the action of other neuromuscular blocking agents. Therefore, it should be used with caution in patients receiving such agents).
No products indexed under this heading.

Cisatracurium Besylate (Clindamycin has been shown to have neuromuscular blocking properties that may enhance the action of other neuromuscular blocking agents. Therefore, it should be used with caution in patients receiving such agents). Products include:
Nimbex Injection 494

Doxacurium Chloride (Clindamycin has been shown to have neuromuscular blocking properties that may enhance the action of other neuromuscular blocking agents. Therefore, it should be used with caution in patients receiving such agents).
No products indexed under this heading.

Metocurine Iodide (Clindamycin has been shown to have neuromuscular blocking properties that may enhance the action of other neuromuscular blocking agents. Therefore, it should be used with caution in patients receiving such agents).
No products indexed under this heading.

Mivacurium Chloride (Clindamycin has been shown to have neuromuscular blocking properties that may enhance the action of other neuromuscular blocking agents. Therefore, it should be used with caution in patients receiving such agents). Products include:
Mivacron Injection 489

Pancuronium Bromide (Clindamycin has been shown to have neuromuscular blocking properties that may enhance the action of other neuromuscular blocking agents. Therefore, it should be used with caution in patients receiving such agents).
No products indexed under this heading.

Rapacuronium Bromide (Clindamycin has been shown to have neuromuscular blocking properties that may enhance the action of other neuromuscular blocking agents. Therefore, it should be used with caution in patients receiving such agents).
No products indexed under this heading.

Rocuronium Bromide (Clindamycin has been shown to have neuromuscular blocking properties that may enhance the action of other neuromuscular blocking agents. Therefore, it should be used with caution in patients receiving such agents). Products include:
Zemuron Injection 2363

Succinylcholine Chloride (Clindamycin has been shown to have neuromuscular blocking properties that may enhance the action of other neuromuscular blocking agents. Therefore, it should be used with caution in patients receiving such agents).
No products indexed under this heading.

Vecuronium Bromide (Clindamycin has been shown to have neuromuscular blocking properties that may enhance the action of other neuromuscular blocking agents. Therefore, it should be used with caution in patients receiving such agents).
No products indexed under this heading.

CLINDETS PLEDGETS

(Clindamycin Phosphate) 3212

May interact with neuromuscular blocking agents. Compounds in these categories include:

Atracurium Besylate (Clindamycin has neuromuscular blocking properties and it may enhance the neuromuscular blocking agents).
No products indexed under this heading.

Cisatracurium Besylate (Clindamycin has neuromuscular blocking properties and it may enhance the neuromuscular blocking agents). Products include:
Nimbex Injection 494

Doxacurium Chloride (Clindamycin has neuromuscular blocking properties and it may enhance the neuromuscular blocking agents).
No products indexed under this heading.

Metocurine Iodide (Clindamycin has neuromuscular blocking properties and it may enhance the neuromuscular blocking agents).
No products indexed under this heading.

Mivacurium Chloride (Clindamycin has neuromuscular blocking properties and it may enhance the neuromuscular blocking agents). Products include:
Mivacron Injection 489

Pancuronium Bromide (Clindamycin has neuromuscular blocking properties and it may enhance the neuromuscular blocking agents).
No products indexed under this heading.

Rapacuronium Bromide (Clindamycin has neuromuscular blocking properties and it may enhance the neuromuscular blocking agents).
No products indexed under this heading.

Rocuronium Bromide (Clindamycin has neuromuscular blocking properties and it may enhance the neuromuscular blocking agents). Products include:
Zemuron Injection 2363

Succinylcholine Chloride (Clindamycin has neuromuscular blocking properties and it may enhance the neuromuscular blocking agents).
No products indexed under this heading.

Vecuronium Bromide (Clindamycin has neuromuscular blocking properties and it may enhance the neuromuscular blocking agents).
No products indexed under this heading.

CLINORIL TABLETS

(Sulindac) 1899

May interact with ACE inhibitors, angiotensin-II receptor antagonists, oral anticoagulants, diuretics, oral hypoglycemic agents, lithium preparations, non-steroidal anti-inflammatory agents, and certain other agents. Compounds in these categories include:

Acarbose (Special attention should be paid to patients taking higher doses than those recommended and to patients with renal or metabolic impairment). Products include:
Precose Tablets 776

Amiloride Hydrochloride (Sulindac can reduce the natriuretic effect of furosemide and thiazides in some patients. This response has been attributed to inhibition of renal prostaglandin synthesis. During concomitant therapy with NSAIDs, the patient should be observed closely for signs of renal failure, as well as to assure diuretic efficacy). Products include:
Midamor Tablets 2000
Moduretic Tablets 2003

Anisindione (Special attention should be paid to patients taking higher doses than those recommended and to patients with renal or metabolic impairment). Products include:
Miradon Tablets 3056

Aspirin (Increased gastrointestinal reactions). Products include:
Aggrenox Capsules 855
Bayer, Aspirin Regimen 606
Bayer Aspirin Tablets 3515
BC Powder 612
BC Allergy Sinus Cold Powder 612
Arthritis Strength BC Powder 612
BC Sinus Cold Powder 612
Ecotrin Enteric Coated Aspirin Low, Regular and Maximum Strength Tablets 1627
Goody's Body Pain Formula Powder 621
Goody's Extra Strength Headache Powder 621
Goody's Extra Strength Pain Relief Tablets 621
Percodan Tablets 1115
St. Joseph 81 mg Aspirin Chewable and Enteric Coated Tablets 1841

Aspirin, Enteric Coated (Increased gastrointestinal reactions).
No products indexed under this heading.

Benazepril Hydrochloride (Reports suggest that NSAIDs may diminish the antihypertensive effect of ACE-inhibitors and angiotensin II antagonists. These interactions should be given consideration in patients taking NSAIDs concomitantly with ACE-inhibitors or angiotensin II antagonists. In some patients with compromised renal function, the co-administration of an NSAID and an ACE-inhibitor or an angiotensin II antagonist may result in further deterioration of renal function, including possible acute renal failure, which is usually reversible). Products include:
Lotensin Tablets 2232
Lotensin HCT Tablets 2235
Lotrel Capsules 2238

Bendroflumethiazide (Sulindac can reduce the natriuretic effect of furosemide and thiazides in some patients. This response has been attributed to inhibition of renal prostaglandin synthesis. During concomitant therapy with NSAIDs, the patient should be observed closely for signs of renal failure, as well as to assure diuretic efficacy).
No products indexed under this heading.

Bumetanide (Sulindac can reduce the natriuretic effect of furosemide and thiazides in some patients. This response has been attributed to inhibition of renal prostaglandin synthesis. During concomitant therapy with NSAIDs, the patient should be observed closely for signs of renal failure, as well as to assure diuretic efficacy).
No products indexed under this heading.

Candesartan Cilexetil (Reports suggest that NSAIDs may diminish the antihypertensive effect of ACE-inhibitors and angiotensin II antagonists. These interactions should be given consideration in patients taking NSAIDs concomitantly with ACE-inhibitors or angiotensin II antagonists. In some patients with compromised renal function, the co-administration of an NSAID and an ACE-inhibitor or an angiotensin II antagonist may result in further deterioration of renal function, including possible acute renal failure, which is usually reversible). Products include:
Atacand Tablets 634
Atacand HCT 637

Captopril (Reports suggest that NSAIDs may diminish the antihypertensive effect of ACE-inhibitors and angiotensin II antagonists. These interactions should be given consideration in patients taking NSAIDs concomitantly with ACE-inhibitors or angiotensin II antagonists. In some patients with compromised renal function, the co-administration of an NSAID and an ACE-inhibitor or an angiotensin II antagonist may result in further deterioration of renal function, including possible acute renal failure, which is usually reversible). Products include:
Captopril Tablets 2114

Celecoxib (Concomitant use is not recommended due to the increased possibility of gastrointestinal toxicity, with little or no increase in efficacy). Products include:
Celebrex Capsules 3130

Chlorothiazide (Sulindac can reduce the natriuretic effect of furosemide and thiazides in some patients. This response has been attributed to inhibition of renal prostaglandin synthesis. During concomitant therapy with NSAIDs, the patient should be observed closely for signs of renal failure, as well as to assure diuretic efficacy). Products include:
Aldoclor Tablets 1881
Diuril Oral 1936

Chlorothiazide Sodium (Sulindac can reduce the natriuretic effect of furosemide and thiazides in some patients. This response has been attributed to inhibition of renal prostaglandin synthesis. During concomitant therapy with NSAIDs, the patient should be observed closely for signs of renal failure, as well as to assure diuretic efficacy). Products include:

Diuril Sodium Intravenous 1934

Chlorpropamide (Special attention should be paid to patients taking higher doses than those recommended and to patients with renal or metabolic impairment).

No products indexed under this heading.

Chlorthalidone (Sulindac can reduce the natriuretic effect of furosemide and thiazides in some patients. This response has been attributed to inhibition of renal prostaglandin synthesis. During concomitant therapy with NSAIDs, the patient should be observed closely for signs of renal failure, as well as to assure diuretic efficacy). Products include:

Clorpres Tablets 2139

Cyclosporine (Increased cyclosporine-induced toxicity). Products include:

Gengraf Capsules 458
Neoral Soft Gelatin Capsules 2247
Neoral Oral Solution 2247
Restasis Ophthalmic Emulsion 570
Sandimmune 2259

Diclofenac Potassium (Concomitant use is not recommended due to the increased possibility of gastrointestinal toxicity, with little or no increase in efficacy). Products include:

Cataflam Tablets 2173

Diclofenac Sodium (Concomitant use is not recommended due to the increased possibility of gastrointestinal toxicity, with little or no increase in efficacy). Products include:

Arthrotec Tablets 3126
Voltaren Ophthalmic Solution 2300
Voltaren Tablets 2298
Voltaren-XR Tablets 2301

Dicumarol (Special attention should be paid to patients taking higher doses than those recommended and to patients with renal or metabolic impairment).

No products indexed under this heading.

Diflunisal (Decreased plasma levels of sulindac). Products include:

Dolobid Tablets 1937

DMSO (Reduced efficacy of sulindac; peripheral neuropathy).

No products indexed under this heading.

Enalapril Maleate (Reports suggest that NSAIDs may diminish the antihypertensive effect of ACE-inhibitors and angiotensin II antagonists. These interactions should be given consideration in patients taking NSAIDs concomitantly with ACE-inhibitors or angiotensin II antagonists. In some patients with compromised renal function, the co-administration of an NSAID and an ACE-inhibitor or an angiotensin II antagonist may result in further deterioration of renal function, including possible acute renal failure, which is usually reversible). Products include:

Vaseretic Tablets 2073
Vasotec I.V. Injection 2076

Enalaprilat (Reports suggest that NSAIDs may diminish the antihypertensive effect of ACE-inhibitors and angiotensin II antagonists. These interactions should be given consideration in patients taking NSAIDs concomitantly with ACE-inhibitors or angiotensin II antagonists. In some patients with compromised renal function, the co-administration of an NSAID and an ACE-inhibitor or an angiotensin II antagonist may result in further deterioration of renal function, including possible acute renal failure, which is usually reversible).

No products indexed under this heading.

Eprosartan Mesylate (Reports suggest that NSAIDs may diminish the antihypertensive effect of ACE-inhibitors and angiotensin II antagonists. These interactions should be given consideration in patients taking NSAIDs concomitantly with ACE-inhibitors or angiotensin II antagonists. In some patients with compromised renal function, the co-administration of an NSAID and an ACE-inhibitor or an angiotensin II antagonist may result in further deterioration of renal function, including possible acute renal failure, which is usually reversible). Products include:

Teveten Tablets 1707
Teveten HCT Tablets 1710

Ethacrynic Acid (Sulindac can reduce the natriuretic effect of furosemide and thiazides in some patients. This response has been attributed to inhibition of renal prostaglandin synthesis. During concomitant therapy with NSAIDs, the patient should be observed closely for signs of renal failure, as well as to assure diuretic efficacy). Products include:

Edecrin Tablets 1941

Etodolac (Concomitant use is not recommended due to the increased possibility of gastrointestinal toxicity, with little or no increase in efficacy).

No products indexed under this heading.

Fenoprofen Calcium (Concomitant use is not recommended due to the increased possibility of gastrointestinal toxicity, with little or no increase in efficacy). Products include:

Nalfon Capsules 2504

Flurbiprofen (Concomitant use is not recommended due to the increased possibility of gastrointestinal toxicity, with little or no increase in efficacy).

No products indexed under this heading.

Fosinopril Sodium (Reports suggest that NSAIDs may diminish the antihypertensive effect of ACE-inhibitors and angiotensin II antagonists. These interactions should be given consideration in patients taking NSAIDs concomitantly with ACE-inhibitors or angiotensin II antagonists. In some patients with compromised renal function, the co-administration of an NSAID and an ACE-inhibitor or an angiotensin II antagonist may result in further deterioration of renal function, including possible acute renal failure, which is usually reversible).

No products indexed under this heading.

Furosemide (Clinoril may blunt the renal response to I.V. furosemide). Products include:

Furosemide Tablets 2117

Glimepiride (Special attention should be paid to patients taking higher doses than those recommended and to patients with renal or metabolic impairment). Products include:

Amaryl Tablets 2864

Glipizide (Special attention should be paid to patients taking higher doses than those recommended and to patients with renal or metabolic impairment).

No products indexed under this heading.

Glyburide (Special attention should be paid to patients taking higher doses than those recommended and to patients with renal or metabolic impairment).

No products indexed under this heading.

Hydrochlorothiazide (Sulindac can reduce the natriuretic effect of furosemide and thiazides in some patients. This response has been attributed to inhibition of renal prostaglandin synthesis. During concomitant therapy with NSAIDs, the patient should be observed closely for signs of renal failure, as well as to assure diuretic efficacy). Products include:

Aldoril Tablets 1884
Atacand HCT 637
Avalide Tablets 2889
Avalide Tablets 922
Benicar HCT Tablets 2852
Diovan HCT Tablets 2195
Dyazide Capsules 1389
Hyzaar 1964
Lotensin HCT Tablets 2235
Maxzide 2150
Micardis HCT Tablets 886
Moduretic Tablets 2003
Prinzide Tablets 2033
Teveten HCT Tablets 1710
Timolide Tablets 2056
Uniretic Tablets 3114
Vaseretic Tablets 2073
Zestoretic Tablets 701

Hydroflumethiazide (Sulindac can reduce the natriuretic effect of furosemide and thiazides in some patients. This response has been attributed to inhibition of renal prostaglandin synthesis. During concomitant therapy with NSAIDs, the patient should be observed closely for signs of renal failure, as well as to assure diuretic efficacy).

No products indexed under this heading.

Ibuprofen (Concomitant use is not recommended due to the increased possibility of gastrointestinal toxicity, with little or no increase in efficacy). Products include:

Advil Allergy Sinus Caplets .... ▣ 737
Advil .... ▣ 737
Children's Advil Suspension .... ▣ 742
Children's Advil Chewable Tablets .. ▣ 741
Advil Cold & Sinus .... ▣ 739
Advil Flu & Body Ache Caplets .... ▣ 739
Children's Advil Cold Suspension ... ▣ 741
Infants' Advil Concentrated Drops .. ▣ 743
Junior Strength Advil Swallow Tablets .... ▣ 740
Advil Migraine Liquigels .... ▣ 740
Advil Multi-Symptom Cold Caplets .... ▣ 738
Combunox Tablets 1183
Children's Motrin Oral Suspension and Chewable Tablets 1837
Children's Motrin Cold Non-Staining Dye-Free Oral Suspension 1838
Children's Motrin Cold Oral Suspension 1838
Children's Motrin Non-Staining Dye-Free Oral Suspension 1837
Motrin Cold & Sinus Caplets 1836
Motrin IB Tablets and Caplets 1836
Infants' Motrin Concentrated Drops 1837
Infants' Motrin Non-Staining Dye-Free Drops 1837
Junior Strength Motrin Caplets and Chewable Tablets 1837
Vicoprofen Tablets 533

Indapamide (Sulindac can reduce the natriuretic effect of furosemide and thiazides in some patients. This response has been attributed to inhibition of renal prostaglandin synthesis. During concomitant therapy with NSAIDs, the patient should be observed closely for signs of renal failure, as well as to assure diuretic efficacy). Products include:

Indapamide Tablets 2119

Indomethacin (Concomitant use is not recommended due to the increased possibility of gastrointestinal toxicity, with little or no increase in efficacy). Products include:

Indocin 1968

Indomethacin Sodium Trihydrate (Concomitant use is not recommended due to the increased possibility of gastrointestinal toxicity, with little or no increase in efficacy). Products include:

Indocin I.V. 1973

Irbesartan (Reports suggest that NSAIDs may diminish the antihypertensive effect of ACE-inhibitors and angiotensin II antagonists. These interactions should be given consideration in patients taking NSAIDs concomitantly with ACE-inhibitors or angiotensin II antagonists. In some patients with compromised renal function, the co-administration of an NSAID and an ACE-inhibitor or an angiotensin II antagonist may result in further deterioration of renal function, including possible acute renal failure, which is usually reversible). Products include:

Avalide Tablets 922
Avalide Tablets 2889
Avapro Tablets 925
Avapro Tablets 2886

Ketoprofen (Concomitant use is not recommended due to the increased possibility of gastrointestinal toxicity, with little or no increase in efficacy).

No products indexed under this heading.

Ketorolac Tromethamine (Concomitant use is not recommended due to the increased possibility of gastrointestinal toxicity, with little or no increase in efficacy). Products include:

Acular Ophthalmic Solution 561
Acular LS Ophthalmic Solution 562

Lisinopril (Reports suggest that NSAIDs may diminish the antihypertensive effect of ACE-inhibitors and angiotensin II antagonists. These interactions should be given consideration in patients taking NSAIDs concomitantly with ACE-inhibitors or angiotensin II antagonists. In some patients with compromised renal function, the co-administration of an NSAID and an ACE-inhibitor or an angiotensin II antagonist may result in further deterioration of renal function, including possible acute renal failure, which is usually reversible). Products include:

Prinivil Tablets 2029
Prinzide Tablets 2033
Zestoretic Tablets 701
Zestril Tablets 704

Lithium (NSAIDs have produced an elevation of plasma lithium levels and a reduction in renal lithium clearance. The mean minimum lithium concentration increased 15% and the renal clearance was decreased by approximately 20%. These effects have been attributed to inhibition of renal prostaglandin synthesis by the NSAID. Thus, when NSAIDs

and lithium are administered concurrently, subject should be observed carefully for signs of lithium toxicity).
No products indexed under this heading.

Lithium Carbonate (NSAIDs have produced an elevation of plasma lithium levels and a reduction in renal lithium clearance. The mean minimum lithium concentration increased 15% and the renal clearance was decreased by approximately 20%. These effects have been attributed to inhibition of renal prostaglandin synthesis by the NSAID. Thus, when NSAIDs and lithium are administered concurrently, subject should be observed carefully for signs of lithium toxicity). Products include:
Eskalith **1406**
Lithobid Tablets **1670**

Lithium Citrate (NSAIDs have produced an elevation of plasma lithium levels and a reduction in renal lithium clearance. The mean minimum lithium concentration increased 15% and the renal clearance was decreased by approximately 20%. These effects have been attributed to inhibition of renal prostaglandin synthesis by the NSAID. Thus, when NSAIDs and lithium are administered concurrently, subject should be observed carefully for signs of lithium toxicity).
No products indexed under this heading.

Losartan Potassium (Reports suggest that NSAIDs may diminish the antihypertensive effect of ACE-inhibitors and angiotensin II antagonists. These interactions should be given consideration in patients taking NSAIDs concomitantly with ACE-inhibitors or angiotensin II antagonists. In some patients with compromised renal function, the co-administration of an NSAID and an ACE-inhibitor or an angiotensin II antagonist may result in further deterioration of renal function, including possible acute renal failure, which is usually reversible). Products include:
Cozaar Tablets **1913**
Hyzaar **1964**

Meclofenamate Sodium (Concomitant use is not recommended due to the increased possibility of gastrointestinal toxicity, with little or no increase in efficacy).
No products indexed under this heading.

Mefenamic Acid (Concomitant use is not recommended due to the increased possibility of gastrointestinal toxicity, with little or no increase in efficacy).
No products indexed under this heading.

Meloxicam (Concomitant use is not recommended due to the increased possibility of gastrointestinal toxicity, with little or no increase in efficacy). Products include:
Mobic Oral Suspension **893**
Mobic Tablets **893**

Metformin Hydrochloride (Special attention should be paid to patients taking higher doses than those recommended and to patients with renal or metabolic impairment). Products include:
ActoPlus Met Tablets **3219**
Avandamet Tablets **1343**
Fortamet Extended-Release Tablets **1156**

Methotrexate Sodium (Decreased tubular secretion of methotrexate and potentiation of its toxicity).
No products indexed under this heading.

Methyclothiazide (Sulindac can reduce the natriuretic effect of furosemide and thiazides in some patients. This response has been attributed to inhibition of renal prostaglandin synthesis. During concomitant therapy with NSAIDs, the patient should be observed closely for signs of renal failure, as well as to assure diuretic efficacy).
No products indexed under this heading.

Metolazone (Sulindac can reduce the natriuretic effect of furosemide and thiazides in some patients. This response has been attributed to inhibition of renal prostaglandin synthesis. During concomitant therapy with NSAIDs, the patient should be observed closely for signs of renal failure, as well as to assure diuretic efficacy).
No products indexed under this heading.

Miglitol (Special attention should be paid to patients taking higher doses than those recommended and to patients with renal or metabolic impairment).
No products indexed under this heading.

Moexipril Hydrochloride (Reports suggest that NSAIDs may diminish the antihypertensive effect of ACE-inhibitors and angiotensin II antagonists. These interactions should be given consideration in patients taking NSAIDs concomitantly with ACE-inhibitors or angiotensin II antagonists. In some patients with compromised renal function, the co-administration of an NSAID and an ACE-inhibitor or an angiotensin II antagonist may result in further deterioration of renal function, including possible acute renal failure, which is usually reversible). Products include:
Uniretic Tablets **3114**
Univasc Tablets **3118**

Nabumetone (Concomitant use is not recommended due to the increased possibility of gastrointestinal toxicity, with little or no increase in efficacy). Products include:
Relafen Tablets **1523**

Naproxen (Concomitant use is not recommended due to the increased possibility of gastrointestinal toxicity, with little or no increase in efficacy). Products include:
EC-Naprosyn Delayed-Release Tablets **2769**
Naprosyn Suspension **2769**
Naprosyn Tablets **2769**
Prevacid NapraPAC **3277**

Naproxen Sodium (Concomitant use is not recommended due to the increased possibility of gastrointestinal toxicity, with little or no increase in efficacy). Products include:
Aleve Tablets, Caplets and Gelcaps **605**
Anaprox Tablets **2769**
Anaprox DS Tablets **2769**

Oxaprozin (Concomitant use is not recommended due to the increased possibility of gastrointestinal toxicity, with little or no increase in efficacy).
No products indexed under this heading.

Perindopril Erbumine (Reports suggest that NSAIDs may diminish the antihypertensive effect of ACE-inhibitors and angiotensin II antagonists. These interactions should be given consideration in patients taking NSAIDs concomitantly with ACE-inhibitors or angiotensin II antagonists. In some patients with compromised renal function, the co-administration of an NSAID and an ACE-inhibitor or an angiotensin II antagonist may result in further deterioration of renal function, including possible acute renal failure, which is usually reversible). Products include:
Aceon Tablets (2 mg, 4 mg, 8 mg) **3191**

Phenylbutazone (Concomitant use is not recommended due to the increased possibility of gastrointestinal toxicity, with little or no increase in efficacy).
No products indexed under this heading.

Pioglitazone Hydrochloride (Special attention should be paid to patients taking higher doses than those recommended and to patients with renal or metabolic impairment). Products include:
ActoPlus Met Tablets **3219**
Actos Tablets **3224**

Piroxicam (Concomitant use is not recommended due to the increased possibility of gastrointestinal toxicity, with little or no increase in efficacy).
No products indexed under this heading.

Polythiazide (Sulindac can reduce the natriuretic effect of furosemide and thiazides in some patients. This response has been attributed to inhibition of renal prostaglandin synthesis. During concomitant therapy with NSAIDs, the patient should be observed closely for signs of renal failure, as well as to assure diuretic efficacy).
No products indexed under this heading.

Probenecid (Increased plasma levels of sulindac; modest reduction in uricosuric action of probenecid).
No products indexed under this heading.

Quinapril Hydrochloride (Reports suggest that NSAIDs may diminish the antihypertensive effect of ACE-inhibitors and angiotensin II antagonists. These interactions should be given consideration in patients taking NSAIDs concomitantly with ACE-inhibitors or angiotensin II antagonists. In some patients with compromised renal function, the co-administration of an NSAID and an ACE-inhibitor or an angiotensin II antagonist may result in further deterioration of renal function, including possible acute renal failure, which is usually reversible).
No products indexed under this heading.

Ramipril (Reports suggest that NSAIDs may diminish the antihypertensive effect of ACE-inhibitors and angiotensin II antagonists. These interactions should be given consideration in patients taking NSAIDs concomitantly with ACE-inhibitors or angiotensin II antagonists. In some patients with compromised renal function, the co-administration of an NSAID and an ACE-inhibitor or an angiotensin II antagonist may result in further deterioration of renal function, including possible acute renal failure, which is usually reversible). Products include:
Altace Capsules **1673**

Repaglinide (Special attention should be paid to patients taking higher doses than those recommended and to patients with renal or metabolic impairment). Products include:
Prandin Tablets (0.5, 1, and 2 mg) **2337**

Rofecoxib (Concomitant use is not recommended due to the increased possibility of gastrointestinal toxicity, with little or no increase in efficacy).
No products indexed under this heading.

Rosiglitazone Maleate (Special attention should be paid to patients taking higher doses than those recommended and to patients with renal or metabolic impairment). Products include:
Avandamet Tablets **1343**
Avandia Tablets **1348**

Spirapril Hydrochloride (Reports suggest that NSAIDs may diminish the antihypertensive effect of ACE-inhibitors and angiotensin II antagonists. These interactions should be given consideration in patients taking NSAIDs concomitantly with ACE-inhibitors or angiotensin II antagonists. In some patients with compromised renal function, the co-administration of an NSAID and an ACE-inhibitor or an angiotensin II antagonist may result in further deterioration of renal function, including possible acute renal failure, which is usually reversible).
No products indexed under this heading.

Spironolactone (Sulindac can reduce the natriuretic effect of furosemide and thiazides in some patients. This response has been attributed to inhibition of renal prostaglandin synthesis. During concomitant therapy with NSAIDs, the patient should be observed closely for signs of renal failure, as well as to assure diuretic efficacy).
No products indexed under this heading.

Telmisartan (Reports suggest that NSAIDs may diminish the antihypertensive effect of ACE-inhibitors and angiotensin II antagonists. These interactions should be given consideration in patients taking NSAIDs concomitantly with ACE-inhibitors or angiotensin II antagonists. In some patients with compromised renal function, the co-administration of an NSAID and an ACE-inhibitor or an angiotensin II antagonist may result in further deterioration of renal function, including possible acute renal failure, which is usually reversible). Products include:
Micardis Tablets **884**
Micardis HCT Tablets **886**

Tolazamide (Special attention should be paid to patients taking higher doses than those recommended and to patients with renal or metabolic impairment).
No products indexed under this heading.

Tolbutamide (Special attention should be paid to patients taking higher doses than those recommended and to patients with renal or metabolic impairment).
No products indexed under this heading.

Tolmetin Sodium (Concomitant use is not recommended due to the increased possibility of gastrointestinal toxicity, with little or no increase in efficacy).
No products indexed under this heading.

Torsemide (Sulindac can reduce the natriuretic effect of furosemide and thiazides in some patients. This response has been attributed to inhibition of renal prostaglandin synthesis. During concomitant therapy with NSAIDs, the patient should be observed closely for signs of renal failure, as well as to assure diuretic efficacy).
No products indexed under this heading.

Trandolapril (Reports suggest that NSAIDs may diminish the antihypertensive effect of ACE-inhibitors and angiotensin II antagonists. These interactions should be given consideration in patients taking NSAIDs concomitantly with ACE-inhibitors or angiotensin II antagonists. In some patients with compromised renal function, the co-administration of an NSAID and an ACE-inhibitor or an angiotensin II antagonist may result in further deterioration of renal function, including possible acute renal failure, which is usually reversible). Products include:

Mavik Tablets 482
Tarka Tablets 519

Triamterene (Sulindac can reduce the natriuretic effect of furosemide and thiazides in some patients. This response has been attributed to inhibition of renal prostaglandin synthesis. During concomitant therapy with NSAIDs, the patient should be observed closely for signs of renal failure, as well as to assure diuretic efficacy). Products include:

Dyazide Capsules 1389
Dyrenium Capsules 3390
Maxzide 2150

Troglitazone (Special attention should be paid to patients taking higher doses than those recommended and to patients with renal or metabolic impairment).
No products indexed under this heading.

Valdecoxib (Concomitant use is not recommended due to the increased possibility of gastrointestinal toxicity, with little or no increase in efficacy).
No products indexed under this heading.

Valsartan (Reports suggest that NSAIDs may diminish the antihypertensive effect of ACE-inhibitors and angiotensin II antagonists. These interactions should be given consideration in patients taking NSAIDs concomitantly with ACE-inhibitors or angiotensin II antagonists. In some patients with compromised renal function, the co-administration of an NSAID and an ACE-inhibitor or an angiotensin II antagonist may result in further deterioration of renal function, including possible acute renal failure, which is usually reversible). Products include:

Diovan HCT Tablets 2195
Diovan Tablets 2191

Warfarin Sodium (Special attention should be paid to patients taking higher doses than those recommended and to patients with renal or metabolic impairment). Products include:

Coumadin for Injection 932
Coumadin Tablets 932

Food Interactions

Food, unspecified (The peak plasma concentrations of biologically active sulfide metabolite is delayed slightly in the presence of food).

CLOBEVATE GEL

(Clobetasol Propionate) 3213
None cited in PDR database.

CLOBEX SHAMPOO

(Clobetasol Propionate) 1209
None cited in PDR database.

CLOBEX LOTION

(Clobetasol Propionate) 1208
None cited in PDR database.

CLOLAR FOR INTRAVENOUS INFUSION

(Clofarabine) 1264
None cited in PDR database.

CLORPACTIN WCS-90

(Sodium Oxychlorosene) 1636
None cited in PDR database.

CLORPRES TABLETS

(Chlorthalidone, Clonidine Hydrochloride) 2139
May interact with antihypertensives, barbiturates, beta blockers, cardiac glycosides, oral hypoglycemic agents, hypnotics and sedatives, insulin, lithium preparations, narcotic analgesics, tricyclic antidepressants, and certain other agents. Compounds in these categories include:

Acarbose (Chlorthalidone causes hyperglycemia; higher dosage of oral hypoglycemic agents may be required). Products include:

Precose Tablets 776

Acebutolol Hydrochloride (Chlorthalidone may add to or potentiate the action of other antihypertensives; if therapy is to be discontinued in patients receiving clonidine and beta blockers concurrently, beta blockers should be discontinued several days before the gradual withdrawal of clonidine).
No products indexed under this heading.

Alfentanil Hydrochloride (Orthostatic hypotension may be aggravated by narcotics; orthostatic hypotension may be aggravated by barbiturates).
No products indexed under this heading.

Amitriptyline Hydrochloride (Co-administration of clonidine with tricyclic antidepressants may result in reduced effect of clonidine, necessitating an increase in dosage; concurrent use enhances the manifestation of corneal lesions in rats).
No products indexed under this heading.

Amlodipine Besylate (Chlorthalidone may add to or potentiate the action of other antihypertensives). Products include:

Caduet Tablets 2507
Lotrel Capsules 2238
Norvasc Tablets 2529

Amoxapine (Co-administration of clonidine with tricyclic antidepressants may result in reduced effect of clonidine, necessitating an increase in dosage).
No products indexed under this heading.

Aprobarbital (Clonidine may enhance the CNS-depressive effects of barbiturates; orthostatic hypotension may be aggravated by barbiturates).
No products indexed under this heading.

Atenolol (Chlorthalidone may add to or potentiate the action of other antihypertensives; if therapy is to be discontinued in patients receiving clonidine and beta blockers concurrently, beta blockers should be discontinued several days before the gradual withdrawal of clonidine). Products include:

Tenormin I.V. Injection 698
Tenormin Tablets 695

Benazepril Hydrochloride (Chlorthalidone may add to or potentiate the action of other antihypertensives). Products include:

Lotensin Tablets 2232
Lotensin HCT Tablets 2235
Lotrel Capsules 2238

Bendroflumethiazide (Chlorthalidone may add to or potentiate the action of other antihypertensives).
No products indexed under this heading.

Betaxolol Hydrochloride (Chlorthalidone may add to or potentiate the action of other antihypertensives; if therapy is to be discontinued in patients receiving clonidine and beta blockers concurrently, beta blockers should be discontinued several days before the gradual withdrawal of clonidine). Products include:

Betoptic S Ophthalmic Suspension 554

Bisoprolol Fumarate (Chlorthalidone may add to or potentiate the action of other antihypertensives; if therapy is to be discontinued in patients receiving clonidine and beta blockers concurrently, beta blockers should be discontinued several days before the gradual withdrawal of clonidine).
No products indexed under this heading.

Buprenorphine Hydrochloride (Orthostatic hypotension may be aggravated by narcotics; orthostatic hypotension may be aggravated by barbiturates). Products include:

Buprenex Injectable 2718
Suboxone Tablets 2719
Subutex Tablets 2719

Butabarbital (Clonidine may enhance the CNS-depressive effects of barbiturates; orthostatic hypotension may be aggravated by barbiturates).
No products indexed under this heading.

Butalbital (Clonidine may enhance the CNS-depressive effects of barbiturates; orthostatic hypotension may be aggravated by barbiturates). Products include:

Sedapap Tablets 50 mg/650 mg 2098

Candesartan Cilexetil (Chlorthalidone may add to or potentiate the action of other antihypertensives). Products include:

Atacand Tablets 634
Atacand HCT 637

Captopril (Chlorthalidone may add to or potentiate the action of other antihypertensives). Products include:

Captopril Tablets 2114

Carteolol Hydrochloride (Chlorthalidone may add to or potentiate the action of other antihypertensives; if therapy is to be discontinued in patients receiving clonidine and beta blockers concurrently, beta blockers should be discontinued several days before the gradual withdrawal of clonidine). Products include:

Carteolol Hydrochloride Ophthalmic Solution USP, 1% .... ⊙246

Chlorothiazide (Chlorthalidone may add to or potentiate the action of other antihypertensives). Products include:

Aldoclor Tablets 1881
Diuril Oral 1936

Chlorothiazide Sodium (Chlorthalidone may add to or potentiate the action of other antihypertensives). Products include:

Diuril Sodium Intravenous 1934

Chlorpropamide (Chlorthalidone causes hyperglycemia; higher dosage of oral hypoglycemic agents may be required).
No products indexed under this heading.

Clomipramine Hydrochloride (Co-administration of clonidine with tricyclic antidepressants may result in reduced effect of clonidine, necessitating an increase in dosage).
No products indexed under this heading.

Clonidine (Chlorthalidone may add to or potentiate the action of other antihypertensives). Products include:

Catapres-TTS 875

Codeine Phosphate (Orthostatic hypotension may be aggravated by narcotics; orthostatic hypotension may be aggravated by barbiturates). Products include:

Tylenol with Codeine 2461

Deserpidine (Chlorthalidone may add to or potentiate the action of other antihypertensives).
No products indexed under this heading.

Desipramine Hydrochloride (Co-administration of clonidine with tricyclic antidepressants may result in reduced effect of clonidine, necessitating an increase in dosage).
No products indexed under this heading.

Deslanoside (Digitalis therapy may exaggerate the metabolic effects of hypokalemia especially with reference to myocardial activity).
No products indexed under this heading.

Dezocine (Orthostatic hypotension may be aggravated by narcotics; orthostatic hypotension may be aggravated by barbiturates).
No products indexed under this heading.

Diazoxide (Chlorthalidone may add to or potentiate the action of other antihypertensives). Products include:

Hyperstat I.V. Injection 3031

Digitalis Glycoside Preparations (Digitalis therapy may exaggerate the metabolic effects of hypokalemia especially with reference to myocardial activity).

Digitoxin (Digitalis therapy may exaggerate the metabolic effects of hypokalemia especially with reference to myocardial activity).
No products indexed under this heading.

Digoxin (Digitalis therapy may exaggerate the metabolic effects of hypokalemia especially with reference to myocardial activity). Products include:

Digitek Tablets ... 2146
Lanoxicaps Capsules ... 1458
Lanoxin Injection ... 1462
Lanoxin Tablets ... 1468
Lanoxin Injection Pediatric ... 1465

Diltiazem Hydrochloride (Chlorthalidone may add to or potentiate the action of other antihypertensives). Products include:
Cardizem LA Extended Release Tablets ... 1699
Tiazac Capsules ... 1204

Doxazosin Mesylate (Chlorthalidone may add to or potentiate the action of other antihypertensives).
No products indexed under this heading.

Doxepin Hydrochloride (Co-administration of clonidine with tricyclic antidepressants may result in reduced effect of clonidine, necessitating an increase in dosage).
No products indexed under this heading.

Enalapril Maleate (Chlorthalidone may add to or potentiate the action of other antihypertensives). Products include:
Vaseretic Tablets ... 2073
Vasotec I.V. Injection ... 2076

Enalaprilat (Chlorthalidone may add to or potentiate the action of other antihypertensives).
No products indexed under this heading.

Eprosartan Mesylate (Chlorthalidone may add to or potentiate the action of other antihypertensives). Products include:
Teveten Tablets ... 1707
Teveten HCT Tablets ... 1710

Esmolol Hydrochloride (Chlorthalidone may add to or potentiate the action of other antihypertensives; if therapy is to be discontinued in patients receiving clonidine and beta blockers concurrently, beta blockers should be discontinued several days before the gradual withdrawal of clonidine). Products include:
Brevibloc Concentrate ... 766
Brevibloc Injection ... 766
Brevibloc Double Strength Injection ... 766
Brevibloc Premixed Injection ... 766
Brevibloc Double Strength Premixed Injection ... 766

Estazolam (Clonidine may enhance the CNS-depressive effects of other sedatives). Products include:
ProSom Tablets ... 512

Ethchlorvynol (Clonidine may enhance the CNS-depressive effects of other sedatives).
No products indexed under this heading.

Ethinamate (Clonidine may enhance the CNS-depressive effects of other sedatives).
No products indexed under this heading.

Felodipine (Chlorthalidone may add to or potentiate the action of other antihypertensives). Products include:
Plendil Extended-Release Tablets ... 651

Fentanyl (Orthostatic hypotension may be aggravated by narcotics; orthostatic hypotension may be aggravated by barbiturates). Products include:
Duragesic Transdermal System ... 2448

Fentanyl Citrate (Orthostatic hypotension may be aggravated by narcotics; orthostatic hypotension may be aggravated by barbiturates). Products include:
Actiq ... 993

Flurazepam Hydrochloride (Clonidine may enhance the CNS-depressive effects of other sedatives). Products include:
Dalmane Capsules ... 3343

Fosinopril Sodium (Chlorthalidone may add to or potentiate the action of other antihypertensives).
No products indexed under this heading.

Furosemide (Chlorthalidone may add to or potentiate the action of other antihypertensives). Products include:
Furosemide Tablets ... 2117

Glimepiride (Chlorthalidone causes hyperglycemia; higher dosage of oral hypoglycemic agents may be required). Products include:
Amaryl Tablets ... 2864

Glipizide (Chlorthalidone causes hyperglycemia; higher dosage of oral hypoglycemic agents may be required).
No products indexed under this heading.

Glutethimide (Clonidine may enhance the CNS-depressive effects of other sedatives).
No products indexed under this heading.

Glyburide (Chlorthalidone causes hyperglycemia; higher dosage of oral hypoglycemic agents may be required).
No products indexed under this heading.

Guanabenz Acetate (Chlorthalidone may add to or potentiate the action of other antihypertensives).
No products indexed under this heading.

Guanethidine Monosulfate (Chlorthalidone may add to or potentiate the action of other antihypertensives).
No products indexed under this heading.

Hydralazine Hydrochloride (Chlorthalidone may add to or potentiate the action of other antihypertensives). Products include:
BiDil Tablets ... 2161

Hydrochlorothiazide (Chlorthalidone may add to or potentiate the action of other antihypertensives). Products include:
Aldoril Tablets ... 1884
Atacand HCT ... 637
Avalide Tablets ... 2889
Avalide Tablets ... 922
Benicar HCT Tablets ... 2852
Diovan HCT Tablets ... 2195
Dyazide Capsules ... 1389
Hyzaar ... 1964
Lotensin HCT Tablets ... 2235
Maxzide ... 2150
Micardis HCT Tablets ... 886
Moduretic Tablets ... 2003
Prinzide Tablets ... 2033
Teveten HCT Tablets ... 1710
Timolide Tablets ... 2056
Uniretic Tablets ... 3114
Vaseretic Tablets ... 2073
Zestoretic Tablets ... 701

Hydrocodone Bitartrate (Orthostatic hypotension may be aggravated by narcotics; orthostatic hypotension may be aggravated by barbiturates). Products include:
Hycodan ... 1104
Hycomine Compound Tablets ... 1105
Hycotuss Expectorant Syrup ... 1106
Lortab ... 3315
Lortab Elixir ... 3312
Vicodin Tablets ... 530
Vicodin ES Tablets ... 531
Vicodin HP Tablets ... 532
Vicoprofen Tablets ... 533
Zydone Tablets ... 1118

Hydrocodone Polistirex (Orthostatic hypotension may be aggravated by narcotics; orthostatic hypotension may be aggravated by barbiturates). Products include:
Tussionex Pennkinetic Extended-Release Suspension ... 3322

Hydroflumethiazide (Chlorthalidone may add to or potentiate the action of other antihypertensives).
No products indexed under this heading.

Hydromorphone Hydrochloride (Orthostatic hypotension may be aggravated by narcotics; orthostatic hypotension may be aggravated by barbiturates). Products include:
Dilaudid ... 439
Dilaudid Oral Liquid ... 443
Dilaudid Non-Sterile Powder ... 439
Dilaudid Rectal Suppositories ... 439
Dilaudid Tablets ... 439
Dilaudid Tablets - 8 mg ... 443
Dilaudid-HP ... 441

Imipramine Hydrochloride (Co-administration of clonidine with tricyclic antidepressants may result in reduced effect of clonidine, necessitating an increase in dosage).
No products indexed under this heading.

Imipramine Pamoate (Co-administration of clonidine with tricyclic antidepressants may result in reduced effect of clonidine, necessitating an increase in dosage).
No products indexed under this heading.

Indapamide (Chlorthalidone may add to or potentiate the action of other antihypertensives). Products include:
Indapamide Tablets ... 2119

Insulin, Human, Zinc Suspension (Chlorthalidone causes hyperglycemia; insulin requirements may be increased, decreased, or unchanged). Products include:
Humulin L, 100 Units ... 1763
Humulin U, 100 Units ... 1770

Insulin, Human NPH (Chlorthalidone causes hyperglycemia; insulin requirements may be increased, decreased, or unchanged). Products include:
Humulin N, 100 Units ... 1764
Humulin N Pen ... 1765
Novolin N Human Insulin 10 ml Vials ... 2322
Novolin N InnoLet ... 2322
Novolin N PenFill 3 ml Cartridges ... 2325
Novolin R InnoLet ... 2322

Insulin, Human Regular (Chlorthalidone causes hyperglycemia; insulin requirements may be increased, decreased, or unchanged). Products include:
Humulin R (U-500) ... 1768
Humulin R, 100 Units ... 1767
Novolin R Human Insulin 10 ml Vials ... 2322
Novolin R PenFill ... 2325

Insulin, Human Regular and Human NPH Mixture (Chlorthalidone causes hyperglycemia; insulin requirements may be increased, decreased, or unchanged). Products include:
Humulin 50/50, 100 Units ... 1760
Humulin 70/30 Pen ... 1761
Novolin 70/30 Human Insulin 10 ml Vials ... 2321
Novolin 70/30 InnoLet ... 2322
Novolin 70/30 PenFill 3 ml Cartridges ... 2325

Insulin, NPH (Chlorthalidone causes hyperglycemia; insulin requirements may be increased, decreased, or unchanged).
No products indexed under this heading.

Insulin, Regular (Chlorthalidone causes hyperglycemia; insulin requirements may be increased, decreased, or unchanged).
No products indexed under this heading.

Insulin, Zinc Crystals (Chlorthalidone causes hyperglycemia; insulin requirements may be increased, decreased, or unchanged).
No products indexed under this heading.

Insulin, Zinc Suspension (Chlorthalidone causes hyperglycemia; insulin requirements may be increased, decreased, or unchanged).
No products indexed under this heading.

Insulin Aspart, Human Regular (Chlorthalidone causes hyperglycemia; insulin requirements may be increased, decreased, or unchanged). Products include:
NovoLog Injection ... 2326

Insulin glargine (Chlorthalidone causes hyperglycemia; insulin requirements may be increased, decreased, or unchanged). Products include:
Lantus Injection ... 2925

Insulin Lispro, Human (Chlorthalidone causes hyperglycemia; insulin requirements may be increased, decreased, or unchanged). Products include:
Humalog-Pen ... 1751
Humalog Mix 75/25-Pen ... 1754

Insulin Lispro Protamine, Human (Chlorthalidone causes hyperglycemia; insulin requirements may be increased, decreased, or unchanged). Products include:
Humalog Mix 75/25-Pen ... 1754

Irbesartan (Chlorthalidone may add to or potentiate the action of other antihypertensives). Products include:
Avalide Tablets ... 922
Avalide Tablets ... 2889
Avapro Tablets ... 925
Avapro Tablets ... 2886

Isradipine (Chlorthalidone may add to or potentiate the action of other antihypertensives). Products include:
DynaCirc CR Tablets ... 2726

Labetalol Hydrochloride (Chlorthalidone may add to or potentiate the action of other antihypertensives; if therapy is to be discontinued in patients receiving clonidine and beta blockers concurrently, beta blockers should be discontinued several days before the gradual withdrawal of clonidine).
No products indexed under this heading.

Levobunolol Hydrochloride (Chlorthalidone may add to or potentiate the action of other antihypertensives; if therapy is to be discontinued in patients receiving clonidine and beta blockers concurrently, beta blockers should be discontinued several days before the gradual withdrawal of clonidine). Products include:
Betagan Ophthalmic Solution, USP ... ⊙217

Levorphanol Tartrate (Orthostatic hypotension may be aggravated by narcotics; orthostatic hypotension may be aggravated by barbiturates).
No products indexed under this heading.

Lisinopril (Chlorthalidone may add to or potentiate the action of other antihypertensives). Products include:
Prinivil Tablets ... 2029
Prinzide Tablets ... 2033
Zestoretic Tablets ... 701
Zestril Tablets ... 704

Lithium (Chlorthalidone reduces renal clearance of lithium, increasing the risk of lithium toxicity).
No products indexed under this heading.

Lithium Carbonate (Chlorthalidone reduces renal clearance of lithium, increasing the risk of lithium toxicity). Products include:
Eskalith ... 1406
Lithobid Tablets ... 1670

Lithium Citrate (Chlorthalidone reduces renal clearance of lithium, increasing the risk of lithium toxicity).
No products indexed under this heading.

Lorazepam (Clonidine may enhance the CNS-depressive effects of other sedatives).
No products indexed under this heading.

Losartan Potassium (Chlorthalidone may add to or potentiate the action of other antihypertensives). Products include:
Cozaar Tablets ... 1913
Hyzaar ... 1964

Maprotiline Hydrochloride (Co-administration of clonidine with tricyclic antidepressants may result in reduced effect of clonidine, necessitating an increase in dosage).
No products indexed under this heading.

Mecamylamine Hydrochloride (Chlorthalidone may add to or potentiate the action of other antihypertensives). Products include:
Inversine Tablets ... 3286

Meperidine Hydrochloride (Orthostatic hypotension may be aggravated by narcotics; orthostatic hypotension may be aggravated by barbiturates).
No products indexed under this heading.

Mephobarbital (Clonidine may enhance the CNS-depressive effects of barbiturates; orthostatic hypotension may be aggravated by barbiturates). Products include:
Mebaral Tablets, USP ... 2483

Metformin Hydrochloride (Chlorthalidone causes hyperglycemia; higher dosage of oral hypoglycemic agents may be required). Products include:
ActoPlus Met Tablets ... 3219
Avandamet Tablets ... 1343
Fortamet Extended-Release Tablets ... 1156

Methadone Hydrochloride (Orthostatic hypotension may be aggravated by narcotics; orthostatic hypotension may be aggravated by barbiturates).
No products indexed under this heading.

Methyclothiazide (Chlorthalidone may add to or potentiate the action of other antihypertensives).
No products indexed under this heading.

Methyldopa (Chlorthalidone may add to or potentiate the action of other antihypertensives). Products include:
Aldoclor Tablets ... 1881
Aldoril Tablets ... 1884

Methyldopate Hydrochloride (Chlorthalidone may add to or potentiate the action of other antihypertensives).
No products indexed under this heading.

Metipranolol Hydrochloride (Chlorthalidone may add to or potentiate the action of other antihypertensives; if therapy is to be discontinued in patients receiving clonidine and beta blockers concurrently, beta blockers should be discontinued several days before the gradual withdrawal of clonidine).
No products indexed under this heading.

Metolazone (Chlorthalidone may add to or potentiate the action of other antihypertensives).
No products indexed under this heading.

Metoprolol Succinate (Chlorthalidone may add to or potentiate the action of other antihypertensives; if therapy is to be discontinued in patients receiving clonidine and beta blockers concurrently, beta blockers should be discontinued several days before the gradual withdrawal of clonidine). Products include:
Toprol-XL Tablets ... 660

Metoprolol Tartrate (Chlorthalidone may add to or potentiate the action of other antihypertensives; if therapy is to be discontinued in patients receiving clonidine and beta blockers concurrently, beta blockers should be discontinued several days before the gradual withdrawal of clonidine).
No products indexed under this heading.

Metyrosine (Chlorthalidone may add to or potentiate the action of other antihypertensives). Products include:
Demser Capsules ... 1933

Mibefradil Dihydrochloride (Chlorthalidone may add to or potentiate the action of other antihypertensives).
No products indexed under this heading.

Midazolam Hydrochloride (Clonidine may enhance the CNS-depressive effects of other sedatives).
No products indexed under this heading.

Miglitol (Chlorthalidone causes hyperglycemia; higher dosage of oral hypoglycemic agents may be required).
No products indexed under this heading.

Minoxidil (Chlorthalidone may add to or potentiate the action of other antihypertensives). Products include:
Men's Rogaine Extra Strength Topical Solution, Ocean Rush Scent and Original Unscented ... ▣ 706
Women's Rogaine Topical Solution, Spring Bloom Scent and Original Unscented ... ▣ 707

Moexipril Hydrochloride (Chlorthalidone may add to or potentiate the action of other antihypertensives). Products include:
Uniretic Tablets ... 3114
Univasc Tablets ... 3118

Morphine Sulfate (Orthostatic hypotension may be aggravated by narcotics; orthostatic hypotension may be aggravated by barbiturates). Products include:
Avinza Capsules ... 1714
Kadian Capsules ... 572
MS Contin Tablets ... 2703

Nadolol (Chlorthalidone may add to or potentiate the action of other antihypertensives; if therapy is to be discontinued in patients receiving clonidine and beta blockers concurrently, beta blockers should be discontinued several days before the gradual withdrawal of clonidine). Products include:
Nadolol Tablets ... 2121

Nicardipine Hydrochloride (Chlorthalidone may add to or potentiate the action of other antihypertensives). Products include:
Cardene I.V. ... 1129

Nifedipine (Chlorthalidone may add to or potentiate the action of other antihypertensives). Products include:
Adalat CC Tablets ... 2978

Nisoldipine (Chlorthalidone may add to or potentiate the action of other antihypertensives). Products include:
Sular Tablets ... 1163

Nitroglycerin (Chlorthalidone may add to or potentiate the action of other antihypertensives). Products include:
Nitro-Dur Transdermal Infusion System ... 3060
Nitrolingual Pumpspray ... 1161

Norepinephrine Bitartrate (Chlorthalidone may decrease arterial responsiveness to norepinephrine).
No products indexed under this heading.

Nortriptyline Hydrochloride (Co-administration of clonidine with tricyclic antidepressants may result in reduced effect of clonidine, necessitating an increase in dosage).
No products indexed under this heading.

Oxycodone Hydrochloride (Orthostatic hypotension may be aggravated by narcotics; orthostatic hypotension may be aggravated by barbiturates). Products include:
Combunox Tablets ... 1183
OxyContin Tablets ... 2699
OxyFast Oral Concentrate Solution ... 2704
OxyIR Capsules ... 2704
Percocet Tablets ... 1114
Percodan Tablets ... 1115

Penbutolol Sulfate (Chlorthalidone may add to or potentiate the action of other antihypertensives; if therapy is to be discontinued in patients receiving clonidine and beta blockers concurrently, beta blockers should be discontinued several days before the gradual withdrawal of clonidine).
No products indexed under this heading.

Pentobarbital Sodium (Clonidine may enhance the CNS-depressive effects of barbiturates; orthostatic hypotension may be aggravated by barbiturates). Products include:
Nembutal Sodium Solution, USP ... 2484

Perindopril Erbumine (Chlorthalidone may add to or potentiate the action of other antihypertensives). Products include:
Aceon Tablets (2 mg, 4 mg, 8 mg) ... 3191

Phenobarbital (Clonidine may enhance the CNS-depressive effects of barbiturates; orthostatic hypotension may be aggravated by barbiturates).
No products indexed under this heading.

Phenoxybenzamine Hydrochloride (Chlorthalidone may add to or potentiate the action of other antihypertensives). Products include:
Dibenzyline Capsules ... 3390

Phentolamine Mesylate (Chlorthalidone may add to or potentiate the action of other antihypertensives).
No products indexed under this heading.

Pindolol (Chlorthalidone may add to or potentiate the action of other antihypertensives; if therapy is to be discontinued in patients receiving clonidine and beta blockers concurrently, beta blockers should be discontinued several days before the gradual withdrawal of clonidine).
No products indexed under this heading.

Pioglitazone Hydrochloride (Chlorthalidone causes hyperglycemia; higher dosage of oral hypoglycemic agents may be required). Products include:
ActoPlus Met Tablets ... 3219
Actos Tablets ... 3224

Polythiazide (Chlorthalidone may add to or potentiate the action of other antihypertensives).
No products indexed under this heading.

Prazosin Hydrochloride (Chlorthalidone may add to or potentiate the action of other antihypertensives).
No products indexed under this heading.

Propofol (Clonidine may enhance the CNS-depressive effects of other sedatives). Products include:
Diprivan Injectable Emulsion ... 676

Propoxyphene Hydrochloride (Orthostatic hypotension may be aggravated by narcotics; orthostatic hypotension may be aggravated by barbiturates).
No products indexed under this heading.

Propoxyphene Napsylate (Orthostatic hypotension may be aggravated by narcotics; orthostatic hypotension may be aggravated by barbiturates). Products include:
Darvocet A 500 Tablets ... 3497

Propranolol Hydrochloride (Chlorthalidone may add to or potentiate the action of other antihypertensives; if therapy is to be discontinued in patients receiving clonidine and beta blockers concurrently, beta blockers should be discontinued several days before the gradual withdrawal of clonidine). Products include:
Inderal LA Long-Acting Capsules ... 3421
InnoPran XL Capsules ... 2728

Protriptyline Hydrochloride (Co-administration of clonidine with tricyclic antidepressants may result in reduced effect of clonidine, necessitating an increase in dosage). Products include:
Vivactil Tablets ... 2350

Quazepam (Clonidine may enhance the CNS-depressive effects of other sedatives).
No products indexed under this heading.

Quinapril Hydrochloride (Chlorthalidone may add to or potentiate the action of other antihypertensives).
No products indexed under this heading.

Ramipril (Chlorthalidone may add to or potentiate the action of other antihypertensives). Products include:
Altace Capsules 1673

Rauwolfia Serpentina (Chlorthalidone may add to or potentiate the action of other antihypertensives).
No products indexed under this heading.

Remifentanil Hydrochloride (Orthostatic hypotension may be aggravated by narcotics; orthostatic hypotension may be aggravated by barbiturates).
No products indexed under this heading.

Repaglinide (Chlorthalidone causes hyperglycemia; higher dosage of oral hypoglycemic agents may be required). Products include:
Prandin Tablets (0.5, 1, and 2 mg) 2337

Rescinnamine (Chlorthalidone may add to or potentiate the action of other antihypertensives).
No products indexed under this heading.

Reserpine (Chlorthalidone may add to or potentiate the action of other antihypertensives).
No products indexed under this heading.

Rosiglitazone Maleate (Chlorthalidone causes hyperglycemia; higher dosage of oral hypoglycemic agents may be required). Products include:
Avandamet Tablets 1343
Avandia Tablets 1348

Secobarbital Sodium (Clonidine may enhance the CNS-depressive effects of barbiturates; orthostatic hypotension may be aggravated by barbiturates).
No products indexed under this heading.

Sodium Nitroprusside (Chlorthalidone may add to or potentiate the action of other antihypertensives).
No products indexed under this heading.

Sotalol Hydrochloride (Chlorthalidone may add to or potentiate the action of other antihypertensives; if therapy is to be discontinued in patients receiving clonidine and beta blockers concurrently, beta blockers should be discontinued several days before the gradual withdrawal of clonidine).
No products indexed under this heading.

Spirapril Hydrochloride (Chlorthalidone may add to or potentiate the action of other antihypertensives).
No products indexed under this heading.

Sufentanil Citrate (Orthostatic hypotension may be aggravated by narcotics; orthostatic hypotension may be aggravated by barbiturates).
No products indexed under this heading.

Telmisartan (Chlorthalidone may add to or potentiate the action of other antihypertensives). Products include:
Micardis Tablets 884
Micardis HCT Tablets 886

Temazepam (Clonidine may enhance the CNS-depressive effects of other sedatives).
No products indexed under this heading.

Terazosin Hydrochloride (Chlorthalidone may add to or potentiate the action of other antihypertensives). Products include:
Hytrin Capsules 469

Thiamylal Sodium (Clonidine may enhance the CNS-depressive effects of barbiturates; orthostatic hypotension may be aggravated by barbiturates).
No products indexed under this heading.

Timolol Hemihydrate (Chlorthalidone may add to or potentiate the action of other antihypertensives; if therapy is to be discontinued in patients receiving clonidine and beta blockers concurrently, beta blockers should be discontinued several days before the gradual withdrawal of clonidine). Products include:
Betimol Ophthalmic Solution 3371
Betimol Ophthalmic Solution ⊙283

Timolol Maleate (Chlorthalidone may add to or potentiate the action of other antihypertensives; if therapy is to be discontinued in patients receiving clonidine and beta blockers concurrently, beta blockers should be discontinued several days before the gradual withdrawal of clonidine). Products include:
Blocadren Tablets 1891
Cosopt Sterile Ophthalmic Solution 1910
Timolide Tablets 2056
Timoptic in Ocudose 2061
Timoptic Sterile Ophthalmic Solution 2058
Timoptic-XE Sterile Ophthalmic Gel Forming Solution 2062

Tolazamide (Chlorthalidone causes hyperglycemia; higher dosage of oral hypoglycemic agents may be required).
No products indexed under this heading.

Tolbutamide (Chlorthalidone causes hyperglycemia; higher dosage of oral hypoglycemic agents may be required).
No products indexed under this heading.

Torsemide (Chlorthalidone may add to or potentiate the action of other antihypertensives).
No products indexed under this heading.

Trandolapril (Chlorthalidone may add to or potentiate the action of other antihypertensives). Products include:
Mavik Tablets 482
Tarka Tablets 519

Triazolam (Clonidine may enhance the CNS-depressive effects of other sedatives).
No products indexed under this heading.

Trimethaphan Camsylate (Chlorthalidone may add to or potentiate the action of other antihypertensives).
No products indexed under this heading.

Trimipramine Maleate (Co-administration of clonidine with tricyclic antidepressants may result in reduced effect of clonidine, necessitating an increase in dosage). Products include:
Surmontil Capsules 2347

Troglitazone (Chlorthalidone causes hyperglycemia; higher dosage of oral hypoglycemic agents may be required).
No products indexed under this heading.

Tubocurarine Chloride (Chlorthalidone may increase responsiveness to tubocurarine).
No products indexed under this heading.

Valsartan (Chlorthalidone may add to or potentiate the action of other antihypertensives). Products include:
Diovan HCT Tablets 2195
Diovan Tablets 2191

Verapamil Hydrochloride (Chlorthalidone may add to or potentiate the action of other antihypertensives). Products include:
Covera-HS Tablets 3135
Tarka Tablets 519
Verelan PM Capsules 3120

Zaleplon (Clonidine may enhance the CNS-depressive effects of other sedatives). Products include:
Sonata Capsules 1686

Zolpidem Tartrate (Clonidine may enhance the CNS-depressive effects of other sedatives). Products include:
Ambien Tablets 2867

Food Interactions

Alcohol (Clonidine may enhance the CNS-depressive effects of alcohol; orthostatic hypotension may be aggravated by alcohol).

CLOZAPINE TABLETS

(Clozapine) 2141

May interact with anticholinergics, antihypertensives, benzodiazepines, central nervous system depressants, antidepressant drugs, erythromycin, phenytoin, psychotropics, quinidine, and certain other agents. Compounds in these categories include:

Acebutolol Hydrochloride (Clozapine causes orthostatic hypotension and may potentiate hypotensive effects of antihypertensive drugs).
No products indexed under this heading.

Alfentanil Hydrochloride (Clozapine induces drowsiness and sedation in a significant number of patients; caution is advised with concomitant use).
No products indexed under this heading.

Alprazolam (Co-administration with benzodiazepines or other psychotropic agents may be accompanied by orthostatic hypotension leading to profound collapse and respiratory and/or cardiac arrest; caution is advised if used concurrently). Products include:
Niravam Orally Disintegrating Tablets 3106
Xanax XR Tablets 2655

Amitriptyline Hydrochloride (Concomitant use of clozapine with other drugs metabolized by CYP4502D6 may require lower than usual doses for either drug).
No products indexed under this heading.

Amlodipine Besylate (Clozapine causes orthostatic hypotension and may potentiate hypotensive effects of antihypertensive drugs). Products include:
Caduet Tablets 2507
Lotrel Capsules 2238
Norvasc Tablets 2529

Amoxapine (Concomitant use of clozapine with other drugs metabolized by CYP4502D6 may require lower than usual doses for either drug).
No products indexed under this heading.

Aprobarbital (Clozapine induces drowsiness and sedation in a significant number of patients; caution is advised with concomitant use).
No products indexed under this heading.

Atenolol (Clozapine causes orthostatic hypotension and may potentiate hypotensive effects of antihypertensive drugs). Products include:
Tenormin I.V. Injection 698
Tenormin Tablets 695

Atropine Sulfate (Clozapine may potentiate anticholinergic effects).
No products indexed under this heading.

Belladonna Alkaloids (Clozapine may potentiate anticholinergic effects). Products include:
Hyland's Teething Tablets 736

Benazepril Hydrochloride (Clozapine causes orthostatic hypotension and may potentiate hypotensive effects of antihypertensive drugs). Products include:
Lotensin Tablets 2232
Lotensin HCT Tablets 2235
Lotrel Capsules 2238

Bendroflumethiazide (Clozapine causes orthostatic hypotension and may potentiate hypotensive effects of antihypertensive drugs).
No products indexed under this heading.

Benztropine Mesylate (Clozapine may potentiate anticholinergic effects). Products include:
Cogentin Injection 1903

Betaxolol Hydrochloride (Clozapine causes orthostatic hypotension and may potentiate hypotensive effects of antihypertensive drugs). Products include:
Betoptic S Ophthalmic Suspension 554

Biperiden Hydrochloride (Clozapine may potentiate anticholinergic effects).
No products indexed under this heading.

Bisoprolol Fumarate (Clozapine causes orthostatic hypotension and may potentiate hypotensive effects of antihypertensive drugs).
No products indexed under this heading.

Bone Marrow Depressants, unspecified (Increases the risk and/or severity of bone marrow suppression).
No products indexed under this heading.

Buprenorphine Hydrochloride (Clozapine induces drowsiness and sedation in a significant number of patients; caution is advised with concomitant use). Products include:
Buprenex Injectable 2718
Suboxone Tablets 2719
Subutex Tablets 2719

Bupropion Hydrochloride (Concomitant use of clozapine with other

drugs metabolized by CYP4502D6 may require lower than usual doses for either drug). Products include:
Wellbutrin Tablets 1579
Wellbutrin SR Sustained-Release Tablets 1583
Wellbutrin XL Extended-Release Tablets 1588
Zyban Sustained-Release Tablets 1620

Buspirone Hydrochloride (Co-administration with benzodiazepines or other psychotropic agents may be accompanied by orthostatic hypotension leading to profound collapse and respiratory and/or cardiac arrest; caution is advised if used concurrently).
No products indexed under this heading.

Butabarbital (Clozapine induces drowsiness and sedation in a significant number of patients; caution is advised with concomitant use).
No products indexed under this heading.

Butalbital (Clozapine induces drowsiness and sedation in a significant number of patients; caution is advised with concomitant use). Products include:
Sedapap Tablets 50 mg/650 mg 2098

Caffeine (May increase plasma levels of clozapine, potentially resulting in adverse effects). Products include:
Athena Hair System Shampoo .... ▣767
BC Powder .... ▣612
Arthritis Strength BC Powder .... ▣612
Goody's Extra Strength Headache Powder .... ▣621
Goody's Extra Strength Pain Relief Tablets .... ▣621
Hycomine Compound Tablets 1105
Spartan Hair System Shampoo .... ▣767
Vivarin .... ▣639

Caffeine Citrate (May increase plasma levels of clozapine, potentially resulting in adverse effects). Products include:
Cafcit 1854

Candesartan Cilexetil (Clozapine causes orthostatic hypotension and may potentiate hypotensive effects of antihypertensive drugs). Products include:
Atacand Tablets 634
Atacand HCT 637

Captopril (Clozapine causes orthostatic hypotension and may potentiate hypotensive effects of antihypertensive drugs). Products include:
Captopril Tablets 2114

Carbamazepine (Concomitant use is not recommended; discontinuation of concomitant carbamazepine administration may result in increase in clozapine levels). Products include:
Carbatrol Capsules 3174
Equetro Extended-Release Capsules 3178
Tegretol/Tegretol-XR 2278

Carteolol Hydrochloride (Clozapine causes orthostatic hypotension and may potentiate hypotensive effects of antihypertensive drugs). Products include:
Carteolol Hydrochloride Ophthalmic Solution USP, 1% .... ⊙246

Chlordiazepoxide (Co-administration with benzodiazepines or other psychotropic agents may be accompanied by orthostatic hypotension leading to profound collapse and respiratory and/or cardiac arrest; caution is advised if used concurrently).
No products indexed under this heading.

Chlordiazepoxide Hydrochloride (Co-administration with benzodiazepines or other psychotropic agents may be accompanied by orthostatic hypotension leading to profound collapse and respiratory and/or cardiac arrest; caution is advised if used concurrently). Products include:
Librium Capsules 3349

Chlorothiazide (Clozapine causes orthostatic hypotension and may potentiate hypotensive effects of antihypertensive drugs). Products include:
Aldoclor Tablets 1881
Diuril Oral 1936

Chlorothiazide Sodium (Clozapine causes orthostatic hypotension and may potentiate hypotensive effects of antihypertensive drugs). Products include:
Diuril Sodium Intravenous 1934

Chlorpromazine (Co-administration with benzodiazepines or other psychotropic agents may be accompanied by orthostatic hypotension leading to profound collapse and respiratory and/or cardiac arrest; caution is advised if used concurrently).
No products indexed under this heading.

Chlorpromazine Hydrochloride (Co-administration with benzodiazepines or other psychotropic agents may be accompanied by orthostatic hypotension leading to profound collapse and respiratory and/or cardiac arrest; caution is advised if used concurrently).
No products indexed under this heading.

Chlorprothixene (Co-administration with benzodiazepines or other psychotropic agents may be accompanied by orthostatic hypotension leading to profound collapse and respiratory and/or cardiac arrest; caution is advised if used concurrently).
No products indexed under this heading.

Chlorprothixene Hydrochloride (Co-administration with benzodiazepines or other psychotropic agents may be accompanied by orthostatic hypotension leading to profound collapse and respiratory and/or cardiac arrest; caution is advised if used concurrently).
No products indexed under this heading.

Chlorprothixene Lactate (Clozapine induces drowsiness and sedation in a significant number of patients; caution is advised with concomitant use).
No products indexed under this heading.

Chlorthalidone (Clozapine causes orthostatic hypotension and may potentiate hypotensive effects of antihypertensive drugs). Products include:
Clorpres Tablets 2139

Cimetidine (May increase plasma levels of clozapine, potentially resulting in adverse effects). Products include:
Tagamet HB 200 Tablets .... ▣637
Tagamet Tablets 1547

Cimetidine Hydrochloride (May increase plasma levels of clozapine, potentially resulting in adverse effects).
No products indexed under this heading.

Citalopram Hydrobromide (Concomitant use of clozapine with other drugs metabolized by CYP4502D6 may require lower than usual doses for either drug). Products include:
Celexa 1177

Clidinium Bromide (Clozapine may potentiate anticholinergic effects).
No products indexed under this heading.

Clonidine (Clozapine causes orthostatic hypotension and may potentiate hypotensive effects of antihypertensive drugs). Products include:
Catapres-TTS 875

Clonidine Hydrochloride (Clozapine causes orthostatic hypotension and may potentiate hypotensive effects of antihypertensive drugs). Products include:
Catapres Tablets 874
Clorpres Tablets 2139

Clorazepate Dipotassium (Co-administration with benzodiazepines or other psychotropic agents may be accompanied by orthostatic hypotension leading to profound collapse and respiratory and/or cardiac arrest; caution is advised if used concurrently). Products include:
Tranxene 2488

Codeine Phosphate (Clozapine induces drowsiness and sedation in a significant number of patients; caution is advised with concomitant use). Products include:
Tylenol with Codeine 2461

Deserpidine (Clozapine causes orthostatic hypotension and may potentiate hypotensive effects of antihypertensive drugs).
No products indexed under this heading.

Desflurane (Clozapine induces drowsiness and sedation in a significant number of patients; caution is advised with concomitant use). Products include:
Suprane Liquid for Inhalation 770

Desipramine Hydrochloride (Concomitant use of clozapine with other drugs metabolized by CYP4502D6 may require lower than usual doses for either drug).
No products indexed under this heading.

Dezocine (Clozapine induces drowsiness and sedation in a significant number of patients; caution is advised with concomitant use).
No products indexed under this heading.

Diazepam (Co-administration with benzodiazepines or other psychotropic agents may be accompanied by orthostatic hypotension leading to profound collapse and respiratory and/or cardiac arrest; caution is advised if used concurrently). Products include:
Diastat Rectal Delivery System 3344
Valium Tablets 2822

Diazoxide (Clozapine causes orthostatic hypotension and may potentiate hypotensive effects of antihypertensive drugs). Products include:
Hyperstat I.V. Injection 3031

Dicyclomine Hydrochloride (Clozapine may potentiate anticholinergic effects). Products include:
Bentyl Capsules 724
Bentyl Injection 724
Bentyl Syrup 724
Bentyl Tablets 724

Diltiazem Hydrochloride (Clozapine causes orthostatic hypotension and may potentiate hypotensive effects of antihypertensive drugs). Products include:
Cardizem LA Extended Release Tablets 1699
Tiazac Capsules 1204

Doxazosin Mesylate (Clozapine causes orthostatic hypotension and may potentiate hypotensive effects of antihypertensive drugs).
No products indexed under this heading.

Doxepin Hydrochloride (Concomitant use of clozapine with other drugs metabolized by CYP4502D6 may require lower than usual doses for either drug).
No products indexed under this heading.

Droperidol (Co-administration with benzodiazepines or other psychotropic agents may be accompanied by orthostatic hypotension leading to profound collapse and respiratory and/or cardiac arrest; caution is advised if used concurrently).
No products indexed under this heading.

Enalapril Maleate (Clozapine causes orthostatic hypotension and may potentiate hypotensive effects of antihypertensive drugs). Products include:
Vaseretic Tablets 2073
Vasotec I.V. Injection 2076

Enalaprilat (Clozapine causes orthostatic hypotension and may potentiate hypotensive effects of antihypertensive drugs).
No products indexed under this heading.

Encainide Hydrochloride (Concomitant use of clozapine with other drugs metabolized by CYP4502D6 may require lower than usual doses for either drug).
No products indexed under this heading.

Enflurane (Clozapine induces drowsiness and sedation in a significant number of patients; caution is advised with concomitant use).
No products indexed under this heading.

Epinephrine (The administration of epinephrine should be avoided in the treatment of clozapine-induced hypotension because of a possible reverse epinephrine effect). Products include:
EpiPen 1061
Primatene Mist .... ▣749

Epinephrine Hydrochloride (The administration of epinephrine should be avoided in the treatment of clozapine-induced hypotension because of a possible reverse epinephrine effect).
No products indexed under this heading.

Eprosartan Mesylate (Clozapine causes orthostatic hypotension and

may potentiate hypotensive effects of antihypertensive drugs). Products include:
Teveten Tablets 1707
Teveten HCT Tablets 1710

Erythromycin (May increase plasma levels of clozapine, potentially resulting in adverse effects). Products include:
Erygel Topical Gel 2096
Ery-Tab Tablets 447
Erythromycin Base Filmtab Tablets 454
Erythromycin Delayed-Release Capsules, USP 456
PCE Dispertab Tablets 510

Erythromycin Estolate (May increase plasma levels of clozapine, potentially resulting in adverse effects).
No products indexed under this heading.

Erythromycin Ethylsuccinate (May increase plasma levels of clozapine, potentially resulting in adverse effects). Products include:
E.E.S. 449
EryPed 445

Erythromycin Gluceptate (May increase plasma levels of clozapine, potentially resulting in adverse effects).
No products indexed under this heading.

Erythromycin Lactobionate (May increase plasma levels of clozapine, potentially resulting in adverse effects).
No products indexed under this heading.

Erythromycin Stearate (May increase plasma levels of clozapine, potentially resulting in adverse effects). Products include:
Erythrocin Stearate Filmtab Tablets 452

Escitalopram Oxalate (Concomitant use of clozapine with other drugs metabolized by CYP4502D6 may require lower than usual doses for either drug). Products include:
Lexapro Oral Solution 1193
Lexapro Tablets 1193

Esmolol Hydrochloride (Clozapine causes orthostatic hypotension and may potentiate hypotensive effects of antihypertensive drugs). Products include:
Brevibloc Concentrate 766
Brevibloc Injection 766
Brevibloc Double Strength Injection 766
Brevibloc Premixed Injection 766
Brevibloc Double Strength Premixed Injection 766

Estazolam (Co-administration with benzodiazepines or other psychotropic agents may be accompanied by orthostatic hypotension leading to profound collapse and respiratory and/or cardiac arrest; caution is advised if used concurrently). Products include:
ProSom Tablets 512

Ethanol (Clozapine induces drowsiness and sedation in a significant number of patients; caution is advised with concomitant use).
No products indexed under this heading.

Ethchlorvynol (Clozapine induces drowsiness and sedation in a significant number of patients; caution is advised with concomitant use).
No products indexed under this heading.

Ethinamate (Clozapine induces drowsiness and sedation in a significant number of patients; caution is advised with concomitant use).
No products indexed under this heading.

Ethyl Alcohol (Clozapine induces drowsiness and sedation in a significant number of patients; caution is advised with concomitant use).
No products indexed under this heading.

Felodipine (Clozapine causes orthostatic hypotension and may potentiate hypotensive effects of antihypertensive drugs). Products include:
Plendil Extended-Release Tablets 651

Fentanyl (Clozapine induces drowsiness and sedation in a significant number of patients; caution is advised with concomitant use). Products include:
Duragesic Transdermal System 2448

Fentanyl Citrate (Clozapine induces drowsiness and sedation in a significant number of patients; caution is advised with concomitant use). Products include:
Actiq 993

Flecainide Acetate (Concomitant use of clozapine with other drugs metabolized by CYP4502D6 may require lower than usual doses for either drug). Products include:
Tambocor Tablets 1824

Fluoxetine Hydrochloride (Co-administration in schizophrenic patients has resulted in elevated mean trough concentrations of clozapine and its metabolites by less than two-fold compared to baseline concentrations; a reduced clozapine dose should be considered). Products include:
Prozac Pulvules and Liquid 1771
Symbyax Capsules 1788

Fluphenazine Decanoate (Co-administration with benzodiazepines or other psychotropic agents may be accompanied by orthostatic hypotension leading to profound collapse and respiratory and/or cardiac arrest; caution is advised if used concurrently).
No products indexed under this heading.

Fluphenazine Enanthate (Co-administration with benzodiazepines or other psychotropic agents may be accompanied by orthostatic hypotension leading to profound collapse and respiratory and/or cardiac arrest; caution is advised if used concurrently).
No products indexed under this heading.

Fluphenazine Hydrochloride (Co-administration with benzodiazepines or other psychotropic agents may be accompanied by orthostatic hypotension leading to profound collapse and respiratory and/or cardiac arrest; caution is advised if used concurrently).
No products indexed under this heading.

Flurazepam Hydrochloride (Co-administration with benzodiazepines or other psychotropic agents may be accompanied by orthostatic hypotension leading to profound collapse and respiratory and/or cardiac arrest; caution is advised if used concurrently). Products include:
Dalmane Capsules 3343

Fluvoxamine Maleate (Co-administration in schizophrenic patients has resulted in elevated mean trough concentrations of clozapine and its metabolites by about three-fold compared to baseline concentrations; a reduced clozapine dose should be considered).
No products indexed under this heading.

Fosinopril Sodium (Clozapine causes orthostatic hypotension and may potentiate hypotensive effects of antihypertensive drugs).
No products indexed under this heading.

Fosphenytoin Sodium (May decrease clozapine plasma levels resulting in a decrease in effectiveness of a previously effective clozapine dose).
No products indexed under this heading.

Furosemide (Clozapine causes orthostatic hypotension and may potentiate hypotensive effects of antihypertensive drugs). Products include:
Furosemide Tablets 2117

Glutethimide (Clozapine induces drowsiness and sedation in a significant number of patients; caution is advised with concomitant use).
No products indexed under this heading.

Glycopyrrolate (Clozapine may potentiate anticholinergic effects).
No products indexed under this heading.

Guanabenz Acetate (Clozapine causes orthostatic hypotension and may potentiate hypotensive effects of antihypertensive drugs).
No products indexed under this heading.

Guanethidine Monosulfate (Clozapine causes orthostatic hypotension and may potentiate hypotensive effects of antihypertensive drugs).
No products indexed under this heading.

Halazepam (Co-administration with benzodiazepines or other psychotropic agents may be accompanied by orthostatic hypotension leading to profound collapse and respiratory and/or cardiac arrest; caution is advised if used concurrently).
No products indexed under this heading.

Haloperidol (Co-administration with benzodiazepines or other psychotropic agents may be accompanied by orthostatic hypotension leading to profound collapse and respiratory and/or cardiac arrest; caution is advised if used concurrently).
No products indexed under this heading.

Haloperidol Decanoate (Co-administration with benzodiazepines or other psychotropic agents may be accompanied by orthostatic hypotension leading to profound collapse and respiratory and/or cardiac arrest; caution is advised if used concurrently).
No products indexed under this heading.

Hydralazine Hydrochloride (Clozapine causes orthostatic hypotension and may potentiate hypotensive effects of antihypertensive drugs). Products include:
BiDil Tablets 2161

Hydrochlorothiazide (Clozapine causes orthostatic hypotension and may potentiate hypotensive effects of antihypertensive drugs). Products include:
Aldoril Tablets 1884
Atacand HCT 637
Avalide Tablets 2889
Avalide Tablets 922
Benicar HCT Tablets 2852
Diovan HCT Tablets 2195
Dyazide Capsules 1389
Hyzaar 1964
Lotensin HCT Tablets 2235
Maxzide 2150
Micardis HCT Tablets 886
Moduretic Tablets 2003
Prinzide Tablets 2033
Teveten HCT Tablets 1710
Timolide Tablets 2056
Uniretic Tablets 3114
Vaseretic Tablets 2073
Zestoretic Tablets 701

Hydrocodone Bitartrate (Clozapine induces drowsiness and sedation in a significant number of patients; caution is advised with concomitant use). Products include:
Hycodan 1104
Hycomine Compound Tablets 1105
Hycotuss Expectorant Syrup 1106
Lortab 3315
Lortab Elixir 3312
Vicodin Tablets 530
Vicodin ES Tablets 531
Vicodin HP Tablets 532
Vicoprofen Tablets 533
Zydone Tablets 1118

Hydrocodone Polistirex (Clozapine induces drowsiness and sedation in a significant number of patients; caution is advised with concomitant use). Products include:
Tussionex Pennkinetic Extended-Release Suspension 3322

Hydroflumethiazide (Clozapine causes orthostatic hypotension and may potentiate hypotensive effects of antihypertensive drugs).
No products indexed under this heading.

Hydromorphone Hydrochloride (Clozapine induces drowsiness and sedation in a significant number of patients; caution is advised with concomitant use). Products include:
Dilaudid 439
Dilaudid Oral Liquid 443
Dilaudid Non-Sterile Powder 439
Dilaudid Rectal Suppositories 439
Dilaudid Tablets 439
Dilaudid Tablets - 8 mg 443
Dilaudid-HP 441

Hydroxyzine Hydrochloride (Co-administration with benzodiazepines or other psychotropic agents may be accompanied by orthostatic hypotension leading to profound collapse and respiratory and/or cardiac arrest; caution is advised if used concurrently).
No products indexed under this heading.

Hyoscyamine (Clozapine may potentiate anticholinergic effects).
No products indexed under this heading.

Hyoscyamine Sulfate (Clozapine may potentiate anticholinergic effects).
No products indexed under this heading.

Imipramine Hydrochloride (Concomitant use of clozapine with other drugs metabolized by CYP4502D6 may require lower than usual doses for either drug).
No products indexed under this heading.

Imipramine Pamoate (Concomitant use of clozapine with other drugs metabolized by CYP4502D6 may require lower than usual doses for either drug).
No products indexed under this heading.

Indapamide (Clozapine causes orthostatic hypotension and may potentiate hypotensive effects of antihypertensive drugs). Products include:
Indapamide Tablets 2119

Ipratropium Bromide (Clozapine may potentiate anticholinergic effects). Products include:
Atrovent HFA Inhalation Aerosol 872
Atrovent Inhalation Solution 868
Atrovent Nasal Spray 0.03% 869
Atrovent Nasal Spray 0.06% 870
Combivent Inhalation Aerosol 878
DuoNeb Inhalation Solution 1058

Irbesartan (Clozapine causes orthostatic hypotension and may potentiate hypotensive effects of antihypertensive drugs). Products include:
Avalide Tablets 922
Avalide Tablets 2889
Avapro Tablets 925
Avapro Tablets 2886

Isocarboxazid (Concomitant use of clozapine with other drugs metabolized by CYP4502D6 may require lower than usual doses for either drug).
No products indexed under this heading.

Isoflurane (Clozapine induces drowsiness and sedation in a significant number of patients; caution is advised with concomitant use).
No products indexed under this heading.

Isradipine (Clozapine causes orthostatic hypotension and may potentiate hypotensive effects of antihypertensive drugs). Products include:
DynaCirc CR Tablets 2726

Ketamine Hydrochloride (Clozapine induces drowsiness and sedation in a significant number of patients; caution is advised with concomitant use).
No products indexed under this heading.

Labetalol Hydrochloride (Clozapine causes orthostatic hypotension and may potentiate hypotensive effects of antihypertensive drugs).
No products indexed under this heading.

Levomethadyl Acetate Hydrochloride (Clozapine induces drowsiness and sedation in a significant number of patients; caution is advised with concomitant use).
No products indexed under this heading.

Levorphanol Tartrate (Clozapine induces drowsiness and sedation in a significant number of patients; caution is advised with concomitant use).
No products indexed under this heading.

Lisinopril (Clozapine causes orthostatic hypotension and may potentiate hypotensive effects of antihypertensive drugs). Products include:
Prinivil Tablets 2029
Prinzide Tablets 2033
Zestoretic Tablets 701
Zestril Tablets 704

Lithium Carbonate (Co-administration with benzodiazepines or other psychotropic agents may be accompanied by orthostatic hypotension leading to profound collapse and respiratory and/or cardiac arrest; caution is advised if used concurrently). Products include:
Eskalith 1406
Lithobid Tablets 1670

Lithium Citrate (Co-administration with benzodiazepines or other psychotropic agents may be accompanied by orthostatic hypotension leading to profound collapse and respiratory and/or cardiac arrest; caution is advised if used concurrently).
No products indexed under this heading.

Lorazepam (Co-administration with benzodiazepines or other psychotropic agents may be accompanied by orthostatic hypotension leading to profound collapse and respiratory and/or cardiac arrest; caution is advised if used concurrently).
No products indexed under this heading.

Losartan Potassium (Clozapine causes orthostatic hypotension and may potentiate hypotensive effects of antihypertensive drugs). Products include:
Cozaar Tablets 1913
Hyzaar 1964

Loxapine Hydrochloride (Co-administration with benzodiazepines or other psychotropic agents may be accompanied by orthostatic hypotension leading to profound collapse and respiratory and/or cardiac arrest; caution is advised if used concurrently).
No products indexed under this heading.

Loxapine Succinate (Co-administration with benzodiazepines or other psychotropic agents may be accompanied by orthostatic hypotension leading to profound collapse and respiratory and/or cardiac arrest; caution is advised if used concurrently).
No products indexed under this heading.

Maprotiline Hydrochloride (Concomitant use of clozapine with other drugs metabolized by CYP4502D6 may require lower than usual doses for either drug).
No products indexed under this heading.

Mecamylamine Hydrochloride (Clozapine causes orthostatic hypotension and may potentiate hypotensive effects of antihypertensive drugs). Products include:
Inversine Tablets 3286

Mepenzolate Bromide (Clozapine may potentiate anticholinergic effects).
No products indexed under this heading.

Meperidine Hydrochloride (Clozapine induces drowsiness and sedation in a significant number of patients; caution is advised with concomitant use).
No products indexed under this heading.

Mephobarbital (Clozapine induces drowsiness and sedation in a significant number of patients; caution is advised with concomitant use). Products include:
Mebaral Tablets, USP 2483

Meprobamate (Co-administration with benzodiazepines or other psychotropic agents may be accompanied by orthostatic hypotension leading to profound collapse and respiratory and/or cardiac arrest; caution is advised if used concurrently).
No products indexed under this heading.

Mesoridazine Besylate (Co-administration with benzodiazepines or other psychotropic agents may be accompanied by orthostatic hypotension leading to profound collapse and respiratory and/or cardiac arrest; caution is advised if used concurrently).
No products indexed under this heading.

Methadone Hydrochloride (Clozapine induces drowsiness and sedation in a significant number of patients; caution is advised with concomitant use).
No products indexed under this heading.

Methohexital Sodium (Clozapine induces drowsiness and sedation in a significant number of patients; caution is advised with concomitant use).
No products indexed under this heading.

Methotrimeprazine (Clozapine induces drowsiness and sedation in a significant number of patients; caution is advised with concomitant use).
No products indexed under this heading.

Methoxyflurane (Clozapine induces drowsiness and sedation in a significant number of patients; caution is advised with concomitant use).
No products indexed under this heading.

Methyclothiazide (Clozapine causes orthostatic hypotension and may potentiate hypotensive effects of antihypertensive drugs).
No products indexed under this heading.

Methyldopa (Clozapine causes orthostatic hypotension and may potentiate hypotensive effects of antihypertensive drugs). Products include:
Aldoclor Tablets 1881
Aldoril Tablets 1884

Methyldopate Hydrochloride (Clozapine causes orthostatic hypotension and may potentiate hypotensive effects of antihypertensive drugs).
No products indexed under this heading.

Metolazone (Clozapine causes orthostatic hypotension and may potentiate hypotensive effects of antihypertensive drugs).
No products indexed under this heading.

Metoprolol Succinate (Clozapine causes orthostatic hypotension and may potentiate hypotensive effects of antihypertensive drugs). Products include:
Toprol-XL Tablets 660

Metoprolol Tartrate (Clozapine causes orthostatic hypotension and may potentiate hypotensive effects of antihypertensive drugs).
No products indexed under this heading.

Metyrosine (Clozapine causes orthostatic hypotension and may potentiate hypotensive effects of antihypertensive drugs). Products include:
Demser Capsules 1933

Mibefradil Dihydrochloride (Clozapine causes orthostatic hypotension and may potentiate hypotensive effects of antihypertensive drugs).
No products indexed under this heading.

Midazolam Hydrochloride (Co-administration with benzodiazepines or other psychotropic agents may be accompanied by orthostatic hypotension leading to profound collapse and respiratory and/or cardiac arrest; caution is advised if used concurrently).
No products indexed under this heading.

Minoxidil (Clozapine causes orthostatic hypotension and may potentiate hypotensive effects of antihypertensive drugs). Products include:
Men's Rogaine Extra Strength Topical Solution, Ocean Rush Scent and Original Unscented ..... ▣706
Women's Rogaine Topical Solution, Spring Bloom Scent and Original Unscented .... ▣707

Mirtazapine (Concomitant use of clozapine with other drugs metabolized by CYP4502D6 may require lower than usual doses for either drug).
No products indexed under this heading.

Moexipril Hydrochloride (Clozapine causes orthostatic hypotension and may potentiate hypotensive effects of antihypertensive drugs). Products include:
Uniretic Tablets 3114
Univasc Tablets 3118

Molindone Hydrochloride (Co-administration with benzodiazepines or other psychotropic agents may be accompanied by orthostatic hypotension leading to profound collapse and respiratory and/or cardiac arrest; caution is advised if used concurrently). Products include:
Moban Tablets 1108

Morphine Sulfate (Clozapine induces drowsiness and sedation in a significant number of patients; caution is advised with concomitant use). Products include:
Avinza Capsules 1714
Kadian Capsules 572
MS Contin Tablets 2703

Nadolol (Clozapine causes orthostatic hypotension and may potentiate hypotensive effects of antihypertensive drugs). Products include:
Nadolol Tablets 2121

Nefazodone Hydrochloride (Concomitant use of clozapine with other drugs metabolized by CYP4502D6 may require lower than usual doses for either drug).
No products indexed under this heading.

Nicardipine Hydrochloride (Clozapine causes orthostatic hypotension and may potentiate hypotensive effects of antihypertensive drugs). Products include:
Cardene I.V. 1129

Nicotine (May decrease clozapine plasma levels resulting in a decrease in effectiveness of a previously effective clozapine dose). Products include:

Nicoderm CQ Patch 1629
NicoDerm CQ Clear Patch 627
Nicotrol Inhaler 2594
Nicotrol NS 2596

Nicotine Polacrilex (May decrease clozapine plasma levels resulting in a decrease in effectiveness of a previously effective clozapine dose). Products include:
Commit Lozenges 1625
Nicorette Gum 1632

Nifedipine (Clozapine causes orthostatic hypotension and may potentiate hypotensive effects of antihypertensive drugs). Products include:
Adalat CC Tablets 2978

Nisoldipine (Clozapine causes orthostatic hypotension and may potentiate hypotensive effects of antihypertensive drugs). Products include:
Sular Tablets 1163

Nitroglycerin (Clozapine causes orthostatic hypotension and may potentiate hypotensive effects of antihypertensive drugs). Products include:
Nitro-Dur Transdermal Infusion System........ 3060
Nitrolingual Pumpspray 1161

Nortriptyline Hydrochloride (Concomitant use of clozapine with other drugs metabolized by CYP4502D6 may require lower than usual doses for either drug).
No products indexed under this heading.

Olanzapine (Co-administration with benzodiazepines or other psychotropic agents may be accompanied by orthostatic hypotension leading to profound collapse and respiratory and/or cardiac arrest; caution is advised if used concurrently). Products include:
Symbyax Capsules 1788
Zyprexa Tablets 1798
Zyprexa IntraMuscular 1798
Zyprexa ZYDIS Orally Disintegrating Tablets........ 1798

Oxazepam (Co-administration with benzodiazepines or other psychotropic agents may be accompanied by orthostatic hypotension leading to profound collapse and respiratory and/or cardiac arrest; caution is advised if used concurrently).
No products indexed under this heading.

Oxybutynin Chloride (Clozapine may potentiate anticholinergic effects). Products include:
Ditropan XL Extended Release Tablets 2391

Oxycodone Hydrochloride (Clozapine induces drowsiness and sedation in a significant number of patients; caution is advised with concomitant use). Products include:
Combunox Tablets 1183
OxyContin Tablets 2699
OxyFast Oral Concentrate Solution........ 2704
OxyIR Capsules 2704
Percocet Tablets 1114
Percodan Tablets 1115

Paroxetine Hydrochloride (Co-administration in schizophrenic patients has resulted in elevated mean trough concentrations of clozapine and its metabolites by less than two-fold compared to baseline concentrations; a reduced clozapine dose should be considered). Products include:
Paxil CR Controlled-Release Tablets 1509
Paxil 1501

Penbutolol Sulfate (Clozapine causes orthostatic hypotension and may potentiate hypotensive effects of antihypertensive drugs).
No products indexed under this heading.

Pentobarbital Sodium (Clozapine induces drowsiness and sedation in a significant number of patients; caution is advised with concomitant use). Products include:
Nembutal Sodium Solution, USP 2484

Perindopril Erbumine (Clozapine causes orthostatic hypotension and may potentiate hypotensive effects of antihypertensive drugs). Products include:
Aceon Tablets (2 mg, 4 mg, 8 mg)........ 3191

Perphenazine (Co-administration with benzodiazepines or other psychotropic agents may be accompanied by orthostatic hypotension leading to profound collapse and respiratory and/or cardiac arrest; caution is advised if used concurrently).
No products indexed under this heading.

Phenelzine Sulfate (Concomitant use of clozapine with other drugs metabolized by CYP4502D6 may require lower than usual doses for either drug).
No products indexed under this heading.

Phenobarbital (Clozapine induces drowsiness and sedation in a significant number of patients; caution is advised with concomitant use).
No products indexed under this heading.

Phenoxybenzamine Hydrochloride (Clozapine causes orthostatic hypotension and may potentiate hypotensive effects of antihypertensive drugs). Products include:
Dibenzyline Capsules 3390

Phentolamine Mesylate (Clozapine causes orthostatic hypotension and may potentiate hypotensive effects of antihypertensive drugs).
No products indexed under this heading.

Phenytoin (May decrease clozapine plasma levels resulting in a decrease in effectiveness of a previously effective clozapine dose).
No products indexed under this heading.

Phenytoin Sodium (May decrease clozapine plasma levels resulting in a decrease in effectiveness of a previously effective clozapine dose). Products include:
Phenytek Capsules 2153

Pindolol (Clozapine causes orthostatic hypotension and may potentiate hypotensive effects of antihypertensive drugs).
No products indexed under this heading.

Polythiazide (Clozapine causes orthostatic hypotension and may potentiate hypotensive effects of antihypertensive drugs).
No products indexed under this heading.

Prazepam (Co-administration with benzodiazepines or other psychotropic agents may be accompanied by orthostatic hypotension leading to profound collapse and respiratory and/or cardiac arrest; caution is advised if used concurrently).
No products indexed under this heading.

Prazosin Hydrochloride (Clozapine causes orthostatic hypotension and may potentiate hypotensive effects of antihypertensive drugs).
No products indexed under this heading.

Prochlorperazine (Co-administration with benzodiazepines or other psychotropic agents may be accompanied by orthostatic hypotension leading to profound collapse and respiratory and/or cardiac arrest; caution is advised if used concurrently).
No products indexed under this heading.

Procyclidine Hydrochloride (Clozapine may potentiate anticholinergic effects).
No products indexed under this heading.

Promethazine Hydrochloride (Co-administration with benzodiazepines or other psychotropic agents may be accompanied by orthostatic hypotension leading to profound collapse and respiratory and/or cardiac arrest; caution is advised if used concurrently). Products include:
Phenergan 3438

Propantheline Bromide (Clozapine may potentiate anticholinergic effects).
No products indexed under this heading.

Propofol (Clozapine induces drowsiness and sedation in a significant number of patients; caution is advised with concomitant use). Products include:
Diprivan Injectable Emulsion 676

Propoxyphene Hydrochloride (Clozapine induces drowsiness and sedation in a significant number of patients; caution is advised with concomitant use).
No products indexed under this heading.

Propoxyphene Napsylate (Clozapine induces drowsiness and sedation in a significant number of patients; caution is advised with concomitant use). Products include:
Darvocet A 500 Tablets 3497

Propranolol Hydrochloride (Clozapine causes orthostatic hypotension and may potentiate hypotensive effects of antihypertensive drugs). Products include:
Inderal LA Long-Acting Capsules 3421
InnoPran XL Capsules 2728

Protriptyline Hydrochloride (Concomitant use of clozapine with other drugs metabolized by CYP4502D6 may require lower than usual doses for either drug). Products include:
Vivactil Tablets 2350

Quazepam (Co-administration with benzodiazepines or other psychotropic agents may be accompanied by orthostatic hypotension leading to profound collapse and respiratory and/or cardiac arrest; caution is advised if used concurrently).
No products indexed under this heading.

Quetiapine Fumarate (Co-administration with benzodiazepines or other psychotropic agents may be accompanied by orthostatic hypotension leading to profound collapse and respiratory and/or cardiac arrest; caution is advised if used concurrently). Products include:
Seroquel Tablets 691

Quinapril Hydrochloride (Clozapine causes orthostatic hypotension and may potentiate hypotensive effects of antihypertensive drugs).
No products indexed under this heading.

Quinidine (Co-administration of drugs that inhibit CYP4502D6, such as quinidine, should be approached with caution).
No products indexed under this heading.

Quinidine Gluconate (Co-administration of drugs that inhibit CYP4502D6, such as quinidine, should be approached with caution).
No products indexed under this heading.

Quinidine Hydrochloride (Co-administration of drugs that inhibit CYP4502D6, such as quinidine, should be approached with caution).
No products indexed under this heading.

Quinidine Polygalacturonate (Co-administration of drugs that inhibit CYP4502D6, such as quinidine, should be approached with caution).
No products indexed under this heading.

Quinidine Sulfate (Co-administration of drugs that inhibit CYP4502D6, such as quinidine, should be approached with caution).
No products indexed under this heading.

Ramipril (Clozapine causes orthostatic hypotension and may potentiate hypotensive effects of antihypertensive drugs). Products include:
Altace Capsules 1673

Rauwolfia Serpentina (Clozapine causes orthostatic hypotension and may potentiate hypotensive effects of antihypertensive drugs).
No products indexed under this heading.

Remifentanil Hydrochloride (Clozapine induces drowsiness and sedation in a significant number of patients; caution is advised with concomitant use).
No products indexed under this heading.

Rescinnamine (Clozapine causes orthostatic hypotension and may potentiate hypotensive effects of antihypertensive drugs).
No products indexed under this heading.

Reserpine (Clozapine causes orthostatic hypotension and may potentiate hypotensive effects of antihypertensive drugs).
No products indexed under this heading.

Rifampin (May decrease clozapine plasma levels resulting in a decrease in effectiveness of a previously effective clozapine dose).
No products indexed under this heading.

Risperidone (Co-administration with benzodiazepines or other psychotropic agents may be accompanied by orthostatic hypotension leading to profound collapse and respiratory and/or cardiac arrest; caution is advised if used concurrently). Products include:
Risperdal Consta Long-Acting Injection 1664
Risperdal M-Tab Orally Disintegrating Tablets........ 1658
Risperdal 1658

Scopolamine (Clozapine may potentiate anticholinergic effects). Products include:
- Transderm Scōp Transdermal Therapeutic System 2166

Scopolamine Hydrobromide (Clozapine may potentiate anticholinergic effects).
- No products indexed under this heading.

Secobarbital Sodium (Clozapine induces drowsiness and sedation in a significant number of patients; caution is advised with concomitant use).
- No products indexed under this heading.

Sertraline Hydrochloride (Co-administration in schizophrenic patients has resulted in elevated mean trough concentrations of clozapine and its metabolites by less than two-fold compared to baseline concentrations; a reduced clozapine dose should be considered). Products include:
- Zoloft 2581

Sevoflurane (Clozapine induces drowsiness and sedation in a significant number of patients; caution is advised with concomitant use). Products include:
- Ultane Liquid for Inhalation 526

Sodium Nitroprusside (Clozapine causes orthostatic hypotension and may potentiate hypotensive effects of antihypertensive drugs).
- No products indexed under this heading.

Sodium Oxybate (Clozapine induces drowsiness and sedation in a significant number of patients; caution is advised with concomitant use).
- No products indexed under this heading.

Sotalol Hydrochloride (Clozapine causes orthostatic hypotension and may potentiate hypotensive effects of antihypertensive drugs).
- No products indexed under this heading.

Spirapril Hydrochloride (Clozapine causes orthostatic hypotension and may potentiate hypotensive effects of antihypertensive drugs).
- No products indexed under this heading.

Sufentanil Citrate (Clozapine induces drowsiness and sedation in a significant number of patients; caution is advised with concomitant use).
- No products indexed under this heading.

Telmisartan (Clozapine causes orthostatic hypotension and may potentiate hypotensive effects of antihypertensive drugs). Products include:
- Micardis Tablets 884
- Micardis HCT Tablets 886

Temazepam (Co-administration with benzodiazepines or other psychotropic agents may be accompanied by orthostatic hypotension leading to profound collapse and respiratory and/or cardiac arrest; caution is advised if used concurrently).
- No products indexed under this heading.

Terazosin Hydrochloride (Clozapine causes orthostatic hypotension and may potentiate hypotensive effects of antihypertensive drugs). Products include:
- Hytrin Capsules 469

Thiamylal Sodium (Clozapine induces drowsiness and sedation in a significant number of patients; caution is advised with concomitant use).
- No products indexed under this heading.

Thioridazine Hydrochloride (Co-administration with benzodiazepines or other psychotropic agents may be accompanied by orthostatic hypotension leading to profound collapse and respiratory and/or cardiac arrest; caution is advised if used concurrently). Products include:
- Thioridazine Hydrochloride Tablets 2122

Thiothixene (Co-administration with benzodiazepines or other psychotropic agents may be accompanied by orthostatic hypotension leading to profound collapse and respiratory and/or cardiac arrest; caution is advised if used concurrently). Products include:
- Thiothixene Capsules 2124

Timolol Maleate (Clozapine causes orthostatic hypotension and may potentiate hypotensive effects of antihypertensive drugs). Products include:
- Blocadren Tablets 1891
- Cosopt Sterile Ophthalmic Solution 1910
- Timolide Tablets 2056
- Timoptic in Ocudose 2061
- Timoptic Sterile Ophthalmic Solution 2058
- Timoptic-XE Sterile Ophthalmic Gel Forming Solution 2062

Tolterodine Tartrate (Clozapine may potentiate anticholinergic effects). Products include:
- Detrol Tablets 2626
- Detrol LA Capsules 2629

Torsemide (Clozapine causes orthostatic hypotension and may potentiate hypotensive effects of antihypertensive drugs).
- No products indexed under this heading.

Trandolapril (Clozapine causes orthostatic hypotension and may potentiate hypotensive effects of antihypertensive drugs). Products include:
- Mavik Tablets 482
- Tarka Tablets 519

Tranylcypromine Sulfate (Concomitant use of clozapine with other drugs metabolized by CYP4502D6 may require lower than usual doses for either drug). Products include:
- Parnate Tablets 1499

Trazodone Hydrochloride (Concomitant use of clozapine with other drugs metabolized by CYP4502D6 may require lower than usual doses for either drug).
- No products indexed under this heading.

Triazolam (Co-administration with benzodiazepines or other psychotropic agents may be accompanied by orthostatic hypotension leading to profound collapse and respiratory and/or cardiac arrest; caution is advised if used concurrently).
- No products indexed under this heading.

Tridihexethyl Chloride (Clozapine may potentiate anticholinergic effects).
- No products indexed under this heading.

Trifluoperazine Hydrochloride (Co-administration with benzodiazepines or other psychotropic agents may be accompanied by orthostatic hypotension leading to profound collapse and respiratory and/or cardiac arrest; caution is advised if used concurrently).
- No products indexed under this heading.

Trihexyphenidyl Hydrochloride (Clozapine may potentiate anticholinergic effects).
- No products indexed under this heading.

Trimethaphan Camsylate (Clozapine causes orthostatic hypotension and may potentiate hypotensive effects of antihypertensive drugs).
- No products indexed under this heading.

Trimipramine Maleate (Concomitant use of clozapine with other drugs metabolized by CYP4502D6 may require lower than usual doses for either drug). Products include:
- Surmontil Capsules 2347

Valsartan (Clozapine causes orthostatic hypotension and may potentiate hypotensive effects of antihypertensive drugs). Products include:
- Diovan HCT Tablets 2195
- Diovan Tablets 2191

Venlafaxine Hydrochloride (Concomitant use of clozapine with other drugs metabolized by CYP4502D6 may require lower than usual doses for either drug). Products include:
- Effexor Tablets 3405
- Effexor XR Capsules 3411

Verapamil Hydrochloride (Clozapine causes orthostatic hypotension and may potentiate hypotensive effects of antihypertensive drugs). Products include:
- Covera-HS Tablets 3135
- Tarka Tablets 519
- Verelan PM Capsules 3120

Zaleplon (Clozapine induces drowsiness and sedation in a significant number of patients; caution is advised with concomitant use). Products include:
- Sonata Capsules 1686

Ziprasidone Hydrochloride (Co-administration with benzodiazepines or other psychotropic agents may be accompanied by orthostatic hypotension leading to profound collapse and respiratory and/or cardiac arrest; caution is advised if used concurrently). Products include:
- Geodon Capsules 2514

Zolpidem Tartrate (Clozapine induces drowsiness and sedation in a significant number of patients; caution is advised with concomitant use). Products include:
- Ambien Tablets 2867

Food Interactions

Alcohol (Clozapine induces drowsiness and sedation in a significant number of patients; caution is advised with concomitant use).

CLOZARIL TABLETS

(Clozapine) 2174

May interact with anticholinergics, antihypertensives, benzodiazepines, central nervous system depressants, antidepressant drugs, erythromycin, general anesthetics, phenothiazines, phenytoin, psychotropics, quinidine, and certain other agents. Compounds in these categories include:

Acebutolol Hydrochloride (Clozapine may potentiate the hypotensive effects of antihypertensive drugs).
- No products indexed under this heading.

Alfentanil Hydrochloride (Given the primary CNS effect of clozapine, caution is advised in using it concomitantly with CNS-active drugs).
- No products indexed under this heading.

Alprazolam (Co-administration with benzodiazepines or other psychotropic agents may be accompanied by orthostatic hypotension leading to profound collapse and respiratory and/or cardiac arrest; caution is advised if used concurrently). Products include:
- Niravam Orally Disintegrating Tablets 3106
- Xanax XR Tablets 2655

Amitriptyline Hydrochloride (Concomitant use of clozapine with other drugs metabolized by CYP4502D6 may require lower than usual doses for either drug).
- No products indexed under this heading.

Amlodipine Besylate (Clozapine may potentiate the hypotensive effects of antihypertensive drugs). Products include:
- Caduet Tablets 2507
- Lotrel Capsules 2238
- Norvasc Tablets 2529

Amoxapine (Concomitant use of clozapine with other drugs metabolized by CYP4502D6 may require lower than usual doses for either drug).
- No products indexed under this heading.

Aprobarbital (Given the primary CNS effect of clozapine, caution is advised in using it concomitantly with CNS-active drugs).
- No products indexed under this heading.

Atenolol (Clozapine may potentiate the hypotensive effects of antihypertensive drugs). Products include:
- Tenormin I.V. Injection 698
- Tenormin Tablets 695

Atropine Sulfate (Clozapine may potentiate anticholinergic effects).
- No products indexed under this heading.

Belladonna Alkaloids (Clozapine may potentiate anticholinergic effects). Products include:
- Hyland's Teething Tablets .... ▣736

Benazepril Hydrochloride (Clozapine may potentiate the hypotensive effects of antihypertensive drugs). Products include:
- Lotensin Tablets 2232
- Lotensin HCT Tablets 2235
- Lotrel Capsules 2238

Bendroflumethiazide (Clozapine may potentiate the hypotensive effects of antihypertensive drugs).
- No products indexed under this heading.

Benztropine Mesylate (Clozapine may potentiate anticholinergic effects). Products include:
Cogentin Injection 1903

Betaxolol Hydrochloride (Clozapine may potentiate the hypotensive effects of antihypertensive drugs). Products include:
Betoptic S Ophthalmic Suspension.................................. 554

Biperiden Hydrochloride (Clozapine may potentiate anticholinergic effects).
No products indexed under this heading.

Bisoprolol Fumarate (Clozapine may potentiate the hypotensive effects of antihypertensive drugs).
No products indexed under this heading.

Bone Marrow Depressants, unspecified (Clozapine should not be used with agents having a well-known potential to suppress bone-marrow function. Co-administration may increase the risk and/or severity of bone marrow suppression).
No products indexed under this heading.

Buprenorphine Hydrochloride (Given the primary CNS effect of clozapine, caution is advised in using it concomitantly with CNS-active drugs). Products include:
Buprenex Injectable 2718
Suboxone Tablets 2719
Subutex Tablets 2719

Bupropion Hydrochloride (Concomitant use of clozapine with other drugs metabolized by CYP4502D6 may require lower than usual doses for either drug). Products include:
Wellbutrin Tablets 1579
Wellbutrin SR Sustained-Release Tablets... 1583
Wellbutrin XL Extended-Release Tablets... 1588
Zyban Sustained-Release Tablets 1620

Buspirone Hydrochloride (Co-administration with benzodiazepines or other psychotropic agents may be accompanied by orthostatic hypotension leading to profound collapse and respiratory and/or cardiac arrest; caution is advised if used concurrently).
No products indexed under this heading.

Butabarbital (Given the primary CNS effect of clozapine, caution is advised in using it concomitantly with CNS-active drugs).
No products indexed under this heading.

Butalbital (Given the primary CNS effect of clozapine, caution is advised in using it concomitantly with CNS-active drugs). Products include:
Sedapap Tablets 50 mg/650 mg 2098

Caffeine (May increase plasma levels of clozapine, potentially resulting in adverse effects). Products include:
Athena Hair System Shampoo 767
BC Powder 612
Arthritis Strength BC Powder 612
Goody's Extra Strength Headache Powder....................... 621
Goody's Extra Strength Pain Relief Tablets............................. 621
Hycomine Compound Tablets 1105
Spartan Hair System Shampoo 767
Vivarin 639

Caffeine Citrate (May increase plasma levels of clozapine, potentially resulting in adverse effects). Products include:
Cafcit 1854

Candesartan Cilexetil (Clozapine may potentiate the hypotensive effects of antihypertensive drugs). Products include:
Atacand Tablets 634
Atacand HCT 637

Captopril (Clozapine may potentiate the hypotensive effects of antihypertensive drugs). Products include:
Captopril Tablets 2114

Carbamazepine (Concomitant use is not recommended; discontinuation of concomitant carbamazepine administration may result in increase in clozapine levels). Products include:
Carbatrol Capsules 3174
Equetro Extended-Release Capsules...................................... 3178
Tegretol/Tegretol-XR 2278

Carteolol Hydrochloride (Clozapine may potentiate the hypotensive effects of antihypertensive drugs). Products include:
Carteolol Hydrochloride Ophthalmic Solution USP, 1%....... ⊙ 246

Chlordiazepoxide (Co-administration with benzodiazepines or other psychotropic agents may be accompanied by orthostatic hypotension leading to profound collapse and respiratory and/or cardiac arrest; caution is advised if used concurrently).
No products indexed under this heading.

Chlordiazepoxide Hydrochloride (Co-administration with benzodiazepines or other psychotropic agents may be accompanied by orthostatic hypotension leading to profound collapse and respiratory and/or cardiac arrest; caution is advised if used concurrently). Products include:
Librium Capsules 3349

Chlorothiazide (Clozapine may potentiate the hypotensive effects of antihypertensive drugs). Products include:
Aldoclor Tablets 1881
Diuril Oral 1936

Chlorothiazide Sodium (Clozapine may potentiate the hypotensive effects of antihypertensive drugs). Products include:
Diuril Sodium Intravenous 1934

Chlorpromazine (Co-administration with benzodiazepines or other psychotropic agents may be accompanied by orthostatic hypotension leading to profound collapse and respiratory and/or cardiac arrest; caution is advised if used concurrently).
No products indexed under this heading.

Chlorpromazine Hydrochloride (Co-administration with benzodiazepines or other psychotropic agents may be accompanied by orthostatic hypotension leading to profound collapse and respiratory and/or cardiac arrest; caution is advised if used concurrently).
No products indexed under this heading.

Chlorprothixene (Co-administration with benzodiazepines or other psychotropic agents may be accompanied by orthostatic hypotension leading to profound collapse and respiratory and/or cardiac arrest; caution is advised if used concurrently).
No products indexed under this heading.

Chlorprothixene Hydrochloride (Co-administration with benzodiazepines or other psychotropic agents may be accompanied by orthostatic hypotension leading to profound collapse and respiratory and/or cardiac arrest; caution is advised if used concurrently).
No products indexed under this heading.

Chlorprothixene Lactate (Given the primary CNS effect of clozapine, caution is advised in using it concomitantly with CNS-active drugs).
No products indexed under this heading.

Chlorthalidone (Clozapine may potentiate the hypotensive effects of antihypertensive drugs). Products include:
Clorpres Tablets 2139

Cimetidine (May increase plasma levels of clozapine, potentially resulting in adverse effects). Products include:
Tagamet HB 200 Tablets 637
Tagamet Tablets 1547

Cimetidine Hydrochloride (May increase plasma levels of clozapine, potentially resulting in adverse effects).
No products indexed under this heading.

Citalopram Hydrobromide (May increase plasma levels of clozaril, potentially resulting in adverse effects). Products include:
Celexa 1177

Clidinium Bromide (Clozapine may potentiate anticholinergic effects).
No products indexed under this heading.

Clonidine (Clozapine may potentiate the hypotensive effects of antihypertensive drugs). Products include:
Catapres-TTS 875

Clonidine Hydrochloride (Clozapine may potentiate the hypotensive effects of antihypertensive drugs). Products include:
Catapres Tablets 874
Clorpres Tablets 2139

Clorazepate Dipotassium (Co-administration with benzodiazepines or other psychotropic agents may be accompanied by orthostatic hypotension leading to profound collapse and respiratory and/or cardiac arrest; caution is advised if used concurrently). Products include:
Tranxene 2488

Codeine Phosphate (Given the primary CNS effect of clozapine, caution is advised in using it concomitantly with CNS-active drugs). Products include:
Tylenol with Codeine 2461

Deserpidine (Clozapine may potentiate the hypotensive effects of antihypertensive drugs).
No products indexed under this heading.

Desflurane (Given the primary CNS effect of clozapine, caution is advised in using it concomitantly with CNS-active drugs). Products include:
Suprane Liquid for Inhalation 770

Desipramine Hydrochloride (Concomitant use of clozapine with other drugs metabolized by CYP4502D6 may require lower than usual doses for either drug).
No products indexed under this heading.

Dezocine (Given the primary CNS effect of clozapine, caution is advised in using it concomitantly with CNS-active drugs).
No products indexed under this heading.

Diazepam (Co-administration with benzodiazepines or other psychotropic agents may be accompanied by orthostatic hypotension leading to profound collapse and respiratory and/or cardiac arrest; caution is advised if used concurrently). Products include:
Diastat Rectal Delivery System 3344
Valium Tablets 2822

Diazoxide (Clozapine may potentiate the hypotensive effects of antihypertensive drugs). Products include:
Hyperstat I.V. Injection 3031

Dicyclomine Hydrochloride (Clozapine may potentiate anticholinergic effects). Products include:
Bentyl Capsules 724
Bentyl Injection 724
Bentyl Syrup 724
Bentyl Tablets 724

Diltiazem Hydrochloride (Clozapine may potentiate the hypotensive effects of antihypertensive drugs). Products include:
Cardizem LA Extended Release Tablets... 1699
Tiazac Capsules 1204

Doxazosin Mesylate (Clozapine may potentiate the hypotensive effects of antihypertensive drugs).
No products indexed under this heading.

Doxepin Hydrochloride (Concomitant use of clozapine with other drugs metabolized by CYP4502D6 may require lower than usual doses for either drug).
No products indexed under this heading.

Droperidol (Co-administration with benzodiazepines or other psychotropic agents may be accompanied by orthostatic hypotension leading to profound collapse and respiratory and/or cardiac arrest; caution is advised if used concurrently).
No products indexed under this heading.

Enalapril Maleate (Clozapine may potentiate the hypotensive effects of antihypertensive drugs). Products include:
Vaseretic Tablets 2073
Vasotec I.V. Injection 2076

Enalaprilat (Clozapine may potentiate the hypotensive effects of antihypertensive drugs).
No products indexed under this heading.

Encainide Hydrochloride (Concomitant use of clozapine with other drugs metabolized by CYP4502D6 may require lower than usual doses for either drug).
No products indexed under this heading.

Enflurane (Given the primary CNS effect of clozapine, caution is advised in using it concomitantly with CNS-active drugs).
No products indexed under this heading.

Epinephrine (The administration of epinephrine should be avoided in the treatment of clozapine-induced hypotension because of a possible reverse epinephrine effect). Products include:
EpiPen 1061

Primatene Mist ▣ 749

Epinephrine Hydrochloride (The administration of epinephrine should be avoided in the treatment of clozapine-induced hypotension because of a possible reverse epinephrine effect).
No products indexed under this heading.

Eprosartan Mesylate (Clozapine may potentiate the hypotensive effects of antihypertensive drugs). Products include:
Teveten Tablets 1707
Teveten HCT Tablets 1710

Erythromycin (May increase plasma levels of clozapine, potentially resulting in adverse effects). Products include:
Erygel Topical Gel 2096
Ery-Tab Tablets 447
Erythromycin Base Filmtab Tablets 454
Erythromycin Delayed-Release Capsules, USP 456
PCE Dispertab Tablets 510

Erythromycin Estolate (May increase plasma levels of clozapine, potentially resulting in adverse effects).
No products indexed under this heading.

Erythromycin Ethylsuccinate (May increase plasma levels of clozapine, potentially resulting in adverse effects). Products include:
E.E.S. 449
EryPed 445

Erythromycin Gluceptate (May increase plasma levels of clozapine, potentially resulting in adverse effects).
No products indexed under this heading.

Erythromycin Lactobionate (May increase plasma levels of clozapine, potentially resulting in adverse effects).
No products indexed under this heading.

Erythromycin Stearate (May increase plasma levels of clozapine, potentially resulting in adverse effects). Products include:
Erythrocin Stearate Filmtab Tablets 452

Escitalopram Oxalate (Concomitant use of clozapine with other drugs metabolized by CYP4502D6 may require lower than usual doses for either drug). Products include:
Lexapro Oral Solution 1193
Lexapro Tablets 1193

Esmolol Hydrochloride (Clozapine may potentiate the hypotensive effects of antihypertensive drugs). Products include:
Brevibloc Concentrate 766
Brevibloc Injection 766
Brevibloc Double Strength Injection 766
Brevibloc Premixed Injection 766
Brevibloc Double Strength Premixed Injection 766

Estazolam (Co-administration with benzodiazepines or other psychotropic agents may be accompanied by orthostatic hypotension leading to profound collapse and respiratory and/or cardiac arrest; caution is advised if used concurrently). Products include:
ProSom Tablets 512

Ethanol (Given the primary CNS effect of clozapine, caution is advised in using it concomitantly with CNS-active drugs).
No products indexed under this heading.

Ethchlorvynol (Given the primary CNS effect of clozapine, caution is advised in using it concomitantly with CNS-active drugs).
No products indexed under this heading.

Ethinamate (Given the primary CNS effect of clozapine, caution is advised in using it concomitantly with CNS-active drugs).
No products indexed under this heading.

Ethyl Alcohol (Given the primary CNS effect of clozapine, caution is advised in using it concomitantly with CNS-active drugs).
No products indexed under this heading.

Felodipine (Clozapine may potentiate the hypotensive effects of antihypertensive drugs). Products include:
Plendil Extended-Release Tablets 651

Fentanyl (Given the primary CNS effect of clozapine, caution is advised in using it concomitantly with CNS-active drugs). Products include:
Duragesic Transdermal System 2448

Fentanyl Citrate (Given the primary CNS effect of clozapine, caution is advised in using it concomitantly with CNS-active drugs). Products include:
Actiq 993

Flecainide Acetate (Concomitant use of clozapine with other drugs metabolized by CYP4502D6 may require lower than usual doses for either drug). Products include:
Tambocor Tablets 1824

Fluoxetine Hydrochloride (Co-administration in schizophrenic patients has resulted in elevated mean trough concentrations of clozapine and its metabolites by less than two-fold compared to baseline concentrations; a reduced clozapine dose should be considered). Products include:
Prozac Pulvules and Liquid 1771
Symbyax Capsules 1788

Fluphenazine Decanoate (Co-administration with benzodiazepines or other psychotropic agents may be accompanied by orthostatic hypotension leading to profound collapse and respiratory and/or cardiac arrest; caution is advised if used concurrently).
No products indexed under this heading.

Fluphenazine Enanthate (Co-administration with benzodiazepines or other psychotropic agents may be accompanied by orthostatic hypotension leading to profound collapse and respiratory and/or cardiac arrest; caution is advised if used concurrently).
No products indexed under this heading.

Fluphenazine Hydrochloride (Co-administration with benzodiazepines or other psychotropic agents may be accompanied by orthostatic hypotension leading to profound collapse and respiratory and/or cardiac arrest; caution is advised if used concurrently).
No products indexed under this heading.

Flurazepam Hydrochloride (Co-administration with benzodiazepines or other psychotropic agents may be accompanied by orthostatic hypotension leading to profound collapse and respiratory and/or cardiac arrest; caution is advised if used concurrently). Products include:
Dalmane Capsules 3343

Fluvoxamine Maleate (Co-administration in schizophrenic patients has resulted in elevated mean trough concentrations of clozapine and its metabolites by about three-fold compared to baseline concentrations; a reduced clozapine dose should be considered).
No products indexed under this heading.

Fosinopril Sodium (Clozapine may potentiate the hypotensive effects of antihypertensive drugs).
No products indexed under this heading.

Fosphenytoin Sodium (May decrease clozapine plasma levels resulting in a decrease in effectiveness of a previously effective clozapine dose).
No products indexed under this heading.

Furosemide (Clozapine may potentiate the hypotensive effects of antihypertensive drugs). Products include:
Furosemide Tablets 2117

Glutethimide (Given the primary CNS effect of clozapine, caution is advised in using it concomitantly with CNS-active drugs).
No products indexed under this heading.

Glycopyrrolate (Clozapine may potentiate anticholinergic effects).
No products indexed under this heading.

Guanabenz Acetate (Clozapine may potentiate the hypotensive effects of antihypertensive drugs).
No products indexed under this heading.

Guanethidine Monosulfate (Clozapine may potentiate the hypotensive effects of antihypertensive drugs).
No products indexed under this heading.

Halazepam (Co-administration with benzodiazepines or other psychotropic agents may be accompanied by orthostatic hypotension leading to profound collapse and respiratory and/or cardiac arrest; caution is advised if used concurrently).
No products indexed under this heading.

Haloperidol (Co-administration with benzodiazepines or other psychotropic agents may be accompanied by orthostatic hypotension leading to profound collapse and respiratory and/or cardiac arrest; caution is advised if used concurrently).
No products indexed under this heading.

Haloperidol Decanoate (Co-administration with benzodiazepines or other psychotropic agents may be accompanied by orthostatic hypotension leading to profound collapse and respiratory and/or cardiac arrest; caution is advised if used concurrently).
No products indexed under this heading.

Hydralazine Hydrochloride (Clozapine may potentiate the hypotensive effects of antihypertensive drugs). Products include:
BiDil Tablets 2161

Hydrochlorothiazide (Clozapine may potentiate the hypotensive effects of antihypertensive drugs). Products include:
Aldoril Tablets 1884
Atacand HCT 637
Avalide Tablets 2889
Avalide Tablets 922
Benicar HCT Tablets 2852
Diovan HCT Tablets 2195
Dyazide Capsules 1389
Hyzaar 1964
Lotensin HCT Tablets 2235
Maxzide 2150
Micardis HCT Tablets 886
Moduretic Tablets 2003
Prinzide Tablets 2033
Teveten HCT Tablets 1710
Timolide Tablets 2056
Uniretic Tablets 3114
Vaseretic Tablets 2073
Zestoretic Tablets 701

Hydrocodone Bitartrate (Given the primary CNS effect of clozapine, caution is advised in using it concomitantly with CNS-active drugs). Products include:
Hycodan 1104
Hycomine Compound Tablets 1105
Hycotuss Expectorant Syrup 1106
Lortab 3315
Lortab Elixir 3312
Vicodin Tablets 530
Vicodin ES Tablets 531
Vicodin HP Tablets 532
Vicoprofen Tablets 533
Zydone Tablets 1118

Hydrocodone Polistirex (Given the primary CNS effect of clozapine, caution is advised in using it concomitantly with CNS-active drugs). Products include:
Tussionex Pennkinetic Extended-Release Suspension 3322

Hydroflumethiazide (Clozapine may potentiate the hypotensive effects of antihypertensive drugs).
No products indexed under this heading.

Hydromorphone Hydrochloride (Given the primary CNS effect of clozapine, caution is advised in using it concomitantly with CNS-active drugs). Products include:
Dilaudid 439
Dilaudid Oral Liquid 443
Dilaudid Non-Sterile Powder 439
Dilaudid Rectal Suppositories 439
Dilaudid Tablets 439
Dilaudid Tablets - 8 mg 443
Dilaudid-HP 441

Hydroxyzine Hydrochloride (Co-administration with benzodiazepines or other psychotropic agents may be accompanied by orthostatic hypotension leading to profound collapse and respiratory and/or cardiac arrest; caution is advised if used concurrently).
No products indexed under this heading.

Hyoscyamine (Clozapine may potentiate anticholinergic effects).
No products indexed under this heading.

Hyoscyamine Sulfate (Clozapine may potentiate anticholinergic effects).
No products indexed under this heading.

Imipramine Hydrochloride (Concomitant use of clozapine with other drugs metabolized by CYP4502D6 may require lower than usual doses for either drug).
No products indexed under this heading.

Imipramine Pamoate (Concomitant use of clozapine with other drugs metabolized by CYP4502D6 may require lower than usual doses for either drug).
No products indexed under this heading.

Indapamide (Clozapine may potentiate the hypotensive effects of antihypertensive drugs). Products include:
Indapamide Tablets 2119

Ipratropium Bromide (Clozapine may potentiate anticholinergic effects). Products include:
Atrovent HFA Inhalation Aerosol 872
Atrovent Inhalation Solution 868
Atrovent Nasal Spray 0.03% 869
Atrovent Nasal Spray 0.06% 870
Combivent Inhalation Aerosol 878
DuoNeb Inhalation Solution 1058

Irbesartan (Clozapine may potentiate the hypotensive effects of antihypertensive drugs). Products include:
Avalide Tablets 922
Avalide Tablets 2889
Avapro Tablets 925
Avapro Tablets 2886

Isocarboxazid (Concomitant use of clozapine with other drugs metabolized by CYP4502D6 may require lower than usual doses for either drug).
No products indexed under this heading.

Isoflurane (Given the primary CNS effect of clozapine, caution is advised in using it concomitantly with CNS-active drugs).
No products indexed under this heading.

Isradipine (Clozapine may potentiate the hypotensive effects of antihypertensive drugs). Products include:
DynaCirc CR Tablets 2726

Ketamine Hydrochloride (Given the primary CNS effect of clozapine, caution is advised in using it concomitantly with CNS-active drugs).
No products indexed under this heading.

Labetalol Hydrochloride (Clozapine may potentiate the hypotensive effects of antihypertensive drugs).
No products indexed under this heading.

Levomethadyl Acetate Hydrochloride (Given the primary CNS effect of clozapine, caution is advised in using it concomitantly with CNS-active drugs).
No products indexed under this heading.

Levorphanol Tartrate (Given the primary CNS effect of clozapine, caution is advised in using it concomitantly with CNS-active drugs).
No products indexed under this heading.

Lisinopril (Clozapine may potentiate the hypotensive effects of antihypertensive drugs). Products include:
Prinivil Tablets 2029
Prinzide Tablets 2033
Zestoretic Tablets 701
Zestril Tablets 704

Lithium Carbonate (Co-administration with benzodiazepines or other psychotropic agents may be accompanied by orthostatic hypotension leading to profound collapse and respiratory and/or cardiac arrest; caution is advised if used concurrently). Products include:
Eskalith 1406
Lithobid Tablets 1670

Lithium Citrate (Co-administration with benzodiazepines or other psychotropic agents may be accompanied by orthostatic hypotension leading to profound collapse and respiratory and/or cardiac arrest; caution is advised if used concurrently).
No products indexed under this heading.

Lorazepam (Co-administration with benzodiazepines or other psychotropic agents may be accompanied by orthostatic hypotension leading to profound collapse and respiratory and/or cardiac arrest; caution is advised if used concurrently).
No products indexed under this heading.

Losartan Potassium (Clozapine may potentiate the hypotensive effects of antihypertensive drugs). Products include:
Cozaar Tablets 1913
Hyzaar 1964

Loxapine Hydrochloride (Co-administration with benzodiazepines or other psychotropic agents may be accompanied by orthostatic hypotension leading to profound collapse and respiratory and/or cardiac arrest; caution is advised if used concurrently).
No products indexed under this heading.

Loxapine Succinate (Co-administration with benzodiazepines or other psychotropic agents may be accompanied by orthostatic hypotension leading to profound collapse and respiratory and/or cardiac arrest; caution is advised if used concurrently).
No products indexed under this heading.

Maprotiline Hydrochloride (Concomitant use of clozapine with other drugs metabolized by CYP4502D6 may require lower than usual doses for either drug).
No products indexed under this heading.

Mecamylamine Hydrochloride (Clozapine may potentiate the hypotensive effects of antihypertensive drugs). Products include:
Inversine Tablets 3286

Mepenzolate Bromide (Clozapine may potentiate anticholinergic effects).
No products indexed under this heading.

Meperidine Hydrochloride (Given the primary CNS effect of clozapine, caution is advised in using it concomitantly with CNS-active drugs).
No products indexed under this heading.

Mephobarbital (Given the primary CNS effect of clozapine, caution is advised in using it concomitantly with CNS-active drugs). Products include:
Mebaral Tablets, USP 2483

Meprobamate (Co-administration with benzodiazepines or other psychotropic agents may be accompanied by orthostatic hypotension leading to profound collapse and respiratory and/or cardiac arrest; caution is advised if used concurrently).
No products indexed under this heading.

Mesoridazine Besylate (Co-administration with benzodiazepines or other psychotropic agents may be accompanied by orthostatic hypotension leading to profound collapse and respiratory and/or cardiac arrest; caution is advised if used concurrently).
No products indexed under this heading.

Methadone Hydrochloride (Given the primary CNS effect of clozapine, caution is advised in using it concomitantly with CNS-active drugs).
No products indexed under this heading.

Methohexital Sodium (Given the primary CNS effect of clozapine, caution is advised in using it concomitantly with CNS-active drugs).
No products indexed under this heading.

Methotrimeprazine (Given the primary CNS effect of clozapine, caution is advised in using it concomitantly with CNS-active drugs).
No products indexed under this heading.

Methoxyflurane (Given the primary CNS effect of clozapine, caution is advised in using it concomitantly with CNS-active drugs).
No products indexed under this heading.

Methyclothiazide (Clozapine may potentiate the hypotensive effects of antihypertensive drugs).
No products indexed under this heading.

Methyldopa (Clozapine may potentiate the hypotensive effects of antihypertensive drugs). Products include:
Aldoclor Tablets 1881
Aldoril Tablets 1884

Methyldopate Hydrochloride (Clozapine may potentiate the hypotensive effects of antihypertensive drugs).
No products indexed under this heading.

Metolazone (Clozapine may potentiate the hypotensive effects of antihypertensive drugs).
No products indexed under this heading.

Metoprolol Succinate (Clozapine may potentiate the hypotensive effects of antihypertensive drugs). Products include:
Toprol-XL Tablets 660

Metoprolol Tartrate (Clozapine may potentiate the hypotensive effects of antihypertensive drugs).
No products indexed under this heading.

Metyrosine (Clozapine may potentiate the hypotensive effects of antihypertensive drugs). Products include:
Demser Capsules 1933

Mibefradil Dihydrochloride (Clozapine may potentiate the hypotensive effects of antihypertensive drugs).
No products indexed under this heading.

Midazolam Hydrochloride (Co-administration with benzodiazepines or other psychotropic agents may be accompanied by orthostatic hypotension leading to profound collapse and respiratory and/or cardiac arrest; caution is advised if used concurrently).
No products indexed under this heading.

Minoxidil (Clozapine may potentiate the hypotensive effects of antihypertensive drugs). Products include:
Men's Rogaine Extra Strength Topical Solution, Ocean Rush Scent and Original Unscented 706
Women's Rogaine Topical Solution, Spring Bloom Scent and Original Unscented 707

Mirtazapine (Concomitant use of clozapine with other drugs metabolized by CYP4502D6 may require lower than usual doses for either drug).
No products indexed under this heading.

Moexipril Hydrochloride (Clozapine may potentiate the hypotensive effects of antihypertensive drugs). Products include:
Uniretic Tablets 3114
Univasc Tablets 3118

Molindone Hydrochloride (Co-administration with benzodiazepines or other psychotropic agents may be accompanied by orthostatic hypotension leading to profound collapse and respiratory and/or cardiac arrest; caution is advised if used concurrently). Products include:
Moban Tablets 1108

Morphine Sulfate (Given the primary CNS effect of clozapine, caution is advised in using it concomitantly with CNS-active drugs). Products include:
Avinza Capsules 1714
Kadian Capsules 572
MS Contin Tablets 2703

Nadolol (Clozapine may potentiate the hypotensive effects of antihypertensive drugs). Products include:
Nadolol Tablets 2121

Nefazodone Hydrochloride (Concomitant use of clozapine with other drugs metabolized by CYP4502D6 may require lower than usual doses for either drug).
No products indexed under this heading.

Nicardipine Hydrochloride (Clozapine may potentiate the hypotensive effects of antihypertensive drugs). Products include:
Cardene I.V. 1129

Nicotine (May decrease clozapine plasma levels resulting in a decrease in effectiveness of a previously effective clozapine dose). Products include:
Nicoderm CQ Patch 1629
NicoDerm CQ Clear Patch 627
Nicotrol Inhaler 2594
Nicotrol NS 2596

Nicotine Polacrilex (May decrease clozapine plasma levels resulting in a decrease in effectiveness of a previously effective clozapine dose). Products include:
Commit Lozenges 1625
Nicorette Gum 1632

Nifedipine (Clozapine may potentiate the hypotensive effects of antihypertensive drugs). Products include:
Adalat CC Tablets 2978

Nisoldipine (Clozapine may potentiate the hypotensive effects of antihypertensive drugs). Products include:
Sular Tablets ... 1163

Nitroglycerin (Clozapine may potentiate the hypotensive effects of antihypertensive drugs). Products include:
Nitro-Dur Transdermal Infusion System ... 3060
Nitrolingual Pumpspray ... 1161

Nortriptyline Hydrochloride (Concomitant use of clozapine with other drugs metabolized by CYP4502D6 may require lower than usual doses for either drug).
No products indexed under this heading.

Olanzapine (Co-administration with benzodiazepines or other psychotropic agents may be accompanied by orthostatic hypotension leading to profound collapse and respiratory and/or cardiac arrest; caution is advised if used concurrently).
Products include:
Symbyax Capsules ... 1788
Zyprexa Tablets ... 1798
Zyprexa IntraMuscular ... 1798
Zyprexa ZYDIS Orally Disintegrating Tablets ... 1798

Oxazepam (Co-administration with benzodiazepines or other psychotropic agents may be accompanied by orthostatic hypotension leading to profound collapse and respiratory and/or cardiac arrest; caution is advised if used concurrently).
No products indexed under this heading.

Oxybutynin Chloride (Clozapine may potentiate anticholinergic effects). Products include:
Ditropan XL Extended Release Tablets ... 2391

Oxycodone Hydrochloride (Given the primary CNS effect of clozapine, caution is advised in using it concomitantly with CNS-active drugs).
Products include:
Combunox Tablets ... 1183
OxyContin Tablets ... 2699
OxyFast Oral Concentrate Solution ... 2704
OxyIR Capsules ... 2704
Percocet Tablets ... 1114
Percodan Tablets ... 1115

Paroxetine Hydrochloride (Co-administration in schizophrenic patients has resulted in elevated mean trough concentrations of clozapine and its metabolites by less than two-fold compared to baseline concentrations; a reduced clozapine dose should be considered).
Products include:
Paxil CR Controlled-Release Tablets ... 1509
Paxil ... 1501

Penbutolol Sulfate (Clozapine may potentiate the hypotensive effects of antihypertensive drugs).
No products indexed under this heading.

Pentobarbital Sodium (Given the primary CNS effect of clozapine, caution is advised in using it concomitantly with CNS-active drugs).
Products include:
Nembutal Sodium Solution, USP ... 2484

Perindopril Erbumine (Clozapine may potentiate the hypotensive effects of antihypertensive drugs).
Products include:
Aceon Tablets (2 mg, 4 mg, 8 mg) ... 3191

Perphenazine (Co-administration with benzodiazepines or other psychotropic agents may be accompanied by orthostatic hypotension leading to profound collapse and respiratory and/or cardiac arrest; caution is advised if used concurrently).
No products indexed under this heading.

Phenelzine Sulfate (Concomitant use of clozapine with other drugs metabolized by CYP4502D6 may require lower than usual doses for either drug).
No products indexed under this heading.

Phenobarbital (Given the primary CNS effect of clozapine, caution is advised in using it concomitantly with CNS-active drugs).
No products indexed under this heading.

Phenoxybenzamine Hydrochloride (Clozapine may potentiate the hypotensive effects of antihypertensive drugs). Products include:
Dibenzyline Capsules ... 3390

Phentolamine Mesylate (Clozapine may potentiate the hypotensive effects of antihypertensive drugs).
No products indexed under this heading.

Phenytoin (May decrease clozapine plasma levels resulting in a decrease in effectiveness of a previously effective clozapine dose).
No products indexed under this heading.

Phenytoin Sodium (May decrease clozapine plasma levels resulting in a decrease in effectiveness of a previously effective clozapine dose).
Products include:
Phenytek Capsules ... 2153

Pindolol (Clozapine may potentiate the hypotensive effects of antihypertensive drugs).
No products indexed under this heading.

Polythiazide (Clozapine may potentiate the hypotensive effects of antihypertensive drugs).
No products indexed under this heading.

Prazepam (Co-administration with benzodiazepines or other psychotropic agents may be accompanied by orthostatic hypotension leading to profound collapse and respiratory and/or cardiac arrest; caution is advised if used concurrently).
No products indexed under this heading.

Prazosin Hydrochloride (Clozapine may potentiate the hypotensive effects of antihypertensive drugs).
No products indexed under this heading.

Prochlorperazine (Co-administration with benzodiazepines or other psychotropic agents may be accompanied by orthostatic hypotension leading to profound collapse and respiratory and/or cardiac arrest; caution is advised if used concurrently).
No products indexed under this heading.

Procyclidine Hydrochloride (Clozapine may potentiate anticholinergic effects).
No products indexed under this heading.

Promethazine Hydrochloride (Co-administration with benzodiazepines or other psychotropic agents may be accompanied by orthostatic hypotension leading to profound collapse and respiratory and/or cardiac arrest; caution is advised if used concurrently). Products include:
Phenergan ... 3438

Propafenone Hydrochloride (Concomitant use of clozapine with other drugs metabolized by CYP4502D6 may require lower than usual doses for either drug).
Products include:
Rythmol SR Capsules ... 2736

Propantheline Bromide (Clozapine may potentiate anticholinergic effects).
No products indexed under this heading.

Propofol (Given the primary CNS effect of clozapine, caution is advised in using it concomitantly with CNS-active drugs). Products include:
Diprivan Injectable Emulsion ... 676

Propoxyphene Hydrochloride (Given the primary CNS effect of clozapine, caution is advised in using it concomitantly with CNS-active drugs).
No products indexed under this heading.

Propoxyphene Napsylate (Given the primary CNS effect of clozapine, caution is advised in using it concomitantly with CNS-active drugs).
Products include:
Darvocet A 500 Tablets ... 3497

Propranolol Hydrochloride (Clozapine may potentiate the hypotensive effects of antihypertensive drugs). Products include:
Inderal LA Long-Acting Capsules ... 3421
InnoPran XL Capsules ... 2728

Protriptyline Hydrochloride (Concomitant use of clozapine with other drugs metabolized by CYP4502D6 may require lower than usual doses for either drug). Products include:
Vivactil Tablets ... 2350

Quazepam (Co-administration with benzodiazepines or other psychotropic agents may be accompanied by orthostatic hypotension leading to profound collapse and respiratory and/or cardiac arrest; caution is advised if used concurrently).
No products indexed under this heading.

Quetiapine Fumarate (Co-administration with benzodiazepines or other psychotropic agents may be accompanied by orthostatic hypotension leading to profound collapse and respiratory and/or cardiac arrest; caution is advised if used concurrently). Products include:
Seroquel Tablets ... 691

Quinapril Hydrochloride (Clozapine may potentiate the hypotensive effects of antihypertensive drugs).
No products indexed under this heading.

Quinidine (Co-administration of drugs that inhibit CYP4502D6, such as quinidine, should be approached with caution).
No products indexed under this heading.

Quinidine Gluconate (Co-administration of drugs that inhibit CYP4502D6, such as quinidine, should be approached with caution).
No products indexed under this heading.

Quinidine Hydrochloride (Co-administration of drugs that inhibit CYP4502D6, such as quinidine, should be approached with caution).
No products indexed under this heading.

Quinidine Polygalacturonate (Co-administration of drugs that inhibit CYP4502D6, such as quinidine, should be approached with caution).
No products indexed under this heading.

Quinidine Sulfate (Co-administration of drugs that inhibit CYP4502D6, such as quinidine, should be approached with caution).
No products indexed under this heading.

Ramipril (Clozapine may potentiate the hypotensive effects of antihypertensive drugs). Products include:
Altace Capsules ... 1673

Rauwolfia Serpentina (Clozapine may potentiate the hypotensive effects of antihypertensive drugs).
No products indexed under this heading.

Remifentanil Hydrochloride (Given the primary CNS effect of clozapine, caution is advised in using it concomitantly with CNS-active drugs).
No products indexed under this heading.

Rescinnamine (Clozapine may potentiate the hypotensive effects of antihypertensive drugs).
No products indexed under this heading.

Reserpine (Clozapine may potentiate the hypotensive effects of antihypertensive drugs).
No products indexed under this heading.

Rifampin (May decrease clozapine plasma levels resulting in a decrease in effectiveness of a previously effective clozapine dose).
No products indexed under this heading.

Risperidone (Co-administration with benzodiazepines or other psychotropic agents may be accompanied by orthostatic hypotension leading to profound collapse and respiratory and/or cardiac arrest; caution is advised if used concurrently).
Products include:
Risperdal Consta Long-Acting Injection ... 1664
Risperdal M-Tab Orally Disintegrating Tablets ... 1658
Risperdal ... 1658

Scopolamine (Clozapine may potentiate anticholinergic effects).
Products include:
Transderm Scōp Transdermal Therapeutic System ... 2166

Scopolamine Hydrobromide (Clozapine may potentiate anticholinergic effects).
No products indexed under this heading.

Secobarbital Sodium (Given the primary CNS effect of clozapine, caution is advised in using it concomitantly with CNS-active drugs).
No products indexed under this heading.

Sertraline Hydrochloride (Co-administration in schizophrenic patients has resulted in elevated mean trough concentrations of clozapine and its metabolites by less than two-fold compared to baseline concentrations; a reduced clozapine dose should be considered).
Products include:

Zoloft 2581

Sevoflurane (Given the primary CNS effect of clozapine, caution is advised in using it concomitantly with CNS-active drugs). Products include:
Ultane Liquid for Inhalation 526

Sodium Nitroprusside (Clozapine may potentiate the hypotensive effects of antihypertensive drugs).
No products indexed under this heading.

Sodium Oxybate (Given the primary CNS effect of clozapine, caution is advised in using it concomitantly with CNS-active drugs).
No products indexed under this heading.

Sotalol Hydrochloride (Clozapine may potentiate the hypotensive effects of antihypertensive drugs).
No products indexed under this heading.

Spirapril Hydrochloride (Clozapine may potentiate the hypotensive effects of antihypertensive drugs).
No products indexed under this heading.

Sufentanil Citrate (Given the primary CNS effect of clozapine, caution is advised in using it concomitantly with CNS-active drugs).
No products indexed under this heading.

Telmisartan (Clozapine may potentiate the hypotensive effects of antihypertensive drugs). Products include:
Micardis Tablets 884
Micardis HCT Tablets 886

Temazepam (Co-administration with benzodiazepines or other psychotropic agents may be accompanied by orthostatic hypotension leading to profound collapse and respiratory and/or cardiac arrest; caution is advised if used concurrently).
No products indexed under this heading.

Terazosin Hydrochloride (Clozapine may potentiate the hypotensive effects of antihypertensive drugs). Products include:
Hytrin Capsules 469

Thiamylal Sodium (Given the primary CNS effect of clozapine, caution is advised in using it concomitantly with CNS-active drugs).
No products indexed under this heading.

Thioridazine Hydrochloride (Co-administration with benzodiazepines or other psychotropic agents may be accompanied by orthostatic hypotension leading to profound collapse and respiratory and/or cardiac arrest; caution is advised if used concurrently). Products include:
Thioridazine Hydrochloride Tablets 2122

Thiothixene (Co-administration with benzodiazepines or other psychotropic agents may be accompanied by orthostatic hypotension leading to profound collapse and respiratory and/or cardiac arrest; caution is advised if used concurrently). Products include:
Thiothixene Capsules 2124

Timolol Maleate (Clozapine may potentiate the hypotensive effects of antihypertensive drugs). Products include:
Blocadren Tablets 1891
Cosopt Sterile Ophthalmic Solution 1910
Timolide Tablets 2056
Timoptic in Ocudose 2061
Timoptic Sterile Ophthalmic Solution 2058
Timoptic-XE Sterile Ophthalmic Gel Forming Solution 2062

Tolterodine Tartrate (Clozapine may potentiate anticholinergic effects). Products include:
Detrol Tablets 2626
Detrol LA Capsules 2629

Torsemide (Clozapine may potentiate the hypotensive effects of antihypertensive drugs).
No products indexed under this heading.

Trandolapril (Clozapine may potentiate the hypotensive effects of antihypertensive drugs). Products include:
Mavik Tablets 482
Tarka Tablets 519

Tranylcypromine Sulfate (Concomitant use of clozapine with other drugs metabolized by CYP4502D6 may require lower than usual doses for either drug). Products include:
Parnate Tablets 1499

Trazodone Hydrochloride (Concomitant use of clozapine with other drugs metabolized by CYP4502D6 may require lower than usual doses for either drug).
No products indexed under this heading.

Triazolam (Co-administration with benzodiazepines or other psychotropic agents may be accompanied by orthostatic hypotension leading to profound collapse and respiratory and/or cardiac arrest; caution is advised if used concurrently).
No products indexed under this heading.

Tridihexethyl Chloride (Clozapine may potentiate anticholinergic effects).
No products indexed under this heading.

Trifluoperazine Hydrochloride (Co-administration with benzodiazepines or other psychotropic agents may be accompanied by orthostatic hypotension leading to profound collapse and respiratory and/or cardiac arrest; caution is advised if used concurrently).
No products indexed under this heading.

Trihexyphenidyl Hydrochloride (Clozapine may potentiate anticholinergic effects).
No products indexed under this heading.

Trimethaphan Camsylate (Clozapine may potentiate the hypotensive effects of antihypertensive drugs).
No products indexed under this heading.

Trimipramine Maleate (Concomitant use of clozapine with other drugs metabolized by CYP4502D6 may require lower than usual doses for either drug). Products include:
Surmontil Capsules 2347

Valsartan (Clozapine may potentiate the hypotensive effects of antihypertensive drugs). Products include:
Diovan HCT Tablets 2195
Diovan Tablets 2191

Venlafaxine Hydrochloride (Concomitant use of clozapine with other drugs metabolized by CYP4502D6 may require lower than usual doses for either drug). Products include:
Effexor Tablets 3405
Effexor XR Capsules 3411

Verapamil Hydrochloride (Clozapine may potentiate the hypotensive effects of antihypertensive drugs). Products include:
Covera-HS Tablets 3135
Tarka Tablets 519
Verelan PM Capsules 3120

Zaleplon (Given the primary CNS effect of clozapine, caution is advised in using it concomitantly with CNS-active drugs). Products include:
Sonata Capsules 1686

Ziprasidone Hydrochloride (Co-administration with benzodiazepines or other psychotropic agents may be accompanied by orthostatic hypotension leading to profound collapse and respiratory and/or cardiac arrest; caution is advised if used concurrently). Products include:
Geodon Capsules 2514

Zolpidem Tartrate (Given the primary CNS effect of clozapine, caution is advised in using it concomitantly with CNS-active drugs). Products include:
Ambien Tablets 2867

Food Interactions

Alcohol (Given the primary CNS effect of clozapine, caution is advised in using it concomitantly with alcohol).

CM PLEX CREAM

(Cetyl Myristate, Cetyl Myristoleate, Fatty Acids) 3328
None cited in PDR database.

CM PLEX SOFTGELS

(Cetyl Myristate, Cetyl Myristoleate, Fatty Acids) 3328
None cited in PDR database.

COGENTIN INJECTION

(Benztropine Mesylate) 1903
May interact with anticholinergics, dopamine antagonists, belladona products, butyrophenones, phenothiazines, and tricyclic antidepressants. Compounds in these categories include:

Amitriptyline Hydrochloride (Potential for paralytic ileus, hyperthermia and heat stroke).
No products indexed under this heading.

Amoxapine (Potential for paralytic ileus, hyperthermia and heat stroke).
No products indexed under this heading.

Atropine Sulfate (Potential for paralytic ileus, hyperthermia and heat stroke).
No products indexed under this heading.

Belladonna Alkaloids (Potential for paralytic ileus, hyperthermia and heat stroke). Products include:
Hyland's Teething Tablets 736

Biperiden Hydrochloride (Potential for paralytic ileus, hyperthermia and heat stroke).
No products indexed under this heading.

Chlorpromazine (Potential for paralytic ileus, hyperthermia and heat stroke).
No products indexed under this heading.

Chlorpromazine Hydrochloride (Potential for paralytic ileus, hyperthermia and heat stroke).
No products indexed under this heading.

Clidinium Bromide (Potential for paralytic ileus, hyperthermia and heat stroke).
No products indexed under this heading.

Clomipramine Hydrochloride (Potential for paralytic ileus, hyperthermia and heat stroke).
No products indexed under this heading.

Clozapine (Potential for paralytic ileus, hyperthermia and heat stroke). Products include:
Clozapine Tablets 2141
Clozaril Tablets 2174
FazaClo Orally Disintegrating Tablets 547

Desipramine Hydrochloride (Potential for paralytic ileus, hyperthermia and heat stroke).
No products indexed under this heading.

Dicyclomine Hydrochloride (Potential for paralytic ileus, hyperthermia and heat stroke). Products include:
Bentyl Capsules 724
Bentyl Injection 724
Bentyl Syrup 724
Bentyl Tablets 724

Doxepin Hydrochloride (Potential for paralytic ileus, hyperthermia and heat stroke).
No products indexed under this heading.

Fluphenazine Decanoate (Potential for paralytic ileus, hyperthermia and heat stroke).
No products indexed under this heading.

Fluphenazine Enanthate (Potential for paralytic ileus, hyperthermia and heat stroke).
No products indexed under this heading.

Fluphenazine Hydrochloride (Potential for paralytic ileus, hyperthermia and heat stroke).
No products indexed under this heading.

Glycopyrrolate (Potential for paralytic ileus, hyperthermia and heat stroke).
No products indexed under this heading.

Haloperidol (Potential for paralytic ileus, hyperthermia and heat stroke).
No products indexed under this heading.

Haloperidol Decanoate (Potential for paralytic ileus, hyperthermia and heat stroke).
No products indexed under this heading.

Hyoscyamine (Potential for paralytic ileus, hyperthermia and heat stroke).
No products indexed under this heading.

Hyoscyamine Sulfate (Potential for paralytic ileus, hyperthermia and heat stroke).
No products indexed under this heading.

Imipramine Hydrochloride (Potential for paralytic ileus, hyperthermia and heat stroke).
No products indexed under this heading.

Imipramine Pamoate (Potential for paralytic ileus, hyperthermia and heat stroke).
No products indexed under this heading.

Ipratropium Bromide (Potential for paralytic ileus, hyperthermia and heat stroke). Products include:

Atrovent HFA Inhalation Aerosol 872
Atrovent Inhalation Solution 868
Atrovent Nasal Spray 0.03% 869
Atrovent Nasal Spray 0.06% 870
Combivent Inhalation Aerosol 878
DuoNeb Inhalation Solution 1058

Maprotiline Hydrochloride (Potential for paralytic ileus, hyperthermia and heat stroke).
No products indexed under this heading.

Mepenzolate Bromide (Potential for paralytic ileus, hyperthermia and heat stroke).
No products indexed under this heading.

Mesoridazine Besylate (Potential for paralytic ileus, hyperthermia and heat stroke).
No products indexed under this heading.

Methotrimeprazine (Potential for paralytic ileus, hyperthermia and heat stroke).
No products indexed under this heading.

Metoclopramide Hydrochloride (Potential for paralytic ileus, hyperthermia and heat stroke).
No products indexed under this heading.

Nortriptyline Hydrochloride (Potential for paralytic ileus, hyperthermia and heat stroke).
No products indexed under this heading.

Olanzapine (Potential for paralytic ileus, hyperthermia and heat stroke). Products include:
Symbyax Capsules 1788
Zyprexa Tablets 1798
Zyprexa IntraMuscular 1798
Zyprexa ZYDIS Orally Disintegrating Tablets 1798

Oxybutynin Chloride (Potential for paralytic ileus, hyperthermia and heat stroke). Products include:
Ditropan XL Extended Release Tablets 2391

Perphenazine (Potential for paralytic ileus, hyperthermia and heat stroke).
No products indexed under this heading.

Pimozide (Potential for paralytic ileus, hyperthermia and heat stroke). Products include:
Orap Tablets 1220

Prochlorperazine (Potential for paralytic ileus, hyperthermia and heat stroke).
No products indexed under this heading.

Procyclidine Hydrochloride (Potential for paralytic ileus, hyperthermia and heat stroke).
No products indexed under this heading.

Promethazine Hydrochloride (Potential for paralytic ileus, hyperthermia and heat stroke). Products include:
Phenergan 3438

Propantheline Bromide (Potential for paralytic ileus, hyperthermia and heat stroke).
No products indexed under this heading.

Protriptyline Hydrochloride (Potential for paralytic ileus, hyperthermia and heat stroke). Products include:
Vivactil Tablets 2350

Quetiapine Fumarate (Potential for paralytic ileus, hyperthermia and heat stroke). Products include:
Seroquel Tablets 691

Scopolamine (Potential for paralytic ileus, hyperthermia and heat stroke). Products include:
Transderm Scōp Transdermal Therapeutic System 2166

Scopolamine Hydrobromide (Potential for paralytic ileus, hyperthermia and heat stroke).
No products indexed under this heading.

Thioridazine Hydrochloride (Potential for paralytic ileus, hyperthermia and heat stroke). Products include:
Thioridazine Hydrochloride Tablets 2122

Tolterodine Tartrate (Potential for paralytic ileus, hyperthermia and heat stroke). Products include:
Detrol Tablets 2626
Detrol LA Capsules 2629

Tridihexethyl Chloride (Potential for paralytic ileus, hyperthermia and heat stroke).
No products indexed under this heading.

Trifluoperazine Hydrochloride (Potential for paralytic ileus, hyperthermia and heat stroke).
No products indexed under this heading.

Trihexyphenidyl Hydrochloride (Potential for paralytic ileus, hyperthermia and heat stroke).
No products indexed under this heading.

Trimipramine Maleate (Potential for paralytic ileus, hyperthermia and heat stroke). Products include:
Surmontil Capsules 2347

COLACE CAPSULES 50 MG

(Docusate Sodium) 2715
May interact with:

Mineral Oil (Do not use laxative products if you are presently taking mineral oil, unless told to do so by a doctor). Products include:
Fleet Mineral Oil Enema 1170
Lubriderm Advanced Therapy Moisturizing Lotion..................... ■702
Mineral Oil 2716
Preparation H Ointment .... ■747
Refresh P.M. Lubricant Eye Ointment.................................... ⊙239
Tucks Hemorrhoidal Ointment .... ■711

COLACE CAPSULES 100 MG

(Docusate Sodium) 2715
May interact with:

Mineral Oil (Do not use laxative products if you are presently taking mineral oil, unless told to do so by a doctor). Products include:
Fleet Mineral Oil Enema 1170
Lubriderm Advanced Therapy Moisturizing Lotion..................... ■702
Mineral Oil 2716
Preparation H Ointment .... ■747
Refresh P.M. Lubricant Eye Ointment.................................... ⊙239
Tucks Hemorrhoidal Ointment .... ■711

COLACE GLYCERIN SUPPOSITORIES, USP 1.2 GRAMS - INFANTS AND CHILDREN

(Glycerin) 2715
None cited in PDR database.

COLACE GLYCERIN SUPPOSITORIES, USP 2.1 GRAMS - ADULTS AND CHILDREN

(Glycerin) 2716
None cited in PDR database.

COLACE LIQUID 1% SOLUTION

(Docusate Sodium) 2716
May interact with:

Mineral Oil (Do not use laxative products if you are presently taking mineral oil, unless told to do so by a doctor). Products include:
Fleet Mineral Oil Enema 1170
Lubriderm Advanced Therapy Moisturizing Lotion..................... ■702
Mineral Oil 2716
Preparation H Ointment .... ■747
Refresh P.M. Lubricant Eye Ointment.................................... ⊙239
Tucks Hemorrhoidal Ointment .... ■711

COLACE SYRUP

(Docusate Sodium) 2716
May interact with:

Mineral Oil (Co-administration with mineral oil is not recommended). Products include:
Fleet Mineral Oil Enema 1170
Lubriderm Advanced Therapy Moisturizing Lotion..................... ■702
Mineral Oil 2716
Preparation H Ointment .... ■747
Refresh P.M. Lubricant Eye Ointment.................................... ⊙239
Tucks Hemorrhoidal Ointment .... ■711

COLAZAL CAPSULES

(Balsalazide Disodium) 2845
May interact with:

Antibiotics, unspecified (Use of orally administered antibiotics could, theoretically, interfere with the release of mesalamine in the colon).
No products indexed under this heading.

COLYTE WITH FLAVOR PACKS FOR ORAL SOLUTION

(Polyethylene Glycol, Potassium Chloride, Sodium Bicarbonate, Sodium Chloride, Sodium Sulfate)....... 3102
May interact with:

Oral Medications, unspecified (Those administered within one hour of Colyte usage may be flushed from the gastrointestinal tract and not absorbed).
No products indexed under this heading.

COMBIPATCH TRANSDERMAL SYSTEM

(Estradiol, Norethindrone Acetate) 2180
May interact with cytochrome p450 3a4 inducers (selected) and cytochrome p450 3a4 inhibitors (selected). Compounds in these categories include:

Acetazolamide (Studies have shown that estrogens are metabolized partially by cytochrome P4503A. Inhibitors of CYP3A4 may increase concentrations of estrogens and in side effects).
No products indexed under this heading.

Allium sativum (Studies have shown that estrogens are metabolized partially by cytochrome P4503A. Inducers of CYP3A4 may reduce plasma concentrations of estrogens, possibly resulting in a decrease in therapeutic effects, and/or changes in the uterine bleeding profile).
No products indexed under this heading.

Amiodarone Hydrochloride (Studies have shown that estrogens are metabolized partially by cytochrome P4503A. Inhibitors of CYP3A4 may increase concentrations of estrogens and in side effects). Products include:
Pacerone Tablets 3337

Amprenavir (Studies have shown that estrogens are metabolized partially by cytochrome P4503A. Inhibitors of CYP3A4 may increase concentrations of estrogens and in side effects). Products include:
Agenerase Capsules 1299
Agenerase Oral Solution 1304

Anastrozole (Studies have shown that estrogens are metabolized partially by cytochrome P4503A. Inhibitors of CYP3A4 may increase concentrations of estrogens and in side effects). Products include:
Arimidex Tablets 665

Aprepitant (Studies have shown that estrogens are metabolized partially by cytochrome P4503A. Inducers of CYP3A4 may reduce plasma concentrations of estrogens, possibly resulting in a decrease in therapeutic effects, and/or changes in the uterine bleeding profile). Products include:
Emend Capsules 1944

Betamethasone Acetate (Studies have shown that estrogens are metabolized partially by cytochrome P4503A. Inducers of CYP3A4 may reduce plasma concentrations of estrogens, possibly resulting in a decrease in therapeutic effects, and/or changes in the uterine bleeding profile).
No products indexed under this heading.

Betamethasone Sodium Phosphate (Studies have shown that estrogens are metabolized partially by cytochrome P4503A. Inducers of CYP3A4 may reduce plasma concentrations of estrogens, possibly resulting in a decrease in therapeutic effects, and/or changes in the uterine bleeding profile).
No products indexed under this heading.

Carbamazepine (Studies have shown that estrogens are metabolized partially by cytochrome P4503A. Inducers of CYP3A4 may reduce plasma concentrations of

estrogens, possibly resulting in a decrease in therapeutic effects, and/or changes in the uterine bleeding profile). Products include:
Carbatrol Capsules 3174
Equetro Extended-Release Capsules 3178
Tegretol/Tegretol-XR 2278

Cimetidine (Studies have shown that estrogens are metabolized partially by cytochrome P4503A. Inhibitors of CYP3A4 may increase concentrations of estrogens and in side effects). Products include:
Tagamet HB 200 Tablets 637
Tagamet Tablets 1547

Cimetidine Hydrochloride (Studies have shown that estrogens are metabolized partially by cytochrome P4503A. Inhibitors of CYP3A4 may increase concentrations of estrogens and in side effects).
No products indexed under this heading.

Ciprofloxacin (Studies have shown that estrogens are metabolized partially by cytochrome P4503A. Inhibitors of CYP3A4 may increase concentrations of estrogens and in side effects). Products include:
Cipro I.V. 2998
Cipro I.V. Pharmacy Bulk Package ... 3509
Cipro Oral Suspension 2991
Cipro XR Tablets 3004
Ciprodex Otic Suspension 555

Ciprofloxacin Hydrochloride (Studies have shown that estrogens are metabolized partially by cytochrome P4503A. Inducers of CYP3A4 may reduce plasma concentrations of estrogens, possibly resulting in a decrease in therapeutic effects, and/or changes in the uterine bleeding profile). Products include:
Ciloxan Ophthalmic Ointment 554
Cipro Tablets 2991

Cisplatin (Studies have shown that estrogens are metabolized partially by cytochrome P4503A. Inducers of CYP3A4 may reduce plasma concentrations of estrogens, possibly resulting in a decrease in therapeutic effects, and/or changes in the uterine bleeding profile).
No products indexed under this heading.

Clarithromycin (Studies have shown that estrogens are metabolized partially by cytochrome P4503A. Inhibitors of CYP3A4 may increase concentrations of estrogens and in side effects). Products include:
Biaxin/Biaxin XL 402
PREVPAC 3281

Clotrimazole (Studies have shown that estrogens are metabolized partially by cytochrome P4503A. Inhibitors of CYP3A4 may increase concentrations of estrogens and in side effects). Products include:
Lotrimin 3053
Lotrisone 3054

Cortisone Acetate (Studies have shown that estrogens are metabolized partially by cytochrome P4503A. Inducers of CYP3A4 may reduce plasma concentrations of estrogens, possibly resulting in a decrease in therapeutic effects, and/or changes in the uterine bleeding profile).
No products indexed under this heading.

Cyclosporine (Studies have shown that estrogens are metabolized partially by cytochrome P4503A. Inhibitors of CYP3A4 may increase concentrations of estrogens and in side effects). Products include:
Gengraf Capsules 458
Neoral Soft Gelatin Capsules 2247
Neoral Oral Solution 2247
Restasis Ophthalmic Emulsion 570
Sandimmune 2259

Dalfopristin (Studies have shown that estrogens are metabolized partially by cytochrome P4503A. Inhibitors of CYP3A4 may increase concentrations of estrogens and in side effects). Products include:
Synercid I.V. 1690

Danazol (Studies have shown that estrogens are metabolized partially by cytochrome P4503A. Inhibitors of CYP3A4 may increase concentrations of estrogens and in side effects).
No products indexed under this heading.

Delavirdine Mesylate (Studies have shown that estrogens are metabolized partially by cytochrome P4503A. Inhibitors of CYP3A4 may increase concentrations of estrogens and in side effects). Products include:
Rescriptor Tablets 2535

Dexamethasone (Studies have shown that estrogens are metabolized partially by cytochrome P4503A. Inducers of CYP3A4 may reduce plasma concentrations of estrogens, possibly resulting in a decrease in therapeutic effects, and/or changes in the uterine bleeding profile). Products include:
Ciprodex Otic Suspension 555
Decadron Tablets 1929
TobraDex Ophthalmic Ointment 558
TobraDex Ophthalmic Suspension ... 558

Dexamethasone Acetate (Studies have shown that estrogens are metabolized partially by cytochrome P4503A. Inducers of CYP3A4 may reduce plasma concentrations of estrogens, possibly resulting in a decrease in therapeutic effects, and/or changes in the uterine bleeding profile).
No products indexed under this heading.

Dexamethasone Sodium Phosphate (Studies have shown that estrogens are metabolized partially by cytochrome P4503A. Inducers of CYP3A4 may reduce plasma concentrations of estrogens, possibly resulting in a decrease in therapeutic effects, and/or changes in the uterine bleeding profile). Products include:
Decadron Phosphate Injection 1931

Diltiazem Hydrochloride (Studies have shown that estrogens are metabolized partially by cytochrome P4503A. Inhibitors of CYP3A4 may increase concentrations of estrogens and in side effects). Products include:
Cardizem LA Extended Release Tablets 1699
Tiazac Capsules 1204

Diltiazem Maleate (Studies have shown that estrogens are metabolized partially by cytochrome P4503A. Inhibitors of CYP3A4 may increase concentrations of estrogens and in side effects).
No products indexed under this heading.

Doxorubicin Hydrochloride (Studies have shown that estrogens are metabolized partially by cytochrome P4503A. Inducers of CYP3A4 may reduce plasma concentrations of estrogens, possibly resulting in a decrease in therapeutic effects, and/or changes in the uterine bleeding profile). Products include:
Adriamycin for Injection, USP 786
Adriamycin Injection, USP 786

Efavirenz (Studies have shown that estrogens are metabolized partially by cytochrome P4503A. Inducers of CYP3A4 may reduce plasma concentrations of estrogens, possibly resulting in a decrease in therapeutic effects, and/or changes in the uterine bleeding profile). Products include:
Sustiva Capsules 957

Erythromycin (Studies have shown that estrogens are metabolized partially by cytochrome P4503A. Inhibitors of CYP3A4 may increase concentrations of estrogens and in side effects). Products include:
Erygel Topical Gel 2096
Ery-Tab Tablets 447
Erythromycin Base Filmtab Tablets 454
Erythromycin Delayed-Release Capsules, USP 456
PCE Dispertab Tablets 510

Erythromycin Estolate (Studies have shown that estrogens are metabolized partially by cytochrome P4503A. Inhibitors of CYP3A4 may increase concentrations of estrogens and in side effects).
No products indexed under this heading.

Erythromycin Ethylsuccinate (Studies have shown that estrogens are metabolized partially by cytochrome P4503A. Inhibitors of CYP3A4 may increase concentrations of estrogens and in side effects). Products include:
E.E.S. 449
EryPed 445

Erythromycin Gluceptate (Studies have shown that estrogens are metabolized partially by cytochrome P4503A. Inhibitors of CYP3A4 may increase concentrations of estrogens and in side effects).
No products indexed under this heading.

Erythromycin Lactobionate (Studies have shown that estrogens are metabolized partially by cytochrome P4503A. Inhibitors of CYP3A4 may increase concentrations of estrogens and in side effects).
No products indexed under this heading.

Erythromycin Stearate (Studies have shown that estrogens are metabolized partially by cytochrome P4503A. Inhibitors of CYP3A4 may increase concentrations of estrogens and in side effects). Products include:
Erythrocin Stearate Filmtab Tablets 452

Esomeprazole Magnesium (Studies have shown that estrogens are metabolized partially by cytochrome P4503A. Inhibitors of CYP3A4 may increase concentrations of estrogens and in side effects). Products include:
Nexium Delayed-Release Capsules 645

Ethosuximide (Studies have shown that estrogens are metabolized partially by cytochrome P4503A. Inducers of CYP3A4 may reduce plasma concentrations of estrogens, possibly resulting in a decrease in therapeutic effects, and/or changes in the uterine bleeding profile).
No products indexed under this heading.

Felbamate (Studies have shown that estrogens are metabolized partially by cytochrome P4503A. Inducers of CYP3A4 may reduce plasma concentrations of estrogens, possibly resulting in a decrease in therapeutic effects, and/or changes in the uterine bleeding profile).
No products indexed under this heading.

Fluconazole (Studies have shown that estrogens are metabolized partially by cytochrome P4503A. Inhibitors of CYP3A4 may increase concentrations of estrogens and in side effects).
No products indexed under this heading.

Fludrocortisone Acetate (Studies have shown that estrogens are metabolized partially by cytochrome P4503A. Inducers of CYP3A4 may reduce plasma concentrations of estrogens, possibly resulting in a decrease in therapeutic effects, and/or changes in the uterine bleeding profile).
No products indexed under this heading.

Fluoxetine Hydrochloride (Studies have shown that estrogens are metabolized partially by cytochrome P4503A. Inhibitors of CYP3A4 may increase concentrations of estrogens and in side effects). Products include:
Prozac Pulvules and Liquid 1771
Symbyax Capsules 1788

Fluvoxamine Maleate (Studies have shown that estrogens are metabolized partially by cytochrome P4503A. Inhibitors of CYP3A4 may increase concentrations of estrogens and in side effects).
No products indexed under this heading.

Fosamprenavir Calcium (Studies have shown that estrogens are metabolized partially by cytochrome P4503A. Inhibitors of CYP3A4 may increase concentrations of estrogens and in side effects). Products include:
Lexiva Tablets 1473

Fosphenytoin Sodium (Studies have shown that estrogens are metabolized partially by cytochrome P4503A. Inducers of CYP3A4 may reduce plasma concentrations of estrogens, possibly resulting in a decrease in therapeutic effects, and/or changes in the uterine bleeding profile).
No products indexed under this heading.

Garlic Extract (Studies have shown that estrogens are metabolized partially by cytochrome P4503A. Inducers of CYP3A4 may reduce plasma concentrations of estrogens, possibly resulting in a decrease in therapeutic effects, and/or changes in the uterine bleeding profile).
No products indexed under this heading.

Garlic Oil (Studies have shown that estrogens are metabolized partially by cytochrome P4503A. Inducers of CYP3A4 may reduce plasma concentrations of estrogens, possibly resulting in a decrease in therapeutic effects, and/or changes in the uterine bleeding profile).
No products indexed under this heading.

Hydrocortisone (Studies have shown that estrogens are metabolized partially by cytochrome P4503A. Inducers of CYP3A4 may reduce plasma concentrations of estrogens, possibly resulting in a decrease in therapeutic effects, and/or changes in the uterine bleeding profile). Products include:
Cortizone•5 Ointment ▣ 699
Cortizone•10 Creme ▣ 699
Cortizone•10 Ointment ▣ 699
Cortizone•10 Plus Creme ▣ 700
Cortizone•10 Maximum Strength Quick Shot Spray ▣ 700
Hydrocortone Tablets 1963
Preparation H Hydrocortisone Cream ▣ 748

Hydrocortisone Acetate (Studies have shown that estrogens are metabolized partially by cytochrome P4503A. Inducers of CYP3A4 may reduce plasma concentrations of estrogens, possibly resulting in a decrease in therapeutic effects, and/or changes in the uterine bleeding profile). Products include:
Analpram-HC 1136
Pramosone 1139
ProctoFoam-HC 3113
Tucks Anti-Itch Ointment ▣ 712
U-cort 1% Cream 3289

Hydrocortisone Butyrate (Studies have shown that estrogens are metabolized partially by cytochrome P4503A. Inducers of CYP3A4 may reduce plasma concentrations of estrogens, possibly resulting in a decrease in therapeutic effects, and/or changes in the uterine bleeding profile). Products include:
Locoid 1138
Locoid Lipocream Cream 1138

Hydrocortisone Cypionate (Studies have shown that estrogens are metabolized partially by cytochrome P4503A. Inducers of CYP3A4 may reduce plasma concentrations of estrogens, possibly resulting in a decrease in therapeutic effects, and/or changes in the uterine bleeding profile).
No products indexed under this heading.

Hydrocortisone Hemisuccinate (Studies have shown that estrogens are metabolized partially by cytochrome P4503A. Inducers of CYP3A4 may reduce plasma concentrations of estrogens, possibly resulting in a decrease in therapeutic effects, and/or changes in the uterine bleeding profile).
No products indexed under this heading.

Hydrocortisone Probutate (Studies have shown that estrogens are metabolized partially by cytochrome P4503A. Inducers of CYP3A4 may reduce plasma concentrations of estrogens, possibly resulting in a decrease in therapeutic effects, and/or changes in the uterine bleeding profile). Products include:
Pandel Cream, 0.1% 1017

Hydrocortisone Sodium Phosphate (Studies have shown that estrogens are metabolized partially by cytochrome P4503A. Inducers of CYP3A4 may reduce plasma concentrations of estrogens, possibly resulting in a decrease in therapeutic effects, and/or changes in the uterine bleeding profile).
No products indexed under this heading.

Hydrocortisone Sodium Succinate (Studies have shown that estrogens are metabolized partially by cytochrome P4503A. Inducers of CYP3A4 may reduce plasma concentrations of estrogens, possibly resulting in a decrease in therapeutic effects, and/or changes in the uterine bleeding profile).
No products indexed under this heading.

Hydrocortisone Valerate (Studies have shown that estrogens are metabolized partially by cytochrome P4503A. Inducers of CYP3A4 may reduce plasma concentrations of estrogens, possibly resulting in a decrease in therapeutic effects, and/or changes in the uterine bleeding profile).
No products indexed under this heading.

Hypericum (Studies have shown that estrogens are metabolized partially by cytochrome P4503A. Inducers of CYP3A4 may reduce plasma concentrations of estrogens, possibly resulting in a decrease in therapeutic effects, and/or changes in the uterine bleeding profile).
No products indexed under this heading.

Hypericum Perforatum (Studies have shown that estrogens are metabolized partially by cytochrome P4503A. Inducers of CYP3A4 may reduce plasma concentrations of estrogens, possibly resulting in a decrease in therapeutic effects, and/or changes in the uterine bleeding profile).
No products indexed under this heading.

Indinavir Sulfate (Studies have shown that estrogens are metabolized partially by cytochrome P4503A. Inhibitors of CYP3A4 may increase concentrations of estrogens and in side effects). Products include:
Crixivan Capsules 1918

Isoniazid (Studies have shown that estrogens are metabolized partially by cytochrome P4503A. Inhibitors of CYP3A4 may increase concentrations of estrogens and in side effects).
No products indexed under this heading.

Itraconazole (Studies have shown that estrogens are metabolized partially by cytochrome P4503A. Inhibitors of CYP3A4 may increase concentrations of estrogens and in side effects).
No products indexed under this heading.

Ketoconazole (Studies have shown that estrogens are metabolized partially by cytochrome P4503A. Inhibitors of CYP3A4 may increase concentrations of estrogens and in side effects). Products include:
Nizoral A-D Shampoo, 1% 1839
Nizoral 2% Shampoo 1838

Lopinavir (Studies have shown that estrogens are metabolized partially by cytochrome P4503A. Inhibitors of CYP3A4 may increase concentrations of estrogens and in side effects). Products include:
Kaletra 474

Loratadine (Studies have shown that estrogens are metabolized partially by cytochrome P4503A. Inhibitors of CYP3A4 may increase concentrations of estrogens and in side effects). Products include:
Alavert Allergy & Sinus D-12 Hour Tablets ▣ 743
Alavert ▣ 743
Children's Claritin 24 Hour Non-Drowsy Allergy Syrup ▣ 732
Claritin Non-Drowsy 24 Hour Tablets ▣ 731
Non-Drowsy Claritin Hives Relief Tablets ▣ 733
Claritin Reditabs 24 Hour Non-Drowsy Tablets ▣ 732
Claritin-D Non-Drowsy 12 Hour Tablets ▣ 731
Claritin-D Non-Drowsy 24 Hour Tablets ▣ 731
Children's Dimetapp ND Non-Drowsy Allergy Syrup ▣ 746
Triaminic Allerchews ▣ 684

Mephenytoin (Studies have shown that estrogens are metabolized partially by cytochrome P4503A. Inducers of CYP3A4 may reduce plasma concentrations of estrogens, possibly resulting in a decrease in therapeutic effects, and/or changes in the uterine bleeding profile).
No products indexed under this heading.

Methsuximide (Studies have shown that estrogens are metabolized partially by cytochrome P4503A. Inducers of CYP3A4 may reduce plasma concentrations of estrogens, possibly resulting in a decrease in therapeutic effects, and/or changes in the uterine bleeding profile).
No products indexed under this heading.

Methylprednisolone (Studies have shown that estrogens are metabolized partially by cytochrome P4503A. Inducers of CYP3A4 may reduce plasma concentrations of estrogens, possibly resulting in a decrease in therapeutic effects, and/or changes in the uterine bleeding profile).
No products indexed under this heading.

Methylprednisolone Acetate (Studies have shown that estrogens are metabolized partially by cytochrome P4503A. Inducers of CYP3A4 may reduce plasma concentrations of estrogens, possibly resulting in a decrease in therapeutic effects, and/or changes in the uterine bleeding profile). Products include:
Depo-Medrol Injectable Suspension 2615
Depo-Medrol Single-Dose Vial 2617

Methylprednisolone Sodium Succinate (Studies have shown that estrogens are metabolized partially by cytochrome P4503A. Inducers of CYP3A4 may reduce plasma concentrations of estrogens, possibly resulting in a decrease in therapeutic effects, and/or changes in the uterine bleeding profile).
No products indexed under this heading.

Metronidazole (Studies have shown that estrogens are metabolized partially by cytochrome P4503A. Inhibitors of CYP3A4 may increase concentrations of estrogens and in side effects). Products include:
Metrogel 1% 1212
MetroGel-Vaginal Gel 1822
Noritate Cream, 1% 1051

Metronidazole Benzoate (Studies have shown that estrogens are metabolized partially by cytochrome P4503A. Inhibitors of CYP3A4 may increase concentrations of estrogens and in side effects).
No products indexed under this heading.

Metronidazole Hydrochloride (Studies have shown that estrogens are metabolized partially by cytochrome P4503A. Inhibitors of CYP3A4 may increase concentrations of estrogens and in side effects).
No products indexed under this heading.

Miconazole (Studies have shown that estrogens are metabolized partially by cytochrome P4503A. Inhibitors of CYP3A4 may increase concentrations of estrogens and in side effects).
No products indexed under this heading.

Miconazole Nitrate (Studies have shown that estrogens are metabolized partially by cytochrome P4503A. Inhibitors of CYP3A4 may increase concentrations of estrogens and in side effects). Products include:
Desenex ▣ 674
Desenex Jock Itch Spray Powder ▣ 674

Modafinil (Studies have shown that estrogens are metabolized partially by cytochrome P4503A. Inducers of CYP3A4 may reduce plasma concentrations of estrogens, possibly resulting in a decrease in therapeutic effects, and/or changes in the uterine bleeding profile). Products include:
Provigil Tablets 1002

Nefazodone Hydrochloride (Studies have shown that estrogens are metabolized partially by cytochrome P4503A. Inhibitors of CYP3A4 may increase concentrations of estrogens and in side effects).
No products indexed under this heading.

Nelfinavir Mesylate (Studies have shown that estrogens are metabolized partially by cytochrome P4503A. Inhibitors of CYP3A4 may increase concentrations of estrogens and in side effects). Products include:
Viracept 2556

Nevirapine (Studies have shown that estrogens are metabolized partially by cytochrome P4503A. Inducers of CYP3A4 may reduce plasma concentrations of estrogens, possibly resulting in a decrease in therapeutic effects, and/or changes in the uterine bleeding profile). Products include:
Viramune Oral Suspension 903
Viramune Tablets 903

Niacinamide (Studies have shown that estrogens are metabolized partially by cytochrome P4503A. Inhibitors of CYP3A4 may increase concentrations of estrogens and in side effects).
No products indexed under this heading.

Nicotinamide (Studies have shown that estrogens are metabolized partially by cytochrome P4503A. Inhibitors of CYP3A4 may increase concentrations of estrogens and in side effects). Products include:
Nicomide Tablets 3190

Nifedipine (Studies have shown that estrogens are metabolized partially by cytochrome P4503A. Inhibitors of CYP3A4 may increase concentrations of estrogens and in side effects). Products include:
Adalat CC Tablets 2978

Norfloxacin (Studies have shown that estrogens are metabolized partially by cytochrome P4503A. Inhibitors of CYP3A4 may increase concentrations of estrogens and in side effects). Products include:
Noroxin Tablets 2009

Omeprazole (Studies have shown that estrogens are metabolized partially by cytochrome P4503A. Inhibitors of CYP3A4 may increase concentrations of estrogens and in side effects). Products include:
Zegerid Powder for Oral Solution 2972

Oxcarbazepine (Studies have shown that estrogens are metabolized partially by cytochrome P4503A. Inducers of CYP3A4 may reduce plasma concentrations of estrogens, possibly resulting in a decrease in therapeutic effects, and/or changes in the uterine bleeding profile). Products include:
Trileptal Oral Suspension 2281
Trileptal Tablets 2281

Paroxetine Hydrochloride (Studies have shown that estrogens are metabolized partially by cytochrome P4503A. Inhibitors of CYP3A4 may increase concentrations of estrogens and in side effects). Products include:
Paxil CR Controlled-Release Tablets 1509
Paxil 1501

Phenobarbital (Studies have shown that estrogens are metabolized partially by cytochrome P4503A. Inducers of CYP3A4 may reduce plasma concentrations of estrogens, possibly resulting in a decrease in therapeutic effects, and/or changes in the uterine bleeding profile).
No products indexed under this heading.

Phenobarbital Sodium (Studies have shown that estrogens are metabolized partially by cytochrome P4503A. Inducers of CYP3A4 may reduce plasma concentrations of estrogens, possibly resulting in a decrease in therapeutic effects, and/or changes in the uterine bleeding profile).
No products indexed under this heading.

Phenytoin (Studies have shown that estrogens are metabolized partially by cytochrome P4503A. Inducers of CYP3A4 may reduce plasma concentrations of estrogens, possibly resulting in a decrease in therapeutic effects, and/or changes in the uterine bleeding profile).
No products indexed under this heading.

Phenytoin Sodium (Studies have shown that estrogens are metabolized partially by cytochrome P4503A. Inducers of CYP3A4 may reduce plasma concentrations of estrogens, possibly resulting in a decrease in therapeutic effects, and/or changes in the uterine bleeding profile). Products include:
Phenytek Capsules 2153

Prednisolone Acetate (Studies have shown that estrogens are metabolized partially by cytochrome P4503A. Inducers of CYP3A4 may reduce plasma concentrations of estrogens, possibly resulting in a decrease in therapeutic effects, and/or changes in the uterine bleeding profile). Products include:
Blephamide Ophthalmic Ointment 563
Blephamide Ophthalmic Suspension 564
Poly-Pred Liquifilm Ophthalmic Suspension .... ⊙231
Pred Forte Ophthalmic Suspension .... ⊙233
Pred Mild Sterile Ophthalmic Suspension .... ⊙236
Pred-G Ophthalmic Suspension .... ⊙234
Pred-G Sterile Ophthalmic Ointment .... ⊙235

Prednisolone Sodium Phosphate (Studies have shown that estrogens are metabolized partially by cytochrome P4503A. Inducers of CYP3A4 may reduce plasma concentrations of estrogens, possibly resulting in a decrease in therapeutic effects, and/or changes in the uterine bleeding profile). Products include:
Pediapred Oral Solution 3319

Prednisolone Tebutate (Studies have shown that estrogens are metabolized partially by cytochrome P4503A. Inducers of CYP3A4 may reduce plasma concentrations of estrogens, possibly resulting in a decrease in therapeutic effects, and/or changes in the uterine bleeding profile).
No products indexed under this heading.

Prednisone (Studies have shown that estrogens are metabolized partially by cytochrome P4503A. Inducers of CYP3A4 may reduce plasma concentrations of estrogens, possibly resulting in a decrease in therapeutic effects, and/or changes in the uterine bleeding profile).
No products indexed under this heading.

Primidone (Studies have shown that estrogens are metabolized partially by cytochrome P4503A. Inducers of CYP3A4 may reduce plasma concentrations of estrogens, possibly resulting in a decrease in therapeutic effects, and/or changes in the uterine bleeding profile).
No products indexed under this heading.

Propoxyphene Hydrochloride (Studies have shown that estrogens are metabolized partially by cytochrome P4503A. Inhibitors of CYP3A4 may increase concentrations of estrogens and in side effects).
No products indexed under this heading.

Propoxyphene Napsylate (Studies have shown that estrogens are metabolized partially by cytochrome P4503A. Inhibitors of CYP3A4 may increase concentrations of estrogens and in side effects). Products include:
Darvocet A 500 Tablets 3497

Quinidine (Studies have shown that estrogens are metabolized partially by cytochrome P4503A. Inhibitors of CYP3A4 may increase concentrations of estrogens and in side effects).
No products indexed under this heading.

Quinidine Hydrochloride (Studies have shown that estrogens are metabolized partially by cytochrome P4503A. Inhibitors of CYP3A4 may increase concentrations of estrogens and in side effects).
No products indexed under this heading.

Quinidine Polygalacturonate (Studies have shown that estrogens are metabolized partially by cytochrome P4503A. Inhibitors of CYP3A4 may increase concentrations of estrogens and in side effects).
No products indexed under this heading.

Quinidine Sulfate (Studies have shown that estrogens are metabolized partially by cytochrome P4503A. Inhibitors of CYP3A4 may increase concentrations of estrogens and in side effects).
No products indexed under this heading.

Quinine (Studies have shown that estrogens are metabolized partially by cytochrome P4503A. Inhibitors of CYP3A4 may increase concentrations of estrogens and in side effects).
No products indexed under this heading.

Quinine Sulfate (Studies have shown that estrogens are metabolized partially by cytochrome P4503A. Inhibitors of CYP3A4 may increase concentrations of estrogens and in side effects).
No products indexed under this heading.

Quinupristin (Studies have shown that estrogens are metabolized partially by cytochrome P4503A. Inhibitors of CYP3A4 may increase concentrations of estrogens and in side effects). Products include:
Synercid I.V. 1690

Ranitidine Bismuth Citrate (Studies have shown that estrogens are metabolized partially by cytochrome P4503A. Inhibitors of CYP3A4 may increase concentrations of estrogens and in side effects).
No products indexed under this heading.

Ranitidine Hydrochloride (Studies have shown that estrogens are metabolized partially by cytochrome P4503A. Inhibitors of CYP3A4 may increase concentrations of estrogens and in side effects). Products include:
Zantac 1597
Zantac Injection 1593
Zantac 75 Tablets 715
Zantac 150 Maximum Strength Tablets 715
Zantac Injection Pharmacy Bulk Package 1595

Rifabutin (Studies have shown that estrogens are metabolized partially by cytochrome P4503A. Inducers of CYP3A4 may reduce plasma concentrations of estrogens, possibly resulting in a decrease in therapeutic effects, and/or changes in the uterine bleeding profile).
No products indexed under this heading.

Rifampicin (Studies have shown that estrogens are metabolized partially by cytochrome P4503A. Inducers of CYP3A4 may reduce plasma concentrations of estrogens, possibly resulting in a decrease in therapeutic effects, and/or changes in the uterine bleeding profile).
No products indexed under this heading.

Rifampin (Studies have shown that estrogens are metabolized partially by cytochrome P4503A. Inducers of CYP3A4 may reduce plasma concentrations of estrogens, possibly resulting in a decrease in therapeutic effects, and/or changes in the uterine bleeding profile).
No products indexed under this heading.

Rifapentine (Studies have shown that estrogens are metabolized partially by cytochrome P4503A. Inducers of CYP3A4 may reduce plasma concentrations of estrogens, possibly resulting in a decrease in therapeutic effects, and/or changes in the uterine bleeding profile).
No products indexed under this heading.

Ritonavir (Studies have shown that estrogens are metabolized partially by cytochrome P4503A. Inhibitors of CYP3A4 may increase concentrations of estrogens and in side effects). Products include:
Kaletra 474
Norvir 499

Saquinavir (Studies have shown that estrogens are metabolized partially by cytochrome P4503A. Inhibitors of CYP3A4 may increase concentrations of estrogens and in side effects).
No products indexed under this heading.

Saquinavir Mesylate (Studies have shown that estrogens are metabolized partially by cytochrome P4503A. Inhibitors of CYP3A4 may increase concentrations of estrogens and in side effects). Products include:
Invirase 2776

Sertraline Hydrochloride (Studies have shown that estrogens are metabolized partially by cytochrome P4503A. Inhibitors of CYP3A4 may increase concentrations of estrogens and in side effects). Products include:
Zoloft 2581

Sulfinpyrazone (Studies have shown that estrogens are metabolized partially by cytochrome P4503A. Inducers of CYP3A4 may reduce plasma concentrations of estrogens, possibly resulting in a decrease in therapeutic effects, and/or changes in the uterine bleeding profile).
No products indexed under this heading.

Telithromycin (Studies have shown that estrogens are metabolized partially by cytochrome P4503A. Inhibitors of CYP3A4 may increase concentrations of estrogens and in side effects). Products include:
Ketek Tablets 2920

Theophylline (Studies have shown that estrogens are metabolized partially by cytochrome P4503A. Inducers of CYP3A4 may reduce plasma concentrations of estrogens, possibly resulting in a decrease in therapeutic effects, and/or changes in the uterine bleeding profile).
No products indexed under this heading.

Triamcinolone (Studies have shown that estrogens are metabolized partially by cytochrome P4503A. Inducers of CYP3A4 may reduce plasma concentrations of estrogens, possibly resulting in a decrease in therapeutic effects, and/or changes in the uterine bleeding profile).
No products indexed under this heading.

Triamcinolone Acetonide (Studies have shown that estrogens are metabolized partially by cytochrome P4503A. Inducers of CYP3A4 may reduce plasma concentrations of estrogens, possibly resulting in a decrease in therapeutic effects, and/or changes in the uterine bleeding profile). Products include:
Azmacort Inhalation Aerosol **1701**
Nasacort HFA Inhalation Aerosol **2939**
Nasacort AQ Nasal Spray **2937**

Triamcinolone Diacetate (Studies have shown that estrogens are metabolized partially by cytochrome P4503A. Inducers of CYP3A4 may reduce plasma concentrations of estrogens, possibly resulting in a decrease in therapeutic effects, and/or changes in the uterine bleeding profile).
No products indexed under this heading.

Triamcinolone Hexacetonide (Studies have shown that estrogens are metabolized partially by cytochrome P4503A. Inducers of CYP3A4 may reduce plasma concentrations of estrogens, possibly resulting in a decrease in therapeutic effects, and/or changes in the uterine bleeding profile).
No products indexed under this heading.

Troglitazone (Studies have shown that estrogens are metabolized partially by cytochrome P4503A. Inducers of CYP3A4 may reduce plasma concentrations of estrogens, possibly resulting in a decrease in therapeutic effects, and/or changes in the uterine bleeding profile).
No products indexed under this heading.

Troleandomycin (Studies have shown that estrogens are metabolized partially by cytochrome P4503A. Inhibitors of CYP3A4 may increase concentrations of estrogens and in side effects).
No products indexed under this heading.

Valproate Sodium (Studies have shown that estrogens are metabolized partially by cytochrome P4503A. Inhibitors of CYP3A4 may increase concentrations of estrogens and in side effects). Products include:
Depacon Injection **412**

Verapamil Hydrochloride (Studies have shown that estrogens are metabolized partially by cytochrome P4503A. Inhibitors of CYP3A4 may increase concentrations of estrogens and in side effects). Products include:
Covera-HS Tablets **3135**
Tarka Tablets **519**
Verelan PM Capsules **3120**

Voriconazole (Studies have shown that estrogens are metabolized partially by cytochrome P4503A. Inhibitors of CYP3A4 may increase concentrations of estrogens and in side effects). Products include:
VFEND I.V. **2543**
VFEND Oral Suspension **2543**
VFEND Tablets **2543**

Zafirlukast (Studies have shown that estrogens are metabolized partially by cytochrome P4503A. Inhibitors of CYP3A4 may increase concentrations of estrogens and in side effects). Products include:
Accolate Tablets **663**

Zileuton (Studies have shown that estrogens are metabolized partially by cytochrome P4503A. Inhibitors of CYP3A4 may increase concentrations of estrogens and in side effects).
No products indexed under this heading.

Food Interactions

Grapefruit (Studies have shown that estrogens are metabolized partially by cytochrome P4503A. Inhibitors of CYP3A4 may increase concentrations of estrogens and in side effects).

Grapefruit Juice (Studies have shown that estrogens are metabolized partially by cytochrome P4503A. Inhibitors of CYP3A4 may increase concentrations of estrogens and in side effects).

COMBIVENT INHALATION AEROSOL

(Albuterol Sulfate, Ipratropium Bromide) **878**
May interact with anticholinergics, beta blockers, monoamine oxidase inhibitors, potassium-depleting diuretics, sympathomimetics, and tricyclic antidepressants. Compounds in these categories include:

Acebutolol Hydrochloride (Co-administration with beta blockers inhibits the effects of each other).
No products indexed under this heading.

Albuterol (Co-administration with other sympathomimetic agents increases the risk of adverse cardiovascular effects). Products include:
Proventil Inhalation Aerosol **3067**

Amitriptyline Hydrochloride (Co-administration with tricyclic antidepressant can potentiate the action of albuterol on the cardiovascular system).
No products indexed under this heading.

Amoxapine (Co-administration with tricyclic antidepressant can potentiate the action of albuterol on the cardiovascular system).
No products indexed under this heading.

Atenolol (Co-administration with beta blockers inhibits the effects of each other). Products include:
Tenormin I.V. Injection **698**
Tenormin Tablets **695**

Atropine Sulfate (Co-administration has some potential for additive anticholinergic effects; caution is advised).
No products indexed under this heading.

Belladonna Alkaloids (Co-administration has some potential for additive anticholinergic effects; caution is advised). Products include:
Hyland's Teething Tablets .... ▣**736**

Bendroflumethiazide (Co-administration with non-potassium-sparing diuretics can result in acute worsening of ECG changes and/or hypokalemia, especially when recommended dose of the beta agonist is exceeded; clinical significance of this interaction is unknown).
No products indexed under this heading.

Benztropine Mesylate (Co-administration has some potential for additive anticholinergic effects; caution is advised). Products include:
Cogentin Injection **1903**

Betaxolol Hydrochloride (Co-administration with beta blockers inhibits the effects of each other). Products include:
Betoptic S Ophthalmic Suspension................................. **554**

Biperiden Hydrochloride (Co-administration has some potential for additive anticholinergic effects; caution is advised).
No products indexed under this heading.

Bisoprolol Fumarate (Co-administration with beta blockers inhibits the effects of each other).
No products indexed under this heading.

Bumetanide (Co-administration with non-potassium-sparing diuretics can result in acute worsening of ECG changes and/or hypokalemia, especially when recommended dose of the beta agonist is exceeded; clinical significance of this interaction is unknown).
No products indexed under this heading.

Carteolol Hydrochloride (Co-administration with beta blockers inhibits the effects of each other). Products include:
Carteolol Hydrochloride Ophthalmic Solution USP, 1%....... ⊙**246**

Chlorothiazide (Co-administration with non-potassium-sparing diuretics can result in acute worsening of ECG changes and/or hypokalemia, especially when recommended dose of the beta agonist is exceeded; clinical significance of this interaction is unknown). Products include:
Aldoclor Tablets **1881**
Diuril Oral **1936**

Chlorothiazide Sodium (Co-administration with non-potassium-sparing diuretics can result in acute worsening of ECG changes and/or hypokalemia, especially when recommended dose of the beta agonist is exceeded; clinical significance of this interaction is unknown). Products include:
Diuril Sodium Intravenous **1934**

Clidinium Bromide (Co-administration has some potential for additive anticholinergic effects; caution is advised).
No products indexed under this heading.

Clomipramine Hydrochloride (Co-administration with tricyclic antidepressant can potentiate the action of albuterol on the cardiovascular system).
No products indexed under this heading.

Desipramine Hydrochloride (Co-administration with tricyclic antidepressant can potentiate the action of albuterol on the cardiovascular system).
No products indexed under this heading.

Dicyclomine Hydrochloride (Co-administration has some potential for additive anticholinergic effects; caution is advised). Products include:
Bentyl Capsules **724**
Bentyl Injection **724**
Bentyl Syrup **724**
Bentyl Tablets **724**

Dobutamine Hydrochloride (Co-administration with other sympathomimetic agents increases the risk of adverse cardiovascular effects).
No products indexed under this heading.

Dopamine Hydrochloride (Co-administration with other sympathomimetic agents increases the risk of adverse cardiovascular effects).
No products indexed under this heading.

Doxepin Hydrochloride (Co-administration with tricyclic antidepressant can potentiate the action of albuterol on the cardiovascular system).
No products indexed under this heading.

Ephedrine Hydrochloride (Co-administration with other sympathomimetic agents increases the risk of adverse cardiovascular effects). Products include:
Primatene Tablets .... ▣**749**

Ephedrine Sulfate (Co-administration with other sympathomimetic agents increases the risk of adverse cardiovascular effects).
No products indexed under this heading.

Ephedrine Tannate (Co-administration with other sympathomimetic agents increases the risk of adverse cardiovascular effects).
No products indexed under this heading.

Epinephrine (Co-administration with other sympathomimetic agents increases the risk of adverse cardiovascular effects). Products include:
EpiPen **1061**
Primatene Mist .... ▣**749**

Epinephrine Bitartrate (Co-administration with other sympathomimetic agents increases the risk of adverse cardiovascular effects).
No products indexed under this heading.

Epinephrine Hydrochloride (Co-administration with other sympathomimetic agents increases the risk of adverse cardiovascular effects).
No products indexed under this heading.

Esmolol Hydrochloride (Co-administration with beta blockers inhibits the effects of each other). Products include:
Brevibloc Concentrate **766**
Brevibloc Injection **766**
Brevibloc Double Strength Injection.. **766**

Brevibloc Premixed Injection 766
Brevibloc Double Strength Premixed Injection 766

Ethacrynic Acid (Co-administration with non-potassium-sparing diuretics can result in acute worsening of ECG changes and/or hypokalemia, especially when recommended dose of the beta agonist is exceeded; clinical significance of this interaction is unknown). Products include:
Edecrin Tablets 1941

Furosemide (Co-administration with non-potassium-sparing diuretics can result in acute worsening of ECG changes and/or hypokalemia, especially when recommended dose of the beta agonist is exceeded; clinical significance of this interaction is unknown). Products include:
Furosemide Tablets 2117

Glycopyrrolate (Co-administration has some potential for additive anticholinergic effects; caution is advised).
No products indexed under this heading.

Hydrochlorothiazide (Co-administration with non-potassium-sparing diuretics can result in acute worsening of ECG changes and/or hypokalemia, especially when recommended dose of the beta agonist is exceeded; clinical significance of this interaction is unknown).
Products include:
Aldoril Tablets 1884
Atacand HCT 637
Avalide Tablets 2889
Avalide Tablets 922
Benicar HCT Tablets 2852
Diovan HCT Tablets 2195
Dyazide Capsules 1389
Hyzaar 1964
Lotensin HCT Tablets 2235
Maxzide 2150
Micardis HCT Tablets 886
Moduretic Tablets 2003
Prinzide Tablets 2033
Teveten HCT Tablets 1710
Timolide Tablets 2056
Uniretic Tablets 3114
Vaseretic Tablets 2073
Zestoretic Tablets 701

Hydroflumethiazide (Co-administration with non-potassium-sparing diuretics can result in acute worsening of ECG changes and/or hypokalemia, especially when recommended dose of the beta agonist is exceeded; clinical significance of this interaction is unknown).
No products indexed under this heading.

Hyoscyamine (Co-administration has some potential for additive anticholinergic effects; caution is advised).
No products indexed under this heading.

Hyoscyamine Sulfate (Co-administration has some potential for additive anticholinergic effects; caution is advised).
No products indexed under this heading.

Imipramine Hydrochloride (Co-administration with tricyclic antidepressant can potentiate the action of albuterol on the cardiovascular system).
No products indexed under this heading.

Imipramine Pamoate (Co-administration with tricyclic antidepressant can potentiate the action of albuterol on the cardiovascular system).
No products indexed under this heading.

Isocarboxazid (Co-administration with MAO inhibitors can potentiate the action of albuterol on the cardiovascular system).
No products indexed under this heading.

Isoproterenol Hydrochloride (Co-administration with other sympathomimetic agents increases the risk of adverse cardiovascular effects).
No products indexed under this heading.

Isoproterenol Sulfate (Co-administration with other sympathomimetic agents increases the risk of adverse cardiovascular effects).
No products indexed under this heading.

Labetalol Hydrochloride (Co-administration with beta blockers inhibits the effects of each other).
No products indexed under this heading.

Levalbuterol Hydrochloride (Co-administration with other sympathomimetic agents increases the risk of adverse cardiovascular effects).
Products include:
Xopenex Inhalation Solution 3143
Xopenex Inhalation Solution Concentrate 3147

Levobunolol Hydrochloride (Co-administration with beta blockers inhibits the effects of each other).
Products include:
Betagan Ophthalmic Solution, USP.. ⊙217

Maprotiline Hydrochloride (Co-administration with tricyclic antidepressant can potentiate the action of albuterol on the cardiovascular system).
No products indexed under this heading.

Mepenzolate Bromide (Co-administration has some potential for additive anticholinergic effects; caution is advised).
No products indexed under this heading.

Metaproterenol Sulfate (Co-administration with other sympathomimetic agents increases the risk of adverse cardiovascular effects).
Products include:
Alupent Inhalation Aerosol 858

Metaraminol Bitartrate (Co-administration with other sympathomimetic agents increases the risk of adverse cardiovascular effects).
Products include:
Aramine Injection 1889

Methoxamine Hydrochloride (Co-administration with other sympathomimetic agents increases the risk of adverse cardiovascular effects).
No products indexed under this heading.

Methyclothiazide (Co-administration with non-potassium-sparing diuretics can result in acute worsening of ECG changes and/or hypokalemia, especially when recommended dose of the beta agonist is exceeded; clinical significance of this interaction is unknown).
No products indexed under this heading.

Metipranolol Hydrochloride (Co-administration with beta blockers inhibits the effects of each other).
No products indexed under this heading.

Metoprolol Succinate (Co-administration with beta blockers inhibits the effects of each other).
Products include:
Toprol-XL Tablets 660

Metoprolol Tartrate (Co-administration with beta blockers inhibits the effects of each other).
No products indexed under this heading.

Moclobemide (Co-administration with MAO inhibitors can potentiate the action of albuterol on the cardiovascular system).
No products indexed under this heading.

Nadolol (Co-administration with beta blockers inhibits the effects of each other). Products include:
Nadolol Tablets 2121

Norepinephrine Bitartrate (Co-administration with other sympathomimetic agents increases the risk of adverse cardiovascular effects).
No products indexed under this heading.

Nortriptyline Hydrochloride (Co-administration with tricyclic antidepressant can potentiate the action of albuterol on the cardiovascular system).
No products indexed under this heading.

Oxybutynin Chloride (Co-administration has some potential for additive anticholinergic effects; caution is advised). Products include:
Ditropan XL Extended Release Tablets 2391

Pargyline Hydrochloride (Co-administration with MAO inhibitors can potentiate the action of albuterol on the cardiovascular system).
No products indexed under this heading.

Penbutolol Sulfate (Co-administration with beta blockers inhibits the effects of each other).
No products indexed under this heading.

Phenelzine Sulfate (Co-administration with MAO inhibitors can potentiate the action of albuterol on the cardiovascular system).
No products indexed under this heading.

Phenylephrine Bitartrate (Co-administration with other sympathomimetic agents increases the risk of adverse cardiovascular effects).
No products indexed under this heading.

Phenylephrine Hydrochloride (Co-administration with other sympathomimetic agents increases the risk of adverse cardiovascular effects).
Products include:
Alacol DM Syrup 739
Hycomine Compound Tablets 1105
Preparation H Maximum Strength Cream .... ▣747
Preparation H Cooling Gel .... ▣747
Preparation H .... ▣747
Sudafed PE Tablets .... ▣711
Vicks Sinex Nasal Spray and Ultra Fine Mist for Sinus Relief............... 2677
Zicam Concentrated Cough Mist for Kids Plus D Cool Cherry......... ▣643
Zicam Concentrated Cough Mist Plus D Cool Cherry...................... ▣642

Phenylephrine Tannate (Co-administration with other sympathomimetic agents increases the risk of adverse cardiovascular effects).
No products indexed under this heading.

Phenylpropanolamine Hydrochloride (Co-administration with other sympathomimetic agents increases the risk of adverse cardiovascular effects).
No products indexed under this heading.

Pindolol (Co-administration with beta blockers inhibits the effects of each other).
No products indexed under this heading.

Pirbuterol Acetate (Co-administration with other sympathomimetic agents increases the risk of adverse cardiovascular effects).
Products include:
Maxair Autohaler 1820

Polythiazide (Co-administration with non-potassium-sparing diuretics can result in acute worsening of ECG changes and/or hypokalemia, especially when recommended dose of the beta agonist is exceeded; clinical significance of this interaction is unknown).
No products indexed under this heading.

Procarbazine Hydrochloride (Co-administration with MAO inhibitors can potentiate the action of albuterol on the cardiovascular system).
Products include:
Matulane Capsules 3188

Procyclidine Hydrochloride (Co-administration has some potential for additive anticholinergic effects; caution is advised).
No products indexed under this heading.

Propantheline Bromide (Co-administration has some potential for additive anticholinergic effects; caution is advised).
No products indexed under this heading.

Propranolol Hydrochloride (Co-administration with beta blockers inhibits the effects of each other).
Products include:
Inderal LA Long-Acting Capsules 3421
InnoPran XL Capsules 2728

Protriptyline Hydrochloride (Co-administration with tricyclic antidepressant can potentiate the action of albuterol on the cardiovascular system). Products include:
Vivactil Tablets 2350

Pseudoephedrine Hydrochloride (Co-administration with other sympathomimetic agents increases the risk of adverse cardiovascular effects).
Products include:
Advil Allergy Sinus Caplets .... ▣737
Advil Cold & Sinus .... ▣739
Advil Flu & Body Ache Caplets .... ▣739
Children's Advil Cold Suspension ... ▣741
Advil Multi-Symptom Cold Caplets..................................... ▣738
Allegra-D 12 Hour Extended-Release Tablets............ 2860
Allegra-D 24 Hour Extended-Release Tablets............ 2862
Balamine DM 739
BC Cold Powder .... ▣612
Benadryl Allergy & Cold Tablets ..... ▣692
Benadryl Allergy & Sinus Headache Caplets & Gelcaps...... ▣693
Children's Benadryl Allergy & Cold Fastmelt Tablets................. ▣695

Benadryl Maximum Strength Severe Allergy & Sinus Headache Caplets .... ■□694
Children's Benadryl D Allergy & Sinus Fastmelt Tablets .... ■□694
Children's Benadryl D Liquid Medication .... ■□693
Benadryl D Tablets .... ■□694
Contac Non-Drowsy 12 Hour Cold Caplets .... ■□614
Contac Non-Drowsy Timed Release 12 Hour Cold Caplets .... ■□615
Contac Severe Cold and Flu Caplets Maximum Strength .... ■□615
Contac Severe Cold and Flu Caplets Non-Drowsy .... ■□615
Children's Dimetapp Cold & Allergy Elixir .... ■□745
Children's Dimetapp DM Cold & Cough Elixir .... ■□745
Children's Dimetapp Long Acting Cough Plus Cold Syrup .... ■□746
Dimetapp Infant Drops Decongestant Plus Cough .... ■□746
Children's Motrin Cold Non-Staining Dye-Free Oral Suspension 1838
Children's Motrin Cold Oral Suspension 1838
Motrin Cold & Sinus Caplets 1836
PediaCare Decongestant & Cough Infant Drops .... ■□705
PediaCare Decongestant Infants' Drops .... ■□705
PediaCare Long-Acting Cough Plus Cold Liquid .... ■□704
PediaCare Multi-Symptom Cold Liquid .... ■□704
PediaCare NightRest Cough & Cold Liquid .... ■□704
Robitussin Allergy & Cough Syrup .... ■□750
Robitussin CF Liquid .... ■□755
Robitussin Cough & Cold Liquid-filled Capsules .... ■□750
Robitussin Cough, Cold & Flu Liquid-filled Capsules .... ■□750
Robitussin Cough & Cold Infant Drops .... ■□755
Robitussin Flu Liquid .... ■□752
Robitussin Maximum Strength Cough & Cold Liquid .... ■□754
Robitussin PE Syrup .... ■□753
Robitussin Pediatric Cough & Cold Liquid .... ■□754
Robitussin PM Cough & Cold Liquid .... ■□752
Robitussin Severe Congestion Liquid-filled Capsules .... ■□751
Simply Stuffy Liquid 1841
Singlet Caplets .... ■□636
Sudafed 12 Hour Caplets .... ■□708
Sudafed 24 Hour Tablets .... ■□709
Sudafed Nasal Decongestant Tablets .... ■□709
Sudafed Severe Cold .... ■□710
Sudafed Non-Drying Sinus Liquid Caps .... ■□709
Sudafed Sinus & Allergy Tablets .... ■□710
Sudafed Sinus Headache .... ■□711
TheraFlu Cold & Cough Hot Liquid .... ■□680
TheraFlu Cold & Sore Throat Hot Liquid .... ■□680
TheraFlu Flu & Chest Congestion Non-Drowsy Hot Liquid .... ■□681
TheraFlu Flu & Sore Throat Hot Liquid .... ■□681
TheraFlu Severe Cold Non-Drowsy Hot Liquid .... ■□683
TheraFlu Severe Cold & Cough Hot Liquid .... ■□683
TheraFlu Severe Cold Caplets .... ■□679
TheraFlu Severe Cold Hot Liquid .... ■□682
TheraFlu Severe Cold Non-Drowsy Caplets .... ■□679
Triaminic Chest & Nasal Congestion Liquid .... ■□685
Triaminic Cold & Allergy Liquid .... ■□685
Triaminic Cold & Cough Liquid .... ■□685
Triaminic Cough Liquid .... ■□687
Triaminic Cough & Nasal Congestion Liquid .... ■□687
Triaminic Cough & Sore Throat Liquid .... ■□687
Triaminic Flu, Cough & Fever Liquid .... ■□685
Triaminic Night Time Cough & Cold Liquid .... ■□685
Triaminic Allergy Runny Nose & Congestion Softchews .... ■□688
Triaminic Cold & Cough Softchews .... ■□688
Triaminic Cough & Sore Throat Softchews .... ■□689
Tylenol Sinus NightTime Caplets .... ■□663
Children's Tylenol Plus Cold & Allergy Suspension Liquid 1850
Children's Tylenol Plus Cold NightTime Suspension Liquid 1851
Children's Tylenol Plus Cold & Cough Suspension Liquid and Chewable Tablets 1851
Children's Tylenol Plus Cold Chewable Tablets 1851
Children's Tylenol Plus Cold Daytime Non-Drowsy Suspension Liquid 1851
Children's Tylenol Plus Flu Suspension Liquid 1853
Concentrated Tylenol Infants' Drops Plus Cold 1851
Concentrated Tylenol Infants' Drops Plus Cold and Cough 1851
Tylenol Cold & Flu Severe Daytime Liquid with Cool Bust 1846
Tylenol Cold & Flu Severe NightTime Liquid with Cool Burst 1846
Tylenol Cold Severe Congestion Non-Drowsy Caplets with Cool Burst 1846
Tylenol Allergy Complete Night Time Caplets 1844
Tylenol Allergy Complete Multi-Symptom Caplets and Gelcaps with Cool Burst 1844
Tylenol Flu NightTime Gelcaps 1846
Tylenol Flu Day Non-Drowsy Gelcaps 1846
Concentrated Tylenol Infants' Drops Plus Cold Nasal Congestant, Fever Reducer & Pain Reliever .... ■□668
Concentrated Tylenol Infants' Drops Plus Cold & Cough Nasal Decongestant, Fever Reducer & Pain Reliever .... ■□668
Multi-Symptom Tylenol Cold Night Time Caplets 1845
Multi-Symptom Tylenol Cold Day Non-Drowsy Caplets and Gelcaps 1845
Tylenol Sinus Day Non-Drowsy 1848
Tylenol Sinus Night Time Caplets 1848
Tylenol Sinus Severe Congestion Caplets with Cool Burst 1848
Vicks 44D Cough & Head Congestion Relief 2676
Vicks 44D Cough & Head Congestion Relief Liquid .... ■□721
Vicks 44M Cough, Cold & Flu Relief 2676
Pediatric Vicks 44m Cough & Cold Relief 2673
Vicks DayQuil LiquiCaps/Liquid Multi-Symptom Cold/Flu Relief .... ■□723
Vicks DayQuil Multi-Symptom Cold/Flu Relief LiquiCaps 2675
Vicks DayQuil Multi-Symptom Cold/Flu Relief Liquid 2675
Children's Vicks NyQuil Cold/Cough Relief 2671
Vicks NyQuil LiquiCaps 2677
Vicks NyQuil LiquiCaps/Liquid Multi-Symptom Cold/Flu Relief .... ■□725
Vicks NyQuil Liquid 2677
Zyrtec-D 12 Hour Extended Release Tablets 2591

Pseudoephedrine Sulfate (Co-administration with other sympathomimetic agents increases the risk of adverse cardiovascular effects). Products include:
Alavert Allergy & Sinus D-12 Hour Tablets .... ■□743
Clarinex-D 24-Hour Extended-Release Tablets 3012
Claritin-D Non-Drowsy 12 Hour Tablets .... ■□731
Claritin-D Non-Drowsy 24 Hour Tablets .... ■□731

Salmeterol Xinafoate (Co-administration with other sympathomimetic agents increases the risk of adverse cardiovascular effects). Products include:
Advair Diskus 100/50 1291
Advair Diskus 250/50 1291
Advair Diskus 500/50 1291
Serevent Diskus 1540

Scopolamine (Co-administration has some potential for additive anticholinergic effects; caution is advised). Products include:
Transderm Scōp Transdermal Therapeutic System 2166

Scopolamine Hydrobromide (Co-administration has some potential for additive anticholinergic effects; caution is advised).
No products indexed under this heading.

Selegiline Hydrochloride (Co-administration with MAO inhibitors can potentiate the action of albuterol on the cardiovascular system). Products include:
Eldepryl Capsules 3209

Sotalol Hydrochloride (Co-administration with beta blockers inhibits the effects of each other).
No products indexed under this heading.

Terbutaline Sulfate (Co-administration with other sympathomimetic agents increases the risk of adverse cardiovascular effects).
No products indexed under this heading.

Timolol Hemihydrate (Co-administration with beta blockers inhibits the effects of each other). Products include:
Betimol Ophthalmic Solution 3371
Betimol Ophthalmic Solution .... ⊙283

Timolol Maleate (Co-administration with beta blockers inhibits the effects of each other). Products include:
Blocadren Tablets 1891
Cosopt Sterile Ophthalmic Solution 1910
Timolide Tablets 2056
Timoptic in Ocudose 2061
Timoptic Sterile Ophthalmic Solution 2058
Timoptic-XE Sterile Ophthalmic Gel Forming Solution 2062

Tolterodine Tartrate (Co-administration has some potential for additive anticholinergic effects; caution is advised). Products include:
Detrol Tablets 2626
Detrol LA Capsules 2629

Torsemide (Co-administration with non-potassium-sparing diuretics can result in acute worsening of ECG changes and/or hypokalemia, especially when recommended dose of the beta agonist is exceeded; clinical significance of this interaction is unknown).
No products indexed under this heading.

Tranylcypromine Sulfate (Co-administration with MAO inhibitors can potentiate the action of albuterol on the cardiovascular system). Products include:
Parnate Tablets 1499

Tridihexethyl Chloride (Co-administration has some potential for additive anticholinergic effects; caution is advised).
No products indexed under this heading.

Trihexyphenidyl Hydrochloride (Co-administration has some potential for additive anticholinergic effects; caution is advised).
No products indexed under this heading.

Trimipramine Maleate (Co-administration with tricyclic antidepressant can potentiate the action of albuterol on the cardiovascular system). Products include:
Surmontil Capsules 2347

COMBIVIR TABLETS

(Lamivudine, Zidovudine) 1373

May interact with cytotoxic drugs and certain other agents. Compounds in these categories include:

Bleomycin Sulfate (May increase the hematologic toxicity of zidovudine).
No products indexed under this heading.

Bone Marrow Depressants, unspecified (May increase the hematologic toxicity of zidovudine).
No products indexed under this heading.

Cyclophosphamide (May increase the hematologic toxicity of zidovudine).
No products indexed under this heading.

Daunorubicin Hydrochloride (May increase the hematologic toxicity of zidovudine). Products include:
Cerubidine for Injection 788

Doxorubicin Hydrochloride (Co-administration should be avoided since an antagonistic relationship with zidovudine has been demonstrated in vitro; may increase the hematologic toxicity of zidovudine). Products include:
Adriamycin for Injection, USP 786
Adriamycin Injection, USP 786

Epirubicin Hydrochloride (May increase the hematologic toxicity of zidovudine). Products include:
Ellence Injection 2632

Fluorouracil (May increase the hematologic toxicity of zidovudine). Products include:
Carac Cream, 0.5% 1048
Efudex 3348

Ganciclovir Sodium (May increase the hematologic toxicity of zidovudine). Products include:
Cytovene-IV 2763

Hydroxyurea (May increase the hematologic toxicity of zidovudine).
No products indexed under this heading.

Interferon alfa-2a, Recombinant (May increase the hematologic toxicity of zidovudine). Products include:
Roferon-A Injection 2805

Interferon alfa-2b, Recombinant (May increase the hematologic toxicity of zidovudine). Products include:
Intron A for Injection 3038
Rebetron Combination Therapy 3078

Methotrexate Sodium (May increase the hematologic toxicity of zidovudine).
No products indexed under this heading.

Mitotane (May increase the hematologic toxicity of zidovudine).
No products indexed under this heading.

Mitoxantrone Hydrochloride (May increase the hematologic toxicity of zidovudine). Products include:

Novantrone for Injection Concentrate 3158

Procarbazine Hydrochloride (May increase the hematologic toxicity of zidovudine). Products include:

Matulane Capsules 3188

Ribavirin (Co-administration should be avoided since an antagonistic relationship with zidovudine has been demonstrated in vitro). Products include:

Copegus Tablets 2759
Rebetol 3073
Rebetron Combination Therapy 3078
Ribavirin, USP Capsules 3083
Virazole for Inhalation Solution 3365

Stavudine (Co-administration should be avoided since an antagonistic relationship with zidovudine has been demonstrated in vitro). Products include:

Zerit 971

Sulfamethoxazole (Co-administration with TMP/SMX has been shown to increase lamivudine exposure).

No products indexed under this heading.

Tamoxifen Citrate (May increase the hematologic toxicity of zidovudine).

No products indexed under this heading.

Trimethoprim (Co-administration with TMP/SMX has been shown to increase lamivudine exposure).

No products indexed under this heading.

Vincristine Sulfate (May increase the hematologic toxicity of zidovudine).

No products indexed under this heading.

Zalacitabine (Lamivudine and zalacitabine may inhibit the intracellular phosphorylation of one another; combination therapy is not recommended).

No products indexed under this heading.

COMBUNOX TABLETS

(Ibuprofen, Oxycodone Hydrochloride) 1183

May interact with ACE inhibitors, anticholinergics, central nervous system depressants, anticoagulants, diuretics, general anesthetics, hypnotics and sedatives, monoamine oxidase inhibitors, mixed agonist/antagonist opioid analgesics, narcotic analgesics, neuromuscular blocking agents, phenothiazines, thiazides, tranquilizers, and certain other agents. Compounds in these categories include:

Alfentanil Hydrochloride (Patients receiving other CNS depressants (including alcohol) concomitantly with oxycodone may exhibit an additive CNS depression. Interactive effects resulting in respiratory depression, hypotension, profound sedation, or coma may result if these drugs are taken in combination with the usual dosage of oxycodone. When such combined therapy is contemplated, the dose of one or both agents should be reduced).

No products indexed under this heading.

Alprazolam (Patients receiving other CNS depressants (including alcohol) concomitantly with oxycodone may exhibit an additive CNS depression. Interactive effects resulting in respiratory depression, hypotension, profound sedation, or coma may result if these drugs are taken in combination with the usual dosage of oxycodone. When such combined therapy is contemplated, the dose of one or both agents should be reduced). Products include:

Niravam Orally Disintegrating Tablets 3106
Xanax XR Tablets 2655

Amiloride Hydrochloride (Ibuprofen has been shown to reduce the natriuretic effect of furosemide and thiazides in some patients. This response has been attributed to inhibition of renal prostaglandin synthesis. During concomitant therapy with Combunox the patient should be observed closely for signs of renal failure, as well as diuretic efficacy). Products include:

Midamor Tablets 2000
Moduretic Tablets 2003

Anisindione (Ibuprofen, like other NSAIDs, can inhibit platelet aggregation but the effect is quantitatively less and of shorter duration than that seen with aspirin. Ibuprofen has been shown to prolong bleeding time in normal subjects. Because this prolonged bleeding effect may be exaggerated in patients with underlying hemostatic defects, Combunox should be used with caution in persons on anticoagulant therapy). Products include:

Miradon Tablets 3056

Aprobarbital (Patients receiving other CNS depressants (including alcohol) concomitantly with oxycodone may exhibit an additive CNS depression. Interactive effects resulting in respiratory depression, hypotension, profound sedation, or coma may result if these drugs are taken in combination with the usual dosage of oxycodone. When such combined therapy is contemplated, the dose of one or both agents should be reduced).

No products indexed under this heading.

Ardeparin Sodium (Ibuprofen, like other NSAIDs, can inhibit platelet aggregation but the effect is quantitatively less and of shorter duration than that seen with aspirin. Ibuprofen has been shown to prolong bleeding time in normal subjects. Because this prolonged bleeding effect may be exaggerated in patients with underlying hemostatic defects, Combunox should be used with caution in persons on anticoagulant therapy).

No products indexed under this heading.

Aspirin (As with other products containing NSAIDs, concomitant administration of Combunox and aspirin is not generally recommended because of the potential of increased adverse effects. Combunox should not be given to patients who have experienced asthma, urticaria, or allergic-type reactions after taking aspirin). Products include:

Aggrenox Capsules 855
Bayer, Aspirin Regimen 606
Bayer Aspirin Tablets 3515
BC Powder 612
BC Allergy Sinus Cold Powder 612
Arthritis Strength BC Powder 612
BC Sinus Cold Powder 612
Ecotrin Enteric Coated Aspirin Low, Regular and Maximum Strength Tablets 1627
Goody's Body Pain Formula Powder 621
Goody's Extra Strength Headache Powder 621
Goody's Extra Strength Pain Relief Tablets 621
Percodan Tablets 1115
St. Joseph 81 mg Aspirin Chewable and Enteric Coated Tablets 1841

Aspirin, Enteric Coated (As with other products containing NSAIDs, concomitant administration of Combunox and aspirin is not generally recommended because of the potential of increased adverse effects. Combunox should not be given to patients who have experienced asthma, urticaria, or allergic-type reactions after taking aspirin).

No products indexed under this heading.

Aspirin Buffered (As with other products containing NSAIDs, concomitant administration of Combunox and aspirin is not generally recommended because of the potential of increased adverse effects. Combunox should not be given to patients who have experienced asthma, urticaria, or allergic-type reactions after taking aspirin).

No products indexed under this heading.

Atracurium Besylate (Oxycodone, as well as other opioid analgesics, may enhance the neuromuscular blocking action of skeletal muscle relaxants and produce an increased degree of respiratory depression).

No products indexed under this heading.

Atropine Sulfate (The concurrent use of anticholinergics with oxycodone preparations may produce paralytic ileus).

No products indexed under this heading.

Belladonna Alkaloids (The concurrent use of anticholinergics with oxycodone preparations may produce paralytic ileus). Products include:

Hyland's Teething Tablets 736

Benazepril Hydrochloride (Reports suggest that NSAIDs may diminish the antihypertensive effect of ACE-inhibitors. This interaction should be given consideration in patients taking Combunox concomitantly with ACE-inhibitors). Products include:

Lotensin Tablets 2232
Lotensin HCT Tablets 2235
Lotrel Capsules 2238

Bendroflumethiazide (Ibuprofen has been shown to reduce the natriuretic effect of furosemide and thiazides in some patients. This response has been attributed to inhibition of renal prostaglandin synthesis. During concomitant therapy with Combunox the patient should be observed closely for signs of renal failure, as well as diuretic efficacy).

No products indexed under this heading.

Benztropine Mesylate (The concurrent use of anticholinergics with oxycodone preparations may produce paralytic ileus). Products include:

Cogentin Injection 1903

Biperiden Hydrochloride (The concurrent use of anticholinergics with oxycodone preparations may produce paralytic ileus).

No products indexed under this heading.

Bumetanide (Ibuprofen has been shown to reduce the natriuretic effect of furosemide and thiazides in some patients. This response has been attributed to inhibition of renal prostaglandin synthesis. During concomitant therapy with Combunox the patient should be observed closely for signs of renal failure, as well as diuretic efficacy).

No products indexed under this heading.

Buprenorphine Hydrochloride (Patients receiving other CNS depressants (including alcohol) concomitantly with oxycodone may exhibit an additive CNS depression. Interactive effects resulting in respiratory depression, hypotension, profound sedation, or coma may result if these drugs are taken in combination with the usual dosage of oxycodone. When such combined therapy is contemplated, the dose of one or both agents should be reduced). Products include:

Buprenex Injectable 2718
Suboxone Tablets 2719
Subutex Tablets 2719

Buspirone Hydrochloride (Patients receiving other CNS depressants (including alcohol) concomitantly with oxycodone may exhibit an additive CNS depression. Interactive effects resulting in respiratory depression, hypotension, profound sedation, or coma may result if these drugs are taken in combination with the usual dosage of oxycodone. When such combined therapy is contemplated, the dose of one or both agents should be reduced).

No products indexed under this heading.

Butabarbital (Patients receiving other CNS depressants (including alcohol) concomitantly with oxycodone may exhibit an additive CNS depression. Interactive effects resulting in respiratory depression, hypotension, profound sedation, or coma may result if these drugs are taken in combination with the usual dosage of oxycodone. When such combined therapy is contemplated, the dose of one or both agents should be reduced).

No products indexed under this heading.

Butalbital (Patients receiving other CNS depressants (including alcohol) concomitantly with oxycodone may exhibit an additive CNS depression. Interactive effects resulting in respiratory depression, hypotension, profound sedation, or coma may result if these drugs are taken in combination with the usual dosage of oxycodone. When such combined therapy is contemplated, the dose of one or both agents should be reduced). Products include:

Sedapap Tablets 50 mg/650 mg 2098

Butorphanol Tartrate (Agonist/antagonist analgesics (eg., pentazocine, nalbuphine, butorphanol and buprenorphine) should be administered with caution to patients who have received or are receiving a course of therapy with a pure opioid agonist analgesic such as oxycodone. In this situation, mixed agonist/antagonist analgesics may reduce the analgesic effect of oxycodone and/or may precipitate withdrawal symptoms in these patients).

No products indexed under this heading.

Captopril (Reports suggest that NSAIDs may diminish the antihypertensive effect of ACE-inhibitors. This interaction should be given consideration in patients taking Combunox concomitantly with ACE-inhibitors). Products include:

Captopril Tablets **2114**

Chlordiazepoxide (Patients receiving other CNS depressants (including alcohol) concomitantly with oxycodone may exhibit an additive CNS depression. Interactive effects resulting in respiratory depression, hypotension, profound sedation, or coma may result if these drugs are taken in combination with the usual dosage of oxycodone. When such combined therapy is contemplated, the dose of one or both agents should be reduced).

No products indexed under this heading.

Chlordiazepoxide Hydrochloride (Patients receiving other CNS depressants (including alcohol) concomitantly with oxycodone may exhibit an additive CNS depression. Interactive effects resulting in respiratory depression, hypotension, profound sedation, or coma may result if these drugs are taken in combination with the usual dosage of oxycodone. When such combined therapy is contemplated, the dose of one or both agents should be reduced). Products include:

Librium Capsules **3349**

Chlorothiazide (Ibuprofen has been shown to reduce the natriuretic effect of furosemide and thiazides in some patients. This response has been attributed to inhibition of renal prostaglandin synthesis. During concomitant therapy with Combunox the patient should be observed closely for signs of renal failure, as well as diuretic efficacy). Products include:

Aldoclor Tablets **1881**
Diuril Oral **1936**

Chlorothiazide Sodium (Ibuprofen has been shown to reduce the natriuretic effect of furosemide and thiazides in some patients. This response has been attributed to inhibition of renal prostaglandin synthesis. During concomitant therapy with Combunox the patient should be observed closely for signs of renal failure, as well as diuretic efficacy). Products include:

Diuril Sodium Intravenous **1934**

Chlorpromazine (Patients receiving other CNS depressants (including alcohol) concomitantly with oxycodone may exhibit an additive CNS depression. Interactive effects resulting in respiratory depression, hypotension, profound sedation, or coma may result if these drugs are taken in combination with the usual dosage of oxycodone. When such combined therapy is contemplated, the dose of one or both agents should be reduced).

No products indexed under this heading.

Chlorpromazine Hydrochloride (Patients receiving other CNS depressants (including alcohol) concomitantly with oxycodone may exhibit an additive CNS depression. Interactive effects resulting in respiratory depression, hypotension, profound sedation, or coma may result if these drugs are taken in combination with the usual dosage of oxycodone. When such combined therapy is contemplated, the dose of one or both agents should be reduced).

No products indexed under this heading.

Chlorprothixene (Patients receiving other CNS depressants (including alcohol) concomitantly with oxycodone may exhibit an additive CNS depression. Interactive effects resulting in respiratory depression, hypotension, profound sedation, or coma may result if these drugs are taken in combination with the usual dosage of oxycodone. When such combined therapy is contemplated, the dose of one or both agents should be reduced).

No products indexed under this heading.

Chlorprothixene Hydrochloride (Patients receiving other CNS depressants (including alcohol) concomitantly with oxycodone may exhibit an additive CNS depression. Interactive effects resulting in respiratory depression, hypotension, profound sedation, or coma may result if these drugs are taken in combination with the usual dosage of oxycodone. When such combined therapy is contemplated, the dose of one or both agents should be reduced).

No products indexed under this heading.

Chlorprothixene Lactate (Patients receiving other CNS depressants (including alcohol) concomitantly with oxycodone may exhibit an additive CNS depression. Interactive effects resulting in respiratory depression, hypotension, profound sedation, or coma may result if these drugs are taken in combination with the usual dosage of oxycodone. When such combined therapy is contemplated, the dose of one or both agents should be reduced).

No products indexed under this heading.

Chlorthalidone (Ibuprofen has been shown to reduce the natriuretic effect of furosemide and thiazides in some patients. This response has been attributed to inhibition of renal prostaglandin synthesis. During concomitant therapy with Combunox the patient should be observed closely for signs of renal failure, as well as diuretic efficacy). Products include:

Clorpres Tablets **2139**

Cisatracurium Besylate (Oxycodone, as well as other opioid analgesics, may enhance the neuromuscular blocking action of skeletal muscle relaxants and produce an increased degree of respiratory depression). Products include:

Nimbex Injection **494**

Clidinium Bromide (The concurrent use of anticholinergics with oxycodone preparations may produce paralytic ileus).

No products indexed under this heading.

Clorazepate Dipotassium (Patients receiving other CNS depressants (including alcohol) concomitantly with oxycodone may exhibit an additive CNS depression. Interactive effects resulting in respiratory depression, hypotension, profound sedation, or coma may result if these drugs are taken in combination with the usual dosage of oxycodone. When such combined therapy is contemplated, the dose of one or both agents should be reduced). Products include:

Tranxene **2488**

Clozapine (Patients receiving other CNS depressants (including alcohol) concomitantly with oxycodone may exhibit an additive CNS depression. Interactive effects resulting in respiratory depression, hypotension, profound sedation, or coma may result if these drugs are taken in combination with the usual dosage of oxycodone. When such combined therapy is contemplated, the dose of one or both agents should be reduced). Products include:

Clozapine Tablets **2141**
Clozaril Tablets **2174**
FazaClo Orally Disintegrating Tablets **547**

Codeine Phosphate (Patients receiving other CNS depressants (including alcohol) concomitantly with oxycodone may exhibit an additive CNS depression. Interactive effects resulting in respiratory depression, hypotension, profound sedation, or coma may result if these drugs are taken in combination with the usual dosage of oxycodone. When such combined therapy is contemplated, the dose of one or both agents should be reduced). Products include:

Tylenol with Codeine **2461**

Dalteparin Sodium (Ibuprofen, like other NSAIDs, can inhibit platelet aggregation but the effect is quantitatively less and of shorter duration than that seen with aspirin. Ibuprofen has been shown to prolong bleeding time in normal subjects. Because this prolonged bleeding effect may be exaggerated in patients with underlying hemostatic defects, Combunox should be used with caution in persons on anticoagulant therapy). Products include:

Fragmin Injection **2638**

Danaparoid Sodium (Ibuprofen, like other NSAIDs, can inhibit platelet aggregation but the effect is quantitatively less and of shorter duration than that seen with aspirin. Ibuprofen has been shown to prolong bleeding time in normal subjects. Because this prolonged bleeding effect may be exaggerated in patients with underlying hemostatic defects, Combunox should be used with caution in persons on anticoagulant therapy).

No products indexed under this heading.

Desflurane (Patients receiving other CNS depressants (including alcohol) concomitantly with oxycodone may exhibit an additive CNS depression. Interactive effects resulting in respiratory depression, hypotension, profound sedation, or coma may result if these drugs are taken in combination with the usual dosage of oxycodone. When such combined therapy is contemplated, the dose of one or both agents should be reduced). Products include:

Suprane Liquid for Inhalation **770**

Dezocine (Patients receiving other CNS depressants (including alcohol) concomitantly with oxycodone may exhibit an additive CNS depression. Interactive effects resulting in respiratory depression, hypotension, profound sedation, or coma may result if these drugs are taken in combination with the usual dosage of oxycodone. When such combined therapy is contemplated, the dose of one or both agents should be reduced).

No products indexed under this heading.

Diazepam (Patients receiving other CNS depressants (including alcohol) concomitantly with oxycodone may exhibit an additive CNS depression. Interactive effects resulting in respiratory depression, hypotension, profound sedation, or coma may result if these drugs are taken in combination with the usual dosage of oxycodone. When such combined therapy is contemplated, the dose of one or both agents should be reduced). Products include:

Diastat Rectal Delivery System **3344**
Valium Tablets **2822**

Dicumarol (Ibuprofen, like other NSAIDs, can inhibit platelet aggregation but the effect is quantitatively less and of shorter duration than that seen with aspirin. Ibuprofen has been shown to prolong bleeding time in normal subjects. Because this prolonged bleeding effect may be exaggerated in patients with underlying hemostatic defects, Combunox should be used with caution in persons on anticoagulant therapy).

No products indexed under this heading.

Dicyclomine Hydrochloride (The concurrent use of anticholinergics with oxycodone preparations may produce paralytic ileus). Products include:

Bentyl Capsules **724**
Bentyl Injection **724**
Bentyl Syrup **724**
Bentyl Tablets **724**

Doxacurium Chloride (Oxycodone, as well as other opioid analgesics, may enhance the neuromuscular blocking action of skeletal muscle relaxants and produce an increased degree of respiratory depression).

No products indexed under this heading.

Droperidol (Patients receiving other CNS depressants (including alcohol) concomitantly with oxycodone may exhibit an additive CNS depression. Interactive effects resulting in respiratory depression, hypotension, profound sedation, or coma may result if these drugs are taken in combination with the usual dosage of oxycodone. When such combined therapy is contemplated, the dose of one or both agents should be reduced).

No products indexed under this heading.

Enalapril Maleate (Reports suggest that NSAIDs may diminish the antihypertensive effect of ACE-inhibitors. This interaction should be given consideration in patients taking Combunox concomitantly with ACE-inhibitors). Products include:

Vaseretic Tablets **2073**
Vasotec I.V. Injection **2076**

Enalaprilat (Reports suggest that NSAIDs may diminish the antihypertensive effect of ACE-inhibitors. This interaction should be given consideration in patients taking Combunox concomitantly with ACE-inhibitors).

No products indexed under this heading.

Enflurane (Patients receiving other CNS depressants (including alcohol) concomitantly with oxycodone may exhibit an additive CNS depression. Interactive effects resulting in respiratory depression, hypotension, pro-

found sedation, or coma may result if these drugs are taken in combination with the usual dosage of oxycodone. When such combined therapy is contemplated, the dose of one or both agents should be reduced).
No products indexed under this heading.

Enoxaparin Sodium (Ibuprofen, like other NSAIDs, can inhibit platelet aggregation but the effect is quantitatively less and of shorter duration than that seen with aspirin. Ibuprofen has been shown to prolong bleeding time in normal subjects. Because this prolonged bleeding effect may be exaggerated in patients with underlying hemostatic defects, Combunox should be used with caution in persons on anticoagulant therapy). Products include:
Lovenox Injection **2931**

Estazolam (Patients receiving other CNS depressants (including alcohol) concomitantly with oxycodone may exhibit an additive CNS depression. Interactive effects resulting in respiratory depression, hypotension, profound sedation, or coma may result if these drugs are taken in combination with the usual dosage of oxycodone. When such combined therapy is contemplated, the dose of one or both agents should be reduced). Products include:
ProSom Tablets **512**

Ethacrynic Acid (Ibuprofen has been shown to reduce the natriuretic effect of furosemide and thiazides in some patients. This response has been attributed to inhibition of renal prostaglandin synthesis. During concomitant therapy with Combunox the patient should be observed closely for signs of renal failure, as well as diuretic efficacy). Products include:
Edecrin Tablets **1941**

Ethanol (Patients receiving other CNS depressants (including alcohol) concomitantly with oxycodone may exhibit an additive CNS depression. Interactive effects resulting in respiratory depression, hypotension, profound sedation, or coma may result if these drugs are taken in combination with the usual dosage of oxycodone. When such combined therapy is contemplated, the dose of one or both agents should be reduced).
No products indexed under this heading.

Ethchlorvynol (Patients receiving other CNS depressants (including alcohol) concomitantly with oxycodone may exhibit an additive CNS depression. Interactive effects resulting in respiratory depression, hypotension, profound sedation, or coma may result if these drugs are taken in combination with the usual dosage of oxycodone. When such combined therapy is contemplated, the dose of one or both agents should be reduced).
No products indexed under this heading.

Ethinamate (Patients receiving other CNS depressants (including alcohol) concomitantly with oxycodone may exhibit an additive CNS depression. Interactive effects resulting in respiratory depression, hypotension, profound sedation, or coma may result if these drugs are taken in combination with the usual dosage of oxycodone. When such combined therapy is contemplated, the dose of one or both agents should be reduced).
No products indexed under this heading.

Ethyl Alcohol (Patients receiving other CNS depressants (including alcohol) concomitantly with oxycodone may exhibit an additive CNS depression. Interactive effects resulting in respiratory depression, hypotension, profound sedation, or coma may result if these drugs are taken in combination with the usual dosage of oxycodone. When such combined therapy is contemplated, the dose of one or both agents should be reduced).
No products indexed under this heading.

Fentanyl (Patients receiving other CNS depressants (including alcohol) concomitantly with oxycodone may exhibit an additive CNS depression. Interactive effects resulting in respiratory depression, hypotension, profound sedation, or coma may result if these drugs are taken in combination with the usual dosage of oxycodone. When such combined therapy is contemplated, the dose of one or both agents should be reduced). Products include:
Duragesic Transdermal System **2448**

Fentanyl Citrate (Patients receiving other CNS depressants (including alcohol) concomitantly with oxycodone may exhibit an additive CNS depression. Interactive effects resulting in respiratory depression, hypotension, profound sedation, or coma may result if these drugs are taken in combination with the usual dosage of oxycodone. When such combined therapy is contemplated, the dose of one or both agents should be reduced). Products include:
Actiq **993**

Fluphenazine Decanoate (Patients receiving other CNS depressants (including alcohol) concomitantly with oxycodone may exhibit an additive CNS depression. Interactive effects resulting in respiratory depression, hypotension, profound sedation, or coma may result if these drugs are taken in combination with the usual dosage of oxycodone. When such combined therapy is contemplated, the dose of one or both agents should be reduced).
No products indexed under this heading.

Fluphenazine Enanthate (Patients receiving other CNS depressants (including alcohol) concomitantly with oxycodone may exhibit an additive CNS depression. Interactive effects resulting in respiratory depression, hypotension, profound sedation, or coma may result if these drugs are taken in combination with the usual dosage of oxycodone. When such combined therapy is contemplated, the dose of one or both agents should be reduced).
No products indexed under this heading.

Fluphenazine Hydrochloride (Patients receiving other CNS depressants (including alcohol) concomitantly with oxycodone may exhibit an additive CNS depression. Interactive effects resulting in respiratory depression, hypotension, profound sedation, or coma may result if these drugs are taken in combination with the usual dosage of oxycodone. When such combined therapy is contemplated, the dose of one or both agents should be reduced).
No products indexed under this heading.

Flurazepam Hydrochloride (Patients receiving other CNS depressants (including alcohol) concomitantly with oxycodone may exhibit an additive CNS depression. Interactive effects resulting in respiratory depression, hypotension, profound sedation, or coma may result if these drugs are taken in combination with the usual dosage of oxycodone. When such combined therapy is contemplated, the dose of one or both agents should be reduced). Products include:
Dalmane Capsules **3343**

Fondaparinux Sodium (Ibuprofen, like other NSAIDs, can inhibit platelet aggregation but the effect is quantitatively less and of shorter duration than that seen with aspirin. Ibuprofen has been shown to prolong bleeding time in normal subjects. Because this prolonged bleeding effect may be exaggerated in patients with underlying hemostatic defects, Combunox should be used with caution in persons on anticoagulant therapy). Products include:
Arixtra Injection **1325**

Fosinopril Sodium (Reports suggest that NSAIDs may diminish the antihypertensive effect of ACE-inhibitors. This interaction should be given consideration in patients taking Combunox concomitantly with ACE-inhibitors).
No products indexed under this heading.

Furosemide (Ibuprofen has been shown to reduce the natriuretic effect of furosemide and thiazides in some patients. This response has been attributed to inhibition of renal prostaglandin synthesis. During concomitant therapy with Combunox the patient should be observed closely for signs of renal failure, as well as diuretic efficacy). Products include:
Furosemide Tablets **2117**

Glutethimide (Patients receiving other CNS depressants (including alcohol) concomitantly with oxycodone may exhibit an additive CNS depression. Interactive effects resulting in respiratory depression, hypotension, profound sedation, or coma may result if these drugs are taken in combination with the usual dosage of oxycodone. When such combined therapy is contemplated, the dose of one or both agents should be reduced).
No products indexed under this heading.

Glycopyrrolate (The concurrent use of anticholinergics with oxycodone preparations may produce paralytic ileus).
No products indexed under this heading.

Haloperidol (Patients receiving other CNS depressants (including alcohol) concomitantly with oxycodone may exhibit an additive CNS depression. Interactive effects resulting in respiratory depression, hypotension, profound sedation, or coma may result if these drugs are taken in combination with the usual dosage of oxycodone. When such combined therapy is contemplated, the dose of one or both agents should be reduced).
No products indexed under this heading.

Haloperidol Decanoate (Patients receiving other CNS depressants (including alcohol) concomitantly with oxycodone may exhibit an additive CNS depression. Interactive effects resulting in respiratory depression, hypotension, profound sedation, or coma may result if these drugs are taken in combination with the usual dosage of oxycodone. When such combined therapy is contemplated, the dose of one or both agents should be reduced).
No products indexed under this heading.

Heparin Calcium (Ibuprofen, like other NSAIDs, can inhibit platelet aggregation but the effect is quantitatively less and of shorter duration than that seen with aspirin. Ibuprofen has been shown to prolong bleeding time in normal subjects. Because this prolonged bleeding effect may be exaggerated in patients with underlying hemostatic defects, Combunox should be used with caution in persons on anticoagulant therapy).
No products indexed under this heading.

Heparin Sodium (Ibuprofen, like other NSAIDs, can inhibit platelet aggregation but the effect is quantitatively less and of shorter duration than that seen with aspirin. Ibuprofen has been shown to prolong bleeding time in normal subjects. Because this prolonged bleeding effect may be exaggerated in patients with underlying hemostatic defects, Combunox should be used with caution in persons on anticoagulant therapy).
No products indexed under this heading.

Hydrochlorothiazide (Ibuprofen has been shown to reduce the natriuretic effect of furosemide and thiazides in some patients. This response has been attributed to inhibition of renal prostaglandin synthesis. During concomitant therapy with Combunox the patient should be observed closely for signs of renal failure, as well as diuretic efficacy). Products include:
Aldoril Tablets **1884**
Atacand HCT **637**
Avalide Tablets **2889**
Avalide Tablets **922**
Benicar HCT Tablets **2852**
Diovan HCT Tablets **2195**
Dyazide Capsules **1389**
Hyzaar **1964**
Lotensin HCT Tablets **2235**
Maxzide **2150**
Micardis HCT Tablets **886**
Moduretic Tablets **2003**
Prinzide Tablets **2033**
Teveten HCT Tablets **1710**
Timolide Tablets **2056**
Uniretic Tablets **3114**
Vaseretic Tablets **2073**
Zestoretic Tablets **701**

Hydrocodone Bitartrate (Patients receiving other CNS depressants (including alcohol) concomitantly with oxycodone may exhibit an additive CNS depression. Interactive effects resulting in respiratory depression, hypotension, profound sedation, or coma may result if these drugs are taken in combination with the usual dosage of oxycodone. When such combined therapy is contemplated, the dose of one or both agents should be reduced). Products include:

Hycodan **1104**
Hycomine Compound Tablets **1105**
Hycotuss Expectorant Syrup **1106**
Lortab **3315**
Lortab Elixir **3312**
Vicodin Tablets **530**
Vicodin ES Tablets **531**
Vicodin HP Tablets **532**
Vicoprofen Tablets **533**
Zydone Tablets **1118**

Hydrocodone Polistirex (Patients receiving other CNS depressants (including alcohol) concomitantly with oxycodone may exhibit an additive CNS depression. Interactive effects resulting in respiratory depression, hypotension, profound sedation, or coma may result if these drugs are taken in combination with the usual dosage of oxycodone. When such combined therapy is contemplated, the dose of one or both agents should be reduced). Products include:
Tussionex Pennkinetic Extended-Release Suspension **3322**

Hydroflumethiazide (Ibuprofen has been shown to reduce the natriuretic effect of furosemide and thiazides in some patients. This response has been attributed to inhibition of renal prostaglandin synthesis. During concomitant therapy with Combunox the patient should be observed closely for signs of renal failure, as well as diuretic efficacy).
No products indexed under this heading.

Hydromorphone Hydrochloride (Patients receiving other CNS depressants (including alcohol) concomitantly with oxycodone may exhibit an additive CNS depression. Interactive effects resulting in respiratory depression, hypotension, profound sedation, or coma may result if these drugs are taken in combination with the usual dosage of oxycodone. When such combined therapy is contemplated, the dose of one or both agents should be reduced). Products include:
Dilaudid **439**
Dilaudid Oral Liquid **443**
Dilaudid Non-Sterile Powder **439**
Dilaudid Rectal Suppositories **439**
Dilaudid Tablets **439**
Dilaudid Tablets - 8 mg **443**
Dilaudid-HP **441**

Hydroxyzine Hydrochloride (Patients receiving other CNS depressants (including alcohol) concomitantly with oxycodone may exhibit an additive CNS depression. Interactive effects resulting in respiratory depression, hypotension, profound sedation, or coma may result if these drugs are taken in combination with the usual dosage of oxycodone. When such combined therapy is contemplated, the dose of one or both agents should be reduced).
No products indexed under this heading.

Hyoscyamine (The concurrent use of anticholinergics with oxycodone preparations may produce paralytic ileus).
No products indexed under this heading.

Hyoscyamine Sulfate (The concurrent use of anticholinergics with oxycodone preparations may produce paralytic ileus).
No products indexed under this heading.

Indapamide (Ibuprofen has been shown to reduce the natriuretic effect of furosemide and thiazides in some patients. This response has been attributed to inhibition of renal prostaglandin synthesis. During concomitant therapy with Combunox the patient should be observed closely for signs of renal failure, as well as diuretic efficacy). Products include:
Indapamide Tablets **2119**

Ipratropium Bromide (The concurrent use of anticholinergics with oxycodone preparations may produce paralytic ileus). Products include:
Atrovent HFA Inhalation Aerosol **872**
Atrovent Inhalation Solution **868**
Atrovent Nasal Spray 0.03% **869**
Atrovent Nasal Spray 0.06% **870**
Combivent Inhalation Aerosol **878**
DuoNeb Inhalation Solution **1058**

Isocarboxazid (Monoamine oxidase inhibitors (MAOIs) have been reported to intensify the effects of at least one opioid drug causing anxiety, confusion and significant depression of respiration or coma. The use of oxycodone is not recommended for patients taking MAOIs or within 14 days of stopping such treatment).
No products indexed under this heading.

Isoflurane (Patients receiving other CNS depressants (including alcohol) concomitantly with oxycodone may exhibit an additive CNS depression. Interactive effects resulting in respiratory depression, hypotension, profound sedation, or coma may result if these drugs are taken in combination with the usual dosage of oxycodone. When such combined therapy is contemplated, the dose of one or both agents should be reduced).
No products indexed under this heading.

Ketamine Hydrochloride (Patients receiving other CNS depressants (including alcohol) concomitantly with oxycodone may exhibit an additive CNS depression. Interactive effects resulting in respiratory depression, hypotension, profound sedation, or coma may result if these drugs are taken in combination with the usual dosage of oxycodone. When such combined therapy is contemplated, the dose of one or both agents should be reduced).
No products indexed under this heading.

Levomethadyl Acetate Hydrochloride (Patients receiving other CNS depressants (including alcohol) concomitantly with oxycodone may exhibit an additive CNS depression. Interactive effects resulting in respiratory depression, hypotension, profound sedation, or coma may result if these drugs are taken in combination with the usual dosage of oxycodone. When such combined therapy is contemplated, the dose of one or both agents should be reduced).
No products indexed under this heading.

Levorphanol Tartrate (Patients receiving other CNS depressants (including alcohol) concomitantly with oxycodone may exhibit an additive CNS depression. Interactive effects resulting in respiratory depression, hypotension, profound sedation, or coma may result if these drugs are taken in combination with the usual dosage of oxycodone. When such combined therapy is contemplated, the dose of one or both agents should be reduced).
No products indexed under this heading.

Lisinopril (Reports suggest that NSAIDs may diminish the antihypertensive effect of ACE-inhibitors. This interaction should be given consideration in patients taking Combunox concomitantly with ACE-inhibitors). Products include:
Prinivil Tablets **2029**
Prinzide Tablets **2033**
Zestoretic Tablets **701**
Zestril Tablets **704**

Lithium (Ibuprofen has been shown to elevate plasma lithium concentration and reduce renal lithium clearance. This effect has been attributed to inhibition of renal prostaglandin synthesis by ibuprofen. Thus, when Combunox and lithium are administered concurrently, patients should be observed for signs of lithium toxicity).
No products indexed under this heading.

Lithium Carbonate (Ibuprofen has been shown to elevate plasma lithium concentration and reduce renal lithium clearance. This effect has been attributed to inhibition of renal prostaglandin synthesis by ibuprofen. Thus, when Combunox and lithium are administered concurrently, patients should be observed for signs of lithium toxicity). Products include:
Eskalith **1406**
Lithobid Tablets **1670**

Lithium Citrate (Ibuprofen has been shown to elevate plasma lithium concentration and reduce renal lithium clearance. This effect has been attributed to inhibition of renal prostaglandin synthesis by ibuprofen. Thus, when Combunox and lithium are administered concurrently, patients should be observed for signs of lithium toxicity).
No products indexed under this heading.

Lorazepam (Patients receiving other CNS depressants (including alcohol) concomitantly with oxycodone may exhibit an additive CNS depression. Interactive effects resulting in respiratory depression, hypotension, profound sedation, or coma may result if these drugs are taken in combination with the usual dosage of oxycodone. When such combined therapy is contemplated, the dose of one or both agents should be reduced).
No products indexed under this heading.

Low Molecular Weight Heparins (Ibuprofen, like other NSAIDs, can inhibit platelet aggregation but the effect is quantitatively less and of shorter duration than that seen with aspirin. Ibuprofen has been shown to prolong bleeding time in normal subjects. Because this prolonged bleeding effect may be exaggerated in patients with underlying hemostatic defects, Combunox should be used with caution in persons on anticoagulant therapy).
No products indexed under this heading.

Loxapine Hydrochloride (Patients receiving other CNS depressants (including alcohol) concomitantly with oxycodone may exhibit an additive CNS depression. Interactive effects resulting in respiratory depression, hypotension, profound sedation, or coma may result if these drugs are taken in combination with the usual dosage of oxycodone. When such combined therapy is contemplated, the dose of one or both agents should be reduced).
No products indexed under this heading.

Loxapine Succinate (Patients receiving other CNS depressants (including alcohol) concomitantly with oxycodone may exhibit an additive CNS depression. Interactive effects resulting in respiratory depression, hypotension, profound sedation, or coma may result if these drugs are taken in combination with the usual dosage of oxycodone. When such combined therapy is contemplated, the dose of one or both agents should be reduced).
No products indexed under this heading.

Mepenzolate Bromide (The concurrent use of anticholinergics with oxycodone preparations may produce paralytic ileus).
No products indexed under this heading.

Meperidine Hydrochloride (Patients receiving other CNS depressants (including alcohol) concomitantly with oxycodone may exhibit an additive CNS depression. Interactive effects resulting in respiratory depression, hypotension, profound sedation, or coma may result if these drugs are taken in combination with the usual dosage of oxycodone. When such combined therapy is contemplated, the dose of one or both agents should be reduced).
No products indexed under this heading.

Mephobarbital (Patients receiving other CNS depressants (including alcohol) concomitantly with oxycodone may exhibit an additive CNS depression. Interactive effects resulting in respiratory depression, hypotension, profound sedation, or coma may result if these drugs are taken in combination with the usual dosage of oxycodone. When such combined therapy is contemplated, the dose of one or both agents should be reduced). Products include:
Mebaral Tablets, USP **2483**

Meprobamate (Patients receiving other CNS depressants (including alcohol) concomitantly with oxycodone may exhibit an additive CNS depression. Interactive effects resulting in respiratory depression, hypotension, profound sedation, or coma may result if these drugs are taken in combination with the usual dosage of oxycodone. When such combined therapy is contemplated, the dose of one or both agents should be reduced).
No products indexed under this heading.

Mesoridazine Besylate (Patients receiving other CNS depressants (including alcohol) concomitantly with oxycodone may exhibit an additive CNS depression. Interactive effects resulting in respiratory depression, hypotension, profound sedation, or coma may result if these drugs are taken in combination with the usual dosage of oxycodone. When such combined therapy is contemplated, the dose of one

or both agents should be reduced).
No products indexed under this heading.

Methadone Hydrochloride (Patients receiving other CNS depressants (including alcohol) concomitantly with oxycodone may exhibit an additive CNS depression. Interactive effects resulting in respiratory depression, hypotension, profound sedation, or coma may result if these drugs are taken in combination with the usual dosage of oxycodone. When such combined therapy is contemplated, the dose of one or both agents should be reduced).
No products indexed under this heading.

Methohexital Sodium (Patients receiving other CNS depressants (including alcohol) concomitantly with oxycodone may exhibit an additive CNS depression. Interactive effects resulting in respiratory depression, hypotension, profound sedation, or coma may result if these drugs are taken in combination with the usual dosage of oxycodone. When such combined therapy is contemplated, the dose of one or both agents should be reduced).
No products indexed under this heading.

Methotrexate (Ibuprofen, as well as other NSAIDs, has been reported to competitively inhibit methotrexate accumulation in rabbit kidney slices. This may indicate that ibuprofen could enhance the toxicity of methotrexate. Caution should be used when Combunox is administered concomitantly with methotrexate).
No products indexed under this heading.

Methotrexate Sodium (Ibuprofen, as well as other NSAIDs, has been reported to competitively inhibit methotrexate accumulation in rabbit kidney slices. This may indicate that ibuprofen could enhance the toxicity of methotrexate. Caution should be used when Combunox is administered concomitantly with methotrexate).
No products indexed under this heading.

Methotrimeprazine (Patients receiving other CNS depressants (including alcohol) concomitantly with oxycodone may exhibit an additive CNS depression. Interactive effects resulting in respiratory depression, hypotension, profound sedation, or coma may result if these drugs are taken in combination with the usual dosage of oxycodone. When such combined therapy is contemplated, the dose of one or both agents should be reduced).
No products indexed under this heading.

Methoxyflurane (Patients receiving other CNS depressants (including alcohol) concomitantly with oxycodone may exhibit an additive CNS depression. Interactive effects resulting in respiratory depression, hypotension, profound sedation, or coma may result if these drugs are taken in combination with the usual dosage of oxycodone. When such combined therapy is contemplated, the dose of one or both agents should be reduced).
No products indexed under this heading.

Methyclothiazide (Ibuprofen has been shown to reduce the natriuretic effect of furosemide and thiazides in some patients. This response has been attributed to inhibition of renal prostaglandin synthesis. During concomitant therapy with Combunox the patient should be observed closely for signs of renal failure, as well as diuretic efficacy).
No products indexed under this heading.

Metocurine Iodide (Oxycodone, as well as other opioid analgesics, may enhance the neuromuscular blocking action of skeletal muscle relaxants and produce an increased degree of respiratory depression).
No products indexed under this heading.

Metolazone (Ibuprofen has been shown to reduce the natriuretic effect of furosemide and thiazides in some patients. This response has been attributed to inhibition of renal prostaglandin synthesis. During concomitant therapy with Combunox the patient should be observed closely for signs of renal failure, as well as diuretic efficacy).
No products indexed under this heading.

Midazolam Hydrochloride (Patients receiving other CNS depressants (including alcohol) concomitantly with oxycodone may exhibit an additive CNS depression. Interactive effects resulting in respiratory depression, hypotension, profound sedation, or coma may result if these drugs are taken in combination with the usual dosage of oxycodone. When such combined therapy is contemplated, the dose of one or both agents should be reduced).
No products indexed under this heading.

Mivacurium Chloride (Oxycodone, as well as other opioid analgesics, may enhance the neuromuscular blocking action of skeletal muscle relaxants and produce an increased degree of respiratory depression). Products include:
Mivacron Injection 489

Moclobemide (Monoamine oxidase inhibitors (MAOIs) have been reported to intensify the effects of at least one opioid drug causing anxiety, confusion and significant depression of respiration or coma. The use of oxycodone is not recommended for patients taking MAOIs or within 14 days of stopping such treatment).
No products indexed under this heading.

Moexipril Hydrochloride (Reports suggest that NSAIDs may diminish the antihypertensive effect of ACE-inhibitors. This interaction should be given consideration in patients taking Combunox concomitantly with ACE-inhibitors). Products include:
Uniretic Tablets 3114
Univasc Tablets 3118

Molindone Hydrochloride (Patients receiving other CNS depressants (including alcohol) concomitantly with oxycodone may exhibit an additive CNS depression. Interactive effects resulting in respiratory depression, hypotension, profound sedation, or coma may result if these drugs are taken in combination with the usual dosage of oxycodone. When such combined therapy is contemplated, the dose of one or both agents should be reduced). Products include:
Moban Tablets 1108

Morphine Sulfate (Patients receiving other CNS depressants (including alcohol) concomitantly with oxycodone may exhibit an additive CNS depression. Interactive effects resulting in respiratory depression, hypotension, profound sedation, or coma may result if these drugs are taken in combination with the usual dosage of oxycodone. When such combined therapy is contemplated, the dose of one or both agents should be reduced). Products include:
Avinza Capsules 1714
Kadian Capsules 572
MS Contin Tablets 2703

Nalbuphine Hydrochloride (Agonist/antagonist analgesics (eg., pentazocine, nalbuphine, butorphanol and buprenorphine) should be administered with caution to patients who have received or are receiving a course of therapy with a pure opioid agonist analgesic such as oxycodone. In this situation, mixed agonist/antagonist analgesics may reduce the analgesic effect of oxycodone and/or may precipitate withdrawal symptoms in these patients). Products include:
Nubain Injection 1111

Olanzapine (Patients receiving other CNS depressants (including alcohol) concomitantly with oxycodone may exhibit an additive CNS depression. Interactive effects resulting in respiratory depression, hypotension, profound sedation, or coma may result if these drugs are taken in combination with the usual dosage of oxycodone. When such combined therapy is contemplated, the dose of one or both agents should be reduced). Products include:
Symbyax Capsules 1788
Zyprexa Tablets 1798
Zyprexa IntraMuscular 1798
Zyprexa ZYDIS Orally Disintegrating Tablets 1798

Oxazepam (Patients receiving other CNS depressants (including alcohol) concomitantly with oxycodone may exhibit an additive CNS depression. Interactive effects resulting in respiratory depression, hypotension, profound sedation, or coma may result if these drugs are taken in combination with the usual dosage of oxycodone. When such combined therapy is contemplated, the dose of one or both agents should be reduced).
No products indexed under this heading.

Oxybutynin Chloride (The concurrent use of anticholinergics with oxycodone preparations may produce paralytic ileus). Products include:
Ditropan XL Extended Release Tablets 2391

Pancuronium Bromide (Oxycodone, as well as other opioid analgesics, may enhance the neuromuscular blocking action of skeletal muscle relaxants and produce an increased degree of respiratory depression).
No products indexed under this heading.

Pargyline Hydrochloride (Monoamine oxidase inhibitors (MAOIs) have been reported to intensify the effects of at least one opioid drug causing anxiety, confusion and significant depression of respiration or coma. The use of oxycodone is not recommended for patients taking MAOIs or within 14 days of stopping such treatment).
No products indexed under this heading.

Pentazocine Hydrochloride (Agonist/antagonist analgesics (eg., pentazocine, nalbuphine, butorphanol and buprenorphine) should be administered with caution to patients who have received or are receiving a course of therapy with a pure opioid agonist analgesic such as oxycodone. In this situation, mixed agonist/antagonist analgesics may reduce the analgesic effect of oxycodone and/or may precipitate withdrawal symptoms in these patients).
No products indexed under this heading.

Pentazocine Lactate (Agonist/antagonist analgesics (eg., pentazocine, nalbuphine, butorphanol and buprenorphine) should be administered with caution to patients who have received or are receiving a course of therapy with a pure opioid agonist analgesic such as oxycodone. In this situation, mixed agonist/antagonist analgesics may reduce the analgesic effect of oxycodone and/or may precipitate withdrawal symptoms in these patients).
No products indexed under this heading.

Pentobarbital Sodium (Patients receiving other CNS depressants (including alcohol) concomitantly with oxycodone may exhibit an additive CNS depression. Interactive effects resulting in respiratory depression, hypotension, profound sedation, or coma may result if these drugs are taken in combination with the usual dosage of oxycodone. When such combined therapy is contemplated, the dose of one or both agents should be reduced). Products include:
Nembutal Sodium Solution, USP 2484

Perindopril Erbumine (Reports suggest that NSAIDs may diminish the antihypertensive effect of ACE-inhibitors. This interaction should be given consideration in patients taking Combunox concomitantly with ACE-inhibitors). Products include:
Aceon Tablets (2 mg, 4 mg, 8 mg) 3191

Perphenazine (Patients receiving other CNS depressants (including alcohol) concomitantly with oxycodone may exhibit an additive CNS depression. Interactive effects resulting in respiratory depression, hypotension, profound sedation, or coma may result if these drugs are taken in combination with the usual dosage of oxycodone. When such combined therapy is contemplated, the dose of one or both agents should be reduced).
No products indexed under this heading.

Phenelzine Sulfate (Monoamine oxidase inhibitors (MAOIs) have been reported to intensify the effects of at least one opioid drug causing anxiety, confusion and significant depression of respiration or coma. The use of oxycodone is not recommended for patients taking MAOIs or within 14 days of stopping such treatment).

No products indexed under this heading.

Phenobarbital (Patients receiving other CNS depressants (including alcohol) concomitantly with oxycodone may exhibit an additive CNS depression. Interactive effects resulting in respiratory depression, hypotension, profound sedation, or coma may result if these drugs are taken in combination with the usual dosage of oxycodone. When such combined therapy is contemplated, the dose of one or both agents should be reduced).

No products indexed under this heading.

Polythiazide (Ibuprofen has been shown to reduce the natriuretic effect of furosemide and thiazides in some patients. This response has been attributed to inhibition of renal prostaglandin synthesis. During concomitant therapy with Combunox the patient should be observed closely for signs of renal failure, as well as diuretic efficacy).

No products indexed under this heading.

Prazepam (Patients receiving other CNS depressants (including alcohol) concomitantly with oxycodone may exhibit an additive CNS depression. Interactive effects resulting in respiratory depression, hypotension, profound sedation, or coma may result if these drugs are taken in combination with the usual dosage of oxycodone. When such combined therapy is contemplated, the dose of one or both agents should be reduced).

No products indexed under this heading.

Procarbazine Hydrochloride (Monoamine oxidase inhibitors (MAOIs) have been reported to intensify the effects of at least one opioid drug causing anxiety, confusion and significant depression of respiration or coma. The use of oxycodone is not recommended for patients taking MAOIs or within 14 days of stopping such treatment). Products include:

Matulane Capsules 3188

Prochlorperazine (Patients receiving other CNS depressants (including alcohol) concomitantly with oxycodone may exhibit an additive CNS depression. Interactive effects resulting in respiratory depression, hypotension, profound sedation, or coma may result if these drugs are taken in combination with the usual dosage of oxycodone. When such combined therapy is contemplated, the dose of one or both agents should be reduced).

No products indexed under this heading.

Procyclidine Hydrochloride (The concurrent use of anticholinergics with oxycodone preparations may produce paralytic ileus).

No products indexed under this heading.

Promethazine Hydrochloride (Patients receiving other CNS depressants (including alcohol) concomitantly with oxycodone may exhibit an additive CNS depression. Interactive effects resulting in respiratory depression, hypotension, profound sedation, or coma may result if these drugs are taken in combination with the usual dosage of oxycodone. When such combined therapy is contemplated, the dose of one or both agents should be reduced). Products include:

Phenergan 3438

Propantheline Bromide (The concurrent use of anticholinergics with oxycodone preparations may produce paralytic ileus).

No products indexed under this heading.

Propofol (Patients receiving other CNS depressants (including alcohol) concomitantly with oxycodone may exhibit an additive CNS depression. Interactive effects resulting in respiratory depression, hypotension, profound sedation, or coma may result if these drugs are taken in combination with the usual dosage of oxycodone. When such combined therapy is contemplated, the dose of one or both agents should be reduced). Products include:

Diprivan Injectable Emulsion 676

Propoxyphene Hydrochloride (Patients receiving other CNS depressants (including alcohol) concomitantly with oxycodone may exhibit an additive CNS depression. Interactive effects resulting in respiratory depression, hypotension, profound sedation, or coma may result if these drugs are taken in combination with the usual dosage of oxycodone. When such combined therapy is contemplated, the dose of one or both agents should be reduced).

No products indexed under this heading.

Propoxyphene Napsylate (Patients receiving other CNS depressants (including alcohol) concomitantly with oxycodone may exhibit an additive CNS depression. Interactive effects resulting in respiratory depression, hypotension, profound sedation, or coma may result if these drugs are taken in combination with the usual dosage of oxycodone. When such combined therapy is contemplated, the dose of one or both agents should be reduced). Products include:

Darvocet A 500 Tablets 3497

Quazepam (Patients receiving other CNS depressants (including alcohol) concomitantly with oxycodone may exhibit an additive CNS depression. Interactive effects resulting in respiratory depression, hypotension, profound sedation, or coma may result if these drugs are taken in combination with the usual dosage of oxycodone. When such combined therapy is contemplated, the dose of one or both agents should be reduced).

No products indexed under this heading.

Quetiapine Fumarate (Patients receiving other CNS depressants (including alcohol) concomitantly with oxycodone may exhibit an additive CNS depression. Interactive effects resulting in respiratory depression, hypotension, profound sedation, or coma may result if these drugs are taken in combination with the usual dosage of oxycodone. When such combined therapy is contemplated, the dose of one or both agents should be reduced). Products include:

Seroquel Tablets 691

Quinapril Hydrochloride (Reports suggest that NSAIDs may diminish the antihypertensive effect of ACE-inhibitors. This interaction should be given consideration in patients taking Combunox concomitantly with ACE-inhibitors).

No products indexed under this heading.

Ramipril (Reports suggest that NSAIDs may diminish the antihypertensive effect of ACE-inhibitors. This interaction should be given consideration in patients taking Combunox concomitantly with ACE-inhibitors). Products include:

Altace Capsules 1673

Rapacuronium Bromide (Oxycodone, as well as other opioid analgesics, may enhance the neuromuscular blocking action of skeletal muscle relaxants and produce an increased degree of respiratory depression).

No products indexed under this heading.

Remifentanil Hydrochloride (Patients receiving other CNS depressants (including alcohol) concomitantly with oxycodone may exhibit an additive CNS depression. Interactive effects resulting in respiratory depression, hypotension, profound sedation, or coma may result if these drugs are taken in combination with the usual dosage of oxycodone. When such combined therapy is contemplated, the dose of one or both agents should be reduced).

No products indexed under this heading.

Risperidone (Patients receiving other CNS depressants (including alcohol) concomitantly with oxycodone may exhibit an additive CNS depression. Interactive effects resulting in respiratory depression, hypotension, profound sedation, or coma may result if these drugs are taken in combination with the usual dosage of oxycodone. When such combined therapy is contemplated, the dose of one or both agents should be reduced). Products include:

Risperdal Consta Long-Acting Injection 1664
Risperdal M-Tab Orally Disintegrating Tablets 1658
Risperdal 1658

Rocuronium Bromide (Oxycodone, as well as other opioid analgesics, may enhance the neuromuscular blocking action of skeletal muscle relaxants and produce an increased degree of respiratory depression). Products include:

Zemuron Injection 2363

Scopolamine (The concurrent use of anticholinergics with oxycodone preparations may produce paralytic ileus). Products include:

Transderm Scōp Transdermal Therapeutic System 2166

Scopolamine Hydrobromide (The concurrent use of anticholinergics with oxycodone preparations may produce paralytic ileus).

No products indexed under this heading.

Secobarbital Sodium (Patients receiving other CNS depressants (including alcohol) concomitantly with oxycodone may exhibit an additive CNS depression. Interactive effects resulting in respiratory depression, hypotension, profound sedation, or coma may result if these drugs are taken in combination with the usual dosage of oxycodone. When such combined therapy is contemplated, the dose of one or both agents should be reduced).

No products indexed under this heading.

Selegiline Hydrochloride (Monoamine oxidase inhibitors (MAOIs) have been reported to intensify the effects of at least one opioid drug causing anxiety, confusion and significant depression of respiration or coma. The use of oxycodone is not recommended for patients taking MAOIs or within 14 days of stopping such treatment). Products include:

Eldepryl Capsules 3209

Sevoflurane (Patients receiving other CNS depressants (including alcohol) concomitantly with oxycodone may exhibit an additive CNS depression. Interactive effects resulting in respiratory depression, hypotension, profound sedation, or coma may result if these drugs are taken in combination with the usual dosage of oxycodone. When such combined therapy is contemplated, the dose of one or both agents should be reduced). Products include:

Ultane Liquid for Inhalation 526

Sodium Oxybate (Patients receiving other CNS depressants (including alcohol) concomitantly with oxycodone may exhibit an additive CNS depression. Interactive effects resulting in respiratory depression, hypotension, profound sedation, or coma may result if these drugs are taken in combination with the usual dosage of oxycodone. When such combined therapy is contemplated, the dose of one or both agents should be reduced).

No products indexed under this heading.

Spirapril Hydrochloride (Reports suggest that NSAIDs may diminish the antihypertensive effect of ACE-inhibitors. This interaction should be given consideration in patients taking Combunox concomitantly with ACE-inhibitors).

No products indexed under this heading.

Spironolactone (Ibuprofen has been shown to reduce the natriuretic effect of furosemide and thiazides in some patients. This response has been attributed to inhibition of renal prostaglandin synthesis. During concomitant therapy with Combunox the patient should be observed closely for signs of renal failure, as well as diuretic efficacy).

No products indexed under this heading.

Succinylcholine Chloride (Oxycodone, as well as other opioid analgesics, may enhance the neuromuscular blocking action of skeletal muscle relaxants and produce an increased degree of respiratory depression).

No products indexed under this heading.

Sufentanil Citrate (Patients receiving other CNS depressants (includ-

ing alcohol) concomitantly with oxycodone may exhibit an additive CNS depression. Interactive effects resulting in respiratory depression, hypotension, profound sedation, or coma may result if these drugs are taken in combination with the usual dosage of oxycodone. When such combined therapy is contemplated, the dose of one or both agents should be reduced).
No products indexed under this heading.

Temazepam (Patients receiving other CNS depressants (including alcohol) concomitantly with oxycodone may exhibit an additive CNS depression. Interactive effects resulting in respiratory depression, hypotension, profound sedation, or coma may result if these drugs are taken in combination with the usual dosage of oxycodone. When such combined therapy is contemplated, the dose of one or both agents should be reduced).
No products indexed under this heading.

Thiamylal Sodium (Patients receiving other CNS depressants (including alcohol) concomitantly with oxycodone may exhibit an additive CNS depression. Interactive effects resulting in respiratory depression, hypotension, profound sedation, or coma may result if these drugs are taken in combination with the usual dosage of oxycodone. When such combined therapy is contemplated, the dose of one or both agents should be reduced).
No products indexed under this heading.

Thioridazine Hydrochloride (Patients receiving other CNS depressants (including alcohol) concomitantly with oxycodone may exhibit an additive CNS depression. Interactive effects resulting in respiratory depression, hypotension, profound sedation, or coma may result if these drugs are taken in combination with the usual dosage of oxycodone. When such combined therapy is contemplated, the dose of one or both agents should be reduced). Products include:
Thioridazine Hydrochloride Tablets **2122**

Thiothixene (Patients receiving other CNS depressants (including alcohol) concomitantly with oxycodone may exhibit an additive CNS depression. Interactive effects resulting in respiratory depression, hypotension, profound sedation, or coma may result if these drugs are taken in combination with the usual dosage of oxycodone. When such combined therapy is contemplated, the dose of one or both agents should be reduced). Products include:
Thiothixene Capsules **2124**

Tinzaparin Sodium (Ibuprofen, like other NSAIDs, can inhibit platelet aggregation but the effect is quantitatively less and of shorter duration than that seen with aspirin. Ibuprofen has been shown to prolong bleeding time in normal subjects. Because this prolonged bleeding effect may be exaggerated in patients with underlying hemostatic defects, Combunox should be used with caution in persons on anticoagulant therapy).
No products indexed under this heading.

Tolterodine Tartrate (The concurrent use of anticholinergics with oxycodone preparations may produce paralytic ileus). Products include:
Detrol Tablets **2626**
Detrol LA Capsules **2629**

Torsemide (Ibuprofen has been shown to reduce the natriuretic effect of furosemide and thiazides in some patients. This response has been attributed to inhibition of renal prostaglandin synthesis. During concomitant therapy with Combunox the patient should be observed closely for signs of renal failure, as well as diuretic efficacy).
No products indexed under this heading.

Trandolapril (Reports suggest that NSAIDs may diminish the antihypertensive effect of ACE-inhibitors. This interaction should be given consideration in patients taking Combunox concomitantly with ACE-inhibitors). Products include:
Mavik Tablets **482**
Tarka Tablets **519**

Tranylcypromine Sulfate (Monoamine oxidase inhibitors (MAOIs) have been reported to intensify the effects of at least one opioid drug causing anxiety, confusion and significant depression of respiration or coma. The use of oxycodone is not recommended for patients taking MAOIs or within 14 days of stopping such treatment). Products include:
Parnate Tablets **1499**

Triamterene (Ibuprofen has been shown to reduce the natriuretic effect of furosemide and thiazides in some patients. This response has been attributed to inhibition of renal prostaglandin synthesis. During concomitant therapy with Combunox the patient should be observed closely for signs of renal failure, as well as diuretic efficacy). Products include:
Dyazide Capsules **1389**
Dyrenium Capsules **3390**
Maxzide **2150**

Triazolam (Patients receiving other CNS depressants (including alcohol) concomitantly with oxycodone may exhibit an additive CNS depression. Interactive effects resulting in respiratory depression, hypotension, profound sedation, or coma may result if these drugs are taken in combination with the usual dosage of oxycodone. When such combined therapy is contemplated, the dose of one or both agents should be reduced).
No products indexed under this heading.

Tridihexethyl Chloride (The concurrent use of anticholinergics with oxycodone preparations may produce paralytic ileus).
No products indexed under this heading.

Trifluoperazine Hydrochloride (Patients receiving other CNS depressants (including alcohol) concomitantly with oxycodone may exhibit an additive CNS depression. Interactive effects resulting in respiratory depression, hypotension, profound sedation, or coma may result if these drugs are taken in combination with the usual dosage of oxycodone. When such combined therapy is contemplated, the dose of one or both agents should be reduced).
No products indexed under this heading.

Trihexyphenidyl Hydrochloride (The concurrent use of anticholinergics with oxycodone preparations may produce paralytic ileus).
No products indexed under this heading.

Vecuronium Bromide (Oxycodone, as well as other opioid analgesics, may enhance the neuromuscular blocking action of skeletal muscle relaxants and produce an increased degree of respiratory depression).
No products indexed under this heading.

Warfarin Sodium (Ibuprofen, like other NSAIDs, can inhibit platelet aggregation but the effect is quantitatively less and of shorter duration than that seen with aspirin. Ibuprofen has been shown to prolong bleeding time in normal subjects. Because this prolonged bleeding effect may be exaggerated in patients with underlying hemostatic defects, Combunox should be used with caution in persons on anticoagulant therapy. The effects of warfarin and NSAIDs on GI bleeding are synergistic, such that users of both drugs together have a greater risk of serious GI bleeding than users of either drug alone). Products include:
Coumadin for Injection **932**
Coumadin Tablets **932**

Zaleplon (Patients receiving other CNS depressants (including alcohol) concomitantly with oxycodone may exhibit an additive CNS depression. Interactive effects resulting in respiratory depression, hypotension, profound sedation, or coma may result if these drugs are taken in combination with the usual dosage of oxycodone. When such combined therapy is contemplated, the dose of one or both agents should be reduced). Products include:
Sonata Capsules **1686**

Ziprasidone Hydrochloride (Patients receiving other CNS depressants (including alcohol) concomitantly with oxycodone may exhibit an additive CNS depression. Interactive effects resulting in respiratory depression, hypotension, profound sedation, or coma may result if these drugs are taken in combination with the usual dosage of oxycodone. When such combined therapy is contemplated, the dose of one or both agents should be reduced). Products include:
Geodon Capsules **2514**

Zolpidem Tartrate (Patients receiving other CNS depressants (including alcohol) concomitantly with oxycodone may exhibit an additive CNS depression. Interactive effects resulting in respiratory depression, hypotension, profound sedation, or coma may result if these drugs are taken in combination with the usual dosage of oxycodone. When such combined therapy is contemplated, the dose of one or both agents should be reduced). Products include:
Ambien Tablets **2867**

Food Interactions

Alcohol (Patients receiving other CNS depressants (including alcohol) concomitantly with oxycodone may exhibit an additive CNS depression. Interactive effects resulting in respiratory depression, hypotension, profound sedation, or coma may result if these drugs are taken in combination with the usual dosage of oxycodone. When such combined therapy is contemplated, the dose of one or both agents should be reduced).

COMMIT LOZENGES

(Nicotine Polacrilex) **1625**
May interact with asthma medications and antidepressant drugs. Compounds in these categories include:

Albuterol (Concurrent use with prescription asthma medications should be undertaken under physician's or pharmacist's supervision because the dose may need to be adjusted). Products include:
Proventil Inhalation Aerosol **3067**

Albuterol Sulfate (Concurrent use with prescription asthma medications should be undertaken under physician's or pharmacist's supervision because the dose may need to be adjusted). Products include:
AccuNeb Inhalation Solution **1055**
Combivent Inhalation Aerosol **878**
DuoNeb Inhalation Solution **1058**
Proventil Inhalation Solution 0.083% **3069**
Proventil HFA Inhalation Aerosol **3071**
Ventolin HFA Inhalation Aerosol **1576**
VoSpire Extended-Release Tablets **2352**

Amitriptyline Hydrochloride (Concurrent use with antidepressant medications should be undertaken under physician's or pharmacist's supervision because the dose may need to be adjusted).
No products indexed under this heading.

Amoxapine (Concurrent use with antidepressant medications should be undertaken under physician's or pharmacist's supervision because the dose may need to be adjusted).
No products indexed under this heading.

Bitolterol Mesylate (Concurrent use with prescription asthma medications should be undertaken under physician's or pharmacist's supervision because the dose may need to be adjusted).
No products indexed under this heading.

Bupropion Hydrochloride (Concurrent use with antidepressant medications should be undertaken under physician's or pharmacist's supervision because the dose may need to be adjusted). Products include:
Wellbutrin Tablets **1579**
Wellbutrin SR Sustained-Release Tablets **1583**
Wellbutrin XL Extended-Release Tablets **1588**
Zyban Sustained-Release Tablets **1620**

Citalopram Hydrobromide (Concurrent use with antidepressant medications should be undertaken under physician's or pharmacist's supervision because the dose may need to be adjusted). Products include:
Celexa **1177**

Desipramine Hydrochloride (Concurrent use with antidepressant medications should be undertaken under physician's or pharmacist's supervision because the dose may need to be adjusted).
No products indexed under this heading.

Doxepin Hydrochloride (Concurrent use with antidepressant medications should be undertaken under physician's or pharmacist's supervision because the dose may need to be adjusted).
No products indexed under this heading.

Ephedrine Hydrochloride (Concurrent use with prescription asthma medications should be undertaken under physician's or pharmacist's supervision because the dose may need to be adjusted). Products include:
Primatene Tablets .... ▣ 749

Ephedrine Sulfate (Concurrent use with prescription asthma medications should be undertaken under physician's or pharmacist's supervision because the dose may need to be adjusted).
No products indexed under this heading.

Ephedrine Tannate (Concurrent use with prescription asthma medications should be undertaken under physician's or pharmacist's supervision because the dose may need to be adjusted).
No products indexed under this heading.

Epinephrine (Concurrent use with prescription asthma medications should be undertaken under physician's or pharmacist's supervision because the dose may need to be adjusted). Products include:
EpiPen 1061
Primatene Mist .... ▣ 749

Epinephrine Bitartrate (Concurrent use with prescription asthma medications should be undertaken under physician's or pharmacist's supervision because the dose may need to be adjusted).
No products indexed under this heading.

Epinephrine Hydrochloride (Concurrent use with prescription asthma medications should be undertaken under physician's or pharmacist's supervision because the dose may need to be adjusted).
No products indexed under this heading.

Escitalopram Oxalate (Concurrent use with antidepressant medications should be undertaken under physician's or pharmacist's supervision because the dose may need to be adjusted). Products include:
Lexapro Oral Solution 1193
Lexapro Tablets 1193

Fluoxetine Hydrochloride (Concurrent use with antidepressant medications should be undertaken under physician's or pharmacist's supervision because the dose may need to be adjusted). Products include:
Prozac Pulvules and Liquid 1771
Symbyax Capsules 1788

Imipramine Hydrochloride (Concurrent use with antidepressant medications should be undertaken under physician's or pharmacist's supervision because the dose may need to be adjusted).
No products indexed under this heading.

Imipramine Pamoate (Concurrent use with antidepressant medications should be undertaken under physician's or pharmacist's supervision because the dose may need to be adjusted).
No products indexed under this heading.

Isocarboxazid (Concurrent use with antidepressant medications should be undertaken under physician's or pharmacist's supervision because the dose may need to be adjusted).
No products indexed under this heading.

Isoetharine (Concurrent use with prescription asthma medications should be undertaken under physician's or pharmacist's supervision because the dose may need to be adjusted).
No products indexed under this heading.

Isoproterenol Hydrochloride (Concurrent use with prescription asthma medications should be undertaken under physician's or pharmacist's supervision because the dose may need to be adjusted).
No products indexed under this heading.

Isoproterenol Sulfate (Concurrent use with prescription asthma medications should be undertaken under physician's or pharmacist's supervision because the dose may need to be adjusted).
No products indexed under this heading.

Levalbuterol Hydrochloride (Concurrent use with prescription asthma medications should be undertaken under physician's or pharmacist's supervision because the dose may need to be adjusted). Products include:
Xopenex Inhalation Solution 3143
Xopenex Inhalation Solution Concentrate 3147

Maprotiline Hydrochloride (Concurrent use with antidepressant medications should be undertaken under physician's or pharmacist's supervision because the dose may need to be adjusted).
No products indexed under this heading.

Metaproterenol Sulfate (Concurrent use with prescription asthma medications should be undertaken under physician's or pharmacist's supervision because the dose may need to be adjusted). Products include:
Alupent Inhalation Aerosol 858

Mirtazapine (Concurrent use with antidepressant medications should be undertaken under physician's or pharmacist's supervision because the dose may need to be adjusted).
No products indexed under this heading.

Nefazodone Hydrochloride (Concurrent use with antidepressant medications should be undertaken under physician's or pharmacist's supervision because the dose may need to be adjusted).
No products indexed under this heading.

Nortriptyline Hydrochloride (Concurrent use with antidepressant medications should be undertaken under physician's or pharmacist's supervision because the dose may need to be adjusted).
No products indexed under this heading.

Paroxetine Hydrochloride (Concurrent use with antidepressant medications should be undertaken under physician's or pharmacist's supervision because the dose may need to be adjusted). Products include:
Paxil CR Controlled-Release Tablets 1509
Paxil 1501

Phenelzine Sulfate (Concurrent use with antidepressant medications should be undertaken under physician's or pharmacist's supervision because the dose may need to be adjusted).
No products indexed under this heading.

Pirbuterol Acetate (Concurrent use with prescription asthma medications should be undertaken under physician's or pharmacist's supervision because the dose may need to be adjusted). Products include:
Maxair Autohaler 1820

Protriptyline Hydrochloride (Concurrent use with antidepressant medications should be undertaken under physician's or pharmacist's supervision because the dose may need to be adjusted). Products include:
Vivactil Tablets 2350

Salmeterol Xinafoate (Concurrent use with prescription asthma medications should be undertaken under physician's or pharmacist's supervision because the dose may need to be adjusted). Products include:
Advair Diskus 100/50 1291
Advair Diskus 250/50 1291
Advair Diskus 500/50 1291
Serevent Diskus 1540

Sertraline Hydrochloride (Concurrent use with antidepressant medications should be undertaken under physician's or pharmacist's supervision because the dose may need to be adjusted). Products include:
Zoloft 2581

Terbutaline Sulfate (Concurrent use with prescription asthma medications should be undertaken under physician's or pharmacist's supervision because the dose may need to be adjusted).
No products indexed under this heading.

Tranylcypromine Sulfate (Concurrent use with antidepressant medications should be undertaken under physician's or pharmacist's supervision because the dose may need to be adjusted). Products include:
Parnate Tablets 1499

Trazodone Hydrochloride (Concurrent use with antidepressant medications should be undertaken under physician's or pharmacist's supervision because the dose may need to be adjusted).
No products indexed under this heading.

Trimipramine Maleate (Concurrent use with antidepressant medications should be undertaken under physician's or pharmacist's supervision because the dose may need to be adjusted). Products include:
Surmontil Capsules 2347

Venlafaxine Hydrochloride (Concurrent use with antidepressant medications should be undertaken under physician's or pharmacist's supervision because the dose may need to be adjusted). Products include:
Effexor Tablets 3405
Effexor XR Capsules 3411

COMTAN TABLETS

(Entacapone) 2186

May interact with central nervous system depressants, drugs metabolized by Catechol-O-methyltransferase, erythromycin, nonselective MAO inhibitors, and certain other agents. Compounds in these categories include:

Alfentanil Hydrochloride (Possible additive sedative effects).
No products indexed under this heading.

Alprazolam (Possible additive sedative effects). Products include:
Niravam Orally Disintegrating Tablets 3106
Xanax XR Tablets 2655

Ampicillin Sodium (As most entacapone excretion is via bile, co-administration with drugs known to interfere with biliary excretion, glucuronidation, and intestinal beta-glucuronidation, such as ampicillin, requires caution).
No products indexed under this heading.

Apomorphine (Co-administration of drugs that are metabolized by catechol-O-methyltransferase (COMT) may result in increased heart rates, possibly arrhythmias, and excessive changes in blood pressure).
No products indexed under this heading.

Aprobarbital (Possible additive sedative effects).
No products indexed under this heading.

Bitolterol Mesylate (Co-administration of drugs that are metabolized by catechol-O-methyltransferase (COMT) may result in increased heart rates, possibly arrhythmias, and excessive changes in blood pressure).
No products indexed under this heading.

Buprenorphine Hydrochloride (Possible additive sedative effects). Products include:
Buprenex Injectable 2718
Suboxone Tablets 2719
Subutex Tablets 2719

Buspirone Hydrochloride (Possible additive sedative effects).
No products indexed under this heading.

Butabarbital (Possible additive sedative effects).
No products indexed under this heading.

Butalbital (Possible additive sedative effects). Products include:
Sedapap Tablets 50 mg/650 mg 2098

Chloramphenicol Sodium Succinate (As most entacapone excretion is via bile, co-administration with drugs known to interfere with biliary excretion, glucuronidation, and intestinal beta-glucuronidation, such as chloramphenicol, requires caution).
No products indexed under this heading.

Chlordiazepoxide (Possible additive sedative effects).
No products indexed under this heading.

Chlordiazepoxide Hydrochloride (Possible additive sedative effects). Products include:
Librium Capsules 3349

Chlorpromazine (Possible additive sedative effects).
No products indexed under this heading.

Chlorpromazine Hydrochloride (Possible additive sedative effects).
No products indexed under this heading.

Chlorprothixene (Possible additive sedative effects).
No products indexed under this heading.

Chlorprothixene Hydrochloride (Possible additive sedative effects).
No products indexed under this heading.

Chlorprothixene Lactate (Possible additive sedative effects).
No products indexed under this heading.

Cholestyramine (As most entacapone excretion is via bile, co-administration with drugs known to interfere with biliary excretion, glucuronidation, and intestinal beta-glucuronidation, such as cholestyramine, requires caution).
No products indexed under this heading.

Clorazepate Dipotassium (Possible additive sedative effects). Products include:
Tranxene 2488

Clozapine (Possible additive sedative effects). Products include:
Clozapine Tablets 2141
Clozaril Tablets 2174
FazaClo Orally Disintegrating Tablets 547

Codeine Phosphate (Possible additive sedative effects). Products include:
Tylenol with Codeine 2461

Desflurane (Possible additive sedative effects). Products include:
Suprane Liquid for Inhalation 770

Dezocine (Possible additive sedative effects).
No products indexed under this heading.

Diazepam (Possible additive sedative effects). Products include:
Diastat Rectal Delivery System 3344
Valium Tablets 2822

Dobutamine Hydrochloride (Co-administration of drugs that are metabolized by catechol-O-methyltransferase (COMT) may result in increased heart rates, possibly arrhythmias, and excessive changes in blood pressure).
No products indexed under this heading.

Dopamine Hydrochloride (Co-administration of drugs that are metabolized by catechol-O-methyltransferase (COMT) may result in increased heart rates, possibly arrhythmias, and excessive changes in blood pressure).
No products indexed under this heading.

Droperidol (Possible additive sedative effects).
No products indexed under this heading.

Enflurane (Possible additive sedative effects).
No products indexed under this heading.

Epinephrine (Co-administration of drugs that are metabolized by catechol-O-methyltransferase (COMT) may result in increased heart rates, possibly arrhythmias, and excessive changes in blood pressure; concurrent use of epinephrine infusion has resulted in a case report of ventricular tachycardia). Products include:
EpiPen 1061
Primatene Mist .... ▣749

Epinephrine Bitartrate (Co-administration of drugs that are metabolized by catechol-O-methyltransferase (COMT) may result in increased heart rates, possibly arrhythmias, and excessive changes in blood pressure; concurrent use of epinephrine infusion has resulted in a case report of ventricular tachycardia).
No products indexed under this heading.

Epinephrine Hydrochloride (Co-administration of drugs that are metabolized by catechol-O-methyltransferase (COMT) may result in increased heart rates, possibly arrhythmias, and excessive changes in blood pressure; concurrent use of epinephrine infusion has resulted in a case report of ventricular tachycardia).
No products indexed under this heading.

Erythromycin (As most entacapone excretion is via bile, co-administration with drugs known to interfere with biliary excretion, glucuronidation, and intestinal beta-glucuronidation, such as erythromycin, requires caution). Products include:
Erygel Topical Gel 2096
Ery-Tab Tablets 447
Erythromycin Base Filmtab Tablets 454
Erythromycin Delayed-Release Capsules, USP 456
PCE Dispertab Tablets 510

Erythromycin Estolate (As most entacapone excretion is via bile, co-administration with drugs known to interfere with biliary excretion, glucuronidation, and intestinal beta-glucuronidation, such as erythromycin, requires caution).
No products indexed under this heading.

Erythromycin Ethylsuccinate (As most entacapone excretion is via bile, co-administration with drugs known to interfere with biliary excretion, glucuronidation, and intestinal beta-glucuronidation, such as erythromycin, requires caution). Products include:
E.E.S. 449
EryPed 445

Erythromycin Gluceptate (As most entacapone excretion is via bile, co-administration with drugs known to interfere with biliary excretion, glucuronidation, and intestinal beta-glucuronidation, such as erythromycin, requires caution).
No products indexed under this heading.

Erythromycin Lactobionate (As most entacapone excretion is via bile, co-administration with drugs known to interfere with biliary excretion, glucuronidation, and intestinal beta-glucuronidation, such as erythromycin, requires caution).
No products indexed under this heading.

Erythromycin Stearate (As most entacapone excretion is via bile, co-administration with drugs known to interfere with biliary excretion, glucuronidation, and intestinal beta-glucuronidation, such as erythromycin, requires caution). Products include:
Erythrocin Stearate Filmtab Tablets 452

Estazolam (Possible additive sedative effects). Products include:
ProSom Tablets 512

Ethanol (Possible additive sedative effects).
No products indexed under this heading.

Ethchlorvynol (Possible additive sedative effects).
No products indexed under this heading.

Ethinamate (Possible additive sedative effects).
No products indexed under this heading.

Ethyl Alcohol (Possible additive sedative effects).
No products indexed under this heading.

Fentanyl (Possible additive sedative effects). Products include:
Duragesic Transdermal System 2448

Fentanyl Citrate (Possible additive sedative effects). Products include:
Actiq 993

Fluphenazine Decanoate (Possible additive sedative effects).
No products indexed under this heading.

Fluphenazine Enanthate (Possible additive sedative effects).
No products indexed under this heading.

Fluphenazine Hydrochloride (Possible additive sedative effects).
No products indexed under this heading.

Flurazepam Hydrochloride (Possible additive sedative effects). Products include:
Dalmane Capsules 3343

Glutethimide (Possible additive sedative effects).
No products indexed under this heading.

Haloperidol (Possible additive sedative effects).
No products indexed under this heading.

Haloperidol Decanoate (Possible additive sedative effects).
No products indexed under this heading.

Hydrocodone Bitartrate (Possible additive sedative effects). Products include:
Hycodan 1104
Hycomine Compound Tablets 1105
Hycotuss Expectorant Syrup 1106
Lortab 3315
Lortab Elixir 3312
Vicodin Tablets 530
Vicodin ES Tablets 531
Vicodin HP Tablets 532
Vicoprofen Tablets 533
Zydone Tablets 1118

Hydrocodone Polistirex (Possible additive sedative effects). Products include:
Tussionex Pennkinetic Extended-Release Suspension 3322

Hydromorphone Hydrochloride (Possible additive sedative effects). Products include:
Dilaudid 439
Dilaudid Oral Liquid 443
Dilaudid Non-Sterile Powder 439
Dilaudid Rectal Suppositories 439
Dilaudid Tablets 439
Dilaudid Tablets - 8 mg 443
Dilaudid-HP 441

Hydroxyzine Hydrochloride (Possible additive sedative effects).
No products indexed under this heading.

Isocarboxazid (Co-administration of non-selective MAO inhibitors with entacapone would result in inhibition of the majority of the pathways responsible for normal catecholamine metabolism; concurrent use should be avoided).
No products indexed under this heading.

Isoetharine (Co-administration of drugs that are metabolized by catechol-O-methyltransferase (COMT) may result in increased heart rates, possibly arrhythmias, and excessive changes in blood pressure).
No products indexed under this heading.

Isoflurane (Possible additive sedative effects).
No products indexed under this heading.

Isoproterenol Hydrochloride (Co-administration of drugs that are metabolized by catechol-O-methyltransferase (COMT) may result in increased heart rates, possibly arrhythmias, and excessive changes in blood pressure).
No products indexed under this heading.

Isoproterenol Sulfate (Co-administration of drugs that are metabolized by catechol-O-methyltransferase (COMT) may result in increased heart rates, possibly arrhythmias, and excessive changes in blood pressure).
No products indexed under this heading.

Ketamine Hydrochloride (Possible additive sedative effects).
No products indexed under this heading.

Levodopa (Entacapone enhances levodopa bioavailability and, therefore, might be expected to increase the occurence of orthostatic hypotension). Products include:
Parcopa Orally Disintegrating Tablets 3111
Stalevo Tablets 2270

Levomethadyl Acetate Hydrochloride (Possible additive sedative effects).
No products indexed under this heading.

Levorphanol Tartrate (Possible additive sedative effects).
No products indexed under this heading.

Lorazepam (Possible additive sedative effects).
No products indexed under this heading.

Loxapine Hydrochloride (Possible additive sedative effects).
No products indexed under this heading.

Loxapine Succinate (Possible additive sedative effects).
No products indexed under this heading.

Meperidine Hydrochloride (Possible additive sedative effects).
No products indexed under this heading.

Mephobarbital (Possible additive sedative effects). Products include:
Mebaral Tablets, USP **2483**

Meprobamate (Possible additive sedative effects).
No products indexed under this heading.

Mesoridazine Besylate (Possible additive sedative effects).
No products indexed under this heading.

Methadone Hydrochloride (Possible additive sedative effects).
No products indexed under this heading.

Methohexital Sodium (Possible additive sedative effects).
No products indexed under this heading.

Methotrimeprazine (Possible additive sedative effects).
No products indexed under this heading.

Methoxyflurane (Possible additive sedative effects).
No products indexed under this heading.

Methyldopa (Co-administration of drugs that are metabolized by catechol-O-methyltransferase (COMT) may result in increased heart rates, possibly arrhythmias, and excessive changes in blood pressure). Products include:
Aldoclor Tablets **1881**
Aldoril Tablets **1884**

Midazolam Hydrochloride (Possible additive sedative effects).
No products indexed under this heading.

Molindone Hydrochloride (Possible additive sedative effects).
Products include:
Moban Tablets **1108**

Morphine Sulfate (Possible additive sedative effects). Products include:
Avinza Capsules **1714**
Kadian Capsules **572**
MS Contin Tablets **2703**

Norepinephrine Bitartrate (Co-administration of drugs that are metabolized by catechol-O-methyltransferase (COMT) may result in increased heart rates, possibly arrhythmias, and excessive changes in blood pressure).
No products indexed under this heading.

Olanzapine (Possible additive sedative effects). Products include:
Symbyax Capsules **1788**
Zyprexa Tablets **1798**
Zyprexa IntraMuscular **1798**
Zyprexa ZYDIS Orally Disintegrating Tablets **1798**

Oxazepam (Possible additive sedative effects).
No products indexed under this heading.

Oxycodone Hydrochloride (Possible additive sedative effects).
Products include:
Combunox Tablets **1183**
OxyContin Tablets **2699**
OxyFast Oral Concentrate Solution **2704**
OxyIR Capsules **2704**
Percocet Tablets **1114**
Percodan Tablets **1115**

Pargyline Hydrochloride (Co-administration of non-selective MAO inhibitors with entacapone would result in inhibition of the majority of the pathways responsible for normal catecholamine metabolism; concurrent use should be avoided).
No products indexed under this heading.

Pentobarbital Sodium (Possible additive sedative effects). Products include:
Nembutal Sodium Solution, USP **2484**

Perphenazine (Possible additive sedative effects).
No products indexed under this heading.

Phenelzine Sulfate (Co-administration of non-selective MAO inhibitors with entacapone would result in inhibition of the majority of the pathways responsible for normal catecholamine metabolism; concurrent use should be avoided).
No products indexed under this heading.

Phenobarbital (Possible additive sedative effects).
No products indexed under this heading.

Prazepam (Possible additive sedative effects).
No products indexed under this heading.

Probenecid (As most entacapone excretion is via bile, co-administration with drugs known to interfere with biliary excretion, glucuronidation, and intestinal beta-glucuronidation, such as probenecid, requires caution).
No products indexed under this heading.

Procarbazine Hydrochloride (Co-administration of non-selective MAO inhibitors with entacapone would result in inhibition of the majority of the pathways responsible for normal catecholamine metabolism; concurrent use should be avoided).
Products include:
Matulane Capsules **3188**

Prochlorperazine (Possible additive sedative effects).
No products indexed under this heading.

Promethazine Hydrochloride (Possible additive sedative effects).
Products include:
Phenergan **3438**

Propofol (Possible additive sedative effects). Products include:
Diprivan Injectable Emulsion **676**

Propoxyphene Hydrochloride (Possible additive sedative effects).
No products indexed under this heading.

Propoxyphene Napsylate (Possible additive sedative effects).
Products include:
Darvocet A 500 Tablets **3497**

Quazepam (Possible additive sedative effects).
No products indexed under this heading.

Quetiapine Fumarate (Possible additive sedative effects). Products include:
Seroquel Tablets **691**

Remifentanil Hydrochloride (Possible additive sedative effects).
No products indexed under this heading.

Rifampin (As most entacapone excretion is via bile, co-administration with drugs known to interfere with biliary excretion, glucuronidation, and intestinal beta-glucuronidation, such as rifampin, requires caution).
No products indexed under this heading.

Risperidone (Possible additive sedative effects). Products include:
Risperdal Consta Long-Acting Injection **1664**
Risperdal M-Tab Orally Disintegrating Tablets **1658**
Risperdal **1658**

Secobarbital Sodium (Possible additive sedative effects).
No products indexed under this heading.

Sevoflurane (Possible additive sedative effects). Products include:
Ultane Liquid for Inhalation **526**

Sufentanil Citrate (Possible additive sedative effects).
No products indexed under this heading.

Temazepam (Possible additive sedative effects).
No products indexed under this heading.

Thiamylal Sodium (Possible additive sedative effects).
No products indexed under this heading.

Thioridazine Hydrochloride (Possible additive sedative effects).
Products include:
Thioridazine Hydrochloride Tablets **2122**

Thiothixene (Possible additive sedative effects). Products include:
Thiothixene Capsules **2124**

Tranylcypromine Sulfate (Co-administration of non-selective MAO inhibitors with entacapone would result in inhibition of the majority of the pathways responsible for normal catecholamine metabolism; concurrent use should be avoided).
Products include:
Parnate Tablets **1499**

Triazolam (Possible additive sedative effects).
No products indexed under this heading.

Trifluoperazine Hydrochloride (Possible additive sedative effects).
No products indexed under this heading.

Zaleplon (Possible additive sedative effects). Products include:
Sonata Capsules **1686**

Ziprasidone Hydrochloride (Possible additive sedative effects).
Products include:
Geodon Capsules **2514**

Zolpidem Tartrate (Possible additive sedative effects). Products include:
Ambien Tablets **2867**

Food Interactions

Alcohol (Possible additive sedative effects).

COMVAX

(Haemophilus B Conjugate Vaccine, Hepatitis B Vaccine, Recombinant) **1904**
May interact with immunosuppressive agents. Compounds in these categories include:

Azathioprine (Deferral of immunization may be considered in individuals receiving immunosuppresive therapy). Products include:
Azasan Tablets **2844**

Basiliximab (Deferral of immunization may be considered in individuals receiving immunosuppresive therapy). Products include:
Simulect for Injection **2268**

Cyclosporine (Deferral of immunization may be considered in individuals receiving immunosuppresive therapy). Products include:
Gengraf Capsules **458**
Neoral Soft Gelatin Capsules **2247**
Neoral Oral Solution **2247**
Restasis Ophthalmic Emulsion **570**
Sandimmune **2259**

Muromonab-CD3 (Deferral of immunization may be considered in individuals receiving immunosuppresive therapy). Products include:
Orthoclone OKT3 Sterile Solution **2370**

Mycophenolate Mofetil (Deferral of immunization may be considered in individuals receiving immunosuppresive therapy). Products include:
CellCept Capsules **2751**
CellCept Oral Suspension **2751**
CellCept Tablets **2751**

Sirolimus (Deferral of immunization may be considered in individuals receiving immunosuppresive therapy). Products include:
Rapamune Oral Solution and Tablets **3472**

Tacrolimus (Deferral of immunization may be considered in individuals receiving immunosuppresive therapy). Products include:
Prograf Capsules and Injection **624**
Protopic Ointment **629**

CONCERTA EXTENDED-RELEASE TABLETS

(Methylphenidate Hydrochloride) **1828**
May interact with oral anticoagulants, monoamine oxidase inhibitors, phenytoin, selective serotonin reuptake inhibitors, tricyclic antidepressants, vasopressors, and certain other agents. Compounds in these categories include:

Amitriptyline Hydrochloride (Methylphenidate may inhibit the metabolism of certain tricyclic antidepressants; downward dosage adjustment of tricyclic antidepressants may be required).
No products indexed under this heading.

Amoxapine (Methylphenidate may inhibit the metabolism of certain tricyclic antidepressants; downward dosage adjustment of tricyclic antidepressants may be required).
No products indexed under this heading.

Anisindione (Methylphenidate may inhibit the metabolism of coumarin anticoagulants; downward dosage adjustment of anticoagulants may be required). Products include:

Miradon Tablets ... 3056

Citalopram Hydrobromide (Methylphenidate may inhibit the metabolism of certain selective serotonin reuptake inhibitors; downward dosage adjustment of these drugs may be required). Products include:
Celexa ... 1177

Clomipramine Hydrochloride (Methylphenidate may inhibit the metabolism of certain tricyclic antidepressants; downward dosage adjustment of tricyclic antidepressants may be required).
No products indexed under this heading.

Desipramine Hydrochloride (Methylphenidate may inhibit the metabolism of certain tricyclic antidepressants; downward dosage adjustment of tricyclic antidepressants may be required).
No products indexed under this heading.

Dicumarol (Methylphenidate may inhibit the metabolism of coumarin anticoagulants; downward dosage adjustment of anticoagulants may be required).
No products indexed under this heading.

Dobutamine (Methylphenidate causes a rise in blood pressure; co-administration with other pressor agents should be undertaken with caution).
No products indexed under this heading.

Dobutamine Hydrochloride (Methylphenidate causes a rise in blood pressure; co-administration with other pressor agents should be undertaken with caution).
No products indexed under this heading.

Dopamine Hydrochloride (Methylphenidate causes a rise in blood pressure; co-administration with other pressor agents should be undertaken with caution).
No products indexed under this heading.

Doxepin Hydrochloride (Methylphenidate may inhibit the metabolism of certain tricyclic antidepressants; downward dosage adjustment of tricyclic antidepressants may be required).
No products indexed under this heading.

Ephedrine Sulfate (Methylphenidate causes a rise in blood pressure; co-administration with other pressor agents should be undertaken with caution).
No products indexed under this heading.

Epinephrine Bitartrate (Methylphenidate causes a rise in blood pressure; co-administration with other pressor agents should be undertaken with caution).
No products indexed under this heading.

Epinephrine Hydrochloride (Methylphenidate causes a rise in blood pressure; co-administration with other pressor agents should be undertaken with caution).
No products indexed under this heading.

Escitalopram Oxalate (Methylphenidate may inhibit the metabolism of certain selective serotonin reuptake inhibitors; downward dosage adjustment of these drugs may be required). Products include:
Lexapro Oral Solution ... 1193
Lexapro Tablets ... 1193

Fluoxetine Hydrochloride (Methylphenidate may inhibit the metabolism of certain selective serotonin reuptake inhibitors; downward dosage adjustment of these drugs may be required). Products include:
Prozac Pulvules and Liquid ... 1771
Symbyax Capsules ... 1788

Fluvoxamine Maleate (Methylphenidate may inhibit the metabolism of certain selective serotonin reuptake inhibitors; downward dosage adjustment of these drugs may be required).
No products indexed under this heading.

Fosphenytoin Sodium (Methylphenidate may inhibit the metabolism of phenytoin; downward dosage adjustment of phenytoin may be required).
No products indexed under this heading.

Imipramine Hydrochloride (Methylphenidate may inhibit the metabolism of certain tricyclic antidepressants; downward dosage adjustment of tricyclic antidepressants may be required).
No products indexed under this heading.

Imipramine Pamoate (Methylphenidate may inhibit the metabolism of certain tricyclic antidepressants; downward dosage adjustment of tricyclic antidepressants may be required).
No products indexed under this heading.

Isocarboxazid (Co-administration with MAO inhibitors may result in hypertensive crises; concurrent and/or sequential use is contraindicated).
No products indexed under this heading.

Isoproterenol Hydrochloride (Methylphenidate causes a rise in blood pressure; co-administration with other pressor agents should be undertaken with caution).
No products indexed under this heading.

Isoproterenol Sulfate (Methylphenidate causes a rise in blood pressure; co-administration with other pressor agents should be undertaken with caution).
No products indexed under this heading.

Maprotiline Hydrochloride (Methylphenidate may inhibit the metabolism of certain tricyclic antidepressants; downward dosage adjustment of tricyclic antidepressants may be required).
No products indexed under this heading.

Mephentermine Sulfate (Methylphenidate causes a rise in blood pressure; co-administration with other pressor agents should be undertaken with caution).
No products indexed under this heading.

Metaraminol Bitartrate (Methylphenidate causes a rise in blood pressure; co-administration with other pressor agents should be undertaken with caution). Products include:
Aramine Injection ... 1889

Methoxamine Hydrochloride (Methylphenidate causes a rise in blood pressure; co-administration with other pressor agents should be undertaken with caution).
No products indexed under this heading.

Moclobemide (Co-administration with MAO inhibitors may result in hypertensive crises; concurrent and/or sequential use is contraindicated).
No products indexed under this heading.

Norepinephrine Bitartrate (Methylphenidate causes a rise in blood pressure; co-administration with other pressor agents should be undertaken with caution).
No products indexed under this heading.

Nortriptyline Hydrochloride (Methylphenidate may inhibit the metabolism of certain tricyclic antidepressants; downward dosage adjustment of tricyclic antidepressants may be required).
No products indexed under this heading.

Pargyline Hydrochloride (Co-administration with MAO inhibitors may result in hypertensive crises; concurrent and/or sequential use is contraindicated).
No products indexed under this heading.

Paroxetine Hydrochloride (Methylphenidate may inhibit the metabolism of certain selective serotonin reuptake inhibitors; downward dosage adjustment of these drugs may be required). Products include:
Paxil CR Controlled-Release Tablets ... 1509
Paxil ... 1501

Phenelzine Sulfate (Co-administration with MAO inhibitors may result in hypertensive crises; concurrent and/or sequential use is contraindicated).
No products indexed under this heading.

Phenobarbital (Methylphenidate may inhibit the metabolism of phenobarbital; downward dosage adjustment of phenobarbital may be required).
No products indexed under this heading.

Phenylephrine Hydrochloride (Methylphenidate causes a rise in blood pressure; co-administration with other pressor agents should be undertaken with caution). Products include:
Alacol DM Syrup ... 739
Hycomine Compound Tablets ... 1105
Preparation H Maximum Strength Cream ... 747
Preparation H Cooling Gel ... 747
Preparation H ... 747
Sudafed PE Tablets ... 711
Vicks Sinex Nasal Spray and Ultra Fine Mist for Sinus Relief ... 2677
Zicam Concentrated Cough Mist for Kids Plus D Cool Cherry ... 643
Zicam Concentrated Cough Mist Plus D Cool Cherry ... 642

Phenytoin (Methylphenidate may inhibit the metabolism of phenytoin; downward dosage adjustment of phenytoin may be required).
No products indexed under this heading.

Phenytoin Sodium (Methylphenidate may inhibit the metabolism of phenytoin; downward dosage adjustment of phenytoin may be required). Products include:
Phenytek Capsules ... 2153

Primidone (Methylphenidate may inhibit the metabolism of primidone; downward dosage adjustment of primidone may be required).
No products indexed under this heading.

Procarbazine Hydrochloride (Co-administration with MAO inhibitors may result in hypertensive crises; concurrent and/or sequential use is contraindicated). Products include:
Matulane Capsules ... 3188

Protriptyline Hydrochloride (Methylphenidate may inhibit the metabolism of certain tricyclic antidepressants; downward dosage adjustment of tricyclic antidepressants may be required). Products include:
Vivactil Tablets ... 2350

Selegiline Hydrochloride (Co-administration with MAO inhibitors may result in hypertensive crises; concurrent and/or sequential use is contraindicated). Products include:
Eldepryl Capsules ... 3209

Sertraline Hydrochloride (Methylphenidate may inhibit the metabolism of certain selective serotonin reuptake inhibitors; downward dosage adjustment of these drugs may be required). Products include:
Zoloft ... 2581

Tranylcypromine Sulfate (Co-administration with MAO inhibitors may result in hypertensive crises; concurrent and/or sequential use is contraindicated). Products include:
Parnate Tablets ... 1499

Trimipramine Maleate (Methylphenidate may inhibit the metabolism of certain tricyclic antidepressants; downward dosage adjustment of tricyclic antidepressants may be required). Products include:
Surmontil Capsules ... 2347

Warfarin Sodium (Methylphenidate may inhibit the metabolism of coumarin anticoagulants; downward dosage adjustment of anticoagulants may be required). Products include:
Coumadin for Injection ... 932
Coumadin Tablets ... 932

CONTAC NON-DROWSY 12 HOUR COLD CAPLETS

(Pseudoephedrine Hydrochloride) ... 614
May interact with monoamine oxidase inhibitors. Compounds in these categories include:

Isocarboxazid (Concurrent and/or sequential use with MAO inhibitors is not recommended).
No products indexed under this heading.

Moclobemide (Concurrent and/or sequential use with MAO inhibitors is not recommended).
No products indexed under this heading.

Pargyline Hydrochloride (Concurrent and/or sequential use with MAO inhibitors is not recommended).
No products indexed under this heading.

Phenelzine Sulfate (Concurrent and/or sequential use with MAO inhibitors is not recommended).
No products indexed under this heading.

Procarbazine Hydrochloride (Concurrent and/or sequential use with MAO inhibitors is not recommended). Products include:

Matulane Capsules 3188

Selegiline Hydrochloride (Concurrent and/or sequential use with MAO inhibitors is not recommended). Products include:

Eldepryl Capsules 3209

Tranylcypromine Sulfate (Concurrent and/or sequential use with MAO inhibitors is not recommended). Products include:

Parnate Tablets 1499

CONTAC NON-DROWSY TIMED RELEASE 12 HOUR COLD CAPLETS

(Pseudoephedrine Hydrochloride) ..... ▣615

See Contac Non-Drowsy 12 Hour Cold Caplets

CONTAC SEVERE COLD AND FLU CAPLETS MAXIMUM STRENGTH

(Acetaminophen, Chlorpheniramine Maleate, Dextromethorphan Hydrobromide, Pseudoephedrine Hydrochloride)....... ▣615

May interact with hypnotics and sedatives, monoamine oxidase inhibitors, tranquilizers, and certain other agents. Compounds in these categories include:

Alprazolam (May increase drowsiness effect; concurrent use should be avoided). Products include:

Niravam Orally Disintegrating Tablets 3106
Xanax XR Tablets 2655

Buspirone Hydrochloride (May increase drowsiness effect; concurrent use should be avoided).

No products indexed under this heading.

Chlordiazepoxide (May increase drowsiness effect; concurrent use should be avoided).

No products indexed under this heading.

Chlordiazepoxide Hydrochloride (May increase drowsiness effect; concurrent use should be avoided). Products include:

Librium Capsules 3349

Chlorpromazine (May increase drowsiness effect; concurrent use should be avoided).

No products indexed under this heading.

Chlorpromazine Hydrochloride (May increase drowsiness effect; concurrent use should be avoided).

No products indexed under this heading.

Chlorprothixene (May increase drowsiness effect; concurrent use should be avoided).

No products indexed under this heading.

Chlorprothixene Hydrochloride (May increase drowsiness effect; concurrent use should be avoided).

No products indexed under this heading.

Clorazepate Dipotassium (May increase drowsiness effect; concurrent use should be avoided). Products include:

Tranxene 2488

Diazepam (May increase drowsiness effect; concurrent use should be avoided). Products include:

Diastat Rectal Delivery System 3344
Valium Tablets 2822

Droperidol (May increase drowsiness effect; concurrent use should be avoided).

No products indexed under this heading.

Estazolam (May increase drowsiness effect; concurrent use should be avoided). Products include:

ProSom Tablets 512

Ethchlorvynol (May increase drowsiness effect; concurrent use should be avoided).

No products indexed under this heading.

Ethinamate (May increase drowsiness effect; concurrent use should be avoided).

No products indexed under this heading.

Fluphenazine Decanoate (May increase drowsiness effect; concurrent use should be avoided).

No products indexed under this heading.

Fluphenazine Enanthate (May increase drowsiness effect; concurrent use should be avoided).

No products indexed under this heading.

Fluphenazine Hydrochloride (May increase drowsiness effect; concurrent use should be avoided).

No products indexed under this heading.

Flurazepam Hydrochloride (May increase drowsiness effect; concurrent use should be avoided). Products include:

Dalmane Capsules 3343

Glutethimide (May increase drowsiness effect; concurrent use should be avoided).

No products indexed under this heading.

Haloperidol (May increase drowsiness effect; concurrent use should be avoided).

No products indexed under this heading.

Haloperidol Decanoate (May increase drowsiness effect; concurrent use should be avoided).

No products indexed under this heading.

Hydroxyzine Hydrochloride (May increase drowsiness effect; concurrent use should be avoided).

No products indexed under this heading.

Isocarboxazid (Concurrent and/or sequential use is not recommended unless directed by a doctor).

No products indexed under this heading.

Lorazepam (May increase drowsiness effect; concurrent use should be avoided).

No products indexed under this heading.

Loxapine Hydrochloride (May increase drowsiness effect; concurrent use should be avoided).

No products indexed under this heading.

Loxapine Succinate (May increase drowsiness effect; concurrent use should be avoided).

No products indexed under this heading.

Meprobamate (May increase drowsiness effect; concurrent use should be avoided).

No products indexed under this heading.

Mesoridazine Besylate (May increase drowsiness effect; concurrent use should be avoided).

No products indexed under this heading.

Midazolam Hydrochloride (May increase drowsiness effect; concurrent use should be avoided).

No products indexed under this heading.

Moclobemide (Concurrent and/or sequential use is not recommended unless directed by a doctor).

No products indexed under this heading.

Molindone Hydrochloride (May increase drowsiness effect; concurrent use should be avoided). Products include:

Moban Tablets 1108

Oxazepam (May increase drowsiness effect; concurrent use should be avoided).

No products indexed under this heading.

Pargyline Hydrochloride (Concurrent and/or sequential use is not recommended unless directed by a doctor).

No products indexed under this heading.

Perphenazine (May increase drowsiness effect; concurrent use should be avoided).

No products indexed under this heading.

Phenelzine Sulfate (Concurrent and/or sequential use is not recommended unless directed by a doctor).

No products indexed under this heading.

Prazepam (May increase drowsiness effect; concurrent use should be avoided).

No products indexed under this heading.

Procarbazine Hydrochloride (Concurrent and/or sequential use is not recommended unless directed by a doctor). Products include:

Matulane Capsules 3188

Prochlorperazine (May increase drowsiness effect; concurrent use should be avoided).

No products indexed under this heading.

Promethazine Hydrochloride (May increase drowsiness effect; concurrent use should be avoided). Products include:

Phenergan 3438

Propofol (May increase drowsiness effect; concurrent use should be avoided). Products include:

Diprivan Injectable Emulsion 676

Quazepam (May increase drowsiness effect; concurrent use should be avoided).

No products indexed under this heading.

Secobarbital Sodium (May increase drowsiness effect; concurrent use should be avoided).

No products indexed under this heading.

Selegiline Hydrochloride (Concurrent and/or sequential use is not recommended unless directed by a doctor). Products include:

Eldepryl Capsules 3209

Temazepam (May increase drowsiness effect; concurrent use should be avoided).

No products indexed under this heading.

Thioridazine Hydrochloride (May increase drowsiness effect; concurrent use should be avoided). Products include:

Thioridazine Hydrochloride Tablets 2122

Thiothixene (May increase drowsiness effect; concurrent use should be avoided). Products include:

Thiothixene Capsules 2124

Tranylcypromine Sulfate (Concurrent and/or sequential use is not recommended unless directed by a doctor). Products include:

Parnate Tablets 1499

Triazolam (May increase drowsiness effect; concurrent use should be avoided).

No products indexed under this heading.

Trifluoperazine Hydrochloride (May increase drowsiness effect; concurrent use should be avoided).

No products indexed under this heading.

Zaleplon (May increase drowsiness effect; concurrent use should be avoided). Products include:

Sonata Capsules 1686

Zolpidem Tartrate (May increase drowsiness effect; concurrent use should be avoided). Products include:

Ambien Tablets 2867

Food Interactions

Alcohol (May increase drowsiness effect; concurrent use should be avoided).

CONTAC SEVERE COLD AND FLU CAPLETS NON-DROWSY

(Acetaminophen, Dextromethorphan Hydrobromide, Pseudoephedrine Hydrochloride)....... ▣615

See Contac Severe Cold and Flu Caplets Maximum Strength

COPAXONE FOR INJECTION

(Glatiramer Acetate) 3292

None cited in PDR database.

COPEGUS TABLETS

(Ribavirin) 2759

May interact with nucleoside analogue reverse transcriptase inhibitors and certain other agents. Compounds in these categories include:

Didanosine (Co-administration of ribavirin and didanosine is not recommended. Reports of fatal kepatic failure, as well as peripheral neuropathy, pancreatitis, and symptomatic hyperlactatemia/lactic acidosis have been reported).

No products indexed under this heading.

Lamivudine (Co-administration of ribavirin and nucleoside analogue reverse transcriptase inhibitors should be closely monitored for treatment associated toxicities. In addition, dose reduction or discontinuation of ribavirin or both should also be considered if worsening of toxicities are observed). Products include:

Combivir Tablets 1373
Epivir 1394
Epivir-HBV 1398
Epzicom Tablets 1402
Trizivir Tablets 1565

Stavudine (Ribavirin can antagonize the in-vitro antiviral activity of stavudine against HIV. Therefore, concom-

itant use of ribavirin with stavudine should be avoided). Products include:
- Zerit ... 971

Zalcitabine (Co-administration of ribavirin and nucleoside analogue reverse transcriptase inhibitors should be closely monitored for treatment associated toxicities. In addition, dose reduction or discontinuation of ribavirin or both should also be considered if worsening of toxicities are observed).
- No products indexed under this heading.

Zidovudine (Ribavirin can antagonize the in-vitro antiviral activity of zidovudine against HIV. Therefore, concomitant use of ribavirin with zidovudine should be avoided). Products include:
- Combivir Tablets ... 1373
- Retrovir ... 1533
- Retrovir IV Infusion ... 1537
- Trizivir Tablets ... 1565

COQUINONE CAPSULES

(Coenzyme Q-10, Lipoic Acid) ... 3343
None cited in PDR database.

CORDYMAX CS-4 CAPSULES

(Herbals, Multiple) ... 2669
May interact with oral anticoagulants and monoamine oxidase inhibitors. Compounds in these categories include:

Anisindione (Concurrent use with anticoagulants requires consultation with a physician). Products include:
- Miradon Tablets ... 3056

Dicumarol (Concurrent use with anticoagulants requires consultation with a physician).
- No products indexed under this heading.

Isocarboxazid (Concurrent use with MAO inhibitors requires consultation with a physician).
- No products indexed under this heading.

Moclobemide (Concurrent use with MAO inhibitors requires consultation with a physician).
- No products indexed under this heading.

Pargyline Hydrochloride (Concurrent use with MAO inhibitors requires consultation with a physician).
- No products indexed under this heading.

Phenelzine Sulfate (Concurrent use with MAO inhibitors requires consultation with a physician).
- No products indexed under this heading.

Procarbazine Hydrochloride (Concurrent use with MAO inhibitors requires consultation with a physician). Products include:
- Matulane Capsules ... 3188

Selegiline Hydrochloride (Concurrent use with MAO inhibitors requires consultation with a physician). Products include:
- Eldepryl Capsules ... 3209

Tranylcypromine Sulfate (Concurrent use with MAO inhibitors requires consultation with a physician). Products include:
- Parnate Tablets ... 1499

Warfarin Sodium (Concurrent use with anticoagulants requires consultation with a physician). Products include:
- Coumadin for Injection ... 932
- Coumadin Tablets ... 932

COREG TABLETS

(Carvedilol) ... 1376
May interact with catecholamine depleting drugs, cytochrome p450 2d6 inhibitors (selected), epinephrine-containing products, oral hypoglycemic agents, insulin, monoamine oxidase inhibitors, quinidine, and certain other agents. Compounds in these categories include:

Acarbose (Beta-blockers may mask some of the manifestations of hypoglycemia, particularly tachycardia; nonselective beta-blockers may potentiate insulin-induced hypoglycemia and delay recovery of serum glucose levels; in congestive heart failure patients with diabetes, carvedilol therapy may lead to worsening of hyperglycemia, which responds to intensification of hypoglycemia). Products include:
- Precose Tablets ... 776

Amiodarone Hydrochloride (Interactions of carvedilol with strong inhibitors of CYP2D6, such as quinidine, have not been studied, but these drugs would be expected to increase blood levels of the R(+) enantiomer of carvedilol. Analysis of side effects showed that poor 2D6 metabolizers had a higher rate of dizziness during up-titration, presumably resulting from vasodilating effects of the higher concentrations of the alpha-blocking R(+) enantiomer). Products include:
- Pacerone Tablets ... 3337

Amitriptyline Hydrochloride (Interactions of carvedilol with strong inhibitors of CYP2D6, such as quinidine, have not been studied, but these drugs would be expected to increase blood levels of the R(+) enantiomer of carvedilol. Analysis of side effects showed that poor 2D6 metabolizers had a higher rate of dizziness during up-titration, presumably resulting from vasodilating effects of the higher concentrations of the alpha-blocking R(+) enantiomer).
- No products indexed under this heading.

Amoxapine (Interactions of carvedilol with strong inhibitors of CYP2D6, such as quinidine, have not been studied, but these drugs would be expected to increase blood levels of the R(+) enantiomer of carvedilol. Analysis of side effects showed that poor 2D6 metabolizers had a higher rate of dizziness during up-titration, presumably resulting from vasodilating effects of the higher concentrations of the alpha-blocking R(+) enantiomer).
- No products indexed under this heading.

Bupropion Hydrochloride (Interactions of carvedilol with strong inhibitors of CYP2D6, such as quinidine, have not been studied, but these drugs would be expected to increase blood levels of the R(+) enantiomer of carvedilol. Analysis of side effects showed that poor 2D6 metabolizers had a higher rate of dizziness during up-titration, presumably resulting from vasodilating effects of the higher concentrations of the alpha-blocking R(+) enantiomer). Products include:
- Wellbutrin Tablets ... 1579
- Wellbutrin SR Sustained-Release Tablets ... 1583
- Wellbutrin XL Extended-Release Tablets ... 1588
- Zyban Sustained-Release Tablets ... 1620

Celecoxib (Interactions of carvedilol with strong inhibitors of CYP2D6, such as quinidine, have not been studied, but these drugs would be expected to increase blood levels of the R(+) enantiomer of carvedilol. Analysis of side effects showed that poor 2D6 metabolizers had a higher rate of dizziness during up-titration, presumably resulting from vasodilating effects of the higher concentrations of the alpha-blocking R(+) enantiomer). Products include:
- Celebrex Capsules ... 3130

Chloroquine Hydrochloride (Interactions of carvedilol with strong inhibitors of CYP2D6, such as quinidine, have not been studied, but these drugs would be expected to increase blood levels of the R(+) enantiomer of carvedilol. Analysis of side effects showed that poor 2D6 metabolizers had a higher rate of dizziness during up-titration, presumably resulting from vasodilating effects of the higher concentrations of the alpha-blocking R(+) enantiomer).
- No products indexed under this heading.

Chloroquine Phosphate (Interactions of carvedilol with strong inhibitors of CYP2D6, such as quinidine, have not been studied, but these drugs would be expected to increase blood levels of the R(+) enantiomer of carvedilol. Analysis of side effects showed that poor 2D6 metabolizers had a higher rate of dizziness during up-titration, presumably resulting from vasodilating effects of the higher concentrations of the alpha-blocking R(+) enantiomer).
- No products indexed under this heading.

Chlorpheniramine (Interactions of carvedilol with strong inhibitors of CYP2D6, such as quinidine, have not been studied, but these drugs would be expected to increase blood levels of the R(+) enantiomer of carvedilol. Analysis of side effects showed that poor 2D6 metabolizers had a higher rate of dizziness during up-titration, presumably resulting from vasodilating effects of the higher concentrations of the alpha-blocking R(+) enantiomer).
- No products indexed under this heading.

Chlorpheniramine Maleate (Interactions of carvedilol with strong inhibitors of CYP2D6, such as quinidine, have not been studied, but these drugs would be expected to increase blood levels of the R(+) enantiomer of carvedilol. Analysis of side effects showed that poor 2D6 metabolizers had a higher rate of dizziness during up-titration, presumably resulting from vasodilating effects of the higher concentrations of the alpha-blocking R(+) enantiomer). Products include:
- Advil Allergy Sinus Caplets ... 737
- Advil Multi-Symptom Cold Caplets ... 738
- BC Allergy Sinus Cold Powder ... 612
- Contac Severe Cold and Flu Caplets Maximum Strength ... 615
- Hycomine Compound Tablets ... 1105
- PediaCare Multi-Symptom Cold Liquid ... 704
- PediaCare NightRest Cough & Cold Liquid ... 704
- Robitussin Flu Liquid ... 752
- Robitussin PM Cough & Cold Liquid ... 752
- Singlet Caplets ... 636
- Sudafed Sinus & Allergy Tablets ... 710
- TheraFlu Cold & Cough Hot Liquid ... 680
- TheraFlu Cold & Sore Throat Hot Liquid ... 680
- TheraFlu Flu & Sore Throat Hot Liquid ... 681
- TheraFlu Severe Cold & Cough Hot Liquid ... 683
- TheraFlu Severe Cold Caplets ... 679
- TheraFlu Severe Cold Hot Liquid ... 682
- Triaminic Cold & Allergy Liquid ... 685
- Triaminic Cold & Cough Liquid ... 685
- Triaminic Flu, Cough & Fever Liquid ... 685
- Triaminic Night Time Cough & Cold Liquid ... 685
- Triaminic Allergy Runny Nose & Congestion Softchews ... 688
- Triaminic Cold & Cough Softchews ... 688
- Children's Tylenol Plus Cold NightTime Suspension Liquid ... 1851
- Children's Tylenol Plus Cold & Cough Suspension Liquid and Chewable Tablets ... 1851
- Children's Tylenol Plus Cold Chewable Tablets ... 1851
- Children's Tylenol Plus Flu Suspension Liquid ... 1853
- Tylenol Allergy Complete Multi-Symptom Caplets and Gelcaps with Cool Burst ... 1844
- Multi-Symptom Tylenol Cold Night Time Caplets ... 1845
- Vicks 44M Cough, Cold & Flu Relief ... 2676
- Pediatric Vicks 44m Cough & Cold Relief ... 2673
- Children's Vicks NyQuil Cold/Cough Relief ... 2671

Chlorpheniramine Polistirex (Interactions of carvedilol with strong inhibitors of CYP2D6, such as quinidine, have not been studied, but these drugs would be expected to increase blood levels of the R(+) enantiomer of carvedilol. Analysis of side effects showed that poor 2D6 metabolizers had a higher rate of dizziness during up-titration, presumably resulting from vasodilating effects of the higher concentrations of the alpha-blocking R(+) enantiomer). Products include:
- Tussionex Pennkinetic Extended-Release Suspension ... 3322

Chlorpheniramine Tannate (Interactions of carvedilol with strong inhibitors of CYP2D6, such as quinidine, have not been studied, but these drugs would be expected to increase blood levels of the R(+) enantiomer of carvedilol. Analysis of side effects showed that poor 2D6 metabolizers had a higher rate of dizziness during up-titration, presumably resulting from vasodilating effects of the higher concentrations of the alpha-blocking R(+) enantiomer).
- No products indexed under this heading.

Chlorpropamide (Beta-blockers may mask some of the manifestations of hypoglycemia, particularly tachycardia; nonselective beta-blockers may potentiate insulin-induced hypoglycemia and delay recovery of serum glucose levels; in congestive heart failure patients with diabetes, carvedilol therapy may lead to worsening of hyperglycemia, which responds to intensification of hypoglycemia).
- No products indexed under this heading.

Cimetidine (Carvedilol undergoes substantial oxidative metabolism; co-administration has resulted in increased steady-state AUC of carvedilol by about 30% with no change in Cmax). Products include:

Tagamet HB 200 Tablets .... ▣637
Tagamet Tablets 1547

Cimetidine Hydrochloride (Carvedilol undergoes substantial oxidative metabolism; co-administration has resulted in increased steady-state AUC of carvedilol by about 30% with no change in Cmax).

No products indexed under this heading.

Citalopram Hydrobromide (Interactions of carvedilol with strong inhibitors of CYP2D6, such as quinidine, have not been studied, but these drugs would be expected to increase blood levels of the R(+) enantiomer of carvedilol. Analysis of side effects showed that poor 2D6 metabolizers had a higher rate of dizziness during up-titration, presumably resulting from vasodilating effects of the higher concentrations of the alpha-blocking R(+) enantiomer). Products include:

Celexa 1177

Clomipramine Hydrochloride (Interactions of carvedilol with strong inhibitors of CYP2D6, such as quinidine, have not been studied, but these drugs would be expected to increase blood levels of the R(+) enantiomer of carvedilol. Analysis of side effects showed that poor 2D6 metabolizers had a higher rate of dizziness during up-titration, presumably resulting from vasodilating effects of the higher concentrations of the alpha-blocking R(+) enantiomer).

No products indexed under this heading.

Clonidine (Co-administration of clonidine with agents with β-blocking properties may potentiate blood pressure- and heart rate-lowering effects). Products include:

Catapres-TTS 875

Clonidine Hydrochloride (Co-administration of clonidine with agents with β-blocking properties may potentiate blood pressure- and heart rate-lowering effects). Products include:

Catapres Tablets 874
Clorpres Tablets 2139

Cocaine Hydrochloride (Interactions of carvedilol with strong inhibitors of CYP2D6, such as quinidine, have not been studied, but these drugs would be expected to increase blood levels of the R(+) enantiomer of carvedilol. Analysis of side effects showed that poor 2D6 metabolizers had a higher rate of dizziness during up-titration, presumably resulting from vasodilating effects of the higher concentrations of the alpha-blocking R(+) enantiomer).

No products indexed under this heading.

Cyclosporine (Co-administration in renal transplant patients has resulted in a modest increase in mean trough cyclosporine concentrations; dose of cyclosporine may need to be reduced in some patients). Products include:

Gengraf Capsules 458
Neoral Soft Gelatin Capsules 2247
Neoral Oral Solution 2247
Restasis Ophthalmic Emulsion 570
Sandimmune 2259

Deserpidine (Patients receiving agents with beta-blocking properties and a drug that may deplete catecholamines should be observed closely for signs of hypotension and/or severe bradycardia).

No products indexed under this heading.

Desipramine Hydrochloride (Interactions of carvedilol with strong inhibitors of CYP2D6, such as quinidine, have not been studied, but these drugs would be expected to increase blood levels of the R(+) enantiomer of carvedilol. Analysis of side effects showed that poor 2D6 metabolizers had a higher rate of dizziness during up-titration, presumably resulting from vasodilating effects of the higher concentrations of the alpha-blocking R(+) enantiomer).

No products indexed under this heading.

Digoxin (Co-administration increases digoxin concentraton by 15%. Both digoxin and carvedilol slow AV conduction. Therefore, increased monitoring of digoxin is recommended when initiating, adjusting or discontinuing carvedilol). Products include:

Digitek Tablets 2146
Lanoxicaps Capsules 1458
Lanoxin Injection 1462
Lanoxin Tablets 1468
Lanoxin Injection Pediatric 1465

Diltiazem Hydrochloride (Co-administration has resulted in isolated cases of conduction disturbances, rarely with hemodynamic. Monitoring of ECG and blood pressure is recommended). Products include:

Cardizem LA Extended Release Tablets 1699
Tiazac Capsules 1204

Diphenhydramine (Interactions of carvedilol with strong inhibitors of CYP2D6, such as quinidine, have not been studied, but these drugs would be expected to increase blood levels of the R(+) enantiomer of carvedilol. Analysis of side effects showed that poor 2D6 metabolizers had a higher rate of dizziness during up-titration, presumably resulting from vasodilating effects of the higher concentrations of the alpha-blocking R(+) enantiomer). Products include:

Tylenol Sore Throat NightTime Liquid with Cool Burst 1849

Diphenhydramine Hydrochloride (Interactions of carvedilol with strong inhibitors of CYP2D6, such as quinidine, have not been studied, but these drugs would be expected to increase blood levels of the R(+) enantiomer of carvedilol. Analysis of side effects showed that poor 2D6 metabolizers had a higher rate of dizziness during up-titration, presumably resulting from vasodilating effects of the higher concentrations of the alpha-blocking R(+) enantiomer). Products include:

Benadryl Allergy & Cold Tablets ..... ▣692
Benadryl Allergy .... ▣691
Benadryl Allergy & Sinus Headache Caplets & Gelcaps...... ▣693
Children's Benadryl Allergy Liquid ... ▣695
Children's Benadryl Dye-Free Allergy Liquid .... ▣695
Benadryl Dye-Free Allergy Liqui-Gels Softgels .... ▣692
Benadryl Itch Relief Stick Extra Strength .... ▣696
Benadryl Itch Stopping Cream Extra Strength .... ▣697
Benadryl Itch Stopping Gel Extra Strength .... ▣697
Benadryl Itch Stopping Spray Extra Strength .... ▣697
Benadryl Maximum Strength Severe Allergy & Sinus Headache Caplets...................... ▣694
Children's Benadryl D Liquid Medication..................................... ▣693
Benadryl D Tablets .... ▣694
Nytol QuickCaps Caplets .... ▣635
Maximum Strength Nytol QuickGels Softgels .... ▣635
Simply Sleep Caplets 1841
Sominex Original Formula Tablets .. ▣637
TheraFlu Thin Strips Multi Symptom...................................... ▣684
Triaminic Thin Strips Cough & Runny Nose .... ▣690
Children's Tylenol Plus Cold & Allergy Suspension Liquid 1850
Tylenol Allergy Complete Night Time Caplets 1844
Tylenol Severe Allergy Caplets 1844
Tylenol Flu NightTime Gelcaps 1846
Extra Strength Tylenol PM Caplets, Geltabs, Gelcaps and Liquid 1847
Unisom Maximum Strength SleepGels .... ▣712

Doxepin Hydrochloride (Interactions of carvedilol with strong inhibitors of CYP2D6, such as quinidine, have not been studied, but these drugs would be expected to increase blood levels of the R(+) enantiomer of carvedilol. Analysis of side effects showed that poor 2D6 metabolizers had a higher rate of dizziness during up-titration, presumably resulting from vasodilating effects of the higher concentrations of the alpha-blocking R(+) enantiomer).

No products indexed under this heading.

Epinephrine (Patients on beta-blocker therapy and with a history of severe anaphylactic reactions to a variety of allergens may be unresponsive to the usual doses of epinephrine used to treat allergic reactions). Products include:

EpiPen 1061
Primatene Mist .... ▣749

Epinephrine Bitartrate (Patients on beta-blocker therapy and with a history of severe anaphylactic reactions to a variety of allergens may be unresponsive to the usual doses of epinephrine used to treat allergic reactions).

No products indexed under this heading.

Epinephrine Hydrochloride (Potential for unresponsiveness to the usual dose of epinephrine used to treat allergic reactions).

No products indexed under this heading.

Escitalopram Oxalate (Interactions of carvedilol with strong inhibitors of CYP2D6, such as quinidine, have not been studied, but these drugs would be expected to increase blood levels of the R(+) enantiomer of carvedilol. Analysis of side effects showed that poor 2D6 metabolizers had a higher rate of dizziness during up-titration, presumably resulting from vasodilating effects of the higher concentrations of the alpha-blocking R(+) enantiomer). Products include:

Lexapro Oral Solution 1193
Lexapro Tablets 1193

Fluoxetine (Interactions of carvedilol with strong inhibitors of CYP2D6, such as quinidine, have not been studied, but these drugs would be expected to increase blood levels of the R(+) enantiomer of carvedilol. Analysis of side effects showed that poor 2D6 metabolizers had a higher rate of dizziness during up-titration, presumably resulting from vasodilating effects of the higher concentrations of the alpha-blocking R(+) enantiomer).

No products indexed under this heading.

Fluoxetine Hydrochloride (Interactions of carvedilol with strong inhibitors of CYP2D6, such as fluoxetine, have not been studied, but these drugs would be expected to increase blood levels of the R(+) enantiomer of carvedilol. Analysis of side effects showed that poor 2D6 metabolizers had a higher rate of dizziness during up-titration, presumably resulting from vasodilating effects of the higher concentrations of the alpha-blocking R(+) enantiomer). Products include:

Prozac Pulvules and Liquid 1771
Symbyax Capsules 1788

Fluphenazine Decanoate (Interactions of carvedilol with strong inhibitors of CYP2D6, such as quinidine, have not been studied, but these drugs would be expected to increase blood levels of the R(+) enantiomer of carvedilol. Analysis of side effects showed that poor 2D6 metabolizers had a higher rate of dizziness during up-titration, presumably resulting from vasodilating effects of the higher concentrations of the alpha-blocking R(+) enantiomer).

No products indexed under this heading.

Fluphenazine Enanthate (Interactions of carvedilol with strong inhibitors of CYP2D6, such as quinidine, have not been studied, but these drugs would be expected to increase blood levels of the R(+) enantiomer of carvedilol. Analysis of side effects showed that poor 2D6 metabolizers had a higher rate of dizziness during up-titration, presumably resulting from vasodilating effects of the higher concentrations of the alpha-blocking R(+) enantiomer).

No products indexed under this heading.

Fluphenazine Hydrochloride (Interactions of carvedilol with strong inhibitors of CYP2D6, such as quinidine, have not been studied, but these drugs would be expected to increase blood levels of the R(+) enantiomer of carvedilol. Analysis of side effects showed that poor 2D6 metabolizers had a higher rate of dizziness during up-titration, presumably resulting from vasodilating effects of the higher concentrations of the alpha-blocking R(+) enantiomer).

No products indexed under this heading.

Fluvoxamine Maleate (Interactions of carvedilol with strong inhibitors of CYP2D6, such as quinidine, have not been studied, but these drugs would be expected to increase blood levels of the R(+) enantiomer of carvedilol. Analysis of side effects showed that poor 2D6 metabolizers had a higher rate of

dizziness during up-titration, presumably resulting from vasodilating effects of the higher concentrations of the alpha-blocking R(+) enantiomer).
No products indexed under this heading.

Glimepiride (Beta-blockers may mask some of the manifestations of hypoglycemia, particularly tachycardia; nonselective beta-blockers may potentiate insulin-induced hypoglycemia and delay recovery of serum glucose levels; in congestive heart failure patients with diabetes, carvedilol therapy may lead to worsening of hyperglycemia, which responds to intensification of hypoglycemia). Products include:
Amaryl Tablets **2864**

Glipizide (Beta-blockers may mask some of the manifestations of hypoglycemia, particularly tachycardia; nonselective beta-blockers may potentiate insulin-induced hypoglycemia and delay recovery of serum glucose levels; in congestive heart failure patients with diabetes, carvedilol therapy may lead to worsening of hyperglycemia, which responds to intensification of hypoglycemia).
No products indexed under this heading.

Glyburide (Beta-blockers may mask some of the manifestations of hypoglycemia, particularly tachycardia; nonselective beta-blockers may potentiate insulin-induced hypoglycemia and delay recovery of serum glucose levels; in congestive heart failure patients with diabetes, carvedilol therapy may lead to worsening of hyperglycemia, which responds to intensification of hypoglycemia).
No products indexed under this heading.

Guanethidine Monosulfate (Patients receiving agents with beta-blocking properties and a drug that may deplete catecholamines should be observed closely for signs of hypotension and/or severe bradycardia).
No products indexed under this heading.

Halofantrine Hydrochloride (Interactions of carvedilol with strong inhibitors of CYP2D6, such as quinidine, have not been studied, but these drugs would be expected to increase blood levels of the R(+) enantiomer of carvedilol. Analysis of side effects showed that poor 2D6 metabolizers had a higher rate of dizziness during up-titration, presumably resulting from vasodilating effects of the higher concentrations of the alpha-blocking R(+) enantiomer).
No products indexed under this heading.

Haloperidol (Interactions of carvedilol with strong inhibitors of CYP2D6, such as quinidine, have not been studied, but these drugs would be expected to increase blood levels of the R(+) enantiomer of carvedilol. Analysis of side effects showed that poor 2D6 metabolizers had a higher rate of dizziness during up-titration, presumably resulting from vasodilating effects of the higher concentrations of the alpha-blocking R(+) enantiomer).
No products indexed under this heading.

Haloperidol Decanoate (Interactions of carvedilol with strong inhibitors of CYP2D6, such as quinidine, have not been studied, but these drugs would be expected to increase blood levels of the R(+) enantiomer of carvedilol. Analysis of side effects showed that poor 2D6 metabolizers had a higher rate of dizziness during up-titration, presumably resulting from vasodilating effects of the higher concentrations of the alpha-blocking R(+) enantiomer).
No products indexed under this heading.

Hydroxychloroquine Sulfate (Interactions of carvedilol with strong inhibitors of CYP2D6, such as quinidine, have not been studied, but these drugs would be expected to increase blood levels of the R(+) enantiomer of carvedilol. Analysis of side effects showed that poor 2D6 metabolizers had a higher rate of dizziness during up-titration, presumably resulting from vasodilating effects of the higher concentrations of the alpha-blocking R(+) enantiomer).
No products indexed under this heading.

Imatinib Mesylate (Interactions of carvedilol with strong inhibitors of CYP2D6, such as quinidine, have not been studied, but these drugs would be expected to increase blood levels of the R(+) enantiomer of carvedilol. Analysis of side effects showed that poor 2D6 metabolizers had a higher rate of dizziness during up-titration, presumably resulting from vasodilating effects of the higher concentrations of the alpha-blocking R(+) enantiomer). Products include:
Gleevec Tablets **2221**

Imipramine Hydrochloride (Interactions of carvedilol with strong inhibitors of CYP2D6, such as quinidine, have not been studied, but these drugs would be expected to increase blood levels of the R(+) enantiomer of carvedilol. Analysis of side effects showed that poor 2D6 metabolizers had a higher rate of dizziness during up-titration, presumably resulting from vasodilating effects of the higher concentrations of the alpha-blocking R(+) enantiomer).
No products indexed under this heading.

Imipramine Pamoate (Interactions of carvedilol with strong inhibitors of CYP2D6, such as quinidine, have not been studied, but these drugs would be expected to increase blood levels of the R(+) enantiomer of carvedilol. Analysis of side effects showed that poor 2D6 metabolizers had a higher rate of dizziness during up-titration, presumably resulting from vasodilating effects of the higher concentrations of the alpha-blocking R(+) enantiomer).
No products indexed under this heading.

Insulin, Human, Zinc Suspension (Beta-blockers may mask some of the manifestations of hypoglycemia, particularly tachycardia; nonselective beta-blockers may potentiate insulin-induced hypoglycemia and delay recovery of serum glucose levels; in congestive heart failure patients with diabetes, carvedilol therapy may lead to worsening of hyperglycemia, which responds to intensification of hypoglycemia). Products include:
Humulin L, 100 Units **1763**
Humulin U, 100 Units **1770**

Insulin, Human NPH (Beta-blockers may mask some of the manifestations of hypoglycemia, particularly tachycardia; nonselective beta-blockers may potentiate insulin-induced hypoglycemia and delay recovery of serum glucose levels; in congestive heart failure patients with diabetes, carvedilol therapy may lead to worsening of hyperglycemia, which responds to intensification of hypoglycemia). Products include:
Humulin N, 100 Units **1764**
Humulin N Pen **1765**
Novolin N Human Insulin 10 ml Vials **2322**
Novolin N InnoLet **2322**
Novolin N PenFill 3 ml Cartridges **2325**
Novolin R InnoLet **2322**

Insulin, Human Regular (Beta-blockers may mask some of the manifestations of hypoglycemia, particularly tachycardia; nonselective beta-blockers may potentiate insulin-induced hypoglycemia and delay recovery of serum glucose levels; in congestive heart failure patients with diabetes, carvedilol therapy may lead to worsening of hyperglycemia, which responds to intensification of hypoglycemia). Products include:
Humulin R (U-500) **1768**
Humulin R, 100 Units **1767**
Novolin R Human Insulin 10 ml Vials **2322**
Novolin R PenFill **2325**

Insulin, Human Regular and Human NPH Mixture (Beta-blockers may mask some of the manifestations of hypoglycemia, particularly tachycardia; nonselective beta-blockers may potentiate insulin-induced hypoglycemia and delay recovery of serum glucose levels; in congestive heart failure patients with diabetes, carvedilol therapy may lead to worsening of hyperglycemia, which responds to intensification of hypoglycemia). Products include:
Humulin 50/50, 100 Units **1760**
Humulin 70/30 Pen **1761**
Novolin 70/30 Human Insulin 10 ml Vials **2321**
Novolin 70/30 InnoLet **2322**
Novolin 70/30 PenFill 3 ml Cartridges **2325**

Insulin, NPH (Beta-blockers may mask some of the manifestations of hypoglycemia, particularly tachycardia; nonselective beta-blockers may potentiate insulin-induced hypoglycemia and delay recovery of serum glucose levels; in congestive heart failure patients with diabetes, carvedilol therapy may lead to worsening of hyperglycemia, which responds to intensification of hypoglycemia).
No products indexed under this heading.

Insulin, Regular (Beta-blockers may mask some of the manifestations of hypoglycemia, particularly tachycardia; nonselective beta-blockers may potentiate insulin-induced hypoglycemia and delay recovery of serum glucose levels; in congestive heart failure patients with diabetes, carvedilol therapy may lead to worsening of hyperglycemia, which responds to intensification of hypoglycemia).
No products indexed under this heading.

Insulin, Zinc Crystals (Beta-blockers may mask some of the manifestations of hypoglycemia, particularly tachycardia; nonselective beta-blockers may potentiate insulin-induced hypoglycemia and delay recovery of serum glucose levels; in congestive heart failure patients with diabetes, carvedilol therapy may lead to worsening of hyperglycemia, which responds to intensification of hypoglycemia).
No products indexed under this heading.

Insulin, Zinc Suspension (Beta-blockers may mask some of the manifestations of hypoglycemia, particularly tachycardia; nonselective beta-blockers may potentiate insulin-induced hypoglycemia and delay recovery of serum glucose levels; in congestive heart failure patients with diabetes, carvedilol therapy may lead to worsening of hyperglycemia, which responds to intensification of hypoglycemia).
No products indexed under this heading.

Insulin Aspart, Human Regular (Beta-blockers may mask some of the manifestations of hypoglycemia, particularly tachycardia; nonselective beta-blockers may potentiate insulin-induced hypoglycemia and delay recovery of serum glucose levels; in congestive heart failure patients with diabetes, carvedilol therapy may lead to worsening of hyperglycemia, which responds to intensification of hypoglycemia). Products include:
NovoLog Injection **2326**

Insulin glargine (Beta-blockers may mask some of the manifestations of hypoglycemia, particularly tachycardia; nonselective beta-blockers may potentiate insulin-induced hypoglycemia and delay recovery of serum glucose levels; in congestive heart failure patients with diabetes, carvedilol therapy may lead to worsening of hyperglycemia, which responds to intensification of hypoglycemia). Products include:
Lantus Injection **2925**

Insulin Lispro, Human (Beta-blockers may mask some of the manifestations of hypoglycemia, particularly tachycardia; nonselective beta-blockers may potentiate insulin-induced hypoglycemia and delay recovery of serum glucose levels; in congestive heart failure patients with diabetes, carvedilol therapy may lead to worsening of hyperglycemia, which responds to intensification of hypoglycemia). Products include:
Humalog-Pen **1751**
Humalog Mix 75/25-Pen **1754**

Insulin Lispro Protamine, Human (Beta-blockers may mask some of the manifestations of hypoglycemia, particularly tachycardia; nonselective beta-blockers may potentiate insulin-induced hypoglycemia and delay recovery of serum glucose levels; in congestive heart failure patients with diabetes, carvedilol therapy may lead to worsening of hyperglycemia, which responds to intensification of hypoglycemia). Products include:
Humalog Mix 75/25-Pen **1754**

Isocarboxazid (Patients receiving agents with beta-blocking properties and a drug that may deplete catecholamines should be observed closely for signs of hypotension and/or severe bradycardia).
No products indexed under this heading.

Maprotiline Hydrochloride (Interactions of carvedilol with strong inhibitors of CYP2D6, such as quinidine, have not been studied, but these drugs would be expected to increase blood levels of the R(+) enantiomer of carvedilol. Analysis of side effects showed that poor 2D6 metabolizers had a higher rate of dizziness during up-titration, presumably resulting from vasodilating effects of the higher concentrations of the alpha-blocking R(+) enantiomer).
No products indexed under this heading.

Metformin Hydrochloride (Beta-blockers may mask some of the manifestations of hypoglycemia, particularly tachycardia; nonselective beta-blockers may potentiate insulin-induced hypoglycemia and delay recovery of serum glucose levels; in congestive heart failure patients with diabetes, carvedilol therapy may lead to worsening of hyperglycemia, which responds to intensification of hypoglycemia). Products include:
ActoPlus Met Tablets 3219
Avandamet Tablets 1343
Fortamet Extended-Release Tablets 1156

Methadone Hydrochloride (Interactions of carvedilol with strong inhibitors of CYP2D6, such as quinidine, have not been studied, but these drugs would be expected to increase blood levels of the R(+) enantiomer of carvedilol. Analysis of side effects showed that poor 2D6 metabolizers had a higher rate of dizziness during up-titration, presumably resulting from vasodilating effects of the higher concentrations of the alpha-blocking R(+) enantiomer).
No products indexed under this heading.

Mibefradil Dihydrochloride (Interactions of carvedilol with strong inhibitors of CYP2D6, such as quinidine, have not been studied, but these drugs would be expected to increase blood levels of the R(+) enantiomer of carvedilol. Analysis of side effects showed that poor 2D6 metabolizers had a higher rate of dizziness during up-titration, presumably resulting from vasodilating effects of the higher concentrations of the alpha-blocking R(+) enantiomer).
No products indexed under this heading.

Miglitol (Beta-blockers may mask some of the manifestations of hypoglycemia, particularly tachycardia; nonselective beta-blockers may potentiate insulin-induced hypoglycemia and delay recovery of serum glucose levels; in congestive heart failure patients with diabetes, carvedilol therapy may lead to worsening of hyperglycemia, which responds to intensification of hypoglycemia).
No products indexed under this heading.

Moclobemide (Patients receiving agents with beta-blocking properties and a drug that may deplete catecholamines should be observed closely for signs of hypotension and/or severe bradycardia).
No products indexed under this heading.

Nortriptyline Hydrochloride (Interactions of carvedilol with strong inhibitors of CYP2D6, such as quinidine, have not been studied, but these drugs would be expected to increase blood levels of the R(+) enantiomer of carvedilol. Analysis of side effects showed that poor 2D6 metabolizers had a higher rate of dizziness during up-titration, presumably resulting from vasodilating effects of the higher concentrations of the alpha-blocking R(+) enantiomer).
No products indexed under this heading.

Pargyline Hydrochloride (Patients receiving agents with beta-blocking properties and a drug that may deplete catecholamines should be observed closely for signs of hypotension and/or severe bradycardia).
No products indexed under this heading.

Paroxetine Hydrochloride (Interactions of carvedilol with strong inhibitors of CYP2D6, such as paroxetine, have not been studied, but these drugs would be expected to increase blood levels of the R(+) enantiomer of carvedilol. Analysis of side effects showed that poor 2D6 metabolizers had a higher rate of dizziness during up-titration, presumably resulting from vasodilating effects of the higher concentrations of the alpha-blocking R(+) enantiomer). Products include:
Paxil CR Controlled-Release Tablets 1509
Paxil 1501

Perphenazine (Interactions of carvedilol with strong inhibitors of CYP2D6, such as quinidine, have not been studied, but these drugs would be expected to increase blood levels of the R(+) enantiomer of carvedilol. Analysis of side effects showed that poor 2D6 metabolizers had a higher rate of dizziness during up-titration, presumably resulting from vasodilating effects of the higher concentrations of the alpha-blocking R(+) enantiomer).
No products indexed under this heading.

Phenelzine Sulfate (Patients receiving agents with beta-blocking properties and a drug that may deplete catecholamines should be observed closely for signs of hypotension and/or severe bradycardia).
No products indexed under this heading.

Pioglitazone Hydrochloride (Beta-blockers may mask some of the manifestations of hypoglycemia, particularly tachycardia; nonselective beta-blockers may potentiate insulin-induced hypoglycemia and delay recovery of serum glucose levels; in congestive heart failure patients with diabetes, carvedilol therapy may lead to worsening of hyperglycemia, which responds to intensification of hypoglycemia). Products include:
ActoPlus Met Tablets 3219
Actos Tablets 3224

Procarbazine Hydrochloride (Patients receiving agents with beta-blocking properties and a drug that may deplete catecholamines should be observed closely for signs of hypotension and/or severe bradycardia). Products include:
Matulane Capsules 3188

Propafenone Hydrochloride (Interactions of carvedilol with strong inhibitors of CYP2D6, such as propafenone, have not been studied, but these drugs would be expected to increase blood levels of the R(+) enantiomer of carvedilol. Analysis of side effects showed that poor 2D6 metabolizers had a higher rate of dizziness during up-titration, presumably resulting from vasodilating effects of the higher concentrations of the alpha-blocking R(+) enantiomer). Products include:
Rythmol SR Capsules 2736

Propoxyphene Hydrochloride (Interactions of carvedilol with strong inhibitors of CYP2D6, such as quinidine, have not been studied, but these drugs would be expected to increase blood levels of the R(+) enantiomer of carvedilol. Analysis of side effects showed that poor 2D6 metabolizers had a higher rate of dizziness during up-titration, presumably resulting from vasodilating effects of the higher concentrations of the alpha-blocking R(+) enantiomer).
No products indexed under this heading.

Propoxyphene Napsylate (Interactions of carvedilol with strong inhibitors of CYP2D6, such as quinidine, have not been studied, but these drugs would be expected to increase blood levels of the R(+) enantiomer of carvedilol. Analysis of side effects showed that poor 2D6 metabolizers had a higher rate of dizziness during up-titration, presumably resulting from vasodilating effects of the higher concentrations of the alpha-blocking R(+) enantiomer). Products include:
Darvocet A 500 Tablets 3497

Protriptyline Hydrochloride (Interactions of carvedilol with strong inhibitors of CYP2D6, such as quinidine, have not been studied, but these drugs would be expected to increase blood levels of the R(+) enantiomer of carvedilol. Analysis of side effects showed that poor 2D6 metabolizers had a higher rate of dizziness during up-titration, presumably resulting from vasodilating effects of the higher concentrations of the alpha-blocking R(+) enantiomer). Products include:
Vivactil Tablets 2350

Quinacrine Hydrochloride (Interactions of carvedilol with strong inhibitors of CYP2D6, such as quinidine, have not been studied, but these drugs would be expected to increase blood levels of the R(+) enantiomer of carvedilol. Analysis of side effects showed that poor 2D6 metabolizers had a higher rate of dizziness during up-titration, presumably resulting from vasodilating effects of the higher concentrations of the alpha-blocking R(+) enantiomer).
No products indexed under this heading.

Quinidine (Co-administration of carvedilol with strong inhibitors of CYP2D6, such as quinidine, have not been studied, but quinidine would be expected to increase blood levels).
No products indexed under this heading.

Quinidine Gluconate (Co-administration of carvedilol with strong inhibitors of CYP2D6, such as quinidine, have not been studied, but quinidine would be expected to increase blood levels).
No products indexed under this heading.

Quinidine Hydrochloride (Co-administration of carvedilol with strong inhibitors of CYP2D6, such as quinidine, have not been studied, but quinidine would be expected to increase blood levels).
No products indexed under this heading.

Quinidine Polygalacturonate (Co-administration of carvedilol with strong inhibitors of CYP2D6, such as quinidine, have not been studied, but quinidine would be expected to increase blood levels).
No products indexed under this heading.

Quinidine Sulfate (Co-administration of carvedilol with strong inhibitors of CYP2D6, such as quinidine, have not been studied, but quinidine would be expected to increase blood levels).
No products indexed under this heading.

Ranitidine Bismuth Citrate (Interactions of carvedilol with strong inhibitors of CYP2D6, such as quinidine, have not been studied, but these drugs would be expected to increase blood levels of the R(+) enantiomer of carvedilol. Analysis of side effects showed that poor 2D6 metabolizers had a higher rate of dizziness during up-titration, presumably resulting from vasodilating effects of the higher concentrations of the alpha-blocking R(+) enantiomer).
No products indexed under this heading.

Ranitidine Hydrochloride (Interactions of carvedilol with strong inhibitors of CYP2D6, such as quinidine, have not been studied, but these drugs would be expected to increase blood levels of the R(+) enantiomer of carvedilol. Analysis of side effects showed that poor 2D6 metabolizers had a higher rate of dizziness during up-titration, presumably resulting from vasodilating effects of the higher concentrations of the alpha-blocking R(+) enantiomer). Products include:
Zantac 1597
Zantac Injection 1593
Zantac 75 Tablets .... ▣715
Zantac 150 Maximum Strength Tablets .... ▣715
Zantac Injection Pharmacy Bulk Package 1595

Rauwolfia Serpentina (Patients receiving agents with beta-blocking properties and a drug that may deplete catecholamines should be observed closely for signs of hypotension and/or severe bradycardia).
No products indexed under this heading.

Repaglinide (Beta-blockers may mask some of the manifestations of hypoglycemia, particularly tachycardia; nonselective beta-blockers may potentiate insulin-induced hypoglycemia and delay recovery of serum glucose levels; in congestive heart failure patients with diabetes, carvedilol therapy may lead to worsening of hyperglycemia, which responds to intensification of hypoglycemia). Products include:
- Prandin Tablets (0.5, 1, and 2 mg) **2337**

Rescinnamine (Patients receiving agents with beta-blocking properties and a drug that may deplete catecholamines should be observed closely for signs of hypotension and/or severe bradycardia).
- No products indexed under this heading.

Reserpine (Co-administration of agents with beta-blocking properties and a drug that can deplete catecholamines, such as reserpine, may result in hypotension and/or severe bradycardia).
- No products indexed under this heading.

Rifampin (Carvedilol undergoes substantial oxidative metabolism, co-administration has resulted in decreased AUC and Cmax of carvedilol by about 70%).
- No products indexed under this heading.

Ritonavir (Interactions of carvedilol with strong inhibitors of CYP2D6, such as quinidine, have not been studied, but these drugs would be expected to increase blood levels of the R(+) enantiomer of carvedilol. Analysis of side effects showed that poor 2D6 metabolizers had a higher rate of dizziness during up-titration, presumably resulting from vasodilating effects of the higher concentrations of the alpha-blocking R(+) enantiomer). Products include:
- Kaletra **474**
- Norvir **499**

Rosiglitazone Maleate (Beta-blockers may mask some of the manifestations of hypoglycemia, particularly tachycardia; nonselective beta-blockers may potentiate insulin-induced hypoglycemia and delay recovery of serum glucose levels; in congestive heart failure patients with diabetes, carvedilol therapy may lead to worsening of hyperglycemia, which responds to intensification of hypoglycemia). Products include:
- Avandamet Tablets **1343**
- Avandia Tablets **1348**

Selegiline Hydrochloride (Patients receiving agents with beta-blocking properties and a drug that may deplete catecholamines should be observed closely for signs of hypotension and/or severe bradycardia). Products include:
- Eldepryl Capsules **3209**

Sertraline Hydrochloride (Interactions of carvedilol with strong inhibitors of CYP2D6, such as quinidine, have not been studied, but these drugs would be expected to increase blood levels of the R(+) enantiomer of carvedilol. Analysis of side effects showed that poor 2D6 metabolizers had a higher rate of dizziness during up-titration, presumably resulting from vasodilating effects of the higher concentrations of the alpha-blocking R(+) enantiomer). Products include:
- Zoloft **2581**

Terbinafine Hydrochloride (Interactions of carvedilol with strong inhibitors of CYP2D6, such as quinidine, have not been studied, but these drugs would be expected to increase blood levels of the R(+) enantiomer of carvedilol. Analysis of side effects showed that poor 2D6 metabolizers had a higher rate of dizziness during up-titration, presumably resulting from vasodilating effects of the higher concentrations of the alpha-blocking R(+) enantiomer). Products include:
- Lamisil AT Creams (Athlete's Foot & Jock Itch) .... **▣676**
- Lamisil Tablets **2226**

Thioridazine Hydrochloride (Interactions of carvedilol with strong inhibitors of CYP2D6, such as quinidine, have not been studied, but these drugs would be expected to increase blood levels of the R(+) enantiomer of carvedilol. Analysis of side effects showed that poor 2D6 metabolizers had a higher rate of dizziness during up-titration, presumably resulting from vasodilating effects of the higher concentrations of the alpha-blocking R(+) enantiomer). Products include:
- Thioridazine Hydrochloride Tablets **2122**

Tolazamide (Beta-blockers may mask some of the manifestations of hypoglycemia, particularly tachycardia; nonselective beta-blockers may potentiate insulin-induced hypoglycemia and delay recovery of serum glucose levels; in congestive heart failure patients with diabetes, carvedilol therapy may lead to worsening of hyperglycemia, which responds to intensification of hypoglycemia).
- No products indexed under this heading.

Tolbutamide (Beta-blockers may mask some of the manifestations of hypoglycemia, particularly tachycardia; nonselective beta-blockers may potentiate insulin-induced hypoglycemia and delay recovery of serum glucose levels; in congestive heart failure patients with diabetes, carvedilol therapy may lead to worsening of hyperglycemia, which responds to intensification of hypoglycemia).
- No products indexed under this heading.

Tranylcypromine Sulfate (Patients receiving agents with beta-blocking properties and a drug that may deplete catecholamines should be observed closely for signs of hypotension and/or severe bradycardia). Products include:
- Parnate Tablets **1499**

Trimipramine Maleate (Interactions of carvedilol with strong inhibitors of CYP2D6, such as quinidine, have not been studied, but these drugs would be expected to increase blood levels of the R(+) enantiomer of carvedilol. Analysis of side effects showed that poor 2D6 metabolizers had a higher rate of dizziness during up-titration, presumably resulting from vasodilating effects of the higher concentrations of the alpha-blocking R(+) enantiomer). Products include:
- Surmontil Capsules **2347**

Troglitazone (Beta-blockers may mask some of the manifestations of hypoglycemia, particularly tachycardia; nonselective beta-blockers may potentiate insulin-induced hypoglycemia and delay recovery of serum glucose levels; in congestive heart failure patients with diabetes, carvedilol therapy may lead to worsening of hyperglycemia, which responds to intensification of hypoglycemia).
- No products indexed under this heading.

Verapamil Hydrochloride (Co-administration has resulted in isolated cases of conduction disturbances, rarely with hemodynamic. Monitoring of ECG and blood pressure is recommended). Products include:
- Covera-HS Tablets **3135**
- Tarka Tablets **519**
- Verelan PM Capsules **3120**

Food Interactions

Food, unspecified (When carvedilol is administered with food, the rate of absorption is slowed, as evidenced by a delay in the time to reach peak plasma levels, with no significant difference in extent of bioavailability; patients should be instructed to take Coreg with food in order to minimize the risk of hypotension).

CORTIZONE•5 OINTMENT
(Hydrocortisone) .... ▣699
None cited in PDR database.

CORTIZONE•10 CREME
(Hydrocortisone) .... ▣699
None cited in PDR database.

CORTIZONE•10 OINTMENT
(Hydrocortisone) .... ▣699
None cited in PDR database.

CORTIZONE•10 PLUS CREME
(Hydrocortisone) .... ▣700
None cited in PDR database.

CORTIZONE•10 MAXIMUM STRENGTH QUICK SHOT SPRAY
(Hydrocortisone) .... ▣700
None cited in PDR database.

COSMEGEN FOR INJECTION
(Dactinomycin) **1907**
May interact with vaccines, live. Compounds in these categories include:

BCG Vaccine (Live virus vaccines should not be administered during drug therapy with dactinomycin).
- No products indexed under this heading.

Measles, Mumps & Rubella Virus Vaccine, Live (Live virus vaccines should not be administered during drug therapy with dactinomycin). Products include:
- M-M-R II **1980**

Measles & Rubella Virus Vaccine Live (Live virus vaccines should not be administered during drug therapy with dactinomycin).
- No products indexed under this heading.

Measles Virus Vaccine Live (Live virus vaccines should not be administered during drug therapy with dactinomycin). Products include:
- Attenuvax **1889**

Mumps Virus Vaccine, Live (Live virus vaccines should not be administered during drug therapy with dactinomycin). Products include:
- Mumpsvax **2005**

Poliovirus Vaccine, Live, Oral, Trivalent, Types 1,2,3 (Sabin) (Live virus vaccines should not be administered during drug therapy with dactinomycin).
- No products indexed under this heading.

Rotavirus Vaccine, Live, Oral, Tetravalent (Live virus vaccines should not be administered during drug therapy with dactinomycin).
- No products indexed under this heading.

Rubella & Mumps Virus Vaccine Live (Live virus vaccines should not be administered during drug therapy with dactinomycin).
- No products indexed under this heading.

Rubella Virus Vaccine Live (Live virus vaccines should not be administered during drug therapy with dactinomycin). Products include:
- Meruvax II **1994**

Smallpox Vaccine (Live virus vaccines should not be administered during drug therapy with dactinomycin).
- No products indexed under this heading.

Typhoid Vaccine (Live virus vaccines should not be administered during drug therapy with dactinomycin).
- No products indexed under this heading.

Varicella Virus Vaccine Live (Live virus vaccines should not be administered during drug therapy with dactinomycin). Products include:
- Varivax **2070**

Yellow Fever Vaccine (Live virus vaccines should not be administered during drug therapy with dactinomycin).
- No products indexed under this heading.

COSOPT STERILE OPHTHALMIC SOLUTION
(Dorzolamide Hydrochloride, Timolol Maleate) **1910**
May interact with beta blockers, carbonic anhydrase inhibitors, calcium channel blockers, cardiac glycosides, quinidine, salicylates, and certain other agents. Compounds in these categories include:

Acebutolol Hydrochloride (Co-administration of oral beta-adrenergic blockers and Cosopt may result in potential additive effects of beta-blockade, both systemic and on intraocular pressure).
- No products indexed under this heading.

Acetazolamide (Co-administration with oral carbonic anhydrase inhibitor may result in additive carbonic anhydrase inhibition).
- No products indexed under this heading.

Amlodipine Besylate (Co-administration of beta-adrenergic blockers and calcium channel blockers may result in possible atrioventricular conduction disturbances, left ventricular failure, and hypotension). Products include:

Caduet Tablets 2507
Lotrel Capsules 2238
Norvasc Tablets 2529

Aspirin (Potential for acid-base and electrolyte disturbances with high-dose salicylate therapy). Products include:
Aggrenox Capsules 855
Bayer, Aspirin Regimen .... ▣606
Bayer Aspirin Tablets 3515
BC Powder .... ▣612
BC Allergy Sinus Cold Powder .... ▣612
Arthritis Strength BC Powder .... ▣612
BC Sinus Cold Powder .... ▣612
Ecotrin Enteric Coated Aspirin Low, Regular and Maximum Strength Tablets 1627
Goody's Body Pain Formula Powder .... ▣621
Goody's Extra Strength Headache Powder .... ▣621
Goody's Extra Strength Pain Relief Tablets .... ▣621
Percodan Tablets 1115
St. Joseph 81 mg Aspirin Chewable and Enteric Coated Tablets 1841

Aspirin, Enteric Coated (Potential for acid-base and electrolyte disturbances with high-dose salicylate therapy).
No products indexed under this heading.

Aspirin Buffered (Potential for acid-base and electrolyte disturbances with high-dose salicylate therapy).
No products indexed under this heading.

Atenolol (Co-administration of oral beta-adrenergic blockers and Cosopt may result in potential additive effects of beta-blockade, both systemic and on intraocular pressure). Products include:
Tenormin I.V. Injection 698
Tenormin Tablets 695

Bepridil Hydrochloride (Co-administration of beta-adrenergic blockers and calcium channel blockers may result in possible atrioventricular conduction disturbances, left ventricular failure, and hypotension).
No products indexed under this heading.

Betaxolol Hydrochloride (Co-administration of oral beta-adrenergic blockers and Cosopt may result in potential additive effects of beta-blockade, both systemic and on intraocular pressure; the concomitant use of two topical beta-adrenergic agents is not recommended). Products include:
Betoptic S Ophthalmic Suspension 554

Carteolol Hydrochloride (Co-administration of oral beta-adrenergic blockers and Cosopt may result in potential additive effects of beta-blockade, both systemic and on intraocular pressure; the concomitant use of two topical beta-adrenergic agents is not recommended). Products include:
Carteolol Hydrochloride Ophthalmic Solution USP, 1% .... ⊙246

Choline Magnesium Trisalicylate (Potential for acid-base and electrolyte disturbances with high-dose salicylate therapy).
No products indexed under this heading.

Clonidine (Oral beta-adrenergic blocking agents may exacerbate the rebound hypertension which can follow withdrawal of clonidine; there have been no reports of exacerbation of rebound hypertension with ophthalmic timolol). Products include:
Catapres-TTS 875

Clonidine Hydrochloride (Oral beta-adrenergic blocking agents may exacerbate the rebound hypertension which can follow withdrawal of clonidine; there have been no reports of exacerbation of rebound hypertension with ophthalmic timolol). Products include:
Catapres Tablets 874
Clorpres Tablets 2139

Deslanoside (The concomitant use of beta-adrenergic blocking agents with digitalis and calcium antagonists may have additive effects in prolonging atrioventricular conduction time).
No products indexed under this heading.

Dichlorphenamide (Co-administration with oral carbonic anhydrase inhibitor may result in additive carbonic anhydrase inhibition). Products include:
Daranide Tablets 1928

Diflunisal (Potential for acid-base and electrolyte disturbances with high-dose salicylate therapy). Products include:
Dolobid Tablets 1937

Digitalis Glycoside Preparations (The concomitant use of beta-adrenergic blocking agents with digitalis and calcium antagonists may have additive effects in prolonging atrioventricular conduction time).
No products indexed under this heading.

Digitoxin (The concomitant use of beta-adrenergic blocking agents with digitalis and calcium antagonists may have additive effects in prolonging atrioventricular conduction time).
No products indexed under this heading.

Digoxin (The concomitant use of beta-adrenergic blocking agents with digitalis and calcium antagonists may have additive effects in prolonging atrioventricular conduction time). Products include:
Digitek Tablets 2146
Lanoxicaps Capsules 1458
Lanoxin Injection 1462
Lanoxin Tablets 1468
Lanoxin Injection Pediatric 1465

Diltiazem Hydrochloride (Co-administration of beta-adrenergic blockers and calcium channel blockers may result in possible atrioventricular conduction disturbances, left ventricular failure, and hypotension). Products include:
Cardizem LA Extended Release Tablets 1699
Tiazac Capsules 1204

Epinephrine (Patients with a history of atopy or anaphylactic reactions to a variety of allergens may be unresponsive to the usual dose of injectable epinephrine used to treat allergic reactions). Products include:
EpiPen 1061
Primatene Mist .... ▣749

Epinephrine Hydrochloride (Patients with a history of atopy or anaphylactic reactions to a variety of allergens may be unresponsive to the usual dose of injectable epinephrine used to treat allergic reactions).
No products indexed under this heading.

Felodipine (Co-administration of beta-adrenergic blockers and calcium channel blockers may result in possible atrioventricular conduction disturbances, left ventricular failure, and hypotension). Products include:
Plendil Extended-Release Tablets 651

Isradipine (Co-administration of beta-adrenergic blockers and calcium channel blockers may result in possible atrioventricular conduction disturbances, left ventricular failure, and hypotension). Products include:
DynaCirc CR Tablets 2726

Levobunolol Hydrochloride (Co-administration of oral beta-adrenergic blockers and Cosopt may result in potential additive effects of beta-blockade, both systemic and on intraocular pressure; the concomitant use of two topical beta-adrenergic agents is not recommended). Products include:
Betagan Ophthalmic Solution, USP .... ⊙217

Magnesium Salicylate (Potential for acid-base and electrolyte disturbances with high-dose salicylate therapy).
No products indexed under this heading.

Methazolamide (Co-administration with oral carbonic anhydrase inhibitor may result in additive carbonic anhydrase inhibition).
No products indexed under this heading.

Metipranolol Hydrochloride (Co-administration of oral beta-adrenergic blockers and Cosopt may result in potential additive effects of beta-blockade, both systemic and on intraocular pressure; the concomitant use of two topical beta-adrenergic agents is not recommended).
No products indexed under this heading.

Mibefradil Dihydrochloride (Co-administration of beta-adrenergic blockers and calcium channel blockers may result in possible atrioventricular conduction disturbances, left ventricular failure, and hypotension).
No products indexed under this heading.

Nicardipine Hydrochloride (Co-administration of beta-adrenergic blockers and calcium channel blockers may result in possible atrioventricular conduction disturbances, left ventricular failure, and hypotension). Products include:
Cardene I.V. 1129

Nifedipine (Co-administration of beta-adrenergic blockers and calcium channel blockers may result in possible atrioventricular conduction disturbances, left ventricular failure, and hypotension). Products include:
Adalat CC Tablets 2978

Nimodipine (Co-administration of beta-adrenergic blockers and calcium channel blockers may result in possible atrioventricular conduction disturbances, left ventricular failure, and hypotension). Products include:
Nimotop Capsules 774

Nisoldipine (Co-administration of beta-adrenergic blockers and calcium channel blockers may result in possible atrioventricular conduction disturbances, left ventricular failure, and hypotension). Products include:
Sular Tablets 1163

Quinidine (Potentiated systemic beta-blockade has been reported during combined treatment with quinidine and timolol).
No products indexed under this heading.

Quinidine Gluconate (Potentiated systemic beta-blockade has been reported during combined treatment with quinidine and timolol).
No products indexed under this heading.

Quinidine Hydrochloride (Potentiated systemic beta-blockade has been reported during combined treatment with quinidine and timolol).
No products indexed under this heading.

Quinidine Polygalacturonate (Potentiated systemic beta-blockade has been reported during combined treatment with quinidine and timolol).
No products indexed under this heading.

Quinidine Sulfate (Potentiated systemic beta-blockade has been reported during combined treatment with quinidine and timolol).
No products indexed under this heading.

Reserpine (Co-administration of catecholamine-depleting drugs and beta-adrenergic blocker may result in possible additive effects and the production of hypotension and/or marked bradycardia).
No products indexed under this heading.

Salsalate (Potential for acid-base and electrolyte disturbances with high-dose salicylate therapy).
No products indexed under this heading.

Timolol Hemihydrate (Co-administration of oral beta-adrenergic blockers and Cosopt may result in potential additive effects of beta-blockade, both systemic and on intraocular pressure; the concomitant use of two topical beta-adrenergic agents is not recommended). Products include:
Betimol Ophthalmic Solution 3371
Betimol Ophthalmic Solution .... ⊙283

Verapamil Hydrochloride (Co-administration of beta-adrenergic blockers and calcium channel blockers may result in possible atrioventricular conduction disturbances, left ventricular failure, and hypotension). Products include:
Covera-HS Tablets 3135
Tarka Tablets 519
Verelan PM Capsules 3120

COUMADIN FOR INJECTION

(Warfarin Sodium) 932

See Coumadin Tablets

COUMADIN TABLETS

(Warfarin Sodium) 932

May interact with 5-lipoxygenase inhibitors, oral aminoglycosides, androgens, antacids, antihistamines, antiandrogens, barbiturates, corticosteroids, diuretics, erythromycin, fluoroquinolone antibiotics, inhalant anesthetics, leukotriene receptor antagonists, monoamine oxidase inhibitors, narcotic analgesics, nonsteroidal anti-inflammatory agents, oral contraceptives, pyrazolon derivatives, salicylates, selective serotonin reuptake inhibitors, sulfonamides, thyroid preparations, and certain other agents. Compounds in these categories include:

Acetaminophen (May be responsible for increased prothrombin time response). Products include:

Benadryl Allergy & Cold Tablets ... ▣692
Benadryl Allergy & Sinus Headache Caplets & Gelcaps ... ▣693
Benadryl Maximum Strength Severe Allergy & Sinus Headache Caplets ... ▣694
Contac Severe Cold and Flu Caplets Maximum Strength ... ▣615
Contac Severe Cold and Flu Caplets Non-Drowsy ... ▣615
Darvocet A 500 Tablets ... 3497
Goody's Body Pain Formula Powder ... ▣621
Goody's Extra Strength Headache Powder ... ▣621
Goody's Extra Strength Pain Relief Tablets ... ▣621
Goody's PM Powder ... ▣622
Hycomine Compound Tablets ... 1105
Lortab ... 3315
Lortab Elixir ... 3312
Percocet Tablets ... 1114
Robitussin Cough, Cold & Flu Liquid-filled Capsules ... ▣750
Robitussin Flu Liquid ... ▣752
Sedapap Tablets 50 mg/650 mg ... 2098
Singlet Caplets ... ▣636
Sudafed Severe Cold ... ▣710
Sudafed Sinus Headache ... ▣711
TheraFlu Cold & Cough Hot Liquid ... ▣680
TheraFlu Cold & Sore Throat Hot Liquid ... ▣680
TheraFlu Flu & Chest Congestion Non-Drowsy Hot Liquid ... ▣681
TheraFlu Flu & Sore Throat Hot Liquid ... ▣681
TheraFlu Severe Cold Non-Drowsy Hot Liquid ... ▣683
TheraFlu Severe Cold & Cough Hot Liquid ... ▣683
TheraFlu Severe Cold Caplets ... ▣679
TheraFlu Severe Cold Hot Liquid ... ▣682
TheraFlu Severe Cold Non-Drowsy Caplets ... ▣679
Triaminic Cough & Sore Throat Liquid ... ▣687
Triaminic Flu, Cough & Fever Liquid ... ▣685
Triaminic Cough & Sore Throat Softchews ... ▣689
Tylenol 8 Hour Extended Release Geltabs and Caplets ... 1843
Tylenol Sinus NightTime Caplets ... ▣663
Children's Tylenol Suspension Liquid and Meltaways ... 1850
Children's Tylenol Plus Cold & Allergy Suspension Liquid ... 1850
Children's Tylenol Plus Cold NightTime Suspension Liquid ... 1851
Children's Tylenol Plus Cold & Cough Suspension Liquid and Chewable Tablets ... 1851
Children's Tylenol Plus Cold Chewable Tablets ... 1851
Children's Tylenol Plus Cold Daytime Non-Drowsy Suspension Liquid ... 1851
Children's Tylenol Plus Flu Suspension Liquid ... 1853
Concentrated Tylenol Infants' Drops Plus Cold ... 1851
Concentrated Tylenol Infants' Drops Plus Cold and Cough ... 1851
Concentrated Tylenol Infants' Drops ... 1850
Junior Tylenol Meltaways ... 1850
Tylenol Cold & Flu Severe Daytime Liquid with Cool Bust ... 1846
Tylenol Cold & Flu Severe NightTime Liquid with Cool Burst ... 1846
Tylenol Cold Severe Congestion Non-Drowsy Caplets with Cool Burst ... 1846
Tylenol Cough & Sore Throat Daytime Liquid with Cool Burst ... 1849
Tylenol Cough & Sore Throat NightTime Liquid with Cool Burst ... 1849
Tylenol ... 1843
Extra Strength Tylenol Rapid Release Gels ... 1843
Tylenol ... 1843
Tylenol Allergy Complete Night Time Caplets ... 1844
Tylenol Allergy Complete Multi-Symptom Caplets and Gelcaps with Cool Burst ... 1844
Tylenol Severe Allergy Caplets ... 1844
Tylenol Flu NightTime Gelcaps ... 1846
Tylenol Flu Day Non-Drowsy Gelcaps ... 1846
Concentrated Tylenol Infants' Drops Plus Cold Nasal Congestant, Fever Reducer & Pain Reliever ... ▣668
Concentrated Tylenol Infants' Drops Plus Cold & Cough Nasal Decongestant, Fever Reducer & Pain Reliever ... ▣668
Multi-Symptom Tylenol Cold Night Time Caplets ... 1845
Multi-Symptom Tylenol Cold Day Non-Drowsy Caplets and Gelcaps ... 1845
Extra Strength Tylenol PM Caplets, Geltabs, Gelcaps and Liquid ... 1847
Tylenol Sinus Day Non-Drowsy ... 1848
Tylenol Sinus Night Time Caplets ... 1848
Tylenol Sinus Severe Congestion Caplets with Cool Burst ... 1848
Tylenol Sore Throat Daytime Liquid with Cool Burst ... 1849
Tylenol Sore Throat NightTime Liquid with Cool Burst ... 1849
Tylenol with Codeine ... 2461
Women's Tylenol Menstrual Relief Caplets ... 1849
Ultracet Tablets ... 2462
Vicks 44M Cough, Cold & Flu Relief ... 2676
Vicks DayQuil LiquiCaps/Liquid Multi-Symptom Cold/Flu Relief ... ▣723
Vicks DayQuil Multi-Symptom Cold/Flu Relief LiquiCaps ... 2675
Vicks DayQuil Multi-Symptom Cold/Flu Relief Liquid ... 2675
Vicks NyQuil LiquiCaps ... 2677
Vicks NyQuil LiquiCaps/Liquid Multi-Symptom Cold/Flu Relief ... ▣725
Vicks NyQuil Liquid ... 2677
Vicodin Tablets ... 530
Vicodin ES Tablets ... 531
Vicodin HP Tablets ... 532
Zydone Tablets ... 1118

Achillea millefolium (Co-administration with botanicals with coagulant properties, such as yarrow, may affect the anticoagulant effects of warfarin).
No products indexed under this heading.

Acrivastine (Decreased prothrombin time response).
No products indexed under this heading.

ACTH (Decreased prothrombin time response).
No products indexed under this heading.

Agrimonia eupatoria (Co-administration with botanicals that contain salicylate and/or have antiplatelet properties, such as agrimony, may result in increased anticoagulant effects; agrimony contains salicylate and has coagulant properties).
No products indexed under this heading.

Alatrofloxacin Mesylate (Increased prothrombin time response).
No products indexed under this heading.

Alfentanil Hydrochloride (Increased prothrombin time response with prolonged use).
No products indexed under this heading.

Allium cepa (Co-administration with botanicals that contain salicylate and/or have antiplatelet or fibrinolytic properties, such as onion, may result in increased anticoagulant effects). Products include:
Mederma for Kids Topical Gel ... 2097
Mederma Topical Gel ... 2096

Allium sativum (Co-administration is associated most often with increases in the effects of warfarin; garlic may cause bleeding events when taken alone and may have anticoagulant, antiplatelet, and/or fibrinolytic properties).
No products indexed under this heading.

Allopurinol (Increased prothrombin time response).
No products indexed under this heading.

Aloe Gel (Co-administration with botanicals that contain salicylate and/or have antiplatelet properties, such as aloe gel, may result in increased anticoagulant effects).
No products indexed under this heading.

Alteplase (Increased prothrombin time response). Products include:
Activase I.V. ... 1225
Cathflo Activase ... 1232

Aluminum Carbonate (Decreased prothrombin time response).
No products indexed under this heading.

Aluminum Hydroxide (Decreased prothrombin time response). Products include:
Gaviscon Regular Strength Liquid ... ▣620
Gaviscon Regular Strength Tablets ... ▣619
Gaviscon Extra Strength Liquid ... ▣620
Gaviscon Extra Strength Tablets ... ▣619
Maalox Max Maximum Strength Antacid/Anti-Gas Liquid ... 2165
Maalox Regular Strength Antacid/Antigas Liquid ... 2164

Amiloride Hydrochloride (Decreased or increased prothrombin time response). Products include:
Midamor Tablets ... 2000
Moduretic Tablets ... 2003

Aminoglutethimide (Decreased prothrombin time response).
No products indexed under this heading.

p-Aminosalicylic Acid (Increased prothrombin time response).
No products indexed under this heading.

Amiodarone Hydrochloride (Increased prothrombin time response). Products include:
Pacerone Tablets ... 3337

Amobarbital (Decreased prothrombin time response).
No products indexed under this heading.

Aniseed (Co-administration with botanicals that contain coumarins, such as aniseed, may result in increased anticoagulant effects).
No products indexed under this heading.

Anistreplase (Increased prothrombin time response).
No products indexed under this heading.

Antibiotics, unspecified (Decreased or increased prothrombin time response).
No products indexed under this heading.

Antipyrine (Increased prothrombin time response).
No products indexed under this heading.

Apium graveolens (Co-administration with botanicals that contain coumarins, such as celery, may result in increased anticoagulant effects).
No products indexed under this heading.

Aprobarbital (Decreased prothrombin time response).
No products indexed under this heading.

Ardeparin Sodium (Co-administration has resulted in cases of venous limb ischemia, necrosis, and gangrene in patients with heparin-induced thrombocytopenia and deep venous thrombosis when heparin treatment was discontinued and warfarin therapy was started or continued; sequelae have included amputation of the involved area and/or death).
No products indexed under this heading.

Armoracia rusticana (Co-administration with botanicals that contain coumarins, such as horseradish, may result in increased anticoagulant effects).
No products indexed under this heading.

Arnica montana (Co-administration with botanicals that contain coumarins, such as arnica, may result in increased anticoagulant effects). Products include:
SinEcch Capsules ... ▣758
Zeel Solution ... 1639

Aspen (Co-administration with botanicals that contain salicylate and/or have antiplatelet properties, such as aspen, may result in increased anticoagulant effects).
No products indexed under this heading.

Aspirin (Increased prothrombin time response; caution should be observed when used concurrently). Products include:
Aggrenox Capsules ... 855
Bayer, Aspirin Regimen ... ▣606
Bayer Aspirin Tablets ... 3515
BC Powder ... ▣612
BC Allergy Sinus Cold Powder ... ▣612
Arthritis Strength BC Powder ... ▣612
BC Sinus Cold Powder ... ▣612
Ecotrin Enteric Coated Aspirin Low, Regular and Maximum Strength Tablets ... 1627
Goody's Body Pain Formula Powder ... ▣621
Goody's Extra Strength Headache Powder ... ▣621
Goody's Extra Strength Pain Relief Tablets ... ▣621
Percodan Tablets ... 1115
St. Joseph 81 mg Aspirin Chewable and Enteric Coated Tablets ... 1841

Aspirin, Enteric Coated (Increased prothrombin time response; caution should be observed when used concurrently).
No products indexed under this heading.

Aspirin Buffered (Increased prothrombin time response; caution should be observed when used concurrently).
No products indexed under this heading.

Astemizole (Decreased prothrombin time response).
No products indexed under this heading.

Atorvastatin Calcium (Decreased prothrombin time response). Products include:

Caduet Tablets 2507
Lipitor Tablets 2495

Azatadine Maleate (Decreased prothrombin time response).
No products indexed under this heading.

Azathioprine (Decreased prothrombin time response). Products include:
Azasan Tablets 2844

Azithromycin Dihydrate (Increased prothrombin time response). Products include:
Zithromax 2568
Zithromax for IV Infusion 2573
Zithromax for Oral Suspension, 300 mg, 600 mg, 900 mg, 1200 mg 2561
Zithromax Tablets, 250 mg, 500 mg 2561
Zithromax Tri-Pak 2561
Zithromax Z-Pak 2568

Bendroflumethiazide (Decreased or increased prothrombin time response).
No products indexed under this heading.

Betamethasone Acetate (Decreased or increased prothrombin time response).
No products indexed under this heading.

Betamethasone Sodium Phosphate (Decreased or increased prothrombin time response).
No products indexed under this heading.

Bicalutamide (May be responsible, alone or in combination, for increased prothrombin time/international normalized ratio (PT/INR) response). Products include:
Casodex Tablets 670

Black Cohosh (Co-administration with botanicals that contain salicylate and/or have antiplatelet properties, such as black cohosh, may result in increased anticoagulant effects). Products include:
Remifemin Menopause Tablets .... ▣766

Bromelains (Co-administration is associated most often with increases in the effects of warfarin).
No products indexed under this heading.

Bromodiphenhydramine Hydrochloride (Decreased prothrombin time response).
No products indexed under this heading.

Brompheniramine Maleate (Decreased prothrombin time response). Products include:
Alacol DM Syrup 739
Children's Dimetapp Cold & Allergy Elixir .... ▣745
Children's Dimetapp DM Cold & Cough Elixir .... ▣745
Robitussin Allergy & Cough Syrup .. ▣750

Buchu (Co-administration with botanicals that contain coumarins, such as buchu, may result in increased anticoagulant effects).
No products indexed under this heading.

Bumetanide (Decreased or increased prothrombin time response).
No products indexed under this heading.

Buprenorphine Hydrochloride (Increased prothrombin time response with prolonged use). Products include:
Buprenex Injectable 2718
Suboxone Tablets 2719
Subutex Tablets 2719

Butabarbital (Decreased prothrombin time response).
No products indexed under this heading.

Butalbital (Decreased prothrombin time response). Products include:
Sedapap Tablets 50 mg/650 mg 2098

Capecitabine (Increased prothrombin time response). Products include:
Xeloda Tablets 2825

Capsicum annuum (Co-administration with botanicals that contain coumarins, such as capsicum, may result in increased anticoagulant effects; capsicum also has fibrinolytic properties).
No products indexed under this heading.

Carbamazepine (Decreased prothrombin time response). Products include:
Carbatrol Capsules 3174
Equetro Extended-Release Capsules 3178
Tegretol/Tegretol-XR 2278

Cassia angustifolia (Co-administration with botanicals that contain coumarins, such as cassia, may result in increased anticoagulant effects).
No products indexed under this heading.

Cassia fistula (Co-administration with botanicals that contain coumarins, such as cassia, may result in increased anticoagulant effects).
No products indexed under this heading.

Cassia senna (Co-administration with botanicals that contain coumarins, such as cassia, may result in increased anticoagulant effects).
No products indexed under this heading.

Cefamandole Nafate (Increased prothrombin time response).
No products indexed under this heading.

Cefazolin Sodium (Increased prothrombin time response). Products include:
Ancef for Injection 1318

Cefoperazone Sodium (Increased prothrombin time response).
No products indexed under this heading.

Cefotetan (Increased prothrombin time response).
No products indexed under this heading.

Cefoxitin Sodium (Increased prothrombin time response). Products include:
Mefoxin for Injection 1987
Mefoxin Premixed Intravenous Solution 1990

Ceftriaxone Sodium (Increased prothrombin time response). Products include:
Rocephin Injectable Vials, ADD-Vantage, Galaxy, Bulk 2801

Celecoxib (Increased prothrombin time response; caution should be observed when used concurrently). Products include:
Celebrex Capsules 3130

Cerivastatin Sodium (May be responsible, alone or in combination, for increased prothrombin time/international normalized ratio (PT/INR) response).
No products indexed under this heading.

Cetirizine Hydrochloride (Decreased prothrombin time response). Products include:
Zyrtec Chewable Tablets 2589
Zyrtec 2589
Zyrtec-D 12 Hour Extended Release Tablets 2591

Chenodiol (Increased prothrombin time response).
No products indexed under this heading.

Chloral Hydrate (Decreased or increased prothrombin time response).
No products indexed under this heading.

Chloramphenicol (Increased prothrombin time response).
No products indexed under this heading.

Chloramphenicol Palmitate (Increased prothrombin time response).
No products indexed under this heading.

Chloramphenicol Sodium Succinate (Increased prothrombin time response).
No products indexed under this heading.

Chlordiazepoxide (Decreased prothrombin time response).
No products indexed under this heading.

Chlordiazepoxide Hydrochloride (Decreased prothrombin time response). Products include:
Librium Capsules 3349

Chlorothiazide (Decreased or increased prothrombin time response). Products include:
Aldoclor Tablets 1881
Diuril Oral 1936

Chlorothiazide Sodium (Decreased or increased prothrombin time response). Products include:
Diuril Sodium Intravenous 1934

Chlorpheniramine Maleate (Decreased prothrombin time response). Products include:
Advil Allergy Sinus Caplets .... ▣737
Advil Multi-Symptom Cold Caplets .... ▣738
BC Allergy Sinus Cold Powder .... ▣612
Contac Severe Cold and Flu Caplets Maximum Strength .... ▣615
Hycomine Compound Tablets 1105
PediaCare Multi-Symptom Cold Liquid .... ▣704
PediaCare NightRest Cough & Cold Liquid .... ▣704
Robitussin Flu Liquid .... ▣752
Robitussin PM Cough & Cold Liquid .... ▣752
Singlet Caplets .... ▣636
Sudafed Sinus & Allergy Tablets ..... ▣710
TheraFlu Cold & Cough Hot Liquid .... ▣680
TheraFlu Cold & Sore Throat Hot Liquid .... ▣680
TheraFlu Flu & Sore Throat Hot Liquid .... ▣681
TheraFlu Severe Cold & Cough Hot Liquid .... ▣683
TheraFlu Severe Cold Caplets .... ▣679
TheraFlu Severe Cold Hot Liquid .... ▣682
Triaminic Cold & Allergy Liquid .... ▣685
Triaminic Cold & Cough Liquid .... ▣685
Triaminic Flu, Cough & Fever Liquid .... ▣685
Triaminic Night Time Cough & Cold Liquid .... ▣685
Triaminic Allergy Runny Nose & Congestion Softchews .... ▣688
Triaminic Cold & Cough Softchews .... ▣688
Children's Tylenol Plus Cold NightTime Suspension Liquid 1851
Children's Tylenol Plus Cold & Cough Suspension Liquid and Chewable Tablets 1851
Children's Tylenol Plus Cold Chewable Tablets 1851
Children's Tylenol Plus Flu Suspension Liquid 1853
Tylenol Allergy Complete Multi-Symptom Caplets and Gelcaps with Cool Burst 1844
Multi-Symptom Tylenol Cold Night Time Caplets 1845
Vicks 44M Cough, Cold & Flu Relief 2676
Pediatric Vicks 44m Cough & Cold Relief 2673
Children's Vicks NyQuil Cold/Cough Relief 2671

Chlorpheniramine Polistirex (Decreased prothrombin time response). Products include:
Tussionex Pennkinetic Extended-Release Suspension 3322

Chlorpheniramine Tannate (Decreased prothrombin time response).
No products indexed under this heading.

Chlorpropamide (Increased prothrombin time response; accumulation of chlorpropamide).
No products indexed under this heading.

Chlorthalidone (Decreased or increased prothrombin time response). Products include:
Clorpres Tablets 2139

Cholestyramine (Decreased or increased prothrombin time response).
No products indexed under this heading.

Choline Magnesium Trisalicylate (Increased prothrombin time response; caution should be observed when used concurrently).
No products indexed under this heading.

Cimetidine (Increased prothrombin time response). Products include:
Tagamet HB 200 Tablets .... ▣637
Tagamet Tablets 1547

Cimetidine Hydrochloride (Increased prothrombin time response).
No products indexed under this heading.

Ciprofloxacin (Increased prothrombin time response). Products include:
Cipro I.V. 2998
Cipro I.V. Pharmacy Bulk Package ... 3509
Cipro Oral Suspension 2991
Cipro XR Tablets 3004
Ciprodex Otic Suspension 555

Ciprofloxacin Hydrochloride (Increased prothrombin time response). Products include:
Ciloxan Ophthalmic Ointment 554
Cipro Tablets 2991

Cisapride (Increased prothrombin time response).
No products indexed under this heading.

Citalopram Hydrobromide (Increased prothrombin time response). Products include:
Celexa 1177

Clarithromycin (Increased prothrombin time response). Products include:
Biaxin/Biaxin XL 402
PREVPAC 3281

Clemastine Fumarate (Decreased prothrombin time response).
No products indexed under this heading.

Clofibrate (Increased prothrombin time response).
No products indexed under this heading.

Clozapine (May be responsible, alone or in combination, for decreased prothrombin time/international normalized ratio (PT/INR) response). Products include:
- Clozapine Tablets 2141
- Clozaril Tablets 2174
- FazaClo Orally Disintegrating Tablets 547

Codeine Phosphate (Increased prothrombin time response with prolonged use). Products include:
- Tylenol with Codeine 2461

Coenzyme Q-10 (Co-administration is associated most often with decreases in the effects of warfarin). Products include:
- Cardio Essentials Capsules 3328
- CoQuinone Capsules 3343

Cortisone Acetate (Decreased or increased prothrombin time response).
No products indexed under this heading.

Cyclophosphamide (Increased or decreased prothrombin time response).
No products indexed under this heading.

Cyproheptadine Hydrochloride (Decreased prothrombin time response).
No products indexed under this heading.

Dalteparin Sodium (Co-administration has resulted in cases of venous limb ischemia, necrosis, and gangrene in patients with heparin-induced thrombocytopenia and deep venous thrombosis when heparin treatment was discontinued and warfarin therapy was started or continued; sequelae have included amputation of the involved area and/or death). Products include:
- Fragmin Injection 2638

Danazol (Increased prothrombin time response).
No products indexed under this heading.

Danshen (Increased prothrombin time response).
No products indexed under this heading.

Daucus carota (Co-administration with botanicals that contain coumarins, such as wild carrots, may result in increased anticoagulant effects).
No products indexed under this heading.

Desflurane (Increased prothrombin time response). Products include:
- Suprane Liquid for Inhalation 770

Desogestrel (Decreased prothrombin time response). Products include:
- Ortho-Cept Tablets 2395

Dexamethasone (Decreased or increased prothrombin time response). Products include:
- Ciprodex Otic Suspension 555
- Decadron Tablets 1929
- TobraDex Ophthalmic Ointment 558
- TobraDex Ophthalmic Suspension 558

Dexamethasone Acetate (Decreased or increased prothrombin time response).
No products indexed under this heading.

Dexamethasone Sodium Phosphate (Decreased or increased prothrombin time response). Products include:
- Decadron Phosphate Injection 1931

Dexchlorpheniramine Maleate (Decreased prothrombin time response).
No products indexed under this heading.

Dextrans (Low Molecular Weight) (Increased prothrombin time response).
No products indexed under this heading.

Dextrothyroxine Sodium (Increased prothrombin time response).
No products indexed under this heading.

Dezocine (Increased prothrombin time response with prolonged use).
No products indexed under this heading.

Diazoxide (Increased prothrombin time response). Products include:
- Hyperstat I.V. Injection 3031

Diclofenac Potassium (Increased prothrombin time response; caution should be observed when used concurrently). Products include:
- Cataflam Tablets 2173

Diclofenac Sodium (Increased prothrombin time response; caution should be observed when used concurrently). Products include:
- Arthrotec Tablets 3126
- Voltaren Ophthalmic Solution 2300
- Voltaren Tablets 2298
- Voltaren-XR Tablets 2301

Dicloxacillin Sodium (Decreased prothrombin time response).
No products indexed under this heading.

Dicumarol (Increased prothrombin time response).
No products indexed under this heading.

Diflunisal (Increased prothrombin time response; caution should be observed when used concurrently). Products include:
- Dolobid Tablets 1937

Diphenhydramine Citrate (Decreased prothrombin time response). Products include:
- Children's Benadryl Allergy & Cold Fastmelt Tablets 695
- Children's Benadryl D Allergy & Sinus Fastmelt Tablets 694
- Children's Benadryl Allergy Fastmelt Tablets 696
- Goody's PM Powder 622

Diphenhydramine Hydrochloride (Decreased prothrombin time response). Products include:
- Benadryl Allergy & Cold Tablets 692
- Benadryl Allergy 691
- Benadryl Allergy & Sinus Headache Caplets & Gelcaps 693
- Children's Benadryl Allergy Liquid 695
- Children's Benadryl Dye-Free Allergy Liquid 695
- Benadryl Dye-Free Allergy Liqui-Gels Softgels 692
- Benadryl Itch Relief Stick Extra Strength 696
- Benadryl Itch Stopping Cream Extra Strength 697
- Benadryl Itch Stopping Gel Extra Strength 697
- Benadryl Itch Stopping Spray Extra Strength 697
- Benadryl Maximum Strength Severe Allergy & Sinus Headache Caplets 694
- Children's Benadryl D Liquid Medication 693
- Benadryl D Tablets 694
- Nytol QuickCaps Caplets 635
- Maximum Strength Nytol QuickGels Softgels 635
- Simply Sleep Caplets 1841
- Sominex Original Formula Tablets 637
- TheraFlu Thin Strips Multi Symptom 684
- Triaminic Thin Strips Cough & Runny Nose 690
- Children's Tylenol Plus Cold & Allergy Suspension Liquid 1850
- Tylenol Allergy Complete Night Time Caplets 1844
- Tylenol Severe Allergy Caplets 1844
- Tylenol Flu NightTime Gelcaps 1846
- Extra Strength Tylenol PM Caplets, Geltabs, Gelcaps and Liquid 1847
- Unisom Maximum Strength SleepGels 712

Diphenylpyraline Hydrochloride (Decreased prothrombin time response).
No products indexed under this heading.

Dipteryx odorata (Co-administration with botanicals that contain coumarins, such as tonka beans, may result in increased anticoagulant effects).
No products indexed under this heading.

Disulfiram (Increased prothrombin time response). Products include:
- Antabuse Tablets 2343

Divalproex Sodium (Increased prothrombin time response). Products include:
- Depakote Sprinkle Capsules 422
- Depakote Tablets 427
- Depakote ER Tablets 433

Dong Quai (Co-administration with botanicals that contain coumarins, such as dong quai (angelica), may result in increased anticoagulant effects).
No products indexed under this heading.

Doxycycline Calcium (Increased prothrombin time response).
No products indexed under this heading.

Doxycycline Hyclate (Increased prothrombin time response).
No products indexed under this heading.

Doxycycline Monohydrate (Increased prothrombin time response).
No products indexed under this heading.

Enflurane (Increased prothrombin time response).
No products indexed under this heading.

Enoxacin (Increased prothrombin time response).
No products indexed under this heading.

Enoxaparin Sodium (Co-administration has resulted in cases of venous limb ischemia, necrosis, and gangrene in patients with heparin-induced thrombocytopenia and deep venous thrombosis when heparin treatment was discontinued and warfarin therapy was started or continued; sequelae have included amputation of the involved area and/or death). Products include:
- Lovenox Injection 2931

Erythromycin (Increased prothrombin time response). Products include:
- Erygel Topical Gel 2096
- Ery-Tab Tablets 447
- Erythromycin Base Filmtab Tablets 454
- Erythromycin Delayed-Release Capsules, USP 456
- PCE Dispertab Tablets 510

Erythromycin Estolate (Increased prothrombin time response).
No products indexed under this heading.

Erythromycin Ethylsuccinate (Increased prothrombin time response). Products include:
- E.E.S. 449
- EryPed 445

Erythromycin Gluceptate (Increased prothrombin time response).
No products indexed under this heading.

Erythromycin Lactobionate (Increased prothrombin time response).
No products indexed under this heading.

Erythromycin Stearate (Increased prothrombin time response). Products include:
- Erythrocin Stearate Filmtab Tablets 452

Escitalopram Oxalate (Increased prothrombin time response). Products include:
- Lexapro Oral Solution 1193
- Lexapro Tablets 1193

Ethacrynic Acid (Decreased or increased prothrombin time response). Products include:
- Edecrin Tablets 1941

Ethchlorvynol (Decreased prothrombin time response).
No products indexed under this heading.

Ethinyl Estradiol (Decreased prothrombin time response). Products include:
- Alesse-28 Tablets 3392
- Lo/Ovral-28 Tablets 3423
- NuvaRing 2357
- Ortho-Cept Tablets 2395
- Ortho-Cyclen/Ortho Tri-Cyclen 2414
- Ortho Evra Transdermal System 2402
- Ortho Tri-Cyclen Lo Tablets 2421
- Seasonale Tablets 1073
- Triphasil-28 Tablets 3483
- Yasmin 28 Tablets 818

Ethynodiol Diacetate (Decreased prothrombin time response).
No products indexed under this heading.

Etodolac (Increased prothrombin time response; caution should be observed when used concurrently).
No products indexed under this heading.

Fenofibrate (Increased prothrombin time response). Products include:
- Antara Capsules 2723
- Lofibra Capsules 1217
- Tricor Tablets 523
- Triglide Tablets 1165

Fenoprofen Calcium (Increased prothrombin time response; caution should be observed when used concurrently). Products include:
- Nalfon Capsules 2504

Fentanyl (Increased prothrombin time response with prolonged use). Products include:
- Duragesic Transdermal System 2448

Fentanyl Citrate (Increased prothrombin time response with prolonged use). Products include:
- Actiq 993

Ferula foetida (Co-administration with botanicals that contain coumarins, such as asafoetida, may result in increased anticoagulant effects).
No products indexed under this heading.

Fexofenadine Hydrochloride (Decreased prothrombin time response). Products include:
Allegra ... 2857
Allegra-D 12 Hour Extended-Release Tablets ... 2860
Allegra-D 24 Hour Extended-Release Tablets ... 2862

Filipendula ulmaria (Co-administration with botanicals that contain coumarins and salicylate, such as meadowsweet, may result in increased anticoagulant effects).
No products indexed under this heading.

Fluconazole (Increased prothrombin time response).
No products indexed under this heading.

Fludrocortisone Acetate (Decreased or increased prothrombin time response).
No products indexed under this heading.

Fluorouracil (Increased prothrombin time response). Products include:
Carac Cream, 0.5% ... 1048
Efudex ... 3348

Fluoxetine Hydrochloride (Increased prothrombin time response). Products include:
Prozac Pulvules and Liquid ... 1771
Symbyax Capsules ... 1788

Fluoxymesterone (Increased prothrombin time response).
No products indexed under this heading.

Flurbiprofen (Increased prothrombin time response; caution should be observed when used concurrently).
No products indexed under this heading.

Flutamide (May be responsible, alone or in combination, for increased prothrombin time/international normalized ratio (PT/INR) response). Products include:
Eulexin Capsules ... 3023

Fluvastatin Sodium (Increased prothrombin time response). Products include:
Lescol Capsules ... 2227
Lescol ... 2730
Lescol XL Tablets ... 2227

Fluvoxamine Maleate (Increased prothrombin time response).
No products indexed under this heading.

Fosphenytoin Sodium (Accumulation of phenytoin; decreased or increased prothrombin time response).
No products indexed under this heading.

Fucus vesiculosus (Concurrent use may result in increased anticoagulant effects).
No products indexed under this heading.

Furosemide (Decreased or increased prothrombin time response). Products include:
Furosemide Tablets ... 2117

Galium odoratum (Co-administration with botanicals that contain coumarins, such as sweet woodruff, may result in increased anticoagulant effects).
No products indexed under this heading.

Garlic Extract (Co-administration is associated most often with increases in the effects of warfarin; garlic may cause bleeding events when taken alone and may have anti-coagulant, antiplatelet, and/or fibrinolytic properties).
No products indexed under this heading.

Garlic Oil (Co-administration is associated most often with increases in the effects of warfarin; garlic may cause bleeding events when taken alone and may have anti-coagulant, antiplatelet, and/or fibrinolytic properties).
No products indexed under this heading.

Gaultheria procumbens (Co-administration with botanicals that contain salicylate and/or have antiplatelet properties, such as wintergreen, may result in increased anticoagulant effects).
No products indexed under this heading.

Gefitinib (Increased prothrombin time response). Products include:
Iressa Tablets ... 684

Gemfibrozil (May be responsible, alone or in combination, for increased prothrombin time/international normalized ratio (PT/INR) response).
No products indexed under this heading.

Ginger (Co-administration with botanicals that contain salicylate and/or have antiplatelet properties, such as ginger, may result in increased anticoagulant effects).
No products indexed under this heading.

Ginkgo biloba (Co-administration is associated most often with increases in the effects of warfarin; Gingko biloba may cause bleeding events when taken alone and may have anticoagulant, antiplatelet, and/or fibrinolytic properties).
No products indexed under this heading.

Ginseng (Co-administration with botanicals that contain salicylate and/or have antiplatelet properties, such as ginseng (Panax) may result in increased anticoagulant effects).
No products indexed under this heading.

Glipizide (Increased prothrombin time response).
No products indexed under this heading.

Glucagon (Increased prothrombin time response). Products include:
GlucaGen for Injection ... 790
Glucagon for Injection Vials and Emergency Kit ... 1749

Glutethimide (Decreased prothrombin time response).
No products indexed under this heading.

Glyburide (Increased prothrombin time response).
No products indexed under this heading.

Grepafloxacin Hydrochloride (Increased prothrombin time response).
No products indexed under this heading.

Griseofulvin (Decreased prothrombin time response). Products include:
Grifulvin V Tablets Microsize and Oral Suspension Microsize ... 2384
Gris-PEG Tablets ... 2504

Haloperidol (Decreased prothrombin time response).
No products indexed under this heading.

Haloperidol Decanoate (Decreased prothrombin time response).
No products indexed under this heading.

Halothane (Increased prothrombin time response).
No products indexed under this heading.

Heparin Sodium (Co-administration has resulted in cases of venous limb ischemia, necrosis, and gangrene in patients with heparin-induced thrombocytopenia and deep venous thrombosis when heparin treatment was discontinued and warfarin therapy was started or continued; sequelae have included amputation of the involved area and/or death).
No products indexed under this heading.

Hepatotoxic Drugs, unspecified (Increased prothrombin time response).
No products indexed under this heading.

Horse Chestnut Seed Extract (Co-administration with botanicals that contain coumarins, such as horse chestnut, may result in increased anticoagulant effects).
No products indexed under this heading.

Hydrastis canadensis (Co-administration with botanicals with coagulant properties, such as goldenseal, may affect the anticoagulant effects of warfarin).
No products indexed under this heading.

Hydrochlorothiazide (Decreased or increased prothrombin time response). Products include:
Aldoril Tablets ... 1884
Atacand HCT ... 637
Avalide Tablets ... 2889
Avalide Tablets ... 922
Benicar HCT Tablets ... 2852
Diovan HCT Tablets ... 2195
Dyazide Capsules ... 1389
Hyzaar ... 1964
Lotensin HCT Tablets ... 2235
Maxzide ... 2150
Micardis HCT Tablets ... 886
Moduretic Tablets ... 2003
Prinzide Tablets ... 2033
Teveten HCT Tablets ... 1710
Timolide Tablets ... 2056
Uniretic Tablets ... 3114
Vaseretic Tablets ... 2073
Zestoretic Tablets ... 701

Hydrocodone Bitartrate (Increased prothrombin time response with prolonged use). Products include:
Hycodan ... 1104
Hycomine Compound Tablets ... 1105
Hycotuss Expectorant Syrup ... 1106
Lortab ... 3315
Lortab Elixir ... 3312
Vicodin Tablets ... 530
Vicodin ES Tablets ... 531
Vicodin HP Tablets ... 532
Vicoprofen Tablets ... 533
Zydone Tablets ... 1118

Hydrocodone Polistirex (Increased prothrombin time response with prolonged use). Products include:
Tussionex Pennkinetic Extended-Release Suspension ... 3322

Hydrocortisone (Decreased or increased prothrombin time response). Products include:
Cortizone•5 Ointment ... ▣699
Cortizone•10 Creme ... ▣699
Cortizone•10 Ointment ... ▣699
Cortizone•10 Plus Creme ... ▣700
Cortizone•10 Maximum Strength Quick Shot Spray ... ▣700
Hydrocortone Tablets ... 1963
Preparation H Hydrocortisone Cream ... ▣748

Hydrocortisone Acetate (Decreased or increased prothrombin time response). Products include:
Analpram-HC ... 1136
Pramosone ... 1139
ProctoFoam-HC ... 3113
Tucks Anti-Itch Ointment ... ▣712
U-cort 1% Cream ... 3289

Hydrocortisone Sodium Phosphate (Decreased or increased prothrombin time response).
No products indexed under this heading.

Hydrocortisone Sodium Succinate (Decreased or increased prothrombin time response).
No products indexed under this heading.

Hydroflumethiazide (Decreased or increased prothrombin time response).
No products indexed under this heading.

Hydromorphone Hydrochloride (Increased prothrombin time response with prolonged use). Products include:
Dilaudid ... 439
Dilaudid Oral Liquid ... 443
Dilaudid Non-Sterile Powder ... 439
Dilaudid Rectal Suppositories ... 439
Dilaudid Tablets ... 439
Dilaudid Tablets - 8 mg ... 443
Dilaudid-HP ... 441

Hypericum (Co-administration is associated most often with decreases in the effects of warfarin).
No products indexed under this heading.

Ibuprofen (Increased prothrombin time response; caution should be observed when used concurrently). Products include:
Advil Allergy Sinus Caplets ... ▣737
Advil ... ▣737
Children's Advil Suspension ... ▣742
Children's Advil Chewable Tablets ... ▣741
Advil Cold & Sinus ... ▣739
Advil Flu & Body Ache Caplets ... ▣739
Children's Advil Cold Suspension ... ▣741
Infants' Advil Concentrated Drops ... ▣743
Junior Strength Advil Swallow Tablets ... ▣740
Advil Migraine Liquigels ... ▣740
Advil Multi-Symptom Cold Caplets ... ▣738
Combunox Tablets ... 1183
Children's Motrin Oral Suspension and Chewable Tablets ... 1837
Children's Motrin Cold Non-Staining Dye-Free Oral Suspension ... 1838
Children's Motrin Cold Oral Suspension ... 1838
Children's Motrin Non-Staining Dye-Free Oral Suspension ... 1837
Motrin Cold & Sinus Caplets ... 1836
Motrin IB Tablets and Caplets ... 1836
Infants' Motrin Concentrated Drops ... 1837
Infants' Motrin Non-Staining Dye-Free Drops ... 1837
Junior Strength Motrin Caplets and Chewable Tablets ... 1837
Vicoprofen Tablets ... 533

Ifosfamide (Increased prothrombin time response).
No products indexed under this heading.

Indapamide (Decreased or increased prothrombin time response). Products include:
Indapamide Tablets **2119**

Indomethacin (Increased prothrombin time response; caution should be observed when used concurrently). Products include:
Indocin **1968**

Indomethacin Sodium Trihydrate (Increased prothrombin time response; caution should be observed when used concurrently). Products include:
Indocin I.V. **1973**

Influenza Virus Vaccine (Increased prothrombin time response). Products include:
Flumist Vaccine **1872**

Inositol Nicotinate (Co-administration with botanicals that contain salicylate and/or have antiplatelet properties, such as inositol nicotinate, may result in increased anticoagulant effects).
No products indexed under this heading.

Isocarboxazid (Increased prothrombin time response).
No products indexed under this heading.

Isoflurane (Increased prothrombin time response).
No products indexed under this heading.

Itraconazole (Increased prothrombin time response).
No products indexed under this heading.

Kanamycin Sulfate (Increased prothrombin time response with oral aminoglycosides).
No products indexed under this heading.

Ketoprofen (Increased prothrombin time response; caution should be observed when used concurrently).
No products indexed under this heading.

Ketorolac Tromethamine (Increased prothrombin time response; caution should be observed when used concurrently). Products include:
Acular Ophthalmic Solution **561**
Acular LS Ophthalmic Solution **562**

Lansoprazole (Increased prothrombin time response). Products include:
Prevacid Delayed-Release Capsules **3268**
Prevacid for Delayed-Release Oral Suspension **3268**
Prevacid I.V. for Injection **3274**
Prevacid NapraPAC **3277**
Prevacid SoluTab Delayed-Release Orally Disintegrating Tablets **3268**
PREVPAC **3281**

Levamisole Hydrochloride (Increased prothrombin time response).
No products indexed under this heading.

Levonorgestrel (Decreased prothrombin time response). Products include:
Alesse-28 Tablets **3392**
Climara Pro Transdermal System **800**
Mirena Intrauterine System **810**
Plan B Tablets **1068**
Seasonale Tablets **1073**
Triphasil-28 Tablets **3483**

Levorphanol Tartrate (Increased prothrombin time response with prolonged use).
No products indexed under this heading.

Levothyroxine Sodium (Decreased or increased prothrombin time response). Products include:
Levothroid Tablets **1189**
Levoxyl Tablets **1680**
Synthroid Tablets **515**
Unithroid Tablets **3521**

Licorice (Co-administration with botanicals that contain coumarins, such as licorice, may result in increased anticoagulant effects; licorice also has antiplatelet properties).
No products indexed under this heading.

Liothyronine Sodium (Decreased or increased prothrombin time response). Products include:
Cytomel Tablets **1678**

Liotrix (Decreased or increased prothrombin time response). Products include:
Thyrolar **1203**

Lomefloxacin Hydrochloride (Increased prothrombin time response).
No products indexed under this heading.

Loratadine (Decreased prothrombin time response). Products include:
Alavert Allergy & Sinus D-12 Hour Tablets .... ▣**743**
Alavert .... ▣**743**
Children's Claritin 24 Hour Non-Drowsy Allergy Syrup .... ▣**732**
Claritin Non-Drowsy 24 Hour Tablets .... ▣**731**
Non-Drowsy Claritin Hives Relief Tablets .... ▣**733**
Claritin Reditabs 24 Hour Non-Drowsy Tablets .... ▣**732**
Claritin-D Non-Drowsy 12 Hour Tablets .... ▣**731**
Claritin-D Non-Drowsy 24 Hour Tablets .... ▣**731**
Children's Dimetapp ND Non-Drowsy Allergy Syrup .... ▣**746**
Triaminic Allerchews .... ▣**684**

Lovastatin (Increased prothrombin time response). Products include:
Advicor Tablets **1694**
Altoprev Extended-Release Tablets **1151**
Mevacor Tablets **1996**

Magaldrate (Decreased prothrombin time response).
No products indexed under this heading.

Magnesium Hydroxide (Decreased prothrombin time response). Products include:
Maalox Max Maximum Strength Antacid/Anti-Gas Liquid **2165**
Maalox Regular Strength Antacid/Antigas Liquid **2164**
Pepcid Complete Chewable Tablets **1672**
Rolaids Tablets .... ▣**707**
Extra Strength Rolaids Tablets .... ▣**707**
Rolaids Multi-Symptom Antacid & Antigas Tablets .... ▣**708**

Magnesium Oxide (Decreased prothrombin time response). Products include:
Beelith Tablets **784**
PremCal Light, Regular, and Extra Strength Tablets .... ▣**762**

Magnesium Salicylate (Increased prothrombin time response; caution should be observed when used concurrently).
No products indexed under this heading.

Matricaria recutita (Co-administration with botanicals that contain coumarins, such as chamomile, may result in increased anticoagulant effects).
No products indexed under this heading.

Meclofenamate Sodium (Increased prothrombin time response; caution should be observed when used concurrently).
No products indexed under this heading.

Medicago sativa (Co-administration with botanicals that contain coumarins, such as alfalfa, may result in increased anticoagulant effects).
No products indexed under this heading.

Mefenamic Acid (Increased prothrombin time response; caution should be observed when used concurrently).
No products indexed under this heading.

Melilotus officinalis (Co-administration with botanicals that contain coumarins, such as sweet clover, may result in increased anticoagulant effects).
No products indexed under this heading.

Meloxicam (Increased prothrombin time response; caution should be observed when used concurrently). Products include:
Mobic Oral Suspension **893**
Mobic Tablets **893**

Menyanthes trifoliata (Co-administration with botanicals that contain coumarins, such as bogbean, may result in increased anticoagulant effects).
No products indexed under this heading.

Meperidine Hydrochloride (Increased prothrombin time response with prolonged use).
No products indexed under this heading.

Mephobarbital (Decreased prothrombin time response). Products include:
Mebaral Tablets, USP **2483**

Meprobamate (Decreased prothrombin time response).
No products indexed under this heading.

Mercaptopurine (Decreased prothrombin time response). Products include:
Purinethol Tablets **1222**

Mestranol (Decreased prothrombin time response).
No products indexed under this heading.

Methadone Hydrochloride (Increased prothrombin time response with prolonged use).
No products indexed under this heading.

Methdilazine Hydrochloride (Decreased prothrombin time response).
No products indexed under this heading.

Methimazole (Increased or decreased prothrombin time response).
No products indexed under this heading.

Methoxyflurane (Increased or decreased prothrombin time response).
No products indexed under this heading.

Methyclothiazide (Decreased or increased prothrombin time response).
No products indexed under this heading.

Methyl Salicylate (Increased prothrombin time response with topical methyl salicylate ointment). Products include:
BenGay External Analgesic Products .... ▣**698**
Thera-Gesic Creme **2108**
Thera-Gesic Plus Creme .... ▣**673**

Methyldopa (Increased prothrombin time response). Products include:
Aldoclor Tablets **1881**
Aldoril Tablets **1884**

Methyldopate Hydrochloride (Increased prothrombin time response).
No products indexed under this heading.

Methylphenidate Hydrochloride (Increased prothrombin time response). Products include:
Concerta Extended-Release Tablets **1828**
Metadate CD Capsules **3316**
Ritalin **2254**
Ritalin LA Capsules **2255**

Methylprednisolone Acetate (Decreased or increased prothrombin time response). Products include:
Depo-Medrol Injectable Suspension **2615**
Depo-Medrol Single-Dose Vial **2617**

Methylprednisolone Sodium Succinate (Decreased or increased prothrombin time response).
No products indexed under this heading.

Methyltestosterone (Increased prothrombin time response). Products include:
Estratest Tablets **3196**
Estratest H.S. Tablets **3196**

Metolazone (Decreased or increased prothrombin time response).
No products indexed under this heading.

Metronidazole (Increased prothrombin time response). Products include:
Metrogel 1% **1212**
MetroGel-Vaginal Gel **1822**
Noritate Cream, 1% **1051**

Metronidazole Hydrochloride (Increased prothrombin time response).
No products indexed under this heading.

Miconazole (Increased prothrombin time response).
No products indexed under this heading.

Mistletoe (Co-administration with botanicals with coagulant properties, such as mistletoe, may affect the anticoagulant effects of warfarin).
No products indexed under this heading.

Moclobemide (Increased prothrombin time response).
No products indexed under this heading.

Montelukast Sodium (May be responsible, alone or in combination,

for increased prothrombin time/ international normalized ratio (PT/ INR) response). Products include:
Singulair 2047

Moricizine Hydrochloride (Decreased or increased prothrombin time response).
No products indexed under this heading.

Morphine Sulfate (Increased prothrombin time response with prolonged use). Products include:
Avinza Capsules 1714
Kadian Capsules 572
MS Contin Tablets 2703

Moxifloxacin Hydrochloride (Increased prothrombin time response). Products include:
Avelox 2984
Vigamox Ophthalmic Solution 560

Nabumetone (Increased prothrombin time response; caution should be observed when used concurrently). Products include:
Relafen Tablets 1523

Nafcillin Sodium (Decreased prothrombin time response).
No products indexed under this heading.

Nalidixic Acid (Increased prothrombin time response).
No products indexed under this heading.

Naproxen (Increased prothrombin time response; caution should be observed when used concurrently). Products include:
EC-Naprosyn Delayed-Release Tablets 2769
Naprosyn Suspension 2769
Naprosyn Tablets 2769
Prevacid NapraPAC 3277

Naproxen Sodium (Increased prothrombin time response; caution should be observed when used concurrently). Products include:
Aleve Tablets, Caplets and Gelcaps .... ▣605
Anaprox Tablets 2769
Anaprox DS Tablets 2769

Neomycin, oral (Increased prothrombin time response with oral aminoglycosides).
No products indexed under this heading.

Nettle (Co-administration with botanicals that contain coumarins, such as nettle, may result in increased anticoagulant effects).
No products indexed under this heading.

Nilutamide (May be responsible, alone or in combination, for increased prothrombin time/ international normalized ratio (PT/ INR) response).
No products indexed under this heading.

Norethindrone (Decreased prothrombin time response). Products include:
Ortho Micronor Tablets 2411

Norethynodrel (Decreased prothrombin time response).
No products indexed under this heading.

Norfloxacin (Increased prothrombin time response). Products include:
Noroxin Tablets 2009

Norgestimate (Decreased prothrombin time response). Products include:
Ortho-Cyclen/Ortho Tri-Cyclen 2414
Ortho Tri-Cyclen Lo Tablets 2421
Prefest Tablets 1069

Norgestrel (Decreased prothrombin time response). Products include:
Lo/Ovral-28 Tablets 3423

Ofloxacin (Increased prothrombin time response). Products include:
Floxin Otic Singles 1045
Floxin Otic Solution 1043

Olsalazine Sodium (Increased prothrombin time response).
No products indexed under this heading.

Omeprazole (Increased prothrombin time response). Products include:
Zegerid Powder for Oral Solution 2972

Oxandrolone (Increased prothrombin time response). Products include:
Oxandrin Tablets 2977

Oxaprozin (Increased prothrombin time response; caution should be observed when used concurrently).
No products indexed under this heading.

Oxycodone Hydrochloride (Increased prothrombin time response with prolonged use). Products include:
Combunox Tablets 1183
OxyContin Tablets 2699
OxyFast Oral Concentrate Solution 2704
OxyIR Capsules 2704
Percocet Tablets 1114
Percodan Tablets 1115

Oxymetholone (Increased prothrombin time response). Products include:
Anadrol-50 Tablets 3329

Oxyphenbutazone (Increased prothrombin time response).
No products indexed under this heading.

Pantoprazole Sodium (Increased prothrombin time response). Products include:
Protonix I.V. 3468
Protonix Tablets 3465

Paraldehyde (Decreased prothrombin time response).
No products indexed under this heading.

Pargyline Hydrochloride (Increased prothrombin time response).
No products indexed under this heading.

Paromomycin Sulfate (Increased prothrombin time response with oral aminoglycosides).
No products indexed under this heading.

Paroxetine Hydrochloride (Increased prothrombin time response). Products include:
Paxil CR Controlled-Release Tablets 1509
Paxil 1501

Passiflora incarnata (Co-administration with botanicals that contain coumarins, such as passion flower, may result in increased anticoagulant effects).
No products indexed under this heading.

Pau d'arco (Concurrent use may result in increased anticoagulant effects).
No products indexed under this heading.

Penicillin G Potassium (Increased prothrombin time response with intravenous penicillin G).
No products indexed under this heading.

Penicillin G Sodium (Increased prothrombin time response with intravenous penicillin G).
No products indexed under this heading.

Pentobarbital Sodium (Decreased prothrombin time response). Products include:
Nembutal Sodium Solution, USP 2484

Pentoxifylline (Increased prothrombin time response).
No products indexed under this heading.

Petroselinum crispum (Co-administration with botanicals that contain coumarins, such as parsley, may result in increased anticoagulant effects).
No products indexed under this heading.

Peumus boldus (Co-administration with botanicals that contain coumarins, such as boldo, may result in increased anticoagulant effects).
No products indexed under this heading.

Phenelzine Sulfate (Increased prothrombin time response).
No products indexed under this heading.

Phenobarbital (Decreased prothrombin time response; accumulation of phenobarbital).
No products indexed under this heading.

Phenylbutazone (Increased prothrombin time response; caution should be observed when used concurrently).
No products indexed under this heading.

Phenytoin (Accumulation of phenytoin; decreased or increased prothrombin time response).
No products indexed under this heading.

Phenytoin Sodium (Accumulation of phenytoin; decreased or increased prothrombin time response). Products include:
Phenytek Capsules 2153

Phytonadione (Decreased prothrombin time response).
No products indexed under this heading.

Piperacillin Sodium (Increased prothrombin time response). Products include:
Zosyn 3492

Piroxicam (Increased prothrombin time response; caution should be observed when used concurrently).
No products indexed under this heading.

Policosanol (Co-administration with botanicals that contain salicylate and/or have antiplatelet properties, such as policosanol, may result in increased anticoagulant effects).
No products indexed under this heading.

Polythiazide (Decreased or increased prothrombin time response).
No products indexed under this heading.

Populus species (Co-administration with botanicals that contain salicylate and/or have antiplatelet properties, such as poplar, may result in increased anticoagulant effects).
No products indexed under this heading.

Prednisolone Acetate (Decreased or increased prothrombin time response). Products include:
Blephamide Ophthalmic Ointment 563
Blephamide Ophthalmic Suspension 564
Poly-Pred Liquifilm Ophthalmic Suspension .... ⊙231
Pred Forte Ophthalmic Suspension .... ⊙233
Pred Mild Sterile Ophthalmic Suspension .... ⊙236
Pred-G Ophthalmic Suspension .... ⊙234
Pred-G Sterile Ophthalmic Ointment .... ⊙235

Prednisolone Sodium Phosphate (Decreased or increased prothrombin time response). Products include:
Pediapred Oral Solution 3319

Prednisolone Tebutate (Decreased or increased prothrombin time response).
No products indexed under this heading.

Prednisone (Decreased or increased prothrombin time response).
No products indexed under this heading.

Prickly Ash (Co-administration with botanicals that contain coumarins, such as prickly ash, may result in increased anticoagulant effects).
No products indexed under this heading.

Primidone (Decreased prothrombin time response).
No products indexed under this heading.

Procarbazine Hydrochloride (Increased prothrombin time response). Products include:
Matulane Capsules 3188

Promethazine Hydrochloride (Decreased prothrombin time response). Products include:
Phenergan 3438

Propafenone Hydrochloride (Increased prothrombin time response). Products include:
Rythmol SR Capsules 2736

Propoxyphene Hydrochloride (Increased prothrombin time response with prolonged use).
No products indexed under this heading.

Propoxyphene Napsylate (Increased prothrombin time response with prolonged use). Products include:
Darvocet A 500 Tablets 3497

Propranolol Hydrochloride (Increased prothrombin time response). Products include:
Inderal LA Long-Acting Capsules 3421
InnoPran XL Capsules 2728

Propylthiouracil (Increased or decreased prothrombin time response).
No products indexed under this heading.

Pyrazolones (Increased prothrombin time response).
No products indexed under this heading.

Pyrilamine Maleate (Decreased prothrombin time response).
No products indexed under this heading.

Pyrilamine Tannate (Decreased prothrombin time response).
No products indexed under this heading.

Quassia amara (Co-administration with botanicals that contain coumarins, such as quassia, may result in increased anticoagulant effects).
No products indexed under this heading.

Quinidine Gluconate (Increased prothrombin time response).
No products indexed under this heading.

Quinidine Polygalacturonate (Increased prothrombin time response).
No products indexed under this heading.

Quinidine Sulfate (Increased prothrombin time response).
No products indexed under this heading.

Quinine Sulfate (Increased prothrombin time response).
No products indexed under this heading.

Raloxifene Hydrochloride (May be responsible, alone or in combination, for decreased prothrombin time/international normalized ratio (PT/INR) response). Products include:
Evista Tablets **1735**

Ranitidine Hydrochloride (Decreased or increased prothrombin time response). Products include:
Zantac **1597**
Zantac Injection **1593**
Zantac 75 Tablets **715**
Zantac 150 Maximum Strength Tablets **715**
Zantac Injection Pharmacy Bulk Package **1595**

Remifentanil Hydrochloride (Increased prothrombin time response with prolonged use).
No products indexed under this heading.

Rifampin (Decreased prothrombin time response).
No products indexed under this heading.

Rofecoxib (Increased prothrombin time response; caution should be observed when used concurrently).
No products indexed under this heading.

Salsalate (Increased prothrombin time response; caution should be observed when used concurrently).
No products indexed under this heading.

Sarsaparilla, German (Co-administration with botanicals that contain salicylate and/or have antiplatelet properties, such as German sarsaparilla, may result in increased anticoagulant effects).
No products indexed under this heading.

Secobarbital Sodium (Decreased prothrombin time response).
No products indexed under this heading.

Selegiline Hydrochloride (Increased prothrombin time response). Products include:
Eldepryl Capsules **3209**

Senega (Co-administration with botanicals that contain salicylate and/or have antiplatelet properties, such as senega, may result in increased anticoagulant effects).
No products indexed under this heading.

Sertraline Hydrochloride (Increased prothrombin time response). Products include:
Zoloft **2581**

Simvastatin (Increased prothrombin time response). Products include:
Vytorin 10/10 Tablets **2084**
Vytorin 10/10 Tablets **3092**
Vytorin 10/20 Tablets **2084**
Vytorin 10/20 Tablets **3092**
Vytorin 10/40 Tablets **3092**
Vytorin 10/40 Tablets **2084**
Vytorin 10/80 Tablets **2084**
Vytorin 10/80 Tablets **3092**
Zocor Tablets **2078**

Sodium Bicarbonate (Decreased prothrombin time response). Products include:
Ceo-Two Evacuant Suppository **607**
Colyte with Flavor Packs for Oral Solution **3102**
HalfLytely and Bisacodyl Tablets Bowel Prep Kit with Flavors Packs **915**
TriLyte with Flavor Packs for Oral Solution **3114**

Spironolactone (Decreased or increased prothrombin time response).
No products indexed under this heading.

Stanozolol (Increased prothrombin time response).
No products indexed under this heading.

Streptokinase (Concurrent use is not recommended and may be hazardous; increased prothrombin time response).
No products indexed under this heading.

Sucralfate (Decreased prothrombin time response). Products include:
Carafate Suspension **727**
Carafate Tablets **728**

Sufentanil Citrate (Increased prothrombin time response with prolonged use).
No products indexed under this heading.

Sulfacytine (Increased prothrombin time response).
No products indexed under this heading.

Sulfamethizole (Increased prothrombin time response).
No products indexed under this heading.

Sulfamethoxazole (Increased prothrombin time response).
No products indexed under this heading.

Sulfasalazine (Increased prothrombin time response).
No products indexed under this heading.

Sulfinpyrazone (Increased prothrombin time response).
No products indexed under this heading.

Sulfisoxazole (Increased prothrombin time response).
No products indexed under this heading.

Sulfisoxazole Acetyl (Increased prothrombin time response).
No products indexed under this heading.

Sulfisoxazole Diolamine (Increased prothrombin time response).
No products indexed under this heading.

Sulindac (Increased prothrombin time response; caution should be observed when used concurrently). Products include:
Clinoril Tablets **1899**

Syzygium aromaticum (Co-administration with botanicals that contain salicylate and/or have antiplatelet properties, such as clove, may result in increased anticoagulant effects).
No products indexed under this heading.

Tamarindus indica (Co-administration with botanicals that contain salicylate and/or have antiplatelet properties, such as tamarind, may result in increased anticoagulant effects).
No products indexed under this heading.

Tamoxifen Citrate (Increased prothrombin time response).
No products indexed under this heading.

Tanacetum parthenium (Co-administration with botanicals that contain salicylate and/or have antiplatelet properties, such as feverfew, may result in increased anticoagulant effects).
No products indexed under this heading.

Taraxacum officinale (Co-administration with botanicals that contain coumarins, such as dandelion, may result in increased anticoagulant effects; dandelion also has antiplatelet properties).
No products indexed under this heading.

Terfenadine (Decreased prothrombin time response).
No products indexed under this heading.

Tetracycline Hydrochloride (Increased prothrombin time response).
No products indexed under this heading.

Thiamylal Sodium (Decreased prothrombin time response).
No products indexed under this heading.

Thyroglobulin (Decreased or increased prothrombin time response).
No products indexed under this heading.

Thyroid (Decreased or increased prothrombin time response).
No products indexed under this heading.

Thyroxine (Decreased or increased prothrombin time response).
No products indexed under this heading.

Thyroxine Sodium (Decreased or increased prothrombin time response).
No products indexed under this heading.

Ticarcillin Disodium (Increased prothrombin time response). Products include:
Timentin ADD-Vantage **1556**
Timentin Injection Galaxy Container **1559**
Timentin IV Infusion **1553**
Timentin Pharmacy Bulk Package **1562**

Ticlopidine Hydrochloride (Concomitant administration may be associated with cholestatic hepatitis; increased prothrombin time response). Products include:
Ticlid Tablets **2813**

Tolazamide (Increased prothrombin time response).
No products indexed under this heading.

Tolbutamide (Increased prothrombin time response; accumulation of tolbutamide).
No products indexed under this heading.

Tolmetin Sodium (Increased prothrombin time response; caution should be observed when used concurrently).
No products indexed under this heading.

Torsemide (Decreased or increased prothrombin time response).
No products indexed under this heading.

Tramadol Hydrochloride (Increased prothrombin time response). Products include:
Ultracet Tablets **2462**

Tranylcypromine Sulfate (Increased prothrombin time response). Products include:
Parnate Tablets **1499**

Trazodone Hydrochloride (Decreased prothrombin time response).
No products indexed under this heading.

Triamcinolone (Decreased or increased prothrombin time response).
No products indexed under this heading.

Triamcinolone Acetonide (Decreased or increased prothrombin time response). Products include:
Azmacort Inhalation Aerosol **1701**
Nasacort HFA Inhalation Aerosol **2939**
Nasacort AQ Nasal Spray **2937**

Triamcinolone Diacetate (Decreased or increased prothrombin time response).
No products indexed under this heading.

Triamcinolone Hexacetonide (Decreased or increased prothrombin time response).
No products indexed under this heading.

Triamterene (Decreased or increased prothrombin time response). Products include:
Dyazide Capsules **1389**
Dyrenium Capsules **3390**
Maxzide **2150**

Trifolium pratense (Co-administration with botanicals that contain coumarins, such as red clover, may result in increased anticoagulant effects).
No products indexed under this heading.

Trigonella foenum-graecum (Co-administration with botanicals that contain coumarins, such as fenugreek, may result in increased anticoagulant effects).
No products indexed under this heading.

Trimeprazine Tartrate (Decreased prothrombin time response).
No products indexed under this heading.

Trimethoprim (Increased prothrombin time response).
No products indexed under this heading.

Tripelennamine Hydrochloride (Decreased prothrombin time response).
No products indexed under this heading.

IMPORTANT NOTE: Always consult each drug listing in the patient's regimen for possible interactions.

Triprolidine Hydrochloride (Decreased prothrombin time response).
No products indexed under this heading.

Trovafloxacin Mesylate (Increased prothrombin time response).
No products indexed under this heading.

Urokinase (Concurrent use is not recommended and may be hazardous).
No products indexed under this heading.

Valdecoxib (Increased prothrombin time response; caution should be observed when used concurrently).
No products indexed under this heading.

Valproic Acid (Increased prothrombin time response). Products include:
Depakene **417**

Viburnum prunifolium (Co-administration with botanicals that contain salicylate and/or have antiplatelet properties, such as black haw, may result in increased anticoagulant effects).
No products indexed under this heading.

Vitamin C (Decreased prothrombin time response (with high dose)). Products include:
Chromagen Forte Soft Gelatin Capsules **3296**
Halls Defense Sugarfree Vitamin C Drops .... ▣**611**
Niferex-150 Forte Capsules **3299**
Peridin-C Tablets .... ▣**761**
Repliva 21/7 Tablets **3301**

Vitamin E (Increased prothrombin time response). Products include:
MarineOmega Softgel Capsules **2669**
Unique E Vitamin E Concentrate Capsules .... ▣**602**

Wild Lettuce (Co-administration with botanicals that contain coumarins, such as wild lettuce, may result in increased anticoagulant effects).
No products indexed under this heading.

Willow (Co-administration with botanicals that contain salicylate and/or have antiplatelet properties, such as willow, may result in increased anticoagulant effects).
No products indexed under this heading.

Zafirlukast (May be responsible, alone or in combination, for increased prothrombin time/international normalized ratio (PT/INR) response). Products include:
Accolate Tablets **663**

Zileuton (May be responsible, alone or in combination, for increased prothrombin time/international normalized ratio (PT/INR) response).
No products indexed under this heading.

Food Interactions

Alcohol (Decreased or increased prothrombin time response).

Diet high in vitamin K (Decreased prothrombin time).

Vegetables, green leafy (Large amounts of green leafy vegetables may affect warfarin therapy).

COVERA-HS TABLETS

(Verapamil Hydrochloride) **3135**
May interact with ACE inhibitors, antihypertensives, beta blockers, cytochrome p450 3a4 inducers (selected), cytochrome p450 3a4 inhibitors (selected), diuretics, cardiac glycosides, inhalant anesthetics, lithium preparations, nondepolarizing neuromuscular blocking agents, vasodilators, xanthines, and certain other agents. Compounds in these categories include:

Acebutolol Hydrochloride (Concomitant therapy may result in additive negative effects on heart rate, atrioventricular conduction and/or cardiac contractility; excessive bradycardia and AV block, including complete heart block).
No products indexed under this heading.

Acetazolamide (Clinically significant interactions have been reported with inhibitors of CYP3A4 causing elevation of plasma levels of verapamil while inducers of CYP3A4 have caused a lowering of plasma levels of verapamil).
No products indexed under this heading.

Allium sativum (Clinically significant interactions have been reported with inhibitors of CYP3A4 causing elevation of plasma levels of verapamil while inducers of CYP3A4 have caused a lowering of plasma levels of verapamil).
No products indexed under this heading.

Amiloride Hydrochloride (Possible additive effect on lowering of blood pressure). Products include:
Midamor Tablets **2000**
Moduretic Tablets **2003**

Aminophylline (Verapamil may inhibit the clearance and increase plasma levels of theophylline).
No products indexed under this heading.

Amiodarone Hydrochloride (Clinically significant interactions have been reported with inhibitors of CYP3A4 causing elevation of plasma levels of verapamil while inducers of CYP3A4 have caused a lowering of plasma levels of verapamil). Products include:
Pacerone Tablets **3337**

Amlodipine Besylate (Possible additive effect on lowering of blood pressure). Products include:
Caduet Tablets **2507**
Lotrel Capsules **2238**
Norvasc Tablets **2529**

Amprenavir (Clinically significant interactions have been reported with inhibitors of CYP3A4 causing elevation of plasma levels of verapamil while inducers of CYP3A4 have caused a lowering of plasma levels of verapamil). Products include:
Agenerase Capsules **1299**
Agenerase Oral Solution **1304**

Amyl Nitrite (Possible additive effect on lowering of blood pressure).
No products indexed under this heading.

Anastrozole (Clinically significant interactions have been reported with inhibitors of CYP3A4 causing elevation of plasma levels of verapamil while inducers of CYP3A4 have caused a lowering of plasma levels of verapamil). Products include:
Arimidex Tablets **665**

Aprepitant (Clinically significant interactions have been reported with inhibitors of CYP3A4 causing elevation of plasma levels of verapamil while inducers of CYP3A4 have caused a lowering of plasma levels of verapamil). Products include:
Emend Capsules **1944**

Aspirin (In a few reported cases, co-administration of verapamil with aspirin has led to increased bleeding times greater than observed with aspirin alone). Products include:
Aggrenox Capsules **855**
Bayer, Aspirin Regimen .... ▣**606**
Bayer Aspirin Tablets **3515**
BC Powder .... ▣**612**
BC Allergy Sinus Cold Powder .... ▣**612**
Arthritis Strength BC Powder .... ▣**612**
BC Sinus Cold Powder .... ▣**612**
Ecotrin Enteric Coated Aspirin Low, Regular and Maximum Strength Tablets **1627**
Goody's Body Pain Formula Powder .... ▣**621**
Goody's Extra Strength Headache Powder .... ▣**621**
Goody's Extra Strength Pain Relief Tablets .... ▣**621**
Percodan Tablets **1115**
St. Joseph 81 mg Aspirin Chewable and Enteric Coated Tablets **1841**

Atenolol (Concomitant therapy may result in additive negative effects on heart rate, atrioventricular conduction and/or cardiac contractility; excessive bradycardia and AV block, including complete heart block; a variable effect on atenolol clearance has been observed with concomitant use). Products include:
Tenormin I.V. Injection **698**
Tenormin Tablets **695**

Atracurium Besylate (Verapamil may potentiate the activity of neuromuscular blocking agents).
No products indexed under this heading.

Benazepril Hydrochloride (Possible additive effect on lowering of blood pressure). Products include:
Lotensin Tablets **2232**
Lotensin HCT Tablets **2235**
Lotrel Capsules **2238**

Bendroflumethiazide (Possible additive effect on lowering of blood pressure).
No products indexed under this heading.

Betamethasone Acetate (Clinically significant interactions have been reported with inhibitors of CYP3A4 causing elevation of plasma levels of verapamil while inducers of CYP3A4 have caused a lowering of plasma levels of verapamil).
No products indexed under this heading.

Betamethasone Sodium Phosphate (Clinically significant interactions have been reported with inhibitors of CYP3A4 causing elevation of plasma levels of verapamil while inducers of CYP3A4 have caused a lowering of plasma levels of verapamil).
No products indexed under this heading.

Betaxolol Hydrochloride (Concomitant therapy may result in additive negative effects on heart rate, atrioventricular conduction and/or cardiac contractility; excessive bradycardia and AV block, including complete heart block). Products include:
Betoptic S Ophthalmic Suspension **554**

Bisoprolol Fumarate (Concomitant therapy may result in additive negative effects on heart rate, atrioventricular conduction and/or cardiac contractility; excessive bradycardia and AV block, including complete heart block).
No products indexed under this heading.

Bumetanide (Possible additive effect on lowering of blood pressure).
No products indexed under this heading.

Candesartan Cilexetil (Possible additive effect on lowering of blood pressure). Products include:
Atacand Tablets **634**
Atacand HCT **637**

Captopril (Possible additive effect on lowering of blood pressure). Products include:
Captopril Tablets **2114**

Carbamazepine (Co-administration may increase carbamazepine concentrations and this may produce side effects such as diplopia, headache, ataxia, or dizziness). Products include:
Carbatrol Capsules **3174**
Equetro Extended-Release Capsules **3178**
Tegretol/Tegretol-XR **2278**

Carteolol Hydrochloride (Concomitant therapy may result in additive negative effects on heart rate, atrioventricular conduction and/or cardiac contractility; excessive bradycardia and AV block, including complete heart block). Products include:
Carteolol Hydrochloride Ophthalmic Solution USP, 1% .... ⊙**246**

Chlorothiazide (Possible additive effect on lowering of blood pressure). Products include:
Aldoclor Tablets **1881**
Diuril Oral **1936**

Chlorothiazide Sodium (Possible additive effect on lowering of blood pressure). Products include:
Diuril Sodium Intravenous **1934**

Chlorthalidone (Possible additive effect on lowering of blood pressure). Products include:
Clorpres Tablets **2139**

Cimetidine (Variable results on verapamil clearance). Products include:
Tagamet HB 200 Tablets .... ▣**637**
Tagamet Tablets **1547**

Cimetidine Hydrochloride (Variable results on verapamil clearance).
No products indexed under this heading.

Ciprofloxacin (Clinically significant interactions have been reported with inhibitors of CYP3A4 causing elevation of plasma levels of verapamil while inducers of CYP3A4 have caused a lowering of plasma levels of verapamil). Products include:
Cipro I.V. **2998**
Cipro I.V. Pharmacy Bulk Package **3509**
Cipro Oral Suspension **2991**
Cipro XR Tablets **3004**
Ciprodex Otic Suspension **555**

Ciprofloxacin Hydrochloride (Clinically significant interactions have been reported with inhibitors of CYP3A4 causing elevation of plasma levels of verapamil while inducers of CYP3A4 have caused a lowering of plasma levels of verapamil). Products include:
Ciloxan Ophthalmic Ointment **554**
Cipro Tablets **2991**

Cisatracurium Besylate (Verapamil may potentiate the activity of neuromuscular blocking agents). Products include:
Nimbex Injection 494

Cisplatin (Clinically significant interactions have been reported with inhibitors of CYP3A4 causing elevation of plasma levels of verapamil while inducers of CYP3A4 have caused a lowering of plasma levels of verapamil).
No products indexed under this heading.

Clarithromycin (Clinically significant interactions have been reported with inhibitors of CYP3A4 causing elevation of plasma levels of verapamil while inducers of CYP3A4 have caused a lowering of plasma levels of verapamil). Products include:
Biaxin/Biaxin XL 402
PREVPAC 3281

Clonidine (Possible additive effect on lowering of blood pressure). Products include:
Catapres-TTS 875

Clonidine Hydrochloride (Possible additive effect on lowering of blood pressure). Products include:
Catapres Tablets 874
Clorpres Tablets 2139

Clotrimazole (Clinically significant interactions have been reported with inhibitors of CYP3A4 causing elevation of plasma levels of verapamil while inducers of CYP3A4 have caused a lowering of plasma levels of verapamil). Products include:
Lotrimin 3053
Lotrisone 3054

Cortisone Acetate (Clinically significant interactions have been reported with inhibitors of CYP3A4 causing elevation of plasma levels of verapamil while inducers of CYP3A4 have caused a lowering of plasma levels of verapamil).
No products indexed under this heading.

Cyclosporine (Increased serum levels of cyclosporine). Products include:
Gengraf Capsules 458
Neoral Soft Gelatin Capsules 2247
Neoral Oral Solution 2247
Restasis Ophthalmic Emulsion 570
Sandimmune 2259

Dalfopristin (Clinically significant interactions have been reported with inhibitors of CYP3A4 causing elevation of plasma levels of verapamil while inducers of CYP3A4 have caused a lowering of plasma levels of verapamil). Products include:
Synercid I.V. 1690

Danazol (Clinically significant interactions have been reported with inhibitors of CYP3A4 causing elevation of plasma levels of verapamil while inducers of CYP3A4 have caused a lowering of plasma levels of verapamil).
No products indexed under this heading.

Delavirdine Mesylate (Clinically significant interactions have been reported with inhibitors of CYP3A4 causing elevation of plasma levels of verapamil while inducers of CYP3A4 have caused a lowering of plasma levels of verapamil). Products include:
Rescriptor Tablets 2535

Deserpidine (Possible additive effect on lowering of blood pressure).
No products indexed under this heading.

Desflurane (Potential for excessive cardiovascular depression). Products include:
Suprane Liquid for Inhalation 770

Deslanoside (Chronic verapamil treatment can increase serum digoxin levels by 50% to 75% and this can result in digitalis toxicity).
No products indexed under this heading.

Dexamethasone (Clinically significant interactions have been reported with inhibitors of CYP3A4 causing elevation of plasma levels of verapamil while inducers of CYP3A4 have caused a lowering of plasma levels of verapamil). Products include:
Ciprodex Otic Suspension 555
Decadron Tablets 1929
TobraDex Ophthalmic Ointment 558
TobraDex Ophthalmic Suspension 558

Dexamethasone Acetate (Clinically significant interactions have been reported with inhibitors of CYP3A4 causing elevation of plasma levels of verapamil while inducers of CYP3A4 have caused a lowering of plasma levels of verapamil).
No products indexed under this heading.

Dexamethasone Sodium Phosphate (Clinically significant interactions have been reported with inhibitors of CYP3A4 causing elevation of plasma levels of verapamil while inducers of CYP3A4 have caused a lowering of plasma levels of verapamil). Products include:
Decadron Phosphate Injection 1931

Diazoxide (Possible additive effect on lowering of blood pressure). Products include:
Hyperstat I.V. Injection 3031

Digitalis Glycoside Preparations (Chronic verapamil treatment can increase serum digoxin levels by 50% to 75% and this can result in digitalis toxicity).
No products indexed under this heading.

Digitoxin (Chronic verapamil treatment can increase serum digoxin levels by 50% to 75% and this can result in digitalis toxicity).
No products indexed under this heading.

Digoxin (Chronic verapamil treatment can increase serum digoxin levels by 50% to 75% and this can result in digitalis toxicity). Products include:
Digitek Tablets 2146
Lanoxicaps Capsules 1458
Lanoxin Injection 1462
Lanoxin Tablets 1468
Lanoxin Injection Pediatric 1465

Diltiazem Hydrochloride (Possible additive effect on lowering of blood pressure). Products include:
Cardizem LA Extended Release Tablets 1699
Tiazac Capsules 1204

Diltiazem Maleate (Clinically significant interactions have been reported with inhibitors of CYP3A4 causing elevation of plasma levels of verapamil while inducers of CYP3A4 have caused a lowering of plasma levels of verapamil).
No products indexed under this heading.

Disopyramide Phosphate (Concurrent use within 48 hours before or 24 hours after verapamil administration is not recommended).
No products indexed under this heading.

Doxazosin Mesylate (Possible additive effect on lowering of blood pressure).
No products indexed under this heading.

Doxorubicin Hydrochloride (Clinically significant interactions have been reported with inhibitors of CYP3A4 causing elevation of plasma levels of verapamil while inducers of CYP3A4 have caused a lowering of plasma levels of verapamil). Products include:
Adriamycin for Injection, USP 786
Adriamycin Injection, USP 786

Dyphylline (Verapamil may inhibit the clearance and increase plasma levels of theophylline).
No products indexed under this heading.

Efavirenz (Clinically significant interactions have been reported with inhibitors of CYP3A4 causing elevation of plasma levels of verapamil while inducers of CYP3A4 have caused a lowering of plasma levels of verapamil). Products include:
Sustiva Capsules 957

Enalapril Maleate (Possible additive effect on lowering of blood pressure). Products include:
Vaseretic Tablets 2073
Vasotec I.V. Injection 2076

Enalaprilat (Possible additive effect on lowering of blood pressure).
No products indexed under this heading.

Enflurane (Potential for excessive cardiovascular depression).
No products indexed under this heading.

Epoprostenol Sodium (Possible additive effect on lowering of blood pressure). Products include:
Flolan for Injection 1408

Eprosartan Mesylate (Possible additive effect on lowering of blood pressure). Products include:
Teveten Tablets 1707
Teveten HCT Tablets 1710

Erythromycin (Clinically significant interactions have been reported with inhibitors of CYP3A4 causing elevation of plasma levels of verapamil while inducers of CYP3A4 have caused a lowering of plasma levels of verapamil). Products include:
Erygel Topical Gel 2096
Ery-Tab Tablets 447
Erythromycin Base Filmtab Tablets 454
Erythromycin Delayed-Release Capsules, USP 456
PCE Dispertab Tablets 510

Erythromycin Estolate (Clinically significant interactions have been reported with inhibitors of CYP3A4 causing elevation of plasma levels of verapamil while inducers of CYP3A4 have caused a lowering of plasma levels of verapamil).
No products indexed under this heading.

Erythromycin Ethylsuccinate (Clinically significant interactions have been reported with inhibitors of CYP3A4 causing elevation of plasma levels of verapamil while inducers of CYP3A4 have caused a lowering of plasma levels of verapamil). Products include:
E.E.S. 449
EryPed 445

Erythromycin Gluceptate (Clinically significant interactions have been reported with inhibitors of CYP3A4 causing elevation of plasma levels of verapamil while inducers of CYP3A4 have caused a lowering of plasma levels of verapamil).
No products indexed under this heading.

Erythromycin Lactobionate (Clinically significant interactions have been reported with inhibitors of CYP3A4 causing elevation of plasma levels of verapamil while inducers of CYP3A4 have caused a lowering of plasma levels of verapamil).
No products indexed under this heading.

Erythromycin Stearate (Clinically significant interactions have been reported with inhibitors of CYP3A4 causing elevation of plasma levels of verapamil while inducers of CYP3A4 have caused a lowering of plasma levels of verapamil). Products include:
Erythrocin Stearate Filmtab Tablets 452

Esmolol Hydrochloride (Concomitant therapy may result in additive negative effects on heart rate, atrioventricular conduction and/or cardiac contractility; excessive bradycardia and AV block, including complete heart block). Products include:
Brevibloc Concentrate 766
Brevibloc Injection 766
Brevibloc Double Strength Injection 766
Brevibloc Premixed Injection 766
Brevibloc Double Strength Premixed Injection 766

Esomeprazole Magnesium (Clinically significant interactions have been reported with inhibitors of CYP3A4 causing elevation of plasma levels of verapamil while inducers of CYP3A4 have caused a lowering of plasma levels of verapamil). Products include:
Nexium Delayed-Release Capsules 645

Ethacrynic Acid (Possible additive effect on lowering of blood pressure). Products include:
Edecrin Tablets 1941

Ethaverine Hydrochloride (Possible additive effect on lowering of blood pressure).
No products indexed under this heading.

Ethosuximide (Clinically significant interactions have been reported with inhibitors of CYP3A4 causing elevation of plasma levels of verapamil while inducers of CYP3A4 have caused a lowering of plasma levels of verapamil).
No products indexed under this heading.

Felbamate (Clinically significant interactions have been reported with inhibitors of CYP3A4 causing elevation of plasma levels of verapamil while inducers of CYP3A4 have caused a lowering of plasma levels of verapamil).
No products indexed under this heading.

Felodipine (Possible additive effect on lowering of blood pressure). Products include:
Plendil Extended-Release Tablets 651

Flecainide Acetate (Potential for additive effects on myocardial contractility, AV conduction, and repolarization). Products include:
Tambocor Tablets 1824

Fluconazole (Clinically significant interactions have been reported with inhibitors of CYP3A4 causing elevation of plasma levels of verapamil while inducers of CYP3A4 have caused a lowering of plasma levels of verapamil).
No products indexed under this heading.

Fludrocortisone Acetate (Clinically significant interactions have been reported with inhibitors of CYP3A4 causing elevation of plasma levels of verapamil while inducers of CYP3A4 have caused a lowering of plasma levels of verapamil).
No products indexed under this heading.

Fluoxetine Hydrochloride (Clinically significant interactions have been reported with inhibitors of CYP3A4 causing elevation of plasma levels of verapamil while inducers of CYP3A4 have caused a lowering of plasma levels of verapamil). Products include:
Prozac Pulvules and Liquid 1771
Symbyax Capsules 1788

Fluvoxamine Maleate (Clinically significant interactions have been reported with inhibitors of CYP3A4 causing elevation of plasma levels of verapamil while inducers of CYP3A4 have caused a lowering of plasma levels of verapamil).
No products indexed under this heading.

Fosamprenavir Calcium (Clinically significant interactions have been reported with inhibitors of CYP3A4 causing elevation of plasma levels of verapamil while inducers of CYP3A4 have caused a lowering of plasma levels of verapamil). Products include:
Lexiva Tablets 1473

Fosinopril Sodium (Possible additive effect on lowering of blood pressure).
No products indexed under this heading.

Fosphenytoin Sodium (Clinically significant interactions have been reported with inhibitors of CYP3A4 causing elevation of plasma levels of verapamil while inducers of CYP3A4 have caused a lowering of plasma levels of verapamil).
No products indexed under this heading.

Furosemide (Possible additive effect on lowering of blood pressure). Products include:
Furosemide Tablets 2117

Garlic Extract (Clinically significant interactions have been reported with inhibitors of CYP3A4 causing elevation of plasma levels of verapamil while inducers of CYP3A4 have caused a lowering of plasma levels of verapamil).
No products indexed under this heading.

Garlic Oil (Clinically significant interactions have been reported with inhibitors of CYP3A4 causing elevation of plasma levels of verapamil while inducers of CYP3A4 have caused a lowering of plasma levels of verapamil).
No products indexed under this heading.

Guanabenz Acetate (Possible additive effect on lowering of blood pressure).
No products indexed under this heading.

Guanethidine Monosulfate (Possible additive effect on lowering of blood pressure).
No products indexed under this heading.

Halothane (Potential for excessive cardiovascular depression).
No products indexed under this heading.

Hydralazine Hydrochloride (Possible additive effect on lowering of blood pressure). Products include:
BiDil Tablets 2161

Hydrochlorothiazide (Possible additive effect on lowering of blood pressure). Products include:
Aldoril Tablets 1884
Atacand HCT 637
Avalide Tablets 2889
Avalide Tablets 922
Benicar HCT Tablets 2852
Diovan HCT Tablets 2195
Dyazide Capsules 1389
Hyzaar 1964
Lotensin HCT Tablets 2235
Maxzide 2150
Micardis HCT Tablets 886
Moduretic Tablets 2003
Prinzide Tablets 2033
Teveten HCT Tablets 1710
Timolide Tablets 2056
Uniretic Tablets 3114
Vaseretic Tablets 2073
Zestoretic Tablets 701

Hydrocortisone (Clinically significant interactions have been reported with inhibitors of CYP3A4 causing elevation of plasma levels of verapamil while inducers of CYP3A4 have caused a lowering of plasma levels of verapamil). Products include:
Cortizone•5 Ointment .... ▣699
Cortizone•10 Creme .... ▣699
Cortizone•10 Ointment .... ▣699
Cortizone•10 Plus Creme .... ▣700
Cortizone•10 Maximum Strength Quick Shot Spray .... ▣700
Hydrocortone Tablets 1963
Preparation H Hydrocortisone Cream .... ▣748

Hydrocortisone Acetate (Clinically significant interactions have been reported with inhibitors of CYP3A4 causing elevation of plasma levels of verapamil while inducers of CYP3A4 have caused a lowering of plasma levels of verapamil). Products include:
Analpram-HC 1136
Pramosone 1139
ProctoFoam-HC 3113
Tucks Anti-Itch Ointment .... ▣712
U-cort 1% Cream 3289

Hydrocortisone Butyrate (Clinically significant interactions have been reported with inhibitors of CYP3A4 causing elevation of plasma levels of verapamil while inducers of CYP3A4 have caused a lowering of plasma levels of verapamil). Products include:
Locoid 1138
Locoid Lipocream Cream 1138

Hydrocortisone Cypionate (Clinically significant interactions have been reported with inhibitors of CYP3A4 causing elevation of plasma levels of verapamil while inducers of CYP3A4 have caused a lowering of plasma levels of verapamil).
No products indexed under this heading.

Hydrocortisone Hemisuccinate (Clinically significant interactions have been reported with inhibitors of CYP3A4 causing elevation of plasma levels of verapamil while inducers of CYP3A4 have caused a lowering of plasma levels of verapamil).
No products indexed under this heading.

Hydrocortisone Probutate (Clinically significant interactions have been reported with inhibitors of CYP3A4 causing elevation of plasma levels of verapamil while inducers of CYP3A4 have caused a lowering of plasma levels of verapamil). Products include:
Pandel Cream, 0.1% 1017

Hydrocortisone Sodium Phosphate (Clinically significant interactions have been reported with inhibitors of CYP3A4 causing elevation of plasma levels of verapamil while inducers of CYP3A4 have caused a lowering of plasma levels of verapamil).
No products indexed under this heading.

Hydrocortisone Sodium Succinate (Clinically significant interactions have been reported with inhibitors of CYP3A4 causing elevation of plasma levels of verapamil while inducers of CYP3A4 have caused a lowering of plasma levels of verapamil).
No products indexed under this heading.

Hydrocortisone Valerate (Clinically significant interactions have been reported with inhibitors of CYP3A4 causing elevation of plasma levels of verapamil while inducers of CYP3A4 have caused a lowering of plasma levels of verapamil).
No products indexed under this heading.

Hydroflumethiazide (Possible additive effect on lowering of blood pressure).
No products indexed under this heading.

Hypericum (Clinically significant interactions have been reported with inhibitors of CYP3A4 causing elevation of plasma levels of verapamil while inducers of CYP3A4 have caused a lowering of plasma levels of verapamil).
No products indexed under this heading.

Hypericum Perforatum (Clinically significant interactions have been reported with inhibitors of CYP3A4 causing elevation of plasma levels of verapamil while inducers of CYP3A4 have caused a lowering of plasma levels of verapamil).
No products indexed under this heading.

Indapamide (Possible additive effect on lowering of blood pressure). Products include:
Indapamide Tablets 2119

Indinavir Sulfate (Clinically significant interactions have been reported with inhibitors of CYP3A4 causing elevation of plasma levels of verapamil while inducers of CYP3A4 have caused a lowering of plasma levels of verapamil). Products include:
Crixivan Capsules 1918

Irbesartan (Possible additive effect on lowering of blood pressure). Products include:
Avalide Tablets 922
Avalide Tablets 2889
Avapro Tablets 925
Avapro Tablets 2886

Isoflurane (Potential for excessive cardiovascular depression).
No products indexed under this heading.

Isoniazid (Clinically significant interactions have been reported with inhibitors of CYP3A4 causing elevation of plasma levels of verapamil while inducers of CYP3A4 have caused a lowering of plasma levels of verapamil).
No products indexed under this heading.

Isosorbide Dinitrate (Possible additive effect on lowering of blood pressure). Products include:
BiDil Tablets 2161

Isosorbide Mononitrate (Possible additive effect on lowering of blood pressure). Products include:
Imdur Tablets 3032

Isoxsuprine Hydrochloride (Possible additive effect on lowering of blood pressure).
No products indexed under this heading.

Isradipine (Possible additive effect on lowering of blood pressure). Products include:
DynaCirc CR Tablets 2726

Itraconazole (Clinically significant interactions have been reported with inhibitors of CYP3A4 causing elevation of plasma levels of verapamil while inducers of CYP3A4 have caused a lowering of plasma levels of verapamil).
No products indexed under this heading.

Ketoconazole (Clinically significant interactions have been reported with inhibitors of CYP3A4 causing elevation of plasma levels of verapamil while inducers of CYP3A4 have caused a lowering of plasma levels of verapamil). Products include:
Nizoral A-D Shampoo, 1% 1839
Nizoral 2% Shampoo 1838

Labetalol Hydrochloride (Concomitant therapy may result in additive negative effects on heart rate, atrioventricular conduction and/or cardiac contractility; excessive bradycardia and AV block, including complete heart block).
No products indexed under this heading.

Levobunolol Hydrochloride (Concomitant therapy may result in additive negative effects on heart rate, atrioventricular conduction and/or cardiac contractility; excessive bradycardia and AV block, including complete heart block). Products include:
Betagan Ophthalmic Solution, USP .... ⊙217

Lisinopril (Possible additive effect on lowering of blood pressure). Products include:
Prinivil Tablets 2029
Prinzide Tablets 2033
Zestoretic Tablets 701
Zestril Tablets 704

Lithium (Co-administration has resulted in increased sensitivity to the effects of lithium neurotoxicity; lithium levels have been observed sometimes to increase, decrease, or remain unchanged).
No products indexed under this heading.

Lithium Carbonate (Co-administration has resulted in increased sensitivity to the effects of

lithium neurotoxicity; lithium levels have been observed sometimes to increase, decrease, or remain unchanged). Products include:
- Eskalith 1406
- Lithobid Tablets 1670

Lithium Citrate (Co-administration has resulted in increased sensitivity to the effects of lithium neurotoxicity; lithium levels have been observed sometimes to increase, decrease, or remain unchanged).
No products indexed under this heading.

Lopinavir (Clinically significant interactions have been reported with inhibitors of CYP3A4 causing elevation of plasma levels of verapamil while inducers of CYP3A4 have caused a lowering of plasma levels of verapamil). Products include:
- Kaletra 474

Loratadine (Clinically significant interactions have been reported with inhibitors of CYP3A4 causing elevation of plasma levels of verapamil while inducers of CYP3A4 have caused a lowering of plasma levels of verapamil). Products include:
- Alavert Allergy & Sinus D-12 Hour Tablets 743
- Alavert 743
- Children's Claritin 24 Hour Non-Drowsy Allergy Syrup 732
- Claritin Non-Drowsy 24 Hour Tablets 731
- Non-Drowsy Claritin Hives Relief Tablets 733
- Claritin Reditabs 24 Hour Non-Drowsy Tablets 732
- Claritin-D Non-Drowsy 12 Hour Tablets 731
- Claritin-D Non-Drowsy 24 Hour Tablets 731
- Children's Dimetapp ND Non-Drowsy Allergy Syrup 746
- Triaminic Allerchews 684

Losartan Potassium (Possible additive effect on lowering of blood pressure). Products include:
- Cozaar Tablets 1913
- Hyzaar 1964

Mecamylamine Hydrochloride (Possible additive effect on lowering of blood pressure). Products include:
- Inversine Tablets 3286

Mephenytoin (Clinically significant interactions have been reported with inhibitors of CYP3A4 causing elevation of plasma levels of verapamil while inducers of CYP3A4 have caused a lowering of plasma levels of verapamil).
No products indexed under this heading.

Methoxyflurane (Potential for excessive cardiovascular depression).
No products indexed under this heading.

Methsuximide (Clinically significant interactions have been reported with inhibitors of CYP3A4 causing elevation of plasma levels of verapamil while inducers of CYP3A4 have caused a lowering of plasma levels of verapamil).
No products indexed under this heading.

Methyclothiazide (Possible additive effect on lowering of blood pressure).
No products indexed under this heading.

Methyldopa (Possible additive effect on lowering of blood pressure). Products include:
- Aldoclor Tablets 1881
- Aldoril Tablets 1884

Methyldopate Hydrochloride (Possible additive effect on lowering of blood pressure).
No products indexed under this heading.

Methylprednisolone (Clinically significant interactions have been reported with inhibitors of CYP3A4 causing elevation of plasma levels of verapamil while inducers of CYP3A4 have caused a lowering of plasma levels of verapamil).
No products indexed under this heading.

Methylprednisolone Acetate (Clinically significant interactions have been reported with inhibitors of CYP3A4 causing elevation of plasma levels of verapamil while inducers of CYP3A4 have caused a lowering of plasma levels of verapamil). Products include:
- Depo-Medrol Injectable Suspension 2615
- Depo-Medrol Single-Dose Vial 2617

Methylprednisolone Sodium Succinate (Clinically significant interactions have been reported with inhibitors of CYP3A4 causing elevation of plasma levels of verapamil while inducers of CYP3A4 have caused a lowering of plasma levels of verapamil).
No products indexed under this heading.

Metipranolol Hydrochloride (Concomitant therapy may result in additive negative effects on heart rate, atrioventricular conduction and/or cardiac contractility; excessive bradycardia and AV block, including complete heart block).
No products indexed under this heading.

Metocurine Iodide (Verapamil may potentiate the activity of neuromuscular blocking agents).
No products indexed under this heading.

Metolazone (Possible additive effect on lowering of blood pressure).
No products indexed under this heading.

Metoprolol Succinate (Concomitant therapy may result in additive negative effects on heart rate, atrioventricular conduction and/or cardiac contractility; excessive bradycardia and AV block, including complete heart block; a decrease in metoprolol clearance has been observed with concomitant use). Products include:
- Toprol-XL Tablets 660

Metoprolol Tartrate (Concomitant therapy may result in additive negative effects on heart rate, atrioventricular conduction and/or cardiac contractility; excessive bradycardia and AV block, including complete heart block; a decrease in metoprolol clearance has been observed with concomitant use).
No products indexed under this heading.

Metronidazole (Clinically significant interactions have been reported with inhibitors of CYP3A4 causing elevation of plasma levels of verapamil while inducers of CYP3A4 have caused a lowering of plasma levels of verapamil). Products include:
- Metrogel 1% 1212
- MetroGel-Vaginal Gel 1822
- Noritate Cream, 1% 1051

Metronidazole Benzoate (Clinically significant interactions have been reported with inhibitors of CYP3A4 causing elevation of plasma levels of verapamil while inducers of CYP3A4 have caused a lowering of plasma levels of verapamil).
No products indexed under this heading.

Metronidazole Hydrochloride (Clinically significant interactions have been reported with inhibitors of CYP3A4 causing elevation of plasma levels of verapamil while inducers of CYP3A4 have caused a lowering of plasma levels of verapamil).
No products indexed under this heading.

Metyrosine (Possible additive effect on lowering of blood pressure). Products include:
- Demser Capsules 1933

Mibefradil Dihydrochloride (Possible additive effect on lowering of blood pressure).
No products indexed under this heading.

Miconazole (Clinically significant interactions have been reported with inhibitors of CYP3A4 causing elevation of plasma levels of verapamil while inducers of CYP3A4 have caused a lowering of plasma levels of verapamil).
No products indexed under this heading.

Miconazole Nitrate (Clinically significant interactions have been reported with inhibitors of CYP3A4 causing elevation of plasma levels of verapamil while inducers of CYP3A4 have caused a lowering of plasma levels of verapamil). Products include:
- Desenex 674
- Desenex Jock Itch Spray Powder 674

Minoxidil (Possible additive effect on lowering of blood pressure). Products include:
- Men's Rogaine Extra Strength Topical Solution, Ocean Rush Scent and Original Unscented 706
- Women's Rogaine Topical Solution, Spring Bloom Scent and Original Unscented 707

Mivacurium Chloride (Verapamil may potentiate the activity of neuromuscular blocking agents). Products include:
- Mivacron Injection 489

Modafinil (Clinically significant interactions have been reported with inhibitors of CYP3A4 causing elevation of plasma levels of verapamil while inducers of CYP3A4 have caused a lowering of plasma levels of verapamil). Products include:
- Provigil Tablets 1002

Moexipril Hydrochloride (Possible additive effect on lowering of blood pressure). Products include:
- Uniretic Tablets 3114
- Univasc Tablets 3118

Nadolol (Concomitant therapy may result in additive negative effects on heart rate, atrioventricular conduction and/or cardiac contractility; excessive bradycardia and AV block, including complete heart block). Products include:
- Nadolol Tablets 2121

Nefazodone Hydrochloride (Clinically significant interactions have been reported with inhibitors of CYP3A4 causing elevation of plasma levels of verapamil while inducers of CYP3A4 have caused a lowering of plasma levels of verapamil).
No products indexed under this heading.

Nelfinavir Mesylate (Clinically significant interactions have been reported with inhibitors of CYP3A4 causing elevation of plasma levels of verapamil while inducers of CYP3A4 have caused a lowering of plasma levels of verapamil). Products include:
- Viracept 2556

Nevirapine (Clinically significant interactions have been reported with inhibitors of CYP3A4 causing elevation of plasma levels of verapamil while inducers of CYP3A4 have caused a lowering of plasma levels of verapamil). Products include:
- Viramune Oral Suspension 903
- Viramune Tablets 903

Niacinamide (Clinically significant interactions have been reported with inhibitors of CYP3A4 causing elevation of plasma levels of verapamil while inducers of CYP3A4 have caused a lowering of plasma levels of verapamil).
No products indexed under this heading.

Nicardipine Hydrochloride (Possible additive effect on lowering of blood pressure). Products include:
- Cardene I.V. 1129

Nicotinamide (Clinically significant interactions have been reported with inhibitors of CYP3A4 causing elevation of plasma levels of verapamil while inducers of CYP3A4 have caused a lowering of plasma levels of verapamil). Products include:
- Nicomide Tablets 3190

Nifedipine (Possible additive effect on lowering of blood pressure). Products include:
- Adalat CC Tablets 2978

Nisoldipine (Possible additive effect on lowering of blood pressure). Products include:
- Sular Tablets 1163

Nitroglycerin (Possible additive effect on lowering of blood pressure). Products include:
- Nitro-Dur Transdermal Infusion System 3060
- Nitrolingual Pumpspray 1161

Nitroglycerin, long-acting formulations (Possible additive effect on lowering of blood pressure).
No products indexed under this heading.

Nitroglycerin Intravenous (Possible additive effect on lowering of blood pressure).
No products indexed under this heading.

Norfloxacin (Clinically significant interactions have been reported with inhibitors of CYP3A4 causing elevation of plasma levels of verapamil while inducers of CYP3A4 have caused a lowering of plasma levels of verapamil). Products include:
- Noroxin Tablets 2009

Omeprazole (Clinically significant interactions have been reported with inhibitors of CYP3A4 causing elevation of plasma levels of verapamil while inducers of CYP3A4 have caused a lowering of plasma levels of verapamil). Products include:

Zegerid Powder for Oral Solution 2972

Oxcarbazepine (Clinically significant interactions have been reported with inhibitors of CYP3A4 causing elevation of plasma levels of verapamil while inducers of CYP3A4 have caused a lowering of plasma levels of verapamil). Products include:

Trileptal Oral Suspension 2281
Trileptal Tablets 2281

Pancuronium Bromide (Verapamil may potentiate the activity of neuromuscular blocking agents).

No products indexed under this heading.

Papaverine (Possible additive effect on lowering of blood pressure).

No products indexed under this heading.

Papaverine Hydrochloride (Possible additive effect on lowering of blood pressure).

No products indexed under this heading.

Paroxetine Hydrochloride (Clinically significant interactions have been reported with inhibitors of CYP3A4 causing elevation of plasma levels of verapamil while inducers of CYP3A4 have caused a lowering of plasma levels of verapamil). Products include:

Paxil CR Controlled-Release Tablets 1509
Paxil 1501

Penbutolol Sulfate (Concomitant therapy may result in additive negative effects on heart rate, atrioventricular conduction and/or cardiac contractility; excessive bradycardia and AV block, including complete heart block).

No products indexed under this heading.

Perindopril Erbumine (Possible additive effect on lowering of blood pressure). Products include:

Aceon Tablets (2 mg, 4 mg, 8 mg) 3191

Phenobarbital (May increase verapamil clearance).

No products indexed under this heading.

Phenobarbital Sodium (Clinically significant interactions have been reported with inhibitors of CYP3A4 causing elevation of plasma levels of verapamil while inducers of CYP3A4 have caused a lowering of plasma levels of verapamil).

No products indexed under this heading.

Phenoxybenzamine Hydrochloride (Possible additive effect on lowering of blood pressure). Products include:

Dibenzyline Capsules 3390

Phentolamine Mesylate (Possible additive effect on lowering of blood pressure).

No products indexed under this heading.

Phenytoin (Clinically significant interactions have been reported with inhibitors of CYP3A4 causing elevation of plasma levels of verapamil while inducers of CYP3A4 have caused a lowering of plasma levels of verapamil).

No products indexed under this heading.

Phenytoin Sodium (Clinically significant interactions have been reported with inhibitors of CYP3A4 causing elevation of plasma levels of verapamil while inducers of CYP3A4 have caused a lowering of plasma levels of verapamil). Products include:

Phenytek Capsules 2153

Pindolol (Concomitant therapy may result in additive negative effects on heart rate, atrioventricular conduction and/or cardiac contractility; excessive bradycardia and AV block, including complete heart block).

No products indexed under this heading.

Polythiazide (Possible additive effect on lowering of blood pressure).

No products indexed under this heading.

Prazosin Hydrochloride (Possible additive effect on lowering of blood pressure).

No products indexed under this heading.

Prednisolone Acetate (Clinically significant interactions have been reported with inhibitors of CYP3A4 causing elevation of plasma levels of verapamil while inducers of CYP3A4 have caused a lowering of plasma levels of verapamil). Products include:

Blephamide Ophthalmic Ointment 563
Blephamide Ophthalmic Suspension.................................. 564
Poly-Pred Liquifilm Ophthalmic Suspension .... ⊙231
Pred Forte Ophthalmic Suspension .... ⊙233
Pred Mild Sterile Ophthalmic Suspension .... ⊙236
Pred-G Ophthalmic Suspension ...... ⊙234
Pred-G Sterile Ophthalmic Ointment .... ⊙235

Prednisolone Sodium Phosphate (Clinically significant interactions have been reported with inhibitors of CYP3A4 causing elevation of plasma levels of verapamil while inducers of CYP3A4 have caused a lowering of plasma levels of verapamil). Products include:

Pediapred Oral Solution 3319

Prednisolone Tebutate (Clinically significant interactions have been reported with inhibitors of CYP3A4 causing elevation of plasma levels of verapamil while inducers of CYP3A4 have caused a lowering of plasma levels of verapamil).

No products indexed under this heading.

Prednisone (Clinically significant interactions have been reported with inhibitors of CYP3A4 causing elevation of plasma levels of verapamil while inducers of CYP3A4 have caused a lowering of plasma levels of verapamil).

No products indexed under this heading.

Primidone (Clinically significant interactions have been reported with inhibitors of CYP3A4 causing elevation of plasma levels of verapamil while inducers of CYP3A4 have caused a lowering of plasma levels of verapamil).

No products indexed under this heading.

Propoxyphene Hydrochloride (Clinically significant interactions have been reported with inhibitors of CYP3A4 causing elevation of plasma levels of verapamil while inducers of CYP3A4 have caused a lowering of plasma levels of verapamil).

No products indexed under this heading.

Propoxyphene Napsylate (Clinically significant interactions have been reported with inhibitors of CYP3A4 causing elevation of plasma levels of verapamil while inducers of CYP3A4 have caused a lowering of plasma levels of verapamil). Products include:

Darvocet A 500 Tablets 3497

Propranolol Hydrochloride (Concomitant therapy may result in additive negative effects on heart rate, atrioventricular conduction and/or cardiac contractility; excessive bradycardia and AV block, including complete heart block; a decrease in propranolol clearance has been observed with concomitant use). Products include:

Inderal LA Long-Acting Capsules 3421
InnoPran XL Capsules 2728

Quinapril Hydrochloride (Possible additive effect on lowering of blood pressure).

No products indexed under this heading.

Quinidine (Clinically significant interactions have been reported with inhibitors of CYP3A4 causing elevation of plasma levels of verapamil while inducers of CYP3A4 have caused a lowering of plasma levels of verapamil).

No products indexed under this heading.

Quinidine Gluconate (Concomitant use may result in significant hypertension; verapamil significantly counteracts the effects of quinidine on AV conduction; potential for increased quinidine levels with co-administration).

No products indexed under this heading.

Quinidine Hydrochloride (Clinically significant interactions have been reported with inhibitors of CYP3A4 causing elevation of plasma levels of verapamil while inducers of CYP3A4 have caused a lowering of plasma levels of verapamil).

No products indexed under this heading.

Quinidine Polygalacturonate (Concomitant use may result in significant hypertension; verapamil significantly counteracts the effects of quinidine on AV conduction; potential for increased quinidine levels with co-administration).

No products indexed under this heading.

Quinidine Sulfate (Concomitant use may result in significant hypertension; verapamil significantly counteracts the effects of quinidine on AV conduction; potential for increased quinidine levels with co-administration).

No products indexed under this heading.

Quinine (Clinically significant interactions have been reported with inhibitors of CYP3A4 causing elevation of plasma levels of verapamil while inducers of CYP3A4 have caused a lowering of plasma levels of verapamil).

No products indexed under this heading.

Quinine Sulfate (Clinically significant interactions have been reported with inhibitors of CYP3A4 causing elevation of plasma levels of verapamil while inducers of CYP3A4 have caused a lowering of plasma levels of verapamil).

No products indexed under this heading.

Quinupristin (Clinically significant interactions have been reported with inhibitors of CYP3A4 causing elevation of plasma levels of verapamil while inducers of CYP3A4 have caused a lowering of plasma levels of verapamil). Products include:

Synercid I.V. 1690

Ramipril (Possible additive effect on lowering of blood pressure). Products include:

Altace Capsules 1673

Ranitidine Bismuth Citrate (Clinically significant interactions have been reported with inhibitors of CYP3A4 causing elevation of plasma levels of verapamil while inducers of CYP3A4 have caused a lowering of plasma levels of verapamil).

No products indexed under this heading.

Ranitidine Hydrochloride (Clinically significant interactions have been reported with inhibitors of CYP3A4 causing elevation of plasma levels of verapamil while inducers of CYP3A4 have caused a lowering of plasma levels of verapamil). Products include:

Zantac 1597
Zantac Injection 1593
Zantac 75 Tablets .... ▣715
Zantac 150 Maximum Strength Tablets.. ▣715
Zantac Injection Pharmacy Bulk Package.. 1595

Rapacuronium Bromide (Verapamil may potentiate the activity of neuromuscular blocking agents).

No products indexed under this heading.

Rauwolfia Serpentina (Possible additive effect on lowering of blood pressure).

No products indexed under this heading.

Rescinnamine (Possible additive effect on lowering of blood pressure).

No products indexed under this heading.

Reserpine (Possible additive effect on lowering of blood pressure).

No products indexed under this heading.

Rifabutin (Clinically significant interactions have been reported with inhibitors of CYP3A4 causing elevation of plasma levels of verapamil while inducers of CYP3A4 have caused a lowering of plasma levels of verapamil).

No products indexed under this heading.

Rifampicin (Clinically significant interactions have been reported with inhibitors of CYP3A4 causing elevation of plasma levels of verapamil while inducers of CYP3A4 have caused a lowering of plasma levels of verapamil).

No products indexed under this heading.

Rifampin (Therapy with rifampin may markedly reduce oral verapamil bioavailability).

No products indexed under this heading.

Rifapentine (Clinically significant interactions have been reported with inhibitors of CYP3A4 causing elevation of plasma levels of verapamil while inducers of CYP3A4 have caused a lowering of plasma levels of verapamil).
No products indexed under this heading.

Ritonavir (Clinically significant interactions have been reported with inhibitors of CYP3A4 causing elevation of plasma levels of verapamil while inducers of CYP3A4 have caused a lowering of plasma levels of verapamil). Products include:
Kaletra ... 474
Norvir ... 499

Rocuronium Bromide (Verapamil may potentiate the activity of neuromuscular blocking agents). Products include:
Zemuron Injection ... 2363

Saquinavir (Clinically significant interactions have been reported with inhibitors of CYP3A4 causing elevation of plasma levels of verapamil while inducers of CYP3A4 have caused a lowering of plasma levels of verapamil).
No products indexed under this heading.

Saquinavir Mesylate (Clinically significant interactions have been reported with inhibitors of CYP3A4 causing elevation of plasma levels of verapamil while inducers of CYP3A4 have caused a lowering of plasma levels of verapamil). Products include:
Invirase ... 2776

Sertraline Hydrochloride (Clinically significant interactions have been reported with inhibitors of CYP3A4 causing elevation of plasma levels of verapamil while inducers of CYP3A4 have caused a lowering of plasma levels of verapamil). Products include:
Zoloft ... 2581

Sodium Nitroprusside (Possible additive effect on lowering of blood pressure).
No products indexed under this heading.

Sotalol Hydrochloride (Concomitant therapy may result in additive negative effects on heart rate, atrioventricular conduction and/or cardiac contractility; excessive bradycardia and AV block, including complete heart block).
No products indexed under this heading.

Spirapril Hydrochloride (Possible additive effect on lowering of blood pressure).
No products indexed under this heading.

Spironolactone (Possible additive effect on lowering of blood pressure).
No products indexed under this heading.

Sulfinpyrazone (Clinically significant interactions have been reported with inhibitors of CYP3A4 causing elevation of plasma levels of verapamil while inducers of CYP3A4 have caused a lowering of plasma levels of verapamil).
No products indexed under this heading.

Telithromycin (Clinically significant interactions have been reported with inhibitors of CYP3A4 causing elevation of plasma levels of verapamil while inducers of CYP3A4 have caused a lowering of plasma levels of verapamil). Products include:
Ketek Tablets ... 2920

Telmisartan (Possible additive effect on lowering of blood pressure). Products include:
Micardis Tablets ... 884
Micardis HCT Tablets ... 886

Terazosin Hydrochloride (Possible additive effect on lowering of blood pressure). Products include:
Hytrin Capsules ... 469

Theophylline (Verapamil may inhibit the clearance and increase plasma levels of theophylline).
No products indexed under this heading.

Theophylline Anhydrous (Verapamil may inhibit the clearance and increase plasma levels of theophylline). Products include:
Uniphyl Tablets ... 2708

Theophylline Calcium Salicylate (Verapamil may inhibit the clearance and increase plasma levels of theophylline).
No products indexed under this heading.

Theophylline Dihydroxypropyl (Glyceryl) (Verapamil may inhibit the clearance and increase plasma levels of theophylline).
No products indexed under this heading.

Theophylline Ethylenediamine (Verapamil may inhibit the clearance and increase plasma levels of theophylline).
No products indexed under this heading.

Theophylline Sodium Glycinate (Verapamil may inhibit the clearance and increase plasma levels of theophylline).
No products indexed under this heading.

Timolol Hemihydrate (Concomitant therapy may result in additive negative effects on heart rate, atrioventricular conduction and/or cardiac contractility; excessive bradycardia and AV block, including complete heart block; one case of asymptomatic bradycardia with a wandering atrial pacemaker has been observed with timolol eye drops and oral verapamil). Products include:
Betimol Ophthalmic Solution ... 3371
Betimol Ophthalmic Solution ... ⊙ 283

Timolol Maleate (Concomitant therapy may result in additive negative effects on heart rate, atrioventricular conduction and/or cardiac contractility; excessive bradycardia and AV block, including complete heart block; one case of asymptomatic bradycardia with a wandering atrial pacemaker has been observed with timolol eye drops and oral verapamil). Products include:
Blocadren Tablets ... 1891
Cosopt Sterile Ophthalmic Solution ... 1910
Timolide Tablets ... 2056
Timoptic in Ocudose ... 2061
Timoptic Sterile Ophthalmic Solution ... 2058
Timoptic-XE Sterile Ophthalmic Gel Forming Solution ... 2062

Tolazoline Hydrochloride (Possible additive effect on lowering of blood pressure).
No products indexed under this heading.

Torsemide (Possible additive effect on lowering of blood pressure).
No products indexed under this heading.

Trandolapril (Possible additive effect on lowering of blood pressure). Products include:
Mavik Tablets ... 482
Tarka Tablets ... 519

Triamcinolone (Clinically significant interactions have been reported with inhibitors of CYP3A4 causing elevation of plasma levels of verapamil while inducers of CYP3A4 have caused a lowering of plasma levels of verapamil).
No products indexed under this heading.

Triamcinolone Acetonide (Clinically significant interactions have been reported with inhibitors of CYP3A4 causing elevation of plasma levels of verapamil while inducers of CYP3A4 have caused a lowering of plasma levels of verapamil). Products include:
Azmacort Inhalation Aerosol ... 1701
Nasacort HFA Inhalation Aerosol ... 2939
Nasacort AQ Nasal Spray ... 2937

Triamcinolone Diacetate (Clinically significant interactions have been reported with inhibitors of CYP3A4 causing elevation of plasma levels of verapamil while inducers of CYP3A4 have caused a lowering of plasma levels of verapamil).
No products indexed under this heading.

Triamcinolone Hexacetonide (Clinically significant interactions have been reported with inhibitors of CYP3A4 causing elevation of plasma levels of verapamil while inducers of CYP3A4 have caused a lowering of plasma levels of verapamil).
No products indexed under this heading.

Triamterene (Possible additive effect on lowering of blood pressure). Products include:
Dyazide Capsules ... 1389
Dyrenium Capsules ... 3390
Maxzide ... 2150

Trimethaphan Camsylate (Possible additive effect on lowering of blood pressure).
No products indexed under this heading.

Troglitazone (Clinically significant interactions have been reported with inhibitors of CYP3A4 causing elevation of plasma levels of verapamil while inducers of CYP3A4 have caused a lowering of plasma levels of verapamil).
No products indexed under this heading.

Troleandomycin (Clinically significant interactions have been reported with inhibitors of CYP3A4 causing elevation of plasma levels of verapamil while inducers of CYP3A4 have caused a lowering of plasma levels of verapamil).
No products indexed under this heading.

Valproate Sodium (Clinically significant interactions have been reported with inhibitors of CYP3A4 causing elevation of plasma levels of verapamil while inducers of CYP3A4 have caused a lowering of plasma levels of verapamil). Products include:
Depacon Injection ... 412

Valsartan (Possible additive effect on lowering of blood pressure). Products include:
Diovan HCT Tablets ... 2195
Diovan Tablets ... 2191

Vecuronium Bromide (Verapamil may potentiate the activity of neuromuscular blocking agents).
No products indexed under this heading.

Voriconazole (Clinically significant interactions have been reported with inhibitors of CYP3A4 causing elevation of plasma levels of verapamil while inducers of CYP3A4 have caused a lowering of plasma levels of verapamil). Products include:
VFEND I.V. ... 2543
VFEND Oral Suspension ... 2543
VFEND Tablets ... 2543

Zafirlukast (Clinically significant interactions have been reported with inhibitors of CYP3A4 causing elevation of plasma levels of verapamil while inducers of CYP3A4 have caused a lowering of plasma levels of verapamil). Products include:
Accolate Tablets ... 663

Zileuton (Clinically significant interactions have been reported with inhibitors of CYP3A4 causing elevation of plasma levels of verapamil while inducers of CYP3A4 have caused a lowering of plasma levels of verapamil).
No products indexed under this heading.

Food Interactions

Alcohol (Verapamil may increase blood alcohol concentrations and prolong its effect).

Grapefruit (Clinically significant interactions have been reported with inhibitors of CYP3A4 causing elevation of plasma levels of verapamil while inducers of CYP3A4 have caused a lowering of plasma levels of verapamil).

Grapefruit Juice (Grapefruit juice may significantly increase concentrations of verapamil).

COZAAR TABLETS

(Losartan Potassium) ... 1913
May interact with non-steroidal anti-inflammatory agents, potassium preparations, potassium sparing diuretics, and certain other agents. Compounds in these categories include:

Amiloride Hydrochloride (Concomitant use with potassium-sparing diuretics may lead to hyperkalemia). Products include:
Midamor Tablets ... 2000
Moduretic Tablets ... 2003

Celecoxib (Concomitant use may diminish the antihypertensive effects of losartan). Products include:
Celebrex Capsules ... 3130

Cimetidine (Co-administration leads to an increase of about 18% in AUC of losartan with no effect on pharmacokinetics of its active metabolites). Products include:
Tagamet HB 200 Tablets ... ▣ 637
Tagamet Tablets ... 1547

Cimetidine Hydrochloride (Co-administration leads to an increase of about 18% in AUC of losartan with no effect on pharmacokinetics of its active metabolites).
No products indexed under this heading.

Diclofenac Potassium (Concomitant use may diminish the antihypertensive effects of losartan). Products include:
Cataflam Tablets ... 2173

Diclofenac Sodium (Concomitant use may diminish the antihypertensive effects of losartan). Products include:

- Arthrotec Tablets 3126
- Voltaren Ophthalmic Solution 2300
- Voltaren Tablets 2298
- Voltaren-XR Tablets 2301

Etodolac (Concomitant use may diminish the antihypertensive effects of losartan).

No products indexed under this heading.

Fenoprofen Calcium (Concomitant use may diminish the antihypertensive effects of losartan). Products include:

- Nalfon Capsules 2504

Flurbiprofen (Concomitant use may diminish the antihypertensive effects of losartan).

No products indexed under this heading.

Gestodene (In vitro studies show significant inhibition of the formation of the active metabolite by inhibitors of P450 3A4 such as gestodene; pharmacodynamic consequences of concomitant use is undefined).

No products indexed under this heading.

Ibuprofen (Concomitant use may diminish the antihypertensive effects of losartan). Products include:

- Advil Allergy Sinus Caplets .... ▣737
- Advil .... ▣737
- Children's Advil Suspension .... ▣742
- Children's Advil Chewable Tablets .... ▣741
- Advil Cold & Sinus .... ▣739
- Advil Flu & Body Ache Caplets .... ▣739
- Children's Advil Cold Suspension .... ▣741
- Infants' Advil Concentrated Drops .... ▣743
- Junior Strength Advil Swallow Tablets .... ▣740
- Advil Migraine Liquigels .... ▣740
- Advil Multi-Symptom Cold Caplets .... ▣738
- Combunox Tablets 1183
- Children's Motrin Oral Suspension and Chewable Tablets 1837
- Children's Motrin Cold Non-Staining Dye-Free Oral Suspension 1838
- Children's Motrin Cold Oral Suspension 1838
- Children's Motrin Non-Staining Dye-Free Oral Suspension 1837
- Motrin Cold & Sinus Caplets 1836
- Motrin IB Tablets and Caplets 1836
- Infants' Motrin Concentrated Drops 1837
- Infants' Motrin Non-Staining Dye-Free Drops 1837
- Junior Strength Motrin Caplets and Chewable Tablets 1837
- Vicoprofen Tablets 533

Indomethacin (Antihypertensive effect of losartan may be blunted by indomethacin). Products include:

- Indocin 1968

Indomethacin Sodium Trihydrate (Antihypertensive effect of losartan may be blunted by indomethacin). Products include:

- Indocin I.V. 1973

Ketoconazole (In vitro studies show significant inhibition of the formation of the active metabolite by inhibitors of P450 3A4 such as ketoconazole or complete inhibition by the combination of ketoconazole and sulfaphenazole; pharmacodynamic consequences of concomitant use is undefined). Products include:

- Nizoral A-D Shampoo, 1% 1839
- Nizoral 2% Shampoo 1838

Ketoprofen (Concomitant use may diminish the antihypertensive effects of losartan).

No products indexed under this heading.

Ketorolac Tromethamine (Concomitant use may diminish the antihypertensive effects of losartan). Products include:

- Acular Ophthalmic Solution 561
- Acular LS Ophthalmic Solution 562

Meclofenamate Sodium (Concomitant use may diminish the antihypertensive effects of losartan).

No products indexed under this heading.

Mefenamic Acid (Concomitant use may diminish the antihypertensive effects of losartan).

No products indexed under this heading.

Meloxicam (Concomitant use may diminish the antihypertensive effects of losartan). Products include:

- Mobic Oral Suspension 893
- Mobic Tablets 893

Nabumetone (Concomitant use may diminish the antihypertensive effects of losartan). Products include:

- Relafen Tablets 1523

Naproxen (Concomitant use may diminish the antihypertensive effects of losartan). Products include:

- EC-Naprosyn Delayed-Release Tablets 2769
- Naprosyn Suspension 2769
- Naprosyn Tablets 2769
- Prevacid NapraPAC 3277

Naproxen Sodium (Concomitant use may diminish the antihypertensive effects of losartan). Products include:

- Aleve Tablets, Caplets and Gelcaps .... ▣605
- Anaprox Tablets 2769
- Anaprox DS Tablets 2769

Oxaprozin (Concomitant use may diminish the antihypertensive effects of losartan).

No products indexed under this heading.

Phenobarbital (Co-administration leads to a reduction of about 20% in AUC of losartan and that of its active metabolites).

No products indexed under this heading.

Phenylbutazone (Concomitant use may diminish the antihypertensive effects of losartan).

No products indexed under this heading.

Piroxicam (Concomitant use may diminish the antihypertensive effects of losartan).

No products indexed under this heading.

Potassium Acid Phosphate (Concomitant use with potassium supplements or salt substitute containing potassium may lead to hyperkalemia; patients should be advised to avoid these potassium-containing preparations). Products include:

- K-Phos Original (Sodium Free) Tablets 785

Potassium Bicarbonate (Concomitant use with potassium supplements or salt substitute containing potassium may lead to hyperkalemia; patients should be advised to avoid these potassium-containing preparations).

No products indexed under this heading.

Potassium Chloride (Concomitant use with potassium supplements or salt substitute containing potassium may lead to hyperkalemia; patients should be advised to avoid these potassium-containing preparations). Products include:

- Colyte with Flavor Packs for Oral Solution 3102
- HalfLytely and Bisacodyl Tablets Bowel Prep Kit with Flavors Packs 915
- K-Dur Extended-Relase Tablets 3047
- K-Lor Powder Packets 472
- K-Tab Filmtab Tablets 473
- TriLyte with Flavor Packs for Oral Solution 3114

Potassium Citrate (Concomitant use with potassium supplements or salt substitute containing potassium may lead to hyperkalemia; patients should be advised to avoid these potassium-containing preparations). Products include:

- Urocit-K Tablets 2109

Potassium Gluconate (Concomitant use with potassium supplements or salt substitute containing potassium may lead to hyperkalemia; patients should be advised to avoid these potassium-containing preparations).

No products indexed under this heading.

Potassium Phosphate (Concomitant use with potassium supplements or salt substitute containing potassium may lead to hyperkalemia; patients should be advised to avoid these potassium-containing preparations). Products include:

- K-Phos Neutral Tablets 785

Rofecoxib (Concomitant use may diminish the antihypertensive effects of losartan).

No products indexed under this heading.

Salt Substitutes (Concomitant use with salt substitutes may lead to hyperkalemia).

No products indexed under this heading.

Spironolactone (Concomitant use with potassium-sparing diuretics may lead to hyperkalemia).

No products indexed under this heading.

Sulfaphenazole (In vitro studies show significant inhibition of the formation of the active metabolite by inhibitors of P450 3A4 such as sulfaphenazole; pharmacodynamic consequences of concomitant use is undefined).

No products indexed under this heading.

Sulindac (Concomitant use may diminish the antihypertensive effects of losartan). Products include:

- Clinoril Tablets 1899

Tolmetin Sodium (Concomitant use may diminish the antihypertensive effects of losartan).

No products indexed under this heading.

Triamterene (Concomitant use with potassium-sparing diuretics may lead to hyperkalemia). Products include:

- Dyazide Capsules 1389
- Dyrenium Capsules 3390
- Maxzide 2150

Troleandomycin (In vitro studies show significant inhibition of the formation of the active metabolite by inhibitors of P450 3A4 such as troleandomycin; pharmacodynamic consequences of concomitant use is undefined).

No products indexed under this heading.

Valdecoxib (Concomitant use may diminish the antihypertensive effects of losartan).

No products indexed under this heading.

Food Interactions

Meal, unspecified (Meal slows absorption and decreases Cmax, but has minor effects on losartan AUC or on the AUC of the metabolite).

CREON 5 CAPSULES

(Pancrelipase) 3195

Food Interactions

Food having a pH greater than 5.5 (Can dissolve the protective coating resulting in early release of enzymes, irritation of oral mucosa, and/or loss of enzyme activity).

CREON 10 CAPSULES

(Pancrelipase) 3195

See Creon 5 Capsules

CREON 20 CAPSULES

(Pancrelipase) 3196

See Creon 5 Capsules

CRESTOR TABLETS

(Rosuvastatin Calcium) 672

May interact with oral anticoagulants, erythromycin, fibrates, oral contraceptives, and certain other agents. Compounds in these categories include:

Anisindione (Co-administration of rosuvastatin to patients on stable warfarin therapy resulted in clinically significant rises in INR. In patients taking coumarin anticoagulants and rosuvastatin concomitantly, INR should be monitored). Products include:

- Miradon Tablets 3056

Antacids, unspecified (Co-administration of an antacid (aluminum and magnesium hydroxide combination) with rosuvastatin resulted in a decrease in plasma concentrations of rosuvastatin by 54%. However, when the antacid was given 2 hours after rosuvastatin, there were no clinically significant changes in plasma concentrations of rosuvastatin).

No products indexed under this heading.

Cimetidine (Caution should be exercised if any HMG-CoA reductase inhibitor is administered concomitantly with drugs that may decrease the levels or activity of endogenous steroid hormones, such as cimetidine). Products include:

- Tagamet HB 200 Tablets .... ▣637
- Tagamet Tablets 1547

Cimetidine Hydrochloride (Caution should be exercised if any HMG-CoA reductase inhibitor is administered concomitantly with drugs that may decrease the levels or activity of endogenous steroid hormones, such as cimetidine).

No products indexed under this heading.

Clofibrate (The risk of myopathy during treatment with rosuvastatin may be increased with concurrent administration of other lipid-lowering therapies. The benefit of further alterations in lipid levels by the combined use of rosuvastatin with fibrates should be carefully weighed against the potential risks of this combination).
No products indexed under this heading.

Cyclosporine (Co-administration of cyclosporine with rosuvastatin resulted in no significant changes in cyclosporine concentrations. However, Cmax and AUC of rosuvastatin increased 11- and 7-fold, respectively, compared with historical data in healthy subjects. These increases are considered to be clinically significant. The risk of myopathy during treatment with rosuvastatin may be increased with concurrent administration of cyclosporine). Products include:
Gengraf Capsules **458**
Neoral Soft Gelatin Capsules **2247**
Neoral Oral Solution **2247**
Restasis Ophthalmic Emulsion **570**
Sandimmune **2259**

Desogestrel (Co-administration of oral contraceptives (ethinyl estradiol and norgestrel) with rosuvastatin resulted in an increase in plasma concentrations of ethinyl estradiol and norgestrel by 26% and 34%, respectively). Products include:
Ortho-Cept Tablets **2395**

Dicumarol (Co-administration of rosuvastatin to patients on stable warfarin therapy resulted in clinically significant rises in INR. In patients taking coumarin anticoagulants and rosuvastatin concomitantly, INR should be monitored).
No products indexed under this heading.

Erythromycin (Co-administration of erythromycin and rosuvastatin decreased AUC and Cmax of rosuvastatin by 20% and 31%, respectively. These reductions are not considered clinically significant). Products include:
Erygel Topical Gel **2096**
Ery-Tab Tablets **447**
Erythromycin Base Filmtab Tablets **454**
Erythromycin Delayed-Release Capsules, USP............................. **456**
PCE Dispertab Tablets **510**

Erythromycin Estolate (Co-administration of erythromycin and rosuvastatin decreased AUC and Cmax of rosuvastatin by 20% and 31%, respectively. These reductions are not considered clinically significant).
No products indexed under this heading.

Erythromycin Ethylsuccinate (Co-administration of erythromycin and rosuvastatin decreased AUC and Cmax of rosuvastatin by 20% and 31%, respectively. These reductions are not considered clinically significant). Products include:
E.E.S. **449**
EryPed **445**

Erythromycin Gluceptate (Co-administration of erythromycin and rosuvastatin decreased AUC and Cmax of rosuvastatin by 20% and 31%, respectively. These reductions are not considered clinically significant).
No products indexed under this heading.

Erythromycin Lactobionate (Co-administration of erythromycin and rosuvastatin decreased AUC and Cmax of rosuvastatin by 20% and 31%, respectively. These reductions are not considered clinically significant).
No products indexed under this heading.

Erythromycin Stearate (Co-administration of erythromycin and rosuvastatin decreased AUC and Cmax of rosuvastatin by 20% and 31%, respectively. These reductions are not considered clinically significant). Products include:
Erythrocin Stearate Filmtab Tablets **452**

Ethinyl Estradiol (Co-administration of oral contraceptives (ethinyl estradiol and norgestrel) with rosuvastatin resulted in an increase in plasma concentrations of ethinyl estradiol and norgestrel by 26% and 34%, respectively). Products include:
Alesse-28 Tablets **3392**
Lo/Ovral-28 Tablets **3423**
NuvaRing **2357**
Ortho-Cept Tablets **2395**
Ortho-Cyclen/Ortho Tri-Cyclen **2414**
Ortho Evra Transdermal System **2402**
Ortho Tri-Cyclen Lo Tablets **2421**
Seasonale Tablets **1073**
Triphasil-28 Tablets **3483**
Yasmin 28 Tablets **818**

Ethynodiol Diacetate (Co-administration of oral contraceptives (ethinyl estradiol and norgestrel) with rosuvastatin resulted in an increase in plasma concentrations of ethinyl estradiol and norgestrel by 26% and 34%, respectively).
No products indexed under this heading.

Fenofibrate (The risk of myopathy during treatment with rosuvastatin may be increased with concurrent administration of other lipid-lowering therapies. The benefit of further alterations in lipid levels by the combined use of rosuvastatin with fibrates should be carefully weighed against the potential risks of this combination). Products include:
Antara Capsules **2723**
Lofibra Capsules **1217**
Tricor Tablets **523**
Triglide Tablets **1165**

Fluconazole (Co-administration of fluconazole with rosuvastatin resulted in a 14% increase in AUC of rosuvastatin. This increase is not considered clinically significant).
No products indexed under this heading.

Gemfibrozil (Co-administration of gemfibrozil with rosuvastatin resulted in a 90% and 120% increase for AUC and Cmax of rosuvastatin, respectively. This increase is considered to be clinically significant; combination therapy with rosuvastatin and gemfibrozil should generally be avoided).
No products indexed under this heading.

Itraconazole (Itraconazole resulted in a 39% and 28% increase in AUC of rosuvastatin after 10mg and 80mg dosing, respectively. These increases are not considered clinically significant).
No products indexed under this heading.

Ketoconazole (Caution should be exercised if any HMG-CoA reductase inhibitor is administered concomitantly with drugs that may decrease the levels or activity of endogenous steroid hormones, such as ketoconazole). Products include:
Nizoral A-D Shampoo, 1% **1839**
Nizoral 2% Shampoo **1838**

Levonorgestrel (Co-administration of oral contraceptives (ethinyl estradiol and norgestrel) with rosuvastatin resulted in an increase in plasma concentrations of ethinyl estradiol and norgestrel by 26% and 34%, respectively). Products include:
Alesse-28 Tablets **3392**
Climara Pro Transdermal System **800**
Mirena Intrauterine System **810**
Plan B Tablets **1068**
Seasonale Tablets **1073**
Triphasil-28 Tablets **3483**

Mestranol (Co-administration of oral contraceptives (ethinyl estradiol and norgestrel) with rosuvastatin resulted in an increase in plasma concentrations of ethinyl estradiol and norgestrel by 26% and 34%, respectively).
No products indexed under this heading.

Niacin (The risk of myopathy during treatment with rosuvastatin may be increased with concurrent administration of other lipid-lowering therapies. The benefit of further alterations in lipid levels by the combined use of rosuvastatin with niacin should be carefully weighed against the potential risks of this combination). Products include:
Advicor Tablets **1694**
Niaspan Extended-Release Tablets **1703**

Niacinamide (The risk of myopathy during treatment with rosuvastatin may be increased with concurrent administration of other lipid-lowering therapies. The benefit of further alterations in lipid levels by the combined use of rosuvastatin with niacin should be carefully weighed against the potential risks of this combination).
No products indexed under this heading.

Norethindrone (Co-administration of oral contraceptives (ethinyl estradiol and norgestrel) with rosuvastatin resulted in an increase in plasma concentrations of ethinyl estradiol and norgestrel by 26% and 34%, respectively). Products include:
Ortho Micronor Tablets **2411**

Norethynodrel (Co-administration of oral contraceptives (ethinyl estradiol and norgestrel) with rosuvastatin resulted in an increase in plasma concentrations of ethinyl estradiol and norgestrel by 26% and 34%, respectively).
No products indexed under this heading.

Norgestimate (Co-administration of oral contraceptives (ethinyl estradiol and norgestrel) with rosuvastatin resulted in an increase in plasma concentrations of ethinyl estradiol and norgestrel by 26% and 34%, respectively). Products include:
Ortho-Cyclen/Ortho Tri-Cyclen **2414**
Ortho Tri-Cyclen Lo Tablets **2421**
Prefest Tablets **1069**

Norgestrel (Co-administration of oral contraceptives (ethinyl estradiol and norgestrel) with rosuvastatin resulted in an increase in plasma concentrations of ethinyl estradiol and norgestrel by 26% and 34%, respectively). Products include:
Lo/Ovral-28 Tablets **3423**

Spironolactone (Caution should be exercised if any HMG-CoA reductase inhibitor is administered concomitantly with drugs that may decrease the levels or activity of endogenous steroid hormones, such as spironolactone).
No products indexed under this heading.

Warfarin Sodium (Co-administration of rosuvastatin to patients on stable warfarin therapy resulted in clinically significant rises in INR. In patients taking coumarin anticoagulants and rosuvastatin concomitantly, INR should be monitored). Products include:
Coumadin for Injection **932**
Coumadin Tablets **932**

CRIXIVAN CAPSULES

(Indinavir Sulfate) **1918**

May interact with calcium channel blockers, dexamethasone, ergot-containing drugs, phenytoin, and certain other agents. Compounds in these categories include:

Amiodarone Hydrochloride (Inhibition of CYP3A4 by indinavir could result in elevated plasma concentrations of amiodarone potentially causing serious or life-threatening reactions; co-administration is contraindicated). Products include:
Pacerone Tablets **3337**

Amlodipine Besylate (Co-administration of calcium channel blockers with indinavir may result in increased plasma concentrations of the dihydropyridine calcium channel blockers which could increase or prolong their therapeutic and adverse effects. Caution is warranted and clinical monitoring is recommended). Products include:
Caduet Tablets **2507**
Lotrel Capsules **2238**
Norvasc Tablets **2529**

Astemizole (Inhibition of CYP3A4 by indinavir could result in elevated plasma concentrations of astemizole potentially causing serious or life-threatening reactions; co-administration is contraindicated).
No products indexed under this heading.

Atazanavir (Both indinavir sulfate and atazanavir are associated with indirect (unconjugated) hyperbilirubinemia. Combinations of these drugs have not been studied and co-administration of indinavir sulfate and atazanavir is not recommended).
No products indexed under this heading.

Atazanavir sulfate (Both indinavir sulfate and atazanavir are associated with indirect (unconjugated) hyperbilirubinemia. Combinations of these drugs have not been studied and coadministration of indinavir sulfate and atazanavir is not recommended). Products include:
Reyataz Capsules **948**

Atorvastatin Calcium (Co-administration of indinavir and atorvastatin may lead to increased astorvastatin concentrations. The risk of myopathy, including rhabdomyolysis, may be increased when protease inhibitors, including indinavir, are used in combination with HMG-CoA inhibitors that are metabolized by the CYP3A4 pathway. Use lowest possible dose of atorvastatin with careful monitoring, or consider HMG-CoA reduuctase inhibitors that are

not primarily metabolized by CYP3A, such as pravastatin, fluvastatin, or rosuvastain in combination with indinavir). Products include:

Caduet Tablets 2507
Lipitor Tablets 2495

Bepridil Hydrochloride (Co-administration may lead to increased bepridil concentrations. Caution is warranted and therapeutic concentration monitoring is recommended for antiarrhythmics when co-administered with indinavir).

No products indexed under this heading.

Carbamazepine (Could diminish plasma concentrations of indinavir because carbamazepine is an inducer of P450 3A4; caution is advised if co-administered). Products include:

Carbatrol Capsules 3174
Equetro Extended-Release Capsules 3178
Tegretol/Tegretol-XR 2278

Cerivastatin Sodium (The risk of myopathy including rhabdomyolysis may be increased when protease inhibitors, including indinavir, are used in combination with HMG-CoA inhibitors that are metabolized by the CYP3A4 pathway).

No products indexed under this heading.

Cisapride (Inhibition of CYP3A4 by indinavir could result in elevated plasma concentrations of amiodarone, potentially causing serious or life-threatening reactions; co-administration is contraindicated).

No products indexed under this heading.

Clarithromycin (Co-administration of indinavir and clarithromycin may lead to increased clarithromycin and indinvair concentrations. The appropriate doses for this combination, with respect to safety and efficacy, have not been established). Products include:

Biaxin/Biaxin XL 402
PREVPAC 3281

Cyclosporine (Co-administration of indinavir and cyclosporine may lead to increased cyclosporine concentrations). Products include:

Gengraf Capsules 458
Neoral Soft Gelatin Capsules 2247
Neoral Oral Solution 2247
Restasis Ophthalmic Emulsion 570
Sandimmune 2259

Delavirdine Mesylate (Co-administration results in inhibition of indinavir metabolism producing an increase in indinavir concentrations; a reduction of indinavir dosage should be considered when used concurrently). Products include:

Rescriptor Tablets 2535

Dexamethasone (Could diminish plasma concentrations of indinavir because dexamethasone is an inducer of P450 3A4; caution is advised if co-administered). Products include:

Ciprodex Otic Suspension 555
Decadron Tablets 1929
TobraDex Ophthalmic Ointment 558
TobraDex Ophthalmic Suspension ... 558

Dexamethasone Acetate (Could diminish plasma concentrations of indinavir because dexamethasone is an inducer of P450 3A4; caution is advised if co-administered).

No products indexed under this heading.

Dexamethasone Sodium Phosphate (Could diminish plasma concentrations of indinavir because dexamethasone is an inducer of P450 3A4; caution is advised if co-administered). Products include:

Decadron Phosphate Injection 1931

Didanosine (Gastric acid rapidly degrades didanosine and a normal (acidic) gastric pH may be necessary for the optimum absorption of indinavir; if administered concomitantly, they should be administered at least one hour apart on an empty stomach).

No products indexed under this heading.

Dihydroergotamine Mesylate (Inhibition of CYP3A4 by indinavir could result in elevated plasma concentrations of ergot derivatives, potentially causing serious or life-threatening reactions; co-administration is contraindicated). Products include:

Migranal Nasal Spray 3350

Diltiazem Hydrochloride (Co-administration of calcium channel blockers with indinavir may result in increased plasma concentrations of the dihydropyridine calcium channel blockers which could increase or prolong their therapeutic and adverse effects. Caution is warranted and clinical monitoring is recommended). Products include:

Cardizem LA Extended Release Tablets 1699
Tiazac Capsules 1204

Efavirenz (Co-administration results in a decrease in the plasma concentrations of indinavir; a dosage increase of indinavir is recommended when used concurrently). Products include:

Sustiva Capsules 957

Ergonovine Maleate (Inhibition of CYP3A4 by indinavir could result in elevated plasma concentrations of ergot derivatives, potentially causing serious or life-threatening reactions; co-administration is contraindicated).

No products indexed under this heading.

Ergotamine Tartrate (Inhibition of CYP3A4 by indinavir could result in elevated plasma concentrations of ergot derivatives, potentially causing serious or life-threatening reactions; co-administration is contraindicated).

No products indexed under this heading.

Ethinyl Estradiol (Co-administration with Ortho-Novum 1/35 has resulted in an increase in ethinyl estradiol AUC). Products include:

Alesse-28 Tablets 3392
Lo/Ovral-28 Tablets 3423
NuvaRing 2357
Ortho-Cept Tablets 2395
Ortho-Cyclen/Ortho Tri-Cyclen 2414
Ortho Evra Transdermal System 2402
Ortho Tri-Cyclen Lo Tablets 2421
Seasonale Tablets 1073
Triphasil-28 Tablets 3483
Yasmin 28 Tablets 818

Felodipine (Co-administration of calcium channel blockers with indinavir may result in increased plasma concentrations of the dihydropyridine calcium channel blockers which could increase or prolong their therapeutic and adverse effects. Caution is warranted and clinical monitoring is recommended). Products include:

Plendil Extended-Release Tablets 651

Fluconazole (Co-administration has resulted in a 19% ± 33% decrease in indinavir AUC).

No products indexed under this heading.

Fluticasone Propionate (Concomitant use of fluticasone propionate and indinavir sulfate may increase plasma concentrations of fluticasone propionate; co-administer with caution. Consider alternatives to fluticasone propionate, particularly for long-term use). Products include:

Advair Diskus 100/50 1291
Advair Diskus 250/50 1291
Advair Diskus 500/50 1291
Cutivate Cream 1381
Cutivate Lotion 0.05% 1383
Cutivate Ointment 1384
Flonase Nasal Spray 1412
Flovent Diskus 100 mcg 1418
Flovent Diskus 50 mcg 1415

Fluticasone Propionate HFA (Concomitant use of fluticasone propionate and indinavir sulfate may increase plasma concentrations of fluticasone propionate; co-administer with caution. Consider alternatives to fluticasone propionate, particularly for long-term use). Products include:

Flovent HFA 1418

Fosphenytoin Sodium (Could diminish plasma concentrations of indinavir because phenytoin is an inducer of P450 3A4; caution is advised if co-administered).

No products indexed under this heading.

Hypericum (Co-administration of indinavir and St. John's Wort (hypericum perforatum) or products containing St. John's Wort has been shown to substantially decrease indinavir concentrations and may lead to loss of virologic response and possible resistance to indinavir or to the class of protease inhibitors; co-administration is not recommended).

No products indexed under this heading.

Isoniazid (Co-administration has resulted in a 13% ± 15% increase in isoniazid AUC).

No products indexed under this heading.

Isradipine (Co-administration of calcium channel blockers with indinavir may result in increased plasma concentrations of the dihydropyridine calcium channel blockers which could increase or prolong their therapeutic and adverse effects. Caution is warranted and clinical monitoring is recommended). Products include:

DynaCirc CR Tablets 2726

Itraconazole (Co-administration of indinavir and itraconzole may lead to increased indinvair concentrations. Dose reduction of indinavir to 600 mg every 8 hours is recommended when administering itraconzole concomitantly).

No products indexed under this heading.

Ketoconazole (Co-administration of indinavir and ketoconazole may lead to increased indinvair concentrations. Dose reduction of indinavir to 600 mg every 8 hours is recommended when administering ketoconazole concomitantly). Products include:

Nizoral A-D Shampoo, 1% 1839
Nizoral 2% Shampoo 1838

Lidocaine (Co-administration may lead to increased lidocaine concentrations. Caution is warranted and therapeutic concentration monitoring is recommended for antiarrhythmics when co-administered with indinavir). Products include:

Lidoderm Patch 1107

Lidocaine Hydrochloride (Co-administration may lead to increased lidocaine concentrations. Caution is warranted and therapeutic concentration monitoring is recommended for antiarrhythmics when co-administered with indinavir).

No products indexed under this heading.

Lovastatin (The risk of myopathy including rhabdomyolysis may be increased when protease inhibitors, including indinavir, are used in combination with HMG-CoA inhibitors that are metabolized by the CYP3A4 pathway; concomitant use is not recommended). Products include:

Advicor Tablets 1694
Altoprev Extended-Release Tablets 1151
Mevacor Tablets 1996

Methylergonovine Maleate (Inhibition of CYP3A4 by indinavir could result in elevated plasma concentrations of ergot derivatives, potentially causing serious or life-threatening reactions; co-administration is contraindicated).

No products indexed under this heading.

Methysergide Maleate (Inhibition of CYP3A4 by indinavir could result in elevated plasma concentrations of ergot derivatives, potentially causing serious or life-threatening reactions; co-administration is contraindicated).

No products indexed under this heading.

Mibefradil Dihydrochloride (Co-administration of calcium channel blockers with indinavir may result in increased plasma concentrations of the dihydropyridine calcium channel blockers which could increase or prolong their therapeutic and adverse effects. Caution is warranted and clinical monitoring is recommended).

No products indexed under this heading.

Midazolam Hydrochloride (Inhibition of CYP3A4 by indinavir could result in elevated plasma concentrations of midazolam potentially causing serious or life-threatening reactions; co-administration is contraindicated).

No products indexed under this heading.

Nelfinavir Mesylate (Co-administration of indinavir and nelfinavir may lead to increased indinavir concentrations. The appropriate doses for this combination, with respect to safety and efficacy, have not been established). Products include:

Viracept 2556

Nevirapine (Co-administration of indinavir and nevirapine may lead to decreased indinavir concentrations. The appropriate doses for this combination, with respect to saftey and efficacy, have not been established). Products include:

Viramune Oral Suspension 903
Viramune Tablets 903

Nicardipine Hydrochloride (Co-administration of calcium channel blockers with indinavir may result in increased plasma concentrations of the dihydropyridine calcium channel blockers which could increase or

prolong their therapeutic and adverse effects. Caution is warranted and clinical monitoring is recommended). Products include:
Cardene I.V. 1129
Nifedipine (Co-administration of calcium channel blockers with indinavir may result in increased plasma concentrations of the dihydropyridine calcium channel blockers which could increase or prolong their therapeutic and adverse effects. Caution is warranted and clinical monitoring is recommended). Products include:
Adalat CC Tablets 2978
Nimodipine (Co-administration of calcium channel blockers with indinavir may result in increased plasma concentrations of the dihydropyridine calcium channel blockers which could increase or prolong their therapeutic and adverse effects. Caution is warranted and clinical monitoring is recommended). Products include:
Nimotop Capsules 774
Nisoldipine (Co-administration of calcium channel blockers with indinavir may result in increased plasma concentrations of the dihydropyridine calcium channel blockers which could increase or prolong their therapeutic and adverse effects. Caution is warranted and clinical monitoring is recommended). Products include:
Sular Tablets 1163
Norethindrone (Co-administration with Ortho-Novum 1/35 has resulted in an increase in norethindrone AUC). Products include:
Ortho Micronor Tablets 2411
Phenobarbital (Could diminish plasma concentrations of indinavir because phenobarbital is an inducer of P450 3A4; caution is advised if co-administered).
No products indexed under this heading.
Phenytoin (Could diminish plasma concentrations of indinavir because phenytoin is an inducer of P450 3A4; caution is advised if co-administered).
No products indexed under this heading.
Phenytoin Sodium (Could diminish plasma concentrations of indinavir because phenytoin is an inducer of P450 3A4; caution is advised if co-administered). Products include:
Phenytek Capsules 2153
Pimozide (Inhibition of CYP3A4 by indinavir could result in elevated plasma concentrations of pimozide potentially causing serious or life-threatening reactions; co-administration is contraindicated). Products include:
Orap Tablets 1220
Quinidine (Co-administration of indinavir and quinidine may lead to increased quinidine concentrations. Caution is warranted and therapeutic concentration monitoring is recommended for antiarrhythmics when co-administered with indinavir).
No products indexed under this heading.
Quinidine Gluconate (Co-administration of indinavir and quinidine may lead to increased quinidine concentrations. Caution is warranted and therapeutic concentration monitoring is recommended for antiarrhythmics when co-administered with indinavir).
No products indexed under this heading.
Quinidine Hydrochloride (Co-administration of indinavir and quinidine may lead to increased quinidine concentrations. Caution is warranted and therapeutic concentration monitoring is recommended for antiarrhythmics when co-administered with indinavir).
No products indexed under this heading.
Quinidine Polygalacturonate (Co-administration of indinavir and quinidine lead to increased quinidine, concentrations. Caution is warranted and therapeutic concentration monitoring is recommended for antiarrhythmics when co-administered with indinavir).
No products indexed under this heading.
Quinidine Sulfate (Co-administration of indinavir and quinidine lead to increased quinidine, concentrations. Caution is warranted and therapeutic concentration monitoring is recommended for antiarrhythmics when co-administered with indinavir).
No products indexed under this heading.
Rifabutin (Co-administration of indinavir and rifabutin may lead to decreased indinavir and increased rifabutin concentrations. Dose reduction of rifabutin to half the standard dose and a dose increase of indinavir to 1000 mg (three 333-mg capsules) every 8 hours are recommended when rifabutin and indinavir are co-administered).
No products indexed under this heading.
Rifampin (Markedly diminishes plasma concentrations of indinavir because rifampin is a potent inducer of P450 3A4; co-administration is not recommended).
No products indexed under this heading.
Ritonavir (Co-administration of indinavir and ritonavir may lead to increased indinavir and ritonavir concentrations. The appropriate doses for this combination, with respect to saftey and efficacy, have not been established. Preliminary clinical data suggest that the incidence of nephrolithiasis is higher in patients receiving indinavir in combination with ritonavir than those receiving indinavir 800 mg q8h). Products include:
Kaletra 474
Norvir 499
Saquinavir (Co-administration of indinavir and saquinavir may lead to increased saquinavir concentrations).
No products indexed under this heading.
Saquinavir Mesylate (Co-administration of indinavir and saquinavir may lead to increased saquinavir concentrations). Products include:
Invirase 2776
Sildenafil Citrate (Co-administration has resulted in increased sildenafil AUC by 340%; this may result in an increase in sildenafil-associated adverse events, including hypotension, priapism, and visual changes; based on this result the dose of sildenafil should not exceed 25 mg in a 48-hour period). Products include:
Revatio Tablets 2541
Viagra Tablets 2552
Simvastatin (The risk of myopathy including rhabdomyolysis may be increased when protease inhibitors, including indinavir, are used in combination with HMG-CoA inhibitors that are metabolized by the CYP3A4 pathway; concomitant use is not recommended). Products include:
Vytorin 10/10 Tablets 2084
Vytorin 10/10 Tablets 3092
Vytorin 10/20 Tablets 2084
Vytorin 10/20 Tablets 3092
Vytorin 10/40 Tablets 3092
Vytorin 10/40 Tablets 2084
Vytorin 10/80 Tablets 2084
Vytorin 10/80 Tablets 3092
Zocor Tablets 2078
Sirolimus (Co-administration of indinavir and sirolimus may lead to increased sirolimus concentrations). Products include:
Rapamune Oral Solution and Tablets 3472
Stavudine (Co-administration has resulted in a 25% ± 26% increase in stavudine AUC and no change in indinavir AUC; co-administration does not require dose modification). Products include:
Zerit 971
Tacrolimus (Co-administration of indinavir and tacrolimus may lead to increased tacrolimus concentrations). Products include:
Prograf Capsules and Injection 624
Protopic Ointment 629
Tadalafil (Co-administration of indinavir and tadalafil is expected to substantially increase plasma concentrations of tadalafil and may result in an increase in adverse events. Tadalafil dose should not exceed a maximum of 10 mg in a 72-hour period in patients receiving concomitant indinavir therapy). Products include:
Cialis Tablets 1806
Terfenadine (Inhibition of CYP3A4 by indinavir could result in elevated plasma concentrations of terfenadine potentially causing serious or life-threatening reactions; co-administration is contraindicated).
No products indexed under this heading.
Trazodone Hydrochloride (Concomitant use of trazodone hydrochloride and indinavir sulfate may increase plasma concentrations of trazodone. If trazodone is used with a CYP3A4 inhibitor such as indinavir sulfate, the combinatin should be used with caution and a lower dose of trazodone should be considered).
No products indexed under this heading.
Triazolam (Inhibition of CYP3A4 by indinavir could result in elevated plasma concentrations of triazolam potentially causing serious or life-threatening reactions; co-administration is contraindicated).
No products indexed under this heading.
Trimethoprim (Co-administration with trimethoprim/sulfamethoxazole tablets has resulted in a 19% ± 31% increase in trimethoprim AUC).
No products indexed under this heading.
Vardenafil Hydrochloride (Co-administration of indinavir and vardenafil is expected to substantially increase plasma concentrations of vardenafil and may result in an increase in adverse events. Vardenafil dose should not exceed a maximum of 2.5 mg in a 24-hour period in patient receiving concomitant indinavir therapy). Products include:
Levitra Tablets 3048
Venlafaxine Hydrochloride (In a study, venlafaxine administered under steady-state conditions at 150 mg/day resulted in a 28% decrease in the AUC of a single 800 mg oral dose of indinavir and a 36% decrease in indinavir Cmax. Indinavir did not affect the pharmacokinetics of venlafaxine). Products include:
Effexor Tablets 3405
Effexor XR Capsules 3411
Verapamil Hydrochloride (Co-administration of calcium channel blockers with indinavir may result in increased plasma concentrations of the dihydropyridine calcium channel blockers which could increase or prolong their therapeutic and adverse effects. Caution is warranted and clinical monitoring is recommended). Products include:
Covera-HS Tablets 3135
Tarka Tablets 519
Verelan PM Capsules 3120
Zidovudine (Co-administration has resulted in a 13% ± 48% increase in indinavir AUC and a 17% +/- 23% increase in zidovudine AUC; co-administration does not require dose modification). Products include:
Combivir Tablets 1373
Retrovir 1533
Retrovir IV Infusion 1537
Trizivir Tablets 1565

Food Interactions

Food, unspecified (Co-administration with a meal high in calories, fat, and protein has resulted in a 77% ± 8% reduction in AUC and an 84% ± 7% reduction in Cmax; administer without food 1 hour before or 2 hours after a meal).
Grapefruit Juice (Potential for decrease in indinavir AUC).

CROLOM CROMOLYN SODIUM STERILE OPHTHALMIC SOLUTION USP 4%

(Cromolyn Sodium) .... ⊙248
None cited in PDR database.

CUBICIN FOR INJECTION

(Daptomycin) 1038
May interact with HMG-CoA reductase inhibitors. Compounds in these categories include:

Atorvastatin Calcium (Experience with co-administration of HMG-CoA reductase inhibitors and Cubicin is limited, therefore, considerations should be given to temporarily suspending use of HMG-CoA reductase inhibitors in patients recieving Cubicin). Products include:
Caduet Tablets 2507
Lipitor Tablets 2495
Cerivastatin Sodium (Experience with co-administration of HMG-CoA reductase inhibitors and Cubicin is limited, therefore, considerations should be given to temporarily suspending use of HMG-CoA reductase inhibitors in patients recieving Cubicin).
No products indexed under this heading.
Fluvastatin Sodium (Experience with co-administration of HMG-CoA reductase inhibitors and Cubicin is limited, therefore, considerations should be given to temporarily sus-

pending use of HMG-CoA reductase inhibitors in patients recieving Cubicin). Products include:
- Lescol Capsules 2227
- Lescol 2730
- Lescol XL Tablets 2227

Lovastatin (Experience with co-administration of HMG-CoA reductase inhibitors and Cubicin is limited, therefore, considerations should be given to temporarily suspending use of HMG-CoA reductase inhibitors in patients recieving Cubicin). Products include:
- Advicor Tablets 1694
- Altoprev Extended-Release Tablets 1151
- Mevacor Tablets 1996

Pravastatin Sodium (Experience with co-administration of HMG-CoA reductase inhibitors and Cubicin is limited, therefore, considerations should be given to temporarily suspending use of HMG-CoA reductase inhibitors in patients recieving Cubicin). Products include:
- Pravachol Tablets 943

Simvastatin (Experience with co-administration of HMG-CoA reductase inhibitors and Cubicin is limited, therefore, considerations should be given to temporarily suspending use of HMG-CoA reductase inhibitors in patients recieving Cubicin). Products include:
- Vytorin 10/10 Tablets 2084
- Vytorin 10/10 Tablets 3092
- Vytorin 10/20 Tablets 2084
- Vytorin 10/20 Tablets 3092
- Vytorin 10/40 Tablets 3092
- Vytorin 10/40 Tablets 2084
- Vytorin 10/80 Tablets 2084
- Vytorin 10/80 Tablets 3092
- Zocor Tablets 2078

Tobramycin Sulfate (Mean Cmax and AUC 0-8 of daptomycin increased when administered with tobramycin, and the mean Cmax and AUC 0-8 of tobramycin decreased when administered with daptomycin. Therefore, caution is warranted when daptomycin is co-administered with tobramycin).
No products indexed under this heading.

CUPRIMINE CAPSULES

(Penicillamine) 1925

May interact with antacids, antimalarials, cytotoxic drugs, iron containing oral preparations, and certain other agents. Compounds in these categories include:

Aluminum Carbonate (Antacids reduce the absorption of penicillamine. In all patients receiving penicillamine, it is important that penicillamine be given at least one hour apart from any antacid. This permits maximum strength absorption and reduces the likelihood of inactivation by metal binding in the gastrointestinal tract).
No products indexed under this heading.

Aluminum Hydroxide (Antacids reduce the absorption of penicillamine. In all patients receiving penicillamine, it is important that penicillamine be given at least one hour apart from any antacid. This permits maximum strength absorption and reduces the likelihood of inactivation by metal binding in the gastrointestinal tract). Products include:
- Gaviscon Regular Strength Liquid .. ■620
- Gaviscon Regular Strength Tablets .... ■619
- Gaviscon Extra Strength Liquid .... ■620
- Gaviscon Extra Strength Tablets .... ■619
- Maalox Max Maximum Strength Antacid/Anti-Gas Liquid 2165
- Maalox Regular Strength Antacid/Antigas Liquid 2164

Auranofin (Concurrent use not recommended).
No products indexed under this heading.

Aurothioglucose (Concurrent use not recommended).
No products indexed under this heading.

Bleomycin Sulfate (Concurrent use not recommended).
No products indexed under this heading.

Chloroquine Hydrochloride (Concurrent use not recommended).
No products indexed under this heading.

Chloroquine Phosphate (Concurrent use not recommended).
No products indexed under this heading.

Cyclophosphamide (Concurrent use not recommended).
No products indexed under this heading.

Daunorubicin Hydrochloride (Concurrent use not recommended). Products include:
- Cerubidine for Injection 788

Doxorubicin Hydrochloride (Concurrent use not recommended). Products include:
- Adriamycin for Injection, USP 786
- Adriamycin Injection, USP 786

Epirubicin Hydrochloride (Concurrent use not recommended). Products include:
- Ellence Injection 2632

Ferrous Fumarate (In all patients receiving penicillamine, it is important that penicillamine be given at least one hour apart from any iron-containing preparation. This permits maximum aborption and reduces the likelihood of inactivation by metal binding in the gastrointestinal tract). Products include:
- Chromagen Forte Soft Gelatin Capsules 3296
- Ferretts Tablets .... ■773
- Repliva 21/7 Tablets 3301

Ferrous Gluconate (In all patients receiving penicillamine, it is important that penicillamine be given at least one hour apart from any iron-containing preparation. This permits maximum aborption and reduces the likelihood of inactivation by metal binding in the gastrointestinal tract).
No products indexed under this heading.

Ferrous Sulfate (In all patients receiving penicillamine, it is important that penicillamine be given at least one hour apart from any iron-containing preparation. This permits maximum aborption and reduces the likelihood of inactivation by metal binding in the gastrointestinal tract). Products include:
- Feosol Tablets 1629
- Slow Fe Iron Tablets .... ■772
- Slow Fe with Folic Acid Tablets .... ■773

Fluorouracil (Concurrent use not recommended). Products include:
- Carac Cream, 0.5% 1048
- Efudex 3348

Hydroxychloroquine Sulfate (Concurrent use not recommended).
No products indexed under this heading.

Hydroxyurea (Concurrent use not recommended).
No products indexed under this heading.

Iron (In all patients receiving penicillamine, it is important that penicillamine be given at least one hour apart from any iron-containing preparation. This permits maximum aborption and reduces the likelihood of inactivation by metal binding in the gastrointestinal tract). Products include:
- Chromagen Forte Soft Gelatin Capsules 3296
- Ferretts IPS Liquid .... ■773
- OptiNate 1162
- Repliva 21/7 Tablets 3301

Magaldrate (Antacids reduce the absorption of penicillamine. In all patients receiving penicillamine, it is important that penicillamine be given at least one hour apart from any antacid. This permits maximum strength absorption and reduces the likelihood of inactivation by metal binding in the gastrointestinal tract).
No products indexed under this heading.

Magnesium Hydroxide (Antacids reduce the absorption of penicillamine. In all patients receiving penicillamine, it is important that penicillamine be given at least one hour apart from any antacid. This permits maximum strength absorption and reduces the likelihood of inactivation by metal binding in the gastrointestinal tract). Products include:
- Maalox Max Maximum Strength Antacid/Anti-Gas Liquid 2165
- Maalox Regular Strength Antacid/Antigas Liquid 2164
- Pepcid Complete Chewable Tablets 1672
- Rolaids Tablets .... ■707
- Extra Strength Rolaids Tablets .... ■707
- Rolaids Multi-Symptom Antacid & Antigas Tablets .... ■708

Magnesium Oxide (Antacids reduce the absorption of penicillamine. In all patients receiving penicillamine, it is important that penicillamine be given at least one hour apart from any antacid. This permits maximum strength absorption and reduces the likelihood of inactivation by metal binding in the gastrointestinal tract). Products include:
- Beelith Tablets 784
- PremCal Light, Regular, and Extra Strength Tablets .... ■762

Mefloquine Hydrochloride (Concurrent use not recommended). Products include:
- Lariam Tablets 2790

Methotrexate Sodium (Concurrent use not recommended).
No products indexed under this heading.

Mineral Supplements (Block response).
No products indexed under this heading.

Mitotane (Concurrent use not recommended).
No products indexed under this heading.

Mitoxantrone Hydrochloride (Concurrent use not recommended). Products include:
- Novantrone for Injection Concentrate 3158

Oxyphenbutazone (Concurrent use not recommended).
No products indexed under this heading.

Phenylbutazone (Concurrent use not recommended).
No products indexed under this heading.

Polysaccharide Iron Complex (In all patients receiving penicillamine, it is important that penicillamine be given at least one hour apart from any iron-containing preparation. This permits maximum aborption and reduces the likelihood of inactivation by metal binding in the gastrointestinal tract). Products include:
- Niferex-150 Forte Capsules 3299
- Nu-Iron 150 Capsules 2098

Procarbazine Hydrochloride (Concurrent use not recommended). Products include:
- Matulane Capsules 3188

Pyridoxine (Penicillamine increases pyridoxine requirement).
No products indexed under this heading.

Pyrimethamine (Concurrent use not recommended). Products include:
- Daraprim Tablets 1385

Sodium Bicarbonate (Antacids reduce the absorption of penicillamine. In all patients receiving penicillamine, it is important that penicillamine be given at least one hour apart from any antacid. This permits maximum strength absorption and reduces the likelihood of inactivation by metal binding in the gastrointestinal tract). Products include:
- Ceo-Two Evacuant Suppository .... ■607
- Colyte with Flavor Packs for Oral Solution 3102
- HalfLytely and Bisacodyl Tablets Bowel Prep Kit with Flavors Packs 915
- TriLyte with Flavor Packs for Oral Solution 3114

Tamoxifen Citrate (Concurrent use not recommended).
No products indexed under this heading.

Vincristine Sulfate (Concurrent use not recommended).
No products indexed under this heading.

Zinc-Containing Multivitamins (In all patients receiving penicillamine, it is important that penicillamine be given at least one hour apart from any iron-containing preparation. This permits maximim absorption and reduces the likelihood of inactivation by metal binding in the gastrointestinal tract).
No products indexed under this heading.

Zinc Gluconate (In all patients receiving penicillamine, it is important that penicillamine be given at least one hour apart from any iron-containing preparation. This permits maximim absorption and reduces the likelihood of inactivation by metal binding in the gastrointestinal tract).
No products indexed under this heading.

Zinc Sulfate (In all patients receiving penicillamine, it is important that penicillamine be given at least one hour apart from any iron-containing preparation. This permits maximim absorption and reduces the likelihood of inactivation by metal binding in the gastrointestinal tract). Products include:
- Athena Hair System Shampoo .... ■767
- Spartan Hair System Shampoo .... ■767
- Visine A.C. Seasonal Itching and Redness Relief Drops .... ⊙278

Zinc-220 Capsules 576

Food Interactions

Dairy products (In all patients receiving penicillamine, it is important that penicillamine be given at least one hour apart from milk. This permits maximim absorption and reduces the likelihood of inactivation by metal binding in the gastrointestinal tract).

Food, unspecified (Food reduces the absorption of penicillamine. In all patients receiving penicillamine, it is important that penicillamine be given on an empty stomach, at least one hour before meals or two hours after meals. This permits maximum absorption and reduces the likelihood of inactivation by metal binding in the gastrointestinal tract).

CUROSURF INTRATRACHEAL SUSPENSION

(Poractant alfa) 1057
None cited in PDR database.

CUSTODIOL HTK SOLUTION

(Electrolyte Solution) 2344
None cited in PDR database.

CUTIVATE CREAM

(Fluticasone Propionate) 1381
None cited in PDR database.

CUTIVATE LOTION 0.05%

(Fluticasone Propionate) 1383
None cited in PDR database.

CUTIVATE OINTMENT

(Fluticasone Propionate) 1384
None cited in PDR database.

CYMBALTA DELAYED-RELEASE CAPSULES

(Duloxetine Hydrochloride) 1729

May interact with central nervous system depressants, central nervous system stimulants, cytochrome p450 1a2 inhibitors (selected), cytochrome p450 2d6 inhibitors (selected), cytochrome p450 2d6 substrates (selected), drugs that reduce gastric acidity, monoamine oxidase inhibitors, phenothiazines, quinolones, tricyclic antidepressants, and certain other agents. Compounds in these categories include:

Alatrofloxacin Mesylate (Some quinolones, inhibitors of CYP1A2, would be expected to increase the AUC and Cmax of duloxetine; co-administration should be avoided).
No products indexed under this heading.

Alfentanil Hydrochloride (Given the primary CNS effects of duloxetine, it should be used with caution when it is taken in combination with or substituted for other centrally acting drugs, including those with a similar mechanism of action).
No products indexed under this heading.

Alprazolam (Given the primary CNS effects of duloxetine, it should be used with caution when it is taken in combination with or substituted for other centrally acting drugs, including those with a similar mechanism of action). Products include:
Niravam Orally Disintegrating Tablets 3106
Xanax XR Tablets 2655

Aluminum Carbonate (Duloxetine has an enteric coating that resists dissolution until reaching a segment of the gastrointestinal tract where the pH exceeds 5.5. Drugs that raise the gastrointestinal pH may lead to an earlier release of duloxetine).
No products indexed under this heading.

Aluminum Hydroxide (Duloxetine has an enteric coating that resists dissolution until reaching a segment of the gastrointestinal tract where the pH exceeds 5.5. Drugs that raise the gastrointestinal pH may lead to an earlier release of duloxetine). Products include:
Gaviscon Regular Strength Liquid .. 620
Gaviscon Regular Strength Tablets.. 619
Gaviscon Extra Strength Liquid 620
Gaviscon Extra Strength Tablets 619
Maalox Max Maximum Strength Antacid/Anti-Gas Liquid................ 2165
Maalox Regular Strength Antacid/Antigas Liquid................. 2164

Amiodarone Hydrochloride (Because CYP2D6 is involved in duloxetine metabolism, concomitant use of duloxetine with potent inhibitors of CYP2D6 would be expected to, and does, result in higher concentrations of duloxetine). Products include:
Pacerone Tablets 3337

Amitriptyline Hydrochloride (Because CYP2D6 is involved in duloxetine metabolism, concomitant use of duloxetine with potent inhibitors of CYP2D6 would be expected to, and does, result in higher concentrations of duloxetine).
No products indexed under this heading.

Amoxapine (Because CYP2D6 is involved in duloxetine metabolism, concomitant use of duloxetine with potent inhibitors of CYP2D6 would be expected to, and does, result in higher concentrations of duloxetine).
No products indexed under this heading.

Amphetamine Aspartate (Duloxetine is a moderate inhibitor of CYP2D6. Co-administration of duloxetine with other drugs that are extensively metabolized by this isoenzyme, and which have a narrow therapeutic window, should be approached with caution). Products include:
Adderall Tablets 3168
Adderall XR Capsules 3169

Amphetamine Aspartate Monohydrate (Duloxetine is a moderate inhibitor of CYP2D6. Co-administration of duloxetine with other drugs that are extensively metabolized by this isoenzyme, and which have a narrow therapeutic window, should be approached with caution).
No products indexed under this heading.

Amphetamine Resins (Given the primary CNS effects of duloxetine, it should be used with caution when it is taken in combination with or substituted for other centrally acting drugs, including those with a similar mechanism of action).
No products indexed under this heading.

Amphetamine Sulfate (Duloxetine is a moderate inhibitor of CYP2D6. Co-administration of duloxetine with other drugs that are extensively metabolized by this isoenzyme, and which have a narrow therapeutic window, should be approached with caution). Products include:
Adderall Tablets 3168
Adderall XR Capsules 3169

Anastrozole (Concomitant use of duloxetine with fluvoxamine, an inhibitor of CYP1A2, results in approximately a 6-fold increase in AUC and about a 2.5-fold increase in Cmax of duloxetine. Since duloxetine is metabolized in part by CYP1A2, concomitant use of duloxetine with other inhibitors of CYP1A2, would be expected to have the same effects; these combinations should be avoided). Products include:
Arimidex Tablets 665

Aprobarbital (Given the primary CNS effects of duloxetine, it should be used with caution when it is taken in combination with or substituted for other centrally acting drugs, including those with a similar mechanism of action).
No products indexed under this heading.

Atomoxetine Hydrochloride (Duloxetine is a moderate inhibitor of CYP2D6. Co-administration of duloxetine with other drugs that are extensively metabolized by this isoenzyme, and which have a narrow therapeutic window, should be approached with caution). Products include:
Strattera Capsules 1784

Bisoprolol Fumarate (Duloxetine is a moderate inhibitor of CYP2D6. Co-administration of duloxetine with other drugs that are extensively metabolized by this isoenzyme, and which have a narrow therapeutic window, should be approached with caution).
No products indexed under this heading.

Buprenorphine Hydrochloride (Given the primary CNS effects of duloxetine, it should be used with caution when it is taken in combination with or substituted for other centrally acting drugs, including those with a similar mechanism of action). Products include:
Buprenex Injectable 2718
Suboxone Tablets 2719
Subutex Tablets 2719

Bupropion Hydrochloride (Because CYP2D6 is involved in duloxetine metabolism, concomitant use of duloxetine with potent inhibitors of CYP2D6 would be expected to, and does, result in higher concentrations of duloxetine). Products include:
Wellbutrin Tablets 1579
Wellbutrin SR Sustained-Release Tablets 1583
Wellbutrin XL Extended-Release Tablets 1588
Zyban Sustained-Release Tablets 1620

Buspirone Hydrochloride (Given the primary CNS effects of duloxetine, it should be used with caution when it is taken in combination with or substituted for other centrally acting drugs, including those with a similar mechanism of action).
No products indexed under this heading.

Butabarbital (Given the primary CNS effects of duloxetine, it should be used with caution when it is taken in combination with or substituted for other centrally acting drugs, including those with a similar mechanism of action).
No products indexed under this heading.

Butalbital (Given the primary CNS effects of duloxetine, it should be used with caution when it is taken in combination with or substituted for other centrally acting drugs, including those with a similar mechanism of action). Products include:
Sedapap Tablets 50 mg/650 mg 2098

Captopril (Duloxetine is a moderate inhibitor of CYP2D6. Co-administration of duloxetine with other drugs that are extensively metabolized by this isoenzyme, and which have a narrow therapeutic window, should be approached with caution). Products include:
Captopril Tablets 2114

Carvedilol (Duloxetine is a moderate inhibitor of CYP2D6. Co-administration of duloxetine with other drugs that are extensively metabolized by this isoenzyme, and which have a narrow therapeutic window, should be approached with caution). Products include:
Coreg Tablets 1376

Celecoxib (Because CYP2D6 is involved in duloxetine metabolism, concomitant use of duloxetine with potent inhibitors of CYP2D6 would be expected to, and does, result in higher concentrations of duloxetine). Products include:
Celebrex Capsules 3130

Cevimeline Hydrochloride (Duloxetine is a moderate inhibitor of CYP2D6. Co-administration of duloxetine with other drugs that are extensively metabolized by this isoenzyme, and which have a narrow therapeutic window, should be approached with caution). Products include:
Evoxac Capsules 1042

Chlordiazepoxide (Given the primary CNS effects of duloxetine, it should be used with caution when it is taken in combination with or substituted for other centrally acting drugs, including those with a similar mechanism of action).
No products indexed under this heading.

Chlordiazepoxide Hydrochloride (Given the primary CNS effects of duloxetine, it should be used with caution when it is taken in combination with or substituted for other centrally acting drugs, including those with a similar mechanism of action). Products include:
Librium Capsules 3349

Chloroquine Hydrochloride (Because CYP2D6 is involved in duloxetine metabolism, concomitant use of duloxetine with potent inhibitors of CYP2D6 would be expected to, and does, result in higher concentrations of duloxetine).
No products indexed under this heading.

Chloroquine Phosphate (Because CYP2D6 is involved in duloxetine metabolism, concomitant use of duloxetine with potent inhibitors of CYP2D6 would be expected to, and does, result in higher concentrations of duloxetine).
No products indexed under this heading.

Chlorpheniramine (Because CYP2D6 is involved in duloxetine metabolism, concomitant use of duloxetine with potent inhibitors of CYP2D6 would be expected to, and does, result in higher concentrations of duloxetine).
No products indexed under this heading.

Chlorpheniramine Maleate (Because CYP2D6 is involved in duloxetine metabolism, concomitant use of duloxetine with potent inhibitors of CYP2D6 would be expected to, and does, result in higher concentrations of duloxetine). Products include:
Advil Allergy Sinus Caplets .... ▣737
Advil Multi-Symptom Cold Caplets .... ▣738
BC Allergy Sinus Cold Powder .... ▣612
Contac Severe Cold and Flu Caplets Maximum Strength .... ▣615
Hycomine Compound Tablets 1105
PediaCare Multi-Symptom Cold Liquid .... ▣704
PediaCare NightRest Cough & Cold Liquid .... ▣704
Robitussin Flu Liquid .... ▣752
Robitussin PM Cough & Cold Liquid .... ▣752
Singlet Caplets .... ▣636
Sudafed Sinus & Allergy Tablets ..... ▣710
TheraFlu Cold & Cough Hot Liquid .... ▣680
TheraFlu Cold & Sore Throat Hot Liquid .... ▣680
TheraFlu Flu & Sore Throat Hot Liquid .... ▣681
TheraFlu Severe Cold & Cough Hot Liquid .... ▣683
TheraFlu Severe Cold Caplets .... ▣679
TheraFlu Severe Cold Hot Liquid .... ▣682
Triaminic Cold & Allergy Liquid .... ▣685
Triaminic Cold & Cough Liquid .... ▣685
Triaminic Flu, Cough & Fever Liquid .... ▣685
Triaminic Night Time Cough & Cold Liquid .... ▣685
Triaminic Allergy Runny Nose & Congestion Softchews .... ▣688
Triaminic Cold & Cough Softchews .... ▣688
Children's Tylenol Plus Cold NightTime Suspension Liquid 1851
Children's Tylenol Plus Cold & Cough Suspension Liquid and Chewable Tablets 1851
Children's Tylenol Plus Cold Chewable Tablets 1851
Children's Tylenol Plus Flu Suspension Liquid 1853
Tylenol Allergy Complete Multi-Symptom Caplets and Gelcaps with Cool Burst 1844
Multi-Symptom Tylenol Cold Night Time Caplets 1845
Vicks 44M Cough, Cold & Flu Relief 2676
Pediatric Vicks 44m Cough & Cold Relief 2673
Children's Vicks NyQuil Cold/Cough Relief 2671

Chlorpheniramine Polistirex (Because CYP2D6 is involved in duloxetine metabolism, concomitant use of duloxetine with potent inhibitors of CYP2D6 would be expected to, and does, result in higher concentrations of duloxetine). Products include:
Tussionex Pennkinetic Extended-Release Suspension 3322

Chlorpheniramine Tannate (Because CYP2D6 is involved in duloxetine metabolism, concomitant use of duloxetine with potent inhibitors of CYP2D6 would be expected to, and does, result in higher concentrations of duloxetine).
No products indexed under this heading.

Chlorpromazine (Duloxetine is a moderate inhibitor of CYP2D6. Co-administration of duloxetine with other drugs that are extensively metabolized by this isoenzyme, and which have a narrow therapeutic window, should be approached with caution).
No products indexed under this heading.

Chlorpromazine Hydrochloride (Duloxetine is a moderate inhibitor of CYP2D6. Co-administration of duloxetine with other drugs that are extensively metabolized by this isoenzyme, and which have a narrow therapeutic window, should be approached with caution).
No products indexed under this heading.

Chlorpropamide (Duloxetine is a moderate inhibitor of CYP2D6. Co-administration of duloxetine with other drugs that are extensively metabolized by this isoenzyme, and which have a narrow therapeutic window, should be approached with caution).
No products indexed under this heading.

Chlorprothixene (Given the primary CNS effects of duloxetine, it should be used with caution when it is taken in combination with or substituted for other centrally acting drugs, including those with a similar mechanism of action).
No products indexed under this heading.

Chlorprothixene Hydrochloride (Given the primary CNS effects of duloxetine, it should be used with caution when it is taken in combination with or substituted for other centrally acting drugs, including those with a similar mechanism of action).
No products indexed under this heading.

Chlorprothixene Lactate (Given the primary CNS effects of duloxetine, it should be used with caution when it is taken in combination with or substituted for other centrally acting drugs, including those with a similar mechanism of action).
No products indexed under this heading.

Cimetidine (Because CYP2D6 is involved in duloxetine metabolism, concomitant use of duloxetine with potent inhibitors of CYP2D6 would be expected to, and does, result in higher concentrations of duloxetine). Products include:
Tagamet HB 200 Tablets .... ▣637
Tagamet Tablets 1547

Cimetidine Hydrochloride (Because CYP2D6 is involved in duloxetine metabolism, concomitant use of duloxetine with potent inhibitors of CYP2D6 would be expected to, and does, result in higher concentrations of duloxetine).
No products indexed under this heading.

Ciprofloxacin (Some quinolones, inhibitors of CYP1A2, would be expected to increase the AUC and Cmax of duloxetine; co-administration should be avoided). Products include:
Cipro I.V. 2998
Cipro I.V. Pharmacy Bulk Package ... 3509
Cipro Oral Suspension 2991
Cipro XR Tablets 3004
Ciprodex Otic Suspension 555

Ciprofloxacin Hydrochloride (Some quinolones, inhibitors of CYP1A2, would be expected to increase the AUC and Cmax of duloxetine; co-administration should be avoided). Products include:
Ciloxan Ophthalmic Ointment 554
Cipro Tablets 2991

Citalopram Hydrobromide (Because CYP2D6 is involved in duloxetine metabolism, concomitant use of duloxetine with potent inhibitors of CYP2D6 would be expected to, and does, result in higher concentrations of duloxetine). Products include:
Celexa 1177

Clarithromycin (Concomitant use of duloxetine with fluvoxamine, an inhibitor of CYP1A2, results in approximately a 6-fold increase in AUC and about a 2.5-fold increase in Cmax of duloxetine. Since duloxetine is metabolized in part by CYP1A2, concomitant use of duloxetine with other inhibitors of CYP1A2, would be expected to have the same effects; these combinations should be avoided). Products include:
Biaxin/Biaxin XL 402
PREVPAC 3281

Clomipramine Hydrochloride (Because CYP2D6 is involved in duloxetine metabolism, concomitant use of duloxetine with potent inhibitors of CYP2D6 would be expected to, and does, result in higher concentrations of duloxetine).
No products indexed under this heading.

Clorazepate Dipotassium (Given the primary CNS effects of duloxetine, it should be used with caution when it is taken in combination with or substituted for other centrally acting drugs, including those with a similar mechanism of action). Products include:
Tranxene 2488

Clozapine (Duloxetine is a moderate inhibitor of CYP2D6. Co-administration of duloxetine with other drugs that are extensively metabolized by this isoenzyme, and which have a narrow therapeutic window, should be approached with caution). Products include:
Clozapine Tablets 2141
Clozaril Tablets 2174
FazaClo Orally Disintegrating Tablets 547

Cocaine Hydrochloride (Because CYP2D6 is involved in duloxetine metabolism, concomitant use of duloxetine with potent inhibitors of CYP2D6 would be expected to, and does, result in higher concentrations of duloxetine).
No products indexed under this heading.

Codeine Phosphate (Duloxetine is a moderate inhibitor of CYP2D6. Co-administration of duloxetine with other drugs that are extensively metabolized by this isoenzyme, and which have a narrow therapeutic window, should be approached with caution). Products include:
Tylenol with Codeine 2461

Codeine Sulfate (Duloxetine is a moderate inhibitor of CYP2D6. Co-administration of duloxetine with other drugs that are extensively metabolized by this isoenzyme, and which have a narrow therapeutic window, should be approached with caution).
No products indexed under this heading.

Cyclobenzaprine Hydrochloride (Duloxetine is a moderate inhibitor of CYP2D6. Co-administration of duloxetine with other drugs that are extensively metabolized by this isoenzyme, and which have a narrow therapeutic window, should be approached with caution). Products include:
Flexeril Tablets 1832

Desflurane (Given the primary CNS effects of duloxetine, it should be used with caution when it is taken in combination with or substituted for other centrally acting drugs, including those with a similar mechanism of action). Products include:
Suprane Liquid for Inhalation 770

Desipramine Hydrochloride (Because CYP2D6 is involved in duloxetine metabolism, concomitant use of duloxetine with potent inhibitors of CYP2D6 would be expected to, and does, result in higher concentrations of duloxetine).
No products indexed under this heading.

Desogestrel (Concomitant use of duloxetine with fluvoxamine, an inhibitor of CYP1A2, results in approximately a 6-fold increase in AUC and about a 2.5-fold increase in Cmax of duloxetine. Since duloxetine is metabolized in part by CYP1A2, concomitant use of duloxetine with other inhibitors of CYP1A2, would be expected to have the same effects; these combinations should be avoided). Products include:
Ortho-Cept Tablets 2395

Dexfenfluramine Hydrochloride (Duloxetine is a moderate inhibitor of CYP2D6. Co-administration of duloxetine with other drugs that are extensively metabolized by this isoenzyme, and which have a narrow therapeutic window, should be approached with caution).
No products indexed under this heading.

Dextroamphetamine Sulfate (Given the primary CNS effects of duloxetine, it should be used with caution when it is taken in combination with or substituted for other centrally acting drugs, including those with a similar mechanism of action). Products include:
Adderall Tablets 3168
Adderall XR Capsules 3169
Dexedrine 1386
DextroStat Tablets 3177

Dextromethorphan Hydrobromide (Duloxetine is a moderate inhibitor of CYP2D6. Co-administration of duloxetine with other drugs that are extensively metabolized by this isoenzyme, and which have a narrow therapeutic window, should be approached with caution). Products include:
Alacol DM Syrup 739
Balamine DM 739
Contac Severe Cold and Flu Caplets Maximum Strength .... ▣615
Contac Severe Cold and Flu Caplets Non-Drowsy .... ▣615
Children's Dimetapp DM Cold & Cough Elixir .... ▣745

Children's Dimetapp Long Acting Cough Plus Cold Syrup................ 746
Dimetapp Infant Drops Decongestant Plus Cough........... 746
Mucinex DM Tablets....................... 602
PediaCare Decongestant & Cough Infant Drops..................... 705
PediaCare Freezer Pops Long-Acting Cough-Glacier Grape and Polar Berry Blue......... 706
PediaCare Long-Acting Cough Infant Drops............................. 705
PediaCare Long-Acting Cough Plus Cold Liquid......................... 704
PediaCare Multi-Symptom Cold Liquid... 704
PediaCare NightRest Cough & Cold Liquid................................ 704
Robitussin Allergy & Cough Syrup .. 750
Robitussin CF Liquid...................... 755
Robitussin Cough & Cold Liquid-filled Capsules.................. 750
Robitussin Cough, Cold & Flu Liquid-filled Capsules.................. 750
Robitussin Cough & Cold Infant Drops... 755
Robitussin DM Infant Drops............ 753
Robitussin DM Liquid...................... 753
Robitussin Flu Liquid...................... 752
Robitussin Maximum Strength Cough Liquid............................. 754
Robitussin Maximum Strength Cough & Cold Liquid.................. 754
Robitussin Pediatric Cough Liquid... 754
Robitussin Pediatric Cough & Cold Liquid................................. 754
Robitussin PM Cough & Cold Liquid... 752
Robitussin Sugar Free Cough Liquid... 753
Simply Cough Liquid........................ 1840
Sudafed Severe Cold......................... 710
TheraFlu Cold & Cough Hot Liquid... 680
TheraFlu Flu & Chest Congestion Non-Drowsy Hot Liquid................ 681
TheraFlu Severe Cold Non-Drowsy Hot Liquid................ 683
TheraFlu Severe Cold & Cough Hot Liquid.................................. 683
TheraFlu Severe Cold Caplets......... 679
TheraFlu Severe Cold Hot Liquid 682
TheraFlu Severe Cold Non-Drowsy Caplets.................... 679
TheraFlu Thin Strips Long Acting Cough.. 684
Triaminic Cold & Cough Liquid 685
Triaminic Cough Liquid.................. 687
Triaminic Cough & Nasal Congestion Liquid....................... 687
Triaminic Cough & Sore Throat Liquid... 687
Triaminic Flu, Cough & Fever Liquid... 685
Triaminic Night Time Cough & Cold Liquid................................ 685
Triaminic Cold & Cough Softchews................................. 688
Triaminic Cough & Sore Throat Softchews................................. 689
Triaminic Thin Strips Long Acting Cough.. 689
Children's Tylenol Plus Cold & Cough Suspension Liquid and Chewable Tablets........................ 1851
Children's Tylenol Plus Flu Suspension Liquid....................... 1853
Concentrated Tylenol Infants' Drops Plus Cold and Cough.......... 1851
Tylenol Cold & Flu Severe Daytime Liquid with Cool Bust....... 1846
Tylenol Cold & Flu Severe NightTime Liquid with Cool Burst... 1846
Tylenol Cold Severe Congestion Non-Drowsy Caplets with Cool Burst... 1846
Tylenol Cough & Sore Throat Daytime Liquid with Cool Burst...... 1849
Tylenol Cough & Sore Throat NightTime Liquid with Cool Burst... 1849
Tylenol Flu Day Non-Drowsy Gelcaps....................................... 1846
Concentrated Tylenol Infants' Drops Plus Cold & Cough Nasal Decongestant, Fever Reducer & Pain Reliever............. 668
Multi-Symptom Tylenol Cold Night Time Caplets............................... 1845
Multi-Symptom Tylenol Cold Day Non-Drowsy Caplets and Gelcaps.. 1845
Vicks 44 Cough Relief.................... 2675
Vicks 44D Cough & Head Congestion Relief......................... 2676
Vicks 44D Cough & Head Congestion Relief Liquid............. 721
Vicks 44E Cough & Chest Congestion Relief......................... 2676
Pediatric Vicks 44e Cough & Chest Congestion Relief Liquid...... 2673
Vicks 44M Cough, Cold & Flu Relief.. 2676
Pediatric Vicks 44m Cough & Cold Relief.................................. 2673
Vicks DayQuil LiquiCaps/Liquid Multi-Symptom Cold/Flu Relief..... 723
Vicks DayQuil Multi-Symptom Cold/Flu Relief LiquiCaps............. 2675
Vicks DayQuil Multi-Symptom Cold/Flu Relief Liquid................... 2675
Children's Vicks NyQuil Cold/Cough Relief....................... 2671
Vicks NyQuil Cough Liquid.............. 2677
Vicks NyQuil LiquiCaps................... 2677
Vicks NyQuil LiquiCaps/Liquid Multi-Symptom Cold/Flu Relief..... 725
Vicks NyQuil Liquid......................... 2677
Zicam Concentrated Cough Mist for Kids Cool Cherry.................... 643
Zicam Concentrated Cough Mist for Kids Plus D Cool Cherry......... 643
Zicam Concentrated Cough Mist Nite-Cool Cherry........................ 642
Zicam Concentrated Cough Mist Plus D Cool Cherry..................... 642
Zicam Concentrated Cough Mist-Honey Lemon & Cool Cherry.. 642

Dextromethorphan Polistirex (Duloxetine is a moderate inhibitor of CYP2D6. Co-administration of duloxetine with other drugs that are extensively metabolized by this isoenzyme, and which have a narrow therapeutic window, should be approached with caution). Products include:

Delsym Extended-Release Suspension.................................. 611
Delsym 12 Hour Cough Suppressant for Children............ 611

Dezocine (Given the primary CNS effects of duloxetine, it should be used with caution when it is taken in combination with or substituted for other centrally acting drugs, including those with a similar mechanism of action).

No products indexed under this heading.

Diazepam (Given the primary CNS effects of duloxetine, it should be used with caution when it is taken in combination with or substituted for other centrally acting drugs, including those with a similar mechanism of action). Products include:

Diastat Rectal Delivery System........ 3344
Valium Tablets................................ 2822

Diphenhydramine (Because CYP2D6 is involved in duloxetine metabolism, concomitant use of duloxetine with potent inhibitors of CYP2D6 would be expected to, and does, result in higher concentrations of duloxetine). Products include:

Tylenol Sore Throat NightTime Liquid with Cool Burst.................. 1849

Diphenhydramine Hydrochloride (Because CYP2D6 is involved in duloxetine metabolism, concomitant use of duloxetine with potent inhibitors of CYP2D6 would be expected to, and does, result in higher concentrations of duloxetine). Products include:

Benadryl Allergy & Cold Tablets 692
Benadryl Allergy 691
Benadryl Allergy & Sinus Headache Caplets & Gelcaps...... 693
Children's Benadryl Allergy Liquid... 695
Children's Benadryl Dye-Free Allergy Liquid.............................. 695
Benadryl Dye-Free Allergy Liqui-Gels Softgels...................... 692
Benadryl Itch Relief Stick Extra Strength.................................... 696
Benadryl Itch Stopping Cream Extra Strength............................ 697
Benadryl Itch Stopping Gel Extra Strength.................................... 697
Benadryl Itch Stopping Spray Extra Strength............................ 697
Benadryl Maximum Strength Severe Allergy & Sinus Headache Caplets....................... 694
Children's Benadryl D Liquid Medication.................................. 693
Benadryl D Tablets.......................... 694
Nytol QuickCaps Caplets 635
Maximum Strength Nytol QuickGels Softgels..................... 635
Simply Sleep Caplets...................... 1841
Sominex Original Formula Tablets .. 637
TheraFlu Thin Strips Multi Symptom................................... 684
Triaminic Thin Strips Cough & Runny Nose................................ 690
Children's Tylenol Plus Cold & Allergy Suspension Liquid............ 1850
Tylenol Allergy Complete Night Time Caplets.............................. 1844
Tylenol Severe Allergy Caplets......... 1844
Tylenol Flu NightTime Gelcaps......... 1846
Extra Strength Tylenol PM Caplets, Geltabs, Gelcaps and Liquid... 1847
Unisom Maximum Strength SleepGels................................... 712

Dolasetron Mesylate (Duloxetine is a moderate inhibitor of CYP2D6. Co-administration of duloxetine with other drugs that are extensively metabolized by this isoenzyme, and which have a narrow therapeutic window, should be approached with caution). Products include:

Anzemet Injection........................... 2871
Anzemet Tablets 2874

Donepezil Hydrochloride (Duloxetine is a moderate inhibitor of CYP2D6. Co-administration of duloxetine with other drugs that are extensively metabolized by this isoenzyme, and which have a narrow therapeutic window, should be approached with caution). Products include:

Aricept Tablets................................ 1086
Aricept ODT Tablets 1086

Doxepin Hydrochloride (Because CYP2D6 is involved in duloxetine metabolism, concomitant use of duloxetine with potent inhibitors of CYP2D6 would be expected to, and does, result in higher concentrations of duloxetine).

No products indexed under this heading.

Droperidol (Given the primary CNS effects of duloxetine, it should be used with caution when it is taken in combination with or substituted for other centrally acting drugs, including those with a similar mechanism of action).

No products indexed under this heading.

Encainide Hydrochloride (Duloxetine is a moderate inhibitor of CYP2D6. Co-administration of duloxetine with other drugs that are extensively metabolized by this isoenzyme, and which have a narrow therapeutic window, should be approached with caution).

No products indexed under this heading.

Enflurane (Given the primary CNS effects of duloxetine, it should be used with caution when it is taken in combination with or substituted for other centrally acting drugs, including those with a similar mechanism of action).

No products indexed under this heading.

Enoxacin (Some quinolones, inhibitors of CYP1A2, would be expected to increase the AUC and Cmax of duloxetine; co-administration should be avoided).

No products indexed under this heading.

Escitalopram Oxalate (Because CYP2D6 is involved in duloxetine metabolism, concomitant use of duloxetine with potent inhibitors of CYP2D6 would be expected to, and does, result in higher concentrations of duloxetine). Products include:

Lexapro Oral Solution..................... 1193
Lexapro Tablets 1193

Esomeprazole Magnesium (Duloxetine has an enteric coating that resists dissolution until reaching a segment of the gastrointestinal tract where the pH exceeds 5.5. Drugs that raise the gastrointestinal pH may lead to an earlier release of duloxetine). Products include:

Nexium Delayed-Release Capsules.................................... 645

Estazolam (Given the primary CNS effects of duloxetine, it should be used with caution when it is taken in combination with or substituted for other centrally acting drugs, including those with a similar mechanism of action). Products include:

ProSom Tablets.............................. 512

Ethanol (Given the primary CNS effects of duloxetine, it should be used with caution when it is taken in combination with or substituted for other centrally acting drugs, including those with a similar mechanism of action).

No products indexed under this heading.

Ethchlorvynol (Given the primary CNS effects of duloxetine, it should be used with caution when it is taken in combination with or substituted for other centrally acting drugs, including those with a similar mechanism of action).

No products indexed under this heading.

Ethinamate (Given the primary CNS effects of duloxetine, it should be used with caution when it is taken in combination with or substituted for other centrally acting drugs, including those with a similar mechanism of action).

No products indexed under this heading.

Ethinyl Estradiol (Concomitant use of duloxetine with fluvoxamine, an inhibitor of CYP1A2, results in approximately a 6-fold increase in AUC and about a 2.5-fold increase in Cmax of duloxetine. Since duloxetine is metabolized in part by CYP1A2,

concomitant use of duloxetine with other inhibitors of CYP1A2, would be expected to have the same effects; these combinations should be avoided). Products include:

Alesse-28 Tablets ... 3392
Lo/Ovral-28 Tablets ... 3423
NuvaRing ... 2357
Ortho-Cept Tablets ... 2395
Ortho-Cyclen/Ortho Tri-Cyclen ... 2414
Ortho Evra Transdermal System ... 2402
Ortho Tri-Cyclen Lo Tablets ... 2421
Seasonale Tablets ... 1073
Triphasil-28 Tablets ... 3483
Yasmin 28 Tablets ... 818

Ethyl Alcohol (Given the primary CNS effects of duloxetine, it should be used with caution when it is taken in combination with or substituted for other centrally acting drugs, including those with a similar mechanism of action).

No products indexed under this heading.

Famotidine (Duloxetine has an enteric coating that resists dissolution until reaching a segment of the gastrointestinal tract where the pH exceeds 5.5. Drugs that raise the gastrointestinal pH may lead to an earlier release of duloxetine). Products include:

Pepcid AC Chewable Tablets ... 1672
Pepcid AC Gelcaps ... 1672
Pepcid AC Tablets ... 1672
Maximum Strength Pepcid AC Tablets ... 1672
Pepcid Complete Chewable Tablets ... 1672
Pepcid Injection ... 2017
Pepcid ... 2014

Fentanyl (Duloxetine is a moderate inhibitor of CYP2D6. Co-administration of duloxetine with other drugs that are extensively metabolized by this isoenzyme, and which have a narrow therapeutic window, should be approached with caution). Products include:

Duragesic Transdermal System ... 2448

Fentanyl Citrate (Duloxetine is a moderate inhibitor of CYP2D6. Co-administration of duloxetine with other drugs that are extensively metabolized by this isoenzyme, and which have a narrow therapeutic window, should be approached with caution). Products include:

Actiq ... 993

Flecainide Acetate (Duloxetine is a moderate inhibitor of CYP2D6. Co-administration of duloxetine with other drugs that are extensively metabolized by this isoenzyme, and which have a narrow therapeutic window, should be approached with caution). Products include:

Tambocor Tablets ... 1824

Fluoxetine (Because CYP2D6 is involved in duloxetine metabolism, concomitant use of duloxetine with potent inhibitors of CYP2D6 would be expected to, and does, result in higher concentrations of duloxetine).

No products indexed under this heading.

Fluoxetine Hydrochloride (Because CYP2D6 is involved in duloxetine metabolism, concomitant use of duloxetine with potent inhibitors of CYP2D6 would be expected to, and does, result in higher concentrations of duloxetine). Products include:

Prozac Pulvules and Liquid ... 1771
Symbyax Capsules ... 1788

Fluphenazine Decanoate (Because CYP2D6 is involved in duloxetine metabolism, concomitant use of duloxetine with potent inhibitors of CYP2D6 would be expected to, and does, result in higher concentrations of duloxetine).

No products indexed under this heading.

Fluphenazine Enanthate (Because CYP2D6 is involved in duloxetine metabolism, concomitant use of duloxetine with potent inhibitors of CYP2D6 would be expected to, and does, result in higher concentrations of duloxetine).

No products indexed under this heading.

Fluphenazine Hydrochloride (Because CYP2D6 is involved in duloxetine metabolism, concomitant use of duloxetine with potent inhibitors of CYP2D6 would be expected to, and does, result in higher concentrations of duloxetine).

No products indexed under this heading.

Flurazepam Hydrochloride (Given the primary CNS effects of duloxetine, it should be used with caution when it is taken in combination with or substituted for other centrally acting drugs, including those with a similar mechanism of action). Products include:

Dalmane Capsules ... 3343

Fluvoxamine (Concomitant use of duloxetine with fluvoxamine, an inhibitor of CYP1A2, results in approximately a 6-fold increase in AUC and about a 2.5-fold increase in Cmax of duloxetine; co-administration should be avoided).

No products indexed under this heading.

Fluvoxamine Maleate (Concomitant use of duloxetine with fluvoxamine, an inhibitor of CYP1A2, results in approximately a 6-fold increase in AUC and about a 2.5-fold increase in Cmax of duloxetine; co-administration should be avoided).

No products indexed under this heading.

Formoterol Fumarate (Duloxetine is a moderate inhibitor of CYP2D6. Co-administration of duloxetine with other drugs that are extensively metabolized by this isoenzyme, and which have a narrow therapeutic window, should be approached with caution). Products include:

Foradil Aerolizer ... 3024

Galantamine Hydrobromide (Duloxetine is a moderate inhibitor of CYP2D6. Co-administration of duloxetine with other drugs that are extensively metabolized by this isoenzyme, and which have a narrow therapeutic window, should be approached with caution). Products include:

Razadyne ER Extended-Release Capsules ... 2434
Razadyne ... 2434

Gatifloxacin (Concomitant use of duloxetine with fluvoxamine, an inhibitor of CYP1A2, results in approximately a 6-fold increase in AUC and about a 2.5-fold increase in Cmax of duloxetine. Since duloxetine is metabolized in part by CYP1A2, concomitant use of duloxetine with other inhibitors of CYP1A2, would be expected to have the same effects; these combinations should be avoided). Products include:

Tequin Injection ... 964
Tequin Tablets ... 964
Zymar Ophthalmic Solution ... 571

Gemifloxacin Mesylate (Concomitant use of duloxetine with fluvoxamine, an inhibitor of CYP1A2, results in approximately a 6-fold increase in AUC and about a 2.5-fold increase in Cmax of duloxetine. Since duloxetine is metabolized in part by CYP1A2, concomitant use of duloxetine with other inhibitors of CYP1A2, would be expected to have the same effects; these combinations should be avoided). Products include:

Factive Tablets ... 2464

Glutethimide (Given the primary CNS effects of duloxetine, it should be used with caution when it is taken in combination with or substituted for other centrally acting drugs, including those with a similar mechanism of action).

No products indexed under this heading.

Grepafloxacin Hydrochloride (Some quinolones, inhibitors of CYP1A2, would be expected to increase the AUC and Cmax of duloxetine; co-administration should be avoided).

No products indexed under this heading.

Halofantrine Hydrochloride (Because CYP2D6 is involved in duloxetine metabolism, concomitant use of duloxetine with potent inhibitors of CYP2D6 would be expected to, and does, result in higher concentrations of duloxetine).

No products indexed under this heading.

Haloperidol (Because CYP2D6 is involved in duloxetine metabolism, concomitant use of duloxetine with potent inhibitors of CYP2D6 would be expected to, and does, result in higher concentrations of duloxetine).

No products indexed under this heading.

Haloperidol Decanoate (Because CYP2D6 is involved in duloxetine metabolism, concomitant use of duloxetine with potent inhibitors of CYP2D6 would be expected to, and does, result in higher concentrations of duloxetine).

No products indexed under this heading.

Hydrocodone Bitartrate (Duloxetine is a moderate inhibitor of CYP2D6. Co-administration of duloxetine with other drugs that are extensively metabolized by this isoenzyme, and which have a narrow therapeutic window, should be approached with caution). Products include:

Hycodan ... 1104
Hycomine Compound Tablets ... 1105
Hycotuss Expectorant Syrup ... 1106
Lortab ... 3315
Lortab Elixir ... 3312
Vicodin Tablets ... 530
Vicodin ES Tablets ... 531
Vicodin HP Tablets ... 532
Vicoprofen Tablets ... 533
Zydone Tablets ... 1118

Hydrocodone Polistirex (Given the primary CNS effects of duloxetine, it should be used with caution when it is taken in combination with or substituted for other centrally acting drugs, including those with a similar mechanism of action). Products include:

Tussionex Pennkinetic Extended-Release Suspension ... 3322

Hydromorphone Hydrochloride (Given the primary CNS effects of duloxetine, it should be used with caution when it is taken in combination with or substituted for other centrally acting drugs, including those with a similar mechanism of action). Products include:

Dilaudid ... 439
Dilaudid Oral Liquid ... 443
Dilaudid Non-Sterile Powder ... 439
Dilaudid Rectal Suppositories ... 439
Dilaudid Tablets ... 439
Dilaudid Tablets - 8 mg ... 443
Dilaudid-HP ... 441

Hydroxychloroquine Sulfate (Because CYP2D6 is involved in duloxetine metabolism, concomitant use of duloxetine with potent inhibitors of CYP2D6 would be expected to, and does, result in higher concentrations of duloxetine).

No products indexed under this heading.

Hydroxyzine Hydrochloride (Given the primary CNS effects of duloxetine, it should be used with caution when it is taken in combination with or substituted for other centrally acting drugs, including those with a similar mechanism of action).

No products indexed under this heading.

Imatinib Mesylate (Because CYP2D6 is involved in duloxetine metabolism, concomitant use of duloxetine with potent inhibitors of CYP2D6 would be expected to, and does, result in higher concentrations of duloxetine). Products include:

Gleevec Tablets ... 2221

Imipramine Hydrochloride (Because CYP2D6 is involved in duloxetine metabolism, concomitant use of duloxetine with potent inhibitors of CYP2D6 would be expected to, and does, result in higher concentrations of duloxetine).

No products indexed under this heading.

Imipramine Pamoate (Because CYP2D6 is involved in duloxetine metabolism, concomitant use of duloxetine with potent inhibitors of CYP2D6 would be expected to, and does, result in higher concentrations of duloxetine).

No products indexed under this heading.

Indoramin Hydrochloride (Duloxetine is a moderate inhibitor of CYP2D6. Co-administration of duloxetine with other drugs that are extensively metabolized by this isoenzyme, and which have a narrow therapeutic window, should be approached with caution).

No products indexed under this heading.

Isocarboxazid (There have been reports of serious, sometimes fatal, reactions in patients receiving a serotonin reuptake inhibitor in combination with a monoamine oxidase inhibitor (MAOI). These reactions have also been reported in patients who have recently discontinued serotonin reuptake inhibitors and are started on an MAOI. Therefore, duloxetine use is contraindicated in combination with an MAOI, or within at least 14 days of discontinuing treatment with an MAOI. Based on the half-life of duloxetine, at least 5 days should be allowed after stopping duloxetine before starting an MAOI).

No products indexed under this heading.

Isoflurane (Given the primary CNS effects of duloxetine, it should be used with caution when it is taken in combination with or substituted for other centrally acting drugs, including those with a similar mechanism of action).
No products indexed under this heading.

Isoniazid (Concomitant use of duloxetine with fluvoxamine, an inhibitor of CYP1A2, results in approximately a 6-fold increase in AUC and about a 2.5-fold increase in Cmax of duloxetine. Since duloxetine is metabolized in part by CYP1A2, concomitant use of duloxetine with other inhibitors of CYP1A2, would be expected to have the same effects; these combinations should be avoided).
No products indexed under this heading.

Ketamine Hydrochloride (Given the primary CNS effects of duloxetine, it should be used with caution when it is taken in combination with or substituted for other centrally acting drugs, including those with a similar mechanism of action).
No products indexed under this heading.

Ketoconazole (Concomitant use of duloxetine with fluvoxamine, an inhibitor of CYP1A2, results in approximately a 6-fold increase in AUC and about a 2.5-fold increase in Cmax of duloxetine. Since duloxetine is metabolized in part by CYP1A2, concomitant use of duloxetine with other inhibitors of CYP1A2, would be expected to have the same effects; these combinations should be avoided). Products include:
Nizoral A-D Shampoo, 1% 1839
Nizoral 2% Shampoo 1838

Labetalol Hydrochloride (Duloxetine is a moderate inhibitor of CYP2D6. Co-administration of duloxetine with other drugs that are extensively metabolized by this isoenzyme, and which have a narrow therapeutic window, should be approached with caution).
No products indexed under this heading.

Lansoprazole (Duloxetine has an enteric coating that resists dissolution until reaching a segment of the gastrointestinal tract where the pH exceeds 5.5. Drugs that raise the gastrointestinal pH may lead to an earlier release of duloxetine). Products include:
Prevacid Delayed-Release Capsules 3268
Prevacid for Delayed-Release Oral Suspension 3268
Prevacid I.V. for Injection 3274
Prevacid NapraPAC 3277
Prevacid SoluTab Delayed-Release Orally Disintegrating Tablets 3268
PREVPAC 3281

Levofloxacin (Concomitant use of duloxetine with fluvoxamine, an inhibitor of CYP1A2, results in approximately a 6-fold increase in AUC and about a 2.5-fold increase in Cmax of duloxetine. Since duloxetine is metabolized in part by CYP1A2, concomitant use of duloxetine with other inhibitors of CYP1A2, would be expected to have the same effects; these combinations should be avoided). Products include:
Levaquin in 5% Dextrose Injection 2453
Levaquin 2453
Quixin Ophthalmic Solution 3373

Levomethadyl Acetate Hydrochloride (Given the primary CNS effects of duloxetine, it should be used with caution when it is taken in combination with or substituted for other centrally acting drugs, including those with a similar mechanism of action).
No products indexed under this heading.

Levonorgestrel (Concomitant use of duloxetine with fluvoxamine, an inhibitor of CYP1A2, results in approximately a 6-fold increase in AUC and about a 2.5-fold increase in Cmax of duloxetine. Since duloxetine is metabolized in part by CYP1A2, concomitant use of duloxetine with other inhibitors of CYP1A2, would be expected to have the same effects; these combinations should be avoided). Products include:
Alesse-28 Tablets 3392
Climara Pro Transdermal System 800
Mirena Intrauterine System 810
Plan B Tablets 1068
Seasonale Tablets 1073
Triphasil-28 Tablets 3483

Levorphanol Tartrate (Given the primary CNS effects of duloxetine, it should be used with caution when it is taken in combination with or substituted for other centrally acting drugs, including those with a similar mechanism of action).
No products indexed under this heading.

Lidocaine (Duloxetine is a moderate inhibitor of CYP2D6. Co-administration of duloxetine with other drugs that are extensively metabolized by this isoenzyme, and which have a narrow therapeutic window, should be approached with caution). Products include:
Lidoderm Patch 1107

Lidocaine Hydrochloride (Duloxetine is a moderate inhibitor of CYP2D6. Co-administration of duloxetine with other drugs that are extensively metabolized by this isoenzyme, and which have a narrow therapeutic window, should be approached with caution).
No products indexed under this heading.

Lomefloxacin Hydrochloride (Some quinolones, inhibitors of CYP1A2, would be expected to increase the AUC and Cmax of duloxetine; co-administration should be avoided).
No products indexed under this heading.

Lorazepam (Given the primary CNS effects of duloxetine, it should be used with caution when it is taken in combination with or substituted for other centrally acting drugs, including those with a similar mechanism of action).
No products indexed under this heading.

Loxapine Hydrochloride (Given the primary CNS effects of duloxetine, it should be used with caution when it is taken in combination with or substituted for other centrally acting drugs, including those with a similar mechanism of action).
No products indexed under this heading.

Loxapine Succinate (Given the primary CNS effects of duloxetine, it should be used with caution when it is taken in combination with or substituted for other centrally acting drugs, including those with a similar mechanism of action).
No products indexed under this heading.

Magnesium Hydroxide (Duloxetine has an enteric coating that resists dissolution until reaching a segment of the gastrointestinal tract where the pH exceeds 5.5. Drugs that raise the gastrointestinal pH may lead to an earlier release of duloxetine). Products include:
Maalox Max Maximum Strength Antacid/Anti-Gas Liquid................. 2165
Maalox Regular Strength Antacid/Antigas Liquid................. 2164
Pepcid Complete Chewable Tablets 1672
Rolaids Tablets 707
Extra Strength Rolaids Tablets 707
Rolaids Multi-Symptom Antacid & Antigas Tablets 708

Maprotiline Hydrochloride (Because CYP2D6 is involved in duloxetine metabolism, concomitant use of duloxetine with potent inhibitors of CYP2D6 would be expected to, and does, result in higher concentrations of duloxetine).
No products indexed under this heading.

Meperidine Hydrochloride (Duloxetine is a moderate inhibitor of CYP2D6. Co-administration of duloxetine with other drugs that are extensively metabolized by this isoenzyme, and which have a narrow therapeutic window, should be approached with caution).
No products indexed under this heading.

Mephobarbital (Given the primary CNS effects of duloxetine, it should be used with caution when it is taken in combination with or substituted for other centrally acting drugs, including those with a similar mechanism of action). Products include:
Mebaral Tablets, USP 2483

Meprobamate (Given the primary CNS effects of duloxetine, it should be used with caution when it is taken in combination with or substituted for other centrally acting drugs, including those with a similar mechanism of action).
No products indexed under this heading.

Mesoridazine Besylate (Duloxetine is a moderate inhibitor of CYP2D6. Co-administration of duloxetine with other drugs that are extensively metabolized by this isoenzyme, and which have a narrow therapeutic window, should be approached with caution).
No products indexed under this heading.

Mestranol (Concomitant use of duloxetine with fluvoxamine, an inhibitor of CYP1A2, results in approximately a 6-fold increase in AUC and about a 2.5-fold increase in Cmax of duloxetine. Since duloxetine is metabolized in part by CYP1A2, concomitant use of duloxetine with other inhibitors of CYP1A2, would be expected to have the same effects; these combinations should be avoided).
No products indexed under this heading.

Methadone Hydrochloride (Because CYP2D6 is involved in duloxetine metabolism, concomitant use of duloxetine with potent inhibitors of CYP2D6 would be expected to, and does, result in higher concentrations of duloxetine).
No products indexed under this heading.

Methamphetamine Hydrochloride (Duloxetine is a moderate inhibitor of CYP2D6. Co-administration of duloxetine with other drugs that are extensively metabolized by this isoenzyme, and which have a narrow therapeutic window, should be approached with caution). Products include:
Desoxyn Tablets, USP 2482

Methohexital Sodium (Given the primary CNS effects of duloxetine, it should be used with caution when it is taken in combination with or substituted for other centrally acting drugs, including those with a similar mechanism of action).
No products indexed under this heading.

Methotrimeprazine (Duloxetine is a moderate inhibitor of CYP2D6. Co-administration of duloxetine with other drugs that are extensively metabolized by this isoenzyme, and which have a narrow therapeutic window, should be approached with caution).
No products indexed under this heading.

Methoxsalen (Concomitant use of duloxetine with fluvoxamine, an inhibitor of CYP1A2, results in approximately a 6-fold increase in AUC and about a 2.5-fold increase in Cmax of duloxetine. Since duloxetine is metabolized in part by CYP1A2, concomitant use of duloxetine with other inhibitors of CYP1A2, would be expected to have the same effects; these combinations should be avoided). Products include:
Oxsoralen Lotion 1% 3354
Oxsoralen-Ultra Capsules 3354

Methoxyflurane (Given the primary CNS effects of duloxetine, it should be used with caution when it is taken in combination with or substituted for other centrally acting drugs, including those with a similar mechanism of action).
No products indexed under this heading.

Methylphenidate Hydrochloride (Given the primary CNS effects of duloxetine, it should be used with caution when it is taken in combination with or substituted for other centrally acting drugs, including those with a similar mechanism of action). Products include:
Concerta Extended-Release Tablets 1828
Metadate CD Capsules 3316
Ritalin 2254
Ritalin LA Capsules 2255

Metoprolol Succinate (Duloxetine is a moderate inhibitor of CYP2D6. Co-administration of duloxetine with other drugs that are extensively metabolized by this isoenzyme, and which have a narrow therapeutic window, should be approached with caution). Products include:
Toprol-XL Tablets 660

Metoprolol Tartrate (Duloxetine is a moderate inhibitor of CYP2D6. Co-administration of duloxetine with other drugs that are extensively metabolized by this isoenzyme, and which have a narrow therapeutic window, should be approached with caution).
No products indexed under this heading.

Mexiletine Hydrochloride (Duloxetine is a moderate inhibitor of CYP2D6. Co-administration of duloxetine with other drugs that are extensively metabolized by this isoenzyme, and which have a narrow therapeutic window, should be approached with caution).
No products indexed under this heading.

Mibefradil Dihydrochloride (Because CYP2D6 is involved in duloxetine metabolism, concomitant use of duloxetine with potent inhibitors of CYP2D6 would be expected to, and does, result in higher concentrations of duloxetine).
No products indexed under this heading.

Midazolam Hydrochloride (Given the primary CNS effects of duloxetine, it should be used with caution when it is taken in combination with or substituted for other centrally acting drugs, including those with a similar mechanism of action).
No products indexed under this heading.

Mirtazapine (Duloxetine is a moderate inhibitor of CYP2D6. Co-administration of duloxetine with other drugs that are extensively metabolized by this isoenzyme, and which have a narrow therapeutic window, should be approached with caution).
No products indexed under this heading.

Moclobemide (There have been reports of serious, sometimes fatal, reactions in patients receiving a serotonin reuptake inhibitor in combination with a monoamine oxidase inhibitor (MAOI). These reactions have also been reported in patients who have recently discontinued serotonin reuptake inhibitors and are started on an MAOI. Therefore, duloxetine use is contraindicated in combination with an MAOI, or within at least 14 days of discontinuing treatment with an MAOI. Based on the half-life of duloxetine, at least 5 days should be allowed after stopping duloxetine before starting an MAOI).
No products indexed under this heading.

Molindone Hydrochloride (Given the primary CNS effects of duloxetine, it should be used with caution when it is taken in combination with or substituted for other centrally acting drugs, including those with a similar mechanism of action). Products include:
Moban Tablets 1108

Morphine Sulfate (Duloxetine is a moderate inhibitor of CYP2D6. Co-administration of duloxetine with other drugs that are extensively metabolized by this isoenzyme, and which have a narrow therapeutic window, should be approached with caution). Products include:
Avinza Capsules 1714
Kadian Capsules 572
MS Contin Tablets 2703

Moxifloxacin Hydrochloride (Some quinolones, inhibitors of CYP1A2, would be expected to increase the AUC and Cmax of duloxetine; co-administration should be avoided). Products include:
Avelox 2984
Vigamox Ophthalmic Solution 560

Nalidixic Acid (Concomitant use of duloxetine with fluvoxamine, an inhibitor of CYP1A2, results in approximately a 6-fold increase in AUC and about a 2.5-fold increase in Cmax of duloxetine. Since duloxetine is metabolized in part by CYP1A2, concomitant use of duloxetine with other inhibitors of CYP1A2, would be expected to have the same effects; these combinations should be avoided).
No products indexed under this heading.

Nelfinavir Mesylate (Duloxetine is a moderate inhibitor of CYP2D6. Co-administration of duloxetine with other drugs that are extensively metabolized by this isoenzyme, and which have a narrow therapeutic window, should be approached with caution). Products include:
Viracept 2556

Nizatidine (Duloxetine has an enteric coating that resists dissolution until reaching a segment of the gastrointestinal tract where the pH exceeds 5.5. Drugs that raise the gastrointestinal pH may lead to an earlier release of duloxetine). Products include:
Axid Oral Solution 913

Norethindrone (Concomitant use of duloxetine with fluvoxamine, an inhibitor of CYP1A2, results in approximately a 6-fold increase in AUC and about a 2.5-fold increase in Cmax of duloxetine. Since duloxetine is metabolized in part by CYP1A2, concomitant use of duloxetine with other inhibitors of CYP1A2, would be expected to have the same effects; these combinations should be avoided). Products include:
Ortho Micronor Tablets 2411

Norfloxacin (Some quinolones, inhibitors of CYP1A2, would be expected to increase the AUC and Cmax of duloxetine; co-administration should be avoided). Products include:
Noroxin Tablets 2009

Norgestrel (Concomitant use of duloxetine with fluvoxamine, an inhibitor of CYP1A2, results in approximately a 6-fold increase in AUC and about a 2.5-fold increase in Cmax of duloxetine. Since duloxetine is metabolized in part by CYP1A2, concomitant use of duloxetine with other inhibitors of CYP1A2, would be expected to have the same effects; these combinations should be avoided). Products include:
Lo/Ovral-28 Tablets 3423

Nortriptyline Hydrochloride (Because CYP2D6 is involved in duloxetine metabolism, concomitant use of duloxetine with potent inhibitors of CYP2D6 would be expected to, and does, result in higher concentrations of duloxetine).
No products indexed under this heading.

Ofloxacin (Some quinolones, inhibitors of CYP1A2, would be expected to increase the AUC and Cmax of duloxetine; co-administration should be avoided). Products include:
Floxin Otic Singles 1045
Floxin Otic Solution 1043

Olanzapine (Duloxetine is a moderate inhibitor of CYP2D6. Co-administration of duloxetine with other drugs that are extensively metabolized by this isoenzyme, and which have a narrow therapeutic window, should be approached with caution). Products include:
Symbyax Capsules 1788
Zyprexa Tablets 1798
Zyprexa IntraMuscular 1798
Zyprexa ZYDIS Orally Disintegrating Tablets 1798

Omeprazole (Duloxetine is a moderate inhibitor of CYP2D6. Co-administration of duloxetine with other drugs that are extensively metabolized by this isoenzyme, and which have a narrow therapeutic window, should be approached with caution). Products include:
Zegerid Powder for Oral Solution 2972

Ondansetron (Duloxetine is a moderate inhibitor of CYP2D6. Co-administration of duloxetine with other drugs that are extensively metabolized by this isoenzyme, and which have a narrow therapeutic window, should be approached with caution). Products include:
Zofran ODT Orally Disintegrating Tablets 1613

Ondansetron Hydrochloride (Duloxetine is a moderate inhibitor of CYP2D6. Co-administration of duloxetine with other drugs that are extensively metabolized by this isoenzyme, and which have a narrow therapeutic window, should be approached with caution). Products include:
Zofran Injection 1607
Zofran 1613

Oxazepam (Given the primary CNS effects of duloxetine, it should be used with caution when it is taken in combination with or substituted for other centrally acting drugs, including those with a similar mechanism of action).
No products indexed under this heading.

Oxycodone Hydrochloride (Duloxetine is a moderate inhibitor of CYP2D6. Co-administration of duloxetine with other drugs that are extensively metabolized by this isoenzyme, and which have a narrow therapeutic window, should be approached with caution). Products include:
Combunox Tablets 1183
OxyContin Tablets 2699
OxyFast Oral Concentrate Solution 2704
OxyIR Capsules 2704
Percocet Tablets 1114
Percodan Tablets 1115

Paclitaxel (Duloxetine is a moderate inhibitor of CYP2D6. Co-administration of duloxetine with other drugs that are extensively metabolized by this isoenzyme, and which have a narrow therapeutic window, should be approached with caution).
No products indexed under this heading.

Pargyline Hydrochloride (There have been reports of serious, sometimes fatal, reactions in patients receiving a serotonin reuptake inhibitor in combination with a monoamine oxidase inhibitor (MAOI). These reactions have also been reported in patients who have recently discontinued serotonin reuptake inhibitors and are started on an MAOI. Therefore, duloxetine use is contraindicated in combination with an MAOI, or within at least 14 days of discontinuing treatment with an MAOI. Based on the half-life of duloxetine, at least 5 days should be allowed after stopping duloxetine before starting an MAOI).
No products indexed under this heading.

Paroxetine Hydrochloride (Paroxetine (20mg qd) increased the concentration of duloxetine (40mg qd) by about 60% and greater degrees of inhibition are expected with higher doses of paroxetine). Products include:
Paxil CR Controlled-Release Tablets 1509
Paxil 1501

Pemoline (Given the primary CNS effects of duloxetine, it should be used with caution when it is taken in combination with or substituted for other centrally acting drugs, including those with a similar mechanism of action).
No products indexed under this heading.

Pentobarbital Sodium (Given the primary CNS effects of duloxetine, it should be used with caution when it is taken in combination with or substituted for other centrally acting drugs, including those with a similar mechanism of action). Products include:
Nembutal Sodium Solution, USP 2484

Perphenazine (Because CYP2D6 is involved in duloxetine metabolism, concomitant use of duloxetine with potent inhibitors of CYP2D6 would be expected to, and does, result in higher concentrations of duloxetine).
No products indexed under this heading.

Phenelzine Sulfate (There have been reports of serious, sometimes fatal, reactions in patients receiving a serotonin reuptake inhibitor in combination with a monoamine oxidase inhibitor (MAOI). These reactions have also been reported in patients who have recently discontinued serotonin reuptake inhibitors and are started on an MAOI. Therefore, duloxetine use is contraindicated in combination with an MAOI, or within at least 14 days of discontinuing treatment with an MAOI. Based on the half-life of duloxetine, at least 5 days should be allowed after stopping duloxetine before starting an MAOI).
No products indexed under this heading.

Phenobarbital (Given the primary CNS effects of duloxetine, it should be used with caution when it is taken in combination with or substituted for other centrally acting drugs, including those with a similar mechanism of action).
No products indexed under this heading.

Pindolol (Duloxetine is a moderate inhibitor of CYP2D6. Co-administration of duloxetine with other drugs that are extensively metabolized by this isoenzyme, and which have a narrow therapeutic window, should be approached with caution).
No products indexed under this heading.

Prazepam (Given the primary CNS effects of duloxetine, it should be used with caution when it is taken in combination with or substituted for other centrally acting drugs, including those with a similar mechanism of action).

No products indexed under this heading.

Procarbazine Hydrochloride (There have been reports of serious, sometimes fatal, reactions in patients receiving a serotonin reuptake inhibitor in combination with a monoamine oxidase inhibitor (MAOI). These reactions have also been reported in patients who have recently discontinued serotonin reuptake inhibitors and are started on an MAOI. Therefore, duloxetine use is contraindicated in combination with an MAOI, or within at least 14 days of discontinuing treatment with an MAOI. Based on the half-life of duloxetine, at least 5 days should be allowed after stopping duloxetine before starting an MAOI). Products include:

Matulane Capsules 3188

Prochlorperazine (Duloxetine is a moderate inhibitor of CYP2D6. Co-administration of duloxetine with other drugs that are extensively metabolized by this isoenzyme, and which have a narrow therapeutic window, should be approached with caution).

No products indexed under this heading.

Promethazine Hydrochloride (Duloxetine is a moderate inhibitor of CYP2D6. Co-administration of duloxetine with other drugs that are extensively metabolized by this isoenzyme, and which have a narrow therapeutic window, should be approached with caution). Products include:

Phenergan 3438

Propafenone Hydrochloride (Duloxetine is a moderate inhibitor of CYP2D6. Co-administration of duloxetine with other drugs that are extensively metabolized by this isoenzyme, and which have a narrow therapeutic window, should be approached with caution). Products include:

Rythmol SR Capsules 2736

Propofol (Given the primary CNS effects of duloxetine, it should be used with caution when it is taken in combination with or substituted for other centrally acting drugs, including those with a similar mechanism of action). Products include:

Diprivan Injectable Emulsion 676

Propoxyphene Hydrochloride (Because CYP2D6 is involved in duloxetine metabolism, concomitant use of duloxetine with potent inhibitors of CYP2D6 would be expected to, and does, result in higher concentrations of duloxetine).

No products indexed under this heading.

Propoxyphene Napsylate (Because CYP2D6 is involved in duloxetine metabolism, concomitant use of duloxetine with potent inhibitors of CYP2D6 would be expected to, and does, result in higher concentrations of duloxetine). Products include:

Darvocet A 500 Tablets 3497

Propranolol Hydrochloride (Duloxetine is a moderate inhibitor of CYP2D6. Co-administration of duloxetine with other drugs that are extensively metabolized by this isoenzyme, and which have a narrow therapeutic window, should be approached with caution). Products include:

Inderal LA Long-Acting Capsules 3421
InnoPran XL Capsules 2728

Protriptyline Hydrochloride (Because CYP2D6 is involved in duloxetine metabolism, concomitant use of duloxetine with potent inhibitors of CYP2D6 would be expected to, and does, result in higher concentrations of duloxetine). Products include:

Vivactil Tablets 2350

Quazepam (Given the primary CNS effects of duloxetine, it should be used with caution when it is taken in combination with or substituted for other centrally acting drugs, including those with a similar mechanism of action).

No products indexed under this heading.

Quetiapine Fumarate (Duloxetine is a moderate inhibitor of CYP2D6. Co-administration of duloxetine with other drugs that are extensively metabolized by this isoenzyme, and which have a narrow therapeutic window, should be approached with caution). Products include:

Seroquel Tablets 691

Quinacrine Hydrochloride (Because CYP2D6 is involved in duloxetine metabolism, concomitant use of duloxetine with potent inhibitors of CYP2D6 would be expected to, and does, result in higher concentrations of duloxetine).

No products indexed under this heading.

Quinidine Gluconate (Because CYP2D6 is involved in duloxetine metabolism, concomitant use of duloxetine with potent inhibitors of CYP2D6 would be expected to, and does, result in higher concentrations of duloxetine).

No products indexed under this heading.

Quinidine Hydrochloride (Because CYP2D6 is involved in duloxetine metabolism, concomitant use of duloxetine with potent inhibitors of CYP2D6 would be expected to, and does, result in higher concentrations of duloxetine).

No products indexed under this heading.

Quinidine Polygalacturonate (Because CYP2D6 is involved in duloxetine metabolism, concomitant use of duloxetine with potent inhibitors of CYP2D6 would be expected to, and does, result in higher concentrations of duloxetine).

No products indexed under this heading.

Quinidine Sulfate (Because CYP2D6 is involved in duloxetine metabolism, concomitant use of duloxetine with potent inhibitors of CYP2D6 would be expected to, and does, result in higher concentrations of duloxetine).

No products indexed under this heading.

Rabeprazole Sodium (Duloxetine has an enteric coating that resists dissolution until reaching a segment of the gastrointestinal tract where the pH exceeds 5.5. Drugs that raise the gastrointestinal pH may lead to an earlier release of duloxetine). Products include:

Aciphex Tablets 1081

Ranitidine Bismuth Citrate (Because CYP2D6 is involved in duloxetine metabolism, concomitant use of duloxetine with potent inhibitors of CYP2D6 would be expected to, and does, result in higher concentrations of duloxetine).

No products indexed under this heading.

Ranitidine Hydrochloride (Because CYP2D6 is involved in duloxetine metabolism, concomitant use of duloxetine with potent inhibitors of CYP2D6 would be expected to, and does, result in higher concentrations of duloxetine). Products include:

Zantac 1597
Zantac Injection 1593
Zantac 75 Tablets 715
Zantac 150 Maximum Strength Tablets 715
Zantac Injection Pharmacy Bulk Package 1595

Remifentanil Hydrochloride (Given the primary CNS effects of duloxetine, it should be used with caution when it is taken in combination with or substituted for other centrally acting drugs, including those with a similar mechanism of action).

No products indexed under this heading.

Risperidone (Duloxetine is a moderate inhibitor of CYP2D6. Co-administration of duloxetine with other drugs that are extensively metabolized by this isoenzyme, and which have a narrow therapeutic window, should be approached with caution). Products include:

Risperdal Consta Long-Acting Injection 1664
Risperdal M-Tab Orally Disintegrating Tablets 1658
Risperdal 1658

Ritonavir (Because CYP2D6 is involved in duloxetine metabolism, concomitant use of duloxetine with potent inhibitors of CYP2D6 would be expected to, and does, result in higher concentrations of duloxetine). Products include:

Kaletra 474
Norvir 499

Secobarbital Sodium (Given the primary CNS effects of duloxetine, it should be used with caution when it is taken in combination with or substituted for other centrally acting drugs, including those with a similar mechanism of action).

No products indexed under this heading.

Selegiline Hydrochloride (There have been reports of serious, sometimes fatal, reactions in patients receiving a serotonin reuptake inhibitor in combination with a monoamine oxidase inhibitor (MAOI). These reactions have also been reported in patients who have recently discontinued serotonin reuptake inhibitors and are started on an MAOI. Therefore, duloxetine use is contraindicated in combination with an MAOI, or within at least 14 days of discontinuing treatment with an MAOI. Based on the half-life of duloxetine, at least 5 days should be allowed after stopping duloxetine before starting an MAOI). Products include:

Eldepryl Capsules 3209

Sertraline Hydrochloride (Because CYP2D6 is involved in duloxetine metabolism, concomitant use of duloxetine with potent inhibitors of CYP2D6 would be expected to, and does, result in higher concentrations of duloxetine). Products include:

Zoloft 2581

Sevoflurane (Given the primary CNS effects of duloxetine, it should be used with caution when it is taken in combination with or substituted for other centrally acting drugs, including those with a similar mechanism of action). Products include:

Ultane Liquid for Inhalation 526

Sodium Oxybate (Given the primary CNS effects of duloxetine, it should be used with caution when it is taken in combination with or substituted for other centrally acting drugs, including those with a similar mechanism of action).

No products indexed under this heading.

Sparfloxacin (Concomitant use of duloxetine with fluvoxamine, an inhibitor of CYP1A2, results in approximately a 6-fold increase in AUC and about a 2.5-fold increase in Cmax of duloxetine. Since duloxetine is metabolized in part by CYP1A2, concomitant use of duloxetine with other inhibitors of CYP1A2, would be expected to have the same effects; these combinations should be avoided).

No products indexed under this heading.

Sufentanil Citrate (Given the primary CNS effects of duloxetine, it should be used with caution when it is taken in combination with or substituted for other centrally acting drugs, including those with a similar mechanism of action).

No products indexed under this heading.

Tacrine Hydrochloride (Concomitant use of duloxetine with fluvoxamine, an inhibitor of CYP1A2, results in approximately a 6-fold increase in AUC and about a 2.5-fold increase in Cmax of duloxetine. Since duloxetine is metabolized in part by CYP1A2, concomitant use of duloxetine with other inhibitors of CYP1A2, would be expected to have the same effects; these combinations should be avoided).

No products indexed under this heading.

Tamoxifen Citrate (Duloxetine is a moderate inhibitor of CYP2D6. Co-administration of duloxetine with other drugs that are extensively metabolized by this isoenzyme, and which have a narrow therapeutic window, should be approached with caution).

No products indexed under this heading.

Temazepam (Given the primary CNS effects of duloxetine, it should be used with caution when it is taken in combination with or substituted for other centrally acting drugs, including those with a similar mechanism of action).

No products indexed under this heading.

Teniposide (Duloxetine is a moderate inhibitor of CYP2D6. Co-administration of duloxetine with other drugs that are extensively metabolized by this isoenzyme, and which have a narrow therapeutic window, should be approached with caution).
No products indexed under this heading.

Terbinafine Hydrochloride (Because CYP2D6 is involved in duloxetine metabolism, concomitant use of duloxetine with potent inhibitors of CYP2D6 would be expected to, and does, result in higher concentrations of duloxetine). Products include:
Lamisil AT Creams (Athlete's Foot & Jock Itch) .... ▣ 676
Lamisil Tablets 2226

Testosterone (Duloxetine is a moderate inhibitor of CYP2D6. Co-administration of duloxetine with other drugs that are extensively metabolized by this isoenzyme, and which have a narrow therapeutic window, should be approached with caution). Products include:
AndroGel 3330
Striant Mucoadhesive 1022
Testim 1% Gel 722

Testosterone Cypionate (Duloxetine is a moderate inhibitor of CYP2D6. Co-administration of duloxetine with other drugs that are extensively metabolized by this isoenzyme, and which have a narrow therapeutic window, should be approached with caution).
No products indexed under this heading.

Testosterone Enanthate (Duloxetine is a moderate inhibitor of CYP2D6. Co-administration of duloxetine with other drugs that are extensively metabolized by this isoenzyme, and which have a narrow therapeutic window, should be approached with caution). Products include:
Delatestryl Injection 2976

Testosterone Propionate (Duloxetine is a moderate inhibitor of CYP2D6. Co-administration of duloxetine with other drugs that are extensively metabolized by this isoenzyme, and which have a narrow therapeutic window, should be approached with caution).
No products indexed under this heading.

Thiamylal Sodium (Given the primary CNS effects of duloxetine, it should be used with caution when it is taken in combination with or substituted for other centrally acting drugs, including those with a similar mechanism of action).
No products indexed under this heading.

Thioridazine (Duloxetine is a moderate inhibitor of CYP2D6. Co-administration of duloxetine with other drugs that are extensively metabolized by this isoenzyme, and which have a narrow therapeutic window, should be approached with caution. Because of the risk of serious ventricular arrhythmias and sudden death potentially associated with elevated plasma levels of thioridazine, duloxetine and thioridazine should not be coadministered).
No products indexed under this heading.

Thioridazine Hydrochloride (Duloxetine is a moderate inhibitor of CYP2D6. Co-administration of duloxetine with other drugs that are extensively metabolized by this isoenzyme, and which have a narrow therapeutic window, should be approached with caution. Because of the risk of serious ventricular arrhythmias and sudden death potentially associated with elevated plasma levels of thioridazine, duloxetine and thioridazine should not be coadministered). Products include:
Thioridazine Hydrochloride Tablets 2122

Thiothixene (Given the primary CNS effects of duloxetine, it should be used with caution when it is taken in combination with or substituted for other centrally acting drugs, including those with a similar mechanism of action). Products include:
Thiothixene Capsules 2124

Ticlopidine Hydrochloride (Concomitant use of duloxetine with fluvoxamine, an inhibitor of CYP1A2, results in approximately a 6-fold increase in AUC and about a 2.5-fold increase in Cmax of duloxetine. Since duloxetine is metabolized in part by CYP1A2, concomitant use of duloxetine with other inhibitors of CYP1A2, would be expected to have the same effects; these combinations should be avoided). Products include:
Ticlid Tablets 2813

Timolol Maleate (Duloxetine is a moderate inhibitor of CYP2D6. Co-administration of duloxetine with other drugs that are extensively metabolized by this isoenzyme, and which have a narrow therapeutic window, should be approached with caution). Products include:
Blocadren Tablets 1891
Cosopt Sterile Ophthalmic Solution 1910
Timolide Tablets 2056
Timoptic in Ocudose 2061
Timoptic Sterile Ophthalmic Solution 2058
Timoptic-XE Sterile Ophthalmic Gel Forming Solution 2062

Tolterodine Tartrate (Duloxetine is a moderate inhibitor of CYP2D6. Co-administration of duloxetine with other drugs that are extensively metabolized by this isoenzyme, and which have a narrow therapeutic window, should be approached with caution). Products include:
Detrol Tablets 2626
Detrol LA Capsules 2629

Tramadol Hydrochloride (Duloxetine is a moderate inhibitor of CYP2D6. Co-administration of duloxetine with other drugs that are extensively metabolized by this isoenzyme, and which have a narrow therapeutic window, should be approached with caution). Products include:
Ultracet Tablets 2462

Tranylcypromine Sulfate (There have been reports of serious, sometimes fatal, reactions in patients receiving a serotonin reuptake inhibitor in combination with a monoamine oxidase inhibitor (MAOI). These reactions have also been reported in patients who have recently discontinued serotonin reuptake inhibitors and are started on an MAOI. Therefore, duloxetine use is contraindicated in combination with an MAOI, or within at least 14 days of discontinuing treatment with an MAOI. Based on the half-life of duloxetine, at least 5 days should be allowed after stopping duloxetine before starting an MAOI). Products include:
Parnate Tablets 1499

Trazodone Hydrochloride (Duloxetine is a moderate inhibitor of CYP2D6. Co-administration of duloxetine with other drugs that are extensively metabolized by this isoenzyme, and which have a narrow therapeutic window, should be approached with caution).
No products indexed under this heading.

Triazolam (Duloxetine is a moderate inhibitor of CYP2D6. Co-administration of duloxetine with other drugs that are extensively metabolized by this isoenzyme, and which have a narrow therapeutic window, should be approached with caution).
No products indexed under this heading.

Trifluoperazine Hydrochloride (Duloxetine is a moderate inhibitor of CYP2D6. Co-administration of duloxetine with other drugs that are extensively metabolized by this isoenzyme, and which have a narrow therapeutic window, should be approached with caution).
No products indexed under this heading.

Trimipramine Maleate (Because CYP2D6 is involved in duloxetine metabolism, concomitant use of duloxetine with potent inhibitors of CYP2D6 would be expected to, and does, result in higher concentrations of duloxetine). Products include:
Surmontil Capsules 2347

Troleandomycin (Concomitant use of duloxetine with fluvoxamine, an inhibitor of CYP1A2, results in approximately a 6-fold increase in AUC and about a 2.5-fold increase in Cmax of duloxetine. Since duloxetine is metabolized in part by CYP1A2, concomitant use of duloxetine with other inhibitors of CYP1A2, would be expected to have the same effects; these combinations should be avoided).
No products indexed under this heading.

Trovafloxacin Mesylate (Some quinolones, inhibitors of CYP1A2, would be expected to increase the AUC and Cmax of duloxetine; co-administration should be avoided).
No products indexed under this heading.

Venlafaxine Hydrochloride (Duloxetine is a moderate inhibitor of CYP2D6. Co-administration of duloxetine with other drugs that are extensively metabolized by this isoenzyme, and which have a narrow therapeutic window, should be approached with caution). Products include:
Effexor Tablets 3405
Effexor XR Capsules 3411

Vinblastine Sulfate (Duloxetine is a moderate inhibitor of CYP2D6. Co-administration of duloxetine with other drugs that are extensively metabolized by this isoenzyme, and which have a narrow therapeutic window, should be approached with caution).
No products indexed under this heading.

Zaleplon (Given the primary CNS effects of duloxetine, it should be used with caution when it is taken in combination with or substituted for other centrally acting drugs, including those with a similar mechanism of action). Products include:
Sonata Capsules 1686

Zileuton (Concomitant use of duloxetine with fluvoxamine, an inhibitor of CYP1A2, results in approximately a 6-fold increase in AUC and about a 2.5-fold increase in Cmax of duloxetine. Since duloxetine is metabolized in part by CYP1A2, concomitant use of duloxetine with other inhibitors of CYP1A2, would be expected to have the same effects; these combinations should be avoided).
No products indexed under this heading.

Ziprasidone Hydrochloride (Given the primary CNS effects of duloxetine, it should be used with caution when it is taken in combination with or substituted for other centrally acting drugs, including those with a similar mechanism of action). Products include:
Geodon Capsules 2514

Zolpidem Tartrate (Given the primary CNS effects of duloxetine, it should be used with caution when it is taken in combination with or substituted for other centrally acting drugs, including those with a similar mechanism of action). Products include:
Ambien Tablets 2867

Zonisamide (Duloxetine is a moderate inhibitor of CYP2D6. Co-administration of duloxetine with other drugs that are extensively metabolized by this isoenzyme, and which have a narrow therapeutic window, should be approached with caution). Products include:
Zonegran Capsules 1089

Food Interactions

Alcohol (Use of duloxetine concomitantly with heavy alcohol intake may be associated with severe liver injury; therefore, duloxetine should ordinarily not be prescribed for patients with substantial alcohol use).

Grapefruit Juice (Concomitant use of duloxetine with fluvoxamine, an inhibitor of CYP1A2, results in approximately a 6-fold increase in AUC and about a 2.5-fold increase in Cmax of duloxetine. Since duloxetine is metabolized in part by CYP1A2, concomitant use of duloxetine with other inhibitors of CYP1A2, would be expected to have the same effects; these combinations should be avoided).

CYTOGAM INTRAVENOUS

(Cytomegalovirus Immune Globulin) ... 1866
May interact with:

Measles, Mumps & Rubella Virus Vaccine, Live (May interfere with the immune response to live virus vaccine). Products include:
M-M-R II 1980

CYTOMEL TABLETS

(Liothyronine Sodium) 1678
May interact with oral anticoagulants, estrogens, cardiac glycosides, oral hypoglycemic agents, insulin, tricyclic antidepressants, and certain other agents. Compounds in these categories include:

Acarbose (Initiating thyroid replacement therapy may cause increases in oral hypoglycemic requirements). Products include:
Precose Tablets 776

Amitriptyline Hydrochloride (Use of thyroid hormones may increase receptor sensitivity and enhance antidepressant activity; transient cardiac arrhythmias; thyroid hormone activity may also be enhanced).
No products indexed under this heading.

Amoxapine (Use of thyroid hormones may increase receptor sensitivity and enhance antidepressant activity; transient cardiac arrhythmias; thyroid hormone activity may also be enhanced).
No products indexed under this heading.

Anisindione (Thyroid hormones appear to increase catabolism of vitamin K-dependent clotting factor; if oral anticoagulants are also given compensatory increases in clotting factor synthesis are impaired). Products include:
Miradon Tablets 3056

Chlorotrianisene (Estrogens tend to increase serum thyroxine-binding globulin in a patient with a nonfunctioning thyroid gland who is receiving thyroid replacement therapy; patients without functioning thyroid gland who are on thyroid replacement therapy may need to increase their thyroid dose if estrogens or estrogen-containing oral contraceptives are given).
No products indexed under this heading.

Chlorpropamide (Initiating thyroid replacement therapy may cause increases in oral hypoglycemic requirements).
No products indexed under this heading.

Cholestyramine (Binds both T4 and T3 in the intestine thus impairing absorption of thyroid hormones; 4 to 5 hours should elapse between administration of thyroid hormone and cholestyramine).
No products indexed under this heading.

Clomipramine Hydrochloride (Use of thyroid hormones may increase receptor sensitivity and enhance antidepressant activity; transient cardiac arrhythmias; thyroid hormone activity may also be enhanced).
No products indexed under this heading.

Desipramine Hydrochloride (Use of thyroid hormones may increase receptor sensitivity and enhance antidepressant activity; transient cardiac arrhythmias; thyroid hormone activity may also be enhanced).
No products indexed under this heading.

Deslanoside (Thyroid preparations may potentiate the toxic effects of digitalis; thyroid hormone increase metabolic rate which requires an increase in digitalis dosage).
No products indexed under this heading.

Dicumarol (Thyroid hormones appear to increase catabolism of vitamin K-dependent clotting factor; if oral anticoagulants are also given compensatory increases in clotting factor synthesis are impaired).
No products indexed under this heading.

Dienestrol (Estrogens tend to increase serum thyroxine-binding globulin in a patient with a nonfunctioning thyroid gland who is receiving thyroid replacement therapy; patients without functioning thyroid gland who are on thyroid replacement therapy may need to increase their thyroid dose if estrogens or estrogen-containing oral contraceptives are given).
No products indexed under this heading.

Diethylstilbestrol (Estrogens tend to increase serum thyroxine-binding globulin in a patient with a nonfunctioning thyroid gland who is receiving thyroid replacement therapy; patients without functioning thyroid gland who are on thyroid replacement therapy may need to increase their thyroid dose if estrogens or estrogen-containing oral contraceptives are given).
No products indexed under this heading.

Digitalis Glycoside Preparations (Thyroid preparations may potentiate the toxic effects of digitalis; thyroid hormone increase metabolic rate which requires an increase in digitalis dosage).
No products indexed under this heading.

Digitoxin (Thyroid preparations may potentiate the toxic effects of digitalis; thyroid hormone increase metabolic rate which requires an increase in digitalis dosage).
No products indexed under this heading.

Digoxin (Thyroid preparations may potentiate the toxic effects of digitalis; thyroid hormone increase metabolic rate which requires an increase in digitalis dosage). Products include:
Digitek Tablets 2146
Lanoxicaps Capsules 1458
Lanoxin Injection 1462
Lanoxin Tablets 1468
Lanoxin Injection Pediatric 1465

Doxepin Hydrochloride (Use of thyroid hormones may increase receptor sensitivity and enhance antidepressant activity; transient cardiac arrhythmias; thyroid hormone activity may also be enhanced).
No products indexed under this heading.

Epinephrine (Thyroxine increases the adrenergic effect of catecholamines, such as epinephrine). Products include:
EpiPen 1061
Primatene Mist 749

Epinephrine Bitartrate (Thyroxine increases the adrenergic effect of catecholamines, such as epinephrine).
No products indexed under this heading.

Epinephrine Hydrochloride (Thyroxine increases the adrenergic effect of catecholamines, such as epinephrine).
No products indexed under this heading.

Estradiol (Estrogens tend to increase serum thyroxine-binding globulin in a patient with a nonfunctioning thyroid gland who is receiving thyroid replacement therapy; patients without functioning thyroid gland who are on thyroid replacement therapy may need to increase their thyroid dose if estrogens or estrogen-containing oral contraceptives are given). Products include:
Activella Tablets 2311
Climara Transdermal System 795
Climara Pro Transdermal System 800
CombiPatch Transdermal System 2180
Estrogel 0.06% 3200
Menostar Transdermal System 805
Prefest Tablets 1069
Vagifem Tablets 2340
Vivelle Transdermal System 2288
Vivelle-Dot Transdermal System 2293

Estrogens, Conjugated (Estrogens tend to increase serum thyroxine-binding globulin in a patient with a nonfunctioning thyroid gland who is receiving thyroid replacement therapy; patients without functioning thyroid gland who are on thyroid replacement therapy may need to increase their thyroid dose if estrogens or estrogen-containing oral contraceptives are given). Products include:
Premarin Intravenous 3440
Premarin Tablets 3443
Premarin Vaginal Cream 3449
Premphase Tablets 3452
Prempro Tablets 3452

Estrogens, Esterified (Estrogens tend to increase serum thyroxine-binding globulin in a patient with a nonfunctioning thyroid gland who is receiving thyroid replacement therapy; patients without functioning thyroid gland who are on thyroid replacement therapy may need to increase their thyroid dose if estrogens or estrogen-containing oral contraceptives are given). Products include:
Estratest Tablets 3196
Estratest H.S. Tablets 3196

Estropipate (Estrogens tend to increase serum thyroxine-binding globulin in a patient with a nonfunctioning thyroid gland who is receiving thyroid replacement therapy; patients without functioning thyroid gland who are on thyroid replacement therapy may need to increase their thyroid dose if estrogens or estrogen-containing oral contraceptives are given).
No products indexed under this heading.

Ethinyl Estradiol (Estrogens tend to increase serum thyroxine-binding globulin in a patient with a nonfunctioning thyroid gland who is receiving thyroid replacement therapy; patients without functioning thyroid gland who are on thyroid replacement therapy may need to increase their thyroid dose if estrogens or estrogen-containing oral contraceptives are given). Products include:
Alesse-28 Tablets 3392
Lo/Ovral-28 Tablets 3423
NuvaRing 2357
Ortho-Cept Tablets 2395
Ortho-Cyclen/Ortho Tri-Cyclen 2414
Ortho Evra Transdermal System 2402
Ortho Tri-Cyclen Lo Tablets 2421
Seasonale Tablets 1073
Triphasil-28 Tablets 3483
Yasmin 28 Tablets 818

Glimepiride (Initiating thyroid replacement therapy may cause increases in oral hypoglycemic requirements). Products include:
Amaryl Tablets 2864

Glipizide (Initiating thyroid replacement therapy may cause increases in oral hypoglycemic requirements).
No products indexed under this heading.

Glyburide (Initiating thyroid replacement therapy may cause increases in oral hypoglycemic requirements).
No products indexed under this heading.

Imipramine Hydrochloride (Use of thyroid hormones may increase receptor sensitivity and enhance antidepressant activity; transient cardiac arrhythmias; thyroid hormone activity may also be enhanced).
No products indexed under this heading.

Imipramine Pamoate (Use of thyroid hormones may increase receptor sensitivity and enhance antidepressant activity; transient cardiac arrhythmias; thyroid hormone activity may also be enhanced).
No products indexed under this heading.

Insulin, Human, Zinc Suspension (Initiating thyroid replacement therapy may cause increases in insulin requirements). Products include:
Humulin L, 100 Units 1763
Humulin U, 100 Units 1770

Insulin, Human NPH (Initiating thyroid replacement therapy may cause increases in insulin requirements). Products include:
Humulin N, 100 Units 1764
Humulin N Pen 1765
Novolin N Human Insulin 10 ml Vials 2322
Novolin N InnoLet 2322
Novolin N PenFill 3 ml Cartridges 2325
Novolin R InnoLet 2322

Insulin, Human Regular (Initiating thyroid replacement therapy may cause increases in insulin requirements). Products include:
Humulin R (U-500) 1768
Humulin R, 100 Units 1767
Novolin R Human Insulin 10 ml Vials 2322
Novolin R PenFill 2325

Insulin, Human Regular and Human NPH Mixture (Initiating thyroid replacement therapy may cause increases in insulin requirements). Products include:
Humulin 50/50, 100 Units 1760
Humulin 70/30 Pen 1761
Novolin 70/30 Human Insulin 10 ml Vials 2321
Novolin 70/30 InnoLet 2322
Novolin 70/30 PenFill 3 ml Cartridges 2325

Insulin, NPH (Initiating thyroid replacement therapy may cause increases in insulin requirements).
No products indexed under this heading.

Insulin, Regular (Initiating thyroid replacement therapy may cause increases in insulin requirements).
No products indexed under this heading.

Insulin, Zinc Crystals (Initiating thyroid replacement therapy may cause increases in insulin requirements).
No products indexed under this heading.

Insulin, Zinc Suspension (Initiating thyroid replacement therapy may cause increases in insulin requirements).
No products indexed under this heading.

Insulin Aspart, Human Regular (Initiating thyroid replacement therapy may cause increases in insulin requirements). Products include:
NovoLog Injection 2326

IMPORTANT NOTE: Always consult each drug listing in the patient's regimen for possible interactions.

Insulin glargine (Initiating thyroid replacement therapy may cause increases in insulin requirements). Products include:
- Lantus Injection 2925

Insulin Lispro, Human (Initiating thyroid replacement therapy may cause increases in insulin requirements). Products include:
- Humalog-Pen 1751
- Humalog Mix 75/25-Pen 1754

Insulin Lispro Protamine, Human (Initiating thyroid replacement therapy may cause increases in insulin requirements). Products include:
- Humalog Mix 75/25-Pen 1754

Ketamine Hydrochloride (Co-administration may cause hypertension and tachycardia).
No products indexed under this heading.

Maprotiline Hydrochloride (Use of thyroid hormones may increase receptor sensitivity and enhance antidepressant activity; transient cardiac arrhythmias; thyroid hormone activity may also be enhanced).
No products indexed under this heading.

Metformin Hydrochloride (Initiating thyroid replacement therapy may cause increases in oral hypoglycemic requirements). Products include:
- ActoPlus Met Tablets 3219
- Avandamet Tablets 1343
- Fortamet Extended-Release Tablets 1156

Miglitol (Initiating thyroid replacement therapy may cause increases in oral hypoglycemic requirements).
No products indexed under this heading.

Norepinephrine Hydrochloride (Thyroxine increases the adrenergic effect of catecholamines, such as norepinephrine).
No products indexed under this heading.

Nortriptyline Hydrochloride (Use of thyroid hormones may increase receptor sensitivity and enhance antidepressant activity; transient cardiac arrhythmias; thyroid hormone activity may also be enhanced).
No products indexed under this heading.

Pioglitazone Hydrochloride (Initiating thyroid replacement therapy may cause increases in oral hypoglycemic requirements). Products include:
- ActoPlus Met Tablets 3219
- Actos Tablets 3224

Polyestradiol Phosphate (Estrogens tend to increase serum thyroxine-binding globulin in a patient with a nonfunctioning thyroid gland who is receiving thyroid replacement therapy; patients without functioning thyroid gland who are on thyroid replacement therapy may need to increase their thyroid dose if estrogens or estrogen-containing oral contraceptives are given).
No products indexed under this heading.

Protriptyline Hydrochloride (Use of thyroid hormones may increase receptor sensitivity and enhance antidepressant activity; transient cardiac arrhythmias; thyroid hormone activity may also be enhanced). Products include:
- Vivactil Tablets 2350

Quinestrol (Estrogens tend to increase serum thyroxine-binding globulin in a patient with a nonfunctioning thyroid gland who is receiving thyroid replacement therapy; patients without functioning thyroid gland who are on thyroid replacement therapy may need to increase their thyroid dose if estrogens or estrogen-containing oral contraceptives are given).
No products indexed under this heading.

Repaglinide (Initiating thyroid replacement therapy may cause increases in oral hypoglycemic requirements). Products include:
- Prandin Tablets (0.5, 1, and 2 mg) 2337

Rosiglitazone Maleate (Initiating thyroid replacement therapy may cause increases in oral hypoglycemic requirements). Products include:
- Avandamet Tablets 1343
- Avandia Tablets 1348

Tolazamide (Initiating thyroid replacement therapy may cause increases in oral hypoglycemic requirements).
No products indexed under this heading.

Tolbutamide (Initiating thyroid replacement therapy may cause increases in oral hypoglycemic requirements).
No products indexed under this heading.

Trimipramine Maleate (Use of thyroid hormones may increase receptor sensitivity and enhance antidepressant activity; transient cardiac arrhythmias; thyroid hormone activity may also be enhanced). Products include:
- Surmontil Capsules 2347

Troglitazone (Initiating thyroid replacement therapy may cause increases in oral hypoglycemic requirements).
No products indexed under this heading.

Warfarin Sodium (Thyroid hormones appear to increase catabolism of vitamin K-dependent clotting factor; if oral anticoagulants are also given compensatory increases in clotting factor synthesis are impaired). Products include:
- Coumadin for Injection 932
- Coumadin Tablets 932

CYTOVENE CAPSULES

(Ganciclovir) 2763

May interact with nucleoside analogues, drugs inhibiting replication of cell populations of bone marrow, spermatogonia, and germinal layers, and certain other agents. Compounds in these categories include:

Acyclovir (Potential for additive toxicity). Products include:
- Zovirax 1616
- Zovirax Cream 853
- Zovirax Ointment 854

Acyclovir Sodium (Potential for additive toxicity). Products include:
- Zovirax for Injection 1618

Amphotericin B (Potential for additive toxicity; increases in serum creatinine and may result in increased nephrotoxicity).
No products indexed under this heading.

Cilastatin Sodium (Co-administration results in generalized seizures). Products include:
- Primaxin I.M. 2022
- Primaxin I.V. 2024

Cyclosporine (Increases in serum creatinine and may result in increased nephrotoxicity). Products include:
- Gengraf Capsules 458
- Neoral Soft Gelatin Capsules 2247
- Neoral Oral Solution 2247
- Restasis Ophthalmic Emulsion 570
- Sandimmune 2259

Dapsone (Potential for additive toxicity). Products include:
- Dapsone Tablets USP 1656

Didanosine (When administered concurrently or 2 hours prior to oral Cytovene, the steady-state didanosine AUC 0-12 increased 111 ± 114%; a decrease in ganciclovir steady-state AUC of 21 ±- 17%).
No products indexed under this heading.

Doxorubicin Hydrochloride (Potential for additive toxicity). Products include:
- Adriamycin for Injection, USP 786
- Adriamycin Injection, USP 786

Flucytosine (Potential for additive toxicity).
No products indexed under this heading.

Imipenem (Co-administration results in generalized seizures). Products include:
- Primaxin I.M. 2022
- Primaxin I.V. 2024

Pentamidine Isethionate (Potential for additive toxicity).
No products indexed under this heading.

Probenecid (Increases AUC 0-8 53 ± 91%, decreases renal clearance 22 ± 20%).
No products indexed under this heading.

Sulfamethoxazole (Potential for additive toxicity).
No products indexed under this heading.

Trimethoprim (Potential for additive toxicity).
No products indexed under this heading.

Vinblastine Sulfate (Potential for additive toxicity).
No products indexed under this heading.

Vincristine Sulfate (Potential for additive toxicity).
No products indexed under this heading.

Zidovudine (Man steady-state ganciclovir AUC 0-8 decreases 17 ± 25% in presence of zidovudine; steady-state zidovudine AUC 0-4 increases 19 ± 27%; both have potential to cause anemia and neutropenia). Products include:
- Combivir Tablets 1373
- Retrovir 1533
- Retrovir IV Infusion 1537
- Trizivir Tablets 1565

Food Interactions

Meal, unspecified (Meal containing 46.5% fat increases the steady-state AUC of oral Cytovene by 22% ± 22% and significant prolongation of time Tmax and a higher Cmax; patients should take Cytovene Capsules with food to maximize bioavailability).

CYTOVENE-IV

(Ganciclovir Sodium) 2763

See Cytovene Capsules

DAILY COMPLETE LIQUID

(Aloe vera, Amino Acid Preparations, Antioxidants, Herbals with Vitamins & Minerals) ...... ▣ 760

None cited in PDR database.

DALMANE CAPSULES

(Flurazepam Hydrochloride) 3343

None cited in PDR database.

DANTRIUM CAPSULES

(Dantrolene Sodium) 2690

May interact with calcium channel blockers, central nervous system depressants, estrogens, hypnotics and sedatives, tranquilizers, and certain other agents. Compounds in these categories include:

Alfentanil Hydrochloride (Co-administration may result in increased drowsiness; caution should be exercised).
No products indexed under this heading.

Alprazolam (Co-administration may result in increased drowsiness; caution should be exercised). Products include:
- Niravam Orally Disintegrating Tablets 3106
- Xanax XR Tablets 2655

Amlodipine Besylate (Due to interaction between verapamil and dantrolene, combination of dantrolene and calcium channel blockers is not recommended during the management of malignant hyperthermia). Products include:
- Caduet Tablets 2507
- Lotrel Capsules 2238
- Norvasc Tablets 2529

Aprobarbital (Co-administration may result in increased drowsiness; caution should be exercised).
No products indexed under this heading.

Bepridil Hydrochloride (Due to interaction between verapamil and dantrolene, combination of dantrolene and calcium channel blockers is not recommended during the management of malignant hyperthermia).
No products indexed under this heading.

Buprenorphine Hydrochloride (Co-administration may result in increased drowsiness; caution should be exercised). Products include:
- Buprenex Injectable 2718
- Suboxone Tablets 2719
- Subutex Tablets 2719

Buspirone Hydrochloride (Co-administration may result in increased drowsiness; caution should be exercised).
No products indexed under this heading.

Butabarbital (Co-administration may result in increased drowsiness; caution should be exercised).
No products indexed under this heading.

Butalbital (Co-administration may result in increased drowsiness; caution should be exercised). Products include:
- Sedapap Tablets 50 mg/650 mg 2098

Chlordiazepoxide (Co-administration may result in increased drowsiness; caution should be exercised).
No products indexed under this heading.

Chlordiazepoxide Hydrochloride (Co-administration may result in

increased drowsiness; caution should be exercised). Products include:
Librium Capsules ... 3349

Chlorotrianisene (Hepatotoxicity has occurred more often in women over 35 years of age receiving concomitant estrogen therapy).
No products indexed under this heading.

Chlorpromazine (Co-administration may result in increased drowsiness; caution should be exercised).
No products indexed under this heading.

Chlorpromazine Hydrochloride (Co-administration may result in increased drowsiness; caution should be exercised).
No products indexed under this heading.

Chlorprothixene (Co-administration may result in increased drowsiness; caution should be exercised).
No products indexed under this heading.

Chlorprothixene Hydrochloride (Co-administration may result in increased drowsiness; caution should be exercised).
No products indexed under this heading.

Chlorprothixene Lactate (Co-administration may result in increased drowsiness; caution should be exercised).
No products indexed under this heading.

Clorazepate Dipotassium (Co-administration may result in increased drowsiness; caution should be exercised). Products include:
Tranxene ... 2488

Clozapine (Co-administration may result in increased drowsiness; caution should be exercised). Products include:
Clozapine Tablets ... 2141
Clozaril Tablets ... 2174
FazaClo Orally Disintegrating Tablets ... 547

Codeine Phosphate (Co-administration may result in increased drowsiness; caution should be exercised). Products include:
Tylenol with Codeine ... 2461

Desflurane (Co-administration may result in increased drowsiness; caution should be exercised). Products include:
Suprane Liquid for Inhalation ... 770

Dezocine (Co-administration may result in increased drowsiness; caution should be exercised).
No products indexed under this heading.

Diazepam (Co-administration may result in increased drowsiness; caution should be exercised). Products include:
Diastat Rectal Delivery System ... 3344
Valium Tablets ... 2822

Dienestrol (Hepatotoxicity has occurred more often in women over 35 years of age receiving concomitant estrogen therapy).
No products indexed under this heading.

Diethylstilbestrol (Hepatotoxicity has occurred more often in women over 35 years of age receiving concomitant estrogen therapy).
No products indexed under this heading.

Diltiazem Hydrochloride (Due to interaction between verapamil and dantrolene, combination of dantrolene and calcium channel blockers is not recommended during the management of malignant hyperthermia). Products include:
Cardizem LA Extended Release Tablets ... 1699
Tiazac Capsules ... 1204

Droperidol (Co-administration may result in increased drowsiness; caution should be exercised).
No products indexed under this heading.

Enflurane (Co-administration may result in increased drowsiness; caution should be exercised).
No products indexed under this heading.

Estazolam (Co-administration may result in increased drowsiness; caution should be exercised). Products include:
ProSom Tablets ... 512

Estradiol (Hepatotoxicity has occurred more often in women over 35 years of age receiving concomitant estrogen therapy). Products include:
Activella Tablets ... 2311
Climara Transdermal System ... 795
Climara Pro Transdermal System ... 800
CombiPatch Transdermal System ... 2180
Estrogel 0.06% ... 3200
Menostar Transdermal System ... 805
Prefest Tablets ... 1069
Vagifem Tablets ... 2340
Vivelle Transdermal System ... 2288
Vivelle-Dot Transdermal System ... 2293

Estrogens, Conjugated (Hepatotoxicity has occurred more often in women over 35 years of age receiving concomitant estrogen therapy). Products include:
Premarin Intravenous ... 3440
Premarin Tablets ... 3443
Premarin Vaginal Cream ... 3449
Premphase Tablets ... 3452
Prempro Tablets ... 3452

Estrogens, Esterified (Hepatotoxicity has occurred more often in women over 35 years of age receiving concomitant estrogen therapy). Products include:
Estratest Tablets ... 3196
Estratest H.S. Tablets ... 3196

Estropipate (Hepatotoxicity has occurred more often in women over 35 years of age receiving concomitant estrogen therapy).
No products indexed under this heading.

Ethanol (Co-administration may result in increased drowsiness; caution should be exercised).
No products indexed under this heading.

Ethchlorvynol (Co-administration may result in increased drowsiness; caution should be exercised).
No products indexed under this heading.

Ethinamate (Co-administration may result in increased drowsiness; caution should be exercised).
No products indexed under this heading.

Ethinyl Estradiol (Hepatotoxicity has occurred more often in women over 35 years of age receiving concomitant estrogen therapy). Products include:
Alesse-28 Tablets ... 3392
Lo/Ovral-28 Tablets ... 3423
NuvaRing ... 2357
Ortho-Cept Tablets ... 2395
Ortho-Cyclen/Ortho Tri-Cyclen ... 2414
Ortho Evra Transdermal System ... 2402
Ortho Tri-Cyclen Lo Tablets ... 2421
Seasonale Tablets ... 1073
Triphasil-28 Tablets ... 3483
Yasmin 28 Tablets ... 818

Ethyl Alcohol (Co-administration may result in increased drowsiness; caution should be exercised).
No products indexed under this heading.

Felodipine (Due to interaction between verapamil and dantrolene, combination of dantrolene and calcium channel blockers is not recommended during the management of malignant hyperthermia). Products include:
Plendil Extended-Release Tablets ... 651

Fentanyl (Co-administration may result in increased drowsiness; caution should be exercised). Products include:
Duragesic Transdermal System ... 2448

Fentanyl Citrate (Co-administration may result in increased drowsiness; caution should be exercised). Products include:
Actiq ... 993

Fluphenazine Decanoate (Co-administration may result in increased drowsiness; caution should be exercised).
No products indexed under this heading.

Fluphenazine Enanthate (Co-administration may result in increased drowsiness; caution should be exercised).
No products indexed under this heading.

Fluphenazine Hydrochloride (Co-administration may result in increased drowsiness; caution should be exercised).
No products indexed under this heading.

Flurazepam Hydrochloride (Co-administration may result in increased drowsiness; caution should be exercised). Products include:
Dalmane Capsules ... 3343

Glutethimide (Co-administration may result in increased drowsiness; caution should be exercised).
No products indexed under this heading.

Haloperidol (Co-administration may result in increased drowsiness; caution should be exercised).
No products indexed under this heading.

Haloperidol Decanoate (Co-administration may result in increased drowsiness; caution should be exercised).
No products indexed under this heading.

Hydrocodone Bitartrate (Co-administration may result in increased drowsiness; caution should be exercised). Products include:
Hycodan ... 1104
Hycomine Compound Tablets ... 1105
Hycotuss Expectorant Syrup ... 1106
Lortab ... 3315
Lortab Elixir ... 3312
Vicodin Tablets ... 530
Vicodin ES Tablets ... 531
Vicodin HP Tablets ... 532
Vicoprofen Tablets ... 533
Zydone Tablets ... 1118

Hydrocodone Polistirex (Co-administration may result in increased drowsiness; caution should be exercised). Products include:
Tussionex Pennkinetic Extended-Release Suspension ... 3322

Hydromorphone Hydrochloride (Co-administration may result in increased drowsiness; caution should be exercised). Products include:
Dilaudid ... 439
Dilaudid Oral Liquid ... 443
Dilaudid Non-Sterile Powder ... 439
Dilaudid Rectal Suppositories ... 439
Dilaudid Tablets ... 439
Dilaudid Tablets - 8 mg ... 443
Dilaudid-HP ... 441

Hydroxyzine Hydrochloride (Co-administration may result in increased drowsiness; caution should be exercised).
No products indexed under this heading.

Isoflurane (Co-administration may result in increased drowsiness; caution should be exercised).
No products indexed under this heading.

Isradipine (Due to interaction between verapamil and dantrolene, combination of dantrolene and calcium channel blockers is not recommended during the management of malignant hyperthermia). Products include:
DynaCirc CR Tablets ... 2726

Ketamine Hydrochloride (Co-administration may result in increased drowsiness; caution should be exercised).
No products indexed under this heading.

Levomethadyl Acetate Hydrochloride (Co-administration may result in increased drowsiness; caution should be exercised).
No products indexed under this heading.

Levorphanol Tartrate (Co-administration may result in increased drowsiness; caution should be exercised).
No products indexed under this heading.

Lorazepam (Co-administration may result in increased drowsiness; caution should be exercised).
No products indexed under this heading.

Loxapine Hydrochloride (Co-administration may result in increased drowsiness; caution should be exercised).
No products indexed under this heading.

Loxapine Succinate (Co-administration may result in increased drowsiness; caution should be exercised).
No products indexed under this heading.

Meperidine Hydrochloride (Co-administration may result in increased drowsiness; caution should be exercised).
No products indexed under this heading.

Mephobarbital (Co-administration may result in increased drowsiness; caution should be exercised). Products include:
Mebaral Tablets, USP ... 2483

Meprobamate (Co-administration may result in increased drowsiness; caution should be exercised).
No products indexed under this heading.

Mesoridazine Besylate (Co-administration may result in increased drowsiness; caution should be exercised).
No products indexed under this heading.

Methadone Hydrochloride (Co-administration may result in increased drowsiness; caution should be exercised).
No products indexed under this heading.

Methohexital Sodium (Co-administration may result in increased drowsiness; caution should be exercised).
No products indexed under this heading.

Methotrimeprazine (Co-administration may result in increased drowsiness; caution should be exercised).
No products indexed under this heading.

Methoxyflurane (Co-administration may result in increased drowsiness; caution should be exercised).
No products indexed under this heading.

Mibefradil Dihydrochloride (Due to interaction between verapamil and dantrolene, combination of dantrolene and calcium channel blockers is not recommended during the management of malignant hyperthermia).
No products indexed under this heading.

Midazolam Hydrochloride (Co-administration may result in increased drowsiness; caution should be exercised).
No products indexed under this heading.

Molindone Hydrochloride (Co-administration may result in increased drowsiness; caution should be exercised). Products include:
Moban Tablets 1108

Morphine Sulfate (Co-administration may result in increased drowsiness; caution should be exercised). Products include:
Avinza Capsules 1714
Kadian Capsules 572
MS Contin Tablets 2703

Nicardipine Hydrochloride (Due to interaction between verapamil and dantrolene, combination of dantrolene and calcium channel blockers is not recommended during the management of malignant hyperthermia). Products include:
Cardene I.V. 1129

Nifedipine (Due to interaction between verapamil and dantrolene, combination of dantrolene and calcium channel blockers is not recommended during the management of malignant hyperthermia). Products include:
Adalat CC Tablets 2978

Nimodipine (Due to interaction between verapamil and dantrolene, combination of dantrolene and calcium channel blockers is not recommended during the management of malignant hyperthermia). Products include:
Nimotop Capsules 774

Nisoldipine (Due to interaction between verapamil and dantrolene, combination of dantrolene and calcium channel blockers is not recommended during the management of malignant hyperthermia). Products include:
Sular Tablets 1163

Olanzapine (Co-administration may result in increased drowsiness; caution should be exercised). Products include:
Symbyax Capsules 1788
Zyprexa Tablets 1798
Zyprexa IntraMuscular 1798
Zyprexa ZYDIS Orally Disintegrating Tablets 1798

Oxazepam (Co-administration may result in increased drowsiness; caution should be exercised).
No products indexed under this heading.

Oxycodone Hydrochloride (Co-administration may result in increased drowsiness; caution should be exercised). Products include:
Combunox Tablets 1183
OxyContin Tablets 2699
OxyFast Oral Concentrate Solution 2704
OxyIR Capsules 2704
Percocet Tablets 1114
Percodan Tablets 1115

Pentobarbital Sodium (Co-administration may result in increased drowsiness; caution should be exercised). Products include:
Nembutal Sodium Solution, USP 2484

Perphenazine (Co-administration may result in increased drowsiness; caution should be exercised).
No products indexed under this heading.

Phenobarbital (Co-administration may result in increased drowsiness; caution should be exercised).
No products indexed under this heading.

Polyestradiol Phosphate (Hepatotoxicity has occurred more often in women over 35 years of age receiving concomitant estrogen therapy).
No products indexed under this heading.

Prazepam (Co-administration may result in increased drowsiness; caution should be exercised).
No products indexed under this heading.

Prochlorperazine (Co-administration may result in increased drowsiness; caution should be exercised).
No products indexed under this heading.

Promethazine Hydrochloride (Co-administration may result in increased drowsiness; caution should be exercised). Products include:
Phenergan 3438

Propofol (Co-administration may result in increased drowsiness; caution should be exercised). Products include:
Diprivan Injectable Emulsion 676

Propoxyphene Hydrochloride (Co-administration may result in increased drowsiness; caution should be exercised).
No products indexed under this heading.

Propoxyphene Napsylate (Co-administration may result in increased drowsiness; caution should be exercised). Products include:
Darvocet A 500 Tablets 3497

Quazepam (Co-administration may result in increased drowsiness; caution should be exercised).
No products indexed under this heading.

Quetiapine Fumarate (Co-administration may result in increased drowsiness; caution should be exercised). Products include:
Seroquel Tablets 691

Quinestrol (Hepatotoxicity has occurred more often in women over 35 years of age receiving concomitant estrogen therapy).
No products indexed under this heading.

Remifentanil Hydrochloride (Co-administration may result in increased drowsiness; caution should be exercised).
No products indexed under this heading.

Risperidone (Co-administration may result in increased drowsiness; caution should be exercised). Products include:
Risperdal Consta Long-Acting Injection 1664
Risperdal M-Tab Orally Disintegrating Tablets 1658
Risperdal 1658

Secobarbital Sodium (Co-administration may result in increased drowsiness; caution should be exercised).
No products indexed under this heading.

Sevoflurane (Co-administration may result in increased drowsiness; caution should be exercised). Products include:
Ultane Liquid for Inhalation 526

Sufentanil Citrate (Co-administration may result in increased drowsiness; caution should be exercised).
No products indexed under this heading.

Temazepam (Co-administration may result in increased drowsiness; caution should be exercised).
No products indexed under this heading.

Thiamylal Sodium (Co-administration may result in increased drowsiness; caution should be exercised).
No products indexed under this heading.

Thioridazine Hydrochloride (Co-administration may result in increased drowsiness; caution should be exercised). Products include:
Thioridazine Hydrochloride Tablets 2122

Thiothixene (Co-administration may result in increased drowsiness; caution should be exercised). Products include:
Thiothixene Capsules 2124

Triazolam (Co-administration may result in increased drowsiness; caution should be exercised).
No products indexed under this heading.

Trifluoperazine Hydrochloride (Co-administration may result in increased drowsiness; caution should be exercised).
No products indexed under this heading.

Vecuronium Bromide (Co-administration may result in potentiation of vecuronium-induced neuromuscular block).
No products indexed under this heading.

Verapamil Hydrochloride (Simultaneous use has resulted in rare cases of cardiovascular collapse). Products include:
Covera-HS Tablets 3135
Tarka Tablets 519
Verelan PM Capsules 3120

Zaleplon (Co-administration may result in increased drowsiness; caution should be exercised). Products include:
Sonata Capsules 1686

Ziprasidone Hydrochloride (Co-administration may result in increased drowsiness; caution should be exercised). Products include:
Geodon Capsules 2514

Zolpidem Tartrate (Co-administration may result in increased drowsiness; caution should be exercised). Products include:
Ambien Tablets 2867

Food Interactions

Alcohol (Co-administration may result in increased drowsiness; caution should be exercised).

DANTRIUM INTRAVENOUS

(Dantrolene Sodium) 2691
May interact with:

Clofibrate (Reduces binding of dantrolene to plasma proteins).
No products indexed under this heading.

Tolbutamide (Increases binding of dantrolene to plasma proteins).
No products indexed under this heading.

Vecuronium Bromide (Administration of dantrolene may potentiate vecuronium-induced neuromuscular block).
No products indexed under this heading.

Verapamil Hydrochloride (The combination of therapeutic doses of intravenous dantrolene sodium and verapamil in halothane/alpha-chloralose anesthetized swine has resulted in ventricular fibrillation and cardiovascular collapse in association with hyperkalemia; it is recommended that this combination should not be used during the management of malignant hyperthermia crisis until the human data is available). Products include:
Covera-HS Tablets 3135
Tarka Tablets 519
Verelan PM Capsules 3120

Warfarin Sodium (Reduces binding of dantrolene to plasma proteins). Products include:
Coumadin for Injection 932
Coumadin Tablets 932

DAPSONE TABLETS USP

(Dapsone) 1656
May interact with:

Pyrimethamine (Agranulocytosis; increased likelihood of hematological reactions). Products include:
Daraprim Tablets 1385

Rifampin (Lowered Dapsone levels).
No products indexed under this heading.

Trimethoprim (Mutual interaction between Dapsone and trimethoprim in which each raises the level of the other about 1.5 times).
No products indexed under this heading.

DAPTACEL

(Diphtheria & Tetanus Toxoids and Acellular Pertussis Vaccine Adsorbed) **2964**
May interact with alkylating agents, antimetabolites, antineoplastics, corticosteroids, oral anticoagulants, and cytotoxic drugs. Compounds in these categories include:

Altretamine (May reduce the immune response to vaccine). Products include:
Hexalen Capsules **2101**

Anastrozole (May reduce the immune response to vaccine). Products include:
Arimidex Tablets **665**

Anisindione (Intra-muscular injection should be used with caution in patients on anticoagulant therapy). Products include:
Miradon Tablets **3056**

Asparaginase (May reduce the immune response to vaccine). Products include:
Elspar for Injection **1943**

Betamethasone Acetate (May reduce the immune response to vaccine when corticosteroids are used in greater than physiologic doses).
No products indexed under this heading.

Betamethasone Sodium Phosphate (May reduce the immune response to vaccine when corticosteroids are used in greater than physiologic doses).
No products indexed under this heading.

Bicalutamide (May reduce the immune response to vaccine). Products include:
Casodex Tablets **670**

Bleomycin Sulfate (May reduce the immune response to vaccine).
No products indexed under this heading.

Busulfan (May reduce the immune response to vaccine). Products include:
I.V. Busulfex **1125**
Myleran Tablets **1492**

Capecitabine (Immunosuppressive therapies may reduce the immune response to vaccines). Products include:
Xeloda Tablets **2825**

Carboplatin (May reduce the immune response to vaccine).
No products indexed under this heading.

Carmustine (BCNU) (May reduce the immune response to vaccine).
No products indexed under this heading.

Chlorambucil (May reduce the immune response to vaccine). Products include:
Leukeran Tablets **1472**

Cisplatin (May reduce the immune response to vaccine).
No products indexed under this heading.

Cladribine (Immunosuppressive therapies may reduce the immune response to vaccines). Products include:
Leustatin Injection **2368**

Cortisone Acetate (May reduce the immune response to vaccine when corticosteroids are used in greater than physiologic doses).
No products indexed under this heading.

Cyclophosphamide (May reduce the immune response to vaccine).
No products indexed under this heading.

Cytarabine (Immunosuppressive therapies may reduce the immune response to vaccines).
No products indexed under this heading.

Dacarbazine (May reduce the immune response to vaccine).
No products indexed under this heading.

Daunorubicin Citrate (May reduce the immune response to vaccine).
No products indexed under this heading.

Daunorubicin Hydrochloride (May reduce the immune response to vaccine). Products include:
Cerubidine for Injection **788**

Denileukin Diftitox (May reduce the immune response to vaccine). Products include:
Ontak Vials **1717**

Dexamethasone (May reduce the immune response to vaccine when corticosteroids are used in greater than physiologic doses). Products include:
Ciprodex Otic Suspension **555**
Decadron Tablets **1929**
TobraDex Ophthalmic Ointment **558**
TobraDex Ophthalmic Suspension ... **558**

Dexamethasone Acetate (May reduce the immune response to vaccine when corticosteroids are used in greater than physiologic doses).
No products indexed under this heading.

Dexamethasone Sodium Phosphate (May reduce the immune response to vaccine when corticosteroids are used in greater than physiologic doses). Products include:
Decadron Phosphate Injection **1931**

Dicumarol (Intra-muscular injection should be used with caution in patients on anticoagulant therapy).
No products indexed under this heading.

Docetaxel (May reduce the immune response to vaccine). Products include:
Taxotere Injection Concentrate **2947**

Doxorubicin Hydrochloride (May reduce the immune response to vaccine). Products include:
Adriamycin for Injection, USP **786**
Adriamycin Injection, USP **786**

Epirubicin Hydrochloride (May reduce the immune response to vaccine). Products include:
Ellence Injection **2632**

Estramustine Phosphate Sodium (May reduce the immune response to vaccine). Products include:
Emcyt Capsules **3137**

Etoposide (May reduce the immune response to vaccine).
No products indexed under this heading.

Exemestane (May reduce the immune response to vaccine). Products include:
Aromasin Tablets **2600**

Floxuridine (May reduce the immune response to vaccine).
No products indexed under this heading.

Fludarabine Phosphate (Immunosuppressive therapies may reduce the immune response to vaccines).
No products indexed under this heading.

Fludrocortisone Acetate (May reduce the immune response to vaccine when corticosteroids are used in greater than physiologic doses).
No products indexed under this heading.

Fluorouracil (May reduce the immune response to vaccine). Products include:
Carac Cream, 0.5% **1048**
Efudex **3348**

Flutamide (May reduce the immune response to vaccine). Products include:
Eulexin Capsules **3023**

Gemcitabine Hydrochloride (May reduce the immune response to vaccine). Products include:
Gemzar for Injection **1743**

Hydrocortisone (May reduce the immune response to vaccine when corticosteroids are used in greater than physiologic doses). Products include:
Cortizone•5 Ointment **699**
Cortizone•10 Creme **699**
Cortizone•10 Ointment **699**
Cortizone•10 Plus Creme **700**
Cortizone•10 Maximum Strength Quick Shot Spray **700**
Hydrocortone Tablets **1963**
Preparation H Hydrocortisone Cream **748**

Hydrocortisone Acetate (May reduce the immune response to vaccine when corticosteroids are used in greater than physiologic doses). Products include:
Analpram-HC **1136**
Pramosone **1139**
ProctoFoam-HC **3113**
Tucks Anti-Itch Ointment **712**
U-cort 1% Cream **3289**

Hydrocortisone Sodium Phosphate (May reduce the immune response to vaccine when corticosteroids are used in greater than physiologic doses).
No products indexed under this heading.

Hydrocortisone Sodium Succinate (May reduce the immune response to vaccine when corticosteroids are used in greater than physiologic doses).
No products indexed under this heading.

Hydroxyurea (May reduce the immune response to vaccine).
No products indexed under this heading.

Idarubicin Hydrochloride (May reduce the immune response to vaccine). Products include:
Idamycin PFS Injection **2645**

Ifosfamide (May reduce the immune response to vaccine).
No products indexed under this heading.

Interferon alfa-2a, Recombinant (May reduce the immune response to vaccine). Products include:
Roferon-A Injection **2805**

Interferon alfa-2b, Recombinant (May reduce the immune response to vaccine). Products include:
Intron A for Injection **3038**
Rebetron Combination Therapy **3078**

Irinotecan Hydrochloride (May reduce the immune response to vaccine). Products include:
Camptosar Injection **2602**

Levamisole Hydrochloride (May reduce the immune response to vaccine).
No products indexed under this heading.

Lomustine (CCNU) (May reduce the immune response to vaccine).
No products indexed under this heading.

Mechlorethamine Hydrochloride (May reduce the immune response to vaccine). Products include:
Mustargen for Injection **2007**

Megestrol Acetate (May reduce the immune response to vaccine). Products include:
Megace ES Oral Suspension **2492**

Melphalan (May reduce the immune response to vaccine). Products include:
Alkeran Tablets **977**

Mercaptopurine (May reduce the immune response to vaccine). Products include:
Purinethol Tablets **1222**

Methotrexate (Immunosuppressive therapies may reduce the immune response to vaccines).
No products indexed under this heading.

Methotrexate Sodium (May reduce the immune response to vaccine).
No products indexed under this heading.

Methylprednisolone Acetate (May reduce the immune response to vaccine when corticosteroids are used in greater than physiologic doses). Products include:
Depo-Medrol Injectable Suspension **2615**
Depo-Medrol Single-Dose Vial **2617**

Methylprednisolone Sodium Succinate (May reduce the immune response to vaccine when corticosteroids are used in greater than physiologic doses).
No products indexed under this heading.

Mitomycin (Mitomycin-C) (May reduce the immune response to vaccine).
No products indexed under this heading.

Mitotane (May reduce the immune response to vaccine).
No products indexed under this heading.

Mitoxantrone Hydrochloride (May reduce the immune response to vaccine). Products include:
Novantrone for Injection Concentrate **3158**

Oxaliplatin (May reduce the immune response to vaccine). Products include:
Eloxatin for Injection **2908**

Paclitaxel (May reduce the immune response to vaccine).
No products indexed under this heading.

Pentostatin (Immunosuppressive therapies may reduce the immune response to vaccines). Products include:
Nipent for Injection **3216**

Prednisolone Acetate (May reduce the immune response to vaccine when corticosteroids are used in greater than physiologic doses). Products include:

Blephamide Ophthalmic Ointment 563
Blephamide Ophthalmic Suspension 564
Poly-Pred Liquifilm Ophthalmic Suspension .... ⊙231
Pred Forte Ophthalmic Suspension .... ⊙233
Pred Mild Sterile Ophthalmic Suspension .... ⊙236
Pred-G Ophthalmic Suspension .... ⊙234
Pred-G Sterile Ophthalmic Ointment .... ⊙235

Prednisolone Sodium Phosphate (May reduce the immune response to vaccine when corticosteroids are used in greater than physiologic doses). Products include:
Pediapred Oral Solution 3319

Prednisolone Tebutate (May reduce the immune response to vaccine when corticosteroids are used in greater than physiologic doses).
No products indexed under this heading.

Prednisone (May reduce the immune response to vaccine when corticosteroids are used in greater than physiologic doses).
No products indexed under this heading.

Procarbazine Hydrochloride (May reduce the immune response to vaccine). Products include:
Matulane Capsules 3188

Streptozocin (May reduce the immune response to vaccine).
No products indexed under this heading.

Tamoxifen Citrate (May reduce the immune response to vaccine).
No products indexed under this heading.

Teniposide (May reduce the immune response to vaccine).
No products indexed under this heading.

Thioguanine (May reduce the immune response to vaccine). Products include:
Tabloid Tablets 1545

Thiotepa (May reduce the immune response to vaccine).
No products indexed under this heading.

Topotecan Hydrochloride (May reduce the immune response to vaccine). Products include:
Hycamtin for Injection 1427

Toremifene Citrate (May reduce the immune response to vaccine).
No products indexed under this heading.

Triamcinolone (May reduce the immune response to vaccine when corticosteroids are used in greater than physiologic doses).
No products indexed under this heading.

Triamcinolone Acetonide (May reduce the immune response to vaccine when corticosteroids are used in greater than physiologic doses). Products include:
Azmacort Inhalation Aerosol 1701
Nasacort HFA Inhalation Aerosol 2939
Nasacort AQ Nasal Spray 2937

Triamcinolone Diacetate (May reduce the immune response to vaccine when corticosteroids are used in greater than physiologic doses).
No products indexed under this heading.

Triamcinolone Hexacetonide (May reduce the immune response to vaccine when corticosteroids are used in greater than physiologic doses).
No products indexed under this heading.

Valrubicin (May reduce the immune response to vaccine).
No products indexed under this heading.

Vincristine Sulfate (May reduce the immune response to vaccine).
No products indexed under this heading.

Vinorelbine Tartrate (May reduce the immune response to vaccine). Products include:
Navelbine Injection 1494

Warfarin Sodium (Intra-muscular injection should be used with caution in patients on anticoagulant therapy). Products include:
Coumadin for Injection 932
Coumadin Tablets 932

DARANIDE TABLETS

(Dichlorphenamide) 1928
May interact with corticosteroids and certain other agents. Compounds in these categories include:

ACTH (Hypokalemia may develop).
No products indexed under this heading.

Aspirin (Concomitant high-dose aspirin may produce anorexia, tachypnea, lethargy and coma). Products include:
Aggrenox Capsules 855
Bayer, Aspirin Regimen .... ■606
Bayer Aspirin Tablets 3515
BC Powder .... ■612
BC Allergy Sinus Cold Powder .... ■612
Arthritis Strength BC Powder .... ■612
BC Sinus Cold Powder .... ■612
Ecotrin Enteric Coated Aspirin Low, Regular and Maximum Strength Tablets 1627
Goody's Body Pain Formula Powder .... ■621
Goody's Extra Strength Headache Powder .... ■621
Goody's Extra Strength Pain Relief Tablets .... ■621
Percodan Tablets 1115
St. Joseph 81 mg Aspirin Chewable and Enteric Coated Tablets 1841

Aspirin, Enteric Coated (Concomitant high-dose aspirin may produce anorexia, tachypnea, lethargy and coma).
No products indexed under this heading.

Betamethasone Acetate (Hypokalemia may develop).
No products indexed under this heading.

Betamethasone Sodium Phosphate (Hypokalemia may develop).
No products indexed under this heading.

Cortisone Acetate (Hypokalemia may develop).
No products indexed under this heading.

Dexamethasone (Hypokalemia may develop). Products include:
Ciprodex Otic Suspension 555
Decadron Tablets 1929
TobraDex Ophthalmic Ointment 558
TobraDex Ophthalmic Suspension 558

Dexamethasone Acetate (Hypokalemia may develop).
No products indexed under this heading.

Dexamethasone Sodium Phosphate (Hypokalemia may develop). Products include:
Decadron Phosphate Injection 1931

Fludrocortisone Acetate (Hypokalemia may develop).
No products indexed under this heading.

Hydrocortisone (Hypokalemia may develop). Products include:
Cortizone•5 Ointment .... ■699
Cortizone•10 Creme .... ■699
Cortizone•10 Ointment .... ■699
Cortizone•10 Plus Creme .... ■700
Cortizone•10 Maximum Strength Quick Shot Spray .... ■700
Hydrocortone Tablets 1963
Preparation H Hydrocortisone Cream .... ■748

Hydrocortisone Acetate (Hypokalemia may develop). Products include:
Analpram-HC 1136
Pramosone 1139
ProctoFoam-HC 3113
Tucks Anti-Itch Ointment .... ■712
U-cort 1% Cream 3289

Hydrocortisone Sodium Phosphate (Hypokalemia may develop).
No products indexed under this heading.

Hydrocortisone Sodium Succinate (Hypokalemia may develop).
No products indexed under this heading.

Methylprednisolone Acetate (Hypokalemia may develop). Products include:
Depo-Medrol Injectable Suspension 2615
Depo-Medrol Single-Dose Vial 2617

Methylprednisolone Sodium Succinate (Hypokalemia may develop).
No products indexed under this heading.

Prednisolone Acetate (Hypokalemia may develop). Products include:
Blephamide Ophthalmic Ointment 563
Blephamide Ophthalmic Suspension 564
Poly-Pred Liquifilm Ophthalmic Suspension .... ⊙231
Pred Forte Ophthalmic Suspension .... ⊙233
Pred Mild Sterile Ophthalmic Suspension .... ⊙236
Pred-G Ophthalmic Suspension .... ⊙234
Pred-G Sterile Ophthalmic Ointment .... ⊙235

Prednisolone Sodium Phosphate (Hypokalemia may develop). Products include:
Pediapred Oral Solution 3319

Prednisolone Tebutate (Hypokalemia may develop).
No products indexed under this heading.

Prednisone (Hypokalemia may develop).
No products indexed under this heading.

Triamcinolone (Hypokalemia may develop).
No products indexed under this heading.

Triamcinolone Acetonide (Hypokalemia may develop). Products include:
Azmacort Inhalation Aerosol 1701
Nasacort HFA Inhalation Aerosol 2939
Nasacort AQ Nasal Spray 2937

Triamcinolone Diacetate (Hypokalemia may develop).
No products indexed under this heading.

Triamcinolone Hexacetonide (Hypokalemia may develop).
No products indexed under this heading.

DARAPRIM TABLETS

(Pyrimethamine) 1385
May interact with cytotoxic drugs, dihydrofolate reductase inhibitors, agents associated with myelosuppression, phenytoin, sulfonamides, and certain other agents. Compounds in these categories include:

Altretamine (The concomitant use of other antifolic drugs or agents associated with myelosuppression including cytostatic agents while the patient is receiving pyrimethamine, may increase the risk of bone marrow suppression). Products include:
Hexalen Capsules 2101

Bendroflumethiazide (Co-administration of other antifolic drugs, such as sulfonamides, may increase the risk of bone marrow suppression; potential for hypersensitivity reactions such as Stevens-Johnson syndrome, toxic epidermal necrolysis, erythema multiforme, and anaphylaxis).
No products indexed under this heading.

Bleomycin Sulfate (The concomitant use of other antifolic drugs or agents associated with myelosuppression including cytostatic agents while the patient is receiving pyrimethamine, may increase the risk of bone marrow suppression).
No products indexed under this heading.

Busulfan (The concomitant use of other antifolic drugs or agents associated with myelosuppression including cytostatic agents while the patient is receiving pyrimethamine, may increase the risk of bone marrow suppression). Products include:
I.V. Busulfex 1125
Myleran Tablets 1492

Chlorambucil (The concomitant use of other antifolic drugs or agents associated with myelosuppression including cytostatic agents while the patient is receiving pyrimethamine, may increase the risk of bone marrow suppression). Products include:
Leukeran Tablets 1472

Chlorothiazide (Co-administration of other antifolic drugs, such as sulfonamides, may increase the risk of bone marrow suppression; potential for hypersensitivity reactions such as Stevens-Johnson syndrome, toxic epidermal necrolysis, erythema multiforme, and anaphylaxis). Products include:
Aldoclor Tablets 1881
Diuril Oral 1936

Chlorothiazide Sodium (Co-administration of other antifolic drugs, such as sulfonamides, may increase the risk of bone marrow suppression; potential for hypersensitivity reactions such as Stevens-Johnson syndrome, toxic epidermal necrolysis, erythema multiforme, and anaphylaxis). Products include:
Diuril Sodium Intravenous 1934

Chlorpropamide (Co-administration of other antifolic drugs, such as sulfonamides, may increase the risk of bone marrow suppression; potential for hypersensitivity reactions such as Stevens-Johnson syndrome, toxic epidermal necrolysis, erythema multiforme, and anaphylaxis).
No products indexed under this heading.

Cladribine (The concomitant use of other antifolic drugs or agents associated with myelosuppression including cytostatic agents while the patient is receiving pyrimethamine, may increase the risk of bone marrow suppression). Products include:
Leustatin Injection 2368

Cyclophosphamide (The concomitant use of other antifolic drugs or agents associated with myelosuppression including cytostatic agents while the patient is receiving pyrimethamine, may increase the risk of bone marrow suppression).
No products indexed under this heading.

Daunorubicin Citrate Liposome (The concomitant use of other antifolic drugs or agents associated with myelosuppression including cytostatic agents while the patient is receiving pyrimethamine, may increase the risk of bone marrow suppression).
No products indexed under this heading.

Daunorubicin Hydrochloride (The concomitant use of other antifolic drugs or agents associated with myelosuppression including cytostatic agents while the patient is receiving pyrimethamine, may increase the risk of bone marrow suppression). Products include:
Cerubidine for Injection 788

Dexrazoxane (The concomitant use of other antifolic drugs or agents associated with myelosuppression including cytostatic agents while the patient is receiving pyrimethamine, may increase the risk of bone marrow suppression). Products include:
Zinecard for Injection 2659

Doxorubicin Hydrochloride (The concomitant use of other antifolic drugs or agents associated with myelosuppression including cytostatic agents while the patient is receiving pyrimethamine, may increase the risk of bone marrow suppression). Products include:
Adriamycin for Injection, USP 786
Adriamycin Injection, USP 786

Doxorubicin Hydrochloride Liposome (The concomitant use of other antifolic drugs or agents associated with myelosuppression including cytostatic agents while the patient is receiving pyrimethamine, may increase the risk of bone marrow suppression). Products include:
Doxil Injection 3302

Epirubicin Hydrochloride (The concomitant use of other antifolic drugs or agents associated with myelosuppression including cytostatic agents while the patient is receiving pyrimethamine, may increase the risk of bone marrow suppression). Products include:
Ellence Injection 2632

Fludarabine Phosphate (The concomitant use of other antifolic drugs or agents associated with myelosuppression including cytostatic agents while the patient is receiving pyrimethamine, may increase the risk of bone marrow suppression).
No products indexed under this heading.

Fluorouracil (The concomitant use of other antifolic drugs or agents associated with myelosuppression including cytostatic agents while the patient is receiving pyrimethamine, may increase the risk of bone marrow suppression). Products include:
Carac Cream, 0.5% 1048
Efudex 3348

Fosphenytoin Sodium (Co-administration with agents that affect folate levels, such as phenytoin, should be undertaken with caution).
No products indexed under this heading.

Gemcitabine Hydrochloride (The concomitant use of other antifolic drugs or agents associated with myelosuppression including cytostatic agents while the patient is receiving pyrimethamine, may increase the risk of bone marrow suppression). Products include:
Gemzar for Injection 1743

Gemtuzumab Ozogamicin (The concomitant use of other antifolic drugs or agents associated with myelosuppression including cytostatic agents while the patient is receiving pyrimethamine, may increase the risk of bone marrow suppression). Products include:
Mylotarg for Injection 3429

Glipizide (Co-administration of other antifolic drugs, such as sulfonamides, may increase the risk of bone marrow suppression; potential for hypersensitivity reactions such as Stevens-Johnson syndrome, toxic epidermal necrolysis, erythema multiforme, and anaphylaxis).
No products indexed under this heading.

Glyburide (Co-administration of other antifolic drugs, such as sulfonamides, may increase the risk of bone marrow suppression; potential for hypersensitivity reactions such as Stevens-Johnson syndrome, toxic epidermal necrolysis, erythema multiforme, and anaphylaxis).
No products indexed under this heading.

Hydrochlorothiazide (Co-administration of other antifolic drugs, such as sulfonamides, may increase the risk of bone marrow suppression; potential for hypersensitivity reactions such as Stevens-Johnson syndrome, toxic epidermal necrolysis, erythema multiforme, and anaphylaxis). Products include:
Aldoril Tablets 1884
Atacand HCT 637
Avalide Tablets 2889
Avalide Tablets 922
Benicar HCT Tablets 2852
Diovan HCT Tablets 2195
Dyazide Capsules 1389
Hyzaar 1964
Lotensin HCT Tablets 2235
Maxzide 2150
Micardis HCT Tablets 886
Moduretic Tablets 2003
Prinzide Tablets 2033
Teveten HCT Tablets 1710
Timolide Tablets 2056
Uniretic Tablets 3114
Vaseretic Tablets 2073
Zestoretic Tablets 701

Hydroflumethiazide (Co-administration of other antifolic drugs, such as sulfonamides, may increase the risk of bone marrow suppression; potential for hypersensitivity reactions such as Stevens-Johnson syndrome, toxic epidermal necrolysis, erythema multiforme, and anaphylaxis).
No products indexed under this heading.

Hydroxyurea (The concomitant use of other antifolic drugs or agents associated with myelosuppression including cytostatic agents while the patient is receiving pyrimethamine, may increase the risk of bone marrow suppression).
No products indexed under this heading.

Idarubicin Hydrochloride (The concomitant use of other antifolic drugs or agents associated with myelosuppression including cytostatic agents while the patient is receiving pyrimethamine, may increase the risk of bone marrow suppression). Products include:
Idamycin PFS Injection 2645

Interferon alfa-2a, Recombinant (The concomitant use of other antifolic drugs or agents associated with myelosuppression including cytostatic agents while the patient is receiving pyrimethamine, may increase the risk of bone marrow suppression). Products include:
Roferon-A Injection 2805

Irinotecan Hydrochloride (The concomitant use of other antifolic drugs or agents associated with myelosuppression including cytostatic agents while the patient is receiving pyrimethamine, may increase the risk of bone marrow suppression). Products include:
Camptosar Injection 2602

Lamotrigine (The concomitant use of other antifolic drugs, while the patient is receiving pyrimethamine, may increase the risk of bone marrow suppression). Products include:
Lamictal 1449

Lorazepam (Concomitant therapy may result in mild hepatotoxicity).
No products indexed under this heading.

Melphalan Hydrochloride (The concomitant use of other antifolic drugs or agents associated with myelosuppression including cytostatic agents while the patient is receiving pyrimethamine, may increase the risk of bone marrow suppression). Products include:
Alkeran for Injection 976

Mercaptopurine (The concomitant use of other antifolic drugs or agents associated with myelosuppression including cytostatic agents while the patient is receiving pyrimethamine, may increase the risk of bone marrow suppression). Products include:
Purinethol Tablets 1222

Methotrexate Sodium (The concomitant use of other antifolic drugs or agents associated with myelosuppression including cytostatic agents while the patient is receiving pyrimethamine, may increase the risk of bone marrow suppression).
No products indexed under this heading.

Methyclothiazide (Co-administration of other antifolic drugs, such as sulfonamides, may increase the risk of bone marrow suppression; potential for hypersensitivity reactions such as Stevens-Johnson syndrome, toxic epidermal necrolysis, erythema multiforme, and anaphylaxis).
No products indexed under this heading.

Mitotane (The concomitant use of other antifolic drugs or agents associated with myelosuppression including cytostatic agents while the patient is receiving pyrimethamine, may increase the risk of bone marrow suppression).
No products indexed under this heading.

Mitoxantrone Hydrochloride (The concomitant use of other antifolic drugs or agents associated with myelosuppression including cytostatic agents while the patient is receiving pyrimethamine, may increase the risk of bone marrow suppression). Products include:
Novantrone for Injection Concentrate 3158

Phenytoin (Co-administration with agents that affect folate levels, such as phenytoin, should be undertaken with caution).
No products indexed under this heading.

Phenytoin Sodium (Co-administration with agents that affect folate levels, such as phenytoin, should be undertaken with caution). Products include:
Phenytek Capsules 2153

Polythiazide (Co-administration of other antifolic drugs, such as sulfonamides, may increase the risk of bone marrow suppression; potential for hypersensitivity reactions such as Stevens-Johnson syndrome, toxic epidermal necrolysis, erythema multiforme, and anaphylaxis).
No products indexed under this heading.

Procarbazine Hydrochloride (The concomitant use of other antifolic drugs or agents associated with myelosuppression including cytostatic agents while the patient is receiving pyrimethamine, may increase the risk of bone marrow suppression). Products include:
Matulane Capsules 3188

Proguanil (May increase risk of bone marrow suppression).
No products indexed under this heading.

Sulfacytine (Co-administration of other antifolic drugs, such as sulfonamides, may increase the risk of bone marrow suppression; potential for hypersensitivity reactions such as Stevens-Johnson syndrome, toxic epidermal necrolysis, erythema multiforme, and anaphylaxis).
No products indexed under this heading.

Sulfamethizole (Co-administration of other antifolic drugs, such as sulfonamides, may increase the risk of bone marrow suppression; potential for hypersensitivity reactions such as Stevens-Johnson syndrome, toxic epidermal necrolysis, erythema multiforme, and anaphylaxis).
No products indexed under this heading.

Sulfamethoxazole (Co-administration of other antifolic drugs, such as sulfonamides, may increase the risk of bone marrow suppression; potential for hypersensitivity reactions such as Stevens-Johnson syndrome, toxic epidermal necrolysis, erythema multiforme, and anaphylaxis).
No products indexed under this heading.

Sulfasalazine (Co-administration of other antifolic drugs, such as sulfonamides, may increase the risk of bone marrow suppression; potential for hypersensitivity reactions such as Stevens-Johnson syndrome, toxic epidermal necrolysis, erythema multiforme, and anaphylaxis).
No products indexed under this heading.

Sulfinpyrazone (Co-administration of other antifolic drugs, such as sulfonamides, may increase the risk of bone marrow suppression; potential for hypersensitivity reactions such as Stevens-Johnson syndrome, toxic epidermal necrolysis, erythema multiforme, and anaphylaxis).
No products indexed under this heading.

Sulfisoxazole (Co-administration of other antifolic drugs, such as sulfonamides, may increase the risk of bone marrow suppression; potential for hypersensitivity reactions such as Stevens-Johnson syndrome, toxic epidermal necrolysis, erythema multiforme, and anaphylaxis).
No products indexed under this heading.

Sulfisoxazole Acetyl (Co-administration of other antifolic drugs, such as sulfonamides, may increase the risk of bone marrow suppression; potential for hypersensitivity reactions such as Stevens-Johnson syndrome, toxic epidermal necrolysis, erythema multiforme, and anaphylaxis).
No products indexed under this heading.

Sulfisoxazole Diolamine (Co-administration of other antifolic drugs, such as sulfonamides, may increase the risk of bone marrow suppression; potential for hypersensitivity reactions such as Stevens-Johnson syndrome, toxic epidermal necrolysis, erythema multiforme, and anaphylaxis).
No products indexed under this heading.

Tamoxifen Citrate (The concomitant use of other antifolic drugs or agents associated with myelosuppression including cytostatic agents while the patient is receiving pyrimethamine, may increase the risk of bone marrow suppression).
No products indexed under this heading.

Temozolomide (The concomitant use of other antifolic drugs or agents associated with myelosuppression including cytostatic agents while the patient is receiving pyrimethamine, may increase the risk of bone marrow suppression). Products include:
Temodar Capsules 3088

Thioguanine (The concomitant use of other antifolic drugs or agents associated with myelosuppression including cytostatic agents while the patient is receiving pyrimethamine, may increase the risk of bone marrow suppression). Products include:
Tabloid Tablets 1545

Tolazamide (Co-administration of other antifolic drugs, such as sulfonamides, may increase the risk of bone marrow suppression; potential for hypersensitivity reactions such as Stevens-Johnson syndrome, toxic epidermal necrolysis, erythema multiforme, and anaphylaxis).
No products indexed under this heading.

Tolbutamide (Co-administration of other antifolic drugs, such as sulfonamides, may increase the risk of bone marrow suppression; potential for hypersensitivity reactions such as Stevens-Johnson syndrome, toxic epidermal necrolysis, erythema multiforme, and anaphylaxis).
No products indexed under this heading.

Trimethoprim (Co-administration of other antifolic drugs, such as sulfonamides or trimethoprim-sulfamethoxazole combinations, may increase the risk of bone marrow suppression; potential for hypersensitivity reactions such as Stevens-Johnson syndrome, toxic epidermal necrolysis, erythema multiforme, and anaphylaxis).
No products indexed under this heading.

Trimetrexate Glucuronate (The concomitant use of other antifolic drugs, while the patient is receiving pyrimethamine, may increase the risk of bone marrow suppression).
No products indexed under this heading.

Vincristine Sulfate (The concomitant use of other antifolic drugs or agents associated with myelosuppression including cytostatic agents while the patient is receiving pyrimethamine, may increase the risk of bone marrow suppression).
No products indexed under this heading.

Vinorelbine Tartrate (The concomitant use of other antifolic drugs or agents associated with myelosuppression including cytostatic agents while the patient is receiving pyrimethamine, may increase the risk of bone marrow suppression). Products include:
Navelbine Injection 1494

Zidovudine (May increase risk of bone marrow suppression). Products include:
Combivir Tablets 1373
Retrovir 1533
Retrovir IV Infusion 1537
Trizivir Tablets 1565

DARVOCET A 500 TABLETS

(Acetaminophen, Propoxyphene Napsylate) 3497
May interact with central nervous system depressants, oral anticoagulants, antidepressant drugs, anticonvulsants, and certain other agents. Compounds in these categories include:

Alfentanil Hydrochloride (Co-administration with CNS depressants results in additive CNS depressant effects).
No products indexed under this heading.

Alprazolam (Co-administration with CNS depressants results in additive CNS depressant effects). Products include:
Niravam Orally Disintegrating Tablets 3106
Xanax XR Tablets 2655

Amitriptyline Hydrochloride (Propoxyphene may slow the metabolism of antidepressants leading to higher serum levels of antidepressants).
No products indexed under this heading.

Amoxapine (Propoxyphene may slow the metabolism of antidepressants leading to higher serum levels of antidepressants).
No products indexed under this heading.

Anisindione (Propoxyphene may slow the metabolism of anticoagulants leading to higher serum levels of anticoagulants). Products include:
Miradon Tablets 3056

Aprobarbital (Co-administration with CNS depressants results in additive CNS depressant effects).
No products indexed under this heading.

Buprenorphine Hydrochloride (Co-administration with CNS depressants results in additive CNS depressant effects). Products include:
Buprenex Injectable 2718
Suboxone Tablets 2719
Subutex Tablets 2719

Bupropion Hydrochloride (Propoxyphene may slow the metabolism of antidepressants leading to higher serum levels of antidepressants). Products include:
Wellbutrin Tablets 1579
Wellbutrin SR Sustained-Release Tablets 1583
Wellbutrin XL Extended-Release Tablets 1588
Zyban Sustained-Release Tablets 1620

Buspirone Hydrochloride (Co-administration with CNS depressants results in additive CNS depressant effects).
No products indexed under this heading.

Butabarbital (Co-administration with CNS depressants results in additive CNS depressant effects).
No products indexed under this heading.

Butalbital (Co-administration with CNS depressants results in additive CNS depressant effects). Products include:
Sedapap Tablets 50 mg/650 mg 2098

Carbamazepine (Co-administration has resulted in severe neurologic signs, including coma). Products include:
Carbatrol Capsules 3174
Equetro Extended-Release Capsules 3178
Tegretol/Tegretol-XR 2278

Chlordiazepoxide (Co-administration with CNS depressants results in additive CNS depressant effects).
No products indexed under this heading.

Chlordiazepoxide Hydrochloride (Co-administration with CNS depressants results in additive CNS depressant effects). Products include:
Librium Capsules 3349

Chlorpromazine (Co-administration with CNS depressants results in additive CNS depressant effects).
No products indexed under this heading.

Chlorpromazine Hydrochloride (Co-administration with CNS depressants results in additive CNS depressant effects).
No products indexed under this heading.

Chlorprothixene (Co-administration with CNS depressants results in additive CNS depressant effects).
No products indexed under this heading.

Chlorprothixene Hydrochloride (Co-administration with CNS depressants results in additive CNS depressant effects).
No products indexed under this heading.

Chlorprothixene Lactate (Co-administration with CNS depressants results in additive CNS depressant effects).
No products indexed under this heading.

Citalopram Hydrobromide (Propoxyphene may slow the metabolism of antidepressants leading to higher serum levels of antidepressants). Products include:
Celexa 1177

Clorazepate Dipotassium (Co-administration with CNS depressants results in additive CNS depressant effects). Products include:
Tranxene 2488

Clozapine (Co-administration with CNS depressants results in additive CNS depressant effects). Products include:
Clozapine Tablets 2141
Clozaril Tablets 2174
FazaClo Orally Disintegrating Tablets 547

Codeine Phosphate (Co-administration with CNS depressants results in additive CNS depressant effects). Products include:
Tylenol with Codeine 2461

Desflurane (Co-administration with CNS depressants results in additive CNS depressant effects). Products include:
Suprane Liquid for Inhalation 770

Desipramine Hydrochloride (Propoxyphene may slow the metabolism of antidepressants leading to higher serum levels of antidepressants).
No products indexed under this heading.

Dezocine (Co-administration with CNS depressants results in additive CNS depressant effects).
No products indexed under this heading.

Diazepam (Co-administration with CNS depressants results in additive CNS depressant effects). Products include:
Diastat Rectal Delivery System 3344
Valium Tablets 2822

Dicumarol (Propoxyphene may slow the metabolism of anticoagulants leading to higher serum levels of anticoagulants).
No products indexed under this heading.

Divalproex Sodium (Propoxyphene may slow the metabolism of anticonvulsants leading to higher serum levels of anticonvulsants). Products include:
Depakote Sprinkle Capsules 422
Depakote Tablets 427
Depakote ER Tablets 433

Doxepin Hydrochloride (Propoxyphene may slow the metabolism of antidepressants leading to higher serum levels of antidepressants).
No products indexed under this heading.

Droperidol (Co-administration with CNS depressants results in additive CNS depressant effects).
No products indexed under this heading.

Enflurane (Co-administration with CNS depressants results in additive CNS depressant effects).
No products indexed under this heading.

Estazolam (Co-administration with CNS depressants results in additive CNS depressant effects). Products include:
ProSom Tablets **512**

Ethanol (Co-administration with CNS depressants results in additive CNS depressant effects).
No products indexed under this heading.

Ethchlorvynol (Co-administration with CNS depressants results in additive CNS depressant effects).
No products indexed under this heading.

Ethinamate (Co-administration with CNS depressants results in additive CNS depressant effects).
No products indexed under this heading.

Ethosuximide (Propoxyphene may slow the metabolism of anticonvulsants leading to higher serum levels of anticonvulsants).
No products indexed under this heading.

Ethotoin (Propoxyphene may slow the metabolism of anticonvulsants leading to higher serum levels of anticonvulsants). Products include:
Peganone Tablets, USP **2487**

Ethyl Alcohol (Co-administration with CNS depressants results in additive CNS depressant effects).
No products indexed under this heading.

Felbamate (Propoxyphene may slow the metabolism of anticonvulsants leading to higher serum levels of anticonvulsants).
No products indexed under this heading.

Fentanyl (Co-administration with CNS depressants results in additive CNS depressant effects). Products include:
Duragesic Transdermal System **2448**

Fentanyl Citrate (Co-administration with CNS depressants results in additive CNS depressant effects). Products include:
Actiq **993**

Fluoxetine Hydrochloride (Propoxyphene may slow the metabolism of antidepressants leading to higher serum levels of antidepressants). Products include:
Prozac Pulvules and Liquid **1771**
Symbyax Capsules **1788**

Fluphenazine Decanoate (Co-administration with CNS depressants results in additive CNS depressant effects).
No products indexed under this heading.

Fluphenazine Enanthate (Co-administration with CNS depressants results in additive CNS depressant effects).
No products indexed under this heading.

Fluphenazine Hydrochloride (Co-administration with CNS depressants results in additive CNS depressant effects).
No products indexed under this heading.

Flurazepam Hydrochloride (Co-administration with CNS depressants results in additive CNS depressant effects). Products include:
Dalmane Capsules **3343**

Fosphenytoin (Propoxyphene may slow the metabolism of anticonvulsants leading to higher serum levels of anticonvulsants).
No products indexed under this heading.

Fosphenytoin Sodium (Propoxyphene may slow the metabolism of anticonvulsants leading to higher serum levels of anticonvulsants).
No products indexed under this heading.

Gabapentin (Propoxyphene may slow the metabolism of anticonvulsants leading to higher serum levels of anticonvulsants). Products include:
Neurontin Capsules **2498**
Neurontin Oral Solution **2498**
Neurontin Tablets **2498**

Glutethimide (Co-administration with CNS depressants results in additive CNS depressant effects).
No products indexed under this heading.

Haloperidol (Co-administration with CNS depressants results in additive CNS depressant effects).
No products indexed under this heading.

Haloperidol Decanoate (Co-administration with CNS depressants results in additive CNS depressant effects).
No products indexed under this heading.

Hydrocodone Bitartrate (Co-administration with CNS depressants results in additive CNS depressant effects). Products include:
Hycodan **1104**
Hycomine Compound Tablets **1105**
Hycotuss Expectorant Syrup **1106**
Lortab **3315**
Lortab Elixir **3312**
Vicodin Tablets **530**
Vicodin ES Tablets **531**
Vicodin HP Tablets **532**
Vicoprofen Tablets **533**
Zydone Tablets **1118**

Hydrocodone Polistirex (Co-administration with CNS depressants results in additive CNS depressant effects). Products include:
Tussionex Pennkinetic Extended-Release Suspension **3322**

Hydromorphone Hydrochloride (Co-administration with CNS depressants results in additive CNS depressant effects). Products include:
Dilaudid **439**
Dilaudid Oral Liquid **443**
Dilaudid Non-Sterile Powder **439**
Dilaudid Rectal Suppositories **439**
Dilaudid Tablets **439**
Dilaudid Tablets - 8 mg **443**
Dilaudid-HP **441**

Hydroxyzine Hydrochloride (Co-administration with CNS depressants results in additive CNS depressant effects).
No products indexed under this heading.

Imipramine Hydrochloride (Propoxyphene may slow the metabolism of antidepressants leading to higher serum levels of antidepressants).
No products indexed under this heading.

Imipramine Pamoate (Propoxyphene may slow the metabolism of antidepressants leading to higher serum levels of antidepressants).
No products indexed under this heading.

Isocarboxazid (Propoxyphene may slow the metabolism of antidepressants leading to higher serum levels of antidepressants).
No products indexed under this heading.

Isoflurane (Co-administration with CNS depressants results in additive CNS depressant effects).
No products indexed under this heading.

Ketamine Hydrochloride (Co-administration with CNS depressants results in additive CNS depressant effects).
No products indexed under this heading.

Lamotrigine (Propoxyphene may slow the metabolism of anticonvulsants leading to higher serum levels of anticonvulsants). Products include:
Lamictal **1449**

Levetiracetam (Propoxyphene may slow the metabolism of anticonvulsants leading to higher serum levels of anticonvulsants). Products include:
Keppra Oral Solution **3307**
Keppra Tablets **3307**

Levomethadyl Acetate Hydrochloride (Co-administration with CNS depressants results in additive CNS depressant effects).
No products indexed under this heading.

Levorphanol Tartrate (Co-administration with CNS depressants results in additive CNS depressant effects).
No products indexed under this heading.

Lorazepam (Co-administration with CNS depressants results in additive CNS depressant effects).
No products indexed under this heading.

Loxapine Hydrochloride (Co-administration with CNS depressants results in additive CNS depressant effects).
No products indexed under this heading.

Loxapine Succinate (Co-administration with CNS depressants results in additive CNS depressant effects).
No products indexed under this heading.

Maprotiline Hydrochloride (Propoxyphene may slow the metabolism of antidepressants leading to higher serum levels of antidepressants).
No products indexed under this heading.

Meperidine Hydrochloride (Co-administration with CNS depressants results in additive CNS depressant effects).
No products indexed under this heading.

Mephenytoin (Propoxyphene may slow the metabolism of anticonvulsants leading to higher serum levels of anticonvulsants).
No products indexed under this heading.

Mephobarbital (Co-administration with CNS depressants results in additive CNS depressant effects). Products include:
Mebaral Tablets, USP **2483**

Meprobamate (Co-administration with CNS depressants results in additive CNS depressant effects).
No products indexed under this heading.

Mesoridazine Besylate (Co-administration with CNS depressants results in additive CNS depressant effects).
No products indexed under this heading.

Methadone Hydrochloride (Co-administration with CNS depressants results in additive CNS depressant effects).
No products indexed under this heading.

Methohexital Sodium (Co-administration with CNS depressants results in additive CNS depressant effects).
No products indexed under this heading.

Methotrimeprazine (Co-administration with CNS depressants results in additive CNS depressant effects).
No products indexed under this heading.

Methoxyflurane (Co-administration with CNS depressants results in additive CNS depressant effects).
No products indexed under this heading.

Methsuximide (Propoxyphene may slow the metabolism of anticonvulsants leading to higher serum levels of anticonvulsants).
No products indexed under this heading.

Midazolam Hydrochloride (Co-administration with CNS depressants results in additive CNS depressant effects).
No products indexed under this heading.

Mirtazapine (Propoxyphene may slow the metabolism of antidepressants leading to higher serum levels of antidepressants).
No products indexed under this heading.

Molindone Hydrochloride (Co-administration with CNS depressants results in additive CNS depressant effects). Products include:
Moban Tablets **1108**

Morphine Sulfate (Co-administration with CNS depressants results in additive CNS depressant effects). Products include:
Avinza Capsules **1714**
Kadian Capsules **572**
MS Contin Tablets **2703**

Nefazodone Hydrochloride (Propoxyphene may slow the metabolism of antidepressants leading to higher serum levels of antidepressants).
No products indexed under this heading.

Nortriptyline Hydrochloride (Propoxyphene may slow the metabolism of antidepressants leading to higher serum levels of antidepressants).
No products indexed under this heading.

Olanzapine (Co-administration with CNS depressants results in additive CNS depressant effects). Products include:
Symbyax Capsules 1788
Zyprexa Tablets 1798
Zyprexa IntraMuscular 1798
Zyprexa ZYDIS Orally Disintegrating Tablets 1798

Oxazepam (Co-administration with CNS depressants results in additive CNS depressant effects).
No products indexed under this heading.

Oxcarbazepine (Propoxyphene may slow the metabolism of anticonvulsants leading to higher serum levels of anticonvulsants). Products include:
Trileptal Oral Suspension 2281
Trileptal Tablets 2281

Oxycodone Hydrochloride (Co-administration with CNS depressants results in additive CNS depressant effects). Products include:
Combunox Tablets 1183
OxyContin Tablets 2699
OxyFast Oral Concentrate Solution 2704
OxyIR Capsules 2704
Percocet Tablets 1114
Percodan Tablets 1115

Paramethadione (Propoxyphene may slow the metabolism of anticonvulsants leading to higher serum levels of anticonvulsants).
No products indexed under this heading.

Paroxetine Hydrochloride (Propoxyphene may slow the metabolism of antidepressants leading to higher serum levels of antidepressants). Products include:
Paxil CR Controlled-Release Tablets 1509
Paxil 1501

Pentobarbital Sodium (Co-administration with CNS depressants results in additive CNS depressant effects). Products include:
Nembutal Sodium Solution, USP 2484

Perphenazine (Co-administration with CNS depressants results in additive CNS depressant effects).
No products indexed under this heading.

Phenacemide (Propoxyphene may slow the metabolism of anticonvulsants leading to higher serum levels of anticonvulsants).
No products indexed under this heading.

Phenelzine Sulfate (Propoxyphene may slow the metabolism of antidepressants leading to higher serum levels of antidepressants).
No products indexed under this heading.

Phenobarbital (Propoxyphene may slow the metabolism of anticonvulsants leading to higher serum levels of anticonvulsants).
No products indexed under this heading.

Phensuximide (Propoxyphene may slow the metabolism of anticonvulsants leading to higher serum levels of anticonvulsants).
No products indexed under this heading.

Phenytoin (Propoxyphene may slow the metabolism of anticonvulsants leading to higher serum levels of anticonvulsants).
No products indexed under this heading.

Phenytoin Sodium (Propoxyphene may slow the metabolism of anticonvulsants leading to higher serum levels of anticonvulsants). Products include:
Phenytek Capsules 2153

Prazepam (Co-administration with CNS depressants results in additive CNS depressant effects).
No products indexed under this heading.

Primidone (Propoxyphene may slow the metabolism of anticonvulsants leading to higher serum levels of anticonvulsants).
No products indexed under this heading.

Prochlorperazine (Co-administration with CNS depressants results in additive CNS depressant effects).
No products indexed under this heading.

Promethazine Hydrochloride (Co-administration with CNS depressants results in additive CNS depressant effects). Products include:
Phenergan 3438

Propofol (Co-administration with CNS depressants results in additive CNS depressant effects). Products include:
Diprivan Injectable Emulsion 676

Propoxyphene Napsylate (Co-administration with CNS depressants results in additive CNS depressant effects). Products include:
Darvocet A 500 Tablets 3497

Protriptyline Hydrochloride (Propoxyphene may slow the metabolism of antidepressants leading to higher serum levels of antidepressants). Products include:
Vivactil Tablets 2350

Quazepam (Co-administration with CNS depressants results in additive CNS depressant effects).
No products indexed under this heading.

Quetiapine Fumarate (Co-administration with CNS depressants results in additive CNS depressant effects). Products include:
Seroquel Tablets 691

Remifentanil Hydrochloride (Co-administration with CNS depressants results in additive CNS depressant effects).
No products indexed under this heading.

Risperidone (Co-administration with CNS depressants results in additive CNS depressant effects). Products include:
Risperdal Consta Long-Acting Injection 1664
Risperdal M-Tab Orally Disintegrating Tablets 1658
Risperdal 1658

Secobarbital Sodium (Co-administration with CNS depressants results in additive CNS depressant effects).
No products indexed under this heading.

Sertraline Hydrochloride (Propoxyphene may slow the metabolism of antidepressants leading to higher serum levels of antidepressants). Products include:
Zoloft 2581

Sevoflurane (Co-administration with CNS depressants results in additive CNS depressant effects). Products include:
Ultane Liquid for Inhalation 526

Sufentanil Citrate (Co-administration with CNS depressants results in additive CNS depressant effects).
No products indexed under this heading.

Temazepam (Co-administration with CNS depressants results in additive CNS depressant effects).
No products indexed under this heading.

Thiamylal Sodium (Co-administration with CNS depressants results in additive CNS depressant effects).
No products indexed under this heading.

Thioridazine Hydrochloride (Co-administration with CNS depressants results in additive CNS depressant effects). Products include:
Thioridazine Hydrochloride Tablets 2122

Thiothixene (Co-administration with CNS depressants results in additive CNS depressant effects). Products include:
Thiothixene Capsules 2124

Tiagabine Hydrochloride (Propoxyphene may slow the metabolism of anticonvulsants leading to higher serum levels of anticonvulsants). Products include:
Gabitril Tablets 998

Topiramate (Propoxyphene may slow the metabolism of anticonvulsants leading to higher serum levels of anticonvulsants). Products include:
Topamax Sprinkle Capsules 2438
Topamax Tablets 2438

Tranylcypromine Sulfate (Propoxyphene may slow the metabolism of antidepressants leading to higher serum levels of antidepressants). Products include:
Parnate Tablets 1499

Trazodone Hydrochloride (Propoxyphene may slow the metabolism of antidepressants leading to higher serum levels of antidepressants).
No products indexed under this heading.

Triazolam (Co-administration with CNS depressants results in additive CNS depressant effects).
No products indexed under this heading.

Trifluoperazine Hydrochloride (Co-administration with CNS depressants results in additive CNS depressant effects).
No products indexed under this heading.

Trimethadione (Propoxyphene may slow the metabolism of anticonvulsants leading to higher serum levels of anticonvulsants).
No products indexed under this heading.

Trimipramine Maleate (Propoxyphene may slow the metabolism of antidepressants leading to higher serum levels of antidepressants). Products include:
Surmontil Capsules 2347

Valproate Sodium (Propoxyphene may slow the metabolism of anticonvulsants leading to higher serum levels of anticonvulsants). Products include:
Depacon Injection 412

Valproic Acid (Propoxyphene may slow the metabolism of anticonvulsants leading to higher serum levels of anticonvulsants). Products include:
Depakene 417

Venlafaxine Hydrochloride (Propoxyphene may slow the metabolism of antidepressants leading to higher serum levels of antidepressants). Products include:
Effexor Tablets 3405
Effexor XR Capsules 3411

Warfarin Sodium (Propoxyphene may slow the metabolism of anticoagulants leading to higher serum levels of anticoagulants). Products include:
Coumadin for Injection 932
Coumadin Tablets 932

Zaleplon (Co-administration with CNS depressants results in additive CNS depressant effects). Products include:
Sonata Capsules 1686

Ziprasidone Hydrochloride (Co-administration with CNS depressants results in additive CNS depressant effects). Products include:
Geodon Capsules 2514

Zolpidem Tartrate (Co-administration with CNS depressants results in additive CNS depressant effects). Products include:
Ambien Tablets 2867

Zonisamide (Propoxyphene may slow the metabolism of anticonvulsants leading to higher serum levels of anticonvulsants). Products include:
Zonegran Capsules 1089

Food Interactions

Alcohol (Additive CNS depressant effects).

DDAVP INJECTION 4 MCG/ML

(Desmopressin Acetate) 2893

May interact with vasopressors. Compounds in these categories include:

Dobutamine (Co-administration with other pressor agents may result in possible additive pressor activity).
No products indexed under this heading.

Dobutamine Hydrochloride (Co-administration with other pressor agents may result in possible additive pressor activity).
No products indexed under this heading.

Dopamine Hydrochloride (Co-administration with other pressor agents may result in possible additive pressor activity).
No products indexed under this heading.

Ephedrine Sulfate (Co-administration with other pressor agents may result in possible additive pressor activity).
No products indexed under this heading.

Epinephrine Bitartrate (Co-administration with other pressor agents may result in possible additive pressor activity).
No products indexed under this heading.

Epinephrine Hydrochloride (Co-administration with other pressor agents may result in possible additive pressor activity).
No products indexed under this heading.

Isoproterenol Hydrochloride (Co-administration with other pressor agents may result in possible additive pressor activity).
No products indexed under this heading.

Isoproterenol Sulfate (Co-administration with other pressor agents may result in possible additive pressor activity).
No products indexed under this heading.

Mephentermine Sulfate (Co-administration with other pressor agents may result in possible additive pressor activity).
No products indexed under this heading.

Metaraminol Bitartrate (Co-administration with other pressor agents may result in possible additive pressor activity). Products include:
- Aramine Injection 1889

Methoxamine Hydrochloride (Co-administration with other pressor agents may result in possible additive pressor activity).
No products indexed under this heading.

Norepinephrine Bitartrate (Co-administration with other pressor agents may result in possible additive pressor activity).
No products indexed under this heading.

Phenylephrine Hydrochloride (Co-administration with other pressor agents may result in possible additive pressor activity). Products include:
- Alacol DM Syrup 739
- Hycomine Compound Tablets 1105
- Preparation H Maximum Strength Cream 747
- Preparation H Cooling Gel 747
- Preparation H 747
- Sudafed PE Tablets 711
- Vicks Sinex Nasal Spray and Ultra Fine Mist for Sinus Relief............... 2677
- Zicam Concentrated Cough Mist for Kids Plus D Cool Cherry......... 643
- Zicam Concentrated Cough Mist Plus D Cool Cherry...................... 642

DDAVP NASAL SPRAY

(Desmopressin Acetate) 2894
See DDAVP Injection 4 mcg/mL

DDAVP TABLETS

(Desmopressin Acetate) 2895
May interact with vasopressors. Compounds in these categories include:

Dobutamine (Although the pressor activity of DDAVP is very low, large doses of DDAVP tablets should be used with other vasopressor agents only with careful patient monitoring).
No products indexed under this heading.

Dobutamine Hydrochloride (Although the pressor activity of DDAVP is very low, large doses of DDAVP tablets should be used with other vasopressor agents only with careful patient monitoring).
No products indexed under this heading.

Dopamine Hydrochloride (Although the pressor activity of DDAVP is very low, large doses of DDAVP tablets should be used with other vasopressor agents only with careful patient monitoring).
No products indexed under this heading.

Ephedrine Sulfate (Although the pressor activity of DDAVP is very low, large doses of DDAVP tablets should be used with other vasopressor agents only with careful patient monitoring).
No products indexed under this heading.

Epinephrine Bitartrate (Although the pressor activity of DDAVP is very low, large doses of DDAVP tablets should be used with other vasopressor agents only with careful patient monitoring).
No products indexed under this heading.

Epinephrine Hydrochloride (Although the pressor activity of DDAVP is very low, large doses of DDAVP tablets should be used with other vasopressor agents only with careful patient monitoring).
No products indexed under this heading.

Isoproterenol Hydrochloride (Although the pressor activity of DDAVP is very low, large doses of DDAVP tablets should be used with other vasopressor agents only with careful patient monitoring).
No products indexed under this heading.

Isoproterenol Sulfate (Although the pressor activity of DDAVP is very low, large doses of DDAVP tablets should be used with other vasopressor agents only with careful patient monitoring).
No products indexed under this heading.

Mephentermine Sulfate (Although the pressor activity of DDAVP is very low, large doses of DDAVP tablets should be used with other vasopressor agents only with careful patient monitoring).
No products indexed under this heading.

Metaraminol Bitartrate (Although the pressor activity of DDAVP is very low, large doses of DDAVP tablets should be used with other vasopressor agents only with careful patient monitoring). Products include:
- Aramine Injection 1889

Methoxamine Hydrochloride (Although the pressor activity of DDAVP is very low, large doses of DDAVP tablets should be used with other vasopressor agents only with careful patient monitoring).
No products indexed under this heading.

Norepinephrine Bitartrate (Although the pressor activity of DDAVP is very low, large doses of DDAVP tablets should be used with other vasopressor agents only with careful patient monitoring).
No products indexed under this heading.

Phenylephrine Hydrochloride (Although the pressor activity of DDAVP is very low, large doses of DDAVP tablets should be used with other vasopressor agents only with careful patient monitoring). Products include:
- Alacol DM Syrup 739
- Hycomine Compound Tablets 1105
- Preparation H Maximum Strength Cream 747
- Preparation H Cooling Gel 747
- Preparation H 747
- Sudafed PE Tablets 711
- Vicks Sinex Nasal Spray and Ultra Fine Mist for Sinus Relief.............. 2677
- Zicam Concentrated Cough Mist for Kids Plus D Cool Cherry......... 643
- Zicam Concentrated Cough Mist Plus D Cool Cherry...................... 642

DDS-ACIDOPHILUS CAPSULES, TABLETS, AND POWDER

(Lactobacillus Acidophilus) 736
None cited in PDR database.

DEBROX DROPS

(Carbamide Peroxide) 616
None cited in PDR database.

DECADRON PHOSPHATE INJECTION

(Dexamethasone Sodium Phosphate)... 1931
May interact with oral anticoagulants, erythromycin, oral hypoglycemic agents, insulin, phenytoin, potassium-depleting diuretics, and certain other agents. Compounds in these categories include:

Acarbose (Potential for increased requirements of oral hypoglycemic agents). Products include:
- Precose Tablets 776

Anisindione (Potential for altered response to coumarin anticoagulants). Products include:
- Miradon Tablets 3056

Aspirin (Aspirin should be used cautiously in conjunction with corticosteroids in hypoprothrombinemia). Products include:
- Aggrenox Capsules 855
- Bayer, Aspirin Regimen 606
- Bayer Aspirin Tablets 3515
- BC Powder 612
- BC Allergy Sinus Cold Powder 612
- Arthritis Strength BC Powder 612
- BC Sinus Cold Powder 612
- Ecotrin Enteric Coated Aspirin Low, Regular and Maximum Strength Tablets.......................... 1627
- Goody's Body Pain Formula Powder... 621
- Goody's Extra Strength Headache Powder....................... 621
- Goody's Extra Strength Pain Relief Tablets 621
- Percodan Tablets 1115
- St. Joseph 81 mg Aspirin Chewable and Enteric Coated Tablets.. 1841

Bendroflumethiazide (Co-administration may result in hypokalemia).
No products indexed under this heading.

Bumetanide (Co-administration may result in hypokalemia).
No products indexed under this heading.

Carbamazepine (CYP450 3A4 enzyme inducers, such as carbamazepine, may enhance the metabolic clearance of corticosteroids resulting in decreased blood levels and lessened physiologic activity, thus requiring an increase in corticosteroid dosage). Products include:
- Carbatrol Capsules 3174
- Equetro Extended-Release Capsules.. 3178
- Tegretol/Tegretol-XR 2278

Chlorothiazide (Co-administration may result in hypokalemia). Products include:
- Aldoclor Tablets 1881
- Diuril Oral 1936

Chlorothiazide Sodium (Co-administration may result in hypokalemia). Products include:
- Diuril Sodium Intravenous 1934

Chlorpropamide (Potential for increased requirements of oral hypoglycemic agents).
No products indexed under this heading.

Dicumarol (Potential for altered response to coumarin anticoagulants).
No products indexed under this heading.

Ephedrine Hydrochloride (May enhance the metabolic clearance of corticosteroids resulting in decreased blood levels and lessened physiologic activity, thus requiring an increase in corticosteroid dosage). Products include:
- Primatene Tablets 749

Ephedrine Sulfate (May enhance the metabolic clearance of corticosteroids resulting in decreased blood levels and lessened physiologic activity, thus requiring an increase in corticosteroid dosage).
No products indexed under this heading.

Ephedrine Tannate (May enhance the metabolic clearance of corticosteroids resulting in decreased blood levels and lessened physiologic activity, thus requiring an increase in corticosteroid dosage).
No products indexed under this heading.

Erythromycin (CYP450 3A4 enzyme inhibitors, such as erythromycin, has the potential to result in increased plasma levels of dexamethasone; dexamethasone is a moderate inducer of CYP3A4 and may increase erythromycin clearance resulting in decreased plasma concentrations of erythromycin). Products include:
- Erygel Topical Gel 2096
- Ery-Tab Tablets 447
- Erythromycin Base Filmtab Tablets 454
- Erythromycin Delayed-Release Capsules, USP............................... 456
- PCE Dispertab Tablets 510

Erythromycin Estolate (CYP450 3A4 enzyme inhibitors, such as erythromycin, has the potential to result in increased plasma levels of dexamethasone; dexamethasone is a moderate inducer of CYP3A4 and may increase erythromycin clearance resulting in decreased plasma concentrations of erythromycin).
No products indexed under this heading.

Erythromycin Ethylsuccinate (CYP450 3A4 enzyme inhibitors, such as erythromycin, has the potential to result in increased plasma levels of dexamethasone; dexamethasone is a moderate inducer of CYP3A4 and may increase erythromycin clearance resulting in decreased plasma concentrations of erythromycin). Products include:
- E.E.S. 449
- EryPed 445

Erythromycin Gluceptate (CYP450 3A4 enzyme inhibitors, such as erythromycin, has the potential to result in increased plasma levels of dexamethasone; dexamethasone is a moderate inducer of CYP3A4 and may increase erythromycin clearance resulting in decreased plasma concentrations of erythromycin).
No products indexed under this heading.

Erythromycin Lactobionate (CYP450 3A4 enzyme inhibitors, such as erythromycin, has the potential to result in increased plasma levels of dexamethasone; dexamethasone is a moderate inducer of CYP3A4 and may increase erythromycin clearance resulting in decreased plasma concentrations of erythromycin).
No products indexed under this heading.

Erythromycin Stearate (CYP450 3A4 enzyme inhibitors, such as erythromycin, has the potential to result in increased plasma levels of dexamethasone; dexamethasone is a moderate inducer of CYP3A4 and may increase erythromycin clearance resulting in decreased plasma concentrations of erythromycin). Products include:
Erythrocin Stearate Filmtab Tablets **452**

Ethacrynic Acid (Co-administration may result in hypokalemia). Products include:
Edecrin Tablets **1941**

Fosphenytoin Sodium (CYP450 3A4 enzyme inducers, such as phenytoin, may enhance the metabolic clearance of corticosteroids resulting in decreased blood levels and lessened physiologic activity, thus requiring an increase in corticosteroid dosage; there have been reports of both increases and decreases in phenytoin levels with dexamethasone co-administration, leading to alterations in seizure control).
No products indexed under this heading.

Furosemide (Co-administration may result in hypokalemia). Products include:
Furosemide Tablets **2117**

Glimepiride (Potential for increased requirements of oral hypoglycemic agents). Products include:
Amaryl Tablets **2864**

Glipizide (Potential for increased requirements of oral hypoglycemic agents).
No products indexed under this heading.

Glyburide (Potential for increased requirements of oral hypoglycemic agents).
No products indexed under this heading.

Hydrochlorothiazide (Co-administration may result in hypokalemia). Products include:
Aldoril Tablets **1884**
Atacand HCT **637**
Avalide Tablets **2889**
Avalide Tablets **922**
Benicar HCT Tablets **2852**
Diovan HCT Tablets **2195**
Dyazide Capsules **1389**
Hyzaar **1964**
Lotensin HCT Tablets **2235**
Maxzide **2150**
Micardis HCT Tablets **886**
Moduretic Tablets **2003**
Prinzide Tablets **2033**
Teveten HCT Tablets **1710**
Timolide Tablets **2056**
Uniretic Tablets **3114**
Vaseretic Tablets **2073**
Zestoretic Tablets **701**

Hydroflumethiazide (Co-administration may result in hypokalemia).
No products indexed under this heading.

Indinavir Sulfate (Dexamethasone is a moderate inducer of CYP3A4 and may increase indinavir clearance resulting in decreased plasma concentrations of indinavir). Products include:
Crixivan Capsules **1918**

Insulin, Human, Zinc Suspension (Potential for increased requirements of insulin). Products include:
Humulin L, 100 Units **1763**
Humulin U, 100 Units **1770**

Insulin, Human NPH (Potential for increased requirements of insulin). Products include:
Humulin N, 100 Units **1764**
Humulin N Pen **1765**
Novolin N Human Insulin 10 ml Vials **2322**
Novolin N InnoLet **2322**
Novolin N PenFill 3 ml Cartridges **2325**
Novolin R InnoLet **2322**

Insulin, Human Regular (Potential for increased requirements of insulin). Products include:
Humulin R (U-500) **1768**
Humulin R, 100 Units **1767**
Novolin R Human Insulin 10 ml Vials **2322**
Novolin R PenFill **2325**

Insulin, Human Regular and Human NPH Mixture (Potential for increased requirements of insulin). Products include:
Humulin 50/50, 100 Units **1760**
Humulin 70/30 Pen **1761**
Novolin 70/30 Human Insulin 10 ml Vials **2321**
Novolin 70/30 InnoLet **2322**
Novolin 70/30 PenFill 3 ml Cartridges **2325**

Insulin, NPH (Potential for increased requirements of insulin).
No products indexed under this heading.

Insulin, Regular (Potential for increased requirements of insulin).
No products indexed under this heading.

Insulin, Zinc Crystals (Potential for increased requirements of insulin).
No products indexed under this heading.

Insulin, Zinc Suspension (Potential for increased requirements of insulin).
No products indexed under this heading.

Insulin Aspart, Human Regular (Potential for increased requirements of insulin). Products include:
NovoLog Injection **2326**

Insulin glargine (Potential for increased requirements of insulin). Products include:
Lantus Injection **2925**

Insulin Lispro, Human (Potential for increased requirements of insulin). Products include:
Humalog-Pen **1751**
Humalog Mix 75/25-Pen **1754**

Insulin Lispro Protamine, Human (Potential for increased requirements of insulin). Products include:
Humalog Mix 75/25-Pen **1754**

Ketoconazole (CYP450 3A4 enzyme inhibitors, such as ketoconazole, have the potential to result in increased plasma levels of dexamethasone). Products include:
Nizoral A-D Shampoo, 1% **1839**
Nizoral 2% Shampoo **1838**

Live Virus Vaccines (Co-administration is contraindicated in patients receiving immunosuppressive doses of corticosteroids).
No products indexed under this heading.

Metformin Hydrochloride (Potential for increased requirements of oral hypoglycemic agents). Products include:
ActoPlus Met Tablets **3219**
Avandamet Tablets **1343**
Fortamet Extended-Release Tablets **1156**

Methyclothiazide (Co-administration may result in hypokalemia).
No products indexed under this heading.

Miglitol (Potential for increased requirements of oral hypoglycemic agents).
No products indexed under this heading.

Phenobarbital (CYP450 3A4 enzyme inducers, such as phenobarbital, may enhance the metabolic clearance of corticosteroids resulting in decreased blood levels and lessened physiologic activity, thus requiring an increase in corticosteroid dosage).
No products indexed under this heading.

Phenytoin (CYP450 3A4 enzyme inducers, such as phenytoin, may enhance the metabolic clearance of corticosteroids resulting in decreased blood levels and lessened physiologic activity, thus requiring an increase in corticosteroid dosage; there have been reports of both increases and decreases in phenytoin levels with dexamethasone co-administration, leading to alterations in seizure control).
No products indexed under this heading.

Phenytoin Sodium (CYP450 3A4 enzyme inducers, such as phenytoin, may enhance the metabolic clearance of corticosteroids resulting in decreased blood levels and lessened physiologic activity, thus requiring an increase in corticosteroid dosage; there have been reports of both increases and decreases in phenytoin levels with dexamethasone co-administration, leading to alterations in seizure control). Products include:
Phenytek Capsules **2153**

Pioglitazone Hydrochloride (Potential for increased requirements of oral hypoglycemic agents). Products include:
ActoPlus Met Tablets **3219**
Actos Tablets **3224**

Polythiazide (Co-administration may result in hypokalemia).
No products indexed under this heading.

Repaglinide (Potential for increased requirements of oral hypoglycemic agents). Products include:
Prandin Tablets (0.5, 1, and 2 mg) **2337**

Rifampin (CYP450 3A4 enzyme inducers, such as rifampin, may enhance the metabolic clearance of corticosteroids resulting in decreased blood levels and lessened physiologic activity, thus requiring an increase in corticosteroid dosage).
No products indexed under this heading.

Rosiglitazone Maleate (Potential for increased requirements of oral hypoglycemic agents). Products include:
Avandamet Tablets **1343**
Avandia Tablets **1348**

Thalidomide (Co-administration has resulted in toxic epidermal necrolysis). Products include:
Thalomid Capsules **979**

Tolazamide (Potential for increased requirements of oral hypoglycemic agents).
No products indexed under this heading.

Tolbutamide (Potential for increased requirements of oral hypoglycemic agents).
No products indexed under this heading.

Torsemide (Co-administration may result in hypokalemia).
No products indexed under this heading.

Troglitazone (Potential for increased requirements of oral hypoglycemic agents).
No products indexed under this heading.

Warfarin Sodium (Potential for altered response to coumarin anticoagulants). Products include:
Coumadin for Injection **932**
Coumadin Tablets **932**

DECADRON TABLETS

(Dexamethasone) **1929**

May interact with anticholinesterase drugs, barbiturates, oral anticoagulants, cytochrome p450 3a4 inducers (selected), cytochrome p450 3a4 inhibitors (selected), cytochrome p450 3a4 substrates (selected), estrogens, cardiac glycosides, oral hypoglycemic agents, insulin, macrolide antibiotics, nonsteroidal anti-inflammatory agents, oral contraceptives, phenytoin, potassium-depleting diuretics, vaccines, live, and certain other agents. Compounds in these categories include:

Acarbose (Because corticosteroids may increase blood glucose concentrations, dosage adjustments of antidiabetic agents may be required). Products include:
Precose Tablets **776**

Acetazolamide (Drugs which inhibit cytochrome P450 3A4 enzyme activity have the potential to result in increased plasma concentrations of corticosteroids).
No products indexed under this heading.

Alfentanil Hydrochloride (Dexamethasone is a moderate inducer of the cytochrome P450 3A4 enzyme system. Co-administration with other drugs that are metabolized by CYP 3A4 may increase their clearance, resulting in decreased plasma concentrations).
No products indexed under this heading.

Allium sativum (Drugs which induce cytochrome P450 3A4 enzyme activity may enhance the metabolism of corticosteroids and require that the dosage of the corticosteroid be increased).

No products indexed under this heading.

Alprazolam (Dexamethasone is a moderate inducer of the cytochrome P450 3A4 enzyme system. Co-administration with other drugs that are metabolized by CYP 3A4 may increase their clearance, resulting in decreased plasma concentrations). Products include:

Niravam Orally Disintegrating Tablets 3106
Xanax XR Tablets 2655

Aminoglutethimide (Aminoglutethimide may diminish adrenal suppression by corticosteroids).

No products indexed under this heading.

Amiodarone Hydrochloride (Drugs which inhibit cytochrome P450 3A4 enzyme activity have the potential to result in increased plasma concentrations of corticosteroids). Products include:

Pacerone Tablets 3337

Amitriptyline Hydrochloride (Dexamethasone is a moderate inducer of the cytochrome P450 3A4 enzyme system. Co-administration with other drugs that are metabolized by CYP 3A4 may increase their clearance, resulting in decreased plasma concentrations).

No products indexed under this heading.

Amlodipine Besylate (Dexamethasone is a moderate inducer of the cytochrome P450 3A4 enzyme system. Co-administration with other drugs that are metabolized by CYP 3A4 may increase their clearance, resulting in decreased plasma concentrations). Products include:

Caduet Tablets 2507
Lotrel Capsules 2238
Norvasc Tablets 2529

Amphotericin B (When corticosteroids are administered with potassium-depleting agents (eg, amphotericin B), patients should be observed closely for development of hypokalemia. In addition, there have been cases reported in which concomitant use of amphotericin B and hydrocortisone was followed by cardiac enlargement and congestive heart failure).

No products indexed under this heading.

Amphotericin B, liposomal (When corticosteroids are administered with potassium-depleting agents (eg, amphotericin B), patients should be observed closely for development of hypokalemia. In addition, there have been cases reported in which concomitant use of amphotericin B and hydrocortisone was followed by cardiac enlargement and congestive heart failure). Products include:

AmBisome for Injection 615

Amphotericin B Cholesteryl Sulfate (When corticosteroids are administered with potassium-depleting agents (eg, amphotericin B), patients should be observed closely for development of hypokalemia. In addition, there have been cases reported in which concomitant use of amphotericin B and hydrocortisone was followed by cardiac enlargement and congestive heart failure).

No products indexed under this heading.

Amphotericin B Lipid Complex (When corticosteroids are administered with potassium-depleting agents (eg, amphotericin B), patients should be observed closely for development of hypokalemia. In addition, there have been cases reported in which concomitant use of amphotericin B and hydrocortisone was followed by cardiac enlargement and congestive heart failure). Products include:

Abelcet Injection 1119

Amprenavir (Drugs which inhibit cytochrome P450 3A4 enzyme activity have the potential to result in increased plasma concentrations of corticosteroids). Products include:

Agenerase Capsules 1299
Agenerase Oral Solution 1304

Anastrozole (Drugs which inhibit cytochrome P450 3A4 enzyme activity have the potential to result in increased plasma concentrations of corticosteroids). Products include:

Arimidex Tablets 665

Anisindione (Co-administration of corticosteroids and warfarin usually results in inhibition of response to warfarin, although there have been some conflicting reports. Therefore, coagulation indices should be monitored frequently to maintain the desired anticoagulant effect). Products include:

Miradon Tablets 3056

Aprepitant (Drugs which inhibit cytochrome P450 3A4 enzyme activity have the potential to result in increased plasma concentrations of corticosteroids). Products include:

Emend Capsules 1944

Aprobarbital (Drugs which induce cytochrome P450 3A4 enzyme activity (eg, barbiturates) may enhance the metabolism of corticosteroids and require that the dosage of the corticosteroid be increased).

No products indexed under this heading.

Astemizole (Dexamethasone is a moderate inducer of the cytochrome P450 3A4 enzyme system. Co-administration with other drugs that are metabolized by CYP 3A4 may increase their clearance, resulting in decreased plasma concentrations).

No products indexed under this heading.

Atorvastatin Calcium (Dexamethasone is a moderate inducer of the cytochrome P450 3A4 enzyme system. Co-administration with other drugs that are metabolized by CYP 3A4 may increase their clearance, resulting in decreased plasma concentrations). Products include:

Caduet Tablets 2507
Lipitor Tablets 2495

Azithromycin Dihydrate (Macrolide antibiotics have been reported to cause a significant decrease in corticosteroid clearance. Drugs which inhibit cytochrome P450 3A4 enzyme activity (eg, macrolide antibiotics) have the potential to result in increased plasma concentrations of corticosteroids. Dexamethasone is a moderate inducer of the cytochrome P450 3A4 enzyme system. Co-administration with other drugs that are metabolized by CYP 3A4 (eg, erythromycin) may increase their clearance, resulting in decreased plasma concentrations). Products include:

Zithromax 2568
Zithromax for IV Infusion 2573
Zithromax for Oral Suspension, 300 mg, 600 mg, 900 mg, 1200 mg 2561
Zithromax Tablets, 250 mg, 500 mg 2561
Zithromax Tri-Pak 2561
Zithromax Z-Pak 2568

BCG Vaccine (Patients on corticosteroid therapy may exhibit a diminished response to toxoids and live or inactivated vaccines due to inhibition of antibody response. Corticosteroids may also potentiate the replication of some organisms contained in live attenuated vaccines. Routine administration of vaccines or toxoids should be deferred until corticosteroid therapy is discontinued if possible. Administration of live or live, attenuated vaccines is contraindicated in patients receiving immunosuppressive doses of corticosteroids).

No products indexed under this heading.

Belladonna Ergotamine (Dexamethasone is a moderate inducer of the cytochrome P450 3A4 enzyme system. Co-administration with other drugs that are metabolized by CYP 3A4 may increase their clearance, resulting in decreased plasma concentrations).

No products indexed under this heading.

Bendroflumethiazide (When corticosteroids are administered with potassium-depleting agents (eg, diuretics), patients should be observed closely for development of hypokalemia).

No products indexed under this heading.

Betamethasone Acetate (Drugs which induce cytochrome P450 3A4 enzyme activity may enhance the metabolism of corticosteroids and require that the dosage of the corticosteroid be increased).

No products indexed under this heading.

Betamethasone Sodium Phosphate (Drugs which induce cytochrome P450 3A4 enzyme activity may enhance the metabolism of corticosteroids and require that the dosage of the corticosteroid be increased).

No products indexed under this heading.

Bumetanide (When corticosteroids are administered with potassium-depleting agents (eg, diuretics), patients should be observed closely for development of hypokalemia).

No products indexed under this heading.

Buspirone Hydrochloride (Dexamethasone is a moderate inducer of the cytochrome P450 3A4 enzyme system. Co-administration with other drugs that are metabolized by CYP 3A4 may increase their clearance, resulting in decreased plasma concentrations).

No products indexed under this heading.

Busulfan (Dexamethasone is a moderate inducer of the cytochrome P450 3A4 enzyme system. Co-administration with other drugs that are metabolized by CYP 3A4 may increase their clearance, resulting in decreased plasma concentrations). Products include:

I.V. Busulfex 1125
Myleran Tablets 1492

Butabarbital (Drugs which induce cytochrome P450 3A4 enzyme activity (eg, barbiturates) may enhance the metabolism of corticosteroids and require that the dosage of the corticosteroid be increased).

No products indexed under this heading.

Butalbital (Drugs which induce cytochrome P450 3A4 enzyme activity (eg, barbiturates) may enhance the metabolism of corticosteroids and require that the dosage of the corticosteroid be increased). Products include:

Sedapap Tablets 50 mg/650 mg 2098

Carbamazepine (Dexamethasone is a moderate inducer of the cytochrome P450 3A4 enzyme system. Co-administration with other drugs that are metabolized by CYP 3A4 may increase their clearance, resulting in decreased plasma concentrations). Products include:

Carbatrol Capsules 3174
Equetro Extended-Release Capsules 3178
Tegretol/Tegretol-XR 2278

Celecoxib (Concomitant use of nonsteroidal anti-inflammatory agents and corticosteroids increases the risk of gastrointestinal side effects). Products include:

Celebrex Capsules 3130

Cerivastatin Sodium (Dexamethasone is a moderate inducer of the cytochrome P450 3A4 enzyme system. Co-administration with other drugs that are metabolized by CYP 3A4 may increase their clearance, resulting in decreased plasma concentrations).

No products indexed under this heading.

Chlorothiazide (When corticosteroids are administered with potassium-depleting agents (eg, diuretics), patients should be observed closely for development of hypokalemia). Products include:

Aldoclor Tablets 1881
Diuril Oral 1936

Chlorothiazide Sodium (When corticosteroids are administered with potassium-depleting agents (eg, diuretics), patients should be observed closely for development of hypokalemia). Products include:

Diuril Sodium Intravenous 1934

Chlorotrianisene (Estrogens may decrease the hepatic metabolism of certain corticosteroids, thereby increasing their effect).

No products indexed under this heading.

Chlorpheniramine (Dexamethasone is a moderate inducer of the cytochrome P450 3A4 enzyme system. Co-administration with other drugs that are metabolized by CYP 3A4 may increase their clearance, resulting in decreased plasma concentrations).
No products indexed under this heading.

Chlorpheniramine Maleate (Dexamethasone is a moderate inducer of the cytochrome P450 3A4 enzyme system. Co-administration with other drugs that are metabolized by CYP 3A4 may increase their clearance, resulting in decreased plasma concentrations). Products include:
Advil Allergy Sinus Caplets .... ▣737
Advil Multi-Symptom Cold Caplets .... ▣738
BC Allergy Sinus Cold Powder .... ▣612
Contac Severe Cold and Flu Caplets Maximum Strength .... ▣615
Hycomine Compound Tablets 1105
PediaCare Multi-Symptom Cold Liquid .... ▣704
PediaCare NightRest Cough & Cold Liquid .... ▣704
Robitussin Flu Liquid .... ▣752
Robitussin PM Cough & Cold Liquid .... ▣752
Singlet Caplets .... ▣636
Sudafed Sinus & Allergy Tablets .... ▣710
TheraFlu Cold & Cough Hot Liquid .... ▣680
TheraFlu Cold & Sore Throat Hot Liquid .... ▣680
TheraFlu Flu & Sore Throat Hot Liquid .... ▣681
TheraFlu Severe Cold & Cough Hot Liquid .... ▣683
TheraFlu Severe Cold Caplets .... ▣679
TheraFlu Severe Cold Hot Liquid .... ▣682
Triaminic Cold & Allergy Liquid .... ▣685
Triaminic Cold & Cough Liquid .... ▣685
Triaminic Flu, Cough & Fever Liquid .... ▣685
Triaminic Night Time Cough & Cold Liquid .... ▣685
Triaminic Allergy Runny Nose & Congestion Softchews .... ▣688
Triaminic Cold & Cough Softchews .... ▣688
Children's Tylenol Plus Cold NightTime Suspension Liquid 1851
Children's Tylenol Plus Cold & Cough Suspension Liquid and Chewable Tablets 1851
Children's Tylenol Plus Cold Chewable Tablets 1851
Children's Tylenol Plus Flu Suspension Liquid 1853
Tylenol Allergy Complete Multi-Symptom Caplets and Gelcaps with Cool Burst 1844
Multi-Symptom Tylenol Cold Night Time Caplets 1845
Vicks 44M Cough, Cold & Flu Relief 2676
Pediatric Vicks 44m Cough & Cold Relief 2673
Children's Vicks NyQuil Cold/Cough Relief 2671

Chlorpheniramine Polistirex (Dexamethasone is a moderate inducer of the cytochrome P450 3A4 enzyme system. Co-administration with other drugs that are metabolized by CYP 3A4 may increase their clearance, resulting in decreased plasma concentrations). Products include:
Tussionex Pennkinetic Extended-Release Suspension 3322

Chlorpheniramine Tannate (Dexamethasone is a moderate inducer of the cytochrome P450 3A4 enzyme system. Co-administration with other drugs that are metabolized by CYP 3A4 may increase their clearance, resulting in decreased plasma concentrations).
No products indexed under this heading.

Chlorpropamide (Because corticosteroids may increase blood glucose concentrations, dosage adjustments of antidiabetic agents may be required).
No products indexed under this heading.

Cholestyramine (Cholestyramine may increase the clearance of corticosteroids).
No products indexed under this heading.

Cimetidine (Drugs which inhibit cytochrome P450 3A4 enzyme activity have the potential to result in increased plasma concentrations of corticosteroids). Products include:
Tagamet HB 200 Tablets .... ▣637
Tagamet Tablets 1547

Cimetidine Hydrochloride (Drugs which inhibit cytochrome P450 3A4 enzyme activity have the potential to result in increased plasma concentrations of corticosteroids).
No products indexed under this heading.

Ciprofloxacin (Drugs which inhibit cytochrome P450 3A4 enzyme activity have the potential to result in increased plasma concentrations of corticosteroids). Products include:
Cipro I.V. 2998
Cipro I.V. Pharmacy Bulk Package ... 3509
Cipro Oral Suspension 2991
Cipro XR Tablets 3004
Ciprodex Otic Suspension 555

Ciprofloxacin Hydrochloride (Drugs which induce cytochrome P450 3A4 enzyme activity may enhance the metabolism of corticosteroids and require that the dosage of the corticosteroid be increased). Products include:
Ciloxan Ophthalmic Ointment 554
Cipro Tablets 2991

Cisapride (Dexamethasone is a moderate inducer of the cytochrome P450 3A4 enzyme system. Co-administration with other drugs that are metabolized by CYP 3A4 may increase their clearance, resulting in decreased plasma concentrations).
No products indexed under this heading.

Cisplatin (Drugs which induce cytochrome P450 3A4 enzyme activity may enhance the metabolism of corticosteroids and require that the dosage of the corticosteroid be increased).
No products indexed under this heading.

Clarithromycin (Macrolide antibiotics have been reported to cause a significant decrease in corticosteroid clearance. Drugs which inhibit cytochrome P450 3A4 enzyme activity (eg, macrolide antibiotics) have the potential to result in increased plasma concentrations of corticosteroids. Dexamethasone is a moderate inducer of the cytochrome P450 3A4 enzyme system. Co-administration with other drugs that are metabolized by CYP 3A4 (eg, erythromycin) may increase their clearance, resulting in decreased plasma concentrations). Products include:
Biaxin/Biaxin XL 402
PREVPAC 3281

Clotrimazole (Drugs which inhibit cytochrome P450 3A4 enzyme activity have the potential to result in increased plasma concentrations of corticosteroids). Products include:
Lotrimin 3053
Lotrisone 3054

Cortisone Acetate (Drugs which induce cytochrome P450 3A4 enzyme activity may enhance the metabolism of corticosteroids and require that the dosage of the corticosteroid be increased).
No products indexed under this heading.

Cyclosporine (Increased activity of both cyclosporine and corticosteroids may occur when the two are used concurrently. Convulsions have been reported with this concurrent use). Products include:
Gengraf Capsules 458
Neoral Soft Gelatin Capsules 2247
Neoral Oral Solution 2247
Restasis Ophthalmic Emulsion 570
Sandimmune 2259

Dalfopristin (Drugs which inhibit cytochrome P450 3A4 enzyme activity have the potential to result in increased plasma concentrations of corticosteroids). Products include:
Synercid I.V. 1690

Danazol (Drugs which inhibit cytochrome P450 3A4 enzyme activity have the potential to result in increased plasma concentrations of corticosteroids).
No products indexed under this heading.

Delavirdine Mesylate (Drugs which inhibit cytochrome P450 3A4 enzyme activity have the potential to result in increased plasma concentrations of corticosteroids). Products include:
Rescriptor Tablets 2535

Deslanoside (Patients on digitalis glycosides may be at increased risk of arrhythmias due to hypokalemia).
No products indexed under this heading.

Desogestrel (Estrogens may decrease the hepatic metabolism of certain corticosteroids, thereby increasing their effect). Products include:
Ortho-Cept Tablets 2395

Dexamethasone Acetate (Drugs which induce cytochrome P450 3A4 enzyme activity may enhance the metabolism of corticosteroids and require that the dosage of the corticosteroid be increased).
No products indexed under this heading.

Dexamethasone Sodium Phosphate (Drugs which induce cytochrome P450 3A4 enzyme activity may enhance the metabolism of corticosteroids and require that the dosage of the corticosteroid be increased). Products include:
Decadron Phosphate Injection 1931

Diazepam (Dexamethasone is a moderate inducer of the cytochrome P450 3A4 enzyme system. Co-administration with other drugs that are metabolized by CYP 3A4 may increase their clearance, resulting in decreased plasma concentrations). Products include:
Diastat Rectal Delivery System 3344
Valium Tablets 2822

Diclofenac Potassium (Concomitant use of non-steroidal anti-inflammatory agents and corticosteroids increases the risk of gastrointestinal side effects). Products include:
Cataflam Tablets 2173

Diclofenac Sodium (Concomitant use of non-steroidal anti-inflammatory agents and corticosteroids increases the risk of gastrointestinal side effects). Products include:
Arthrotec Tablets 3126
Voltaren Ophthalmic Solution 2300
Voltaren Tablets 2298
Voltaren-XR Tablets 2301

Dicumarol (Co-administration of corticosteroids and warfarin usually results in inhibition of response to warfarin, although there have been some conflicting reports. Therefore, coagulation indices should be monitored frequently to maintain the desired anticoagulant effect).
No products indexed under this heading.

Dienestrol (Estrogens may decrease the hepatic metabolism of certain corticosteroids, thereby increasing their effect).
No products indexed under this heading.

Diethylstilbestrol (Estrogens may decrease the hepatic metabolism of certain corticosteroids, thereby increasing their effect).
No products indexed under this heading.

Digitalis Glycoside Preparations (Patients on digitalis glycosides may be at increased risk of arrhythmias due to hypokalemia).
No products indexed under this heading.

Digitoxin (Patients on digitalis glycosides may be at increased risk of arrhythmias due to hypokalemia).
No products indexed under this heading.

Digoxin (Patients on digitalis glycosides may be at increased risk of arrhythmias due to hypokalemia). Products include:
Digitek Tablets 2146
Lanoxicaps Capsules 1458
Lanoxin Injection 1462
Lanoxin Tablets 1468
Lanoxin Injection Pediatric 1465

Dihydroergotamine Mesylate (Dexamethasone is a moderate inducer of the cytochrome P450 3A4 enzyme system. Co-administration with other drugs that are metabolized by CYP 3A4 may increase their clearance, resulting in decreased plasma concentrations). Products include:
Migranal Nasal Spray 3350

Diltiazem Hydrochloride (Drugs which inhibit cytochrome P450 3A4 enzyme activity have the potential to result in increased plasma concentrations of corticosteroids). Products include:
Cardizem LA Extended Release Tablets 1699
Tiazac Capsules 1204

Diltiazem Maleate (Drugs which inhibit cytochrome P450 3A4 enzyme activity have the potential to result in increased plasma concentrations of corticosteroids).
No products indexed under this heading.

Dirithromycin (Macrolide antibiotics have been reported to cause a significant decrease in corticosteroid clearance. Drugs which inhibit cytochrome P450 3A4 enzyme activity (eg, macrolide antibiotics) have the potential to result in increased plasma concentrations of corticosteroids. Dexamethasone is a moderate inducer of the cytochrome P450 3A4 enzyme system. Co-administration with other drugs that are metabolized by CYP 3A4 (eg, erythromycin) may increase their clearance, resulting in decreased plasma concentrations).
No products indexed under this heading.

Disopyramide (Dexamethasone is a moderate inducer of the cytochrome P450 3A4 enzyme system. Co-administration with other drugs that are metabolized by CYP 3A4 may increase their clearance, resulting in decreased plasma concentrations).
No products indexed under this heading.

Disopyramide Phosphate (Dexamethasone is a moderate inducer of the cytochrome P450 3A4 enzyme system. Co-administration with other drugs that are metabolized by CYP 3A4 may increase their clearance, resulting in decreased plasma concentrations).
No products indexed under this heading.

Disulfiram (Dexamethasone is a moderate inducer of the cytochrome P450 3A4 enzyme system. Co-administration with other drugs that are metabolized by CYP 3A4 may increase their clearance, resulting in decreased plasma concentrations). Products include:
Antabuse Tablets **2343**

Donepezil Hydrochloride (Concomitant use of anticholinesterase agents and corticosteroids may produce severe weakness in patients with myasthenia gravis. If possible, anticholinesterase agents should be withdrawn at least 24 hours before initiating corticosteroid therapy). Products include:
Aricept Tablets **1086**
Aricept ODT Tablets **1086**

Doxorubicin Hydrochloride (Dexamethasone is a moderate inducer of the cytochrome P450 3A4 enzyme system. Co-administration with other drugs that are metabolized by CYP 3A4 may increase their clearance, resulting in decreased plasma concentrations). Products include:
Adriamycin for Injection, USP **786**
Adriamycin Injection, USP **786**

Dronabinol (Dexamethasone is a moderate inducer of the cytochrome P450 3A4 enzyme system. Co-administration with other drugs that are metabolized by CYP 3A4 may increase their clearance, resulting in decreased plasma concentrations). Products include:
Marinol Capsules **3334**

Efavirenz (Drugs which inhibit cytochrome P450 3A4 enzyme activity have the potential to result in increased plasma concentrations of corticosteroids). Products include:
Sustiva Capsules **957**

Ephedrine Hydrochloride (Ephedrine may enhance the metabolic clearance of corticosteroids, resulting in decreased blood levels and lessened physiologic activity, thus requiring an increase in corticosteroid dosage). Products include:
Primatene Tablets **749**

Ephedrine Sulfate (Ephedrine may enhance the metabolic clearance of corticosteroids, resulting in decreased blood levels and lessened physiologic activity, thus requiring an increase in corticosteroid dosage).
No products indexed under this heading.

Ephedrine Tannate (Ephedrine may enhance the metabolic clearance of corticosteroids, resulting in decreased blood levels and lessened physiologic activity, thus requiring an increase in corticosteroid dosage).
No products indexed under this heading.

Ergotamine Tartrate (Dexamethasone is a moderate inducer of the cytochrome P450 3A4 enzyme system. Co-administration with other drugs that are metabolized by CYP 3A4 may increase their clearance, resulting in decreased plasma concentrations).
No products indexed under this heading.

Erythromycin (Macrolide antibiotics have been reported to cause a significant decrease in corticosteroid clearance. Drugs which inhibit cytochrome P450 3A4 enzyme activity (eg, macrolide antibiotics) have the potential to result in increased plasma concentrations of corticosteroids. Dexamethasone is a moderate inducer of the cytochrome P450 3A4 enzyme system. Co-administration with other drugs that are metabolized by CYP 3A4 (eg, erythromycin) may increase their clearance, resulting in decreased plasma concentrations). Products include:
Erygel Topical Gel **2096**
Ery-Tab Tablets **447**
Erythromycin Base Filmtab Tablets **454**
Erythromycin Delayed-Release Capsules, USP **456**
PCE Dispertab Tablets **510**

Erythromycin Estolate (Macrolide antibiotics have been reported to cause a significant decrease in corticosteroid clearance. Drugs which inhibit cytochrome P450 3A4 enzyme activity (eg, macrolide antibiotics) have the potential to result in increased plasma concentrations of corticosteroids. Dexamethasone is a moderate inducer of the cytochrome P450 3A4 enzyme system. Co-administration with other drugs that are metabolized by CYP 3A4 (eg, erythromycin) may increase their clearance, resulting in decreased plasma concentrations).
No products indexed under this heading.

Erythromycin Ethylsuccinate (Macrolide antibiotics have been reported to cause a significant decrease in corticosteroid clearance. Drugs which inhibit cytochrome P450 3A4 enzyme activity (eg, macrolide antibiotics) have the potential to result in increased plasma concentrations of corticosteroids. Dexamethasone is a moderate inducer of the cytochrome P450 3A4 enzyme system. Co-administration with other drugs that are metabolized by CYP 3A4 (eg, erythromycin) may increase their clearance, resulting in decreased plasma concentrations). Products include:
E.E.S. **449**
EryPed **445**

Erythromycin Gluceptate (Macrolide antibiotics have been reported to cause a significant decrease in corticosteroid clearance. Drugs which inhibit cytochrome P450 3A4 enzyme activity (eg, macrolide antibiotics) have the potential to result in increased plasma concentrations of corticosteroids. Dexamethasone is a moderate inducer of the cytochrome P450 3A4 enzyme system. Co-administration with other drugs that are metabolized by CYP 3A4 (eg, erythromycin) may increase their clearance, resulting in decreased plasma concentrations).
No products indexed under this heading.

Erythromycin Lactobionate (Drugs which inhibit cytochrome P450 3A4 enzyme activity have the potential to result in increased plasma concentrations of corticosteroids).
No products indexed under this heading.

Erythromycin Stearate (Macrolide antibiotics have been reported to cause a significant decrease in corticosteroid clearance. Drugs which inhibit cytochrome P450 3A4 enzyme activity (eg, macrolide antibiotics) have the potential to result in increased plasma concentrations of corticosteroids. Dexamethasone is a moderate inducer of the cytochrome P450 3A4 enzyme system. Co-administration with other drugs that are metabolized by CYP 3A4 (eg, erythromycin) may increase their clearance, resulting in decreased plasma concentrations). Products include:
Erythrocin Stearate Filmtab Tablets **452**

Esomeprazole Magnesium (Drugs which inhibit cytochrome P450 3A4 enzyme activity have the potential to result in increased plasma concentrations of corticosteroids). Products include:
Nexium Delayed-Release Capsules **645**

Estradiol (Estrogens may decrease the hepatic metabolism of certain corticosteroids, thereby increasing their effect). Products include:
Activella Tablets **2311**
Climara Transdermal System **795**
Climara Pro Transdermal System **800**
CombiPatch Transdermal System **2180**
Estrogel 0.06% **3200**
Menostar Transdermal System **805**
Prefest Tablets **1069**
Vagifem Tablets **2340**
Vivelle Transdermal System **2288**
Vivelle-Dot Transdermal System **2293**

Estradiol Benzoate (Dexamethasone is a moderate inducer of the cytochrome P450 3A4 enzyme system. Co-administration with other drugs that are metabolized by CYP 3A4 may increase their clearance, resulting in decreased plasma concentrations).
No products indexed under this heading.

Estradiol Cypionate (Dexamethasone is a moderate inducer of the cytochrome P450 3A4 enzyme system. Co-administration with other drugs that are metabolized by CYP 3A4 may increase their clearance, resulting in decreased plasma concentrations).
No products indexed under this heading.

Estradiol Valerate (Dexamethasone is a moderate inducer of the cytochrome P450 3A4 enzyme system. Co-administration with other drugs that are metabolized by CYP 3A4 may increase their clearance, resulting in decreased plasma concentrations).
No products indexed under this heading.

Estrogens, Conjugated (Estrogens may decrease the hepatic metabolism of certain corticosteroids, thereby increasing their effect). Products include:
Premarin Intravenous **3440**
Premarin Tablets **3443**
Premarin Vaginal Cream **3449**
Premphase Tablets **3452**
Prempro Tablets **3452**

Estrogens, Esterified (Estrogens may decrease the hepatic metabolism of certain corticosteroids, thereby increasing their effect). Products include:
Estratest Tablets **3196**
Estratest H.S. Tablets **3196**

Estropipate (Estrogens may decrease the hepatic metabolism of certain corticosteroids, thereby increasing their effect).
No products indexed under this heading.

Ethacrynic Acid (When corticosteroids are administered with potassium-depleting agents (eg, diuretics), patients should be observed closely for development of hypokalemia). Products include:
Edecrin Tablets **1941**

Ethinyl Estradiol (Estrogens may decrease the hepatic metabolism of certain corticosteroids, thereby increasing their effect). Products include:
Alesse-28 Tablets **3392**
Lo/Ovral-28 Tablets **3423**
NuvaRing **2357**
Ortho-Cept Tablets **2395**
Ortho-Cyclen/Ortho Tri-Cyclen **2414**
Ortho Evra Transdermal System **2402**
Ortho Tri-Cyclen Lo Tablets **2421**
Seasonale Tablets **1073**
Triphasil-28 Tablets **3483**
Yasmin 28 Tablets **818**

Ethosuximide (Dexamethasone is a moderate inducer of the cytochrome P450 3A4 enzyme system. Co-administration with other drugs that are metabolized by CYP 3A4 may increase their clearance, resulting in decreased plasma concentrations).
No products indexed under this heading.

Ethynodiol Diacetate (Estrogens may decrease the hepatic metabolism of certain corticosteroids, thereby increasing their effect).
No products indexed under this heading.

Etodolac (Concomitant use of nonsteroidal anti-inflammatory agents and corticosteroids increases the risk of gastrointestinal side effects).
No products indexed under this heading.

Etoposide (Dexamethasone is a moderate inducer of the cytochrome P450 3A4 enzyme system. Co-administration with other drugs that are metabolized by CYP 3A4 may increase their clearance, resulting in decreased plasma concentrations).
No products indexed under this heading.

Etoposide Phosphate (Dexamethasone is a moderate inducer of the cytochrome P450 3A4 enzyme system. Co-administration with other drugs that are metabolized by CYP 3A4 may increase their clearance, resulting in decreased plasma concentrations).
No products indexed under this heading.

Felbamate (Drugs which induce cytochrome P450 3A4 enzyme activity may enhance the metabolism of corticosteroids and require that the dosage of the corticosteroid be increased).
No products indexed under this heading.

Felodipine (Dexamethasone is a moderate inducer of the cytochrome P450 3A4 enzyme system. Co-administration with other drugs that are metabolized by CYP 3A4 may increase their clearance, resulting in decreased plasma concentrations). Products include:
Plendil Extended-Release Tablets 651

Fenoprofen Calcium (Concomitant use of non-steroidal anti-inflammatory agents and corticosteroids increases the risk of gastrointestinal side effects). Products include:
Nalfon Capsules 2504

Fentanyl (Dexamethasone is a moderate inducer of the cytochrome P450 3A4 enzyme system. Co-administration with other drugs that are metabolized by CYP 3A4 may increase their clearance, resulting in decreased plasma concentrations). Products include:
Duragesic Transdermal System 2448

Fentanyl Citrate (Dexamethasone is a moderate inducer of the cytochrome P450 3A4 enzyme system. Co-administration with other drugs that are metabolized by CYP 3A4 may increase their clearance, resulting in decreased plasma concentrations). Products include:
Actiq 993

Fluconazole (Drugs which inhibit cytochrome P450 3A4 enzyme activity have the potential to result in increased plasma concentrations of corticosteroids).
No products indexed under this heading.

Fludrocortisone Acetate (Drugs which induce cytochrome P450 3A4 enzyme activity may enhance the metabolism of corticosteroids and require that the dosage of the corticosteroid be increased).
No products indexed under this heading.

Fluoxetine Hydrochloride (Drugs which inhibit cytochrome P450 3A4 enzyme activity have the potential to result in increased plasma concentrations of corticosteroids). Products include:
Prozac Pulvules and Liquid 1771
Symbyax Capsules 1788

Flurbiprofen (Concomitant use of non-steroidal anti-inflammatory agents and corticosteroids increases the risk of gastrointestinal side effects).
No products indexed under this heading.

Fluvoxamine Maleate (Drugs which inhibit cytochrome P450 3A4 enzyme activity have the potential to result in increased plasma concentrations of corticosteroids).
No products indexed under this heading.

Fosamprenavir Calcium (Drugs which inhibit cytochrome P450 3A4 enzyme activity have the potential to result in increased plasma concentrations of corticosteroids). Products include:
Lexiva Tablets 1473

Fosphenytoin Sodium (Drugs which induce cytochrome P450 3A4 enzyme activity (eg, phenytoin) may enhance the metabolism of corticosteroids and require that the dosage of the corticosteroid be increased. In post-marketing experience, there have been reports of both increases and decreases in phenytoin levels with dexamethsone co-administration, leading to alterations in seizure control).
No products indexed under this heading.

Furosemide (When corticosteroids are administered with potassium-depleting agents (eg, diuretics), patients should be observed closely for development of hypokalemia). Products include:
Furosemide Tablets 2117

Galantamine Hydrobromide (Concomitant use of anticholinesterase agents and corticosteroids may produce severe weakness in patients with myasthenia gravis. If possible, anticholinesterase agents should be withdrawn at least 24 hours before initiating corticosteroid therapy). Products include:
Razadyne ER Extended-Release Capsules 2434
Razadyne 2434

Garlic Extract (Drugs which induce cytochrome P450 3A4 enzyme activity may enhance the metabolism of corticosteroids and require that the dosage of the corticosteroid be increased).
No products indexed under this heading.

Garlic Oil (Drugs which induce cytochrome P450 3A4 enzyme activity may enhance the metabolism of corticosteroids and require that the dosage of the corticosteroid be increased).
No products indexed under this heading.

Glimepiride (Because corticosteroids may increase blood glucose concentrations, dosage adjustments of antidiabetic agents may be required). Products include:
Amaryl Tablets 2864

Glipizide (Because corticosteroids may increase blood glucose concentrations, dosage adjustments of antidiabetic agents may be required).
No products indexed under this heading.

Glyburide (Because corticosteroids may increase blood glucose concentrations, dosage adjustments of antidiabetic agents may be required).
No products indexed under this heading.

Haloperidol (Dexamethasone is a moderate inducer of the cytochrome P450 3A4 enzyme system. Co-administration with other drugs that are metabolized by CYP 3A4 may increase their clearance, resulting in decreased plasma concentrations).
No products indexed under this heading.

Haloperidol Decanoate (Dexamethasone is a moderate inducer of the cytochrome P450 3A4 enzyme system. Co-administration with other drugs that are metabolized by CYP 3A4 may increase their clearance, resulting in decreased plasma concentrations).
No products indexed under this heading.

Haloperidol Lactate (Dexamethasone is a moderate inducer of the cytochrome P450 3A4 enzyme system. Co-administration with other drugs that are metabolized by CYP 3A4 may increase their clearance, resulting in decreased plasma concentrations).
No products indexed under this heading.

Hydrochlorothiazide (When corticosteroids are administered with potassium-depleting agents (eg, diuretics), patients should be observed closely for development of hypokalemia). Products include:
Aldoril Tablets 1884
Atacand HCT 637
Avalide Tablets 2889
Avalide Tablets 922
Benicar HCT Tablets 2852
Diovan HCT Tablets 2195
Dyazide Capsules 1389
Hyzaar 1964
Lotensin HCT Tablets 2235
Maxzide 2150
Micardis HCT Tablets 886
Moduretic Tablets 2003
Prinzide Tablets 2033
Teveten HCT Tablets 1710
Timolide Tablets 2056
Uniretic Tablets 3114
Vaseretic Tablets 2073
Zestoretic Tablets 701

Hydrocortisone (Drugs which induce cytochrome P450 3A4 enzyme activity may enhance the metabolism of corticosteroids and require that the dosage of the corticosteroid be increased). Products include:
Cortizone•5 Ointment .... ▣699
Cortizone•10 Creme .... ▣699
Cortizone•10 Ointment .... ▣699
Cortizone•10 Plus Creme .... ▣700
Cortizone•10 Maximum Strength Quick Shot Spray .... ▣700
Hydrocortone Tablets 1963
Preparation H Hydrocortisone Cream .... ▣748

Hydrocortisone Acetate (Drugs which induce cytochrome P450 3A4 enzyme activity may enhance the metabolism of corticosteroids and require that the dosage of the corticosteroid be increased). Products include:
Analpram-HC 1136
Pramosone 1139
ProctoFoam-HC 3113
Tucks Anti-Itch Ointment .... ▣712
U-cort 1% Cream 3289

Hydrocortisone Butyrate (Drugs which induce cytochrome P450 3A4 enzyme activity may enhance the metabolism of corticosteroids and require that the dosage of the corticosteroid be increased). Products include:
Locoid 1138
Locoid Lipocream Cream 1138

Hydrocortisone Cypionate (Drugs which induce cytochrome P450 3A4 enzyme activity may enhance the metabolism of corticosteroids and require that the dosage of the corticosteroid be increased).
No products indexed under this heading.

Hydrocortisone Hemisuccinate (Drugs which induce cytochrome P450 3A4 enzyme activity may enhance the metabolism of corticosteroids and require that the dosage of the corticosteroid be increased).
No products indexed under this heading.

Hydrocortisone Probutate (Drugs which induce cytochrome P450 3A4 enzyme activity may enhance the metabolism of corticosteroids and require that the dosage of the corticosteroid be increased). Products include:
Pandel Cream, 0.1% 1017

Hydrocortisone Sodium Phosphate (Drugs which induce cytochrome P450 3A4 enzyme activity may enhance the metabolism of corticosteroids and require that the dosage of the corticosteroid be increased).
No products indexed under this heading.

Hydrocortisone Sodium Succinate (Drugs which induce cytochrome P450 3A4 enzyme activity may enhance the metabolism of corticosteroids and require that the dosage of the corticosteroid be increased).
No products indexed under this heading.

Hydrocortisone Valerate (Drugs which induce cytochrome P450 3A4 enzyme activity may enhance the metabolism of corticosteroids and require that the dosage of the corticosteroid be increased).
No products indexed under this heading.

Hydroflumethiazide (When corticosteroids are administered with potassium-depleting agents (eg, diuretics), patients should be observed closely for development of hypokalemia).
No products indexed under this heading.

Hypericum (Drugs which induce cytochrome P450 3A4 enzyme activity may enhance the metabolism of corticosteroids and require that the dosage of the corticosteroid be increased).
No products indexed under this heading.

Hypericum Perforatum (Drugs which induce cytochrome P450 3A4 enzyme activity may enhance the metabolism of corticosteroids and require that the dosage of the corticosteroid be increased).
No products indexed under this heading.

Ibuprofen (Concomitant use of non-steroidal anti-inflammatory agents and corticosteroids increases the risk of gastrointestinal side effects). Products include:
Advil Allergy Sinus Caplets .... ▣737

Advil 737
Children's Advil Suspension 742
Children's Advil Chewable Tablets .. 741
Advil Cold & Sinus 739
Advil Flu & Body Ache Caplets 739
Children's Advil Cold Suspension ... 741
Infants' Advil Concentrated Drops .. 743
Junior Strength Advil Swallow Tablets.. 740
Advil Migraine Liquigels 740
Advil Multi-Symptom Cold Caplets.. 738
Combunox Tablets 1183
Children's Motrin Oral Suspension and Chewable Tablets.................. 1837
Children's Motrin Cold Non-Staining Dye-Free Oral Suspension.................................. 1838
Children's Motrin Cold Oral Suspension.................................. 1838
Children's Motrin Non-Staining Dye-Free Oral Suspension............. 1837
Motrin Cold & Sinus Caplets 1836
Motrin IB Tablets and Caplets 1836
Infants' Motrin Concentrated Drops... 1837
Infants' Motrin Non-Staining Dye-Free Drops............................ 1837
Junior Strength Motrin Caplets and Chewable Tablets.................. 1837
Vicoprofen Tablets 533

Indinavir Sulfate (Drugs which inhibit cytochrome P450 3A4 enzyme activity have the potential to result in increased plasma concentrations of corticosteroids). Products include:
Crixivan Capsules 1918

Indomethacin (Concomitant use of non-steroidal anti-inflammatory agents and corticosteroids increases the risk of gastrointestinal side effects). Products include:
Indocin 1968

Indomethacin Sodium Trihydrate (Concomitant use of non-steroidal anti-inflammatory agents and corticosteroids increases the risk of gastrointestinal side effects). Products include:
Indocin I.V. 1973

Insulin, Human, Zinc Suspension (Because corticosteroids may increase blood glucose concentrations, dosage adjustments of antidiabetic agents may be required). Products include:
Humulin L, 100 Units 1763
Humulin U, 100 Units 1770

Insulin, Human NPH (Because corticosteroids may increase blood glucose concentrations, dosage adjustments of antidiabetic agents may be required). Products include:
Humulin N, 100 Units 1764
Humulin N Pen 1765
Novolin N Human Insulin 10 ml Vials... 2322
Novolin N InnoLet 2322
Novolin N PenFill 3 ml Cartridges 2325
Novolin R InnoLet 2322

Insulin, Human Regular (Because corticosteroids may increase blood glucose concentrations, dosage adjustments of antidiabetic agents may be required). Products include:
Humulin R (U-500) 1768
Humulin R, 100 Units 1767
Novolin R Human Insulin 10 ml Vials... 2322
Novolin R PenFill 2325

Insulin, Human Regular and Human NPH Mixture (Because corticosteroids may increase blood glucose concentrations, dosage adjustments of antidiabetic agents may be required). Products include:
Humulin 50/50, 100 Units 1760
Humulin 70/30 Pen 1761
Novolin 70/30 Human Insulin 10 ml Vials.................................. 2321
Novolin 70/30 InnoLet 2322
Novolin 70/30 PenFill 3 ml Cartridges.................................. 2325

Insulin, NPH (Because corticosteroids may increase blood glucose concentrations, dosage adjustments of antidiabetic agents may be required).
No products indexed under this heading.

Insulin, Regular (Because corticosteroids may increase blood glucose concentrations, dosage adjustments of antidiabetic agents may be required).
No products indexed under this heading.

Insulin, Zinc Crystals (Because corticosteroids may increase blood glucose concentrations, dosage adjustments of antidiabetic agents may be required).
No products indexed under this heading.

Insulin, Zinc Suspension (Because corticosteroids may increase blood glucose concentrations, dosage adjustments of antidiabetic agents may be required).
No products indexed under this heading.

Insulin Aspart, Human Regular (Because corticosteroids may increase blood glucose concentrations, dosage adjustments of antidiabetic agents may be required). Products include:
NovoLog Injection 2326

Insulin glargine (Because corticosteroids may increase blood glucose concentrations, dosage adjustments of antidiabetic agents may be required). Products include:
Lantus Injection 2925

Insulin Lispro, Human (Because corticosteroids may increase blood glucose concentrations, dosage adjustments of antidiabetic agents may be required). Products include:
Humalog-Pen 1751
Humalog Mix 75/25-Pen 1754

Insulin Lispro Protamine, Human (Because corticosteroids may increase blood glucose concentrations, dosage adjustments of antidiabetic agents may be required). Products include:
Humalog Mix 75/25-Pen 1754

Isoniazid (Serum concentrations of isoniazid may be decreased).
No products indexed under this heading.

Isradipine (Dexamethasone is a moderate inducer of the cytochrome P450 3A4 enzyme system. Co-administration with other drugs that are metabolized by CYP 3A4 may increase their clearance, resulting in decreased plasma concentrations). Products include:
DynaCirc CR Tablets 2726

Itraconazole (Drugs which inhibit cytochrome P450 3A4 enzyme activity have the potential to result in increased plasma concentrations of corticosteroids).
No products indexed under this heading.

Ketoconazole (Drugs which inhibit cytochrome P450 3A4 enzyme activity (eg, ketoconazole) have the potential to result in increased plasma concentrations of corticosteroids. Ketoconazole has been reported to decrease the metabolism of certain corticosteroids by up to 60%, leading to increased risk of corticosteroid side effects. In addition, ketoconazole alone can inhibit adrenal corticosteroid synthesis and may cause adrenal insufficiency during corticosteroid withdrawal). Products include:
Nizoral A-D Shampoo, 1% 1839
Nizoral 2% Shampoo 1838

Ketoprofen (Concomitant use of non-steroidal anti-inflammatory agents and corticosteroids increases the risk of gastrointestinal side effects).
No products indexed under this heading.

Ketorolac Tromethamine (Concomitant use of non-steroidal anti-inflammatory agents and corticosteroids increases the risk of gastrointestinal side effects). Products include:
Acular Ophthalmic Solution 561
Acular LS Ophthalmic Solution 562

Levonorgestrel (Estrogens may decrease the hepatic metabolism of certain corticosteroids, thereby increasing their effect). Products include:
Alesse-28 Tablets 3392
Climara Pro Transdermal System 800
Mirena Intrauterine System 810
Plan B Tablets 1068
Seasonale Tablets 1073
Triphasil-28 Tablets 3483

Lidocaine (Dexamethasone is a moderate inducer of the cytochrome P450 3A4 enzyme system. Co-administration with other drugs that are metabolized by CYP 3A4 may increase their clearance, resulting in decreased plasma concentrations). Products include:
Lidoderm Patch 1107

Lidocaine Hydrochloride (Dexamethasone is a moderate inducer of the cytochrome P450 3A4 enzyme system. Co-administration with other drugs that are metabolized by CYP 3A4 may increase their clearance, resulting in decreased plasma concentrations).
No products indexed under this heading.

Lopinavir (Drugs which inhibit cytochrome P450 3A4 enzyme activity have the potential to result in increased plasma concentrations of corticosteroids). Products include:
Kaletra 474

Loratadine (Drugs which inhibit cytochrome P450 3A4 enzyme activity have the potential to result in increased plasma concentrations of corticosteroids). Products include:
Alavert Allergy & Sinus D-12 Hour Tablets.. 743
Alavert 743
Children's Claritin 24 Hour Non-Drowsy Allergy Syrup........... 732
Claritin Non-Drowsy 24 Hour Tablets.. 731
Non-Drowsy Claritin Hives Relief Tablets.. 733
Claritin Reditabs 24 Hour Non-Drowsy Tablets.................... 732
Claritin-D Non-Drowsy 12 Hour Tablets.. 731
Claritin-D Non-Drowsy 24 Hour Tablets.. 731
Children's Dimetapp ND Non-Drowsy Allergy Syrup........... 746
Triaminic Allerchews 684

Lovastatin (Dexamethasone is a moderate inducer of the cytochrome P450 3A4 enzyme system. Co-administration with other drugs that are metabolized by CYP 3A4 may increase their clearance, resulting in decreased plasma concentrations). Products include:
Advicor Tablets 1694
Altoprev Extended-Release Tablets... 1151
Mevacor Tablets 1996

Measles, Mumps & Rubella Virus Vaccine, Live (Patients on corticosteroid therapy may exhibit a diminished response to toxoids and live or inactivated vaccines due to inhibition of antibody response. Corticosteroids may also potentiate the replication of some organisms contained in live attenuated vaccines. Routine administration of vaccines or toxoids should be deferred until corticosteroid therapy is discontinued if possible. Administration of live or live, attenuated vaccines is contraindicated in patients receiving immunosuppressive doses of corticosteroids). Products include:
M-M-R II 1980

Measles & Rubella Virus Vaccine Live (Patients on corticosteroid therapy may exhibit a diminished response to toxoids and live or inactivated vaccines due to inhibition of antibody response. Corticosteroids may also potentiate the replication of some organisms contained in live attenuated vaccines. Routine administration of vaccines or toxoids should be deferred until corticosteroid therapy is discontinued if possible. Administration of live or live, attenuated vaccines is contraindicated in patients receiving immunosuppressive doses of corticosteroids).
No products indexed under this heading.

Measles Virus Vaccine Live (Patients on corticosteroid therapy may exhibit a diminished response to toxoids and live or inactivated vaccines due to inhibition of antibody response. Corticosteroids may also potentiate the replication of some organisms contained in live attenuated vaccines. Routine administration of vaccines or toxoids should be deferred until corticosteroid therapy is discontinued if possible. Administration of live or live, attenuated vaccines is contraindicated in patients receiving immunosuppressive doses of corticosteroids). Products include:
Attenuvax 1889

Meclofenamate Sodium (Concomitant use of non-steroidal anti-inflammatory agents and corticosteroids increases the risk of gastrointestinal side effects).
No products indexed under this heading.

Mefenamic Acid (Concomitant use of non-steroidal anti-inflammatory agents and corticosteroids increases the risk of gastrointestinal side effects).
No products indexed under this heading.

Meloxicam (Concomitant use of non-steroidal anti-inflammatory agents and corticosteroids increases the risk of gastrointestinal side effects). Products include:
Mobic Oral Suspension 893
Mobic Tablets 893

Mephenytoin (Drugs which induce cytochrome P450 3A4 enzyme activity may enhance the metabolism of corticosteroids and require that the dosage of the corticosteroid be increased).
No products indexed under this heading.

Mephobarbital (Drugs which induce cytochrome P450 3A4 enzyme activity (eg, barbiturates) may enhance the metabolism of corticosteroids and require that the dosage of the corticosteroid be increased). Products include:
Mebaral Tablets, USP **2483**

Mestranol (Estrogens may decrease the hepatic metabolism of certain corticosteroids, thereby increasing their effect).
No products indexed under this heading.

Metformin Hydrochloride (Because corticosteroids may increase blood glucose concentrations, dosage adjustments of antidiabetic agents may be required). Products include:
ActoPlus Met Tablets **3219**
Avandamet Tablets **1343**
Fortamet Extended-Release Tablets **1156**

Methadone Hydrochloride (Dexamethasone is a moderate inducer of the cytochrome P450 3A4 enzyme system. Co-administration with other drugs that are metabolized by CYP 3A4 may increase their clearance, resulting in decreased plasma concentrations).
No products indexed under this heading.

Methsuximide (Drugs which induce cytochrome P450 3A4 enzyme activity may enhance the metabolism of corticosteroids and require that the dosage of the corticosteroid be increased).
No products indexed under this heading.

Methyclothiazide (When corticosteroids are administered with potassium-depleting agents (eg, diuretics), patients should be observed closely for development of hypokalemia).
No products indexed under this heading.

Methylprednisolone (Drugs which induce cytochrome P450 3A4 enzyme activity may enhance the metabolism of corticosteroids and require that the dosage of the corticosteroid be increased).
No products indexed under this heading.

Methylprednisolone Acetate (Drugs which induce cytochrome P450 3A4 enzyme activity may enhance the metabolism of corticosteroids and require that the dosage of the corticosteroid be increased). Products include:
Depo-Medrol Injectable Suspension **2615**
Depo-Medrol Single-Dose Vial **2617**

Methylprednisolone Sodium Succinate (Drugs which induce cytochrome P450 3A4 enzyme activity may enhance the metabolism of corticosteroids and require that the dosage of the corticosteroid be increased).
No products indexed under this heading.

Metronidazole (Drugs which inhibit cytochrome P450 3A4 enzyme activity have the potential to result in increased plasma concentrations of corticosteroids). Products include:
Metrogel 1% **1212**
MetroGel-Vaginal Gel **1822**
Noritate Cream, 1% **1051**

Metronidazole Benzoate (Drugs which inhibit cytochrome P450 3A4 enzyme activity have the potential to result in increased plasma concentrations of corticosteroids).
No products indexed under this heading.

Metronidazole Hydrochloride (Drugs which inhibit cytochrome P450 3A4 enzyme activity have the potential to result in increased plasma concentrations of corticosteroids).
No products indexed under this heading.

Miconazole (Drugs which inhibit cytochrome P450 3A4 enzyme activity have the potential to result in increased plasma concentrations of corticosteroids).
No products indexed under this heading.

Miconazole Nitrate (Drugs which inhibit cytochrome P450 3A4 enzyme activity have the potential to result in increased plasma concentrations of corticosteroids). Products include:
Desenex .... ▣ **674**
Desenex Jock Itch Spray Powder .... ▣ **674**

Midazolam Hydrochloride (Dexamethasone is a moderate inducer of the cytochrome P450 3A4 enzyme system. Co-administration with other drugs that are metabolized by CYP 3A4 may increase their clearance, resulting in decreased plasma concentrations).
No products indexed under this heading.

Miglitol (Because corticosteroids may increase blood glucose concentrations, dosage adjustments of antidiabetic agents may be required).
No products indexed under this heading.

Modafinil (Drugs which induce cytochrome P450 3A4 enzyme activity may enhance the metabolism of corticosteroids and require that the dosage of the corticosteroid be increased). Products include:
Provigil Tablets **1002**

Mumps Virus Vaccine, Live (Patients on corticosteroid therapy may exhibit a diminished response to toxoids and live or inactivated vaccines due to inhibition of antibody response. Corticosteroids may also potentiate the replication of some organisms contained in live attenuated vaccines. Routine administration of vaccines or toxoids should be deferred until corticosteroid therapy is discontinued if possible. Administration of live or live, attenuated vaccines is contraindicated in patients receiving immunosuppressive doses of corticosteroids). Products include:
Mumpsvax **2005**

Nabumetone (Concomitant use of non-steroidal anti-inflammatory agents and corticosteroids increases the risk of gastrointestinal side effects). Products include:
Relafen Tablets **1523**

Naproxen (Concomitant use of non-steroidal anti-inflammatory agents and corticosteroids increases the risk of gastrointestinal side effects). Products include:
EC-Naprosyn Delayed-Release Tablets **2769**
Naprosyn Suspension **2769**
Naprosyn Tablets **2769**
Prevacid NapraPAC **3277**

Naproxen Sodium (Concomitant use of non-steroidal anti-inflammatory agents and corticosteroids increases the risk of gastrointestinal side effects). Products include:
Aleve Tablets, Caplets and Gelcaps .... ▣ **605**
Anaprox Tablets **2769**
Anaprox DS Tablets **2769**

Nefazodone Hydrochloride (Drugs which inhibit cytochrome P450 3A4 enzyme activity have the potential to result in increased plasma concentrations of corticosteroids).
No products indexed under this heading.

Nelfinavir Mesylate (Drugs which inhibit cytochrome P450 3A4 enzyme activity have the potential to result in increased plasma concentrations of corticosteroids). Products include:
Viracept **2556**

Neostigmine Bromide (Concomitant use of anticholinesterase agents and corticosteroids may produce severe weakness in patients with myasthenia gravis. If possible, anticholinesterase agents should be withdrawn at least 24 hours before initiating corticosteroid therapy).
No products indexed under this heading.

Neostigmine Methylsulfate (Concomitant use of anticholinesterase agents and corticosteroids may produce severe weakness in patients with myasthenia gravis. If possible, anticholinesterase agents should be withdrawn at least 24 hours before initiating corticosteroid therapy).
No products indexed under this heading.

Nevirapine (Drugs which inhibit cytochrome P450 3A4 enzyme activity have the potential to result in increased plasma concentrations of corticosteroids). Products include:
Viramune Oral Suspension **903**
Viramune Tablets **903**

Niacinamide (Drugs which inhibit cytochrome P450 3A4 enzyme activity have the potential to result in increased plasma concentrations of corticosteroids).
No products indexed under this heading.

Nicardipine Hydrochloride (Dexamethasone is a moderate inducer of the cytochrome P450 3A4 enzyme system. Co-administration with other drugs that are metabolized by CYP 3A4 may increase their clearance, resulting in decreased plasma concentrations). Products include:
Cardene I.V. **1129**

Nicotinamide (Drugs which inhibit cytochrome P450 3A4 enzyme activity have the potential to result in increased plasma concentrations of corticosteroids). Products include:
Nicomide Tablets **3190**

Nifedipine (Drugs which inhibit cytochrome P450 3A4 enzyme activity have the potential to result in increased plasma concentrations of corticosteroids). Products include:
Adalat CC Tablets **2978**

Nimodipine (Dexamethasone is a moderate inducer of the cytochrome P450 3A4 enzyme system. Co-administration with other drugs that are metabolized by CYP 3A4 may increase their clearance, resulting in decreased plasma concentrations). Products include:
Nimotop Capsules **774**

Nisoldipine (Dexamethasone is a moderate inducer of the cytochrome P450 3A4 enzyme system. Co-administration with other drugs that are metabolized by CYP 3A4 may increase their clearance, resulting in decreased plasma concentrations). Products include:
Sular Tablets **1163**

Nitrendipine (Dexamethasone is a moderate inducer of the cytochrome P450 3A4 enzyme system. Co-administration with other drugs that are metabolized by CYP 3A4 may increase their clearance, resulting in decreased plasma concentrations).
No products indexed under this heading.

Norethindrone (Estrogens may decrease the hepatic metabolism of certain corticosteroids, thereby increasing their effect). Products include:
Ortho Micronor Tablets **2411**

Norethindrone Acetate (Dexamethasone is a moderate inducer of the cytochrome P450 3A4 enzyme system. Co-administration with other drugs that are metabolized by CYP 3A4 may increase their clearance, resulting in decreased plasma concentrations). Products include:
Activella Tablets **2311**
Aygestin Tablets **1062**
CombiPatch Transdermal System **2180**

Norethynodrel (Estrogens may decrease the hepatic metabolism of certain corticosteroids, thereby increasing their effect).
No products indexed under this heading.

Norfloxacin (Drugs which inhibit cytochrome P450 3A4 enzyme activity have the potential to result in increased plasma concentrations of corticosteroids). Products include:
Noroxin Tablets **2009**

Norgestimate (Estrogens may decrease the hepatic metabolism of certain corticosteroids, thereby increasing their effect). Products include:
Ortho-Cyclen/Ortho Tri-Cyclen **2414**
Ortho Tri-Cyclen Lo Tablets **2421**
Prefest Tablets **1069**

Norgestrel (Estrogens may decrease the hepatic metabolism of certain corticosteroids, thereby increasing their effect). Products include:
Lo/Ovral-28 Tablets **3423**

Omeprazole (Drugs which inhibit cytochrome P450 3A4 enzyme activity have the potential to result in increased plasma concentrations of corticosteroids). Products include:
Zegerid Powder for Oral Solution..... **2972**

Ondansetron (Dexamethasone is a moderate inducer of the cytochrome P450 3A4 enzyme system. Co-administration with other drugs that are metabolized by CYP 3A4 may increase their clearance, resulting in decreased plasma concentrations). Products include:
Zofran ODT Orally Disintegrating Tablets **1613**

Ondansetron Hydrochloride (Dexamethasone is a moderate inducer of the cytochrome P450 3A4 enzyme system. Co-administration with other drugs that are metabolized by CYP 3A4 may increase their clearance, resulting in decreased plasma concentrations). Products include:

Zofran Injection **1607**
Zofran **1613**

Oxaprozin (Concomitant use of non-steroidal anti-inflammatory agents and corticosteroids increases the risk of gastrointestinal side effects).

No products indexed under this heading.

Oxcarbazepine (Drugs which induce cytochrome P450 3A4 enzyme activity may enhance the metabolism of corticosteroids and require that the dosage of the corticosteroid be increased). Products include:

Trileptal Oral Suspension **2281**
Trileptal Tablets **2281**

Paclitaxel (Dexamethasone is a moderate inducer of the cytochrome P450 3A4 enzyme system. Co-administration with other drugs that are metabolized by CYP 3A4 may increase their clearance, resulting in decreased plasma concentrations).

No products indexed under this heading.

Paroxetine Hydrochloride (Drugs which inhibit cytochrome P450 3A4 enzyme activity have the potential to result in increased plasma concentrations of corticosteroids). Products include:

Paxil CR Controlled-Release Tablets **1509**
Paxil **1501**

Pentobarbital Sodium (Drugs which induce cytochrome P450 3A4 enzyme activity (eg, barbiturates) may enhance the metabolism of corticosteroids and require that the dosage of the corticosteroid be increased). Products include:

Nembutal Sodium Solution, USP **2484**

Phenobarbital (Drugs which induce cytochrome P450 3A4 enzyme activity (eg, barbiturates) may enhance the metabolism of corticosteroids and require that the dosage of the corticosteroid be increased).

No products indexed under this heading.

Phenobarbital Sodium (Drugs which induce cytochrome P450 3A4 enzyme activity may enhance the metabolism of corticosteroids and require that the dosage of the corticosteroid be increased).

No products indexed under this heading.

Phenylbutazone (Concomitant use of non-steroidal anti-inflammatory agents and corticosteroids increases the risk of gastrointestinal side effects).

No products indexed under this heading.

Phenytoin (Drugs which induce cytochrome P450 3A4 enzyme activity (eg, phenytoin) may enhance the metabolism of corticosteroids and require that the dosage of the corticosteroid be increased. In post-marketing experience, there have been reports of both increases and decreases in phenytoin levels with dexamethsone co-administration, leading to alterations in seizure control).

No products indexed under this heading.

Phenytoin Sodium (Drugs which induce cytochrome P450 3A4 enzyme activity (eg, phenytoin) may enhance the metabolism of corticosteroids and require that the dosage of the corticosteroid be increased. In post-marketing experience, there have been reports of both increases and decreases in phenytoin levels with dexamethsone co-administration, leading to alterations in seizure control). Products include:

Phenytek Capsules **2153**

Pimozide (Dexamethasone is a moderate inducer of the cytochrome P450 3A4 enzyme system. Co-administration with other drugs that are metabolized by CYP 3A4 may increase their clearance, resulting in decreased plasma concentrations). Products include:

Orap Tablets **1220**

Pioglitazone Hydrochloride (Because corticosteroids may increase blood glucose concentrations, dosage adjustments of antidiabetic agents may be required). Products include:

ActoPlus Met Tablets **3219**
Actos Tablets **3224**

Piroxicam (Concomitant use of non-steroidal anti-inflammatory agents and corticosteroids increases the risk of gastrointestinal side effects).

No products indexed under this heading.

Poliovirus Vaccine, Live, Oral, Trivalent, Types 1,2,3 (Sabin) (Patients on corticosteroid therapy may exhibit a diminished response to toxoids and live or inactivated vaccines due to inhibition of antibody response. Corticosteroids may also potentiate the replication of some organisms contained in live attenuated vaccines. Routine administration of vaccines or toxoids should be deferred until corticosteroid therapy is discontinued if possible. Administration of live or live, attenuated vaccines is contraindicated in patients receiving immunosuppressive doses of corticosteroids).

No products indexed under this heading.

Polyestradiol Phosphate (Estrogens may decrease the hepatic metabolism of certain corticosteroids, thereby increasing their effect).

No products indexed under this heading.

Polythiazide (When corticosteroids are administered with potassium-depleting agents (eg, diuretics), patients should be observed closely for development of hypokalemia).

No products indexed under this heading.

Prednisolone Acetate (Drugs which induce cytochrome P450 3A4 enzyme activity may enhance the metabolism of corticosteroids and require that the dosage of the corticosteroid be increased). Products include:

Blephamide Ophthalmic Ointment **563**
Blephamide Ophthalmic Suspension **564**
Poly-Pred Liquifilm Ophthalmic Suspension .... ⊙**231**
Pred Forte Ophthalmic Suspension .... ⊙**233**
Pred Mild Sterile Ophthalmic Suspension .... ⊙**236**
Pred-G Ophthalmic Suspension ...... ⊙**234**
Pred-G Sterile Ophthalmic Ointment .... ⊙**235**

Prednisolone Sodium Phosphate (Drugs which induce cytochrome P450 3A4 enzyme activity may enhance the metabolism of corticosteroids and require that the dosage of the corticosteroid be increased). Products include:

Pediapred Oral Solution **3319**

Prednisolone Tebutate (Drugs which induce cytochrome P450 3A4 enzyme activity may enhance the metabolism of corticosteroids and require that the dosage of the corticosteroid be increased).

No products indexed under this heading.

Prednisone (Drugs which induce cytochrome P450 3A4 enzyme activity may enhance the metabolism of corticosteroids and require that the dosage of the corticosteroid be increased).

No products indexed under this heading.

Primidone (Drugs which induce cytochrome P450 3A4 enzyme activity may enhance the metabolism of corticosteroids and require that the dosage of the corticosteroid be increased).

No products indexed under this heading.

Propoxyphene Hydrochloride (Drugs which inhibit cytochrome P450 3A4 enzyme activity have the potential to result in increased plasma concentrations of corticosteroids).

No products indexed under this heading.

Propoxyphene Napsylate (Drugs which inhibit cytochrome P450 3A4 enzyme activity have the potential to result in increased plasma concentrations of corticosteroids). Products include:

Darvocet A 500 Tablets **3497**

Pyridostigmine Bromide (Concomitant use of anticholinesterase agents and corticosteroids may produce severe weakness in patients with myasthenia gravis. If possible, anticholinesterase agents should be withdrawn at least 24 hours before initiating corticosteroid therapy).

No products indexed under this heading.

Quinestrol (Estrogens may decrease the hepatic metabolism of certain corticosteroids, thereby increasing their effect).

No products indexed under this heading.

Quinidine (Drugs which inhibit cytochrome P450 3A4 enzyme activity have the potential to result in increased plasma concentrations of corticosteroids).

No products indexed under this heading.

Quinidine Gluconate (Dexamethasone is a moderate inducer of the cytochrome P450 3A4 enzyme system. Co-administration with other drugs that are metabolized by CYP 3A4 may increase their clearance, resulting in decreased plasma concentrations).

No products indexed under this heading.

Quinidine Hydrochloride (Drugs which inhibit cytochrome P450 3A4 enzyme activity have the potential to result in increased plasma concentrations of corticosteroids).

No products indexed under this heading.

Quinidine Polygalacturonate (Drugs which inhibit cytochrome P450 3A4 enzyme activity have the potential to result in increased plasma concentrations of corticosteroids).

No products indexed under this heading.

Quinidine Sulfate (Drugs which inhibit cytochrome P450 3A4 enzyme activity have the potential to result in increased plasma concentrations of corticosteroids).

No products indexed under this heading.

Quinine (Drugs which inhibit cytochrome P450 3A4 enzyme activity have the potential to result in increased plasma concentrations of corticosteroids).

No products indexed under this heading.

Quinine Sulfate (Drugs which inhibit cytochrome P450 3A4 enzyme activity have the potential to result in increased plasma concentrations of corticosteroids).

No products indexed under this heading.

Quinupristin (Drugs which inhibit cytochrome P450 3A4 enzyme activity have the potential to result in increased plasma concentrations of corticosteroids). Products include:

Synercid I.V. **1690**

Ranitidine Bismuth Citrate (Drugs which inhibit cytochrome P450 3A4 enzyme activity have the potential to result in increased plasma concentrations of corticosteroids).

No products indexed under this heading.

Ranitidine Hydrochloride (Drugs which inhibit cytochrome P450 3A4 enzyme activity have the potential to result in increased plasma concentrations of corticosteroids). Products include:

Zantac **1597**
Zantac Injection **1593**
Zantac 75 Tablets **715**
Zantac 150 Maximum Strength Tablets **715**
Zantac Injection Pharmacy Bulk Package **1595**

Repaglinide (Because corticosteroids may increase blood glucose concentrations, dosage adjustments of antidiabetic agents may be required). Products include:

Prandin Tablets (0.5, 1, and 2 mg) **2337**

Rifabutin (Dexamethasone is a moderate inducer of the cytochrome P450 3A4 enzyme system. Co-administration with other drugs that are metabolized by CYP 3A4 may increase their clearance, resulting in decreased plasma concentrations).
No products indexed under this heading.

Rifampicin (Drugs which induce cytochrome P450 3A4 enzyme activity may enhance the metabolism of corticosteroids and require that the dosage of the corticosteroid be increased).
No products indexed under this heading.

Rifampin (Drugs which induce cytochrome P450 3A4 enzyme activity may enhance the metabolism of corticosteroids and require that the dosage of the corticosteroid be increased).
No products indexed under this heading.

Rifapentine (Drugs which induce cytochrome P450 3A4 enzyme activity may enhance the metabolism of corticosteroids and require that the dosage of the corticosteroid be increased).
No products indexed under this heading.

Ritonavir (Drugs which inhibit cytochrome P450 3A4 enzyme activity have the potential to result in increased plasma concentrations of corticosteroids). Products include:
Kaletra 474
Norvir 499

Rivastigmine Tartrate (Concomitant use of anticholinesterase agents and corticosteroids may produce severe weakness in patients with myasthenia gravis. If possible, anticholinesterase agents should be withdrawn at least 24 hours before initiating corticosteroid therapy). Products include:
Exelon Capsules 2204

Rofecoxib (Concomitant use of nonsteroidal anti-inflammatory agents and corticosteroids increases the risk of gastrointestinal side effects).
No products indexed under this heading.

Rosiglitazone Maleate (Because corticosteroids may increase blood glucose concentrations, dosage adjustments of antidiabetic agents may be required). Products include:
Avandamet Tablets 1343
Avandia Tablets 1348

Rotavirus Vaccine, Live, Oral, Tetravalent (Patients on corticosteroid therapy may exhibit a diminished response to toxoids and live or inactivated vaccines due to inhibition of antibody response. Corticosteroids may also potentiate the replication of some organisms contained in live attenuated vaccines. Routine administration of vaccines or toxoids should be deferred until corticosteroid therapy is discontinued if possible. Administration of live or live, attenuated vaccines is contraindicated in patients receiving immunosuppressive doses of corticosteroids).
No products indexed under this heading.

Rubella & Mumps Virus Vaccine Live (Patients on corticosteroid therapy may exhibit a diminished response to toxoids and live or inactivated vaccines due to inhibition of antibody response. Corticosteroids may also potentiate the replication of some organisms contained in live attenuated vaccines. Routine administration of vaccines or toxoids should be deferred until corticosteroid therapy is discontinued if possible. Administration of live or live, attenuated vaccines is contraindicated in patients receiving immunosuppressive doses of corticosteroids).
No products indexed under this heading.

Rubella Virus Vaccine Live (Patients on corticosteroid therapy may exhibit a diminished response to toxoids and live or inactivated vaccines due to inhibition of antibody response. Corticosteroids may also potentiate the replication of some organisms contained in live attenuated vaccines. Routine administration of vaccines or toxoids should be deferred until corticosteroid therapy is discontinued if possible. Administration of live or live, attenuated vaccines is contraindicated in patients receiving immunosuppressive doses of corticosteroids). Products include:
Meruvax II 1994

Saquinavir (Drugs which inhibit cytochrome P450 3A4 enzyme activity have the potential to result in increased plasma concentrations of corticosteroids).
No products indexed under this heading.

Saquinavir Mesylate (Drugs which inhibit cytochrome P450 3A4 enzyme activity have the potential to result in increased plasma concentrations of corticosteroids). Products include:
Invirase 2776

Secobarbital Sodium (Drugs which induce cytochrome P450 3A4 enzyme activity (eg, barbiturates) may enhance the metabolism of corticosteroids and require that the dosage of the corticosteroid be increased).
No products indexed under this heading.

Sertraline Hydrochloride (Drugs which inhibit cytochrome P450 3A4 enzyme activity have the potential to result in increased plasma concentrations of corticosteroids). Products include:
Zoloft 2581

Sildenafil Citrate (Dexamethasone is a moderate inducer of the cytochrome P450 3A4 enzyme system. Co-administration with other drugs that are metabolized by CYP 3A4 may increase their clearance, resulting in decreased plasma concentrations). Products include:
Revatio Tablets 2541
Viagra Tablets 2552

Simvastatin (Dexamethasone is a moderate inducer of the cytochrome P450 3A4 enzyme system. Co-administration with other drugs that are metabolized by CYP 3A4 may increase their clearance, resulting in decreased plasma concentrations). Products include:
Vytorin 10/10 Tablets 2084
Vytorin 10/10 Tablets 3092
Vytorin 10/20 Tablets 2084
Vytorin 10/20 Tablets 3092
Vytorin 10/40 Tablets 3092
Vytorin 10/40 Tablets 2084
Vytorin 10/80 Tablets 2084
Vytorin 10/80 Tablets 3092
Zocor Tablets 2078

Sirolimus (Dexamethasone is a moderate inducer of the cytochrome P450 3A4 enzyme system. Co-administration with other drugs that are metabolized by CYP 3A4 may increase their clearance, resulting in decreased plasma concentrations). Products include:
Rapamune Oral Solution and Tablets 3472

Smallpox Vaccine (Patients on corticosteroid therapy may exhibit a diminished response to toxoids and live or inactivated vaccines due to inhibition of antibody response. Corticosteroids may also potentiate the replication of some organisms contained in live attenuated vaccines. Routine administration of vaccines or toxoids should be deferred until corticosteroid therapy is discontinued if possible. Administration of live or live, attenuated vaccines is contraindicated in patients receiving immunosuppressive doses of corticosteroids).
No products indexed under this heading.

Sulfinpyrazone (Drugs which induce cytochrome P450 3A4 enzyme activity may enhance the metabolism of corticosteroids and require that the dosage of the corticosteroid be increased).
No products indexed under this heading.

Sulindac (Concomitant use of nonsteroidal anti-inflammatory agents and corticosteroids increases the risk of gastrointestinal side effects). Products include:
Clinoril Tablets 1899

Tacrine Hydrochloride (Concomitant use of anticholinesterase agents and corticosteroids may produce severe weakness in patients with myasthenia gravis. If possible, anticholinesterase agents should be withdrawn at least 24 hours before initiating corticosteroid therapy).
No products indexed under this heading.

Tacrolimus (Dexamethasone is a moderate inducer of the cytochrome P450 3A4 enzyme system. Co-administration with other drugs that are metabolized by CYP 3A4 may increase their clearance, resulting in decreased plasma concentrations). Products include:
Prograf Capsules and Injection 624
Protopic Ointment 629

Tamoxifen Citrate (Dexamethasone is a moderate inducer of the cytochrome P450 3A4 enzyme system. Co-administration with other drugs that are metabolized by CYP 3A4 may increase their clearance, resulting in decreased plasma concentrations).
No products indexed under this heading.

Telithromycin (Drugs which inhibit cytochrome P450 3A4 enzyme activity have the potential to result in increased plasma concentrations of corticosteroids). Products include:
Ketek Tablets 2920

Thalidomide (Co-administration with thalidomide should be employed cautiously, as toxic epidermal necrolysis has been reported with concomitant use). Products include:
Thalomid Capsules 979

Theophylline (Drugs which induce cytochrome P450 3A4 enzyme activity may enhance the metabolism of corticosteroids and require that the dosage of the corticosteroid be increased).
No products indexed under this heading.

Thiamylal Sodium (Drugs which induce cytochrome P450 3A4 enzyme activity (eg, barbiturates) may enhance the metabolism of corticosteroids and require that the dosage of the corticosteroid be increased).
No products indexed under this heading.

Tiagabine Hydrochloride (Dexamethasone is a moderate inducer of the cytochrome P450 3A4 enzyme system. Co-administration with other drugs that are metabolized by CYP 3A4 may increase their clearance, resulting in decreased plasma concentrations). Products include:
Gabitril Tablets 998

Tolazamide (Because corticosteroids may increase blood glucose concentrations, dosage adjustments of antidiabetic agents may be required).
No products indexed under this heading.

Tolbutamide (Because corticosteroids may increase blood glucose concentrations, dosage adjustments of antidiabetic agents may be required).
No products indexed under this heading.

Tolmetin Sodium (Concomitant use of non-steroidal anti-inflammatory agents and corticosteroids increases the risk of gastrointestinal side effects).
No products indexed under this heading.

Tolterodine Tartrate (Dexamethasone is a moderate inducer of the cytochrome P450 3A4 enzyme system. Co-administration with other drugs that are metabolized by CYP 3A4 may increase their clearance, resulting in decreased plasma concentrations). Products include:
Detrol Tablets 2626
Detrol LA Capsules 2629

Torsemide (When corticosteroids are administered with potassium-depleting agents (eg, diuretics), patients should be observed closely for development of hypokalemia).
No products indexed under this heading.

Trazodone Hydrochloride (Dexamethasone is a moderate inducer of the cytochrome P450 3A4 enzyme system. Co-administration with other drugs that are metabolized by CYP 3A4 may increase their clearance, resulting in decreased plasma concentrations).
No products indexed under this heading.

Triamcinolone (Drugs which induce cytochrome P450 3A4 enzyme activity may enhance the metabolism of corticosteroids and require that the dosage of the corticosteroid be increased).
No products indexed under this heading.

Triamcinolone Acetonide (Drugs which induce cytochrome P450 3A4 enzyme activity may enhance the metabolism of corticosteroids and

require that the dosage of the corticosteroid be increased). Products include:
- Azmacort Inhalation Aerosol 1701
- Nasacort HFA Inhalation Aerosol 2939
- Nasacort AQ Nasal Spray 2937

Triamcinolone Diacetate (Drugs which induce cytochrome P450 3A4 enzyme activity may enhance the metabolism of corticosteroids and require that the dosage of the corticosteroid be increased).
No products indexed under this heading.

Triamcinolone Hexacetonide (Drugs which induce cytochrome P450 3A4 enzyme activity may enhance the metabolism of corticosteroids and require that the dosage of the corticosteroid be increased).
No products indexed under this heading.

Triazolam (Dexamethasone is a moderate inducer of the cytochrome P450 3A4 enzyme system. Co-administration with other drugs that are metabolized by CYP 3A4 may increase their clearance, resulting in decreased plasma concentrations).
No products indexed under this heading.

Troglitazone (Because corticosteroids may increase blood glucose concentrations, dosage adjustments of antidiabetic agents may be required).
No products indexed under this heading.

Troleandomycin (Macrolide antibiotics have been reported to cause a significant decrease in corticosteroid clearance. Drugs which inhibit cytochrome P450 3A4 enzyme activity (eg, macrolide antibiotics) have the potential to result in increased plasma concentrations of corticosteroids. Dexamethasone is a moderate inducer of the cytochrome P450 3A4 enzyme system. Co-administration with other drugs that are metabolized by CYP 3A4 (eg, erythromycin) may increase their clearance, resulting in decreased plasma concentrations).
No products indexed under this heading.

Typhoid Vaccine (Patients on corticosteroid therapy may exhibit a diminished response to toxoids and live or inactivated vaccines due to inhibition of antibody response. Corticosteroids may also potentiate the replication of some organisms contained in live attenuated vaccines. Routine administration of vaccines or toxoids should be deferred until corticosteroid therapy is discontinued if possible. Administration of live or live, attenuated vaccines is contraindicated in patients receiving immunosuppressive doses of corticosteroids).
No products indexed under this heading.

Valdecoxib (Concomitant use of non-steroidal anti-inflammatory agents and corticosteroids increases the risk of gastrointestinal side effects).
No products indexed under this heading.

Valproate Sodium (Drugs which inhibit cytochrome P450 3A4 enzyme activity have the potential to result in increased plasma concentrations of corticosteroids). Products include:
- Depacon Injection 412

Varicella Virus Vaccine Live (Patients on corticosteroid therapy may exhibit a diminished response to toxoids and live or inactivated vaccines due to inhibition of antibody response. Corticosteroids may also potentiate the replication of some organisms contained in live attenuated vaccines. Routine administration of vaccines or toxoids should be deferred until corticosteroid therapy is discontinued if possible. Administration of live or live, attenuated vaccines is contraindicated in patients receiving immunosuppressive doses of corticosteroids). Products include:
- Varivax 2070

Verapamil Hydrochloride (Drugs which inhibit cytochrome P450 3A4 enzyme activity have the potential to result in increased plasma concentrations of corticosteroids). Products include:
- Covera-HS Tablets 3135
- Tarka Tablets 519
- Verelan PM Capsules 3120

Vinblastine Sulfate (Dexamethasone is a moderate inducer of the cytochrome P450 3A4 enzyme system. Co-administration with other drugs that are metabolized by CYP 3A4 may increase their clearance, resulting in decreased plasma concentrations).
No products indexed under this heading.

Vincristine Sulfate (Dexamethasone is a moderate inducer of the cytochrome P450 3A4 enzyme system. Co-administration with other drugs that are metabolized by CYP 3A4 may increase their clearance, resulting in decreased plasma concentrations).
No products indexed under this heading.

Voriconazole (Drugs which inhibit cytochrome P450 3A4 enzyme activity have the potential to result in increased plasma concentrations of corticosteroids). Products include:
- VFEND I.V. 2543
- VFEND Oral Suspension 2543
- VFEND Tablets 2543

Warfarin Sodium (Co-administration of corticosteroids and warfarin usually results in inhibition of response to warfarin, although there have been some conflicting reports. Therefore, coagulation indices should be monitored frequently to maintain the desired anticoagulant effect). Products include:
- Coumadin for Injection 932
- Coumadin Tablets 932

Yellow Fever Vaccine (Patients on corticosteroid therapy may exhibit a diminished response to toxoids and live or inactivated vaccines due to inhibition of antibody response. Corticosteroids may also potentiate the replication of some organisms contained in live attenuated vaccines. Routine administration of vaccines or toxoids should be deferred until corticosteroid therapy is discontinued if possible. Administration of live or live, attenuated vaccines is contraindicated in patients receiving immunosuppressive doses of corticosteroids).
No products indexed under this heading.

Zafirlukast (Drugs which inhibit cytochrome P450 3A4 enzyme activity have the potential to result in increased plasma concentrations of corticosteroids). Products include:
- Accolate Tablets 663

Zileuton (Drugs which inhibit cytochrome P450 3A4 enzyme activity have the potential to result in increased plasma concentrations of corticosteroids).
No products indexed under this heading.

Food Interactions

Grapefruit (Drugs which inhibit cytochrome P450 3A4 enzyme activity have the potential to result in increased plasma concentrations of corticosteroids).

Grapefruit Juice (Drugs which inhibit cytochrome P450 3A4 enzyme activity have the potential to result in increased plasma concentrations of corticosteroids).

DELATESTRYL INJECTION

(Testosterone Enanthate) 2976
May interact with corticosteroids, oral anticoagulants, oral hypoglycemic agents, insulin, and certain other agents. Compounds in these categories include:

Acarbose (In diabetic patients, the metabolic effects of androgens may decrease blood glucose and, therefore, antidiabetic drug requirements). Products include:
- Precose Tablets 776

ACTH (Co-administration of testosterone with ACTH may enhance edema formation).
No products indexed under this heading.

Anisindione (Co-administration of C-17 substituted derivatives of testosterone have been reported to decrease the anticoagulant requirements; concomitant therapy has resulted in bleeding). Products include:
- Miradon Tablets 3056

Betamethasone Acetate (Co-administration of testosterone with corticosteroids may enhance edema formation).
No products indexed under this heading.

Betamethasone Sodium Phosphate (Co-administration of testosterone with corticosteroids may enhance edema formation).
No products indexed under this heading.

Chlorpropamide (In diabetic patients, the metabolic effects of androgens may decrease blood glucose and, therefore, antidiabetic drug requirements).
No products indexed under this heading.

Cortisone Acetate (Co-administration of testosterone with corticosteroids may enhance edema formation).
No products indexed under this heading.

Dexamethasone (Co-administration of testosterone with corticosteroids may enhance edema formation). Products include:
- Ciprodex Otic Suspension 555
- Decadron Tablets 1929
- TobraDex Ophthalmic Ointment 558
- TobraDex Ophthalmic Suspension ... 558

Dexamethasone Acetate (Co-administration of testosterone with corticosteroids may enhance edema formation).
No products indexed under this heading.

Dexamethasone Sodium Phosphate (Co-administration of testosterone with corticosteroids may enhance edema formation). Products include:
- Decadron Phosphate Injection 1931

Dicumarol (Co-administration of C-17 substituted derivatives of testosterone have been reported to decrease the anticoagulant requirements; concomitant therapy has resulted in bleeding).
No products indexed under this heading.

Fludrocortisone Acetate (Co-administration of testosterone with corticosteroids may enhance edema formation).
No products indexed under this heading.

Glimepiride (In diabetic patients, the metabolic effects of androgens may decrease blood glucose and, therefore, antidiabetic drug requirements). Products include:
- Amaryl Tablets 2864

Glipizide (In diabetic patients, the metabolic effects of androgens may decrease blood glucose and, therefore, antidiabetic drug requirements).
No products indexed under this heading.

Glyburide (In diabetic patients, the metabolic effects of androgens may decrease blood glucose and, therefore, antidiabetic drug requirements).
No products indexed under this heading.

Hydrocortisone (Co-administration of testosterone with corticosteroids may enhance edema formation). Products include:
- Cortizone•5 Ointment 699
- Cortizone•10 Creme 699
- Cortizone•10 Ointment 699
- Cortizone•10 Plus Creme 700
- Cortizone•10 Maximum Strength Quick Shot Spray 700
- Hydrocortone Tablets 1963
- Preparation H Hydrocortisone Cream 748

Hydrocortisone Acetate (Co-administration of testosterone with corticosteroids may enhance edema formation). Products include:
- Analpram-HC 1136
- Pramosone 1139
- ProctoFoam-HC 3113
- Tucks Anti-Itch Ointment 712
- U-cort 1% Cream 3289

Hydrocortisone Sodium Phosphate (Co-administration of testosterone with corticosteroids may enhance edema formation).
No products indexed under this heading.

Hydrocortisone Sodium Succinate (Co-administration of testosterone with corticosteroids may enhance edema formation).
No products indexed under this heading.

Insulin, Human, Zinc Suspension (In diabetic patients, the metabolic effects of androgens may decrease blood glucose and, therefore, insulin requirements). Products include:
- Humulin L, 100 Units 1763
- Humulin U, 100 Units 1770

Insulin, Human NPH (In diabetic patients, the metabolic effects of androgens may decrease blood glucose and, therefore, insulin requirements). Products include:
Humulin N, 100 Units 1764
Humulin N Pen 1765
Novolin N Human Insulin 10 ml Vials 2322
Novolin N InnoLet 2322
Novolin N PenFill 3 ml Cartridges 2325
Novolin R InnoLet 2322

Insulin, Human Regular (In diabetic patients, the metabolic effects of androgens may decrease blood glucose and, therefore, insulin requirements). Products include:
Humulin R (U-500) 1768
Humulin R, 100 Units 1767
Novolin R Human Insulin 10 ml Vials 2322
Novolin R PenFill 2325

Insulin, Human Regular and Human NPH Mixture (In diabetic patients, the metabolic effects of androgens may decrease blood glucose and, therefore, insulin requirements). Products include:
Humulin 50/50, 100 Units 1760
Humulin 70/30 Pen 1761
Novolin 70/30 Human Insulin 10 ml Vials 2321
Novolin 70/30 InnoLet 2322
Novolin 70/30 PenFill 3 ml Cartridges 2325

Insulin, NPH (In diabetic patients, the metabolic effects of androgens may decrease blood glucose and, therefore, insulin requirements).
No products indexed under this heading.

Insulin, Regular (In diabetic patients, the metabolic effects of androgens may decrease blood glucose and, therefore, insulin requirements).
No products indexed under this heading.

Insulin, Zinc Crystals (In diabetic patients, the metabolic effects of androgens may decrease blood glucose and, therefore, insulin requirements).
No products indexed under this heading.

Insulin, Zinc Suspension (In diabetic patients, the metabolic effects of androgens may decrease blood glucose and, therefore, insulin requirements).
No products indexed under this heading.

Insulin Aspart, Human Regular (In diabetic patients, the metabolic effects of androgens may decrease blood glucose and, therefore, insulin requirements). Products include:
NovoLog Injection 2326

Insulin glargine (In diabetic patients, the metabolic effects of androgens may decrease blood glucose and, therefore, insulin requirements). Products include:
Lantus Injection 2925

Insulin Lispro, Human (In diabetic patients, the metabolic effects of androgens may decrease blood glucose and, therefore, insulin requirements). Products include:
Humalog-Pen 1751
Humalog Mix 75/25-Pen 1754

Insulin Lispro Protamine, Human (In diabetic patients, the metabolic effects of androgens may decrease blood glucose and, therefore, insulin requirements). Products include:
Humalog Mix 75/25-Pen 1754

Metformin Hydrochloride (In diabetic patients, the metabolic effects of androgens may decrease blood glucose and, therefore, antidiabetic drug requirements). Products include:
ActoPlus Met Tablets 3219
Avandamet Tablets 1343
Fortamet Extended-Release Tablets 1156

Methylprednisolone Acetate (Co-administration of testosterone with corticosteroids may enhance edema formation). Products include:
Depo-Medrol Injectable Suspension 2615
Depo-Medrol Single-Dose Vial 2617

Methylprednisolone Sodium Succinate (Co-administration of testosterone with corticosteroids may enhance edema formation).
No products indexed under this heading.

Miglitol (In diabetic patients, the metabolic effects of androgens may decrease blood glucose and, therefore, antidiabetic drug requirements).
No products indexed under this heading.

Oxyphenbutazone (Co-administration of androgens and oxyphenbutazone may result in elevated serum levels of oxyphenbutazone).
No products indexed under this heading.

Pioglitazone Hydrochloride (In diabetic patients, the metabolic effects of androgens may decrease blood glucose and, therefore, antidiabetic drug requirements). Products include:
ActoPlus Met Tablets 3219
Actos Tablets 3224

Prednisolone Acetate (Co-administration of testosterone with corticosteroids may enhance edema formation). Products include:
Blephamide Ophthalmic Ointment 563
Blephamide Ophthalmic Suspension 564
Poly-Pred Liquifilm Ophthalmic Suspension .... ⊙231
Pred Forte Ophthalmic Suspension .... ⊙233
Pred Mild Sterile Ophthalmic Suspension .... ⊙236
Pred-G Ophthalmic Suspension ...... ⊙234
Pred-G Sterile Ophthalmic Ointment .... ⊙235

Prednisolone Sodium Phosphate (Co-administration of testosterone with corticosteroids may enhance edema formation). Products include:
Pediapred Oral Solution 3319

Prednisolone Tebutate (Co-administration of testosterone with corticosteroids may enhance edema formation).
No products indexed under this heading.

Prednisone (Co-administration of testosterone with corticosteroids may enhance edema formation).
No products indexed under this heading.

Repaglinide (In diabetic patients, the metabolic effects of androgens may decrease blood glucose and, therefore, antidiabetic drug requirements). Products include:
Prandin Tablets (0.5, 1, and 2 mg) 2337

Rosiglitazone Maleate (In diabetic patients, the metabolic effects of androgens may decrease blood glucose and, therefore, antidiabetic drug requirements). Products include:
Avandamet Tablets 1343
Avandia Tablets 1348

Tolazamide (In diabetic patients, the metabolic effects of androgens may decrease blood glucose and, therefore, antidiabetic drug requirements).
No products indexed under this heading.

Tolbutamide (In diabetic patients, the metabolic effects of androgens may decrease blood glucose and, therefore, antidiabetic drug requirements).
No products indexed under this heading.

Triamcinolone (Co-administration of testosterone with corticosteroids may enhance edema formation).
No products indexed under this heading.

Triamcinolone Acetonide (Co-administration of testosterone with corticosteroids may enhance edema formation). Products include:
Azmacort Inhalation Aerosol 1701
Nasacort HFA Inhalation Aerosol 2939
Nasacort AQ Nasal Spray 2937

Triamcinolone Diacetate (Co-administration of testosterone with corticosteroids may enhance edema formation).
No products indexed under this heading.

Triamcinolone Hexacetonide (Co-administration of testosterone with corticosteroids may enhance edema formation).
No products indexed under this heading.

Troglitazone (In diabetic patients, the metabolic effects of androgens may decrease blood glucose and, therefore, antidiabetic drug requirements).
No products indexed under this heading.

Warfarin Sodium (Co-administration of C-17 substituted derivatives of testosterone have been reported to decrease the anticoagulant requirements; concomitant therapy has resulted in bleeding). Products include:
Coumadin for Injection 932
Coumadin Tablets 932

DELSYM EXTENDED-RELEASE SUSPENSION

(Dextromethorphan Polistirex) .... ▣611
May interact with monoamine oxidase inhibitors. Compounds in these categories include:

Isocarboxazid (Concurrent and/or sequential use is not recommended).
No products indexed under this heading.

Moclobemide (Concurrent and/or sequential use is not recommended).
No products indexed under this heading.

Pargyline Hydrochloride (Concurrent and/or sequential use is not recommended).
No products indexed under this heading.

Phenelzine Sulfate (Concurrent and/or sequential use is not recommended).
No products indexed under this heading.

Procarbazine Hydrochloride (Concurrent and/or sequential use is not recommended). Products include:
Matulane Capsules 3188

Selegiline Hydrochloride (Concurrent and/or sequential use is not recommended). Products include:
Eldepryl Capsules 3209

Tranylcypromine Sulfate (Concurrent and/or sequential use is not recommended). Products include:
Parnate Tablets 1499

DELSYM 12 HOUR COUGH SUPPRESSANT FOR CHILDREN

(Dextromethorphan Polistirex) .... ▣611
See Delsym Extended-Release Suspension

DEMSER CAPSULES

(Metyrosine) 1933
May interact with central nervous system depressants, phenothiazines, and certain other agents. Compounds in these categories include:

Alfentanil Hydrochloride (Additive sedative effects).
No products indexed under this heading.

Alprazolam (Additive sedative effects). Products include:
Niravam Orally Disintegrating Tablets 3106
Xanax XR Tablets 2655

Aprobarbital (Additive sedative effects).
No products indexed under this heading.

Buprenorphine Hydrochloride (Additive sedative effects). Products include:
Buprenex Injectable 2718
Suboxone Tablets 2719
Subutex Tablets 2719

Buspirone Hydrochloride (Additive sedative effects).
No products indexed under this heading.

Butabarbital (Additive sedative effects).
No products indexed under this heading.

Butalbital (Additive sedative effects). Products include:
Sedapap Tablets 50 mg/650 mg 2098

Chlordiazepoxide (Additive sedative effects).
No products indexed under this heading.

Chlordiazepoxide Hydrochloride (Additive sedative effects). Products include:
Librium Capsules 3349

Chlorpromazine (Possible potentiation of extrapyramidal effects; additive sedative effects).
No products indexed under this heading.

Chlorpromazine Hydrochloride (Possible potentiation of extrapyramidal effects; additive sedative effects).
No products indexed under this heading.

Chlorprothixene (Additive sedative effects).
No products indexed under this heading.

Chlorprothixene Hydrochloride (Additive sedative effects).
No products indexed under this heading.

Chlorprothixene Lactate (Additive sedative effects).
No products indexed under this heading.

Clorazepate Dipotassium (Additive sedative effects). Products include:
Tranxene 2488

Clozapine (Additive sedative effects). Products include:
Clozapine Tablets 2141
Clozaril Tablets 2174
FazaClo Orally Disintegrating Tablets 547

Codeine Phosphate (Additive sedative effects). Products include:
Tylenol with Codeine 2461

Desflurane (Additive sedative effects). Products include:
Suprane Liquid for Inhalation 770

Dezocine (Additive sedative effects).
No products indexed under this heading.

Diazepam (Additive sedative effects). Products include:
Diastat Rectal Delivery System 3344
Valium Tablets 2822

Droperidol (Additive sedative effects).
No products indexed under this heading.

Enflurane (Additive sedative effects).
No products indexed under this heading.

Estazolam (Additive sedative effects). Products include:
ProSom Tablets 512

Ethanol (Additive sedative effects).
No products indexed under this heading.

Ethchlorvynol (Additive sedative effects).
No products indexed under this heading.

Ethinamate (Additive sedative effects).
No products indexed under this heading.

Ethyl Alcohol (Additive sedative effects).
No products indexed under this heading.

Fentanyl (Additive sedative effects). Products include:
Duragesic Transdermal System 2448

Fentanyl Citrate (Additive sedative effects). Products include:
Actiq 993

Fluphenazine Decanoate (Possible potentiation of extrapyramidal effects; additive sedative effects).
No products indexed under this heading.

Fluphenazine Enanthate (Possible potentiation of extrapyramidal effects; additive sedative effects).
No products indexed under this heading.

Fluphenazine Hydrochloride (Possible potentiation of extrapyramidal effects; additive sedative effects).
No products indexed under this heading.

Flurazepam Hydrochloride (Additive sedative effects). Products include:
Dalmane Capsules 3343

Glutethimide (Additive sedative effects).
No products indexed under this heading.

Haloperidol (Possible potentiation of extrapyramidal effects; additive sedative effects).
No products indexed under this heading.

Haloperidol Decanoate (Possible potentiation of extrapyramidal effects; additive sedative effects).
No products indexed under this heading.

Hydrocodone Bitartrate (Additive sedative effects). Products include:
Hycodan 1104
Hycomine Compound Tablets 1105
Hycotuss Expectorant Syrup 1106
Lortab 3315
Lortab Elixir 3312
Vicodin Tablets 530
Vicodin ES Tablets 531
Vicodin HP Tablets 532
Vicoprofen Tablets 533
Zydone Tablets 1118

Hydrocodone Polistirex (Additive sedative effects). Products include:
Tussionex Pennkinetic Extended-Release Suspension 3322

Hydromorphone Hydrochloride (Additive sedative effects). Products include:
Dilaudid 439
Dilaudid Oral Liquid 443
Dilaudid Non-Sterile Powder 439
Dilaudid Rectal Suppositories 439
Dilaudid Tablets 439
Dilaudid Tablets - 8 mg 443
Dilaudid-HP 441

Hydroxyzine Hydrochloride (Additive sedative effects).
No products indexed under this heading.

Isoflurane (Additive sedative effects).
No products indexed under this heading.

Ketamine Hydrochloride (Additive sedative effects).
No products indexed under this heading.

Levomethadyl Acetate Hydrochloride (Additive sedative effects).
No products indexed under this heading.

Levorphanol Tartrate (Additive sedative effects).
No products indexed under this heading.

Lorazepam (Additive sedative effects).
No products indexed under this heading.

Loxapine Hydrochloride (Additive sedative effects).
No products indexed under this heading.

Loxapine Succinate (Additive sedative effects).
No products indexed under this heading.

Meperidine Hydrochloride (Additive sedative effects).
No products indexed under this heading.

Mephobarbital (Additive sedative effects). Products include:
Mebaral Tablets, USP 2483

Meprobamate (Additive sedative effects).
No products indexed under this heading.

Mesoridazine Besylate (Possible potentiation of extrapyramidal effects; additive sedative effects).
No products indexed under this heading.

Methadone Hydrochloride (Additive sedative effects).
No products indexed under this heading.

Methohexital Sodium (Additive sedative effects).
No products indexed under this heading.

Methotrimeprazine (Possible potentiation of extrapyramidal effects; additive sedative effects).
No products indexed under this heading.

Methoxyflurane (Additive sedative effects).
No products indexed under this heading.

Midazolam Hydrochloride (Additive sedative effects).
No products indexed under this heading.

Molindone Hydrochloride (Additive sedative effects). Products include:
Moban Tablets 1108

Morphine Sulfate (Additive sedative effects). Products include:
Avinza Capsules 1714
Kadian Capsules 572
MS Contin Tablets 2703

Olanzapine (Additive sedative effects). Products include:
Symbyax Capsules 1788
Zyprexa Tablets 1798
Zyprexa IntraMuscular 1798
Zyprexa ZYDIS Orally Disintegrating Tablets 1798

Oxazepam (Additive sedative effects).
No products indexed under this heading.

Oxycodone Hydrochloride (Additive sedative effects). Products include:
Combunox Tablets 1183
OxyContin Tablets 2699
OxyFast Oral Concentrate Solution 2704
OxyIR Capsules 2704
Percocet Tablets 1114
Percodan Tablets 1115

Pentobarbital Sodium (Additive sedative effects). Products include:
Nembutal Sodium Solution, USP 2484

Perphenazine (Possible potentiation of extrapyramidal effects of perphenazine; additive sedative effects).
No products indexed under this heading.

Phenobarbital (Additive sedative effects).
No products indexed under this heading.

Prazepam (Additive sedative effects).
No products indexed under this heading.

Prochlorperazine (Possible potentiation of extrapyramidal effects; additive sedative effects).
No products indexed under this heading.

Promethazine Hydrochloride (Possible potentiation of extrapyramidal effects; additive sedative effects). Products include:
Phenergan 3438

Propofol (Additive sedative effects). Products include:
Diprivan Injectable Emulsion 676

Propoxyphene Hydrochloride (Additive sedative effects).
No products indexed under this heading.

Propoxyphene Napsylate (Additive sedative effects). Products include:
Darvocet A 500 Tablets 3497

Quazepam (Additive sedative effects).
No products indexed under this heading.

Quetiapine Fumarate (Additive sedative effects). Products include:
Seroquel Tablets 691

Remifentanil Hydrochloride (Additive sedative effects).
No products indexed under this heading.

Risperidone (Additive sedative effects). Products include:
Risperdal Consta Long-Acting Injection 1664
Risperdal M-Tab Orally Disintegrating Tablets 1658
Risperdal 1658

Secobarbital Sodium (Additive sedative effects).
No products indexed under this heading.

Sevoflurane (Additive sedative effects). Products include:
Ultane Liquid for Inhalation 526

Sufentanil Citrate (Additive sedative effects).
No products indexed under this heading.

Temazepam (Additive sedative effects).
No products indexed under this heading.

Thiamylal Sodium (Additive sedative effects).
No products indexed under this heading.

Thioridazine Hydrochloride (Possible potentiation of extrapyramidal effects; additive sedative effects). Products include:
Thioridazine Hydrochloride Tablets 2122

Thiothixene (Additive sedative effects). Products include:
Thiothixene Capsules 2124

Triazolam (Additive sedative effects).
No products indexed under this heading.

Trifluoperazine Hydrochloride (Possible potentiation of extrapyramidal effects; additive sedative effects).
No products indexed under this heading.

Zaleplon (Additive sedative effects). Products include:
Sonata Capsules 1686

Ziprasidone Hydrochloride (Additive sedative effects). Products include:
Geodon Capsules 2514

Zolpidem Tartrate (Additive sedative effects). Products include:
Ambien Tablets 2867

Food Interactions

Alcohol (Additive sedative effects).

DENAVIR CREAM

(Penciclovir) 2163
None cited in PDR database.

IMPORTANT NOTE: Always consult each drug listing in the patient's regimen for possible interactions.

DEPACON INJECTION
(Valproate Sodium) 412
May interact with central nervous system depressants, phenytoin, and certain other agents. Compounds in these categories include:

Alfentanil Hydrochloride (Co-administration may result in additive CNS depression).
No products indexed under this heading.

Alprazolam (Co-administration may result in additive CNS depression). Products include:
Niravam Orally Disintegrating Tablets 3106
Xanax XR Tablets 2655

Amitriptyline Hydrochloride (Co-administration has resulted in a 21% decrease in plasma clearance of amitriptyline; this interaction is likely to be clinically unimportant).
No products indexed under this heading.

Aprobarbital (Co-administration may result in additive CNS depression).
No products indexed under this heading.

Aspirin (Co-administration has resulted in decreased protein binding and an inhibition of metabolism of valproate). Products include:
Aggrenox Capsules 855
Bayer, Aspirin Regimen .... ▣606
Bayer Aspirin Tablets 3515
BC Powder .... ▣612
BC Allergy Sinus Cold Powder .... ▣612
Arthritis Strength BC Powder .... ▣612
BC Sinus Cold Powder .... ▣612
Ecotrin Enteric Coated Aspirin Low, Regular and Maximum Strength Tablets 1627
Goody's Body Pain Formula Powder .... ▣621
Goody's Extra Strength Headache Powder .... ▣621
Goody's Extra Strength Pain Relief Tablets .... ▣621
Percodan Tablets 1115
St. Joseph 81 mg Aspirin Chewable and Enteric Coated Tablets 1841

Buprenorphine Hydrochloride (Co-administration may result in additive CNS depression). Products include:
Buprenex Injectable 2718
Suboxone Tablets 2719
Subutex Tablets 2719

Buspirone Hydrochloride (Co-administration may result in additive CNS depression).
No products indexed under this heading.

Butabarbital (Co-administration may result in additive CNS depression).
No products indexed under this heading.

Butalbital (Co-administration may result in additive CNS depression). Products include:
Sedapap Tablets 50 mg/650 mg 2098

Carbamazepine (Can double the clearance of valproate; co-administration has resulted in decreased carbamazepine and increased carbamazepine 10,11-epoxide serum levels). Products include:
Carbatrol Capsules 3174
Equetro Extended-Release Capsules 3178
Tegretol/Tegretol-XR 2278

Chlordiazepoxide (Co-administration may result in additive CNS depression).
No products indexed under this heading.

Chlordiazepoxide Hydrochloride (Co-administration may result in additive CNS depression). Products include:
Librium Capsules 3349

Chlorpromazine (Co-administration has resulted in a 15% increase in trough plasma levels of valproate; concurrent use may result in additive CNS depression).
No products indexed under this heading.

Chlorpromazine Hydrochloride (Co-administration has resulted in a 15% increase in trough plasma levels of valproate; concurrent use may result in additive CNS depression).
No products indexed under this heading.

Chlorprothixene (Co-administration may result in additive CNS depression).
No products indexed under this heading.

Chlorprothixene Hydrochloride (Co-administration may result in additive CNS depression).
No products indexed under this heading.

Chlorprothixene Lactate (Co-administration may result in additive CNS depression).
No products indexed under this heading.

Clonazepam (Co-administration may induce absence status in patients with a history of absence-type seizures). Products include:
Klonopin 2782

Clorazepate Dipotassium (Co-administration may result in additive CNS depression). Products include:
Tranxene 2488

Clozapine (Co-administration may result in additive CNS depression). Products include:
Clozapine Tablets 2141
Clozaril Tablets 2174
FazaClo Orally Disintegrating Tablets 547

Codeine Phosphate (Co-administration may result in additive CNS depression). Products include:
Tylenol with Codeine 2461

Desflurane (Co-administration may result in additive CNS depression). Products include:
Suprane Liquid for Inhalation 770

Dezocine (Co-administration may result in additive CNS depression).
No products indexed under this heading.

Diazepam (Valproate displaces diazepam from its plasma albumin binding sites and inhibits its metabolism; plasma clearance and volume of distribution for free diazepam may be reduced; concurrent use may result in additive CNS depression). Products include:
Diastat Rectal Delivery System 3344
Valium Tablets 2822

Droperidol (Co-administration may result in additive CNS depression).
No products indexed under this heading.

Enflurane (Co-administration may result in additive CNS depression).
No products indexed under this heading.

Estazolam (Co-administration may result in additive CNS depression). Products include:
ProSom Tablets 512

Ethanol (Co-administration may result in additive CNS depression).
No products indexed under this heading.

Ethchlorvynol (Co-administration may result in additive CNS depression).
No products indexed under this heading.

Ethinamate (Co-administration may result in additive CNS depression).
No products indexed under this heading.

Ethosuximide (Valproate inhibits the metabolism of ethosuximide).
No products indexed under this heading.

Ethyl Alcohol (Co-administration may result in additive CNS depression).
No products indexed under this heading.

Felbamate (Co-administration has resulted in an increase in mean valproate peak concentration; a reduction in valproate dosage may be necessary).
No products indexed under this heading.

Fentanyl (Co-administration may result in additive CNS depression). Products include:
Duragesic Transdermal System 2448

Fentanyl Citrate (Co-administration may result in additive CNS depression). Products include:
Actiq 993

Fluphenazine Decanoate (Co-administration may result in additive CNS depression).
No products indexed under this heading.

Fluphenazine Enanthate (Co-administration may result in additive CNS depression).
No products indexed under this heading.

Fluphenazine Hydrochloride (Co-administration may result in additive CNS depression).
No products indexed under this heading.

Flurazepam Hydrochloride (Co-administration may result in additive CNS depression). Products include:
Dalmane Capsules 3343

Fosphenytoin Sodium (Can double the clearance of valproate; valproate displaces phenytoin from its plasma albumin binding sites and inhibits its hepatic metabolism; co-administration has resulted in breakthrough seizures).
No products indexed under this heading.

Glutethimide (Co-administration may result in additive CNS depression).
No products indexed under this heading.

Haloperidol (Co-administration may result in additive CNS depression).
No products indexed under this heading.

Haloperidol Decanoate (Co-administration may result in additive CNS depression).
No products indexed under this heading.

Hydrocodone Bitartrate (Co-administration may result in additive CNS depression). Products include:
Hycodan 1104
Hycomine Compound Tablets 1105
Hycotuss Expectorant Syrup 1106
Lortab 3315
Lortab Elixir 3312
Vicodin Tablets 530
Vicodin ES Tablets 531
Vicodin HP Tablets 532
Vicoprofen Tablets 533
Zydone Tablets 1118

Hydrocodone Polistirex (Co-administration may result in additive CNS depression). Products include:
Tussionex Pennkinetic Extended-Release Suspension 3322

Hydromorphone Hydrochloride (Co-administration may result in additive CNS depression). Products include:
Dilaudid 439
Dilaudid Oral Liquid 443
Dilaudid Non-Sterile Powder 439
Dilaudid Rectal Suppositories 439
Dilaudid Tablets 439
Dilaudid Tablets - 8 mg 443
Dilaudid-HP 441

Hydroxyzine Hydrochloride (Co-administration may result in additive CNS depression).
No products indexed under this heading.

Isoflurane (Co-administration may result in additive CNS depression).
No products indexed under this heading.

Ketamine Hydrochloride (Co-administration may result in additive CNS depression).
No products indexed under this heading.

Lamotrigine (Co-administration has resulted in increased elimination half-life of lamotrigine, and serious skin reactions, such as Stevens-Johnson syndrome and toxic epidermal necrolysis; the dose of lamotrigine should be reduced if used concurrently). Products include:
Lamictal 1449

Levomethadyl Acetate Hydrochloride (Co-administration may result in additive CNS depression).
No products indexed under this heading.

Levorphanol Tartrate (Co-administration may result in additive CNS depression).
No products indexed under this heading.

Lorazepam (Co-administration was accompanied by a 17% decrease in the plasma clearance of lorazepam; this pharmacokinetic interaction is likely to be clinically unimportant; concurrent use may result in additive CNS depression).
No products indexed under this heading.

Loxapine Hydrochloride (Co-administration may result in additive CNS depression).
No products indexed under this heading.

Loxapine Succinate (Co-administration may result in additive CNS depression).
No products indexed under this heading.

Meperidine Hydrochloride (Co-administration may result in additive CNS depression).
No products indexed under this heading.

Mephobarbital (Co-administration may result in additive CNS depression). Products include:
Mebaral Tablets, USP 2483

Meprobamate (Co-administration may result in additive CNS depression).
No products indexed under this heading.

Meropenem (Sub-therapeutic valproic acid levels have been reported when meropenem was co-administered). Products include:
Merrem I.V. 687

Mesoridazine Besylate (Co-administration may result in additive CNS depression).
No products indexed under this heading.

Methadone Hydrochloride (Co-administration may result in additive CNS depression).
No products indexed under this heading.

Methohexital Sodium (Co-administration may result in additive CNS depression).
No products indexed under this heading.

Methotrimeprazine (Co-administration may result in additive CNS depression).
No products indexed under this heading.

Methoxyflurane (Co-administration may result in additive CNS depression).
No products indexed under this heading.

Midazolam Hydrochloride (Co-administration may result in additive CNS depression).
No products indexed under this heading.

Molindone Hydrochloride (Co-administration may result in additive CNS depression). Products include:
Moban Tablets 1108

Morphine Sulfate (Co-administration may result in additive CNS depression). Products include:
Avinza Capsules 1714
Kadian Capsules 572
MS Contin Tablets 2703

Nortriptyline Hydrochloride (Co-administration has resulted in a 34% decrease in the net clearance of nortriptyline; this interaction is likely to be clinically unimportant).
No products indexed under this heading.

Olanzapine (Co-administration may result in additive CNS depression). Products include:
Symbyax Capsules 1788
Zyprexa Tablets 1798
Zyprexa IntraMuscular 1798
Zyprexa ZYDIS Orally Disintegrating Tablets 1798

Oxazepam (Co-administration may result in additive CNS depression).
No products indexed under this heading.

Oxycodone Hydrochloride (Co-administration may result in additive CNS depression). Products include:
Combunox Tablets 1183
OxyContin Tablets 2699
OxyFast Oral Concentrate Solution 2704
OxyIR Capsules 2704
Percocet Tablets 1114
Percodan Tablets 1115

Pentobarbital Sodium (Co-administration may result in additive CNS depression). Products include:
Nembutal Sodium Solution, USP 2484

Perphenazine (Co-administration may result in additive CNS depression).
No products indexed under this heading.

Phenobarbital (Can double the clearance of valproate; co-administration has resulted in inhibition of the metabolism of phenobarbital resulting in increased half-life and decreased plasma clearance; concurrent use may result in additive CNS depression).
No products indexed under this heading.

Phenytoin (Can double the clearance of valproate; valproate displaces phenytoin from its plasma albumin binding sites and inhibits its hepatic metabolism; co-administration has resulted in breakthrough seizures).
No products indexed under this heading.

Phenytoin Sodium (Can double the clearance of valproate; valproate displaces phenytoin from its plasma albumin binding sites and inhibits its hepatic metabolism; co-administration has resulted in breakthrough seizures). Products include:
Phenytek Capsules 2153

Prazepam (Co-administration may result in additive CNS depression).
No products indexed under this heading.

Primidone (Can double the clearance of valproate; primidone is metabolized to a barbiturate; therefore, co-administration may result in inhibition of the metabolism of primidone resulting in increased half-life and decreased plasma clearance).
No products indexed under this heading.

Prochlorperazine (Co-administration may result in additive CNS depression).
No products indexed under this heading.

Promethazine Hydrochloride (Co-administration may result in additive CNS depression). Products include:
Phenergan 3438

Propofol (Co-administration may result in additive CNS depression). Products include:
Diprivan Injectable Emulsion 676

Propoxyphene Hydrochloride (Co-administration may result in additive CNS depression).
No products indexed under this heading.

Propoxyphene Napsylate (Co-administration may result in additive CNS depression). Products include:
Darvocet A 500 Tablets 3497

Quazepam (Co-administration may result in additive CNS depression).
No products indexed under this heading.

Quetiapine Fumarate (Co-administration may result in additive CNS depression). Products include:
Seroquel Tablets 691

Remifentanil Hydrochloride (Co-administration may result in additive CNS depression).
No products indexed under this heading.

Rifampin (Co-administration has resulted in a 40% increase in oral clearance of valproate).
No products indexed under this heading.

Risperidone (Co-administration may result in additive CNS depression). Products include:
Risperdal Consta Long-Acting Injection 1664
Risperdal M-Tab Orally Disintegrating Tablets 1658
Risperdal 1658

Secobarbital Sodium (Co-administration may result in additive CNS depression).
No products indexed under this heading.

Sevoflurane (Co-administration may result in additive CNS depression). Products include:
Ultane Liquid for Inhalation 526

Sufentanil Citrate (Co-administration may result in additive CNS depression).
No products indexed under this heading.

Temazepam (Co-administration may result in additive CNS depression).
No products indexed under this heading.

Thiamylal Sodium (Co-administration may result in additive CNS depression).
No products indexed under this heading.

Thioridazine Hydrochloride (Co-administration may result in additive CNS depression). Products include:
Thioridazine Hydrochloride Tablets 2122

Thiothixene (Co-administration may result in additive CNS depression). Products include:
Thiothixene Capsules 2124

Tolbutamide (Co-administration in in vitro studies has resulted in an increase in unbound fraction of tolbutamide; the clinical relevance of this displacement is unknown).
No products indexed under this heading.

Triazolam (Co-administration may result in additive CNS depression).
No products indexed under this heading.

Trifluoperazine Hydrochloride (Co-administration may result in additive CNS depression).
No products indexed under this heading.

Warfarin Sodium (In an *in vitro* study, valproate increased the unbound fraction of warfarin by up to 32.6%; therapeutic relevance of this is unknown). Products include:
Coumadin for Injection 932
Coumadin Tablets 932

Zaleplon (Co-administration may result in additive CNS depression). Products include:
Sonata Capsules 1686

Ziprasidone Hydrochloride (Co-administration may result in additive CNS depression). Products include:
Geodon Capsules 2514

Zolpidem Tartrate (Co-administration may result in additive CNS depression). Products include:
Ambien Tablets 2867

Food Interactions

Alcohol (Co-administration may result in additive CNS depression).

DEPAKENE CAPSULES

(Valproic Acid) 417

May interact with central nervous system depressants, phenytoin, and certain other agents. Compounds in these categories include:

Alfentanil Hydrochloride (Valproate produces CNS depression, especially when combined with another CNS depressant).
No products indexed under this heading.

Alprazolam (Valproate produces CNS depression, especially when combined with another CNS depressant). Products include:
Niravam Orally Disintegrating Tablets 3106
Xanax XR Tablets 2655

Amitriptyline Hydrochloride (Co-administration has resulted in a decrease in plasma clearance of amitriptyline; rare postmarketing reports of increased amitriptyline levels).
No products indexed under this heading.

Aprobarbital (Valproate produces CNS depression, especially when combined with another CNS depressant).
No products indexed under this heading.

Aspirin (Co-administration has resulted in a decrease in protein binding and an inhibition of metabolism of valproate; valproate free fraction was increased 4-fold in the presence of aspirin compared to valproate alone). Products include:
Aggrenox Capsules 855
Bayer, Aspirin Regimen 606
Bayer Aspirin Tablets 3515
BC Powder 612
BC Allergy Sinus Cold Powder 612
Arthritis Strength BC Powder 612
BC Sinus Cold Powder 612
Ecotrin Enteric Coated Aspirin Low, Regular and Maximum Strength Tablets 1627
Goody's Body Pain Formula Powder 621
Goody's Extra Strength Headache Powder 621
Goody's Extra Strength Pain Relief Tablets 621
Percodan Tablets 1115
St. Joseph 81 mg Aspirin Chewable and Enteric Coated Tablets 1841

Buprenorphine Hydrochloride (Valproate produces CNS depression, especially when combined with another CNS depressant). Products include:
Buprenex Injectable 2718
Suboxone Tablets 2719
Subutex Tablets 2719

Buspirone Hydrochloride (Valproate produces CNS depression, especially when combined with another CNS depressant).
No products indexed under this heading.

Butabarbital (Valproate produces CNS depression, especially when combined with another CNS depressant).
No products indexed under this heading.

Butalbital (Valproate produces CNS depression, especially when combined with another CNS depressant). Products include:
Sedapap Tablets 50 mg/650 mg 2098

Carbamazepine (Co-administration has resulted in decreased serum levels of carbamazepine and

increased serum levels of carbamazepine 10, 11-epoxide; drugs that affect the levels of expression of hepatic enzymes, particularly those that elevate levels of glucuronosyltransferases, such as carbamazepine, may increase the clearance of valproate). Products include:

Carbatrol Capsules **3174**
Equetro Extended-Release Capsules **3178**
Tegretol/Tegretol-XR **2278**

Chlordiazepoxide (Valproate produces CNS depression, especially when combined with another CNS depressant).
No products indexed under this heading.

Chlordiazepoxide Hydrochloride (Valproate produces CNS depression, especially when combined with another CNS depressant). Products include:
Librium Capsules **3349**

Chlorpromazine (Co-administration has resulted in an increase in trough plasma levels of valproate).
No products indexed under this heading.

Chlorpromazine Hydrochloride (Co-administration has resulted in an increase in trough plasma levels of valproate).
No products indexed under this heading.

Chlorprothixene (Valproate produces CNS depression, especially when combined with another CNS depressant).
No products indexed under this heading.

Chlorprothixene Hydrochloride (Valproate produces CNS depression, especially when combined with another CNS depressant).
No products indexed under this heading.

Chlorprothixene Lactate (Valproate produces CNS depression, especially when combined with another CNS depressant).
No products indexed under this heading.

Clonazepam (Co-administration may induce absence status in patients with a history of absence type seizures). Products include:
Klonopin **2782**

Clorazepate Dipotassium (Valproate produces CNS depression, especially when combined with another CNS depressant). Products include:
Tranxene **2488**

Clozapine (Valproate produces CNS depression, especially when combined with another CNS depressant). Products include:
Clozapine Tablets **2141**
Clozaril Tablets **2174**
FazaClo Orally Disintegrating Tablets **547**

Codeine Phosphate (Valproate produces CNS depression, especially when combined with another CNS depressant). Products include:
Tylenol with Codeine **2461**

Desflurane (Valproate produces CNS depression, especially when combined with another CNS depressant). Products include:
Suprane Liquid for Inhalation **770**

Dezocine (Valproate produces CNS depression, especially when combined with another CNS depressant).
No products indexed under this heading.

Diazepam (Co-administration increases the free fraction of diazepam by 90% in healthy volunteers; plasma clearance and volume of distribution for diazepam were reduced by 25% and 20%, respectively, in the presence of valproate). Products include:
Diastat Rectal Delivery System **3344**
Valium Tablets **2822**

Droperidol (Valproate produces CNS depression, especially when combined with another CNS depressant).
No products indexed under this heading.

Enflurane (Valproate produces CNS depression, especially when combined with another CNS depressant).
No products indexed under this heading.

Estazolam (Valproate produces CNS depression, especially when combined with another CNS depressant). Products include:
ProSom Tablets **512**

Ethanol (Valproate produces CNS depression, especially when combined with another CNS depressant).
No products indexed under this heading.

Ethchlorvynol (Valproate produces CNS depression, especially when combined with another CNS depressant).
No products indexed under this heading.

Ethinamate (Valproate produces CNS depression, especially when combined with another CNS depressant).
No products indexed under this heading.

Ethosuximide (Valproate inhibits the metabolism of ethosuximide; co-administration was accompanied by a 25% increase in elimination half-life of ethosuximide and a 15% decrease in its total clearance as compared to ethosuximide alone).
No products indexed under this heading.

Ethyl Alcohol (Valproate produces CNS depression, especially when combined with another CNS depressant).
No products indexed under this heading.

Felbamate (Co-administration has resulted in an increase in mean valproate peak concentration).
No products indexed under this heading.

Fentanyl (Valproate produces CNS depression, especially when combined with another CNS depressant). Products include:
Duragesic Transdermal System **2448**

Fentanyl Citrate (Valproate produces CNS depression, especially when combined with another CNS depressant). Products include:
Actiq **993**

Fluphenazine Decanoate (Valproate produces CNS depression, especially when combined with another CNS depressant).
No products indexed under this heading.

Fluphenazine Enanthate (Valproate produces CNS depression, especially when combined with another CNS depressant).
No products indexed under this heading.

Fluphenazine Hydrochloride (Valproate produces CNS depression, especially when combined with another CNS depressant).
No products indexed under this heading.

Flurazepam Hydrochloride (Valproate produces CNS depression, especially when combined with another CNS depressant). Products include:
Dalmane Capsules **3343**

Fosphenytoin Sodium (Co-administration with drugs that affect the levels of expression of hepatic enzymes, particularly those that elevate levels of glucuronosyltransferases, such as phenytoin, may increase the clearance of valproate; valproate displaces phenytoin from its plasma binding sites and inhibits its hepatic metabolism; concurrent use has resulted in breakthrough seizures).
No products indexed under this heading.

Glutethimide (Valproate produces CNS depression, especially when combined with another CNS depressant).
No products indexed under this heading.

Haloperidol (Valproate produces CNS depression, especially when combined with another CNS depressant).
No products indexed under this heading.

Haloperidol Decanoate (Valproate produces CNS depression, especially when combined with another CNS depressant).
No products indexed under this heading.

Hydrocodone Bitartrate (Valproate produces CNS depression, especially when combined with another CNS depressant). Products include:
Hycodan **1104**
Hycomine Compound Tablets **1105**
Hycotuss Expectorant Syrup **1106**
Lortab **3315**
Lortab Elixir **3312**
Vicodin Tablets **530**
Vicodin ES Tablets **531**
Vicodin HP Tablets **532**
Vicoprofen Tablets **533**
Zydone Tablets **1118**

Hydrocodone Polistirex (Valproate produces CNS depression, especially when combined with another CNS depressant). Products include:
Tussionex Pennkinetic Extended-Release Suspension **3322**

Hydromorphone Hydrochloride (Valproate produces CNS depression, especially when combined with another CNS depressant). Products include:
Dilaudid **439**
Dilaudid Oral Liquid **443**
Dilaudid Non-Sterile Powder **439**
Dilaudid Rectal Suppositories **439**
Dilaudid Tablets **439**
Dilaudid Tablets - 8 mg **443**
Dilaudid-HP **441**

Hydroxyzine Hydrochloride (Valproate produces CNS depression, especially when combined with another CNS depressant).
No products indexed under this heading.

Isoflurane (Valproate produces CNS depression, especially when combined with another CNS depressant).
No products indexed under this heading.

Ketamine Hydrochloride (Valproate produces CNS depression, especially when combined with another CNS depressant).
No products indexed under this heading.

Lamotrigine (Co-administration has resulted in increased elimination half-life of lamotrigine from 26 to 72 hours and serious skin reactions, such as Stevens-Johnson syndrome and toxic epidermal necrolysis). Products include:
Lamictal **1449**

Levomethadyl Acetate Hydrochloride (Valproate produces CNS depression, especially when combined with another CNS depressant).
No products indexed under this heading.

Levorphanol Tartrate (Valproate produces CNS depression, especially when combined with another CNS depressant).
No products indexed under this heading.

Lorazepam (Co-administration was accompanied by a 17% decrease in the plasma clearance of lorazepam).
No products indexed under this heading.

Loxapine Hydrochloride (Valproate produces CNS depression, especially when combined with another CNS depressant).
No products indexed under this heading.

Loxapine Succinate (Valproate produces CNS depression, especially when combined with another CNS depressant).
No products indexed under this heading.

Meperidine Hydrochloride (Valproate produces CNS depression, especially when combined with another CNS depressant).
No products indexed under this heading.

Mephobarbital (Valproate produces CNS depression, especially when combined with another CNS depressant). Products include:
Mebaral Tablets, USP **2483**

Meprobamate (Valproate produces CNS depression, especially when combined with another CNS depressant).
No products indexed under this heading.

Meropenem (Sub-therapeutic valproic acid levels have been reported when meropenem was co-administered). Products include:
Merrem I.V. **687**

Mesoridazine Besylate (Valproate produces CNS depression, especially when combined with another CNS depressant).
No products indexed under this heading.

Methadone Hydrochloride (Valproate produces CNS depression, especially when combined with another CNS depressant).
No products indexed under this heading.

Methohexital Sodium (Valproate produces CNS depression, especially when combined with another CNS depressant).
No products indexed under this heading.

Methotrimeprazine (Valproate produces CNS depression, especially when combined with another CNS depressant).
No products indexed under this heading.

Methoxyflurane (Valproate produces CNS depression, especially when combined with another CNS depressant).
No products indexed under this heading.

Midazolam Hydrochloride (Valproate produces CNS depression, especially when combined with another CNS depressant).
No products indexed under this heading.

Molindone Hydrochloride (Valproate produces CNS depression, especially when combined with another CNS depressant). Products include:
Moban Tablets 1108

Morphine Sulfate (Valproate produces CNS depression, especially when combined with another CNS depressant). Products include:
Avinza Capsules 1714
Kadian Capsules 572
MS Contin Tablets 2703

Nortriptyline Hydrochloride (Co-administration has resulted in a decrease in the net clearance of nortriptyline).
No products indexed under this heading.

Olanzapine (Valproate produces CNS depression, especially when combined with another CNS depressant). Products include:
Symbyax Capsules 1788
Zyprexa Tablets 1798
Zyprexa IntraMuscular 1798
Zyprexa ZYDIS Orally Disintegrating Tablets 1798

Oxazepam (Valproate produces CNS depression, especially when combined with another CNS depressant).
No products indexed under this heading.

Oxycodone Hydrochloride (Valproate produces CNS depression, especially when combined with another CNS depressant). Products include:
Combunox Tablets 1183
OxyContin Tablets 2699
OxyFast Oral Concentrate Solution 2704
OxyIR Capsules 2704
Percocet Tablets 1114
Percodan Tablets 1115

Pentobarbital Sodium (Valproate produces CNS depression, especially when combined with another CNS depressant). Products include:
Nembutal Sodium Solution, USP 2484

Perphenazine (Valproate produces CNS depression, especially when combined with another CNS depressant).
No products indexed under this heading.

Phenobarbital (Co-administration with drugs that affect the levels of expression of hepatic enzymes, particularly those that elevate levels of glucuronosyltransferases, such as phenobarbital, may increase the clearance of valproate; valproate inhibits the metabolism of phenobarbital; co-administration has resulted in an increase in half-life and decrease in plasma clearance of phenobarbital; all patients should be monitored for neurological toxicity because of severe CNS depression).
No products indexed under this heading.

Phenytoin (Co-administration with drugs that affect the levels of expression of hepatic enzymes, particularly those that elevate levels of glucuronosyltransferases, such as phenytoin, may increase the clearance of valproate; valproate displaces phenytoin from its plasma binding sites and inhibits its hepatic metabolism; concurrent use has resulted in breakthrough seizures).
No products indexed under this heading.

Phenytoin Sodium (Co-administration with drugs that affect the levels of expression of hepatic enzymes, particularly those that elevate levels of glucuronosyltransferases, such as phenytoin, may increase the clearance of valproate; valproate displaces phenytoin from its plasma binding sites and inhibits its hepatic metabolism; concurrent use has resulted in breakthrough seizures). Products include:
Phenytek Capsules 2153

Prazepam (Valproate produces CNS depression, especially when combined with another CNS depressant).
No products indexed under this heading.

Primidone (Co-administraion may result in severe CNS depression because primidone is metabolized to a barbiturate; potential for same interaction as phenobarbital and valproate).
No products indexed under this heading.

Prochlorperazine (Valproate produces CNS depression, especially when combined with another CNS depressant).
No products indexed under this heading.

Promethazine Hydrochloride (Valproate produces CNS depression, especially when combined with another CNS depressant). Products include:
Phenergan 3438

Propofol (Valproate produces CNS depression, especially when combined with another CNS depressant). Products include:
Diprivan Injectable Emulsion 676

Propoxyphene Hydrochloride (Valproate produces CNS depression, especially when combined with another CNS depressant).
No products indexed under this heading.

Propoxyphene Napsylate (Valproate produces CNS depression, especially when combined with another CNS depressant). Products include:
Darvocet A 500 Tablets 3497

Quazepam (Valproate produces CNS depression, especially when combined with another CNS depressant).
No products indexed under this heading.

Quetiapine Fumarate (Valproate produces CNS depression, especially when combined with another CNS depressant). Products include:
Seroquel Tablets 691

Remifentanil Hydrochloride (Valproate produces CNS depression, especially when combined with another CNS depressant).
No products indexed under this heading.

Rifampin (Co-administration has resulted in an increase in the oral clearance of valproate).
No products indexed under this heading.

Risperidone (Valproate produces CNS depression, especially when combined with another CNS depressant). Products include:
Risperdal Consta Long-Acting Injection 1664
Risperdal M-Tab Orally Disintegrating Tablets 1658
Risperdal 1658

Secobarbital Sodium (Valproate produces CNS depression, especially when combined with another CNS depressant).
No products indexed under this heading.

Sevoflurane (Valproate produces CNS depression, especially when combined with another CNS depressant). Products include:
Ultane Liquid for Inhalation 526

Sufentanil Citrate (Valproate produces CNS depression, especially when combined with another CNS depressant).
No products indexed under this heading.

Temazepam (Valproate produces CNS depression, especially when combined with another CNS depressant).
No products indexed under this heading.

Thiamylal Sodium (Valproate produces CNS depression, especially when combined with another CNS depressant).
No products indexed under this heading.

Thioridazine Hydrochloride (Valproate produces CNS depression, especially when combined with another CNS depressant). Products include:
Thioridazine Hydrochloride Tablets 2122

Thiothixene (Valproate produces CNS depression, especially when combined with another CNS depressant). Products include:
Thiothixene Capsules 2124

Tolbutamide (Co-administration in in vitro experiments has resulted in increased unbound fraction of tolbutamide).
No products indexed under this heading.

Triazolam (Valproate produces CNS depression, especially when combined with another CNS depressant).
No products indexed under this heading.

Trifluoperazine Hydrochloride (Valproate produces CNS depression, especially when combined with another CNS depressant).
No products indexed under this heading.

Warfarin Sodium (Co-administration in in vitro experiments has resulted in increased unbound fraction of warfarin). Products include:
Coumadin for Injection 932
Coumadin Tablets 932

Zaleplon (Valproate produces CNS depression, especially when combined with another CNS depressant). Products include:
Sonata Capsules 1686

Zidovudine (Co-administration has resulted in decreased clearance of zidovudine; the half-life of zidovudine was unaffected). Products include:
Combivir Tablets 1373
Retrovir 1533
Retrovir IV Infusion 1537
Trizivir Tablets 1565

Ziprasidone Hydrochloride (Valproate produces CNS depression, especially when combined with another CNS depressant). Products include:
Geodon Capsules 2514

Zolpidem Tartrate (Valproate produces CNS depression, especially when combined with another CNS depressant). Products include:
Ambien Tablets 2867

Food Interactions

Alcohol (Valproate produces CNS depression, especially when combined with another CNS depressant, such as alcohol).

DEPAKENE SYRUP

(Valproic Acid) 417
See Depakene Capsules

DEPAKOTE SPRINKLE CAPSULES

(Divalproex Sodium) 422
See Depakote Tablets

DEPAKOTE TABLETS

(Divalproex Sodium) 427
May interact with central nervous system depressants, phenytoin, and certain other agents. Compounds in these categories include:

Alfentanil Hydrochloride (Valproate produces CNS depression, especially when combined with another CNS depressant).
No products indexed under this heading.

Alprazolam (Valproate produces CNS depression, especially when combined with another CNS depressant). Products include:
Niravam Orally Disintegrating Tablets 3106
Xanax XR Tablets 2655

Amitriptyline Hydrochloride (Co-administration has resulted in a decrease in plasma clearance of amitriptyline; rare postmarketing reports of increased amitriptyline levels).
No products indexed under this heading.

Aprobarbital (Valproate produces CNS depression, especially when combined with another CNS depressant).
No products indexed under this heading.

Aspirin (Co-administration has resulted in a decrease in protein

binding and an inhibition of metabolism of valproate; valproate free fraction was increased 4-fold in the presence of aspirin compared to valproate alone). Products include:

- Aggrenox Capsules 855
- Bayer, Aspirin Regimen ..... ▣ 606
- Bayer Aspirin Tablets 3515
- BC Powder ..... ▣ 612
- BC Allergy Sinus Cold Powder ..... ▣ 612
- Arthritis Strength BC Powder ..... ▣ 612
- BC Sinus Cold Powder ..... ▣ 612
- Ecotrin Enteric Coated Aspirin Low, Regular and Maximum Strength Tablets 1627
- Goody's Body Pain Formula Powder ..... ▣ 621
- Goody's Extra Strength Headache Powder ..... ▣ 621
- Goody's Extra Strength Pain Relief Tablets ..... ▣ 621
- Percodan Tablets 1115
- St. Joseph 81 mg Aspirin Chewable and Enteric Coated Tablets 1841

Buprenorphine Hydrochloride (Valproate produces CNS depression, especially when combined with another CNS depressant). Products include:

- Buprenex Injectable 2718
- Suboxone Tablets 2719
- Subutex Tablets 2719

Buspirone Hydrochloride (Valproate produces CNS depression, especially when combined with another CNS depressant).

No products indexed under this heading.

Butabarbital (Valproate produces CNS depression, especially when combined with another CNS depressant).

No products indexed under this heading.

Butalbital (Valproate produces CNS depression, especially when combined with another CNS depressant). Products include:

- Sedapap Tablets 50 mg/650 mg 2098

Carbamazepine (Co-administration has resulted in decreased serum levels of carbamazepine and increased serum levels of carbamazepine 10,11-epoxide; drugs that affect the levels of expression of hepatic enzymes, particularly those that elevate levels of glucuronosyltransferases, such as carbamazepine, may increase the clearance of valproate). Products include:

- Carbatrol Capsules 3174
- Equetro Extended-Release Capsules 3178
- Tegretol/Tegretol-XR 2278

Chlordiazepoxide (Valproate produces CNS depression, especially when combined with another CNS depressant).

No products indexed under this heading.

Chlordiazepoxide Hydrochloride (Valproate produces CNS depression, especially when combined with another CNS depressant). Products include:

- Librium Capsules 3349

Chlorpromazine (Co-administration has resulted in an increase in trough plasma levels of valproate).

No products indexed under this heading.

Chlorpromazine Hydrochloride (Co-administration has resulted in an increase in trough plasma levels of valproate).

No products indexed under this heading.

Chlorprothixene (Valproate produces CNS depression, especially when combined with another CNS depressant).

No products indexed under this heading.

Chlorprothixene Hydrochloride (Valproate produces CNS depression, especially when combined with another CNS depressant).

No products indexed under this heading.

Chlorprothixene Lactate (Valproate produces CNS depression, especially when combined with another CNS depressant).

No products indexed under this heading.

Clonazepam (Co-administration may induce absence status in patients with a history of absence type seizures). Products include:

- Klonopin 2782

Clorazepate Dipotassium (Valproate produces CNS depression, especially when combined with another CNS depressant). Products include:

- Tranxene 2488

Clozapine (Valproate produces CNS depression, especially when combined with another CNS depressant). Products include:

- Clozapine Tablets 2141
- Clozaril Tablets 2174
- FazaClo Orally Disintegrating Tablets 547

Codeine Phosphate (Valproate produces CNS depression, especially when combined with another CNS depressant). Products include:

- Tylenol with Codeine 2461

Desflurane (Valproate produces CNS depression, especially when combined with another CNS depressant). Products include:

- Suprane Liquid for Inhalation 770

Dezocine (Valproate produces CNS depression, especially when combined with another CNS depressant).

No products indexed under this heading.

Diazepam (Co-administration increases the free fraction of diazepam by 90% in healthy volunteers; plasma clearance and volume of distribution for diazepam were reduced by 25% and 20%, respectively, in the presence of valproate). Products include:

- Diastat Rectal Delivery System 3344
- Valium Tablets 2822

Droperidol (Valproate produces CNS depression, especially when combined with another CNS depressant).

No products indexed under this heading.

Enflurane (Valproate produces CNS depression, especially when combined with another CNS depressant).

No products indexed under this heading.

Estazolam (Valproate produces CNS depression, especially when combined with another CNS depressant). Products include:

- ProSom Tablets 512

Ethanol (Valproate produces CNS depression, especially when combined with another CNS depressant).

No products indexed under this heading.

Ethchlorvynol (Valproate produces CNS depression, especially when combined with another CNS depressant).

No products indexed under this heading.

Ethinamate (Valproate produces CNS depression, especially when combined with another CNS depressant).

No products indexed under this heading.

Ethosuximide (Valproate inhibits the metabolism of ethosuximide; co-administration was accompanied by a 25% increase in elimination half-life of ethosuximide and a 15% decrease in its total clearance as compared to ethosuximide alone).

No products indexed under this heading.

Ethyl Alcohol (Valproate produces CNS depression, especially when combined with another CNS depressant).

No products indexed under this heading.

Felbamate (Co-administration has resulted in an increase in mean valproate peak concentration).

No products indexed under this heading.

Fentanyl (Valproate produces CNS depression, especially when combined with another CNS depressant). Products include:

- Duragesic Transdermal System 2448

Fentanyl Citrate (Valproate produces CNS depression, especially when combined with another CNS depressant). Products include:

- Actiq 993

Fluphenazine Decanoate (Valproate produces CNS depression, especially when combined with another CNS depressant).

No products indexed under this heading.

Fluphenazine Enanthate (Valproate produces CNS depression, especially when combined with another CNS depressant).

No products indexed under this heading.

Fluphenazine Hydrochloride (Valproate produces CNS depression, especially when combined with another CNS depressant).

No products indexed under this heading.

Flurazepam Hydrochloride (Valproate produces CNS depression, especially when combined with another CNS depressant). Products include:

- Dalmane Capsules 3343

Fosphenytoin Sodium (Co-administration with drugs that affect the levels of expression of hepatic enzymes, particularly those that elevate levels of glucuronosyltransferases, such as phenytoin, may increase the clearance of valproate; valproate displaces phenytoin from its plasma binding sites and inhibits its hepatic metabolism; concurrent use has resulted in breakthrough seizures).

No products indexed under this heading.

Glutethimide (Valproate produces CNS depression, especially when combined with another CNS depressant).

No products indexed under this heading.

Haloperidol (Valproate produces CNS depression, especially when combined with another CNS depressant).

No products indexed under this heading.

Haloperidol Decanoate (Valproate produces CNS depression, especially when combined with another CNS depressant).

No products indexed under this heading.

Hydrocodone Bitartrate (Valproate produces CNS depression, especially when combined with another CNS depressant). Products include:

- Hycodan 1104
- Hycomine Compound Tablets 1105
- Hycotuss Expectorant Syrup 1106
- Lortab 3315
- Lortab Elixir 3312
- Vicodin Tablets 530
- Vicodin ES Tablets 531
- Vicodin HP Tablets 532
- Vicoprofen Tablets 533
- Zydone Tablets 1118

Hydrocodone Polistirex (Valproate produces CNS depression, especially when combined with another CNS depressant). Products include:

- Tussionex Pennkinetic Extended-Release Suspension 3322

Hydromorphone Hydrochloride (Valproate produces CNS depression, especially when combined with another CNS depressant). Products include:

- Dilaudid 439
- Dilaudid Oral Liquid 443
- Dilaudid Non-Sterile Powder 439
- Dilaudid Rectal Suppositories 439
- Dilaudid Tablets 439
- Dilaudid Tablets - 8 mg 443
- Dilaudid-HP 441

Hydroxyzine Hydrochloride (Valproate produces CNS depression, especially when combined with another CNS depressant).

No products indexed under this heading.

Isoflurane (Valproate produces CNS depression, especially when combined with another CNS depressant).

No products indexed under this heading.

Ketamine Hydrochloride (Valproate produces CNS depression, especially when combined with another CNS depressant).

No products indexed under this heading.

Lamotrigine (Co-administration has resulted in increased elimination half-life of lamotrigine from 26 to 72 hours and serious skin reactions, such as Stevens-Johnson syndrome and toxic epidermal necrolysis). Products include:

- Lamictal 1449

Levomethadyl Acetate Hydrochloride (Valproate produces CNS depression, especially when combined with another CNS depressant).

No products indexed under this heading.

Levorphanol Tartrate (Valproate produces CNS depression, especially when combined with another CNS depressant).

No products indexed under this heading.

Lorazepam (Co-administration was accompanied by a 17% decrease in the plasma clearance of lorazepam).
No products indexed under this heading.

Loxapine Hydrochloride (Valproate produces CNS depression, especially when combined with another CNS depressant).
No products indexed under this heading.

Loxapine Succinate (Valproate produces CNS depression, especially when combined with another CNS depressant).
No products indexed under this heading.

Meperidine Hydrochloride (Valproate produces CNS depression, especially when combined with another CNS depressant).
No products indexed under this heading.

Mephobarbital (Valproate produces CNS depression, especially when combined with another CNS depressant). Products include:
Mebaral Tablets, USP **2483**

Meprobamate (Valproate produces CNS depression, especially when combined with another CNS depressant).
No products indexed under this heading.

Meropenem (Sub-therapeutic valproic acid levels have been reported when meropenem was co-administered). Products include:
Merrem I.V. **687**

Mesoridazine Besylate (Valproate produces CNS depression, especially when combined with another CNS depressant).
No products indexed under this heading.

Methadone Hydrochloride (Valproate produces CNS depression, especially when combined with another CNS depressant).
No products indexed under this heading.

Methohexital Sodium (Valproate produces CNS depression, especially when combined with another CNS depressant).
No products indexed under this heading.

Methotrimeprazine (Valproate produces CNS depression, especially when combined with another CNS depressant).
No products indexed under this heading.

Methoxyflurane (Valproate produces CNS depression, especially when combined with another CNS depressant).
No products indexed under this heading.

Midazolam Hydrochloride (Valproate produces CNS depression, especially when combined with another CNS depressant).
No products indexed under this heading.

Molindone Hydrochloride (Valproate produces CNS depression, especially when combined with another CNS depressant). Products include:
Moban Tablets **1108**

Morphine Sulfate (Valproate produces CNS depression, especially when combined with another CNS depressant). Products include:
Avinza Capsules **1714**
Kadian Capsules **572**
MS Contin Tablets **2703**

Nortriptyline Hydrochloride (Co-administration has resulted in a decrease in the net clearance of nortriptyline).
No products indexed under this heading.

Olanzapine (Valproate produces CNS depression, especially when combined with another CNS depressant). Products include:
Symbyax Capsules **1788**
Zyprexa Tablets **1798**
Zyprexa IntraMuscular **1798**
Zyprexa ZYDIS Orally Disintegrating Tablets.................. **1798**

Oxazepam (Valproate produces CNS depression, especially when combined with another CNS depressant).
No products indexed under this heading.

Oxycodone Hydrochloride (Valproate produces CNS depression, especially when combined with another CNS depressant). Products include:
Combunox Tablets **1183**
OxyContin Tablets **2699**
OxyFast Oral Concentrate Solution....................................... **2704**
OxyIR Capsules **2704**
Percocet Tablets **1114**
Percodan Tablets **1115**

Pentobarbital Sodium (Valproate produces CNS depression, especially when combined with another CNS depressant). Products include:
Nembutal Sodium Solution, USP **2484**

Perphenazine (Valproate produces CNS depression, especially when combined with another CNS depressant).
No products indexed under this heading.

Phenobarbital (Co-administration with drugs that affect the levels of expression of hepatic enzymes, particularly those that elevate levels of glucuronosyltransferases, such as phenobarbital, may increase the clearance of valproate; valproate inhibits the metabolism of phenobarbital; co-administration has resulted in an increase in half-life and a decrease in plasma clearance of phenobarbital; all patients should be monitored for neurological toxicity because of severe CNS depression).
No products indexed under this heading.

Phenytoin (Co-administration with drugs that affect the levels of expression of hepatic enzymes, particularly those that elevate levels of glucuronosyltransferases, such as phenytoin, may increase the clearance of valproate; valproate displaces phenytoin from its plasma binding sites and inhibits its hepatic metabolism; concurrent use has resulted in breakthrough seizures).
No products indexed under this heading.

Phenytoin Sodium (Co-administration with drugs that affect the levels of expression of hepatic enzymes, particularly those that elevate levels of glucuronosyltransferases, such as phenytoin, may increase the clearance of valproate; valproate displaces phenytoin from its plasma binding sites and inhibits its hepatic metabolism; concurrent use has resulted in breakthrough seizures). Products include:
Phenytek Capsules **2153**

Prazepam (Valproate produces CNS depression, especially when combined with another CNS depressant).
No products indexed under this heading.

Primidone (Co-administration may result in severe CNS depression because primidone is metabolized to a barbiturate; potential for same interaction as phenobarbital and valproate).
No products indexed under this heading.

Prochlorperazine (Valproate produces CNS depression, especially when combined with another CNS depressant).
No products indexed under this heading.

Promethazine Hydrochloride (Valproate produces CNS depression, especially when combined with another CNS depressant). Products include:
Phenergan **3438**

Propofol (Valproate produces CNS depression, especially when combined with another CNS depressant). Products include:
Diprivan Injectable Emulsion **676**

Propoxyphene Hydrochloride (Valproate produces CNS depression, especially when combined with another CNS depressant).
No products indexed under this heading.

Propoxyphene Napsylate (Valproate produces CNS depression, especially when combined with another CNS depressant). Products include:
Darvocet A 500 Tablets **3497**

Quazepam (Valproate produces CNS depression, especially when combined with another CNS depressant).
No products indexed under this heading.

Quetiapine Fumarate (Valproate produces CNS depression, especially when combined with another CNS depressant). Products include:
Seroquel Tablets **691**

Remifentanil Hydrochloride (Valproate produces CNS depression, especially when combined with another CNS depressant).
No products indexed under this heading.

Rifampin (Co-administration has resulted in an increase in the oral clearance of valproate).
No products indexed under this heading.

Risperidone (Valproate produces CNS depression, especially when combined with another CNS depressant). Products include:
Risperdal Consta Long-Acting Injection.. **1664**
Risperdal M-Tab Orally Disintegrating Tablets.................. **1658**
Risperdal **1658**

Secobarbital Sodium (Valproate produces CNS depression, especially when combined with another CNS depressant).
No products indexed under this heading.

Sevoflurane (Valproate produces CNS depression, especially when combined with another CNS depressant). Products include:
Ultane Liquid for Inhalation **526**

Sufentanil Citrate (Valproate produces CNS depression, especially when combined with another CNS depressant).
No products indexed under this heading.

Temazepam (Valproate produces CNS depression, especially when combined with another CNS depressant).
No products indexed under this heading.

Thiamylal Sodium (Valproate produces CNS depression, especially when combined with another CNS depressant).
No products indexed under this heading.

Thioridazine Hydrochloride (Valproate produces CNS depression, especially when combined with another CNS depressant). Products include:
Thioridazine Hydrochloride Tablets.. **2122**

Thiothixene (Valproate produces CNS depression, especially when combined with another CNS depressant). Products include:
Thiothixene Capsules **2124**

Tolbutamide (Co-administration in in vitro experiments has resulted in increased unbound fraction of tolbutamide).
No products indexed under this heading.

Triazolam (Valproate produces CNS depression, especially when combined with another CNS depressant).
No products indexed under this heading.

Trifluoperazine Hydrochloride (Valproate produces CNS depression, especially when combined with another CNS depressant).
No products indexed under this heading.

Warfarin Sodium (Co-administration in in vitro experiments has resulted in increased unbound fraction of warfarin). Products include:
Coumadin for Injection **932**
Coumadin Tablets **932**

Zaleplon (Valproate produces CNS depression, especially when combined with another CNS depressant). Products include:
Sonata Capsules **1686**

Zidovudine (Co-administration has resulted in decreased clearance of zidovudine; the half-life of zidovudine was unaffected). Products include:
Combivir Tablets **1373**
Retrovir **1533**
Retrovir IV Infusion **1537**
Trizivir Tablets **1565**

Ziprasidone Hydrochloride (Valproate produces CNS depression, especially when combined with another CNS depressant). Products include:
Geodon Capsules **2514**

Zolpidem Tartrate (Valproate produces CNS depression, especially when combined with another CNS depressant). Products include:
Ambien Tablets **2867**

Food Interactions

Alcohol (Valproate produces CNS depression, especially when combined with another CNS depressant, such as alcohol).

IMPORTANT NOTE: Always consult each drug listing in the patient's regimen for possible interactions.

DEPAKOTE ER TABLETS
(Divalproex Sodium) 433
See Depakote Tablets

DEPOCYT INJECTION
(Cytarabine Liposome) 1121
May interact with cytotoxic drugs. Compounds in these categories include:

Bleomycin Sulfate (Co-administration of intrathecal cytarabine and other cytotoxic agents administered intrathecally may enhance neurotoxicity).
No products indexed under this heading.

Cyclophosphamide (Co-administration of intrathecal cytarabine and other cytotoxic agents administered intrathecally may enhance neurotoxicity).
No products indexed under this heading.

Daunorubicin Hydrochloride (Co-administration of intrathecal cytarabine and other cytotoxic agents administered intrathecally may enhance neurotoxicity). Products include:
Cerubidine for Injection 788

Doxorubicin Hydrochloride (Co-administration of intrathecal cytarabine and other cytotoxic agents administered intrathecally may enhance neurotoxicity). Products include:
Adriamycin for Injection, USP 786
Adriamycin Injection, USP 786

Epirubicin Hydrochloride (Co-administration of intrathecal cytarabine and other cytotoxic agents administered intrathecally may enhance neurotoxicity). Products include:
Ellence Injection 2632

Fluorouracil (Co-administration of intrathecal cytarabine and other cytotoxic agents administered intrathecally may enhance neurotoxicity). Products include:
Carac Cream, 0.5% 1048
Efudex 3348

Hydroxyurea (Co-administration of intrathecal cytarabine and other cytotoxic agents administered intrathecally may enhance neurotoxicity).
No products indexed under this heading.

Methotrexate Sodium (Co-administration of intrathecal cytarabine and other cytotoxic agents administered intrathecally may enhance neurotoxicity).
No products indexed under this heading.

Mitotane (Co-administration of intrathecal cytarabine and other cytotoxic agents administered intrathecally may enhance neurotoxicity).
No products indexed under this heading.

Mitoxantrone Hydrochloride (Co-administration of intrathecal cytarabine and other cytotoxic agents administered intrathecally may enhance neurotoxicity). Products include:
Novantrone for Injection Concentrate 3158

Procarbazine Hydrochloride (Co-administration of intrathecal cytarabine and other cytotoxic agents administered intrathecally may enhance neurotoxicity). Products include:
Matulane Capsules 3188

Tamoxifen Citrate (Co-administration of intrathecal cytarabine and other cytotoxic agents administered intrathecally may enhance neurotoxicity).
No products indexed under this heading.

Vincristine Sulfate (Co-administration of intrathecal cytarabine and other cytotoxic agents administered intrathecally may enhance neurotoxicity).
No products indexed under this heading.

DEPODUR EXTENDED-RELEASE INJECTION
(Morphine sulfate, liposomal) 1098
May interact with central nervous system depressants, general anesthetics, hypnotics and sedatives, monoamine oxidase inhibitors, neuromuscular blocking agents, phenothiazines, tranquilizers, and certain other agents. Compounds in these categories include:

Alfentanil Hydrochloride (The concurrent use of other central nervous system (CNS) depressants increases the risk of respiratory depression, hypotension, profound sedation or coma. Use with caution and with vigilant monitoring in patients taking these agents).
No products indexed under this heading.

Alprazolam (The concurrent use of other central nervous system (CNS) depressants, including tranquilizers, increases the risk of respiratory depression, hypotension, profound sedation or coma. Use with caution and with vigilant monitoring in patients taking these agents). Products include:
Niravam Orally Disintegrating Tablets 3106
Xanax XR Tablets 2655

Aprobarbital (The concurrent use of other central nervous system (CNS) depressants increases the risk of respiratory depression, hypotension, profound sedation or coma. Use with caution and with vigilant monitoring in patients taking these agents).
No products indexed under this heading.

Atracurium Besylate (Respiratory depression associated with morphine may delay recovery of spontaneous pulmonary ventilation when neuromuscular blocking agents are co-administered).
No products indexed under this heading.

Buprenorphine Hydrochloride (The concurrent use of other central nervous system (CNS) depressants increases the risk of respiratory depression, hypotension, profound sedation or coma. Use with caution and with vigilant monitoring in patients taking these agents). Products include:
Buprenex Injectable 2718
Suboxone Tablets 2719
Subutex Tablets 2719

Buspirone Hydrochloride (The concurrent use of other central nervous system (CNS) depressants, including tranquilizers, increases the risk of respiratory depression, hypotension, profound sedation or coma. Use with caution and with vigilant monitoring in patients taking these agents).
No products indexed under this heading.

Butabarbital (The concurrent use of other central nervous system (CNS) depressants increases the risk of respiratory depression, hypotension, profound sedation or coma. Use with caution and with vigilant monitoring in patients taking these agents).
No products indexed under this heading.

Butalbital (The concurrent use of other central nervous system (CNS) depressants increases the risk of respiratory depression, hypotension, profound sedation or coma. Use with caution and with vigilant monitoring in patients taking these agents). Products include:
Sedapap Tablets 50 mg/650 mg 2098

Chlordiazepoxide (The concurrent use of other central nervous system (CNS) depressants, including tranquilizers, increases the risk of respiratory depression, hypotension, profound sedation or coma. Use with caution and with vigilant monitoring in patients taking these agents).
No products indexed under this heading.

Chlordiazepoxide Hydrochloride (The concurrent use of other central nervous system (CNS) depressants, including tranquilizers, increases the risk of respiratory depression, hypotension, profound sedation or coma. Use with caution and with vigilant monitoring in patients taking these agents). Products include:
Librium Capsules 3349

Chlorpromazine (The concurrent use of other central nervous system (CNS) depressants, including phenothiazines, increases the risk of respiratory depression, hypotension, profound sedation or coma. Use with caution and with vigilant monitoring in patients taking these agents).
No products indexed under this heading.

Chlorpromazine Hydrochloride (The concurrent use of other central nervous system (CNS) depressants, including phenothiazines, increases the risk of respiratory depression, hypotension, profound sedation or coma. Use with caution and with vigilant monitoring in patients taking these agents).
No products indexed under this heading.

Chlorprothixene (The concurrent use of other central nervous system (CNS) depressants, including tranquilizers, increases the risk of respiratory depression, hypotension, profound sedation or coma. Use with caution and with vigilant monitoring in patients taking these agents).
No products indexed under this heading.

Chlorprothixene Hydrochloride (The concurrent use of other central nervous system (CNS) depressants, including tranquilizers, increases the risk of respiratory depression, hypotension, profound sedation or coma. Use with caution and with vigilant monitoring in patients taking these agents).
No products indexed under this heading.

Chlorprothixene Lactate (The concurrent use of other central nervous system (CNS) depressants increases the risk of respiratory depression, hypotension, profound sedation or coma. Use with caution and with vigilant monitoring in patients taking these agents).
No products indexed under this heading.

Cisatracurium Besylate (Respiratory depression associated with morphine may delay recovery of spontaneous pulmonary ventilation when neuromuscular blocking agents are co-administered). Products include:
Nimbex Injection 494

Clorazepate Dipotassium (The concurrent use of other central nervous system (CNS) depressants, including tranquilizers, increases the risk of respiratory depression, hypotension, profound sedation or coma. Use with caution and with vigilant monitoring in patients taking these agents). Products include:
Tranxene 2488

Clozapine (The concurrent use of other central nervous system (CNS) depressants increases the risk of respiratory depression, hypotension, profound sedation or coma. Use with caution and with vigilant monitoring in patients taking these agents). Products include:
Clozapine Tablets 2141
Clozaril Tablets 2174
FazaClo Orally Disintegrating Tablets 547

Codeine Phosphate (The concurrent use of other central nervous system (CNS) depressants increases the risk of respiratory depression, hypotension, profound sedation or coma. Use with caution and with vigilant monitoring in patients taking these agents). Products include:
Tylenol with Codeine 2461

Desflurane (The concurrent use of other central nervous system (CNS) depressants increases the risk of respiratory depression, hypotension, profound sedation or coma. Use with caution and with vigilant monitoring in patients taking these agents). Products include:
Suprane Liquid for Inhalation 770

Dezocine (The concurrent use of other central nervous system (CNS) depressants increases the risk of respiratory depression, hypotension, profound sedation or coma. Use with caution and with vigilant monitoring in patients taking these agents).
No products indexed under this heading.

Diazepam (The concurrent use of other central nervous system (CNS) depressants, including tranquilizers, increases the risk of respiratory depression, hypotension, profound sedation or coma. Use with caution and with vigilant monitoring in patients taking these agents). Products include:
Diastat Rectal Delivery System 3344

Valium Tablets 2822

Doxacurium Chloride (Respiratory depression associated with morphine may delay recovery of spontaneous pulmonary ventilation when neuromuscular blocking agents are co-administered).
No products indexed under this heading.

Droperidol (The concurrent use of other central nervous system (CNS) depressants, including droperidol, increases the risk of respiratory depression, hypotension, profound sedation or coma. Use with caution and with vigilant monitoring in patients taking these agents).
No products indexed under this heading.

Enflurane (The concurrent use of other central nervous system (CNS) depressants increases the risk of respiratory depression, hypotension, profound sedation or coma. Use with caution and with vigilant monitoring in patients taking these agents).
No products indexed under this heading.

Estazolam (The concurrent use of other central nervous system (CNS) depressants, including sedatives and hypnotics, increases the risk of respiratory depression, hypotension, profound sedation or coma. Use with caution and with vigilant monitoring in patients taking these agents). Products include:
ProSom Tablets 512

Ethanol (The concurrent use of other central nervous system (CNS) depressants increases the risk of respiratory depression, hypotension, profound sedation or coma. Use with caution and with vigilant monitoring in patients taking these agents).
No products indexed under this heading.

Ethchlorvynol (The concurrent use of other central nervous system (CNS) depressants, including sedatives and hypnotics, increases the risk of respiratory depression, hypotension, profound sedation or coma. Use with caution and with vigilant monitoring in patients taking these agents).
No products indexed under this heading.

Ethinamate (The concurrent use of other central nervous system (CNS) depressants, including sedatives and hypnotics, increases the risk of respiratory depression, hypotension, profound sedation or coma. Use with caution and with vigilant monitoring in patients taking these agents).
No products indexed under this heading.

Ethyl Alcohol (The concurrent use of other central nervous system (CNS) depressants increases the risk of respiratory depression, hypotension, profound sedation or coma. Use with caution and with vigilant monitoring in patients taking these agents).
No products indexed under this heading.

Fentanyl (The concurrent use of other central nervous system (CNS) depressants increases the risk of respiratory depression, hypotension, profound sedation or coma. Use with caution and with vigilant monitoring in patients taking these agents). Products include:
Duragesic Transdermal System 2448

Fentanyl Citrate (The concurrent use of other central nervous system (CNS) depressants increases the risk of respiratory depression, hypotension, profound sedation or coma. Use with caution and with vigilant monitoring in patients taking these agents). Products include:
Actiq 993

Fluphenazine Decanoate (The concurrent use of other central nervous system (CNS) depressants, including phenothiazines, increases the risk of respiratory depression, hypotension, profound sedation or coma. Use with caution and with vigilant monitoring in patients taking these agents).
No products indexed under this heading.

Fluphenazine Enanthate (The concurrent use of other central nervous system (CNS) depressants, including phenothiazines, increases the risk of respiratory depression, hypotension, profound sedation or coma. Use with caution and with vigilant monitoring in patients taking these agents).
No products indexed under this heading.

Fluphenazine Hydrochloride (The concurrent use of other central nervous system (CNS) depressants, including phenothiazines, increases the risk of respiratory depression, hypotension, profound sedation or coma. Use with caution and with vigilant monitoring in patients taking these agents).
No products indexed under this heading.

Flurazepam Hydrochloride (The concurrent use of other central nervous system (CNS) depressants, including sedatives and hypnotics, increases the risk of respiratory depression, hypotension, profound sedation or coma. Use with caution and with vigilant monitoring in patients taking these agents). Products include:
Dalmane Capsules 3343

Glutethimide (The concurrent use of other central nervous system (CNS) depressants, including sedatives and hypnotics, increases the risk of respiratory depression, hypotension, profound sedation or coma. Use with caution and with vigilant monitoring in patients taking these agents).
No products indexed under this heading.

Haloperidol (The concurrent use of other central nervous system (CNS) depressants, including tranquilizers, increases the risk of respiratory depression, hypotension, profound sedation or coma. Use with caution and with vigilant monitoring in patients taking these agents).
No products indexed under this heading.

Haloperidol Decanoate (The concurrent use of other central nervous system (CNS) depressants, including tranquilizers, increases the risk of respiratory depression, hypotension, profound sedation or coma. Use with caution and with vigilant monitoring in patients taking these agents).
No products indexed under this heading.

Hydrocodone Bitartrate (The concurrent use of other central nervous system (CNS) depressants increases the risk of respiratory depression, hypotension, profound sedation or coma. Use with caution and with vigilant monitoring in patients taking these agents). Products include:
Hycodan 1104
Hycomine Compound Tablets 1105
Hycotuss Expectorant Syrup 1106
Lortab 3315
Lortab Elixir 3312
Vicodin Tablets 530
Vicodin ES Tablets 531
Vicodin HP Tablets 532
Vicoprofen Tablets 533
Zydone Tablets 1118

Hydrocodone Polistirex (The concurrent use of other central nervous system (CNS) depressants increases the risk of respiratory depression, hypotension, profound sedation or coma. Use with caution and with vigilant monitoring in patients taking these agents). Products include:
Tussionex Pennkinetic Extended-Release Suspension 3322

Hydromorphone Hydrochloride (The concurrent use of other central nervous system (CNS) depressants increases the risk of respiratory depression, hypotension, profound sedation or coma. Use with caution and with vigilant monitoring in patients taking these agents). Products include:
Dilaudid 439
Dilaudid Oral Liquid 443
Dilaudid Non-Sterile Powder 439
Dilaudid Rectal Suppositories 439
Dilaudid Tablets 439
Dilaudid Tablets - 8 mg 443
Dilaudid-HP 441

Hydroxyzine Hydrochloride (The concurrent use of other central nervous system (CNS) depressants, including tranquilizers, increases the risk of respiratory depression, hypotension, profound sedation or coma. Use with caution and with vigilant monitoring in patients taking these agents).
No products indexed under this heading.

Isocarboxazid (MAOIs markedly potentiate the action of morphine. DepoDur should not be used in patients taking MAOIs, or within 14 days of stopping such treatment).
No products indexed under this heading.

Isoflurane (The concurrent use of other central nervous system (CNS) depressants increases the risk of respiratory depression, hypotension, profound sedation or coma. Use with caution and with vigilant monitoring in patients taking these agents).
No products indexed under this heading.

Ketamine Hydrochloride (The concurrent use of other central nervous system (CNS) depressants increases the risk of respiratory depression, hypotension, profound sedation or coma. Use with caution and with vigilant monitoring in patients taking these agents).
No products indexed under this heading.

Levomethadyl Acetate Hydrochloride (The concurrent use of other central nervous system (CNS) depressants increases the risk of respiratory depression, hypotension, profound sedation or coma. Use with caution and with vigilant monitoring in patients taking these agents).
No products indexed under this heading.

Levorphanol Tartrate (The concurrent use of other central nervous system (CNS) depressants increases the risk of respiratory depression, hypotension, profound sedation or coma. Use with caution and with vigilant monitoring in patients taking these agents).
No products indexed under this heading.

Lorazepam (The concurrent use of other central nervous system (CNS) depressants, including sedatives and hypnotics, increases the risk of respiratory depression, hypotension, profound sedation or coma. Use with caution and with vigilant monitoring in patients taking these agents).
No products indexed under this heading.

Loxapine Hydrochloride (The concurrent use of other central nervous system (CNS) depressants, including tranquilizers, increases the risk of respiratory depression, hypotension, profound sedation or coma. Use with caution and with vigilant monitoring in patients taking these agents).
No products indexed under this heading.

Loxapine Succinate (The concurrent use of other central nervous system (CNS) depressants, including tranquilizers, increases the risk of respiratory depression, hypotension, profound sedation or coma. Use with caution and with vigilant monitoring in patients taking these agents).
No products indexed under this heading.

Meperidine Hydrochloride (The concurrent use of other central nervous system (CNS) depressants increases the risk of respiratory depression, hypotension, profound sedation or coma. Use with caution and with vigilant monitoring in patients taking these agents).
No products indexed under this heading.

Mephobarbital (The concurrent use of other central nervous system (CNS) depressants increases the risk of respiratory depression, hypotension, profound sedation or coma. Use with caution and with vigilant monitoring in patients taking these agents). Products include:
Mebaral Tablets, USP 2483

Meprobamate (The concurrent use of other central nervous system (CNS) depressants, including tranquilizers, increases the risk of respiratory depression, hypotension, profound sedation or coma. Use with caution and with vigilant monitoring in patients taking these agents).
No products indexed under this heading.

Mesoridazine Besylate (The concurrent use of other central nervous system (CNS) depressants, including phenothiazines, increases the risk of respiratory depression, hypotension, profound sedation or coma. Use with caution and with vigilant monitoring in patients taking these agents).
No products indexed under this heading.

Methadone Hydrochloride (The concurrent use of other central nervous system (CNS) depressants increases the risk of respiratory depression, hypotension, profound sedation or coma. Use with caution and with vigilant monitoring in patients taking these agents).
No products indexed under this heading.

Methohexital Sodium (The concurrent use of other central nervous system (CNS) depressants increases the risk of respiratory depression, hypotension, profound sedation or coma. Use with caution and with vigilant monitoring in patients taking these agents).
No products indexed under this heading.

Methotrimeprazine (The concurrent use of other central nervous system (CNS) depressants, including phenothiazines, increases the risk of respiratory depression, hypotension, profound sedation or coma. Use with caution and with vigilant monitoring in patients taking these agents).
No products indexed under this heading.

Methoxyflurane (The concurrent use of other central nervous system (CNS) depressants increases the risk of respiratory depression, hypotension, profound sedation or coma. Use with caution and with vigilant monitoring in patients taking these agents).
No products indexed under this heading.

Metocurine Iodide (Respiratory depression associated with morphine may delay recovery of spontaneous pulmonary ventilation when neuromuscular blocking agents are co-administered).
No products indexed under this heading.

Midazolam Hydrochloride (The concurrent use of other central nervous system (CNS) depressants, including sedatives and hypnotics, increases the risk of respiratory depression, hypotension, profound sedation or coma. Use with caution and with vigilant monitoring in patients taking these agents).
No products indexed under this heading.

Mivacurium Chloride (Respiratory depression associated with morphine may delay recovery of spontaneous pulmonary ventilation when neuromuscular blocking agents are co-administered). Products include:
Mivacron Injection 489

Moclobemide (MAOIs markedly potentiate the action of morphine. DepoDur should not be used in patients taking MAOIs, or within 14 days of stopping such treatment).
No products indexed under this heading.

Molindone Hydrochloride (The concurrent use of other central nervous system (CNS) depressants, including tranquilizers, increases the risk of respiratory depression, hypotension, profound sedation or coma. Use with caution and with vigilant monitoring in patients taking these agents). Products include:
Moban Tablets 1108

Morphine Sulfate (The concurrent use of other central nervous system (CNS) depressants increases the risk of respiratory depression, hypotension, profound sedation or coma. Use with caution and with vigilant monitoring in patients taking these agents). Products include:
Avinza Capsules 1714
Kadian Capsules 572
MS Contin Tablets 2703

Olanzapine (The concurrent use of other central nervous system (CNS) depressants increases the risk of respiratory depression, hypotension, profound sedation or coma. Use with caution and with vigilant monitoring in patients taking these agents).
Products include:
Symbyax Capsules 1788
Zyprexa Tablets 1798
Zyprexa IntraMuscular 1798
Zyprexa ZYDIS Orally Disintegrating Tablets 1798

Oxazepam (The concurrent use of other central nervous system (CNS) depressants, including tranquilizers, increases the risk of respiratory depression, hypotension, profound sedation or coma. Use with caution and with vigilant monitoring in patients taking these agents).
No products indexed under this heading.

Oxycodone Hydrochloride (The concurrent use of other central nervous system (CNS) depressants increases the risk of respiratory depression, hypotension, profound sedation or coma. Use with caution and with vigilant monitoring in patients taking these agents).
Products include:
Combunox Tablets 1183
OxyContin Tablets 2699
OxyFast Oral Concentrate Solution 2704
OxyIR Capsules 2704
Percocet Tablets 1114
Percodan Tablets 1115

Pancuronium Bromide (Respiratory depression associated with morphine may delay recovery of spontaneous pulmonary ventilation when neuromuscular blocking agents are co-administered).
No products indexed under this heading.

Pargyline Hydrochloride (MAOIs markedly potentiate the action of morphine. DepoDur should not be used in patients taking MAOIs, or within 14 days of stopping such treatment).
No products indexed under this heading.

Pentobarbital Sodium (The concurrent use of other central nervous system (CNS) depressants increases the risk of respiratory depression, hypotension, profound sedation or coma. Use with caution and with vigilant monitoring in patients taking these agents). Products include:
Nembutal Sodium Solution, USP 2484

Perphenazine (The concurrent use of other central nervous system (CNS) depressants, including phenothiazines, increases the risk of respiratory depression, hypotension, profound sedation or coma. Use with caution and with vigilant monitoring in patients taking these agents).
No products indexed under this heading.

Phenelzine Sulfate (MAOIs markedly potentiate the action of morphine. DepoDur should not be used in patients taking MAOIs, or within 14 days of stopping such treatment).
No products indexed under this heading.

Phenobarbital (The concurrent use of other central nervous system (CNS) depressants increases the risk of respiratory depression, hypotension, profound sedation or coma. Use with caution and with vigilant monitoring in patients taking these agents).
No products indexed under this heading.

Prazepam (The concurrent use of other central nervous system (CNS) depressants, including tranquilizers, increases the risk of respiratory depression, hypotension, profound sedation or coma. Use with caution and with vigilant monitoring in patients taking these agents).
No products indexed under this heading.

Procarbazine Hydrochloride (MAOIs markedly potentiate the action of morphine. DepoDur should not be used in patients taking MAOIs, or within 14 days of stopping such treatment). Products include:
Matulane Capsules 3188

Prochlorperazine (The concurrent use of other central nervous system (CNS) depressants, including phenothiazines, increases the risk of respiratory depression, hypotension, profound sedation or coma. Use with caution and with vigilant monitoring in patients taking these agents).
No products indexed under this heading.

Promethazine Hydrochloride (The concurrent use of other central nervous system (CNS) depressants, including phenothiazines, increases the risk of respiratory depression, hypotension, profound sedation or coma. Use with caution and with vigilant monitoring in patients taking these agents). Products include:
Phenergan 3438

Propofol (The concurrent use of other central nervous system (CNS) depressants, including sedatives and hypnotics, increases the risk of respiratory depression, hypotension, profound sedation or coma. Use with caution and with vigilant monitoring in patients taking these agents).
Products include:
Diprivan Injectable Emulsion 676

Propoxyphene Hydrochloride (The concurrent use of other central nervous system (CNS) depressants increases the risk of respiratory depression, hypotension, profound sedation or coma. Use with caution and with vigilant monitoring in patients taking these agents).
No products indexed under this heading.

Propoxyphene Napsylate (The concurrent use of other central nervous system (CNS) depressants increases the risk of respiratory depression, hypotension, profound sedation or coma. Use with caution and with vigilant monitoring in patients taking these agents).
Products include:
Darvocet A 500 Tablets 3497

Quazepam (The concurrent use of other central nervous system (CNS) depressants, including sedatives and hypnotics, increases the risk of respiratory depression, hypotension, profound sedation or coma. Use with caution and with vigilant monitoring in patients taking these agents).
No products indexed under this heading.

Quetiapine Fumarate (The concurrent use of other central nervous system (CNS) depressants increases the risk of respiratory depression, hypotension, profound sedation or coma. Use with caution and with vigilant monitoring in patients taking these agents). Products include:
Seroquel Tablets 691

Rapacuronium Bromide (Respiratory depression associated with morphine may delay recovery of spontaneous pulmonary ventilation when neuromuscular blocking agents are co-administered).
No products indexed under this heading.

Remifentanil Hydrochloride (The concurrent use of other central nervous system (CNS) depressants increases the risk of respiratory depression, hypotension, profound sedation or coma. Use with caution and with vigilant monitoring in patients taking these agents).
No products indexed under this heading.

Risperidone (The concurrent use of other central nervous system (CNS) depressants increases the risk of respiratory depression, hypotension, profound sedation or coma. Use with caution and with vigilant monitoring in patients taking these agents).
Products include:
Risperdal Consta Long-Acting Injection 1664
Risperdal M-Tab Orally Disintegrating Tablets 1658
Risperdal 1658

Rocuronium Bromide (Respiratory depression associated with morphine may delay recovery of spontaneous pulmonary ventilation when neuromuscular blocking agents are co-administered). Products include:
Zemuron Injection 2363

Secobarbital Sodium (The concurrent use of other central nervous system (CNS) depressants, including sedatives and hypnotics, increases the risk of respiratory depression, hypotension, profound sedation or coma. Use with caution and with vigilant monitoring in patients taking these agents).
No products indexed under this heading.

Selegiline Hydrochloride (MAOIs markedly potentiate the action of morphine. DepoDur should not be used in patients taking MAOIs, or within 14 days of stopping such treatment). Products include:
Eldepryl Capsules 3209

Sevoflurane (The concurrent use of other central nervous system (CNS) depressants increases the risk of respiratory depression, hypotension, profound sedation or coma. Use with caution and with vigilant monitoring in patients taking these agents).
Products include:
Ultane Liquid for Inhalation 526

Sodium Oxybate (The concurrent use of other central nervous system (CNS) depressants increases the risk of respiratory depression, hypotension, profound sedation or coma. Use with caution and with vigilant monitoring in patients taking these agents).
No products indexed under this heading.

Succinylcholine Chloride (Respiratory depression associated with morphine may delay recovery of spontaneous pulmonary ventilation when neuromuscular blocking agents are co-administered).
No products indexed under this heading.

Sufentanil Citrate (The concurrent use of other central nervous system (CNS) depressants increases the risk of respiratory depression, hypotension, profound sedation or coma. Use with caution and with vigilant monitoring in patients taking these agents).
No products indexed under this heading.

Temazepam (The concurrent use of other central nervous system (CNS) depressants, including sedatives and hypnotics, increases the risk of respiratory depression, hypotension, profound sedation or coma. Use with caution and with vigilant monitoring in patients taking these agents).
No products indexed under this heading.

Thiamylal Sodium (The concurrent use of other central nervous system (CNS) depressants increases the risk of respiratory depression, hypotension, profound sedation or coma. Use with caution and with vigilant monitoring in patients taking these agents).
No products indexed under this heading.

Thioridazine Hydrochloride (The concurrent use of other central nervous system (CNS) depressants, including phenothiazines, increases the risk of respiratory depression, hypotension, profound sedation or coma. Use with caution and with vigilant monitoring in patients taking these agents). Products include:
Thioridazine Hydrochloride Tablets 2122

Thiothixene (The concurrent use of other central nervous system (CNS) depressants, including tranquilizers, increases the risk of respiratory depression, hypotension, profound sedation or coma. Use with caution and with vigilant monitoring in patients taking these agents). Products include:
Thiothixene Capsules 2124

Tranylcypromine Sulfate (MAOIs markedly potentiate the action of morphine. DepoDur should not be used in patients taking MAOIs, or within 14 days of stopping such treatment). Products include:
Parnate Tablets 1499

Triazolam (The concurrent use of other central nervous system (CNS) depressants, including sedatives and hypnotics, increases the risk of respiratory depression, hypotension, profound sedation or coma. Use with caution and with vigilant monitoring in patients taking these agents).
No products indexed under this heading.

Trifluoperazine Hydrochloride (The concurrent use of other central nervous system (CNS) depressants, including phenothiazines, increases the risk of respiratory depression, hypotension, profound sedation or coma. Use with caution and with vigilant monitoring in patients taking these agents).
No products indexed under this heading.

Vecuronium Bromide (Respiratory depression associated with morphine may delay recovery of spontaneous pulmonary ventilation when neuromuscular blocking agents are co-administered).
No products indexed under this heading.

Zaleplon (The concurrent use of other central nervous system (CNS) depressants, including sedatives and hypnotics, increases the risk of respiratory depression, hypotension, profound sedation or coma. Use with caution and with vigilant monitoring in patients taking these agents). Products include:
Sonata Capsules 1686

Ziprasidone Hydrochloride (The concurrent use of other central nervous system (CNS) depressants increases the risk of respiratory depression, hypotension, profound sedation or coma. Use with caution and with vigilant monitoring in patients taking these agents). Products include:
Geodon Capsules 2514

Zolpidem Tartrate (The concurrent use of other central nervous system (CNS) depressants, including sedatives and hypnotics, increases the risk of respiratory depression, hypotension, profound sedation or coma. Use with caution and with vigilant monitoring in patients taking these agents). Products include:
Ambien Tablets 2867

Food Interactions

Alcohol (The concurrent use of other central nervous system (CNS) depressants, including alcohol, increases the risk of respiratory depression, hypotension, profound sedation or coma. Use with caution and with vigilant monitoring in patients taking these agents).

DEPO-MEDROL INJECTABLE SUSPENSION

(Methylprednisolone Acetate) 2615
May interact with oral anticoagulants, phenytoin, killed/inactivated vaccines, vaccines, live, and certain other agents. Compounds in these categories include:

Anisindione (The effect of methylprednisolone on oral anticoagulants is variable; there are reports of enhanced as well as diminished effects of anticoagulants when given concurrently with corticosteroids). Products include:
Miradon Tablets 3056

Aspirin (Methylprednisolone may increase the clearance of chronic high dose aspirin resulting in decreased salicylate serum levels or increased risk of salicylate toxicity when methylprednisolone is withdrawn; aspirin should be used cautiously in conjunction withcorticosteroids in patients suffering from hypoprothrombinemia). Products include:
Aggrenox Capsules 855
Bayer, Aspirin Regimen 606
Bayer Aspirin Tablets 3515
BC Powder 612
BC Allergy Sinus Cold Powder 612
Arthritis Strength BC Powder 612
BC Sinus Cold Powder 612
Ecotrin Enteric Coated Aspirin Low, Regular and Maximum Strength Tablets 1627
Goody's Body Pain Formula Powder 621
Goody's Extra Strength Headache Powder 621
Goody's Extra Strength Pain Relief Tablets 621
Percodan Tablets 1115
St. Joseph 81 mg Aspirin Chewable and Enteric Coated Tablets 1841

BCG Vaccine (Administration of live or live, attenuated vaccines is contraindicated in patients receiving immunosuppressive doses of corticosteroids).
No products indexed under this heading.

Cyclosporine (Co-administration results in mutual inhibition of metabolism, therefore, it is possible that adverse events associated with the individual use of either drug may be more apt to occur; convulsions have been reported with concurrent use). Products include:
Gengraf Capsules 458
Neoral Soft Gelatin Capsules 2247
Neoral Oral Solution 2247
Restasis Ophthalmic Emulsion 570
Sandimmune 2259

Dicumarol (The effect of methylprednisolone on oral anticoagulants is variable; there are reports of enhanced as well as diminished effects of anticoagulants when given concurrently with corticosteroids).
No products indexed under this heading.

Diphtheria & Tetanus Toxoids and Acellular Pertussis Vaccine Adsorbed, Hepatitis B (recombinant) and Inactivated Poliovirus Vaccine Combined (Killed or inactivated vaccines may be administered to patients receiving immunosuppressive doses of corticosteroids; however, the response to such vaccines may be diminished).
No products indexed under this heading.

Fosphenytoin Sodium (Co-administration with drugs that induce hepatic metabolism, such as phenytoin, may increase the clearance of methylprednisolone and may require increases in methylprednisolone dose to achieve the desired response).
No products indexed under this heading.

Hepatitis A Vaccine, Inactivated (Killed or inactivated vaccines may be administered to patients receiving immunosuppressive doses of corticosteroids; however, the response to such vaccines may be diminished). Products include:
Havrix Vaccine 1425
Twinrix Vaccine 1571
Vaqta 2067

Influenza Virus Vaccine (Killed or inactivated vaccines may be administered to patients receiving immunosuppressive doses of corticosteroids; however, the response to such vaccines may be diminished). Products include:
Flumist Vaccine 1872

Japanese Encephalitis Vaccine Inactivated (Killed or inactivated vaccines may be administered to patients receiving immunosuppressive doses of corticosteroids; however, the response to such vaccines may be diminished).
No products indexed under this heading.

Ketoconazole (Co-administration with drugs that inhibit the metabolism of methylprednisolone, such as ketoconazole, may decrease the clearance of methylprednisolone and may require dose titration to avoid steroid toxicity). Products include:
Nizoral A-D Shampoo, 1% 1839
Nizoral 2% Shampoo 1838

Measles, Mumps & Rubella Virus Vaccine, Live (Administration of live or live, attenuated vaccines is contraindicated in patients receiving immunosuppressive doses of corticosteroids). Products include:
M-M-R II 1980

Measles & Rubella Virus Vaccine Live (Administration of live or live, attenuated vaccines is contraindicated in patients receiving immunosuppressive doses of corticosteroids).
No products indexed under this heading.

Measles Virus Vaccine Live (Administration of live or live, attenuated vaccines is contraindicated in patients receiving immunosuppressive doses of corticosteroids). Products include:
Attenuvax 1889

Mumps Virus Vaccine, Live (Administration of live or live, attenuated vaccines is contraindicated in patients receiving immunosuppressive doses of corticosteroids). Products include:
Mumpsvax 2005

Phenobarbital (Co-administration with drugs that induce hepatic metabolism, such as phenobarbital, may increase the clearance of methylprednisolone and may require increases in methylprednisolone dose to achieve the desired response).
No products indexed under this heading.

Phenytoin (Co-administration with drugs that induce hepatic metabolism, such as phenytoin, may increase the clearance of methylprednisolone and may require increases in methylprednisolone dose to achieve the desired response).
No products indexed under this heading.

Phenytoin Sodium (Co-administration with drugs that induce hepatic metabolism, such as phenytoin, may increase the clearance of methylprednisolone and may require increases in methylprednisolone dose to achieve the desired response). Products include:
Phenytek Capsules 2153

Poliovirus Vaccine, Live, Oral, Trivalent, Types 1,2,3 (Sabin) (Administration of live or live, attenuated vaccines is contraindicated in patients receiving immunosuppressive doses of corticosteroids).
No products indexed under this heading.

Poliovirus Vaccine Inactivated, Trivalent Types 1,2,3 (Killed or inactivated vaccines may be administered to patients receiving immunosuppressive doses of corticosteroids; however, the response to such vaccines may be diminished). Products include:
Pediarix Vaccine 1518

Rifampin (Co-administration with drugs that induce hepatic metabolism, such as rifampin, may increase the clearance of methylprednisolone and may require increases in methylprednisolone dose to achieve the desired response).
No products indexed under this heading.

Rotavirus Vaccine, Live, Oral, Tetravalent (Administration of live or live, attenuated vaccines is contraindicated in patients receiving immunosuppressive doses of corticosteroids).
No products indexed under this heading.

Rubella & Mumps Virus Vaccine Live (Administration of live or live, attenuated vaccines is contraindicated in patients receiving immunosuppressive doses of corticosteroids).
No products indexed under this heading.

Rubella Virus Vaccine Live (Administration of live or live, attenuated vaccines is contraindicated in patients receiving immunosuppressive doses of corticosteroids). Products include:
Meruvax II 1994

Smallpox Vaccine (Administration of live or live, attenuated vaccines is contraindicated in patients receiving immunosuppressive doses of corticosteroids).
No products indexed under this heading.

Troleandomycin (Co-administration with drugs that inhibit the metabolism of methylprednisolone, such as troleandomycin, may decrease the clearance of methylprednisolone and may require dose titration to avoid steroid toxicity).
No products indexed under this heading.

Typhoid Vaccine (Administration of live or live, attenuated vaccines is contraindicated in patients receiving immunosuppressive doses of corticosteroids).
No products indexed under this heading.

Varicella Virus Vaccine Live (Administration of live or live, attenuated vaccines is contraindicated in patients receiving immunosuppressive doses of corticosteroids). Products include:
Varivax 2070

Warfarin Sodium (The effect of methylprednisolone on oral anticoagulants is variable; there are reports of enhanced as well as diminished effects of anticoagulants when given concurrently with corticosteroids). Products include:
Coumadin for Injection 932
Coumadin Tablets 932

Yellow Fever Vaccine (Administration of live or live, attenuated vaccines is contraindicated in patients receiving immunosuppressive doses of corticosteroids).
No products indexed under this heading.

DEPO-MEDROL SINGLE-DOSE VIAL

(Methylprednisolone Acetate) 2617
May interact with oral anticoagulants, hepatic microsomal enzyme inducers, killed/inactivated vaccines, vaccines, live, and certain other agents. Compounds in these categories include:

Anisindione (There are reports of enhanced as well as diminished effects of anticoagulant when given concurrently with corticosteroids. Therefore, coagulation indices should be monitored to maintain the desired anticoagulant effect). Products include:
Miradon Tablets 3056

Aspirin (Methylprednisolone may increase the clearance of chronic high dose aspirin. This could lead to decreased salicylate serum levels or increase the risk of salicylate toxicity when methylprednisolone is withdrawn. Aspirin should be used cautiously in conjunction with corticosteroids in patients suffering from hypoprothrombinemia). Products include:
Aggrenox Capsules 855
Bayer, Aspirin Regimen .... ▣606
Bayer Aspirin Tablets 3515
BC Powder .... ▣612
BC Allergy Sinus Cold Powder .... ▣612
Arthritis Strength BC Powder .... ▣612
BC Sinus Cold Powder .... ▣612
Ecotrin Enteric Coated Aspirin Low, Regular and Maximum Strength Tablets 1627
Goody's Body Pain Formula Powder .... ▣621
Goody's Extra Strength Headache Powder .... ▣621
Goody's Extra Strength Pain Relief Tablets .... ▣621
Percodan Tablets 1115
St. Joseph 81 mg Aspirin Chewable and Enteric Coated Tablets 1841

BCG Vaccine (Administration of live or live, attenuated vaccines is contraindicated in patients receiving immunosuppressive doses of corticosteroids).
No products indexed under this heading.

Carbamazepine (Drugs that induce hepatic enzymes such as phenobarbital, phenytoin and rifampin may increase the clearance of methylprednisolone and may require increases in methylprednisolone dose to achieve the desired response). Products include:
Carbatrol Capsules 3174
Equetro Extended-Release Capsules 3178
Tegretol/Tegretol-XR 2278

Chlorpropamide (Drugs that induce hepatic enzymes such as phenobarbital, phenytoin and rifampin may increase the clearance of methylprednisolone and may require increases in methylprednisolone dose to achieve the desired response).
No products indexed under this heading.

Cyclosporine (Mutual inhibition of metabolism occurs with concurrent use of cyclosporine and methylprednisolone; therefore, it is possible that adverse events associated with the individual use of either drug may be more apt to occur. Convulsions have been reported with concurrent use of methylprednisolone and cyclosporine). Products include:
Gengraf Capsules 458
Neoral Soft Gelatin Capsules 2247
Neoral Oral Solution 2247
Restasis Ophthalmic Emulsion 570
Sandimmune 2259

Dicumarol (There are reports of enhanced as well as diminished effects of anticoagulant when given concurrently with corticosteroids. Therefore, coagulation indices should be monitored to maintain the desired anticoagulant effect).
No products indexed under this heading.

Diphtheria & Tetanus Toxoids and Acellular Pertussis Vaccine Adsorbed, Hepatitis B (recombinant) and Inactivated Poliovirus Vaccine Combined (Killed or inactivated vaccines may be administered to patients receiving immunosuppressive doses of corticosteroids; however, the response to such vaccines may be diminished).
No products indexed under this heading.

Ethanol (Drugs that induce hepatic enzymes such as phenobarbital, phenytoin and rifampin may increase the clearance of methylprednisolone and may require increases in methylprednisolone dose to achieve the desired response).
No products indexed under this heading.

Fosphenytoin Sodium (Drugs that induce hepatic enzymes such as phenobarbital, phenytoin and rifampin may increase the clearance of methylprednisolone and may require increases in methylprednisolone dose to achieve the desired response).
No products indexed under this heading.

Glipizide (Drugs that induce hepatic enzymes such as phenobarbital, phenytoin and rifampin may increase the clearance of methylprednisolone and may require increases in methylprednisolone dose to achieve the desired response).
No products indexed under this heading.

Glyburide (Drugs that induce hepatic enzymes such as phenobarbital, phenytoin and rifampin may increase the clearance of methylprednisolone and may require increases in methylprednisolone dose to achieve the desired response).
No products indexed under this heading.

Hepatitis A Vaccine, Inactivated (Killed or inactivated vaccines may be administered to patients receiving immunosuppressive doses of corticosteroids; however, the response to such vaccines may be diminished). Products include:
Havrix Vaccine 1425
Twinrix Vaccine 1571
Vaqta 2067

Influenza Virus Vaccine (Killed or inactivated vaccines may be administered to patients receiving immunosuppressive doses of corticosteroids; however, the response to such vaccines may be diminished). Products include:
Flumist Vaccine 1872

Japanese Encephalitis Vaccine Inactivated (Killed or inactivated vaccines may be administered to patients receiving immunosuppressive doses of corticosteroids; however, the response to such vaccines may be diminished).
No products indexed under this heading.

Ketoconazole (Drugs such as ketoconazole may inhibit the metabolism of methylprednisolone and decrease its clearance; therefore, the dose of methylprednisolone should be titrated to avoid steroid toxicity). Products include:
Nizoral A-D Shampoo, 1% 1839
Nizoral 2% Shampoo 1838

Measles, Mumps & Rubella Virus Vaccine, Live (Administration of live or live, attenuated vaccines is contraindicated in patients receiving immunosuppressive doses of corticosteroids). Products include:
M-M-R II 1980

Measles & Rubella Virus Vaccine Live (Administration of live or live, attenuated vaccines is contraindicated in patients receiving immunosuppressive doses of corticosteroids).
No products indexed under this heading.

Measles Virus Vaccine Live (Administration of live or live, attenuated vaccines is contraindicated in patients receiving immunosuppressive doses of corticosteroids). Products include:
Attenuvax 1889

Mumps Virus Vaccine, Live (Administration of live or live, attenuated vaccines is contraindicated in patients receiving immunosuppressive doses of corticosteroids). Products include:
Mumpsvax 2005

Phenobarbital (Drugs that induce hepatic enzymes such as phenobarbital, phenytoin and rifampin may increase the clearance of methylprednisolone and may require increases in methylprednisolone dose to achieve the desired response).
No products indexed under this heading.

Phenylbutazone (Drugs that induce hepatic enzymes such as phenobarbital, phenytoin and rifampin may increase the clearance of methylprednisolone and may require increases in methylprednisolone dose to achieve the desired response).
No products indexed under this heading.

Phenytoin (Drugs that induce hepatic enzymes such as phenobarbital, phenytoin and rifampin may increase the clearance of methylprednisolone and may require increases in methylprednisolone dose to achieve the desired response).
No products indexed under this heading.

Phenytoin Sodium (Drugs that induce hepatic enzymes such as phenobarbital, phenytoin and rifampin may increase the clearance of methylprednisolone and may require increases in methylprednisolone dose to achieve the desired response). Products include:
Phenytek Capsules 2153

Poliovirus Vaccine, Live, Oral, Trivalent, Types 1,2,3 (Sabin) (Administration of live or live, attenuated vaccines is contraindicated in patients receiving immunosuppressive doses of corticosteroids).
No products indexed under this heading.

Poliovirus Vaccine Inactivated, Trivalent Types 1,2,3 (Killed or inactivated vaccines may be administered to patients receiving immunosuppressive doses of corticosteroids; however, the response to such vaccines may be diminished). Products include:
Pediarix Vaccine 1518

Rifampin (Drugs that induce hepatic enzymes such as phenobarbital, phenytoin and rifampin may increase the clearance of methylprednisolone and may require increases in methylprednisolone dose to achieve the desired response).
No products indexed under this heading.

Rifapentine (Drugs that induce hepatic enzymes such as phenobarbital, phenytoin and rifampin may increase the clearance of methylprednisolone and may require increases in methylprednisolone dose to achieve the desired response).
No products indexed under this heading.

Rotavirus Vaccine, Live, Oral, Tetravalent (Administration of live or live, attenuated vaccines is contraindicated in patients receiving immunosuppressive doses of corticosteroids).
No products indexed under this heading.

Rubella & Mumps Virus Vaccine Live (Administration of live or live, attenuated vaccines is contraindicated in patients receiving immunosuppressive doses of corticosteroids).
No products indexed under this heading.

Rubella Virus Vaccine Live (Administration of live or live, attenuated vaccines is contraindicated in patients receiving immunosuppressive doses of corticosteroids). Products include:
Meruvax II 1994

Smallpox Vaccine (Administration of live or live, attenuated vaccines is contraindicated in patients receiving immunosuppressive doses of corticosteroids).
No products indexed under this heading.

Tolazamide (Drugs that induce hepatic enzymes such as phenobarbital, phenytoin and rifampin may increase the clearance of methylprednisolone and may require increases in methylprednisolone dose to achieve the desired response).
No products indexed under this heading.

Tolbutamide (Drugs that induce hepatic enzymes such as phenobarbital, phenytoin and rifampin may increase the clearance of methylprednisolone and may require increases in methylprednisolone dose to achieve the desired response).
No products indexed under this heading.

Troleandomycin (Drugs such as troleandomycin may inhibit the metabolism of methylprednisolone and decrease its clearance; therefore, the dose of methylprednisolone should be titrated to avoid steroid toxicity).
No products indexed under this heading.

Typhoid Vaccine (Administration of live or live, attenuated vaccines is contraindicated in patients receiving immunosuppressive doses of corticosteroids).
No products indexed under this heading.

Varicella Virus Vaccine Live (Administration of live or live, attenuated vaccines is contraindicated in patients receiving immunosuppressive doses of corticosteroids). Products include:
Varivax 2070

Warfarin Sodium (There are reports of enhanced as well as diminished effects of anticoagulant when given concurrently with corticosteroids. Therefore, coagulation indices should be monitored to maintain the desired anticoagulant effect). Products include:
Coumadin for Injection 932
Coumadin Tablets 932

Yellow Fever Vaccine (Administration of live or live, attenuated vaccines is contraindicated in patients receiving immunosuppressive doses of corticosteroids).
No products indexed under this heading.

DEPO-PROVERA CONTRACEPTIVE INJECTION

(Medroxyprogesterone Acetate) 2619
May interact with:

Aminoglutethimide (Aminoglutethimide may significantly depress the serum concentrations of medroxyprogesterone acetate).
No products indexed under this heading.

DEPO-SUBQ PROVERA 104 INJECTABLE SUSPENSION

(Medroxyprogesterone Acetate) 2622
May interact with:

Aminoglutethimide (Aminoglutethimide may significantly decrease the serum concentrations of medroxyprogesterone acetate).
No products indexed under this heading.

DESENEX LIQUID SPRAY

(Miconazole Nitrate) 674
None cited in PDR database.

DESENEX SHAKE POWDER

(Miconazole Nitrate) 674
None cited in PDR database.

DESENEX SPRAY POWDER

(Miconazole Nitrate) 674
None cited in PDR database.

DESENEX JOCK ITCH SPRAY POWDER

(Miconazole Nitrate) 674
None cited in PDR database.

DESFERAL VIALS

(Deferoxamine Mesylate) 2190
May interact with:

Aluminum Hydroxide (Treatment with Desferal in the presence of aluminum overload may result in decreased serum calcium and aggravation of hyperparathyroidism). Products include:
Gaviscon Regular Strength Liquid 620
Gaviscon Regular Strength Tablets 619
Gaviscon Extra Strength Liquid 620
Gaviscon Extra Strength Tablets 619
Maalox Max Maximum Strength Antacid/Anti-Gas Liquid 2165
Maalox Regular Strength Antacid/Antigas Liquid 2164

Gallium-67 (Imaging results may be distorted because of the rapid urinary excretion of Desferal-bound gallium-67).
No products indexed under this heading.

Prochlorperazine (Co-administration may lead to temporary impairment of consciousness).
No products indexed under this heading.

Vitamin C (Co-administration with high doses of vitamin C (more than 500 mg daily in adults) in patients with severe chronic iron overload has resulted in impairment of cardiac function; vitamin C supplements should not be given to patients with cardiac failure; as an adjuvant to iron chelation therapy, vitamin C in doses up to 200 mg/day for adults may be given in divided doses). Products include:
Chromagen Forte Soft Gelatin Capsules 3296
Halls Defense Sugarfree Vitamin C Drops 611
Niferex-150 Forte Capsules 3299
Peridin-C Tablets 761
Repliva 21/7 Tablets 3301

DESITIN CREAMY OINTMENT

(Zinc Oxide) 700
None cited in PDR database.

DESITIN OINTMENT

(Zinc Oxide) 700
None cited in PDR database.

DESMOPRESSIN ACETATE INJECTION

(Desmopressin Acetate) 1143
See Desmopressin Acetate Rhinal Tube

DESMOPRESSIN ACETATE RHINAL TUBE

(Desmopressin Acetate) 1144
May interact with vasopressors. Compounds in these categories include:

Dobutamine (The pressor activity of desmopressin is very low, use of large doses of desmopressin with pressor agents should only be done with careful monitoring).
No products indexed under this heading.

Dobutamine Hydrochloride (The pressor activity of desmopressin is very low, use of large doses of desmopressin with pressor agents should only be done with careful monitoring).
No products indexed under this heading.

Dopamine Hydrochloride (The pressor activity of desmopressin is very low, use of large doses of desmopressin with pressor agents should only be done with careful monitoring).
No products indexed under this heading.

Ephedrine Sulfate (The pressor activity of desmopressin is very low, use of large doses of desmopressin with pressor agents should only be done with careful monitoring).
No products indexed under this heading.

Epinephrine Bitartrate (The pressor activity of desmopressin is very low, use of large doses of desmopressin with pressor agents should only be done with careful monitoring).
No products indexed under this heading.

Epinephrine Hydrochloride (The pressor activity of desmopressin is very low, use of large doses of desmopressin with pressor agents should only be done with careful monitoring).
No products indexed under this heading.

Isoproterenol Hydrochloride (The pressor activity of desmopressin is very low, use of large doses of desmopressin with pressor agents should only be done with careful monitoring).
No products indexed under this heading.

Isoproterenol Sulfate (The pressor activity of desmopressin is very low, use of large doses of desmopressin with pressor agents should only be done with careful monitoring).
No products indexed under this heading.

Mephentermine Sulfate (The pressor activity of desmopressin is very low, use of large doses of desmopressin with pressor agents should only be done with careful monitoring).
No products indexed under this heading.

Metaraminol Bitartrate (The pressor activity of desmopressin is very low, use of large doses of desmopressin with pressor agents should only be done with careful monitoring). Products include:
Aramine Injection 1889

Methoxamine Hydrochloride (The pressor activity of desmopressin is very low, use of large doses of desmopressin with pressor agents should only be done with careful monitoring).
No products indexed under this heading.

Norepinephrine Bitartrate (The pressor activity of desmopressin is very low, use of large doses of desmopressin with pressor agents should only be done with careful monitoring).
No products indexed under this heading.

Phenylephrine Hydrochloride (The pressor activity of desmopressin is very low, use of large doses of desmopressin with pressor agents should only be done with careful monitoring). Products include:
Alacol DM Syrup 739
Hycomine Compound Tablets 1105
Preparation H Maximum Strength Cream 747
Preparation H Cooling Gel 747
Preparation H 747
Sudafed PE Tablets 711
Vicks Sinex Nasal Spray and Ultra Fine Mist for Sinus Relief 2677
Zicam Concentrated Cough Mist for Kids Plus D Cool Cherry 643
Zicam Concentrated Cough Mist Plus D Cool Cherry 642

DESOXYN TABLETS, USP
(Methamphetamine Hydrochloride) 2482
May interact with insulin, monoamine oxidase inhibitors, phenothiazines, tricyclic antidepressants, and certain other agents. Compounds in these categories include:

Amitriptyline Hydrochloride (Co-administration of tricyclic antidepressants and indirect-acting sympathomimetic amines such as amphetamines should be closely supervised and dosage carefully adjusted).
No products indexed under this heading.

Amoxapine (Co-administration of tricyclic antidepressants and indirect-acting sympathomimetic amines such as amphetamines should be closely supervised and dosage carefully adjusted).
No products indexed under this heading.

Chlorpromazine (May antagonize the CNS stimulant action of the amphetamine).
No products indexed under this heading.

Chlorpromazine Hydrochloride (May antagonize the CNS stimulant action of the amphetamine).
No products indexed under this heading.

Clomipramine Hydrochloride (Co-administration of tricyclic antidepressants and indirect-acting sympathomimetic amines such as amphetamines should be closely supervised and dosage carefully adjusted).
No products indexed under this heading.

Desipramine Hydrochloride (Co-administration of tricyclic antidepressants and indirect-acting sympathomimetic amines such as amphetamines should be closely supervised and dosage carefully adjusted).
No products indexed under this heading.

Doxepin Hydrochloride (Co-administration of tricyclic antidepressants and indirect-acting sympathomimetic amines such as amphetamines should be closely supervised and dosage carefully adjusted).
No products indexed under this heading.

Fluphenazine Decanoate (May antagonize the CNS stimulant action of the amphetamine).
No products indexed under this heading.

Fluphenazine Enanthate (May antagonize the CNS stimulant action of the amphetamine).
No products indexed under this heading.

Fluphenazine Hydrochloride (May antagonize the CNS stimulant action of the amphetamine).
No products indexed under this heading.

Guanethidine Monosulfate (Decreased hypotensive effect).
No products indexed under this heading.

Imipramine Hydrochloride (Co-administration of tricyclic antidepressants and indirect-acting sympathomimetic amines such as amphetamines should be closely supervised and dosage carefully adjusted).
No products indexed under this heading.

Imipramine Pamoate (Co-administration of tricyclic antidepressants and indirect-acting sympathomimetic amines such as amphetamines should be closely supervised and dosage carefully adjusted).
No products indexed under this heading.

Insulin, Human, Zinc Suspension (Insulin requirement in diabetics may be altered). Products include:
Humulin L, 100 Units 1763
Humulin U, 100 Units 1770

Insulin, Human NPH (Insulin requirement in diabetics may be altered). Products include:
Humulin N, 100 Units 1764
Humulin N Pen 1765
Novolin N Human Insulin 10 ml Vials 2322
Novolin N InnoLet 2322
Novolin N PenFill 3 ml Cartridges 2325
Novolin R InnoLet 2322

Insulin, Human Regular (Insulin requirement in diabetics may be altered). Products include:
Humulin R (U-500) 1768
Humulin R, 100 Units 1767
Novolin R Human Insulin 10 ml Vials 2322
Novolin R PenFill 2325

Insulin, Human Regular and Human NPH Mixture (Insulin requirement in diabetics may be altered). Products include:
Humulin 50/50, 100 Units 1760
Humulin 70/30 Pen 1761
Novolin 70/30 Human Insulin 10 ml Vials 2321
Novolin 70/30 InnoLet 2322
Novolin 70/30 PenFill 3 ml Cartridges 2325

Insulin, NPH (Insulin requirement in diabetics may be altered).
No products indexed under this heading.

Insulin, Regular (Insulin requirement in diabetics may be altered).
No products indexed under this heading.

Insulin, Zinc Crystals (Insulin requirement in diabetics may be altered).
No products indexed under this heading.

Insulin, Zinc Suspension (Insulin requirement in diabetics may be altered).
No products indexed under this heading.

Insulin Aspart, Human Regular (Insulin requirement in diabetics may be altered). Products include:
NovoLog Injection 2326

Insulin glargine (Insulin requirement in diabetics may be altered). Products include:
Lantus Injection 2925

Insulin Lispro, Human (Insulin requirement in diabetics may be altered). Products include:
Humalog-Pen 1751
Humalog Mix 75/25-Pen 1754

Insulin Lispro Protamine, Human (Insulin requirement in diabetics may be altered). Products include:
Humalog Mix 75/25-Pen 1754

Isocarboxazid (Co-administration may result in hypertensive crises; concurrent and/or sequential use is contraindicated).
No products indexed under this heading.

Maprotiline Hydrochloride (Co-administration of tricyclic antidepressants and indirect-acting sympathomimetic amines such as amphetamines should be closely supervised and dosage carefully adjusted).
No products indexed under this heading.

Mesoridazine Besylate (May antagonize the CNS stimulant action of the amphetamine).
No products indexed under this heading.

Methotrimeprazine (May antagonize the CNS stimulant action of the amphetamine).
No products indexed under this heading.

Moclobemide (Co-administration may result in hypertensive crises; concurrent and/or sequential use is contraindicated).
No products indexed under this heading.

Nortriptyline Hydrochloride (Co-administration of tricyclic antidepressants and indirect-acting sympathomimetic amines such as amphetamines should be closely supervised and dosage carefully adjusted).
No products indexed under this heading.

Pargyline Hydrochloride (Co-administration may result in hypertensive crises; concurrent and/or sequential use is contraindicated).
No products indexed under this heading.

Perphenazine (May antagonize the CNS stimulant action of the amphetamine).
No products indexed under this heading.

Phenelzine Sulfate (Co-administration may result in hypertensive crises; concurrent and/or sequential use is contraindicated).
No products indexed under this heading.

Procarbazine Hydrochloride (Co-administration may result in hypertensive crises; concurrent and/or sequential use is contraindicated). Products include:
Matulane Capsules 3188

Prochlorperazine (May antagonize the CNS stimulant action of the amphetamine).
No products indexed under this heading.

Promethazine Hydrochloride (May antagonize the CNS stimulant action of the amphetamine). Products include:
Phenergan 3438

Protriptyline Hydrochloride (Co-administration of tricyclic antidepressants and indirect-acting sympathomimetic amines such as amphetamines should be closely supervised and dosage carefully adjusted). Products include:
Vivactil Tablets 2350

Selegiline Hydrochloride (Co-administration may result in hypertensive crises; concurrent and/or sequential use is contraindicated). Products include:
Eldepryl Capsules 3209

Thioridazine Hydrochloride (May antagonize the CNS stimulant action of the amphetamine). Products include:
Thioridazine Hydrochloride Tablets 2122

Tranylcypromine Sulfate (Co-administration may result in hypertensive crises; concurrent and/or sequential use is contraindicated). Products include:
Parnate Tablets 1499

Trifluoperazine Hydrochloride (May antagonize the CNS stimulant action of the amphetamine).
No products indexed under this heading.

Trimipramine Maleate (Co-administration of tricyclic antidepressants and indirect-acting sympathomimetic amines such as amphetamines should be closely supervised and dosage carefully adjusted). Products include:
Surmontil Capsules 2347

DETROL TABLETS
(Tolterodine Tartrate) 2626
See Detrol LA Capsules

DETROL LA CAPSULES
(Tolterodine Tartrate) 2629
May interact with erythromycin and certain other agents. Compounds in these categories include:

Clarithromycin (Co-administration with other potent inhibitors of CYP3A4, such as clarithromycin, may lead to increase of tolterodine plasma concentrations; for patients receiving concomitant erythromycin, the recommended dose of Detrol LA is 2 mg). Products include:
Biaxin/Biaxin XL 402
PREVPAC 3281

Cyclosporine (Co-administration with other potent inhibitors of CYP3A4, such as cyclosporine, may lead to increase of tolterodine plasma concentrations; for patients receiving concomitant cyclosporine, the recommended dose of Detrol LA is 2 mg). Products include:
Gengraf Capsules 458
Neoral Soft Gelatin Capsules 2247
Neoral Oral Solution 2247
Restasis Ophthalmic Emulsion 570
Sandimmune 2259

Erythromycin (Co-administration with other potent inhibitors of CYP3A4, such as erythromycin, may lead to increase of tolterodine plasma concentrations; for patients receiving concomitant erythromycin, the recommended dose of Detrol LA is 2 mg). Products include:
Erygel Topical Gel 2096
Ery-Tab Tablets 447
Erythromycin Base Filmtab Tablets 454
Erythromycin Delayed-Release Capsules, USP 456
PCE Dispertab Tablets 510

Erythromycin Estolate (Co-administration with other potent inhibitors of CYP3A4, such as erythromycin, may lead to increase of tolterodine plasma concentrations; for patients receiving concomitant erythromycin, the recommended dose of Detrol LA is 2 mg).
No products indexed under this heading.

Erythromycin Ethylsuccinate (Co-administration with other potent inhibitors of CYP3A4, such as erythromycin, may lead to increase of

tolterodine plasma concentrations; for patients receiving concomitant erythromycin, the recommended dose of Detrol LA is 2 mg). Products include:

E.E.S. 449
EryPed 445

Erythromycin Gluceptate (Co-administration with other potent inhibitors of CYP3A4, such as erythromycin, may lead to increase of tolterodine plasma concentrations; for patients receiving concomitant erythromycin, the recommended dose of Detrol LA is 2 mg).

No products indexed under this heading.

Erythromycin Lactobionate (Co-administration with other potent inhibitors of CYP3A4, such as erythromycin, may lead to increase of tolterodine plasma concentrations; for patients receiving concomitant erythromycin, the recommended dose of Detrol LA is 2 mg).

No products indexed under this heading.

Erythromycin Stearate (Co-administration with other potent inhibitors of CYP3A4, such as erythromycin, may lead to increase of tolterodine plasma concentrations; for patients receiving concomitant erythromycin, the recommended dose of Detrol LA is 2 mg). Products include:

Erythrocin Stearate Filmtab Tablets 452

Fluoxetine Hydrochloride (Co-administration with a potent inhibitor of CYP2D6, such as fluoxetine, significantly inhibits the metabolism of tolterodine immediate release formulation in extensive metabolizers, resulting in a 4.8-fold increase in tolterodine AUC; the sums of unbound serum concentrations of tolterodine and the 5-hydroxymethyl metabolite are only 25% higher during the interaction; no dose adjustment is required). Products include:

Prozac Pulvules and Liquid 1771
Symbyax Capsules 1788

Itraconazole (Co-administration with other potent inhibitors of CYP3A4, such as itraconazole, may lead to increase of tolterodine plasma concentrations; for patients receiving concomitant itraconazole, the recommended dose of Detrol LA is 2 mg).

No products indexed under this heading.

Ketoconazole (Co-administration of ketoconazole, an inhibitor of CYP3A4, significantly increased plasma concentrations of tolterodine to subjects who were poor metabolizers; for patients receiving concomitant ketoconazole, the recommended dose of Detrol LA is 2 mg). Products include:

Nizoral A-D Shampoo, 1% 1839
Nizoral 2% Shampoo 1838

Miconazole (Co-administration with other potent inhibitors of CYP3A4, such as miconazole, may lead to increase of tolterodine plasma concentrations; for patients receiving concomitant miconazole, the recommended dose of Detrol LA is 2 mg).

No products indexed under this heading.

Vinblastine Sulfate (Co-administration with other potent inhibitors of CYP3A4, such as vinblastine, may lead to increase of tolterodine plasma concentrations; for patients receiving concomitant vinblastine, the recommended dose of Detrol LA is 2 mg).

No products indexed under this heading.

DEXEDRINE SPANSULE CAPSULES

(Dextroamphetamine Sulfate) 1386

May interact with antihistamines, antihypertensives, beta blockers, monoamine oxidase inhibitors, phenytoin, thiazides, tricyclic antidepressants, urinary alkalinizing agents, veratrum alkaloids, and certain other agents. Compounds in these categories include:

Acebutolol Hydrochloride (Amphetamine may antagonize the hypotensive effects of antihypertensives; adrenergic blockers are inhibited by amphetamines).

No products indexed under this heading.

Acetazolamide (Increases the concentration of the non-ionized species of the amphetamine molecule, thereby decreasing urinary excretion; increases amphetamines blood levels and thereby potentiates the actions of amphetamines).

No products indexed under this heading.

Acetazolamide Sodium (Increases the concentration of the non-ionized species of the amphetamine molecule, thereby decreasing urinary excretion; increases amphetamines blood levels and thereby potentiates the actions of amphetamines).

No products indexed under this heading.

Acrivastine (Amphetamines may counteract the sedative effect of antihistamine).

No products indexed under this heading.

Amitriptyline Hydrochloride (Enhanced activity of tricyclic or sympathomimetics; possible increases in the brain concentration of d-amphetamine in the brain; cardiovascular effect may be potentiated).

No products indexed under this heading.

Amlodipine Besylate (Amphetamine may antagonize the hypotensive effects of antihypertensives). Products include:

Caduet Tablets 2507
Lotrel Capsules 2238
Norvasc Tablets 2529

Ammonium Chloride (Increases the concentration of the ionized species of the amphetamine molecule, thereby increasing urinary excretion; lowers amphetamines blood levels and efficacy).

No products indexed under this heading.

Amoxapine (Enhanced activity of tricyclic or sympathomimetics; possible increases in the brain concentration of d-amphetamine in the brain; cardiovascular effect may be potentiated).

No products indexed under this heading.

Astemizole (Amphetamines may counteract the sedative effect of antihistamine).

No products indexed under this heading.

Atenolol (Amphetamine may antagonize the hypotensive effects of antihypertensives; adrenergic blockers are inhibited by amphetamines). Products include:

Tenormin I.V. Injection 698
Tenormin Tablets 695

Azatadine Maleate (Amphetamines may counteract the sedative effect of antihistamine).

No products indexed under this heading.

Benazepril Hydrochloride (Amphetamine may antagonize the hypotensive effects of antihypertensives). Products include:

Lotensin Tablets 2232
Lotensin HCT Tablets 2235
Lotrel Capsules 2238

Bendroflumethiazide (Increases the concentration of the non-ionized species of the amphetamine molecule, thereby decreasing urinary excretion; increases amphetamines blood levels and thereby potentiates the actions of amphetamines).

No products indexed under this heading.

Betaxolol Hydrochloride (Amphetamine may antagonize the hypotensive effects of antihypertensives; adrenergic blockers are inhibited by amphetamines). Products include:

Betoptic S Ophthalmic Suspension 554

Bisoprolol Fumarate (Amphetamine may antagonize the hypotensive effects of antihypertensives; adrenergic blockers are inhibited by amphetamines).

No products indexed under this heading.

Bromodiphenhydramine Hydrochloride (Amphetamines may counteract the sedative effect of antihistamine).

No products indexed under this heading.

Brompheniramine Maleate (Amphetamines may counteract the sedative effect of antihistamine). Products include:

Alacol DM Syrup 739
Children's Dimetapp Cold & Allergy Elixir 745
Children's Dimetapp DM Cold & Cough Elixir 745
Robitussin Allergy & Cough Syrup 750

Candesartan Cilexetil (Amphetamine may antagonize the hypotensive effects of antihypertensives). Products include:

Atacand Tablets 634
Atacand HCT 637

Captopril (Amphetamine may antagonize the hypotensive effects of antihypertensives). Products include:

Captopril Tablets 2114

Carteolol Hydrochloride (Amphetamine may antagonize the hypotensive effects of antihypertensives; adrenergic blockers are inhibited by amphetamines). Products include:

Carteolol Hydrochloride Ophthalmic Solution USP, 1% .... ⊙ 246

Cetirizine Hydrochloride (Amphetamines may counteract the sedative effect of antihistamine). Products include:

Zyrtec Chewable Tablets 2589
Zyrtec 2589
Zyrtec-D 12 Hour Extended Release Tablets 2591

Chlorothiazide (Increases the concentration of the non-ionized species of the amphetamine molecule, thereby decreasing urinary excretion; increases amphetamines blood levels and thereby potentiates the actions of amphetamines). Products include:

Aldoclor Tablets 1881
Diuril Oral 1936

Chlorothiazide Sodium (Increases the concentration of the non-ionized species of the amphetamine molecule, thereby decreasing urinary excretion; increases amphetamines blood levels and thereby potentiates the actions of amphetamines). Products include:

Diuril Sodium Intravenous 1934

Chlorpheniramine Maleate (Amphetamines may counteract the sedative effect of antihistamine). Products include:

Advil Allergy Sinus Caplets 737
Advil Multi-Symptom Cold Caplets 738
BC Allergy Sinus Cold Powder 612
Contac Severe Cold and Flu Caplets Maximum Strength 615
Hycomine Compound Tablets 1105
PediaCare Multi-Symptom Cold Liquid 704
PediaCare NightRest Cough & Cold Liquid 704
Robitussin Flu Liquid 752
Robitussin PM Cough & Cold Liquid 752
Singlet Caplets 636
Sudafed Sinus & Allergy Tablets 710
TheraFlu Cold & Cough Hot Liquid 680
TheraFlu Cold & Sore Throat Hot Liquid 680
TheraFlu Flu & Sore Throat Hot Liquid 681
TheraFlu Severe Cold & Cough Hot Liquid 683
TheraFlu Severe Cold Caplets 679
TheraFlu Severe Cold Hot Liquid 682
Triaminic Cold & Allergy Liquid 685
Triaminic Cold & Cough Liquid 685
Triaminic Flu, Cough & Fever Liquid 685
Triaminic Night Time Cough & Cold Liquid 685
Triaminic Allergy Runny Nose & Congestion Softchews 688
Triaminic Cold & Cough Softchews 688
Children's Tylenol Plus Cold NightTime Suspension Liquid 1851
Children's Tylenol Plus Cold & Cough Suspension Liquid and Chewable Tablets 1851
Children's Tylenol Plus Cold Chewable Tablets 1851
Children's Tylenol Plus Flu Suspension Liquid 1853
Tylenol Allergy Complete Multi-Symptom Caplets and Gelcaps with Cool Burst 1844
Multi-Symptom Tylenol Cold Night Time Caplets 1845
Vicks 44M Cough, Cold & Flu Relief 2676
Pediatric Vicks 44m Cough & Cold Relief 2673
Children's Vicks NyQuil Cold/Cough Relief 2671

Chlorpheniramine Polistirex (Amphetamines may counteract the sedative effect of antihistamine). Products include:

Tussionex Pennkinetic Extended-Release Suspension 3322

Chlorpheniramine Tannate (Amphetamines may counteract the sedative effect of antihistamine).

No products indexed under this heading.

IMPORTANT NOTE: Always consult each drug listing in the patient's regimen for possible interactions.

Chlorpromazine (Blocks dopamine and norepinephrine reuptake resulting in inhibition of central stimulating effects).
No products indexed under this heading.

Chlorpromazine Hydrochloride (Blocks dopamine and norepinephrine reuptake resulting in inhibition of central stimulating effects).
No products indexed under this heading.

Chlorthalidone (Amphetamine may antagonize the hypotensive effects of antihypertensives). Products include:
- Clorpres Tablets 2139

Clemastine Fumarate (Amphetamines may counteract the sedative effect of antihistamine).
No products indexed under this heading.

Clomipramine Hydrochloride (Enhanced activity of tricyclic or sympathomimetics; possible increases in the brain concentration of d-amphetamine in the brain; cardiovascular effect may be potentiated).
No products indexed under this heading.

Clonidine (Amphetamine may antagonize the hypotensive effects of antihypertensives). Products include:
- Catapres-TTS 875

Clonidine Hydrochloride (Amphetamine may antagonize the hypotensive effects of antihypertensives). Products include:
- Catapres Tablets 874
- Clorpres Tablets 2139

Cryptenamine Preparations (Amphetamines inhibit the hypotensive effect of veratrum alkaloids).
No products indexed under this heading.

Cyproheptadine Hydrochloride (Amphetamines may counteract the sedative effect of antihistamine).
No products indexed under this heading.

Deserpidine (Amphetamine may antagonize the hypotensive effects of antihypertensives).
No products indexed under this heading.

Desipramine Hydrochloride (Enhanced activity of tricyclic or sympathomimetics; possible increases in the brain concentration of d-amphetamine in the brain; cardiovascular effect may be potentiated).
No products indexed under this heading.

Dexchlorpheniramine Maleate (Amphetamines may counteract the sedative effect of antihistamine).
No products indexed under this heading.

Diazoxide (Amphetamine may antagonize the hypotensive effects of antihypertensives). Products include:
- Hyperstat I.V. Injection 3031

Diltiazem Hydrochloride (Amphetamine may antagonize the hypotensive effects of antihypertensives). Products include:
- Cardizem LA Extended Release Tablets 1699
- Tiazac Capsules 1204

Diphenhydramine Citrate (Amphetamines may counteract the sedative effect of antihistamine). Products include:
- Children's Benadryl Allergy & Cold Fastmelt Tablets .... ▣695
- Children's Benadryl D Allergy & Sinus Fastmelt Tablets .... ▣694
- Children's Benadryl Allergy Fastmelt Tablets .... ▣696
- Goody's PM Powder .... ▣622

Diphenhydramine Hydrochloride (Amphetamines may counteract the sedative effect of antihistamine). Products include:
- Benadryl Allergy & Cold Tablets .... ▣692
- Benadryl Allergy .... ▣691
- Benadryl Allergy & Sinus Headache Caplets & Gelcaps .... ▣693
- Children's Benadryl Allergy Liquid .... ▣695
- Children's Benadryl Dye-Free Allergy Liquid .... ▣695
- Benadryl Dye-Free Allergy Liqui-Gels Softgels .... ▣692
- Benadryl Itch Relief Stick Extra Strength .... ▣696
- Benadryl Itch Stopping Cream Extra Strength .... ▣697
- Benadryl Itch Stopping Gel Extra Strength .... ▣697
- Benadryl Itch Stopping Spray Extra Strength .... ▣697
- Benadryl Maximum Strength Severe Allergy & Sinus Headache Caplets .... ▣694
- Children's Benadryl D Liquid Medication .... ▣693
- Benadryl D Tablets .... ▣694
- Nytol QuickCaps Caplets .... ▣635
- Maximum Strength Nytol QuickGels Softgels .... ▣635
- Simply Sleep Caplets 1841
- Sominex Original Formula Tablets .... ▣637
- TheraFlu Thin Strips Multi Symptom .... ▣684
- Triaminic Thin Strips Cough & Runny Nose .... ▣690
- Children's Tylenol Plus Cold & Allergy Suspension Liquid 1850
- Tylenol Allergy Complete Night Time Caplets 1844
- Tylenol Severe Allergy Caplets 1844
- Tylenol Flu NightTime Gelcaps 1846
- Extra Strength Tylenol PM Caplets, Geltabs, Gelcaps and Liquid 1847
- Unisom Maximum Strength SleepGels .... ▣712

Diphenylpyraline Hydrochloride (Amphetamines may counteract the sedative effect of antihistamine).
No products indexed under this heading.

Doxazosin Mesylate (Amphetamine may antagonize the hypotensive effects of antihypertensives).
No products indexed under this heading.

Doxepin Hydrochloride (Enhanced activity of tricyclic or sympathomimetics; possible increases in the brain concentration of d-amphetamine in the brain; cardiovascular effect may be potentiated).
No products indexed under this heading.

Enalapril Maleate (Amphetamine may antagonize the hypotensive effects of antihypertensives). Products include:
- Vaseretic Tablets 2073
- Vasotec I.V. Injection 2076

Enalaprilat (Amphetamine may antagonize the hypotensive effects of antihypertensives).
No products indexed under this heading.

Eprosartan Mesylate (Amphetamine may antagonize the hypotensive effects of antihypertensives). Products include:
- Teveten Tablets 1707
- Teveten HCT Tablets 1710

Esmolol Hydrochloride (Amphetamine may antagonize the hypotensive effects of antihypertensives; adrenergic blockers are inhibited by amphetamines). Products include:
- Brevibloc Concentrate 766
- Brevibloc Injection 766
- Brevibloc Double Strength Injection 766
- Brevibloc Premixed Injection 766
- Brevibloc Double Strength Premixed Injection 766

Ethosuximide (Amphetamine may delay intestinal absorption of ethosuximide).
No products indexed under this heading.

Felodipine (Amphetamine may antagonize the hypotensive effects of antihypertensives). Products include:
- Plendil Extended-Release Tablets 651

Fexofenadine Hydrochloride (Amphetamines may counteract the sedative effect of antihistamine). Products include:
- Allegra 2857
- Allegra-D 12 Hour Extended-Release Tablets 2860
- Allegra-D 24 Hour Extended-Release Tablets 2862

Fosinopril Sodium (Amphetamine may antagonize the hypotensive effects of antihypertensives).
No products indexed under this heading.

Fosphenytoin Sodium (Amphetamine delays intestinal absorption of phenytoin; co-administration may produce synergestic anticonvulsant action).
No products indexed under this heading.

Furosemide (Amphetamine may antagonize the hypotensive effects of antihypertensives). Products include:
- Furosemide Tablets 2117

Glutamic Acid Hydrochloride (Lowers absorption of amphetamines).
No products indexed under this heading.

Guanabenz Acetate (Amphetamine may antagonize the hypotensive effects of antihypertensives).
No products indexed under this heading.

Guanethidine Monosulfate (Lowers absorption of amphetamines).
No products indexed under this heading.

Haloperidol (Blocks dopamine and norepinephrine reuptake resulting in inhibition of central stimulating effects).
No products indexed under this heading.

Haloperidol Decanoate (Blocks dopamine and norepinephrine reuptake resulting in inhibition of central stimulating effects).
No products indexed under this heading.

Hydralazine Hydrochloride (Amphetamine may antagonize the hypotensive effects of antihypertensives). Products include:
- BiDil Tablets 2161

Hydrochlorothiazide (Increases the concentration of the non-ionized species of the amphetamine molecule, thereby decreasing urinary excretion; increases amphetamines blood levels and thereby potentiates the actions of amphetamines). Products include:
- Aldoril Tablets 1884
- Atacand HCT 637
- Avalide Tablets 2889
- Avalide Tablets 922
- Benicar HCT Tablets 2852
- Diovan HCT Tablets 2195
- Dyazide Capsules 1389
- Hyzaar 1964
- Lotensin HCT Tablets 2235
- Maxzide 2150
- Micardis HCT Tablets 886
- Moduretic Tablets 2003
- Prinzide Tablets 2033
- Teveten HCT Tablets 1710
- Timolide Tablets 2056
- Uniretic Tablets 3114
- Vaseretic Tablets 2073
- Zestoretic Tablets 701

Hydroflumethiazide (Increases the concentration of the non-ionized species of the amphetamine molecule, thereby decreasing urinary excretion; increases amphetamines blood levels and thereby potentiates the actions of amphetamines).
No products indexed under this heading.

Imipramine Hydrochloride (Enhanced activity of tricyclic or sympathomimetics; possible increases in the brain concentration of d-amphetamine in the brain; cardiovascular effect may be potentiated).
No products indexed under this heading.

Imipramine Pamoate (Enhanced activity of tricyclic or sympathomimetics; possible increases in the brain concentration of d-amphetamine in the brain; cardiovascular effect may be potentiated).
No products indexed under this heading.

Indapamide (Amphetamine may antagonize the hypotensive effects of antihypertensives). Products include:
- Indapamide Tablets 2119

Irbesartan (Amphetamine may antagonize the hypotensive effects of antihypertensives). Products include:
- Avalide Tablets 922
- Avalide Tablets 2889
- Avapro Tablets 925
- Avapro Tablets 2886

Isocarboxazid (Concurrent and/or sequential use with MAO inhibitors is contraindicated; hypertensive crisis may occur).
No products indexed under this heading.

Isradipine (Amphetamine may antagonize the hypotensive effects of antihypertensives). Products include:
- DynaCirc CR Tablets 2726

Labetalol Hydrochloride (Amphetamine may antagonize the hypotensive effects of antihypertensives; adrenergic blockers are inhibited by amphetamines).
No products indexed under this heading.

Levobunolol Hydrochloride (Amphetamine may antagonize the hypotensive effects of antihypertensives; adrenergic blockers are inhibited by amphetamines). Products include:
- Betagan Ophthalmic Solution, USP .... ⊙217

(▣ Described in PDR For Nonprescription Drugs)

(⊙ Described in PDR For Ophthalmic Medicines™)

Lisinopril (Amphetamine may antagonize the hypotensive effects of antihypertensives). Products include:
- Prinivil Tablets 2029
- Prinzide Tablets 2033
- Zestoretic Tablets 701
- Zestril Tablets 704

Lithium Carbonate (Inhibits stimulatory effects of amphetamines). Products include:
- Eskalith 1406
- Lithobid Tablets 1670

Loratadine (Amphetamines may counteract the sedative effect of antihistamine). Products include:
- Alavert Allergy & Sinus D-12 Hour Tablets 743
- Alavert 743
- Children's Claritin 24 Hour Non-Drowsy Allergy Syrup 732
- Claritin Non-Drowsy 24 Hour Tablets 731
- Non-Drowsy Claritin Hives Relief Tablets 733
- Claritin Reditabs 24 Hour Non-Drowsy Tablets 732
- Claritin-D Non-Drowsy 12 Hour Tablets 731
- Claritin-D Non-Drowsy 24 Hour Tablets 731
- Children's Dimetapp ND Non-Drowsy Allergy Syrup 746
- Triaminic Allerchews 684

Losartan Potassium (Amphetamine may antagonize the hypotensive effects of antihypertensives). Products include:
- Cozaar Tablets 1913
- Hyzaar 1964

Maprotiline Hydrochloride (Enhanced activity of tricyclic or sympathomimetics; possible increases in the brain concentration of d-amphetamine in the brain; cardiovascular effect may be potentiated).
No products indexed under this heading.

Mecamylamine Hydrochloride (Amphetamine may antagonize the hypotensive effects of antihypertensives). Products include:
- Inversine Tablets 3286

Meperidine Hydrochloride (Amphetamine potentiates the analgesic effect of meperidine).
No products indexed under this heading.

Methdilazine Hydrochloride (Amphetamines may counteract the sedative effect of antihistamine).
No products indexed under this heading.

Methenamine (Acidifying agents used in methenamine therapy increases the urinary excretion and reduces the efficacy of amphetamine).
No products indexed under this heading.

Methenamine Hippurate (Acidifying agents used in methenamine therapy increases the urinary excretion and reduces the efficacy of amphetamine).
No products indexed under this heading.

Methenamine Mandelate (Acidifying agents used in methenamine therapy increases the urinary excretion and reduces the efficacy of amphetamine). Products include:
- Uroqid-Acid No. 2 Tablets 785

Methyclothiazide (Increases the concentration of the non-ionized species of the amphetamine molecule, thereby decreasing urinary excretion; increases amphetamines blood levels and thereby potentiates the actions of amphetamines).
No products indexed under this heading.

Methyldopa (Amphetamine may antagonize the hypotensive effects of antihypertensives). Products include:
- Aldoclor Tablets 1881
- Aldoril Tablets 1884

Methyldopate Hydrochloride (Amphetamine may antagonize the hypotensive effects of antihypertensives).
No products indexed under this heading.

Metipranolol Hydrochloride (Amphetamine may antagonize the hypotensive effects of antihypertensives; adrenergic blockers are inhibited by amphetamines).
No products indexed under this heading.

Metolazone (Amphetamine may antagonize the hypotensive effects of antihypertensives).
No products indexed under this heading.

Metoprolol Succinate (Amphetamine may antagonize the hypotensive effects of antihypertensives; adrenergic blockers are inhibited by amphetamines). Products include:
- Toprol-XL Tablets 660

Metoprolol Tartrate (Amphetamine may antagonize the hypotensive effects of antihypertensives; adrenergic blockers are inhibited by amphetamines).
No products indexed under this heading.

Metyrosine (Amphetamine may antagonize the hypotensive effects of antihypertensives). Products include:
- Demser Capsules 1933

Mibefradil Dihydrochloride (Amphetamine may antagonize the hypotensive effects of antihypertensives).
No products indexed under this heading.

Minoxidil (Amphetamine may antagonize the hypotensive effects of antihypertensives). Products include:
- Men's Rogaine Extra Strength Topical Solution, Ocean Rush Scent and Original Unscented 706
- Women's Rogaine Topical Solution, Spring Bloom Scent and Original Unscented 707

Moclobemide (Concurrent and/or sequential use with MAO inhibitors is contraindicated; hypertensive crisis may occur).
No products indexed under this heading.

Moexipril Hydrochloride (Amphetamine may antagonize the hypotensive effects of antihypertensives). Products include:
- Uniretic Tablets 3114
- Univasc Tablets 3118

Nadolol (Amphetamine may antagonize the hypotensive effects of antihypertensives; adrenergic blockers are inhibited by amphetamines). Products include:
- Nadolol Tablets 2121

Nicardipine Hydrochloride (Amphetamine may antagonize the hypotensive effects of antihypertensives). Products include:
- Cardene I.V. 1129

Nifedipine (Amphetamine may antagonize the hypotensive effects of antihypertensives). Products include:
- Adalat CC Tablets 2978

Nisoldipine (Amphetamine may antagonize the hypotensive effects of antihypertensives). Products include:
- Sular Tablets 1163

Nitroglycerin (Amphetamine may antagonize the hypotensive effects of antihypertensives). Products include:
- Nitro-Dur Transdermal Infusion System 3060
- Nitrolingual Pumpspray 1161

Norepinephrine Hydrochloride (Enhances adenergic effect of norepinephrine).
No products indexed under this heading.

Nortriptyline Hydrochloride (Enhanced activity of tricyclic or sympathomimetics; possible increases in the brain concentration of d-amphetamine in the brain; cardiovascular effect may be potentiated).
No products indexed under this heading.

Pargyline Hydrochloride (Concurrent and/or sequential use with MAO inhibitors is contraindicated; hypertensive crisis may occur).
No products indexed under this heading.

Penbutolol Sulfate (Amphetamine may antagonize the hypotensive effects of antihypertensives; adrenergic blockers are inhibited by amphetamines).
No products indexed under this heading.

Perindopril Erbumine (Amphetamine may antagonize the hypotensive effects of antihypertensives). Products include:
- Aceon Tablets (2 mg, 4 mg, 8 mg) 3191

Phenelzine Sulfate (Concurrent and/or sequential use with MAO inhibitors is contraindicated; hypertensive crisis may occur).
No products indexed under this heading.

Phenobarbital (Amphetamine delays intestinal absorption of phenobarbital; co-administration may produce synergistic anticonvulsant action).
No products indexed under this heading.

Phenoxybenzamine Hydrochloride (Amphetamine may antagonize the hypotensive effects of antihypertensives). Products include:
- Dibenzyline Capsules 3390

Phentolamine Mesylate (Amphetamine may antagonize the hypotensive effects of antihypertensives).
No products indexed under this heading.

Phenytoin (Amphetamine delays intestinal absorption of phenytoin; co-administration may produce synergistic anticonvulsant action).
No products indexed under this heading.

Phenytoin Sodium (Amphetamine delays intestinal absorption of phenytoin; co-administration may produce synergistic anticonvulsant action). Products include:
- Phenytek Capsules 2153

Pindolol (Amphetamine may antagonize the hypotensive effects of antihypertensives; adrenergic blockers are inhibited by amphetamines).
No products indexed under this heading.

Polythiazide (Increases the concentration of the non-ionized species of the amphetamine molecule, thereby decreasing urinary excretion; increases amphetamines blood levels and thereby potentiates the actions of amphetamines).
No products indexed under this heading.

Potassium Citrate (Increases the concentration of the non-ionized species of the amphetamine molecule, thereby decreasing urinary excretion; increases amphetamines blood levels and thereby potentiates the actions of amphetamines). Products include:
- Urocit-K Tablets 2109

Prazosin Hydrochloride (Amphetamine may antagonize the hypotensive effects of antihypertensives).
No products indexed under this heading.

Procarbazine Hydrochloride (Concurrent and/or sequential use with MAO inhibitors is contraindicated; hypertensive crisis may occur). Products include:
- Matulane Capsules 3188

Promethazine Hydrochloride (Amphetamines may counteract the sedative effect of antihistamine). Products include:
- Phenergan 3438

Propoxyphene Hydrochloride (In cases of propoxyphene overdosage, amphetamine CNS stimulation is potentiated and fatal convulsions can occur).
No products indexed under this heading.

Propoxyphene Napsylate (In cases of propoxyphene overdosage, amphetamine CNS stimulation is potentiated and fatal convulsions can occur). Products include:
- Darvocet A 500 Tablets 3497

Propranolol Hydrochloride (Amphetamine may antagonize the hypotensive effects of antihypertensives; adrenergic blockers are inhibited by amphetamines). Products include:
- Inderal LA Long-Acting Capsules 3421
- InnoPran XL Capsules 2728

Protriptyline Hydrochloride (Enhanced activity of tricyclic or sympathomimetics; possible increases in the brain concentration of d-amphetamine in the brain; cardiovascular effect may be potentiated). Products include:
- Vivactil Tablets 2350

Pyrilamine Maleate (Amphetamines may counteract the sedative effect of antihistamine).
No products indexed under this heading.

Pyrilamine Tannate (Amphetamines may counteract the sedative effect of antihistamine).
No products indexed under this heading.

IMPORTANT NOTE: Always consult each drug listing in the patient's regimen for possible interactions.

Quinapril Hydrochloride (Amphetamine may antagonize the hypotensive effects of antihypertensives).
No products indexed under this heading.

Ramipril (Amphetamine may antagonize the hypotensive effects of antihypertensives). Products include:
Altace Capsules 1673

Rauwolfia Serpentina (Amphetamine may antagonize the hypotensive effects of antihypertensives).
No products indexed under this heading.

Rescinnamine (Amphetamine may antagonize the hypotensive effects of antihypertensives).
No products indexed under this heading.

Reserpine (Lowers absorption of amphetamines).
No products indexed under this heading.

Selegiline Hydrochloride (Concurrent and/or sequential use with MAO inhibitors is contraindicated; hypertensive crisis may occur). Products include:
Eldepryl Capsules 3209

Sodium Acid Phosphate (Increases the concentration of the ionized species of the amphetamine molecule, thereby increasing urinary excretion; lowers amphetamines blood levels and efficacy). Products include:
Uroqid-Acid No. 2 Tablets 785

Sodium Bicarbonate (Increases absorption of amphetamines). Products include:
Ceo-Two Evacuant Suppository ...... ▣ 607
Colyte with Flavor Packs for Oral Solution 3102
HalfLytely and Bisacodyl Tablets Bowel Prep Kit with Flavors Packs 915
TriLyte with Flavor Packs for Oral Solution 3114

Sodium Citrate (Increases the concentration of the non-ionized species of the amphetamine molecule, thereby decreasing urinary excretion; increases amphetamines blood levels and thereby potentiates the actions of amphetamines).
No products indexed under this heading.

Sodium Nitroprusside (Amphetamine may antagonize the hypotensive effects of antihypertensives).
No products indexed under this heading.

Sotalol Hydrochloride (Amphetamine may antagonize the hypotensive effects of antihypertensives; adrenergic blockers are inhibited by amphetamines).
No products indexed under this heading.

Spirapril Hydrochloride (Amphetamine may antagonize the hypotensive effects of antihypertensives).
No products indexed under this heading.

Telmisartan (Amphetamine may antagonize the hypotensive effects of antihypertensives). Products include:
Micardis Tablets 884
Micardis HCT Tablets 886

Terazosin Hydrochloride (Amphetamine may antagonize the hypotensive effects of antihypertensives). Products include:
Hytrin Capsules 469

Terfenadine (Amphetamines may counteract the sedative effect of antihistamine).
No products indexed under this heading.

Timolol Hemihydrate (Amphetamine may antagonize the hypotensive effects of antihypertensives; adrenergic blockers are inhibited by amphetamines). Products include:
Betimol Ophthalmic Solution 3371
Betimol Ophthalmic Solution .... ⊙ 283

Timolol Maleate (Amphetamine may antagonize the hypotensive effects of antihypertensives; adrenergic blockers are inhibited by amphetamines). Products include:
Blocadren Tablets 1891
Cosopt Sterile Ophthalmic Solution 1910
Timolide Tablets 2056
Timoptic in Ocudose 2061
Timoptic Sterile Ophthalmic Solution 2058
Timoptic-XE Sterile Ophthalmic Gel Forming Solution 2062

Torsemide (Amphetamine may antagonize the hypotensive effects of antihypertensives).
No products indexed under this heading.

Trandolapril (Amphetamine may antagonize the hypotensive effects of antihypertensives). Products include:
Mavik Tablets 482
Tarka Tablets 519

Tranylcypromine Sulfate (Concurrent and/or sequential use with MAO inhibitors is contraindicated; hypertensive crisis may occur). Products include:
Parnate Tablets 1499

Trimeprazine Tartrate (Amphetamines may counteract the sedative effect of antihistamine).
No products indexed under this heading.

Trimethaphan Camsylate (Amphetamine may antagonize the hypotensive effects of antihypertensives).
No products indexed under this heading.

Trimipramine Maleate (Enhanced activity of tricyclic or sympathomimetics; possible increases in the brain concentration of d-amphetamine in the brain; cardiovascular effect may be potentiated). Products include:
Surmontil Capsules 2347

Tripelennamine Hydrochloride (Amphetamines may counteract the sedative effect of antihistamine).
No products indexed under this heading.

Triprolidine Hydrochloride (Amphetamines may counteract the sedative effect of antihistamine).
No products indexed under this heading.

Valsartan (Amphetamine may antagonize the hypotensive effects of antihypertensives). Products include:
Diovan HCT Tablets 2195
Diovan Tablets 2191

Verapamil Hydrochloride (Amphetamine may antagonize the hypotensive effects of antihypertensives). Products include:
Covera-HS Tablets 3135
Tarka Tablets 519
Verelan PM Capsules 3120

Vitamin C (Lowers absorption of amphetamines). Products include:
Chromagen Forte Soft Gelatin Capsules 3296
Halls Defense Sugarfree Vitamin C Drops .... ▣ 611
Niferex-150 Forte Capsules 3299
Peridin-C Tablets .... ▣ 761
Repliva 21/7 Tablets 3301

Food Interactions

Fruit juices, unspecified (Lowers absorption of amphetamines).

DEXEDRINE TABLETS

(Dextroamphetamine Sulfate) 1386
See Dexedrine Spansule Capsules

DEXTROSTAT TABLETS

(Dextroamphetamine Sulfate) 3177
May interact with alpha adrenergic blockers, antihistamines, antihypertensives, beta blockers, monoamine oxidase inhibitors, sympathomimetics, thiazides, tricyclic antidepressants, urinary alkalinizing agents, veratrum alkaloids, and certain other agents. Compounds in these categories include:

Acebutolol Hydrochloride (Adrenergic blockers are inhibited by amphetamines; amphetamines may antagonize the hypotensive effects of antihypertensives).
No products indexed under this heading.

Acetazolamide (Increases the concentration of the non-ionized species of the amphetamine molecule thereby decreasing urinary excretion; increases blood levels and potentiates the action of amphetamines).
No products indexed under this heading.

Acetazolamide Sodium (Increases the concentration of the non-ionized species of the amphetamine molecule thereby decreasing urinary excretion; increases blood levels and potentiates the action of amphetamines).
No products indexed under this heading.

Acrivastine (Amphetamines may counteract the sedative effect of antihistamines).
No products indexed under this heading.

Albuterol (Enhanced activity of sympathomimetics). Products include:
Proventil Inhalation Aerosol 3067

Albuterol Sulfate (Enhanced activity of sympathomimetics). Products include:
AccuNeb Inhalation Solution 1055
Combivent Inhalation Aerosol 878
DuoNeb Inhalation Solution 1058
Proventil Inhalation Solution 0.083% 3069
Proventil HFA Inhalation Aerosol 3071
Ventolin HFA Inhalation Aerosol 1576
VoSpire Extended-Release Tablets ... 2352

Amitriptyline Hydrochloride (Enhanced activity of tricyclic antidepressants; cardiovascular effects can be potentiated).
No products indexed under this heading.

Amlodipine Besylate (Amphetamines may antagonize the hypotensive effects of antihypertensives). Products include:
Caduet Tablets 2507
Lotrel Capsules 2238
Norvasc Tablets 2529

Ammonium Chloride (Increases the concentration of ionized species of the amphetamine molecule thereby increasing urinary excretion; lowers blood levels and efficacy of amphetamines).
No products indexed under this heading.

Amoxapine (Enhanced activity of tricyclic antidepressants; cardiovascular effects can be potentiated).
No products indexed under this heading.

Astemizole (Amphetamines may counteract the sedative effect of antihistamines).
No products indexed under this heading.

Atenolol (Adrenergic blockers are inhibited by amphetamines; amphetamines may antagonize the hypotensive effects of antihypertensives). Products include:
Tenormin I.V. Injection 698
Tenormin Tablets 695

Azatadine Maleate (Amphetamines may counteract the sedative effect of antihistamines).
No products indexed under this heading.

Benazepril Hydrochloride (Amphetamines may antagonize the hypotensive effects of antihypertensives). Products include:
Lotensin Tablets 2232
Lotensin HCT Tablets 2235
Lotrel Capsules 2238

Bendroflumethiazide (Some thiazide diuretics increase concentration of the non-ionized species of the amphetamine molecule thereby decreasing urinary excretion; increases blood levels and potentiates the action of amphetamines; amphetamines may antagonize the hypotensive effects of antihypertensives).
No products indexed under this heading.

Betaxolol Hydrochloride (Adrenergic blockers are inhibited by amphetamines; amphetamines may antagonize the hypotensive effects of antihypertensives). Products include:
Betoptic S Ophthalmic Suspension................................. 554

Bisoprolol Fumarate (Adrenergic blockers are inhibited by amphetamines; amphetamines may antagonize the hypotensive effects of antihypertensives).
No products indexed under this heading.

Bromodiphenhydramine Hydrochloride (Amphetamines may counteract the sedative effect of antihistamines).
No products indexed under this heading.

Brompheniramine Maleate (Amphetamines may counteract the sedative effect of antihistamines). Products include:
Alacol DM Syrup 739
Children's Dimetapp Cold & Allergy Elixir .... ▣ 745
Children's Dimetapp DM Cold & Cough Elixir .... ▣ 745
Robitussin Allergy & Cough Syrup .. ▣ 750

Candesartan Cilexetil (Amphetamines may antagonize the hypotensive effects of antihypertensives). Products include:
Atacand Tablets 634
Atacand HCT 637

Captopril (Amphetamines may antagonize the hypotensive effects of antihypertensives). Products include:
Captopril Tablets 2114

Carteolol Hydrochloride (Adrenergic blockers are inhibited by amphetamines; amphetamines may antagonize the hypotensive effects of antihypertensives). Products include:
Carteolol Hydrochloride Ophthalmic Solution USP, 1%..... ⊙ 246

Cetirizine Hydrochloride (Amphetamines may counteract the sedative effect of antihistamines). Products include:
Zyrtec Chewable Tablets 2589
Zyrtec 2589
Zyrtec-D 12 Hour Extended Release Tablets 2591

Chlorothiazide (Some thiazide diuretics increase concentration of the non-ionized species of the amphetamine molecule thereby decreasing urinary excretion; increases blood levels and potentiates the action of amphetamines; amphetamines may antagonize the hypotensive effects of antihypertensives). Products include:
Aldoclor Tablets 1881
Diuril Oral 1936

Chlorothiazide Sodium (Some thiazide diuretics increase concentration of the non-ionized species of the amphetamine molecule thereby decreasing urinary excretion; increases blood levels and potentiates the action of amphetamines; amphetamines may antagonize the hypotensive effects of antihypertensives). Products include:
Diuril Sodium Intravenous 1934

Chlorpheniramine Maleate (Amphetamines may counteract the sedative effect of antihistamines). Products include:
Advil Allergy Sinus Caplets ..... ▣ 737
Advil Multi-Symptom Cold Caplets ..... ▣ 738
BC Allergy Sinus Cold Powder ..... ▣ 612
Contac Severe Cold and Flu Caplets Maximum Strength ..... ▣ 615
Hycomine Compound Tablets 1105
PediaCare Multi-Symptom Cold Liquid ..... ▣ 704
PediaCare NightRest Cough & Cold Liquid ..... ▣ 704
Robitussin Flu Liquid ..... ▣ 752
Robitussin PM Cough & Cold Liquid ..... ▣ 752
Singlet Caplets ..... ▣ 636
Sudafed Sinus & Allergy Tablets ..... ▣ 710
TheraFlu Cold & Cough Hot Liquid ..... ▣ 680
TheraFlu Cold & Sore Throat Hot Liquid ..... ▣ 680
TheraFlu Flu & Sore Throat Hot Liquid ..... ▣ 681
TheraFlu Severe Cold & Cough Hot Liquid ..... ▣ 683
TheraFlu Severe Cold Caplets ..... ▣ 679
TheraFlu Severe Cold Hot Liquid ..... ▣ 682
Triaminic Cold & Allergy Liquid ..... ▣ 685
Triaminic Cold & Cough Liquid ..... ▣ 685
Triaminic Flu, Cough & Fever Liquid ..... ▣ 685
Triaminic Night Time Cough & Cold Liquid ..... ▣ 685
Triaminic Allergy Runny Nose & Congestion Softchews ..... ▣ 688
Triaminic Cold & Cough Softchews ..... ▣ 688
Children's Tylenol Plus Cold NightTime Suspension Liquid 1851
Children's Tylenol Plus Cold & Cough Suspension Liquid and Chewable Tablets 1851
Children's Tylenol Plus Cold Chewable Tablets 1851
Children's Tylenol Plus Flu Suspension Liquid 1853
Tylenol Allergy Complete Multi-Symptom Caplets and Gelcaps with Cool Burst 1844
Multi-Symptom Tylenol Cold Night Time Caplets 1845
Vicks 44M Cough, Cold & Flu Relief 2676
Pediatric Vicks 44m Cough & Cold Relief 2673
Children's Vicks NyQuil Cold/Cough Relief 2671

Chlorpheniramine Polistirex (Amphetamines may counteract the sedative effect of antihistamines). Products include:
Tussionex Pennkinetic Extended-Release Suspension 3322

Chlorpheniramine Tannate (Amphetamines may counteract the sedative effect of antihistamines).
No products indexed under this heading.

Chlorpromazine (Inhibits central stimulant effects of amphetamines).
No products indexed under this heading.

Chlorpromazine Hydrochloride (Inhibits central stimulant effects of amphetamines).
No products indexed under this heading.

Chlorthalidone (Amphetamines may antagonize the hypotensive effects of antihypertensives). Products include:
Clorpres Tablets 2139

Clemastine Fumarate (Amphetamines may counteract the sedative effect of antihistamines).
No products indexed under this heading.

Clomipramine Hydrochloride (Enhanced activity of tricyclic antidepressants; cardiovascular effects can be potentiated).
No products indexed under this heading.

Clonidine (Amphetamines may antagonize the hypotensive effects of antihypertensives). Products include:
Catapres-TTS 875

Clonidine Hydrochloride (Amphetamines may antagonize the hypotensive effects of antihypertensives). Products include:
Catapres Tablets 874
Clorpres Tablets 2139

Cryptenamine Preparations (Amphetamines may inhibit the hypotensive effects of veratrum alkaloids).
No products indexed under this heading.

Cyproheptadine Hydrochloride (Amphetamines may counteract the sedative effect of antihistamines).
No products indexed under this heading.

Deserpidine (Amphetamines may antagonize the hypotensive effects of antihypertensives).
No products indexed under this heading.

Desipramine Hydrochloride (Enhanced activity of tricyclic antidepressants; cardiovascular effects can be potentiated).
No products indexed under this heading.

Dexchlorpheniramine Maleate (Amphetamines may counteract the sedative effect of antihistamines).
No products indexed under this heading.

Diazoxide (Amphetamines may antagonize the hypotensive effects of antihypertensives). Products include:
Hyperstat I.V. Injection 3031

Diltiazem Hydrochloride (Amphetamines may antagonize the hypotensive effects of antihypertensives). Products include:
Cardizem LA Extended Release Tablets 1699
Tiazac Capsules 1204

Diphenhydramine Citrate (Amphetamines may counteract the sedative effect of antihistamines). Products include:
Children's Benadryl Allergy & Cold Fastmelt Tablets ..... ▣ 695
Children's Benadryl D Allergy & Sinus Fastmelt Tablets ..... ▣ 694
Children's Benadryl Allergy Fastmelt Tablets ..... ▣ 696
Goody's PM Powder ..... ▣ 622

Diphenhydramine Hydrochloride (Amphetamines may counteract the sedative effect of antihistamines). Products include:
Benadryl Allergy & Cold Tablets ..... ▣ 692
Benadryl Allergy ..... ▣ 691
Benadryl Allergy & Sinus Headache Caplets & Gelcaps ..... ▣ 693
Children's Benadryl Allergy Liquid ..... ▣ 695
Children's Benadryl Dye-Free Allergy Liquid ..... ▣ 695
Benadryl Dye-Free Allergy Liqui-Gels Softgels ..... ▣ 692
Benadryl Itch Relief Stick Extra Strength ..... ▣ 696
Benadryl Itch Stopping Cream Extra Strength ..... ▣ 697
Benadryl Itch Stopping Gel Extra Strength ..... ▣ 697
Benadryl Itch Stopping Spray Extra Strength ..... ▣ 697
Benadryl Maximum Strength Severe Allergy & Sinus Headache Caplets ..... ▣ 694
Children's Benadryl D Liquid Medication ..... ▣ 693
Benadryl D Tablets ..... ▣ 694
Nytol QuickCaps Caplets ..... ▣ 635
Maximum Strength Nytol QuickGels Softgels ..... ▣ 635
Simply Sleep Caplets 1841
Sominex Original Formula Tablets ..... ▣ 637
TheraFlu Thin Strips Multi Symptom ..... ▣ 684
Triaminic Thin Strips Cough & Runny Nose ..... ▣ 690
Children's Tylenol Plus Cold & Allergy Suspension Liquid 1850
Tylenol Allergy Complete Night Time Caplets 1844
Tylenol Severe Allergy Caplets 1844
Tylenol Flu NightTime Gelcaps 1846
Extra Strength Tylenol PM Caplets, Geltabs, Gelcaps and Liquid 1847
Unisom Maximum Strength SleepGels ..... ▣ 712

Diphenylpyraline Hydrochloride (Amphetamines may counteract the sedative effect of antihistamines).
No products indexed under this heading.

Dobutamine Hydrochloride (Enhanced activity of sympathomimetics).
No products indexed under this heading.

Dopamine Hydrochloride (Enhanced activity of sympathomimetics).
No products indexed under this heading.

Doxazosin Mesylate (Adrenergic blockers are inhibited by amphetamines; amphetamines may antagonize the hypotensive effects of antihypertensives).
No products indexed under this heading.

Doxepin Hydrochloride (Enhanced activity of tricyclic antidepressants; cardiovascular effects can be potentiated).
No products indexed under this heading.

Enalapril Maleate (Amphetamines may antagonize the hypotensive effects of antihypertensives). Products include:
Vaseretic Tablets 2073
Vasotec I.V. Injection 2076

Enalaprilat (Amphetamines may antagonize the hypotensive effects of antihypertensives).
No products indexed under this heading.

Ephedrine Hydrochloride (Enhanced activity of sympathomimetics). Products include:
Primatene Tablets ..... ▣ 749

Ephedrine Sulfate (Enhanced activity of sympathomimetics).
No products indexed under this heading.

Ephedrine Tannate (Enhanced activity of sympathomimetics).
No products indexed under this heading.

Epinephrine (Enhanced activity of sympathomimetics). Products include:
EpiPen 1061
Primatene Mist ..... ▣ 749

Epinephrine Bitartrate (Enhanced activity of sympathomimetics).
No products indexed under this heading.

Epinephrine Hydrochloride (Enhanced activity of sympathomimetics).
No products indexed under this heading.

Eprosartan Mesylate (Amphetamines may antagonize the hypotensive effects of antihypertensives). Products include:
Teveten Tablets 1707
Teveten HCT Tablets 1710

Esmolol Hydrochloride (Adrenergic blockers are inhibited by amphetamines; amphetamines may antagonize the hypotensive effects of antihypertensives). Products include:
Brevibloc Concentrate 766
Brevibloc Injection 766
Brevibloc Double Strength Injection 766
Brevibloc Premixed Injection 766
Brevibloc Double Strength Premixed Injection 766

Ethosuximide (Delayed intestinal absorption of ethosuximide).
No products indexed under this heading.

Felodipine (Amphetamines may antagonize the hypotensive effects of antihypertensives). Products include:
Plendil Extended-Release Tablets 651

Fexofenadine Hydrochloride (Amphetamines may counteract the sedative effect of antihistamines). Products include:
Allegra 2857
Allegra-D 12 Hour Extended-Release Tablets 2860
Allegra-D 24 Hour Extended-Release Tablets 2862

Fosinopril Sodium (Amphetamines may antagonize the hypotensive effects of antihypertensives).
No products indexed under this heading.

IMPORTANT NOTE: Always consult each drug listing in the patient's regimen for possible interactions.

Fosphenytoin Sodium (Co-administration may produce synergistic anticonvulsant action).
No products indexed under this heading.

Furosemide (Amphetamines may antagonize the hypotensive effects of antihypertensives). Products include:
Furosemide Tablets 2117

Glutamic Acid Hydrochloride (Lowers absorption of amphetamines by acting as gastrointestinal acidifying agent).
No products indexed under this heading.

Guanabenz Acetate (Amphetamines may antagonize the hypotensive effects of antihypertensives).
No products indexed under this heading.

Guanethidine Monosulfate (Lowers absorption of amphetamines by acting as gastrointestinal acidifying agent; amphetamines may antagonize the hypotensive effects of antihypertensives).
No products indexed under this heading.

Haloperidol (Inhibits central stimulant effects of amphetamines).
No products indexed under this heading.

Haloperidol Decanoate (Inhibits central stimulant effects of amphetamines).
No products indexed under this heading.

Hydralazine Hydrochloride (Amphetamines may antagonize the hypotensive effects of antihypertensives). Products include:
BiDil Tablets 2161

Hydrochlorothiazide (Some thiazide diuretics increase concentration of the non-ionized species of the amphetamine molecule thereby decreasing urinary excretion; increases blood levels and potentiates the action of amphetamines; amphetamines may antagonize the hypotensive effects of antihypertensives). Products include:
Aldoril Tablets 1884
Atacand HCT 637
Avalide Tablets 2889
Avalide Tablets 922
Benicar HCT Tablets 2852
Diovan HCT Tablets 2195
Dyazide Capsules 1389
Hyzaar 1964
Lotensin HCT Tablets 2235
Maxzide 2150
Micardis HCT Tablets 886
Moduretic Tablets 2003
Prinzide Tablets 2033
Teveten HCT Tablets 1710
Timolide Tablets 2056
Uniretic Tablets 3114
Vaseretic Tablets 2073
Zestoretic Tablets 701

Hydroflumethiazide (Some thiazide diuretics increase concentration of the non-ionized species of the amphetamine molecule thereby decreasing urinary excretion; increases blood levels and potentiates the action of amphetamines; amphetamines may antagonize the hypotensive effects of antihypertensives).
No products indexed under this heading.

Imipramine Hydrochloride (Enhanced activity of tricyclic antidepressants; cardiovascular effects can be potentiated).
No products indexed under this heading.

Imipramine Pamoate (Enhanced activity of tricyclic antidepressants; cardiovascular effects can be potentiated).
No products indexed under this heading.

Indapamide (Amphetamines may antagonize the hypotensive effects of antihypertensives). Products include:
Indapamide Tablets 2119

Irbesartan (Amphetamines may antagonize the hypotensive effects of antihypertensives). Products include:
Avalide Tablets 922
Avalide Tablets 2889
Avapro Tablets 925
Avapro Tablets 2886

Isocarboxazid (Potential for hypertensive crisis; slows amphetamine metabolism; concurrent and/or sequential use is contraindicated).
No products indexed under this heading.

Isoproterenol Hydrochloride (Enhanced activity of sympathomimetics).
No products indexed under this heading.

Isoproterenol Sulfate (Enhanced activity of sympathomimetics).
No products indexed under this heading.

Isradipine (Amphetamines may antagonize the hypotensive effects of antihypertensives). Products include:
DynaCirc CR Tablets 2726

Labetalol Hydrochloride (Adrenergic blockers are inhibited by amphetamines; amphetamines may antagonize the hypotensive effects of antihypertensives).
No products indexed under this heading.

Levalbuterol Hydrochloride (Enhanced activity of sympathomimetics). Products include:
Xopenex Inhalation Solution 3143
Xopenex Inhalation Solution Concentrate 3147

Levobunolol Hydrochloride (Adrenergic blockers are inhibited by amphetamines; amphetamines may antagonize the hypotensive effects of antihypertensives). Products include:
Betagan Ophthalmic Solution, USP .... ⊙217

Lisinopril (Amphetamines may antagonize the hypotensive effects of antihypertensives). Products include:
Prinivil Tablets 2029
Prinzide Tablets 2033
Zestoretic Tablets 701
Zestril Tablets 704

Lithium Carbonate (Inhibits stimulatory effects of amphetamines). Products include:
Eskalith 1406
Lithobid Tablets 1670

Loratadine (Amphetamines may counteract the sedative effect of antihistamines). Products include:
Alavert Allergy & Sinus D-12 Hour Tablets .... ▣743
Alavert .... ▣743
Children's Claritin 24 Hour Non-Drowsy Allergy Syrup .... ▣732
Claritin Non-Drowsy 24 Hour Tablets .... ▣731
Non-Drowsy Claritin Hives Relief Tablets .... ▣733
Claritin Reditabs 24 Hour Non-Drowsy Tablets .... ▣732
Claritin-D Non-Drowsy 12 Hour Tablets .... ▣731
Claritin-D Non-Drowsy 24 Hour Tablets .... ▣731
Children's Dimetapp ND Non-Drowsy Allergy Syrup .... ▣746
Triaminic Allerchews .... ▣684

Losartan Potassium (Amphetamines may antagonize the hypotensive effects of antihypertensives). Products include:
Cozaar Tablets 1913
Hyzaar 1964

Maprotiline Hydrochloride (Enhanced activity of tricyclic antidepressants; cardiovascular effects can be potentiated).
No products indexed under this heading.

Mecamylamine Hydrochloride (Amphetamines may antagonize the hypotensive effects of antihypertensives). Products include:
Inversine Tablets 3286

Meperidine Hydrochloride (Analgesic effect of meperidine potentiated).
No products indexed under this heading.

Metaproterenol Sulfate (Enhanced activity of sympathomimetics). Products include:
Alupent Inhalation Aerosol 858

Metaraminol Bitartrate (Enhanced activity of sympathomimetics). Products include:
Aramine Injection 1889

Methdilazine Hydrochloride (Amphetamines may counteract the sedative effect of antihistamines).
No products indexed under this heading.

Methenamine (Increases urinary excretion and efficacy is reduced by acidifying agents used in methenamine therapy).
No products indexed under this heading.

Methenamine Hippurate (Increases urinary excretion and efficacy is reduced by acidifying agents used in methenamine therapy).
No products indexed under this heading.

Methenamine Mandelate (Increases urinary excretion and efficacy is reduced by acidifying agents used in methenamine therapy). Products include:
Uroqid-Acid No. 2 Tablets 785

Methoxamine Hydrochloride (Enhanced activity of sympathomimetics).
No products indexed under this heading.

Methyclothiazide (Some thiazide diuretics increase concentration of the non-ionized species of the amphetamine molecule thereby decreasing urinary excretion; increases blood levels and potentiates the action of amphetamines; amphetamines may antagonize the hypotensive effects of antihypertensives).
No products indexed under this heading.

Methyldopa (Amphetamines may antagonize the hypotensive effects of antihypertensives). Products include:
Aldoclor Tablets 1881
Aldoril Tablets 1884

Methyldopate Hydrochloride (Amphetamines may antagonize the hypotensive effects of antihypertensives).
No products indexed under this heading.

Metipranolol Hydrochloride (Adrenergic blockers are inhibited by amphetamines; amphetamines may antagonize the hypotensive effects of antihypertensives).
No products indexed under this heading.

Metolazone (Amphetamines may antagonize the hypotensive effects of antihypertensives).
No products indexed under this heading.

Metoprolol Succinate (Adrenergic blockers are inhibited by amphetamines; amphetamines may antagonize the hypotensive effects of antihypertensives). Products include:
Toprol-XL Tablets 660

Metoprolol Tartrate (Adrenergic blockers are inhibited by amphetamines; amphetamines may antagonize the hypotensive effects of antihypertensives).
No products indexed under this heading.

Metyrosine (Amphetamines may antagonize the hypotensive effects of antihypertensives). Products include:
Demser Capsules 1933

Mibefradil Dihydrochloride (Amphetamines may antagonize the hypotensive effects of antihypertensives).
No products indexed under this heading.

Minoxidil (Amphetamines may antagonize the hypotensive effects of antihypertensives). Products include:
Men's Rogaine Extra Strength Topical Solution, Ocean Rush Scent and Original Unscented ..... ▣706
Women's Rogaine Topical Solution, Spring Bloom Scent and Original Unscented .... ▣707

Moclobemide (Potential for hypertensive crisis; slows amphetamine metabolism; concurrent and/or sequential use is contraindicated).
No products indexed under this heading.

Moexipril Hydrochloride (Amphetamines may antagonize the hypotensive effects of antihypertensives). Products include:
Uniretic Tablets 3114
Univasc Tablets 3118

Nadolol (Adrenergic blockers are inhibited by amphetamines; amphetamines may antagonize the hypotensive effects of antihypertensives). Products include:
Nadolol Tablets 2121

Nicardipine Hydrochloride (Amphetamines may antagonize the hypotensive effects of antihypertensives). Products include:
Cardene I.V. 1129

Nifedipine (Amphetamines may antagonize the hypotensive effects of antihypertensives). Products include:
Adalat CC Tablets 2978

Nisoldipine (Amphetamines may antagonize the hypotensive effects of antihypertensives). Products include:

Sular Tablets 1163

Nitroglycerin (Amphetamines may antagonize the hypotensive effects of antihypertensives). Products include:

Nitro-Dur Transdermal Infusion System 3060
Nitrolingual Pumpspray 1161

Norepinephrine Bitartrate (Enhanced activity of sympathomimetics).

No products indexed under this heading.

Norepinephrine Hydrochloride (Enhanced adrenergic effect of norepinephrine).

No products indexed under this heading.

Nortriptyline Hydrochloride (Enhanced activity of tricyclic antidepressants; cardiovascular effects can be potentiated).

No products indexed under this heading.

Pargyline Hydrochloride (Potential for hypertensive crisis; slows amphetamine metabolism; concurrent and/or sequential use is contraindicated).

No products indexed under this heading.

Penbutolol Sulfate (Adrenergic blockers are inhibited by amphetamines; amphetamines may antagonize the hypotensive effects of antihypertensives).

No products indexed under this heading.

Perindopril Erbumine (Amphetamines may antagonize the hypotensive effects of antihypertensives). Products include:

Aceon Tablets (2 mg, 4 mg, 8 mg) 3191

Phenelzine Sulfate (Potential for hypertensive crisis; slows amphetamine metabolism; concurrent and/or sequential use is contraindicated).

No products indexed under this heading.

Phenobarbital (Delayed intestinal absorption of phenobarbital; synergistic anticonvulsant action may be produced).

No products indexed under this heading.

Phenoxybenzamine Hydrochloride (Amphetamines may antagonize the hypotensive effects of antihypertensives). Products include:

Dibenzyline Capsules 3390

Phentolamine Mesylate (Amphetamines may antagonize the hypotensive effects of antihypertensives).

No products indexed under this heading.

Phenylephrine Bitartrate (Enhanced activity of sympathomimetics).

No products indexed under this heading.

Phenylephrine Hydrochloride (Enhanced activity of sympathomimetics). Products include:

Alacol DM Syrup 739
Hycomine Compound Tablets 1105
Preparation H Maximum Strength Cream 747
Preparation H Cooling Gel 747
Preparation H 747
Sudafed PE Tablets 711
Vicks Sinex Nasal Spray and Ultra Fine Mist for Sinus Relief 2677
Zicam Concentrated Cough Mist for Kids Plus D Cool Cherry 643
Zicam Concentrated Cough Mist Plus D Cool Cherry 642

Phenylephrine Tannate (Enhanced activity of sympathomimetics).

No products indexed under this heading.

Phenylpropanolamine Hydrochloride (Enhanced activity of sympathomimetics).

No products indexed under this heading.

Phenytoin (Delayed intestinal absorption of phenobarbital; synergistic anticonvulsant action may be produced).

No products indexed under this heading.

Phenytoin Sodium (Delayed intestinal absorption of phenobarbital; synergistic anticonvulsant action may be produced). Products include:

Phenytek Capsules 2153

Pindolol (Adrenergic blockers are inhibited by amphetamines; amphetamines may antagonize the hypotensive effects of antihypertensives).

No products indexed under this heading.

Pirbuterol Acetate (Enhanced activity of sympathomimetics). Products include:

Maxair Autohaler 1820

Polythiazide (Some thiazide diuretics increase concentration of the non-ionized species of the amphetamine molecule thereby decreasing urinary excretion; increases blood levels and potentiates the action of amphetamines; amphetamines may antagonize the hypotensive effects of antihypertensives).

No products indexed under this heading.

Potassium Citrate (Increases the concentration of the non-ionized species of the amphetamine molecule thereby decreasing urinary excretion; increases blood levels and potentiates the action of amphetamines). Products include:

Urocit-K Tablets 2109

Prazosin Hydrochloride (Adrenergic blockers are inhibited by amphetamines; amphetamines may antagonize the hypotensive effects of antihypertensives).

No products indexed under this heading.

Procarbazine Hydrochloride (Potential for hypertensive crisis; slows amphetamine metabolism; concurrent and/or sequential use is contraindicated). Products include:

Matulane Capsules 3188

Promethazine Hydrochloride (Amphetamines may counteract the sedative effect of antihistamines). Products include:

Phenergan 3438

Propoxyphene Hydrochloride (In cases of propoxyphene overdosage, amphetamine CNS stimulation is potentiated and fatal convulsions can occur).

No products indexed under this heading.

Propoxyphene Napsylate (In cases of propoxyphene overdosage, amphetamine CNS stimulation is potentiated and fatal convulsions can occur). Products include:

Darvocet A 500 Tablets 3497

Propranolol Hydrochloride (Adrenergic blockers are inhibited by amphetamines; amphetamines may antagonize the hypotensive effects of antihypertensives). Products include:

Inderal LA Long-Acting Capsules 3421
InnoPran XL Capsules 2728

Protriptyline Hydrochloride (Enhanced activity of tricyclic antidepressants; cardiovascular effects can be potentiated). Products include:

Vivactil Tablets 2350

Pseudoephedrine Hydrochloride (Enhanced activity of sympathomimetics). Products include:

Advil Allergy Sinus Caplets 737
Advil Cold & Sinus 739
Advil Flu & Body Ache Caplets 739
Children's Advil Cold Suspension 741
Advil Multi-Symptom Cold Caplets 738
Allegra-D 12 Hour Extended-Release Tablets 2860
Allegra-D 24 Hour Extended-Release Tablets 2862
Balamine DM 739
BC Cold Powder 612
Benadryl Allergy & Cold Tablets 692
Benadryl Allergy & Sinus Headache Caplets & Gelcaps 693
Children's Benadryl Allergy & Cold Fastmelt Tablets 695
Benadryl Maximum Strength Severe Allergy & Sinus Headache Caplets 694
Children's Benadryl D Allergy & Sinus Fastmelt Tablets 694
Children's Benadryl D Liquid Medication 693
Benadryl D Tablets 694
Contac Non-Drowsy 12 Hour Cold Caplets 614
Contac Non-Drowsy Timed Release 12 Hour Cold Caplets 615
Contac Severe Cold and Flu Caplets Maximum Strength 615
Contac Severe Cold and Flu Caplets Non-Drowsy 615
Children's Dimetapp Cold & Allergy Elixir 745
Children's Dimetapp DM Cold & Cough Elixir 745
Children's Dimetapp Long Acting Cough Plus Cold Syrup 746
Dimetapp Infant Drops Decongestant Plus Cough 746
Children's Motrin Cold Non-Staining Dye-Free Oral Suspension 1838
Children's Motrin Cold Oral Suspension 1838
Motrin Cold & Sinus Caplets 1836
PediaCare Decongestant & Cough Infant Drops 705
PediaCare Decongestant Infants' Drops 705
PediaCare Long-Acting Cough Plus Cold Liquid 704
PediaCare Multi-Symptom Cold Liquid 704
PediaCare NightRest Cough & Cold Liquid 704
Robitussin Allergy & Cough Syrup 750
Robitussin CF Liquid 755
Robitussin Cough & Cold Liquid-filled Capsules 750
Robitussin Cough, Cold & Flu Liquid-filled Capsules 750
Robitussin Cough & Cold Infant Drops 755
Robitussin Flu Liquid 752
Robitussin Maximum Strength Cough & Cold Liquid 754
Robitussin PE Syrup 753
Robitussin Pediatric Cough & Cold Liquid 754
Robitussin PM Cough & Cold Liquid 752
Robitussin Severe Congestion Liquid-filled Capsules 751
Simply Stuffy Liquid 1841
Singlet Caplets 636
Sudafed 12 Hour Caplets 708
Sudafed 24 Hour Tablets 709
Sudafed Nasal Decongestant Tablets 709
Sudafed Severe Cold 710
Sudafed Non-Drying Sinus Liquid Caps 709
Sudafed Sinus & Allergy Tablets 710
Sudafed Sinus Headache 711
TheraFlu Cold & Cough Hot Liquid 680
TheraFlu Cold & Sore Throat Hot Liquid 680
TheraFlu Flu & Chest Congestion Non-Drowsy Hot Liquid 681
TheraFlu Flu & Sore Throat Hot Liquid 681
TheraFlu Severe Cold Non-Drowsy Hot Liquid 683
TheraFlu Severe Cold & Cough Hot Liquid 683
TheraFlu Severe Cold Caplets 679
TheraFlu Severe Cold Hot Liquid 682
TheraFlu Severe Cold Non-Drowsy Caplets 679
Triaminic Chest & Nasal Congestion Liquid 685
Triaminic Cold & Allergy Liquid 685
Triaminic Cold & Cough Liquid 685
Triaminic Cough Liquid 687
Triaminic Cough & Nasal Congestion Liquid 687
Triaminic Cough & Sore Throat Liquid 687
Triaminic Flu, Cough & Fever Liquid 685
Triaminic Night Time Cough & Cold Liquid 685
Triaminic Allergy Runny Nose & Congestion Softchews 688
Triaminic Cold & Cough Softchews 688
Triaminic Cough & Sore Throat Softchews 689
Tylenol Sinus NightTime Caplets 663
Children's Tylenol Plus Cold & Allergy Suspension Liquid 1850
Children's Tylenol Plus Cold NightTime Suspension Liquid 1851
Children's Tylenol Plus Cold & Cough Suspension Liquid and Chewable Tablets 1851
Children's Tylenol Plus Cold Chewable Tablets 1851
Children's Tylenol Plus Cold Daytime Non-Drowsy Suspension Liquid 1851
Children's Tylenol Plus Flu Suspension Liquid 1853
Concentrated Tylenol Infants' Drops Plus Cold 1851
Concentrated Tylenol Infants' Drops Plus Cold and Cough 1851
Tylenol Cold & Flu Severe Daytime Liquid with Cool Burst 1846
Tylenol Cold & Flu Severe NightTime Liquid with Cool Burst 1846
Tylenol Cold Severe Congestion Non-Drowsy Caplets with Cool Burst 1846
Tylenol Allergy Complete Night Time Caplets 1844
Tylenol Allergy Complete Multi-Symptom Caplets and Gelcaps with Cool Burst 1844
Tylenol Flu NightTime Gelcaps 1846
Tylenol Flu Day Non-Drowsy Gelcaps 1846
Concentrated Tylenol Infants' Drops Plus Cold Nasal Congestant, Fever Reducer & Pain Reliever 668
Concentrated Tylenol Infants' Drops Plus Cold & Cough Nasal Decongestant, Fever Reducer & Pain Reliever 668
Multi-Symptom Tylenol Cold Night Time Caplets 1845
Multi-Symptom Tylenol Cold Day Non-Drowsy Caplets and Gelcaps 1845
Tylenol Sinus Day Non-Drowsy 1848
Tylenol Sinus Night Time Caplets 1848
Tylenol Sinus Severe Congestion Caplets with Cool Burst 1848
Vicks 44D Cough & Head Congestion Relief 2676
Vicks 44D Cough & Head Congestion Relief Liquid 721
Vicks 44M Cough, Cold & Flu Relief 2676

IMPORTANT NOTE: Always consult each drug listing in the patient's regimen for possible interactions.

Pediatric Vicks 44m Cough & Cold Relief 2673
Vicks DayQuil LiquiCaps/Liquid Multi-Symptom Cold/Flu Relief .... ▣ 723
Vicks DayQuil Multi-Symptom Cold/Flu Relief LiquiCaps 2675
Vicks DayQuil Multi-Symptom Cold/Flu Relief Liquid 2675
Children's Vicks NyQuil Cold/Cough Relief 2671
Vicks NyQuil LiquiCaps 2677
Vicks NyQuil LiquiCaps/Liquid Multi-Symptom Cold/Flu Relief .... ▣ 725
Vicks NyQuil Liquid 2677
Zyrtec-D 12 Hour Extended Release Tablets 2591

Pseudoephedrine Sulfate (Enhanced activity of sympathomimetics). Products include:
Alavert Allergy & Sinus D-12 Hour Tablets .... ▣ 743
Clarinex-D 24-Hour Extended-Release Tablets 3012
Claritin-D Non-Drowsy 12 Hour Tablets .... ▣ 731
Claritin-D Non-Drowsy 24 Hour Tablets .... ▣ 731

Pyrilamine Maleate (Amphetamines may counteract the sedative effect of antihistamines).
No products indexed under this heading.

Pyrilamine Tannate (Amphetamines may counteract the sedative effect of antihistamines).
No products indexed under this heading.

Quinapril Hydrochloride (Amphetamines may antagonize the hypotensive effects of antihypertensives).
No products indexed under this heading.

Ramipril (Amphetamines may antagonize the hypotensive effects of antihypertensives). Products include:
Altace Capsules 1673

Rauwolfia Serpentina (Amphetamines may antagonize the hypotensive effects of antihypertensives).
No products indexed under this heading.

Rescinnamine (Amphetamines may antagonize the hypotensive effects of antihypertensives).
No products indexed under this heading.

Reserpine (Lowers absorption of amphetamines by acting as gastrointestinal acidifying agent; amphetamines may antagonize the hypotensive effects of antihypertensives).
No products indexed under this heading.

Salmeterol Xinafoate (Enhanced activity of sympathomimetics). Products include:
Advair Diskus 100/50 1291
Advair Diskus 250/50 1291
Advair Diskus 500/50 1291
Serevent Diskus 1540

Selegiline Hydrochloride (Potential for hypertensive crisis; slows amphetamine metabolism; concurrent and/or sequential use is contraindicated). Products include:
Eldepryl Capsules 3209

Sodium Acid Phosphate (Increases the concentration of ionized species of the amphetamine molecule thereby increasing urinary excretion; lowers blood levels and efficacy of amphetamines). Products include:
Uroqid-Acid No. 2 Tablets 785

Sodium Bicarbonate (Increases absorption of amphetamines; increases blood levels and potentiates the action of amphetamines). Products include:
Ceo-Two Evacuant Suppository .... ▣ 607
Colyte with Flavor Packs for Oral Solution 3102
HalfLytely and Bisacodyl Tablets Bowel Prep Kit with Flavors Packs 915
TriLyte with Flavor Packs for Oral Solution 3114

Sodium Citrate (Increases the concentration of the non-ionized species of the amphetamine molecule thereby decreasing urinary excretion; increases blood levels and potentiates the action of amphetamines).
No products indexed under this heading.

Sodium Nitroprusside (Amphetamines may antagonize the hypotensive effects of antihypertensives).
No products indexed under this heading.

Sotalol Hydrochloride (Adrenergic blockers are inhibited by amphetamines; amphetamines may antagonize the hypotensive effects of antihypertensives).
No products indexed under this heading.

Spirapril Hydrochloride (Amphetamines may antagonize the hypotensive effects of antihypertensives).
No products indexed under this heading.

Tamsulosin Hydrochloride (Adrenergic blockers are inhibited by amphetamines; amphetamines may antagonize the hypotensive effects of antihypertensives). Products include:
Flomax Capsules 881

Telmisartan (Amphetamines may antagonize the hypotensive effects of antihypertensives). Products include:
Micardis Tablets 884
Micardis HCT Tablets 886

Terazosin Hydrochloride (Adrenergic blockers are inhibited by amphetamines; amphetamines may antagonize the hypotensive effects of antihypertensives). Products include:
Hytrin Capsules 469

Terbutaline Sulfate (Enhanced activity of sympathomimetics).
No products indexed under this heading.

Terfenadine (Amphetamines may counteract the sedative effect of antihistamines).
No products indexed under this heading.

Timolol Hemihydrate (Adrenergic blockers are inhibited by amphetamines; amphetamines may antagonize the hypotensive effects of antihypertensives). Products include:
Betimol Ophthalmic Solution 3371
Betimol Ophthalmic Solution .... ⊙ 283

Timolol Maleate (Adrenergic blockers are inhibited by amphetamines; amphetamines may antagonize the hypotensive effects of antihypertensives). Products include:
Blocadren Tablets 1891
Cosopt Sterile Ophthalmic Solution 1910
Timolide Tablets 2056
Timoptic in Ocudose 2061
Timoptic Sterile Ophthalmic Solution 2058
Timoptic-XE Sterile Ophthalmic Gel Forming Solution 2062

Torsemide (Amphetamines may antagonize the hypotensive effects of antihypertensives).
No products indexed under this heading.

Trandolapril (Amphetamines may antagonize the hypotensive effects of antihypertensives). Products include:
Mavik Tablets 482
Tarka Tablets 519

Tranylcypromine Sulfate (Potential for hypertensive crisis; slows amphetamine metabolism; concurrent and/or sequential use is contraindicated). Products include:
Parnate Tablets 1499

Trimeprazine Tartrate (Amphetamines may counteract the sedative effect of antihistamines).
No products indexed under this heading.

Trimethaphan Camsylate (Amphetamines may antagonize the hypotensive effects of antihypertensives).
No products indexed under this heading.

Trimipramine Maleate (Enhanced activity of tricyclic antidepressants; cardiovascular effects can be potentiated). Products include:
Surmontil Capsules 2347

Tripelennamine Hydrochloride (Amphetamines may counteract the sedative effect of antihistamines).
No products indexed under this heading.

Triprolidine Hydrochloride (Amphetamines may counteract the sedative effect of antihistamines).
No products indexed under this heading.

Valsartan (Amphetamines may antagonize the hypotensive effects of antihypertensives). Products include:
Diovan HCT Tablets 2195
Diovan Tablets 2191

Verapamil Hydrochloride (Amphetamines may antagonize the hypotensive effects of antihypertensives). Products include:
Covera-HS Tablets 3135
Tarka Tablets 519
Verelan PM Capsules 3120

Vitamin C (Lowers absorption of amphetamines by acting as gastrointestinal acidifying agent). Products include:
Chromagen Forte Soft Gelatin Capsules 3296
Halls Defense Sugarfree Vitamin C Drops .... ▣ 611
Niferex-150 Forte Capsules 3299
Peridin-C Tablets .... ▣ 761
Repliva 21/7 Tablets 3301

Food Interactions

Fruit juices, unspecified (Lowers absorption of amphetamines by acting as gastrointestinal acidifying agent).

DIASTAT RECTAL DELIVERY SYSTEM

(Diazepam) 3344
May interact with barbiturates, central nervous system depressants, cytochrome p450 2c19 inducers (selected), cytochrome p450 2c19 inhibitors (selected), cytochrome p450 2c19 substrates (selected), cytochrome p450 3a4 inducers (selected), cytochrome p450 3a4 inhibitors (selected), cytochrome p450 3a4 substrates (selected), antidepressant drugs, dexamethasone, monoamine oxidase inhibitors, narcotic analgesics, phenothiazines, phenytoin, quinidine, valproate, xanthines, and certain other agents. Compounds in these categories include:

Acetazolamide (Studies suggest that CYP2C19 and CYP3A4 are the principal enzymes involved in the initial oxidative metabolism of diazepam. Therefore, potential interactions may occur when diazepam is given concurrently with agents that affect CYP2C19 and CYP3A4 activity. Potential inhibitors of CYP3A4 could decrease the rate of diazepam elimination).
No products indexed under this heading.

Alfentanil Hydrochloride (Potential for synergistic CNS-depressant effect).
No products indexed under this heading.

Allium sativum (Studies suggest that CYP2C19 and CYP3A4 are the principal enzymes involved in the initial oxidative metabolism of diazepam. Therefore, potential interactions may occur when diazepam is given concurrently with agents that affect CYP2C19 and CYP3A4 activity. Potential inducers of CYP3A4 could increase the rate of diazepam elimination).
No products indexed under this heading.

Alprazolam (Potential for synergistic CNS-depressant effect). Products include:
Niravam Orally Disintegrating Tablets 3106
Xanax XR Tablets 2655

Aminophylline (Diazepam is a substrate of CYP2C19 and CYP3A4, it is possible that diazepam may interfere with the metabolism of drugs which are substrates for CYP3A4, such as theophylline).
No products indexed under this heading.

Amiodarone Hydrochloride (Studies suggest that CYP2C19 and CYP3A4 are the principal enzymes involved in the initial oxidative metabolism of diazepam. Therefore, potential interactions may occur when diazepam is given concurrently with agents that affect CYP2C19 and CYP3A4 activity. Potential inhibitors of CYP3A4 could decrease the rate of diazepam elimination). Products include:
Pacerone Tablets 3337

Amitriptyline Hydrochloride (Potential for synergistic CNS-depressant effect).
No products indexed under this heading.

Amlodipine Besylate (There are no reports as to which isoenzymes could be inhibited or induced by diazepam. But based on the fact that diazepam is a substrate for CYP2C19 and CYP3A4, it is possible

that diazepam may interfere with the metabolism of drugs which are substrates for CYP2C19 and CYP3A4 leading to a potential drug-drug interaction). Products include:

- Caduet Tablets 2507
- Lotrel Capsules 2238
- Norvasc Tablets 2529

Amoxapine (Potential for synergistic CNS-depressant effect).

No products indexed under this heading.

Amprenavir (Studies suggest that CYP2C19 and CYP3A4 are the principal enzymes involved in the initial oxidative metabolism of diazepam. Therefore, potential interactions may occur when diazepam is given concurrently with agents that affect CYP2C19 and CYP3A4 activity. Potential inhibitors of CYP3A4 could decrease the rate of diazepam elimination). Products include:

- Agenerase Capsules 1299
- Agenerase Oral Solution 1304

Anastrozole (Studies suggest that CYP2C19 and CYP3A4 are the principal enzymes involved in the initial oxidative metabolism of diazepam. Therefore, potential interactions may occur when diazepam is given concurrently with agents that affect CYP2C19 and CYP3A4 activity. Potential inhibitors of CYP3A4 could decrease the rate of diazepam elimination). Products include:

- Arimidex Tablets 665

Aprepitant (Studies suggest that CYP2C19 and CYP3A4 are the principal enzymes involved in the initial oxidative metabolism of diazepam. Therefore, potential interactions may occur when diazepam is given concurrently with agents that affect CYP2C19 and CYP3A4 activity. Potential inhibitors of CYP3A4 could decrease the rate of diazepam elimination). Products include:

- Emend Capsules 1944

Aprobarbital (Potential for synergistic CNS-depressant effect).

No products indexed under this heading.

Astemizole (There are no reports as to which isoenzymes could be inhibited or induced by diazepam. But based on the fact that diazepam is a substrate for CYP2C19 and CYP3A4, it is possible that diazepam may interfere with the metabolism of drugs which are substrates for CYP2C19 and CYP3A4 leading to a potential drug-drug interaction).

No products indexed under this heading.

Atorvastatin Calcium (There are no reports as to which isoenzymes could be inhibited or induced by diazepam. But based on the fact that diazepam is a substrate for CYP2C19 and CYP3A4, it is possible that diazepam may interfere with the metabolism of drugs which are substrates for CYP2C19 and CYP3A4 leading to a potential drug-drug interaction). Products include:

- Caduet Tablets 2507
- Lipitor Tablets 2495

Belladonna Ergotamine (There are no reports as to which isoenzymes could be inhibited or induced by diazepam. But based on the fact that diazepam is a substrate for CYP2C19 and CYP3A4, it is possible that diazepam may interfere with the metabolism of drugs which are substrates for CYP2C19 and CYP3A4 leading to a potential drug-drug interaction).

No products indexed under this heading.

Betamethasone Acetate (Studies suggest that CYP2C19 and CYP3A4 are the principal enzymes involved in the initial oxidative metabolism of diazepam. Therefore, potential interactions may occur when diazepam is given concurrently with agents that affect CYP2C19 and CYP3A4 activity. Potential inducers of CYP3A4 could increase the rate of diazepam elimination).

No products indexed under this heading.

Betamethasone Sodium Phosphate (Studies suggest that CYP2C19 and CYP3A4 are the principal enzymes involved in the initial oxidative metabolism of diazepam. Therefore, potential interactions may occur when diazepam is given concurrently with agents that affect CYP2C19 and CYP3A4 activity. Potential inducers of CYP3A4 could increase the rate of diazepam elimination).

No products indexed under this heading.

Buprenorphine Hydrochloride (Potential for synergistic CNS-depressant effect). Products include:

- Buprenex Injectable 2718
- Suboxone Tablets 2719
- Subutex Tablets 2719

Bupropion Hydrochloride (Potential for synergistic CNS-depressant effect). Products include:

- Wellbutrin Tablets 1579
- Wellbutrin SR Sustained-Release Tablets 1583
- Wellbutrin XL Extended-Release Tablets 1588
- Zyban Sustained-Release Tablets 1620

Buspirone Hydrochloride (Potential for synergistic CNS-depressant effect).

No products indexed under this heading.

Busulfan (There are no reports as to which isoenzymes could be inhibited or induced by diazepam. But based on the fact that diazepam is a substrate for CYP2C19 and CYP3A4, it is possible that diazepam may interfere with the metabolism of drugs which are substrates for CYP2C19 and CYP3A4 leading to a potential drug-drug interaction). Products include:

- I.V. Busulfex 1125
- Myleran Tablets 1492

Butabarbital (Potential for synergistic CNS-depressant effect).

No products indexed under this heading.

Butalbital (Potential for synergistic CNS-depressant effect). Products include:

- Sedapap Tablets 50 mg/650 mg 2098

Carbamazepine (Inducers of CYP3A4, such as carbamazepine, could increase the rate of elimination of diazepam). Products include:

- Carbatrol Capsules 3174
- Equetro Extended-Release Capsules 3178
- Tegretol/Tegretol-XR 2278

Carisoprodol (There are no reports as to which isoenzymes could be inhibited or induced by diazepam. But based on the fact that diazepam is a substrate for CYP2C19 and CYP3A4, it is possible that diazepam may interfere with the metabolism of drugs which are substrates for CYP2C19 and CYP3A4 leading to a potential drug-drug interaction).

No products indexed under this heading.

Cerivastatin Sodium (There are no reports as to which isoenzymes could be inhibited or induced by diazepam. But based on the fact that diazepam is a substrate for CYP2C19 and CYP3A4, it is possible that diazepam may interfere with the metabolism of drugs which are substrates for CYP2C19 and CYP3A4 leading to a potential drug-drug interaction).

No products indexed under this heading.

Chlordiazepoxide (Potential for synergistic CNS-depressant effect).

No products indexed under this heading.

Chlordiazepoxide Hydrochloride (Potential for synergistic CNS-depressant effect). Products include:

- Librium Capsules 3349

Chlorpheniramine (There are no reports as to which isoenzymes could be inhibited or induced by diazepam. But based on the fact that diazepam is a substrate for CYP2C19 and CYP3A4, it is possible that diazepam may interfere with the metabolism of drugs which are substrates for CYP2C19 and CYP3A4 leading to a potential drug-drug interaction).

No products indexed under this heading.

Chlorpheniramine Maleate (There are no reports as to which isoenzymes could be inhibited or induced by diazepam. But based on the fact that diazepam is a substrate for CYP2C19 and CYP3A4, it is possible that diazepam may interfere with the metabolism of drugs which are substrates for CYP2C19 and CYP3A4 leading to a potential drug-drug interaction). Products include:

- Advil Allergy Sinus Caplets 737
- Advil Multi-Symptom Cold Caplets 738
- BC Allergy Sinus Cold Powder 612
- Contac Severe Cold and Flu Caplets Maximum Strength 615
- Hycomine Compound Tablets 1105
- PediaCare Multi-Symptom Cold Liquid 704
- PediaCare NightRest Cough & Cold Liquid 704
- Robitussin Flu Liquid 752
- Robitussin PM Cough & Cold Liquid 752
- Singlet Caplets 636
- Sudafed Sinus & Allergy Tablets 710
- TheraFlu Cold & Cough Hot Liquid 680
- TheraFlu Cold & Sore Throat Hot Liquid 680
- TheraFlu Flu & Sore Throat Hot Liquid 681
- TheraFlu Severe Cold & Cough Hot Liquid 683
- TheraFlu Severe Cold Caplets 679
- TheraFlu Severe Cold Hot Liquid 682
- Triaminic Cold & Allergy Liquid 685
- Triaminic Cold & Cough Liquid 685
- Triaminic Flu, Cough & Fever Liquid 685
- Triaminic Night Time Cough & Cold Liquid 685
- Triaminic Allergy Runny Nose & Congestion Softchews 688
- Triaminic Cold & Cough Softchews 688
- Children's Tylenol Plus Cold NightTime Suspension Liquid 1851
- Children's Tylenol Plus Cold & Cough Suspension Liquid and Chewable Tablets 1851
- Children's Tylenol Plus Cold Chewable Tablets 1851
- Children's Tylenol Plus Flu Suspension Liquid 1853
- Tylenol Allergy Complete Multi-Symptom Caplets and Gelcaps with Cool Burst 1844
- Multi-Symptom Tylenol Cold Night Time Caplets 1845
- Vicks 44M Cough, Cold & Flu Relief 2676
- Pediatric Vicks 44m Cough & Cold Relief 2673
- Children's Vicks NyQuil Cold/Cough Relief 2671

Chlorpheniramine Polistirex (There are no reports as to which isoenzymes could be inhibited or induced by diazepam. But based on the fact that diazepam is a substrate for CYP2C19 and CYP3A4, it is possible that diazepam may interfere with the metabolism of drugs which are substrates for CYP2C19 and CYP3A4 leading to a potential drug-drug interaction). Products include:

- Tussionex Pennkinetic Extended-Release Suspension 3322

Chlorpheniramine Tannate (There are no reports as to which isoenzymes could be inhibited or induced by diazepam. But based on the fact that diazepam is a substrate for CYP2C19 and CYP3A4, it is possible that diazepam may interfere with the metabolism of drugs which are substrates for CYP2C19 and CYP3A4 leading to a potential drug-drug interaction).

No products indexed under this heading.

Chlorpromazine (Potential for synergistic CNS-depressant effect).

No products indexed under this heading.

Chlorpromazine Hydrochloride (Potential for synergistic CNS-depressant effect).

No products indexed under this heading.

Chlorprothixene (Potential for synergistic CNS-depressant effect).

No products indexed under this heading.

Chlorprothixene Hydrochloride (Potential for synergistic CNS-depressant effect).

No products indexed under this heading.

Chlorprothixene Lactate (Potential for synergistic CNS-depressant effect).

No products indexed under this heading.

Cilostazol (There are no reports as to which isoenzymes could be inhibited or induced by diazepam. But based on the fact that diazepam is a substrate for CYP2C19 and CYP3A4, it is possible that diazepam may interfere with the metabolism of drugs which are substrates for CYP2C19 and CYP3A4 leading to a potential drug-drug interaction). Products include:

- Pletal Tablets 2478

Cimetidine (Potential inhibitors of CYP2C19, such as cimetidine, could decrease the rate of diazepam elimination). Products include:
- Tagamet HB 200 Tablets ... ▣ 637
- Tagamet Tablets ... **1547**

Cimetidine Hydrochloride (Potential inhibitors of CYP2C19, such as cimetidine, could decrease the rate of diazepam elimination).
No products indexed under this heading.

Ciprofloxacin (Studies suggest that CYP2C19 and CYP3A4 are the principal enzymes involved in the initial oxidative metabolism of diazepam. Therefore, potential interactions may occur when diazepam is given concurrently with agents that affect CYP2C19 and CYP3A4 activity. Potential inhibitors of CYP3A4 could decrease the rate of diazepam elimination). Products include:
- Cipro I.V. ... **2998**
- Cipro I.V. Pharmacy Bulk Package ... **3509**
- Cipro Oral Suspension ... **2991**
- Cipro XR Tablets ... **3004**
- Ciprodex Otic Suspension ... **555**

Ciprofloxacin Hydrochloride (Studies suggest that CYP2C19 and CYP3A4 are the principal enzymes involved in the initial oxidative metabolism of diazepam. Therefore, potential interactions may occur when diazepam is given concurrently with agents that affect CYP2C19 and CYP3A4 activity. Potential inducers of CYP3A4 could increase the rate of diazepam elimination). Products include:
- Ciloxan Ophthalmic Ointment ... **554**
- Cipro Tablets ... **2991**

Cisapride (There are no reports as to which isoenzymes could be inhibited or induced by diazepam. But based on the fact that diazepam is a substrate for CYP2C19 and CYP3A4, it is possible that diazepam may interfere with the metabolism of drugs which are substrates for CYP2C19 and CYP3A4 leading to a potential drug-drug interaction).
No products indexed under this heading.

Cisplatin (Studies suggest that CYP2C19 and CYP3A4 are the principal enzymes involved in the initial oxidative metabolism of diazepam. Therefore, potential interactions may occur when diazepam is given concurrently with agents that affect CYP2C19 and CYP3A4 activity. Potential inducers of CYP3A4 could increase the rate of diazepam elimination).
No products indexed under this heading.

Citalopram Hydrobromide (Potential for synergistic CNS-depressant effect). Products include:
- Celexa ... **1177**

Clarithromycin (Studies suggest that CYP2C19 and CYP3A4 are the principal enzymes involved in the initial oxidative metabolism of diazepam. Therefore, potential interactions may occur when diazepam is given concurrently with agents that affect CYP2C19 and CYP3A4 activity. Potential inhibitors of CYP3A4 could decrease the rate of diazepam elimination). Products include:
- Biaxin/Biaxin XL ... **402**
- PREVPAC ... **3281**

Clomipramine Hydrochloride (There are no reports as to which isoenzymes could be inhibited or induced by diazepam. But based on the fact that diazepam is a substrate for CYP2C19 and CYP3A4, it is possible that diazepam may interfere with the metabolism of drugs which are substrates for CYP2C19 and CYP3A4 leading to a potential drug-drug interaction).
No products indexed under this heading.

Clorazepate Dipotassium (Potential for synergistic CNS-depressant effect). Products include:
- Tranxene ... **2488**

Clotrimazole (Potential inhibitors of CYP3A4, such as clotrimazole, could decrease the rate of diazepam elimination). Products include:
- Lotrimin ... **3053**
- Lotrisone ... **3054**

Clozapine (Potential for synergistic CNS-depressant effect). Products include:
- Clozapine Tablets ... **2141**
- Clozaril Tablets ... **2174**
- FazaClo Orally Disintegrating Tablets ... **547**

Codeine Phosphate (Potential for synergistic CNS-depressant effect). Products include:
- Tylenol with Codeine ... **2461**

Cortisone Acetate (Studies suggest that CYP2C19 and CYP3A4 are the principal enzymes involved in the initial oxidative metabolism of diazepam. Therefore, potential interactions may occur when diazepam is given concurrently with agents that affect CYP2C19 and CYP3A4 activity. Potential inducers of CYP3A4 could increase the rate of diazepam elimination).
No products indexed under this heading.

Cyclophosphamide (There are no reports as to which isoenzymes could be inhibited or induced by diazepam. But based on the fact that diazepam is a substrate for CYP2C19 and CYP3A4, it is possible that diazepam may interfere with the metabolism of drugs which are substrates for CYP2C19 and CYP3A4 leading to a potential drug-drug interaction).
No products indexed under this heading.

Cyclosporine (Diazepam is a substrate of CYP2C19 and CYP3A4, it is possible that diazepam may interfere with the metabolism of drugs which are substrates for CYP3A4, such as cyclosporine). Products include:
- Gengraf Capsules ... **458**
- Neoral Soft Gelatin Capsules ... **2247**
- Neoral Oral Solution ... **2247**
- Restasis Ophthalmic Emulsion ... **570**
- Sandimmune ... **2259**

Dalfopristin (Studies suggest that CYP2C19 and CYP3A4 are the principal enzymes involved in the initial oxidative metabolism of diazepam. Therefore, potential interactions may occur when diazepam is given concurrently with agents that affect CYP2C19 and CYP3A4 activity. Potential inhibitors of CYP3A4 could decrease the rate of diazepam elimination). Products include:
- Synercid I.V. ... **1690**

Danazol (Studies suggest that CYP2C19 and CYP3A4 are the principal enzymes involved in the initial oxidative metabolism of diazepam. Therefore, potential interactions may occur when diazepam is given concurrently with agents that affect CYP2C19 and CYP3A4 activity. Potential inhibitors of CYP3A4 could decrease the rate of diazepam elimination).
No products indexed under this heading.

Delavirdine Mesylate (Studies suggest that CYP2C19 and CYP3A4 are the principal enzymes involved in the initial oxidative metabolism of diazepam. Therefore, potential interactions may occur when diazepam is given concurrently with agents that affect CYP2C19 and CYP3A4 activity. Potential inhibitors of CYP2C19 could decrease the rate of diazepam elimination). Products include:
- Rescriptor Tablets ... **2535**

Desflurane (Potential for synergistic CNS-depressant effect). Products include:
- Suprane Liquid for Inhalation ... **770**

Desipramine Hydrochloride (Potential for synergistic CNS-depressant effect).
No products indexed under this heading.

Desogestrel (Studies suggest that CYP2C19 and CYP3A4 are the principal enzymes involved in the initial oxidative metabolism of diazepam. Therefore, potential interactions may occur when diazepam is given concurrently with agents that affect CYP2C19 and CYP3A4 activity. Potential inhibitors of CYP2C19 could decrease the rate of diazepam elimination). Products include:
- Ortho-Cept Tablets ... **2395**

Dexamethasone (Potential inducers of CYP3A4, such as dexamethasone, could increase the rate of elimination of diazepam). Products include:
- Ciprodex Otic Suspension ... **555**
- Decadron Tablets ... **1929**
- TobraDex Ophthalmic Ointment ... **558**
- TobraDex Ophthalmic Suspension ... **558**

Dexamethasone Acetate (Potential inducers of CYP3A4, such as dexamethasone, could increase the rate of elimination of diazepam).
No products indexed under this heading.

Dexamethasone Sodium Phosphate (Potential inducers of CYP3A4, such as dexamethasone, could increase the rate of elimination of diazepam). Products include:
- Decadron Phosphate Injection ... **1931**

Dextromethorphan (There are no reports as to which isoenzymes could be inhibited or induced by diazepam. But based on the fact that diazepam is a substrate for CYP2C19 and CYP3A4, it is possible that diazepam may interfere with the metabolism of drugs which are substrates for CYP2C19 and CYP3A4 leading to a potential drug-drug interaction).
No products indexed under this heading.

Dextromethorphan Hydrobromide (There are no reports as to which isoenzymes could be inhibited or induced by diazepam. But based on the fact that diazepam is a substrate for CYP2C19 and CYP3A4, it is possible that diazepam may interfere with the metabolism of drugs which are substrates for CYP2C19 and CYP3A4 leading to a potential drug-drug interaction). Products include:
- Alacol DM Syrup ... **739**
- Balamine DM ... **739**
- Contac Severe Cold and Flu Caplets Maximum Strength ... ▣ 615
- Contac Severe Cold and Flu Caplets Non-Drowsy ... ▣ 615
- Children's Dimetapp DM Cold & Cough Elixir ... ▣ 745
- Children's Dimetapp Long Acting Cough Plus Cold Syrup ... ▣ 746
- Dimetapp Infant Drops Decongestant Plus Cough ... ▣ 746
- Mucinex DM Tablets ... ▣ 602
- PediaCare Decongestant & Cough Infant Drops ... ▣ 705
- PediaCare Freezer Pops Long-Acting Cough-Glacier Grape and Polar Berry Blue ... ▣ 706
- PediaCare Long-Acting Cough Infant Drops ... ▣ 705
- PediaCare Long-Acting Cough Plus Cold Liquid ... ▣ 704
- PediaCare Multi-Symptom Cold Liquid ... ▣ 704
- PediaCare NightRest Cough & Cold Liquid ... ▣ 704
- Robitussin Allergy & Cough Syrup ... ▣ 750
- Robitussin CF Liquid ... ▣ 755
- Robitussin Cough & Cold Liquid-filled Capsules ... ▣ 750
- Robitussin Cough, Cold & Flu Liquid-filled Capsules ... ▣ 750
- Robitussin Cough & Cold Infant Drops ... ▣ 755
- Robitussin DM Infant Drops ... ▣ 753
- Robitussin DM Liquid ... ▣ 753
- Robitussin Flu Liquid ... ▣ 752
- Robitussin Maximum Strength Cough Liquid ... ▣ 754
- Robitussin Maximum Strength Cough & Cold Liquid ... ▣ 754
- Robitussin Pediatric Cough Liquid ... ▣ 754
- Robitussin Pediatric Cough & Cold Liquid ... ▣ 754
- Robitussin PM Cough & Cold Liquid ... ▣ 752
- Robitussin Sugar Free Cough Liquid ... ▣ 753
- Simply Cough Liquid ... **1840**
- Sudafed Severe Cold ... ▣ 710
- TheraFlu Cold & Cough Hot Liquid ... ▣ 680
- TheraFlu Flu & Chest Congestion Non-Drowsy Hot Liquid ... ▣ 681
- TheraFlu Severe Cold Non-Drowsy Hot Liquid ... ▣ 683
- TheraFlu Severe Cold & Cough Hot Liquid ... ▣ 683
- TheraFlu Severe Cold Caplets ... ▣ 679
- TheraFlu Severe Cold Hot Liquid ... ▣ 682
- TheraFlu Severe Cold Non-Drowsy Caplets ... ▣ 679
- TheraFlu Thin Strips Long Acting Cough ... ▣ 684
- Triaminic Cold & Cough Liquid ... ▣ 685
- Triaminic Cough Liquid ... ▣ 687
- Triaminic Cough & Nasal Congestion Liquid ... ▣ 687
- Triaminic Cough & Sore Throat Liquid ... ▣ 687
- Triaminic Flu, Cough & Fever Liquid ... ▣ 685
- Triaminic Night Time Cough & Cold Liquid ... ▣ 685
- Triaminic Cold & Cough Softchews ... ▣ 688
- Triaminic Cough & Sore Throat Softchews ... ▣ 689
- Triaminic Thin Strips Long Acting Cough ... ▣ 689
- Children's Tylenol Plus Cold & Cough Suspension Liquid and Chewable Tablets ... **1851**
- Children's Tylenol Plus Flu Suspension Liquid ... **1853**
- Concentrated Tylenol Infants' Drops Plus Cold and Cough ... **1851**
- Tylenol Cold & Flu Severe Daytime Liquid with Cool Burst ... **1846**

Tylenol Cold & Flu Severe NightTime Liquid with Cool Burst 1846
Tylenol Cold Severe Congestion Non-Drowsy Caplets with Cool Burst 1846
Tylenol Cough & Sore Throat Daytime Liquid with Cool Burst 1849
Tylenol Cough & Sore Throat NightTime Liquid with Cool Burst 1849
Tylenol Flu Day Non-Drowsy Gelcaps 1846
Concentrated Tylenol Infants' Drops Plus Cold & Cough Nasal Decongestant, Fever Reducer & Pain Reliever 668
Multi-Symptom Tylenol Cold Night Time Caplets 1845
Multi-Symptom Tylenol Cold Day Non-Drowsy Caplets and Gelcaps 1845
Vicks 44 Cough Relief 2675
Vicks 44D Cough & Head Congestion Relief 2676
Vicks 44D Cough & Head Congestion Relief Liquid 721
Vicks 44E Cough & Chest Congestion Relief 2676
Pediatric Vicks 44e Cough & Chest Congestion Relief Liquid 2673
Vicks 44M Cough, Cold & Flu Relief 2676
Pediatric Vicks 44m Cough & Cold Relief 2673
Vicks DayQuil LiquiCaps/Liquid Multi-Symptom Cold/Flu Relief 723
Vicks DayQuil Multi-Symptom Cold/Flu Relief LiquiCaps 2675
Vicks DayQuil Multi-Symptom Cold/Flu Relief Liquid 2675
Children's Vicks NyQuil Cold/Cough Relief 2671
Vicks NyQuil Cough Liquid 2677
Vicks NyQuil LiquiCaps 2677
Vicks NyQuil LiquiCaps/Liquid Multi-Symptom Cold/Flu Relief 725
Vicks NyQuil Liquid 2677
Zicam Concentrated Cough Mist for Kids Cool Cherry 643
Zicam Concentrated Cough Mist for Kids Plus D Cool Cherry 643
Zicam Concentrated Cough Mist Nite-Cool Cherry 642
Zicam Concentrated Cough Mist Plus D Cool Cherry 642
Zicam Concentrated Cough Mist-Honey Lemon & Cool Cherry 642

Dezocine (Potential for synergistic CNS-depressant effect).
No products indexed under this heading.

Dihydroergotamine Mesylate (There are no reports as to which isoenzymes could be inhibited or induced by diazepam. But based on the fact that diazepam is a substrate for CYP2C19 and CYP3A4, it is possible that diazepam may interfere with the metabolism of drugs which are substrates for CYP2C19 and CYP3A4 leading to a potential drug-drug interaction). Products include:
Migranal Nasal Spray 3350

Diltiazem Hydrochloride (Studies suggest that CYP2C19 and CYP3A4 are the principal enzymes involved in the initial oxidative metabolism of diazepam. Therefore, potential interactions may occur when diazepam is given concurrently with agents that affect CYP2C19 and CYP3A4 activity. Potential inhibitors of CYP3A4 could decrease the rate of diazepam elimination). Products include:
Cardizem LA Extended Release Tablets 1699
Tiazac Capsules 1204

Diltiazem Maleate (Studies suggest that CYP2C19 and CYP3A4 are the principal enzymes involved in the initial oxidative metabolism of diazepam. Therefore, potential interactions may occur when diazepam is given concurrently with agents that affect CYP2C19 and CYP3A4 activity. Potential inhibitors of CYP3A4 could decrease the rate of diazepam elimination).
No products indexed under this heading.

Disopyramide (There are no reports as to which isoenzymes could be inhibited or induced by diazepam. But based on the fact that diazepam is a substrate for CYP2C19 and CYP3A4, it is possible that diazepam may interfere with the metabolism of drugs which are substrates for CYP2C19 and CYP3A4 leading to a potential drug-drug interaction).
No products indexed under this heading.

Disopyramide Phosphate (There are no reports as to which isoenzymes could be inhibited or induced by diazepam. But based on the fact that diazepam is a substrate for CYP2C19 and CYP3A4, it is possible that diazepam may interfere with the metabolism of drugs which are substrates for CYP2C19 and CYP3A4 leading to a potential drug-drug interaction).
No products indexed under this heading.

Disulfiram (There are no reports as to which isoenzymes could be inhibited or induced by diazepam. But based on the fact that diazepam is a substrate for CYP2C19 and CYP3A4, it is possible that diazepam may interfere with the metabolism of drugs which are substrates for CYP2C19 and CYP3A4 leading to a potential drug-drug interaction). Products include:
Antabuse Tablets 2343

Divalproex Sodium (Valproate may potentiate the CNS-depressant effect). Products include:
Depakote Sprinkle Capsules 422
Depakote Tablets 427
Depakote ER Tablets 433

Doxepin Hydrochloride (Potential for synergistic CNS-depressant effect).
No products indexed under this heading.

Doxorubicin Hydrochloride (Studies suggest that CYP2C19 and CYP3A4 are the principal enzymes involved in the initial oxidative metabolism of diazepam. Therefore, potential interactions may occur when diazepam is given concurrently with agents that affect CYP2C19 and CYP3A4 activity. Potential inducers of CYP3A4 could increase the rate of diazepam elimination). Products include:
Adriamycin for Injection, USP 786
Adriamycin Injection, USP 786

Dronabinol (There are no reports as to which isoenzymes could be inhibited or induced by diazepam. But based on the fact that diazepam is a substrate for CYP2C19 and CYP3A4, it is possible that diazepam may interfere with the metabolism of drugs which are substrates for CYP2C19 and CYP3A4 leading to a potential drug-drug interaction). Products include:
Marinol Capsules 3334

Droperidol (Potential for synergistic CNS-depressant effect).
No products indexed under this heading.

Dyphylline (Diazepam is a substrate of CYP2C19 and CYP3A4, it is possible that diazepam may interfere with the metabolism of drugs which are substrates for CYP3A4, such as theophylline).
No products indexed under this heading.

Efavirenz (Studies suggest that CYP2C19 and CYP3A4 are the principal enzymes involved in the initial oxidative metabolism of diazepam. Therefore, potential interactions may occur when diazepam is given concurrently with agents that affect CYP2C19 and CYP3A4 activity. Potential inhibitors of CYP2C19 could decrease the rate of diazepam elimination). Products include:
Sustiva Capsules 957

Enflurane (Potential for synergistic CNS-depressant effect).
No products indexed under this heading.

Ergotamine Tartrate (There are no reports as to which isoenzymes could be inhibited or induced by diazepam. But based on the fact that diazepam is a substrate for CYP2C19 and CYP3A4, it is possible that diazepam may interfere with the metabolism of drugs which are substrates for CYP2C19 and CYP3A4 leading to a potential drug-drug interaction).
No products indexed under this heading.

Erythromycin (Studies suggest that CYP2C19 and CYP3A4 are the principal enzymes involved in the initial oxidative metabolism of diazepam. Therefore, potential interactions may occur when diazepam is given concurrently with agents that affect CYP2C19 and CYP3A4 activity. Potential inhibitors of CYP3A4 could decrease the rate of diazepam elimination). Products include:
Erygel Topical Gel 2096
Ery-Tab Tablets 447
Erythromycin Base Filmtab Tablets 454
Erythromycin Delayed-Release Capsules, USP 456
PCE Dispertab Tablets 510

Erythromycin Estolate (Studies suggest that CYP2C19 and CYP3A4 are the principal enzymes involved in the initial oxidative metabolism of diazepam. Therefore, potential interactions may occur when diazepam is given concurrently with agents that affect CYP2C19 and CYP3A4 activity. Potential inhibitors of CYP3A4 could decrease the rate of diazepam elimination).
No products indexed under this heading.

Erythromycin Ethylsuccinate (Studies suggest that CYP2C19 and CYP3A4 are the principal enzymes involved in the initial oxidative metabolism of diazepam. Therefore, potential interactions may occur when diazepam is given concurrently with agents that affect CYP2C19 and CYP3A4 activity. Potential inhibitors of CYP3A4 could decrease the rate of diazepam elimination). Products include:
E.E.S. 449
EryPed 445

Erythromycin Gluceptate (Studies suggest that CYP2C19 and CYP3A4 are the principal enzymes involved in the initial oxidative metabolism of diazepam. Therefore, potential interactions may occur when diazepam is given concurrently with agents that affect CYP2C19 and CYP3A4 activity. Potential inhibitors of CYP3A4 could decrease the rate of diazepam elimination).
No products indexed under this heading.

Erythromycin Lactobionate (Studies suggest that CYP2C19 and CYP3A4 are the principal enzymes involved in the initial oxidative metabolism of diazepam. Therefore, potential interactions may occur when diazepam is given concurrently with agents that affect CYP2C19 and CYP3A4 activity. Potential inhibitors of CYP3A4 could decrease the rate of diazepam elimination).
No products indexed under this heading.

Erythromycin Stearate (Studies suggest that CYP2C19 and CYP3A4 are the principal enzymes involved in the initial oxidative metabolism of diazepam. Therefore, potential interactions may occur when diazepam is given concurrently with agents that affect CYP2C19 and CYP3A4 activity. Potential inhibitors of CYP3A4 could decrease the rate of diazepam elimination). Products include:
Erythrocin Stearate Filmtab Tablets 452

Escitalopram Oxalate (Potential for synergistic CNS-depressant effect). Products include:
Lexapro Oral Solution 1193
Lexapro Tablets 1193

Esomeprazole Magnesium (Studies suggest that CYP2C19 and CYP3A4 are the principal enzymes involved in the initial oxidative metabolism of diazepam. Therefore, potential interactions may occur when diazepam is given concurrently with agents that affect CYP2C19 and CYP3A4 activity. Potential inhibitors of CYP3A4 could decrease the rate of diazepam elimination). Products include:
Nexium Delayed-Release Capsules 645

Estazolam (Potential for synergistic CNS-depressant effect). Products include:
ProSom Tablets 512

Estradiol (There are no reports as to which isoenzymes could be inhibited or induced by diazepam. But based on the fact that diazepam is a substrate for CYP2C19 and CYP3A4, it is possible that diazepam may interfere with the metabolism of drugs which are substrates for CYP2C19 and CYP3A4 leading to a potential drug-drug interaction). Products include:
Activella Tablets 2311
Climara Transdermal System 795
Climara Pro Transdermal System 800
CombiPatch Transdermal System 2180
Estrogel 0.06% 3200
Menostar Transdermal System 805
Prefest Tablets 1069
Vagifem Tablets 2340
Vivelle Transdermal System 2288
Vivelle-Dot Transdermal System 2293

IMPORTANT NOTE: Always consult each drug listing in the patient's regimen for possible interactions.

Estradiol Benzoate (There are no reports as to which isoenzymes could be inhibited or induced by diazepam. But based on the fact that diazepam is a substrate for CYP2C19 and CYP3A4, it is possible that diazepam may interfere with the metabolism of drugs which are substrates for CYP2C19 and CYP3A4 leading to a potential drug-drug interaction).

No products indexed under this heading.

Estradiol Cypionate (There are no reports as to which isoenzymes could be inhibited or induced by diazepam. But based on the fact that diazepam is a substrate for CYP2C19 and CYP3A4, it is possible that diazepam may interfere with the metabolism of drugs which are substrates for CYP2C19 and CYP3A4 leading to a potential drug-drug interaction).

No products indexed under this heading.

Estradiol Valerate (There are no reports as to which isoenzymes could be inhibited or induced by diazepam. But based on the fact that diazepam is a substrate for CYP2C19 and CYP3A4, it is possible that diazepam may interfere with the metabolism of drugs which are substrates for CYP2C19 and CYP3A4 leading to a potential drug-drug interaction).

No products indexed under this heading.

Ethanol (Potential for synergistic CNS-depressant effect).

No products indexed under this heading.

Ethchlorvynol (Potential for synergistic CNS-depressant effect).

No products indexed under this heading.

Ethinamate (Potential for synergistic CNS-depressant effect).

No products indexed under this heading.

Ethinyl Estradiol (Studies suggest that CYP2C19 and CYP3A4 are the principal enzymes involved in the initial oxidative metabolism of diazepam. Therefore, potential interactions may occur when diazepam is given concurrently with agents that affect CYP2C19 and CYP3A4 activity. Potential inhibitors of CYP2C19 could decrease the rate of diazepam elimination). Products include:

Alesse-28 Tablets 3392
Lo/Ovral-28 Tablets 3423
NuvaRing 2357
Ortho-Cept Tablets 2395
Ortho-Cyclen/Ortho Tri-Cyclen 2414
Ortho Evra Transdermal System 2402
Ortho Tri-Cyclen Lo Tablets 2421
Seasonale Tablets 1073
Triphasil-28 Tablets 3483
Yasmin 28 Tablets 818

Ethosuximide (Studies suggest that CYP2C19 and CYP3A4 are the principal enzymes involved in the initial oxidative metabolism of diazepam. Therefore, potential interactions may occur when diazepam is given concurrently with agents that affect CYP2C19 and CYP3A4 activity. Potential inducers of CYP3A4 could increase the rate of diazepam elimination).

No products indexed under this heading.

Ethotoin (There are no reports as to which isoenzymes could be inhibited or induced by diazepam. But based on the fact that diazepam is a substrate for CYP2C19 and CYP3A4, it is possible that diazepam may interfere with the metabolism of drugs which are substrates for CYP2C19 and CYP3A4 leading to a potential drug-drug interaction). Products include:

Peganone Tablets, USP 2487

Ethyl Alcohol (Potential for synergistic CNS-depressant effect).

No products indexed under this heading.

Ethynodiol Diacetate (Studies suggest that CYP2C19 and CYP3A4 are the principal enzymes involved in the initial oxidative metabolism of diazepam. Therefore, potential interactions may occur when diazepam is given concurrently with agents that affect CYP2C19 and CYP3A4 activity. Potential inhibitors of CYP2C19 could decrease the rate of diazepam elimination).

No products indexed under this heading.

Etoposide (There are no reports as to which isoenzymes could be inhibited or induced by diazepam. But based on the fact that diazepam is a substrate for CYP2C19 and CYP3A4, it is possible that diazepam may interfere with the metabolism of drugs which are substrates for CYP2C19 and CYP3A4 leading to a potential drug-drug interaction).

No products indexed under this heading.

Etoposide Phosphate (There are no reports as to which isoenzymes could be inhibited or induced by diazepam. But based on the fact that diazepam is a substrate for CYP2C19 and CYP3A4, it is possible that diazepam may interfere with the metabolism of drugs which are substrates for CYP2C19 and CYP3A4 leading to a potential drug-drug interaction).

No products indexed under this heading.

Felbamate (Studies suggest that CYP2C19 and CYP3A4 are the principal enzymes involved in the initial oxidative metabolism of diazepam. Therefore, potential interactions may occur when diazepam is given concurrently with agents that affect CYP2C19 and CYP3A4 activity. Potential inhibitors of CYP2C19 could decrease the rate of diazepam elimination).

No products indexed under this heading.

Felodipine (There are no reports as to which isoenzymes could be inhibited or induced by diazepam. But based on the fact that diazepam is a substrate for CYP2C19 and CYP3A4, it is possible that diazepam may interfere with the metabolism of drugs which are substrates for CYP2C19 and CYP3A4 leading to a potential drug-drug interaction). Products include:

Plendil Extended-Release Tablets 651

Fentanyl (Potential for synergistic CNS-depressant effect). Products include:

Duragesic Transdermal System 2448

Fentanyl Citrate (Potential for synergistic CNS-depressant effect). Products include:

Actiq 993

Fluconazole (Studies suggest that CYP2C19 and CYP3A4 are the principal enzymes involved in the initial oxidative metabolism of diazepam. Therefore, potential interactions may occur when diazepam is given concurrently with agents that affect CYP2C19 and CYP3A4 activity. Potential inhibitors of CYP3A4 could decrease the rate of diazepam elimination).

No products indexed under this heading.

Fludrocortisone Acetate (Studies suggest that CYP2C19 and CYP3A4 are the principal enzymes involved in the initial oxidative metabolism of diazepam. Therefore, potential interactions may occur when diazepam is given concurrently with agents that affect CYP2C19 and CYP3A4 activity. Potential inducers of CYP3A4 could increase the rate of diazepam elimination).

No products indexed under this heading.

Fluoxetine (Studies suggest that CYP2C19 and CYP3A4 are the principal enzymes involved in the initial oxidative metabolism of diazepam. Therefore, potential interactions may occur when diazepam is given concurrently with agents that affect CYP2C19 and CYP3A4 activity. Potential inhibitors of CYP2C19 could decrease the rate of diazepam elimination).

No products indexed under this heading.

Fluoxetine Hydrochloride (Potential for synergistic CNS-depressant effect). Products include:

Prozac Pulvules and Liquid 1771
Symbyax Capsules 1788

Fluphenazine Decanoate (Potential for synergistic CNS-depressant effect).

No products indexed under this heading.

Fluphenazine Enanthate (Potential for synergistic CNS-depressant effect).

No products indexed under this heading.

Fluphenazine Hydrochloride (Potential for synergistic CNS-depressant effect).

No products indexed under this heading.

Flurazepam Hydrochloride (Potential for synergistic CNS-depressant effect). Products include:

Dalmane Capsules 3343

Fluvastatin Sodium (Studies suggest that CYP2C19 and CYP3A4 are the principal enzymes involved in the initial oxidative metabolism of diazepam. Therefore, potential interactions may occur when diazepam is given concurrently with agents that affect CYP2C19 and CYP3A4 activity. Potential inhibitors of CYP2C19 could decrease the rate of diazepam elimination). Products include:

Lescol Capsules 2227
Lescol 2730
Lescol XL Tablets 2227

Fluvoxamine (Studies suggest that CYP2C19 and CYP3A4 are the principal enzymes involved in the initial oxidative metabolism of diazepam. Therefore, potential interactions may occur when diazepam is given concurrently with agents that affect CYP2C19 and CYP3A4 activity. Potential inhibitors of CYP2C19 could decrease the rate of diazepam elimination).

No products indexed under this heading.

Fluvoxamine Maleate (Studies suggest that CYP2C19 and CYP3A4 are the principal enzymes involved in the initial oxidative metabolism of diazepam. Therefore, potential interactions may occur when diazepam is given concurrently with agents that affect CYP2C19 and CYP3A4 activity. Potential inhibitors of CYP2C19 could decrease the rate of diazepam elimination).

No products indexed under this heading.

Formoterol Fumarate (There are no reports as to which isoenzymes could be inhibited or induced by diazepam. But based on the fact that diazepam is a substrate for CYP2C19 and CYP3A4, it is possible that diazepam may interfere with the metabolism of drugs which are substrates for CYP2C19 and CYP3A4 leading to a potential drug-drug interaction). Products include:

Foradil Aerolizer 3024

Fosamprenavir Calcium (Studies suggest that CYP2C19 and CYP3A4 are the principal enzymes involved in the initial oxidative metabolism of diazepam. Therefore, potential interactions may occur when diazepam is given concurrently with agents that affect CYP2C19 and CYP3A4 activity. Potential inhibitors of CYP3A4 could decrease the rate of diazepam elimination). Products include:

Lexiva Tablets 1473

Fosphenytoin (There are no reports as to which isoenzymes could be inhibited or induced by diazepam. But based on the fact that diazepam is a substrate for CYP2C19 and CYP3A4, it is possible that diazepam may interfere with the metabolism of drugs which are substrates for CYP2C19 and CYP3A4 leading to a potential drug-drug interaction).

No products indexed under this heading.

Fosphenytoin Sodium (Inducers of CYP3A4, such as phenytoin, could increase the rate of elimination of diazepam).

No products indexed under this heading.

Gabapentin (There are no reports as to which isoenzymes could be inhibited or induced by diazepam. But based on the fact that diazepam is a substrate for CYP2C19 and CYP3A4, it is possible that diazepam may interfere with the metabolism of drugs which are substrates for CYP2C19 and CYP3A4 leading to a potential drug-drug interaction). Products include:

Neurontin Capsules 2498
Neurontin Oral Solution 2498
Neurontin Tablets 2498

Garlic Extract (Studies suggest that CYP2C19 and CYP3A4 are the principal enzymes involved in the initial oxidative metabolism of diazepam. Therefore, potential interactions may occur when diazepam is given concurrently with agents that affect CYP2C19 and CYP3A4 activity. Potential inducers of CYP3A4 could increase the rate of diazepam elimination).
No products indexed under this heading.

Garlic Oil (Studies suggest that CYP2C19 and CYP3A4 are the principal enzymes involved in the initial oxidative metabolism of diazepam. Therefore, potential interactions may occur when diazepam is given concurrently with agents that affect CYP2C19 and CYP3A4 activity. Potential inducers of CYP3A4 could increase the rate of diazepam elimination).
No products indexed under this heading.

Glutethimide (Potential for synergistic CNS-depressant effect).
No products indexed under this heading.

Haloperidol (Potential for synergistic CNS-depressant effect).
No products indexed under this heading.

Haloperidol Decanoate (Potential for synergistic CNS-depressant effect).
No products indexed under this heading.

Haloperidol Lactate (There are no reports as to which isoenzymes could be inhibited or induced by diazepam. But based on the fact that diazepam is a substrate for CYP2C19 and CYP3A4, it is possible that diazepam may interfere with the metabolism of drugs which are substrates for CYP2C19 and CYP3A4 leading to a potential drug-drug interaction).
No products indexed under this heading.

Hydrocodone Bitartrate (Potential for synergistic CNS-depressant effect). Products include:
Hycodan 1104
Hycomine Compound Tablets 1105
Hycotuss Expectorant Syrup 1106
Lortab 3315
Lortab Elixir 3312
Vicodin Tablets 530
Vicodin ES Tablets 531
Vicodin HP Tablets 532
Vicoprofen Tablets 533
Zydone Tablets 1118

Hydrocodone Polistirex (Potential for synergistic CNS-depressant effect). Products include:
Tussionex Pennkinetic Extended-Release Suspension 3322

Hydrocortisone (Studies suggest that CYP2C19 and CYP3A4 are the principal enzymes involved in the initial oxidative metabolism of diazepam. Therefore, potential interactions may occur when diazepam is given concurrently with agents that affect CYP2C19 and CYP3A4 activity. Potential inducers of CYP3A4 could increase the rate of diazepam elimination). Products include:
Cortizone•5 Ointment 699
Cortizone•10 Creme 699
Cortizone•10 Ointment 699
Cortizone•10 Plus Creme 700
Cortizone•10 Maximum Strength Quick Shot Spray 700
Hydrocortone Tablets 1963
Preparation H Hydrocortisone Cream 748

Hydrocortisone Acetate (Studies suggest that CYP2C19 and CYP3A4 are the principal enzymes involved in the initial oxidative metabolism of diazepam. Therefore, potential interactions may occur when diazepam is given concurrently with agents that affect CYP2C19 and CYP3A4 activity. Potential inducers of CYP3A4 could increase the rate of diazepam elimination). Products include:
Analpram-HC 1136
Pramosone 1139
ProctoFoam-HC 3113
Tucks Anti-Itch Ointment 712
U-cort 1% Cream 3289

Hydrocortisone Butyrate (Studies suggest that CYP2C19 and CYP3A4 are the principal enzymes involved in the initial oxidative metabolism of diazepam. Therefore, potential interactions may occur when diazepam is given concurrently with agents that affect CYP2C19 and CYP3A4 activity. Potential inducers of CYP3A4 could increase the rate of diazepam elimination). Products include:
Locoid 1138
Locoid Lipocream Cream 1138

Hydrocortisone Cypionate (Studies suggest that CYP2C19 and CYP3A4 are the principal enzymes involved in the initial oxidative metabolism of diazepam. Therefore, potential interactions may occur when diazepam is given concurrently with agents that affect CYP2C19 and CYP3A4 activity. Potential inducers of CYP3A4 could increase the rate of diazepam elimination).
No products indexed under this heading.

Hydrocortisone Hemisuccinate (Studies suggest that CYP2C19 and CYP3A4 are the principal enzymes involved in the initial oxidative metabolism of diazepam. Therefore, potential interactions may occur when diazepam is given concurrently with agents that affect CYP2C19 and CYP3A4 activity. Potential inducers of CYP3A4 could increase the rate of diazepam elimination).
No products indexed under this heading.

Hydrocortisone Probutate (Studies suggest that CYP2C19 and CYP3A4 are the principal enzymes involved in the initial oxidative metabolism of diazepam. Therefore, potential interactions may occur when diazepam is given concurrently with agents that affect CYP2C19 and CYP3A4 activity. Potential inducers of CYP3A4 could increase the rate of diazepam elimination). Products include:
Pandel Cream, 0.1% 1017

Hydrocortisone Sodium Phosphate (Studies suggest that CYP2C19 and CYP3A4 are the principal enzymes involved in the initial oxidative metabolism of diazepam. Therefore, potential interactions may occur when diazepam is given concurrently with agents that affect CYP2C19 and CYP3A4 activity. Potential inducers of CYP3A4 could increase the rate of diazepam elimination).
No products indexed under this heading.

Hydrocortisone Sodium Succinate (Studies suggest that CYP2C19 and CYP3A4 are the principal enzymes involved in the initial oxidative metabolism of diazepam. Therefore, potential interactions may occur when diazepam is given concurrently with agents that affect CYP2C19 and CYP3A4 activity. Potential inducers of CYP3A4 could increase the rate of diazepam elimination).
No products indexed under this heading.

Hydrocortisone Valerate (Studies suggest that CYP2C19 and CYP3A4 are the principal enzymes involved in the initial oxidative metabolism of diazepam. Therefore, potential interactions may occur when diazepam is given concurrently with agents that affect CYP2C19 and CYP3A4 activity. Potential inducers of CYP3A4 could increase the rate of diazepam elimination).
No products indexed under this heading.

Hydromorphone Hydrochloride (Potential for synergistic CNS-depressant effect). Products include:
Dilaudid 439
Dilaudid Oral Liquid 443
Dilaudid Non-Sterile Powder 439
Dilaudid Rectal Suppositories 439
Dilaudid Tablets 439
Dilaudid Tablets - 8 mg 443
Dilaudid-HP 441

Hydroxyzine Hydrochloride (Potential for synergistic CNS-depressant effect).
No products indexed under this heading.

Hypericum (Studies suggest that CYP2C19 and CYP3A4 are the principal enzymes involved in the initial oxidative metabolism of diazepam. Therefore, potential interactions may occur when diazepam is given concurrently with agents that affect CYP2C19 and CYP3A4 activity. Potential inducers of CYP3A4 could increase the rate of diazepam elimination).
No products indexed under this heading.

Hypericum Perforatum (Studies suggest that CYP2C19 and CYP3A4 are the principal enzymes involved in the initial oxidative metabolism of diazepam. Therefore, potential interactions may occur when diazepam is given concurrently with agents that affect CYP2C19 and CYP3A4 activity. Potential inducers of CYP3A4 could increase the rate of diazepam elimination).
No products indexed under this heading.

Imipramine Hydrochloride (Diazepam is a substrate of CYP2C19 and CYP3A4, it is possible that diazepam may interfere with the metabolism of drugs which are substrates for CYP2C19, such as imipramine; potential for synergistic CNS-depressant effect).
No products indexed under this heading.

Imipramine Pamoate (Diazepam is a substrate of CYP2C19 and CYP3A4, it is possible that diazepam may interfere with the metabolism of drugs which are substrates for CYP2C19, such as imipramine; potential for synergistic CNS-depressant effect).
No products indexed under this heading.

Indinavir Sulfate (Studies suggest that CYP2C19 and CYP3A4 are the principal enzymes involved in the initial oxidative metabolism of diazepam. Therefore, potential interactions may occur when diazepam is given concurrently with agents that affect CYP2C19 and CYP3A4 activity. Potential inhibitors of CYP3A4 could decrease the rate of diazepam elimination). Products include:
Crixivan Capsules 1918

Indomethacin (Studies suggest that CYP2C19 and CYP3A4 are the principal enzymes involved in the initial oxidative metabolism of diazepam. Therefore, potential interactions may occur when diazepam is given concurrently with agents that affect CYP2C19 and CYP3A4 activity. Potential inhibitors of CYP2C19 could decrease the rate of diazepam elimination). Products include:
Indocin 1968

Indomethacin Sodium Trihydrate (Studies suggest that CYP2C19 and CYP3A4 are the principal enzymes involved in the initial oxidative metabolism of diazepam. Therefore, potential interactions may occur when diazepam is given concurrently with agents that affect CYP2C19 and CYP3A4 activity. Potential inhibitors of CYP2C19 could decrease the rate of diazepam elimination). Products include:
Indocin I.V. 1973

Isocarboxazid (Potential for synergistic CNS-depressant effect).
No products indexed under this heading.

Isoflurane (Potential for synergistic CNS-depressant effect).
No products indexed under this heading.

Isoniazid (Studies suggest that CYP2C19 and CYP3A4 are the principal enzymes involved in the initial oxidative metabolism of diazepam. Therefore, potential interactions may occur when diazepam is given concurrently with agents that affect CYP2C19 and CYP3A4 activity. Potential inhibitors of CYP2C19 could decrease the rate of diazepam elimination).
No products indexed under this heading.

Isradipine (There are no reports as to which isoenzymes could be inhibited or induced by diazepam. But based on the fact that diazepam is a substrate for CYP2C19 and CYP3A4, it is possible that diazepam may interfere with the metabolism of drugs which are substrates for CYP2C19 and CYP3A4 leading to a potential drug-drug interaction). Products include:
DynaCirc CR Tablets 2726

Itraconazole (Studies suggest that CYP2C19 and CYP3A4 are the principal enzymes involved in the initial oxidative metabolism of diazepam. Therefore, potential interactions may occur when diazepam is given concurrently with agents that affect CYP2C19 and CYP3A4 activity. Potential inhibitors of CYP3A4 could decrease the rate of diazepam elimination).
No products indexed under this heading.

Ketamine Hydrochloride (Potential for synergistic CNS-depressant effect).
No products indexed under this heading.

Ketoconazole (Potential inhibitors of CYP3A4, such as ketoconazole, could decrease the rate of diazepam elimination). Products include:
- Nizoral A-D Shampoo, 1% 1839
- Nizoral 2% Shampoo 1838

Lamotrigine (There are no reports as to which isoenzymes could be inhibited or induced by diazepam. But based on the fact that diazepam is a substrate for CYP2C19 and CYP3A4, it is possible that diazepam may interfere with the metabolism of drugs which are substrates for CYP2C19 and CYP3A4 leading to a potential drug-drug interaction). Products include:
- Lamictal 1449

Lansoprazole (Studies suggest that CYP2C19 and CYP3A4 are the principal enzymes involved in the initial oxidative metabolism of diazepam. Therefore, potential interactions may occur when diazepam is given concurrently with agents that affect CYP2C19 and CYP3A4 activity. Potential inhibitors of CYP2C19 could decrease the rate of diazepam elimination). Products include:
- Prevacid Delayed-Release Capsules 3268
- Prevacid for Delayed-Release Oral Suspension 3268
- Prevacid I.V. for Injection 3274
- Prevacid NapraPAC 3277
- Prevacid SoluTab Delayed-Release Orally Disintegrating Tablets.................. 3268
- PREVPAC 3281

Letrozole (Studies suggest that CYP2C19 and CYP3A4 are the principal enzymes involved in the initial oxidative metabolism of diazepam. Therefore, potential interactions may occur when diazepam is given concurrently with agents that affect CYP2C19 and CYP3A4 activity. Potential inhibitors of CYP2C19 could decrease the rate of diazepam elimination). Products include:
- Femara Tablets 2210

Levetiracetam (There are no reports as to which isoenzymes could be inhibited or induced by diazepam. But based on the fact that diazepam is a substrate for CYP2C19 and CYP3A4, it is possible that diazepam may interfere with the metabolism of drugs which are substrates for CYP2C19 and CYP3A4 leading to a potential drug-drug interaction). Products include:
- Keppra Oral Solution 3307
- Keppra Tablets 3307

Levomethadyl Acetate Hydrochloride (Potential for synergistic CNS-depressant effect).
No products indexed under this heading.

Levonorgestrel (Studies suggest that CYP2C19 and CYP3A4 are the principal enzymes involved in the initial oxidative metabolism of diazepam. Therefore, potential interactions may occur when diazepam is given concurrently with agents that affect CYP2C19 and CYP3A4 activity. Potential inhibitors of CYP2C19 could decrease the rate of diazepam elimination). Products include:
- Alesse-28 Tablets 3392
- Climara Pro Transdermal System 800
- Mirena Intrauterine System 810
- Plan B Tablets 1068
- Seasonale Tablets 1073
- Triphasil-28 Tablets 3483

Levorphanol Tartrate (Potential for synergistic CNS-depressant effect).
No products indexed under this heading.

Lidocaine (There are no reports as to which isoenzymes could be inhibited or induced by diazepam. But based on the fact that diazepam is a substrate for CYP2C19 and CYP3A4, it is possible that diazepam may interfere with the metabolism of drugs which are substrates for CYP2C19 and CYP3A4 leading to a potential drug-drug interaction). Products include:
- Lidoderm Patch 1107

Lidocaine Hydrochloride (There are no reports as to which isoenzymes could be inhibited or induced by diazepam. But based on the fact that diazepam is a substrate for CYP2C19 and CYP3A4, it is possible that diazepam may interfere with the metabolism of drugs which are substrates for CYP2C19 and CYP3A4 leading to a potential drug-drug interaction).
No products indexed under this heading.

Lopinavir (Studies suggest that CYP2C19 and CYP3A4 are the principal enzymes involved in the initial oxidative metabolism of diazepam. Therefore, potential interactions may occur when diazepam is given concurrently with agents that affect CYP2C19 and CYP3A4 activity. Potential inhibitors of CYP3A4 could decrease the rate of diazepam elimination). Products include:
- Kaletra 474

Loratadine (Studies suggest that CYP2C19 and CYP3A4 are the principal enzymes involved in the initial oxidative metabolism of diazepam. Therefore, potential interactions may occur when diazepam is given concurrently with agents that affect CYP2C19 and CYP3A4 activity. Potential inhibitors of CYP3A4 could decrease the rate of diazepam elimination). Products include:
- Alavert Allergy & Sinus D-12 Hour Tablets.. ▣743
- Alavert .... ▣743
- Children's Claritin 24 Hour Non-Drowsy Allergy Syrup........... ▣732
- Claritin Non-Drowsy 24 Hour Tablets.. ▣731
- Non-Drowsy Claritin Hives Relief Tablets.. ▣733
- Claritin Reditabs 24 Hour Non-Drowsy Tablets.................... ▣732
- Claritin-D Non-Drowsy 12 Hour Tablets.. ▣731
- Claritin-D Non-Drowsy 24 Hour Tablets.. ▣731
- Children's Dimetapp ND Non-Drowsy Allergy Syrup........... ▣746
- Triaminic Allerchews .... ▣684

Lorazepam (Potential for synergistic CNS-depressant effect).
No products indexed under this heading.

Lovastatin (There are no reports as to which isoenzymes could be inhibited or induced by diazepam. But based on the fact that diazepam is a substrate for CYP2C19 and CYP3A4, it is possible that diazepam may interfere with the metabolism of drugs which are substrates for CYP2C19 and CYP3A4 leading to a potential drug-drug interaction). Products include:
- Advicor Tablets 1694
- Altoprev Extended-Release Tablets.. 1151
- Mevacor Tablets 1996

Loxapine Hydrochloride (Potential for synergistic CNS-depressant effect).
No products indexed under this heading.

Loxapine Succinate (Potential for synergistic CNS-depressant effect).
No products indexed under this heading.

Maprotiline Hydrochloride (Potential for synergistic CNS-depressant effect).
No products indexed under this heading.

Meperidine Hydrochloride (Potential for synergistic CNS-depressant effect).
No products indexed under this heading.

Mephenytoin (Studies suggest that CYP2C19 and CYP3A4 are the principal enzymes involved in the initial oxidative metabolism of diazepam. Therefore, potential interactions may occur when diazepam is given concurrently with agents that affect CYP2C19 and CYP3A4 activity. Potential inducers of CYP3A4 could increase the rate of diazepam elimination).
No products indexed under this heading.

Mephobarbital (Potential for synergistic CNS-depressant effect). Products include:
- Mebaral Tablets, USP 2483

Meprobamate (Potential for synergistic CNS-depressant effect).
No products indexed under this heading.

Mesoridazine Besylate (Potential for synergistic CNS-depressant effect).
No products indexed under this heading.

Mestranol (Studies suggest that CYP2C19 and CYP3A4 are the principal enzymes involved in the initial oxidative metabolism of diazepam. Therefore, potential interactions may occur when diazepam is given concurrently with agents that affect CYP2C19 and CYP3A4 activity. Potential inhibitors of CYP2C19 could decrease the rate of diazepam elimination).
No products indexed under this heading.

Methadone Hydrochloride (Potential for synergistic CNS-depressant effect).
No products indexed under this heading.

Methohexital Sodium (Potential for synergistic CNS-depressant effect).
No products indexed under this heading.

Methotrimeprazine (Potential for synergistic CNS-depressant effect).
No products indexed under this heading.

Methoxyflurane (Potential for synergistic CNS-depressant effect).
No products indexed under this heading.

Methsuximide (Studies suggest that CYP2C19 and CYP3A4 are the principal enzymes involved in the initial oxidative metabolism of diazepam. Therefore, potential interactions may occur when diazepam is given concurrently with agents that affect CYP2C19 and CYP3A4 activity. Potential inducers of CYP3A4 could increase the rate of diazepam elimination).
No products indexed under this heading.

Methylprednisolone (Studies suggest that CYP2C19 and CYP3A4 are the principal enzymes involved in the initial oxidative metabolism of diazepam. Therefore, potential interactions may occur when diazepam is given concurrently with agents that affect CYP2C19 and CYP3A4 activity. Potential inducers of CYP3A4 could increase the rate of diazepam elimination).
No products indexed under this heading.

Methylprednisolone Acetate (Studies suggest that CYP2C19 and CYP3A4 are the principal enzymes involved in the initial oxidative metabolism of diazepam. Therefore, potential interactions may occur when diazepam is given concurrently with agents that affect CYP2C19 and CYP3A4 activity. Potential inducers of CYP3A4 could increase the rate of diazepam elimination). Products include:
- Depo-Medrol Injectable Suspension 2615
- Depo-Medrol Single-Dose Vial 2617

Methylprednisolone Sodium Succinate (Studies suggest that CYP2C19 and CYP3A4 are the principal enzymes involved in the initial oxidative metabolism of diazepam. Therefore, potential interactions may occur when diazepam is given concurrently with agents that affect CYP2C19 and CYP3A4 activity. Potential inducers of CYP3A4 could increase the rate of diazepam elimination).
No products indexed under this heading.

Metronidazole (Studies suggest that CYP2C19 and CYP3A4 are the principal enzymes involved in the initial oxidative metabolism of diazepam. Therefore, potential interactions may occur when diazepam is given concurrently with agents that affect CYP2C19 and CYP3A4 activity. Potential inhibitors of CYP3A4 could decrease the rate of diazepam elimination). Products include:
- Metrogel 1% 1212
- MetroGel-Vaginal Gel 1822
- Noritate Cream, 1% 1051

Metronidazole Benzoate (Studies suggest that CYP2C19 and CYP3A4 are the principal enzymes involved in the initial oxidative metabolism of diazepam. Therefore, potential interactions may occur when diazepam is given concurrently with agents that affect CYP2C19 and CYP3A4 activity. Potential inhibitors of CYP3A4 could decrease the rate of diazepam elimination).
No products indexed under this heading.

Metronidazole Hydrochloride (Studies suggest that CYP2C19 and CYP3A4 are the principal enzymes involved in the initial oxidative metabolism of diazepam. Therefore, potential interactions may occur when diazepam is given concurrently with agents that affect CYP2C19 and CYP3A4 activity. Potential inhibitors of CYP3A4 could decrease the rate of diazepam elimination).
No products indexed under this heading.

Miconazole (Studies suggest that CYP2C19 and CYP3A4 are the principal enzymes involved in the initial oxidative metabolism of diazepam. Therefore, potential interactions may occur when diazepam is given concurrently with agents that affect CYP2C19 and CYP3A4 activity. Potential inhibitors of CYP3A4 could decrease the rate of diazepam elimination).
No products indexed under this heading.

Miconazole Nitrate (Studies suggest that CYP2C19 and CYP3A4 are the principal enzymes involved in the initial oxidative metabolism of diazepam. Therefore, potential interactions may occur when diazepam is given concurrently with agents that affect CYP2C19 and CYP3A4 activity. Potential inhibitors of CYP3A4 could decrease the rate of diazepam elimination). Products include:
Desenex 674
Desenex Jock Itch Spray Powder ... 674

Midazolam Hydrochloride (Potential for synergistic CNS-depressant effect).
No products indexed under this heading.

Mirtazapine (Potential for synergistic CNS-depressant effect).
No products indexed under this heading.

Moclobemide (Potential for synergistic CNS-depressant effect).
No products indexed under this heading.

Modafinil (Studies suggest that CYP2C19 and CYP3A4 are the principal enzymes involved in the initial oxidative metabolism of diazepam. Therefore, potential interactions may occur when diazepam is given concurrently with agents that affect CYP2C19 and CYP3A4 activity. Potential inhibitors of CYP2C19 could decrease the rate of diazepam elimination). Products include:
Provigil Tablets 1002

Molindone Hydrochloride (Potential for synergistic CNS-depressant effect). Products include:
Moban Tablets 1108

Morphine Sulfate (Potential for synergistic CNS-depressant effect). Products include:
Avinza Capsules 1714
Kadian Capsules 572
MS Contin Tablets 2703

Nefazodone Hydrochloride (Potential for synergistic CNS-depressant effect).
No products indexed under this heading.

Nelfinavir Mesylate (Studies suggest that CYP2C19 and CYP3A4 are the principal enzymes involved in the initial oxidative metabolism of diazepam. Therefore, potential interactions may occur when diazepam is given concurrently with agents that affect CYP2C19 and CYP3A4 activity. Potential inhibitors of CYP3A4 could decrease the rate of diazepam elimination). Products include:
Viracept 2556

Nevirapine (Studies suggest that CYP2C19 and CYP3A4 are the principal enzymes involved in the initial oxidative metabolism of diazepam. Therefore, potential interactions may occur when diazepam is given concurrently with agents that affect CYP2C19 and CYP3A4 activity. Potential inhibitors of CYP3A4 could decrease the rate of diazepam elimination). Products include:
Viramune Oral Suspension 903
Viramune Tablets 903

Niacinamide (Studies suggest that CYP2C19 and CYP3A4 are the principal enzymes involved in the initial oxidative metabolism of diazepam. Therefore, potential interactions may occur when diazepam is given concurrently with agents that affect CYP2C19 and CYP3A4 activity. Potential inhibitors of CYP3A4 could decrease the rate of diazepam elimination).
No products indexed under this heading.

Nicardipine Hydrochloride (There are no reports as to which isoenzymes could be inhibited or induced by diazepam. But based on the fact that diazepam is a substrate for CYP2C19 and CYP3A4, it is possible that diazepam may interfere with the metabolism of drugs which are substrates for CYP2C19 and CYP3A4 leading to a potential drug-drug interaction). Products include:
Cardene I.V. 1129

Nicotinamide (Studies suggest that CYP2C19 and CYP3A4 are the principal enzymes involved in the initial oxidative metabolism of diazepam. Therefore, potential interactions may occur when diazepam is given concurrently with agents that affect CYP2C19 and CYP3A4 activity. Potential inhibitors of CYP3A4 could decrease the rate of diazepam elimination). Products include:
Nicomide Tablets 3190

Nifedipine (Studies suggest that CYP2C19 and CYP3A4 are the principal enzymes involved in the initial oxidative metabolism of diazepam. Therefore, potential interactions may occur when diazepam is given concurrently with agents that affect CYP2C19 and CYP3A4 activity. Potential inhibitors of CYP3A4 could decrease the rate of diazepam elimination). Products include:
Adalat CC Tablets 2978

Nilutamide (There are no reports as to which isoenzymes could be inhibited or induced by diazepam. But based on the fact that diazepam is a substrate for CYP2C19 and CYP3A4, it is possible that diazepam may interfere with the metabolism of drugs which are substrates for CYP2C19 and CYP3A4 leading to a potential drug-drug interaction).
No products indexed under this heading.

Nimodipine (There are no reports as to which isoenzymes could be inhibited or induced by diazepam. But based on the fact that diazepam is a substrate for CYP2C19 and CYP3A4, it is possible that diazepam may interfere with the metabolism of drugs which are substrates for CYP2C19 and CYP3A4 leading to a potential drug-drug interaction). Products include:
Nimotop Capsules 774

Nisoldipine (There are no reports as to which isoenzymes could be inhibited or induced by diazepam. But based on the fact that diazepam is a substrate for CYP2C19 and CYP3A4, it is possible that diazepam may interfere with the metabolism of drugs which are substrates for CYP2C19 and CYP3A4 leading to a potential drug-drug interaction). Products include:
Sular Tablets 1163

Nitrendipine (There are no reports as to which isoenzymes could be inhibited or induced by diazepam. But based on the fact that diazepam is a substrate for CYP2C19 and CYP3A4, it is possible that diazepam may interfere with the metabolism of drugs which are substrates for CYP2C19 and CYP3A4 leading to a potential drug-drug interaction).
No products indexed under this heading.

Norethindrone (Studies suggest that CYP2C19 and CYP3A4 are the principal enzymes involved in the initial oxidative metabolism of diazepam. Therefore, potential interactions may occur when diazepam is given concurrently with agents that affect CYP2C19 and CYP3A4 activity. Potential inhibitors of CYP2C19 could decrease the rate of diazepam elimination). Products include:
Ortho Micronor Tablets 2411

Norethindrone Acetate (Studies suggest that CYP2C19 and CYP3A4 are the principal enzymes involved in the initial oxidative metabolism of diazepam. Therefore, potential interactions may occur when diazepam is given concurrently with agents that affect CYP2C19 and CYP3A4 activity. Potential inducers of CYP2C19 could increase the rate of diazepam elimination). Products include:
Activella Tablets 2311
Aygestin Tablets 1062
CombiPatch Transdermal System 2180

Norethynodrel (Studies suggest that CYP2C19 and CYP3A4 are the principal enzymes involved in the initial oxidative metabolism of diazepam. Therefore, potential interactions may occur when diazepam is given concurrently with agents that affect CYP2C19 and CYP3A4 activity. Potential inhibitors of CYP2C19 could decrease the rate of diazepam elimination).
No products indexed under this heading.

Norfloxacin (Studies suggest that CYP2C19 and CYP3A4 are the principal enzymes involved in the initial oxidative metabolism of diazepam. Therefore, potential interactions may occur when diazepam is given concurrently with agents that affect CYP2C19 and CYP3A4 activity. Potential inhibitors of CYP3A4 could decrease the rate of diazepam elimination). Products include:
Noroxin Tablets 2009

Norgestimate (Studies suggest that CYP2C19 and CYP3A4 are the principal enzymes involved in the initial oxidative metabolism of diazepam. Therefore, potential interactions may occur when diazepam is given concurrently with agents that affect CYP2C19 and CYP3A4 activity. Potential inhibitors of CYP2C19 could decrease the rate of diazepam elimination). Products include:
Ortho-Cyclen/Ortho Tri-Cyclen 2414
Ortho Tri-Cyclen Lo Tablets 2421
Prefest Tablets 1069

Norgestrel (Studies suggest that CYP2C19 and CYP3A4 are the principal enzymes involved in the initial oxidative metabolism of diazepam. Therefore, potential interactions may occur when diazepam is given concurrently with agents that affect CYP2C19 and CYP3A4 activity. Potential inhibitors of CYP2C19 could decrease the rate of diazepam elimination). Products include:
Lo/Ovral-28 Tablets 3423

Nortriptyline Hydrochloride (Potential for synergistic CNS-depressant effect).
No products indexed under this heading.

Olanzapine (Potential for synergistic CNS-depressant effect). Products include:
Symbyax Capsules 1788
Zyprexa Tablets 1798
Zyprexa IntraMuscular 1798
Zyprexa ZYDIS Orally Disintegrating Tablets 1798

Omeprazole (Diazepam is a substrate of CYP2C19 and CYP3A4, it is possible that diazepam may interfere with the metabolism of drugs which are substrates for CYP2C19, such as omeprazole). Products include:
Zegerid Powder for Oral Solution 2972

Ondansetron (There are no reports as to which isoenzymes could be inhibited or induced by diazepam. But based on the fact that diazepam is a substrate for CYP2C19 and CYP3A4, it is possible that diazepam may interfere with the metabolism of drugs which are substrates for CYP2C19 and CYP3A4 leading to a potential drug-drug interaction). Products include:
Zofran ODT Orally Disintegrating Tablets 1613

Ondansetron Hydrochloride (There are no reports as to which isoenzymes could be inhibited or induced by diazepam. But based on the fact that diazepam is a substrate for CYP2C19 and CYP3A4, it is possible that diazepam may interfere with the metabolism of drugs which are substrates for CYP2C19 and CYP3A4 leading to a potential drug-drug interaction). Products include:
Zofran Injection 1607
Zofran 1613

Oxazepam (Potential for synergistic CNS-depressant effect).
No products indexed under this heading.

Oxcarbazepine (Studies suggest that CYP2C19 and CYP3A4 are the principal enzymes involved in the initial oxidative metabolism of diazepam. Therefore, potential interactions may occur when diazepam is given concurrently with agents that affect CYP2C19 and CYP3A4 activity. Potential inhibitors of CYP2C19 could decrease the rate of diazepam elimination). Products include:
Trileptal Oral Suspension 2281
Trileptal Tablets 2281

Oxycodone Hydrochloride (Potential for synergistic CNS-depressant effect). Products include:
Combunox Tablets 1183
OxyContin Tablets 2699

IMPORTANT NOTE: Always consult each drug listing in the patient's regimen for possible interactions.

OxyFast Oral Concentrate Solution 2704
OxyIR Capsules 2704
Percocet Tablets 1114
Percodan Tablets 1115

Paclitaxel (Diazepam is a substrate of CYP2C19 and CYP3A4, it is possible that diazepam may interfere with the metabolism of drugs which are substrates for CYP3A4, such as paclitaxel).
No products indexed under this heading.

Pantoprazole Sodium (There are no reports as to which isoenzymes could be inhibited or induced by diazepam. But based on the fact that diazepam is a substrate for CYP2C19 and CYP3A4, it is possible that diazepam may interfere with the metabolism of drugs which are substrates for CYP2C19 and CYP3A4 leading to a potential drug-drug interaction). Products include:
Protonix I.V. 3468
Protonix Tablets 3465

Paramethadione (There are no reports as to which isoenzymes could be inhibited or induced by diazepam. But based on the fact that diazepam is a substrate for CYP2C19 and CYP3A4, it is possible that diazepam may interfere with the metabolism of drugs which are substrates for CYP2C19 and CYP3A4 leading to a potential drug-drug interaction).
No products indexed under this heading.

Pargyline Hydrochloride (Potential for synergistic CNS-depressant effect).
No products indexed under this heading.

Paroxetine Hydrochloride (Potential for synergistic CNS-depressant effect). Products include:
Paxil CR Controlled-Release Tablets 1509
Paxil 1501

Pentamidine Isethionate (There are no reports as to which isoenzymes could be inhibited or induced by diazepam. But based on the fact that diazepam is a substrate for CYP2C19 and CYP3A4, it is possible that diazepam may interfere with the metabolism of drugs which are substrates for CYP2C19 and CYP3A4 leading to a potential drug-drug interaction).
No products indexed under this heading.

Pentobarbital Sodium (Potential for synergistic CNS-depressant effect). Products include:
Nembutal Sodium Solution, USP 2484

Perphenazine (Potential for synergistic CNS-depressant effect).
No products indexed under this heading.

Phenacemide (There are no reports as to which isoenzymes could be inhibited or induced by diazepam. But based on the fact that diazepam is a substrate for CYP2C19 and CYP3A4, it is possible that diazepam may interfere with the metabolism of drugs which are substrates for CYP2C19 and CYP3A4 leading to a potential drug-drug interaction).
No products indexed under this heading.

Phenelzine Sulfate (Potential for synergistic CNS-depressant effect).
No products indexed under this heading.

Phenobarbital (Potential inducers of CYP3A4, such as phenobarbital, could increase the rate of elimination of diazepam; potential for synergistic CNS-depressant effect).
No products indexed under this heading.

Phenobarbital Sodium (Studies suggest that CYP2C19 and CYP3A4 are the principal enzymes involved in the initial oxidative metabolism of diazepam. Therefore, potential interactions may occur when diazepam is given concurrently with agents that affect CYP2C19 and CYP3A4 activity. Potential inducers of CYP2C19 could increase the rate of diazepam elimination).
No products indexed under this heading.

Phensuximide (There are no reports as to which isoenzymes could be inhibited or induced by diazepam. But based on the fact that diazepam is a substrate for CYP2C19 and CYP3A4, it is possible that diazepam may interfere with the metabolism of drugs which are substrates for CYP2C19 and CYP3A4 leading to a potential drug-drug interaction).
No products indexed under this heading.

Phenytoin (Inducers of CYP3A4, such as phenytoin, could increase the rate of elimination of diazepam).
No products indexed under this heading.

Phenytoin Sodium (Inducers of CYP3A4, such as phenytoin, could increase the rate of elimination of diazepam). Products include:
Phenytek Capsules 2153

Pimozide (There are no reports as to which isoenzymes could be inhibited or induced by diazepam. But based on the fact that diazepam is a substrate for CYP2C19 and CYP3A4, it is possible that diazepam may interfere with the metabolism of drugs which are substrates for CYP2C19 and CYP3A4 leading to a potential drug-drug interaction). Products include:
Orap Tablets 1220

Polyestradiol Phosphate (There are no reports as to which isoenzymes could be inhibited or induced by diazepam. But based on the fact that diazepam is a substrate for CYP2C19 and CYP3A4, it is possible that diazepam may interfere with the metabolism of drugs which are substrates for CYP2C19 and CYP3A4 leading to a potential drug-drug interaction).
No products indexed under this heading.

Prazepam (Potential for synergistic CNS-depressant effect).
No products indexed under this heading.

Prednisolone Acetate (Studies suggest that CYP2C19 and CYP3A4 are the principal enzymes involved in the initial oxidative metabolism of diazepam. Therefore, potential interactions may occur when diazepam is given concurrently with agents that affect CYP2C19 and CYP3A4 activity. Potential inducers of CYP3A4 could increase the rate of diazepam elimination). Products include:
Blephamide Ophthalmic Ointment 563
Blephamide Ophthalmic Suspension 564
Poly-Pred Liquifilm Ophthalmic Suspension .... ⊙ 231
Pred Forte Ophthalmic Suspension .... ⊙ 233
Pred Mild Sterile Ophthalmic Suspension .... ⊙ 236
Pred-G Ophthalmic Suspension .... ⊙ 234
Pred-G Sterile Ophthalmic Ointment .... ⊙ 235

Prednisolone Sodium Phosphate (Studies suggest that CYP2C19 and CYP3A4 are the principal enzymes involved in the initial oxidative metabolism of diazepam. Therefore, potential interactions may occur when diazepam is given concurrently with agents that affect CYP2C19 and CYP3A4 activity. Potential inducers of CYP3A4 could increase the rate of diazepam elimination). Products include:
Pediapred Oral Solution 3319

Prednisolone Tebutate (Studies suggest that CYP2C19 and CYP3A4 are the principal enzymes involved in the initial oxidative metabolism of diazepam. Therefore, potential interactions may occur when diazepam is given concurrently with agents that affect CYP2C19 and CYP3A4 activity. Potential inducers of CYP3A4 could increase the rate of diazepam elimination).
No products indexed under this heading.

Prednisone (Studies suggest that CYP2C19 and CYP3A4 are the principal enzymes involved in the initial oxidative metabolism of diazepam. Therefore, potential interactions may occur when diazepam is given concurrently with agents that affect CYP2C19 and CYP3A4 activity. Potential inducers of CYP2C19 could increase the rate of diazepam elimination).
No products indexed under this heading.

Primidone (Studies suggest that CYP2C19 and CYP3A4 are the principal enzymes involved in the initial oxidative metabolism of diazepam. Therefore, potential interactions may occur when diazepam is given concurrently with agents that affect CYP2C19 and CYP3A4 activity. Potential inducers of CYP3A4 could increase the rate of diazepam elimination).
No products indexed under this heading.

Procarbazine Hydrochloride (Potential for synergistic CNS-depressant effect). Products include:
Matulane Capsules 3188

Prochlorperazine (Potential for synergistic CNS-depressant effect).
No products indexed under this heading.

Progesterone (There are no reports as to which isoenzymes could be inhibited or induced by diazepam. But based on the fact that diazepam is a substrate for CYP2C19 and CYP3A4, it is possible that diazepam may interfere with the metabolism of drugs which are substrates for CYP2C19 and CYP3A4 leading to a potential drug-drug interaction). Products include:
Prochieve 4% Gel 1018
Prochieve 8% Gel 1018
Prometrium Capsules (100 mg, 200 mg) 3205

Proguanil Hydrochloride (There are no reports as to which isoenzymes could be inhibited or induced by diazepam. But based on the fact that diazepam is a substrate for CYP2C19 and CYP3A4, it is possible that diazepam may interfere with the metabolism of drugs which are substrates for CYP2C19 and CYP3A4 leading to a potential drug-drug interaction). Products include:
Malarone Tablets 1484
Malarone Pediatric Tablets 1484

Promethazine Hydrochloride (Potential for synergistic CNS-depressant effect). Products include:
Phenergan 3438

Propofol (Potential for synergistic CNS-depressant effect). Products include:
Diprivan Injectable Emulsion 676

Propoxyphene Hydrochloride (Potential for synergistic CNS-depressant effect).
No products indexed under this heading.

Propoxyphene Napsylate (Potential for synergistic CNS-depressant effect). Products include:
Darvocet A 500 Tablets 3497

Propranolol Hydrochloride (Diazepam is a substrate of CYP2C19 and CYP3A4; it is possible that diazepam may interfere with the metabolism of drugs which are substrates for CYP2C19, such as propranolol). Products include:
Inderal LA Long-Acting Capsules 3421
InnoPran XL Capsules 2728

Protriptyline Hydrochloride (Potential for synergistic CNS-depressant effect). Products include:
Vivactil Tablets 2350

Quazepam (Potential for synergistic CNS-depressant effect).
No products indexed under this heading.

Quetiapine Fumarate (Potential for synergistic CNS-depressant effect). Products include:
Seroquel Tablets 691

Quinidine (Potential inhibitors of CYP2C19, such as quinidine, could decrease the rate of diazepam elimination).
No products indexed under this heading.

Quinidine Gluconate (Potential inhibitors of CYP2C19, such as quinidine, could decrease the rate of diazepam elimination).
No products indexed under this heading.

Quinidine Hydrochloride (Potential inhibitors of CYP2C19, such as quinidine, could decrease the rate of diazepam elimination).
No products indexed under this heading.

Quinidine Polygalacturonate (Potential inhibitors of CYP2C19, such as quinidine, could decrease the rate of diazepam elimination).
No products indexed under this heading.

Quinidine Sulfate (Potential inhibitors of CYP2C19, such as quinidine, could decrease the rate of diazepam elimination).
No products indexed under this heading.

Quinine (Studies suggest that CYP2C19 and CYP3A4 are the principal enzymes involved in the initial oxidative metabolism of diazepam. Therefore, potential interactions may occur when diazepam is given concurrently with agents that affect CYP2C19 and CYP3A4 activity. Potential inhibitors of CYP3A4 could decrease the rate of diazepam elimination).
No products indexed under this heading.

Quinine Sulfate (Studies suggest that CYP2C19 and CYP3A4 are the principal enzymes involved in the initial oxidative metabolism of diazepam. Therefore, potential interactions may occur when diazepam is given concurrently with agents that affect CYP2C19 and CYP3A4 activity. Potential inhibitors of CYP3A4 could decrease the rate of diazepam elimination).
No products indexed under this heading.

Quinupristin (Studies suggest that CYP2C19 and CYP3A4 are the principal enzymes involved in the initial oxidative metabolism of diazepam. Therefore, potential interactions may occur when diazepam is given concurrently with agents that affect CYP2C19 and CYP3A4 activity. Potential inhibitors of CYP3A4 could decrease the rate of diazepam elimination). Products include:
Synercid I.V. 1690

Rabeprazole Sodium (There are no reports as to which isoenzymes could be inhibited or induced by diazepam. But based on the fact that diazepam is a substrate for CYP2C19 and CYP3A4, it is possible that diazepam may interfere with the metabolism of drugs which are substrates for CYP2C19 and CYP3A4 leading to a potential drug-drug interaction). Products include:
Aciphex Tablets 1081

Ranitidine Bismuth Citrate (Studies suggest that CYP2C19 and CYP3A4 are the principal enzymes involved in the initial oxidative metabolism of diazepam. Therefore, potential interactions may occur when diazepam is given concurrently with agents that affect CYP2C19 and CYP3A4 activity. Potential inhibitors of CYP3A4 could decrease the rate of diazepam elimination).
No products indexed under this heading.

Ranitidine Hydrochloride (Studies suggest that CYP2C19 and CYP3A4 are the principal enzymes involved in the initial oxidative metabolism of diazepam. Therefore, potential interactions may occur when diazepam is given concurrently with agents that affect CYP2C19 and CYP3A4 activity. Potential inhibitors of CYP3A4 could decrease the rate of diazepam elimination). Products include:
Zantac 1597
Zantac Injection 1593
Zantac 75 Tablets .... ◙715
Zantac 150 Maximum Strength Tablets .... ◙715
Zantac Injection Pharmacy Bulk Package 1595

Remifentanil Hydrochloride (Potential for synergistic CNS-depressant effect).
No products indexed under this heading.

Rifabutin (Studies suggest that CYP2C19 and CYP3A4 are the principal enzymes involved in the initial oxidative metabolism of diazepam. Therefore, potential interactions may occur when diazepam is given concurrently with agents that affect CYP2C19 and CYP3A4 activity. Potential inducers of CYP3A4 could increase the rate of diazepam elimination).
No products indexed under this heading.

Rifampicin (Studies suggest that CYP2C19 and CYP3A4 are the principal enzymes involved in the initial oxidative metabolism of diazepam. Therefore, potential interactions may occur when diazepam is given concurrently with agents that affect CYP2C19 and CYP3A4 activity. Potential inducers of CYP3A4 could increase the rate of diazepam elimination).
No products indexed under this heading.

Rifampin (Inducers of CYP3A4, such as rifampin, could increase the rate of elimination of diazepam).
No products indexed under this heading.

Rifapentine (Studies suggest that CYP2C19 and CYP3A4 are the principal enzymes involved in the initial oxidative metabolism of diazepam. Therefore, potential interactions may occur when diazepam is given concurrently with agents that affect CYP2C19 and CYP3A4 activity. Potential inducers of CYP3A4 could increase the rate of diazepam elimination).
No products indexed under this heading.

Risperidone (Potential for synergistic CNS-depressant effect). Products include:
Risperdal Consta Long-Acting Injection 1664
Risperdal M-Tab Orally Disintegrating Tablets 1658
Risperdal 1658

Ritonavir (Studies suggest that CYP2C19 and CYP3A4 are the principal enzymes involved in the initial oxidative metabolism of diazepam. Therefore, potential interactions may occur when diazepam is given concurrently with agents that affect CYP2C19 and CYP3A4 activity. Potential inhibitors of CYP2C19 could decrease the rate of diazepam elimination). Products include:
Kaletra 474
Norvir 499

Saquinavir (Studies suggest that CYP2C19 and CYP3A4 are the principal enzymes involved in the initial oxidative metabolism of diazepam. Therefore, potential interactions may occur when diazepam is given concurrently with agents that affect CYP2C19 and CYP3A4 activity. Potential inhibitors of CYP3A4 could decrease the rate of diazepam elimination).
No products indexed under this heading.

Saquinavir Mesylate (Studies suggest that CYP2C19 and CYP3A4 are the principal enzymes involved in the initial oxidative metabolism of diazepam. Therefore, potential interactions may occur when diazepam is given concurrently with agents that affect CYP2C19 and CYP3A4 activity. Potential inhibitors of CYP3A4 could decrease the rate of diazepam elimination). Products include:
Invirase 2776

Secobarbital Sodium (Potential for synergistic CNS-depressant effect).
No products indexed under this heading.

Selegiline Hydrochloride (Potential for synergistic CNS-depressant effect). Products include:
Eldepryl Capsules 3209

Sertraline Hydrochloride (Potential for synergistic CNS-depressant effect). Products include:
Zoloft 2581

Sevoflurane (Potential for synergistic CNS-depressant effect). Products include:
Ultane Liquid for Inhalation 526

Sildenafil Citrate (There are no reports as to which isoenzymes could be inhibited or induced by diazepam. But based on the fact that diazepam is a substrate for CYP2C19 and CYP3A4, it is possible that diazepam may interfere with the metabolism of drugs which are substrates for CYP2C19 and CYP3A4 leading to a potential drug-drug interaction). Products include:
Revatio Tablets 2541
Viagra Tablets 2552

Simvastatin (There are no reports as to which isoenzymes could be inhibited or induced by diazepam. But based on the fact that diazepam is a substrate for CYP2C19 and CYP3A4, it is possible that diazepam may interfere with the metabolism of drugs which are substrates for CYP2C19 and CYP3A4 leading to a potential drug-drug interaction). Products include:
Vytorin 10/10 Tablets 2084
Vytorin 10/10 Tablets 3092
Vytorin 10/20 Tablets 2084
Vytorin 10/20 Tablets 3092
Vytorin 10/40 Tablets 3092
Vytorin 10/40 Tablets 2084
Vytorin 10/80 Tablets 2084
Vytorin 10/80 Tablets 3092
Zocor Tablets 2078

Sirolimus (There are no reports as to which isoenzymes could be inhibited or induced by diazepam. But based on the fact that diazepam is a substrate for CYP2C19 and CYP3A4, it is possible that diazepam may interfere with the metabolism of drugs which are substrates for CYP2C19 and CYP3A4 leading to a potential drug-drug interaction). Products include:
Rapamune Oral Solution and Tablets 3472

Sodium Oxybate (Potential for synergistic CNS-depressant effect).
No products indexed under this heading.

Sufentanil Citrate (Potential for synergistic CNS-depressant effect).
No products indexed under this heading.

Sulfaphenazole (Studies suggest that CYP2C19 and CYP3A4 are the principal enzymes involved in the initial oxidative metabolism of diazepam. Therefore, potential interactions may occur when diazepam is given concurrently with agents that affect CYP2C19 and CYP3A4 activity. Potential inhibitors of CYP2C19 could decrease the rate of diazepam elimination).
No products indexed under this heading.

Sulfinpyrazone (Studies suggest that CYP2C19 and CYP3A4 are the principal enzymes involved in the initial oxidative metabolism of diazepam. Therefore, potential interactions may occur when diazepam is given concurrently with agents that affect CYP2C19 and CYP3A4 activity. Potential inducers of CYP3A4 could increase the rate of diazepam elimination).
No products indexed under this heading.

Tacrolimus (There are no reports as to which isoenzymes could be inhibited or induced by diazepam. But based on the fact that diazepam is a substrate for CYP2C19 and CYP3A4, it is possible that diazepam may interfere with the metabolism of drugs which are substrates for CYP2C19 and CYP3A4 leading to a potential drug-drug interaction). Products include:
Prograf Capsules and Injection 624
Protopic Ointment 629

Tamoxifen Citrate (There are no reports as to which isoenzymes could be inhibited or induced by diazepam. But based on the fact that diazepam is a substrate for CYP2C19 and CYP3A4, it is possible that diazepam may interfere with the metabolism of drugs which are substrates for CYP2C19 and CYP3A4 leading to a potential drug-drug interaction).
No products indexed under this heading.

Telithromycin (Studies suggest that CYP2C19 and CYP3A4 are the principal enzymes involved in the initial oxidative metabolism of diazepam. Therefore, potential interactions may occur when diazepam is given concurrently with agents that affect CYP2C19 and CYP3A4 activity. Potential inhibitors of CYP3A4 could decrease the rate of diazepam elimination). Products include:
Ketek Tablets 2920

Telmisartan (Studies suggest that CYP2C19 and CYP3A4 are the principal enzymes involved in the initial oxidative metabolism of diazepam. Therefore, potential interactions may occur when diazepam is given concurrently with agents that affect CYP2C19 and CYP3A4 activity. Potential inhibitors of CYP2C19 could decrease the rate of diazepam elimination). Products include:
Micardis Tablets 884
Micardis HCT Tablets 886

Temazepam (Potential for synergistic CNS-depressant effect).
No products indexed under this heading.

Teniposide (There are no reports as to which isoenzymes could be inhibited or induced by diazepam. But based on the fact that diazepam is a substrate for CYP2C19 and CYP3A4, it is possible that diazepam may interfere with the metabolism of drugs which are substrates for CYP2C19 and CYP3A4 leading to a potential drug-drug interaction).
No products indexed under this heading.

Terfenadine (Diazepam is a substrate of CYP2C19 and CYP3A4; it is possible that diazepam may interfere with the metabolism of drugs which are substrates for CYP3A4, such as terfenadine).
No products indexed under this heading.

Theophylline (Diazepam is a substrate of CYP2C19 and CYP3A4, it is possible that diazepam may interfere with the metabolism of drugs which are substrates for CYP3A4, such as theophylline).
No products indexed under this heading.

Theophylline Anhydrous (Diazepam is a substrate of CYP2C19 and CYP3A4, it is possible that diazepam may interfere with the metabolism of drugs which are substrates for CYP3A4, such as theophylline). Products include:
Uniphyl Tablets 2708

Theophylline Calcium Salicylate (Diazepam is a substrate of CYP2C19 and CYP3A4, it is possible that diazepam may interfere with the metabolism of drugs which are substrates for CYP3A4, such as theophylline).
No products indexed under this heading.

Theophylline Dihydroxypropyl (Glyceryl) (Diazepam is a substrate of CYP2C19 and CYP3A4, it is possible that diazepam may interfere with the metabolism of drugs which are substrates for CYP3A4, such as theophylline).
No products indexed under this heading.

Theophylline Ethylenediamine (Diazepam is a substrate of CYP2C19 and CYP3A4, it is possible that diazepam may interfere with the metabolism of drugs which are substrates for CYP3A4, such as theophylline).
No products indexed under this heading.

Theophylline Sodium Glycinate (Diazepam is a substrate of CYP2C19 and CYP3A4, it is possible that diazepam may interfere with the metabolism of drugs which are substrates for CYP3A4, such as theophylline).
No products indexed under this heading.

Thiamylal Sodium (Potential for synergistic CNS-depressant effect).
No products indexed under this heading.

Thioridazine (There are no reports as to which isoenzymes could be inhibited or induced by diazepam. But based on the fact that diazepam is a substrate for CYP2C19 and CYP3A4, it is possible that diazepam may interfere with the metabolism of drugs which are substrates for CYP2C19 and CYP3A4 leading to a potential drug-drug interaction).
No products indexed under this heading.

Thioridazine Hydrochloride (Potential for synergistic CNS-depressant effect). Products include:
Thioridazine Hydrochloride Tablets 2122

Thiothixene (Potential for synergistic CNS-depressant effect). Products include:
Thiothixene Capsules 2124

Tiagabine Hydrochloride (There are no reports as to which isoenzymes could be inhibited or induced by diazepam. But based on the fact that diazepam is a substrate for CYP2C19 and CYP3A4, it is possible that diazepam may interfere with the metabolism of drugs which are substrates for CYP2C19 and CYP3A4 leading to a potential drug-drug interaction). Products include:
Gabitril Tablets 998

Ticlopidine Hydrochloride (Studies suggest that CYP2C19 and CYP3A4 are the principal enzymes involved in the initial oxidative metabolism of diazepam. Therefore, potential interactions may occur when diazepam is given concurrently with agents that affect CYP2C19 and CYP3A4 activity. Potential inhibitors of CYP2C19 could decrease the rate of diazepam elimination). Products include:
Ticlid Tablets 2813

Tolbutamide (Studies suggest that CYP2C19 and CYP3A4 are the principal enzymes involved in the initial oxidative metabolism of diazepam. Therefore, potential interactions may occur when diazepam is given concurrently with agents that affect CYP2C19 and CYP3A4 activity. Potential inhibitors of CYP2C19 could decrease the rate of diazepam elimination).
No products indexed under this heading.

Tolbutamide Sodium (Studies suggest that CYP2C19 and CYP3A4 are the principal enzymes involved in the initial oxidative metabolism of diazepam. Therefore, potential interactions may occur when diazepam is given concurrently with agents that affect CYP2C19 and CYP3A4 activity. Potential inhibitors of CYP2C19 could decrease the rate of diazepam elimination).
No products indexed under this heading.

Tolterodine Tartrate (There are no reports as to which isoenzymes could be inhibited or induced by diazepam. But based on the fact that diazepam is a substrate for CYP2C19 and CYP3A4, it is possible that diazepam may interfere with the metabolism of drugs which are substrates for CYP2C19 and CYP3A4 leading to a potential drug-drug interaction). Products include:
Detrol Tablets 2626
Detrol LA Capsules 2629

Topiramate (Studies suggest that CYP2C19 and CYP3A4 are the principal enzymes involved in the initial oxidative metabolism of diazepam. Therefore, potential interactions may occur when diazepam is given concurrently with agents that affect CYP2C19 and CYP3A4 activity. Potential inhibitors of CYP2C19 could decrease the rate of diazepam elimination). Products include:
Topamax Sprinkle Capsules 2438
Topamax Tablets 2438

Tranylcypromine Sulfate (Potential inhibitors of CYP2C19, such as tranylcypromine, could decrease the rate of diazepam elimination; potential for synergistic CNS-depressant effect). Products include:
Parnate Tablets 1499

Trazodone Hydrochloride (Potential for synergistic CNS-depressant effect).
No products indexed under this heading.

Triamcinolone (Studies suggest that CYP2C19 and CYP3A4 are the principal enzymes involved in the initial oxidative metabolism of diazepam. Therefore, potential interactions may occur when diazepam is given concurrently with agents that affect CYP2C19 and CYP3A4 activity. Potential inducers of CYP3A4 could increase the rate of diazepam elimination).
No products indexed under this heading.

Triamcinolone Acetonide (Studies suggest that CYP2C19 and CYP3A4 are the principal enzymes involved in the initial oxidative metabolism of diazepam. Therefore, potential interactions may occur when diazepam is given concurrently with agents that affect CYP2C19 and CYP3A4 activity. Potential inducers of CYP3A4 could increase the rate of diazepam elimination). Products include:
Azmacort Inhalation Aerosol 1701
Nasacort HFA Inhalation Aerosol 2939
Nasacort AQ Nasal Spray 2937

Triamcinolone Diacetate (Studies suggest that CYP2C19 and CYP3A4 are the principal enzymes involved in the initial oxidative metabolism of diazepam. Therefore, potential interactions may occur when diazepam is given concurrently with agents that affect CYP2C19 and CYP3A4 activity. Potential inducers of CYP3A4 could increase the rate of diazepam elimination).
No products indexed under this heading.

Triamcinolone Hexacetonide (Studies suggest that CYP2C19 and CYP3A4 are the principal enzymes involved in the initial oxidative metabolism of diazepam. Therefore, potential interactions may occur when diazepam is given concurrently with agents that affect CYP2C19 and CYP3A4 activity. Potential inducers of CYP3A4 could increase the rate of diazepam elimination).
No products indexed under this heading.

Triazolam (Potential for synergistic CNS-depressant effect).
No products indexed under this heading.

Trifluoperazine Hydrochloride (Potential for synergistic CNS-depressant effect).
No products indexed under this heading.

Trimethadione (There are no reports as to which isoenzymes could be inhibited or induced by diazepam. But based on the fact that diazepam is a substrate for CYP2C19 and CYP3A4, it is possible that diazepam may interfere with the metabolism of drugs which are substrates for CYP2C19 and CYP3A4 leading to a potential drug-drug interaction).
No products indexed under this heading.

Trimipramine Maleate (Potential for synergistic CNS-depressant effect). Products include:
Surmontil Capsules 2347

Troglitazone (Studies suggest that CYP2C19 and CYP3A4 are the principal enzymes involved in the initial oxidative metabolism of diazepam. Therefore, potential interactions may occur when diazepam is given concurrently with agents that affect CYP2C19 and CYP3A4 activity. Potential inhibitors of CYP3A4 could decrease the rate of diazepam elimination).
No products indexed under this heading.

Troleandomycin (Potential inhibitors of CYP3A4, such as troleandomycin, could decrease the rate of diazepam elimination).
No products indexed under this heading.

Valproate Sodium (Valproate may potentiate the CNS-depressant effect). Products include:
Depacon Injection 412

Valproic Acid (Valproate may potentiate the CNS-depressant effect). Products include:
Depakene 417

Venlafaxine Hydrochloride (Potential for synergistic CNS-depressant effect). Products include:
Effexor Tablets 3405
Effexor XR Capsules 3411

Verapamil Hydrochloride (Studies suggest that CYP2C19 and CYP3A4 are the principal enzymes involved in the initial oxidative metabolism of diazepam. Therefore, potential interactions may occur when diazepam is given concurrently with agents that affect CYP2C19 and CYP3A4 activity. Potential inhibitors of CYP3A4 could decrease the rate of diazepam elimination). Products include:
Covera-HS Tablets 3135
Tarka Tablets 519
Verelan PM Capsules 3120

Vinblastine Sulfate (There are no reports as to which isoenzymes could be inhibited or induced by diazepam. But based on the fact that diazepam is a substrate for CYP2C19 and CYP3A4, it is possible that diazepam may interfere with the metabolism of drugs which are substrates for CYP2C19 and CYP3A4 leading to a potential drug-drug interaction).
No products indexed under this heading.

Vincristine Sulfate (There are no reports as to which isoenzymes could be inhibited or induced by diazepam. But based on the fact that diazepam is a substrate for CYP2C19 and CYP3A4, it is possible that diazepam may interfere with the metabolism of drugs which are substrates for CYP2C19 and CYP3A4 leading to a potential drug-drug interaction).
No products indexed under this heading.

Voriconazole (Studies suggest that CYP2C19 and CYP3A4 are the principal enzymes involved in the initial oxidative metabolism of diazepam. Therefore, potential interactions may occur when diazepam is given concurrently with agents that affect CYP2C19 and CYP3A4 activity. Potential inhibitors of CYP2C19 could decrease the rate of diazepam elimination). Products include:
VFEND I.V. 2543
VFEND Oral Suspension 2543
VFEND Tablets 2543

Warfarin Sodium (Diazepam is a substrate of CYP2C19 and CYP3A4, it is possible that diazepam may interfere with the metabolism of drugs which are substrates for CYP3A4, such as warfarin). Products include:

- Coumadin for Injection ... **932**
- Coumadin Tablets ... **932**

Zafirlukast (Studies suggest that CYP2C19 and CYP3A4 are the principal enzymes involved in the initial oxidative metabolism of diazepam. Therefore, potential interactions may occur when diazepam is given concurrently with agents that affect CYP2C19 and CYP3A4 activity. Potential inhibitors of CYP3A4 could decrease the rate of diazepam elimination). Products include:

- Accolate Tablets ... **663**

Zaleplon (Potential for synergistic CNS-depressant effect). Products include:

- Sonata Capsules ... **1686**

Zileuton (Studies suggest that CYP2C19 and CYP3A4 are the principal enzymes involved in the initial oxidative metabolism of diazepam. Therefore, potential interactions may occur when diazepam is given concurrently with agents that affect CYP2C19 and CYP3A4 activity. Potential inhibitors of CYP3A4 could decrease the rate of diazepam elimination).

No products indexed under this heading.

Ziprasidone Hydrochloride (Potential for synergistic CNS-depressant effect). Products include:

- Geodon Capsules ... **2514**

Zolpidem Tartrate (Potential for synergistic CNS-depressant effect). Products include:

- Ambien Tablets ... **2867**

Zonisamide (There are no reports as to which isoenzymes could be inhibited or induced by diazepam. But based on the fact that diazepam is a substrate for CYP2C19 and CYP3A4, it is possible that diazepam may interfere with the metabolism of drugs which are substrates for CYP2C19 and CYP3A4 leading to a potential drug-drug interaction). Products include:

- Zonegran Capsules ... **1089**

Food Interactions

Alcohol (Potential for synergistic CNS-depressant effect).

Grapefruit (Studies suggest that CYP2C19 and CYP3A4 are the principal enzymes involved in the initial oxidative metabolism of diazepam. Therefore, potential interactions may occur when diazepam is given concurrently with agents that affect CYP2C19 and CYP3A4 activity. Potential inhibitors of CYP3A4 could decrease the rate of diazepam elimination).

Grapefruit Juice (Studies suggest that CYP2C19 and CYP3A4 are the principal enzymes involved in the initial oxidative metabolism of diazepam. Therefore, potential interactions may occur when diazepam is given concurrently with agents that affect CYP2C19 and CYP3A4 activity. Potential inhibitors of CYP3A4 could decrease the rate of diazepam elimination).

DIBENZYLINE CAPSULES

(Phenoxybenzamine Hydrochloride) ... **3390**
May interact with:

Alpha and Beta Adrenergic Stimulators (Exaggerated hypotensive response; tachycardia).

No products indexed under this heading.

Epinephrine (Exaggerated hypotensive response; tachycardia). Products include:

- EpiPen ... **1061**
- Primatene Mist ... **749**

Epinephrine Bitartrate (Exaggerated hypotensive response; tachycardia).

No products indexed under this heading.

Norepinephrine Bitartrate (Hyperthermia production of levarterenol blocked by dibenzyline).

No products indexed under this heading.

Reserpine (Hypothermia production of reserpine blocked by dibenzyline).

No products indexed under this heading.

DIDRONEL TABLETS

(Etidronate Disodium) ... **2693**
May interact with:

Warfarin Sodium (Co-administration has resulted in isolated reports of increase in prothrombin time without clinically significant sequelae). Products include:

- Coumadin for Injection ... **932**
- Coumadin Tablets ... **932**

DIFFERIN CREAM

(Adapalene) ... **1210**
See Differin Gel

DIFFERIN GEL

(Adapalene) ... **1211**
May interact with:

Resorcinol (Increased potential for local irritation).

No products indexed under this heading.

Salicylic Acid (Increased potential for local irritation).

No products indexed under this heading.

Sulfur (Increased potential for local irritation). Products include:

- Avar Cleanser ... **3189**
- Avar Gel ... **3189**
- Avar Green ... **3189**
- Avar-e Emollient Cream ... **3189**
- Avar-e Green Cream ... **3189**
- Plexion ... **1863**
- Rosac Cream with Sunscreens ... **3216**
- Zeel Solution ... **1639**
- Zicam Allergy Relief Nasal Pump ...

DIGIBIND FOR INJECTION

(Digoxin Immune Fab (Ovine)) ... **1388**
None cited in PDR database.

DIGITEK TABLETS

(Digoxin) ... **2146**
May interact with antacids, beta blockers, calcium channel blockers, corticosteroids, macrolide antibiotics, potassium-depleting diuretics, quinidine, sympathomimetics, tetracyclines, thyroid preparations, and certain other agents. Compounds in these categories include:

Acebutolol Hydrochloride (Co-administration of digoxin and beta blockers may result in the additive effects on AV node conduction).

No products indexed under this heading.

Albuterol (Co-administration of digoxin and sympathomimetics increases the risk of cardiac arrhythmias). Products include:

- Proventil Inhalation Aerosol ... **3067**

Albuterol Sulfate (Co-administration of digoxin and sympathomimetics increases the risk of cardiac arrhythmias). Products include:

- AccuNeb Inhalation Solution ... **1055**
- Combivent Inhalation Aerosol ... **878**
- DuoNeb Inhalation Solution ... **1058**
- Proventil Inhalation Solution 0.083% ... **3069**
- Proventil HFA Inhalation Aerosol ... **3071**
- Ventolin HFA Inhalation Aerosol ... **1576**
- VoSpire Extended-Release Tablets ... **2352**

Alprazolam (Co-administration of digoxin with alprazolam raises the serum digoxin concentration due to reduction in clearance and/or in volume of distribution of the drug with implication that digitalis toxicity may result). Products include:

- Niravam Orally Disintegrating Tablets ... **3106**
- Xanax XR Tablets ... **2655**

Aluminum Carbonate (Antacids may interfere with intestinal digoxin absorption resulting in unexpectedly low serum concentrations).

No products indexed under this heading.

Aluminum Hydroxide (Antacids may interfere with intestinal digoxin absorption resulting in unexpectedly low serum concentrations). Products include:

- Gaviscon Regular Strength Liquid ... **620**
- Gaviscon Regular Strength Tablets ... **619**
- Gaviscon Extra Strength Liquid ... **620**
- Gaviscon Extra Strength Tablets ... **619**
- Maalox Max Maximum Strength Antacid/Anti-Gas Liquid ... **2165**
- Maalox Regular Strength Antacid/Antigas Liquid ... **2164**

Amiodarone Hydrochloride (Co-administration of digoxin with verapamil raises the serum digoxin concentration due to reduction in clearance and/or in volume of distribution of the drug with implication that digitalis toxicity may result). Products include:

- Pacerone Tablets ... **3337**

Amlodipine Besylate (Co-administration of digoxin and calcium channel blockers may result in the additive effects on AV node conduction). Products include:

- Caduet Tablets ... **2507**
- Lotrel Capsules ... **2238**
- Norvasc Tablets ... **2529**

Amphotericin B (Can cause hypokalemia or hypomagnesemia and potassium or magnesium depletion can sensitize the myocardium to digoxin resulting in digitalis toxicity).

No products indexed under this heading.

Anticancer Drugs, unspecified (Certain anticancer drugs may interfere with intestinal digoxin absorption resulting in unexpectedly low serum concentrations).

No products indexed under this heading.

Atenolol (Co-administration of digoxin and beta blockers may result in the additive effects on AV node conduction). Products include:

- Tenormin I.V. Injection ... **698**
- Tenormin Tablets ... **695**

Azithromycin Dihydrate (Co-administration with erythromycin and other macrolide antibiotics may increase digoxin absorption in patients with inactivate digoxin by bacterial metabolism in the lower intestine, so that digitalis intoxication may result). Products include:

- Zithromax ... **2568**
- Zithromax for IV Infusion ... **2573**
- Zithromax for Oral Suspension, 300 mg, 600 mg, 900 mg, 1200 mg ... **2561**
- Zithromax Tablets, 250 mg, 500 mg ... **2561**
- Zithromax Tri-Pak ... **2561**
- Zithromax Z-Pak ... **2568**

Bendroflumethiazide (Potassium-depleting diuretics can cause hypokalemia and co-administration can result in digitalis toxicity).

No products indexed under this heading.

Bepridil Hydrochloride (Co-administration of digoxin and calcium channel blockers may result in the additive effects on AV node conduction).

No products indexed under this heading.

Betamethasone Acetate (Corticosteroids can cause hypokalemia or hypomagnesemia and potassium or magnesium depletion can sensitize the myocardium to digoxin resulting in digitalis toxicity).

No products indexed under this heading.

Betamethasone Sodium Phosphate (Corticosteroids can cause hypokalemia or hypomagnesemia and potassium or magnesium depletion can sensitize the myocardium to digoxin resulting in digitalis toxicity).

No products indexed under this heading.

Betaxolol Hydrochloride (Co-administration of digoxin and beta blockers may result in the additive effects on AV node conduction). Products include:

- Betoptic S Ophthalmic Suspension ... **554**

Bisoprolol Fumarate (Co-administration of digoxin and beta blockers may result in the additive effects on AV node conduction).

No products indexed under this heading.

Bumetanide (Potassium-depleting diuretics can cause hypokalemia and co-administration can result in digitalis toxicity).

No products indexed under this heading.

Calcium, intravenous (Co-administration with calcium, particularly if administered rapidly by the intravenous route may produce serious arrhythmias in digitalized patients).

No products indexed under this heading.

Carteolol Hydrochloride (Co-administration of digoxin and beta blockers may result in the additive effects on AV node conduction). Products include:

- Carteolol Hydrochloride Ophthalmic Solution USP, 1% ... ⊙**246**

Chlorothiazide (Potassium-depleting diuretics can cause hypokalemia and co-administration can result in digitalis toxicity). Products include:

- Aldoclor Tablets ... **1881**
- Diuril Oral ... **1936**

Chlorothiazide Sodium (Potassium-depleting diuretics can

cause hypokalemia and co-administration can result in digitalis toxicity). Products include:
Diuril Sodium Intravenous 1934

Cholestyramine (May interfere with intestinal digoxin absorption resulting in unexpectedly low serum concentrations).
No products indexed under this heading.

Clarithromycin (Co-administration with erythromycin and other macrolide antibiotics may increase digoxin absorption in patients with inactivate digoxin by bacterial metabolism in the lower intestine, so that digitalis intoxication may result). Products include:
Biaxin/Biaxin XL 402
PREVPAC 3281

Cortisone Acetate (Corticosteroids can cause hypokalemia or hypomagnesemia and potassium or magnesium depletion can sensitize the myocardium to digoxin resulting in digitalis toxicity).
No products indexed under this heading.

Demeclocycline Hydrochloride (Co-administration with tetracyclines may increase digoxin absorption in patients with inactivate digoxin by bacterial metabolism in the lower intestine, so that digitalis intoxication may result).
No products indexed under this heading.

Dexamethasone (Corticosteroids can cause hypokalemia or hypomagnesemia and potassium or magnesium depletion can sensitize the myocardium to digoxin resulting in digitalis toxicity). Products include:
Ciprodex Otic Suspension 555
Decadron Tablets 1929
TobraDex Ophthalmic Ointment 558
TobraDex Ophthalmic Suspension ... 558

Dexamethasone Acetate (Corticosteroids can cause hypokalemia or hypomagnesemia and potassium or magnesium depletion can sensitize the myocardium to digoxin resulting in digitalis toxicity).
No products indexed under this heading.

Dexamethasone Sodium Phosphate (Corticosteroids can cause hypokalemia or hypomagnesemia and potassium or magnesium depletion can sensitize the myocardium to digoxin resulting in digitalis toxicity). Products include:
Decadron Phosphate Injection 1931

Diltiazem Hydrochloride (Co-administration of digoxin and calcium channel blockers may result in the additive effects on AV node conduction). Products include:
Cardizem LA Extended Release Tablets 1699
Tiazac Capsules 1204

Diphenoxylate Hydrochloride (Decreases gut motility and may increase digoxin absorption).
No products indexed under this heading.

Dirithromycin (Co-administration with erythromycin and other macrolide antibiotics may increase digoxin absorption in patients with inactivate digoxin by bacterial metabolism in the lower intestine, so that digitalis intoxication may result).
No products indexed under this heading.

Dobutamine Hydrochloride (Co-administration of digoxin and sympathomimetics increases the risk of cardiac arrhythmias).
No products indexed under this heading.

Dopamine Hydrochloride (Co-administration of digoxin and sympathomimetics increases the risk of cardiac arrhythmias).
No products indexed under this heading.

Doxycycline Calcium (Co-administration with tetracyclines may increase digoxin absorption in patients with inactivate digoxin by bacterial metabolism in the lower intestine, so that digitalis intoxication may result).
No products indexed under this heading.

Doxycycline Hyclate (Co-administration with tetracyclines may increase digoxin absorption in patients with inactivate digoxin by bacterial metabolism in the lower intestine, so that digitalis intoxication may result).
No products indexed under this heading.

Doxycycline Monohydrate (Co-administration with tetracyclines may increase digoxin absorption in patients with inactivate digoxin by bacterial metabolism in the lower intestine, so that digitalis intoxication may result).
No products indexed under this heading.

Ephedrine Hydrochloride (Co-administration of digoxin and sympathomimetics increases the risk of cardiac arrhythmias). Products include:
Primatene Tablets .... ▣749

Ephedrine Sulfate (Co-administration of digoxin and sympathomimetics increases the risk of cardiac arrhythmias).
No products indexed under this heading.

Ephedrine Tannate (Co-administration of digoxin and sympathomimetics increases the risk of cardiac arrhythmias).
No products indexed under this heading.

Epinephrine (Co-administration of digoxin and sympathomimetics increases the risk of cardiac arrhythmias). Products include:
EpiPen 1061
Primatene Mist .... ▣749

Epinephrine Bitartrate (Co-administration of digoxin and sympathomimetics increases the risk of cardiac arrhythmias).
No products indexed under this heading.

Epinephrine Hydrochloride (Co-administration of digoxin and sympathomimetics increases the risk of cardiac arrhythmias).
No products indexed under this heading.

Erythromycin (Co-administration with erythromycin and other macrolide antibiotics may increase digoxin absorption in patients with inactivate digoxin by bacterial metabolism in the lower intestine, so that digitalis intoxication may result). Products include:
Erygel Topical Gel 2096
Ery-Tab Tablets 447
Erythromycin Base Filmtab Tablets 454
Erythromycin Delayed-Release Capsules, USP.............................. 456
PCE Dispertab Tablets 510

Erythromycin Estolate (Co-administration with erythromycin and other macrolide antibiotics may increase digoxin absorption in patients with inactivate digoxin by bacterial metabolism in the lower intestine, so that digitalis intoxication may result).
No products indexed under this heading.

Erythromycin Ethylsuccinate (Co-administration with erythromycin and other macrolide antibiotics may increase digoxin absorption in patients with inactivate digoxin by bacterial metabolism in the lower intestine, so that digitalis intoxication may result). Products include:
E.E.S. 449
EryPed 445

Erythromycin Gluceptate (Co-administration with erythromycin and other macrolide antibiotics may increase digoxin absorption in patients with inactivate digoxin by bacterial metabolism in the lower intestine, so that digitalis intoxication may result).
No products indexed under this heading.

Erythromycin Stearate (Co-administration with erythromycin and other macrolide antibiotics may increase digoxin absorption in patients with inactivate digoxin by bacterial metabolism in the lower intestine, so that digitalis intoxication may result). Products include:
Erythrocin Stearate Filmtab Tablets 452

Esmolol Hydrochloride (Co-administration of digoxin and beta blockers may result in the additive effects on AV node conduction). Products include:
Brevibloc Concentrate 766
Brevibloc Injection 766
Brevibloc Double Strength Injection.. 766
Brevibloc Premixed Injection 766
Brevibloc Double Strength Premixed Injection 766

Ethacrynic Acid (Potassium-depleting diuretics can cause hypokalemia and co-administration can result in digitalis toxicity). Products include:
Edecrin Tablets 1941

Felodipine (Co-administration of digoxin and calcium channel blockers may result in the additive effects on AV node conduction). Products include:
Plendil Extended-Release Tablets 651

Fludrocortisone Acetate (Corticosteroids can cause hypokalemia or hypomagnesemia and potassium or magnesium depletion can sensitize the myocardium to digoxin resulting in digitalis toxicity).
No products indexed under this heading.

Furosemide (Potassium-depleting diuretics can cause hypokalemia and co-administration can result in digitalis toxicity). Products include:
Furosemide Tablets 2117

Hydrochlorothiazide (Potassium-depleting diuretics can cause hypokalemia and co-administration can result in digitalis toxicity). Products include:
Aldoril Tablets 1884
Atacand HCT 637
Avalide Tablets 2889
Avalide Tablets 922
Benicar HCT Tablets 2852
Diovan HCT Tablets 2195
Dyazide Capsules 1389
Hyzaar 1964
Lotensin HCT Tablets 2235
Maxzide 2150
Micardis HCT Tablets 886
Moduretic Tablets 2003
Prinzide Tablets 2033
Teveten HCT Tablets 1710
Timolide Tablets 2056
Uniretic Tablets 3114
Vaseretic Tablets 2073
Zestoretic Tablets 701

Hydrocortisone (Corticosteroids can cause hypokalemia or hypomagnesemia and potassium or magnesium depletion can sensitize the myocardium to digoxin resulting in digitalis toxicity). Products include:
Cortizone•5 Ointment .... ▣699
Cortizone•10 Creme .... ▣699
Cortizone•10 Ointment .... ▣699
Cortizone•10 Plus Creme .... ▣700
Cortizone•10 Maximum Strength Quick Shot Spray...................... ▣700
Hydrocortone Tablets 1963
Preparation H Hydrocortisone Cream .... ▣748

Hydrocortisone Acetate (Corticosteroids can cause hypokalemia or hypomagnesemia and potassium or magnesium depletion can sensitize the myocardium to digoxin resulting in digitalis toxicity). Products include:
Analpram-HC 1136
Pramosone 1139
ProctoFoam-HC 3113
Tucks Anti-Itch Ointment .... ▣712
U-cort 1% Cream 3289

Hydrocortisone Sodium Phosphate (Corticosteroids can cause hypokalemia or hypomagnesemia and potassium or magnesium depletion can sensitize the myocardium to digoxin resulting in digitalis toxicity).
No products indexed under this heading.

Hydrocortisone Sodium Succinate (Corticosteroids can cause hypokalemia or hypomagnesemia and potassium or magnesium depletion can sensitize the myocardium to digoxin resulting in digitalis toxicity).
No products indexed under this heading.

Hydroflumethiazide (Potassium-depleting diuretics can cause hypokalemia and co-administration can result in digitalis toxicity).
No products indexed under this heading.

Indomethacin (Co-administration of digoxin with indomethacin raises the serum digoxin concentration due to reduction in clearance and/or in volume of distribution of the drug with implication that digitalis toxicity may result). Products include:
Indocin 1968

Indomethacin Sodium Trihydrate (Co-administration of digoxin with indomethacin raises the serum digoxin concentration due to reduction in clearance and/or in volume of distribution of the drug with implication that digitalis toxicity may result). Products include:
Indocin I.V. 1973

Isoproterenol Hydrochloride (Co-administration of digoxin and sympathomimetics increases the risk of cardiac arrhythmias).
No products indexed under this heading.

Isoproterenol Sulfate (Co-administration of digoxin and sympathomimetics increases the risk of cardiac arrhythmias).
No products indexed under this heading.

Isradipine (Co-administration of digoxin and calcium channel blockers may result in the additive effects on AV node conduction). Products include:
DynaCirc CR Tablets 2726

Itraconazole (Co-administration of digoxin with itraconazole raises the serum digoxin concentration due to reduction in clearance and/or in volume of distribution of the drug with implication that digitalis toxicity may result).
No products indexed under this heading.

Kaolin (May interfere with intestinal digoxin absorption resulting in unexpectedly low serum concentrations).
No products indexed under this heading.

Labetalol Hydrochloride (Co-administration of digoxin and beta blockers may result in the additive effects on AV node conduction).
No products indexed under this heading.

Levalbuterol Hydrochloride (Co-administration of digoxin and sympathomimetics increases the risk of cardiac arrhythmias). Products include:
Xopenex Inhalation Solution 3143
Xopenex Inhalation Solution Concentrate 3147

Levobunolol Hydrochloride (Co-administration of digoxin and beta blockers may result in the additive effects on AV node conduction). Products include:
Betagan Ophthalmic Solution, USP .... ⊙217

Levothyroxine Sodium (Thyroid administration to a digitalized, hypothyroid patient may increase the dose requirement of digoxin). Products include:
Levothroid Tablets 1189
Levoxyl Tablets 1680
Synthroid Tablets 515
Unithroid Tablets 3521

Liothyronine Sodium (Thyroid administration to a digitalized, hypothyroid patient may increase the dose requirement of digoxin). Products include:
Cytomel Tablets 1678

Liotrix (Thyroid administration to a digitalized, hypothyroid patient may increase the dose requirement of digoxin). Products include:
Thyrolar 1203

Magaldrate (Antacids may interfere with intestinal digoxin absorption resulting in unexpectedly low serum concentrations).
No products indexed under this heading.

Magnesium Hydroxide (Antacids may interfere with intestinal digoxin absorption resulting in unexpectedly low serum concentrations). Products include:
Maalox Max Maximum Strength Antacid/Anti-Gas Liquid 2165
Maalox Regular Strength Antacid/Antigas Liquid 2164
Pepcid Complete Chewable Tablets 1672
Rolaids Tablets .... ▣707
Extra Strength Rolaids Tablets .... ▣707
Rolaids Multi-Symptom Antacid & Antigas Tablets .... ▣708

Magnesium Oxide (Antacids may interfere with intestinal digoxin absorption resulting in unexpectedly low serum concentrations). Products include:
Beelith Tablets 784
PremCal Light, Regular, and Extra Strength Tablets .... ▣762

Metaproterenol Sulfate (Co-administration of digoxin and sympathomimetics increases the risk of cardiac arrhythmias). Products include:
Alupent Inhalation Aerosol 858

Metaraminol Bitartrate (Co-administration of digoxin and sympathomimetics increases the risk of cardiac arrhythmias). Products include:
Aramine Injection 1889

Methacycline Hydrochloride (Co-administration with tetracyclines may increase digoxin absorption in patients with inactivate digoxin by bacterial metabolism in the lower intestine, so that digitalis intoxication may result).
No products indexed under this heading.

Methoxamine Hydrochloride (Co-administration of digoxin and sympathomimetics increases the risk of cardiac arrhythmias).
No products indexed under this heading.

Methyclothiazide (Potassium-depleting diuretics can cause hypokalemia and co-administration can result in digitalis toxicity).
No products indexed under this heading.

Methylprednisolone Acetate (Corticosteroids can cause hypokalemia or hypomagnesemia and potassium or magnesium depletion can sensitize the myocardium to digoxin resulting in digitalis toxicity). Products include:
Depo-Medrol Injectable Suspension 2615
Depo-Medrol Single-Dose Vial 2617

Methylprednisolone Sodium Succinate (Corticosteroids can cause hypokalemia or hypomagnesemia and potassium or magnesium depletion can sensitize the myocardium to digoxin resulting in digitalis toxicity).
No products indexed under this heading.

Metipranolol Hydrochloride (Co-administration of digoxin and beta blockers may result in the additive effects on AV node conduction).
No products indexed under this heading.

Metoclopramide Hydrochloride (May interfere with intestinal digoxin absorption resulting in unexpectedly low serum concentrations).
No products indexed under this heading.

Metoprolol Succinate (Co-administration of digoxin and beta blockers may result in the additive effects on AV node conduction). Products include:
Toprol-XL Tablets 660

Metoprolol Tartrate (Co-administration of digoxin and beta blockers may result in the additive effects on AV node conduction).
No products indexed under this heading.

Mibefradil Dihydrochloride (Co-administration of digoxin and calcium channel blockers may result in the additive effects on AV node conduction).
No products indexed under this heading.

Minocycline Hydrochloride (Co-administration with tetracyclines may increase digoxin absorption in patients with inactivate digoxin by bacterial metabolism in the lower intestine, so that digitalis intoxication may result). Products include:
Dynacin Tablets 1859

Nadolol (Co-administration of digoxin and beta blockers may result in the additive effects on AV node conduction). Products include:
Nadolol Tablets 2121

Neomycin, oral (May interfere with intestinal digoxin absorption resulting in unexpectedly low serum concentrations).
No products indexed under this heading.

Nicardipine Hydrochloride (Co-administration of digoxin and calcium channel blockers may result in the additive effects on AV node conduction). Products include:
Cardene I.V. 1129

Nifedipine (Co-administration of digoxin and calcium channel blockers may result in the additive effects on AV node conduction). Products include:
Adalat CC Tablets 2978

Nimodipine (Co-administration of digoxin and calcium channel blockers may result in the additive effects on AV node conduction). Products include:
Nimotop Capsules 774

Nisoldipine (Co-administration of digoxin and calcium channel blockers may result in the additive effects on AV node conduction). Products include:
Sular Tablets 1163

Norepinephrine Bitartrate (Co-administration of digoxin and sympathomimetics increases the risk of cardiac arrhythmias).
No products indexed under this heading.

Oxytetracycline Hydrochloride (Co-administration with tetracyclines may increase digoxin absorption in patients with inactivate digoxin by bacterial metabolism in the lower intestine, so that digitalis intoxication may result).
No products indexed under this heading.

Pectin (May interfere with intestinal digoxin absorption resulting in unexpectedly low serum concentrations). Products include:
Halls Fruit Breezers Pectin Throat Drops .... ▣609
Halls Plus Cough Drops .... ▣609

Penbutolol Sulfate (Co-administration of digoxin and beta blockers may result in the additive effects on AV node conduction).
No products indexed under this heading.

Penicillamine (Co-administration has resulted in inconsistent reports regarding the effects of penicillamine on serum digoxin concentration). Products include:
Cuprimine Capsules 1925

Phenylephrine Bitartrate (Co-administration of digoxin and sympathomimetics increases the risk of cardiac arrhythmias).
No products indexed under this heading.

Phenylephrine Hydrochloride (Co-administration of digoxin and sympathomimetics increases the risk of cardiac arrhythmias). Products include:
Alacol DM Syrup 739
Hycomine Compound Tablets 1105
Preparation H Maximum Strength Cream .... ▣747
Preparation H Cooling Gel .... ▣747
Preparation H .... ▣747
Sudafed PE Tablets .... ▣711
Vicks Sinex Nasal Spray and Ultra Fine Mist for Sinus Relief 2677
Zicam Concentrated Cough Mist for Kids Plus D Cool Cherry .... ▣643
Zicam Concentrated Cough Mist Plus D Cool Cherry .... ▣642

Phenylephrine Tannate (Co-administration of digoxin and sympathomimetics increases the risk of cardiac arrhythmias).
No products indexed under this heading.

Phenylpropanolamine Hydrochloride (Co-administration of digoxin and sympathomimetics increases the risk of cardiac arrhythmias).
No products indexed under this heading.

Pindolol (Co-administration of digoxin and beta blockers may result in the additive effects on AV node conduction).
No products indexed under this heading.

Pirbuterol Acetate (Co-administration of digoxin and sympathomimetics increases the risk of cardiac arrhythmias). Products include:
Maxair Autohaler 1820

Polythiazide (Potassium-depleting diuretics can cause hypokalemia and co-administration can result in digitalis toxicity).
No products indexed under this heading.

Prednisolone Acetate (Corticosteroids can cause hypokalemia or hypomagnesemia and potassium or magnesium depletion can sensitize the myocardium to digoxin resulting in digitalis toxicity). Products include:
Blephamide Ophthalmic Ointment 563
Blephamide Ophthalmic Suspension 564
Poly-Pred Liquifilm Ophthalmic Suspension .... ⊙231
Pred Forte Ophthalmic Suspension .... ⊙233
Pred Mild Sterile Ophthalmic Suspension .... ⊙236
Pred-G Ophthalmic Suspension .... ⊙234
Pred-G Sterile Ophthalmic Ointment .... ⊙235

Prednisolone Sodium Phosphate (Corticosteroids can cause hypokalemia or hypomagnesemia and potassium or magnesium depletion can sensitize the myocardium to digoxin resulting in digitalis toxicity). Products include:
Pediapred Oral Solution 3319

Prednisolone Tebutate (Corticosteroids can cause hypokalemia or hypomagnesemia and potassium or magnesium depletion can sensitize the myocardium to digoxin resulting in digitalis toxicity).
No products indexed under this heading.

IMPORTANT NOTE: Always consult each drug listing in the patient's regimen for possible interactions.

Prednisone (Corticosteroids can cause hypokalemia or hypomagnesemia and potassium or magnesium depletion can sensitize the myocardium to digoxin resulting in digitalis toxicity).
No products indexed under this heading.

Propafenone Hydrochloride (Co-administration of digoxin with propafenone raises the serum digoxin concentration due to reduction in clearance and/or in volume of distribution of the drug with implication that digitalis toxicity may result). Products include:
Rythmol SR Capsules 2736

Propantheline Bromide (Decreases gut motility and may increase digoxin absorption).
No products indexed under this heading.

Propranolol Hydrochloride (Co-administration of digoxin and beta blockers may result in the additive effects on AV node conduction). Products include:
Inderal LA Long-Acting Capsules 3421
InnoPran XL Capsules 2728

Pseudoephedrine Hydrochloride (Co-administration of digoxin and sympathomimetics increases the risk of cardiac arrhythmias). Products include:
Advil Allergy Sinus Caplets .... ▣ 737
Advil Cold & Sinus .... ▣ 739
Advil Flu & Body Ache Caplets .... ▣ 739
Children's Advil Cold Suspension ... ▣ 741
Advil Multi-Symptom Cold Caplets .... ▣ 738
Allegra-D 12 Hour Extended-Release Tablets 2860
Allegra-D 24 Hour Extended-Release Tablets 2862
Balamine DM 739
BC Cold Powder .... ▣ 612
Benadryl Allergy & Cold Tablets ..... ▣ 692
Benadryl Allergy & Sinus Headache Caplets & Gelcaps ...... ▣ 693
Children's Benadryl Allergy & Cold Fastmelt Tablets .... ▣ 695
Benadryl Maximum Strength Severe Allergy & Sinus Headache Caplets .... ▣ 694
Children's Benadryl D Allergy & Sinus Fastmelt Tablets .... ▣ 694
Children's Benadryl D Liquid Medication .... ▣ 693
Benadryl D Tablets .... ▣ 694
Contac Non-Drowsy 12 Hour Cold Caplets .... ▣ 614
Contac Non-Drowsy Timed Release 12 Hour Cold Caplets .... ▣ 615
Contac Severe Cold and Flu Caplets Maximum Strength .... ▣ 615
Contac Severe Cold and Flu Caplets Non-Drowsy .... ▣ 615
Children's Dimetapp Cold & Allergy Elixir .... ▣ 745
Children's Dimetapp DM Cold & Cough Elixir .... ▣ 745
Children's Dimetapp Long Acting Cough Plus Cold Syrup .... ▣ 746
Dimetapp Infant Drops Decongestant Plus Cough .... ▣ 746
Children's Motrin Cold Non-Staining Dye-Free Oral Suspension 1838
Children's Motrin Cold Oral Suspension 1838
Motrin Cold & Sinus Caplets 1836
PediaCare Decongestant & Cough Infant Drops .... ▣ 705
PediaCare Decongestant Infants' Drops .... ▣ 705
PediaCare Long-Acting Cough Plus Cold Liquid .... ▣ 704
PediaCare Multi-Symptom Cold Liquid .... ▣ 704
PediaCare NightRest Cough & Cold Liquid .... ▣ 704
Robitussin Allergy & Cough Syrup .. ▣ 750
Robitussin CF Liquid .... ▣ 755
Robitussin Cough & Cold Liquid-filled Capsules .... ▣ 750
Robitussin Cough, Cold & Flu Liquid-filled Capsules .... ▣ 750
Robitussin Cough & Cold Infant Drops .... ▣ 755
Robitussin Flu Liquid .... ▣ 752
Robitussin Maximum Strength Cough & Cold Liquid .... ▣ 754
Robitussin PE Syrup .... ▣ 753
Robitussin Pediatric Cough & Cold Liquid .... ▣ 754
Robitussin PM Cough & Cold Liquid .... ▣ 752
Robitussin Severe Congestion Liquid-filled Capsules .... ▣ 751
Simply Stuffy Liquid 1841
Singlet Caplets .... ▣ 636
Sudafed 12 Hour Caplets .... ▣ 708
Sudafed 24 Hour Tablets .... ▣ 709
Sudafed Nasal Decongestant Tablets .... ▣ 709
Sudafed Severe Cold .... ▣ 710
Sudafed Non-Drying Sinus Liquid Caps .... ▣ 709
Sudafed Sinus & Allergy Tablets ..... ▣ 710
Sudafed Sinus Headache .... ▣ 711
TheraFlu Cold & Cough Hot Liquid .... ▣ 680
TheraFlu Cold & Sore Throat Hot Liquid .... ▣ 680
TheraFlu Flu & Chest Congestion Non-Drowsy Hot Liquid .... ▣ 681
TheraFlu Flu & Sore Throat Hot Liquid .... ▣ 681
TheraFlu Severe Cold Non-Drowsy Hot Liquid .... ▣ 683
TheraFlu Severe Cold & Cough Hot Liquid .... ▣ 683
TheraFlu Severe Cold Caplets .... ▣ 679
TheraFlu Severe Cold Hot Liquid .... ▣ 682
TheraFlu Severe Cold Non-Drowsy Caplets .... ▣ 679
Triaminic Chest & Nasal Congestion Liquid .... ▣ 685
Triaminic Cold & Allergy Liquid .... ▣ 685
Triaminic Cold & Cough Liquid .... ▣ 685
Triaminic Cough Liquid .... ▣ 687
Triaminic Cough & Nasal Congestion Liquid .... ▣ 687
Triaminic Cough & Sore Throat Liquid .... ▣ 687
Triaminic Flu, Cough & Fever Liquid .... ▣ 685
Triaminic Night Time Cough & Cold Liquid .... ▣ 685
Triaminic Allergy Runny Nose & Congestion Softchews .... ▣ 688
Triaminic Cold & Cough Softchews .... ▣ 688
Triaminic Cough & Sore Throat Softchews .... ▣ 689
Tylenol Sinus NightTime Caplets .... ▣ 663
Children's Tylenol Plus Cold & Allergy Suspension Liquid 1850
Children's Tylenol Plus Cold NightTime Suspension Liquid 1851
Children's Tylenol Plus Cold & Cough Suspension Liquid and Chewable Tablets 1851
Children's Tylenol Plus Cold Chewable Tablets 1851
Children's Tylenol Plus Cold Daytime Non-Drowsy Suspension Liquid 1851
Children's Tylenol Plus Flu Suspension Liquid 1853
Concentrated Tylenol Infants' Drops Plus Cold 1851
Concentrated Tylenol Infants' Drops Plus Cold and Cough 1851
Tylenol Cold & Flu Severe Daytime Liquid with Cool Bust....... 1846
Tylenol Cold & Flu Severe NightTime Liquid with Cool Burst 1846
Tylenol Cold Severe Congestion Non-Drowsy Caplets with Cool Burst 1846
Tylenol Allergy Complete Night Time Caplets 1844
Tylenol Allergy Complete Multi-Symptom Caplets and Gelcaps with Cool Burst 1844
Tylenol Flu NightTime Gelcaps 1846
Tylenol Flu Day Non-Drowsy Gelcaps 1846
Concentrated Tylenol Infants' Drops Plus Cold Nasal Congestant, Fever Reducer & Pain Reliever .... ▣ 668
Concentrated Tylenol Infants' Drops Plus Cold & Cough Nasal Decongestant, Fever Reducer & Pain Reliever .... ▣ 668
Multi-Symptom Tylenol Cold Night Time Caplets 1845
Multi-Symptom Tylenol Cold Day Non-Drowsy Caplets and Gelcaps 1845
Tylenol Sinus Day Non-Drowsy 1848
Tylenol Sinus Night Time Caplets 1848
Tylenol Sinus Severe Congestion Caplets with Cool Burst 1848
Vicks 44D Cough & Head Congestion Relief 2676
Vicks 44D Cough & Head Congestion Relief Liquid .... ▣ 721
Vicks 44M Cough, Cold & Flu Relief 2676
Pediatric Vicks 44m Cough & Cold Relief 2673
Vicks DayQuil LiquiCaps/Liquid Multi-Symptom Cold/Flu Relief..... ▣ 723
Vicks DayQuil Multi-Symptom Cold/Flu Relief LiquiCaps 2675
Vicks DayQuil Multi-Symptom Cold/Flu Relief Liquid 2675
Children's Vicks NyQuil Cold/Cough Relief 2671
Vicks NyQuil LiquiCaps 2677
Vicks NyQuil LiquiCaps/Liquid Multi-Symptom Cold/Flu Relief..... ▣ 725
Vicks NyQuil Liquid 2677
Zyrtec-D 12 Hour Extended Release Tablets 2591

Pseudoephedrine Sulfate (Co-administration of digoxin and sympathomimetics increases the risk of cardiac arrhythmias). Products include:
Alavert Allergy & Sinus D-12 Hour Tablets .... ▣ 743
Clarinex-D 24-Hour Extended-Release Tablets 3012
Claritin-D Non-Drowsy 12 Hour Tablets .... ▣ 731
Claritin-D Non-Drowsy 24 Hour Tablets .... ▣ 731

Quinidine (Co-administration of digoxin with quinidine raises the serum digoxin concentration due to reduction in clearance and/or in volume of distribution of the drug with implication that digitalis toxicity may result).
No products indexed under this heading.

Quinidine Gluconate (Co-administration of digoxin with quinidine raises the serum digoxin concentration due to reduction in clearance and/or in volume of distribution of the drug with implication that digitalis toxicity may result).
No products indexed under this heading.

Quinidine Hydrochloride (Co-administration of digoxin with quinidine raises the serum digoxin concentration due to reduction in clearance and/or in volume of distribution of the drug with implication that digitalis toxicity may result).
No products indexed under this heading.

Quinidine Polygalacturonate (Co-administration of digoxin with quinidine raises the serum digoxin concentration due to reduction in clearance and/or in volume of distribution of the drug with implication that digitalis toxicity may result).
No products indexed under this heading.

Quinidine Sulfate (Co-administration of digoxin with quinidine raises the serum digoxin concentration due to reduction in clearance and/or in volume of distribution of the drug with implication that digitalis toxicity may result).
No products indexed under this heading.

Quinine (Co-administration has resulted in inconsistent reports regarding the effects of quinine on serum digoxin concentration).
No products indexed under this heading.

Rifampin (May decrease serum digoxin concentration, especially in patients with renal dysfunction, by increasing the non-renal clearance of digoxin).
No products indexed under this heading.

Salmeterol Xinafoate (Co-administration of digoxin and sympathomimetics increases the risk of cardiac arrhythmias). Products include:
Advair Diskus 100/50 1291
Advair Diskus 250/50 1291
Advair Diskus 500/50 1291
Serevent Diskus 1540

Sodium Bicarbonate (Antacids may interfere with intestinal digoxin absorption resulting in unexpectedly low serum concentrations). Products include:
Ceo-Two Evacuant Suppository ...... ▣ 607
Colyte with Flavor Packs for Oral Solution 3102
HalfLytely and Bisacodyl Tablets Bowel Prep Kit with Flavors Packs 915
TriLyte with Flavor Packs for Oral Solution 3114

Sotalol Hydrochloride (Co-administration of digoxin and beta blockers may result in the additive effects on AV node conduction).
No products indexed under this heading.

Spironolactone (Co-administration of digoxin with spironolactone raises the serum digoxin concentration due to reduction in clearance and/or in volume of distribution of the drug with implication that digitalis toxicity may result).
No products indexed under this heading.

Succinylcholine Chloride (May cause sudden extrusion of potassium from muscle cells, and may thereby cause arrhythmias in digitalized patients).
No products indexed under this heading.

Sulfasalazine (May interfere with intestinal digoxin absorption resulting in unexpectedly low serum concentrations).
No products indexed under this heading.

Terbutaline Sulfate (Co-administration of digoxin and sympathomimetics increases the risk of cardiac arrhythmias).
No products indexed under this heading.

Tetracycline Hydrochloride (Co-administration with tetracyclines may increase digoxin absorption in patients with inactivate digoxin by bacterial metabolism in the lower intestine, so that digitalis intoxication may result).
No products indexed under this heading.

Thyroglobulin (Thyroid administration to a digitalized, hypothyroid patient may increase the dose requirement of digoxin).
No products indexed under this heading.

Thyroid (Thyroid administration to a digitalized, hypothyroid patient may increase the dose requirement of digoxin).
No products indexed under this heading.

Thyroxine (Thyroid administration to a digitalized, hypothyroid patient may increase the dose requirement of digoxin).
No products indexed under this heading.

Thyroxine Sodium (Thyroid administration to a digitalized, hypothyroid patient may increase the dose requirement of digoxin).
No products indexed under this heading.

Timolol Hemihydrate (Co-administration of digoxin and beta blockers may result in the additive effects on AV node conduction). Products include:
Betimol Ophthalmic Solution 3371
Betimol Ophthalmic Solution .... ⊙283

Timolol Maleate (Co-administration of digoxin and beta blockers may result in the additive effects on AV node conduction). Products include:
Blocadren Tablets 1891
Cosopt Sterile Ophthalmic Solution 1910
Timolide Tablets 2056
Timoptic in Ocudose 2061
Timoptic Sterile Ophthalmic Solution 2058
Timoptic-XE Sterile Ophthalmic Gel Forming Solution 2062

Torsemide (Potassium-depleting diuretics can cause hypokalemia and co-administration can result in digitalis toxicity).
No products indexed under this heading.

Triamcinolone (Corticosteroids can cause hypokalemia or hypomagnesemia and potassium or magnesium depletion can sensitize the myocardium to digoxin resulting in digitalis toxicity).
No products indexed under this heading.

Triamcinolone Acetonide (Corticosteroids can cause hypokalemia or hypomagnesemia and potassium or magnesium depletion can sensitize the myocardium to digoxin resulting in digitalis toxicity). Products include:
Azmacort Inhalation Aerosol 1701
Nasacort HFA Inhalation Aerosol 2939
Nasacort AQ Nasal Spray 2937

Triamcinolone Diacetate (Corticosteroids can cause hypokalemia or hypomagnesemia and potassium or magnesium depletion can sensitize the myocardium to digoxin resulting in digitalis toxicity).
No products indexed under this heading.

Triamcinolone Hexacetonide (Corticosteroids can cause hypokalemia or hypomagnesemia and potassium or magnesium depletion can sensitize the myocardium to digoxin resulting in digitalis toxicity).
No products indexed under this heading.

Troleandomycin (Co-administration with erythromycin and other macrolide antibiotics may increase digoxin absorption in patients with inactivate digoxin by bacterial metabolism in the lower intestine, so that digitalis intoxication may result).
No products indexed under this heading.

Verapamil Hydrochloride (Co-administration of digoxin with verapamil raises the serum digoxin concentration due to reduction in clearance and/or in volume of distribution of the drug with implication that digitalis toxicity may result). Products include:
Covera-HS Tablets 3135
Tarka Tablets 519
Verelan PM Capsules 3120

Food Interactions

Meal, high in bran fiber (The amount of digoxin from an oral dose may be reduced when taken with meal high in bran fiber).

Meal, unspecified (Slows the rate of absorption).

DILAUDID AMPULES

(Hydromorphone Hydrochloride) 439
May interact with central nervous system depressants, neuromuscular blocking agents, tricyclic antidepressants, and certain other agents. Compounds in these categories include:

Alfentanil Hydrochloride (Additive CNS depression).
No products indexed under this heading.

Alprazolam (Additive CNS depression). Products include:
Niravam Orally Disintegrating Tablets 3106
Xanax XR Tablets 2655

Amitriptyline Hydrochloride (Additive CNS depression).
No products indexed under this heading.

Amoxapine (Additive CNS depression).
No products indexed under this heading.

Aprobarbital (Additive CNS depression).
No products indexed under this heading.

Atracurium Besylate (Opioid analgesics including Dilaudid may enhance the action of neuromuscular blocking agents and produce an excessive degree of respiratory depression).
No products indexed under this heading.

Buprenorphine Hydrochloride (Additive CNS depression). Products include:
Buprenex Injectable 2718
Suboxone Tablets 2719
Subutex Tablets 2719

Buspirone Hydrochloride (Additive CNS depression).
No products indexed under this heading.

Butabarbital (Additive CNS depression).
No products indexed under this heading.

Butalbital (Additive CNS depression). Products include:
Sedapap Tablets 50 mg/650 mg 2098

Chlordiazepoxide (Additive CNS depression).
No products indexed under this heading.

Chlordiazepoxide Hydrochloride (Additive CNS depression). Products include:
Librium Capsules 3349

Chlorpromazine (Additive CNS depression).
No products indexed under this heading.

Chlorpromazine Hydrochloride (Additive CNS depression).
No products indexed under this heading.

Chlorprothixene (Additive CNS depression).
No products indexed under this heading.

Chlorprothixene Hydrochloride (Additive CNS depression).
No products indexed under this heading.

Chlorprothixene Lactate (Additive CNS depression).
No products indexed under this heading.

Cisatracurium Besylate (Opioid analgesics including Dilaudid may enhance the action of neuromuscular blocking agents and produce an excessive degree of respiratory depression). Products include:
Nimbex Injection 494

Clomipramine Hydrochloride (Additive CNS depression).
No products indexed under this heading.

Clorazepate Dipotassium (Additive CNS depression). Products include:
Tranxene 2488

Clozapine (Additive CNS depression). Products include:
Clozapine Tablets 2141
Clozaril Tablets 2174
FazaClo Orally Disintegrating Tablets 547

Codeine Phosphate (Additive CNS depression). Products include:
Tylenol with Codeine 2461

Desflurane (Additive CNS depression). Products include:
Suprane Liquid for Inhalation 770

Desipramine Hydrochloride (Additive CNS depression).
No products indexed under this heading.

Dezocine (Additive CNS depression).
No products indexed under this heading.

Diazepam (Additive CNS depression). Products include:
Diastat Rectal Delivery System 3344
Valium Tablets 2822

Doxacurium Chloride (Opioid analgesics including Dilaudid may enhance the action of neuromuscular blocking agents and produce an excessive degree of respiratory depression).
No products indexed under this heading.

Doxepin Hydrochloride (Additive CNS depression).
No products indexed under this heading.

Droperidol (Additive CNS depression).
No products indexed under this heading.

Enflurane (Additive CNS depression).
No products indexed under this heading.

Estazolam (Additive CNS depression). Products include:
ProSom Tablets 512

Ethanol (Additive CNS depression).
No products indexed under this heading.

Ethchlorvynol (Additive CNS depression).
No products indexed under this heading.

Ethinamate (Additive CNS depression).
No products indexed under this heading.

Ethyl Alcohol (Additive CNS depression).
No products indexed under this heading.

Fentanyl (Additive CNS depression). Products include:
Duragesic Transdermal System 2448

Fentanyl Citrate (Additive CNS depression). Products include:
Actiq 993

Fluphenazine Decanoate (Additive CNS depression).
No products indexed under this heading.

Fluphenazine Enanthate (Additive CNS depression).
No products indexed under this heading.

Fluphenazine Hydrochloride (Additive CNS depression).
No products indexed under this heading.

Flurazepam Hydrochloride (Additive CNS depression). Products include:
Dalmane Capsules 3343

Glutethimide (Additive CNS depression).
No products indexed under this heading.

Haloperidol (Additive CNS depression).
No products indexed under this heading.

Haloperidol Decanoate (Additive CNS depression).
No products indexed under this heading.

Hydrocodone Bitartrate (Additive CNS depression). Products include:
Hycodan 1104
Hycomine Compound Tablets 1105
Hycotuss Expectorant Syrup 1106
Lortab 3315
Lortab Elixir 3312
Vicodin Tablets 530
Vicodin ES Tablets 531
Vicodin HP Tablets 532
Vicoprofen Tablets 533
Zydone Tablets 1118

Hydrocodone Polistirex (Additive CNS depression). Products include:
Tussionex Pennkinetic Extended-Release Suspension 3322

Hydroxyzine Hydrochloride (Additive CNS depression).
No products indexed under this heading.

Imipramine Hydrochloride (Additive CNS depression).
No products indexed under this heading.

Imipramine Pamoate (Additive CNS depression).
No products indexed under this heading.

Isoflurane (Additive CNS depression).
No products indexed under this heading.

Ketamine Hydrochloride (Additive CNS depression).
No products indexed under this heading.

IMPORTANT NOTE: Always consult each drug listing in the patient's regimen for possible interactions.

Levomethadyl Acetate Hydrochloride (Additive CNS depression).
No products indexed under this heading.

Levorphanol Tartrate (Additive CNS depression).
No products indexed under this heading.

Lorazepam (Additive CNS depression).
No products indexed under this heading.

Loxapine Hydrochloride (Additive CNS depression).
No products indexed under this heading.

Loxapine Succinate (Additive CNS depression).
No products indexed under this heading.

Maprotiline Hydrochloride (Additive CNS depression).
No products indexed under this heading.

Meperidine Hydrochloride (Additive CNS depression).
No products indexed under this heading.

Mephobarbital (Additive CNS depression). Products include:
Mebaral Tablets, USP **2483**

Meprobamate (Additive CNS depression).
No products indexed under this heading.

Mesoridazine Besylate (Additive CNS depression).
No products indexed under this heading.

Methadone Hydrochloride (Additive CNS depression).
No products indexed under this heading.

Methohexital Sodium (Additive CNS depression).
No products indexed under this heading.

Methotrimeprazine (Additive CNS depression).
No products indexed under this heading.

Methoxyflurane (Additive CNS depression).
No products indexed under this heading.

Metocurine Iodide (Opioid analgesics including Dilaudid may enhance the action of neuromuscular blocking agents and produce an excessive degree of respiratory depression).
No products indexed under this heading.

Midazolam Hydrochloride (Additive CNS depression).
No products indexed under this heading.

Mivacurium Chloride (Opioid analgesics including Dilaudid may enhance the action of neuromuscular blocking agents and produce an excessive degree of respiratory depression). Products include:
Mivacron Injection **489**

Molindone Hydrochloride (Additive CNS depression). Products include:
Moban Tablets **1108**

Morphine Sulfate (Additive CNS depression). Products include:
Avinza Capsules **1714**
Kadian Capsules **572**
MS Contin Tablets **2703**

Nortriptyline Hydrochloride (Additive CNS depression).
No products indexed under this heading.

Olanzapine (Additive CNS depression). Products include:
Symbyax Capsules **1788**
Zyprexa Tablets **1798**
Zyprexa IntraMuscular **1798**
Zyprexa ZYDIS Orally Disintegrating Tablets **1798**

Oxazepam (Additive CNS depression).
No products indexed under this heading.

Oxycodone Hydrochloride (Additive CNS depression). Products include:
Combunox Tablets **1183**
OxyContin Tablets **2699**
OxyFast Oral Concentrate Solution **2704**
OxyIR Capsules **2704**
Percocet Tablets **1114**
Percodan Tablets **1115**

Pancuronium Bromide (Opioid analgesics including Dilaudid may enhance the action of neuromuscular blocking agents and produce an excessive degree of respiratory depression).
No products indexed under this heading.

Pentobarbital Sodium (Additive CNS depression). Products include:
Nembutal Sodium Solution, USP **2484**

Perphenazine (Additive CNS depression).
No products indexed under this heading.

Phenobarbital (Additive CNS depression).
No products indexed under this heading.

Prazepam (Additive CNS depression).
No products indexed under this heading.

Prochlorperazine (Additive CNS depression).
No products indexed under this heading.

Promethazine Hydrochloride (Additive CNS depression). Products include:
Phenergan **3438**

Propofol (Additive CNS depression). Products include:
Diprivan Injectable Emulsion **676**

Propoxyphene Hydrochloride (Additive CNS depression).
No products indexed under this heading.

Propoxyphene Napsylate (Additive CNS depression). Products include:
Darvocet A 500 Tablets **3497**

Protriptyline Hydrochloride (Additive CNS depression). Products include:
Vivactil Tablets **2350**

Quazepam (Additive CNS depression).
No products indexed under this heading.

Quetiapine Fumarate (Additive CNS depression). Products include:
Seroquel Tablets **691**

Rapacuronium Bromide (Opioid analgesics including Dilaudid may enhance the action of neuromuscular blocking agents and produce an excessive degree of respiratory depression).
No products indexed under this heading.

Remifentanil Hydrochloride (Additive CNS depression).
No products indexed under this heading.

Risperidone (Additive CNS depression). Products include:
Risperdal Consta Long-Acting Injection **1664**
Risperdal M-Tab Orally Disintegrating Tablets **1658**
Risperdal **1658**

Rocuronium Bromide (Opioid analgesics including Dilaudid may enhance the action of neuromuscular blocking agents and produce an excessive degree of respiratory depression). Products include:
Zemuron Injection **2363**

Secobarbital Sodium (Additive CNS depression).
No products indexed under this heading.

Sevoflurane (Additive CNS depression). Products include:
Ultane Liquid for Inhalation **526**

Sodium Oxybate (Additive CNS depression).
No products indexed under this heading.

Succinylcholine Chloride (Opioid analgesics including Dilaudid may enhance the action of neuromuscular blocking agents and produce an excessive degree of respiratory depression).
No products indexed under this heading.

Sufentanil Citrate (Additive CNS depression).
No products indexed under this heading.

Temazepam (Additive CNS depression).
No products indexed under this heading.

Thiamylal Sodium (Additive CNS depression).
No products indexed under this heading.

Thioridazine Hydrochloride (Additive CNS depression). Products include:
Thioridazine Hydrochloride Tablets **2122**

Thiothixene (Additive CNS depression). Products include:
Thiothixene Capsules **2124**

Triazolam (Additive CNS depression).
No products indexed under this heading.

Trifluoperazine Hydrochloride (Additive CNS depression).
No products indexed under this heading.

Trimipramine Maleate (Additive CNS depression). Products include:
Surmontil Capsules **2347**

Vecuronium Bromide (Opioid analgesics including Dilaudid may enhance the action of neuromuscular blocking agents and produce an excessive degree of respiratory depression).
No products indexed under this heading.

Zaleplon (Additive CNS depression). Products include:
Sonata Capsules **1686**

Ziprasidone Hydrochloride (Additive CNS depression). Products include:
Geodon Capsules **2514**

Zolpidem Tartrate (Additive CNS depression). Products include:
Ambien Tablets **2867**

Food Interactions

Alcohol (Additive CNS depression).

DILAUDID MULTIPLE DOSE VIALS

(Hydromorphone Hydrochloride) **439**
See Dilaudid Ampules

DILAUDID ORAL LIQUID

(Hydromorphone Hydrochloride) **443**
May interact with central nervous system depressants, general anesthetics, hypnotics and sedatives, neuromuscular blocking agents, phenothiazines, tranquilizers, and certain other agents. Compounds in these categories include:

Alfentanil Hydrochloride (May produce additive depressant effects; respiratory depression, hypotension and profound sedation or coma may occur; the dose of one or both agents should be reduced).
No products indexed under this heading.

Alprazolam (May produce additive depressant effects; respiratory depression, hypotension and profound sedation or coma may occur; the dose of one or both agents should be reduced). Products include:
Niravam Orally Disintegrating Tablets **3106**
Xanax XR Tablets **2655**

Aprobarbital (May produce additive depressant effects; respiratory depression, hypotension and profound sedation or coma may occur; the dose of one or both agents should be reduced).
No products indexed under this heading.

Atracurium Besylate (Enhanced action of neuromuscular blocking agents and produce an excessive degree of respiratory depression).
No products indexed under this heading.

Buprenorphine Hydrochloride (May produce additive depressant effects; respiratory depression, hypotension and profound sedation or coma may occur; the dose of one or both agents should be reduced). Products include:
Buprenex Injectable **2718**
Suboxone Tablets **2719**
Subutex Tablets **2719**

Buspirone Hydrochloride (May produce additive depressant effects; respiratory depression, hypotension and profound sedation or coma may occur; the dose of one or both agents should be reduced).
No products indexed under this heading.

Butabarbital (May produce additive depressant effects; respiratory depression, hypotension and profound sedation or coma may occur; the dose of one or both agents should be reduced).
No products indexed under this heading.

Butalbital (May produce additive depressant effects; respiratory depression, hypotension and profound sedation or coma may occur; the dose of one or both agents should be reduced). Products include:
Sedapap Tablets 50 mg/650 mg **2098**

Chlordiazepoxide (May produce additive depressant effects; respiratory depression, hypotension and profound sedation or coma may occur; the dose of one or both agents should be reduced).
No products indexed under this heading.

Chlordiazepoxide Hydrochloride (May produce additive depressant effects; respiratory depression, hypotension and profound sedation or coma may occur; the dose of one or both agents should be reduced). Products include:
Librium Capsules 3349

Chlorpromazine (May produce additive depressant effects; respiratory depression, hypotension and profound sedation or coma may occur; the dose of one or both agents should be reduced).
No products indexed under this heading.

Chlorpromazine Hydrochloride (May produce additive depressant effects; respiratory depression, hypotension and profound sedation or coma may occur; the dose of one or both agents should be reduced).
No products indexed under this heading.

Chlorprothixene (May produce additive depressant effects; respiratory depression, hypotension and profound sedation or coma may occur; the dose of one or both agents should be reduced).
No products indexed under this heading.

Chlorprothixene Hydrochloride (May produce additive depressant effects; respiratory depression, hypotension and profound sedation or coma may occur; the dose of one or both agents should be reduced).
No products indexed under this heading.

Chlorprothixene Lactate (May produce additive depressant effects; respiratory depression, hypotension and profound sedation or coma may occur; the dose of one or both agents should be reduced).
No products indexed under this heading.

Cisatracurium Besylate (Enhanced action of neuromuscular blocking agents and produce an excessive degree of respiratory depression). Products include:
Nimbex Injection 494

Clorazepate Dipotassium (May produce additive depressant effects; respiratory depression, hypotension and profound sedation or coma may occur; the dose of one or both agents should be reduced). Products include:
Tranxene 2488

Clozapine (May produce additive depressant effects; respiratory depression, hypotension and profound sedation or coma may occur; the dose of one or both agents should be reduced). Products include:
Clozapine Tablets 2141
Clozaril Tablets 2174
FazaClo Orally Disintegrating Tablets 547

Codeine Phosphate (May produce additive depressant effects; respiratory depression, hypotension and profound sedation or coma may occur; the dose of one or both agents should be reduced). Products include:
Tylenol with Codeine 2461

Desflurane (May produce additive depressant effects; respiratory depression, hypotension and profound sedation or coma may occur; the dose of one or both agents should be reduced). Products include:
Suprane Liquid for Inhalation 770

Dezocine (May produce additive depressant effects; respiratory depression, hypotension and profound sedation or coma may occur; the dose of one or both agents should be reduced).
No products indexed under this heading.

Diazepam (May produce additive depressant effects; respiratory depression, hypotension and profound sedation or coma may occur; the dose of one or both agents should be reduced). Products include:
Diastat Rectal Delivery System 3344
Valium Tablets 2822

Doxacurium Chloride (Enhanced action of neuromuscular blocking agents and produce an excessive degree of respiratory depression).
No products indexed under this heading.

Droperidol (May produce additive depressant effects; respiratory depression, hypotension and profound sedation or coma may occur; the dose of one or both agents should be reduced).
No products indexed under this heading.

Enflurane (May produce additive depressant effects; respiratory depression, hypotension and profound sedation or coma may occur; the dose of one or both agents should be reduced).
No products indexed under this heading.

Estazolam (May produce additive depressant effects; respiratory depression, hypotension and profound sedation or coma may occur; the dose of one or both agents should be reduced). Products include:
ProSom Tablets 512

Ethanol (May produce additive depressant effects; respiratory depression, hypotension and profound sedation or coma may occur; the dose of one or both agents should be reduced).
No products indexed under this heading.

Ethchlorvynol (May produce additive depressant effects; respiratory depression, hypotension and profound sedation or coma may occur; the dose of one or both agents should be reduced).
No products indexed under this heading.

Ethinamate (May produce additive depressant effects; respiratory depression, hypotension and profound sedation or coma may occur; the dose of one or both agents should be reduced).
No products indexed under this heading.

Ethyl Alcohol (May produce additive depressant effects; respiratory depression, hypotension and profound sedation or coma may occur; the dose of one or both agents should be reduced).
No products indexed under this heading.

Fentanyl (May produce additive depressant effects; respiratory depression, hypotension and profound sedation or coma may occur; the dose of one or both agents should be reduced). Products include:
Duragesic Transdermal System 2448

Fentanyl Citrate (May produce additive depressant effects; respiratory depression, hypotension and profound sedation or coma may occur; the dose of one or both agents should be reduced). Products include:
Actiq 993

Fluphenazine Decanoate (May produce additive depressant effects; respiratory depression, hypotension and profound sedation or coma may occur; the dose of one or both agents should be reduced).
No products indexed under this heading.

Fluphenazine Enanthate (May produce additive depressant effects; respiratory depression, hypotension and profound sedation or coma may occur; the dose of one or both agents should be reduced).
No products indexed under this heading.

Fluphenazine Hydrochloride (May produce additive depressant effects; respiratory depression, hypotension and profound sedation or coma may occur; the dose of one or both agents should be reduced).
No products indexed under this heading.

Flurazepam Hydrochloride (May produce additive depressant effects; respiratory depression, hypotension and profound sedation or coma may occur; the dose of one or both agents should be reduced). Products include:
Dalmane Capsules 3343

Glutethimide (May produce additive depressant effects; respiratory depression, hypotension and profound sedation or coma may occur; the dose of one or both agents should be reduced).
No products indexed under this heading.

Haloperidol (May produce additive depressant effects; respiratory depression, hypotension and profound sedation or coma may occur; the dose of one or both agents should be reduced).
No products indexed under this heading.

Haloperidol Decanoate (May produce additive depressant effects; respiratory depression, hypotension and profound sedation or coma may occur; the dose of one or both agents should be reduced).
No products indexed under this heading.

Hydrocodone Bitartrate (May produce additive depressant effects; respiratory depression, hypotension and profound sedation or coma may occur; the dose of one or both agents should be reduced). Products include:
Hycodan 1104
Hycomine Compound Tablets 1105
Hycotuss Expectorant Syrup 1106
Lortab 3315
Lortab Elixir 3312
Vicodin Tablets 530
Vicodin ES Tablets 531
Vicodin HP Tablets 532
Vicoprofen Tablets 533
Zydone Tablets 1118

Hydrocodone Polistirex (May produce additive depressant effects; respiratory depression, hypotension and profound sedation or coma may occur; the dose of one or both agents should be reduced). Products include:
Tussionex Pennkinetic Extended-Release Suspension 3322

Hydroxyzine Hydrochloride (May produce additive depressant effects; respiratory depression, hypotension and profound sedation or coma may occur; the dose of one or both agents should be reduced).
No products indexed under this heading.

Isoflurane (May produce additive depressant effects; respiratory depression, hypotension and profound sedation or coma may occur; the dose of one or both agents should be reduced).
No products indexed under this heading.

Ketamine Hydrochloride (May produce additive depressant effects; respiratory depression, hypotension and profound sedation or coma may occur; the dose of one or both agents should be reduced).
No products indexed under this heading.

Levomethadyl Acetate Hydrochloride (May produce additive depressant effects; respiratory depression, hypotension and profound sedation or coma may occur; the dose of one or both agents should be reduced).
No products indexed under this heading.

Levorphanol Tartrate (May produce additive depressant effects; respiratory depression, hypotension and profound sedation or coma may occur; the dose of one or both agents should be reduced).
No products indexed under this heading.

Lorazepam (May produce additive depressant effects; respiratory depression, hypotension and profound sedation or coma may occur; the dose of one or both agents should be reduced).
No products indexed under this heading.

Loxapine Hydrochloride (May produce additive depressant effects; respiratory depression, hypotension and profound sedation or coma may occur; the dose of one or both agents should be reduced).
No products indexed under this heading.

Loxapine Succinate (May produce additive depressant effects; respiratory depression, hypotension and profound sedation or coma may occur; the dose of one or both agents should be reduced).
No products indexed under this heading.

Meperidine Hydrochloride (May produce additive depressant effects; respiratory depression, hypotension and profound sedation or coma may occur; the dose of one or both agents should be reduced).
No products indexed under this heading.

Mephobarbital (May produce additive depressant effects; respiratory depression, hypotension and profound sedation or coma may occur; the dose of one or both agents should be reduced). Products include:
Mebaral Tablets, USP 2483

Meprobamate (May produce additive depressant effects; respiratory depression, hypotension and profound sedation or coma may occur; the dose of one or both agents should be reduced).
No products indexed under this heading.

Mesoridazine Besylate (May produce additive depressant effects; respiratory depression, hypotension and profound sedation or coma may occur; the dose of one or both agents should be reduced).
No products indexed under this heading.

Methadone Hydrochloride (May produce additive depressant effects; respiratory depression, hypotension and profound sedation or coma may occur; the dose of one or both agents should be reduced).
No products indexed under this heading.

Methohexital Sodium (May produce additive depressant effects; respiratory depression, hypotension and profound sedation or coma may occur; the dose of one or both agents should be reduced).
No products indexed under this heading.

Methotrimeprazine (May produce additive depressant effects; respiratory depression, hypotension and profound sedation or coma may occur; the dose of one or both agents should be reduced).
No products indexed under this heading.

Methoxyflurane (May produce additive depressant effects; respiratory depression, hypotension and profound sedation or coma may occur; the dose of one or both agents should be reduced).
No products indexed under this heading.

Metocurine Iodide (Enhanced action of neuromuscular blocking agents and produce an excessive degree of respiratory depression).
No products indexed under this heading.

Midazolam Hydrochloride (May produce additive depressant effects; respiratory depression, hypotension and profound sedation or coma may occur; the dose of one or both agents should be reduced).
No products indexed under this heading.

Mivacurium Chloride (Enhanced action of neuromuscular blocking agents and produce an excessive degree of respiratory depression). Products include:
Mivacron Injection 489

Molindone Hydrochloride (May produce additive depressant effects; respiratory depression, hypotension and profound sedation or coma may occur; the dose of one or both agents should be reduced). Products include:
Moban Tablets 1108

Morphine Sulfate (May produce additive depressant effects; respiratory depression, hypotension and profound sedation or coma may occur; the dose of one or both agents should be reduced). Products include:
Avinza Capsules 1714
Kadian Capsules 572
MS Contin Tablets 2703

Olanzapine (May produce additive depressant effects; respiratory depression, hypotension and profound sedation or coma may occur; the dose of one or both agents should be reduced). Products include:
Symbyax Capsules 1788
Zyprexa Tablets 1798
Zyprexa IntraMuscular 1798
Zyprexa ZYDIS Orally Disintegrating Tablets 1798

Oxazepam (May produce additive depressant effects; respiratory depression, hypotension and profound sedation or coma may occur; the dose of one or both agents should be reduced).
No products indexed under this heading.

Oxycodone Hydrochloride (May produce additive depressant effects; respiratory depression, hypotension and profound sedation or coma may occur; the dose of one or both agents should be reduced). Products include:
Combunox Tablets 1183
OxyContin Tablets 2699
OxyFast Oral Concentrate Solution 2704
OxyIR Capsules 2704
Percocet Tablets 1114
Percodan Tablets 1115

Pancuronium Bromide (Enhanced action of neuromuscular blocking agents and produce an excessive degree of respiratory depression).
No products indexed under this heading.

Pentobarbital Sodium (May produce additive depressant effects; respiratory depression, hypotension and profound sedation or coma may occur; the dose of one or both agents should be reduced). Products include:
Nembutal Sodium Solution, USP 2484

Perphenazine (May produce additive depressant effects; respiratory depression, hypotension and profound sedation or coma may occur; the dose of one or both agents should be reduced).
No products indexed under this heading.

Phenobarbital (May produce additive depressant effects; respiratory depression, hypotension and profound sedation or coma may occur; the dose of one or both agents should be reduced).
No products indexed under this heading.

Prazepam (May produce additive depressant effects; respiratory depression, hypotension and profound sedation or coma may occur; the dose of one or both agents should be reduced).
No products indexed under this heading.

Prochlorperazine (May produce additive depressant effects; respiratory depression, hypotension and profound sedation or coma may occur; the dose of one or both agents should be reduced).
No products indexed under this heading.

Promethazine Hydrochloride (May produce additive depressant effects; respiratory depression, hypotension and profound sedation or coma may occur; the dose of one or both agents should be reduced). Products include:
Phenergan 3438

Propofol (May produce additive depressant effects; respiratory depression, hypotension and profound sedation or coma may occur; the dose of one or both agents should be reduced). Products include:
Diprivan Injectable Emulsion 676

Propoxyphene Hydrochloride (May produce additive depressant effects; respiratory depression, hypotension and profound sedation or coma may occur; the dose of one or both agents should be reduced).
No products indexed under this heading.

Propoxyphene Napsylate (May produce additive depressant effects; respiratory depression, hypotension and profound sedation or coma may occur; the dose of one or both agents should be reduced). Products include:
Darvocet A 500 Tablets 3497

Quazepam (May produce additive depressant effects; respiratory depression, hypotension and profound sedation or coma may occur; the dose of one or both agents should be reduced).
No products indexed under this heading.

Quetiapine Fumarate (May produce additive depressant effects; respiratory depression, hypotension and profound sedation or coma may occur; the dose of one or both agents should be reduced). Products include:
Seroquel Tablets 691

Rapacuronium Bromide (Enhanced action of neuromuscular blocking agents and produce an excessive degree of respiratory depression).
No products indexed under this heading.

Remifentanil Hydrochloride (May produce additive depressant effects; respiratory depression, hypotension and profound sedation or coma may occur; the dose of one or both agents should be reduced).
No products indexed under this heading.

Risperidone (May produce additive depressant effects; respiratory depression, hypotension and profound sedation or coma may occur; the dose of one or both agents should be reduced). Products include:
Risperdal Consta Long-Acting Injection 1664
Risperdal M-Tab Orally Disintegrating Tablets 1658
Risperdal 1658

Rocuronium Bromide (Enhanced action of neuromuscular blocking agents and produce an excessive degree of respiratory depression). Products include:
Zemuron Injection 2363

Secobarbital Sodium (May produce additive depressant effects; respiratory depression, hypotension and profound sedation or coma may occur; the dose of one or both agents should be reduced).
No products indexed under this heading.

Sevoflurane (May produce additive depressant effects; respiratory depression, hypotension and profound sedation or coma may occur; the dose of one or both agents should be reduced). Products include:
Ultane Liquid for Inhalation 526

Succinylcholine Chloride (Enhanced action of neuromuscular blocking agents and produce an excessive degree of respiratory depression).
No products indexed under this heading.

Sufentanil Citrate (May produce additive depressant effects; respiratory depression, hypotension and profound sedation or coma may occur; the dose of one or both agents should be reduced).
No products indexed under this heading.

Temazepam (May produce additive depressant effects; respiratory depression, hypotension and profound sedation or coma may occur; the dose of one or both agents should be reduced).
No products indexed under this heading.

Thiamylal Sodium (May produce additive depressant effects; respiratory depression, hypotension and profound sedation or coma may occur; the dose of one or both agents should be reduced).
No products indexed under this heading.

Thioridazine Hydrochloride (May produce additive depressant effects; respiratory depression, hypotension and profound sedation or coma may occur; the dose of one or both agents should be reduced). Products include:
Thioridazine Hydrochloride Tablets 2122

Thiothixene (May produce additive depressant effects; respiratory depression, hypotension and profound sedation or coma may occur; the dose of one or both agents should be reduced). Products include:
Thiothixene Capsules 2124

Triazolam (May produce additive depressant effects; respiratory depression, hypotension and profound sedation or coma may occur; the dose of one or both agents should be reduced).
No products indexed under this heading.

Trifluoperazine Hydrochloride (May produce additive depressant effects; respiratory depression, hypotension and profound sedation or coma may occur; the dose of one or both agents should be reduced).
No products indexed under this heading.

Vecuronium Bromide (Enhanced action of neuromuscular blocking agents and produce an excessive degree of respiratory depression).
No products indexed under this heading.

Zaleplon (May produce additive depressant effects; respiratory depression, hypotension and profound sedation or coma may occur; the dose of one or both agents should be reduced). Products include:
Sonata Capsules 1686

Ziprasidone Hydrochloride (May produce additive depressant effects; respiratory depression, hypotension and profound sedation or coma may occur; the dose of one or both agents should be reduced). Products include:
Geodon Capsules 2514

Zolpidem Tartrate (May produce additive depressant effects; respiratory depression, hypotension and profound sedation or coma may occur; the dose of one or both agents should be reduced). Products include:
Ambien Tablets 2867

Food Interactions

Alcohol (May exhibit an additive CNS depression).

DILAUDID NON-STERILE POWDER

(Hydromorphone Hydrochloride) 439
See Dilaudid Ampules

DILAUDID RECTAL SUPPOSITORIES

(Hydromorphone Hydrochloride) 439
See Dilaudid Ampules

DILAUDID TABLETS

(Hydromorphone Hydrochloride) 439
See Dilaudid Ampules

DILAUDID TABLETS - 8 MG

(Hydromorphone Hydrochloride) 443
See Dilaudid Oral Liquid

DILAUDID-HP INJECTION

(Hydromorphone Hydrochloride) 441
See Dilaudid Oral Liquid

DILAUDID-HP LYOPHILIZED POWDER 250 MG

(Hydromorphone Hydrochloride) 441
See Dilaudid Oral Liquid

CHILDREN'S DIMETAPP COLD & ALLERGY ELIXIR

(Brompheniramine Maleate, Pseudoephedrine Hydrochloride)....... 745
May interact with hypnotics and sedatives, monoamine oxidase inhibitors, tranquilizers, and certain other agents. Compounds in these categories include:

Alprazolam (May increase drowsiness effect). Products include:
Niravam Orally Disintegrating Tablets 3106
Xanax XR Tablets 2655

Buspirone Hydrochloride (May increase drowsiness effect).
No products indexed under this heading.

Chlordiazepoxide (May increase drowsiness effect).
No products indexed under this heading.

Chlordiazepoxide Hydrochloride (May increase drowsiness effect). Products include:
Librium Capsules 3349

Chlorpromazine (May increase drowsiness effect).
No products indexed under this heading.

Chlorpromazine Hydrochloride (May increase drowsiness effect).
No products indexed under this heading.

Chlorprothixene (May increase drowsiness effect).
No products indexed under this heading.

Chlorprothixene Hydrochloride (May increase drowsiness effect).
No products indexed under this heading.

Clorazepate Dipotassium (May increase drowsiness effect). Products include:
Tranxene 2488

Diazepam (May increase drowsiness effect). Products include:
Diastat Rectal Delivery System 3344
Valium Tablets 2822

Droperidol (May increase drowsiness effect).
No products indexed under this heading.

Estazolam (May increase drowsiness effect). Products include:
ProSom Tablets 512

Ethchlorvynol (May increase drowsiness effect).
No products indexed under this heading.

Ethinamate (May increase drowsiness effect).
No products indexed under this heading.

Fluphenazine Decanoate (May increase drowsiness effect).
No products indexed under this heading.

Fluphenazine Enanthate (May increase drowsiness effect).
No products indexed under this heading.

Fluphenazine Hydrochloride (May increase drowsiness effect).
No products indexed under this heading.

Flurazepam Hydrochloride (May increase drowsiness effect). Products include:
Dalmane Capsules 3343

Glutethimide (May increase drowsiness effect).
No products indexed under this heading.

Haloperidol (May increase drowsiness effect).
No products indexed under this heading.

Haloperidol Decanoate (May increase drowsiness effect).
No products indexed under this heading.

Hydroxyzine Hydrochloride (May increase drowsiness effect).
No products indexed under this heading.

Isocarboxazid (Concurrent and/or sequential use with MAO inhibitors is not recommended).
No products indexed under this heading.

Lorazepam (May increase drowsiness effect).
No products indexed under this heading.

Loxapine Hydrochloride (May increase drowsiness effect).
No products indexed under this heading.

Loxapine Succinate (May increase drowsiness effect).
No products indexed under this heading.

Meprobamate (May increase drowsiness effect).
No products indexed under this heading.

Mesoridazine Besylate (May increase drowsiness effect).
No products indexed under this heading.

Midazolam Hydrochloride (May increase drowsiness effect).
No products indexed under this heading.

Moclobemide (Concurrent and/or sequential use with MAO inhibitors is not recommended).
No products indexed under this heading.

Molindone Hydrochloride (May increase drowsiness effect). Products include:
Moban Tablets 1108

Oxazepam (May increase drowsiness effect).
No products indexed under this heading.

Pargyline Hydrochloride (Concurrent and/or sequential use with MAO inhibitors is not recommended).
No products indexed under this heading.

Perphenazine (May increase drowsiness effect).
No products indexed under this heading.

Phenelzine Sulfate (Concurrent and/or sequential use with MAO inhibitors is not recommended).
No products indexed under this heading.

Prazepam (May increase drowsiness effect).
No products indexed under this heading.

Procarbazine Hydrochloride (Concurrent and/or sequential use with MAO inhibitors is not recommended). Products include:
Matulane Capsules 3188

Prochlorperazine (May increase drowsiness effect).
No products indexed under this heading.

Promethazine Hydrochloride (May increase drowsiness effect). Products include:
Phenergan 3438

Propofol (May increase drowsiness effect). Products include:
Diprivan Injectable Emulsion 676

Quazepam (May increase drowsiness effect).
No products indexed under this heading.

Secobarbital Sodium (May increase drowsiness effect).
No products indexed under this heading.

Selegiline Hydrochloride (Concurrent and/or sequential use with MAO inhibitors is not recommended). Products include:
Eldepryl Capsules 3209

Temazepam (May increase drowsiness effect).
No products indexed under this heading.

Thioridazine Hydrochloride (May increase drowsiness effect). Products include:
Thioridazine Hydrochloride Tablets 2122

Thiothixene (May increase drowsiness effect). Products include:
Thiothixene Capsules 2124

Tranylcypromine Sulfate (Concurrent and/or sequential use with MAO inhibitors is not recommended). Products include:
Parnate Tablets 1499

Triazolam (May increase drowsiness effect).
No products indexed under this heading.

Trifluoperazine Hydrochloride (May increase drowsiness effect).
No products indexed under this heading.

Zaleplon (May increase drowsiness effect). Products include:
Sonata Capsules 1686

Zolpidem Tartrate (May increase drowsiness effect). Products include:
Ambien Tablets 2867

Food Interactions

Alcohol (May increase drowsiness effect).

CHILDREN'S DIMETAPP DM COLD & COUGH ELIXIR

(Brompheniramine Maleate, Dextromethorphan Hydrobromide, Pseudoephedrine Hydrochloride)....... 745
May interact with hypnotics and sedatives, monoamine oxidase inhibitors, tranquilizers, and certain other agents. Compounds in these categories include:

Alprazolam (Increases drowsiness effect). Products include:
Niravam Orally Disintegrating Tablets 3106
Xanax XR Tablets 2655

Buspirone Hydrochloride (Increases drowsiness effect).
No products indexed under this heading.

Chlordiazepoxide (Increases drowsiness effect).
No products indexed under this heading.

Chlordiazepoxide Hydrochloride (Increases drowsiness effect). Products include:
Librium Capsules 3349

Chlorpromazine (Increases drowsiness effect).
No products indexed under this heading.

Chlorpromazine Hydrochloride (Increases drowsiness effect).
No products indexed under this heading.

Chlorprothixene (Increases drowsiness effect).
No products indexed under this heading.

Chlorprothixene Hydrochloride (Increases drowsiness effect).
No products indexed under this heading.

Clorazepate Dipotassium (Increases drowsiness effect). Products include:
Tranxene 2488

Diazepam (Increases drowsiness effect). Products include:
Diastat Rectal Delivery System 3344
Valium Tablets 2822

Droperidol (Increases drowsiness effect).
No products indexed under this heading.

Estazolam (Increases drowsiness effect). Products include:

ProSom Tablets 512

Ethchlorvynol (Increases drowsiness effect).
No products indexed under this heading.

Ethinamate (Increases drowsiness effect).
No products indexed under this heading.

Fluphenazine Decanoate (Increases drowsiness effect).
No products indexed under this heading.

Fluphenazine Enanthate (Increases drowsiness effect).
No products indexed under this heading.

Fluphenazine Hydrochloride (Increases drowsiness effect).
No products indexed under this heading.

Flurazepam Hydrochloride (Increases drowsiness effect). Products include:
Dalmane Capsules 3343

Glutethimide (Increases drowsiness effect).
No products indexed under this heading.

Haloperidol (Increases drowsiness effect).
No products indexed under this heading.

Haloperidol Decanoate (Increases drowsiness effect).
No products indexed under this heading.

Hydroxyzine Hydrochloride (Increases drowsiness effect).
No products indexed under this heading.

Isocarboxazid (Concurrent and/or sequential use with MAO inhibitors is contraindicated).
No products indexed under this heading.

Lorazepam (Increases drowsiness effect).
No products indexed under this heading.

Loxapine Hydrochloride (Increases drowsiness effect).
No products indexed under this heading.

Loxapine Succinate (Increases drowsiness effect).
No products indexed under this heading.

Meprobamate (Increases drowsiness effect).
No products indexed under this heading.

Mesoridazine Besylate (Increases drowsiness effect).
No products indexed under this heading.

Midazolam Hydrochloride (Increases drowsiness effect).
No products indexed under this heading.

Moclobemide (Concurrent and/or sequential use with MAO inhibitors is contraindicated).
No products indexed under this heading.

Molindone Hydrochloride (Increases drowsiness effect). Products include:
Moban Tablets 1108

Oxazepam (Increases drowsiness effect).
No products indexed under this heading.

Pargyline Hydrochloride (Concurrent and/or sequential use with MAO inhibitors is contraindicated).
No products indexed under this heading.

Perphenazine (Increases drowsiness effect).
No products indexed under this heading.

Phenelzine Sulfate (Concurrent and/or sequential use with MAO inhibitors is contraindicated).
No products indexed under this heading.

Prazepam (Increases drowsiness effect).
No products indexed under this heading.

Procarbazine Hydrochloride (Concurrent and/or sequential use with MAO inhibitors is contraindicated). Products include:
Matulane Capsules 3188

Prochlorperazine (Increases drowsiness effect).
No products indexed under this heading.

Promethazine Hydrochloride (Increases drowsiness effect). Products include:
Phenergan 3438

Propofol (Increases drowsiness effect). Products include:
Diprivan Injectable Emulsion 676

Quazepam (Increases drowsiness effect).
No products indexed under this heading.

Secobarbital Sodium (Increases drowsiness effect).
No products indexed under this heading.

Selegiline Hydrochloride (Concurrent and/or sequential use with MAO inhibitors is contraindicated). Products include:
Eldepryl Capsules 3209

Temazepam (Increases drowsiness effect).
No products indexed under this heading.

Thioridazine Hydrochloride (Increases drowsiness effect). Products include:
Thioridazine Hydrochloride Tablets 2122

Thiothixene (Increases drowsiness effect). Products include:
Thiothixene Capsules 2124

Tranylcypromine Sulfate (Concurrent and/or sequential use with MAO inhibitors is contraindicated). Products include:
Parnate Tablets 1499

Triazolam (Increases drowsiness effect).
No products indexed under this heading.

Trifluoperazine Hydrochloride (Increases drowsiness effect).
No products indexed under this heading.

Zaleplon (Increases drowsiness effect). Products include:
Sonata Capsules 1686

Zolpidem Tartrate (Increases drowsiness effect). Products include:
Ambien Tablets 2867

Food Interactions

Alcohol (Increases drowsiness effect; avoid concurrent use).

CHILDREN'S DIMETAPP LONG ACTING COUGH PLUS COLD SYRUP

(Dextromethorphan Hydrobromide, Pseudoephedrine Hydrochloride) .... ▣ 746
May interact with monoamine oxidase inhibitors. Compounds in these categories include:

Isocarboxazid (Do not use while taking, or for up to two weeks after stopping, MAO inhibitors).
No products indexed under this heading.

Moclobemide (Do not use while taking, or for up to two weeks after stopping, MAO inhibitors).
No products indexed under this heading.

Pargyline Hydrochloride (Do not use while taking, or for up to two weeks after stopping, MAO inhibitors).
No products indexed under this heading.

Phenelzine Sulfate (Do not use while taking, or for up to two weeks after stopping, MAO inhibitors).
No products indexed under this heading.

Procarbazine Hydrochloride (Do not use while taking, or for up to two weeks after stopping, MAO inhibitors). Products include:
Matulane Capsules 3188

Selegiline Hydrochloride (Do not use while taking, or for up to two weeks after stopping, MAO inhibitors). Products include:
Eldepryl Capsules 3209

Tranylcypromine Sulfate (Do not use while taking, or for up to two weeks after stopping, MAO inhibitors). Products include:
Parnate Tablets 1499

CHILDREN'S DIMETAPP ND NON-DROWSY ALLERGY SYRUP

(Loratadine) .... ▣ 746
None cited in PDR database.

DIMETAPP INFANT DROPS DECONGESTANT PLUS COUGH

(Dextromethorphan Hydrobromide, Pseudoephedrine Hydrochloride) .... ▣ 746
May interact with monoamine oxidase inhibitors. Compounds in these categories include:

Isocarboxazid (Concurrent and/or sequential use with MAO inhibitors is not recommended).
No products indexed under this heading.

Moclobemide (Concurrent and/or sequential use with MAO inhibitors is not recommended).
No products indexed under this heading.

Pargyline Hydrochloride (Concurrent and/or sequential use with MAO inhibitors is not recommended).
No products indexed under this heading.

Phenelzine Sulfate (Concurrent and/or sequential use with MAO inhibitors is not recommended).
No products indexed under this heading.

Procarbazine Hydrochloride (Concurrent and/or sequential use with MAO inhibitors is not recommended). Products include:
Matulane Capsules 3188

Selegiline Hydrochloride (Concurrent and/or sequential use with MAO inhibitors is not recommended). Products include:
Eldepryl Capsules 3209

Tranylcypromine Sulfate (Concurrent and/or sequential use with MAO inhibitors is not recommended). Products include:
Parnate Tablets 1499

DIOVAN HCT TABLETS

(Hydrochlorothiazide, Valsartan) 2195
May interact with antihypertensives, barbiturates, corticosteroids, cardiac glycosides, oral hypoglycemic agents, insulin, lithium preparations, narcotic analgesics, nondepolarizing neuromuscular blocking agents, nonsteroidal anti-inflammatory agents, potassium preparations, and certain other agents. Compounds in these categories include:

Acarbose (Dosage adjustment of the antidiabetic drug may be required). Products include:
Precose Tablets 776

Acebutolol Hydrochloride (Co-administration with other antihypertensives may result in additive effect or potentiation).
No products indexed under this heading.

ACTH (Co-administration of thiazide diuretics and ACTH may intensify electrolyte depletion, particularly hypokalemia).
No products indexed under this heading.

Alfentanil Hydrochloride (Co-administration of thiazide diuretics and narcotics may result in potentiation of orthostatic hypotension).
No products indexed under this heading.

Amlodipine Besylate (Co-administration with other antihypertensives may result in additive effect or potentiation). Products include:
Caduet Tablets 2507
Lotrel Capsules 2238
Norvasc Tablets 2529

Aprobarbital (Co-administration of thiazide diuretics and barbiturates may result in potentiation of orthostatic hypotension).
No products indexed under this heading.

Atenolol (Co-administration with other antihypertensives may result in additive effect or potentiation). Products include:
Tenormin I.V. Injection 698
Tenormin Tablets 695

Atracurium Besylate (Co-administration of thiazide diuretics and nondepolarizing skeletal muscle relaxants increases responsiveness to the muscle relaxants).
No products indexed under this heading.

Benazepril Hydrochloride (Co-administration with other antihypertensives may result in additive effect or potentiation). Products include:
Lotensin Tablets 2232
Lotensin HCT Tablets 2235
Lotrel Capsules 2238

Bendroflumethiazide (Co-administration with other antihypertensives may result in additive effect or potentiation).
No products indexed under this heading.

Betamethasone Acetate (Co-administration of thiazide diuretics and corticosteroids may intensify electrolyte depletion, particularly hypokalemia).
No products indexed under this heading.

Betamethasone Sodium Phosphate (Co-administration of thiazide diuretics and corticosteroids may intensify electrolyte depletion, particularly hypokalemia).
No products indexed under this heading.

Betaxolol Hydrochloride (Co-administration with other antihypertensives may result in additive effect or potentiation). Products include:
Betoptic S Ophthalmic Suspension.... 554

Bisoprolol Fumarate (Co-administration with other antihypertensives may result in additive effect or potentiation).
No products indexed under this heading.

Buprenorphine Hydrochloride (Co-administration of thiazide diuretics and narcotics may result in potentiation of orthostatic hypotension). Products include:
Buprenex Injectable.... 2718
Suboxone Tablets.... 2719
Subutex Tablets.... 2719

Butabarbital (Co-administration of thiazide diuretics and barbiturates may result in potentiation of orthostatic hypotension).
No products indexed under this heading.

Butalbital (Co-administration of thiazide diuretics and barbiturates may result in potentiation of orthostatic hypotension). Products include:
Sedapap Tablets 50 mg/650 mg.... 2098

Candesartan Cilexetil (Co-administration with other antihypertensives may result in additive effect or potentiation). Products include:
Atacand Tablets.... 634
Atacand HCT.... 637

Captopril (Co-administration with other antihypertensives may result in additive effect or potentiation). Products include:
Captopril Tablets.... 2114

Carteolol Hydrochloride (Co-administration with other antihypertensives may result in additive effect or potentiation). Products include:
Carteolol Hydrochloride Ophthalmic Solution USP, 1%.... ⊙246

Celecoxib (Co-administration of thiazide diuretics and non-steroidal anti-inflammatory agents can reduce the diuretic, natiuretic, and antihypertensive effects). Products include:
Celebrex Capsules.... 3130

Chlorothiazide (Co-administration with other antihypertensives may result in additive effect or potentiation). Products include:
Aldoclor Tablets.... 1881
Diuril Oral.... 1936

Chlorothiazide Sodium (Co-administration with other antihypertensives may result in additive effect or potentiation). Products include:
Diuril Sodium Intravenous.... 1934

Chlorpropamide (Dosage adjustment of the antidiabetic drug may be required).
No products indexed under this heading.

Chlorthalidone (Co-administration with other antihypertensives may result in additive effect or potentiation). Products include:
Clorpres Tablets.... 2139

Cholestyramine (Absorption of hydrochlorothiazide is impaired in the presence of anionic exchange resins, such as cholestyramine resulting in binding of the hydrochlorothiazide resulting in reduced absorption from GI tract by 85%).
No products indexed under this heading.

Cisatracurium Besylate (Co-administration of thiazide diuretics and nondepolarizing skeletal muscle relaxants increases responsiveness to the muscle relaxants). Products include:
Nimbex Injection.... 494

Clonidine (Co-administration with other antihypertensives may result in additive effect or potentiation). Products include:
Catapres-TTS.... 875

Clonidine Hydrochloride (Co-administration with other antihypertensives may result in additive effect or potentiation). Products include:
Catapres Tablets.... 874
Clorpres Tablets.... 2139

Codeine Phosphate (Co-administration of thiazide diuretics and narcotics may result in potentiation of orthostatic hypotension). Products include:
Tylenol with Codeine.... 2461

Colestipol Hydrochloride (Absorption of hydrochlorothiazide is impaired in the presence of anionic exchange resins, such as colestipol resulting in binding of the hydrochlorothiazide resulting in reduced absorption from GI tract by 43%).
No products indexed under this heading.

Cortisone Acetate (Co-administration of thiazide diuretics and corticosteroids may intensify electrolyte depletion, particularly hypokalemia).
No products indexed under this heading.

Deserpidine (Co-administration with other antihypertensives may result in additive effect or potentiation).
No products indexed under this heading.

Deslanoside (Hypokalemia induced by thiazides may cause cardiac arrhythmia and may sensitize or exaggerate the response of the heart to the toxic effects of digitalis, such as increased ventricular irritability).
No products indexed under this heading.

Dexamethasone (Co-administration of thiazide diuretics and corticosteroids may intensify electrolyte depletion, particularly hypokalemia). Products include:
Ciprodex Otic Suspension.... 555
Decadron Tablets.... 1929
TobraDex Ophthalmic Ointment.... 558
TobraDex Ophthalmic Suspension.... 558

Dexamethasone Acetate (Co-administration of thiazide diuretics and corticosteroids may intensify electrolyte depletion, particularly hypokalemia).
No products indexed under this heading.

Dexamethasone Sodium Phosphate (Co-administration of thiazide diuretics and corticosteroids may intensify electrolyte depletion, particularly hypokalemia). Products include:
Decadron Phosphate Injection.... 1931

Dezocine (Co-administration of thiazide diuretics and narcotics may result in potentiation of orthostatic hypotension).
No products indexed under this heading.

Diazoxide (Co-administration with other antihypertensives may result in additive effect or potentiation). Products include:
Hyperstat I.V. Injection.... 3031

Diclofenac Potassium (Co-administration of thiazide diuretics and non-steroidal anti-inflammatory agents can reduce the diuretic, natiuretic, and antihypertensive effects). Products include:
Cataflam Tablets.... 2173

Diclofenac Sodium (Co-administration of thiazide diuretics and non-steroidal anti-inflammatory agents can reduce the diuretic, natiuretic, and antihypertensive effects). Products include:
Arthrotec Tablets.... 3126
Voltaren Ophthalmic Solution.... 2300
Voltaren Tablets.... 2298
Voltaren-XR Tablets.... 2301

Digitalis Glycoside Preparations (Hypokalemia induced by thiazides may cause cardiac arrhythmia and may sensitize or exaggerate the response of the heart to the toxic effects of digitalis, such as increased ventricular irritability).
No products indexed under this heading.

Digitoxin (Hypokalemia induced by thiazides may cause cardiac arrhythmia and may sensitize or exaggerate the response of the heart to the toxic effects of digitalis, such as increased ventricular irritability).
No products indexed under this heading.

Digoxin (Hypokalemia induced by thiazides may cause cardiac arrhythmia and may sensitize or exaggerate the response of the heart to the toxic effects of digitalis, such as increased ventricular irritability). Products include:
Digitek Tablets.... 2146
Lanoxicaps Capsules.... 1458
Lanoxin Injection.... 1462
Lanoxin Tablets.... 1468
Lanoxin Injection Pediatric.... 1465

Diltiazem Hydrochloride (Co-administration with other antihypertensives may result in additive effect or potentiation). Products include:
Cardizem LA Extended Release Tablets.... 1699
Tiazac Capsules.... 1204

Doxazosin Mesylate (Co-administration with other antihypertensives may result in additive effect or potentiation).
No products indexed under this heading.

Enalapril Maleate (Co-administration with other antihypertensives may result in additive effect or potentiation). Products include:
Vaseretic Tablets.... 2073
Vasotec I.V. Injection.... 2076

Enalaprilat (Co-administration with other antihypertensives may result in additive effect or potentiation).
No products indexed under this heading.

Eprosartan Mesylate (Co-administration with other antihypertensives may result in additive effect or potentiation). Products include:
Teveten Tablets.... 1707
Teveten HCT Tablets.... 1710

Esmolol Hydrochloride (Co-administration with other antihypertensives may result in additive effect or potentiation). Products include:
Brevibloc Concentrate.... 766
Brevibloc Injection.... 766
Brevibloc Double Strength Injection.... 766
Brevibloc Premixed Injection.... 766
Brevibloc Double Strength Premixed Injection.... 766

Etodolac (Co-administration of thiazide diuretics and non-steroidal anti-inflammatory agents can reduce the diuretic, natiuretic, and antihypertensive effects).
No products indexed under this heading.

Felodipine (Co-administration with other antihypertensives may result in additive effect or potentiation). Products include:
Plendil Extended-Release Tablets.... 651

Fenoprofen Calcium (Co-administration of thiazide diuretics and non-steroidal anti-inflammatory agents can reduce the diuretic, natiuretic, and antihypertensive effects). Products include:
Nalfon Capsules.... 2504

Fentanyl (Co-administration of thiazide diuretics and narcotics may result in potentiation of orthostatic hypotension). Products include:
Duragesic Transdermal System.... 2448

Fentanyl Citrate (Co-administration of thiazide diuretics and narcotics may result in potentiation of orthostatic hypotension). Products include:
Actiq.... 993

Fludrocortisone Acetate (Co-administration of thiazide diuretics and corticosteroids may intensify electrolyte depletion, particularly hypokalemia).
No products indexed under this heading.

Flurbiprofen (Co-administration of thiazide diuretics and non-steroidal anti-inflammatory agents can reduce the diuretic, natiuretic, and antihypertensive effects).
No products indexed under this heading.

Fosinopril Sodium (Co-administration with other antihypertensives may result in additive effect or potentiation).
No products indexed under this heading.

Furosemide (Co-administration with other antihypertensives may result in additive effect or potentiation). Products include:
Furosemide Tablets.... 2117

Glimepiride (Dosage adjustment of the antidiabetic drug may be required). Products include:
Amaryl Tablets.... 2864

Glipizide (Dosage adjustment of the antidiabetic drug may be required).
No products indexed under this heading.

Glyburide (Dosage adjustment of the antidiabetic drug may be required).
No products indexed under this heading.

IMPORTANT NOTE: Always consult each drug listing in the patient's regimen for possible interactions.

Guanabenz Acetate (Co-administration with other antihypertensives may result in additive effect or potentiation).
No products indexed under this heading.

Guanethidine Monosulfate (Co-administration with other antihypertensives may result in additive effect or potentiation).
No products indexed under this heading.

Hydralazine Hydrochloride (Co-administration with other antihypertensives may result in additive effect or potentiation). Products include:
BiDil Tablets 2161

Hydrocodone Bitartrate (Co-administration of thiazide diuretics and narcotics may result in potentiation of orthostatic hypotension). Products include:
Hycodan 1104
Hycomine Compound Tablets 1105
Hycotuss Expectorant Syrup 1106
Lortab 3315
Lortab Elixir 3312
Vicodin Tablets 530
Vicodin ES Tablets 531
Vicodin HP Tablets 532
Vicoprofen Tablets 533
Zydone Tablets 1118

Hydrocodone Polistirex (Co-administration of thiazide diuretics and narcotics may result in potentiation of orthostatic hypotension). Products include:
Tussionex Pennkinetic Extended-Release Suspension 3322

Hydrocortisone (Co-administration of thiazide diuretics and corticosteroids may intensify electrolyte depletion, particularly hypokalemia). Products include:
Cortizone•5 Ointment .... ▣699
Cortizone•10 Creme .... ▣699
Cortizone•10 Ointment .... ▣699
Cortizone•10 Plus Creme .... ▣700
Cortizone•10 Maximum Strength Quick Shot Spray .... ▣700
Hydrocortone Tablets 1963
Preparation H Hydrocortisone Cream .... ▣748

Hydrocortisone Acetate (Co-administration of thiazide diuretics and corticosteroids may intensify electrolyte depletion, particularly hypokalemia). Products include:
Analpram-HC 1136
Pramosone 1139
ProctoFoam-HC 3113
Tucks Anti-Itch Ointment .... ▣712
U-cort 1% Cream 3289

Hydrocortisone Sodium Phosphate (Co-administration of thiazide diuretics and corticosteroids may intensify electrolyte depletion, particularly hypokalemia).
No products indexed under this heading.

Hydrocortisone Sodium Succinate (Co-administration of thiazide diuretics and corticosteroids may intensify electrolyte depletion, particularly hypokalemia).
No products indexed under this heading.

Hydroflumethiazide (Co-administration with other antihypertensives may result in additive effect or potentiation).
No products indexed under this heading.

Hydromorphone Hydrochloride (Co-administration of thiazide diuretics and narcotics may result in potentiation of orthostatic hypotension). Products include:
Dilaudid 439
Dilaudid Oral Liquid 443
Dilaudid Non-Sterile Powder 439
Dilaudid Rectal Suppositories 439
Dilaudid Tablets 439
Dilaudid Tablets - 8 mg 443
Dilaudid-HP 441

Ibuprofen (Co-administration of thiazide diuretics and non-steroidal anti-inflammatory agents can reduce the diuretic, natiuretic, and antihypertensive effects). Products include:
Advil Allergy Sinus Caplets .... ▣737
Advil .... ▣737
Children's Advil Suspension .... ▣742
Children's Advil Chewable Tablets .... ▣741
Advil Cold & Sinus .... ▣739
Advil Flu & Body Ache Caplets .... ▣739
Children's Advil Cold Suspension .... ▣741
Infants' Advil Concentrated Drops .... ▣743
Junior Strength Advil Swallow Tablets .... ▣740
Advil Migraine Liquigels .... ▣740
Advil Multi-Symptom Cold Caplets .... ▣738
Combunox Tablets 1183
Children's Motrin Oral Suspension and Chewable Tablets 1837
Children's Motrin Cold Non-Staining Dye-Free Oral Suspension 1838
Children's Motrin Cold Oral Suspension 1838
Children's Motrin Non-Staining Dye-Free Oral Suspension 1837
Motrin Cold & Sinus Caplets 1836
Motrin IB Tablets and Caplets 1836
Infants' Motrin Concentrated Drops 1837
Infants' Motrin Non-Staining Dye-Free Drops 1837
Junior Strength Motrin Caplets and Chewable Tablets 1837
Vicoprofen Tablets 533

Indapamide (Co-administration with other antihypertensives may result in additive effect or potentiation). Products include:
Indapamide Tablets 2119

Indomethacin (Co-administration of thiazide diuretics and non-steroidal anti-inflammatory agents can reduce the diuretic, natiuretic, and antihypertensive effects). Products include:
Indocin 1968

Indomethacin Sodium Trihydrate (Co-administration of thiazide diuretics and non-steroidal anti-inflammatory agents can reduce the diuretic, natiuretic, and antihypertensive effects). Products include:
Indocin I.V. 1973

Insulin, Human, Zinc Suspension (Dosage adjustment of the antidiabetic drug may be required). Products include:
Humulin L, 100 Units 1763
Humulin U, 100 Units 1770

Insulin, Human NPH (Dosage adjustment of the antidiabetic drug may be required). Products include:
Humulin N, 100 Units 1764
Humulin N Pen 1765
Novolin N Human Insulin 10 ml Vials 2322
Novolin N InnoLet 2322
Novolin N PenFill 3 ml Cartridges 2325
Novolin R InnoLet 2322

Insulin, Human Regular (Dosage adjustment of the antidiabetic drug may be required). Products include:
Humulin R (U-500) 1768
Humulin R, 100 Units 1767
Novolin R Human Insulin 10 ml Vials 2322
Novolin R PenFill 2325

Insulin, Human Regular and Human NPH Mixture (Dosage adjustment of the antidiabetic drug may be required). Products include:
Humulin 50/50, 100 Units 1760
Humulin 70/30 Pen 1761
Novolin 70/30 Human Insulin 10 ml Vials 2321
Novolin 70/30 InnoLet 2322
Novolin 70/30 PenFill 3 ml Cartridges 2325

Insulin, NPH (Dosage adjustment of the antidiabetic drug may be required).
No products indexed under this heading.

Insulin, Regular (Dosage adjustment of the antidiabetic drug may be required).
No products indexed under this heading.

Insulin, Zinc Crystals (Dosage adjustment of the antidiabetic drug may be required).
No products indexed under this heading.

Insulin, Zinc Suspension (Dosage adjustment of the antidiabetic drug may be required).
No products indexed under this heading.

Insulin Aspart, Human Regular (Dosage adjustment of the antidiabetic drug may be required). Products include:
NovoLog Injection 2326

Insulin glargine (Dosage adjustment of the antidiabetic drug may be required). Products include:
Lantus Injection 2925

Insulin Lispro, Human (Dosage adjustment of the antidiabetic drug may be required). Products include:
Humalog-Pen 1751
Humalog Mix 75/25-Pen 1754

Insulin Lispro Protamine, Human (Dosage adjustment of the antidiabetic drug may be required). Products include:
Humalog Mix 75/25-Pen 1754

Irbesartan (Co-administration with other antihypertensives may result in additive effect or potentiation). Products include:
Avalide Tablets 922
Avalide Tablets 2889
Avapro Tablets 925
Avapro Tablets 2886

Isradipine (Co-administration with other antihypertensives may result in additive effect or potentiation). Products include:
DynaCirc CR Tablets 2726

Ketoprofen (Co-administration of thiazide diuretics and non-steroidal anti-inflammatory agents can reduce the diuretic, natiuretic, and antihypertensive effects).
No products indexed under this heading.

Ketorolac Tromethamine (Co-administration of thiazide diuretics and non-steroidal anti-inflammatory agents can reduce the diuretic, natiuretic, and antihypertensive effects). Products include:
Acular Ophthalmic Solution 561
Acular LS Ophthalmic Solution 562

Labetalol Hydrochloride (Co-administration with other antihypertensives may result in additive effect or potentiation).
No products indexed under this heading.

Levorphanol Tartrate (Co-administration of thiazide diuretics and narcotics may result in potentiation of orthostatic hypotension).
No products indexed under this heading.

Lisinopril (Co-administration with other antihypertensives may result in additive effect or potentiation). Products include:
Prinivil Tablets 2029
Prinzide Tablets 2033
Zestoretic Tablets 701
Zestril Tablets 704

Lithium (Diuretics reduce the renal clearance of lithium and add a high risk of lithium toxicity; concurrent use should be avoided).
No products indexed under this heading.

Lithium Carbonate (Diuretics reduce the renal clearance of lithium and add a high risk of lithium toxicity; concurrent use should be avoided). Products include:
Eskalith 1406
Lithobid Tablets 1670

Lithium Citrate (Diuretics reduce the renal clearance of lithium and add a high risk of lithium toxicity; concurrent use should be avoided).
No products indexed under this heading.

Losartan Potassium (Co-administration with other antihypertensives may result in additive effect or potentiation). Products include:
Cozaar Tablets 1913
Hyzaar 1964

Mecamylamine Hydrochloride (Co-administration with other antihypertensives may result in additive effect or potentiation). Products include:
Inversine Tablets 3286

Meclofenamate Sodium (Co-administration of thiazide diuretics and non-steroidal anti-inflammatory agents can reduce the diuretic, natiuretic, and antihypertensive effects).
No products indexed under this heading.

Mefenamic Acid (Co-administration of thiazide diuretics and non-steroidal anti-inflammatory agents can reduce the diuretic, natiuretic, and antihypertensive effects).
No products indexed under this heading.

Meloxicam (Co-administration of thiazide diuretics and non-steroidal anti-inflammatory agents can reduce the diuretic, natiuretic, and antihypertensive effects). Products include:
Mobic Oral Suspension 893
Mobic Tablets 893

Meperidine Hydrochloride (Co-administration of thiazide diuretics and narcotics may result in potentiation of orthostatic hypotension).
No products indexed under this heading.

Mephobarbital (Co-administration of thiazide diuretics and barbiturates may result in potentiation of orthostatic hypotension). Products include:
Mebaral Tablets, USP 2483

Metformin Hydrochloride (Dosage adjustment of the antidiabetic drug may be required). Products include:
ActoPlus Met Tablets 3219
Avandamet Tablets 1343
Fortamet Extended-Release Tablets 1156

Methadone Hydrochloride (Co-administration of thiazide diuretics and narcotics may result in potentiation of orthostatic hypotension).
No products indexed under this heading.

Methyclothiazide (Co-administration with other antihypertensives may result in additive effect or potentiation).
No products indexed under this heading.

Methyldopa (Co-administration with other antihypertensives may result in additive effect or potentiation). Products include:
Aldoclor Tablets 1881
Aldoril Tablets 1884

Methyldopate Hydrochloride (Co-administration with other antihypertensives may result in additive effect or potentiation).
No products indexed under this heading.

Methylprednisolone Acetate (Co-administration of thiazide diuretics and corticosteroids may intensify electrolyte depletion, particularly hypokalemia). Products include:
Depo-Medrol Injectable Suspension 2615
Depo-Medrol Single-Dose Vial 2617

Methylprednisolone Sodium Succinate (Co-administration of thiazide diuretics and corticosteroids may intensify electrolyte depletion, particularly hypokalemia).
No products indexed under this heading.

Metocurine Iodide (Co-administration of thiazide diuretics and nondepolarizing skeletal muscle relaxants increases responsiveness to the muscle relaxants).
No products indexed under this heading.

Metolazone (Co-administration with other antihypertensives may result in additive effect or potentiation).
No products indexed under this heading.

Metoprolol Succinate (Co-administration with other antihypertensives may result in additive effect or potentiation). Products include:
Toprol-XL Tablets 660

Metoprolol Tartrate (Co-administration with other antihypertensives may result in additive effect or potentiation).
No products indexed under this heading.

Metyrosine (Co-administration with other antihypertensives may result in additive effect or potentiation). Products include:
Demser Capsules 1933

Mibefradil Dihydrochloride (Co-administration with other antihypertensives may result in additive effect or potentiation).
No products indexed under this heading.

Miglitol (Dosage adjustment of the antidiabetic drug may be required).
No products indexed under this heading.

Minoxidil (Co-administration with other antihypertensives may result in additive effect or potentiation). Products include:
Men's Rogaine Extra Strength Topical Solution, Ocean Rush Scent and Original Unscented 706
Women's Rogaine Topical Solution, Spring Bloom Scent and Original Unscented 707

Mivacurium Chloride (Co-administration of thiazide diuretics and nondepolarizing skeletal muscle relaxants increases responsiveness to the muscle relaxants). Products include:
Mivacron Injection 489

Moexipril Hydrochloride (Co-administration with other antihypertensives may result in additive effect or potentiation). Products include:
Uniretic Tablets 3114
Univasc Tablets 3118

Morphine Sulfate (Co-administration of thiazide diuretics and narcotics may result in potentiation of orthostatic hypotension). Products include:
Avinza Capsules 1714
Kadian Capsules 572
MS Contin Tablets 2703

Nabumetone (Co-administration of thiazide diuretics and non-steroidal anti-inflammatory agents can reduce the diuretic, natiuretic, and antihypertensive effects). Products include:
Relafen Tablets 1523

Nadolol (Co-administration with other antihypertensives may result in additive effect or potentiation). Products include:
Nadolol Tablets 2121

Naproxen (Co-administration of thiazide diuretics and non-steroidal anti-inflammatory agents can reduce the diuretic, natiuretic, and antihypertensive effects). Products include:
EC-Naprosyn Delayed-Release Tablets 2769
Naprosyn Suspension 2769
Naprosyn Tablets 2769
Prevacid NapraPAC 3277

Naproxen Sodium (Co-administration of thiazide diuretics and non-steroidal anti-inflammatory agents can reduce the diuretic, natiuretic, and antihypertensive effects). Products include:
Aleve Tablets, Caplets and Gelcaps 605
Anaprox Tablets 2769
Anaprox DS Tablets 2769

Nicardipine Hydrochloride (Co-administration with other antihypertensives may result in additive effect or potentiation). Products include:
Cardene I.V. 1129

Nifedipine (Co-administration with other antihypertensives may result in additive effect or potentiation). Products include:
Adalat CC Tablets 2978

Nisoldipine (Co-administration with other antihypertensives may result in additive effect or potentiation). Products include:
Sular Tablets 1163

Nitroglycerin (Co-administration with other antihypertensives may result in additive effect or potentiation). Products include:
Nitro-Dur Transdermal Infusion System 3060
Nitrolingual Pumpspray 1161

Norepinephrine Bitartrate (Possible decreased response to pressor amines but not sufficient to preclude their use).
No products indexed under this heading.

Oxaprozin (Co-administration of thiazide diuretics and non-steroidal anti-inflammatory agents can reduce the diuretic, natiuretic, and antihypertensive effects).
No products indexed under this heading.

Oxycodone Hydrochloride (Co-administration of thiazide diuretics and narcotics may result in potentiation of orthostatic hypotension). Products include:
Combunox Tablets 1183
OxyContin Tablets 2699
OxyFast Oral Concentrate Solution 2704
OxyIR Capsules 2704
Percocet Tablets 1114
Percodan Tablets 1115

Pancuronium Bromide (Co-administration of thiazide diuretics and nondepolarizing skeletal muscle relaxants increases responsiveness to the muscle relaxants).
No products indexed under this heading.

Penbutolol Sulfate (Co-administration with other antihypertensives may result in additive effect or potentiation).
No products indexed under this heading.

Pentobarbital Sodium (Co-administration of thiazide diuretics and barbiturates may result in potentiation of orthostatic hypotension). Products include:
Nembutal Sodium Solution, USP 2484

Perindopril Erbumine (Co-administration with other antihypertensives may result in additive effect or potentiation). Products include:
Aceon Tablets (2 mg, 4 mg, 8 mg) 3191

Phenobarbital (Co-administration of thiazide diuretics and barbiturates may result in potentiation of orthostatic hypotension).
No products indexed under this heading.

Phenoxybenzamine Hydrochloride (Co-administration with other antihypertensives may result in additive effect or potentiation). Products include:
Dibenzyline Capsules 3390

Phentolamine Mesylate (Co-administration with other antihypertensives may result in additive effect or potentiation).
No products indexed under this heading.

Phenylbutazone (Co-administration of thiazide diuretics and non-steroidal anti-inflammatory agents can reduce the diuretic, natiuretic, and antihypertensive effects).
No products indexed under this heading.

Pindolol (Co-administration with other antihypertensives may result in additive effect or potentiation).
No products indexed under this heading.

Pioglitazone Hydrochloride (Dosage adjustment of the antidiabetic drug may be required). Products include:
ActoPlus Met Tablets 3219
Actos Tablets 3224

Piroxicam (Co-administration of thiazide diuretics and non-steroidal anti-inflammatory agents can reduce the diuretic, natiuretic, and antihypertensive effects).
No products indexed under this heading.

Polythiazide (Co-administration with other antihypertensives may result in additive effect or potentiation).
No products indexed under this heading.

Potassium Acid Phosphate (Concurrent use with potassium salt substitutes or potassium supplements should be avoided unless directed by a prescriber). Products include:
K-Phos Original (Sodium Free) Tablets 785

Potassium Bicarbonate (Concurrent use with potassium salt substitutes or potassium supplements should be avoided unless directed by a prescriber).
No products indexed under this heading.

Potassium Chloride (Concurrent use with potassium salt substitutes or potassium supplements should be avoided unless directed by a prescriber). Products include:
Colyte with Flavor Packs for Oral Solution 3102
HalfLytely and Bisacodyl Tablets Bowel Prep Kit with Flavors Packs 915
K-Dur Extended-Relase Tablets 3047
K-Lor Powder Packets 472
K-Tab Filmtab Tablets 473
TriLyte with Flavor Packs for Oral Solution 3114

Potassium Citrate (Concurrent use with potassium salt substitutes or potassium supplements should be avoided unless directed by a prescriber). Products include:
Urocit-K Tablets 2109

Potassium Gluconate (Concurrent use with potassium salt substitutes or potassium supplements should be avoided unless directed by a prescriber).
No products indexed under this heading.

Potassium Phosphate (Concurrent use with potassium salt substitutes or potassium supplements should be avoided unless directed by a prescriber). Products include:
K-Phos Neutral Tablets 785

Prazosin Hydrochloride (Co-administration with other antihypertensives may result in additive effect or potentiation).
No products indexed under this heading.

Prednisolone Acetate (Co-administration of thiazide diuretics and corticosteroids may intensify electrolyte depletion, particularly hypokalemia). Products include:
Blephamide Ophthalmic Ointment 563
Blephamide Ophthalmic Suspension 564
Poly-Pred Liquifilm Ophthalmic Suspension .... ⊙231
Pred Forte Ophthalmic Suspension .... ⊙233
Pred Mild Sterile Ophthalmic Suspension .... ⊙236
Pred-G Ophthalmic Suspension .... ⊙234
Pred-G Sterile Ophthalmic Ointment .... ⊙235

Prednisolone Sodium Phosphate (Co-administration of thiazide diuretics and corticosteroids may intensify electrolyte depletion, particularly hypokalemia). Products include:
Pediapred Oral Solution 3319

Prednisolone Tebutate (Co-administration of thiazide diuretics and corticosteroids may intensify electrolyte depletion, particularly hypokalemia).
No products indexed under this heading.

Prednisone (Co-administration of thiazide diuretics and corticosteroids may intensify electrolyte depletion, particularly hypokalemia).
No products indexed under this heading.

IMPORTANT NOTE: Always consult each drug listing in the patient's regimen for possible interactions.

Propoxyphene Hydrochloride (Co-administration of thiazide diuretics and narcotics may result in potentiation of orthostatic hypotension).
No products indexed under this heading.

Propoxyphene Napsylate (Co-administration of thiazide diuretics and narcotics may result in potentiation of orthostatic hypotension). Products include:
Darvocet A 500 Tablets 3497

Propranolol Hydrochloride (Co-administration with other antihypertensives may result in additive effect or potentiation). Products include:
Inderal LA Long-Acting Capsules 3421
InnoPran XL Capsules 2728

Quinapril Hydrochloride (Co-administration with other antihypertensives may result in additive effect or potentiation).
No products indexed under this heading.

Ramipril (Co-administration with other antihypertensives may result in additive effect or potentiation). Products include:
Altace Capsules 1673

Rapacuronium Bromide (Co-administration of thiazide diuretics and nondepolarizing skeletal muscle relaxants increases responsiveness to the muscle relaxants).
No products indexed under this heading.

Rauwolfia Serpentina (Co-administration with other antihypertensives may result in additive effect or potentiation).
No products indexed under this heading.

Remifentanil Hydrochloride (Co-administration of thiazide diuretics and narcotics may result in potentiation of orthostatic hypotension).
No products indexed under this heading.

Repaglinide (Dosage adjustment of the antidiabetic drug may be required). Products include:
Prandin Tablets (0.5, 1, and 2 mg) 2337

Rescinnamine (Co-administration with other antihypertensives may result in additive effect or potentiation).
No products indexed under this heading.

Reserpine (Co-administration with other antihypertensives may result in additive effect or potentiation).
No products indexed under this heading.

Rocuronium Bromide (Co-administration of thiazide diuretics and nondepolarizing skeletal muscle relaxants increases responsiveness to the muscle relaxants). Products include:
Zemuron Injection 2363

Rofecoxib (Co-administration of thiazide diuretics and non-steroidal anti-inflammatory agents can reduce the diuretic, natiuretic, and antihypertensive effects).
No products indexed under this heading.

Rosiglitazone Maleate (Dosage adjustment of the antidiabetic drug may be required). Products include:
Avandamet Tablets 1343
Avandia Tablets 1348

Secobarbital Sodium (Co-administration of thiazide diuretics and barbiturates may result in potentiation of orthostatic hypotension).
No products indexed under this heading.

Sodium Nitroprusside (Co-administration with other antihypertensives may result in additive effect or potentiation).
No products indexed under this heading.

Sotalol Hydrochloride (Co-administration with other antihypertensives may result in additive effect or potentiation).
No products indexed under this heading.

Spirapril Hydrochloride (Co-administration with other antihypertensives may result in additive effect or potentiation).
No products indexed under this heading.

Sufentanil Citrate (Co-administration of thiazide diuretics and narcotics may result in potentiation of orthostatic hypotension).
No products indexed under this heading.

Sulindac (Co-administration of thiazide diuretics and non-steroidal anti-inflammatory agents can reduce the diuretic, natiuretic, and antihypertensive effects). Products include:
Clinoril Tablets 1899

Telmisartan (Co-administration with other antihypertensives may result in additive effect or potentiation). Products include:
Micardis Tablets 884
Micardis HCT Tablets 886

Terazosin Hydrochloride (Co-administration with other antihypertensives may result in additive effect or potentiation). Products include:
Hytrin Capsules 469

Thiamylal Sodium (Co-administration of thiazide diuretics and barbiturates may result in potentiation of orthostatic hypotension).
No products indexed under this heading.

Timolol Maleate (Co-administration with other antihypertensives may result in additive effect or potentiation). Products include:
Blocadren Tablets 1891
Cosopt Sterile Ophthalmic Solution 1910
Timolide Tablets 2056
Timoptic in Ocudose 2061
Timoptic Sterile Ophthalmic Solution 2058
Timoptic-XE Sterile Ophthalmic Gel Forming Solution 2062

Tolazamide (Dosage adjustment of the antidiabetic drug may be required).
No products indexed under this heading.

Tolbutamide (Dosage adjustment of the antidiabetic drug may be required).
No products indexed under this heading.

Tolmetin Sodium (Co-administration of thiazide diuretics and non-steroidal anti-inflammatory agents can reduce the diuretic, natiuretic, and antihypertensive effects).
No products indexed under this heading.

Torsemide (Co-administration with other antihypertensives may result in additive effect or potentiation).
No products indexed under this heading.

Trandolapril (Co-administration with other antihypertensives may result in additive effect or potentiation). Products include:
Mavik Tablets 482
Tarka Tablets 519

Triamcinolone (Co-administration of thiazide diuretics and corticosteroids may intensify electrolyte depletion, particularly hypokalemia).
No products indexed under this heading.

Triamcinolone Acetonide (Co-administration of thiazide diuretics and corticosteroids may intensify electrolyte depletion, particularly hypokalemia). Products include:
Azmacort Inhalation Aerosol 1701
Nasacort HFA Inhalation Aerosol 2939
Nasacort AQ Nasal Spray 2937

Triamcinolone Diacetate (Co-administration of thiazide diuretics and corticosteroids may intensify electrolyte depletion, particularly hypokalemia).
No products indexed under this heading.

Triamcinolone Hexacetonide (Co-administration of thiazide diuretics and corticosteroids may intensify electrolyte depletion, particularly hypokalemia).
No products indexed under this heading.

Trimethaphan Camsylate (Co-administration with other antihypertensives may result in additive effect or potentiation).
No products indexed under this heading.

Troglitazone (Dosage adjustment of the antidiabetic drug may be required).
No products indexed under this heading.

Tubocurarine Chloride (Co-administration of thiazide diuretics and nondepolarizing skeletal muscle relaxants increases responsiveness to the muscle relaxants).
No products indexed under this heading.

Valdecoxib (Co-administration of thiazide diuretics and non-steroidal anti-inflammatory agents can reduce the diuretic, natiuretic, and antihypertensive effects).
No products indexed under this heading.

Vecuronium Bromide (Co-administration of thiazide diuretics and nondepolarizing skeletal muscle relaxants increases responsiveness to the muscle relaxants).
No products indexed under this heading.

Verapamil Hydrochloride (Co-administration with other antihypertensives may result in additive effect or potentiation). Products include:
Covera-HS Tablets 3135
Tarka Tablets 519
Verelan PM Capsules 3120

Food Interactions

Alcohol (Co-administration of thiazide diuretics and alcohol may result in potentiation of orthostatic hypotension).

DIOVAN TABLETS

(Valsartan) 2191
May interact with potassium preparations, potassium sparing diuretics, and certain other agents. Compounds in these categories include:

Amiloride Hydrochloride (Concurrent use may lead to hyperkalemia; potential for increase in serum creatinine in heart failure patients if used concurrently). Products include:
Midamor Tablets 2000
Moduretic Tablets 2003

Atenolol (Combination therapy is more antihypertensive than either component, but does not lower the heart rate more than atenolol alone). Products include:
Tenormin I.V. Injection 698
Tenormin Tablets 695

Potassium Acid Phosphate (Concurrent use may lead to hyperkalemia; potential for increase in serum creatinine in heart failure patients if used concurrently). Products include:
K-Phos Original (Sodium Free) Tablets 785

Potassium Bicarbonate (Concurrent use may lead to hyperkalemia; potential for increase in serum creatinine in heart failure patients if used concurrently).
No products indexed under this heading.

Potassium Chloride (Concurrent use may lead to hyperkalemia; potential for increase in serum creatinine in heart failure patients if used concurrently). Products include:
Colyte with Flavor Packs for Oral Solution 3102
HalfLytely and Bisacodyl Tablets Bowel Prep Kit with Flavors Packs 915
K-Dur Extended-Release Tablets 3047
K-Lor Powder Packets 472
K-Tab Filmtab Tablets 473
TriLyte with Flavor Packs for Oral Solution 3114

Potassium Citrate (Concurrent use may lead to hyperkalemia; potential for increase in serum creatinine in heart failure patients if used concurrently). Products include:
Urocit-K Tablets 2109

Potassium Gluconate (Concurrent use may lead to hyperkalemia; potential for increase in serum creatinine in heart failure patients if used concurrently).
No products indexed under this heading.

Potassium Phosphate (Concurrent use may lead to hyperkalemia; potential for increase in serum creatinine in heart failure patients if used concurrently). Products include:
K-Phos Neutral Tablets 785

Salt Substitutes (Concurrent use may lead to hyperkalemia; potential for increase in serum creatinine in heart failure patients if used concurrently).
No products indexed under this heading.

Spironolactone (Concurrent use may lead to hyperkalemia; potential for increase in serum creatinine in heart failure patients if used concurrently).
No products indexed under this heading.

Triamterene (Concurrent use may lead to hyperkalemia; potential for increase in serum creatinine in heart failure patients if used concurrently). Products include:

Dyazide Capsules **1389**
Dyrenium Capsules **3390**
Maxzide **2150**

Food Interactions

Food, unspecified (Decreases the exposure (as measured by AUC) to valsartan about 40% and peak plasma concentration by about 50%).

DIPRIVAN INJECTABLE EMULSION

(Propofol) **676**

May interact with barbiturates, benzodiazepines, hypnotics and sedatives, inhalant anesthetics, narcotic analgesics, and certain other agents. Compounds in these categories include:

Alfentanil Hydrochloride (Increases anesthetic or sedative effects; may also result in pronounced decreases in systolic, diastolic, and mean arterial pressure and cardiac output).
No products indexed under this heading.

Alprazolam (Increases anesthetic or sedative effects; may also result in pronounced decreases in systolic, diastolic, and mean arterial pressure and cardiac output). Products include:
Niravam Orally Disintegrating Tablets **3106**
Xanax XR Tablets **2655**

Aprobarbital (Increases anesthetic or sedative effects; may also result in pronounced decreases in systolic, diastolic, and mean arterial pressure and cardiac output).
No products indexed under this heading.

Buprenorphine Hydrochloride (Increases anesthetic or sedative effects; may also result in pronounced decreases in systolic, diastolic, and mean arterial pressure and cardiac output). Products include:
Buprenex Injectable **2718**
Suboxone Tablets **2719**
Subutex Tablets **2719**

Butabarbital (Increases anesthetic or sedative effects; may also result in pronounced decreases in systolic, diastolic, and mean arterial pressure and cardiac output).
No products indexed under this heading.

Butalbital (Increases anesthetic or sedative effects; may also result in pronounced decreases in systolic, diastolic, and mean arterial pressure and cardiac output). Products include:
Sedapap Tablets 50 mg/650 mg **2098**

Chloral Hydrate (Increases anesthetic or sedative effects; may also result in pronounced decreases in systolic, diastolic, and mean arterial pressure and cardiac output).
No products indexed under this heading.

Chlordiazepoxide (Increases anesthetic or sedative effects; may also result in pronounced decreases in systolic, diastolic, and mean arterial pressure and cardiac output).
No products indexed under this heading.

Chlordiazepoxide Hydrochloride (Increases anesthetic or sedative effects; may also result in pronounced decreases in systolic, diastolic, and mean arterial pressure and cardiac output). Products include:
Librium Capsules **3349**

Clonazepam (Increases anesthetic or sedative effects; may also result in pronounced decreases in systolic, diastolic, and mean arterial pressure and cardiac output). Products include:
Klonopin **2782**

Clorazepate Dipotassium (Increases anesthetic or sedative effects; may also result in pronounced decreases in systolic, diastolic, and mean arterial pressure and cardiac output). Products include:
Tranxene **2488**

Codeine Phosphate (Increases anesthetic or sedative effects; may also result in pronounced decreases in systolic, diastolic, and mean arterial pressure and cardiac output). Products include:
Tylenol with Codeine **2461**

Desflurane (Increases anesthetic or sedative and cardiorespiratory effects). Products include:
Suprane Liquid for Inhalation **770**

Dezocine (Increases anesthetic or sedative effects; may also result in pronounced decreases in systolic, diastolic, and mean arterial pressure and cardiac output).
No products indexed under this heading.

Diazepam (Increases anesthetic or sedative effects; may also result in pronounced decreases in systolic, diastolic, and mean arterial pressure and cardiac output). Products include:
Diastat Rectal Delivery System **3344**
Valium Tablets **2822**

Droperidol (Increases anesthetic or sedative effects; may also result in pronounced decreases in systolic, diastolic, and mean arterial pressure and cardiac output).
No products indexed under this heading.

Enflurane (Increases anesthetic or sedative and cardiorespiratory effects).
No products indexed under this heading.

Estazolam (Increases anesthetic or sedative effects; may also result in pronounced decreases in systolic, diastolic, and mean arterial pressure and cardiac output). Products include:
ProSom Tablets **512**

Ethchlorvynol (Increases anesthetic or sedative effects; may also result in pronounced decreases in systolic, diastolic, and mean arterial pressure and cardiac output).
No products indexed under this heading.

Ethinamate (Increases anesthetic or sedative effects; may also result in pronounced decreases in systolic, diastolic, and mean arterial pressure and cardiac output).
No products indexed under this heading.

Fentanyl (Co-administration in pediatric patients may result in serious bradycardia; increases anesthetic or sedative effects; may also result in pronounced decreases in systolic, diastolic, and mean arterial pressure and cardiac output). Products include:
Duragesic Transdermal System **2448**

Fentanyl Citrate (Co-administration in pediatric patients may result in serious bradycardia; increases anesthetic or sedative effects; may also result in pronounced decreases in systolic, diastolic, and mean arterial pressure and cardiac output). Products include:
Actiq **993**

Flurazepam Hydrochloride (Increases anesthetic or sedative effects; may also result in pronounced decreases in systolic, diastolic, and mean arterial pressure and cardiac output). Products include:
Dalmane Capsules **3343**

Glutethimide (Increases anesthetic or sedative effects; may also result in pronounced decreases in systolic, diastolic, and mean arterial pressure and cardiac output).
No products indexed under this heading.

Halazepam (Increases anesthetic or sedative effects; may also result in pronounced decreases in systolic, diastolic, and mean arterial pressure and cardiac output).
No products indexed under this heading.

Halothane (Increases anesthetic or sedative and cardiorespiratory effects).
No products indexed under this heading.

Hydrocodone Bitartrate (Increases anesthetic or sedative effects; may also result in pronounced decreases in systolic, diastolic, and mean arterial pressure and cardiac output). Products include:
Hycodan **1104**
Hycomine Compound Tablets **1105**
Hycotuss Expectorant Syrup **1106**
Lortab **3315**
Lortab Elixir **3312**
Vicodin Tablets **530**
Vicodin ES Tablets **531**
Vicodin HP Tablets **532**
Vicoprofen Tablets **533**
Zydone Tablets **1118**

Hydrocodone Polistirex (Increases anesthetic or sedative effects; may also result in pronounced decreases in systolic, diastolic, and mean arterial pressure and cardiac output). Products include:
Tussionex Pennkinetic Extended-Release Suspension **3322**

Hydromorphone Hydrochloride (Increases anesthetic or sedative effects; may also result in pronounced decreases in systolic, diastolic, and mean arterial pressure and cardiac output). Products include:
Dilaudid **439**
Dilaudid Oral Liquid **443**
Dilaudid Non-Sterile Powder **439**
Dilaudid Rectal Suppositories **439**
Dilaudid Tablets **439**
Dilaudid Tablets - 8 mg **443**
Dilaudid-HP **441**

Isoflurane (Increases anesthetic or sedative and cardiorespiratory effects).
No products indexed under this heading.

Levorphanol Tartrate (Increases anesthetic or sedative effects; may also result in pronounced decreases in systolic, diastolic, and mean arterial pressure and cardiac output).
No products indexed under this heading.

Lorazepam (Increases anesthetic or sedative effects; may also result in pronounced decreases in systolic, diastolic, and mean arterial pressure and cardiac output).
No products indexed under this heading.

Meperidine Hydrochloride (Increases anesthetic or sedative effects; may also result in pronounced decreases in systolic, diastolic, and mean arterial pressure and cardiac output).
No products indexed under this heading.

Mephobarbital (Increases anesthetic or sedative effects; may also result in pronounced decreases in systolic, diastolic, and mean arterial pressure and cardiac output). Products include:
Mebaral Tablets, USP **2483**

Methadone Hydrochloride (Increases anesthetic or sedative effects; may also result in pronounced decreases in systolic, diastolic, and mean arterial pressure and cardiac output).
No products indexed under this heading.

Methoxyflurane (Increases anesthetic or sedative and cardiorespiratory effects).
No products indexed under this heading.

Midazolam Hydrochloride (Increases anesthetic or sedative effects; may also result in pronounced decreases in systolic, diastolic, and mean arterial pressure and cardiac output).
No products indexed under this heading.

Morphine Sulfate (Increases anesthetic or sedative effects; may also result in pronounced decreases in systolic, diastolic, and mean arterial pressure and cardiac output). Products include:
Avinza Capsules **1714**
Kadian Capsules **572**
MS Contin Tablets **2703**

Nitrous Oxide (Rate of administration requires adjustment).
No products indexed under this heading.

Oxazepam (Increases anesthetic or sedative effects; may also result in pronounced decreases in systolic, diastolic, and mean arterial pressure and cardiac output).
No products indexed under this heading.

Oxycodone Hydrochloride (Increases anesthetic or sedative effects; may also result in pronounced decreases in systolic, diastolic, and mean arterial pressure and cardiac output). Products include:
Combunox Tablets **1183**
OxyContin Tablets **2699**
OxyFast Oral Concentrate Solution **2704**
OxyIR Capsules **2704**
Percocet Tablets **1114**
Percodan Tablets **1115**

Pentobarbital Sodium (Increases anesthetic or sedative effects; may also result in pronounced decreases in systolic, diastolic, and mean arterial pressure and cardiac output). Products include:
Nembutal Sodium Solution, USP **2484**

Phenobarbital (Increases anesthetic or sedative effects; may also result in pronounced decreases in systolic, diastolic, and mean arterial pressure and cardiac output).
No products indexed under this heading.

Prazepam (Increases anesthetic or sedative effects; may also result in pronounced decreases in systolic, diastolic, and mean arterial pressure and cardiac output).
No products indexed under this heading.

Propoxyphene Hydrochloride (Increases anesthetic or sedative effects; may also result in pronounced decreases in systolic, diastolic, and mean arterial pressure and cardiac output).
No products indexed under this heading.

Propoxyphene Napsylate (Increases anesthetic or sedative effects; may also result in pronounced decreases in systolic, diastolic, and mean arterial pressure and cardiac output). Products include:
Darvocet A 500 Tablets 3497

Quazepam (Increases anesthetic or sedative effects; may also result in pronounced decreases in systolic, diastolic, and mean arterial pressure and cardiac output).
No products indexed under this heading.

Remifentanil Hydrochloride (Increases anesthetic or sedative effects; may also result in pronounced decreases in systolic, diastolic, and mean arterial pressure and cardiac output).
No products indexed under this heading.

Secobarbital Sodium (Increases anesthetic or sedative effects; may also result in pronounced decreases in systolic, diastolic, and mean arterial pressure and cardiac output).
No products indexed under this heading.

Sufentanil Citrate (Increases anesthetic or sedative effects; may also result in pronounced decreases in systolic, diastolic, and mean arterial pressure and cardiac output).
No products indexed under this heading.

Temazepam (Increases anesthetic or sedative effects; may also result in pronounced decreases in systolic, diastolic, and mean arterial pressure and cardiac output).
No products indexed under this heading.

Thiamylal Sodium (Increases anesthetic or sedative effects; may also result in pronounced decreases in systolic, diastolic, and mean arterial pressure and cardiac output).
No products indexed under this heading.

Triazolam (Increases anesthetic or sedative effects; may also result in pronounced decreases in systolic, diastolic, and mean arterial pressure and cardiac output).
No products indexed under this heading.

Zaleplon (Increases anesthetic or sedative effects; may also result in pronounced decreases in systolic, diastolic, and mean arterial pressure and cardiac output). Products include:
Sonata Capsules 1686

Zolpidem Tartrate (Increases anesthetic or sedative effects; may also result in pronounced decreases in systolic, diastolic, and mean arterial pressure and cardiac output). Products include:
Ambien Tablets 2867

DIPROLENE GEL 0.05%

(Betamethasone Dipropionate) 3015
None cited in PDR database.

DIPROLENE LOTION 0.05%

(Betamethasone Dipropionate) 3016
None cited in PDR database.

DIPROLENE OINTMENT 0.05%

(Betamethasone Dipropionate) 3017
None cited in PDR database.

DIPROLENE AF CREAM 0.05%

(Betamethasone Dipropionate) 3014
None cited in PDR database.

DIPROSONE CREAM, USP 0.05%

(Betamethasone Dipropionate) 3018
None cited in PDR database.

DITROPAN XL EXTENDED RELEASE TABLETS

(Oxybutynin Chloride) 2391
May interact with anticholinergics, bisphosphonates, erythromycin, and certain other agents. Compounds in these categories include:

Alendronate Sodium (Concurrent use with drugs that can cause or exacerbate esophagitis, such as biphosphonates, should be undertaken with caution). Products include:
Fosamax 1949
Fosamax Plus D Tablets 1956

Atropine Sulfate (Co-administration of oxybutynin with other anticholinergic drugs may increase the frequency and/or severity of anticholinergic side effects such as dry mouth, constipation, drowsiness and others).
No products indexed under this heading.

Belladonna Alkaloids (Co-administration of oxybutynin with other anticholinergic drugs may increase the frequency and/or severity of anticholinergic side effects such as dry mouth, constipation, drowsiness and others). Products include:
Hyland's Teething Tablets .... ▣736

Benztropine Mesylate (Co-administration of oxybutynin with other anticholinergic drugs may increase the frequency and/or severity of anticholinergic side effects such as dry mouth, constipation, drowsiness and others). Products include:
Cogentin Injection 1903

Biperiden Hydrochloride (Co-administration of oxybutynin with other anticholinergic drugs may increase the frequency and/or severity of anticholinergic side effects such as dry mouth, constipation, drowsiness and others).
No products indexed under this heading.

Cisapride (Co-administration of cisapride with anticholinergic agents would be expected to compromise the beneficial effects of cisapride).
No products indexed under this heading.

Clarithromycin (Clarythromycin, a CYP3A4 inhibitor, may alter mean pharmacokinetic parameters (ie, Cmax, AUC). The clinical relevance of such potential interaction is not known; caution should be used when co-administered). Products include:
Biaxin/Biaxin XL 402
PREVPAC 3281

Clidinium Bromide (Co-administration of oxybutynin with other anticholinergic drugs may increase the frequency and/or severity of anticholinergic side effects such as dry mouth, constipation, drowsiness and others).
No products indexed under this heading.

Dicyclomine Hydrochloride (Co-administration of oxybutynin with other anticholinergic drugs may increase the frequency and/or severity of anticholinergic side effects such as dry mouth, constipation, drowsiness and others). Products include:
Bentyl Capsules 724
Bentyl Injection 724
Bentyl Syrup 724
Bentyl Tablets 724

Erythromycin (Erythromycin, a CYP3A4 inhibitor, may alter mean pharmacokinetic parameters (ie, Cmax, AUC). The clinical relevance of such potential interaction is not known, caution should be used when co-administered). Products include:
Erygel Topical Gel 2096
Ery-Tab Tablets 447
Erythromycin Base Filmtab Tablets 454
Erythromycin Delayed-Release Capsules, USP 456
PCE Dispertab Tablets 510

Erythromycin Estolate (Erythromycin, a CYP3A4 inhibitor, may alter mean pharmacokinetic parameters (ie, Cmax, AUC). The clinical relevance of such potential interaction is not known, caution should be used when co-administered).
No products indexed under this heading.

Erythromycin Ethylsuccinate (Erythromycin, a CYP3A4 inhibitor, may alter mean pharmacokinetic parameters (ie, Cmax, AUC). The clinical relevance of such potential interaction is not known, caution should be used when co-administered). Products include:
E.E.S. 449
EryPed 445

Erythromycin Gluceptate (Erythromycin, a CYP3A4 inhibitor, may alter mean pharmacokinetic parameters (ie, Cmax, AUC). The clinical relevance of such potential interaction is not known, caution should be used when co-administered).
No products indexed under this heading.

Erythromycin Lactobionate (Erythromycin, a CYP3A4 inhibitor, may alter mean pharmacokinetic parameters (ie, Cmax, AUC). The clinical relevance of such potential interaction is not known, caution should be used when co-administered).
No products indexed under this heading.

Erythromycin Stearate (Erythromycin, a CYP3A4 inhibitor, may alter mean pharmacokinetic parameters (ie, Cmax, AUC). The clinical relevance of such potential interaction is not known, caution should be used when co-administered). Products include:
Erythrocin Stearate Filmtab Tablets 452

Etidronate Disodium (Concurrent use with drugs that can cause or exacerbate esophagitis, such as biphosphonates, should be undertaken with caution). Products include:
Didronel Tablets 2693

Glycopyrrolate (Co-administration of oxybutynin with other anticholinergic drugs may increase the frequency and/or severity of anticholinergic side effects such as dry mouth, constipation, drowsiness and others).
No products indexed under this heading.

Hyoscyamine (Co-administration of oxybutynin with other anticholinergic drugs may increase the frequency and/or severity of anticholinergic side effects such as dry mouth, constipation, drowsiness and others).
No products indexed under this heading.

Hyoscyamine Sulfate (Co-administration of oxybutynin with other anticholinergic drugs may increase the frequency and/or severity of anticholinergic side effects such as dry mouth, constipation, drowsiness and others).
No products indexed under this heading.

Ipratropium Bromide (Co-administration of oxybutynin with other anticholinergic drugs may increase the frequency and/or severity of anticholinergic side effects such as dry mouth, constipation, drowsiness and others). Products include:
Atrovent HFA Inhalation Aerosol 872
Atrovent Inhalation Solution 868
Atrovent Nasal Spray 0.03% 869
Atrovent Nasal Spray 0.06% 870
Combivent Inhalation Aerosol 878
DuoNeb Inhalation Solution 1058

Itraconazole (Itraconazole, a CYP3A4 inhibitor, may alter mean pharmacokinetic parameters (ie, Cmax, AUC). The clinical relevance of such potential interaction is not known; caution should be used when co-administered).
No products indexed under this heading.

Ketoconazole (Mean oxybutynin plasma concentrations were approximately 2-fold higher when oxybutynin was administered with ketoconazole, a potent CYP3A4 inhibitor). Products include:
Nizoral A-D Shampoo, 1% 1839
Nizoral 2% Shampoo 1838

Mepenzolate Bromide (Co-administration of oxybutynin with other anticholinergic drugs may increase the frequency and/or severity of anticholinergic side effects such as dry mouth, constipation, drowsiness and others).
No products indexed under this heading.

Miconazole (Miconazole, a CYP3A4 inhibitor, may alter mean pharmacokinetic parameters (ie, Cmax, AUC). The clinical relevance of such potential interaction is not known; caution should be used when co-administered).
No products indexed under this heading.

Oxybutynin Chloride (Co-administration of oxybutynin with other anticholinergic drugs may increase the frequency and/or severity of anticholinergic side effects such as dry mouth, constipation, drowsiness and others). Products include:
Ditropan XL Extended Release Tablets 2391

Procyclidine Hydrochloride (Co-administration of oxybutynin with other anticholinergic drugs may increase the frequency and/or severity of anticholinergic side effects such as dry mouth, constipation, drowsiness and others).
No products indexed under this heading.

Propantheline Bromide (Co-administration of oxybutynin with other anticholinergic drugs may increase the frequency and/or severity of anticholinergic side effects such as dry mouth, constipation, drowsiness and others).
No products indexed under this heading.

Risedronate Sodium (Concurrent use with drugs that can cause or exacerbate esophagitis, such as biphosphonates, should be undertaken with caution). Products include:
Actonel Tablets 2679
Actonel with Calcium Tablets 2684

Scopolamine (Co-administration of oxybutynin with other anticholinergic drugs may increase the frequency and/or severity of anticholinergic side effects such as dry mouth, constipation, drowsiness and others). Products include:
Transderm Scōp Transdermal Therapeutic System 2166

Scopolamine Hydrobromide (Co-administration of oxybutynin with other anticholinergic drugs may increase the frequency and/or severity of anticholinergic side effects such as dry mouth, constipation, drowsiness and others).
No products indexed under this heading.

Tiludronate Disodium (Concurrent use with drugs that can cause or exacerbate esophagitis, such as biphosphonates, should be undertaken with caution).
No products indexed under this heading.

Tolterodine Tartrate (Co-administration of oxybutynin with other anticholinergic drugs may increase the frequency and/or severity of anticholinergic side effects such as dry mouth, constipation, drowsiness and others). Products include:
Detrol Tablets 2626
Detrol LA Capsules 2629

Tridihexethyl Chloride (Co-administration of oxybutynin with other anticholinergic drugs may increase the frequency and/or severity of anticholinergic side effects such as dry mouth, constipation, drowsiness and others).
No products indexed under this heading.

Trihexyphenidyl Hydrochloride (Co-administration of oxybutynin with other anticholinergic drugs may increase the frequency and/or severity of anticholinergic side effects such as dry mouth, constipation, drowsiness and others).
No products indexed under this heading.

Food Interactions

Alcohol (Enhances the drowsiness effect caused by anticholinergic agents such as oxybutynin).

DIURIL ORAL SUSPENSION

(Chlorothiazide) 1936

May interact with antihypertensives, barbiturates, bile acid sequestering agents, corticosteroids, cardiac glycosides, oral hypoglycemic agents, insulin, lithium preparations, narcotic analgesics, nondepolarizing neuromuscular blocking agents, non-steroidal anti-inflammatory agents, and certain other agents. Compounds in these categories include:

Acarbose (Thiazide-induced hyperglycemia may require dosage adjustment of hypoglycemic agents). Products include:
Precose Tablets 776

Acebutolol Hydrochloride (Concurrent use with other antihypertensive agents may result in additive effect or potentiation).
No products indexed under this heading.

ACTH (Intensified electrolyte depletion particularly hypokalemia).
No products indexed under this heading.

Alfentanil Hydrochloride (Potentiation of orthostatic hypotension may occur).
No products indexed under this heading.

Amlodipine Besylate (Concurrent use with other antihypertensive agents may result in additive effect or potentiation). Products include:
Caduet Tablets 2507
Lotrel Capsules 2238
Norvasc Tablets 2529

Aprobarbital (Potentiation of orthostatic hypotension may occur).
No products indexed under this heading.

Atenolol (Concurrent use with other antihypertensive agents may result in additive effect or potentiation). Products include:
Tenormin I.V. Injection 698
Tenormin Tablets 695

Atracurium Besylate (Possible increased responsiveness to the muscle relaxants).
No products indexed under this heading.

Benazepril Hydrochloride (Concurrent use with other antihypertensive agents may result in additive effect or potentiation). Products include:
Lotensin Tablets 2232
Lotensin HCT Tablets 2235
Lotrel Capsules 2238

Bendroflumethiazide (Concurrent use with other antihypertensive agents may result in additive effect or potentiation).
No products indexed under this heading.

Betamethasone Acetate (Intensified electrolyte depletion particularly hypokalemia).
No products indexed under this heading.

Betamethasone Sodium Phosphate (Intensified electrolyte depletion particularly hypokalemia).
No products indexed under this heading.

Betaxolol Hydrochloride (Concurrent use with other antihypertensive agents may result in additive effect or potentiation). Products include:
Betoptic S Ophthalmic Suspension.................................. 554

Bisoprolol Fumarate (Concurrent use with other antihypertensive agents may result in additive effect or potentiation).
No products indexed under this heading.

Buprenorphine Hydrochloride (Potentiation of orthostatic hypotension may occur). Products include:
Buprenex Injectable 2718
Suboxone Tablets 2719
Subutex Tablets 2719

Butabarbital (Potentiation of orthostatic hypotension may occur).
No products indexed under this heading.

Butalbital (Potentiation of orthostatic hypotension may occur). Products include:
Sedapap Tablets 50 mg/650 mg 2098

Candesartan Cilexetil (Concurrent use with other antihypertensive agents may result in additive effect or potentiation). Products include:
Atacand Tablets 634
Atacand HCT 637

Captopril (Concurrent use with other antihypertensive agents may result in additive effect or potentiation). Products include:
Captopril Tablets 2114

Carteolol Hydrochloride (Concurrent use with other antihypertensive agents may result in additive effect or potentiation). Products include:
Carteolol Hydrochloride Ophthalmic Solution USP, 1%....... ⊙246

Celecoxib (Reduces diuretic, natriuretic, and antihypertensive effects). Products include:
Celebrex Capsules 3130

Chlorothiazide Sodium (Concurrent use with other antihypertensive agents may result in additive effect or potentiation). Products include:
Diuril Sodium Intravenous 1934

Chlorpropamide (Thiazide-induced hyperglycemia may require dosage adjustment of hypoglycemic agents).
No products indexed under this heading.

Chlorthalidone (Concurrent use with other antihypertensive agents may result in additive effect or potentiation). Products include:
Clorpres Tablets 2139

Cholestyramine (Resins have potential to bind thiazide diuretics and reduce their absorption from the gastrointestinal tract).
No products indexed under this heading.

Cisatracurium Besylate (Possible increased responsiveness to the muscle relaxants). Products include:
Nimbex Injection 494

Clonidine (Concurrent use with other antihypertensive agents may result in additive effect or potentiation). Products include:
Catapres-TTS 875

Clonidine Hydrochloride (Concurrent use with other antihypertensive agents may result in additive effect or potentiation). Products include:
Catapres Tablets 874
Clorpres Tablets 2139

Codeine Phosphate (Potentiation of orthostatic hypotension may occur). Products include:
Tylenol with Codeine 2461

Colesevelam Hydrochloride (Resins have potential to bind thiazide diuretics and reduce their absorption from the gastrointestinal tract). Products include:
WelChol Tablets 2855

Colestipol Hydrochloride (Resins have potential to bind thiazide diuretics and reduce their absorption from the gastrointestinal tract).
No products indexed under this heading.

Cortisone Acetate (Intensified electrolyte depletion particularly hypokalemia).
No products indexed under this heading.

Deserpidine (Concurrent use with other antihypertensive agents may result in additive effect or potentiation).
No products indexed under this heading.

Deslanoside (Thiazide-induced hypokalemia may sensitize or exaggerate the response of the heart to the toxic effects of digitalis).
No products indexed under this heading.

Dexamethasone (Intensified electrolyte depletion particularly hypokalemia). Products include:
Ciprodex Otic Suspension 555
Decadron Tablets 1929
TobraDex Ophthalmic Ointment 558
TobraDex Ophthalmic Suspension ... 558

Dexamethasone Acetate (Intensified electrolyte depletion particularly hypokalemia).
No products indexed under this heading.

Dexamethasone Sodium Phosphate (Intensified electrolyte depletion particularly hypokalemia). Products include:
Decadron Phosphate Injection 1931

Dezocine (Potentiation of orthostatic hypotension may occur).
No products indexed under this heading.

Diazoxide (Concurrent use with other antihypertensive agents may result in additive effect or potentiation). Products include:
Hyperstat I.V. Injection 3031

Diclofenac Potassium (Reduces diuretic, natriuretic, and antihypertensive effects). Products include:
Cataflam Tablets 2173

Diclofenac Sodium (Reduces diuretic, natriuretic, and antihypertensive effects). Products include:
Arthrotec Tablets 3126
Voltaren Ophthalmic Solution 2300
Voltaren Tablets 2298
Voltaren-XR Tablets 2301

Digitalis Glycoside Preparations (Thiazide-induced hypokalemia may sensitize or exaggerate the response of the heart to the toxic effects of digitalis).
No products indexed under this heading.

Digitoxin (Thiazide-induced hypokalemia may sensitize or exaggerate the response of the heart to the toxic effects of digitalis).
No products indexed under this heading.

Digoxin (Thiazide-induced hypokalemia may sensitize or exaggerate the response of the heart to the toxic effects of digitalis). Products include:
Digitek Tablets ... **2146**
Lanoxicaps Capsules ... **1458**
Lanoxin Injection ... **1462**
Lanoxin Tablets ... **1468**
Lanoxin Injection Pediatric ... **1465**

Diltiazem Hydrochloride (Concurrent use with other antihypertensive agents may result in additive effect or potentiation). Products include:
Cardizem LA Extended Release Tablets ... **1699**
Tiazac Capsules ... **1204**

Doxazosin Mesylate (Concurrent use with other antihypertensive agents may result in additive effect or potentiation).
No products indexed under this heading.

Enalapril Maleate (Concurrent use with other antihypertensive agents may result in additive effect or potentiation). Products include:
Vaseretic Tablets ... **2073**
Vasotec I.V. Injection ... **2076**

Enalaprilat (Concurrent use with other antihypertensive agents may result in additive effect or potentiation).
No products indexed under this heading.

Eprosartan Mesylate (Concurrent use with other antihypertensive agents may result in additive effect or potentiation). Products include:
Teveten Tablets ... **1707**
Teveten HCT Tablets ... **1710**

Esmolol Hydrochloride (Concurrent use with other antihypertensive agents may result in additive effect or potentiation). Products include:
Brevibloc Concentrate ... **766**
Brevibloc Injection ... **766**
Brevibloc Double Strength Injection ... **766**
Brevibloc Premixed Injection ... **766**
Brevibloc Double Strength Premixed Injection ... **766**

Etodolac (Reduces diuretic, natriuretic, and antihypertensive effects).
No products indexed under this heading.

Felodipine (Concurrent use with other antihypertensive agents may result in additive effect or potentiation). Products include:
Plendil Extended-Release Tablets ... **651**

Fenoprofen Calcium (Reduces diuretic, natriuretic, and antihypertensive effects). Products include:
Nalfon Capsules ... **2504**

Fentanyl (Potentiation of orthostatic hypotension may occur). Products include:
Duragesic Transdermal System ... **2448**

Fentanyl Citrate (Potentiation of orthostatic hypotension may occur). Products include:
Actiq ... **993**

Fludrocortisone Acetate (Intensified electrolyte depletion particularly hypokalemia).
No products indexed under this heading.

Flurbiprofen (Reduces diuretic, natriuretic, and antihypertensive effects).
No products indexed under this heading.

Fosinopril Sodium (Concurrent use with other antihypertensive agents may result in additive effect or potentiation).
No products indexed under this heading.

Furosemide (Concurrent use with other antihypertensive agents may result in additive effect or potentiation). Products include:
Furosemide Tablets ... **2117**

Glimepiride (Thiazide-induced hyperglycemia may require dosage adjustment of hypoglycemic agents). Products include:
Amaryl Tablets ... **2864**

Glipizide (Thiazide-induced hyperglycemia may require dosage adjustment of hypoglycemic agents).
No products indexed under this heading.

Glyburide (Thiazide-induced hyperglycemia may require dosage adjustment of hypoglycemic agents).
No products indexed under this heading.

Guanabenz Acetate (Concurrent use with other antihypertensive agents may result in additive effect or potentiation).
No products indexed under this heading.

Guanethidine Monosulfate (Concurrent use with other antihypertensive agents may result in additive effect or potentiation).
No products indexed under this heading.

Hydralazine Hydrochloride (Concurrent use with other antihypertensive agents may result in additive effect or potentiation). Products include:
BiDil Tablets ... **2161**

Hydrochlorothiazide (Concurrent use with other antihypertensive agents may result in additive effect or potentiation). Products include:
Aldoril Tablets ... **1884**
Atacand HCT ... **637**
Avalide Tablets ... **2889**
Avalide Tablets ... **922**
Benicar HCT Tablets ... **2852**
Diovan HCT Tablets ... **2195**
Dyazide Capsules ... **1389**
Hyzaar ... **1964**
Lotensin HCT Tablets ... **2235**
Maxzide ... **2150**
Micardis HCT Tablets ... **886**
Moduretic Tablets ... **2003**
Prinzide Tablets ... **2033**
Teveten HCT Tablets ... **1710**
Timolide Tablets ... **2056**
Uniretic Tablets ... **3114**
Vaseretic Tablets ... **2073**
Zestoretic Tablets ... **701**

Hydrocodone Bitartrate (Potentiation of orthostatic hypotension may occur). Products include:
Hycodan ... **1104**
Hycomine Compound Tablets ... **1105**
Hycotuss Expectorant Syrup ... **1106**
Lortab ... **3315**
Lortab Elixir ... **3312**
Vicodin Tablets ... **530**
Vicodin ES Tablets ... **531**
Vicodin HP Tablets ... **532**
Vicoprofen Tablets ... **533**
Zydone Tablets ... **1118**

Hydrocodone Polistirex (Potentiation of orthostatic hypotension may occur). Products include:
Tussionex Pennkinetic Extended-Release Suspension ... **3322**

Hydrocortisone (Intensified electrolyte depletion particularly hypokalemia). Products include:
Cortizone•5 Ointment ... ■**699**
Cortizone•10 Creme ... ■**699**
Cortizone•10 Ointment ... ■**699**
Cortizone•10 Plus Creme ... ■**700**
Cortizone•10 Maximum Strength Quick Shot Spray ... ■**700**
Hydrocortone Tablets ... **1963**
Preparation H Hydrocortisone Cream ... ■**748**

Hydrocortisone Acetate (Intensified electrolyte depletion particularly hypokalemia). Products include:
Analpram-HC ... **1136**
Pramosone ... **1139**
ProctoFoam-HC ... **3113**
Tucks Anti-Itch Ointment ... ■**712**
U-cort 1% Cream ... **3289**

Hydrocortisone Sodium Phosphate (Intensified electrolyte depletion particularly hypokalemia).
No products indexed under this heading.

Hydrocortisone Sodium Succinate (Intensified electrolyte depletion particularly hypokalemia).
No products indexed under this heading.

Hydroflumethiazide (Concurrent use with other antihypertensive agents may result in additive effect or potentiation).
No products indexed under this heading.

Hydromorphone Hydrochloride (Potentiation of orthostatic hypotension may occur). Products include:
Dilaudid ... **439**
Dilaudid Oral Liquid ... **443**
Dilaudid Non-Sterile Powder ... **439**
Dilaudid Rectal Suppositories ... **439**
Dilaudid Tablets ... **439**
Dilaudid Tablets - 8 mg ... **443**
Dilaudid-HP ... **441**

Ibuprofen (Reduces diuretic, natriuretic, and antihypertensive effects). Products include:
Advil Allergy Sinus Caplets ... ■**737**
Advil ... ■**737**
Children's Advil Suspension ... ■**742**
Children's Advil Chewable Tablets ... ■**741**
Advil Cold & Sinus ... ■**739**
Advil Flu & Body Ache Caplets ... ■**739**
Children's Advil Cold Suspension ... ■**741**
Infants' Advil Concentrated Drops ... ■**743**
Junior Strength Advil Swallow Tablets ... ■**740**
Advil Migraine Liquigels ... ■**740**
Advil Multi-Symptom Cold Caplets ... ■**738**
Combunox Tablets ... **1183**
Children's Motrin Oral Suspension and Chewable Tablets ... **1837**
Children's Motrin Cold Non-Staining Dye-Free Oral Suspension ... **1838**
Children's Motrin Cold Oral Suspension ... **1838**
Children's Motrin Non-Staining Dye-Free Oral Suspension ... **1837**
Motrin Cold & Sinus Caplets ... **1836**
Motrin IB Tablets and Caplets ... **1836**
Infants' Motrin Concentrated Drops ... **1837**
Infants' Motrin Non-Staining Dye-Free Drops ... **1837**
Junior Strength Motrin Caplets and Chewable Tablets ... **1837**
Vicoprofen Tablets ... **533**

Indapamide (Concurrent use with other antihypertensive agents may result in additive effect or potentiation). Products include:
Indapamide Tablets ... **2119**

Indomethacin (Reduces diuretic, natriuretic, and antihypertensive effects). Products include:
Indocin ... **1968**

Indomethacin Sodium Trihydrate (Reduces diuretic, natriuretic, and antihypertensive effects). Products include:
Indocin I.V. ... **1973**

Insulin, Human, Zinc Suspension (Thiazide-induce hyperglycemia may require dosage adjustment of hypoglycemic agents). Products include:
Humulin L, 100 Units ... **1763**
Humulin U, 100 Units ... **1770**

Insulin, Human NPH (Thiazide-induce hyperglycemia may require dosage adjustment of hypoglycemic agents). Products include:
Humulin N, 100 Units ... **1764**
Humulin N Pen ... **1765**
Novolin N Human Insulin 10 ml Vials ... **2322**
Novolin N InnoLet ... **2322**
Novolin N PenFill 3 ml Cartridges ... **2325**
Novolin R InnoLet ... **2322**

Insulin, Human Regular (Thiazide-induce hyperglycemia may require dosage adjustment of hypoglycemic agents). Products include:
Humulin R (U-500) ... **1768**
Humulin R, 100 Units ... **1767**
Novolin R Human Insulin 10 ml Vials ... **2322**
Novolin R PenFill ... **2325**

Insulin, Human Regular and Human NPH Mixture (Thiazide-induce hyperglycemia may require dosage adjustment of hypoglycemic agents). Products include:
Humulin 50/50, 100 Units ... **1760**
Humulin 70/30 Pen ... **1761**
Novolin 70/30 Human Insulin 10 ml Vials ... **2321**
Novolin 70/30 InnoLet ... **2322**
Novolin 70/30 PenFill 3 ml Cartridges ... **2325**

Insulin, NPH (Thiazide-induce hyperglycemia may require dosage adjustment of hypoglycemic agents).
No products indexed under this heading.

Insulin, Regular (Thiazide-induce hyperglycemia may require dosage adjustment of hypoglycemic agents).
No products indexed under this heading.

Insulin, Zinc Crystals (Thiazide-induce hyperglycemia may require dosage adjustment of hypoglycemic agents).
No products indexed under this heading.

Insulin, Zinc Suspension (Thiazide-induce hyperglycemia may require dosage adjustment of hypoglycemic agents).
No products indexed under this heading.

Insulin Aspart, Human Regular (Thiazide-induce hyperglycemia may require dosage adjustment of hypoglycemic agents). Products include:
NovoLog Injection ... **2326**

Insulin glargine (Thiazide-induce hyperglycemia may require dosage adjustment of hypoglycemic agents). Products include:
Lantus Injection ... **2925**

Insulin Lispro, Human (Thiazide-induce hyperglycemia may require dosage adjustment of hypoglycemic agents). Products include:
Humalog-Pen ... **1751**
Humalog Mix 75/25-Pen ... **1754**

Insulin Lispro Protamine, Human (Thiazide-induce hyperglycemia may

require dosage adjustment of hypoglycemic agents). Products include:
- Humalog Mix 75/25-Pen 1754

Irbesartan (Concurrent use with other antihypertensive agents may result in additive effect or potentiation). Products include:
- Avalide Tablets 922
- Avalide Tablets 2889
- Avapro Tablets 925
- Avapro Tablets 2886

Isradipine (Concurrent use with other antihypertensive agents may result in additive effect or potentiation). Products include:
- DynaCirc CR Tablets 2726

Ketoprofen (Reduces diuretic, natriuretic, and antihypertensive effects).
No products indexed under this heading.

Ketorolac Tromethamine (Reduces diuretic, natriuretic, and antihypertensive effects). Products include:
- Acular Ophthalmic Solution 561
- Acular LS Ophthalmic Solution 562

Labetalol Hydrochloride (Concurrent use with other antihypertensive agents may result in additive effect or potentiation).
No products indexed under this heading.

Levorphanol Tartrate (Potentiation of orthostatic hypotension may occur).
No products indexed under this heading.

Lisinopril (Concurrent use with other antihypertensive agents may result in additive effect or potentiation). Products include:
- Prinivil Tablets 2029
- Prinzide Tablets 2033
- Zestoretic Tablets 701
- Zestril Tablets 704

Lithium (Diuretics reduce the renal clearance of lithium and this may lead to lithium toxicity).
No products indexed under this heading.

Lithium Carbonate (Diuretics reduce the renal clearance of lithium and this may lead to lithium toxicity). Products include:
- Eskalith 1406
- Lithobid Tablets 1670

Lithium Citrate (Diuretics reduce the renal clearance of lithium and this may lead to lithium toxicity).
No products indexed under this heading.

Losartan Potassium (Concurrent use with other antihypertensive agents may result in additive effect or potentiation). Products include:
- Cozaar Tablets 1913
- Hyzaar 1964

Mecamylamine Hydrochloride (Concurrent use with other antihypertensive agents may result in additive effect or potentiation). Products include:
- Inversine Tablets 3286

Meclofenamate Sodium (Reduces diuretic, natriuretic, and antihypertensive effects).
No products indexed under this heading.

Mefenamic Acid (Reduces diuretic, natriuretic, and antihypertensive effects).
No products indexed under this heading.

Meloxicam (Reduces diuretic, natriuretic, and antihypertensive effects). Products include:
- Mobic Oral Suspension 893
- Mobic Tablets 893

Meperidine Hydrochloride (Potentiation of orthostatic hypotension may occur).
No products indexed under this heading.

Mephobarbital (Potentiation of orthostatic hypotension may occur). Products include:
- Mebaral Tablets, USP 2483

Metformin Hydrochloride (Thiazide-induced hyperglycemia may require dosage adjustment of hypoglycemic agents). Products include:
- ActoPlus Met Tablets 3219
- Avandamet Tablets 1343
- Fortamet Extended-Release Tablets 1156

Methadone Hydrochloride (Potentiation of orthostatic hypotension may occur).
No products indexed under this heading.

Methyclothiazide (Concurrent use with other antihypertensive agents may result in additive effect or potentiation).
No products indexed under this heading.

Methyldopa (Concurrent use with other antihypertensive agents may result in additive effect or potentiation). Products include:
- Aldoclor Tablets 1881
- Aldoril Tablets 1884

Methyldopate Hydrochloride (Concurrent use with other antihypertensive agents may result in additive effect or potentiation).
No products indexed under this heading.

Methylprednisolone Acetate (Intensified electrolyte depletion particularly hypokalemia). Products include:
- Depo-Medrol Injectable Suspension 2615
- Depo-Medrol Single-Dose Vial 2617

Methylprednisolone Sodium Succinate (Intensified electrolyte depletion particularly hypokalemia).
No products indexed under this heading.

Metipranolol Hydrochloride (Concurrent use with other antihypertensive agents may result in additive effect or potentiation).
No products indexed under this heading.

Metocurine Iodide (Possible increased responsiveness to the muscle relaxants).
No products indexed under this heading.

Metolazone (Concurrent use with other antihypertensive agents may result in additive effect or potentiation).
No products indexed under this heading.

Metoprolol Succinate (Concurrent use with other antihypertensive agents may result in additive effect or potentiation). Products include:
- Toprol-XL Tablets 660

Metoprolol Tartrate (Concurrent use with other antihypertensive agents may result in additive effect or potentiation).
No products indexed under this heading.

Metyrosine (Concurrent use with other antihypertensive agents may result in additive effect or potentiation). Products include:
- Demser Capsules 1933

Mibefradil Dihydrochloride (Concurrent use with other antihypertensive agents may result in additive effect or potentiation).
No products indexed under this heading.

Miglitol (Thiazide-induced hyperglycemia may require dosage adjustment of hypoglycemic agents).
No products indexed under this heading.

Minoxidil (Concurrent use with other antihypertensive agents may result in additive effect or potentiation). Products include:
- Men's Rogaine Extra Strength Topical Solution, Ocean Rush Scent and Original Unscented 706
- Women's Rogaine Topical Solution, Spring Bloom Scent and Original Unscented 707

Mivacurium Chloride (Possible increased responsiveness to the muscle relaxants). Products include:
- Mivacron Injection 489

Moexipril Hydrochloride (Concurrent use with other antihypertensive agents may result in additive effect or potentiation). Products include:
- Uniretic Tablets 3114
- Univasc Tablets 3118

Morphine Sulfate (Potentiation of orthostatic hypotension may occur). Products include:
- Avinza Capsules 1714
- Kadian Capsules 572
- MS Contin Tablets 2703

Nabumetone (Reduces diuretic, natriuretic, and antihypertensive effects). Products include:
- Relafen Tablets 1523

Nadolol (Concurrent use with other antihypertensive agents may result in additive effect or potentiation). Products include:
- Nadolol Tablets 2121

Naproxen (Reduces diuretic, natriuretic, and antihypertensive effects). Products include:
- EC-Naprosyn Delayed-Release Tablets 2769
- Naprosyn Suspension 2769
- Naprosyn Tablets 2769
- Prevacid NapraPAC 3277

Naproxen Sodium (Reduces diuretic, natriuretic, and antihypertensive effects). Products include:
- Aleve Tablets, Caplets and Gelcaps 605
- Anaprox Tablets 2769
- Anaprox DS Tablets 2769

Nicardipine Hydrochloride (Concurrent use with other antihypertensive agents may result in additive effect or potentiation). Products include:
- Cardene I.V. 1129

Nifedipine (Concurrent use with other antihypertensive agents may result in additive effect or potentiation). Products include:
- Adalat CC Tablets 2978

Nisoldipine (Concurrent use with other antihypertensive agents may result in additive effect or potentiation). Products include:
- Sular Tablets 1163

Nitroglycerin (Concurrent use with other antihypertensive agents may result in additive effect or potentiation). Products include:
- Nitro-Dur Transdermal Infusion System 3060
- Nitrolingual Pumpspray 1161

Norepinephrine Hydrochloride (Decreased arterial responsiveness to pressor amine).
No products indexed under this heading.

Oxaprozin (Reduces diuretic, natriuretic, and antihypertensive effects).
No products indexed under this heading.

Oxycodone Hydrochloride (Potentiation of orthostatic hypotension may occur). Products include:
- Combunox Tablets 1183
- OxyContin Tablets 2699
- OxyFast Oral Concentrate Solution 2704
- OxyIR Capsules 2704
- Percocet Tablets 1114
- Percodan Tablets 1115

Pancuronium Bromide (Possible increased responsiveness to the muscle relaxants).
No products indexed under this heading.

Penbutolol Sulfate (Concurrent use with other antihypertensive agents may result in additive effect or potentiation).
No products indexed under this heading.

Pentobarbital Sodium (Potentiation of orthostatic hypotension may occur). Products include:
- Nembutal Sodium Solution, USP 2484

Perindopril Erbumine (Concurrent use with other antihypertensive agents may result in additive effect or potentiation). Products include:
- Aceon Tablets (2 mg, 4 mg, 8 mg) 3191

Phenobarbital (Potentiation of orthostatic hypotension may occur).
No products indexed under this heading.

Phenoxybenzamine Hydrochloride (Concurrent use with other antihypertensive agents may result in additive effect or potentiation). Products include:
- Dibenzyline Capsules 3390

Phentolamine Mesylate (Concurrent use with other antihypertensive agents may result in additive effect or potentiation).
No products indexed under this heading.

Phenylbutazone (Reduces diuretic, natriuretic, and antihypertensive effects).
No products indexed under this heading.

Pindolol (Concurrent use with other antihypertensive agents may result in additive effect or potentiation).
No products indexed under this heading.

Pioglitazone Hydrochloride (Thiazide-induced hyperglycemia may require dosage adjustment of hypoglycemic agents). Products include:
- ActoPlus Met Tablets 3219
- Actos Tablets 3224

Piroxicam (Reduces diuretic, natriuretic, and antihypertensive effects).
No products indexed under this heading.

Polythiazide (Concurrent use with other antihypertensive agents may result in additive effect or potentiation).
No products indexed under this heading.

Prazosin Hydrochloride (Concurrent use with other antihypertensive agents may result in additive effect or potentiation).
No products indexed under this heading.

Prednisolone Acetate (Intensified electrolyte depletion particularly hypokalemia). Products include:
Blephamide Ophthalmic Ointment 563
Blephamide Ophthalmic Suspension 564
Poly-Pred Liquifilm Ophthalmic Suspension .... ⊙231
Pred Forte Ophthalmic Suspension .... ⊙233
Pred Mild Sterile Ophthalmic Suspension .... ⊙236
Pred-G Ophthalmic Suspension .... ⊙234
Pred-G Sterile Ophthalmic Ointment .... ⊙235

Prednisolone Sodium Phosphate (Intensified electrolyte depletion particularly hypokalemia). Products include:
Pediapred Oral Solution 3319

Prednisolone Tebutate (Intensified electrolyte depletion particularly hypokalemia).
No products indexed under this heading.

Prednisone (Intensified electrolyte depletion particularly hypokalemia).
No products indexed under this heading.

Propoxyphene Hydrochloride (Potentiation of orthostatic hypotension may occur).
No products indexed under this heading.

Propoxyphene Napsylate (Potentiation of orthostatic hypotension may occur). Products include:
Darvocet A 500 Tablets 3497

Propranolol Hydrochloride (Concurrent use with other antihypertensive agents may result in additive effect or potentiation). Products include:
Inderal LA Long-Acting Capsules 3421
InnoPran XL Capsules 2728

Quinapril Hydrochloride (Concurrent use with other antihypertensive agents may result in additive effect or potentiation).
No products indexed under this heading.

Ramipril (Concurrent use with other antihypertensive agents may result in additive effect or potentiation). Products include:
Altace Capsules 1673

Rapacuronium Bromide (Possible increased responsiveness to the muscle relaxants).
No products indexed under this heading.

Rauwolfia Serpentina (Concurrent use with other antihypertensive agents may result in additive effect or potentiation).
No products indexed under this heading.

Remifentanil Hydrochloride (Potentiation of orthostatic hypotension may occur).
No products indexed under this heading.

Repaglinide (Thiazide-induced hyperglycemia may require dosage adjustment of hypoglycemic agents). Products include:
Prandin Tablets (0.5, 1, and 2 mg) 2337

Rescinnamine (Concurrent use with other antihypertensive agents may result in additive effect or potentiation).
No products indexed under this heading.

Reserpine (Concurrent use with other antihypertensive agents may result in additive effect or potentiation).
No products indexed under this heading.

Rocuronium Bromide (Possible increased responsiveness to the muscle relaxants). Products include:
Zemuron Injection 2363

Rofecoxib (Reduces diuretic, natriuretic, and antihypertensive effects).
No products indexed under this heading.

Rosiglitazone Maleate (Thiazide-induced hyperglycemia may require dosage adjustment of hypoglycemic agents). Products include:
Avandamet Tablets 1343
Avandia Tablets 1348

Secobarbital Sodium (Potentiation of orthostatic hypotension may occur).
No products indexed under this heading.

Sodium Nitroprusside (Concurrent use with other antihypertensive agents may result in additive effect or potentiation).
No products indexed under this heading.

Sotalol Hydrochloride (Concurrent use with other antihypertensive agents may result in additive effect or potentiation).
No products indexed under this heading.

Spirapril Hydrochloride (Concurrent use with other antihypertensive agents may result in additive effect or potentiation).
No products indexed under this heading.

Sufentanil Citrate (Potentiation of orthostatic hypotension may occur).
No products indexed under this heading.

Sulindac (Reduces diuretic, natriuretic, and antihypertensive effects). Products include:
Clinoril Tablets 1899

Telmisartan (Concurrent use with other antihypertensive agents may result in additive effect or potentiation). Products include:
Micardis Tablets 884
Micardis HCT Tablets 886

Terazosin Hydrochloride (Concurrent use with other antihypertensive agents may result in additive effect or potentiation). Products include:
Hytrin Capsules 469

Thiamylal Sodium (Potentiation of orthostatic hypotension may occur).
No products indexed under this heading.

Timolol Maleate (Concurrent use with other antihypertensive agents may result in additive effect or potentiation). Products include:
Blocadren Tablets 1891
Cosopt Sterile Ophthalmic Solution 1910
Timolide Tablets 2056
Timoptic in Ocudose 2061
Timoptic Sterile Ophthalmic Solution 2058
Timoptic-XE Sterile Ophthalmic Gel Forming Solution 2062

Tolazamide (Thiazide-induced hyperglycemia may require dosage adjustment of hypoglycemic agents).
No products indexed under this heading.

Tolbutamide (Thiazide-induced hyperglycemia may require dosage adjustment of hypoglycemic agents).
No products indexed under this heading.

Tolmetin Sodium (Reduces diuretic, natriuretic, and antihypertensive effects).
No products indexed under this heading.

Torsemide (Concurrent use with other antihypertensive agents may result in additive effect or potentiation).
No products indexed under this heading.

Trandolapril (Concurrent use with other antihypertensive agents may result in additive effect or potentiation). Products include:
Mavik Tablets 482
Tarka Tablets 519

Triamcinolone (Intensified electrolyte depletion particularly hypokalemia).
No products indexed under this heading.

Triamcinolone Acetonide (Intensified electrolyte depletion particularly hypokalemia). Products include:
Azmacort Inhalation Aerosol 1701
Nasacort HFA Inhalation Aerosol 2939
Nasacort AQ Nasal Spray 2937

Triamcinolone Diacetate (Intensified electrolyte depletion particularly hypokalemia).
No products indexed under this heading.

Triamcinolone Hexacetonide (Intensified electrolyte depletion particularly hypokalemia).
No products indexed under this heading.

Trimethaphan Camsylate (Concurrent use with other antihypertensive agents may result in additive effect or potentiation).
No products indexed under this heading.

Troglitazone (Thiazide-induced hyperglycemia may require dosage adjustment of hypoglycemic agents).
No products indexed under this heading.

Tubocurarine Chloride (Possible increased responsiveness to the muscle relaxants).
No products indexed under this heading.

Valdecoxib (Reduces diuretic, natriuretic, and antihypertensive effects).
No products indexed under this heading.

Valsartan (Concurrent use with other antihypertensive agents may result in additive effect or potentiation). Products include:
Diovan HCT Tablets 2195
Diovan Tablets 2191

Vecuronium Bromide (Possible increased responsiveness to the muscle relaxants).
No products indexed under this heading.

Verapamil Hydrochloride (Concurrent use with other antihypertensive agents may result in additive effect or potentiation). Products include:
Covera-HS Tablets 3135
Tarka Tablets 519
Verelan PM Capsules 3120

Food Interactions

Alcohol (Potentiation of orthostatic hypotension may occur).

DIURIL TABLETS

(Chlorothiazide) 1936
See Diuril Oral Suspension

DIURIL SODIUM INTRAVENOUS

(Chlorothiazide Sodium) 1934
May interact with antihypertensives, barbiturates, corticosteroids, cardiac glycosides, oral hypoglycemic agents, insulin, lithium preparations, narcotic analgesics, nondepolarizing neuromuscular blocking agents, nonsteroidal anti-inflammatory agents, and certain other agents. Compounds in these categories include:

Acarbose (Thiazide-induced hyperglycemia may require dosage adjustment of hypoglycemic agents). Products include:
Precose Tablets 776

Acebutolol Hydrochloride (Concurrent use with other antihypertensive agents may result in additive effect or potentiation).
No products indexed under this heading.

ACTH (Intensified electrolyte depletion particularly hypokalemia).
No products indexed under this heading.

Alfentanil Hydrochloride (Potentiation of orthostatic hypotension may occur).
No products indexed under this heading.

Amlodipine Besylate (Concurrent use with other antihypertensive agents may result in additive effect or potentiation). Products include:
Caduet Tablets 2507
Lotrel Capsules 2238
Norvasc Tablets 2529

Aprobarbital (Potentiation of orthostatic hypotension may occur).
No products indexed under this heading.

Atenolol (Concurrent use with other antihypertensive agents may result in additive effect or potentiation). Products include:
Tenormin I.V. Injection 698
Tenormin Tablets 695

Atracurium Besylate (Possible increased responsiveness to the muscle relaxants).
No products indexed under this heading.

Benazepril Hydrochloride (Concurrent use with other antihypertensive agents may result in additive effect or potentiation). Products include:
Lotensin Tablets 2232
Lotensin HCT Tablets 2235
Lotrel Capsules 2238

Bendroflumethiazide (Concurrent use with other antihypertensive agents may result in additive effect or potentiation).
No products indexed under this heading.

Betamethasone Acetate (Intensified electrolyte depletion particularly hypokalemia).
No products indexed under this heading.

Betamethasone Sodium Phosphate (Intensified electrolyte depletion particularly hypokalemia).
No products indexed under this heading.

Betaxolol Hydrochloride (Concurrent use with other antihypertensive agents may result in additive effect or potentiation). Products include:
Betoptic S Ophthalmic Suspension 554

Bisoprolol Fumarate (Concurrent use with other antihypertensive agents may result in additive effect or potentiation).
No products indexed under this heading.

Buprenorphine Hydrochloride (Potentiation of orthostatic hypotension may occur). Products include:
Buprenex Injectable 2718
Suboxone Tablets 2719
Subutex Tablets 2719

Butabarbital (Potentiation of orthostatic hypotension may occur).
No products indexed under this heading.

Butalbital (Potentiation of orthostatic hypotension may occur). Products include:
Sedapap Tablets 50 mg/650 mg 2098

Candesartan Cilexetil (Concurrent use with other antihypertensive agents may result in additive effect or potentiation). Products include:
Atacand Tablets 634
Atacand HCT 637

Captopril (Concurrent use with other antihypertensive agents may result in additive effect or potentiation). Products include:
Captopril Tablets 2114

Carteolol Hydrochloride (Concurrent use with other antihypertensive agents may result in additive effect or potentiation). Products include:
Carteolol Hydrochloride Ophthalmic Solution USP, 1% .... ⊙246

Celecoxib (Reduces diuretic, natriuretic, and antihypertensive effects). Products include:
Celebrex Capsules 3130

Chlorothiazide (Concurrent use with other antihypertensive agents may result in additive effect or potentiation). Products include:
Aldoclor Tablets 1881
Diuril Oral 1936

Chlorpropamide (Thiazide-induced hyperglycemia may require dosage adjustment of hypoglycemic agents).
No products indexed under this heading.

Chlorthalidone (Concurrent use with other antihypertensive agents may result in additive effect or potentiation). Products include:
Clorpres Tablets 2139

Cisatracurium Besylate (Possible increased responsiveness to the muscle relaxants). Products include:
Nimbex Injection 494

Clonidine (Concurrent use with other antihypertensive agents may result in additive effect or potentiation). Products include:
Catapres-TTS 875

Clonidine Hydrochloride (Concurrent use with other antihypertensive agents may result in additive effect or potentiation). Products include:
Catapres Tablets 874
Clorpres Tablets 2139

Codeine Phosphate (Potentiation of orthostatic hypotension may occur). Products include:
Tylenol with Codeine 2461

Cortisone Acetate (Intensified electrolyte depletion particularly hypokalemia).
No products indexed under this heading.

Deserpidine (Concurrent use with other antihypertensive agents may result in additive effect or potentiation).
No products indexed under this heading.

Deslanoside (Thiazide-induced hypokalemia may sensitize or exaggerate the response of the heart to the toxic effects of digitalis).
No products indexed under this heading.

Dexamethasone (Intensified electrolyte depletion particularly hypokalemia). Products include:
Ciprodex Otic Suspension 555
Decadron Tablets 1929
TobraDex Ophthalmic Ointment 558
TobraDex Ophthalmic Suspension 558

Dexamethasone Acetate (Intensified electrolyte depletion particularly hypokalemia).
No products indexed under this heading.

Dexamethasone Sodium Phosphate (Intensified electrolyte depletion particularly hypokalemia). Products include:
Decadron Phosphate Injection 1931

Dezocine (Potentiation of orthostatic hypotension may occur).
No products indexed under this heading.

Diazoxide (Concurrent use with other antihypertensive agents may result in additive effect or potentiation). Products include:
Hyperstat I.V. Injection 3031

Diclofenac Potassium (Reduces diuretic, natriuretic, and antihypertensive effects). Products include:
Cataflam Tablets 2173

Diclofenac Sodium (Reduces diuretic, natriuretic, and antihypertensive effects). Products include:
Arthrotec Tablets 3126
Voltaren Ophthalmic Solution 2300
Voltaren Tablets 2298
Voltaren-XR Tablets 2301

Digitalis Glycoside Preparations (Thiazide-induced hypokalemia may sensitize or exaggerate the response of the heart to the toxic effects of digitalis).
No products indexed under this heading.

Digitoxin (Thiazide-induced hypokalemia may sensitize or exaggerate the response of the heart to the toxic effects of digitalis).
No products indexed under this heading.

Digoxin (Thiazide-induced hypokalemia may sensitize or exaggerate the response of the heart to the toxic effects of digitalis). Products include:
Digitek Tablets 2146
Lanoxicaps Capsules 1458
Lanoxin Injection 1462
Lanoxin Tablets 1468
Lanoxin Injection Pediatric 1465

Diltiazem Hydrochloride (Concurrent use with other antihypertensive agents may result in additive effect or potentiation). Products include:
Cardizem LA Extended Release Tablets 1699
Tiazac Capsules 1204

Doxazosin Mesylate (Concurrent use with other antihypertensive agents may result in additive effect or potentiation).
No products indexed under this heading.

Enalapril Maleate (Concurrent use with other antihypertensive agents may result in additive effect or potentiation). Products include:
Vaseretic Tablets 2073
Vasotec I.V. Injection 2076

Enalaprilat (Concurrent use with other antihypertensive agents may result in additive effect or potentiation).
No products indexed under this heading.

Eprosartan Mesylate (Concurrent use with other antihypertensive agents may result in additive effect or potentiation). Products include:
Teveten Tablets 1707
Teveten HCT Tablets 1710

Esmolol Hydrochloride (Concurrent use with other antihypertensive agents may result in additive effect or potentiation). Products include:
Brevibloc Concentrate 766
Brevibloc Injection 766
Brevibloc Double Strength Injection 766
Brevibloc Premixed Injection 766
Brevibloc Double Strength Premixed Injection 766

Etodolac (Reduces diuretic, natriuretic, and antihypertensive effects).
No products indexed under this heading.

Felodipine (Concurrent use with other antihypertensive agents may result in additive effect or potentiation). Products include:
Plendil Extended-Release Tablets 651

Fenoprofen Calcium (Reduces diuretic, natriuretic, and antihypertensive effects). Products include:
Nalfon Capsules 2504

Fentanyl (Potentiation of orthostatic hypotension may occur). Products include:
Duragesic Transdermal System 2448

Fentanyl Citrate (Potentiation of orthostatic hypotension may occur). Products include:
Actiq 993

Fludrocortisone Acetate (Intensified electrolyte depletion particularly hypokalemia).
No products indexed under this heading.

Flurbiprofen (Reduces diuretic, natriuretic, and antihypertensive effects).
No products indexed under this heading.

Fosinopril Sodium (Concurrent use with other antihypertensive agents may result in additive effect or potentiation).
No products indexed under this heading.

Furosemide (Concurrent use with other antihypertensive agents may result in additive effect or potentiation). Products include:
Furosemide Tablets 2117

Glimepiride (Thiazide-induced hyperglycemia may require dosage adjustment of hypoglycemic agents). Products include:
Amaryl Tablets 2864

Glipizide (Thiazide-induced hyperglycemia may require dosage adjustment of hypoglycemic agents).
No products indexed under this heading.

Glyburide (Thiazide-induced hyperglycemia may require dosage adjustment of hypoglycemic agents).
No products indexed under this heading.

Guanabenz Acetate (Concurrent use with other antihypertensive agents may result in additive effect or potentiation).
No products indexed under this heading.

Guanethidine Monosulfate (Concurrent use with other antihypertensive agents may result in additive effect or potentiation).
No products indexed under this heading.

Hydralazine Hydrochloride (Concurrent use with other antihypertensive agents may result in additive effect or potentiation). Products include:
BiDil Tablets 2161

Hydrochlorothiazide (Concurrent use with other antihypertensive agents may result in additive effect or potentiation). Products include:
Aldoril Tablets 1884
Atacand HCT 637
Avalide Tablets 2889
Avalide Tablets 922
Benicar HCT Tablets 2852
Diovan HCT Tablets 2195
Dyazide Capsules 1389
Hyzaar 1964
Lotensin HCT Tablets 2235
Maxzide 2150
Micardis HCT Tablets 886
Moduretic Tablets 2003
Prinzide Tablets 2033
Teveten HCT Tablets 1710
Timolide Tablets 2056
Uniretic Tablets 3114
Vaseretic Tablets 2073
Zestoretic Tablets 701

Hydrocodone Bitartrate (Potentiation of orthostatic hypotension may occur). Products include:
Hycodan 1104
Hycomine Compound Tablets 1105
Hycotuss Expectorant Syrup 1106
Lortab 3315
Lortab Elixir 3312
Vicodin Tablets 530
Vicodin ES Tablets 531
Vicodin HP Tablets 532
Vicoprofen Tablets 533
Zydone Tablets 1118

Hydrocodone Polistirex (Potentiation of orthostatic hypotension may occur). Products include:
Tussionex Pennkinetic Extended-Release Suspension 3322

Hydrocortisone (Intensified electrolyte depletion particularly hypokalemia). Products include:
Cortizone•5 Ointment .... ▣699
Cortizone•10 Creme .... ▣699
Cortizone•10 Ointment .... ▣699
Cortizone•10 Plus Creme .... ▣700
Cortizone•10 Maximum Strength Quick Shot Spray .... ▣700
Hydrocortone Tablets 1963
Preparation H Hydrocortisone Cream .... ▣748

Hydrocortisone Acetate (Intensified electrolyte depletion particularly hypokalemia). Products include:
Analpram-HC 1136
Pramosone 1139
ProctoFoam-HC 3113
Tucks Anti-Itch Ointment .... ▣712
U-cort 1% Cream 3289

Hydrocortisone Sodium Phosphate (Intensified electrolyte depletion particularly hypokalemia).
No products indexed under this heading.

Hydrocortisone Sodium Succinate (Intensified electrolyte depletion particularly hypokalemia).
No products indexed under this heading.

Hydroflumethiazide (Concurrent use with other antihypertensive agents may result in additive effect or potentiation).
No products indexed under this heading.

Hydromorphone Hydrochloride (Potentiation of orthostatic hypotension may occur). Products include:
Dilaudid 439
Dilaudid Oral Liquid 443
Dilaudid Non-Sterile Powder 439
Dilaudid Rectal Suppositories 439
Dilaudid Tablets 439
Dilaudid Tablets - 8 mg 443
Dilaudid-HP 441

Ibuprofen (Reduces diuretic, natriuretic, and antihypertensive effects). Products include:
Advil Allergy Sinus Caplets .... ▣737
Advil .... ▣737
Children's Advil Suspension .... ▣742
Children's Advil Chewable Tablets .... ▣741
Advil Cold & Sinus .... ▣739
Advil Flu & Body Ache Caplets .... ▣739
Children's Advil Cold Suspension .... ▣741
Infants' Advil Concentrated Drops .... ▣743
Junior Strength Advil Swallow Tablets .... ▣740
Advil Migraine Liquigels .... ▣740
Advil Multi-Symptom Cold Caplets .... ▣738
Combunox Tablets 1183
Children's Motrin Oral Suspension and Chewable Tablets 1837
Children's Motrin Cold Non-Staining Dye-Free Oral Suspension 1838
Children's Motrin Cold Oral Suspension 1838
Children's Motrin Non-Staining Dye-Free Oral Suspension 1837
Motrin Cold & Sinus Caplets 1836
Motrin IB Tablets and Caplets 1836
Infants' Motrin Concentrated Drops 1837
Infants' Motrin Non-Staining Dye-Free Drops 1837
Junior Strength Motrin Caplets and Chewable Tablets 1837
Vicoprofen Tablets 533

Indapamide (Concurrent use with other antihypertensive agents may result in additive effect or potentiation). Products include:
Indapamide Tablets 2119

Indomethacin (Reduces diuretic, natriuretic, and antihypertensive effects). Products include:
Indocin 1968

Indomethacin Sodium Trihydrate (Reduces diuretic, natriuretic, and antihypertensive effects). Products include:
Indocin I.V. 1973

Insulin, Human, Zinc Suspension (Thiazide-induced hyperglycemia may require dosage adjustment of hypoglycemic agents). Products include:
Humulin L, 100 Units 1763
Humulin U, 100 Units 1770

Insulin, Human NPH (Thiazide-induced hyperglycemia may require dosage adjustment of hypoglycemic agents). Products include:
Humulin N, 100 Units 1764
Humulin N Pen 1765
Novolin N Human Insulin 10 ml Vials 2322
Novolin N InnoLet 2322
Novolin N PenFill 3 ml Cartridges 2325
Novolin R InnoLet 2322

Insulin, Human Regular (Thiazide-induced hyperglycemia may require dosage adjustment of hypoglycemic agents). Products include:
Humulin R (U-500) 1768
Humulin R, 100 Units 1767
Novolin R Human Insulin 10 ml Vials 2322
Novolin R PenFill 2325

Insulin, Human Regular and Human NPH Mixture (Thiazide-induced hyperglycemia may require dosage adjustment of hypoglycemic agents). Products include:
Humulin 50/50, 100 Units 1760
Humulin 70/30 Pen 1761
Novolin 70/30 Human Insulin 10 ml Vials 2321
Novolin 70/30 InnoLet 2322
Novolin 70/30 PenFill 3 ml Cartridges 2325

Insulin, NPH (Thiazide-induced hyperglycemia may require dosage adjustment of hypoglycemic agents).
No products indexed under this heading.

Insulin, Regular (Thiazide-induced hyperglycemia may require dosage adjustment of hypoglycemic agents).
No products indexed under this heading.

Insulin, Zinc Crystals (Thiazide-induced hyperglycemia may require dosage adjustment of hypoglycemic agents).
No products indexed under this heading.

Insulin, Zinc Suspension (Thiazide-induced hyperglycemia may require dosage adjustment of hypoglycemic agents).
No products indexed under this heading.

Insulin Aspart, Human Regular (Thiazide-induced hyperglycemia may require dosage adjustment of hypoglycemic agents). Products include:
NovoLog Injection 2326

Insulin glargine (Thiazide-induced hyperglycemia may require dosage adjustment of hypoglycemic agents). Products include:
Lantus Injection 2925

Insulin Lispro, Human (Thiazide-induced hyperglycemia may require dosage adjustment of hypoglycemic agents). Products include:
Humalog-Pen 1751
Humalog Mix 75/25-Pen 1754

Insulin Lispro Protamine, Human (Thiazide-induced hyperglycemia may require dosage adjustment of hypoglycemic agents). Products include:
Humalog Mix 75/25-Pen 1754

Irbesartan (Concurrent use with other antihypertensive agents may result in additive effect or potentiation). Products include:
Avalide Tablets 922
Avalide Tablets 2889
Avapro Tablets 925
Avapro Tablets 2886

Isradipine (Concurrent use with other antihypertensive agents may result in additive effect or potentiation). Products include:
DynaCirc CR Tablets 2726

Ketoprofen (Reduces diuretic, natriuretic, and antihypertensive effects).
No products indexed under this heading.

Ketorolac Tromethamine (Reduces diuretic, natriuretic, and antihypertensive effects). Products include:
Acular Ophthalmic Solution 561
Acular LS Ophthalmic Solution 562

Labetalol Hydrochloride (Concurrent use with other antihypertensive agents may result in additive effect or potentiation).
No products indexed under this heading.

Levobunolol Hydrochloride (Concurrent use with other antihypertensive agents may result in additive effect or potentiation). Products include:
Betagan Ophthalmic Solution, USP .... ⊙217

Levorphanol Tartrate (Potentiation of orthostatic hypotension may occur).
No products indexed under this heading.

Lisinopril (Concurrent use with other antihypertensive agents may result in additive effect or potentiation). Products include:
Prinivil Tablets 2029
Prinzide Tablets 2033
Zestoretic Tablets 701
Zestril Tablets 704

Lithium (Diuretics reduce the renal clearance of lithium and this may lead to lithium toxicity).
No products indexed under this heading.

Lithium Carbonate (Diuretics reduce the renal clearance of lithium and this may lead to lithium toxicity). Products include:
Eskalith 1406
Lithobid Tablets 1670

Lithium Citrate (Diuretics reduce the renal clearance of lithium and this may lead to lithium toxicity).
No products indexed under this heading.

Losartan Potassium (Concurrent use with other antihypertensive agents may result in additive effect or potentiation). Products include:
Cozaar Tablets 1913
Hyzaar 1964

Mecamylamine Hydrochloride (Concurrent use with other antihypertensive agents may result in additive effect or potentiation). Products include:
Inversine Tablets 3286

Meclofenamate Sodium (Reduces diuretic, natriuretic, and antihypertensive effects).
No products indexed under this heading.

Mefenamic Acid (Reduces diuretic, natriuretic, and antihypertensive effects).
No products indexed under this heading.

Meloxicam (Reduces diuretic, natriuretic, and antihypertensive effects). Products include:
Mobic Oral Suspension 893
Mobic Tablets 893

Meperidine Hydrochloride (Potentiation of orthostatic hypotension may occur).
No products indexed under this heading.

Mephobarbital (Potentiation of orthostatic hypotension may occur). Products include:
Mebaral Tablets, USP 2483

Metformin Hydrochloride (Thiazide-induced hyperglycemia may require dosage adjustment of hypoglycemic agents). Products include:
ActoPlus Met Tablets 3219
Avandamet Tablets 1343
Fortamet Extended-Release Tablets 1156

Methadone Hydrochloride (Potentiation of orthostatic hypotension may occur).
No products indexed under this heading.

Methyclothiazide (Concurrent use with other antihypertensive agents may result in additive effect or potentiation).
No products indexed under this heading.

Methyldopa (Concurrent use with other antihypertensive agents may result in additive effect or potentiation). Products include:
Aldoclor Tablets 1881
Aldoril Tablets 1884

Methyldopate Hydrochloride (Concurrent use with other antihypertensive agents may result in additive effect or potentiation).
No products indexed under this heading.

Methylprednisolone Acetate (Intensified electrolyte depletion particularly hypokalemia). Products include:
Depo-Medrol Injectable Suspension 2615
Depo-Medrol Single-Dose Vial 2617

Methylprednisolone Sodium Succinate (Intensified electrolyte depletion particularly hypokalemia).
No products indexed under this heading.

Metipranolol Hydrochloride (Concurrent use with other antihypertensive agents may result in additive effect or potentiation).
No products indexed under this heading.

Metocurine Iodide (Possible increased responsiveness to the muscle relaxants).
No products indexed under this heading.

Metolazone (Concurrent use with other antihypertensive agents may result in additive effect or potentiation).
No products indexed under this heading.

Metoprolol Succinate (Concurrent use with other antihypertensive agents may result in additive effect or potentiation). Products include:
Toprol-XL Tablets 660

Metoprolol Tartrate (Concurrent use with other antihypertensive agents may result in additive effect or potentiation).
No products indexed under this heading.

Metyrosine (Concurrent use with other antihypertensive agents may result in additive effect or potentiation). Products include:
Demser Capsules 1933

Mibefradil Dihydrochloride (Concurrent use with other antihypertensive agents may result in additive effect or potentiation).
No products indexed under this heading.

Miglitol (Thiazide-induced hyperglycemia may require dosage adjustment of hypoglycemic agents).
No products indexed under this heading.

Minoxidil (Concurrent use with other antihypertensive agents may result in additive effect or potentiation). Products include:

Men's Rogaine Extra Strength Topical Solution, Ocean Rush Scent and Original Unscented 706
Women's Rogaine Topical Solution, Spring Bloom Scent and Original Unscented 707

Mivacurium Chloride (Possible increased responsiveness to the muscle relaxants). Products include:
Mivacron Injection 489

Moexipril Hydrochloride (Concurrent use with other antihypertensive agents may result in additive effect or potentiation). Products include:
Uniretic Tablets 3114
Univasc Tablets 3118

Morphine Sulfate (Potentiation of orthostatic hypotension may occur). Products include:
Avinza Capsules 1714
Kadian Capsules 572
MS Contin Tablets 2703

Nabumetone (Reduces diuretic, natriuretic, and antihypertensive effects). Products include:
Relafen Tablets 1523

Nadolol (Concurrent use with other antihypertensive agents may result in additive effect or potentiation). Products include:
Nadolol Tablets 2121

Naproxen (Reduces diuretic, natriuretic, and antihypertensive effects). Products include:
EC-Naprosyn Delayed-Release Tablets 2769
Naprosyn Suspension 2769
Naprosyn Tablets 2769
Prevacid NapraPAC 3277

Naproxen Sodium (Reduces diuretic, natriuretic, and antihypertensive effects). Products include:
Aleve Tablets, Caplets and Gelcaps 605
Anaprox Tablets 2769
Anaprox DS Tablets 2769

Nicardipine Hydrochloride (Concurrent use with other antihypertensive agents may result in additive effect or potentiation). Products include:
Cardene I.V. 1129

Nifedipine (Concurrent use with other antihypertensive agents may result in additive effect or potentiation). Products include:
Adalat CC Tablets 2978

Nisoldipine (Concurrent use with other antihypertensive agents may result in additive effect or potentiation). Products include:
Sular Tablets 1163

Nitroglycerin (Concurrent use with other antihypertensive agents may result in additive effect or potentiation). Products include:
Nitro-Dur Transdermal Infusion System.. 3060
Nitrolingual Pumpspray 1161

Norepinephrine Hydrochloride (Decreased arterial responsiveness to pressor amine).
No products indexed under this heading.

Oxaprozin (Reduces diuretic, natriuretic, and antihypertensive effects).
No products indexed under this heading.

Oxycodone Hydrochloride (Potentiation of orthostatic hypotension may occur). Products include:
Combunox Tablets 1183
OxyContin Tablets 2699
OxyFast Oral Concentrate Solution 2704
OxyIR Capsules 2704
Percocet Tablets 1114
Percodan Tablets 1115

Pancuronium Bromide (Possible increased responsiveness to the muscle relaxants).
No products indexed under this heading.

Penbutolol Sulfate (Concurrent use with other antihypertensive agents may result in additive effect or potentiation).
No products indexed under this heading.

Pentobarbital Sodium (Potentiation of orthostatic hypotension may occur). Products include:
Nembutal Sodium Solution, USP 2484

Perindopril Erbumine (Concurrent use with other antihypertensive agents may result in additive effect or potentiation). Products include:
Aceon Tablets (2 mg, 4 mg, 8 mg) 3191

Phenobarbital (Potentiation of orthostatic hypotension may occur).
No products indexed under this heading.

Phenoxybenzamine Hydrochloride (Concurrent use with other antihypertensive agents may result in additive effect or potentiation). Products include:
Dibenzyline Capsules 3390

Phentolamine Mesylate (Concurrent use with other antihypertensive agents may result in additive effect or potentiation).
No products indexed under this heading.

Phenylbutazone (Reduces diuretic, natriuretic, and antihypertensive effects).
No products indexed under this heading.

Pindolol (Concurrent use with other antihypertensive agents may result in additive effect or potentiation).
No products indexed under this heading.

Pioglitazone Hydrochloride (Thiazide-induced hyperglycemia may require dosage adjustment of hypoglycemic agents). Products include:
ActoPlus Met Tablets 3219
Actos Tablets 3224

Piroxicam (Reduces diuretic, natriuretic, and antihypertensive effects).
No products indexed under this heading.

Polythiazide (Concurrent use with other antihypertensive agents may result in additive effect or potentiation).
No products indexed under this heading.

Prazosin Hydrochloride (Concurrent use with other antihypertensive agents may result in additive effect or potentiation).
No products indexed under this heading.

Prednisolone Acetate (Intensified electrolyte depletion particularly hypokalemia). Products include:
Blephamide Ophthalmic Ointment 563
Blephamide Ophthalmic Suspension................................. 564
Poly-Pred Liquifilm Ophthalmic Suspension .... ⊙231
Pred Forte Ophthalmic Suspension .... ⊙233
Pred Mild Sterile Ophthalmic Suspension .... ⊙236
Pred-G Ophthalmic Suspension ...... ⊙234
Pred-G Sterile Ophthalmic Ointment.................................. ⊙235

Prednisolone Sodium Phosphate (Intensified electrolyte depletion particularly hypokalemia). Products include:
Pediapred Oral Solution 3319

Prednisolone Tebutate (Intensified electrolyte depletion particularly hypokalemia).
No products indexed under this heading.

Prednisone (Intensified electrolyte depletion particularly hypokalemia).
No products indexed under this heading.

Propoxyphene Hydrochloride (Potentiation of orthostatic hypotension may occur).
No products indexed under this heading.

Propoxyphene Napsylate (Potentiation of orthostatic hypotension may occur). Products include:
Darvocet A 500 Tablets 3497

Propranolol Hydrochloride (Concurrent use with other antihypertensive agents may result in additive effect or potentiation). Products include:
Inderal LA Long-Acting Capsules 3421
InnoPran XL Capsules 2728

Quinapril Hydrochloride (Concurrent use with other antihypertensive agents may result in additive effect or potentiation).
No products indexed under this heading.

Ramipril (Concurrent use with other antihypertensive agents may result in additive effect or potentiation). Products include:
Altace Capsules 1673

Rapacuronium Bromide (Possible increased responsiveness to the muscle relaxants).
No products indexed under this heading.

Rauwolfia Serpentina (Concurrent use with other antihypertensive agents may result in additive effect or potentiation).
No products indexed under this heading.

Remifentanil Hydrochloride (Potentiation of orthostatic hypotension may occur).
No products indexed under this heading.

Repaglinide (Thiazide-induced hyperglycemia may require dosage adjustment of hypoglycemic agents). Products include:
Prandin Tablets (0.5, 1, and 2 mg).. 2337

Rescinnamine (Concurrent use with other antihypertensive agents may result in additive effect or potentiation).
No products indexed under this heading.

Reserpine (Concurrent use with other antihypertensive agents may result in additive effect or potentiation).
No products indexed under this heading.

Rocuronium Bromide (Possible increased responsiveness to the muscle relaxants). Products include:
Zemuron Injection 2363

Rofecoxib (Reduces diuretic, natriuretic, and antihypertensive effects).
No products indexed under this heading.

Rosiglitazone Maleate (Thiazide-induced hyperglycemia may require dosage adjustment of hypoglycemic agents). Products include:
Avandamet Tablets 1343
Avandia Tablets 1348

Secobarbital Sodium (Potentiation of orthostatic hypotension may occur).
No products indexed under this heading.

Sodium Nitroprusside (Concurrent use with other antihypertensive agents may result in additive effect or potentiation).
No products indexed under this heading.

Sotalol Hydrochloride (Concurrent use with other antihypertensive agents may result in additive effect or potentiation).
No products indexed under this heading.

Spirapril Hydrochloride (Concurrent use with other antihypertensive agents may result in additive effect or potentiation).
No products indexed under this heading.

Sufentanil Citrate (Potentiation of orthostatic hypotension may occur).
No products indexed under this heading.

Sulindac (Reduces diuretic, natriuretic, and antihypertensive effects). Products include:
Clinoril Tablets 1899

Telmisartan (Concurrent use with other antihypertensive agents may result in additive effect or potentiation). Products include:
Micardis Tablets 884
Micardis HCT Tablets 886

Terazosin Hydrochloride (Concurrent use with other antihypertensive agents may result in additive effect or potentiation). Products include:
Hytrin Capsules 469

Thiamylal Sodium (Potentiation of orthostatic hypotension may occur).
No products indexed under this heading.

Timolol Maleate (Concurrent use with other antihypertensive agents may result in additive effect or potentiation). Products include:
Blocadren Tablets 1891
Cosopt Sterile Ophthalmic Solution.. 1910
Timolide Tablets 2056
Timoptic in Ocudose 2061
Timoptic Sterile Ophthalmic Solution.. 2058
Timoptic-XE Sterile Ophthalmic Gel Forming Solution.................... 2062

Tolazamide (Thiazide-induced hyperglycemia may require dosage adjustment of hypoglycemic agents).
No products indexed under this heading.

Tolbutamide (Thiazide-induced hyperglycemia may require dosage adjustment of hypoglycemic agents).
No products indexed under this heading.

Tolmetin Sodium (Reduces diuretic, natriuretic, and antihypertensive effects).
No products indexed under this heading.

Torsemide (Concurrent use with other antihypertensive agents may result in additive effect or potentiation).
No products indexed under this heading.

IMPORTANT NOTE: Always consult each drug listing in the patient's regimen for possible interactions.

Trandolapril (Concurrent use with other antihypertensive agents may result in additive effect or potentiation). Products include:
- Mavik Tablets ... 482
- Tarka Tablets ... 519

Triamcinolone (Intensified electrolyte depletion particularly hypokalemia).
- No products indexed under this heading.

Triamcinolone Acetonide (Intensified electrolyte depletion particularly hypokalemia). Products include:
- Azmacort Inhalation Aerosol ... 1701
- Nasacort HFA Inhalation Aerosol ... 2939
- Nasacort AQ Nasal Spray ... 2937

Triamcinolone Diacetate (Intensified electrolyte depletion particularly hypokalemia).
- No products indexed under this heading.

Triamcinolone Hexacetonide (Intensified electrolyte depletion particularly hypokalemia).
- No products indexed under this heading.

Trimethaphan Camsylate (Concurrent use with other antihypertensive agents may result in additive effect or potentiation).
- No products indexed under this heading.

Troglitazone (Thiazide-induced hyperglycemia may require dosage adjustment of hypoglycemic agents).
- No products indexed under this heading.

Tubocurarine Chloride (Possible increased responsiveness to the muscle relaxants).
- No products indexed under this heading.

Valdecoxib (Reduces diuretic, natriuretic, and antihypertensive effects).
- No products indexed under this heading.

Valsartan (Concurrent use with other antihypertensive agents may result in additive effect or potentiation). Products include:
- Diovan HCT Tablets ... 2195
- Diovan Tablets ... 2191

Vecuronium Bromide (Possible increased responsiveness to the muscle relaxants).
- No products indexed under this heading.

Verapamil Hydrochloride (Concurrent use with other antihypertensive agents may result in additive effect or potentiation). Products include:
- Covera-HS Tablets ... 3135
- Tarka Tablets ... 519
- Verelan PM Capsules ... 3120

Food Interactions

Alcohol (Potentiation of orthostatic hypotension may occur).

DOLOBID TABLETS

(Diflunisal) ... 1937

May interact with antacids, aspirin-acetylsalicylic acid, oral anticoagulants, lithium preparations, non-steroidal anti-inflammatory agents, thiazides, and certain other agents. Compounds in these categories include:

Acetaminophen (Concomitant administraton of diflunisal and acetaminophen has resulted in an approximate 50% increase in plasma levels of acetaminophen. Acetaminophen had no effect on plasma levels of diflunisal. Since acetaminophen in high doses has been associated with hepatotoxicity, concomitant administration of diflunisal and acetaminophen should be used cautiously, with careful monitoring of patients). Products include:
- Benadryl Allergy & Cold Tablets ... ◙692
- Benadryl Allergy & Sinus Headache Caplets & Gelcaps ... ◙693
- Benadryl Maximum Strength Severe Allergy & Sinus Headache Caplets ... ◙694
- Contac Severe Cold and Flu Caplets Maximum Strength ... ◙615
- Contac Severe Cold and Flu Caplets Non-Drowsy ... ◙615
- Darvocet A 500 Tablets ... 3497
- Goody's Body Pain Formula Powder ... ◙621
- Goody's Extra Strength Headache Powder ... ◙621
- Goody's Extra Strength Pain Relief Tablets ... ◙621
- Goody's PM Powder ... ◙622
- Hycomine Compound Tablets ... 1105
- Lortab ... 3315
- Lortab Elixir ... 3312
- Percocet Tablets ... 1114
- Robitussin Cough, Cold & Flu Liquid-filled Capsules ... ◙750
- Robitussin Flu Liquid ... ◙752
- Sedapap Tablets 50 mg/650 mg ... 2098
- Singlet Caplets ... ◙636
- Sudafed Severe Cold ... ◙710
- Sudafed Sinus Headache ... ◙711
- TheraFlu Cold & Cough Hot Liquid ... ◙680
- TheraFlu Cold & Sore Throat Hot Liquid ... ◙680
- TheraFlu Flu & Chest Congestion Non-Drowsy Hot Liquid ... ◙681
- TheraFlu Flu & Sore Throat Hot Liquid ... ◙681
- TheraFlu Severe Cold Non-Drowsy Hot Liquid ... ◙683
- TheraFlu Severe Cold & Cough Hot Liquid ... ◙683
- TheraFlu Severe Cold Caplets ... ◙679
- TheraFlu Severe Cold Hot Liquid ... ◙682
- TheraFlu Severe Cold Non-Drowsy Caplets ... ◙679
- Triaminic Cough & Sore Throat Liquid ... ◙687
- Triaminic Flu, Cough & Fever Liquid ... ◙685
- Triaminic Cough & Sore Throat Softchews ... ◙689
- Tylenol 8 Hour Extended Release Geltabs and Caplets ... 1843
- Tylenol Sinus NightTime Caplets ... ◙663
- Children's Tylenol Suspension Liquid and Meltaways ... 1850
- Children's Tylenol Plus Cold & Allergy Suspension Liquid ... 1850
- Children's Tylenol Plus Cold NightTime Suspension Liquid ... 1851
- Children's Tylenol Plus Cold & Cough Suspension Liquid and Chewable Tablets ... 1851
- Children's Tylenol Plus Cold Chewable Tablets ... 1851
- Children's Tylenol Plus Cold Daytime Non-Drowsy Suspension Liquid ... 1851
- Children's Tylenol Plus Flu Suspension Liquid ... 1853
- Concentrated Tylenol Infants' Drops Plus Cold ... 1851
- Concentrated Tylenol Infants' Drops Plus Cold and Cough ... 1851
- Concentrated Tylenol Infants' Drops ... 1850
- Junior Tylenol Meltaways ... 1850
- Tylenol Cold & Flu Severe Daytime Liquid with Cool Bust ... 1846
- Tylenol Cold & Flu Severe NightTime Liquid with Cool Burst ... 1846
- Tylenol Cold Severe Congestion Non-Drowsy Caplets with Cool Burst ... 1846
- Tylenol Cough & Sore Throat Daytime Liquid with Cool Burst ... 1849
- Tylenol Cough & Sore Throat NightTime Liquid with Cool Burst ... 1849
- Tylenol ... 1843
- Extra Strength Tylenol Rapid Release Gels ... 1843
- Tylenol ... 1843
- Tylenol Allergy Complete Night Time Caplets ... 1844
- Tylenol Allergy Complete Multi-Symptom Caplets and Gelcaps with Cool Burst ... 1844
- Tylenol Severe Allergy Caplets ... 1844
- Tylenol Flu NightTime Gelcaps ... 1846
- Tylenol Flu Day Non-Drowsy Gelcaps ... 1846
- Concentrated Tylenol Infants' Drops Plus Cold Nasal Congestant, Fever Reducer & Pain Reliever ... ◙668
- Concentrated Tylenol Infants' Drops Plus Cold & Cough Nasal Decongestant, Fever Reducer & Pain Reliever ... ◙668
- Multi-Symptom Tylenol Cold Night Time Caplets ... 1845
- Multi-Symptom Tylenol Cold Day Non-Drowsy Caplets and Gelcaps ... 1845
- Extra Strength Tylenol PM Caplets, Geltabs, Gelcaps and Liquid ... 1847
- Tylenol Sinus Day Non-Drowsy ... 1848
- Tylenol Sinus Night Time Caplets ... 1848
- Tylenol Sinus Severe Congestion Caplets with Cool Burst ... 1848
- Tylenol Sore Throat Daytime Liquid with Cool Burst ... 1849
- Tylenol Sore Throat NightTime Liquid with Cool Burst ... 1849
- Tylenol with Codeine ... 2461
- Women's Tylenol Menstrual Relief Caplets ... 1849
- Ultracet Tablets ... 2462
- Vicks 44M Cough, Cold & Flu Relief ... 2676
- Vicks DayQuil LiquiCaps/Liquid Multi-Symptom Cold/Flu Relief ... ◙723
- Vicks DayQuil Multi-Symptom Cold/Flu Relief LiquiCaps ... 2675
- Vicks DayQuil Multi-Symptom Cold/Flu Relief Liquid ... 2675
- Vicks NyQuil LiquiCaps ... 2677
- Vicks NyQuil LiquiCaps/Liquid Multi-Symptom Cold/Flu Relief ... ◙725
- Vicks NyQuil Liquid ... 2677
- Vicodin Tablets ... 530
- Vicodin ES Tablets ... 531
- Vicodin HP Tablets ... 532
- Zydone Tablets ... 1118

Aluminum Carbonate (Concomitant administration of antacids may reduce plasma levels of diflunisal. This effect is small with occasional doses of antacids, but may be clinically significant when antacids are used on a continuous schedule).
- No products indexed under this heading.

Aluminum Hydroxide (Concomitant administration of antacids may reduce plasma levels of diflunisal. This effect is small with occasional doses of antacids, but may be clinically significant when antacids are used on a continuous schedule). Products include:
- Gaviscon Regular Strength Liquid ... ◙620
- Gaviscon Regular Strength Tablets ... ◙619
- Gaviscon Extra Strength Liquid ... ◙620
- Gaviscon Extra Strength Tablets ... ◙619
- Maalox Max Maximum Strength Antacid/Anti-Gas Liquid ... 2165
- Maalox Regular Strength Antacid/Antigas Liquid ... 2164

Anisindione (In normal volunteers, the concomitant administration of diflunisal and warfarin, acenocoumarol or phenprocoumon resulted in prolongation of prothrombin time. This may occur because diflunisal competitively displaces coumarins from protein binding sites. Accordingly, when diflunisal is administered with oral anticoagulants, the prothrombin time should be closely monitored during, and for several days after, concomitant drug administration. Adjustment of dosage of oral anticoagulants may be required. The effects of warfarin and NSAIDs on GI bleeding are synergistic, such that users of both drugs together have a risk of serious GI bleeding higher than users of either drug alone). Products include:
- Miradon Tablets ... 3056

Aspirin (When diflunisal is administered with aspirin, its protein binding is reduced, although the clearance of free diflunisal is not altered. The clinical significance of this interaction is not known, however, as with other NSAIDs, concomitant administrationof diflunisal and aspirin is not generally recommended because of the potential of increased adverse effects). Products include:
- Aggrenox Capsules ... 855
- Bayer, Aspirin Regimen ... ◙606
- Bayer Aspirin Tablets ... 3515
- BC Powder ... ◙612
- BC Allergy Sinus Cold Powder ... ◙612
- Arthritis Strength BC Powder ... ◙612
- BC Sinus Cold Powder ... ◙612
- Ecotrin Enteric Coated Aspirin Low, Regular and Maximum Strength Tablets ... 1627
- Goody's Body Pain Formula Powder ... ◙621
- Goody's Extra Strength Headache Powder ... ◙621
- Goody's Extra Strength Pain Relief Tablets ... ◙621
- Percodan Tablets ... 1115
- St. Joseph 81 mg Aspirin Chewable and Enteric Coated Tablets ... 1841

Aspirin, Enteric Coated (When diflunisal is administered with aspirin, its protein binding is reduced, although the clearance of free diflunisal is not altered. The clinical significance of this interaction is not known, however, as with other NSAIDs, concomitant administrationof diflunisal and aspirin is not generally recommended because of the potential of increased adverse effects).
- No products indexed under this heading.

Aspirin Buffered (When diflunisal is administered with aspirin, its protein binding is reduced, although the clearance of free diflunisal is not altered. The clinical significance of this interaction is not known, however, as with other NSAIDs, concomitant administrationof diflunisal and aspirin is not generally recommended because of the potential of increased adverse effects).
- No products indexed under this heading.

Bendroflumethiazide (Clinical studies, as well as post-marketing observations, have shown that diflunisal can reduce the natriuretic effect of thiazides in some patients. This response has been attributed to inhibition of renal prostaglandin synthesis. In normal volunteers, concomitant administration of diflunisal and hydrochlorothiazide (HCTZ) resulted in significantly increased plasma levels of HCTZ. Diflunisal also decreased the hyperuricemic effect of HCTZ. During concomitant therapy with NSAIDs, the patients shouldbe observed closely for signs of renal failure, as well as to assure diuretic efficacy).
- No products indexed under this heading.

Celecoxib (The concomitant use of diflunisal and other NSAIDs is not

recommended due to the increased possibility of gastrointestinal toxicity, with little or no increase in efficacy). Products include:

Celebrex Capsules 3130

Chlorothiazide (Clinical studies, as well as post-marketing observations, have shown that diflunisal can reduce the natriuretic effect of thiazides in some patients. This response has been attributed to inhibition of renal prostaglandin synthesis. In normal volunteers, concomitant administration of diflunisal and hydrochlorothiazide (HCTZ) resulted in significantly increased plasma levels of HCTZ. Diflunisal also decreased the hyperiuricemic effect of HCTZ. During concomitant therapy with NSAIDs, the patients shouldbe observed closely for signs of renal failure, as well as to assure diuretic efficacy). Products include:

Aldoclor Tablets 1881
Diuril Oral 1936

Chlorothiazide Sodium (Clinical studies, as well as post-marketing observations, have shown that diflunisal can reduce the natriuretic effect of thiazides in some patients. This response has been attributed to inhibition of renal prostaglandin synthesis. In normal volunteers, concomitant administration of diflunisal and hydrochlorothiazide (HCTZ) resulted in significantly increased plasma levels of HCTZ. Diflunisal also decreased the hyperiuricemic effect of HCTZ. During concomitant therapy with NSAIDs, the patients shouldbe observed closely for signs of renal failure, as well as to assure diuretic efficacy). Products include:

Diuril Sodium Intravenous 1934

Cyclosporine (Administration of non-steroidal anti-inflamatory drugs concomitantly with cyclosporine has been associated with an increase in cyclosporine-induced toxicity, possibly due to decreased synthesis of renal prostacyclin. NSAIDs should be used with caution in patients taking cyclosporine, and renal function should be carefully monitored). Products include:

Gengraf Capsules 458
Neoral Soft Gelatin Capsules 2247
Neoral Oral Solution 2247
Restasis Ophthalmic Emulsion 570
Sandimmune 2259

Diclofenac Potassium (The concomitant use of diflunisal and other NSAIDs is not recommended due to the increased possibility of gastrointestinal toxicity, with little or no increase in efficacy). Products include:

Cataflam Tablets 2173

Diclofenac Sodium (The concomitant use of diflunisal and other NSAIDs is not recommended due to the increased possibility of gastrointestinal toxicity, with little or no increase in efficacy). Products include:

Arthrotec Tablets 3126
Voltaren Ophthalmic Solution 2300
Voltaren Tablets 2298
Voltaren-XR Tablets 2301

Dicumarol (In normal volunteers, the concomitant administration of diflunisal and warfarin, acenocoumarol or phenprocoumon resulted in prolongation of prothrombin time. This may occur because diflunisal competitively displaces coumarins from protein binding sites. Accordingly, when diflunisal is administered with oral anticoagulants, the prothrombin time should be closely monitored during, and for several days after, concomitant drug administration. Adjustment of dosage of oral anticoagulants may be required. The effects of warfarin and NSAIDs on GI bleeding are synergistic, such that users of both drugs together have a risk of serious GI bleeding higher than users of either drug alone).

No products indexed under this heading.

Etodolac (The concomitant use of diflunisal and other NSAIDs is not recommended due to the increased possibility of gastrointestinal toxicity, with little or no increase in efficacy).

No products indexed under this heading.

Fenoprofen Calcium (The concomitant use of diflunisal and other NSAIDs is not recommended due to the increased possibility of gastrointestinal toxicity, with little or no increase in efficacy). Products include:

Nalfon Capsules 2504

Flurbiprofen (The concomitant use of diflunisal and other NSAIDs is not recommended due to the increased possibility of gastrointestinal toxicity, with little or no increase in efficacy).

No products indexed under this heading.

Furosemide (Decreased hyperuricemic effect). Products include:

Furosemide Tablets 2117

Hydrochlorothiazide (Decreased hyperuricemic effect; increased plasma levels). Products include:

Aldoril Tablets 1884
Atacand HCT 637
Avalide Tablets 2889
Avalide Tablets 922
Benicar HCT Tablets 2852
Diovan HCT Tablets 2195
Dyazide Capsules 1389
Hyzaar 1964
Lotensin HCT Tablets 2235
Maxzide 2150
Micardis HCT Tablets 886
Moduretic Tablets 2003
Prinzide Tablets 2033
Teveten HCT Tablets 1710
Timolide Tablets 2056
Uniretic Tablets 3114
Vaseretic Tablets 2073
Zestoretic Tablets 701

Hydroflumethiazide (Clinical studies, as well as post-marketing observations, have shown that diflunisal can reduce the natriuretic effect of thiazides in some patients. This response has been attributed to inhibition of renal prostaglandin synthesis. In normal volunteers, concomitant administration of diflunisal and hydrochlorothiazide (HCTZ) resulted in significantly increased plasma levels of HCTZ. Diflunisal also decreased the hyperiuricemic effect of HCTZ. During concomitant therapy with NSAIDs, the patients shouldbe observed closely for signs of renal failure, as well as to assure diuretic efficacy).

No products indexed under this heading.

Ibuprofen (The concomitant use of diflunisal and other NSAIDs is not recommended due to the increased possibility of gastrointestinal toxicity, with little or no increase in efficacy). Products include:

Advil Allergy Sinus Caplets 737
Advil 737
Children's Advil Suspension 742
Children's Advil Chewable Tablets 741
Advil Cold & Sinus 739
Advil Flu & Body Ache Caplets 739
Children's Advil Cold Suspension 741
Infants' Advil Concentrated Drops 743
Junior Strength Advil Swallow Tablets 740
Advil Migraine Liquigels 740
Advil Multi-Symptom Cold Caplets 738
Combunox Tablets 1183
Children's Motrin Oral Suspension and Chewable Tablets 1837
Children's Motrin Cold Non-Staining Dye-Free Oral Suspension 1838
Children's Motrin Cold Oral Suspension 1838
Children's Motrin Non-Staining Dye-Free Oral Suspension 1837
Motrin Cold & Sinus Caplets 1836
Motrin IB Tablets and Caplets 1836
Infants' Motrin Concentrated Drops 1837
Infants' Motrin Non-Staining Dye-Free Drops 1837
Junior Strength Motrin Caplets and Chewable Tablets 1837
Vicoprofen Tablets 533

Indomethacin (The administration of diflunisal to normal volunteers receiving indomethacin decreased the renal clearance and significantly increased the plasma levels of indomethacin. In some patients the combined use of indomethacin and diflunisal has been associated with fatal gastrointestinal hemorrhage. Therefore, indomethacin and diflunisal should not be used concomitantly). Products include:

Indocin 1968

Indomethacin Sodium Trihydrate (The administration of diflunisal to normal volunteers receiving indomethacin decreased the renal clearance and significantly increased the plasma levels of indomethacin. In some patients the combined use of indomethacin and diflunisal has been associated with fatal gastrointestinal hemorrhage. Therefore, indomethacin and diflunisal should not be used concomitantly). Products include:

Indocin I.V. 1973

Ketoprofen (The concomitant use of diflunisal and other NSAIDs is not recommended due to the increased possibility of gastrointestinal toxicity, with little or no increase in efficacy).

No products indexed under this heading.

Ketorolac Tromethamine (The concomitant use of diflunisal and other NSAIDs is not recommended due to the increased possibility of gastrointestinal toxicity, with little or no increase in efficacy). Products include:

Acular Ophthalmic Solution 561
Acular LS Ophthalmic Solution 562

Lithium (NSAIDs have produced an elevation of plasma lithium levels and a reduction in renal lithium clearance. The mean minimum lithium concentration increased 15% and the renal clearance was decreased by approximately 20%. These effects have been attributed to the inhibition of renal prostaglandin synthesis by the NSAID. Thus, when NSAIDs and lithium are administered concurrently, subjects should be observed carefully for signs of lithium toxicity).

No products indexed under this heading.

Lithium Carbonate (NSAIDs have produced an elevation of plasma lithium levels and a reduction in renal lithium clearance. The mean minimum lithium concentration increased 15% and the renal clearance was decreased by approximately 20%. These effects have been attributed to the inhibition of renal prostaglandin synthesis by the NSAID. Thus, when NSAIDs and lithium are administered concurrently, subjects should be observed carefully for signs of lithium toxicity). Products include:

Eskalith 1406
Lithobid Tablets 1670

Lithium Citrate (NSAIDs have produced an elevation of plasma lithium levels and a reduction in renal lithium clearance. The mean minimum lithium concentration increased 15% and the renal clearance was decreased by approximately 20%. These effects have been attributed to the inhibition of renal prostaglandin synthesis by the NSAID. Thus, when NSAIDs and lithium are administered concurrently, subjects should be observed carefully for signs of lithium toxicity).

No products indexed under this heading.

Magaldrate (Concomitant administration of antacids may reduce plasma levels of diflunisal. This effect is small with occasional doses of antacids, but may be clinically significant when antacids are used on a continuous schedule).

No products indexed under this heading.

Magnesium Hydroxide (Concomitant administration of antacids may reduce plasma levels of diflunisal. This effect is small with occasional doses of antacids, but may be clinically significant when antacids are used on a continuous schedule). Products include:

Maalox Max Maximum Strength Antacid/Anti-Gas Liquid 2165
Maalox Regular Strength Antacid/Antigas Liquid 2164
Pepcid Complete Chewable Tablets 1672
Rolaids Tablets 707
Extra Strength Rolaids Tablets 707
Rolaids Multi-Symptom Antacid & Antigas Tablets 708

Magnesium Oxide (Concomitant administration of antacids may reduce plasma levels of diflunisal. This effect is small with occasional doses of antacids, but may be clinically significant when antacids are used on a continuous schedule). Products include:

Beelith Tablets 784
PremCal Light, Regular, and Extra Strength Tablets 762

Meclofenamate Sodium (The concomitant use of diflunisal and other NSAIDs is not recommended due to the increased possibility of gastrointestinal toxicity, with little or no increase in efficacy).

No products indexed under this heading.

Mefenamic Acid (The concomitant use of diflunisal and other NSAIDs is not recommended due to the increased possibility of gastrointestinal toxicity, with little or no increase in efficacy).

No products indexed under this heading.

Meloxicam (The concomitant use of diflunisal and other NSAIDs is not recommended due to the increased

possibility of gastrointestinal toxicity, with little or no increase in efficacy). Products include:

Mobic Oral Suspension 893
Mobic Tablets 893

Methotrexate Sodium (NSAIDs have been reported to competitively inhibit methotrexate accumulation in rabbit kidney slices. This may indicate that they could enhance the toxicity of methotrexate. Caution should be used when NSAIDs are administered concomitantly with methotrexate).
No products indexed under this heading.

Methyclothiazide (Clinical studies, as well as post-marketing observations, have shown that diflunisal can reduce the natriuretic effect of thiazides in some patients. This response has been attributed to inhibition of renal prostaglandin synthesis. In normal volunteers, concomitant administration of diflunisal and hydrochlorothiazide (HCTZ) resulted in significantly increased plasma levels of HCTZ. Diflunisal also decreased the hyperiuricemic effect of HCTZ. During concomitant therapy with NSAIDs, the patients shouldbe observed closely for signs of renal failure, as well as to assure diuretic efficacy).
No products indexed under this heading.

Nabumetone (The concomitant use of diflunisal and other NSAIDs is not recommended due to the increased possibility of gastrointestinal toxicity, with little or no increase in efficacy). Products include:

Relafen Tablets 1523

Naproxen (The concomitant administration of diflunisal and naproxen in normal volunteers had no effect on plasma levels of naproxen, but significantly decreased the urinary excretion of naproxen and its glucuronide metabolite. Naproxen had no effect on plasma levels of diflunisal). Products include:

EC-Naprosyn Delayed-Release Tablets 2769
Naprosyn Suspension 2769
Naprosyn Tablets 2769
Prevacid NapraPAC 3277

Naproxen Sodium (The concomitant administration of diflunisal and naproxen in normal volunteers had no effect on plasma levels of naproxen, but significantly decreased the urinary excretion of naproxen and its glucuronide metabolite. Naproxen had no effect on plasma levels of diflunisal). Products include:

Aleve Tablets, Caplets and Gelcaps .... ▣ 605
Anaprox Tablets 2769
Anaprox DS Tablets 2769

Nephrotoxic Drugs (Overt renal decompensation).
No products indexed under this heading.

Oxaprozin (The concomitant use of diflunisal and other NSAIDs is not recommended due to the increased possibility of gastrointestinal toxicity, with little or no increase in efficacy).
No products indexed under this heading.

Phenprocoumon (Prolonged prothrombin time).
No products indexed under this heading.

Phenylbutazone (The concomitant use of diflunisal and other NSAIDs is not recommended due to the increased possibility of gastrointestinal toxicity, with little or no increase in efficacy).
No products indexed under this heading.

Piroxicam (The concomitant use of diflunisal and other NSAIDs is not recommended due to the increased possibility of gastrointestinal toxicity, with little or no increase in efficacy).
No products indexed under this heading.

Polythiazide (Clinical studies, as well as post-marketing observations, have shown that diflunisal can reduce the natriuretic effect of thiazides in some patients. This response has been attributed to inhibition of renal prostaglandin synthesis. In normal volunteers, concomitant administration of diflunisal and hydrochlorothiazide (HCTZ) resulted in significantly increased plasma levels of HCTZ. Diflunisal also decreased the hyperiuricemic effect of HCTZ. During concomitant therapy with NSAIDs, the patients shouldbe observed closely for signs of renal failure, as well as to assure diuretic efficacy).
No products indexed under this heading.

Rofecoxib (The concomitant use of diflunisal and other NSAIDs is not recommended due to the increased possibility of gastrointestinal toxicity, with little or no increase in efficacy).
No products indexed under this heading.

Sodium Bicarbonate (Concomitant administration of antacids may reduce plasma levels of diflunisal. This effect is small with occasional doses of antacids, but may be clinically significant when antacids are used on a continuous schedule). Products include:

Ceo-Two Evacuant Suppository ...... ▣ 607
Colyte with Flavor Packs for Oral Solution 3102
HalfLytely and Bisacodyl Tablets Bowel Prep Kit with Flavors Packs 915
TriLyte with Flavor Packs for Oral Solution 3114

Sulindac (The concomitant administration of diflunisal and sulindac in normal volunteers resulted in lowering of the plasma levels of the active sulindac sulfide metabolite by approximately one-third). Products include:

Clinoril Tablets 1899

Tolmetin Sodium (The concomitant use of diflunisal and other NSAIDs is not recommended due to the increased possibility of gastrointestinal toxicity, with little or no increase in efficacy).
No products indexed under this heading.

Valdecoxib (The concomitant use of diflunisal and other NSAIDs is not recommended due to the increased possibility of gastrointestinal toxicity, with little or no increase in efficacy).
No products indexed under this heading.

Warfarin Sodium (In normal volunteers, the concomitant administration of diflunisal and warfarin, acenocoumarol or phenprocoumon resulted in prolongation of prothrombin time. This may occur because diflunisal competitively displaces coumarins from protein binding sites. Accordingly, when diflunisal is administered with oral anticoagulants, the prothrombin time should be closely monitored during, and for several days after, concomitant drug administration. Adjustment of dosage of oral anticoagulants may be required. The effects of warfarin and NSAIDs on GI bleeding are synergistic, such that users of both drugs together have a risk of serious GI bleeding higher than users of either drug alone). Products include:

Coumadin for Injection 932
Coumadin Tablets 932

DOSTINEX TABLETS

(Cabergoline) 2631
May interact with dopamine D2 antagonists. Compounds in these categories include:

Chlorpromazine (Cabergoline is a dopamine receptor antagonist with a high affinity for D2 receptors; concurrent use with dopamine D2-antagonists is not recommended).
No products indexed under this heading.

Chlorpromazine Hydrochloride (Cabergoline is a dopamine receptor antagonist with a high affinity for D2 receptors; concurrent use with dopamine D2-antagonists is not recommended).
No products indexed under this heading.

Chlorprothixene (Cabergoline is a dopamine receptor antagonist with a high affinity for D2 receptors; concurrent use with dopamine D2-antagonists is not recommended).
No products indexed under this heading.

Chlorprothixene Hydrochloride (Cabergoline is a dopamine receptor antagonist with a high affinity for D2 receptors; concurrent use with dopamine D2-antagonists is not recommended).
No products indexed under this heading.

Fluphenazine Decanoate (Cabergoline is a dopamine receptor antagonist with a high affinity for D2 receptors; concurrent use with dopamine D2-antagonists is not recommended).
No products indexed under this heading.

Fluphenazine Enanthate (Cabergoline is a dopamine receptor antagonist with a high affinity for D2 receptors; concurrent use with dopamine D2-antagonists is not recommended).
No products indexed under this heading.

Fluphenazine Hydrochloride (Cabergoline is a dopamine receptor antagonist with a high affinity for D2 receptors; concurrent use with dopamine D2-antagonists is not recommended).
No products indexed under this heading.

Haloperidol (Cabergoline is a dopamine receptor antagonist with a high affinity for D2 receptors; concurrent use with dopamine D2-antagonists is not recommended).
No products indexed under this heading.

Haloperidol Decanoate (Cabergoline is a dopamine receptor antagonist with a high affinity for D2 receptors; concurrent use with dopamine D2-antagonists is not recommended).
No products indexed under this heading.

Loxapine Hydrochloride (Cabergoline is a dopamine receptor antagonist with a high affinity for D2 receptors; concurrent use with dopamine D2-antagonists is not recommended).
No products indexed under this heading.

Loxapine Succinate (Cabergoline is a dopamine receptor antagonist with a high affinity for D2 receptors; concurrent use with dopamine D2-antagonists is not recommended).
No products indexed under this heading.

Mesoridazine Besylate (Cabergoline is a dopamine receptor antagonist with a high affinity for D2 receptors; concurrent use with dopamine D2-antagonists is not recommended).
No products indexed under this heading.

Methotrimeprazine (Cabergoline is a dopamine receptor antagonist with a high affinity for D2 receptors; concurrent use with dopamine D2-antagonists is not recommended).
No products indexed under this heading.

Metoclopramide Hydrochloride (Cabergoline is a dopamine receptor antagonist with a high affinity for D2 receptors; concurrent use with dopamine D2-antagonists is not recommended).
No products indexed under this heading.

Molindone Hydrochloride (Cabergoline is a dopamine receptor antagonist with a high affinity for D2 receptors; concurrent use with dopamine D2-antagonists is not recommended). Products include:

Moban Tablets 1108

Perphenazine (Cabergoline is a dopamine receptor antagonist with a high affinity for D2 receptors; concurrent use with dopamine D2-antagonists is not recommended).
No products indexed under this heading.

Prochlorperazine (Cabergoline is a dopamine receptor antagonist with a high affinity for D2 receptors; concurrent use with dopamine D2-antagonists is not recommended).
No products indexed under this heading.

Promethazine Hydrochloride (Cabergoline is a dopamine receptor antagonist with a high affinity for D2 receptors; concurrent use with dopamine D2-antagonists is not recommended). Products include:

Phenergan 3438

Quetiapine Fumarate (Cabergoline is a dopamine receptor antagonist with a high affinity for D2 receptors; concurrent use with dopamine D2-antagonists is not recommended). Products include:

Seroquel Tablets 691

Risperidone (Cabergoline is a dopamine receptor antagonist with a

high affinity for D2 receptors; concurrent use with dopamine D2-antagonists is not recommended). Products include:
Risperdal Consta Long-Acting Injection 1664
Risperdal M-Tab Orally Disintegrating Tablets 1658
Risperdal 1658

Thioridazine Hydrochloride (Cabergoline is a dopamine receptor antagonist with a high affinity for D2 receptors; concurrent use with dopamine D2-antagonists is not recommended). Products include:
Thioridazine Hydrochloride Tablets 2122

Thiothixene (Cabergoline is a dopamine receptor antagonist with a high affinity for D2 receptors; concurrent use with dopamine D2-antagonists is not recommended). Products include:
Thiothixene Capsules 2124

Trifluoperazine Hydrochloride (Cabergoline is a dopamine receptor antagonist with a high affinity for D2 receptors; concurrent use with dopamine D2-antagonists is not recommended).
No products indexed under this heading.

DOVONEX CREAM 0.005%

(Calcipotriene) 3374
None cited in PDR database.

DOVONEX OINTMENT 0.005%

(Calcipotriene) 3375
None cited in PDR database.

DOVONEX SCALP SOLUTION 0.005%

(Calcipotriene) 3375
None cited in PDR database.

DOXIL INJECTION

(Doxorubicin Hydrochloride Liposome) 3302
May interact with antineoplastics and certain other agents. Compounds in these categories include:

Altretamine (Co-administration with the conventional formulation of doxorubicin results in potentiation of the toxicity of other anticancer therapies; this interaction may occur with Doxil). Products include:
Hexalen Capsules 2101

Anastrozole (Co-administration with the conventional formulation of doxorubicin results in potentiation of the toxicity of other anticancer therapies; this interaction may occur with Doxil). Products include:
Arimidex Tablets 665

Asparaginase (Co-administration with the conventional formulation of doxorubicin results in potentiation of the toxicity of other anticancer therapies; this interaction may occur with Doxil). Products include:
Elspar for Injection 1943

Bicalutamide (Co-administration with the conventional formulation of doxorubicin results in potentiation of the toxicity of other anticancer therapies; this interaction may occur with Doxil). Products include:
Casodex Tablets 670

Bleomycin Sulfate (Co-administration with the conventional formulation of doxorubicin results in potentiation of the toxicity of other anticancer therapies; this interaction may occur with Doxil).
No products indexed under this heading.

Busulfan (Co-administration with the conventional formulation of doxorubicin results in potentiation of the toxicity of other anticancer therapies; this interaction may occur with Doxil). Products include:
I.V. Busulfex 1125
Myleran Tablets 1492

Carboplatin (Co-administration with the conventional formulation of doxorubicin results in potentiation of the toxicity of other anticancer therapies; this interaction may occur with Doxil).
No products indexed under this heading.

Carmustine (BCNU) (Co-administration with the conventional formulation of doxorubicin results in potentiation of the toxicity of other anticancer therapies; this interaction may occur with Doxil).
No products indexed under this heading.

Chlorambucil (Co-administration with the conventional formulation of doxorubicin results in potentiation of the toxicity of other anticancer therapies; this interaction may occur with Doxil). Products include:
Leukeran Tablets 1472

Cisplatin (Co-administration with the conventional formulation of doxorubicin results in potentiation of the toxicity of other anticancer therapies; this interaction may occur with Doxil).
No products indexed under this heading.

Cyclophosphamide (Co-administration of conventional formulation of doxorubicin with cyclophosphamide has resulted in exacerbation of cyclophosphamide-induced hemorrhagic cystitis; cardiac toxicity may occur at lower cumulative doses in patients who are receiving cyclophosphamide).
No products indexed under this heading.

Cyclosporine (Co-administration of conventional formulation of doxorubicin may result in increases in AUC for both doxorubicin and doxorubicinol possibly due to a decrease in clearance of parent drug and a decrease in metabolism of doxorubicin; potential for more profound and prolonged hematologic toxicity is associated with combined use; coma and seizures have also been reported). Products include:
Gengraf Capsules 458
Neoral Soft Gelatin Capsules 2247
Neoral Oral Solution 2247
Restasis Ophthalmic Emulsion 570
Sandimmune 2259

Dacarbazine (Co-administration with the conventional formulation of doxorubicin results in potentiation of the toxicity of other anticancer therapies; this interaction may occur with Doxil).
No products indexed under this heading.

Daunorubicin Citrate (Co-administration with the conventional formulation of doxorubicin results in potentiation of the toxicity of other anticancer therapies; this interaction may occur with Doxil).
No products indexed under this heading.

Daunorubicin Hydrochloride (Co-administration with the conventional formulation of doxorubicin results in potentiation of the toxicity of other anticancer therapies; this interaction may occur with Doxil). Products include:
Cerubidine for Injection 788

Denileukin Diftitox (Co-administration with the conventional formulation of doxorubicin results in potentiation of the toxicity of other anticancer therapies; this interaction may occur with Doxil). Products include:
Ontak Vials 1717

Docetaxel (Co-administration with the conventional formulation of doxorubicin results in potentiation of the toxicity of other anticancer therapies; this interaction may occur with Doxil). Products include:
Taxotere Injection Concentrate 2947

Epirubicin Hydrochloride (Co-administration with the conventional formulation of doxorubicin results in potentiation of the toxicity of other anticancer therapies; this interaction may occur with Doxil). Products include:
Ellence Injection 2632

Estramustine Phosphate Sodium (Co-administration with the conventional formulation of doxorubicin results in potentiation of the toxicity of other anticancer therapies; this interaction may occur with Doxil). Products include:
Emcyt Capsules 3137

Etoposide (Co-administration with the conventional formulation of doxorubicin results in potentiation of the toxicity of other anticancer therapies; this interaction may occur with Doxil).
No products indexed under this heading.

Exemestane (Co-administration with the conventional formulation of doxorubicin results in potentiation of the toxicity of other anticancer therapies; this interaction may occur with Doxil). Products include:
Aromasin Tablets 2600

Floxuridine (Co-administration with the conventional formulation of doxorubicin results in potentiation of the toxicity of other anticancer therapies; this interaction may occur with Doxil).
No products indexed under this heading.

Fluorouracil (Co-administration with the conventional formulation of doxorubicin results in potentiation of the toxicity of other anticancer therapies; this interaction may occur with Doxil). Products include:
Carac Cream, 0.5% 1048
Efudex 3348

Flutamide (Co-administration with the conventional formulation of doxorubicin results in potentiation of the toxicity of other anticancer therapies; this interaction may occur with Doxil). Products include:
Eulexin Capsules 3023

Gemcitabine Hydrochloride (Co-administration with the conventional formulation of doxorubicin results in potentiation of the toxicity of other anticancer therapies; this interaction may occur with Doxil). Products include:
Gemzar for Injection 1743

Hydroxyurea (Co-administration with the conventional formulation of doxorubicin results in potentiation of the toxicity of other anticancer therapies; this interaction may occur with Doxil).
No products indexed under this heading.

Idarubicin Hydrochloride (Co-administration with the conventional formulation of doxorubicin results in potentiation of the toxicity of other anticancer therapies; this interaction may occur with Doxil). Products include:
Idamycin PFS Injection 2645

Ifosfamide (Co-administration with the conventional formulation of doxorubicin results in potentiation of the toxicity of other anticancer therapies; this interaction may occur with Doxil).
No products indexed under this heading.

Interferon alfa-2a, Recombinant (Co-administration with the conventional formulation of doxorubicin results in potentiation of the toxicity of other anticancer therapies; this interaction may occur with Doxil). Products include:
Roferon-A Injection 2805

Interferon alfa-2b, Recombinant (Co-administration with the conventional formulation of doxorubicin results in potentiation of the toxicity of other anticancer therapies; this interaction may occur with Doxil). Products include:
Intron A for Injection 3038
Rebetron Combination Therapy 3078

Irinotecan Hydrochloride (Co-administration with the conventional formulation of doxorubicin results in potentiation of the toxicity of other anticancer therapies; this interaction may occur with Doxil). Products include:
Camptosar Injection 2602

Levamisole Hydrochloride (Co-administration with the conventional formulation of doxorubicin results in potentiation of the toxicity of other anticancer therapies; this interaction may occur with Doxil).
No products indexed under this heading.

Lomustine (CCNU) (Co-administration with the conventional formulation of doxorubicin results in potentiation of the toxicity of other anticancer therapies; this interaction may occur with Doxil).
No products indexed under this heading.

Mechlorethamine Hydrochloride (Co-administration with the conventional formulation of doxorubicin results in potentiation of the toxicity of other anticancer therapies; this interaction may occur with Doxil). Products include:
Mustargen for Injection 2007

Medroxyprogesterone Acetate (Co-administration of intravenous progesterone to patients with advanced malignancies at high doses with conventional formulation of fixed doxorubicin dose via bolus enhances doxorubicin-induced neu-

tropenia and thrombocytopenia; this interaction may occur with Doxil). Products include:

Depo-Provera Contraceptive Injection **2619**
depo-subQ provera 104 Injectable Suspension.................. **2622**
Premphase Tablets **3452**
Prempro Tablets **3452**

Megestrol Acetate (Co-administration with the conventional formulation of doxorubicin results in potentiation of the toxicity of other anticancer therapies; this interaction may occur with Doxil). Products include:

Megace ES Oral Suspension **2492**

Melphalan (Co-administration with the conventional formulation of doxorubicin results in potentiation of the toxicity of other anticancer therapies; this interaction may occur with Doxil). Products include:

Alkeran Tablets **977**

Mercaptopurine (Co-administration of conventional formulation of doxorubicin with 6-mercaptopurine has resulted in enhancement of hepatotoxicity of 6-mercaptopurine). Products include:

Purinethol Tablets **1222**

Methotrexate Sodium (Co-administration with the conventional formulation of doxorubicin results in potentiation of the toxicity of other anticancer therapies; this interaction may occur with Doxil).

No products indexed under this heading.

Mitomycin (Mitomycin-C) (Co-administration with the conventional formulation of doxorubicin results in potentiation of the toxicity of other anticancer therapies; this interaction may occur with Doxil).

No products indexed under this heading.

Mitotane (Co-administration with the conventional formulation of doxorubicin results in potentiation of the toxicity of other anticancer therapies; this interaction may occur with Doxil).

No products indexed under this heading.

Mitoxantrone Hydrochloride (Co-administration with the conventional formulation of doxorubicin results in potentiation of the toxicity of other anticancer therapies; this interaction may occur with Doxil). Products include:

Novantrone for Injection Concentrate **3158**

Paclitaxel (Administration of paclitaxel infused over 24 hours followed by conventional formulation of doxorubicin administered over 48 hours resulted in a significant decrease in doxorubicin clearance with more profound neutropenic and stomatitis episodes than the reverse sequence of administration; this interaction may occur with Doxil).

No products indexed under this heading.

Phenobarbital (Co-administration with the conventional formulation of doxorubicin results in increased elimination of doxorubicin; this interaction may occur with Doxil).

No products indexed under this heading.

Phenytoin (Co-administration with the conventional formulation of doxorubicin results in decreased phenytoin levels; this interaction may occur with Doxil).

No products indexed under this heading.

Phenytoin Sodium (Co-administration with the conventional formulation of doxorubicin results in decreased phenytoin levels; this interaction may occur with Doxil). Products include:

Phenytek Capsules **2153**

Procarbazine Hydrochloride (Co-administration with the conventional formulation of doxorubicin results in potentiation of the toxicity of other anticancer therapies; this interaction may occur with Doxil). Products include:

Matulane Capsules **3188**

Progesterone (Co-administration of intravenous progesterone to patients with advanced malignancies at high doses with conventional formulation of fixed doxorubicin dose via bolus enhances doxorubicin-induced neutropenia and thrombocytopenia; this interaction may occur with Doxil). Products include:

Prochieve 4% Gel **1018**
Prochieve 8% Gel **1018**
Prometrium Capsules (100 mg, 200 mg).. **3205**

Streptozocin (Co-administration with the conventional formulation of doxorubicin results in inhibition of hepatic metabolism; this interaction may occur with Doxil).

No products indexed under this heading.

Tamoxifen Citrate (Co-administration with the conventional formulation of doxorubicin results in potentiation of the toxicity of other anticancer therapies; this interaction may occur with Doxil).

No products indexed under this heading.

Teniposide (Co-administration with the conventional formulation of doxorubicin results in potentiation of the toxicity of other anticancer therapies; this interaction may occur with Doxil).

No products indexed under this heading.

Thioguanine (Co-administration with the conventional formulation of doxorubicin results in potentiation of the toxicity of other anticancer therapies; this interaction may occur with Doxil). Products include:

Tabloid Tablets **1545**

Thiotepa (Co-administration with the conventional formulation of doxorubicin results in potentiation of the toxicity of other anticancer therapies; this interaction may occur with Doxil).

No products indexed under this heading.

Topotecan Hydrochloride (Co-administration with the conventional formulation of doxorubicin results in potentiation of the toxicity of other anticancer therapies; this interaction may occur with Doxil). Products include:

Hycamtin for Injection **1427**

Toremifene Citrate (Co-administration with the conventional formulation of doxorubicin results in potentiation of the toxicity of other anticancer therapies; this interaction may occur with Doxil).

No products indexed under this heading.

Valrubicin (Co-administration with the conventional formulation of doxorubicin results in potentiation of the toxicity of other anticancer therapies; this interaction may occur with Doxil).

No products indexed under this heading.

Verapamil Hydrochloride (Co-administration of conventional formulation of doxorubicin in animal studies has resulted in higher initial peak concentrations of doxorubicin in the heart with a higher incidence and severity of degenerative changes in cardiac tissue resulting in a shorter survival; this interaction may occur with Doxil). Products include:

Covera-HS Tablets **3135**
Tarka Tablets **519**
Verelan PM Capsules **3120**

Vincristine Sulfate (Co-administration with the conventional formulation of doxorubicin results in potentiation of the toxicity of other anticancer therapies; this interaction may occur with Doxil).

No products indexed under this heading.

Vinorelbine Tartrate (Co-administration with the conventional formulation of doxorubicin results in potentiation of the toxicity of other anticancer therapies; this interaction may occur with Doxil). Products include:

Navelbine Injection **1494**

DRYSOL SOLUTION

(Aluminum Chloride) **2506**
None cited in PDR database.

DUAC TOPICAL GEL

(Benzoyl Peroxide, Clindamycin) **3214**
May interact with:

Concomitant Topical Acne Therapy (Possible cumulative irritancy effect may occur, especially with the use of peeling, desquamating, or abrasive agents).

No products indexed under this heading.

DULCOLAX STOOL SOFTENER

(Docusate Sodium) .... ■**608**
None cited in PDR database.

DULCOLAX SUPPOSITORIES

(Bisacodyl) .... ■**608**
None cited in PDR database.

DULCOLAX TABLETS

(Bisacodyl) .... ■**607**
May interact with antacids and certain other agents. Compounds in these categories include:

Aluminum Carbonate (Dulcolax should not be taken within one hour of taking an antacid).

No products indexed under this heading.

Aluminum Hydroxide (Dulcolax should not be taken within one hour of taking an antacid). Products include:

Gaviscon Regular Strength Liquid .. ■**620**
Gaviscon Regular Strength Tablets.. ■**619**
Gaviscon Extra Strength Liquid ...... ■**620**
Gaviscon Extra Strength Tablets .... ■**619**
Maalox Max Maximum Strength Antacid/Anti-Gas Liquid................ **2165**
Maalox Regular Strength Antacid/Antigas Liquid................. **2164**

Magaldrate (Dulcolax should not be taken within one hour of taking an antacid).

No products indexed under this heading.

Magnesium Hydroxide (Dulcolax should not be taken within one hour of taking an antacid). Products include:

Maalox Max Maximum Strength Antacid/Anti-Gas Liquid................ **2165**
Maalox Regular Strength Antacid/Antigas Liquid................. **2164**
Pepcid Complete Chewable Tablets... **1672**
Rolaids Tablets .... ■**707**
Extra Strength Rolaids Tablets .... ■**707**
Rolaids Multi-Symptom Antacid & Antigas Tablets .... ■**708**

Magnesium Oxide (Dulcolax should not be taken within one hour of taking an antacid). Products include:

Beelith Tablets **784**
PremCal Light, Regular, and Extra Strength Tablets................ ■**762**

Sodium Bicarbonate (Dulcolax should not be taken within one hour of taking an antacid). Products include:

Ceo-Two Evacuant Suppository ...... ■**607**
Colyte with Flavor Packs for Oral Solution.. **3102**
HalfLytely and Bisacodyl Tablets Bowel Prep Kit with Flavors Packs... **915**
TriLyte with Flavor Packs for Oral Solution.. **3114**

Food Interactions

Dairy products (Dulcolax should not be taken within one hour of taking milk).

DUONEB INHALATION SOLUTION

(Albuterol Sulfate, Ipratropium Bromide).. **1058**
May interact with anticholinergics, beta blockers, monoamine oxidase inhibitors, potassium-depleting diuretics, sympathomimetics, and tricyclic antidepressants. Compounds in these categories include:

Acebutolol Hydrochloride (Co-administration with beta blockers inhibits the effects of each other).

No products indexed under this heading.

Albuterol (Co-administration with other sympathomimetic agents increases the risk of adverse cardiovascular effects). Products include:

Proventil Inhalation Aerosol **3067**

Amitriptyline Hydrochloride (Co-administration with tricyclic antidepressants can potentiate the action of albuterol on the cardiovascular system).

No products indexed under this heading.

Amoxapine (Co-administration with tricyclic antidepressants can potentiate the action of albuterol on the cardiovascular system).

No products indexed under this heading.

Atenolol (Co-administration with beta blockers inhibits the effects of each other). Products include:

Tenormin I.V. Injection **698**
Tenormin Tablets **695**

Atropine Sulfate (Co-administration has some potential for additive anticholinergic effects; caution is advised).
No products indexed under this heading.

Belladonna Alkaloids (Co-administration has some potential for additive anticholinergic effects; caution is advised). Products include:
Hyland's Teething Tablets 736

Bendroflumethiazide (Co-administration with non-potassium sparing diuretics can result in acute worsening of ECG changes and/or hypokalemia, especially when recommended dose of the beta agonist is exceeded; clinical significance of this interaction is unknown).
No products indexed under this heading.

Benztropine Mesylate (Co-administration has some potential for additive anticholinergic effects; caution is advised). Products include:
Cogentin Injection 1903

Betaxolol Hydrochloride (Co-administration with beta blockers inhibits the effects of each other). Products include:
Betoptic S Ophthalmic Suspension.................................. 554

Biperiden Hydrochloride (Co-administration has some potential for additive anticholinergic effects; caution is advised).
No products indexed under this heading.

Bisoprolol Fumarate (Co-administration with beta blockers inhibits the effects of each other).
No products indexed under this heading.

Bumetanide (Co-administration with non-potassium sparing diuretics can result in acute worsening of ECG changes and/or hypokalemia, especially when recommended dose of the beta agonist is exceeded; clinical significance of this interaction is unknown).
No products indexed under this heading.

Carteolol Hydrochloride (Co-administration with beta blockers inhibits the effects of each other). Products include:
Carteolol Hydrochloride Ophthalmic Solution USP, 1%....... ⊙246

Chlorothiazide (Co-administration with non-potassium sparing diuretics can result in acute worsening of ECG changes and/or hypokalemia, especially when recommended dose of the beta agonist is exceeded; clinical significance of this interaction is unknown). Products include:
Aldoclor Tablets 1881
Diuril Oral 1936

Chlorothiazide Sodium (Co-administration with non-potassium sparing diuretics can result in acute worsening of ECG changes and/or hypokalemia, especially when recommended dose of the beta agonist is exceeded; clinical significance of this interaction is unknown). Products include:
Diuril Sodium Intravenous 1934

Clidinium Bromide (Co-administration has some potential for additive anticholinergic effects; caution is advised).
No products indexed under this heading.

Clomipramine Hydrochloride (Co-administration with tricyclic antidepressants can potentiate the action of albuterol on the cardiovascular system).
No products indexed under this heading.

Desipramine Hydrochloride (Co-administration with tricyclic antidepressants can potentiate the action of albuterol on the cardiovascular system).
No products indexed under this heading.

Dicyclomine Hydrochloride (Co-administration has some potential for additive anticholinergic effects; caution is advised). Products include:
Bentyl Capsules 724
Bentyl Injection 724
Bentyl Syrup 724
Bentyl Tablets 724

Dobutamine Hydrochloride (Co-administration with other sympathomimetic agents increases the risk of adverse cardiovascular effects).
No products indexed under this heading.

Dopamine Hydrochloride (Co-administration with other sympathomimetic agents increases the risk of adverse cardiovascular effects).
No products indexed under this heading.

Doxepin Hydrochloride (Co-administration with tricyclic antidepressants can potentiate the action of albuterol on the cardiovascular system).
No products indexed under this heading.

Ephedrine Hydrochloride (Co-administration with other sympathomimetic agents increases the risk of adverse cardiovascular effects). Products include:
Primatene Tablets 749

Ephedrine Sulfate (Co-administration with other sympathomimetic agents increases the risk of adverse cardiovascular effects).
No products indexed under this heading.

Ephedrine Tannate (Co-administration with other sympathomimetic agents increases the risk of adverse cardiovascular effects).
No products indexed under this heading.

Epinephrine (Co-administration with other sympathomimetic agents increases the risk of adverse cardiovascular effects). Products include:
EpiPen 1061
Primatene Mist 749

Epinephrine Bitartrate (Co-administration with other sympathomimetic agents increases the risk of adverse cardiovascular effects).
No products indexed under this heading.

Epinephrine Hydrochloride (Co-administration with other sympathomimetic agents increases the risk of adverse cardiovascular effects).
No products indexed under this heading.

Esmolol Hydrochloride (Co-administration with beta blockers inhibits the effects of each other). Products include:
Brevibloc Concentrate 766
Brevibloc Injection 766
Brevibloc Double Strength Injection.. 766
Brevibloc Premixed Injection 766
Brevibloc Double Strength Premixed Injection 766

Ethacrynic Acid (Co-administration with non-potassium sparing diuretics can result in acute worsening of ECG changes and/or hypokalemia, especially when recommended dose of the beta agonist is exceeded; clinical significance of this interaction is unknown). Products include:
Edecrin Tablets 1941

Furosemide (Co-administration with non-potassium sparing diuretics can result in acute worsening of ECG changes and/or hypokalemia, especially when recommended dose of the beta agonist is exceeded; clinical significance of this interaction is unknown). Products include:
Furosemide Tablets 2117

Glycopyrrolate (Co-administration has some potential for additive anticholinergic effects; caution is advised).
No products indexed under this heading.

Hydrochlorothiazide (Co-administration with non-potassium sparing diuretics can result in acute worsening of ECG changes and/or hypokalemia, especially when recommended dose of the beta agonist is exceeded; clinical significance of this interaction is unknown). Products include:
Aldoril Tablets 1884
Atacand HCT 637
Avalide Tablets 2889
Avalide Tablets 922
Benicar HCT Tablets 2852
Diovan HCT Tablets 2195
Dyazide Capsules 1389
Hyzaar 1964
Lotensin HCT Tablets 2235
Maxzide 2150
Micardis HCT Tablets 886
Moduretic Tablets 2003
Prinzide Tablets 2033
Teveten HCT Tablets 1710
Timolide Tablets 2056
Uniretic Tablets 3114
Vaseretic Tablets 2073
Zestoretic Tablets 701

Hydroflumethiazide (Co-administration with non-potassium sparing diuretics can result in acute worsening of ECG changes and/or hypokalemia, especially when recommended dose of the beta agonist is exceeded; clinical significance of this interaction is unknown).
No products indexed under this heading.

Hyoscyamine (Co-administration has some potential for additive anticholinergic effects; caution is advised).
No products indexed under this heading.

Hyoscyamine Sulfate (Co-administration has some potential for additive anticholinergic effects; caution is advised).
No products indexed under this heading.

Imipramine Hydrochloride (Co-administration with tricyclic antidepressants can potentiate the action of albuterol on the cardiovascular system).
No products indexed under this heading.

Imipramine Pamoate (Co-administration with tricyclic antidepressants can potentiate the action of albuterol on the cardiovascular system).
No products indexed under this heading.

Isocarboxazid (Co-administration with MAO inhibitors can potentiate the action of albuterol on the cardiovascular system).
No products indexed under this heading.

Isoproterenol Hydrochloride (Co-administration with other sympathomimetic agents increases the risk of adverse cardiovascular effects).
No products indexed under this heading.

Isoproterenol Sulfate (Co-administration with other sympathomimetic agents increases the risk of adverse cardiovascular effects).
No products indexed under this heading.

Labetalol Hydrochloride (Co-administration with beta blockers inhibits the effects of each other).
No products indexed under this heading.

Levalbuterol Hydrochloride (Co-administration with other sympathomimetic agents increases the risk of adverse cardiovascular effects). Products include:
Xopenex Inhalation Solution 3143
Xopenex Inhalation Solution Concentrate 3147

Levobunolol Hydrochloride (Co-administration with beta blockers inhibits the effects of each other). Products include:
Betagan Ophthalmic Solution, USP.. ⊙217

Maprotiline Hydrochloride (Co-administration with tricyclic antidepressants can potentiate the action of albuterol on the cardiovascular system).
No products indexed under this heading.

Mepenzolate Bromide (Co-administration has some potential for additive anticholinergic effects; caution is advised).
No products indexed under this heading.

Metaproterenol Sulfate (Co-administration with other sympathomimetic agents increases the risk of adverse cardiovascular effects). Products include:
Alupent Inhalation Aerosol 858

Metaraminol Bitartrate (Co-administration with other sympathomimetic agents increases the risk of adverse cardiovascular effects). Products include:
Aramine Injection 1889

Methoxamine Hydrochloride (Co-administration with other sympathomimetic agents increases the risk of adverse cardiovascular effects).
No products indexed under this heading.

Methyclothiazide (Co-administration with non-potassium sparing diuretics can result in acute worsening of ECG changes and/or hypokalemia, especially when recommended dose of the beta agonist is exceeded; clinical significance of this interaction is unknown).
No products indexed under this heading.

Metipranolol Hydrochloride (Co-administration with beta blockers inhibits the effects of each other).
No products indexed under this heading.

Metoprolol Succinate (Co-administration with beta blockers inhibits the effects of each other). Products include:
Toprol-XL Tablets 660

Metoprolol Tartrate (Co-administration with beta blockers inhibits the effects of each other).
No products indexed under this heading.

Moclobemide (Co-administration with MAO inhibitors can potentiate the action of albuterol on the cardiovascular system).
No products indexed under this heading.

Nadolol (Co-administration with beta blockers inhibits the effects of each other). Products include:
Nadolol Tablets 2121

Norepinephrine Bitartrate (Co-administration with other sympathomimetic agents increases the risk of adverse cardiovascular effects).
No products indexed under this heading.

Nortriptyline Hydrochloride (Co-administration with tricyclic antidepressants can potentiate the action of albuterol on the cardiovascular system).
No products indexed under this heading.

Oxybutynin Chloride (Co-administration has some potential for additive anticholinergic effects; caution is advised). Products include:
Ditropan XL Extended Release Tablets 2391

Pargyline Hydrochloride (Co-administration with MAO inhibitors can potentiate the action of albuterol on the cardiovascular system).
No products indexed under this heading.

Penbutolol Sulfate (Co-administration with beta blockers inhibits the effects of each other).
No products indexed under this heading.

Phenelzine Sulfate (Co-administration with MAO inhibitors can potentiate the action of albuterol on the cardiovascular system).
No products indexed under this heading.

Phenylephrine Bitartrate (Co-administration with other sympathomimetic agents increases the risk of adverse cardiovascular effects).
No products indexed under this heading.

Phenylephrine Hydrochloride (Co-administration with other sympathomimetic agents increases the risk of adverse cardiovascular effects). Products include:
Alacol DM Syrup 739
Hycomine Compound Tablets 1105
Preparation H Maximum Strength Cream .... ■ 747
Preparation H Cooling Gel .... ■ 747
Preparation H .... ■ 747
Sudafed PE Tablets .... ■ 711
Vicks Sinex Nasal Spray and Ultra Fine Mist for Sinus Relief 2677
Zicam Concentrated Cough Mist for Kids Plus D Cool Cherry .... ■ 643
Zicam Concentrated Cough Mist Plus D Cool Cherry .... ■ 642

Phenylephrine Tannate (Co-administration with other sympathomimetic agents increases the risk of adverse cardiovascular effects).
No products indexed under this heading.

Phenylpropanolamine Hydrochloride (Co-administration with other sympathomimetic agents increases the risk of adverse cardiovascular effects).
No products indexed under this heading.

Pindolol (Co-administration with beta blockers inhibits the effects of each other).
No products indexed under this heading.

Pirbuterol Acetate (Co-administration with other sympathomimetic agents increases the risk of adverse cardiovascular effects). Products include:
Maxair Autohaler 1820

Polythiazide (Co-administration with non-potassium sparing diuretics can result in acute worsening of ECG changes and/or hypokalemia, especially when recommended dose of the beta agonist is exceeded; clinical significance of this interaction is unknown).
No products indexed under this heading.

Procarbazine Hydrochloride (Co-administration with MAO inhibitors can potentiate the action of albuterol on the cardiovascular system). Products include:
Matulane Capsules 3188

Procyclidine Hydrochloride (Co-administration has some potential for additive anticholinergic effects; caution is advised).
No products indexed under this heading.

Propantheline Bromide (Co-administration has some potential for additive anticholinergic effects; caution is advised).
No products indexed under this heading.

Propranolol Hydrochloride (Co-administration with beta blockers inhibits the effects of each other). Products include:
Inderal LA Long-Acting Capsules 3421
InnoPran XL Capsules 2728

Protriptyline Hydrochloride (Co-administration with tricyclic antidepressants can potentiate the action of albuterol on the cardiovascular system). Products include:
Vivactil Tablets 2350

Pseudoephedrine Hydrochloride (Co-administration with other sympathomimetic agents increases the risk of adverse cardiovascular effects). Products include:
Advil Allergy Sinus Caplets .... ■ 737
Advil Cold & Sinus .... ■ 739
Advil Flu & Body Ache Caplets .... ■ 739
Children's Advil Cold Suspension .... ■ 741
Advil Multi-Symptom Cold Caplets .... ■ 738
Allegra-D 12 Hour Extended-Release Tablets 2860
Allegra-D 24 Hour Extended-Release Tablets 2862
Balamine DM 739
BC Cold Powder .... ■ 612
Benadryl Allergy & Cold Tablets .... ■ 692
Benadryl Allergy & Sinus Headache Caplets & Gelcaps .... ■ 693
Children's Benadryl Allergy & Cold Fastmelt Tablets .... ■ 695
Benadryl Maximum Strength Severe Allergy & Sinus Headache Caplets .... ■ 694
Children's Benadryl D Allergy & Sinus Fastmelt Tablets .... ■ 694
Children's Benadryl D Liquid Medication .... ■ 693
Benadryl D Tablets .... ■ 694
Contac Non-Drowsy 12 Hour Cold Caplets .... ■ 614
Contac Non-Drowsy Timed Release 12 Hour Cold Caplets .... ■ 615
Contac Severe Cold and Flu Caplets Maximum Strength .... ■ 615
Contac Severe Cold and Flu Caplets Non-Drowsy .... ■ 615
Children's Dimetapp Cold & Allergy Elixir .... ■ 745
Children's Dimetapp DM Cold & Cough Elixir .... ■ 745
Children's Dimetapp Long Acting Cough Plus Cold Syrup .... ■ 746
Dimetapp Infant Drops Decongestant Plus Cough .... ■ 746
Children's Motrin Cold Non-Staining Dye-Free Oral Suspension 1838
Children's Motrin Cold Oral Suspension 1838
Motrin Cold & Sinus Caplets 1836
PediaCare Decongestant & Cough Infant Drops .... ■ 705
PediaCare Decongestant Infants' Drops .... ■ 705
PediaCare Long-Acting Cough Plus Cold Liquid .... ■ 704
PediaCare Multi-Symptom Cold Liquid .... ■ 704
PediaCare NightRest Cough & Cold Liquid .... ■ 704
Robitussin Allergy & Cough Syrup .... ■ 750
Robitussin CF Liquid .... ■ 755
Robitussin Cough & Cold Liquid-filled Capsules .... ■ 750
Robitussin Cough, Cold & Flu Liquid-filled Capsules .... ■ 750
Robitussin Cough & Cold Infant Drops .... ■ 755
Robitussin Flu Liquid .... ■ 752
Robitussin Maximum Strength Cough & Cold Liquid .... ■ 754
Robitussin PE Syrup .... ■ 753
Robitussin Pediatric Cough & Cold Liquid .... ■ 754
Robitussin PM Cough & Cold Liquid .... ■ 752
Robitussin Severe Congestion Liquid-filled Capsules .... ■ 751
Simply Stuffy Liquid 1841
Singlet Caplets .... ■ 636
Sudafed 12 Hour Caplets .... ■ 708
Sudafed 24 Hour Tablets .... ■ 709
Sudafed Nasal Decongestant Tablets .... ■ 709
Sudafed Severe Cold .... ■ 710
Sudafed Non-Drying Sinus Liquid Caps .... ■ 709
Sudafed Sinus & Allergy Tablets .... ■ 710
Sudafed Sinus Headache .... ■ 711
TheraFlu Cold & Cough Hot Liquid .... ■ 680
TheraFlu Cold & Sore Throat Hot Liquid .... ■ 680
TheraFlu Flu & Chest Congestion Non-Drowsy Hot Liquid .... ■ 681
TheraFlu Flu & Sore Throat Hot Liquid .... ■ 681
TheraFlu Severe Cold Non-Drowsy Hot Liquid .... ■ 683
TheraFlu Severe Cold & Cough Hot Liquid .... ■ 683
TheraFlu Severe Cold Caplets .... ■ 679
TheraFlu Severe Cold Hot Liquid .... ■ 682
TheraFlu Severe Cold Non-Drowsy Caplets .... ■ 679
Triaminic Chest & Nasal Congestion Liquid .... ■ 685
Triaminic Cold & Allergy Liquid .... ■ 685
Triaminic Cold & Cough Liquid .... ■ 685
Triaminic Cough Liquid .... ■ 687
Triaminic Cough & Nasal Congestion Liquid .... ■ 687
Triaminic Cough & Sore Throat Liquid .... ■ 687
Triaminic Flu, Cough & Fever Liquid .... ■ 685
Triaminic Night Time Cough & Cold Liquid .... ■ 685
Triaminic Allergy Runny Nose & Congestion Softchews .... ■ 688
Triaminic Cold & Cough Softchews .... ■ 688
Triaminic Cough & Sore Throat Softchews .... ■ 689
Tylenol Sinus NightTime Caplets .... ■ 663
Children's Tylenol Plus Cold & Allergy Suspension Liquid 1850
Children's Tylenol Plus Cold NightTime Suspension Liquid 1851
Children's Tylenol Plus Cold & Cough Suspension Liquid and Chewable Tablets 1851
Children's Tylenol Plus Cold Chewable Tablets 1851
Children's Tylenol Plus Cold Daytime Non-Drowsy Suspension Liquid 1851
Children's Tylenol Plus Flu Suspension Liquid 1853
Concentrated Tylenol Infants' Drops Plus Cold 1851
Concentrated Tylenol Infants' Drops Plus Cold and Cough 1851
Tylenol Cold & Flu Severe Daytime Liquid with Cool Burst 1846
Tylenol Cold & Flu Severe NightTime Liquid with Cool Burst 1846
Tylenol Cold Severe Congestion Non-Drowsy Caplets with Cool Burst 1846
Tylenol Allergy Complete Night Time Caplets 1844
Tylenol Allergy Complete Multi-Symptom Caplets and Gelcaps with Cool Burst 1844
Tylenol Flu NightTime Gelcaps 1846
Tylenol Flu Day Non-Drowsy Gelcaps 1846
Concentrated Tylenol Infants' Drops Plus Cold Nasal Congestant, Fever Reducer & Pain Reliever .... ■ 668
Concentrated Tylenol Infants' Drops Plus Cold & Cough Nasal Decongestant, Fever Reducer & Pain Reliever .... ■ 668
Multi-Symptom Tylenol Cold Night Time Caplets 1845
Multi-Symptom Tylenol Cold Day Non-Drowsy Caplets and Gelcaps 1845
Tylenol Sinus Day Non-Drowsy 1848
Tylenol Sinus Night Time Caplets 1848
Tylenol Sinus Severe Congestion Caplets with Cool Burst 1848
Vicks 44D Cough & Head Congestion Relief 2676
Vicks 44D Cough & Head Congestion Relief Liquid .... ■ 721
Vicks 44M Cough, Cold & Flu Relief 2676
Pediatric Vicks 44m Cough & Cold Relief 2673
Vicks DayQuil LiquiCaps/Liquid Multi-Symptom Cold/Flu Relief .... ■ 723
Vicks DayQuil Multi-Symptom Cold/Flu Relief LiquiCaps 2675
Vicks DayQuil Multi-Symptom Cold/Flu Relief Liquid 2675
Children's Vicks NyQuil Cold/Cough Relief 2671
Vicks NyQuil LiquiCaps 2677
Vicks NyQuil LiquiCaps/Liquid Multi-Symptom Cold/Flu Relief .... ■ 725
Vicks NyQuil Liquid 2677
Zyrtec-D 12 Hour Extended Release Tablets 2591

Pseudoephedrine Sulfate (Co-administration with other sympathomimetic agents increases the risk of adverse cardiovascular effects). Products include:
Alavert Allergy & Sinus D-12 Hour Tablets .... ■ 743
Clarinex-D 24-Hour Extended-Release Tablets 3012
Claritin-D Non-Drowsy 12 Hour Tablets .... ■ 731
Claritin-D Non-Drowsy 24 Hour Tablets .... ■ 731

Salmeterol Xinafoate (Co-administration with other sympatho-

mimetic agents increases the risk of adverse cardiovascular effects). Products include:

Advair Diskus 100/50 .... **1291**
Advair Diskus 250/50 .... **1291**
Advair Diskus 500/50 .... **1291**
Serevent Diskus **1540**

Scopolamine (Co-administration has some potential for additive anticholinergic effects; caution is advised). Products include:

Transderm Scōp Transdermal Therapeutic System **2166**

Scopolamine Hydrobromide (Co-administration has some potential for additive anticholinergic effects; caution is advised).

No products indexed under this heading.

Selegiline Hydrochloride (Co-administration with MAO inhibitors can potentiate the action of albuterol on the cardiovascular system). Products include:

Eldepryl Capsules **3209**

Sotalol Hydrochloride (Co-administration with beta blockers inhibits the effects of each other).

No products indexed under this heading.

Terbutaline Sulfate (Co-administration with other sympathomimetic agents increases the risk of adverse cardiovascular effects).

No products indexed under this heading.

Timolol Hemihydrate (Co-administration with beta blockers inhibits the effects of each other). Products include:

Betimol Ophthalmic Solution **3371**
Betimol Ophthalmic Solution .... ⊙**283**

Timolol Maleate (Co-administration with beta blockers inhibits the effects of each other). Products include:

Blocadren Tablets **1891**
Cosopt Sterile Ophthalmic Solution.. **1910**
Timolide Tablets **2056**
Timoptic in Ocudose **2061**
Timoptic Sterile Ophthalmic Solution.. **2058**
Timoptic-XE Sterile Ophthalmic Gel Forming Solution **2062**

Tolterodine Tartrate (Co-administration has some potential for additive anticholinergic effects; caution is advised). Products include:

Detrol Tablets **2626**
Detrol LA Capsules **2629**

Torsemide (Co-administration with non-potassium sparing diuretics can result in acute worsening of ECG changes and/or hypokalemia, especially when recommended dose of the beta agonist is exceeded; clinical significance of this interaction is unknown).

No products indexed under this heading.

Tranylcypromine Sulfate (Co-administration with MAO inhibitors can potentiate the action of albuterol on the cardiovascular system). Products include:

Parnate Tablets **1499**

Tridihexethyl Chloride (Co-administration has some potential for additive anticholinergic effects; caution is advised).

No products indexed under this heading.

Trihexyphenidyl Hydrochloride (Co-administration has some potential for additive anticholinergic effects; caution is advised).

No products indexed under this heading.

Trimipramine Maleate (Co-administration with tricyclic antidepressants can potentiate the action of albuterol on the cardiovascular system). Products include:

Surmontil Capsules **2347**

DURAGESIC TRANSDERMAL SYSTEM

(Fentanyl) **2448**

May interact with central nervous system depressants, cytochrome p450 3a4 inducers (selected), cytochrome p450 3a4 inhibitors (selected), cytochrome p450 3a4 inhibitors, potent, general anesthetics, hypnotics and sedatives, monoamine oxidase inhibitors, narcotic analgesics, phenothiazines, skeletal muscle relaxants, tranquilizers, and certain other agents. Compounds in these categories include:

Acetazolamide (The concurrent use of CYP3A4 inhibitors with transdermal fentanyl may result in an increase in fentanyl plasma concentrations, which could increase or prolong adverse drug effects and may cause serious respiratory depression. In this situation, special patient care and observation are appropriate).

No products indexed under this heading.

Alfentanil Hydrochloride (The concomitant use of fentanyl with other CNS depressants, including other opioids, may cause respiratory depression, hypotension, and profound sedation or potentially result in coma. When such combined therapy is contemplated, the dose of one or both agents should be significantly reduced).

No products indexed under this heading.

Allium sativum (Fentanyl is metabolized mainly via the human cytochrome P450 3A4 isoenzyme system (CYP3A4). Co-administration with agents that induce CYP 3A4 activity may reduce the efficacy of fentanyl).

No products indexed under this heading.

Alprazolam (The concomitant use of fentanyl with other CNS depressants, including tranquilizers, may cause respiratory depression, hypotension, and profound sedation or potentially result in coma. When such combined therapy is contemplated, the dose of one or both agents should be significantly reduced). Products include:

Niravam Orally Disintegrating Tablets **3106**
Xanax XR Tablets **2655**

Amiodarone Hydrochloride (The concurrent use of CYP3A4 inhibitors with transdermal fentanyl may result in an increase in fentanyl plasma concentrations, which could increase or prolong adverse drug effects and may cause serious respiratory depression. In this situation, special patient care and observation are appropriate). Products include:

Pacerone Tablets **3337**

Amprenavir (The concurrent use of CYP3A4 inhibitors with transdermal fentanyl may result in an increase in fentanyl plasma concentrations, which could increase or prolong adverse drug effects and may cause serious respiratory depression. In this situation, special patient care and observation are appropriate). Products include:

Agenerase Capsules **1299**
Agenerase Oral Solution **1304**

Anastrozole (The concurrent use of CYP3A4 inhibitors with transdermal fentanyl may result in an increase in fentanyl plasma concentrations, which could increase or prolong adverse drug effects and may cause serious respiratory depression. In this situation, special patient care and observation are appropriate). Products include:

Arimidex Tablets **665**

Aprepitant (The concurrent use of CYP3A4 inhibitors with transdermal fentanyl may result in an increase in fentanyl plasma concentrations, which could increase or prolong adverse drug effects and may cause serious respiratory depression. In this situation, special patient care and observation are appropriate). Products include:

Emend Capsules **1944**

Aprobarbital (The comcomitant use of fentanyl with other CNS depressants may cause respiratory depression, hypotension, and profound sedation or potentially result in coma. When such combined therapy is contemplated, the dose of one or both agents should be significantly reduced).

No products indexed under this heading.

Atazanavir sulfate (The concomitant use of fentanyl with potent cytochrome P450 3A4 inhibitors may result in an increase in fentanyl plasma concentrations, which could increase or prolong adverse drug effects and may cause potentially fatal respiratory depression. Patients receiving fentanyl and potent CYP3A4 inhibitors should be carefully monitored for an extended period of time and dosage adjustments should be made if warranted). Products include:

Reyataz Capsules **948**

Baclofen (The concomitant use of fentanyl with other CNS depressants, including skeletal muscle relaxants, may cause respiratory depression, hypotension, and profound sedation or potentially result in coma. When such combined therapy is contemplated, the dose of one or both agents should be significantly reduced).

No products indexed under this heading.

Betamethasone Acetate (Fentanyl is metabolized mainly via the human cytochrome P450 3A4 isoenzyme system (CYP3A4). Co-administration with agents that induce CYP 3A4 activity may reduce the efficacy of fentanyl).

No products indexed under this heading.

Betamethasone Sodium Phosphate (Fentanyl is metabolized mainly via the human cytochrome P450 3A4 isoenzyme system (CYP3A4). Co-administration with agents that induce CYP 3A4 activity may reduce the efficacy of fentanyl).

No products indexed under this heading.

Buprenorphine Hydrochloride (The concomitant use of fentanyl with other CNS depressants, including other opioids, may cause respiratory depression, hypotension, and profound sedation or potentially result in coma. When such combined therapy is contemplated, the dose of one or both agents should be significantly reduced). Products include:

Buprenex Injectable **2718**
Suboxone Tablets **2719**
Subutex Tablets **2719**

Buspirone Hydrochloride (The concomitant use of fentanyl with other CNS depressants, including tranquilizers, may cause respiratory depression, hypotension, and profound sedation or potentially result in coma. When such combined therapy is contemplated, the dose of one or both agents should be significantly reduced).

No products indexed under this heading.

Butabarbital (The comcomitant use of fentanyl with other CNS depressants may cause respiratory depression, hypotension, and profound sedation or potentially result in coma. When such combined therapy is contemplated, the dose of one or both agents should be significantly reduced).

No products indexed under this heading.

Butalbital (The comcomitant use of fentanyl with other CNS depressants may cause respiratory depression, hypotension, and profound sedation or potentially result in coma. When such combined therapy is contemplated, the dose of one or both agents should be significantly reduced). Products include:

Sedapap Tablets 50 mg/650 mg **2098**

Carbamazepine (Fentanyl is metabolized mainly via the human cytochrome P450 3A4 isoenzyme system (CYP3A4). Co-administration with agents that induce CYP 3A4 activity may reduce the efficacy of fentanyl). Products include:

Carbatrol Capsules **3174**
Equetro Extended-Release Capsules **3178**
Tegretol/Tegretol-XR **2278**

Carisoprodol (The concomitant use of fentanyl with other CNS depressants, including skeletal muscle relaxants, may cause respiratory depression, hypotension, and profound sedation or potentially result in coma. When such combined therapy is contemplated, the dose of one or both agents should be significantly reduced).

No products indexed under this heading.

Chlordiazepoxide (The concomitant use of fentanyl with other CNS depressants, including tranquilizers, may cause respiratory depression, hypotension, and profound sedation or potentially result in coma. When such combined therapy is contemplated, the dose of one or both agents should be significantly reduced).

No products indexed under this heading.

Chlordiazepoxide Hydrochloride (The concomitant use of fentanyl with other CNS depressants, including tranquilizers, may cause respiratory depression, hypotension, and profound sedation or potentially result in coma. When such combined

therapy is contemplated, the dose of one or both agents should be significantly reduced). Products include:

Librium Capsules 3349

Chlorpromazine (The concomitant use of fentanyl with other CNS depressants, including phenothiazines, may cause respiratory depression, hypotension, and profound sedation or potentially result in coma. When such combined therapy is contemplated, the dose of one or both agents should be significantly reduced).

No products indexed under this heading.

Chlorpromazine Hydrochloride (The concomitant use of fentanyl with other CNS depressants, including phenothiazines, may cause respiratory depression, hypotension, and profound sedation or potentially result in coma. When such combined therapy is contemplated, the dose of one or both agents should be significantly reduced).

No products indexed under this heading.

Chlorprothixene (The concomitant use of fentanyl with other CNS depressants, including tranquilizers, may cause respiratory depression, hypotension, and profound sedation or potentially result in coma. When such combined therapy is contemplated, the dose of one or both agents should be significantly reduced).

No products indexed under this heading.

Chlorprothixene Hydrochloride (The concomitant use of fentanyl with other CNS depressants, including tranquilizers, may cause respiratory depression, hypotension, and profound sedation or potentially result in coma. When such combined therapy is contemplated, the dose of one or both agents should be significantly reduced).

No products indexed under this heading.

Chlorprothixene Lactate (The comcomitant use of fentanyl with other CNS depressants may cause respiratory depression, hypotension, and profound sedation or potentially result in coma. When such combined therapy is contemplated, the dose of one or both agents should be significantly reduced).

No products indexed under this heading.

Chlorzoxazone (The concomitant use of fentanyl with other CNS depressants, including skeletal muscle relaxants, may cause respiratory depression, hypotension, and profound sedation or potentially result in coma. When such combined therapy is contemplated, the dose of one or both agents should be significantly reduced).

No products indexed under this heading.

Cimetidine (The concurrent use of CYP3A4 inhibitors with transdermal fentanyl may result in an increase in fentanyl plasma concentrations, which could increase or prolong adverse drug effects and may cause serious respiratory depression. In this situation, special patient care and observation are appropriate). Products include:

Tagamet HB 200 Tablets .... ▣ 637
Tagamet Tablets 1547

Cimetidine Hydrochloride (The concurrent use of CYP3A4 inhibitors with transdermal fentanyl may result in an increase in fentanyl plasma concentrations, which could increase or prolong adverse drug effects and may cause serious respiratory depression. In this situation, special patient care and observation are appropriate).

No products indexed under this heading.

Ciprofloxacin (The concurrent use of CYP3A4 inhibitors with transdermal fentanyl may result in an increase in fentanyl plasma concentrations, which could increase or prolong adverse drug effects and may cause serious respiratory depression. In this situation, special patient care and observation are appropriate). Products include:

Cipro I.V. 2998
Cipro I.V. Pharmacy Bulk Package ... 3509
Cipro Oral Suspension 2991
Cipro XR Tablets 3004
Ciprodex Otic Suspension 555

Ciprofloxacin Hydrochloride (Fentanyl is metabolized mainly via the human cytochrome P450 3A4 isoenzyme system (CYP3A4). Co-administration with agents that induce CYP 3A4 activity may reduce the efficacy of fentanyl). Products include:

Ciloxan Ophthalmic Ointment 554
Cipro Tablets 2991

Cisplatin (Fentanyl is metabolized mainly via the human cytochrome P450 3A4 isoenzyme system (CYP3A4). Co-administration with agents that induce CYP 3A4 activity may reduce the efficacy of fentanyl).

No products indexed under this heading.

Clarithromycin (The concurrent use of CYP3A4 inhibitors with transdermal fentanyl may result in an increase in fentanyl plasma concentrations, which could increase or prolong adverse drug effects and may cause serious respiratory depression. In this situation, special patient care and observation are appropriate). Products include:

Biaxin/Biaxin XL 402
PREVPAC 3281

Clorazepate Dipotassium (The concomitant use of fentanyl with other CNS depressants, including tranquilizers, may cause respiratory depression, hypotension, and profound sedation or potentially result in coma. When such combined therapy is contemplated, the dose of one or both agents should be significantly reduced). Products include:

Tranxene 2488

Clotrimazole (The concurrent use of CYP3A4 inhibitors with transdermal fentanyl may result in an increase in fentanyl plasma concentrations, which could increase or prolong adverse drug effects and may cause serious respiratory depression. In this situation, special patient care and observation are appropriate). Products include:

Lotrimin 3053
Lotrisone 3054

Clozapine (The comcomitant use of fentanyl with other CNS depressants may cause respiratory depression, hypotension, and profound sedation or potentially result in coma. When such combined therapy is contemplated, the dose of one or both agents should be significantly reduced). Products include:

Clozapine Tablets 2141
Clozaril Tablets 2174
FazaClo Orally Disintegrating Tablets 547

Codeine Phosphate (The concomitant use of fentanyl with other CNS depressants, including other opioids, may cause respiratory depression, hypotension, and profound sedation or potentially result in coma. When such combined therapy is contemplated, the dose of one or both agents should be significantly reduced). Products include:

Tylenol with Codeine 2461

Cortisone Acetate (Fentanyl is metabolized mainly via the human cytochrome P450 3A4 isoenzyme system (CYP3A4). Co-administration with agents that induce CYP 3A4 activity may reduce the efficacy of fentanyl).

No products indexed under this heading.

Cyclobenzaprine Hydrochloride (The concomitant use of fentanyl with other CNS depressants, including skeletal muscle relaxants, may cause respiratory depression, hypotension, and profound sedation or potentially result in coma. When such combined therapy is contemplated, the dose of one or both agents should be significantly reduced). Products include:

Flexeril Tablets 1832

Cyclosporine (The concurrent use of CYP3A4 inhibitors with transdermal fentanyl may result in an increase in fentanyl plasma concentrations, which could increase or prolong adverse drug effects and may cause serious respiratory depression. In this situation, special patient care and observation are appropriate). Products include:

Gengraf Capsules 458
Neoral Soft Gelatin Capsules 2247
Neoral Oral Solution 2247
Restasis Ophthalmic Emulsion 570
Sandimmune 2259

Dalfopristin (The concurrent use of CYP3A4 inhibitors with transdermal fentanyl may result in an increase in fentanyl plasma concentrations, which could increase or prolong adverse drug effects and may cause serious respiratory depression. In this situation, special patient care and observation are appropriate). Products include:

Synercid I.V. 1690

Danazol (The concurrent use of CYP3A4 inhibitors with transdermal fentanyl may result in an increase in fentanyl plasma concentrations, which could increase or prolong adverse drug effects and may cause serious respiratory depression. In this situation, special patient care and observation are appropriate).

No products indexed under this heading.

Dantrolene Sodium (The concomitant use of fentanyl with other CNS depressants, including skeletal muscle relaxants, may cause respiratory depression, hypotension, and profound sedation or potentially result in coma. When such combined therapy is contemplated, the dose of one or both agents should be significantly reduced). Products include:

Dantrium Capsules 2690
Dantrium Intravenous 2691

Delavirdine Mesylate (The concurrent use of CYP3A4 inhibitors with transdermal fentanyl may result in an increase in fentanyl plasma concentrations, which could increase or prolong adverse drug effects and may cause serious respiratory depression. In this situation, special patient care and observation are appropriate). Products include:

Rescriptor Tablets 2535

Desflurane (The comcomitant use of fentanyl with other CNS depressants may cause respiratory depression, hypotension, and profound sedation or potentially result in coma. When such combined therapy is contemplated, the dose of one or both agents should be significantly reduced). Products include:

Suprane Liquid for Inhalation 770

Dexamethasone (Fentanyl is metabolized mainly via the human cytochrome P450 3A4 isoenzyme system (CYP3A4). Co-administration with agents that induce CYP 3A4 activity may reduce the efficacy of fentanyl). Products include:

Ciprodex Otic Suspension 555
Decadron Tablets 1929
TobraDex Ophthalmic Ointment 558
TobraDex Ophthalmic Suspension ... 558

Dexamethasone Acetate (Fentanyl is metabolized mainly via the human cytochrome P450 3A4 isoenzyme system (CYP3A4). Co-administration with agents that induce CYP 3A4 activity may reduce the efficacy of fentanyl).

No products indexed under this heading.

Dexamethasone Sodium Phosphate (Fentanyl is metabolized mainly via the human cytochrome P450 3A4 isoenzyme system (CYP3A4). Co-administration with agents that induce CYP 3A4 activity may reduce the efficacy of fentanyl). Products include:

Decadron Phosphate Injection 1931

Dezocine (The concomitant use of fentanyl with other CNS depressants, including other opioids, may cause respiratory depression, hypotension, and profound sedation or potentially result in coma. When such combined therapy is contemplated, the dose of one or both agents should be significantly reduced).

No products indexed under this heading.

Diazepam (The concomitant use of fentanyl with other CNS depressants, including tranquilizers, may cause respiratory depression, hypotension, and profound sedation or potentially result in coma. When such combined therapy is contemplated, the dose of one or both agents should be significantly reduced). Products include:

Diastat Rectal Delivery System 3344
Valium Tablets 2822

Diltiazem Hydrochloride (The concurrent use of CYP3A4 inhibitors with transdermal fentanyl may result in an increase in fentanyl plasma concentrations, which could increase or prolong adverse drug effects and may cause serious respiratory depression. In this situation, special patient care and observation are appropriate). Products include:

Cardizem LA Extended Release Tablets 1699
Tiazac Capsules 1204

Diltiazem Maleate (The concurrent use of CYP3A4 inhibitors with transdermal fentanyl may result in an increase in fentanyl plasma concentrations, which could increase or prolong adverse drug effects and may cause serious respiratory depression. In this situation, special patient care and observation are appropriate).
No products indexed under this heading.

Doxorubicin Hydrochloride (Fentanyl is metabolized mainly via the human cytochrome P450 3A4 isoenzyme system (CYP3A4). Co-administration with agents that induce CYP 3A4 activity may reduce the efficacy of fentanyl). Products include:
Adriamycin for Injection, USP 786
Adriamycin Injection, USP 786

Droperidol (The concomitant use of fentanyl with other CNS depressants, including tranquilizers, may cause respiratory depression, hypotension, and profound sedation or potentially result in coma. When such combined therapy is contemplated, the dose of one or both agents should be significantly reduced).
No products indexed under this heading.

Efavirenz (The concurrent use of CYP3A4 inhibitors with transdermal fentanyl may result in an increase in fentanyl plasma concentrations, which could increase or prolong adverse drug effects and may cause serious respiratory depression. In this situation, special patient care and observation are appropriate). Products include:
Sustiva Capsules 957

Enflurane (The comcomitant use of fentanyl with other CNS depressants may cause respiratory depression, hypotension, and profound sedation or potentially result in coma. When such combined therapy is contemplated, the dose of one or both agents should be significantly reduced).
No products indexed under this heading.

Erythromycin (The concurrent use of CYP3A4 inhibitors with transdermal fentanyl may result in an increase in fentanyl plasma concentrations, which could increase or prolong adverse drug effects and may cause serious respiratory depression. In this situation, special patient care and observation are appropriate). Products include:
Erygel Topical Gel 2096
Ery-Tab Tablets 447
Erythromycin Base Filmtab Tablets 454
Erythromycin Delayed-Release Capsules, USP.............................. 456
PCE Dispertab Tablets 510

Erythromycin Estolate (The concurrent use of CYP3A4 inhibitors with transdermal fentanyl may result in an increase in fentanyl plasma concentrations, which could increase or prolong adverse drug effects and may cause serious respiratory depression. In this situation, special patient care and observation are appropriate).
No products indexed under this heading.

Erythromycin Ethylsuccinate (The concurrent use of CYP3A4 inhibitors with transdermal fentanyl may result in an increase in fentanyl plasma concentrations, which could increase or prolong adverse drug effects and may cause serious respiratory depression. In this situation, special patient care and observation are appropriate). Products include:
E.E.S. 449
EryPed 445

Erythromycin Gluceptate (The concurrent use of CYP3A4 inhibitors with transdermal fentanyl may result in an increase in fentanyl plasma concentrations, which could increase or prolong adverse drug effects and may cause serious respiratory depression. In this situation, special patient care and observation are appropriate).
No products indexed under this heading.

Erythromycin Lactobionate (The concurrent use of CYP3A4 inhibitors with transdermal fentanyl may result in an increase in fentanyl plasma concentrations, which could increase or prolong adverse drug effects and may cause serious respiratory depression. In this situation, special patient care and observation are appropriate).
No products indexed under this heading.

Erythromycin Stearate (The concurrent use of CYP3A4 inhibitors with transdermal fentanyl may result in an increase in fentanyl plasma concentrations, which could increase or prolong adverse drug effects and may cause serious respiratory depression. In this situation, special patient care and observation are appropriate). Products include:
Erythrocin Stearate Filmtab Tablets 452

Esomeprazole Magnesium (The concurrent use of CYP3A4 inhibitors with transdermal fentanyl may result in an increase in fentanyl plasma concentrations, which could increase or prolong adverse drug effects and may cause serious respiratory depression. In this situation, special patient care and observation are appropriate). Products include:
Nexium Delayed-Release Capsules 645

Estazolam (The concomitant use of fentanyl with other CNS depressants, including sedatives and hypnotics, may cause respiratory depression, hypotension, and profound sedation or potentially result in coma. When such combined therapy is contemplated, the dose of one or both agents should be significantly reduced). Products include:
ProSom Tablets 512

Ethanol (The comcomitant use of fentanyl with other CNS depressants may cause respiratory depression, hypotension, and profound sedation or potentially result in coma. When such combined therapy is contemplated, the dose of one or both agents should be significantly reduced).
No products indexed under this heading.

Ethchlorvynol (The concomitant use of fentanyl with other CNS depressants, including sedatives and hypnotics, may cause respiratory depression, hypotension, and profound sedation or potentially result in coma. When such combined therapy is contemplated, the dose of one or both agents should be significantly reduced).
No products indexed under this heading.

Ethinamate (The concomitant use of fentanyl with other CNS depressants, including sedatives and hypnotics, may cause respiratory depression, hypotension, and profound sedation or potentially result in coma. When such combined therapy is contemplated, the dose of one or both agents should be significantly reduced).
No products indexed under this heading.

Ethosuximide (Fentanyl is metabolized mainly via the human cytochrome P450 3A4 isoenzyme system (CYP3A4). Co-administration with agents that induce CYP 3A4 activity may reduce the efficacy of fentanyl).
No products indexed under this heading.

Ethyl Alcohol (The comcomitant use of fentanyl with other CNS depressants may cause respiratory depression, hypotension, and profound sedation or potentially result in coma. When such combined therapy is contemplated, the dose of one or both agents should be significantly reduced).
No products indexed under this heading.

Felbamate (Fentanyl is metabolized mainly via the human cytochrome P450 3A4 isoenzyme system (CYP3A4). Co-administration with agents that induce CYP 3A4 activity may reduce the efficacy of fentanyl).
No products indexed under this heading.

Fentanyl Citrate (The concomitant use of fentanyl with other CNS depressants, including other opioids, may cause respiratory depression, hypotension, and profound sedation or potentially result in coma. When such combined therapy is contemplated, the dose of one or both agents should be significantly reduced). Products include:
Actiq 993

Fluconazole (The concurrent use of CYP3A4 inhibitors with transdermal fentanyl may result in an increase in fentanyl plasma concentrations, which could increase or prolong adverse drug effects and may cause serious respiratory depression. In this situation, special patient care and observation are appropriate).
No products indexed under this heading.

Fludrocortisone Acetate (Fentanyl is metabolized mainly via the human cytochrome P450 3A4 isoenzyme system (CYP3A4). Co-administration with agents that induce CYP 3A4 activity may reduce the efficacy of fentanyl).
No products indexed under this heading.

Fluoxetine Hydrochloride (The concurrent use of CYP3A4 inhibitors with transdermal fentanyl may result in an increase in fentanyl plasma concentrations, which could increase or prolong adverse drug effects and may cause serious respiratory depression. In this situation, special patient care and observation are appropriate). Products include:
Prozac Pulvules and Liquid 1771
Symbyax Capsules 1788

Fluphenazine Decanoate (The concomitant use of fentanyl with other CNS depressants, including phenothiazines, may cause respiratory depression, hypotension, and profound sedation or potentially result in coma. When such combined therapy is contemplated, the dose of one or both agents should be significantly reduced).
No products indexed under this heading.

Fluphenazine Enanthate (The concomitant use of fentanyl with other CNS depressants, including phenothiazines, may cause respiratory depression, hypotension, and profound sedation or potentially result in coma. When such combined therapy is contemplated, the dose of one or both agents should be significantly reduced).
No products indexed under this heading.

Fluphenazine Hydrochloride (The concomitant use of fentanyl with other CNS depressants, including phenothiazines, may cause respiratory depression, hypotension, and profound sedation or potentially result in coma. When such combined therapy is contemplated, the dose of one or both agents should be significantly reduced).
No products indexed under this heading.

Flurazepam Hydrochloride (The concomitant use of fentanyl with other CNS depressants, including sedatives and hypnotics, may cause respiratory depression, hypotension, and profound sedation or potentially result in coma. When such combined therapy is contemplated, the dose of one or both agents should be significantly reduced). Products include:
Dalmane Capsules 3343

Fluvoxamine Maleate (The concurrent use of CYP3A4 inhibitors with transdermal fentanyl may result in an increase in fentanyl plasma concentrations, which could increase or prolong adverse drug effects and may cause serious respiratory depression. In this situation, special patient care and observation are appropriate).
No products indexed under this heading.

Fosamprenavir Calcium (The concurrent use of CYP3A4 inhibitors with transdermal fentanyl may result in an increase in fentanyl plasma concentrations, which could increase or prolong adverse drug effects and may cause serious respiratory depression. In this situation, special patient care and observation are appropriate). Products include:
Lexiva Tablets 1473

Fosphenytoin Sodium (Fentanyl is metabolized mainly via the human cytochrome P450 3A4 isoenzyme system (CYP3A4). Co-administration with agents that induce CYP 3A4 activity may reduce the efficacy of fentanyl).
No products indexed under this heading.

Garlic Extract (Fentanyl is metabolized mainly via the human cytochrome P450 3A4 isoenzyme system (CYP3A4). Co-administration with agents that induce CYP 3A4 activity may reduce the efficacy of fentanyl).
No products indexed under this heading.

Garlic Oil (Fentanyl is metabolized mainly via the human cytochrome P450 3A4 isoenzyme system (CYP3A4). Co-administration with agents that induce CYP 3A4 activity may reduce the efficacy of fentanyl).
No products indexed under this heading.

Glutethimide (The concomitant use of fentanyl with other CNS depressants, including sedatives and hypnotics, may cause respiratory depression, hypotension, and profound sedation or potentially result in coma. When such combined therapy is contemplated, the dose of one or both agents should be significantly reduced).
No products indexed under this heading.

Haloperidol (The concomitant use of fentanyl with other CNS depressants, including tranquilizers, may cause respiratory depression, hypotension, and profound sedation or potentially result in coma. When such combined therapy is contemplated, the dose of one or both agents should be significantly reduced).
No products indexed under this heading.

Haloperidol Decanoate (The concomitant use of fentanyl with other CNS depressants, including tranquilizers, may cause respiratory depression, hypotension, and profound sedation or potentially result in coma. When such combined therapy is contemplated, the dose of one or both agents should be significantly reduced).
No products indexed under this heading.

Hydrocodone Bitartrate (The concomitant use of fentanyl with other CNS depressants, including other opioids, may cause respiratory depression, hypotension, and profound sedation or potentially result in coma. When such combined therapy is contemplated, the dose of one or both agents should be significantly reduced). Products include:
- Hycodan 1104
- Hycomine Compound Tablets 1105
- Hycotuss Expectorant Syrup 1106
- Lortab 3315
- Lortab Elixir 3312
- Vicodin Tablets 530
- Vicodin ES Tablets 531
- Vicodin HP Tablets 532
- Vicoprofen Tablets 533
- Zydone Tablets 1118

Hydrocodone Polistirex (The concomitant use of fentanyl with other CNS depressants, including other opioids, may cause respiratory depression, hypotension, and profound sedation or potentially result in coma. When such combined therapy is contemplated, the dose of one or both agents should be significantly reduced). Products include:
- Tussionex Pennkinetic Extended-Release Suspension 3322

Hydrocortisone (Fentanyl is metabolized mainly via the human cytochrome P450 3A4 isoenzyme system (CYP3A4). Co-administration with agents that induce CYP 3A4 activity may reduce the efficacy of fentanyl). Products include:
- Cortizone•5 Ointment .... ▣ 699
- Cortizone•10 Creme .... ▣ 699
- Cortizone•10 Ointment .... ▣ 699
- Cortizone•10 Plus Creme .... ▣ 700
- Cortizone•10 Maximum Strength Quick Shot Spray .... ▣ 700
- Hydrocortone Tablets 1963
- Preparation H Hydrocortisone Cream .... ▣ 748

Hydrocortisone Acetate (Fentanyl is metabolized mainly via the human cytochrome P450 3A4 isoenzyme system (CYP3A4). Co-administration with agents that induce CYP 3A4 activity may reduce the efficacy of fentanyl). Products include:
- Analpram-HC 1136
- Pramosone 1139
- ProctoFoam-HC 3113
- Tucks Anti-Itch Ointment .... ▣ 712
- U-cort 1% Cream 3289

Hydrocortisone Butyrate (Fentanyl is metabolized mainly via the human cytochrome P450 3A4 isoenzyme system (CYP3A4). Co-administration with agents that induce CYP 3A4 activity may reduce the efficacy of fentanyl). Products include:
- Locoid 1138
- Locoid Lipocream Cream 1138

Hydrocortisone Cypionate (Fentanyl is metabolized mainly via the human cytochrome P450 3A4 isoenzyme system (CYP3A4). Co-administration with agents that induce CYP 3A4 activity may reduce the efficacy of fentanyl).
No products indexed under this heading.

Hydrocortisone Hemisuccinate (Fentanyl is metabolized mainly via the human cytochrome P450 3A4 isoenzyme system (CYP3A4). Co-administration with agents that induce CYP 3A4 activity may reduce the efficacy of fentanyl).
No products indexed under this heading.

Hydrocortisone Probutate (Fentanyl is metabolized mainly via the human cytochrome P450 3A4 isoenzyme system (CYP3A4). Co-administration with agents that induce CYP 3A4 activity may reduce the efficacy of fentanyl). Products include:
- Pandel Cream, 0.1% 1017

Hydrocortisone Sodium Phosphate (Fentanyl is metabolized mainly via the human cytochrome P450 3A4 isoenzyme system (CYP3A4). Co-administration with agents that induce CYP 3A4 activity may reduce the efficacy of fentanyl).
No products indexed under this heading.

Hydrocortisone Sodium Succinate (Fentanyl is metabolized mainly via the human cytochrome P450 3A4 isoenzyme system (CYP3A4). Co-administration with agents that induce CYP 3A4 activity may reduce the efficacy of fentanyl).
No products indexed under this heading.

Hydrocortisone Valerate (Fentanyl is metabolized mainly via the human cytochrome P450 3A4 isoenzyme system (CYP3A4). Co-administration with agents that induce CYP 3A4 activity may reduce the efficacy of fentanyl).
No products indexed under this heading.

Hydromorphone Hydrochloride (The concomitant use of fentanyl with other CNS depressants, including other opioids, may cause respiratory depression, hypotension, and profound sedation or potentially result in coma. When such combined therapy is contemplated, the dose of one or both agents should be significantly reduced). Products include:
- Dilaudid 439
- Dilaudid Oral Liquid 443
- Dilaudid Non-Sterile Powder 439
- Dilaudid Rectal Suppositories 439
- Dilaudid Tablets 439
- Dilaudid Tablets - 8 mg 443
- Dilaudid-HP 441

Hydroxyzine Hydrochloride (The concomitant use of fentanyl with other CNS depressants, including tranquilizers, may cause respiratory depression, hypotension, and profound sedation or potentially result in coma. When such combined therapy is contemplated, the dose of one or both agents should be significantly reduced).
No products indexed under this heading.

Hypericum (Fentanyl is metabolized mainly via the human cytochrome P450 3A4 isoenzyme system (CYP3A4). Co-administration with agents that induce CYP 3A4 activity may reduce the efficacy of fentanyl).
No products indexed under this heading.

Indinavir Sulfate (The concurrent use of CYP3A4 inhibitors with transdermal fentanyl may result in an increase in fentanyl plasma concentrations, which could increase or prolong adverse drug effects and may cause serious respiratory depression. In this situation, special patient care and observation are appropriate). Products include:
- Crixivan Capsules 1918

Isocarboxazid (Fentanyl is not recommended for use in patients who have received monoamine oxidase (MAO) inhibitors within 14 days because severe and unpredictable potentiation by MAO inhibitors has been reported with opioid analgesics).
No products indexed under this heading.

Isoflurane (The comcomitant use of fentanyl with other CNS depressants may cause respiratory depression, hypotension, and profound sedation or potentially result in coma. When such combined therapy is contemplated, the dose of one or both agents should be significantly reduced).
No products indexed under this heading.

Isoniazid (The concurrent use of CYP3A4 inhibitors with transdermal fentanyl may result in an increase in fentanyl plasma concentrations, which could increase or prolong adverse drug effects and may cause serious respiratory depression. In this situation, special patient care and observation are appropriate).
No products indexed under this heading.

Itraconazole (The concurrent use of CYP3A4 inhibitors with transdermal fentanyl may result in an increase in fentanyl plasma concentrations, which could increase or prolong adverse drug effects and may cause serious respiratory depression. In this situation, special patient care and observation are appropriate).
No products indexed under this heading.

Ketamine Hydrochloride (The comcomitant use of fentanyl with other CNS depressants may cause respiratory depression, hypotension, and profound sedation or potentially result in coma. When such combined therapy is contemplated, the dose of one or both agents should be significantly reduced).
No products indexed under this heading.

Ketoconazole (The concurrent use of CYP3A4 inhibitors with transdermal fentanyl may result in an increase in fentanyl plasma concentrations, which could increase or prolong adverse drug effects and may cause serious respiratory depression. In this situation, special patient care and observation are appropriate). Products include:
- Nizoral A-D Shampoo, 1% 1839
- Nizoral 2% Shampoo 1838

Levomethadyl Acetate Hydrochloride (The comcomitant use of fentanyl with other CNS depressants may cause respiratory depression, hypotension, and profound sedation or potentially result in coma. When such combined therapy is contemplated, the dose of one or both agents should be significantly reduced).
No products indexed under this heading.

Levorphanol Tartrate (The concomitant use of fentanyl with other CNS depressants, including other opioids, may cause respiratory depression, hypotension, and profound sedation or potentially result in coma. When such combined therapy is contemplated, the dose of one or both agents should be significantly reduced).
No products indexed under this heading.

Lopinavir (The concurrent use of CYP3A4 inhibitors with transdermal fentanyl may result in an increase in fentanyl plasma concentrations, which could increase or prolong adverse drug effects and may cause serious respiratory depression. In this situation, special patient care and observation are appropriate). Products include:
- Kaletra 474

Loratadine (The concurrent use of CYP3A4 inhibitors with transdermal fentanyl may result in an increase in fentanyl plasma concentrations, which could increase or prolong adverse drug effects and may cause

serious respiratory depression. In this situation, special patient care and observation are appropriate). Products include:

- Alavert Allergy & Sinus D-12 Hour Tablets 743
- Alavert 743
- Children's Claritin 24 Hour Non-Drowsy Allergy Syrup 732
- Claritin Non-Drowsy 24 Hour Tablets 731
- Non-Drowsy Claritin Hives Relief Tablets 733
- Claritin Reditabs 24 Hour Non-Drowsy Tablets 732
- Claritin-D Non-Drowsy 12 Hour Tablets 731
- Claritin-D Non-Drowsy 24 Hour Tablets 731
- Children's Dimetapp ND Non-Drowsy Allergy Syrup 746
- Triaminic Allerchews 684

Lorazepam (The concomitant use of fentanyl with other CNS depressants, including sedatives and hypnotics, may cause respiratory depression, hypotension, and profound sedation or potentially result in coma. When such combined therapy is contemplated, the dose of one or both agents should be significantly reduced).
No products indexed under this heading.

Loxapine Hydrochloride (The concomitant use of fentanyl with other CNS depressants, including tranquilizers, may cause respiratory depression, hypotension, and profound sedation or potentially result in coma. When such combined therapy is contemplated, the dose of one or both agents should be significantly reduced).
No products indexed under this heading.

Loxapine Succinate (The concomitant use of fentanyl with other CNS depressants, including tranquilizers, may cause respiratory depression, hypotension, and profound sedation or potentially result in coma. When such combined therapy is contemplated, the dose of one or both agents should be significantly reduced).
No products indexed under this heading.

Meperidine Hydrochloride (The concomitant use of fentanyl with other CNS depressants, including other opioids, may cause respiratory depression, hypotension, and profound sedation or potentially result in coma. When such combined therapy is contemplated, the dose of one or both agents should be significantly reduced).
No products indexed under this heading.

Mephenytoin (Fentanyl is metabolized mainly via the human cytochrome P450 3A4 isoenzyme system (CYP3A4). Co-administration with agents that induce CYP 3A4 activity may reduce the efficacy of fentanyl).
No products indexed under this heading.

Mephobarbital (The comcomitant use of fentanyl with other CNS depressants may cause respiratory depression, hypotension, and profound sedation or potentially result in coma. When such combined therapy is contemplated, the dose of one or both agents should be significantly reduced). Products include:

- Mebaral Tablets, USP 2483

Meprobamate (The concomitant use of fentanyl with other CNS depressants, including tranquilizers, may cause respiratory depression, hypotension, and profound sedation or potentially result in coma. When such combined therapy is contemplated, the dose of one or both agents should be significantly reduced).
No products indexed under this heading.

Mesoridazine Besylate (The concomitant use of fentanyl with other CNS depressants, including phenothiazines, may cause respiratory depression, hypotension, and profound sedation or potentially result in coma. When such combined therapy is contemplated, the dose of one or both agents should be significantly reduced).
No products indexed under this heading.

Metaxalone (The concomitant use of fentanyl with other CNS depressants, including skeletal muscle relaxants, may cause respiratory depression, hypotension, and profound sedation or potentially result in coma. When such combined therapy is contemplated, the dose of one or both agents should be significantly reduced). Products include:

- Skelaxin Tablets 1685

Methadone Hydrochloride (The concomitant use of fentanyl with other CNS depressants, including other opioids, may cause respiratory depression, hypotension, and profound sedation or potentially result in coma. When such combined therapy is contemplated, the dose of one or both agents should be significantly reduced).
No products indexed under this heading.

Methocarbamol (The concomitant use of fentanyl with other CNS depressants, including skeletal muscle relaxants, may cause respiratory depression, hypotension, and profound sedation or potentially result in coma. When such combined therapy is contemplated, the dose of one or both agents should be significantly reduced).
No products indexed under this heading.

Methohexital Sodium (The concomitant use of fentanyl with other CNS depressants may cause respiratory depression, hypotension, and profound sedation or potentially result in coma. When such combined therapy is contemplated, the dose of one or both agents should be significantly reduced).
No products indexed under this heading.

Methotrimeprazine (The concomitant use of fentanyl with other CNS depressants, including phenothiazines, may cause respiratory depression, hypotension, and profound sedation or potentially result in coma. When such combined therapy is contemplated, the dose of one or both agents should be significantly reduced).
No products indexed under this heading.

Methoxyflurane (The comcomitant use of fentanyl with other CNS depressants may cause respiratory depression, hypotension, and profound sedation or potentially result in coma. When such combined therapy is contemplated, the dose of one or both agents should be significantly reduced).
No products indexed under this heading.

Methsuximide (Fentanyl is metabolized mainly via the human cytochrome P450 3A4 isoenzyme system (CYP3A4). Co-administration with agents that induce CYP 3A4 activity may reduce the efficacy of fentanyl).
No products indexed under this heading.

Methylprednisolone (Fentanyl is metabolized mainly via the human cytochrome P450 3A4 isoenzyme system (CYP3A4). Co-administration with agents that induce CYP 3A4 activity may reduce the efficacy of fentanyl).
No products indexed under this heading.

Methylprednisolone Acetate (Fentanyl is metabolized mainly via the human cytochrome P450 3A4 isoenzyme system (CYP3A4). Co-administration with agents that induce CYP 3A4 activity may reduce the efficacy of fentanyl). Products include:

- Depo-Medrol Injectable Suspension 2615
- Depo-Medrol Single-Dose Vial 2617

Methylprednisolone Sodium Succinate (Fentanyl is metabolized mainly via the human cytochrome P450 3A4 isoenzyme system (CYP3A4). Co-administration with agents that induce CYP 3A4 activity may reduce the efficacy of fentanyl).
No products indexed under this heading.

Metronidazole (The concurrent use of CYP3A4 inhibitors with transdermal fentanyl may result in an increase in fentanyl plasma concentrations, which could increase or prolong adverse drug effects and may cause serious respiratory depression. In this situation, special patient care and observation are appropriate). Products include:

- Metrogel 1% 1212
- MetroGel-Vaginal Gel 1822
- Noritate Cream, 1% 1051

Metronidazole Benzoate (The concurrent use of CYP3A4 inhibitors with transdermal fentanyl may result in an increase in fentanyl plasma concentrations, which could increase or prolong adverse drug effects and may cause serious respiratory depression. In this situation, special patient care and observation are appropriate).
No products indexed under this heading.

Metronidazole Hydrochloride (The concurrent use of CYP3A4 inhibitors with transdermal fentanyl may result in an increase in fentanyl plasma concentrations, which could increase or prolong adverse drug effects and may cause serious respiratory depression. In this situation, special patient care and observation are appropriate).
No products indexed under this heading.

Miconazole (The concurrent use of CYP3A4 inhibitors with transdermal fentanyl may result in an increase in fentanyl plasma concentrations, which could increase or prolong adverse drug effects and may cause serious respiratory depression. In this situation, special patient care and observation are appropriate).
No products indexed under this heading.

Miconazole Nitrate (The concurrent use of CYP3A4 inhibitors with transdermal fentanyl may result in an increase in fentanyl plasma concentrations, which could increase or prolong adverse drug effects and may cause serious respiratory depression. In this situation, special patient care and observation are appropriate). Products include:

- Desenex 674
- Desenex Jock Itch Spray Powder 674

Midazolam Hydrochloride (The concomitant use of fentanyl with other CNS depressants, including sedatives and hypnotics, may cause respiratory depression, hypotension, and profound sedation or potentially result in coma. When such combined therapy is contemplated, the dose of one or both agents should be significantly reduced).
No products indexed under this heading.

Moclobemide (Fentanyl is not recommended for use in patients who have received monoamine oxidase (MAO) inhibitors within 14 days because severe and unpredictable potentiation by MAO inhibitors has been reported with opioid analgesics).
No products indexed under this heading.

Modafinil (Fentanyl is metabolized mainly via the human cytochrome P450 3A4 isoenzyme system (CYP3A4). Co-administration with agents that induce CYP 3A4 activity may reduce the efficacy of fentanyl). Products include:

- Provigil Tablets 1002

Molindone Hydrochloride (The concomitant use of fentanyl with other CNS depressants, including tranquilizers, may cause respiratory depression, hypotension, and profound sedation or potentially result in coma. When such combined therapy is contemplated, the dose of one or both agents should be significantly reduced). Products include:

- Moban Tablets 1108

Morphine Sulfate (The concomitant use of fentanyl with other CNS depressants, including other opioids, may cause respiratory depression, hypotension, and profound sedation or potentially result in coma. When such combined therapy is contemplated, the dose of one or both agents should be significantly reduced). Products include:

- Avinza Capsules 1714
- Kadian Capsules 572
- MS Contin Tablets 2703

Nefazodone Hydrochloride (The concurrent use of CYP3A4 inhibitors with transdermal fentanyl may result in an increase in fentanyl plasma concentrations, which could increase or prolong adverse drug effects and may cause serious respiratory depression. In this situation, special patient care and observation are appropriate).
No products indexed under this heading.

Nelfinavir Mesylate (The concurrent use of CYP3A4 inhibitors with transdermal fentanyl may result in an increase in fentanyl plasma concentrations, which could increase or prolong adverse drug effects and may cause serious respiratory depression. In this situation, special patient care and observation are appropriate). Products include:

Viracept 2556

Nevirapine (The concurrent use of CYP3A4 inhibitors with transdermal fentanyl may result in an increase in fentanyl plasma concentrations, which could increase or prolong adverse drug effects and may cause serious respiratory depression. In this situation, special patient care and observation are appropriate). Products include:

Viramune Oral Suspension 903
Viramune Tablets 903

Niacinamide (The concurrent use of CYP3A4 inhibitors with transdermal fentanyl may result in an increase in fentanyl plasma concentrations, which could increase or prolong adverse drug effects and may cause serious respiratory depression. In this situation, special patient care and observation are appropriate).

No products indexed under this heading.

Nicotinamide (The concurrent use of CYP3A4 inhibitors with transdermal fentanyl may result in an increase in fentanyl plasma concentrations, which could increase or prolong adverse drug effects and may cause serious respiratory depression. In this situation, special patient care and observation are appropriate). Products include:

Nicomide Tablets 3190

Nifedipine (The concurrent use of CYP3A4 inhibitors with transdermal fentanyl may result in an increase in fentanyl plasma concentrations, which could increase or prolong adverse drug effects and may cause serious respiratory depression. In this situation, special patient care and observation are appropriate). Products include:

Adalat CC Tablets 2978

Norfloxacin (The concurrent use of CYP3A4 inhibitors with transdermal fentanyl may result in an increase in fentanyl plasma concentrations, which could increase or prolong adverse drug effects and may cause serious respiratory depression. In this situation, special patient care and observation are appropriate). Products include:

Noroxin Tablets 2009

Olanzapine (The comcomitant use of fentanyl with other CNS depressants may cause respiratory depression, hypotension, and profound sedation or potentially result in coma. When such combined therapy is contemplated, the dose of one or both agents should be significantly reduced). Products include:

Symbyax Capsules 1788
Zyprexa Tablets 1798
Zyprexa IntraMuscular 1798
Zyprexa ZYDIS Orally Disintegrating Tablets 1798

Omeprazole (The concurrent use of CYP3A4 inhibitors with transdermal fentanyl may result in an increase in fentanyl plasma concentrations, which could increase or prolong adverse drug effects and may cause serious respiratory depression. In this situation, special patient care and observation are appropriate). Products include:

Zegerid Powder for Oral Solution 2972

Orphenadrine Citrate (The concomitant use of fentanyl with other CNS depressants, including skeletal muscle relaxants, may cause respiratory depression, hypotension, and profound sedation or potentially result in coma. When such combined therapy is contemplated, the dose of one or both agents should be significantly reduced). Products include:

Norflex Injection 1824

Oxazepam (The concomitant use of fentanyl with other CNS depressants, including tranquilizers, may cause respiratory depression, hypotension, and profound sedation or potentially result in coma. When such combined therapy is contemplated, the dose of one or both agents should be significantly reduced).

No products indexed under this heading.

Oxcarbazepine (Fentanyl is metabolized mainly via the human cytochrome P450 3A4 isoenzyme system (CYP3A4). Co-administration with agents that induce CYP 3A4 activity may reduce the efficacy of fentanyl). Products include:

Trileptal Oral Suspension 2281
Trileptal Tablets 2281

Oxycodone Hydrochloride (The concomitant use of fentanyl with other CNS depressants, including other opioids, may cause respiratory depression, hypotension, and profound sedation or potentially result in coma. When such combined therapy is contemplated, the dose of one or both agents should be significantly reduced). Products include:

Combunox Tablets 1183
OxyContin Tablets 2699
OxyFast Oral Concentrate Solution 2704
OxyIR Capsules 2704
Percocet Tablets 1114
Percodan Tablets 1115

Pargyline Hydrochloride (Fentanyl is not recommended for use in patients who have received monoamine oxidase (MAO) inhibitors within 14 days because severe and unpredictable potentiation by MAO inhibitors has been reported with opioid analgesics).

No products indexed under this heading.

Paroxetine Hydrochloride (The concurrent use of CYP3A4 inhibitors with transdermal fentanyl may result in an increase in fentanyl plasma concentrations, which could increase or prolong adverse drug effects and may cause serious respiratory depression. In this situation, special patient care and observation are appropriate). Products include:

Paxil CR Controlled-Release Tablets 1509
Paxil 1501

Pentobarbital Sodium (The comcomitant use of fentanyl with other CNS depressants may cause respiratory depression, hypotension, and profound sedation or potentially result in coma. When such combined therapy is contemplated, the dose of one or both agents should be significantly reduced). Products include:

Nembutal Sodium Solution, USP 2484

Perphenazine (The concomitant use of fentanyl with other CNS depressants, including phenothiazines, may cause respiratory depression, hypotension, and profound sedation or potentially result in coma. When such combined therapy is contemplated, the dose of one or both agents should be significantly reduced).

No products indexed under this heading.

Phenelzine Sulfate (Fentanyl is not recommended for use in patients who have received monoamine oxidase (MAO) inhibitors within 14 days because severe and unpredictable potentiation by MAO inhibitors has been reported with opioid analgesics).

No products indexed under this heading.

Phenobarbital (The comcomitant use of fentanyl with other CNS depressants may cause respiratory depression, hypotension, and profound sedation or potentially result in coma. When such combined therapy is contemplated, the dose of one or both agents should be significantly reduced).

No products indexed under this heading.

Phenobarbital Sodium (Fentanyl is metabolized mainly via the human cytochrome P450 3A4 isoenzyme system (CYP3A4). Co-administration with agents that induce CYP 3A4 activity may reduce the efficacy of fentanyl).

No products indexed under this heading.

Phenytoin (Fentanyl is metabolized mainly via the human cytochrome P450 3A4 isoenzyme system (CYP3A4). Co-administration with agents that induce CYP 3A4 activity may reduce the efficacy of fentanyl).

No products indexed under this heading.

Phenytoin Sodium (Fentanyl is metabolized mainly via the human cytochrome P450 3A4 isoenzyme system (CYP3A4). Co-administration with agents that induce CYP 3A4 activity may reduce the efficacy of fentanyl). Products include:

Phenytek Capsules 2153

Prazepam (The concomitant use of fentanyl with other CNS depressants, including tranquilizers, may cause respiratory depression, hypotension, and profound sedation or potentially result in coma. When such combined therapy is contemplated, the dose of one or both agents should be significantly reduced).

No products indexed under this heading.

Prednisolone Acetate (Fentanyl is metabolized mainly via the human cytochrome P450 3A4 isoenzyme system (CYP3A4). Co-administration with agents that induce CYP 3A4 activity may reduce the efficacy of fentanyl). Products include:

Blephamide Ophthalmic Ointment 563
Blephamide Ophthalmic Suspension 564
Poly-Pred Liquifilm Ophthalmic Suspension .... ⊙ 231
Pred Forte Ophthalmic Suspension .... ⊙ 233
Pred Mild Sterile Ophthalmic Suspension .... ⊙ 236
Pred-G Ophthalmic Suspension .... ⊙ 234
Pred-G Sterile Ophthalmic Ointment .... ⊙ 235

Prednisolone Sodium Phosphate (Fentanyl is metabolized mainly via the human cytochrome P450 3A4 isoenzyme system (CYP3A4). Co-administration with agents that induce CYP 3A4 activity may reduce the efficacy of fentanyl). Products include:

Pediapred Oral Solution 3319

Prednisolone Tebutate (Fentanyl is metabolized mainly via the human cytochrome P450 3A4 isoenzyme system (CYP3A4). Co-administration with agents that induce CYP 3A4 activity may reduce the efficacy of fentanyl).

No products indexed under this heading.

Prednisone (Fentanyl is metabolized mainly via the human cytochrome P450 3A4 isoenzyme system (CYP3A4). Co-administration with agents that induce CYP 3A4 activity may reduce the efficacy of fentanyl).

No products indexed under this heading.

Primidone (Fentanyl is metabolized mainly via the human cytochrome P450 3A4 isoenzyme system (CYP3A4). Co-administration with agents that induce CYP 3A4 activity may reduce the efficacy of fentanyl).

No products indexed under this heading.

Procarbazine Hydrochloride (Fentanyl is not recommended for use in patients who have received monoamine oxidase (MAO) inhibitors within 14 days because severe and unpredictable potentiation by MAO inhibitors has been reported with opioid analgesics). Products include:

Matulane Capsules 3188

Prochlorperazine (The concomitant use of fentanyl with other CNS depressants, including phenothiazines, may cause respiratory depression, hypotension, and profound sedation or potentially result in coma. When such combined therapy is contemplated, the dose of one or both agents should be significantly reduced).

No products indexed under this heading.

Propofol (The concomitant use of fentanyl with other CNS depressants, including sedatives and hypnotics, may cause respiratory depression, hypotension, and profound sedation or potentially result in coma. When such combined therapy is contemplated, the dose of one or both agents should be significantly reduced). Products include:

Diprivan Injectable Emulsion 676

Propoxyphene Hydrochloride (The concomitant use of fentanyl with other CNS depressants, including other opioids, may cause respiratory depression, hypotension, and profound sedation or potentially result in coma. When such combined therapy is contemplated, the dose of one or both agents should be significantly reduced).

No products indexed under this heading.

Propoxyphene Napsylate (The concomitant use of fentanyl with other CNS depressants, including other opioids, may cause respiratory depression, hypotension, and profound sedation or potentially result in

coma. When such combined therapy is contemplated, the dose of one or both agents should be significantly reduced). Products include:
Darvocet A 500 Tablets 3497

Quazepam (The concomitant use of fentanyl with other CNS depressants, including sedatives and hypnotics, may cause respiratory depression, hypotension, and profound sedation or potentially result in coma. When such combined therapy is contemplated, the dose of one or both agents should be significantly reduced).
No products indexed under this heading.

Quetiapine Fumarate (The comcomitant use of fentanyl with other CNS depressants may cause respiratory depression, hypotension, and profound sedation or potentially result in coma. When such combined therapy is contemplated, the dose of one or both agents should be significantly reduced). Products include:
Seroquel Tablets 691

Quinidine (The concurrent use of CYP3A4 inhibitors with transdermal fentanyl may result in an increase in fentanyl plasma concentrations, which could increase or prolong adverse drug effects and may cause serious respiratory depression. In this situation, special patient care and observation are appropriate).
No products indexed under this heading.

Quinidine Hydrochloride (The concurrent use of CYP3A4 inhibitors with transdermal fentanyl may result in an increase in fentanyl plasma concentrations, which could increase or prolong adverse drug effects and may cause serious respiratory depression. In this situation, special patient care and observation are appropriate).
No products indexed under this heading.

Quinidine Polygalacturonate (The concurrent use of CYP3A4 inhibitors with transdermal fentanyl may result in an increase in fentanyl plasma concentrations, which could increase or prolong adverse drug effects and may cause serious respiratory depression. In this situation, special patient care and observation are appropriate).
No products indexed under this heading.

Quinidine Sulfate (The concurrent use of CYP3A4 inhibitors with transdermal fentanyl may result in an increase in fentanyl plasma concentrations, which could increase or prolong adverse drug effects and may cause serious respiratory depression. In this situation, special patient care and observation are appropriate).
No products indexed under this heading.

Quinine (The concurrent use of CYP3A4 inhibitors with transdermal fentanyl may result in an increase in fentanyl plasma concentrations, which could increase or prolong adverse drug effects and may cause serious respiratory depression. In this situation, special patient care and observation are appropriate).
No products indexed under this heading.

Quinine Sulfate (The concurrent use of CYP3A4 inhibitors with transdermal fentanyl may result in an increase in fentanyl plasma concentrations, which could increase or prolong adverse drug effects and may cause serious respiratory depression. In this situation, special patient care and observation are appropriate).
No products indexed under this heading.

Quinupristin (The concurrent use of CYP3A4 inhibitors with transdermal fentanyl may result in an increase in fentanyl plasma concentrations, which could increase or prolong adverse drug effects and may cause serious respiratory depression. In this situation, special patient care and observation are appropriate). Products include:
Synercid I.V. 1690

Ranitidine Bismuth Citrate (The concurrent use of CYP3A4 inhibitors with transdermal fentanyl may result in an increase in fentanyl plasma concentrations, which could increase or prolong adverse drug effects and may cause serious respiratory depression. In this situation, special patient care and observation are appropriate).
No products indexed under this heading.

Ranitidine Hydrochloride (The concurrent use of CYP3A4 inhibitors with transdermal fentanyl may result in an increase in fentanyl plasma concentrations, which could increase or prolong adverse drug effects and may cause serious respiratory depression. In this situation, special patient care and observation are appropriate). Products include:
Zantac 1597
Zantac Injection 1593
Zantac 75 Tablets .... ▣715
Zantac 150 Maximum Strength Tablets .... ▣715
Zantac Injection Pharmacy Bulk Package 1595

Remifentanil Hydrochloride (The concomitant use of fentanyl with other CNS depressants, including other opioids, may cause respiratory depression, hypotension, and profound sedation or potentially result in coma. When such combined therapy is contemplated, the dose of one or both agents should be significantly reduced).
No products indexed under this heading.

Rifabutin (Fentanyl is metabolized mainly via the human cytochrome P450 3A4 isoenzyme system (CYP3A4). Co-administration with agents that induce CYP 3A4 activity may reduce the efficacy of fentanyl).
No products indexed under this heading.

Rifampicin (Fentanyl is metabolized mainly via the human cytochrome P450 3A4 isoenzyme system (CYP3A4). Co-administration with agents that induce CYP 3A4 activity may reduce the efficacy of fentanyl).
No products indexed under this heading.

Rifampin (Fentanyl is metabolized mainly via the human cytochrome P450 3A4 isoenzyme system (CYP3A4). Co-administration with agents that induce CYP 3A4 activity may reduce the efficacy of fentanyl).
No products indexed under this heading.

Rifapentine (Fentanyl is metabolized mainly via the human cytochrome P450 3A4 isoenzyme system (CYP3A4). Co-administration with agents that induce CYP 3A4 activity may reduce the efficacy of fentanyl).
No products indexed under this heading.

Risperidone (The comcomitant use of fentanyl with other CNS depressants may cause respiratory depression, hypotension, and profound sedation or potentially result in coma. When such combined therapy is contemplated, the dose of one or both agents should be significantly reduced). Products include:
Risperdal Consta Long-Acting Injection 1664
Risperdal M-Tab Orally Disintegrating Tablets 1658
Risperdal 1658

Ritonavir (The concurrent use of CYP3A4 inhibitors with transdermal fentanyl may result in an increase in fentanyl plasma concentrations, which could increase or prolong adverse drug effects and may cause serious respiratory depression. In this situation, special patient care and observation are appropriate). Products include:
Kaletra 474
Norvir 499

Saquinavir (The concurrent use of CYP3A4 inhibitors with transdermal fentanyl may result in an increase in fentanyl plasma concentrations, which could increase or prolong adverse drug effects and may cause serious respiratory depression. In this situation, special patient care and observation are appropriate).
No products indexed under this heading.

Saquinavir Mesylate (The concurrent use of CYP3A4 inhibitors with transdermal fentanyl may result in an increase in fentanyl plasma concentrations, which could increase or prolong adverse drug effects and may cause serious respiratory depression. In this situation, special patient care and observation are appropriate). Products include:
Invirase 2776

Secobarbital Sodium (The concomitant use of fentanyl with other CNS depressants, including sedatives and hypnotics, may cause respiratory depression, hypotension, and profound sedation or potentially result in coma. When such combined therapy is contemplated, the dose of one or both agents should be significantly reduced).
No products indexed under this heading.

Selegiline Hydrochloride (Fentanyl is not recommended for use in patients who have received monoamine oxidase (MAO) inhibitors within 14 days because severe and unpredictable potentiation by MAO inhibitors has been reported with opioid analgesics). Products include:
Eldepryl Capsules 3209

Sertraline Hydrochloride (The concurrent use of CYP3A4 inhibitors with transdermal fentanyl may result in an increase in fentanyl plasma concentrations, which could increase or prolong adverse drug effects and may cause serious respiratory depression. In this situation, special patient care and observation are appropriate). Products include:
Zoloft 2581

Sevoflurane (The comcomitant use of fentanyl with other CNS depressants may cause respiratory depression, hypotension, and profound sedation or potentially result in coma. When such combined therapy is contemplated, the dose of one or both agents should be significantly reduced). Products include:
Ultane Liquid for Inhalation 526

Sufentanil Citrate (The concomitant use of fentanyl with other CNS depressants, including other opioids, may cause respiratory depression, hypotension, and profound sedation or potentially result in coma. When such combined therapy is contemplated, the dose of one or both agents should be significantly reduced).
No products indexed under this heading.

Sulfinpyrazone (Fentanyl is metabolized mainly via the human cytochrome P450 3A4 isoenzyme system (CYP3A4). Co-administration with agents that induce CYP 3A4 activity may reduce the efficacy of fentanyl).
No products indexed under this heading.

Telithromycin (The concurrent use of CYP3A4 inhibitors with transdermal fentanyl may result in an increase in fentanyl plasma concentrations, which could increase or prolong adverse drug effects and may cause serious respiratory depression. In this situation, special patient care and observation are appropriate). Products include:
Ketek Tablets 2920

Temazepam (The concomitant use of fentanyl with other CNS depressants, including sedatives and hypnotics, may cause respiratory depression, hypotension, and profound sedation or potentially result in coma. When such combined therapy is contemplated, the dose of one or both agents should be significantly reduced).
No products indexed under this heading.

Theophylline (Fentanyl is metabolized mainly via the human cytochrome P450 3A4 isoenzyme system (CYP3A4). Co-administration with agents that induce CYP 3A4 activity may reduce the efficacy of fentanyl).
No products indexed under this heading.

Thiamylal Sodium (The comcomitant use of fentanyl with other CNS depressants may cause respiratory depression, hypotension, and profound sedation or potentially result in coma. When such combined therapy is contemplated, the dose of one or both agents should be significantly reduced).
No products indexed under this heading.

Thioridazine Hydrochloride (The concomitant use of fentanyl with other CNS depressants, including phenothiazines, may cause respiratory depression, hypotension, and profound sedation or potentially result in coma. When such combined therapy is contemplated, the dose of one or both agents should be significantly reduced). Products include:
Thioridazine Hydrochloride Tablets 2122

Thiothixene (The concomitant use of fentanyl with other CNS depressants, including tranquilizers, may cause respiratory depression, hypotension, and profound sedation or potentially result in coma. When such combined therapy is contemplated, the dose of one or both agents should be significantly reduced). Products include:
Thiothixene Capsules **2124**

Tranylcypromine Sulfate (Fentanyl is not recommended for use in patients who have received monoamine oxidase (MAO) inhibitors within 14 days because severe and unpredictable potentiation by MAO inhibitors has been reported with opioid analgesics). Products include:
Parnate Tablets **1499**

Triamcinolone (Fentanyl is metabolized mainly via the human cytochrome P450 3A4 isoenzyme system (CYP3A4). Co-administration with agents that induce CYP 3A4 activity may reduce the efficacy of fentanyl).
No products indexed under this heading.

Triamcinolone Acetonide (Fentanyl is metabolized mainly via the human cytochrome P450 3A4 isoenzyme system (CYP3A4). Co-administration with agents that induce CYP 3A4 activity may reduce the efficacy of fentanyl). Products include:
Azmacort Inhalation Aerosol **1701**
Nasacort HFA Inhalation Aerosol **2939**
Nasacort AQ Nasal Spray **2937**

Triamcinolone Diacetate (Fentanyl is metabolized mainly via the human cytochrome P450 3A4 isoenzyme system (CYP3A4). Co-administration with agents that induce CYP 3A4 activity may reduce the efficacy of fentanyl).
No products indexed under this heading.

Triamcinolone Hexacetonide (Fentanyl is metabolized mainly via the human cytochrome P450 3A4 isoenzyme system (CYP3A4). Co-administration with agents that induce CYP 3A4 activity may reduce the efficacy of fentanyl).
No products indexed under this heading.

Triazolam (The concomitant use of fentanyl with other CNS depressants, including sedatives and hypnotics, may cause respiratory depression, hypotension, and profound sedation or potentially result in coma. When such combined therapy is contemplated, the dose of one or both agents should be significantly reduced).
No products indexed under this heading.

Trifluoperazine Hydrochloride (The concomitant use of fentanyl with other CNS depressants, including phenothiazines, may cause respiratory depression, hypotension, and profound sedation or potentially result in coma. When such combined therapy is contemplated, the dose of one or both agents should be significantly reduced).
No products indexed under this heading.

Troglitazone (The concurrent use of CYP3A4 inhibitors with transdermal fentanyl may result in an increase in fentanyl plasma concentrations, which could increase or prolong adverse drug effects and may cause serious respiratory depression. In this situation, special patient care and observation are appropriate).
No products indexed under this heading.

Troleandomycin (The concurrent use of CYP3A4 inhibitors with transdermal fentanyl may result in an increase in fentanyl plasma concentrations, which could increase or prolong adverse drug effects and may cause serious respiratory depression. In this situation, special patient care and observation are appropriate).
No products indexed under this heading.

Valproate Sodium (The concurrent use of CYP3A4 inhibitors with transdermal fentanyl may result in an increase in fentanyl plasma concentrations, which could increase or prolong adverse drug effects and may cause serious respiratory depression. In this situation, special patient care and observation are appropriate). Products include:
Depacon Injection **412**

Verapamil Hydrochloride (The concurrent use of CYP3A4 inhibitors with transdermal fentanyl may result in an increase in fentanyl plasma concentrations, which could increase or prolong adverse drug effects and may cause serious respiratory depression. In this situation, special patient care and observation are appropriate). Products include:
Covera-HS Tablets **3135**
Tarka Tablets **519**
Verelan PM Capsules **3120**

Voriconazole (The concurrent use of CYP3A4 inhibitors with transdermal fentanyl may result in an increase in fentanyl plasma concentrations, which could increase or prolong adverse drug effects and may cause serious respiratory depression. In this situation, special patient care and observation are appropriate). Products include:
VFEND I.V. **2543**
VFEND Oral Suspension **2543**
VFEND Tablets **2543**

Zafirlukast (The concurrent use of CYP3A4 inhibitors with transdermal fentanyl may result in an increase in fentanyl plasma concentrations, which could increase or prolong adverse drug effects and may cause serious respiratory depression. In this situation, special patient care and observation are appropriate). Products include:
Accolate Tablets **663**

Zaleplon (The concomitant use of fentanyl with other CNS depressants, including sedatives and hypnotics, may cause respiratory depression, hypotension, and profound sedation or potentially result in coma. When such combined therapy is contemplated, the dose of one or both agents should be significantly reduced). Products include:
Sonata Capsules **1686**

Zileuton (The concurrent use of CYP3A4 inhibitors with transdermal fentanyl may result in an increase in fentanyl plasma concentrations, which could increase or prolong adverse drug effects and may cause serious respiratory depression. In this situation, special patient care and observation are appropriate).
No products indexed under this heading.

Ziprasidone Hydrochloride (The comcomitant use of fentanyl with other CNS depressants may cause respiratory depression, hypotension, and profound sedation or potentially result in coma. When such combined therapy is contemplated, the dose of one or both agents should be significantly reduced). Products include:
Geodon Capsules **2514**

Zolpidem Tartrate (The concomitant use of fentanyl with other CNS depressants, including sedatives and hypnotics, may cause respiratory depression, hypotension, and profound sedation or potentially result in coma. When such combined therapy is contemplated, the dose of one or both agents should be significantly reduced). Products include:
Ambien Tablets **2867**

Food Interactions

Alcohol (The concomitant use of fentanyl with other CNS depressants, including alcohol, may cause respiratory depression, hypotension, and profound sedation or potentially result in coma. When such combined therapy is contemplated, the dose of one or both agents should be significantly reduced).

Grapefruit (The concurrent use of CYP3A4 inhibitors with transdermal fentanyl may result in an increase in fentanyl plasma concentrations, which could increase or prolong adverse drug effects and may cause serious respiratory depression. In this situation, special patient care and observation are appropriate).

Grapefruit Juice (The concurrent use of CYP3A4 inhibitors with transdermal fentanyl may result in an increase in fentanyl plasma concentrations, which could increase or prolong adverse drug effects and may cause serious respiratory depression. In this situation, special patient care and observation are appropriate).

DYAZIDE CAPSULES

(Hydrochlorothiazide, Triamterene) **1389**
May interact with ACE inhibitors, antihypertensives, corticosteroids, oral anticoagulants, antigout agents, oral hypoglycemic agents, insulin, lithium preparations, nondepolarizing neuromuscular blocking agents, nonsteroidal anti-inflammatory agents, potassium preparations, potassium sparing diuretics, and certain other agents. Compounds in these categories include:

Acarbose (Increased risk of severe hyponatremia). Products include:
Precose Tablets **776**

Acebutolol Hydrochloride (May add to potentiate the action of other hypertensives).
No products indexed under this heading.

ACTH (May intensify electrolyte imbalance, particularly hypokalemia).
No products indexed under this heading.

Allopurinol (Dyazide may raise the level of blood uric acid; may require dosage adjustment of antigout agent).
No products indexed under this heading.

Amiloride Hydrochloride (Concurrent use is contraindicated). Products include:
Midamor Tablets **2000**
Moduretic Tablets **2003**

Amlodipine Besylate (May add to potentiate the action of other hypertensives). Products include:
Caduet Tablets **2507**
Lotrel Capsules **2238**
Norvasc Tablets **2529**

Amphotericin B (May intensify electrolyte imbalance, particularly hypokalemia).
No products indexed under this heading.

Anisindione (Effects of oral anticoagulants may be decreased). Products include:
Miradon Tablets **3056**

Atenolol (May add to potentiate the action of other hypertensives). Products include:
Tenormin I.V. Injection **698**
Tenormin Tablets **695**

Atracurium Besylate (Increased paralyzing effect).
No products indexed under this heading.

Benazepril Hydrochloride (May add to potentiate the action of other hypertensives; increased risk of hyperkalemia). Products include:
Lotensin Tablets **2232**
Lotensin HCT Tablets **2235**
Lotrel Capsules **2238**

Bendroflumethiazide (May add to potentiate the action of other hypertensives).
No products indexed under this heading.

Betamethasone Acetate (May intensify electrolyte imbalance, particularly hypokalemia).
No products indexed under this heading.

Betamethasone Sodium Phosphate (May intensify electrolyte imbalance, particularly hypokalemia).
No products indexed under this heading.

Betaxolol Hydrochloride (May add to potentiate the action of other hypertensives). Products include:
Betoptic S Ophthalmic Suspension................................ **554**

Bisoprolol Fumarate (May add to potentiate the action of other hypertensives).
No products indexed under this heading.

Blood, whole (Concurrent use of whole blood from blood bank with triamterene may result in hyperkalemia, especially in patients with renal insufficiency).
No products indexed under this heading.

Candesartan Cilexetil (May add to potentiate the action of other hypertensives). Products include:
Atacand Tablets **634**
Atacand HCT **637**

Captopril (May add to potentiate the action of other hypertensives; increased risk of hyperkalemia). Products include:
Captopril Tablets **2114**

Carteolol Hydrochloride (May add to potentiate the action of other hypertensives). Products include:
- Carteolol Hydrochloride Ophthalmic Solution USP, 1% 246

Celecoxib (Potential for acute renal failure). Products include:
- Celebrex Capsules 3130

Chlorothiazide (May add to potentiate the action of other hypertensives). Products include:
- Aldoclor Tablets 1881
- Diuril Oral 1936

Chlorothiazide Sodium (May add to potentiate the action of other hypertensives). Products include:
- Diuril Sodium Intravenous 1934

Chlorpropamide (Increased risk of severe hyponatremia).
No products indexed under this heading.

Chlorthalidone (May add to potentiate the action of other hypertensives). Products include:
- Clorpres Tablets 2139

Cisatracurium Besylate (Increased paralyzing effect). Products include:
- Nimbex Injection 494

Clonidine (May add to potentiate the action of other hypertensives). Products include:
- Catapres-TTS 875

Clonidine Hydrochloride (May add to potentiate the action of other hypertensives). Products include:
- Catapres Tablets 874
- Clorpres Tablets 2139

Cortisone Acetate (May intensify electrolyte imbalance, particularly hypokalemia).
No products indexed under this heading.

Deserpidine (May add to potentiate the action of other hypertensives).
No products indexed under this heading.

Dexamethasone (May intensify electrolyte imbalance, particularly hypokalemia). Products include:
- Ciprodex Otic Suspension 555
- Decadron Tablets 1929
- TobraDex Ophthalmic Ointment 558
- TobraDex Ophthalmic Suspension 558

Dexamethasone Acetate (May intensify electrolyte imbalance, particularly hypokalemia).
No products indexed under this heading.

Dexamethasone Sodium Phosphate (May intensify electrolyte imbalance, particularly hypokalemia). Products include:
- Decadron Phosphate Injection 1931

Diazoxide (May add to potentiate the action of other hypertensives). Products include:
- Hyperstat I.V. Injection 3031

Diclofenac Potassium (Potential for acute renal failure). Products include:
- Cataflam Tablets 2173

Diclofenac Sodium (Potential for acute renal failure). Products include:
- Arthrotec Tablets 3126
- Voltaren Ophthalmic Solution 2300
- Voltaren Tablets 2298
- Voltaren-XR Tablets 2301

Dicumarol (Effects of oral anticoagulants may be decreased).
No products indexed under this heading.

Diltiazem Hydrochloride (May add to potentiate the action of other hypertensives). Products include:
- Cardizem LA Extended Release Tablets 1699
- Tiazac Capsules 1204

Doxazosin Mesylate (May add to potentiate the action of other hypertensives).
No products indexed under this heading.

Enalapril Maleate (May add to potentiate the action of other hypertensives; increased risk of hyperkalemia). Products include:
- Vaseretic Tablets 2073
- Vasotec I.V. Injection 2076

Enalaprilat (May add to potentiate the action of other hypertensives; increased risk of hyperkalemia).
No products indexed under this heading.

Eprosartan Mesylate (May add to potentiate the action of other hypertensives). Products include:
- Teveten Tablets 1707
- Teveten HCT Tablets 1710

Esmolol Hydrochloride (May add to potentiate the action of other hypertensives). Products include:
- Brevibloc Concentrate 766
- Brevibloc Injection 766
- Brevibloc Double Strength Injection 766
- Brevibloc Premixed Injection 766
- Brevibloc Double Strength Premixed Injection 766

Etodolac (Potential for acute renal failure).
No products indexed under this heading.

Felodipine (May add to potentiate the action of other hypertensives). Products include:
- Plendil Extended-Release Tablets 651

Fenoprofen Calcium (Potential for acute renal failure). Products include:
- Nalfon Capsules 2504

Fludrocortisone Acetate (May intensify electrolyte imbalance, particularly hypokalemia).
No products indexed under this heading.

Flurbiprofen (Potential for acute renal failure).
No products indexed under this heading.

Fosinopril Sodium (May add to potentiate the action of other hypertensives; increased risk of hyperkalemia).
No products indexed under this heading.

Furosemide (May add to potentiate the action of other hypertensives). Products include:
- Furosemide Tablets 2117

Glimepiride (Thiazides may cause hyperglycemia and glycosuria; dosage alteration of oral antidiabetic agents may be required). Products include:
- Amaryl Tablets 2864

Glipizide (Thiazides may cause hyperglycemia and glycosuria; dosage alteration of oral antidiabetic agents may be required).
No products indexed under this heading.

Glyburide (Thiazides may cause hyperglycemia and glycosuria; dosage alteration of oral antidiabetic agents may be required).
No products indexed under this heading.

Guanabenz Acetate (May add to potentiate the action of other hypertensives).
No products indexed under this heading.

Guanethidine Monosulfate (May add to potentiate the action of other hypertensives).
No products indexed under this heading.

Hydralazine Hydrochloride (May add to potentiate the action of other hypertensives). Products include:
- BiDil Tablets 2161

Hydrocortisone (May intensify electrolyte imbalance, particularly hypokalemia). Products include:
- Cortizone•5 Ointment 699
- Cortizone•10 Creme 699
- Cortizone•10 Ointment 699
- Cortizone•10 Plus Creme 700
- Cortizone•10 Maximum Strength Quick Shot Spray 700
- Hydrocortone Tablets 1963
- Preparation H Hydrocortisone Cream 748

Hydrocortisone Acetate (May intensify electrolyte imbalance, particularly hypokalemia). Products include:
- Analpram-HC 1136
- Pramosone 1139
- ProctoFoam-HC 3113
- Tucks Anti-Itch Ointment 712
- U-cort 1% Cream 3289

Hydrocortisone Sodium Phosphate (May intensify electrolyte imbalance, particularly hypokalemia).
No products indexed under this heading.

Hydrocortisone Sodium Succinate (May intensify electrolyte imbalance, particularly hypokalemia).
No products indexed under this heading.

Hydroflumethiazide (May add to potentiate the action of other hypertensives).
No products indexed under this heading.

Ibuprofen (Potential for acute renal failure). Products include:
- Advil Allergy Sinus Caplets 737
- Advil 737
- Children's Advil Suspension 742
- Children's Advil Chewable Tablets 741
- Advil Cold & Sinus 739
- Advil Flu & Body Ache Caplets 739
- Children's Advil Cold Suspension 741
- Infants' Advil Concentrated Drops 743
- Junior Strength Advil Swallow Tablets 740
- Advil Migraine Liquigels 740
- Advil Multi-Symptom Cold Caplets 738
- Combunox Tablets 1183
- Children's Motrin Oral Suspension and Chewable Tablets 1837
- Children's Motrin Cold Non-Staining Dye-Free Oral Suspension 1838
- Children's Motrin Cold Oral Suspension 1838
- Children's Motrin Non-Staining Dye-Free Oral Suspension 1837
- Motrin Cold & Sinus Caplets 1836
- Motrin IB Tablets and Caplets 1836
- Infants' Motrin Concentrated Drops 1837
- Infants' Motrin Non-Staining Dye-Free Drops 1837
- Junior Strength Motrin Caplets and Chewable Tablets 1837
- Vicoprofen Tablets 533

Indapamide (May add to potentiate the action of other hypertensives). Products include:
- Indapamide Tablets 2119

Indomethacin (Potential for acute renal failure). Products include:
- Indocin 1968

Indomethacin Sodium Trihydrate (Potential for acute renal failure). Products include:
- Indocin I.V. 1973

Insulin, Human, Zinc Suspension (Thiazides may cause hyperglycemia, glycosuria and alter insulin requirements in diabetes; diabetes mellitus may become manifest during thiazide administration). Products include:
- Humulin L, 100 Units 1763
- Humulin U, 100 Units 1770

Insulin, Human NPH (Thiazides may cause hyperglycemia, glycosuria and alter insulin requirements in diabetes; diabetes mellitus may become manifest during thiazide administration). Products include:
- Humulin N, 100 Units 1764
- Humulin N Pen 1765
- Novolin N Human Insulin 10 ml Vials 2322
- Novolin N InnoLet 2322
- Novolin N PenFill 3 ml Cartridges 2325
- Novolin R InnoLet 2322

Insulin, Human Regular (Thiazides may cause hyperglycemia, glycosuria and alter insulin requirements in diabetes; diabetes mellitus may become manifest during thiazide administration). Products include:
- Humulin R (U-500) 1768
- Humulin R, 100 Units 1767
- Novolin R Human Insulin 10 ml Vials 2322
- Novolin R PenFill 2325

Insulin, Human Regular and Human NPH Mixture (Thiazides may cause hyperglycemia, glycosuria and alter insulin requirements in diabetes; diabetes mellitus may become manifest during thiazide administration). Products include:
- Humulin 50/50, 100 Units 1760
- Humulin 70/30 Pen 1761
- Novolin 70/30 Human Insulin 10 ml Vials 2321
- Novolin 70/30 InnoLet 2322
- Novolin 70/30 PenFill 3 ml Cartridges 2325

Insulin, NPH (Thiazides may cause hyperglycemia, glycosuria and alter insulin requirements in diabetes; diabetes mellitus may become manifest during thiazide administration).
No products indexed under this heading.

Insulin, Regular (Thiazides may cause hyperglycemia, glycosuria and alter insulin requirements in diabetes; diabetes mellitus may become manifest during thiazide administration).
No products indexed under this heading.

Insulin, Zinc Crystals (Thiazides may cause hyperglycemia, glycosuria and alter insulin requirements in diabetes; diabetes mellitus may become manifest during thiazide administration).
No products indexed under this heading.

Insulin, Zinc Suspension (Thiazides may cause hyperglycemia, glycosuria and alter insulin requirements in diabetes; diabetes mellitus may become manifest during thiazide administration).
No products indexed under this heading.

Insulin Aspart, Human Regular (Thiazides may cause hyperglycemia, glycosuria and alter insulin requirements in diabetes; diabetes

IMPORTANT NOTE: Always consult each drug listing in the patient's regimen for possible interactions.

mellitus may become manifest during thiazide administration). Products include:
NovoLog Injection 2326

Insulin glargine (Thiazides may cause hyperglycemia, glycosuria and alter insulin requirements in diabetes; diabetes mellitus may become manifest during thiazide administration). Products include:
Lantus Injection 2925

Insulin Lispro, Human (Thiazides may cause hyperglycemia, glycosuria and alter insulin requirements in diabetes; diabetes mellitus may become manifest during thiazide administration). Products include:
Humalog-Pen 1751
Humalog Mix 75/25-Pen 1754

Insulin Lispro Protamine, Human (Thiazides may cause hyperglycemia, glycosuria and alter insulin requirements in diabetes; diabetes mellitus may become manifest during thiazide administration). Products include:
Humalog Mix 75/25-Pen 1754

Irbesartan (May add to potentiate the action of other hypertensives). Products include:
Avalide Tablets 922
Avalide Tablets 2889
Avapro Tablets 925
Avapro Tablets 2886

Isradipine (May add to potentiate the action of other hypertensives). Products include:
DynaCirc CR Tablets 2726

Ketoprofen (Potential for acute renal failure).
No products indexed under this heading.

Ketorolac Tromethamine (Potential for acute renal failure). Products include:
Acular Ophthalmic Solution 561
Acular LS Ophthalmic Solution 562

Labetalol Hydrochloride (May add to potentiate the action of other hypertensives).
No products indexed under this heading.

Laxatives, unspecified (Interferes with the potassium-retaining effects of triamterene; chronic or overuse of laxatives may reduce serum potassium).
No products indexed under this heading.

Lisinopril (May add to potentiate the action of other hypertensives; increased risk of hyperkalemia). Products include:
Prinivil Tablets 2029
Prinzide Tablets 2033
Zestoretic Tablets 701
Zestril Tablets 704

Lithium (Reduced renal clearance and increased risk of lithium toxicity).
No products indexed under this heading.

Lithium Carbonate (Reduced renal clearance and increased risk of lithium toxicity). Products include:
Eskalith 1406
Lithobid Tablets 1670

Lithium Citrate (Reduced renal clearance and increased risk of lithium toxicity).
No products indexed under this heading.

Losartan Potassium (May add to potentiate the action of other hypertensives). Products include:
Cozaar Tablets 1913

Hyzaar 1964

Mecamylamine Hydrochloride (May add to potentiate the action of other hypertensives). Products include:
Inversine Tablets 3286

Meclofenamate Sodium (Potential for acute renal failure).
No products indexed under this heading.

Mefenamic Acid (Potential for acute renal failure).
No products indexed under this heading.

Meloxicam (Potential for acute renal failure). Products include:
Mobic Oral Suspension 893
Mobic Tablets 893

Metformin Hydrochloride (Increased risk of severe hyponatremia). Products include:
ActoPlus Met Tablets 3219
Avandamet Tablets 1343
Fortamet Extended-Release Tablets 1156

Methenamine (Decreased effectiveness of methenamine due to alkalinization of urine).
No products indexed under this heading.

Methenamine Hippurate (Decreased effectiveness of methenamine due to alkalinization of urine).
No products indexed under this heading.

Methenamine Mandelate (Decreased effectiveness of methenamine due to alkalinization of urine). Products include:
Uroqid-Acid No. 2 Tablets 785

Methyclothiazide (May add to potentiate the action of other hypertensives).
No products indexed under this heading.

Methyldopa (May add to potentiate the action of other hypertensives). Products include:
Aldoclor Tablets 1881
Aldoril Tablets 1884

Methyldopate Hydrochloride (May add to potentiate the action of other hypertensives).
No products indexed under this heading.

Methylprednisolone Acetate (May intensify electrolyte imbalance, particularly hypokalemia). Products include:
Depo-Medrol Injectable Suspension 2615
Depo-Medrol Single-Dose Vial 2617

Methylprednisolone Sodium Succinate (May intensify electrolyte imbalance, particularly hypokalemia).
No products indexed under this heading.

Metocurine Iodide (Increased paralyzing effect).
No products indexed under this heading.

Metolazone (May add to potentiate the action of other hypertensives).
No products indexed under this heading.

Metoprolol Succinate (May add to potentiate the action of other hypertensives). Products include:
Toprol-XL Tablets 660

Metoprolol Tartrate (May add to potentiate the action of other hypertensives).
No products indexed under this heading.

Metyrosine (May add to potentiate the action of other hypertensives). Products include:
Demser Capsules 1933

Mibefradil Dihydrochloride (May add to potentiate the action of other hypertensives).
No products indexed under this heading.

Miglitol (Thiazides may cause hyperglycemia and glycosuria; dosage alteration of oral antidiabetic agents may be required).
No products indexed under this heading.

Minoxidil (May add to potentiate the action of other hypertensives). Products include:
Men's Rogaine Extra Strength Topical Solution, Ocean Rush Scent and Original Unscented ..... ▣ 706
Women's Rogaine Topical Solution, Spring Bloom Scent and Original Unscented .... ▣ 707

Mivacurium Chloride (Increased paralyzing effect). Products include:
Mivacron Injection 489

Moexipril Hydrochloride (May add to potentiate the action of other hypertensives; increased risk of hyperkalemia). Products include:
Uniretic Tablets 3114
Univasc Tablets 3118

Nabumetone (Potential for acute renal failure). Products include:
Relafen Tablets 1523

Nadolol (May add to potentiate the action of other hypertensives). Products include:
Nadolol Tablets 2121

Naproxen (Potential for acute renal failure). Products include:
EC-Naprosyn Delayed-Release Tablets 2769
Naprosyn Suspension 2769
Naprosyn Tablets 2769
Prevacid NapraPAC 3277

Naproxen Sodium (Potential for acute renal failure). Products include:
Aleve Tablets, Caplets and Gelcaps .... ▣ 605
Anaprox Tablets 2769
Anaprox DS Tablets 2769

Nicardipine Hydrochloride (May add to potentiate the action of other hypertensives). Products include:
Cardene I.V. 1129

Nifedipine (May add to potentiate the action of other hypertensives). Products include:
Adalat CC Tablets 2978

Nisoldipine (May add to potentiate the action of other hypertensives). Products include:
Sular Tablets 1163

Nitroglycerin (May add to potentiate the action of other hypertensives). Products include:
Nitro-Dur Transdermal Infusion System 3060
Nitrolingual Pumpspray 1161

Norepinephrine Bitartrate (Decreased arterial responsiveness to norepinephrine).
No products indexed under this heading.

Oxaprozin (Potential for acute renal failure).
No products indexed under this heading.

Pancuronium Bromide (Increased paralyzing effect).
No products indexed under this heading.

Penbutolol Sulfate (May add to potentiate the action of other hypertensives).
No products indexed under this heading.

Penicillin G Potassium (Concurrent use of parenteral penicillin G potassium with triamterene may result in hyperkalemia, especially in patients with renal insufficiency).
No products indexed under this heading.

Perindopril Erbumine (May add to potentiate the action of other hypertensives; increased risk of hyperkalemia). Products include:
Aceon Tablets (2 mg, 4 mg, 8 mg) 3191

Phenoxybenzamine Hydrochloride (May add to potentiate the action of other hypertensives). Products include:
Dibenzyline Capsules 3390

Phentolamine Mesylate (May add to potentiate the action of other hypertensives).
No products indexed under this heading.

Phenylbutazone (Potential for acute renal failure).
No products indexed under this heading.

Pindolol (May add to potentiate the action of other hypertensives).
No products indexed under this heading.

Pioglitazone Hydrochloride (Thiazides may cause hyperglycemia and glycosuria; dosage alteration of oral antidiabetic agents may be required). Products include:
ActoPlus Met Tablets 3219
Actos Tablets 3224

Piroxicam (Potential for acute renal failure).
No products indexed under this heading.

Polythiazide (May add to potentiate the action of other hypertensives).
No products indexed under this heading.

Potassium Acid Phosphate (Potential for hyperkalemia; concomitant use should be avoided). Products include:
K-Phos Original (Sodium Free) Tablets 785

Potassium Bicarbonate (Potential for hyperkalemia; concomitant use should be avoided).
No products indexed under this heading.

Potassium Chloride (Potential for hyperkalemia; concomitant use should be avoided). Products include:
Colyte with Flavor Packs for Oral Solution 3102
HalfLytely and Bisacodyl Tablets Bowel Prep Kit with Flavors Packs 915
K-Dur Extended-Relase Tablets 3047
K-Lor Powder Packets 472
K-Tab Filmtab Tablets 473
TriLyte with Flavor Packs for Oral Solution 3114

Potassium Citrate (Potential for hyperkalemia; concomitant use should be avoided). Products include:
Urocit-K Tablets 2109

Potassium Gluconate (Potential for hyperkalemia; concomitant use should be avoided).
No products indexed under this heading.

Potassium Phosphate (Potential for hyperkalemia; concomitant use should be avoided). Products include:
- K-Phos Neutral Tablets 785

Prazosin Hydrochloride (May add to potentiate the action of other hypertensives).
- No products indexed under this heading.

Prednisolone Acetate (May intensify electrolyte imbalance, particularly hypokalemia). Products include:
- Blephamide Ophthalmic Ointment 563
- Blephamide Ophthalmic Suspension 564
- Poly-Pred Liquifilm Ophthalmic Suspension .... ⊙231
- Pred Forte Ophthalmic Suspension .... ⊙233
- Pred Mild Sterile Ophthalmic Suspension .... ⊙236
- Pred-G Ophthalmic Suspension ...... ⊙234
- Pred-G Sterile Ophthalmic Ointment .... ⊙235

Prednisolone Sodium Phosphate (May intensify electrolyte imbalance, particularly hypokalemia). Products include:
- Pediapred Oral Solution 3319

Prednisolone Tebutate (May intensify electrolyte imbalance, particularly hypokalemia).
- No products indexed under this heading.

Prednisone (May intensify electrolyte imbalance, particularly hypokalemia).
- No products indexed under this heading.

Probenecid (Dyazide may raise the level of blood uric acid; may require dosage adjustment of antigout agent).
- No products indexed under this heading.

Propranolol Hydrochloride (May add to potentiate the action of other hypertensives). Products include:
- Inderal LA Long-Acting Capsules 3421
- InnoPran XL Capsules 2728

Quinapril Hydrochloride (May add to potentiate the action of other hypertensives; increased risk of hyperkalemia).
- No products indexed under this heading.

Ramipril (May add to potentiate the action of other hypertensives; increased risk of hyperkalemia). Products include:
- Altace Capsules 1673

Rapacuronium Bromide (Increased paralyzing effect).
- No products indexed under this heading.

Rauwolfia Serpentina (May add to potentiate the action of other hypertensives).
- No products indexed under this heading.

Repaglinide (Thiazides may cause hyperglycemia and glycosuria; dosage alteration of oral antidiabetic agents may be required). Products include:
- Prandin Tablets (0.5, 1, and 2 mg) 2337

Rescinnamine (May add to potentiate the action of other hypertensives).
- No products indexed under this heading.

Reserpine (May add to potentiate the action of other hypertensives).
- No products indexed under this heading.

Rocuronium Bromide (Increased paralyzing effect). Products include:
- Zemuron Injection 2363

Rofecoxib (Potential for acute renal failure).
- No products indexed under this heading.

Rosiglitazone Maleate (Thiazides may cause hyperglycemia and glycosuria; dosage alteration of oral antidiabetic agents may be required). Products include:
- Avandamet Tablets 1343
- Avandia Tablets 1348

Salt Substitutes (Concurrent use of salt substitues with triamterene may result in hyperkalemia, especially in patients with renal insufficiency).
- No products indexed under this heading.

Sodium Nitroprusside (May add to potentiate the action of other hypertensives).
- No products indexed under this heading.

Sodium Polystyrene Sulfonate (May result in fluid retention).
- No products indexed under this heading.

Sotalol Hydrochloride (May add to potentiate the action of other hypertensives).
- No products indexed under this heading.

Spirapril Hydrochloride (May add to potentiate the action of other hypertensives; increased risk of hyperkalemia).
- No products indexed under this heading.

Spironolactone (Concurrent use is contraindicated).
- No products indexed under this heading.

Sulfinpyrazone (Dyazide may raise the level of blood uric acid; may require dosage adjustment of antigout agent).
- No products indexed under this heading.

Sulindac (Potential for acute renal failure). Products include:
- Clinoril Tablets 1899

Telmisartan (May add to potentiate the action of other hypertensives). Products include:
- Micardis Tablets 884
- Micardis HCT Tablets 886

Terazosin Hydrochloride (May add to potentiate the action of other hypertensives). Products include:
- Hytrin Capsules 469

Timolol Maleate (May add to potentiate the action of other hypertensives). Products include:
- Blocadren Tablets 1891
- Cosopt Sterile Ophthalmic Solution 1910
- Timolide Tablets 2056
- Timoptic in Ocudose 2061
- Timoptic Sterile Ophthalmic Solution 2058
- Timoptic-XE Sterile Ophthalmic Gel Forming Solution 2062

Tolazamide (Thiazides may cause hyperglycemia and glycosuria; dosage alteration of oral antidiabetic agents may be required).
- No products indexed under this heading.

Tolbutamide (Thiazides may cause hyperglycemia and glycosuria; dosage alteration of oral antidiabetic agents may be required).
- No products indexed under this heading.

Tolmetin Sodium (Potential for acute renal failure).
- No products indexed under this heading.

Torsemide (May add to potentiate the action of other hypertensives).
- No products indexed under this heading.

Trandolapril (May add to potentiate the action of other hypertensives; increased risk of hyperkalemia). Products include:
- Mavik Tablets 482
- Tarka Tablets 519

Triamcinolone (May intensify electrolyte imbalance, particularly hypokalemia).
- No products indexed under this heading.

Triamcinolone Acetonide (May intensify electrolyte imbalance, particularly hypokalemia). Products include:
- Azmacort Inhalation Aerosol 1701
- Nasacort HFA Inhalation Aerosol 2939
- Nasacort AQ Nasal Spray 2937

Triamcinolone Diacetate (May intensify electrolyte imbalance, particularly hypokalemia).
- No products indexed under this heading.

Triamcinolone Hexacetonide (May intensify electrolyte imbalance, particularly hypokalemia).
- No products indexed under this heading.

Trimethaphan Camsylate (May add to potentiate the action of other hypertensives).
- No products indexed under this heading.

Troglitazone (Thiazides may cause hyperglycemia and glycosuria; dosage alteration of oral antidiabetic agents may be required).
- No products indexed under this heading.

Tubocurarine Chloride (Increased paralyzing effect).
- No products indexed under this heading.

Valdecoxib (Potential for acute renal failure).
- No products indexed under this heading.

Valsartan (May add to potentiate the action of other hypertensives). Products include:
- Diovan HCT Tablets 2195
- Diovan Tablets 2191

Vecuronium Bromide (Increased paralyzing effect).
- No products indexed under this heading.

Verapamil Hydrochloride (May add to potentiate the action of other hypertensives). Products include:
- Covera-HS Tablets 3135
- Tarka Tablets 519
- Verelan PM Capsules 3120

Warfarin Sodium (Effects of oral anticoagulants may be decreased). Products include:
- Coumadin for Injection 932
- Coumadin Tablets 932

Food Interactions

Milk, low fat (Concurrent use of low-salt milk with triamterene may result in hyperkalemia, especially in patients with renal insufficiency).

DYNACIN TABLETS

(Minocycline Hydrochloride) 1859

May interact with antacids containing aluminum, calcium and magnesium, anticoagulants, iron containing oral preparations, oral contraceptives, penicillins, and certain other agents. Compounds in these categories include:

Aluminum Carbonate (Absorption of tetracyclines is impaired by antacids containing aluminum, calcium or magnesium, and iron-containing preparations).
- No products indexed under this heading.

Aluminum Hydroxide (Absorption of tetracyclines is impaired by antacids containing aluminum, calcium or magnesium, and iron-containing preparations). Products include:
- Gaviscon Regular Strength Liquid .. 620
- Gaviscon Regular Strength Tablets 619
- Gaviscon Extra Strength Liquid 620
- Gaviscon Extra Strength Tablets 619
- Maalox Max Maximum Strength Antacid/Anti-Gas Liquid 2165
- Maalox Regular Strength Antacid/Antigas Liquid 2164

Amoxicillin (Since bacteriostatic drugs may interfere with the bactericidal action of penicillin, it is advisable to avoid giving tetracycline-class drugs in conjunction with penicillin). Products include:
- Amoxil Capsules 1315
- Amoxil Chewable Tablets 1315
- Amoxil Pediatric Drops for Oral Suspension 1315
- Amoxil Powder for Oral Suspension 1315
- Amoxil Tablets 1315
- Augmentin 1331
- Augmentin Tablets 1334
- Augmentin XR Extended-Release Tablets 1340
- Augmentin ES-600 Powder for Oral Suspension 1337
- PREVPAC 3281

Amoxicillin Trihydrate (Since bacteriostatic drugs may interfere with the bactericidal action of penicillin, it is advisable to avoid giving tetracycline-class drugs in conjunction with penicillin).
- No products indexed under this heading.

Ampicillin (Since bacteriostatic drugs may interfere with the bactericidal action of penicillin, it is advisable to avoid giving tetracycline-class drugs in conjunction with penicillin).
- No products indexed under this heading.

Ampicillin Sodium (Since bacteriostatic drugs may interfere with the bactericidal action of penicillin, it is advisable to avoid giving tetracycline-class drugs in conjunction with penicillin).
- No products indexed under this heading.

Ampicillin Trihydrate (Since bacteriostatic drugs may interfere with the bactericidal action of penicillin, it is advisable to avoid giving tetracycline-class drugs in conjunction with penicillin).
- No products indexed under this heading.

Anisindione (Because tetracyclines have been shown to depress plasma prothrombin activity, patients who are on anticoagulant therapy may require downward adjustment of their anticoagulant dosage). Products include:

Miradon Tablets 3056

Ardeparin Sodium (Because tetracyclines have been shown to depress plasma prothrombin activity, patients who are on anticoagulant therapy may require downward adjustment of their anticoagulant dosage).
No products indexed under this heading.

Azlocillin Sodium (Since bacteriostatic drugs may interfere with the bactericidal action of penicillin, it is advisable to avoid giving tetracycline-class drugs in conjunction with penicillin).
No products indexed under this heading.

Bacampicillin Hydrochloride (Since bacteriostatic drugs may interfere with the bactericidal action of penicillin, it is advisable to avoid giving tetracycline-class drugs in conjunction with penicillin).
No products indexed under this heading.

Carbenicillin Disodium (Since bacteriostatic drugs may interfere with the bactericidal action of penicillin, it is advisable to avoid giving tetracycline-class drugs in conjunction with penicillin).
No products indexed under this heading.

Carbenicillin Indanyl Sodium (Since bacteriostatic drugs may interfere with the bactericidal action of penicillin, it is advisable to avoid giving tetracycline-class drugs in conjunction with penicillin).
No products indexed under this heading.

Dalteparin Sodium (Because tetracyclines have been shown to depress plasma prothrombin activity, patients who are on anticoagulant therapy may require downward adjustment of their anticoagulant dosage). Products include:
Fragmin Injection 2638

Danaparoid Sodium (Because tetracyclines have been shown to depress plasma prothrombin activity, patients who are on anticoagulant therapy may require downward adjustment of their anticoagulant dosage).
No products indexed under this heading.

Desogestrel (Concurrent use of tetracyclines with oral contraceptives may render oral contraceptives less effective). Products include:
Ortho-Cept Tablets 2395

Dicloxacillin Sodium (Since bacteriostatic drugs may interfere with the bactericidal action of penicillin, it is advisable to avoid giving tetracycline-class drugs in conjunction with penicillin).
No products indexed under this heading.

Dicumarol (Because tetracyclines have been shown to depress plasma prothrombin activity, patients who are on anticoagulant therapy may require downward adjustment of their anticoagulant dosage).
No products indexed under this heading.

Enoxaparin Sodium (Because tetracyclines have been shown to depress plasma prothrombin activity, patients who are on anticoagulant therapy may require downward adjustment of their anticoagulant dosage). Products include:
Lovenox Injection 2931

Ethinyl Estradiol (Concurrent use of tetracyclines with oral contraceptives may render oral contraceptives less effective). Products include:
Alesse-28 Tablets 3392
Lo/Ovral-28 Tablets 3423
NuvaRing 2357
Ortho-Cept Tablets 2395
Ortho-Cyclen/Ortho Tri-Cyclen 2414
Ortho Evra Transdermal System 2402
Ortho Tri-Cyclen Lo Tablets 2421
Seasonale Tablets 1073
Triphasil-28 Tablets 3483
Yasmin 28 Tablets 818

Ethynodiol Diacetate (Concurrent use of tetracyclines with oral contraceptives may render oral contraceptives less effective).
No products indexed under this heading.

Ferrous Fumarate (Absorption of tetracyclines is impaired by antacids containing aluminum, calcium or magnesium, and iron-containing preparations). Products include:
Chromagen Forte Soft Gelatin Capsules 3296
Ferretts Tablets .... ▣773
Repliva 21/7 Tablets 3301

Ferrous Gluconate (Absorption of tetracyclines is impaired by antacids containing aluminum, calcium or magnesium, and iron-containing preparations).
No products indexed under this heading.

Ferrous Sulfate (Absorption of tetracyclines is impaired by antacids containing aluminum, calcium or magnesium, and iron-containing preparations). Products include:
Feosol Tablets 1629
Slow Fe Iron Tablets .... ▣772
Slow Fe with Folic Acid Tablets .... ▣773

Fondaparinux Sodium (Because tetracyclines have been shown to depress plasma prothrombin activity, patients who are on anticoagulant therapy may require downward adjustment of their anticoagulant dosage). Products include:
Arixtra Injection 1325

Heparin Calcium (Because tetracyclines have been shown to depress plasma prothrombin activity, patients who are on anticoagulant therapy may require downward adjustment of their anticoagulant dosage).
No products indexed under this heading.

Heparin Sodium (Because tetracyclines have been shown to depress plasma prothrombin activity, patients who are on anticoagulant therapy may require downward adjustment of their anticoagulant dosage).
No products indexed under this heading.

Iron (Absorption of tetracyclines is impaired by antacids containing aluminum, calcium or magnesium, and iron-containing preparations). Products include:
Chromagen Forte Soft Gelatin Capsules 3296
Ferretts IPS Liquid .... ▣773
OptiNate 1162
Repliva 21/7 Tablets 3301

Levonorgestrel (Concurrent use of tetracyclines with oral contraceptives may render oral contraceptives less effective). Products include:
Alesse-28 Tablets 3392
Climara Pro Transdermal System 800
Mirena Intrauterine System 810
Plan B Tablets 1068
Seasonale Tablets 1073
Triphasil-28 Tablets 3483

Low Molecular Weight Heparins (Because tetracyclines have been shown to depress plasma prothrombin activity, patients who are on anticoagulant therapy may require downward adjustment of their anticoagulant dosage).
No products indexed under this heading.

Magaldrate (Absorption of tetracyclines is impaired by antacids containing aluminum, calcium or magnesium, and iron-containing preparations).
No products indexed under this heading.

Magnesium Hydroxide (Absorption of tetracyclines is impaired by antacids containing aluminum, calcium or magnesium, and iron-containing preparations). Products include:
Maalox Max Maximum Strength Antacid/Anti-Gas Liquid 2165
Maalox Regular Strength Antacid/Antigas Liquid 2164
Pepcid Complete Chewable Tablets 1672
Rolaids Tablets .... ▣707
Extra Strength Rolaids Tablets .... ▣707
Rolaids Multi-Symptom Antacid & Antigas Tablets .... ▣708

Magnesium Oxide (Absorption of tetracyclines is impaired by antacids containing aluminum, calcium or magnesium, and iron-containing preparations). Products include:
Beelith Tablets 784
PremCal Light, Regular, and Extra Strength Tablets .... ▣762

Mestranol (Concurrent use of tetracyclines with oral contraceptives may render oral contraceptives less effective).
No products indexed under this heading.

Methoxyflurane (Concurrent use of tetracycline and methoxyflurane has been reported to result in fatal renal toxicity).
No products indexed under this heading.

Mezlocillin Sodium (Since bacteriostatic drugs may interfere with the bactericidal action of penicillin, it is advisable to avoid giving tetracycline-class drugs in conjunction with penicillin).
No products indexed under this heading.

Nafcillin Sodium (Since bacteriostatic drugs may interfere with the bactericidal action of penicillin, it is advisable to avoid giving tetracycline-class drugs in conjunction with penicillin).
No products indexed under this heading.

Norethindrone (Concurrent use of tetracyclines with oral contraceptives may render oral contraceptives less effective). Products include:
Ortho Micronor Tablets 2411

Norethynodrel (Concurrent use of tetracyclines with oral contraceptives may render oral contraceptives less effective).
No products indexed under this heading.

Norgestimate (Concurrent use of tetracyclines with oral contraceptives may render oral contraceptives less effective). Products include:
Ortho-Cyclen/Ortho Tri-Cyclen 2414
Ortho Tri-Cyclen Lo Tablets 2421
Prefest Tablets 1069

Norgestrel (Concurrent use of tetracyclines with oral contraceptives may render oral contraceptives less effective). Products include:
Lo/Ovral-28 Tablets 3423

Penicillin G Benzathine (Since bacteriostatic drugs may interfere with the bactericidal action of penicillin, it is advisable to avoid giving tetracycline-class drugs in conjunction with penicillin).
No products indexed under this heading.

Penicillin G Potassium (Since bacteriostatic drugs may interfere with the bactericidal action of penicillin, it is advisable to avoid giving tetracycline-class drugs in conjunction with penicillin).
No products indexed under this heading.

Penicillin G Procaine (Since bacteriostatic drugs may interfere with the bactericidal action of penicillin, it is advisable to avoid giving tetracycline-class drugs in conjunction with penicillin).
No products indexed under this heading.

Penicillin G Sodium (Since bacteriostatic drugs may interfere with the bactericidal action of penicillin, it is advisable to avoid giving tetracycline-class drugs in conjunction with penicillin).
No products indexed under this heading.

Penicillin V Potassium (Since bacteriostatic drugs may interfere with the bactericidal action of penicillin, it is advisable to avoid giving tetracycline-class drugs in conjunction with penicillin).
No products indexed under this heading.

Polysaccharide Iron Complex (Absorption of tetracyclines is impaired by antacids containing aluminum, calcium or magnesium, and iron-containing preparations). Products include:
Niferex-150 Forte Capsules 3299
Nu-Iron 150 Capsules 2098

Ticarcillin Disodium (Since bacteriostatic drugs may interfere with the bactericidal action of penicillin, it is advisable to avoid giving tetracycline-class drugs in conjunction with penicillin). Products include:
Timentin ADD-Vantage 1556
Timentin Injection Galaxy Container 1559
Timentin IV Infusion 1553
Timentin Pharmacy Bulk Package 1562

Tinzaparin Sodium (Because tetracyclines have been shown to depress plasma prothrombin activity, patients who are on anticoagulant therapy may require downward adjustment of their anticoagulant dosage).
No products indexed under this heading.

Warfarin Sodium (Because tetracyclines have been shown to depress plasma prothrombin activity, patients who are on anticoagulant therapy may require downward adjustment of their anticoagulant dosage). Products include:
Coumadin for Injection 932
Coumadin Tablets 932

DYNACIRC CR TABLETS

(Isradipine) 2726
May interact with:

Cimetidine (Co-administration has resulted in increase in isradipine mean peak plasma concentrations and significant increase in the AUC). Products include:
Tagamet HB 200 Tablets 637
Tagamet Tablets 1547

Cimetidine Hydrochloride (Co-administration has resulted in increase in isradipine mean peak plasma concentrations and significant increase in the AUC).
No products indexed under this heading.

Fentanyl (Severe hypotension has been reported during fentanyl anesthesia with concomitant use of beta-blocker and a calcium channel blocker). Products include:
Duragesic Transdermal System 2448

Fentanyl Citrate (Severe hypotension has been reported during fentanyl anesthesia with concomitant use of beta-blocker and a calcium channel blocker). Products include:
Actiq 993

Hydrochlorothiazide (Additive antihypertensive effect). Products include:
Aldoril Tablets 1884
Atacand HCT 637
Avalide Tablets 2889
Avalide Tablets 922
Benicar HCT Tablets 2852
Diovan HCT Tablets 2195
Dyazide Capsules 1389
Hyzaar 1964
Lotensin HCT Tablets 2235
Maxzide 2150
Micardis HCT Tablets 886
Moduretic Tablets 2003
Prinzide Tablets 2033
Teveten HCT Tablets 1710
Timolide Tablets 2056
Uniretic Tablets 3114
Vaseretic Tablets 2073
Zestoretic Tablets 701

Propranolol Hydrochloride (Co-administration has resulted in a small effect on the rate but no effect on the extent of isradipine bioavailability; significant increases in AUC and Cmax and decreases in tmax of propranolol were noted). Products include:
Inderal LA Long-Acting Capsules 3421
InnoPran XL Capsules 2728

Rifampin (Co-administration has resulted in increased metabolism and higher clearance of isradipine; a reduction in isradipine levels to below the detectable limits has been noted).
No products indexed under this heading.

DYRENIUM CAPSULES

(Triamterene) 3390
May interact with ACE inhibitors, anesthetics, antihypertensives, diuretics, oral hypoglycemic agents, lithium preparations, nondepolarizing neuromuscular blocking agents, potassium preparations, preanesthetic medications, potassium sparing diuretics, and certain other agents. Compounds in these categories include:

Acarbose (Triamterene may raise blood glucose levels; for adult onset diabetes, dosage adjustments of hypoglycemic agents may be necessary during and after therapy). Products include:
Precose Tablets 776

Acebutolol Hydrochloride (The effects of antihypertensive agents may be potentiated when given concurrently).
No products indexed under this heading.

Alfentanil Hydrochloride (The effects of anesthetics may be potentiated when given concurrently).
No products indexed under this heading.

Amiloride Hydrochloride (Co-administration with other potassium-sparing agents has resulted in fatalities; these agents should not be given concomitantly). Products include:
Midamor Tablets 2000
Moduretic Tablets 2003

Amlodipine Besylate (The effects of antihypertensive agents may be potentiated when given concurrently). Products include:
Caduet Tablets 2507
Lotrel Capsules 2238
Norvasc Tablets 2529

Atenolol (The effects of antihypertensive agents may be potentiated when given concurrently). Products include:
Tenormin I.V. Injection 698
Tenormin Tablets 695

Atracurium Besylate (The effects of nondepolarizing skeletal muscle relaxants may be potentiated when given concurrently).
No products indexed under this heading.

Benazepril Hydrochloride (Co-administration with potassium-sparing agents and angiotensin-coverting enzyme inhibitors increases the risk of hyperkalemia). Products include:
Lotensin Tablets 2232
Lotensin HCT Tablets 2235
Lotrel Capsules 2238

Bendroflumethiazide (The effects of other diuretics may be potentiated when given concurrently).
No products indexed under this heading.

Betaxolol Hydrochloride (The effects of antihypertensive agents may be potentiated when given concurrently). Products include:
Betoptic S Ophthalmic Suspension 554

Bisoprolol Fumarate (The effects of antihypertensive agents may be potentiated when given concurrently).
No products indexed under this heading.

Blood, whole (Co-administration with blood from blood banks may promote serum potassium accumulation and possibly result in hyperkalemia).
No products indexed under this heading.

Bumetanide (The effects of other diuretics may be potentiated when given concurrently).
No products indexed under this heading.

Candesartan Cilexetil (The effects of antihypertensive agents may be potentiated when given concurrently). Products include:
Atacand Tablets 634
Atacand HCT 637

Captopril (Co-administration with potassium-sparing agents and angiotensin-coverting enzyme inhibitors increases the risk of hyperkalemia). Products include:
Captopril Tablets 2114

Carteolol Hydrochloride (The effects of antihypertensive agents may be potentiated when given concurrently). Products include:
Carteolol Hydrochloride Ophthalmic Solution USP, 1% ..... ⊙ 246

Chlorothiazide (The effects of other diuretics may be potentiated when given concurrently). Products include:
Aldoclor Tablets 1881
Diuril Oral 1936

Chlorothiazide Sodium (The effects of other diuretics may be potentiated when given concurrently). Products include:
Diuril Sodium Intravenous 1934

Chlorpropamide (Triamterene may raise blood glucose levels; for adult onset diabetes, dosage adjustments of hypoglycemic agents may be necessary during and after therapy; increased risk of severe hyponatremia with concurrent use).
No products indexed under this heading.

Chlorthalidone (The effects of other diuretics may be potentiated when given concurrently). Products include:
Clorpres Tablets 2139

Cisatracurium Besylate (The effects of nondepolarizing skeletal muscle relaxants may be potentiated when given concurrently). Products include:
Nimbex Injection 494

Clonidine (The effects of antihypertensive agents may be potentiated when given concurrently). Products include:
Catapres-TTS 875

Clonidine Hydrochloride (The effects of antihypertensive agents may be potentiated when given concurrently). Products include:
Catapres Tablets 874
Clorpres Tablets 2139

Deserpidine (The effects of antihypertensive agents may be potentiated when given concurrently).
No products indexed under this heading.

Diazepam (The effects of preanesthetic agents may be potentiated when given concurrently). Products include:
Diastat Rectal Delivery System 3344
Valium Tablets 2822

Diazoxide (The effects of antihypertensive agents may be potentiated when given concurrently). Products include:
Hyperstat I.V. Injection 3031

Diltiazem Hydrochloride (The effects of antihypertensive agents may be potentiated when given concurrently). Products include:
Cardizem LA Extended Release Tablets 1699
Tiazac Capsules 1204

Doxazosin Mesylate (The effects of antihypertensive agents may be potentiated when given concurrently).
No products indexed under this heading.

Droperidol (The effects of preanesthetic agents may be potentiated when given concurrently).
No products indexed under this heading.

Enalapril Maleate (Co-administration with potassium-sparing agents and angiotensin-coverting enzyme inhibitors increases the risk of hyperkalemia). Products include:
Vaseretic Tablets 2073
Vasotec I.V. Injection 2076

Enalaprilat (Co-administration with potassium-sparing agents and angiotensin-coverting enzyme inhibitors increases the risk of hyperkalemia).
No products indexed under this heading.

Enflurane (The effects of anesthetics may be potentiated when given concurrently).
No products indexed under this heading.

Eprosartan Mesylate (The effects of antihypertensive agents may be potentiated when given concurrently). Products include:
Teveten Tablets 1707
Teveten HCT Tablets 1710

Esmolol Hydrochloride (The effects of antihypertensive agents may be potentiated when given concurrently). Products include:
Brevibloc Concentrate 766
Brevibloc Injection 766
Brevibloc Double Strength Injection 766
Brevibloc Premixed Injection 766
Brevibloc Double Strength Premixed Injection 766

Ethacrynic Acid (The effects of other diuretics may be potentiated when given concurrently). Products include:
Edecrin Tablets 1941

Felodipine (The effects of antihypertensive agents may be potentiated when given concurrently). Products include:
Plendil Extended-Release Tablets 651

Fentanyl Citrate (The effects of anesthetics may be potentiated when given concurrently). Products include:
Actiq 993

Fosinopril Sodium (Co-administration with potassium-sparing agents and angiotensin-coverting enzyme inhibitors increases the risk of hyperkalemia).
No products indexed under this heading.

Furosemide (The effects of other diuretics may be potentiated when given concurrently). Products include:
Furosemide Tablets 2117

Glimepiride (Triamterene may raise blood glucose levels; for adult onset diabetes, dosage adjustments of hypoglycemic agents may be necessary during and after therapy). Products include:
Amaryl Tablets 2864

Glipizide (Triamterene may raise blood glucose levels; for adult onset diabetes, dosage adjustments of hypoglycemic agents may be necessary during and after therapy).
No products indexed under this heading.

Glyburide (Triamterene may raise blood glucose levels; for adult onset diabetes, dosage adjustments of hypoglycemic agents may be necessary during and after therapy).
No products indexed under this heading.

Guanabenz Acetate (The effects of antihypertensive agents may be potentiated when given concurrently).
No products indexed under this heading.

Guanethidine Monosulfate (The effects of antihypertensive agents may be potentiated when given concurrently).
No products indexed under this heading.

Halothane (The effects of anesthetics may be potentiated when given concurrently).
No products indexed under this heading.

Hydralazine Hydrochloride (The effects of antihypertensive agents may be potentiated when given concurrently). Products include:
BiDil Tablets ... **2161**

Hydrochlorothiazide (The effects of other diuretics may be potentiated when given concurrently). Products include:
Aldoril Tablets ... **1884**
Atacand HCT ... **637**
Avalide Tablets ... **2889**
Avalide Tablets ... **922**
Benicar HCT Tablets ... **2852**
Diovan HCT Tablets ... **2195**
Dyazide Capsules ... **1389**
Hyzaar ... **1964**
Lotensin HCT Tablets ... **2235**
Maxzide ... **2150**
Micardis HCT Tablets ... **886**
Moduretic Tablets ... **2003**
Prinzide Tablets ... **2033**
Teveten HCT Tablets ... **1710**
Timolide Tablets ... **2056**
Uniretic Tablets ... **3114**
Vaseretic Tablets ... **2073**
Zestoretic Tablets ... **701**

Hydroflumethiazide (The effects of other diuretics may be potentiated when given concurrently).
No products indexed under this heading.

Hydroxyzine Hydrochloride (The effects of pre-anesthetic agents may be potentiated when given concurrently).
No products indexed under this heading.

Indapamide (The effects of other diuretics may be potentiated when given concurrently). Products include:
Indapamide Tablets ... **2119**

Indomethacin (Co-administration has resulted in acute renal failure). Products include:
Indocin ... **1968**

Irbesartan (The effects of antihypertensive agents may be potentiated when given concurrently). Products include:
Avalide Tablets ... **922**
Avalide Tablets ... **2889**
Avapro Tablets ... **925**
Avapro Tablets ... **2886**

Isoflurane (The effects of anesthetics may be potentiated when given concurrently).
No products indexed under this heading.

Isradipine (The effects of antihypertensive agents may be potentiated when given concurrently). Products include:
DynaCirc CR Tablets ... **2726**

Ketamine Hydrochloride (The effects of anesthetics may be potentiated when given concurrently).
No products indexed under this heading.

Labetalol Hydrochloride (The effects of antihypertensive agents may be potentiated when given concurrently).
No products indexed under this heading.

Lisinopril (Co-administration with potassium-sparing agents and angiotensin-coverting enzyme inhibitors increases the risk of hyperkalemia). Products include:
Prinivil Tablets ... **2029**
Prinzide Tablets ... **2033**
Zestoretic Tablets ... **701**
Zestril Tablets ... **704**

Lithium (Co-administration of lithium and diuretics results in diuretic-induced sodium loss that may reduce renal clearance of lithium and increase serum lithium levels with risk of lithium toxicity).
No products indexed under this heading.

Lithium Carbonate (Co-administration of lithium and diuretics results in diuretic-induced sodium loss that may reduce renal clearance of lithium and increase serum lithium levels with risk of lithium toxicity). Products include:
Eskalith ... **1406**
Lithobid Tablets ... **1670**

Lithium Citrate (Co-administration of lithium and diuretics results in diuretic-induced sodium loss that may reduce renal clearance of lithium and increase serum lithium levels with risk of lithium toxicity).
No products indexed under this heading.

Lorazepam (The effects of pre-anesthetic agents may be potentiated when given concurrently).
No products indexed under this heading.

Losartan Potassium (The effects of antihypertensive agents may be potentiated when given concurrently). Products include:
Cozaar Tablets ... **1913**
Hyzaar ... **1964**

Mecamylamine Hydrochloride (The effects of antihypertensive agents may be potentiated when given concurrently). Products include:
Inversine Tablets ... **3286**

Meperidine Hydrochloride (The effects of pre-anesthetic agents may be potentiated when given concurrently).
No products indexed under this heading.

Metformin Hydrochloride (Triamterene may raise blood glucose levels; for adult onset diabetes, dosage adjustments of hypoglycemic agents may be necessary during and after therapy). Products include:
ActoPlus Met Tablets ... **3219**
Avandamet Tablets ... **1343**
Fortamet Extended-Release Tablets ... **1156**

Methohexital Sodium (The effects of anesthetics may be potentiated when given concurrently).
No products indexed under this heading.

Methyclothiazide (The effects of other diuretics may be potentiated when given concurrently).
No products indexed under this heading.

Methyldopa (The effects of antihypertensive agents may be potentiated when given concurrently). Products include:
Aldoclor Tablets ... **1881**
Aldoril Tablets ... **1884**

Methyldopate Hydrochloride (The effects of antihypertensive agents may be potentiated when given concurrently).
No products indexed under this heading.

Metocurine Iodide (The effects of nondepolarizing skeletal muscle relaxants may be potentiated when given concurrently).
No products indexed under this heading.

Metolazone (The effects of other diuretics may be potentiated when given concurrently).
No products indexed under this heading.

Metoprolol Succinate (The effects of antihypertensive agents may be potentiated when given concurrently). Products include:
Toprol-XL Tablets ... **660**

Metoprolol Tartrate (The effects of antihypertensive agents may be potentiated when given concurrently).
No products indexed under this heading.

Metyrosine (The effects of antihypertensive agents may be potentiated when given concurrently). Products include:
Demser Capsules ... **1933**

Mibefradil Dihydrochloride (The effects of antihypertensive agents may be potentiated when given concurrently).
No products indexed under this heading.

Midazolam Hydrochloride (The effects of anesthetics may be potentiated when given concurrently).
No products indexed under this heading.

Miglitol (Triamterene may raise blood glucose levels; for adult onset diabetes, dosage adjustments of hypoglycemic agents may be necessary during and after therapy).
No products indexed under this heading.

Minoxidil (The effects of antihypertensive agents may be potentiated when given concurrently). Products include:
Men's Rogaine Extra Strength Topical Solution, Ocean Rush Scent and Original Unscented ... ▣ **706**
Women's Rogaine Topical Solution, Spring Bloom Scent and Original Unscented ... ▣ **707**

Mivacurium Chloride (The effects of nondepolarizing skeletal muscle relaxants may be potentiated when given concurrently). Products include:
Mivacron Injection ... **489**

Moexipril Hydrochloride (Co-administration with potassium-sparing agents and angiotensin-coverting enzyme inhibitors increases the risk of hyperkalemia). Products include:
Uniretic Tablets ... **3114**
Univasc Tablets ... **3118**

Morphine Sulfate (The effects of pre-anesthetic agents may be potentiated when given concurrently). Products include:
Avinza Capsules ... **1714**
Kadian Capsules ... **572**
MS Contin Tablets ... **2703**

Nadolol (The effects of antihypertensive agents may be potentiated when given concurrently). Products include:
Nadolol Tablets ... **2121**

Nicardipine Hydrochloride (The effects of antihypertensive agents may be potentiated when given concurrently). Products include:
Cardene I.V. ... **1129**

Nifedipine (The effects of antihypertensive agents may be potentiated when given concurrently). Products include:
Adalat CC Tablets ... **2978**

Nisoldipine (The effects of antihypertensive agents may be potentiated when given concurrently). Products include:
Sular Tablets ... **1163**

Nitroglycerin (The effects of antihypertensive agents may be potentiated when given concurrently). Products include:
Nitro-Dur Transdermal Infusion System ... **3060**
Nitrolingual Pumpspray ... **1161**

Pancuronium Bromide (The effects of nondepolarizing skeletal muscle relaxants may be potentiated when given concurrently).
No products indexed under this heading.

Penbutolol Sulfate (The effects of antihypertensive agents may be potentiated when given concurrently).
No products indexed under this heading.

Penicillin G Potassium (Co-administration may promote serum potassium accumulation and possibly result in hyperkalemia).
No products indexed under this heading.

Pentobarbital Sodium (The effects of pre-anesthetic agents may be potentiated when given concurrently). Products include:
Nembutal Sodium Solution, USP ... **2484**

Perindopril Erbumine (Co-administration with potassium-sparing agents and angiotensin-coverting enzyme inhibitors increases the risk of hyperkalemia). Products include:
Aceon Tablets (2 mg, 4 mg, 8 mg) ... **3191**

Phenoxybenzamine Hydrochloride (The effects of antihypertensive agents may be potentiated when given concurrently). Products include:
Dibenzyline Capsules ... **3390**

Phentolamine Mesylate (The effects of antihypertensive agents may be potentiated when given concurrently).
No products indexed under this heading.

Pindolol (The effects of antihypertensive agents may be potentiated when given concurrently).
No products indexed under this heading.

Pioglitazone Hydrochloride (Triamterene may raise blood glucose levels; for adult onset diabetes, dosage adjustments of hypoglycemic agents may be necessary during and after therapy). Products include:
ActoPlus Met Tablets ... **3219**
Actos Tablets ... **3224**

Polythiazide (The effects of other diuretics may be potentiated when given concurrently).
No products indexed under this heading.

Potassium Acid Phosphate (Co-administration with dietary potassium supplements increases the risk of hyperkalemia; concurrent use is contraindicated). Products include:
K-Phos Original (Sodium Free) Tablets 785

Potassium Bicarbonate (Co-administration with dietary potassium supplements increases the risk of hyperkalemia; concurrent use is contraindicated).
No products indexed under this heading.

Potassium Chloride (Co-administration with dietary potassium supplements increases the risk of hyperkalemia; concurrent use is contraindicated). Products include:
Colyte with Flavor Packs for Oral Solution 3102
HalfLytely and Bisacodyl Tablets Bowel Prep Kit with Flavors Packs 915
K-Dur Extended-Relase Tablets 3047
K-Lor Powder Packets 472
K-Tab Filmtab Tablets 473
TriLyte with Flavor Packs for Oral Solution 3114

Potassium Citrate (Co-administration with dietary potassium supplements increases the risk of hyperkalemia; concurrent use is contraindicated). Products include:
Urocit-K Tablets 2109

Potassium Gluconate (Co-administration with dietary potassium supplements increases the risk of hyperkalemia; concurrent use is contraindicated).
No products indexed under this heading.

Potassium Phosphate (Co-administration with dietary potassium supplements increases the risk of hyperkalemia; concurrent use is contraindicated). Products include:
K-Phos Neutral Tablets 785

Prazosin Hydrochloride (The effects of antihypertensive agents may be potentiated when given concurrently).
No products indexed under this heading.

Promethazine Hydrochloride (The effects of pre-anesthetic agents may be potentiated when given concurrently). Products include:
Phenergan 3438

Propofol (The effects of anesthetics may be potentiated when given concurrently). Products include:
Diprivan Injectable Emulsion 676

Propranolol Hydrochloride (The effects of antihypertensive agents may be potentiated when given concurrently). Products include:
Inderal LA Long-Acting Capsules 3421
InnoPran XL Capsules 2728

Quinapril Hydrochloride (Co-administration with potassium-sparing agents and angiotensin-coverting enzyme inhibitors increases the risk of hyperkalemia).
No products indexed under this heading.

Ramipril (Co-administration with potassium-sparing agents and angiotensin-coverting enzyme inhibitors increases the risk of hyperkalemia). Products include:
Altace Capsules 1673

Rapacuronium Bromide (The effects of nondepolarizing skeletal muscle relaxants may be potentiated when given concurrently).
No products indexed under this heading.

Rauwolfia Serpentina (The effects of antihypertensive agents may be potentiated when given concurrently).
No products indexed under this heading.

Remifentanil Hydrochloride (The effects of anesthetics may be potentiated when given concurrently).
No products indexed under this heading.

Repaglinide (Triamterene may raise blood glucose levels; for adult onset diabetes, dosage adjustments of hypoglycemic agents may be necessary during and after therapy). Products include:
Prandin Tablets (0.5, 1, and 2 mg) 2337

Rescinnamine (The effects of antihypertensive agents may be potentiated when given concurrently).
No products indexed under this heading.

Reserpine (The effects of antihypertensive agents may be potentiated when given concurrently).
No products indexed under this heading.

Rocuronium Bromide (The effects of nondepolarizing skeletal muscle relaxants may be potentiated when given concurrently). Products include:
Zemuron Injection 2363

Rosiglitazone Maleate (Triamterene may raise blood glucose levels; for adult onset diabetes, dosage adjustments of hypoglycemic agents may be necessary during and after therapy). Products include:
Avandamet Tablets 1343
Avandia Tablets 1348

Secobarbital Sodium (The effects of pre-anesthetic agents may be potentiated when given concurrently).
No products indexed under this heading.

Sodium Nitroprusside (The effects of antihypertensive agents may be potentiated when given concurrently).
No products indexed under this heading.

Sotalol Hydrochloride (The effects of antihypertensive agents may be potentiated when given concurrently).
No products indexed under this heading.

Spirapril Hydrochloride (Co-administration with potassium-sparing agents and angiotensin-coverting enzyme inhibitors increases the risk of hyperkalemia).
No products indexed under this heading.

Spironolactone (Co-administration with other potassium-sparing agents has resulted in fatalities; these agents should not be given concomitantly).
No products indexed under this heading.

Sufentanil Citrate (The effects of anesthetics may be potentiated when given concurrently).
No products indexed under this heading.

Telmisartan (The effects of antihypertensive agents may be potentiated when given concurrently). Products include:
Micardis Tablets 884
Micardis HCT Tablets 886

Terazosin Hydrochloride (The effects of antihypertensive agents may be potentiated when given concurrently). Products include:
Hytrin Capsules 469

Thiamylal Sodium (The effects of anesthetics may be potentiated when given concurrently).
No products indexed under this heading.

Timolol Maleate (The effects of antihypertensive agents may be potentiated when given concurrently). Products include:
Blocadren Tablets 1891
Cosopt Sterile Ophthalmic Solution 1910
Timolide Tablets 2056
Timoptic in Ocudose 2061
Timoptic Sterile Ophthalmic Solution 2058
Timoptic-XE Sterile Ophthalmic Gel Forming Solution 2062

Tolazamide (Triamterene may raise blood glucose levels; for adult onset diabetes, dosage adjustments of hypoglycemic agents may be necessary during and after therapy).
No products indexed under this heading.

Tolbutamide (Triamterene may raise blood glucose levels; for adult onset diabetes, dosage adjustments of hypoglycemic agents may be necessary during and after therapy).
No products indexed under this heading.

Torsemide (The effects of other diuretics may be potentiated when given concurrently).
No products indexed under this heading.

Trandolapril (Co-administration with potassium-sparing agents and angiotensin-coverting enzyme inhibitors increases the risk of hyperkalemia). Products include:
Mavik Tablets 482
Tarka Tablets 519

Trimethaphan Camsylate (The effects of antihypertensive agents may be potentiated when given concurrently).
No products indexed under this heading.

Troglitazone (Triamterene may raise blood glucose levels; for adult onset diabetes, dosage adjustments of hypoglycemic agents may be necessary during and after therapy).
No products indexed under this heading.

Valsartan (The effects of antihypertensive agents may be potentiated when given concurrently). Products include:
Diovan HCT Tablets 2195
Diovan Tablets 2191

Vecuronium Bromide (The effects of nondepolarizing skeletal muscle relaxants may be potentiated when given concurrently).
No products indexed under this heading.

Verapamil Hydrochloride (The effects of antihypertensive agents may be potentiated when given concurrently). Products include:
Covera-HS Tablets 3135
Tarka Tablets 519
Verelan PM Capsules 3120

Food Interactions

Milk, low salt (Co-administration may promote serum potassium accumulation and possibly result in hyperkalemia).

EC-NAPROSYN DELAYED-RELEASE TABLETS

(Naproxen) 2769

May interact with ACE inhibitors, antacids containing aluminum, calcium and magnesium, beta blockers, oral anticoagulants, histamine H_2-receptor antagonists, hydantoin anticonvulsants, lithium preparations, sulfonylureas, and certain other agents. Compounds in these categories include:

Acebutolol Hydrochloride (Reduced antihypertensive effect of beta blockers).
No products indexed under this heading.

Aluminum Carbonate (Due to the gastric pH elevating effects of intensive antacids therapy, concomitant administration of EC-Naprosyn is not recommended).
No products indexed under this heading.

Aluminum Hydroxide (Due to the gastric pH elevating effects of intensive antacids therapy, concomitant administration of EC-Naprosyn is not recommended). Products include:
Gaviscon Regular Strength Liquid 620
Gaviscon Regular Strength Tablets 619
Gaviscon Extra Strength Liquid 620
Gaviscon Extra Strength Tablets 619
Maalox Max Maximum Strength Antacid/Anti-Gas Liquid 2165
Maalox Regular Strength Antacid/Antigas Liquid 2164

Anisindione (Short-term studies have failed to show any significant effect of concurrent use on prothrombin time; caution is advised since interactions have been seen with other NSAIDs). Products include:
Miradon Tablets 3056

Aspirin (Naproxen is displaced from its binding sites during the concomitant administration of aspirin resulting in lower plasma concentrations and peak plasma levels; concurrent use is not recommended). Products include:
Aggrenox Capsules 855
Bayer, Aspirin Regimen 606
Bayer Aspirin Tablets 3515
BC Powder 612
BC Allergy Sinus Cold Powder 612
Arthritis Strength BC Powder 612
BC Sinus Cold Powder 612
Ecotrin Enteric Coated Aspirin Low, Regular and Maximum Strength Tablets 1627
Goody's Body Pain Formula Powder 621
Goody's Extra Strength Headache Powder 621
Goody's Extra Strength Pain Relief Tablets 621
Percodan Tablets 1115
St. Joseph 81 mg Aspirin Chewable and Enteric Coated Tablets 1841

Atenolol (Reduced antihypertensive effect of beta blockers). Products include:
Tenormin I.V. Injection 698
Tenormin Tablets 695

Benazepril Hydrochloride (Reports suggest that NSAIDs may diminish the antihypertensive effect of ACE-inhibitors. The use of NSAIDs

IMPORTANT NOTE: Always consult each drug listing in the patient's regimen for possible interactions.

in patiens who are receiving ACE-inhibitors may potentiate renal dise states). Products include:
- Lotensin Tablets 2232
- Lotensin HCT Tablets 2235
- Lotrel Capsules 2238

Betaxolol Hydrochloride (Reduced antihypertensive effect of beta blockers). Products include:
- Betoptic S Ophthalmic Suspension.......... 554

Bisoprolol Fumarate (Reduced antihypertensive effect of beta blockers).
- No products indexed under this heading.

Captopril (Reports suggest that NSAIDs may diminish the antihypertensive effect of ACE-inhibitors. The use of NSAIDs in patiens who are receiving ACE-inhibitors may potentiate renal dise states). Products include:
- Captopril Tablets 2114

Carteolol Hydrochloride (Reduced antihypertensive effect of beta blockers). Products include:
- Carteolol Hydrochloride Ophthalmic Solution USP, 1%.......... ⊙246

Chlorpropamide (Potential for sulfonylurea toxicity).
- No products indexed under this heading.

Cimetidine (Due to the gastric pH elevating effects of H_2-blockers concomitant administration of EC-Naprosyn is not recommended). Products include:
- Tagamet HB 200 Tablets .... ■637
- Tagamet Tablets 1547

Cimetidine Hydrochloride (Due to the gastric pH elevating effects of H_2-blockers concomitant administration of EC-Naprosyn is not recommended).
- No products indexed under this heading.

Dicumarol (Short-term studies have failed to show any significant effect of concurrent use on prothrombin time; caution is advised since interactions have been seen with other NSAIDs).
- No products indexed under this heading.

Enalapril Maleate (Reports suggest that NSAIDs may diminish the antihypertensive effect of ACE-inhibitors. The use of NSAIDs in patiens who are receiving ACE-inhibitors may potentiate renal dise states). Products include:
- Vaseretic Tablets 2073
- Vasotec I.V. Injection 2076

Enalaprilat (Reports suggest that NSAIDs may diminish the antihypertensive effect of ACE-inhibitors. The use of NSAIDs in patiens who are receiving ACE-inhibitors may potentiate renal dise states).
- No products indexed under this heading.

Esmolol Hydrochloride (Reduced antihypertensive effect of beta blockers). Products include:
- Brevibloc Concentrate 766
- Brevibloc Injection 766
- Brevibloc Double Strength Injection.......... 766
- Brevibloc Premixed Injection 766
- Brevibloc Double Strength Premixed Injection 766

Ethotoin (Potential for hydantoin toxicity). Products include:
- Peganone Tablets, USP 2487

Famotidine (Due to the gastric pH elevating effects of H_2-blockers concomitant administration of EC-Naprosyn is not recommended). Products include:
- Pepcid AC Chewable Tablets 1672
- Pepcid AC Gelcaps 1672
- Pepcid AC Tablets 1672
- Maximum Strength Pepcid AC Tablets 1672
- Pepcid Complete Chewable Tablets 1672
- Pepcid Injection 2017
- Pepcid 2014

Fosinopril Sodium (Reports suggest that NSAIDs may diminish the antihypertensive effect of ACE-inhibitors. The use of NSAIDs in patiens who are receiving ACE-inhibitors may potentiate renal dise states).
- No products indexed under this heading.

Fosphenytoin Sodium (Potential for hydantoin toxicity).
- No products indexed under this heading.

Furosemide (Inhibition of natriuretic effect of furosemide). Products include:
- Furosemide Tablets 2117

Glimepiride (Potential for sulfonylurea toxicity). Products include:
- Amaryl Tablets 2864

Glipizide (Potential for sulfonylurea toxicity).
- No products indexed under this heading.

Glyburide (Potential for sulfonylurea toxicity).
- No products indexed under this heading.

Labetalol Hydrochloride (Reduced antihypertensive effect of beta blockers).
- No products indexed under this heading.

Levobunolol Hydrochloride (Reduced antihypertensive effect of beta blockers). Products include:
- Betagan Ophthalmic Solution, USP.......... ⊙217

Lisinopril (Reports suggest that NSAIDs may diminish the antihypertensive effect of ACE-inhibitors. The use of NSAIDs in patiens who are receiving ACE-inhibitors may potentiate renal dise states). Products include:
- Prinivil Tablets 2029
- Prinzide Tablets 2033
- Zestoretic Tablets 701
- Zestril Tablets 704

Lithium (Inhibition of lithium renal clearance leading to increase in plasma lithium concentrations).
- No products indexed under this heading.

Lithium Carbonate (Inhibition of lithium renal clearance leading to increase in plasma lithium concentrations). Products include:
- Eskalith 1406
- Lithobid Tablets 1670

Lithium Citrate (Inhibition of lithium renal clearance leading to increase in plasma lithium concentrations).
- No products indexed under this heading.

Magaldrate (Due to the gastric pH elevating effects of intensive antacids therapy, concomitant administration of EC-Naprosyn is not recommended).
- No products indexed under this heading.

Magnesium Hydroxide (Due to the gastric pH elevating effects of intensive antacids therapy, concomitant administration of EC-Naprosyn is not recommended). Products include:
- Maalox Max Maximum Strength Antacid/Anti-Gas Liquid.......... 2165
- Maalox Regular Strength Antacid/Antigas Liquid.......... 2164
- Pepcid Complete Chewable Tablets 1672
- Rolaids Tablets .... ■707
- Extra Strength Rolaids Tablets .... ■707
- Rolaids Multi-Symptom Antacid & Antigas Tablets .... ■708

Magnesium Oxide (Due to the gastric pH elevating effects of intensive antacids therapy, concomitant administration of EC-Naprosyn is not recommended). Products include:
- Beelith Tablets 784
- PremCal Light, Regular, and Extra Strength Tablets.......... ■762

Mephenytoin (Potential for hydantoin toxicity).
- No products indexed under this heading.

Methotrexate Sodium (Potential for reduced tubular secretion of methotrexate and possible increased methotrexate toxicity as shown in animal model; caution is recommended).
- No products indexed under this heading.

Metipranolol Hydrochloride (Reduced antihypertensive effect of beta blockers).
- No products indexed under this heading.

Metoprolol Succinate (Reduced antihypertensive effect of beta blockers). Products include:
- Toprol-XL Tablets 660

Metoprolol Tartrate (Reduced antihypertensive effect of beta blockers).
- No products indexed under this heading.

Moexipril Hydrochloride (Reports suggest that NSAIDs may diminish the antihypertensive effect of ACE-inhibitors. The use of NSAIDs in patiens who are receiving ACE-inhibitors may potentiate renal dise states). Products include:
- Uniretic Tablets 3114
- Univasc Tablets 3118

Nadolol (Reduced antihypertensive effect of beta blockers). Products include:
- Nadolol Tablets 2121

Naproxen Sodium (Concurrent use of naproxen or naproxen sodium in any dosage form is not recommended since they all circulate in the plasma as the naproxen anion). Products include:
- Aleve Tablets, Caplets and Gelcaps.......... ■605
- Anaprox Tablets 2769
- Anaprox DS Tablets 2769

Nizatidine (Due to the gastric pH elevating effects of H_2-blockers concomitant administration of EC-Naprosyn is not recommended). Products include:
- Axid Oral Solution 913

Penbutolol Sulfate (Reduced antihypertensive effect of beta blockers).
- No products indexed under this heading.

Perindopril Erbumine (Reports suggest that NSAIDs may diminish the antihypertensive effect of ACE-inhibitors. The use of NSAIDs in patiens who are receiving ACE-inhibitors may potentiate renal dise states). Products include:
- Aceon Tablets (2 mg, 4 mg, 8 mg).......... 3191

Phenytoin (Potential for hydantoin toxicity).
- No products indexed under this heading.

Phenytoin Sodium (Potential for hydantoin toxicity). Products include:
- Phenytek Capsules 2153

Pindolol (Reduced antihypertensive effect of beta blockers).
- No products indexed under this heading.

Probenecid (Probenecid given concurrently increases naproxen anion plasma levels and extends its plasma half-life significantly).
- No products indexed under this heading.

Propranolol Hydrochloride (Reduced antihypertensive effect of beta blockers). Products include:
- Inderal LA Long-Acting Capsules 3421
- InnoPran XL Capsules 2728

Quinapril Hydrochloride (Reports suggest that NSAIDs may diminish the antihypertensive effect of ACE-inhibitors. The use of NSAIDs in patiens who are receiving ACE-inhibitors may potentiate renal dise states).
- No products indexed under this heading.

Ramipril (Reports suggest that NSAIDs may diminish the antihypertensive effect of ACE-inhibitors. The use of NSAIDs in patiens who are receiving ACE-inhibitors may potentiate renal dise states). Products include:
- Altace Capsules 1673

Ranitidine Bismuth Citrate (Due to the gastric pH elevating effects of H_2-blockers concomitant administration of EC-Naprosyn is not recommended).
- No products indexed under this heading.

Ranitidine Hydrochloride (Due to the gastric pH elevating effects of H_2-blockers concomitant administration of EC-Naprosyn is not recommended). Products include:
- Zantac 1597
- Zantac Injection 1593
- Zantac 75 Tablets .... ■715
- Zantac 150 Maximum Strength Tablets.......... ■715
- Zantac Injection Pharmacy Bulk Package 1595

Sotalol Hydrochloride (Reduced antihypertensive effect of beta blockers).
- No products indexed under this heading.

Spirapril Hydrochloride (Reports suggest that NSAIDs may diminish the antihypertensive effect of ACE-inhibitors. The use of NSAIDs in patiens who are receiving ACE-inhibitors may potentiate renal dise states).
- No products indexed under this heading.

Sucralfate (Due to the gastric pH elevating effects of sucralfate, concomitant administration of EC-Naprosyn is not recommended). Products include:
- Carafate Suspension 727
- Carafate Tablets 728

Sulfamethoxazole (Potential for sulfonamide toxicity).
- No products indexed under this heading.

Sulfisoxazole Acetyl (Potential for sulfonamide toxicity).
No products indexed under this heading.

Timolol Hemihydrate (Reduced antihypertensive effect of beta blockers). Products include:
Betimol Ophthalmic Solution 3371
Betimol Ophthalmic Solution .... ⊙283

Timolol Maleate (Reduced antihypertensive effect of beta blockers). Products include:
Blocadren Tablets 1891
Cosopt Sterile Ophthalmic Solution.. 1910
Timolide Tablets 2056
Timoptic in Ocudose 2061
Timoptic Sterile Ophthalmic Solution.. 2058
Timoptic-XE Sterile Ophthalmic Gel Forming Solution 2062

Tolazamide (Potential for sulfonylurea toxicity).
No products indexed under this heading.

Tolbutamide (Potential for sulfonylurea toxicity).
No products indexed under this heading.

Trandolapril (Co-administration of NSAIDs and ACE inhibitors may potentiate renal disease states). Products include:
Mavik Tablets 482
Tarka Tablets 519

Warfarin Sodium (Short-term studies have failed to show any significant effect of concurrent use on prothrombin time; caution is advised since interactions have been seen with other NSAIDs). Products include:
Coumadin for Injection 932
Coumadin Tablets 932

Food Interactions

Food, unspecified (The presence of food prolonged the time the EC-Naprosyn remained in the stomach, time to first detectable serum naproxen levels, and time to maximal naproxen levels (Tmax), but did not affect peak naproxen levels (Cmax)).

ECOTRIN ENTERIC COATED ASPIRIN LOW, REGULAR AND MAXIMUM STRENGTH TABLETS

(Aspirin) 1627

May interact with ACE inhibitors, beta blockers, anticoagulants, diuretics, oral hypoglycemic agents, non-steroidal anti-inflammatory agents, phenytoin, valproate, and certain other agents. Compounds in these categories include:

Acarbose (Moderate doses of aspirin may increase the effectiveness of oral hypoglycemic drugs, leading to hypoglycemia). Products include:
Precose Tablets 776

Acebutolol Hydrochloride (Co-administration of beta blockers with aspirin may diminish the hypotensive effects of beta blockers due to inhibition of renal prostaglandins, leading to decreased renal blood flow, and salt and fluid retention).
No products indexed under this heading.

Acetazolamide (Co-administration can lead to high serum concentrations of acetazolamide (and toxicity) due to competition at the renal tubule for secretion).
No products indexed under this heading.

Acetazolamide Sodium (Co-administration can lead to high serum concentrations of acetazolamide (and toxicity) due to competition at the renal tubule for secretion).
No products indexed under this heading.

Amiloride Hydrochloride (Co-administration of diuretics with aspirin may diminish the effectiveness of diuretics due to inhibition of renal prostaglandins, leading to decreased renal blood flow, and salt and fluid retention). Products include:
Midamor Tablets 2000
Moduretic Tablets 2003

Anisindione (Patients on anticoagulant therapy are at increased risk for bleeding). Products include:
Miradon Tablets 3056

Ardeparin Sodium (Patients on anticoagulant therapy are at increased risk for bleeding).
No products indexed under this heading.

Atenolol (Co-administration of beta blockers with aspirin may diminish the hypotensive effects of beta blockers due to inhibition of renal prostaglandins, leading to decreased renal blood flow, and salt and fluid retention). Products include:
Tenormin I.V. Injection 698
Tenormin Tablets 695

Benazepril Hydrochloride (Co-administration of aspirin with ACE inhibitors may result in hyponatremic and hypotensive effects of ACE inhibitors due to aspirin's direct effect on the renin-angiotensin conversion pathway). Products include:
Lotensin Tablets 2232
Lotensin HCT Tablets 2235
Lotrel Capsules 2238

Bendroflumethiazide (Co-administration of diuretics with aspirin may diminish the effectiveness of diuretics due to inhibition of renal prostaglandins, leading to decreased renal blood flow, and salt and fluid retention).
No products indexed under this heading.

Betaxolol Hydrochloride (Co-administration of beta blockers with aspirin may diminish the hypotensive effects of beta blockers due to inhibition of renal prostaglandins, leading to decreased renal blood flow, and salt and fluid retention). Products include:
Betoptic S Ophthalmic Suspension................................. 554

Bisoprolol Fumarate (Co-administration of beta blockers with aspirin may diminish the hypotensive effects of beta blockers due to inhibition of renal prostaglandins, leading to decreased renal blood flow, and salt and fluid retention).
No products indexed under this heading.

Bumetanide (Co-administration of diuretics with aspirin may diminish the effectiveness of diuretics due to inhibition of renal prostaglandins, leading to decreased renal blood flow, and salt and fluid retention).
No products indexed under this heading.

Captopril (Co-administration of aspirin with ACE inhibitors may result in hyponatremic and hypotensive effects of ACE inhibitors due to aspirin's direct effect on the renin-angiotensin conversion pathway). Products include:
Captopril Tablets 2114

Carteolol Hydrochloride (Co-administration of beta blockers with aspirin may diminish the hypotensive effects of beta blockers due to inhibition of renal prostaglandins, leading to decreased renal blood flow, and salt and fluid retention). Products include:
Carteolol Hydrochloride Ophthalmic Solution USP, 1%....... ⊙246

Celecoxib (Co-administration may increase bleeding or lead to decreased renal function). Products include:
Celebrex Capsules 3130

Chlorothiazide (Co-administration of diuretics with aspirin may diminish the effectiveness of diuretics due to inhibition of renal prostaglandins, leading to decreased renal blood flow, and salt and fluid retention). Products include:
Aldoclor Tablets 1881
Diuril Oral 1936

Chlorothiazide Sodium (Co-administration of diuretics with aspirin may diminish the effectiveness of diuretics due to inhibition of renal prostaglandins, leading to decreased renal blood flow, and salt and fluid retention). Products include:
Diuril Sodium Intravenous 1934

Chlorpropamide (Moderate doses of aspirin may increase the effectiveness of oral hypoglycemic drugs, leading to hypoglycemia).
No products indexed under this heading.

Chlorthalidone (Co-administration of diuretics with aspirin may diminish the effectiveness of diuretics due to inhibition of renal prostaglandins, leading to decreased renal blood flow, and salt and fluid retention). Products include:
Clorpres Tablets 2139

Dalteparin Sodium (Patients on anticoagulant therapy are at increased risk for bleeding). Products include:
Fragmin Injection 2638

Danaparoid Sodium (Patients on anticoagulant therapy are at increased risk for bleeding).
No products indexed under this heading.

Diclofenac Potassium (Co-administration may increase bleeding or lead to decreased renal function). Products include:
Cataflam Tablets 2173

Diclofenac Sodium (Co-administration may increase bleeding or lead to decreased renal function). Products include:
Arthrotec Tablets 3126
Voltaren Ophthalmic Solution 2300
Voltaren Tablets 2298
Voltaren-XR Tablets 2301

Dicumarol (Patients on anticoagulant therapy are at increased risk for bleeding).
No products indexed under this heading.

Divalproex Sodium (Salicylate can displace protein-bound valproic acid leading to an increase in serum valproic acid levels). Products include:
Depakote Sprinkle Capsules 422
Depakote Tablets 427
Depakote ER Tablets 433

Enalapril Maleate (Co-administration of aspirin with ACE inhibitors may result in hyponatremic and hypotensive effects of ACE inhibitors due to aspirin's direct effect on the renin-angiotensin conversion pathway). Products include:
Vaseretic Tablets 2073
Vasotec I.V. Injection 2076

Enalaprilat (Co-administration of aspirin with ACE inhibitors may result in hyponatremic and hypotensive effects of ACE inhibitors due to aspirin's direct effect on the renin-angiotensin conversion pathway).
No products indexed under this heading.

Enoxaparin Sodium (Patients on anticoagulant therapy are at increased risk for bleeding). Products include:
Lovenox Injection 2931

Esmolol Hydrochloride (Co-administration of beta blockers with aspirin may diminish the hypotensive effects of beta blockers due to inhibition of renal prostaglandins, leading to decreased renal blood flow, and salt and fluid retention). Products include:
Brevibloc Concentrate 766
Brevibloc Injection 766
Brevibloc Double Strength Injection.. 766
Brevibloc Premixed Injection 766
Brevibloc Double Strength Premixed Injection 766

Ethacrynic Acid (Co-administration of diuretics with aspirin may diminish the effectiveness of diuretics due to inhibition of renal prostaglandins, leading to decreased renal blood flow, and salt and fluid retention). Products include:
Edecrin Tablets 1941

Etodolac (Co-administration may increase bleeding or lead to decreased renal function).
No products indexed under this heading.

Fenoprofen Calcium (Co-administration may increase bleeding or lead to decreased renal function). Products include:
Nalfon Capsules 2504

Flurbiprofen (Co-administration may increase bleeding or lead to decreased renal function).
No products indexed under this heading.

Fondaparinux Sodium (Patients on anticoagulant therapy are at increased risk for bleeding). Products include:
Arixtra Injection 1325

Fosinopril Sodium (Co-administration of aspirin with ACE inhibitors may result in hyponatremic and hypotensive effects of ACE inhibitors due to aspirin's direct effect on the renin-angiotensin conversion pathway).
No products indexed under this heading.

Fosphenytoin Sodium (Salicylate can displace protein-bound phenytoin leading to a decrease in the total concentration of phenytoin).
No products indexed under this heading.

Furosemide (Co-administration of diuretics with aspirin may diminish the effectiveness of diuretics due to inhibition of renal prostaglandins, leading to decreased renal blood flow, and salt and fluid retention). Products include:

Furosemide Tablets 2117

Glimepiride (Moderate doses of aspirin may increase the effectiveness of oral hypoglycemic drugs, leading to hypoglycemia). Products include:

Amaryl Tablets 2864

Glipizide (Moderate doses of aspirin may increase the effectiveness of oral hypoglycemic drugs, leading to hypoglycemia).

No products indexed under this heading.

Glyburide (Moderate doses of aspirin may increase the effectiveness of oral hypoglycemic drugs, leading to hypoglycemia).

No products indexed under this heading.

Heparin Calcium (Patients on anticoagulant therapy are at increased risk for bleeding).

No products indexed under this heading.

Heparin Sodium (Patients on anticoagulant therapy are at increased risk for bleeding).

No products indexed under this heading.

Hydrochlorothiazide (Co-administration of diuretics with aspirin may diminish the effectiveness of diuretics due to inhibition of renal prostaglandins, leading to decreased renal blood flow, and salt and fluid retention). Products include:

Aldoril Tablets 1884
Atacand HCT 637
Avalide Tablets 2889
Avalide Tablets 922
Benicar HCT Tablets 2852
Diovan HCT Tablets 2195
Dyazide Capsules 1389
Hyzaar 1964
Lotensin HCT Tablets 2235
Maxzide 2150
Micardis HCT Tablets 886
Moduretic Tablets 2003
Prinzide Tablets 2033
Teveten HCT Tablets 1710
Timolide Tablets 2056
Uniretic Tablets 3114
Vaseretic Tablets 2073
Zestoretic Tablets 701

Hydroflumethiazide (Co-administration of diuretics with aspirin may diminish the effectiveness of diuretics due to inhibition of renal prostaglandins, leading to decreased renal blood flow, and salt and fluid retention).

No products indexed under this heading.

Ibuprofen (Co-administration may increase bleeding or lead to decreased renal function). Products include:

Advil Allergy Sinus Caplets .... ▣737
Advil .... ▣737
Children's Advil Suspension .... ▣742
Children's Advil Chewable Tablets .... ▣741
Advil Cold & Sinus .... ▣739
Advil Flu & Body Ache Caplets .... ▣739
Children's Advil Cold Suspension .... ▣741
Infants' Advil Concentrated Drops .... ▣743
Junior Strength Advil Swallow Tablets .... ▣740
Advil Migraine Liquigels .... ▣740
Advil Multi-Symptom Cold Caplets .... ▣738
Combunox Tablets 1183
Children's Motrin Oral Suspension and Chewable Tablets 1837
Children's Motrin Cold Non-Staining Dye-Free Oral Suspension 1838
Children's Motrin Cold Oral Suspension 1838
Children's Motrin Non-Staining Dye-Free Oral Suspension 1837
Motrin Cold & Sinus Caplets 1836
Motrin IB Tablets and Caplets 1836
Infants' Motrin Concentrated Drops 1837
Infants' Motrin Non-Staining Dye-Free Drops 1837
Junior Strength Motrin Caplets and Chewable Tablets 1837
Vicoprofen Tablets 533

Indapamide (Co-administration of diuretics with aspirin may diminish the effectiveness of diuretics due to inhibition of renal prostaglandins, leading to decreased renal blood flow, and salt and fluid retention). Products include:

Indapamide Tablets 2119

Indomethacin (Co-administration may increase bleeding or lead to decreased renal function). Products include:

Indocin 1968

Indomethacin Sodium Trihydrate (Co-administration may increase bleeding or lead to decreased renal function). Products include:

Indocin I.V. 1973

Ketoprofen (Co-administration may increase bleeding or lead to decreased renal function).

No products indexed under this heading.

Ketorolac Tromethamine (Co-administration may increase bleeding or lead to decreased renal function). Products include:

Acular Ophthalmic Solution 561
Acular LS Ophthalmic Solution 562

Labetalol Hydrochloride (Co-administration of beta blockers with aspirin may diminish the hypotensive effects of beta blockers due to inhibition of renal prostaglandins, leading to decreased renal blood flow, and salt and fluid retention).

No products indexed under this heading.

Levobunolol Hydrochloride (Co-administration of beta blockers with aspirin may diminish the hypotensive effects of beta blockers due to inhibition of renal prostaglandins, leading to decreased renal blood flow, and salt and fluid retention). Products include:

Betagan Ophthalmic Solution, USP .... ⊙217

Lisinopril (Co-administration of aspirin with ACE inhibitors may result in hyponatremic and hypotensive effects of ACE inhibitors due to aspirin's direct effect on the renin-angiotensin conversion pathway). Products include:

Prinivil Tablets 2029
Prinzide Tablets 2033
Zestoretic Tablets 701
Zestril Tablets 704

Low Molecular Weight Heparins (Patients on anticoagulant therapy are at increased risk for bleeding).

No products indexed under this heading.

Meclofenamate Sodium (Co-administration may increase bleeding or lead to decreased renal function).

No products indexed under this heading.

Mefenamic Acid (Co-administration may increase bleeding or lead to decreased renal function).

No products indexed under this heading.

Meloxicam (Co-administration may increase bleeding or lead to decreased renal function). Products include:

Mobic Oral Suspension 893
Mobic Tablets 893

Metformin Hydrochloride (Moderate doses of aspirin may increase the effectiveness of oral hypoglycemic drugs, leading to hypoglycemia). Products include:

ActoPlus Met Tablets 3219
Avandamet Tablets 1343
Fortamet Extended-Release Tablets 1156

Methotrexate Sodium (Salicylate can inhibit renal clearance of methotrexate, leading to bone marrow toxicity, especially in the elderly or renal impaired).

No products indexed under this heading.

Methyclothiazide (Co-administration of diuretics with aspirin may diminish the effectiveness of diuretics due to inhibition of renal prostaglandins, leading to decreased renal blood flow, and salt and fluid retention).

No products indexed under this heading.

Metipranolol Hydrochloride (Co-administration of beta blockers with aspirin may diminish the hypotensive effects of beta blockers due to inhibition of renal prostaglandins, leading to decreased renal blood flow, and salt and fluid retention).

No products indexed under this heading.

Metolazone (Co-administration of diuretics with aspirin may diminish the effectiveness of diuretics due to inhibition of renal prostaglandins, leading to decreased renal blood flow, and salt and fluid retention).

No products indexed under this heading.

Metoprolol Succinate (Co-administration of beta blockers with aspirin may diminish the hypotensive effects of beta blockers due to inhibition of renal prostaglandins, leading to decreased renal blood flow, and salt and fluid retention). Products include:

Toprol-XL Tablets 660

Metoprolol Tartrate (Co-administration of beta blockers with aspirin may diminish the hypotensive effects of beta blockers due to inhibition of renal prostaglandins, leading to decreased renal blood flow, and salt and fluid retention).

No products indexed under this heading.

Miglitol (Moderate doses of aspirin may increase the effectiveness of oral hypoglycemic drugs, leading to hypoglycemia).

No products indexed under this heading.

Moexipril Hydrochloride (Co-administration of aspirin with ACE inhibitors may result in hyponatremic and hypotensive effects of ACE inhibitors due to aspirin's direct effect on the renin-angiotensin conversion pathway). Products include:

Uniretic Tablets 3114
Univasc Tablets 3118

Nabumetone (Co-administration may increase bleeding or lead to decreased renal function). Products include:

Relafen Tablets 1523

Nadolol (Co-administration of beta blockers with aspirin may diminish the hypotensive effects of beta blockers due to inhibition of renal prostaglandins, leading to decreased renal blood flow, and salt and fluid retention). Products include:

Nadolol Tablets 2121

Naproxen (Co-administration may increase bleeding or lead to decreased renal function). Products include:

EC-Naprosyn Delayed-Release Tablets 2769
Naprosyn Suspension 2769
Naprosyn Tablets 2769
Prevacid NapraPAC 3277

Naproxen Sodium (Co-administration may increase bleeding or lead to decreased renal function). Products include:

Aleve Tablets, Caplets and Gelcaps .... ▣605
Anaprox Tablets 2769
Anaprox DS Tablets 2769

Oxaprozin (Co-administration may increase bleeding or lead to decreased renal function).

No products indexed under this heading.

Penbutolol Sulfate (Co-administration of beta blockers with aspirin may diminish the hypotensive effects of beta blockers due to inhibition of renal prostaglandins, leading to decreased renal blood flow, and salt and fluid retention).

No products indexed under this heading.

Perindopril Erbumine (Co-administration of aspirin with ACE inhibitors may result in hyponatremic and hypotensive effects of ACE inhibitors due to aspirin's direct effect on the renin-angiotensin conversion pathway). Products include:

Aceon Tablets (2 mg, 4 mg, 8 mg) 3191

Phenylbutazone (Co-administration may increase bleeding or lead to decreased renal function).

No products indexed under this heading.

Phenytoin (Salicylate can displace protein-bound phenytoin leading to a decrease in the total concentration of phenytoin).

No products indexed under this heading.

Phenytoin Sodium (Salicylate can displace protein-bound phenytoin leading to a decrease in the total concentration of phenytoin). Products include:

Phenytek Capsules 2153

Pindolol (Co-administration of beta blockers with aspirin may diminish the hypotensive effects of beta blockers due to inhibition of renal prostaglandins, leading to decreased renal blood flow, and salt and fluid retention).

No products indexed under this heading.

Pioglitazone Hydrochloride (Moderate doses of aspirin may increase the effectiveness of oral hypoglycemic drugs, leading to hypoglycemia). Products include:

ActoPlus Met Tablets 3219
Actos Tablets 3224

Piroxicam (Co-administration may increase bleeding or lead to decreased renal function).

No products indexed under this heading.

Polythiazide (Co-administration of diuretics with aspirin may diminish the effectiveness of diuretics due to inhibition of renal prostaglandins, leading to decreased renal blood flow, and salt and fluid retention).
No products indexed under this heading.

Probenecid (Salicylate can antagonize the uricosuric action of uricosuric agents).
No products indexed under this heading.

Propranolol Hydrochloride (Co-administration of beta blockers with aspirin may diminish the hypotensive effects of beta blockers due to inhibition of renal prostaglandins, leading to decreased renal blood flow, and salt and fluid retention).
Products include:
Inderal LA Long-Acting Capsules 3421
InnoPran XL Capsules 2728

Quinapril Hydrochloride (Co-administration of aspirin with ACE inhibitors may result in hyponatremic and hypotensive effects of ACE inhibitors due to aspirin's direct effect on the renin-angiotensin conversion pathway).
No products indexed under this heading.

Ramipril (Co-administration of aspirin with ACE inhibitors may result in hyponatremic and hypotensive effects of ACE inhibitors due to aspirin's direct effect on the renin-angiotensin conversion pathway).
Products include:
Altace Capsules 1673

Repaglinide (Moderate doses of aspirin may increase the effectiveness of oral hypoglycemic drugs, leading to hypoglycemia). Products include:
Prandin Tablets (0.5, 1, and 2 mg).. 2337

Rofecoxib (Co-administration may increase bleeding or lead to decreased renal function).
No products indexed under this heading.

Rosiglitazone Maleate (Moderate doses of aspirin may increase the effectiveness of oral hypoglycemic drugs, leading to hypoglycemia).
Products include:
Avandamet Tablets 1343
Avandia Tablets 1348

Sotalol Hydrochloride (Co-administration of beta blockers with aspirin may diminish the hypotensive effects of beta blockers due to inhibition of renal prostaglandins, leading to decreased renal blood flow, and salt and fluid retention).
No products indexed under this heading.

Spirapril Hydrochloride (Co-administration of aspirin with ACE inhibitors may result in hyponatremic and hypotensive effects of ACE inhibitors due to aspirin's direct effect on the renin-angiotensin conversion pathway).
No products indexed under this heading.

Spironolactone (Co-administration of diuretics with aspirin may diminish the effectiveness of diuretics due to inhibition of renal prostaglandins, leading to decreased renal blood flow, and salt and fluid retention).
No products indexed under this heading.

Sulfinpyrazone (Salicylate can antagonize the uricosuric action of uricosuric agents).
No products indexed under this heading.

Sulindac (Co-administration may increase bleeding or lead to decreased renal function). Products include:
Clinoril Tablets 1899

Timolol Hemihydrate (Co-administration of beta blockers with aspirin may diminish the hypotensive effects of beta blockers due to inhibition of renal prostaglandins, leading to decreased renal blood flow, and salt and fluid retention).
Products include:
Betimol Ophthalmic Solution 3371
Betimol Ophthalmic Solution .... ⊙283

Timolol Maleate (Co-administration of beta blockers with aspirin may diminish the hypotensive effects of beta blockers due to inhibition of renal prostaglandins, leading to decreased renal blood flow, and salt and fluid retention). Products include:
Blocadren Tablets 1891
Cosopt Sterile Ophthalmic Solution.. 1910
Timolide Tablets 2056
Timoptic in Ocudose 2061
Timoptic Sterile Ophthalmic Solution.. 2058
Timoptic-XE Sterile Ophthalmic Gel Forming Solution 2062

Tinzaparin Sodium (Patients on anticoagulant therapy are at increased risk for bleeding).
No products indexed under this heading.

Tolazamide (Moderate doses of aspirin may increase the effectiveness of oral hypoglycemic drugs, leading to hypoglycemia).
No products indexed under this heading.

Tolbutamide (Moderate doses of aspirin may increase the effectiveness of oral hypoglycemic drugs, leading to hypoglycemia).
No products indexed under this heading.

Tolmetin Sodium (Co-administration may increase bleeding or lead to decreased renal function).
No products indexed under this heading.

Torsemide (Co-administration of diuretics with aspirin may diminish the effectiveness of diuretics due to inhibition of renal prostaglandins, leading to decreased renal blood flow, and salt and fluid retention).
No products indexed under this heading.

Trandolapril (Co-administration of aspirin with ACE inhibitors may result in hyponatremic and hypotensive effects of ACE inhibitors due to aspirin's direct effect on the renin-angiotensin conversion pathway).
Products include:
Mavik Tablets 482
Tarka Tablets 519

Triamterene (Co-administration of diuretics with aspirin may diminish the effectiveness of diuretics due to inhibition of renal prostaglandins, leading to decreased renal blood flow, and salt and fluid retention).
Products include:
Dyazide Capsules 1389
Dyrenium Capsules 3390
Maxzide 2150

Troglitazone (Moderate doses of aspirin may increase the effectiveness of oral hypoglycemic drugs, leading to hypoglycemia).
No products indexed under this heading.

Valdecoxib (Co-administration may increase bleeding or lead to decreased renal function).
No products indexed under this heading.

Valproate Sodium (Salicylate can displace protein-bound valproic acid leading to an increase in serum valproic acid levels). Products include:
Depacon Injection 412

Valproic Acid (Salicylate can displace protein-bound valproic acid leading to an increase in serum valproic acid levels). Products include:
Depakene 417

Warfarin Sodium (Aspirin can displace warfarin from protein binding sites, leading to prolongation of both the prothrombin time and the bleeding time). Products include:
Coumadin for Injection 932
Coumadin Tablets 932

Food Interactions

Alcohol (Chronic heavy alcohol users, 3 or more drinks per day, in combination with analgesic/antipyretic drug products containing aspirin increases the risk of adverse GI events, including stomach bleeding).

EDECRIN TABLETS

(Ethacrynic Acid) 1941
See Edecrin Sodium Intravenous

EDECRIN SODIUM INTRAVENOUS

(Ethacrynate Sodium) 1941
May interact with aminoglycosides, cephalosporins, cardiac glycosides, non-steroidal anti-inflammatory agents, and certain other agents. Compounds in these categories include:

Amikacin Sulfate (Increased ototoxic potential of aminoglycosides).
No products indexed under this heading.

Cefaclor (Increased ototoxic potential of cephalosporins).
No products indexed under this heading.

Cefadroxil (Increased ototoxic potential of cephalosporins).
No products indexed under this heading.

Cefamandole Nafate (Increased ototoxic potential of cephalosporins).
No products indexed under this heading.

Cefazolin Sodium (Increased ototoxic potential of cephalosporins).
Products include:
Ancef for Injection 1318

Cefdinir (Increased ototoxic potential of cephalosporins). Products include:
Omnicef Capsules 506
Omnicef for Oral Suspension 506

Cefepime Hydrochloride (Increased ototoxic potential of cephalosporins). Products include:
Maxipime for Injection 1093

Cefixime (Increased ototoxic potential of cephalosporins). Products include:
Suprax 1811

Cefmetazole Sodium (Increased ototoxic potential of cephalosporins).
No products indexed under this heading.

Cefonicid Sodium (Increased ototoxic potential of cephalosporins).
No products indexed under this heading.

Cefoperazone Sodium (Increased ototoxic potential of cephalosporins).
No products indexed under this heading.

Ceforanide (Increased ototoxic potential of cephalosporins).
No products indexed under this heading.

Cefotaxime Sodium (Increased ototoxic potential of cephalosporins).
No products indexed under this heading.

Cefotetan (Increased ototoxic potential of cephalosporins).
No products indexed under this heading.

Cefoxitin Sodium (Increased ototoxic potential of cephalosporins).
Products include:
Mefoxin for Injection 1987
Mefoxin Premixed Intravenous Solution 1990

Cefpodoxime Proxetil (Increased ototoxic potential of cephalosporins). Products include:
Vantin Tablets and Oral Suspension 2650

Cefprozil (Increased ototoxic potential of cephalosporins).
No products indexed under this heading.

Ceftazidime (Increased ototoxic potential of cephalosporins).
Products include:
Fortaz for Injection 1422

Ceftizoxime Sodium (Increased ototoxic potential of cephalosporins).
No products indexed under this heading.

Ceftriaxone Sodium (Increased ototoxic potential of cephalosporins). Products include:
Rocephin Injectable Vials, ADD-Vantage, Galaxy, Bulk........... 2801

Cefuroxime Axetil (Increased ototoxic potential of cephalosporins).
Products include:
Ceftin 1369

Cefuroxime Sodium (Increased ototoxic potential of cephalosporins).
No products indexed under this heading.

Celecoxib (Reduces diuretic, natriuretic, and antihypertensive effects).
Products include:
Celebrex Capsules 3130

Cephalexin (Increased ototoxic potential of cephalosporins).
No products indexed under this heading.

Cephalothin Sodium (Increased ototoxic potential of cephalosporins).
No products indexed under this heading.

Cephapirin Sodium (Increased ototoxic potential of cephalosporins).
No products indexed under this heading.

IMPORTANT NOTE: Always consult each drug listing in the patient's regimen for possible interactions.

Cephradine (Increased ototoxic potential of cephalosporins).
No products indexed under this heading.

Deslanoside (Excessive potassium loss may precipitate digitalis toxicity).
No products indexed under this heading.

Diclofenac Potassium (Reduces diuretic, natriuretic, and antihypertensive effects). Products include:
Cataflam Tablets **2173**

Diclofenac Sodium (Reduces diuretic, natriuretic, and antihypertensive effects). Products include:
Arthrotec Tablets **3126**
Voltaren Ophthalmic Solution **2300**
Voltaren Tablets **2298**
Voltaren-XR Tablets **2301**

Digitalis Glycoside Preparations (Excessive potassium loss may precipitate digitalis toxicity).
No products indexed under this heading.

Digitoxin (Excessive potassium loss may precipitate digitalis toxicity).
No products indexed under this heading.

Digoxin (Excessive potassium loss may precipitate digitalis toxicity). Products include:
Digitek Tablets **2146**
Lanoxicaps Capsules **1458**
Lanoxin Injection **1462**
Lanoxin Tablets **1468**
Lanoxin Injection Pediatric **1465**

Etodolac (Reduces diuretic, natriuretic, and antihypertensive effects).
No products indexed under this heading.

Fenoprofen Calcium (Reduces diuretic, natriuretic, and antihypertensive effects). Products include:
Nalfon Capsules **2504**

Flurbiprofen (Reduces diuretic, natriuretic, and antihypertensive effects).
No products indexed under this heading.

Gentamicin Sulfate (Increased ototoxic potential of aminoglycosides). Products include:
Garamycin Injectable **3028**
Genoptic Sterile Ophthalmic Solution.......... ⊙ **227**
Pred-G Ophthalmic Suspension .... ⊙ **234**
Pred-G Sterile Ophthalmic Ointment.......... ⊙ **235**

Ibuprofen (Reduces diuretic, natriuretic, and antihypertensive effects). Products include:
Advil Allergy Sinus Caplets .... ▣ **737**
Advil .... ▣ **737**
Children's Advil Suspension .... ▣ **742**
Children's Advil Chewable Tablets .. ▣ **741**
Advil Cold & Sinus .... ▣ **739**
Advil Flu & Body Ache Caplets .... ▣ **739**
Children's Advil Cold Suspension .... ▣ **741**
Infants' Advil Concentrated Drops .. ▣ **743**
Junior Strength Advil Swallow Tablets.......... ▣ **740**
Advil Migraine Liquigels .... ▣ **740**
Advil Multi-Symptom Cold Caplets.......... ▣ **738**
Combunox Tablets **1183**
Children's Motrin Oral Suspension and Chewable Tablets.......... **1837**
Children's Motrin Cold Non-Staining Dye-Free Oral Suspension **1838**
Children's Motrin Cold Oral Suspension **1838**
Children's Motrin Non-Staining Dye-Free Oral Suspension.......... **1837**
Motrin Cold & Sinus Caplets **1836**
Motrin IB Tablets and Caplets **1836**
Infants' Motrin Concentrated Drops.......... **1837**
Infants' Motrin Non-Staining Dye-Free Drops.......... **1837**
Junior Strength Motrin Caplets and Chewable Tablets.......... **1837**
Vicoprofen Tablets **533**

Indomethacin (Reduces diuretic, natriuretic, and antihypertensive effects). Products include:
Indocin **1968**

Indomethacin Sodium Trihydrate (Reduces diuretic, natriuretic, and antihypertensive effects). Products include:
Indocin I.V. **1973**

Isoproterenol Hydrochloride (Careful adjustment of dosages required).
No products indexed under this heading.

Kanamycin Sulfate (Increased ototoxic potential of aminoglycosides).
No products indexed under this heading.

Ketoprofen (Reduces diuretic, natriuretic, and antihypertensive effects).
No products indexed under this heading.

Ketorolac Tromethamine (Reduces diuretic, natriuretic, and antihypertensive effects). Products include:
Acular Ophthalmic Solution **561**
Acular LS Ophthalmic Solution **562**

Lithium Carbonate (High risk of lithium toxicity). Products include:
Eskalith **1406**
Lithobid Tablets **1670**

Lithium Citrate (High risk of lithium toxicity).
No products indexed under this heading.

Loracarbef (Increased ototoxic potential of cephalosporins).
No products indexed under this heading.

Meclofenamate Sodium (Reduces diuretic, natriuretic, and antihypertensive effects).
No products indexed under this heading.

Mefenamic Acid (Reduces diuretic, natriuretic, and antihypertensive effects).
No products indexed under this heading.

Meloxicam (Reduces diuretic, natriuretic, and antihypertensive effects). Products include:
Mobic Oral Suspension **893**
Mobic Tablets **893**

Nabumetone (Reduces diuretic, natriuretic, and antihypertensive effects). Products include:
Relafen Tablets **1523**

Naproxen (Reduces diuretic, natriuretic, and antihypertensive effects). Products include:
EC-Naprosyn Delayed-Release Tablets **2769**
Naprosyn Suspension **2769**
Naprosyn Tablets **2769**
Prevacid NapraPAC **3277**

Naproxen Sodium (Reduces diuretic, natriuretic, and antihypertensive effects). Products include:
Aleve Tablets, Caplets and Gelcaps.......... ▣ **605**
Anaprox Tablets **2769**
Anaprox DS Tablets **2769**

Oxaprozin (Reduces diuretic, natriuretic, and antihypertensive effects).
No products indexed under this heading.

Phenylbutazone (Reduces diuretic, natriuretic, and antihypertensive effects).
No products indexed under this heading.

Piroxicam (Reduces diuretic, natriuretic, and antihypertensive effects).
No products indexed under this heading.

Rofecoxib (Reduces diuretic, natriuretic, and antihypertensive effects).
No products indexed under this heading.

Streptomycin Sulfate (Increased ototoxic potential of aminoglycosides).
No products indexed under this heading.

Sulindac (Reduces diuretic, natriuretic, and antihypertensive effects). Products include:
Clinoril Tablets **1899**

Tobramycin (Increased ototoxic potential of aminoglycosides). Products include:
TOBI Solution for Inhalation **1015**
TobraDex Ophthalmic Ointment **558**
TobraDex Ophthalmic Suspension **558**
Zylet Ophthalmic Suspension **3508**

Tobramycin Sulfate (Increased ototoxic potential of aminoglycosides).
No products indexed under this heading.

Tolmetin Sodium (Reduces diuretic, natriuretic, and antihypertensive effects).
No products indexed under this heading.

Valdecoxib (Reduces diuretic, natriuretic, and antihypertensive effects).
No products indexed under this heading.

Warfarin Sodium (Warfarin displaced from plasma protein; reduction in warfarin dosage may be required). Products include:
Coumadin for Injection **932**
Coumadin Tablets **932**

EDEX INJECTION

(Alprostadil) **3103**
May interact with:

Heparin Calcium (The pharmacodynamic interaction between heparin and alprostadil intravenous infusion was investigated. The results indicate significant changes in partial thromboplastin time (140% increase) and thrombin time (120% increase). Therefore, caution should be exercised with concomitant administration of heparin and alprostadil).
No products indexed under this heading.

Heparin Sodium (The pharmacodynamic interaction between heparin and alprostadil intravenous infusion was investigated. The results indicate significant changes in partial thromboplastin time (140% increase) and thrombin time (120% increase). Therefore, caution should be exercised with concomitant administration of heparin and alprostadil).
No products indexed under this heading.

E.E.S. 200 LIQUID

(Erythromycin Ethylsuccinate) **449**
See E.E.S. 400 Filmtab Tablets

E.E.S. 400 LIQUID

(Erythromycin Ethylsuccinate) **449**
See E.E.S. 400 Filmtab Tablets

E.E.S. 400 FILMTAB TABLETS

(Erythromycin Ethylsuccinate) **449**
May interact with oral anticoagulants, HMG-CoA reductase inhibitors, phenytoin, triazolobenzodiazepines, valproate, xanthines, and certain other agents. Compounds in these categories include:

Alfentanil Hydrochloride (Concurrent use of erythromycin in patients receiving drugs metabolized by the cytochrome P450 system may be associated with elevation in serum levels of alfentanil).
No products indexed under this heading.

Alprazolam (Erythromycin has been reported to decrease the clearance of triazolam and midazolam; may increase the pharmacologic effect of these benzodiazepines). Products include:
Niravam Orally Disintegrating Tablets.......... **3106**
Xanax XR Tablets **2655**

Aminophylline (Co-administration in patients who are receiving high doses of theophylline may be associated with an increase in serum theophylline levels and potential theophylline toxicity).
No products indexed under this heading.

Anisindione (Co-administration has resulted in increased anticoagulant effects). Products include:
Miradon Tablets **3056**

Astemizole (Concurrent use of erythromycin in patients receiving astemizole has been reported to significantly alter the metabolism of astemizole; rare cases of cardiovascular adverse events, including prolonged QT interval, cardiac arrest, torsade de pointes, and other ventricular arrhythmias have been reported; co-administration is contraindicated).
No products indexed under this heading.

Atorvastatin Calcium (Erythromycin has been reported to increase concentrations of HMG-CoA reductase inhibitors (e.g. lovastatin and simvastatin); rare reports of rhabdomyolysis have been reported in patients taking these drugs concomitantly). Products include:
Caduet Tablets **2507**
Lipitor Tablets **2495**

Bromocriptine Mesylate (Concurrent use of erythromycin in patients receiving drugs metabolized by the cytochrome P450 system may be associated with elevation in serum levels of bromocriptine).
No products indexed under this heading.

Carbamazepine (Concurrent use of erythromycin in patients receiving drugs metabolized by the cytochrome P450 system may be associated with elevation in serum levels of carbamazepine). Products include:
Carbatrol Capsules **3174**
Equetro Extended-Release Capsules.......... **3178**
Tegretol/Tegretol-XR **2278**

Cerivastatin Sodium (Erythromycin has been reported to increase concentrations of HMG-CoA reductase inhibitors (e.g. lovastatin and simvastatin); rare reports of rhabdomyolysis have been reported in patients taking these drugs concomitantly).
No products indexed under this heading.

Cisapride (Concurrent use of erythromycin in patients receiving cisapride has been reported to inhibit the metabolism of cisapride; cases of cardiovascular adverse events, including prolonged QT interval, torsade de pointes, ventricular tachycardia, and ventricular fibrillation have been reported; co-administration is contraindicated).
No products indexed under this heading.

Cyclosporine (Concurrent use of erythromycin in patients receiving drugs metabolized by the cytochrome P450 system may be associated with elevation in serum levels of cyclosporine). Products include:
Gengraf Capsules 458
Neoral Soft Gelatin Capsules 2247
Neoral Oral Solution 2247
Restasis Ophthalmic Emulsion 570
Sandimmune 2259

Dicumarol (Co-administration has resulted in increased anticoagulant effects).
No products indexed under this heading.

Digoxin (Co-administration has been reported to result in elevated digoxin serum levels). Products include:
Digitek Tablets 2146
Lanoxicaps Capsules 1458
Lanoxin Injection 1462
Lanoxin Tablets 1468
Lanoxin Injection Pediatric 1465

Dihydroergotamine Mesylate (Co-administration has been associated in some patients with acute ergot toxicity characterized by severe peripheral vasospasm and dysesthesia). Products include:
Migranal Nasal Spray 3350

Disopyramide Phosphate (Concurrent use of erythromycin in patients receiving drugs metabolized by the cytochrome P450 system may be associated with elevation in serum levels of disopyramide).
No products indexed under this heading.

Divalproex Sodium (There have been reports of interactions of erythromycin with drugs not thought to be metabolized by CYP3A, including valproate). Products include:
Depakote Sprinkle Capsules 422
Depakote Tablets 427
Depakote ER Tablets 433

Dyphylline (Co-administration in patients who are receiving high doses of theophylline may be associated with an increase in serum theophylline levels and potential theophylline toxicity).
No products indexed under this heading.

Ergotamine Tartrate (Co-administration has been associated in some patients with acute ergot toxicity characterized by severe peripheral vasospasm and dysesthesia).
No products indexed under this heading.

Fluvastatin Sodium (Erythromycin has been reported to increase concentrations of HMG-CoA reductase inhibitors (e.g. lovastatin and simvastatin); rare reports of rhabdomyolysis have been reported in patients taking these drugs concomitantly). Products include:
Lescol Capsules 2227
Lescol 2730
Lescol XL Tablets 2227

Fosphenytoin Sodium (There have been reports of interactions of erythromycin with drugs not thought to be metabolized by CYP3A, including phenytoin).
No products indexed under this heading.

Hexobarbital (There have been reports of interactions of erythromycin with drugs not thought to be metabolized by CYP3A, including hexobarbital).
No products indexed under this heading.

Lovastatin (Erythromycin has been reported to increase concentrations of HMG-CoA reductase inhibitors (e.g. lovastatin and simvastatin); rare reports of rhabdomyolysis have been reported in patients taking these drugs concomitantly). Products include:
Advicor Tablets 1694
Altoprev Extended-Release Tablets 1151
Mevacor Tablets 1996

Midazolam Hydrochloride (Erythromycin has been reported to decrease the clearance of triazolam and midazolam; may increase the pharmacologic effect of these benzodiazepines).
No products indexed under this heading.

Phenytoin (There have been reports of interactions of erythromycin with drugs not thought to be metabolized by CYP3A, including phenytoin).
No products indexed under this heading.

Phenytoin Sodium (There have been reports of interactions of erythromycin with drugs not thought to be metabolized by CYP3A, including phenytoin). Products include:
Phenytek Capsules 2153

Pimozide (Concurrent use of erythromycin in patients receiving drugs metabolized by the cytochrome P450 system may be associated with elevation in serum levels of pimozide; co-administration is contraindicated). Products include:
Orap Tablets 1220

Pravastatin Sodium (Erythromycin has been reported to increase concentrations of HMG-CoA reductase inhibitors (e.g. lovastatin and simvastatin); rare reports of rhabdomyolysis have been reported in patients taking these drugs concomitantly). Products include:
Pravachol Tablets 943

Sildenafil Citrate (Erythromycin has been reported to increase the systemic exposure (AUC) of sildenafil). Products include:
Revatio Tablets 2541
Viagra Tablets 2552

Simvastatin (Erythromycin has been reported to increase concentrations of HMG-CoA reductase inhibitors (e.g. lovastatin and simvastatin); rare reports of rhabdomyolysis have been reported in patients taking these drugs concomitantly). Products include:
Vytorin 10/10 Tablets 2084
Vytorin 10/10 Tablets 3092
Vytorin 10/20 Tablets 2084
Vytorin 10/20 Tablets 3092
Vytorin 10/40 Tablets 3092
Vytorin 10/40 Tablets 2084
Vytorin 10/80 Tablets 2084
Vytorin 10/80 Tablets 3092
Zocor Tablets 2078

Tacrolimus (Concurrent use of erythromycin in patients receiving drugs metabolized by the cytochrome P450 system may be associated with elevation in serum levels of tacrolimus). Products include:
Prograf Capsules and Injection 624
Protopic Ointment 629

Terfenadine (Concurrent use of erythromycin in patients receiving terfenadine has been reported to significantly alter the metabolism of terfenadine; rare cases of cardiovascular adverse events, including prolonged QT interval, cardiac arrest, torsade de pointes, other ventricular arrhythmias, and death have been reported; co-administration is contraindicated).
No products indexed under this heading.

Theophylline (Co-administration in patients who are receiving high doses of theophylline may be associated with an increase in serum theophylline levels and potential theophylline toxicity).
No products indexed under this heading.

Theophylline Anhydrous (Co-administration in patients who are receiving high doses of theophylline may be associated with an increase in serum theophylline levels and potential theophylline toxicity). Products include:
Uniphyl Tablets 2708

Theophylline Calcium Salicylate (Co-administration in patients who are receiving high doses of theophylline may be associated with an increase in serum theophylline levels and potential theophylline toxicity).
No products indexed under this heading.

Theophylline Dihydroxypropyl (Glyceryl) (Co-administration in patients who are receiving high doses of theophylline may be associated with an increase in serum theophylline levels and potential theophylline toxicity).
No products indexed under this heading.

Theophylline Ethylenediamine (Co-administration in patients who are receiving high doses of theophylline may be associated with an increase in serum theophylline levels and potential theophylline toxicity).
No products indexed under this heading.

Theophylline Sodium Glycinate (Co-administration in patients who are receiving high doses of theophylline may be associated with an increase in serum theophylline levels and potential theophylline toxicity).
No products indexed under this heading.

Triazolam (Erythromycin has been reported to decrease the clearance of triazolam and, thus, may increase the pharmacologic effect of the benzodiazepine).
No products indexed under this heading.

Valproate Sodium (There have been reports of interactions of erythromycin with drugs not thought to be metabolized by CYP3A, including valproate). Products include:
Depacon Injection 412

Valproic Acid (There have been reports of interactions of erythromycin with drugs not thought to be metabolized by CYP3A, including valproate). Products include:
Depakene 417

Warfarin Sodium (Co-administration has resulted in increased anticoagulant effects). Products include:
Coumadin for Injection 932
Coumadin Tablets 932

E.E.S. GRANULES

(Erythromycin Ethylsuccinate) 449
See E.E.S. 400 Filmtab Tablets

EFFEXOR TABLETS

(Venlafaxine Hydrochloride) 3405
See Effexor XR Capsules

EFFEXOR XR CAPSULES

(Venlafaxine Hydrochloride) 3411

May interact with 5HT1-receptor agonists, central nervous system depressants, central nervous system stimulants, monoamine oxidase inhibitors, quinidine, selective serotonin reuptake inhibitors, and certain other agents. Compounds in these categories include:

Alfentanil Hydrochloride (Caution is advised if the concomitant administration of venlafaxine and CNS-active drugs is required).
No products indexed under this heading.

Alprazolam (Caution is advised if the concomitant administration of venlafaxine and CNS-active drugs is required). Products include:
Niravam Orally Disintegrating Tablets 3106
Xanax XR Tablets 2655

Amphetamine Resins (Caution is advised if the concomitant administration of venlafaxine and CNS-active drugs is required).
No products indexed under this heading.

Aprobarbital (Caution is advised if the concomitant administration of venlafaxine and CNS-active drugs is required).
No products indexed under this heading.

Buprenorphine Hydrochloride (Caution is advised if the concomitant administration of venlafaxine and CNS-active drugs is required). Products include:
Buprenex Injectable 2718
Suboxone Tablets 2719
Subutex Tablets 2719

Buspirone Hydrochloride (Caution is advised if the concomitant administration of venlafaxine and CNS-active drugs is required).
No products indexed under this heading.

Butabarbital (Caution is advised if the concomitant administration of venlafaxine and CNS-active drugs is required).
No products indexed under this heading.

Butalbital (Caution is advised if the concomitant administration of venlafaxine and CNS-active drugs is required). Products include:
Sedapap Tablets 50 mg/650 mg 2098

Chlordiazepoxide (Caution is advised if the concomitant administration of venlafaxine and CNS-active drugs is required).
No products indexed under this heading.

Chlordiazepoxide Hydrochloride (Caution is advised if the concomitant administration of venlafaxine and CNS-active drugs is required). Products include:
Librium Capsules 3349

Chlorpromazine (Caution is advised if the concomitant administration of venlafaxine and CNS-active drugs is required).
No products indexed under this heading.

Chlorpromazine Hydrochloride (Caution is advised if the concomitant administration of venlafaxine and CNS-active drugs is required).
No products indexed under this heading.

Chlorprothixene (Caution is advised if the concomitant administration of venlafaxine and CNS-active drugs is required).
No products indexed under this heading.

Chlorprothixene Hydrochloride (Caution is advised if the concomitant administration of venlafaxine and CNS-active drugs is required).
No products indexed under this heading.

Chlorprothixene Lactate (Caution is advised if the concomitant administration of venlafaxine and CNS-active drugs is required).
No products indexed under this heading.

Cimetidine (Co-administration in a steady-state study for both drugs has resulted in inhibition of first-pass metabolism of venlafaxine; the oral clearance of venlafaxine was reduced by 43% and AUC and Cmax were increased by about 60%). Products include:
Tagamet HB 200 Tablets .... ▣637
Tagamet Tablets 1547

Cimetidine Hydrochloride (Co-administration in a steady-state study for both drugs has resulted in inhibition of first-pass metabolism of venlafaxine; the oral clearance of venlafaxine was reduced by 43% and AUC and Cmax were increased by about 60%).
No products indexed under this heading.

Citalopram Hydrobromide (Based on the mechanism of action of venlafaxine and the potential for serotonin syndrome, caution is advised when velafaxine is co-administered with other drugs that may affect the serotonergic neurotransmitter systems, such as serotonin reuptake inhibitors). Products include:
Celexa 1177

Clorazepate Dipotassium (Caution is advised if the concomitant administration of venlafaxine and CNS-active drugs is required). Products include:
Tranxene 2488

Clozapine (There have been reports of elevated clozapine levels that were temporarily associated with adverse events including seizures, following the addition of venlafaxine). Products include:
Clozapine Tablets 2141
Clozaril Tablets 2174
FazaClo Orally Disintegrating Tablets 547

Codeine Phosphate (Caution is advised if the concomitant administration of venlafaxine and CNS-active drugs is required). Products include:
Tylenol with Codeine 2461

Desflurane (Caution is advised if the concomitant administration of venlafaxine and CNS-active drugs is required). Products include:
Suprane Liquid for Inhalation 770

Desipramine Hydrochloride (Co-administration has resulted in increased desipramine AUC, Cmax, and Cmin by 35%; the 2-OH-desipramine AUC's increased by at least 2.5- to 4.5-fold; the clinical significance of this elevation is unknown).
No products indexed under this heading.

Dextroamphetamine Sulfate (Caution is advised if the concomitant administration of venlafaxine and CNS-active drugs is required). Products include:
Adderall Tablets 3168
Adderall XR Capsules 3169
Dexedrine 1386
DextroStat Tablets 3177

Dezocine (Caution is advised if the concomitant administration of venlafaxine and CNS-active drugs is required).
No products indexed under this heading.

Diazepam (Caution is advised if the concomitant administration of venlafaxine and CNS-active drugs is required). Products include:
Diastat Rectal Delivery System 3344
Valium Tablets 2822

3-Diphenylacrylate (Based on the mechanism of action of venlafaxine and the potential for serotonin syndrome, caution is advised when velafaxine is co-administered with other drugs that may affect the serotonergic neurotransmitter systems, such as triptans).
No products indexed under this heading.

Droperidol (Caution is advised if the concomitant administration of venlafaxine and CNS-active drugs is required).
No products indexed under this heading.

Enflurane (Caution is advised if the concomitant administration of venlafaxine and CNS-active drugs is required).
No products indexed under this heading.

Escitalopram Oxalate (Based on the mechanism of action of venlafaxine and the potential for serotonin syndrome, caution is advised when velafaxine is co-administered with other drugs that may affect the serotonergic neurotransmitter systems, such as serotonin reuptake inhibitors). Products include:
Lexapro Oral Solution 1193
Lexapro Tablets 1193

Estazolam (Caution is advised if the concomitant administration of venlafaxine and CNS-active drugs is required). Products include:
ProSom Tablets 512

Ethanol (Caution is advised if the concomitant administration of venlafaxine and CNS-active drugs is required).
No products indexed under this heading.

Ethchlorvynol (Caution is advised if the concomitant administration of venlafaxine and CNS-active drugs is required).
No products indexed under this heading.

Ethinamate (Caution is advised if the concomitant administration of venlafaxine and CNS-active drugs is required).
No products indexed under this heading.

Ethyl Alcohol (Caution is advised if the concomitant administration of venlafaxine and CNS-active drugs is required).
No products indexed under this heading.

Fentanyl (Caution is advised if the concomitant administration of venlafaxine and CNS-active drugs is required). Products include:
Duragesic Transdermal System 2448

Fentanyl Citrate (Caution is advised if the concomitant administration of venlafaxine and CNS-active drugs is required). Products include:
Actiq 993

Fluoxetine Hydrochloride (Based on the mechanism of action of venlafaxine and the potential for serotonin syndrome, caution is advised when velafaxine is co-administered with other drugs that may affect the serotonergic neurotransmitter systems, such as serotonin reuptake inhibitors). Products include:
Prozac Pulvules and Liquid 1771
Symbyax Capsules 1788

Fluphenazine Decanoate (Caution is advised if the concomitant administration of venlafaxine and CNS-active drugs is required).
No products indexed under this heading.

Fluphenazine Enanthate (Caution is advised if the concomitant administration of venlafaxine and CNS-active drugs is required).
No products indexed under this heading.

Fluphenazine Hydrochloride (Caution is advised if the concomitant administration of venlafaxine and CNS-active drugs is required).
No products indexed under this heading.

Flurazepam Hydrochloride (Caution is advised if the concomitant administration of venlafaxine and CNS-active drugs is required). Products include:
Dalmane Capsules 3343

Fluvoxamine Maleate (Based on the mechanism of action of venlafaxine and the potential for serotonin syndrome, caution is advised when velafaxine is co-administered with other drugs that may affect the serotonergic neurotransmitter systems, such as serotonin reuptake inhibitors).
No products indexed under this heading.

Glutethimide (Caution is advised if the concomitant administration of venlafaxine and CNS-active drugs is required).
No products indexed under this heading.

Haloperidol (Venlafaxine administered under steady-state conditions in healthy subjects decreased total oral-dose clearance of a single dose of haloperidol by 42%, which resulted in a 70% increase in haloperidol AUC and an 88% increase in Cmax).
No products indexed under this heading.

Haloperidol Decanoate (Venlafaxine administered under steady-state conditions in healthy subjects decreased total oral-dose clearance of a single dose of haloperidol by 42%, which resulted in a 70% increase in haloperidol AUC and an 88% increase in Cmax).
No products indexed under this heading.

Hydrocodone Bitartrate (Caution is advised if the concomitant administration of venlafaxine and CNS-active drugs is required). Products include:
Hycodan 1104
Hycomine Compound Tablets 1105
Hycotuss Expectorant Syrup 1106
Lortab 3315
Lortab Elixir 3312
Vicodin Tablets 530
Vicodin ES Tablets 531
Vicodin HP Tablets 532
Vicoprofen Tablets 533
Zydone Tablets 1118

Hydrocodone Polistirex (Caution is advised if the concomitant administration of venlafaxine and CNS-active drugs is required). Products include:
Tussionex Pennkinetic Extended-Release Suspension 3322

Hydromorphone Hydrochloride (Caution is advised if the concomitant administration of venlafaxine and CNS-active drugs is required). Products include:
Dilaudid 439
Dilaudid Oral Liquid 443
Dilaudid Non-Sterile Powder 439
Dilaudid Rectal Suppositories 439
Dilaudid Tablets 439
Dilaudid Tablets - 8 mg 443
Dilaudid-HP 441

Hydroxyzine Hydrochloride (Caution is advised if the concomitant administration of venlafaxine and CNS-active drugs is required).
No products indexed under this heading.

Indinavir Sulfate (Co-administration has resulted in a 28% decrease in the AUC and 36% decrease in the indinavir Cmax; the clinical significance of these findings is unknown). Products include:
Crixivan Capsules 1918

Isocarboxazid (Adverse reactions, some of which were serious, have been reported in patients who have recently been discontinued from an MAO inhibitor and started on venlafaxine, or who have recently had venlafaxine therapy discontinued prior to initiation of an MAO inhibitor; concurrent and/or sequential use is contraindicated).
No products indexed under this heading.

Isoflurane (Caution is advised if the concomitant administration of venlafaxine and CNS-active drugs is required).
No products indexed under this heading.

Ketamine Hydrochloride (Caution is advised if the concomitant administration of venlafaxine and CNS-active drugs is required).
No products indexed under this heading.

Levomethadyl Acetate Hydrochloride (Caution is advised if the concomitant administration of venlafaxine and CNS-active drugs is required).
No products indexed under this heading.

Levorphanol Tartrate (Caution is advised if the concomitant administration of venlafaxine and CNS-active drugs is required).
No products indexed under this heading.

Lithium Carbonate (Based on the mechanism of action of venlafaxine and the potential for serotonin syndrome, caution is advised when velafaxine is co-administered with other drugs that may affect the serotonergic neurotransmitter systems, such as lithium). Products include:
Eskalith **1406**
Lithobid Tablets **1670**

Lithium Citrate (Based on the mechanism of action of venlafaxine and the potential for serotonin syndrome, caution is advised when velafaxine is co-administered with other drugs that may affect the serotonergic neurotransmitter systems, such as lithium).
No products indexed under this heading.

Lorazepam (Caution is advised if the concomitant administration of venlafaxine and CNS-active drugs is required).
No products indexed under this heading.

Loxapine Hydrochloride (Caution is advised if the concomitant administration of venlafaxine and CNS-active drugs is required).
No products indexed under this heading.

Loxapine Succinate (Caution is advised if the concomitant administration of venlafaxine and CNS-active drugs is required).
No products indexed under this heading.

Meperidine Hydrochloride (Caution is advised if the concomitant administration of venlafaxine and CNS-active drugs is required).
No products indexed under this heading.

Mephobarbital (Caution is advised if the concomitant administration of venlafaxine and CNS-active drugs is required). Products include:
Mebaral Tablets, USP **2483**

Meprobamate (Caution is advised if the concomitant administration of venlafaxine and CNS-active drugs is required).
No products indexed under this heading.

Mesoridazine Besylate (Caution is advised if the concomitant administration of venlafaxine and CNS-active drugs is required).
No products indexed under this heading.

Methadone Hydrochloride (Caution is advised if the concomitant administration of venlafaxine and CNS-active drugs is required).
No products indexed under this heading.

Methamphetamine Hydrochloride (Caution is advised if the concomitant administration of venlafaxine and CNS-active drugs is required). Products include:
Desoxyn Tablets, USP **2482**

Methohexital Sodium (Caution is advised if the concomitant administration of venlafaxine and CNS-active drugs is required).
No products indexed under this heading.

Methotrimeprazine (Caution is advised if the concomitant administration of venlafaxine and CNS-active drugs is required).
No products indexed under this heading.

Methoxyflurane (Caution is advised if the concomitant administration of venlafaxine and CNS-active drugs is required).
No products indexed under this heading.

Methylphenidate Hydrochloride (Caution is advised if the concomitant administration of venlafaxine and CNS-active drugs is required). Products include:
Concerta Extended-Release Tablets **1828**
Metadate CD Capsules **3316**
Ritalin **2254**
Ritalin LA Capsules **2255**

Midazolam Hydrochloride (Caution is advised if the concomitant administration of venlafaxine and CNS-active drugs is required).
No products indexed under this heading.

Moclobemide (Adverse reactions, some of which were serious, have been reported in patients who have recently been discontinued from an MAO inhibitor and started on venlafaxine, or who have recently had venlafaxine therapy discontinued prior to initiation of an MAO inhibitor; concurrent and/or sequential use is contraindicated).
No products indexed under this heading.

Molindone Hydrochloride (Caution is advised if the concomitant administration of venlafaxine and CNS-active drugs is required). Products include:
Moban Tablets **1108**

Morphine Sulfate (Caution is advised if the concomitant administration of venlafaxine and CNS-active drugs is required). Products include:
Avinza Capsules **1714**
Kadian Capsules **572**
MS Contin Tablets **2703**

Naratriptan Hydrochloride (Based on the mechanism of action of venlafaxine and the potential for serotonin syndrome, caution is advised when velafaxine is co-administered with other drugs that may affect the serotonergic neurotransmitter systems, such as triptans). Products include:
Amerge Tablets **1312**

Olanzapine (Caution is advised if the concomitant administration of venlafaxine and CNS-active drugs is required). Products include:
Symbyax Capsules **1788**
Zyprexa Tablets **1798**
Zyprexa IntraMuscular **1798**
Zyprexa ZYDIS Orally Disintegrating Tablets **1798**

Oxazepam (Caution is advised if the concomitant administration of venlafaxine and CNS-active drugs is required).
No products indexed under this heading.

Oxycodone Hydrochloride (Caution is advised if the concomitant administration of venlafaxine and CNS-active drugs is required). Products include:
Combunox Tablets **1183**
OxyContin Tablets **2699**
OxyFast Oral Concentrate Solution **2704**
OxyIR Capsules **2704**
Percocet Tablets **1114**
Percodan Tablets **1115**

Pargyline Hydrochloride (Adverse reactions, some of which were serious, have been reported in patients who have recently been discontinued from an MAO inhibitor and started on venlafaxine, or who have recently had venlafaxine therapy discontinued prior to initiation of an MAO inhibitor; concurrent and/or sequential use is contraindicated).
No products indexed under this heading.

Paroxetine Hydrochloride (Based on the mechanism of action of venlafaxine and the potential for serotonin syndrome, caution is advised when velafaxine is co-administered with other drugs that may affect the serotonergic neurotransmitter systems, such as serotonin reuptake inhibitors). Products include:
Paxil CR Controlled-Release Tablets **1509**
Paxil **1501**

Pemoline (Caution is advised if the concomitant administration of venlafaxine and CNS-active drugs is required).
No products indexed under this heading.

Pentobarbital Sodium (Caution is advised if the concomitant administration of venlafaxine and CNS-active drugs is required). Products include:
Nembutal Sodium Solution, USP **2484**

Perphenazine (Caution is advised if the concomitant administration of venlafaxine and CNS-active drugs is required).
No products indexed under this heading.

Phenelzine Sulfate (Adverse reactions, some of which were serious, have been reported in patients who have recently been discontinued from an MAO inhibitor and started on venlafaxine, or who have recently had venlafaxine therapy discontinued prior to initiation of an MAO inhibitor; concurrent and/or sequential use is contraindicated).
No products indexed under this heading.

Phenobarbital (Caution is advised if the concomitant administration of venlafaxine and CNS-active drugs is required).
No products indexed under this heading.

Prazepam (Caution is advised if the concomitant administration of venlafaxine and CNS-active drugs is required).
No products indexed under this heading.

Procarbazine Hydrochloride (Adverse reactions, some of which were serious, have been reported in patients who have recently been discontinued from an MAO inhibitor and started on venlafaxine, or who have recently had venlafaxine therapy discontinued prior to initiation of an MAO inhibitor; concurrent and/or sequential use is contraindicated). Products include:
Matulane Capsules **3188**

Prochlorperazine (Caution is advised if the concomitant administration of venlafaxine and CNS-active drugs is required).
No products indexed under this heading.

Promethazine Hydrochloride (Caution is advised if the concomitant administration of venlafaxine and CNS-active drugs is required). Products include:
Phenergan **3438**

Propofol (Caution is advised if the concomitant administration of venlafaxine and CNS-active drugs is required). Products include:
Diprivan Injectable Emulsion **676**

Propoxyphene Hydrochloride (Caution is advised if the concomitant administration of venlafaxine and CNS-active drugs is required).
No products indexed under this heading.

Propoxyphene Napsylate (Caution is advised if the concomitant administration of venlafaxine and CNS-active drugs is required). Products include:
Darvocet A 500 Tablets **3497**

Quazepam (Caution is advised if the concomitant administration of venlafaxine and CNS-active drugs is required).
No products indexed under this heading.

Quetiapine Fumarate (Caution is advised if the concomitant administration of venlafaxine and CNS-active drugs is required). Products include:
Seroquel Tablets **691**

Quinidine (Venlafaxine is metabolized to its active metabolite, ODV, by CYP2D6; therefore, the potential exists for a drug interaction between the inhibitors of CYP2D6, such as quinidine and venlafaxine, resulting in increased plasma concentrations of venlafaxine and decreased concentrations of the active metabolite).
No products indexed under this heading.

Quinidine Gluconate (Venlafaxine is metabolized to its active metabolite, ODV, by CYP2D6; therefore, the potential exists for a drug interaction between the inhibitors of CYP2D6, such as quinidine and venlafaxine, resulting in increased plasma concentrations of venlafaxine and decreased concentrations of the active metabolite).
No products indexed under this heading.

Quinidine Hydrochloride (Venlafaxine is metabolized to its active metabolite, ODV, by CYP2D6; therefore, the potential exists for a drug interaction between the inhibitors of CYP2D6, such as quinidine and venlafaxine, resulting in increased plasma concentrations of venlafaxine and decreased concentrations of the active metabolite).
No products indexed under this heading.

Quinidine Polygalacturonate (Venlafaxine is metabolized to its active metabolite, ODV, by CYP2D6; therefore, the potential exists for a drug interaction between the inhibitors of CYP2D6, such as quinidine and venlafaxine, resulting in increased plasma concentrations of venlafaxine and decreased concentrations of the active metabolite).
No products indexed under this heading.

Quinidine Sulfate (Venlafaxine is metabolized to its active metabolite, ODV, by CYP2D6; therefore, the potential exists for a drug interaction between the inhibitors of CYP2D6, such as quinidine and venlafaxine, resulting in increased plasma concentrations of venlafaxine and decreased concentrations of the active metabolite).
No products indexed under this heading.

Remifentanil Hydrochloride (Caution is advised if the concomitant administration of venlafaxine and CNS-active drugs is required).
No products indexed under this heading.

Risperidone (Venlafaxine slightly inhibits the CYP2D6-mediated metabolism of risperidone resulting in an approximate 32% increase in risperidone AUC). Products include:
Risperdal Consta Long-Acting Injection **1664**
Risperdal M-Tab Orally Disintegrating Tablets **1658**
Risperdal **1658**

Rizatriptan Benzoate (Based on the mechanism of action of venlafaxine and the potential for serotonin syndrome, caution is advised when velafaxine is co-administered with other drugs that may affect the serotonergic neurotransmitter systems, such as triptans). Products include:
Maxalt Tablets **1983**
Maxalt-MLT Orally Disintegrating Tablets **1983**

Secobarbital Sodium (Caution is advised if the concomitant administration of venlafaxine and CNS-active drugs is required).
No products indexed under this heading.

Selegiline Hydrochloride (Adverse reactions, some of which were serious, have been reported in patients who have recently been discontinued from an MAO inhibitor and started on venlafaxine, or who have recently had venlafaxine therapy discontinued prior to initiation of an MAO inhibitor; concurrent and/or sequential use is contraindicated). Products include:
Eldepryl Capsules **3209**

Sertraline Hydrochloride (Based on the mechanism of action of venlafaxine and the potential for serotonin syndrome, caution is advised when velafaxine is co-administered with other drugs that may affect the serotonergic neurotransmitter systems, such as serotonin reuptake inhibitors). Products include:
Zoloft **2581**

Sevoflurane (Caution is advised if the concomitant administration of venlafaxine and CNS-active drugs is required). Products include:
Ultane Liquid for Inhalation **526**

Sodium Oxybate (Caution is advised if the concomitant administration of venlafaxine and CNS-active drugs is required).
No products indexed under this heading.

Sufentanil Citrate (Caution is advised if the concomitant administration of venlafaxine and CNS-active drugs is required).
No products indexed under this heading.

Sumatriptan (Based on the mechanism of action of venlafaxine and the potential for serotonin syndrome, caution is advised when velafaxine is co-administered with other drugs that may affect the serotonergic neurotransmitter systems, such as triptans). Products include:
Imitrex Nasal Spray **1435**

Sumatriptan Succinate (Based on the mechanism of action of venlafaxine and the potential for serotonin syndrome, caution is advised when velafaxine is co-administered with other drugs that may affect the serotonergic neurotransmitter systems, such as triptans). Products include:
Imitrex Injection **1431**
Imitrex Tablets **1440**

Temazepam (Caution is advised if the concomitant administration of venlafaxine and CNS-active drugs is required).
No products indexed under this heading.

Thiamylal Sodium (Caution is advised if the concomitant administration of venlafaxine and CNS-active drugs is required).
No products indexed under this heading.

Thioridazine Hydrochloride (Caution is advised if the concomitant administration of venlafaxine and CNS-active drugs is required). Products include:
Thioridazine Hydrochloride Tablets **2122**

Thiothixene (Caution is advised if the concomitant administration of venlafaxine and CNS-active drugs is required). Products include:
Thiothixene Capsules **2124**

Tranylcypromine Sulfate (Adverse reactions, some of which were serious, have been reported in patients who have recently been discontinued from an MAO inhibitor and started on venlafaxine, or who have recently had venlafaxine therapy discontinued prior to initiation of an MAO inhibitor; concurrent and/or sequential use is contraindicated). Products include:
Parnate Tablets **1499**

Triazolam (Caution is advised if the concomitant administration of venlafaxine and CNS-active drugs is required).
No products indexed under this heading.

Trifluoperazine Hydrochloride (Caution is advised if the concomitant administration of venlafaxine and CNS-active drugs is required).
No products indexed under this heading.

Warfarin Sodium (There have been reports of increases in prothrombin time, partial thromboplastin time, or INR when venlafaxine was given to patients receiving warfarin therapy). Products include:
Coumadin for Injection **932**
Coumadin Tablets **932**

Zaleplon (Caution is advised if the concomitant administration of venlafaxine and CNS-active drugs is required). Products include:
Sonata Capsules **1686**

Ziprasidone Hydrochloride (Caution is advised if the concomitant administration of venlafaxine and CNS-active drugs is required). Products include:
Geodon Capsules **2514**

Zolmitriptan (Based on the mechanism of action of venlafaxine and the potential for serotonin syndrome, caution is advised when velafaxine is co-administered with other drugs that may affect the serotonergic neurotransmitter systems, such as triptans). Products include:
Zomig Nasal Spray **718**
Zomig Tablets **714**
Zomig-ZMT Tablets **714**

Zolpidem Tartrate (Caution is advised if the concomitant administration of venlafaxine and CNS-active drugs is required). Products include:
Ambien Tablets **2867**

Food Interactions

Alcohol (Co-administration of venlafaxine as a stable regimen did not exaggerate the psychomotor and psychometric effects of alcohol; however, patients should be advised to avoid alcohol while taking venlafaxine).

EFUDEX TOPICAL CREAM

(Fluorouracil) **3348**
None cited in PDR database.

EFUDEX TOPICAL SOLUTIONS

(Fluorouracil) **3348**
None cited in PDR database.

ELDEPRYL CAPSULES

(Selegiline Hydrochloride) **3209**
May interact with narcotic analgesics, selective serotonin reuptake inhibitors, tricyclic antidepressants, and certain other agents. Compounds in these categories include:

Alfentanil Hydrochloride (Contraindication warning for meperidine is extended to other opioids).
No products indexed under this heading.

Amitriptyline Hydrochloride (Co-administraton has resulted in severe CNS toxicity associated with hyperpyrexia and fatality; concurrent use in some patients may result in hypertension, syncope, asystole, diaphoresis seizures, changes in behavioral and mental status, and muscular rigidity; concurrent and/or sequential use is not recommended).
No products indexed under this heading.

Amoxapine (Co-administration may result in hypertension, syncope, asystole, diaphoresis seizures, changes in behavioral and mental status, and muscular rigidity; concurrent and/or sequential use is not recommended).
No products indexed under this heading.

Buprenorphine Hydrochloride (Contraindication warning for meperidine is extended to other opioids). Products include:
Buprenex Injectable **2718**
Suboxone Tablets **2719**
Subutex Tablets **2719**

Citalopram Hydrobromide (Potential for serious, sometimes fatal, reactions including hyperthermia, rigidity, myoclonus, autonomic instability, extreme agitation progressing to delirium and coma; concurrent and/or sequential use is not recommended). Products include:
Celexa **1177**

Clomipramine Hydrochloride (Co-administration may result in hypertension, syncope, asystole, diaphoresis seizures, changes in behavioral and mental status, and muscular rigidity; concurrent and/or sequential use is not recommended).
No products indexed under this heading.

Codeine Phosphate (Contraindication warning for meperidine is extended to other opioids). Products include:
Tylenol with Codeine **2461**

Desipramine Hydrochloride (Co-administration may result in hypertension, syncope, asystole, diaphoresis seizures, changes in behavioral and mental status, and muscular rigidity; concurrent and/or sequential use is not recommended).
No products indexed under this heading.

Dezocine (Contraindication warning for meperidine is extended to other opioids).
No products indexed under this heading.

Doxepin Hydrochloride (Co-administration may result in hypertension, syncope, asystole, diaphoresis seizures, changes in behavioral and mental status, and muscular rigidity; concurrent and/or sequential use is not recommended).
No products indexed under this heading.

Ephedrine Hydrochloride (Co-administration has resulted in one case of hypertensive crisis). Products include:
Primatene Tablets .... ▣ **749**

Ephedrine Sulfate (Co-administration has resulted in one case of hypertensive crisis).
No products indexed under this heading.

Ephedrine Tannate (Co-administration has resulted in one case of hypertensive crisis).
No products indexed under this heading.

Fentanyl (Contraindication warning for meperidine is extended to other opioids). Products include:
Duragesic Transdermal System **2448**

Fentanyl Citrate (Contraindication warning for meperidine is extended to other opioids). Products include:
Actiq **993**

Fluoxetine Hydrochloride (Co-administration has resulted in serious, sometimes fatal, reactions including hyperthermia, rigidity, myoclonus, autonomic instability, extreme agitation progressing to delirium and coma; concurrent and/or sequential use is not recommended; because of long half-life of fluoxetine, at least 5 weeks or longer should elapse between discontinuation of fluoxetine and initiation of Eldepryl). Products include:
Prozac Pulvules and Liquid **1771**
Symbyax Capsules **1788**

Fluvoxamine Maleate (Potential for serious, sometimes fatal, reactions including hyperthermia, rigidity, myoclonus, autonomic instability, extreme agitation progressing to delirium and coma; concurrent and/or sequential use is not recommended).
No products indexed under this heading.

Hydrocodone Bitartrate (Contraindication warning for meperidine is extended to other opioids). Products include:
Hycodan 1104
Hycomine Compound Tablets 1105
Hycotuss Expectorant Syrup 1106
Lortab 3315
Lortab Elixir 3312
Vicodin Tablets 530
Vicodin ES Tablets 531
Vicodin HP Tablets 532
Vicoprofen Tablets 533
Zydone Tablets 1118

Hydrocodone Polistirex (Contraindication warning for meperidine is extended to other opioids). Products include:
Tussionex Pennkinetic Extended-Release Suspension 3322

Hydromorphone Hydrochloride (Contraindication warning for meperidine is extended to other opioids). Products include:
Dilaudid 439
Dilaudid Oral Liquid 443
Dilaudid Non-Sterile Powder 439
Dilaudid Rectal Suppositories 439
Dilaudid Tablets 439
Dilaudid Tablets - 8 mg 443
Dilaudid-HP 441

Imipramine Hydrochloride (Co-administration may result in hypertension, syncope, asystole, diaphoresis seizures, changes in behavioral and mental status, and muscular rigidity; concurrent and/or sequential use is not recommended).
No products indexed under this heading.

Imipramine Pamoate (Co-administration may result in hypertension, syncope, asystole, diaphoresis seizures, changes in behavioral and mental status, and muscular rigidity; concurrent and/or sequential use is not recommended).
No products indexed under this heading.

Levodopa (Co-administration in some patients may exacerbate levodopa-associated side effects). Products include:
Parcopa Orally Disintegrating Tablets 3111
Stalevo Tablets 2270

Levorphanol Tartrate (Contraindication warning for meperidine is extended to other opioids).
No products indexed under this heading.

Maprotiline Hydrochloride (Co-administration may result in hypertension, syncope, asystole, diaphoresis seizures, changes in behavioral and mental status, and muscular rigidity; concurrent and/or sequential use is not recommended).
No products indexed under this heading.

Meperidine Hydrochloride (Co-administration has resulted in stupor, muscular rigidity, severe agitation, hallucination, and hyperpyrexia; concurrent use is contraindicated).
No products indexed under this heading.

Methadone Hydrochloride (Contraindication warning for meperidine is extended to other opioids).
No products indexed under this heading.

Morphine Sulfate (Contraindication warning for meperidine is extended to other opioids). Products include:
Avinza Capsules 1714
Kadian Capsules 572
MS Contin Tablets 2703

Nortriptyline Hydrochloride (Co-administration may result in hypertension, syncope, asystole, diaphoresis seizures, changes in behavioral and mental status, and muscular rigidity; concurrent and/or sequential use is not recommended).
No products indexed under this heading.

Oxycodone Hydrochloride (Contraindication warning for meperidine is extended to other opioids). Products include:
Combunox Tablets 1183
OxyContin Tablets 2699
OxyFast Oral Concentrate Solution 2704
OxyIR Capsules 2704
Percocet Tablets 1114
Percodan Tablets 1115

Paroxetine Hydrochloride (Potential for serious, sometimes fatal, reactions including hyperthermia, rigidity, myoclonus, autonomic instability, extreme agitation progressing to delirium and coma; concurrent and/or sequential use is not recommended). Products include:
Paxil CR Controlled-Release Tablets 1509
Paxil 1501

Propoxyphene Hydrochloride (Contraindication warning for meperidine is extended to other opioids).
No products indexed under this heading.

Propoxyphene Napsylate (Contraindication warning for meperidine is extended to other opioids). Products include:
Darvocet A 500 Tablets 3497

Protriptyline Hydrochloride (Co-administration has resulted in tremors, agitation, and restlessness followed by unresponsiveness and fatality; concurrent use in some patients may result in hypertension, syncope, asystole, diaphoresis seizures, changes in behavioral and mental status, and muscular rigidity; concurrent and/or sequential use is not recommended). Products include:
Vivactil Tablets 2350

Sertraline Hydrochloride (Potential for serious, sometimes fatal, reactions including hyperthermia, rigidity, myoclonus, autonomic instability, extreme agitation progressing to delirium and coma; concurrent and/or sequential use is not recommended). Products include:
Zoloft 2581

Sufentanil Citrate (Contraindication warning for meperidine is extended to other opioids).
No products indexed under this heading.

Trimipramine Maleate (Co-administration may result in hypertension, syncope, asystole, diaphoresis seizures, changes in behavioral and mental status, and muscular rigidity; concurrent and/or sequential use is not recommended). Products include:
Surmontil Capsules 2347

Venlafaxine Hydrochloride (Potential for serious, sometimes fatal, reactions including hyperthermia, rigidity, myoclonus, autonomic instability, extreme agitation progressing to delirium and coma; concurrent and/or sequential use is not recommended). Products include:
Effexor Tablets 3405
Effexor XR Capsules 3411

Food Interactions

Food, unspecified (The bioavailability of selegiline is increased 3 to 4 fold when it is taken with food).

ELDERTONIC
(Vitamins with Minerals) 2096
None cited in PDR database.

ELESTAT OPHTHALMIC SOLUTION
(Epinastine Hydrochloride) 1643
None cited in PDR database.

ELIDEL CREAM 1%
(Pimecrolimus) 2198
None cited in PDR database.

ELIGARD 7.5 MG
(Leuprolide Acetate) 2896
None cited in PDR database.

ELIGARD 22.5 MG
(Leuprolide Acetate) 2899
None cited in PDR database.

ELIGARD 30 MG
(Leuprolide Acetate) 2901
None cited in PDR database.

ELIGARD 45 MG
(Leuprolide Acetate) 2904
None cited in PDR database.

ELITEK
(Rasburicase) 2906
None cited in PDR database.

ELLENCE INJECTION
(Epirubicin Hydrochloride) 2632
May interact with calcium channel blockers, cytotoxic drugs, and certain other agents. Compounds in these categories include:

Amlodipine Besylate (Co-administration with other cardioactive agents that cause heart failure, such as calcium channel blockers, requires close monitoring of cardiac function throughout treatment). Products include:
Caduet Tablets 2507
Lotrel Capsules 2238
Norvasc Tablets 2529

Bepridil Hydrochloride (Co-administration with other cardioactive agents that cause heart failure, such as calcium channel blockers, requires close monitoring of cardiac function throughout treatment).
No products indexed under this heading.

Bleomycin Sulfate (Combination therapy with other cytotoxic drugs may show on-treatment additive toxicity, especially hematologic and gastrointestinal effects).
No products indexed under this heading.

Cimetidine (Co-administration increases the AUC of epirubicin by 50%; cimetidine treatment should be stopped during treatment with Ellence). Products include:
Tagamet HB 200 Tablets 637
Tagamet Tablets 1547

Cimetidine Hydrochloride (Co-administration increases the AUC of epirubicin by 50%; cimetidine treatment should be stopped during treatment with Ellence).
No products indexed under this heading.

Cyclophosphamide (Combination therapy with other cytotoxic drugs may show on-treatment additive toxicity, especially hematologic and gastrointestinal effects).
No products indexed under this heading.

Daunorubicin Hydrochloride (Combination therapy with other cytotoxic drugs may show on-treatment additive toxicity, especially hematologic and gastrointestinal effects). Products include:
Cerubidine for Injection 788

Diltiazem Hydrochloride (Co-administration with other cardioactive agents that cause heart failure, such as calcium channel blockers, requires close monitoring of cardiac function throughout treatment). Products include:
Cardizem LA Extended Release Tablets 1699
Tiazac Capsules 1204

Doxorubicin Hydrochloride (Combination therapy with other cytotoxic drugs may show on-treatment additive toxicity, especially hematologic and gastrointestinal effects). Products include:
Adriamycin for Injection, USP 786
Adriamycin Injection, USP 786

Felodipine (Co-administration with other cardioactive agents that cause heart failure, such as calcium channel blockers, requires close monitoring of cardiac function throughout treatment). Products include:
Plendil Extended-Release Tablets 651

Fluorouracil (Combination therapy with other cytotoxic drugs may show on-treatment additive toxicity, especially hematologic and gastrointestinal effects). Products include:
Carac Cream, 0.5% 1048
Efudex 3348

Hydroxyurea (Combination therapy with other cytotoxic drugs may show on-treatment additive toxicity, especially hematologic and gastrointestinal effects).
No products indexed under this heading.

Isradipine (Co-administration with other cardioactive agents that cause heart failure, such as calcium channel blockers, requires close monitoring of cardiac function throughout treatment). Products include:
DynaCirc CR Tablets 2726

Methotrexate Sodium (Combination therapy with other cytotoxic drugs may show on-treatment additive toxicity, especially hematologic and gastrointestinal effects).
No products indexed under this heading.

Mibefradil Dihydrochloride (Co-administration with other cardioactive agents that cause heart failure, such as calcium channel blockers, requires close monitoring of cardiac function throughout treatment).
No products indexed under this heading.

Mitotane (Combination therapy with other cytotoxic drugs may show on-treatment additive toxicity, especially hematologic and gastrointestinal effects).
No products indexed under this heading.

Mitoxantrone Hydrochloride (Combination therapy with other cytotoxic drugs may show on-treatment additive toxicity, especially hematologic and gastrointestinal effects). Products include:
Novantrone for Injection Concentrate 3158

Nicardipine Hydrochloride (Co-administration with other cardioactive agents that cause heart failure, such as calcium channel blockers, requires close monitoring of cardiac function throughout treatment). Products include:
Cardene I.V. 1129

Nifedipine (Co-administration with other cardioactive agents that cause heart failure, such as calcium channel blockers, requires close monitoring of cardiac function throughout treatment). Products include:
Adalat CC Tablets 2978

Nimodipine (Co-administration with other cardioactive agents that cause heart failure, such as calcium channel blockers, requires close monitoring of cardiac function throughout treatment). Products include:
Nimotop Capsules 774

Nisoldipine (Co-administration with other cardioactive agents that cause heart failure, such as calcium channel blockers, requires close monitoring of cardiac function throughout treatment). Products include:
Sular Tablets 1163

Procarbazine Hydrochloride (Combination therapy with other cytotoxic drugs may show on-treatment additive toxicity, especially hematologic and gastrointestinal effects). Products include:
Matulane Capsules 3188

Tamoxifen Citrate (Combination therapy with other cytotoxic drugs may show on-treatment additive toxicity, especially hematologic and gastrointestinal effects).
No products indexed under this heading.

Verapamil Hydrochloride (Co-administration with other cardioactive agents that cause heart failure, such as calcium channel blockers, requires close monitoring of cardiac function throughout treatment). Products include:
Covera-HS Tablets 3135
Tarka Tablets 519
Verelan PM Capsules 3120

Vincristine Sulfate (Combination therapy with other cytotoxic drugs may show on-treatment additive toxicity, especially hematologic and gastrointestinal effects).
No products indexed under this heading.

ELMIRON CAPSULES

(Pentosan Polysulfate Sodium) 2393
May interact with anticoagulants, thrombolytics, and certain other agents. Compounds in these categories include:

Alteplase (Pentosan polysulfate sodium is a weak anticoagulant and bleeding complications of ecchymosis, epistaxis and gum hemorrhage have been reported with its use; caution should be exercised in patients with increased risk of bleeding due to other concomitant therapies, such as thrombolytics). Products include:
Activase I.V. 1225
Cathflo Activase 1232

Anisindione (Pentosan polysulfate sodium is a weak anticoagulant and bleeding complications of ecchymosis, epistaxis and gum hemorrhage have been reported with its use; caution should be exercised in patients with increased risk of bleeding due to other concomitant therapies, such as anticoagulants). Products include:
Miradon Tablets 3056

Anistreplase (Pentosan polysulfate sodium is a weak anticoagulant and bleeding complications of ecchymosis, epistaxis and gum hemorrhage have been reported with its use; caution should be exercised in patients with increased risk of bleeding due to other concomitant therapies, such as thrombolytics).
No products indexed under this heading.

Ardeparin Sodium (Pentosan polysulfate sodium is a weak anticoagulant and bleeding complications of ecchymosis, epistaxis and gum hemorrhage have been reported with its use; caution should be exercised in patients with increased risk of bleeding due to other concomitant therapies, such as anticoagulants).
No products indexed under this heading.

Aspirin (Pentosan polysulfate sodium is a weak anticoagulant and bleeding complications of ecchymosis, epistaxis and gum hemorrhage have been reported with its use; caution should be exercised in patients with increased risk of bleeding due to other concomitant therapies, such as high dose aspirin). Products include:
Aggrenox Capsules 855
Bayer, Aspirin Regimen .... ▣606
Bayer Aspirin Tablets 3515
BC Powder .... ▣612
BC Allergy Sinus Cold Powder .... ▣612
Arthritis Strength BC Powder .... ▣612
BC Sinus Cold Powder .... ▣612
Ecotrin Enteric Coated Aspirin Low, Regular and Maximum Strength Tablets 1627
Goody's Body Pain Formula Powder .... ▣621
Goody's Extra Strength Headache Powder .... ▣621
Goody's Extra Strength Pain Relief Tablets .... ▣621
Percodan Tablets 1115
St. Joseph 81 mg Aspirin Chewable and Enteric Coated Tablets 1841

Dalteparin Sodium (Pentosan polysulfate sodium is a weak anticoagulant and bleeding complications of ecchymosis, epistaxis and gum hemorrhage have been reported with its use; caution should be exercised in patients with increased risk of bleeding due to other concomitant therapies, such as anticoagulants). Products include:
Fragmin Injection 2638

Danaparoid Sodium (Pentosan polysulfate sodium is a weak anticoagulant and bleeding complications of ecchymosis, epistaxis and gum hemorrhage have been reported with its use; caution should be exercised in patients with increased risk of bleeding due to other concomitant therapies, such as anticoagulants).
No products indexed under this heading.

Dicumarol (Pentosan polysulfate sodium is a weak anticoagulant and bleeding complications of ecchymosis, epistaxis and gum hemorrhage have been reported with its use; caution should be exercised in patients with increased risk of bleeding due to other concomitant therapies, such as anticoagulants).
No products indexed under this heading.

Enoxaparin Sodium (Pentosan polysulfate sodium is a weak anticoagulant and bleeding complications of ecchymosis, epistaxis and gum hemorrhage have been reported with its use; caution should be exercised in patients with increased risk of bleeding due to other concomitant therapies, such as anticoagulants). Products include:
Lovenox Injection 2931

Fondaparinux Sodium (Pentosan polysulfate sodium is a weak anticoagulant and bleeding complications of ecchymosis, epistaxis and gum hemorrhage have been reported with its use; caution should be exercised in patients with increased risk of bleeding due to other concomitant therapies, such as anticoagulants). Products include:
Arixtra Injection 1325

Heparin Calcium (Pentosan polysulfate sodium is a weak anticoagulant and bleeding complications of ecchymosis, epistaxis and gum hemorrhage have been reported with its use; caution should be exercised in patients with increased risk of bleeding due to other concomitant therapies, such as anticoagulants).
No products indexed under this heading.

Heparin Sodium (Pentosan polysulfate sodium is a weak anticoagulant and bleeding complications of ecchymosis, epistaxis and gum hemorrhage have been reported with its use; caution should be exercised in patients with increased risk of bleeding due to other concomitant therapies, such as anticoagulants).
No products indexed under this heading.

Low Molecular Weight Heparins (Pentosan polysulfate sodium is a weak anticoagulant and bleeding complications of ecchymosis, epistaxis and gum hemorrhage have been reported with its use; caution should be exercised in patients with increased risk of bleeding due to other concomitant therapies, such as anticoagulants).
No products indexed under this heading.

Reteplase (Pentosan polysulfate sodium is a weak anticoagulant and bleeding complications of ecchymosis, epistaxis and gum hemorrhage have been reported with its use; caution should be exercised in patients with increased risk of bleeding due to other concomitant therapies, such as thrombolytics). Products include:
Retavase 1131

Streptokinase (Pentosan polysulfate sodium is a weak anticoagulant and bleeding complications of ecchymosis, epistaxis and gum hemorrhage have been reported with its use; caution should be exercised in patients with increased risk of bleeding due to other concomitant therapies, such as thrombolytics).
No products indexed under this heading.

Tinzaparin Sodium (Pentosan polysulfate sodium is a weak anticoagulant and bleeding complications of ecchymosis, epistaxis and gum hemorrhage have been reported with its use; caution should be exercised in patients with increased risk of bleeding due to other concomitant therapies, such as anticoagulants).
No products indexed under this heading.

Urokinase (Pentosan polysulfate sodium is a weak anticoagulant and bleeding complications of ecchymosis, epistaxis and gum hemorrhage have been reported with its use; caution should be exercised in patients with increased risk of bleeding due to other concomitant therapies, such as thrombolytics).
No products indexed under this heading.

Warfarin Sodium (Pentosan polysulfate sodium is a weak anticoagulant and bleeding complications of ecchymosis, epistaxis and gum hemorrhage have been reported with its use; caution should be exercised in patients with increased risk of bleeding due to other concomitant therapies, such as anticoagulants). Products include:
Coumadin for Injection 932
Coumadin Tablets 932

ELOCON CREAM 0.1%

(Mometasone Furoate) 3019
None cited in PDR database.

ELOCON LOTION 0.1%

(Mometasone Furoate) 3020
None cited in PDR database.

ELOCON OINTMENT 0.1%

(Mometasone Furoate) 3021
None cited in PDR database.

ELOXATIN FOR INJECTION

(Oxaliplatin) 2908
May interact with anticoagulants and certain other agents. Compounds in these categories include:

Anisindione (Prolongation of prothrombin time and of INR occasionally associated with hemorrhage in patients receiving anticoagulants has been reported with oxaliplatin plus 5-FU/LV). Products include:
Miradon Tablets 3056

Ardeparin Sodium (Prolongation of prothrombin time and of INR occasionally associated with hemorrhage in patients receiving anticoagulants has been reported with oxaliplatin plus 5-FU/LV).
No products indexed under this heading.

Dalteparin Sodium (Prolongation of prothrombin time and of INR occasionally associated with hemorrhage in patients receiving anticoagulants has been reported with oxaliplatin plus 5-FU/LV). Products include:
Fragmin Injection 2638

Danaparoid Sodium (Prolongation of prothrombin time and of INR occasionally associated with hemorrhage in patients receiving anticoagulants has been reported with oxaliplatin plus 5-FU/LV).
No products indexed under this heading.

Dicumarol (Prolongation of prothrombin time and of INR occasionally associated with hemorrhage in patients receiving anticoagulants has been reported with oxaliplatin plus 5-FU/LV).
No products indexed under this heading.

Enoxaparin Sodium (Prolongation of prothrombin time and of INR occasionally associated with hemorrhage in patients receiving anticoagulants has been reported with oxaliplatin plus 5-FU/LV). Products include:
Lovenox Injection 2931

Fondaparinux Sodium (Prolongation of prothrombin time and of INR occasionally associated with hemorrhage in patients receiving anticoagulants has been reported with oxaliplatin plus 5-FU/LV). Products include:
Arixtra Injection 1325

Heparin Calcium (Prolongation of prothrombin time and of INR occasionally associated with hemorrhage in patients receiving anticoagulants has been reported with oxaliplatin plus 5-FU/LV).
No products indexed under this heading.

Heparin Sodium (Prolongation of prothrombin time and of INR occasionally associated with hemorrhage in patients receiving anticoagulants has been reported with oxaliplatin plus 5-FU/LV).
No products indexed under this heading.

Low Molecular Weight Heparins (Prolongation of prothrombin time and of INR occasionally associated with hemorrhage in patients receiving anticoagulants has been reported with oxaliplatin plus 5-FU/LV).
No products indexed under this heading.

Nephrotoxic Drugs (Co-administration with nephrotoxic drugs may decrease renal clearance although this has not been studied).
No products indexed under this heading.

Tinzaparin Sodium (Prolongation of prothrombin time and of INR occasionally associated with hemorrhage in patients receiving anticoagulants has been reported with oxaliplatin plus 5-FU/LV).
No products indexed under this heading.

Warfarin Sodium (Prolongation of prothrombin time and of INR occasionally associated with hemorrhage in patients receiving anticoagulants has been reported with oxaliplatin plus 5-FU/LV). Products include:
Coumadin for Injection 932
Coumadin Tablets 932

ELSPAR FOR INJECTION

(Asparaginase) 1943
May interact with:

Methotrexate Sodium (Tissue culture and animal studies indicate that asparaginase can diminish or abolish the effect of methotrexate on malignant cells).
No products indexed under this heading.

Prednisone (The administration of asparaginase intravenously and concurrently with or immediately before a course of prednisone may be associated with increased toxicity).
No products indexed under this heading.

Vincristine Sulfate (The administration of asparaginase intravenously and concurrently with or immediately before a course of prednisone may be associated with increased toxicity).
No products indexed under this heading.

EMCYT CAPSULES

(Estramustine Phosphate Sodium) 3137
May interact with calcium preparations and certain other agents. Compounds in these categories include:

Calcium Carbonate (Calcium-rich drugs may impair the absorption of estramustine). Products include:
Actonel with Calcium Tablets 2684
Caltrate 600 PLUS Chewables 779
Caltrate 600 PLUS Tablets 779
Caltrate 600 + D Tablets 779
Encora Capsules 3298
Encora AM Tablets 3298
Encora PM Tablets 3298
Gas-X with Maalox 675
Maalox Regular Strength Antacid Tablets 2166
Quick Dissolve Maalox Max Maximum Strength Antacid/Antigas Tablets 2165
Maalox Max Quick Dissolve Maximum Strength Chewable Tablets 678
Os-Cal Chewable Tablets 765
Pepcid Complete Chewable Tablets 1672
PremCal Light, Regular, and Extra Strength Tablets 762
Rolaids Tablets 707
Extra Strength Rolaids Softchews 708
Extra Strength Rolaids Tablets 707
Rolaids Multi-Symptom Antacid & Antigas Tablets 708
Tums 639

Calcium Chloride (Calcium-rich drugs may impair the absorption of estramustine).
No products indexed under this heading.

Calcium Citrate (Calcium-rich drugs may impair the absorption of estramustine). Products include:
Active Calcium Tablets 3342
Citracal Tablets 2108

Calcium Glubionate (Calcium-rich drugs may impair the absorption of estramustine).
No products indexed under this heading.

Food Interactions

Dairy products (Calcium-rich foods may impair the absorption of estramustine).

Food, calcium-rich (Calcium-rich foods may impair the absorption of estramustine).

EMEND CAPSULES

(Aprepitant) 1944
May interact with benzodiazepine that are metabolized by CYP3A4, cytochrome p450 3a4 inducers (selected), cytochrome p450 3a4 inhibitors (selected), dexamethasone, methylprednisolone, oral contraceptives, phenytoin, and certain other agents. Compounds in these categories include:

Acetazolamide (Co-administration of EMEND with drugs that inhibit CYP3A4 activity may result in increased plasma concentrations of aprepitant and should be approached with caution).
No products indexed under this heading.

Allium sativum (Co-administration of EMEND with drugs that strongly induce CYP3A4 activity may result in reduced plasma concentrations of aprepitant that may result in decreased efficacy of EMEND).
No products indexed under this heading.

Alprazolam (The potential effects of increased plasma concentrations of midazolam or other benzodiazepines metabolized via CYP3A4 (alprazolam, triazolam) should be considered when co-administering these agents with EMEND). Products include:
Niravam Orally Disintegrating Tablets 3106
Xanax XR Tablets 2655

Amiodarone Hydrochloride (Co-administration of EMEND with drugs that inhibit CYP3A4 activity may result in increased plasma concentrations of aprepitant and should be approached with caution). Products include:
Pacerone Tablets 3337

Amprenavir (Co-administration of EMEND with drugs that inhibit CYP3A4 activity may result in increased plasma concentrations of aprepitant and should be approached with caution). Products include:
Agenerase Capsules 1299
Agenerase Oral Solution 1304

Anastrozole (Co-administration of EMEND with drugs that inhibit CYP3A4 activity may result in increased plasma concentrations of aprepitant and should be approached with caution). Products include:
Arimidex Tablets 665

Astemizole (EMEND is a moderate CYP3A4 inhibitor; concurrent use with EMEND could result in elevated plasma concentrations of astemizole, potentially causing serious or life-threatening reactions, and is contraindicated).
No products indexed under this heading.

Betamethasone Acetate (Co-administration of EMEND with drugs that strongly induce CYP3A4 activity may result in reduced plasma concentrations of aprepitant that may result in decreased efficacy of EMEND).
No products indexed under this heading.

Betamethasone Sodium Phosphate (Co-administration of EMEND with drugs that strongly induce CYP3A4 activity may result in reduced plasma concentrations of aprepitant that may result in decreased efficacy of EMEND).
No products indexed under this heading.

Carbamazepine (Co-administration of EMEND with drugs that strongly induce CYP3A4 activity may result in reduced plasma concentrations of aprepitant that may result in decreased efficacy of EMEND). Products include:
Carbatrol Capsules 3174
Equetro Extended-Release Capsules 3178
Tegretol/Tegretol-XR 2278

Cimetidine (Co-administration of EMEND with drugs that inhibit CYP3A4 activity may result in increased plasma concentrations of aprepitant and should be approached with caution). Products include:
Tagamet HB 200 Tablets 637
Tagamet Tablets 1547

Cimetidine Hydrochloride (Co-administration of EMEND with drugs that inhibit CYP3A4 activity may result in increased plasma concentrations of aprepitant and should be approached with caution).
No products indexed under this heading.

Ciprofloxacin (Co-administration of EMEND with drugs that inhibit CYP3A4 activity may result in increased plasma concentrations of aprepitant and should be approached with caution). Products include:
Cipro I.V. 2998
Cipro I.V. Pharmacy Bulk Package 3509
Cipro Oral Suspension 2991
Cipro XR Tablets 3004
Ciprodex Otic Suspension 555

Ciprofloxacin Hydrochloride (Co-administration of EMEND with drugs that strongly induce CYP3A4 activity may result in reduced plasma concentrations of aprepitant that may result in decreased efficacy of EMEND). Products include:
Ciloxan Ophthalmic Ointment 554
Cipro Tablets 2991

Cisapride (EMEND is a moderate CYP3A4 inhibitor; concurrent use with EMEND could result in elevated plasma concentrations of cisapride, potentially causing serious or life-threatening reactions, and is contraindicated).
No products indexed under this heading.

Cisplatin (Co-administration of EMEND with drugs that strongly induce CYP3A4 activity may result in reduced plasma concentrations of aprepitant that may result in decreased efficacy of EMEND).
No products indexed under this heading.

Clarithromycin (Co-administration of EMEND with drugs that inhibit CYP3A4 activity may result in increased plasma concentrations of aprepitant and should be approached with caution). Products include:
Biaxin/Biaxin XL 402
PREVPAC 3281

Clotrimazole (Co-administration of EMEND with drugs that inhibit CYP3A4 activity may result in increased plasma concentrations of aprepitant and should be approached with caution). Products include:
Lotrimin 3053
Lotrisone 3054

Cortisone Acetate (Co-administration of EMEND with drugs that strongly induce CYP3A4 activity may result in reduced plasma concentrations of aprepitant that may result in decreased efficacy of EMEND).
No products indexed under this heading.

Cyclosporine (Co-administration of EMEND with drugs that inhibit CYP3A4 activity may result in increased plasma concentrations of aprepitant and should be approached with caution). Products include:
Gengraf Capsules 458
Neoral Soft Gelatin Capsules 2247

Neoral Oral Solution 2247
Restasis Ophthalmic Emulsion 570
Sandimmune 2259

Dalfopristin (Co-administration of EMEND with drugs that inhibit CYP3A4 activity may result in increased plasma concentrations of aprepitant and should be approached with caution). Products include:
Synercid I.V. 1690

Danazol (Co-administration of EMEND with drugs that inhibit CYP3A4 activity may result in increased plasma concentrations of aprepitant and should be approached with caution).
No products indexed under this heading.

Delavirdine Mesylate (Co-administration of EMEND with drugs that inhibit CYP3A4 activity may result in increased plasma concentrations of aprepitant and should be approached with caution). Products include:
Rescriptor Tablets 2535

Desogestrel (The co-administration of aprepitant may reduce the efficacy of hormonal contraceptives during and for 28 days after administration of the last dose of aprepitant. Alternative or back-up methods of contraception should be used during treatment with aprepitant and for one month following the last dose of aprepitant). Products include:
Ortho-Cept Tablets 2395

Dexamethasone (The oral dexamethasone doses should be reduced by approximately 50% when co-administered with EMEND, to achieve exposures of dexamethasone similar to those obtained when it is given without EMEND). Products include:
Ciprodex Otic Suspension 555
Decadron Tablets 1929
TobraDex Ophthalmic Ointment 558
TobraDex Ophthalmic Suspension 558

Dexamethasone Acetate (The oral dexamethasone doses should be reduced by approximately 50% when co-administered with EMEND, to achieve exposures of dexamethasone similar to those obtained when it is given without EMEND).
No products indexed under this heading.

Dexamethasone Sodium Phosphate (The oral dexamethasone doses should be reduced by approximately 50% when co-administered with EMEND, to achieve exposures of dexamethasone similar to those obtained when it is given without EMEND). Products include:
Decadron Phosphate Injection 1931

Diazepam (The potential effects of increased plasma concentrations of midazolam or other benzodiazepines metabolized via CYP3A4 (alprazolam, triazolam) should be considered when co-administering these agents with EMEND). Products include:
Diastat Rectal Delivery System 3344
Valium Tablets 2822

Diltiazem Hydrochloride (Co-administration of EMEND with drugs that inhibit CYP3A4 activity may result in increased plasma concentrations of aprepitant and should be approached with caution). Products include:
Cardizem LA Extended Release Tablets 1699
Tiazac Capsules 1204

Diltiazem Maleate (Co-administration of EMEND with drugs that inhibit CYP3A4 activity may result in increased plasma concentrations of aprepitant and should be approached with caution).
No products indexed under this heading.

Doxorubicin Hydrochloride (Co-administration of EMEND with drugs that strongly induce CYP3A4 activity may result in reduced plasma concentrations of aprepitant that may result in decreased efficacy of EMEND). Products include:
Adriamycin for Injection, USP 786
Adriamycin Injection, USP 786

Efavirenz (Co-administration of EMEND with drugs that inhibit CYP3A4 activity may result in increased plasma concentrations of aprepitant and should be approached with caution). Products include:
Sustiva Capsules 957

Erythromycin (Co-administration of EMEND with drugs that inhibit CYP3A4 activity may result in increased plasma concentrations of aprepitant and should be approached with caution). Products include:
Erygel Topical Gel 2096
Ery-Tab Tablets 447
Erythromycin Base Filmtab Tablets 454
Erythromycin Delayed-Release Capsules, USP 456
PCE Dispertab Tablets 510

Erythromycin Estolate (Co-administration of EMEND with drugs that inhibit CYP3A4 activity may result in increased plasma concentrations of aprepitant and should be approached with caution).
No products indexed under this heading.

Erythromycin Ethylsuccinate (Co-administration of EMEND with drugs that inhibit CYP3A4 activity may result in increased plasma concentrations of aprepitant and should be approached with caution). Products include:
E.E.S. 449
EryPed 445

Erythromycin Gluceptate (Co-administration of EMEND with drugs that inhibit CYP3A4 activity may result in increased plasma concentrations of aprepitant and should be approached with caution).
No products indexed under this heading.

Erythromycin Lactobionate (Co-administration of EMEND with drugs that inhibit CYP3A4 activity may result in increased plasma concentrations of aprepitant and should be approached with caution).
No products indexed under this heading.

Erythromycin Stearate (Co-administration of EMEND with drugs that inhibit CYP3A4 activity may result in increased plasma concentrations of aprepitant and should be approached with caution). Products include:
Erythrocin Stearate Filmtab Tablets 452

Esomeprazole Magnesium (Co-administration of EMEND with drugs that inhibit CYP3A4 activity may result in increased plasma concentrations of aprepitant and should be approached with caution). Products include:
Nexium Delayed-Release Capsules 645

Ethinyl Estradiol (The co-administration of aprepitant may reduce the efficacy of hormonal contraceptives during and for 28 days after administration of the last dose of aprepitant. Alternative or back-up methods of contraception should be used during treatment with aprepitant and for one month following the last dose of aprepitant). Products include:
Alesse-28 Tablets 3392
Lo/Ovral-28 Tablets 3423
NuvaRing 2357
Ortho-Cept Tablets 2395
Ortho-Cyclen/Ortho Tri-Cyclen 2414
Ortho Evra Transdermal System 2402
Ortho Tri-Cyclen Lo Tablets 2421
Seasonale Tablets 1073
Triphasil-28 Tablets 3483
Yasmin 28 Tablets 818

Ethosuximide (Co-administration of EMEND with drugs that strongly induce CYP3A4 activity may result in reduced plasma concentrations of aprepitant that may result in decreased efficacy of EMEND).
No products indexed under this heading.

Ethynodiol Diacetate (The co-administration of aprepitant may reduce the efficacy of hormonal contraceptives during and for 28 days after administration of the last dose of aprepitant. Alternative or back-up methods of contraception should be used during treatment with aprepitant and for one month following the last dose of aprepitant).
No products indexed under this heading.

Etoposide (Particular caution and careful monitoring are advised in patients receiving chemotherapy agents metabolized primarily by CYP3A4, like etoposide).
No products indexed under this heading.

Felbamate (Co-administration of EMEND with drugs that strongly induce CYP3A4 activity may result in reduced plasma concentrations of aprepitant that may result in decreased efficacy of EMEND).
No products indexed under this heading.

Fluconazole (Co-administration of EMEND with drugs that inhibit CYP3A4 activity may result in increased plasma concentrations of aprepitant and should be approached with caution).
No products indexed under this heading.

Fludrocortisone Acetate (Co-administration of EMEND with drugs that strongly induce CYP3A4 activity may result in reduced plasma concentrations of aprepitant that may result in decreased efficacy of EMEND).
No products indexed under this heading.

Fluoxetine Hydrochloride (Co-administration of EMEND with drugs that inhibit CYP3A4 activity may result in increased plasma concentrations of aprepitant and should be approached with caution). Products include:
Prozac Pulvules and Liquid 1771
Symbyax Capsules 1788

Fluvoxamine Maleate (Co-administration of EMEND with drugs that inhibit CYP3A4 activity may result in increased plasma concentrations of aprepitant and should be approached with caution).
No products indexed under this heading.

Fosamprenavir Calcium (Co-administration of EMEND with drugs that inhibit CYP3A4 activity may result in increased plasma concentrations of aprepitant and should be approached with caution). Products include:
Lexiva Tablets 1473

Fosphenytoin Sodium (Aprepitant is an inducer of CYP2C9; co-administration has been shown to induce the metabolism of tolbutamide, which is metabolized through CYP2C9).
No products indexed under this heading.

Garlic Extract (Co-administration of EMEND with drugs that strongly induce CYP3A4 activity may result in reduced plasma concentrations of aprepitant that may result in decreased efficacy of EMEND).
No products indexed under this heading.

Garlic Oil (Co-administration of EMEND with drugs that strongly induce CYP3A4 activity may result in reduced plasma concentrations of aprepitant that may result in decreased efficacy of EMEND).
No products indexed under this heading.

Hydrocortisone (Co-administration of EMEND with drugs that strongly induce CYP3A4 activity may result in reduced plasma concentrations of aprepitant that may result in decreased efficacy of EMEND). Products include:
Cortizone•5 Ointment .... ▣699
Cortizone•10 Creme .... ▣699
Cortizone•10 Ointment .... ▣699
Cortizone•10 Plus Creme .... ▣700
Cortizone•10 Maximum Strength Quick Shot Spray .... ▣700
Hydrocortone Tablets 1963
Preparation H Hydrocortisone Cream .... ▣748

Hydrocortisone Acetate (Co-administration of EMEND with drugs that strongly induce CYP3A4 activity may result in reduced plasma concentrations of aprepitant that may result in decreased efficacy of EMEND). Products include:
Analpram-HC 1136
Pramosone 1139
ProctoFoam-HC 3113
Tucks Anti-Itch Ointment .... ▣712
U-cort 1% Cream 3289

Hydrocortisone Butyrate (Co-administration of EMEND with drugs that strongly induce CYP3A4 activity may result in reduced plasma concentrations of aprepitant that may result in decreased efficacy of EMEND). Products include:
Locoid 1138
Locoid Lipocream Cream 1138

Hydrocortisone Cypionate (Co-administration of EMEND with drugs that strongly induce CYP3A4 activity may result in reduced plasma concentrations of aprepitant that may result in decreased efficacy of EMEND).
No products indexed under this heading.

Hydrocortisone Hemisuccinate (Co-administration of EMEND with drugs that strongly induce CYP3A4 activity may result in reduced plasma concentrations of aprepitant that may result in decreased efficacy of EMEND).
No products indexed under this heading.

Hydrocortisone Probutate (Co-administration of EMEND with drugs that strongly induce CYP3A4 activity may result in reduced plasma concentrations of aprepitant that may result in decreased efficacy of EMEND). Products include:
Pandel Cream, 0.1% **1017**

Hydrocortisone Sodium Phosphate (Co-administration of EMEND with drugs that strongly induce CYP3A4 activity may result in reduced plasma concentrations of aprepitant that may result in decreased efficacy of EMEND).
No products indexed under this heading.

Hydrocortisone Sodium Succinate (Co-administration of EMEND with drugs that strongly induce CYP3A4 activity may result in reduced plasma concentrations of aprepitant that may result in decreased efficacy of EMEND).
No products indexed under this heading.

Hydrocortisone Valerate (Co-administration of EMEND with drugs that strongly induce CYP3A4 activity may result in reduced plasma concentrations of aprepitant that may result in decreased efficacy of EMEND).
No products indexed under this heading.

Hypericum (Co-administration of EMEND with drugs that strongly induce CYP3A4 activity may result in reduced plasma concentrations of aprepitant that may result in decreased efficacy of EMEND).
No products indexed under this heading.

Hypericum Perforatum (Co-administration of EMEND with drugs that strongly induce CYP3A4 activity may result in reduced plasma concentrations of aprepitant that may result in decreased efficacy of EMEND).
No products indexed under this heading.

Ifosfamide (Particular caution and careful monitoring are advised in patients receiving chemotherapy agents metabolized primarily by CYP3A4, like ifosfamide).
No products indexed under this heading.

Imatinib Mesylate (Particular caution and careful monitoring are advised in patients receiving chemotherapy agents metabolized primarily by CYP3A4, like imatinib). Products include:
Gleevec Tablets **2221**

Indinavir Sulfate (Co-administration of EMEND with drugs that inhibit CYP3A4 activity may result in increased plasma concentrations of aprepitant and should be approached with caution). Products include:
Crixivan Capsules **1918**

Irinotecan Hydrochloride (Particular caution and careful monitoring are advised in patients receiving chemotherapy agents metabolized primarily by CYP3A4, like irinotecan). Products include:
Camptosar Injection **2602**

Isoniazid (Co-administration of EMEND with drugs that inhibit CYP3A4 activity may result in increased plasma concentrations of aprepitant and should be approached with caution).
No products indexed under this heading.

Itraconazole (Co-administration of EMEND with drugs that inhibit CYP3A4 activity may result in increased plasma concentrations of aprepitant and should be approached with caution).
No products indexed under this heading.

Ketoconazole (Co-administration of EMEND with drugs that inhibit CYP3A4 activity may result in increased plasma concentrations of aprepitant and should be approached with caution). Products include:
Nizoral A-D Shampoo, 1% **1839**
Nizoral 2% Shampoo **1838**

Levonorgestrel (The co-administration of aprepitant may reduce the efficacy of hormonal contraceptives during and for 28 days after administration of the last dose of aprepitant. Alternative or back-up methods of contraception should be used during treatment with aprepitant and for one month following the last dose of aprepitant). Products include:
Alesse-28 Tablets **3392**
Climara Pro Transdermal System **800**
Mirena Intrauterine System **810**
Plan B Tablets **1068**
Seasonale Tablets **1073**
Triphasil-28 Tablets **3483**

Lopinavir (Co-administration of EMEND with drugs that inhibit CYP3A4 activity may result in increased plasma concentrations of aprepitant and should be approached with caution). Products include:
Kaletra **474**

Loratadine (Co-administration of EMEND with drugs that inhibit CYP3A4 activity may result in increased plasma concentrations of aprepitant and should be approached with caution). Products include:
Alavert Allergy & Sinus D-12 Hour Tablets...................................... **743**
Alavert **743**
Children's Claritin 24 Hour Non-Drowsy Allergy Syrup **732**
Claritin Non-Drowsy 24 Hour Tablets...................................... **731**
Non-Drowsy Claritin Hives Relief Tablets...................................... **733**
Claritin Reditabs 24 Hour Non-Drowsy Tablets **732**
Claritin-D Non-Drowsy 12 Hour Tablets...................................... **731**
Claritin-D Non-Drowsy 24 Hour Tablets...................................... **731**
Children's Dimetapp ND Non-Drowsy Allergy Syrup **746**
Triaminic Allerchews **684**

Mephenytoin (Co-administration of EMEND with drugs that strongly induce CYP3A4 activity may result in reduced plasma concentrations of aprepitant that may result in decreased efficacy of EMEND).
No products indexed under this heading.

Mestranol (The co-administration of aprepitant may reduce the efficacy of hormonal contraceptives during and for 28 days after administration of the last dose of aprepitant. Alternative or back-up methods of contraception should be used during treatment with aprepitant and for one month following the last dose of aprepitant).
No products indexed under this heading.

Methsuximide (Co-administration of EMEND with drugs that strongly induce CYP3A4 activity may result in reduced plasma concentrations of aprepitant that may result in decreased efficacy of EMEND).
No products indexed under this heading.

Methylprednisolone (The IV methylprednisolone doses should be reduced by approximately 25% and the oral methylprednisolone dose should be reduced by approximately 50% when co-administered with EMEND, to achieve exposures of dexamethasone similar to those obtained when it is given without EMEND).
No products indexed under this heading.

Methylprednisolone Acetate (The IV methylprednisolone doses should be reduced by approximately 25% and the oral methylprednisolone dose should be reduced by approximately 50% when co-administered with EMEND, to achieve exposures of dexamethasone similar to those obtained when it is given without EMEND). Products include:
Depo-Medrol Injectable Suspension **2615**
Depo-Medrol Single-Dose Vial **2617**

Methylprednisolone Sodium Succinate (The IV methylprednisolone doses should be reduced by approximately 25% and the oral methylprednisolone dose should be reduced by approximately 50% when co-administered with EMEND, to achieve exposures of dexamethasone similar to those obtained when it is given without EMEND).
No products indexed under this heading.

Metronidazole (Co-administration of EMEND with drugs that inhibit CYP3A4 activity may result in increased plasma concentrations of aprepitant and should be approached with caution). Products include:
Metrogel 1% **1212**
MetroGel-Vaginal Gel **1822**
Noritate Cream, 1% **1051**

Metronidazole Benzoate (Co-administration of EMEND with drugs that inhibit CYP3A4 activity may result in increased plasma concentrations of aprepitant and should be approached with caution).
No products indexed under this heading.

Metronidazole Hydrochloride (Co-administration of EMEND with drugs that inhibit CYP3A4 activity may result in increased plasma concentrations of aprepitant and should be approached with caution).
No products indexed under this heading.

Miconazole (Co-administration of EMEND with drugs that inhibit CYP3A4 activity may result in increased plasma concentrations of aprepitant and should be approached with caution).
No products indexed under this heading.

Miconazole Nitrate (Co-administration of EMEND with drugs that inhibit CYP3A4 activity may result in increased plasma concentrations of aprepitant and should be approached with caution). Products include:
Desenex **674**
Desenex Jock Itch Spray Powder ... **674**

Midazolam Hydrochloride (The potential effects of increased plasma concentrations of midazolam or other benzodiazepines metabolized via CYP3A4 (alprazolam, triazolam) should be considered when co-administering these agents with EMEND).
No products indexed under this heading.

Modafinil (Co-administration of EMEND with drugs that strongly induce CYP3A4 activity may result in reduced plasma concentrations of aprepitant that may result in decreased efficacy of EMEND). Products include:
Provigil Tablets **1002**

Nefazodone Hydrochloride (Co-administration of EMEND with drugs that inhibit CYP3A4 activity may result in increased plasma concentrations of aprepitant and should be approached with caution).
No products indexed under this heading.

Nelfinavir Mesylate (Co-administration of EMEND with drugs that inhibit CYP3A4 activity may result in increased plasma concentrations of aprepitant and should be approached with caution). Products include:
Viracept **2556**

Nevirapine (Co-administration of EMEND with drugs that inhibit CYP3A4 activity may result in increased plasma concentrations of aprepitant and should be approached with caution). Products include:
Viramune Oral Suspension **903**
Viramune Tablets **903**

Niacinamide (Co-administration of EMEND with drugs that inhibit CYP3A4 activity may result in increased plasma concentrations of aprepitant and should be approached with caution).
No products indexed under this heading.

Nicotinamide (Co-administration of EMEND with drugs that inhibit CYP3A4 activity may result in increased plasma concentrations of aprepitant and should be approached with caution). Products include:
Nicomide Tablets **3190**

Nifedipine (Co-administration of EMEND with drugs that inhibit CYP3A4 activity may result in increased plasma concentrations of aprepitant and should be approached with caution). Products include:
Adalat CC Tablets **2978**

Norethindrone (The co-administration of aprepitant may reduce the efficacy of hormonal con-

traceptives during and for 28 days after administration of the last dose of aprepitant. Alternative or back-up methods of contraception should be used during treatment with aprepitant and for one month following the last dose of aprepitant). Products include:

Ortho Micronor Tablets **2411**

Norethynodrel (The co-administration of aprepitant may reduce the efficacy of hormonal contraceptives during and for 28 days after administration of the last dose of aprepitant. Alternative or back-up methods of contraception should be used during treatment with aprepitant and for one month following the last dose of aprepitant).

No products indexed under this heading.

Norfloxacin (Co-administration of EMEND with drugs that inhibit CYP3A4 activity may result in increased plasma concentrations of aprepitant and should be approached with caution). Products include:

Noroxin Tablets **2009**

Norgestimate (The co-administration of aprepitant may reduce the efficacy of hormonal contraceptives during and for 28 days after administration of the last dose of aprepitant. Alternative or back-up methods of contraception should be used during treatment with aprepitant and for one month following the last dose of aprepitant). Products include:

Ortho-Cyclen/Ortho Tri-Cyclen **2414**
Ortho Tri-Cyclen Lo Tablets **2421**
Prefest Tablets **1069**

Norgestrel (The co-administration of aprepitant may reduce the efficacy of hormonal contraceptives during and for 28 days after administration of the last dose of aprepitant. Alternative or back-up methods of contraception should be used during treatment with aprepitant and for one month following the last dose of aprepitant). Products include:

Lo/Ovral-28 Tablets **3423**

Omeprazole (Co-administration of EMEND with drugs that inhibit CYP3A4 activity may result in increased plasma concentrations of aprepitant and should be approached with caution). Products include:

Zegerid Powder for Oral Solution **2972**

Oxcarbazepine (Co-administration of EMEND with drugs that strongly induce CYP3A4 activity may result in reduced plasma concentrations of aprepitant that may result in decreased efficacy of EMEND). Products include:

Trileptal Oral Suspension **2281**
Trileptal Tablets **2281**

Paclitaxel (Particular caution and careful monitoring are advised in patients receiving chemotherapy agents metabolized primarily by CYP3A4, like paclitaxel).

No products indexed under this heading.

Paroxetine Hydrochloride (Co-administration resulted in a decrease in AUC by approximately 25% and Cmax by approximately 20% of both aprepitant and paroxetine). Products include:

Paxil CR Controlled-Release Tablets **1509**
Paxil **1501**

Phenobarbital (Co-administration of EMEND with drugs that strongly induce CYP3A4 activity may result in reduced plasma concentrations of aprepitant that may result in decreased efficacy of EMEND).

No products indexed under this heading.

Phenobarbital Sodium (Co-administration of EMEND with drugs that strongly induce CYP3A4 activity may result in reduced plasma concentrations of aprepitant that may result in decreased efficacy of EMEND).

No products indexed under this heading.

Phenytoin (Aprepitant is an inducer of CYP2C9; co-administration has been shown to induce the metabolism of tolbutamide, which is metabolized through CYP2C9).

No products indexed under this heading.

Phenytoin Sodium (Aprepitant is an inducer of CYP2C9; co-administration has been shown to induce the metabolism of tolbutamide, which is metabolized through CYP2C9). Products include:

Phenytek Capsules **2153**

Pimozide (EMEND is a moderate CYP3A4 inhibitor; concurrent use with EMEND could result in elevated plasma concentrations of pimozide, potentially causing serious or life-threatening reactions, and is contraindicated). Products include:

Orap Tablets **1220**

Prednisolone Acetate (Co-administration of EMEND with drugs that strongly induce CYP3A4 activity may result in reduced plasma concentrations of aprepitant that may result in decreased efficacy of EMEND). Products include:

Blephamide Ophthalmic Ointment **563**
Blephamide Ophthalmic Suspension **564**
Poly-Pred Liquifilm Ophthalmic Suspension .... ⊙ **231**
Pred Forte Ophthalmic Suspension .... ⊙ **233**
Pred Mild Sterile Ophthalmic Suspension .... ⊙ **236**
Pred-G Ophthalmic Suspension .... ⊙ **234**
Pred-G Sterile Ophthalmic Ointment .... ⊙ **235**

Prednisolone Sodium Phosphate (Co-administration of EMEND with drugs that strongly induce CYP3A4 activity may result in reduced plasma concentrations of aprepitant that may result in decreased efficacy of EMEND). Products include:

Pediapred Oral Solution **3319**

Prednisolone Tebutate (Co-administration of EMEND with drugs that strongly induce CYP3A4 activity may result in reduced plasma concentrations of aprepitant that may result in decreased efficacy of EMEND).

No products indexed under this heading.

Prednisone (Co-administration of EMEND with drugs that strongly induce CYP3A4 activity may result in reduced plasma concentrations of aprepitant that may result in decreased efficacy of EMEND).

No products indexed under this heading.

Primidone (Co-administration of EMEND with drugs that strongly induce CYP3A4 activity may result in reduced plasma concentrations of aprepitant that may result in decreased efficacy of EMEND).

No products indexed under this heading.

Propoxyphene Hydrochloride (Co-administration of EMEND with drugs that inhibit CYP3A4 activity may result in increased plasma concentrations of aprepitant and should be approached with caution).

No products indexed under this heading.

Propoxyphene Napsylate (Co-administration of EMEND with drugs that inhibit CYP3A4 activity may result in increased plasma concentrations of aprepitant and should be approached with caution). Products include:

Darvocet A 500 Tablets **3497**

Quinidine (Co-administration of EMEND with drugs that inhibit CYP3A4 activity may result in increased plasma concentrations of aprepitant and should be approached with caution).

No products indexed under this heading.

Quinidine Hydrochloride (Co-administration of EMEND with drugs that inhibit CYP3A4 activity may result in increased plasma concentrations of aprepitant and should be approached with caution).

No products indexed under this heading.

Quinidine Polygalacturonate (Co-administration of EMEND with drugs that inhibit CYP3A4 activity may result in increased plasma concentrations of aprepitant and should be approached with caution).

No products indexed under this heading.

Quinidine Sulfate (Co-administration of EMEND with drugs that inhibit CYP3A4 activity may result in increased plasma concentrations of aprepitant and should be approached with caution).

No products indexed under this heading.

Quinine (Co-administration of EMEND with drugs that inhibit CYP3A4 activity may result in increased plasma concentrations of aprepitant and should be approached with caution).

No products indexed under this heading.

Quinine Sulfate (Co-administration of EMEND with drugs that inhibit CYP3A4 activity may result in increased plasma concentrations of aprepitant and should be approached with caution).

No products indexed under this heading.

Quinupristin (Co-administration of EMEND with drugs that inhibit CYP3A4 activity may result in increased plasma concentrations of aprepitant and should be approached with caution). Products include:

Synercid I.V. **1690**

Ranitidine Bismuth Citrate (Co-administration of EMEND with drugs that inhibit CYP3A4 activity may result in increased plasma concentrations of aprepitant and should be approached with caution).

No products indexed under this heading.

Ranitidine Hydrochloride (Co-administration of EMEND with drugs that inhibit CYP3A4 activity may result in increased plasma concentrations of aprepitant and should be approached with caution). Products include:

Zantac **1597**
Zantac Injection **1593**
Zantac 75 Tablets .... ▣ **715**
Zantac 150 Maximum Strength Tablets .... ▣ **715**
Zantac Injection Pharmacy Bulk Package **1595**

Rifabutin (Co-administration of EMEND with drugs that strongly induce CYP3A4 activity may result in reduced plasma concentrations of aprepitant that may result in decreased efficacy of EMEND).

No products indexed under this heading.

Rifampicin (Co-administration of EMEND with drugs that strongly induce CYP3A4 activity may result in reduced plasma concentrations of aprepitant that may result in decreased efficacy of EMEND).

No products indexed under this heading.

Rifampin (Co-administration of EMEND with drugs that strongly induce CYP3A4 activity may result in reduced plasma concentrations of aprepitant that may result in decreased efficacy of EMEND).

No products indexed under this heading.

Rifapentine (Co-administration of EMEND with drugs that strongly induce CYP3A4 activity may result in reduced plasma concentrations of aprepitant that may result in decreased efficacy of EMEND).

No products indexed under this heading.

Ritonavir (Co-administration of EMEND with drugs that inhibit CYP3A4 activity may result in increased plasma concentrations of aprepitant and should be approached with caution). Products include:

Kaletra **474**
Norvir **499**

Saquinavir (Co-administration of EMEND with drugs that inhibit CYP3A4 activity may result in increased plasma concentrations of aprepitant and should be approached with caution).

No products indexed under this heading.

Saquinavir Mesylate (Co-administration of EMEND with drugs that inhibit CYP3A4 activity may result in increased plasma concentrations of aprepitant and should be approached with caution). Products include:

Invirase **2776**

Sertraline Hydrochloride (Co-administration of EMEND with drugs that inhibit CYP3A4 activity may result in increased plasma concentrations of aprepitant and should be approached with caution). Products include:

Zoloft **2581**

Sulfinpyrazone (Co-administration of EMEND with drugs that strongly induce CYP3A4 activity may result in reduced plasma concentrations of aprepitant that may result in decreased efficacy of EMEND).
No products indexed under this heading.

Telithromycin (Co-administration of EMEND with drugs that inhibit CYP3A4 activity may result in increased plasma concentrations of aprepitant and should be approached with caution). Products include:
Ketek Tablets 2920

Terfenadine (EMEND is a moderate CYP3A4 inhibitor; concurrent use with EMEND could result in elevated plasma concentrations of terfenadine, potentially causing serious or life-threatening reactions, and is contraindicated).
No products indexed under this heading.

Theophylline (Co-administration of EMEND with drugs that strongly induce CYP3A4 activity may result in reduced plasma concentrations of aprepitant that may result in decreased efficacy of EMEND).
No products indexed under this heading.

Tolbutamide (Aprepitant is an inducer of CYP2C9; co-administration has been shown to induce the metabolism of tolbutamide, which is metabolized through CYP2C9).
No products indexed under this heading.

Triamcinolone (Co-administration of EMEND with drugs that strongly induce CYP3A4 activity may result in reduced plasma concentrations of aprepitant that may result in decreased efficacy of EMEND).
No products indexed under this heading.

Triamcinolone Acetonide (Co-administration of EMEND with drugs that strongly induce CYP3A4 activity may result in reduced plasma concentrations of aprepitant that may result in decreased efficacy of EMEND). Products include:
Azmacort Inhalation Aerosol 1701
Nasacort HFA Inhalation Aerosol 2939
Nasacort AQ Nasal Spray 2937

Triamcinolone Diacetate (Co-administration of EMEND with drugs that strongly induce CYP3A4 activity may result in reduced plasma concentrations of aprepitant that may result in decreased efficacy of EMEND).
No products indexed under this heading.

Triamcinolone Hexacetonide (Co-administration of EMEND with drugs that strongly induce CYP3A4 activity may result in reduced plasma concentrations of aprepitant that may result in decreased efficacy of EMEND).
No products indexed under this heading.

Triazolam (The potential effects of increased plasma concentrations of midazolam or other benzodiazepines metabolized via CYP3A4 (alprazolam, triazolam) should be considered when co-administering these agents with EMEND).
No products indexed under this heading.

Troglitazone (Co-administration of EMEND with drugs that inhibit CYP3A4 activity may result in increased plasma concentrations of aprepitant and should be approached with caution).
No products indexed under this heading.

Troleandomycin (Co-administration of EMEND with drugs that inhibit CYP3A4 activity may result in increased plasma concentrations of aprepitant and should be approached with caution).
No products indexed under this heading.

Valproate Sodium (Co-administration of EMEND with drugs that inhibit CYP3A4 activity may result in increased plasma concentrations of aprepitant and should be approached with caution). Products include:
Depacon Injection 412

Verapamil Hydrochloride (Co-administration of EMEND with drugs that inhibit CYP3A4 activity may result in increased plasma concentrations of aprepitant and should be approached with caution). Products include:
Covera-HS Tablets 3135
Tarka Tablets 519
Verelan PM Capsules 3120

Vinblastine Sulfate (Particular caution and careful monitoring are advised in patients receiving chemotherapy agents metabolized primarily by CYP3A4, like vinblastine).
No products indexed under this heading.

Vincristine Sulfate (Particular caution and careful monitoring are advised in patients receiving chemotherapy agents metabolized primarily by CYP3A4, like vincristine).
No products indexed under this heading.

Vinorelbine Tartrate (Particular caution and careful monitoring are advised in patients receiving chemotherapy agents metabolized primarily by CYP3A4, like vinorelbine). Products include:
Navelbine Injection 1494

Voriconazole (Co-administration of EMEND with drugs that inhibit CYP3A4 activity may result in increased plasma concentrations of aprepitant and should be approached with caution). Products include:
VFEND I.V. 2543
VFEND Oral Suspension 2543
VFEND Tablets 2543

Warfarin Sodium (Aprepitant is an inducer of CYP2C9; co-administration has been shown to induce the metabolism of S(-) warfarin, which is metabolized through CYP2C9; may result in a clinically significant decrease in INR of prothrombin time). Products include:
Coumadin for Injection 932
Coumadin Tablets 932

Zafirlukast (Co-administration of EMEND with drugs that inhibit CYP3A4 activity may result in increased plasma concentrations of aprepitant and should be approached with caution). Products include:
Accolate Tablets 663

Zileuton (Co-administration of EMEND with drugs that inhibit CYP3A4 activity may result in increased plasma concentrations of aprepitant and should be approached with caution).
No products indexed under this heading.

Food Interactions

Grapefruit (Co-administration of EMEND with drugs that inhibit CYP3A4 activity may result in increased plasma concentrations of aprepitant and should be approached with caution).

Grapefruit Juice (Co-administration of EMEND with drugs that inhibit CYP3A4 activity may result in increased plasma concentrations of aprepitant and should be approached with caution).

EMTRIVA CAPSULES

(Emtricitabine) 1272
None cited in PDR database.

ENABLEX EXTENDED-RELEASE TABLETS

(Darifenacin) 2201
May interact with anticholinergics, cytochrome p450 2d6 substrates (selected), cytochrome p450 3a4 inhibitors, potent, and certain other agents. Compounds in these categories include:

Amitriptyline Hydrochloride (Caution should be taken when darifenacin is used concomitantly with medications that are predominantly metabolized by CYP2D6 and which have a narrow therapeutic window).
No products indexed under this heading.

Amphetamine Aspartate (Caution should be taken when darifenacin is used concomitantly with medications that are predominantly metabolized by CYP2D6 and which have a narrow therapeutic window). Products include:
Adderall Tablets 3168
Adderall XR Capsules 3169

Amphetamine Aspartate Monohydrate (Caution should be taken when darifenacin is used concomitantly with medications that are predominantly metabolized by CYP2D6 and which have a narrow therapeutic window).
No products indexed under this heading.

Amphetamine Sulfate (Caution should be taken when darifenacin is used concomitantly with medications that are predominantly metabolized by CYP2D6 and which have a narrow therapeutic window). Products include:
Adderall Tablets 3168
Adderall XR Capsules 3169

Amprenavir (The daily dose of darifenacin should not exceed 7.5 mg when co-administered with potent CYP3A4 inhibitors). Products include:
Agenerase Capsules 1299
Agenerase Oral Solution 1304

Atazanavir (The daily dose of darifenacin should not exceed 7.5 mg when co-administered with potent CYP3A4 inhibitors).
No products indexed under this heading.

Atazanavir sulfate (The daily dose of darifenacin should not exceed 7.5 mg when co-administered with potent CYP3A4 inhibitors). Products include:
Reyataz Capsules 948

Atomoxetine Hydrochloride (Caution should be taken when darifenacin is used concomitantly with medications that are predominantly metabolized by CYP2D6 and which have a narrow therapeutic window). Products include:
Strattera Capsules 1784

Atropine Sulfate (The concomitant use of darifenacin with other anticholinergic agents may increase the frequency and/or severity of dry mouth, constipation, blurred vision and other anticholinergic pharmacolgical effects. Anticholinergic agents may potentially alter the absorption of some concomitantly administered drugs due to effects on gastrointestinal motility).
No products indexed under this heading.

Belladonna Alkaloids (The concomitant use of darifenacin with other anticholinergic agents may increase the frequency and/or severity of dry mouth, constipation, blurred vision and other anticholinergic pharmacolgical effects. Anticholinergic agents may potentially alter the absorption of some concomitantly administered drugs due to effects on gastrointestinal motility). Products include:
Hyland's Teething Tablets 736

Benztropine Mesylate (The concomitant use of darifenacin with other anticholinergic agents may increase the frequency and/or severity of dry mouth, constipation, blurred vision and other anticholinergic pharmacolgical effects. Anticholinergic agents may potentially alter the absorption of some concomitantly administered drugs due to effects on gastrointestinal motility). Products include:
Cogentin Injection 1903

Biperiden Hydrochloride (The concomitant use of darifenacin with other anticholinergic agents may increase the frequency and/or severity of dry mouth, constipation, blurred vision and other anticholinergic pharmacolgical effects. Anticholinergic agents may potentially alter the absorption of some concomitantly administered drugs due to effects on gastrointestinal motility).
No products indexed under this heading.

Bisoprolol Fumarate (Caution should be taken when darifenacin is used concomitantly with medications that are predominantly metabolized by CYP2D6 and which have a narrow therapeutic window).
No products indexed under this heading.

Captopril (Caution should be taken when darifenacin is used concomitantly with medications that are predominantly metabolized by CYP2D6 and which have a narrow therapeutic window). Products include:
Captopril Tablets 2114

Carvedilol (Caution should be taken when darifenacin is used concomitantly with medications that are predominantly metabolized by CYP2D6 and which have a narrow therapeutic window). Products include:
Coreg Tablets 1376

Cevimeline Hydrochloride (Caution should be taken when darifenacin is used concomitantly with medi-

cations that are predominantly metabolized by CYP2D6 and which have a narrow therapeutic window). Products include:
Evoxac Capsules 1042

Chlorpromazine (Caution should be taken when darifenacin is used concomitantly with medications that are predominantly metabolized by CYP2D6 and which have a narrow therapeutic window).
No products indexed under this heading.

Chlorpromazine Hydrochloride (Caution should be taken when darifenacin is used concomitantly with medications that are predominantly metabolized by CYP2D6 and which have a narrow therapeutic window).
No products indexed under this heading.

Chlorpropamide (Caution should be taken when darifenacin is used concomitantly with medications that are predominantly metabolized by CYP2D6 and which have a narrow therapeutic window).
No products indexed under this heading.

Clarithromycin (The daily dose of darifenacin should not exceed 7.5 mg when co-administered with potent CYP3A4 inhibitors). Products include:
Biaxin/Biaxin XL 402
PREVPAC 3281

Clidinium Bromide (The concomitant use of darifenacin with other anticholinergic agents may increase the frequency and/or severity of dry mouth, constipation, blurred vision and other anticholinergic pharmacolgical effects. Anticholinergic agents may potentially alter the absorption of some concomitantly administered drugs due to effects on gastrointestinal motility).
No products indexed under this heading.

Clomipramine Hydrochloride (Caution should be taken when darifenacin is used concomitantly with medications that are predominantly metabolized by CYP2D6 and which have a narrow therapeutic window).
No products indexed under this heading.

Clozapine (Caution should be taken when darifenacin is used concomitantly with medications that are predominantly metabolized by CYP2D6 and which have a narrow therapeutic window). Products include:
Clozapine Tablets 2141
Clozaril Tablets 2174
FazaClo Orally Disintegrating Tablets 547

Codeine Phosphate (Caution should be taken when darifenacin is used concomitantly with medications that are predominantly metabolized by CYP2D6 and which have a narrow therapeutic window). Products include:
Tylenol with Codeine 2461

Codeine Sulfate (Caution should be taken when darifenacin is used concomitantly with medications that are predominantly metabolized by CYP2D6 and which have a narrow therapeutic window).
No products indexed under this heading.

Cyclobenzaprine Hydrochloride (Caution should be taken when darifenacin is used concomitantly with medications that are predominantly metabolized by CYP2D6 and which have a narrow therapeutic window). Products include:
Flexeril Tablets 1832

Desipramine Hydrochloride (Caution should be taken when darifenacin is used concomitantly with medications that are predominantly metabolized by CYP2D6 and which have a narrow therapeutic window).
No products indexed under this heading.

Dexfenfluramine Hydrochloride (Caution should be taken when darifenacin is used concomitantly with medications that are predominantly metabolized by CYP2D6 and which have a narrow therapeutic window).
No products indexed under this heading.

Dextromethorphan Hydrobromide (Caution should be taken when darifenacin is used concomitantly with medications that are predominantly metabolized by CYP2D6 and which have a narrow therapeutic window). Products include:
Alacol DM Syrup 739
Balamine DM 739
Contac Severe Cold and Flu Caplets Maximum Strength .... ▣ 615
Contac Severe Cold and Flu Caplets Non-Drowsy .... ▣ 615
Children's Dimetapp DM Cold & Cough Elixir .... ▣ 745
Children's Dimetapp Long Acting Cough Plus Cold Syrup .... ▣ 746
Dimetapp Infant Drops Decongestant Plus Cough .... ▣ 746
Mucinex DM Tablets .... ▣ 602
PediaCare Decongestant & Cough Infant Drops .... ▣ 705
PediaCare Freezer Pops Long-Acting Cough-Glacier Grape and Polar Berry Blue .... ▣ 706
PediaCare Long-Acting Cough Infant Drops .... ▣ 705
PediaCare Long-Acting Cough Plus Cold Liquid .... ▣ 704
PediaCare Multi-Symptom Cold Liquid .... ▣ 704
PediaCare NightRest Cough & Cold Liquid .... ▣ 704
Robitussin Allergy & Cough Syrup .... ▣ 750
Robitussin CF Liquid .... ▣ 755
Robitussin Cough & Cold Liquid-filled Capsules .... ▣ 750
Robitussin Cough, Cold & Flu Liquid-filled Capsules .... ▣ 750
Robitussin Cough & Cold Infant Drops .... ▣ 755
Robitussin DM Infant Drops .... ▣ 753
Robitussin DM Liquid .... ▣ 753
Robitussin Flu Liquid .... ▣ 752
Robitussin Maximum Strength Cough Liquid .... ▣ 754
Robitussin Maximum Strength Cough & Cold Liquid .... ▣ 754
Robitussin Pediatric Cough Liquid .... ▣ 754
Robitussin Pediatric Cough & Cold Liquid .... ▣ 754
Robitussin PM Cough & Cold Liquid .... ▣ 752
Robitussin Sugar Free Cough Liquid .... ▣ 753
Simply Cough Liquid 1840
Sudafed Severe Cold .... ▣ 710
TheraFlu Cold & Cough Hot Liquid .... ▣ 680
TheraFlu Flu & Chest Congestion Non-Drowsy Hot Liquid .... ▣ 681
TheraFlu Severe Cold Non-Drowsy Hot Liquid .... ▣ 683
TheraFlu Severe Cold & Cough Hot Liquid .... ▣ 683
TheraFlu Severe Cold Caplets .... ▣ 679
TheraFlu Severe Cold Hot Liquid .... ▣ 682
TheraFlu Severe Cold Non-Drowsy Caplets .... ▣ 679
TheraFlu Thin Strips Long Acting Cough .... ▣ 684
Triaminic Cold & Cough Liquid .... ▣ 685
Triaminic Cough Liquid .... ▣ 687
Triaminic Cough & Nasal Congestion Liquid .... ▣ 687
Triaminic Cough & Sore Throat Liquid .... ▣ 687
Triaminic Flu, Cough & Fever Liquid .... ▣ 685
Triaminic Night Time Cough & Cold Liquid .... ▣ 685
Triaminic Cold & Cough Softchews .... ▣ 688
Triaminic Cough & Sore Throat Softchews .... ▣ 689
Triaminic Thin Strips Long Acting Cough .... ▣ 689
Children's Tylenol Plus Cold & Cough Suspension Liquid and Chewable Tablets 1851
Children's Tylenol Plus Flu Suspension Liquid 1853
Concentrated Tylenol Infants' Drops Plus Cold and Cough 1851
Tylenol Cold & Flu Severe Daytime Liquid with Cool Bust 1846
Tylenol Cold & Flu Severe NightTime Liquid with Cool Burst 1846
Tylenol Cold Severe Congestion Non-Drowsy Caplets with Cool Burst 1846
Tylenol Cough & Sore Throat Daytime Liquid with Cool Burst 1849
Tylenol Cough & Sore Throat NightTime Liquid with Cool Burst 1849
Tylenol Flu Day Non-Drowsy Gelcaps 1846
Concentrated Tylenol Infants' Drops Plus Cold & Cough Nasal Decongestant, Fever Reducer & Pain Reliever .... ▣ 668
Multi-Symptom Tylenol Cold Night Time Caplets 1845
Multi-Symptom Tylenol Cold Day Non-Drowsy Caplets and Gelcaps 1845
Vicks 44 Cough Relief 2675
Vicks 44D Cough & Head Congestion Relief 2676
Vicks 44D Cough & Head Congestion Relief Liquid .... ▣ 721
Vicks 44E Cough & Chest Congestion Relief 2676
Pediatric Vicks 44e Cough & Chest Congestion Relief Liquid 2673
Vicks 44M Cough, Cold & Flu Relief 2676
Pediatric Vicks 44m Cough & Cold Relief 2673
Vicks DayQuil LiquiCaps/Liquid Multi-Symptom Cold/Flu Relief .... ▣ 723
Vicks DayQuil Multi-Symptom Cold/Flu Relief LiquiCaps 2675
Vicks DayQuil Multi-Symptom Cold/Flu Relief Liquid 2675
Children's Vicks NyQuil Cold/Cough Relief 2671
Vicks NyQuil Cough Liquid 2677
Vicks NyQuil LiquiCaps 2677
Vicks NyQuil LiquiCaps/Liquid Multi-Symptom Cold/Flu Relief .... ▣ 725
Vicks NyQuil Liquid 2677
Zicam Concentrated Cough Mist for Kids Cool Cherry .... ▣ 643
Zicam Concentrated Cough Mist for Kids Plus D Cool Cherry .... ▣ 643
Zicam Concentrated Cough Mist Nite-Cool Cherry .... ▣ 642
Zicam Concentrated Cough Mist Plus D Cool Cherry .... ▣ 642
Zicam Concentrated Cough Mist-Honey Lemon & Cool Cherry .... ▣ 642

Dextromethorphan Polistirex (Caution should be taken when darifenacin is used concomitantly with medications that are predominantly metabolized by CYP2D6 and which have a narrow therapeutic window). Products include:
Delsym Extended-Release Suspension .... ▣ 611
Delsym 12 Hour Cough Suppressant for Children .... ▣ 611

Dicyclomine Hydrochloride (The concomitant use of darifenacin with other anticholinergic agents may increase the frequency and/or severity of dry mouth, constipation, blurred vision and other anticholinergic pharmacolgical effects. Anticholinergic agents may potentially alter the absorption of some concomitantly administered drugs due to effects on gastrointestinal motility). Products include:
Bentyl Capsules 724
Bentyl Injection 724
Bentyl Syrup 724
Bentyl Tablets 724

Digoxin (Darifenacin (30 mg daily) co-administered with digoxin (0.25 mg) at steady state resulted in a 16% increase in digoxin exposure. Routine therapeutic drug monitoring for digoxin should be continued). Products include:
Digitek Tablets 2146
Lanoxicaps Capsules 1458
Lanoxin Injection 1462
Lanoxin Tablets 1468
Lanoxin Injection Pediatric 1465

Dolasetron Mesylate (Caution should be taken when darifenacin is used concomitantly with medications that are predominantly metabolized by CYP2D6 and which have a narrow therapeutic window). Products include:
Anzemet Injection 2871
Anzemet Tablets 2874

Donepezil Hydrochloride (Caution should be taken when darifenacin is used concomitantly with medications that are predominantly metabolized by CYP2D6 and which have a narrow therapeutic window). Products include:
Aricept Tablets 1086
Aricept ODT Tablets 1086

Doxepin Hydrochloride (Caution should be taken when darifenacin is used concomitantly with medications that are predominantly metabolized by CYP2D6 and which have a narrow therapeutic window).
No products indexed under this heading.

Encainide Hydrochloride (Caution should be taken when darifenacin is used concomitantly with medications that are predominantly metabolized by CYP2D6 and which have a narrow therapeutic window).
No products indexed under this heading.

Fentanyl (Caution should be taken when darifenacin is used concomitantly with medications that are predominantly metabolized by CYP2D6 and which have a narrow therapeutic window). Products include:
Duragesic Transdermal System 2448

Fentanyl Citrate (Caution should be taken when darifenacin is used concomitantly with medications that are predominantly metabolized by CYP2D6 and which have a narrow therapeutic window). Products include:
Actiq 993

Flecainide Acetate (Caution should be taken when darifenacin is used concomitantly with medications that are predominantly metabolized by CYP2D6 and which have a narrow therapeutic window). Products include:
Tambocor Tablets 1824

Fluoxetine (Caution should be taken when darifenacin is used concomitantly with medications that are predominantly metabolized by CYP2D6 and which have a narrow therapeutic window).
No products indexed under this heading.

Fluoxetine Hydrochloride (Caution should be taken when darifenacin is used concomitantly with medications that are predominantly metabolized by CYP2D6 and which have a narrow therapeutic window). Products include:
Prozac Pulvules and Liquid 1771
Symbyax Capsules 1788

Fluphenazine Decanoate (Caution should be taken when darifenacin is used concomitantly with medications that are predominantly metabolized by CYP2D6 and which have a narrow therapeutic window).
No products indexed under this heading.

Fluphenazine Enanthate (Caution should be taken when darifenacin is used concomitantly with medications that are predominantly metabolized by CYP2D6 and which have a narrow therapeutic window).
No products indexed under this heading.

Fluphenazine Hydrochloride (Caution should be taken when darifenacin is used concomitantly with medications that are predominantly metabolized by CYP2D6 and which have a narrow therapeutic window).
No products indexed under this heading.

Fluvoxamine Maleate (Caution should be taken when darifenacin is used concomitantly with medications that are predominantly metabolized by CYP2D6 and which have a narrow therapeutic window).
No products indexed under this heading.

Formoterol Fumarate (Caution should be taken when darifenacin is used concomitantly with medications that are predominantly metabolized by CYP2D6 and which have a narrow therapeutic window). Products include:
Foradil Aerolizer 3024

Fosamprenavir Calcium (The daily dose of darifenacin should not exceed 7.5 mg when co-administered with potent CYP3A4 inhibitors). Products include:
Lexiva Tablets 1473

Galantamine Hydrobromide (Caution should be taken when darifenacin is used concomitantly with medications that are predominantly metabolized by CYP2D6 and which have a narrow therapeutic window). Products include:
Razadyne ER Extended-Release Capsules 2434
Razadyne 2434

Glycopyrrolate (The concomitant use of darifenacin with other anticholinergic agents may increase the frequency and/or severity of dry mouth, constipation, blurred vision and other anticholinergic pharmacolgical effects. Anticholinergic agents may potentially alter the absorption of some concomitantly administered drugs due to effects on gastrointestinal motility).
No products indexed under this heading.

Haloperidol (Caution should be taken when darifenacin is used concomitantly with medications that are predominantly metabolized by CYP2D6 and which have a narrow therapeutic window).
No products indexed under this heading.

Haloperidol Decanoate (Caution should be taken when darifenacin is used concomitantly with medications that are predominantly metabolized by CYP2D6 and which have a narrow therapeutic window).
No products indexed under this heading.

Hydrocodone Bitartrate (Caution should be taken when darifenacin is used concomitantly with medications that are predominantly metabolized by CYP2D6 and which have a narrow therapeutic window). Products include:
Hycodan 1104
Hycomine Compound Tablets 1105
Hycotuss Expectorant Syrup 1106
Lortab 3315
Lortab Elixir 3312
Vicodin Tablets 530
Vicodin ES Tablets 531
Vicodin HP Tablets 532
Vicoprofen Tablets 533
Zydone Tablets 1118

Hyoscyamine (The concomitant use of darifenacin with other anticholinergic agents may increase the frequency and/or severity of dry mouth, constipation, blurred vision and other anticholinergic pharmacolgical effects. Anticholinergic agents may potentially alter the absorption of some concomitantly administered drugs due to effects on gastrointestinal motility).
No products indexed under this heading.

Hyoscyamine Sulfate (The concomitant use of darifenacin with other anticholinergic agents may increase the frequency and/or severity of dry mouth, constipation, blurred vision and other anticholinergic pharmacolgical effects. Anticholinergic agents may potentially alter the absorption of some concomitantly administered drugs due to effects on gastrointestinal motility).
No products indexed under this heading.

Imipramine Hydrochloride (The mean Cmax and AUC of imipramine, a CYP2D6 substrate, were increased 57% and 70%, respectively, in the presence of steady state darifenacin 30 mg once daily. This was accompanied by a 3.6 fold increase in the mean Cmax and AUC of desipramine, the active metabolite of imipramine. Caution should be taken when darifenacin is used concomitantly with medications that are predominantly metabolized by CYP2D6 and which have a narrow therapeutic window).
No products indexed under this heading.

Imipramine Pamoate (The mean Cmax and AUC of imipramine, a CYP2D6 substrate, were increased 57% and 70%, respectively, in the presence of steady state darifenacin 30 mg once daily. This was accompanied by a 3.6 fold increase in the mean Cmax and AUC of desipramine, the active metabolite of imipramine. Caution should be taken when darifenacin is used concomitantly with medications that are predominantly metabolized by CYP2D6 and which have a narrow therapeutic window).
No products indexed under this heading.

Indinavir Sulfate (The daily dose of darifenacin should not exceed 7.5 mg when co-administered with potent CYP3A4 inhibitors). Products include:
Crixivan Capsules 1918

Indoramin Hydrochloride (Caution should be taken when darifenacin is used concomitantly with medications that are predominantly metabolized by CYP2D6 and which have a narrow therapeutic window).
No products indexed under this heading.

Ipratropium Bromide (The concomitant use of darifenacin with other anticholinergic agents may increase the frequency and/or severity of dry mouth, constipation, blurred vision and other anticholinergic pharmacolgical effects. Anticholinergic agents may potentially alter the absorption of some concomitantly administered drugs due to effects on gastrointestinal motility). Products include:
Atrovent HFA Inhalation Aerosol 872
Atrovent Inhalation Solution 868
Atrovent Nasal Spray 0.03% 869
Atrovent Nasal Spray 0.06% 870
Combivent Inhalation Aerosol 878
DuoNeb Inhalation Solution 1058

Itraconazole (The daily dose of darifenacin should not exceed 7.5 mg when co-administered with potent CYP3A4 inhibitors).
No products indexed under this heading.

Ketoconazole (The daily dose of darifenacin should not exceed 7.5 mg when co-administered with potent CYP3A4 inhibitors). Products include:
Nizoral A-D Shampoo, 1% 1839
Nizoral 2% Shampoo 1838

Labetalol Hydrochloride (Caution should be taken when darifenacin is used concomitantly with medications that are predominantly metabolized by CYP2D6 and which have a narrow therapeutic window).
No products indexed under this heading.

Lidocaine (Caution should be taken when darifenacin is used concomitantly with medications that are predominantly metabolized by CYP2D6 and which have a narrow therapeutic window). Products include:
Lidoderm Patch 1107

Lidocaine Hydrochloride (Caution should be taken when darifenacin is used concomitantly with medications that are predominantly metabolized by CYP2D6 and which have a narrow therapeutic window).
No products indexed under this heading.

Lopinavir (The daily dose of darifenacin should not exceed 7.5 mg when co-administered with potent CYP3A4 inhibitors). Products include:
Kaletra 474

Maprotiline Hydrochloride (Caution should be taken when darifenacin is used concomitantly with medications that are predominantly metabolized by CYP2D6 and which have a narrow therapeutic window).
No products indexed under this heading.

Mepenzolate Bromide (The concomitant use of darifenacin with other anticholinergic agents may increase the frequency and/or severity of dry mouth, constipation, blurred vision and other anticholinergic pharmacolgical effects. Anticholinergic agents may potentially alter the absorption of some concomitantly administered drugs due to effects on gastrointestinal motility).
No products indexed under this heading.

Meperidine Hydrochloride (Caution should be taken when darifenacin is used concomitantly with medications that are predominantly metabolized by CYP2D6 and which have a narrow therapeutic window).
No products indexed under this heading.

Methadone Hydrochloride (Caution should be taken when darifenacin is used concomitantly with medications that are predominantly metabolized by CYP2D6 and which have a narrow therapeutic window).
No products indexed under this heading.

Methamphetamine Hydrochloride (Caution should be taken when darifenacin is used concomitantly with medications that are predominantly metabolized by CYP2D6 and which have a narrow therapeutic window). Products include:
Desoxyn Tablets, USP 2482

Metoprolol Succinate (Caution should be taken when darifenacin is used concomitantly with medications that are predominantly metabolized by CYP2D6 and which have a narrow therapeutic window). Products include:
Toprol-XL Tablets 660

Metoprolol Tartrate (Caution should be taken when darifenacin is used concomitantly with medications that are predominantly metabolized by CYP2D6 and which have a narrow therapeutic window).
No products indexed under this heading.

Mexiletine Hydrochloride (Caution should be taken when darifenacin is used concomitantly with medications that are predominantly metabolized by CYP2D6 and which have a narrow therapeutic window).
No products indexed under this heading.

Midazolam Hydrochloride (Darifenacin (30 mg daily) co-administered with a single oral dose of midazolam 7.5 mg resulted in a 17% increase in midazolam exposure).
No products indexed under this heading.

Mirtazapine (Caution should be taken when darifenacin is used concomitantly with medications that are predominantly metabolized by CYP2D6 and which have a narrow therapeutic window).
No products indexed under this heading.

Morphine Sulfate (Caution should be taken when darifenacin is used concomitantly with medications that are predominantly metabolized by CYP2D6 and which have a narrow therapeutic window). Products include:
Avinza Capsules 1714
Kadian Capsules 572
MS Contin Tablets 2703

Nefazodone Hydrochloride (The daily dose of darifenacin should not exceed 7.5 mg when co-administered with potent CYP3A4 inhibitors).
No products indexed under this heading.

Nelfinavir Mesylate (The daily dose of darifenacin should not exceed 7.5 mg when co-administered with potent CYP3A4 inhibitors). Products include:
Viracept 2556

Nortriptyline Hydrochloride (Caution should be taken when darifenacin is used concomitantly with medications that are predominantly metabolized by CYP2D6 and which have a narrow therapeutic window).
No products indexed under this heading.

Olanzapine (Caution should be taken when darifenacin is used concomitantly with medications that are predominantly metabolized by CYP2D6 and which have a narrow therapeutic window). Products include:
Symbyax Capsules 1788
Zyprexa Tablets 1798
Zyprexa IntraMuscular 1798
Zyprexa ZYDIS Orally Disintegrating Tablets 1798

Omeprazole (Caution should be taken when darifenacin is used concomitantly with medications that are predominantly metabolized by CYP2D6 and which have a narrow therapeutic window). Products include:
Zegerid Powder for Oral Solution 2972

Ondansetron (Caution should be taken when darifenacin is used concomitantly with medications that are predominantly metabolized by CYP2D6 and which have a narrow therapeutic window). Products include:
Zofran ODT Orally Disintegrating Tablets 1613

Ondansetron Hydrochloride (Caution should be taken when darifenacin is used concomitantly with medications that are predominantly metabolized by CYP2D6 and which have a narrow therapeutic window). Products include:
Zofran Injection 1607
Zofran 1613

Oxybutynin Chloride (The concomitant use of darifenacin with other anticholinergic agents may increase the frequency and/or severity of dry mouth, constipation, blurred vision and other anticholinergic pharmacolgical effects. Anticholinergic agents may potentially alter the absorption of some concomitantly administered drugs due to effects on gastrointestinal motility). Products include:
Ditropan XL Extended Release Tablets 2391

Oxycodone Hydrochloride (Caution should be taken when darifenacin is used concomitantly with medications that are predominantly metabolized by CYP2D6 and which have a narrow therapeutic window). Products include:
Combunox Tablets 1183
OxyContin Tablets 2699
OxyFast Oral Concentrate Solution 2704
OxyIR Capsules 2704
Percocet Tablets 1114
Percodan Tablets 1115

Paclitaxel (Caution should be taken when darifenacin is used concomitantly with medications that are predominantly metabolized by CYP2D6 and which have a narrow therapeutic window).
No products indexed under this heading.

Paroxetine Hydrochloride (Caution should be taken when darifenacin is used concomitantly with medications that are predominantly metabolized by CYP2D6 and which have a narrow therapeutic window). Products include:
Paxil CR Controlled-Release Tablets 1509
Paxil 1501

Pindolol (Caution should be taken when darifenacin is used concomitantly with medications that are predominantly metabolized by CYP2D6 and which have a narrow therapeutic window).
No products indexed under this heading.

Procyclidine Hydrochloride (The concomitant use of darifenacin with other anticholinergic agents may increase the frequency and/or severity of dry mouth, constipation, blurred vision and other anticholinergic pharmacolgical effects. Anticholinergic agents may potentially alter the absorption of some concomitantly administered drugs due to effects on gastrointestinal motility).
No products indexed under this heading.

Propafenone Hydrochloride (Caution should be taken when darifenacin is used concomitantly with medications that are predominantly metabolized by CYP2D6 and which have a narrow therapeutic window). Products include:
Rythmol SR Capsules 2736

Propantheline Bromide (The concomitant use of darifenacin with other anticholinergic agents may increase the frequency and/or severity of dry mouth, constipation, blurred vision and other anticholinergic pharmacolgical effects. Anticholinergic agents may potentially alter the absorption of some concomitantly administered drugs due to effects on gastrointestinal motility).
No products indexed under this heading.

Propoxyphene Hydrochloride (Caution should be taken when darifenacin is used concomitantly with medications that are predominantly metabolized by CYP2D6 and which have a narrow therapeutic window).
No products indexed under this heading.

Propoxyphene Napsylate (Caution should be taken when darifenacin is used concomitantly with medications that are predominantly metabolized by CYP2D6 and which have a narrow therapeutic window). Products include:
Darvocet A 500 Tablets 3497

Propranolol Hydrochloride (Caution should be taken when darifenacin is used concomitantly with medications that are predominantly metabolized by CYP2D6 and which have a narrow therapeutic window). Products include:
Inderal LA Long-Acting Capsules 3421
InnoPran XL Capsules 2728

Quetiapine Fumarate (Caution should be taken when darifenacin is used concomitantly with medications that are predominantly metabolized by CYP2D6 and which have a narrow therapeutic window). Products include:
Seroquel Tablets 691

Quinidine Gluconate (Caution should be taken when darifenacin is used concomitantly with medications that are predominantly metabolized by CYP2D6 and which have a narrow therapeutic window).
No products indexed under this heading.

Quinidine Hydrochloride (Caution should be taken when darifenacin is used concomitantly with medications that are predominantly metabolized by CYP2D6 and which have a narrow therapeutic window).
No products indexed under this heading.

Quinidine Polygalacturonate (Caution should be taken when darifenacin is used concomitantly with medications that are predominantly metabolized by CYP2D6 and which have a narrow therapeutic window).
No products indexed under this heading.

Quinidine Sulfate (Caution should be taken when darifenacin is used concomitantly with medications that are predominantly metabolized by CYP2D6 and which have a narrow therapeutic window).
No products indexed under this heading.

Risperidone (Caution should be taken when darifenacin is used concomitantly with medications that are predominantly metabolized by CYP2D6 and which have a narrow therapeutic window). Products include:
Risperdal Consta Long-Acting Injection 1664
Risperdal M-Tab Orally Disintegrating Tablets 1658
Risperdal 1658

Ritonavir (The daily dose of darifenacin should not exceed 7.5 mg when co-administered with potent CYP3A4 inhibitors). Products include:
Kaletra 474
Norvir 499

Saquinavir (The daily dose of darifenacin should not exceed 7.5 mg when co-administered with potent CYP3A4 inhibitors).
No products indexed under this heading.

Saquinavir Mesylate (The daily dose of darifenacin should not exceed 7.5 mg when co-administered with potent CYP3A4 inhibitors). Products include:
Invirase 2776

Scopolamine (The concomitant use of darifenacin with other anticholinergic agents may increase the frequency and/or severity of dry mouth, constipation, blurred vision and other anticholinergic pharmacolgical effects. Anticholinergic agents may potentially alter the absorption of some concomitantly administered drugs due to effects on gastrointestinal motility). Products include:
Transderm Scōp Transdermal Therapeutic System 2166

Scopolamine Hydrobromide (The concomitant use of darifenacin with other anticholinergic agents may increase the frequency and/or severity of dry mouth, constipation, blurred vision and other anticholinergic pharmacolgical effects. Anticholinergic agents may potentially alter the absorption of some concomitantly administered drugs due to effects on gastrointestinal motility).
No products indexed under this heading.

Tamoxifen Citrate (Caution should be taken when darifenacin is used concomitantly with medications that are predominantly metabolized by CYP2D6 and which have a narrow therapeutic window).
No products indexed under this heading.

Telithromycin (The daily dose of darifenacin should not exceed 7.5 mg when co-administered with potent CYP3A4 inhibitors). Products include:
Ketek Tablets 2920

Teniposide (Caution should be taken when darifenacin is used concomitantly with medications that are predominantly metabolized by CYP2D6 and which have a narrow therapeutic window).
No products indexed under this heading.

Testosterone (Caution should be taken when darifenacin is used concomitantly with medications that are predominantly metabolized by CYP2D6 and which have a narrow therapeutic window). Products include:
AndroGel 3330
Striant Mucoadhesive 1022
Testim 1% Gel 722

Testosterone Cypionate (Caution should be taken when darifenacin is used concomitantly with medications that are predominantly metabolized by CYP2D6 and which have a narrow therapeutic window).
No products indexed under this heading.

Testosterone Enanthate (Caution should be taken when darifenacin is used concomitantly with medications that are predominantly metabolized by CYP2D6 and which have a narrow therapeutic window). Products include:
Delatestryl Injection 2976

Testosterone Propionate (Caution should be taken when darifenacin is used concomitantly with medications that are predominantly metabolized by CYP2D6 and which have a narrow therapeutic window).
No products indexed under this heading.

Thioridazine (Caution should be taken when darifenacin is used concomitantly with medications that are predominantly metabolized by CYP2D6 and which have a narrow therapeutic window).
No products indexed under this heading.

Thioridazine Hydrochloride (Caution should be taken when darifenacin is used concomitantly with medications that are predominantly metabolized by CYP2D6 and which have a narrow therapeutic window). Products include:
- Thioridazine Hydrochloride Tablets 2122

Timolol Maleate (Caution should be taken when darifenacin is used concomitantly with medications that are predominantly metabolized by CYP2D6 and which have a narrow therapeutic window). Products include:
- Blocadren Tablets 1891
- Cosopt Sterile Ophthalmic Solution 1910
- Timolide Tablets 2056
- Timoptic in Ocudose 2061
- Timoptic Sterile Ophthalmic Solution 2058
- Timoptic-XE Sterile Ophthalmic Gel Forming Solution 2062

Tolterodine Tartrate (Caution should be taken when darifenacin is used concomitantly with medications that are predominantly metabolized by CYP2D6 and which have a narrow therapeutic window). Products include:
- Detrol Tablets 2626
- Detrol LA Capsules 2629

Tramadol Hydrochloride (Caution should be taken when darifenacin is used concomitantly with medications that are predominantly metabolized by CYP2D6 and which have a narrow therapeutic window). Products include:
- Ultracet Tablets 2462

Trazodone Hydrochloride (Caution should be taken when darifenacin is used concomitantly with medications that are predominantly metabolized by CYP2D6 and which have a narrow therapeutic window).
No products indexed under this heading.

Triazolam (Caution should be taken when darifenacin is used concomitantly with medications that are predominantly metabolized by CYP2D6 and which have a narrow therapeutic window).
No products indexed under this heading.

Tridihexethyl Chloride (The concomitant use of darifenacin with other anticholinergic agents may increase the frequency and/or severity of dry mouth, constipation, blurred vision and other anticholinergic pharmacolgical effects. Anticholinergic agents may potentially alter the absorption of some concomitantly administered drugs due to effects on gastrointestinal motility).
No products indexed under this heading.

Trihexyphenidyl Hydrochloride (The concomitant use of darifenacin with other anticholinergic agents may increase the frequency and/or severity of dry mouth, constipation, blurred vision and other anticholinergic pharmacolgical effects. Anticholinergic agents may potentially alter the absorption of some concomitantly administered drugs due to effects on gastrointestinal motility).
No products indexed under this heading.

Trimipramine Maleate (Caution should be taken when darifenacin is used concomitantly with medications that are predominantly metabolized by CYP2D6 and which have a narrow therapeutic window). Products include:
- Surmontil Capsules 2347

Troleandomycin (The daily dose of darifenacin should not exceed 7.5 mg when co-administered with potent CYP3A4 inhibitors).
No products indexed under this heading.

Venlafaxine Hydrochloride (Caution should be taken when darifenacin is used concomitantly with medications that are predominantly metabolized by CYP2D6 and which have a narrow therapeutic window). Products include:
- Effexor Tablets 3405
- Effexor XR Capsules 3411

Vinblastine Sulfate (Caution should be taken when darifenacin is used concomitantly with medications that are predominantly metabolized by CYP2D6 and which have a narrow therapeutic window).
No products indexed under this heading.

Voriconazole (The daily dose of darifenacin should not exceed 7.5 mg when co-administered with potent CYP3A4 inhibitors). Products include:
- VFEND I.V. 2543
- VFEND Oral Suspension 2543
- VFEND Tablets 2543

Zonisamide (Caution should be taken when darifenacin is used concomitantly with medications that are predominantly metabolized by CYP2D6 and which have a narrow therapeutic window). Products include:
- Zonegran Capsules 1089

ENBREL FOR INJECTION
(Etanercept) 580
May interact with:

Anakinra (Co-administration results in a 7% rate of serious infections and 2% of the patients develop neutropenia). Products include:
- Kineret Injection 594

Sulfasalazine (Co-administration results in a mild decrease in mean neutrophil count).
No products indexed under this heading.

ENCORA CAPSULES
(Calcium Carbonate, Fatty Acids, Folic Acid, Vitamins, Multiple) 3298
None cited in PDR database.

ENCORA AM TABLETS
(Calcium Carbonate, Fatty Acids, Folic Acid, Vitamins, Multiple) 3298
See Encora Capsules

ENCORA PM TABLETS
(Calcium Carbonate, Fatty Acids, Folic Acid, Vitamins, Multiple) 3298
See Encora Capsules

ENGERIX-B VACCINE
(Hepatitis B Vaccine, Recombinant) ... 1391
None cited in PDR database.

ENTOCORT EC CAPSULES
(Budesonide) 2694
May interact with cytochrome p450 3a4 inducers (selected), cytochrome p450 3a4 inhibitors (selected), erythromycin, and certain other agents. Compounds in these categories include:

Acetazolamide (Co-administration with known inhibitors of CYP3A4 may increase the plasma levels of budesonide several-fold).
No products indexed under this heading.

Allium sativum (Induction of CYP3A4 can result in the lowering of budesonide plasma levels).
No products indexed under this heading.

Amiodarone Hydrochloride (Co-administration with known inhibitors of CYP3A4 may increase the plasma levels of budesonide several-fold). Products include:
- Pacerone Tablets 3337

Amprenavir (Co-administration with known inhibitors of CYP3A4 may increase the plasma levels of budesonide several-fold). Products include:
- Agenerase Capsules 1299
- Agenerase Oral Solution 1304

Anastrozole (Co-administration with known inhibitors of CYP3A4 may increase the plasma levels of budesonide several-fold). Products include:
- Arimidex Tablets 665

Aprepitant (Co-administration with known inhibitors of CYP3A4 may increase the plasma levels of budesonide several-fold). Products include:
- Emend Capsules 1944

Betamethasone Acetate (Induction of CYP3A4 can result in the lowering of budesonide plasma levels).
No products indexed under this heading.

Betamethasone Sodium Phosphate (Induction of CYP3A4 can result in the lowering of budesonide plasma levels).
No products indexed under this heading.

Carbamazepine (Induction of CYP3A4 can result in the lowering of budesonide plasma levels). Products include:
- Carbatrol Capsules 3174
- Equetro Extended-Release Capsules 3178
- Tegretol/Tegretol-XR 2278

Cimetidine (Co-administration with known inhibitors of CYP3A4 may increase the plasma levels of budesonide several-fold). Products include:
- Tagamet HB 200 Tablets 637
- Tagamet Tablets 1547

Cimetidine Hydrochloride (Co-administration with known inhibitors of CYP3A4 may increase the plasma levels of budesonide several-fold).
No products indexed under this heading.

Ciprofloxacin (Co-administration with known inhibitors of CYP3A4 may increase the plasma levels of budesonide several-fold). Products include:
- Cipro I.V. 2998
- Cipro I.V. Pharmacy Bulk Package ... 3509
- Cipro Oral Suspension 2991
- Cipro XR Tablets 3004
- Ciprodex Otic Suspension 555

Ciprofloxacin Hydrochloride (Induction of CYP3A4 can result in the lowering of budesonide plasma levels). Products include:
- Ciloxan Ophthalmic Ointment 554
- Cipro Tablets 2991

Cisplatin (Induction of CYP3A4 can result in the lowering of budesonide plasma levels).
No products indexed under this heading.

Clarithromycin (Co-administration with known inhibitors of CYP3A4 may increase the plasma levels of budesonide several-fold). Products include:
- Biaxin/Biaxin XL 402
- PREVPAC 3281

Clotrimazole (Co-administration with known inhibitors of CYP3A4 may increase the plasma levels of budesonide several-fold). Products include:
- Lotrimin 3053
- Lotrisone 3054

Cortisone Acetate (Induction of CYP3A4 can result in the lowering of budesonide plasma levels).
No products indexed under this heading.

Cyclosporine (Co-administration with known inhibitors of CYP3A4 may increase the plasma levels of budesonide several-fold). Products include:
- Gengraf Capsules 458
- Neoral Soft Gelatin Capsules 2247
- Neoral Oral Solution 2247
- Restasis Ophthalmic Emulsion 570
- Sandimmune 2259

Dalfopristin (Co-administration with known inhibitors of CYP3A4 may increase the plasma levels of budesonide several-fold). Products include:
- Synercid I.V. 1690

Danazol (Co-administration with known inhibitors of CYP3A4 may increase the plasma levels of budesonide several-fold).
No products indexed under this heading.

Delavirdine Mesylate (Co-administration with known inhibitors of CYP3A4 may increase the plasma levels of budesonide several-fold). Products include:
- Rescriptor Tablets 2535

Dexamethasone (Induction of CYP3A4 can result in the lowering of budesonide plasma levels). Products include:
- Ciprodex Otic Suspension 555
- Decadron Tablets 1929
- TobraDex Ophthalmic Ointment 558
- TobraDex Ophthalmic Suspension ... 558

Dexamethasone Acetate (Induction of CYP3A4 can result in the lowering of budesonide plasma levels).
No products indexed under this heading.

Dexamethasone Sodium Phosphate (Induction of CYP3A4 can result in the lowering of budesonide plasma levels). Products include:
- Decadron Phosphate Injection 1931

Diltiazem Hydrochloride (Co-administration with known inhibitors of CYP3A4 may increase the plasma levels of budesonide several-fold). Products include:
- Cardizem LA Extended Release Tablets 1699
- Tiazac Capsules 1204

Diltiazem Maleate (Co-administration with known inhibitors of CYP3A4 may increase the plasma levels of budesonide several-fold).
No products indexed under this heading.

Doxorubicin Hydrochloride (Induction of CYP3A4 can result in the lowering of budesonide plasma levels). Products include:
- Adriamycin for Injection, USP 786
- Adriamycin Injection, USP 786

Efavirenz (Co-administration with known inhibitors of CYP3A4 may increase the plasma levels of budesonide several-fold). Products include:
- Sustiva Capsules 957

Erythromycin (Co-administration with known inhibitors of CYP3A4 may cause rise in systemic exposure to oral budesonide; reduction in budesonide dosage should be considered). Products include:
- Erygel Topical Gel 2096
- Ery-Tab Tablets 447
- Erythromycin Base Filmtab Tablets 454
- Erythromycin Delayed-Release Capsules, USP 456
- PCE Dispertab Tablets 510

Erythromycin Estolate (Co-administration with known inhibitors of CYP3A4 may cause rise in systemic exposure to oral budesonide; reduction in budesonide dosage should be considered).
No products indexed under this heading.

Erythromycin Ethylsuccinate (Co-administration with known inhibitors of CYP3A4 may cause rise in systemic exposure to oral budesonide; reduction in budesonide dosage should be considered). Products include:
- E.E.S. 449
- EryPed 445

Erythromycin Gluceptate (Co-administration with known inhibitors of CYP3A4 may cause rise in systemic exposure to oral budesonide; reduction in budesonide dosage should be considered).
No products indexed under this heading.

Erythromycin Lactobionate (Co-administration with known inhibitors of CYP3A4 may cause rise in systemic exposure to oral budesonide; reduction in budesonide dosage should be considered).
No products indexed under this heading.

Erythromycin Stearate (Co-administration with known inhibitors of CYP3A4 may cause rise in systemic exposure to oral budesonide; reduction in budesonide dosage should be considered). Products include:
- Erythrocin Stearate Filmtab Tablets 452

Esomeprazole Magnesium (Co-administration with known inhibitors of CYP3A4 may increase the plasma levels of budesonide several-fold). Products include:
- Nexium Delayed-Release Capsules 645

Ethosuximide (Induction of CYP3A4 can result in the lowering of budesonide plasma levels).
No products indexed under this heading.

Felbamate (Induction of CYP3A4 can result in the lowering of budesonide plasma levels).
No products indexed under this heading.

Fluconazole (Co-administration with known inhibitors of CYP3A4 may increase the plasma levels of budesonide several-fold).
No products indexed under this heading.

Fludrocortisone Acetate (Induction of CYP3A4 can result in the lowering of budesonide plasma levels).
No products indexed under this heading.

Fluoxetine Hydrochloride (Co-administration with known inhibitors of CYP3A4 may increase the plasma levels of budesonide several-fold). Products include:
- Prozac Pulvules and Liquid 1771
- Symbyax Capsules 1788

Fluvoxamine Maleate (Co-administration with known inhibitors of CYP3A4 may increase the plasma levels of budesonide several-fold).
No products indexed under this heading.

Fosamprenavir Calcium (Co-administration with known inhibitors of CYP3A4 may increase the plasma levels of budesonide several-fold). Products include:
- Lexiva Tablets 1473

Fosphenytoin Sodium (Induction of CYP3A4 can result in the lowering of budesonide plasma levels).
No products indexed under this heading.

Garlic Extract (Induction of CYP3A4 can result in the lowering of budesonide plasma levels).
No products indexed under this heading.

Garlic Oil (Induction of CYP3A4 can result in the lowering of budesonide plasma levels).
No products indexed under this heading.

Hydrocortisone (Induction of CYP3A4 can result in the lowering of budesonide plasma levels). Products include:
- Cortizone•5 Ointment .... ■□699
- Cortizone•10 Creme .... ■□699
- Cortizone•10 Ointment .... ■□699
- Cortizone•10 Plus Creme .... ■□700
- Cortizone•10 Maximum Strength Quick Shot Spray .... ■□700
- Hydrocortone Tablets 1963
- Preparation H Hydrocortisone Cream .... ■□748

Hydrocortisone Acetate (Induction of CYP3A4 can result in the lowering of budesonide plasma levels). Products include:
- Analpram-HC 1136
- Pramosone 1139
- ProctoFoam-HC 3113
- Tucks Anti-Itch Ointment .... ■□712
- U-cort 1% Cream 3289

Hydrocortisone Butyrate (Induction of CYP3A4 can result in the lowering of budesonide plasma levels). Products include:
- Locoid 1138
- Locoid Lipocream Cream 1138

Hydrocortisone Cypionate (Induction of CYP3A4 can result in the lowering of budesonide plasma levels).
No products indexed under this heading.

Hydrocortisone Hemisuccinate (Induction of CYP3A4 can result in the lowering of budesonide plasma levels).
No products indexed under this heading.

Hydrocortisone Probutate (Induction of CYP3A4 can result in the lowering of budesonide plasma levels). Products include:
- Pandel Cream, 0.1% 1017

Hydrocortisone Sodium Phosphate (Induction of CYP3A4 can result in the lowering of budesonide plasma levels).
No products indexed under this heading.

Hydrocortisone Sodium Succinate (Induction of CYP3A4 can result in the lowering of budesonide plasma levels).
No products indexed under this heading.

Hydrocortisone Valerate (Induction of CYP3A4 can result in the lowering of budesonide plasma levels).
No products indexed under this heading.

Hypericum (Induction of CYP3A4 can result in the lowering of budesonide plasma levels).
No products indexed under this heading.

Hypericum Perforatum (Induction of CYP3A4 can result in the lowering of budesonide plasma levels).
No products indexed under this heading.

Indinavir Sulfate (Co-administration with known inhibitors of CYP3A4 may cause rise in systemic exposure to oral budesonide; reduction in budesonide dosage should be considered). Products include:
- Crixivan Capsules 1918

Isoniazid (Co-administration with known inhibitors of CYP3A4 may increase the plasma levels of budesonide several-fold).
No products indexed under this heading.

Itraconazole (Co-administration with known inhibitors of CYP3A4 may cause rise in systemic exposure to oral budesonide; reduction in budesonide dosage should be considered).
No products indexed under this heading.

Ketoconazole (Co-administration caused an eight-fold increase of the systemic exposure to oral budesonide; reduction in budesonide dosage should be considered). Products include:
- Nizoral A-D Shampoo, 1% 1839
- Nizoral 2% Shampoo 1838

Lopinavir (Co-administration with known inhibitors of CYP3A4 may increase the plasma levels of budesonide several-fold). Products include:
- Kaletra 474

Loratadine (Co-administration with known inhibitors of CYP3A4 may increase the plasma levels of budesonide several-fold). Products include:
- Alavert Allergy & Sinus D-12 Hour Tablets .... ■□743
- Alavert .... ■□743
- Children's Claritin 24 Hour Non-Drowsy Allergy Syrup .... ■□732
- Claritin Non-Drowsy 24 Hour Tablets .... ■□731
- Non-Drowsy Claritin Hives Relief Tablets .... ■□733
- Claritin Reditabs 24 Hour Non-Drowsy Tablets .... ■□732
- Claritin-D Non-Drowsy 12 Hour Tablets .... ■□731
- Claritin-D Non-Drowsy 24 Hour Tablets .... ■□731
- Children's Dimetapp ND Non-Drowsy Allergy Syrup .... ■□746
- Triaminic Allerchews .... ■□684

Mephenytoin (Induction of CYP3A4 can result in the lowering of budesonide plasma levels).
No products indexed under this heading.

Methsuximide (Induction of CYP3A4 can result in the lowering of budesonide plasma levels).
No products indexed under this heading.

Methylprednisolone (Induction of CYP3A4 can result in the lowering of budesonide plasma levels).
No products indexed under this heading.

Methylprednisolone Acetate (Induction of CYP3A4 can result in the lowering of budesonide plasma levels). Products include:
- Depo-Medrol Injectable Suspension 2615
- Depo-Medrol Single-Dose Vial 2617

Methylprednisolone Sodium Succinate (Induction of CYP3A4 can result in the lowering of budesonide plasma levels).
No products indexed under this heading.

Metronidazole (Co-administration with known inhibitors of CYP3A4 may increase the plasma levels of budesonide several-fold). Products include:
- Metrogel 1% 1212
- MetroGel-Vaginal Gel 1822
- Noritate Cream, 1% 1051

Metronidazole Benzoate (Co-administration with known inhibitors of CYP3A4 may increase the plasma levels of budesonide several-fold).
No products indexed under this heading.

Metronidazole Hydrochloride (Co-administration with known inhibitors of CYP3A4 may increase the plasma levels of budesonide several-fold).
No products indexed under this heading.

Miconazole (Co-administration with known inhibitors of CYP3A4 may increase the plasma levels of budesonide several-fold).
No products indexed under this heading.

Miconazole Nitrate (Co-administration with known inhibitors of CYP3A4 may increase the plasma levels of budesonide several-fold). Products include:
- Desenex .... ■□674
- Desenex Jock Itch Spray Powder .... ■□674

Modafinil (Induction of CYP3A4 can result in the lowering of budesonide plasma levels). Products include:
- Provigil Tablets 1002

Nefazodone Hydrochloride (Co-administration with known inhibitors of CYP3A4 may increase the plasma levels of budesonide several-fold).
No products indexed under this heading.

Nelfinavir Mesylate (Co-administration with known inhibitors of CYP3A4 may increase the plasma levels of budesonide several-fold). Products include:
- Viracept 2556

Nevirapine (Co-administration with known inhibitors of CYP3A4 may increase the plasma levels of budesonide several-fold). Products include:
- Viramune Oral Suspension 903
- Viramune Tablets 903

Niacinamide (Co-administration with known inhibitors of CYP3A4 may increase the plasma levels of budesonide several-fold).
No products indexed under this heading.

Nicotinamide (Co-administration with known inhibitors of CYP3A4 may increase the plasma levels of budesonide several-fold). Products include:
Nicomide Tablets 3190

Nifedipine (Co-administration with known inhibitors of CYP3A4 may increase the plasma levels of budesonide several-fold). Products include:
Adalat CC Tablets 2978

Norfloxacin (Co-administration with known inhibitors of CYP3A4 may increase the plasma levels of budesonide several-fold). Products include:
Noroxin Tablets 2009

Omeprazole (Co-administration with known inhibitors of CYP3A4 may increase the plasma levels of budesonide several-fold). Products include:
Zegerid Powder for Oral Solution 2972

Oxcarbazepine (Induction of CYP3A4 can result in the lowering of budesonide plasma levels). Products include:
Trileptal Oral Suspension 2281
Trileptal Tablets 2281

Paroxetine Hydrochloride (Co-administration with known inhibitors of CYP3A4 may increase the plasma levels of budesonide several-fold). Products include:
Paxil CR Controlled-Release Tablets 1509
Paxil 1501

Phenobarbital (Induction of CYP3A4 can result in the lowering of budesonide plasma levels).
No products indexed under this heading.

Phenobarbital Sodium (Induction of CYP3A4 can result in the lowering of budesonide plasma levels).
No products indexed under this heading.

Phenytoin (Induction of CYP3A4 can result in the lowering of budesonide plasma levels).
No products indexed under this heading.

Phenytoin Sodium (Induction of CYP3A4 can result in the lowering of budesonide plasma levels). Products include:
Phenytek Capsules 2153

Prednisolone Acetate (Induction of CYP3A4 can result in the lowering of budesonide plasma levels). Products include:
Blephamide Ophthalmic Ointment 563
Blephamide Ophthalmic Suspension 564
Poly-Pred Liquifilm Ophthalmic Suspension .... ⊙231
Pred Forte Ophthalmic Suspension .... ⊙233
Pred Mild Sterile Ophthalmic Suspension .... ⊙236
Pred-G Ophthalmic Suspension ...... ⊙234
Pred-G Sterile Ophthalmic Ointment .... ⊙235

Prednisolone Sodium Phosphate (Induction of CYP3A4 can result in the lowering of budesonide plasma levels). Products include:
Pediapred Oral Solution 3319

Prednisolone Tebutate (Induction of CYP3A4 can result in the lowering of budesonide plasma levels).
No products indexed under this heading.

Prednisone (Induction of CYP3A4 can result in the lowering of budesonide plasma levels).
No products indexed under this heading.

Primidone (Induction of CYP3A4 can result in the lowering of budesonide plasma levels).
No products indexed under this heading.

Propoxyphene Hydrochloride (Co-administration with known inhibitors of CYP3A4 may increase the plasma levels of budesonide several-fold).
No products indexed under this heading.

Propoxyphene Napsylate (Co-administration with known inhibitors of CYP3A4 may increase the plasma levels of budesonide several-fold). Products include:
Darvocet A 500 Tablets 3497

Quinidine (Co-administration with known inhibitors of CYP3A4 may increase the plasma levels of budesonide several-fold).
No products indexed under this heading.

Quinidine Hydrochloride (Co-administration with known inhibitors of CYP3A4 may increase the plasma levels of budesonide several-fold).
No products indexed under this heading.

Quinidine Polygalacturonate (Co-administration with known inhibitors of CYP3A4 may increase the plasma levels of budesonide several-fold).
No products indexed under this heading.

Quinidine Sulfate (Co-administration with known inhibitors of CYP3A4 may increase the plasma levels of budesonide several-fold).
No products indexed under this heading.

Quinine (Co-administration with known inhibitors of CYP3A4 may increase the plasma levels of budesonide several-fold).
No products indexed under this heading.

Quinine Sulfate (Co-administration with known inhibitors of CYP3A4 may increase the plasma levels of budesonide several-fold).
No products indexed under this heading.

Quinupristin (Co-administration with known inhibitors of CYP3A4 may increase the plasma levels of budesonide several-fold). Products include:
Synercid I.V. 1690

Ranitidine Bismuth Citrate (Co-administration with known inhibitors of CYP3A4 may increase the plasma levels of budesonide several-fold).
No products indexed under this heading.

Ranitidine Hydrochloride (Co-administration with known inhibitors of CYP3A4 may increase the plasma levels of budesonide several-fold). Products include:
Zantac 1597
Zantac Injection 1593
Zantac 75 Tablets .... ▣715
Zantac 150 Maximum Strength Tablets .... ▣715
Zantac Injection Pharmacy Bulk Package 1595

Rifabutin (Induction of CYP3A4 can result in the lowering of budesonide plasma levels).
No products indexed under this heading.

Rifampicin (Induction of CYP3A4 can result in the lowering of budesonide plasma levels).
No products indexed under this heading.

Rifampin (Induction of CYP3A4 can result in the lowering of budesonide plasma levels).
No products indexed under this heading.

Rifapentine (Induction of CYP3A4 can result in the lowering of budesonide plasma levels).
No products indexed under this heading.

Ritonavir (Co-administration with known inhibitors of CYP3A4 may cause rise in systemic exposure to oral budesonide; reduction in budesonide dosage should be considered). Products include:
Kaletra 474
Norvir 499

Saquinavir (Co-administration with known inhibitors of CYP3A4 may cause rise in systemic exposure to oral budesonide; reduction in budesonide dosage should be considered).
No products indexed under this heading.

Saquinavir Mesylate (Co-administration with known inhibitors of CYP3A4 may cause rise in systemic exposure to oral budesonide; reduction in budesonide dosage should be considered). Products include:
Invirase 2776

Sertraline Hydrochloride (Co-administration with known inhibitors of CYP3A4 may increase the plasma levels of budesonide several-fold). Products include:
Zoloft 2581

Sulfinpyrazone (Induction of CYP3A4 can result in the lowering of budesonide plasma levels).
No products indexed under this heading.

Telithromycin (Co-administration with known inhibitors of CYP3A4 may increase the plasma levels of budesonide several-fold). Products include:
Ketek Tablets 2920

Theophylline (Induction of CYP3A4 can result in the lowering of budesonide plasma levels).
No products indexed under this heading.

Triamcinolone (Induction of CYP3A4 can result in the lowering of budesonide plasma levels).
No products indexed under this heading.

Triamcinolone Acetonide (Induction of CYP3A4 can result in the lowering of budesonide plasma levels). Products include:
Azmacort Inhalation Aerosol 1701
Nasacort HFA Inhalation Aerosol 2939
Nasacort AQ Nasal Spray 2937

Triamcinolone Diacetate (Induction of CYP3A4 can result in the lowering of budesonide plasma levels).
No products indexed under this heading.

Triamcinolone Hexacetonide (Induction of CYP3A4 can result in the lowering of budesonide plasma levels).
No products indexed under this heading.

Troglitazone (Co-administration with known inhibitors of CYP3A4 may increase the plasma levels of budesonide several-fold).
No products indexed under this heading.

Troleandomycin (Co-administration with known inhibitors of CYP3A4 may increase the plasma levels of budesonide several-fold).
No products indexed under this heading.

Valproate Sodium (Co-administration with known inhibitors of CYP3A4 may increase the plasma levels of budesonide several-fold). Products include:
Depacon Injection 412

Verapamil Hydrochloride (Co-administration with known inhibitors of CYP3A4 may increase the plasma levels of budesonide several-fold). Products include:
Covera-HS Tablets 3135
Tarka Tablets 519
Verelan PM Capsules 3120

Voriconazole (Co-administration with known inhibitors of CYP3A4 may increase the plasma levels of budesonide several-fold). Products include:
VFEND I.V. 2543
VFEND Oral Suspension 2543
VFEND Tablets 2543

Zafirlukast (Co-administration with known inhibitors of CYP3A4 may increase the plasma levels of budesonide several-fold). Products include:
Accolate Tablets 663

Zileuton (Co-administration with known inhibitors of CYP3A4 may increase the plasma levels of budesonide several-fold).
No products indexed under this heading.

Food Interactions

Grapefruit (Concurrent use with extensive intake of grapefruit juice has caused rise in systemic exposure of budesonide by two-fold; ingestion of grapefruit should be avoided).

Grapefruit Juice (Concurrent use with extensive intake of grapefruit juice has caused rise in systemic exposure of budesonide by two-fold; ingestion of grapefruit juice should be avoided).

EPIPEN AUTO-INJECTOR

(Epinephrine) 1061
May interact with cardiac glycosides, monoamine oxidase inhibitors, quinidine, tricyclic antidepressants, and certain other agents. Compounds in these categories include:

Amitriptyline Hydrochloride (Co-administration with tricyclic antidepressants may potentiate the effects of epinephrine).
No products indexed under this heading.

Amoxapine (Co-administration with tricyclic antidepressants may potentiate the effects of epinephrine).
No products indexed under this heading.

IMPORTANT NOTE: Always consult each drug listing in the patient's regimen for possible interactions.

Clomipramine Hydrochloride (Co-administration with tricylcic antidepressants may potentiate the effects of epinephrine).
  No products indexed under this heading.

Desipramine Hydrochloride (Co-administration with tricylcic antidepressants may potentiate the effects of epinephrine).
  No products indexed under this heading.

Deslanoside (Co-administration with drugs that may sensitize the heart to arrhythmias, such as digitalis, is not recommended).
  No products indexed under this heading.

Digitalis Glycoside Preparations (Co-administration with drugs that may sensitize the heart to arrhythmias, such as digitalis, is not recommended).
  No products indexed under this heading.

Digitoxin (Co-administration with drugs that may sensitize the heart to arrhythmias, such as digitalis, is not recommended).
  No products indexed under this heading.

Digoxin (Co-administration with drugs that may sensitize the heart to arrhythmias, such as digitalis, is not recommended). Products include:
  Digitek Tablets **2146**
  Lanoxicaps Capsules **1458**
  Lanoxin Injection **1462**
  Lanoxin Tablets **1468**
  Lanoxin Injection Pediatric **1465**

Doxepin Hydrochloride (Co-administration with tricylcic antidepressants may potentiate the effects of epinephrine).
  No products indexed under this heading.

Imipramine Hydrochloride (Co-administration with tricylcic antidepressants may potentiate the effects of epinephrine).
  No products indexed under this heading.

Imipramine Pamoate (Co-administration with tricylcic antidepressants may potentiate the effects of epinephrine).
  No products indexed under this heading.

Isocarboxazid (Co-administration with MAO inhibitors may potentiate the effects of epinephrine).
  No products indexed under this heading.

Maprotiline Hydrochloride (Co-administration with tricylcic antidepressants may potentiate the effects of epinephrine).
  No products indexed under this heading.

Mercurial Diuretics (Co-administration with drugs that may sensitize the heart to arrhythmias, such as mercurial diuretics, is not recommended).
  No products indexed under this heading.

Moclobemide (Co-administration with MAO inhibitors may potentiate the effects of epinephrine).
  No products indexed under this heading.

Nortriptyline Hydrochloride (Co-administration with tricylcic antidepressants may potentiate the effects of epinephrine).
  No products indexed under this heading.

Pargyline Hydrochloride (Co-administration with MAO inhibitors may potentiate the effects of epinephrine).
  No products indexed under this heading.

Phenelzine Sulfate (Co-administration with MAO inhibitors may potentiate the effects of epinephrine).
  No products indexed under this heading.

Procarbazine Hydrochloride (Co-administration with MAO inhibitors may potentiate the effects of epinephrine). Products include:
  Matulane Capsules **3188**

Protriptyline Hydrochloride (Co-administration with tricylcic antidepressants may potentiate the effects of epinephrine). Products include:
  Vivactil Tablets **2350**

Quinidine (Co-administration with drugs that may sensitize the heart to arrhythmias, such as quinidine, is not recommended).
  No products indexed under this heading.

Quinidine Gluconate (Co-administration with drugs that may sensitize the heart to arrhythmias, such as quinidine, is not recommended).
  No products indexed under this heading.

Quinidine Hydrochloride (Co-administration with drugs that may sensitize the heart to arrhythmias, such as quinidine, is not recommended).
  No products indexed under this heading.

Quinidine Polygalacturonate (Co-administration with drugs that may sensitize the heart to arrhythmias, such as quinidine, is not recommended).
  No products indexed under this heading.

Quinidine Sulfate (Co-administration with drugs that may sensitize the heart to arrhythmias, such as quinidine, is not recommended).
  No products indexed under this heading.

Selegiline Hydrochloride (Co-administration with MAO inhibitors may potentiate the effects of epinephrine). Products include:
  Eldepryl Capsules **3209**

Tranylcypromine Sulfate (Co-administration with MAO inhibitors may potentiate the effects of epinephrine). Products include:
  Parnate Tablets **1499**

Trimipramine Maleate (Co-administration with tricylcic antidepressants may potentiate the effects of epinephrine). Products include:
  Surmontil Capsules **2347**

EPIPEN JR. AUTO-INJECTOR

(Epinephrine) **1061**
See EpiPen Auto-Injector

EPIVIR ORAL SOLUTION

(Lamivudine) **1394**
See Epivir Tablets

EPIVIR TABLETS

(Lamivudine) **1394**
May interact with cationic drugs that are eliminated by renal tubular and certain other agents. Compounds in these categories include:

Amiloride Hydrochloride (Lamivudine is predominantly eliminated in the urine by active organic secretion; therefore, the possibility of interactions with other drugs whose main route of elimination is active renal secretion via the organic cationic transport system should be considered). Products include:
  Midamor Tablets **2000**
  Moduretic Tablets **2003**

Digoxin (Lamivudine is predominantly eliminated in the urine by active organic secretion; therefore, the possibility of interactions with other drugs whose main route of elimination is active renal secretion via the organic cationic transport system should be considered). Products include:
  Digitek Tablets **2146**
  Lanoxicaps Capsules **1458**
  Lanoxin Injection **1462**
  Lanoxin Tablets **1468**
  Lanoxin Injection Pediatric **1465**

Morphine Sulfate (Lamivudine is predominantly eliminated in the urine by active organic secretion; therefore, the possibility of interactions with other drugs whose main route of elimination is active renal secretion via the organic cationic transport system should be considered). Products include:
  Avinza Capsules **1714**
  Kadian Capsules **572**
  MS Contin Tablets **2703**

Procainamide Hydrochloride (Lamivudine is predominantly eliminated in the urine by active organic secretion; therefore, the possibility of interactions with other drugs whose main route of elimination is active renal secretion via the organic cationic transport system should be considered).
  No products indexed under this heading.

Quinidine Gluconate (Lamivudine is predominantly eliminated in the urine by active organic secretion; therefore, the possibility of interactions with other drugs whose main route of elimination is active renal secretion via the organic cationic transport system should be considered).
  No products indexed under this heading.

Quinidine Polygalacturonate (Lamivudine is predominantly eliminated in the urine by active organic secretion; therefore, the possibility of interactions with other drugs whose main route of elimination is active renal secretion via the organic cationic transport system should be considered).
  No products indexed under this heading.

Quinidine Sulfate (Lamivudine is predominantly eliminated in the urine by active organic secretion; therefore, the possibility of interactions with other drugs whose main route of elimination is active renal secretion via the organic cationic transport system should be considered).
  No products indexed under this heading.

Quinine Sulfate (Lamivudine is predominantly eliminated in the urine by active organic secretion; therefore, the possibility of interactions with other drugs whose main route of elimination is active renal secretion via the organic cationic transport system should be considered).
  No products indexed under this heading.

Ranitidine Hydrochloride (Lamivudine is predominantly eliminated in the urine by active organic secretion; therefore, the possibility of interactions with other drugs whose main route of elimination is active renal secretion via the organic cationic transport system should be considered). Products include:
  Zantac **1597**
  Zantac Injection **1593**
  Zantac 75 Tablets .... ▣**715**
  Zantac 150 Maximum Strength Tablets .... ▣**715**
  Zantac Injection Pharmacy Bulk Package **1595**

Sulfamethoxazole (Co-administration of lamivudine with 160 mg of trimethoprim and 800 mg of sulfamethoxazole once daily has been shown to increase lamivudine exposure (AUC); the effect of higher doses of TMP/SMX on lamivudine pharmacokinetics has not been investigated; no change in dose of either drug is recommended).
  No products indexed under this heading.

Triamterene (Lamivudine is predominantly eliminated in the urine by active organic secretion; therefore, the possibility of interactions with other drugs whose main route of elimination is active renal secretion via the organic cationic transport system should be considered). Products include:
  Dyazide Capsules **1389**
  Dyrenium Capsules **3390**
  Maxzide **2150**

Trimethoprim (Co-administration of lamivudine with 160 mg of trimethoprim and 800 mg of sulfamethoxazole once daily has been shown to increase lamivudine exposure (AUC); the effect of higher doses of TMP/SMX on lamivudine pharmacokinetics has not been investigated; no change in dose of either drug is recommended).
  No products indexed under this heading.

Trimethoprim Sulfate (Lamivudine is predominantly eliminated in the urine by active organic secretion; therefore, the possibility of interactions with other drugs whose main route of elimination is active renal secretion via the organic cationic transport system should be considered). Products include:
  Polytrim Ophthalmic Solution **570**

Vancomycin Hydrochloride (Lamivudine is predominantly eliminated in the urine by active organic secretion; therefore, the possibility of interactions with other drugs whose main route of elimination is active renal secretion via the organic cationic transport system should be considered). Products include:
  Vancocin HCl Capsules, USP **3370**

Zalcitabine (Lamivudine and zalcitabine may inhibit the intracellular phosphorylation of one another; concurrent use is not recommended).
  No products indexed under this heading.

Food Interactions

Food, unspecified (Absorption of lamivudine was slower in the fed state compared with fasted state; there was no significant difference in systemic exposure in the fed state and fasted states; Epivir may be given with or without food).

EPIVIR-HBV ORAL SOLUTION

(Lamivudine) 1398

See Epivir-HBV Tablets

EPIVIR-HBV TABLETS

(Lamivudine) 1398

May interact with cationic drugs that are eliminated by renal tubular and certain other agents. Compounds in these categories include:

Amiloride Hydrochloride (Lamivudine is predominantly eliminated in the urine by active organic secretion; therefore, the possibility of interactions with other drugs whose main route of elimination is active renal secretion via the organic cationic transport system should be considered). Products include:

- Midamor Tablets 2000
- Moduretic Tablets 2003

Digoxin (Lamivudine is predominantly eliminated in the urine by active organic secretion; therefore, the possibility of interactions with other drugs whose main route of elimination is active renal secretion via the organic cationic transport system should be considered). Products include:

- Digitek Tablets 2146
- Lanoxicaps Capsules 1458
- Lanoxin Injection 1462
- Lanoxin Tablets 1468
- Lanoxin Injection Pediatric 1465

Morphine Sulfate (Lamivudine is predominantly eliminated in the urine by active organic secretion; therefore, the possibility of interactions with other drugs whose main route of elimination is active renal secretion via the organic cationic transport system should be considered). Products include:

- Avinza Capsules 1714
- Kadian Capsules 572
- MS Contin Tablets 2703

Procainamide Hydrochloride (Lamivudine is predominantly eliminated in the urine by active organic secretion; therefore, the possibility of interactions with other drugs whose main route of elimination is active renal secretion via the organic cationic transport system should be considered).

No products indexed under this heading.

Quinidine Gluconate (Lamivudine is predominantly eliminated in the urine by active organic secretion; therefore, the possibility of interactions with other drugs whose main route of elimination is active renal secretion via the organic cationic transport system should be considered).

No products indexed under this heading.

Quinidine Polygalacturonate (Lamivudine is predominantly eliminated in the urine by active organic secretion; therefore, the possibility of interactions with other drugs whose main route of elimination is active renal secretion via the organic cationic transport system should be considered).

No products indexed under this heading.

Quinidine Sulfate (Lamivudine is predominantly eliminated in the urine by active organic secretion; therefore, the possibility of interactions with other drugs whose main route of elimination is active renal secretion via the organic cationic transport system should be considered).

No products indexed under this heading.

Quinine Sulfate (Lamivudine is predominantly eliminated in the urine by active organic secretion; therefore, the possibility of interactions with other drugs whose main route of elimination is active renal secretion via the organic cationic transport system should be considered).

No products indexed under this heading.

Ranitidine Hydrochloride (Lamivudine is predominantly eliminated in the urine by active organic secretion; therefore, the possibility of interactions with other drugs whose main route of elimination is active renal secretion via the organic cationic transport system should be considered). Products include:

- Zantac 1597
- Zantac Injection 1593
- Zantac 75 Tablets 715
- Zantac 150 Maximum Strength Tablets 715
- Zantac Injection Pharmacy Bulk Package 1595

Sulfamethoxazole (Co-administration of lamivudine with 160 mg of trimethoprim and 800 mg of sulfamethoxazole once daily has been shown to increase lamivudine exposure (AUC); the effect of higher doses of TMP/SMX on lamivudine pharmacokinetics has not been investigated; no change in dose of either drug is recommended).

No products indexed under this heading.

Triamterene (Lamivudine is predominantly eliminated in the urine by active organic secretion; therefore, the possibility of interactions with other drugs whose main route of elimination is active renal secretion via the organic cationic transport system should be considered). Products include:

- Dyazide Capsules 1389
- Dyrenium Capsules 3390
- Maxzide 2150

Trimethoprim (Co-administration of lamivudine with 160 mg of trimethoprim and 800 mg of sulfamethoxazole once daily has been shown to increase lamivudine exposure (AUC); the effect of higher doses of TMP/SMX on lamivudine pharmacokinetics has not been investigated; no change in dose of either drug is recommended).

No products indexed under this heading.

Trimethoprim Sulfate (Lamivudine is predominantly eliminated in the urine by active organic secretion; therefore, the possibility of interactions with other drugs whose main route of elimination is active renal secretion via the organic cationic transport system should be considered). Products include:

- Polytrim Ophthalmic Solution 570

Vancomycin Hydrochloride (Lamivudine is predominantly eliminated in the urine by active organic secretion; therefore, the possibility of interactions with other drugs whose main route of elimination is active renal secretion via the organic cationic transport system should be considered). Products include:

- Vancocin HCl Capsules, USP 3370

Zalacitabine (Lamivudine and zalcitabine may inhibit the intracellular phosphorylation of one another; co-administration is not recommended).

No products indexed under this heading.

EPOGEN FOR INJECTION

(Epoetin Alfa) 586

None cited in PDR database.

EPZICOM TABLETS

(Abacavir Sulfate, Lamivudine) 1402

May interact with:

Ethanol (Ethanol decreased the elimination of abacavir causing an increase in overall exposure).

No products indexed under this heading.

Methadone Hydrochloride (Co-administration in patients on methadone-maintenance therapy had increased methadone clearance by 22%. This alteration will not result in a methadone dose modification in the majority of patients; however, an increased methadone dose may be required in a small number of patients).

No products indexed under this heading.

Nelfinavir Mesylate (Co-administration of lamivudine with nelfinavir has been shown to increase the AUC of lamivudine by 10%). Products include:

- Viracept 2556

Sulfamethoxazole (Co-administration of lamivudine with 160mg of trimethoprim and 800mg of sulfamethoxazole once daily has been shown to increase lamivudine exposure (AUC). The effect of higher doses of TMP/SMX on lamivudine pharmacokinetics has not been investigated; no change in dose of either drug is recommended).

No products indexed under this heading.

Trimethoprim (Co-administration of lamivudine with 160mg of trimethoprim and 800mg of sulfamethoxazole once daily has been shown to increase lamivudine exposure (AUC). The effect of higher doses of TMP/SMX on lamivudine pharmacokinetics has not been investigated; no change in dose of either drug is recommended).

No products indexed under this heading.

Zalcitabine (Lamivudine and zalcitabine may inhibit the intracellular phosphorylation of one another; concurrent use is not recommended).

No products indexed under this heading.

EQUETRO EXTENDED-RELEASE CAPSULES

(Carbamazepine) 3178

May interact with antimalarials, central nervous system depressants, cytochrome p450 1a2 substrates (selected), cytochrome p450 3a4 inducers (selected), cytochrome p450 3a4 inhibitors (selected), cytochrome p450 3a4 substrates (selected), oral contraceptives, phenytoin, and certain other agents. Compounds in these categories include:

Acetaminophen (Carbamazepine is known to induce CYP1A2 and CYP3A4. Therefore, the potential exists for interaction between carbamazepine and any agent metabolized by one (or more) of these enzymes. Agents that are metabolized by CYP1A2 and CYP3A4 may have decreased plasma levels when administered concomitantly with carbamazepine. Thus, if a patient has been titrated to a stable dosage on one of the agents in these categories, and then begins a course of treatment with carbamazepine, it is reasonable to expect that a dose increase for the concomitant agent may be necessary). Products include:

- Benadryl Allergy & Cold Tablets 692
- Benadryl Allergy & Sinus Headache Caplets & Gelcaps...... 693
- Benadryl Maximum Strength Severe Allergy & Sinus Headache Caplets...................... 694
- Contac Severe Cold and Flu Caplets Maximum Strength......... 615
- Contac Severe Cold and Flu Caplets Non-Drowsy................... 615
- Darvocet A 500 Tablets 3497
- Goody's Body Pain Formula Powder 621
- Goody's Extra Strength Headache Powder.......................... 621
- Goody's Extra Strength Pain Relief Tablets 621
- Goody's PM Powder 622
- Hycomine Compound Tablets 1105
- Lortab 3315
- Lortab Elixir 3312
- Percocet Tablets 1114
- Robitussin Cough, Cold & Flu Liquid-filled Capsules.................. 750
- Robitussin Flu Liquid 752
- Sedapap Tablets 50 mg/650 mg 2098
- Singlet Caplets 636
- Sudafed Severe Cold 710
- Sudafed Sinus Headache 711
- TheraFlu Cold & Cough Hot Liquid 680
- TheraFlu Cold & Sore Throat Hot Liquid 680
- TheraFlu Flu & Chest Congestion Non-Drowsy Hot Liquid............... 681
- TheraFlu Flu & Sore Throat Hot Liquid 681
- TheraFlu Severe Cold Non-Drowsy Hot Liquid............... 683
- TheraFlu Severe Cold & Cough Hot Liquid 683
- TheraFlu Severe Cold Caplets 679
- TheraFlu Severe Cold Hot Liquid 682
- TheraFlu Severe Cold Non-Drowsy Caplets.................. 679
- Triaminic Cough & Sore Throat Liquid 687
- Triaminic Flu, Cough & Fever Liquid 685
- Triaminic Cough & Sore Throat Softchews 689
- Tylenol 8 Hour Extended Release Geltabs and Caplets 1843
- Tylenol Sinus NightTime Caplets 663
- Children's Tylenol Suspension Liquid and Meltaways.................. 1850
- Children's Tylenol Plus Cold & Allergy Suspension Liquid............ 1850
- Children's Tylenol Plus Cold NightTime Suspension Liquid........ 1851
- Children's Tylenol Plus Cold & Cough Suspension Liquid and Chewable Tablets 1851
- Children's Tylenol Plus Cold Chewable Tablets 1851
- Children's Tylenol Plus Cold Daytime Non-Drowsy Suspension Liquid 1851
- Children's Tylenol Plus Flu Suspension Liquid 1853
- Concentrated Tylenol Infants' Drops Plus Cold.......................... 1851
- Concentrated Tylenol Infants' Drops Plus Cold and Cough......... 1851
- Concentrated Tylenol Infants' Drops.. 1850
- Junior Tylenol Meltaways 1850
- Tylenol Cold & Flu Severe Daytime Liquid with Cool Bust....... 1846

Tylenol Cold & Flu Severe NightTime Liquid with Cool Burst 1846
Tylenol Cold Severe Congestion Non-Drowsy Caplets with Cool Burst 1846
Tylenol Cough & Sore Throat Daytime Liquid with Cool Burst 1849
Tylenol Cough & Sore Throat NightTime Liquid with Cool Burst 1849
Tylenol 1843
Extra Strength Tylenol Rapid Release Gels 1843
Tylenol 1843
Tylenol Allergy Complete Night Time Caplets 1844
Tylenol Allergy Complete Multi-Symptom Caplets and Gelcaps with Cool Burst 1844
Tylenol Severe Allergy Caplets 1844
Tylenol Flu NightTime Gelcaps 1846
Tylenol Flu Day Non-Drowsy Gelcaps 1846
Concentrated Tylenol Infants' Drops Plus Cold Nasal Congestant, Fever Reducer & Pain Reliever .... ▣668
Concentrated Tylenol Infants' Drops Plus Cold & Cough Nasal Decongestant, Fever Reducer & Pain Reliever .... ▣668
Multi-Symptom Tylenol Cold Night Time Caplets 1845
Multi-Symptom Tylenol Cold Day Non-Drowsy Caplets and Gelcaps 1845
Extra Strength Tylenol PM Caplets, Geltabs, Gelcaps and Liquid 1847
Tylenol Sinus Day Non-Drowsy 1848
Tylenol Sinus Night Time Caplets 1848
Tylenol Sinus Severe Congestion Caplets with Cool Burst 1848
Tylenol Sore Throat Daytime Liquid with Cool Burst 1849
Tylenol Sore Throat NightTime Liquid with Cool Burst 1849
Tylenol with Codeine 2461
Women's Tylenol Menstrual Relief Caplets 1849
Ultracet Tablets 2462
Vicks 44M Cough, Cold & Flu Relief 2676
Vicks DayQuil LiquiCaps/Liquid Multi-Symptom Cold/Flu Relief .... ▣723
Vicks DayQuil Multi-Symptom Cold/Flu Relief LiquiCaps 2675
Vicks DayQuil Multi-Symptom Cold/Flu Relief Liquid 2675
Vicks NyQuil LiquiCaps 2677
Vicks NyQuil LiquiCaps/Liquid Multi-Symptom Cold/Flu Relief .... ▣725
Vicks NyQuil Liquid 2677
Vicodin Tablets 530
Vicodin ES Tablets 531
Vicodin HP Tablets 532
Zydone Tablets 1118

Acetazolamide (Carbamazepine is metabolized mainly by CYP3A4 the active carbamazepine 10,11-epoxide, which is futher metabolized to the trans-diol by epoxide hydrolase. Therefore, the potential exists for interaction between carbamazepine and any agent that inhibits CYP3A4 and/or epoxide hydrolase. Agents that are CYP3A4 inhibitors may increase the plasma levels of carbamazepine. Thus, if a patient has been titrated to a stable dosage of carbamazepine, and then begins a course of treatment with a CYP3A4 or epoxide hydrolase inhibitor, it is reasonable to expect that a dose reduction for carbamazepine may be necessary).

No products indexed under this heading.

Alatrofloxacin Mesylate (Carbamazepine is known to induce CYP1A2 and CYP3A4. Therefore, the potential exists for interaction between carbamazepine and any agent metabolized by one (or more) of these enzymes. Agents that are metabolized by CYP1A2 and CYP3A4 may have decreased plasma levels when administered concomitantly with carbamazepine. Thus, if a patient has been titrated to a stable dosage on one of the agents in these categories, and then begins a course of treatment with carbamazepine, it is reasonable to expect that a dose increase for the concomitant agent may be necessary).

No products indexed under this heading.

Alfentanil Hydrochloride (Carbamazepine is known to induce CYP1A2 and CYP3A4. Therefore, the potential exists for interaction between carbamazepine and any agent metabolized by one (or more) of these enzymes. Agents that are metabolized by CYP1A2 and CYP3A4 may have decreased plasma levels when administered concomitantly with carbamazepine. Thus, if a patient has been titrated to a stable dosage on one of the agents in these categories, and then begins a course of treatment with carbamazepine, it is reasonable to expect that a dose increase for the concomitant agent may be necessary).

No products indexed under this heading.

Allium sativum (Carbamazepine is metabolized by CYP3A4. Therefore, the potential exists for interaction between carbamazepine and any agent that induces CYP3A4. Agents that are CYP3A4 inducers may decrease plasma levels of carbamazepine. Thus, if a patient has been titrated to a stable dosage on carbamazepine, and then begins a course of treatment with a CYP3A4 inducers, it is reasonable to expect that a dose increase for carbamazepine may be necessary).

No products indexed under this heading.

Alprazolam (Carbamazepine is known to induce CYP1A2 and CYP3A4. Therefore, the potential exists for interaction between carbamazepine and any agent metabolized by one (or more) of these enzymes. Agents that are metabolized by CYP1A2 and CYP3A4 may have decreased plasma levels when administered concomitantly with carbamazepine. Thus, if a patient has been titrated to a stable dosage on one of the agents in these categories, and then begins a course of treatment with carbamazepine, it is reasonable to expect that a dose increase for the concomitant agent may be necessary). Products include:

Niravam Orally Disintegrating Tablets 3106
Xanax XR Tablets 2655

Amiodarone Hydrochloride (Carbamazepine is metabolized mainly by CYP3A4 the active carbamazepine 10,11-epoxide, which is futher metabolized to the trans-diol by epoxide hydrolase. Therefore, the potential exists for interaction between carbamazepine and any agent that inhibits CYP3A4 and/or epoxide hydrolase. Agents that are CYP3A4 inhibitors may increase the plasma levels of carbamazepine. Thus, if a patient has been titrated to a stable dosage of carbamazepine, and then begins a course of treatment with a CYP3A4 or epoxide hydrolase inhibitor, it is reasonable to expect that a dose reduction for carbamazepine may be necessary). Products include:

Pacerone Tablets 3337

Amitriptyline Hydrochloride (Carbamazepine is known to induce CYP1A2 and CYP3A4. Therefore, the potential exists for interaction between carbamazepine and any agent metabolized by one (or more) of these enzymes. Agents that are metabolized by CYP1A2 and CYP3A4 may have decreased plasma levels when administered concomitantly with carbamazepine. Thus, if a patient has been titrated to a stable dosage on one of the agents in these categories, and then begins a course of treatment with carbamazepine, it is reasonable to expect that a dose increase for the concomitant agent may be necessary).

No products indexed under this heading.

Amlodipine Besylate (Carbamazepine is known to induce CYP1A2 and CYP3A4. Therefore, the potential exists for interaction between carbamazepine and any agent metabolized by one (or more) of these enzymes. Agents that are metabolized by CYP1A2 and CYP3A4 may have decreased plasma levels when administered concomitantly with carbamazepine. Thus, if a patient has been titrated to a stable dosage on one of the agents in these categories, and then begins a course of treatment with carbamazepine, it is reasonable to expect that a dose increase for the concomitant agent may be necessary). Products include:

Caduet Tablets 2507
Lotrel Capsules 2238
Norvasc Tablets 2529

Amoxapine (Carbamazepine is known to induce CYP1A2 and CYP3A4. Therefore, the potential exists for interaction between carbamazepine and any agent metabolized by one (or more) of these enzymes. Agents that are metabolized by CYP1A2 and CYP3A4 may have decreased plasma levels when administered concomitantly with carbamazepine. Thus, if a patient has been titrated to a stable dosage on one of the agents in these categories, and then begins a course of treatment with carbamazepine, it is reasonable to expect that a dose increase for the concomitant agent may be necessary).

No products indexed under this heading.

Amprenavir (Carbamazepine is metabolized mainly by CYP3A4 the active carbamazepine 10,11-epoxide, which is futher metabolized to the trans-diol by epoxide hydrolase. Therefore, the potential exists for interaction between carbamazepine and any agent that inhibits CYP3A4 and/or epoxide hydrolase. Agents that are CYP3A4 inhibitors may increase the plasma levels of carbamazepine. Thus, if a patient has been titrated to a stable dosage of carbamazepine, and then begins a course of treatment with a CYP3A4 or epoxide hydrolase inhibitor, it is reasonable to expect that a dose reduction for carbamazepine may be necessary). Products include:

Agenerase Capsules 1299
Agenerase Oral Solution 1304

Anagrelide Hydrochloride (Carbamazepine is known to induce CYP1A2 and CYP3A4. Therefore, the potential exists for interaction between carbamazepine and any agent metabolized by one (or more) of these enzymes. Agents that are metabolized by CYP1A2 and CYP3A4 may have decreased plasma levels when administered concomitantly with carbamazepine. Thus, if a patient has been titrated to a stable dosage on one of the agents in these categories, and then begins a course of treatment with carbamazepine, it is reasonable to expect that a dose increase for the concomitant agent may be necessary). Products include:

Agrylin Capsules 3172

Anastrozole (Carbamazepine is metabolized mainly by CYP3A4 the active carbamazepine 10,11-epoxide, which is futher metabolized to the trans-diol by epoxide hydrolase. Therefore, the potential exists for interaction between carbamazepine and any agent that inhibits CYP3A4 and/or epoxide hydrolase. Agents that are CYP3A4 inhibitors may increase the plasma levels of carbamazepine. Thus, if a patient has been titrated to a stable dosage of carbamazepine, and then begins a course of treatment with a CYP3A4 or epoxide hydrolase inhibitor, it is reasonable to expect that a dose reduction for carbamazepine may be necessary). Products include:

Arimidex Tablets 665

Aprepitant (Carbamazepine is metabolized mainly by CYP3A4 the active carbamazepine 10,11-epoxide, which is futher metabolized to the trans-diol by epoxide hydrolase. Therefore, the potential exists for interaction between carbamazepine and any agent that inhibits CYP3A4 and/or epoxide hydrolase. Agents that are CYP3A4 inhibitors may increase the plasma levels of carbamazepine. Thus, if a patient has been titrated to a stable dosage of carbamazepine, and then begins a course of treatment with a CYP3A4 or epoxide hydrolase inhibitor, it is reasonable to expect that a dose reduction for carbamazepine may be necessary). Products include:

Emend Capsules 1944

Aprobarbital (Because of its primary CNS effect, caution should be used when carbamazepine is taken with other centrally-acting drugs).

No products indexed under this heading.

Astemizole (Carbamazepine is known to induce CYP1A2 and CYP3A4. Therefore, the potential exists for interaction between carbamazepine and any agent metabolized by one (or more) of these enzymes. Agents that are metabolized by CYP1A2 and CYP3A4 may have decreased plasma levels when administered concomitantly with carbamazepine. Thus, if a patient has been titrated to a stable dosage on one of the agents in these categories, and then begins a course of treatment with carbamazepine, it is

reasonable to expect that a dose increase for the concomitant agent may be necessary).

No products indexed under this heading.

Atorvastatin Calcium (Carbamazepine is known to induce CYP1A2 and CYP3A4. Therefore, the potential exists for interaction between carbamazepine and any agent metabolized by one (or more) of these enzymes. Agents that are metabolized by CYP1A2 and CYP3A4 may have decreased plasma levels when administered concomitantly with carbamazepine. Thus, if a patient has been titrated to a stable dosage on one of the agents in these categories, and then begins a course of treatment with carbamazepine, it is reasonable to expect that a dose increase for the concomitant agent may be necessary). Products include:

Caduet Tablets **2507**
Lipitor Tablets **2495**

Belladonna Ergotamine (Carbamazepine is known to induce CYP1A2 and CYP3A4. Therefore, the potential exists for interaction between carbamazepine and any agent metabolized by one (or more) of these enzymes. Agents that are metabolized by CYP1A2 and CYP3A4 may have decreased plasma levels when administered concomitantly with carbamazepine. Thus, if a patient has been titrated to a stable dosage on one of the agents in these categories, and then begins a course of treatment with carbamazepine, it is reasonable to expect that a dose increase for the concomitant agent may be necessary).

No products indexed under this heading.

Betamethasone Acetate (Carbamazepine is metabolized by CYP3A4. Therefore, the potential exists for interaction between carbamazepine and any agent that induces CYP3A4. Agents that are CYP3A4 inducers may decrease plasma levels of carbamazepine. Thus, if a patient has been titrated to a stable dosage on carbamazepine, and then begins a course of treatment with a CYP3A4 inducers, it is reasonable to expect that a dose increase for carbamazepine may be necessary).

No products indexed under this heading.

Betamethasone Sodium Phosphate (Carbamazepine is metabolized by CYP3A4. Therefore, the potential exists for interaction between carbamazepine and any agent that induces CYP3A4. Agents that are CYP3A4 inducers may decrease plasma levels of carbamazepine. Thus, if a patient has been titrated to a stable dosage on carbamazepine, and then begins a course of treatment with a CYP3A4 inducers, it is reasonable to expect that a dose increase for carbamazepine may be necessary).

No products indexed under this heading.

Buprenorphine Hydrochloride (Because of its primary CNS effect, caution should be used when carbamazepine is taken with other centrally-acting drugs). Products include:

Buprenex Injectable **2718**
Suboxone Tablets **2719**
Subutex Tablets **2719**

Buspirone Hydrochloride (Carbamazepine is known to induce CYP1A2 and CYP3A4. Therefore, the potential exists for interaction between carbamazepine and any agent metabolized by one (or more) of these enzymes. Agents that are metabolized by CYP1A2 and CYP3A4 may have decreased plasma levels when administered concomitantly with carbamazepine. Thus, if a patient has been titrated to a stable dosage on one of the agents in these categories, and then begins a course of treatment with carbamazepine, it is reasonable to expect that a dose increase for the concomitant agent may be necessary).

No products indexed under this heading.

Busulfan (Carbamazepine is known to induce CYP1A2 and CYP3A4. Therefore, the potential exists for interaction between carbamazepine and any agent metabolized by one (or more) of these enzymes. Agents that are metabolized by CYP1A2 and CYP3A4 may have decreased plasma levels when administered concomitantly with carbamazepine. Thus, if a patient has been titrated to a stable dosage on one of the agents in these categories, and then begins a course of treatment with carbamazepine, it is reasonable to expect that a dose increase for the concomitant agent may be necessary). Products include:

I.V. Busulfex **1125**
Myleran Tablets **1492**

Butabarbital (Because of its primary CNS effect, caution should be used when carbamazepine is taken with other centrally-acting drugs).

No products indexed under this heading.

Butalbital (Because of its primary CNS effect, caution should be used when carbamazepine is taken with other centrally-acting drugs). Products include:

Sedapap Tablets 50 mg/650 mg **2098**

Caffeine (Carbamazepine is known to induce CYP1A2 and CYP3A4. Therefore, the potential exists for interaction between carbamazepine and any agent metabolized by one (or more) of these enzymes. Agents that are metabolized by CYP1A2 and CYP3A4 may have decreased plasma levels when administered concomitantly with carbamazepine. Thus, if a patient has been titrated to a stable dosage on one of the agents in these categories, and then begins a course of treatment with carbamazepine, it is reasonable to expect that a dose increase for the concomitant agent may be necessary). Products include:

Athena Hair System Shampoo **767**
BC Powder **612**
Arthritis Strength BC Powder **612**
Goody's Extra Strength Headache Powder **621**
Goody's Extra Strength Pain Relief Tablets **621**
Hycomine Compound Tablets **1105**
Spartan Hair System Shampoo **767**
Vivarin **639**

Caffeine Anhydrous (Carbamazepine is known to induce CYP1A2 and CYP3A4. Therefore, the potential exists for interaction between carbamazepine and any agent metabolized by one (or more) of these enzymes. Agents that are metabolized by CYP1A2 and CYP3A4 may have decreased plasma levels when administered concomitantly with carbamazepine. Thus, if a patient has been titrated to a stable dosage on one of the agents in these categories, and then begins a course of treatment with carbamazepine, it is reasonable to expect that a dose increase for the concomitant agent may be necessary).

No products indexed under this heading.

Cerivastatin Sodium (Carbamazepine is known to induce CYP1A2 and CYP3A4. Therefore, the potential exists for interaction between carbamazepine and any agent metabolized by one (or more) of these enzymes. Agents that are metabolized by CYP1A2 and CYP3A4 may have decreased plasma levels when administered concomitantly with carbamazepine. Thus, if a patient has been titrated to a stable dosage on one of the agents in these categories, and then begins a course of treatment with carbamazepine, it is reasonable to expect that a dose increase for the concomitant agent may be necessary).

No products indexed under this heading.

Chlordiazepoxide (Carbamazepine is known to induce CYP1A2 and CYP3A4. Therefore, the potential exists for interaction between carbamazepine and any agent metabolized by one (or more) of these enzymes. Agents that are metabolized by CYP1A2 and CYP3A4 may have decreased plasma levels when administered concomitantly with carbamazepine. Thus, if a patient has been titrated to a stable dosage on one of the agents in these categories, and then begins a course of treatment with carbamazepine, it is reasonable to expect that a dose increase for the concomitant agent may be necessary).

No products indexed under this heading.

Chlordiazepoxide Hydrochloride (Carbamazepine is known to induce CYP1A2 and CYP3A4. Therefore, the potential exists for interaction between carbamazepine and any agent metabolized by one (or more) of these enzymes. Agents that are metabolized by CYP1A2 and CYP3A4 may have decreased plasma levels when administered concomitantly with carbamazepine. Thus, if a patient has been titrated to a stable dosage on one of the agents in these categories, and then begins a course of treatment with carbamazepine, it is reasonable to expect that a dose increase for the concomitant agent may be necessary). Products include:

Librium Capsules **3349**

Chloroquine Hydrochloride (Antimalarial drugs, such as chloroquine and mefloquine, may antagonize the activity of carbamazepine).

No products indexed under this heading.

Chloroquine Phosphate (Antimalarial drugs, such as chloroquine and mefloquine, may antagonize the activity of carbamazepine).

No products indexed under this heading.

Chlorpheniramine (Carbamazepine is known to induce CYP1A2 and CYP3A4. Therefore, the potential exists for interaction between carbamazepine and any agent metabolized by one (or more) of these enzymes. Agents that are metabolized by CYP1A2 and CYP3A4 may have decreased plasma levels when administered concomitantly with carbamazepine. Thus, if a patient has been titrated to a stable dosage on one of the agents in these categories, and then begins a course of treatment with carbamazepine, it is reasonable to expect that a dose increase for the concomitant agent may be necessary).

No products indexed under this heading.

Chlorpheniramine Maleate (Carbamazepine is known to induce CYP1A2 and CYP3A4. Therefore, the potential exists for interaction between carbamazepine and any agent metabolized by one (or more) of these enzymes. Agents that are metabolized by CYP1A2 and CYP3A4 may have decreased plasma levels when administered concomitantly with carbamazepine. Thus, if a patient has been titrated to a stable dosage on one of the agents in these categories, and then begins a course of treatment with carbamazepine, it is reasonable to expect that a dose increase for the concomitant agent may be necessary). Products include:

Advil Allergy Sinus Caplets **737**
Advil Multi-Symptom Cold Caplets **738**
BC Allergy Sinus Cold Powder **612**
Contac Severe Cold and Flu Caplets Maximum Strength **615**
Hycomine Compound Tablets **1105**
PediaCare Multi-Symptom Cold Liquid **704**
PediaCare NightRest Cough & Cold Liquid **704**
Robitussin Flu Liquid **752**
Robitussin PM Cough & Cold Liquid **752**
Singlet Caplets **636**
Sudafed Sinus & Allergy Tablets **710**
TheraFlu Cold & Cough Hot Liquid **680**
TheraFlu Cold & Sore Throat Hot Liquid **680**
TheraFlu Flu & Sore Throat Hot Liquid **681**
TheraFlu Severe Cold & Cough Hot Liquid **683**
TheraFlu Severe Cold Caplets **679**
TheraFlu Severe Cold Hot Liquid **682**
Triaminic Cold & Allergy Liquid **685**
Triaminic Cold & Cough Liquid **685**
Triaminic Flu, Cough & Fever Liquid **685**
Triaminic Night Time Cough & Cold Liquid **685**
Triaminic Allergy Runny Nose & Congestion Softchews **688**
Triaminic Cold & Cough Softchews **688**
Children's Tylenol Plus Cold NightTime Suspension Liquid **1851**
Children's Tylenol Plus Cold & Cough Suspension Liquid and Chewable Tablets **1851**
Children's Tylenol Plus Cold Chewable Tablets **1851**
Children's Tylenol Plus Flu Suspension Liquid **1853**
Tylenol Allergy Complete Multi-Symptom Caplets and Gelcaps with Cool Burst **1844**
Multi-Symptom Tylenol Cold Night Time Caplets **1845**
Vicks 44M Cough, Cold & Flu Relief **2676**
Pediatric Vicks 44m Cough & Cold Relief **2673**

Children's Vicks NyQuil Cold/Cough Relief 2671

Chlorpheniramine Polistirex (Carbamazepine is known to induce CYP1A2 and CYP3A4. Therefore, the potential exists for interaction between carbamazepine and any agent metabolized by one (or more) of these enzymes. Agents that are metabolized by CYP1A2 and CYP3A4 may have decreased plasma levels when administered concomitantly with carbamazepine. Thus, if a patient has been titrated to a stable dosage on one of the agents in these categories, and then begins a course of treatment with carbamazepine, it is reasonable to expect that a dose increase for the concomitant agent may be necessary). Products include:

Tussionex Pennkinetic Extended-Release Suspension 3322

Chlorpheniramine Tannate (Carbamazepine is known to induce CYP1A2 and CYP3A4. Therefore, the potential exists for interaction between carbamazepine and any agent metabolized by one (or more) of these enzymes. Agents that are metabolized by CYP1A2 and CYP3A4 may have decreased plasma levels when administered concomitantly with carbamazepine. Thus, if a patient has been titrated to a stable dosage on one of the agents in these categories, and then begins a course of treatment with carbamazepine, it is reasonable to expect that a dose increase for the concomitant agent may be necessary).

No products indexed under this heading.

Chlorpromazine (Because of its primary CNS effect, caution should be used when carbamazepine is taken with other centrally-acting drugs).

No products indexed under this heading.

Chlorpromazine Hydrochloride (Because of its primary CNS effect, caution should be used when carbamazepine is taken with other centrally-acting drugs).

No products indexed under this heading.

Chlorprothixene (Because of its primary CNS effect, caution should be used when carbamazepine is taken with other centrally-acting drugs).

No products indexed under this heading.

Chlorprothixene Hydrochloride (Because of its primary CNS effect, caution should be used when carbamazepine is taken with other centrally-acting drugs).

No products indexed under this heading.

Chlorprothixene Lactate (Because of its primary CNS effect, caution should be used when carbamazepine is taken with other centrally-acting drugs).

No products indexed under this heading.

Cimetidine (Carbamazepine is metabolized mainly by CYP3A4 the active carbamazepine 10,11-epoxide, which is futher metabolized to the trans-diol by epoxide hydrolase. Therefore, the potential exists for interaction between carbamazepine and any agent that inhibits CYP3A4 and/or epoxide hydrolase. Agents that are CYP3A4 inhibitors may increase the plasma levels of carbamazepine. Thus, if a patient has been titrated to a stable dosage of carbamazepine, and then begins a course of treatment with a CYP3A4 or epoxide hydrolase inhibitor, it is reasonable to expect that a dose reduction for carbamazepine may be necessary). Products include:

Tagamet HB 200 Tablets .... ▣ 637
Tagamet Tablets 1547

Cimetidine Hydrochloride (Carbamazepine is metabolized mainly by CYP3A4 the active carbamazepine 10,11-epoxide, which is futher metabolized to the trans-diol by epoxide hydrolase. Therefore, the potential exists for interaction between carbamazepine and any agent that inhibits CYP3A4 and/or epoxide hydrolase. Agents that are CYP3A4 inhibitors may increase the plasma levels of carbamazepine. Thus, if a patient has been titrated to a stable dosage of carbamazepine, and then begins a course of treatment with a CYP3A4 or epoxide hydrolase inhibitor, it is reasonable to expect that a dose reduction for carbamazepine may be necessary).

No products indexed under this heading.

Ciprofloxacin (Carbamazepine is metabolized mainly by CYP3A4 the active carbamazepine 10,11-epoxide, which is futher metabolized to the trans-diol by epoxide hydrolase. Therefore, the potential exists for interaction between carbamazepine and any agent that inhibits CYP3A4 and/or epoxide hydrolase. Agents that are CYP3A4 inhibitors may increase the plasma levels of carbamazepine. Thus, if a patient has been titrated to a stable dosage of carbamazepine, and then begins a course of treatment with a CYP3A4 or epoxide hydrolase inhibitor, it is reasonable to expect that a dose reduction for carbamazepine may be necessary). Products include:

Cipro I.V. 2998
Cipro I.V. Pharmacy Bulk Package ... 3509
Cipro Oral Suspension 2991
Cipro XR Tablets 3004
Ciprodex Otic Suspension 555

Ciprofloxacin Hydrochloride (Carbamazepine is metabolized by CYP3A4. Therefore, the potential exists for interaction between carbamazepine and any agent that induces CYP3A4. Agents that are CYP3A4 inducers may decrease plasma levels of carbamazepine. Thus, if a patient has been titrated to a stable dosage on carbamazepine, and then begins a course of treatment with a CYP3A4 inducers, it is reasonable to expect that a dose increase for carbamazepine may be necessary). Products include:

Ciloxan Ophthalmic Ointment 554
Cipro Tablets 2991

Cisapride (Carbamazepine is known to induce CYP1A2 and CYP3A4. Therefore, the potential exists for interaction between carbamazepine and any agent metabolized by one (or more) of these enzymes. Agents that are metabolized by CYP1A2 and CYP3A4 may have decreased plasma levels when administered concomitantly with carbamazepine. Thus, if a patient has been titrated to a stable dosage on one of the agents in these categories, and then begins a course of treatment with carbamazepine, it is reasonable to expect that a dose increase for the concomitant agent may be necessary).

No products indexed under this heading.

Cisplatin (Carbamazepine is metabolized by CYP3A4. Therefore, the potential exists for interaction between carbamazepine and any agent that induces CYP3A4. Agents that are CYP3A4 inducers may decrease plasma levels of carbamazepine. Thus, if a patient has been titrated to a stable dosage on carbamazepine, and then begins a course of treatment with a CYP3A4 inducers, it is reasonable to expect that a dose increase for carbamazepine may be necessary).

No products indexed under this heading.

Clarithromycin (Carbamazepine is metabolized mainly by CYP3A4 the active carbamazepine 10,11-epoxide, which is futher metabolized to the trans-diol by epoxide hydrolase. Therefore, the potential exists for interaction between carbamazepine and any agent that inhibits CYP3A4 and/or epoxide hydrolase. Agents that are CYP3A4 inhibitors may increase the plasma levels of carbamazepine. Thus, if a patient has been titrated to a stable dosage of carbamazepine, and then begins a course of treatment with a CYP3A4 or epoxide hydrolase inhibitor, it is reasonable to expect that a dose reduction for carbamazepine may be necessary). Products include:

Biaxin/Biaxin XL 402
PREVPAC 3281

Clomipramine Hydrochloride (Carbamazepine increases the plasma levels of clomipramine HCl).

No products indexed under this heading.

Clopidogrel Bisulfate (Carbamazepine is known to induce CYP1A2 and CYP3A4. Therefore, the potential exists for interaction between carbamazepine and any agent metabolized by one (or more) of these enzymes. Agents that are metabolized by CYP1A2 and CYP3A4 may have decreased plasma levels when administered concomitantly with carbamazepine. Thus, if a patient has been titrated to a stable dosage on one of the agents in these categories, and then begins a course of treatment with carbamazepine, it is reasonable to expect that a dose increase for the concomitant agent may be necessary). Products include:

Plavix Tablets 940
Plavix Tablets 2942

Clorazepate Dipotassium (Because of its primary CNS effect, caution should be used when carbamazepine is taken with other centrally-acting drugs). Products include:

Tranxene 2488

Clotrimazole (Carbamazepine is metabolized mainly by CYP3A4 the active carbamazepine 10,11-epoxide, which is futher metabolized to the trans-diol by epoxide hydrolase. Therefore, the potential exists for interaction between carbamazepine and any agent that inhibits CYP3A4 and/or epoxide hydrolase. Agents that are CYP3A4 inhibitors may increase the plasma levels of carbamazepine. Thus, if a patient has been titrated to a stable dosage of carbamazepine, and then begins a course of treatment with a CYP3A4 or epoxide hydrolase inhibitor, it is reasonable to expect that a dose reduction for carbamazepine may be necessary). Products include:

Lotrimin 3053
Lotrisone 3054

Clozapine (Carbamazepine is known to induce CYP1A2 and CYP3A4. Therefore, the potential exists for interaction between carbamazepine and any agent metabolized by one (or more) of these enzymes. Agents that are metabolized by CYP1A2 and CYP3A4 may have decreased plasma levels when administered concomitantly with carbamazepine. Thus, if a patient has been titrated to a stable dosage on one of the agents in these categories, and then begins a course of treatment with carbamazepine, it is reasonable to expect that a dose increase for the concomitant agent may be necessary). Products include:

Clozapine Tablets 2141
Clozaril Tablets 2174
FazaClo Orally Disintegrating Tablets 547

Codeine Phosphate (Because of its primary CNS effect, caution should be used when carbamazepine is taken with other centrally-acting drugs). Products include:

Tylenol with Codeine 2461

Cortisone Acetate (Carbamazepine is metabolized by CYP3A4. Therefore, the potential exists for interaction between carbamazepine and any agent that induces CYP3A4. Agents that are CYP3A4 inducers may decrease plasma levels of carbamazepine. Thus, if a patient has been titrated to a stable dosage on carbamazepine, and then begins a course of treatment with a CYP3A4 inducers, it is reasonable to expect that a dose increase for carbamazepine may be necessary).

No products indexed under this heading.

Cyclobenzaprine (Carbamazepine is known to induce CYP1A2 and CYP3A4. Therefore, the potential exists for interaction between carbamazepine and any agent metabolized by one (or more) of these enzymes. Agents that are metabolized by CYP1A2 and CYP3A4 may have decreased plasma levels when administered concomitantly with carbamazepine. Thus, if a patient has been titrated to a stable dosage on one of the agents in these categories, and then begins a course of treatment with carbamazepine, it is reasonable to expect that a dose increase for the concomitant agent may be necessary).

No products indexed under this heading.

Cyclobenzaprine Hydrochloride (Carbamazepine is known to induce CYP1A2 and CYP3A4. Therefore, the potential exists for interaction between carbamazepine and any agent metabolized by one (or more) of these enzymes. Agents that are metabolized by CYP1A2 and CYP3A4 may have decreased plas-

ma levels when administered concomitantly with carbamazepine. Thus, if a patient has been titrated to a stable dosage on one of the agents in these categories, and then begins a course of treatment with carbamazepine, it is reasonable to expect that a dose increase for the concomitant agent may be necessary). Products include:

Flexeril Tablets **1832**

Cyclosporine (Carbamazepine is metabolized mainly by CYP3A4 the active carbamazepine 10,11-epoxide, which is futher metabolized to the trans-diol by epoxide hydrolase. Therefore, the potential exists for interaction between carbamazepine and any agent that inhibits CYP3A4 and/or epoxide hydrolase. Agents that are CYP3A4 inhibitors may increase the plasma levels of carbamazepine. Thus, if a patient has been titrated to a stable dosage of carbamazepine, and then begins a course of treatment with a CYP3A4 or epoxide hydrolase inhibitor, it is reasonable to expect that a dose reduction for carbamazepine may be necessary). Products include:

Gengraf Capsules **458**
Neoral Soft Gelatin Capsules **2247**
Neoral Oral Solution **2247**
Restasis Ophthalmic Emulsion **570**
Sandimmune **2259**

Dalfopristin (Carbamazepine is metabolized mainly by CYP3A4 the active carbamazepine 10,11-epoxide, which is futher metabolized to the trans-diol by epoxide hydrolase. Therefore, the potential exists for interaction between carbamazepine and any agent that inhibits CYP3A4 and/or epoxide hydrolase. Agents that are CYP3A4 inhibitors may increase the plasma levels of carbamazepine. Thus, if a patient has been titrated to a stable dosage of carbamazepine, and then begins a course of treatment with a CYP3A4 or epoxide hydrolase inhibitor, it is reasonable to expect that a dose reduction for carbamazepine may be necessary). Products include:

Synercid I.V. **1690**

Danazol (Carbamazepine is metabolized mainly by CYP3A4 the active carbamazepine 10,11-epoxide, which is futher metabolized to the trans-diol by epoxide hydrolase. Therefore, the potential exists for interaction between carbamazepine and any agent that inhibits CYP3A4 and/or epoxide hydrolase. Agents that are CYP3A4 inhibitors may increase the plasma levels of carbamazepine. Thus, if a patient has been titrated to a stable dosage of carbamazepine, and then begins a course of treatment with a CYP3A4 or epoxide hydrolase inhibitor, it is reasonable to expect that a dose reduction for carbamazepine may be necessary).

No products indexed under this heading.

Delavirdine Mesylate (Carbamazepine is metabolized mainly by CYP3A4 the active carbamazepine 10,11-epoxide, which is futher metabolized to the trans-diol by epoxide hydrolase. Therefore, the potential exists for interaction between carbamazepine and any agent that inhibits CYP3A4 and/or epoxide hydrolase. Agents that are CYP3A4 inhibitors may increase the plasma levels of carbamazepine. Thus, if a patient has been titrated to a stable dosage of carbamazepine, and then begins a course of treatment with a CYP3A4 or epoxide hydrolase inhibitor, it is reasonable to expect that a dose reduction for carbamazepine may be necessary). Products include:

Rescriptor Tablets **2535**

Desflurane (Because of its primary CNS effect, caution should be used when carbamazepine is taken with other centrally-acting drugs). Products include:

Suprane Liquid for Inhalation **770**

Desipramine Hydrochloride (Carbamazepine is known to induce CYP1A2 and CYP3A4. Therefore, the potential exists for interaction between carbamazepine and any agent metabolized by one (or more) of these enzymes. Agents that are metabolized by CYP1A2 and CYP3A4 may have decreased plasma levels when administered concomitantly with carbamazepine. Thus, if a patient has been titrated to a stable dosage on one of the agents in these categories, and then begins a course of treatment with carbamazepine, it is reasonable to expect that a dose increase for the concomitant agent may be necessary).

No products indexed under this heading.

Desogestrel (Carbamazepine is known to induce CYP1A2 and CYP3A4. Therefore, the potential exists for interaction between carbamazepine and any agent metabolized by one (or more) of these enzymes. Agents that are metabolized by CYP1A2 or CYP3A4 may have decreased plasma levels when administered concomitantly with carbamazepine. Breakthrough bleeding has been reported among patients receiving concomitant oral contraceptives and their reliability may be adversely affected). Products include:

Ortho-Cept Tablets **2395**

Dexamethasone (Carbamazepine is metabolized by CYP3A4. Therefore, the potential exists for interaction between carbamazepine and any agent that induces CYP3A4. Agents that are CYP3A4 inducers may decrease plasma levels of carbamazepine. Thus, if a patient has been titrated to a stable dosage on carbamazepine, and then begins a course of treatment with a CYP3A4 inducers, it is reasonable to expect that a dose increase for carbamazepine may be necessary). Products include:

Ciprodex Otic Suspension **555**
Decadron Tablets **1929**
TobraDex Ophthalmic Ointment **558**
TobraDex Ophthalmic Suspension ... **558**

Dexamethasone Acetate (Carbamazepine is metabolized by CYP3A4. Therefore, the potential exists for interaction between carbamazepine and any agent that induces CYP3A4. Agents that are CYP3A4 inducers may decrease plasma levels of carbamazepine. Thus, if a patient has been titrated to a stable dosage on carbamazepine, and then begins a course of treatment with a CYP3A4 inducers, it is reasonable to expect that a dose increase for carbamazepine may be necessary).

No products indexed under this heading.

Dexamethasone Sodium Phosphate (Carbamazepine is metabolized by CYP3A4. Therefore, the potential exists for interaction between carbamazepine and any agent that induces CYP3A4. Agents that are CYP3A4 inducers may decrease plasma levels of carbamazepine. Thus, if a patient has been titrated to a stable dosage on carbamazepine, and then begins a course of treatment with a CYP3A4 inducers, it is reasonable to expect that a dose increase for carbamazepine may be necessary). Products include:

Decadron Phosphate Injection **1931**

Dezocine (Because of its primary CNS effect, caution should be used when carbamazepine is taken with other centrally-acting drugs).

No products indexed under this heading.

Diazepam (Carbamazepine is known to induce CYP1A2 and CYP3A4. Therefore, the potential exists for interaction between carbamazepine and any agent metabolized by one (or more) of these enzymes. Agents that are metabolized by CYP1A2 and CYP3A4 may have decreased plasma levels when administered concomitantly with carbamazepine. Thus, if a patient has been titrated to a stable dosage on one of the agents in these categories, and then begins a course of treatment with carbamazepine, it is reasonable to expect that a dose increase for the concomitant agent may be necessary). Products include:

Diastat Rectal Delivery System **3344**
Valium Tablets **2822**

Dihydroergotamine Mesylate (Carbamazepine is known to induce CYP1A2 and CYP3A4. Therefore, the potential exists for interaction between carbamazepine and any agent metabolized by one (or more) of these enzymes. Agents that are metabolized by CYP1A2 and CYP3A4 may have decreased plasma levels when administered concomitantly with carbamazepine. Thus, if a patient has been titrated to a stable dosage on one of the agents in these categories, and then begins a course of treatment with carbamazepine, it is reasonable to expect that a dose increase for the concomitant agent may be necessary). Products include:

Migranal Nasal Spray **3350**

Diltiazem Hydrochloride (Carbamazepine is metabolized mainly by CYP3A4 the active carbamazepine 10,11-epoxide, which is futher metabolized to the trans-diol by epoxide hydrolase. Therefore, the potential exists for interaction between carbamazepine and any agent that inhibits CYP3A4 and/or epoxide hydrolase. Agents that are CYP3A4 inhibitors may increase the plasma levels of carbamazepine. Thus, if a patient has been titrated to a stable dosage of carbamazepine, and then begins a course of treatment with a CYP3A4 or epoxide hydrolase inhibitor, it is reasonable to expect that a dose reduction for carbamazepine may be necessary). Products include:

Cardizem LA Extended Release Tablets **1699**
Tiazac Capsules **1204**

Diltiazem Maleate (Carbamazepine is metabolized mainly by CYP3A4 the active carbamazepine 10,11-epoxide, which is futher metabolized to the trans-diol by epoxide hydrolase. Therefore, the potential exists for interaction between carbamazepine and any agent that inhibits CYP3A4 and/or epoxide hydrolase. Agents that are CYP3A4 inhibitors may increase the plasma levels of carbamazepine. Thus, if a patient has been titrated to a stable dosage of carbamazepine, and then begins a course of treatment with a CYP3A4 or epoxide hydrolase inhibitor, it is reasonable to expect that a dose reduction for carbamazepine may be necessary).

No products indexed under this heading.

Disopyramide (Carbamazepine is known to induce CYP1A2 and CYP3A4. Therefore, the potential exists for interaction between carbamazepine and any agent metabolized by one (or more) of these enzymes. Agents that are metabolized by CYP1A2 and CYP3A4 may have decreased plasma levels when administered concomitantly with carbamazepine. Thus, if a patient has been titrated to a stable dosage on one of the agents in these categories, and then begins a course of treatment with carbamazepine, it is reasonable to expect that a dose increase for the concomitant agent may be necessary).

No products indexed under this heading.

Disopyramide Phosphate (Carbamazepine is known to induce CYP1A2 and CYP3A4. Therefore, the potential exists for interaction between carbamazepine and any agent metabolized by one (or more) of these enzymes. Agents that are metabolized by CYP1A2 and CYP3A4 may have decreased plasma levels when administered concomitantly with carbamazepine. Thus, if a patient has been titrated to a stable dosage on one of the agents in these categories, and then begins a course of treatment with carbamazepine, it is reasonable to expect that a dose increase for the concomitant agent may be necessary).

No products indexed under this heading.

Disulfiram (Carbamazepine is known to induce CYP1A2 and CYP3A4. Therefore, the potential exists for interaction between carbamazepine and any agent metabolized by one (or more) of these enzymes. Agents that are metabolized by CYP1A2 and CYP3A4 may have decreased plasma levels when administered concomitantly with carbamazepine. Thus, if a patient has been titrated to a stable dosage on one of the agents in these categories, and then begins a course of treatment with carbamazepine, it is reasonable to expect that a dose increase for the concomitant agent may be necessary). Products include:

Antabuse Tablets **2343**

Doxepin Hydrochloride (Carbamazepine is known to induce CYP1A2 and CYP3A4. Therefore, the poten-

tial exists for interaction between carbamazepine and any agent metabolized by one (or more) of these enzymes. Agents that are metabolized by CYP1A2 and CYP3A4 may have decreased plasma levels when administered concomitantly with carbamazepine. Thus, if a patient has been titrated to a stable dosage on one of the agents in these categories, and then begins a course of treatment with carbamazepine, it is reasonable to expect that a dose increase for the concomitant agent may be necessary).

No products indexed under this heading.

Doxorubicin Hydrochloride (Carbamazepine is metabolized by CYP3A4. Therefore, the potential exists for interaction between carbamazepine and any agent that induces CYP3A4. Agents that are CYP3A4 inducers may decrease plasma levels of carbamazepine. Thus, if a patient has been titrated to a stable dosage on carbamazepine, and then begins a course of treatment with a CYP3A4 inducers, it is reasonable to expect that a dose increase for carbamazepine may be necessary). Products include:

Adriamycin for Injection, USP 786
Adriamycin Injection, USP 786

Dronabinol (Carbamazepine is known to induce CYP1A2 and CYP3A4. Therefore, the potential exists for interaction between carbamazepine and any agent metabolized by one (or more) of these enzymes. Agents that are metabolized by CYP1A2 and CYP3A4 may have decreased plasma levels when administered concomitantly with carbamazepine. Thus, if a patient has been titrated to a stable dosage on one of the agents in these categories, and then begins a course of treatment with carbamazepine, it is reasonable to expect that a dose increase for the concomitant agent may be necessary). Products include:

Marinol Capsules 3334

Droperidol (Because of its primary CNS effect, caution should be used when carbamazepine is taken with other centrally-acting drugs).

No products indexed under this heading.

Efavirenz (Carbamazepine is metabolized mainly by CYP3A4 the active carbamazepine 10,11-epoxide, which is futher metabolized to the trans-diol by epoxide hydrolase. Therefore, the potential exists for interaction between carbamazepine and any agent that inhibits CYP3A4 and/or epoxide hydrolase. Agents that are CYP3A4 inhibitors may increase the plasma levels of carbamazepine. Thus, if a patient has been titrated to a stable dosage of carbamazepine, and then begins a course of treatment with a CYP3A4 or epoxide hydrolase inhibitor, it is reasonable to expect that a dose reduction for carbamazepine may be necessary). Products include:

Sustiva Capsules 957

Enflurane (Because of its primary CNS effect, caution should be used when carbamazepine is taken with other centrally-acting drugs).

No products indexed under this heading.

Enoxacin (Carbamazepine is known to induce CYP1A2 and CYP3A4. Therefore, the potential exists for interaction between carbamazepine and any agent metabolized by one (or more) of these enzymes. Agents that are metabolized by CYP1A2 and CYP3A4 may have decreased plasma levels when administered concomitantly with carbamazepine. Thus, if a patient has been titrated to a stable dosage on one of the agents in these categories, and then begins a course of treatment with carbamazepine, it is reasonable to expect that a dose increase for the concomitant agent may be necessary).

No products indexed under this heading.

Ergotamine Tartrate (Carbamazepine is known to induce CYP1A2 and CYP3A4. Therefore, the potential exists for interaction between carbamazepine and any agent metabolized by one (or more) of these enzymes. Agents that are metabolized by CYP1A2 and CYP3A4 may have decreased plasma levels when administered concomitantly with carbamazepine. Thus, if a patient has been titrated to a stable dosage on one of the agents in these categories, and then begins a course of treatment with carbamazepine, it is reasonable to expect that a dose increase for the concomitant agent may be necessary).

No products indexed under this heading.

Erythromycin (Carbamazepine is metabolized mainly by CYP3A4 the active carbamazepine 10,11-epoxide, which is futher metabolized to the trans-diol by epoxide hydrolase. Therefore, the potential exists for interaction between carbamazepine and any agent that inhibits CYP3A4 and/or epoxide hydrolase. Agents that are CYP3A4 inhibitors may increase the plasma levels of carbamazepine. Thus, if a patient has been titrated to a stable dosage of carbamazepine, and then begins a course of treatment with a CYP3A4 or epoxide hydrolase inhibitor, it is reasonable to expect that a dose reduction for carbamazepine may be necessary). Products include:

Erygel Topical Gel 2096
Ery-Tab Tablets 447
Erythromycin Base Filmtab Tablets 454
Erythromycin Delayed-Release Capsules, USP 456
PCE Dispertab Tablets 510

Erythromycin Estolate (Carbamazepine is metabolized mainly by CYP3A4 the active carbamazepine 10,11-epoxide, which is futher metabolized to the trans-diol by epoxide hydrolase. Therefore, the potential exists for interaction between carbamazepine and any agent that inhibits CYP3A4 and/or epoxide hydrolase. Agents that are CYP3A4 inhibitors may increase the plasma levels of carbamazepine. Thus, if a patient has been titrated to a stable dosage of carbamazepine, and then begins a course of treatment with a CYP3A4 or epoxide hydrolase inhibitor, it is reasonable to expect that a dose reduction for carbamazepine may be necessary).

No products indexed under this heading.

Erythromycin Ethylsuccinate (Carbamazepine is metabolized mainly by CYP3A4 the active carbamazepine 10,11-epoxide, which is futher metabolized to the trans-diol by epoxide hydrolase. Therefore, the potential exists for interaction between carbamazepine and any agent that inhibits CYP3A4 and/or epoxide hydrolase. Agents that are CYP3A4 inhibitors may increase the plasma levels of carbamazepine. Thus, if a patient has been titrated to a stable dosage of carbamazepine, and then begins a course of treatment with a CYP3A4 or epoxide hydrolase inhibitor, it is reasonable to expect that a dose reduction for carbamazepine may be necessary). Products include:

E.E.S. 449
EryPed 445

Erythromycin Gluceptate (Carbamazepine is metabolized mainly by CYP3A4 the active carbamazepine 10,11-epoxide, which is futher metabolized to the trans-diol by epoxide hydrolase. Therefore, the potential exists for interaction between carbamazepine and any agent that inhibits CYP3A4 and/or epoxide hydrolase. Agents that are CYP3A4 inhibitors may increase the plasma levels of carbamazepine. Thus, if a patient has been titrated to a stable dosage of carbamazepine, and then begins a course of treatment with a CYP3A4 or epoxide hydrolase inhibitor, it is reasonable to expect that a dose reduction for carbamazepine may be necessary).

No products indexed under this heading.

Erythromycin Lactobionate (Carbamazepine is metabolized mainly by CYP3A4 the active carbamazepine 10,11-epoxide, which is futher metabolized to the trans-diol by epoxide hydrolase. Therefore, the potential exists for interaction between carbamazepine and any agent that inhibits CYP3A4 and/or epoxide hydrolase. Agents that are CYP3A4 inhibitors may increase the plasma levels of carbamazepine. Thus, if a patient has been titrated to a stable dosage of carbamazepine, and then begins a course of treatment with a CYP3A4 or epoxide hydrolase inhibitor, it is reasonable to expect that a dose reduction for carbamazepine may be necessary).

No products indexed under this heading.

Erythromycin Stearate (Carbamazepine is metabolized mainly by CYP3A4 the active carbamazepine 10,11-epoxide, which is futher metabolized to the trans-diol by epoxide hydrolase. Therefore, the potential exists for interaction between carbamazepine and any agent that inhibits CYP3A4 and/or epoxide hydrolase. Agents that are CYP3A4 inhibitors may increase the plasma levels of carbamazepine. Thus, if a patient has been titrated to a stable dosage of carbamazepine, and then begins a course of treatment with a CYP3A4 or epoxide hydrolase inhibitor, it is reasonable to expect that a dose reduction for carbamazepine may be necessary). Products include:

Erythrocin Stearate Filmtab Tablets 452

Esomeprazole Magnesium (Carbamazepine is metabolized mainly by CYP3A4 the active carbamazepine 10,11-epoxide, which is futher metabolized to the trans-diol by epoxide hydrolase. Therefore, the potential exists for interaction between carbamazepine and any agent that inhibits CYP3A4 and/or epoxide hydrolase. Agents that are CYP3A4 inhibitors may increase the plasma levels of carbamazepine. Thus, if a patient has been titrated to a stable dosage of carbamazepine, and then begins a course of treatment with a CYP3A4 or epoxide hydrolase inhibitor, it is reasonable to expect that a dose reduction for carbamazepine may be necessary). Products include:

Nexium Delayed-Release Capsules 645

Estazolam (Because of its primary CNS effect, caution should be used when carbamazepine is taken with other centrally-acting drugs). Products include:

ProSom Tablets 512

Estradiol (Carbamazepine is known to induce CYP1A2 and CYP3A4. Therefore, the potential exists for interaction between carbamazepine and any agent metabolized by one (or more) of these enzymes. Agents that are metabolized by CYP1A2 and CYP3A4 may have decreased plasma levels when administered concomitantly with carbamazepine. Thus, if a patient has been titrated to a stable dosage on one of the agents in these categories, and then begins a course of treatment with carbamazepine, it is reasonable to expect that a dose increase for the concomitant agent may be necessary). Products include:

Activella Tablets 2311
Climara Transdermal System 795
Climara Pro Transdermal System 800
CombiPatch Transdermal System 2180
Estrogel 0.06% 3200
Menostar Transdermal System 805
Prefest Tablets 1069
Vagifem Tablets 2340
Vivelle Transdermal System 2288
Vivelle-Dot Transdermal System 2293

Estradiol Benzoate (Carbamazepine is known to induce CYP1A2 and CYP3A4. Therefore, the potential exists for interaction between carbamazepine and any agent metabolized by one (or more) of these enzymes. Agents that are metabolized by CYP1A2 and CYP3A4 may have decreased plasma levels when administered concomitantly with carbamazepine. Thus, if a patient has been titrated to a stable dosage on one of the agents in these categories, and then begins a course of treatment with carbamazepine, it is reasonable to expect that a dose increase for the concomitant agent may be necessary).

No products indexed under this heading.

Estradiol Cypionate (Carbamazepine is known to induce CYP1A2 and CYP3A4. Therefore, the potential exists for interaction between carbamazepine and any agent metabolized by one (or more) of these enzymes. Agents that are metabolized by CYP1A2 and CYP3A4 may have decreased plasma levels when administered concomitantly with carbamazepine. Thus, if a patient has been titrated to a stable dosage on one of the agents in these categories, and then begins a course of treatment with carbamazepine, it is

reasonable to expect that a dose increase for the concomitant agent may be necessary).
No products indexed under this heading.

Estradiol Valerate (Carbamazepine is known to induce CYP1A2 and CYP3A4. Therefore, the potential exists for interaction between carbamazepine and any agent metabolized by one (or more) of these enzymes. Agents that are metabolized by CYP1A2 and CYP3A4 may have decreased plasma levels when administered concomitantly with carbamazepine. Thus, if a patient has been titrated to a stable dosage on one of the agents in these categories, and then begins a course of treatment with carbamazepine, it is reasonable to expect that a dose increase for the concomitant agent may be necessary).
No products indexed under this heading.

Ethanol (Because of its primary CNS effect, caution should be used when carbamazepine is taken with alcohol).
No products indexed under this heading.

Ethchlorvynol (Because of its primary CNS effect, caution should be used when carbamazepine is taken with other centrally-acting drugs).
No products indexed under this heading.

Ethinamate (Because of its primary CNS effect, caution should be used when carbamazepine is taken with other centrally-acting drugs).
No products indexed under this heading.

Ethinyl Estradiol (Carbamazepine is known to induce CYP1A2 and CYP3A4. Therefore, the potential exists for interaction between carbamazepine and any agent metabolized by one (or more) of these enzymes. Agents that are metabolized by CYP1A2 or CYP3A4 may have decreased plasma levels when administered concomitantly with carbamazepine. Breakthrough bleeding has been reported among patients receiving concomitant oral contraceptives and their reliability may be adversely affected). Products include:
Alesse-28 Tablets **3392**
Lo/Ovral-28 Tablets **3423**
NuvaRing **2357**
Ortho-Cept Tablets **2395**
Ortho-Cyclen/Ortho Tri-Cyclen **2414**
Ortho Evra Transdermal System **2402**
Ortho Tri-Cyclen Lo Tablets **2421**
Seasonale Tablets **1073**
Triphasil-28 Tablets **3483**
Yasmin 28 Tablets **818**

Ethosuximide (Carbamazepine is metabolized by CYP3A4. Therefore, the potential exists for interaction between carbamazepine and any agent that induces CYP3A4. Agents that are CYP3A4 inducers may decrease plasma levels of carbamazepine. Thus, if a patient has been titrated to a stable dosage on carbamazepine, and then begins a course of treatment with a CYP3A4 inducers, it is reasonable to expect that a dose increase for carbamazepine may be necessary).
No products indexed under this heading.

Ethyl Alcohol (Because of its primary CNS effect, caution should be used when carbamazepine is taken with other centrally-acting drugs).
No products indexed under this heading.

Ethynodiol Diacetate (Carbamazepine is known to induce CYP1A2 and CYP3A4. Therefore, the potential exists for interaction between carbamazepine and any agent metabolized by one (or more) of these enzymes. Agents that are metabolized by CYP1A2 or CYP3A4 may have decreased plasma levels when administered concomitantly with carbamazepine. Breakthrough bleeding has been reported among patients receiving concomitant oral contraceptives and their reliability may be adversely affected).
No products indexed under this heading.

Etoposide (Carbamazepine is known to induce CYP1A2 and CYP3A4. Therefore, the potential exists for interaction between carbamazepine and any agent metabolized by one (or more) of these enzymes. Agents that are metabolized by CYP1A2 and CYP3A4 may have decreased plasma levels when administered concomitantly with carbamazepine. Thus, if a patient has been titrated to a stable dosage on one of the agents in these categories, and then begins a course of treatment with carbamazepine, it is reasonable to expect that a dose increase for the concomitant agent may be necessary).
No products indexed under this heading.

Etoposide Phosphate (Carbamazepine is known to induce CYP1A2 and CYP3A4. Therefore, the potential exists for interaction between carbamazepine and any agent metabolized by one (or more) of these enzymes. Agents that are metabolized by CYP1A2 and CYP3A4 may have decreased plasma levels when administered concomitantly with carbamazepine. Thus, if a patient has been titrated to a stable dosage on one of the agents in these categories, and then begins a course of treatment with carbamazepine, it is reasonable to expect that a dose increase for the concomitant agent may be necessary).
No products indexed under this heading.

Felbamate (Carbamazepine is metabolized by CYP3A4. Therefore, the potential exists for interaction between carbamazepine and any agent that induces CYP3A4. Agents that are CYP3A4 inducers may decrease plasma levels of carbamazepine. Thus, if a patient has been titrated to a stable dosage on carbamazepine, and then begins a course of treatment with a CYP3A4 inducers, it is reasonable to expect that a dose increase for carbamazepine may be necessary).
No products indexed under this heading.

Felodipine (Carbamazepine is known to induce CYP1A2 and CYP3A4. Therefore, the potential exists for interaction between carbamazepine and any agent metabolized by one (or more) of these enzymes. Agents that are metabolized by CYP1A2 and CYP3A4 may have decreased plasma levels when administered concomitantly with carbamazepine. Thus, if a patient has been titrated to a stable dosage on one of the agents in these categories, and then begins a course of treatment with carbamazepine, it is reasonable to expect that a dose increase for the concomitant agent may be necessary). Products include:
Plendil Extended-Release Tablets **651**

Fentanyl (Carbamazepine is known to induce CYP1A2 and CYP3A4. Therefore, the potential exists for interaction between carbamazepine and any agent metabolized by one (or more) of these enzymes. Agents that are metabolized by CYP1A2 and CYP3A4 may have decreased plasma levels when administered concomitantly with carbamazepine. Thus, if a patient has been titrated to a stable dosage on one of the agents in these categories, and then begins a course of treatment with carbamazepine, it is reasonable to expect that a dose increase for the concomitant agent may be necessary). Products include:
Duragesic Transdermal System **2448**

Fentanyl Citrate (Carbamazepine is known to induce CYP1A2 and CYP3A4. Therefore, the potential exists for interaction between carbamazepine and any agent metabolized by one (or more) of these enzymes. Agents that are metabolized by CYP1A2 and CYP3A4 may have decreased plasma levels when administered concomitantly with carbamazepine. Thus, if a patient has been titrated to a stable dosage on one of the agents in these categories, and then begins a course of treatment with carbamazepine, it is reasonable to expect that a dose increase for the concomitant agent may be necessary). Products include:
Actiq **993**

Fluconazole (Carbamazepine is metabolized mainly by CYP3A4 the active carbamazepine 10,11-epoxide, which is futher metabolized to the trans-diol by epoxide hydrolase. Therefore, the potential exists for interaction between carbamazepine and any agent that inhibits CYP3A4 and/or epoxide hydrolase. Agents that are CYP3A4 inhibitors may increase the plasma levels of carbamazepine. Thus, if a patient has been titrated to a stable dosage of carbamazepine, and then begins a course of treatment with a CYP3A4 or epoxide hydrolase inhibitor, it is reasonable to expect that a dose reduction for carbamazepine may be necessary).
No products indexed under this heading.

Fludrocortisone Acetate (Carbamazepine is metabolized by CYP3A4. Therefore, the potential exists for interaction between carbamazepine and any agent that induces CYP3A4. Agents that are CYP3A4 inducers may decrease plasma levels of carbamazepine. Thus, if a patient has been titrated to a stable dosage on carbamazepine, and then begins a course of treatment with a CYP3A4 inducers, it is reasonable to expect that a dose increase for carbamazepine may be necessary).
No products indexed under this heading.

Fluoxetine Hydrochloride (Carbamazepine is metabolized mainly by CYP3A4 the active carbamazepine 10,11-epoxide, which is futher metabolized to the trans-diol by epoxide hydrolase. Therefore, the potential exists for interaction between carbamazepine and any agent that inhibits CYP3A4 and/or epoxide hydrolase. Agents that are CYP3A4 inhibitors may increase the plasma levels of carbamazepine. Thus, if a patient has been titrated to a stable dosage of carbamazepine, and then begins a course of treatment with a CYP3A4 or epoxide hydrolase inhibitor, it is reasonable to expect that a dose reduction for carbamazepine may be necessary). Products include:
Prozac Pulvules and Liquid **1771**
Symbyax Capsules **1788**

Fluphenazine Decanoate (Because of its primary CNS effect, caution should be used when carbamazepine is taken with other centrally-acting drugs).
No products indexed under this heading.

Fluphenazine Enanthate (Because of its primary CNS effect, caution should be used when carbamazepine is taken with other centrally-acting drugs).
No products indexed under this heading.

Fluphenazine Hydrochloride (Because of its primary CNS effect, caution should be used when carbamazepine is taken with other centrally-acting drugs).
No products indexed under this heading.

Flurazepam Hydrochloride (Because of its primary CNS effect, caution should be used when carbamazepine is taken with other centrally-acting drugs). Products include:
Dalmane Capsules **3343**

Flutamide (Carbamazepine is known to induce CYP1A2 and CYP3A4. Therefore, the potential exists for interaction between carbamazepine and any agent metabolized by one (or more) of these enzymes. Agents that are metabolized by CYP1A2 and CYP3A4 may have decreased plasma levels when administered concomitantly with carbamazepine. Thus, if a patient has been titrated to a stable dosage on one of the agents in these categories, and then begins a course of treatment with carbamazepine, it is reasonable to expect that a dose increase for the concomitant agent may be necessary). Products include:
Eulexin Capsules **3023**

Fluticasone Propionate (Carbamazepine is known to induce CYP1A2 and CYP3A4. Therefore, the potential exists for interaction between carbamazepine and any agent metabolized by one (or more) of these enzymes. Agents that are metabolized by CYP1A2 and CYP3A4 may have decreased plasma levels when administered concomitantly with carbamazepine. Thus, if a patient has been titrated to a stable dosage on one of the agents in these categories, and then begins a course of treatment with

carbamazepine, it is reasonable to expect that a dose increase for the concomitant agent may be necessary). Products include:

Advair Diskus 100/50 1291
Advair Diskus 250/50 1291
Advair Diskus 500/50 1291
Cutivate Cream 1381
Cutivate Lotion 0.05% 1383
Cutivate Ointment 1384
Flonase Nasal Spray 1412
Flovent Diskus 100 mcg 1418
Flovent Diskus 50 mcg 1415

Fluvoxamine Maleate (Carbamazepine is metabolized mainly by CYP3A4 the active carbamazepine 10,11-epoxide, which is futher metabolized to the trans-diol by epoxide hydrolase. Therefore, the potential exists for interaction between carbamazepine and any agent that inhibits CYP3A4 and/or epoxide hydrolase. Agents that are CYP3A4 inhibitors may increase the plasma levels of carbamazepine. Thus, if a patient has been titrated to a stable dosage of carbamazepine, and then begins a course of treatment with a CYP3A4 or epoxide hydrolase inhibitor, it is reasonable to expect that a dose reduction for carbamazepine may be necessary).
No products indexed under this heading.

Fosamprenavir Calcium (Carbamazepine is metabolized mainly by CYP3A4 the active carbamazepine 10,11-epoxide, which is futher metabolized to the trans-diol by epoxide hydrolase. Therefore, the potential exists for interaction between carbamazepine and any agent that inhibits CYP3A4 and/or epoxide hydrolase. Agents that are CYP3A4 inhibitors may increase the plasma levels of carbamazepine. Thus, if a patient has been titrated to a stable dosage of carbamazepine, and then begins a course of treatment with a CYP3A4 or epoxide hydrolase inhibitor, it is reasonable to expect that a dose reduction for carbamazepine may be necessary). Products include:

Lexiva Tablets 1473

Fosphenytoin Sodium (Carbamazepine is metabolized by CYP3A4. Therefore, the potential exists for interaction between carbamazepine and any agent that induces CYP3A4. Agents that are CYP3A4 inducers may decrease plasma levels of carbamazepine. Thus, if a patient has been titrated to a stable dosage on carbamazepine, and then begins a course of treatment with a CYP3A4 inducers, it is reasonable to expect that a dose increase for carbamazepine may be necessary).
No products indexed under this heading.

Garlic Extract (Carbamazepine is metabolized by CYP3A4. Therefore, the potential exists for interaction between carbamazepine and any agent that induces CYP3A4. Agents that are CYP3A4 inducers may decrease plasma levels of carbamazepine. Thus, if a patient has been titrated to a stable dosage on carbamazepine, and then begins a course of treatment with a CYP3A4 inducers, it is reasonable to expect that a dose increase for carbamazepine may be necessary).
No products indexed under this heading.

Garlic Oil (Carbamazepine is metabolized by CYP3A4. Therefore, the potential exists for interaction between carbamazepine and any agent that induces CYP3A4. Agents that are CYP3A4 inducers may decrease plasma levels of carbamazepine. Thus, if a patient has been titrated to a stable dosage on carbamazepine, and then begins a course of treatment with a CYP3A4 inducers, it is reasonable to expect that a dose increase for carbamazepine may be necessary).
No products indexed under this heading.

Glutethimide (Because of its primary CNS effect, caution should be used when carbamazepine is taken with other centrally-acting drugs).
No products indexed under this heading.

Grepafloxacin Hydrochloride (Carbamazepine is known to induce CYP1A2 and CYP3A4. Therefore, the potential exists for interaction between carbamazepine and any agent metabolized by one (or more) of these enzymes. Agents that are metabolized by CYP1A2 and CYP3A4 may have decreased plasma levels when administered concomitantly with carbamazepine. Thus, if a patient has been titrated to a stable dosage on one of the agents in these categories, and then begins a course of treatment with carbamazepine, it is reasonable to expect that a dose increase for the concomitant agent may be necessary).
No products indexed under this heading.

Haloperidol (Carbamazepine is known to induce CYP1A2 and CYP3A4. Therefore, the potential exists for interaction between carbamazepine and any agent metabolized by one (or more) of these enzymes. Agents that are metabolized by CYP1A2 and CYP3A4 may have decreased plasma levels when administered concomitantly with carbamazepine. Thus, if a patient has been titrated to a stable dosage on one of the agents in these categories, and then begins a course of treatment with carbamazepine, it is reasonable to expect that a dose increase for the concomitant agent may be necessary).
No products indexed under this heading.

Haloperidol Decanoate (Carbamazepine is known to induce CYP1A2 and CYP3A4. Therefore, the potential exists for interaction between carbamazepine and any agent metabolized by one (or more) of these enzymes. Agents that are metabolized by CYP1A2 and CYP3A4 may have decreased plasma levels when administered concomitantly with carbamazepine. Thus, if a patient has been titrated to a stable dosage on one of the agents in these categories, and then begins a course of treatment with carbamazepine, it is reasonable to expect that a dose increase for the concomitant agent may be necessary).
No products indexed under this heading.

Haloperidol Lactate (Carbamazepine is known to induce CYP1A2 and CYP3A4. Therefore, the potential exists for interaction between carbamazepine and any agent metabolized by one (or more) of these enzymes. Agents that are metabolized by CYP1A2 and CYP3A4 may have decreased plasma levels when administered concomitantly with carbamazepine. Thus, if a patient has been titrated to a stable dosage on one of the agents in these categories, and then begins a course of treatment with carbamazepine, it is reasonable to expect that a dose increase for the concomitant agent may be necessary).
No products indexed under this heading.

Hydrocodone Bitartrate (Because of its primary CNS effect, caution should be used when carbamazepine is taken with other centrally-acting drugs). Products include:

Hycodan 1104
Hycomine Compound Tablets 1105
Hycotuss Expectorant Syrup 1106
Lortab 3315
Lortab Elixir 3312
Vicodin Tablets 530
Vicodin ES Tablets 531
Vicodin HP Tablets 532
Vicoprofen Tablets 533
Zydone Tablets 1118

Hydrocodone Polistirex (Because of its primary CNS effect, caution should be used when carbamazepine is taken with other centrally-acting drugs). Products include:

Tussionex Pennkinetic Extended-Release Suspension 3322

Hydrocortisone (Carbamazepine is metabolized by CYP3A4. Therefore, the potential exists for interaction between carbamazepine and any agent that induces CYP3A4. Agents that are CYP3A4 inducers may decrease plasma levels of carbamazepine. Thus, if a patient has been titrated to a stable dosage on carbamazepine, and then begins a course of treatment with a CYP3A4 inducers, it is reasonable to expect that a dose increase for carbamazepine may be necessary). Products include:

Cortizone•5 Ointment .... ▣699
Cortizone•10 Creme .... ▣699
Cortizone•10 Ointment .... ▣699
Cortizone•10 Plus Creme .... ▣700
Cortizone•10 Maximum Strength Quick Shot Spray .... ▣700
Hydrocortone Tablets 1963
Preparation H Hydrocortisone Cream .... ▣748

Hydrocortisone Acetate (Carbamazepine is metabolized by CYP3A4. Therefore, the potential exists for interaction between carbamazepine and any agent that induces CYP3A4. Agents that are CYP3A4 inducers may decrease plasma levels of carbamazepine. Thus, if a patient has been titrated to a stable dosage on carbamazepine, and then begins a course of treatment with a CYP3A4 inducers, it is reasonable to expect that a dose increase for carbamazepine may be necessary). Products include:

Analpram-HC 1136
Pramosone 1139
ProctoFoam-HC 3113
Tucks Anti-Itch Ointment .... ▣712
U-cort 1% Cream 3289

Hydrocortisone Butyrate (Carbamazepine is metabolized by CYP3A4. Therefore, the potential exists for interaction between carbamazepine and any agent that induces CYP3A4. Agents that are CYP3A4 inducers may decrease plasma levels of carbamazepine. Thus, if a patient has been titrated to a stable dosage on carbamazepine, and then begins a course of treatment with a CYP3A4 inducers, it is reasonable to expect that a dose increase for carbamazepine may be necessary). Products include:

Locoid 1138
Locoid Lipocream Cream 1138

Hydrocortisone Cypionate (Carbamazepine is metabolized by CYP3A4. Therefore, the potential exists for interaction between carbamazepine and any agent that induces CYP3A4. Agents that are CYP3A4 inducers may decrease plasma levels of carbamazepine. Thus, if a patient has been titrated to a stable dosage on carbamazepine, and then begins a course of treatment with a CYP3A4 inducers, it is reasonable to expect that a dose increase for carbamazepine may be necessary).
No products indexed under this heading.

Hydrocortisone Hemisuccinate (Carbamazepine is metabolized by CYP3A4. Therefore, the potential exists for interaction between carbamazepine and any agent that induces CYP3A4. Agents that are CYP3A4 inducers may decrease plasma levels of carbamazepine. Thus, if a patient has been titrated to a stable dosage on carbamazepine, and then begins a course of treatment with a CYP3A4 inducers, it is reasonable to expect that a dose increase for carbamazepine may be necessary).
No products indexed under this heading.

Hydrocortisone Probutate (Carbamazepine is metabolized by CYP3A4. Therefore, the potential exists for interaction between carbamazepine and any agent that induces CYP3A4. Agents that are CYP3A4 inducers may decrease plasma levels of carbamazepine. Thus, if a patient has been titrated to a stable dosage on carbamazepine, and then begins a course of treatment with a CYP3A4 inducers, it is reasonable to expect that a dose increase for carbamazepine may be necessary). Products include:

Pandel Cream, 0.1% 1017

Hydrocortisone Sodium Phosphate (Carbamazepine is metabolized by CYP3A4. Therefore, the potential exists for interaction between carbamazepine and any agent that induces CYP3A4. Agents that are CYP3A4 inducers may decrease plasma levels of carbamazepine. Thus, if a patient has been titrated to a stable dosage on carbamazepine, and then begins a course of treatment with a CYP3A4 inducers, it is reasonable to expect that a dose increase for carbamazepine may be necessary).
No products indexed under this heading.

Hydrocortisone Sodium Succinate (Carbamazepine is metabolized by CYP3A4. Therefore, the potential exists for interaction between carbamazepine and any agent that induces CYP3A4. Agents that are CYP3A4 inducers may decrease plasma levels of carbamazepine. Thus, if a patient has been titrated to a stable dosage on carbamazepine, and then begins a course of treat-

ment with a CYP3A4 inducers, it is reasonable to expect that a dose increase for carbamazepine may be necessary).
No products indexed under this heading.

Hydrocortisone Valerate (Carbamazepine is metabolized by CYP3A4. Therefore, the potential exists for interaction between carbamazepine and any agent that induces CYP3A4. Agents that are CYP3A4 inducers may decrease plasma levels of carbamazepine. Thus, if a patient has been titrated to a stable dosage on carbamazepine, and then begins a course of treatment with a CYP3A4 inducers, it is reasonable to expect that a dose increase for carbamazepine may be necessary).
No products indexed under this heading.

Hydromorphone Hydrochloride (Because of its primary CNS effect, caution should be used when carbamazepine is taken with other centrally-acting drugs). Products include:

Dilaudid 439
Dilaudid Oral Liquid 443
Dilaudid Non-Sterile Powder 439
Dilaudid Rectal Suppositories 439
Dilaudid Tablets 439
Dilaudid Tablets - 8 mg 443
Dilaudid-HP 441

Hydroxyzine Hydrochloride (Because of its primary CNS effect, caution should be used when carbamazepine is taken with other centrally-acting drugs).
No products indexed under this heading.

Hypericum (Carbamazepine is metabolized by CYP3A4. Therefore, the potential exists for interaction between carbamazepine and any agent that induces CYP3A4. Agents that are CYP3A4 inducers may decrease plasma levels of carbamazepine. Thus, if a patient has been titrated to a stable dosage on carbamazepine, and then begins a course of treatment with a CYP3A4 inducers, it is reasonable to expect that a dose increase for carbamazepine may be necessary).
No products indexed under this heading.

Hypericum Perforatum (Carbamazepine is metabolized by CYP3A4. Therefore, the potential exists for interaction between carbamazepine and any agent that induces CYP3A4. Agents that are CYP3A4 inducers may decrease plasma levels of carbamazepine. Thus, if a patient has been titrated to a stable dosage on carbamazepine, and then begins a course of treatment with a CYP3A4 inducers, it is reasonable to expect that a dose increase for carbamazepine may be necessary).
No products indexed under this heading.

Imipramine Hydrochloride (Carbamazepine is known to induce CYP1A2 and CYP3A4. Therefore, the potential exists for interaction between carbamazepine and any agent metabolized by one (or more) of these enzymes. Agents that are metabolized by CYP1A2 and CYP3A4 may have decreased plasma levels when administered concomitantly with carbamazepine. Thus, if a patient has been titrated to a stable dosage on one of the agents in these categories, and then begins a course of treatment with carbamazepine, it is reasonable to expect that a dose increase for the concomitant agent may be necessary).
No products indexed under this heading.

Imipramine Pamoate (Carbamazepine is known to induce CYP1A2 and CYP3A4. Therefore, the potential exists for interaction between carbamazepine and any agent metabolized by one (or more) of these enzymes. Agents that are metabolized by CYP1A2 and CYP3A4 may have decreased plasma levels when administered concomitantly with carbamazepine. Thus, if a patient has been titrated to a stable dosage on one of the agents in these categories, and then begins a course of treatment with carbamazepine, it is reasonable to expect that a dose increase for the concomitant agent may be necessary).
No products indexed under this heading.

Indinavir Sulfate (Carbamazepine is metabolized mainly by CYP3A4 the active carbamazepine 10,11-epoxide, which is futher metabolized to the trans-diol by epoxide hydrolase. Therefore, the potential exists for interaction between carbamazepine and any agent that inhibits CYP3A4 and/or epoxide hydrolase. Agents that are CYP3A4 inhibitors may increase the plasma levels of carbamazepine. Thus, if a patient has been titrated to a stable dosage of carbamazepine, and then begins a course of treatment with a CYP3A4 or epoxide hydrolase inhibitor, it is reasonable to expect that a dose reduction for carbamazepine may be necessary). Products include:

Crixivan Capsules 1918

Isoflurane (Because of its primary CNS effect, caution should be used when carbamazepine is taken with other centrally-acting drugs).
No products indexed under this heading.

Isoniazid (Carbamazepine is metabolized mainly by CYP3A4 the active carbamazepine 10,11-epoxide, which is futher metabolized to the trans-diol by epoxide hydrolase. Therefore, the potential exists for interaction between carbamazepine and any agent that inhibits CYP3A4 and/or epoxide hydrolase. Agents that are CYP3A4 inhibitors may increase the plasma levels of carbamazepine. Thus, if a patient has been titrated to a stable dosage of carbamazepine, and then begins a course of treatment with a CYP3A4 or epoxide hydrolase inhibitor, it is reasonable to expect that a dose reduction for carbamazepine may be necessary).
No products indexed under this heading.

Isradipine (Carbamazepine is known to induce CYP1A2 and CYP3A4. Therefore, the potential exists for interaction between carbamazepine and any agent metabolized by one (or more) of these enzymes. Agents that are metabolized by CYP1A2 and CYP3A4 may have decreased plasma levels when administered concomitantly with carbamazepine. Thus, if a patient has been titrated to a stable dosage on one of the agents in these categories, and then begins a course of treatment with carbamazepine, it is reasonable to expect that a dose increase for the concomitant agent may be necessary). Products include:

DynaCirc CR Tablets 2726

Itraconazole (Carbamazepine is metabolized mainly by CYP3A4 the active carbamazepine 10,11-epoxide, which is futher metabolized to the trans-diol by epoxide hydrolase. Therefore, the potential exists for interaction between carbamazepine and any agent that inhibits CYP3A4 and/or epoxide hydrolase. Agents that are CYP3A4 inhibitors may increase the plasma levels of carbamazepine. Thus, if a patient has been titrated to a stable dosage of carbamazepine, and then begins a course of treatment with a CYP3A4 or epoxide hydrolase inhibitor, it is reasonable to expect that a dose reduction for carbamazepine may be necessary).
No products indexed under this heading.

Ketamine Hydrochloride (Because of its primary CNS effect, caution should be used when carbamazepine is taken with other centrally-acting drugs).
No products indexed under this heading.

Ketoconazole (Carbamazepine is metabolized mainly by CYP3A4 the active carbamazepine 10,11-epoxide, which is futher metabolized to the trans-diol by epoxide hydrolase. Therefore, the potential exists for interaction between carbamazepine and any agent that inhibits CYP3A4 and/or epoxide hydrolase. Agents that are CYP3A4 inhibitors may increase the plasma levels of carbamazepine. Thus, if a patient has been titrated to a stable dosage of carbamazepine, and then begins a course of treatment with a CYP3A4 or epoxide hydrolase inhibitor, it is reasonable to expect that a dose reduction for carbamazepine may be necessary). Products include:

Nizoral A-D Shampoo, 1% 1839
Nizoral 2% Shampoo 1838

Levobupivacaine Hydrochloride (Carbamazepine is known to induce CYP1A2 and CYP3A4. Therefore, the potential exists for interaction between carbamazepine and any agent metabolized by one (or more) of these enzymes. Agents that are metabolized by CYP1A2 and CYP3A4 may have decreased plasma levels when administered concomitantly with carbamazepine. Thus, if a patient has been titrated to a stable dosage on one of the agents in these categories, and then begins a course of treatment with carbamazepine, it is reasonable to expect that a dose increase for the concomitant agent may be necessary).
No products indexed under this heading.

Levomethadyl Acetate Hydrochloride (Because of its primary CNS effect, caution should be used when carbamazepine is taken with other centrally-acting drugs).
No products indexed under this heading.

Levonorgestrel (Carbamazepine is known to induce CYP1A2 and CYP3A4. Therefore, the potential exists for interaction between carbamazepine and any agent metabolized by one (or more) of these enzymes. Agents that are metabolized by CYP1A2 or CYP3A4 may have decreased plasma levels when administered concomitantly with carbamazepine. Breakthrough bleeding has been reported among patients receiving concomitant oral contraceptives and their reliability may be adversely affected). Products include:

Alesse-28 Tablets 3392
Climara Pro Transdermal System 800
Mirena Intrauterine System 810
Plan B Tablets 1068
Seasonale Tablets 1073
Triphasil-28 Tablets 3483

Levorphanol Tartrate (Because of its primary CNS effect, caution should be used when carbamazepine is taken with other centrally-acting drugs).
No products indexed under this heading.

Lidocaine (Carbamazepine is known to induce CYP1A2 and CYP3A4. Therefore, the potential exists for interaction between carbamazepine and any agent metabolized by one (or more) of these enzymes. Agents that are metabolized by CYP1A2 and CYP3A4 may have decreased plasma levels when administered concomitantly with carbamazepine. Thus, if a patient has been titrated to a stable dosage on one of the agents in these categories, and then begins a course of treatment with carbamazepine, it is reasonable to expect that a dose increase for the concomitant agent may be necessary). Products include:

Lidoderm Patch 1107

Lidocaine Hydrochloride (Carbamazepine is known to induce CYP1A2 and CYP3A4. Therefore, the potential exists for interaction between carbamazepine and any agent metabolized by one (or more) of these enzymes. Agents that are metabolized by CYP1A2 and CYP3A4 may have decreased plasma levels when administered concomitantly with carbamazepine. Thus, if a patient has been titrated to a stable dosage on one of the agents in these categories, and then begins a course of treatment with carbamazepine, it is reasonable to expect that a dose increase for the concomitant agent may be necessary).
No products indexed under this heading.

Lithium (Concomitant administration of carbamazepine and lithium may increase the risk of neurotoxic side effects).
No products indexed under this heading.

Lithium Carbonate (Concomitant administration of carbamazepine and lithium may increase the risk of neurotoxic side effects). Products include:

Eskalith 1406
Lithobid Tablets 1670

Lithium Citrate (Concomitant administration of carbamazepine and lithium may increase the risk of neurotoxic side effects).
No products indexed under this heading.

Lomefloxacin Hydrochloride (Carbamazepine is known to induce CYP1A2 and CYP3A4. Therefore, the potential exists for interaction between carbamazepine and any agent metabolized by one (or more) of these enzymes. Agents that are metabolized by CYP1A2 and CYP3A4 may have decreased plasma levels when administered concomitantly with carbamazepine. Thus, if a patient has been titrated to a stable dosage on one of the agents in these categories, and then begins a course of treatment with carbamazepine, it is reasonable to expect that a dose increase for the concomitant agent may be necessary).
No products indexed under this heading.

Lopinavir (Carbamazepine is metabolized mainly by CYP3A4 the active carbamazepine 10,11-epoxide, which is futher metabolized to the trans-diol by epoxide hydrolase. Therefore, the potential exists for interaction between carbamazepine and any agent that inhibits CYP3A4 and/or epoxide hydrolase. Agents that are CYP3A4 inhibitors may increase the plasma levels of carbamazepine. Thus, if a patient has been titrated to a stable dosage of carbamazepine, and then begins a course of treatment with a CYP3A4 or epoxide hydrolase inhibitor, it is reasonable to expect that a dose reduction for carbamazepine may be necessary). Products include:
Kaletra 474

Loratadine (Carbamazepine is metabolized mainly by CYP3A4 the active carbamazepine 10,11-epoxide, which is futher metabolized to the trans-diol by epoxide hydrolase. Therefore, the potential exists for interaction between carbamazepine and any agent that inhibits CYP3A4 and/or epoxide hydrolase. Agents that are CYP3A4 inhibitors may increase the plasma levels of carbamazepine. Thus, if a patient has been titrated to a stable dosage of carbamazepine, and then begins a course of treatment with a CYP3A4 or epoxide hydrolase inhibitor, it is reasonable to expect that a dose reduction for carbamazepine may be necessary). Products include:
Alavert Allergy & Sinus D-12 Hour Tablets .... ■743
Alavert .... ■743
Children's Claritin 24 Hour Non-Drowsy Allergy Syrup .... ■732
Claritin Non-Drowsy 24 Hour Tablets .... ■731
Non-Drowsy Claritin Hives Relief Tablets .... ■733
Claritin Reditabs 24 Hour Non-Drowsy Tablets .... ■732
Claritin-D Non-Drowsy 12 Hour Tablets .... ■731
Claritin-D Non-Drowsy 24 Hour Tablets .... ■731
Children's Dimetapp ND Non-Drowsy Allergy Syrup .... ■746
Triaminic Allerchews .... ■684

Lorazepam (Because of its primary CNS effect, caution should be used when carbamazepine is taken with other centrally-acting drugs).
No products indexed under this heading.

Lovastatin (Carbamazepine is known to induce CYP1A2 and CYP3A4. Therefore, the potential exists for interaction between carbamazepine and any agent metabolized by one (or more) of these enzymes. Agents that are metabolized by CYP1A2 and CYP3A4 may have decreased plasma levels when administered concomitantly with carbamazepine. Thus, if a patient has been titrated to a stable dosage on one of the agents in these categories, and then begins a course of treatment with carbamazepine, it is reasonable to expect that a dose increase for the concomitant agent may be necessary). Products include:
Advicor Tablets 1694
Altoprev Extended-Release Tablets 1151
Mevacor Tablets 1996

Loxapine Hydrochloride (Because of its primary CNS effect, caution should be used when carbamazepine is taken with other centrally-acting drugs).
No products indexed under this heading.

Loxapine Succinate (Because of its primary CNS effect, caution should be used when carbamazepine is taken with other centrally-acting drugs).
No products indexed under this heading.

Maprotiline Hydrochloride (Carbamazepine is known to induce CYP1A2 and CYP3A4. Therefore, the potential exists for interaction between carbamazepine and any agent metabolized by one (or more) of these enzymes. Agents that are metabolized by CYP1A2 and CYP3A4 may have decreased plasma levels when administered concomitantly with carbamazepine. Thus, if a patient has been titrated to a stable dosage on one of the agents in these categories, and then begins a course of treatment with carbamazepine, it is reasonable to expect that a dose increase for the concomitant agent may be necessary).
No products indexed under this heading.

Mefloquine Hydrochloride (Antimalarial drugs, such as chloroquine and mefloquine, may antagonize the activity of carbamazepine). Products include:
Lariam Tablets 2790

Meperidine Hydrochloride (Because of its primary CNS effect, caution should be used when carbamazepine is taken with other centrally-acting drugs).
No products indexed under this heading.

Mephenytoin (Carbamazepine is metabolized by CYP3A4. Therefore, the potential exists for interaction between carbamazepine and any agent that induces CYP3A4. Agents that are CYP3A4 inducers may decrease plasma levels of carbamazepine. Thus, if a patient has been titrated to a stable dosage on carbamazepine, and then begins a course of treatment with a CYP3A4 inducers, it is reasonable to expect that a dose increase for carbamazepine may be necessary).
No products indexed under this heading.

Mephobarbital (Because of its primary CNS effect, caution should be used when carbamazepine is taken with other centrally-acting drugs). Products include:
Mebaral Tablets, USP 2483

Meprobamate (Because of its primary CNS effect, caution should be used when carbamazepine is taken with other centrally-acting drugs).
No products indexed under this heading.

Mesoridazine Besylate (Because of its primary CNS effect, caution should be used when carbamazepine is taken with other centrally-acting drugs).
No products indexed under this heading.

Mestranol (Carbamazepine is known to induce CYP1A2 and CYP3A4. Therefore, the potential exists for interaction between carbamazepine and any agent metabolized by one (or more) of these enzymes. Agents that are metabolized by CYP1A2 or CYP3A4 may have decreased plasma levels when administered concomitantly with carbamazepine. Breakthrough bleeding has been reported among patients receiving concomitant oral contraceptives and their reliability may be adversely affected).
No products indexed under this heading.

Methadone Hydrochloride (Carbamazepine is known to induce CYP1A2 and CYP3A4. Therefore, the potential exists for interaction between carbamazepine and any agent metabolized by one (or more) of these enzymes. Agents that are metabolized by CYP1A2 and CYP3A4 may have decreased plasma levels when administered concomitantly with carbamazepine. Thus, if a patient has been titrated to a stable dosage on one of the agents in these categories, and then begins a course of treatment with carbamazepine, it is reasonable to expect that a dose increase for the concomitant agent may be necessary).
No products indexed under this heading.

Methohexital Sodium (Because of its primary CNS effect, caution should be used when carbamazepine is taken with other centrally-acting drugs).
No products indexed under this heading.

Methotrimeprazine (Because of its primary CNS effect, caution should be used when carbamazepine is taken with other centrally-acting drugs).
No products indexed under this heading.

Methoxyflurane (Because of its primary CNS effect, caution should be used when carbamazepine is taken with other centrally-acting drugs).
No products indexed under this heading.

Methsuximide (Carbamazepine is metabolized by CYP3A4. Therefore, the potential exists for interaction between carbamazepine and any agent that induces CYP3A4. Agents that are CYP3A4 inducers may decrease plasma levels of carbamazepine. Thus, if a patient has been titrated to a stable dosage on carbamazepine, and then begins a course of treatment with a CYP3A4 inducers, it is reasonable to expect that a dose increase for carbamazepine may be necessary).
No products indexed under this heading.

Methylprednisolone (Carbamazepine is metabolized by CYP3A4. Therefore, the potential exists for interaction between carbamazepine and any agent that induces CYP3A4. Agents that are CYP3A4 inducers may decrease plasma levels of carbamazepine. Thus, if a patient has been titrated to a stable dosage on carbamazepine, and then begins a course of treatment with a CYP3A4 inducers, it is reasonable to expect that a dose increase for carbamazepine may be necessary).
No products indexed under this heading.

Methylprednisolone Acetate (Carbamazepine is metabolized by CYP3A4. Therefore, the potential exists for interaction between carbamazepine and any agent that induces CYP3A4. Agents that are CYP3A4 inducers may decrease plasma levels of carbamazepine. Thus, if a patient has been titrated to a stable dosage on carbamazepine, and then begins a course of treatment with a CYP3A4 inducers, it is reasonable to expect that a dose increase for carbamazepine may be necessary). Products include:
Depo-Medrol Injectable Suspension 2615
Depo-Medrol Single-Dose Vial 2617

Methylprednisolone Sodium Succinate (Carbamazepine is metabolized by CYP3A4. Therefore, the potential exists for interaction between carbamazepine and any agent that induces CYP3A4. Agents that are CYP3A4 inducers may decrease plasma levels of carbamazepine. Thus, if a patient has been titrated to a stable dosage on carbamazepine, and then begins a course of treatment with a CYP3A4 inducers, it is reasonable to expect that a dose increase for carbamazepine may be necessary).
No products indexed under this heading.

Metronidazole (Carbamazepine is metabolized mainly by CYP3A4 the active carbamazepine 10,11-epoxide, which is futher metabolized to the trans-diol by epoxide hydrolase. Therefore, the potential exists for interaction between carbamazepine and any agent that inhibits CYP3A4 and/or epoxide hydrolase. Agents that are CYP3A4 inhibitors may increase the plasma levels of carbamazepine. Thus, if a patient has been titrated to a stable dosage of carbamazepine, and then begins a course of treatment with a CYP3A4 or epoxide hydrolase inhibitor, it is reasonable to expect that a dose reduction for carbamazepine may be necessary). Products include:
Metrogel 1% 1212
MetroGel-Vaginal Gel 1822
Noritate Cream, 1% 1051

Metronidazole Benzoate (Carbamazepine is metabolized mainly

by CYP3A4 the active carbamazepine 10,11-epoxide, which is futher metabolized to the trans-diol by epoxide hydrolase. Therefore, the potential exists for interaction between carbamazepine and any agent that inhibits CYP3A4 and/or epoxide hydrolase. Agents that are CYP3A4 inhibitors may increase the plasma levels of carbamazepine. Thus, if a patient has been titrated to a stable dosage of carbamazepine, and then begins a course of treatment with a CYP3A4 or epoxide hydrolase inhibitor, it is reasonable to expect that a dose reduction for carbamazepine may be necessary).

No products indexed under this heading.

Metronidazole Hydrochloride (Carbamazepine is metabolized mainly by CYP3A4 the active carbamazepine 10,11-epoxide, which is futher metabolized to the trans-diol by epoxide hydrolase. Therefore, the potential exists for interaction between carbamazepine and any agent that inhibits CYP3A4 and/or epoxide hydrolase. Agents that are CYP3A4 inhibitors may increase the plasma levels of carbamazepine. Thus, if a patient has been titrated to a stable dosage of carbamazepine, and then begins a course of treatment with a CYP3A4 or epoxide hydrolase inhibitor, it is reasonable to expect that a dose reduction for carbamazepine may be necessary).

No products indexed under this heading.

Mexiletine Hydrochloride (Carbamazepine is known to induce CYP1A2 and CYP3A4. Therefore, the potential exists for interaction between carbamazepine and any agent metabolized by one (or more) of these enzymes. Agents that are metabolized by CYP1A2 and CYP3A4 may have decreased plasma levels when administered concomitantly with carbamazepine. Thus, if a patient has been titrated to a stable dosage on one of the agents in these categories, and then begins a course of treatment with carbamazepine, it is reasonable to expect that a dose increase for the concomitant agent may be necessary).

No products indexed under this heading.

Miconazole (Carbamazepine is metabolized mainly by CYP3A4 the active carbamazepine 10,11-epoxide, which is futher metabolized to the trans-diol by epoxide hydrolase. Therefore, the potential exists for interaction between carbamazepine and any agent that inhibits CYP3A4 and/or epoxide hydrolase. Agents that are CYP3A4 inhibitors may increase the plasma levels of carbamazepine. Thus, if a patient has been titrated to a stable dosage of carbamazepine, and then begins a course of treatment with a CYP3A4 or epoxide hydrolase inhibitor, it is reasonable to expect that a dose reduction for carbamazepine may be necessary).

No products indexed under this heading.

Miconazole Nitrate (Carbamazepine is metabolized mainly by CYP3A4 the active carbamazepine 10,11-epoxide, which is futher metabolized to the trans-diol by epoxide hydrolase. Therefore, the potential exists for interaction between carbamazepine and any agent that inhibits CYP3A4 and/or epoxide hydrolase. Agents that are CYP3A4 inhibitors may increase the plasma levels of carbamazepine. Thus, if a patient has been titrated to a stable dosage of carbamazepine, and then begins a course of treatment with a CYP3A4 or epoxide hydrolase inhibitor, it is reasonable to expect that a dose reduction for carbamazepine may be necessary). Products include:

Desenex 674
Desenex Jock Itch Spray Powder 674

Midazolam Hydrochloride (Carbamazepine is known to induce CYP1A2 and CYP3A4. Therefore, the potential exists for interaction between carbamazepine and any agent metabolized by one (or more) of these enzymes. Agents that are metabolized by CYP1A2 and CYP3A4 may have decreased plasma levels when administered concomitantly with carbamazepine. Thus, if a patient has been titrated to a stable dosage on one of the agents in these categories, and then begins a course of treatment with carbamazepine, it is reasonable to expect that a dose increase for the concomitant agent may be necessary).

No products indexed under this heading.

Mirtazapine (Carbamazepine is known to induce CYP1A2 and CYP3A4. Therefore, the potential exists for interaction between carbamazepine and any agent metabolized by one (or more) of these enzymes. Agents that are metabolized by CYP1A2 and CYP3A4 may have decreased plasma levels when administered concomitantly with carbamazepine. Thus, if a patient has been titrated to a stable dosage on one of the agents in these categories, and then begins a course of treatment with carbamazepine, it is reasonable to expect that a dose increase for the concomitant agent may be necessary).

No products indexed under this heading.

Modafinil (Carbamazepine is metabolized by CYP3A4. Therefore, the potential exists for interaction between carbamazepine and any agent that induces CYP3A4. Agents that are CYP3A4 inducers may decrease plasma levels of carbamazepine. Thus, if a patient has been titrated to a stable dosage on carbamazepine, and then begins a course of treatment with a CYP3A4 inducers, it is reasonable to expect that a dose increase for carbamazepine may be necessary). Products include:

Provigil Tablets 1002

Molindone Hydrochloride (Because of its primary CNS effect, caution should be used when carbamazepine is taken with other centrally-acting drugs). Products include:

Moban Tablets 1108

Morphine Sulfate (Because of its primary CNS effect, caution should be used when carbamazepine is taken with other centrally-acting drugs). Products include:

Avinza Capsules 1714
Kadian Capsules 572
MS Contin Tablets 2703

Moxifloxacin Hydrochloride (Carbamazepine is known to induce CYP1A2 and CYP3A4. Therefore, the potential exists for interaction between carbamazepine and any agent metabolized by one (or more) of these enzymes. Agents that are metabolized by CYP1A2 and CYP3A4 may have decreased plasma levels when administered concomitantly with carbamazepine. Thus, if a patient has been titrated to a stable dosage on one of the agents in these categories, and then begins a course of treatment with carbamazepine, it is reasonable to expect that a dose increase for the concomitant agent may be necessary). Products include:

Avelox 2984
Vigamox Ophthalmic Solution 560

Nafcillin Sodium (Carbamazepine is known to induce CYP1A2 and CYP3A4. Therefore, the potential exists for interaction between carbamazepine and any agent metabolized by one (or more) of these enzymes. Agents that are metabolized by CYP1A2 and CYP3A4 may have decreased plasma levels when administered concomitantly with carbamazepine. Thus, if a patient has been titrated to a stable dosage on one of the agents in these categories, and then begins a course of treatment with carbamazepine, it is reasonable to expect that a dose increase for the concomitant agent may be necessary).

No products indexed under this heading.

Naproxen (Carbamazepine is known to induce CYP1A2 and CYP3A4. Therefore, the potential exists for interaction between carbamazepine and any agent metabolized by one (or more) of these enzymes. Agents that are metabolized by CYP1A2 and CYP3A4 may have decreased plasma levels when administered concomitantly with carbamazepine. Thus, if a patient has been titrated to a stable dosage on one of the agents in these categories, and then begins a course of treatment with carbamazepine, it is reasonable to expect that a dose increase for the concomitant agent may be necessary). Products include:

EC-Naprosyn Delayed-Release Tablets 2769
Naprosyn Suspension 2769
Naprosyn Tablets 2769
Prevacid NapraPAC 3277

Naproxen Sodium (Carbamazepine is known to induce CYP1A2 and CYP3A4. Therefore, the potential exists for interaction between carbamazepine and any agent metabolized by one (or more) of these enzymes. Agents that are metabolized by CYP1A2 and CYP3A4 may have decreased plasma levels when administered concomitantly with carbamazepine. Thus, if a patient has been titrated to a stable dosage on one of the agents in these categories, and then begins a course of treatment with carbamazepine, it is reasonable to expect that a dose increase for the concomitant agent may be necessary). Products include:

Aleve Tablets, Caplets and Gelcaps 605
Anaprox Tablets 2769
Anaprox DS Tablets 2769

Nefazodone Hydrochloride (Carbamazepine is metabolized mainly by CYP3A4 the active carbamazepine 10,11-epoxide, which is futher metabolized to the trans-diol by epoxide hydrolase. Therefore, the potential exists for interaction between carbamazepine and any agent that inhibits CYP3A4 and/or epoxide hydrolase. Agents that are CYP3A4 inhibitors may increase the plasma levels of carbamazepine. Thus, if a patient has been titrated to a stable dosage of carbamazepine, and then begins a course of treatment with a CYP3A4 or epoxide hydrolase inhibitor, it is reasonable to expect that a dose reduction for carbamazepine may be necessary).

No products indexed under this heading.

Nelfinavir Mesylate (Carbamazepine is metabolized mainly by CYP3A4 the active carbamazepine 10,11-epoxide, which is futher metabolized to the trans-diol by epoxide hydrolase. Therefore, the potential exists for interaction between carbamazepine and any agent that inhibits CYP3A4 and/or epoxide hydrolase. Agents that are CYP3A4 inhibitors may increase the plasma levels of carbamazepine. Thus, if a patient has been titrated to a stable dosage of carbamazepine, and then begins a course of treatment with a CYP3A4 or epoxide hydrolase inhibitor, it is reasonable to expect that a dose reduction for carbamazepine may be necessary). Products include:

Viracept 2556

Nevirapine (Carbamazepine is metabolized mainly by CYP3A4 the active carbamazepine 10,11-epoxide, which is futher metabolized to the trans-diol by epoxide hydrolase. Therefore, the potential exists for interaction between carbamazepine and any agent that inhibits CYP3A4 and/or epoxide hydrolase. Agents that are CYP3A4 inhibitors may increase the plasma levels of carbamazepine. Thus, if a patient has been titrated to a stable dosage of carbamazepine, and then begins a course of treatment with a CYP3A4 or epoxide hydrolase inhibitor, it is reasonable to expect that a dose reduction for carbamazepine may be necessary). Products include:

Viramune Oral Suspension 903
Viramune Tablets 903

Niacinamide (Carbamazepine is metabolized mainly by CYP3A4 the active carbamazepine 10,11-epoxide, which is futher metabolized to the trans-diol by epoxide hydrolase. Therefore, the potential exists for interaction between carbamazepine and any agent that inhibits CYP3A4 and/or epoxide hydrolase. Agents that are CYP3A4 inhibitors may increase the plasma levels of carbamazepine. Thus, if a patient has been titrated to a stable dosage of carbamazepine, and then begins a course of treatment with a CYP3A4 or epoxide hydrolase inhibitor, it is reasonable to expect that a dose reduction for carbamazepine may be necessary).

No products indexed under this heading.

Nicardipine Hydrochloride (Carbamazepine is known to induce CYP1A2 and CYP3A4. Therefore, the

potential exists for interaction between carbamazepine and any agent metabolized by one (or more) of these enzymes. Agents that are metabolized by CYP1A2 and CYP3A4 may have decreased plasma levels when administered concomitantly with carbamazepine. Thus, if a patient has been titrated to a stable dosage on one of the agents in these categories, and then begins a course of treatment with carbamazepine, it is reasonable to expect that a dose increase for the concomitant agent may be necessary). Products include:

Cardene I.V. 1129

Nicotinamide (Carbamazepine is metabolized mainly by CYP3A4 the active carbamazepine 10,11-epoxide, which is futher metabolized to the trans-diol by epoxide hydrolase. Therefore, the potential exists for interaction between carbamazepine and any agent that inhibits CYP3A4 and/or epoxide hydrolase. Agents that are CYP3A4 inhibitors may increase the plasma levels of carbamazepine. Thus, if a patient has been titrated to a stable dosage of carbamazepine, and then begins a course of treatment with a CYP3A4 or epoxide hydrolase inhibitor, it is reasonable to expect that a dose reduction for carbamazepine may be necessary). Products include:

Nicomide Tablets 3190

Nicotine Polacrilex (Carbamazepine is known to induce CYP1A2 and CYP3A4. Therefore, the potential exists for interaction between carbamazepine and any agent metabolized by one (or more) of these enzymes. Agents that are metabolized by CYP1A2 and CYP3A4 may have decreased plasma levels when administered concomitantly with carbamazepine. Thus, if a patient has been titrated to a stable dosage on one of the agents in these categories, and then begins a course of treatment with carbamazepine, it is reasonable to expect that a dose increase for the concomitant agent may be necessary). Products include:

Commit Lozenges 1625

Nicorette Gum 1632

Nicotine Salicylate (Carbamazepine is known to induce CYP1A2 and CYP3A4. Therefore, the potential exists for interaction between carbamazepine and any agent metabolized by one (or more) of these enzymes. Agents that are metabolized by CYP1A2 and CYP3A4 may have decreased plasma levels when administered concomitantly with carbamazepine. Thus, if a patient has been titrated to a stable dosage on one of the agents in these categories, and then begins a course of treatment with carbamazepine, it is reasonable to expect that a dose increase for the concomitant agent may be necessary).

No products indexed under this heading.

Nicotine Sulfate (Carbamazepine is known to induce CYP1A2 and CYP3A4. Therefore, the potential exists for interaction between carbamazepine and any agent metabolized by one (or more) of these enzymes. Agents that are metabolized by CYP1A2 and CYP3A4 may have decreased plasma levels when administered concomitantly with carbamazepine. Thus, if a patient has been titrated to a stable dosage on one of the agents in these categories, and then begins a course of treatment with carbamazepine, it is reasonable to expect that a dose increase for the concomitant agent may be necessary).

No products indexed under this heading.

Nifedipine (Carbamazepine is metabolized mainly by CYP3A4 the active carbamazepine 10,11-epoxide, which is futher metabolized to the trans-diol by epoxide hydrolase. Therefore, the potential exists for interaction between carbamazepine and any agent that inhibits CYP3A4 and/or epoxide hydrolase. Agents that are CYP3A4 inhibitors may increase the plasma levels of carbamazepine. Thus, if a patient has been titrated to a stable dosage of carbamazepine, and then begins a course of treatment with a CYP3A4 or epoxide hydrolase inhibitor, it is reasonable to expect that a dose reduction for carbamazepine may be necessary). Products include:

Adalat CC Tablets 2978

Nimodipine (Carbamazepine is known to induce CYP1A2 and CYP3A4. Therefore, the potential exists for interaction between carbamazepine and any agent metabolized by one (or more) of these enzymes. Agents that are metabolized by CYP1A2 and CYP3A4 may have decreased plasma levels when administered concomitantly with carbamazepine. Thus, if a patient has been titrated to a stable dosage on one of the agents in these categories, and then begins a course of treatment with carbamazepine, it is reasonable to expect that a dose increase for the concomitant agent may be necessary). Products include:

Nimotop Capsules 774

Nisoldipine (Carbamazepine is known to induce CYP1A2 and CYP3A4. Therefore, the potential exists for interaction between carbamazepine and any agent metabolized by one (or more) of these enzymes. Agents that are metabolized by CYP1A2 and CYP3A4 may have decreased plasma levels when administered concomitantly with carbamazepine. Thus, if a patient has been titrated to a stable dosage on one of the agents in these categories, and then begins a course of treatment with carbamazepine, it is reasonable to expect that a dose increase for the concomitant agent may be necessary). Products include:

Sular Tablets 1163

Nitrendipine (Carbamazepine is known to induce CYP1A2 and CYP3A4. Therefore, the potential exists for interaction between carbamazepine and any agent metabolized by one (or more) of these enzymes. Agents that are metabolized by CYP1A2 and CYP3A4 may have decreased plasma levels when administered concomitantly with carbamazepine. Thus, if a patient has been titrated to a stable dosage on one of the agents in these categories, and then begins a course of treatment with carbamazepine, it is reasonable to expect that a dose increase for the concomitant agent may be necessary).

No products indexed under this heading.

Norethindrone (Carbamazepine is known to induce CYP1A2 and CYP3A4. Therefore, the potential exists for interaction between carbamazepine and any agent metabolized by one (or more) of these enzymes. Agents that are metabolized by CYP1A2 or CYP3A4 may have decreased plasma levels when administered concomitantly with carbamazepine. Breakthrough bleeding has been reported among patients receiving concomitant oral contraceptives and their reliability may be adversely affected). Products include:

Ortho Micronor Tablets 2411

Norethindrone Acetate (Carbamazepine is known to induce CYP1A2 and CYP3A4. Therefore, the potential exists for interaction between carbamazepine and any agent metabolized by one (or more) of these enzymes. Agents that are metabolized by CYP1A2 and CYP3A4 may have decreased plasma levels when administered concomitantly with carbamazepine. Thus, if a patient has been titrated to a stable dosage on one of the agents in these categories, and then begins a course of treatment with carbamazepine, it is reasonable to expect that a dose increase for the concomitant agent may be necessary). Products include:

Activella Tablets 2311

Aygestin Tablets 1062

CombiPatch Transdermal System 2180

Norethynodrel (Carbamazepine is known to induce CYP1A2 and CYP3A4. Therefore, the potential exists for interaction between carbamazepine and any agent metabolized by one (or more) of these enzymes. Agents that are metabolized by CYP1A2 or CYP3A4 may have decreased plasma levels when administered concomitantly with carbamazepine. Breakthrough bleeding has been reported among patients receiving concomitant oral contraceptives and their reliability may be adversely affected).

No products indexed under this heading.

Norfloxacin (Carbamazepine is metabolized mainly by CYP3A4 the active carbamazepine 10,11-epoxide, which is futher metabolized to the trans-diol by epoxide hydrolase. Therefore, the potential exists for interaction between carbamazepine and any agent that inhibits CYP3A4 and/or epoxide hydrolase. Agents that are CYP3A4 inhibitors may increase the plasma levels of carbamazepine. Thus, if a patient has been titrated to a stable dosage of carbamazepine, and then begins a course of treatment with a CYP3A4 or epoxide hydrolase inhibitor, it is reasonable to expect that a dose reduction for carbamazepine may be necessary). Products include:

Noroxin Tablets 2009

Norgestimate (Carbamazepine is known to induce CYP1A2 and CYP3A4. Therefore, the potential exists for interaction between carbamazepine and any agent metabolized by one (or more) of these enzymes. Agents that are metabolized by CYP1A2 or CYP3A4 may have decreased plasma levels when administered concomitantly with carbamazepine. Breakthrough bleeding has been reported among patients receiving concomitant oral contraceptives and their reliability may be adversely affected). Products include:

Ortho-Cyclen/Ortho Tri-Cyclen 2414

Ortho Tri-Cyclen Lo Tablets 2421

Prefest Tablets 1069

Norgestrel (Carbamazepine is known to induce CYP1A2 and CYP3A4. Therefore, the potential exists for interaction between carbamazepine and any agent metabolized by one (or more) of these enzymes. Agents that are metabolized by CYP1A2 or CYP3A4 may have decreased plasma levels when administered concomitantly with carbamazepine. Breakthrough bleeding has been reported among patients receiving concomitant oral contraceptives and their reliability may be adversely affected). Products include:

Lo/Ovral-28 Tablets 3423

Nortriptyline Hydrochloride (Carbamazepine is known to induce CYP1A2 and CYP3A4. Therefore, the potential exists for interaction between carbamazepine and any agent metabolized by one (or more) of these enzymes. Agents that are metabolized by CYP1A2 and CYP3A4 may have decreased plasma levels when administered concomitantly with carbamazepine. Thus, if a patient has been titrated to a stable dosage on one of the agents in these categories, and then begins a course of treatment with carbamazepine, it is reasonable to expect that a dose increase for the concomitant agent may be necessary).

No products indexed under this heading.

Ofloxacin (Carbamazepine is known to induce CYP1A2 and CYP3A4. Therefore, the potential exists for interaction between carbamazepine and any agent metabolized by one (or more) of these enzymes. Agents that are metabolized by CYP1A2 and CYP3A4 may have decreased plasma levels when administered concomitantly with carbamazepine. Thus, if a patient has been titrated to a stable dosage on one of the agents in these categories, and then begins a course of treatment with carbamazepine, it is reasonable to expect that a dose increase for the concomitant agent may be necessary). Products include:

Floxin Otic Singles 1045

Floxin Otic Solution 1043

Olanzapine (Carbamazepine is known to induce CYP1A2 and CYP3A4. Therefore, the potential exists for interaction between carbamazepine and any agent metabolized by one (or more) of these enzymes. Agents that are metabolized by CYP1A2 and CYP3A4 may have decreased plasma levels when administered concomitantly with carbamazepine. Thus, if a patient has been titrated to a stable dosage on one of the agents in these categories, and then begins a course of treatment with carbamazepine, it is reasonable to expect that a dose

increase for the concomitant agent may be necessary). Products include:

- Symbyax Capsules 1788
- Zyprexa Tablets 1798
- Zyprexa IntraMuscular 1798
- Zyprexa ZYDIS Orally Disintegrating Tablets 1798

Omeprazole (Carbamazepine is metabolized mainly by CYP3A4 the active carbamazepine 10,11-epoxide, which is futher metabolized to the trans-diol by epoxide hydrolase. Therefore, the potential exists for interaction between carbamazepine and any agent that inhibits CYP3A4 and/or epoxide hydrolase. Agents that are CYP3A4 inhibitors may increase the plasma levels of carbamazepine. Thus, if a patient has been titrated to a stable dosage of carbamazepine, and then begins a course of treatment with a CYP3A4 or epoxide hydrolase inhibitor, it is reasonable to expect that a dose reduction for carbamazepine may be necessary). Products include:

- Zegerid Powder for Oral Solution 2972

Ondansetron (Carbamazepine is known to induce CYP1A2 and CYP3A4. Therefore, the potential exists for interaction between carbamazepine and any agent metabolized by one (or more) of these enzymes. Agents that are metabolized by CYP1A2 and CYP3A4 may have decreased plasma levels when administered concomitantly with carbamazepine. Thus, if a patient has been titrated to a stable dosage on one of the agents in these categories, and then begins a course of treatment with carbamazepine, it is reasonable to expect that a dose increase for the concomitant agent may be necessary). Products include:

- Zofran ODT Orally Disintegrating Tablets 1613

Ondansetron Hydrochloride (Carbamazepine is known to induce CYP1A2 and CYP3A4. Therefore, the potential exists for interaction between carbamazepine and any agent metabolized by one (or more) of these enzymes. Agents that are metabolized by CYP1A2 and CYP3A4 may have decreased plasma levels when administered concomitantly with carbamazepine. Thus, if a patient has been titrated to a stable dosage on one of the agents in these categories, and then begins a course of treatment with carbamazepine, it is reasonable to expect that a dose increase for the concomitant agent may be necessary). Products include:

- Zofran Injection 1607
- Zofran 1613

Oxazepam (Because of its primary CNS effect, caution should be used when carbamazepine is taken with other centrally-acting drugs).

No products indexed under this heading.

Oxcarbazepine (Carbamazepine is metabolized by CYP3A4. Therefore, the potential exists for interaction between carbamazepine and any agent that induces CYP3A4. Agents that are CYP3A4 inducers may decrease plasma levels of carbamazepine. Thus, if a patient has been titrated to a stable dosage on carbamazepine, and then begins a course of treatment with a CYP3A4 inducers, it is reasonable to expect that a dose increase for carbamazepine may be necessary). Products include:

- Trileptal Oral Suspension 2281
- Trileptal Tablets 2281

Oxycodone Hydrochloride (Because of its primary CNS effect, caution should be used when carbamazepine is taken with other centrally-acting drugs). Products include:

- Combunox Tablets 1183
- OxyContin Tablets 2699
- OxyFast Oral Concentrate Solution 2704
- OxyIR Capsules 2704
- Percocet Tablets 1114
- Percodan Tablets 1115

Paclitaxel (Carbamazepine is known to induce CYP1A2 and CYP3A4. Therefore, the potential exists for interaction between carbamazepine and any agent metabolized by one (or more) of these enzymes. Agents that are metabolized by CYP1A2 and CYP3A4 may have decreased plasma levels when administered concomitantly with carbamazepine. Thus, if a patient has been titrated to a stable dosage on one of the agents in these categories, and then begins a course of treatment with carbamazepine, it is reasonable to expect that a dose increase for the concomitant agent may be necessary).

No products indexed under this heading.

Paroxetine Hydrochloride (Carbamazepine is metabolized mainly by CYP3A4 the active carbamazepine 10,11-epoxide, which is futher metabolized to the trans-diol by epoxide hydrolase. Therefore, the potential exists for interaction between carbamazepine and any agent that inhibits CYP3A4 and/or epoxide hydrolase. Agents that are CYP3A4 inhibitors may increase the plasma levels of carbamazepine. Thus, if a patient has been titrated to a stable dosage of carbamazepine, and then begins a course of treatment with a CYP3A4 or epoxide hydrolase inhibitor, it is reasonable to expect that a dose reduction for carbamazepine may be necessary). Products include:

- Paxil CR Controlled-Release Tablets 1509
- Paxil 1501

Pentobarbital Sodium (Because of its primary CNS effect, caution should be used when carbamazepine is taken with other centrally-acting drugs). Products include:

- Nembutal Sodium Solution, USP 2484

Perphenazine (Because of its primary CNS effect, caution should be used when carbamazepine is taken with other centrally-acting drugs).

No products indexed under this heading.

Phenobarbital (Carbamazepine is metabolized by CYP3A4. Therefore, the potential exists for interaction between carbamazepine and any agent that induces CYP3A4. Agents that are CYP3A4 inducers may decrease plasma levels of carbamazepine. Thus, if a patient has been titrated to a stable dosage on carbamazepine, and then begins a course of treatment with a CYP3A4 inducers, it is reasonable to expect that a dose increase for carbamazepine may be necessary).

No products indexed under this heading.

Phenobarbital Sodium (Carbamazepine is metabolized by CYP3A4. Therefore, the potential exists for interaction between carbamazepine and any agent that induces CYP3A4. Agents that are CYP3A4 inducers may decrease plasma levels of carbamazepine. Thus, if a patient has been titrated to a stable dosage on carbamazepine, and then begins a course of treatment with a CYP3A4 inducers, it is reasonable to expect that a dose increase for carbamazepine may be necessary).

No products indexed under this heading.

Phenytoin (Carbamazepine is metabolized by CYP3A4. Therefore, the potential exists for interaction between carbamazepine and any agent that induces CYP3A4. Agents that are CYP3A4 inducers may decrease plasma levels of carbamazepine. Thus, if a patient has been titrated to a stable dosage on carbamazepine, and then begins a course of treatment with a CYP3A4 inducers, it is reasonable to expect that a dose increase for carbamazepine may be necessary).

No products indexed under this heading.

Phenytoin Sodium (Carbamazepine is metabolized by CYP3A4. Therefore, the potential exists for interaction between carbamazepine and any agent that induces CYP3A4. Agents that are CYP3A4 inducers may decrease plasma levels of carbamazepine. Thus, if a patient has been titrated to a stable dosage on carbamazepine, and then begins a course of treatment with a CYP3A4 inducers, it is reasonable to expect that a dose increase for carbamazepine may be necessary). Products include:

- Phenytek Capsules 2153

Pimozide (Carbamazepine is known to induce CYP1A2 and CYP3A4. Therefore, the potential exists for interaction between carbamazepine and any agent metabolized by one (or more) of these enzymes. Agents that are metabolized by CYP1A2 and CYP3A4 may have decreased plasma levels when administered concomitantly with carbamazepine. Thus, if a patient has been titrated to a stable dosage on one of the agents in these categories, and then begins a course of treatment with carbamazepine, it is reasonable to expect that a dose increase for the concomitant agent may be necessary). Products include:

- Orap Tablets 1220

Polyestradiol Phosphate (Carbamazepine is known to induce CYP1A2 and CYP3A4. Therefore, the potential exists for interaction between carbamazepine and any agent metabolized by one (or more) of these enzymes. Agents that are metabolized by CYP1A2 and CYP3A4 may have decreased plasma levels when administered concomitantly with carbamazepine. Thus, if a patient has been titrated to a stable dosage on one of the agents in these categories, and then begins a course of treatment with carbamazepine, it is reasonable to expect that a dose increase for the concomitant agent may be necessary).

No products indexed under this heading.

Prazepam (Because of its primary CNS effect, caution should be used when carbamazepine is taken with other centrally-acting drugs).

No products indexed under this heading.

Prednisolone Acetate (Carbamazepine is metabolized by CYP3A4. Therefore, the potential exists for interaction between carbamazepine and any agent that induces CYP3A4. Agents that are CYP3A4 inducers may decrease plasma levels of carbamazepine. Thus, if a patient has been titrated to a stable dosage on carbamazepine, and then begins a course of treatment with a CYP3A4 inducers, it is reasonable to expect that a dose increase for carbamazepine may be necessary). Products include:

- Blephamide Ophthalmic Ointment 563
- Blephamide Ophthalmic Suspension 564
- Poly-Pred Liquifilm Ophthalmic Suspension .... ⊙231
- Pred Forte Ophthalmic Suspension .... ⊙233
- Pred Mild Sterile Ophthalmic Suspension .... ⊙236
- Pred-G Ophthalmic Suspension ...... ⊙234
- Pred-G Sterile Ophthalmic Ointment .... ⊙235

Prednisolone Sodium Phosphate (Carbamazepine is metabolized by CYP3A4. Therefore, the potential exists for interaction between carbamazepine and any agent that induces CYP3A4. Agents that are CYP3A4 inducers may decrease plasma levels of carbamazepine. Thus, if a patient has been titrated to a stable dosage on carbamazepine, and then begins a course of treatment with a CYP3A4 inducers, it is reasonable to expect that a dose increase for carbamazepine may be necessary). Products include:

- Pediapred Oral Solution 3319

Prednisolone Tebutate (Carbamazepine is metabolized by CYP3A4. Therefore, the potential exists for interaction between carbamazepine and any agent that induces CYP3A4. Agents that are CYP3A4 inducers may decrease plasma levels of carbamazepine. Thus, if a patient has been titrated to a stable dosage on carbamazepine, and then begins a course of treatment with a CYP3A4 inducers, it is reasonable to expect that a dose increase for carbamazepine may be necessary).

No products indexed under this heading.

Prednisone (Carbamazepine is metabolized by CYP3A4. Therefore, the potential exists for interaction between carbamazepine and any agent that induces CYP3A4. Agents that are CYP3A4 inducers may decrease plasma levels of carbamazepine. Thus, if a patient has been titrated to a stable dosage on carbamazepine, and then begins a course of treatment with a CYP3A4 inducers, it is reasonable to expect that a dose increase for carbamazepine may be necessary).

No products indexed under this heading.

Primidone (Carbamazepine increases the plasma levels of primidone).

No products indexed under this heading.

Prochlorperazine (Because of its primary CNS effect, caution should be used when carbamazepine is taken with other centrally-acting drugs).
No products indexed under this heading.

Promethazine Hydrochloride (Because of its primary CNS effect, caution should be used when carbamazepine is taken with other centrally-acting drugs). Products include:
Phenergan 3438

Propafenone Hydrochloride (Carbamazepine is known to induce CYP1A2 and CYP3A4. Therefore, the potential exists for interaction between carbamazepine and any agent metabolized by one (or more) of these enzymes. Agents that are metabolized by CYP1A2 and CYP3A4 may have decreased plasma levels when administered concomitantly with carbamazepine. Thus, if a patient has been titrated to a stable dosage on one of the agents in these categories, and then begins a course of treatment with carbamazepine, it is reasonable to expect that a dose increase for the concomitant agent may be necessary). Products include:
Rythmol SR Capsules 2736

Propofol (Because of its primary CNS effect, caution should be used when carbamazepine is taken with other centrally-acting drugs). Products include:
Diprivan Injectable Emulsion 676

Propoxyphene Hydrochloride (Carbamazepine is metabolized mainly by CYP3A4 the active carbamazepine 10,11-epoxide, which is futher metabolized to the trans-diol by epoxide hydrolase. Therefore, the potential exists for interaction between carbamazepine and any agent that inhibits CYP3A4 and/or epoxide hydrolase. Agents that are CYP3A4 inhibitors may increase the plasma levels of carbamazepine. Thus, if a patient has been titrated to a stable dosage of carbamazepine, and then begins a course of treatment with a CYP3A4 or epoxide hydrolase inhibitor, it is reasonable to expect that a dose reduction for carbamazepine may be necessary).
No products indexed under this heading.

Propoxyphene Napsylate (Carbamazepine is metabolized mainly by CYP3A4 the active carbamazepine 10,11-epoxide, which is futher metabolized to the trans-diol by epoxide hydrolase. Therefore, the potential exists for interaction between carbamazepine and any agent that inhibits CYP3A4 and/or epoxide hydrolase. Agents that are CYP3A4 inhibitors may increase the plasma levels of carbamazepine. Thus, if a patient has been titrated to a stable dosage of carbamazepine, and then begins a course of treatment with a CYP3A4 or epoxide hydrolase inhibitor, it is reasonable to expect that a dose reduction for carbamazepine may be necessary). Products include:
Darvocet A 500 Tablets 3497

Propranolol Hydrochloride (Carbamazepine is known to induce CYP1A2 and CYP3A4. Therefore, the potential exists for interaction between carbamazepine and any agent metabolized by one (or more) of these enzymes. Agents that are metabolized by CYP1A2 and CYP3A4 may have decreased plasma levels when administered concomitantly with carbamazepine. Thus, if a patient has been titrated to a stable dosage on one of the agents in these categories, and then begins a course of treatment with carbamazepine, it is reasonable to expect that a dose increase for the concomitant agent may be necessary). Products include:
Inderal LA Long-Acting Capsules 3421
InnoPran XL Capsules 2728

Protriptyline Hydrochloride (Carbamazepine is known to induce CYP1A2 and CYP3A4. Therefore, the potential exists for interaction between carbamazepine and any agent metabolized by one (or more) of these enzymes. Agents that are metabolized by CYP1A2 and CYP3A4 may have decreased plasma levels when administered concomitantly with carbamazepine. Thus, if a patient has been titrated to a stable dosage on one of the agents in these categories, and then begins a course of treatment with carbamazepine, it is reasonable to expect that a dose increase for the concomitant agent may be necessary). Products include:
Vivactil Tablets 2350

Pyrimethamine (Anti-malarial drugs, such as chloroquine and mefloquine, may antagonize the activity of carbamazepine). Products include:
Daraprim Tablets 1385

Quazepam (Because of its primary CNS effect, caution should be used when carbamazepine is taken with other centrally-acting drugs).
No products indexed under this heading.

Quetiapine Fumarate (Because of its primary CNS effect, caution should be used when carbamazepine is taken with other centrally-acting drugs). Products include:
Seroquel Tablets 691

Quinidine (Carbamazepine is metabolized mainly by CYP3A4 the active carbamazepine 10,11-epoxide, which is futher metabolized to the trans-diol by epoxide hydrolase. Therefore, the potential exists for interaction between carbamazepine and any agent that inhibits CYP3A4 and/or epoxide hydrolase. Agents that are CYP3A4 inhibitors may increase the plasma levels of carbamazepine. Thus, if a patient has been titrated to a stable dosage of carbamazepine, and then begins a course of treatment with a CYP3A4 or epoxide hydrolase inhibitor, it is reasonable to expect that a dose reduction for carbamazepine may be necessary).
No products indexed under this heading.

Quinidine Gluconate (Carbamazepine is known to induce CYP1A2 and CYP3A4. Therefore, the potential exists for interaction between carbamazepine and any agent metabolized by one (or more) of these enzymes. Agents that are metabolized by CYP1A2 and CYP3A4 may have decreased plasma levels when administered concomitantly with carbamazepine. Thus, if a patient has been titrated to a stable dosage on one of the agents in these categories, and then begins a course of treatment with carbamazepine, it is reasonable to expect that a dose increase for the concomitant agent may be necessary).
No products indexed under this heading.

Quinidine Hydrochloride (Carbamazepine is metabolized mainly by CYP3A4 the active carbamazepine 10,11-epoxide, which is futher metabolized to the trans-diol by epoxide hydrolase. Therefore, the potential exists for interaction between carbamazepine and any agent that inhibits CYP3A4 and/or epoxide hydrolase. Agents that are CYP3A4 inhibitors may increase the plasma levels of carbamazepine. Thus, if a patient has been titrated to a stable dosage of carbamazepine, and then begins a course of treatment with a CYP3A4 or epoxide hydrolase inhibitor, it is reasonable to expect that a dose reduction for carbamazepine may be necessary).
No products indexed under this heading.

Quinidine Polygalacturonate (Carbamazepine is metabolized mainly by CYP3A4 the active carbamazepine 10,11-epoxide, which is futher metabolized to the trans-diol by epoxide hydrolase. Therefore, the potential exists for interaction between carbamazepine and any agent that inhibits CYP3A4 and/or epoxide hydrolase. Agents that are CYP3A4 inhibitors may increase the plasma levels of carbamazepine. Thus, if a patient has been titrated to a stable dosage of carbamazepine, and then begins a course of treatment with a CYP3A4 or epoxide hydrolase inhibitor, it is reasonable to expect that a dose reduction for carbamazepine may be necessary).
No products indexed under this heading.

Quinidine Sulfate (Carbamazepine is metabolized mainly by CYP3A4 the active carbamazepine 10,11-epoxide, which is futher metabolized to the trans-diol by epoxide hydrolase. Therefore, the potential exists for interaction between carbamazepine and any agent that inhibits CYP3A4 and/or epoxide hydrolase. Agents that are CYP3A4 inhibitors may increase the plasma levels of carbamazepine. Thus, if a patient has been titrated to a stable dosage of carbamazepine, and then begins a course of treatment with a CYP3A4 or epoxide hydrolase inhibitor, it is reasonable to expect that a dose reduction for carbamazepine may be necessary).
No products indexed under this heading.

Quinine (Carbamazepine is metabolized mainly by CYP3A4 the active carbamazepine 10,11-epoxide, which is futher metabolized to the trans-diol by epoxide hydrolase. Therefore, the potential exists for interaction between carbamazepine and any agent that inhibits CYP3A4 and/or epoxide hydrolase. Agents that are CYP3A4 inhibitors may increase the plasma levels of carbamazepine. Thus, if a patient has been titrated to a stable dosage of carbamazepine, and then begins a course of treatment with a CYP3A4 or epoxide hydrolase inhibitor, it is reasonable to expect that a dose reduction for carbamazepine may be necessary).
No products indexed under this heading.

Quinine Sulfate (Carbamazepine is metabolized mainly by CYP3A4 the active carbamazepine 10,11-epoxide, which is futher metabolized to the trans-diol by epoxide hydrolase. Therefore, the potential exists for interaction between carbamazepine and any agent that inhibits CYP3A4 and/or epoxide hydrolase. Agents that are CYP3A4 inhibitors may increase the plasma levels of carbamazepine. Thus, if a patient has been titrated to a stable dosage of carbamazepine, and then begins a course of treatment with a CYP3A4 or epoxide hydrolase inhibitor, it is reasonable to expect that a dose reduction for carbamazepine may be necessary).
No products indexed under this heading.

Quinupristin (Carbamazepine is metabolized mainly by CYP3A4 the active carbamazepine 10,11-epoxide, which is futher metabolized to the trans-diol by epoxide hydrolase. Therefore, the potential exists for interaction between carbamazepine and any agent that inhibits CYP3A4 and/or epoxide hydrolase. Agents that are CYP3A4 inhibitors may increase the plasma levels of carbamazepine. Thus, if a patient has been titrated to a stable dosage of carbamazepine, and then begins a course of treatment with a CYP3A4 or epoxide hydrolase inhibitor, it is reasonable to expect that a dose reduction for carbamazepine may be necessary). Products include:
Synercid I.V. 1690

Ranitidine Bismuth Citrate (Carbamazepine is metabolized mainly by CYP3A4 the active carbamazepine 10,11-epoxide, which is futher metabolized to the trans-diol by epoxide hydrolase. Therefore, the potential exists for interaction between carbamazepine and any agent that inhibits CYP3A4 and/or epoxide hydrolase. Agents that are CYP3A4 inhibitors may increase the plasma levels of carbamazepine. Thus, if a patient has been titrated to a stable dosage of carbamazepine, and then begins a course of treatment with a CYP3A4 or epoxide hydrolase inhibitor, it is reasonable to expect that a dose reduction for carbamazepine may be necessary).
No products indexed under this heading.

Ranitidine Hydrochloride (Carbamazepine is metabolized mainly by CYP3A4 the active carbamazepine 10,11-epoxide, which is futher metabolized to the trans-diol by epoxide hydrolase. Therefore, the potential exists for interaction between carbamazepine and any agent that inhibits CYP3A4 and/or epoxide hydrolase. Agents that are CYP3A4 inhibitors may increase the plasma levels of carbamazepine. Thus, if a patient has been titrated to a stable dosage of carbamazepine, and then begins a course of treatment with a CYP3A4 or epoxide hydrolase inhibitor, it is reasonable to expect that a dose reduction for carbamazepine may be necessary). Products include:
Zantac 1597
Zantac Injection 1593

Zantac 75 Tablets 715
Zantac 150 Maximum Strength Tablets 715
Zantac Injection Pharmacy Bulk Package 1595

Remifentanil Hydrochloride (Because of its primary CNS effect, caution should be used when carbamazepine is taken with other centrally-acting drugs).
No products indexed under this heading.

Rifabutin (Carbamazepine is metabolized by CYP3A4. Therefore, the potential exists for interaction between carbamazepine and any agent that induces CYP3A4. Agents that are CYP3A4 inducers may decrease plasma levels of carbamazepine. Thus, if a patient has been titrated to a stable dosage on carbamazepine, and then begins a course of treatment with a CYP3A4 inducers, it is reasonable to expect that a dose increase for carbamazepine may be necessary).
No products indexed under this heading.

Rifampicin (Carbamazepine is metabolized by CYP3A4. Therefore, the potential exists for interaction between carbamazepine and any agent that induces CYP3A4. Agents that are CYP3A4 inducers may decrease plasma levels of carbamazepine. Thus, if a patient has been titrated to a stable dosage on carbamazepine, and then begins a course of treatment with a CYP3A4 inducers, it is reasonable to expect that a dose increase for carbamazepine may be necessary).
No products indexed under this heading.

Rifampin (Carbamazepine is metabolized by CYP3A4. Therefore, the potential exists for interaction between carbamazepine and any agent that induces CYP3A4. Agents that are CYP3A4 inducers may decrease plasma levels of carbamazepine. Thus, if a patient has been titrated to a stable dosage on carbamazepine, and then begins a course of treatment with a CYP3A4 inducers, it is reasonable to expect that a dose increase for carbamazepine may be necessary).
No products indexed under this heading.

Rifapentine (Carbamazepine is metabolized by CYP3A4. Therefore, the potential exists for interaction between carbamazepine and any agent that induces CYP3A4. Agents that are CYP3A4 inducers may decrease plasma levels of carbamazepine. Thus, if a patient has been titrated to a stable dosage on carbamazepine, and then begins a course of treatment with a CYP3A4 inducers, it is reasonable to expect that a dose increase for carbamazepine may be necessary).
No products indexed under this heading.

Riluzole (Carbamazepine is known to induce CYP1A2 and CYP3A4. Therefore, the potential exists for interaction between carbamazepine and any agent metabolized by one (or more) of these enzymes. Agents that are metabolized by CYP1A2 and CYP3A4 may have decreased plasma levels when administered concomitantly with carbamazepine. Thus, if a patient has been titrated to a stable dosage on one of the agents in these categories, and then begins a course of treatment with carbamazepine, it is reasonable to expect that a dose increase for the concomitant agent may be necessary). Products include:
Rilutek Tablets 2945

Risperidone (Because of its primary CNS effect, caution should be used when carbamazepine is taken with other centrally-acting drugs). Products include:
Risperdal Consta Long-Acting Injection 1664
Risperdal M-Tab Orally Disintegrating Tablets 1658
Risperdal 1658

Ritonavir (Carbamazepine is metabolized mainly by CYP3A4 the active carbamazepine 10,11-epoxide, which is futher metabolized to the trans-diol by epoxide hydrolase. Therefore, the potential exists for interaction between carbamazepine and any agent that inhibits CYP3A4 and/or epoxide hydrolase. Agents that are CYP3A4 inhibitors may increase the plasma levels of carbamazepine. Thus, if a patient has been titrated to a stable dosage of carbamazepine, and then begins a course of treatment with a CYP3A4 or epoxide hydrolase inhibitor, it is reasonable to expect that a dose reduction for carbamazepine may be necessary). Products include:
Kaletra 474
Norvir 499

Ropinirole Hydrochloride (Carbamazepine is known to induce CYP1A2 and CYP3A4. Therefore, the potential exists for interaction between carbamazepine and any agent metabolized by one (or more) of these enzymes. Agents that are metabolized by CYP1A2 and CYP3A4 may have decreased plasma levels when administered concomitantly with carbamazepine. Thus, if a patient has been titrated to a stable dosage on one of the agents in these categories, and then begins a course of treatment with carbamazepine, it is reasonable to expect that a dose increase for the concomitant agent may be necessary). Products include:
Requip Tablets 1528

Ropivacaine Hydrochloride (Carbamazepine is known to induce CYP1A2 and CYP3A4. Therefore, the potential exists for interaction between carbamazepine and any agent metabolized by one (or more) of these enzymes. Agents that are metabolized by CYP1A2 and CYP3A4 may have decreased plasma levels when administered concomitantly with carbamazepine. Thus, if a patient has been titrated to a stable dosage on one of the agents in these categories, and then begins a course of treatment with carbamazepine, it is reasonable to expect that a dose increase for the concomitant agent may be necessary). Products include:
Naropin Injection 640

Saquinavir (Carbamazepine is metabolized mainly by CYP3A4 the active carbamazepine 10,11-epoxide, which is futher metabolized to the trans-diol by epoxide hydrolase. Therefore, the potential exists for interaction between carbamazepine and any agent that inhibits CYP3A4 and/or epoxide hydrolase. Agents that are CYP3A4 inhibitors may increase the plasma levels of carbamazepine. Thus, if a patient has been titrated to a stable dosage of carbamazepine, and then begins a course of treatment with a CYP3A4 or epoxide hydrolase inhibitor, it is reasonable to expect that a dose reduction for carbamazepine may be necessary).
No products indexed under this heading.

Saquinavir Mesylate (Carbamazepine is metabolized mainly by CYP3A4 the active carbamazepine 10,11-epoxide, which is futher metabolized to the trans-diol by epoxide hydrolase. Therefore, the potential exists for interaction between carbamazepine and any agent that inhibits CYP3A4 and/or epoxide hydrolase. Agents that are CYP3A4 inhibitors may increase the plasma levels of carbamazepine. Thus, if a patient has been titrated to a stable dosage of carbamazepine, and then begins a course of treatment with a CYP3A4 or epoxide hydrolase inhibitor, it is reasonable to expect that a dose reduction for carbamazepine may be necessary). Products include:
Invirase 2776

Secobarbital Sodium (Because of its primary CNS effect, caution should be used when carbamazepine is taken with other centrally-acting drugs).
No products indexed under this heading.

Sertraline Hydrochloride (Carbamazepine is metabolized mainly by CYP3A4 the active carbamazepine 10,11-epoxide, which is futher metabolized to the trans-diol by epoxide hydrolase. Therefore, the potential exists for interaction between carbamazepine and any agent that inhibits CYP3A4 and/or epoxide hydrolase. Agents that are CYP3A4 inhibitors may increase the plasma levels of carbamazepine. Thus, if a patient has been titrated to a stable dosage of carbamazepine, and then begins a course of treatment with a CYP3A4 or epoxide hydrolase inhibitor, it is reasonable to expect that a dose reduction for carbamazepine may be necessary). Products include:
Zoloft 2581

Sevoflurane (Because of its primary CNS effect, caution should be used when carbamazepine is taken with other centrally-acting drugs). Products include:
Ultane Liquid for Inhalation 526

Sildenafil Citrate (Carbamazepine is known to induce CYP1A2 and CYP3A4. Therefore, the potential exists for interaction between carbamazepine and any agent metabolized by one (or more) of these enzymes. Agents that are metabolized by CYP1A2 and CYP3A4 may have decreased plasma levels when administered concomitantly with carbamazepine. Thus, if a patient has been titrated to a stable dosage on one of the agents in these categories, and then begins a course of treatment with carbamazepine, it is reasonable to expect that a dose increase for the concomitant agent may be necessary). Products include:
Revatio Tablets 2541
Viagra Tablets 2552

Simvastatin (Carbamazepine is known to induce CYP1A2 and CYP3A4. Therefore, the potential exists for interaction between carbamazepine and any agent metabolized by one (or more) of these enzymes. Agents that are metabolized by CYP1A2 and CYP3A4 may have decreased plasma levels when administered concomitantly with carbamazepine. Thus, if a patient has been titrated to a stable dosage on one of the agents in these categories, and then begins a course of treatment with carbamazepine, it is reasonable to expect that a dose increase for the concomitant agent may be necessary). Products include:
Vytorin 10/10 Tablets 2084
Vytorin 10/10 Tablets 3092
Vytorin 10/20 Tablets 2084
Vytorin 10/20 Tablets 3092
Vytorin 10/40 Tablets 3092
Vytorin 10/40 Tablets 2084
Vytorin 10/80 Tablets 2084
Vytorin 10/80 Tablets 3092
Zocor Tablets 2078

Sirolimus (Carbamazepine is known to induce CYP1A2 and CYP3A4. Therefore, the potential exists for interaction between carbamazepine and any agent metabolized by one (or more) of these enzymes. Agents that are metabolized by CYP1A2 and CYP3A4 may have decreased plasma levels when administered concomitantly with carbamazepine. Thus, if a patient has been titrated to a stable dosage on one of the agents in these categories, and then begins a course of treatment with carbamazepine, it is reasonable to expect that a dose increase for the concomitant agent may be necessary). Products include:
Rapamune Oral Solution and Tablets 3472

Sodium Oxybate (Because of its primary CNS effect, caution should be used when carbamazepine is taken with other centrally-acting drugs).
No products indexed under this heading.

Sufentanil Citrate (Because of its primary CNS effect, caution should be used when carbamazepine is taken with other centrally-acting drugs).
No products indexed under this heading.

Sulfinpyrazone (Carbamazepine is metabolized by CYP3A4. Therefore, the potential exists for interaction between carbamazepine and any agent that induces CYP3A4. Agents that are CYP3A4 inducers may decrease plasma levels of carbamazepine. Thus, if a patient has been titrated to a stable dosage on carbamazepine, and then begins a course of treatment with a CYP3A4 inducers, it is reasonable to expect that a dose increase for carbamazepine may be necessary).
No products indexed under this heading.

Tacrine Hydrochloride (Carbamazepine is known to induce CYP1A2 and CYP3A4. Therefore, the potential exists for interaction between carbamazepine and any agent metabolized by one (or more) of these enzymes. Agents that are metabolized by CYP1A2 and CYP3A4 may have decreased plasma levels when administered concomitantly with carbamazepine.

Thus, if a patient has been titrated to a stable dosage on one of the agents in these categories, and then begins a course of treatment with carbamazepine, it is reasonable to expect that a dose increase for the concomitant agent may be necessary).

No products indexed under this heading.

Tacrolimus (Carbamazepine is known to induce CYP1A2 and CYP3A4. Therefore, the potential exists for interaction between carbamazepine and any agent metabolized by one (or more) of these enzymes. Agents that are metabolized by CYP1A2 and CYP3A4 may have decreased plasma levels when administered concomitantly with carbamazepine. Thus, if a patient has been titrated to a stable dosage on one of the agents in these categories, and then begins a course of treatment with carbamazepine, it is reasonable to expect that a dose increase for the concomitant agent may be necessary). Products include:

Prograf Capsules and Injection **624**
Protopic Ointment **629**

Tamoxifen Citrate (Carbamazepine is known to induce CYP1A2 and CYP3A4. Therefore, the potential exists for interaction between carbamazepine and any agent metabolized by one (or more) of these enzymes. Agents that are metabolized by CYP1A2 and CYP3A4 may have decreased plasma levels when administered concomitantly with carbamazepine. Thus, if a patient has been titrated to a stable dosage on one of the agents in these categories, and then begins a course of treatment with carbamazepine, it is reasonable to expect that a dose increase for the concomitant agent may be necessary).

No products indexed under this heading.

Telithromycin (Carbamazepine is metabolized mainly by CYP3A4 the active carbamazepine 10,11-epoxide, which is futher metabolized to the trans-diol by epoxide hydrolase. Therefore, the potential exists for interaction between carbamazepine and any agent that inhibits CYP3A4 and/or epoxide hydrolase. Agents that are CYP3A4 inhibitors may increase the plasma levels of carbamazepine. Thus, if a patient has been titrated to a stable dosage of carbamazepine, and then begins a course of treatment with a CYP3A4 or epoxide hydrolase inhibitor, it is reasonable to expect that a dose reduction for carbamazepine may be necessary). Products include:

Ketek Tablets **2920**

Temazepam (Because of its primary CNS effect, caution should be used when carbamazepine is taken with other centrally-acting drugs).

No products indexed under this heading.

Theophylline (Carbamazepine is metabolized by CYP3A4. Therefore, the potential exists for interaction between carbamazepine and any agent that induces CYP3A4. Agents that are CYP3A4 inducers may decrease plasma levels of carbamazepine. Thus, if a patient has been titrated to a stable dosage on carbamazepine, and then begins a course of treatment with a CYP3A4 inducers, it is reasonable to expect that a dose increase for carbamazepine may be necessary).

No products indexed under this heading.

Theophylline Anhydrous (Carbamazepine is known to induce CYP1A2 and CYP3A4. Therefore, the potential exists for interaction between carbamazepine and any agent metabolized by one (or more) of these enzymes. Agents that are metabolized by CYP1A2 and CYP3A4 may have decreased plasma levels when administered concomitantly with carbamazepine. Thus, if a patient has been titrated to a stable dosage on one of the agents in these categories, and then begins a course of treatment with carbamazepine, it is reasonable to expect that a dose increase for the concomitant agent may be necessary). Products include:

Uniphyl Tablets **2708**

Thiamylal Sodium (Because of its primary CNS effect, caution should be used when carbamazepine is taken with other centrally-acting drugs).

No products indexed under this heading.

Thioridazine Hydrochloride (Because of its primary CNS effect, caution should be used when carbamazepine is taken with other centrally-acting drugs). Products include:

Thioridazine Hydrochloride Tablets **2122**

Thiothixene (Because of its primary CNS effect, caution should be used when carbamazepine is taken with other centrally-acting drugs). Products include:

Thiothixene Capsules **2124**

Tiagabine Hydrochloride (Carbamazepine is known to induce CYP1A2 and CYP3A4. Therefore, the potential exists for interaction between carbamazepine and any agent metabolized by one (or more) of these enzymes. Agents that are metabolized by CYP1A2 and CYP3A4 may have decreased plasma levels when administered concomitantly with carbamazepine. Thus, if a patient has been titrated to a stable dosage on one of the agents in these categories, and then begins a course of treatment with carbamazepine, it is reasonable to expect that a dose increase for the concomitant agent may be necessary). Products include:

Gabitril Tablets **998**

Tolterodine Tartrate (Carbamazepine is known to induce CYP1A2 and CYP3A4. Therefore, the potential exists for interaction between carbamazepine and any agent metabolized by one (or more) of these enzymes. Agents that are metabolized by CYP1A2 and CYP3A4 may have decreased plasma levels when administered concomitantly with carbamazepine. Thus, if a patient has been titrated to a stable dosage on one of the agents in these categories, and then begins a course of treatment with carbamazepine, it is reasonable to expect that a dose increase for the concomitant agent may be necessary). Products include:

Detrol Tablets **2626**
Detrol LA Capsules **2629**

Trazodone Hydrochloride (Carbamazepine is known to induce CYP1A2 and CYP3A4. Therefore, the potential exists for interaction between carbamazepine and any agent metabolized by one (or more) of these enzymes. Agents that are metabolized by CYP1A2 and CYP3A4 may have decreased plasma levels when administered concomitantly with carbamazepine. Thus, if a patient has been titrated to a stable dosage on one of the agents in these categories, and then begins a course of treatment with carbamazepine, it is reasonable to expect that a dose increase for the concomitant agent may be necessary).

No products indexed under this heading.

Triamcinolone (Carbamazepine is metabolized by CYP3A4. Therefore, the potential exists for interaction between carbamazepine and any agent that induces CYP3A4. Agents that are CYP3A4 inducers may decrease plasma levels of carbamazepine. Thus, if a patient has been titrated to a stable dosage on carbamazepine, and then begins a course of treatment with a CYP3A4 inducers, it is reasonable to expect that a dose increase for carbamazepine may be necessary).

No products indexed under this heading.

Triamcinolone Acetonide (Carbamazepine is metabolized by CYP3A4. Therefore, the potential exists for interaction between carbamazepine and any agent that induces CYP3A4. Agents that are CYP3A4 inducers may decrease plasma levels of carbamazepine. Thus, if a patient has been titrated to a stable dosage on carbamazepine, and then begins a course of treatment with a CYP3A4 inducers, it is reasonable to expect that a dose increase for carbamazepine may be necessary). Products include:

Azmacort Inhalation Aerosol **1701**
Nasacort HFA Inhalation Aerosol **2939**
Nasacort AQ Nasal Spray **2937**

Triamcinolone Diacetate (Carbamazepine is metabolized by CYP3A4. Therefore, the potential exists for interaction between carbamazepine and any agent that induces CYP3A4. Agents that are CYP3A4 inducers may decrease plasma levels of carbamazepine. Thus, if a patient has been titrated to a stable dosage on carbamazepine, and then begins a course of treatment with a CYP3A4 inducers, it is reasonable to expect that a dose increase for carbamazepine may be necessary).

No products indexed under this heading.

Triamcinolone Hexacetonide (Carbamazepine is metabolized by CYP3A4. Therefore, the potential exists for interaction between carbamazepine and any agent that induces CYP3A4. Agents that are CYP3A4 inducers may decrease plasma levels of carbamazepine. Thus, if a patient has been titrated to a stable dosage on carbamazepine, and then begins a course of treatment with a CYP3A4 inducers, it is reasonable to expect that a dose increase for carbamazepine may be necessary).

No products indexed under this heading.

Triazolam (Carbamazepine is known to induce CYP1A2 and CYP3A4. Therefore, the potential exists for interaction between carbamazepine and any agent metabolized by one (or more) of these enzymes. Agents that are metabolized by CYP1A2 and CYP3A4 may have decreased plasma levels when administered concomitantly with carbamazepine. Thus, if a patient has been titrated to a stable dosage on one of the agents in these categories, and then begins a course of treatment with carbamazepine, it is reasonable to expect that a dose increase for the concomitant agent may be necessary).

No products indexed under this heading.

Trifluoperazine Hydrochloride (Because of its primary CNS effect, caution should be used when carbamazepine is taken with other centrally-acting drugs).

No products indexed under this heading.

Trimethaphan Camsylate (Carbamazepine is known to induce CYP1A2 and CYP3A4. Therefore, the potential exists for interaction between carbamazepine and any agent metabolized by one (or more) of these enzymes. Agents that are metabolized by CYP1A2 and CYP3A4 may have decreased plasma levels when administered concomitantly with carbamazepine. Thus, if a patient has been titrated to a stable dosage on one of the agents in these categories, and then begins a course of treatment with carbamazepine, it is reasonable to expect that a dose increase for the concomitant agent may be necessary).

No products indexed under this heading.

Trimipramine Maleate (Carbamazepine is known to induce CYP1A2 and CYP3A4. Therefore, the potential exists for interaction between carbamazepine and any agent metabolized by one (or more) of these enzymes. Agents that are metabolized by CYP1A2 and CYP3A4 may have decreased plasma levels when administered concomitantly with carbamazepine. Thus, if a patient has been titrated to a stable dosage on one of the agents in these categories, and then begins a course of treatment with carbamazepine, it is reasonable to expect that a dose increase for the concomitant agent may be necessary). Products include:

Surmontil Capsules **2347**

Troglitazone (Carbamazepine is metabolized mainly by CYP3A4 the active carbamazepine 10,11-epoxide, which is futher metabolized to the trans-diol by epoxide hydrolase. Therefore, the potential exists for interaction between carbamazepine and any agent that inhibits CYP3A4 and/or epoxide hydrolase. Agents that are CYP3A4 inhibitors may increase the plasma levels of carbamazepine. Thus, if a patient has been titrated to a stable dosage of carbamazepine, and then begins a course of treatment with a CYP3A4 or epoxide hydrolase inhibitor, it is reasonable

to expect that a dose reduction for carbamazepine may be necessary).
No products indexed under this heading.

Troleandomycin (Carbamazepine is metabolized mainly by CYP3A4 the active carbamazepine 10,11-epoxide, which is futher metabolized to the trans-diol by epoxide hydrolase. Therefore, the potential exists for interaction between carbamazepine and any agent that inhibits CYP3A4 and/or epoxide hydrolase. Agents that are CYP3A4 inhibitors may increase the plasma levels of carbamazepine. Thus, if a patient has been titrated to a stable dosage of carbamazepine, and then begins a course of treatment with a CYP3A4 or epoxide hydrolase inhibitor, it is reasonable to expect that a dose reduction for carbamazepine may be necessary).
No products indexed under this heading.

Trovafloxacin Mesylate (Carbamazepine is known to induce CYP1A2 and CYP3A4. Therefore, the potential exists for interaction between carbamazepine and any agent metabolized by one (or more) of these enzymes. Agents that are metabolized by CYP1A2 and CYP3A4 may have decreased plasma levels when administered concomitantly with carbamazepine. Thus, if a patient has been titrated to a stable dosage on one of the agents in these categories, and then begins a course of treatment with carbamazepine, it is reasonable to expect that a dose increase for the concomitant agent may be necessary).
No products indexed under this heading.

Valproate Sodium (Carbamazepine is metabolized mainly by CYP3A4 the active carbamazepine 10,11-epoxide, which is futher metabolized to the trans-diol by epoxide hydrolase. Therefore, the potential exists for interaction between carbamazepine and any agent that inhibits CYP3A4 and/or epoxide hydrolase. Agents that are CYP3A4 inhibitors may increase the plasma levels of carbamazepine. Thus, if a patient has been titrated to a stable dosage of carbamazepine, and then begins a course of treatment with a CYP3A4 or epoxide hydrolase inhibitor, it is reasonable to expect that a dose reduction for carbamazepine may be necessary). Products include:
Depacon Injection ... 412

Verapamil Hydrochloride (Carbamazepine is metabolized mainly by CYP3A4 the active carbamazepine 10,11-epoxide, which is futher metabolized to the trans-diol by epoxide hydrolase. Therefore, the potential exists for interaction between carbamazepine and any agent that inhibits CYP3A4 and/or epoxide hydrolase. Agents that are CYP3A4 inhibitors may increase the plasma levels of carbamazepine. Thus, if a patient has been titrated to a stable dosage of carbamazepine, and then begins a course of treatment with a CYP3A4 or epoxide hydrolase inhibitor, it is reasonable to expect that a dose reduction for carbamazepine may be necessary). Products include:
Covera-HS Tablets ... 3135
Tarka Tablets ... 519
Verelan PM Capsules ... 3120

Vinblastine Sulfate (Carbamazepine is known to induce CYP1A2 and CYP3A4. Therefore, the potential exists for interaction between carbamazepine and any agent metabolized by one (or more) of these enzymes. Agents that are metabolized by CYP1A2 and CYP3A4 may have decreased plasma levels when administered concomitantly with carbamazepine. Thus, if a patient has been titrated to a stable dosage on one of the agents in these categories, and then begins a course of treatment with carbamazepine, it is reasonable to expect that a dose increase for the concomitant agent may be necessary).
No products indexed under this heading.

Vincristine Sulfate (Carbamazepine is known to induce CYP1A2 and CYP3A4. Therefore, the potential exists for interaction between carbamazepine and any agent metabolized by one (or more) of these enzymes. Agents that are metabolized by CYP1A2 and CYP3A4 may have decreased plasma levels when administered concomitantly with carbamazepine. Thus, if a patient has been titrated to a stable dosage on one of the agents in these categories, and then begins a course of treatment with carbamazepine, it is reasonable to expect that a dose increase for the concomitant agent may be necessary).
No products indexed under this heading.

Voriconazole (Carbamazepine is metabolized mainly by CYP3A4 the active carbamazepine 10,11-epoxide, which is futher metabolized to the trans-diol by epoxide hydrolase. Therefore, the potential exists for interaction between carbamazepine and any agent that inhibits CYP3A4 and/or epoxide hydrolase. Agents that are CYP3A4 inhibitors may increase the plasma levels of carbamazepine. Thus, if a patient has been titrated to a stable dosage of carbamazepine, and then begins a course of treatment with a CYP3A4 or epoxide hydrolase inhibitor, it is reasonable to expect that a dose reduction for carbamazepine may be necessary). Products include:
VFEND I.V. ... 2543
VFEND Oral Suspension ... 2543
VFEND Tablets ... 2543

Warfarin Sodium (Carbamazepine is known to induce CYP1A2 and CYP3A4. Therefore, the potential exists for interaction between carbamazepine and any agent metabolized by one (or more) of these enzymes. Agents that are metabolized by CYP1A2 or CYP3A4 may have decreased plasma levels when administered concomitantly with carbamazepine. Thus, if a patient has been titrated to a stable dosage on one of the agents in these categories, and then begins a course of treatment with carbamazepine, it is reasonable to expect that a dose increase for the concomitant agent may be necessary. Therefore, warfarin's anticoagulant effect may be reduced in the presence of carbamazepine and dosage adjustment may). Products include:
Coumadin for Injection ... 932
Coumadin Tablets ... 932

Zafirlukast (Carbamazepine is metabolized mainly by CYP3A4 the active carbamazepine 10,11-epoxide, which is futher metabolized to the trans-diol by epoxide hydrolase. Therefore, the potential exists for interaction between carbamazepine and any agent that inhibits CYP3A4 and/or epoxide hydrolase. Agents that are CYP3A4 inhibitors may increase the plasma levels of carbamazepine. Thus, if a patient has been titrated to a stable dosage of carbamazepine, and then begins a course of treatment with a CYP3A4 or epoxide hydrolase inhibitor, it is reasonable to expect that a dose reduction for carbamazepine may be necessary). Products include:
Accolate Tablets ... 663

Zaleplon (Because of its primary CNS effect, caution should be used when carbamazepine is taken with other centrally-acting drugs). Products include:
Sonata Capsules ... 1686

Zileuton (Carbamazepine is metabolized mainly by CYP3A4 the active carbamazepine 10,11-epoxide, which is futher metabolized to the trans-diol by epoxide hydrolase. Therefore, the potential exists for interaction between carbamazepine and any agent that inhibits CYP3A4 and/or epoxide hydrolase. Agents that are CYP3A4 inhibitors may increase the plasma levels of carbamazepine. Thus, if a patient has been titrated to a stable dosage of carbamazepine, and then begins a course of treatment with a CYP3A4 or epoxide hydrolase inhibitor, it is reasonable to expect that a dose reduction for carbamazepine may be necessary).
No products indexed under this heading.

Ziprasidone Hydrochloride (Because of its primary CNS effect, caution should be used when carbamazepine is taken with other centrally-acting drugs). Products include:
Geodon Capsules ... 2514

Zolmitriptan (Carbamazepine is known to induce CYP1A2 and CYP3A4. Therefore, the potential exists for interaction between carbamazepine and any agent metabolized by one (or more) of these enzymes. Agents that are metabolized by CYP1A2 and CYP3A4 may have decreased plasma levels when administered concomitantly with carbamazepine. Thus, if a patient has been titrated to a stable dosage on one of the agents in these categories, and then begins a course of treatment with carbamazepine, it is reasonable to expect that a dose increase for the concomitant agent may be necessary). Products include:
Zomig Nasal Spray ... 718
Zomig Tablets ... 714
Zomig-ZMT Tablets ... 714

Zolpidem Tartrate (Because of its primary CNS effect, caution should be used when carbamazepine is taken with other centrally-acting drugs). Products include:
Ambien Tablets ... 2867

Food Interactions

Alcohol (Because of its primary CNS effect, caution should be used when carbamazepine is taken with alcohol).

Grapefruit (Carbamazepine is metabolized mainly by CYP3A4 the active carbamazepine 10,11-epoxide, which is futher metabolized to the trans-diol by epoxide hydrolase. Therefore, the potential exists for interaction between carbamazepine and any agent that inhibits CYP3A4 and/or epoxide hydrolase. Agents that are CYP3A4 inhibitors may increase the plasma levels of carbamazepine. Thus, if a patient has been titrated to a stable dosage of carbamazepine, and then begins a course of treatment with a CYP3A4 or epoxide hydrolase inhibitor, it is reasonable to expect that a dose reduction for carbamazepine may be necessary).

Grapefruit Juice (Carbamazepine is metabolized mainly by CYP3A4 the active carbamazepine 10,11-epoxide, which is futher metabolized to the trans-diol by epoxide hydrolase. Therefore, the potential exists for interaction between carbamazepine and any agent that inhibits CYP3A4 and/or epoxide hydrolase. Agents that are CYP3A4 inhibitors may increase the plasma levels of carbamazepine. Thus, if a patient has been titrated to a stable dosage of carbamazepine, and then begins a course of treatment with a CYP3A4 or epoxide hydrolase inhibitor, it is reasonable to expect that a dose reduction for carbamazepine may be necessary).

ERBITUX
(Cetuximab) ... 937
None cited in PDR database.

ERTACZO CREAM, 2%
(Sertaconazole Nitrate) ... 2383
None cited in PDR database.

ERYGEL TOPICAL GEL
(Erythromycin) ... 2096
May interact with peeling/desquamating agents. Compounds in these categories include:

Acitretin (Concomitant topical acne therapy should be used with caution because a possible cumulative irritancy may occur, especially with the use of peeling, desquamating or abrasive agents). Products include:
Soriatane Capsules ... 1028

Adapalene (Concomitant topical acne therapy should be used with caution because a possible cumulative irritancy may occur, especially with the use of peeling, desquamating or abrasive agents). Products include:
Differin Cream ... 1210
Differin Gel ... 1211

Azelaic Acid (Concomitant topical acne therapy should be used with caution because a possible cumulative irritancy may occur, especially with the use of peeling, desquamating or abrasive agents). Products include:
Athena Hair System Shampoo ... 767
Finacea Gel ... 1644
Spartan Hair System Shampoo ... 767

Benzoyl Peroxide (Concomitant topical acne therapy should be used with caution because a possible cumulative irritancy may occur, especially with the use of peeling, desquamating or abrasive agents). Products include:
Benzaclin Topical Gel ... 1046
Brevoxyl ... 3212
Brevoxyl ... 3211
Clinac BPO 7 Gel USP ... 1137
Duac Topical Gel ... 3214
Triaz ... 1864

Triaz Pads 1864

Calcipotriene (Concomitant topical acne therapy should be used with caution because a possible cumulative irritancy may occur, especially with the use of peeling, desquamating or abrasive agents). Products include:
- Dovonex Cream 0.005% 3374
- Dovonex Ointment 0.005% 3375
- Dovonex Scalp Solution 0.005% 3375

Clindamycin, Topical (Concomitant topical acne therapy should be used with caution because a possible cumulative irritancy may occur, especially with the use of peeling, desquamating or abrasive agents).
No products indexed under this heading.

Clindamycin Phosphate (Concomitant topical acne therapy should be used with caution because a possible cumulative irritancy may occur, especially with the use of peeling, desquamating or abrasive agents). Products include:
- Benzaclin Topical Gel 1046
- Clindagel 1207
- Clindesse Vaginal Cream 3296
- Clindets Pledgets 3212
- Evoclin Foam, 1% 1025

Clotrimazole, Topical (Concomitant topical acne therapy should be used with caution because a possible cumulative irritancy may occur, especially with the use of peeling, desquamating or abrasive agents).
No products indexed under this heading.

Coal Tar (Concomitant topical acne therapy should be used with caution because a possible cumulative irritancy may occur, especially with the use of peeling, desquamating or abrasive agents). Products include:
- Tegrin Dandruff Shampoo - Extra Conditioning .... ▣637
- Tegrin Dandruff Shampoo - Fresh Herbal .... ▣638
- Tegrin Skin Cream .... ▣638

Erythromycin, Topical (Concomitant topical acne therapy should be used with caution because a possible cumulative irritancy may occur, especially with the use of peeling, desquamating or abrasive agents).
No products indexed under this heading.

Fluorouracil, Topical (Concomitant topical acne therapy should be used with caution because a possible cumulative irritancy may occur, especially with the use of peeling, desquamating or abrasive agents).
No products indexed under this heading.

Hydroquinone (Concomitant topical acne therapy should be used with caution because a possible cumulative irritancy may occur, especially with the use of peeling, desquamating or abrasive agents). Products include:
- Claripel Cream 3212
- Lustra Cream 3287
- Lustra-AF Cream 3287
- Lustra-Ultra Cream 3287
- Tri-Luma Cream 1213

Isotretinoin (Concomitant topical acne therapy should be used with caution because a possible cumulative irritancy may occur, especially with the use of peeling, desquamating or abrasive agents). Products include:
- Accutane Capsules 2740
- Amnesteem Capsules 2126

Mequinol (Concomitant topical acne therapy should be used with caution because a possible cumulative irritancy may occur, especially with the use of peeling, desquamating or abrasive agents). Products include:
- Solage Topical Solution 740

Podofilox (Concomitant topical acne therapy should be used with caution because a possible cumulative irritancy may occur, especially with the use of peeling, desquamating or abrasive agents).
No products indexed under this heading.

Salicylic Acid (Concomitant topical acne therapy should be used with caution because a possible cumulative irritancy may occur, especially with the use of peeling, desquamating or abrasive agents).
No products indexed under this heading.

Sulfur Preparations (Concomitant topical acne therapy should be used with caution because a possible cumulative irritancy may occur, especially with the use of peeling, desquamating or abrasive agents).
No products indexed under this heading.

Tazarotene (Concomitant topical acne therapy should be used with caution because a possible cumulative irritancy may occur, especially with the use of peeling, desquamating or abrasive agents).
No products indexed under this heading.

Tretinoin (Concomitant topical acne therapy should be used with caution because a possible cumulative irritancy may occur, especially with the use of peeling, desquamating or abrasive agents). Products include:
- Avita Cream 2136
- Avita Gel 2138
- Renova 0.02% Cream 2384
- Renova 0.05% Cream 2387
- Retin-A Micro 0.1%/0.04% 2388
- Solage Topical Solution 740
- Tri-Luma Cream 1213
- Vesanoid Capsules 2823

Zalcitabine (Concomitant topical acne therapy should be used with caution because a possible cumulative irritancy may occur, especially with the use of peeling, desquamating or abrasive agents).
No products indexed under this heading.

ERYPED 200 & ERYPED 400

(Erythromycin Ethylsuccinate) 445

See EryPed Drops

ERYPED DROPS

(Erythromycin Ethylsuccinate) 445

May interact with oral anticoagulants, HMG-CoA reductase inhibitors, phenytoin, triazolobenzodiazepines, valproate, xanthines, and certain other agents. Compounds in these categories include:

Alfentanil Hydrochloride (Concurrent use of erythromycin in patients receiving drugs metabolized by the cytochrome P450 system may be associated with elevation in serum levels of alfentanil).
No products indexed under this heading.

Alprazolam (Erythromycin has been reported to decrease the clearance of triazolam and midazolam; may increase the pharmacologic effect of these benzodiazepines). Products include:
- Niravam Orally Disintegrating Tablets 3106
- Xanax XR Tablets 2655

Aminophylline (Co-administration in patients who are receiving high doses of theophylline may be associated with an increase in serum theophylline levels and potential theophylline toxicity).
No products indexed under this heading.

Anisindione (Co-administration has resulted in increased anticoagulant effects). Products include:
- Miradon Tablets 3056

Astemizole (Concurrent use of erythromycin in patients receiving drugs metabolized by the cytochrome P450 system may be associated with elevation in serum levels of astemizole; co-administration is contraindicated).
No products indexed under this heading.

Atorvastatin Calcium (Erythromycin has been reported to increase concentrations of HMG-CoA reductase inhibitors (e.g. lovastatin and simvastatin); rare reports of rhabdomyolysis have been reported in patients taking these drugs concomitantly). Products include:
- Caduet Tablets 2507
- Lipitor Tablets 2495

Bromocriptine Mesylate (Concurrent use of erythromycin in patients receiving drugs metabolized by the cytochrome P450 system may be associated with elevation in serum levels of bromocriptine).
No products indexed under this heading.

Carbamazepine (Concurrent use of erythromycin in patients receiving drugs metabolized by the cytochrome P450 system may be associated with elevation in serum levels of carbamazepine). Products include:
- Carbatrol Capsules 3174
- Equetro Extended-Release Capsules 3178
- Tegretol/Tegretol-XR 2278

Cerivastatin Sodium (Erythromycin has been reported to increase concentrations of HMG-CoA reductase inhibitors (e.g. lovastatin and simvastatin); rare reports of rhabdomyolysis have been reported in patients taking these drugs concomitantly).
No products indexed under this heading.

Cisapride (Post-marketing reports have shown concurrent use of erythromycin and cisapride may result in QT prolongation, cardiac arrhythmias, ventricular tachycardia, ventricular fibrillation, and torsade de pointes; most likely due to the inhibition of hepatic metabolism of cisapride by erythromycin; co-administration is contraindicated).
No products indexed under this heading.

Cyclosporine (Concurrent use of erythromycin in patients receiving drugs metabolized by the cytochrome P450 system may be associated with elevation in serum levels of cyclosporine). Products include:
- Gengraf Capsules 458
- Neoral Soft Gelatin Capsules 2247
- Neoral Oral Solution 2247
- Restasis Ophthalmic Emulsion .... ⊙570
- Sandimmune 2259

Dicumarol (Co-administration has resulted in increased anticoagulant effects).
No products indexed under this heading.

Digoxin (Co-administration has been reported to result in elevated digoxin serum levels). Products include:
- Digitek Tablets 2146
- Lanoxicaps Capsules 1458
- Lanoxin Injection 1462
- Lanoxin Tablets 1468
- Lanoxin Injection Pediatric 1465

Dihydroergotamine Mesylate (Co-administration has been associated in some patients with acute ergot toxicity characterized by severe peripheral vasospasm and dysesthesia). Products include:
- Migranal Nasal Spray 3350

Disopyramide Phosphate (Concurrent use of erythromycin in patients receiving drugs metabolized by the cytochrome P450 system may be associated with elevation in serum levels of disopyramide).
No products indexed under this heading.

Divalproex Sodium (There have been reports of interactions of erythromycin with drugs not thought to be metabolized by CYP3A, including valproate). Products include:
- Depakote Sprinkle Capsules 422
- Depakote Tablets 427
- Depakote ER Tablets 433

Dyphylline (Co-administration in patients who are receiving high doses of theophylline may be associated with an increase in serum theophylline levels and potential theophylline toxicity).
No products indexed under this heading.

Ergotamine Tartrate (Co-administration has been associated in some patients with acute ergot toxicity characterized by severe peripheral vasospasm and dysesthesia).
No products indexed under this heading.

Fluvastatin Sodium (Erythromycin has been reported to increase concentrations of HMG-CoA reductase inhibitors (e.g. lovastatin and simvastatin); rare reports of rhabdomyolysis have been reported in patients taking these drugs concomitantly). Products include:
- Lescol Capsules 2227
- Lescol 2730
- Lescol XL Tablets 2227

Fosphenytoin Sodium (There have been reports of interactions of erythromycin with drugs not thought to be metabolized by CYP3A, including phenytoin).
No products indexed under this heading.

Hexobarbital (There have been reports of interactions of erythromycin with drugs not thought to be metabolized by CYP3A, including hexobarbital).
No products indexed under this heading.

Lovastatin (Erythromycin has been reported to increase concentrations of HMG-CoA reductase inhibitors (e.g. lovastatin and simvastatin); rare reports of rhabdomyolysis have been reported in patients taking these drugs concomitantly). Products include:

Advicor Tablets 1694
Altoprev Extended-Release Tablets 1151
Mevacor Tablets 1996

Midazolam Hydrochloride (Erythromycin has been reported to decrease the clearance of triazolam and midazolam; may increase the pharmacologic effect of these benzodiazepines).
No products indexed under this heading.

Phenytoin (There have been reports of interactions of erythromycin with drugs not thought to be metabolized by CYP3A, including phenytoin).
No products indexed under this heading.

Phenytoin Sodium (There have been reports of interactions of erythromycin with drugs not thought to be metabolized by CYP3A, including phenytoin). Products include:
Phenytek Capsules 2153

Pimozide (Concurrent use of erythromycin in patients receiving drugs metabolized by the cytochrome P450 system may be associated with elevation in serum levels of pimozide; co-administration is contraindicated). Products include:
Orap Tablets 1220

Pravastatin Sodium (Erythromycin has been reported to increase concentrations of HMG-CoA reductase inhibitors (e.g. lovastatin and simvastatin); rare reports of rhabdomyolysis have been reported in patients taking these drugs concomitantly). Products include:
Pravachol Tablets 943

Sildenafil Citrate (Erythromycin has been reported to increase the systemic exposure (AUC) of sildenafil). Products include:
Revatio Tablets 2541
Viagra Tablets 2552

Simvastatin (Erythromycin has been reported to increase concentrations of HMG-CoA reductase inhibitors (e.g. lovastatin and simvastatin); rare reports of rhabdomyolysis have been reported in patients taking these drugs concomitantly). Products include:
Vytorin 10/10 Tablets 2084
Vytorin 10/10 Tablets 3092
Vytorin 10/20 Tablets 2084
Vytorin 10/20 Tablets 3092
Vytorin 10/40 Tablets 3092
Vytorin 10/40 Tablets 2084
Vytorin 10/80 Tablets 2084
Vytorin 10/80 Tablets 3092
Zocor Tablets 2078

Tacrolimus (Concurrent use of erythromycin in patients receiving drugs metabolized by the cytochrome P450 system may be associated with elevation in serum levels of tacrolimus). Products include:
Prograf Capsules and Injection 624
Protopic Ointment 629

Terfenadine (Erythromycin has been reported to significantly alter the metabolism of the nonsedating antihistamine terfenadine when taken concomitantly; rare cases of electrocardiographic QT/QTc interval prolongation, cardiac arrest, torsade de pointes, and other ventricular arrhythmias have been observed; co-administration is contraindicated).
No products indexed under this heading.

Theophylline (Co-administration in patients who are receiving high doses of theophylline may be associated with an increase in serum theophylline levels and potential theophylline toxicity).
No products indexed under this heading.

Theophylline Anhydrous (Co-administration in patients who are receiving high doses of theophylline may be associated with an increase in serum theophylline levels and potential theophylline toxicity). Products include:
Uniphyl Tablets 2708

Theophylline Calcium Salicylate (Co-administration in patients who are receiving high doses of theophylline may be associated with an increase in serum theophylline levels and potential theophylline toxicity).
No products indexed under this heading.

Theophylline Dihydroxypropyl (Glyceryl) (Co-administration in patients who are receiving high doses of theophylline may be associated with an increase in serum theophylline levels and potential theophylline toxicity).
No products indexed under this heading.

Theophylline Ethylenediamine (Co-administration in patients who are receiving high doses of theophylline may be associated with an increase in serum theophylline levels and potential theophylline toxicity).
No products indexed under this heading.

Theophylline Sodium Glycinate (Co-administration in patients who are receiving high doses of theophylline may be associated with an increase in serum theophylline levels and potential theophylline toxicity).
No products indexed under this heading.

Triazolam (Erythromycin has been reported to decrease the clearance of triazolam and midazolam; may increase the pharmacologic effect of these benzodiazepines).
No products indexed under this heading.

Valproate Sodium (There have been reports of interactions of erythromycin with drugs not thought to be metabolized by CYP3A, including valproate). Products include:
Depacon Injection 412

Valproic Acid (There have been reports of interactions of erythromycin with drugs not thought to be metabolized by CYP3A, including valproate). Products include:
Depakene 417

Warfarin Sodium (Co-administration has resulted in increased anticoagulant effects). Products include:
Coumadin for Injection 932
Coumadin Tablets 932

ERYPED CHEWABLE TABLETS

(Erythromycin Ethylsuccinate) 445
See EryPed Drops

ERY-TAB TABLETS

(Erythromycin) 447
May interact with oral anticoagulants, phenytoin, valproate, xanthines, and certain other agents. Compounds in these categories include:

Alfentanil Hydrochloride (Concurrent use of erythromycin in patients receiving drugs metabolized by the cytochrome P450 system may be associated with elevation in serum levels of alfentanil).
No products indexed under this heading.

Aminophylline (Co-administration in patients who are receiving high doses of theophylline may be associated with an increase in serum theophylline levels and potential theophylline toxicity).
No products indexed under this heading.

Anisindione (Co-administration has resulted in increased anticoagulant effects; these effects may be pronounced in the elderly). Products include:
Miradon Tablets 3056

Astemizole (Concurrent use of erythromycin in patients receiving astemizole has been reported to significantly alter the metabolism of astemizole; rare cases of cardiovascular adverse events, including prolonged QT interval, cardiac arrest, torsade de pointes, and other ventricular arrhythmias have been reported; co-administration is contraindicated).
No products indexed under this heading.

Bromocriptine Mesylate (Concurrent use of erythromycin in patients receiving drugs metabolized by the cytochrome P450 system may be associated with elevation in serum levels of bromocriptine).
No products indexed under this heading.

Carbamazepine (Concurrent use of erythromycin in patients receiving drugs metabolized by the cytochrome P450 system may be associated with elevation in serum levels of carbamazepine). Products include:
Carbatrol Capsules 3174
Equetro Extended-Release Capsules 3178
Tegretol/Tegretol-XR 2278

Cisapride (Concurrent use of erythromycin in patients receiving cisapride has been reported to inhibit the metabolism of cisapride; cases of cardiovascular adverse events, including prolonged QT interval, cardiac arrest, torsade de pointes, ventricular tachycardia,ventricular fibrillation and fatalities have been reported; co-administration is contraindicated).
No products indexed under this heading.

Cyclosporine (Concurrent use of erythromycin in patients receiving drugs metabolized by the cytochrome P450 system may be associated with elevation in serum levels of cyclosporine). Products include:
Gengraf Capsules 458
Neoral Soft Gelatin Capsules 2247
Neoral Oral Solution 2247
Restasis Ophthalmic Emulsion 570
Sandimmune 2259

Dicumarol (Co-administration has resulted in increased anticoagulant effects; these effects may be pronounced in the elderly).
No products indexed under this heading.

Digoxin (Co-administration has been reported to result in elevated digoxin serum levels). Products include:
Digitek Tablets 2146
Lanoxicaps Capsules 1458
Lanoxin Injection 1462
Lanoxin Tablets 1468
Lanoxin Injection Pediatric 1465

Dihydroergotamine Mesylate (Co-administration has been associated in some patients with acute ergot toxicity characterized by severe peripheral vasospasm and dysethesia). Products include:
Migranal Nasal Spray 3350

Disopyramide Phosphate (Concurrent use of erythromycin in patients receiving drugs metabolized by the cytochrome P450 system may be associated with elevation in serum levels of disopyramide).
No products indexed under this heading.

Divalproex Sodium (Concurrent use of erythromycin in patients receiving drugs metabolized by the cytochrome P450 system may be associated with elevation in serum levels of valproate). Products include:
Depakote Sprinkle Capsules 422
Depakote Tablets 427
Depakote ER Tablets 433

Dyphylline (Co-administration in patients who are receiving high doses of theophylline may be associated with an increase in serum theophylline levels and potential theophylline toxicity).
No products indexed under this heading.

Ergotamine Tartrate (Co-administration has been associated in some patients with acute ergot toxicity characterized by severe peripheral vasospasm and dysethesia).
No products indexed under this heading.

Fosphenytoin Sodium (Concurrent use of erythromycin in patients receiving drugs metabolized by the cytochrome P450 system may be associated with elevation in serum levels of phenytoin).
No products indexed under this heading.

Hexobarbital (Concurrent use of erythromycin in patients receiving drugs metabolized by the cytochrome P450 system may be associated with elevation in serum levels of hexobarbital).
No products indexed under this heading.

Lovastatin (Concurrent use of erythromycin in patients receiving drugs metabolized by the cytochrome P450 system may be associated with elevation in serum levels of lovastatin). Products include:
Advicor Tablets 1694
Altoprev Extended-Release Tablets 1151
Mevacor Tablets 1996

Midazolam Hydrochloride (Erythromycin has been reported to decrease clearance of midazolam and, thus, may increase the pharmacologic effect of the benzodiazepines).
No products indexed under this heading.

Phenytoin (Concurrent use of erythromycin in patients receiving drugs metabolized by the cytochrome P450 system may be associated with elevation in serum levels of phenytoin).
No products indexed under this heading.

Phenytoin Sodium (Concurrent use of erythromycin in patients receiving drugs metabolized by the cytochrome P450 system may be associated with elevation in serum levels of phenytoin). Products include:
Phenytek Capsules 2153

Tacrolimus (Concurrent use of erythromycin in patients receiving drugs metabolized by the cytochrome P450 system may be associated with elevation in serum levels of tacrolimus). Products include:
Prograf Capsules and Injection 624
Protopic Ointment 629

Terfenadine (Concurrent use of erythromycin in patients receiving terfenadine has been reported to significantly alter the metabolism of terfenadine; rare cases of cardiovascular adverse events, including prolonged QT interval, cardiac arrest, torsade de pointes, other ventricular arrhythmias, and death have been reported; co-administration is contraindicated).
No products indexed under this heading.

Theophylline (Co-administration in patients who are receiving high doses of theophylline may be associated with an increase in serum theophylline levels and potential theophylline toxicity).
No products indexed under this heading.

Theophylline Anhydrous (Co-administration in patients who are receiving high doses of theophylline may be associated with an increase in serum theophylline levels and potential theophylline toxicity). Products include:
Uniphyl Tablets 2708

Theophylline Calcium Salicylate (Co-administration in patients who are receiving high doses of theophylline may be associated with an increase in serum theophylline levels and potential theophylline toxicity).
No products indexed under this heading.

Theophylline Dihydroxypropyl (Glyceryl) (Co-administration in patients who are receiving high doses of theophylline may be associated with an increase in serum theophylline levels and potential theophylline toxicity).
No products indexed under this heading.

Theophylline Ethylenediamine (Co-administration in patients who are receiving high doses of theophylline may be associated with an increase in serum theophylline levels and potential theophylline toxicity).
No products indexed under this heading.

Theophylline Sodium Glycinate (Co-administration in patients who are receiving high doses of theophylline may be associated with an increase in serum theophylline levels and potential theophylline toxicity).
No products indexed under this heading.

Triazolam (Erythromycin has been reported to decrease clearance of triazolam and, thus, may increase the pharmacologic effect of the benzodiazepines).
No products indexed under this heading.

Valproate Sodium (Concurrent use of erythromycin in patients receiving drugs metabolized by the cytochrome P450 system may be associated with elevation in serum levels of valproate). Products include:
Depacon Injection 412

Valproic Acid (Concurrent use of erythromycin in patients receiving drugs metabolized by the cytochrome P450 system may be associated with elevation in serum levels of valproate). Products include:
Depakene 417

Warfarin Sodium (Co-administration has resulted in increased anticoagulant effects; these effects may be pronounced in the elderly). Products include:
Coumadin for Injection 932
Coumadin Tablets 932

ERYTHROCIN STEARATE FILMTAB TABLETS

(Erythromycin Stearate) 452

May interact with oral anticoagulants, HMG-CoA reductase inhibitors, phenytoin, valproate, xanthines, and certain other agents. Compounds in these categories include:

Alfentanil Hydrochloride (Potential for elevated serum alfentanil levels).
No products indexed under this heading.

Aminophylline (Co-administration in patients who are receiving high doses of theophylline may be associated with an increase in serum theophylline levels and potential theophylline toxicity).
No products indexed under this heading.

Anisindione (Co-administration has been reported to result in increased anticoagulant effects). Products include:
Miradon Tablets 3056

Astemizole (Co-administration has produced a significant alteration in astemizole metabolism resulting in rare cases of serious cardiovascular adverse events, including QT prolongation, cardiac arrest, torsade de pointes and death; concurrent use is contraindicated).
No products indexed under this heading.

Atorvastatin Calcium (Co-administration has been reported to increase concentrations of HMG-CoA reductase inhibitors. Rare reports of rhabdomyolysis have also been reported during concurrent therapy). Products include:
Caduet Tablets 2507
Lipitor Tablets 2495

Bromocriptine Mesylate (Potential for elevated serum bromocriptine levels).
No products indexed under this heading.

Carbamazepine (Potential for elevated serum carbamazepine levels). Products include:
Carbatrol Capsules 3174
Equetro Extended-Release Capsules 3178
Tegretol/Tegretol-XR 2278

Cerivastatin Sodium (Co-administration has been reported to increase concentrations of HMG-CoA reductase inhibitors. Rare reports of rhabdomyolysis have also been reported during concurrent therapy).
No products indexed under this heading.

Cilostazol (Potential for elevated serum cilostazol levels). Products include:
Pletal Tablets 2478

Cisapride (Co-administration has produced an inhibition of hepatic metabolism of cisapride metabolism resulting in QT prolongation, cardiac arrhythmias, ventricular tachycardia, ventricular fibrillation, and torsade de pointes; concurrent use is contraindicated).
No products indexed under this heading.

Cyclosporine (Potential for elevated serum cyclosporine levels). Products include:
Gengraf Capsules 458
Neoral Soft Gelatin Capsules 2247
Neoral Oral Solution 2247
Restasis Ophthalmic Emulsion 570
Sandimmune 2259

Dicumarol (Co-administration has been reported to result in increased anticoagulant effects).
No products indexed under this heading.

Digoxin (Co-administration has been reported to result in elevated digoxin serum levels). Products include:
Digitek Tablets 2146
Lanoxicaps Capsules 1458
Lanoxin Injection 1462
Lanoxin Tablets 1468
Lanoxin Injection Pediatric 1465

Dihydroergotamine Mesylate (Co-administration has been reported to result in acute ergot toxicity characterized by severe peripheral vasospasm and dysesthesia). Products include:
Migranal Nasal Spray 3350

Disopyramide Phosphate (Potential for elevated serum disopyramide levels).
No products indexed under this heading.

Divalproex Sodium (Potential for elevated serum valproate levels). Products include:
Depakote Sprinkle Capsules 422
Depakote Tablets 427
Depakote ER Tablets 433

Dyphylline (Co-administration in patients who are receiving high doses of theophylline may be associated with an increase in serum theophylline levels and potential theophylline toxicity).
No products indexed under this heading.

Ergotamine Tartrate (Co-administration has been reported to result in acute ergot toxicity characterized by severe peripheral vasospasm and dysesthesia).
No products indexed under this heading.

Fluvastatin Sodium (Co-administration has been reported to increase concentrations of HMG-CoA reductase inhibitors. Rare reports of rhabdomyolysis have also been reported during concurrent therapy). Products include:
Lescol Capsules 2227
Lescol 2730
Lescol XL Tablets 2227

Fosphenytoin Sodium (Potential for elevated serum phenytoin levels).
No products indexed under this heading.

Hexobarbital (Potential for elevated serum hexobarbital levels).
No products indexed under this heading.

Lovastatin (Co-administration has been reported to increase concentrations of HMG-CoA reductase inhibitors. Rare reports of rhabdomyolysis have also been reported during concurrent therapy). Products include:
Advicor Tablets 1694
Altoprev Extended-Release Tablets 1151
Mevacor Tablets 1996

Methylprednisolone (Potential for elevated serum methylprednisolone levels).
No products indexed under this heading.

Methylprednisolone Acetate (Potential for elevated serum methylprednisolone levels). Products include:
Depo-Medrol Injectable Suspension 2615
Depo-Medrol Single-Dose Vial 2617

Methylprednisolone Sodium Succinate (Potential for elevated serum methylprednisolone levels).
No products indexed under this heading.

Midazolam Hydrochloride (Erythromycin has been reported to decrease the clearance of midazolam and may increase the pharmacologic effect of the benzodiazepine).
No products indexed under this heading.

Phenytoin (Potential for elevated serum phenytoin levels).
No products indexed under this heading.

Phenytoin Sodium (Potential for elevated serum phenytoin levels). Products include:
Phenytek Capsules 2153

Pimozide (Concurrent use is contraindicated). Products include:
Orap Tablets 1220

Pravastatin Sodium (Co-administration has been reported to increase concentrations of HMG-CoA reductase inhibitors. Rare reports of rhabdomyolysis have also been reported during concurrent therapy). Products include:
Pravachol Tablets 943

Quinidine (Potential for elevated serum quinidine levels).
No products indexed under this heading.

Quinidine Gluconate (Potential for elevated serum quinidine levels).
No products indexed under this heading.

Quinidine Hydrochloride (Potential for elevated serum quinidine levels).
No products indexed under this heading.

Quinidine Polygalacturonate (Potential for elevated serum quinidine levels).
No products indexed under this heading.

Quinidine Sulfate (Potential for elevated serum quinidine levels).
No products indexed under this heading.

Rifabutin (Potential for elevated serum rifabutin levels).
No products indexed under this heading.

Sildenafil Citrate (Co-administration has been reported to increase the systemic exposure (AUC) of sildenafil; reduction of sildenafil dosage should be considered). Products include:
Revatio Tablets 2541
Viagra Tablets 2552

Simvastatin (Co-administration has been reported to increase concentrations of HMG-CoA reductase inhibitors. Rare reports of rhabdomyolysis have also been reported during concurrent therapy). Products include:
Vytorin 10/10 Tablets 2084
Vytorin 10/10 Tablets 3092
Vytorin 10/20 Tablets 2084
Vytorin 10/20 Tablets 3092
Vytorin 10/40 Tablets 3092
Vytorin 10/40 Tablets 2084
Vytorin 10/80 Tablets 2084
Vytorin 10/80 Tablets 3092
Zocor Tablets 2078

Tacrolimus (Potential for elevated serum tacrolimus levels). Products include:
Prograf Capsules and Injection 624
Protopic Ointment 629

Terfenadine (Co-administration has produced a significant alteration in terfenadine metabolism resulting in rare cases of serious cardiovascular adverse events, including QT prolongation, cardiac arrest, torsade de pointes and death; concurrent use is contraindicated).
No products indexed under this heading.

Theophylline (Co-administration in patients who are receiving high doses of theophylline may be associated with an increase in serum theophylline levels and potential theophylline toxicity).
No products indexed under this heading.

Theophylline Anhydrous (Co-administration in patients who are receiving high doses of theophylline may be associated with an increase in serum theophylline levels and potential theophylline toxicity). Products include:
Uniphyl Tablets 2708

Theophylline Calcium Salicylate (Co-administration in patients who are receiving high doses of theophylline may be associated with an increase in serum theophylline levels and potential theophylline toxicity).
No products indexed under this heading.

Theophylline Dihydroxypropyl (Glyceryl) (Co-administration in patients who are receiving high doses of theophylline may be associated with an increase in serum theophylline levels and potential theophylline toxicity).
No products indexed under this heading.

Theophylline Ethylenediamine (Co-administration in patients who are receiving high doses of theophylline may be associated with an increase in serum theophylline levels and potential theophylline toxicity).
No products indexed under this heading.

Theophylline Sodium Glycinate (Co-administration in patients who are receiving high doses of theophylline may be associated with an increase in serum theophylline levels and potential theophylline toxicity).
No products indexed under this heading.

Triazolam (Erythromycin has been reported to decrease the clearance of triazolam and may increase the pharmacologic effect of the benzodiazepine).
No products indexed under this heading.

Valproate Sodium (Potential for elevated serum valproate levels). Products include:
Depacon Injection 412

Valproic Acid (Potential for elevated serum valproate levels). Products include:
Depakene 417

Vinblastine Sulfate (Potential for elevated serum vinblastine levels).
No products indexed under this heading.

Warfarin Sodium (Co-administration has been reported to result in increased anticoagulant effects). Products include:
Coumadin for Injection 932
Coumadin Tablets 932

ERYTHROMYCIN BASE FILMTAB TABLETS

(Erythromycin) 454
May interact with oral anticoagulants, phenytoin, valproate, xanthines, and certain other agents. Compounds in these categories include:

Alfentanil Hydrochloride (Potential for elevated serum alfentanil levels).
No products indexed under this heading.

Aminophylline (Co-administration in patients who are receiving high doses of theophylline may be associated with an increase in serum theophylline levels and potential theophylline toxicity).
No products indexed under this heading.

Anisindione (Co-administration has been reported to result in increased anticoagulant effects). Products include:
Miradon Tablets 3056

Astemizole (Co-administration has produced a significant alteration in astemizole metabolism resulting in rare cases of serious cardiovascular adverse events, including QT prolongation, cardiac arrest, torsade de pointes and death; concurrent use is contraindicated).
No products indexed under this heading.

Bromocriptine Mesylate (Potential for elevated serum bromocriptine levels).
No products indexed under this heading.

Carbamazepine (Potential for elevated serum carbamazepine levels). Products include:
Carbatrol Capsules 3174
Equetro Extended-Release Capsules 3178
Tegretol/Tegretol-XR 2278

Cisapride (Co-administration has produced an inhibition of hepatic metabolism of cisapride metabolism resulting in QT prolongation, cardiac arrhythmias, ventricular fibrillation, and torsade de pointes; concurrent use is contraindicated).
No products indexed under this heading.

Cyclosporine (Potential for elevated serum cyclosporine levels). Products include:
Gengraf Capsules 458
Neoral Soft Gelatin Capsules 2247
Neoral Oral Solution 2247
Restasis Ophthalmic Emulsion 570
Sandimmune 2259

Dicumarol (Co-administration has been reported to result in increased anticoagulant effects).
No products indexed under this heading.

Digoxin (Co-administration has been reported to result in elevated digoxin serum levels). Products include:
Digitek Tablets 2146
Lanoxicaps Capsules 1458
Lanoxin Injection 1462
Lanoxin Tablets 1468
Lanoxin Injection Pediatric 1465

Dihydroergotamine Mesylate (Co-administration has been reported to result in acute ergot toxicity characterized by severe peripheral vasospasm and dysesthesia). Products include:
Migranal Nasal Spray 3350

Disopyramide Phosphate (Potential for elevated serum disopyramide levels).
No products indexed under this heading.

Divalproex Sodium (Potential for elevated serum valproate levels). Products include:
Depakote Sprinkle Capsules 422
Depakote Tablets 427
Depakote ER Tablets 433

Dyphylline (Co-administration in patients who are receiving high doses of theophylline may be associated with an increase in serum theophylline levels and potential theophylline toxicity).
No products indexed under this heading.

Ergotamine Tartrate (Co-administration has been reported to result in acute ergot toxicity characterized by severe peripheral vasospasm and dysesthesia).
No products indexed under this heading.

Fosphenytoin Sodium (Potential for elevated serum phenytoin levels).
No products indexed under this heading.

Hexobarbital (Potential for elevated serum hexobarbital levels).
No products indexed under this heading.

Lovastatin (Potential for elevated serum lovastatin levels). Products include:
Advicor Tablets 1694
Altoprev Extended-Release Tablets 1151
Mevacor Tablets 1996

Midazolam Hydrochloride (Erythromycin has been reported to decrease the clearance of midazolam and may increase the pharmacologic effect of benzodiazepine).
No products indexed under this heading.

Phenytoin (Potential for elevated serum phenytoin levels).
No products indexed under this heading.

Phenytoin Sodium (Potential for elevated serum phenytoin levels). Products include:
Phenytek Capsules 2153

Tacrolimus (Potential for elevated serum tacrolimus levels). Products include:
Prograf Capsules and Injection 624
Protopic Ointment 629

Terfenadine (Co-administration has produced a significant alteration in terfenadine metabolism resulting in rare cases of serious cardiovascular events, including QT prolongation, cardiac arrest, torsade de pointes and death; concurrent use is contraindicated).
No products indexed under this heading.

Theophylline (Co-administration in patients who are receiving high doses of theophylline may be associated with an increase in serum theophylline levels and potential theophylline toxicity).
No products indexed under this heading.

Theophylline Anhydrous (Co-administration in patients who are receiving high doses of theophylline may be associated with an increase in serum theophylline levels and potential theophylline toxicity). Products include:
Uniphyl Tablets 2708

Theophylline Calcium Salicylate (Co-administration in patients who are receiving high doses of theophylline may be associated with an increase in serum theophylline levels and potential theophylline toxicity).
No products indexed under this heading.

Theophylline Dihydroxypropyl (Glyceryl) (Co-administration in patients who are receiving high doses of theophylline may be associated with an increase in serum theophylline levels and potential theophylline toxicity).
No products indexed under this heading.

Theophylline Ethylenediamine (Co-administration in patients who are receiving high doses of theophylline may be associated with an increase in serum theophylline levels and potential theophylline toxicity).
No products indexed under this heading.

Theophylline Sodium Glycinate (Co-administration in patients who are receiving high doses of theophylline may be associated with an increase in serum theophylline levels and potential theophylline toxicity).
No products indexed under this heading.

Triazolam (Erythromycin has been reported to decrease the clearance of triazolam and may increase the pharmacologic effect of the benzodiazepine).
No products indexed under this heading.

Valproate Sodium (Potential for elevated serum valproate levels). Products include:
Depacon Injection 412

Valproic Acid (Potential for elevated serum valproate levels). Products include:

Depakene 417

Warfarin Sodium (Co-administration has been reported to result in increased anticoagulant effects). Products include:

Coumadin for Injection 932
Coumadin Tablets 932

ERYTHROMYCIN DELAYED-RELEASE CAPSULES, USP

(Erythromycin) 456

May interact with oral anticoagulants, cytochrome p450 3a substrates (selected), HMG-CoA reductase inhibitors, xanthines, and certain other agents. Compounds in these categories include:

Alfentanil Hydrochloride (Co-administration of erythromycin and a drug primarily matabolized by CYP3A, like alfentanil, may be associated with elevation in drug concentrations that could increase or prolong both the therapeutic and adverse effects of alfentanil).

No products indexed under this heading.

Alprazolam (Erythromycin is a substrate and inhibitor of the 3A isoform subfamily of the cytochrome p450 enzyme system (CYP3A). Co-administration of erythromycin and a drug primarily metabolized by CYP3A may be associated with elevations in drug concentrations that could increase or prolong both the therapeutic and adverse effects of the concomitant drug). Products include:

Niravam Orally Disintegrating Tablets 3106
Xanax XR Tablets 2655

Aminophylline (Concomitant administration with high doses of theophylline may be associated with increased theophylline levels and potential toxicity).

No products indexed under this heading.

Amitriptyline Hydrochloride (Erythromycin is a substrate and inhibitor of the 3A isoform subfamily of the cytochrome p450 enzyme system (CYP3A). Co-administration of erythromycin and a drug primarily metabolized by CYP3A may be associated with elevations in drug concentrations that could increase or prolong both the therapeutic and adverse effects of the concomitant drug).

No products indexed under this heading.

Amlodipine Besylate (Erythromycin is a substrate and inhibitor of the 3A isoform subfamily of the cytochrome p450 enzyme system (CYP3A). Co-administration of erythromycin and a drug primarily metabolized by CYP3A may be associated with elevations in drug concentrations that could increase or prolong both the therapeutic and adverse effects of the concomitant drug). Products include:

Caduet Tablets 2507
Lotrel Capsules 2238
Norvasc Tablets 2529

Anisindione (Increased anticoagulant effects). Products include:

Miradon Tablets 3056

Aprepitant (Erythromycin is a substrate and inhibitor of the 3A isoform subfamily of the cytochrome p450 enzyme system (CYP3A). Co-administration of erythromycin and a drug primarily metabolized by CYP3A may be associated with elevations in drug concentrations that could increase or prolong both the therapeutic and adverse effects of the concomitant drug). Products include:

Emend Capsules 1944

Astemizole (Co-administration is contraindicated).

No products indexed under this heading.

Atorvastatin Calcium (Erythromycin is a substrate and inhibitor of the 3A isoform subfamily of the cytochrome p450 enzyme system (CYP3A). Co-administration of erythromycin and a drug primarily metabolized by CYP3A may be associated with elevations in drug concentrations that could increase or prolong both the therapeutic and adverse effects of the concomitant drug). Products include:

Caduet Tablets 2507
Lipitor Tablets 2495

Bromocriptine Mesylate (Co-administration of erythromycin and a drug primarily matabolized by CYP3A, like bromocriptine, may be associated with elevation in drug concentrations that could increase or prolong both the therapeutic and adverse effects of bromocriptine).

No products indexed under this heading.

Buspirone Hydrochloride (Erythromycin is a substrate and inhibitor of the 3A isoform subfamily of the cytochrome p450 enzyme system (CYP3A). Co-administration of erythromycin and a drug primarily metabolized by CYP3A may be associated with elevations in drug concentrations that could increase or prolong both the therapeutic and adverse effects of the concomitant drug).

No products indexed under this heading.

Busulfan (Erythromycin is a substrate and inhibitor of the 3A isoform subfamily of the cytochrome p450 enzyme system (CYP3A). Co-administration of erythromycin and a drug primarily metabolized by CYP3A may be associated with elevations in drug concentrations that could increase or prolong both the therapeutic and adverse effects of the concomitant drug). Products include:

I.V. Busulfex 1125
Myleran Tablets 1492

Carbamazepine (Elevations in serum erythromycin and carbamazepine concentration). Products include:

Carbatrol Capsules 3174
Equetro Extended-Release Capsules 3178
Tegretol/Tegretol-XR 2278

Cerivastatin Sodium (Erythromycin is a substrate and inhibitor of the 3A isoform subfamily of the cytochrome p450 enzyme system (CYP3A). Co-administration of erythromycin and a drug primarily metabolized by CYP3A may be associated with elevations in drug concentrations that could increase or prolong both the therapeutic and adverse effects of the concomitant drug).

No products indexed under this heading.

Chlorpheniramine (Erythromycin is a substrate and inhibitor of the 3A isoform subfamily of the cytochrome p450 enzyme system (CYP3A). Co-administration of erythromycin and a drug primarily metabolized by CYP3A may be associated with elevations in drug concentrations that could increase or prolong both the therapeutic and adverse effects of the concomitant drug).

No products indexed under this heading.

Chlorpheniramine Maleate (Erythromycin is a substrate and inhibitor of the 3A isoform subfamily of the cytochrome p450 enzyme system (CYP3A). Co-administration of erythromycin and a drug primarily metabolized by CYP3A may be associated with elevations in drug concentrations that could increase or prolong both the therapeutic and adverse effects of the concomitant drug). Products include:

Advil Allergy Sinus Caplets .... ▣737
Advil Multi-Symptom Cold Caplets .... ▣738
BC Allergy Sinus Cold Powder .... ▣612
Contac Severe Cold and Flu Caplets Maximum Strength .... ▣615
Hycomine Compound Tablets 1105
PediaCare Multi-Symptom Cold Liquid .... ▣704
PediaCare NightRest Cough & Cold Liquid .... ▣704
Robitussin Flu Liquid .... ▣752
Robitussin PM Cough & Cold Liquid .... ▣752
Singlet Caplets .... ▣636
Sudafed Sinus & Allergy Tablets .... ▣710
TheraFlu Cold & Cough Hot Liquid .... ▣680
TheraFlu Cold & Sore Throat Hot Liquid .... ▣680
TheraFlu Flu & Sore Throat Hot Liquid .... ▣681
TheraFlu Severe Cold & Cough Hot Liquid .... ▣683
TheraFlu Severe Cold Caplets .... ▣679
TheraFlu Severe Cold Hot Liquid .... ▣682
Triaminic Cold & Allergy Liquid .... ▣685
Triaminic Cold & Cough Liquid .... ▣685
Triaminic Flu, Cough & Fever Liquid .... ▣685
Triaminic Night Time Cough & Cold Liquid .... ▣685
Triaminic Allergy Runny Nose & Congestion Softchews .... ▣688
Triaminic Cold & Cough Softchews .... ▣688
Children's Tylenol Plus Cold NightTime Suspension Liquid 1851
Children's Tylenol Plus Cold & Cough Suspension Liquid and Chewable Tablets 1851
Children's Tylenol Plus Cold Chewable Tablets 1851
Children's Tylenol Plus Flu Suspension Liquid 1853
Tylenol Allergy Complete Multi-Symptom Caplets and Gelcaps with Cool Burst 1844
Multi-Symptom Tylenol Cold Night Time Caplets 1845
Vicks 44M Cough, Cold & Flu Relief 2676
Pediatric Vicks 44m Cough & Cold Relief 2673
Children's Vicks NyQuil Cold/Cough Relief 2671

Chlorpheniramine Polistirex (Erythromycin is a substrate and inhibitor of the 3A isoform subfamily of the cytochrome p450 enzyme system (CYP3A). Co-administration of erythromycin and a drug primarily metabolized by CYP3A may be associated with elevations in drug concentrations that could increase or prolong both the therapeutic and adverse effects of the concomitant drug). Products include:

Tussionex Pennkinetic Extended-Release Suspension 3322

Chlorpheniramine Tannate (Erythromycin is a substrate and inhibitor of the 3A isoform subfamily of the cytochrome p450 enzyme system (CYP3A). Co-administration of erythromycin and a drug primarily metabolized by CYP3A may be associated with elevations in drug concentrations that could increase or prolong both the therapeutic and adverse effects of the concomitant drug).

No products indexed under this heading.

Cilostazol (Co-administration of erythromycin and a drug primarily matabolized by CYP3A, like cilostazol, may be associated with elevation in drug concentrations that could increase or prolong both the therapeutic and adverse effects of cilostazol). Products include:

Pletal Tablets 2478

Cisapride (Co-administration is contraindicated).

No products indexed under this heading.

Clarithromycin (Erythromycin is a substrate and inhibitor of the 3A isoform subfamily of the cytochrome p450 enzyme system (CYP3A). Co-administration of erythromycin and a drug primarily metabolized by CYP3A may be associated with elevations in drug concentrations that could increase or prolong both the therapeutic and adverse effects of the concomitant drug). Products include:

Biaxin/Biaxin XL 402
PREVPAC 3281

Cyclosporine (Elevations in serum erythromycin and cyclosporine concentration). Products include:

Gengraf Capsules 458
Neoral Soft Gelatin Capsules 2247
Neoral Oral Solution 2247
Restasis Ophthalmic Emulsion 570
Sandimmune 2259

Desogestrel (Erythromycin is a substrate and inhibitor of the 3A isoform subfamily of the cytochrome p450 enzyme system (CYP3A). Co-administration of erythromycin and a drug primarily metabolized by CYP3A may be associated with elevations in drug concentrations that could increase or prolong both the therapeutic and adverse effects of the concomitant drug). Products include:

Ortho-Cept Tablets 2395

Dexamethasone (Erythromycin is a substrate and inhibitor of the 3A isoform subfamily of the cytochrome p450 enzyme system (CYP3A). Co-administration of erythromycin and a drug primarily metabolized by CYP3A may be associated with elevations in drug concentrations that could increase or prolong both the therapeutic and adverse effects of the concomitant drug). Products include:

Ciprodex Otic Suspension 555
Decadron Tablets 1929
TobraDex Ophthalmic Ointment 558
TobraDex Ophthalmic Suspension 558

Dexamethasone Acetate (Erythromycin is a substrate and inhibitor of the 3A isoform subfamily of the cytochrome p450 enzyme system (CYP3A). Co-administration of erythromycin and a drug primarily metabolized by CYP3A may be associated with elevations in drug concentrations that could increase or prolong both the therapeutic and adverse effects of the concomitant drug).
No products indexed under this heading.

Dexamethasone Phosphate (Erythromycin is a substrate and inhibitor of the 3A isoform subfamily of the cytochrome p450 enzyme system (CYP3A). Co-administration of erythromycin and a drug primarily metabolized by CYP3A may be associated with elevations in drug concentrations that could increase or prolong both the therapeutic and adverse effects of the concomitant drug).
No products indexed under this heading.

Dexamethasone Sodium (Erythromycin is a substrate and inhibitor of the 3A isoform subfamily of the cytochrome p450 enzyme system (CYP3A). Co-administration of erythromycin and a drug primarily metabolized by CYP3A may be associated with elevations in drug concentrations that could increase or prolong both the therapeutic and adverse effects of the concomitant drug).
No products indexed under this heading.

Dexamethasone Sodium Phosphate (Erythromycin is a substrate and inhibitor of the 3A isoform subfamily of the cytochrome p450 enzyme system (CYP3A). Co-administration of erythromycin and a drug primarily metabolized by CYP3A may be associated with elevations in drug concentrations that could increase or prolong both the therapeutic and adverse effects of the concomitant drug). Products include:
Decadron Phosphate Injection **1931**

Diazepam (Erythromycin is a substrate and inhibitor of the 3A isoform subfamily of the cytochrome p450 enzyme system (CYP3A). Co-administration of erythromycin and a drug primarily metabolized by CYP3A may be associated with elevations in drug concentrations that could increase or prolong both the therapeutic and adverse effects of the concomitant drug). Products include:
Diastat Rectal Delivery System **3344**
Valium Tablets **2822**

Dicumarol (Increased anticoagulant effects).
No products indexed under this heading.

Digoxin (Elevated digoxin serum levels). Products include:
Digitek Tablets **2146**
Lanoxicaps Capsules **1458**
Lanoxin Injection **1462**
Lanoxin Tablets **1468**
Lanoxin Injection Pediatric **1465**

Dihydroergotamine Mesylate (Potential for acute ergot toxicity characterized by severe peripheral vasospasm and dysesthesia). Products include:
Migranal Nasal Spray **3350**

Diltiazem Hydrochloride (Erythromycin is a substrate and inhibitor of the 3A isoform subfamily of the cytochrome p450 enzyme system (CYP3A). Co-administration of erythromycin and a drug primarily metabolized by CYP3A may be associated with elevations in drug concentrations that could increase or prolong both the therapeutic and adverse effects of the concomitant drug). Products include:
Cardizem LA Extended Release Tablets **1699**
Tiazac Capsules **1204**

Diltiazem Maleate (Erythromycin is a substrate and inhibitor of the 3A isoform subfamily of the cytochrome p450 enzyme system (CYP3A). Co-administration of erythromycin and a drug primarily metabolized by CYP3A may be associated with elevations in drug concentrations that could increase or prolong both the therapeutic and adverse effects of the concomitant drug).
No products indexed under this heading.

Disopyramide (Co-administration of erythromycin and a drug primarily matabolized by CYP3A, like disopyramide, may be associated with elevation in drug concentrations that could increase or prolong both the therapeutic and adverse effects of disopyramide).
No products indexed under this heading.

Disopyramide Phosphate (Co-administration of erythromycin and a drug primarily matabolized by CYP3A, like disopyramide, may be associated with elevation in drug concentrations that could increase or prolong both the therapeutic and adverse effects of disopyramide).
No products indexed under this heading.

Doxorubicin Hydrochloride (Erythromycin is a substrate and inhibitor of the 3A isoform subfamily of the cytochrome p450 enzyme system (CYP3A). Co-administration of erythromycin and a drug primarily metabolized by CYP3A may be associated with elevations in drug concentrations that could increase or prolong both the therapeutic and adverse effects of the concomitant drug). Products include:
Adriamycin for Injection, USP **786**
Adriamycin Injection, USP **786**

Dronabinol (Erythromycin is a substrate and inhibitor of the 3A isoform subfamily of the cytochrome p450 enzyme system (CYP3A). Co-administration of erythromycin and a drug primarily metabolized by CYP3A may be associated with elevations in drug concentrations that could increase or prolong both the therapeutic and adverse effects of the concomitant drug). Products include:
Marinol Capsules **3334**

Dyphylline (Concomitant administration with high doses of theophylline may be associated with increased theophylline levels and potential toxicity).
No products indexed under this heading.

Ergotamine Tartrate (Potential for acute ergot toxicity characterized by severe peripheral vasospasm and dysesthesia).
No products indexed under this heading.

Erythromycin Estolate (Erythromycin is a substrate and inhibitor of the 3A isoform subfamily of the cytochrome p450 enzyme system (CYP3A). Co-administration of erythromycin and a drug primarily metabolized by CYP3A may be associated with elevations in drug concentrations that could increase or prolong both the therapeutic and adverse effects of the concomitant drug).
No products indexed under this heading.

Erythromycin Ethylsuccinate (Erythromycin is a substrate and inhibitor of the 3A isoform subfamily of the cytochrome p450 enzyme system (CYP3A). Co-administration of erythromycin and a drug primarily metabolized by CYP3A may be associated with elevations in drug concentrations that could increase or prolong both the therapeutic and adverse effects of the concomitant drug). Products include:
E.E.S. **449**
EryPed **445**

Erythromycin Gluceptate (Erythromycin is a substrate and inhibitor of the 3A isoform subfamily of the cytochrome p450 enzyme system (CYP3A). Co-administration of erythromycin and a drug primarily metabolized by CYP3A may be associated with elevations in drug concentrations that could increase or prolong both the therapeutic and adverse effects of the concomitant drug).
No products indexed under this heading.

Erythromycin Lactobionate (Erythromycin is a substrate and inhibitor of the 3A isoform subfamily of the cytochrome p450 enzyme system (CYP3A). Co-administration of erythromycin and a drug primarily metabolized by CYP3A may be associated with elevations in drug concentrations that could increase or prolong both the therapeutic and adverse effects of the concomitant drug).
No products indexed under this heading.

Erythromycin Stearate (Erythromycin is a substrate and inhibitor of the 3A isoform subfamily of the cytochrome p450 enzyme system (CYP3A). Co-administration of erythromycin and a drug primarily metabolized by CYP3A may be associated with elevations in drug concentrations that could increase or prolong both the therapeutic and adverse effects of the concomitant drug). Products include:
Erythrocin Stearate Filmtab Tablets **452**

Estrogen (Erythromycin is a substrate and inhibitor of the 3A isoform subfamily of the cytochrome p450 enzyme system (CYP3A). Co-administration of erythromycin and a drug primarily metabolized by CYP3A may be associated with elevations in drug concentrations that could increase or prolong both the therapeutic and adverse effects of the concomitant drug).
No products indexed under this heading.

Estrogens, Conjugated (Erythromycin is a substrate and inhibitor of the 3A isoform subfamily of the cytochrome p450 enzyme system (CYP3A). Co-administration of erythromycin and a drug primarily metabolized by CYP3A may be associated with elevations in drug concentrations that could increase or prolong both the therapeutic and adverse effects of the concomitant drug). Products include:
Premarin Intravenous **3440**
Premarin Tablets **3443**
Premarin Vaginal Cream **3449**
Premphase Tablets **3452**
Prempro Tablets **3452**

Estrogens, Conjugated, Synthetic A (Erythromycin is a substrate and inhibitor of the 3A isoform subfamily of the cytochrome p450 enzyme system (CYP3A). Co-administration of erythromycin and a drug primarily metabolized by CYP3A may be associated with elevations in drug concentrations that could increase or prolong both the therapeutic and adverse effects of the concomitant drug). Products include:
Cenestin Tablets, 0.45mg, 0.625mg, 0.9mg, 1.25mg.......... **1063**
Cenestin Tablets, 0.3mg **1063**

Estrogens, Esterified (Erythromycin is a substrate and inhibitor of the 3A isoform subfamily of the cytochrome p450 enzyme system (CYP3A). Co-administration of erythromycin and a drug primarily metabolized by CYP3A may be associated with elevations in drug concentrations that could increase or prolong both the therapeutic and adverse effects of the concomitant drug). Products include:
Estratest Tablets **3196**
Estratest H.S. Tablets **3196**

Ethinyl Estradiol (Erythromycin is a substrate and inhibitor of the 3A isoform subfamily of the cytochrome p450 enzyme system (CYP3A). Co-administration of erythromycin and a drug primarily metabolized by CYP3A may be associated with elevations in drug concentrations that could increase or prolong both the therapeutic and adverse effects of the concomitant drug). Products include:
Alesse-28 Tablets **3392**
Lo/Ovral-28 Tablets **3423**
NuvaRing **2357**
Ortho-Cept Tablets **2395**
Ortho-Cyclen/Ortho Tri-Cyclen **2414**
Ortho Evra Transdermal System **2402**
Ortho Tri-Cyclen Lo Tablets **2421**
Seasonale Tablets **1073**
Triphasil-28 Tablets **3483**
Yasmin 28 Tablets **818**

Ethosuximide (Erythromycin is a substrate and inhibitor of the 3A isoform subfamily of the cytochrome p450 enzyme system (CYP3A). Co-administration of erythromycin and a drug primarily metabolized by CYP3A may be associated with elevations in drug concentrations that could increase or prolong both the therapeutic and adverse effects of the concomitant drug).
No products indexed under this heading.

Ethynodiol Diacetate (Erythromycin is a substrate and inhibitor of the 3A isoform subfamily of the cytochrome p450 enzyme system (CYP3A). Co-administration of erythromycin and a drug primarily metabolized by CYP3A may be associated with elevations in drug concentrations that could increase or prolong both the therapeutic and adverse effects of the concomitant drug).
No products indexed under this heading.

Etoposide (Erythromycin is a substrate and inhibitor of the 3A isoform subfamily of the cytochrome p450 enzyme system (CYP3A). Co-administration of erythromycin and a drug primarily metabolized by CYP3A may be associated with elevations in drug concentrations that could increase or prolong both the therapeutic and adverse effects of the concomitant drug).
No products indexed under this heading.

Etoposide Phosphate (Erythromycin is a substrate and inhibitor of the 3A isoform subfamily of the cytochrome p450 enzyme system (CYP3A). Co-administration of erythromycin and a drug primarily metabolized by CYP3A may be associated with elevations in drug concentrations that could increase or prolong both the therapeutic and adverse effects of the concomitant drug).
No products indexed under this heading.

Felodipine (Erythromycin is a substrate and inhibitor of the 3A isoform subfamily of the cytochrome p450 enzyme system (CYP3A). Co-administration of erythromycin and a drug primarily metabolized by CYP3A may be associated with elevations in drug concentrations that could increase or prolong both the therapeutic and adverse effects of the concomitant drug). Products include:
Plendil Extended-Release Tablets 651

Fentanyl (Erythromycin is a substrate and inhibitor of the 3A isoform subfamily of the cytochrome p450 enzyme system (CYP3A). Co-administration of erythromycin and a drug primarily metabolized by CYP3A may be associated with elevations in drug concentrations that could increase or prolong both the therapeutic and adverse effects of the concomitant drug). Products include:
Duragesic Transdermal System 2448

Fentanyl Citrate (Erythromycin is a substrate and inhibitor of the 3A isoform subfamily of the cytochrome p450 enzyme system (CYP3A). Co-administration of erythromycin and a drug primarily metabolized by CYP3A may be associated with elevations in drug concentrations that could increase or prolong both the therapeutic and adverse effects of the concomitant drug). Products include:
Actiq 993

Fluvastatin Sodium (Erythromycin has been reported to increase concentrations of HMG-CoA reductase inhibitors (e.g., lovastatin and simvastatin); rare reports of rhabdomyolysis have been reported in patients taking these drugs concomitantly). Products include:
Lescol Capsules 2227
Lescol 2730
Lescol XL Tablets 2227

Glyburide (Erythromycin is a substrate and inhibitor of the 3A isoform subfamily of the cytochrome p450 enzyme system (CYP3A). Co-administration of erythromycin and a drug primarily metabolized by CYP3A may be associated with elevations in drug concentrations that could increase or prolong both the therapeutic and adverse effects of the concomitant drug).
No products indexed under this heading.

Haloperidol (Erythromycin is a substrate and inhibitor of the 3A isoform subfamily of the cytochrome p450 enzyme system (CYP3A). Co-administration of erythromycin and a drug primarily metabolized by CYP3A may be associated with elevations in drug concentrations that could increase or prolong both the therapeutic and adverse effects of the concomitant drug).
No products indexed under this heading.

Haloperidol Decanoate (Erythromycin is a substrate and inhibitor of the 3A isoform subfamily of the cytochrome p450 enzyme system (CYP3A). Co-administration of erythromycin and a drug primarily metabolized by CYP3A may be associated with elevations in drug concentrations that could increase or prolong both the therapeutic and adverse effects of the concomitant drug).
No products indexed under this heading.

Hexobarbital (There have been reportd of interactions of erythromyin with drugs not thought to be metaboilzed by CYP3A, including hexobarbital).
No products indexed under this heading.

Imipramine Hydrochloride (Erythromycin is a substrate and inhibitor of the 3A isoform subfamily of the cytochrome p450 enzyme system (CYP3A). Co-administration of erythromycin and a drug primarily metabolized by CYP3A may be associated with elevations in drug concentrations that could increase or prolong both the therapeutic and adverse effects of the concomitant drug).
No products indexed under this heading.

Imipramine Pamoate (Erythromycin is a substrate and inhibitor of the 3A isoform subfamily of the cytochrome p450 enzyme system (CYP3A). Co-administration of erythromycin and a drug primarily metabolized by CYP3A may be associated with elevations in drug concentrations that could increase or prolong both the therapeutic and adverse effects of the concomitant drug).
No products indexed under this heading.

Indinavir Sulfate (Erythromycin is a substrate and inhibitor of the 3A isoform subfamily of the cytochrome p450 enzyme system (CYP3A). Co-administration of erythromycin and a drug primarily metabolized by CYP3A may be associated with elevations in drug concentrations that could increase or prolong both the therapeutic and adverse effects of the concomitant drug). Products include:
Crixivan Capsules 1918

Isradipine (Erythromycin is a substrate and inhibitor of the 3A isoform subfamily of the cytochrome p450 enzyme system (CYP3A). Co-administration of erythromycin and a drug primarily metabolized by CYP3A may be associated with elevations in drug concentrations that could increase or prolong both the therapeutic and adverse effects of the concomitant drug). Products include:
DynaCirc CR Tablets 2726

Itraconazole (Erythromycin is a substrate and inhibitor of the 3A isoform subfamily of the cytochrome p450 enzyme system (CYP3A). Co-administration of erythromycin and a drug primarily metabolized by CYP3A may be associated with elevations in drug concentrations that could increase or prolong both the therapeutic and adverse effects of the concomitant drug).
No products indexed under this heading.

Ketoconazole (Erythromycin is a substrate and inhibitor of the 3A isoform subfamily of the cytochrome p450 enzyme system (CYP3A). Co-administration of erythromycin and a drug primarily metabolized by CYP3A may be associated with elevations in drug concentrations that could increase or prolong both the therapeutic and adverse effects of the concomitant drug). Products include:
Nizoral A-D Shampoo, 1% 1839
Nizoral 2% Shampoo 1838

Levonorgestrel (Erythromycin is a substrate and inhibitor of the 3A isoform subfamily of the cytochrome p450 enzyme system (CYP3A). Co-administration of erythromycin and a drug primarily metabolized by CYP3A may be associated with elevations in drug concentrations that could increase or prolong both the therapeutic and adverse effects of the concomitant drug). Products include:
Alesse-28 Tablets 3392
Climara Pro Transdermal System 800
Mirena Intrauterine System 810
Plan B Tablets 1068
Seasonale Tablets 1073
Triphasil-28 Tablets 3483

Lidocaine (Erythromycin is a substrate and inhibitor of the 3A isoform subfamily of the cytochrome p450 enzyme system (CYP3A). Co-administration of erythromycin and a drug primarily metabolized by CYP3A may be associated with elevations in drug concentrations that could increase or prolong both the therapeutic and adverse effects of the concomitant drug). Products include:
Lidoderm Patch 1107

Lidocaine Hydrochloride (Erythromycin is a substrate and inhibitor of the 3A isoform subfamily of the cytochrome p450 enzyme system (CYP3A). Co-administration of erythromycin and a drug primarily metabolized by CYP3A may be associated with elevations in drug concentrations that could increase or prolong both the therapeutic and adverse effects of the concomitant drug).
No products indexed under this heading.

Lovastatin (Erythromycin has been reported to increase concentrations of HMG-CoA reductase inhibitors. Rare reports of rhabdomyolysis have been reported in patients taking these drugs concomitantly). Products include:
Advicor Tablets 1694
Altoprev Extended-Release Tablets 1151
Mevacor Tablets 1996

Mestranol (Erythromycin is a substrate and inhibitor of the 3A isoform subfamily of the cytochrome p450 enzyme system (CYP3A). Co-administration of erythromycin and a drug primarily metabolized by CYP3A may be associated with elevations in drug concentrations that could increase or prolong both the therapeutic and adverse effects of the concomitant drug).
No products indexed under this heading.

Methadone Hydrochloride (Erythromycin is a substrate and inhibitor of the 3A isoform subfamily of the cytochrome p450 enzyme system (CYP3A). Co-administration of erythromycin and a drug primarily metabolized by CYP3A may be associated with elevations in drug concentrations that could increase or prolong both the therapeutic and adverse effects of the concomitant drug).
No products indexed under this heading.

Methylprednisolone (Co-administration of erythromycin and a drug primarily matabolized by CYP3A, like methylprednisolone, may be associated with elevation in drug concentrations that could increase or prolong both the therapeutic and adverse effects of methylprednisolone).
No products indexed under this heading.

Methylprednisolone Acetate (Co-administration of erythromycin and a drug primarily matabolized by CYP3A, like methylprednisolone, may be associated with elevation in drug concentrations that could increase or prolong both the therapeutic and adverse effects of methylprednisolone). Products include:
Depo-Medrol Injectable Suspension 2615
Depo-Medrol Single-Dose Vial 2617

Methylprednisolone Sodium Succinate (Co-administration of erythromycin and a drug primarily matabolized by CYP3A, like methylprednisolone, may be associated with elevation in drug concentrations that could increase or prolong both the therapeutic and adverse effects of methylprednisolone).
No products indexed under this heading.

Midazolam Hydrochloride (Decreased clearance of midazolam, and thus, may increase the pharmacologic effect of midazolam).
No products indexed under this heading.

Nefazodone Hydrochloride (Erythromycin is a substrate and inhibitor of the 3A isoform subfamily of the cytochrome p450 enzyme system (CYP3A). Co-administration of erythromycin and a drug primarily metabolized by CYP3A may be associated with elevations in drug concentrations that could increase or prolong both the therapeutic and adverse effects of the concomitant drug).
No products indexed under this heading.

Nelfinavir Mesylate (Erythromycin is a substrate and inhibitor of the 3A isoform subfamily of the cytochrome p450 enzyme system (CYP3A). Co-administration of erythromycin and a drug primarily metabolized by CYP3A may be associated with elevations in drug concentrations

that could increase or prolong both the therapeutic and adverse effects of the concomitant drug). Products include:
Viracept 2556

Nicardipine (Erythromycin is a substrate and inhibitor of the 3A isoform subfamily of the cytochrome p450 enzyme system (CYP3A). Co-administration of erythromycin and a drug primarily metabolized by CYP3A may be associated with elevations in drug concentrations that could increase or prolong both the therapeutic and adverse effects of the concomitant drug).
No products indexed under this heading.

Nicardipine Hydrochloride (Erythromycin is a substrate and inhibitor of the 3A isoform subfamily of the cytochrome p450 enzyme system (CYP3A). Co-administration of erythromycin and a drug primarily metabolized by CYP3A may be associated with elevations in drug concentrations that could increase or prolong both the therapeutic and adverse effects of the concomitant drug). Products include:
Cardene I.V. 1129

Nifedipine (Erythromycin is a substrate and inhibitor of the 3A isoform subfamily of the cytochrome p450 enzyme system (CYP3A). Co-administration of erythromycin and a drug primarily metabolized by CYP3A may be associated with elevations in drug concentrations that could increase or prolong both the therapeutic and adverse effects of the concomitant drug). Products include:
Adalat CC Tablets 2978

Nimodipine (Erythromycin is a substrate and inhibitor of the 3A isoform subfamily of the cytochrome p450 enzyme system (CYP3A). Co-administration of erythromycin and a drug primarily metabolized by CYP3A may be associated with elevations in drug concentrations that could increase or prolong both the therapeutic and adverse effects of the concomitant drug). Products include:
Nimotop Capsules 774

Nisoldipine (Erythromycin is a substrate and inhibitor of the 3A isoform subfamily of the cytochrome p450 enzyme system (CYP3A). Co-administration of erythromycin and a drug primarily metabolized by CYP3A may be associated with elevations in drug concentrations that could increase or prolong both the therapeutic and adverse effects of the concomitant drug). Products include:
Sular Tablets 1163

Norethindrone (Erythromycin is a substrate and inhibitor of the 3A isoform subfamily of the cytochrome p450 enzyme system (CYP3A). Co-administration of erythromycin and a drug primarily metabolized by CYP3A may be associated with elevations in drug concentrations that could increase or prolong both the therapeutic and adverse effects of the concomitant drug). Products include:
Ortho Micronor Tablets 2411

Norgestrel (Erythromycin is a substrate and inhibitor of the 3A isoform subfamily of the cytochrome p450 enzyme system (CYP3A). Co-administration of erythromycin and a drug primarily metabolized by CYP3A may be associated with elevations in drug concentrations that could increase or prolong both the therapeutic and adverse effects of the concomitant drug). Products include:
Lo/Ovral-28 Tablets 3423

Ondansetron Hydrochloride (Erythromycin is a substrate and inhibitor of the 3A isoform subfamily of the cytochrome p450 enzyme system (CYP3A). Co-administration of erythromycin and a drug primarily metabolized by CYP3A may be associated with elevations in drug concentrations that could increase or prolong both the therapeutic and adverse effects of the concomitant drug). Products include:
Zofran Injection 1607
Zofran 1613

Paclitaxel (Erythromycin is a substrate and inhibitor of the 3A isoform subfamily of the cytochrome p450 enzyme system (CYP3A). Co-administration of erythromycin and a drug primarily metabolized by CYP3A may be associated with elevations in drug concentrations that could increase or prolong both the therapeutic and adverse effects of the concomitant drug).
No products indexed under this heading.

Phenytoin (There have been reports of interaction of erythromycin with drugs not thought to be metabolized by CYP3A, including phenytoin).
No products indexed under this heading.

Phenytoin Sodium (There have been reports of interaction of erythromycin with drugs not thought to be metabolized by CYP3A, including phenytoin). Products include:
Phenytek Capsules 2153

Pimozide (Co-administration is contraindicated). Products include:
Orap Tablets 1220

Pravastatin Sodium (Erythromycin has been reported to increase concentrations of HMG-CoA reductase inhibitors (e.g., lovastatin and simvastatin); rare reports of rhabdomyolysis have been reported in patients taking these drugs concomitantly). Products include:
Pravachol Tablets 943

Quinidine (Co-administration of erythromycin and a drug primarily matabolized by CYP3A, like quinidine, may be associated with elevation in drug concentrations that could increase or prolong both the therapeutic and adverse effects of quinidine).
No products indexed under this heading.

Quinidine Gluconate (Co-administration of erythromycin and a drug primarily matabolized by CYP3A, like quinidine, may be associated with elevation in drug concentrations that could increase or prolong both the therapeutic and adverse effects of quinidine).
No products indexed under this heading.

Quinidine Hydrochloride (Co-administration of erythromycin and a drug primarily matabolized by CYP3A, like quinidine, may be associated with elevation in drug concentrations that could increase or prolong both the therapeutic and adverse effects of quinidine).
No products indexed under this heading.

Quinidine Polygalacturonate (Co-administration of erythromycin and a drug primarily matabolized by CYP3A, like quinidine, may be associated with elevation in drug concentrations that could increase or prolong both the therapeutic and adverse effects of quinidine).
No products indexed under this heading.

Quinidine Sulfate (Co-administration of erythromycin and a drug primarily matabolized by CYP3A, like quinidine, may be associated with elevation in drug concentrations that could increase or prolong both the therapeutic and adverse effects of quinidine).
No products indexed under this heading.

Quinine (Erythromycin is a substrate and inhibitor of the 3A isoform subfamily of the cytochrome p450 enzyme system (CYP3A). Co-administration of erythromycin and a drug primarily metabolized by CYP3A may be associated with elevations in drug concentrations that could increase or prolong both the therapeutic and adverse effects of the concomitant drug).
No products indexed under this heading.

Quinine Sulfate (Erythromycin is a substrate and inhibitor of the 3A isoform subfamily of the cytochrome p450 enzyme system (CYP3A). Co-administration of erythromycin and a drug primarily metabolized by CYP3A may be associated with elevations in drug concentrations that could increase or prolong both the therapeutic and adverse effects of the concomitant drug).
No products indexed under this heading.

Rifabutin (Co-administration of erythromycin and a drug primarily matabolized by CYP3A, like rifabutin, may be associated with elevation in drug concentrations that could increase or prolong both the therapeutic and adverse effects of rifabutin).
No products indexed under this heading.

Ritonavir (Erythromycin is a substrate and inhibitor of the 3A isoform subfamily of the cytochrome p450 enzyme system (CYP3A). Co-administration of erythromycin and a drug primarily metabolized by CYP3A may be associated with elevations in drug concentrations that could increase or prolong both the therapeutic and adverse effects of the concomitant drug). Products include:
Kaletra 474
Norvir 499

Saquinavir (Erythromycin is a substrate and inhibitor of the 3A isoform subfamily of the cytochrome p450 enzyme system (CYP3A). Co-administration of erythromycin and a drug primarily metabolized by CYP3A may be associated with elevations in drug concentrations that could increase or prolong both the therapeutic and adverse effects of the concomitant drug).
No products indexed under this heading.

Saquinavir Mesylate (Erythromycin is a substrate and inhibitor of the 3A isoform subfamily of the cytochrome p450 enzyme system (CYP3A). Co-administration of erythromycin and a drug primarily metabolized by CYP3A may be associated with elevations in drug concentrations that could increase or prolong both the therapeutic and adverse effects of the concomitant drug). Products include:
Invirase 2776

Sertraline Hydrochloride (Erythromycin is a substrate and inhibitor of the 3A isoform subfamily of the cytochrome p450 enzyme system (CYP3A). Co-administration of erythromycin and a drug primarily metabolized by CYP3A may be associated with elevations in drug concentrations that could increase or prolong both the therapeutic and adverse effects of the concomitant drug). Products include:
Zoloft 2581

Sildenafil Citrate (Erythromycin has been reported to increase the systemic exposure (AUC) of sildenafil; should consider reduction of sildenafil dosage). Products include:
Revatio Tablets 2541
Viagra Tablets 2552

Simvastatin (Erythromycin has been reported to increase concentrations of HMG-CoA reductase inhibitors. Rare reports of rhabdomyolysis have been reported in patients taking these drugs concomitantly). Products include:
Vytorin 10/10 Tablets 2084
Vytorin 10/10 Tablets 3092
Vytorin 10/20 Tablets 2084
Vytorin 10/20 Tablets 3092
Vytorin 10/40 Tablets 3092
Vytorin 10/40 Tablets 2084
Vytorin 10/80 Tablets 2084
Vytorin 10/80 Tablets 3092
Zocor Tablets 2078

Sirolimus (Erythromycin is a substrate and inhibitor of the 3A isoform subfamily of the cytochrome p450 enzyme system (CYP3A). Co-administration of erythromycin and a drug primarily metabolized by CYP3A may be associated with elevations in drug concentrations that could increase or prolong both the therapeutic and adverse effects of the concomitant drug). Products include:
Rapamune Oral Solution and Tablets 3472

Tacrolimus (Co-administration of erythromycin and a drug primarily matabolized by CYP3A, like tacrolimus, may be associated with elevation in drug concentrations that could increase or prolong both the therapeutic and adverse effects of tacrolimus). Products include:
Prograf Capsules and Injection 624
Protopic Ointment 629

Tamoxifen Citrate (Erythromycin is a substrate and inhibitor of the 3A isoform subfamily of the cytochrome p450 enzyme system (CYP3A). Co-administration of erythromycin and a drug primarily metabolized by CYP3A may be associated with elevations in drug concentrations that could increase or prolong both the therapeutic and adverse effects of the concomitant drug).
No products indexed under this heading.

Terfenadine (Potential for altered terfenadine metabolism. Co-administration is contraindicated).
No products indexed under this heading.

Testosterone (Erythromycin is a substrate and inhibitor of the 3A isoform subfamily of the cytochrome p450 enzyme system (CYP3A). Co-administration of erythromycin and a drug primarily metabolized by CYP3A may be associated with elevations in drug concentrations that could increase or prolong both the therapeutic and adverse effects of the concomitant drug). Products include:
AndroGel **3330**
Striant Mucoadhesive **1022**
Testim 1% Gel **722**

Testosterone Cypionate (Erythromycin is a substrate and inhibitor of the 3A isoform subfamily of the cytochrome p450 enzyme system (CYP3A). Co-administration of erythromycin and a drug primarily metabolized by CYP3A may be associated with elevations in drug concentrations that could increase or prolong both the therapeutic and adverse effects of the concomitant drug).
No products indexed under this heading.

Testosterone Enanthate (Erythromycin is a substrate and inhibitor of the 3A isoform subfamily of the cytochrome p450 enzyme system (CYP3A). Co-administration of erythromycin and a drug primarily metabolized by CYP3A may be associated with elevations in drug concentrations that could increase or prolong both the therapeutic and adverse effects of the concomitant drug). Products include:
Delatestryl Injection **2976**

Testosterone Propionate (Erythromycin is a substrate and inhibitor of the 3A isoform subfamily of the cytochrome p450 enzyme system (CYP3A). Co-administration of erythromycin and a drug primarily metabolized by CYP3A may be associated with elevations in drug concentrations that could increase or prolong both the therapeutic and adverse effects of the concomitant drug).
No products indexed under this heading.

Theophylline (Concomitant administration with high doses of theophylline may be associated with increased theophylline levels and potential toxicity).
No products indexed under this heading.

Theophylline Anhydrous (Concomitant administration with high doses of theophylline may be associated with increased theophylline levels and potential toxicity). Products include:
Uniphyl Tablets **2708**

Theophylline Calcium Salicylate (Concomitant administration with high doses of theophylline may be associated with increased theophylline levels and potential toxicity).
No products indexed under this heading.

Theophylline Dihydroxypropyl (Glyceryl) (Concomitant administration with high doses of theophylline may be associated with increased theophylline levels and potential toxicity).
No products indexed under this heading.

Theophylline Ethylenediamine (Concomitant administration with high doses of theophylline may be associated with increased theophylline levels and potential toxicity).
No products indexed under this heading.

Theophylline Sodium Glycinate (Concomitant administration with high doses of theophylline may be associated with increased theophylline levels and potential toxicity).
No products indexed under this heading.

Tiagabine Hydrochloride (Erythromycin is a substrate and inhibitor of the 3A isoform subfamily of the cytochrome p450 enzyme system (CYP3A). Co-administration of erythromycin and a drug primarily metabolized by CYP3A may be associated with elevations in drug concentrations that could increase or prolong both the therapeutic and adverse effects of the concomitant drug). Products include:
Gabitril Tablets **998**

Tolterodine Tartrate (Erythromycin is a substrate and inhibitor of the 3A isoform subfamily of the cytochrome p450 enzyme system (CYP3A). Co-administration of erythromycin and a drug primarily metabolized by CYP3A may be associated with elevations in drug concentrations that could increase or prolong both the therapeutic and adverse effects of the concomitant drug). Products include:
Detrol Tablets **2626**
Detrol LA Capsules **2629**

Trazodone Hydrochloride (Erythromycin is a substrate and inhibitor of the 3A isoform subfamily of the cytochrome p450 enzyme system (CYP3A). Co-administration of erythromycin and a drug primarily metabolized by CYP3A may be associated with elevations in drug concentrations that could increase or prolong both the therapeutic and adverse effects of the concomitant drug).
No products indexed under this heading.

Triazolam (Decreased clearance of triazolam, and thus, may increase the pharmacologic effect of triazolam).
No products indexed under this heading.

Valproate Sodium (There have been reports of interaction of erythromycin with drugs not thought to be metabolized by CYP3A, including valproate). Products include:
Depacon Injection **412**

Venlafaxine Hydrochloride (Erythromycin is a substrate and inhibitor of the 3A isoform subfamily of the cytochrome p450 enzyme system (CYP3A). Co-administration of erythromycin and a drug primarily metabolized by CYP3A may be associated with elevations in drug concentrations that could increase or prolong both the therapeutic and adverse effects of the concomitant drug). Products include:
Effexor Tablets **3405**
Effexor XR Capsules **3411**

Verapamil Hydrochloride (Erythromycin is a substrate and inhibitor of the 3A isoform subfamily of the cytochrome p450 enzyme system (CYP3A). Co-administration of erythromycin and a drug primarily metabolized by CYP3A may be associated with elevations in drug concentrations that could increase or prolong both the therapeutic and adverse effects of the concomitant drug). Products include:
Covera-HS Tablets **3135**
Tarka Tablets **519**
Verelan PM Capsules **3120**

Vinblastine Sulfate (Co-administration of erythromycin and a drug primarily matabolized by CYP3A, like vinblastine, may be associated with elevation in drug concentrations that could increase or prolong both the therapeutic and adverse effects of vinblastine).
No products indexed under this heading.

Vincristine Sulfate (Erythromycin is a substrate and inhibitor of the 3A isoform subfamily of the cytochrome p450 enzyme system (CYP3A). Co-administration of erythromycin and a drug primarily metabolized by CYP3A may be associated with elevations in drug concentrations that could increase or prolong both the therapeutic and adverse effects of the concomitant drug).
No products indexed under this heading.

Warfarin Sodium (Erythromycin is a substrate and inhibitor of the 3A isoform subfamily of the cytochrome p450 enzyme system (CYP3A). Co-administration of erythromycin and a drug primarily metabolized by CYP3A may be associated with elevations in drug concentrations that could increase or prolong both the therapeutic and adverse effects of the concomitant drug). Products include:
Coumadin for Injection **932**
Coumadin Tablets **932**

Food Interactions

Food, unspecified (Lowers the blood levels of systemically available erythromycin).

ESKALITH CAPSULES

(Lithium Carbonate) **1406**
May interact with ACE inhibitors, angiotensin-II receptor antagonists, calcium channel blockers, diuretics, antipsychotic agents, neuromuscular blocking agents, non-steroidal anti-inflammatory agents, phenytoin, selective serotonin reuptake inhibitors, urinary alkalinizing agents, xanthines, and certain other agents. Compounds in these categories include:

Acetazolamide (Lowers serum lithium concentrations by increasing urinary lithium excretion).
No products indexed under this heading.

Acetazolamide Sodium (Lowers serum lithium concentrations by increasing urinary lithium excretion).
No products indexed under this heading.

Amiloride Hydrochloride (Diuretic-induced sodium loss may reduce the renal clearance of lithium and increase serum lithium levels with risk of lithium toxicity). Products include:
Midamor Tablets **2000**
Moduretic Tablets **2003**

Aminophylline (Lowers serum lithium concentrations by increasing urinary lithium excretion).
No products indexed under this heading.

Amlodipine Besylate (Increases the risk of neurotoxicity). Products include:
Caduet Tablets **2507**
Lotrel Capsules **2238**
Norvasc Tablets **2529**

Aripiprazole (Potential for an encephalopathic syndrome with possible irreversible brain damage with co-administration of lithium with a neuroleptic). Products include:
Abilify Tablets **2472**
Abilify Tablets **916**

Atracurium Besylate (Lithium may prolong the effect of neuromuscular blocking agents).
No products indexed under this heading.

Benazepril Hydrochloride (May substantially increase steady-state plasma lithium levels resulting in lithium toxicity). Products include:
Lotensin Tablets **2232**
Lotensin HCT Tablets **2235**
Lotrel Capsules **2238**

Bendroflumethiazide (Diuretic-induced sodium loss may reduce the renal clearance of lithium and increase serum lithium levels with risk of lithium toxicity).
No products indexed under this heading.

Bepridil Hydrochloride (Increases the risk of neurotoxicity).
No products indexed under this heading.

Bumetanide (Diuretic-induced sodium loss may reduce the renal clearance of lithium and increase serum lithium levels with risk of lithium toxicity).
No products indexed under this heading.

Candesartan Cilexetil (May substantially increase steady-state plasma lithium levels resulting in lithium toxicity). Products include:
Atacand Tablets **634**
Atacand HCT **637**

Captopril (May substantially increase steady-state plasma lithium levels resulting in lithium toxicity). Products include:
Captopril Tablets **2114**

Carbamazepine (Effect of co-administration not specified in the current prescribing information). Products include:
Carbatrol Capsules **3174**
Equetro Extended-Release Capsules **3178**
Tegretol/Tegretol-XR **2278**

Celecoxib (Co-administration has resulted in increased mean steady-state plasma lithium levels by 17%). Products include:
Celebrex Capsules **3130**

Chlorothiazide (Diuretic-induced sodium loss may reduce the renal clearance of lithium and increase serum lithium levels with risk of lithium toxicity). Products include:
Aldoclor Tablets **1881**
Diuril Oral **1936**

Chlorothiazide Sodium (Diuretic-induced sodium loss may reduce the renal clearance of lithium and increase serum lithium levels with risk of lithium toxicity). Products include:
- Diuril Sodium Intravenous ... **1934**

Chlorpromazine (Potential for an encephalopathic syndrome with possible irreversible brain damage with co-administration of lithium with a neuroleptic).
- No products indexed under this heading.

Chlorpromazine Hydrochloride (Potential for an encephalopathic syndrome with possible irreversible brain damage with co-administration of lithium with a neuroleptic).
- No products indexed under this heading.

Chlorprothixene (Potential for an encephalopathic syndrome with possible irreversible brain damage with co-administration of lithium with a neuroleptic).
- No products indexed under this heading.

Chlorprothixene Hydrochloride (Potential for an encephalopathic syndrome with possible irreversible brain damage with co-administration of lithium with a neuroleptic).
- No products indexed under this heading.

Chlorthalidone (Diuretic-induced sodium loss may reduce the renal clearance of lithium and increase serum lithium levels with risk of lithium toxicity). Products include:
- Clorpres Tablets ... **2139**

Cisatracurium Besylate (Lithium may prolong the effect of neuromuscular blocking agents). Products include:
- Nimbex Injection ... **494**

Citalopram Hydrobromide (Co-administration with selective serotonin reuptake inhibitors has been reported to result in diarrhea, confusion, tremor, dizziness and agitation). Products include:
- Celexa ... **1177**

Clozapine (Potential for an encephalopathic syndrome with possible irreversible brain damage with co-administration of lithium with a neuroleptic). Products include:
- Clozapine Tablets ... **2141**
- Clozaril Tablets ... **2174**
- FazaClo Orally Disintegrating Tablets ... **547**

Diclofenac Potassium (Lithium-indomethacin-type interaction may occur with other nonsteroidal anti-inflammatory agents; potential for increase in steady-state plasma lithium levels). Products include:
- Cataflam Tablets ... **2173**

Diclofenac Sodium (Lithium-indomethacin-type interaction may occur with other nonsteroidal anti-inflammatory agents; potential for increase in steady-state plasma lithium levels). Products include:
- Arthrotec Tablets ... **3126**
- Voltaren Ophthalmic Solution ... **2300**
- Voltaren Tablets ... **2298**
- Voltaren-XR Tablets ... **2301**

Diltiazem Hydrochloride (Increases the risk of neurotoxicity). Products include:
- Cardizem LA Extended Release Tablets ... **1699**
- Tiazac Capsules ... **1204**

Doxacurium Chloride (Lithium may prolong the effect of neuromuscular blocking agents).
- No products indexed under this heading.

Dyphylline (Lowers serum lithium concentrations by increasing urinary lithium excretion).
- No products indexed under this heading.

Enalapril Maleate (May substantially increase steady-state plasma lithium levels resulting in lithium toxicity). Products include:
- Vaseretic Tablets ... **2073**
- Vasotec I.V. Injection ... **2076**

Enalaprilat (May substantially increase steady-state plasma lithium levels resulting in lithium toxicity).
- No products indexed under this heading.

Eprosartan Mesylate (May substantially increase steady-state plasma lithium levels resulting in lithium toxicity). Products include:
- Teveten Tablets ... **1707**
- Teveten HCT Tablets ... **1710**

Escitalopram Oxalate (Co-administration with selective serotonin reuptake inhibitors has been reported to result in diarrhea, confusion, tremor, dizziness and agitation). Products include:
- Lexapro Oral Solution ... **1193**
- Lexapro Tablets ... **1193**

Ethacrynic Acid (Diuretic-induced sodium loss may reduce the renal clearance of lithium and increase serum lithium levels with risk of lithium toxicity). Products include:
- Edecrin Tablets ... **1941**

Etodolac (Lithium-indomethacin-type interaction may occur with other nonsteroidal anti-inflammatory agents; potential for increase in steady-state plasma lithium levels).
- No products indexed under this heading.

Felodipine (Increases the risk of neurotoxicity). Products include:
- Plendil Extended-Release Tablets ... **651**

Fenoprofen Calcium (Lithium-indomethacin-type interaction may occur with other nonsteroidal anti-inflammatory agents; potential for increase in steady-state plasma lithium levels). Products include:
- Nalfon Capsules ... **2504**

Fluoxetine Hydrochloride (Co-administration with selective serotonin reuptake inhibitors has been reported to result in diarrhea, confusion, tremor, dizziness and agitation). Products include:
- Prozac Pulvules and Liquid ... **1771**
- Symbyax Capsules ... **1788**

Fluphenazine Decanoate (Potential for an encephalopathic syndrome with possible irreversible brain damage with co-administration of lithium with a neuroleptic).
- No products indexed under this heading.

Fluphenazine Enanthate (Potential for an encephalopathic syndrome with possible irreversible brain damage with co-administration of lithium with a neuroleptic).
- No products indexed under this heading.

Fluphenazine Hydrochloride (Potential for an encephalopathic syndrome with possible irreversible brain damage with co-administration of lithium with a neuroleptic).
- No products indexed under this heading.

Flurbiprofen (Lithium-indomethacin-type interaction may occur with other nonsteroidal anti-inflammatory agents; potential for increase in steady-state plasma lithium levels).
- No products indexed under this heading.

Fluvoxamine Maleate (Co-administration with selective serotonin reuptake inhibitors has been reported to result in diarrhea, confusion, tremor, dizziness and agitation).
- No products indexed under this heading.

Fosinopril Sodium (May substantially increase steady-state plasma lithium levels resulting in lithium toxicity).
- No products indexed under this heading.

Fosphenytoin Sodium (Effect of co-administration not specified in the current prescribing information).
- No products indexed under this heading.

Furosemide (Diuretic-induced sodium loss may reduce the renal clearance of lithium and increase serum lithium levels with risk of lithium toxicity). Products include:
- Furosemide Tablets ... **2117**

Haloperidol (Potential for an encephalopathic syndrome with possible irreversible brain damage with co-administration of lithium with a neuroleptic).
- No products indexed under this heading.

Haloperidol Decanoate (Potential for an encephalopathic syndrome with possible irreversible brain damage with co-administration of lithium with a neuroleptic).
- No products indexed under this heading.

Hydrochlorothiazide (Diuretic-induced sodium loss may reduce the renal clearance of lithium and increase serum lithium levels with risk of lithium toxicity). Products include:
- Aldoril Tablets ... **1884**
- Atacand HCT ... **637**
- Avalide Tablets ... **2889**
- Avalide Tablets ... **922**
- Benicar HCT Tablets ... **2852**
- Diovan HCT Tablets ... **2195**
- Dyazide Capsules ... **1389**
- Hyzaar ... **1964**
- Lotensin HCT Tablets ... **2235**
- Maxzide ... **2150**
- Micardis HCT Tablets ... **886**
- Moduretic Tablets ... **2003**
- Prinzide Tablets ... **2033**
- Teveten HCT Tablets ... **1710**
- Timolide Tablets ... **2056**
- Uniretic Tablets ... **3114**
- Vaseretic Tablets ... **2073**
- Zestoretic Tablets ... **701**

Hydroflumethiazide (Diuretic-induced sodium loss may reduce the renal clearance of lithium and increase serum lithium levels with risk of lithium toxicity).
- No products indexed under this heading.

Ibuprofen (Lithium-indomethacin-type interaction may occur with other nonsteroidal anti-inflammatory agents; potential for increase in steady-state plasma lithium levels). Products include:
- Advil Allergy Sinus Caplets ... ■**737**
- Advil ... ■**737**
- Children's Advil Suspension ... ■**742**
- Children's Advil Chewable Tablets ... ■**741**
- Advil Cold & Sinus ... ■**739**
- Advil Flu & Body Ache Caplets ... ■**739**
- Children's Advil Cold Suspension ... ■**741**
- Infants' Advil Concentrated Drops ... ■**743**
- Junior Strength Advil Swallow Tablets ... ■**740**
- Advil Migraine Liquigels ... ■**740**
- Advil Multi-Symptom Cold Caplets ... ■**738**
- Combunox Tablets ... **1183**
- Children's Motrin Oral Suspension and Chewable Tablets ... **1837**
- Children's Motrin Cold Non-Staining Dye-Free Oral Suspension ... **1838**
- Children's Motrin Cold Oral Suspension ... **1838**
- Children's Motrin Non-Staining Dye-Free Oral Suspension ... **1837**
- Motrin Cold & Sinus Caplets ... **1836**
- Motrin IB Tablets and Caplets ... **1836**
- Infants' Motrin Concentrated Drops ... **1837**
- Infants' Motrin Non-Staining Dye-Free Drops ... **1837**
- Junior Strength Motrin Caplets and Chewable Tablets ... **1837**
- Vicoprofen Tablets ... **533**

Indapamide (Diuretic-induced sodium loss may reduce the renal clearance of lithium and increase serum lithium levels with risk of lithium toxicity). Products include:
- Indapamide Tablets ... **2119**

Indomethacin (Co-administration has resulted in significant increase in steady state plasma lithium levels with risk of lithium toxicity). Products include:
- Indocin ... **1968**

Indomethacin Sodium Trihydrate (Co-administration has resulted in significant increase in steady-state plasma lithium levels with risk of lithium toxicity). Products include:
- Indocin I.V. ... **1973**

Irbesartan (May substantially increase steady-state plasma lithium levels resulting in lithium toxicity). Products include:
- Avalide Tablets ... **922**
- Avalide Tablets ... **2889**
- Avapro Tablets ... **925**
- Avapro Tablets ... **2886**

Isradipine (Increases the risk of neurotoxicity). Products include:
- DynaCirc CR Tablets ... **2726**

Ketoprofen (Lithium-indomethacin-type interaction may occur with other nonsteroidal anti-inflammatory agents; potential for increase in steady-state plasma lithium levels).
- No products indexed under this heading.

Ketorolac Tromethamine (Lithium-indomethacin-type interaction may occur with other nonsteroidal anti-inflammatory agents; potential for increase in steady-state plasma lithium levels). Products include:
- Acular Ophthalmic Solution ... **561**
- Acular LS Ophthalmic Solution ... **562**

Lisinopril (May substantially increase steady-state plasma lithium levels resulting in lithium toxicity). Products include:
- Prinivil Tablets ... **2029**
- Prinzide Tablets ... **2033**
- Zestoretic Tablets ... **701**
- Zestril Tablets ... **704**

Lithium Citrate (Potential for an encephalopathic syndrome with possible irreversible brain damage with co-administration of lithium with a neuroleptic).
- No products indexed under this heading.

Losartan Potassium (May substantially increase steady-state plasma lithium levels resulting in lithium toxicity). Products include:
- Cozaar Tablets **1913**
- Hyzaar **1964**

Loxapine Hydrochloride (Potential for an encephalopathic syndrome with possible irreversible brain damage with co-administration of lithium with a neuroleptic).
- No products indexed under this heading.

Loxapine Succinate (Potential for an encephalopathic syndrome with possible irreversible brain damage with co-administration of lithium with a neuroleptic).
- No products indexed under this heading.

Meclofenamate Sodium (Lithium-indomethacin-type interaction may occur with other nonsteroidal anti-inflammatory agents; potential for increase in steady-state plasma lithium levels).
- No products indexed under this heading.

Mefenamic Acid (Lithium-indomethacin-type interaction may occur with other nonsteroidal anti-inflammatory agents; potential for increase in steady-state plasma lithium levels).
- No products indexed under this heading.

Meloxicam (Lithium-indomethacin-type interaction may occur with other nonsteroidal anti-inflammatory agents; potential for increase in steady-state plasma lithium levels). Products include:
- Mobic Oral Suspension **893**
- Mobic Tablets **893**

Mesoridazine Besylate (Potential for an encephalopathic syndrome with possible irreversible brain damage with co-administration of lithium with a neuroleptic).
- No products indexed under this heading.

Methotrimeprazine (Potential for an encephalopathic syndrome with possible irreversible brain damage with co-administration of lithium with a neuroleptic).
- No products indexed under this heading.

Methyclothiazide (Diuretic-induced sodium loss may reduce the renal clearance of lithium and increase serum lithium levels with risk of lithium toxicity).
- No products indexed under this heading.

Methyldopa (Effect of co-administration not specified in the current prescribing information). Products include:
- Aldoclor Tablets **1881**
- Aldoril Tablets **1884**

Metocurine Iodide (Lithium may prolong the effect of neuromuscular blocking agents).
- No products indexed under this heading.

Metolazone (Diuretic-induced sodium loss may reduce the renal clearance of lithium and increase serum lithium levels with risk of lithium toxicity).
- No products indexed under this heading.

Metronidazole (May provoke lithium toxicity due to reduced renal clearance). Products include:
- Metrogel 1% **1212**
- MetroGel-Vaginal Gel **1822**
- Noritate Cream, 1% **1051**

Metronidazole Hydrochloride (May provoke lithium toxicity due to reduced renal clearance).
- No products indexed under this heading.

Mibefradil Dihydrochloride (Increases the risk of neurotoxicity).
- No products indexed under this heading.

Mivacurium Chloride (Lithium may prolong the effect of neuromuscular blocking agents). Products include:
- Mivacron Injection **489**

Moexipril Hydrochloride (May substantially increase steady-state plasma lithium levels resulting in lithium toxicity). Products include:
- Uniretic Tablets **3114**
- Univasc Tablets **3118**

Molindone Hydrochloride (Potential for an encephalopathic syndrome with possible irreversible brain damage with co-administration of lithium with a neuroleptic). Products include:
- Moban Tablets **1108**

Nabumetone (Lithium-indomethacin-type interaction may occur with other nonsteroidal anti-inflammatory agents; potential for increase in steady-state plasma lithium levels). Products include:
- Relafen Tablets **1523**

Naproxen (Lithium-indomethacin-type interaction may occur with other nonsteroidal anti-inflammatory agents; potential for increase in steady-state plasma lithium levels). Products include:
- EC-Naprosyn Delayed-Release Tablets **2769**
- Naprosyn Suspension **2769**
- Naprosyn Tablets **2769**
- Prevacid NapraPAC **3277**

Naproxen Sodium (Lithium-indomethacin-type interaction may occur with other nonsteroidal anti-inflammatory agents; potential for increase in steady-state plasma lithium levels). Products include:
- Aleve Tablets, Caplets and Gelcaps .... ■**605**
- Anaprox Tablets **2769**
- Anaprox DS Tablets **2769**

Nicardipine Hydrochloride (Increases the risk of neurotoxicity). Products include:
- Cardene I.V. **1129**

Nifedipine (Increases the risk of neurotoxicity). Products include:
- Adalat CC Tablets **2978**

Nimodipine (Increases the risk of neurotoxicity). Products include:
- Nimotop Capsules **774**

Nisoldipine (Increases the risk of neurotoxicity). Products include:
- Sular Tablets **1163**

Olanzapine (Potential for an encephalopathic syndrome with possible irreversible brain damage with co-administration of lithium with a neuroleptic). Products include:
- Symbyax Capsules **1788**
- Zyprexa Tablets **1798**
- Zyprexa IntraMuscular **1798**
- Zyprexa ZYDIS Orally Disintegrating Tablets **1798**

Oxaprozin (Lithium-indomethacin-type interaction may occur with other nonsteroidal anti-inflammatory agents; potential for increase in steady-state plasma lithium levels).
- No products indexed under this heading.

Pancuronium Bromide (Lithium may prolong the effect of neuromuscular blocking agents).
- No products indexed under this heading.

Paroxetine Hydrochloride (Co-administration with selective serotonin reuptake inhibitors has been reported to result in diarrhea, confusion, tremor, dizziness and agitation). Products include:
- Paxil CR Controlled-Release Tablets **1509**
- Paxil **1501**

Perindopril Erbumine (May substantially increase steady-state plasma lithium levels resulting in lithium toxicity). Products include:
- Aceon Tablets (2 mg, 4 mg, 8 mg) **3191**

Perphenazine (Potential for an encephalopathic syndrome with possible irreversible brain damage with co-administration of lithium with a neuroleptic).
- No products indexed under this heading.

Phenylbutazone (Lithium-indomethacin-type interaction may occur with other nonsteroidal anti-inflammatory agents; potential for increase in steady-state plasma lithium levels).
- No products indexed under this heading.

Phenytoin (Effect of co-administration not specified in the current prescribing information).
- No products indexed under this heading.

Phenytoin Sodium (Effect of co-administration not specified in the current prescribing information). Products include:
- Phenytek Capsules **2153**

Pimozide (Potential for an encephalopathic syndrome with possible irreversible brain damage with co-administration of lithium with a neuroleptic). Products include:
- Orap Tablets **1220**

Piroxicam (Co-administration has resulted in significant increase in steady-state plasma lithium levels with risk of lithium toxicity).
- No products indexed under this heading.

Polythiazide (Diuretic-induced sodium loss may reduce the renal clearance of lithium and increase serum lithium levels with risk of lithium toxicity).
- No products indexed under this heading.

Potassium Citrate (Lowers serum lithium concentrations by increasing urinary lithium excretion). Products include:
- Urocit-K Tablets **2109**

Prochlorperazine (Potential for an encephalopathic syndrome with possible irreversible brain damage with co-administration of lithium with a neuroleptic).
- No products indexed under this heading.

Promethazine Hydrochloride (Potential for an encephalopathic syndrome with possible irreversible brain damage with co-administration of lithium with a neuroleptic). Products include:
- Phenergan **3438**

Quetiapine Fumarate (Potential for an encephalopathic syndrome with possible irreversible brain damage with co-administration of lithium with a neuroleptic). Products include:
- Seroquel Tablets **691**

Quinapril Hydrochloride (May substantially increase steady-state plasma lithium levels resulting in lithium toxicity).
- No products indexed under this heading.

Ramipril (May substantially increase steady-state plasma lithium levels resulting in lithium toxicity). Products include:
- Altace Capsules **1673**

Rapacuronium Bromide (Lithium may prolong the effect of neuromuscular blocking agents).
- No products indexed under this heading.

Risperidone (Potential for an encephalopathic syndrome with possible irreversible brain damage with co-administration of lithium with a neuroleptic). Products include:
- Risperdal Consta Long-Acting Injection **1664**
- Risperdal M-Tab Orally Disintegrating Tablets **1658**
- Risperdal **1658**

Rocuronium Bromide (Lithium may prolong the effect of neuromuscular blocking agents). Products include:
- Zemuron Injection **2363**

Rofecoxib (Lithium-indomethacin-type interaction may occur with other nonsteroidal anti-inflammatory agents; potential for increase in steady-state plasma lithium levels).
- No products indexed under this heading.

Sertraline Hydrochloride (Co-administration with selective serotonin reuptake inhibitors has been reported to result in diarrhea, confusion, tremor, dizziness and agitation). Products include:
- Zoloft **2581**

Sodium Bicarbonate (Systemic sodium bicarbonate lowers serum lithium concentrations by increasing urinary lithium excretion). Products include:
- Ceo-Two Evacuant Suppository .... ■**607**
- Colyte with Flavor Packs for Oral Solution **3102**
- HalfLytely and Bisacodyl Tablets Bowel Prep Kit with Flavors Packs **915**
- TriLyte with Flavor Packs for Oral Solution **3114**

Sodium Citrate (Lowers serum lithium concentrations by increasing urinary lithium excretion).
- No products indexed under this heading.

Spirapril Hydrochloride (May substantially increase steady-state plasma lithium levels resulting in lithium toxicity).
- No products indexed under this heading.

Spironolactone (Diuretic-induced sodium loss may reduce the renal clearance of lithium and increase serum lithium levels with risk of lithium toxicity).
- No products indexed under this heading.

Succinylcholine Chloride (Lithium may prolong the effect of neuromuscular blocking agents).
- No products indexed under this heading.

Sulindac (Lithium-indomethacin-type interaction may occur with other nonsteroidal anti-inflammatory

agents; potential for increase in steady-state plasma lithium levels). Products include:

Clinoril Tablets 1899

Telmisartan (May substantially increase steady-state plasma lithium levels resulting in lithium toxicity). Products include:

Micardis Tablets 884
Micardis HCT Tablets 886

Theophylline (Lowers serum lithium concentrations by increasing urinary lithium excretion).

No products indexed under this heading.

Theophylline Anhydrous (Lowers serum lithium concentrations by increasing urinary lithium excretion). Products include:

Uniphyl Tablets 2708

Theophylline Calcium Salicylate (Lowers serum lithium concentrations by increasing urinary lithium excretion).

No products indexed under this heading.

Theophylline Dihydroxypropyl (Glyceryl) (Lowers serum lithium concentrations by increasing urinary lithium excretion).

No products indexed under this heading.

Theophylline Ethylenediamine (Lowers serum lithium concentrations by increasing urinary lithium excretion).

No products indexed under this heading.

Theophylline Sodium Glycinate (Lowers serum lithium concentrations by increasing urinary lithium excretion).

No products indexed under this heading.

Thioridazine Hydrochloride (Potential for an encephalopathic syndrome with possible irreversible brain damage with co-administration of lithium with a neuroleptic). Products include:

Thioridazine Hydrochloride Tablets 2122

Thiothixene (Potential for an encephalopathic syndrome with possible irreversible brain damage with co-administration of lithium with a neuroleptic). Products include:

Thiothixene Capsules 2124

Tolmetin Sodium (Lithium-indomethacin-type interaction may occur with other nonsteroidal anti-inflammatory agents; potential for increase in steady-state plasma lithium levels).

No products indexed under this heading.

Torsemide (Diuretic-induced sodium loss may reduce the renal clearance of lithium and increase serum lithium levels with risk of lithium toxicity).

No products indexed under this heading.

Trandolapril (May substantially increase steady-state plasma lithium levels resulting in lithium toxicity). Products include:

Mavik Tablets 482
Tarka Tablets 519

Triamterene (Diuretic-induced sodium loss may reduce the renal clearance of lithium and increase serum lithium levels with risk of lithium toxicity). Products include:

Dyazide Capsules 1389
Dyrenium Capsules 3390
Maxzide 2150

Trifluoperazine Hydrochloride (Potential for an encephalopathic syndrome with possible irreversible brain damage with co-administration of lithium with a neuroleptic).

No products indexed under this heading.

Urea (Systemic administration of urea with lithium therapy can lower serum lithium concentration by increasing urinary lithium excretion). Products include:

Accuzyme Debriding Ointment 1636
Accuzyme Spray 1637
Panafil Ointment 1637
Panafil Spray 1637
U-Kera Cream 3290
Ultralytic 2 Cream 20% 1651
Ultralytic 2 Foam 20% 1652

Valdecoxib (Lithium-indomethacin-type interaction may occur with other nonsteroidal anti-inflammatory agents; potential for increase in steady-state plasma lithium levels).

No products indexed under this heading.

Valsartan (May substantially increase steady-state plasma lithium levels resulting in lithium toxicity). Products include:

Diovan HCT Tablets 2195
Diovan Tablets 2191

Vecuronium Bromide (Lithium may prolong the effect of neuromuscular blocking agents).

No products indexed under this heading.

Verapamil Hydrochloride (Increases the risk of neurotoxicity). Products include:

Covera-HS Tablets 3135
Tarka Tablets 519
Verelan PM Capsules 3120

Ziprasidone Hydrochloride (Potential for an encephalopathic syndrome with possible irreversible brain damage with co-administration of lithium with a neuroleptic). Products include:

Geodon Capsules 2514

ESKALITH CR CONTROLLED-RELEASE TABLETS

(Lithium Carbonate) 1406
See Eskalith Capsules

ESTRATEST TABLETS

(Estrogens, Esterified, Methyltestosterone)........................... 3196
See Estratest H.S. Tablets

ESTRATEST H.S. TABLETS

(Estrogens, Esterified, Methyltestosterone)........................... 3196
May interact with oral anticoagulants, cytochrome p450 3a4 inducers (selected), cytochrome p450 3a4 inhibitors (selected), insulin, and certain other agents. Compounds in these categories include:

Acetazolamide (Co-administration with inhibitors of CYP3A4 may increase plasma concentrations of estrogens and may result in side effects).

No products indexed under this heading.

Allium sativum (Co-administration with inducers of CYP3A4 may reduce plasma concentrations of estrogens, possibly resulting in a decrease in therapeutic effects and/or changes in uterine bleeding profile).

No products indexed under this heading.

Amiodarone Hydrochloride (Co-administration with inhibitors of CYP3A4 may increase plasma concentrations of estrogens and may result in side effects). Products include:

Pacerone Tablets 3337

Amprenavir (Co-administration with inhibitors of CYP3A4 may increase plasma concentrations of estrogens and may result in side effects). Products include:

Agenerase Capsules 1299
Agenerase Oral Solution 1304

Anastrozole (Co-administration with inhibitors of CYP3A4 may increase plasma concentrations of estrogens and may result in side effects). Products include:

Arimidex Tablets 665

Anisindione (Decreased anticoagulant requirements). Products include:

Miradon Tablets 3056

Aprepitant (Co-administration with inducers of CYP3A4 may reduce plasma concentrations of estrogens, possibly resulting in a decrease in therapeutic effects and/or changes in uterine bleeding profile). Products include:

Emend Capsules 1944

Betamethasone Acetate (Co-administration with inducers of CYP3A4 may reduce plasma concentrations of estrogens, possibly resulting in a decrease in therapeutic effects and/or changes in uterine bleeding profile).

No products indexed under this heading.

Betamethasone Sodium Phosphate (Co-administration with inducers of CYP3A4 may reduce plasma concentrations of estrogens, possibly resulting in a decrease in therapeutic effects and/or changes in uterine bleeding profile).

No products indexed under this heading.

Carbamazepine (Co-administration with inducers of CYP3A4 may reduce plasma concentrations of estrogens, possibly resulting in a decrease in therapeutic effects and/or changes in uterine bleeding profile). Products include:

Carbatrol Capsules 3174
Equetro Extended-Release Capsules.. 3178
Tegretol/Tegretol-XR 2278

Cimetidine (Co-administration with inhibitors of CYP3A4 may increase plasma concentrations of estrogens and may result in side effects). Products include:

Tagamet HB 200 Tablets .... ▣637
Tagamet Tablets 1547

Cimetidine Hydrochloride (Co-administration with inhibitors of CYP3A4 may increase plasma concentrations of estrogens and may result in side effects).

No products indexed under this heading.

Ciprofloxacin (Co-administration with inhibitors of CYP3A4 may increase plasma concentrations of estrogens and may result in side effects). Products include:

Cipro I.V. 2998
Cipro I.V. Pharmacy Bulk Package ... 3509
Cipro Oral Suspension 2991
Cipro XR Tablets 3004
Ciprodex Otic Suspension 555

Ciprofloxacin Hydrochloride (Co-administration with inducers of CYP3A4 may reduce plasma concentrations of estrogens, possibly resulting in a decrease in therapeutic effects and/or changes in uterine bleeding profile). Products include:

Ciloxan Ophthalmic Ointment 554
Cipro Tablets 2991

Cisplatin (Co-administration with inducers of CYP3A4 may reduce plasma concentrations of estrogens, possibly resulting in a decrease in therapeutic effects and/or changes in uterine bleeding profile).

No products indexed under this heading.

Clarithromycin (Co-administration with inhibitors of CYP3A4 may increase plasma concentrations of estrogens and may result in side effects). Products include:

Biaxin/Biaxin XL 402
PREVPAC 3281

Clotrimazole (Co-administration with inhibitors of CYP3A4 may increase plasma concentrations of estrogens and may result in side effects). Products include:

Lotrimin 3053
Lotrisone 3054

Cortisone Acetate (Co-administration with inducers of CYP3A4 may reduce plasma concentrations of estrogens, possibly resulting in a decrease in therapeutic effects and/or changes in uterine bleeding profile).

No products indexed under this heading.

Cyclosporine (Co-administration with inhibitors of CYP3A4 may increase plasma concentrations of estrogens and may result in side effects). Products include:

Gengraf Capsules 458
Neoral Soft Gelatin Capsules 2247
Neoral Oral Solution 2247
Restasis Ophthalmic Emulsion 570
Sandimmune 2259

Dalfopristin (Co-administration with inhibitors of CYP3A4 may increase plasma concentrations of estrogens and may result in side effects). Products include:

Synercid I.V. 1690

Danazol (Co-administration with inhibitors of CYP3A4 may increase plasma concentrations of estrogens and may result in side effects).

No products indexed under this heading.

Delavirdine Mesylate (Co-administration with inhibitors of CYP3A4 may increase plasma concentrations of estrogens and may result in side effects). Products include:

Rescriptor Tablets 2535

Dexamethasone (Co-administration with inducers of CYP3A4 may reduce plasma concentrations of estrogens, possibly resulting in a decrease in therapeutic effects and/or changes in uterine bleeding profile). Products include:

Ciprodex Otic Suspension 555
Decadron Tablets 1929
TobraDex Ophthalmic Ointment 558
TobraDex Ophthalmic Suspension ... 558

Dexamethasone Acetate (Co-administration with inducers of CYP3A4 may reduce plasma concentrations of estrogens, possibly resulting in a decrease in therapeutic effects and/or changes in uterine bleeding profile).

No products indexed under this heading.

Dexamethasone Sodium Phosphate (Co-administration with inducers of CYP3A4 may reduce plasma concentrations of estrogens, possibly resulting in a decrease in therapeutic effects and/or changes in uterine bleeding profile). Products include:
Decadron Phosphate Injection 1931

Dicumarol (Decreased anticoagulant requirements).
No products indexed under this heading.

Diltiazem Hydrochloride (Co-administration with inhibitors of CYP3A4 may increase plasma concentrations of estrogens and may result in side effects). Products include:
Cardizem LA Extended Release Tablets 1699
Tiazac Capsules 1204

Diltiazem Maleate (Co-administration with inhibitors of CYP3A4 may increase plasma concentrations of estrogens and may result in side effects).
No products indexed under this heading.

Doxorubicin Hydrochloride (Co-administration with inducers of CYP3A4 may reduce plasma concentrations of estrogens, possibly resulting in a decrease in therapeutic effects and/or changes in uterine bleeding profile). Products include:
Adriamycin for Injection, USP 786
Adriamycin Injection, USP 786

Efavirenz (Co-administration with inducers of CYP3A4 may reduce plasma concentrations of estrogens, possibly resulting in a decrease in therapeutic effects and/or changes in uterine bleeding profile). Products include:
Sustiva Capsules 957

Erythromycin (Co-administration with inhibitors of CYP3A4 may increase plasma concentrations of estrogens and may result in side effects). Products include:
Erygel Topical Gel 2096
Ery-Tab Tablets 447
Erythromycin Base Filmtab Tablets 454
Erythromycin Delayed-Release Capsules, USP 456
PCE Dispertab Tablets 510

Erythromycin Estolate (Co-administration with inhibitors of CYP3A4 may increase plasma concentrations of estrogens and may result in side effects).
No products indexed under this heading.

Erythromycin Ethylsuccinate (Co-administration with inhibitors of CYP3A4 may increase plasma concentrations of estrogens and may result in side effects). Products include:
E.E.S. 449
EryPed 445

Erythromycin Gluceptate (Co-administration with inhibitors of CYP3A4 may increase plasma concentrations of estrogens and may result in side effects).
No products indexed under this heading.

Erythromycin Lactobionate (Co-administration with inhibitors of CYP3A4 may increase plasma concentrations of estrogens and may result in side effects).
No products indexed under this heading.

Erythromycin Stearate (Co-administration with inhibitors of CYP3A4 may increase plasma concentrations of estrogens and may result in side effects). Products include:
Erythrocin Stearate Filmtab Tablets 452

Esomeprazole Magnesium (Co-administration with inhibitors of CYP3A4 may increase plasma concentrations of estrogens and may result in side effects). Products include:
Nexium Delayed-Release Capsules 645

Ethosuximide (Co-administration with inducers of CYP3A4 may reduce plasma concentrations of estrogens, possibly resulting in a decrease in therapeutic effects and/or changes in uterine bleeding profile).
No products indexed under this heading.

Felbamate (Co-administration with inducers of CYP3A4 may reduce plasma concentrations of estrogens, possibly resulting in a decrease in therapeutic effects and/or changes in uterine bleeding profile).
No products indexed under this heading.

Fluconazole (Co-administration with inhibitors of CYP3A4 may increase plasma concentrations of estrogens and may result in side effects).
No products indexed under this heading.

Fludrocortisone Acetate (Co-administration with inducers of CYP3A4 may reduce plasma concentrations of estrogens, possibly resulting in a decrease in therapeutic effects and/or changes in uterine bleeding profile).
No products indexed under this heading.

Fluoxetine Hydrochloride (Co-administration with inhibitors of CYP3A4 may increase plasma concentrations of estrogens and may result in side effects). Products include:
Prozac Pulvules and Liquid 1771
Symbyax Capsules 1788

Fluvoxamine Maleate (Co-administration with inhibitors of CYP3A4 may increase plasma concentrations of estrogens and may result in side effects).
No products indexed under this heading.

Fosamprenavir Calcium (Co-administration with inhibitors of CYP3A4 may increase plasma concentrations of estrogens and may result in side effects). Products include:
Lexiva Tablets 1473

Fosphenytoin Sodium (Co-administration with inducers of CYP3A4 may reduce plasma concentrations of estrogens, possibly resulting in a decrease in therapeutic effects and/or changes in uterine bleeding profile).
No products indexed under this heading.

Garlic Extract (Co-administration with inducers of CYP3A4 may reduce plasma concentrations of estrogens, possibly resulting in a decrease in therapeutic effects and/or changes in uterine bleeding profile).
No products indexed under this heading.

Garlic Oil (Co-administration with inducers of CYP3A4 may reduce plasma concentrations of estrogens, possibly resulting in a decrease in therapeutic effects and/or changes in uterine bleeding profile).
No products indexed under this heading.

Hydrocortisone (Co-administration with inducers of CYP3A4 may reduce plasma concentrations of estrogens, possibly resulting in a decrease in therapeutic effects and/or changes in uterine bleeding profile). Products include:
Cortizone•5 Ointment .... ▣699
Cortizone•10 Creme .... ▣699
Cortizone•10 Ointment .... ▣699
Cortizone•10 Plus Creme .... ▣700
Cortizone•10 Maximum Strength Quick Shot Spray .... ▣700
Hydrocortone Tablets 1963
Preparation H Hydrocortisone Cream .... ▣748

Hydrocortisone Acetate (Co-administration with inducers of CYP3A4 may reduce plasma concentrations of estrogens, possibly resulting in a decrease in therapeutic effects and/or changes in uterine bleeding profile). Products include:
Analpram-HC 1136
Pramosone 1139
ProctoFoam-HC 3113
Tucks Anti-Itch Ointment .... ▣712
U-cort 1% Cream 3289

Hydrocortisone Butyrate (Co-administration with inducers of CYP3A4 may reduce plasma concentrations of estrogens, possibly resulting in a decrease in therapeutic effects and/or changes in uterine bleeding profile). Products include:
Locoid 1138
Locoid Lipocream Cream 1138

Hydrocortisone Cypionate (Co-administration with inducers of CYP3A4 may reduce plasma concentrations of estrogens, possibly resulting in a decrease in therapeutic effects and/or changes in uterine bleeding profile).
No products indexed under this heading.

Hydrocortisone Hemisuccinate (Co-administration with inducers of CYP3A4 may reduce plasma concentrations of estrogens, possibly resulting in a decrease in therapeutic effects and/or changes in uterine bleeding profile).
No products indexed under this heading.

Hydrocortisone Probutate (Co-administration with inducers of CYP3A4 may reduce plasma concentrations of estrogens, possibly resulting in a decrease in therapeutic effects and/or changes in uterine bleeding profile). Products include:
Pandel Cream, 0.1% 1017

Hydrocortisone Sodium Phosphate (Co-administration with inducers of CYP3A4 may reduce plasma concentrations of estrogens, possibly resulting in a decrease in therapeutic effects and/or changes in uterine bleeding profile).
No products indexed under this heading.

Hydrocortisone Sodium Succinate (Co-administration with inducers of CYP3A4 may reduce plasma concentrations of estrogens, possibly resulting in a decrease in therapeutic effects and/or changes in uterine bleeding profile).
No products indexed under this heading.

Hydrocortisone Valerate (Co-administration with inducers of CYP3A4 may reduce plasma concentrations of estrogens, possibly resulting in a decrease in therapeutic effects and/or changes in uterine bleeding profile).
No products indexed under this heading.

Hypericum (Co-administration with inducers of CYP3A4 may reduce plasma concentrations of estrogens, possibly resulting in a decrease in therapeutic effects and/or changes in uterine bleeding profile).
No products indexed under this heading.

Hypericum Perforatum (Co-administration with inducers of CYP3A4 may reduce plasma concentrations of estrogens, possibly resulting in a decrease in therapeutic effects and/or changes in uterine bleeding profile).
No products indexed under this heading.

Indinavir Sulfate (Co-administration with inhibitors of CYP3A4 may increase plasma concentrations of estrogens and may result in side effects). Products include:
Crixivan Capsules 1918

Insulin, Human, Zinc Suspension (Decreased blood glucose and insulin requirements). Products include:
Humulin L, 100 Units 1763
Humulin U, 100 Units 1770

Insulin, Human NPH (Decreased blood glucose and insulin requirements). Products include:
Humulin N, 100 Units 1764
Humulin N Pen 1765
Novolin N Human Insulin 10 ml Vials 2322
Novolin N InnoLet 2322
Novolin N PenFill 3 ml Cartridges 2325
Novolin R InnoLet 2322

Insulin, Human Regular (Decreased blood glucose and insulin requirements). Products include:
Humulin R (U-500) 1768
Humulin R, 100 Units 1767
Novolin R Human Insulin 10 ml Vials 2322
Novolin R PenFill 2325

Insulin, Human Regular and Human NPH Mixture (Decreased blood glucose and insulin requirements). Products include:
Humulin 50/50, 100 Units 1760
Humulin 70/30 Pen 1761
Novolin 70/30 Human Insulin 10 ml Vials 2321
Novolin 70/30 InnoLet 2322
Novolin 70/30 PenFill 3 ml Cartridges 2325

Insulin, NPH (Decreased blood glucose and insulin requirements).
No products indexed under this heading.

Insulin, Regular (Decreased blood glucose and insulin requirements).
No products indexed under this heading.

Insulin, Zinc Crystals (Decreased blood glucose and insulin requirements).
No products indexed under this heading.

Insulin, Zinc Suspension (Decreased blood glucose and insulin requirements).
No products indexed under this heading.

Insulin Aspart, Human Regular (Decreased blood glucose and insulin requirements). Products include:
NovoLog Injection 2326

Insulin glargine (Decreased blood glucose and insulin requirements). Products include:
Lantus Injection 2925

Insulin Lispro, Human (Decreased blood glucose and insulin requirements). Products include:
Humalog-Pen 1751
Humalog Mix 75/25-Pen 1754

Insulin Lispro Protamine, Human (Decreased blood glucose and insulin requirements). Products include:
Humalog Mix 75/25-Pen 1754

Isoniazid (Co-administration with inhibitors of CYP3A4 may increase plasma concentrations of estrogens and may result in side effects).
No products indexed under this heading.

Itraconazole (Co-administration with inhibitors of CYP3A4 may increase plasma concentrations of estrogens and may result in side effects).
No products indexed under this heading.

Ketoconazole (Co-administration with inhibitors of CYP3A4 may increase plasma concentrations of estrogens and may result in side effects). Products include:
Nizoral A-D Shampoo, 1% 1839
Nizoral 2% Shampoo 1838

Lopinavir (Co-administration with inhibitors of CYP3A4 may increase plasma concentrations of estrogens and may result in side effects). Products include:
Kaletra 474

Loratadine (Co-administration with inhibitors of CYP3A4 may increase plasma concentrations of estrogens and may result in side effects). Products include:
Alavert Allergy & Sinus D-12 Hour Tablets 743
Alavert 743
Children's Claritin 24 Hour Non-Drowsy Allergy Syrup 732
Claritin Non-Drowsy 24 Hour Tablets 731
Non-Drowsy Claritin Hives Relief Tablets 733
Claritin Reditabs 24 Hour Non-Drowsy Tablets 732
Claritin-D Non-Drowsy 12 Hour Tablets 731
Claritin-D Non-Drowsy 24 Hour Tablets 731
Children's Dimetapp ND Non-Drowsy Allergy Syrup 746
Triaminic Allerchews 684

Mephenytoin (Co-administration with inducers of CYP3A4 may reduce plasma concentrations of estrogens, possibly resulting in a decrease in therapeutic effects and/or changes in uterine bleeding profile).
No products indexed under this heading.

Methsuximide (Co-administration with inducers of CYP3A4 may reduce plasma concentrations of estrogens, possibly resulting in a decrease in therapeutic effects and/or changes in uterine bleeding profile).
No products indexed under this heading.

Methylprednisolone (Co-administration with inducers of CYP3A4 may reduce plasma concentrations of estrogens, possibly resulting in a decrease in therapeutic effects and/or changes in uterine bleeding profile).
No products indexed under this heading.

Methylprednisolone Acetate (Co-administration with inducers of CYP3A4 may reduce plasma concentrations of estrogens, possibly resulting in a decrease in therapeutic effects and/or changes in uterine bleeding profile). Products include:
Depo-Medrol Injectable Suspension 2615
Depo-Medrol Single-Dose Vial 2617

Methylprednisolone Sodium Succinate (Co-administration with inducers of CYP3A4 may reduce plasma concentrations of estrogens, possibly resulting in a decrease in therapeutic effects and/or changes in uterine bleeding profile).
No products indexed under this heading.

Metronidazole (Co-administration with inhibitors of CYP3A4 may increase plasma concentrations of estrogens and may result in side effects). Products include:
Metrogel 1% 1212
MetroGel-Vaginal Gel 1822
Noritate Cream, 1% 1051

Metronidazole Benzoate (Co-administration with inhibitors of CYP3A4 may increase plasma concentrations of estrogens and may result in side effects).
No products indexed under this heading.

Metronidazole Hydrochloride (Co-administration with inhibitors of CYP3A4 may increase plasma concentrations of estrogens and may result in side effects).
No products indexed under this heading.

Miconazole (Co-administration with inhibitors of CYP3A4 may increase plasma concentrations of estrogens and may result in side effects).
No products indexed under this heading.

Miconazole Nitrate (Co-administration with inhibitors of CYP3A4 may increase plasma concentrations of estrogens and may result in side effects). Products include:
Desenex 674
Desenex Jock Itch Spray Powder 674

Modafinil (Co-administration with inducers of CYP3A4 may reduce plasma concentrations of estrogens, possibly resulting in a decrease in therapeutic effects and/or changes in uterine bleeding profile). Products include:
Provigil Tablets 1002

Nefazodone Hydrochloride (Co-administration with inhibitors of CYP3A4 may increase plasma concentrations of estrogens and may result in side effects).
No products indexed under this heading.

Nelfinavir Mesylate (Co-administration with inhibitors of CYP3A4 may increase plasma concentrations of estrogens and may result in side effects). Products include:
Viracept 2556

Nevirapine (Co-administration with inducers of CYP3A4 may reduce plasma concentrations of estrogens, possibly resulting in a decrease in therapeutic effects and/or changes in uterine bleeding profile). Products include:
Viramune Oral Suspension 903
Viramune Tablets 903

Niacinamide (Co-administration with inhibitors of CYP3A4 may increase plasma concentrations of estrogens and may result in side effects).
No products indexed under this heading.

Nicotinamide (Co-administration with inhibitors of CYP3A4 may increase plasma concentrations of estrogens and may result in side effects). Products include:
Nicomide Tablets 3190

Nifedipine (Co-administration with inhibitors of CYP3A4 may increase plasma concentrations of estrogens and may result in side effects). Products include:
Adalat CC Tablets 2978

Norfloxacin (Co-administration with inhibitors of CYP3A4 may increase plasma concentrations of estrogens and may result in side effects). Products include:
Noroxin Tablets 2009

Omeprazole (Co-administration with inhibitors of CYP3A4 may increase plasma concentrations of estrogens and may result in side effects). Products include:
Zegerid Powder for Oral Solution 2972

Oxcarbazepine (Co-administration with inducers of CYP3A4 may reduce plasma concentrations of estrogens, possibly resulting in a decrease in therapeutic effects and/or changes in uterine bleeding profile). Products include:
Trileptal Oral Suspension 2281
Trileptal Tablets 2281

Oxyphenbutazone (Concurrent use may result in elevated serum levels of oxyphenbutazone).
No products indexed under this heading.

Paroxetine Hydrochloride (Co-administration with inhibitors of CYP3A4 may increase plasma concentrations of estrogens and may result in side effects). Products include:
Paxil CR Controlled-Release Tablets 1509
Paxil 1501

Phenobarbital (Co-administration with inducers of CYP3A4 may reduce plasma concentrations of estrogens, possibly resulting in a decrease in therapeutic effects and/or changes in uterine bleeding profile).
No products indexed under this heading.

Phenobarbital Sodium (Co-administration with inducers of CYP3A4 may reduce plasma concentrations of estrogens, possibly resulting in a decrease in therapeutic effects and/or changes in uterine bleeding profile).
No products indexed under this heading.

Phenytoin (Co-administration with inducers of CYP3A4 may reduce plasma concentrations of estrogens, possibly resulting in a decrease in therapeutic effects and/or changes in uterine bleeding profile).
No products indexed under this heading.

Phenytoin Sodium (Co-administration with inducers of CYP3A4 may reduce plasma concentrations of estrogens, possibly resulting in a decrease in therapeutic effects and/or changes in uterine bleeding profile). Products include:
Phenytek Capsules 2153

Prednisolone Acetate (Co-administration with inducers of CYP3A4 may reduce plasma concentrations of estrogens, possibly resulting in a decrease in therapeutic effects and/or changes in uterine bleeding profile). Products include:
Blephamide Ophthalmic Ointment 563
Blephamide Ophthalmic Suspension 564
Poly-Pred Liquifilm Ophthalmic Suspension .... ⊙ 231
Pred Forte Ophthalmic Suspension .... ⊙ 233
Pred Mild Sterile Ophthalmic Suspension .... ⊙ 236
Pred-G Ophthalmic Suspension .... ⊙ 234
Pred-G Sterile Ophthalmic Ointment .... ⊙ 235

Prednisolone Sodium Phosphate (Co-administration with inducers of CYP3A4 may reduce plasma concentrations of estrogens, possibly resulting in a decrease in therapeutic effects and/or changes in uterine bleeding profile). Products include:
Pediapred Oral Solution 3319

Prednisolone Tebutate (Co-administration with inducers of CYP3A4 may reduce plasma concentrations of estrogens, possibly resulting in a decrease in therapeutic effects and/or changes in uterine bleeding profile).
No products indexed under this heading.

Prednisone (Co-administration with inducers of CYP3A4 may reduce plasma concentrations of estrogens, possibly resulting in a decrease in therapeutic effects and/or changes in uterine bleeding profile).
No products indexed under this heading.

Primidone (Co-administration with inducers of CYP3A4 may reduce plasma concentrations of estrogens, possibly resulting in a decrease in therapeutic effects and/or changes in uterine bleeding profile).
No products indexed under this heading.

Propoxyphene Hydrochloride (Co-administration with inhibitors of CYP3A4 may increase plasma concentrations of estrogens and may result in side effects).
No products indexed under this heading.

Propoxyphene Napsylate (Co-administration with inhibitors of CYP3A4 may increase plasma concentrations of estrogens and may result in side effects). Products include:
Darvocet A 500 Tablets 3497

Quinidine (Co-administration with inhibitors of CYP3A4 may increase plasma concentrations of estrogens and may result in side effects).
No products indexed under this heading.

Quinidine Hydrochloride (Co-administration with inhibitors of CYP3A4 may increase plasma concentrations of estrogens and may result in side effects).
No products indexed under this heading.

Quinidine Polygalacturonate (Co-administration with inhibitors of CYP3A4 may increase plasma concentrations of estrogens and may result in side effects).
No products indexed under this heading.

Quinidine Sulfate (Co-administration with inhibitors of CYP3A4 may increase plasma concentrations of estrogens and may result in side effects).
No products indexed under this heading.

Quinine (Co-administration with inhibitors of CYP3A4 may increase plasma concentrations of estrogens and may result in side effects).
No products indexed under this heading.

Quinine Sulfate (Co-administration with inhibitors of CYP3A4 may increase plasma concentrations of estrogens and may result in side effects).
No products indexed under this heading.

Quinupristin (Co-administration with inhibitors of CYP3A4 may increase plasma concentrations of estrogens and may result in side effects). Products include:
Synercid I.V. 1690

Ranitidine Bismuth Citrate (Co-administration with inhibitors of CYP3A4 may increase plasma concentrations of estrogens and may result in side effects).
No products indexed under this heading.

Ranitidine Hydrochloride (Co-administration with inhibitors of CYP3A4 may increase plasma concentrations of estrogens and may result in side effects). Products include:
Zantac 1597
Zantac Injection 1593
Zantac 75 Tablets .... ▣715
Zantac 150 Maximum Strength Tablets .... ▣715
Zantac Injection Pharmacy Bulk Package.................................... 1595

Rifabutin (Co-administration with inducers of CYP3A4 may reduce plasma concentrations of estrogens, possibly resulting in a decrease in therapeutic effects and/or changes in uterine bleeding profile).
No products indexed under this heading.

Rifampicin (Co-administration with inducers of CYP3A4 may reduce plasma concentrations of estrogens, possibly resulting in a decrease in therapeutic effects and/or changes in uterine bleeding profile).
No products indexed under this heading.

Rifampin (Co-administration with inducers of CYP3A4 may reduce plasma concentrations of estrogens, possibly resulting in a decrease in therapeutic effects and/or changes in uterine bleeding profile).
No products indexed under this heading.

Rifapentine (Co-administration with inducers of CYP3A4 may reduce plasma concentrations of estrogens, possibly resulting in a decrease in therapeutic effects and/or changes in uterine bleeding profile).
No products indexed under this heading.

Ritonavir (Co-administration with inhibitors of CYP3A4 may increase plasma concentrations of estrogens and may result in side effects). Products include:
Kaletra 474
Norvir 499

Saquinavir (Co-administration with inhibitors of CYP3A4 may increase plasma concentrations of estrogens and may result in side effects).
No products indexed under this heading.

Saquinavir Mesylate (Co-administration with inhibitors of CYP3A4 may increase plasma concentrations of estrogens and may result in side effects). Products include:
Invirase 2776

Sertraline Hydrochloride (Co-administration with inhibitors of CYP3A4 may increase plasma concentrations of estrogens and may result in side effects). Products include:
Zoloft 2581

Sulfinpyrazone (Co-administration with inducers of CYP3A4 may reduce plasma concentrations of estrogens, possibly resulting in a decrease in therapeutic effects and/or changes in uterine bleeding profile).
No products indexed under this heading.

Telithromycin (Co-administration with inhibitors of CYP3A4 may increase plasma concentrations of estrogens and may result in side effects). Products include:
Ketek Tablets 2920

Theophylline (Co-administration with inducers of CYP3A4 may reduce plasma concentrations of estrogens, possibly resulting in a decrease in therapeutic effects and/or changes in uterine bleeding profile).
No products indexed under this heading.

Triamcinolone (Co-administration with inducers of CYP3A4 may reduce plasma concentrations of estrogens, possibly resulting in a decrease in therapeutic effects and/or changes in uterine bleeding profile).
No products indexed under this heading.

Triamcinolone Acetonide (Co-administration with inducers of CYP3A4 may reduce plasma concentrations of estrogens, possibly resulting in a decrease in therapeutic effects and/or changes in uterine bleeding profile). Products include:
Azmacort Inhalation Aerosol 1701
Nasacort HFA Inhalation Aerosol 2939
Nasacort AQ Nasal Spray 2937

Triamcinolone Diacetate (Co-administration with inducers of CYP3A4 may reduce plasma concentrations of estrogens, possibly resulting in a decrease in therapeutic effects and/or changes in uterine bleeding profile).
No products indexed under this heading.

Triamcinolone Hexacetonide (Co-administration with inducers of CYP3A4 may reduce plasma concentrations of estrogens, possibly resulting in a decrease in therapeutic effects and/or changes in uterine bleeding profile).
No products indexed under this heading.

Troglitazone (Co-administration with inducers of CYP3A4 may reduce plasma concentrations of estrogens, possibly resulting in a decrease in therapeutic effects and/or changes in uterine bleeding profile).
No products indexed under this heading.

Troleandomycin (Co-administration with inhibitors of CYP3A4 may increase plasma concentrations of estrogens and may result in side effects).
No products indexed under this heading.

Valproate Sodium (Co-administration with inhibitors of CYP3A4 may increase plasma concentrations of estrogens and may result in side effects). Products include:
Depacon Injection 412

Verapamil Hydrochloride (Co-administration with inhibitors of CYP3A4 may increase plasma concentrations of estrogens and may result in side effects). Products include:
Covera-HS Tablets 3135
Tarka Tablets 519
Verelan PM Capsules 3120

Voriconazole (Co-administration with inhibitors of CYP3A4 may increase plasma concentrations of estrogens and may result in side effects). Products include:
VFEND I.V. 2543
VFEND Oral Suspension 2543
VFEND Tablets 2543

Warfarin Sodium (Decreased anticoagulant requirements). Products include:
Coumadin for Injection 932
Coumadin Tablets 932

Zafirlukast (Co-administration with inhibitors of CYP3A4 may increase plasma concentrations of estrogens and may result in side effects). Products include:
Accolate Tablets 663

Zileuton (Co-administration with inhibitors of CYP3A4 may increase plasma concentrations of estrogens and may result in side effects).
No products indexed under this heading.

Food Interactions

Grapefruit (Co-administration with inhibitors of CYP3A4 may increase plasma concentrations of estrogens and may result in side effects).

Grapefruit Juice (Co-administration with inhibitors of CYP3A4 may increase plasma concentrations of estrogens and may result in side effects).

ESTROGEL 0.06%

(Estradiol) 3200
May interact with erythromycin. Compounds in these categories include:

Carbamazepine (Inducers of CYP3A4, such as carbamazepine, may reduce plasma concentrations of estrogens, possibly resulting in a decrease in therapeutic effects and/or changes in uterine bleeding profile). Products include:
Carbatrol Capsules 3174
Equetro Extended-Release Capsules.. 3178
Tegretol/Tegretol-XR 2278

Clarithromycin (Inhibitors of CYP3A4, such as clarithromycin, may increase plasma concentrations of estrogens and may result in side effects). Products include:
Biaxin/Biaxin XL 402
PREVPAC 3281

Erythromycin (Inhibitors of CYP3A4, such as erythromycin, may increase plasma concentrations of estrogens and may result in side effects). Products include:
Erygel Topical Gel 2096
Ery-Tab Tablets 447
Erythromycin Base Filmtab Tablets... 454
Erythromycin Delayed-Release Capsules, USP.............................. 456
PCE Dispertab Tablets 510

Erythromycin Estolate (Inhibitors of CYP3A4, such as erythromycin, may increase plasma concentrations of estrogens and may result in side effects).
No products indexed under this heading.

Erythromycin Ethylsuccinate (Inhibitors of CYP3A4, such as erythromycin, may increase plasma concentrations of estrogens and may result in side effects). Products include:
E.E.S. 449
EryPed 445

Erythromycin Gluceptate (Inhibitors of CYP3A4, such as erythromycin, may increase plasma concentrations of estrogens and may result in side effects).
No products indexed under this heading.

Erythromycin Lactobionate (Inhibitors of CYP3A4, such as erythromycin, may increase plasma concentrations of estrogens and may result in side effects).
No products indexed under this heading.

Erythromycin Stearate (Inhibitors of CYP3A4, such as erythromycin, may increase plasma concentrations of estrogens and may result in side effects). Products include:

Erythrocin Stearate Filmtab Tablets ... 452

Hypericum Perforatum (Inducers of CYP3A4, such as St. John's Wort preparations (Hypericum perforatum), may reduce plasma concentrations of estrogens, possibly resulting in a decrease in therapeutic effects and/or changes in uterine bleeding profile).
No products indexed under this heading.

Itraconazole (Inhibitors of CYP3A4, such as itraconazole, may increase plasma concentrations of estrogens and may result in side effects).
No products indexed under this heading.

Ketoconazole (Inhibitors of CYP3A4, such as ketoconazole, may increase plasma concentrations of estrogens and may result in side effects). Products include:
Nizoral A-D Shampoo, 1% ... 1839
Nizoral 2% Shampoo ... 1838

Phenobarbital (Inducers of CYP3A4, such as phenobarbital, may reduce plasma concentrations of estrogens, possibly resulting in a decrease in therapeutic effects and/or changes in uterine bleeding profile).
No products indexed under this heading.

Phenobarbital Sodium (Inducers of CYP3A4, such as phenobarbital, may reduce plasma concentrations of estrogens, possibly resulting in a decrease in therapeutic effects and/or changes in uterine bleeding profile).
No products indexed under this heading.

Rifampin (Inducers of CYP3A4, such as rifampin, may reduce plasma concentrations of estrogens, possibly resulting in a decrease in therapeutic effects and/or changes in uterine bleeding profile).
No products indexed under this heading.

Ritonavir (Inhibitors of CYP3A4, such as ritonavir, may increase plasma concentrations of estrogens and may result in side effects). Products include:
Kaletra ... 474
Norvir ... 499

Food Interactions

Grapefruit Juice (Inhibitors of CYP3A4, such as grapefruit juice, may increase plasma concentrations of estrogens and may result in side effects).

ETHYOL FOR INJECTION
(Amifostine) ... 1869
May interact with antihypertensives. Compounds in these categories include:

Acebutolol Hydrochloride (Amifostine produces transient hypotension; caution is advised if it is used with other antihypertensive agents).
No products indexed under this heading.

Amlodipine Besylate (Amifostine produces transient hypotension; caution is advised if it is used with other antihypertensive agents). Products include:
Caduet Tablets ... 2507
Lotrel Capsules ... 2238
Norvasc Tablets ... 2529

Atenolol (Amifostine produces transient hypotension; caution is advised if it is used with other antihypertensive agents). Products include:
Tenormin I.V. Injection ... 698
Tenormin Tablets ... 695

Benazepril Hydrochloride (Amifostine produces transient hypotension; caution is advised if it is used with other antihypertensive agents). Products include:
Lotensin Tablets ... 2232
Lotensin HCT Tablets ... 2235
Lotrel Capsules ... 2238

Bendroflumethiazide (Amifostine produces transient hypotension; caution is advised if it is used with other antihypertensive agents).
No products indexed under this heading.

Betaxolol Hydrochloride (Amifostine produces transient hypotension; caution is advised if it is used with other antihypertensive agents). Products include:
Betoptic S Ophthalmic Suspension ... 554

Bisoprolol Fumarate (Amifostine produces transient hypotension; caution is advised if it is used with other antihypertensive agents).
No products indexed under this heading.

Candesartan Cilexetil (Amifostine produces transient hypotension; caution is advised if it is used with other antihypertensive agents). Products include:
Atacand Tablets ... 634
Atacand HCT ... 637

Captopril (Amifostine produces transient hypotension; caution is advised if it is used with other antihypertensive agents). Products include:
Captopril Tablets ... 2114

Carteolol Hydrochloride (Amifostine produces transient hypotension; caution is advised if it is used with other antihypertensive agents). Products include:
Carteolol Hydrochloride Ophthalmic Solution USP, 1% ... ⊙246

Chlorothiazide (Amifostine produces transient hypotension; caution is advised if it is used with other antihypertensive agents). Products include:
Aldoclor Tablets ... 1881
Diuril Oral ... 1936

Chlorothiazide Sodium (Amifostine produces transient hypotension; caution is advised if it is used with other antihypertensive agents). Products include:
Diuril Sodium Intravenous ... 1934

Chlorthalidone (Amifostine produces transient hypotension; caution is advised if it is used with other antihypertensive agents). Products include:
Clorpres Tablets ... 2139

Clonidine (Amifostine produces transient hypotension; caution is advised if it is used with other antihypertensive agents). Products include:
Catapres-TTS ... 875

Clonidine Hydrochloride (Amifostine produces transient hypotension; caution is advised if it is used with other antihypertensive agents). Products include:
Catapres Tablets ... 874
Clorpres Tablets ... 2139

Deserpidine (Amifostine produces transient hypotension; caution is advised if it is used with other antihypertensive agents).
No products indexed under this heading.

Diazoxide (Amifostine produces transient hypotension; caution is advised if it is used with other antihypertensive agents). Products include:
Hyperstat I.V. Injection ... 3031

Diltiazem Hydrochloride (Amifostine produces transient hypotension; caution is advised if it is used with other antihypertensive agents). Products include:
Cardizem LA Extended Release Tablets ... 1699
Tiazac Capsules ... 1204

Doxazosin Mesylate (Amifostine produces transient hypotension; caution is advised if it is used with other antihypertensive agents).
No products indexed under this heading.

Enalapril Maleate (Amifostine produces transient hypotension; caution is advised if it is used with other antihypertensive agents). Products include:
Vaseretic Tablets ... 2073
Vasotec I.V. Injection ... 2076

Enalaprilat (Amifostine produces transient hypotension; caution is advised if it is used with other antihypertensive agents).
No products indexed under this heading.

Eprosartan Mesylate (Amifostine produces transient hypotension; caution is advised if it is used with other antihypertensive agents). Products include:
Teveten Tablets ... 1707
Teveten HCT Tablets ... 1710

Esmolol Hydrochloride (Amifostine produces transient hypotension; caution is advised if it is used with other antihypertensive agents). Products include:
Brevibloc Concentrate ... 766
Brevibloc Injection ... 766
Brevibloc Double Strength Injection ... 766
Brevibloc Premixed Injection ... 766
Brevibloc Double Strength Premixed Injection ... 766

Felodipine (Amifostine produces transient hypotension; caution is advised if it is used with other antihypertensive agents). Products include:
Plendil Extended-Release Tablets ... 651

Fosinopril Sodium (Amifostine produces transient hypotension; caution is advised if it is used with other antihypertensive agents).
No products indexed under this heading.

Furosemide (Amifostine produces transient hypotension; caution is advised if it is used with other antihypertensive agents). Products include:
Furosemide Tablets ... 2117

Guanabenz Acetate (Amifostine produces transient hypotension; caution is advised if it is used with other antihypertensive agents).
No products indexed under this heading.

Guanethidine Monosulfate (Amifostine produces transient hypotension; caution is advised if it is used with other antihypertensive agents).
No products indexed under this heading.

Hydralazine Hydrochloride (Amifostine produces transient hypotension; caution is advised if it is used with other antihypertensive agents). Products include:
BiDil Tablets ... 2161

Hydrochlorothiazide (Amifostine produces transient hypotension; caution is advised if it is used with other antihypertensive agents). Products include:
Aldoril Tablets ... 1884
Atacand HCT ... 637
Avalide Tablets ... 2889
Avalide Tablets ... 922
Benicar HCT Tablets ... 2852
Diovan HCT Tablets ... 2195
Dyazide Capsules ... 1389
Hyzaar ... 1964
Lotensin HCT Tablets ... 2235
Maxzide ... 2150
Micardis HCT Tablets ... 886
Moduretic Tablets ... 2003
Prinzide Tablets ... 2033
Teveten HCT Tablets ... 1710
Timolide Tablets ... 2056
Uniretic Tablets ... 3114
Vaseretic Tablets ... 2073
Zestoretic Tablets ... 701

Hydroflumethiazide (Amifostine produces transient hypotension; caution is advised if it is used with other antihypertensive agents).
No products indexed under this heading.

Indapamide (Amifostine produces transient hypotension; caution is advised if it is used with other antihypertensive agents). Products include:
Indapamide Tablets ... 2119

Irbesartan (Amifostine produces transient hypotension; caution is advised if it is used with other antihypertensive agents). Products include:
Avalide Tablets ... 922
Avalide Tablets ... 2889
Avapro Tablets ... 925
Avapro Tablets ... 2886

Isradipine (Amifostine produces transient hypotension; caution is advised if it is used with other antihypertensive agents). Products include:
DynaCirc CR Tablets ... 2726

Labetalol Hydrochloride (Amifostine produces transient hypotension; caution is advised if it is used with other antihypertensive agents).
No products indexed under this heading.

Lisinopril (Amifostine produces transient hypotension; caution is advised if it is used with other antihypertensive agents). Products include:
Prinivil Tablets ... 2029
Prinzide Tablets ... 2033
Zestoretic Tablets ... 701
Zestril Tablets ... 704

Losartan Potassium (Amifostine produces transient hypotension; caution is advised if it is used with other antihypertensive agents). Products include:
Cozaar Tablets ... 1913
Hyzaar ... 1964

Mecamylamine Hydrochloride (Amifostine produces transient hypo-

tension; caution is advised if it is used with other antihypertensive agents). Products include:
Inversine Tablets 3286

Methyclothiazide (Amifostine produces transient hypotension; caution is advised if it is used with other antihypertensive agents).
No products indexed under this heading.

Methyldopa (Amifostine produces transient hypotension; caution is advised if it is used with other antihypertensive agents). Products include:
Aldoclor Tablets 1881
Aldoril Tablets 1884

Methyldopate Hydrochloride (Amifostine produces transient hypotension; caution is advised if it is used with other antihypertensive agents).
No products indexed under this heading.

Metolazone (Amifostine produces transient hypotension; caution is advised if it is used with other antihypertensive agents).
No products indexed under this heading.

Metoprolol Succinate (Amifostine produces transient hypotension; caution is advised if it is used with other antihypertensive agents). Products include:
Toprol-XL Tablets 660

Metoprolol Tartrate (Amifostine produces transient hypotension; caution is advised if it is used with other antihypertensive agents).
No products indexed under this heading.

Metyrosine (Amifostine produces transient hypotension; caution is advised if it is used with other antihypertensive agents). Products include:
Demser Capsules 1933

Mibefradil Dihydrochloride (Amifostine produces transient hypotension; caution is advised if it is used with other antihypertensive agents).
No products indexed under this heading.

Minoxidil (Amifostine produces transient hypotension; caution is advised if it is used with other antihypertensive agents). Products include:
Men's Rogaine Extra Strength Topical Solution, Ocean Rush Scent and Original Unscented ..... ▣ 706
Women's Rogaine Topical Solution, Spring Bloom Scent and Original Unscented .... ▣ 707

Moexipril Hydrochloride (Amifostine produces transient hypotension; caution is advised if it is used with other antihypertensive agents). Products include:
Uniretic Tablets 3114
Univasc Tablets 3118

Nadolol (Amifostine produces transient hypotension; caution is advised if it is used with other antihypertensive agents). Products include:
Nadolol Tablets 2121

Nicardipine Hydrochloride (Amifostine produces transient hypotension; caution is advised if it is used with other antihypertensive agents). Products include:
Cardene I.V. 1129

Nifedipine (Amifostine produces transient hypotension; caution is advised if it is used with other antihypertensive agents). Products include:
Adalat CC Tablets 2978

Nisoldipine (Amifostine produces transient hypotension; caution is advised if it is used with other antihypertensive agents). Products include:
Sular Tablets 1163

Nitroglycerin (Amifostine produces transient hypotension; caution is advised if it is used with other antihypertensive agents). Products include:
Nitro-Dur Transdermal Infusion System 3060
Nitrolingual Pumpspray 1161

Penbutolol Sulfate (Amifostine produces transient hypotension; caution is advised if it is used with other antihypertensive agents).
No products indexed under this heading.

Perindopril Erbumine (Amifostine produces transient hypotension; caution is advised if it is used with other antihypertensive agents). Products include:
Aceon Tablets (2 mg, 4 mg, 8 mg) 3191

Phenoxybenzamine Hydrochloride (Amifostine produces transient hypotension; caution is advised if it is used with other antihypertensive agents). Products include:
Dibenzyline Capsules 3390

Phentolamine Mesylate (Amifostine produces transient hypotension; caution is advised if it is used with other antihypertensive agents).
No products indexed under this heading.

Pindolol (Amifostine produces transient hypotension; caution is advised if it is used with other antihypertensive agents).
No products indexed under this heading.

Polythiazide (Amifostine produces transient hypotension; caution is advised if it is used with other antihypertensive agents).
No products indexed under this heading.

Prazosin Hydrochloride (Amifostine produces transient hypotension; caution is advised if it is used with other antihypertensive agents).
No products indexed under this heading.

Propranolol Hydrochloride (Amifostine produces transient hypotension; caution is advised if it is used with other antihypertensive agents). Products include:
Inderal LA Long-Acting Capsules 3421
InnoPran XL Capsules 2728

Quinapril Hydrochloride (Amifostine produces transient hypotension; caution is advised if it is used with other antihypertensive agents).
No products indexed under this heading.

Ramipril (Amifostine produces transient hypotension; caution is advised if it is used with other antihypertensive agents). Products include:
Altace Capsules 1673

Rauwolfia Serpentina (Amifostine produces transient hypotension; caution is advised if it is used with other antihypertensive agents).
No products indexed under this heading.

Rescinnamine (Amifostine produces transient hypotension; caution is advised if it is used with other antihypertensive agents).
No products indexed under this heading.

Reserpine (Amifostine produces transient hypotension; caution is advised if it is used with other antihypertensive agents).
No products indexed under this heading.

Sodium Nitroprusside (Amifostine produces transient hypotension; caution is advised if it is used with other antihypertensive agents).
No products indexed under this heading.

Sotalol Hydrochloride (Amifostine produces transient hypotension; caution is advised if it is used with other antihypertensive agents).
No products indexed under this heading.

Spirapril Hydrochloride (Amifostine produces transient hypotension; caution is advised if it is used with other antihypertensive agents).
No products indexed under this heading.

Telmisartan (Amifostine produces transient hypotension; caution is advised if it is used with other antihypertensive agents). Products include:
Micardis Tablets 884
Micardis HCT Tablets 886

Terazosin Hydrochloride (Amifostine produces transient hypotension; caution is advised if it is used with other antihypertensive agents). Products include:
Hytrin Capsules 469

Timolol Maleate (Amifostine produces transient hypotension; caution is advised if it is used with other antihypertensive agents). Products include:
Blocadren Tablets 1891
Cosopt Sterile Ophthalmic Solution 1910
Timolide Tablets 2056
Timoptic in Ocudose 2061
Timoptic Sterile Ophthalmic Solution 2058
Timoptic-XE Sterile Ophthalmic Gel Forming Solution 2062

Torsemide (Amifostine produces transient hypotension; caution is advised if it is used with other antihypertensive agents).
No products indexed under this heading.

Trandolapril (Amifostine produces transient hypotension; caution is advised if it is used with other antihypertensive agents). Products include:
Mavik Tablets 482
Tarka Tablets 519

Trimethaphan Camsylate (Amifostine produces transient hypotension; caution is advised if it is used with other antihypertensive agents).
No products indexed under this heading.

Valsartan (Amifostine produces transient hypotension; caution is advised if it is used with other antihypertensive agents). Products include:
Diovan HCT Tablets 2195
Diovan Tablets 2191

Verapamil Hydrochloride (Amifostine produces transient hypotension; caution is advised if it is used with other antihypertensive agents). Products include:
Covera-HS Tablets 3135
Tarka Tablets 519
Verelan PM Capsules 3120

EULEXIN CAPSULES

(Flutamide) 3023
May interact with:

Warfarin Sodium (Increases in prothrombin time have been noted in patients receiving long-term warfarin therapy after flutamide was initiated). Products include:
Coumadin for Injection 932
Coumadin Tablets 932

EVISTA TABLETS

(Raloxifene Hydrochloride) 1735
May interact with:

Cholestyramine (Co-administration causes a 60% reduction in the absorption and enterohepatic cycling of raloxifene; concurrent use should be avoided).
No products indexed under this heading.

Diazepam (Raloxifene might affect the protein binding of other highly protein-bound drugs such as diazepam; caution should be exercised). Products include:
Diastat Rectal Delivery System 3344
Valium Tablets 2822

Diazoxide (Raloxifene might affect the protein binding of other highly protein-bound drugs such as diazoxide; caution should be exercised). Products include:
Hyperstat I.V. Injection 3031

Lidocaine Hydrochloride (Raloxifene might affect the protein binding of other highly protein-bound drugs such as lidocaine; caution should be exercised).
No products indexed under this heading.

Warfarin Sodium (Co-administration has resulted in a 10% decrease in prothrombin time in single-dose studies; if used concurrently, prothrombin time should be monitored). Products include:
Coumadin for Injection 932
Coumadin Tablets 932

Food Interactions

Food, unspecified (Administration of raloxifene with a standardized, high fat meal increases the absorption of raloxifene, but does not lead to clinically meaningful changes in systemic exposure; Evista can be administered without regard to meals).

EVOCLIN FOAM, 1%

(Clindamycin Phosphate) 1025
May interact with neuromuscular blocking agents and certain other agents. Compounds in these categories include:

Atracurium Besylate (Clindamycin has been shown to have neuromuscular blocking properties that may enhance the action of other neuromuscular blocking agents; therefore, it should be used with caution in patients receiving such agents).
No products indexed under this heading.

Cisatracurium Besylate (Clindamycin has been shown to have neuromuscular blocking properties that may enhance the action of other neuromuscular blocking agents;

therefore, it should be used with caution in patients receiving such agents). Products include:
Nimbex Injection 494

Doxacurium Chloride (Clindamycin has been shown to have neuromuscular blocking properties that may enhance the action of other neuromuscular blocking agents; therefore, it should be used with caution in patients receiving such agents).
No products indexed under this heading.

Metocurine Iodide (Clindamycin has been shown to have neuromuscular blocking properties that may enhance the action of other neuromuscular blocking agents; therefore, it should be used with caution in patients receiving such agents).
No products indexed under this heading.

Mivacurium Chloride (Clindamycin has been shown to have neuromuscular blocking properties that may enhance the action of other neuromuscular blocking agents; therefore, it should be used with caution in patients receiving such agents). Products include:
Mivacron Injection 489

Pancuronium Bromide (Clindamycin has been shown to have neuromuscular blocking properties that may enhance the action of other neuromuscular blocking agents; therefore, it should be used with caution in patients receiving such agents).
No products indexed under this heading.

Rapacuronium Bromide (Clindamycin has been shown to have neuromuscular blocking properties that may enhance the action of other neuromuscular blocking agents; therefore, it should be used with caution in patients receiving such agents).
No products indexed under this heading.

Rocuronium Bromide (Clindamycin has been shown to have neuromuscular blocking properties that may enhance the action of other neuromuscular blocking agents; therefore, it should be used with caution in patients receiving such agents). Products include:
Zemuron Injection 2363

Succinylcholine Chloride (Clindamycin has been shown to have neuromuscular blocking properties that may enhance the action of other neuromuscular blocking agents; therefore, it should be used with caution in patients receiving such agents).
No products indexed under this heading.

Vecuronium Bromide (Clindamycin has been shown to have neuromuscular blocking properties that may enhance the action of other neuromuscular blocking agents; therefore, it should be used with caution in patients receiving such agents).
No products indexed under this heading.

EVOXAC CAPSULES

(Cevimeline Hydrochloride) 1042
May interact with antimuscarinic drugs, beta blockers, cytochrome p450 2d6 inhibitors (selected), cytochrome p450 3a4 inhibitors (selected), parasympathomimetics, and certain other agents. Compounds in these categories include:

Acebutolol Hydrochloride (Possibility of conduction disturbances; co-administration with beta adrenergic antagonists requires caution).
No products indexed under this heading.

Acetazolamide (Drugs which inhibit CYP3A3/4 also inhibit the metabolism of cevimeline).
No products indexed under this heading.

Amiodarone Hydrochloride (Co-administration with drugs which inhibit CYP2D6, such as amiodarone, may inhibit the metabolism of cevimeline resulting in a higher risk of adverse events). Products include:
Pacerone Tablets 3337

Amitriptyline Hydrochloride (Drugs which inhibit CYP2D6 also inhibit the metabolism of cevimeline. Cevimeline should be used with caution in individuals known or suspected to be deficient in CYP2D6 activity, as they may be at a higher risk of adverse events).
No products indexed under this heading.

Amoxapine (Drugs which inhibit CYP2D6 also inhibit the metabolism of cevimeline. Cevimeline should be used with caution in individuals known or suspected to be deficient in CYP2D6 activity, as they may be at a higher risk of adverse events).
No products indexed under this heading.

Amprenavir (Drugs which inhibit CYP3A3/4 also inhibit the metabolism of cevimeline). Products include:
Agenerase Capsules 1299
Agenerase Oral Solution 1304

Anastrozole (Drugs which inhibit CYP3A3/4 also inhibit the metabolism of cevimeline). Products include:
Arimidex Tablets 665

Aprepitant (Drugs which inhibit CYP3A3/4 also inhibit the metabolism of cevimeline). Products include:
Emend Capsules 1944

Atenolol (Possibility of conduction disturbances; co-administration with beta adrenergic antagonists requires caution). Products include:
Tenormin I.V. Injection 698
Tenormin Tablets 695

Atropine Sulfate (Cevimeline might interfere with the desirable antimuscarinic effects of drugs used concomitantly).
No products indexed under this heading.

Belladonna Alkaloids (Cevimeline might interfere with the desirable antimuscarinic effects of drugs used concomitantly). Products include:
Hyland's Teething Tablets 736

Betaxolol Hydrochloride (Possibility of conduction disturbances; co-administration with beta adrenergic antagonists requires caution). Products include:
Betoptic S Ophthalmic Suspension............................... 554

Bisoprolol Fumarate (Possibility of conduction disturbances; co-administration with beta adrenergic antagonists requires caution).
No products indexed under this heading.

Bupropion Hydrochloride (Drugs which inhibit CYP2D6 also inhibit the metabolism of cevimeline. Cevimeline should be used with caution in individuals known or suspected to be deficient in CYP2D6 activity, as they may be at a higher risk of adverse events). Products include:
Wellbutrin Tablets 1579
Wellbutrin SR Sustained-Release Tablets 1583
Wellbutrin XL Extended-Release Tablets 1588
Zyban Sustained-Release Tablets 1620

Carteolol Hydrochloride (Possibility of conduction disturbances; co-administration with beta adrenergic antagonists requires caution). Products include:
Carteolol Hydrochloride Ophthalmic Solution USP, 1%....... ⊙246

Celecoxib (Drugs which inhibit CYP2D6 also inhibit the metabolism of cevimeline. Cevimeline should be used with caution in individuals known or suspected to be deficient in CYP2D6 activity, as they may be at a higher risk of adverse events). Products include:
Celebrex Capsules 3130

Chloroquine Hydrochloride (Drugs which inhibit CYP2D6 also inhibit the metabolism of cevimeline. Cevimeline should be used with caution in individuals known or suspected to be deficient in CYP2D6 activity, as they may be at a higher risk of adverse events).
No products indexed under this heading.

Chloroquine Phosphate (Drugs which inhibit CYP2D6 also inhibit the metabolism of cevimeline. Cevimeline should be used with caution in individuals known or suspected to be deficient in CYP2D6 activity, as they may be at a higher risk of adverse events).
No products indexed under this heading.

Chlorpheniramine (Drugs which inhibit CYP2D6 also inhibit the metabolism of cevimeline. Cevimeline should be used with caution in individuals known or suspected to be deficient in CYP2D6 activity, as they may be at a higher risk of adverse events).
No products indexed under this heading.

Chlorpheniramine Maleate (Drugs which inhibit CYP2D6 also inhibit the metabolism of cevimeline. Cevimeline should be used with caution in individuals known or suspected to be deficient in CYP2D6 activity, as they may be at a higher risk of adverse events). Products include:
Advil Allergy Sinus Caplets 737
Advil Multi-Symptom Cold Caplets.. 738
BC Allergy Sinus Cold Powder 612
Contac Severe Cold and Flu Caplets Maximum Strength......... 615
Hycomine Compound Tablets 1105
PediaCare Multi-Symptom Cold Liquid 704
PediaCare NightRest Cough & Cold Liquid................................ 704
Robitussin Flu Liquid 752
Robitussin PM Cough & Cold Liquid 752
Singlet Caplets 636
Sudafed Sinus & Allergy Tablets 710
TheraFlu Cold & Cough Hot Liquid 680
TheraFlu Cold & Sore Throat Hot Liquid 680
TheraFlu Flu & Sore Throat Hot Liquid 681
TheraFlu Severe Cold & Cough Hot Liquid 683
TheraFlu Severe Cold Caplets 679
TheraFlu Severe Cold Hot Liquid 682
Triaminic Cold & Allergy Liquid 685
Triaminic Cold & Cough Liquid 685
Triaminic Flu, Cough & Fever Liquid 685
Triaminic Night Time Cough & Cold Liquid................................. 685
Triaminic Allergy Runny Nose & Congestion Softchews............... 688
Triaminic Cold & Cough Softchews 688
Children's Tylenol Plus Cold NightTime Suspension Liquid........ 1851
Children's Tylenol Plus Cold & Cough Suspension Liquid and Chewable Tablets 1851
Children's Tylenol Plus Cold Chewable Tablets........................ 1851
Children's Tylenol Plus Flu Suspension Liquid 1853
Tylenol Allergy Complete Multi-Symptom Caplets and Gelcaps with Cool Burst............... 1844
Multi-Symptom Tylenol Cold Night Time Caplets.............................. 1845
Vicks 44M Cough, Cold & Flu Relief.. 2676
Pediatric Vicks 44m Cough & Cold Relief.................................. 2673
Children's Vicks NyQuil Cold/Cough Relief....................... 2671

Chlorpheniramine Polistirex (Drugs which inhibit CYP2D6 also inhibit the metabolism of cevimeline. Cevimeline should be used with caution in individuals known or suspected to be deficient in CYP2D6 activity, as they may be at a higher risk of adverse events). Products include:
Tussionex Pennkinetic Extended-Release Suspension...... 3322

Chlorpheniramine Tannate (Drugs which inhibit CYP2D6 also inhibit the metabolism of cevimeline. Cevimeline should be used with caution in individuals known or suspected to be deficient in CYP2D6 activity, as they may be at a higher risk of adverse events).
No products indexed under this heading.

Cimetidine (Co-administration with drugs which inhibit CYP2D6, such as cimetidine, may inhibit the metabolism of cevimeline resulting in a higher risk of adverse events). Products include:
Tagamet HB 200 Tablets 637
Tagamet Tablets 1547

Cimetidine Hydrochloride (Co-administration with drugs which inhibit CYP2D6, such as cimetidine, may inhibit the metabolism of cevimeline resulting in a higher risk of adverse events).
No products indexed under this heading.

Ciprofloxacin (Drugs which inhibit CYP3A3/4 also inhibit the metabolism of cevimeline). Products include:
Cipro I.V. 2998
Cipro I.V. Pharmacy Bulk Package ... 3509
Cipro Oral Suspension 2991
Cipro XR Tablets 3004
Ciprodex Otic Suspension 555

Citalopram Hydrobromide (Drugs which inhibit CYP2D6 also inhibit the metabolism of cevimeline. Cevime-

line should be used with caution in individuals known or suspected to be deficient in CYP2D6 activity, as they may be at a higher risk of adverse events). Products include:
- Celexa 1177

Clarithromycin (Co-administration with drugs which inhibit CYP3A3/4, such as clarithromycin, may inhibit the metabolism of cevimeline resulting in a higher risk of adverse events). Products include:
- Biaxin/Biaxin XL 402
- PREVPAC 3281

Clidinium Bromide (Cevimeline might interfere with the desirable antimuscarinic effects of drugs used concomitantly).
- No products indexed under this heading.

Clomipramine Hydrochloride (Drugs which inhibit CYP2D6 also inhibit the metabolism of cevimeline. Cevimeline should be used with caution in individuals known or suspected to be deficient in CYP2D6 activity, as they may be at a higher risk of adverse events).
- No products indexed under this heading.

Clotrimazole (Drugs which inhibit CYP3A3/4 also inhibit the metabolism of cevimeline). Products include:
- Lotrimin 3053
- Lotrisone 3054

Cocaine Hydrochloride (Drugs which inhibit CYP2D6 also inhibit the metabolism of cevimeline. Cevimeline should be used with caution in individuals known or suspected to be deficient in CYP2D6 activity, as they may be at a higher risk of adverse events).
- No products indexed under this heading.

Cyclosporine (Drugs which inhibit CYP3A3/4 also inhibit the metabolism of cevimeline). Products include:
- Gengraf Capsules 458
- Neoral Soft Gelatin Capsules 2247
- Neoral Oral Solution 2247
- Restasis Ophthalmic Emulsion 570
- Sandimmune 2259

Dalfopristin (Drugs which inhibit CYP3A3/4 also inhibit the metabolism of cevimeline). Products include:
- Synercid I.V. 1690

Danazol (Drugs which inhibit CYP3A3/4 also inhibit the metabolism of cevimeline).
- No products indexed under this heading.

Delavirdine Mesylate (Drugs which inhibit CYP3A3/4 also inhibit the metabolism of cevimeline). Products include:
- Rescriptor Tablets 2535

Desipramine Hydrochloride (Drugs which inhibit CYP2D6 also inhibit the metabolism of cevimeline. Cevimeline should be used with caution in individuals known or suspected to be deficient in CYP2D6 activity, as they may be at a higher risk of adverse events).
- No products indexed under this heading.

Dicyclomine Hydrochloride (Cevimeline might interfere with the desirable antimuscarinic effects of drugs used concomitantly). Products include:
- Bentyl Capsules 724
- Bentyl Injection 724
- Bentyl Syrup 724
- Bentyl Tablets 724

Diltiazem Hydrochloride (Co-administration with drugs which inhibit CYP3A3/4, such as diltiazem, may inhibit the metabolism of cevimeline resulting in a higher risk of adverse events). Products include:
- Cardizem LA Extended Release Tablets 1699
- Tiazac Capsules 1204

Diltiazem Maleate (Drugs which inhibit CYP3A3/4 also inhibit the metabolism of cevimeline).
- No products indexed under this heading.

Diphenhydramine (Drugs which inhibit CYP2D6 also inhibit the metabolism of cevimeline. Cevimeline should be used with caution in individuals known or suspected to be deficient in CYP2D6 activity, as they may be at a higher risk of adverse events). Products include:
- Tylenol Sore Throat NightTime Liquid with Cool Burst.................. 1849

Diphenhydramine Hydrochloride (Drugs which inhibit CYP2D6 also inhibit the metabolism of cevimeline. Cevimeline should be used with caution in individuals known or suspected to be deficient in CYP2D6 activity, as they may be at a higher risk of adverse events). Products include:
- Benadryl Allergy & Cold Tablets ..... ▣692
- Benadryl Allergy .... ▣691
- Benadryl Allergy & Sinus Headache Caplets & Gelcaps...... ▣693
- Children's Benadryl Allergy Liquid ... ▣695
- Children's Benadryl Dye-Free Allergy Liquid .... ▣695
- Benadryl Dye-Free Allergy Liqui-Gels Softgels .... ▣692
- Benadryl Itch Relief Stick Extra Strength .... ▣696
- Benadryl Itch Stopping Cream Extra Strength............................ ▣697
- Benadryl Itch Stopping Gel Extra Strength .... ▣697
- Benadryl Itch Stopping Spray Extra Strength .... ▣697
- Benadryl Maximum Strength Severe Allergy & Sinus Headache Caplets........................... ▣694
- Children's Benadryl D Liquid Medication.................................. ▣693
- Benadryl D Tablets .... ▣694
- Nytol QuickCaps Caplets .... ▣635
- Maximum Strength Nytol QuickGels Softgels .... ▣635
- Simply Sleep Caplets 1841
- Sominex Original Formula Tablets .. ▣637
- TheraFlu Thin Strips Multi Symptom...................................... ▣684
- Triaminic Thin Strips Cough & Runny Nose .... ▣690
- Children's Tylenol Plus Cold & Allergy Suspension Liquid............ 1850
- Tylenol Allergy Complete Night Time Caplets.............................. 1844
- Tylenol Severe Allergy Caplets 1844
- Tylenol Flu NightTime Gelcaps 1846
- Extra Strength Tylenol PM Caplets, Geltabs, Gelcaps and Liquid 1847
- Unisom Maximum Strength SleepGels.................................. ▣712

Doxepin Hydrochloride (Drugs which inhibit CYP2D6 also inhibit the metabolism of cevimeline. Cevimeline should be used with caution in individuals known or suspected to be deficient in CYP2D6 activity, as they may be at a higher risk of adverse events).
- No products indexed under this heading.

Edrophonium Chloride (Co-administration with parasympathomimetic drugs can be expected to have additive effects).
- No products indexed under this heading.

Efavirenz (Drugs which inhibit CYP3A3/4 also inhibit the metabolism of cevimeline). Products include:
- Sustiva Capsules 957

Erythromycin (Drugs which inhibit CYP3A3/4 also inhibit the metabolism of cevimeline). Products include:
- Erygel Topical Gel 2096
- Ery-Tab Tablets 447
- Erythromycin Base Filmtab Tablets 454
- Erythromycin Delayed-Release Capsules, USP.............................. 456
- PCE Dispertab Tablets 510

Erythromycin Estolate (Drugs which inhibit CYP3A3/4 also inhibit the metabolism of cevimeline).
- No products indexed under this heading.

Erythromycin Ethylsuccinate (Drugs which inhibit CYP3A3/4 also inhibit the metabolism of cevimeline). Products include:
- E.E.S. 449
- EryPed 445

Erythromycin Gluceptate (Drugs which inhibit CYP3A3/4 also inhibit the metabolism of cevimeline).
- No products indexed under this heading.

Erythromycin Lactobionate (Drugs which inhibit CYP3A3/4 also inhibit the metabolism of cevimeline).
- No products indexed under this heading.

Erythromycin Stearate (Drugs which inhibit CYP3A3/4 also inhibit the metabolism of cevimeline). Products include:
- Erythrocin Stearate Filmtab Tablets 452

Escitalopram Oxalate (Drugs which inhibit CYP2D6 also inhibit the metabolism of cevimeline. Cevimeline should be used with caution in individuals known or suspected to be deficient in CYP2D6 activity, as they may be at a higher risk of adverse events). Products include:
- Lexapro Oral Solution 1193
- Lexapro Tablets 1193

Esmolol Hydrochloride (Possibility of conduction disturbances; co-administration with beta adrenergic antagonists requires caution). Products include:
- Brevibloc Concentrate 766
- Brevibloc Injection 766
- Brevibloc Double Strength Injection....................................... 766
- Brevibloc Premixed Injection 766
- Brevibloc Double Strength Premixed Injection........................ 766

Esomeprazole Magnesium (Drugs which inhibit CYP3A3/4 also inhibit the metabolism of cevimeline). Products include:
- Nexium Delayed-Release Capsules....................................... 645

Fluconazole (Drugs which inhibit CYP3A3/4 also inhibit the metabolism of cevimeline).
- No products indexed under this heading.

Fluoxetine (Drugs which inhibit CYP2D6 also inhibit the metabolism of cevimeline. Cevimeline should be used with caution in individuals known or suspected to be deficient in CYP2D6 activity, as they may be at a higher risk of adverse events).
- No products indexed under this heading.

Fluoxetine Hydrochloride (Co-administration with drugs which inhibit CYP2D6, such as fluoxetine, may inhibit the metabolism of cevimeline resulting in a higher risk of adverse events). Products include:
- Prozac Pulvules and Liquid 1771
- Symbyax Capsules 1788

Fluphenazine Decanoate (Drugs which inhibit CYP2D6 also inhibit the metabolism of cevimeline. Cevimeline should be used with caution in individuals known or suspected to be deficient in CYP2D6 activity, as they may be at a higher risk of adverse events).
- No products indexed under this heading.

Fluphenazine Enanthate (Drugs which inhibit CYP2D6 also inhibit the metabolism of cevimeline. Cevimeline should be used with caution in individuals known or suspected to be deficient in CYP2D6 activity, as they may be at a higher risk of adverse events).
- No products indexed under this heading.

Fluphenazine Hydrochloride (Drugs which inhibit CYP2D6 also inhibit the metabolism of cevimeline. Cevimeline should be used with caution in individuals known or suspected to be deficient in CYP2D6 activity, as they may be at a higher risk of adverse events).
- No products indexed under this heading.

Fluvoxamine Maleate (Drugs which inhibit CYP2D6 also inhibit the metabolism of cevimeline. Cevimeline should be used with caution in individuals known or suspected to be deficient in CYP2D6 activity, as they may be at a higher risk of adverse events).
- No products indexed under this heading.

Fosamprenavir Calcium (Drugs which inhibit CYP3A3/4 also inhibit the metabolism of cevimeline). Products include:
- Lexiva Tablets 1473

Glycopyrrolate (Cevimeline might interfere with the desirable antimuscarinic effects of drugs used concomitantly).
- No products indexed under this heading.

Halofantrine Hydrochloride (Drugs which inhibit CYP2D6 also inhibit the metabolism of cevimeline. Cevimeline should be used with caution in individuals known or suspected to be deficient in CYP2D6 activity, as they may be at a higher risk of adverse events).
- No products indexed under this heading.

Haloperidol (Drugs which inhibit CYP2D6 also inhibit the metabolism of cevimeline. Cevimeline should be used with caution in individuals known or suspected to be deficient in CYP2D6 activity, as they may be at a higher risk of adverse events).
No products indexed under this heading.

Haloperidol Decanoate (Drugs which inhibit CYP2D6 also inhibit the metabolism of cevimeline. Cevimeline should be used with caution in individuals known or suspected to be deficient in CYP2D6 activity, as they may be at a higher risk of adverse events).
No products indexed under this heading.

Hydroxychloroquine Sulfate (Drugs which inhibit CYP2D6 also inhibit the metabolism of cevimeline. Cevimeline should be used with caution in individuals known or suspected to be deficient in CYP2D6 activity, as they may be at a higher risk of adverse events).
No products indexed under this heading.

Hyoscyamine (Cevimeline might interfere with the desirable antimuscarinic effects of drugs used concomitantly).
No products indexed under this heading.

Hyoscyamine Sulfate (Cevimeline might interfere with the desirable antimuscarinic effects of drugs used concomitantly).
No products indexed under this heading.

Imatinib Mesylate (Drugs which inhibit CYP2D6 also inhibit the metabolism of cevimeline. Cevimeline should be used with caution in individuals known or suspected to be deficient in CYP2D6 activity, as they may be at a higher risk of adverse events). Products include:
Gleevec Tablets 2221

Imipramine Hydrochloride (Drugs which inhibit CYP2D6 also inhibit the metabolism of cevimeline. Cevimeline should be used with caution in individuals known or suspected to be deficient in CYP2D6 activity, as they may be at a higher risk of adverse events).
No products indexed under this heading.

Imipramine Pamoate (Drugs which inhibit CYP2D6 also inhibit the metabolism of cevimeline. Cevimeline should be used with caution in individuals known or suspected to be deficient in CYP2D6 activity, as they may be at a higher risk of adverse events).
No products indexed under this heading.

Indinavir Sulfate (Co-administration with drugs which inhibit CYP3A3/4, such as indinavir, may inhibit the metabolism of cevimeline resulting in a higher risk of adverse events). Products include:
Crixivan Capsules 1918

Ipratropium Bromide (Cevimeline might interfere with the desirable antimuscarinic effects of drugs used concomitantly). Products include:
Atrovent HFA Inhalation Aerosol 872
Atrovent Inhalation Solution 868
Atrovent Nasal Spray 0.03% 869
Atrovent Nasal Spray 0.06% 870
Combivent Inhalation Aerosol 878
DuoNeb Inhalation Solution 1058

Isoniazid (Drugs which inhibit CYP3A3/4 also inhibit the metabolism of cevimeline).
No products indexed under this heading.

Itraconazole (Co-administration with drugs which inhibit CYP3A3/4, such as itraconazole, may inhibit the metabolism of cevimeline resulting in a higher risk of adverse events).
No products indexed under this heading.

Ketoconazole (Co-administration with drugs which inhibit CYP3A3/4, such as ketoconazole, may inhibit the metabolism of cevimeline resulting in a higher risk of adverse events). Products include:
Nizoral A-D Shampoo, 1% 1839
Nizoral 2% Shampoo 1838

Labetalol Hydrochloride (Possibility of conduction disturbances; co-administration with beta adrenergic antagonists requires caution).
No products indexed under this heading.

Levobunolol Hydrochloride (Possibility of conduction disturbances; co-administration with beta adrenergic antagonists requires caution). Products include:
Betagan Ophthalmic Solution, USP .... ⊙217

Lopinavir (Drugs which inhibit CYP3A3/4 also inhibit the metabolism of cevimeline). Products include:
Kaletra 474

Loratadine (Drugs which inhibit CYP3A3/4 also inhibit the metabolism of cevimeline). Products include:
Alavert Allergy & Sinus D-12 Hour Tablets 743
Alavert 743
Children's Claritin 24 Hour Non-Drowsy Allergy Syrup 732
Claritin Non-Drowsy 24 Hour Tablets 731
Non-Drowsy Claritin Hives Relief Tablets 733
Claritin Reditabs 24 Hour Non-Drowsy Tablets 732
Claritin-D Non-Drowsy 12 Hour Tablets 731
Claritin-D Non-Drowsy 24 Hour Tablets 731
Children's Dimetapp ND Non-Drowsy Allergy Syrup 746
Triaminic Allerchews 684

Maprotiline Hydrochloride (Drugs which inhibit CYP2D6 also inhibit the metabolism of cevimeline. Cevimeline should be used with caution in individuals known or suspected to be deficient in CYP2D6 activity, as they may be at a higher risk of adverse events).
No products indexed under this heading.

Mepenzolate Bromide (Cevimeline might interfere with the desirable antimuscarinic effects of drugs used concomitantly).
No products indexed under this heading.

Methadone Hydrochloride (Drugs which inhibit CYP2D6 also inhibit the metabolism of cevimeline. Cevimeline should be used with caution in individuals known or suspected to be deficient in CYP2D6 activity, as they may be at a higher risk of adverse events).
No products indexed under this heading.

Metipranolol Hydrochloride (Possibility of conduction disturbances; co-administration with beta adrenergic antagonists requires caution).
No products indexed under this heading.

Metoprolol Succinate (Possibility of conduction disturbances; co-administration with beta adrenergic antagonists requires caution). Products include:
Toprol-XL Tablets 660

Metoprolol Tartrate (Possibility of conduction disturbances; co-administration with beta adrenergic antagonists requires caution).
No products indexed under this heading.

Metronidazole (Drugs which inhibit CYP3A3/4 also inhibit the metabolism of cevimeline). Products include:
Metrogel 1% 1212
MetroGel-Vaginal Gel 1822
Noritate Cream, 1% 1051

Metronidazole Benzoate (Drugs which inhibit CYP3A3/4 also inhibit the metabolism of cevimeline).
No products indexed under this heading.

Metronidazole Hydrochloride (Drugs which inhibit CYP3A3/4 also inhibit the metabolism of cevimeline).
No products indexed under this heading.

Mibefradil Dihydrochloride (Drugs which inhibit CYP2D6 also inhibit the metabolism of cevimeline. Cevimeline should be used with caution in individuals known or suspected to be deficient in CYP2D6 activity, as they may be at a higher risk of adverse events).
No products indexed under this heading.

Miconazole (Drugs which inhibit CYP3A3/4 also inhibit the metabolism of cevimeline).
No products indexed under this heading.

Miconazole Nitrate (Drugs which inhibit CYP3A3/4 also inhibit the metabolism of cevimeline). Products include:
Desenex 674
Desenex Jock Itch Spray Powder ... 674

Moclobemide (Drugs which inhibit CYP2D6 also inhibit the metabolism of cevimeline. Cevimeline should be used with caution in individuals known or suspected to be deficient in CYP2D6 activity, as they may be at a higher risk of adverse events).
No products indexed under this heading.

Nadolol (Possibility of conduction disturbances; co-administration with beta adrenergic antagonists requires caution). Products include:
Nadolol Tablets 2121

Nefazodone Hydrochloride (Co-administration with drugs which inhibit CYP3A3/4, such as nefazodone, may inhibit the metabolism of cevimeline resulting in a higher risk of adverse events).
No products indexed under this heading.

Nelfinavir Mesylate (Co-administration with drugs which inhibit CYP3A3/4, such as nelfinavir, may inhibit the metabolism of cevimeline resulting in a higher risk of adverse events). Products include:
Viracept 2556

Neostigmine Bromide (Co-administration with parasympathomimetic drugs can be expected to have additive effects).
No products indexed under this heading.

Neostigmine Methylsulfate (Co-administration with parasympathomimetic drugs can be expected to have additive effects).
No products indexed under this heading.

Nevirapine (Drugs which inhibit CYP3A3/4 also inhibit the metabolism of cevimeline). Products include:
Viramune Oral Suspension 903
Viramune Tablets 903

Niacinamide (Drugs which inhibit CYP3A3/4 also inhibit the metabolism of cevimeline).
No products indexed under this heading.

Nicotinamide (Drugs which inhibit CYP3A3/4 also inhibit the metabolism of cevimeline). Products include:
Nicomide Tablets 3190

Nifedipine (Drugs which inhibit CYP3A3/4 also inhibit the metabolism of cevimeline). Products include:
Adalat CC Tablets 2978

Norfloxacin (Drugs which inhibit CYP3A3/4 also inhibit the metabolism of cevimeline). Products include:
Noroxin Tablets 2009

Nortriptyline Hydrochloride (Drugs which inhibit CYP2D6 also inhibit the metabolism of cevimeline. Cevimeline should be used with caution in individuals known or suspected to be deficient in CYP2D6 activity, as they may be at a higher risk of adverse events).
No products indexed under this heading.

Omeprazole (Drugs which inhibit CYP3A3/4 also inhibit the metabolism of cevimeline). Products include:
Zegerid Powder for Oral Solution 2972

Oxyphenonium Bromide (Cevimeline might interfere with the desirable antimuscarinic effects of drugs used concomitantly).
No products indexed under this heading.

Paroxetine Hydrochloride (Co-administration with drugs which inhibit CYP2D6, such as paroxetine, may inhibit the metabolism of cevimeline resulting in a higher risk of adverse events). Products include:
Paxil CR Controlled-Release Tablets 1509
Paxil 1501

Penbutolol Sulfate (Possibility of conduction disturbances; co-administration with beta adrenergic antagonists requires caution).
No products indexed under this heading.

Perphenazine (Drugs which inhibit CYP2D6 also inhibit the metabolism of cevimeline. Cevimeline should be used with caution in individuals known or suspected to be deficient in CYP2D6 activity, as they may be at a higher risk of adverse events).
No products indexed under this heading.

Pindolol (Possibility of conduction disturbances; co-administration with beta adrenergic antagonists requires caution).
No products indexed under this heading.

Propafenone Hydrochloride (Drugs which inhibit CYP2D6 also inhibit the metabolism of cevimeline. Cevimeline should be used with caution in individuals known or suspected to be deficient in CYP2D6 activity, as they may be at a higher risk of adverse events). Products include:
Rythmol SR Capsules ... 2736

Propantheline Bromide (Cevimeline might interfere with the desirable antimuscarinic effects of drugs used concomitantly).
No products indexed under this heading.

Propoxyphene Hydrochloride (Drugs which inhibit CYP2D6 also inhibit the metabolism of cevimeline. Cevimeline should be used with caution in individuals known or suspected to be deficient in CYP2D6 activity, as they may be at a higher risk of adverse events).
No products indexed under this heading.

Propoxyphene Napsylate (Drugs which inhibit CYP2D6 also inhibit the metabolism of cevimeline. Cevimeline should be used with caution in individuals known or suspected to be deficient in CYP2D6 activity, as they may be at a higher risk of adverse events). Products include:
Darvocet A 500 Tablets ... 3497

Propranolol Hydrochloride (Possibility of conduction disturbances; co-administration with beta adrenergic antagonists requires caution). Products include:
Inderal LA Long-Acting Capsules ... 3421
InnoPran XL Capsules ... 2728

Protriptyline Hydrochloride (Drugs which inhibit CYP2D6 also inhibit the metabolism of cevimeline. Cevimeline should be used with caution in individuals known or suspected to be deficient in CYP2D6 activity, as they may be at a higher risk of adverse events). Products include:
Vivactil Tablets ... 2350

Pyridostigmine Bromide (Co-administration with parasympathomimetic drugs can be expected to have additive effects).
No products indexed under this heading.

Quinacrine Hydrochloride (Drugs which inhibit CYP2D6 also inhibit the metabolism of cevimeline. Cevimeline should be used with caution in individuals known or suspected to be deficient in CYP2D6 activity, as they may be at a higher risk of adverse events).
No products indexed under this heading.

Quinidine (Drugs which inhibit CYP3A3/4 also inhibit the metabolism of cevimeline).
No products indexed under this heading.

Quinidine Gluconate (Drugs which inhibit CYP2D6 also inhibit the metabolism of cevimeline. Cevimeline should be used with caution in individuals known or suspected to be deficient in CYP2D6 activity, as they may be at a higher risk of adverse events).
No products indexed under this heading.

Quinidine Hydrochloride (Drugs which inhibit CYP2D6 also inhibit the metabolism of cevimeline. Cevimeline should be used with caution in individuals known or suspected to be deficient in CYP2D6 activity, as they may be at a higher risk of adverse events).
No products indexed under this heading.

Quinidine Polygalacturonate (Drugs which inhibit CYP2D6 also inhibit the metabolism of cevimeline. Cevimeline should be used with caution in individuals known or suspected to be deficient in CYP2D6 activity, as they may be at a higher risk of adverse events).
No products indexed under this heading.

Quinidine Sulfate (Drugs which inhibit CYP2D6 also inhibit the metabolism of cevimeline. Cevimeline should be used with caution in individuals known or suspected to be deficient in CYP2D6 activity, as they may be at a higher risk of adverse events).
No products indexed under this heading.

Quinine (Drugs which inhibit CYP3A3/4 also inhibit the metabolism of cevimeline).
No products indexed under this heading.

Quinine Sulfate (Drugs which inhibit CYP3A3/4 also inhibit the metabolism of cevimeline).
No products indexed under this heading.

Quinupristin (Drugs which inhibit CYP3A3/4 also inhibit the metabolism of cevimeline). Products include:
Synercid I.V. ... 1690

Ranitidine Bismuth Citrate (Drugs which inhibit CYP2D6 also inhibit the metabolism of cevimeline. Cevimeline should be used with caution in individuals known or suspected to be deficient in CYP2D6 activity, as they may be at a higher risk of adverse events).
No products indexed under this heading.

Ranitidine Hydrochloride (Drugs which inhibit CYP2D6 also inhibit the metabolism of cevimeline. Cevimeline should be used with caution in individuals known or suspected to be deficient in CYP2D6 activity, as they may be at a higher risk of adverse events). Products include:
Zantac ... 1597
Zantac Injection ... 1593
Zantac 75 Tablets ... ▣715
Zantac 150 Maximum Strength Tablets ... ▣715
Zantac Injection Pharmacy Bulk Package ... 1595

Ritonavir (Co-administration with drugs which inhibit CYP2D6 and/or CYP3A3/4, such as ritonavir, may inhibit the metabolism of cevimeline resulting in a higher risk of adverse events). Products include:
Kaletra ... 474
Norvir ... 499

Saquinavir (Drugs which inhibit CYP3A3/4 also inhibit the metabolism of cevimeline).
No products indexed under this heading.

Saquinavir Mesylate (Drugs which inhibit CYP3A3/4 also inhibit the metabolism of cevimeline). Products include:
Invirase ... 2776

Scopolamine (Cevimeline might interfere with the desirable antimuscarinic effects of drugs used concomitantly). Products include:
Transderm Scōp Transdermal Therapeutic System ... 2166

Scopolamine Hydrobromide (Cevimeline might interfere with the desirable antimuscarinic effects of drugs used concomitantly).
No products indexed under this heading.

Sertraline Hydrochloride (Co-administration with drugs which inhibit CYP2D6, such as sertraline, may inhibit the metabolism of cevimeline resulting in a higher risk of adverse events). Products include:
Zoloft ... 2581

Sotalol Hydrochloride (Possibility of conduction disturbances; co-administration with beta adrenergic antagonists requires caution).
No products indexed under this heading.

Telithromycin (Drugs which inhibit CYP3A3/4 also inhibit the metabolism of cevimeline). Products include:
Ketek Tablets ... 2920

Terbinafine Hydrochloride (Drugs which inhibit CYP2D6 also inhibit the metabolism of cevimeline. Cevimeline should be used with caution in individuals known or suspected to be deficient in CYP2D6 activity, as they may be at a higher risk of adverse events). Products include:
Lamisil AT Creams (Athlete's Foot & Jock Itch) ... ▣676
Lamisil Tablets ... 2226

Thioridazine Hydrochloride (Drugs which inhibit CYP2D6 also inhibit the metabolism of cevimeline. Cevimeline should be used with caution in individuals known or suspected to be deficient in CYP2D6 activity, as they may be at a higher risk of adverse events). Products include:
Thioridazine Hydrochloride Tablets ... 2122

Timolol Hemihydrate (Possibility of conduction disturbances; co-administration with beta adrenergic antagonists requires caution). Products include:
Betimol Ophthalmic Solution ... 3371
Betimol Ophthalmic Solution ... ⊙283

Timolol Maleate (Possibility of conduction disturbances; co-administration with beta adrenergic antagonists requires caution). Products include:
Blocadren Tablets ... 1891
Cosopt Sterile Ophthalmic Solution ... 1910
Timolide Tablets ... 2056
Timoptic in Ocudose ... 2061
Timoptic Sterile Ophthalmic Solution ... 2058
Timoptic-XE Sterile Ophthalmic Gel Forming Solution ... 2062

Tolterodine Tartrate (Cevimeline might interfere with the desirable antimuscarinic effects of drugs used concomitantly). Products include:
Detrol Tablets ... 2626
Detrol LA Capsules ... 2629

Tridihexethyl Chloride (Cevimeline might interfere with the desirable antimuscarinic effects of drugs used concomitantly).
No products indexed under this heading.

Trimipramine Maleate (Drugs which inhibit CYP2D6 also inhibit the metabolism of cevimeline. Cevimeline should be used with caution in individuals known or suspected to be deficient in CYP2D6 activity, as they may be at a higher risk of adverse events). Products include:
Surmontil Capsules ... 2347

Troglitazone (Drugs which inhibit CYP3A3/4 also inhibit the metabolism of cevimeline).
No products indexed under this heading.

Troleandomycin (Drugs which inhibit CYP3A3/4 also inhibit the metabolism of cevimeline).
No products indexed under this heading.

Valproate Sodium (Drugs which inhibit CYP3A3/4 also inhibit the metabolism of cevimeline). Products include:
Depacon Injection ... 412

Verapamil Hydrochloride (Co-administration with drugs which inhibit CYP3A3/4, such as verapamil, may inhibit the metabolism of cevimeline resulting in a higher risk of adverse events). Products include:
Covera-HS Tablets ... 3135
Tarka Tablets ... 519
Verelan PM Capsules ... 3120

Voriconazole (Drugs which inhibit CYP3A3/4 also inhibit the metabolism of cevimeline). Products include:
VFEND I.V. ... 2543
VFEND Oral Suspension ... 2543
VFEND Tablets ... 2543

Zafirlukast (Drugs which inhibit CYP3A3/4 also inhibit the metabolism of cevimeline). Products include:
Accolate Tablets ... 663

Zileuton (Drugs which inhibit CYP3A3/4 also inhibit the metabolism of cevimeline).
No products indexed under this heading.

Food Interactions

Food, unspecified (Co-administration with food decreases the rate of absorption, with a fasting Tmax of 1.53 hours and a Tmax of 2.86 hours after a meal; the peak concentration is reduced by 17.3%).

Grapefruit (Drugs which inhibit CYP3A3/4 also inhibit the metabolism of cevimeline).

Grapefruit Juice (Co-administration with drugs which inhibit CYP3A3/4, such as grapefruit juice, may inhibit the metabolism of cevimeline resulting in a higher risk of adverse events).

EXELON CAPSULES

(Rivastigmine Tartrate) ... 2204
May interact with anticholinergics and certain other agents. Compounds in these categories include:

Atropine Sulfate (Rivastigmine, a cholinesterase inhibitor, has the potential to interfere with the activity of anticholinergic medications).
No products indexed under this heading.

Belladonna Alkaloids (Rivastigmine, a cholinesterase inhibitor, has the potential to interfere with the activity of anticholinergic medications). Products include:
Hyland's Teething Tablets ... ▣736

Benztropine Mesylate (Rivastigmine, a cholinesterase inhibitor, has

the potential to interfere with the activity of anticholinergic medications). Products include:
- Cogentin Injection 1903

Bethanechol Chloride (Co-administration with cholinergic agonist, such as bethanechol, can be expected to result in a synergistic effect). Products include:
- Urecholine Tablets 2349

Biperiden Hydrochloride (Rivastigmine, a cholinesterase inhibitor, has the potential to interfere with the activity of anticholinergic medications).
No products indexed under this heading.

Clidinium Bromide (Rivastigmine, a cholinesterase inhibitor, has the potential to interfere with the activity of anticholinergic medications).
No products indexed under this heading.

Dicyclomine Hydrochloride (Rivastigmine, a cholinesterase inhibitor, has the potential to interfere with the activity of anticholinergic medications). Products include:
- Bentyl Capsules 724
- Bentyl Injection 724
- Bentyl Syrup 724
- Bentyl Tablets 724

Glycopyrrolate (Rivastigmine, a cholinesterase inhibitor, has the potential to interfere with the activity of anticholinergic medications).
No products indexed under this heading.

Hyoscyamine (Rivastigmine, a cholinesterase inhibitor, has the potential to interfere with the activity of anticholinergic medications).
No products indexed under this heading.

Hyoscyamine Sulfate (Rivastigmine, a cholinesterase inhibitor, has the potential to interfere with the activity of anticholinergic medications).
No products indexed under this heading.

Ipratropium Bromide (Rivastigmine, a cholinesterase inhibitor, has the potential to interfere with the activity of anticholinergic medications). Products include:
- Atrovent HFA Inhalation Aerosol 872
- Atrovent Inhalation Solution 868
- Atrovent Nasal Spray 0.03% 869
- Atrovent Nasal Spray 0.06% 870
- Combivent Inhalation Aerosol 878
- DuoNeb Inhalation Solution 1058

Mepenzolate Bromide (Rivastigmine, a cholinesterase inhibitor, has the potential to interfere with the activity of anticholinergic medications).
No products indexed under this heading.

Oxybutynin Chloride (Rivastigmine, a cholinesterase inhibitor, has the potential to interfere with the activity of anticholinergic medications). Products include:
- Ditropan XL Extended Release Tablets 2391

Procyclidine Hydrochloride (Rivastigmine, a cholinesterase inhibitor, has the potential to interfere with the activity of anticholinergic medications).
No products indexed under this heading.

Propantheline Bromide (Rivastigmine, a cholinesterase inhibitor, has the potential to interfere with the activity of anticholinergic medications).
No products indexed under this heading.

Scopolamine (Rivastigmine, a cholinesterase inhibitor, has the potential to interfere with the activity of anticholinergic medications). Products include:
- Transderm Scōp Transdermal Therapeutic System 2166

Scopolamine Hydrobromide (Rivastigmine, a cholinesterase inhibitor, has the potential to interfere with the activity of anticholinergic medications).
No products indexed under this heading.

Succinylcholine Chloride (Co-administration with succinylcholine can be expected to result in a synergistic effect).
No products indexed under this heading.

Tolterodine Tartrate (Rivastigmine, a cholinesterase inhibitor, has the potential to interfere with the activity of anticholinergic medications). Products include:
- Detrol Tablets 2626
- Detrol LA Capsules 2629

Tridihexethyl Chloride (Rivastigmine, a cholinesterase inhibitor, has the potential to interfere with the activity of anticholinergic medications).
No products indexed under this heading.

Trihexyphenidyl Hydrochloride (Rivastigmine, a cholinesterase inhibitor, has the potential to interfere with the activity of anticholinergic medications).
No products indexed under this heading.

Food Interactions

Food, unspecified (Co-administration with food delays absorption (tmax) by 90 minutes, lowers Cmax by approximately 30% and increases AUC by approximately 30%).

EX•LAX CHOCOLATED LAXATIVE PIECES

(Sennosides) .... ▣674
None cited in PDR database.

EX•LAX REGULAR STRENGTH PILLS

(Sennosides) .... ▣674
None cited in PDR database.

EX•LAX MAXIMUM STRENGTH PILLS

(Sennosides) .... ▣674
None cited in PDR database.

EXPERIENCE CAPSULES

(Herbals, Multiple, Psyllium Preparations) .... ▣760
None cited in PDR database.

FABRAZYME FOR INTRAVENOUS INFUSION

(Agalsidase beta) 1267
None cited in PDR database.

FACTIVE TABLETS

(Gemifloxacin Mesylate) 2464
May interact with antacids containing aluminum, calcium and magnesium, corticosteroids, iron containing oral preparations, and certain other agents. Compounds in these categories include:

Aluminum Carbonate (Aluminum- and/or magnesium-containing antacids, ferrous sulfate (iron), multivitamin preparations containing zinc or other metal cations should not be taken within 3 hours before or 2 hours after taking Factive tablets).
No products indexed under this heading.

Aluminum Hydroxide (Aluminum- and/or magnesium-containing antacids, ferrous sulfate (iron), multivitamin preparations containing zinc or other metal cations should not be taken within 3 hours before or 2 hours after taking Factive tablets). Products include:
- Gaviscon Regular Strength Liquid .... ▣620
- Gaviscon Regular Strength Tablets .... ▣619
- Gaviscon Extra Strength Liquid .... ▣620
- Gaviscon Extra Strength Tablets .... ▣619
- Maalox Max Maximum Strength Antacid/Anti-Gas Liquid 2165
- Maalox Regular Strength Antacid/Antigas Liquid 2164

Betamethasone Acetate (Tendon ruptures have been reported in patients receiving quinolones. Post-marketing surveillance reports indicate that this risk may be increased in patients receiving concomitant corticosteroids, especially the elderly).
No products indexed under this heading.

Betamethasone Sodium Phosphate (Tendon ruptures have been reported in patients receiving quinolones. Post-marketing surveillance reports indicate that this risk may be increased in patients receiving concomitant corticosteroids, especially the elderly).
No products indexed under this heading.

Cortisone Acetate (Tendon ruptures have been reported in patients receiving quinolones. Post-marketing surveillance reports indicate that this risk may be increased in patients receiving concomitant corticosteroids, especially the elderly).
No products indexed under this heading.

Dexamethasone (Tendon ruptures have been reported in patients receiving quinolones. Post-marketing surveillance reports indicate that this risk may be increased in patients receiving concomitant corticosteroids, especially the elderly). Products include:
- Ciprodex Otic Suspension 555
- Decadron Tablets 1929
- TobraDex Ophthalmic Ointment 558
- TobraDex Ophthalmic Suspension 558

Dexamethasone Acetate (Tendon ruptures have been reported in patients receiving quinolones. Post-marketing surveillance reports indicate that this risk may be increased in patients receiving concomitant corticosteroids, especially the elderly).
No products indexed under this heading.

Dexamethasone Sodium Phosphate (Tendon ruptures have been reported in patients receiving quinolones. Post-marketing surveillance reports indicate that this risk may be increased in patients receiving concomitant corticosteroids, especially the elderly). Products include:
- Decadron Phosphate Injection 1931

Didanosine (Videx (didanosine) chewable/buffered tablets or the pediatric powder for oral solution should not be taken within 3 hours before or 2 hours after taking Factive tablets).
No products indexed under this heading.

Ferrous Fumarate (Aluminum- and/or magnesium-containing antacids, ferrous sulfate (iron), multivitamin preparations containing zinc or other metal cations should not be taken within 3 hours before or 2 hours after taking Factive tablets). Products include:
- Chromagen Forte Soft Gelatin Capsules 3296
- Ferretts Tablets .... ▣773
- Repliva 21/7 Tablets 3301

Ferrous Gluconate (Aluminum- and/or magnesium-containing antacids, ferrous sulfate (iron), multivitamin preparations containing zinc or other metal cations should not be taken within 3 hours before or 2 hours after taking Factive tablets).
No products indexed under this heading.

Ferrous Sulfate (Aluminum- and/or magnesium-containing antacids, ferrous sulfate (iron), multivitamin preparations containing zinc or other metal cations should not be taken within 3 hours before or 2 hours after taking Factive tablets). Products include:
- Feosol Tablets 1629
- Slow Fe Iron Tablets .... ▣772
- Slow Fe with Folic Acid Tablets .... ▣773

Fludrocortisone Acetate (Tendon ruptures have been reported in patients receiving quinolones. Post-marketing surveillance reports indicate that this risk may be increased in patients receiving concomitant corticosteroids, especially the elderly).
No products indexed under this heading.

Hydrocortisone (Tendon ruptures have been reported in patients receiving quinolones. Post-marketing surveillance reports indicate that this risk may be increased in patients receiving concomitant corticosteroids, especially the elderly). Products include:
- Cortizone•5 Ointment .... ▣699
- Cortizone•10 Creme .... ▣699
- Cortizone•10 Ointment .... ▣699
- Cortizone•10 Plus Creme .... ▣700
- Cortizone•10 Maximum Strength Quick Shot Spray .... ▣700
- Hydrocortone Tablets 1963
- Preparation H Hydrocortisone Cream .... ▣748

Hydrocortisone Acetate (Tendon ruptures have been reported in patients receiving quinolones. Post-marketing surveillance reports indicate that this risk may be increased in patients receiving concomitant corticosteroids, especially the elderly). Products include:
- Analpram-HC 1136
- Pramosone 1139
- ProctoFoam-HC 3113
- Tucks Anti-Itch Ointment .... ▣712
- U-cort 1% Cream 3289

IMPORTANT NOTE: Always consult each drug listing in the patient's regimen for possible interactions.

Hydrocortisone Sodium Phosphate (Tendon ruptures have been reported in patients receiving quinolones. Post-marketing surveillance reports indicate that this risk may be increased in patients receiving concomitant corticosteroids, especially the elderly).
No products indexed under this heading.

Hydrocortisone Sodium Succinate (Tendon ruptures have been reported in patients receiving quinolones. Post-marketing surveillance reports indicate that this risk may be increased in patients receiving concomitant corticosteroids, especially the elderly).
No products indexed under this heading.

Iron (Aluminum- and/or magnesium-containing antacids, ferrous sulfate (iron), multivitamin preparations containing zinc or other metal cations should not be taken within 3 hours before or 2 hours after taking Factive tablets). Products include:
Chromagen Forte Soft Gelatin Capsules 3296
Ferretts IPS Liquid ..... ■ 773
OptiNate 1162
Repliva 21/7 Tablets 3301

Magaldrate (Aluminum- and/or magnesium-containing antacids, ferrous sulfate (iron), multivitamin preparations containing zinc or other metal cations should not be taken within 3 hours before or 2 hours after taking Factive tablets).
No products indexed under this heading.

Magnesium Hydroxide (Aluminum- and/or magnesium-containing antacids, ferrous sulfate (iron), multivitamin preparations containing zinc or other metal cations should not be taken within 3 hours before or 2 hours after taking Factive tablets). Products include:
Maalox Max Maximum Strength Antacid/Anti-Gas Liquid 2165
Maalox Regular Strength Antacid/Antigas Liquid 2164
Pepcid Complete Chewable Tablets 1672
Rolaids Tablets ..... ■ 707
Extra Strength Rolaids Tablets ..... ■ 707
Rolaids Multi-Symptom Antacid & Antigas Tablets ..... ■ 708

Magnesium Oxide (Aluminum- and/or magnesium-containing antacids, ferrous sulfate (iron), multivitamin preparations containing zinc or other metal cations should not be taken within 3 hours before or 2 hours after taking Factive tablets). Products include:
Beelith Tablets 784
PremCal Light, Regular, and Extra Strength Tablets ..... ■ 762

Methylprednisolone Acetate (Tendon ruptures have been reported in patients receiving quinolones. Post-marketing surveillance reports indicate that this risk may be increased in patients receiving concomitant corticosteroids, especially the elderly). Products include:
Depo-Medrol Injectable Suspension 2615
Depo-Medrol Single-Dose Vial 2617

Methylprednisolone Sodium Succinate (Tendon ruptures have been reported in patients receiving quinolones. Post-marketing surveillance reports indicate that this risk may be increased in patients receiving concomitant corticosteroids, especially the elderly).
No products indexed under this heading.

Polysaccharide Iron Complex (Aluminum- and/or magnesium-containing antacids, ferrous sulfate (iron), multivitamin preparations containing zinc or other metal cations should not be taken within 3 hours before or 2 hours after taking Factive tablets). Products include:
Niferex-150 Forte Capsules 3299
Nu-Iron 150 Capsules 2098

Prednisolone Acetate (Tendon ruptures have been reported in patients receiving quinolones. Post-marketing surveillance reports indicate that this risk may be increased in patients receiving concomitant corticosteroids, especially the elderly). Products include:
Blephamide Ophthalmic Ointment 563
Blephamide Ophthalmic Suspension 564
Poly-Pred Liquifilm Ophthalmic Suspension ..... ⊙ 231
Pred Forte Ophthalmic Suspension ..... ⊙ 233
Pred Mild Sterile Ophthalmic Suspension ..... ⊙ 236
Pred-G Ophthalmic Suspension ..... ⊙ 234
Pred-G Sterile Ophthalmic Ointment ..... ⊙ 235

Prednisolone Sodium Phosphate (Tendon ruptures have been reported in patients receiving quinolones. Post-marketing surveillance reports indicate that this risk may be increased in patients receiving concomitant corticosteroids, especially the elderly). Products include:
Pediapred Oral Solution 3319

Prednisolone Tebutate (Tendon ruptures have been reported in patients receiving quinolones. Post-marketing surveillance reports indicate that this risk may be increased in patients receiving concomitant corticosteroids, especially the elderly).
No products indexed under this heading.

Prednisone (Tendon ruptures have been reported in patients receiving quinolones. Post-marketing surveillance reports indicate that this risk may be increased in patients receiving concomitant corticosteroids, especially the elderly).
No products indexed under this heading.

Probenecid (Concomitant administration of Factive with probenecid resulted in a 45% increase in systemic exposure to gemifloxacin).
No products indexed under this heading.

Sucralfate (When sucralfate (2g) was administered 3 hours prior to gemifloxacin, the oral bioavailability of gemifloxacin was significantly reduced (53% decrease in AUC; 69% decrease in Cmax); gemifloxacin should be taken at least 2 hours before sucralfate). Products include:
Carafate Suspension 727
Carafate Tablets 728

Triamcinolone (Tendon ruptures have been reported in patients receiving quinolones. Post-marketing surveillance reports indicate that this risk may be increased in patients receiving concomitant corticosteroids, especially the elderly).
No products indexed under this heading.

Triamcinolone Acetonide (Tendon ruptures have been reported in patients receiving quinolones. Post-marketing surveillance reports indicate that this risk may be increased in patients receiving concomitant corticosteroids, especially the elderly). Products include:
Azmacort Inhalation Aerosol 1701
Nasacort HFA Inhalation Aerosol 2939
Nasacort AQ Nasal Spray 2937

Triamcinolone Diacetate (Tendon ruptures have been reported in patients receiving quinolones. Post-marketing surveillance reports indicate that this risk may be increased in patients receiving concomitant corticosteroids, especially the elderly).
No products indexed under this heading.

Triamcinolone Hexacetonide (Tendon ruptures have been reported in patients receiving quinolones. Post-marketing surveillance reports indicate that this risk may be increased in patients receiving concomitant corticosteroids, especially the elderly).
No products indexed under this heading.

Warfarin Sodium (Gemifloxacin had no significant effect on warfarin-induced anticoagulant activity; because some quinolones have been reported to enhance the anticoagulant effects of warfarin or its derivatives in patients, the prothrombin time or other suitable coagulation test should be closely monitored). Products include:
Coumadin for Injection 932
Coumadin Tablets 932

FAMVIR TABLETS

(Famciclovir) 2207
May interact with:

Probenecid (Concurrent use may result in increased plasma concentration of penciclovir).
No products indexed under this heading.

Food Interactions

Meal, unspecified (Penciclovir Cmax decreased approximately 50% and Tmax was delayed by 1.5 hours when a capsule formulation of famciclovir was administered with food; there is no effect on the extent of availability (AUC) of penciclovir).

FASLODEX INJECTION

(Fulvestrant) 682
None cited in PDR database.

FAZACLO ORALLY DISINTEGRATING TABLETS

(Clozapine) 547
May interact with anticholinergics, antihypertensives, benzodiazepines, central nervous system depressants, antidepressant drugs, erythromycin, general anesthetics, phenothiazines, phenytoin, psychotropics, quinidine, and certain other agents. Compounds in these categories include:

Acebutolol Hydrochloride (Clozapine may potentiate the hypotensive effects of antihypertensive drugs).
No products indexed under this heading.

Alfentanil Hydrochloride (Given the primary CNS effect of clozapine, caution is advised in using it concomitantly with CNS-active drugs).
No products indexed under this heading.

Alprazolam (Co-administration with benzodiazepines or other psychotropic agents may be accompanied by orthostatic hypotension leading to profound collapse and respiratory and/or cardiac arrest; caution is advised if used concurrently). Products include:
Niravam Orally Disintegrating Tablets 3106
Xanax XR Tablets 2655

Amitriptyline Hydrochloride (Concomitant use of clozapine with other drugs metabolized by CYP4502D6 may require lower than usual doses for either drug).
No products indexed under this heading.

Amlodipine Besylate (Clozapine may potentiate the hypotensive effects of antihypertensive drugs). Products include:
Caduet Tablets 2507
Lotrel Capsules 2238
Norvasc Tablets 2529

Amoxapine (Concomitant use of clozapine with other drugs metabolized by CYP4502D6 may require lower than usual doses for either drug).
No products indexed under this heading.

Aprobarbital (Given the primary CNS effect of clozapine, caution is advised in using it concomitantly with CNS-active drugs).
No products indexed under this heading.

Atenolol (Clozapine may potentiate the hypotensive effects of antihypertensive drugs). Products include:
Tenormin I.V. Injection 698
Tenormin Tablets 695

Atropine Sulfate (Clozapine may potentiate anticholinergic effects).
No products indexed under this heading.

Belladonna Alkaloids (Clozapine may potentiate anticholinergic effects). Products include:
Hyland's Teething Tablets ..... ■ 736

Benazepril Hydrochloride (Clozapine may potentiate the hypotensive effects of antihypertensive drugs). Products include:
Lotensin Tablets 2232
Lotensin HCT Tablets 2235
Lotrel Capsules 2238

Bendroflumethiazide (Clozapine may potentiate the hypotensive effects of antihypertensive drugs).
No products indexed under this heading.

Benztropine Mesylate (Clozapine may potentiate anticholinergic effects). Products include:
Cogentin Injection 1903

Betaxolol Hydrochloride (Clozapine may potentiate the hypotensive effects of antihypertensive drugs). Products include:
Betoptic S Ophthalmic Suspension 554

Biperiden Hydrochloride (Clozapine may potentiate anticholinergic effects).
No products indexed under this heading.

Bisoprolol Fumarate (Clozapine may potentiate the hypotensive effects of antihypertensive drugs).
No products indexed under this heading.

Bone Marrow Depressants, unspecified (Clozapine should not be used with agents having a well-known potential to suppress bone-marrow function. Co-administration may increase the risk and/or severity of bone marrow suppression).
No products indexed under this heading.

Buprenorphine Hydrochloride (Given the primary CNS effect of clozapine, caution is advised in using it concomitantly with CNS-active drugs). Products include:
Buprenex Injectable **2718**
Suboxone Tablets **2719**
Subutex Tablets **2719**

Bupropion Hydrochloride (Concomitant use of clozapine with other drugs metabolized by CYP4502D6 may require lower than usual doses for either drug). Products include:
Wellbutrin Tablets **1579**
Wellbutrin SR Sustained-Release Tablets **1583**
Wellbutrin XL Extended-Release Tablets **1588**
Zyban Sustained-Release Tablets **1620**

Buspirone Hydrochloride (Co-administration with benzodiazepines or other psychotropic agents may be accompanied by orthostatic hypotension leading to profound collapse and respiratory and/or cardiac arrest; caution is advised if used concurrently).
No products indexed under this heading.

Butabarbital (Given the primary CNS effect of clozapine, caution is advised in using it concomitantly with CNS-active drugs).
No products indexed under this heading.

Butalbital (Given the primary CNS effect of clozapine, caution is advised in using it concomitantly with CNS-active drugs). Products include:
Sedapap Tablets 50 mg/650 mg **2098**

Caffeine (May increase plasma levels of clozapine, potentially resulting in adverse effects). Products include:
Athena Hair System Shampoo .... ■□ **767**
BC Powder .... ■□ **612**
Arthritis Strength BC Powder .... ■□ **612**
Goody's Extra Strength Headache Powder........ ■□ **621**
Goody's Extra Strength Pain Relief Tablets........ ■□ **621**
Hycomine Compound Tablets **1105**
Spartan Hair System Shampoo ...... ■□ **767**
Vivarin .... ■□ **639**

Caffeine Citrate (May increase plasma levels of clozapine, potentially resulting in adverse effects). Products include:
Cafcit **1854**

Candesartan Cilexetil (Clozapine may potentiate the hypotensive effects of antihypertensive drugs). Products include:
Atacand Tablets **634**
Atacand HCT **637**

Captopril (Clozapine may potentiate the hypotensive effects of antihypertensive drugs). Products include:
Captopril Tablets **2114**

Carbamazepine (Concomitant use is not recommended; discontinuation of concomitant carbamazepine administration may result in increase in clozapine levels). Products include:
Carbatrol Capsules **3174**
Equetro Extended-Release Capsules........ **3178**
Tegretol/Tegretol-XR **2278**

Carteolol Hydrochloride (Clozapine may potentiate the hypotensive effects of antihypertensive drugs). Products include:
Carteolol Hydrochloride Ophthalmic Solution USP, 1%....... ⊙ **246**

Chlordiazepoxide (Co-administration with benzodiazepines or other psychotropic agents may be accompanied by orthostatic hypotension leading to profound collapse and respiratory and/or cardiac arrest; caution is advised if used concurrently).
No products indexed under this heading.

Chlordiazepoxide Hydrochloride (Co-administration with benzodiazepines or other psychotropic agents may be accompanied by orthostatic hypotension leading to profound collapse and respiratory and/or cardiac arrest; caution is advised if used concurrently). Products include:
Librium Capsules **3349**

Chlorothiazide (Clozapine may potentiate the hypotensive effects of antihypertensive drugs). Products include:
Aldoclor Tablets **1881**
Diuril Oral **1936**

Chlorothiazide Sodium (Clozapine may potentiate the hypotensive effects of antihypertensive drugs). Products include:
Diuril Sodium Intravenous **1934**

Chlorpromazine (Co-administration with benzodiazepines or other psychotropic agents may be accompanied by orthostatic hypotension leading to profound collapse and respiratory and/or cardiac arrest; caution is advised if used concurrently).
No products indexed under this heading.

Chlorpromazine Hydrochloride (Co-administration with benzodiazepines or other psychotropic agents may be accompanied by orthostatic hypotension leading to profound collapse and respiratory and/or cardiac arrest; caution is advised if used concurrently).
No products indexed under this heading.

Chlorprothixene (Co-administration with benzodiazepines or other psychotropic agents may be accompanied by orthostatic hypotension leading to profound collapse and respiratory and/or cardiac arrest; caution is advised if used concurrently).
No products indexed under this heading.

Chlorprothixene Hydrochloride (Co-administration with benzodiazepines or other psychotropic agents may be accompanied by orthostatic hypotension leading to profound collapse and respiratory and/or cardiac arrest; caution is advised if used concurrently).
No products indexed under this heading.

Chlorprothixene Lactate (Given the primary CNS effect of clozapine, caution is advised in using it concomitantly with CNS-active drugs).
No products indexed under this heading.

Chlorthalidone (Clozapine may potentiate the hypotensive effects of antihypertensive drugs). Products include:
Clorpres Tablets **2139**

Cimetidine (May increase plasma levels of clozapine, potentially resulting in adverse effects). Products include:
Tagamet HB 200 Tablets .... ■□ **637**
Tagamet Tablets **1547**

Cimetidine Hydrochloride (May increase plasma levels of clozapine, potentially resulting in adverse effects).
No products indexed under this heading.

Citalopram Hydrobromide (Concomitant use of clozapine with other drugs metabolized by CYP4502D6 may require lower than usual doses for either drug). Products include:
Celexa **1177**

Clidinium Bromide (Clozapine may potentiate anticholinergic effects).
No products indexed under this heading.

Clonidine (Clozapine may potentiate the hypotensive effects of antihypertensive drugs). Products include:
Catapres-TTS **875**

Clonidine Hydrochloride (Clozapine may potentiate the hypotensive effects of antihypertensive drugs). Products include:
Catapres Tablets **874**
Clorpres Tablets **2139**

Clorazepate Dipotassium (Co-administration with benzodiazepines or other psychotropic agents may be accompanied by orthostatic hypotension leading to profound collapse and respiratory and/or cardiac arrest; caution is advised if used concurrently). Products include:
Tranxene **2488**

Codeine Phosphate (Given the primary CNS effect of clozapine, caution is advised in using it concomitantly with CNS-active drugs). Products include:
Tylenol with Codeine **2461**

Deserpidine (Clozapine may potentiate the hypotensive effects of antihypertensive drugs).
No products indexed under this heading.

Desflurane (Given the primary CNS effect of clozapine, caution is advised in using it concomitantly with CNS-active drugs). Products include:
Suprane Liquid for Inhalation **770**

Desipramine Hydrochloride (Concomitant use of clozapine with other drugs metabolized by CYP4502D6 may require lower than usual doses for either drug).
No products indexed under this heading.

Dezocine (Given the primary CNS effect of clozapine, caution is advised in using it concomitantly with CNS-active drugs).
No products indexed under this heading.

Diazepam (Co-administration with benzodiazepines or other psychotropic agents may be accompanied by orthostatic hypotension leading to profound collapse and respiratory and/or cardiac arrest; caution is advised if used concurrently). Products include:
Diastat Rectal Delivery System **3344**
Valium Tablets **2822**

Diazoxide (Clozapine may potentiate the hypotensive effects of antihypertensive drugs). Products include:
Hyperstat I.V. Injection **3031**

Dicyclomine Hydrochloride (Clozapine may potentiate anticholinergic effects). Products include:
Bentyl Capsules **724**
Bentyl Injection **724**
Bentyl Syrup **724**
Bentyl Tablets **724**

Diltiazem Hydrochloride (Clozapine may potentiate the hypotensive effects of antihypertensive drugs). Products include:
Cardizem LA Extended Release Tablets **1699**
Tiazac Capsules **1204**

Doxazosin Mesylate (Clozapine may potentiate the hypotensive effects of antihypertensive drugs).
No products indexed under this heading.

Doxepin Hydrochloride (Concomitant use of clozapine with other drugs metabolized by CYP4502D6 may require lower than usual doses for either drug).
No products indexed under this heading.

Droperidol (Co-administration with benzodiazepines or other psychotropic agents may be accompanied by orthostatic hypotension leading to profound collapse and respiratory and/or cardiac arrest; caution is advised if used concurrently).
No products indexed under this heading.

Enalapril Maleate (Clozapine may potentiate the hypotensive effects of antihypertensive drugs). Products include:
Vaseretic Tablets **2073**
Vasotec I.V. Injection **2076**

Enalaprilat (Clozapine may potentiate the hypotensive effects of antihypertensive drugs).
No products indexed under this heading.

Encainide Hydrochloride (Concomitant use of clozapine with other drugs metabolized by CYP4502D6 may require lower than usual doses for either drug).
No products indexed under this heading.

Enflurane (Given the primary CNS effect of clozapine, caution is advised in using it concomitantly with CNS-active drugs).
No products indexed under this heading.

Epinephrine (The administration of epinephrine should be avoided in the treatment of clozapine-induced hypotension because of a possible reverse epinephrine effect). Products include:
EpiPen **1061**
Primatene Mist .... ■□ **749**

Epinephrine Hydrochloride (The administration of epinephrine should be avoided in the treatment of clozapine-induced hypotension because of a possible reverse epinephrine effect).
No products indexed under this heading.

Eprosartan Mesylate (Clozapine may potentiate the hypotensive effects of antihypertensive drugs). Products include:
Teveten Tablets **1707**
Teveten HCT Tablets **1710**

Erythromycin (May increase plasma levels of clozapine, potentially resulting in adverse effects). Products include:
Erygel Topical Gel **2096**
Ery-Tab Tablets **447**

IMPORTANT NOTE: Always consult each drug listing in the patient's regimen for possible interactions.

Erythromycin Base Filmtab Tablets 454
Erythromycin Delayed-Release Capsules, USP 456
PCE Dispertab Tablets 510

Erythromycin Estolate (May increase plasma levels of clozapine, potentially resulting in adverse effects).
No products indexed under this heading.

Erythromycin Ethylsuccinate (May increase plasma levels of clozapine, potentially resulting in adverse effects). Products include:
E.E.S. 449
EryPed 445

Erythromycin Gluceptate (May increase plasma levels of clozapine, potentially resulting in adverse effects).
No products indexed under this heading.

Erythromycin Lactobionate (May increase plasma levels of clozapine, potentially resulting in adverse effects).
No products indexed under this heading.

Erythromycin Stearate (May increase plasma levels of clozapine, potentially resulting in adverse effects). Products include:
Erythrocin Stearate Filmtab Tablets 452

Escitalopram Oxalate (Concomitant use of clozapine with other drugs metabolized by CYP4502D6 may require lower than usual doses for either drug). Products include:
Lexapro Oral Solution 1193
Lexapro Tablets 1193

Esmolol Hydrochloride (Clozapine may potentiate the hypotensive effects of antihypertensive drugs). Products include:
Brevibloc Concentrate 766
Brevibloc Injection 766
Brevibloc Double Strength Injection 766
Brevibloc Premixed Injection 766
Brevibloc Double Strength Premixed Injection 766

Estazolam (Co-administration with benzodiazepines or other psychotropic agents may be accompanied by orthostatic hypotension leading to profound collapse and respiratory and/or cardiac arrest; caution is advised if used concurrently). Products include:
ProSom Tablets 512

Ethanol (Given the primary CNS effect of clozapine, caution is advised in using it concomitantly with CNS-active drugs).
No products indexed under this heading.

Ethchlorvynol (Given the primary CNS effect of clozapine, caution is advised in using it concomitantly with CNS-active drugs).
No products indexed under this heading.

Ethinamate (Given the primary CNS effect of clozapine, caution is advised in using it concomitantly with CNS-active drugs).
No products indexed under this heading.

Ethyl Alcohol (Given the primary CNS effect of clozapine, caution is advised in using it concomitantly with CNS-active drugs).
No products indexed under this heading.

Felodipine (Clozapine may potentiate the hypotensive effects of antihypertensive drugs). Products include:
Plendil Extended-Release Tablets 651

Fentanyl (Given the primary CNS effect of clozapine, caution is advised in using it concomitantly with CNS-active drugs). Products include:
Duragesic Transdermal System 2448

Fentanyl Citrate (Given the primary CNS effect of clozapine, caution is advised in using it concomitantly with CNS-active drugs). Products include:
Actiq 993

Flecainide Acetate (Concomitant use of clozapine with other drugs metabolized by CYP4502D6 may require lower than usual doses for either drug). Products include:
Tambocor Tablets 1824

Fluoxetine Hydrochloride (Co-administration in schizophrenic patients has resulted in elevated mean trough concentrations of clozapine and its metabolites by less than two-fold compared to baseline concentrations; a reduced clozapine dose should be considered). Products include:
Prozac Pulvules and Liquid 1771
Symbyax Capsules 1788

Fluphenazine Decanoate (Co-administration with benzodiazepines or other psychotropic agents may be accompanied by orthostatic hypotension leading to profound collapse and respiratory and/or cardiac arrest; caution is advised if used concurrently).
No products indexed under this heading.

Fluphenazine Enanthate (Co-administration with benzodiazepines or other psychotropic agents may be accompanied by orthostatic hypotension leading to profound collapse and respiratory and/or cardiac arrest; caution is advised if used concurrently).
No products indexed under this heading.

Fluphenazine Hydrochloride (Co-administration with benzodiazepines or other psychotropic agents may be accompanied by orthostatic hypotension leading to profound collapse and respiratory and/or cardiac arrest; caution is advised if used concurrently).
No products indexed under this heading.

Flurazepam Hydrochloride (Co-administration with benzodiazepines or other psychotropic agents may be accompanied by orthostatic hypotension leading to profound collapse and respiratory and/or cardiac arrest; caution is advised if used concurrently). Products include:
Dalmane Capsules 3343

Fluvoxamine Maleate (Co-administration in schizophrenic patients has resulted in elevated mean trough concentrations of clozapine and its metabolites by about three-fold compared to baseline concentrations; a reduced clozapine dose should be considered).
No products indexed under this heading.

Fosinopril Sodium (Clozapine may potentiate the hypotensive effects of antihypertensive drugs).
No products indexed under this heading.

Fosphenytoin Sodium (May decrease clozapine plasma levels resulting in a decrease in effectiveness of a previously effective clozapine dose).
No products indexed under this heading.

Furosemide (Clozapine may potentiate the hypotensive effects of antihypertensive drugs). Products include:
Furosemide Tablets 2117

Glutethimide (Given the primary CNS effect of clozapine, caution is advised in using it concomitantly with CNS-active drugs).
No products indexed under this heading.

Glycopyrrolate (Clozapine may potentiate anticholinergic effects).
No products indexed under this heading.

Guanabenz Acetate (Clozapine may potentiate the hypotensive effects of antihypertensive drugs).
No products indexed under this heading.

Guanethidine Monosulfate (Clozapine may potentiate the hypotensive effects of antihypertensive drugs).
No products indexed under this heading.

Halazepam (Co-administration with benzodiazepines or other psychotropic agents may be accompanied by orthostatic hypotension leading to profound collapse and respiratory and/or cardiac arrest; caution is advised if used concurrently).
No products indexed under this heading.

Haloperidol (Co-administration with benzodiazepines or other psychotropic agents may be accompanied by orthostatic hypotension leading to profound collapse and respiratory and/or cardiac arrest; caution is advised if used concurrently).
No products indexed under this heading.

Haloperidol Decanoate (Co-administration with benzodiazepines or other psychotropic agents may be accompanied by orthostatic hypotension leading to profound collapse and respiratory and/or cardiac arrest; caution is advised if used concurrently).
No products indexed under this heading.

Hydralazine Hydrochloride (Clozapine may potentiate the hypotensive effects of antihypertensive drugs). Products include:
BiDil Tablets 2161

Hydrochlorothiazide (Clozapine may potentiate the hypotensive effects of antihypertensive drugs). Products include:
Aldoril Tablets 1884
Atacand HCT 637
Avalide Tablets 2889
Avalide Tablets 922
Benicar HCT Tablets 2852
Diovan HCT Tablets 2195
Dyazide Capsules 1389
Hyzaar 1964
Lotensin HCT Tablets 2235
Maxzide 2150
Micardis HCT Tablets 886
Moduretic Tablets 2003
Prinzide Tablets 2033
Teveten HCT Tablets 1710
Timolide Tablets 2056
Uniretic Tablets 3114
Vaseretic Tablets 2073
Zestoretic Tablets 701

Hydrocodone Bitartrate (Given the primary CNS effect of clozapine, caution is advised in using it concomitantly with CNS-active drugs). Products include:
Hycodan 1104
Hycomine Compound Tablets 1105
Hycotuss Expectorant Syrup 1106
Lortab 3315
Lortab Elixir 3312
Vicodin Tablets 530
Vicodin ES Tablets 531
Vicodin HP Tablets 532
Vicoprofen Tablets 533
Zydone Tablets 1118

Hydrocodone Polistirex (Given the primary CNS effect of clozapine, caution is advised in using it concomitantly with CNS-active drugs). Products include:
Tussionex Pennkinetic Extended-Release Suspension 3322

Hydroflumethiazide (Clozapine may potentiate the hypotensive effects of antihypertensive drugs).
No products indexed under this heading.

Hydromorphone Hydrochloride (Given the primary CNS effect of clozapine, caution is advised in using it concomitantly with CNS-active drugs). Products include:
Dilaudid 439
Dilaudid Oral Liquid 443
Dilaudid Non-Sterile Powder 439
Dilaudid Rectal Suppositories 439
Dilaudid Tablets 439
Dilaudid Tablets - 8 mg 443
Dilaudid-HP 441

Hydroxyzine Hydrochloride (Co-administration with benzodiazepines or other psychotropic agents may be accompanied by orthostatic hypotension leading to profound collapse and respiratory and/or cardiac arrest; caution is advised if used concurrently).
No products indexed under this heading.

Hyoscyamine (Clozapine may potentiate anticholinergic effects).
No products indexed under this heading.

Hyoscyamine Sulfate (Clozapine may potentiate anticholinergic effects).
No products indexed under this heading.

Imipramine Hydrochloride (Concomitant use of clozapine with other drugs metabolized by CYP4502D6 may require lower than usual doses for either drug).
No products indexed under this heading.

Imipramine Pamoate (Concomitant use of clozapine with other drugs metabolized by CYP4502D6 may require lower than usual doses for either drug).
No products indexed under this heading.

Indapamide (Clozapine may potentiate the hypotensive effects of antihypertensive drugs). Products include:
Indapamide Tablets 2119

Ipratropium Bromide (Clozapine may potentiate anticholinergic effects). Products include:
Atrovent HFA Inhalation Aerosol 872
Atrovent Inhalation Solution 868
Atrovent Nasal Spray 0.03% 869
Atrovent Nasal Spray 0.06% 870
Combivent Inhalation Aerosol 878
DuoNeb Inhalation Solution 1058

Irbesartan (Clozapine may potentiate the hypotensive effects of antihypertensive drugs). Products include:

Avalide Tablets ... 922
Avalide Tablets ... 2889
Avapro Tablets ... 925
Avapro Tablets ... 2886

Isocarboxazid (Concomitant use of clozapine with other drugs metabolized by CYP4502D6 may require lower than usual doses for either drug).

No products indexed under this heading.

Isoflurane (Given the primary CNS effect of clozapine, caution is advised in using it concomitantly with CNS-active drugs).

No products indexed under this heading.

Isradipine (Clozapine may potentiate the hypotensive effects of antihypertensive drugs). Products include:

DynaCirc CR Tablets ... 2726

Ketamine Hydrochloride (Given the primary CNS effect of clozapine, caution is advised in using it concomitantly with CNS-active drugs).

No products indexed under this heading.

Labetalol Hydrochloride (Clozapine may potentiate the hypotensive effects of antihypertensive drugs).

No products indexed under this heading.

Levomethadyl Acetate Hydrochloride (Given the primary CNS effect of clozapine, caution is advised in using it concomitantly with CNS-active drugs).

No products indexed under this heading.

Levorphanol Tartrate (Given the primary CNS effect of clozapine, caution is advised in using it concomitantly with CNS-active drugs).

No products indexed under this heading.

Lisinopril (Clozapine may potentiate the hypotensive effects of antihypertensive drugs). Products include:

Prinivil Tablets ... 2029
Prinzide Tablets ... 2033
Zestoretic Tablets ... 701
Zestril Tablets ... 704

Lithium Carbonate (Co-administration with benzodiazepines or other psychotropic agents may be accompanied by orthostatic hypotension leading to profound collapse and respiratory and/or cardiac arrest; caution is advised if used concurrently). Products include:

Eskalith ... 1406
Lithobid Tablets ... 1670

Lithium Citrate (Co-administration with benzodiazepines or other psychotropic agents may be accompanied by orthostatic hypotension leading to profound collapse and respiratory and/or cardiac arrest; caution is advised if used concurrently).

No products indexed under this heading.

Lorazepam (Co-administration with benzodiazepines or other psychotropic agents may be accompanied by orthostatic hypotension leading to profound collapse and respiratory and/or cardiac arrest; caution is advised if used concurrently).

No products indexed under this heading.

Losartan Potassium (Clozapine may potentiate the hypotensive effects of antihypertensive drugs). Products include:

Cozaar Tablets ... 1913
Hyzaar ... 1964

Loxapine Hydrochloride (Co-administration with benzodiazepines or other psychotropic agents may be accompanied by orthostatic hypotension leading to profound collapse and respiratory and/or cardiac arrest; caution is advised if used concurrently).

No products indexed under this heading.

Loxapine Succinate (Co-administration with benzodiazepines or other psychotropic agents may be accompanied by orthostatic hypotension leading to profound collapse and respiratory and/or cardiac arrest; caution is advised if used concurrently).

No products indexed under this heading.

Maprotiline Hydrochloride (Concomitant use of clozapine with other drugs metabolized by CYP4502D6 may require lower than usual doses for either drug).

No products indexed under this heading.

Mecamylamine Hydrochloride (Clozapine may potentiate the hypotensive effects of antihypertensive drugs). Products include:

Inversine Tablets ... 3286

Mepenzolate Bromide (Clozapine may potentiate anticholinergic effects).

No products indexed under this heading.

Meperidine Hydrochloride (Given the primary CNS effect of clozapine, caution is advised in using it concomitantly with CNS-active drugs).

No products indexed under this heading.

Mephobarbital (Given the primary CNS effect of clozapine, caution is advised in using it concomitantly with CNS-active drugs). Products include:

Mebaral Tablets, USP ... 2483

Meprobamate (Co-administration with benzodiazepines or other psychotropic agents may be accompanied by orthostatic hypotension leading to profound collapse and respiratory and/or cardiac arrest; caution is advised if used concurrently).

No products indexed under this heading.

Mesoridazine Besylate (Co-administration with benzodiazepines or other psychotropic agents may be accompanied by orthostatic hypotension leading to profound collapse and respiratory and/or cardiac arrest; caution is advised if used concurrently).

No products indexed under this heading.

Methadone Hydrochloride (Given the primary CNS effect of clozapine, caution is advised in using it concomitantly with CNS-active drugs).

No products indexed under this heading.

Methohexital Sodium (Given the primary CNS effect of clozapine, caution is advised in using it concomitantly with CNS-active drugs).

No products indexed under this heading.

Methotrimeprazine (Given the primary CNS effect of clozapine, caution is advised in using it concomitantly with CNS-active drugs).

No products indexed under this heading.

Methoxyflurane (Given the primary CNS effect of clozapine, caution is advised in using it concomitantly with CNS-active drugs).

No products indexed under this heading.

Methyclothiazide (Clozapine may potentiate the hypotensive effects of antihypertensive drugs).

No products indexed under this heading.

Methyldopa (Clozapine may potentiate the hypotensive effects of antihypertensive drugs). Products include:

Aldoclor Tablets ... 1881
Aldoril Tablets ... 1884

Methyldopate Hydrochloride (Clozapine may potentiate the hypotensive effects of antihypertensive drugs).

No products indexed under this heading.

Metolazone (Clozapine may potentiate the hypotensive effects of antihypertensive drugs).

No products indexed under this heading.

Metoprolol Succinate (Clozapine may potentiate the hypotensive effects of antihypertensive drugs). Products include:

Toprol-XL Tablets ... 660

Metoprolol Tartrate (Clozapine may potentiate the hypotensive effects of antihypertensive drugs).

No products indexed under this heading.

Metyrosine (Clozapine may potentiate the hypotensive effects of antihypertensive drugs). Products include:

Demser Capsules ... 1933

Mibefradil Dihydrochloride (Clozapine may potentiate the hypotensive effects of antihypertensive drugs).

No products indexed under this heading.

Midazolam Hydrochloride (Co-administration with benzodiazepines or other psychotropic agents may be accompanied by orthostatic hypotension leading to profound collapse and respiratory and/or cardiac arrest; caution is advised if used concurrently).

No products indexed under this heading.

Minoxidil (Clozapine may potentiate the hypotensive effects of antihypertensive drugs). Products include:

Men's Rogaine Extra Strength Topical Solution, Ocean Rush Scent and Original Unscented ... ■ 706
Women's Rogaine Topical Solution, Spring Bloom Scent and Original Unscented ... ■ 707

Mirtazapine (Concomitant use of clozapine with other drugs metabolized by CYP4502D6 may require lower than usual doses for either drug).

No products indexed under this heading.

Moexipril Hydrochloride (Clozapine may potentiate the hypotensive effects of antihypertensive drugs). Products include:

Uniretic Tablets ... 3114
Univasc Tablets ... 3118

Molindone Hydrochloride (Co-administration with benzodiazepines or other psychotropic agents may be accompanied by orthostatic hypotension leading to profound collapse and respiratory and/or cardiac arrest; caution is advised if used concurrently). Products include:

Moban Tablets ... 1108

Morphine Sulfate (Given the primary CNS effect of clozapine, caution is advised in using it concomitantly with CNS-active drugs). Products include:

Avinza Capsules ... 1714
Kadian Capsules ... 572
MS Contin Tablets ... 2703

Nadolol (Clozapine may potentiate the hypotensive effects of antihypertensive drugs). Products include:

Nadolol Tablets ... 2121

Nefazodone Hydrochloride (Concomitant use of clozapine with other drugs metabolized by CYP4502D6 may require lower than usual doses for either drug).

No products indexed under this heading.

Nicardipine Hydrochloride (Clozapine may potentiate the hypotensive effects of antihypertensive drugs). Products include:

Cardene I.V. ... 1129

Nicotine (May decrease clozapine plasma levels resulting in a decrease in effectiveness of a previously effective clozapine dose). Products include:

Nicoderm CQ Patch ... 1629
NicoDerm CQ Clear Patch ... ■ 627
Nicotrol Inhaler ... 2594
Nicotrol NS ... 2596

Nicotine Polacrilex (May decrease clozapine plasma levels resulting in a decrease in effectiveness of a previously effective clozapine dose). Products include:

Commit Lozenges ... 1625
Nicorette Gum ... 1632

Nifedipine (Clozapine may potentiate the hypotensive effects of antihypertensive drugs). Products include:

Adalat CC Tablets ... 2978

Nisoldipine (Clozapine may potentiate the hypotensive effects of antihypertensive drugs). Products include:

Sular Tablets ... 1163

Nitroglycerin (Clozapine may potentiate the hypotensive effects of antihypertensive drugs). Products include:

Nitro-Dur Transdermal Infusion System ... 3060
Nitrolingual Pumpspray ... 1161

Nortriptyline Hydrochloride (Concomitant use of clozapine with other drugs metabolized by CYP4502D6 may require lower than usual doses for either drug).

No products indexed under this heading.

Olanzapine (Co-administration with benzodiazepines or other psychotropic agents may be accompanied by orthostatic hypotension leading to profound collapse and respiratory and/or cardiac arrest; caution is advised if used concurrently). Products include:

Symbyax Capsules ... 1788
Zyprexa Tablets ... 1798
Zyprexa IntraMuscular ... 1798
Zyprexa ZYDIS Orally Disintegrating Tablets ... 1798

Oxazepam (Co-administration with benzodiazepines or other psychotropic agents may be accompanied by orthostatic hypotension leading to profound collapse and respiratory and/or cardiac arrest; caution is advised if used concurrently).
No products indexed under this heading.

Oxybutynin Chloride (Clozapine may potentiate anticholinergic effects). Products include:
Ditropan XL Extended Release Tablets 2391

Oxycodone Hydrochloride (Given the primary CNS effect of clozapine, caution is advised in using it concomitantly with CNS-active drugs). Products include:
Combunox Tablets 1183
OxyContin Tablets 2699
OxyFast Oral Concentrate Solution 2704
OxyIR Capsules 2704
Percocet Tablets 1114
Percodan Tablets 1115

Paroxetine Hydrochloride (Co-administration in schizophrenic patients has resulted in elevated mean trough concentrations of clozapine and its metabolites by less than two-fold compared to baseline concentrations; a reduced clozapine dose should be considered). Products include:
Paxil CR Controlled-Release Tablets 1509
Paxil 1501

Penbutolol Sulfate (Clozapine may potentiate the hypotensive effects of antihypertensive drugs).
No products indexed under this heading.

Pentobarbital Sodium (Given the primary CNS effect of clozapine, caution is advised in using it concomitantly with CNS-active drugs). Products include:
Nembutal Sodium Solution, USP 2484

Perindopril Erbumine (Clozapine may potentiate the hypotensive effects of antihypertensive drugs). Products include:
Aceon Tablets (2 mg, 4 mg, 8 mg) 3191

Perphenazine (Co-administration with benzodiazepines or other psychotropic agents may be accompanied by orthostatic hypotension leading to profound collapse and respiratory and/or cardiac arrest; caution is advised if used concurrently).
No products indexed under this heading.

Phenelzine Sulfate (Concomitant use of clozapine with other drugs metabolized by CYP4502D6 may require lower than usual doses for either drug).
No products indexed under this heading.

Phenobarbital (Given the primary CNS effect of clozapine, caution is advised in using it concomitantly with CNS-active drugs).
No products indexed under this heading.

Phenoxybenzamine Hydrochloride (Clozapine may potentiate the hypotensive effects of antihypertensive drugs). Products include:
Dibenzyline Capsules 3390

Phentolamine Mesylate (Clozapine may potentiate the hypotensive effects of antihypertensive drugs).
No products indexed under this heading.

Phenytoin (May decrease clozapine plasma levels resulting in a decrease in effectiveness of a previously effective clozapine dose).
No products indexed under this heading.

Phenytoin Sodium (May decrease clozapine plasma levels resulting in a decrease in effectiveness of a previously effective clozapine dose). Products include:
Phenytek Capsules 2153

Pindolol (Clozapine may potentiate the hypotensive effects of antihypertensive drugs).
No products indexed under this heading.

Polythiazide (Clozapine may potentiate the hypotensive effects of antihypertensive drugs).
No products indexed under this heading.

Prazepam (Co-administration with benzodiazepines or other psychotropic agents may be accompanied by orthostatic hypotension leading to profound collapse and respiratory and/or cardiac arrest; caution is advised if used concurrently).
No products indexed under this heading.

Prazosin Hydrochloride (Clozapine may potentiate the hypotensive effects of antihypertensive drugs).
No products indexed under this heading.

Prochlorperazine (Co-administration with benzodiazepines or other psychotropic agents may be accompanied by orthostatic hypotension leading to profound collapse and respiratory and/or cardiac arrest; caution is advised if used concurrently).
No products indexed under this heading.

Procyclidine Hydrochloride (Clozapine may potentiate anticholinergic effects).
No products indexed under this heading.

Promethazine Hydrochloride (Co-administration with benzodiazepines or other psychotropic agents may be accompanied by orthostatic hypotension leading to profound collapse and respiratory and/or cardiac arrest; caution is advised if used concurrently). Products include:
Phenergan 3438

Propafenone Hydrochloride (Concomitant use of clozapine with other drugs metabolized by CYP4502D6 may require lower than usual doses for either drug). Products include:
Rythmol SR Capsules 2736

Propantheline Bromide (Clozapine may potentiate anticholinergic effects).
No products indexed under this heading.

Propofol (Given the primary CNS effect of clozapine, caution is advised in using it concomitantly with CNS-active drugs). Products include:
Diprivan Injectable Emulsion 676

Propoxyphene Hydrochloride (Given the primary CNS effect of clozapine, caution is advised in using it concomitantly with CNS-active drugs).
No products indexed under this heading.

Propoxyphene Napsylate (Given the primary CNS effect of clozapine, caution is advised in using it concomitantly with CNS-active drugs). Products include:
Darvocet A 500 Tablets 3497

Propranolol Hydrochloride (Clozapine may potentiate the hypotensive effects of antihypertensive drugs). Products include:
Inderal LA Long-Acting Capsules 3421
InnoPran XL Capsules 2728

Protriptyline Hydrochloride (Concomitant use of clozapine with other drugs metabolized by CYP4502D6 may require lower than usual doses for either drug). Products include:
Vivactil Tablets 2350

Quazepam (Co-administration with benzodiazepines or other psychotropic agents may be accompanied by orthostatic hypotension leading to profound collapse and respiratory and/or cardiac arrest; caution is advised if used concurrently).
No products indexed under this heading.

Quetiapine Fumarate (Co-administration with benzodiazepines or other psychotropic agents may be accompanied by orthostatic hypotension leading to profound collapse and respiratory and/or cardiac arrest; caution is advised if used concurrently). Products include:
Seroquel Tablets 691

Quinapril Hydrochloride (Clozapine may potentiate the hypotensive effects of antihypertensive drugs).
No products indexed under this heading.

Quinidine (Co-administration of drugs that inhibit CYP4502D6, such as quinidine, should be approached with caution).
No products indexed under this heading.

Quinidine Gluconate (Co-administration of drugs that inhibit CYP4502D6, such as quinidine, should be approached with caution).
No products indexed under this heading.

Quinidine Hydrochloride (Co-administration of drugs that inhibit CYP4502D6, such as quinidine, should be approached with caution).
No products indexed under this heading.

Quinidine Polygalacturonate (Co-administration of drugs that inhibit CYP4502D6, such as quinidine, should be approached with caution).
No products indexed under this heading.

Quinidine Sulfate (Co-administration of drugs that inhibit CYP4502D6, such as quinidine, should be approached with caution).
No products indexed under this heading.

Ramipril (Clozapine may potentiate the hypotensive effects of antihypertensive drugs). Products include:
Altace Capsules 1673

Rauwolfia Serpentina (Clozapine may potentiate the hypotensive effects of antihypertensive drugs).
No products indexed under this heading.

Remifentanil Hydrochloride (Given the primary CNS effect of clozapine, caution is advised in using it concomitantly with CNS-active drugs).
No products indexed under this heading.

Rescinnamine (Clozapine may potentiate the hypotensive effects of antihypertensive drugs).
No products indexed under this heading.

Reserpine (Clozapine may potentiate the hypotensive effects of antihypertensive drugs).
No products indexed under this heading.

Rifampin (May decrease clozapine plasma levels resulting in a decrease in effectiveness of a previously effective clozapine dose).
No products indexed under this heading.

Risperidone (Co-administration with benzodiazepines or other psychotropic agents may be accompanied by orthostatic hypotension leading to profound collapse and respiratory and/or cardiac arrest; caution is advised if used concurrently). Products include:
Risperdal Consta Long-Acting Injection 1664
Risperdal M-Tab Orally Disintegrating Tablets 1658
Risperdal 1658

Scopolamine (Clozapine may potentiate anticholinergic effects). Products include:
Transderm Scōp Transdermal Therapeutic System 2166

Scopolamine Hydrobromide (Clozapine may potentiate anticholinergic effects).
No products indexed under this heading.

Secobarbital Sodium (Given the primary CNS effect of clozapine, caution is advised in using it concomitantly with CNS-active drugs).
No products indexed under this heading.

Sertraline Hydrochloride (Co-administration in schizophrenic patients has resulted in elevated mean trough concentrations of clozapine and its metabolites by less than two-fold compared to baseline concentrations; a reduced clozapine dose should be considered). Products include:
Zoloft 2581

Sevoflurane (Given the primary CNS effect of clozapine, caution is advised in using it concomitantly with CNS-active drugs). Products include:
Ultane Liquid for Inhalation 526

Sodium Nitroprusside (Clozapine may potentiate the hypotensive effects of antihypertensive drugs).
No products indexed under this heading.

Sodium Oxybate (Given the primary CNS effect of clozapine, caution is advised in using it concomitantly with CNS-active drugs).
No products indexed under this heading.

Sotalol Hydrochloride (Clozapine may potentiate the hypotensive effects of antihypertensive drugs).
No products indexed under this heading.

Spirapril Hydrochloride (Clozapine may potentiate the hypotensive effects of antihypertensive drugs).
No products indexed under this heading.

Sufentanil Citrate (Given the primary CNS effect of clozapine, caution is advised in using it concomitantly with CNS-active drugs).
No products indexed under this heading.

Telmisartan (Clozapine may potentiate the hypotensive effects of antihypertensive drugs). Products include:
Micardis Tablets 884
Micardis HCT Tablets 886

Temazepam (Co-administration with benzodiazepines or other psychotropic agents may be accompanied by orthostatic hypotension leading to profound collapse and respiratory and/or cardiac arrest; caution is advised if used concurrently).
No products indexed under this heading.

Terazosin Hydrochloride (Clozapine may potentiate the hypotensive effects of antihypertensive drugs). Products include:
Hytrin Capsules 469

Thiamylal Sodium (Given the primary CNS effect of clozapine, caution is advised in using it concomitantly with CNS-active drugs).
No products indexed under this heading.

Thioridazine Hydrochloride (Co-administration with benzodiazepines or other psychotropic agents may be accompanied by orthostatic hypotension leading to profound collapse and respiratory and/or cardiac arrest; caution is advised if used concurrently). Products include:
Thioridazine Hydrochloride Tablets 2122

Thiothixene (Co-administration with benzodiazepines or other psychotropic agents may be accompanied by orthostatic hypotension leading to profound collapse and respiratory and/or cardiac arrest; caution is advised if used concurrently). Products include:
Thiothixene Capsules 2124

Timolol Maleate (Clozapine may potentiate the hypotensive effects of antihypertensive drugs). Products include:
Blocadren Tablets 1891
Cosopt Sterile Ophthalmic Solution 1910
Timolide Tablets 2056
Timoptic in Ocudose 2061
Timoptic Sterile Ophthalmic Solution 2058
Timoptic-XE Sterile Ophthalmic Gel Forming Solution 2062

Tolterodine Tartrate (Clozapine may potentiate anticholinergic effects). Products include:
Detrol Tablets 2626
Detrol LA Capsules 2629

Torsemide (Clozapine may potentiate the hypotensive effects of antihypertensive drugs).
No products indexed under this heading.

Trandolapril (Clozapine may potentiate the hypotensive effects of antihypertensive drugs). Products include:
Mavik Tablets 482
Tarka Tablets 519

Tranylcypromine Sulfate (Concomitant use of clozapine with other drugs metabolized by CYP4502D6 may require lower than usual doses for either drug). Products include:
Parnate Tablets 1499

Trazodone Hydrochloride (Concomitant use of clozapine with other drugs metabolized by CYP4502D6 may require lower than usual doses for either drug).
No products indexed under this heading.

Triazolam (Co-administration with benzodiazepines or other psychotropic agents may be accompanied by orthostatic hypotension leading to profound collapse and respiratory and/or cardiac arrest; caution is advised if used concurrently).
No products indexed under this heading.

Tridihexethyl Chloride (Clozapine may potentiate anticholinergic effects).
No products indexed under this heading.

Trifluoperazine Hydrochloride (Co-administration with benzodiazepines or other psychotropic agents may be accompanied by orthostatic hypotension leading to profound collapse and respiratory and/or cardiac arrest; caution is advised if used concurrently).
No products indexed under this heading.

Trihexyphenidyl Hydrochloride (Clozapine may potentiate anticholinergic effects).
No products indexed under this heading.

Trimethaphan Camsylate (Clozapine may potentiate the hypotensive effects of antihypertensive drugs).
No products indexed under this heading.

Trimipramine Maleate (Concomitant use of clozapine with other drugs metabolized by CYP4502D6 may require lower than usual doses for either drug). Products include:
Surmontil Capsules 2347

Valsartan (Clozapine may potentiate the hypotensive effects of antihypertensive drugs). Products include:
Diovan HCT Tablets 2195
Diovan Tablets 2191

Venlafaxine Hydrochloride (Concomitant use of clozapine with other drugs metabolized by CYP4502D6 may require lower than usual doses for either drug). Products include:
Effexor Tablets 3405
Effexor XR Capsules 3411

Verapamil Hydrochloride (Clozapine may potentiate the hypotensive effects of antihypertensive drugs). Products include:
Covera-HS Tablets 3135
Tarka Tablets 519
Verelan PM Capsules 3120

Zaleplon (Given the primary CNS effect of clozapine, caution is advised in using it concomitantly with CNS-active drugs). Products include:
Sonata Capsules 1686

Ziprasidone Hydrochloride (Co-administration with benzodiazepines or other psychotropic agents may be accompanied by orthostatic hypotension leading to profound collapse and respiratory and/or cardiac arrest; caution is advised if used concurrently). Products include:
Geodon Capsules 2514

Zolpidem Tartrate (Given the primary CNS effect of clozapine, caution is advised in using it concomitantly with CNS-active drugs). Products include:
Ambien Tablets 2867

Food Interactions

Alcohol (Given the primary CNS effect of clozapine, caution is advised in using it concomitantly with alcohol).

FEIBA VH

(Anti-Inhibitor Coagulant Complex) 749
None cited in PDR database.

FEMARA TABLETS

(Letrozole) 2210
May interact with:

Tamoxifen Citrate (Co-administration of Femara and tamoxifen 20 mg daily resulted in a reduction of letrozole plasma levels of 38% on average. Clinical experience in the second-line breast cancer pivotal trials indicates that the therapeutic effect of Femara therapy is not impaired if Femara is administered immediately after tamoxifen).
No products indexed under this heading.

FEOSOL CAPLETS

(Iron Carbonyl) 1629
May interact with fluoroquinolone antibiotics and tetracyclines. Compounds in these categories include:

Alatrofloxacin Mesylate (Oral iron products interfere with absorption of certain antibiotics; these products should not be taken within two hours of each other).
No products indexed under this heading.

Ciprofloxacin (Oral iron products interfere with absorption of certain antibiotics; these products should not be taken within two hours of each other). Products include:
Cipro I.V. 2998
Cipro I.V. Pharmacy Bulk Package 3509
Cipro Oral Suspension 2991
Cipro XR Tablets 3004
Ciprodex Otic Suspension 555

Ciprofloxacin Hydrochloride (Oral iron products interfere with absorption of certain antibiotics; these products should not be taken within two hours of each other). Products include:
Ciloxan Ophthalmic Ointment 554
Cipro Tablets 2991

Demeclocycline Hydrochloride (Oral iron products interfere with absorption of certain antibiotics; these products should not be taken within two hours of each other).
No products indexed under this heading.

Doxycycline Calcium (Oral iron products interfere with absorption of certain antibiotics; these products should not be taken within two hours of each other).
No products indexed under this heading.

Doxycycline Hyclate (Oral iron products interfere with absorption of certain antibiotics; these products should not be taken within two hours of each other).
No products indexed under this heading.

Doxycycline Monohydrate (Oral iron products interfere with absorption of certain antibiotics; these products should not be taken within two hours of each other).
No products indexed under this heading.

Enoxacin (Oral iron products interfere with absorption of certain antibiotics; these products should not be taken within two hours of each other).
No products indexed under this heading.

Grepafloxacin Hydrochloride (Oral iron products interfere with absorption of certain antibiotics; these products should not be taken within two hours of each other).
No products indexed under this heading.

Lomefloxacin Hydrochloride (Oral iron products interfere with absorption of certain antibiotics; these products should not be taken within two hours of each other).
No products indexed under this heading.

Methacycline Hydrochloride (Oral iron products interfere with absorption of certain antibiotics; these products should not be taken within two hours of each other).
No products indexed under this heading.

Minocycline Hydrochloride (Oral iron products interfere with absorption of certain antibiotics; these products should not be taken within two hours of each other). Products include:
Dynacin Tablets 1859

Moxifloxacin Hydrochloride (Oral iron products interfere with absorption of certain antibiotics; these products should not be taken within two hours of each other). Products include:
Avelox 2984
Vigamox Ophthalmic Solution 560

Norfloxacin (Oral iron products interfere with absorption of certain antibiotics; these products should not be taken within two hours of each other). Products include:
Noroxin Tablets 2009

Ofloxacin (Oral iron products interfere with absorption of certain antibiotics; these products should not be taken within two hours of each other). Products include:
Floxin Otic Singles 1045
Floxin Otic Solution 1043

Oxytetracycline Hydrochloride (Oral iron products interfere with absorption of certain antibiotics; these products should not be taken within two hours of each other).
No products indexed under this heading.

Tetracycline Hydrochloride (Oral iron products interfere with absorption of certain antibiotics; these products should not be taken within two hours of each other).
No products indexed under this heading.

Trovafloxacin Mesylate (Oral iron products interfere with absorption of certain antibiotics; these products should not be taken within two hours of each other).
No products indexed under this heading.

FEOSOL TABLETS

(Ferrous Sulfate) 1629
See Feosol Caplets

FERRETTS IPS LIQUID

(Iron) ..... ■□773
None cited in PDR database.

FERRETTS TABLETS

(Ferrous Fumarate) ..... ■□773
None cited in PDR database.

FERRLECIT INJECTION
(Sodium Ferric Gluconate) 3379
May interact with ACE inhibitors and iron containing oral preparations. Compounds in these categories include:

Benazepril Hydrochloride (Co-administration with ACE inhibitors has resulted in increased incidence of both drug intolerance or suspected allergic events). Products include:
Lotensin Tablets 2232
Lotensin HCT Tablets 2235
Lotrel Capsules 2238

Captopril (Co-administration with ACE inhibitors has resulted in increased incidence of both drug intolerance or suspected allergic events). Products include:
Captopril Tablets 2114

Enalapril Maleate (Co-administration with ACE inhibitors has resulted in increased incidence of both drug intolerance or suspected allergic events). Products include:
Vaseretic Tablets 2073
Vasotec I.V. Injection 2076

Enalaprilat (Co-administration with ACE inhibitors has resulted in increased incidence of both drug intolerance or suspected allergic events).
No products indexed under this heading.

Ferrous Fumarate (Like other parenteral iron preparations, sodium ferric gluconate complex may be expected to reduce the absorption of concomitantly administered oral iron preparations). Products include:
Chromagen Forte Soft Gelatin Capsules 3296
Ferretts Tablets .... ■773
Repliva 21/7 Tablets 3301

Ferrous Gluconate (Like other parenteral iron preparations, sodium ferric gluconate complex may be expected to reduce the absorption of concomitantly administered oral iron preparations).
No products indexed under this heading.

Ferrous Sulfate (Like other parenteral iron preparations, sodium ferric gluconate complex may be expected to reduce the absorption of concomitantly administered oral iron preparations). Products include:
Feosol Tablets 1629
Slow Fe Iron Tablets .... ■772
Slow Fe with Folic Acid Tablets .... ■773

Fosinopril Sodium (Co-administration with ACE inhibitors has resulted in increased incidence of both drug intolerance or suspected allergic events).
No products indexed under this heading.

Iron (Like other parenteral iron preparations, sodium ferric gluconate complex may be expected to reduce the absorption of concomitantly administered oral iron preparations). Products include:
Chromagen Forte Soft Gelatin Capsules 3296
Ferretts IPS Liquid .... ■773
OptiNate 1162
Repliva 21/7 Tablets 3301

Lisinopril (Co-administration with ACE inhibitors has resulted in increased incidence of both drug intolerance or suspected allergic events). Products include:
Prinivil Tablets 2029
Prinzide Tablets 2033
Zestoretic Tablets 701
Zestril Tablets 704

Moexipril Hydrochloride (Co-administration with ACE inhibitors has resulted in increased incidence of both drug intolerance or suspected allergic events). Products include:
Uniretic Tablets 3114
Univasc Tablets 3118

Perindopril Erbumine (Co-administration with ACE inhibitors has resulted in increased incidence of both drug intolerance or suspected allergic events). Products include:
Aceon Tablets (2 mg, 4 mg, 8 mg) 3191

Polysaccharide Iron Complex (Like other parenteral iron preparations, sodium ferric gluconate complex may be expected to reduce the absorption of concomitantly administered oral iron preparations). Products include:
Niferex-150 Forte Capsules 3299
Nu-Iron 150 Capsules 2098

Quinapril Hydrochloride (Co-administration with ACE inhibitors has resulted in increased incidence of both drug intolerance or suspected allergic events).
No products indexed under this heading.

Ramipril (Co-administration with ACE inhibitors has resulted in increased incidence of both drug intolerance or suspected allergic events). Products include:
Altace Capsules 1673

Spirapril Hydrochloride (Co-administration with ACE inhibitors has resulted in increased incidence of both drug intolerance or suspected allergic events).
No products indexed under this heading.

Trandolapril (Co-administration with ACE inhibitors has resulted in increased incidence of both drug intolerance or suspected allergic events). Products include:
Mavik Tablets 482
Tarka Tablets 519

FIBERCON CAPLETS
(Calcium Polycarbophil) .... ■747
May interact with tetracyclines. Compounds in these categories include:

Demeclocycline Hydrochloride (Fibercon should be taken at least one hour before or two hours after you have taken any form of tetracycline).
No products indexed under this heading.

Doxycycline Calcium (Fibercon should be taken at least one hour before or two hours after you have taken any form of tetracycline).
No products indexed under this heading.

Doxycycline Hyclate (Fibercon should be taken at least one hour before or two hours after you have taken any form of tetracycline).
No products indexed under this heading.

Doxycycline Monohydrate (Fibercon should be taken at least one hour before or two hours after you have taken any form of tetracycline).
No products indexed under this heading.

Methacycline Hydrochloride (Fibercon should be taken at least one hour before or two hours after you have taken any form of tetracycline).
No products indexed under this heading.

Minocycline Hydrochloride (Fibercon should be taken at least one hour before or two hours after you have taken any form of tetracycline). Products include:
Dynacin Tablets 1859

Oxytetracycline Hydrochloride (Fibercon should be taken at least one hour before or two hours after you have taken any form of tetracycline).
No products indexed under this heading.

Tetracycline Hydrochloride (Fibercon should be taken at least one hour before or two hours after you have taken any form of tetracycline).
No products indexed under this heading.

FINACEA GEL
(Azelaic Acid) 1644
None cited in PDR database.

FLEET BISACODYL LAXATIVES
(Bisacodyl) 1169
None cited in PDR database.

FLEET ENEMA
(Sodium Phosphate) 1169
May interact with:

Diuretics, Unspecified (Effect not specified).
No products indexed under this heading.

FLEET ENEMA FOR CHILDREN
(Sodium Phosphate) 1169
See Fleet Enema

FLEET GLYCERIN LAXATIVES
(Glycerin) 1168
None cited in PDR database.

FLEET MINERAL OIL ENEMA
(Mineral Oil) 1170
None cited in PDR database.

FLEET PHOSPHO-SODA
(Sodium Phosphate) 1170
See Fleet Prep Kits

FLEET PHOSPHO-SODA ACCU-PREP
(Glycerin, Pramoxine Hydrochloride, Sodium Phosphate)..... 1171
May interact with antacids, diuretics, drugs that prolong the QT interval, and certain other agents. Compounds in these categories include:

Aluminum Carbonate (Concurrent use within one hour should be avoided).
No products indexed under this heading.

Aluminum Hydroxide (Concurrent use within one hour should be avoided). Products include:
Gaviscon Regular Strength Liquid .. ■620
Gaviscon Regular Strength Tablets.. ■619
Gaviscon Extra Strength Liquid ...... ■620
Gaviscon Extra Strength Tablets .... ■619
Maalox Max Maximum Strength Antacid/Anti-Gas Liquid................ 2165
Maalox Regular Strength Antacid/Antigas Liquid................... 2164

Amiloride Hydrochloride (Electrolyte disturbances are a risk associated with this product; concurrent use in patients taking agents known to disturb electrolyte balance requires caution). Products include:
Midamor Tablets 2000
Moduretic Tablets 2003

Amiodarone Hydrochloride (Electrolyte disturbances are a risk associated with this product; concurrent use in patients taking agents known to disturb electrolyte balance requires caution). Products include:
Pacerone Tablets 3337

Amitriptyline Hydrochloride (Electrolyte disturbances are a risk associated with this product; concurrent use in patients taking agents known to disturb electrolyte balance requires caution).
No products indexed under this heading.

Amoxapine (Electrolyte disturbances are a risk associated with this product; concurrent use in patients taking agents known to disturb electrolyte balance requires caution).
No products indexed under this heading.

Astemizole (Electrolyte disturbances are a risk associated with this product; concurrent use in patients taking agents known to disturb electrolyte balance requires caution).
No products indexed under this heading.

Bendroflumethiazide (Electrolyte disturbances are a risk associated with this product; concurrent use in patients taking agents known to disturb electrolyte balance requires caution).
No products indexed under this heading.

Bretylium Tosylate (Electrolyte disturbances are a risk associated with this product; concurrent use in patients taking agents known to disturb electrolyte balance requires caution).
No products indexed under this heading.

Bumetanide (Electrolyte disturbances are a risk associated with this product; concurrent use in patients taking agents known to disturb electrolyte balance requires caution).
No products indexed under this heading.

Chlorothiazide (Electrolyte disturbances are a risk associated with this product; concurrent use in patients taking agents known to disturb electrolyte balance requires caution). Products include:
Aldoclor Tablets 1881
Diuril Oral 1936

Chlorothiazide Sodium (Electrolyte disturbances are a risk associated with this product; concurrent use in patients taking agents known to disturb electrolyte balance requires caution). Products include:
Diuril Sodium Intravenous 1934

Chlorpromazine (Electrolyte disturbances are a risk associated with this product; concurrent use in patients taking agents known to disturb electrolyte balance requires caution).
No products indexed under this heading.

Chlorpromazine Hydrochloride (Electrolyte disturbances are a risk associated with this product; concurrent use in patients taking agents known to disturb electrolyte balance requires caution).
No products indexed under this heading.

Chlorthalidone (Electrolyte disturbances are a risk associated with this product; concurrent use in patients taking agents known to disturb electrolyte balance requires caution). Products include:
Clorpres Tablets 2139

Clomipramine Hydrochloride (Electrolyte disturbances are a risk associated with this product; concurrent use in patients taking agents known to disturb electrolyte balance requires caution).
No products indexed under this heading.

Desipramine Hydrochloride (Electrolyte disturbances are a risk associated with this product; concurrent use in patients taking agents known to disturb electrolyte balance requires caution).
No products indexed under this heading.

Disopyramide Phosphate (Electrolyte disturbances are a risk associated with this product; concurrent use in patients taking agents known to disturb electrolyte balance requires caution).
No products indexed under this heading.

Dofetilide (Electrolyte disturbances are a risk associated with this product; concurrent use in patients taking agents known to disturb electrolyte balance requires caution).
No products indexed under this heading.

Doxepin Hydrochloride (Electrolyte disturbances are a risk associated with this product; concurrent use in patients taking agents known to disturb electrolyte balance requires caution).
No products indexed under this heading.

Ethacrynic Acid (Electrolyte disturbances are a risk associated with this product; concurrent use in patients taking agents known to disturb electrolyte balance requires caution). Products include:
Edecrin Tablets 1941

Flecainide Acetate (Electrolyte disturbances are a risk associated with this product; concurrent use in patients taking agents known to disturb electrolyte balance requires caution). Products include:
Tambocor Tablets 1824

Fluphenazine Decanoate (Electrolyte disturbances are a risk associated with this product; concurrent use in patients taking agents known to disturb electrolyte balance requires caution).
No products indexed under this heading.

Fluphenazine Enanthate (Electrolyte disturbances are a risk associated with this product; concurrent use in patients taking agents known to disturb electrolyte balance requires caution).
No products indexed under this heading.

Fluphenazine Hydrochloride (Electrolyte disturbances are a risk associated with this product; concurrent use in patients taking agents known to disturb electrolyte balance requires caution).
No products indexed under this heading.

Furosemide (Electrolyte disturbances are a risk associated with this product; concurrent use in patients taking agents known to disturb electrolyte balance requires caution). Products include:
Furosemide Tablets 2117

Hydrochlorothiazide (Electrolyte disturbances are a risk associated with this product; concurrent use in patients taking agents known to disturb electrolyte balance requires caution). Products include:
Aldoril Tablets 1884
Atacand HCT 637
Avalide Tablets 2889
Avalide Tablets 922
Benicar HCT Tablets 2852
Diovan HCT Tablets 2195
Dyazide Capsules 1389
Hyzaar 1964
Lotensin HCT Tablets 2235
Maxzide 2150
Micardis HCT Tablets 886
Moduretic Tablets 2003
Prinzide Tablets 2033
Teveten HCT Tablets 1710
Timolide Tablets 2056
Uniretic Tablets 3114
Vaseretic Tablets 2073
Zestoretic Tablets 701

Hydroflumethiazide (Electrolyte disturbances are a risk associated with this product; concurrent use in patients taking agents known to disturb electrolyte balance requires caution).
No products indexed under this heading.

Imipramine Hydrochloride (Electrolyte disturbances are a risk associated with this product; concurrent use in patients taking agents known to disturb electrolyte balance requires caution).
No products indexed under this heading.

Imipramine Pamoate (Electrolyte disturbances are a risk associated with this product; concurrent use in patients taking agents known to disturb electrolyte balance requires caution).
No products indexed under this heading.

Indapamide (Electrolyte disturbances are a risk associated with this product; concurrent use in patients taking agents known to disturb electrolyte balance requires caution). Products include:
Indapamide Tablets 2119

Lidocaine Hydrochloride (Electrolyte disturbances are a risk associated with this product; concurrent use in patients taking agents known to disturb electrolyte balance requires caution).
No products indexed under this heading.

Magaldrate (Concurrent use within one hour should be avoided).
No products indexed under this heading.

Magnesium Hydroxide (Concurrent use within one hour should be avoided). Products include:
Maalox Max Maximum Strength Antacid/Anti-Gas Liquid 2165
Maalox Regular Strength Antacid/Antigas Liquid 2164
Pepcid Complete Chewable Tablets 1672
Rolaids Tablets .... ▣ 707
Extra Strength Rolaids Tablets .... ▣ 707
Rolaids Multi-Symptom Antacid & Antigas Tablets .... ▣ 708

Magnesium Oxide (Concurrent use within one hour should be avoided). Products include:
Beelith Tablets 784
PremCal Light, Regular, and Extra Strength Tablets .... ▣ 762

Maprotiline Hydrochloride (Electrolyte disturbances are a risk associated with this product; concurrent use in patients taking agents known to disturb electrolyte balance requires caution).
No products indexed under this heading.

Mesoridazine Besylate (Electrolyte disturbances are a risk associated with this product; concurrent use in patients taking agents known to disturb electrolyte balance requires caution).
No products indexed under this heading.

Methyclothiazide (Electrolyte disturbances are a risk associated with this product; concurrent use in patients taking agents known to disturb electrolyte balance requires caution).
No products indexed under this heading.

Metolazone (Electrolyte disturbances are a risk associated with this product; concurrent use in patients taking agents known to disturb electrolyte balance requires caution).
No products indexed under this heading.

Mexiletine Hydrochloride (Electrolyte disturbances are a risk associated with this product; concurrent use in patients taking agents known to disturb electrolyte balance requires caution).
No products indexed under this heading.

Nortriptyline Hydrochloride (Electrolyte disturbances are a risk associated with this product; concurrent use in patients taking agents known to disturb electrolyte balance requires caution).
No products indexed under this heading.

Perphenazine (Electrolyte disturbances are a risk associated with this product; concurrent use in patients taking agents known to disturb electrolyte balance requires caution).
No products indexed under this heading.

Polythiazide (Electrolyte disturbances are a risk associated with this product; concurrent use in patients taking agents known to disturb electrolyte balance requires caution).
No products indexed under this heading.

Procainamide Hydrochloride (Electrolyte disturbances are a risk associated with this product; concurrent use in patients taking agents known to disturb electrolyte balance requires caution).
No products indexed under this heading.

Prochlorperazine (Electrolyte disturbances are a risk associated with this product; concurrent use in patients taking agents known to disturb electrolyte balance requires caution).
No products indexed under this heading.

Promethazine Hydrochloride (Electrolyte disturbances are a risk associated with this product; concurrent use in patients taking agents known to disturb electrolyte balance requires caution). Products include:
Phenergan 3438

Propafenone Hydrochloride (Electrolyte disturbances are a risk associated with this product; concurrent use in patients taking agents known to disturb electrolyte balance requires caution). Products include:
Rythmol SR Capsules 2736

Protriptyline Hydrochloride (Electrolyte disturbances are a risk associated with this product; concurrent use in patients taking agents known to disturb electrolyte balance requires caution). Products include:
Vivactil Tablets 2350

Quinidine Gluconate (Electrolyte disturbances are a risk associated with this product; concurrent use in patients taking agents known to disturb electrolyte balance requires caution).
No products indexed under this heading.

Quinidine Polygalacturonate (Electrolyte disturbances are a risk associated with this product; concurrent use in patients taking agents known to disturb electrolyte balance requires caution).
No products indexed under this heading.

Quinidine Sulfate (Electrolyte disturbances are a risk associated with this product; concurrent use in patients taking agents known to disturb electrolyte balance requires caution).
No products indexed under this heading.

Sodium Bicarbonate (Concurrent use within one hour should be avoided). Products include:
Ceo-Two Evacuant Suppository .... ▣ 607
Colyte with Flavor Packs for Oral Solution 3102
HalfLytely and Bisacodyl Tablets Bowel Prep Kit with Flavors Packs 915
TriLyte with Flavor Packs for Oral Solution 3114

Spironolactone (Electrolyte disturbances are a risk associated with this product; concurrent use in patients taking agents known to disturb electrolyte balance requires caution).
No products indexed under this heading.

Thioridazine Hydrochloride (Electrolyte disturbances are a risk associated with this product; concurrent use in patients taking agents known to disturb electrolyte balance requires caution). Products include:
Thioridazine Hydrochloride Tablets 2122

IMPORTANT NOTE: Always consult each drug listing in the patient's regimen for possible interactions.

Tocainide Hydrochloride (Electrolyte disturbances are a risk associated with this product; concurrent use in patients taking agents known to disturb electrolyte balance requires caution).
No products indexed under this heading.

Torsemide (Electrolyte disturbances are a risk associated with this product; concurrent use in patients taking agents known to disturb electrolyte balance requires caution).
No products indexed under this heading.

Triamterene (Electrolyte disturbances are a risk associated with this product; concurrent use in patients taking agents known to disturb electrolyte balance requires caution).
Products include:
Dyazide Capsules 1389
Dyrenium Capsules 3390
Maxzide 2150

Trifluoperazine Hydrochloride (Electrolyte disturbances are a risk associated with this product; concurrent use in patients taking agents known to disturb electrolyte balance requires caution).
No products indexed under this heading.

Trimipramine Maleate (Electrolyte disturbances are a risk associated with this product; concurrent use in patients taking agents known to disturb electrolyte balance requires caution). Products include:
Surmontil Capsules 2347

Ziprasidone Hydrochloride (Electrolyte disturbances are a risk associated with this product; concurrent use in patients taking agents known to disturb electrolyte balance requires caution). Products include:
Geodon Capsules 2514

Food Interactions

Dairy products (Concurrent use within one hour should be avoided).

FLEET PREP KITS

(Bisacodyl, Sodium Phosphate) 1172
May interact with antacids, diuretics, drugs that prolong the QT interval, and certain other agents. Compounds in these categories include:

Aluminum Carbonate (Concurrent use within one hour should be avoided).
No products indexed under this heading.

Aluminum Hydroxide (Concurrent use within one hour should be avoided). Products include:
Gaviscon Regular Strength Liquid .. ▣620
Gaviscon Regular Strength Tablets.. ▣619
Gaviscon Extra Strength Liquid ...... ▣620
Gaviscon Extra Strength Tablets .... ▣619
Maalox Max Maximum Strength Antacid/Anti-Gas Liquid................ 2165
Maalox Regular Strength Antacid/Antigas Liquid................. 2164

Amiloride Hydrochloride (Electrolyte disturbances are a risk associated with this product; concurrent use in patients taking agents known to disturb electrolyte balance requires caution). Products include:
Midamor Tablets 2000
Moduretic Tablets 2003

Amiodarone Hydrochloride (Electrolyte disturbances are a risk associated with this product; concurrent use in patients taking agents known to prolong QT interval requires caution). Products include:
Pacerone Tablets 3337

Amitriptyline Hydrochloride (Electrolyte disturbances are a risk associated with this product; concurrent use in patients taking agents known to prolong QT interval requires caution).
No products indexed under this heading.

Amoxapine (Electrolyte disturbances are a risk associated with this product; concurrent use in patients taking agents known to prolong QT interval requires caution).
No products indexed under this heading.

Astemizole (Electrolyte disturbances are a risk associated with this product; concurrent use in patients taking agents known to prolong QT interval requires caution).
No products indexed under this heading.

Bendroflumethiazide (Electrolyte disturbances are a risk associated with this product; concurrent use in patients taking agents known to disturb electrolyte balance requires caution).
No products indexed under this heading.

Bretylium Tosylate (Electrolyte disturbances are a risk associated with this product; concurrent use in patients taking agents known to prolong QT interval requires caution).
No products indexed under this heading.

Bumetanide (Electrolyte disturbances are a risk associated with this product; concurrent use in patients taking agents known to disturb electrolyte balance requires caution).
No products indexed under this heading.

Chlorothiazide (Electrolyte disturbances are a risk associated with this product; concurrent use in patients taking agents known to disturb electrolyte balance requires caution).
Products include:
Aldoclor Tablets 1881
Diuril Oral 1936

Chlorothiazide Sodium (Electrolyte disturbances are a risk associated with this product; concurrent use in patients taking agents known to disturb electrolyte balance requires caution). Products include:
Diuril Sodium Intravenous 1934

Chlorpromazine (Electrolyte disturbances are a risk associated with this product; concurrent use in patients taking agents known to prolong QT interval requires caution).
No products indexed under this heading.

Chlorpromazine Hydrochloride (Electrolyte disturbances are a risk associated with this product; concurrent use in patients taking agents known to prolong QT interval requires caution).
No products indexed under this heading.

Chlorthalidone (Electrolyte disturbances are a risk associated with this product; concurrent use in patients taking agents known to disturb electrolyte balance requires caution).
Products include:
Clorpres Tablets 2139

Clomipramine Hydrochloride (Electrolyte disturbances are a risk associated with this product; concurrent use in patients taking agents known to prolong QT interval requires caution).
No products indexed under this heading.

Desipramine Hydrochloride (Electrolyte disturbances are a risk associated with this product; concurrent use in patients taking agents known to prolong QT interval requires caution).
No products indexed under this heading.

Disopyramide Phosphate (Electrolyte disturbances are a risk associated with this product; concurrent use in patients taking agents known to prolong QT interval requires caution).
No products indexed under this heading.

Dofetilide (Electrolyte disturbances are a risk associated with this product; concurrent use in patients taking agents known to prolong QT interval requires caution).
No products indexed under this heading.

Doxepin Hydrochloride (Electrolyte disturbances are a risk associated with this product; concurrent use in patients taking agents known to prolong QT interval requires caution).
No products indexed under this heading.

Ethacrynic Acid (Electrolyte disturbances are a risk associated with this product; concurrent use in patients taking agents known to disturb electrolyte balance requires caution). Products include:
Edecrin Tablets 1941

Flecainide Acetate (Electrolyte disturbances are a risk associated with this product; concurrent use in patients taking agents known to prolong QT interval requires caution).
Products include:
Tambocor Tablets 1824

Fluphenazine Decanoate (Electrolyte disturbances are a risk associated with this product; concurrent use in patients taking agents known to prolong QT interval requires caution).
No products indexed under this heading.

Fluphenazine Enanthate (Electrolyte disturbances are a risk associated with this product; concurrent use in patients taking agents known to prolong QT interval requires caution).
No products indexed under this heading.

Fluphenazine Hydrochloride (Electrolyte disturbances are a risk associated with this product; concurrent use in patients taking agents known to prolong QT interval requires caution).
No products indexed under this heading.

Furosemide (Electrolyte disturbances are a risk associated with this product; concurrent use in patients taking agents known to disturb electrolyte balance requires caution).
Products include:
Furosemide Tablets 2117

Hydrochlorothiazide (Electrolyte disturbances are a risk associated with this product; concurrent use in patients taking agents known to disturb electrolyte balance requires caution). Products include:
Aldoril Tablets 1884
Atacand HCT 637
Avalide Tablets 2889
Avalide Tablets 922
Benicar HCT Tablets 2852
Diovan HCT Tablets 2195
Dyazide Capsules 1389
Hyzaar 1964
Lotensin HCT Tablets 2235
Maxzide 2150
Micardis HCT Tablets 886
Moduretic Tablets 2003
Prinzide Tablets 2033
Teveten HCT Tablets 1710
Timolide Tablets 2056
Uniretic Tablets 3114
Vaseretic Tablets 2073
Zestoretic Tablets 701

Hydroflumethiazide (Electrolyte disturbances are a risk associated with this product; concurrent use in patients taking agents known to disturb electrolyte balance requires caution).
No products indexed under this heading.

Imipramine Hydrochloride (Electrolyte disturbances are a risk associated with this product; concurrent use in patients taking agents known to prolong QT interval requires caution).
No products indexed under this heading.

Imipramine Pamoate (Electrolyte disturbances are a risk associated with this product; concurrent use in patients taking agents known to prolong QT interval requires caution).
No products indexed under this heading.

Indapamide (Electrolyte disturbances are a risk associated with this product; concurrent use in patients taking agents known to disturb electrolyte balance requires caution).
Products include:
Indapamide Tablets 2119

Lidocaine Hydrochloride (Electrolyte disturbances are a risk associated with this product; concurrent use in patients taking agents known to prolong QT interval requires caution).
No products indexed under this heading.

Magaldrate (Concurrent use within one hour should be avoided).
No products indexed under this heading.

Magnesium Hydroxide (Concurrent use within one hour should be avoided). Products include:
Maalox Max Maximum Strength Antacid/Anti-Gas Liquid................ 2165
Maalox Regular Strength Antacid/Antigas Liquid................. 2164
Pepcid Complete Chewable Tablets.. 1672
Rolaids Tablets .... ▣707
Extra Strength Rolaids Tablets .... ▣707
Rolaids Multi-Symptom Antacid & Antigas Tablets .... ▣708

Magnesium Oxide (Concurrent use within one hour should be avoided). Products include:
Beelith Tablets 784
PremCal Light, Regular, and Extra Strength Tablets................. ▣762

Maprotiline Hydrochloride (Electrolyte disturbances are a risk associated with this product; concurrent use in patients taking agents known to prolong QT interval requires caution).
No products indexed under this heading.

Mesoridazine Besylate (Electrolyte disturbances are a risk associated with this product; concurrent use in patients taking agents known to prolong QT interval requires caution).
No products indexed under this heading.

Methyclothiazide (Electrolyte disturbances are a risk associated with this product; concurrent use in patients taking agents known to disturb electrolyte balance requires caution).
No products indexed under this heading.

Metolazone (Electrolyte disturbances are a risk associated with this product; concurrent use in patients taking agents known to disturb electrolyte balance requires caution).
No products indexed under this heading.

Mexiletine Hydrochloride (Electrolyte disturbances are a risk associated with this product; concurrent use in patients taking agents known to prolong QT interval requires caution).
No products indexed under this heading.

Nortriptyline Hydrochloride (Electrolyte disturbances are a risk associated with this product; concurrent use in patients taking agents known to prolong QT interval requires caution).
No products indexed under this heading.

Perphenazine (Electrolyte disturbances are a risk associated with this product; concurrent use in patients taking agents known to prolong QT interval requires caution).
No products indexed under this heading.

Polythiazide (Electrolyte disturbances are a risk associated with this product; concurrent use in patients taking agents known to disturb electrolyte balance requires caution).
No products indexed under this heading.

Procainamide Hydrochloride (Electrolyte disturbances are a risk associated with this product; concurrent use in patients taking agents known to prolong QT interval requires caution).
No products indexed under this heading.

Prochlorperazine (Electrolyte disturbances are a risk associated with this product; concurrent use in patients taking agents known to prolong QT interval requires caution).
No products indexed under this heading.

Promethazine Hydrochloride (Electrolyte disturbances are a risk associated with this product; concurrent use in patients taking agents known to prolong QT interval requires caution). Products include:
Phenergan 3438

Propafenone Hydrochloride (Electrolyte disturbances are a risk associated with this product; concurrent use in patients taking agents known to prolong QT interval requires caution). Products include:
Rythmol SR Capsules 2736

Protriptyline Hydrochloride (Electrolyte disturbances are a risk associated with this product; concurrent use in patients taking agents known to prolong QT interval requires caution). Products include:
Vivactil Tablets 2350

Quinidine Gluconate (Electrolyte disturbances are a risk associated with this product; concurrent use in patients taking agents known to prolong QT interval requires caution).
No products indexed under this heading.

Quinidine Polygalacturonate (Electrolyte disturbances are a risk associated with this product; concurrent use in patients taking agents known to prolong QT interval requires caution).
No products indexed under this heading.

Quinidine Sulfate (Electrolyte disturbances are a risk associated with this product; concurrent use in patients taking agents known to prolong QT interval requires caution).
No products indexed under this heading.

Sodium Bicarbonate (Concurrent use within one hour should be avoided). Products include:
Ceo-Two Evacuant Suppository 607
Colyte with Flavor Packs for Oral Solution 3102
HalfLytely and Bisacodyl Tablets Bowel Prep Kit with Flavors Packs 915
TriLyte with Flavor Packs for Oral Solution 3114

Spironolactone (Electrolyte disturbances are a risk associated with this product; concurrent use in patients taking agents known to disturb electrolyte balance requires caution).
No products indexed under this heading.

Thioridazine Hydrochloride (Electrolyte disturbances are a risk associated with this product; concurrent use in patients taking agents known to prolong QT interval requires caution). Products include:
Thioridazine Hydrochloride Tablets 2122

Tocainide Hydrochloride (Electrolyte disturbances are a risk associated with this product; concurrent use in patients taking agents known to prolong QT interval requires caution).
No products indexed under this heading.

Torsemide (Electrolyte disturbances are a risk associated with this product; concurrent use in patients taking agents known to disturb electrolyte balance requires caution).
No products indexed under this heading.

Triamterene (Electrolyte disturbances are a risk associated with this product; concurrent use in patients taking agents known to disturb electrolyte balance requires caution). Products include:
Dyazide Capsules 1389
Dyrenium Capsules 3390
Maxzide 2150

Trifluoperazine Hydrochloride (Electrolyte disturbances are a risk associated with this product; concurrent use in patients taking agents known to prolong QT interval requires caution).
No products indexed under this heading.

Trimipramine Maleate (Electrolyte disturbances are a risk associated with this product; concurrent use in patients taking agents known to prolong QT interval requires caution). Products include:
Surmontil Capsules 2347

Ziprasidone Hydrochloride (Electrolyte disturbances are a risk associated with this product; concurrent use in patients taking agents known to prolong QT interval requires caution). Products include:
Geodon Capsules 2514

Food Interactions

Dairy products (Concurrent use within one hour should be avoided).

FLEXERIL TABLETS

(Cyclobenzaprine Hydrochloride) 1832

May interact with anticholinergics, barbiturates, central nervous system depressants, monoamine oxidase inhibitors, and certain other agents. Compounds in these categories include:

Alfentanil Hydrochloride (Co-administration results in enhanced effects).
No products indexed under this heading.

Alprazolam (Co-administration results in enhanced effects). Products include:
Niravam Orally Disintegrating Tablets 3106
Xanax XR Tablets 2655

Aprobarbital (Co-administration results in enhanced effects).
No products indexed under this heading.

Atropine Sulfate (Caution is advised when co-administered due to cyclobenzaprine-induced atropine-like actions).
No products indexed under this heading.

Belladonna Alkaloids (Caution is advised when co-administered due to cyclobenzaprine-induced atropine-like actions). Products include:
Hyland's Teething Tablets 736

Benztropine Mesylate (Caution is advised when co-administered due to cyclobenzaprine-induced atropine-like actions). Products include:
Cogentin Injection 1903

Biperiden Hydrochloride (Caution is advised when co-administered due to cyclobenzaprine-induced atropine-like actions).
No products indexed under this heading.

Buprenorphine Hydrochloride (Co-administration results in enhanced effects). Products include:
Buprenex Injectable 2718
Suboxone Tablets 2719
Subutex Tablets 2719

Buspirone Hydrochloride (Co-administration results in enhanced effects).
No products indexed under this heading.

Butabarbital (Co-administration results in enhanced effects).
No products indexed under this heading.

Butalbital (Co-administration results in enhanced effects). Products include:
Sedapap Tablets 50 mg/650 mg 2098

Chlordiazepoxide (Co-administration results in enhanced effects).
No products indexed under this heading.

Chlordiazepoxide Hydrochloride (Co-administration results in enhanced effects). Products include:
Librium Capsules 3349

Chlorpromazine (Co-administration results in enhanced effects).
No products indexed under this heading.

Chlorpromazine Hydrochloride (Co-administration results in enhanced effects).
No products indexed under this heading.

Chlorprothixene (Co-administration results in enhanced effects).
No products indexed under this heading.

Chlorprothixene Hydrochloride (Co-administration results in enhanced effects).
No products indexed under this heading.

Chlorprothixene Lactate (Co-administration results in enhanced effects).
No products indexed under this heading.

Clidinium Bromide (Caution is advised when co-administered due to cyclobenzaprine-induced atropine-like actions).
No products indexed under this heading.

Clorazepate Dipotassium (Co-administration results in enhanced effects). Products include:
Tranxene 2488

Clozapine (Co-administration results in enhanced effects). Products include:
Clozapine Tablets 2141
Clozaril Tablets 2174
FazaClo Orally Disintegrating Tablets 547

Codeine Phosphate (Co-administration results in enhanced effects). Products include:
Tylenol with Codeine 2461

Desflurane (Co-administration results in enhanced effects). Products include:
Suprane Liquid for Inhalation 770

Dezocine (Co-administration results in enhanced effects).
No products indexed under this heading.

Diazepam (Co-administration results in enhanced effects). Products include:
Diastat Rectal Delivery System 3344
Valium Tablets 2822

Dicyclomine Hydrochloride (Caution is advised when co-administered due to cyclobenzaprine-induced atropine-like actions). Products include:
Bentyl Capsules 724
Bentyl Injection 724
Bentyl Syrup 724
Bentyl Tablets 724

Droperidol (Co-administration results in enhanced effects).
No products indexed under this heading.

Enflurane (Co-administration results in enhanced effects).
No products indexed under this heading.

Estazolam (Co-administration results in enhanced effects). Products include:
ProSom Tablets 512

Ethanol (Co-administration results in enhanced effects).
No products indexed under this heading.

IMPORTANT NOTE: Always consult each drug listing in the patient's regimen for possible interactions.

Ethchlorvynol (Co-administration results in enhanced effects).
No products indexed under this heading.

Ethinamate (Co-administration results in enhanced effects).
No products indexed under this heading.

Ethyl Alcohol (Co-administration results in enhanced effects).
No products indexed under this heading.

Fentanyl (Co-administration results in enhanced effects). Products include:
Duragesic Transdermal System 2448

Fentanyl Citrate (Co-administration results in enhanced effects). Products include:
Actiq 993

Fluphenazine Decanoate (Co-administration results in enhanced effects).
No products indexed under this heading.

Fluphenazine Enanthate (Co-administration results in enhanced effects).
No products indexed under this heading.

Fluphenazine Hydrochloride (Co-administration results in enhanced effects).
No products indexed under this heading.

Flurazepam Hydrochloride (Co-administration results in enhanced effects). Products include:
Dalmane Capsules 3343

Glutethimide (Co-administration results in enhanced effects).
No products indexed under this heading.

Glycopyrrolate (Caution is advised when co-administered due to cyclobenzaprine-induced atropine-like actions).
No products indexed under this heading.

Guanethidine Monosulfate (Cyclobenzaprine is closely related to tricyclic antidepressants and potential exists for cyclobenzaprine to block antihypertensive effects).
No products indexed under this heading.

Haloperidol (Co-administration results in enhanced effects).
No products indexed under this heading.

Haloperidol Decanoate (Co-administration results in enhanced effects).
No products indexed under this heading.

Hydrocodone Bitartrate (Co-administration results in enhanced effects). Products include:
Hycodan 1104
Hycomine Compound Tablets 1105
Hycotuss Expectorant Syrup 1106
Lortab 3315
Lortab Elixir 3312
Vicodin Tablets 530
Vicodin ES Tablets 531
Vicodin HP Tablets 532
Vicoprofen Tablets 533
Zydone Tablets 1118

Hydrocodone Polistirex (Co-administration results in enhanced effects). Products include:
Tussionex Pennkinetic Extended-Release Suspension 3322

Hydromorphone Hydrochloride (Co-administration results in enhanced effects). Products include:
Dilaudid 439
Dilaudid Oral Liquid 443
Dilaudid Non-Sterile Powder 439
Dilaudid Rectal Suppositories 439
Dilaudid Tablets 439
Dilaudid Tablets - 8 mg 443
Dilaudid-HP 441

Hydroxyzine Hydrochloride (Co-administration results in enhanced effects).
No products indexed under this heading.

Hyoscyamine (Caution is advised when co-administered due to cyclobenzaprine-induced atropine-like actions).
No products indexed under this heading.

Hyoscyamine Sulfate (Caution is advised when co-administered due to cyclobenzaprine-induced atropine-like actions).
No products indexed under this heading.

Ipratropium Bromide (Caution is advised when co-administered due to cyclobenzaprine-induced atropine-like actions). Products include:
Atrovent HFA Inhalation Aerosol 872
Atrovent Inhalation Solution 868
Atrovent Nasal Spray 0.03% 869
Atrovent Nasal Spray 0.06% 870
Combivent Inhalation Aerosol 878
DuoNeb Inhalation Solution 1058

Isocarboxazid (Cyclobenzaprine is closely related to tricyclic antidepressants and hyperpyretic crises, severe convulsions and death have occurred in patients taking these agents concurrently; cyclobenzaprine may interact in the same fashion with MAO inhibitors; hence,concurrent and/or sequential use is contraindicated).
No products indexed under this heading.

Isoflurane (Co-administration results in enhanced effects).
No products indexed under this heading.

Ketamine Hydrochloride (Co-administration results in enhanced effects).
No products indexed under this heading.

Levomethadyl Acetate Hydrochloride (Co-administration results in enhanced effects).
No products indexed under this heading.

Levorphanol Tartrate (Co-administration results in enhanced effects).
No products indexed under this heading.

Lorazepam (Co-administration results in enhanced effects).
No products indexed under this heading.

Loxapine Hydrochloride (Co-administration results in enhanced effects).
No products indexed under this heading.

Loxapine Succinate (Co-administration results in enhanced effects).
No products indexed under this heading.

Mepenzolate Bromide (Caution is advised when co-administered due to cyclobenzaprine-induced atropine-like actions).
No products indexed under this heading.

Meperidine Hydrochloride (Co-administration results in enhanced effects).
No products indexed under this heading.

Mephobarbital (Co-administration results in enhanced effects). Products include:
Mebaral Tablets, USP 2483

Meprobamate (Co-administration results in enhanced effects).
No products indexed under this heading.

Mesoridazine Besylate (Co-administration results in enhanced effects).
No products indexed under this heading.

Methadone Hydrochloride (Co-administration results in enhanced effects).
No products indexed under this heading.

Methohexital Sodium (Co-administration results in enhanced effects).
No products indexed under this heading.

Methotrimeprazine (Co-administration results in enhanced effects).
No products indexed under this heading.

Methoxyflurane (Co-administration results in enhanced effects).
No products indexed under this heading.

Midazolam Hydrochloride (Co-administration results in enhanced effects).
No products indexed under this heading.

Moclobemide (Cyclobenzaprine is closely related to tricyclic antidepressants and hyperpyretic crises, severe convulsions and death have occurred in patients taking these agents concurrently; cyclobenzaprine may interact in the same fashion with MAO inhibitors; hence,concurrent and/or sequential use is contraindicated).
No products indexed under this heading.

Molindone Hydrochloride (Co-administration results in enhanced effects). Products include:
Moban Tablets 1108

Morphine Sulfate (Co-administration results in enhanced effects). Products include:
Avinza Capsules 1714
Kadian Capsules 572
MS Contin Tablets 2703

Olanzapine (Co-administration results in enhanced effects). Products include:
Symbyax Capsules 1788
Zyprexa Tablets 1798
Zyprexa IntraMuscular 1798
Zyprexa ZYDIS Orally Disintegrating Tablets 1798

Oxazepam (Co-administration results in enhanced effects).
No products indexed under this heading.

Oxybutynin Chloride (Caution is advised when co-administered due to cyclobenzaprine-induced atropine-like actions). Products include:
Ditropan XL Extended Release Tablets 2391

Oxycodone Hydrochloride (Co-administration results in enhanced effects). Products include:
Combunox Tablets 1183
OxyContin Tablets 2699
OxyFast Oral Concentrate Solution 2704
OxyIR Capsules 2704
Percocet Tablets 1114
Percodan Tablets 1115

Pargyline Hydrochloride (Cyclobenzaprine is closely related to tricyclic antidepressants and hyperpyretic crises, severe convulsions and death have occurred in patients taking these agents concurrently; cyclobenzaprine may interact in the same fashion with MAO inhibitors; hence,concurrent and/or sequential use is contraindicated).
No products indexed under this heading.

Pentobarbital Sodium (Co-administration results in enhanced effects). Products include:
Nembutal Sodium Solution, USP 2484

Perphenazine (Co-administration results in enhanced effects).
No products indexed under this heading.

Phenelzine Sulfate (Cyclobenzaprine is closely related to tricyclic antidepressants and hyperpyretic crises, severe convulsions and death have occurred in patients taking these agents concurrently; cyclobenzaprine may interact in the same fashion with MAO inhibitors; hence,concurrent and/or sequential use is contraindicated).
No products indexed under this heading.

Phenobarbital (Co-administration results in enhanced effects).
No products indexed under this heading.

Prazepam (Co-administration results in enhanced effects).
No products indexed under this heading.

Procarbazine Hydrochloride (Cyclobenzaprine is closely related to tricyclic antidepressants and hyperpyretic crises, severe convulsions and death have occurred in patients taking these agents concurrently; cyclobenzaprine may interact in the same fashion with MAO inhibitors; hence,concurrent and/or sequential use is contraindicated). Products include:
Matulane Capsules 3188

Prochlorperazine (Co-administration results in enhanced effects).
No products indexed under this heading.

Procyclidine Hydrochloride (Caution is advised when co-administered due to cyclobenzaprine-induced atropine-like actions).
No products indexed under this heading.

Promethazine Hydrochloride (Co-administration results in enhanced effects). Products include:
Phenergan 3438

Propantheline Bromide (Caution is advised when co-administered due to cyclobenzaprine-induced atropine-like actions).
No products indexed under this heading.

Propofol (Co-administration results in enhanced effects). Products include:
Diprivan Injectable Emulsion 676

Propoxyphene Hydrochloride (Co-administration results in enhanced effects).
No products indexed under this heading.

Propoxyphene Napsylate (Co-administration results in enhanced effects). Products include:
Darvocet A 500 Tablets 3497

Quazepam (Co-administration results in enhanced effects).
No products indexed under this heading.

Quetiapine Fumarate (Co-administration results in enhanced effects). Products include:
Seroquel Tablets 691

Remifentanil Hydrochloride (Co-administration results in enhanced effects).
No products indexed under this heading.

Risperidone (Co-administration results in enhanced effects). Products include:
Risperdal Consta Long-Acting Injection 1664
Risperdal M-Tab Orally Disintegrating Tablets 1658
Risperdal 1658

Scopolamine (Caution is advised when co-administered due to cyclobenzaprine-induced atropine-like actions). Products include:
Transderm Scōp Transdermal Therapeutic System 2166

Scopolamine Hydrobromide (Caution is advised when co-administered due to cyclobenzaprine-induced atropine-like actions).
No products indexed under this heading.

Secobarbital Sodium (Co-administration results in enhanced effects).
No products indexed under this heading.

Selegiline Hydrochloride (Cyclobenzaprine is closely related to tricyclic antidepressants and hyperpyretic crises, severe convulsions and death have occurred in patients taking these agents concurrently; cyclobenzaprine may interact in the same fashion with MAO inhibitors; hence,concurrent and/or sequential use is contraindicated). Products include:
Eldepryl Capsules 3209

Sevoflurane (Co-administration results in enhanced effects). Products include:
Ultane Liquid for Inhalation 526

Sodium Oxybate (Co-administration results in enhanced effects).
No products indexed under this heading.

Sufentanil Citrate (Co-administration results in enhanced effects).
No products indexed under this heading.

Temazepam (Co-administration results in enhanced effects).
No products indexed under this heading.

Thiamylal Sodium (Co-administration results in enhanced effects).
No products indexed under this heading.

Thioridazine Hydrochloride (Co-administration results in enhanced effects). Products include:
Thioridazine Hydrochloride Tablets 2122

Thiothixene (Co-administration results in enhanced effects). Products include:
Thiothixene Capsules 2124

Tolterodine Tartrate (Caution is advised when co-administered due to cyclobenzaprine-induced atropine-like actions). Products include:
Detrol Tablets 2626
Detrol LA Capsules 2629

Tramadol Hydrochloride (Cyclobenzaprine is closely related to tricyclic antidepressants; hence, it may enhance the seizure risk in patients taking tramadol). Products include:
Ultracet Tablets 2462

Tranylcypromine Sulfate (Cyclobenzaprine is closely related to tricyclic antidepressants and hyperpyretic crises, severe convulsions and death have occurred in patients taking these agents concurrently; cyclobenzaprine may interact in the same fashion with MAO inhibitors; hence,concurrent and/or sequential use is contraindicated). Products include:
Parnate Tablets 1499

Triazolam (Co-administration results in enhanced effects).
No products indexed under this heading.

Tridihexethyl Chloride (Caution is advised when co-administered due to cyclobenzaprine-induced atropine-like actions).
No products indexed under this heading.

Trifluoperazine Hydrochloride (Co-administration results in enhanced effects).
No products indexed under this heading.

Trihexyphenidyl Hydrochloride (Caution is advised when co-administered due to cyclobenzaprine-induced atropine-like actions).
No products indexed under this heading.

Zaleplon (Co-administration results in enhanced effects). Products include:
Sonata Capsules 1686

Ziprasidone Hydrochloride (Co-administration results in enhanced effects). Products include:
Geodon Capsules 2514

Zolpidem Tartrate (Co-administration results in enhanced effects). Products include:
Ambien Tablets 2867

Food Interactions

Alcohol (Concurrent use results in enhanced effects).

FLOLAN FOR INJECTION

(Epoprostenol Sodium) 1408
May interact with antihypertensives, oral anticoagulants, diuretics, platelet inhibitors, vasodilators, and certain other agents. Compounds in these categories include:

Acebutolol Hydrochloride (Additional reductions in blood pressure may occur).
No products indexed under this heading.

Amiloride Hydrochloride (Additional reductions in blood pressure may occur). Products include:
Midamor Tablets 2000
Moduretic Tablets 2003

Amlodipine Besylate (Additional reductions in blood pressure may occur). Products include:
Caduet Tablets 2507
Lotrel Capsules 2238
Norvasc Tablets 2529

Amyl Nitrite (Additional reductions in blood pressure may occur).
No products indexed under this heading.

Anisindione (Potential for increased risk of bleeding). Products include:
Miradon Tablets 3056

Aspirin (Potential for increased risk of bleeding). Products include:
Aggrenox Capsules 855
Bayer, Aspirin Regimen 606
Bayer Aspirin Tablets 3515
BC Powder 612
BC Allergy Sinus Cold Powder 612
Arthritis Strength BC Powder 612
BC Sinus Cold Powder 612
Ecotrin Enteric Coated Aspirin Low, Regular and Maximum Strength Tablets 1627
Goody's Body Pain Formula Powder 621
Goody's Extra Strength Headache Powder 621
Goody's Extra Strength Pain Relief Tablets 621
Percodan Tablets 1115
St. Joseph 81 mg Aspirin Chewable and Enteric Coated Tablets 1841

Aspirin, Enteric Coated (Potential for increased risk of bleeding).
No products indexed under this heading.

Aspirin Buffered (Potential for increased risk of bleeding).
No products indexed under this heading.

Atenolol (Additional reductions in blood pressure may occur). Products include:
Tenormin I.V. Injection 698
Tenormin Tablets 695

Azlocillin Sodium (Potential for increased risk of bleeding).
No products indexed under this heading.

Benazepril Hydrochloride (Additional reductions in blood pressure may occur). Products include:
Lotensin Tablets 2232
Lotensin HCT Tablets 2235
Lotrel Capsules 2238

Bendroflumethiazide (Additional reductions in blood pressure may occur).
No products indexed under this heading.

Betaxolol Hydrochloride (Additional reductions in blood pressure may occur). Products include:
Betoptic S Ophthalmic Suspension 554

Bisoprolol Fumarate (Additional reductions in blood pressure may occur).
No products indexed under this heading.

Bumetanide (Additional reductions in blood pressure may occur).
No products indexed under this heading.

Candesartan Cilexetil (Additional reductions in blood pressure may occur). Products include:
Atacand Tablets 634
Atacand HCT 637

Captopril (Additional reductions in blood pressure may occur). Products include:
Captopril Tablets 2114

Carbenicillin Indanyl Sodium (Potential for increased risk of bleeding).
No products indexed under this heading.

Carteolol Hydrochloride (Additional reductions in blood pressure may occur). Products include:
Carteolol Hydrochloride Ophthalmic Solution USP, 1% .... ⊙ 246

Chlorothiazide (Additional reductions in blood pressure may occur). Products include:
Aldoclor Tablets 1881
Diuril Oral 1936

Chlorothiazide Sodium (Additional reductions in blood pressure may occur). Products include:
Diuril Sodium Intravenous 1934

Chlorthalidone (Additional reductions in blood pressure may occur). Products include:
Clorpres Tablets 2139

Choline Magnesium Trisalicylate (Potential for increased risk of bleeding).
No products indexed under this heading.

Clonidine (Additional reductions in blood pressure may occur). Products include:
Catapres-TTS 875

Clonidine Hydrochloride (Additional reductions in blood pressure may occur). Products include:
Catapres Tablets 874
Clorpres Tablets 2139

Clopidogrel Bisulfate (Potential for increased risk of bleeding). Products include:
Plavix Tablets 940
Plavix Tablets 2942

Deserpidine (Additional reductions in blood pressure may occur).
No products indexed under this heading.

Diazoxide (Additional reductions in blood pressure may occur). Products include:
Hyperstat I.V. Injection 3031

Diclofenac Potassium (Potential for increased risk of bleeding). Products include:
Cataflam Tablets 2173

Diclofenac Sodium (Potential for increased risk of bleeding). Products include:
Arthrotec Tablets 3126
Voltaren Ophthalmic Solution 2300
Voltaren Tablets 2298
Voltaren-XR Tablets 2301

Dicumarol (Potential for increased risk of bleeding).
No products indexed under this heading.

Diflunisal (Potential for increased risk of bleeding). Products include:
Dolobid Tablets 1937

Digoxin (Co-administration of epoprostenol with digoxin in patients with congestive heart failure has resulted in decreased apparent oral clearance values of digoxin by 15%; patients on digoxin may show elevations of digoxin concentrations after initiation of epoprostenol therapy, which may be clinically significant in patients prone to digoxin toxicity). Products include:
Digitek Tablets 2146
Lanoxicaps Capsules 1458
Lanoxin Injection 1462
Lanoxin Tablets 1468
Lanoxin Injection Pediatric 1465

IMPORTANT NOTE: Always consult each drug listing in the patient's regimen for possible interactions.

Diltiazem Hydrochloride (Additional reductions in blood pressure may occur). Products include:
Cardizem LA Extended Release Tablets 1699
Tiazac Capsules 1204

Dipyridamole (Potential for increased risk of bleeding). Products include:
Aggrenox Capsules 855
Persantine Tablets 898

Doxazosin Mesylate (Additional reductions in blood pressure may occur).
No products indexed under this heading.

Enalapril Maleate (Additional reductions in blood pressure may occur). Products include:
Vaseretic Tablets 2073
Vasotec I.V. Injection 2076

Enalaprilat (Additional reductions in blood pressure may occur).
No products indexed under this heading.

Eprosartan Mesylate (Additional reductions in blood pressure may occur). Products include:
Teveten Tablets 1707
Teveten HCT Tablets 1710

Esmolol Hydrochloride (Additional reductions in blood pressure may occur). Products include:
Brevibloc Concentrate 766
Brevibloc Injection 766
Brevibloc Double Strength Injection 766
Brevibloc Premixed Injection 766
Brevibloc Double Strength Premixed Injection 766

Ethacrynic Acid (Additional reductions in blood pressure may occur). Products include:
Edecrin Tablets 1941

Ethaverine Hydrochloride (Additional reductions in blood pressure may occur).
No products indexed under this heading.

Felodipine (Additional reductions in blood pressure may occur). Products include:
Plendil Extended-Release Tablets 651

Fenoprofen Calcium (Potential for increased risk of bleeding). Products include:
Nalfon Capsules 2504

Flurbiprofen (Potential for increased risk of bleeding).
No products indexed under this heading.

Fosinopril Sodium (Additional reductions in blood pressure may occur).
No products indexed under this heading.

Furosemide (Co-administration in patients with congestive heart failure receiving furosemide apparent oral clearance values for furosemide were decreased by 13% on the second day of therapy and had returned to baseline values by day 87). Products include:
Furosemide Tablets 2117

Guanabenz Acetate (Additional reductions in blood pressure may occur).
No products indexed under this heading.

Guanethidine Monosulfate (Additional reductions in blood pressure may occur).
No products indexed under this heading.

Hydralazine Hydrochloride (Additional reductions in blood pressure may occur). Products include:
BiDil Tablets 2161

Hydrochlorothiazide (Additional reductions in blood pressure may occur). Products include:
Aldoril Tablets 1884
Atacand HCT 637
Avalide Tablets 2889
Avalide Tablets 922
Benicar HCT Tablets 2852
Diovan HCT Tablets 2195
Dyazide Capsules 1389
Hyzaar 1964
Lotensin HCT Tablets 2235
Maxzide 2150
Micardis HCT Tablets 886
Moduretic Tablets 2003
Prinzide Tablets 2033
Teveten HCT Tablets 1710
Timolide Tablets 2056
Uniretic Tablets 3114
Vaseretic Tablets 2073
Zestoretic Tablets 701

Hydroflumethiazide (Additional reductions in blood pressure may occur).
No products indexed under this heading.

Ibuprofen (Potential for increased risk of bleeding). Products include:
Advil Allergy Sinus Caplets ..... ▣737
Advil ..... ▣737
Children's Advil Suspension ..... ▣742
Children's Advil Chewable Tablets ..... ▣741
Advil Cold & Sinus ..... ▣739
Advil Flu & Body Ache Caplets ..... ▣739
Children's Advil Cold Suspension ..... ▣741
Infants' Advil Concentrated Drops ..... ▣743
Junior Strength Advil Swallow Tablets ..... ▣740
Advil Migraine Liquigels ..... ▣740
Advil Multi-Symptom Cold Caplets ..... ▣738
Combunox Tablets 1183
Children's Motrin Oral Suspension and Chewable Tablets 1837
Children's Motrin Cold Non-Staining Dye-Free Oral Suspension 1838
Children's Motrin Cold Oral Suspension 1838
Children's Motrin Non-Staining Dye-Free Oral Suspension 1837
Motrin Cold & Sinus Caplets 1836
Motrin IB Tablets and Caplets 1836
Infants' Motrin Concentrated Drops 1837
Infants' Motrin Non-Staining Dye-Free Drops 1837
Junior Strength Motrin Caplets and Chewable Tablets 1837
Vicoprofen Tablets 533

Indapamide (Additional reductions in blood pressure may occur). Products include:
Indapamide Tablets 2119

Indomethacin (Potential for increased risk of bleeding). Products include:
Indocin 1968

Indomethacin Sodium Trihydrate (Potential for increased risk of bleeding). Products include:
Indocin I.V. 1973

Irbesartan (Additional reductions in blood pressure may occur). Products include:
Avalide Tablets 922
Avalide Tablets 2889
Avapro Tablets 925
Avapro Tablets 2886

Isosorbide Dinitrate (Additional reductions in blood pressure may occur). Products include:
BiDil Tablets 2161

Isosorbide Mononitrate (Additional reductions in blood pressure may occur). Products include:
Imdur Tablets 3032

Isoxsuprine Hydrochloride (Additional reductions in blood pressure may occur).
No products indexed under this heading.

Isradipine (Additional reductions in blood pressure may occur). Products include:
DynaCirc CR Tablets 2726

Ketoprofen (Potential for increased risk of bleeding).
No products indexed under this heading.

Labetalol Hydrochloride (Additional reductions in blood pressure may occur).
No products indexed under this heading.

Lisinopril (Additional reductions in blood pressure may occur). Products include:
Prinivil Tablets 2029
Prinzide Tablets 2033
Zestoretic Tablets 701
Zestril Tablets 704

Losartan Potassium (Additional reductions in blood pressure may occur). Products include:
Cozaar Tablets 1913
Hyzaar 1964

Magnesium Salicylate (Potential for increased risk of bleeding).
No products indexed under this heading.

Mecamylamine Hydrochloride (Additional reductions in blood pressure may occur). Products include:
Inversine Tablets 3286

Meclofenamate Sodium (Potential for increased risk of bleeding).
No products indexed under this heading.

Mefenamic Acid (Potential for increased risk of bleeding).
No products indexed under this heading.

Methyclothiazide (Additional reductions in blood pressure may occur).
No products indexed under this heading.

Methyldopa (Additional reductions in blood pressure may occur). Products include:
Aldoclor Tablets 1881
Aldoril Tablets 1884

Methyldopate Hydrochloride (Additional reductions in blood pressure may occur).
No products indexed under this heading.

Metolazone (Additional reductions in blood pressure may occur).
No products indexed under this heading.

Metoprolol Succinate (Additional reductions in blood pressure may occur). Products include:
Toprol-XL Tablets 660

Metoprolol Tartrate (Additional reductions in blood pressure may occur).
No products indexed under this heading.

Metyrosine (Additional reductions in blood pressure may occur). Products include:
Demser Capsules 1933

Mezlocillin Sodium (Potential for increased risk of bleeding).
No products indexed under this heading.

Mibefradil Dihydrochloride (Additional reductions in blood pressure may occur).
No products indexed under this heading.

Minoxidil (Additional reductions in blood pressure may occur). Products include:
Men's Rogaine Extra Strength Topical Solution, Ocean Rush Scent and Original Unscented ..... ▣706
Women's Rogaine Topical Solution, Spring Bloom Scent and Original Unscented ..... ▣707

Moexipril Hydrochloride (Additional reductions in blood pressure may occur). Products include:
Uniretic Tablets 3114
Univasc Tablets 3118

Nadolol (Additional reductions in blood pressure may occur). Products include:
Nadolol Tablets 2121

Nafcillin Sodium (Potential for increased risk of bleeding).
No products indexed under this heading.

Naproxen (Potential for increased risk of bleeding). Products include:
EC-Naprosyn Delayed-Release Tablets 2769
Naprosyn Suspension 2769
Naprosyn Tablets 2769
Prevacid NapraPAC 3277

Naproxen Sodium (Potential for increased risk of bleeding). Products include:
Aleve Tablets, Caplets and Gelcaps ..... ▣605
Anaprox Tablets 2769
Anaprox DS Tablets 2769

Nicardipine Hydrochloride (Additional reductions in blood pressure may occur). Products include:
Cardene I.V. 1129

Nifedipine (Additional reductions in blood pressure may occur). Products include:
Adalat CC Tablets 2978

Nisoldipine (Additional reductions in blood pressure may occur). Products include:
Sular Tablets 1163

Nitroglycerin (Additional reductions in blood pressure may occur). Products include:
Nitro-Dur Transdermal Infusion System 3060
Nitrolingual Pumpspray 1161

Nitroglycerin, long-acting formulations (Additional reductions in blood pressure may occur).
No products indexed under this heading.

Nitroglycerin Intravenous (Additional reductions in blood pressure may occur).
No products indexed under this heading.

Papaverine (Additional reductions in blood pressure may occur).
No products indexed under this heading.

Papaverine Hydrochloride (Additional reductions in blood pressure may occur).
No products indexed under this heading.

Penbutolol Sulfate (Additional reductions in blood pressure may occur).
No products indexed under this heading.

Penicillin G Benzathine (Potential for increased risk of bleeding).
No products indexed under this heading.

Penicillin G Procaine (Potential for increased risk of bleeding).
No products indexed under this heading.

Perindopril Erbumine (Additional reductions in blood pressure may occur). Products include:
Aceon Tablets (2 mg, 4 mg, 8 mg) 3191

Phenoxybenzamine Hydrochloride (Additional reductions in blood pressure may occur). Products include:
Dibenzyline Capsules 3390

Phentolamine Mesylate (Additional reductions in blood pressure may occur).
No products indexed under this heading.

Phenylbutazone (Potential for increased risk of bleeding).
No products indexed under this heading.

Pindolol (Additional reductions in blood pressure may occur).
No products indexed under this heading.

Piroxicam (Potential for increased risk of bleeding).
No products indexed under this heading.

Polythiazide (Additional reductions in blood pressure may occur).
No products indexed under this heading.

Prazosin Hydrochloride (Additional reductions in blood pressure may occur).
No products indexed under this heading.

Propranolol Hydrochloride (Additional reductions in blood pressure may occur). Products include:
Inderal LA Long-Acting Capsules 3421
InnoPran XL Capsules 2728

Quinapril Hydrochloride (Additional reductions in blood pressure may occur).
No products indexed under this heading.

Ramipril (Additional reductions in blood pressure may occur). Products include:
Altace Capsules 1673

Rauwolfia Serpentina (Additional reductions in blood pressure may occur).
No products indexed under this heading.

Rescinnamine (Additional reductions in blood pressure may occur).
No products indexed under this heading.

Reserpine (Additional reductions in blood pressure may occur).
No products indexed under this heading.

Salsalate (Potential for increased risk of bleeding).
No products indexed under this heading.

Sodium Nitroprusside (Additional reductions in blood pressure may occur).
No products indexed under this heading.

Sotalol Hydrochloride (Additional reductions in blood pressure may occur).
No products indexed under this heading.

Spirapril Hydrochloride (Additional reductions in blood pressure may occur).
No products indexed under this heading.

Spironolactone (Additional reductions in blood pressure may occur).
No products indexed under this heading.

Sulindac (Potential for increased risk of bleeding). Products include:
Clinoril Tablets 1899

Telmisartan (Additional reductions in blood pressure may occur). Products include:
Micardis Tablets 884
Micardis HCT Tablets 886

Terazosin Hydrochloride (Additional reductions in blood pressure may occur). Products include:
Hytrin Capsules 469

Ticarcillin Disodium (Potential for increased risk of bleeding). Products include:
Timentin ADD-Vantage 1556
Timentin Injection Galaxy Container 1559
Timentin IV Infusion 1553
Timentin Pharmacy Bulk Package 1562

Ticlopidine Hydrochloride (Potential for increased risk of bleeding). Products include:
Ticlid Tablets 2813

Timolol Maleate (Additional reductions in blood pressure may occur). Products include:
Blocadren Tablets 1891
Cosopt Sterile Ophthalmic Solution 1910
Timolide Tablets 2056
Timoptic in Ocudose 2061
Timoptic Sterile Ophthalmic Solution 2058
Timoptic-XE Sterile Ophthalmic Gel Forming Solution 2062

Tolazoline Hydrochloride (Additional reductions in blood pressure may occur).
No products indexed under this heading.

Tolmetin Sodium (Potential for increased risk of bleeding).
No products indexed under this heading.

Torsemide (Additional reductions in blood pressure may occur).
No products indexed under this heading.

Trandolapril (Additional reductions in blood pressure may occur). Products include:
Mavik Tablets 482
Tarka Tablets 519

Triamterene (Additional reductions in blood pressure may occur). Products include:
Dyazide Capsules 1389
Dyrenium Capsules 3390
Maxzide 2150

Trimethaphan Camsylate (Additional reductions in blood pressure may occur).
No products indexed under this heading.

Valsartan (Additional reductions in blood pressure may occur). Products include:
Diovan HCT Tablets 2195
Diovan Tablets 2191

Verapamil Hydrochloride (Additional reductions in blood pressure may occur). Products include:
Covera-HS Tablets 3135
Tarka Tablets 519
Verelan PM Capsules 3120

Warfarin Sodium (Potential for increased risk of bleeding). Products include:
Coumadin for Injection 932
Coumadin Tablets 932

Food Interactions

Alcohol (Additional reductions in blood pressure may occur).

FLOMAX CAPSULES

(Tamsulosin Hydrochloride) 881

May interact with alpha adrenergic blockers and certain other agents. Compounds in these categories include:

Cimetidine (Co-administration with highest recommended dose of cimetidine has resulted in a significant decrease (26%) in the clearance of tamsulosin which resulted in a moderate increase in tamsulosin AUC (44%)). Products include:
Tagamet HB 200 Tablets 637
Tagamet Tablets 1547

Cimetidine Hydrochloride (Co-administration with highest recommended dose of cimetidine has resulted in a significant decrease (26%) in the clearance of tamsulosin which resulted in a moderate increase in tamsulosin AUC (44%)).
No products indexed under this heading.

Doxazosin Mesylate (The pharmacokinetic and pharmacodynamic interactions between tamsulosin and other alpha-adrenergic blockers have not been determined, however, interactions may be expected and co-administration should be avoided).
No products indexed under this heading.

Furosemide (Co-administration produces an 11% to 12% reduction in tamsulosin Cmax and AUC; these changes are expected to be clinically insignificant). Products include:
Furosemide Tablets 2117

Prazosin Hydrochloride (The pharmacokinetic and pharmacodynamic interactions between tamsulosin and other alpha-adrenergic blockers have not been determined, however, interactions may be expected and co-administration should be avoided).
No products indexed under this heading.

Terazosin Hydrochloride (The pharmacokinetic and pharmacodynamic interactions between tamsulosin and other alpha-adrenergic blockers have not been determined, however, interactions may be expected and co-administration should be avoided). Products include:
Hytrin Capsules 469

Warfarin Sodium (Results from *in vitro* and *in vivo* interaction studies are inconclusive, therefore, caution should be exercised with concomitant use). Products include:
Coumadin for Injection 932
Coumadin Tablets 932

Food Interactions

Food, unspecified (Tmax is reached by 4 to 5 hours under fasting conditions and by 6 to 7 hours when tamsulosin is administered with food; taking tamsulosin under fasted conditions results in a 30% increase in AUC and 40% to 70% increase in Cmax compared to fed conditions; Flomax should be taken approximately 30 minutes following the meal).

FLONASE NASAL SPRAY

(Fluticasone Propionate) 1412

May interact with cytochrome p450 3a4 inhibitors (selected) and certain other agents. Compounds in these categories include:

Acetazolamide (Caution should be exercised when potent cytochrome P450 3A4 inhibitors are co-administered with fluticasone propionate).
No products indexed under this heading.

Amiodarone Hydrochloride (Caution should be exercised when potent cytochrome P450 3A4 inhibitors are co-administered with fluticasone propionate). Products include:
Pacerone Tablets 3337

Amprenavir (Caution should be exercised when potent cytochrome P450 3A4 inhibitors are co-administered with fluticasone propionate). Products include:
Agenerase Capsules 1299
Agenerase Oral Solution 1304

Anastrozole (Caution should be exercised when potent cytochrome P450 3A4 inhibitors are co-administered with fluticasone propionate). Products include:
Arimidex Tablets 665

Aprepitant (Caution should be exercised when potent cytochrome P450 3A4 inhibitors are co-administered with fluticasone propionate). Products include:
Emend Capsules 1944

Cimetidine (Caution should be exercised when potent cytochrome P450 3A4 inhibitors are co-administered with fluticasone propionate). Products include:
Tagamet HB 200 Tablets 637
Tagamet Tablets 1547

Cimetidine Hydrochloride (Caution should be exercised when potent cytochrome P450 3A4 inhibitors are co-administered with fluticasone propionate).
No products indexed under this heading.

Ciprofloxacin (Caution should be exercised when potent cytochrome P450 3A4 inhibitors are co-administered with fluticasone propionate). Products include:
Cipro I.V. 2998
Cipro I.V. Pharmacy Bulk Package 3509
Cipro Oral Suspension 2991
Cipro XR Tablets 3004
Ciprodex Otic Suspension 555

Clarithromycin (Caution should be exercised when potent cytochrome P450 3A4 inhibitors are co-administered with fluticasone propionate). Products include:
Biaxin/Biaxin XL 402
PREVPAC 3281

Clotrimazole (Caution should be exercised when potent cytochrome P450 3A4 inhibitors are co-administered with fluticasone propionate). Products include:
Lotrimin 3053
Lotrisone 3054

Cyclosporine (Caution should be exercised when potent cytochrome P450 3A4 inhibitors are co-administered with fluticasone propionate). Products include:
Gengraf Capsules 458
Neoral Soft Gelatin Capsules 2247
Neoral Oral Solution 2247
Restasis Ophthalmic Emulsion 570
Sandimmune 2259

Dalfopristin (Caution should be exercised when potent cytochrome P450 3A4 inhibitors are co-administered with fluticasone propionate). Products include:
Synercid I.V. 1690

Danazol (Caution should be exercised when potent cytochrome P450 3A4 inhibitors are co-administered with fluticasone propionate).
No products indexed under this heading.

Delavirdine Mesylate (Caution should be exercised when potent cytochrome P450 3A4 inhibitors are co-administered with fluticasone propionate). Products include:
Rescriptor Tablets 2535

Diltiazem Hydrochloride (Caution should be exercised when potent cytochrome P450 3A4 inhibitors are co-administered with fluticasone propionate). Products include:
Cardizem LA Extended Release Tablets 1699
Tiazac Capsules 1204

Diltiazem Maleate (Caution should be exercised when potent cytochrome P450 3A4 inhibitors are co-administered with fluticasone propionate).
No products indexed under this heading.

Efavirenz (Caution should be exercised when potent cytochrome P450 3A4 inhibitors are co-administered with fluticasone propionate).
Products include:
Sustiva Capsules 957

Erythromycin (Caution should be exercised when potent cytochrome P450 3A4 inhibitors are co-administered with fluticasone propionate). Products include:
Erygel Topical Gel 2096
Ery-Tab Tablets 447
Erythromycin Base Filmtab Tablets 454
Erythromycin Delayed-Release Capsules, USP 456
PCE Dispertab Tablets 510

Erythromycin Estolate (Caution should be exercised when potent cytochrome P450 3A4 inhibitors are co-administered with fluticasone propionate).
No products indexed under this heading.

Erythromycin Ethylsuccinate (Caution should be exercised when potent cytochrome P450 3A4 inhibitors are co-administered with fluticasone propionate). Products include:
E.E.S. 449
EryPed 445

Erythromycin Gluceptate (Caution should be exercised when potent cytochrome P450 3A4 inhibitors are co-administered with fluticasone propionate).
No products indexed under this heading.

Erythromycin Lactobionate (Caution should be exercised when potent cytochrome P450 3A4 inhibitors are co-administered with fluticasone propionate).
No products indexed under this heading.

Erythromycin Stearate (Caution should be exercised when potent cytochrome P450 3A4 inhibitors are co-administered with fluticasone propionate). Products include:
Erythrocin Stearate Filmtab Tablets 452

Esomeprazole Magnesium (Caution should be exercised when potent cytochrome P450 3A4 inhibitors are co-administered with fluticasone propionate). Products include:
Nexium Delayed-Release Capsules 645

Fluconazole (Caution should be exercised when potent cytochrome P450 3A4 inhibitors are co-administered with fluticasone propionate).
No products indexed under this heading.

Fluoxetine Hydrochloride (Caution should be exercised when potent cytochrome P450 3A4 inhibitors are co-administered with fluticasone propionate). Products include:
Prozac Pulvules and Liquid 1771
Symbyax Capsules 1788

Fluvoxamine Maleate (Caution should be exercised when potent cytochrome P450 3A4 inhibitors are co-administered with fluticasone propionate).
No products indexed under this heading.

Fosamprenavir Calcium (Caution should be exercised when potent cytochrome P450 3A4 inhibitors are co-administered with fluticasone propionate). Products include:
Lexiva Tablets 1473

Indinavir Sulfate (Caution should be exercised when potent cytochrome P450 3A4 inhibitors are co-administered with fluticasone propionate). Products include:
Crixivan Capsules 1918

Isoniazid (Caution should be exercised when potent cytochrome P450 3A4 inhibitors are co-administered with fluticasone propionate).
No products indexed under this heading.

Itraconazole (Caution should be exercised when potent cytochrome P450 3A4 inhibitors are co-administered with fluticasone propionate).
No products indexed under this heading.

Ketoconazole (Fluticasone propionate is a substrate of cytochrome P450 3A4. Co-administration with ketoconazole resulted in increased plasma fluticasone propionate exposure, a reduction in plasma cortisol AUC, and no effect on urinary excretion of cortisol. Caution should be exercised when potent cytochrome P450 3A inhibitors are co-administered with fluticasone propionate). Products include:
Nizoral A-D Shampoo, 1% 1839
Nizoral 2% Shampoo 1838

Lopinavir (Caution should be exercised when potent cytochrome P450 3A4 inhibitors are co-administered with fluticasone propionate).
Products include:
Kaletra 474

Loratadine (Caution should be exercised when potent cytochrome P450 3A4 inhibitors are co-administered with fluticasone propionate).
Products include:
Alavert Allergy & Sinus D-12 Hour Tablets .... ▣ 743
Alavert .... ▣ 743
Children's Claritin 24 Hour Non-Drowsy Allergy Syrup .... ▣ 732
Claritin Non-Drowsy 24 Hour Tablets .... ▣ 731
Non-Drowsy Claritin Hives Relief Tablets .... ▣ 733
Claritin Reditabs 24 Hour Non-Drowsy Tablets .... ▣ 732
Claritin-D Non-Drowsy 12 Hour Tablets .... ▣ 731
Claritin-D Non-Drowsy 24 Hour Tablets .... ▣ 731
Children's Dimetapp ND Non-Drowsy Allergy Syrup .... ▣ 746
Triaminic Allerchews .... ▣ 684

Metronidazole (Caution should be exercised when potent cytochrome P450 3A4 inhibitors are co-administered with fluticasone propionate). Products include:
Metrogel 1% 1212
MetroGel-Vaginal Gel 1822
Noritate Cream, 1% 1051

Metronidazole Benzoate (Caution should be exercised when potent cytochrome P450 3A4 inhibitors are co-administered with fluticasone propionate).
No products indexed under this heading.

Metronidazole Hydrochloride (Caution should be exercised when potent cytochrome P450 3A4 inhibitors are co-administered with fluticasone propionate).
No products indexed under this heading.

Miconazole (Caution should be exercised when potent cytochrome P450 3A4 inhibitors are co-administered with fluticasone propionate).
No products indexed under this heading.

Miconazole Nitrate (Caution should be exercised when potent cytochrome P450 3A4 inhibitors are co-administered with fluticasone propionate). Products include:
Desenex .... ▣ 674
Desenex Jock Itch Spray Powder .... ▣ 674

Nefazodone Hydrochloride (Caution should be exercised when potent cytochrome P450 3A4 inhibitors are co-administered with fluticasone propionate).
No products indexed under this heading.

Nelfinavir Mesylate (Caution should be exercised when potent cytochrome P450 3A4 inhibitors are co-administered with fluticasone propionate). Products include:
Viracept 2556

Nevirapine (Caution should be exercised when potent cytochrome P450 3A4 inhibitors are co-administered with fluticasone propionate). Products include:
Viramune Oral Suspension 903
Viramune Tablets 903

Niacinamide (Caution should be exercised when potent cytochrome P450 3A4 inhibitors are co-administered with fluticasone propionate).
No products indexed under this heading.

Nicotinamide (Caution should be exercised when potent cytochrome P450 3A4 inhibitors are co-administered with fluticasone propionate). Products include:
Nicomide Tablets 3190

Nifedipine (Caution should be exercised when potent cytochrome P450 3A4 inhibitors are co-administered with fluticasone propionate).
Products include:
Adalat CC Tablets 2978

Norfloxacin (Caution should be exercised when potent cytochrome P450 3A4 inhibitors are co-administered with fluticasone propionate). Products include:
Noroxin Tablets 2009

Omeprazole (Caution should be exercised when potent cytochrome P450 3A4 inhibitors are co-administered with fluticasone propionate). Products include:
Zegerid Powder for Oral Solution 2972

Paroxetine Hydrochloride (Caution should be exercised when potent cytochrome P450 3A4 inhibitors are co-administered with fluticasone propionate). Products include:
Paxil CR Controlled-Release Tablets 1509
Paxil 1501

Propoxyphene Hydrochloride (Caution should be exercised when potent cytochrome P450 3A4 inhibitors are co-administered with fluticasone propionate).
No products indexed under this heading.

Propoxyphene Napsylate (Caution should be exercised when potent cytochrome P450 3A4 inhibitors are co-administered with fluticasone propionate). Products include:
Darvocet A 500 Tablets 3497

Quinidine (Caution should be exercised when potent cytochrome P450 3A4 inhibitors are co-administered with fluticasone propionate).
No products indexed under this heading.

Quinidine Hydrochloride (Caution should be exercised when potent cytochrome P450 3A4 inhibitors are co-administered with fluticasone propionate).
No products indexed under this heading.

Quinidine Polygalacturonate (Caution should be exercised when potent cytochrome P450 3A4 inhibitors are co-administered with fluticasone propionate).
No products indexed under this heading.

Quinidine Sulfate (Caution should be exercised when potent cytochrome P450 3A4 inhibitors are co-administered with fluticasone propionate).
No products indexed under this heading.

Quinine (Caution should be exercised when potent cytochrome P450 3A4 inhibitors are co-administered with fluticasone propionate).
No products indexed under this heading.

Quinine Sulfate (Caution should be exercised when potent cytochrome P450 3A4 inhibitors are co-administered with fluticasone propionate).
No products indexed under this heading.

Quinupristin (Caution should be exercised when potent cytochrome P450 3A4 inhibitors are co-administered with fluticasone propionate). Products include:
Synercid I.V. 1690

Ranitidine Bismuth Citrate (Caution should be exercised when potent cytochrome P450 3A4 inhibitors are co-administered with fluticasone propionate).
No products indexed under this heading.

Ranitidine Hydrochloride (Caution should be exercised when potent

cytochrome P450 3A4 inhibitors are co-administered with fluticasone propionate). Products include:
- Zantac 1597
- Zantac Injection 1593
- Zantac 75 Tablets 715
- Zantac 150 Maximum Strength Tablets 715
- Zantac Injection Pharmacy Bulk Package 1595

Ritonavir (Fluticasone propionate is a substrate of cytochrome P450 3A4. A drug interaction study has shown that ritonavir (a highly potent cytochrome P450 3A4 inhibitor) can significantly increase plasma fluticasone propionate exposure, resulting in significantly reduced serum cortisol concentrations. Therefore, co-administration of fluticasone propionate and ritonavir is not recommended unless the potential benefit to the patient outweighs the risk of systemic corticosteroid side effects). Products include:
- Kaletra 474
- Norvir 499

Saquinavir (Caution should be exercised when potent cytochrome P450 3A4 inhibitors are co-administered with fluticasone propionate).
No products indexed under this heading.

Saquinavir Mesylate (Caution should be exercised when potent cytochrome P450 3A4 inhibitors are co-administered with fluticasone propionate). Products include:
- Invirase 2776

Sertraline Hydrochloride (Caution should be exercised when potent cytochrome P450 3A4 inhibitors are co-administered with fluticasone propionate). Products include:
- Zoloft 2581

Telithromycin (Caution should be exercised when potent cytochrome P450 3A4 inhibitors are co-administered with fluticasone propionate). Products include:
- Ketek Tablets 2920

Troglitazone (Caution should be exercised when potent cytochrome P450 3A4 inhibitors are co-administered with fluticasone propionate).
No products indexed under this heading.

Troleandomycin (Caution should be exercised when potent cytochrome P450 3A4 inhibitors are co-administered with fluticasone propionate).
No products indexed under this heading.

Valproate Sodium (Caution should be exercised when potent cytochrome P450 3A4 inhibitors are co-administered with fluticasone propionate). Products include:
- Depacon Injection 412

Verapamil Hydrochloride (Caution should be exercised when potent cytochrome P450 3A4 inhibitors are co-administered with fluticasone propionate). Products include:
- Covera-HS Tablets 3135
- Tarka Tablets 519
- Verelan PM Capsules 3120

Voriconazole (Caution should be exercised when potent cytochrome P450 3A4 inhibitors are co-administered with fluticasone propionate). Products include:
- VFEND I.V. 2543
- VFEND Oral Suspension 2543
- VFEND Tablets 2543

Zafirlukast (Caution should be exercised when potent cytochrome P450 3A4 inhibitors are co-administered with fluticasone propionate). Products include:
- Accolate Tablets 663

Zileuton (Caution should be exercised when potent cytochrome P450 3A4 inhibitors are co-administered with fluticasone propionate).
No products indexed under this heading.

Food Interactions

Grapefruit (Caution should be exercised when potent cytochrome P450 3A4 inhibitors are co-administered with fluticasone propionate).

Grapefruit Juice (Caution should be exercised when potent cytochrome P450 3A4 inhibitors are co-administered with fluticasone propionate).

FLOVENT DISKUS 50 MCG

(Fluticasone Propionate) 1415
May interact with cytochrome p450 3a4 inhibitors, potent and certain other agents. Compounds in these categories include:

Amprenavir (Caution should be exercised when potent cytochrome P450 3A4 inhibitors are co-administered with fluticasone. Interactions with ritonavir and ketoconazole, both potent CYP3A4 inhibitors, have resulted in increased fluticasone exposure). Products include:
- Agenerase Capsules 1299
- Agenerase Oral Solution 1304

Atazanavir (Caution should be exercised when potent cytochrome P450 3A4 inhibitors are co-administered with fluticasone. Interactions with ritonavir and ketoconazole, both potent CYP3A4 inhibitors, have resulted in increased fluticasone exposure).
No products indexed under this heading.

Atazanavir sulfate (Caution should be exercised when potent cytochrome P450 3A4 inhibitors are co-administered with fluticasone. Interactions with ritonavir and ketoconazole, both potent CYP3A4 inhibitors, have resulted in increased fluticasone exposure). Products include:
- Reyataz Capsules 948

Clarithromycin (Caution should be exercised when potent cytochrome P450 3A4 inhibitors are co-administered with fluticasone. Interactions with ritonavir and ketoconazole, both potent CYP3A4 inhibitors, have resulted in increased fluticasone exposure). Products include:
- Biaxin/Biaxin XL 402
- PREVPAC 3281

Fosamprenavir Calcium (Caution should be exercised when potent cytochrome P450 3A4 inhibitors are co-administered with fluticasone. Interactions with ritonavir and ketoconazole, both potent CYP3A4 inhibitors, have resulted in increased fluticasone exposure). Products include:
- Lexiva Tablets 1473

Indinavir Sulfate (Caution should be exercised when potent cytochrome P450 3A4 inhibitors are co-administered with fluticasone. Interactions with ritonavir and ketoconazole, both potent CYP3A4 inhibitors, have resulted in increased fluticasone exposure). Products include:
- Crixivan Capsules 1918

Itraconazole (Caution should be exercised when potent cytochrome P450 3A4 inhibitors are co-administered with fluticasone. Interactions with ritonavir and ketoconazole, both potent CYP3A4 inhibitors, have resulted in increased fluticasone exposure).
No products indexed under this heading.

Ketoconazole (Co-administration of a single dose of fluticasone (1000 mcg) with multiple doses of ketoconazole (200 mg) to steady state has resulted in increased mean fluticasone concentrations, a reduction in plasma cortisol AUC, and no effect on urinary excretion ofcortisol). Products include:
- Nizoral A-D Shampoo, 1% 1839
- Nizoral 2% Shampoo 1838

Lopinavir (Caution should be exercised when potent cytochrome P450 3A4 inhibitors are co-administered with fluticasone. Interactions with ritonavir and ketoconazole, both potent CYP3A4 inhibitors, have resulted in increased fluticasone exposure). Products include:
- Kaletra 474

Nefazodone Hydrochloride (Caution should be exercised when potent cytochrome P450 3A4 inhibitors are co-administered with fluticasone. Interactions with ritonavir and ketoconazole, both potent CYP3A4 inhibitors, have resulted in increased fluticasone exposure).
No products indexed under this heading.

Nelfinavir Mesylate (Caution should be exercised when potent cytochrome P450 3A4 inhibitors are co-administered with fluticasone. Interactions with ritonavir and ketoconazole, both potent CYP3A4 inhibitors, have resulted in increased fluticasone exposure). Products include:
- Viracept 2556

Ritonavir (Ritonavir can significantly increase plasma fluticasone exposure, resulting in significantly reduced serum cortisol concentrations. Cushing syndrome and adrenal suppression have been reported; therefore, co-administration is not recommended unless the potential benefit outweighs the risks). Products include:
- Kaletra 474
- Norvir 499

Saquinavir (Caution should be exercised when potent cytochrome P450 3A4 inhibitors are co-administered with fluticasone. Interactions with ritonavir and ketoconazole, both potent CYP3A4 inhibitors, have resulted in increased fluticasone exposure).
No products indexed under this heading.

Saquinavir Mesylate (Caution should be exercised when potent cytochrome P450 3A4 inhibitors are co-administered with fluticasone. Interactions with ritonavir and ketoconazole, both potent CYP3A4 inhibitors, have resulted in increased fluticasone exposure). Products include:
- Invirase 2776

Telithromycin (Caution should be exercised when potent cytochrome P450 3A4 inhibitors are co-administered with fluticasone. Interactions with ritonavir and ketoconazole, both potent CYP3A4 inhibitors, have resulted in increased fluticasone exposure). Products include:
- Ketek Tablets 2920

Troleandomycin (Caution should be exercised when potent cytochrome P450 3A4 inhibitors are co-administered with fluticasone. Interactions with ritonavir and ketoconazole, both potent CYP3A4 inhibitors, have resulted in increased fluticasone exposure).
No products indexed under this heading.

Voriconazole (Caution should be exercised when potent cytochrome P450 3A4 inhibitors are co-administered with fluticasone. Interactions with ritonavir and ketoconazole, both potent CYP3A4 inhibitors, have resulted in increased fluticasone exposure). Products include:
- VFEND I.V. 2543
- VFEND Oral Suspension 2543
- VFEND Tablets 2543

FLOVENT HFA 44 MCG INHALATION AEROSOL

(Fluticasone Propionate HFA) 1418
May interact with:

Ketoconazole (Co-administration of a single dose of fluticasone (1000 mcg) with multiple doses of ketoconazole (200 mg) to steady state has resulted in increased mean plasma fluticasone exposure, a reduction in plasma cortisol AUC, and no effect on urinary excretion of cortisol). Products include:
- Nizoral A-D Shampoo, 1% 1839
- Nizoral 2% Shampoo 1838

Ritonavir (Ritonavir can significantly increase plasma fluticasone exposure, resulting in significantly reduced serum cortisol concentrations. Cushing syndrome and adrenal suppression have been reported; therefore, co-administration is not recommended unless the potential benefit outweighs the risks). Products include:
- Kaletra 474
- Norvir 499

FLOVENT HFA 110 MCG INHALATION AEROSOL

(Fluticasone Propionate HFA) 1418
See Flovent HFA 44 mcg Inhalation Aerosol

FLOVENT HFA 220 MCG INHALATION AEROSOL

(Fluticasone Propionate HFA) 1418
See Flovent HFA 44 mcg Inhalation Aerosol

FLOXIN OTIC SINGLES

(Ofloxacin) 1045
None cited in PDR database.

FLOXIN OTIC SOLUTION

(Ofloxacin) 1043
None cited in PDR database.

FLUMADINE SYRUP

(Rimantadine Hydrochloride) 1186
See Flumadine Tablets

FLUMADINE TABLETS

(Rimantadine Hydrochloride) 1186
May interact with:

Acetaminophen (Coadministration reduces the peak concentration and AUC values for rimantadine). Products include:

Benadryl Allergy & Cold Tablets ..... ▣692
Benadryl Allergy & Sinus Headache Caplets & Gelcaps ..... ▣693
Benadryl Maximum Strength Severe Allergy & Sinus Headache Caplets ..... ▣694
Contac Severe Cold and Flu Caplets Maximum Strength ..... ▣615
Contac Severe Cold and Flu Caplets Non-Drowsy ..... ▣615
Darvocet A 500 Tablets 3497
Goody's Body Pain Formula Powder ..... ▣621
Goody's Extra Strength Headache Powder ..... ▣621
Goody's Extra Strength Pain Relief Tablets ..... ▣621
Goody's PM Powder ..... ▣622
Hycomine Compound Tablets 1105
Lortab 3315
Lortab Elixir 3312
Percocet Tablets 1114
Robitussin Cough, Cold & Flu Liquid-filled Capsules ..... ▣750
Robitussin Flu Liquid ..... ▣752
Sedapap Tablets 50 mg/650 mg 2098
Singlet Caplets ..... ▣636
Sudafed Severe Cold ..... ▣710
Sudafed Sinus Headache ..... ▣711
TheraFlu Cold & Cough Hot Liquid ..... ▣680
TheraFlu Cold & Sore Throat Hot Liquid ..... ▣680
TheraFlu Flu & Chest Congestion Non-Drowsy Hot Liquid ..... ▣681
TheraFlu Flu & Sore Throat Hot Liquid ..... ▣681
TheraFlu Severe Cold Non-Drowsy Hot Liquid ..... ▣683
TheraFlu Severe Cold & Cough Hot Liquid ..... ▣683
TheraFlu Severe Cold Caplets ..... ▣679
TheraFlu Severe Cold Hot Liquid ..... ▣682
TheraFlu Severe Cold Non-Drowsy Caplets ..... ▣679
Triaminic Cough & Sore Throat Liquid ..... ▣687
Triaminic Flu, Cough & Fever Liquid ..... ▣685
Triaminic Cough & Sore Throat Softchews ..... ▣689
Tylenol 8 Hour Extended Release Geltabs and Caplets 1843
Tylenol Sinus NightTime Caplets ..... ▣663
Children's Tylenol Suspension Liquid and Meltaways 1850
Children's Tylenol Plus Cold & Allergy Suspension Liquid 1850
Children's Tylenol Plus Cold NightTime Suspension Liquid 1851
Children's Tylenol Plus Cold & Cough Suspension Liquid and Chewable Tablets 1851
Children's Tylenol Plus Cold Chewable Tablets 1851
Children's Tylenol Plus Cold Daytime Non-Drowsy Suspension Liquid 1851
Children's Tylenol Plus Flu Suspension Liquid 1853
Concentrated Tylenol Infants' Drops Plus Cold 1851
Concentrated Tylenol Infants' Drops Plus Cold and Cough 1851
Concentrated Tylenol Infants' Drops 1850
Junior Tylenol Meltaways 1850
Tylenol Cold & Flu Severe Daytime Liquid with Cool Bust 1846
Tylenol Cold & Flu Severe NightTime Liquid with Cool Burst 1846
Tylenol Cold Severe Congestion Non-Drowsy Caplets with Cool Burst 1846
Tylenol Cough & Sore Throat Daytime Liquid with Cool Burst 1849
Tylenol Cough & Sore Throat NightTime Liquid with Cool Burst 1849
Tylenol 1843
Extra Strength Tylenol Rapid Release Gels 1843
Tylenol 1843
Tylenol Allergy Complete Night Time Caplets 1844
Tylenol Allergy Complete Multi-Symptom Caplets and Gelcaps with Cool Burst 1844
Tylenol Severe Allergy Caplets 1844
Tylenol Flu NightTime Gelcaps 1846
Tylenol Flu Day Non-Drowsy Gelcaps 1846
Concentrated Tylenol Infants' Drops Plus Cold Nasal Congestant, Fever Reducer & Pain Reliever ..... ▣668
Concentrated Tylenol Infants' Drops Plus Cold & Cough Nasal Decongestant, Fever Reducer & Pain Reliever ..... ▣668
Multi-Symptom Tylenol Cold Night Time Caplets 1845
Multi-Symptom Tylenol Cold Day Non-Drowsy Caplets and Gelcaps 1845
Extra Strength Tylenol PM Caplets, Geltabs, Gelcaps and Liquid 1847
Tylenol Sinus Day Non-Drowsy 1848
Tylenol Sinus Night Time Caplets 1848
Tylenol Sinus Severe Congestion Caplets with Cool Burst 1848
Tylenol Sore Throat Daytime Liquid with Cool Burst 1849
Tylenol Sore Throat NightTime Liquid with Cool Burst 1849
Tylenol with Codeine 2461
Women's Tylenol Menstrual Relief Caplets 1849
Ultracet Tablets 2462
Vicks 44M Cough, Cold & Flu Relief 2676
Vicks DayQuil LiquiCaps/Liquid Multi-Symptom Cold/Flu Relief ..... ▣723
Vicks DayQuil Multi-Symptom Cold/Flu Relief LiquiCaps 2675
Vicks DayQuil Multi-Symptom Cold/Flu Relief Liquid 2675
Vicks NyQuil LiquiCaps 2677
Vicks NyQuil LiquiCaps/Liquid Multi-Symptom Cold/Flu Relief ..... ▣725
Vicks NyQuil Liquid 2677
Vicodin Tablets 530
Vicodin ES Tablets 531
Vicodin HP Tablets 532
Zydone Tablets 1118

Aspirin (Coadministration reduces the peak concentration and AUC values for rimantadine). Products include:
Aggrenox Capsules 855
Bayer, Aspirin Regimen ..... ▣606
Bayer Aspirin Tablets 3515
BC Powder ..... ▣612
BC Allergy Sinus Cold Powder ..... ▣612
Arthritis Strength BC Powder ..... ▣612
BC Sinus Cold Powder ..... ▣612
Ecotrin Enteric Coated Aspirin Low, Regular and Maximum Strength Tablets 1627
Goody's Body Pain Formula Powder ..... ▣621
Goody's Extra Strength Headache Powder ..... ▣621
Goody's Extra Strength Pain Relief Tablets ..... ▣621
Percodan Tablets 1115
St. Joseph 81 mg Aspirin Chewable and Enteric Coated Tablets 1841

Cimetidine (Potential for reduced clearance of total rimantadine). Products include:
Tagamet HB 200 Tablets ..... ▣637
Tagamet Tablets 1547

Cimetidine Hydrochloride (Potential for reduced clearance of total rimantadine).
No products indexed under this heading.

FLUMIST VACCINE

(Influenza Virus Vaccine) 1872
May interact with alkylating agents, antivirals active against influenza, antimetabolites, corticosteroids, immunosuppressive agents, killed/inactivated vaccines, vaccines, live, and certain other agents. Compounds in these categories include:

Amantadine Hydrochloride (Based upon the potential for interference between Influenza Virus Vaccine Live, Intranasal and antiviral compounds that are active against influenza A and/or B viruses, it is advisable not to administer Influenza Virus Vaccine Live, Intranasal until 48 hours after the cessation of antiviral therapy. Antiviral agents should not be administered until two weeks after administration of Influenza Virus Vaccine Live, Intranasal unless medically indicated). Products include:
Symmetrel 1115

Aspirin (Influenza Virus Vaccine Live, Intranasal is contraindicated in children and adolescents receiving aspirin therapy or aspirin-containing therapy, because of the association of Reye syndrome with aspirin and wild-type influenza infection). Products include:
Aggrenox Capsules 855
Bayer, Aspirin Regimen ..... ▣606
Bayer Aspirin Tablets 3515
BC Powder ..... ▣612
BC Allergy Sinus Cold Powder ..... ▣612
Arthritis Strength BC Powder ..... ▣612
BC Sinus Cold Powder ..... ▣612
Ecotrin Enteric Coated Aspirin Low, Regular and Maximum Strength Tablets 1627
Goody's Body Pain Formula Powder ..... ▣621
Goody's Extra Strength Headache Powder ..... ▣621
Goody's Extra Strength Pain Relief Tablets ..... ▣621
Percodan Tablets 1115
St. Joseph 81 mg Aspirin Chewable and Enteric Coated Tablets 1841

Azathioprine (Influenza Virus Vaccine Live, Intranasal is contraindicated in patients who have altered or compressed immune status as a consequence of immunosuppressive therapies). Products include:
Azasan Tablets 2844

Basiliximab (Influenza Virus Vaccine Live, Intranasal is contraindicated in patients who have altered or compressed immune status as a consequence of immunosuppressive therapies). Products include:
Simulect for Injection 2268

BCG Vaccine (The safety and immunogenicity of FluMist, when administered concurrently with other vaccines, have not been determined. Studies of FluMist in healthy individuals excluded subjects who received any live virus vaccine within one month of enrollment and anyinactivated or subunit vaccine within two weeks of enrollment. Therefore, healthcare providers should consider the risks and benefits of concurrent administration of FluMist with other vaccines).
No products indexed under this heading.

Betamethasone Acetate (Influenza Virus Vaccine Live, Intranasal is contraindicated in patients who may be immunosuppressed or have altered or compromised immune status as a consequence of treatment with systemic corticosteroids).
No products indexed under this heading.

Betamethasone Sodium Phosphate (Influenza Virus Vaccine Live, Intranasal is contraindicated in patients who may be immunosuppressed or have altered or compromised immune status as a consequence of treatment with systemic corticosteroids).
No products indexed under this heading.

Busulfan (Influenza Virus Vaccine Live, Intranasal is contraindicated in patients who may be immunosuppressed or have altered or compromised immune status as a consequence of treatment with alkylating drugs). Products include:
I.V. Busulfex 1125
Myleran Tablets 1492

Capecitabine (Influenza Virus Vaccine Live, Intranasal is contraindicated in patients who may be immunosuppressed or have altered or compromised immune status as a consequence of treatment with antimetabolites). Products include:
Xeloda Tablets 2825

Carmustine (BCNU) (Influenza Virus Vaccine Live, Intranasal is contraindicated in patients who may be immunosuppressed or have altered or compromised immune status as a consequence of treatment with alkylating drugs).
No products indexed under this heading.

Chlorambucil (Influenza Virus Vaccine Live, Intranasal is contraindicated in patients who may be immunosuppressed or have altered or compromised immune status as a consequence of treatment with alkylating drugs). Products include:
Leukeran Tablets 1472

Cladribine (Influenza Virus Vaccine Live, Intranasal is contraindicated in patients who may be immunosuppressed or have altered or compromised immune status as a consequence of treatment with antimetabolites). Products include:
Leustatin Injection 2368

Cortisone Acetate (Influenza Virus Vaccine Live, Intranasal is contraindicated in patients who may be immunosuppressed or have altered or compromised immune status as a consequence of treatment with systemic corticosteroids).
No products indexed under this heading.

Cyclophosphamide (Influenza Virus Vaccine Live, Intranasal is contraindicated in patients who may be immunosuppressed or have altered or compromised immune status as a consequence of treatment with alkylating drugs).
No products indexed under this heading.

Cyclosporine (Influenza Virus Vaccine Live, Intranasal is contraindicated in patients who have altered or compressed immune status as a consequence of immunosuppressive therapies). Products include:
Gengraf Capsules 458
Neoral Soft Gelatin Capsules 2247
Neoral Oral Solution 2247
Restasis Ophthalmic Emulsion 570
Sandimmune 2259

Cytarabine (Influenza Virus Vaccine Live, Intranasal is contraindicated in patients who may be immunosuppressed or have altered or compromised immune status as a consequence of treatment with antimetabolites).
No products indexed under this heading.

Dacarbazine (Influenza Virus Vaccine Live, Intranasal is contraindicated in patients who may be immunosuppressed or have altered or compromised immune status as a consequence of treatment with alkylating drugs).
No products indexed under this heading.

Dexamethasone (Influenza Virus Vaccine Live, Intranasal is contraindicated in patients who may be immunosuppressed or have altered or compromised immune status as a consequence of treatment with systemic corticosteroids). Products include:
Ciprodex Otic Suspension **555**
Decadron Tablets **1929**
TobraDex Ophthalmic Ointment **558**
TobraDex Ophthalmic Suspension ... **558**

Dexamethasone Acetate (Influenza Virus Vaccine Live, Intranasal is contraindicated in patients who may be immunosuppressed or have altered or compromised immune status as a consequence of treatment with systemic corticosteroids).
No products indexed under this heading.

Dexamethasone Sodium Phosphate (Influenza Virus Vaccine Live, Intranasal is contraindicated in patients who may be immunosuppressed or have altered or compromised immune status as a consequence of treatment with systemic corticosteroids). Products include:
Decadron Phosphate Injection **1931**

Diphtheria & Tetanus Toxoids and Acellular Pertussis Vaccine Adsorbed, Hepatitis B (recombinant) and Inactivated Poliovirus Vaccine Combined (The safety and immunogenicity of FluMist, when administered concurrently with other vaccines, have not been determined. Studies of FluMist in healthy individuals excluded subjects who received any live virus vaccine within one month of enrollment and anyinactivated or subunit vaccine within two weeks of enrollment. Therefore, healthcare providers should consider the risks and benefits of concurrent administration of FluMist with other vaccines).
No products indexed under this heading.

Estramustine Phosphate Sodium (Influenza Virus Vaccine Live, Intranasal is contraindicated in patients who may be immunosuppressed or have altered or compromised immune status as a consequence of treatment with alkylating drugs). Products include:
Emcyt Capsules **3137**

Floxuridine (Influenza Virus Vaccine Live, Intranasal is contraindicated in patients who may be immunosuppressed or have altered or compromised immune status as a consequence of treatment with antimetabolites).
No products indexed under this heading.

Fludarabine Phosphate (Influenza Virus Vaccine Live, Intranasal is contraindicated in patients who may be immunosuppressed or have altered or compromised immune status as a consequence of treatment with antimetabolites).
No products indexed under this heading.

Fludrocortisone Acetate (Influenza Virus Vaccine Live, Intranasal is contraindicated in patients who may be immunosuppressed or have altered or compromised immune status as a consequence of treatment with systemic corticosteroids).
No products indexed under this heading.

Fluorouracil (Influenza Virus Vaccine Live, Intranasal is contraindicated in patients who may be immunosuppressed or have altered or compromised immune status as a consequence of treatment with antimetabolites). Products include:
Carac Cream, 0.5% **1048**
Efudex **3348**

Gemcitabine Hydrochloride (Influenza Virus Vaccine Live, Intranasal is contraindicated in patients who may be immunosuppressed or have altered or compromised immune status as a consequence of treatment with antimetabolites). Products include:
Gemzar for Injection **1743**

Hepatitis A Vaccine, Inactivated (The safety and immunogenicity of FluMist, when administered concurrently with other vaccines, have not been determined. Studies of FluMist in healthy individuals excluded subjects who received any live virus vaccine within one month of enrollment and anyinactivated or subunit vaccine within two weeks of enrollment. Therefore, healthcare providers should consider the risks and benefits of concurrent administration of FluMist with other vaccines). Products include:
Havrix Vaccine **1425**
Twinrix Vaccine **1571**
Vaqta **2067**

Hydrocortisone (Influenza Virus Vaccine Live, Intranasal is contraindicated in patients who may be immunosuppressed or have altered or compromised immune status as a consequence of treatment with systemic corticosteroids). Products include:
Cortizone•5 Ointment **699**
Cortizone•10 Creme **699**
Cortizone•10 Ointment **699**
Cortizone•10 Plus Creme **700**
Cortizone•10 Maximum Strength Quick Shot Spray **700**
Hydrocortone Tablets **1963**
Preparation H Hydrocortisone Cream **748**

Hydrocortisone Acetate (Influenza Virus Vaccine Live, Intranasal is contraindicated in patients who may be immunosuppressed or have altered or compromised immune status as a consequence of treatment with systemic corticosteroids). Products include:
Analpram-HC **1136**
Pramosone **1139**
ProctoFoam-HC **3113**
Tucks Anti-Itch Ointment **712**
U-cort 1% Cream **3289**

Hydrocortisone Sodium Phosphate (Influenza Virus Vaccine Live, Intranasal is contraindicated in patients who may be immunosuppressed or have altered or compromised immune status as a consequence of treatment with systemic corticosteroids).
No products indexed under this heading.

Hydrocortisone Sodium Succinate (Influenza Virus Vaccine Live, Intranasal is contraindicated in patients who may be immunosuppressed or have altered or compromised immune status as a consequence of treatment with systemic corticosteroids).
No products indexed under this heading.

Japanese Encephalitis Vaccine Inactivated (The safety and immunogenicity of FluMist, when administered concurrently with other vaccines, have not been determined. Studies of FluMist in healthy individuals excluded subjects who received any live virus vaccine within one month of enrollment and anyinactivated or subunit vaccine within two weeks of enrollment. Therefore, healthcare providers should consider the risks and benefits of concurrent administration of FluMist with other vaccines).
No products indexed under this heading.

Lomustine (CCNU) (Influenza Virus Vaccine Live, Intranasal is contraindicated in patients who may be immunosuppressed or have altered or compromised immune status as a consequence of treatment with alkylating drugs).
No products indexed under this heading.

Measles, Mumps & Rubella Virus Vaccine, Live (The safety and immunogenicity of FluMist, when administered concurrently with other vaccines, have not been determined. Studies of FluMist in healthy individuals excluded subjects who received any live virus vaccine within one month of enrollment and anyinactivated or subunit vaccine within two weeks of enrollment. Therefore, healthcare providers should consider the risks and benefits of concurrent administration of FluMist with other vaccines). Products include:
M-M-R II **1980**

Measles & Rubella Virus Vaccine Live (The safety and immunogenicity of FluMist, when administered concurrently with other vaccines, have not been determined. Studies of FluMist in healthy individuals excluded subjects who received any live virus vaccine within one month of enrollment and anyinactivated or subunit vaccine within two weeks of enrollment. Therefore, healthcare providers should consider the risks and benefits of concurrent administration of FluMist with other vaccines).
No products indexed under this heading.

Measles Virus Vaccine Live (The safety and immunogenicity of FluMist, when administered concurrently with other vaccines, have not been determined. Studies of FluMist in healthy individuals excluded subjects who received any live virus vaccine within one month of enrollment and anyinactivated or subunit vaccine within two weeks of enrollment. Therefore, healthcare providers should consider the risks and benefits of concurrent administration of FluMist with other vaccines). Products include:
Attenuvax **1889**

Mechlorethamine Hydrochloride (Influenza Virus Vaccine Live, Intranasal is contraindicated in patients who may be immunosuppressed or have altered or compromised immune status as a consequence of treatment with alkylating drugs). Products include:
Mustargen for Injection **2007**

Melphalan (Influenza Virus Vaccine Live, Intranasal is contraindicated in patients who may be immunosuppressed or have altered or compromised immune status as a consequence of treatment with alkylating drugs). Products include:
Alkeran Tablets **977**

Mercaptopurine (Influenza Virus Vaccine Live, Intranasal is contraindicated in patients who may be immunosuppressed or have altered or compromised immune status as a consequence of treatment with antimetabolites). Products include:
Purinethol Tablets **1222**

Methotrexate (Influenza Virus Vaccine Live, Intranasal is contraindicated in patients who may be immunosuppressed or have altered or compromised immune status as a consequence of treatment with antimetabolites).
No products indexed under this heading.

Methylprednisolone Acetate (Influenza Virus Vaccine Live, Intranasal is contraindicated in patients who may be immunosuppressed or have altered or compromised immune status as a consequence of treatment with systemic corticosteroids). Products include:
Depo-Medrol Injectable Suspension **2615**
Depo-Medrol Single-Dose Vial **2617**

Methylprednisolone Sodium Succinate (Influenza Virus Vaccine Live, Intranasal is contraindicated in patients who may be immunosuppressed or have altered or compromised immune status as a consequence of treatment with systemic corticosteroids).
No products indexed under this heading.

Mumps Virus Vaccine, Live (The safety and immunogenicity of FluMist, when administered concurrently with other vaccines, have not been determined. Studies of FluMist in healthy individuals excluded subjects who received any live virus vaccine within one month of enrollment and anyinactivated or subunit vaccine within two weeks of enrollment. Therefore, healthcare providers should consider the risks and benefits of concurrent administration of FluMist with other vaccines). Products include:
Mumpsvax **2005**

Muromonab-CD3 (Influenza Virus Vaccine Live, Intranasal is contraindicated in patients who have altered or compressed immune status as a consequence of immunosuppressive therapies). Products include:
Orthoclone OKT3 Sterile Solution **2370**

Mycophenolate Mofetil (Influenza Virus Vaccine Live, Intranasal is contraindicated in patients who have altered or compressed immune status as a consequence of immunosuppressive therapies). Products include:
CellCept Capsules **2751**
CellCept Oral Suspension **2751**
CellCept Tablets **2751**

Oseltamivir Phosphate (Based upon the potential for interference

between Influenza Virus Vaccine Live, Intranasal and antiviral compounds that are active against influenza A and/or B viruses, it is advisable not to administer Influenza Virus Vaccine Live, Intranasal until 48 hours after the cessation of antiviral therapy. Antiviral agents should not be administered until two weeks after administration of Influenza Virus Vaccine Live, Intranasal unless medically indicated). Products include:

Tamiflu Capsules 2810
Tamiflu Oral Suspension 2810

Pentostatin (Influenza Virus Vaccine Live, Intranasal is contraindicated in patients who may be immunosuppressed or have altered or compromised immune status as a consequence of treatment with antimetabolites). Products include:

Nipent for Injection 3216

Poliovirus Vaccine, Live, Oral, Trivalent, Types 1,2,3 (Sabin) (The safety and immunogenicity of FluMist, when administered concurrently with other vaccines, have not been determined. Studies of FluMist in healthy individuals excluded subjects who received any live virus vaccine within one month of enrollment and anyinactivated or subunit vaccine within two weeks of enrollment. Therefore, healthcare providers should consider the risks and benefits of concurrent administration of FluMist with other vaccines).

No products indexed under this heading.

Poliovirus Vaccine Inactivated, Trivalent Types 1,2,3 (The safety and immunogenicity of FluMist, when administered concurrently with other vaccines, have not been determined. Studies of FluMist in healthy individuals excluded subjects who received any live virus vaccine within one month of enrollment and anyinactivated or subunit vaccine within two weeks of enrollment. Therefore, healthcare providers should consider the risks and benefits of concurrent administration of FluMist with other vaccines). Products include:

Pediarix Vaccine 1518

Prednisolone Acetate (Influenza Virus Vaccine Live, Intranasal is contraindicated in patients who may be immunosuppressed or have altered or compromised immune status as a consequence of treatment with systemic corticosteroids). Products include:

Blephamide Ophthalmic Ointment 563
Blephamide Ophthalmic Suspension.................................. 564
Poly-Pred Liquifilm Ophthalmic Suspension .... ⊙231
Pred Forte Ophthalmic Suspension .... ⊙233
Pred Mild Sterile Ophthalmic Suspension .... ⊙236
Pred-G Ophthalmic Suspension ...... ⊙234
Pred-G Sterile Ophthalmic Ointment.................................... ⊙235

Prednisolone Sodium Phosphate (Influenza Virus Vaccine Live, Intranasal is contraindicated in patients who may be immunosuppressed or have altered or compromised immune status as a consequence of treatment with systemic corticosteroids). Products include:

Pediapred Oral Solution 3319

Prednisolone Tebutate (Influenza Virus Vaccine Live, Intranasal is contraindicated in patients who may be immunosuppressed or have altered or compromised immune status as a consequence of treatment with systemic corticosteroids).

No products indexed under this heading.

Prednisone (Influenza Virus Vaccine Live, Intranasal is contraindicated in patients who may be immunosuppressed or have altered or compromised immune status as a consequence of treatment with systemic corticosteroids).

No products indexed under this heading.

Rimantadine Hydrochloride (Based upon the potential for interference between Influenza Virus Vaccine Live, Intranasal and antiviral compounds that are active against influenza A and/or B viruses, it is advisable not to administer Influenza Virus Vaccine Live, Intranasal until 48 hours after the cessation of antiviral therapy. Antiviral agents should not be administered until two weeks after administration of Influenza Virus Vaccine Live, Intranasal unless medically indicated). Products include:

Flumadine 1186

Rotavirus Vaccine, Live, Oral, Tetravalent (The safety and immunogenicity of FluMist, when administered concurrently with other vaccines, have not been determined. Studies of FluMist in healthy individuals excluded subjects who received any live virus vaccine within one month of enrollment and anyinactivated or subunit vaccine within two weeks of enrollment. Therefore, healthcare providers should consider the risks and benefits of concurrent administration of FluMist with other vaccines).

No products indexed under this heading.

Rubella & Mumps Virus Vaccine Live (The safety and immunogenicity of FluMist, when administered concurrently with other vaccines, have not been determined. Studies of FluMist in healthy individuals excluded subjects who received any live virus vaccine within one month of enrollment and anyinactivated or subunit vaccine within two weeks of enrollment. Therefore, healthcare providers should consider the risks and benefits of concurrent administration of FluMist with other vaccines).

No products indexed under this heading.

Rubella Virus Vaccine Live (The safety and immunogenicity of FluMist, when administered concurrently with other vaccines, have not been determined. Studies of FluMist in healthy individuals excluded subjects who received any live virus vaccine within one month of enrollment and anyinactivated or subunit vaccine within two weeks of enrollment. Therefore, healthcare providers should consider the risks and benefits of concurrent administration of FluMist with other vaccines). Products include:

Meruvax II 1994

Sirolimus (Influenza Virus Vaccine Live, Intranasal is contraindicated in patients who have altered or compressed immune status as a consequence of immunosuppressive therapies). Products include:

Rapamune Oral Solution and Tablets 3472

Smallpox Vaccine (The safety and immunogenicity of FluMist, when administered concurrently with other vaccines, have not been determined. Studies of FluMist in healthy individuals excluded subjects who received any live virus vaccine within one month of enrollment and anyinactivated or subunit vaccine within two weeks of enrollment. Therefore, healthcare providers should consider the risks and benefits of concurrent administration of FluMist with other vaccines).

No products indexed under this heading.

Tacrolimus (Influenza Virus Vaccine Live, Intranasal is contraindicated in patients who have altered or compressed immune status as a consequence of immunosuppressive therapies). Products include:

Prograf Capsules and Injection 624
Protopic Ointment 629

Thioguanine (Influenza Virus Vaccine Live, Intranasal is contraindicated in patients who may be immunosuppressed or have altered or compromised immune status as a consequence of treatment with antimetabolites). Products include:

Tabloid Tablets 1545

Thiotepa (Influenza Virus Vaccine Live, Intranasal is contraindicated in patients who may be immunosuppressed or have altered or compromised immune status as a consequence of treatment with alkylating drugs).

No products indexed under this heading.

Triamcinolone (Influenza Virus Vaccine Live, Intranasal is contraindicated in patients who may be immunosuppressed or have altered or compromised immune status as a consequence of treatment with systemic corticosteroids).

No products indexed under this heading.

Triamcinolone Acetonide (Influenza Virus Vaccine Live, Intranasal is contraindicated in patients who may be immunosuppressed or have altered or compromised immune status as a consequence of treatment with systemic corticosteroids). Products include:

Azmacort Inhalation Aerosol 1701
Nasacort HFA Inhalation Aerosol 2939
Nasacort AQ Nasal Spray 2937

Triamcinolone Diacetate (Influenza Virus Vaccine Live, Intranasal is contraindicated in patients who may be immunosuppressed or have altered or compromised immune status as a consequence of treatment with systemic corticosteroids).

No products indexed under this heading.

Triamcinolone Hexacetonide (Influenza Virus Vaccine Live, Intranasal is contraindicated in patients who may be immunosuppressed or have altered or compromised immune status as a consequence of treatment with systemic corticosteroids).

No products indexed under this heading.

Typhoid Vaccine (The safety and immunogenicity of FluMist, when administered concurrently with other vaccines, have not been determined. Studies of FluMist in healthy individuals excluded subjects who received any live virus vaccine within one month of enrollment and anyinactivated or subunit vaccine within two weeks of enrollment. Therefore, healthcare providers should consider the risks and benefits of concurrent administration of FluMist with other vaccines).

No products indexed under this heading.

Varicella Virus Vaccine Live (The safety and immunogenicity of FluMist, when administered concurrently with other vaccines, have not been determined. Studies of FluMist in healthy individuals excluded subjects who received any live virus vaccine within one month of enrollment and anyinactivated or subunit vaccine within two weeks of enrollment. Therefore, healthcare providers should consider the risks and benefits of concurrent administration of FluMist with other vaccines). Products include:

Varivax 2070

Yellow Fever Vaccine (The safety and immunogenicity of FluMist, when administered concurrently with other vaccines, have not been determined. Studies of FluMist in healthy individuals excluded subjects who received any live virus vaccine within one month of enrollment and anyinactivated or subunit vaccine within two weeks of enrollment. Therefore, healthcare providers should consider the risks and benefits of concurrent administration of FluMist with other vaccines).

No products indexed under this heading.

Zanamivir (Based upon the potential for interference between Influenza Virus Vaccine Live, Intranasal and antiviral compounds that are active against influenza A and/or B viruses, it is advisable not to administer Influenza Virus Vaccine Live, Intranasal until 48 hours after the cessation of antiviral therapy. Antiviral agents should not be administered until two weeks after administration of Influenza Virus Vaccine Live, Intranasal unless medically indicated). Products include:

Relenza Rotadisk 1525

FLUORESCITE INJECTION

(Fluorescein Sodium) .... ⊙207
None cited in PDR database.

FLUOR-I-STRIP A.T. OPHTHALMIC STRIPS 1 MG

(Fluorescein Sodium) .... ⊙249
None cited in PDR database.

FLUOR-I-STRIP OPHTHALMIC STRIPS 9 MG

(Fluorescein Sodium) .... ⊙249
None cited in PDR database.

FML OPHTHALMIC OINTMENT

(Fluorometholone) .... ⊙225
None cited in PDR database.

FML OPHTHALMIC SUSPENSION

(Fluorometholone) .... ⊙224
None cited in PDR database.

FML FORTE OPHTHALMIC SUSPENSION
(Fluorometholone) .... ⊙223
None cited in PDR database.

FML-S LIQUIFILM STERILE OPHTHALMIC SUSPENSION
(Fluorometholone, Sulfacetamide Sodium) .... ⊙226
May interact with silver preparations. Compounds in these categories include:

Silver Acetate (Sulfacetamide preparations are incompatible with silver preparations).
No products indexed under this heading.

Silver Nitrate (Sulfacetamide preparations are incompatible with silver preparations).
No products indexed under this heading.

Silver Sulfadiazine (Sulfacetamide preparations are incompatible with silver preparations).
No products indexed under this heading.

FOCALIN TABLETS
(Dexmethylphenidate Hydrochloride) 2214
May interact with antihypertensives, oral anticoagulants, monoamine oxidase inhibitors, phenytoin, selective serotonin reuptake inhibitors, tricyclic antidepressants, vasopressors, and certain other agents. Compounds in these categories include:

Acebutolol Hydrochloride (Methylphenidate may decrease the effectiveness of antihypertensive drugs).
No products indexed under this heading.

Amitriptyline Hydrochloride (Racemic methylphenidate may inhibit the metabolism of tricyclic antidepressants).
No products indexed under this heading.

Amlodipine Besylate (Methylphenidate may decrease the effectiveness of antihypertensive drugs). Products include:
Caduet Tablets 2507
Lotrel Capsules 2238
Norvasc Tablets 2529

Amoxapine (Racemic methylphenidate may inhibit the metabolism of tricyclic antidepressants).
No products indexed under this heading.

Anisindione (Racemic methylphenidate may inhibit the metabolism of coumarin anticoagulants). Products include:
Miradon Tablets 3056

Atenolol (Methylphenidate may decrease the effectiveness of antihypertensive drugs). Products include:
Tenormin I.V. Injection 698
Tenormin Tablets 695

Benazepril Hydrochloride (Methylphenidate may decrease the effectiveness of antihypertensive drugs). Products include:
Lotensin Tablets 2232
Lotensin HCT Tablets 2235
Lotrel Capsules 2238

Bendroflumethiazide (Methylphenidate may decrease the effectiveness of antihypertensive drugs).
No products indexed under this heading.

Betaxolol Hydrochloride (Methylphenidate may decrease the effectiveness of antihypertensive drugs). Products include:
Betoptic S Ophthalmic Suspension 554

Bisoprolol Fumarate (Methylphenidate may decrease the effectiveness of antihypertensive drugs).
No products indexed under this heading.

Candesartan Cilexetil (Methylphenidate may decrease the effectiveness of antihypertensive drugs). Products include:
Atacand Tablets 634
Atacand HCT 637

Captopril (Methylphenidate may decrease the effectiveness of antihypertensive drugs). Products include:
Captopril Tablets 2114

Carteolol Hydrochloride (Methylphenidate may decrease the effectiveness of antihypertensive drugs). Products include:
Carteolol Hydrochloride Ophthalmic Solution USP, 1% .... ⊙246

Chlorothiazide (Methylphenidate may decrease the effectiveness of antihypertensive drugs). Products include:
Aldoclor Tablets 1881
Diuril Oral 1936

Chlorothiazide Sodium (Methylphenidate may decrease the effectiveness of antihypertensive drugs). Products include:
Diuril Sodium Intravenous 1934

Chlorthalidone (Methylphenidate may decrease the effectiveness of antihypertensive drugs). Products include:
Clorpres Tablets 2139

Citalopram Hydrobromide (Racemic methylphenidate may inhibit the metabolism of selective serotonin reuptake inhibitors). Products include:
Celexa 1177

Clomipramine Hydrochloride (Racemic methylphenidate may inhibit the metabolism of tricyclic antidepressants).
No products indexed under this heading.

Clonidine (Co-administration has resulted in serious adverse events). Products include:
Catapres-TTS 875

Clonidine Hydrochloride (Co-administration has resulted in serious adverse events). Products include:
Catapres Tablets 874
Clorpres Tablets 2139

Deserpidine (Methylphenidate may decrease the effectiveness of antihypertensive drugs).
No products indexed under this heading.

Desipramine Hydrochloride (Racemic methylphenidate may inhibit the metabolism of tricyclic antidepressants).
No products indexed under this heading.

Diazoxide (Methylphenidate may decrease the effectiveness of antihypertensive drugs). Products include:
Hyperstat I.V. Injection 3031

Dicumarol (Racemic methylphenidate may inhibit the metabolism of coumarin anticoagulants).
No products indexed under this heading.

Diltiazem Hydrochloride (Methylphenidate may decrease the effectiveness of antihypertensive drugs). Products include:
Cardizem LA Extended Release Tablets 1699
Tiazac Capsules 1204

Dobutamine (Methylphenidate has potential to increase blood pressure; concurrent use with pressor agents requires caution).
No products indexed under this heading.

Dobutamine Hydrochloride (Methylphenidate has potential to increase blood pressure; concurrent use with pressor agents requires caution).
No products indexed under this heading.

Dopamine Hydrochloride (Methylphenidate has potential to increase blood pressure; concurrent use with pressor agents requires caution).
No products indexed under this heading.

Doxazosin Mesylate (Methylphenidate may decrease the effectiveness of antihypertensive drugs).
No products indexed under this heading.

Doxepin Hydrochloride (Racemic methylphenidate may inhibit the metabolism of tricyclic antidepressants).
No products indexed under this heading.

Enalapril Maleate (Methylphenidate may decrease the effectiveness of antihypertensive drugs). Products include:
Vaseretic Tablets 2073
Vasotec I.V. Injection 2076

Enalaprilat (Methylphenidate may decrease the effectiveness of antihypertensive drugs).
No products indexed under this heading.

Ephedrine Sulfate (Methylphenidate has potential to increase blood pressure; concurrent use with pressor agents requires caution).
No products indexed under this heading.

Epinephrine Bitartrate (Methylphenidate has potential to increase blood pressure; concurrent use with pressor agents requires caution).
No products indexed under this heading.

Epinephrine Hydrochloride (Methylphenidate has potential to increase blood pressure; concurrent use with pressor agents requires caution).
No products indexed under this heading.

Eprosartan Mesylate (Methylphenidate may decrease the effectiveness of antihypertensive drugs). Products include:
Teveten Tablets 1707
Teveten HCT Tablets 1710

Escitalopram Oxalate (Racemic methylphenidate may inhibit the metabolism of selective serotonin reuptake inhibitors). Products include:
Lexapro Oral Solution 1193
Lexapro Tablets 1193

Esmolol Hydrochloride (Methylphenidate may decrease the effectiveness of antihypertensive drugs). Products include:
Brevibloc Concentrate 766
Brevibloc Injection 766
Brevibloc Double Strength Injection 766
Brevibloc Premixed Injection 766
Brevibloc Double Strength Premixed Injection 766

Felodipine (Methylphenidate may decrease the effectiveness of antihypertensive drugs). Products include:
Plendil Extended-Release Tablets 651

Fluoxetine Hydrochloride (Racemic methylphenidate may inhibit the metabolism of selective serotonin reuptake inhibitors). Products include:
Prozac Pulvules and Liquid 1771
Symbyax Capsules 1788

Fluvoxamine Maleate (Racemic methylphenidate may inhibit the metabolism of selective serotonin reuptake inhibitors).
No products indexed under this heading.

Fosinopril Sodium (Methylphenidate may decrease the effectiveness of antihypertensive drugs).
No products indexed under this heading.

Fosphenytoin Sodium (Racemic methylphenidate may inhibit the metabolism of phenytoin).
No products indexed under this heading.

Furosemide (Methylphenidate may decrease the effectiveness of antihypertensive drugs). Products include:
Furosemide Tablets 2117

Guanabenz Acetate (Methylphenidate may decrease the effectiveness of antihypertensive drugs).
No products indexed under this heading.

Guanethidine Monosulfate (Methylphenidate may decrease the effectiveness of antihypertensive drugs).
No products indexed under this heading.

Hydralazine Hydrochloride (Methylphenidate may decrease the effectiveness of antihypertensive drugs). Products include:
BiDil Tablets 2161

Hydrochlorothiazide (Methylphenidate may decrease the effectiveness of antihypertensive drugs). Products include:
Aldoril Tablets 1884
Atacand HCT 637
Avalide Tablets 2889
Avalide Tablets 922
Benicar HCT Tablets 2852
Diovan HCT Tablets 2195
Dyazide Capsules 1389
Hyzaar 1964
Lotensin HCT Tablets 2235
Maxzide 2150
Micardis HCT Tablets 886
Moduretic Tablets 2003
Prinzide Tablets 2033
Teveten HCT Tablets 1710
Timolide Tablets 2056
Uniretic Tablets 3114
Vaseretic Tablets 2073
Zestoretic Tablets 701

Hydroflumethiazide (Methylphenidate may decrease the effectiveness of antihypertensive drugs).
No products indexed under this heading.

Imipramine Hydrochloride (Racemic methylphenidate may inhibit the metabolism of tricyclic antidepressants).
No products indexed under this heading.

Imipramine Pamoate (Racemic methylphenidate may inhibit the metabolism of tricyclic antidepressants).
No products indexed under this heading.

Indapamide (Methylphenidate may decrease the effectiveness of antihypertensive drugs). Products include:
Indapamide Tablets 2119

Irbesartan (Methylphenidate may decrease the effectiveness of antihypertensive drugs). Products include:
Avalide Tablets 922
Avalide Tablets 2889
Avapro Tablets 925
Avapro Tablets 2886

Isocarboxazid (Co-administration with MAO inhibitor may result in hypertensive crises; concurrent and/or sequential use is contraindicated).
No products indexed under this heading.

Isoproterenol Hydrochloride (Methylphenidate has potential to increase blood pressure; concurrent use with pressor agents requires caution).
No products indexed under this heading.

Isoproterenol Sulfate (Methylphenidate has potential to increase blood pressure; concurrent use with pressor agents requires caution).
No products indexed under this heading.

Isradipine (Methylphenidate may decrease the effectiveness of antihypertensive drugs). Products include:
DynaCirc CR Tablets 2726

Labetalol Hydrochloride (Methylphenidate may decrease the effectiveness of antihypertensive drugs).
No products indexed under this heading.

Lisinopril (Methylphenidate may decrease the effectiveness of antihypertensive drugs). Products include:
Prinivil Tablets 2029
Prinzide Tablets 2033
Zestoretic Tablets 701
Zestril Tablets 704

Losartan Potassium (Methylphenidate may decrease the effectiveness of antihypertensive drugs). Products include:
Cozaar Tablets 1913
Hyzaar 1964

Maprotiline Hydrochloride (Racemic methylphenidate may inhibit the metabolism of tricyclic antidepressants).
No products indexed under this heading.

Mecamylamine Hydrochloride (Methylphenidate may decrease the effectiveness of antihypertensive drugs). Products include:
Inversine Tablets 3286

Mephentermine Sulfate (Methylphenidate has potential to increase blood pressure; concurrent use with pressor agents requires caution).
No products indexed under this heading.

Metaraminol Bitartrate (Methylphenidate has potential to increase blood pressure; concurrent use with pressor agents requires caution). Products include:
Aramine Injection 1889

Methoxamine Hydrochloride (Methylphenidate has potential to increase blood pressure; concurrent use with pressor agents requires caution).
No products indexed under this heading.

Methyclothiazide (Methylphenidate may decrease the effectiveness of antihypertensive drugs).
No products indexed under this heading.

Methyldopa (Methylphenidate may decrease the effectiveness of antihypertensive drugs). Products include:
Aldoclor Tablets 1881
Aldoril Tablets 1884

Methyldopate Hydrochloride (Methylphenidate may decrease the effectiveness of antihypertensive drugs).
No products indexed under this heading.

Metolazone (Methylphenidate may decrease the effectiveness of antihypertensive drugs).
No products indexed under this heading.

Metoprolol Succinate (Methylphenidate may decrease the effectiveness of antihypertensive drugs). Products include:
Toprol-XL Tablets 660

Metoprolol Tartrate (Methylphenidate may decrease the effectiveness of antihypertensive drugs).
No products indexed under this heading.

Metyrosine (Methylphenidate may decrease the effectiveness of antihypertensive drugs). Products include:
Demser Capsules 1933

Mibefradil Dihydrochloride (Methylphenidate may decrease the effectiveness of antihypertensive drugs).
No products indexed under this heading.

Minoxidil (Methylphenidate may decrease the effectiveness of antihypertensive drugs). Products include:
Men's Rogaine Extra Strength Topical Solution, Ocean Rush Scent and Original Unscented .... ▣ 706
Women's Rogaine Topical Solution, Spring Bloom Scent and Original Unscented .... ▣ 707

Moclobemide (Co-administration with MAO inhibitor may result in hypertensive crises; concurrent and/or sequential use is contraindicated).
No products indexed under this heading.

Moexipril Hydrochloride (Methylphenidate may decrease the effectiveness of antihypertensive drugs). Products include:
Uniretic Tablets 3114
Univasc Tablets 3118

Nadolol (Methylphenidate may decrease the effectiveness of antihypertensive drugs). Products include:
Nadolol Tablets 2121

Nicardipine Hydrochloride (Methylphenidate may decrease the effectiveness of antihypertensive drugs). Products include:
Cardene I.V. 1129

Nifedipine (Methylphenidate may decrease the effectiveness of antihypertensive drugs). Products include:
Adalat CC Tablets 2978

Nisoldipine (Methylphenidate may decrease the effectiveness of antihypertensive drugs). Products include:
Sular Tablets 1163

Nitroglycerin (Methylphenidate may decrease the effectiveness of antihypertensive drugs). Products include:
Nitro-Dur Transdermal Infusion System 3060
Nitrolingual Pumpspray 1161

Norepinephrine Bitartrate (Methylphenidate has potential to increase blood pressure; concurrent use with pressor agents requires caution).
No products indexed under this heading.

Nortriptyline Hydrochloride (Racemic methylphenidate may inhibit the metabolism of tricyclic antidepressants).
No products indexed under this heading.

Pargyline Hydrochloride (Co-administration with MAO inhibitor may result in hypertensive crises; concurrent and/or sequential use is contraindicated).
No products indexed under this heading.

Paroxetine Hydrochloride (Racemic methylphenidate may inhibit the metabolism of selective serotonin reuptake inhibitors). Products include:
Paxil CR Controlled-Release Tablets 1509
Paxil 1501

Penbutolol Sulfate (Methylphenidate may decrease the effectiveness of antihypertensive drugs).
No products indexed under this heading.

Perindopril Erbumine (Methylphenidate may decrease the effectiveness of antihypertensive drugs). Products include:
Aceon Tablets (2 mg, 4 mg, 8 mg) 3191

Phenelzine Sulfate (Co-administration with MAO inhibitor may result in hypertensive crises; concurrent and/or sequential use is contraindicated).
No products indexed under this heading.

Phenobarbital (Racemic methylphenidate may inhibit the metabolism of phenobarbital).
No products indexed under this heading.

Phenoxybenzamine Hydrochloride (Methylphenidate may decrease the effectiveness of antihypertensive drugs). Products include:
Dibenzyline Capsules 3390

Phentolamine Mesylate (Methylphenidate may decrease the effectiveness of antihypertensive drugs).
No products indexed under this heading.

Phenylephrine Hydrochloride (Methylphenidate has potential to increase blood pressure; concurrent use with pressor agents requires caution). Products include:
Alacol DM Syrup 739
Hycomine Compound Tablets 1105
Preparation H Maximum Strength Cream .... ▣ 747
Preparation H Cooling Gel .... ▣ 747
Preparation H .... ▣ 747
Sudafed PE Tablets .... ▣ 711
Vicks Sinex Nasal Spray and Ultra Fine Mist for Sinus Relief 2677
Zicam Concentrated Cough Mist for Kids Plus D Cool Cherry .... ▣ 643
Zicam Concentrated Cough Mist Plus D Cool Cherry .... ▣ 642

Phenytoin (Racemic methylphenidate may inhibit the metabolism of phenytoin).
No products indexed under this heading.

Phenytoin Sodium (Racemic methylphenidate may inhibit the metabolism of phenytoin). Products include:
Phenytek Capsules 2153

Pindolol (Methylphenidate may decrease the effectiveness of antihypertensive drugs).
No products indexed under this heading.

Polythiazide (Methylphenidate may decrease the effectiveness of antihypertensive drugs).
No products indexed under this heading.

Prazosin Hydrochloride (Methylphenidate may decrease the effectiveness of antihypertensive drugs).
No products indexed under this heading.

Primidone (Racemic methylphenidate may inhibit the metabolism of primidone).
No products indexed under this heading.

Procarbazine Hydrochloride (Co-administration with MAO inhibitor may result in hypertensive crises; concurrent and/or sequential use is contraindicated). Products include:
Matulane Capsules 3188

Propranolol Hydrochloride (Methylphenidate may decrease the effectiveness of antihypertensive drugs). Products include:
Inderal LA Long-Acting Capsules 3421
InnoPran XL Capsules 2728

Protriptyline Hydrochloride (Racemic methylphenidate may inhibit the metabolism of tricyclic antidepressants). Products include:
Vivactil Tablets 2350

Quinapril Hydrochloride (Methylphenidate may decrease the effectiveness of antihypertensive drugs).
No products indexed under this heading.

Ramipril (Methylphenidate may decrease the effectiveness of antihypertensive drugs). Products include:
Altace Capsules 1673

Rauwolfia Serpentina (Methylphenidate may decrease the effectiveness of antihypertensive drugs).
No products indexed under this heading.

Rescinnamine (Methylphenidate may decrease the effectiveness of antihypertensive drugs).
No products indexed under this heading.

Reserpine (Methylphenidate may decrease the effectiveness of antihypertensive drugs).
No products indexed under this heading.

Selegiline Hydrochloride (Co-administration with MAO inhibitor may result in hypertensive crises; concurrent and/or sequential use is contraindicated). Products include:
Eldepryl Capsules 3209

Sertraline Hydrochloride (Racemic methylphenidate may inhibit the metabolism of selective serotonin reuptake inhibitors). Products include:
Zoloft 2581

Sodium Nitroprusside (Methylphenidate may decrease the effectiveness of antihypertensive drugs).
No products indexed under this heading.

Sotalol Hydrochloride (Methylphenidate may decrease the effectiveness of antihypertensive drugs).
No products indexed under this heading.

Spirapril Hydrochloride (Methylphenidate may decrease the effectiveness of antihypertensive drugs).
No products indexed under this heading.

Telmisartan (Methylphenidate may decrease the effectiveness of antihypertensive drugs). Products include:
Micardis Tablets 884
Micardis HCT Tablets 886

Terazosin Hydrochloride (Methylphenidate may decrease the effectiveness of antihypertensive drugs). Products include:
Hytrin Capsules 469

Timolol Maleate (Methylphenidate may decrease the effectiveness of antihypertensive drugs). Products include:
Blocadren Tablets 1891
Cosopt Sterile Ophthalmic Solution 1910
Timolide Tablets 2056
Timoptic in Ocudose 2061
Timoptic Sterile Ophthalmic Solution 2058
Timoptic-XE Sterile Ophthalmic Gel Forming Solution 2062

Torsemide (Methylphenidate may decrease the effectiveness of antihypertensive drugs).
No products indexed under this heading.

Trandolapril (Methylphenidate may decrease the effectiveness of antihypertensive drugs). Products include:
Mavik Tablets 482
Tarka Tablets 519

Tranylcypromine Sulfate (Co-administration with MAO inhibitor may result in hypertensive crises; concurrent and/or sequential use is contraindicated). Products include:
Parnate Tablets 1499

Trimethaphan Camsylate (Methylphenidate may decrease the effectiveness of antihypertensive drugs).
No products indexed under this heading.

Trimipramine Maleate (Racemic methylphenidate may inhibit the metabolism of tricyclic antidepressants). Products include:
Surmontil Capsules 2347

Valsartan (Methylphenidate may decrease the effectiveness of antihypertensive drugs). Products include:
Diovan HCT Tablets 2195
Diovan Tablets 2191

Verapamil Hydrochloride (Methylphenidate may decrease the effectiveness of antihypertensive drugs). Products include:
Covera-HS Tablets 3135
Tarka Tablets 519
Verelan PM Capsules 3120

Warfarin Sodium (Racemic methylphenidate may inhibit the metabolism of coumarin anticoagulants). Products include:
Coumadin for Injection 932
Coumadin Tablets 932

FOCALIN XR CAPSULES

(Dexmethylphenidate Hydrochloride) 2217
May interact with oral anticoagulants, histamine H_2-receptor antagonists, monoamine oxidase inhibitors, phenytoin, proton pump inhibitor, tricyclic antidepressants, vasopressors, and certain other agents. Compounds in these categories include:

Acebutolol Hydrochloride (Methylphenidate may decrease the effectiveness of antihypertensive drugs).
No products indexed under this heading.

Aluminum Carbonate (The effects of gastrointestinal pH alterations on the absorption of dexmethylphenidate from Focalin XR have not been studied. Since the modified release characteristics of Focalin XR are pH dependent, the co-administration of antacids or acid suppressants could alter the release of dexmethylphenidate).
No products indexed under this heading.

Aluminum Hydroxide (The effects of gastrointestinal pH alterations on the absorption of dexmethylphenidate from Focalin XR have not been studied. Since the modified release characteristics of Focalin XR are pH dependent, the co-administration of antacids or acid suppressants could alter the release of dexmethylphenidate). Products include:
Gaviscon Regular Strength Liquid 620
Gaviscon Regular Strength Tablets 619
Gaviscon Extra Strength Liquid 620
Gaviscon Extra Strength Tablets 619
Maalox Max Maximum Strength Antacid/Anti-Gas Liquid 2165
Maalox Regular Strength Antacid/Antigas Liquid 2164

Amitriptyline Hydrochloride (Racemic methylphenidate may inhibit the metabolism of tricyclic antidepressants).
No products indexed under this heading.

Amlodipine Besylate (Methylphenidate may decrease the effectiveness of antihypertensive drugs). Products include:
Caduet Tablets 2507
Lotrel Capsules 2238
Norvasc Tablets 2529

Amoxapine (Racemic methylphenidate may inhibit the metabolism of tricyclic antidepressants).
No products indexed under this heading.

Anisindione (Racemic methylphenidate may inhibit the metabolism of coumarin anticoagulants). Products include:
Miradon Tablets 3056

Atenolol (Methylphenidate may decrease the effectiveness of antihypertensive drugs). Products include:
Tenormin I.V. Injection 698
Tenormin Tablets 695

Benazepril Hydrochloride (Methylphenidate may decrease the effectiveness of antihypertensive drugs). Products include:
Lotensin Tablets 2232
Lotensin HCT Tablets 2235
Lotrel Capsules 2238

Bendroflumethiazide (Methylphenidate may decrease the effectiveness of antihypertensive drugs).
No products indexed under this heading.

Betaxolol Hydrochloride (Methylphenidate may decrease the effectiveness of antihypertensive drugs). Products include:
Betoptic S Ophthalmic Suspension 554

Bisoprolol Fumarate (Methylphenidate may decrease the effectiveness of antihypertensive drugs).
No products indexed under this heading.

Candesartan Cilexetil (Methylphenidate may decrease the effectiveness of antihypertensive drugs). Products include:
Atacand Tablets 634
Atacand HCT 637

Captopril (Methylphenidate may decrease the effectiveness of antihypertensive drugs). Products include:
Captopril Tablets 2114

Carteolol Hydrochloride (Methylphenidate may decrease the effectiveness of antihypertensive drugs). Products include:
Carteolol Hydrochloride Ophthalmic Solution USP, 1% .... ⊙246

Chlorothiazide (Methylphenidate may decrease the effectiveness of antihypertensive drugs). Products include:
Aldoclor Tablets 1881
Diuril Oral 1936

Chlorothiazide Sodium (Methylphenidate may decrease the effectiveness of antihypertensive drugs). Products include:
Diuril Sodium Intravenous 1934

Chlorthalidone (Methylphenidate may decrease the effectiveness of antihypertensive drugs). Products include:
Clorpres Tablets 2139

Cimetidine (The effects of gastrointestinal pH alterations on the absorption of dexmethylphenidate from Focalin XR have not been studied. Since the modified release characteristics of Focalin XR are pH dependent, the co-administration of antacids or acid suppressants could alter the release of dexmethylphenidate). Products include:
Tagamet HB 200 Tablets 637
Tagamet Tablets 1547

Cimetidine Hydrochloride (The effects of gastrointestinal pH alterations on the absorption of dexmethylphenidate from Focalin XR have not been studied. Since the modified release characteristics of Focalin XR are pH dependent, the co-administration of antacids or acid suppressants could alter the release of dexmethylphenidate).
No products indexed under this heading.

Clomipramine Hydrochloride (Racemic methylphenidate may inhibit the metabolism of tricyclic antidepressants).
No products indexed under this heading.

Clonidine (Co-administration has resulted in serious adverse events). Products include:
Catapres-TTS 875

Clonidine Hydrochloride (Co-administration has resulted in serious adverse events). Products include:
Catapres Tablets 874
Clorpres Tablets 2139

Deserpidine (Methylphenidate may decrease the effectiveness of antihypertensive drugs).
No products indexed under this heading.

Desipramine Hydrochloride (Racemic methylphenidate may inhibit the metabolism of tricyclic antidepressants).
No products indexed under this heading.

Diazoxide (Methylphenidate may decrease the effectiveness of antihypertensive drugs). Products include:
Hyperstat I.V. Injection 3031

Dicumarol (Racemic methylphenidate may inhibit the metabolism of coumarin anticoagulants).
No products indexed under this heading.

Diltiazem Hydrochloride (Methylphenidate may decrease the effectiveness of antihypertensive drugs). Products include:
Cardizem LA Extended Release Tablets 1699
Tiazac Capsules 1204

Dobutamine (Methylphenidate has potential to increase blood pressure; concurrent use with pressor agents requires caution).
No products indexed under this heading.

Dobutamine Hydrochloride (Methylphenidate has potential to increase blood pressure; concurrent use with pressor agents requires caution).
No products indexed under this heading.

Dopamine Hydrochloride (Methylphenidate has potential to increase blood pressure; concurrent use with pressor agents requires caution).
No products indexed under this heading.

Doxazosin Mesylate (Methylphenidate may decrease the effectiveness of antihypertensive drugs).
No products indexed under this heading.

Doxepin Hydrochloride (Racemic methylphenidate may inhibit the metabolism of tricyclic antidepressants).
No products indexed under this heading.

Enalapril Maleate (Methylphenidate may decrease the effectiveness of antihypertensive drugs). Products include:
Vaseretic Tablets 2073
Vasotec I.V. Injection 2076

Enalaprilat (Methylphenidate may decrease the effectiveness of antihypertensive drugs).
No products indexed under this heading.

Ephedrine Sulfate (Methylphenidate has potential to increase blood pressure; concurrent use with pressor agents requires caution).
No products indexed under this heading.

Epinephrine Bitartrate (Methylphenidate has potential to increase blood pressure; concurrent use with pressor agents requires caution).
No products indexed under this heading.

Epinephrine Hydrochloride (Methylphenidate has potential to increase blood pressure; concurrent use with pressor agents requires caution).
No products indexed under this heading.

Eprosartan Mesylate (Methylphenidate may decrease the effectiveness of antihypertensive drugs). Products include:
Teveten Tablets 1707
Teveten HCT Tablets 1710

Esmolol Hydrochloride (Methylphenidate may decrease the effectiveness of antihypertensive drugs). Products include:
Brevibloc Concentrate 766
Brevibloc Injection 766
Brevibloc Double Strength Injection 766
Brevibloc Premixed Injection 766
Brevibloc Double Strength Premixed Injection 766

Esomeprazole Magnesium (The effects of gastrointestinal pH alterations on the absorption of dexmethylphenidate from Focalin XR have not been studied. Since the modified release characteristics of Focalin XR are pH dependent, the co-administration of antacids or acid suppressants could alter the release of dexmethylphenidate). Products include:
Nexium Delayed-Release Capsules 645

Famotidine (The effects of gastrointestinal pH alterations on the absorption of dexmethylphenidate from Focalin XR have not been studied. Since the modified release characteristics of Focalin XR are pH dependent, the co-administration of antacids or acid suppressants could alter the release of dexmethylphenidate). Products include:
Pepcid AC Chewable Tablets 1672
Pepcid AC Gelcaps 1672
Pepcid AC Tablets 1672
Maximum Strength Pepcid AC Tablets 1672
Pepcid Complete Chewable Tablets 1672
Pepcid Injection 2017
Pepcid 2014

Felodipine (Methylphenidate may decrease the effectiveness of antihypertensive drugs). Products include:
Plendil Extended-Release Tablets 651

Fosinopril Sodium (Methylphenidate may decrease the effectiveness of antihypertensive drugs).
No products indexed under this heading.

Fosphenytoin Sodium (Racemic methylphenidate may inhibit the metabolism of phenytoin).
No products indexed under this heading.

Furosemide (Methylphenidate may decrease the effectiveness of antihypertensive drugs). Products include:
Furosemide Tablets 2117

Guanabenz Acetate (Methylphenidate may decrease the effectiveness of antihypertensive drugs).
No products indexed under this heading.

Guanethidine Monosulfate (Methylphenidate may decrease the effectiveness of antihypertensive drugs).
No products indexed under this heading.

Hydralazine Hydrochloride (Methylphenidate may decrease the effectiveness of antihypertensive drugs). Products include:
BiDil Tablets 2161

Hydrochlorothiazide (Methylphenidate may decrease the effectiveness of antihypertensive drugs). Products include:
Aldoril Tablets 1884
Atacand HCT 637
Avalide Tablets 2889
Avalide Tablets 922
Benicar HCT Tablets 2852
Diovan HCT Tablets 2195
Dyazide Capsules 1389
Hyzaar 1964
Lotensin HCT Tablets 2235
Maxzide 2150
Micardis HCT Tablets 886
Moduretic Tablets 2003
Prinzide Tablets 2033
Teveten HCT Tablets 1710
Timolide Tablets 2056
Uniretic Tablets 3114
Vaseretic Tablets 2073
Zestoretic Tablets 701

Hydroflumethiazide (Methylphenidate may decrease the effectiveness of antihypertensive drugs).
No products indexed under this heading.

Imipramine Hydrochloride (Racemic methylphenidate may inhibit the metabolism of tricyclic antidepressants).
No products indexed under this heading.

Imipramine Pamoate (Racemic methylphenidate may inhibit the metabolism of tricyclic antidepressants).
No products indexed under this heading.

Indapamide (Methylphenidate may decrease the effectiveness of antihypertensive drugs). Products include:
Indapamide Tablets 2119

Irbesartan (Methylphenidate may decrease the effectiveness of antihypertensive drugs). Products include:
Avalide Tablets 922
Avalide Tablets 2889
Avapro Tablets 925
Avapro Tablets 2886

Isocarboxazid (Co-administration with MAO inhibitor may result in hypertensive crises; concurrent and/or sequential use is contraindicated).
No products indexed under this heading.

Isoproterenol Hydrochloride (Methylphenidate has potential to increase blood pressure; concurrent use with pressor agents requires caution).
No products indexed under this heading.

Isoproterenol Sulfate (Methylphenidate has potential to increase blood pressure; concurrent use with pressor agents requires caution).
No products indexed under this heading.

Isradipine (Methylphenidate may decrease the effectiveness of antihypertensive drugs). Products include:
DynaCirc CR Tablets 2726

Labetalol Hydrochloride (Methylphenidate may decrease the effectiveness of antihypertensive drugs).
No products indexed under this heading.

Lansoprazole (The effects of gastrointestinal pH alterations on the absorption of dexmethylphenidate from Focalin XR have not been studied. Since the modified release characteristics of Focalin XR are pH dependent, the co-administration of antacids or acid suppressants could alter the release of dexmethylphenidate). Products include:
Prevacid Delayed-Release Capsules 3268
Prevacid for Delayed-Release Oral Suspension 3268
Prevacid I.V. for Injection 3274
Prevacid NapraPAC 3277
Prevacid SoluTab Delayed-Release Orally Disintegrating Tablets 3268
PREVPAC 3281

Lisinopril (Methylphenidate may decrease the effectiveness of antihypertensive drugs). Products include:
Prinivil Tablets 2029
Prinzide Tablets 2033
Zestoretic Tablets 701
Zestril Tablets 704

Losartan Potassium (Methylphenidate may decrease the effectiveness of antihypertensive drugs). Products include:
Cozaar Tablets 1913
Hyzaar 1964

Magaldrate (The effects of gastrointestinal pH alterations on the absorption of dexmethylphenidate from Focalin XR have not been studied. Since the modified release characteristics of Focalin XR are pH dependent, the co-administration of antacids or acid suppressants could alter the release of dexmethylphenidate).
No products indexed under this heading.

Magnesium Hydroxide (The effects of gastrointestinal pH alterations on the absorption of dexmethylphenidate from Focalin XR have not been studied. Since the modified release characteristics of Focalin XR are pH dependent, the co-administration of antacids or acid suppressants could alter the release of dexmethylphenidate). Products include:
Maalox Max Maximum Strength Antacid/Anti-Gas Liquid 2165
Maalox Regular Strength Antacid/Antigas Liquid 2164
Pepcid Complete Chewable Tablets 1672
Rolaids Tablets .... ■ 707
Extra Strength Rolaids Tablets .... ■ 707
Rolaids Multi-Symptom Antacid & Antigas Tablets .... ■ 708

Magnesium Oxide (The effects of gastrointestinal pH alterations on the absorption of dexmethylphenidate from Focalin XR have not been studied. Since the modified release characteristics of Focalin XR are pH dependent, the co-administration of antacids or acid suppressants could alter the release of dexmethylphenidate). Products include:
Beelith Tablets 784
PremCal Light, Regular, and Extra Strength Tablets .... ■ 762

Maprotiline Hydrochloride (Racemic methylphenidate may inhibit the metabolism of tricyclic antidepressants).
No products indexed under this heading.

Mecamylamine Hydrochloride (Methylphenidate may decrease the effectiveness of antihypertensive drugs). Products include:
Inversine Tablets 3286

Mephentermine Sulfate (Methylphenidate has potential to increase blood pressure; concurrent use with pressor agents requires caution).
No products indexed under this heading.

Metaraminol Bitartrate (Methylphenidate has potential to increase blood pressure; concurrent use with pressor agents requires caution). Products include:
Aramine Injection 1889

Methoxamine Hydrochloride (Methylphenidate has potential to increase blood pressure; concurrent use with pressor agents requires caution).
No products indexed under this heading.

Methyclothiazide (Methylphenidate may decrease the effectiveness of antihypertensive drugs).
No products indexed under this heading.

Methyldopa (Methylphenidate may decrease the effectiveness of antihypertensive drugs). Products include:
Aldoclor Tablets 1881
Aldoril Tablets 1884

Methyldopate Hydrochloride (Methylphenidate may decrease the effectiveness of antihypertensive drugs).
No products indexed under this heading.

Metolazone (Methylphenidate may decrease the effectiveness of antihypertensive drugs).
No products indexed under this heading.

Metoprolol Succinate (Methylphenidate may decrease the effectiveness of antihypertensive drugs). Products include:
Toprol-XL Tablets 660

Metoprolol Tartrate (Methylphenidate may decrease the effectiveness of antihypertensive drugs).
No products indexed under this heading.

Metyrosine (Methylphenidate may decrease the effectiveness of antihypertensive drugs). Products include:
Demser Capsules 1933

Mibefradil Dihydrochloride (Methylphenidate may decrease the effectiveness of antihypertensive drugs).
No products indexed under this heading.

Minoxidil (Methylphenidate may decrease the effectiveness of antihypertensive drugs). Products include:
Men's Rogaine Extra Strength Topical Solution, Ocean Rush Scent and Original Unscented .... ■ 706
Women's Rogaine Topical Solution, Spring Bloom Scent and Original Unscented .... ■ 707

Moclobemide (Co-administration with MAO inhibitor may result in hypertensive crises; concurrent and/or sequential use is contraindicated).
No products indexed under this heading.

Moexipril Hydrochloride (Methylphenidate may decrease the effectiveness of antihypertensive drugs). Products include:
Uniretic Tablets 3114
Univasc Tablets 3118

Nadolol (Methylphenidate may decrease the effectiveness of antihypertensive drugs). Products include:
Nadolol Tablets 2121

Nicardipine Hydrochloride (Methylphenidate may decrease the effectiveness of antihypertensive drugs). Products include:
Cardene I.V. 1129

Nifedipine (Methylphenidate may decrease the effectiveness of antihypertensive drugs). Products include:
Adalat CC Tablets 2978

Nisoldipine (Methylphenidate may decrease the effectiveness of antihypertensive drugs). Products include:
Sular Tablets 1163

Nitroglycerin (Methylphenidate may decrease the effectiveness of antihypertensive drugs). Products include:
- Nitro-Dur Transdermal Infusion System 3060
- Nitrolingual Pumpspray 1161

Nizatidine (The effects of gastrointestinal pH alterations on the absorption of dexmethylphenidate from Focalin XR have not been studied. Since the modified release characteristics of Focalin XR are pH dependent, the co-administration of antacids or acid suppressants could alter the release of dexmethylphenidate). Products include:
- Axid Oral Solution 913

Norepinephrine Bitartrate (Methylphenidate has potential to increase blood pressure; concurrent use with pressor agents requires caution).
No products indexed under this heading.

Nortriptyline Hydrochloride (Racemic methylphenidate may inhibit the metabolism of tricyclic antidepressants).
No products indexed under this heading.

Omeprazole (The effects of gastrointestinal pH alterations on the absorption of dexmethylphenidate from Focalin XR have not been studied. Since the modified release characteristics of Focalin XR are pH dependent, the co-administration of antacids or acid suppressants could alter the release of dexmethylphenidate). Products include:
- Zegerid Powder for Oral Solution 2972

Pantoprazole Sodium (The effects of gastrointestinal pH alterations on the absorption of dexmethylphenidate from Focalin XR have not been studied. Since the modified release characteristics of Focalin XR are pH dependent, the co-administration of antacids or acid suppressants could alter the release of dexmethylphenidate). Products include:
- Protonix I.V. 3468
- Protonix Tablets 3465

Pargyline Hydrochloride (Co-administration with MAO inhibitor may result in hypertensive crises; concurrent and/or sequential use is contraindicated).
No products indexed under this heading.

Penbutolol Sulfate (Methylphenidate may decrease the effectiveness of antihypertensive drugs).
No products indexed under this heading.

Perindopril Erbumine (Methylphenidate may decrease the effectiveness of antihypertensive drugs). Products include:
- Aceon Tablets (2 mg, 4 mg, 8 mg) 3191

Phenelzine Sulfate (Co-administration with MAO inhibitor may result in hypertensive crises; concurrent and/or sequential use is contraindicated).
No products indexed under this heading.

Phenobarbital (Racemic methylphenidate may inhibit the metabolism of phenobarbital).
No products indexed under this heading.

Phenoxybenzamine Hydrochloride (Methylphenidate may decrease the effectiveness of antihypertensive drugs). Products include:
- Dibenzyline Capsules 3390

Phentolamine Mesylate (Methylphenidate may decrease the effectiveness of antihypertensive drugs).
No products indexed under this heading.

Phenylephrine Hydrochloride (Methylphenidate has potential to increase blood pressure; concurrent use with pressor agents requires caution). Products include:
- Alacol DM Syrup 739
- Hycomine Compound Tablets 1105
- Preparation H Maximum Strength Cream 747
- Preparation H Cooling Gel 747
- Preparation H 747
- Sudafed PE Tablets 711
- Vicks Sinex Nasal Spray and Ultra Fine Mist for Sinus Relief 2677
- Zicam Concentrated Cough Mist for Kids Plus D Cool Cherry 643
- Zicam Concentrated Cough Mist Plus D Cool Cherry 642

Phenytoin (Racemic methylphenidate may inhibit the metabolism of phenytoin).
No products indexed under this heading.

Phenytoin Sodium (Racemic methylphenidate may inhibit the metabolism of phenytoin). Products include:
- Phenytek Capsules 2153

Pindolol (Methylphenidate may decrease the effectiveness of antihypertensive drugs).
No products indexed under this heading.

Polythiazide (Methylphenidate may decrease the effectiveness of antihypertensive drugs).
No products indexed under this heading.

Prazosin Hydrochloride (Methylphenidate may decrease the effectiveness of antihypertensive drugs).
No products indexed under this heading.

Primidone (Racemic methylphenidate may inhibit the metabolism of primidone).
No products indexed under this heading.

Procarbazine Hydrochloride (Co-administration with MAO inhibitor may result in hypertensive crises; concurrent and/or sequential use is contraindicated). Products include:
- Matulane Capsules 3188

Propranolol Hydrochloride (Methylphenidate may decrease the effectiveness of antihypertensive drugs). Products include:
- Inderal LA Long-Acting Capsules 3421
- InnoPran XL Capsules 2728

Protriptyline Hydrochloride (Racemic methylphenidate may inhibit the metabolism of tricyclic antidepressants). Products include:
- Vivactil Tablets 2350

Quinapril Hydrochloride (Methylphenidate may decrease the effectiveness of antihypertensive drugs).
No products indexed under this heading.

Rabeprazole Sodium (The effects of gastrointestinal pH alterations on the absorption of dexmethylphenidate from Focalin XR have not been studied. Since the modified release characteristics of Focalin XR are pH dependent, the co-administration of antacids or acid suppressants could alter the release of dexmethylphenidate). Products include:
- Aciphex Tablets 1081

Ramipril (Methylphenidate may decrease the effectiveness of antihypertensive drugs). Products include:
- Altace Capsules 1673

Ranitidine Bismuth Citrate (The effects of gastrointestinal pH alterations on the absorption of dexmethylphenidate from Focalin XR have not been studied. Since the modified release characteristics of Focalin XR are pH dependent, the co-administration of antacids or acid suppressants could alter the release of dexmethylphenidate).
No products indexed under this heading.

Ranitidine Hydrochloride (The effects of gastrointestinal pH alterations on the absorption of dexmethylphenidate from Focalin XR have not been studied. Since the modified release characteristics of Focalin XR are pH dependent, the co-administration of antacids or acid suppressants could alter the release of dexmethylphenidate). Products include:
- Zantac 1597
- Zantac Injection 1593
- Zantac 75 Tablets 715
- Zantac 150 Maximum Strength Tablets 715
- Zantac Injection Pharmacy Bulk Package 1595

Rauwolfia Serpentina (Methylphenidate may decrease the effectiveness of antihypertensive drugs).
No products indexed under this heading.

Rescinnamine (Methylphenidate may decrease the effectiveness of antihypertensive drugs).
No products indexed under this heading.

Reserpine (Methylphenidate may decrease the effectiveness of antihypertensive drugs).
No products indexed under this heading.

Selegiline Hydrochloride (Co-administration with MAO inhibitor may result in hypertensive crises; concurrent and/or sequential use is contraindicated). Products include:
- Eldepryl Capsules 3209

Sodium Bicarbonate (The effects of gastrointestinal pH alterations on the absorption of dexmethylphenidate from Focalin XR have not been studied. Since the modified release characteristics of Focalin XR are pH dependent, the co-administration of antacids or acid suppressants could alter the release of dexmethylphenidate). Products include:
- Ceo-Two Evacuant Suppository 607
- Colyte with Flavor Packs for Oral Solution 3102
- HalfLytely and Bisacodyl Tablets Bowel Prep Kit with Flavors Packs 915
- TriLyte with Flavor Packs for Oral Solution 3114

Sodium Nitroprusside (Methylphenidate may decrease the effectiveness of antihypertensive drugs).
No products indexed under this heading.

Sotalol Hydrochloride (Methylphenidate may decrease the effectiveness of antihypertensive drugs).
No products indexed under this heading.

Spirapril Hydrochloride (Methylphenidate may decrease the effectiveness of antihypertensive drugs).
No products indexed under this heading.

Telmisartan (Methylphenidate may decrease the effectiveness of antihypertensive drugs). Products include:
- Micardis Tablets 884
- Micardis HCT Tablets 886

Terazosin Hydrochloride (Methylphenidate may decrease the effectiveness of antihypertensive drugs). Products include:
- Hytrin Capsules 469

Timolol Maleate (Methylphenidate may decrease the effectiveness of antihypertensive drugs). Products include:
- Blocadren Tablets 1891
- Cosopt Sterile Ophthalmic Solution 1910
- Timolide Tablets 2056
- Timoptic in Ocudose 2061
- Timoptic Sterile Ophthalmic Solution 2058
- Timoptic-XE Sterile Ophthalmic Gel Forming Solution 2062

Torsemide (Methylphenidate may decrease the effectiveness of antihypertensive drugs).
No products indexed under this heading.

Trandolapril (Methylphenidate may decrease the effectiveness of antihypertensive drugs). Products include:
- Mavik Tablets 482
- Tarka Tablets 519

Tranylcypromine Sulfate (Co-administration with MAO inhibitor may result in hypertensive crises; concurrent and/or sequential use is contraindicated). Products include:
- Parnate Tablets 1499

Trimethaphan Camsylate (Methylphenidate may decrease the effectiveness of antihypertensive drugs).
No products indexed under this heading.

Trimipramine Maleate (Racemic methylphenidate may inhibit the metabolism of tricyclic antidepressants). Products include:
- Surmontil Capsules 2347

Valsartan (Methylphenidate may decrease the effectiveness of antihypertensive drugs). Products include:
- Diovan HCT Tablets 2195
- Diovan Tablets 2191

Verapamil Hydrochloride (Methylphenidate may decrease the effectiveness of antihypertensive drugs). Products include:
- Covera-HS Tablets 3135
- Tarka Tablets 519
- Verelan PM Capsules 3120

Warfarin Sodium (Racemic methylphenidate may inhibit the metabolism of coumarin anticoagulants). Products include:
- Coumadin for Injection 932
- Coumadin Tablets 932

FOLLISTIM AQ CARTRIDGE

(Follitropin Beta) 2354

None cited in PDR database.

FORADIL AEROLIZER
(Formoterol Fumarate) 3024
May interact with beta blockers, diuretics, glucocorticoids, monoamine oxidase inhibitors, and potassium-depleting diuretics. Compounds in these categories include:

Acebutolol Hydrochloride (Co-administration with beta-blockers may inhibit the effect of each other. Beta-blockers not only block the therapeutic effect of beta-agonists, such as formoterol, but may produce severe bronchospasm in patients with asthma).
No products indexed under this heading.

Albuterol (Co-administration with additional adrenergic drugs may potentiate the sympathetic effects of formoterol). Products include:
Proventil Inhalation Aerosol 3067

Albuterol Sulfate (Co-administration with additional adrenergic drugs may potentiate the sympathetic effects of formoterol). Products include:
AccuNeb Inhalation Solution 1055
Combivent Inhalation Aerosol 878
DuoNeb Inhalation Solution 1058
Proventil Inhalation Solution 0.083% 3069
Proventil HFA Inhalation Aerosol 3071
Ventolin HFA Inhalation Aerosol 1576
VoSpire Extended-Release Tablets ... 2352

Amiloride Hydrochloride (Concomitant treatment with diuretics may potentiate any hypokalemic effect of adrenergic agonists). Products include:
Midamor Tablets 2000
Moduretic Tablets 2003

Aminophylline (Co-administration with xanthine derivatives may potentiate hypokalemic effect of adrenergic agonists).
No products indexed under this heading.

Amiodarone Hydrochloride (Co-administration with drugs known to prolong the QTc interval may lead to an increased risk of ventricular arrhythmias; co-administer with extreme caution). Products include:
Pacerone Tablets 3337

Amitriptyline Hydrochloride (Concurrent and/or sequential administration with tricyclic antidepressants may potentiate the action of adrenergic agonists on the cardiovascular system; co-administer with extreme caution).
No products indexed under this heading.

Amoxapine (Concurrent and/or sequential administration with tricyclic antidepressants may potentiate the action of adrenergic agonists on the cardiovascular system; co-administer with extreme caution).
No products indexed under this heading.

Astemizole (Co-administration with drugs known to prolong the QTc interval may lead to an increased risk of ventricular arrhythmias; co-administer with extreme caution).
No products indexed under this heading.

Atenolol (Co-administration with beta-blockers may inhibit the effect of each other. Beta-blockers not only block the therapeutic effect of beta-agonists, such as formoterol, but may produce severe bronchospasm in patients with asthma). Products include:
Tenormin I.V. Injection 698
Tenormin Tablets 695

Bendroflumethiazide (The ECG changes and/or hypokalemia that may result from the administration of non-potassium sparing diuretics can be acutely worsened by beta-agonists, especially when the recommended dose of beta-agonist is exceeded).
No products indexed under this heading.

Betamethasone Acetate (Co-administration with glucocorticosteroids may potentiate hypokalemic effect of adrenergic agonists).
No products indexed under this heading.

Betamethasone Sodium Phosphate (Co-administration with glucocorticosteroids may potentiate hypokalemic effect of adrenergic agonists).
No products indexed under this heading.

Betaxolol Hydrochloride (Co-administration with beta-blockers may inhibit the effect of each other. Beta-blockers not only block the therapeutic effect of beta-agonists, such as formoterol, but may produce severe bronchospasm in patients with asthma). Products include:
Betoptic S Ophthalmic Suspension.................................. 554

Bisoprolol Fumarate (Co-administration with beta-blockers may inhibit the effect of each other. Beta-blockers not only block the therapeutic effect of beta-agonists, such as formoterol, but may produce severe bronchospasm in patients with asthma).
No products indexed under this heading.

Bretylium Tosylate (Co-administration with drugs known to prolong the QTc interval may lead to an increased risk of ventricular arrhythmias; co-administer with extreme caution).
No products indexed under this heading.

Bumetanide (The ECG changes and/or hypokalemia that may result from the administration of non-potassium sparing diuretics can be acutely worsened by beta-agonists, especially when the recommended dose of beta-agonist is exceeded).
No products indexed under this heading.

Carteolol Hydrochloride (Co-administration with beta-blockers may inhibit the effect of each other. Beta-blockers not only block the therapeutic effect of beta-agonists, such as formoterol, but may produce severe bronchospasm in patients with asthma). Products include:
Carteolol Hydrochloride Ophthalmic Solution USP, 1%....... ⊙246

Chlorothiazide (The ECG changes and/or hypokalemia that may result from the administration of non-potassium sparing diuretics can be acutely worsened by beta-agonists, especially when the recommended dose of beta-agonist is exceeded). Products include:
Aldoclor Tablets 1881
Diuril Oral 1936

Chlorothiazide Sodium (The ECG changes and/or hypokalemia that may result from the administration of non-potassium sparing diuretics can be acutely worsened by beta-agonists, especially when the recommended dose of beta-agonist is exceeded). Products include:
Diuril Sodium Intravenous 1934

Chlorpromazine (Co-administration with drugs known to prolong the QTc interval may lead to an increased risk of ventricular arrhythmias; co-administer with extreme caution).
No products indexed under this heading.

Chlorpromazine Hydrochloride (Co-administration with drugs known to prolong the QTc interval may lead to an increased risk of ventricular arrhythmias; co-administer with extreme caution).
No products indexed under this heading.

Chlorthalidone (Concomitant treatment with diuretics may potentiate any hypokalemic effect of adrenergic agonists). Products include:
Clorpres Tablets 2139

Clomipramine Hydrochloride (Concurrent and/or sequential administration with tricyclic antidepressants may potentiate the action of adrenergic agonists on the cardiovascular system; co-administer with extreme caution).
No products indexed under this heading.

Cortisone Acetate (Co-administration with glucocorticosteroids may potentiate hypokalemic effect of adrenergic agonists).
No products indexed under this heading.

Desipramine Hydrochloride (Concurrent and/or sequential administration with tricyclic antidepressants may potentiate the action of adrenergic agonists on the cardiovascular system; co-administer with extreme caution).
No products indexed under this heading.

Dexamethasone (Co-administration with glucocorticosteroids may potentiate hypokalemic effect of adrenergic agonists). Products include:
Ciprodex Otic Suspension 555
Decadron Tablets 1929
TobraDex Ophthalmic Ointment 558
TobraDex Ophthalmic Suspension ... 558

Dexamethasone Acetate (Co-administration with glucocorticosteroids may potentiate hypokalemic effect of adrenergic agonists).
No products indexed under this heading.

Dexamethasone Sodium Phosphate (Co-administration with glucocorticosteroids may potentiate hypokalemic effect of adrenergic agonists). Products include:
Decadron Phosphate Injection 1931

Disopyramide Phosphate (Co-administration with drugs known to prolong the QTc interval may lead to an increased risk of ventricular arrhythmias; co-administer with extreme caution).
No products indexed under this heading.

Dobutamine Hydrochloride (Co-administration with additional adrenergic drugs may potentiate the sympathetic effects of formoterol).
No products indexed under this heading.

Dofetilide (Co-administration with drugs known to prolong the QTc interval may lead to an increased risk of ventricular arrhythmias; co-administer with extreme caution).
No products indexed under this heading.

Dopamine Hydrochloride (Co-administration with additional adrenergic drugs may potentiate the sympathetic effects of formoterol).
No products indexed under this heading.

Doxepin Hydrochloride (Concurrent and/or sequential administration with tricyclic antidepressants may potentiate the action of adrenergic agonists on the cardiovascular system; co-administer with extreme caution).
No products indexed under this heading.

Dyphylline (Co-administration with xanthine derivatives may potentiate hypokalemic effect of adrenergic agonists).
No products indexed under this heading.

Ephedrine Hydrochloride (Co-administration with additional adrenergic drugs may potentiate the sympathetic effects of formoterol). Products include:
Primatene Tablets .... ▣749

Ephedrine Sulfate (Co-administration with additional adrenergic drugs may potentiate the sympathetic effects of formoterol).
No products indexed under this heading.

Ephedrine Tannate (Co-administration with additional adrenergic drugs may potentiate the sympathetic effects of formoterol).
No products indexed under this heading.

Epinephrine (Co-administration with additional adrenergic drugs may potentiate the sympathetic effects of formoterol). Products include:
EpiPen 1061
Primatene Mist .... ▣749

Epinephrine Bitartrate (Co-administration with additional adrenergic drugs may potentiate the sympathetic effects of formoterol).
No products indexed under this heading.

Epinephrine Hydrochloride (Co-administration with additional adrenergic drugs may potentiate the sympathetic effects of formoterol).
No products indexed under this heading.

Esmolol Hydrochloride (Co-administration with beta-blockers may inhibit the effect of each other. Beta-blockers not only block the therapeutic effect of beta-agonists, such as formoterol, but may produce severe bronchospasm in patients with asthma). Products include:
Brevibloc Concentrate 766
Brevibloc Injection 766
Brevibloc Double Strength Injection.. 766
Brevibloc Premixed Injection 766
Brevibloc Double Strength Premixed Injection 766

Ethacrynic Acid (The ECG changes and/or hypokalemia that may result from the administration of non-potassium sparing diuretics can be acutely worsened by beta-agonists,

especially when the recommended dose of beta-agonist is exceeded). Products include:

Edecrin Tablets 1941

Flecainide Acetate (Co-administration with drugs known to prolong the QTc interval may lead to an increased risk of ventricular arrhythmias; co-administer with extreme caution). Products include:

Tambocor Tablets 1824

Fludrocortisone Acetate (Co-administration with glucocorticosteroids may potentiate hypokalemic effect of adrenergic agonists).

No products indexed under this heading.

Fluphenazine Decanoate (Co-administration with drugs known to prolong the QTc interval may lead to an increased risk of ventricular arrhythmias; co-administer with extreme caution).

No products indexed under this heading.

Fluphenazine Enanthate (Co-administration with drugs known to prolong the QTc interval may lead to an increased risk of ventricular arrhythmias; co-administer with extreme caution).

No products indexed under this heading.

Fluphenazine Hydrochloride (Co-administration with drugs known to prolong the QTc interval may lead to an increased risk of ventricular arrhythmias; co-administer with extreme caution).

No products indexed under this heading.

Furosemide (The ECG changes and/or hypokalemia that may result from the administration of non-potassium sparing diuretics can be acutely worsened by beta-agonists, especially when the recommended dose of beta-agonist is exceeded). Products include:

Furosemide Tablets 2117

Hydrochlorothiazide (The ECG changes and/or hypokalemia that may result from the administration of non-potassium sparing diuretics can be acutely worsened by beta-agonists, especially when the recommended dose of beta-agonist is exceeded). Products include:

Aldoril Tablets 1884
Atacand HCT 637
Avalide Tablets 2889
Avalide Tablets 922
Benicar HCT Tablets 2852
Diovan HCT Tablets 2195
Dyazide Capsules 1389
Hyzaar 1964
Lotensin HCT Tablets 2235
Maxzide 2150
Micardis HCT Tablets 886
Moduretic Tablets 2003
Prinzide Tablets 2033
Teveten HCT Tablets 1710
Timolide Tablets 2056
Uniretic Tablets 3114
Vaseretic Tablets 2073
Zestoretic Tablets 701

Hydrocortisone (Co-administration with glucocorticosteroids may potentiate hypokalemic effect of adrenergic agonists). Products include:

Cortizone•5 Ointment 699
Cortizone•10 Creme 699
Cortizone•10 Ointment 699
Cortizone•10 Plus Creme 700
Cortizone•10 Maximum Strength Quick Shot Spray 700
Hydrocortone Tablets 1963
Preparation H Hydrocortisone Cream 748

Hydrocortisone Acetate (Co-administration with glucocorticosteroids may potentiate hypokalemic effect of adrenergic agonists). Products include:

Analpram-HC 1136
Pramosone 1139
ProctoFoam-HC 3113
Tucks Anti-Itch Ointment 712
U-cort 1% Cream 3289

Hydrocortisone Sodium Phosphate (Co-administration with glucocorticosteroids may potentiate hypokalemic effect of adrenergic agonists).

No products indexed under this heading.

Hydrocortisone Sodium Succinate (Co-administration with glucocorticosteroids may potentiate hypokalemic effect of adrenergic agonists).

No products indexed under this heading.

Hydroflumethiazide (The ECG changes and/or hypokalemia that may result from the administration of non-potassium sparing diuretics can be acutely worsened by beta-agonists, especially when the recommended dose of beta-agonist is exceeded).

No products indexed under this heading.

Imipramine Hydrochloride (Concurrent and/or sequential administration with tricyclic antidepressants may potentiate the action of adrenergic agonists on the cardiovascular system; co-administer with extreme caution).

No products indexed under this heading.

Imipramine Pamoate (Concurrent and/or sequential administration with tricyclic antidepressants may potentiate the action of adrenergic agonists on the cardiovascular system; co-administer with extreme caution).

No products indexed under this heading.

Indapamide (Concomitant treatment with diuretics may potentiate any hypokalemic effect of adrenergic agonists). Products include:

Indapamide Tablets 2119

Isocarboxazid (Concurrent and/or sequential administration with MAO inhibitors may potentiate the action of adrenergic agonists on the cardiovascular system; co-administer with extreme caution).

No products indexed under this heading.

Isoproterenol Hydrochloride (Co-administration with additional adrenergic drugs may potentiate the sympathetic effects of formoterol).

No products indexed under this heading.

Isoproterenol Sulfate (Co-administration with additional adrenergic drugs may potentiate the sympathetic effects of formoterol).

No products indexed under this heading.

Labetalol Hydrochloride (Co-administration with beta-blockers may inhibit the effect of each other. Beta-blockers not only block the therapeutic effect of beta-agonists, such as formoterol, but may produce severe bronchospasm in patients with asthma).

No products indexed under this heading.

Levalbuterol Hydrochloride (Co-administration with additional adrenergic drugs may potentiate the sympathetic effects of formoterol). Products include:

Xopenex Inhalation Solution 3143
Xopenex Inhalation Solution Concentrate 3147

Levobunolol Hydrochloride (Co-administration with beta-blockers may inhibit the effect of each other. Beta-blockers not only block the therapeutic effect of beta-agonists, such as formoterol, but may produce severe bronchospasm in patients with asthma). Products include:

Betagan Ophthalmic Solution, USP 217

Lidocaine Hydrochloride (Co-administration with drugs known to prolong the QTc interval may lead to an increased risk of ventricular arrhythmias; co-administer with extreme caution).

No products indexed under this heading.

Maprotiline Hydrochloride (Concurrent and/or sequential administration with tricyclic antidepressants may potentiate the action of adrenergic agonists on the cardiovascular system; co-administer with extreme caution).

No products indexed under this heading.

Mesoridazine Besylate (Co-administration with drugs known to prolong the QTc interval may lead to an increased risk of ventricular arrhythmias; co-administer with extreme caution).

No products indexed under this heading.

Metaproterenol Sulfate (Co-administration with additional adrenergic drugs may potentiate the sympathetic effects of formoterol). Products include:

Alupent Inhalation Aerosol 858

Metaraminol Bitartrate (Co-administration with additional adrenergic drugs may potentiate the sympathetic effects of formoterol). Products include:

Aramine Injection 1889

Methoxamine Hydrochloride (Co-administration with additional adrenergic drugs may potentiate the sympathetic effects of formoterol).

No products indexed under this heading.

Methyclothiazide (The ECG changes and/or hypokalemia that may result from the administration of non-potassium sparing diuretics can be acutely worsened by beta-agonists, especially when the recommended dose of beta-agonist is exceeded).

No products indexed under this heading.

Methylprednisolone Acetate (Co-administration with glucocorticosteroids may potentiate hypokalemic effect of adrenergic agonists). Products include:

Depo-Medrol Injectable Suspension 2615
Depo-Medrol Single-Dose Vial 2617

Methylprednisolone Sodium Succinate (Co-administration with glucocorticosteroids may potentiate hypokalemic effect of adrenergic agonists).

No products indexed under this heading.

Metipranolol Hydrochloride (Co-administration with beta-blockers may inhibit the effect of each other. Beta-blockers not only block the therapeutic effect of beta-agonists, such as formoterol, but may produce severe bronchospasm in patients with asthma).

No products indexed under this heading.

Metolazone (Concomitant treatment with diuretics may potentiate any hypokalemic effect of adrenergic agonists).

No products indexed under this heading.

Metoprolol Succinate (Co-administration with beta-blockers may inhibit the effect of each other. Beta-blockers not only block the therapeutic effect of beta-agonists, such as formoterol, but may produce severe bronchospasm in patients with asthma). Products include:

Toprol-XL Tablets 660

Metoprolol Tartrate (Co-administration with beta-blockers may inhibit the effect of each other. Beta-blockers not only block the therapeutic effect of beta-agonists, such as formoterol, but may produce severe bronchospasm in patients with asthma).

No products indexed under this heading.

Mexiletine Hydrochloride (Co-administration with drugs known to prolong the QTc interval may lead to an increased risk of ventricular arrhythmias; co-administer with extreme caution).

No products indexed under this heading.

Moclobemide (Concurrent and/or sequential administration with MAO inhibitors may potentiate the action of adrenergic agonists on the cardiovascular system; co-administer with extreme caution).

No products indexed under this heading.

Nadolol (Co-administration with beta-blockers may inhibit the effect of each other. Beta-blockers not only block the therapeutic effect of beta-agonists, such as formoterol, but may produce severe bronchospasm in patients with asthma). Products include:

Nadolol Tablets 2121

Norepinephrine Bitartrate (Co-administration with additional adrenergic drugs may potentiate the sympathetic effects of formoterol).

No products indexed under this heading.

Nortriptyline Hydrochloride (Concurrent and/or sequential administration with tricyclic antidepressants may potentiate the action of adrenergic agonists on the cardiovascular system; co-administer with extreme caution).

No products indexed under this heading.

Pargyline Hydrochloride (Concurrent and/or sequential administration with MAO inhibitors may potentiate the action of adrenergic agonists on the cardiovascular system; co-administer with extreme caution).

No products indexed under this heading.

Penbutolol Sulfate (Co-administration with beta-blockers may inhibit the effect of each other. Beta-blockers not only block the therapeutic effect of beta-agonists, such as formoterol, but may produce severe bronchospasm in patients with asthma).
No products indexed under this heading.

Perphenazine (Co-administration with drugs known to prolong the QTc interval may lead to an increased risk of ventricular arrhythmias; co-administer with extreme caution).
No products indexed under this heading.

Phenelzine Sulfate (Concurrent and/or sequential administration with MAO inhibitors may potentiate the action of adrenergic agonists on the cardiovascular system; co-administer with extreme caution).
No products indexed under this heading.

Phenylephrine Bitartrate (Co-administration with additional adrenergic drugs may potentiate the sympathetic effects of formoterol).
No products indexed under this heading.

Phenylephrine Hydrochloride (Co-administration with additional adrenergic drugs may potentiate the sympathetic effects of formoterol). Products include:

- Alacol DM Syrup ... 739
- Hycomine Compound Tablets ... 1105
- Preparation H Maximum Strength Cream ... ▣ 747
- Preparation H Cooling Gel ... ▣ 747
- Preparation H ... ▣ 747
- Sudafed PE Tablets ... ▣ 711
- Vicks Sinex Nasal Spray and Ultra Fine Mist for Sinus Relief ... 2677
- Zicam Concentrated Cough Mist for Kids Plus D Cool Cherry ... ▣ 643
- Zicam Concentrated Cough Mist Plus D Cool Cherry ... ▣ 642

Phenylephrine Tannate (Co-administration with additional adrenergic drugs may potentiate the sympathetic effects of formoterol).
No products indexed under this heading.

Phenylpropanolamine Hydrochloride (Co-administration with additional adrenergic drugs may potentiate the sympathetic effects of formoterol).
No products indexed under this heading.

Pindolol (Co-administration with beta-blockers may inhibit the effect of each other. Beta-blockers not only block the therapeutic effect of beta-agonists, such as formoterol, but may produce severe bronchospasm in patients with asthma).
No products indexed under this heading.

Pirbuterol Acetate (Co-administration with additional adrenergic drugs may potentiate the sympathetic effects of formoterol). Products include:

- Maxair Autohaler ... 1820

Polythiazide (The ECG changes and/or hypokalemia that may result from the administration of non-potassium sparing diuretics can be acutely worsened by beta-agonists, especially when the recommended dose of beta-agonist is exceeded).
No products indexed under this heading.

Prednisolone Acetate (Co-administration with glucocorticosteroids may potentiate hypokalemic effect of adrenergic agonists). Products include:

- Blephamide Ophthalmic Ointment ... 563
- Blephamide Ophthalmic Suspension ... 564
- Poly-Pred Liquifilm Ophthalmic Suspension ... ⊙ 231
- Pred Forte Ophthalmic Suspension ... ⊙ 233
- Pred Mild Sterile Ophthalmic Suspension ... ⊙ 236
- Pred-G Ophthalmic Suspension ... ⊙ 234
- Pred-G Sterile Ophthalmic Ointment ... ⊙ 235

Prednisolone Sodium Phosphate (Co-administration with glucocorticosteroids may potentiate hypokalemic effect of adrenergic agonists). Products include:

- Pediapred Oral Solution ... 3319

Prednisolone Tebutate (Co-administration with glucocorticosteroids may potentiate hypokalemic effect of adrenergic agonists).
No products indexed under this heading.

Prednisone (Co-administration with glucocorticosteroids may potentiate hypokalemic effect of adrenergic agonists).
No products indexed under this heading.

Procainamide Hydrochloride (Co-administration with drugs known to prolong the QTc interval may lead to an increased risk of ventricular arrhythmias; co-administer with extreme caution).
No products indexed under this heading.

Procarbazine Hydrochloride (Concurrent and/or sequential administration with MAO inhibitors may potentiate the action of adrenergic agonists on the cardiovascular system; co-administer with extreme caution). Products include:

- Matulane Capsules ... 3188

Prochlorperazine (Co-administration with drugs known to prolong the QTc interval may lead to an increased risk of ventricular arrhythmias; co-administer with extreme caution).
No products indexed under this heading.

Promethazine Hydrochloride (Co-administration with drugs known to prolong the QTc interval may lead to an increased risk of ventricular arrhythmias; co-administer with extreme caution). Products include:

- Phenergan ... 3438

Propafenone Hydrochloride (Co-administration with drugs known to prolong the QTc interval may lead to an increased risk of ventricular arrhythmias; co-administer with extreme caution). Products include:

- Rythmol SR Capsules ... 2736

Propranolol Hydrochloride (Co-administration with beta-blockers may inhibit the effect of each other. Beta-blockers not only block the therapeutic effect of beta-agonists, such as formoterol, but may produce severe bronchospasm in patients with asthma). Products include:

- Inderal LA Long-Acting Capsules ... 3421
- InnoPran XL Capsules ... 2728

Protriptyline Hydrochloride (Concurrent and/or sequential administration with tricyclic antidepressants may potentiate the action of adrenergic agonists on the cardiovascular system; co-administer with extreme caution). Products include:

- Vivactil Tablets ... 2350

Pseudoephedrine Hydrochloride (Co-administration with additional adrenergic drugs may potentiate the sympathetic effects of formoterol). Products include:

- Advil Allergy Sinus Caplets ... ▣ 737
- Advil Cold & Sinus ... ▣ 739
- Advil Flu & Body Ache Caplets ... ▣ 739
- Children's Advil Cold Suspension ... ▣ 741
- Advil Multi-Symptom Cold Caplets ... ▣ 738
- Allegra-D 12 Hour Extended-Release Tablets ... 2860
- Allegra-D 24 Hour Extended-Release Tablets ... 2862
- Balamine DM ... 739
- BC Cold Powder ... ▣ 612
- Benadryl Allergy & Cold Tablets ... ▣ 692
- Benadryl Allergy & Sinus Headache Caplets & Gelcaps ... ▣ 693
- Children's Benadryl Allergy & Cold Fastmelt Tablets ... ▣ 695
- Benadryl Maximum Strength Severe Allergy & Sinus Headache Caplets ... ▣ 694
- Children's Benadryl D Allergy & Sinus Fastmelt Tablets ... ▣ 694
- Children's Benadryl D Liquid Medication ... ▣ 693
- Benadryl D Tablets ... ▣ 694
- Contac Non-Drowsy 12 Hour Cold Caplets ... ▣ 614
- Contac Non-Drowsy Timed Release 12 Hour Cold Caplets ... ▣ 615
- Contac Severe Cold and Flu Caplets Maximum Strength ... ▣ 615
- Contac Severe Cold and Flu Caplets Non-Drowsy ... ▣ 615
- Children's Dimetapp Cold & Allergy Elixir ... ▣ 745
- Children's Dimetapp DM Cold & Cough Elixir ... ▣ 745
- Children's Dimetapp Long Acting Cough Plus Cold Syrup ... ▣ 746
- Dimetapp Infant Drops Decongestant Plus Cough ... ▣ 746
- Children's Motrin Cold Non-Staining Dye-Free Oral Suspension ... 1838
- Children's Motrin Cold Oral Suspension ... 1838
- Motrin Cold & Sinus Caplets ... 1836
- PediaCare Decongestant & Cough Infant Drops ... ▣ 705
- PediaCare Decongestant Infants' Drops ... ▣ 705
- PediaCare Long-Acting Cough Plus Cold Liquid ... ▣ 704
- PediaCare Multi-Symptom Cold Liquid ... ▣ 704
- PediaCare NightRest Cough & Cold Liquid ... ▣ 704
- Robitussin Allergy & Cough Syrup ... ▣ 750
- Robitussin CF Liquid ... ▣ 755
- Robitussin Cough & Cold Liquid-filled Capsules ... ▣ 750
- Robitussin Cough, Cold & Flu Liquid-filled Capsules ... ▣ 750
- Robitussin Cough & Cold Infant Drops ... ▣ 755
- Robitussin Flu Liquid ... ▣ 752
- Robitussin Maximum Strength Cough & Cold Liquid ... ▣ 754
- Robitussin PE Syrup ... ▣ 753
- Robitussin Pediatric Cough & Cold Liquid ... ▣ 754
- Robitussin PM Cough & Cold Liquid ... ▣ 752
- Robitussin Severe Congestion Liquid-filled Capsules ... ▣ 751
- Simply Stuffy Liquid ... 1841
- Singlet Caplets ... ▣ 636
- Sudafed 12 Hour Caplets ... ▣ 708
- Sudafed 24 Hour Tablets ... ▣ 709
- Sudafed Nasal Decongestant Tablets ... ▣ 709
- Sudafed Severe Cold ... ▣ 710
- Sudafed Non-Drying Sinus Liquid Caps ... ▣ 709
- Sudafed Sinus & Allergy Tablets ... ▣ 710
- Sudafed Sinus Headache ... ▣ 711
- TheraFlu Cold & Cough Hot Liquid ... ▣ 680
- TheraFlu Cold & Sore Throat Hot Liquid ... ▣ 680
- TheraFlu Flu & Chest Congestion Non-Drowsy Hot Liquid ... ▣ 681
- TheraFlu Flu & Sore Throat Hot Liquid ... ▣ 681
- TheraFlu Severe Cold Non-Drowsy Hot Liquid ... ▣ 683
- TheraFlu Severe Cold & Cough Hot Liquid ... ▣ 683
- TheraFlu Severe Cold Caplets ... ▣ 679
- TheraFlu Severe Cold Hot Liquid ... ▣ 682
- TheraFlu Severe Cold Non-Drowsy Caplets ... ▣ 679
- Triaminic Chest & Nasal Congestion Liquid ... ▣ 685
- Triaminic Cold & Allergy Liquid ... ▣ 685
- Triaminic Cold & Cough Liquid ... ▣ 685
- Triaminic Cough Liquid ... ▣ 687
- Triaminic Cough & Nasal Congestion Liquid ... ▣ 687
- Triaminic Cough & Sore Throat Liquid ... ▣ 687
- Triaminic Flu, Cough & Fever Liquid ... ▣ 685
- Triaminic Night Time Cough & Cold Liquid ... ▣ 685
- Triaminic Allergy Runny Nose & Congestion Softchews ... ▣ 688
- Triaminic Cold & Cough Softchews ... ▣ 688
- Triaminic Cough & Sore Throat Softchews ... ▣ 689
- Tylenol Sinus NightTime Caplets ... ▣ 663
- Children's Tylenol Plus Cold & Allergy Suspension Liquid ... 1850
- Children's Tylenol Plus Cold NightTime Suspension Liquid ... 1851
- Children's Tylenol Plus Cold & Cough Suspension Liquid and Chewable Tablets ... 1851
- Children's Tylenol Plus Cold Chewable Tablets ... 1851
- Children's Tylenol Plus Cold Daytime Non-Drowsy Suspension Liquid ... 1851
- Children's Tylenol Plus Flu Suspension Liquid ... 1853
- Concentrated Tylenol Infants' Drops Plus Cold ... 1851
- Concentrated Tylenol Infants' Drops Plus Cold and Cough ... 1851
- Tylenol Cold & Flu Severe Daytime Liquid with Cool Bust ... 1846
- Tylenol Cold & Flu Severe NightTime Liquid with Cool Burst ... 1846
- Tylenol Cold Severe Congestion Non-Drowsy Caplets with Cool Burst ... 1846
- Tylenol Allergy Complete Night Time Caplets ... 1844
- Tylenol Allergy Complete Multi-Symptom Caplets and Gelcaps with Cool Burst ... 1844
- Tylenol Flu NightTime Gelcaps ... 1846
- Tylenol Flu Day Non-Drowsy Gelcaps ... 1846
- Concentrated Tylenol Infants' Drops Plus Cold Nasal Congestant, Fever Reducer & Pain Reliever ... ▣ 668
- Concentrated Tylenol Infants' Drops Plus Cold & Cough Nasal Decongestant, Fever Reducer & Pain Reliever ... ▣ 668
- Multi-Symptom Tylenol Cold Night Time Caplets ... 1845
- Multi-Symptom Tylenol Cold Day Non-Drowsy Caplets and Gelcaps ... 1845
- Tylenol Sinus Day Non-Drowsy ... 1848
- Tylenol Sinus Night Time Caplets ... 1848
- Tylenol Sinus Severe Congestion Caplets with Cool Burst ... 1848
- Vicks 44D Cough & Head Congestion Relief ... 2676
- Vicks 44D Cough & Head Congestion Relief Liquid ... ▣ 721
- Vicks 44M Cough, Cold & Flu Relief ... 2676
- Pediatric Vicks 44m Cough & Cold Relief ... 2673
- Vicks DayQuil LiquiCaps/Liquid Multi-Symptom Cold/Flu Relief ... ▣ 723

Vicks DayQuil Multi-Symptom Cold/Flu Relief LiquiCaps............. 2675
Vicks DayQuil Multi-Symptom Cold/Flu Relief Liquid.................... 2675
Children's Vicks NyQuil Cold/Cough Relief......................... 2671
Vicks NyQuil LiquiCaps 2677
Vicks NyQuil LiquiCaps/Liquid Multi-Symptom Cold/Flu Relief..... 725
Vicks NyQuil Liquid 2677
Zyrtec-D 12 Hour Extended Release Tablets.......................... 2591

Pseudoephedrine Sulfate (Co-administration with additional adrenergic drugs may potentiate the sympathetic effects of formoterol). Products include:
Alavert Allergy & Sinus D-12 Hour Tablets.. 743
Clarinex-D 24-Hour Extended-Release Tablets............ 3012
Claritin-D Non-Drowsy 12 Hour Tablets.. 731
Claritin-D Non-Drowsy 24 Hour Tablets.. 731

Quinidine Gluconate (Co-administration with drugs known to prolong the QTc interval may lead to an increased risk of ventricular arrhythmias; co-administer with extreme caution).
No products indexed under this heading.

Quinidine Polygalacturonate (Co-administration with drugs known to prolong the QTc interval may lead to an increased risk of ventricular arrhythmias; co-administer with extreme caution).
No products indexed under this heading.

Quinidine Sulfate (Co-administration with drugs known to prolong the QTc interval may lead to an increased risk of ventricular arrhythmias; co-administer with extreme caution).
No products indexed under this heading.

Salmeterol Xinafoate (Co-administration with additional adrenergic drugs may potentiate the sympathetic effects of formoterol). Products include:
Advair Diskus 100/50 1291
Advair Diskus 250/50 1291
Advair Diskus 500/50 1291
Serevent Diskus 1540

Selegiline Hydrochloride (Concurrent and/or sequential administration with MAO inhibitors may potentiate the action of adrenergic agonists on the cardiovascular system; co-administer with extreme caution). Products include:
Eldepryl Capsules 3209

Sotalol Hydrochloride (Co-administration with beta-blockers may inhibit the effect of each other. Beta-blockers not only block the therapeutic effect of beta-agonists, such as formoterol, but may produce severe bronchospasm in patients with asthma).
No products indexed under this heading.

Spironolactone (Concomitant treatment with diuretics may potentiate any hypokalemic effect of adrenergic agonists).
No products indexed under this heading.

Terbutaline Sulfate (Co-administration with additional adrenergic drugs may potentiate the sympathetic effects of formoterol).
No products indexed under this heading.

Theophylline (Co-administration with xanthine derivatives may potentiate hypokalemic effect of adrenergic agonists).
No products indexed under this heading.

Theophylline Anhydrous (Co-administration with xanthine derivatives may potentiate hypokalemic effect of adrenergic agonists). Products include:
Uniphyl Tablets 2708

Theophylline Calcium Salicylate (Co-administration with xanthine derivatives may potentiate hypokalemic effect of adrenergic agonists).
No products indexed under this heading.

Theophylline Dihydroxypropyl (Glyceryl) (Co-administration with xanthine derivatives may potentiate hypokalemic effect of adrenergic agonists).
No products indexed under this heading.

Theophylline Ethylenediamine (Co-administration with xanthine derivatives may potentiate hypokalemic effect of adrenergic agonists).
No products indexed under this heading.

Theophylline Sodium Glycinate (Co-administration with xanthine derivatives may potentiate hypokalemic effect of adrenergic agonists).
No products indexed under this heading.

Thioridazine Hydrochloride (Co-administration with drugs known to prolong the QTc interval may lead to an increased risk of ventricular arrhythmias; co-administer with extreme caution). Products include:
Thioridazine Hydrochloride Tablets 2122

Timolol Hemihydrate (Co-administration with beta-blockers may inhibit the effect of each other. Beta-blockers not only block the therapeutic effect of beta-agonists, such as formoterol, but may produce severe bronchospasm in patients with asthma). Products include:
Betimol Ophthalmic Solution 3371
Betimol Ophthalmic Solution .... ⊙ 283

Timolol Maleate (Co-administration with beta-blockers may inhibit the effect of each other. Beta-blockers not only block the therapeutic effect of beta-agonists, such as formoterol, but may produce severe bronchospasm in patients with asthma). Products include:
Blocadren Tablets 1891
Cosopt Sterile Ophthalmic Solution... 1910
Timolide Tablets 2056
Timoptic in Ocudose 2061
Timoptic Sterile Ophthalmic Solution... 2058
Timoptic-XE Sterile Ophthalmic Gel Forming Solution.................. 2062

Tocainide Hydrochloride (Co-administration with drugs known to prolong the QTc interval may lead to an increased risk of ventricular arrhythmias; co-administer with extreme caution).
No products indexed under this heading.

Torsemide (The ECG changes and/or hypokalemia that may result from the administration of non-potassium sparing diuretics can be acutely worsened by beta-agonists, especially when the recommended dose of beta-agonist is exceeded).
No products indexed under this heading.

Tranylcypromine Sulfate (Concurrent and/or sequential administration with MAO inhibitors may potentiate the action of adrenergic agonists on the cardiovascular system; co-administer with extreme caution). Products include:
Parnate Tablets 1499

Triamcinolone (Co-administration with glucocorticosteroids may potentiate hypokalemic effect of adrenergic agonists).
No products indexed under this heading.

Triamcinolone Acetonide (Co-administration with glucocorticosteroids may potentiate hypokalemic effect of adrenergic agonists). Products include:
Azmacort Inhalation Aerosol 1701
Nasacort HFA Inhalation Aerosol 2939
Nasacort AQ Nasal Spray 2937

Triamcinolone Diacetate (Co-administration with glucocorticosteroids may potentiate hypokalemic effect of adrenergic agonists).
No products indexed under this heading.

Triamcinolone Hexacetonide (Co-administration with glucocorticosteroids may potentiate hypokalemic effect of adrenergic agonists).
No products indexed under this heading.

Triamterene (Concomitant treatment with diuretics may potentiate any hypokalemic effect of adrenergic agonists). Products include:
Dyazide Capsules 1389
Dyrenium Capsules 3390
Maxzide 2150

Trifluoperazine Hydrochloride (Co-administration with drugs known to prolong the QTc interval may lead to an increased risk of ventricular arrhythmias; co-administer with extreme caution).
No products indexed under this heading.

Trimipramine Maleate (Concurrent and/or sequential administration with tricyclic antidepressants may potentiate the action of adrenergic agonists on the cardiovascular system; co-administer with extreme caution). Products include:
Surmontil Capsules 2347

Ziprasidone Hydrochloride (Co-administration with drugs known to prolong the QTc interval may lead to an increased risk of ventricular arrhythmias; co-administer with extreme caution). Products include:
Geodon Capsules 2514

FORTAMET EXTENDED-RELEASE TABLETS

(Metformin Hydrochloride) 1156

May interact with cationic drugs that are eliminated by renal tubular, calcium channel blockers, corticosteroids, diuretics, estrogens, oral contraceptives, phenothiazines, phenytoin, radiographic iodinated contrast media, sympathomimetics, thiazides, thyroid preparations, and certain other agents. Compounds in these categories include:

Albuterol (Sympathomimetics tend to produce hyperglycemia and may lead to loss of glycemic control). Products include:
Proventil Inhalation Aerosol 3067

Albuterol Sulfate (Sympathomimetics tend to produce hyperglycemia and may lead to loss of glycemic control). Products include:
AccuNeb Inhalation Solution 1055
Combivent Inhalation Aerosol 878
DuoNeb Inhalation Solution 1058
Proventil Inhalation Solution 0.083%.. 3069
Proventil HFA Inhalation Aerosol 3071
Ventolin HFA Inhalation Aerosol 1576
VoSpire Extended-Release Tablets ... 2352

Amiloride Hydrochloride (Diuretics tend to produce hyperglycemia and may lead to loss of glycemic control). Products include:
Midamor Tablets 2000
Moduretic Tablets 2003

Amlodipine Besylate (Calcium channel blocking drugs tend to produce hyperglycemia and may lead to loss of glycemic control). Products include:
Caduet Tablets 2507
Lotrel Capsules 2238
Norvasc Tablets 2529

Bendroflumethiazide (Thiazides tend to produce hyperglycemia and may lead to loss of glycemic control).
No products indexed under this heading.

Bepridil Hydrochloride (Calcium channel blocking drugs tend to produce hyperglycemia and may lead to loss of glycemic control).
No products indexed under this heading.

Betamethasone Acetate (Corticosteroids tend to produce hyperglycemia and may lead to loss of glycemic control).
No products indexed under this heading.

Betamethasone Sodium Phosphate (Corticosteroids tend to produce hyperglycemia and may lead to loss of glycemic control).
No products indexed under this heading.

Bumetanide (Diuretics tend to produce hyperglycemia and may lead to loss of glycemic control).
No products indexed under this heading.

Chlorothiazide (Thiazides tend to produce hyperglycemia and may lead to loss of glycemic control). Products include:
Aldoclor Tablets 1881
Diuril Oral 1936

Chlorothiazide Sodium (Thiazides tend to produce hyperglycemia and may lead to loss of glycemic control). Products include:
Diuril Sodium Intravenous 1934

Chlorotrianisene (Estrogens tend to produce hyperglycemia and may lead to loss of glycemic control).
No products indexed under this heading.

Chlorpromazine (Phenothiazines tend to produce hyperglycemia and may lead to loss of glycemic control).
No products indexed under this heading.

Chlorpromazine Hydrochloride (Phenothiazines tend to produce hyperglycemia and may lead to loss of glycemic control).
No products indexed under this heading.

Chlorthalidone (Diuretics tend to produce hyperglycemia and may lead to loss of glycemic control). Products include:
Clorpres Tablets 2139

Cimetidine (Co-administration of cimetidine increased peak plasma metformin and whole blood concentrations by 60% and plasma and whole blood metformin AUC by 40%). Products include:
Tagamet HB 200 Tablets .... ▣637
Tagamet Tablets 1547

Cimetidine Hydrochloride (Co-administration of cimetidine increased peak plasma metformin and whole blood concentrations by 60% and plasma and whole blood metformin AUC by 40%).
No products indexed under this heading.

Cortisone Acetate (Corticosteroids tend to produce hyperglycemia and may lead to loss of glycemic control).
No products indexed under this heading.

Desogestrel (Oral contraceptives tend to produce hyperglycemia and may lead to loss of glycemic control). Products include:
Ortho-Cept Tablets 2395

Dexamethasone (Corticosteroids tend to produce hyperglycemia and may lead to loss of glycemic control). Products include:
Ciprodex Otic Suspension 555
Decadron Tablets 1929
TobraDex Ophthalmic Ointment 558
TobraDex Ophthalmic Suspension 558

Dexamethasone Acetate (Corticosteroids tend to produce hyperglycemia and may lead to loss of glycemic control).
No products indexed under this heading.

Dexamethasone Sodium Phosphate (Corticosteroids tend to produce hyperglycemia and may lead to loss of glycemic control). Products include:
Decadron Phosphate Injection 1931

Diatrizoate Meglumine (Intravascular contrast studies with iodinated materials can lead to acute alteration of renal function and have been associated with lactic acidosis in patients receiving metformin. Therefore, discontinue metformin at the time of or prior to the procedure, and for 48 hours subsequent to the procedure until renal function is normal).
No products indexed under this heading.

Diatrizoate Sodium (Intravascular contrast studies with iodinated materials can lead to acute alteration of renal function and have been associated with lactic acidosis in patients receiving metformin. Therefore, discontinue metformin at the time of or prior to the procedure, and for 48 hours subsequent to the procedure until renal function is normal).
No products indexed under this heading.

Dienestrol (Estrogens tend to produce hyperglycemia and may lead to loss of glycemic control).
No products indexed under this heading.

Diethylstilbestrol (Estrogens tend to produce hyperglycemia and may lead to loss of glycemic control).
No products indexed under this heading.

Digoxin (Cationic drugs that are eliminated by renal tubular secretion theoretically have the potential for interaction with metformin by competing for common renal tubular transport system). Products include:
Digitek Tablets 2146
Lanoxicaps Capsules 1458
Lanoxin Injection 1462
Lanoxin Tablets 1468
Lanoxin Injection Pediatric 1465

Diltiazem Hydrochloride (Calcium channel blocking drugs tend to produce hyperglycemia and may lead to loss of glycemic control). Products include:
Cardizem LA Extended Release Tablets 1699
Tiazac Capsules 1204

Dobutamine Hydrochloride (Sympathomimetics tend to produce hyperglycemia and may lead to loss of glycemic control).
No products indexed under this heading.

Dopamine Hydrochloride (Sympathomimetics tend to produce hyperglycemia and may lead to loss of glycemic control).
No products indexed under this heading.

Ephedrine Hydrochloride (Sympathomimetics tend to produce hyperglycemia and may lead to loss of glycemic control). Products include:
Primatene Tablets .... ▣749

Ephedrine Sulfate (Sympathomimetics tend to produce hyperglycemia and may lead to loss of glycemic control).
No products indexed under this heading.

Ephedrine Tannate (Sympathomimetics tend to produce hyperglycemia and may lead to loss of glycemic control).
No products indexed under this heading.

Epinephrine (Sympathomimetics tend to produce hyperglycemia and may lead to loss of glycemic control). Products include:
EpiPen 1061
Primatene Mist .... ▣749

Epinephrine Bitartrate (Sympathomimetics tend to produce hyperglycemia and may lead to loss of glycemic control).
No products indexed under this heading.

Epinephrine Hydrochloride (Sympathomimetics tend to produce hyperglycemia and may lead to loss of glycemic control).
No products indexed under this heading.

Estradiol (Estrogens tend to produce hyperglycemia and may lead to loss of glycemic control). Products include:
Activella Tablets 2311
Climara Transdermal System 795
Climara Pro Transdermal System 800
CombiPatch Transdermal System 2180
Estrogel 0.06% 3200
Menostar Transdermal System 805
Prefest Tablets 1069
Vagifem Tablets 2340
Vivelle Transdermal System 2288
Vivelle-Dot Transdermal System 2293

Estrogens, Conjugated (Estrogens tend to produce hyperglycemia and may lead to loss of glycemic control). Products include:
Premarin Intravenous 3440
Premarin Tablets 3443
Premarin Vaginal Cream 3449
Premphase Tablets 3452
Prempro Tablets 3452

Estrogens, Esterified (Estrogens tend to produce hyperglycemia and may lead to loss of glycemic control). Products include:
Estratest Tablets 3196
Estratest H.S. Tablets 3196

Estropipate (Estrogens tend to produce hyperglycemia and may lead to loss of glycemic control).
No products indexed under this heading.

Ethacrynic Acid (Diuretics tend to produce hyperglycemia and may lead to loss of glycemic control). Products include:
Edecrin Tablets 1941

Ethinyl Estradiol (Estrogens tend to produce hyperglycemia and may lead to loss of glycemic control). Products include:
Alesse-28 Tablets 3392
Lo/Ovral-28 Tablets 3423
NuvaRing 2357
Ortho-Cept Tablets 2395
Ortho-Cyclen/Ortho Tri-Cyclen 2414
Ortho Evra Transdermal System 2402
Ortho Tri-Cyclen Lo Tablets 2421
Seasonale Tablets 1073
Triphasil-28 Tablets 3483
Yasmin 28 Tablets 818

Ethiodized Oil (Intravascular contrast studies with iodinated materials can lead to acute alteration of renal function and have been associated with lactic acidosis in patients receiving metformin. Therefore, discontinue metformin at the time of or prior to the procedure, and for 48 hours subsequent to the procedure until renal function is normal).
No products indexed under this heading.

Ethynodiol Diacetate (Oral contraceptives tend to produce hyperglycemia and may lead to loss of glycemic control).
No products indexed under this heading.

Felodipine (Calcium channel blocking drugs tend to produce hyperglycemia and may lead to loss of glycemic control). Products include:
Plendil Extended-Release Tablets 651

Fludrocortisone Acetate (Corticosteroids tend to produce hyperglycemia and may lead to loss of glycemic control).
No products indexed under this heading.

Fluphenazine Decanoate (Phenothiazines tend to produce hyperglycemia and may lead to loss of glycemic control).
No products indexed under this heading.

Fluphenazine Enanthate (Phenothiazines tend to produce hyperglycemia and may lead to loss of glycemic control).
No products indexed under this heading.

Fluphenazine Hydrochloride (Phenothiazines tend to produce hyperglycemia and may lead to loss of glycemic control).
No products indexed under this heading.

Fosphenytoin Sodium (Phenytoin tends to produce hyperglycemia and may lead to loss of glycemic control).
No products indexed under this heading.

Furosemide (Furosemide increased the metformin plasma and blood Cmax by 22% and blood AUC by 15%, without any significant change in metformin renal clearance. When administered with metformin, the Cmax and AUC of furosemide were 31% and 12% smaller, respectively, and the terminal half-life was decreased by 32%, without any significant change in furosemide renal clearance). Products include:
Furosemide Tablets 2117

Gadopentetate Dimeglumine (Intravascular contrast studies with iodinated materials can lead to acute alteration of renal function and have been associated with lactic acidosis in patients receiving metformin. Therefore, discontinue metformin at the time of or prior to the procedure, and for 48 hours subsequent to the procedure until renal function is normal).
No products indexed under this heading.

Hydrochlorothiazide (Thiazides tend to produce hyperglycemia and may lead to loss of glycemic control). Products include:
Aldoril Tablets 1884
Atacand HCT 637
Avalide Tablets 2889
Avalide Tablets 922
Benicar HCT Tablets 2852
Diovan HCT Tablets 2195
Dyazide Capsules 1389
Hyzaar 1964
Lotensin HCT Tablets 2235
Maxzide 2150
Micardis HCT Tablets 886
Moduretic Tablets 2003
Prinzide Tablets 2033
Teveten HCT Tablets 1710
Timolide Tablets 2056
Uniretic Tablets 3114
Vaseretic Tablets 2073
Zestoretic Tablets 701

Hydrocortisone (Corticosteroids tend to produce hyperglycemia and may lead to loss of glycemic control). Products include:
Cortizone•5 Ointment .... ▣699
Cortizone•10 Creme .... ▣699
Cortizone•10 Ointment .... ▣699
Cortizone•10 Plus Creme .... ▣700
Cortizone•10 Maximum Strength Quick Shot Spray .... ▣700
Hydrocortone Tablets 1963
Preparation H Hydrocortisone Cream .... ▣748

Hydrocortisone Acetate (Corticosteroids tend to produce hyperglycemia and may lead to loss of glycemic control). Products include:
Analpram-HC 1136
Pramosone 1139
ProctoFoam-HC 3113
Tucks Anti-Itch Ointment .... ▣712
U-cort 1% Cream 3289

Hydrocortisone Sodium Phosphate (Corticosteroids tend to produce hyperglycemia and may lead to loss of glycemic control).
No products indexed under this heading.

Hydrocortisone Sodium Succinate (Corticosteroids tend to produce hyperglycemia and may lead to loss of glycemic control).
No products indexed under this heading.

Hydroflumethiazide (Thiazides tend to produce hyperglycemia and may lead to loss of glycemic control).
No products indexed under this heading.

Indapamide (Diuretics tend to produce hyperglycemia and may lead to loss of glycemic control). Products include:
Indapamide Tablets 2119

Iodamide Meglumine (Intravascular contrast studies with iodinated materials can lead to acute alteration of renal function and have been associated with lactic acidosis in patients receiving metformin. Therefore, discontinue metformin at the time of or prior to the procedure, and for 48 hours subsequent to the procedure until renal function is normal).
No products indexed under this heading.

Iohexol (Intravascular contrast studies with iodinated materials can lead to acute alteration of renal function and have been associated with lactic acidosis in patients receiving metformin. Therefore, discontinue metformin at the time of or prior to the procedure, and for 48 hours subsequent to the procedure until renal function is normal).
No products indexed under this heading.

Iopamidol (Intravascular contrast studies with iodinated materials can lead to acute alteration of renal function and have been associated with lactic acidosis in patients receiving metformin. Therefore, discontinue metformin at the time of or prior to the procedure, and for 48 hours subsequent to the procedure until renal function is normal).
No products indexed under this heading.

Iopanoic Acid (Intravascular contrast studies with iodinated materials can lead to acute alteration of renal function and have been associated with lactic acidosis in patients receiving metformin. Therefore, discontinue metformin at the time of or prior to the procedure, and for 48 hours subsequent to the procedure until renal function is normal).
No products indexed under this heading.

Iothalamate Meglumine (Intravascular contrast studies with iodinated materials can lead to acute alteration of renal function and have been associated with lactic acidosis in patients receiving metformin. Therefore, discontinue metformin at the time of or prior to the procedure, and for 48 hours subsequent to the procedure until renal function is normal).
No products indexed under this heading.

Ioxaglate Meglumine (Intravascular contrast studies with iodinated materials can lead to acute alteration of renal function and have been associated with lactic acidosis in patients receiving metformin. Therefore, discontinue metformin at the time of or prior to the procedure, and for 48 hours subsequent to the procedure until renal function is normal).
No products indexed under this heading.

Ioxaglate Sodium (Intravascular contrast studies with iodinated materials can lead to acute alteration of renal function and have been associated with lactic acidosis in patients receiving metformin. Therefore, discontinue metformin at the time of or prior to the procedure, and for 48 hours subsequent to the procedure until renal function is normal).
No products indexed under this heading.

Isoniazid (Isoniazid tends to produce hyperglycemia and may lead to loss of glycemic control).
No products indexed under this heading.

Isoproterenol Hydrochloride (Sympathomimetics tend to produce hyperglycemia and may lead to loss of glycemic control).
No products indexed under this heading.

Isoproterenol Sulfate (Sympathomimetics tend to produce hyperglycemia and may lead to loss of glycemic control).
No products indexed under this heading.

Isradipine (Calcium channel blocking drugs tend to produce hyperglycemia and may lead to loss of glycemic control). Products include:
DynaCirc CR Tablets 2726

Levalbuterol Hydrochloride (Sympathomimetics tend to produce hyperglycemia and may lead to loss of glycemic control). Products include:
Xopenex Inhalation Solution 3143
Xopenex Inhalation Solution Concentrate 3147

Levonorgestrel (Oral contraceptives tend to produce hyperglycemia and may lead to loss of glycemic control). Products include:
Alesse-28 Tablets 3392
Climara Pro Transdermal System 800
Mirena Intrauterine System 810
Plan B Tablets 1068
Seasonale Tablets 1073
Triphasil-28 Tablets 3483

Levothyroxine Sodium (Thyroid products tend to produce hyperglycemia and may lead to loss of glycemic control). Products include:
Levothroid Tablets 1189
Levoxyl Tablets 1680
Synthroid Tablets 515
Unithroid Tablets 3521

Liothyronine Sodium (Thyroid products tend to produce hyperglycemia and may lead to loss of glycemic control). Products include:
Cytomel Tablets 1678

Liotrix (Thyroid products tend to produce hyperglycemia and may lead to loss of glycemic control). Products include:
Thyrolar 1203

Mesoridazine Besylate (Phenothiazines tend to produce hyperglycemia and may lead to loss of glycemic control).
No products indexed under this heading.

Mestranol (Oral contraceptives tend to produce hyperglycemia and may lead to loss of glycemic control).
No products indexed under this heading.

Metaproterenol Sulfate (Sympathomimetics tend to produce hyperglycemia and may lead to loss of glycemic control). Products include:
Alupent Inhalation Aerosol 858

Metaraminol Bitartrate (Sympathomimetics tend to produce hyperglycemia and may lead to loss of glycemic control). Products include:
Aramine Injection 1889

Methotrimeprazine (Phenothiazines tend to produce hyperglycemia and may lead to loss of glycemic control).
No products indexed under this heading.

Methoxamine Hydrochloride (Sympathomimetics tend to produce hyperglycemia and may lead to loss of glycemic control).
No products indexed under this heading.

Methyclothiazide (Thiazides tend to produce hyperglycemia and may lead to loss of glycemic control).
No products indexed under this heading.

Methylprednisolone Acetate (Corticosteroids tend to produce hyperglycemia and may lead to loss of glycemic control). Products include:
Depo-Medrol Injectable Suspension 2615
Depo-Medrol Single-Dose Vial 2617

Methylprednisolone Sodium Succinate (Corticosteroids tend to produce hyperglycemia and may lead to loss of glycemic control).
No products indexed under this heading.

Metolazone (Diuretics tend to produce hyperglycemia and may lead to loss of glycemic control).
No products indexed under this heading.

Mibefradil Dihydrochloride (Calcium channel blocking drugs tend to produce hyperglycemia and may lead to loss of glycemic control).
No products indexed under this heading.

Morphine Sulfate (Cationic drugs that are eliminated by renal tubular secretion theoretically have the potential for interaction with metformin by competing for common renal tubular transport system). Products include:
Avinza Capsules 1714
Kadian Capsules 572
MS Contin Tablets 2703

Nicardipine Hydrochloride (Calcium channel blocking drugs tend to produce hyperglycemia and may lead to loss of glycemic control). Products include:
Cardene I.V. 1129

Nicotinic Acid (Nicotinic acid tends to produce hyperglycemia and may lead to loss of glycemic control).
No products indexed under this heading.

Nifedipine (Co-administration of nifedipine increased plasma metformin Cmax and AUC by 20% and 9%, respectively, and increased the amount excreted in the urine. Nifedipine appears to enhance the absorption of metformin). Products include:
Adalat CC Tablets 2978

Nimodipine (Calcium channel blocking drugs tend to produce hyperglycemia and may lead to loss of glycemic control). Products include:
Nimotop Capsules 774

Nisoldipine (Calcium channel blocking drugs tend to produce hyperglycemia and may lead to loss of glycemic control). Products include:
Sular Tablets 1163

Norepinephrine Bitartrate (Sympathomimetics tend to produce hyperglycemia and may lead to loss of glycemic control).
No products indexed under this heading.

Norethindrone (Oral contraceptives tend to produce hyperglycemia and may lead to loss of glycemic control). Products include:
Ortho Micronor Tablets 2411

Norethynodrel (Oral contraceptives tend to produce hyperglycemia and may lead to loss of glycemic control).
No products indexed under this heading.

Norgestimate (Oral contraceptives tend to produce hyperglycemia and may lead to loss of glycemic control). Products include:
Ortho-Cyclen/Ortho Tri-Cyclen 2414
Ortho Tri-Cyclen Lo Tablets 2421
Prefest Tablets 1069

Norgestrel (Oral contraceptives tend to produce hyperglycemia and may lead to loss of glycemic control). Products include:
Lo/Ovral-28 Tablets 3423

Perphenazine (Phenothiazines tend to produce hyperglycemia and may lead to loss of glycemic control).
No products indexed under this heading.

Phenylephrine Bitartrate (Sympathomimetics tend to produce hyperglycemia and may lead to loss of glycemic control).
No products indexed under this heading.

Phenylephrine Hydrochloride (Sympathomimetics tend to produce hyperglycemia and may lead to loss of glycemic control). Products include:
Alacol DM Syrup 739
Hycomine Compound Tablets 1105
Preparation H Maximum Strength Cream 747
Preparation H Cooling Gel 747
Preparation H 747
Sudafed PE Tablets 711
Vicks Sinex Nasal Spray and Ultra Fine Mist for Sinus Relief............... 2677
Zicam Concentrated Cough Mist for Kids Plus D Cool Cherry......... 643
Zicam Concentrated Cough Mist Plus D Cool Cherry...................... 642

Phenylephrine Tannate (Sympathomimetics tend to produce hyperglycemia and may lead to loss of glycemic control).
No products indexed under this heading.

Phenylpropanolamine Hydrochloride (Sympathomimetics tend to produce hyperglycemia and may lead to loss of glycemic control).
No products indexed under this heading.

Phenytoin (Phenytoin tends to produce hyperglycemia and may lead to loss of glycemic control).
No products indexed under this heading.

Phenytoin Sodium (Phenytoin tends to produce hyperglycemia and may lead to loss of glycemic control). Products include:
Phenytek Capsules 2153

IMPORTANT NOTE: Always consult each drug listing in the patient's regimen for possible interactions.

Pirbuterol Acetate (Sympathomimetics tend to produce hyperglycemia and may lead to loss of glycemic control). Products include:
- Maxair Autohaler 1820

Polyestradiol Phosphate (Estrogens tend to produce hyperglycemia and may lead to loss of glycemic control).
- No products indexed under this heading.

Polythiazide (Thiazides tend to produce hyperglycemia and may lead to loss of glycemic control).
- No products indexed under this heading.

Prednisolone Acetate (Corticosteroids tend to produce hyperglycemia and may lead to loss of glycemic control). Products include:
- Blephamide Ophthalmic Ointment 563
- Blephamide Ophthalmic Suspension 564
- Poly-Pred Liquifilm Ophthalmic Suspension .... ⊙231
- Pred Forte Ophthalmic Suspension .... ⊙233
- Pred Mild Sterile Ophthalmic Suspension .... ⊙236
- Pred-G Ophthalmic Suspension .... ⊙234
- Pred-G Sterile Ophthalmic Ointment .... ⊙235

Prednisolone Sodium Phosphate (Corticosteroids tend to produce hyperglycemia and may lead to loss of glycemic control). Products include:
- Pediapred Oral Solution 3319

Prednisolone Tebutate (Corticosteroids tend to produce hyperglycemia and may lead to loss of glycemic control).
- No products indexed under this heading.

Prednisone (Corticosteroids tend to produce hyperglycemia and may lead to loss of glycemic control).
- No products indexed under this heading.

Procainamide Hydrochloride (Cationic drugs that are eliminated by renal tubular secretion theoretically have the potential for interaction with metformin by competing for common renal tubular transport system).
- No products indexed under this heading.

Prochlorperazine (Phenothiazines tend to produce hyperglycemia and may lead to loss of glycemic control).
- No products indexed under this heading.

Promethazine Hydrochloride (Phenothiazines tend to produce hyperglycemia and may lead to loss of glycemic control). Products include:
- Phenergan 3438

Pseudoephedrine Hydrochloride (Sympathomimetics tend to produce hyperglycemia and may lead to loss of glycemic control). Products include:
- Advil Allergy Sinus Caplets .... ▣737
- Advil Cold & Sinus .... ▣739
- Advil Flu & Body Ache Caplets .... ▣739
- Children's Advil Cold Suspension ... ▣741
- Advil Multi-Symptom Cold Caplets .... ▣738
- Allegra-D 12 Hour Extended-Release Tablets 2860
- Allegra-D 24 Hour Extended-Release Tablets 2862
- Balamine DM 739
- BC Cold Powder .... ▣612
- Benadryl Allergy & Cold Tablets ..... ▣692
- Benadryl Allergy & Sinus Headache Caplets & Gelcaps ...... ▣693
- Children's Benadryl Allergy & Cold Fastmelt Tablets .... ▣695
- Benadryl Maximum Strength Severe Allergy & Sinus Headache Caplets .... ▣694
- Children's Benadryl D Allergy & Sinus Fastmelt Tablets .... ▣694
- Children's Benadryl D Liquid Medication .... ▣693
- Benadryl D Tablets .... ▣694
- Contac Non-Drowsy 12 Hour Cold Caplets .... ▣614
- Contac Non-Drowsy Timed Release 12 Hour Cold Caplets .... ▣615
- Contac Severe Cold and Flu Caplets Maximum Strength .... ▣615
- Contac Severe Cold and Flu Caplets Non-Drowsy .... ▣615
- Children's Dimetapp Cold & Allergy Elixir .... ▣745
- Children's Dimetapp DM Cold & Cough Elixir .... ▣745
- Children's Dimetapp Long Acting Cough Plus Cold Syrup .... ▣746
- Dimetapp Infant Drops Decongestant Plus Cough .... ▣746
- Children's Motrin Cold Non-Staining Dye-Free Oral Suspension 1838
- Children's Motrin Cold Oral Suspension 1838
- Motrin Cold & Sinus Caplets 1836
- PediaCare Decongestant & Cough Infant Drops .... ▣705
- PediaCare Decongestant Infants' Drops .... ▣705
- PediaCare Long-Acting Cough Plus Cold Liquid .... ▣704
- PediaCare Multi-Symptom Cold Liquid .... ▣704
- PediaCare NightRest Cough & Cold Liquid .... ▣704
- Robitussin Allergy & Cough Syrup .. ▣750
- Robitussin CF Liquid .... ▣755
- Robitussin Cough & Cold Liquid-filled Capsules .... ▣750
- Robitussin Cough, Cold & Flu Liquid-filled Capsules .... ▣750
- Robitussin Cough & Cold Infant Drops .... ▣755
- Robitussin Flu Liquid .... ▣752
- Robitussin Maximum Strength Cough & Cold Liquid .... ▣754
- Robitussin PE Syrup .... ▣753
- Robitussin Pediatric Cough & Cold Liquid .... ▣754
- Robitussin PM Cough & Cold Liquid .... ▣752
- Robitussin Severe Congestion Liquid-filled Capsules .... ▣751
- Simply Stuffy Liquid 1841
- Singlet Caplets .... ▣636
- Sudafed 12 Hour Caplets .... ▣708
- Sudafed 24 Hour Tablets .... ▣709
- Sudafed Nasal Decongestant Tablets .... ▣709
- Sudafed Severe Cold .... ▣710
- Sudafed Non-Drying Sinus Liquid Caps .... ▣709
- Sudafed Sinus & Allergy Tablets ..... ▣710
- Sudafed Sinus Headache .... ▣711
- TheraFlu Cold & Cough Hot Liquid .... ▣680
- TheraFlu Cold & Sore Throat Hot Liquid .... ▣680
- TheraFlu Flu & Chest Congestion Non-Drowsy Hot Liquid .... ▣681
- TheraFlu Flu & Sore Throat Hot Liquid .... ▣681
- TheraFlu Severe Cold Non-Drowsy Hot Liquid .... ▣683
- TheraFlu Severe Cold & Cough Hot Liquid .... ▣683
- TheraFlu Severe Cold Caplets .... ▣679
- TheraFlu Severe Cold Hot Liquid .... ▣682
- TheraFlu Severe Cold Non-Drowsy Caplets .... ▣679
- Triaminic Chest & Nasal Congestion Liquid .... ▣685
- Triaminic Cold & Allergy Liquid ...... ▣685
- Triaminic Cold & Cough Liquid ...... ▣685
- Triaminic Cough Liquid .... ▣687
- Triaminic Cough & Nasal Congestion Liquid .... ▣687
- Triaminic Cough & Sore Throat Liquid .... ▣687
- Triaminic Flu, Cough & Fever Liquid .... ▣685
- Triaminic Night Time Cough & Cold Liquid .... ▣685
- Triaminic Allergy Runny Nose & Congestion Softchews .... ▣688
- Triaminic Cold & Cough Softchews .... ▣688
- Triaminic Cough & Sore Throat Softchews .... ▣689
- Tylenol Sinus NightTime Caplets .... ▣663
- Children's Tylenol Plus Cold & Allergy Suspension Liquid 1850
- Children's Tylenol Plus Cold NightTime Suspension Liquid 1851
- Children's Tylenol Plus Cold & Cough Suspension Liquid and Chewable Tablets 1851
- Children's Tylenol Plus Cold Chewable Tablets 1851
- Children's Tylenol Plus Cold Daytime Non-Drowsy Suspension Liquid 1851
- Children's Tylenol Plus Flu Suspension Liquid 1853
- Concentrated Tylenol Infants' Drops Plus Cold 1851
- Concentrated Tylenol Infants' Drops Plus Cold and Cough 1851
- Tylenol Cold & Flu Severe Daytime Liquid with Cool Burst 1846
- Tylenol Cold & Flu Severe NightTime Liquid with Cool Burst 1846
- Tylenol Cold Severe Congestion Non-Drowsy Caplets with Cool Burst 1846
- Tylenol Allergy Complete Night Time Caplets 1844
- Tylenol Allergy Complete Multi-Symptom Caplets and Gelcaps with Cool Burst 1844
- Tylenol Flu NightTime Gelcaps 1846
- Tylenol Flu Day Non-Drowsy Gelcaps 1846
- Concentrated Tylenol Infants' Drops Plus Cold Nasal Congestant, Fever Reducer & Pain Reliever .... ▣668
- Concentrated Tylenol Infants' Drops Plus Cold & Cough Nasal Decongestant, Fever Reducer & Pain Reliever .... ▣668
- Multi-Symptom Tylenol Cold Night Time Caplets 1845
- Multi-Symptom Tylenol Cold Day Non-Drowsy Caplets and Gelcaps 1845
- Tylenol Sinus Day Non-Drowsy 1848
- Tylenol Sinus Night Time Caplets 1848
- Tylenol Sinus Severe Congestion Caplets with Cool Burst 1848
- Vicks 44D Cough & Head Congestion Relief 2676
- Vicks 44D Cough & Head Congestion Relief Liquid .... ▣721
- Vicks 44M Cough, Cold & Flu Relief 2676
- Pediatric Vicks 44m Cough & Cold Relief 2673
- Vicks DayQuil LiquiCaps/Liquid Multi-Symptom Cold/Flu Relief ..... ▣723
- Vicks DayQuil Multi-Symptom Cold/Flu Relief LiquiCaps 2675
- Vicks DayQuil Multi-Symptom Cold/Flu Relief Liquid 2675
- Children's Vicks NyQuil Cold/Cough Relief 2671
- Vicks NyQuil LiquiCaps 2677
- Vicks NyQuil LiquiCaps/Liquid Multi-Symptom Cold/Flu Relief ..... ▣725
- Vicks NyQuil Liquid 2677
- Zyrtec-D 12 Hour Extended Release Tablets 2591

Pseudoephedrine Sulfate (Sympathomimetics tend to produce hyperglycemia and may lead to loss of glycemic control). Products include:
- Alavert Allergy & Sinus D-12 Hour Tablets .... ▣743
- Clarinex-D 24-Hour Extended-Release Tablets 3012
- Claritin-D Non-Drowsy 12 Hour Tablets .... ▣731
- Claritin-D Non-Drowsy 24 Hour Tablets .... ▣731

Quinestrol (Estrogens tend to produce hyperglycemia and may lead to loss of glycemic control).
- No products indexed under this heading.

Quinidine Gluconate (Cationic drugs that are eliminated by renal tubular secretion theoretically have the potential for interaction with metformin by competing for common renal tubular transport system).
- No products indexed under this heading.

Quinidine Polygalacturonate (Cationic drugs that are eliminated by renal tubular secretion theoretically have the potential for interaction with metformin by competing for common renal tubular transport system).
- No products indexed under this heading.

Quinidine Sulfate (Cationic drugs that are eliminated by renal tubular secretion theoretically have the potential for interaction with metformin by competing for common renal tubular transport system).
- No products indexed under this heading.

Quinine Sulfate (Cationic drugs that are eliminated by renal tubular secretion theoretically have the potential for interaction with metformin by competing for common renal tubular transport system).
- No products indexed under this heading.

Ranitidine Hydrochloride (Cationic drugs that are eliminated by renal tubular secretion theoretically have the potential for interaction with metformin by competing for common renal tubular transport system). Products include:
- Zantac 1597
- Zantac Injection 1593
- Zantac 75 Tablets .... ▣715
- Zantac 150 Maximum Strength Tablets .... ▣715
- Zantac Injection Pharmacy Bulk Package 1595

Salmeterol Xinafoate (Sympathomimetics tend to produce hyperglycemia and may lead to loss of glycemic control). Products include:
- Advair Diskus 100/50 1291
- Advair Diskus 250/50 1291
- Advair Diskus 500/50 1291
- Serevent Diskus 1540

Spironolactone (Diuretics tend to produce hyperglycemia and may lead to loss of glycemic control).
- No products indexed under this heading.

Terbutaline Sulfate (Sympathomimetics tend to produce hyperglycemia and may lead to loss of glycemic control).
- No products indexed under this heading.

Thioridazine Hydrochloride (Phenothiazines tend to produce hyperglycemia and may lead to loss of glycemic control). Products include:
- Thioridazine Hydrochloride Tablets 2122

Thyroglobulin (Thyroid products tend to produce hyperglycemia and may lead to loss of glycemic control).
- No products indexed under this heading.

Thyroid (Thyroid products tend to produce hyperglycemia and may lead to loss of glycemic control).
No products indexed under this heading.

Thyroxine (Thyroid products tend to produce hyperglycemia and may lead to loss of glycemic control).
No products indexed under this heading.

Thyroxine Sodium (Thyroid products tend to produce hyperglycemia and may lead to loss of glycemic control).
No products indexed under this heading.

Torsemide (Diuretics tend to produce hyperglycemia and may lead to loss of glycemic control).
No products indexed under this heading.

Triamcinolone (Corticosteroids tend to produce hyperglycemia and may lead to loss of glycemic control).
No products indexed under this heading.

Triamcinolone Acetonide (Corticosteroids tend to produce hyperglycemia and may lead to loss of glycemic control). Products include:
Azmacort Inhalation Aerosol **1701**
Nasacort HFA Inhalation Aerosol **2939**
Nasacort AQ Nasal Spray **2937**

Triamcinolone Diacetate (Corticosteroids tend to produce hyperglycemia and may lead to loss of glycemic control).
No products indexed under this heading.

Triamcinolone Hexacetonide (Corticosteroids tend to produce hyperglycemia and may lead to loss of glycemic control).
No products indexed under this heading.

Triamterene (Diuretics tend to produce hyperglycemia and may lead to loss of glycemic control). Products include:
Dyazide Capsules **1389**
Dyrenium Capsules **3390**
Maxzide **2150**

Trifluoperazine Hydrochloride (Phenothiazines tend to produce hyperglycemia and may lead to loss of glycemic control).
No products indexed under this heading.

Trimethoprim (Cationic drugs that are eliminated by renal tubular secretion theoretically have the potential for interaction with metformin by competing for common renal tubular transport system).
No products indexed under this heading.

Trimethoprim Sulfate (Cationic drugs that are eliminated by renal tubular secretion theoretically have the potential for interaction with metformin by competing for common renal tubular transport system). Products include:
Polytrim Ophthalmic Solution **570**

Tyropanoate Sodium (Intravascular contrast studies with iodinated materials can lead to acute alteration of renal function and have been associated with lactic acidosis in patients receiving metformin. Therefore, discontinue metformin at the time of or prior to the procedure, and for 48 hours subsequent to the procedure until renal function is normal).
No products indexed under this heading.

Vancomycin Hydrochloride (Cationic drugs that are eliminated by renal tubular secretion theoretically have the potential for interaction with metformin by competing for common renal tubular transport system). Products include:
Vancocin HCl Capsules, USP **3370**

Verapamil Hydrochloride (Calcium channel blocking drugs tend to produce hyperglycemia and may lead to loss of glycemic control). Products include:
Covera-HS Tablets **3135**
Tarka Tablets **519**
Verelan PM Capsules **3120**

Food Interactions

Alcohol (Alcohol is known to potentiate the effect of metformin on lactate metabolism; therefore, patients should be warned against excessive acute or chronic intake).

FORTAZ INJECTION
(Ceftazidime Sodium) **1422**
See Fortaz for Injection

FORTAZ FOR INJECTION
(Ceftazidime) **1422**
May interact with aminoglycosides and certain other agents. Compounds in these categories include:

Amikacin Sulfate (Potential for nephrotoxicity following concomitant administration).
No products indexed under this heading.

Chloramphenicol (Possibility of antagonism *"in vivo,"* particularly when bactericidal activity is desired; avoid this combination).
No products indexed under this heading.

Chloramphenicol Palmitate (Possibility of antagonism *"in vivo,"* particularly when bactericidal activity is desired; avoid this combination).
No products indexed under this heading.

Chloramphenicol Sodium Succinate (Possibility of antagonism *"in vivo,"* particularly when bactericidal activity is desired; avoid this combination).
No products indexed under this heading.

Furosemide (Potential for nephrotoxicity following concomitant administration). Products include:
Furosemide Tablets **2117**

Gentamicin Sulfate (Potential for nephrotoxicity following concomitant administration). Products include:
Garamycin Injectable **3028**
Genoptic Sterile Ophthalmic Solution .... ⊙**227**
Pred-G Ophthalmic Suspension ...... ⊙**234**
Pred-G Sterile Ophthalmic Ointment .... ⊙**235**

Kanamycin Sulfate (Potential for nephrotoxicity following concomitant administration).
No products indexed under this heading.

Streptomycin Sulfate (Potential for nephrotoxicity following concomitant administration).
No products indexed under this heading.

Tobramycin (Potential for nephrotoxicity following concomitant administration). Products include:
TOBI Solution for Inhalation **1015**
TobraDex Ophthalmic Ointment **558**
TobraDex Ophthalmic Suspension ... **558**
Zylet Ophthalmic Suspension **3508**

Tobramycin Sulfate (Potential for nephrotoxicity following concomitant administration).
No products indexed under this heading.

FORTEO FOR INJECTION
(Teriparatide) **1739**
May interact with cardiac glycosides. Compounds in these categories include:

Deslanoside (Hypercalcemia may pre-dispose patients to digitalis toxicity. Because teriparatide transiently increases serum calcium, teriparatide should be used with caution in patients taking digitalis).
No products indexed under this heading.

Digitalis Glycoside Preparations (Hypercalcemia may pre-dispose patients to digitalis toxicity. Because teriparatide transiently increases serum calcium, teriparatide should be used with caution in patients taking digitalis).
No products indexed under this heading.

Digitoxin (Hypercalcemia may pre-dispose patients to digitalis toxicity. Because teriparatide transiently increases serum calcium, teriparatide should be used with caution in patients taking digitalis).
No products indexed under this heading.

Digoxin (Hypercalcemia may pre-dispose patients to digitalis toxicity. Because teriparatide transiently increases serum calcium, teriparatide should be used with caution in patients taking digitalis). Products include:
Digitek Tablets **2146**
Lanoxicaps Capsules **1458**
Lanoxin Injection **1462**
Lanoxin Tablets **1468**
Lanoxin Injection Pediatric **1465**

FORTICAL NASAL SPRAY
(Calcitonin-Salmon) **3336**
None cited in PDR database.

FOSAMAX ORAL SOLUTION
(Alendronate Sodium) **1949**
See Fosamax Tablets

FOSAMAX TABLETS
(Alendronate Sodium) **1949**
May interact with antacids containing aluminum, calcium and magnesium, calcium preparations, non-steroidal anti-inflammatory agents, and certain other agents. Compounds in these categories include:

Aluminum Carbonate (May interfere with the absorption of alendronate; patient must wait at least one-half hour after taking alendronate before taking any drug).
No products indexed under this heading.

Aluminum Hydroxide (May interfere with the absorption of alendronate; patient must wait at least one-half hour after taking alendronate before taking any drug). Products include:
Gaviscon Regular Strength Liquid .. **620**
Gaviscon Regular Strength Tablets **619**
Gaviscon Extra Strength Liquid **620**
Gaviscon Extra Strength Tablets **619**
Maalox Max Maximum Strength Antacid/Anti-Gas Liquid **2165**
Maalox Regular Strength Antacid/Antigas Liquid **2164**

Aspirin (Co-administration with doses of alendronate greater than 10 mg/day and aspirin-containing compounds can increase the incidence of gastrointestinal adverse events; one case of anastomotic ulcer with mild hemorrhage has been reported in a patient with history of peptic ulcer disease and gastrectomy on alendronate 10 mg/day plus aspirin). Products include:
Aggrenox Capsules **855**
Bayer, Aspirin Regimen **606**
Bayer Aspirin Tablets **3515**
BC Powder **612**
BC Allergy Sinus Cold Powder **612**
Arthritis Strength BC Powder **612**
BC Sinus Cold Powder **612**
Ecotrin Enteric Coated Aspirin Low, Regular and Maximum Strength Tablets **1627**
Goody's Body Pain Formula Powder **621**
Goody's Extra Strength Headache Powder **621**
Goody's Extra Strength Pain Relief Tablets **621**
Percodan Tablets **1115**
St. Joseph 81 mg Aspirin Chewable and Enteric Coated Tablets **1841**

Aspirin, Enteric Coated (Co-administration with doses of alendronate greater than 10 mg/day and aspirin-containing compounds can increase the incidence of gastrointestinal adverse events; one case of anastomotic ulcer with mild hemorrhage has been reported in a patient with history of peptic ulcer disease and gastrectomy on alendronate 10 mg/day plus aspirin).
No products indexed under this heading.

Aspirin Buffered (Co-administration with doses of alendronate greater than 10 mg/day and aspirin-containing compounds can increase the incidence of gastrointestinal adverse events; one case of anastomotic ulcer with mild hemorrhage has been reported in a patient with history of peptic ulcer disease and gastrectomy on alendronate 10 mg/day plus aspirin).
No products indexed under this heading.

Calcium Carbonate (May interfere with the absorption of alendronate;

patient must wait at least one-half hour after taking alendronate before taking any drug). Products include:
Actonel with Calcium Tablets 2684
Caltrate 600 PLUS Chewables .... ▣779
Caltrate 600 PLUS Tablets .... ▣779
Caltrate 600 + D Tablets .... ▣779
Encora Capsules 3298
Encora AM Tablets 3298
Encora PM Tablets 3298
Gas-X with Maalox .... ▣675
Maalox Regular Strength Antacid Tablets 2166
Quick Dissolve Maalox Max Maximum Strength Antacid/Antigas Tablets 2165
Maalox Max Quick Dissolve Maximum Strength Chewable Tablets .... ▣678
Os-Cal Chewable Tablets .... ▣765
Pepcid Complete Chewable Tablets 1672
PremCal Light, Regular, and Extra Strength Tablets................ ▣762
Rolaids Tablets .... ▣707
Extra Strength Rolaids Softchews .... ▣708
Extra Strength Rolaids Tablets .... ▣707
Rolaids Multi-Symptom Antacid & Antigas Tablets .... ▣708
Tums .... ▣639

Calcium Chloride (May interfere with the absorption of alendronate; patient must wait at least one-half hour after taking alendronate before taking any drug).
No products indexed under this heading.

Calcium Citrate (May interfere with the absorption of alendronate; patient must wait at least one-half hour after taking alendronate before taking any drug). Products include:
Active Calcium Tablets 3342
Citracal Tablets 2108

Calcium Glubionate (May interfere with the absorption of alendronate; patient must wait at least one-half hour after taking alendronate before taking any drug).
No products indexed under this heading.

Celecoxib (Since NSAID use is associated with gastrointestinal irritation, caution should be used during concomitant use; no increase in the incidence of gastrointestinal irritation was reported in clinical trials). Products include:
Celebrex Capsules 3130

Diclofenac Potassium (Since NSAID use is associated with gastrointestinal irritation, caution should be used during concomitant use; no increase in the incidence of gastrointestinal irritation was reported in clinical trials). Products include:
Cataflam Tablets 2173

Diclofenac Sodium (Since NSAID use is associated with gastrointestinal irritation, caution should be used during concomitant use; no increase in the incidence of gastrointestinal irritation was reported in clinical trials). Products include:
Arthrotec Tablets 3126
Voltaren Ophthalmic Solution 2300
Voltaren Tablets 2298
Voltaren-XR Tablets 2301

Etodolac (Since NSAID use is associated with gastrointestinal irritation, caution should be used during concomitant use; no increase in the incidence of gastrointestinal irritation was reported in clinical trials).
No products indexed under this heading.

Fenoprofen Calcium (Since NSAID use is associated with gastrointestinal irritation, caution should be used during concomitant use; no increase in the incidence of gastrointestinal irritation was reported in clinical trials). Products include:
Nalfon Capsules 2504

Flurbiprofen (Since NSAID use is associated with gastrointestinal irritation, caution should be used during concomitant use; no increase in the incidence of gastrointestinal irritation was reported in clinical trials).
No products indexed under this heading.

Ibuprofen (Since NSAID use is associated with gastrointestinal irritation, caution should be used during concomitant use; no increase in the incidence of gastrointestinal irritation was reported in clinical trials). Products include:
Advil Allergy Sinus Caplets .... ▣737
Advil .... ▣737
Children's Advil Suspension .... ▣742
Children's Advil Chewable Tablets .. ▣741
Advil Cold & Sinus .... ▣739
Advil Flu & Body Ache Caplets .... ▣739
Children's Advil Cold Suspension ... ▣741
Infants' Advil Concentrated Drops .. ▣743
Junior Strength Advil Swallow Tablets .... ▣740
Advil Migraine Liquigels .... ▣740
Advil Multi-Symptom Cold Caplets .... ▣738
Combunox Tablets 1183
Children's Motrin Oral Suspension and Chewable Tablets 1837
Children's Motrin Cold Non-Staining Dye-Free Oral Suspension 1838
Children's Motrin Cold Oral Suspension 1838
Children's Motrin Non-Staining Dye-Free Oral Suspension 1837
Motrin Cold & Sinus Caplets 1836
Motrin IB Tablets and Caplets 1836
Infants' Motrin Concentrated Drops 1837
Infants' Motrin Non-Staining Dye-Free Drops 1837
Junior Strength Motrin Caplets and Chewable Tablets 1837
Vicoprofen Tablets 533

Indomethacin (Since NSAID use is associated with gastrointestinal irritation, caution should be used during concomitant use; no increase in the incidence of gastrointestinal irritation was reported in clinical trials). Products include:
Indocin 1968

Indomethacin Sodium Trihydrate (Since NSAID use is associated with gastrointestinal irritation, caution should be used during concomitant use; no increase in the incidence of gastrointestinal irritation was reported in clinical trials). Products include:
Indocin I.V. 1973

Ketoprofen (Since NSAID use is associated with gastrointestinal irritation, caution should be used during concomitant use; no increase in the incidence of gastrointestinal irritation was reported in clinical trials).
No products indexed under this heading.

Ketorolac Tromethamine (Since NSAID use is associated with gastrointestinal irritation, caution should be used during concomitant use; no increase in the incidence of gastrointestinal irritation was reported in clinical trials). Products include:
Acular Ophthalmic Solution 561
Acular LS Ophthalmic Solution 562

Magaldrate (May interfere with the absorption of alendronate; patient must wait at least one-half hour after taking alendronate before taking any drug).
No products indexed under this heading.

Magnesium Hydroxide (May interfere with the absorption of alendronate; patient must wait at least one-half hour after taking alendronate before taking any drug). Products include:
Maalox Max Maximum Strength Antacid/Anti-Gas Liquid................ 2165
Maalox Regular Strength Antacid/Antigas Liquid................. 2164
Pepcid Complete Chewable Tablets 1672
Rolaids Tablets .... ▣707
Extra Strength Rolaids Tablets .... ▣707
Rolaids Multi-Symptom Antacid & Antigas Tablets .... ▣708

Magnesium Oxide (May interfere with the absorption of alendronate; patient must wait at least one-half hour after taking alendronate before taking any drug). Products include:
Beelith Tablets 784
PremCal Light, Regular, and Extra Strength Tablets................ ▣762

Meclofenamate Sodium (Since NSAID use is associated with gastrointestinal irritation, caution should be used during concomitant use; no increase in the incidence of gastrointestinal irritation was reported in clinical trials).
No products indexed under this heading.

Mefenamic Acid (Since NSAID use is associated with gastrointestinal irritation, caution should be used during concomitant use; no increase in the incidence of gastrointestinal irritation was reported in clinical trials).
No products indexed under this heading.

Meloxicam (Since NSAID use is associated with gastrointestinal irritation, caution should be used during concomitant use; no increase in the incidence of gastrointestinal irritation was reported in clinical trials). Products include:
Mobic Oral Suspension 893
Mobic Tablets 893

Nabumetone (Since NSAID use is associated with gastrointestinal irritation, caution should be used during concomitant use; no increase in the incidence of gastrointestinal irritation was reported in clinical trials). Products include:
Relafen Tablets 1523

Naproxen (Since NSAID use is associated with gastrointestinal irritation, caution should be used during concomitant use; no increase in the incidence of gastrointestinal irritation was reported in clinical trials). Products include:
EC-Naprosyn Delayed-Release Tablets 2769
Naprosyn Suspension 2769
Naprosyn Tablets 2769
Prevacid NapraPAC 3277

Naproxen Sodium (Since NSAID use is associated with gastrointestinal irritation, caution should be used during concomitant use; no increase in the incidence of gastrointestinal irritation was reported in clinical trials). Products include:
Aleve Tablets, Caplets and Gelcaps .... ▣605
Anaprox Tablets 2769
Anaprox DS Tablets 2769

Oxaprozin (Since NSAID use is associated with gastrointestinal irritation, caution should be used during concomitant use; no increase in the incidence of gastrointestinal irritation was reported in clinical trials).
No products indexed under this heading.

Phenylbutazone (Since NSAID use is associated with gastrointestinal irritation, caution should be used during concomitant use; no increase in the incidence of gastrointestinal irritation was reported in clinical trials).
No products indexed under this heading.

Piroxicam (Since NSAID use is associated with gastrointestinal irritation, caution should be used during concomitant use; no increase in the incidence of gastrointestinal irritation was reported in clinical trials).
No products indexed under this heading.

Ranitidine Hydrochloride (Intravenous ranitidine has shown to double the bioavailability of oral alendronate; clinical significance of this increased bioavailability and whether similar increases will occur with oral ranitidine are unknown). Products include:
Zantac 1597
Zantac Injection 1593
Zantac 75 Tablets .... ▣715
Zantac 150 Maximum Strength Tablets .... ▣715
Zantac Injection Pharmacy Bulk Package 1595

Rofecoxib (Since NSAID use is associated with gastrointestinal irritation, caution should be used during concomitant use; no increase in the incidence of gastrointestinal irritation was reported in clinical trials).
No products indexed under this heading.

Sulindac (Since NSAID use is associated with gastrointestinal irritation, caution should be used during concomitant use; no increase in the incidence of gastrointestinal irritation was reported in clinical trials). Products include:
Clinoril Tablets 1899

Tolmetin Sodium (Since NSAID use is associated with gastrointestinal irritation, caution should be used during concomitant use; no increase in the incidence of gastrointestinal irritation was reported in clinical trials).
No products indexed under this heading.

Valdecoxib (Since NSAID use is associated with gastrointestinal irritation, caution should be used during concomitant use; no increase in the incidence of gastrointestinal irritation was reported in clinical trials).
No products indexed under this heading.

Food Interactions

Beverages, caffeine-containing (Concomitant administration of alendronate with coffee reduces bioavailability by approximately 60%).

Meal, unspecified (Standardized breakfast decreases bioavailability by approximately 40% when alendronate is administered either one-half or 1 hour before breakfast).

Orange Juice (Concomitant administration of alendronate with orange juice reduces bioavailability by approximately 60%).

FOSAMAX PLUS D TABLETS

(Alendronate Sodium, Cholecalciferol)....................................... 1956

May interact with antacids containing aluminum, calcium and magnesium, aspirin-acetylsalicylic acid, calcium preparations, non-steroidal anti-inflammatory agents, and certain other agents. Compounds in these categories include:

Aluminum Carbonate (Antacids may interfere with the absorption of aledronate. Therefore, patients must wait at least one-half hour after taking aledronate sodium/ cholecalciferol before taking any other oral medications).

No products indexed under this heading.

Aluminum Hydroxide (Antacids may interfere with the absorption of aledronate. Therefore, patients must wait at least one-half hour after taking aledronate sodium/ cholecalciferol before taking any other oral medications). Products include:

- Gaviscon Regular Strength Liquid .. ■620
- Gaviscon Regular Strength Tablets.. ■619
- Gaviscon Extra Strength Liquid ...... ■620
- Gaviscon Extra Strength Tablets .... ■619
- Maalox Max Maximum Strength Antacid/Anti-Gas Liquid................. 2165
- Maalox Regular Strength Antacid/Antigas Liquid................. 2164

Aspirin (Studies have shown an increased incidence of upper gastrointestinal adverse events in patients receiving concomitant therapy with daily doses of aledronate greater than 10 mg and aspirin-containing products). Products include:

- Aggrenox Capsules 855
- Bayer, Aspirin Regimen .... ■606
- Bayer Aspirin Tablets 3515
- BC Powder .... ■612
- BC Allergy Sinus Cold Powder .... ■612
- Arthritis Strength BC Powder .... ■612
- BC Sinus Cold Powder .... ■612
- Ecotrin Enteric Coated Aspirin Low, Regular and Maximum Strength Tablets........................... 1627
- Goody's Body Pain Formula Powder.. ■621
- Goody's Extra Strength Headache Powder....................... ■621
- Goody's Extra Strength Pain Relief Tablets.............................. ■621
- Percodan Tablets............................ 1115
- St. Joseph 81 mg Aspirin Chewable and Enteric Coated Tablets... 1841

Aspirin, Enteric Coated (Studies have shown an increased incidence of upper gastrointestinal adverse events in patients receiving concomitant therapy with daily doses of aledronate greater than 10 mg and aspirin-containing products).

No products indexed under this heading.

Aspirin Buffered (Studies have shown an increased incidence of upper gastrointestinal adverse events in patients receiving concomitant therapy with daily doses of aledronate greater than 10 mg and aspirin-containing products).

No products indexed under this heading.

Calcium Carbonate (Calcium supplements may interfere with the absorption of aledronate. Therefore, patients must wait at least one-half hour after taking aledronate sodium/ cholecalciferol before taking any other oral medications). Products include:

- Actonel with Calcium Tablets 2684
- Caltrate 600 PLUS Chewables .... ■779
- Caltrate 600 PLUS Tablets .... ■779
- Caltrate 600 + D Tablets .... ■779
- Encora Capsules 3298
- Encora AM Tablets 3298
- Encora PM Tablets 3298
- Gas-X with Maalox .... ■675
- Maalox Regular Strength Antacid Tablets... 2166
- Quick Dissolve Maalox Max Maximum Strength Antacid/Antigas Tablets................ 2165
- Maalox Max Quick Dissolve Maximum Strength Chewable Tablets.. ■678
- Os-Cal Chewable Tablets .... ■765
- Pepcid Complete Chewable Tablets 1672
- PremCal Light, Regular, and Extra Strength Tablets................. ■762
- Rolaids Tablets .... ■707
- Extra Strength Rolaids Softchews .... ■708
- Extra Strength Rolaids Tablets .... ■707
- Rolaids Multi-Symptom Antacid & Antigas Tablets.......................... ■708
- Tums .... ■639

Calcium Chloride (Calcium supplements may interfere with the absorption of aledronate. Therefore, patients must wait at least one-half hour after taking aledronate sodium/ cholecalciferol before taking any other oral medications).

No products indexed under this heading.

Calcium Citrate (Calcium supplements may interfere with the absorption of aledronate. Therefore, patients must wait at least one-half hour after taking aledronate sodium/ cholecalciferol before taking any other oral medications). Products include:

- Active Calcium Tablets 3342
- Citracal Tablets 2108

Calcium Glubionate (Calcium supplements may interfere with the absorption of aledronate. Therefore, patients must wait at least one-half hour after taking aledronate sodium/ cholecalciferol before taking any other oral medications).

No products indexed under this heading.

Celecoxib (Since NSAID use is associated with gastrointestinal irritation, caution should be used during concomitant use with aledronate sodium/cholecalciferol. No increase in the incidence of gastrointestinal irritation was reported in clinical trials). Products include:

- Celebrex Capsules 3130

Cholestyramine (Concomitant use with bile acid sequestrants may impair the absorption of vitamin D).

No products indexed under this heading.

Colestipol (Concomitant use with bile acid sequestrants may impair the absorption of vitamin D).

No products indexed under this heading.

Diclofenac Potassium (Since NSAID use is associated with gastrointestinal irritation, caution should be used during concomitant use with aledronate sodium/cholecalciferol. No increase in the incidence of gastrointestinal irritation was reported in clinical trials). Products include:

- Cataflam Tablets 2173

Diclofenac Sodium (Since NSAID use is associated with gastrointestinal irritation, caution should be used during concomitant use with aledronate sodium/cholecalciferol. No increase in the incidence of gastrointestinal irritation was reported in clinical trials). Products include:

- Arthrotec Tablets 3126
- Voltaren Ophthalmic Solution 2300
- Voltaren Tablets 2298
- Voltaren-XR Tablets 2301

Etodolac (Since NSAID use is associated with gastrointestinal irritation, caution should be used during concomitant use with aledronate sodium/cholecalciferol. No increase in the incidence of gastrointestinal irritation was reported in clinical trials).

No products indexed under this heading.

Fenoprofen Calcium (Since NSAID use is associated with gastrointestinal irritation, caution should be used during concomitant use with aledronate sodium/cholecalciferol. No increase in the incidence of gastrointestinal irritation was reported in clinical trials). Products include:

- Nalfon Capsules 2504

Flurbiprofen (Since NSAID use is associated with gastrointestinal irritation, caution should be used during concomitant use with aledronate sodium/cholecalciferol. No increase in the incidence of gastrointestinal irritation was reported in clinical trials).

No products indexed under this heading.

Ibuprofen (Since NSAID use is associated with gastrointestinal irritation, caution should be used during concomitant use with aledronate sodium/cholecalciferol. No increase in the incidence of gastrointestinal irritation was reported in clinical trials). Products include:

- Advil Allergy Sinus Caplets .... ■737
- Advil .... ■737
- Children's Advil Suspension .... ■742
- Children's Advil Chewable Tablets .. ■741
- Advil Cold & Sinus .... ■739
- Advil Flu & Body Ache Caplets .... ■739
- Children's Advil Cold Suspension ... ■741
- Infants' Advil Concentrated Drops .. ■743
- Junior Strength Advil Swallow Tablets.. ■740
- Advil Migraine Liquigels .... ■740
- Advil Multi-Symptom Cold Caplets.. ■738
- Combunox Tablets 1183
- Children's Motrin Oral Suspension and Chewable Tablets................... 1837
- Children's Motrin Cold Non-Staining Dye-Free Oral Suspension 1838
- Children's Motrin Cold Oral Suspension 1838
- Children's Motrin Non-Staining Dye-Free Oral Suspension............. 1837
- Motrin Cold & Sinus Caplets 1836
- Motrin IB Tablets and Caplets 1836
- Infants' Motrin Concentrated Drops.. 1837
- Infants' Motrin Non-Staining Dye-Free Drops........................... 1837
- Junior Strength Motrin Caplets and Chewable Tablets................... 1837
- Vicoprofen Tablets 533

Indomethacin (Since NSAID use is associated with gastrointestinal irritation, caution should be used during concomitant use with aledronate sodium/cholecalciferol. No increase in the incidence of gastrointestinal irritation was reported in clinical trials). Products include:

- Indocin 1968

Indomethacin Sodium Trihydrate (Since NSAID use is associated with gastrointestinal irritation, caution should be used during concomitant use with aledronate sodium/cholecalciferol. No increase in the incidence of gastrointestinal irritation was reported in clinical trials). Products include:

- Indocin I.V. 1973

Ketoprofen (Since NSAID use is associated with gastrointestinal irritation, caution should be used during concomitant use with aledronate sodium/cholecalciferol. No increase in the incidence of gastrointestinal irritation was reported in clinical trials).

No products indexed under this heading.

Ketorolac Tromethamine (Since NSAID use is associated with gastrointestinal irritation, caution should be used during concomitant use with aledronate sodium/cholecalciferol. No increase in the incidence of gastrointestinal irritation was reported in clinical trials). Products include:

- Acular Ophthalmic Solution 561
- Acular LS Ophthalmic Solution 562

Magaldrate (Antacids may interfere with the absorption of aledronate. Therefore, patients must wait at least one-half hour after taking aledronate sodium/cholecalciferol before taking any other oral medications).

No products indexed under this heading.

Magnesium Hydroxide (Antacids may interfere with the absorption of aledronate. Therefore, patients must wait at least one-half hour after taking aledronate sodium/ cholecalciferol before taking any other oral medications). Products include:

- Maalox Max Maximum Strength Antacid/Anti-Gas Liquid................. 2165
- Maalox Regular Strength Antacid/Antigas Liquid................. 2164
- Pepcid Complete Chewable Tablets 1672
- Rolaids Tablets .... ■707
- Extra Strength Rolaids Tablets .... ■707
- Rolaids Multi-Symptom Antacid & Antigas Tablets.......................... ■708

Magnesium Oxide (Antacids may interfere with the absorption of aledronate. Therefore, patients must wait at least one-half hour after taking aledronate sodium/cholecalciferol before taking any other oral medications). Products include:

- Beelith Tablets 784
- PremCal Light, Regular, and Extra Strength Tablets................. ■762

Meclofenamate Sodium (Since NSAID use is associated with gastrointestinal irritation, caution should be used during concomitant use with aledronate sodium/cholecalciferol. No increase in the incidence of gastrointestinal irritation was reported in clinical trials).

No products indexed under this heading.

Mefenamic Acid (Since NSAID use is associated with gastrointestinal irritation, caution should be used during concomitant use with aledronate sodium/cholecalciferol. No increase in the incidence of gastrointestinal irritation was reported in clinical trials).

No products indexed under this heading.

Meloxicam (Since NSAID use is associated with gastrointestinal irritation, caution should be used during concomitant use with aledronate sodium/cholecalciferol. No increase in the incidence of gastrointestinal irritation was reported in clinical trials). Products include:

Mobic Oral Suspension **893**
Mobic Tablets **893**

Nabumetone (Since NSAID use is associated with gastrointestinal irritation, caution should be used during concomitant use with aledronate sodium/cholecalciferol. No increase in the incidence of gastrointestinal irritation was reported in clinical trials). Products include:
Relafen Tablets **1523**

Naproxen (Since NSAID use is associated with gastrointestinal irritation, caution should be used during concomitant use with aledronate sodium/cholecalciferol. No increase in the incidence of gastrointestinal irritation was reported in clinical trials). Products include:
EC-Naprosyn Delayed-Release Tablets **2769**
Naprosyn Suspension **2769**
Naprosyn Tablets **2769**
Prevacid NapraPAC **3277**

Naproxen Sodium (Since NSAID use is associated with gastrointestinal irritation, caution should be used during concomitant use with aledronate sodium/cholecalciferol. No increase in the incidence of gastrointestinal irritation was reported in clinical trials). Products include:
Aleve Tablets, Caplets and Gelcaps .... ■**605**
Anaprox Tablets **2769**
Anaprox DS Tablets **2769**

Orlistat (Concomitant use with orlistat may impair the absorption of vitamin D). Products include:
Xenical Capsules **2834**

Oxaprozin (Since NSAID use is associated with gastrointestinal irritation, caution should be used during concomitant use with aledronate sodium/cholecalciferol. No increase in the incidence of gastrointestinal irritation was reported in clinical trials).
No products indexed under this heading.

Phenylbutazone (Since NSAID use is associated with gastrointestinal irritation, caution should be used during concomitant use with aledronate sodium/cholecalciferol. No increase in the incidence of gastrointestinal irritation was reported in clinical trials).
No products indexed under this heading.

Piroxicam (Since NSAID use is associated with gastrointestinal irritation, caution should be used during concomitant use with aledronate sodium/cholecalciferol. No increase in the incidence of gastrointestinal irritation was reported in clinical trials).
No products indexed under this heading.

Ranitidine Hydrochloride (Intravenous ranitidine was shown to double the bioavailability of oral aledronate. The clinical significance of this increased bioavailability and whether similar increases will occur in patients given oral H2-antagonists is unknown). Products include:
Zantac **1597**
Zantac Injection **1593**
Zantac 75 Tablets .... ■**715**
Zantac 150 Maximum Strength Tablets .... ■**715**
Zantac Injection Pharmacy Bulk Package **1595**

Rofecoxib (Since NSAID use is associated with gastrointestinal irritation, caution should be used during concomitant use with aledronate sodium/cholecalciferol. No increase in the incidence of gastrointestinal irritation was reported in clinical trials).
No products indexed under this heading.

Sulindac (Since NSAID use is associated with gastrointestinal irritation, caution should be used during concomitant use with aledronate sodium/cholecalciferol. No increase in the incidence of gastrointestinal irritation was reported in clinical trials). Products include:
Clinoril Tablets **1899**

Tolmetin Sodium (Since NSAID use is associated with gastrointestinal irritation, caution should be used during concomitant use with aledronate sodium/cholecalciferol. No increase in the incidence of gastrointestinal irritation was reported in clinical trials).
No products indexed under this heading.

Valdecoxib (Since NSAID use is associated with gastrointestinal irritation, caution should be used during concomitant use with aledronate sodium/cholecalciferol. No increase in the incidence of gastrointestinal irritation was reported in clinical trials).
No products indexed under this heading.

Food Interactions

Beverages, caffeine-containing (Concomitant administration of alendronate with coffee reduces bioavailability by approximately 60%).

Meal, unspecified (Bioavailability was decreased (by approximately 40%) when 10 mg alendronate was administered either 0.5 or 1 hour before a standardized breakfast, when compared to dosing 2 hours before eating).

Orange Juice (Concomitant administration of alendronate with orange juice reduces bioavailability by approximately 60%).

FOSRENOL CHEWABLE TABLETS

(Lanthanum Carbonate) **3180**
May interact with antacids. Compounds in these categories include:

Aluminum Carbonate (Avoid administering within 2 hours of antacids).
No products indexed under this heading.

Aluminum Hydroxide (Avoid administering within 2 hours of antacids). Products include:
Gaviscon Regular Strength Liquid .. ■**620**
Gaviscon Regular Strength Tablets .... ■**619**
Gaviscon Extra Strength Liquid ...... ■**620**
Gaviscon Extra Strength Tablets .... ■**619**
Maalox Max Maximum Strength Antacid/Anti-Gas Liquid **2165**
Maalox Regular Strength Antacid/Antigas Liquid **2164**

Magaldrate (Avoid administering within 2 hours of antacids).
No products indexed under this heading.

Magnesium Hydroxide (Avoid administering within 2 hours of antacids). Products include:
Maalox Max Maximum Strength Antacid/Anti-Gas Liquid **2165**
Maalox Regular Strength Antacid/Antigas Liquid **2164**
Pepcid Complete Chewable Tablets **1672**
Rolaids Tablets .... ■**707**
Extra Strength Rolaids Tablets .... ■**707**
Rolaids Multi-Symptom Antacid & Antigas Tablets .... ■**708**

Magnesium Oxide (Avoid administering within 2 hours of antacids). Products include:
Beelith Tablets **784**
PremCal Light, Regular, and Extra Strength Tablets .... ■**762**

Sodium Bicarbonate (Avoid administering within 2 hours of antacids). Products include:
Ceo-Two Evacuant Suppository ...... ■**607**
Colyte with Flavor Packs for Oral Solution **3102**
HalfLytely and Bisacodyl Tablets Bowel Prep Kit with Flavors Packs **915**
TriLyte with Flavor Packs for Oral Solution **3114**

FRAGMIN INJECTION

(Dalteparin Sodium) **2638**
May interact with oral anticoagulants, platelet inhibitors, thrombolytics, and certain other agents. Compounds in these categories include:

Abciximab (Drugs that alter platelet function, such as abciximab, may increase the risk of bleeding). Products include:
ReoPro Vials **1779**

Alteplase (Concomitant use with thrombolytic agents may increase the risk of bleeding). Products include:
Activase I.V. **1225**
Cathflo Activase **1232**

Anisindione (Concomitant use with oral anticoagulants may increase the risk of bleeding). Products include:
Miradon Tablets **3056**

Anistreplase (Concomitant use with thrombolytic agents may increase the risk of bleeding).
No products indexed under this heading.

Aspirin (Concomitant use with platelet inhibitors may increase the risk of bleeding). Products include:
Aggrenox Capsules **855**
Bayer, Aspirin Regimen .... ■**606**
Bayer Aspirin Tablets **3515**
BC Powder .... ■**612**
BC Allergy Sinus Cold Powder .... ■**612**
Arthritis Strength BC Powder .... ■**612**
BC Sinus Cold Powder .... ■**612**
Ecotrin Enteric Coated Aspirin Low, Regular and Maximum Strength Tablets **1627**
Goody's Body Pain Formula Powder .... ■**621**
Goody's Extra Strength Headache Powder .... ■**621**
Goody's Extra Strength Pain Relief Tablets .... ■**621**
Percodan Tablets **1115**
St. Joseph 81 mg Aspirin Chewable and Enteric Coated Tablets **1841**

Aspirin, Enteric Coated (Concomitant use with platelet inhibitors may increase the risk of bleeding).
No products indexed under this heading.

Aspirin Buffered (Concomitant use with platelet inhibitors may increase the risk of bleeding).
No products indexed under this heading.

Azlocillin Sodium (Concomitant use with platelet inhibitors may increase the risk of bleeding).
No products indexed under this heading.

Carbenicillin Indanyl Sodium (Concomitant use with platelet inhibitors may increase the risk of bleeding).
No products indexed under this heading.

Choline Magnesium Trisalicylate (Concomitant use with platelet inhibitors may increase the risk of bleeding).
No products indexed under this heading.

Clopidogrel Bisulfate (Concomitant use with platelet inhibitors may increase the risk of bleeding). Products include:
Plavix Tablets **940**
Plavix Tablets **2942**

Diclofenac Potassium (Concomitant use with platelet inhibitors may increase the risk of bleeding). Products include:
Cataflam Tablets **2173**

Diclofenac Sodium (Concomitant use with platelet inhibitors may increase the risk of bleeding). Products include:
Arthrotec Tablets **3126**
Voltaren Ophthalmic Solution **2300**
Voltaren Tablets **2298**
Voltaren-XR Tablets **2301**

Dicumarol (Concomitant use with oral anticoagulants may increase the risk of bleeding).
No products indexed under this heading.

Diflunisal (Concomitant use with platelet inhibitors may increase the risk of bleeding). Products include:
Dolobid Tablets **1937**

Dipyridamole (Concomitant use with platelet inhibitors may increase the risk of bleeding). Products include:
Aggrenox Capsules **855**
Persantine Tablets **898**

Eptifibatide (Drugs that alter platelet function, such as eptifibatide, may increase the risk of bleeding). Products include:
Integrilin Injection **3034**

Fenoprofen Calcium (Concomitant use with platelet inhibitors may increase the risk of bleeding). Products include:
Nalfon Capsules **2504**

Flurbiprofen (Concomitant use with platelet inhibitors may increase the risk of bleeding).
No products indexed under this heading.

Ibuprofen (Concomitant use with platelet inhibitors may increase the risk of bleeding). Products include:
Advil Allergy Sinus Caplets .... ■**737**
Advil .... ■**737**
Children's Advil Suspension .... ■**742**
Children's Advil Chewable Tablets .. ■**741**
Advil Cold & Sinus .... ■**739**
Advil Flu & Body Ache Caplets .... ■**739**
Children's Advil Cold Suspension ... ■**741**
Infants' Advil Concentrated Drops .. ■**743**
Junior Strength Advil Swallow Tablets .... ■**740**
Advil Migraine Liquigels .... ■**740**
Advil Multi-Symptom Cold Caplets .... ■**738**
Combunox Tablets **1183**
Children's Motrin Oral Suspension and Chewable Tablets **1837**
Children's Motrin Cold Non-Staining Dye-Free Oral Suspension **1838**

Children's Motrin Cold Oral Suspension 1838
Children's Motrin Non-Staining Dye-Free Oral Suspension 1837
Motrin Cold & Sinus Caplets 1836
Motrin IB Tablets and Caplets 1836
Infants' Motrin Concentrated Drops 1837
Infants' Motrin Non-Staining Dye-Free Drops 1837
Junior Strength Motrin Caplets and Chewable Tablets 1837
Vicoprofen Tablets 533

Indomethacin (Concomitant use with platelet inhibitors may increase the risk of bleeding). Products include:
Indocin 1968

Indomethacin Sodium Trihydrate (Concomitant use with platelet inhibitors may increase the risk of bleeding). Products include:
Indocin I.V. 1973

Ketoprofen (Concomitant use with platelet inhibitors may increase the risk of bleeding).
No products indexed under this heading.

Magnesium Salicylate (Concomitant use with platelet inhibitors may increase the risk of bleeding).
No products indexed under this heading.

Meclofenamate Sodium (Concomitant use with platelet inhibitors may increase the risk of bleeding).
No products indexed under this heading.

Mefenamic Acid (Concomitant use with platelet inhibitors may increase the risk of bleeding).
No products indexed under this heading.

Mezlocillin Sodium (Concomitant use with platelet inhibitors may increase the risk of bleeding).
No products indexed under this heading.

Nafcillin Sodium (Concomitant use with platelet inhibitors may increase the risk of bleeding).
No products indexed under this heading.

Naproxen (Concomitant use with platelet inhibitors may increase the risk of bleeding). Products include:
EC-Naprosyn Delayed-Release Tablets 2769
Naprosyn Suspension 2769
Naprosyn Tablets 2769
Prevacid NapraPAC 3277

Naproxen Sodium (Concomitant use with platelet inhibitors may increase the risk of bleeding). Products include:
Aleve Tablets, Caplets and Gelcaps 605
Anaprox Tablets 2769
Anaprox DS Tablets 2769

Penicillin G Benzathine (Concomitant use with platelet inhibitors may increase the risk of bleeding).
No products indexed under this heading.

Penicillin G Procaine (Concomitant use with platelet inhibitors may increase the risk of bleeding).
No products indexed under this heading.

Phenylbutazone (Concomitant use with platelet inhibitors may increase the risk of bleeding).
No products indexed under this heading.

Piroxicam (Concomitant use with platelet inhibitors may increase the risk of bleeding).
No products indexed under this heading.

Reteplase (Concomitant use with thrombolytic agents may increase the risk of bleeding). Products include:
Retavase 1131

Salsalate (Concomitant use with platelet inhibitors may increase the risk of bleeding).
No products indexed under this heading.

Streptokinase (Concomitant use with thrombolytic agents may increase the risk of bleeding).
No products indexed under this heading.

Sulindac (Concomitant use with platelet inhibitors may increase the risk of bleeding). Products include:
Clinoril Tablets 1899

Ticarcillin Disodium (Concomitant use with platelet inhibitors may increase the risk of bleeding). Products include:
Timentin ADD-Vantage 1556
Timentin Injection Galaxy Container 1559
Timentin IV Infusion 1553
Timentin Pharmacy Bulk Package 1562

Ticlopidine Hydrochloride (Concomitant use with platelet inhibitors may increase the risk of bleeding). Products include:
Ticlid Tablets 2813

Tirofiban Hydrochloride (Drugs that alter platelet function, such as tirofiban, may increase the risk of bleeding). Products include:
Aggrastat 1878

Tolmetin Sodium (Concomitant use with platelet inhibitors may increase the risk of bleeding).
No products indexed under this heading.

Urokinase (Concomitant use with thrombolytic agents may increase the risk of bleeding).
No products indexed under this heading.

Warfarin Sodium (Concomitant use with oral anticoagulants may increase the risk of bleeding). Products include:
Coumadin for Injection 932
Coumadin Tablets 932

FROVA TABLETS

(Frovatriptan Succinate) 1101

May interact with 5HT1-receptor agonists, ergot-containing drugs, oral contraceptives, selective serotonin reuptake inhibitors, and certain other agents. Compounds in these categories include:

Citalopram Hydrobromide (Co-administration of 5-HT_1 agonists with selective serotonin reuptake inhibitors (SSRIs) has resulted, rarely, in hyperreflexia, weakness and incoordination). Products include:
Celexa 1177

Desogestrel (Retrospective analysis of pharmacokinetic data indicates that mean C_{max} and AUC of frovatriptan are 30% higher in females taking oral contraceptives). Products include:
Ortho-Cept Tablets 2395

Dihydroergotamine Mesylate (Ergot-containing drugs have been reported to cause prolonged vasospastic reactions; because there is a theoretical basis that these effects may be additive, use of ergot-type agents and frovatriptan within 24 hours is contraindicated). Products include:
Migranal Nasal Spray 3350

3-Diphenylacrylate (Co-administration with other 5-HT_1 agonists within 24 hours of each other is contraindicated).
No products indexed under this heading.

Ergonovine Maleate (Ergot-containing drugs have been reported to cause prolonged vasospastic reactions; because there is a theoretical basis that these effects may be additive, use of ergot-type agents and frovatriptan within 24 hours is contraindicated).
No products indexed under this heading.

Ergotamine Tartrate (Ergot-containing drugs have been reported to cause prolonged vasospastic reactions; because there is a theoretical basis that these effects may be additive, use of ergot-type agents and frovatriptan within 24 hours is contraindicated).
No products indexed under this heading.

Escitalopram Oxalate (Co-administration of 5-HT_1 agonists with selective serotonin reuptake inhibitors (SSRIs) has resulted, rarely, in hyperreflexia, weakness and incoordination). Products include:
Lexapro Oral Solution 1193
Lexapro Tablets 1193

Ethinyl Estradiol (Retrospective analysis of pharmacokinetic data indicates that mean C_{max} and AUC of frovatriptan are 30% higher in females taking oral contraceptives). Products include:
Alesse-28 Tablets 3392
Lo/Ovral-28 Tablets 3423
NuvaRing 2357
Ortho-Cept Tablets 2395
Ortho-Cyclen/Ortho Tri-Cyclen 2414
Ortho Evra Transdermal System 2402
Ortho Tri-Cyclen Lo Tablets 2421
Seasonale Tablets 1073
Triphasil-28 Tablets 3483
Yasmin 28 Tablets 818

Ethynodiol Diacetate (Retrospective analysis of pharmacokinetic data indicates that mean C_{max} and AUC of frovatriptan are 30% higher in females taking oral contraceptives).
No products indexed under this heading.

Fluoxetine Hydrochloride (Co-administration of 5-HT_1 agonists with selective serotonin reuptake inhibitors (SSRIs) has resulted, rarely, in hyperreflexia, weakness and incoordination). Products include:
Prozac Pulvules and Liquid 1771
Symbyax Capsules 1788

Fluvoxamine Maleate (Co-administration of 5-HT_1 agonists with selective serotonin reuptake inhibitors (SSRIs) has resulted, rarely, in hyperreflexia, weakness and incoordination).
No products indexed under this heading.

Levonorgestrel (Retrospective analysis of pharmacokinetic data indicates that mean C_{max} and AUC of frovatriptan are 30% higher in females taking oral contraceptives). Products include:
Alesse-28 Tablets 3392
Climara Pro Transdermal System 800
Mirena Intrauterine System 810
Plan B Tablets 1068
Seasonale Tablets 1073
Triphasil-28 Tablets 3483

Mestranol (Retrospective analysis of pharmacokinetic data indicates that mean C_{max} and AUC of frovatriptan are 30% higher in females taking oral contraceptives).
No products indexed under this heading.

Methylergonovine Maleate (Ergot-containing drugs have been reported to cause prolonged vasospastic reactions; because there is a theoretical basis that these effects may be additive, use of ergot-type agents and frovatriptan within 24 hours is contraindicated).
No products indexed under this heading.

Methysergide Maleate (Ergot-containing drugs have been reported to cause prolonged vasospastic reactions; because there is a theoretical basis that these effects may be additive, use of ergot-type agents and frovatriptan within 24 hours is contraindicated).
No products indexed under this heading.

Naratriptan Hydrochloride (Co-administration with other 5-HT_1 agonists within 24 hours of each other is contraindicated). Products include:
Amerge Tablets 1312

Norethindrone (Retrospective analysis of pharmacokinetic data indicates that mean C_{max4} and AUC of frovatriptan are 30% higher in females taking oral contraceptives). Products include:
Ortho Micronor Tablets 2411

Norethynodrel (Retrospective analysis of pharmacokinetic data indicates that mean C_{max} and AUC of frovatriptan are 30% higher in females taking oral contraceptives).
No products indexed under this heading.

Norgestimate (Retrospective analysis of pharmacokinetic data indicates that mean C_{max} and AUC of frovatriptan are 30% higher in females taking oral contraceptives). Products include:
Ortho-Cyclen/Ortho Tri-Cyclen 2414
Ortho Tri-Cyclen Lo Tablets 2421
Prefest Tablets 1069

Norgestrel (Retrospective analysis of pharmacokinetic data indicates that mean C_{max} and AUC of frovatriptan are 30% higher in females taking oral contraceptives). Products include:
Lo/Ovral-28 Tablets 3423

Paroxetine Hydrochloride (Co-administration of 5-HT_1 agonists with selective serotonin reuptake inhibitors (SSRIs) has resulted, rarely, in hyperreflexia, weakness and incoordination). Products include:
Paxil CR Controlled-Release Tablets 1509
Paxil 1501

Propranolol Hydrochloride (Increases AUC of frovatriptan in males by 60% and in females by 29%; Cmax was increased by 23% in males and 16% in females). Products include:
Inderal LA Long-Acting Capsules 3421
InnoPran XL Capsules 2728

Rizatriptan Benzoate (Co-administration with other 5-HT_1 agonists within 24 hours of each other is contraindicated). Products include:
Maxalt Tablets 1983

IMPORTANT NOTE: Always consult each drug listing in the patient's regimen for possible interactions.

Maxalt-MLT Orally Disintegrating Tablets ... 1983

Sertraline Hydrochloride (Co-administration of 5-HT_1 agonists with selective serotonin reuptake inhibitors (SSRIs) has resulted, rarely, in hyperreflexia, weakness and incoordination). Products include:
Zoloft ... 2581

Sumatriptan (Co-administration with other 5-HT_1 agonists within 24 hours of each other is contraindicated). Products include:
Imitrex Nasal Spray ... 1435

Sumatriptan Succinate (Co-administration with other 5-HT_1 agonists within 24 hours of each other is contraindicated). Products include:
Imitrex Injection ... 1431
Imitrex Tablets ... 1440

Zolmitriptan (Co-administration with other 5-HT_1 agonists within 24 hours of each other is contraindicated). Products include:
Zomig Nasal Spray ... 718
Zomig Tablets ... 714
Zomig-ZMT Tablets ... 714

FUROSEMIDE TABLETS

(Furosemide) ... 2117

May interact with aminoglycosides, antihypertensives, barbiturates, corticosteroids, cardiac glycosides, lithium preparations, narcotic analgesics, non-steroidal anti-inflammatory agents, salicylates, and certain other agents. Compounds in these categories include:

Acebutolol Hydrochloride (Furosemide may add to or potentiate the therapeutic effect of other antihypertensive drugs).
No products indexed under this heading.

ACTH (Co-administration with ACTH may increase the risk of hypokalemia).
No products indexed under this heading.

Alfentanil Hydrochloride (Aggravates orthostatic hypotension).
No products indexed under this heading.

Amikacin Sulfate (Potential for increased risk of ototoxicity with concomitant therapy, especially in the presence of impaired renal function; avoid concurrent use except in presence of life threatening situations).
No products indexed under this heading.

Amlodipine Besylate (Furosemide may add to or potentiate the therapeutic effect of other antihypertensive drugs). Products include:
Caduet Tablets ... 2507
Lotrel Capsules ... 2238
Norvasc Tablets ... 2529

Aprobarbital (Aggravates orthostatic hypotension).
No products indexed under this heading.

Aspirin (Combination of furosemide and aspirin temporarily reduced creatinine clearance in patients with chronic renal insufficiency; co-administration in patients receiving high doses of salicylates may experience salicylate toxicity). Products include:
Aggrenox Capsules ... 855
Bayer, Aspirin Regimen ... ■606
Bayer Aspirin Tablets ... 3515
BC Powder ... ■612
BC Allergy Sinus Cold Powder ... ■612
Arthritis Strength BC Powder ... ■612
BC Sinus Cold Powder ... ■612
Ecotrin Enteric Coated Aspirin Low, Regular and Maximum Strength Tablets ... 1627
Goody's Body Pain Formula Powder ... ■621
Goody's Extra Strength Headache Powder ... ■621
Goody's Extra Strength Pain Relief Tablets ... ■621
Percodan Tablets ... 1115
St. Joseph 81 mg Aspirin Chewable and Enteric Coated Tablets ... 1841

Aspirin, Enteric Coated (Co-administration in patients receiving high doses of salicylates may experience salicylate toxicity).
No products indexed under this heading.

Aspirin Buffered (Co-administration in patients receiving high doses of salicylates may experience salicylate toxicity).
No products indexed under this heading.

Atenolol (Furosemide may add to or potentiate the therapeutic effect of other antihypertensive drugs). Products include:
Tenormin I.V. Injection ... 698
Tenormin Tablets ... 695

Benazepril Hydrochloride (Furosemide may add to or potentiate the therapeutic effect of other antihypertensive drugs). Products include:
Lotensin Tablets ... 2232
Lotensin HCT Tablets ... 2235
Lotrel Capsules ... 2238

Bendroflumethiazide (Furosemide may add to or potentiate the therapeutic effect of other antihypertensive drugs).
No products indexed under this heading.

Betamethasone Acetate (Co-administration with corticosteroids may increase the risk of hypokalemia).
No products indexed under this heading.

Betamethasone Sodium Phosphate (Co-administration with corticosteroids may increase the risk of hypokalemia).
No products indexed under this heading.

Betaxolol Hydrochloride (Furosemide may add to or potentiate the therapeutic effect of other antihypertensive drugs). Products include:
Betoptic S Ophthalmic Suspension ... 554

Bisoprolol Fumarate (Furosemide may add to or potentiate the therapeutic effect of other antihypertensive drugs).
No products indexed under this heading.

Buprenorphine Hydrochloride (Aggravates orthostatic hypotension). Products include:
Buprenex Injectable ... 2718
Suboxone Tablets ... 2719
Subutex Tablets ... 2719

Butabarbital (Aggravates orthostatic hypotension).
No products indexed under this heading.

Butalbital (Aggravates orthostatic hypotension). Products include:
Sedapap Tablets 50 mg/650 mg ... 2098

Candesartan Cilexetil (Furosemide may add to or potentiate the therapeutic effect of other antihypertensive drugs). Products include:
Atacand Tablets ... 634
Atacand HCT ... 637

Captopril (Furosemide may add to or potentiate the therapeutic effect of other antihypertensive drugs). Products include:
Captopril Tablets ... 2114

Carteolol Hydrochloride (Furosemide may add to or potentiate the therapeutic effect of other antihypertensive drugs). Products include:
Carteolol Hydrochloride Ophthalmic Solution USP, 1% ... ⊙246

Celecoxib (Co-administration with NSAIDs has resulted in increased BUN, serum creatinine and serum potassium levels, and weight gain). Products include:
Celebrex Capsules ... 3130

Chlorothiazide (Furosemide may add to or potentiate the therapeutic effect of other antihypertensive drugs). Products include:
Aldoclor Tablets ... 1881
Diuril Oral ... 1936

Chlorothiazide Sodium (Furosemide may add to or potentiate the therapeutic effect of other antihypertensive drugs). Products include:
Diuril Sodium Intravenous ... 1934

Chlorthalidone (Furosemide may add to or potentiate the therapeutic effect of other antihypertensive drugs). Products include:
Clorpres Tablets ... 2139

Choline Magnesium Trisalicylate (Co-administration in patients receiving high doses of salicylates may experience salicylate toxicity).
No products indexed under this heading.

Clonidine (Furosemide may add to or potentiate the therapeutic effect of other antihypertensive drugs). Products include:
Catapres-TTS ... 875

Clonidine Hydrochloride (Furosemide may add to or potentiate the therapeutic effect of other antihypertensive drugs). Products include:
Catapres Tablets ... 874
Clorpres Tablets ... 2139

Codeine Phosphate (Aggravates orthostatic hypotension). Products include:
Tylenol with Codeine ... 2461

Cortisone Acetate (Co-administration with corticosteroids may increase the risk of hypokalemia).
No products indexed under this heading.

Deserpidine (Furosemide may add to or potentiate the therapeutic effect of other antihypertensive drugs).
No products indexed under this heading.

Deslanoside (Concurrent digitalis therapy may exaggerate metabolic effects of hypokalemia, especially myocardial effects).
No products indexed under this heading.

Dexamethasone (Co-administration with corticosteroids may increase the risk of hypokalemia). Products include:
Ciprodex Otic Suspension ... 555
Decadron Tablets ... 1929
TobraDex Ophthalmic Ointment ... 558
TobraDex Ophthalmic Suspension ... 558

Dexamethasone Acetate (Co-administration with corticosteroids may increase the risk of hypokalemia).
No products indexed under this heading.

Dexamethasone Sodium Phosphate (Co-administration with corticosteroids may increase the risk of hypokalemia). Products include:
Decadron Phosphate Injection ... 1931

Dezocine (Aggravates orthostatic hypotension).
No products indexed under this heading.

Diazoxide (Furosemide may add to or potentiate the therapeutic effect of other antihypertensive drugs). Products include:
Hyperstat I.V. Injection ... 3031

Diclofenac Potassium (Co-administration with NSAIDs has resulted in increased BUN, serum creatinine and serum potassium levels, and weight gain). Products include:
Cataflam Tablets ... 2173

Diclofenac Sodium (Co-administration with NSAIDs has resulted in increased BUN, serum creatinine and serum potassium levels, and weight gain). Products include:
Arthrotec Tablets ... 3126
Voltaren Ophthalmic Solution ... 2300
Voltaren Tablets ... 2298
Voltaren-XR Tablets ... 2301

Diflunisal (Co-administration in patients receiving high doses of salicylates may experience salicylate toxicity). Products include:
Dolobid Tablets ... 1937

Digitalis Glycoside Preparations (Concurrent digitalis therapy may exaggerate metabolic effects of hypokalemia, especially myocardial effects).
No products indexed under this heading.

Digitoxin (Concurrent digitalis therapy may exaggerate metabolic effects of hypokalemia, especially myocardial effects).
No products indexed under this heading.

Digoxin (Concurrent digitalis therapy may exaggerate metabolic effects of hypokalemia, especially myocardial effects). Products include:
Digitek Tablets ... 2146
Lanoxicaps Capsules ... 1458
Lanoxin Injection ... 1462
Lanoxin Tablets ... 1468
Lanoxin Injection Pediatric ... 1465

Diltiazem Hydrochloride (Furosemide may add to or potentiate the therapeutic effect of other antihypertensive drugs). Products include:
Cardizem LA Extended Release Tablets ... 1699
Tiazac Capsules ... 1204

Doxazosin Mesylate (Furosemide may add to or potentiate the therapeutic effect of other antihypertensive drugs).
No products indexed under this heading.

Enalapril Maleate (Furosemide may add to or potentiate the therapeutic effect of other antihypertensive drugs). Products include:
Vaseretic Tablets ... 2073
Vasotec I.V. Injection ... 2076

Enalaprilat (Furosemide may add to or potentiate the therapeutic effect of other antihypertensive drugs).
No products indexed under this heading.

(■ Described in PDR For Nonprescription Drugs)

(⊙ Described in PDR For Ophthalmic Medicines™)

Eprosartan Mesylate (Furosemide may add to or potentiate the therapeutic effect of other antihypertensive drugs). Products include:
- Teveten Tablets ... 1707
- Teveten HCT Tablets ... 1710

Esmolol Hydrochloride (Furosemide may add to or potentiate the therapeutic effect of other antihypertensive drugs). Products include:
- Brevibloc Concentrate ... 766
- Brevibloc Injection ... 766
- Brevibloc Double Strength Injection ... 766
- Brevibloc Premixed Injection ... 766
- Brevibloc Double Strength Premixed Injection ... 766

Ethacrynic Acid (Potential for increased risk of ototoxicity with concomitant therapy; concurrent use should be avoided). Products include:
- Edecrin Tablets ... 1941

Etodolac (Co-administration with NSAIDs has resulted in increased BUN, serum creatinine and serum potassium levels, and weight gain).
No products indexed under this heading.

Felodipine (Furosemide may add to or potentiate the therapeutic effect of other antihypertensive drugs). Products include:
- Plendil Extended-Release Tablets ... 651

Fenoprofen Calcium (Co-administration with NSAIDs has resulted in increased BUN, serum creatinine and serum potassium levels, and weight gain). Products include:
- Nalfon Capsules ... 2504

Fentanyl (Aggravates orthostatic hypotension). Products include:
- Duragesic Transdermal System ... 2448

Fentanyl Citrate (Aggravates orthostatic hypotension). Products include:
- Actiq ... 993

Fludrocortisone Acetate (Co-administration with corticosteroids may increase the risk of hypokalemia).
No products indexed under this heading.

Flurbiprofen (Co-administration with NSAIDs has resulted in increased BUN, serum creatinine and serum potassium levels, and weight gain).
No products indexed under this heading.

Fosinopril Sodium (Furosemide may add to or potentiate the therapeutic effect of other antihypertensive drugs).
No products indexed under this heading.

Gentamicin Sulfate (Potential for increased risk of ototoxicity with concomitant therapy, especially in the presence of impaired renal function; avoid concurrent use except in presence of life threatening situations). Products include:
- Garamycin Injectable ... 3028
- Genoptic Sterile Ophthalmic Solution ... ⊙227
- Pred-G Ophthalmic Suspension ... ⊙234
- Pred-G Sterile Ophthalmic Ointment ... ⊙235

Guanabenz Acetate (Furosemide may add to or potentiate the therapeutic effect of other antihypertensive drugs).
No products indexed under this heading.

Guanethidine Monosulfate (Furosemide may add to or potentiate the therapeutic effect of other antihypertensive drugs).
No products indexed under this heading.

Hydralazine Hydrochloride (Furosemide may add to or potentiate the therapeutic effect of other antihypertensive drugs). Products include:
- BiDil Tablets ... 2161

Hydrochlorothiazide (Furosemide may add to or potentiate the therapeutic effect of other antihypertensive drugs). Products include:
- Aldoril Tablets ... 1884
- Atacand HCT ... 637
- Avalide Tablets ... 2889
- Avalide Tablets ... 922
- Benicar HCT Tablets ... 2852
- Diovan HCT Tablets ... 2195
- Dyazide Capsules ... 1389
- Hyzaar ... 1964
- Lotensin HCT Tablets ... 2235
- Maxzide ... 2150
- Micardis HCT Tablets ... 886
- Moduretic Tablets ... 2003
- Prinzide Tablets ... 2033
- Teveten HCT Tablets ... 1710
- Timolide Tablets ... 2056
- Uniretic Tablets ... 3114
- Vaseretic Tablets ... 2073
- Zestoretic Tablets ... 701

Hydrocodone Bitartrate (Aggravates orthostatic hypotension). Products include:
- Hycodan ... 1104
- Hycomine Compound Tablets ... 1105
- Hycotuss Expectorant Syrup ... 1106
- Lortab ... 3315
- Lortab Elixir ... 3312
- Vicodin Tablets ... 530
- Vicodin ES Tablets ... 531
- Vicodin HP Tablets ... 532
- Vicoprofen Tablets ... 533
- Zydone Tablets ... 1118

Hydrocodone Polistirex (Aggravates orthostatic hypotension). Products include:
- Tussionex Pennkinetic Extended-Release Suspension ... 3322

Hydrocortisone (Co-administration with corticosteroids may increase the risk of hypokalemia). Products include:
- Cortizone•5 Ointment ... ■699
- Cortizone•10 Creme ... ■699
- Cortizone•10 Ointment ... ■699
- Cortizone•10 Plus Creme ... ■700
- Cortizone•10 Maximum Strength Quick Shot Spray ... ■700
- Hydrocortone Tablets ... 1963
- Preparation H Hydrocortisone Cream ... ■748

Hydrocortisone Acetate (Co-administration with corticosteroids may increase the risk of hypokalemia). Products include:
- Analpram-HC ... 1136
- Pramosone ... 1139
- ProctoFoam-HC ... 3113
- Tucks Anti-Itch Ointment ... ■712
- U-cort 1% Cream ... 3289

Hydrocortisone Sodium Phosphate (Co-administration with corticosteroids may increase the risk of hypokalemia).
No products indexed under this heading.

Hydrocortisone Sodium Succinate (Co-administration with corticosteroids may increase the risk of hypokalemia).
No products indexed under this heading.

Hydroflumethiazide (Furosemide may add to or potentiate the therapeutic effect of other antihypertensive drugs).
No products indexed under this heading.

Hydromorphone Hydrochloride (Aggravates orthostatic hypotension). Products include:
- Dilaudid ... 439
- Dilaudid Oral Liquid ... 443
- Dilaudid Non-Sterile Powder ... 439
- Dilaudid Rectal Suppositories ... 439
- Dilaudid Tablets ... 439
- Dilaudid Tablets - 8 mg ... 443
- Dilaudid-HP ... 441

Ibuprofen (Co-administration with NSAIDs has resulted in increased BUN, serum creatinine and serum potassium levels, and weight gain). Products include:
- Advil Allergy Sinus Caplets ... ■737
- Advil ... ■737
- Children's Advil Suspension ... ■742
- Children's Advil Chewable Tablets ... ■741
- Advil Cold & Sinus ... ■739
- Advil Flu & Body Ache Caplets ... ■739
- Children's Advil Cold Suspension ... ■741
- Infants' Advil Concentrated Drops ... ■743
- Junior Strength Advil Swallow Tablets ... ■740
- Advil Migraine Liquigels ... ■740
- Advil Multi-Symptom Cold Caplets ... ■738
- Combunox Tablets ... 1183
- Children's Motrin Oral Suspension and Chewable Tablets ... 1837
- Children's Motrin Cold Non-Staining Dye-Free Oral Suspension ... 1838
- Children's Motrin Cold Oral Suspension ... 1838
- Children's Motrin Non-Staining Dye-Free Oral Suspension ... 1837
- Motrin Cold & Sinus Caplets ... 1836
- Motrin IB Tablets and Caplets ... 1836
- Infants' Motrin Concentrated Drops ... 1837
- Infants' Motrin Non-Staining Dye-Free Drops ... 1837
- Junior Strength Motrin Caplets and Chewable Tablets ... 1837
- Vicoprofen Tablets ... 533

Indapamide (Furosemide may add to or potentiate the therapeutic effect of other antihypertensive drugs). Products include:
- Indapamide Tablets ... 2119

Indomethacin (Co-administration may educe the natriuretic and antihypertensive effects of furosemide in some patients by inhibiting prostaglandin synthesis). Products include:
- Indocin ... 1968

Indomethacin Sodium Trihydrate (Co-administration with NSAIDs has resulted in increased BUN, serum creatinine and serum potassium levels, and weight gain). Products include:
- Indocin I.V. ... 1973

Irbesartan (Furosemide may add to or potentiate the therapeutic effect of other antihypertensive drugs). Products include:
- Avalide Tablets ... 922
- Avalide Tablets ... 2889
- Avapro Tablets ... 925
- Avapro Tablets ... 2886

Isradipine (Furosemide may add to or potentiate the therapeutic effect of other antihypertensive drugs). Products include:
- DynaCirc CR Tablets ... 2726

Kanamycin Sulfate (Potential for increased risk of ototoxicity with concomitant therapy, especially in the presence of impaired renal function; avoid concurrent use except in presence of life threatening situations).
No products indexed under this heading.

Ketoprofen (Co-administration with NSAIDs has resulted in increased BUN, serum creatinine and serum potassium levels, and weight gain).
No products indexed under this heading.

Ketorolac Tromethamine (Co-administration with NSAIDs has resulted in increased BUN, serum creatinine and serum potassium levels, and weight gain). Products include:
- Acular Ophthalmic Solution ... 561
- Acular LS Ophthalmic Solution ... 562

Labetalol Hydrochloride (Furosemide may add to or potentiate the therapeutic effect of other antihypertensive drugs).
No products indexed under this heading.

Levorphanol Tartrate (Aggravates orthostatic hypotension).
No products indexed under this heading.

Lisinopril (Furosemide may add to or potentiate the therapeutic effect of other antihypertensive drugs). Products include:
- Prinivil Tablets ... 2029
- Prinzide Tablets ... 2033
- Zestoretic Tablets ... 701
- Zestril Tablets ... 704

Lithium (Diuretics reduce lithium's renal clearance and add a high risk of lithium toxicity).
No products indexed under this heading.

Lithium Carbonate (Diuretics reduce lithium's renal clearance and add a high risk of lithium toxicity). Products include:
- Eskalith ... 1406
- Lithobid Tablets ... 1670

Lithium Citrate (Diuretics reduce lithium's renal clearance and add a high risk of lithium toxicity).
No products indexed under this heading.

Losartan Potassium (Furosemide may add to or potentiate the therapeutic effect of other antihypertensive drugs). Products include:
- Cozaar Tablets ... 1913
- Hyzaar ... 1964

Magnesium Salicylate (Co-administration in patients receiving high doses of salicylates may experience salicylate toxicity).
No products indexed under this heading.

Mecamylamine Hydrochloride (Furosemide may add to or potentiate the therapeutic effect of other antihypertensive drugs). Products include:
- Inversine Tablets ... 3286

Meclofenamate Sodium (Co-administration with NSAIDs has resulted in increased BUN, serum creatinine and serum potassium levels, and weight gain).
No products indexed under this heading.

IMPORTANT NOTE: Always consult each drug listing in the patient's regimen for possible interactions.

Mefenamic Acid (Co-administration with NSAIDs has resulted in increased BUN, serum creatinine and serum potassium levels, and weight gain).
No products indexed under this heading.

Meloxicam (Co-administration with NSAIDs has resulted in increased BUN, serum creatinine and serum potassium levels, and weight gain). Products include:
Mobic Oral Suspension 893
Mobic Tablets 893

Meperidine Hydrochloride (Aggravates orthostatic hypotension).
No products indexed under this heading.

Mephobarbital (Aggravates orthostatic hypotension). Products include:
Mebaral Tablets, USP 2483

Methadone Hydrochloride (Aggravates orthostatic hypotension).
No products indexed under this heading.

Methyclothiazide (Furosemide may add to or potentiate the therapeutic effect of other antihypertensive drugs).
No products indexed under this heading.

Methyldopa (Furosemide may add to or potentiate the therapeutic effect of other antihypertensive drugs). Products include:
Aldoclor Tablets 1881
Aldoril Tablets 1884

Methyldopate Hydrochloride (Furosemide may add to or potentiate the therapeutic effect of other antihypertensive drugs).
No products indexed under this heading.

Methylprednisolone Acetate (Co-administration with corticosteroids may increase the risk of hypokalemia). Products include:
Depo-Medrol Injectable Suspension 2615
Depo-Medrol Single-Dose Vial 2617

Methylprednisolone Sodium Succinate (Co-administration with corticosteroids may increase the risk of hypokalemia).
No products indexed under this heading.

Metolazone (Furosemide may add to or potentiate the therapeutic effect of other antihypertensive drugs).
No products indexed under this heading.

Metoprolol Succinate (Furosemide may add to or potentiate the therapeutic effect of other antihypertensive drugs). Products include:
Toprol-XL Tablets 660

Metoprolol Tartrate (Furosemide may add to or potentiate the therapeutic effect of other antihypertensive drugs).
No products indexed under this heading.

Metyrosine (Furosemide may add to or potentiate the therapeutic effect of other antihypertensive drugs). Products include:
Demser Capsules 1933

Mibefradil Dihydrochloride (Furosemide may add to or potentiate the therapeutic effect of other antihypertensive drugs).
No products indexed under this heading.

Minoxidil (Furosemide may add to or potentiate the therapeutic effect of other antihypertensive drugs). Products include:
Men's Rogaine Extra Strength Topical Solution, Ocean Rush Scent and Original Unscented .... ▣706
Women's Rogaine Topical Solution, Spring Bloom Scent and Original Unscented .... ▣707

Moexipril Hydrochloride (Furosemide may add to or potentiate the therapeutic effect of other antihypertensive drugs). Products include:
Uniretic Tablets 3114
Univasc Tablets 3118

Morphine Sulfate (Aggravates orthostatic hypotension). Products include:
Avinza Capsules 1714
Kadian Capsules 572
MS Contin Tablets 2703

Nabumetone (Co-administration with NSAIDs has resulted in increased BUN, serum creatinine and serum potassium levels, and weight gain). Products include:
Relafen Tablets 1523

Nadolol (Furosemide may add to or potentiate the therapeutic effect of other antihypertensive drugs). Products include:
Nadolol Tablets 2121

Naproxen (Co-administration with NSAIDs has resulted in increased BUN, serum creatinine and serum potassium levels, and weight gain). Products include:
EC-Naprosyn Delayed-Release Tablets 2769
Naprosyn Suspension 2769
Naprosyn Tablets 2769
Prevacid NapraPAC 3277

Naproxen Sodium (Co-administration with NSAIDs has resulted in increased BUN, serum creatinine and serum potassium levels, and weight gain). Products include:
Aleve Tablets, Caplets and Gelcaps .... ▣605
Anaprox Tablets 2769
Anaprox DS Tablets 2769

Nicardipine Hydrochloride (Furosemide may add to or potentiate the therapeutic effect of other antihypertensive drugs). Products include:
Cardene I.V. 1129

Nifedipine (Furosemide may add to or potentiate the therapeutic effect of other antihypertensive drugs). Products include:
Adalat CC Tablets 2978

Nisoldipine (Furosemide may add to or potentiate the therapeutic effect of other antihypertensive drugs). Products include:
Sular Tablets 1163

Nitroglycerin (Furosemide may add to or potentiate the therapeutic effect of other antihypertensive drugs). Products include:
Nitro-Dur Transdermal Infusion System 3060
Nitrolingual Pumpspray 1161

Norepinephrine Bitartrate (Furosemide may decrease arterial responsiveness to norepinephrine).
No products indexed under this heading.

Oxaprozin (Co-administration with NSAIDs has resulted in increased BUN, serum creatinine and serum potassium levels, and weight gain).
No products indexed under this heading.

Oxycodone Hydrochloride (Aggravates orthostatic hypotension). Products include:
Combunox Tablets 1183
OxyContin Tablets 2699
OxyFast Oral Concentrate Solution 2704
OxyIR Capsules 2704
Percocet Tablets 1114
Percodan Tablets 1115

Penbutolol Sulfate (Furosemide may add to or potentiate the therapeutic effect of other antihypertensive drugs).
No products indexed under this heading.

Pentobarbital Sodium (Aggravates orthostatic hypotension). Products include:
Nembutal Sodium Solution, USP 2484

Perindopril Erbumine (Furosemide may add to or potentiate the therapeutic effect of other antihypertensive drugs). Products include:
Aceon Tablets (2 mg, 4 mg, 8 mg) 3191

Phenobarbital (Aggravates orthostatic hypotension).
No products indexed under this heading.

Phenoxybenzamine Hydrochloride (Furosemide may add to or potentiate the therapeutic effect of other antihypertensive drugs). Products include:
Dibenzyline Capsules 3390

Phentolamine Mesylate (Furosemide may add to or potentiate the therapeutic effect of other antihypertensive drugs).
No products indexed under this heading.

Phenylbutazone (Co-administration with NSAIDs has resulted in increased BUN, serum creatinine and serum potassium levels, and weight gain).
No products indexed under this heading.

Pindolol (Furosemide may add to or potentiate the therapeutic effect of other antihypertensive drugs).
No products indexed under this heading.

Piroxicam (Co-administration with NSAIDs has resulted in increased BUN, serum creatinine and serum potassium levels, and weight gain).
No products indexed under this heading.

Polythiazide (Furosemide may add to or potentiate the therapeutic effect of other antihypertensive drugs).
No products indexed under this heading.

Prazosin Hydrochloride (Furosemide may add to or potentiate the therapeutic effect of other antihypertensive drugs).
No products indexed under this heading.

Prednisolone Acetate (Co-administration with corticosteroids may increase the risk of hypokalemia). Products include:
Blephamide Ophthalmic Ointment 563
Blephamide Ophthalmic Suspension 564
Poly-Pred Liquifilm Ophthalmic Suspension .... ⊙231
Pred Forte Ophthalmic Suspension .... ⊙233
Pred Mild Sterile Ophthalmic Suspension .... ⊙236
Pred-G Ophthalmic Suspension .... ⊙234
Pred-G Sterile Ophthalmic Ointment .... ⊙235

Prednisolone Sodium Phosphate (Co-administration with corticosteroids may increase the risk of hypokalemia). Products include:
Pediapred Oral Solution 3319

Prednisolone Tebutate (Co-administration with corticosteroids may increase the risk of hypokalemia).
No products indexed under this heading.

Prednisone (Co-administration with corticosteroids may increase the risk of hypokalemia).
No products indexed under this heading.

Propoxyphene Hydrochloride (Aggravates orthostatic hypotension).
No products indexed under this heading.

Propoxyphene Napsylate (Aggravates orthostatic hypotension). Products include:
Darvocet A 500 Tablets 3497

Propranolol Hydrochloride (Furosemide may add to or potentiate the therapeutic effect of other antihypertensive drugs). Products include:
Inderal LA Long-Acting Capsules 3421
InnoPran XL Capsules 2728

Quinapril Hydrochloride (Furosemide may add to or potentiate the therapeutic effect of other antihypertensive drugs).
No products indexed under this heading.

Ramipril (Furosemide may add to or potentiate the therapeutic effect of other antihypertensive drugs). Products include:
Altace Capsules 1673

Rauwolfia Serpentina (Furosemide may add to or potentiate the therapeutic effect of other antihypertensive drugs).
No products indexed under this heading.

Remifentanil Hydrochloride (Aggravates orthostatic hypotension).
No products indexed under this heading.

Rescinnamine (Furosemide may add to or potentiate the therapeutic effect of other antihypertensive drugs).
No products indexed under this heading.

Reserpine (Furosemide may add to or potentiate the therapeutic effect of other antihypertensive drugs).
No products indexed under this heading.

Rofecoxib (Co-administration with NSAIDs has resulted in increased BUN, serum creatinine and serum potassium levels, and weight gain).
No products indexed under this heading.

Salsalate (Co-administration in patients receiving high doses of salicylates may experience salicylate toxicity).
No products indexed under this heading.

Secobarbital Sodium (Aggravates orthostatic hypotension).
No products indexed under this heading.

Sodium Nitroprusside (Furosemide may add to or potentiate the therapeutic effect of other antihypertensive drugs).
No products indexed under this heading.

Sotalol Hydrochloride (Furosemide may add to or potentiate the therapeutic effect of other antihypertensive drugs).
No products indexed under this heading.

Spirapril Hydrochloride (Furosemide may add to or potentiate the therapeutic effect of other antihypertensive drugs).
No products indexed under this heading.

Streptomycin Sulfate (Potential for increased risk of ototoxicity with concomitant therapy, especially in the presence of impaired renal function; avoid concurrent use except in presence of life threatening situations).
No products indexed under this heading.

Succinylcholine Chloride (Furosemide has a tendency to potentiate the action of succinylcholine).
No products indexed under this heading.

Sucralfate (Simultaneous administration of sucralfate and furosemide may reduce the natriuretic and antihypertensive effects of furosemide; the intake of these two drugs should be separated by at least two hours). Products include:
Carafate Suspension **727**
Carafate Tablets **728**

Sufentanil Citrate (Aggravates orthostatic hypotension).
No products indexed under this heading.

Sulindac (Co-administration with NSAIDs has resulted in increased BUN, serum creatinine and serum potassium levels, and weight gain). Products include:
Clinoril Tablets **1899**

Telmisartan (Furosemide may add to or potentiate the therapeutic effect of other antihypertensive drugs). Products include:
Micardis Tablets **884**
Micardis HCT Tablets **886**

Terazosin Hydrochloride (Furosemide may add to or potentiate the therapeutic effect of other antihypertensive drugs). Products include:
Hytrin Capsules **469**

Thiamylal Sodium (Aggravates orthostatic hypotension).
No products indexed under this heading.

Timolol Maleate (Furosemide may add to or potentiate the therapeutic effect of other antihypertensive drugs). Products include:
Blocadren Tablets **1891**
Cosopt Sterile Ophthalmic Solution **1910**
Timolide Tablets **2056**
Timoptic in Ocudose **2061**
Timoptic Sterile Ophthalmic Solution **2058**
Timoptic-XE Sterile Ophthalmic Gel Forming Solution **2062**

Tobramycin (Potential for increased risk of ototoxicity with concomitant therapy, especially in the presence of impaired renal function; avoid concurrent use except in presence of life threatening situations). Products include:
TOBI Solution for Inhalation **1015**
TobraDex Ophthalmic Ointment **558**
TobraDex Ophthalmic Suspension **558**
Zylet Ophthalmic Suspension **3508**

Tobramycin Sulfate (Potential for increased risk of ototoxicity with concomitant therapy, especially in the presence of impaired renal function; avoid concurrent use except in presence of life threatening situations).
No products indexed under this heading.

Tolmetin Sodium (Co-administration with NSAIDs has resulted in increased BUN, serum creatinine and serum potassium levels, and weight gain).
No products indexed under this heading.

Torsemide (Furosemide may add to or potentiate the therapeutic effect of other antihypertensive drugs).
No products indexed under this heading.

Trandolapril (Furosemide may add to or potentiate the therapeutic effect of other antihypertensive drugs). Products include:
Mavik Tablets **482**
Tarka Tablets **519**

Triamcinolone (Co-administration with corticosteroids may increase the risk of hypokalemia).
No products indexed under this heading.

Triamcinolone Acetonide (Co-administration with corticosteroids may increase the risk of hypokalemia). Products include:
Azmacort Inhalation Aerosol **1701**
Nasacort HFA Inhalation Aerosol **2939**
Nasacort AQ Nasal Spray **2937**

Triamcinolone Diacetate (Co-administration with corticosteroids may increase the risk of hypokalemia).
No products indexed under this heading.

Triamcinolone Hexacetonide (Co-administration with corticosteroids may increase the risk of hypokalemia).
No products indexed under this heading.

Trimethaphan Camsylate (Furosemide may add to or potentiate the therapeutic effect of other antihypertensive drugs).
No products indexed under this heading.

Tubocurarine Chloride (Furosemide has a tendency to antagonize the skeletal muscle relaxing effects of tubocurarine).
No products indexed under this heading.

Valdecoxib (Co-administration with NSAIDs has resulted in increased BUN, serum creatinine and serum potassium levels, and weight gain).
No products indexed under this heading.

Valsartan (Furosemide may add to or potentiate the therapeutic effect of other antihypertensive drugs). Products include:
Diovan HCT Tablets **2195**
Diovan Tablets **2191**

Verapamil Hydrochloride (Furosemide may add to or potentiate the therapeutic effect of other antihypertensive drugs). Products include:
Covera-HS Tablets **3135**
Tarka Tablets **519**
Verelan PM Capsules **3120**

Food Interactions

Alcohol (Aggravates orthostatic hypotension).

FUZEON INJECTION

(Enfuvirtide) **2772**
None cited in PDR database.

GABITRIL TABLETS

(Tiagabine Hydrochloride) **998**
May interact with central nervous system depressants, phenytoin, highly protein bound drugs (selected), valproate, and certain other agents. Compounds in these categories include:

Alfentanil Hydrochloride (Possible additive depressive effects).
No products indexed under this heading.

Alprazolam (Possible additive depressive effects). Products include:
Niravam Orally Disintegrating Tablets **3106**
Xanax XR Tablets **2655**

Amiodarone Hydrochloride (Tiagabine is 96% bound to human plasma protein and therefore has the potential to interact with other highly protein bound compounds. Such an interaction can potentially lead to higher free fractions of either tiagabine or the competing drug). Products include:
Pacerone Tablets **3337**

Amitriptyline Hydrochloride (Tiagabine is 96% bound to human plasma protein and therefore has the potential to interact with other highly protein bound compounds. Such an interaction can potentially lead to higher free fractions of either tiagabine or the competing drug).
No products indexed under this heading.

Aprobarbital (Possible additive depressive effects).
No products indexed under this heading.

Atovaquone (Tiagabine is 96% bound to human plasma protein and therefore has the potential to interact with other highly protein bound compounds. Such an interaction can potentially lead to higher free fractions of either tiagabine or the competing drug). Products include:
Malarone Tablets **1484**
Malarone Pediatric Tablets **1484**
Mepron Suspension **1487**

Buprenorphine Hydrochloride (Possible additive depressive effects). Products include:
Buprenex Injectable **2718**
Suboxone Tablets **2719**
Subutex Tablets **2719**

Buspirone Hydrochloride (Possible additive depressive effects).
No products indexed under this heading.

Butabarbital (Possible additive depressive effects).
No products indexed under this heading.

Butalbital (Possible additive depressive effects). Products include:
Sedapap Tablets 50 mg/650 mg **2098**

Carbamazepine (Population pharmacokinetic analyses indicate that tiagabine clearance is 60% greater in patients taking carbamazepine with or without other enzyme-inducing antiepileptic drugs; tiagabine had no effect on the steady-state plasma concentrations of carbamazepine or its epoxide metabolite in patients with epilepsy). Products include:
Carbatrol Capsules **3174**
Equetro Extended-Release Capsules **3178**
Tegretol/Tegretol-XR **2278**

Cefonicid Sodium (Tiagabine is 96% bound to human plasma protein and therefore has the potential to interact with other highly protein bound compounds. Such an interaction can potentially lead to higher free fractions of either tiagabine or the competing drug).
No products indexed under this heading.

Celecoxib (Tiagabine is 96% bound to human plasma protein and therefore has the potential to interact with other highly protein bound compounds. Such an interaction can potentially lead to higher free fractions of either tiagabine or the competing drug). Products include:
Celebrex Capsules **3130**

Chlordiazepoxide (Possible additive depressive effects).
No products indexed under this heading.

Chlordiazepoxide Hydrochloride (Possible additive depressive effects). Products include:
Librium Capsules **3349**

Chlorpromazine (Possible additive depressive effects).
No products indexed under this heading.

Chlorpromazine Hydrochloride (Possible additive depressive effects).
No products indexed under this heading.

Chlorprothixene (Possible additive depressive effects).
No products indexed under this heading.

Chlorprothixene Hydrochloride (Possible additive depressive effects).
No products indexed under this heading.

Chlorprothixene Lactate (Possible additive depressive effects).
No products indexed under this heading.

Clomipramine Hydrochloride (Tiagabine is 96% bound to human plasma protein and therefore has the potential to interact with other highly protein bound compounds. Such an interaction can potentially lead to higher free fractions of either tiagabine or the competing drug).
No products indexed under this heading.

Clorazepate Dipotassium (Possible additive depressive effects). Products include:
Tranxene **2488**

Clozapine (Possible additive depressive effects). Products include:
Clozapine Tablets **2141**
Clozaril Tablets **2174**
FazaClo Orally Disintegrating Tablets **547**

Codeine Phosphate (Possible additive depressive effects). Products include:
Tylenol with Codeine **2461**

Cyclosporine (Tiagabine is 96% bound to human plasma protein and therefore has the potential to interact with other highly protein bound compounds. Such an interaction can

potentially lead to higher free fractions of either tiagabine or the competing drug). Products include:
Gengraf Capsules 458
Neoral Soft Gelatin Capsules 2247
Neoral Oral Solution 2247
Restasis Ophthalmic Emulsion 570
Sandimmune 2259

Desflurane (Possible additive depressive effects). Products include:
Suprane Liquid for Inhalation 770

Dezocine (Possible additive depressive effects).
No products indexed under this heading.

Diazepam (Possible additive depressive effects). Products include:
Diastat Rectal Delivery System 3344
Valium Tablets 2822

Diclofenac Potassium (Tiagabine is 96% bound to human plasma protein and therefore has the potential to interact with other highly protein bound compounds. Such an interaction can potentially lead to higher free fractions of either tiagabine or the competing drug). Products include:
Cataflam Tablets 2173

Diclofenac Sodium (Tiagabine is 96% bound to human plasma protein and therefore has the potential to interact with other highly protein bound compounds. Such an interaction can potentially lead to higher free fractions of either tiagabine or the competing drug). Products include:
Arthrotec Tablets 3126
Voltaren Ophthalmic Solution 2300
Voltaren Tablets 2298
Voltaren-XR Tablets 2301

Dipyridamole (Tiagabine is 96% bound to human plasma protein and therefore has the potential to interact with other highly protein bound compounds. Such an interaction can potentially lead to higher free fractions of either tiagabine or the competing drug). Products include:
Aggrenox Capsules 855
Persantine Tablets 898

Divalproex Sodium (Co-administration of tiagabine in patients taking valproate chronically had no effect on tiagabine pharmacokinetics, but valproate significantly decreased tiagabine binding in vitro from 96.3% to 94.8% which resulted in an increase of approximately 40% in the tiagabine concentrations; the clinical relevance of this in vitro finding is unknown). Products include:
Depakote Sprinkle Capsules 422
Depakote Tablets 427
Depakote ER Tablets 433

Droperidol (Possible additive depressive effects).
No products indexed under this heading.

Enflurane (Possible additive depressive effects).
No products indexed under this heading.

Estazolam (Possible additive depressive effects). Products include:
ProSom Tablets 512

Ethanol (Possible additive depressive effects).
No products indexed under this heading.

Ethchlorvynol (Possible additive depressive effects).
No products indexed under this heading.

Ethinamate (Possible additive depressive effects).
No products indexed under this heading.

Ethyl Alcohol (Possible additive depressive effects).
No products indexed under this heading.

Fenoprofen Calcium (Tiagabine is 96% bound to human plasma protein and therefore has the potential to interact with other highly protein bound compounds. Such an interaction can potentially lead to higher free fractions of either tiagabine or the competing drug). Products include:
Nalfon Capsules 2504

Fentanyl (Possible additive depressive effects). Products include:
Duragesic Transdermal System 2448

Fentanyl Citrate (Possible additive depressive effects). Products include:
Actiq 993

Fluphenazine Decanoate (Possible additive depressive effects).
No products indexed under this heading.

Fluphenazine Enanthate (Possible additive depressive effects).
No products indexed under this heading.

Fluphenazine Hydrochloride (Possible additive depressive effects).
No products indexed under this heading.

Flurazepam Hydrochloride (Possible additive depressive effects). Products include:
Dalmane Capsules 3343

Flurbiprofen (Tiagabine is 96% bound to human plasma protein and therefore has the potential to interact with other highly protein bound compounds. Such an interaction can potentially lead to higher free fractions of either tiagabine or the competing drug).
No products indexed under this heading.

Fosphenytoin Sodium (Population pharmacokinetic analyses indicate that tiagabine clearance is 60% greater in patients taking phenytoin with or without other enzyme-inducing antiepileptic drugs; tiagabine had no effect on the steady-state plasma concentrations of phenytoin in patients with epilepsy).
No products indexed under this heading.

Glipizide (Tiagabine is 96% bound to human plasma protein and therefore has the potential to interact with other highly protein bound compounds. Such an interaction can potentially lead to higher free fractions of either tiagabine or the competing drug).
No products indexed under this heading.

Glutethimide (Possible additive depressive effects).
No products indexed under this heading.

Haloperidol (Possible additive depressive effects).
No products indexed under this heading.

Haloperidol Decanoate (Possible additive depressive effects).
No products indexed under this heading.

Hydrocodone Bitartrate (Possible additive depressive effects). Products include:
Hycodan 1104
Hycomine Compound Tablets 1105
Hycotuss Expectorant Syrup 1106
Lortab 3315
Lortab Elixir 3312
Vicodin Tablets 530
Vicodin ES Tablets 531
Vicodin HP Tablets 532
Vicoprofen Tablets 533
Zydone Tablets 1118

Hydrocodone Polistirex (Possible additive depressive effects). Products include:
Tussionex Pennkinetic Extended-Release Suspension 3322

Hydromorphone Hydrochloride (Possible additive depressive effects). Products include:
Dilaudid 439
Dilaudid Oral Liquid 443
Dilaudid Non-Sterile Powder 439
Dilaudid Rectal Suppositories 439
Dilaudid Tablets 439
Dilaudid Tablets - 8 mg 443
Dilaudid-HP 441

Hydroxyzine Hydrochloride (Possible additive depressive effects).
No products indexed under this heading.

Ibuprofen (Tiagabine is 96% bound to human plasma protein and therefore has the potential to interact with other highly protein bound compounds. Such an interaction can potentially lead to higher free fractions of either tiagabine or the competing drug). Products include:
Advil Allergy Sinus Caplets .... ▣ 737
Advil .... ▣ 737
Children's Advil Suspension .... ▣ 742
Children's Advil Chewable Tablets .. ▣ 741
Advil Cold & Sinus .... ▣ 739
Advil Flu & Body Ache Caplets .... ▣ 739
Children's Advil Cold Suspension ... ▣ 741
Infants' Advil Concentrated Drops .. ▣ 743
Junior Strength Advil Swallow Tablets .... ▣ 740
Advil Migraine Liquigels .... ▣ 740
Advil Multi-Symptom Cold Caplets .... ▣ 738
Combunox Tablets 1183
Children's Motrin Oral Suspension and Chewable Tablets 1837
Children's Motrin Cold Non-Staining Dye-Free Oral Suspension 1838
Children's Motrin Cold Oral Suspension 1838
Children's Motrin Non-Staining Dye-Free Oral Suspension 1837
Motrin Cold & Sinus Caplets 1836
Motrin IB Tablets and Caplets 1836
Infants' Motrin Concentrated Drops 1837
Infants' Motrin Non-Staining Dye-Free Drops 1837
Junior Strength Motrin Caplets and Chewable Tablets 1837
Vicoprofen Tablets 533

Imipramine Hydrochloride (Tiagabine is 96% bound to human plasma protein and therefore has the potential to interact with other highly protein bound compounds. Such an interaction can potentially lead to higher free fractions of either tiagabine or the competing drug).
No products indexed under this heading.

Imipramine Pamoate (Tiagabine is 96% bound to human plasma protein and therefore has the potential to interact with other highly protein bound compounds. Such an interaction can potentially lead to higher free fractions of either tiagabine or the competing drug).
No products indexed under this heading.

Indomethacin (Tiagabine is 96% bound to human plasma protein and therefore has the potential to interact with other highly protein bound compounds. Such an interaction can potentially lead to higher free fractions of either tiagabine or the competing drug). Products include:
Indocin 1968

Indomethacin Sodium Trihydrate (Tiagabine is 96% bound to human plasma protein and therefore has the potential to interact with other highly protein bound compounds. Such an interaction can potentially lead to higher free fractions of either tiagabine or the competing drug). Products include:
Indocin I.V. 1973

Isoflurane (Possible additive depressive effects).
No products indexed under this heading.

Ketamine Hydrochloride (Possible additive depressive effects).
No products indexed under this heading.

Ketoprofen (Tiagabine is 96% bound to human plasma protein and therefore has the potential to interact with other highly protein bound compounds. Such an interaction can potentially lead to higher free fractions of either tiagabine or the competing drug).
No products indexed under this heading.

Ketorolac Tromethamine (Tiagabine is 96% bound to human plasma protein and therefore has the potential to interact with other highly protein bound compounds. Such an interaction can potentially lead to higher free fractions of either tiagabine or the competing drug). Products include:
Acular Ophthalmic Solution 561
Acular LS Ophthalmic Solution 562

Levomethadyl Acetate Hydrochloride (Possible additive depressive effects).
No products indexed under this heading.

Levorphanol Tartrate (Possible additive depressive effects).
No products indexed under this heading.

Lorazepam (Possible additive depressive effects).
No products indexed under this heading.

Loxapine Hydrochloride (Possible additive depressive effects).
No products indexed under this heading.

Loxapine Succinate (Possible additive depressive effects).
No products indexed under this heading.

Meclofenamate Sodium (Tiagabine is 96% bound to human plasma protein and therefore has the potential to interact with other highly protein bound compounds. Such an interaction can potentially lead to higher free fractions of either tiagabine or the competing drug).
No products indexed under this heading.

Mefenamic Acid (Tiagabine is 96% bound to human plasma protein and therefore has the potential to interact with other highly protein bound compounds. Such an interaction can potentially lead to higher free fractions of either tiagabine or the competing drug).
No products indexed under this heading.

Meperidine Hydrochloride (Possible additive depressive effects).
No products indexed under this heading.

Mephobarbital (Possible additive depressive effects). Products include:
Mebaral Tablets, USP 2483

Meprobamate (Possible additive depressive effects).
No products indexed under this heading.

Mesoridazine Besylate (Possible additive depressive effects).
No products indexed under this heading.

Methadone Hydrochloride (Possible additive depressive effects).
No products indexed under this heading.

Methohexital Sodium (Possible additive depressive effects).
No products indexed under this heading.

Methotrimeprazine (Possible additive depressive effects).
No products indexed under this heading.

Methoxyflurane (Possible additive depressive effects).
No products indexed under this heading.

Midazolam Hydrochloride (Possible additive depressive effects).
No products indexed under this heading.

Molindone Hydrochloride (Possible additive depressive effects). Products include:
Moban Tablets 1108

Morphine Sulfate (Possible additive depressive effects). Products include:
Avinza Capsules 1714
Kadian Capsules 572
MS Contin Tablets 2703

Naproxen (Tiagabine is 96% bound to human plasma protein and therefore has the potential to interact with other highly protein bound compounds. Such an interaction can potentially lead to higher free fractions of either tiagabine or the competing drug). Products include:
EC-Naprosyn Delayed-Release Tablets 2769
Naprosyn Suspension 2769
Naprosyn Tablets 2769
Prevacid NapraPAC 3277

Naproxen Sodium (Tiagabine is 96% bound to human plasma protein and therefore has the potential to interact with other highly protein bound compounds. Such an interaction can potentially lead to higher free fractions of either tiagabine or the competing drug). Products include:
Aleve Tablets, Caplets and Gelcaps 605
Anaprox Tablets 2769
Anaprox DS Tablets 2769

Nortriptyline Hydrochloride (Tiagabine is 96% bound to human plasma protein and therefore has the potential to interact with other highly protein bound compounds. Such an interaction can potentially lead to higher free fractions of either tiagabine or the competing drug).
No products indexed under this heading.

Olanzapine (Possible additive depressive effects). Products include:
Symbyax Capsules 1788
Zyprexa Tablets 1798
Zyprexa IntraMuscular 1798
Zyprexa ZYDIS Orally Disintegrating Tablets.................. 1798

Oxaprozin (Tiagabine is 96% bound to human plasma protein and therefore has the potential to interact with other highly protein bound compounds. Such an interaction can potentially lead to higher free fractions of either tiagabine or the competing drug).
No products indexed under this heading.

Oxazepam (Possible additive depressive effects).
No products indexed under this heading.

Oxycodone Hydrochloride (Possible additive depressive effects). Products include:
Combunox Tablets 1183
OxyContin Tablets 2699
OxyFast Oral Concentrate Solution.. 2704
OxyIR Capsules 2704
Percocet Tablets 1114
Percodan Tablets 1115

Pentobarbital Sodium (Possible additive depressive effects). Products include:
Nembutal Sodium Solution, USP 2484

Perphenazine (Possible additive depressive effects).
No products indexed under this heading.

Phenobarbital (Population pharmacokinetic analyses indicate that tiagabine clearance is 60% greater in patients taking phenobarbital with or without other enzyme-inducing antiepileptic drugs; possible additive depressive effects).
No products indexed under this heading.

Phenylbutazone (Tiagabine is 96% bound to human plasma protein and therefore has the potential to interact with other highly protein bound compounds. Such an interaction can potentially lead to higher free fractions of either tiagabine or the competing drug).
No products indexed under this heading.

Phenytoin (Population pharmacokinetic analyses indicate that tiagabine clearance is 60% greater in patients taking phenytoin with or without other enzyme-inducing antiepileptic drugs; tiagabine had no effect on the steady-state plasma concentrations of phenytoin in patients with epilepsy).
No products indexed under this heading.

Phenytoin Sodium (Population pharmacokinetic analyses indicate that tiagabine clearance is 60% greater in patients taking phenytoin with or without other enzyme-inducing antiepileptic drugs; tiagabine had no effect on the steady-state plasma concentrations of phenytoin in patients with epilepsy). Products include:
Phenytek Capsules 2153

Piroxicam (Tiagabine is 96% bound to human plasma protein and therefore has the potential to interact with other highly protein bound compounds. Such an interaction can potentially lead to higher free fractions of either tiagabine or the competing drug).
No products indexed under this heading.

Prazepam (Possible additive depressive effects).
No products indexed under this heading.

Prochlorperazine (Possible additive depressive effects).
No products indexed under this heading.

Promethazine Hydrochloride (Possible additive depressive effects). Products include:
Phenergan 3438

Propofol (Possible additive depressive effects). Products include:
Diprivan Injectable Emulsion 676

Propoxyphene Hydrochloride (Possible additive depressive effects).
No products indexed under this heading.

Propoxyphene Napsylate (Possible additive depressive effects). Products include:
Darvocet A 500 Tablets 3497

Propranolol Hydrochloride (Tiagabine is 96% bound to human plasma protein and therefore has the potential to interact with other highly protein bound compounds. Such an interaction can potentially lead to higher free fractions of either tiagabine or the competing drug). Products include:
Inderal LA Long-Acting Capsules 3421
InnoPran XL Capsules 2728

Quazepam (Possible additive depressive effects).
No products indexed under this heading.

Quetiapine Fumarate (Possible additive depressive effects). Products include:
Seroquel Tablets 691

Remifentanil Hydrochloride (Possible additive depressive effects).
No products indexed under this heading.

Risperidone (Possible additive depressive effects). Products include:
Risperdal Consta Long-Acting Injection 1664
Risperdal M-Tab Orally Disintegrating Tablets.................. 1658
Risperdal 1658

Secobarbital Sodium (Possible additive depressive effects).
No products indexed under this heading.

Sevoflurane (Possible additive depressive effects). Products include:
Ultane Liquid for Inhalation 526

Sodium Oxybate (Possible additive depressive effects).
No products indexed under this heading.

Sufentanil Citrate (Possible additive depressive effects).
No products indexed under this heading.

Sulindac (Tiagabine is 96% bound to human plasma protein and therefore has the potential to interact with other highly protein bound compounds. Such an interaction can potentially lead to higher free fractions of either tiagabine or the competing drug). Products include:
Clinoril Tablets 1899

Temazepam (Possible additive depressive effects).
No products indexed under this heading.

Thiamylal Sodium (Possible additive depressive effects).
No products indexed under this heading.

Thioridazine Hydrochloride (Possible additive depressive effects). Products include:
Thioridazine Hydrochloride Tablets.. 2122

Thiothixene (Possible additive depressive effects). Products include:
Thiothixene Capsules 2124

Tolbutamide (Tiagabine is 96% bound to human plasma protein and therefore has the potential to interact with other highly protein bound compounds. Such an interaction can potentially lead to higher free fractions of either tiagabine or the competing drug).
No products indexed under this heading.

Tolmetin Sodium (Tiagabine is 96% bound to human plasma protein and therefore has the potential to interact with other highly protein bound compounds. Such an interaction can potentially lead to higher free fractions of either tiagabine or the competing drug).
No products indexed under this heading.

Triazolam (Possible additive depressive effects).
No products indexed under this heading.

Trifluoperazine Hydrochloride (Possible additive depressive effects).
No products indexed under this heading.

Trimipramine Maleate (Tiagabine is 96% bound to human plasma protein and therefore has the potential to interact with other highly protein bound compounds. Such an interaction can potentially lead to higher free fractions of either tiagabine or the competing drug). Products include:
Surmontil Capsules 2347

Valproate Sodium (Coadministration of tiagabine in patients taking valproate chronically had no effect on tiagabine pharmacokinetics, but valproate significantly decreased tiagabine binding in vitro from 96.3% to 94.8% which resulted in an increase of approximately 40% in the tiagabine concentrations; the clinical relevance of this in vitro finding is unknown). Products include:
Depacon Injection 412

Valproic Acid (Co-administration of tiagabine in patients taking valproate chronically had no effect on tiagabine pharmacokinetics, but valproate significantly decreased tiagabine binding in vitro from 96.3% to 94.8% which resulted in an increase of approximately 40% in the tiagabine concentrations; the clinical relevance of this in vitro finding is unknown). Products include:
Depakene 417

Warfarin Sodium (Tiagabine is 96% bound to human plasma protein and therefore has the potential to interact with other highly protein bound compounds. Such an interaction can potentially lead to higher free fractions of either tiagabine or the competing drug). Products include:
Coumadin for Injection 932
Coumadin Tablets 932

Zaleplon (Possible additive depressive effects). Products include:
Sonata Capsules 1686

Ziprasidone Hydrochloride (Possible additive depressive effects). Products include:
Geodon Capsules 2514

Zolpidem Tartrate (Possible additive depressive effects). Products include:
Ambien Tablets 2867

Food Interactions

Alcohol (Possible additive depressive effects).

Food, unspecified (A high fat meal decreases the rate (mean Tmax was prolonged to 2.5 hours, and Cmax was reduced by about 40%) but not the extent (AUC) of tiagabine).

GAMASTAN

(Globulin, Immune (Human)) 3231
None cited in PDR database.

GAMMAGARD LIQUID

(Immune Globulin Intravenous (Human)).. 751
May interact with vaccines, live. Compounds in these categories include:

BCG Vaccine (Antibodies in immune globulin intravenous products may interfere with patient responses to live vaccines, such as those for measles, mumps and rubella).
No products indexed under this heading.

Measles, Mumps & Rubella Virus Vaccine, Live (Antibodies in immune globulin intravenous products may interfere with patient responses to live vaccines, such as those for measles, mumps and rubella). Products include:
M-M-R II 1980

Measles & Rubella Virus Vaccine Live (Antibodies in immune globulin intravenous products may interfere with patient responses to live vaccines, such as those for measles, mumps and rubella).
No products indexed under this heading.

Measles Virus Vaccine Live (Antibodies in immune globulin intravenous products may interfere with patient responses to live vaccines, such as those for measles, mumps and rubella). Products include:
Attenuvax 1889

Mumps Virus Vaccine, Live (Antibodies in immune globulin intravenous products may interfere with patient responses to live vaccines, such as those for measles, mumps and rubella). Products include:
Mumpsvax 2005

Poliovirus Vaccine, Live, Oral, Trivalent, Types 1,2,3 (Sabin) (Antibodies in immune globulin intravenous products may interfere with patient responses to live vaccines, such as those for measles, mumps and rubella).
No products indexed under this heading.

Rotavirus Vaccine, Live, Oral, Tetravalent (Antibodies in immune globulin intravenous products may interfere with patient responses to live vaccines, such as those for measles, mumps and rubella).
No products indexed under this heading.

Rubella & Mumps Virus Vaccine Live (Antibodies in immune globulin intravenous products may interfere with patient responses to live vaccines, such as those for measles, mumps and rubella).
No products indexed under this heading.

Rubella Virus Vaccine Live (Antibodies in immune globulin intravenous products may interfere with patient responses to live vaccines, such as those for measles, mumps and rubella). Products include:
Meruvax II 1994

Smallpox Vaccine (Antibodies in immune globulin intravenous products may interfere with patient responses to live vaccines, such as those for measles, mumps and rubella).
No products indexed under this heading.

Typhoid Vaccine (Antibodies in immune globulin intravenous products may interfere with patient responses to live vaccines, such as those for measles, mumps and rubella).
No products indexed under this heading.

Varicella Virus Vaccine Live (Antibodies in immune globulin intravenous products may interfere with patient responses to live vaccines, such as those for measles, mumps and rubella). Products include:
Varivax 2070

Yellow Fever Vaccine (Antibodies in immune globulin intravenous products may interfere with patient responses to live vaccines, such as those for measles, mumps and rubella).
No products indexed under this heading.

GAMMAGARD S/D

(Immune Globulin Intravenous (Human)).. 754
May interact with vaccines, live. Compounds in these categories include:

BCG Vaccine (Antibodies in immune globulin intravenous products may interfere with patient responses to live vaccines, such as those for measles, mumps and rubella).
No products indexed under this heading.

Measles, Mumps & Rubella Virus Vaccine, Live (Antibodies in immune globulin intravenous products may interfere with patient responses to live vaccines, such as those for measles, mumps and rubella). Products include:
M-M-R II 1980

Measles & Rubella Virus Vaccine Live (Antibodies in immune globulin intravenous products may interfere with patient responses to live vaccines, such as those for measles, mumps and rubella).
No products indexed under this heading.

Measles Virus Vaccine Live (Antibodies in immune globulin intravenous products may interfere with patient responses to live vaccines, such as those for measles, mumps and rubella). Products include:
Attenuvax 1889

Mumps Virus Vaccine, Live (Antibodies in immune globulin intravenous products may interfere with patient responses to live vaccines, such as those for measles, mumps and rubella). Products include:
Mumpsvax 2005

Poliovirus Vaccine, Live, Oral, Trivalent, Types 1,2,3 (Sabin) (Antibodies in immune globulin intravenous products may interfere with patient responses to live vaccines, such as those for measles, mumps and rubella).
No products indexed under this heading.

Rotavirus Vaccine, Live, Oral, Tetravalent (Antibodies in immune globulin intravenous products may interfere with patient responses to live vaccines, such as those for measles, mumps and rubella).
No products indexed under this heading.

Rubella & Mumps Virus Vaccine Live (Antibodies in immune globulin intravenous products may interfere with patient responses to live vaccines, such as those for measles, mumps and rubella).
No products indexed under this heading.

Rubella Virus Vaccine Live (Antibodies in immune globulin intravenous products may interfere with patient responses to live vaccines, such as those for measles, mumps and rubella). Products include:
Meruvax II 1994

Smallpox Vaccine (Antibodies in immune globulin intravenous products may interfere with patient responses to live vaccines, such as those for measles, mumps and rubella).
No products indexed under this heading.

Typhoid Vaccine (Antibodies in immune globulin intravenous products may interfere with patient responses to live vaccines, such as those for measles, mumps and rubella).
No products indexed under this heading.

Varicella Virus Vaccine Live (Antibodies in immune globulin intravenous products may interfere with patient responses to live vaccines, such as those for measles, mumps and rubella). Products include:
Varivax 2070

Yellow Fever Vaccine (Antibodies in immune globulin intravenous products may interfere with patient responses to live vaccines, such as those for measles, mumps and rubella).
No products indexed under this heading.

GAMUNEX IMMUNE GLOBULIN I.V., 10%

(Immune Globulin Intravenous (Human)).. 3232
May interact with:

Measles, Mumps & Rubella Virus Vaccine, Live (Co-administration may interfere with the response to live viral vaccines such as measles. Therefore, use of such vaccines should be deferred until approximately 6 months after Immune Globulin Intravenous (Human) administration). Products include:
M-M-R II 1980

Measles & Rubella Virus Vaccine Live (Co-administration may interfere with the response to live viral vaccines such as measles. Therefore, use of such vaccines should be deferred until approximately 6 months after Immune Globulin Intravenous (Human) administration).
No products indexed under this heading.

Measles Virus Vaccine Live (Co-administration may interfere with the response to live viral vaccines such as measles. Therefore, use of such vaccines should be deferred until approximately 6 months after Immune Globulin Intravenous (Human) administration). Products include:
Attenuvax 1889

Mumps Skin Test Antigen (Co-administration may interfere with the response to live viral vaccines such as mumps. Therefore, use of such vaccines should be deferred until approximately 6 months after Immune Globulin Intravenous (Human) administration).
No products indexed under this heading.

Mumps Virus Vaccine, Live (Co-administration may interfere with the response to live viral vaccines such as mumps. Therefore, use of such vaccines should be deferred until approximately 6 months after Immune Globulin Intravenous (Human) administration). Products include:
Mumpsvax 2005

Rubella & Mumps Virus Vaccine Live (Co-administration may interfere with the response to live viral vaccines such as rubella. Therefore, use of such vaccines should be deferred until approximately 6 months after Immune Globulin Intravenous (Human) administration).
No products indexed under this heading.

Rubella Virus Vaccine Live (Co-administration may interfere with the response to live viral vaccines such as rubella. Therefore, use of such vaccines should be deferred until approximately 6 months after Immune Globulin Intravenous (Human) administration). Products include:
Meruvax II 1994

GARAMYCIN INJECTABLE
(Gentamicin Sulfate) 3028
May interact with aminoglycosides, anesthetics, cephalosporins, neuromuscular blocking agents, and certain other agents. Compounds in these categories include:

Alfentanil Hydrochloride (Increased potential for neuromuscular blockade and respiratory paralysis).
No products indexed under this heading.

Amikacin Sulfate (Concurrent and/or sequential use increases the risk of neurotoxicity and/or nephrotoxicity).
No products indexed under this heading.

Atracurium Besylate (Increased potential for neuromuscular blockade and respiratory paralysis).
No products indexed under this heading.

Carbenicillin Indanyl Sodium (Potential for reduction in gentamicin serum half-life in patients with severe renal impairment receiving concomitant carbenicillin and gentamicin).
No products indexed under this heading.

Cefaclor (Potential for increased nephrotoxicity).
No products indexed under this heading.

Cefadroxil (Potential for increased nephrotoxicity).
No products indexed under this heading.

Cefamandole Nafate (Potential for increased nephrotoxicity).
No products indexed under this heading.

Cefazolin Sodium (Potential for increased nephrotoxicity). Products include:
Ancef for Injection 1318

Cefdinir (Potential for increased nephrotoxicity). Products include:
Omnicef Capsules 506
Omnicef for Oral Suspension 506

Cefepime Hydrochloride (Potential for increased nephrotoxicity). Products include:
Maxipime for Injection 1093

Cefixime (Potential for increased nephrotoxicity). Products include:
Suprax 1811

Cefmetazole Sodium (Potential for increased nephrotoxicity).
No products indexed under this heading.

Cefonicid Sodium (Potential for increased nephrotoxicity).
No products indexed under this heading.

Cefoperazone Sodium (Potential for increased nephrotoxicity).
No products indexed under this heading.

Ceforanide (Potential for increased nephrotoxicity).
No products indexed under this heading.

Cefotaxime Sodium (Potential for increased nephrotoxicity).
No products indexed under this heading.

Cefotetan (Potential for increased nephrotoxicity).
No products indexed under this heading.

Cefoxitin Sodium (Potential for increased nephrotoxicity). Products include:
Mefoxin for Injection 1987
Mefoxin Premixed Intravenous Solution 1990

Cefpodoxime Proxetil (Potential for increased nephrotoxicity). Products include:
Vantin Tablets and Oral Suspension 2650

Cefprozil (Potential for increased nephrotoxicity).
No products indexed under this heading.

Ceftazidime (Potential for increased nephrotoxicity). Products include:
Fortaz for Injection 1422

Ceftizoxime Sodium (Potential for increased nephrotoxicity).
No products indexed under this heading.

Ceftriaxone Sodium (Potential for increased nephrotoxicity). Products include:
Rocephin Injectable Vials, ADD-Vantage, Galaxy, Bulk 2801

Cefuroxime Axetil (Potential for increased nephrotoxicity). Products include:
Ceftin 1369

Cefuroxime Sodium (Potential for increased nephrotoxicity).
No products indexed under this heading.

Cephalexin (Potential for increased nephrotoxicity).
No products indexed under this heading.

Cephaloridine (Concurrent and/or sequential use increases the risk of neurotoxicity and/or nephrotoxicity).
No products indexed under this heading.

Cephalothin Sodium (Potential for increased nephrotoxicity).
No products indexed under this heading.

Cephapirin Sodium (Potential for increased nephrotoxicity).
No products indexed under this heading.

Cephradine (Potential for increased nephrotoxicity).
No products indexed under this heading.

Cisatracurium Besylate (Increased potential for neuromuscular blockade and respiratory paralysis). Products include:
Nimbex Injection 494

Cisplatin (Concurrent and/or sequential use increases the risk of neurotoxicity and/or nephrotoxicity).
No products indexed under this heading.

Colistin Sulfate (Concurrent and/or sequential use increases the risk of neurotoxicity and/or nephrotoxicity).
No products indexed under this heading.

Doxacurium Chloride (Increased potential for neuromuscular blockade and respiratory paralysis).
No products indexed under this heading.

Enflurane (Increased potential for neuromuscular blockade and respiratory paralysis).
No products indexed under this heading.

Ethacrynic Acid (Potential for increased ototoxicity; concurrent use should be avoided). Products include:
Edecrin Tablets 1941

Fentanyl Citrate (Increased potential for neuromuscular blockade and respiratory paralysis). Products include:
Actiq 993

Furosemide (Potential for increased ototoxicity; concurrent use should be avoided). Products include:
Furosemide Tablets 2117

Halothane (Increased potential for neuromuscular blockade and respiratory paralysis).
No products indexed under this heading.

Isoflurane (Increased potential for neuromuscular blockade and respiratory paralysis).
No products indexed under this heading.

Kanamycin Sulfate (Concurrent and/or sequential use increases the risk of neurotoxicity and/or nephrotoxicity).
No products indexed under this heading.

Ketamine Hydrochloride (Increased potential for neuromuscular blockade and respiratory paralysis).
No products indexed under this heading.

Lithium Carbonate (Increased potential for neuromuscular blockade and respiratory paralysis). Products include:
Eskalith 1406
Lithobid Tablets 1670

Lithium Citrate (Increased potential for neuromuscular blockade and respiratory paralysis).
No products indexed under this heading.

Loracarbef (Potential for increased nephrotoxicity).
No products indexed under this heading.

Methohexital Sodium (Increased potential for neuromuscular blockade and respiratory paralysis).
No products indexed under this heading.

Metocurine Iodide (Increased potential for neuromuscular blockade and respiratory paralysis).
No products indexed under this heading.

Midazolam Hydrochloride (Increased potential for neuromuscular blockade and respiratory paralysis).
No products indexed under this heading.

Mivacurium Chloride (Increased potential for neuromuscular blockade and respiratory paralysis). Products include:
Mivacron Injection 489

Neomycin, oral (Concurrent and/or sequential use increases the risk of neurotoxicity and/or nephrotoxicity).
No products indexed under this heading.

Neomycin Sulfate (Concurrent and/or sequential use increases the risk of neurotoxicity and/or nephrotoxicity). Products include:
Poly-Pred Liquifilm Ophthalmic Suspension .... ⊙231

Pancuronium Bromide (Increased potential for neuromuscular blockade and respiratory paralysis).
No products indexed under this heading.

Paromomycin Sulfate (Concurrent and/or sequential use increases the risk of neurotoxicity and/or nephrotoxicity).
No products indexed under this heading.

Polymyxin B Sulfate (Concurrent and/or sequential use increases the risk of neurotoxicity and/or nephrotoxicity). Products include:
Neosporin Ointment 702
Neosporin + Pain Relief Maximum Strength Cream........... 703
Neosporin + Pain Relief Maximum Strength Ointment....... 703
Poly-Pred Liquifilm Ophthalmic Suspension .... ⊙231
Polysporin Ointment 706
Polytrim Ophthalmic Solution 570

Propofol (Increased potential for neuromuscular blockade and respiratory paralysis). Products include:
Diprivan Injectable Emulsion 676

Rapacuronium Bromide (Increased potential for neuromuscular blockade and respiratory paralysis).
No products indexed under this heading.

Remifentanil Hydrochloride (Increased potential for neuromuscular blockade and respiratory paralysis).
No products indexed under this heading.

Rocuronium Bromide (Increased potential for neuromuscular blockade and respiratory paralysis). Products include:
Zemuron Injection 2363

Streptomycin Sulfate (Concurrent and/or sequential use increases the risk of neurotoxicity and/or nephrotoxicity).
No products indexed under this heading.

Succinylcholine Chloride (Increased potential for neuromuscular blockade and respiratory paralysis).
No products indexed under this heading.

Sufentanil Citrate (Increased potential for neuromuscular blockade and respiratory paralysis).
No products indexed under this heading.

Thiamylal Sodium (Increased potential for neuromuscular blockade and respiratory paralysis).
No products indexed under this heading.

Tobramycin (Concurrent and/or sequential use increases the risk of neurotoxicity and/or nephrotoxicity). Products include:
TOBI Solution for Inhalation 1015
TobraDex Ophthalmic Ointment 558
TobraDex Ophthalmic Suspension ... 558
Zylet Ophthalmic Suspension 3508

Tobramycin Sulfate (Concurrent and/or sequential use increases the risk of neurotoxicity and/or nephrotoxicity).
No products indexed under this heading.

Tubocurarine Chloride (Increased potential for neuromuscular blockade and respiratory paralysis).
No products indexed under this heading.

Vancomycin Hydrochloride (Concurrent and/or sequential use increases the risk of neurotoxicity and/or nephrotoxicity). Products include:

Vancocin HCl Capsules, USP 3370

Vecuronium Bromide (Increased potential for neuromuscular blockade and respiratory paralysis).
No products indexed under this heading.

Viomycin (Concurrent and/or sequential use increases the risk of neurotoxicity and/or nephrotoxicity).

GAS-X REGULAR STRENGTH CHEWABLE TABLETS
(Simethicone) .... ▣675
None cited in PDR database.

GAS-X EXTRA STRENGTH CHEWABLE TABLETS
(Simethicone) .... ▣675
None cited in PDR database.

GAS-X EXTRA STRENGTH SOFTGELS
(Simethicone) .... ▣675
None cited in PDR database.

GAS-X MAXIMUM STRENGTH SOFTGELS
(Simethicone) .... ▣675
None cited in PDR database.

GAS-X WITH MAALOX EXTRA STRENGTH CHEWABLE TABLETS
(Calcium Carbonate, Simethicone) ... ▣675
May interact with:

Prescription Drugs, unspecified (Antacids may interact with certain unspecified prescription drugs).
No products indexed under this heading.

GAS-X WITH MAALOX SOFTGELS
(Calcium Carbonate, Simethicone) ... ▣675
See Gas-X with Maalox Extra Strength Chewable Tablets

GAVISCON REGULAR STRENGTH LIQUID
(Aluminum Hydroxide, Magnesium Carbonate) .... ▣620
May interact with:

Prescription Drugs, unspecified (Concurrent use with certain unspecified drugs is not recommended; consult your physicians).
No products indexed under this heading.

GAVISCON REGULAR STRENGTH TABLETS
(Aluminum Hydroxide, Magnesium Trisilicate) .... ▣619
May interact with:

Prescription Drugs, unspecified (Concurrent use with certain unspecified drugs is not recommended; consult your physicians).
No products indexed under this heading.

GAVISCON EXTRA STRENGTH LIQUID
(Aluminum Hydroxide, Magnesium Carbonate) .... ▣620
May interact with:

Prescription Drugs, unspecified (Concurrent use with certain unspecified drugs is not recommended; consult your physicians).
No products indexed under this heading.

GAVISCON EXTRA STRENGTH TABLETS
(Aluminum Hydroxide, Magnesium Carbonate) .... ▣619
May interact with:

Prescription Drugs, unspecified (Concurrent use with certain unspecified drugs is not recommended; consult your physicians).
No products indexed under this heading.

GEMZAR FOR INJECTION
(Gemcitabine Hydrochloride) 1743
None cited in PDR database.

GENGRAF CAPSULES
(Cyclosporine) 458
May interact with erythromycin, immunosuppressive agents, methylprednisolone, non-steroidal anti-inflammatory agents, phenytoin, prednisolone, potassium sparing diuretics, and certain other agents. Compounds in these categories include:

Allopurinol (Cyclosporine is extensively metabolized by CYP450 3A. Substances that inhibit this enzyme could decrease the metabolism and increase cyclosporine concentrations).
No products indexed under this heading.

Amiloride Hydrochloride (Cyclosporine causes hyperkalemia; concurrent use with potassium-sparing diuretics can result in increased risk of hyperkalemia; co-administration should be avoided). Products include:
Midamor Tablets 2000
Moduretic Tablets 2003

Amiodarone Hydrochloride (Cyclosporine is extensively metabolized by CYP450 3A. Substances that inhibit this enzyme could decrease the metabolism and increase cyclosporine concentrations). Products include:
Pacerone Tablets 3337

Amphotericin B (May potentiate renal dysfunction).
No products indexed under this heading.

Azapropazon (May potentiate renal dysfunction).
No products indexed under this heading.

Azathioprine (Co-administration with other immunosuppressive agents increases the possibility of excessive immunosuppression). Products include:
Azasan Tablets 2844

Basiliximab (Co-administration with other immunosuppressive agents increases the possibility of excessive immunosuppression). Products include:
Simulect for Injection 2268

Bromocriptine Mesylate (Cyclosporine is extensively metabolized by CYP450 3A. Substances that inhibit this enzyme could decrease the metabolism and increase cyclosporine concentrations).
No products indexed under this heading.

Carbamazepine (Co-administration with drugs that are inducers of CYP450 3A, such as carbamazepine, could increase metabolism of cyclosporine and decrease its concentrations). Products include:
Carbatrol Capsules 3174
Equetro Extended-Release Capsules 3178
Tegretol/Tegretol-XR 2278

Celecoxib (Cyclosporine can cause nephrotoxicity; clinical status and serum creatinine should be closely monitored when cyclosporine is used with NSAIDs in rheumatoid arthritis patients). Products include:
Celebrex Capsules 3130

Cimetidine (May potentiate renal dysfunction). Products include:
Tagamet HB 200 Tablets .... ▣637
Tagamet Tablets 1547

Cimetidine Hydrochloride (May potentiate renal dysfunction).
No products indexed under this heading.

Clarithromycin (Cyclosporine is extensively metabolized by CYP450 3A. Substances that inhibit this enzyme could decrease the metabolism and increase cyclosporine concentrations). Products include:
Biaxin/Biaxin XL 402
PREVPAC 3281

Colchicine (Cyclosporine is extensively metabolized by CYP450 3A. Substances that inhibit this enzyme could decrease the metabolism and increase cyclosporine concentrations. May potentiate renal dysfunction).
No products indexed under this heading.

Dalfopristin (Cyclosporine is extensively metabolized by CYP450 3A. Substances that inhibit this enzyme could decrease the metabolism and increase cyclosporine concentrations). Products include:
Synercid I.V. 1690

Danazol (Cyclosporine is extensively metabolized by CYP450 3A. Substances that inhibit this enzyme could decrease the metabolism and increase cyclosporine concentrations).
No products indexed under this heading.

Diclofenac Potassium (May potentiate renal dysfunction; potential for doubling of diclofenac blood levels and occasional reports of reversible decreases in renal function have been reported with concurrent use). Products include:
Cataflam Tablets 2173

Diclofenac Sodium (May potentiate renal dysfunction; potential for doubling of diclofenac blood levels and occasional reports of reversible decreases in renal function have been reported with concurrent use). Products include:
Arthrotec Tablets 3126
Voltaren Ophthalmic Solution 2300
Voltaren Tablets 2298
Voltaren-XR Tablets 2301

Digoxin (Co-administration results in reduced clearance of digoxin; decrease in the apparent volume of distribution of digoxin has reported with concurrent use along with digitalis toxicity). Products include:
Digitek Tablets 2146
Lanoxicaps Capsules 1458
Lanoxin Injection 1462
Lanoxin Tablets 1468
Lanoxin Injection Pediatric 1465

Diltiazem Hydrochloride (Cyclosporine is extensively metabolized by CYP450 3A. Substances that inhibit this enzyme could decrease the metabolism and increase cyclosporine concentrations). Products include:
Cardizem LA Extended Release Tablets 1699
Tiazac Capsules 1204

Diltiazem Maleate (Cyclosporine is extensively metabolized by CYP450 3A. Substances that inhibit this enzyme could decrease the metabolism and increase cyclosporine concentrations).
No products indexed under this heading.

Erythromycin (Cyclosporine is extensively metabolized by CYP450 3A. Substances that inhibit this enzyme could decrease the metabolism and increase cyclosporine concentrations). Products include:
Erygel Topical Gel 2096
Ery-Tab Tablets 447
Erythromycin Base Filmtab Tablets 454
Erythromycin Delayed-Release Capsules, USP 456
PCE Dispertab Tablets 510

Erythromycin Estolate (Cyclosporine is extensively metabolized by CYP450 3A. Substances that inhibit this enzyme could decrease the metabolism and increase cyclosporine concentrations).
No products indexed under this heading.

Erythromycin Ethylsuccinate (Cyclosporine is extensively metabolized by CYP450 3A. Substances that inhibit this enzyme could decrease the metabolism and increase cyclosporine concentrations). Products include:
E.E.S. 449
EryPed 445

Erythromycin Gluceptate (Cyclosporine is extensively metabolized by CYP450 3A. Substances that inhibit this enzyme could decrease the metabolism and increase cyclosporine concentrations).
No products indexed under this heading.

Erythromycin Lactobionate (Cyclosporine is extensively metabolized by CYP450 3A. Substances that inhibit this enzyme could decrease the metabolism and increase cyclosporine concentrations).
No products indexed under this heading.

Erythromycin Stearate (Cyclosporine is extensively metabolized by CYP450 3A. Substances that inhibit this enzyme could decrease the metabolism and increase cyclosporine concentrations). Products include:
Erythrocin Stearate Filmtab Tablets 452

Etodolac (Cyclosporine can cause nephrotoxicity; clinical status and serum creatinine should be closely monitored when cyclosporine is used with NSAIDs in rheumatoid arthritis patients).
No products indexed under this heading.

Fenoprofen Calcium (Cyclosporine can cause nephrotoxicity; clinical status and serum creatinine should be closely monitored when cyclosporine is used with NSAIDs in rheumatoid arthritis patients). Products include:
Nalfon Capsules 2504

Fluconazole (Co-administration with drugs that inhibit CYP450 3A, such as fluconazole, could decrease metabolism of cyclosporine and increase its concentrations).
No products indexed under this heading.

Flurbiprofen (Cyclosporine can cause nephrotoxicity; clinical status and serum creatinine should be closely monitored when cyclosporine is used with NSAIDs in rheumatoid arthritis patients).
No products indexed under this heading.

Fosphenytoin Sodium (Co-administration with drugs that are inducers of CYP450 3A, such as phenytoin, could increase metabolism of cyclosporine and decrease its concentrations).
No products indexed under this heading.

Gentamicin Sulfate (May potentiate renal dysfunction). Products include:
Garamycin Injectable 3028
Genoptic Sterile Ophthalmic Solution........ ⊙227
Pred-G Ophthalmic Suspension ...... ⊙234
Pred-G Sterile Ophthalmic Ointment........ ⊙235

Hypericum (Co-administration with drugs that are inducers of CYP450 3A could increase metabolism of cyclosporine and decrease its concentrations. This interaction has been reported to produce a marked reduction in the blood concentrations of cyclosporine, resultingin subtherapeutic levels, rejection of transplant organs, and graft loss).
No products indexed under this heading.

Ibuprofen (Cyclosporine can cause nephrotoxicity; clinical status and serum creatinine should be closely monitored when cyclosporine is used with NSAIDs in rheumatoid arthritis patients). Products include:
Advil Allergy Sinus Caplets .... ▣737
Advil .... ▣737
Children's Advil Suspension .... ▣742
Children's Advil Chewable Tablets .. ▣741
Advil Cold & Sinus .... ▣739
Advil Flu & Body Ache Caplets .... ▣739
Children's Advil Cold Suspension ... ▣741
Infants' Advil Concentrated Drops .. ▣743
Junior Strength Advil Swallow Tablets........ ▣740
Advil Migraine Liquigels .... ▣740
Advil Multi-Symptom Cold Caplets........ ▣738
Combunox Tablets 1183
Children's Motrin Oral Suspension and Chewable Tablets........ 1837
Children's Motrin Cold Non-Staining Dye-Free Oral Suspension........ 1838
Children's Motrin Cold Oral Suspension........ 1838
Children's Motrin Non-Staining Dye-Free Oral Suspension........ 1837
Motrin Cold & Sinus Caplets 1836
Motrin IB Tablets and Caplets 1836
Infants' Motrin Concentrated Drops........ 1837
Infants' Motrin Non-Staining Dye-Free Drops........ 1837
Junior Strength Motrin Caplets and Chewable Tablets........ 1837
Vicoprofen Tablets 533

Indomethacin (Cyclosporine can cause nephrotoxicity; clinical status and serum creatinine should be closely monitored when cyclosporine is used with NSAIDs in rheumatoid arthritis patients). Products include:
Indocin 1968

Indomethacin Sodium Trihydrate (Cyclosporine can cause nephrotoxicity; clinical status and serum creatinine should be closely monitored when cyclosporine is used with NSAIDs in rheumatoid arthritis patients). Products include:
Indocin I.V. 1973

Itraconazole (Co-administration with drugs that inhibit CYP450 3A, such as itraconazole, could decrease metabolism of cyclosporine and increase its concentrations).
No products indexed under this heading.

Ketoconazole (May potentiate renal dysfunction; co-administration with drugs that inhibit CYP4503A, such as ketoconazole, could decrease metabolism of cyclosporine and increase its concentrations). Products include:
Nizoral A-D Shampoo, 1% 1839
Nizoral 2% Shampoo 1838

Ketoprofen (Cyclosporine can cause nephrotoxicity; clinical status and serum creatinine should be closely monitored when cyclosporine is used with NSAIDs in rheumatoid arthritis patients).
No products indexed under this heading.

Ketorolac Tromethamine (Cyclosporine can cause nephrotoxicity; clinical status and serum creatinine should be closely monitored when cyclosporine is used with NSAIDs in rheumatoid arthritis patients). Products include:
Acular Ophthalmic Solution 561
Acular LS Ophthalmic Solution 562

Lovastatin (Co-administration results in reduced clearance of lovastatin; myositis has been reported with concurrent use). Products include:
Advicor Tablets 1694
Altoprev Extended-Release Tablets........ 1151
Mevacor Tablets 1996

Meclofenamate Sodium (Cyclosporine can cause nephrotoxicity; clinical status and serum creatinine should be closely monitored when cyclosporine is used with NSAIDs in rheumatoid arthritis patients).
No products indexed under this heading.

Mefenamic Acid (Cyclosporine can cause nephrotoxicity; clinical status and serum creatinine should be closely monitored when cyclosporine is used with NSAIDs in rheumatoid arthritis patients).
No products indexed under this heading.

Meloxicam (Cyclosporine can cause nephrotoxicity; clinical status and serum creatinine should be closely monitored when cyclosporine is used with NSAIDs in rheumatoid arthritis patients). Products include:
Mobic Oral Suspension 893
Mobic Tablets 893

Melphalan (May potentiate renal dysfunction). Products include:
Alkeran Tablets 977

Methotrexate Sodium (Co-administration in rheumatoid arthritis patients has resulted in increased concentrations (AUC) of methotrexate by approximately 30% and the concentrations of its metabolite, 7-hydroxymethotrexate, were decreased by approximately 80%; the clinical significance of this outcome is not known).
No products indexed under this heading.

Methylprednisolone (Co-administration with drugs that inhibit CYP450 3A such as methylprednisolone, could decrease metabolism of cyclosporine and increase its concentrations; convulsions have been reported with concurrent high dose methylprednisolone).
No products indexed under this heading.

Methylprednisolone Acetate (Co-administration with drugs that inhibit CYP450 3A such as methylprednisolone, could decrease metabolism of cyclosporine and increase its concentrations; convulsions have been reported with concurrent high dose methylprednisolone). Products include:
Depo-Medrol Injectable Suspension 2615
Depo-Medrol Single-Dose Vial 2617

Methylprednisolone Sodium Succinate (Co-administration with drugs that inhibit CYP450 3A such as methylprednisolone, could decrease metabolism of cyclosporine and increase its concentrations; convulsions have been reported with concurrent high dose methylprednisolone).
No products indexed under this heading.

Metoclopramide Hydrochloride (Cyclosporine is extensively metabolized by CYP450 3A. Substances that inhibit this enzyme could decrease the metabolism and increase cyclosporine concentrations).
No products indexed under this heading.

Muromonab-CD3 (Co-administration with other immunosuppressive agents increases the possibility of excessive immunosuppression). Products include:
Orthoclone OKT3 Sterile Solution 2370

Mycophenolate Mofetil (Co-administration with other immunosuppressive agents increases the possibility of excessive immunosuppression). Products include:
CellCept Capsules 2751
CellCept Oral Suspension 2751
CellCept Tablets 2751

Nabumetone (Cyclosporine can cause nephrotoxicity; clinical status and serum creatinine should be closely monitored when cyclosporine is used with NSAIDs in rheumatoid arthritis patients). Products include:
Relafen Tablets 1523

Nafcillin Sodium (Co-administration with drugs that are inducers of CYP450 3A, such as nafcillin, could increase metabolism of cyclosporine and decrease its concentrations).
No products indexed under this heading.

Naproxen (May potentiate renal dysfunction; co-administration is associated with additive decreases in renal function). Products include:
EC-Naprosyn Delayed-Release Tablets........ 2769
Naprosyn Suspension 2769
Naprosyn Tablets 2769
Prevacid NapraPAC 3277

Naproxen Sodium (May potentiate renal dysfunction; co-administration is associated with additive decreases in renal function). Products include:
Aleve Tablets, Caplets and Gelcaps........ ▣605
Anaprox Tablets 2769
Anaprox DS Tablets 2769

Nicardipine Hydrochloride (Cyclosporine is extensively metabolized by CYP450 3A. Substances that inhibit this enzyme could decrease the metabolism and increase cyclosporine concentrations). Products include:
Cardene I.V. 1129

Nifedipine (Co-administration results in frequent episodes of gingival hyperplasia). Products include:
Adalat CC Tablets 2978

Octreotide Acetate (Co-administration with drugs that are inducers of CYP450 3A, such as octreotide, could increase metabolism of cyclosporine and decrease its concentrations). Products include:
Sandostatin Injection 2263
Sandostatin LAR Depot 2264

Orlistat (Co-administration with drugs that are inducers of CYP450 3A could increase metabolism of cyclosporine and decrease its concentrations). Products include:
Xenical Capsules 2834

Oxaprozin (Cyclosporine can cause nephrotoxicity; clinical status and serum creatinine should be closely monitored when cyclosporine is used with NSAIDs in rheumatoid arthritis patients).
No products indexed under this heading.

Phenobarbital (Co-administration with drugs that are inducers of CYP450 3A, such as phenobarbital, could increase metabolism of cyclosporine and decrease its concentrations).
No products indexed under this heading.

Phenylbutazone (Cyclosporine can cause nephrotoxicity; clinical status and serum creatinine should be closely monitored when cyclosporine is used with NSAIDs in rheumatoid arthritis patients).
No products indexed under this heading.

Phenytoin (Co-administration with drugs that are inducers of CYP450 3A, such as phenytoin, could increase metabolism of cyclosporine and decrease its concentrations).
No products indexed under this heading.

Phenytoin Sodium (Co-administration with drugs that are inducers of CYP450 3A, such as phenytoin, could increase metabolism of cyclosporine and decrease its concentrations). Products include:
Phenytek Capsules 2153

Piroxicam (Cyclosporine can cause nephrotoxicity; clinical status and serum creatinine should be closely monitored when cyclosporine is used with NSAIDs in rheumatoid arthritis patients).
No products indexed under this heading.

Prednisolone (Co-administration results in reduced clearance of prednisolone).
No products indexed under this heading.

Prednisolone Acetate (Co-administration results in reduced clearance of prednisolone). Products include:
Blephamide Ophthalmic Ointment 563
Blephamide Ophthalmic Suspension........ 564
Poly-Pred Liquifilm Ophthalmic Suspension........ ⊙231
Pred Forte Ophthalmic Suspension........ ⊙233
Pred Mild Sterile Ophthalmic Suspension........ ⊙236
Pred-G Ophthalmic Suspension ...... ⊙234
Pred-G Sterile Ophthalmic Ointment........ ⊙235

IMPORTANT NOTE: Always consult each drug listing in the patient's regimen for possible interactions.

Prednisolone Sodium Phosphate (Co-administration results in reduced clearance of prednisolone). Products include:
- Pediapred Oral Solution 3319

Prednisolone Tebutate (Co-administration results in reduced clearance of prednisolone).
- No products indexed under this heading.

Quinupristin (Cyclosporine is extensively metabolized by CYP450 3A. Substances that inhibit this enzyme could decrease the metabolism and increase cyclosporine concentrations). Products include:
- Synercid I.V. 1690

Ranitidine Hydrochloride (May potentiate renal dysfunction). Products include:
- Zantac 1597
- Zantac Injection 1593
- Zantac 75 Tablets .... ▣715
- Zantac 150 Maximum Strength Tablets .... ▣715
- Zantac Injection Pharmacy Bulk Package 1595

Rifabutin (Rifabutin is known to increase the metabolism of other drugs metabolized by CYP450 system; cyclosporine is extensively metabolized by CYP450 3A system, therefore, caution should be exercised).
- No products indexed under this heading.

Rifampin (Co-administration with drugs that are inducers of CYP450 3A, such as rifampin, could increase metabolism of cyclosporine and decrease its concentrations).
- No products indexed under this heading.

Rofecoxib (Cyclosporine can cause nephrotoxicity; clinical status and serum creatinine should be closely monitored when cyclosporine is used with NSAIDs in rheumatoid arthritis patients).
- No products indexed under this heading.

Sirolimus (Co-administration with other immunosuppressive agents increases the possibility of excessive immunosuppression). Products include:
- Rapamune Oral Solution and Tablets 3472

Spironolactone (Cyclosporine causes hyperkalemia; concurrent use with potassium-sparing diuretics can result in increased risk of hyperkalemia; co-administration should be avoided).
- No products indexed under this heading.

Sulfamethoxazole (May potentiate renal dysfunction).
- No products indexed under this heading.

Sulindac (May potentiate renal dysfunction; co-administration is associated with additive decreases in renal function). Products include:
- Clinoril Tablets 1899

Tacrolimus (May potentiate renal dysfunction; co-administration with other immunosuppressive agents increases the possibility of excessive immunosuppression). Products include:
- Prograf Capsules and Injection 624
- Protopic Ointment 629

Ticlopidine Hydrochloride (Co-administration with drugs that are inducers of CYP450 3A, such as ticlopidine, could increase metabolism of cyclosporine and decrease its concentrations). Products include:
- Ticlid Tablets 2813

Tobramycin (May potentiate renal dysfunction). Products include:
- TOBI Solution for Inhalation 1015
- TobraDex Ophthalmic Ointment 558
- TobraDex Ophthalmic Suspension ... 558
- Zylet Ophthalmic Suspension 3508

Tobramycin Sulfate (May potentiate renal dysfunction).
- No products indexed under this heading.

Tolmetin Sodium (Cyclosporine can cause nephrotoxicity; clinical status and serum creatinine should be closely monitored when cyclosporine is used with NSAIDs in rheumatoid arthritis patients).
- No products indexed under this heading.

Triamterene (Cyclosporine causes hyperkalemia; concurrent use with potassium-sparing diuretics can result in increased risk of hyperkalemia; co-administration should be avoided). Products include:
- Dyazide Capsules 1389
- Dyrenium Capsules 3390
- Maxzide 2150

Trimethoprim (May potentiate renal dysfunction).
- No products indexed under this heading.

Vaccines (Live) (During treatment with cyclosporine, vaccination may be less effective and the use of live attenuated vaccines should be avoided).
- No products indexed under this heading.

Valdecoxib (Cyclosporine can cause nephrotoxicity; clinical status and serum creatinine should be closely monitored when cyclosporine is used with NSAIDs in rheumatoid arthritis patients).
- No products indexed under this heading.

Vancomycin Hydrochloride (May potentiate renal dysfunction). Products include:
- Vancocin HCl Capsules, USP 3370

Verapamil Hydrochloride (Cyclosporine is extensively metabolized by CYP450 3A. Substances that inhibit this enzyme could decrease the metabolism and increase cyclosporine concentrations). Products include:
- Covera-HS Tablets 3135
- Tarka Tablets 519
- Verelan PM Capsules 3120

Food Interactions

Diet, high-lipid (A high fat meal within one-half hour before cyclosporine administration decreases the AUC by 13% and Cmax by 33%).

Food, unspecified (The administration of food with Gengraf decreases the cyclosporine AUC and Cmax).

Grapefruit (Affects the metabolism of cyclosporine by increasing blood concentration of cyclosporine; concurrent use should be avoided).

Grapefruit Juice (Affects the metabolism of cyclosporine by increasing blood concentration of cyclosporine; concurrent use should be avoided).

GENOPTIC STERILE OPHTHALMIC SOLUTION

(Gentamicin Sulfate) .... ⊙227

None cited in PDR database.

GENOTROPIN LYOPHILIZED POWDER

(Somatropin) 2642

May interact with glucocorticoids and drugs which undergo biotransformation by cytochrome p-450 mixed function oxidase. Compounds in these categories include:

Acarbose (Growth hormone administration may alter the clearance of compounds known to be metabolized by CYP 450 liver enzymes; careful monitoring is advisable). Products include:
- Precose Tablets 776

Acetaminophen (Growth hormone administration may alter the clearance of compounds known to be metabolized by CYP 450 liver enzymes; careful monitoring is advisable). Products include:
- Benadryl Allergy & Cold Tablets ..... ▣692
- Benadryl Allergy & Sinus Headache Caplets & Gelcaps ...... ▣693
- Benadryl Maximum Strength Severe Allergy & Sinus Headache Caplets .... ▣694
- Contac Severe Cold and Flu Caplets Maximum Strength .... ▣615
- Contac Severe Cold and Flu Caplets Non-Drowsy .... ▣615
- Darvocet A 500 Tablets 3497
- Goody's Body Pain Formula Powder .... ▣621
- Goody's Extra Strength Headache Powder .... ▣621
- Goody's Extra Strength Pain Relief Tablets .... ▣621
- Goody's PM Powder .... ▣622
- Hycomine Compound Tablets 1105
- Lortab 3315
- Lortab Elixir 3312
- Percocet Tablets 1114
- Robitussin Cough, Cold & Flu Liquid-filled Capsules .... ▣750
- Robitussin Flu Liquid .... ▣752
- Sedapap Tablets 50 mg/650 mg 2098
- Singlet Caplets .... ▣636
- Sudafed Severe Cold .... ▣710
- Sudafed Sinus Headache .... ▣711
- TheraFlu Cold & Cough Hot Liquid .... ▣680
- TheraFlu Cold & Sore Throat Hot Liquid .... ▣680
- TheraFlu Flu & Chest Congestion Non-Drowsy Hot Liquid .... ▣681
- TheraFlu Flu & Sore Throat Hot Liquid .... ▣681
- TheraFlu Severe Cold Non-Drowsy Hot Liquid .... ▣683
- TheraFlu Severe Cold & Cough Hot Liquid .... ▣683
- TheraFlu Severe Cold Caplets .... ▣679
- TheraFlu Severe Cold Hot Liquid .... ▣682
- TheraFlu Severe Cold Non-Drowsy Caplets .... ▣679
- Triaminic Cough & Sore Throat Liquid .... ▣687
- Triaminic Flu, Cough & Fever Liquid .... ▣685
- Triaminic Cough & Sore Throat Softchews .... ▣689
- Tylenol 8 Hour Extended Release Geltabs and Caplets 1843
- Tylenol Sinus NightTime Caplets .... ▣663
- Children's Tylenol Suspension Liquid and Meltaways 1850
- Children's Tylenol Plus Cold & Allergy Suspension Liquid 1850
- Children's Tylenol Plus Cold NightTime Suspension Liquid 1851
- Children's Tylenol Plus Cold & Cough Suspension Liquid and Chewable Tablets 1851
- Children's Tylenol Plus Cold Chewable Tablets 1851
- Children's Tylenol Plus Cold Daytime Non-Drowsy Suspension Liquid 1851
- Children's Tylenol Plus Flu Suspension Liquid 1853
- Concentrated Tylenol Infants' Drops Plus Cold 1851
- Concentrated Tylenol Infants' Drops Plus Cold and Cough 1851
- Concentrated Tylenol Infants' Drops 1850
- Junior Tylenol Meltaways 1850
- Tylenol Cold & Flu Severe Daytime Liquid with Cool Burst 1846
- Tylenol Cold & Flu Severe NightTime Liquid with Cool Burst 1846
- Tylenol Cold Severe Congestion Non-Drowsy Caplets with Cool Burst 1846
- Tylenol Cough & Sore Throat Daytime Liquid with Cool Burst 1849
- Tylenol Cough & Sore Throat NightTime Liquid with Cool Burst 1849
- Tylenol 1843
- Extra Strength Tylenol Rapid Release Gels 1843
- Tylenol 1843
- Tylenol Allergy Complete Night Time Caplets 1844
- Tylenol Allergy Complete Multi-Symptom Caplets and Gelcaps with Cool Burst 1844
- Tylenol Severe Allergy Caplets 1844
- Tylenol Flu NightTime Gelcaps 1846
- Tylenol Flu Day Non-Drowsy Gelcaps 1846
- Concentrated Tylenol Infants' Drops Plus Cold Nasal Congestant, Fever Reducer & Pain Reliever .... ▣668
- Concentrated Tylenol Infants' Drops Plus Cold & Cough Nasal Decongestant, Fever Reducer & Pain Reliever .... ▣668
- Multi-Symptom Tylenol Cold Night Time Caplets 1845
- Multi-Symptom Tylenol Cold Day Non-Drowsy Caplets and Gelcaps 1845
- Extra Strength Tylenol PM Caplets, Geltabs, Gelcaps and Liquid 1847
- Tylenol Sinus Day Non-Drowsy 1848
- Tylenol Sinus Night Time Caplets 1848
- Tylenol Sinus Severe Congestion Caplets with Cool Burst 1848
- Tylenol Sore Throat Daytime Liquid with Cool Burst 1849
- Tylenol Sore Throat NightTime Liquid with Cool Burst 1849
- Tylenol with Codeine 2461
- Women's Tylenol Menstrual Relief Caplets 1849
- Ultracet Tablets 2462
- Vicks 44M Cough, Cold & Flu Relief 2676
- Vicks DayQuil LiquiCaps/Liquid Multi-Symptom Cold/Flu Relief ..... ▣723
- Vicks DayQuil Multi-Symptom Cold/Flu Relief LiquiCaps 2675
- Vicks DayQuil Multi-Symptom Cold/Flu Relief Liquid 2675
- Vicks NyQuil LiquiCaps 2677
- Vicks NyQuil LiquiCaps/Liquid Multi-Symptom Cold/Flu Relief ..... ▣725
- Vicks NyQuil Liquid 2677
- Vicodin Tablets 530
- Vicodin ES Tablets 531
- Vicodin HP Tablets 532
- Zydone Tablets 1118

Alatrofloxacin Mesylate (Growth hormone administration may alter the clearance of compounds known to be metabolized by CYP 450 liver enzymes; careful monitoring is advisable).
- No products indexed under this heading.

Alfentanil Hydrochloride (Growth hormone administration may alter the clearance of compounds known to be metabolized by CYP 450 liver enzymes; careful monitoring is advisable).
- No products indexed under this heading.

Alprazolam (Growth hormone administration may alter the clearance of compounds known to be

metabolized by CYP 450 liver enzymes; careful monitoring is advisable). Products include:
- Niravam Orally Disintegrating Tablets **3106**
- Xanax XR Tablets **2655**

Aminophylline (Growth hormone administration may alter the clearance of compounds known to be metabolized by CYP 450 liver enzymes; careful monitoring is advisable).
No products indexed under this heading.

Amiodarone Hydrochloride (Growth hormone administration may alter the clearance of compounds known to be metabolized by CYP 450 liver enzymes; careful monitoring is advisable). Products include:
- Pacerone Tablets **3337**

Amitriptyline Hydrochloride (Growth hormone administration may alter the clearance of compounds known to be metabolized by CYP 450 liver enzymes; careful monitoring is advisable).
No products indexed under this heading.

Amlodipine Besylate (Growth hormone administration may alter the clearance of compounds known to be metabolized by CYP 450 liver enzymes; careful monitoring is advisable). Products include:
- Caduet Tablets **2507**
- Lotrel Capsules **2238**
- Norvasc Tablets **2529**

Amoxapine (Growth hormone administration may alter the clearance of compounds known to be metabolized by CYP 450 liver enzymes; careful monitoring is advisable).
No products indexed under this heading.

Amphetamine Aspartate (Growth hormone administration may alter the clearance of compounds known to be metabolized by CYP 450 liver enzymes; careful monitoring is advisable). Products include:
- Adderall Tablets **3168**
- Adderall XR Capsules **3169**

Amphetamine Aspartate Monohydrate (Growth hormone administration may alter the clearance of compounds known to be metabolized by CYP 450 liver enzymes; careful monitoring is advisable).
No products indexed under this heading.

Amphetamine Sulfate (Growth hormone administration may alter the clearance of compounds known to be metabolized by CYP 450 liver enzymes; careful monitoring is advisable). Products include:
- Adderall Tablets **3168**
- Adderall XR Capsules **3169**

Aprepitant (Growth hormone administration may alter the clearance of compounds known to be metabolized by CYP 450 liver enzymes; careful monitoring is advisable). Products include:
- Emend Capsules **1944**

Astemizole (Growth hormone administration may alter the clearance of compounds known to be metabolized by CYP 450 liver enzymes; careful monitoring is advisable).
No products indexed under this heading.

Atomoxetine Hydrochloride (Growth hormone administration may alter the clearance of compounds known to be metabolized by CYP 450 liver enzymes; careful monitoring is advisable). Products include:
- Strattera Capsules **1784**

Atorvastatin Calcium (Growth hormone administration may alter the clearance of compounds known to be metabolized by CYP 450 liver enzymes; careful monitoring is advisable). Products include:
- Caduet Tablets **2507**
- Lipitor Tablets **2495**

Belladonna Ergotamine (Growth hormone administration may alter the clearance of compounds known to be metabolized by CYP 450 liver enzymes; careful monitoring is advisable).
No products indexed under this heading.

Benzphetamine Hydrochloride (Growth hormone administration may alter the clearance of compounds known to be metabolized by CYP 450 liver enzymes; careful monitoring is advisable).
No products indexed under this heading.

Betamethasone Acetate (Concomitant glucocorticoid therapy may inhibit human growth promoting effect).
No products indexed under this heading.

Betamethasone Sodium Phosphate (Concomitant glucocorticoid therapy may inhibit human growth promoting effect).
No products indexed under this heading.

Bisoprolol Fumarate (Growth hormone administration may alter the clearance of compounds known to be metabolized by CYP 450 liver enzymes; careful monitoring is advisable).
No products indexed under this heading.

Buspirone Hydrochloride (Growth hormone administration may alter the clearance of compounds known to be metabolized by CYP 450 liver enzymes; careful monitoring is advisable).
No products indexed under this heading.

Busulfan (Growth hormone administration may alter the clearance of compounds known to be metabolized by CYP 450 liver enzymes; careful monitoring is advisable). Products include:
- I.V. Busulfex **1125**
- Myleran Tablets **1492**

Caffeine (Growth hormone administration may alter the clearance of compounds known to be metabolized by CYP 450 liver enzymes; careful monitoring is advisable). Products include:
- Athena Hair System Shampoo **767**
- BC Powder **612**
- Arthritis Strength BC Powder **612**
- Goody's Extra Strength Headache Powder **621**
- Goody's Extra Strength Pain Relief Tablets **621**
- Hycomine Compound Tablets **1105**
- Spartan Hair System Shampoo **767**
- Vivarin **639**

Caffeine Anhydrous (Growth hormone administration may alter the clearance of compounds known to be metabolized by CYP 450 liver enzymes; careful monitoring is advisable).
No products indexed under this heading.

Caffeine Citrate (Growth hormone administration may alter the clearance of compounds known to be metabolized by CYP 450 liver enzymes; careful monitoring is advisable). Products include:
- Cafcit **1854**

Candesartan Cilexetil (Growth hormone administration may alter the clearance of compounds known to be metabolized by CYP 450 liver enzymes; careful monitoring is advisable). Products include:
- Atacand Tablets **634**
- Atacand HCT **637**

Captopril (Growth hormone administration may alter the clearance of compounds known to be metabolized by CYP 450 liver enzymes; careful monitoring is advisable). Products include:
- Captopril Tablets **2114**

Carbamazepine (Growth hormone administration may alter the clearance of compounds known to be metabolized by CYP 450 liver enzymes; careful monitoring is advisable). Products include:
- Carbatrol Capsules **3174**
- Equetro Extended-Release Capsules **3178**
- Tegretol/Tegretol-XR **2278**

Carisoprodol (Growth hormone administration may alter the clearance of compounds known to be metabolized by CYP 450 liver enzymes; careful monitoring is advisable).
No products indexed under this heading.

Carvedilol (Growth hormone administration may alter the clearance of compounds known to be metabolized by CYP 450 liver enzymes; careful monitoring is advisable). Products include:
- Coreg Tablets **1376**

Celecoxib (Growth hormone administration may alter the clearance of compounds known to be metabolized by CYP 450 liver enzymes; careful monitoring is advisable). Products include:
- Celebrex Capsules **3130**

Cerivastatin Sodium (Growth hormone administration may alter the clearance of compounds known to be metabolized by CYP 450 liver enzymes; careful monitoring is advisable).
No products indexed under this heading.

Cevimeline Hydrochloride (Growth hormone administration may alter the clearance of compounds known to be metabolized by CYP 450 liver enzymes; careful monitoring is advisable). Products include:
- Evoxac Capsules **1042**

Chlordiazepoxide (Growth hormone administration may alter the clearance of compounds known to be metabolized by CYP 450 liver enzymes; careful monitoring is advisable).
No products indexed under this heading.

Chlordiazepoxide Hydrochloride (Growth hormone administration may alter the clearance of compounds known to be metabolized by CYP 450 liver enzymes; careful monitoring is advisable). Products include:
- Librium Capsules **3349**

Chlorpheniramine (Growth hormone administration may alter the clearance of compounds known to be metabolized by CYP 450 liver enzymes; careful monitoring is advisable).
No products indexed under this heading.

Chlorpheniramine Maleate (Growth hormone administration may alter the clearance of compounds known to be metabolized by CYP 450 liver enzymes; careful monitoring is advisable). Products include:
- Advil Allergy Sinus Caplets **737**
- Advil Multi-Symptom Cold Caplets **738**
- BC Allergy Sinus Cold Powder **612**
- Contac Severe Cold and Flu Caplets Maximum Strength **615**
- Hycomine Compound Tablets **1105**
- PediaCare Multi-Symptom Cold Liquid **704**
- PediaCare NightRest Cough & Cold Liquid **704**
- Robitussin Flu Liquid **752**
- Robitussin PM Cough & Cold Liquid **752**
- Singlet Caplets **636**
- Sudafed Sinus & Allergy Tablets **710**
- TheraFlu Cold & Cough Hot Liquid **680**
- TheraFlu Cold & Sore Throat Hot Liquid **680**
- TheraFlu Flu & Sore Throat Hot Liquid **681**
- TheraFlu Severe Cold & Cough Hot Liquid **683**
- TheraFlu Severe Cold Caplets **679**
- TheraFlu Severe Cold Hot Liquid **682**
- Triaminic Cold & Allergy Liquid **685**
- Triaminic Cold & Cough Liquid **685**
- Triaminic Flu, Cough & Fever Liquid **685**
- Triaminic Night Time Cough & Cold Liquid **685**
- Triaminic Allergy Runny Nose & Congestion Softchews **688**
- Triaminic Cold & Cough Softchews **688**
- Children's Tylenol Plus Cold NightTime Suspension Liquid **1851**
- Children's Tylenol Plus Cold & Cough Suspension Liquid and Chewable Tablets **1851**
- Children's Tylenol Plus Cold Chewable Tablets **1851**
- Children's Tylenol Plus Flu Suspension Liquid **1853**
- Tylenol Allergy Complete Multi-Symptom Caplets and Gelcaps with Cool Burst **1844**
- Multi-Symptom Tylenol Cold Night Time Caplets **1845**
- Vicks 44M Cough, Cold & Flu Relief **2676**
- Pediatric Vicks 44m Cough & Cold Relief **2673**
- Children's Vicks NyQuil Cold/Cough Relief **2671**

Chlorpheniramine Polistirex (Growth hormone administration may alter the clearance of compounds known to be metabolized by CYP 450 liver enzymes; careful monitoring is advisable). Products include:
- Tussionex Pennkinetic Extended-Release Suspension **3322**

Chlorpheniramine Tannate (Growth hormone administration may alter the clearance of compounds known to be metabolized by CYP 450 liver enzymes; careful monitoring is advisable).
No products indexed under this heading.

Chlorpromazine (Growth hormone administration may alter the clearance of compounds known to be metabolized by CYP 450 liver enzymes; careful monitoring is advisable).
No products indexed under this heading.

Chlorpromazine Hydrochloride (Growth hormone administration may alter the clearance of compounds known to be metabolized by CYP 450 liver enzymes; careful monitoring is advisable).
No products indexed under this heading.

Chlorpropamide (Growth hormone administration may alter the clearance of compounds known to be metabolized by CYP 450 liver enzymes; careful monitoring is advisable).
No products indexed under this heading.

Cilostazol (Growth hormone administration may alter the clearance of compounds known to be metabolized by CYP 450 liver enzymes; careful monitoring is advisable). Products include:
Pletal Tablets 2478

Cimetidine Hydrochloride (Growth hormone administration may alter the clearance of compounds known to be metabolized by CYP 450 liver enzymes; careful monitoring is advisable).
No products indexed under this heading.

Ciprofloxacin (Growth hormone administration may alter the clearance of compounds known to be metabolized by CYP 450 liver enzymes; careful monitoring is advisable). Products include:
Cipro I.V. 2998
Cipro I.V. Pharmacy Bulk Package ... 3509
Cipro Oral Suspension 2991
Cipro XR Tablets 3004
Ciprodex Otic Suspension 555

Ciprofloxacin Hydrochloride (Growth hormone administration may alter the clearance of compounds known to be metabolized by CYP 450 liver enzymes; careful monitoring is advisable). Products include:
Ciloxan Ophthalmic Ointment 554
Cipro Tablets 2991

Cisapride (Growth hormone administration may alter the clearance of compounds known to be metabolized by CYP 450 liver enzymes; careful monitoring is advisable).
No products indexed under this heading.

Citalopram Hydrobromide (Growth hormone administration may alter the clearance of compounds known to be metabolized by CYP 450 liver enzymes; careful monitoring is advisable). Products include:
Celexa 1177

Clarithromycin (Growth hormone administration may alter the clearance of compounds known to be metabolized by CYP 450 liver enzymes; careful monitoring is advisable). Products include:
Biaxin/Biaxin XL 402
PREVPAC 3281

Clomipramine Hydrochloride (Growth hormone administration may alter the clearance of compounds known to be metabolized by CYP 450 liver enzymes; careful monitoring is advisable).
No products indexed under this heading.

Clopidogrel Hydrogen Sulfate (Growth hormone administration may alter the clearance of compounds known to be metabolized by CYP 450 liver enzymes; careful monitoring is advisable).
No products indexed under this heading.

Clozapine (Growth hormone administration may alter the clearance of compounds known to be metabolized by CYP 450 liver enzymes; careful monitoring is advisable). Products include:
Clozapine Tablets 2141
Clozaril Tablets 2174
FazaClo Orally Disintegrating Tablets 547

Codeine Phosphate (Growth hormone administration may alter the clearance of compounds known to be metabolized by CYP 450 liver enzymes; careful monitoring is advisable). Products include:
Tylenol with Codeine 2461

Codeine Sulfate (Growth hormone administration may alter the clearance of compounds known to be metabolized by CYP 450 liver enzymes; careful monitoring is advisable).
No products indexed under this heading.

Cortisone Acetate (Concomitant glucocorticoid therapy may inhibit human growth promoting effect).
No products indexed under this heading.

Cyclobenzaprine (Growth hormone administration may alter the clearance of compounds known to be metabolized by CYP 450 liver enzymes; careful monitoring is advisable).
No products indexed under this heading.

Cyclobenzaprine Hydrochloride (Growth hormone administration may alter the clearance of compounds known to be metabolized by CYP 450 liver enzymes; careful monitoring is advisable). Products include:
Flexeril Tablets 1832

Cyclophosphamide (Growth hormone administration may alter the clearance of compounds known to be metabolized by CYP 450 liver enzymes; careful monitoring is advisable).
No products indexed under this heading.

Cyclosporine (Growth hormone administration may alter the clearance of compounds known to be metabolized by CYP 450 liver enzymes; careful monitoring is advisable). Products include:
Gengraf Capsules 458
Neoral Soft Gelatin Capsules 2247
Neoral Oral Solution 2247
Restasis Ophthalmic Emulsion 570
Sandimmune 2259

Desipramine Hydrochloride (Growth hormone administration may alter the clearance of compounds known to be metabolized by CYP 450 liver enzymes; careful monitoring is advisable).
No products indexed under this heading.

Desogestrel (Growth hormone administration may alter the clearance of compounds known to be metabolized by CYP 450 liver enzymes; careful monitoring is advisable). Products include:
Ortho-Cept Tablets 2395

Dexamethasone (Concomitant glucocorticoid therapy may inhibit human growth promoting effect). Products include:
Ciprodex Otic Suspension 555
Decadron Tablets 1929
TobraDex Ophthalmic Ointment 558
TobraDex Ophthalmic Suspension 558

Dexamethasone Acetate (Concomitant glucocorticoid therapy may inhibit human growth promoting effect).
No products indexed under this heading.

Dexamethasone Phosphate (Growth hormone administration may alter the clearance of compounds known to be metabolized by CYP 450 liver enzymes; careful monitoring is advisable).
No products indexed under this heading.

Dexamethasone Sodium (Growth hormone administration may alter the clearance of compounds known to be metabolized by CYP 450 liver enzymes; careful monitoring is advisable).
No products indexed under this heading.

Dexamethasone Sodium Phosphate (Concomitant glucocorticoid therapy may inhibit human growth promoting effect). Products include:
Decadron Phosphate Injection 1931

Dexfenfluramine Hydrochloride (Growth hormone administration may alter the clearance of compounds known to be metabolized by CYP 450 liver enzymes; careful monitoring is advisable).
No products indexed under this heading.

Dextromethorphan (Growth hormone administration may alter the clearance of compounds known to be metabolized by CYP 450 liver enzymes; careful monitoring is advisable).
No products indexed under this heading.

Dextromethorphan Hydrobromide (Growth hormone administration may alter the clearance of compounds known to be metabolized by CYP 450 liver enzymes; careful monitoring is advisable). Products include:
Alacol DM Syrup 739
Balamine DM 739
Contac Severe Cold and Flu Caplets Maximum Strength .... ■ 615
Contac Severe Cold and Flu Caplets Non-Drowsy .... ■ 615
Children's Dimetapp DM Cold & Cough Elixir .... ■ 745
Children's Dimetapp Long Acting Cough Plus Cold Syrup .... ■ 746
Dimetapp Infant Drops Decongestant Plus Cough .... ■ 746
Mucinex DM Tablets .... ■ 602
PediaCare Decongestant & Cough Infant Drops .... ■ 705
PediaCare Freezer Pops Long-Acting Cough-Glacier Grape and Polar Berry Blue .... ■ 706
PediaCare Long-Acting Cough Infant Drops .... ■ 705
PediaCare Long-Acting Cough Plus Cold Liquid .... ■ 704
PediaCare Multi-Symptom Cold Liquid .... ■ 704
PediaCare NightRest Cough & Cold Liquid .... ■ 704
Robitussin Allergy & Cough Syrup .. ■ 750
Robitussin CF Liquid .... ■ 755
Robitussin Cough & Cold Liquid-filled Capsules .... ■ 750
Robitussin Cough, Cold & Flu Liquid-filled Capsules .... ■ 750
Robitussin Cough & Cold Infant Drops .... ■ 755
Robitussin DM Infant Drops .... ■ 753
Robitussin DM Liquid .... ■ 753
Robitussin Flu Liquid .... ■ 752
Robitussin Maximum Strength Cough Liquid .... ■ 754
Robitussin Maximum Strength Cough & Cold Liquid .... ■ 754
Robitussin Pediatric Cough Liquid .... ■ 754
Robitussin Pediatric Cough & Cold Liquid .... ■ 754
Robitussin PM Cough & Cold Liquid .... ■ 752
Robitussin Sugar Free Cough Liquid .... ■ 753
Simply Cough Liquid 1840
Sudafed Severe Cold .... ■ 710
TheraFlu Cold & Cough Hot Liquid .... ■ 680
TheraFlu Flu & Chest Congestion Non-Drowsy Hot Liquid .... ■ 681
TheraFlu Severe Cold Non-Drowsy Hot Liquid .... ■ 683
TheraFlu Severe Cold & Cough Hot Liquid .... ■ 683
TheraFlu Severe Cold Caplets .... ■ 679
TheraFlu Severe Cold Hot Liquid .... ■ 682
TheraFlu Severe Cold Non-Drowsy Caplets .... ■ 679
TheraFlu Thin Strips Long Acting Cough .... ■ 684
Triaminic Cold & Cough Liquid .... ■ 685
Triaminic Cough Liquid .... ■ 687
Triaminic Cough & Nasal Congestion Liquid .... ■ 687
Triaminic Cough & Sore Throat Liquid .... ■ 687
Triaminic Flu, Cough & Fever Liquid .... ■ 685
Triaminic Night Time Cough & Cold Liquid .... ■ 685
Triaminic Cold & Cough Softchews .... ■ 688
Triaminic Cough & Sore Throat Softchews .... ■ 689
Triaminic Thin Strips Long Acting Cough .... ■ 689
Children's Tylenol Plus Cold & Cough Suspension Liquid and Chewable Tablets 1851
Children's Tylenol Plus Flu Suspension Liquid 1853
Concentrated Tylenol Infants' Drops Plus Cold and Cough 1851
Tylenol Cold & Flu Severe Daytime Liquid with Cool Bust 1846
Tylenol Cold & Flu Severe NightTime Liquid with Cool Burst 1846
Tylenol Cold Severe Congestion Non-Drowsy Caplets with Cool Burst 1846
Tylenol Cough & Sore Throat Daytime Liquid with Cool Burst 1849
Tylenol Cough & Sore Throat NightTime Liquid with Cool Burst 1849
Tylenol Flu Day Non-Drowsy Gelcaps 1846
Concentrated Tylenol Infants' Drops Plus Cold & Cough Nasal Decongestant, Fever Reducer & Pain Reliever .... ■ 668
Multi-Symptom Tylenol Cold Night Time Caplets 1845
Multi-Symptom Tylenol Cold Day Non-Drowsy Caplets and Gelcaps 1845
Vicks 44 Cough Relief 2675

- Vicks 44D Cough & Head Congestion Relief ... 2676
- Vicks 44D Cough & Head Congestion Relief Liquid ... 721
- Vicks 44E Cough & Chest Congestion Relief ... 2676
- Pediatric Vicks 44e Cough & Chest Congestion Relief Liquid ... 2673
- Vicks 44M Cough, Cold & Flu Relief ... 2676
- Pediatric Vicks 44m Cough & Cold Relief ... 2673
- Vicks DayQuil LiquiCaps/Liquid Multi-Symptom Cold/Flu Relief ... 723
- Vicks DayQuil Multi-Symptom Cold/Flu Relief LiquiCaps ... 2675
- Vicks DayQuil Multi-Symptom Cold/Flu Relief Liquid ... 2675
- Children's Vicks NyQuil Cold/Cough Relief ... 2671
- Vicks NyQuil Cough Liquid ... 2677
- Vicks NyQuil LiquiCaps ... 2677
- Vicks NyQuil LiquiCaps/Liquid Multi-Symptom Cold/Flu Relief ... 725
- Vicks NyQuil Liquid ... 2677
- Zicam Concentrated Cough Mist for Kids Cool Cherry ... 643
- Zicam Concentrated Cough Mist for Kids Plus D Cool Cherry ... 643
- Zicam Concentrated Cough Mist Nite-Cool Cherry ... 642
- Zicam Concentrated Cough Mist Plus D Cool Cherry ... 642
- Zicam Concentrated Cough Mist-Honey Lemon & Cool Cherry ... 642

Dextromethorphan Polistirex (Growth hormone administration may alter the clearance of compounds known to be metabolized by CYP 450 liver enzymes; careful monitoring is advisable). Products include:
- Delsym Extended-Release Suspension ... 611
- Delsym 12 Hour Cough Suppressant for Children ... 611

Diazepam (Growth hormone administration may alter the clearance of compounds known to be metabolized by CYP 450 liver enzymes; careful monitoring is advisable). Products include:
- Diastat Rectal Delivery System ... 3344
- Valium Tablets ... 2822

Diclofenac Potassium (Growth hormone administration may alter the clearance of compounds known to be metabolized by CYP 450 liver enzymes; careful monitoring is advisable). Products include:
- Cataflam Tablets ... 2173

Diclofenac Sodium (Growth hormone administration may alter the clearance of compounds known to be metabolized by CYP 450 liver enzymes; careful monitoring is advisable). Products include:
- Arthrotec Tablets ... 3126
- Voltaren Ophthalmic Solution ... 2300
- Voltaren Tablets ... 2298
- Voltaren-XR Tablets ... 2301

Dihydroergotamine Mesylate (Growth hormone administration may alter the clearance of compounds known to be metabolized by CYP 450 liver enzymes; careful monitoring is advisable). Products include:
- Migranal Nasal Spray ... 3350

Diltiazem Hydrochloride (Growth hormone administration may alter the clearance of compounds known to be metabolized by CYP 450 liver enzymes; careful monitoring is advisable). Products include:
- Cardizem LA Extended Release Tablets ... 1699
- Tiazac Capsules ... 1204

Diltiazem Maleate (Growth hormone administration may alter the clearance of compounds known to be metabolized by CYP 450 liver enzymes; careful monitoring is advisable).
No products indexed under this heading.

Disopyramide (Growth hormone administration may alter the clearance of compounds known to be metabolized by CYP 450 liver enzymes; careful monitoring is advisable).
No products indexed under this heading.

Disopyramide Phosphate (Growth hormone administration may alter the clearance of compounds known to be metabolized by CYP 450 liver enzymes; careful monitoring is advisable).
No products indexed under this heading.

Divalproex Sodium (Growth hormone administration may alter the clearance of compounds known to be metabolized by CYP 450 liver enzymes; careful monitoring is advisable). Products include:
- Depakote Sprinkle Capsules ... 422
- Depakote Tablets ... 427
- Depakote ER Tablets ... 433

Docetaxel (Growth hormone administration may alter the clearance of compounds known to be metabolized by CYP 450 liver enzymes; careful monitoring is advisable). Products include:
- Taxotere Injection Concentrate ... 2947

Dolasetron Mesylate (Growth hormone administration may alter the clearance of compounds known to be metabolized by CYP 450 liver enzymes; careful monitoring is advisable). Products include:
- Anzemet Injection ... 2871
- Anzemet Tablets ... 2874

Donepezil Hydrochloride (Growth hormone administration may alter the clearance of compounds known to be metabolized by CYP 450 liver enzymes; careful monitoring is advisable). Products include:
- Aricept Tablets ... 1086
- Aricept ODT Tablets ... 1086

Doxepin Hydrochloride (Growth hormone administration may alter the clearance of compounds known to be metabolized by CYP 450 liver enzymes; careful monitoring is advisable).
No products indexed under this heading.

Doxorubicin Hydrochloride (Growth hormone administration may alter the clearance of compounds known to be metabolized by CYP 450 liver enzymes; careful monitoring is advisable). Products include:
- Adriamycin for Injection, USP ... 786
- Adriamycin Injection, USP ... 786

Dronabinol (Growth hormone administration may alter the clearance of compounds known to be metabolized by CYP 450 liver enzymes; careful monitoring is advisable). Products include:
- Marinol Capsules ... 3334

Drugs that Undergo Biotransformation by Cytochrome P-450 Mixed Function Oxidase (Growth hormone administration may alter the clearance of compounds known to be metabolized by CYP 450 liver enzymes; careful monitoring is advisable).
No products indexed under this heading.

Dyphylline (Growth hormone administration may alter the clearance of compounds known to be metabolized by CYP 450 liver enzymes; careful monitoring is advisable).
No products indexed under this heading.

Encainide Hydrochloride (Growth hormone administration may alter the clearance of compounds known to be metabolized by CYP 450 liver enzymes; careful monitoring is advisable).
No products indexed under this heading.

Enoxacin (Growth hormone administration may alter the clearance of compounds known to be metabolized by CYP 450 liver enzymes; careful monitoring is advisable).
No products indexed under this heading.

Eprosartan Mesylate (Growth hormone administration may alter the clearance of compounds known to be metabolized by CYP 450 liver enzymes; careful monitoring is advisable). Products include:
- Teveten Tablets ... 1707
- Teveten HCT Tablets ... 1710

Ergotamine Tartrate (Growth hormone administration may alter the clearance of compounds known to be metabolized by CYP 450 liver enzymes; careful monitoring is advisable).
No products indexed under this heading.

Erythromycin (Growth hormone administration may alter the clearance of compounds known to be metabolized by CYP 450 liver enzymes; careful monitoring is advisable). Products include:
- Erygel Topical Gel ... 2096
- Ery-Tab Tablets ... 447
- Erythromycin Base Filmtab Tablets ... 454
- Erythromycin Delayed-Release Capsules, USP ... 456
- PCE Dispertab Tablets ... 510

Erythromycin Estolate (Growth hormone administration may alter the clearance of compounds known to be metabolized by CYP 450 liver enzymes; careful monitoring is advisable).
No products indexed under this heading.

Erythromycin Ethylsuccinate (Growth hormone administration may alter the clearance of compounds known to be metabolized by CYP 450 liver enzymes; careful monitoring is advisable). Products include:
- E.E.S. ... 449
- EryPed ... 445

Erythromycin Gluceptate (Growth hormone administration may alter the clearance of compounds known to be metabolized by CYP 450 liver enzymes; careful monitoring is advisable).
No products indexed under this heading.

Erythromycin Lactobionate (Growth hormone administration may alter the clearance of compounds known to be metabolized by CYP 450 liver enzymes; careful monitoring is advisable).
No products indexed under this heading.

Erythromycin Stearate (Growth hormone administration may alter the clearance of compounds known to be metabolized by CYP 450 liver enzymes; careful monitoring is advisable). Products include:
- Erythrocin Stearate Filmtab Tablets ... 452

Esomeprazole Magnesium (Growth hormone administration may alter the clearance of compounds known to be metabolized by CYP 450 liver enzymes; careful monitoring is advisable). Products include:
- Nexium Delayed-Release Capsules ... 645

Estradiol (Growth hormone administration may alter the clearance of compounds known to be metabolized by CYP 450 liver enzymes; careful monitoring is advisable). Products include:
- Activella Tablets ... 2311
- Climara Transdermal System ... 795
- Climara Pro Transdermal System ... 800
- CombiPatch Transdermal System ... 2180
- Estrogel 0.06% ... 3200
- Menostar Transdermal System ... 805
- Prefest Tablets ... 1069
- Vagifem Tablets ... 2340
- Vivelle Transdermal System ... 2288
- Vivelle-Dot Transdermal System ... 2293

Estradiol Benzoate (Growth hormone administration may alter the clearance of compounds known to be metabolized by CYP 450 liver enzymes; careful monitoring is advisable).
No products indexed under this heading.

Estradiol Cypionate (Growth hormone administration may alter the clearance of compounds known to be metabolized by CYP 450 liver enzymes; careful monitoring is advisable).
No products indexed under this heading.

Estradiol Valerate (Growth hormone administration may alter the clearance of compounds known to be metabolized by CYP 450 liver enzymes; careful monitoring is advisable).
No products indexed under this heading.

Estrogen (Growth hormone administration may alter the clearance of compounds known to be metabolized by CYP 450 liver enzymes; careful monitoring is advisable).
No products indexed under this heading.

Estrogens, Conjugated (Growth hormone administration may alter the clearance of compounds known to be metabolized by CYP 450 liver enzymes; careful monitoring is advisable). Products include:
- Premarin Intravenous ... 3440
- Premarin Tablets ... 3443
- Premarin Vaginal Cream ... 3449
- Premphase Tablets ... 3452
- Prempro Tablets ... 3452

Estrogens, Conjugated, Synthetic A (Growth hormone administration may alter the clearance of compounds known to be metabolized by

CYP 450 liver enzymes; careful monitoring is advisable). Products include:
- Cenestin Tablets, 0.45mg, 0.625mg, 0.9mg, 1.25mg **1063**
- Cenestin Tablets, 0.3mg **1063**

Estrogens, Esterified (Growth hormone administration may alter the clearance of compounds known to be metabolized by CYP 450 liver enzymes; careful monitoring is advisable). Products include:
- Estratest Tablets **3196**
- Estratest H.S. Tablets **3196**

Ethinyl Estradiol (Growth hormone administration may alter the clearance of compounds known to be metabolized by CYP 450 liver enzymes; careful monitoring is advisable). Products include:
- Alesse-28 Tablets **3392**
- Lo/Ovral-28 Tablets **3423**
- NuvaRing **2357**
- Ortho-Cept Tablets **2395**
- Ortho-Cyclen/Ortho Tri-Cyclen **2414**
- Ortho Evra Transdermal System **2402**
- Ortho Tri-Cyclen Lo Tablets **2421**
- Seasonale Tablets **1073**
- Triphasil-28 Tablets **3483**
- Yasmin 28 Tablets **818**

Ethosuximide (Growth hormone administration may alter the clearance of compounds known to be metabolized by CYP 450 liver enzymes; careful monitoring is advisable).
No products indexed under this heading.

Ethotoin (Growth hormone administration may alter the clearance of compounds known to be metabolized by CYP 450 liver enzymes; careful monitoring is advisable). Products include:
- Peganone Tablets, USP **2487**

Ethynodiol Diacetate (Growth hormone administration may alter the clearance of compounds known to be metabolized by CYP 450 liver enzymes; careful monitoring is advisable).
No products indexed under this heading.

Etodolac (Growth hormone administration may alter the clearance of compounds known to be metabolized by CYP 450 liver enzymes; careful monitoring is advisable).
No products indexed under this heading.

Etoposide (Growth hormone administration may alter the clearance of compounds known to be metabolized by CYP 450 liver enzymes; careful monitoring is advisable).
No products indexed under this heading.

Etoposide Phosphate (Growth hormone administration may alter the clearance of compounds known to be metabolized by CYP 450 liver enzymes; careful monitoring is advisable).
No products indexed under this heading.

Felbamate (Growth hormone administration may alter the clearance of compounds known to be metabolized by CYP 450 liver enzymes; careful monitoring is advisable).
No products indexed under this heading.

Felodipine (Growth hormone administration may alter the clearance of compounds known to be metabolized by CYP 450 liver enzymes; careful monitoring is advisable). Products include:
- Plendil Extended-Release Tablets **651**

Fenoprofen Calcium (Growth hormone administration may alter the clearance of compounds known to be metabolized by CYP 450 liver enzymes; careful monitoring is advisable). Products include:
- Nalfon Capsules **2504**

Fentanyl (Growth hormone administration may alter the clearance of compounds known to be metabolized by CYP 450 liver enzymes; careful monitoring is advisable). Products include:
- Duragesic Transdermal System **2448**

Fentanyl Citrate (Growth hormone administration may alter the clearance of compounds known to be metabolized by CYP 450 liver enzymes; careful monitoring is advisable). Products include:
- Actiq **993**

Flecainide Acetate (Growth hormone administration may alter the clearance of compounds known to be metabolized by CYP 450 liver enzymes; careful monitoring is advisable). Products include:
- Tambocor Tablets **1824**

Fludrocortisone Acetate (Concomitant glucocorticoid therapy may inhibit human growth promoting effect).
No products indexed under this heading.

Fluoxetine (Growth hormone administration may alter the clearance of compounds known to be metabolized by CYP 450 liver enzymes; careful monitoring is advisable).
No products indexed under this heading.

Fluoxetine Hydrochloride (Growth hormone administration may alter the clearance of compounds known to be metabolized by CYP 450 liver enzymes; careful monitoring is advisable). Products include:
- Prozac Pulvules and Liquid **1771**
- Symbyax Capsules **1788**

Fluphenazine Decanoate (Growth hormone administration may alter the clearance of compounds known to be metabolized by CYP 450 liver enzymes; careful monitoring is advisable).
No products indexed under this heading.

Fluphenazine Enanthate (Growth hormone administration may alter the clearance of compounds known to be metabolized by CYP 450 liver enzymes; careful monitoring is advisable).
No products indexed under this heading.

Fluphenazine Hydrochloride (Growth hormone administration may alter the clearance of compounds known to be metabolized by CYP 450 liver enzymes; careful monitoring is advisable).
No products indexed under this heading.

Flurbiprofen (Growth hormone administration may alter the clearance of compounds known to be metabolized by CYP 450 liver enzymes; careful monitoring is advisable).
No products indexed under this heading.

Flurbiprofen Sodium (Growth hormone administration may alter the clearance of compounds known to be metabolized by CYP 450 liver enzymes; careful monitoring is advisable). Products include:
- Ocufen Ophthalmic Solution .... ⊙**230**

Flutamide (Growth hormone administration may alter the clearance of compounds known to be metabolized by CYP 450 liver enzymes; careful monitoring is advisable). Products include:
- Eulexin Capsules **3023**

Fluticasone Propionate (Growth hormone administration may alter the clearance of compounds known to be metabolized by CYP 450 liver enzymes; careful monitoring is advisable). Products include:
- Advair Diskus 100/50 .... **1291**
- Advair Diskus 250/50 .... **1291**
- Advair Diskus 500/50 .... **1291**
- Cutivate Cream **1381**
- Cutivate Lotion 0.05% **1383**
- Cutivate Ointment **1384**
- Flonase Nasal Spray **1412**
- Flovent Diskus 100 mcg **1418**
- Flovent Diskus 50 mcg **1415**

Fluvastatin Sodium (Growth hormone administration may alter the clearance of compounds known to be metabolized by CYP 450 liver enzymes; careful monitoring is advisable). Products include:
- Lescol Capsules **2227**
- Lescol **2730**
- Lescol XL Tablets **2227**

Fluvoxamine Maleate (Growth hormone administration may alter the clearance of compounds known to be metabolized by CYP 450 liver enzymes; careful monitoring is advisable).
No products indexed under this heading.

Formoterol Fumarate (Growth hormone administration may alter the clearance of compounds known to be metabolized by CYP 450 liver enzymes; careful monitoring is advisable). Products include:
- Foradil Aerolizer **3024**

Fosphenytoin (Growth hormone administration may alter the clearance of compounds known to be metabolized by CYP 450 liver enzymes; careful monitoring is advisable).
No products indexed under this heading.

Fosphenytoin Sodium (Growth hormone administration may alter the clearance of compounds known to be metabolized by CYP 450 liver enzymes; careful monitoring is advisable).
No products indexed under this heading.

Gabapentin (Growth hormone administration may alter the clearance of compounds known to be metabolized by CYP 450 liver enzymes; careful monitoring is advisable). Products include:
- Neurontin Capsules **2498**
- Neurontin Oral Solution **2498**
- Neurontin Tablets **2498**

Galantamine Hydrobromide (Growth hormone administration may alter the clearance of compounds known to be metabolized by CYP 450 liver enzymes; careful monitoring is advisable). Products include:
- Razadyne ER Extended-Release Capsules **2434**
- Razadyne **2434**

Glimepiride (Growth hormone administration may alter the clearance of compounds known to be metabolized by CYP 450 liver enzymes; careful monitoring is advisable). Products include:
- Amaryl Tablets **2864**

Glipizide (Growth hormone administration may alter the clearance of compounds known to be metabolized by CYP 450 liver enzymes; careful monitoring is advisable).
No products indexed under this heading.

Glyburide (Growth hormone administration may alter the clearance of compounds known to be metabolized by CYP 450 liver enzymes; careful monitoring is advisable).
No products indexed under this heading.

Grepafloxacin Hydrochloride (Growth hormone administration may alter the clearance of compounds known to be metabolized by CYP 450 liver enzymes; careful monitoring is advisable).
No products indexed under this heading.

Haloperidol (Growth hormone administration may alter the clearance of compounds known to be metabolized by CYP 450 liver enzymes; careful monitoring is advisable).
No products indexed under this heading.

Haloperidol Decanoate (Growth hormone administration may alter the clearance of compounds known to be metabolized by CYP 450 liver enzymes; careful monitoring is advisable).
No products indexed under this heading.

Haloperidol Lactate (Growth hormone administration may alter the clearance of compounds known to be metabolized by CYP 450 liver enzymes; careful monitoring is advisable).
No products indexed under this heading.

Hydrocodone Bitartrate (Growth hormone administration may alter the clearance of compounds known to be metabolized by CYP 450 liver enzymes; careful monitoring is advisable). Products include:
- Hycodan **1104**
- Hycomine Compound Tablets **1105**
- Hycotuss Expectorant Syrup **1106**
- Lortab **3315**
- Lortab Elixir **3312**
- Vicodin Tablets **530**
- Vicodin ES Tablets **531**
- Vicodin HP Tablets **532**
- Vicoprofen Tablets **533**
- Zydone Tablets **1118**

Hydrocortisone (Concomitant glucocorticoid therapy may inhibit human growth promoting effect). Products include:
- Cortizone•5 Ointment .... ■**699**
- Cortizone•10 Creme .... ■**699**
- Cortizone•10 Ointment .... ■**699**
- Cortizone•10 Plus Creme .... ■**700**
- Cortizone•10 Maximum Strength Quick Shot Spray .... ■**700**
- Hydrocortone Tablets **1963**
- Preparation H Hydrocortisone Cream .... ■**748**

Hydrocortisone Acetate (Concomitant glucocorticoid therapy may inhibit human growth promoting effect). Products include:
- Analpram-HC **1136**
- Pramosone **1139**
- ProctoFoam-HC **3113**
- Tucks Anti-Itch Ointment .... ■**712**
- U-cort 1% Cream **3289**

Hydrocortisone Sodium Phosphate (Concomitant glucocorticoid therapy may inhibit human growth promoting effect).
No products indexed under this heading.

Hydrocortisone Sodium Succinate (Concomitant glucocorticoid therapy may inhibit human growth promoting effect).
No products indexed under this heading.

Ibuprofen (Growth hormone administration may alter the clearance of compounds known to be metabolized by CYP 450 liver enzymes; careful monitoring is advisable). Products include:
- Advil Allergy Sinus Caplets 737
- Advil 737
- Children's Advil Suspension 742
- Children's Advil Chewable Tablets 741
- Advil Cold & Sinus 739
- Advil Flu & Body Ache Caplets 739
- Children's Advil Cold Suspension 741
- Infants' Advil Concentrated Drops 743
- Junior Strength Advil Swallow Tablets 740
- Advil Migraine Liquigels 740
- Advil Multi-Symptom Cold Caplets 738
- Combunox Tablets 1183
- Children's Motrin Oral Suspension and Chewable Tablets 1837
- Children's Motrin Cold Non-Staining Dye-Free Oral Suspension 1838
- Children's Motrin Cold Oral Suspension 1838
- Children's Motrin Non-Staining Dye-Free Oral Suspension 1837
- Motrin Cold & Sinus Caplets 1836
- Motrin IB Tablets and Caplets 1836
- Infants' Motrin Concentrated Drops 1837
- Infants' Motrin Non-Staining Dye-Free Drops 1837
- Junior Strength Motrin Caplets and Chewable Tablets 1837
- Vicoprofen Tablets 533

Imipramine Hydrochloride (Growth hormone administration may alter the clearance of compounds known to be metabolized by CYP 450 liver enzymes; careful monitoring is advisable).
No products indexed under this heading.

Imipramine Pamoate (Growth hormone administration may alter the clearance of compounds known to be metabolized by CYP 450 liver enzymes; careful monitoring is advisable).
No products indexed under this heading.

Indinavir Sulfate (Growth hormone administration may alter the clearance of compounds known to be metabolized by CYP 450 liver enzymes; careful monitoring is advisable). Products include:
- Crixivan Capsules 1918

Indomethacin (Growth hormone administration may alter the clearance of compounds known to be metabolized by CYP 450 liver enzymes; careful monitoring is advisable). Products include:
- Indocin 1968

Indomethacin Sodium Trihydrate (Growth hormone administration may alter the clearance of compounds known to be metabolized by CYP 450 liver enzymes; careful monitoring is advisable). Products include:
- Indocin I.V. 1973

Indoramin Hydrochloride (Growth hormone administration may alter the clearance of compounds known to be metabolized by CYP 450 liver enzymes; careful monitoring is advisable).
No products indexed under this heading.

Irbesartan (Growth hormone administration may alter the clearance of compounds known to be metabolized by CYP 450 liver enzymes; careful monitoring is advisable). Products include:
- Avalide Tablets 922
- Avalide Tablets 2889
- Avapro Tablets 925
- Avapro Tablets 2886

Isotretinoin (Growth hormone administration may alter the clearance of compounds known to be metabolized by CYP 450 liver enzymes; careful monitoring is advisable). Products include:
- Accutane Capsules 2740
- Amnesteem Capsules 2126

Isradipine (Growth hormone administration may alter the clearance of compounds known to be metabolized by CYP 450 liver enzymes; careful monitoring is advisable). Products include:
- DynaCirc CR Tablets 2726

Itraconazole (Growth hormone administration may alter the clearance of compounds known to be metabolized by CYP 450 liver enzymes; careful monitoring is advisable).
No products indexed under this heading.

Ketoconazole (Growth hormone administration may alter the clearance of compounds known to be metabolized by CYP 450 liver enzymes; careful monitoring is advisable). Products include:
- Nizoral A-D Shampoo, 1% 1839
- Nizoral 2% Shampoo 1838

Ketoprofen (Growth hormone administration may alter the clearance of compounds known to be metabolized by CYP 450 liver enzymes; careful monitoring is advisable).
No products indexed under this heading.

Ketorolac Tromethamine (Growth hormone administration may alter the clearance of compounds known to be metabolized by CYP 450 liver enzymes; careful monitoring is advisable). Products include:
- Acular Ophthalmic Solution 561
- Acular LS Ophthalmic Solution 562

Labetalol Hydrochloride (Growth hormone administration may alter the clearance of compounds known to be metabolized by CYP 450 liver enzymes; careful monitoring is advisable).
No products indexed under this heading.

Lamotrigine (Growth hormone administration may alter the clearance of compounds known to be metabolized by CYP 450 liver enzymes; careful monitoring is advisable). Products include:
- Lamictal 1449

Lansoprazole (Growth hormone administration may alter the clearance of compounds known to be metabolized by CYP 450 liver enzymes; careful monitoring is advisable). Products include:
- Prevacid Delayed-Release Capsules 3268
- Prevacid for Delayed-Release Oral Suspension 3268
- Prevacid I.V. for Injection 3274
- Prevacid NapraPAC 3277
- Prevacid SoluTab Delayed-Release Orally Disintegrating Tablets 3268
- PREVPAC 3281

Levetiracetam (Growth hormone administration may alter the clearance of compounds known to be metabolized by CYP 450 liver enzymes; careful monitoring is advisable). Products include:
- Keppra Oral Solution 3307
- Keppra Tablets 3307

Levobupivacaine Hydrochloride (Growth hormone administration may alter the clearance of compounds known to be metabolized by CYP 450 liver enzymes; careful monitoring is advisable).
No products indexed under this heading.

Levonorgestrel (Growth hormone administration may alter the clearance of compounds known to be metabolized by CYP 450 liver enzymes; careful monitoring is advisable). Products include:
- Alesse-28 Tablets 3392
- Climara Pro Transdermal System 800
- Mirena Intrauterine System 810
- Plan B Tablets 1068
- Seasonale Tablets 1073
- Triphasil-28 Tablets 3483

Lidocaine (Growth hormone administration may alter the clearance of compounds known to be metabolized by CYP 450 liver enzymes; careful monitoring is advisable). Products include:
- Lidoderm Patch 1107

Lidocaine Base (Growth hormone administration may alter the clearance of compounds known to be metabolized by CYP 450 liver enzymes; careful monitoring is advisable).
No products indexed under this heading.

Lidocaine Hydrochloride (Growth hormone administration may alter the clearance of compounds known to be metabolized by CYP 450 liver enzymes; careful monitoring is advisable).
No products indexed under this heading.

Lomefloxacin Hydrochloride (Growth hormone administration may alter the clearance of compounds known to be metabolized by CYP 450 liver enzymes; careful monitoring is advisable).
No products indexed under this heading.

Losartan Potassium (Growth hormone administration may alter the clearance of compounds known to be metabolized by CYP 450 liver enzymes; careful monitoring is advisable). Products include:
- Cozaar Tablets 1913
- Hyzaar 1964

Lovastatin (Growth hormone administration may alter the clearance of compounds known to be metabolized by CYP 450 liver enzymes; careful monitoring is advisable). Products include:
- Advicor Tablets 1694
- Altoprev Extended-Release Tablets 1151
- Mevacor Tablets 1996

Maprotiline Hydrochloride (Growth hormone administration may alter the clearance of compounds known to be metabolized by CYP 450 liver enzymes; careful monitoring is advisable).
No products indexed under this heading.

Meclofenamate Sodium (Growth hormone administration may alter the clearance of compounds known to be metabolized by CYP 450 liver enzymes; careful monitoring is advisable).
No products indexed under this heading.

Mefenamic Acid (Growth hormone administration may alter the clearance of compounds known to be metabolized by CYP 450 liver enzymes; careful monitoring is advisable).
No products indexed under this heading.

Meloxicam (Growth hormone administration may alter the clearance of compounds known to be metabolized by CYP 450 liver enzymes; careful monitoring is advisable). Products include:
- Mobic Oral Suspension 893
- Mobic Tablets 893

Meperidine Hydrochloride (Growth hormone administration may alter the clearance of compounds known to be metabolized by CYP 450 liver enzymes; careful monitoring is advisable).
No products indexed under this heading.

Mephenytoin (Growth hormone administration may alter the clearance of compounds known to be metabolized by CYP 450 liver enzymes; careful monitoring is advisable).
No products indexed under this heading.

Mephobarbital (Growth hormone administration may alter the clearance of compounds known to be metabolized by CYP 450 liver enzymes; careful monitoring is advisable). Products include:
- Mebaral Tablets, USP 2483

Meprobamate (Growth hormone administration may alter the clearance of compounds known to be metabolized by CYP 450 liver enzymes; careful monitoring is advisable).
No products indexed under this heading.

Mestranol (Growth hormone administration may alter the clearance of compounds known to be metabolized by CYP 450 liver enzymes; careful monitoring is advisable).
No products indexed under this heading.

Metformin Hydrochloride (Growth hormone administration may alter the clearance of compounds known to be metabolized by CYP 450 liver enzymes; careful monitoring is advisable). Products include:
- ActoPlus Met Tablets 3219
- Avandamet Tablets 1343
- Fortamet Extended-Release Tablets 1156

Methadone Hydrochloride (Growth hormone administration may alter the clearance of compounds known to be metabolized by CYP 450 liver enzymes; careful monitoring is advisable).
No products indexed under this heading.

Methamphetamine Hydrochloride (Growth hormone administration may alter the clearance of compounds known to be metabolized by CYP 450 liver enzymes; careful monitoring is advisable). Products include:
Desoxyn Tablets, USP 2482

Methsuximide (Growth hormone administration may alter the clearance of compounds known to be metabolized by CYP 450 liver enzymes; careful monitoring is advisable).
No products indexed under this heading.

Methylprednisolone Acetate (Concomitant glucocorticoid therapy may inhibit human growth promoting effect). Products include:
Depo-Medrol Injectable Suspension 2615
Depo-Medrol Single-Dose Vial 2617

Methylprednisolone Sodium Succinate (Concomitant glucocorticoid therapy may inhibit human growth promoting effect).
No products indexed under this heading.

Metoprolol Succinate (Growth hormone administration may alter the clearance of compounds known to be metabolized by CYP 450 liver enzymes; careful monitoring is advisable). Products include:
Toprol-XL Tablets 660

Metoprolol Tartrate (Growth hormone administration may alter the clearance of compounds known to be metabolized by CYP 450 liver enzymes; careful monitoring is advisable).
No products indexed under this heading.

Mexiletine Hydrochloride (Growth hormone administration may alter the clearance of compounds known to be metabolized by CYP 450 liver enzymes; careful monitoring is advisable).
No products indexed under this heading.

Midazolam Hydrochloride (Growth hormone administration may alter the clearance of compounds known to be metabolized by CYP 450 liver enzymes; careful monitoring is advisable).
No products indexed under this heading.

Miglitol (Growth hormone administration may alter the clearance of compounds known to be metabolized by CYP 450 liver enzymes; careful monitoring is advisable).
No products indexed under this heading.

Mirtazapine (Growth hormone administration may alter the clearance of compounds known to be metabolized by CYP 450 liver enzymes; careful monitoring is advisable).
No products indexed under this heading.

Montelukast Sodium (Growth hormone administration may alter the clearance of compounds known to be metabolized by CYP 450 liver enzymes; careful monitoring is advisable). Products include:
Singulair 2047

Morphine Sulfate (Growth hormone administration may alter the clearance of compounds known to be metabolized by CYP 450 liver enzymes; careful monitoring is advisable). Products include:
Avinza Capsules 1714
Kadian Capsules 572
MS Contin Tablets 2703

Moxifloxacin Hydrochloride (Growth hormone administration may alter the clearance of compounds known to be metabolized by CYP 450 liver enzymes; careful monitoring is advisable). Products include:
Avelox 2984
Vigamox Ophthalmic Solution 560

Nabumetone (Growth hormone administration may alter the clearance of compounds known to be metabolized by CYP 450 liver enzymes; careful monitoring is advisable). Products include:
Relafen Tablets 1523

Nafcillin Sodium (Growth hormone administration may alter the clearance of compounds known to be metabolized by CYP 450 liver enzymes; careful monitoring is advisable).
No products indexed under this heading.

Naproxen (Growth hormone administration may alter the clearance of compounds known to be metabolized by CYP 450 liver enzymes; careful monitoring is advisable). Products include:
EC-Naprosyn Delayed-Release Tablets 2769
Naprosyn Suspension 2769
Naprosyn Tablets 2769
Prevacid NapraPAC 3277

Naproxen Sodium (Growth hormone administration may alter the clearance of compounds known to be metabolized by CYP 450 liver enzymes; careful monitoring is advisable). Products include:
Aleve Tablets, Caplets and Gelcaps .... ⊡605
Anaprox Tablets 2769
Anaprox DS Tablets 2769

Nateglinide (Growth hormone administration may alter the clearance of compounds known to be metabolized by CYP 450 liver enzymes; careful monitoring is advisable). Products include:
Starlix Tablets 2276

Nefazodone Hydrochloride (Growth hormone administration may alter the clearance of compounds known to be metabolized by CYP 450 liver enzymes; careful monitoring is advisable).
No products indexed under this heading.

Nelfinavir Mesylate (Growth hormone administration may alter the clearance of compounds known to be metabolized by CYP 450 liver enzymes; careful monitoring is advisable). Products include:
Viracept 2556

Nicardipine (Growth hormone administration may alter the clearance of compounds known to be metabolized by CYP 450 liver enzymes; careful monitoring is advisable).
No products indexed under this heading.

Nicardipine Hydrochloride (Growth hormone administration may alter the clearance of compounds known to be metabolized by CYP 450 liver enzymes; careful monitoring is advisable). Products include:
Cardene I.V. 1129

Nicotine Polacrilex (Growth hormone administration may alter the clearance of compounds known to be metabolized by CYP 450 liver enzymes; careful monitoring is advisable). Products include:
Commit Lozenges 1625
Nicorette Gum 1632

Nicotine Salicylate (Growth hormone administration may alter the clearance of compounds known to be metabolized by CYP 450 liver enzymes; careful monitoring is advisable).
No products indexed under this heading.

Nicotine Sulfate (Growth hormone administration may alter the clearance of compounds known to be metabolized by CYP 450 liver enzymes; careful monitoring is advisable).
No products indexed under this heading.

Nifedipine (Growth hormone administration may alter the clearance of compounds known to be metabolized by CYP 450 liver enzymes; careful monitoring is advisable). Products include:
Adalat CC Tablets 2978

Nilutamide (Growth hormone administration may alter the clearance of compounds known to be metabolized by CYP 450 liver enzymes; careful monitoring is advisable).
No products indexed under this heading.

Nimodipine (Growth hormone administration may alter the clearance of compounds known to be metabolized by CYP 450 liver enzymes; careful monitoring is advisable). Products include:
Nimotop Capsules 774

Nisoldipine (Growth hormone administration may alter the clearance of compounds known to be metabolized by CYP 450 liver enzymes; careful monitoring is advisable). Products include:
Sular Tablets 1163

Nitrendipine (Growth hormone administration may alter the clearance of compounds known to be metabolized by CYP 450 liver enzymes; careful monitoring is advisable).
No products indexed under this heading.

Norethindrone (Growth hormone administration may alter the clearance of compounds known to be metabolized by CYP 450 liver enzymes; careful monitoring is advisable). Products include:
Ortho Micronor Tablets 2411

Norethindrone Acetate (Growth hormone administration may alter the clearance of compounds known to be metabolized by CYP 450 liver enzymes; careful monitoring is advisable). Products include:
Activella Tablets 2311
Aygestin Tablets 1062
CombiPatch Transdermal System 2180

Norfloxacin (Growth hormone administration may alter the clearance of compounds known to be metabolized by CYP 450 liver enzymes; careful monitoring is advisable). Products include:
Noroxin Tablets 2009

Norgestrel (Growth hormone administration may alter the clearance of compounds known to be metabolized by CYP 450 liver enzymes; careful monitoring is advisable). Products include:
Lo/Ovral-28 Tablets 3423

Nortriptyline Hydrochloride (Growth hormone administration may alter the clearance of compounds known to be metabolized by CYP 450 liver enzymes; careful monitoring is advisable).
No products indexed under this heading.

Ofloxacin (Growth hormone administration may alter the clearance of compounds known to be metabolized by CYP 450 liver enzymes; careful monitoring is advisable). Products include:
Floxin Otic Singles 1045
Floxin Otic Solution 1043

Olanzapine (Growth hormone administration may alter the clearance of compounds known to be metabolized by CYP 450 liver enzymes; careful monitoring is advisable). Products include:
Symbyax Capsules 1788
Zyprexa Tablets 1798
Zyprexa IntraMuscular 1798
Zyprexa ZYDIS Orally Disintegrating Tablets 1798

Omeprazole (Growth hormone administration may alter the clearance of compounds known to be metabolized by CYP 450 liver enzymes; careful monitoring is advisable). Products include:
Zegerid Powder for Oral Solution 2972

Ondansetron (Growth hormone administration may alter the clearance of compounds known to be metabolized by CYP 450 liver enzymes; careful monitoring is advisable). Products include:
Zofran ODT Orally Disintegrating Tablets 1613

Ondansetron Hydrochloride (Growth hormone administration may alter the clearance of compounds known to be metabolized by CYP 450 liver enzymes; careful monitoring is advisable). Products include:
Zofran Injection 1607
Zofran 1613

Oxaprozin (Growth hormone administration may alter the clearance of compounds known to be metabolized by CYP 450 liver enzymes; careful monitoring is advisable).
No products indexed under this heading.

Oxcarbazepine (Growth hormone administration may alter the clearance of compounds known to be metabolized by CYP 450 liver enzymes; careful monitoring is advisable). Products include:
Trileptal Oral Suspension 2281
Trileptal Tablets 2281

Oxycodone Hydrochloride (Growth hormone administration may alter the clearance of compounds known to be metabolized by CYP 450 liver enzymes; careful monitoring is advisable). Products include:
Combunox Tablets 1183
OxyContin Tablets 2699
OxyFast Oral Concentrate Solution 2704
OxyIR Capsules 2704
Percocet Tablets 1114

Percodan Tablets 1115

Paclitaxel (Growth hormone administration may alter the clearance of compounds known to be metabolized by CYP 450 liver enzymes; careful monitoring is advisable).
No products indexed under this heading.

Pantoprazole Sodium (Growth hormone administration may alter the clearance of compounds known to be metabolized by CYP 450 liver enzymes; careful monitoring is advisable). Products include:
Protonix I.V. 3468
Protonix Tablets 3465

Paramethadione (Growth hormone administration may alter the clearance of compounds known to be metabolized by CYP 450 liver enzymes; careful monitoring is advisable).
No products indexed under this heading.

Paroxetine Hydrochloride (Growth hormone administration may alter the clearance of compounds known to be metabolized by CYP 450 liver enzymes; careful monitoring is advisable). Products include:
Paxil CR Controlled-Release Tablets 1509
Paxil 1501

Pentamidine Isethionate (Growth hormone administration may alter the clearance of compounds known to be metabolized by CYP 450 liver enzymes; careful monitoring is advisable).
No products indexed under this heading.

Phenacemide (Growth hormone administration may alter the clearance of compounds known to be metabolized by CYP 450 liver enzymes; careful monitoring is advisable).
No products indexed under this heading.

Phenobarbital (Growth hormone administration may alter the clearance of compounds known to be metabolized by CYP 450 liver enzymes; careful monitoring is advisable).
No products indexed under this heading.

Phenobarbital Sodium (Growth hormone administration may alter the clearance of compounds known to be metabolized by CYP 450 liver enzymes; careful monitoring is advisable).
No products indexed under this heading.

Phensuximide (Growth hormone administration may alter the clearance of compounds known to be metabolized by CYP 450 liver enzymes; careful monitoring is advisable).
No products indexed under this heading.

Phenylbutazone (Growth hormone administration may alter the clearance of compounds known to be metabolized by CYP 450 liver enzymes; careful monitoring is advisable).
No products indexed under this heading.

Phenytoin (Growth hormone administration may alter the clearance of compounds known to be metabolized by CYP 450 liver enzymes; careful monitoring is advisable).
No products indexed under this heading.

Phenytoin Sodium (Growth hormone administration may alter the clearance of compounds known to be metabolized by CYP 450 liver enzymes; careful monitoring is advisable). Products include:
Phenytek Capsules 2153

Pimozide (Growth hormone administration may alter the clearance of compounds known to be metabolized by CYP 450 liver enzymes; careful monitoring is advisable). Products include:
Orap Tablets 1220

Pindolol (Growth hormone administration may alter the clearance of compounds known to be metabolized by CYP 450 liver enzymes; careful monitoring is advisable).
No products indexed under this heading.

Pioglitazone Hydrochloride (Growth hormone administration may alter the clearance of compounds known to be metabolized by CYP 450 liver enzymes; careful monitoring is advisable). Products include:
ActoPlus Met Tablets 3219
Actos Tablets 3224

Piroxicam (Growth hormone administration may alter the clearance of compounds known to be metabolized by CYP 450 liver enzymes; careful monitoring is advisable).
No products indexed under this heading.

Polyestradiol Phosphate (Growth hormone administration may alter the clearance of compounds known to be metabolized by CYP 450 liver enzymes; careful monitoring is advisable).
No products indexed under this heading.

Prednisolone Acetate (Concomitant glucocorticoid therapy may inhibit human growth promoting effect). Products include:
Blephamide Ophthalmic Ointment 563
Blephamide Ophthalmic Suspension 564
Poly-Pred Liquifilm Ophthalmic Suspension .... ⊙ 231
Pred Forte Ophthalmic Suspension .... ⊙ 233
Pred Mild Sterile Ophthalmic Suspension .... ⊙ 236
Pred-G Ophthalmic Suspension ...... ⊙ 234
Pred-G Sterile Ophthalmic Ointment .... ⊙ 235

Prednisolone Sodium Phosphate (Concomitant glucocorticoid therapy may inhibit human growth promoting effect). Products include:
Pediapred Oral Solution 3319

Prednisolone Tebutate (Concomitant glucocorticoid therapy may inhibit human growth promoting effect).
No products indexed under this heading.

Prednisone (Concomitant glucocorticoid therapy may inhibit human growth promoting effect).
No products indexed under this heading.

Primidone (Growth hormone administration may alter the clearance of compounds known to be metabolized by CYP 450 liver enzymes; careful monitoring is advisable).
No products indexed under this heading.

Progesterone (Growth hormone administration may alter the clearance of compounds known to be metabolized by CYP 450 liver enzymes; careful monitoring is advisable). Products include:
Prochieve 4% Gel 1018
Prochieve 8% Gel 1018
Prometrium Capsules (100 mg, 200 mg) 3205

Proguanil Hydrochloride (Growth hormone administration may alter the clearance of compounds known to be metabolized by CYP 450 liver enzymes; careful monitoring is advisable). Products include:
Malarone Tablets 1484
Malarone Pediatric Tablets 1484

Propafenone Hydrochloride (Growth hormone administration may alter the clearance of compounds known to be metabolized by CYP 450 liver enzymes; careful monitoring is advisable). Products include:
Rythmol SR Capsules 2736

Propoxyphene Hydrochloride (Growth hormone administration may alter the clearance of compounds known to be metabolized by CYP 450 liver enzymes; careful monitoring is advisable).
No products indexed under this heading.

Propoxyphene Napsylate (Growth hormone administration may alter the clearance of compounds known to be metabolized by CYP 450 liver enzymes; careful monitoring is advisable). Products include:
Darvocet A 500 Tablets 3497

Propranolol Hydrochloride (Growth hormone administration may alter the clearance of compounds known to be metabolized by CYP 450 liver enzymes; careful monitoring is advisable). Products include:
Inderal LA Long-Acting Capsules 3421
InnoPran XL Capsules 2728

Protriptyline Hydrochloride (Growth hormone administration may alter the clearance of compounds known to be metabolized by CYP 450 liver enzymes; careful monitoring is advisable). Products include:
Vivactil Tablets 2350

Quetiapine Fumarate (Growth hormone administration may alter the clearance of compounds known to be metabolized by CYP 450 liver enzymes; careful monitoring is advisable). Products include:
Seroquel Tablets 691

Quinidine Gluconate (Growth hormone administration may alter the clearance of compounds known to be metabolized by CYP 450 liver enzymes; careful monitoring is advisable).
No products indexed under this heading.

Quinidine Hydrochloride (Growth hormone administration may alter the clearance of compounds known to be metabolized by CYP 450 liver enzymes; careful monitoring is advisable).
No products indexed under this heading.

Quinidine Polygalacturonate (Growth hormone administration may alter the clearance of compounds known to be metabolized by CYP 450 liver enzymes; careful monitoring is advisable).
No products indexed under this heading.

Quinidine Sulfate (Growth hormone administration may alter the clearance of compounds known to be metabolized by CYP 450 liver enzymes; careful monitoring is advisable).
No products indexed under this heading.

Quinine (Growth hormone administration may alter the clearance of compounds known to be metabolized by CYP 450 liver enzymes; careful monitoring is advisable).
No products indexed under this heading.

Quinine Sulfate (Growth hormone administration may alter the clearance of compounds known to be metabolized by CYP 450 liver enzymes; careful monitoring is advisable).
No products indexed under this heading.

Rabeprazole Sodium (Growth hormone administration may alter the clearance of compounds known to be metabolized by CYP 450 liver enzymes; careful monitoring is advisable). Products include:
Aciphex Tablets 1081

Repaglinide (Growth hormone administration may alter the clearance of compounds known to be metabolized by CYP 450 liver enzymes; careful monitoring is advisable). Products include:
Prandin Tablets (0.5, 1, and 2 mg) 2337

Rifabutin (Growth hormone administration may alter the clearance of compounds known to be metabolized by CYP 450 liver enzymes; careful monitoring is advisable).
No products indexed under this heading.

Riluzole (Growth hormone administration may alter the clearance of compounds known to be metabolized by CYP 450 liver enzymes; careful monitoring is advisable). Products include:
Rilutek Tablets 2945

Risperidone (Growth hormone administration may alter the clearance of compounds known to be metabolized by CYP 450 liver enzymes; careful monitoring is advisable). Products include:
Risperdal Consta Long-Acting Injection 1664
Risperdal M-Tab Orally Disintegrating Tablets 1658
Risperdal 1658

Ritonavir (Growth hormone administration may alter the clearance of compounds known to be metabolized by CYP 450 liver enzymes; careful monitoring is advisable). Products include:
Kaletra 474
Norvir 499

Rofecoxib (Growth hormone administration may alter the clearance of compounds known to be metabolized by CYP 450 liver enzymes; careful monitoring is advisable).
No products indexed under this heading.

Ropinirole Hydrochloride (Growth hormone administration may alter the clearance of compounds known to be metabolized by CYP 450 liver enzymes; careful monitoring is advisable). Products include:
- Requip Tablets 1528

Ropivacaine Hydrochloride (Growth hormone administration may alter the clearance of compounds known to be metabolized by CYP 450 liver enzymes; careful monitoring is advisable). Products include:
- Naropin Injection 640

Rosiglitazone Maleate (Growth hormone administration may alter the clearance of compounds known to be metabolized by CYP 450 liver enzymes; careful monitoring is advisable). Products include:
- Avandamet Tablets 1343
- Avandia Tablets 1348

Saquinavir (Growth hormone administration may alter the clearance of compounds known to be metabolized by CYP 450 liver enzymes; careful monitoring is advisable).
No products indexed under this heading.

Saquinavir Mesylate (Growth hormone administration may alter the clearance of compounds known to be metabolized by CYP 450 liver enzymes; careful monitoring is advisable). Products include:
- Invirase 2776

Sertraline Hydrochloride (Growth hormone administration may alter the clearance of compounds known to be metabolized by CYP 450 liver enzymes; careful monitoring is advisable). Products include:
- Zoloft 2581

Sildenafil Citrate (Growth hormone administration may alter the clearance of compounds known to be metabolized by CYP 450 liver enzymes; careful monitoring is advisable). Products include:
- Revatio Tablets 2541
- Viagra Tablets 2552

Simvastatin (Growth hormone administration may alter the clearance of compounds known to be metabolized by CYP 450 liver enzymes; careful monitoring is advisable). Products include:
- Vytorin 10/10 Tablets 2084
- Vytorin 10/10 Tablets 3092
- Vytorin 10/20 Tablets 2084
- Vytorin 10/20 Tablets 3092
- Vytorin 10/40 Tablets 3092
- Vytorin 10/40 Tablets 2084
- Vytorin 10/80 Tablets 2084
- Vytorin 10/80 Tablets 3092
- Zocor Tablets 2078

Sirolimus (Growth hormone administration may alter the clearance of compounds known to be metabolized by CYP 450 liver enzymes; careful monitoring is advisable). Products include:
- Rapamune Oral Solution and Tablets 3472

Sulfamethoxazole (Growth hormone administration may alter the clearance of compounds known to be metabolized by CYP 450 liver enzymes; careful monitoring is advisable).
No products indexed under this heading.

Sulindac (Growth hormone administration may alter the clearance of compounds known to be metabolized by CYP 450 liver enzymes; careful monitoring is advisable). Products include:
- Clinoril Tablets 1899

Suprofen (Growth hormone administration may alter the clearance of compounds known to be metabolized by CYP 450 liver enzymes; careful monitoring is advisable).
No products indexed under this heading.

Tacrine Hydrochloride (Growth hormone administration may alter the clearance of compounds known to be metabolized by CYP 450 liver enzymes; careful monitoring is advisable).
No products indexed under this heading.

Tacrolimus (Growth hormone administration may alter the clearance of compounds known to be metabolized by CYP 450 liver enzymes; careful monitoring is advisable). Products include:
- Prograf Capsules and Injection 624
- Protopic Ointment 629

Tamoxifen Citrate (Growth hormone administration may alter the clearance of compounds known to be metabolized by CYP 450 liver enzymes; careful monitoring is advisable).
No products indexed under this heading.

Telmisartan (Growth hormone administration may alter the clearance of compounds known to be metabolized by CYP 450 liver enzymes; careful monitoring is advisable). Products include:
- Micardis Tablets 884
- Micardis HCT Tablets 886

Teniposide (Growth hormone administration may alter the clearance of compounds known to be metabolized by CYP 450 liver enzymes; careful monitoring is advisable).
No products indexed under this heading.

Terfenadine (Growth hormone administration may alter the clearance of compounds known to be metabolized by CYP 450 liver enzymes; careful monitoring is advisable).
No products indexed under this heading.

Testosterone (Growth hormone administration may alter the clearance of compounds known to be metabolized by CYP 450 liver enzymes; careful monitoring is advisable). Products include:
- AndroGel 3330
- Striant Mucoadhesive 1022
- Testim 1% Gel 722

Testosterone Cypionate (Growth hormone administration may alter the clearance of compounds known to be metabolized by CYP 450 liver enzymes; careful monitoring is advisable).
No products indexed under this heading.

Testosterone Enanthate (Growth hormone administration may alter the clearance of compounds known to be metabolized by CYP 450 liver enzymes; careful monitoring is advisable). Products include:
- Delatestryl Injection 2976

Testosterone Propionate (Growth hormone administration may alter the clearance of compounds known to be metabolized by CYP 450 liver enzymes; careful monitoring is advisable).
No products indexed under this heading.

Theophylline (Growth hormone administration may alter the clearance of compounds known to be metabolized by CYP 450 liver enzymes; careful monitoring is advisable).
No products indexed under this heading.

Theophylline Anhydrous (Growth hormone administration may alter the clearance of compounds known to be metabolized by CYP 450 liver enzymes; careful monitoring is advisable). Products include:
- Uniphyl Tablets 2708

Theophylline Sodium Glycinate (Growth hormone administration may alter the clearance of compounds known to be metabolized by CYP 450 liver enzymes; careful monitoring is advisable).
No products indexed under this heading.

Thioridazine (Growth hormone administration may alter the clearance of compounds known to be metabolized by CYP 450 liver enzymes; careful monitoring is advisable).
No products indexed under this heading.

Thioridazine Hydrochloride (Growth hormone administration may alter the clearance of compounds known to be metabolized by CYP 450 liver enzymes; careful monitoring is advisable). Products include:
- Thioridazine Hydrochloride Tablets 2122

Tiagabine Hydrochloride (Growth hormone administration may alter the clearance of compounds known to be metabolized by CYP 450 liver enzymes; careful monitoring is advisable). Products include:
- Gabitril Tablets 998

Timolol Maleate (Growth hormone administration may alter the clearance of compounds known to be metabolized by CYP 450 liver enzymes; careful monitoring is advisable). Products include:
- Blocadren Tablets 1891
- Cosopt Sterile Ophthalmic Solution 1910
- Timolide Tablets 2056
- Timoptic in Ocudose 2061
- Timoptic Sterile Ophthalmic Solution 2058
- Timoptic-XE Sterile Ophthalmic Gel Forming Solution 2062

Tolazamide (Growth hormone administration may alter the clearance of compounds known to be metabolized by CYP 450 liver enzymes; careful monitoring is advisable).
No products indexed under this heading.

Tolbutamide (Growth hormone administration may alter the clearance of compounds known to be metabolized by CYP 450 liver enzymes; careful monitoring is advisable).
No products indexed under this heading.

Tolbutamide Sodium (Growth hormone administration may alter the clearance of compounds known to be metabolized by CYP 450 liver enzymes; careful monitoring is advisable).
No products indexed under this heading.

Tolmetin Sodium (Growth hormone administration may alter the clearance of compounds known to be metabolized by CYP 450 liver enzymes; careful monitoring is advisable).
No products indexed under this heading.

Tolterodine Tartrate (Growth hormone administration may alter the clearance of compounds known to be metabolized by CYP 450 liver enzymes; careful monitoring is advisable). Products include:
- Detrol Tablets 2626
- Detrol LA Capsules 2629

Topiramate (Growth hormone administration may alter the clearance of compounds known to be metabolized by CYP 450 liver enzymes; careful monitoring is advisable). Products include:
- Topamax Sprinkle Capsules 2438
- Topamax Tablets 2438

Torsemide (Growth hormone administration may alter the clearance of compounds known to be metabolized by CYP 450 liver enzymes; careful monitoring is advisable).
No products indexed under this heading.

Tramadol Hydrochloride (Growth hormone administration may alter the clearance of compounds known to be metabolized by CYP 450 liver enzymes; careful monitoring is advisable). Products include:
- Ultracet Tablets 2462

Trazodone Hydrochloride (Growth hormone administration may alter the clearance of compounds known to be metabolized by CYP 450 liver enzymes; careful monitoring is advisable).
No products indexed under this heading.

Tretinoin (Growth hormone administration may alter the clearance of compounds known to be metabolized by CYP 450 liver enzymes; careful monitoring is advisable). Products include:
- Avita Cream 2136
- Avita Gel 2138
- Renova 0.02% Cream 2384
- Renova 0.05% Cream 2387
- Retin-A Micro 0.1%/0.04% 2388
- Solage Topical Solution 740
- Tri-Luma Cream 1213
- Vesanoid Capsules 2823

Triamcinolone (Concomitant glucocorticoid therapy may inhibit human growth promoting effect).
No products indexed under this heading.

Triamcinolone Acetonide (Concomitant glucocorticoid therapy may inhibit human growth promoting effect). Products include:
- Azmacort Inhalation Aerosol 1701
- Nasacort HFA Inhalation Aerosol 2939
- Nasacort AQ Nasal Spray 2937

Triamcinolone Diacetate (Concomitant glucocorticoid therapy may inhibit human growth promoting effect).
No products indexed under this heading.

Triamcinolone Hexacetonide (Concomitant glucocorticoid therapy may inhibit human growth promoting effect).
No products indexed under this heading.

Triazolam (Growth hormone administration may alter the clearance of compounds known to be metabolized by CYP 450 liver enzymes; careful monitoring is advisable).
No products indexed under this heading.

Trimethadione (Growth hormone administration may alter the clearance of compounds known to be metabolized by CYP 450 liver enzymes; careful monitoring is advisable).
No products indexed under this heading.

Trimethaphan Camsylate (Growth hormone administration may alter the clearance of compounds known to be metabolized by CYP 450 liver enzymes; careful monitoring is advisable).
No products indexed under this heading.

Trimipramine Maleate (Growth hormone administration may alter the clearance of compounds known to be metabolized by CYP 450 liver enzymes; careful monitoring is advisable). Products include:
Surmontil Capsules 2347

Troglitazone (Growth hormone administration may alter the clearance of compounds known to be metabolized by CYP 450 liver enzymes; careful monitoring is advisable).
No products indexed under this heading.

Trovafloxacin Mesylate (Growth hormone administration may alter the clearance of compounds known to be metabolized by CYP 450 liver enzymes; careful monitoring is advisable).
No products indexed under this heading.

Valdecoxib (Growth hormone administration may alter the clearance of compounds known to be metabolized by CYP 450 liver enzymes; careful monitoring is advisable).
No products indexed under this heading.

Valproate Sodium (Growth hormone administration may alter the clearance of compounds known to be metabolized by CYP 450 liver enzymes; careful monitoring is advisable). Products include:
Depacon Injection 412

Valproic Acid (Growth hormone administration may alter the clearance of compounds known to be metabolized by CYP 450 liver enzymes; careful monitoring is advisable). Products include:
Depakene 417

Valsartan (Growth hormone administration may alter the clearance of compounds known to be metabolized by CYP 450 liver enzymes; careful monitoring is advisable). Products include:
Diovan HCT Tablets 2195
Diovan Tablets 2191

Venlafaxine Hydrochloride (Growth hormone administration may alter the clearance of compounds known to be metabolized by CYP 450 liver enzymes; careful monitoring is advisable). Products include:
Effexor Tablets 3405
Effexor XR Capsules 3411

Verapamil Hydrochloride (Growth hormone administration may alter the clearance of compounds known to be metabolized by CYP 450 liver enzymes; careful monitoring is advisable). Products include:
Covera-HS Tablets 3135
Tarka Tablets 519
Verelan PM Capsules 3120

Vinblastine Sulfate (Growth hormone administration may alter the clearance of compounds known to be metabolized by CYP 450 liver enzymes; careful monitoring is advisable).
No products indexed under this heading.

Vincristine Sulfate (Growth hormone administration may alter the clearance of compounds known to be metabolized by CYP 450 liver enzymes; careful monitoring is advisable).
No products indexed under this heading.

Vitamin A (Growth hormone administration may alter the clearance of compounds known to be metabolized by CYP 450 liver enzymes; careful monitoring is advisable). Products include:
Visutein Capsules 3328

Vitamin A Acetate (Growth hormone administration may alter the clearance of compounds known to be metabolized by CYP 450 liver enzymes; careful monitoring is advisable).
No products indexed under this heading.

Voriconazole (Growth hormone administration may alter the clearance of compounds known to be metabolized by CYP 450 liver enzymes; careful monitoring is advisable). Products include:
VFEND I.V. 2543
VFEND Oral Suspension 2543
VFEND Tablets 2543

Warfarin Sodium (Growth hormone administration may alter the clearance of compounds known to be metabolized by CYP 450 liver enzymes; careful monitoring is advisable). Products include:
Coumadin for Injection 932
Coumadin Tablets 932

Zafirlukast (Growth hormone administration may alter the clearance of compounds known to be metabolized by CYP 450 liver enzymes; careful monitoring is advisable). Products include:
Accolate Tablets 663

Zileuton (Growth hormone administration may alter the clearance of compounds known to be metabolized by CYP 450 liver enzymes; careful monitoring is advisable).
No products indexed under this heading.

Zolmitriptan (Growth hormone administration may alter the clearance of compounds known to be metabolized by CYP 450 liver enzymes; careful monitoring is advisable). Products include:
Zomig Nasal Spray 718
Zomig Tablets 714
Zomig-ZMT Tablets 714

Zonisamide (Growth hormone administration may alter the clearance of compounds known to be metabolized by CYP 450 liver enzymes; careful monitoring is advisable). Products include:
Zonegran Capsules 1089

Zopiclone (Growth hormone administration may alter the clearance of compounds known to be metabolized by CYP 450 liver enzymes; careful monitoring is advisable).
No products indexed under this heading.

GEODON CAPSULES

(Ziprasidone Hydrochloride) 2514
May interact with antihypertensives, central nervous system depressants, dopamine agonists, erythromycin, potassium-depleting diuretics, quinidine, and certain other agents. Compounds in these categories include:

Acebutolol Hydrochloride (Ziprasidone may induce orthostatic hypotension; co-administration with certain antihypertensive drugs may enhance the hypotensive effects).
No products indexed under this heading.

Alfentanil Hydrochloride (Somnolence was a commonly reported adverse event in patients treated with ziprasidone; concurrent use with other CNS active drugs, such as depressants, should be undertaken with caution).
No products indexed under this heading.

Alprazolam (Somnolence was a commonly reported adverse event in patients treated with ziprasidone; concurrent use with other CNS active drugs, such as depressants, should be undertaken with caution). Products include:
Niravam Orally Disintegrating Tablets 3106
Xanax XR Tablets 2655

Amiodarone Hydrochloride (Ziprasidone produces dose-related prolongation of the QT interval; an additive effect of ziprasidone and other drugs that prolong cannot be excluded; concurrent use is not recommended). Products include:
Pacerone Tablets 3337

Amlodipine Besylate (Ziprasidone may induce orthostatic hypotension; co-administration with certain antihypertensive drugs may enhance the hypotensive effects). Products include:
Caduet Tablets 2507
Lotrel Capsules 2238
Norvasc Tablets 2529

Aprobarbital (Somnolence was a commonly reported adverse event in patients treated with ziprasidone; concurrent use with other CNS active drugs, such as depressants, should be undertaken with caution).
No products indexed under this heading.

Arsenic Trioxide (Ziprasidone produces dose-related prolongation of the QT interval; an additive effect of ziprasidone and other drugs that prolong cannot be excluded; concurrent use is not recommended). Products include:
Trisenox Injection 983

Atenolol (Ziprasidone may induce orthostatic hypotension; co-administration with certain antihypertensive drugs may enhance the hypotensive effects). Products include:
Tenormin I.V. Injection 698
Tenormin Tablets 695

Benazepril Hydrochloride (Ziprasidone may induce orthostatic hypotension; co-administration with certain antihypertensive drugs may enhance the hypotensive effects). Products include:
Lotensin Tablets 2232
Lotensin HCT Tablets 2235
Lotrel Capsules 2238

Bendroflumethiazide (Ziprasidone produces dose-related prolongation of the QT interval; hypokalemia may result from diuretic therapy and this may increase the risk of QT prolongation and arrhythmias; potential for enhanced hypotensive effect if used concurrently).
No products indexed under this heading.

Bepridil Hydrochloride (Ziprasidone produces dose-related prolongation of the QT interval; an additive effect of ziprasidone and other drugs that prolong cannot be excluded; concurrent use is not recommended).
No products indexed under this heading.

Betaxolol Hydrochloride (Ziprasidone may induce orthostatic hypotension; co-administration with certain antihypertensive drugs may enhance the hypotensive effects). Products include:
Betoptic S Ophthalmic Suspension 554

Bisoprolol Fumarate (Ziprasidone may induce orthostatic hypotension; co-administration with certain antihypertensive drugs may enhance the hypotensive effects).
No products indexed under this heading.

Bromocriptine Mesylate (Ziprasidone may antagonize the effects of dopamine agonists).
No products indexed under this heading.

Bumetanide (Ziprasidone produces dose-related prolongation of the QT interval; hypokalemia may result from diuretic therapy and this may increase the risk of QT prolongation and arrhythmias; potential for enhanced hypotensive effect if used concurrently).
No products indexed under this heading.

Buprenorphine Hydrochloride (Somnolence was a commonly reported adverse event in patients treated with ziprasidone; concurrent use with other CNS active drugs, such as depressants, should be undertaken with caution). Products include:
Buprenex Injectable 2718
Suboxone Tablets 2719
Subutex Tablets 2719

Buspirone Hydrochloride (Somnolence was a commonly reported adverse event in patients treated with ziprasidone; concurrent use with other CNS active drugs, such as depressants, should be undertaken with caution).
No products indexed under this heading.

Butabarbital (Somnolence was a commonly reported adverse event in patients treated with ziprasidone; concurrent use with other CNS active drugs, such as depressants, should be undertaken with caution).
No products indexed under this heading.

Butalbital (Somnolence was a commonly reported adverse event in patients treated with ziprasidone; concurrent use with other CNS active drugs, such as depressants, should be undertaken with caution). Products include:
Sedapap Tablets 50 mg/650 mg 2098

Candesartan Cilexetil (Ziprasidone may induce orthostatic hypotension; co-administration with certain antihypertensive drugs may enhance the hypotensive effects). Products include:
Atacand Tablets 634
Atacand HCT 637

Captopril (Ziprasidone may induce orthostatic hypotension; co-administration with certain antihypertensive drugs may enhance the hypotensive effects). Products include:
Captopril Tablets 2114

Carbamazepine (Co-administration with carbamazepine, an inducer of CYP3A4, has resulted in a decrease of approximately 35% in AUC of ziprasidone; this effect may be greater when higher doses of carbamazepine are administered). Products include:
Carbatrol Capsules 3174
Equetro Extended-Release Capsules 3178
Tegretol/Tegretol-XR 2278

Carteolol Hydrochloride (Ziprasidone may induce orthostatic hypotension; co-administration with certain antihypertensive drugs may enhance the hypotensive effects). Products include:
Carteolol Hydrochloride Ophthalmic Solution USP, 1% .... ⊙ 246

Chlordiazepoxide (Somnolence was a commonly reported adverse event in patients treated with ziprasidone; concurrent use with other CNS active drugs, such as depressants, should be undertaken with caution).
No products indexed under this heading.

Chlordiazepoxide Hydrochloride (Somnolence was a commonly reported adverse event in patients treated with ziprasidone; concurrent use with other CNS active drugs, such as depressants, should be undertaken with caution). Products include:
Librium Capsules 3349

Chlorothiazide (Ziprasidone produces dose-related prolongation of the QT interval; hypokalemia may result from diuretic therapy and this may increase the risk of QT prolongation and arrhythmias; potential for enhanced hypotensive effect if used concurrently). Products include:
Aldoclor Tablets 1881
Diuril Oral 1936

Chlorothiazide Sodium (Ziprasidone produces dose-related prolongation of the QT interval; hypokalemia may result from diuretic therapy and this may increase the risk of QT prolongation and arrhythmias; potential for enhanced hypotensive effect if used concurrently). Products include:
Diuril Sodium Intravenous 1934

Chlorpromazine (Ziprasidone produces dose-related prolongation of the QT interval; an additive effect of ziprasidone and other drugs that prolong cannot be excluded; concurrent use is not recommended).
No products indexed under this heading.

Chlorpromazine Hydrochloride (Ziprasidone produces dose-related prolongation of the QT interval; an additive effect of ziprasidone and other drugs that prolong cannot be excluded; concurrent use is not recommended).
No products indexed under this heading.

Chlorprothixene (Somnolence was a commonly reported adverse event in patients treated with ziprasidone; concurrent use with other CNS active drugs, such as depressants, should be undertaken with caution).
No products indexed under this heading.

Chlorprothixene Hydrochloride (Ziprasidone produces dose-related prolongation of the QT interval; an additive effect of ziprasidone and other drugs that prolong cannot be excluded; concurrent use is not recommended).
No products indexed under this heading.

Chlorprothixene Lactate (Somnolence was a commonly reported adverse event in patients treated with ziprasidone; concurrent use with other CNS active drugs, such as depressants, should be undertaken with caution).
No products indexed under this heading.

Chlorthalidone (Ziprasidone may induce orthostatic hypotension; co-administration with certain antihypertensive drugs may enhance the hypotensive effects). Products include:
Clorpres Tablets 2139

Clonidine (Ziprasidone may induce orthostatic hypotension; co-administration with certain antihypertensive drugs may enhance the hypotensive effects). Products include:
Catapres-TTS 875

Clonidine Hydrochloride (Ziprasidone may induce orthostatic hypotension; co-administration with certain antihypertensive drugs may enhance the hypotensive effects). Products include:
Catapres Tablets 874
Clorpres Tablets 2139

Clorazepate Dipotassium (Somnolence was a commonly reported adverse event in patients treated with ziprasidone; concurrent use with other CNS active drugs, such as depressants, should be undertaken with caution). Products include:
Tranxene 2488

Clozapine (Somnolence was a commonly reported adverse event in patients treated with ziprasidone; concurrent use with other CNS active drugs, such as depressants, should be undertaken with caution). Products include:
Clozapine Tablets 2141
Clozaril Tablets 2174
FazaClo Orally Disintegrating Tablets 547

Codeine Phosphate (Somnolence was a commonly reported adverse event in patients treated with ziprasidone; concurrent use with other CNS active drugs, such as depressants, should be undertaken with caution). Products include:
Tylenol with Codeine 2461

Deserpidine (Ziprasidone may induce orthostatic hypotension; co-administration with certain antihypertensive drugs may enhance the hypotensive effects).
No products indexed under this heading.

Desflurane (Somnolence was a commonly reported adverse event in patients treated with ziprasidone; concurrent use with other CNS active drugs, such as depressants, should be undertaken with caution). Products include:
Suprane Liquid for Inhalation 770

Desipramine Hydrochloride (Ziprasidone produces dose-related prolongation of the QT interval; an additive effect of ziprasidone and other drugs that prolong cannot be excluded; concurrent use is not recommended).
No products indexed under this heading.

Dezocine (Somnolence was a commonly reported adverse event in patients treated with ziprasidone; concurrent use with other CNS active drugs, such as depressants, should be undertaken with caution).
No products indexed under this heading.

Diazepam (Somnolence was a commonly reported adverse event in patients treated with ziprasidone; concurrent use with other CNS active drugs, such as depressants, should be undertaken with caution). Products include:
Diastat Rectal Delivery System 3344
Valium Tablets 2822

Diazoxide (Ziprasidone may induce orthostatic hypotension; co-administration with certain antihypertensive drugs may enhance the hypotensive effects). Products include:
Hyperstat I.V. Injection 3031

Diltiazem Hydrochloride (Ziprasidone may induce orthostatic hypotension; co-administration with certain antihypertensive drugs may enhance the hypotensive effects). Products include:
Cardizem LA Extended Release Tablets 1699
Tiazac Capsules 1204

Disopyramide Phosphate (Ziprasidone produces dose-related prolongation of the QT interval; an additive effect of ziprasidone and other drugs that prolong cannot be excluded; concurrent use is not recommended).
No products indexed under this heading.

Dofetilide (Ziprasidone produces dose-related prolongation of the QT interval; an additive effect of ziprasidone and other drugs that prolong cannot be excluded; concurrent use is not recommended).
No products indexed under this heading.

Dolasetron Mesylate (Ziprasidone produces dose-related prolongation of the QT interval; an additive effect of ziprasidone and other drugs that prolong cannot be excluded; concurrent use is not recommended). Products include:
Anzemet Injection 2871
Anzemet Tablets 2874

Dopamine Hydrochloride (Ziprasidone may antagonize the effects of dopamine agonists).
No products indexed under this heading.

Doxazosin Mesylate (Ziprasidone may induce orthostatic hypotension; co-administration with certain antihypertensive drugs may enhance the hypotensive effects).
No products indexed under this heading.

Droperidol (Ziprasidone produces dose-related prolongation of the QT interval; an additive effect of ziprasidone and other drugs that prolong cannot be excluded; concurrent use is not recommended).
No products indexed under this heading.

Enalapril Maleate (Ziprasidone may induce orthostatic hypotension; co-administration with certain antihypertensive drugs may enhance the hypotensive effects). Products include:
Vaseretic Tablets 2073
Vasotec I.V. Injection 2076

Enalaprilat (Ziprasidone may induce orthostatic hypotension; co-administration with certain antihypertensive drugs may enhance the hypotensive effects).
No products indexed under this heading.

Enflurane (Somnolence was a commonly reported adverse event in patients treated with ziprasidone; concurrent use with other CNS active drugs, such as depressants, should be undertaken with caution).
No products indexed under this heading.

Eprosartan Mesylate (Ziprasidone may induce orthostatic hypotension; co-administration with certain antihypertensive drugs may enhance the hypotensive effects). Products include:
Teveten Tablets 1707
Teveten HCT Tablets 1710

Erythromycin (Ziprasidone produces dose-related prolongation of the QT interval; an additive effect of ziprasidone and other drugs that prolong cannot be excluded; concurrent use is not recommended). Products include:
Erygel Topical Gel 2096
Ery-Tab Tablets 447
Erythromycin Base Filmtab Tablets 454
Erythromycin Delayed-Release Capsules, USP 456
PCE Dispertab Tablets 510

Erythromycin Estolate (Ziprasidone produces dose-related prolongation of the QT interval; an additive effect of ziprasidone and other drugs that prolong cannot be excluded; concurrent use is not recommended).
No products indexed under this heading.

Erythromycin Ethylsuccinate (Ziprasidone produces dose-related prolongation of the QT interval; an additive effect of ziprasidone and other drugs that prolong cannot be excluded; concurrent use is not recommended). Products include:
E.E.S. 449
EryPed 445

Erythromycin Gluceptate (Ziprasidone produces dose-related prolongation of the QT interval; an additive effect of ziprasidone and other drugs that prolong cannot be excluded; concurrent use is not recommended).
No products indexed under this heading.

Erythromycin Lactobionate (Ziprasidone produces dose-related prolongation of the QT interval; an additive effect of ziprasidone and other drugs that prolong cannot be excluded; concurrent use is not recommended).
No products indexed under this heading.

Erythromycin Stearate (Ziprasidone produces dose-related prolongation of the QT interval; an additive effect of ziprasidone and other drugs that prolong cannot be excluded; concurrent use is not recommended). Products include:
Erythrocin Stearate Filmtab Tablets 452

Esmolol Hydrochloride (Ziprasidone may induce orthostatic hypotension; co-administration with certain antihypertensive drugs may enhance the hypotensive effects). Products include:
Brevibloc Concentrate 766
Brevibloc Injection 766
Brevibloc Double Strength Injection 766
Brevibloc Premixed Injection 766
Brevibloc Double Strength Premixed Injection 766

Estazolam (Somnolence was a commonly reported adverse event in patients treated with ziprasidone; concurrent use with other CNS active drugs, such as depressants, should be undertaken with caution). Products include:
ProSom Tablets 512

Ethacrynic Acid (Ziprasidone produces dose-related prolongation of the QT interval; hypokalemia may result from diuretic therapy and this may increase the risk of QT prolongation and arrhythmias; potential for enhanced hypotensive effect if used concurrently). Products include:
Edecrin Tablets 1941

Ethanol (Somnolence was a commonly reported adverse event in patients treated with ziprasidone; concurrent use with other CNS active drugs, such as depressants, should be undertaken with caution).
No products indexed under this heading.

Ethchlorvynol (Somnolence was a commonly reported adverse event in patients treated with ziprasidone; concurrent use with other CNS active drugs, such as depressants, should be undertaken with caution).
No products indexed under this heading.

Ethinamate (Somnolence was a commonly reported adverse event in patients treated with ziprasidone; concurrent use with other CNS active drugs, such as depressants, should be undertaken with caution).
No products indexed under this heading.

Ethyl Alcohol (Somnolence was a commonly reported adverse event in patients treated with ziprasidone; concurrent use with other CNS active drugs, such as depressants, should be undertaken with caution).
No products indexed under this heading.

Felodipine (Ziprasidone may induce orthostatic hypotension; co-administration with certain antihypertensive drugs may enhance the hypotensive effects). Products include:
Plendil Extended-Release Tablets 651

Fentanyl (Somnolence was a commonly reported adverse event in patients treated with ziprasidone; concurrent use with other CNS active drugs, such as depressants, should be undertaken with caution). Products include:
Duragesic Transdermal System 2448

Fentanyl Citrate (Somnolence was a commonly reported adverse event in patients treated with ziprasidone; concurrent use with other CNS active drugs, such as depressants, should be undertaken with caution). Products include:
Actiq 993

Flecainide Acetate (Ziprasidone produces dose-related prolongation of the QT interval; an additive effect of ziprasidone and other drugs that prolong cannot be excluded; concurrent use is not recommended). Products include:
Tambocor Tablets 1824

Fluphenazine Decanoate (Somnolence was a commonly reported adverse event in patients treated with ziprasidone; concurrent use with other CNS active drugs, such as depressants, should be undertaken with caution).
No products indexed under this heading.

Fluphenazine Enanthate (Somnolence was a commonly reported adverse event in patients treated with ziprasidone; concurrent use with other CNS active drugs, such as depressants, should be undertaken with caution).
No products indexed under this heading.

Fluphenazine Hydrochloride (Somnolence was a commonly reported adverse event in patients treated with ziprasidone; concurrent use with other CNS active drugs, such as depressants, should be undertaken with caution).
No products indexed under this heading.

Flurazepam Hydrochloride (Somnolence was a commonly reported adverse event in patients treated with ziprasidone; concurrent use with other CNS active drugs, such as depressants, should be undertaken with caution). Products include:
Dalmane Capsules 3343

Fosinopril Sodium (Ziprasidone may induce orthostatic hypotension; co-administration with certain antihypertensive drugs may enhance the hypotensive effects).
No products indexed under this heading.

Furosemide (Ziprasidone produces dose-related prolongation of the QT interval; hypokalemia may result from diuretic therapy and this may increase the risk of QT prolongation and arrhythmias; potential for enhanced hypotensive effect if used concurrently). Products include:
Furosemide Tablets 2117

Gatifloxacin (Ziprasidone produces dose-related prolongation of the QT interval; an additive effect of ziprasidone and other drugs that prolong cannot be excluded; concurrent use is not recommended). Products include:
Tequin Injection 964
Tequin Tablets 964
Zymar Ophthalmic Solution 571

Glutethimide (Somnolence was a commonly reported adverse event in patients treated with ziprasidone; concurrent use with other CNS active drugs, such as depressants, should be undertaken with caution).
No products indexed under this heading.

Guanabenz Acetate (Ziprasidone may induce orthostatic hypotension; co-administration with certain antihypertensive drugs may enhance the hypotensive effects).
No products indexed under this heading.

Guanethidine Monosulfate (Ziprasidone may induce orthostatic hypotension; co-administration with certain antihypertensive drugs may enhance the hypotensive effects).
No products indexed under this heading.

Halofantrine (Ziprasidone produces dose-related prolongation of the QT interval; an additive effect of ziprasidone and other drugs that prolong cannot be excluded; concurrent use is not recommended).
No products indexed under this heading.

Haloperidol (Somnolence was a commonly reported adverse event in patients treated with ziprasidone; concurrent use with other CNS active drugs, such as depressants, should be undertaken with caution).
No products indexed under this heading.

Haloperidol Decanoate (Somnolence was a commonly reported adverse event in patients treated with ziprasidone; concurrent use with other CNS active drugs, such as depressants, should be undertaken with caution).
No products indexed under this heading.

Hydralazine Hydrochloride (Ziprasidone may induce orthostatic hypotension; co-administration with certain antihypertensive drugs may enhance the hypotensive effects). Products include:
BiDil Tablets 2161

Hydrochlorothiazide (Ziprasidone produces dose-related prolongation of the QT interval; hypokalemia may result from diuretic therapy and this may increase the risk of QT prolongation and arrhythmias; potential for enhanced hypotensive effect if used concurrently). Products include:
Aldoril Tablets 1884
Atacand HCT 637
Avalide Tablets 2889
Avalide Tablets 922
Benicar HCT Tablets 2852
Diovan HCT Tablets 2195
Dyazide Capsules 1389
Hyzaar 1964
Lotensin HCT Tablets 2235
Maxzide 2150
Micardis HCT Tablets 886
Moduretic Tablets 2003
Prinzide Tablets 2033
Teveten HCT Tablets 1710
Timolide Tablets 2056
Uniretic Tablets 3114
Vaseretic Tablets 2073
Zestoretic Tablets 701

Hydrocodone Bitartrate (Somnolence was a commonly reported adverse event in patients treated with ziprasidone; concurrent use with other CNS active drugs, such as depressants, should be undertaken with caution). Products include:
Hycodan 1104
Hycomine Compound Tablets 1105
Hycotuss Expectorant Syrup 1106
Lortab 3315
Lortab Elixir 3312
Vicodin Tablets 530
Vicodin ES Tablets 531
Vicodin HP Tablets 532
Vicoprofen Tablets 533
Zydone Tablets 1118

Hydrocodone Polistirex (Somnolence was a commonly reported adverse event in patients treated with ziprasidone; concurrent use with other CNS active drugs, such as depressants, should be undertaken with caution). Products include:
Tussionex Pennkinetic Extended-Release Suspension 3322

Hydroflumethiazide (Ziprasidone produces dose-related prolongation of the QT interval; hypokalemia may result from diuretic therapy and this may increase the risk of QT prolongation and arrhythmias; potential for enhanced hypotensive effect if used concurrently).
No products indexed under this heading.

Hydromorphone Hydrochloride (Somnolence was a commonly reported adverse event in patients treated with ziprasidone; concurrent use with other CNS active drugs, such as depressants, should be undertaken with caution). Products include:
Dilaudid 439
Dilaudid Oral Liquid 443
Dilaudid Non-Sterile Powder 439
Dilaudid Rectal Suppositories 439
Dilaudid Tablets 439
Dilaudid Tablets - 8 mg 443
Dilaudid-HP 441

Hydroxyzine Hydrochloride (Somnolence was a commonly reported adverse event in patients treated with ziprasidone; concurrent use with other CNS active drugs, such as depressants, should be undertaken with caution).
No products indexed under this heading.

Ibutilide Fumarate (Ziprasidone produces dose-related prolongation of the QT interval; an additive effect of ziprasidone and other drugs that prolong cannot be excluded; concurrent use is not recommended).
No products indexed under this heading.

Indapamide (Ziprasidone may induce orthostatic hypotension; co-administration with certain antihypertensive drugs may enhance the hypotensive effects). Products include:
Indapamide Tablets 2119

Irbesartan (Ziprasidone may induce orthostatic hypotension; co-administration with certain antihypertensive drugs may enhance the hypotensive effects). Products include:

Avalide Tablets ... 922
Avalide Tablets ... 2889
Avapro Tablets ... 925
Avapro Tablets ... 2886

Isoflurane (Somnolence was a commonly reported adverse event in patients treated with ziprasidone; concurrent use with other CNS active drugs, such as depressants, should be undertaken with caution).
No products indexed under this heading.

Isradipine (Ziprasidone may induce orthostatic hypotension; co-administration with certain antihypertensive drugs may enhance the hypotensive effects). Products include:
DynaCirc CR Tablets ... 2726

Itraconazole (Co-administration with inhibitors of CYP3A4, such as itraconazole, may result in increased AUC and Cmax of ziprasidone).
No products indexed under this heading.

Ketamine Hydrochloride (Somnolence was a commonly reported adverse event in patients treated with ziprasidone; concurrent use with other CNS active drugs, such as depressants, should be undertaken with caution).
No products indexed under this heading.

Ketoconazole (Co-administration with ketoconazole, a potent inhibitor of CYP3A4, has resulted in increased AUC and Cmax of ziprasidone by about 35-40%). Products include:
Nizoral A-D Shampoo, 1% ... 1839
Nizoral 2% Shampoo ... 1838

Labetalol Hydrochloride (Ziprasidone may induce orthostatic hypotension; co-administration with certain antihypertensive drugs may enhance the hypotensive effects).
No products indexed under this heading.

Levodopa (Ziprasidone may antagonize the effects of levodopa). Products include:
Parcopa Orally Disintegrating Tablets ... 3111
Stalevo Tablets ... 2270

Levomethadyl Acetate Hydrochloride (Ziprasidone produces dose-related prolongation of the QT interval; an additive effect of ziprasidone and other drugs that prolong cannot be excluded; concurrent use is not recommended).
No products indexed under this heading.

Levorphanol Tartrate (Somnolence was a commonly reported adverse event in patients treated with ziprasidone; concurrent use with other CNS active drugs, such as depressants, should be undertaken with caution).
No products indexed under this heading.

Lisinopril (Ziprasidone may induce orthostatic hypotension; co-administration with certain antihypertensive drugs may enhance the hypotensive effects). Products include:
Prinivil Tablets ... 2029
Prinzide Tablets ... 2033
Zestoretic Tablets ... 701
Zestril Tablets ... 704

Lorazepam (Somnolence was a commonly reported adverse event in patients treated with ziprasidone; concurrent use with other CNS active drugs, such as depressants, should be undertaken with caution).
No products indexed under this heading.

Losartan Potassium (Ziprasidone may induce orthostatic hypotension; co-administration with certain antihypertensive drugs may enhance the hypotensive effects). Products include:
Cozaar Tablets ... 1913
Hyzaar ... 1964

Loxapine Hydrochloride (Somnolence was a commonly reported adverse event in patients treated with ziprasidone; concurrent use with other CNS active drugs, such as depressants, should be undertaken with caution).
No products indexed under this heading.

Loxapine Succinate (Somnolence was a commonly reported adverse event in patients treated with ziprasidone; concurrent use with other CNS active drugs, such as depressants, should be undertaken with caution).
No products indexed under this heading.

Mecamylamine Hydrochloride (Ziprasidone may induce orthostatic hypotension; co-administration with certain antihypertensive drugs may enhance the hypotensive effects). Products include:
Inversine Tablets ... 3286

Mefloquine Hydrochloride (Ziprasidone produces dose-related prolongation of the QT interval; an additive effect of ziprasidone and other drugs that prolong cannot be excluded; concurrent use is not recommended). Products include:
Lariam Tablets ... 2790

Meperidine Hydrochloride (Somnolence was a commonly reported adverse event in patients treated with ziprasidone; concurrent use with other CNS active drugs, such as depressants, should be undertaken with caution).
No products indexed under this heading.

Mephobarbital (Somnolence was a commonly reported adverse event in patients treated with ziprasidone; concurrent use with other CNS active drugs, such as depressants, should be undertaken with caution). Products include:
Mebaral Tablets, USP ... 2483

Meprobamate (Somnolence was a commonly reported adverse event in patients treated with ziprasidone; concurrent use with other CNS active drugs, such as depressants, should be undertaken with caution).
No products indexed under this heading.

Mesoridazine Besylate (Ziprasidone produces dose-related prolongation of the QT interval; an additive effect of ziprasidone and other drugs that prolong cannot be excluded; concurrent use is not recommended).
No products indexed under this heading.

Methadone Hydrochloride (Somnolence was a commonly reported adverse event in patients treated with ziprasidone; concurrent use with other CNS active drugs, such as depressants, should be undertaken with caution).
No products indexed under this heading.

Methohexital Sodium (Somnolence was a commonly reported adverse event in patients treated with ziprasidone; concurrent use with other CNS active drugs, such as depressants, should be undertaken with caution).
No products indexed under this heading.

Methotrimeprazine (Somnolence was a commonly reported adverse event in patients treated with ziprasidone; concurrent use with other CNS active drugs, such as depressants, should be undertaken with caution).
No products indexed under this heading.

Methoxyflurane (Somnolence was a commonly reported adverse event in patients treated with ziprasidone; concurrent use with other CNS active drugs, such as depressants, should be undertaken with caution).
No products indexed under this heading.

Methyclothiazide (Ziprasidone produces dose-related prolongation of the QT interval; hypokalemia may result from diuretic therapy and this may increase the risk of QT prolongation and arrhythmias; potential for enhanced hypotensive effect if used concurrently).
No products indexed under this heading.

Methyldopa (Ziprasidone may induce orthostatic hypotension; co-administration with certain antihypertensive drugs may enhance the hypotensive effects). Products include:
Aldoclor Tablets ... 1881
Aldoril Tablets ... 1884

Methyldopate Hydrochloride (Ziprasidone may induce orthostatic hypotension; co-administration with certain antihypertensive drugs may enhance the hypotensive effects).
No products indexed under this heading.

Metolazone (Ziprasidone may induce orthostatic hypotension; co-administration with certain antihypertensive drugs may enhance the hypotensive effects).
No products indexed under this heading.

Metoprolol Succinate (Ziprasidone may induce orthostatic hypotension; co-administration with certain antihypertensive drugs may enhance the hypotensive effects). Products include:
Toprol-XL Tablets ... 660

Metoprolol Tartrate (Ziprasidone may induce orthostatic hypotension; co-administration with certain antihypertensive drugs may enhance the hypotensive effects).
No products indexed under this heading.

Metyrosine (Ziprasidone may induce orthostatic hypotension; co-administration with certain antihypertensive drugs may enhance the hypotensive effects). Products include:
Demser Capsules ... 1933

Mibefradil Dihydrochloride (Ziprasidone may induce orthostatic hypotension; co-administration with certain antihypertensive drugs may enhance the hypotensive effects).
No products indexed under this heading.

Midazolam Hydrochloride (Somnolence was a commonly reported adverse event in patients treated with ziprasidone; concurrent use with other CNS active drugs, such as depressants, should be undertaken with caution).
No products indexed under this heading.

Minoxidil (Ziprasidone may induce orthostatic hypotension; co-administration with certain antihypertensive drugs may enhance the hypotensive effects). Products include:
Men's Rogaine Extra Strength Topical Solution, Ocean Rush Scent and Original Unscented ... ▣ 706
Women's Rogaine Topical Solution, Spring Bloom Scent and Original Unscented ... ▣ 707

Moexipril Hydrochloride (Ziprasidone may induce orthostatic hypotension; co-administration with certain antihypertensive drugs may enhance the hypotensive effects). Products include:
Uniretic Tablets ... 3114
Univasc Tablets ... 3118

Molindone Hydrochloride (Somnolence was a commonly reported adverse event in patients treated with ziprasidone; concurrent use with other CNS active drugs, such as depressants, should be undertaken with caution). Products include:
Moban Tablets ... 1108

Morphine Sulfate (Somnolence was a commonly reported adverse event in patients treated with ziprasidone; concurrent use with other CNS active drugs, such as depressants, should be undertaken with caution). Products include:
Avinza Capsules ... 1714
Kadian Capsules ... 572
MS Contin Tablets ... 2703

Moxifloxacin Hydrochloride (Ziprasidone produces dose-related prolongation of the QT interval; an additive effect of ziprasidone and other drugs that prolong cannot be excluded; concurrent use is not recommended). Products include:
Avelox ... 2984
Vigamox Ophthalmic Solution ... ⊙ 560

Nadolol (Ziprasidone may induce orthostatic hypotension; co-administration with certain antihypertensive drugs may enhance the hypotensive effects). Products include:
Nadolol Tablets ... 2121

Nicardipine Hydrochloride (Ziprasidone may induce orthostatic hypotension; co-administration with certain antihypertensive drugs may enhance the hypotensive effects). Products include:
Cardene I.V. ... 1129

Nifedipine (Ziprasidone may induce orthostatic hypotension; co-administration with certain antihypertensive drugs may enhance the hypotensive effects). Products include:
Adalat CC Tablets ... 2978

Nisoldipine (Ziprasidone may induce orthostatic hypotension; co-administration with certain antihypertensive-

tensive drugs may enhance the hypotensive effects). Products include:
Sular Tablets 1163

Nitroglycerin (Ziprasidone may induce orthostatic hypotension; co-administration with certain antihypertensive drugs may enhance the hypotensive effects). Products include:
Nitro-Dur Transdermal Infusion System.. 3060
Nitrolingual Pumpspray 1161

Olanzapine (Somnolence was a commonly reported adverse event in patients treated with ziprasidone; concurrent use with other CNS active drugs, such as depressants, should be undertaken with caution). Products include:
Symbyax Capsules 1788
Zyprexa Tablets 1798
Zyprexa IntraMuscular 1798
Zyprexa ZYDIS Orally Disintegrating Tablets.................. 1798

Oxazepam (Somnolence was a commonly reported adverse event in patients treated with ziprasidone; concurrent use with other CNS active drugs, such as depressants, should be undertaken with caution).
No products indexed under this heading.

Oxycodone Hydrochloride (Somnolence was a commonly reported adverse event in patients treated with ziprasidone; concurrent use with other CNS active drugs, such as depressants, should be undertaken with caution). Products include:
Combunox Tablets 1183
OxyContin Tablets 2699
OxyFast Oral Concentrate Solution.. 2704
OxyIR Capsules 2704
Percocet Tablets 1114
Percodan Tablets 1115

Penbutolol Sulfate (Ziprasidone may induce orthostatic hypotension; co-administration with certain antihypertensive drugs may enhance the hypotensive effects).
No products indexed under this heading.

Pentamidine Isethionate (Ziprasidone produces dose-related prolongation of the QT interval; an additive effect of ziprasidone and other drugs that prolong cannot be excluded; concurrent use is not recommended).
No products indexed under this heading.

Pentobarbital Sodium (Somnolence was a commonly reported adverse event in patients treated with ziprasidone; concurrent use with other CNS active drugs, such as depressants, should be undertaken with caution). Products include:
Nembutal Sodium Solution, USP 2484

Pergolide Mesylate (Ziprasidone may antagonize the effects of dopamine agonists). Products include:
Permax Tablets 3357

Perindopril Erbumine (Ziprasidone may induce orthostatic hypotension; co-administration with certain antihypertensive drugs may enhance the hypotensive effects). Products include:
Aceon Tablets (2 mg, 4 mg, 8 mg).. 3191

Perphenazine (Somnolence was a commonly reported adverse event in patients treated with ziprasidone; concurrent use with other CNS active drugs, such as depressants, should be undertaken with caution).
No products indexed under this heading.

Phenobarbital (Somnolence was a commonly reported adverse event in patients treated with ziprasidone; concurrent use with other CNS active drugs, such as depressants, should be undertaken with caution).
No products indexed under this heading.

Phenoxybenzamine Hydrochloride (Ziprasidone may induce orthostatic hypotension; co-administration with certain antihypertensive drugs may enhance the hypotensive effects). Products include:
Dibenzyline Capsules 3390

Phentolamine Mesylate (Ziprasidone may induce orthostatic hypotension; co-administration with certain antihypertensive drugs may enhance the hypotensive effects).
No products indexed under this heading.

Pimozide (Ziprasidone produces dose-related prolongation of the QT interval; an additive effect of ziprasidone and other drugs that prolong cannot be excluded; concurrent use is not recommended). Products include:
Orap Tablets 1220

Pindolol (Ziprasidone may induce orthostatic hypotension; co-administration with certain antihypertensive drugs may enhance the hypotensive effects).
No products indexed under this heading.

Polythiazide (Ziprasidone produces dose-related prolongation of the QT interval; hypokalemia may result from diuretic therapy and this may increase the risk of QT prolongation and arrhythmias; potential for enhanced hypotensive effect if used concurrently).
No products indexed under this heading.

Pramipexole Dihydrochloride (Ziprasidone may antagonize the effects of dopamine agonists). Products include:
Mirapex Tablets 889

Prazepam (Somnolence was a commonly reported adverse event in patients treated with ziprasidone; concurrent use with other CNS active drugs, such as depressants, should be undertaken with caution).
No products indexed under this heading.

Prazosin Hydrochloride (Ziprasidone may induce orthostatic hypotension; co-administration with certain antihypertensive drugs may enhance the hypotensive effects).
No products indexed under this heading.

Probucol (Ziprasidone produces dose-related prolongation of the QT interval; an additive effect of ziprasidone and other drugs that prolong cannot be excluded; concurrent use is not recommended).
No products indexed under this heading.

Procainamide Hydrochloride (Ziprasidone produces dose-related prolongation of the QT interval; an additive effect of ziprasidone and other drugs that prolong cannot be excluded; concurrent use is not recommended).
No products indexed under this heading.

Prochlorperazine (Somnolence was a commonly reported adverse event in patients treated with ziprasidone; concurrent use with other CNS active drugs, such as depressants, should be undertaken with caution).
No products indexed under this heading.

Promethazine Hydrochloride (Somnolence was a commonly reported adverse event in patients treated with ziprasidone; concurrent use with other CNS active drugs, such as depressants, should be undertaken with caution). Products include:
Phenergan 3438

Propofol (Somnolence was a commonly reported adverse event in patients treated with ziprasidone; concurrent use with other CNS active drugs, such as depressants, should be undertaken with caution). Products include:
Diprivan Injectable Emulsion 676

Propoxyphene Hydrochloride (Somnolence was a commonly reported adverse event in patients treated with ziprasidone; concurrent use with other CNS active drugs, such as depressants, should be undertaken with caution).
No products indexed under this heading.

Propoxyphene Napsylate (Somnolence was a commonly reported adverse event in patients treated with ziprasidone; concurrent use with other CNS active drugs, such as depressants, should be undertaken with caution). Products include:
Darvocet A 500 Tablets 3497

Propranolol Hydrochloride (Ziprasidone may induce orthostatic hypotension; co-administration with certain antihypertensive drugs may enhance the hypotensive effects). Products include:
Inderal LA Long-Acting Capsules 3421
InnoPran XL Capsules 2728

Quazepam (Somnolence was a commonly reported adverse event in patients treated with ziprasidone; concurrent use with other CNS active drugs, such as depressants, should be undertaken with caution).
No products indexed under this heading.

Quetiapine Fumarate (Somnolence was a commonly reported adverse event in patients treated with ziprasidone; concurrent use with other CNS active drugs, such as depressants, should be undertaken with caution). Products include:
Seroquel Tablets 691

Quinapril Hydrochloride (Ziprasidone may induce orthostatic hypotension; co-administration with certain antihypertensive drugs may enhance the hypotensive effects).
No products indexed under this heading.

Quinidine (Ziprasidone produces dose-related prolongation of the QT interval; an additive effect of ziprasidone and other drugs that prolong cannot be excluded; concurrent use is not recommended).
No products indexed under this heading.

Quinidine Gluconate (Ziprasidone produces dose-related prolongation of the QT interval; an additive effect of ziprasidone and other drugs that prolong cannot be excluded; concurrent use is not recommended).
No products indexed under this heading.

Quinidine Hydrochloride (Ziprasidone produces dose-related prolongation of the QT interval; an additive effect of ziprasidone and other drugs that prolong cannot be excluded; concurrent use is not recommended).
No products indexed under this heading.

Quinidine Polygalacturonate (Ziprasidone produces dose-related prolongation of the QT interval; an additive effect of ziprasidone and other drugs that prolong cannot be excluded; concurrent use is not recommended).
No products indexed under this heading.

Quinidine Sulfate (Ziprasidone produces dose-related prolongation of the QT interval; an additive effect of ziprasidone and other drugs that prolong cannot be excluded; concurrent use is not recommended).
No products indexed under this heading.

Ramipril (Ziprasidone may induce orthostatic hypotension; co-administration with certain antihypertensive drugs may enhance the hypotensive effects). Products include:
Altace Capsules 1673

Rauwolfia Serpentina (Ziprasidone may induce orthostatic hypotension; co-administration with certain antihypertensive drugs may enhance the hypotensive effects).
No products indexed under this heading.

Remifentanil Hydrochloride (Somnolence was a commonly reported adverse event in patients treated with ziprasidone; concurrent use with other CNS active drugs, such as depressants, should be undertaken with caution).
No products indexed under this heading.

Rescinnamine (Ziprasidone may induce orthostatic hypotension; co-administration with certain antihypertensive drugs may enhance the hypotensive effects).
No products indexed under this heading.

Reserpine (Ziprasidone may induce orthostatic hypotension; co-administration with certain antihypertensive drugs may enhance the hypotensive effects).
No products indexed under this heading.

Risperidone (Somnolence was a commonly reported adverse event in patients treated with ziprasidone; concurrent use with other CNS active drugs, such as depressants, should be undertaken with caution). Products include:

Risperdal Consta Long-Acting Injection 1664
Risperdal M-Tab Orally Disintegrating Tablets 1658
Risperdal 1658

Ropinirole Hydrochloride (Ziprasidone may antagonize the effects of dopamine agonists). Products include:
Requip Tablets 1528

Secobarbital Sodium (Somnolence was a commonly reported adverse event in patients treated with ziprasidone; concurrent use with other CNS active drugs, such as depressants, should be undertaken with caution).
No products indexed under this heading.

Sevoflurane (Somnolence was a commonly reported adverse event in patients treated with ziprasidone; concurrent use with other CNS active drugs, such as depressants, should be undertaken with caution). Products include:
Ultane Liquid for Inhalation 526

Sodium Nitroprusside (Ziprasidone may induce orthostatic hypotension; co-administration with certain antihypertensive drugs may enhance the hypotensive effects).
No products indexed under this heading.

Sodium Oxybate (Somnolence was a commonly reported adverse event in patients treated with ziprasidone; concurrent use with other CNS active drugs, such as depressants, should be undertaken with caution).
No products indexed under this heading.

Sotalol Hydrochloride (Ziprasidone produces dose-related prolongation of the QT interval; an additive effect of ziprasidone and other drugs that prolong cannot be excluded; concurrent use is not recommended).
No products indexed under this heading.

Sparfloxacin (Ziprasidone produces dose-related prolongation of the QT interval; an additive effect of ziprasidone and other drugs that prolong cannot be excluded; concurrent use is not recommended).
No products indexed under this heading.

Spirapril Hydrochloride (Ziprasidone may induce orthostatic hypotension; co-administration with certain antihypertensive drugs may enhance the hypotensive effects).
No products indexed under this heading.

Sufentanil Citrate (Somnolence was a commonly reported adverse event in patients treated with ziprasidone; concurrent use with other CNS active drugs, such as depressants, should be undertaken with caution).
No products indexed under this heading.

Tacrolimus (Ziprasidone produces dose-related prolongation of the QT interval; an additive effect of ziprasidone and other drugs that prolong cannot be excluded; concurrent use is not recommended). Products include:
Prograf Capsules and Injection 624
Protopic Ointment 629

Telmisartan (Ziprasidone may induce orthostatic hypotension; co-administration with certain antihypertensive drugs may enhance the hypotensive effects). Products include:
Micardis Tablets 884
Micardis HCT Tablets 886

Temazepam (Somnolence was a commonly reported adverse event in patients treated with ziprasidone; concurrent use with other CNS active drugs, such as depressants, should be undertaken with caution).
No products indexed under this heading.

Terazosin Hydrochloride (Ziprasidone may induce orthostatic hypotension; co-administration with certain antihypertensive drugs may enhance the hypotensive effects). Products include:
Hytrin Capsules 469

Thiamylal Sodium (Somnolence was a commonly reported adverse event in patients treated with ziprasidone; concurrent use with other CNS active drugs, such as depressants, should be undertaken with caution).
No products indexed under this heading.

Thioridazine Hydrochloride (Ziprasidone produces dose-related prolongation of the QT interval; an additive effect of ziprasidone and other drugs that prolong cannot be excluded; concurrent use is not recommended). Products include:
Thioridazine Hydrochloride Tablets 2122

Thiothixene (Somnolence was a commonly reported adverse event in patients treated with ziprasidone; concurrent use with other CNS active drugs, such as depressants, should be undertaken with caution). Products include:
Thiothixene Capsules 2124

Timolol Maleate (Ziprasidone may induce orthostatic hypotension; co-administration with certain antihypertensive drugs may enhance the hypotensive effects). Products include:
Blocadren Tablets 1891
Cosopt Sterile Ophthalmic Solution 1910
Timolide Tablets 2056
Timoptic in Ocudose 2061
Timoptic Sterile Ophthalmic Solution 2058
Timoptic-XE Sterile Ophthalmic Gel Forming Solution 2062

Torsemide (Ziprasidone produces dose-related prolongation of the QT interval; hypokalemia may result from diuretic therapy and this may increase the risk of QT prolongation and arrhythmias; potential for enhanced hypotensive effect if used concurrently).
No products indexed under this heading.

Trandolapril (Ziprasidone may induce orthostatic hypotension; co-administration with certain antihypertensive drugs may enhance the hypotensive effects). Products include:
Mavik Tablets 482
Tarka Tablets 519

Triazolam (Somnolence was a commonly reported adverse event in patients treated with ziprasidone; concurrent use with other CNS active drugs, such as depressants, should be undertaken with caution).
No products indexed under this heading.

Trifluoperazine Hydrochloride (Somnolence was a commonly reported adverse event in patients treated with ziprasidone; concurrent use with other CNS active drugs, such as depressants, should be undertaken with caution).
No products indexed under this heading.

Trimethaphan Camsylate (Ziprasidone may induce orthostatic hypotension; co-administration with certain antihypertensive drugs may enhance the hypotensive effects).
No products indexed under this heading.

Valsartan (Ziprasidone may induce orthostatic hypotension; co-administration with certain antihypertensive drugs may enhance the hypotensive effects). Products include:
Diovan HCT Tablets 2195
Diovan Tablets 2191

Verapamil Hydrochloride (Ziprasidone may induce orthostatic hypotension; co-administration with certain antihypertensive drugs may enhance the hypotensive effects). Products include:
Covera-HS Tablets 3135
Tarka Tablets 519
Verelan PM Capsules 3120

Zaleplon (Somnolence was a commonly reported adverse event in patients treated with ziprasidone; concurrent use with other CNS active drugs, such as depressants, should be undertaken with caution). Products include:
Sonata Capsules 1686

Zolpidem Tartrate (Somnolence was a commonly reported adverse event in patients treated with ziprasidone; concurrent use with other CNS active drugs, such as depressants, should be undertaken with caution). Products include:
Ambien Tablets 2867

Food Interactions

Alcohol (Somnolence was a commonly reported adverse event in patients treated with ziprasidone; concurrent use with alcohol or other CNS active drugs, such as depressants, should be undertaken with caution).

GEODON FOR INJECTION

(Ziprasidone Mesylate) 2514
See Geodon Capsules

GLEEVEC TABLETS

(Imatinib Mesylate) 2221
May interact with calcium channel blockers that are metabolized by CYP3A4, cytochrome p450 2c9 substrates (selected), cytochrome p450 2d6 substrates (selected), cytochrome p450 3a4 inducers (selected), cytochrome p450 3a4 inhibitors (selected), dexamethasone, erythromycin, phenytoin, triazolobenzodiazepines, and certain other agents. Compounds in these categories include:

Acarbose (Imatinib is a potent competitive inhibitor of CYP2C9; therefore, imatinib is likely to increase the blood levels of drugs that are substrates of this enzyme). Products include:
Precose Tablets 776

Acetazolamide (Caution is recommended when administering Gleevec with inhibitors of the CYP3A4 family. Substances that inhibit CYP3A4 activity may decrease metabolism and increase imatinib concentrations. There is a significant increase in exposure to imatinib when Gleevec is co-administered with ketoconazole).
No products indexed under this heading.

Allium sativum (Substances that are inducers of CYP3A4 activity may increase metabolism and decrease imatinib plasma concentrations. Co-medications that induce CYP3A4 may significantly reduce exposure to Gleevec. Dosage of imatinib should be increased by at least 50% and clinical response should be carefully monitored in patients receiving imatinib with potent CYP3A4 inducers).
No products indexed under this heading.

Alprazolam (Imatinib will increase the plasma concentrations of triazolobenzodiazepines by inhibiting CYP3A4). Products include:
Niravam Orally Disintegrating Tablets 3106
Xanax XR Tablets 2655

Amiodarone Hydrochloride (Caution is recommended when administering Gleevec with inhibitors of the CYP3A4 family. Substances that inhibit CYP3A4 activity may decrease metabolism and increase imatinib concentrations. There is a significant increase in exposure to imatinib when Gleevec is co-administered with ketoconazole). Products include:
Pacerone Tablets 3337

Amitriptyline Hydrochloride (Imatinib is a potent competitive inhibitor of CYP2D6; therefore, imatinib is likely to increase the blood levels of drugs that are substrates of this enzyme).
No products indexed under this heading.

Amlodipine Besylate (Imatinib will increase plasma concentration of CYP3A4 metabolized drugs. (e.g., dihydropyridine calcium channel blockers)). Products include:
Caduet Tablets 2507
Lotrel Capsules 2238
Norvasc Tablets 2529

Amphetamine Aspartate (Imatinib is a potent competitive inhibitor of CYP2D6; therefore, imatinib is likely to increase the blood levels of drugs that are substrates of this enzyme). Products include:
Adderall Tablets 3168
Adderall XR Capsules 3169

Amphetamine Aspartate Monohydrate (Imatinib is a potent competitive inhibitor of CYP2D6; therefore, imatinib is likely to increase the blood levels of drugs that are substrates of this enzyme).
No products indexed under this heading.

Amphetamine Sulfate (Imatinib is a potent competitive inhibitor of CYP2D6; therefore, imatinib is likely to increase the blood levels of drugs that are substrates of this enzyme). Products include:
Adderall Tablets 3168
Adderall XR Capsules 3169

Amprenavir (Caution is recommended when administering Gleevec with inhibitors of the CYP3A4 family.

Substances that inhibit CYP3A4 activity may decrease metabolism and increase imatinib concentrations. There is a significant increase in exposure to imatinib when Gleevec is co-administered with ketoconazole). Products include:

Agenerase Capsules 1299
Agenerase Oral Solution 1304

Anastrozole (Caution is recommended when administering Gleevec with inhibitors of the CYP3A4 family. Substances that inhibit CYP3A4 activity may decrease metabolism and increase imatinib concentrations. There is a significant increase in exposure to imatinib when Gleevec is co-administered with ketoconazole). Products include:

Arimidex Tablets 665

Aprepitant (Caution is recommended when administering Gleevec with inhibitors of the CYP3A4 family. Substances that inhibit CYP3A4 activity may decrease metabolism and increase imatinib concentrations. There is a significant increase in exposure to imatinib when Gleevec is co-administered with ketoconazole). Products include:

Emend Capsules 1944

Atomoxetine Hydrochloride (Imatinib is a potent competitive inhibitor of CYP2D6; therefore, imatinib is likely to increase the blood levels of drugs that are substrates of this enzyme). Products include:

Strattera Capsules 1784

Atorvastatin Calcium (Imatinib will increase the plasma concentrations of certain HMG-CoA reductase inhibitors by inhibiting CYP3A4). Products include:

Caduet Tablets 2507
Lipitor Tablets 2495

Betamethasone Acetate (Substances that are inducers of CYP3A4 activity may increase metabolism and decrease imatinib plasma concentrations. Co-medications that induce CYP3A4 may significantly reduce exposure to Gleevec. Dosage of imatinib should be increased by at least 50% and clinical response should be carefully monitored in patients receiving imatinib with potent CYP3A4 inducers).

No products indexed under this heading.

Betamethasone Sodium Phosphate (Substances that are inducers of CYP3A4 activity may increase metabolism and decrease imatinib plasma concentrations. Co-medications that induce CYP3A4 may significantly reduce exposure to Gleevec. Dosage of imatinib should be increased by at least 50% and clinical response should be carefully monitored in patients receiving imatinib with potent CYP3A4 inducers).

No products indexed under this heading.

Bisoprolol Fumarate (Imatinib is a potent competitive inhibitor of CYP2D6; therefore, imatinib is likely to increase the blood levels of drugs that are substrates of this enzyme).

No products indexed under this heading.

Candesartan Cilexetil (Imatinib is a potent competitive inhibitor of CYP2C9; therefore, imatinib is likely to increase the blood levels of drugs that are substrates of this enzyme). Products include:

Atacand Tablets 634
Atacand HCT 637

Captopril (Imatinib is a potent competitive inhibitor of CYP2D6; therefore, imatinib is likely to increase the blood levels of drugs that are substrates of this enzyme). Products include:

Captopril Tablets 2114

Carbamazepine (Co-administration with inducers of CYP3A4, such as carbamazepine, may increase the metabolism and decrease imatinib concentrations). Products include:

Carbatrol Capsules 3174
Equetro Extended-Release Capsules 3178
Tegretol/Tegretol-XR 2278

Carvedilol (Imatinib is a potent competitive inhibitor of CYP2D6; therefore, imatinib is likely to increase the blood levels of drugs that are substrates of this enzyme). Products include:

Coreg Tablets 1376

Celecoxib (Imatinib is a potent competitive inhibitor of CYP2C9; therefore, imatinib is likely to increase the blood levels of drugs that are substrates of this enzyme). Products include:

Celebrex Capsules 3130

Cerivastatin Sodium (Imatinib will increase the plasma concentrations of certain HMG-CoA reductase inhibitors by inhibiting CYP3A4).

No products indexed under this heading.

Cevimeline Hydrochloride (Imatinib is a potent competitive inhibitor of CYP2D6; therefore, imatinib is likely to increase the blood levels of drugs that are substrates of this enzyme). Products include:

Evoxac Capsules 1042

Chlorpromazine (Imatinib is a potent competitive inhibitor of CYP2D6; therefore, imatinib is likely to increase the blood levels of drugs that are substrates of this enzyme).

No products indexed under this heading.

Chlorpromazine Hydrochloride (Imatinib is a potent competitive inhibitor of CYP2D6; therefore, imatinib is likely to increase the blood levels of drugs that are substrates of this enzyme).

No products indexed under this heading.

Chlorpropamide (Imatinib is a potent competitive inhibitor of CYP2D6; therefore, imatinib is likely to increase the blood levels of drugs that are substrates of this enzyme).

No products indexed under this heading.

Cimetidine (Caution is recommended when administering Gleevec with inhibitors of the CYP3A4 family. Substances that inhibit CYP3A4 activity may decrease metabolism and increase imatinib concentrations. There is a significant increase in exposure to imatinib when Gleevec is co-administered with ketoconazole). Products include:

Tagamet HB 200 Tablets 637
Tagamet Tablets 1547

Cimetidine Hydrochloride (Caution is recommended when administering Gleevec with inhibitors of the CYP3A4 family. Substances that inhibit CYP3A4 activity may decrease metabolism and increase imatinib concentrations. There is a significant increase in exposure to imatinib when Gleevec is co-administered with ketoconazole).

No products indexed under this heading.

Ciprofloxacin (Caution is recommended when administering Gleevec with inhibitors of the CYP3A4 family. Substances that inhibit CYP3A4 activity may decrease metabolism and increase imatinib concentrations. There is a significant increase in exposure to imatinib when Gleevec is co-administered with ketoconazole). Products include:

Cipro I.V. 2998
Cipro I.V. Pharmacy Bulk Package 3509
Cipro Oral Suspension 2991
Cipro XR Tablets 3004
Ciprodex Otic Suspension 555

Ciprofloxacin Hydrochloride (Substances that are inducers of CYP3A4 activity may increase metabolism and decrease imatinib plasma concentrations. Co-medications that induce CYP3A4 may significantly reduce exposure to Gleevec. Dosage of imatinib should be increased by at least 50% and clinical response should be carefully monitored in patients receiving imatinib with potent CYP3A4 inducers). Products include:

Ciloxan Ophthalmic Ointment 554
Cipro Tablets 2991

Cisplatin (Substances that are inducers of CYP3A4 activity may increase metabolism and decrease imatinib plasma concentrations. Co-medications that induce CYP3A4 may significantly reduce exposure to Gleevec. Dosage of imatinib should be increased by at least 50% and clinical response should be carefully monitored in patients receiving imatinib with potent CYP3A4 inducers).

No products indexed under this heading.

Clarithromycin (Co-administration with CYP3A4 inhibitors, such as clarithromycin, may decrease the metabolism and increase imatinib concentrations). Products include:

Biaxin/Biaxin XL 402
PREVPAC 3281

Clomipramine Hydrochloride (Imatinib is a potent competitive inhibitor of CYP2D6; therefore, imatinib is likely to increase the blood levels of drugs that are substrates of this enzyme).

No products indexed under this heading.

Clotrimazole (Caution is recommended when administering Gleevec with inhibitors of the CYP3A4 family. Substances that inhibit CYP3A4 activity may decrease metabolism and increase imatinib concentrations. There is a significant increase in exposure to imatinib when Gleevec is co-administered with ketoconazole). Products include:

Lotrimin 3053
Lotrisone 3054

Clozapine (Imatinib is a potent competitive inhibitor of CYP2D6; therefore, imatinib is likely to increase the blood levels of drugs that are substrates of this enzyme). Products include:

Clozapine Tablets 2141
Clozaril Tablets 2174
FazaClo Orally Disintegrating Tablets 547

Codeine Phosphate (Imatinib is a potent competitive inhibitor of CYP2D6; therefore, imatinib is likely to increase the blood levels of drugs that are substrates of this enzyme). Products include:

Tylenol with Codeine 2461

Codeine Sulfate (Imatinib is a potent competitive inhibitor of CYP2D6; therefore, imatinib is likely to increase the blood levels of drugs that are substrates of this enzyme).

No products indexed under this heading.

Cortisone Acetate (Substances that are inducers of CYP3A4 activity may increase metabolism and decrease imatinib plasma concentrations. Co-medications that induce CYP3A4 may significantly reduce exposure to Gleevec. Dosage of imatinib should be increased by at least 50% and clinical response should be carefully monitored in patients receiving imatinib with potent CYP3A4 inducers).

No products indexed under this heading.

Cyclobenzaprine Hydrochloride (Imatinib is a potent competitive inhibitor of CYP2D6; therefore, imatinib is likely to increase the blood levels of drugs that are substrates of this enzyme). Products include:

Flexeril Tablets 1832

Cyclosporine (Particular caution is recommended when administering imatinib with CYP3A4 substrates that have a narrow therapeutic window). Products include:

Gengraf Capsules 458
Neoral Soft Gelatin Capsules 2247
Neoral Oral Solution 2247
Restasis Ophthalmic Emulsion 570
Sandimmune 2259

Dalfopristin (Caution is recommended when administering Gleevec with inhibitors of the CYP3A4 family. Substances that inhibit CYP3A4 activity may decrease metabolism and increase imatinib concentrations. There is a significant increase in exposure to imatinib when Gleevec is co-administered with ketoconazole). Products include:

Synercid I.V. 1690

Danazol (Caution is recommended when administering Gleevec with inhibitors of the CYP3A4 family. Substances that inhibit CYP3A4 activity may decrease metabolism and increase imatinib concentrations. There is a significant increase in exposure to imatinib when Gleevec is co-administered with ketoconazole).

No products indexed under this heading.

Delavirdine Mesylate (Caution is recommended when administering Gleevec with inhibitors of the CYP3A4 family. Substances that inhibit CYP3A4 activity may decrease metabolism and increase imatinib concentrations. There is a significant increase in exposure to imatinib when Gleevec is co-administered with ketoconazole). Products include:

Rescriptor Tablets 2535

Desipramine Hydrochloride (Imatinib is a potent competitive inhibitor of CYP2D6; therefore, imatinib is likely to increase the blood levels of drugs that are substrates of this enzyme).
No products indexed under this heading.

Desogestrel (Imatinib is a potent competitive inhibitor of CYP2C9; therefore, imatinib is likely to increase the blood levels of drugs that are substrates of this enzyme). Products include:
Ortho-Cept Tablets **2395**

Dexamethasone (Co-administration with inducers of CYP3A4, such as dexamethasone, may increase the metabolism and decrease imatinib concentrations). Products include:
Ciprodex Otic Suspension **555**
Decadron Tablets **1929**
TobraDex Ophthalmic Ointment **558**
TobraDex Ophthalmic Suspension ... **558**

Dexamethasone Acetate (Co-administration with inducers of CYP3A4, such as dexamethasone, may increase the metabolism and decrease imatinib concentrations).
No products indexed under this heading.

Dexamethasone Sodium Phosphate (Co-administration with inducers of CYP3A4, such as dexamethasone, may increase the metabolism and decrease imatinib concentrations). Products include:
Decadron Phosphate Injection **1931**

Dexfenfluramine Hydrochloride (Imatinib is a potent competitive inhibitor of CYP2D6; therefore, imatinib is likely to increase the blood levels of drugs that are substrates of this enzyme).
No products indexed under this heading.

Dextromethorphan (Imatinib is a potent competitive inhibitor of CYP2C9; therefore, imatinib is likely to increase the blood levels of drugs that are substrates of this enzyme).
No products indexed under this heading.

Dextromethorphan Hydrobromide (Imatinib is a potent competitive inhibitor of CYP2D6; therefore, imatinib is likely to increase the blood levels of drugs that are substrates of this enzyme). Products include:
Alacol DM Syrup **739**
Balamine DM **739**
Contac Severe Cold and Flu Caplets Maximum Strength .... ▣ **615**
Contac Severe Cold and Flu Caplets Non-Drowsy .... ▣ **615**
Children's Dimetapp DM Cold & Cough Elixir .... ▣ **745**
Children's Dimetapp Long Acting Cough Plus Cold Syrup .... ▣ **746**
Dimetapp Infant Drops Decongestant Plus Cough .... ▣ **746**
Mucinex DM Tablets .... ▣ **602**
PediaCare Decongestant & Cough Infant Drops .... ▣ **705**
PediaCare Freezer Pops Long-Acting Cough-Glacier Grape and Polar Berry Blue .... ▣ **706**
PediaCare Long-Acting Cough Infant Drops .... ▣ **705**
PediaCare Long-Acting Cough Plus Cold Liquid .... ▣ **704**
PediaCare Multi-Symptom Cold Liquid .... ▣ **704**
PediaCare NightRest Cough & Cold Liquid .... ▣ **704**
Robitussin Allergy & Cough Syrup .. ▣ **750**
Robitussin CF Liquid .... ▣ **755**
Robitussin Cough & Cold Liquid-filled Capsules .... ▣ **750**
Robitussin Cough, Cold & Flu Liquid-filled Capsules .... ▣ **750**
Robitussin Cough & Cold Infant Drops .... ▣ **755**
Robitussin DM Infant Drops .... ▣ **753**
Robitussin DM Liquid .... ▣ **753**
Robitussin Flu Liquid .... ▣ **752**
Robitussin Maximum Strength Cough Liquid .... ▣ **754**
Robitussin Maximum Strength Cough & Cold Liquid .... ▣ **754**
Robitussin Pediatric Cough Liquid .... ▣ **754**
Robitussin Pediatric Cough & Cold Liquid .... ▣ **754**
Robitussin PM Cough & Cold Liquid .... ▣ **752**
Robitussin Sugar Free Cough Liquid .... ▣ **753**
Simply Cough Liquid **1840**
Sudafed Severe Cold .... ▣ **710**
TheraFlu Cold & Cough Hot Liquid .... ▣ **680**
TheraFlu Flu & Chest Congestion Non-Drowsy Hot Liquid .... ▣ **681**
TheraFlu Severe Cold Non-Drowsy Hot Liquid .... ▣ **683**
TheraFlu Severe Cold & Cough Hot Liquid .... ▣ **683**
TheraFlu Severe Cold Caplets .... ▣ **679**
TheraFlu Severe Cold Hot Liquid .... ▣ **682**
TheraFlu Severe Cold Non-Drowsy Caplets .... ▣ **679**
TheraFlu Thin Strips Long Acting Cough .... ▣ **684**
Triaminic Cold & Cough Liquid .... ▣ **685**
Triaminic Cough Liquid .... ▣ **687**
Triaminic Cough & Nasal Congestion Liquid .... ▣ **687**
Triaminic Cough & Sore Throat Liquid .... ▣ **687**
Triaminic Flu, Cough & Fever Liquid .... ▣ **685**
Triaminic Night Time Cough & Cold Liquid .... ▣ **685**
Triaminic Cold & Cough Softchews .... ▣ **688**
Triaminic Cough & Sore Throat Softchews .... ▣ **689**
Triaminic Thin Strips Long Acting Cough .... ▣ **689**
Children's Tylenol Plus Cold & Cough Suspension Liquid and Chewable Tablets **1851**
Children's Tylenol Plus Flu Suspension Liquid **1853**
Concentrated Tylenol Infants' Drops Plus Cold and Cough **1851**
Tylenol Cold & Flu Severe Daytime Liquid with Cool Burst **1846**
Tylenol Cold & Flu Severe NightTime Liquid with Cool Burst **1846**
Tylenol Cold Severe Congestion Non-Drowsy Caplets with Cool Burst **1846**
Tylenol Cough & Sore Throat Daytime Liquid with Cool Burst **1849**
Tylenol Cough & Sore Throat NightTime Liquid with Cool Burst **1849**
Tylenol Flu Day Non-Drowsy Gelcaps **1846**
Concentrated Tylenol Infants' Drops Plus Cold & Cough Nasal Decongestant, Fever Reducer & Pain Reliever .... ▣ **668**
Multi-Symptom Tylenol Cold Night Time Caplets **1845**
Multi-Symptom Tylenol Cold Day Non-Drowsy Caplets and Gelcaps **1845**
Vicks 44 Cough Relief **2675**
Vicks 44D Cough & Head Congestion Relief **2676**
Vicks 44D Cough & Head Congestion Relief Liquid .... ▣ **721**
Vicks 44E Cough & Chest Congestion Relief **2676**
Pediatric Vicks 44e Cough & Chest Congestion Relief Liquid **2673**
Vicks 44M Cough, Cold & Flu Relief **2676**
Pediatric Vicks 44m Cough & Cold Relief **2673**
Vicks DayQuil LiquiCaps/Liquid Multi-Symptom Cold/Flu Relief .... ▣ **723**
Vicks DayQuil Multi-Symptom Cold/Flu Relief LiquiCaps **2675**
Vicks DayQuil Multi-Symptom Cold/Flu Relief Liquid **2675**
Children's Vicks NyQuil Cold/Cough Relief **2671**
Vicks NyQuil Cough Liquid **2677**
Vicks NyQuil LiquiCaps **2677**
Vicks NyQuil LiquiCaps/Liquid Multi-Symptom Cold/Flu Relief .... ▣ **725**
Vicks NyQuil Liquid **2677**
Zicam Concentrated Cough Mist for Kids Cool Cherry .... ▣ **643**
Zicam Concentrated Cough Mist for Kids Plus D Cool Cherry .... ▣ **643**
Zicam Concentrated Cough Mist Nite-Cool Cherry .... ▣ **642**
Zicam Concentrated Cough Mist Plus D Cool Cherry .... ▣ **642**
Zicam Concentrated Cough Mist-Honey Lemon & Cool Cherry .... ▣ **642**

Dextromethorphan Polistirex (Imatinib is a potent competitive inhibitor of CYP2D6; therefore, imatinib is likely to increase the blood levels of drugs that are substrates of this enzyme). Products include:
Delsym Extended-Release Suspension .... ▣ **611**
Delsym 12 Hour Cough Suppressant for Children .... ▣ **611**

Diazepam (Imatinib is a potent competitive inhibitor of CYP2C9; therefore, imatinib is likely to increase the blood levels of drugs that are substrates of this enzyme). Products include:
Diastat Rectal Delivery System **3344**
Valium Tablets **2822**

Diclofenac Potassium (Imatinib is a potent competitive inhibitor of CYP2C9; therefore, imatinib is likely to increase the blood levels of drugs that are substrates of this enzyme). Products include:
Cataflam Tablets **2173**

Diclofenac Sodium (Imatinib is a potent competitive inhibitor of CYP2C9; therefore, imatinib is likely to increase the blood levels of drugs that are substrates of this enzyme). Products include:
Arthrotec Tablets **3126**
Voltaren Ophthalmic Solution **2300**
Voltaren Tablets **2298**
Voltaren-XR Tablets **2301**

Diltiazem Hydrochloride (Caution is recommended when administering Gleevec with inhibitors of the CYP3A4 family. Substances that inhibit CYP3A4 activity may decrease metabolism and increase imatinib concentrations. There is a significant increase in exposure to imatinib when Gleevec is co-administered with ketoconazole). Products include:
Cardizem LA Extended Release Tablets **1699**
Tiazac Capsules **1204**

Diltiazem Maleate (Caution is recommended when administering Gleevec with inhibitors of the CYP3A4 family. Substances that inhibit CYP3A4 activity may decrease metabolism and increase imatinib concentrations. There is a significant increase in exposure to imatinib when Gleevec is co-administered with ketoconazole).
No products indexed under this heading.

Dolasetron Mesylate (Imatinib is a potent competitive inhibitor of CYP2D6; therefore, imatinib is likely to increase the blood levels of drugs that are substrates of this enzyme). Products include:
Anzemet Injection **2871**
Anzemet Tablets **2874**

Donepezil Hydrochloride (Imatinib is a potent competitive inhibitor of CYP2D6; therefore, imatinib is likely to increase the blood levels of drugs that are substrates of this enzyme). Products include:
Aricept Tablets **1086**
Aricept ODT Tablets **1086**

Doxepin Hydrochloride (Imatinib is a potent competitive inhibitor of CYP2D6; therefore, imatinib is likely to increase the blood levels of drugs that are substrates of this enzyme).
No products indexed under this heading.

Doxorubicin Hydrochloride (Substances that are inducers of CYP3A4 activity may increase metabolism and decrease imatinib plasma concentrations. Co-medications that induce CYP3A4 may significantly reduce exposure to Gleevec. Dosage of imatinib should be increased by at least 50% and clinical response should be carefully monitored in patients receiving imatinib with potent CYP3A4 inducers). Products include:
Adriamycin for Injection, USP **786**
Adriamycin Injection, USP **786**

Dronabinol (Imatinib is a potent competitive inhibitor of CYP2C9; therefore, imatinib is likely to increase the blood levels of drugs that are substrates of this enzyme). Products include:
Marinol Capsules **3334**

Efavirenz (Caution is recommended when administering Gleevec with inhibitors of the CYP3A4 family. Substances that inhibit CYP3A4 activity may decrease metabolism and increase imatinib concentrations. There is a significant increase in exposure to imatinib when Gleevec is co-administered with ketoconazole). Products include:
Sustiva Capsules **957**

Encainide Hydrochloride (Imatinib is a potent competitive inhibitor of CYP2D6; therefore, imatinib is likely to increase the blood levels of drugs that are substrates of this enzyme).
No products indexed under this heading.

Eprosartan Mesylate (Imatinib is a potent competitive inhibitor of CYP2C9; therefore, imatinib is likely to increase the blood levels of drugs that are substrates of this enzyme). Products include:
Teveten Tablets **1707**
Teveten HCT Tablets **1710**

Erythromycin (Co-administration with CYP3A4 inhibitors, such as erythromycin, may decrease the metabolism and increase imatinib concentrations). Products include:
Erygel Topical Gel **2096**
Ery-Tab Tablets **447**
Erythromycin Base Filmtab Tablets **454**
Erythromycin Delayed-Release Capsules, USP **456**
PCE Dispertab Tablets **510**

Erythromycin Estolate (Co-administration with CYP3A4 inhibitors, such as erythromycin, may decrease the metabolism and increase imatinib concentrations).
No products indexed under this heading.

Erythromycin Ethylsuccinate (Co-administration with CYP3A4 inhibitors, such as erythromycin,

may decrease the metabolism and increase imatinib concentrations). Products include:

E.E.S. 449
EryPed 445

Erythromycin Gluceptate (Co-administration with CYP3A4 inhibitors, such as erythromycin, may decrease the metabolism and increase imatinib concentrations).
No products indexed under this heading.

Erythromycin Lactobionate (Co-administration with CYP3A4 inhibitors, such as erythromycin, may decrease the metabolism and increase imatinib concentrations).
No products indexed under this heading.

Erythromycin Stearate (Co-administration with CYP3A4 inhibitors, such as erythromycin, may decrease the metabolism and increase imatinib concentrations). Products include:

Erythrocin Stearate Filmtab Tablets 452

Esomeprazole Magnesium (Caution is recommended when administering Gleevec with inhibitors of the CYP3A4 family. Substances that inhibit CYP3A4 activity may decrease metabolism and increase imatinib concentrations. There is a significant increase in exposure to imatinib when Gleevec is co-administered with ketoconazole). Products include:

Nexium Delayed-Release Capsules 645

Ethosuximide (Substances that are inducers of CYP3A4 activity may increase metabolism and decrease imatinib plasma concentrations. Co-medications that induce CYP3A4 may significantly reduce exposure to Gleevec. Dosage of imatinib should be increased by at least 50% and clinical response should be carefully monitored in patients receiving imatinib with potent CYP3A4 inducers).
No products indexed under this heading.

Etodolac (Imatinib is a potent competitive inhibitor of CYP2C9; therefore, imatinib is likely to increase the blood levels of drugs that are substrates of this enzyme).
No products indexed under this heading.

Felbamate (Substances that are inducers of CYP3A4 activity may increase metabolism and decrease imatinib plasma concentrations. Co-medications that induce CYP3A4 may significantly reduce exposure to Gleevec. Dosage of imatinib should be increased by at least 50% and clinical response should be carefully monitored in patients receiving imatinib with potent CYP3A4 inducers).
No products indexed under this heading.

Felodipine (Imatinib will increase plasma concentration of CYP3A4 metabolized drugs. (e.g., dihydropyridine calcium channel blockers)). Products include:

Plendil Extended-Release Tablets 651

Fenoprofen Calcium (Imatinib is a potent competitive inhibitor of CYP2C9; therefore, imatinib is likely to increase the blood levels of drugs that are substrates of this enzyme). Products include:

Nalfon Capsules 2504

Fentanyl (Imatinib is a potent competitive inhibitor of CYP2D6; therefore, imatinib is likely to increase the blood levels of drugs that are substrates of this enzyme). Products include:

Duragesic Transdermal System 2448

Fentanyl Citrate (Imatinib is a potent competitive inhibitor of CYP2D6; therefore, imatinib is likely to increase the blood levels of drugs that are substrates of this enzyme). Products include:

Actiq 993

Flecainide Acetate (Imatinib is a potent competitive inhibitor of CYP2D6; therefore, imatinib is likely to increase the blood levels of drugs that are substrates of this enzyme). Products include:

Tambocor Tablets 1824

Fluconazole (Caution is recommended when administering Gleevec with inhibitors of the CYP3A4 family. Substances that inhibit CYP3A4 activity may decrease metabolism and increase imatinib concentrations. There is a significant increase in exposure to imatinib when Gleevec is co-administered with ketoconazole).
No products indexed under this heading.

Fludrocortisone Acetate (Substances that are inducers of CYP3A4 activity may increase metabolism and decrease imatinib plasma concentrations. Co-medications that induce CYP3A4 may significantly reduce exposure to Gleevec. Dosage of imatinib should be increased by at least 50% and clinical response should be carefully monitored in patients receiving imatinib with potent CYP3A4 inducers).
No products indexed under this heading.

Fluoxetine (Imatinib is a potent competitive inhibitor of CYP2D6; therefore, imatinib is likely to increase the blood levels of drugs that are substrates of this enzyme).
No products indexed under this heading.

Fluoxetine Hydrochloride (Caution is recommended when administering Gleevec with inhibitors of the CYP3A4 family. Substances that inhibit CYP3A4 activity may decrease metabolism and increase imatinib concentrations. There is a significant increase in exposure to imatinib when Gleevec is co-administered with ketoconazole). Products include:

Prozac Pulvules and Liquid 1771
Symbyax Capsules 1788

Fluphenazine Decanoate (Imatinib is a potent competitive inhibitor of CYP2D6; therefore, imatinib is likely to increase the blood levels of drugs that are substrates of this enzyme).
No products indexed under this heading.

Fluphenazine Enanthate (Imatinib is a potent competitive inhibitor of CYP2D6; therefore, imatinib is likely to increase the blood levels of drugs that are substrates of this enzyme).
No products indexed under this heading.

Fluphenazine Hydrochloride (Imatinib is a potent competitive inhibitor of CYP2D6; therefore, imatinib is likely to increase the blood levels of drugs that are substrates of this enzyme).
No products indexed under this heading.

Flurbiprofen (Imatinib is a potent competitive inhibitor of CYP2C9; therefore, imatinib is likely to increase the blood levels of drugs that are substrates of this enzyme).
No products indexed under this heading.

Flurbiprofen Sodium (Imatinib is a potent competitive inhibitor of CYP2C9; therefore, imatinib is likely to increase the blood levels of drugs that are substrates of this enzyme). Products include:

Ocufen Ophthalmic Solution .... ⊙ 230

Fluvastatin Sodium (Imatinib is a potent competitive inhibitor of CYP2C9; therefore, imatinib is likely to increase the blood levels of drugs that are substrates of this enzyme). Products include:

Lescol Capsules 2227
Lescol 2730
Lescol XL Tablets 2227

Fluvoxamine Maleate (Caution is recommended when administering Gleevec with inhibitors of the CYP3A4 family. Substances that inhibit CYP3A4 activity may decrease metabolism and increase imatinib concentrations. There is a significant increase in exposure to imatinib when Gleevec is co-administered with ketoconazole).
No products indexed under this heading.

Formoterol Fumarate (Imatinib is a potent competitive inhibitor of CYP2D6; therefore, imatinib is likely to increase the blood levels of drugs that are substrates of this enzyme). Products include:

Foradil Aerolizer 3024

Fosamprenavir Calcium (Caution is recommended when administering Gleevec with inhibitors of the CYP3A4 family. Substances that inhibit CYP3A4 activity may decrease metabolism and increase imatinib concentrations. There is a significant increase in exposure to imatinib when Gleevec is co-administered with ketoconazole). Products include:

Lexiva Tablets 1473

Fosphenytoin Sodium (Co-administration with inducers of CYP3A4, such as phenytoin, may increase the metabolism and decrease imatinib concentrations. Dosage of imatinib should be increased by at least 50% and clinical response should be carefully monitored in patients receiving imatinib with a potent CYP3A4 inducer such as phenytoin).
No products indexed under this heading.

Galantamine Hydrobromide (Imatinib is a potent competitive inhibitor of CYP2D6; therefore, imatinib is likely to increase the blood levels of drugs that are substrates of this enzyme). Products include:

Razadyne ER Extended-Release Capsules 2434
Razadyne 2434

Garlic Extract (Substances that are inducers of CYP3A4 activity may increase metabolism and decrease imatinib plasma concentrations. Co-medications that induce CYP3A4 may significantly reduce exposure to Gleevec. Dosage of imatinib should be increased by at least 50% and clinical response should be carefully monitored in patients receiving imatinib with potent CYP3A4 inducers).
No products indexed under this heading.

Garlic Oil (Substances that are inducers of CYP3A4 activity may increase metabolism and decrease imatinib plasma concentrations. Co-medications that induce CYP3A4 may significantly reduce exposure to Gleevec. Dosage of imatinib should be increased by at least 50% and clinical response should be carefully monitored in patients receiving imatinib with potent CYP3A4 inducers).
No products indexed under this heading.

Glimepiride (Imatinib is a potent competitive inhibitor of CYP2C9; therefore, imatinib is likely to increase the blood levels of drugs that are substrates of this enzyme). Products include:

Amaryl Tablets 2864

Glipizide (Imatinib is a potent competitive inhibitor of CYP2C9; therefore, imatinib is likely to increase the blood levels of drugs that are substrates of this enzyme).
No products indexed under this heading.

Haloperidol (Imatinib is a potent competitive inhibitor of CYP2D6; therefore, imatinib is likely to increase the blood levels of drugs that are substrates of this enzyme).
No products indexed under this heading.

Haloperidol Decanoate (Imatinib is a potent competitive inhibitor of CYP2D6; therefore, imatinib is likely to increase the blood levels of drugs that are substrates of this enzyme).
No products indexed under this heading.

Hydrocodone Bitartrate (Imatinib is a potent competitive inhibitor of CYP2D6; therefore, imatinib is likely to increase the blood levels of drugs that are substrates of this enzyme). Products include:

Hycodan 1104
Hycomine Compound Tablets 1105
Hycotuss Expectorant Syrup 1106
Lortab 3315
Lortab Elixir 3312
Vicodin Tablets 530
Vicodin ES Tablets 531
Vicodin HP Tablets 532
Vicoprofen Tablets 533
Zydone Tablets 1118

Hydrocortisone (Substances that are inducers of CYP3A4 activity may increase metabolism and decrease imatinib plasma concentrations. Co-medications that induce CYP3A4 may significantly reduce exposure to Gleevec. Dosage of imatinib should be increased by at least 50% and clinical response should be carefully monitored in patients receiving imatinib with potent CYP3A4 inducers). Products include:

Cortizone•5 Ointment .... ▣ 699
Cortizone•10 Creme .... ▣ 699
Cortizone•10 Ointment .... ▣ 699
Cortizone•10 Plus Creme .... ▣ 700
Cortizone•10 Maximum Strength Quick Shot Spray .... ▣ 700

Hydrocortone Tablets 1963
Preparation H Hydrocortisone Cream .... ▣748

Hydrocortisone Acetate (Substances that are inducers of CYP3A4 activity may increase metabolism and decrease imatinib plasma concentrations. Co-medications that induce CYP3A4 may significantly reduce exposure to Gleevec. Dosage of imatinib should be increased by at least 50% and clinical response should be carefully monitored in patients receiving imatinib with potent CYP3A4 inducers). Products include:
Analpram-HC 1136
Pramosone 1139
ProctoFoam-HC 3113
Tucks Anti-Itch Ointment .... ▣712
U-cort 1% Cream 3289

Hydrocortisone Butyrate (Substances that are inducers of CYP3A4 activity may increase metabolism and decrease imatinib plasma concentrations. Co-medications that induce CYP3A4 may significantly reduce exposure to Gleevec. Dosage of imatinib should be increased by at least 50% and clinical response should be carefully monitored in patients receiving imatinib with potent CYP3A4 inducers). Products include:
Locoid 1138
Locoid Lipocream Cream 1138

Hydrocortisone Cypionate (Substances that are inducers of CYP3A4 activity may increase metabolism and decrease imatinib plasma concentrations. Co-medications that induce CYP3A4 may significantly reduce exposure to Gleevec. Dosage of imatinib should be increased by at least 50% and clinical response should be carefully monitored in patients receiving imatinib with potent CYP3A4 inducers).
No products indexed under this heading.

Hydrocortisone Hemisuccinate (Substances that are inducers of CYP3A4 activity may increase metabolism and decrease imatinib plasma concentrations. Co-medications that induce CYP3A4 may significantly reduce exposure to Gleevec. Dosage of imatinib should be increased by at least 50% and clinical response should be carefully monitored in patients receiving imatinib with potent CYP3A4 inducers).
No products indexed under this heading.

Hydrocortisone Probutate (Substances that are inducers of CYP3A4 activity may increase metabolism and decrease imatinib plasma concentrations. Co-medications that induce CYP3A4 may significantly reduce exposure to Gleevec. Dosage of imatinib should be increased by at least 50% and clinical response should be carefully monitored in patients receiving imatinib with potent CYP3A4 inducers). Products include:
Pandel Cream, 0.1% 1017

Hydrocortisone Sodium Phosphate (Substances that are inducers of CYP3A4 activity may increase metabolism and decrease imatinib plasma concentrations. Co-medications that induce CYP3A4 may significantly reduce exposure to Gleevec. Dosage of imatinib should be increased by at least 50% and clinical response should be carefully monitored in patients receiving imatinib with potent CYP3A4 inducers).
No products indexed under this heading.

Hydrocortisone Sodium Succinate (Substances that are inducers of CYP3A4 activity may increase metabolism and decrease imatinib plasma concentrations. Co-medications that induce CYP3A4 may significantly reduce exposure to Gleevec. Dosage of imatinib should be increased by at least 50% and clinical response should be carefully monitored in patients receiving imatinib with potent CYP3A4 inducers).
No products indexed under this heading.

Hydrocortisone Valerate (Substances that are inducers of CYP3A4 activity may increase metabolism and decrease imatinib plasma concentrations. Co-medications that induce CYP3A4 may significantly reduce exposure to Gleevec. Dosage of imatinib should be increased by at least 50% and clinical response should be carefully monitored in patients receiving imatinib with potent CYP3A4 inducers).
No products indexed under this heading.

Hypericum (Co-administration with inducers of CYP3A4, such as St. John's Wort, may increase the metabolism and decrease imatinib concentrations).
No products indexed under this heading.

Hypericum Perforatum (Substances that are inducers of CYP3A4 activity may increase metabolism and decrease imatinib plasma concentrations. Co-medications that induce CYP3A4 may significantly reduce exposure to Gleevec. Dosage of imatinib should be increased by at least 50% and clinical response should be carefully monitored in patients receiving imatinib with potent CYP3A4 inducers).
No products indexed under this heading.

Ibuprofen (Imatinib is a potent competitive inhibitor of CYP2C9; therefore, imatinib is likely to increase the blood levels of drugs that are substrates of this enzyme). Products include:
Advil Allergy Sinus Caplets .... ▣737
Advil .... ▣737
Children's Advil Suspension .... ▣742
Children's Advil Chewable Tablets .... ▣741
Advil Cold & Sinus .... ▣739
Advil Flu & Body Ache Caplets .... ▣739
Children's Advil Cold Suspension .... ▣741
Infants' Advil Concentrated Drops .... ▣743
Junior Strength Advil Swallow Tablets .... ▣740
Advil Migraine Liquigels .... ▣740
Advil Multi-Symptom Cold Caplets .... ▣738
Combunox Tablets 1183
Children's Motrin Oral Suspension and Chewable Tablets 1837
Children's Motrin Cold Non-Staining Dye-Free Oral Suspension 1838
Children's Motrin Cold Oral Suspension 1838
Children's Motrin Non-Staining Dye-Free Oral Suspension 1837
Motrin Cold & Sinus Caplets 1836
Motrin IB Tablets and Caplets 1836
Infants' Motrin Concentrated Drops 1837
Infants' Motrin Non-Staining Dye-Free Drops 1837
Junior Strength Motrin Caplets and Chewable Tablets 1837
Vicoprofen Tablets 533

Imipramine Hydrochloride (Imatinib is a potent competitive inhibitor of CYP2D6; therefore, imatinib is likely to increase the blood levels of drugs that are substrates of this enzyme).
No products indexed under this heading.

Imipramine Pamoate (Imatinib is a potent competitive inhibitor of CYP2D6; therefore, imatinib is likely to increase the blood levels of drugs that are substrates of this enzyme).
No products indexed under this heading.

Indinavir Sulfate (Caution is recommended when administering Gleevec with inhibitors of the CYP3A4 family. Substances that inhibit CYP3A4 activity may decrease metabolism and increase imatinib concentrations. There is a significant increase in exposure to imatinib when Gleevec is co-administered with ketoconazole). Products include:
Crixivan Capsules 1918

Indomethacin (Imatinib is a potent competitive inhibitor of CYP2C9; therefore, imatinib is likely to increase the blood levels of drugs that are substrates of this enzyme). Products include:
Indocin 1968

Indomethacin Sodium Trihydrate (Imatinib is a potent competitive inhibitor of CYP2C9; therefore, imatinib is likely to increase the blood levels of drugs that are substrates of this enzyme). Products include:
Indocin I.V. 1973

Indoramin Hydrochloride (Imatinib is a potent competitive inhibitor of CYP2D6; therefore, imatinib is likely to increase the blood levels of drugs that are substrates of this enzyme).
No products indexed under this heading.

Irbesartan (Imatinib is a potent competitive inhibitor of CYP2C9; therefore, imatinib is likely to increase the blood levels of drugs that are substrates of this enzyme). Products include:
Avalide Tablets 922
Avalide Tablets 2889
Avapro Tablets 925
Avapro Tablets 2886

Isoniazid (Caution is recommended when administering Gleevec with inhibitors of the CYP3A4 family. Substances that inhibit CYP3A4 activity may decrease metabolism and increase imatinib concentrations. There is a significant increase in exposure to imatinib when Gleevec is co-administered with ketoconazole).
No products indexed under this heading.

Itraconazole (Co-administration with CYP3A4 inhibitors, such as itraconazole, may decrease the metabolism and increase imatinib concentrations).
No products indexed under this heading.

Ketoconazole (Co-administration with inhibitors of CYP3A4, such as ketoconazole, may decrease the metabolism and increase imatinib concentrations; there is a significant increase in exposure to imatinib when co-administered with ketoconazole). Products include:
Nizoral A-D Shampoo, 1% 1839
Nizoral 2% Shampoo 1838

Ketoprofen (Imatinib is a potent competitive inhibitor of CYP2C9; therefore, imatinib is likely to increase the blood levels of drugs that are substrates of this enzyme).
No products indexed under this heading.

Ketorolac Tromethamine (Imatinib is a potent competitive inhibitor of CYP2C9; therefore, imatinib is likely to increase the blood levels of drugs that are substrates of this enzyme). Products include:
Acular Ophthalmic Solution 561
Acular LS Ophthalmic Solution 562

Labetalol Hydrochloride (Imatinib is a potent competitive inhibitor of CYP2D6; therefore, imatinib is likely to increase the blood levels of drugs that are substrates of this enzyme).
No products indexed under this heading.

Lansoprazole (Imatinib is a potent competitive inhibitor of CYP2C9; therefore, imatinib is likely to increase the blood levels of drugs that are substrates of this enzyme). Products include:
Prevacid Delayed-Release Capsules 3268
Prevacid for Delayed-Release Oral Suspension 3268
Prevacid I.V. for Injection 3274
Prevacid NapraPAC 3277
Prevacid SoluTab Delayed-Release Orally Disintegrating Tablets 3268
PREVPAC 3281

Lidocaine (Imatinib is a potent competitive inhibitor of CYP2D6; therefore, imatinib is likely to increase the blood levels of drugs that are substrates of this enzyme). Products include:
Lidoderm Patch 1107

Lidocaine Hydrochloride (Imatinib is a potent competitive inhibitor of CYP2D6; therefore, imatinib is likely to increase the blood levels of drugs that are substrates of this enzyme).
No products indexed under this heading.

Lopinavir (Caution is recommended when administering Gleevec with inhibitors of the CYP3A4 family. Substances that inhibit CYP3A4 activity may decrease metabolism and increase imatinib concentrations. There is a significant increase in exposure to imatinib when Gleevec is co-administered with ketoconazole). Products include:
Kaletra 474

Loratadine (Caution is recommended when administering Gleevec with inhibitors of the CYP3A4 family. Substances that inhibit CYP3A4 activity may decrease metabolism and increase imatinib concentrations. There is a significant increase in exposure to imatinib when Gleevec is co-administered with ketoconazole). Products include:
Alavert Allergy & Sinus D-12 Hour Tablets .... ▣743
Alavert .... ▣743
Children's Claritin 24 Hour Non-Drowsy Allergy Syrup .... ▣732
Claritin Non-Drowsy 24 Hour Tablets .... ▣731
Non-Drowsy Claritin Hives Relief Tablets .... ▣733
Claritin Reditabs 24 Hour Non-Drowsy Tablets .... ▣732
Claritin-D Non-Drowsy 12 Hour Tablets .... ▣731

Claritin-D Non-Drowsy 24 Hour Tablets 731
Children's Dimetapp ND Non-Drowsy Allergy Syrup 746
Triaminic Allerchews 684

Losartan Potassium (Imatinib is a potent competitive inhibitor of CYP2C9; therefore, imatinib is likely to increase the blood levels of drugs that are substrates of this enzyme). Products include:
Cozaar Tablets **1913**
Hyzaar **1964**

Lovastatin (Imatinib will increase the plasma concentrations of certain HMG-CoA reductase inhibitors by inhibiting CYP3A4). Products include:
Advicor Tablets **1694**
Altoprev Extended-Release Tablets **1151**
Mevacor Tablets **1996**

Maprotiline Hydrochloride (Imatinib is a potent competitive inhibitor of CYP2D6; therefore, imatinib is likely to increase the blood levels of drugs that are substrates of this enzyme).
No products indexed under this heading.

Meclofenamate Sodium (Imatinib is a potent competitive inhibitor of CYP2C9; therefore, imatinib is likely to increase the blood levels of drugs that are substrates of this enzyme).
No products indexed under this heading.

Mefenamic Acid (Imatinib is a potent competitive inhibitor of CYP2C9; therefore, imatinib is likely to increase the blood levels of drugs that are substrates of this enzyme).
No products indexed under this heading.

Meloxicam (Imatinib is a potent competitive inhibitor of CYP2C9; therefore, imatinib is likely to increase the blood levels of drugs that are substrates of this enzyme). Products include:
Mobic Oral Suspension **893**
Mobic Tablets **893**

Meperidine Hydrochloride (Imatinib is a potent competitive inhibitor of CYP2D6; therefore, imatinib is likely to increase the blood levels of drugs that are substrates of this enzyme).
No products indexed under this heading.

Mephenytoin (Substances that are inducers of CYP3A4 activity may increase metabolism and decrease imatinib plasma concentrations. Comedications that induce CYP3A4 may significantly reduce exposure to Gleevec. Dosage of imatinib should be increased by at least 50% and clinical response should be carefully monitored in patients receiving imatinib with potent CYP3A4 inducers).
No products indexed under this heading.

Metformin Hydrochloride (Imatinib is a potent competitive inhibitor of CYP2C9; therefore, imatinib is likely to increase the blood levels of drugs that are substrates of this enzyme). Products include:
ActoPlus Met Tablets **3219**
Avandamet Tablets **1343**
Fortamet Extended-Release Tablets **1156**

Methadone Hydrochloride (Imatinib is a potent competitive inhibitor of CYP2D6; therefore, imatinib is likely to increase the blood levels of drugs that are substrates of this enzyme).
No products indexed under this heading.

Methamphetamine Hydrochloride (Imatinib is a potent competitive inhibitor of CYP2D6; therefore, imatinib is likely to increase the blood levels of drugs that are substrates of this enzyme). Products include:
Desoxyn Tablets, USP **2482**

Methsuximide (Substances that are inducers of CYP3A4 activity may increase metabolism and decrease imatinib plasma concentrations. Comedications that induce CYP3A4 may significantly reduce exposure to Gleevec. Dosage of imatinib should be increased by at least 50% and clinical response should be carefully monitored in patients receiving imatinib with potent CYP3A4 inducers).
No products indexed under this heading.

Methylprednisolone (Substances that are inducers of CYP3A4 activity may increase metabolism and decrease imatinib plasma concentrations. Co-medications that induce CYP3A4 may significantly reduce exposure to Gleevec. Dosage of imatinib should be increased by at least 50% and clinical response should be carefully monitored in patients receiving imatinib with potent CYP3A4 inducers).
No products indexed under this heading.

Methylprednisolone Acetate (Substances that are inducers of CYP3A4 activity may increase metabolism and decrease imatinib plasma concentrations. Comedications that induce CYP3A4 may significantly reduce exposure to Gleevec. Dosage of imatinib should be increased by at least 50% and clinical response should be carefully monitored in patients receiving imatinib with potent CYP3A4 inducers). Products include:
Depo-Medrol Injectable Suspension **2615**
Depo-Medrol Single-Dose Vial **2617**

Methylprednisolone Sodium Succinate (Substances that are inducers of CYP3A4 activity may increase metabolism and decrease imatinib plasma concentrations. Comedications that induce CYP3A4 may significantly reduce exposure to Gleevec. Dosage of imatinib should be increased by at least 50% and clinical response should be carefully monitored in patients receiving imatinib with potent CYP3A4 inducers).
No products indexed under this heading.

Metoprolol Succinate (Imatinib is a potent competitive inhibitor of CYP2D6; therefore, imatinib is likely to increase the blood levels of drugs that are substrates of this enzyme). Products include:
Toprol-XL Tablets **660**

Metoprolol Tartrate (Imatinib is a potent competitive inhibitor of CYP2D6; therefore, imatinib is likely to increase the blood levels of drugs that are substrates of this enzyme).
No products indexed under this heading.

Metronidazole (Caution is recommended when administering Gleevec with inhibitors of the CYP3A4 family. Substances that inhibit CYP3A4 activity may decrease metabolism and increase imatinib concentrations. There is a significant increase in exposure to imatinib when Gleevec is co-administered with ketoconazole). Products include:
Metrogel 1% **1212**
MetroGel-Vaginal Gel **1822**
Noritate Cream, 1% **1051**

Metronidazole Benzoate (Caution is recommended when administering Gleevec with inhibitors of the CYP3A4 family. Substances that inhibit CYP3A4 activity may decrease metabolism and increase imatinib concentrations. There is a significant increase in exposure to imatinib when Gleevec is co-administered with ketoconazole).
No products indexed under this heading.

Metronidazole Hydrochloride (Caution is recommended when administering Gleevec with inhibitors of the CYP3A4 family. Substances that inhibit CYP3A4 activity may decrease metabolism and increase imatinib concentrations. There is a significant increase in exposure to imatinib when Gleevec is co-administered with ketoconazole).
No products indexed under this heading.

Mexiletine Hydrochloride (Imatinib is a potent competitive inhibitor of CYP2D6; therefore, imatinib is likely to increase the blood levels of drugs that are substrates of this enzyme).
No products indexed under this heading.

Miconazole (Caution is recommended when administering Gleevec with inhibitors of the CYP3A4 family. Substances that inhibit CYP3A4 activity may decrease metabolism and increase imatinib concentrations. There is a significant increase in exposure to imatinib when Gleevec is co-administered with ketoconazole).
No products indexed under this heading.

Miconazole Nitrate (Caution is recommended when administering Gleevec with inhibitors of the CYP3A4 family. Substances that inhibit CYP3A4 activity may decrease metabolism and increase imatinib concentrations. There is a significant increase in exposure to imatinib when Gleevec is co-administered with ketoconazole). Products include:
Desenex **674**
Desenex Jock Itch Spray Powder ... **674**

Midazolam Hydrochloride (Imatinib will increase the plasma concentrations of triazolobenzodiazepines by inhibiting CYP3A4).
No products indexed under this heading.

Miglitol (Imatinib is a potent competitive inhibitor of CYP2C9; therefore, imatinib is likely to increase the blood levels of drugs that are substrates of this enzyme).
No products indexed under this heading.

Mirtazapine (Imatinib is a potent competitive inhibitor of CYP2D6; therefore, imatinib is likely to increase the blood levels of drugs that are substrates of this enzyme).
No products indexed under this heading.

Modafinil (Substances that are inducers of CYP3A4 activity may increase metabolism and decrease imatinib plasma concentrations. Comedications that induce CYP3A4 may significantly reduce exposure to Gleevec. Dosage of imatinib should be increased by at least 50% and clinical response should be carefully monitored in patients receiving imatinib with potent CYP3A4 inducers). Products include:
Provigil Tablets **1002**

Montelukast Sodium (Imatinib is a potent competitive inhibitor of CYP2C9; therefore, imatinib is likely to increase the blood levels of drugs that are substrates of this enzyme). Products include:
Singulair **2047**

Morphine Sulfate (Imatinib is a potent competitive inhibitor of CYP2D6; therefore, imatinib is likely to increase the blood levels of drugs that are substrates of this enzyme). Products include:
Avinza Capsules **1714**
Kadian Capsules **572**
MS Contin Tablets **2703**

Nabumetone (Imatinib is a potent competitive inhibitor of CYP2C9; therefore, imatinib is likely to increase the blood levels of drugs that are substrates of this enzyme). Products include:
Relafen Tablets **1523**

Naproxen (Imatinib is a potent competitive inhibitor of CYP2C9; therefore, imatinib is likely to increase the blood levels of drugs that are substrates of this enzyme). Products include:
EC-Naprosyn Delayed-Release Tablets **2769**
Naprosyn Suspension **2769**
Naprosyn Tablets **2769**
Prevacid NapraPAC **3277**

Naproxen Sodium (Imatinib is a potent competitive inhibitor of CYP2C9; therefore, imatinib is likely to increase the blood levels of drugs that are substrates of this enzyme). Products include:
Aleve Tablets, Caplets and Gelcaps **605**
Anaprox Tablets **2769**
Anaprox DS Tablets **2769**

Nateglinide (Imatinib is a potent competitive inhibitor of CYP2C9; therefore, imatinib is likely to increase the blood levels of drugs that are substrates of this enzyme). Products include:
Starlix Tablets **2276**

Nefazodone Hydrochloride (Caution is recommended when administering Gleevec with inhibitors of the CYP3A4 family. Substances that inhibit CYP3A4 activity may decrease metabolism and increase imatinib concentrations. There is a significant increase in exposure to imatinib when Gleevec is co-administered with ketoconazole).
No products indexed under this heading.

Nelfinavir Mesylate (Caution is recommended when administering Gleevec with inhibitors of the CYP3A4 family. Substances that inhibit CYP3A4 activity may decrease metabolism and increase imatinib concentrations. There is a significant increase in exposure to imatinib when Gleevec is co-administered with ketoconazole). Products include:
Viracept **2556**

IMPORTANT NOTE: Always consult each drug listing in the patient's regimen for possible interactions.

Nevirapine (Caution is recommended when administering Gleevec with inhibitors of the CYP3A4 family. Substances that inhibit CYP3A4 activity may decrease metabolism and increase imatinib concentrations. There is a significant increase in exposure to imatinib when Gleevec is co-administered with ketoconazole). Products include:
- Viramune Oral Suspension 903
- Viramune Tablets 903

Niacinamide (Caution is recommended when administering Gleevec with inhibitors of the CYP3A4 family. Substances that inhibit CYP3A4 activity may decrease metabolism and increase imatinib concentrations. There is a significant increase in exposure to imatinib when Gleevec is co-administered with ketoconazole).
- No products indexed under this heading.

Nicotinamide (Caution is recommended when administering Gleevec with inhibitors of the CYP3A4 family. Substances that inhibit CYP3A4 activity may decrease metabolism and increase imatinib concentrations. There is a significant increase in exposure to imatinib when Gleevec is co-administered with ketoconazole). Products include:
- Nicomide Tablets 3190

Nifedipine (Caution is recommended when administering Gleevec with inhibitors of the CYP3A4 family. Substances that inhibit CYP3A4 activity may decrease metabolism and increase imatinib concentrations. There is a significant increase in exposure to imatinib when Gleevec is co-administered with ketoconazole). Products include:
- Adalat CC Tablets 2978

Nisoldipine (Imatinib will increase plasma concentration of CYP3A4 metabolized drugs. (e.g., dihydropyridine calcium channel blockers)). Products include:
- Sular Tablets 1163

Norfloxacin (Caution is recommended when administering Gleevec with inhibitors of the CYP3A4 family. Substances that inhibit CYP3A4 activity may decrease metabolism and increase imatinib concentrations. There is a significant increase in exposure to imatinib when Gleevec is co-administered with ketoconazole). Products include:
- Noroxin Tablets 2009

Nortriptyline Hydrochloride (Imatinib is a potent competitive inhibitor of CYP2D6; therefore, imatinib is likely to increase the blood levels of drugs that are substrates of this enzyme).
- No products indexed under this heading.

Olanzapine (Imatinib is a potent competitive inhibitor of CYP2D6; therefore, imatinib is likely to increase the blood levels of drugs that are substrates of this enzyme). Products include:
- Symbyax Capsules 1788
- Zyprexa Tablets 1798
- Zyprexa IntraMuscular 1798
- Zyprexa ZYDIS Orally Disintegrating Tablets 1798

Omeprazole (Caution is recommended when administering Gleevec with inhibitors of the CYP3A4 family. Substances that inhibit CYP3A4 activity may decrease metabolism and increase imatinib concentrations. There is a significant increase in exposure to imatinib when Gleevec is co-administered with ketoconazole). Products include:
- Zegerid Powder for Oral Solution 2972

Ondansetron (Imatinib is a potent competitive inhibitor of CYP2D6; therefore, imatinib is likely to increase the blood levels of drugs that are substrates of this enzyme). Products include:
- Zofran ODT Orally Disintegrating Tablets 1613

Ondansetron Hydrochloride (Imatinib is a potent competitive inhibitor of CYP2D6; therefore, imatinib is likely to increase the blood levels of drugs that are substrates of this enzyme). Products include:
- Zofran Injection 1607
- Zofran 1613

Oxaprozin (Imatinib is a potent competitive inhibitor of CYP2C9; therefore, imatinib is likely to increase the blood levels of drugs that are substrates of this enzyme).
- No products indexed under this heading.

Oxcarbazepine (Substances that are inducers of CYP3A4 activity may increase metabolism and decrease imatinib plasma concentrations. Co-medications that induce CYP3A4 may significantly reduce exposure to Gleevec. Dosage of imatinib should be increased by at least 50% and clinical response should be carefully monitored in patients receiving imatinib with potent CYP3A4 inducers). Products include:
- Trileptal Oral Suspension 2281
- Trileptal Tablets 2281

Oxycodone Hydrochloride (Imatinib is a potent competitive inhibitor of CYP2D6; therefore, imatinib is likely to increase the blood levels of drugs that are substrates of this enzyme). Products include:
- Combunox Tablets 1183
- OxyContin Tablets 2699
- OxyFast Oral Concentrate Solution 2704
- OxyIR Capsules 2704
- Percocet Tablets 1114
- Percodan Tablets 1115

Paclitaxel (Imatinib is a potent competitive inhibitor of CYP2D6; therefore, imatinib is likely to increase the blood levels of drugs that are substrates of this enzyme).
- No products indexed under this heading.

Paroxetine Hydrochloride (Caution is recommended when administering Gleevec with inhibitors of the CYP3A4 family. Substances that inhibit CYP3A4 activity may decrease metabolism and increase imatinib concentrations. There is a significant increase in exposure to imatinib when Gleevec is co-administered with ketoconazole). Products include:
- Paxil CR Controlled-Release Tablets 1509
- Paxil 1501

Phenobarbital (Co-administration with inducers of CYP3A4, such as phenobarbital, may increase the metabolism and decrease imatinib concentrations).
- No products indexed under this heading.

Phenobarbital Sodium (Substances that are inducers of CYP3A4 activity may increase metabolism and decrease imatinib plasma concentrations. Co-medications that induce CYP3A4 may significantly reduce exposure to Gleevec. Dosage of imatinib should be increased by at least 50% and clinical response should be carefully monitored in patients receiving imatinib with potent CYP3A4 inducers).
- No products indexed under this heading.

Phenylbutazone (Imatinib is a potent competitive inhibitor of CYP2C9; therefore, imatinib is likely to increase the blood levels of drugs that are substrates of this enzyme).
- No products indexed under this heading.

Phenytoin (Co-administration with inducers of CYP3A4, such as phenytoin, may increase the metabolism and decrease imatinib concentrations. Dosage of imatinib should be increased by at least 50% and clinical response should be carefully monitored in patients receiving imatinib with a potent CYP3A4 inducer such as phenytoin).
- No products indexed under this heading.

Phenytoin Sodium (Co-administration with inducers of CYP3A4, such as phenytoin, may increase the metabolism and decrease imatinib concentrations. Dosage of imatinib should be increased by at least 50% and clinical response should be carefully monitored in patients receiving imatinib with a potent CYP3A4 inducer such as phenytoin). Products include:
- Phenytek Capsules 2153

Pimozide (Particular caution is recommended when administering imatinib with CYP3A4 substrates that have a narrow therapeutic window). Products include:
- Orap Tablets 1220

Pindolol (Imatinib is a potent competitive inhibitor of CYP2D6; therefore, imatinib is likely to increase the blood levels of drugs that are substrates of this enzyme).
- No products indexed under this heading.

Pioglitazone Hydrochloride (Imatinib is a potent competitive inhibitor of CYP2C9; therefore, imatinib is likely to increase the blood levels of drugs that are substrates of this enzyme). Products include:
- ActoPlus Met Tablets 3219
- Actos Tablets 3224

Piroxicam (Imatinib is a potent competitive inhibitor of CYP2C9; therefore, imatinib is likely to increase the blood levels of drugs that are substrates of this enzyme).
- No products indexed under this heading.

Prednisolone Acetate (Substances that are inducers of CYP3A4 activity may increase metabolism and decrease imatinib plasma concentrations. Co-medications that induce CYP3A4 may significantly reduce exposure to Gleevec. Dosage of imatinib should be increased by at least 50% and clinical response should be carefully monitored in patients receiving imatinib with potent CYP3A4 inducers). Products include:
- Blephamide Ophthalmic Ointment .... ⊙ 563
- Blephamide Ophthalmic Suspension .... ⊙ 564
- Poly-Pred Liquifilm Ophthalmic Suspension .... ⊙ 231
- Pred Forte Ophthalmic Suspension .... ⊙ 233
- Pred Mild Sterile Ophthalmic Suspension .... ⊙ 236
- Pred-G Ophthalmic Suspension .... ⊙ 234
- Pred-G Sterile Ophthalmic Ointment .... ⊙ 235

Prednisolone Sodium Phosphate (Substances that are inducers of CYP3A4 activity may increase metabolism and decrease imatinib plasma concentrations. Co-medications that induce CYP3A4 may significantly reduce exposure to Gleevec. Dosage of imatinib should be increased by at least 50% and clinical response should be carefully monitored in patients receiving imatinib with potent CYP3A4 inducers). Products include:
- Pediapred Oral Solution 3319

Prednisolone Tebutate (Substances that are inducers of CYP3A4 activity may increase metabolism and decrease imatinib plasma concentrations. Co-medications that induce CYP3A4 may significantly reduce exposure to Gleevec. Dosage of imatinib should be increased by at least 50% and clinical response should be carefully monitored in patients receiving imatinib with potent CYP3A4 inducers).
- No products indexed under this heading.

Prednisone (Substances that are inducers of CYP3A4 activity may increase metabolism and decrease imatinib plasma concentrations. Co-medications that induce CYP3A4 may significantly reduce exposure to Gleevec. Dosage of imatinib should be increased by at least 50% and clinical response should be carefully monitored in patients receiving imatinib with potent CYP3A4 inducers).
- No products indexed under this heading.

Primidone (Substances that are inducers of CYP3A4 activity may increase metabolism and decrease imatinib plasma concentrations. Co-medications that induce CYP3A4 may significantly reduce exposure to Gleevec. Dosage of imatinib should be increased by at least 50% and clinical response should be carefully monitored in patients receiving imatinib with potent CYP3A4 inducers).
- No products indexed under this heading.

Propafenone Hydrochloride (Imatinib is a potent competitive inhibitor of CYP2D6; therefore, imatinib is likely to increase the blood levels of drugs that are substrates of this enzyme). Products include:
- Rythmol SR Capsules 2736

Propoxyphene Hydrochloride (Caution is recommended when administering Gleevec with inhibitors of the CYP3A4 family. Substances that inhibit CYP3A4 activity may decrease metabolism and increase imatinib concentrations. There is a significant increase in exposure to imatinib when Gleevec is co-administered with ketoconazole).
- No products indexed under this heading.

Propoxyphene Napsylate (Caution is recommended when administering Gleevec with inhibitors of the CYP3A4 family. Substances that

inhibit CYP3A4 activity may decrease metabolism and increase imatinib concentrations. There is a significant increase in exposure to imatinib when Gleevec is co-administered with ketoconazole). Products include:

Darvocet A 500 Tablets 3497

Propranolol Hydrochloride (Imatinib is a potent competitive inhibitor of CYP2D6; therefore, imatinib is likely to increase the blood levels of drugs that are substrates of this enzyme). Products include:

Inderal LA Long-Acting Capsules 3421
InnoPran XL Capsules 2728

Quetiapine Fumarate (Imatinib is a potent competitive inhibitor of CYP2D6; therefore, imatinib is likely to increase the blood levels of drugs that are substrates of this enzyme). Products include:

Seroquel Tablets 691

Quinidine (Caution is recommended when administering Gleevec with inhibitors of the CYP3A4 family. Substances that inhibit CYP3A4 activity may decrease metabolism and increase imatinib concentrations. There is a significant increase in exposure to imatinib when Gleevec is co-administered with ketoconazole).

No products indexed under this heading.

Quinidine Gluconate (Imatinib is a potent competitive inhibitor of CYP2D6; therefore, imatinib is likely to increase the blood levels of drugs that are substrates of this enzyme).

No products indexed under this heading.

Quinidine Hydrochloride (Caution is recommended when administering Gleevec with inhibitors of the CYP3A4 family. Substances that inhibit CYP3A4 activity may decrease metabolism and increase imatinib concentrations. There is a significant increase in exposure to imatinib when Gleevec is co-administered with ketoconazole).

No products indexed under this heading.

Quinidine Polygalacturonate (Caution is recommended when administering Gleevec with inhibitors of the CYP3A4 family. Substances that inhibit CYP3A4 activity may decrease metabolism and increase imatinib concentrations. There is a significant increase in exposure to imatinib when Gleevec is co-administered with ketoconazole).

No products indexed under this heading.

Quinidine Sulfate (Caution is recommended when administering Gleevec with inhibitors of the CYP3A4 family. Substances that inhibit CYP3A4 activity may decrease metabolism and increase imatinib concentrations. There is a significant increase in exposure to imatinib when Gleevec is co-administered with ketoconazole).

No products indexed under this heading.

Quinine (Caution is recommended when administering Gleevec with inhibitors of the CYP3A4 family. Substances that inhibit CYP3A4 activity may decrease metabolism and increase imatinib concentrations. There is a significant increase in exposure to imatinib when Gleevec is co-administered with ketoconazole).

No products indexed under this heading.

Quinine Sulfate (Caution is recommended when administering Gleevec with inhibitors of the CYP3A4 family. Substances that inhibit CYP3A4 activity may decrease metabolism and increase imatinib concentrations. There is a significant increase in exposure to imatinib when Gleevec is co-administered with ketoconazole).

No products indexed under this heading.

Quinupristin (Caution is recommended when administering Gleevec with inhibitors of the CYP3A4 family. Substances that inhibit CYP3A4 activity may decrease metabolism and increase imatinib concentrations. There is a significant increase in exposure to imatinib when Gleevec is co-administered with ketoconazole). Products include:

Synercid I.V. 1690

Ranitidine Bismuth Citrate (Caution is recommended when administering Gleevec with inhibitors of the CYP3A4 family. Substances that inhibit CYP3A4 activity may decrease metabolism and increase imatinib concentrations. There is a significant increase in exposure to imatinib when Gleevec is co-administered with ketoconazole).

No products indexed under this heading.

Ranitidine Hydrochloride (Caution is recommended when administering Gleevec with inhibitors of the CYP3A4 family. Substances that inhibit CYP3A4 activity may decrease metabolism and increase imatinib concentrations. There is a significant increase in exposure to imatinib when Gleevec is co-administered with ketoconazole). Products include:

Zantac 1597
Zantac Injection 1593
Zantac 75 Tablets 715
Zantac 150 Maximum Strength Tablets 715
Zantac Injection Pharmacy Bulk Package 1595

Repaglinide (Imatinib is a potent competitive inhibitor of CYP2C9; therefore, imatinib is likely to increase the blood levels of drugs that are substrates of this enzyme). Products include:

Prandin Tablets (0.5, 1, and 2 mg) 2337

Rifabutin (Substances that are inducers of CYP3A4 activity may increase metabolism and decrease imatinib plasma concentrations. Co-medications that induce CYP3A4 may significantly reduce exposure to Gleevec. Dosage of imatinib should be increased by at least 50% and clinical response should be carefully monitored in patients receiving imatinib with potent CYP3A4 inducers).

No products indexed under this heading.

Rifampicin (Substances that are inducers of CYP3A4 activity may increase metabolism and decrease imatinib plasma concentrations. Co-medications that induce CYP3A4 may significantly reduce exposure to Gleevec. Dosage of imatinib should be increased by at least 50% and clinical response should be carefully monitored in patients receiving imatinib with potent CYP3A4 inducers).

No products indexed under this heading.

Rifampin (Co-administration with inducers of CYP3A4, such as rifampin, may increase the metabolism and decrease imatinib concentrations. Dosage of imatinib should be increased by at least 50% and clinical response should be carefully monitored in patients receiving imatinib with a potent CYP3A4 inducer, such as rifampin).

No products indexed under this heading.

Rifapentine (Substances that are inducers of CYP3A4 activity may increase metabolism and decrease imatinib plasma concentrations. Co-medications that induce CYP3A4 may significantly reduce exposure to Gleevec. Dosage of imatinib should be increased by at least 50% and clinical response should be carefully monitored in patients receiving imatinib with potent CYP3A4 inducers).

No products indexed under this heading.

Risperidone (Imatinib is a potent competitive inhibitor of CYP2D6; therefore, imatinib is likely to increase the blood levels of drugs that are substrates of this enzyme). Products include:

Risperdal Consta Long-Acting Injection 1664
Risperdal M-Tab Orally Disintegrating Tablets 1658
Risperdal 1658

Ritonavir (Caution is recommended when administering Gleevec with inhibitors of the CYP3A4 family. Substances that inhibit CYP3A4 activity may decrease metabolism and increase imatinib concentrations. There is a significant increase in exposure to imatinib when Gleevec is co-administered with ketoconazole). Products include:

Kaletra 474
Norvir 499

Rofecoxib (Imatinib is a potent competitive inhibitor of CYP2C9; therefore, imatinib is likely to increase the blood levels of drugs that are substrates of this enzyme).

No products indexed under this heading.

Rosiglitazone Maleate (Imatinib is a potent competitive inhibitor of CYP2C9; therefore, imatinib is likely to increase the blood levels of drugs that are substrates of this enzyme). Products include:

Avandamet Tablets 1343
Avandia Tablets 1348

Saquinavir (Caution is recommended when administering Gleevec with inhibitors of the CYP3A4 family. Substances that inhibit CYP3A4 activity may decrease metabolism and increase imatinib concentrations. There is a significant increase in exposure to imatinib when Gleevec is co-administered with ketoconazole).

No products indexed under this heading.

Saquinavir Mesylate (Caution is recommended when administering Gleevec with inhibitors of the CYP3A4 family. Substances that inhibit CYP3A4 activity may decrease metabolism and increase imatinib concentrations. There is a significant increase in exposure to imatinib when Gleevec is co-administered with ketoconazole). Products include:

Invirase 2776

Sertraline Hydrochloride (Caution is recommended when administering Gleevec with inhibitors of the CYP3A4 family. Substances that inhibit CYP3A4 activity may decrease metabolism and increase imatinib concentrations. There is a significant increase in exposure to imatinib when Gleevec is co-administered with ketoconazole). Products include:

Zoloft 2581

Sildenafil Citrate (Imatinib is a potent competitive inhibitor of CYP2C9; therefore, imatinib is likely to increase the blood levels of drugs that are substrates of this enzyme). Products include:

Revatio Tablets 2541
Viagra Tablets 2552

Simvastatin (Imatinib increases the mean Cmax and AUC of simvastatin 2- and 3.5-fold, respectively by inhibiting CYP3A4). Products include:

Vytorin 10/10 Tablets 2084
Vytorin 10/10 Tablets 3092
Vytorin 10/20 Tablets 2084
Vytorin 10/20 Tablets 3092
Vytorin 10/40 Tablets 3092
Vytorin 10/40 Tablets 2084
Vytorin 10/80 Tablets 2084
Vytorin 10/80 Tablets 3092
Zocor Tablets 2078

Sulfamethoxazole (Imatinib is a potent competitive inhibitor of CYP2C9; therefore, imatinib is likely to increase the blood levels of drugs that are substrates of this enzyme).

No products indexed under this heading.

Sulfinpyrazone (Substances that are inducers of CYP3A4 activity may increase metabolism and decrease imatinib plasma concentrations. Co-medications that induce CYP3A4 may significantly reduce exposure to Gleevec. Dosage of imatinib should be increased by at least 50% and clinical response should be carefully monitored in patients receiving imatinib with potent CYP3A4 inducers).

No products indexed under this heading.

Sulindac (Imatinib is a potent competitive inhibitor of CYP2C9; therefore, imatinib is likely to increase the blood levels of drugs that are substrates of this enzyme). Products include:

Clinoril Tablets 1899

Suprofen (Imatinib is a potent competitive inhibitor of CYP2C9; therefore, imatinib is likely to increase the blood levels of drugs that are substrates of this enzyme).

No products indexed under this heading.

Tamoxifen Citrate (Imatinib is a potent competitive inhibitor of CYP2D6; therefore, imatinib is likely to increase the blood levels of drugs that are substrates of this enzyme).

No products indexed under this heading.

Telithromycin (Caution is recommended when administering Gleevec with inhibitors of the CYP3A4 family. Substances that inhibit CYP3A4 activity may decrease metabolism and increase imatinib concentrations. There is a significant increase in exposure to imatinib when Gleevec is co-administered with ketoconazole). Products include:

Ketek Tablets 2920

Telmisartan (Imatinib is a potent competitive inhibitor of CYP2C9; therefore, imatinib is likely to

increase the blood levels of drugs that are substrates of this enzyme). Products include:
Micardis Tablets 884
Micardis HCT Tablets 886

Teniposide (Imatinib is a potent competitive inhibitor of CYP2D6; therefore, imatinib is likely to increase the blood levels of drugs that are substrates of this enzyme).
No products indexed under this heading.

Testosterone (Imatinib is a potent competitive inhibitor of CYP2D6; therefore, imatinib is likely to increase the blood levels of drugs that are substrates of this enzyme). Products include:
AndroGel 3330
Striant Mucoadhesive 1022
Testim 1% Gel 722

Testosterone Cypionate (Imatinib is a potent competitive inhibitor of CYP2D6; therefore, imatinib is likely to increase the blood levels of drugs that are substrates of this enzyme).
No products indexed under this heading.

Testosterone Enanthate (Imatinib is a potent competitive inhibitor of CYP2D6; therefore, imatinib is likely to increase the blood levels of drugs that are substrates of this enzyme). Products include:
Delatestryl Injection 2976

Testosterone Propionate (Imatinib is a potent competitive inhibitor of CYP2D6; therefore, imatinib is likely to increase the blood levels of drugs that are substrates of this enzyme).
No products indexed under this heading.

Theophylline (Substances that are inducers of CYP3A4 activity may increase metabolism and decrease imatinib plasma concentrations. Co-medications that induce CYP3A4 may significantly reduce exposure to Gleevec. Dosage of imatinib should be increased by at least 50% and clinical response should be carefully monitored in patients receiving imatinib with potent CYP3A4 inducers).
No products indexed under this heading.

Thioridazine (Imatinib is a potent competitive inhibitor of CYP2D6; therefore, imatinib is likely to increase the blood levels of drugs that are substrates of this enzyme).
No products indexed under this heading.

Thioridazine Hydrochloride (Imatinib is a potent competitive inhibitor of CYP2D6; therefore, imatinib is likely to increase the blood levels of drugs that are substrates of this enzyme). Products include:
Thioridazine Hydrochloride Tablets 2122

Timolol Maleate (Imatinib is a potent competitive inhibitor of CYP2D6; therefore, imatinib is likely to increase the blood levels of drugs that are substrates of this enzyme). Products include:
Blocadren Tablets 1891
Cosopt Sterile Ophthalmic Solution 1910
Timolide Tablets 2056
Timoptic in Ocudose 2061
Timoptic Sterile Ophthalmic Solution 2058
Timoptic-XE Sterile Ophthalmic Gel Forming Solution 2062

Tolazamide (Imatinib is a potent competitive inhibitor of CYP2C9; therefore, imatinib is likely to increase the blood levels of drugs that are substrates of this enzyme).
No products indexed under this heading.

Tolbutamide (Imatinib is a potent competitive inhibitor of CYP2C9; therefore, imatinib is likely to increase the blood levels of drugs that are substrates of this enzyme).
No products indexed under this heading.

Tolbutamide Sodium (Imatinib is a potent competitive inhibitor of CYP2C9; therefore, imatinib is likely to increase the blood levels of drugs that are substrates of this enzyme).
No products indexed under this heading.

Tolmetin Sodium (Imatinib is a potent competitive inhibitor of CYP2C9; therefore, imatinib is likely to increase the blood levels of drugs that are substrates of this enzyme).
No products indexed under this heading.

Tolterodine Tartrate (Imatinib is a potent competitive inhibitor of CYP2D6; therefore, imatinib is likely to increase the blood levels of drugs that are substrates of this enzyme). Products include:
Detrol Tablets 2626
Detrol LA Capsules 2629

Torsemide (Imatinib is a potent competitive inhibitor of CYP2C9; therefore, imatinib is likely to increase the blood levels of drugs that are substrates of this enzyme).
No products indexed under this heading.

Tramadol Hydrochloride (Imatinib is a potent competitive inhibitor of CYP2D6; therefore, imatinib is likely to increase the blood levels of drugs that are substrates of this enzyme). Products include:
Ultracet Tablets 2462

Trazodone Hydrochloride (Imatinib is a potent competitive inhibitor of CYP2D6; therefore, imatinib is likely to increase the blood levels of drugs that are substrates of this enzyme).
No products indexed under this heading.

Triamcinolone (Substances that are inducers of CYP3A4 activity may increase metabolism and decrease imatinib plasma concentrations. Co-medications that induce CYP3A4 may significantly reduce exposure to Gleevec. Dosage of imatinib should be increased by at least 50% and clinical response should be carefully monitored in patients receiving imatinib with potent CYP3A4 inducers).
No products indexed under this heading.

Triamcinolone Acetonide (Substances that are inducers of CYP3A4 activity may increase metabolism and decrease imatinib plasma concentrations. Co-medications that induce CYP3A4 may significantly reduce exposure to Gleevec. Dosage of imatinib should be increased by at least 50% and clinical response should be carefully monitored in patients receiving imatinib with potent CYP3A4 inducers). Products include:
Azmacort Inhalation Aerosol 1701
Nasacort HFA Inhalation Aerosol 2939
Nasacort AQ Nasal Spray 2937

Triamcinolone Diacetate (Substances that are inducers of CYP3A4 activity may increase metabolism and decrease imatinib plasma concentrations. Co-medications that induce CYP3A4 may significantly reduce exposure to Gleevec. Dosage of imatinib should be increased by at least 50% and clinical response should be carefully monitored in patients receiving imatinib with potent CYP3A4 inducers).
No products indexed under this heading.

Triamcinolone Hexacetonide (Substances that are inducers of CYP3A4 activity may increase metabolism and decrease imatinib plasma concentrations. Co-medications that induce CYP3A4 may significantly reduce exposure to Gleevec. Dosage of imatinib should be increased by at least 50% and clinical response should be carefully monitored in patients receiving imatinib with potent CYP3A4 inducers).
No products indexed under this heading.

Triazolam (Imatinib is a potent competitive inhibitor of CYP2D6; therefore, imatinib is likely to increase the blood levels of drugs that are substrates of this enzyme).
No products indexed under this heading.

Trimipramine Maleate (Imatinib is a potent competitive inhibitor of CYP2D6; therefore, imatinib is likely to increase the blood levels of drugs that are substrates of this enzyme). Products include:
Surmontil Capsules 2347

Troglitazone (Caution is recommended when administering Gleevec with inhibitors of the CYP3A4 family. Substances that inhibit CYP3A4 activity may decrease metabolism and increase imatinib concentrations. There is a significant increase in exposure to imatinib when Gleevec is co-administered with ketoconazole).
No products indexed under this heading.

Troleandomycin (Caution is recommended when administering Gleevec with inhibitors of the CYP3A4 family. Substances that inhibit CYP3A4 activity may decrease metabolism and increase imatinib concentrations. There is a significant increase in exposure to imatinib when Gleevec is co-administered with ketoconazole).
No products indexed under this heading.

Valdecoxib (Imatinib is a potent competitive inhibitor of CYP2C9; therefore, imatinib is likely to increase the blood levels of drugs that are substrates of this enzyme).
No products indexed under this heading.

Valproate Sodium (Caution is recommended when administering Gleevec with inhibitors of the CYP3A4 family. Substances that inhibit CYP3A4 activity may decrease metabolism and increase imatinib concentrations. There is a significant increase in exposure to imatinib when Gleevec is co-administered with ketoconazole). Products include:
Depacon Injection 412

Valsartan (Imatinib is a potent competitive inhibitor of CYP2C9; therefore, imatinib is likely to increase the blood levels of drugs that are substrates of this enzyme). Products include:
Diovan HCT Tablets 2195
Diovan Tablets 2191

Venlafaxine Hydrochloride (Imatinib is a potent competitive inhibitor of CYP2D6; therefore, imatinib is likely to increase the blood levels of drugs that are substrates of this enzyme). Products include:
Effexor Tablets 3405
Effexor XR Capsules 3411

Verapamil Hydrochloride (Caution is recommended when administering Gleevec with inhibitors of the CYP3A4 family. Substances that inhibit CYP3A4 activity may decrease metabolism and increase imatinib concentrations. There is a significant increase in exposure to imatinib when Gleevec is co-administered with ketoconazole). Products include:
Covera-HS Tablets 3135
Tarka Tablets 519
Verelan PM Capsules 3120

Vinblastine Sulfate (Imatinib is a potent competitive inhibitor of CYP2D6; therefore, imatinib is likely to increase the blood levels of drugs that are substrates of this enzyme).
No products indexed under this heading.

Voriconazole (Caution is recommended when administering Gleevec with inhibitors of the CYP3A4 family. Substances that inhibit CYP3A4 activity may decrease metabolism and increase imatinib concentrations. There is a significant increase in exposure to imatinib when Gleevec is co-administered with ketoconazole). Products include:
VFEND I.V. 2543
VFEND Oral Suspension 2543
VFEND Tablets 2543

Warfarin Sodium (Imatinib is a potent competitive inhibitor of CYP2C9; warfarin is metabolized by CYP2C9; therefore, patients who require anticoagulation should receive low-molecular weight or standard heparin). Products include:
Coumadin for Injection 932
Coumadin Tablets 932

Zafirlukast (Caution is recommended when administering Gleevec with inhibitors of the CYP3A4 family. Substances that inhibit CYP3A4 activity may decrease metabolism and increase imatinib concentrations. There is a significant increase in exposure to imatinib when Gleevec is co-administered with ketoconazole). Products include:
Accolate Tablets 663

Zileuton (Caution is recommended when administering Gleevec with inhibitors of the CYP3A4 family. Substances that inhibit CYP3A4 activity may decrease metabolism and increase imatinib concentrations. There is a significant increase in exposure to imatinib when Gleevec is co-administered with ketoconazole).
No products indexed under this heading.

Zonisamide (Imatinib is a potent competitive inhibitor of CYP2D6; therefore, imatinib is likely to increase the blood levels of drugs that are substrates of this enzyme). Products include:
Zonegran Capsules 1089

Food Interactions

Grapefruit (Caution is recommended when administering Gleevec with inhibitors of the CYP3A4 family. Substances that inhibit CYP3A4 activity may decrease metabolism and increase imatinib concentrations. There is a significant increase in exposure to imatinib when Gleevec is co-administered with ketoconazole).

Grapefruit Juice (Caution is recommended when administering Gleevec with inhibitors of the CYP3A4 family. Substances that inhibit CYP3A4 activity may decrease metabolism and increase imatinib concentrations. There is a significant increase in exposure to imatinib when Gleevec is co-administered with ketoconazole).

GLUCA-BALANCE CAPSULES

(Amino Acid Preparations) 2110
None cited in PDR database.

GLUCAGEN FOR INJECTION

(Glucagon) 790
May interact with beta blockers. Compounds in these categories include:

Acebutolol Hydrochloride (Patients taking beta blockers might be expected to have a greater increase in both pulse and blood pressure).
No products indexed under this heading.

Atenolol (Patients taking beta blockers might be expected to have a greater increase in both pulse and blood pressure). Products include:
Tenormin I.V. Injection 698
Tenormin Tablets 695

Betaxolol Hydrochloride (Patients taking beta blockers might be expected to have a greater increase in both pulse and blood pressure). Products include:
Betoptic S Ophthalmic Suspension.................................. 554

Bisoprolol Fumarate (Patients taking beta blockers might be expected to have a greater increase in both pulse and blood pressure).
No products indexed under this heading.

Carteolol Hydrochloride (Patients taking beta blockers might be expected to have a greater increase in both pulse and blood pressure). Products include:
Carteolol Hydrochloride Ophthalmic Solution USP, 1%....... ⊙246

Esmolol Hydrochloride (Patients taking beta blockers might be expected to have a greater increase in both pulse and blood pressure). Products include:
Brevibloc Concentrate 766
Brevibloc Injection 766
Brevibloc Double Strength Injection.. 766
Brevibloc Premixed Injection 766
Brevibloc Double Strength Premixed Injection 766

Labetalol Hydrochloride (Patients taking beta blockers might be expected to have a greater increase in both pulse and blood pressure).
No products indexed under this heading.

Levobunolol Hydrochloride (Patients taking beta blockers might be expected to have a greater increase in both pulse and blood pressure). Products include:
Betagan Ophthalmic Solution, USP... ⊙217

Metipranolol Hydrochloride (Patients taking beta blockers might be expected to have a greater increase in both pulse and blood pressure).
No products indexed under this heading.

Metoprolol Succinate (Patients taking beta blockers might be expected to have a greater increase in both pulse and blood pressure). Products include:
Toprol-XL Tablets 660

Metoprolol Tartrate (Patients taking beta blockers might be expected to have a greater increase in both pulse and blood pressure).
No products indexed under this heading.

Nadolol (Patients taking beta blockers might be expected to have a greater increase in both pulse and blood pressure). Products include:
Nadolol Tablets 2121

Penbutolol Sulfate (Patients taking beta blockers might be expected to have a greater increase in both pulse and blood pressure).
No products indexed under this heading.

Pindolol (Patients taking beta blockers might be expected to have a greater increase in both pulse and blood pressure).
No products indexed under this heading.

Propranolol Hydrochloride (Patients taking beta blockers might be expected to have a greater increase in both pulse and blood pressure). Products include:
Inderal LA Long-Acting Capsules 3421
InnoPran XL Capsules 2728

Sotalol Hydrochloride (Patients taking beta blockers might be expected to have a greater increase in both pulse and blood pressure).
No products indexed under this heading.

Timolol Hemihydrate (Patients taking beta blockers might be expected to have a greater increase in both pulse and blood pressure). Products include:
Betimol Ophthalmic Solution 3371
Betimol Ophthalmic Solution .... ⊙283

Timolol Maleate (Patients taking beta blockers might be expected to have a greater increase in both pulse and blood pressure). Products include:
Blocadren Tablets 1891
Cosopt Sterile Ophthalmic Solution....................................... 1910
Timolide Tablets 2056
Timoptic in Ocudose 2061
Timoptic Sterile Ophthalmic Solution....................................... 2058
Timoptic-XE Sterile Ophthalmic Gel Forming Solution.................... 2062

GLUCAGON FOR INJECTION VIALS AND EMERGENCY KIT

(Glucagon) 1749
None cited in PDR database.

GLY-OXIDE LIQUID

(Carbamide Peroxide) .... ▣620
None cited in PDR database.

GONAL-F RFF PEN FOR INJECTION

(Follitropin Alfa) 3155
None cited in PDR database.

GOODY'S BODY PAIN FORMULA POWDER

(Acetaminophen, Aspirin) .... ▣621
See Goody's Extra Strength Pain Relief Tablets

GOODY'S EXTRA STRENGTH HEADACHE POWDER

(Acetaminophen, Aspirin, Caffeine)... ▣621
See Goody's Extra Strength Pain Relief Tablets

GOODY'S EXTRA STRENGTH PAIN RELIEF TABLETS

(Acetaminophen, Aspirin, Caffeine)... ▣621
May interact with oral anticoagulants, oral hypoglycemic agents, and certain other agents. Compounds in these categories include:

Acarbose (Concurrent use should be avoided unless directed by a physician). Products include:
Precose Tablets 776

Anisindione (Concurrent use should be avoided unless directed by a physician). Products include:
Miradon Tablets 3056

Chlorpropamide (Concurrent use should be avoided unless directed by a physician).
No products indexed under this heading.

Dicumarol (Concurrent use should be avoided unless directed by a physician).
No products indexed under this heading.

Glimepiride (Concurrent use should be avoided unless directed by a physician). Products include:
Amaryl Tablets 2864

Glipizide (Concurrent use should be avoided unless directed by a physician).
No products indexed under this heading.

Glyburide (Concurrent use should be avoided unless directed by a physician).
No products indexed under this heading.

Metformin Hydrochloride (Concurrent use should be avoided unless directed by a physician). Products include:
ActoPlus Met Tablets 3219
Avandamet Tablets 1343
Fortamet Extended-Release Tablets.. 1156

Miglitol (Concurrent use should be avoided unless directed by a physician).
No products indexed under this heading.

Pioglitazone Hydrochloride (Concurrent use should be avoided unless directed by a physician). Products include:
ActoPlus Met Tablets 3219
Actos Tablets 3224

Repaglinide (Concurrent use should be avoided unless directed by a physician). Products include:
Prandin Tablets (0.5, 1, and 2 mg)... 2337

Rosiglitazone Maleate (Concurrent use should be avoided unless directed by a physician). Products include:
Avandamet Tablets 1343
Avandia Tablets 1348

Tolazamide (Concurrent use should be avoided unless directed by a physician).
No products indexed under this heading.

Tolbutamide (Concurrent use should be avoided unless directed by a physician).
No products indexed under this heading.

Troglitazone (Concurrent use should be avoided unless directed by a physician).
No products indexed under this heading.

Warfarin Sodium (Concurrent use should be avoided unless directed by a physician). Products include:
Coumadin for Injection 932
Coumadin Tablets 932

Food Interactions

Alcohol (Individuals consuming 3 or more alcohol-containing drinks per day should consult their physicians for advice on when and how they should take this product).

GOODY'S PM POWDER

(Acetaminophen, Diphenhydramine Citrate)................. ▣622
May interact with hypnotics and sedatives, tranquilizers, and certain other agents. Compounds in these categories include:

Alprazolam (Concurrent use is not recommended). Products include:
Niravam Orally Disintegrating Tablets.. 3106
Xanax XR Tablets 2655

Buspirone Hydrochloride (Concurrent use is not recommended).
No products indexed under this heading.

Chlordiazepoxide (Concurrent use is not recommended).
No products indexed under this heading.

Chlordiazepoxide Hydrochloride (Concurrent use is not recommended). Products include:
Librium Capsules 3349

Chlorpromazine (Concurrent use is not recommended).
No products indexed under this heading.

Chlorpromazine Hydrochloride (Concurrent use is not recommended).
No products indexed under this heading.

Chlorprothixene (Concurrent use is not recommended).
No products indexed under this heading.

Chlorprothixene Hydrochloride (Concurrent use is not recommended).
No products indexed under this heading.

Clorazepate Dipotassium (Concurrent use is not recommended). Products include:
Tranxene 2488

Diazepam (Concurrent use is not recommended). Products include:
Diastat Rectal Delivery System 3344
Valium Tablets 2822

Diphenhydramine (Concurrent use with other diphenhydramine-containing products is not recommended). Products include:
Tylenol Sore Throat NightTime Liquid with Cool Burst.................. 1849

Diphenhydramine Hydrochloride (Concurrent use with any other prod-

uct containing diphenhydramine, including topical preparations, should be avoided). Products include:

Benadryl Allergy & Cold Tablets ..... ▣692
Benadryl Allergy ..... ▣691
Benadryl Allergy & Sinus Headache Caplets & Gelcaps ..... ▣693
Children's Benadryl Allergy Liquid ... ▣695
Children's Benadryl Dye-Free Allergy Liquid ..... ▣695
Benadryl Dye-Free Allergy Liqui-Gels Softgels ..... ▣692
Benadryl Itch Relief Stick Extra Strength ..... ▣696
Benadryl Itch Stopping Cream Extra Strength ..... ▣697
Benadryl Itch Stopping Gel Extra Strength ..... ▣697
Benadryl Itch Stopping Spray Extra Strength ..... ▣697
Benadryl Maximum Strength Severe Allergy & Sinus Headache Caplets ..... ▣694
Children's Benadryl D Liquid Medication ..... ▣693
Benadryl D Tablets ..... ▣694
Nytol QuickCaps Caplets ..... ▣635
Maximum Strength Nytol QuickGels Softgels ..... ▣635
Simply Sleep Caplets 1841
Sominex Original Formula Tablets .. ▣637
TheraFlu Thin Strips Multi Symptom ..... ▣684
Triaminic Thin Strips Cough & Runny Nose ..... ▣690
Children's Tylenol Plus Cold & Allergy Suspension Liquid 1850
Tylenol Allergy Complete Night Time Caplets 1844
Tylenol Severe Allergy Caplets 1844
Tylenol Flu NightTime Gelcaps 1846
Extra Strength Tylenol PM Caplets, Geltabs, Gelcaps and Liquid 1847
Unisom Maximum Strength SleepGels ..... ▣712

Droperidol (Concurrent use is not recommended).
No products indexed under this heading.

Estazolam (Concurrent use is not recommended). Products include:
ProSom Tablets 512

Ethchlorvynol (Concurrent use is not recommended).
No products indexed under this heading.

Ethinamate (Concurrent use is not recommended).
No products indexed under this heading.

Fluphenazine Decanoate (Concurrent use is not recommended).
No products indexed under this heading.

Fluphenazine Enanthate (Concurrent use is not recommended).
No products indexed under this heading.

Fluphenazine Hydrochloride (Concurrent use is not recommended).
No products indexed under this heading.

Flurazepam Hydrochloride (Concurrent use is not recommended). Products include:
Dalmane Capsules 3343

Glutethimide (Concurrent use is not recommended).
No products indexed under this heading.

Haloperidol (Concurrent use is not recommended).
No products indexed under this heading.

Haloperidol Decanoate (Concurrent use is not recommended).
No products indexed under this heading.

Hydroxyzine Hydrochloride (Concurrent use is not recommended).
No products indexed under this heading.

Lorazepam (Concurrent use is not recommended).
No products indexed under this heading.

Loxapine Hydrochloride (Concurrent use is not recommended).
No products indexed under this heading.

Loxapine Succinate (Concurrent use is not recommended).
No products indexed under this heading.

Meprobamate (Concurrent use is not recommended).
No products indexed under this heading.

Mesoridazine Besylate (Concurrent use is not recommended).
No products indexed under this heading.

Midazolam Hydrochloride (Concurrent use is not recommended).
No products indexed under this heading.

Molindone Hydrochloride (Concurrent use is not recommended). Products include:
Moban Tablets 1108

Oxazepam (Concurrent use is not recommended).
No products indexed under this heading.

Perphenazine (Concurrent use is not recommended).
No products indexed under this heading.

Prazepam (Concurrent use is not recommended).
No products indexed under this heading.

Prochlorperazine (Concurrent use is not recommended).
No products indexed under this heading.

Promethazine Hydrochloride (Concurrent use is not recommended). Products include:
Phenergan 3438

Propofol (Concurrent use is not recommended). Products include:
Diprivan Injectable Emulsion 676

Quazepam (Concurrent use is not recommended).
No products indexed under this heading.

Secobarbital Sodium (Concurrent use is not recommended).
No products indexed under this heading.

Temazepam (Concurrent use is not recommended).
No products indexed under this heading.

Thioridazine Hydrochloride (Concurrent use is not recommended). Products include:
Thioridazine Hydrochloride Tablets 2122

Thiothixene (Concurrent use is not recommended). Products include:
Thiothixene Capsules 2124

Triazolam (Concurrent use is not recommended).
No products indexed under this heading.

Trifluoperazine Hydrochloride (Concurrent use is not recommended).
No products indexed under this heading.

Zaleplon (Concurrent use is not recommended). Products include:
Sonata Capsules 1686

Zolpidem Tartrate (Concurrent use is not recommended). Products include:
Ambien Tablets 2867

Food Interactions

Alcohol (Individuals consuming 3 or more alcohol-containing drinks per day should consult their physicians for advice on when and how they should take this product; avoid alcoholic beverages since diphenhydramine causes drowsiness).

GORDOCHOM SOLUTION

(Chloroxylenol, Undecylenic Acid) 1634
None cited in PDR database.

GRIFULVIN V TABLETS MICROSIZE AND ORAL SUSPENSION MICROSIZE

(Griseofulvin) 2384
May interact with barbiturates, oral anticoagulants, and oral contraceptives. Compounds in these categories include:

Anisindione (Dosage adjustment of anticoagulant may be necessary). Products include:
Miradon Tablets 3056

Aprobarbital (Usually depresses griseofulvin activity; may necessitate dosage increase).
No products indexed under this heading.

Butabarbital (Usually depresses griseofulvin activity; may necessitate dosage increase).
No products indexed under this heading.

Butalbital (Usually depresses griseofulvin activity; may necessitate dosage increase). Products include:
Sedapap Tablets 50 mg/650 mg 2098

Desogestrel (Reduced contraceptive efficacy; increased incidence of breakthrough bleeding). Products include:
Ortho-Cept Tablets 2395

Dicumarol (Dosage adjustment of anticoagulant may be necessary).
No products indexed under this heading.

Ethinyl Estradiol (Reduced contraceptive efficacy; increased incidence of breakthrough bleeding). Products include:
Alesse-28 Tablets 3392
Lo/Ovral-28 Tablets 3423
NuvaRing 2357
Ortho-Cept Tablets 2395
Ortho-Cyclen/Ortho Tri-Cyclen 2414
Ortho Evra Transdermal System 2402
Ortho Tri-Cyclen Lo Tablets 2421
Seasonale Tablets 1073
Triphasil-28 Tablets 3483
Yasmin 28 Tablets 818

Ethynodiol Diacetate (Reduced contraceptive efficacy; increased incidence of breakthrough bleeding).
No products indexed under this heading.

Levonorgestrel (Reduced contraceptive efficacy; increased incidence of breakthrough bleeding). Products include:
Alesse-28 Tablets 3392
Climara Pro Transdermal System 800
Mirena Intrauterine System 810
Plan B Tablets 1068
Seasonale Tablets 1073
Triphasil-28 Tablets 3483

Mephobarbital (Usually depresses griseofulvin activity; may necessitate dosage increase). Products include:
Mebaral Tablets, USP 2483

Mestranol (Reduced contraceptive efficacy; increased incidence of breakthrough bleeding).
No products indexed under this heading.

Norethindrone (Reduced contraceptive efficacy; increased incidence of breakthrough bleeding). Products include:
Ortho Micronor Tablets 2411

Norethynodrel (Reduced contraceptive efficacy; increased incidence of breakthrough bleeding).
No products indexed under this heading.

Norgestimate (Reduced contraceptive efficacy; increased incidence of breakthrough bleeding). Products include:
Ortho-Cyclen/Ortho Tri-Cyclen 2414
Ortho Tri-Cyclen Lo Tablets 2421
Prefest Tablets 1069

Norgestrel (Reduced contraceptive efficacy; increased incidence of breakthrough bleeding). Products include:
Lo/Ovral-28 Tablets 3423

Pentobarbital Sodium (Usually depresses griseofulvin activity; may necessitate dosage increase). Products include:
Nembutal Sodium Solution, USP 2484

Phenobarbital (Usually depresses griseofulvin activity; may necessitate dosage increase).
No products indexed under this heading.

Secobarbital Sodium (Usually depresses griseofulvin activity; may necessitate dosage increase).
No products indexed under this heading.

Thiamylal Sodium (Usually depresses griseofulvin activity; may necessitate dosage increase).
No products indexed under this heading.

Warfarin Sodium (Dosage adjustment of anticoagulant may be necessary). Products include:
Coumadin for Injection 932
Coumadin Tablets 932

GRIS-PEG TABLETS

(Griseofulvin) 2504
May interact with barbiturates, oral contraceptives, and certain other agents. Compounds in these categories include:

Aprobarbital (Barbiturates usually depress griseofulvin activity and co-administration requires a dosage adjustment of the antifungal agent).
No products indexed under this heading.

Butabarbital (Barbiturates usually depress griseofulvin activity and co-administration requires a dosage adjustment of the antifungal agent).
No products indexed under this heading.

Butalbital (Barbiturates usually depress griseofulvin activity and co-administration requires a dosage adjustment of the antifungal agent). Products include:
Sedapap Tablets 50 mg/650 mg 2098

Desogestrel (There have been reports in the literature of possible interactions between griseofulvin and oral contraceptives). Products include:

Ortho-Cept Tablets ... 2395

Ethinyl Estradiol (There have been reports in the literature of possible interactions between griseofulvin and oral contraceptives). Products include:

Alesse-28 Tablets ... 3392
Lo/Ovral-28 Tablets ... 3423
NuvaRing ... 2357
Ortho-Cept Tablets ... 2395
Ortho-Cyclen/Ortho Tri-Cyclen ... 2414
Ortho Evra Transdermal System ... 2402
Ortho Tri-Cyclen Lo Tablets ... 2421
Seasonale Tablets ... 1073
Triphasil-28 Tablets ... 3483
Yasmin 28 Tablets ... 818

Ethynodiol Diacetate (There have been reports in the literature of possible interactions between griseofulvin and oral contraceptives).
No products indexed under this heading.

Levonorgestrel (There have been reports in the literature of possible interactions between griseofulvin and oral contraceptives). Products include:

Alesse-28 Tablets ... 3392
Climara Pro Transdermal System ... 800
Mirena Intrauterine System ... 810
Plan B Tablets ... 1068
Seasonale Tablets ... 1073
Triphasil-28 Tablets ... 3483

Mephobarbital (Barbiturates usually depress griseofulvin activity and co-administration requires a dosage adjustment of the antifungal agent). Products include:

Mebaral Tablets, USP ... 2483

Mestranol (There have been reports in the literature of possible interactions between griseofulvin and oral contraceptives).
No products indexed under this heading.

Norethindrone (There have been reports in the literature of possible interactions between griseofulvin and oral contraceptives). Products include:

Ortho Micronor Tablets ... 2411

Norethynodrel (There have been reports in the literature of possible interactions between griseofulvin and oral contraceptives).
No products indexed under this heading.

Norgestimate (There have been reports in the literature of possible interactions between griseofulvin and oral contraceptives). Products include:

Ortho-Cyclen/Ortho Tri-Cyclen ... 2414
Ortho Tri-Cyclen Lo Tablets ... 2421
Prefest Tablets ... 1069

Norgestrel (There have been reports in the literature of possible interactions between griseofulvin and oral contraceptives). Products include:

Lo/Ovral-28 Tablets ... 3423

Pentobarbital Sodium (Barbiturates usually depress griseofulvin activity and co-administration requires a dosage adjustment of the antifungal agent). Products include:

Nembutal Sodium Solution, USP ... 2484

Phenobarbital (Barbiturates usually depress griseofulvin activity and co-administration requires a dosage adjustment of the antifungal agent).
No products indexed under this heading.

Secobarbital Sodium (Barbiturates usually depress griseofulvin activity and co-administration requires a dosage adjustment of the antifungal agent).
No products indexed under this heading.

Thiamylal Sodium (Barbiturates usually depress griseofulvin activity and co-administration requires a dosage adjustment of the antifungal agent).
No products indexed under this heading.

Warfarin Sodium (Griseofulvin decreases the activity of warfarin-type anticoagulants). Products include:

Coumadin for Injection ... 932
Coumadin Tablets ... 932

Food Interactions

Alcohol (The effects of alcohol may be potentiated by griseofulvin, producing such effects as tachycardia and flushing).

GUANIDINE HYDROCHLORIDE TABLETS

(Guanidine Hydrochloride) ... 3030
None cited in PDR database.

GYNAZOLE-1 VAGINAL CREAM

(Butoconazole Nitrate) ... 3298
None cited in PDR database.

HALFLYTELY AND BISACODYL TABLETS BOWEL PREP KIT WITH FLAVORS PACKS

(Bisacodyl, Polyethylene Glycol, Potassium Chloride, Sodium Bicarbonate, Sodium Chloride) ... 915
May interact with antacids and certain other agents. Compounds in these categories include:

Aluminum Carbonate (Bisacodyl tablets should not be taken within one hour of taking an antacid).
No products indexed under this heading.

Aluminum Hydroxide (Bisacodyl tablets should not be taken within one hour of taking an antacid). Products include:

Gaviscon Regular Strength Liquid ... 620
Gaviscon Regular Strength Tablets ... 619
Gaviscon Extra Strength Liquid ... 620
Gaviscon Extra Strength Tablets ... 619
Maalox Max Maximum Strength Antacid/Anti-Gas Liquid ... 2165
Maalox Regular Strength Antacid/Antigas Liquid ... 2164

Magaldrate (Bisacodyl tablets should not be taken within one hour of taking an antacid).
No products indexed under this heading.

Magnesium Hydroxide (Bisacodyl tablets should not be taken within one hour of taking an antacid). Products include:

Maalox Max Maximum Strength Antacid/Anti-Gas Liquid ... 2165
Maalox Regular Strength Antacid/Antigas Liquid ... 2164
Pepcid Complete Chewable Tablets ... 1672
Rolaids Tablets ... 707
Extra Strength Rolaids Tablets ... 707
Rolaids Multi-Symptom Antacid & Antigas Tablets ... 708

Magnesium Oxide (Bisacodyl tablets should not be taken within one hour of taking an antacid). Products include:

Beelith Tablets ... 784
PremCal Light, Regular, and Extra Strength Tablets ... 762

Oral Medications, unspecified (Oral medication administered within one hour of the start of administration of the solution may be flushed from the gastrointestinal tract and not absorbed).
No products indexed under this heading.

HALLS DEFENSE SUGARFREE VITAMIN C DROPS

(Vitamin C) ... 611
None cited in PDR database.

HALLS DEFENSE MULTIBLEND SUPPLEMENT DROPS

(Echinacea, Herbals with Vitamins) ... 610
None cited in PDR database.

HALLS FRUIT BREEZERS PECTIN THROAT DROPS

(Pectin) ... 609
None cited in PDR database.

HALLS MAX DROPS

(Benzocaine, Menthol) ... 609
None cited in PDR database.

HALLS MENTHO-LYPTUS DROPS

(Menthol) ... 609
None cited in PDR database.

HALLS SUGAR FREE DROPS

(Menthol) ... 610
None cited in PDR database.

HALLS SUGAR FREE SQUARES

(Menthol) ... 610
None cited in PDR database.

HALLS PLUS COUGH DROPS

(Menthol, Pectin) ... 609
None cited in PDR database.

HAVRIX VACCINE

(Hepatitis A Vaccine, Inactivated) ... 1425
May interact with anticoagulants. Compounds in these categories include:

Anisindione (Havrix should be given with caution to individuals on anticoagulant therapy). Products include:

Miradon Tablets ... 3056

Ardeparin Sodium (Havrix should be given with caution to individuals on anticoagulant therapy).
No products indexed under this heading.

Dalteparin Sodium (Havrix should be given with caution to individuals on anticoagulant therapy). Products include:

Fragmin Injection ... 2638

Danaparoid Sodium (Havrix should be given with caution to individuals on anticoagulant therapy).
No products indexed under this heading.

Dicumarol (Havrix should be given with caution to individuals on anticoagulant therapy).
No products indexed under this heading.

Enoxaparin Sodium (Havrix should be given with caution to individuals on anticoagulant therapy). Products include:

Lovenox Injection ... 2931

Fondaparinux Sodium (Havrix should be given with caution to individuals on anticoagulant therapy). Products include:

Arixtra Injection ... 1325

Heparin Calcium (Havrix should be given with caution to individuals on anticoagulant therapy).
No products indexed under this heading.

Heparin Sodium (Havrix should be given with caution to individuals on anticoagulant therapy).
No products indexed under this heading.

Low Molecular Weight Heparins (Havrix should be given with caution to individuals on anticoagulant therapy).
No products indexed under this heading.

Tinzaparin Sodium (Havrix should be given with caution to individuals on anticoagulant therapy).
No products indexed under this heading.

Warfarin Sodium (Havrix should be given with caution to individuals on anticoagulant therapy). Products include:

Coumadin for Injection ... 932
Coumadin Tablets ... 932

HECTOROL CAPSULES

(Doxercalciferol) ... 909
May interact with cytochrome p450 3a4 inhibitors (selected), phenytoin, and certain other agents. Compounds in these categories include:

Acetazolamide (Cytochrome P450 inhibitors may inhibit the 25-hydroxylation of doxercalciferol. Hence, formation of the active doxercalciferol moiety may be hindered).
No products indexed under this heading.

Amiodarone Hydrochloride (Cytochrome P450 inhibitors may inhibit the 25-hydroxylation of doxercalciferol. Hence, formation of the active doxercalciferol moiety may be hindered). Products include:

Pacerone Tablets ... 3337

Amprenavir (Cytochrome P450 inhibitors may inhibit the 25-hydroxylation of doxercalciferol. Hence, formation of the active doxercalciferol moiety may be hindered). Products include:

Agenerase Capsules ... 1299
Agenerase Oral Solution ... 1304

Anastrozole (Cytochrome P450 inhibitors may inhibit the 25-hydroxylation of doxercalciferol. Hence, formation of the active doxercalciferol moiety may be hindered). Products include:

Arimidex Tablets ... 665

Aprepitant (Cytochrome P450 inhibitors may inhibit the 25-hydroxylation of doxercalciferol. Hence, formation of the active doxercalciferol moiety may be hindered). Products include:

Emend Capsules ... 1944

Cholestyramine (Reduces the intestinal absorption of fat-soluble vitamins; therefore, it may impair absorption of doxercalciferol).
No products indexed under this heading.

Cimetidine (Cytochrome P450 inhibitors may inhibit the 25-hydroxylation of doxercalciferol. Hence, formation of the active doxercalciferol moiety may be hindered). Products include:

Tagamet HB 200 Tablets .... ▣637
Tagamet Tablets 1547

Cimetidine Hydrochloride (Cytochrome P450 inhibitors may inhibit the 25-hydroxylation of doxercalciferol. Hence, formation of the active doxercalciferol moiety may be hindered).

No products indexed under this heading.

Ciprofloxacin (Cytochrome P450 inhibitors may inhibit the 25-hydroxylation of doxercalciferol. Hence, formation of the active doxercalciferol moiety may be hindered). Products include:

Cipro I.V. 2998
Cipro I.V. Pharmacy Bulk Package ... 3509
Cipro Oral Suspension 2991
Cipro XR Tablets 3004
Ciprodex Otic Suspension 555

Clarithromycin (Cytochrome P450 inhibitors may inhibit the 25-hydroxylation of doxercalciferol. Hence, formation of the active doxercalciferol moiety may be hindered). Products include:

Biaxin/Biaxin XL 402
PREVPAC 3281

Clotrimazole (Cytochrome P450 inhibitors may inhibit the 25-hydroxylation of doxercalciferol. Hence, formation of the active doxercalciferol moiety may be hindered). Products include:

Lotrimin 3053
Lotrisone 3054

Cyclosporine (Cytochrome P450 inhibitors may inhibit the 25-hydroxylation of doxercalciferol. Hence, formation of the active doxercalciferol moiety may be hindered). Products include:

Gengraf Capsules 458
Neoral Soft Gelatin Capsules 2247
Neoral Oral Solution 2247
Restasis Ophthalmic Emulsion 570
Sandimmune 2259

Dalfopristin (Cytochrome P450 inhibitors may inhibit the 25-hydroxylation of doxercalciferol. Hence, formation of the active doxercalciferol moiety may be hindered). Products include:

Synercid I.V. 1690

Danazol (Cytochrome P450 inhibitors may inhibit the 25-hydroxylation of doxercalciferol. Hence, formation of the active doxercalciferol moiety may be hindered).

No products indexed under this heading.

Delavirdine Mesylate (Cytochrome P450 inhibitors may inhibit the 25-hydroxylation of doxercalciferol. Hence, formation of the active doxercalciferol moiety may be hindered). Products include:

Rescriptor Tablets 2535

Diltiazem Hydrochloride (Cytochrome P450 inhibitors may inhibit the 25-hydroxylation of doxercalciferol. Hence, formation of the active doxercalciferol moiety may be hindered). Products include:

Cardizem LA Extended Release Tablets 1699
Tiazac Capsules 1204

Diltiazem Maleate (Cytochrome P450 inhibitors may inhibit the 25-hydroxylation of doxercalciferol. Hence, formation of the active doxercalciferol moiety may be hindered).

No products indexed under this heading.

Efavirenz (Cytochrome P450 inhibitors may inhibit the 25-hydroxylation of doxercalciferol. Hence, formation of the active doxercalciferol moiety may be hindered). Products include:

Sustiva Capsules 957

Erythromycin (Cytochrome P450 inhibitors may inhibit the 25-hydroxylation of doxercalciferol. Hence, formation of the active doxercalciferol moiety may be hindered). Products include:

Erygel Topical Gel 2096
Ery-Tab Tablets 447
Erythromycin Base Filmtab Tablets 454
Erythromycin Delayed-Release Capsules, USP 456
PCE Dispertab Tablets 510

Erythromycin Estolate (Cytochrome P450 inhibitors may inhibit the 25-hydroxylation of doxercalciferol. Hence, formation of the active doxercalciferol moiety may be hindered).

No products indexed under this heading.

Erythromycin Ethylsuccinate (Cytochrome P450 inhibitors may inhibit the 25-hydroxylation of doxercalciferol. Hence, formation of the active doxercalciferol moiety may be hindered). Products include:

E.E.S. 449
EryPed 445

Erythromycin Gluceptate (Cytochrome P450 inhibitors may inhibit the 25-hydroxylation of doxercalciferol. Hence, formation of the active doxercalciferol moiety may be hindered).

No products indexed under this heading.

Erythromycin Lactobionate (Cytochrome P450 inhibitors may inhibit the 25-hydroxylation of doxercalciferol. Hence, formation of the active doxercalciferol moiety may be hindered).

No products indexed under this heading.

Erythromycin Stearate (Cytochrome P450 inhibitors may inhibit the 25-hydroxylation of doxercalciferol. Hence, formation of the active doxercalciferol moiety may be hindered). Products include:

Erythrocin Stearate Filmtab Tablets 452

Esomeprazole Magnesium (Cytochrome P450 inhibitors may inhibit the 25-hydroxylation of doxercalciferol. Hence, formation of the active doxercalciferol moiety may be hindered). Products include:

Nexium Delayed-Release Capsules 645

Fluconazole (Cytochrome P450 inhibitors may inhibit the 25-hydroxylation of doxercalciferol. Hence, formation of the active doxercalciferol moiety may be hindered).

No products indexed under this heading.

Fluoxetine Hydrochloride (Cytochrome P450 inhibitors may inhibit the 25-hydroxylation of doxercalciferol. Hence, formation of the active doxercalciferol moiety may be hindered). Products include:

Prozac Pulvules and Liquid 1771
Symbyax Capsules 1788

Fluvoxamine Maleate (Cytochrome P450 inhibitors may inhibit the 25-hydroxylation of doxercalciferol. Hence, formation of the active doxercalciferol moiety may be hindered).

No products indexed under this heading.

Fosamprenavir Calcium (Cytochrome P450 inhibitors may inhibit the 25-hydroxylation of doxercalciferol. Hence, formation of the active doxercalciferol moiety may be hindered). Products include:

Lexiva Tablets 1473

Fosphenytoin Sodium (Co-administration with enzyme inhibitors, such as phenytoin, may affect the 25-hydroxylation of Hectorol and may necessitate dosage adjustment).

No products indexed under this heading.

Glutethimide (Co-administration with enzyme inducers, such as glutethimide, may affect the 25-hydroxylation of Hectorol and may necessitate dosage adjustment).

No products indexed under this heading.

Indinavir Sulfate (Cytochrome P450 inhibitors may inhibit the 25-hydroxylation of doxercalciferol. Hence, formation of the active doxercalciferol moiety may be hindered). Products include:

Crixivan Capsules 1918

Isoniazid (Cytochrome P450 inhibitors may inhibit the 25-hydroxylation of doxercalciferol. Hence, formation of the active doxercalciferol moiety may be hindered).

No products indexed under this heading.

Itraconazole (Cytochrome P450 inhibitors may inhibit the 25-hydroxylation of doxercalciferol. Hence, formation of the active doxercalciferol moiety may be hindered).

No products indexed under this heading.

Ketoconazole (Cytochrome P450 inhibitors may inhibit the 25-hydroxylation of doxercalciferol. Hence, formation of the active doxercalciferol moiety may be hindered). Products include:

Nizoral A-D Shampoo, 1% 1839
Nizoral 2% Shampoo 1838

Lopinavir (Cytochrome P450 inhibitors may inhibit the 25-hydroxylation of doxercalciferol. Hence, formation of the active doxercalciferol moiety may be hindered). Products include:

Kaletra 474

Loratadine (Cytochrome P450 inhibitors may inhibit the 25-hydroxylation of doxercalciferol. Hence, formation of the active doxercalciferol moiety may be hindered). Products include:

Alavert Allergy & Sinus D-12 Hour Tablets .... ▣743
Alavert .... ▣743
Children's Claritin 24 Hour Non-Drowsy Allergy Syrup .... ▣732
Claritin Non-Drowsy 24 Hour Tablets .... ▣731
Non-Drowsy Claritin Hives Relief Tablets .... ▣733
Claritin Reditabs 24 Hour Non-Drowsy Tablets .... ▣732
Claritin-D Non-Drowsy 12 Hour Tablets .... ▣731
Claritin-D Non-Drowsy 24 Hour Tablets .... ▣731
Children's Dimetapp ND Non-Drowsy Allergy Syrup .... ▣746
Triaminic Allerchews .... ▣684

Magnesium Hydroxide (Co-administration with magnesium-containing antacids and Hectorol may lead to the development of hypermagnesemia; concurrent use should be avoided). Products include:

Maalox Max Maximum Strength Antacid/Anti-Gas Liquid 2165
Maalox Regular Strength Antacid/Antigas Liquid 2164
Pepcid Complete Chewable Tablets 1672
Rolaids Tablets .... ▣707
Extra Strength Rolaids Tablets .... ▣707
Rolaids Multi-Symptom Antacid & Antigas Tablets .... ▣708

Magnesium Oxide (Co-administration with magnesium-containing antacids and Hectorol may lead to the development of hypermagnesemia; concurrent use should be avoided). Products include:

Beelith Tablets 784
PremCal Light, Regular, and Extra Strength Tablets .... ▣762

Metronidazole (Cytochrome P450 inhibitors may inhibit the 25-hydroxylation of doxercalciferol. Hence, formation of the active doxercalciferol moiety may be hindered). Products include:

Metrogel 1% 1212
MetroGel-Vaginal Gel 1822
Noritate Cream, 1% 1051

Metronidazole Benzoate (Cytochrome P450 inhibitors may inhibit the 25-hydroxylation of doxercalciferol. Hence, formation of the active doxercalciferol moiety may be hindered).

No products indexed under this heading.

Metronidazole Hydrochloride (Cytochrome P450 inhibitors may inhibit the 25-hydroxylation of doxercalciferol. Hence, formation of the active doxercalciferol moiety may be hindered).

No products indexed under this heading.

Miconazole (Cytochrome P450 inhibitors may inhibit the 25-hydroxylation of doxercalciferol. Hence, formation of the active doxercalciferol moiety may be hindered).

No products indexed under this heading.

Miconazole Nitrate (Cytochrome P450 inhibitors may inhibit the 25-hydroxylation of doxercalciferol. Hence, formation of the active doxercalciferol moiety may be hindered). Products include:

Desenex .... ▣674
Desenex Jock Itch Spray Powder ... ▣674

Mineral Oil (The use of mineral oil or other substances that affect absorption of the fat may influence the absorption and availability of Hectorol). Products include:

Fleet Mineral Oil Enema 1170
Lubriderm Advanced Therapy Moisturizing Lotion .... ▣702
Mineral Oil 2716
Preparation H Ointment .... ▣747
Refresh P.M. Lubricant Eye Ointment .... ⊙239
Tucks Hemorrhoidal Ointment .... ▣711

Nefazodone Hydrochloride (Cytochrome P450 inhibitors may inhibit the 25-hydroxylation of doxercalciferol. Hence, formation of the active doxercalciferol moiety may be hindered).
No products indexed under this heading.

Nelfinavir Mesylate (Cytochrome P450 inhibitors may inhibit the 25-hydroxylation of doxercalciferol. Hence, formation of the active doxercalciferol moiety may be hindered). Products include:
Viracept 2556

Nevirapine (Cytochrome P450 inhibitors may inhibit the 25-hydroxylation of doxercalciferol. Hence, formation of the active doxercalciferol moiety may be hindered). Products include:
Viramune Oral Suspension 903
Viramune Tablets 903

Niacinamide (Cytochrome P450 inhibitors may inhibit the 25-hydroxylation of doxercalciferol. Hence, formation of the active doxercalciferol moiety may be hindered).
No products indexed under this heading.

Nicotinamide (Cytochrome P450 inhibitors may inhibit the 25-hydroxylation of doxercalciferol. Hence, formation of the active doxercalciferol moiety may be hindered). Products include:
Nicomide Tablets 3190

Nifedipine (Cytochrome P450 inhibitors may inhibit the 25-hydroxylation of doxercalciferol. Hence, formation of the active doxercalciferol moiety may be hindered). Products include:
Adalat CC Tablets 2978

Norfloxacin (Cytochrome P450 inhibitors may inhibit the 25-hydroxylation of doxercalciferol. Hence, formation of the active doxercalciferol moiety may be hindered). Products include:
Noroxin Tablets 2009

Omeprazole (Cytochrome P450 inhibitors may inhibit the 25-hydroxylation of doxercalciferol. Hence, formation of the active doxercalciferol moiety may be hindered). Products include:
Zegerid Powder for Oral Solution 2972

Paroxetine Hydrochloride (Cytochrome P450 inhibitors may inhibit the 25-hydroxylation of doxercalciferol. Hence, formation of the active doxercalciferol moiety may be hindered). Products include:
Paxil CR Controlled-Release Tablets 1509
Paxil 1501

Phenobarbital (Co-administration with enzyme inducers, such as phenobarbital, may affect the 25-hydroxylation of Hectorol and may necessitate dosage adjustment).
No products indexed under this heading.

Phenytoin (Co-administration with enzyme inhibitors, such as phenytoin, may affect the 25-hydroxylation of Hectorol and may necessitate dosage adjustment).
No products indexed under this heading.

Phenytoin Sodium (Co-administration with enzyme inhibitors, such as phenytoin, may affect the 25-hydroxylation of Hectorol and may necessitate dosage adjustment). Products include:
Phenytek Capsules 2153

Propoxyphene Hydrochloride (Cytochrome P450 inhibitors may inhibit the 25-hydroxylation of doxercalciferol. Hence, formation of the active doxercalciferol moiety may be hindered).
No products indexed under this heading.

Propoxyphene Napsylate (Cytochrome P450 inhibitors may inhibit the 25-hydroxylation of doxercalciferol. Hence, formation of the active doxercalciferol moiety may be hindered). Products include:
Darvocet A 500 Tablets 3497

Quinidine (Cytochrome P450 inhibitors may inhibit the 25-hydroxylation of doxercalciferol. Hence, formation of the active doxercalciferol moiety may be hindered).
No products indexed under this heading.

Quinidine Hydrochloride (Cytochrome P450 inhibitors may inhibit the 25-hydroxylation of doxercalciferol. Hence, formation of the active doxercalciferol moiety may be hindered).
No products indexed under this heading.

Quinidine Polygalacturonate (Cytochrome P450 inhibitors may inhibit the 25-hydroxylation of doxercalciferol. Hence, formation of the active doxercalciferol moiety may be hindered).
No products indexed under this heading.

Quinidine Sulfate (Cytochrome P450 inhibitors may inhibit the 25-hydroxylation of doxercalciferol. Hence, formation of the active doxercalciferol moiety may be hindered).
No products indexed under this heading.

Quinine (Cytochrome P450 inhibitors may inhibit the 25-hydroxylation of doxercalciferol. Hence, formation of the active doxercalciferol moiety may be hindered).
No products indexed under this heading.

Quinine Sulfate (Cytochrome P450 inhibitors may inhibit the 25-hydroxylation of doxercalciferol. Hence, formation of the active doxercalciferol moiety may be hindered).
No products indexed under this heading.

Quinupristin (Cytochrome P450 inhibitors may inhibit the 25-hydroxylation of doxercalciferol. Hence, formation of the active doxercalciferol moiety may be hindered). Products include:
Synercid I.V. 1690

Ranitidine Bismuth Citrate (Cytochrome P450 inhibitors may inhibit the 25-hydroxylation of doxercalciferol. Hence, formation of the active doxercalciferol moiety may be hindered).
No products indexed under this heading.

Ranitidine Hydrochloride (Cytochrome P450 inhibitors may inhibit the 25-hydroxylation of doxercalciferol. Hence, formation of the active doxercalciferol moiety may be hindered). Products include:
Zantac 1597
Zantac Injection 1593
Zantac 75 Tablets 715
Zantac 150 Maximum Strength Tablets 715
Zantac Injection Pharmacy Bulk Package 1595

Ritonavir (Cytochrome P450 inhibitors may inhibit the 25-hydroxylation of doxercalciferol. Hence, formation of the active doxercalciferol moiety may be hindered). Products include:
Kaletra 474
Norvir 499

Saquinavir (Cytochrome P450 inhibitors may inhibit the 25-hydroxylation of doxercalciferol. Hence, formation of the active doxercalciferol moiety may be hindered).
No products indexed under this heading.

Saquinavir Mesylate (Cytochrome P450 inhibitors may inhibit the 25-hydroxylation of doxercalciferol. Hence, formation of the active doxercalciferol moiety may be hindered). Products include:
Invirase 2776

Sertraline Hydrochloride (Cytochrome P450 inhibitors may inhibit the 25-hydroxylation of doxercalciferol. Hence, formation of the active doxercalciferol moiety may be hindered). Products include:
Zoloft 2581

Telithromycin (Cytochrome P450 inhibitors may inhibit the 25-hydroxylation of doxercalciferol. Hence, formation of the active doxercalciferol moiety may be hindered). Products include:
Ketek Tablets 2920

Troglitazone (Cytochrome P450 inhibitors may inhibit the 25-hydroxylation of doxercalciferol. Hence, formation of the active doxercalciferol moiety may be hindered).
No products indexed under this heading.

Troleandomycin (Cytochrome P450 inhibitors may inhibit the 25-hydroxylation of doxercalciferol. Hence, formation of the active doxercalciferol moiety may be hindered).
No products indexed under this heading.

Valproate Sodium (Cytochrome P450 inhibitors may inhibit the 25-hydroxylation of doxercalciferol. Hence, formation of the active doxercalciferol moiety may be hindered). Products include:
Depacon Injection 412

Verapamil Hydrochloride (Cytochrome P450 inhibitors may inhibit the 25-hydroxylation of doxercalciferol. Hence, formation of the active doxercalciferol moiety may be hindered). Products include:
Covera-HS Tablets 3135
Tarka Tablets 519
Verelan PM Capsules 3120

Vitamin D (Pharmacologic doses of Vitamin D and its derivatives should be withheld during doxercalciferol treatment to avoid possible additive effects and hypercalcemia). Products include:
Active Calcium Tablets 3342
Caltrate 600 PLUS Chewables 779
Caltrate 600 PLUS Tablets 779
Caltrate 600 + D Tablets 779
Os-Cal 250 + D Tablets 765
Os-Cal 500 + D Tablets 766

Vitamin D_2 (Pharmacologic doses of Vitamin D and its derivatives should be withheld during doxercalciferol treatment to avoid possible additive effects and hypercalcemia).
No products indexed under this heading.

Voriconazole (Cytochrome P450 inhibitors may inhibit the 25-hydroxylation of doxercalciferol. Hence, formation of the active doxercalciferol moiety may be hindered). Products include:
VFEND I.V. 2543
VFEND Oral Suspension 2543
VFEND Tablets 2543

Zafirlukast (Cytochrome P450 inhibitors may inhibit the 25-hydroxylation of doxercalciferol. Hence, formation of the active doxercalciferol moiety may be hindered). Products include:
Accolate Tablets 663

Zileuton (Cytochrome P450 inhibitors may inhibit the 25-hydroxylation of doxercalciferol. Hence, formation of the active doxercalciferol moiety may be hindered).
No products indexed under this heading.

Food Interactions

Grapefruit (Cytochrome P450 inhibitors may inhibit the 25-hydroxylation of doxercalciferol. Hence, formation of the active doxercalciferol moiety may be hindered).

Grapefruit Juice (Cytochrome P450 inhibitors may inhibit the 25-hydroxylation of doxercalciferol. Hence, formation of the active doxercalciferol moiety may be hindered).

HECTOROL INJECTION

(Doxercalciferol) 911
See Hectorol Capsules

HEMOFIL M

(Antihemophilic Factor (Human)) 757
None cited in PDR database.

HEP-FORTE CAPSULES

(Vitamins with Minerals) 3525
None cited in PDR database.

HEPSERA TABLETS

(Adefovir dipivoxil) 1275
May interact with inhibitors of renal tubular secretion or resorption and certain other agents. Compounds in these categories include:

Ibuprofen (When adefovir was co-administered with ibuprofen, increases in adefovir Cmax (33%), AUC (23%) and urinary recovery were observed. These increases appear to be due to higher oral bioavailability, not a reduction in renal clearance of adefovir). Products include:
Advil Allergy Sinus Caplets 737
Advil 737
Children's Advil Suspension 742
Children's Advil Chewable Tablets 741
Advil Cold & Sinus 739
Advil Flu & Body Ache Caplets 739
Children's Advil Cold Suspension 741
Infants' Advil Concentrated Drops 743
Junior Strength Advil Swallow Tablets 740
Advil Migraine Liquigels 740
Advil Multi-Symptom Cold Caplets 738
Combunox Tablets 1183
Children's Motrin Oral Suspension and Chewable Tablets 1837

Children's Motrin Cold Non-Staining Dye-Free Oral Suspension 1838
Children's Motrin Cold Oral Suspension 1838
Children's Motrin Non-Staining Dye-Free Oral Suspension 1837
Motrin Cold & Sinus Caplets 1836
Motrin IB Tablets and Caplets 1836
Infants' Motrin Concentrated Drops 1837
Infants' Motrin Non-Staining Dye-Free Drops 1837
Junior Strength Motrin Caplets and Chewable Tablets 1837
Vicoprofen Tablets 533

Probenecid (Since adefovir is eliminated by the kidney, co-administration of adefovir with drugs that compete for active tubular secretion may increase serum concentrations of either adefovir and/or these co-administered drugs).
No products indexed under this heading.

Sulfinpyrazone (Since adefovir is eliminated by the kidney, co-administration of adefovir with drugs that compete for active tubular secretion may increase serum concentrations of either adefovir and/or these co-administered drugs).
No products indexed under this heading.

HERCEPTIN I.V.

(Trastuzumab) 1234
May interact with anthracycline antibiotics and their derivatives and certain other agents. Compounds in these categories include:

Cyclophosphamide (The increase and severity of cardiac dysfunction is particularly high in patients who receive trastuzumab in combination with cyclophosphamide).
No products indexed under this heading.

Daunorubicin Hydrochloride (The increase and severity of cardiac dysfunction is particularly high in patients who receive trastuzumab in combination with anthracyclines). Products include:
Cerubidine for Injection 788

Doxorubicin Hydrochloride (The increase and severity of cardiac dysfunction is particularly high in patients who receive trastuzumab in combination with anthracyclines). Products include:
Adriamycin for Injection, USP 786
Adriamycin Injection, USP 786

Epirubicin Hydrochloride (The increase and severity of cardiac dysfunction is particularly high in patients who receive trastuzumab in combination with anthracyclines). Products include:
Ellence Injection 2632

Idarubicin Hydrochloride (The increase and severity of cardiac dysfunction is particularly high in patients who receive trastuzumab in combination with anthracyclines). Products include:
Idamycin PFS Injection 2645

Paclitaxel (Co-administration has resulted in a two-fold decrease in trastuzumab clearance in a non-human primate study and in a 1.5-fold increase in trastuzumab serum levels in clinical studies).
No products indexed under this heading.

HEXALEN CAPSULES

(Altretamine) 2101
May interact with monoamine oxidase inhibitors and certain other agents. Compounds in these categories include:

Cimetidine (Increases altretamine's half-life and toxicity in a rat model). Products include:
Tagamet HB 200 Tablets .... ▣637
Tagamet Tablets 1547

Cimetidine Hydrochloride (Increases altretamine's half-life and toxicity in a rat model).
No products indexed under this heading.

Isocarboxazid (Potential for severe orthostatic hypotension).
No products indexed under this heading.

Moclobemide (Potential for severe orthostatic hypotension).
No products indexed under this heading.

Pargyline Hydrochloride (Potential for severe orthostatic hypotension).
No products indexed under this heading.

Phenelzine Sulfate (Potential for severe orthostatic hypotension).
No products indexed under this heading.

Procarbazine Hydrochloride (Potential for severe orthostatic hypotension). Products include:
Matulane Capsules 3188

Pyridoxine Hydrochloride (May adversely affect response duration; should not be administered with Hexalen and/or Cisplatin).
No products indexed under this heading.

Selegiline Hydrochloride (Potential for severe orthostatic hypotension). Products include:
Eldepryl Capsules 3209

Tranylcypromine Sulfate (Potential for severe orthostatic hypotension). Products include:
Parnate Tablets 1499

HIBTITER

(Haemophilus B Conjugate Vaccine) 3419
May interact with alkylating agents, antimetabolites, anticoagulants, corticosteroids, cytotoxic drugs, immunosuppressive agents, and certain other agents. Compounds in these categories include:

Anisindione (HibTITER should be given with caution to children on anticoagulant therapy). Products include:
Miradon Tablets 3056

Ardeparin Sodium (HibTITER should be given with caution to children on anticoagulant therapy).
No products indexed under this heading.

Azathioprine (Reduces antibody response to active immunization procedures). Products include:
Azasan Tablets 2844

Basiliximab (Reduces antibody response to active immunization procedures). Products include:
Simulect for Injection 2268

Betamethasone Acetate (Reduces antibody response to active immunization procedures).
No products indexed under this heading.

Betamethasone Sodium Phosphate (Reduces antibody response to active immunization procedures).
No products indexed under this heading.

Bleomycin Sulfate (Reduces antibody response to active immunization procedures).
No products indexed under this heading.

Busulfan (Reduces antibody response to active immunization procedures). Products include:
I.V. Busulfex 1125
Myleran Tablets 1492

Capecitabine (Children with impaired immune responsiveness may have reduced antibody response to active immunization procedures. Deferral of administration of vaccine may be considered in individuals receiving immunosuppressive therapy). Products include:
Xeloda Tablets 2825

Carmustine (BCNU) (Reduces antibody response to active immunization procedures).
No products indexed under this heading.

Chlorambucil (Reduces antibody response to active immunization procedures). Products include:
Leukeran Tablets 1472

Cladribine (Children with impaired immune responsiveness may have reduced antibody response to active immunization procedures. Deferral of administration of vaccine may be considered in individuals receiving immunosuppressive therapy). Products include:
Leustatin Injection 2368

Cortisone Acetate (Reduces antibody response to active immunization procedures).
No products indexed under this heading.

Cyclophosphamide (Reduces antibody response to active immunization procedures).
No products indexed under this heading.

Cyclosporine (Reduces antibody response to active immunization procedures). Products include:
Gengraf Capsules 458
Neoral Soft Gelatin Capsules 2247
Neoral Oral Solution 2247
Restasis Ophthalmic Emulsion 570
Sandimmune 2259

Cytarabine (Children with impaired immune responsiveness may have reduced antibody response to active immunization procedures. Deferral of administration of vaccine may be considered in individuals receiving immunosuppressive therapy).
No products indexed under this heading.

Dacarbazine (Reduces antibody response to active immunization procedures).
No products indexed under this heading.

Dalteparin Sodium (HibTITER should be given with caution to children on anticoagulant therapy). Products include:
Fragmin Injection 2638

Danaparoid Sodium (HibTITER should be given with caution to children on anticoagulant therapy).
No products indexed under this heading.

Daunorubicin Hydrochloride (Reduces antibody response to active immunization procedures). Products include:
Cerubidine for Injection 788

Dexamethasone (Reduces antibody response to active immunization procedures). Products include:
Ciprodex Otic Suspension 555
Decadron Tablets 1929
TobraDex Ophthalmic Ointment 558
TobraDex Ophthalmic Suspension 558

Dexamethasone Acetate (Reduces antibody response to active immunization procedures).
No products indexed under this heading.

Dexamethasone Sodium Phosphate (Reduces antibody response to active immunization procedures). Products include:
Decadron Phosphate Injection 1931

Dicumarol (HibTITER should be given with caution to children on anticoagulant therapy).
No products indexed under this heading.

Doxorubicin Hydrochloride (Reduces antibody response to active immunization procedures). Products include:
Adriamycin for Injection, USP 786
Adriamycin Injection, USP 786

Enoxaparin Sodium (HibTITER should be given with caution to children on anticoagulant therapy). Products include:
Lovenox Injection 2931

Epirubicin Hydrochloride (Reduces antibody response to active immunization procedures). Products include:
Ellence Injection 2632

Floxuridine (Children with impaired immune responsiveness may have reduced antibody response to active immunization procedures. Deferral of administration of vaccine may be considered in individuals receiving immunosuppressive therapy).
No products indexed under this heading.

Fludarabine Phosphate (Children with impaired immune responsiveness may have reduced antibody response to active immunization procedures. Deferral of administration of vaccine may be considered in individuals receiving immunosuppressive therapy).
No products indexed under this heading.

Fludrocortisone Acetate (Reduces antibody response to active immunization procedures).
No products indexed under this heading.

Fluorouracil (Reduces antibody response to active immunization procedures). Products include:
Carac Cream, 0.5% 1048
Efudex 3348

Fondaparinux Sodium (HibTITER should be given with caution to children on anticoagulant therapy). Products include:
Arixtra Injection 1325

Gemcitabine Hydrochloride (Children with impaired immune responsiveness may have reduced antibody response to active immunization procedures. Deferral of administration of vaccine may be considered in individuals receiving immunosuppressive therapy). Products include:
Gemzar for Injection 1743

Heparin Calcium (HibTITER should be given with caution to children on anticoagulant therapy).
No products indexed under this heading.

Heparin Sodium (HibTITER should be given with caution to children on anticoagulant therapy).
No products indexed under this heading.

Hydrocortisone (Reduces antibody response to active immunization procedures). Products include:
- Cortizone•5 Ointment 699
- Cortizone•10 Creme 699
- Cortizone•10 Ointment 699
- Cortizone•10 Plus Creme 700
- Cortizone•10 Maximum Strength Quick Shot Spray 700
- Hydrocortone Tablets 1963
- Preparation H Hydrocortisone Cream 748

Hydrocortisone Acetate (Reduces antibody response to active immunization procedures). Products include:
- Analpram-HC 1136
- Pramosone 1139
- ProctoFoam-HC 3113
- Tucks Anti-Itch Ointment 712
- U-cort 1% Cream 3289

Hydrocortisone Sodium Phosphate (Reduces antibody response to active immunization procedures).
No products indexed under this heading.

Hydrocortisone Sodium Succinate (Reduces antibody response to active immunization procedures).
No products indexed under this heading.

Hydroxyurea (Reduces antibody response to active immunization procedures).
No products indexed under this heading.

Immune Globulin Intravenous (Human) (Reduces antibody response to active immunization procedures). Products include:
- Carimune NF 3501
- Gammagard Liquid 751
- Gammagard S/D 754
- Gamunex Immune Globulin I.V., 10% 3232
- Iveegam EN 759

Lomustine (CCNU) (Reduces antibody response to active immunization procedures).
No products indexed under this heading.

Low Molecular Weight Heparins (HibTITER should be given with caution to children on anticoagulant therapy).
No products indexed under this heading.

Mechlorethamine Hydrochloride (Reduces antibody response to active immunization procedures). Products include:
- Mustargen for Injection 2007

Melphalan (Reduces antibody response to active immunization procedures). Products include:
- Alkeran Tablets 977

Mercaptopurine (Children with impaired immune responsiveness may have reduced antibody response to active immunization procedures. Deferral of administration of vaccine may be considered in individuals receiving immunosuppressive therapy). Products include:
- Purinethol Tablets 1222

Methotrexate (Children with impaired immune responsiveness may have reduced antibody response to active immunization procedures. Deferral of administration of vaccine may be considered in individuals receiving immunosuppressive therapy).
No products indexed under this heading.

Methotrexate Sodium (Reduces antibody response to active immunization procedures).
No products indexed under this heading.

Methylprednisolone Acetate (Reduces antibody response to active immunization procedures). Products include:
- Depo-Medrol Injectable Suspension 2615
- Depo-Medrol Single-Dose Vial 2617

Methylprednisolone Sodium Succinate (Reduces antibody response to active immunization procedures).
No products indexed under this heading.

Mitotane (Reduces antibody response to active immunization procedures).
No products indexed under this heading.

Mitoxantrone Hydrochloride (Reduces antibody response to active immunization procedures). Products include:
- Novantrone for Injection Concentrate 3158

Muromonab-CD3 (Reduces antibody response to active immunization procedures). Products include:
- Orthoclone OKT3 Sterile Solution 2370

Mycophenolate Mofetil (Reduces antibody response to active immunization procedures). Products include:
- CellCept Capsules 2751
- CellCept Oral Suspension 2751
- CellCept Tablets 2751

Pentostatin (Children with impaired immune responsiveness may have reduced antibody response to active immunization procedures. Deferral of administration of vaccine may be considered in individuals receiving immunosuppressive therapy). Products include:
- Nipent for Injection 3216

Prednisolone Acetate (Reduces antibody response to active immunization procedures). Products include:
- Blephamide Ophthalmic Ointment 563
- Blephamide Ophthalmic Suspension 564
- Poly-Pred Liquifilm Ophthalmic Suspension .... ⊙231
- Pred Forte Ophthalmic Suspension .... ⊙233
- Pred Mild Sterile Ophthalmic Suspension .... ⊙236
- Pred-G Ophthalmic Suspension .... ⊙234
- Pred-G Sterile Ophthalmic Ointment .... ⊙235

Prednisolone Sodium Phosphate (Reduces antibody response to active immunization procedures). Products include:
- Pediapred Oral Solution 3319

Prednisolone Tebutate (Reduces antibody response to active immunization procedures).
No products indexed under this heading.

Prednisone (Reduces antibody response to active immunization procedures).
No products indexed under this heading.

Procarbazine Hydrochloride (Reduces antibody response to active immunization procedures). Products include:
- Matulane Capsules 3188

Sirolimus (Reduces antibody response to active immunization procedures). Products include:
- Rapamune Oral Solution and Tablets 3472

Tacrolimus (Reduces antibody response to active immunization procedures). Products include:
- Prograf Capsules and Injection 624
- Protopic Ointment 629

Tamoxifen Citrate (Reduces antibody response to active immunization procedures).
No products indexed under this heading.

Thioguanine (Children with impaired immune responsiveness may have reduced antibody response to active immunization procedures. Deferral of administration of vaccine may be considered in individuals receiving immunosuppressive therapy). Products include:
- Tabloid Tablets 1545

Thiotepa (Reduces antibody response to active immunization procedures).
No products indexed under this heading.

Tinzaparin Sodium (HibTITER should be given with caution to children on anticoagulant therapy).
No products indexed under this heading.

Triamcinolone (Reduces antibody response to active immunization procedures).
No products indexed under this heading.

Triamcinolone Acetonide (Reduces antibody response to active immunization procedures). Products include:
- Azmacort Inhalation Aerosol 1701
- Nasacort HFA Inhalation Aerosol 2939
- Nasacort AQ Nasal Spray 2937

Triamcinolone Diacetate (Reduces antibody response to active immunization procedures).
No products indexed under this heading.

Triamcinolone Hexacetonide (Reduces antibody response to active immunization procedures).
No products indexed under this heading.

Vincristine Sulfate (Reduces antibody response to active immunization procedures).
No products indexed under this heading.

Warfarin Sodium (HibTITER should be given with caution to children on anticoagulant therapy). Products include:
- Coumadin for Injection 932
- Coumadin Tablets 932

HMS STERILE OPHTHALMIC SUSPENSION

(Medrysone) .... ⊙228
None cited in PDR database.

HUMALOG-PEN

(Insulin Lispro, Human) 1751
May interact with ACE inhibitors, beta blockers, corticosteroids, estrogens, oral hypoglycemic agents, oral contraceptives, phenothiazines, salicylates, thyroid preparations, and certain other agents. Compounds in these categories include:

Acarbose (Co-administration with drugs with hypoglycemic activity, such as oral hypoglycemic agents, may result in decreased insulin requirements). Products include:
- Precose Tablets 776

Acebutolol Hydrochloride (Co-administration with drugs with hypoglycemic activity, such as beta blockers, may result in decreased insulin requirements; beta blockers may mask the symptoms of hypoglycemia in some patients).
No products indexed under this heading.

Aspirin (Co-administration with drugs with hypoglycemic activity, such as salicylates, may result in decreased insulin requirements). Products include:
- Aggrenox Capsules 855
- Bayer, Aspirin Regimen 606
- Bayer Aspirin Tablets 3515
- BC Powder 612
- BC Allergy Sinus Cold Powder 612
- Arthritis Strength BC Powder 612
- BC Sinus Cold Powder 612
- Ecotrin Enteric Coated Aspirin Low, Regular and Maximum Strength Tablets 1627
- Goody's Body Pain Formula Powder 621
- Goody's Extra Strength Headache Powder 621
- Goody's Extra Strength Pain Relief Tablets 621
- Percodan Tablets 1115
- St. Joseph 81 mg Aspirin Chewable and Enteric Coated Tablets 1841

Aspirin, Enteric Coated (Co-administration with drugs with hypoglycemic activity, such as salicylates, may result in decreased insulin requirements).
No products indexed under this heading.

Aspirin Buffered (Co-administration with drugs with hypoglycemic activity, such as salicylates, may result in decreased insulin requirements).
No products indexed under this heading.

Atenolol (Co-administration with drugs with hypoglycemic activity, such as beta blockers, may result in decreased insulin requirements; beta blockers may mask the symptoms of hypoglycemia in some patients). Products include:
- Tenormin I.V. Injection 698
- Tenormin Tablets 695

Benazepril Hydrochloride (Co-administration with drugs with hypoglycemic activity, such as certain ACE inhibitors, may result in decreased insulin requirements). Products include:
- Lotensin Tablets 2232
- Lotensin HCT Tablets 2235
- Lotrel Capsules 2238

Betamethasone Acetate (Co-administration may result in increased insulin requirements).
No products indexed under this heading.

Betamethasone Sodium Phosphate (Co-administration may result in increased insulin requirements).
No products indexed under this heading.

Betaxolol Hydrochloride (Co-administration with drugs with hypoglycemic activity, such as beta blockers, may result in decreased insulin requirements; beta blockers may mask the symptoms of hypoglycemia in some patients). Products include:
Betoptic S Ophthalmic Suspension 554

Bisoprolol Fumarate (Co-administration with drugs with hypoglycemic activity, such as beta blockers, may result in decreased insulin requirements; beta blockers may mask the symptoms of hypoglycemia in some patients).
No products indexed under this heading.

Captopril (Co-administration with drugs with hypoglycemic activity, such as certain ACE inhibitors, may result in decreased insulin requirements). Products include:
Captopril Tablets 2114

Carteolol Hydrochloride (Co-administration with drugs with hypoglycemic activity, such as beta blockers, may result in decreased insulin requirements; beta blockers may mask the symptoms of hypoglycemia in some patients). Products include:
Carteolol Hydrochloride Ophthalmic Solution USP, 1% .... ⊙246

Chlorotrianisene (Co-administration may result in increased insulin requirements).
No products indexed under this heading.

Chlorpromazine (Co-administration with phenothiazines may result in increased insulin requirements).
No products indexed under this heading.

Chlorpromazine Hydrochloride (Co-administration with phenothiazines may result in increased insulin requirements).
No products indexed under this heading.

Chlorpropamide (Co-administration with drugs with hypoglycemic activity, such as oral hypoglycemic agents, may result in decreased insulin requirements).
No products indexed under this heading.

Choline Magnesium Trisalicylate (Co-administration with drugs with hypoglycemic activity, such as salicylates, may result in decreased insulin requirements).
No products indexed under this heading.

Cortisone Acetate (Co-administration may result in increased insulin requirements).
No products indexed under this heading.

Desogestrel (Co-admininstration with oral contraceptives may result in increased insulin requirements). Products include:
Ortho-Cept Tablets 2395

Dexamethasone (Co-administration may result in increased insulin requirements). Products include:
Ciprodex Otic Suspension 555
Decadron Tablets 1929
TobraDex Ophthalmic Ointment 558
TobraDex Ophthalmic Suspension 558

Dexamethasone Acetate (Co-administration may result in increased insulin requirements).
No products indexed under this heading.

Dexamethasone Sodium Phosphate (Co-administration may result in increased insulin requirements). Products include:
Decadron Phosphate Injection 1931

Dienestrol (Co-administration may result in increased insulin requirements).
No products indexed under this heading.

Diethylstilbestrol (Co-administration may result in increased insulin requirements).
No products indexed under this heading.

Diflunisal (Co-administration with drugs with hypoglycemic activity, such as salicylates, may result in decreased insulin requirements). Products include:
Dolobid Tablets 1937

Enalapril Maleate (Co-administration with drugs with hypoglycemic activity, such as certain ACE inhibitors, may result in decreased insulin requirements). Products include:
Vaseretic Tablets 2073
Vasotec I.V. Injection 2076

Enalaprilat (Co-administration with drugs with hypoglycemic activity, such as certain ACE inhibitors, may result in decreased insulin requirements).
No products indexed under this heading.

Esmolol Hydrochloride (Co-administration with drugs with hypoglycemic activity, such as beta blockers, may result in decreased insulin requirements; beta blockers may mask the symptoms of hypoglycemia in some patients). Products include:
Brevibloc Concentrate 766
Brevibloc Injection 766
Brevibloc Double Strength Injection 766
Brevibloc Premixed Injection 766
Brevibloc Double Strength Premixed Injection 766

Estradiol (Co-administration may result in increased insulin requirements). Products include:
Activella Tablets 2311
Climara Transdermal System 795
Climara Pro Transdermal System 800
CombiPatch Transdermal System 2180
Estrogel 0.06% 3200
Menostar Transdermal System 805
Prefest Tablets 1069
Vagifem Tablets 2340
Vivelle Transdermal System 2288
Vivelle-Dot Transdermal System 2293

Estrogens, Conjugated (Co-administration may result in increased insulin requirements). Products include:
Premarin Intravenous 3440
Premarin Tablets 3443
Premarin Vaginal Cream 3449
Premphase Tablets 3452
Prempro Tablets 3452

Estrogens, Esterified (Co-administration may result in increased insulin requirements). Products include:
Estratest Tablets 3196
Estratest H.S. Tablets 3196

Estropipate (Co-administration may result in increased insulin requirements).
No products indexed under this heading.

Ethinyl Estradiol (Co-administration may result in increased insulin requirements). Products include:
Alesse-28 Tablets 3392
Lo/Ovral-28 Tablets 3423
NuvaRing 2357
Ortho-Cept Tablets 2395
Ortho-Cyclen/Ortho Tri-Cyclen 2414
Ortho Evra Transdermal System 2402
Ortho Tri-Cyclen Lo Tablets 2421
Seasonale Tablets 1073
Triphasil-28 Tablets 3483
Yasmin 28 Tablets 818

Ethynodiol Diacetate (Co-admininstration with oral contraceptives may result in increased insulin requirements).
No products indexed under this heading.

Fludrocortisone Acetate (Co-administration may result in increased insulin requirements).
No products indexed under this heading.

Fluphenazine Decanoate (Co-administration with phenothiazines may result in increased insulin requirements).
No products indexed under this heading.

Fluphenazine Enanthate (Co-administration with phenothiazines may result in increased insulin requirements).
No products indexed under this heading.

Fluphenazine Hydrochloride (Co-administration with phenothiazines may result in increased insulin requirements).
No products indexed under this heading.

Fosinopril Sodium (Co-administration with drugs with hypoglycemic activity, such as certain ACE inhibitors, may result in decreased insulin requirements).
No products indexed under this heading.

Glimepiride (Co-administration with drugs with hypoglycemic activity, such as oral hypoglycemic agents, may result in decreased insulin requirements). Products include:
Amaryl Tablets 2864

Glipizide (Co-administration with drugs with hypoglycemic activity, such as oral hypoglycemic agents, may result in decreased insulin requirements).
No products indexed under this heading.

Glyburide (Co-administration with drugs with hypoglycemic activity, such as oral hypoglycemic agents, may result in decreased insulin requirements).
No products indexed under this heading.

Hydrocortisone (Co-administration may result in increased insulin requirements). Products include:
Cortizone•5 Ointment .... ▣699
Cortizone•10 Creme .... ▣699
Cortizone•10 Ointment .... ▣699
Cortizone•10 Plus Creme .... ▣700
Cortizone•10 Maximum Strength Quick Shot Spray .... ▣700
Hydrocortone Tablets 1963
Preparation H Hydrocortisone Cream .... ▣748

Hydrocortisone Acetate (Co-administration may result in increased insulin requirements). Products include:
Analpram-HC 1136
Pramosone 1139
ProctoFoam-HC 3113
Tucks Anti-Itch Ointment .... ▣712
U-cort 1% Cream 3289

Hydrocortisone Sodium Phosphate (Co-administration may result in increased insulin requirements).
No products indexed under this heading.

Hydrocortisone Sodium Succinate (Co-administration may result in increased insulin requirements).
No products indexed under this heading.

Isoniazid (Co-administration may result in increased insulin requirements).
No products indexed under this heading.

Labetalol Hydrochloride (Co-administration with drugs with hypoglycemic activity, such as beta blockers, may result in decreased insulin requirements; beta blockers may mask the symptoms of hypoglycemia in some patients).
No products indexed under this heading.

Levobunolol Hydrochloride (Co-administration with drugs with hypoglycemic activity, such as beta blockers, may result in decreased insulin requirements; beta blockers may mask the symptoms of hypoglycemia in some patients). Products include:
Betagan Ophthalmic Solution, USP .... ⊙217

Levonorgestrel (Co-admininstration with oral contraceptives may result in increased insulin requirements). Products include:
Alesse-28 Tablets 3392
Climara Pro Transdermal System 800
Mirena Intrauterine System 810
Plan B Tablets 1068
Seasonale Tablets 1073
Triphasil-28 Tablets 3483

Levothyroxine Sodium (Co-administration with thyroid replacement therapy may result in increased insulin requirements). Products include:
Levothroid Tablets 1189
Levoxyl Tablets 1680
Synthroid Tablets 515
Unithroid Tablets 3521

Liothyronine Sodium (Co-administration with thyroid replacement therapy may result in increased insulin requirements). Products include:
Cytomel Tablets 1678

Liotrix (Co-administration with thyroid replacement therapy may result in increased insulin requirements). Products include:
Thyrolar 1203

Lisinopril (Co-administration with drugs with hypoglycemic activity, such as certain ACE inhibitors, may result in decreased insulin requirements). Products include:
Prinivil Tablets 2029
Prinzide Tablets 2033
Zestoretic Tablets 701
Zestril Tablets 704

Magnesium Salicylate (Co-administration with drugs with hypoglycemic activity, such as salicylates, may result in decreased insulin requirements).
No products indexed under this heading.

Mesoridazine Besylate (Co-administration with phenothiazines may result in increased insulin requirements).
No products indexed under this heading.

Mestranol (Co-admininstration with oral contraceptives may result in increased insulin requirements).
No products indexed under this heading.

Metformin Hydrochloride (Co-administration with drugs with hypoglycemic activity, such as oral hypoglycemic agents, may result in decreased insulin requirements).
Products include:
ActoPlus Met Tablets **3219**
Avandamet Tablets **1343**
Fortamet Extended-Release Tablets **1156**

Methotrimeprazine (Co-administration with phenothiazines may result in increased insulin requirements).
No products indexed under this heading.

Methylprednisolone Acetate (Co-administration may result in increased insulin requirements).
Products include:
Depo-Medrol Injectable Suspension **2615**
Depo-Medrol Single-Dose Vial **2617**

Methylprednisolone Sodium Succinate (Co-administration may result in increased insulin requirements).
No products indexed under this heading.

Metipranolol Hydrochloride (Co-administration with drugs with hypoglycemic activity, such as beta blockers, may result in decreased insulin requirements; beta blockers may mask the symptoms of hypoglycemia in some patients).
No products indexed under this heading.

Metoprolol Succinate (Co-administration with drugs with hypoglycemic activity, such as beta blockers, may result in decreased insulin requirements; beta blockers may mask the symptoms of hypoglycemia in some patients). Products include:
Toprol-XL Tablets **660**

Metoprolol Tartrate (Co-administration with drugs with hypoglycemic activity, such as beta blockers, may result in decreased insulin requirements; beta blockers may mask the symptoms of hypoglycemia in some patients).
No products indexed under this heading.

Miglitol (Co-administration with drugs with hypoglycemic activity, such as oral hypoglycemic agents, may result in decreased insulin requirements).
No products indexed under this heading.

Moexipril Hydrochloride (Co-administration with drugs with hypoglycemic activity, such as certain ACE inhibitors, may result in decreased insulin requirements).
Products include:
Uniretic Tablets **3114**
Univasc Tablets **3118**

Nadolol (Co-administration with drugs with hypoglycemic activity, such as beta blockers, may result in decreased insulin requirements; beta blockers may mask the symptoms of hypoglycemia in some patients).
Products include:
Nadolol Tablets **2121**

Niacin (Co-administration may result in increased insulin requirements).
Products include:
Advicor Tablets **1694**
Niaspan Extended-Release Tablets **1703**

Norethindrone (Co-admininstration with oral contraceptives may result in increased insulin requirements).
Products include:
Ortho Micronor Tablets **2411**

Norethynodrel (Co-admininstration with oral contraceptives may result in increased insulin requirements).
No products indexed under this heading.

Norgestimate (Co-admininstration with oral contraceptives may result in increased insulin requirements).
Products include:
Ortho-Cyclen/Ortho Tri-Cyclen **2414**
Ortho Tri-Cyclen Lo Tablets **2421**
Prefest Tablets **1069**

Norgestrel (Co-admininstration with oral contraceptives may result in increased insulin requirements).
Products include:
Lo/Ovral-28 Tablets **3423**

Octreotide Acetate (Co-administration with drugs with hypoglycemic activity, such as inhibitors of pancreatic function, may result in decreased insulin requirements).
Products include:
Sandostatin Injection **2263**
Sandostatin LAR Depot **2264**

Penbutolol Sulfate (Co-administration with drugs with hypoglycemic activity, such as beta blockers, may result in decreased insulin requirements; beta blockers may mask the symptoms of hypoglycemia in some patients).
No products indexed under this heading.

Perindopril Erbumine (Co-administration with drugs with hypoglycemic activity, such as certain ACE inhibitors, may result in decreased insulin requirements).
Products include:
Aceon Tablets (2 mg, 4 mg, 8 mg) **3191**

Perphenazine (Co-administration with phenothiazines may result in increased insulin requirements).
No products indexed under this heading.

Phenelzine Sulfate (Co-administration with drugs with hypoglycemic activity, such as certain MAO inhibitor antidepressants, may result in decreased insulin requirements).
No products indexed under this heading.

Pindolol (Co-administration with drugs with hypoglycemic activity, such as beta blockers, may result in decreased insulin requirements; beta blockers may mask the symptoms of hypoglycemia in some patients).
No products indexed under this heading.

Pioglitazone Hydrochloride (Co-administration with drugs with hypoglycemic activity, such as oral hypoglycemic agents, may result in decreased insulin requirements).
Products include:
ActoPlus Met Tablets **3219**
Actos Tablets **3224**

Polyestradiol Phosphate (Co-administration may result in increased insulin requirements).
No products indexed under this heading.

Prednisolone Acetate (Co-administration may result in increased insulin requirements).
Products include:
Blephamide Ophthalmic Ointment **563**
Blephamide Ophthalmic Suspension **564**
Poly-Pred Liquifilm Ophthalmic Suspension .... ⊙ **231**
Pred Forte Ophthalmic Suspension .... ⊙ **233**
Pred Mild Sterile Ophthalmic Suspension .... ⊙ **236**
Pred-G Ophthalmic Suspension ...... ⊙ **234**
Pred-G Sterile Ophthalmic Ointment .... ⊙ **235**

Prednisolone Sodium Phosphate (Co-administration may result in increased insulin requirements).
Products include:
Pediapred Oral Solution **3319**

Prednisolone Tebutate (Co-administration may result in increased insulin requirements).
No products indexed under this heading.

Prednisone (Co-administration may result in increased insulin requirements).
No products indexed under this heading.

Prochlorperazine (Co-administration with phenothiazines may result in increased insulin requirements).
No products indexed under this heading.

Promethazine Hydrochloride (Co-administration with phenothiazines may result in increased insulin requirements). Products include:
Phenergan **3438**

Propranolol Hydrochloride (Co-administration with drugs with hypoglycemic activity, such as beta blockers, may result in decreased insulin requirements; beta blockers may mask the symptoms of hypoglycemia in some patients). Products include:
Inderal LA Long-Acting Capsules **3421**
InnoPran XL Capsules **2728**

Quinapril Hydrochloride (Co-administration with drugs with hypoglycemic activity, such as certain ACE inhibitors, may result in decreased insulin requirements).
No products indexed under this heading.

Quinestrol (Co-administration may result in increased insulin requirements).
No products indexed under this heading.

Ramipril (Co-administration with drugs with hypoglycemic activity, such as certain ACE inhibitors, may result in decreased insulin requirements). Products include:
Altace Capsules **1673**

Repaglinide (Co-administration with drugs with hypoglycemic activity, such as oral hypoglycemic agents, may result in decreased insulin requirements). Products include:
Prandin Tablets (0.5, 1, and 2 mg) **2337**

Rosiglitazone Maleate (Co-administration with drugs with hypoglycemic activity, such as oral hypoglycemic agents, may result in decreased insulin requirements).
Products include:
Avandamet Tablets **1343**
Avandia Tablets **1348**

Salsalate (Co-administration with drugs with hypoglycemic activity, such as salicylates, may result in decreased insulin requirements).
No products indexed under this heading.

Sotalol Hydrochloride (Co-administration with drugs with hypoglycemic activity, such as beta blockers, may result in decreased insulin requirements; beta blockers may mask the symptoms of hypoglycemia in some patients).
No products indexed under this heading.

Spirapril Hydrochloride (Co-administration with drugs with hypoglycemic activity, such as certain ACE inhibitors, may result in decreased insulin requirements).
No products indexed under this heading.

Sulfacytine (Co-administration with drugs with hypoglycemic activity, such as sulfa antibiotics, may result in decreased insulin requirements).
No products indexed under this heading.

Sulfamethizole (Co-administration with drugs with hypoglycemic activity, such as sulfa antibiotics, may result in decreased insulin requirements).
No products indexed under this heading.

Sulfamethoxazole (Co-administration with drugs with hypoglycemic activity, such as sulfa antibiotics, may result in decreased insulin requirements).
No products indexed under this heading.

Sulfasalazine (Co-administration with drugs with hypoglycemic activity, such as sulfa antibiotics, may result in decreased insulin requirements).
No products indexed under this heading.

Sulfisoxazole (Co-administration with drugs with hypoglycemic activity, such as sulfa antibiotics, may result in decreased insulin requirements).
No products indexed under this heading.

Thioridazine Hydrochloride (Co-administration with phenothiazines may result in increased insulin requirements). Products include:
Thioridazine Hydrochloride Tablets **2122**

Thyroglobulin (Co-administration with thyroid replacement therapy may result in increased insulin requirements).
No products indexed under this heading.

Thyroid (Co-administration with thyroid replacement therapy may result in increased insulin requirements).
No products indexed under this heading.

Thyroxine (Co-administration with thyroid replacement therapy may result in increased insulin requirements).
No products indexed under this heading.

IMPORTANT NOTE: Always consult each drug listing in the patient's regimen for possible interactions.

Thyroxine Sodium (Co-administration with thyroid replacement therapy may result in increased insulin requirements).
No products indexed under this heading.

Timolol Hemihydrate (Co-administration with drugs with hypoglycemic activity, such as beta blockers, may result in decreased insulin requirements; beta blockers may mask the symptoms of hypoglycemia in some patients). Products include:
Betimol Ophthalmic Solution 3371
Betimol Ophthalmic Solution .... ⊙283

Timolol Maleate (Co-administration with drugs with hypoglycemic activity, such as beta blockers, may result in decreased insulin requirements; beta blockers may mask the symptoms of hypoglycemia in some patients). Products include:
Blocadren Tablets 1891
Cosopt Sterile Ophthalmic Solution........................ 1910
Timolide Tablets 2056
Timoptic in Ocudose 2061
Timoptic Sterile Ophthalmic Solution........................ 2058
Timoptic-XE Sterile Ophthalmic Gel Forming Solution 2062

Tolazamide (Co-administration with drugs with hypoglycemic activity, such as oral hypoglycemic agents, may result in decreased insulin requirements).
No products indexed under this heading.

Tolbutamide (Co-administration with drugs with hypoglycemic activity, such as oral hypoglycemic agents, may result in decreased insulin requirements).
No products indexed under this heading.

Trandolapril (Co-administration with drugs with hypoglycemic activity, such as certain ACE inhibitors, may result in decreased insulin requirements). Products include:
Mavik Tablets 482
Tarka Tablets 519

Tranylcypromine Sulfate (Co-administration with drugs with hypoglycemic activity, such as certain MAO inhibitor antidepressants, may result in decreased insulin requirements). Products include:
Parnate Tablets 1499

Triamcinolone (Co-administration may result in increased insulin requirements).
No products indexed under this heading.

Triamcinolone Acetonide (Co-administration may result in increased insulin requirements). Products include:
Azmacort Inhalation Aerosol 1701
Nasacort HFA Inhalation Aerosol 2939
Nasacort AQ Nasal Spray 2937

Triamcinolone Diacetate (Co-administration may result in increased insulin requirements).
No products indexed under this heading.

Triamcinolone Hexacetonide (Co-administration may result in increased insulin requirements).
No products indexed under this heading.

Trifluoperazine Hydrochloride (Co-administration with phenothiazines may result in increased insulin requirements).
No products indexed under this heading.

Troglitazone (Co-administration with drugs with hypoglycemic activity, such as oral hypoglycemic agents, may result in decreased insulin requirements).
No products indexed under this heading.

Food Interactions

Alcohol (Co-administration with drugs with hypoglycemic activity may result in decreased insulin requirements).

HUMALOG MIX 75/25-PEN

(Insulin Lispro, Human, Insulin Lispro Protamine, Human) 1754
See Humalog-Pen

HUMATROPE VIALS AND CARTRIDGES

(Somatropin) 1756
May interact with glucocorticoids, insulin, phenytoin, sex steroids, and certain other agents. Compounds in these categories include:

ACTH (Excessive glucocorticoid therapy will inhibit the growth promoting effect of somatropin; growth hormone administration may alter the clearance of compounds known to be metabolized by cytochrome P450 liver enzymes; such as corticosteroids).
No products indexed under this heading.

Betamethasone Acetate (Excessive glucocorticoid therapy will inhibit the growth promoting effect of somatropin; growth hormone administration may alter the clearance of compounds known to be metabolized by cytochrome P450 liver enzymes; such as corticosteroids).
No products indexed under this heading.

Betamethasone Sodium Phosphate (Excessive glucocorticoid therapy will inhibit the growth promoting effect of somatropin; growth hormone administration may alter the clearance of compounds known to be metabolized by cytochrome P450 liver enzymes; such as corticosteroids).
No products indexed under this heading.

Cortisone Acetate (Excessive glucocorticoid therapy will inhibit the growth promoting effect of somatropin; growth hormone administration may alter the clearance of compounds known to be metabolized by cytochrome P450 liver enzymes; such as corticosteroids).
No products indexed under this heading.

Cyclosporine (Growth hormone administration may alter the clearance of compounds known to be metabolized by cytochrome P450 liver enzymes, such as cyclosporine). Products include:
Gengraf Capsules 458
Neoral Soft Gelatin Capsules 2247
Neoral Oral Solution 2247
Restasis Ophthalmic Emulsion 570
Sandimmune 2259

Desogestrel (Growth hormone administration may alter the clearance of compounds known to be metabolized by cytochrome P450 liver enzymes, such as sex steroids). Products include:
Ortho-Cept Tablets 2395

Dexamethasone (Excessive glucocorticoid therapy will inhibit the growth promoting effect of somatropin; growth hormone administration may alter the clearance of compounds known to be metabolized by cytochrome P450 liver enzymes; such as corticosteroids). Products include:
Ciprodex Otic Suspension 555
Decadron Tablets 1929
TobraDex Ophthalmic Ointment 558
TobraDex Ophthalmic Suspension ... 558

Dexamethasone Acetate (Excessive glucocorticoid therapy will inhibit the growth promoting effect of somatropin; growth hormone administration may alter the clearance of compounds known to be metabolized by cytochrome P450 liver enzymes; such as corticosteroids).
No products indexed under this heading.

Dexamethasone Sodium Phosphate (Excessive glucocorticoid therapy will inhibit the growth promoting effect of somatropin; growth hormone administration may alter the clearance of compounds known to be metabolized by cytochrome P450 liver enzymes; such as corticosteroids). Products include:
Decadron Phosphate Injection 1931

Estradiol (Growth hormone administration may alter the clearance of compounds known to be metabolized by cytochrome P450 liver enzymes, such as sex steroids). Products include:
Activella Tablets 2311
Climara Transdermal System 795
Climara Pro Transdermal System 800
CombiPatch Transdermal System 2180
Estrogel 0.06% 3200
Menostar Transdermal System 805
Prefest Tablets 1069
Vagifem Tablets 2340
Vivelle Transdermal System 2288
Vivelle-Dot Transdermal System 2293

Estrogens, Conjugated (Growth hormone administration may alter the clearance of compounds known to be metabolized by cytochrome P450 liver enzymes, such as sex steroids). Products include:
Premarin Intravenous 3440
Premarin Tablets 3443
Premarin Vaginal Cream 3449
Premphase Tablets 3452
Prempro Tablets 3452

Ethinyl Estradiol (Growth hormone administration may alter the clearance of compounds known to be metabolized by cytochrome P450 liver enzymes, such as sex steroids). Products include:
Alesse-28 Tablets 3392
Lo/Ovral-28 Tablets 3423
NuvaRing 2357
Ortho-Cept Tablets 2395
Ortho-Cyclen/Ortho Tri-Cyclen 2414
Ortho Evra Transdermal System 2402
Ortho Tri-Cyclen Lo Tablets 2421
Seasonale Tablets 1073
Triphasil-28 Tablets 3483
Yasmin 28 Tablets 818

Ethynodiol Diacetate (Growth hormone administration may alter the clearance of compounds known to be metabolized by cytochrome P450 liver enzymes, such as sex steroids).
No products indexed under this heading.

Fludrocortisone Acetate (Excessive glucocorticoid therapy will inhibit the growth promoting effect of somatropin; growth hormone administration may alter the clearance of compounds known to be metabolized by cytochrome P450 liver enzymes; such as corticosteroids).
No products indexed under this heading.

Fluoxymesterone (Growth hormone administration may alter the clearance of compounds known to be metabolized by cytochrome P450 liver enzymes, such as sex steroids).
No products indexed under this heading.

Fosphenytoin Sodium (Growth hormone administration may alter the clearance of compounds known to be metabolized by CYP450 liver enzymes, such as anticonvulsants).
No products indexed under this heading.

Hydrocortisone (Excessive glucocorticoid therapy will inhibit the growth promoting effect of somatropin; growth hormone administration may alter the clearance of compounds known to be metabolized by cytochrome P450 liver enzymes; such as corticosteroids). Products include:
Cortizone•5 Ointment .... ▣699
Cortizone•10 Creme .... ▣699
Cortizone•10 Ointment .... ▣699
Cortizone•10 Plus Creme .... ▣700
Cortizone•10 Maximum Strength Quick Shot Spray .... ▣700
Hydrocortone Tablets 1963
Preparation H Hydrocortisone Cream .... ▣748

Hydrocortisone Acetate (Excessive glucocorticoid therapy will inhibit the growth promoting effect of somatropin; growth hormone administration may alter the clearance of compounds known to be metabolized by cytochrome P450 liver enzymes; such as corticosteroids). Products include:
Analpram-HC 1136
Pramosone 1139
ProctoFoam-HC 3113
Tucks Anti-Itch Ointment .... ▣712
U-cort 1% Cream 3289

Hydrocortisone Sodium Phosphate (Excessive glucocorticoid therapy will inhibit the growth promoting effect of somatropin; growth hormone administration may alter the clearance of compounds known to be metabolized by cytochrome P450 liver enzymes; such as corticosteroids).
No products indexed under this heading.

Hydrocortisone Sodium Succinate (Excessive glucocorticoid therapy will inhibit the growth promoting effect of somatropin; growth hormone administration may alter the clearance of compounds known to be metabolized by cytochrome P450 liver enzymes; such as corticosteroids).
No products indexed under this heading.

Insulin, Human, Zinc Suspension (For diabetics, the insulin dose may require adjustment when somatropin therapy is instituted; growth hormone may induce a state of insulin resistance; patients should be observed for evidence of glucose intolerance). Products include:
Humulin L, 100 Units 1763

Humulin U, 100 Units 1770

Insulin, Human NPH (For diabetics, the insulin dose may require adjustment when somatropin therapy is instituted; growth hormone may induce a state of insulin resistance; patients should be observed for evidence of glucose intolerance). Products include:

Humulin N, 100 Units 1764
Humulin N Pen 1765
Novolin N Human Insulin 10 ml Vials 2322
Novolin N InnoLet 2322
Novolin N PenFill 3 ml Cartridges 2325
Novolin R InnoLet 2322

Insulin, Human Regular (For diabetics, the insulin dose may require adjustment when somatropin therapy is instituted; growth hormone may induce a state of insulin resistance; patients should be observed for evidence of glucose intolerance). Products include:

Humulin R (U-500) 1768
Humulin R, 100 Units 1767
Novolin R Human Insulin 10 ml Vials 2322
Novolin R PenFill 2325

Insulin, Human Regular and Human NPH Mixture (For diabetics, the insulin dose may require adjustment when somatropin therapy is instituted; growth hormone may induce a state of insulin resistance; patients should be observed for evidence of glucose intolerance). Products include:

Humulin 50/50, 100 Units 1760
Humulin 70/30 Pen 1761
Novolin 70/30 Human Insulin 10 ml Vials 2321
Novolin 70/30 InnoLet 2322
Novolin 70/30 PenFill 3 ml Cartridges 2325

Insulin, NPH (For diabetics, the insulin dose may require adjustment when somatropin therapy is instituted; growth hormone may induce a state of insulin resistance; patients should be observed for evidence of glucose intolerance).

No products indexed under this heading.

Insulin, Regular (For diabetics, the insulin dose may require adjustment when somatropin therapy is instituted; growth hormone may induce a state of insulin resistance; patients should be observed for evidence of glucose intolerance).

No products indexed under this heading.

Insulin, Zinc Crystals (For diabetics, the insulin dose may require adjustment when somatropin therapy is instituted; growth hormone may induce a state of insulin resistance; patients should be observed for evidence of glucose intolerance).

No products indexed under this heading.

Insulin, Zinc Suspension (For diabetics, the insulin dose may require adjustment when somatropin therapy is instituted; growth hormone may induce a state of insulin resistance; patients should be observed for evidence of glucose intolerance).

No products indexed under this heading.

Insulin Aspart, Human Regular (For diabetics, the insulin dose may require adjustment when somatropin therapy is instituted; growth hormone may induce a state of insulin resistance; patients should be observed for evidence of glucose intolerance). Products include:

NovoLog Injection 2326

Insulin glargine (For diabetics, the insulin dose may require adjustment when somatropin therapy is instituted; growth hormone may induce a state of insulin resistance; patients should be observed for evidence of glucose intolerance). Products include:

Lantus Injection 2925

Insulin Lispro, Human (For diabetics, the insulin dose may require adjustment when somatropin therapy is instituted; growth hormone may induce a state of insulin resistance; patients should be observed for evidence of glucose intolerance). Products include:

Humalog-Pen 1751
Humalog Mix 75/25-Pen 1754

Insulin Lispro Protamine, Human (For diabetics, the insulin dose may require adjustment when somatropin therapy is instituted; growth hormone may induce a state of insulin resistance; patients should be observed for evidence of glucose intolerance). Products include:

Humalog Mix 75/25-Pen 1754

Levonorgestrel (Growth hormone administration may alter the clearance of compounds known to be metabolized by cytochrome P450 liver enzymes, such as sex steroids). Products include:

Alesse-28 Tablets 3392
Climara Pro Transdermal System 800
Mirena Intrauterine System 810
Plan B Tablets 1068
Seasonale Tablets 1073
Triphasil-28 Tablets 3483

Mestranol (Growth hormone administration may alter the clearance of compounds known to be metabolized by cytochrome P450 liver enzymes, such as sex steroids).

No products indexed under this heading.

Methylprednisolone Acetate (Excessive glucocorticoid therapy will inhibit the growth promoting effect of somatropin; growth hormone administration may alter the clearance of compounds known to be metabolized by cytochrome P450 liver enzymes; such as corticosteroids). Products include:

Depo-Medrol Injectable Suspension 2615
Depo-Medrol Single-Dose Vial 2617

Methylprednisolone Sodium Succinate (Excessive glucocorticoid therapy will inhibit the growth promoting effect of somatropin; growth hormone administration may alter the clearance of compounds known to be metabolized by cytochrome P450 liver enzymes; such as corticosteroids).

No products indexed under this heading.

Methyltestosterone (Growth hormone administration may alter the clearance of compounds known to be metabolized by cytochrome P450 liver enzymes, such as sex steroids). Products include:

Estratest Tablets 3196
Estratest H.S. Tablets 3196

Norethindrone (Growth hormone administration may alter the clearance of compounds known to be metabolized by cytochrome P450 liver enzymes, such as sex steroids). Products include:

Ortho Micronor Tablets 2411

Norethindrone Acetate (Growth hormone administration may alter the clearance of compounds known to be metabolized by cytochrome P450 liver enzymes, such as sex steroids). Products include:

Activella Tablets 2311
Aygestin Tablets 1062
CombiPatch Transdermal System 2180

Norgestimate (Growth hormone administration may alter the clearance of compounds known to be metabolized by cytochrome P450 liver enzymes, such as sex steroids). Products include:

Ortho-Cyclen/Ortho Tri-Cyclen 2414
Ortho Tri-Cyclen Lo Tablets 2421
Prefest Tablets 1069

Phenobarbital (Growth hormone administration may alter the clearance of compounds known to be metabolized by CYP450 liver enzymes, such as anticonvulsants).

No products indexed under this heading.

Phenytoin (Growth hormone administration may alter the clearance of compounds known to be metabolized by CYP450 liver enzymes, such as anticonvulsants).

No products indexed under this heading.

Phenytoin Sodium (Growth hormone administration may alter the clearance of compounds known to be metabolized by CYP450 liver enzymes, such as anticonvulsants). Products include:

Phenytek Capsules 2153

Prednisolone Acetate (Excessive glucocorticoid therapy will inhibit the growth promoting effect of somatropin; growth hormone administration may alter the clearance of compounds known to be metabolized by cytochrome P450 liver enzymes; such as corticosteroids). Products include:

Blephamide Ophthalmic Ointment 563
Blephamide Ophthalmic Suspension 564
Poly-Pred Liquifilm Ophthalmic Suspension .... ⊙231
Pred Forte Ophthalmic Suspension .... ⊙233
Pred Mild Sterile Ophthalmic Suspension .... ⊙236
Pred-G Ophthalmic Suspension .... ⊙234
Pred-G Sterile Ophthalmic Ointment .... ⊙235

Prednisolone Sodium Phosphate (Excessive glucocorticoid therapy will inhibit the growth promoting effect of somatropin; growth hormone administration may alter the clearance of compounds known to be metabolized by cytochrome P450 liver enzymes; such as corticosteroids). Products include:

Pediapred Oral Solution 3319

Prednisolone Tebutate (Excessive glucocorticoid therapy will inhibit the growth promoting effect of somatropin; growth hormone administration may alter the clearance of compounds known to be metabolized by cytochrome P450 liver enzymes; such as corticosteroids).

No products indexed under this heading.

Prednisone (Excessive glucocorticoid therapy will inhibit the growth promoting effect of somatropin; growth hormone administration may alter the clearance of compounds known to be metabolized by cytochrome P450 liver enzymes; such as corticosteroids).

No products indexed under this heading.

Testosterone (Growth hormone administration may alter the clearance of compounds known to be metabolized by cytochrome P450 liver enzymes, such as sex steroids). Products include:

AndroGel 3330
Striant Mucoadhesive 1022
Testim 1% Gel 722

Triamcinolone (Excessive glucocorticoid therapy will inhibit the growth promoting effect of somatropin; growth hormone administration may alter the clearance of compounds known to be metabolized by cytochrome P450 liver enzymes; such as corticosteroids).

No products indexed under this heading.

Triamcinolone Acetonide (Excessive glucocorticoid therapy will inhibit the growth promoting effect of somatropin; growth hormone administration may alter the clearance of compounds known to be metabolized by cytochrome P450 liver enzymes; such as corticosteroids). Products include:

Azmacort Inhalation Aerosol 1701
Nasacort HFA Inhalation Aerosol 2939
Nasacort AQ Nasal Spray 2937

Triamcinolone Diacetate (Excessive glucocorticoid therapy will inhibit the growth promoting effect of somatropin; growth hormone administration may alter the clearance of compounds known to be metabolized by cytochrome P450 liver enzymes; such as corticosteroids).

No products indexed under this heading.

Triamcinolone Hexacetonide (Excessive glucocorticoid therapy will inhibit the growth promoting effect of somatropin; growth hormone administration may alter the clearance of compounds known to be metabolized by cytochrome P450 liver enzymes; such as corticosteroids).

No products indexed under this heading.

HUMIRA INJECTION

(Adalimumab) 464

May interact with:

Anakinra (Concurrent administration of anakinra (an interleukin-1 antagonist) and another TNF-blocking agent has been associated with an increased risk of serious infections, an increased risk of neutropenia and no additional benefit compared to these medicinal agents alone. Therefore, the combination of anakinra with other TNF-blocking agents, including adalimumab, may also result in similar toxicities). Products include:

Kineret Injection 594

Methotrexate (Methotrexate reduced adalimumab apparent clearance after single and multiple dosing by 29% and 44% respectively).

No products indexed under this heading.

Vaccines (Live) (Live vaccines should not be given concurrently with Humira).

No products indexed under this heading.

HUMULIN 50/50, 100 UNITS

(Insulin, Human Regular and Human NPH Mixture) 1760

See Humulin N Pen

HUMULIN 70/30 PEN
(Insulin, Human Regular and Human NPH Mixture).......................... 1761
See Humulin N Pen

HUMULIN L, 100 UNITS
(Insulin, Human, Zinc Suspension) 1763
See Humulin N Pen

HUMULIN N, 100 UNITS
(Insulin, Human NPH) 1764
See Humulin N Pen

HUMULIN R (U-500)
(Insulin, Human Regular) 1768
May interact with beta blockers and oral hypoglycemic agents. Compounds in these categories include:

Acarbose (Concurrent use of oral hypoglycemic agents with Humulin R (U-500) is not recommended since there are no data to support such use). Products include:
Precose Tablets 776

Acebutolol Hydrochloride (Early warning symptoms of hypoglycemia may be different or less pronounced under certain conditions, such as concurrent beta blocker therapy).
No products indexed under this heading.

Atenolol (Early warning symptoms of hypoglycemia may be different or less pronounced under certain conditions, such as concurrent beta blocker therapy). Products include:
Tenormin I.V. Injection 698
Tenormin Tablets 695

Betaxolol Hydrochloride (Early warning symptoms of hypoglycemia may be different or less pronounced under certain conditions, such as concurrent beta blocker therapy). Products include:
Betoptic S Ophthalmic Suspension... 554

Bisoprolol Fumarate (Early warning symptoms of hypoglycemia may be different or less pronounced under certain conditions, such as concurrent beta blocker therapy).
No products indexed under this heading.

Carteolol Hydrochloride (Early warning symptoms of hypoglycemia may be different or less pronounced under certain conditions, such as concurrent beta blocker therapy). Products include:
Carteolol Hydrochloride Ophthalmic Solution USP, 1%....... ⊙246

Chlorpropamide (Concurrent use of oral hypoglycemic agents with Humulin R (U-500) is not recommended since there are no data to support such use).
No products indexed under this heading.

Esmolol Hydrochloride (Early warning symptoms of hypoglycemia may be different or less pronounced under certain conditions, such as concurrent beta blocker therapy). Products include:
Brevibloc Concentrate 766
Brevibloc Injection 766
Brevibloc Double Strength Injection.. 766
Brevibloc Premixed Injection 766
Brevibloc Double Strength Premixed Injection 766

Glimepiride (Concurrent use of oral hypoglycemic agents with Humulin R (U-500) is not recommended since there are no data to support such use). Products include:
Amaryl Tablets 2864

Glipizide (Concurrent use of oral hypoglycemic agents with Humulin R (U-500) is not recommended since there are no data to support such use).
No products indexed under this heading.

Glyburide (Concurrent use of oral hypoglycemic agents with Humulin R (U-500) is not recommended since there are no data to support such use).
No products indexed under this heading.

Labetalol Hydrochloride (Early warning symptoms of hypoglycemia may be different or less pronounced under certain conditions, such as concurrent beta blocker therapy).
No products indexed under this heading.

Levobunolol Hydrochloride (Early warning symptoms of hypoglycemia may be different or less pronounced under certain conditions, such as concurrent beta blocker therapy). Products include:
Betagan Ophthalmic Solution, USP.. ⊙217

Metformin Hydrochloride (Concurrent use of oral hypoglycemic agents with Humulin R (U-500) is not recommended since there are no data to support such use). Products include:
ActoPlus Met Tablets 3219
Avandamet Tablets 1343
Fortamet Extended-Release Tablets 1156

Metipranolol Hydrochloride (Early warning symptoms of hypoglycemia may be different or less pronounced under certain conditions, such as concurrent beta blocker therapy).
No products indexed under this heading.

Metoprolol Succinate (Early warning symptoms of hypoglycemia may be different or less pronounced under certain conditions, such as concurrent beta blocker therapy). Products include:
Toprol-XL Tablets 660

Metoprolol Tartrate (Early warning symptoms of hypoglycemia may be different or less pronounced under certain conditions, such as concurrent beta blocker therapy).
No products indexed under this heading.

Miglitol (Concurrent use of oral hypoglycemic agents with Humulin R (U-500) is not recommended since there are no data to support such use).
No products indexed under this heading.

Nadolol (Early warning symptoms of hypoglycemia may be different or less pronounced under certain conditions, such as concurrent beta blocker therapy). Products include:
Nadolol Tablets 2121

Penbutolol Sulfate (Early warning symptoms of hypoglycemia may be different or less pronounced under certain conditions, such as concurrent beta blocker therapy).
No products indexed under this heading.

Pindolol (Early warning symptoms of hypoglycemia may be different or less pronounced under certain conditions, such as concurrent beta blocker therapy).
No products indexed under this heading.

Pioglitazone Hydrochloride (Concurrent use of oral hypoglycemic agents with Humulin R (U-500) is not recommended since there are no data to support such use). Products include:
ActoPlus Met Tablets 3219
Actos Tablets 3224

Propranolol Hydrochloride (Early warning symptoms of hypoglycemia may be different or less pronounced under certain conditions, such as concurrent beta blocker therapy). Products include:
Inderal LA Long-Acting Capsules 3421
InnoPran XL Capsules 2728

Repaglinide (Concurrent use of oral hypoglycemic agents with Humulin R (U-500) is not recommended since there are no data to support such use). Products include:
Prandin Tablets (0.5, 1, and 2 mg).. 2337

Rosiglitazone Maleate (Concurrent use of oral hypoglycemic agents with Humulin R (U-500) is not recommended since there are no data to support such use). Products include:
Avandamet Tablets 1343
Avandia Tablets 1348

Sotalol Hydrochloride (Early warning symptoms of hypoglycemia may be different or less pronounced under certain conditions, such as concurrent beta blocker therapy).
No products indexed under this heading.

Timolol Hemihydrate (Early warning symptoms of hypoglycemia may be different or less pronounced under certain conditions, such as concurrent beta blocker therapy). Products include:
Betimol Ophthalmic Solution 3371
Betimol Ophthalmic Solution .... ⊙283

Timolol Maleate (Early warning symptoms of hypoglycemia may be different or less pronounced under certain conditions, such as concurrent beta blocker therapy). Products include:
Blocadren Tablets 1891
Cosopt Sterile Ophthalmic Solution.. 1910
Timolide Tablets 2056
Timoptic in Ocudose 2061
Timoptic Sterile Ophthalmic Solution.. 2058
Timoptic-XE Sterile Ophthalmic Gel Forming Solution 2062

Tolazamide (Concurrent use of oral hypoglycemic agents with Humulin R (U-500) is not recommended since there are no data to support such use).
No products indexed under this heading.

Tolbutamide (Concurrent use of oral hypoglycemic agents with Humulin R (U-500) is not recommended since there are no data to support such use).
No products indexed under this heading.

Troglitazone (Concurrent use of oral hypoglycemic agents with Humulin R (U-500) is not recommended since there are no data to support such use).
No products indexed under this heading.

HUMULIN R, 100 UNITS
(Insulin, Human Regular) 1767
See Humulin N Pen

HUMULIN U, 100 UNITS
(Insulin, Human, Zinc Suspension) 1770
See Humulin N Pen

HUMULIN N PEN
(Insulin, Human NPH) 1765
May interact with corticosteroids, oral hypoglycemic agents, oral contraceptives, salicylates, thyroid preparations, and certain other agents. Compounds in these categories include:

Acarbose (Co-administration with drugs with hypoglycemic activity, such as oral hypoglycemic agents, may result in decreased insulin requirements). Products include:
Precose Tablets 776

Aspirin (Co-administration with drugs with hypoglycemic activity, such as salicylates, may result in decreased insulin requirements). Products include:
Aggrenox Capsules 855
Bayer, Aspirin Regimen .... ▣606
Bayer Aspirin Tablets 3515
BC Powder .... ▣612
BC Allergy Sinus Cold Powder .... ▣612
Arthritis Strength BC Powder .... ▣612
BC Sinus Cold Powder .... ▣612
Ecotrin Enteric Coated Aspirin Low, Regular and Maximum Strength Tablets........................... 1627
Goody's Body Pain Formula Powder.. ▣621
Goody's Extra Strength Headache Powder........................... ▣621
Goody's Extra Strength Pain Relief Tablets .... ▣621
Percodan Tablets 1115
St. Joseph 81 mg Aspirin Chewable and Enteric Coated Tablets.. 1841

Aspirin, Enteric Coated (Co-administration with drugs with hypoglycemic activity, such as salicylates, may result in decreased insulin requirements).
No products indexed under this heading.

Aspirin Buffered (Co-administration with drugs with hypoglycemic activity, such as salicylates, may result in decreased insulin requirements).
No products indexed under this heading.

Betamethasone Acetate (Co-administration may result in increased insulin requirements).
No products indexed under this heading.

Betamethasone Sodium Phosphate (Co-administration may result in increased insulin requirements).
No products indexed under this heading.

Chlorpropamide (Co-administration with drugs with hypoglycemic activity, such as oral hypoglycemic agents, may result in decreased insulin requirements).
No products indexed under this heading.

Choline Magnesium Trisalicylate (Co-administration with drugs with hypoglycemic activity, such as salicylates, may result in decreased insulin requirements).
No products indexed under this heading.

Cortisone Acetate (Co-administration may result in increased insulin requirements).
No products indexed under this heading.

Desogestrel (Co-administration with oral contraceptives may result in increased insulin requirements).
Products include:
Ortho-Cept Tablets ... 2395

Dexamethasone (Co-administration may result in increased insulin requirements).
Products include:
Ciprodex Otic Suspension ... 555
Decadron Tablets ... 1929
TobraDex Ophthalmic Ointment ... 558
TobraDex Ophthalmic Suspension ... 558

Dexamethasone Acetate (Co-administration may result in increased insulin requirements).
No products indexed under this heading.

Dexamethasone Sodium Phosphate (Co-administration may result in increased insulin requirements).
Products include:
Decadron Phosphate Injection ... 1931

Diflunisal (Co-administration with drugs with hypoglycemic activity, such as salicylates, may result in decreased insulin requirements).
Products include:
Dolobid Tablets ... 1937

Ethinyl Estradiol (Co-administration with oral contraceptives may result in increased insulin requirements). Products include:
Alesse-28 Tablets ... 3392
Lo/Ovral-28 Tablets ... 3423
NuvaRing ... 2357
Ortho-Cept Tablets ... 2395
Ortho-Cyclen/Ortho Tri-Cyclen ... 2414
Ortho Evra Transdermal System ... 2402
Ortho Tri-Cyclen Lo Tablets ... 2421
Seasonale Tablets ... 1073
Triphasil-28 Tablets ... 3483
Yasmin 28 Tablets ... 818

Ethynodiol Diacetate (Co-administration with oral contraceptives may result in increased insulin requirements).
No products indexed under this heading.

Fludrocortisone Acetate (Co-administration may result in increased insulin requirements).
No products indexed under this heading.

Glimepiride (Co-administration with drugs with hypoglycemic activity, such as oral hypoglycemic agents, may result in decreased insulin requirements). Products include:
Amaryl Tablets ... 2864

Glipizide (Co-administration with drugs with hypoglycemic activity, such as oral hypoglycemic agents, may result in decreased insulin requirements).
No products indexed under this heading.

Glyburide (Co-administration with drugs with hypoglycemic activity, such as oral hypoglycemic agents, may result in decreased insulin requirements).
No products indexed under this heading.

Hydrocortisone (Co-administration may result in increased insulin requirements). Products include:
Cortizone•5 Ointment ... 699
Cortizone•10 Creme ... 699
Cortizone•10 Ointment ... 699
Cortizone•10 Plus Creme ... 700
Cortizone•10 Maximum Strength Quick Shot Spray ... 700
Hydrocortone Tablets ... 1963
Preparation H Hydrocortisone Cream ... 748

Hydrocortisone Acetate (Co-administration may result in increased insulin requirements).
Products include:
Analpram-HC ... 1136
Pramosone ... 1139
ProctoFoam-HC ... 3113
Tucks Anti-Itch Ointment ... 712
U-cort 1% Cream ... 3289

Hydrocortisone Sodium Phosphate (Co-administration may result in increased insulin requirements).
No products indexed under this heading.

Hydrocortisone Sodium Succinate (Co-administration may result in increased insulin requirements).
No products indexed under this heading.

Levonorgestrel (Co-administration with oral contraceptives may result in increased insulin requirements).
Products include:
Alesse-28 Tablets ... 3392
Climara Pro Transdermal System ... 800
Mirena Intrauterine System ... 810
Plan B Tablets ... 1068
Seasonale Tablets ... 1073
Triphasil-28 Tablets ... 3483

Levothyroxine Sodium (Co-administration with thyroid replacement therapy may result in increased insulin requirements). Products include:
Levothroid Tablets ... 1189
Levoxyl Tablets ... 1680
Synthroid Tablets ... 515
Unithroid Tablets ... 3521

Liothyronine Sodium (Co-administration with thyroid replacement therapy may result in increased insulin requirements). Products include:
Cytomel Tablets ... 1678

Liotrix (Co-administration with thyroid replacement therapy may result in increased insulin requirements).
Products include:
Thyrolar ... 1203

Magnesium Salicylate (Co-administration with drugs with hypoglycemic activity, such as salicylates, may result in decreased insulin requirements).
No products indexed under this heading.

Mestranol (Co-administration with oral contraceptives may result in increased insulin requirements).
No products indexed under this heading.

Metformin Hydrochloride (Co-administration with drugs with hypoglycemic activity, such as oral hypoglycemic agents, may result in decreased insulin requirements).
Products include:
ActoPlus Met Tablets ... 3219
Avandamet Tablets ... 1343
Fortamet Extended-Release Tablets ... 1156

Methylprednisolone Acetate (Co-administration may result in increased insulin requirements).
Products include:
Depo-Medrol Injectable Suspension ... 2615
Depo-Medrol Single-Dose Vial ... 2617

Methylprednisolone Sodium Succinate (Co-administration may result in increased insulin requirements).
No products indexed under this heading.

Miglitol (Co-administration with drugs with hypoglycemic activity, such as oral hypoglycemic agents, may result in decreased insulin requirements).
No products indexed under this heading.

Norethindrone (Co-administration with oral contraceptives may result in increased insulin requirements).
Products include:
Ortho Micronor Tablets ... 2411

Norethynodrel (Co-administration with oral contraceptives may result in increased insulin requirements).
No products indexed under this heading.

Norgestimate (Co-administration with oral contraceptives may result in increased insulin requirements).
Products include:
Ortho-Cyclen/Ortho Tri-Cyclen ... 2414
Ortho Tri-Cyclen Lo Tablets ... 2421
Prefest Tablets ... 1069

Norgestrel (Co-administration with oral contraceptives may result in increased insulin requirements).
Products include:
Lo/Ovral-28 Tablets ... 3423

Phenelzine Sulfate (Co-administration with drugs with hypoglycemic activity, such as certain MAO inhibitor antidepressants, may result in decreased insulin requirements).
No products indexed under this heading.

Pioglitazone Hydrochloride (Co-administration with drugs with hypoglycemic activity, such as oral hypoglycemic agents, may result in decreased insulin requirements).
Products include:
ActoPlus Met Tablets ... 3219
Actos Tablets ... 3224

Prednisolone Acetate (Co-administration may result in increased insulin requirements).
Products include:
Blephamide Ophthalmic Ointment ... 563
Blephamide Ophthalmic Suspension ... 564
Poly-Pred Liquifilm Ophthalmic Suspension ... ⊙ 231
Pred Forte Ophthalmic Suspension ... ⊙ 233
Pred Mild Sterile Ophthalmic Suspension ... ⊙ 236
Pred-G Ophthalmic Suspension ... ⊙ 234
Pred-G Sterile Ophthalmic Ointment ... ⊙ 235

Prednisolone Sodium Phosphate (Co-administration may result in increased insulin requirements).
Products include:
Pediapred Oral Solution ... 3319

Prednisolone Tebutate (Co-administration may result in increased insulin requirements).
No products indexed under this heading.

Prednisone (Co-administration may result in increased insulin requirements).
No products indexed under this heading.

Repaglinide (Co-administration with drugs with hypoglycemic activity, such as oral hypoglycemic agents, may result in decreased insulin requirements). Products include:
Prandin Tablets (0.5, 1, and 2 mg) ... 2337

Rosiglitazone Maleate (Co-administration with drugs with hypoglycemic activity, such as oral hypoglycemic agents, may result in decreased insulin requirements).
Products include:
Avandamet Tablets ... 1343
Avandia Tablets ... 1348

Salsalate (Co-administration with drugs with hypoglycemic activity, such as salicylates, may result in decreased insulin requirements).
No products indexed under this heading.

Sulfacytine (Co-administration with drugs with hypoglycemic activity, such as sulfa antibiotics, may result in decreased insulin requirements).
No products indexed under this heading.

Sulfamethizole (Co-administration with drugs with hypoglycemic activity, such as sulfa antibiotics, may result in decreased insulin requirements).
No products indexed under this heading.

Sulfamethoxazole (Co-administration with drugs with hypoglycemic activity, such as sulfa antibiotics, may result in decreased insulin requirements).
No products indexed under this heading.

Sulfasalazine (Co-administration with drugs with hypoglycemic activity, such as sulfa antibiotics, may result in decreased insulin requirements).
No products indexed under this heading.

Sulfisoxazole (Co-administration with drugs with hypoglycemic activity, such as sulfa antibiotics, may result in decreased insulin requirements).
No products indexed under this heading.

Thyroglobulin (Co-administration with thyroid replacement therapy may result in increased insulin requirements).
No products indexed under this heading.

Thyroid (Co-administration with thyroid replacement therapy may result in increased insulin requirements).
No products indexed under this heading.

Thyroxine (Co-administration with thyroid replacement therapy may result in increased insulin requirements).
No products indexed under this heading.

Thyroxine Sodium (Co-administration with thyroid replacement therapy may result in increased insulin requirements).
No products indexed under this heading.

Tolazamide (Co-administration with drugs with hypoglycemic activity, such as oral hypoglycemic agents, may result in decreased insulin requirements).
No products indexed under this heading.

IMPORTANT NOTE: Always consult each drug listing in the patient's regimen for possible interactions.

Tolbutamide (Co-administration with drugs with hypoglycemic activity, such as oral hypoglycemic agents, may result in decreased insulin requirements).
No products indexed under this heading.

Tranylcypromine Sulfate (Co-administration with drugs with hypoglycemic activity, such as certain MAO inhibitor antidepressants, may result in decreased insulin requirements). Products include:
Parnate Tablets 1499

Triamcinolone (Co-administration may result in increased insulin requirements).
No products indexed under this heading.

Triamcinolone Acetonide (Co-administration may result in increased insulin requirements). Products include:
Azmacort Inhalation Aerosol 1701
Nasacort HFA Inhalation Aerosol 2939
Nasacort AQ Nasal Spray 2937

Triamcinolone Diacetate (Co-administration may result in increased insulin requirements).
No products indexed under this heading.

Triamcinolone Hexacetonide (Co-administration may result in increased insulin requirements).
No products indexed under this heading.

Troglitazone (Co-administration with drugs with hypoglycemic activity, such as oral hypoglycemic agents, may result in decreased insulin requirements).
No products indexed under this heading.

HURRICAINE TOPICAL ANESTHETIC AEROSOL SPRAY, 2 OZ. WILD CHERRY

(Benzocaine) 835
None cited in PDR database.

HURRICAINE TOPICAL ANESTHETIC AEROSOL SPRAY KIT, 2 OZ. WILD CHERRY WITH 200 DISPOSABLE EXTENSION TUBES

(Benzocaine) 835
None cited in PDR database.

HURRICAINE TOPICAL ANESTHETIC GEL: 1 OZ. WILD CHERRY, PINA COLADA, WATERMELON, FRESH MINT, 0.18 OZ. WILD CHERRY

(Benzocaine) 835
None cited in PDR database.

HURRICAINE TOPICAL ANESTHETIC GEL, 1 OZ. FRESH MINT, WILD CHERRY, PINA COLADA, WATERMELON, 1/6 OZ. WILD CHERRY

(Benzocaine) .... ▣607
None cited in PDR database.

HURRICAINE TOPICAL ANESTHETIC LIQUID: 1 OZ. WILD CHERRY AND PINA COLADA, SWAB APPLICATOR WILD CHERRY

(Benzocaine) 835
None cited in PDR database.

HURRICAINE TOPICAL ANESTHETIC LIQUID, 1 OZ. WILD CHERRY, PINA COLADA, .25 ML SWAB APPLICATOR WILD CHERRY

(Benzocaine) .... ▣607
None cited in PDR database.

HURRICAINE TOPICAL ANESTHETIC SPRAY EXTENSION TUBES (200)

(Benzocaine) .... ▣607
None cited in PDR database.

HURRICAINE TOPICAL ANESTHETIC SPRAY KIT, 2 OZ. WILD CHERRY

(Benzocaine) .... ▣607
None cited in PDR database.

HURRICAINE TOPICAL ANESTHETIC SPRAY, 2 OZ. WILD CHERRY

(Benzocaine) .... ▣607
None cited in PDR database.

HYALGAN SOLUTION

(Sodium Hyaluronate) 2917
None cited in PDR database.

HYCAMTIN FOR INJECTION

(Topotecan Hydrochloride) 1427
May interact with cytotoxic drugs and certain other agents. Compounds in these categories include:

Bleomycin Sulfate (Greater myelosuppression is also likely to be seen when Hycamtin is used in combination with other cytotoxic agents, thereby necessitating a dose reduction).
No products indexed under this heading.

Carboplatin (Greater myelosuppression is likely to be seen when topotecan hydrochloride is used in combination with other cytotoxic agents, thereby necessitating a dose reduction. However, when combining topotecan hydrochloride with platinum agents (eg, carboplatin),a distinct sequence dependent interaction on myelosuppression has been reported).
No products indexed under this heading.

Cisplatin (Co-administration has resulted in severe myelosuppression; a case of neutropenia and fatal neutropenic sepsis has been reported).
No products indexed under this heading.

Cyclophosphamide (Greater myelosuppression is also likely to be seen when Hycamtin is used in combination with other cytotoxic agents, thereby necessitating a dose reduction).
No products indexed under this heading.

Daunorubicin Hydrochloride (Greater myelosuppression is also likely to be seen when Hycamtin is used in combination with other cytotoxic agents, thereby necessitating a dose reduction). Products include:
Cerubidine for Injection 788

Doxorubicin Hydrochloride (Greater myelosuppression is also likely to be seen when Hycamtin is used in combination with other cytotoxic agents, thereby necessitating a dose reduction). Products include:
Adriamycin for Injection, USP 786
Adriamycin Injection, USP 786

Epirubicin Hydrochloride (Greater myelosuppression is also likely to be seen when Hycamtin is used in combination with other cytotoxic agents, thereby necessitating a dose reduction). Products include:
Ellence Injection 2632

Filgrastim (Concomitant administration of granulocyte colony stimulating factor (G-CSF) can prolong the duration of neutropenia, so if G-CSF is to be used, it should not be initiated until day 6 of the course of therapy, 24 hours after completion of treatment with topotecan hydrochloride). Products include:
Neupogen for Injection 598

Fluorouracil (Greater myelosuppression is also likely to be seen when Hycamtin is used in combination with other cytotoxic agents, thereby necessitating a dose reduction). Products include:
Carac Cream, 0.5% 1048
Efudex 3348

Hydroxyurea (Greater myelosuppression is also likely to be seen when Hycamtin is used in combination with other cytotoxic agents, thereby necessitating a dose reduction).
No products indexed under this heading.

Methotrexate Sodium (Greater myelosuppression is also likely to be seen when Hycamtin is used in combination with other cytotoxic agents, thereby necessitating a dose reduction).
No products indexed under this heading.

Mitotane (Greater myelosuppression is also likely to be seen when Hycamtin is used in combination with other cytotoxic agents, thereby necessitating a dose reduction).
No products indexed under this heading.

Mitoxantrone Hydrochloride (Greater myelosuppression is also likely to be seen when Hycamtin is used in combination with other cytotoxic agents, thereby necessitating a dose reduction). Products include:
Novantrone for Injection Concentrate 3158

Procarbazine Hydrochloride (Greater myelosuppression is also likely to be seen when Hycamtin is used in combination with other cytotoxic agents, thereby necessitating a dose reduction). Products include:
Matulane Capsules 3188

Tamoxifen Citrate (Greater myelosuppression is also likely to be seen when Hycamtin is used in combination with other cytotoxic agents, thereby necessitating a dose reduction).
No products indexed under this heading.

Vincristine Sulfate (Greater myelosuppression is also likely to be seen when Hycamtin is used in combination with other cytotoxic agents, thereby necessitating a dose reduction).
No products indexed under this heading.

HYCODAN SYRUP

(Homatropine Methylbromide, Hydrocodone Bitartrate) 1104
See Hycodan Tablets

HYCODAN TABLETS

(Homatropine Methylbromide, Hydrocodone Bitartrate) 1104
May interact with antihistamines, central nervous system depressants, monoamine oxidase inhibitors, narcotic analgesics, antipsychotic agents, tranquilizers, tricyclic antidepressants, and certain other agents. Compounds in these categories include:

Acrivastine (Exhibits an additive CNS depression).
No products indexed under this heading.

Alfentanil Hydrochloride (Exhibits an additive CNS depression).
No products indexed under this heading.

Alprazolam (Exhibits an additive CNS depression). Products include:
Niravam Orally Disintegrating Tablets 3106
Xanax XR Tablets 2655

Amitriptyline Hydrochloride (Increased effect of either the antidepressant or hydrocodone).
No products indexed under this heading.

Amoxapine (Increased effect of either the antidepressant or hydrocodone).
No products indexed under this heading.

Aprobarbital (Exhibits an additive CNS depression).
No products indexed under this heading.

Aripiprazole (Exhibits an additive CNS depression). Products include:
Abilify Tablets 2472
Abilify Tablets 916

Astemizole (Exhibits an additive CNS depression).
No products indexed under this heading.

Azatadine Maleate (Exhibits an additive CNS depression).
No products indexed under this heading.

Bromodiphenhydramine Hydrochloride (Exhibits an additive CNS depression).
No products indexed under this heading.

Brompheniramine Maleate (Exhibits an additive CNS depression). Products include:
Alacol DM Syrup 739
Children's Dimetapp Cold & Allergy Elixir .... ▣745
Children's Dimetapp DM Cold & Cough Elixir .... ▣745
Robitussin Allergy & Cough Syrup .. ▣750

Buprenorphine Hydrochloride (Exhibits an additive CNS depression). Products include:
Buprenex Injectable 2718
Suboxone Tablets 2719
Subutex Tablets 2719

Buspirone Hydrochloride (Exhibits an additive CNS depression).
No products indexed under this heading.

Butabarbital (Exhibits an additive CNS depression).
No products indexed under this heading.

Butalbital (Exhibits an additive CNS depression). Products include:
Sedapap Tablets 50 mg/650 mg 2098

Cetirizine Hydrochloride (Exhibits an additive CNS depression). Products include:
- Zyrtec Chewable Tablets 2589
- Zyrtec 2589
- Zyrtec-D 12 Hour Extended Release Tablets 2591

Chlordiazepoxide (Exhibits an additive CNS depression).
No products indexed under this heading.

Chlordiazepoxide Hydrochloride (Exhibits an additive CNS depression). Products include:
- Librium Capsules 3349

Chlorpheniramine Maleate (Exhibits an additive CNS depression). Products include:
- Advil Allergy Sinus Caplets 737
- Advil Multi-Symptom Cold Caplets 738
- BC Allergy Sinus Cold Powder 612
- Contac Severe Cold and Flu Caplets Maximum Strength 615
- Hycomine Compound Tablets 1105
- PediaCare Multi-Symptom Cold Liquid 704
- PediaCare NightRest Cough & Cold Liquid 704
- Robitussin Flu Liquid 752
- Robitussin PM Cough & Cold Liquid 752
- Singlet Caplets 636
- Sudafed Sinus & Allergy Tablets 710
- TheraFlu Cold & Cough Hot Liquid 680
- TheraFlu Cold & Sore Throat Hot Liquid 680
- TheraFlu Flu & Sore Throat Hot Liquid 681
- TheraFlu Severe Cold & Cough Hot Liquid 683
- TheraFlu Severe Cold Caplets 679
- TheraFlu Severe Cold Hot Liquid 682
- Triaminic Cold & Allergy Liquid 685
- Triaminic Cold & Cough Liquid 685
- Triaminic Flu, Cough & Fever Liquid 685
- Triaminic Night Time Cough & Cold Liquid 685
- Triaminic Allergy Runny Nose & Congestion Softchews 688
- Triaminic Cold & Cough Softchews 688
- Children's Tylenol Plus Cold NightTime Suspension Liquid 1851
- Children's Tylenol Plus Cold & Cough Suspension Liquid and Chewable Tablets 1851
- Children's Tylenol Plus Cold Chewable Tablets 1851
- Children's Tylenol Plus Flu Suspension Liquid 1853
- Tylenol Allergy Complete Multi-Symptom Caplets and Gelcaps with Cool Burst 1844
- Multi-Symptom Tylenol Cold Night Time Caplets 1845
- Vicks 44M Cough, Cold & Flu Relief 2676
- Pediatric Vicks 44m Cough & Cold Relief 2673
- Children's Vicks NyQuil Cold/Cough Relief 2671

Chlorpheniramine Polistirex (Exhibits an additive CNS depression). Products include:
- Tussionex Pennkinetic Extended-Release Suspension 3322

Chlorpheniramine Tannate (Exhibits an additive CNS depression).
No products indexed under this heading.

Chlorpromazine (Exhibits an additive CNS depression).
No products indexed under this heading.

Chlorpromazine Hydrochloride (Exhibits an additive CNS depression).
No products indexed under this heading.

Chlorprothixene (Exhibits an additive CNS depression).
No products indexed under this heading.

Chlorprothixene Hydrochloride (Exhibits an additive CNS depression).
No products indexed under this heading.

Chlorprothixene Lactate (Exhibits an additive CNS depression).
No products indexed under this heading.

Clemastine Fumarate (Exhibits an additive CNS depression).
No products indexed under this heading.

Clomipramine Hydrochloride (Increased effect of either the antidepressant or hydrocodone).
No products indexed under this heading.

Clorazepate Dipotassium (Exhibits an additive CNS depression). Products include:
- Tranxene 2488

Clozapine (Exhibits an additive CNS depression). Products include:
- Clozapine Tablets 2141
- Clozaril Tablets 2174
- FazaClo Orally Disintegrating Tablets 547

Codeine Phosphate (Exhibits an additive CNS depression). Products include:
- Tylenol with Codeine 2461

Cyproheptadine Hydrochloride (Exhibits an additive CNS depression).
No products indexed under this heading.

Desflurane (Exhibits an additive CNS depression). Products include:
- Suprane Liquid for Inhalation 770

Desipramine Hydrochloride (Increased effect of either the antidepressant or hydrocodone).
No products indexed under this heading.

Dexchlorpheniramine Maleate (Exhibits an additive CNS depression).
No products indexed under this heading.

Dezocine (Exhibits an additive CNS depression).
No products indexed under this heading.

Diazepam (Exhibits an additive CNS depression). Products include:
- Diastat Rectal Delivery System 3344
- Valium Tablets 2822

Diphenhydramine Citrate (Exhibits an additive CNS depression). Products include:
- Children's Benadryl Allergy & Cold Fastmelt Tablets 695
- Children's Benadryl D Allergy & Sinus Fastmelt Tablets 694
- Children's Benadryl Allergy Fastmelt Tablets 696
- Goody's PM Powder 622

Diphenhydramine Hydrochloride (Exhibits an additive CNS depression). Products include:
- Benadryl Allergy & Cold Tablets 692
- Benadryl Allergy 691
- Benadryl Allergy & Sinus Headache Caplets & Gelcaps 693
- Children's Benadryl Allergy Liquid 695
- Children's Benadryl Dye-Free Allergy Liquid 695
- Benadryl Dye-Free Allergy Liqui-Gels Softgels 692
- Benadryl Itch Relief Stick Extra Strength 696
- Benadryl Itch Stopping Cream Extra Strength 697
- Benadryl Itch Stopping Gel Extra Strength 697
- Benadryl Itch Stopping Spray Extra Strength 697
- Benadryl Maximum Strength Severe Allergy & Sinus Headache Caplets 694
- Children's Benadryl D Liquid Medication 693
- Benadryl D Tablets 694
- Nytol QuickCaps Caplets 635
- Maximum Strength Nytol QuickGels Softgels 635
- Simply Sleep Caplets 1841
- Sominex Original Formula Tablets 637
- TheraFlu Thin Strips Multi Symptom 684
- Triaminic Thin Strips Cough & Runny Nose 690
- Children's Tylenol Plus Cold & Allergy Suspension Liquid 1850
- Tylenol Allergy Complete Night Time Caplets 1844
- Tylenol Severe Allergy Caplets 1844
- Tylenol Flu NightTime Gelcaps 1846
- Extra Strength Tylenol PM Caplets, Geltabs, Gelcaps and Liquid 1847
- Unisom Maximum Strength SleepGels 712

Diphenylpyraline Hydrochloride (Exhibits an additive CNS depression).
No products indexed under this heading.

Doxepin Hydrochloride (Increased effect of either the antidepressant or hydrocodone).
No products indexed under this heading.

Droperidol (Exhibits an additive CNS depression).
No products indexed under this heading.

Enflurane (Exhibits an additive CNS depression).
No products indexed under this heading.

Estazolam (Exhibits an additive CNS depression). Products include:
- ProSom Tablets 512

Ethanol (Exhibits an additive CNS depression).
No products indexed under this heading.

Ethchlorvynol (Exhibits an additive CNS depression).
No products indexed under this heading.

Ethinamate (Exhibits an additive CNS depression).
No products indexed under this heading.

Ethyl Alcohol (Exhibits an additive CNS depression).
No products indexed under this heading.

Fentanyl (Exhibits an additive CNS depression). Products include:
- Duragesic Transdermal System 2448

Fentanyl Citrate (Exhibits an additive CNS depression). Products include:
- Actiq 993

Fexofenadine Hydrochloride (Exhibits an additive CNS depression). Products include:
- Allegra 2857
- Allegra-D 12 Hour Extended-Release Tablets 2860
- Allegra-D 24 Hour Extended-Release Tablets 2862

Fluphenazine Decanoate (Exhibits an additive CNS depression).
No products indexed under this heading.

Fluphenazine Enanthate (Exhibits an additive CNS depression).
No products indexed under this heading.

Fluphenazine Hydrochloride (Exhibits an additive CNS depression).
No products indexed under this heading.

Flurazepam Hydrochloride (Exhibits an additive CNS depression). Products include:
- Dalmane Capsules 3343

Glutethimide (Exhibits an additive CNS depression).
No products indexed under this heading.

Haloperidol (Exhibits an additive CNS depression).
No products indexed under this heading.

Haloperidol Decanoate (Exhibits an additive CNS depression).
No products indexed under this heading.

Hydrocodone Polistirex (Exhibits an additive CNS depression). Products include:
- Tussionex Pennkinetic Extended-Release Suspension 3322

Hydromorphone Hydrochloride (Exhibits an additive CNS depression). Products include:
- Dilaudid 439
- Dilaudid Oral Liquid 443
- Dilaudid Non-Sterile Powder 439
- Dilaudid Rectal Suppositories 439
- Dilaudid Tablets 439
- Dilaudid Tablets - 8 mg 443
- Dilaudid-HP 441

Hydroxyzine Hydrochloride (Exhibits an additive CNS depression).
No products indexed under this heading.

Imipramine Hydrochloride (Increased effect of either the antidepressant or hydrocodone).
No products indexed under this heading.

Imipramine Pamoate (Increased effect of either the antidepressant or hydrocodone).
No products indexed under this heading.

Isocarboxazid (May increase the effect of either MAO inhibitor or hydrocodone).
No products indexed under this heading.

Isoflurane (Exhibits an additive CNS depression).
No products indexed under this heading.

Ketamine Hydrochloride (Exhibits an additive CNS depression).
No products indexed under this heading.

Levomethadyl Acetate Hydrochloride (Exhibits an additive CNS depression).
No products indexed under this heading.

Levorphanol Tartrate (Exhibits an additive CNS depression).
No products indexed under this heading.

Lithium Carbonate (Exhibits an additive CNS depression). Products include:
- Eskalith 1406
- Lithobid Tablets 1670

Lithium Citrate (Exhibits an additive CNS depression).
No products indexed under this heading.

Loratadine (Exhibits an additive CNS depression). Products include:
- Alavert Allergy & Sinus D-12 Hour Tablets ■ 743
- Alavert ■ 743
- Children's Claritin 24 Hour Non-Drowsy Allergy Syrup ■ 732
- Claritin Non-Drowsy 24 Hour Tablets ■ 731
- Non-Drowsy Claritin Hives Relief Tablets ■ 733
- Claritin Reditabs 24 Hour Non-Drowsy Tablets ■ 732
- Claritin-D Non-Drowsy 12 Hour Tablets ■ 731
- Claritin-D Non-Drowsy 24 Hour Tablets ■ 731
- Children's Dimetapp ND Non-Drowsy Allergy Syrup ■ 746
- Triaminic Allerchews ■ 684

Lorazepam (Exhibits an additive CNS depression).
No products indexed under this heading.

Loxapine Hydrochloride (Exhibits an additive CNS depression).
No products indexed under this heading.

Loxapine Succinate (Exhibits an additive CNS depression).
No products indexed under this heading.

Maprotiline Hydrochloride (Increased effect of either the antidepressant or hydrocodone).
No products indexed under this heading.

Meperidine Hydrochloride (Exhibits an additive CNS depression).
No products indexed under this heading.

Mephobarbital (Exhibits an additive CNS depression). Products include:
- Mebaral Tablets, USP 2483

Meprobamate (Exhibits an additive CNS depression).
No products indexed under this heading.

Mesoridazine Besylate (Exhibits an additive CNS depression).
No products indexed under this heading.

Methadone Hydrochloride (Exhibits an additive CNS depression).
No products indexed under this heading.

Methdilazine Hydrochloride (Exhibits an additive CNS depression).
No products indexed under this heading.

Methohexital Sodium (Exhibits an additive CNS depression).
No products indexed under this heading.

Methotrimeprazine (Exhibits an additive CNS depression).
No products indexed under this heading.

Methoxyflurane (Exhibits an additive CNS depression).
No products indexed under this heading.

Midazolam Hydrochloride (Exhibits an additive CNS depression).
No products indexed under this heading.

Moclobemide (May increase the effect of either MAO inhibitor or hydrocodone).
No products indexed under this heading.

Molindone Hydrochloride (Exhibits an additive CNS depression). Products include:
- Moban Tablets 1108

Morphine Sulfate (Exhibits an additive CNS depression). Products include:
- Avinza Capsules 1714
- Kadian Capsules 572
- MS Contin Tablets 2703

Nortriptyline Hydrochloride (Increased effect of either the antidepressant or hydrocodone).
No products indexed under this heading.

Olanzapine (Exhibits an additive CNS depression). Products include:
- Symbyax Capsules 1788
- Zyprexa Tablets 1798
- Zyprexa IntraMuscular 1798
- Zyprexa ZYDIS Orally Disintegrating Tablets 1798

Oxazepam (Exhibits an additive CNS depression).
No products indexed under this heading.

Oxycodone Hydrochloride (Exhibits an additive CNS depression). Products include:
- Combunox Tablets 1183
- OxyContin Tablets 2699
- OxyFast Oral Concentrate Solution 2704
- OxyIR Capsules 2704
- Percocet Tablets 1114
- Percodan Tablets 1115

Pargyline Hydrochloride (May increase the effect of either MAO inhibitor or hydrocodone).
No products indexed under this heading.

Pentobarbital Sodium (Exhibits an additive CNS depression). Products include:
- Nembutal Sodium Solution, USP 2484

Perphenazine (Exhibits an additive CNS depression).
No products indexed under this heading.

Phenelzine Sulfate (May increase the effect of either MAO inhibitor or hydrocodone).
No products indexed under this heading.

Phenobarbital (Exhibits an additive CNS depression).
No products indexed under this heading.

Pimozide (Exhibits an additive CNS depression). Products include:
- Orap Tablets 1220

Prazepam (Exhibits an additive CNS depression).
No products indexed under this heading.

Procarbazine Hydrochloride (May increase the effect of either MAO inhibitor or hydrocodone). Products include:
- Matulane Capsules 3188

Prochlorperazine (Exhibits an additive CNS depression).
No products indexed under this heading.

Promethazine Hydrochloride (Exhibits an additive CNS depression). Products include:
- Phenergan 3438

Propofol (Exhibits an additive CNS depression). Products include:
- Diprivan Injectable Emulsion 676

Propoxyphene Hydrochloride (Exhibits an additive CNS depression).
No products indexed under this heading.

Propoxyphene Napsylate (Exhibits an additive CNS depression). Products include:
- Darvocet A 500 Tablets 3497

Protriptyline Hydrochloride (Increased effect of either the antidepressant or hydrocodone). Products include:
- Vivactil Tablets 2350

Pyrilamine Maleate (Exhibits an additive CNS depression).
No products indexed under this heading.

Pyrilamine Tannate (Exhibits an additive CNS depression).
No products indexed under this heading.

Quazepam (Exhibits an additive CNS depression).
No products indexed under this heading.

Quetiapine Fumarate (Exhibits an additive CNS depression). Products include:
- Seroquel Tablets 691

Remifentanil Hydrochloride (Exhibits an additive CNS depression).
No products indexed under this heading.

Risperidone (Exhibits an additive CNS depression). Products include:
- Risperdal Consta Long-Acting Injection 1664
- Risperdal M-Tab Orally Disintegrating Tablets 1658
- Risperdal 1658

Secobarbital Sodium (Exhibits an additive CNS depression).
No products indexed under this heading.

Selegiline Hydrochloride (May increase the effect of either MAO inhibitor or hydrocodone). Products include:
- Eldepryl Capsules 3209

Sevoflurane (Exhibits an additive CNS depression). Products include:
- Ultane Liquid for Inhalation 526

Sodium Oxybate (Exhibits an additive CNS depression).
No products indexed under this heading.

Sufentanil Citrate (Exhibits an additive CNS depression).
No products indexed under this heading.

Temazepam (Exhibits an additive CNS depression).
No products indexed under this heading.

Terfenadine (Exhibits an additive CNS depression).
No products indexed under this heading.

Thiamylal Sodium (Exhibits an additive CNS depression).
No products indexed under this heading.

Thioridazine Hydrochloride (Exhibits an additive CNS depression). Products include:
- Thioridazine Hydrochloride Tablets 2122

Thiothixene (Exhibits an additive CNS depression). Products include:
- Thiothixene Capsules 2124

Tranylcypromine Sulfate (May increase the effect of either MAO inhibitor or hydrocodone). Products include:
- Parnate Tablets 1499

Triazolam (Exhibits an additive CNS depression).
No products indexed under this heading.

Trifluoperazine Hydrochloride (Exhibits an additive CNS depression).
No products indexed under this heading.

Trimeprazine Tartrate (Exhibits an additive CNS depression).
No products indexed under this heading.

Trimipramine Maleate (Increased effect of either the antidepressant or hydrocodone). Products include:
- Surmontil Capsules 2347

Tripelennamine Hydrochloride (Exhibits an additive CNS depression).
No products indexed under this heading.

Triprolidine Hydrochloride (Exhibits an additive CNS depression).
No products indexed under this heading.

Zaleplon (Exhibits an additive CNS depression). Products include:
- Sonata Capsules 1686

Ziprasidone Hydrochloride (Exhibits an additive CNS depression). Products include:
- Geodon Capsules 2514

Zolpidem Tartrate (Exhibits an additive CNS depression). Products include:
- Ambien Tablets 2867

Food Interactions

Alcohol (Exhibits an additive CNS depression).

HYCOMINE COMPOUND TABLETS

(Acetaminophen, Caffeine, Chlorpheniramine Maleate, Hydrocodone Bitartrate, Phenylephrine Hydrochloride) 1105

May interact with beta blockers, central nervous system depressants, general anesthetics, hypnotics and sedatives, monoamine oxidase inhibitors, narcotic analgesics, phenothiazines, sympathomimetics, tranquilizers, and certain other agents. Compounds in these categories include:

Acebutolol Hydrochloride (Concurrent use of phenylephrine with beta blockers may result in hypertensive crises).
No products indexed under this heading.

Albuterol (Additive elevation of blood pressure). Products include:
- Proventil Inhalation Aerosol 3067

Albuterol Sulfate (Additive elevation of blood pressure). Products include:
- AccuNeb Inhalation Solution 1055
- Combivent Inhalation Aerosol 878
- DuoNeb Inhalation Solution 1058
- Proventil Inhalation Solution 0.083% 3069
- Proventil HFA Inhalation Aerosol 3071
- Ventolin HFA Inhalation Aerosol 1576
- VoSpire Extended-Release Tablets 2352

Alfentanil Hydrochloride (Exhibits an additive CNS depression).
No products indexed under this heading.

Alprazolam (Exhibits an additive CNS depression). Products include:
- Niravam Orally Disintegrating Tablets 3106
- Xanax XR Tablets 2655

Aprobarbital (Exhibits an additive CNS depression).
No products indexed under this heading.

Atenolol (Concurrent use of phenylephrine with beta blockers may result in hypertensive crises). Products include:
- Tenormin I.V. Injection 698
- Tenormin Tablets 695

Betaxolol Hydrochloride (Concurrent use of phenylephrine with beta blockers may result in hypertensive crises). Products include:
- Betoptic S Ophthalmic Suspension..... 554

Bisoprolol Fumarate (Concurrent use of phenylephrine with beta blockers may result in hypertensive crises).
- No products indexed under this heading.

Buprenorphine Hydrochloride (Exhibits an additive CNS depression). Products include:
- Buprenex Injectable 2718
- Suboxone Tablets 2719
- Subutex Tablets 2719

Buspirone Hydrochloride (Exhibits an additive CNS depression).
- No products indexed under this heading.

Butabarbital (Exhibits an additive CNS depression).
- No products indexed under this heading.

Butalbital (Exhibits an additive CNS depression). Products include:
- Sedapap Tablets 50 mg/650 mg 2098

Carteolol Hydrochloride (Concurrent use of phenylephrine with beta blockers may result in hypertensive crises). Products include:
- Carteolol Hydrochloride Ophthalmic Solution USP, 1%..... ⊙246

Chlordiazepoxide (Exhibits an additive CNS depression).
- No products indexed under this heading.

Chlordiazepoxide Hydrochloride (Exhibits an additive CNS depression). Products include:
- Librium Capsules 3349

Chlorpromazine (Exhibits an additive CNS depression).
- No products indexed under this heading.

Chlorpromazine Hydrochloride (Exhibits an additive CNS depression).
- No products indexed under this heading.

Chlorprothixene (Exhibits an additive CNS depression).
- No products indexed under this heading.

Chlorprothixene Hydrochloride (Exhibits an additive CNS depression).
- No products indexed under this heading.

Chlorprothixene Lactate (Exhibits an additive CNS depression).
- No products indexed under this heading.

Clorazepate Dipotassium (Exhibits an additive CNS depression). Products include:
- Tranxene 2488

Clozapine (Exhibits an additive CNS depression). Products include:
- Clozapine Tablets 2141
- Clozaril Tablets 2174
- FazaClo Orally Disintegrating Tablets..... 547

Codeine Phosphate (Exhibits an additive CNS depression). Products include:
- Tylenol with Codeine 2461

Desflurane (Exhibits an additive CNS depression). Products include:
- Suprane Liquid for Inhalation 770

Dezocine (Exhibits an additive CNS depression).
- No products indexed under this heading.

Diazepam (Exhibits an additive CNS depression). Products include:
- Diastat Rectal Delivery System 3344
- Valium Tablets 2822

Dobutamine Hydrochloride (Additive elevation of blood pressure).
- No products indexed under this heading.

Dopamine Hydrochloride (Additive elevation of blood pressure).
- No products indexed under this heading.

Droperidol (Exhibits an additive CNS depression).
- No products indexed under this heading.

Enflurane (Exhibits an additive CNS depression).
- No products indexed under this heading.

Ephedrine Hydrochloride (Additive elevation of blood pressure). Products include:
- Primatene Tablets 749

Ephedrine Sulfate (Additive elevation of blood pressure).
- No products indexed under this heading.

Ephedrine Tannate (Additive elevation of blood pressure).
- No products indexed under this heading.

Epinephrine (Additive elevation of blood pressure). Products include:
- EpiPen 1061
- Primatene Mist 749

Epinephrine Bitartrate (Additive elevation of blood pressure).
- No products indexed under this heading.

Epinephrine Hydrochloride (Additive elevation of blood pressure).
- No products indexed under this heading.

Esmolol Hydrochloride (Concurrent use of phenylephrine with beta blockers may result in hypertensive crises). Products include:
- Brevibloc Concentrate 766
- Brevibloc Injection 766
- Brevibloc Double Strength Injection..... 766
- Brevibloc Premixed Injection 766
- Brevibloc Double Strength Premixed Injection 766

Estazolam (Exhibits an additive CNS depression). Products include:
- ProSom Tablets 512

Ethanol (Exhibits an additive CNS depression).
- No products indexed under this heading.

Ethchlorvynol (Exhibits an additive CNS depression).
- No products indexed under this heading.

Ethinamate (Exhibits an additive CNS depression).
- No products indexed under this heading.

Ethyl Alcohol (Exhibits an additive CNS depression).
- No products indexed under this heading.

Fentanyl (Exhibits an additive CNS depression). Products include:
- Duragesic Transdermal System 2448

Fentanyl Citrate (Exhibits an additive CNS depression). Products include:
- Actiq 993

Fluphenazine Decanoate (Exhibits an additive CNS depression).
- No products indexed under this heading.

Fluphenazine Enanthate (Exhibits an additive CNS depression).
- No products indexed under this heading.

Fluphenazine Hydrochloride (Exhibits an additive CNS depression).
- No products indexed under this heading.

Flurazepam Hydrochloride (Exhibits an additive CNS depression). Products include:
- Dalmane Capsules 3343

Glutethimide (Exhibits an additive CNS depression).
- No products indexed under this heading.

Haloperidol (Exhibits an additive CNS depression).
- No products indexed under this heading.

Haloperidol Decanoate (Exhibits an additive CNS depression).
- No products indexed under this heading.

Hydrocodone Polistirex (Exhibits an additive CNS depression). Products include:
- Tussionex Pennkinetic Extended-Release Suspension..... 3322

Hydromorphone Hydrochloride (Exhibits an additive CNS depression). Products include:
- Dilaudid 439
- Dilaudid Oral Liquid 443
- Dilaudid Non-Sterile Powder 439
- Dilaudid Rectal Suppositories 439
- Dilaudid Tablets 439
- Dilaudid Tablets - 8 mg 443
- Dilaudid-HP 441

Hydroxyzine Hydrochloride (Exhibits an additive CNS depression).
- No products indexed under this heading.

Indomethacin (Concurrent use of indomethacin with beta blockers may result in hypertensive crises). Products include:
- Indocin 1968

Isocarboxazid (Co-administration of sympathomimetics and MAO inhibitors may produce an additive elevation of blood pressure leading to hypertensive crises; MAO inhibitors may prolong the anticholinergic effects of antihistamines; concurrent use is contraindicated).
- No products indexed under this heading.

Isoflurane (Exhibits an additive CNS depression).
- No products indexed under this heading.

Isoproterenol Hydrochloride (Additive elevation of blood pressure).
- No products indexed under this heading.

Isoproterenol Sulfate (Additive elevation of blood pressure).
- No products indexed under this heading.

Ketamine Hydrochloride (Exhibits an additive CNS depression).
- No products indexed under this heading.

Labetalol Hydrochloride (Concurrent use of phenylephrine with beta blockers may result in hypertensive crises).
- No products indexed under this heading.

Levalbuterol Hydrochloride (Additive elevation of blood pressure). Products include:
- Xopenex Inhalation Solution 3143
- Xopenex Inhalation Solution Concentrate..... 3147

Levobunolol Hydrochloride (Concurrent use of phenylephrine with beta blockers may result in hypertensive crises). Products include:
- Betagan Ophthalmic Solution, USP..... ⊙217

Levomethadyl Acetate Hydrochloride (Exhibits an additive CNS depression).
- No products indexed under this heading.

Levorphanol Tartrate (Exhibits an additive CNS depression).
- No products indexed under this heading.

Lorazepam (Exhibits an additive CNS depression).
- No products indexed under this heading.

Loxapine Hydrochloride (Exhibits an additive CNS depression).
- No products indexed under this heading.

Loxapine Succinate (Exhibits an additive CNS depression).
- No products indexed under this heading.

Meperidine Hydrochloride (Exhibits an additive CNS depression).
- No products indexed under this heading.

Mephobarbital (Exhibits an additive CNS depression). Products include:
- Mebaral Tablets, USP 2483

Meprobamate (Exhibits an additive CNS depression).
- No products indexed under this heading.

Mesoridazine Besylate (Exhibits an additive CNS depression).
- No products indexed under this heading.

Metaproterenol Sulfate (Additive elevation of blood pressure). Products include:
- Alupent Inhalation Aerosol 858

Metaraminol Bitartrate (Additive elevation of blood pressure). Products include:
- Aramine Injection 1889

Methadone Hydrochloride (Exhibits an additive CNS depression).
- No products indexed under this heading.

Methohexital Sodium (Exhibits an additive CNS depression).
- No products indexed under this heading.

Methotrimeprazine (Exhibits an additive CNS depression).
- No products indexed under this heading.

Methoxamine Hydrochloride (Additive elevation of blood pressure).
- No products indexed under this heading.

Methoxyflurane (Exhibits an additive CNS depression).
- No products indexed under this heading.

IMPORTANT NOTE: Always consult each drug listing in the patient's regimen for possible interactions.

Methyldopa (Concurrent use of methyldopa with beta blockers may result in hypertensive crises). Products include:
- Aldoclor Tablets 1881
- Aldoril Tablets 1884

Metipranolol Hydrochloride (Concurrent use of phenylephrine with beta blockers may result in hypertensive crises).
- No products indexed under this heading.

Metoprolol Succinate (Concurrent use of phenylephrine with beta blockers may result in hypertensive crises). Products include:
- Toprol-XL Tablets 660

Metoprolol Tartrate (Concurrent use of phenylephrine with beta blockers may result in hypertensive crises).
- No products indexed under this heading.

Midazolam Hydrochloride (Exhibits an additive CNS depression).
- No products indexed under this heading.

Moclobemide (Co-administration of sympathomimetics and MAO inhibitors may produce an additive elevation of blood pressure leading to hypertensive crises; MAO inhibitors may prolong the anticholinergic effects of antihistamines; concurrent use is contraindicated).
- No products indexed under this heading.

Molindone Hydrochloride (Exhibits an additive CNS depression). Products include:
- Moban Tablets 1108

Morphine Sulfate (Exhibits an additive CNS depression). Products include:
- Avinza Capsules 1714
- Kadian Capsules 572
- MS Contin Tablets 2703

Nadolol (Concurrent use of phenylephrine with beta blockers may result in hypertensive crises). Products include:
- Nadolol Tablets 2121

Norepinephrine Bitartrate (Additive elevation of blood pressure).
- No products indexed under this heading.

Olanzapine (Exhibits an additive CNS depression). Products include:
- Symbyax Capsules 1788
- Zyprexa Tablets 1798
- Zyprexa IntraMuscular 1798
- Zyprexa ZYDIS Orally Disintegrating Tablets 1798

Oxazepam (Exhibits an additive CNS depression).
- No products indexed under this heading.

Oxycodone Hydrochloride (Exhibits an additive CNS depression). Products include:
- Combunox Tablets 1183
- OxyContin Tablets 2699
- OxyFast Oral Concentrate Solution 2704
- OxyIR Capsules 2704
- Percocet Tablets 1114
- Percodan Tablets 1115

Pargyline Hydrochloride (Co-administration of sympathomimetics and MAO inhibitors may produce an additive elevation of blood pressure leading to hypertensive crises; MAO inhibitors may prolong the anticholinergic effects of antihistamines; concurrent use is contraindicated).
- No products indexed under this heading.

Penbutolol Sulfate (Concurrent use of phenylephrine with beta blockers may result in hypertensive crises).
- No products indexed under this heading.

Pentobarbital Sodium (Exhibits an additive CNS depression). Products include:
- Nembutal Sodium Solution, USP 2484

Perphenazine (Exhibits an additive CNS depression).
- No products indexed under this heading.

Phenelzine Sulfate (Co-administration of sympathomimetics and MAO inhibitors may produce an additive elevation of blood pressure leading to hypertensive crises; MAO inhibitors may prolong the anticholinergic effects of antihistamines; concurrent use is contraindicated).
- No products indexed under this heading.

Phenobarbital (Exhibits an additive CNS depression).
- No products indexed under this heading.

Phenylephrine Bitartrate (Additive elevation of blood pressure).
- No products indexed under this heading.

Phenylephrine Tannate (Additive elevation of blood pressure).
- No products indexed under this heading.

Phenylpropanolamine Hydrochloride (Additive elevation of blood pressure).
- No products indexed under this heading.

Pindolol (Concurrent use of phenylephrine with beta blockers may result in hypertensive crises).
- No products indexed under this heading.

Pirbuterol Acetate (Additive elevation of blood pressure). Products include:
- Maxair Autohaler 1820

Prazepam (Exhibits an additive CNS depression).
- No products indexed under this heading.

Procarbazine Hydrochloride (Co-administration of sympathomimetics and MAO inhibitors may produce an additive elevation of blood pressure leading to hypertensive crises; MAO inhibitors may prolong the anticholinergic effects of antihistamines; concurrent use is contraindicated). Products include:
- Matulane Capsules 3188

Prochlorperazine (Exhibits an additive CNS depression).
- No products indexed under this heading.

Promethazine Hydrochloride (Exhibits an additive CNS depression). Products include:
- Phenergan 3438

Propofol (Exhibits an additive CNS depression). Products include:
- Diprivan Injectable Emulsion 676

Propoxyphene Hydrochloride (Exhibits an additive CNS depression).
- No products indexed under this heading.

Propoxyphene Napsylate (Exhibits an additive CNS depression). Products include:
- Darvocet A 500 Tablets 3497

Propranolol Hydrochloride (Concurrent use of phenylephrine with beta blockers may result in hypertensive crises). Products include:
- Inderal LA Long-Acting Capsules 3421
- InnoPran XL Capsules 2728

Pseudoephedrine Hydrochloride (Additive elevation of blood pressure). Products include:
- Advil Allergy Sinus Caplets ..... ▣737
- Advil Cold & Sinus ..... ▣739
- Advil Flu & Body Ache Caplets ..... ▣739
- Children's Advil Cold Suspension ..... ▣741
- Advil Multi-Symptom Cold Caplets ..... ▣738
- Allegra-D 12 Hour Extended-Release Tablets 2860
- Allegra-D 24 Hour Extended-Release Tablets 2862
- Balamine DM 739
- BC Cold Powder ..... ▣612
- Benadryl Allergy & Cold Tablets ..... ▣692
- Benadryl Allergy & Sinus Headache Caplets & Gelcaps ..... ▣693
- Children's Benadryl Allergy & Cold Fastmelt Tablets ..... ▣695
- Benadryl Maximum Strength Severe Allergy & Sinus Headache Caplets ..... ▣694
- Children's Benadryl D Allergy & Sinus Fastmelt Tablets ..... ▣694
- Children's Benadryl D Liquid Medication ..... ▣693
- Benadryl D Tablets ..... ▣694
- Contac Non-Drowsy 12 Hour Cold Caplets ..... ▣614
- Contac Non-Drowsy Timed Release 12 Hour Cold Caplets ..... ▣615
- Contac Severe Cold and Flu Caplets Maximum Strength ..... ▣615
- Contac Severe Cold and Flu Caplets Non-Drowsy ..... ▣615
- Children's Dimetapp Cold & Allergy Elixir ..... ▣745
- Children's Dimetapp DM Cold & Cough Elixir ..... ▣745
- Children's Dimetapp Long Acting Cough Plus Cold Syrup ..... ▣746
- Dimetapp Infant Drops Decongestant Plus Cough ..... ▣746
- Children's Motrin Cold Non-Staining Dye-Free Oral Suspension 1838
- Children's Motrin Cold Oral Suspension 1838
- Motrin Cold & Sinus Caplets 1836
- PediaCare Decongestant & Cough Infant Drops ..... ▣705
- PediaCare Decongestant Infants' Drops ..... ▣705
- PediaCare Long-Acting Cough Plus Cold Liquid ..... ▣704
- PediaCare Multi-Symptom Cold Liquid ..... ▣704
- PediaCare NightRest Cough & Cold Liquid ..... ▣704
- Robitussin Allergy & Cough Syrup ..... ▣750
- Robitussin CF Liquid ..... ▣755
- Robitussin Cough & Cold Liquid-filled Capsules ..... ▣750
- Robitussin Cough, Cold & Flu Liquid-filled Capsules ..... ▣750
- Robitussin Cough & Cold Infant Drops ..... ▣755
- Robitussin Flu Liquid ..... ▣752
- Robitussin Maximum Strength Cough & Cold Liquid ..... ▣754
- Robitussin PE Syrup ..... ▣753
- Robitussin Pediatric Cough & Cold Liquid ..... ▣754
- Robitussin PM Cough & Cold Liquid ..... ▣752
- Robitussin Severe Congestion Liquid-filled Capsules ..... ▣751
- Simply Stuffy Liquid 1841
- Singlet Caplets ..... ▣636
- Sudafed 12 Hour Caplets ..... ▣708
- Sudafed 24 Hour Tablets ..... ▣709
- Sudafed Nasal Decongestant Tablets ..... ▣709
- Sudafed Severe Cold ..... ▣710
- Sudafed Non-Drying Sinus Liquid Caps ..... ▣709
- Sudafed Sinus & Allergy Tablets ..... ▣710
- Sudafed Sinus Headache ..... ▣711
- TheraFlu Cold & Cough Hot Liquid ..... ▣680
- TheraFlu Cold & Sore Throat Hot Liquid ..... ▣680
- TheraFlu Flu & Chest Congestion Non-Drowsy Hot Liquid ..... ▣681
- TheraFlu Flu & Sore Throat Hot Liquid ..... ▣681
- TheraFlu Severe Cold Non-Drowsy Hot Liquid ..... ▣683
- TheraFlu Severe Cold & Cough Hot Liquid ..... ▣683
- TheraFlu Severe Cold Caplets ..... ▣679
- TheraFlu Severe Cold Hot Liquid ..... ▣682
- TheraFlu Severe Cold Non-Drowsy Caplets ..... ▣679
- Triaminic Chest & Nasal Congestion Liquid ..... ▣685
- Triaminic Cold & Allergy Liquid ..... ▣685
- Triaminic Cold & Cough Liquid ..... ▣685
- Triaminic Cough Liquid ..... ▣687
- Triaminic Cough & Nasal Congestion Liquid ..... ▣687
- Triaminic Cough & Sore Throat Liquid ..... ▣687
- Triaminic Flu, Cough & Fever Liquid ..... ▣685
- Triaminic Night Time Cough & Cold Liquid ..... ▣685
- Triaminic Allergy Runny Nose & Congestion Softchews ..... ▣688
- Triaminic Cold & Cough Softchews ..... ▣688
- Triaminic Cough & Sore Throat Softchews ..... ▣689
- Tylenol Sinus NightTime Caplets ..... ▣663
- Children's Tylenol Plus Cold & Allergy Suspension Liquid 1850
- Children's Tylenol Plus Cold NightTime Suspension Liquid 1851
- Children's Tylenol Plus Cold & Cough Suspension Liquid and Chewable Tablets 1851
- Children's Tylenol Plus Cold Chewable Tablets 1851
- Children's Tylenol Plus Cold Daytime Non-Drowsy Suspension Liquid 1851
- Children's Tylenol Plus Flu Suspension Liquid 1853
- Concentrated Tylenol Infants' Drops Plus Cold 1851
- Concentrated Tylenol Infants' Drops Plus Cold and Cough 1851
- Tylenol Cold & Flu Severe Daytime Liquid with Cool Burst 1846
- Tylenol Cold & Flu Severe NightTime Liquid with Cool Burst 1846
- Tylenol Cold Severe Congestion Non-Drowsy Caplets with Cool Burst 1846
- Tylenol Allergy Complete Night Time Caplets 1844
- Tylenol Allergy Complete Multi-Symptom Caplets and Gelcaps with Cool Burst 1844
- Tylenol Flu NightTime Gelcaps 1846
- Tylenol Flu Day Non-Drowsy Gelcaps 1846
- Concentrated Tylenol Infants' Drops Plus Cold Nasal Congestant, Fever Reducer & Pain Reliever ..... ▣668
- Concentrated Tylenol Infants' Drops Plus Cold & Cough Nasal Decongestant, Fever Reducer & Pain Reliever ..... ▣668
- Multi-Symptom Tylenol Cold Night Time Caplets 1845
- Multi-Symptom Tylenol Cold Day Non-Drowsy Caplets and Gelcaps 1845
- Tylenol Sinus Day Non-Drowsy 1848
- Tylenol Sinus Night Time Caplets 1848
- Tylenol Sinus Severe Congestion Caplets with Cool Burst 1848
- Vicks 44D Cough & Head Congestion Relief 2676
- Vicks 44D Cough & Head Congestion Relief Liquid ..... ▣721
- Vicks 44M Cough, Cold & Flu Relief 2676
- Pediatric Vicks 44m Cough & Cold Relief 2673
- Vicks DayQuil LiquiCaps/Liquid Multi-Symptom Cold/Flu Relief ..... ▣723

Vicks DayQuil Multi-Symptom Cold/Flu Relief LiquiCaps **2675**
Vicks DayQuil Multi-Symptom Cold/Flu Relief Liquid **2675**
Children's Vicks NyQuil Cold/Cough Relief **2671**
Vicks NyQuil LiquiCaps **2677**
Vicks NyQuil LiquiCaps/Liquid Multi-Symptom Cold/Flu Relief **725**
Vicks NyQuil Liquid **2677**
Zyrtec-D 12 Hour Extended Release Tablets **2591**

Pseudoephedrine Sulfate (Additive elevation of blood pressure). Products include:
Alavert Allergy & Sinus D-12 Hour Tablets **743**
Clarinex-D 24-Hour Extended-Release Tablets **3012**
Claritin-D Non-Drowsy 12 Hour Tablets **731**
Claritin-D Non-Drowsy 24 Hour Tablets **731**

Quazepam (Exhibits an additive CNS depression).
No products indexed under this heading.

Quetiapine Fumarate (Exhibits an additive CNS depression). Products include:
Seroquel Tablets **691**

Remifentanil Hydrochloride (Exhibits an additive CNS depression).
No products indexed under this heading.

Risperidone (Exhibits an additive CNS depression). Products include:
Risperdal Consta Long-Acting Injection **1664**
Risperdal M-Tab Orally Disintegrating Tablets **1658**
Risperdal **1658**

Salmeterol Xinafoate (Additive elevation of blood pressure). Products include:
Advair Diskus 100/50 .... **1291**
Advair Diskus 250/50 .... **1291**
Advair Diskus 500/50 .... **1291**
Serevent Diskus **1540**

Secobarbital Sodium (Exhibits an additive CNS depression).
No products indexed under this heading.

Selegiline Hydrochloride (Co-administration of sympathomimetics and MAO inhibitors may produce an additive elevation of blood pressure leading to hypertensive crises; MAO inhibitors may prolong the anticholinergic effects of antihistamines; concurrent use is contraindicated). Products include:
Eldepryl Capsules **3209**

Sevoflurane (Exhibits an additive CNS depression). Products include:
Ultane Liquid for Inhalation **526**

Sodium Oxybate (Exhibits an additive CNS depression).
No products indexed under this heading.

Sotalol Hydrochloride (Concurrent use of phenylephrine with beta blockers may result in hypertensive crises).
No products indexed under this heading.

Sufentanil Citrate (Exhibits an additive CNS depression).
No products indexed under this heading.

Temazepam (Exhibits an additive CNS depression).
No products indexed under this heading.

Terbutaline Sulfate (Additive elevation of blood pressure).
No products indexed under this heading.

Thiamylal Sodium (Exhibits an additive CNS depression).
No products indexed under this heading.

Thioridazine Hydrochloride (Exhibits an additive CNS depression). Products include:
Thioridazine Hydrochloride Tablets **2122**

Thiothixene (Exhibits an additive CNS depression). Products include:
Thiothixene Capsules **2124**

Timolol Hemihydrate (Concurrent use of phenylephrine with beta blockers may result in hypertensive crises). Products include:
Betimol Ophthalmic Solution **3371**
Betimol Ophthalmic Solution .... ⊙**283**

Timolol Maleate (Concurrent use of phenylephrine with beta blockers may result in hypertensive crises). Products include:
Blocadren Tablets **1891**
Cosopt Sterile Ophthalmic Solution **1910**
Timolide Tablets **2056**
Timoptic in Ocudose **2061**
Timoptic Sterile Ophthalmic Solution **2058**
Timoptic-XE Sterile Ophthalmic Gel Forming Solution **2062**

Tranylcypromine Sulfate (Co-administration of sympathomimetics and MAO inhibitors may produce an additive elevation of blood pressure leading to hypertensive crises; MAO inhibitors may prolong the anticholinergic effects of antihistamines; concurrent use is contraindicated). Products include:
Parnate Tablets **1499**

Triazolam (Exhibits an additive CNS depression).
No products indexed under this heading.

Trifluoperazine Hydrochloride (Exhibits an additive CNS depression).
No products indexed under this heading.

Zaleplon (Exhibits an additive CNS depression). Products include:
Sonata Capsules **1686**

Ziprasidone Hydrochloride (Exhibits an additive CNS depression). Products include:
Geodon Capsules **2514**

Zolpidem Tartrate (Exhibits an additive CNS depression). Products include:
Ambien Tablets **2867**

Food Interactions

Alcohol (Exhibits an additive CNS depression).

HYCOTUSS EXPECTORANT SYRUP

(Guaifenesin, Hydrocodone Bitartrate) **1106**

May interact with central nervous system depressants, narcotic analgesics, antipsychotic agents, tranquilizers, and certain other agents. Compounds in these categories include:

Alfentanil Hydrochloride (Exhibits an additive CNS depression).
No products indexed under this heading.

Alprazolam (Exhibits an additive CNS depression). Products include:
Niravam Orally Disintegrating Tablets **3106**
Xanax XR Tablets **2655**

Aprobarbital (Exhibits an additive CNS depression).
No products indexed under this heading.

Aripiprazole (Exhibits an additive CNS depression). Products include:
Abilify Tablets **2472**
Abilify Tablets **916**

Buprenorphine Hydrochloride (Exhibits an additive CNS depression). Products include:
Buprenex Injectable **2718**
Suboxone Tablets **2719**
Subutex Tablets **2719**

Buspirone Hydrochloride (Exhibits an additive CNS depression).
No products indexed under this heading.

Butabarbital (Exhibits an additive CNS depression).
No products indexed under this heading.

Butalbital (Exhibits an additive CNS depression). Products include:
Sedapap Tablets 50 mg/650 mg **2098**

Chlordiazepoxide (Exhibits an additive CNS depression).
No products indexed under this heading.

Chlordiazepoxide Hydrochloride (Exhibits an additive CNS depression). Products include:
Librium Capsules **3349**

Chlorpromazine (Exhibits an additive CNS depression).
No products indexed under this heading.

Chlorpromazine Hydrochloride (Exhibits an additive CNS depression).
No products indexed under this heading.

Chlorprothixene (Exhibits an additive CNS depression).
No products indexed under this heading.

Chlorprothixene Hydrochloride (Exhibits an additive CNS depression).
No products indexed under this heading.

Chlorprothixene Lactate (Exhibits an additive CNS depression).
No products indexed under this heading.

Clorazepate Dipotassium (Exhibits an additive CNS depression). Products include:
Tranxene **2488**

Clozapine (Exhibits an additive CNS depression). Products include:
Clozapine Tablets **2141**
Clozaril Tablets **2174**
FazaClo Orally Disintegrating Tablets **547**

Codeine Phosphate (Exhibits an additive CNS depression). Products include:
Tylenol with Codeine **2461**

Desflurane (Exhibits an additive CNS depression). Products include:
Suprane Liquid for Inhalation **770**

Dezocine (Exhibits an additive CNS depression).
No products indexed under this heading.

Diazepam (Exhibits an additive CNS depression). Products include:
Diastat Rectal Delivery System **3344**
Valium Tablets **2822**

Droperidol (Exhibits an additive CNS depression).
No products indexed under this heading.

Enflurane (Exhibits an additive CNS depression).
No products indexed under this heading.

Estazolam (Exhibits an additive CNS depression). Products include:
ProSom Tablets **512**

Ethanol (Exhibits an additive CNS depression).
No products indexed under this heading.

Ethchlorvynol (Exhibits an additive CNS depression).
No products indexed under this heading.

Ethinamate (Exhibits an additive CNS depression).
No products indexed under this heading.

Ethyl Alcohol (Exhibits an additive CNS depression).
No products indexed under this heading.

Fentanyl (Exhibits an additive CNS depression). Products include:
Duragesic Transdermal System **2448**

Fentanyl Citrate (Exhibits an additive CNS depression). Products include:
Actiq **993**

Fluphenazine Decanoate (Exhibits an additive CNS depression).
No products indexed under this heading.

Fluphenazine Enanthate (Exhibits an additive CNS depression).
No products indexed under this heading.

Fluphenazine Hydrochloride (Exhibits an additive CNS depression).
No products indexed under this heading.

Flurazepam Hydrochloride (Exhibits an additive CNS depression). Products include:
Dalmane Capsules **3343**

Glutethimide (Exhibits an additive CNS depression).
No products indexed under this heading.

Haloperidol (Exhibits an additive CNS depression).
No products indexed under this heading.

Haloperidol Decanoate (Exhibits an additive CNS depression).
No products indexed under this heading.

Hydrocodone Polistirex (Exhibits an additive CNS depression). Products include:
Tussionex Pennkinetic Extended-Release Suspension **3322**

Hydromorphone Hydrochloride (Exhibits an additive CNS depression). Products include:
Dilaudid **439**
Dilaudid Oral Liquid **443**
Dilaudid Non-Sterile Powder **439**
Dilaudid Rectal Suppositories **439**
Dilaudid Tablets **439**
Dilaudid Tablets - 8 mg **443**
Dilaudid-HP **441**

Hydroxyzine Hydrochloride (Exhibits an additive CNS depression).
No products indexed under this heading.

Isoflurane (Exhibits an additive CNS depression).
No products indexed under this heading.

Ketamine Hydrochloride (Exhibits an additive CNS depression).
No products indexed under this heading.

Levomethadyl Acetate Hydrochloride (Exhibits an additive CNS depression).
No products indexed under this heading.

Levorphanol Tartrate (Exhibits an additive CNS depression).
No products indexed under this heading.

Lithium Carbonate (Exhibits an additive CNS depression). Products include:
Eskalith 1406
Lithobid Tablets 1670

Lithium Citrate (Exhibits an additive CNS depression).
No products indexed under this heading.

Lorazepam (Exhibits an additive CNS depression).
No products indexed under this heading.

Loxapine Hydrochloride (Exhibits an additive CNS depression).
No products indexed under this heading.

Loxapine Succinate (Exhibits an additive CNS depression).
No products indexed under this heading.

Meperidine Hydrochloride (Exhibits an additive CNS depression).
No products indexed under this heading.

Mephobarbital (Exhibits an additive CNS depression). Products include:
Mebaral Tablets, USP 2483

Meprobamate (Exhibits an additive CNS depression).
No products indexed under this heading.

Mesoridazine Besylate (Exhibits an additive CNS depression).
No products indexed under this heading.

Methadone Hydrochloride (Exhibits an additive CNS depression).
No products indexed under this heading.

Methohexital Sodium (Exhibits an additive CNS depression).
No products indexed under this heading.

Methotrimeprazine (Exhibits an additive CNS depression).
No products indexed under this heading.

Methoxyflurane (Exhibits an additive CNS depression).
No products indexed under this heading.

Midazolam Hydrochloride (Exhibits an additive CNS depression).
No products indexed under this heading.

Molindone Hydrochloride (Exhibits an additive CNS depression). Products include:
Moban Tablets 1108

Morphine Sulfate (Exhibits an additive CNS depression). Products include:
Avinza Capsules 1714
Kadian Capsules 572
MS Contin Tablets 2703

Olanzapine (Exhibits an additive CNS depression). Products include:
Symbyax Capsules 1788
Zyprexa Tablets 1798
Zyprexa IntraMuscular 1798
Zyprexa ZYDIS Orally Disintegrating Tablets 1798

Oxazepam (Exhibits an additive CNS depression).
No products indexed under this heading.

Oxycodone Hydrochloride (Exhibits an additive CNS depression). Products include:
Combunox Tablets 1183
OxyContin Tablets 2699
OxyFast Oral Concentrate Solution 2704
OxyIR Capsules 2704
Percocet Tablets 1114
Percodan Tablets 1115

Pentobarbital Sodium (Exhibits an additive CNS depression). Products include:
Nembutal Sodium Solution, USP 2484

Perphenazine (Exhibits an additive CNS depression).
No products indexed under this heading.

Phenobarbital (Exhibits an additive CNS depression).
No products indexed under this heading.

Pimozide (Exhibits an additive CNS depression). Products include:
Orap Tablets 1220

Prazepam (Exhibits an additive CNS depression).
No products indexed under this heading.

Prochlorperazine (Exhibits an additive CNS depression).
No products indexed under this heading.

Promethazine Hydrochloride (Exhibits an additive CNS depression). Products include:
Phenergan 3438

Propofol (Exhibits an additive CNS depression). Products include:
Diprivan Injectable Emulsion 676

Propoxyphene Hydrochloride (Exhibits an additive CNS depression).
No products indexed under this heading.

Propoxyphene Napsylate (Exhibits an additive CNS depression). Products include:
Darvocet A 500 Tablets 3497

Quazepam (Exhibits an additive CNS depression).
No products indexed under this heading.

Quetiapine Fumarate (Exhibits an additive CNS depression). Products include:
Seroquel Tablets 691

Remifentanil Hydrochloride (Exhibits an additive CNS depression).
No products indexed under this heading.

Risperidone (Exhibits an additive CNS depression). Products include:
Risperdal Consta Long-Acting Injection 1664
Risperdal M-Tab Orally Disintegrating Tablets 1658
Risperdal 1658

Secobarbital Sodium (Exhibits an additive CNS depression).
No products indexed under this heading.

Sevoflurane (Exhibits an additive CNS depression). Products include:
Ultane Liquid for Inhalation 526

Sodium Oxybate (Exhibits an additive CNS depression).
No products indexed under this heading.

Sufentanil Citrate (Exhibits an additive CNS depression).
No products indexed under this heading.

Temazepam (Exhibits an additive CNS depression).
No products indexed under this heading.

Thiamylal Sodium (Exhibits an additive CNS depression).
No products indexed under this heading.

Thioridazine Hydrochloride (Exhibits an additive CNS depression). Products include:
Thioridazine Hydrochloride Tablets 2122

Thiothixene (Exhibits an additive CNS depression). Products include:
Thiothixene Capsules 2124

Triazolam (Exhibits an additive CNS depression).
No products indexed under this heading.

Trifluoperazine Hydrochloride (Exhibits an additive CNS depression).
No products indexed under this heading.

Zaleplon (Exhibits an additive CNS depression). Products include:
Sonata Capsules 1686

Ziprasidone Hydrochloride (Exhibits an additive CNS depression). Products include:
Geodon Capsules 2514

Zolpidem Tartrate (Exhibits an additive CNS depression). Products include:
Ambien Tablets 2867

Food Interactions

Alcohol (Exhibits an additive CNS depression).

HYDROCORTONE TABLETS
(Hydrocortisone) 1963
May interact with oral anticoagulants, oral hypoglycemic agents, insulin, potassium-depleting diuretics, killed/inactivated vaccines, vaccines, live, and certain other agents. Compounds in these categories include:

Acarbose (Potential for increased requirements of oral hypoglycemic agents). Products include:
Precose Tablets 776

Anisindione (Potential for altered response to coumarin anticoagulants). Products include:
Miradon Tablets 3056

Aspirin (Aspirin should be used cautiously in conjunction with corticosteroids in hypoprothrombinemia). Products include:
Aggrenox Capsules 855
Bayer, Aspirin Regimen .... ▣606
Bayer Aspirin Tablets 3515
BC Powder .... ▣612
BC Allergy Sinus Cold Powder .... ▣612
Arthritis Strength BC Powder .... ▣612
BC Sinus Cold Powder .... ▣612
Ecotrin Enteric Coated Aspirin Low, Regular and Maximum Strength Tablets 1627
Goody's Body Pain Formula Powder .... ▣621
Goody's Extra Strength Headache Powder .... ▣621
Goody's Extra Strength Pain Relief Tablets .... ▣621
Percodan Tablets 1115
St. Joseph 81 mg Aspirin Chewable and Enteric Coated Tablets 1841

BCG Vaccine (Administration of live virus vaccines, including smallpox, is contraindicated in patients receiving immunosuppressive doses of corticosteroids).
No products indexed under this heading.

Bendroflumethiazide (Co-administration may result in hypokalemia).
No products indexed under this heading.

Bumetanide (Co-administration may result in hypokalemia).
No products indexed under this heading.

Chlorothiazide (Co-administration may result in hypokalemia). Products include:
Aldoclor Tablets 1881
Diuril Oral 1936

Chlorothiazide Sodium (Co-administration may result in hypokalemia). Products include:
Diuril Sodium Intravenous 1934

Chlorpropamide (Potential for increased requirements of oral hypoglycemic agents).
No products indexed under this heading.

Dicumarol (Potential for altered response to coumarin anticoagulants).
No products indexed under this heading.

Diphtheria & Tetanus Toxoids and Acellular Pertussis Vaccine Adsorbed, Hepatitis B (recombinant) and Inactivated Poliovirus Vaccine Combined (If inactivated viral or bacterial vaccines are administered to individuals receiving immunosuppressive doses of corticosteroids, the expected serum antibody response may not be obtained. However, immunization procedures may be undertaken in patients whoare receiving corticosteroids as replacement therapy, e.g., for Addison's disease).
No products indexed under this heading.

Ephedrine Hydrochloride (Enhances metabolic clearance of corticosteroids resulting in decreased blood levels and lessened physiologic activity). Products include:
Primatene Tablets .... ▣749

Ephedrine Sulfate (Enhances metabolic clearance of corticosteroids resulting in decreased blood levels and lessened physiologic activity).
No products indexed under this heading.

Ephedrine Tannate (Enhances metabolic clearance of corticosteroids resulting in decreased blood levels and lessened physiologic activity).
No products indexed under this heading.

Ethacrynic Acid (Co-administration may result in hypokalemia). Products include:
Edecrin Tablets 1941

Fosphenytoin Sodium (Enhances metabolic clearance of corticosteroids resulting in decreased blood levels and lessened physiologic activity).
No products indexed under this heading.

Furosemide (Co-administration may result in hypokalemia). Products include:

Furosemide Tablets 2117

Glimepiride (Potential for increased requirements of oral hypoglycemic agents). Products include:

Amaryl Tablets 2864

Glipizide (Potential for increased requirements of oral hypoglycemic agents).

No products indexed under this heading.

Glyburide (Potential for increased requirements of oral hypoglycemic agents).

No products indexed under this heading.

Hepatitis A Vaccine, Inactivated (If inactivated viral or bacterial vaccines are administered to individuals receiving immunosuppressive doses of corticosteroids, the expected serum antibody response may not be obtained. However, immunization procedures may be undertaken in patients whoare receiving corticosteroids as replacement therapy, e.g., for Addison's disease). Products include:

Havrix Vaccine 1425
Twinrix Vaccine 1571
Vaqta 2067

Hydrochlorothiazide (Co-administration may result in hypokalemia). Products include:

Aldoril Tablets 1884
Atacand HCT 637
Avalide Tablets 2889
Avalide Tablets 922
Benicar HCT Tablets 2852
Diovan HCT Tablets 2195
Dyazide Capsules 1389
Hyzaar 1964
Lotensin HCT Tablets 2235
Maxzide 2150
Micardis HCT Tablets 886
Moduretic Tablets 2003
Prinzide Tablets 2033
Teveten HCT Tablets 1710
Timolide Tablets 2056
Uniretic Tablets 3114
Vaseretic Tablets 2073
Zestoretic Tablets 701

Hydroflumethiazide (Co-administration may result in hypokalemia).

No products indexed under this heading.

Influenza Virus Vaccine (If inactivated viral or bacterial vaccines are administered to individuals receiving immunosuppressive doses of corticosteroids, the expected serum antibody response may not be obtained. However, immunization procedures may be undertaken in patients whoare receiving corticosteroids as replacement therapy, e.g., for Addison's disease). Products include:

Flumist Vaccine 1872

Insulin, Human, Zinc Suspension (Potential for increased requirements of insulin). Products include:

Humulin L, 100 Units 1763
Humulin U, 100 Units 1770

Insulin, Human NPH (Potential for increased requirements of insulin). Products include:

Humulin N, 100 Units 1764
Humulin N Pen 1765
Novolin N Human Insulin 10 ml Vials 2322
Novolin N InnoLet 2322
Novolin N PenFill 3 ml Cartridges 2325
Novolin R InnoLet 2322

Insulin, Human Regular (Potential for increased requirements of insulin). Products include:

Humulin R (U-500) 1768
Humulin R, 100 Units 1767
Novolin R Human Insulin 10 ml Vials 2322
Novolin R PenFill 2325

Insulin, Human Regular and Human NPH Mixture (Potential for increased requirements of insulin). Products include:

Humulin 50/50, 100 Units 1760
Humulin 70/30 Pen 1761
Novolin 70/30 Human Insulin 10 ml Vials 2321
Novolin 70/30 InnoLet 2322
Novolin 70/30 PenFill 3 ml Cartridges 2325

Insulin, NPH (Potential for increased requirements of insulin).

No products indexed under this heading.

Insulin, Regular (Potential for increased requirements of insulin).

No products indexed under this heading.

Insulin, Zinc Crystals (Potential for increased requirements of insulin).

No products indexed under this heading.

Insulin, Zinc Suspension (Potential for increased requirements of insulin).

No products indexed under this heading.

Insulin Aspart, Human Regular (Potential for increased requirements of insulin). Products include:

NovoLog Injection 2326

Insulin glargine (Potential for increased requirements of insulin). Products include:

Lantus Injection 2925

Insulin Lispro, Human (Potential for increased requirements of insulin). Products include:

Humalog-Pen 1751
Humalog Mix 75/25-Pen 1754

Insulin Lispro Protamine, Human (Potential for increased requirements of insulin). Products include:

Humalog Mix 75/25-Pen 1754

Japanese Encephalitis Vaccine Inactivated (If inactivated viral or bacterial vaccines are administered to individuals receiving immunosuppressive doses of corticosteroids, the expected serum antibody response may not be obtained. However, immunization procedures may be undertaken in patients whoare receiving corticosteroids as replacement therapy, e.g., for Addison's disease).

No products indexed under this heading.

Ketoconazole (Inhibits adrenal corticosteroid synthesis and may cause cortical insufficiency during corticosteroid withdrawal). Products include:

Nizoral A-D Shampoo, 1% 1839
Nizoral 2% Shampoo 1838

Live Virus Vaccines (Co-administration is contraindicated in patients receiving immunosuppressive doses of corticosteroids).

No products indexed under this heading.

Measles, Mumps & Rubella Virus Vaccine, Live (Administration of live virus vaccines, including smallpox, is contraindicated in patients receiving immunosuppressive doses of corticosteroids). Products include:

M-M-R II 1980

Measles & Rubella Virus Vaccine Live (Administration of live virus vaccines, including smallpox, is contraindicated in patients receiving immunosuppressive doses of corticosteroids).

No products indexed under this heading.

Measles Virus Vaccine Live (Administration of live virus vaccines, including smallpox, is contraindicated in patients receiving immunosuppressive doses of corticosteroids). Products include:

Attenuvax 1889

Metformin Hydrochloride (Potential for increased requirements of oral hypoglycemic agents). Products include:

ActoPlus Met Tablets 3219
Avandamet Tablets 1343
Fortamet Extended-Release Tablets 1156

Methyclothiazide (Co-administration may result in hypokalemia).

No products indexed under this heading.

Miglitol (Potential for increased requirements of oral hypoglycemic agents).

No products indexed under this heading.

Mumps Virus Vaccine, Live (Administration of live virus vaccines, including smallpox, is contraindicated in patients receiving immunosuppressive doses of corticosteroids). Products include:

Mumpsvax 2005

Phenobarbital (Enhances metabolic clearance of corticosteroids resulting in decreased blood levels and lessened physiologic activity).

No products indexed under this heading.

Phenytoin (Enhances metabolic clearance of corticosteroids resulting in decreased blood levels and lessened physiologic activity).

No products indexed under this heading.

Phenytoin Sodium (Enhances metabolic clearance of corticosteroids resulting in decreased blood levels and lessened physiologic activity). Products include:

Phenytek Capsules 2153

Pioglitazone Hydrochloride (Potential for increased requirements of oral hypoglycemic agents). Products include:

ActoPlus Met Tablets 3219
Actos Tablets 3224

Poliovirus Vaccine, Live, Oral, Trivalent, Types 1,2,3 (Sabin) (Administration of live virus vaccines, including smallpox, is contraindicated in patients receiving immunosuppressive doses of corticosteroids).

No products indexed under this heading.

Poliovirus Vaccine Inactivated, Trivalent Types 1,2,3 (If inactivated viral or bacterial vaccines are administered to individuals receiving immunosuppressive doses of corticosteroids, the expected serum antibody response may not be obtained. However, immunization procedures may be undertaken in patients whoare receiving corticosteroids as replacement therapy, e.g., for Addison's disease). Products include:

Pediarix Vaccine 1518

Polythiazide (Co-administration may result in hypokalemia).

No products indexed under this heading.

Repaglinide (Potential for increased requirements of oral hypoglycemic agents). Products include:

Prandin Tablets (0.5, 1, and 2 mg) 2337

Rifampin (Enhances metabolic clearance of corticosteroids resulting in decreased blood levels and lessened physiologic activity).

No products indexed under this heading.

Rosiglitazone Maleate (Potential for increased requirements of oral hypoglycemic agents). Products include:

Avandamet Tablets 1343
Avandia Tablets 1348

Rotavirus Vaccine, Live, Oral, Tetravalent (Administration of live virus vaccines, including smallpox, is contraindicated in patients receiving immunosuppressive doses of corticosteroids).

No products indexed under this heading.

Rubella & Mumps Virus Vaccine Live (Administration of live virus vaccines, including smallpox, is contraindicated in patients receiving immunosuppressive doses of corticosteroids).

No products indexed under this heading.

Rubella Virus Vaccine Live (Administration of live virus vaccines, including smallpox, is contraindicated in patients receiving immunosuppressive doses of corticosteroids). Products include:

Meruvax II 1994

Smallpox Vaccine (Administration of live virus vaccines, including smallpox, is contraindicated in patients receiving immunosuppressive doses of corticosteroids).

No products indexed under this heading.

Tolazamide (Potential for increased requirements of oral hypoglycemic agents).

No products indexed under this heading.

Tolbutamide (Potential for increased requirements of oral hypoglycemic agents).

No products indexed under this heading.

Torsemide (Co-administration may result in hypokalemia).

No products indexed under this heading.

Troglitazone (Potential for increased requirements of oral hypoglycemic agents).

No products indexed under this heading.

Typhoid Vaccine (Administration of live virus vaccines, including smallpox, is contraindicated in patients receiving immunosuppressive doses of corticosteroids).

No products indexed under this heading.

Varicella Virus Vaccine Live (Administration of live virus vaccines, including smallpox, is contraindicated in patients receiving immunosuppressive doses of corticosteroids). Products include:

Varivax 2070

IMPORTANT NOTE: Always consult each drug listing in the patient's regimen for possible interactions.

Warfarin Sodium (Potential for altered response to coumarin anticoagulants). Products include:
Coumadin for Injection 932
Coumadin Tablets 932

Yellow Fever Vaccine (Administration of live virus vaccines, including smallpox, is contraindicated in patients receiving immunosuppressive doses of corticosteroids).
No products indexed under this heading.

HYLAND'S BACKACHE WITH ARNICA CAPLETS

(Homeopathic Formulations) .... ▣733
None cited in PDR database.

HYLAND'S BUMPS 'N BRUISES TABLETS

(Homeopathic Formulations) .... ▣734
None cited in PDR database.

HYLAND'S CALMS FORTE TABLETS AND CAPLETS

(Homeopathic Formulations) .... ▣734
None cited in PDR database.

HYLAND'S COMPLETE FLU CARE TABLETS

(Herbals, Multiple) .... ▣734
None cited in PDR database.

HYLAND'S EARACHE DROPS

(Herbals, Multiple) .... ▣734
None cited in PDR database.

HYLAND'S EARACHE TABLETS

(Homeopathic Formulations) .... ▣734
None cited in PDR database.

HYLAND'S LEG CRAMPS OINTMENT

(Homeopathic Formulations) .... ▣735
None cited in PDR database.

HYLAND'S LEG CRAMPS WITH QUININE TABLETS AND CAPLETS

(Homeopathic Formulations) .... ▣735
None cited in PDR database.

HYLAND'S NERVE TONIC TABLETS AND CAPLETS

(Homeopathic Formulations) .... ▣735
None cited in PDR database.

HYLAND'S SEASONAL ALLERGY TABLETS

(Homeopathic Formulations) .... ▣735
None cited in PDR database.

HYLAND'S TEETHING GEL

(Homeopathic Formulations) .... ▣736
None cited in PDR database.

HYLAND'S TEETHING TABLETS

(Belladonna Alkaloids, Homeopathic Formulations).............. ▣736
None cited in PDR database.

HYPERHEP B S/D

(Hepatitis B Immune Globulin (Human)).. 3237
May interact with:

Vaccines (Live) (May interfere with response. Use should be deferred for 3 months after administration of HyperHep).
No products indexed under this heading.

HYPERRAB

(Rabies Immune Globulin (Human)) 3239
May interact with:

Measles, Mumps & Rubella Virus Vaccine, Live (Interference with the response to live viral vaccines). Products include:
M-M-R II 1980

Measles & Rubella Virus Vaccine Live (Interference with the response to live viral vaccines).
No products indexed under this heading.

Measles Virus Vaccine Live (Interference with the response to live viral vaccines). Products include:
Attenuvax 1889

Mumps Virus Vaccine, Live (Interference with the response to live viral vaccines). Products include:
Mumpsvax 2005

Poliovirus Vaccine, Live, Oral, Trivalent, Types 1,2,3 (Sabin) (Interference with the response to live viral vaccines).
No products indexed under this heading.

Rubella & Mumps Virus Vaccine Live (Interference with the response to live viral vaccines).
No products indexed under this heading.

Rubella Virus Vaccine Live (Interference with the response to live viral vaccines). Products include:
Meruvax II 1994

HYPERRHO S/D FULL DOSE

(Rh_o (D) Immune Globulin (Human)) 3243
May interact with:

Measles, Mumps & Rubella Virus Vaccine, Live (Interference with response to live vaccines). Products include:
M-M-R II 1980

Measles & Rubella Virus Vaccine Live (Interference with response to live vaccines).
No products indexed under this heading.

Measles Virus Vaccine Live (Interference with response to live vaccines). Products include:
Attenuvax 1889

Rubella & Mumps Virus Vaccine Live (Interference with response to live vaccines).
No products indexed under this heading.

Rubella Virus Vaccine Live (Interference with response to live vaccines). Products include:
Meruvax II 1994

HYPERRHO S/D MINI-DOSE

(Rh_o (D) Immune Globulin (Human)) 3241
See HyperRho S/D Full Dose

HYPERSTAT I.V. INJECTION

(Diazoxide) 3031
May interact with antihypertensives, beta blockers, oral anticoagulants, diuretics, and certain other agents. Compounds in these categories include:

Acebutolol Hydrochloride (An undesirable hypotension may result when diazoxide is administered to patients who have received other antihypertensive agents within six hours; do not administer within six hours).
No products indexed under this heading.

Amiloride Hydrochloride (Potentiates the hyperuricemic and antihypertensive effects of diazoxide). Products include:
Midamor Tablets 2000
Moduretic Tablets 2003

Amlodipine Besylate (An undesirable hypotension may result when diazoxide is administered to patients who have received other antihypertensive agents within six hours). Products include:
Caduet Tablets 2507
Lotrel Capsules 2238
Norvasc Tablets 2529

Anisindione (Increased blood levels of coumarin derivatives due to displacement from protein binding sites). Products include:
Miradon Tablets 3056

Atenolol (An undesirable hypotension may result when diazoxide is administered to patients who have received other antihypertensive agents within six hours; do not administer within six hours). Products include:
Tenormin I.V. Injection 698
Tenormin Tablets 695

Benazepril Hydrochloride (An undesirable hypotension may result when diazoxide is administered to patients who have received other antihypertensive agents within six hours). Products include:
Lotensin Tablets 2232
Lotensin HCT Tablets 2235
Lotrel Capsules 2238

Bendroflumethiazide (Potentiates the hyperuricemic and antihypertensive effects of diazoxide).
No products indexed under this heading.

Betaxolol Hydrochloride (An undesirable hypotension may result when diazoxide is administered to patients who have received other antihypertensive agents within six hours; do not administer within six hours). Products include:
Betoptic S Ophthalmic Suspension.................................. 554

Bisoprolol Fumarate (An undesirable hypotension may result when diazoxide is administered to patients who have received other antihypertensive agents within six hours; do not administer within six hours).
No products indexed under this heading.

Bumetanide (Potentiates the hyperuricemic and antihypertensive effects of diazoxide).
No products indexed under this heading.

Candesartan Cilexetil (An undesirable hypotension may result when diazoxide is administered to patients who have received other antihypertensive agents within six hours). Products include:
Atacand Tablets 634
Atacand HCT 637

Captopril (An undesirable hypotension may result when diazoxide is administered to patients who have received other antihypertensive agents within six hours). Products include:
Captopril Tablets 2114

Carteolol Hydrochloride (An undesirable hypotension may result when diazoxide is administered to patients who have received other antihypertensive agents within six hours; do not administer within six hours). Products include:
Carteolol Hydrochloride Ophthalmic Solution USP, 1%....... ⊙246

Chlorothiazide (Potentiates the hyperuricemic and antihypertensive effects of diazoxide). Products include:
Aldoclor Tablets 1881
Diuril Oral 1936

Chlorothiazide Sodium (Potentiates the hyperuricemic and antihypertensive effects of diazoxide). Products include:
Diuril Sodium Intravenous 1934

Chlorthalidone (Potentiates the hyperuricemic and antihypertensive effects of diazoxide). Products include:
Clorpres Tablets 2139

Clonidine (An undesirable hypotension may result when diazoxide is administered to patients who have received other antihypertensive agents within six hours). Products include:
Catapres-TTS 875

Clonidine Hydrochloride (An undesirable hypotension may result when diazoxide is administered to patients who have received other antihypertensive agents within six hours). Products include:
Catapres Tablets 874
Clorpres Tablets 2139

Deserpidine (An undesirable hypotension may result when diazoxide is administered to patients who have received other antihypertensive agents within six hours).
No products indexed under this heading.

Dicumarol (Increased blood levels of coumarin derivatives due to displacement from protein binding sites).
No products indexed under this heading.

Diltiazem Hydrochloride (An undesirable hypotension may result when diazoxide is administered to patients who have received other antihypertensive agents within six hours). Products include:
Cardizem LA Extended Release Tablets 1699
Tiazac Capsules 1204

Doxazosin Mesylate (An undesirable hypotension may result when diazoxide is administered to patients who have received other antihypertensive agents within six hours).
No products indexed under this heading.

Enalapril Maleate (An undesirable hypotension may result when diazoxide is administered to patients who have received other antihypertensive agents within six hours). Products include:
Vaseretic Tablets 2073
Vasotec I.V. Injection 2076

Enalaprilat (An undesirable hypotension may result when diazoxide is administered to patients who have received other antihypertensive agents within six hours).
No products indexed under this heading.

Eprosartan Mesylate (An undesirable hypotension may result when diazoxide is administered to patients who have received other antihypertensive agents within six hours). Products include:
Teveten Tablets 1707
Teveten HCT Tablets 1710

Esmolol Hydrochloride (An undesirable hypotension may result when diazoxide is administered to patients who have received other antihyper-

tensive agents within six hours; do not administer within six hours). Products include:

Brevibloc Concentrate ... 766
Brevibloc Injection ... 766
Brevibloc Double Strength Injection ... 766
Brevibloc Premixed Injection ... 766
Brevibloc Double Strength Premixed Injection ... 766

Ethacrynic Acid (Potentiates the hyperuricemic and antihypertensive effects of diazoxide). Products include:

Edecrin Tablets ... 1941

Felodipine (An undesirable hypotension may result when diazoxide is administered to patients who have received other antihypertensive agents within six hours). Products include:

Plendil Extended-Release Tablets ... 651

Fosinopril Sodium (An undesirable hypotension may result when diazoxide is administered to patients who have received other antihypertensive agents within six hours).

No products indexed under this heading.

Furosemide (Potentiates the hyperuricemic and antihypertensive effects of diazoxide). Products include:

Furosemide Tablets ... 2117

Guanabenz Acetate (An undesirable hypotension may result when diazoxide is administered to patients who have received other antihypertensive agents within six hours).

No products indexed under this heading.

Guanethidine Monosulfate (An undesirable hypotension may result when diazoxide is administered to patients who have received other antihypertensive agents within six hours).

No products indexed under this heading.

Hydralazine Hydrochloride (Co-administration with methyldopa and hydralazine has produced excessive hypotension; do not administer within six hours). Products include:

BiDil Tablets ... 2161

Hydrochlorothiazide (Potentiates the hyperuricemic and antihypertensive effects of diazoxide). Products include:

Aldoril Tablets ... 1884
Atacand HCT ... 637
Avalide Tablets ... 2889
Avalide Tablets ... 922
Benicar HCT Tablets ... 2852
Diovan HCT Tablets ... 2195
Dyazide Capsules ... 1389
Hyzaar ... 1964
Lotensin HCT Tablets ... 2235
Maxzide ... 2150
Micardis HCT Tablets ... 886
Moduretic Tablets ... 2003
Prinzide Tablets ... 2033
Teveten HCT Tablets ... 1710
Timolide Tablets ... 2056
Uniretic Tablets ... 3114
Vaseretic Tablets ... 2073
Zestoretic Tablets ... 701

Hydroflumethiazide (Potentiates the hyperuricemic and antihypertensive effects of diazoxide).

No products indexed under this heading.

Indapamide (Potentiates the hyperuricemic and antihypertensive effects of diazoxide). Products include:

Indapamide Tablets ... 2119

Irbesartan (An undesirable hypotension may result when diazoxide is administered to patients who have received other antihypertensive agents within six hours). Products include:

Avalide Tablets ... 922
Avalide Tablets ... 2889
Avapro Tablets ... 925
Avapro Tablets ... 2886

Isradipine (An undesirable hypotension may result when diazoxide is administered to patients who have received other antihypertensive agents within six hours). Products include:

DynaCirc CR Tablets ... 2726

Labetalol Hydrochloride (An undesirable hypotension may result when diazoxide is administered to patients who have received other antihypertensive agents within six hours; do not administer within six hours).

No products indexed under this heading.

Levobunolol Hydrochloride (An undesirable hypotension may result when diazoxide is administered to patients who have received other antihypertensive agents within six hours; do not administer within six hours). Products include:

Betagan Ophthalmic Solution, USP ... ⊙217

Lisinopril (An undesirable hypotension may result when diazoxide is administered to patients who have received other antihypertensive agents within six hours). Products include:

Prinivil Tablets ... 2029
Prinzide Tablets ... 2033
Zestoretic Tablets ... 701
Zestril Tablets ... 704

Losartan Potassium (An undesirable hypotension may result when diazoxide is administered to patients who have received other antihypertensive agents within six hours). Products include:

Cozaar Tablets ... 1913
Hyzaar ... 1964

Mecamylamine Hydrochloride (An undesirable hypotension may result when diazoxide is administered to patients who have received other antihypertensive agents within six hours). Products include:

Inversine Tablets ... 3286

Methyclothiazide (Potentiates the hyperuricemic and antihypertensive effects of diazoxide).

No products indexed under this heading.

Methyldopa (Co-administration with methyldopa and hydralazine has produced excessive hypotension; do not administer within six hours). Products include:

Aldoclor Tablets ... 1881
Aldoril Tablets ... 1884

Methyldopate Hydrochloride (Co-administration with methyldopa and hydralazine has produced excessive hypotension; do not administer within six hours).

No products indexed under this heading.

Metipranolol Hydrochloride (An undesirable hypotension may result when diazoxide is administered to patients who have received other antihypertensive agents within six hours; do not administer within six hours).

No products indexed under this heading.

Metolazone (Potentiates the hyperuricemic and antihypertensive effects of diazoxide).

No products indexed under this heading.

Metoprolol Succinate (An undesirable hypotension may result when diazoxide is administered to patients who have received other antihypertensive agents within six hours; do not administer within six hours). Products include:

Toprol-XL Tablets ... 660

Metoprolol Tartrate (An undesirable hypotension may result when diazoxide is administered to patients who have received other antihypertensive agents within six hours; do not administer within six hours).

No products indexed under this heading.

Metyrosine (An undesirable hypotension may result when diazoxide is administered to patients who have received other antihypertensive agents within six hours). Products include:

Demser Capsules ... 1933

Mibefradil Dihydrochloride (An undesirable hypotension may result when diazoxide is administered to patients who have received other antihypertensive agents within six hours).

No products indexed under this heading.

Minoxidil (An undesirable hypotension may result when diazoxide is administered to patients who have received other antihypertensive agents within six hours; do not administer within six hours). Products include:

Men's Rogaine Extra Strength Topical Solution, Ocean Rush Scent and Original Unscented ... ▣706
Women's Rogaine Topical Solution, Spring Bloom Scent and Original Unscented ... ▣707

Moexipril Hydrochloride (An undesirable hypotension may result when diazoxide is administered to patients who have received other antihypertensive agents within six hours). Products include:

Uniretic Tablets ... 3114
Univasc Tablets ... 3118

Nadolol (An undesirable hypotension may result when diazoxide is administered to patients who have received other antihypertensive agents within six hours; do not administer within six hours). Products include:

Nadolol Tablets ... 2121

Nicardipine Hydrochloride (An undesirable hypotension may result when diazoxide is administered to patients who have received other antihypertensive agents within six hours). Products include:

Cardene I.V. ... 1129

Nifedipine (An undesirable hypotension may result when diazoxide is administered to patients who have received other antihypertensive agents within six hours). Products include:

Adalat CC Tablets ... 2978

Nisoldipine (An undesirable hypotension may result when diazoxide is administered to patients who have received other antihypertensive agents within six hours). Products include:

Sular Tablets ... 1163

Nitroglycerin (An undesirable hypotension may result when diazoxide is administered to patients who have received other antihypertensive agents within six hours; do not administer within six hours). Products include:

Nitro-Dur Transdermal Infusion System ... 3060
Nitrolingual Pumpspray ... 1161

Papaverine Hydrochloride (An undesirable hypotension may result when diazoxide is administered to patients who have received other antihypertensive agents within six hours; do not administer within six hours).

No products indexed under this heading.

Penbutolol Sulfate (An undesirable hypotension may result when diazoxide is administered to patients who have received other antihypertensive agents within six hours; do not administer within six hours).

No products indexed under this heading.

Perindopril Erbumine (An undesirable hypotension may result when diazoxide is administered to patients who have received other antihypertensive agents within six hours). Products include:

Aceon Tablets (2 mg, 4 mg, 8 mg) ... 3191

Phenoxybenzamine Hydrochloride (An undesirable hypotension may result when diazoxide is administered to patients who have received other antihypertensive agents within six hours). Products include:

Dibenzyline Capsules ... 3390

Phentolamine Mesylate (An undesirable hypotension may result when diazoxide is administered to patients who have received other antihypertensive agents within six hours).

No products indexed under this heading.

Pindolol (An undesirable hypotension may result when diazoxide is administered to patients who have received other antihypertensive agents within six hours; do not administer within six hours).

No products indexed under this heading.

Polythiazide (Potentiates the hyperuricemic and antihypertensive effects of diazoxide).

No products indexed under this heading.

Prazosin Hydrochloride (An undesirable hypotension may result when diazoxide is administered to patients who have received other antihypertensive agents within six hours; do not administer within six hours).

No products indexed under this heading.

Propranolol Hydrochloride (An undesirable hypotension may result when diazoxide is administered to patients who have received other antihypertensive agents within six hours; do not administer within six hours). Products include:

Inderal LA Long-Acting Capsules ... 3421
InnoPran XL Capsules ... 2728

Quinapril Hydrochloride (An undesirable hypotension may result when diazoxide is administered to patients who have received other antihypertensive agents within six hours).

No products indexed under this heading.

Ramipril (An undesirable hypotension may result when diazoxide is administered to patients who have received other antihypertensive agents within six hours). Products include:
Altace Capsules 1673

Rauwolfia Serpentina (An undesirable hypotension may result when diazoxide is administered to patients who have received other antihypertensive agents within six hours).
No products indexed under this heading.

Rescinnamine (An undesirable hypotension may result when diazoxide is administered to patients who have received other antihypertensive agents within six hours).
No products indexed under this heading.

Reserpine (Co-administration with reserpine and hydralazine has produced maternal hypotension and fetal bradycardia in a patient in labor; do not administer within six hours).
No products indexed under this heading.

Sodium Nitroprusside (An undesirable hypotension may result when diazoxide is administered to patients who have received other antihypertensive agents within six hours).
No products indexed under this heading.

Sotalol Hydrochloride (An undesirable hypotension may result when diazoxide is administered to patients who have received other antihypertensive agents within six hours; do not administer within six hours).
No products indexed under this heading.

Spirapril Hydrochloride (An undesirable hypotension may result when diazoxide is administered to patients who have received other antihypertensive agents within six hours).
No products indexed under this heading.

Spironolactone (Potentiates the hyperuricemic and antihypertensive effects of diazoxide).
No products indexed under this heading.

Telmisartan (An undesirable hypotension may result when diazoxide is administered to patients who have received other antihypertensive agents within six hours). Products include:
Micardis Tablets 884
Micardis HCT Tablets 886

Terazosin Hydrochloride (An undesirable hypotension may result when diazoxide is administered to patients who have received other antihypertensive agents within six hours). Products include:
Hytrin Capsules 469

Timolol Hemihydrate (An undesirable hypotension may result when diazoxide is administered to patients who have received other antihypertensive agents within six hours; do not administer within six hours). Products include:
Betimol Ophthalmic Solution 3371
Betimol Ophthalmic Solution .... ⊙283

Timolol Maleate (An undesirable hypotension may result when diazoxide is administered to patients who have received other antihypertensive agents within six hours; do not administer within six hours). Products include:
Blocadren Tablets 1891
Cosopt Sterile Ophthalmic Solution 1910
Timolide Tablets 2056
Timoptic in Ocudose 2061
Timoptic Sterile Ophthalmic Solution 2058
Timoptic-XE Sterile Ophthalmic Gel Forming Solution 2062

Torsemide (Potentiates the hyperuricemic and antihypertensive effects of diazoxide).
No products indexed under this heading.

Trandolapril (An undesirable hypotension may result when diazoxide is administered to patients who have received other antihypertensive agents within six hours). Products include:
Mavik Tablets 482
Tarka Tablets 519

Triamterene (Potentiates the hyperuricemic and antihypertensive effects of diazoxide). Products include:
Dyazide Capsules 1389
Dyrenium Capsules 3390
Maxzide 2150

Trimethaphan Camsylate (An undesirable hypotension may result when diazoxide is administered to patients who have received other antihypertensive agents within six hours).
No products indexed under this heading.

Valsartan (An undesirable hypotension may result when diazoxide is administered to patients who have received other antihypertensive agents within six hours). Products include:
Diovan HCT Tablets 2195
Diovan Tablets 2191

Verapamil Hydrochloride (An undesirable hypotension may result when diazoxide is administered to patients who have received other antihypertensive agents within six hours). Products include:
Covera-HS Tablets 3135
Tarka Tablets 519
Verelan PM Capsules 3120

Warfarin Sodium (Increased blood levels of coumarin derivatives due to displacement from protein binding sites). Products include:
Coumadin for Injection 932
Coumadin Tablets 932

HYPERTET

(Tetanus Immune Globulin (Human)) ... 3245
May interact with:

Vaccines (Live) (May interfere with response. Use should be deferred for 3 months).
No products indexed under this heading.

HYTRIN CAPSULES

(Terazosin Hydrochloride) 469
May interact with antihypertensives and certain other agents. Compounds in these categories include:

Acebutolol Hydrochloride (Possibility of significant hypotension; dosage adjustment may be necessary).
No products indexed under this heading.

Amlodipine Besylate (Possibility of significant hypotension; dosage adjustment may be necessary). Products include:
Caduet Tablets 2507
Lotrel Capsules 2238
Norvasc Tablets 2529

Atenolol (Possibility of significant hypotension; dosage adjustment may be necessary). Products include:
Tenormin I.V. Injection 698
Tenormin Tablets 695

Benazepril Hydrochloride (Possibility of significant hypotension; dosage adjustment may be necessary). Products include:
Lotensin Tablets 2232
Lotensin HCT Tablets 2235
Lotrel Capsules 2238

Bendroflumethiazide (Possibility of significant hypotension; dosage adjustment may be necessary).
No products indexed under this heading.

Betaxolol Hydrochloride (Possibility of significant hypotension; dosage adjustment may be necessary). Products include:
Betoptic S Ophthalmic Suspension 554

Bisoprolol Fumarate (Possibility of significant hypotension; dosage adjustment may be necessary).
No products indexed under this heading.

Candesartan Cilexetil (Possibility of significant hypotension; dosage adjustment may be necessary). Products include:
Atacand Tablets 634
Atacand HCT 637

Captopril (Co-administration increases terazosin's maximum plasma concentrations linearly with dose at steady-state after administration of terazosin plus captopril). Products include:
Captopril Tablets 2114

Carteolol Hydrochloride (Possibility of significant hypotension; dosage adjustment may be necessary). Products include:
Carteolol Hydrochloride Ophthalmic Solution USP, 1% .... ⊙246

Chlorothiazide (Possibility of significant hypotension; dosage adjustment may be necessary). Products include:
Aldoclor Tablets 1881
Diuril Oral 1936

Chlorothiazide Sodium (Possibility of significant hypotension; dosage adjustment may be necessary). Products include:
Diuril Sodium Intravenous 1934

Chlorthalidone (Possibility of significant hypotension; dosage adjustment may be necessary). Products include:
Clorpres Tablets 2139

Clonidine (Possibility of significant hypotension; dosage adjustment may be necessary). Products include:
Catapres-TTS 875

Clonidine Hydrochloride (Possibility of significant hypotension; dosage adjustment may be necessary). Products include:
Catapres Tablets 874
Clorpres Tablets 2139

Deserpidine (Possibility of significant hypotension; dosage adjustment may be necessary).
No products indexed under this heading.

Diazoxide (Possibility of significant hypotension; dosage adjustment may be necessary). Products include:
Hyperstat I.V. Injection 3031

Diltiazem Hydrochloride (Possibility of significant hypotension; dosage adjustment may be necessary). Products include:
Cardizem LA Extended Release Tablets 1699
Tiazac Capsules 1204

Doxazosin Mesylate (Possibility of significant hypotension; dosage adjustment may be necessary).
No products indexed under this heading.

Enalapril Maleate (Possibility of significant hypotension; dosage adjustment may be necessary). Products include:
Vaseretic Tablets 2073
Vasotec I.V. Injection 2076

Enalaprilat (Possibility of significant hypotension; dosage adjustment may be necessary).
No products indexed under this heading.

Eprosartan Mesylate (Possibility of significant hypotension; dosage adjustment may be necessary). Products include:
Teveten Tablets 1707
Teveten HCT Tablets 1710

Esmolol Hydrochloride (Possibility of significant hypotension; dosage adjustment may be necessary). Products include:
Brevibloc Concentrate 766
Brevibloc Injection 766
Brevibloc Double Strength Injection 766
Brevibloc Premixed Injection 766
Brevibloc Double Strength Premixed Injection 766

Felodipine (Possibility of significant hypotension; dosage adjustment may be necessary). Products include:
Plendil Extended-Release Tablets 651

Fosinopril Sodium (Possibility of significant hypotension; dosage adjustment may be necessary).
No products indexed under this heading.

Furosemide (Possibility of significant hypotension; dosage adjustment may be necessary). Products include:
Furosemide Tablets 2117

Guanabenz Acetate (Possibility of significant hypotension; dosage adjustment may be necessary).
No products indexed under this heading.

Guanethidine Monosulfate (Possibility of significant hypotension; dosage adjustment may be necessary).
No products indexed under this heading.

Hydralazine Hydrochloride (Possibility of significant hypotension; dosage adjustment may be necessary). Products include:
BiDil Tablets 2161

Hydrochlorothiazide (Possibility of significant hypotension; dosage adjustment may be necessary). Products include:
Aldoril Tablets 1884
Atacand HCT 637
Avalide Tablets 2889
Avalide Tablets 922
Benicar HCT Tablets 2852
Diovan HCT Tablets 2195
Dyazide Capsules 1389
Hyzaar 1964
Lotensin HCT Tablets 2235
Maxzide 2150
Micardis HCT Tablets 886
Moduretic Tablets 2003

Prinzide Tablets 2033
Teveten HCT Tablets 1710
Timolide Tablets 2056
Uniretic Tablets 3114
Vaseretic Tablets 2073
Zestoretic Tablets 701

Hydroflumethiazide (Possibility of significant hypotension; dosage adjustment may be necessary).
No products indexed under this heading.

Indapamide (Possibility of significant hypotension; dosage adjustment may be necessary). Products include:
Indapamide Tablets 2119

Irbesartan (Possibility of significant hypotension; dosage adjustment may be necessary). Products include:
Avalide Tablets 922
Avalide Tablets 2889
Avapro Tablets 925
Avapro Tablets 2886

Isradipine (Possibility of significant hypotension; dosage adjustment may be necessary). Products include:
DynaCirc CR Tablets 2726

Labetalol Hydrochloride (Possibility of significant hypotension; dosage adjustment may be necessary).
No products indexed under this heading.

Lisinopril (Possibility of significant hypotension; dosage adjustment may be necessary). Products include:
Prinivil Tablets 2029
Prinzide Tablets 2033
Zestoretic Tablets 701
Zestril Tablets 704

Losartan Potassium (Possibility of significant hypotension; dosage adjustment may be necessary). Products include:
Cozaar Tablets 1913
Hyzaar 1964

Mecamylamine Hydrochloride (Possibility of significant hypotension; dosage adjustment may be necessary). Products include:
Inversine Tablets 3286

Methyclothiazide (Possibility of significant hypotension; dosage adjustment may be necessary).
No products indexed under this heading.

Methyldopa (Possibility of significant hypotension; dosage adjustment may be necessary). Products include:
Aldoclor Tablets 1881
Aldoril Tablets 1884

Methyldopate Hydrochloride (Possibility of significant hypotension; dosage adjustment may be necessary).
No products indexed under this heading.

Metipranolol Hydrochloride (Possibility of significant hypotension; dosage adjustment may be necessary).
No products indexed under this heading.

Metolazone (Possibility of significant hypotension; dosage adjustment may be necessary).
No products indexed under this heading.

Metoprolol Succinate (Possibility of significant hypotension; dosage adjustment may be necessary). Products include:
Toprol-XL Tablets 660

Metoprolol Tartrate (Possibility of significant hypotension; dosage adjustment may be necessary).
No products indexed under this heading.

Metyrosine (Possibility of significant hypotension; dosage adjustment may be necessary). Products include:
Demser Capsules 1933

Mibefradil Dihydrochloride (Possibility of significant hypotension; dosage adjustment may be necessary).
No products indexed under this heading.

Minoxidil (Possibility of significant hypotension; dosage adjustment may be necessary). Products include:
Men's Rogaine Extra Strength Topical Solution, Ocean Rush Scent and Original Unscented 706
Women's Rogaine Topical Solution, Spring Bloom Scent and Original Unscented 707

Moexipril Hydrochloride (Possibility of significant hypotension; dosage adjustment may be necessary). Products include:
Uniretic Tablets 3114
Univasc Tablets 3118

Nadolol (Possibility of significant hypotension; dosage adjustment may be necessary). Products include:
Nadolol Tablets 2121

Nicardipine Hydrochloride (Possibility of significant hypotension; dosage adjustment may be necessary). Products include:
Cardene I.V. 1129

Nifedipine (Possibility of significant hypotension; dosage adjustment may be necessary). Products include:
Adalat CC Tablets 2978

Nisoldipine (Possibility of significant hypotension; dosage adjustment may be necessary). Products include:
Sular Tablets 1163

Nitroglycerin (Possibility of significant hypotension; dosage adjustment may be necessary). Products include:
Nitro-Dur Transdermal Infusion System 3060
Nitrolingual Pumpspray 1161

Penbutolol Sulfate (Possibility of significant hypotension; dosage adjustment may be necessary).
No products indexed under this heading.

Perindopril Erbumine (Possibility of significant hypotension; dosage adjustment may be necessary). Products include:
Aceon Tablets (2 mg, 4 mg, 8 mg) 3191

Phenoxybenzamine Hydrochloride (Possibility of significant hypotension; dosage adjustment may be necessary). Products include:
Dibenzyline Capsules 3390

Phentolamine Mesylate (Possibility of significant hypotension; dosage adjustment may be necessary).
No products indexed under this heading.

Pindolol (Possibility of significant hypotension; dosage adjustment may be necessary).
No products indexed under this heading.

Polythiazide (Possibility of significant hypotension; dosage adjustment may be necessary).
No products indexed under this heading.

Prazosin Hydrochloride (Possibility of significant hypotension; dosage adjustment may be necessary).
No products indexed under this heading.

Propranolol Hydrochloride (Possibility of significant hypotension; dosage adjustment may be necessary). Products include:
Inderal LA Long-Acting Capsules 3421
InnoPran XL Capsules 2728

Quinapril Hydrochloride (Possibility of significant hypotension; dosage adjustment may be necessary).
No products indexed under this heading.

Ramipril (Possibility of significant hypotension; dosage adjustment may be necessary). Products include:
Altace Capsules 1673

Rauwolfia Serpentina (Possibility of significant hypotension; dosage adjustment may be necessary).
No products indexed under this heading.

Rescinnamine (Possibility of significant hypotension; dosage adjustment may be necessary).
No products indexed under this heading.

Reserpine (Possibility of significant hypotension; dosage adjustment may be necessary).
No products indexed under this heading.

Sodium Nitroprusside (Possibility of significant hypotension; dosage adjustment may be necessary).
No products indexed under this heading.

Sotalol Hydrochloride (Possibility of significant hypotension; dosage adjustment may be necessary).
No products indexed under this heading.

Spirapril Hydrochloride (Possibility of significant hypotension; dosage adjustment may be necessary).
No products indexed under this heading.

Telmisartan (Possibility of significant hypotension; dosage adjustment may be necessary). Products include:
Micardis Tablets 884
Micardis HCT Tablets 886

Timolol Maleate (Possibility of significant hypotension; dosage adjustment may be necessary). Products include:
Blocadren Tablets 1891
Cosopt Sterile Ophthalmic Solution 1910
Timolide Tablets 2056
Timoptic in Ocudose 2061
Timoptic Sterile Ophthalmic Solution 2058
Timoptic-XE Sterile Ophthalmic Gel Forming Solution 2062

Torsemide (Possibility of significant hypotension; dosage adjustment may be necessary).
No products indexed under this heading.

Trandolapril (Possibility of significant hypotension; dosage adjustment may be necessary). Products include:
Mavik Tablets 482
Tarka Tablets 519

Trimethaphan Camsylate (Possibility of significant hypotension; dosage adjustment may be necessary).
No products indexed under this heading.

Valsartan (Possibility of significant hypotension; dosage adjustment may be necessary). Products include:
Diovan HCT Tablets 2195
Diovan Tablets 2191

Verapamil Hydrochloride (Coadministration increases terazosin's mean AUC0-24 by 11% to 24% with associated increase in Cmax (25%) and Cmin (32%)). Products include:
Covera-HS Tablets 3135
Tarka Tablets 519
Verelan PM Capsules 3120

Food Interactions

Food, unspecified (Delays the time to peak concentration by about 40 minutes; minimal effect on the extent of absorption).

HYZAAR 50-12.5 TABLETS

(Hydrochlorothiazide, Losartan Potassium) 1964

May interact with antihypertensives, barbiturates, corticosteroids, erythromycin, oral hypoglycemic agents, insulin, lithium preparations, narcotic analgesics, nondepolarizing neuromuscular blocking agents, non-steroidal anti-inflammatory agents, potassium preparations, potassium sparing diuretics, and certain other agents. Compounds in these categories include:

Acarbose (Hyperglycemia may occur with thiazide diuretics; dosage adjustment of the antidiabetic drug may be required). Products include:
Precose Tablets 776

Acebutolol Hydrochloride (Additive effect or potentiation of other antihypertensives).
No products indexed under this heading.

ACTH (Potential for intensified electrolyte depletion, particularly hypokalemia).
No products indexed under this heading.

Alfentanil Hydrochloride (Potentiation of orthostatic hypotension).
No products indexed under this heading.

Amiloride Hydrochloride (Concomitant use with potassium-sparing diuretics may lead to hyperkalemia). Products include:
Midamor Tablets 2000
Moduretic Tablets 2003

Amlodipine Besylate (Additive effect or potentiation of other antihypertensives). Products include:
Caduet Tablets 2507
Lotrel Capsules 2238
Norvasc Tablets 2529

Aprobarbital (Potentiation of orthostatic hypotension).
No products indexed under this heading.

Atenolol (Additive effect or potentiation of other antihypertensives). Products include:
Tenormin I.V. Injection 698
Tenormin Tablets 695

Atracurium Besylate (Possible increased responsiveness to the muscle relaxant).
No products indexed under this heading.

Benazepril Hydrochloride (Additive effect or potentiation of other antihypertensives). Products include:

Lotensin Tablets 2232
Lotensin HCT Tablets 2235
Lotrel Capsules 2238

Bendroflumethiazide (Additive effect or potentiation of other antihypertensives).
No products indexed under this heading.

Betamethasone Acetate (Potential for intensified electrolyte depletion, particularly hypokalemia).
No products indexed under this heading.

Betamethasone Sodium Phosphate (Potential for intensified electrolyte depletion, particularly hypokalemia).
No products indexed under this heading.

Betaxolol Hydrochloride (Additive effect or potentiation of other antihypertensives). Products include:
Betoptic S Ophthalmic Suspension 554

Bisoprolol Fumarate (Additive effect or potentiation of other antihypertensives).
No products indexed under this heading.

Buprenorphine Hydrochloride (Potentiation of orthostatic hypotension). Products include:
Buprenex Injectable 2718
Suboxone Tablets 2719
Subutex Tablets 2719

Butabarbital (Potentiation of orthostatic hypotension).
No products indexed under this heading.

Butalbital (Potentiation of orthostatic hypotension). Products include:
Sedapap Tablets 50 mg/650 mg 2098

Candesartan Cilexetil (Additive effect or potentiation of other antihypertensives). Products include:
Atacand Tablets 634
Atacand HCT 637

Captopril (Additive effect or potentiation of other antihypertensives). Products include:
Captopril Tablets 2114

Carteolol Hydrochloride (Additive effect or potentiation of other antihypertensives). Products include:
Carteolol Hydrochloride Ophthalmic Solution USP, 1% .... ⊙246

Celecoxib (Potential reduced diuretic, natriuretic, and antihypertensive effects). Products include:
Celebrex Capsules 3130

Chlorothiazide (Additive effect or potentiation of other antihypertensives). Products include:
Aldoclor Tablets 1881
Diuril Oral 1936

Chlorothiazide Sodium (Additive effect or potentiation of other antihypertensives). Products include:
Diuril Sodium Intravenous 1934

Chlorpropamide (Hyperglycemia may occur with thiazide diuretics; dosage adjustment of the antidiabetic drug may be required).
No products indexed under this heading.

Chlorthalidone (Additive effect or potentiation of other antihypertensives). Products include:
Clorpres Tablets 2139

Cholestyramine (Absorption of hydrochlorothiazide is impaired in the presence of anionic exchange resins; cholestyramine binds hydrochlorothiazide and reduces its absorption from GI tract by up to 85%).
No products indexed under this heading.

Cimetidine (Co-administration led to an increase of about 18% in AUC of losartan but did not affect the pharmacokinetics of its active metabolite). Products include:
Tagamet HB 200 Tablets .... ▪▫637
Tagamet Tablets 1547

Cimetidine Hydrochloride (Co-administration led to an increase of about 18% in AUC of losartan but did not affect the pharmacokinetics of its active metabolite).
No products indexed under this heading.

Cisatracurium Besylate (Possible increased responsiveness to the muscle relaxant). Products include:
Nimbex Injection 494

Clonidine (Additive effect or potentiation of other antihypertensives). Products include:
Catapres-TTS 875

Clonidine Hydrochloride (Additive effect or potentiation of other antihypertensives). Products include:
Catapres Tablets 874
Clorpres Tablets 2139

Codeine Phosphate (Potentiation of orthostatic hypotension). Products include:
Tylenol with Codeine 2461

Colestipol Hydrochloride (Absorption of hydrochlorothiazide is impaired in the presence of anionic exchange resins; cholestyramine binds hydrochlorothiazide and reduces its absorption from GI tract by up to 85%).
No products indexed under this heading.

Cortisone Acetate (Potential for intensified electrolyte depletion, particularly hypokalemia).
No products indexed under this heading.

Deserpidine (Additive effect or potentiation of other antihypertensives).
No products indexed under this heading.

Dexamethasone (Potential for intensified electrolyte depletion, particularly hypokalemia). Products include:
Ciprodex Otic Suspension 555
Decadron Tablets 1929
TobraDex Ophthalmic Ointment 558
TobraDex Ophthalmic Suspension 558

Dexamethasone Acetate (Potential for intensified electrolyte depletion, particularly hypokalemia).
No products indexed under this heading.

Dexamethasone Sodium Phosphate (Potential for intensified electrolyte depletion, particularly hypokalemia). Products include:
Decadron Phosphate Injection 1931

Dezocine (Potentiation of orthostatic hypotension).
No products indexed under this heading.

Diazoxide (Additive effect or potentiation of other antihypertensives). Products include:
Hyperstat I.V. Injection 3031

Diclofenac Potassium (Potential reduced diuretic, natriuretic, and antihypertensive effects). Products include:
Cataflam Tablets 2173

Diclofenac Sodium (Potential reduced diuretic, natriuretic, and antihypertensive effects). Products include:
Arthrotec Tablets 3126
Voltaren Ophthalmic Solution 2300
Voltaren Tablets 2298
Voltaren-XR Tablets 2301

Diltiazem Hydrochloride (Additive effect or potentiation of other antihypertensives). Products include:
Cardizem LA Extended Release Tablets 1699
Tiazac Capsules 1204

Doxazosin Mesylate (Additive effect or potentiation of other antihypertensives).
No products indexed under this heading.

Enalapril Maleate (Additive effect or potentiation of other antihypertensives). Products include:
Vaseretic Tablets 2073
Vasotec I.V. Injection 2076

Enalaprilat (Additive effect or potentiation of other antihypertensives).
No products indexed under this heading.

Eprosartan Mesylate (Additive effect or potentiation of other antihypertensives). Products include:
Teveten Tablets 1707
Teveten HCT Tablets 1710

Erythromycin (Erythromycin increased the AUC of losartan by 30%). Products include:
Erygel Topical Gel 2096
Ery-Tab Tablets 447
Erythromycin Base Filmtab Tablets 454
Erythromycin Delayed-Release Capsules, USP 456
PCE Dispertab Tablets 510

Erythromycin Estolate (Erythromycin increased the AUC of losartan by 30%).
No products indexed under this heading.

Erythromycin Ethylsuccinate (Erythromycin increased the AUC of losartan by 30%). Products include:
E.E.S. 449
EryPed 445

Erythromycin Gluceptate (Erythromycin increased the AUC of losartan by 30%).
No products indexed under this heading.

Erythromycin Lactobionate (Erythromycin increased the AUC of losartan by 30%).
No products indexed under this heading.

Erythromycin Stearate (Erythromycin increased the AUC of losartan by 30%). Products include:
Erythrocin Stearate Filmtab Tablets 452

Esmolol Hydrochloride (Additive effect or potentiation of other antihypertensives). Products include:
Brevibloc Concentrate 766
Brevibloc Injection 766
Brevibloc Double Strength Injection 766
Brevibloc Premixed Injection 766
Brevibloc Double Strength Premixed Injection 766

Etodolac (Potential reduced diuretic, natriuretic, and antihypertensive effects).
No products indexed under this heading.

Felodipine (Additive effect or potentiation of other antihypertensives). Products include:
Plendil Extended-Release Tablets 651

Fenoprofen Calcium (Potential reduced diuretic, natriuretic, and antihypertensive effects). Products include:
Nalfon Capsules 2504

Fentanyl (Potentiation of orthostatic hypotension). Products include:
Duragesic Transdermal System 2448

Fentanyl Citrate (Potentiation of orthostatic hypotension). Products include:
Actiq 993

Fluconazole (Fluconazole decreased the AUC of the active metabolite of losartan by approximately 40%, but increased the AUC of losartan by 70%).
No products indexed under this heading.

Fludrocortisone Acetate (Potential for intensified electrolyte depletion, particularly hypokalemia).
No products indexed under this heading.

Flurbiprofen (Potential reduced diuretic, natriuretic, and antihypertensive effects).
No products indexed under this heading.

Fosinopril Sodium (Additive effect or potentiation of other antihypertensives).
No products indexed under this heading.

Furosemide (Additive effect or potentiation of other antihypertensives). Products include:
Furosemide Tablets 2117

Gestodene (In vitro studies show significant inhibition of the formation of the active metabolite by inhibitors of CYP4503A4, such as gestodene; pharmacodynamic consequences of concomitant use are undefined).
No products indexed under this heading.

Glimepiride (Hyperglycemia may occur with thiazide diuretics; dosage adjustment of the antidiabetic drug may be required). Products include:
Amaryl Tablets 2864

Glipizide (Hyperglycemia may occur with thiazide diuretics; dosage adjustment of the antidiabetic drug may be required).
No products indexed under this heading.

Glyburide (Hyperglycemia may occur with thiazide diuretics; dosage adjustment of the antidiabetic drug may be required).
No products indexed under this heading.

Guanabenz Acetate (Additive effect or potentiation of other antihypertensives).
No products indexed under this heading.

Guanethidine Monosulfate (Additive effect or potentiation of other antihypertensives).
No products indexed under this heading.

Hydralazine Hydrochloride (Additive effect or potentiation of other antihypertensives). Products include:

- BiDil Tablets 2161

Hydrocodone Bitartrate (Potentiation of orthostatic hypotension). Products include:

- Hycodan 1104
- Hycomine Compound Tablets 1105
- Hycotuss Expectorant Syrup 1106
- Lortab 3315
- Lortab Elixir 3312
- Vicodin Tablets 530
- Vicodin ES Tablets 531
- Vicodin HP Tablets 532
- Vicoprofen Tablets 533
- Zydone Tablets 1118

Hydrocodone Polistirex (Potentiation of orthostatic hypotension). Products include:

- Tussionex Pennkinetic Extended-Release Suspension 3322

Hydrocortisone (Potential for intensified electrolyte depletion, particularly hypokalemia). Products include:

- Cortizone•5 Ointment ▣699
- Cortizone•10 Creme ▣699
- Cortizone•10 Ointment ▣699
- Cortizone•10 Plus Creme ▣700
- Cortizone•10 Maximum Strength Quick Shot Spray ▣700
- Hydrocortone Tablets 1963
- Preparation H Hydrocortisone Cream ▣748

Hydrocortisone Acetate (Potential for intensified electrolyte depletion, particularly hypokalemia). Products include:

- Analpram-HC 1136
- Pramosone 1139
- ProctoFoam-HC 3113
- Tucks Anti-Itch Ointment ▣712
- U-cort 1% Cream 3289

Hydrocortisone Sodium Phosphate (Potential for intensified electrolyte depletion, particularly hypokalemia).

No products indexed under this heading.

Hydrocortisone Sodium Succinate (Potential for intensified electrolyte depletion, particularly hypokalemia).

No products indexed under this heading.

Hydroflumethiazide (Additive effect or potentiation of other antihypertensives).

No products indexed under this heading.

Hydromorphone Hydrochloride (Potentiation of orthostatic hypotension). Products include:

- Dilaudid 439
- Dilaudid Oral Liquid 443
- Dilaudid Non-Sterile Powder 439
- Dilaudid Rectal Suppositories 439
- Dilaudid Tablets 439
- Dilaudid Tablets - 8 mg 443
- Dilaudid-HP 441

Ibuprofen (Potential reduced diuretic, natriuretic, and antihypertensive effects). Products include:

- Advil Allergy Sinus Caplets ▣737
- Advil ▣737
- Children's Advil Suspension ▣742
- Children's Advil Chewable Tablets ▣741
- Advil Cold & Sinus ▣739
- Advil Flu & Body Ache Caplets ▣739
- Children's Advil Cold Suspension ▣741
- Infants' Advil Concentrated Drops ▣743
- Junior Strength Advil Swallow Tablets ▣740
- Advil Migraine Liquigels ▣740
- Advil Multi-Symptom Cold Caplets ▣738
- Combunox Tablets 1183
- Children's Motrin Oral Suspension and Chewable Tablets 1837
- Children's Motrin Cold Non-Staining Dye-Free Oral Suspension 1838
- Children's Motrin Cold Oral Suspension 1838
- Children's Motrin Non-Staining Dye-Free Oral Suspension 1837
- Motrin Cold & Sinus Caplets 1836
- Motrin IB Tablets and Caplets 1836
- Infants' Motrin Concentrated Drops 1837
- Infants' Motrin Non-Staining Dye-Free Drops 1837
- Junior Strength Motrin Caplets and Chewable Tablets 1837
- Vicoprofen Tablets 533

Indapamide (Additive effect or potentiation of other antihypertensives). Products include:

- Indapamide Tablets 2119

Indomethacin (Antihypertensive effect of losartan may be blunted by indomethacin). Products include:

- Indocin 1968

Indomethacin Sodium Trihydrate (Antihypertensive effect of losartan may be blunted by indomethacin). Products include:

- Indocin I.V. 1973

Insulin, Human, Zinc Suspension (Hyperglycemia may occur with thiazide diuretics; dosage adjustment of the antidiabetic drug may be required). Products include:

- Humulin L, 100 Units 1763
- Humulin U, 100 Units 1770

Insulin, Human NPH (Hyperglycemia may occur with thiazide diuretics; dosage adjustment of the antidiabetic drug may be required). Products include:

- Humulin N, 100 Units 1764
- Humulin N Pen 1765
- Novolin N Human Insulin 10 ml Vials 2322
- Novolin N InnoLet 2322
- Novolin N PenFill 3 ml Cartridges 2325
- Novolin R InnoLet 2322

Insulin, Human Regular (Hyperglycemia may occur with thiazide diuretics; dosage adjustment of the antidiabetic drug may be required). Products include:

- Humulin R (U-500) 1768
- Humulin R, 100 Units 1767
- Novolin R Human Insulin 10 ml Vials 2322
- Novolin R PenFill 2325

Insulin, Human Regular and Human NPH Mixture (Hyperglycemia may occur with thiazide diuretics; dosage adjustment of the antidiabetic drug may be required). Products include:

- Humulin 50/50, 100 Units 1760
- Humulin 70/30 Pen 1761
- Novolin 70/30 Human Insulin 10 ml Vials 2321
- Novolin 70/30 InnoLet 2322
- Novolin 70/30 PenFill 3 ml Cartridges 2325

Insulin, NPH (Hyperglycemia may occur with thiazide diuretics; dosage adjustment of the antidiabetic drug may be required).

No products indexed under this heading.

Insulin, Regular (Hyperglycemia may occur with thiazide diuretics; dosage adjustment of the antidiabetic drug may be required).

No products indexed under this heading.

Insulin, Zinc Crystals (Hyperglycemia may occur with thiazide diuretics; dosage adjustment of the antidiabetic drug may be required).

No products indexed under this heading.

Insulin, Zinc Suspension (Hyperglycemia may occur with thiazide diuretics; dosage adjustment of the antidiabetic drug may be required).

No products indexed under this heading.

Insulin Aspart, Human Regular (Hyperglycemia may occur with thiazide diuretics; dosage adjustment of the antidiabetic drug may be required). Products include:

- NovoLog Injection 2326

Insulin glargine (Hyperglycemia may occur with thiazide diuretics; dosage adjustment of the antidiabetic drug may be required). Products include:

- Lantus Injection 2925

Insulin Lispro, Human (Hyperglycemia may occur with thiazide diuretics; dosage adjustment of the antidiabetic drug may be required). Products include:

- Humalog-Pen 1751
- Humalog Mix 75/25-Pen 1754

Insulin Lispro Protamine, Human (Hyperglycemia may occur with thiazide diuretics; dosage adjustment of the antidiabetic drug may be required). Products include:

- Humalog Mix 75/25-Pen 1754

Irbesartan (Additive effect or potentiation of other antihypertensives). Products include:

- Avalide Tablets 922
- Avalide Tablets 2889
- Avapro Tablets 925
- Avapro Tablets 2886

Isradipine (Additive effect or potentiation of other antihypertensives). Products include:

- DynaCirc CR Tablets 2726

Ketoconazole (In vitro studies show significant inhibition of the formation of the active metabolite by inhibitors of CYP4503A4, such as ketoconazole or complete inhibition by the combination of ketoconazole and sulfaphenazole; pharmacodynamic consequences of concomitant use are undefined). Products include:

- Nizoral A-D Shampoo, 1% 1839
- Nizoral 2% Shampoo 1838

Ketoprofen (Potential reduced diuretic, natriuretic, and antihypertensive effects).

No products indexed under this heading.

Ketorolac Tromethamine (Potential reduced diuretic, natriuretic, and antihypertensive effects). Products include:

- Acular Ophthalmic Solution 561
- Acular LS Ophthalmic Solution 562

Labetalol Hydrochloride (Additive effect or potentiation of other antihypertensives).

No products indexed under this heading.

Levobunolol Hydrochloride (Additive effect or potentiation of other antihypertensives). Products include:

- Betagan Ophthalmic Solution, USP ⊙217

Levorphanol Tartrate (Potentiation of orthostatic hypotension).

No products indexed under this heading.

Lisinopril (Additive effect or potentiation of other antihypertensives). Products include:

- Prinivil Tablets 2029
- Prinzide Tablets 2033
- Zestoretic Tablets 701
- Zestril Tablets 704

Lithium (Diuretics reduce the renal clearance of lithium and add a high risk of lithium toxicity; concurrent use should be avoided).

No products indexed under this heading.

Lithium Carbonate (Diuretics reduce the renal clearance of lithium and add a high risk of lithium toxicity; concurrent use should be avoided). Products include:

- Eskalith 1406
- Lithobid Tablets 1670

Lithium Citrate (Diuretics reduce the renal clearance of lithium and add a high risk of lithium toxicity; concurrent use should be avoided).

No products indexed under this heading.

Mecamylamine Hydrochloride (Additive effect or potentiation of other antihypertensives). Products include:

- Inversine Tablets 3286

Meclofenamate Sodium (Potential reduced diuretic, natriuretic, and antihypertensive effects).

No products indexed under this heading.

Mefenamic Acid (Potential reduced diuretic, natriuretic, and antihypertensive effects).

No products indexed under this heading.

Meloxicam (Potential reduced diuretic, natriuretic, and antihypertensive effects). Products include:

- Mobic Oral Suspension 893
- Mobic Tablets 893

Meperidine Hydrochloride (Potentiation of orthostatic hypotension).

No products indexed under this heading.

Mephobarbital (Potentiation of orthostatic hypotension). Products include:

- Mebaral Tablets, USP 2483

Metformin Hydrochloride (Hyperglycemia may occur with thiazide diuretics; dosage adjustment of the antidiabetic drug may be required). Products include:

- ActoPlus Met Tablets 3219
- Avandamet Tablets 1343
- Fortamet Extended-Release Tablets 1156

Methadone Hydrochloride (Potentiation of orthostatic hypotension).

No products indexed under this heading.

Methyclothiazide (Additive effect or potentiation of other antihypertensives).

No products indexed under this heading.

Methyldopa (Additive effect or potentiation of other antihypertensives). Products include:

- Aldoclor Tablets 1881
- Aldoril Tablets 1884

Methyldopate Hydrochloride (Additive effect or potentiation of other antihypertensives).

No products indexed under this heading.

Methylprednisolone Acetate (Potential for intensified electrolyte depletion, particularly hypokalemia). Products include:

- Depo-Medrol Injectable Suspension 2615
- Depo-Medrol Single-Dose Vial 2617

Methylprednisolone Sodium Succinate (Potential for intensified electrolyte depletion, particularly hypokalemia).
No products indexed under this heading.

Metipranolol Hydrochloride (Additive effect or potentiation of other antihypertensives).
No products indexed under this heading.

Metocurine Iodide (Possible increased responsiveness to the muscle relaxant).
No products indexed under this heading.

Metolazone (Additive effect or potentiation of other antihypertensives).
No products indexed under this heading.

Metoprolol Succinate (Additive effect or potentiation of other antihypertensives). Products include:
Toprol-XL Tablets ... 660

Metoprolol Tartrate (Additive effect or potentiation of other antihypertensives).
No products indexed under this heading.

Metyrosine (Additive effect or potentiation of other antihypertensives). Products include:
Demser Capsules ... 1933

Mibefradil Dihydrochloride (Additive effect or potentiation of other antihypertensives).
No products indexed under this heading.

Miglitol (Hyperglycemia may occur with thiazide diuretics; dosage adjustment of the antidiabetic drug may be required).
No products indexed under this heading.

Minoxidil (Additive effect or potentiation of other antihypertensives). Products include:
Men's Rogaine Extra Strength Topical Solution, Ocean Rush Scent and Original Unscented ... ▣706
Women's Rogaine Topical Solution, Spring Bloom Scent and Original Unscented ... ▣707

Mivacurium Chloride (Possible increased responsiveness to the muscle relaxant). Products include:
Mivacron Injection ... 489

Moexipril Hydrochloride (Additive effect or potentiation of other antihypertensives). Products include:
Uniretic Tablets ... 3114
Univasc Tablets ... 3118

Morphine Sulfate (Potentiation of orthostatic hypotension). Products include:
Avinza Capsules ... 1714
Kadian Capsules ... 572
MS Contin Tablets ... 2703

Nabumetone (Potential reduced diuretic, natriuretic, and antihypertensive effects). Products include:
Relafen Tablets ... 1523

Nadolol (Additive effect or potentiation of other antihypertensives). Products include:
Nadolol Tablets ... 2121

Naproxen (Potential reduced diuretic, natriuretic, and antihypertensive effects). Products include:
EC-Naprosyn Delayed-Release Tablets ... 2769
Naprosyn Suspension ... 2769
Naprosyn Tablets ... 2769
Prevacid NapraPAC ... 3277

Naproxen Sodium (Potential reduced diuretic, natriuretic, and antihypertensive effects). Products include:
Aleve Tablets, Caplets and Gelcaps ... ▣605
Anaprox Tablets ... 2769
Anaprox DS Tablets ... 2769

Nicardipine Hydrochloride (Additive effect or potentiation of other antihypertensives). Products include:
Cardene I.V. ... 1129

Nifedipine (Additive effect or potentiation of other antihypertensives). Products include:
Adalat CC Tablets ... 2978

Nisoldipine (Additive effect or potentiation of other antihypertensives). Products include:
Sular Tablets ... 1163

Nitroglycerin (Additive effect or potentiation of other antihypertensives). Products include:
Nitro-Dur Transdermal Infusion System ... 3060
Nitrolingual Pumpspray ... 1161

Oxaprozin (Potential reduced diuretic, natriuretic, and antihypertensive effects).
No products indexed under this heading.

Oxycodone Hydrochloride (Potentiation of orthostatic hypotension). Products include:
Combunox Tablets ... 1183
OxyContin Tablets ... 2699
OxyFast Oral Concentrate Solution ... 2704
OxyIR Capsules ... 2704
Percocet Tablets ... 1114
Percodan Tablets ... 1115

Pancuronium Bromide (Possible increased responsiveness to the muscle relaxant).
No products indexed under this heading.

Penbutolol Sulfate (Additive effect or potentiation of other antihypertensives).
No products indexed under this heading.

Pentobarbital Sodium (Potentiation of orthostatic hypotension). Products include:
Nembutal Sodium Solution, USP ... 2484

Perindopril Erbumine (Additive effect or potentiation of other antihypertensives). Products include:
Aceon Tablets (2 mg, 4 mg, 8 mg) ... 3191

Phenobarbital (Co-administration may lead to a reduction of about 20% in AUC of losartan and its active metabolite; potentiation of orthostatic hypotension).
No products indexed under this heading.

Phenoxybenzamine Hydrochloride (Additive effect or potentiation of other antihypertensives). Products include:
Dibenzyline Capsules ... 3390

Phentolamine Mesylate (Additive effect or potentiation of other antihypertensives).
No products indexed under this heading.

Phenylbutazone (Potential reduced diuretic, natriuretic, and antihypertensive effects).
No products indexed under this heading.

Pindolol (Additive effect or potentiation of other antihypertensives).
No products indexed under this heading.

Pioglitazone Hydrochloride (Hyperglycemia may occur with thiazide diuretics; dosage adjustment of the antidiabetic drug may be required). Products include:
ActoPlus Met Tablets ... 3219
Actos Tablets ... 3224

Piroxicam (Potential reduced diuretic, natriuretic, and antihypertensive effects).
No products indexed under this heading.

Polythiazide (Additive effect or potentiation of other antihypertensives).
No products indexed under this heading.

Potassium Acid Phosphate (Concomitant use with potassium supplements may lead to hyperkalemia). Products include:
K-Phos Original (Sodium Free) Tablets ... 785

Potassium Bicarbonate (Concomitant use with potassium supplements may lead to hyperkalemia).
No products indexed under this heading.

Potassium Chloride (Concomitant use with potassium supplements may lead to hyperkalemia). Products include:
Colyte with Flavor Packs for Oral Solution ... 3102
HalfLytely and Bisacodyl Tablets Bowel Prep Kit with Flavors Packs ... 915
K-Dur Extended-Relase Tablets ... 3047
K-Lor Powder Packets ... 472
K-Tab Filmtab Tablets ... 473
TriLyte with Flavor Packs for Oral Solution ... 3114

Potassium Citrate (Concomitant use with potassium supplements may lead to hyperkalemia). Products include:
Urocit-K Tablets ... 2109

Potassium Gluconate (Concomitant use with potassium supplements may lead to hyperkalemia).
No products indexed under this heading.

Potassium Phosphate (Concomitant use with potassium supplements may lead to hyperkalemia). Products include:
K-Phos Neutral Tablets ... 785

Prazosin Hydrochloride (Additive effect or potentiation of other antihypertensives).
No products indexed under this heading.

Prednisolone Acetate (Potential for intensified electrolyte depletion, particularly hypokalemia). Products include:
Blephamide Ophthalmic Ointment ... 563
Blephamide Ophthalmic Suspension ... 564
Poly-Pred Liquifilm Ophthalmic Suspension ... ⊙231
Pred Forte Ophthalmic Suspension ... ⊙233
Pred Mild Sterile Ophthalmic Suspension ... ⊙236
Pred-G Ophthalmic Suspension ... ⊙234
Pred-G Sterile Ophthalmic Ointment ... ⊙235

Prednisolone Sodium Phosphate (Potential for intensified electrolyte depletion, particularly hypokalemia). Products include:
Pediapred Oral Solution ... 3319

Prednisolone Tebutate (Potential for intensified electrolyte depletion, particularly hypokalemia).
No products indexed under this heading.

Prednisone (Potential for intensified electrolyte depletion, particularly hypokalemia).
No products indexed under this heading.

Propoxyphene Hydrochloride (Potentiation of orthostatic hypotension).
No products indexed under this heading.

Propoxyphene Napsylate (Potentiation of orthostatic hypotension). Products include:
Darvocet A 500 Tablets ... 3497

Propranolol Hydrochloride (Additive effect or potentiation of other antihypertensives). Products include:
Inderal LA Long-Acting Capsules ... 3421
InnoPran XL Capsules ... 2728

Quinapril Hydrochloride (Additive effect or potentiation of other antihypertensives).
No products indexed under this heading.

Ramipril (Additive effect or potentiation of other antihypertensives). Products include:
Altace Capsules ... 1673

Rapacuronium Bromide (Possible increased responsiveness to the muscle relaxant).
No products indexed under this heading.

Rauwolfia Serpentina (Additive effect or potentiation of other antihypertensives).
No products indexed under this heading.

Remifentanil Hydrochloride (Potentiation of orthostatic hypotension).
No products indexed under this heading.

Repaglinide (Hyperglycemia may occur with thiazide diuretics; dosage adjustment of the antidiabetic drug may be required). Products include:
Prandin Tablets (0.5, 1, and 2 mg) ... 2337

Rescinnamine (Additive effect or potentiation of other antihypertensives).
No products indexed under this heading.

Reserpine (Additive effect or potentiation of other antihypertensives).
No products indexed under this heading.

Rifampin (Rifampin decreased the concentrations of losartan and its active metabolite).
No products indexed under this heading.

Rocuronium Bromide (Possible increased responsiveness to the muscle relaxant). Products include:
Zemuron Injection ... 2363

Rofecoxib (Potential reduced diuretic, natriuretic, and antihypertensive effects).
No products indexed under this heading.

Rosiglitazone Maleate (Hyperglycemia may occur with thiazide diuretics; dosage adjustment of the antidiabetic drug may be required). Products include:
Avandamet Tablets ... 1343
Avandia Tablets ... 1348

Salt Substitutes (Concomitant use with salt substitutes may lead to hyperkalemia).
No products indexed under this heading.

Secobarbital Sodium (Potentiation of orthostatic hypotension).
No products indexed under this heading.

Sodium Nitroprusside (Additive effect or potentiation of other antihypertensives).
No products indexed under this heading.

Sotalol Hydrochloride (Additive effect or potentiation of other antihypertensives).
No products indexed under this heading.

Spirapril Hydrochloride (Additive effect or potentiation of other antihypertensives).
No products indexed under this heading.

Spironolactone (Concomitant use with potassium-sparing diuretics may lead to hyperkalemia).
No products indexed under this heading.

Sufentanil Citrate (Potentiation of orthostatic hypotension).
No products indexed under this heading.

Sulfaphenazole (In vitro studies show significant inhibition of the formation of the active metabolite by inhibitors of CYP4503A4, such as sulfaphenazole; pharmacodynamic consequences of concomitant use are undefined).
No products indexed under this heading.

Sulindac (Potential reduced diuretic, natriuretic, and antihypertensive effects). Products include:
Clinoril Tablets ... 1899

Telmisartan (Additive effect or potentiation of other antihypertensives). Products include:
Micardis Tablets ... 884
Micardis HCT Tablets ... 886

Terazosin Hydrochloride (Additive effect or potentiation of other antihypertensives). Products include:
Hytrin Capsules ... 469

Thiamylal Sodium (Potentiation of orthostatic hypotension).
No products indexed under this heading.

Timolol Maleate (Additive effect or potentiation of other antihypertensives). Products include:
Blocadren Tablets ... 1891
Cosopt Sterile Ophthalmic Solution ... 1910
Timolide Tablets ... 2056
Timoptic in Ocudose ... 2061
Timoptic Sterile Ophthalmic Solution ... 2058
Timoptic-XE Sterile Ophthalmic Gel Forming Solution ... 2062

Tolazamide (Hyperglycemia may occur with thiazide diuretics; dosage adjustment of the antidiabetic drug may be required).
No products indexed under this heading.

Tolbutamide (Hyperglycemia may occur with thiazide diuretics; dosage adjustment of the antidiabetic drug may be required).
No products indexed under this heading.

Tolmetin Sodium (Potential reduced diuretic, natriuretic, and antihypertensive effects).
No products indexed under this heading.

Torsemide (Additive effect or potentiation of other antihypertensives).
No products indexed under this heading.

Trandolapril (Additive effect or potentiation of other antihypertensives). Products include:
Mavik Tablets ... 482
Tarka Tablets ... 519

Triamcinolone (Potential for intensified electrolyte depletion, particularly hypokalemia).
No products indexed under this heading.

Triamcinolone Acetonide (Potential for intensified electrolyte depletion, particularly hypokalemia). Products include:
Azmacort Inhalation Aerosol ... 1701
Nasacort HFA Inhalation Aerosol ... 2939
Nasacort AQ Nasal Spray ... 2937

Triamcinolone Diacetate (Potential for intensified electrolyte depletion, particularly hypokalemia).
No products indexed under this heading.

Triamcinolone Hexacetonide (Potential for intensified electrolyte depletion, particularly hypokalemia).
No products indexed under this heading.

Triamterene (Concomitant use with potassium-sparing diuretics may lead to hyperkalemia). Products include:
Dyazide Capsules ... 1389
Dyrenium Capsules ... 3390
Maxzide ... 2150

Trimethaphan Camsylate (Additive effect or potentiation of other antihypertensives).
No products indexed under this heading.

Troglitazone (Hyperglycemia may occur with thiazide diuretics; dosage adjustment of the antidiabetic drug may be required).
No products indexed under this heading.

Troleandomycin (In vitro studies show significant inhibition of the formation of the active metabolite by inhibitors of CYP4503A4, such as troleandomycin; pharmacodynamic consequences of concomitant use are undefined).
No products indexed under this heading.

Valdecoxib (Potential reduced diuretic, natriuretic, and antihypertensive effects).
No products indexed under this heading.

Valsartan (Additive effect or potentiation of other antihypertensives). Products include:
Diovan HCT Tablets ... 2195
Diovan Tablets ... 2191

Vecuronium Bromide (Possible increased responsiveness to the muscle relaxant).
No products indexed under this heading.

Verapamil Hydrochloride (Additive effect or potentiation of other antihypertensives). Products include:
Covera-HS Tablets ... 3135
Tarka Tablets ... 519
Verelan PM Capsules ... 3120

Food Interactions

Alcohol (Potentiation of orthostatic hypotension).

Meal, unspecified (Meal slows absorption and decreases Cmax but has minor effects on losartan AUC or on the AUC of the metabolite).

HYZAAR 100-25 TABLETS

(Hydrochlorothiazide, Losartan Potassium) ... 1964
See Hyzaar 50-12.5 Tablets

IDAMYCIN PFS INJECTION

(Idarubicin Hydrochloride) ... 2645
May interact with anthracyclines. Compounds in these categories include:

Daunorubicin Citrate (Previous therapy with anthracyclines is co-factor for increased cardiac toxicity).
No products indexed under this heading.

Daunorubicin Hydrochloride (Previous therapy with anthracyclines is co-factor for increased cardiac toxicity). Products include:
Cerubidine for Injection ... 788

Doxorubicin Hydrochloride (Previous therapy with anthracyclines is co-factor for increased cardiac toxicity). Products include:
Adriamycin for Injection, USP ... 786
Adriamycin Injection, USP ... 786

Epirubicin Hydrochloride (Previous therapy with anthracyclines is co-factor for increased cardiac toxicity). Products include:
Ellence Injection ... 2632

Valrubicin (Previous therapy with anthracyclines is co-factor for increased cardiac toxicity).
No products indexed under this heading.

IMDUR TABLETS

(Isosorbide Mononitrate) ... 3032
May interact with calcium channel blockers, vasodilators, and certain other agents. Compounds in these categories include:

Amlodipine Besylate (Marked symptomatic orthostatic hypotension has been reported when calcium channel blockers and organic nitrates were used in combination). Products include:
Caduet Tablets ... 2507
Lotrel Capsules ... 2238
Norvasc Tablets ... 2529

Amyl Nitrite (Additive vasodilating effects).
No products indexed under this heading.

Bepridil Hydrochloride (Marked symptomatic orthostatic hypotension has been reported when calcium channel blockers and organic nitrates were used in combination).
No products indexed under this heading.

Diazoxide (Additive vasodilating effects). Products include:
Hyperstat I.V. Injection ... 3031

Diltiazem Hydrochloride (Marked symptomatic orthostatic hypotension has been reported when calcium channel blockers and organic nitrates were used in combination). Products include:
Cardizem LA Extended Release Tablets ... 1699
Tiazac Capsules ... 1204

Epoprostenol Sodium (Additive vasodilating effects). Products include:
Flolan for Injection ... 1408

Ethaverine Hydrochloride (Additive vasodilating effects).
No products indexed under this heading.

Felodipine (Marked symptomatic orthostatic hypotension has been reported when calcium channel blockers and organic nitrates were used in combination). Products include:
Plendil Extended-Release Tablets ... 651

Hydralazine Hydrochloride (Additive vasodilating effects). Products include:
BiDil Tablets ... 2161

Isosorbide Dinitrate (Additive vasodilating effects). Products include:
BiDil Tablets ... 2161

Isoxsuprine Hydrochloride (Additive vasodilating effects).
No products indexed under this heading.

Isradipine (Marked symptomatic orthostatic hypotension has been reported when calcium channel blockers and organic nitrates were used in combination). Products include:
DynaCirc CR Tablets ... 2726

Mibefradil Dihydrochloride (Marked symptomatic orthostatic hypotension has been reported when calcium channel blockers and organic nitrates were used in combination).
No products indexed under this heading.

Minoxidil (Additive vasodilating effects). Products include:
Men's Rogaine Extra Strength Topical Solution, Ocean Rush Scent and Original Unscented ... 706
Women's Rogaine Topical Solution, Spring Bloom Scent and Original Unscented ... 707

Nicardipine Hydrochloride (Marked symptomatic orthostatic hypotension has been reported when calcium channel blockers and organic nitrates were used in combination). Products include:
Cardene I.V. ... 1129

Nifedipine (Marked symptomatic orthostatic hypotension has been reported when calcium channel blockers and organic nitrates were used in combination). Products include:
Adalat CC Tablets ... 2978

Nimodipine (Marked symptomatic orthostatic hypotension has been reported when calcium channel blockers and organic nitrates were used in combination). Products include:
Nimotop Capsules ... 774

Nisoldipine (Marked symptomatic orthostatic hypotension has been reported when calcium channel blockers and organic nitrates were used in combination). Products include:
Sular Tablets ... 1163

Nitroglycerin (Additive vasodilating effects). Products include:
Nitro-Dur Transdermal Infusion System ... 3060
Nitrolingual Pumpspray ... 1161

Nitroglycerin, long-acting formulations (Additive vasodilating effects).
No products indexed under this heading.

Nitroglycerin Intravenous (Additive vasodilating effects).
No products indexed under this heading.

Papaverine (Additive vasodilating effects).
No products indexed under this heading.

Papaverine Hydrochloride (Additive vasodilating effects).
No products indexed under this heading.

Sildenafil Citrate (Amplification of the vasodilatory effects of Imdur by sildenafil can result in severe hypotension). Products include:
Revatio Tablets **2541**
Viagra Tablets **2552**

Tolazoline Hydrochloride (Additive vasodilating effects).
No products indexed under this heading.

Verapamil Hydrochloride (Marked symptomatic orthostatic hypotension has been reported when calcium channel blockers and organic nitrates were used in combination). Products include:
Covera-HS Tablets **3135**
Tarka Tablets **519**
Verelan PM Capsules **3120**

Food Interactions

Alcohol (Additive vasodilating effects).

Food, unspecified (May decrease the rate (increase in Tmax) but not the extent (AUC) of absorption).

IMITREX INJECTION

(Sumatriptan Succinate) **1431**
See Imitrex Tablets

IMITREX NASAL SPRAY

(Sumatriptan) **1435**
See Imitrex Tablets

IMITREX TABLETS

(Sumatriptan Succinate) **1440**
May interact with 5HT1-receptor agonists, ergot-containing drugs, nonselective MAO inhibitors, selective serotonin reuptake inhibitors, and certain other agents. Compounds in these categories include:

Citalopram Hydrobromide (Co-administration of sumatriptan with selective serotonin reuptake inhibitors (SSRIs) has resulted, rarely, in hyperreflexia, weakness, and incoordination). Products include:
Celexa **1177**

Dihydroergotamine Mesylate (Ergot-containing drugs have been reported to cause prolonged vasospastic reactions; because there is a theoretical basis that these effects may be additive, use of ergot-type agents and sumatriptan within 24 hours is contraindicated). Products include:
Migranal Nasal Spray **3350**

Ergonovine Maleate (Ergot-containing drugs have been reported to cause prolonged vasospastic reactions; because there is a theoretical basis that these effects may be additive, use of ergot-type agents and sumatriptan within 24 hours is contraindicated).
No products indexed under this heading.

Ergotamine Tartrate (Ergot-containing drugs have been reported to cause prolonged vasospastic reactions; because there is a theoretical basis that these effects may be additive, use of ergot-type agents and sumatriptan within 24 hours is contraindicated).
No products indexed under this heading.

Fluoxetine Hydrochloride (Co-administration of sumatriptan with selective serotonin reuptake inhibitors (SSRIs) has resulted, rarely, in hyperreflexia, weakness, and incoordination). Products include:
Prozac Pulvules and Liquid **1771**
Symbyax Capsules **1788**

Fluvoxamine Maleate (Co-administration of sumatriptan with selective serotonin reuptake inhibitors (SSRIs) has resulted, rarely, in hyperreflexia, weakness, and incoordination).
No products indexed under this heading.

Isocarboxazid (MAO-A inhibitors reduce sumatriptan clearance and significantly increasing systemic exposure; concurrent and/or sequential use is contraindicated).
No products indexed under this heading.

Methylergonovine Maleate (Ergot-containing drugs have been reported to cause prolonged vasospastic reactions; because there is a theoretical basis that these effects may be additive, use of ergot-type agents and sumatriptan within 24 hours is contraindicated).
No products indexed under this heading.

Methysergide Maleate (Ergot-containing drugs have been reported to cause prolonged vasospastic reactions; because there is a theoretical basis that these effects may be additive, use of ergot-type agents and sumatriptan within 24 hours is contraindicated).
No products indexed under this heading.

Naratriptan Hydrochloride (Co-administration with other 5-HT_1 agonists within 24 hours of each other is contraindicated because the vasospastic effects may be additive). Products include:
Amerge Tablets **1312**

Pargyline Hydrochloride (MAO-A inhibitors reduce sumatriptan clearance and significantly increasing systemic exposure; concurrent and/or sequential use is contraindicated).
No products indexed under this heading.

Paroxetine Hydrochloride (Co-administration of sumatriptan with selective serotonin reuptake inhibitors (SSRIs) has resulted, rarely, in hyperreflexia, weakness, and incoordination). Products include:
Paxil CR Controlled-Release Tablets **1509**
Paxil **1501**

Phenelzine Sulfate (MAO-A inhibitors reduce sumatriptan clearance and significantly increasing systemic exposure; concurrent and/or sequential use is contraindicated).
No products indexed under this heading.

Procarbazine Hydrochloride (MAO-A inhibitors reduce sumatriptan clearance and significantly increasing systemic exposure; concurrent and/or sequential use is contraindicated). Products include:
Matulane Capsules **3188**

Rizatriptan Benzoate (Co-administration with other 5-HT1 agonists within 24 hours of each other is contraindicated because the vasospastic effects may be additive). Products include:
Maxalt Tablets **1983**
Maxalt-MLT Orally Disintegrating Tablets **1983**

Sertraline Hydrochloride (Co-administration of sumatriptan with selective serotonin reuptake inhibitors (SSRIs) has resulted, rarely, in hyperreflexia, weakness, and incoordination). Products include:
Zoloft **2581**

Sumatriptan (Co-administration with other 5-HT_1 agonists within 24 hours of each other is contraindicated because the vasospastic effects may be additive). Products include:
Imitrex Nasal Spray **1435**

Tranylcypromine Sulfate (MAO-A inhibitors reduce sumatriptan clearance and significantly increasing systemic exposure; concurrent and/or sequential use is contraindicated). Products include:
Parnate Tablets **1499**

Zolmitriptan (Co-administration with other 5-HT_1 agonists within 24 hours of each other is contraindicated because the vasospastic effects may be additive). Products include:
Zomig Nasal Spray **718**
Zomig Tablets **714**
Zomig-ZMT Tablets **714**

Food Interactions

Food, unspecified (Delays the Tmax slightly by about 0.5 hour with no significant effect on the bioavailability).

IMMUNE[26] BALANCE POWDER SHAKE MIX

(Egg product, hyperimmune) .... ▣**768**
None cited in PDR database.

IMMUNE[26] COMPLETE SUPPORT POWDER SHAKE MIX

(Egg product, hyperimmune) .... ▣**768**
None cited in PDR database.

IMMUNE[26] POWDER, CAPSULES AND CHEWABLE TABLETS

(Egg product, hyperimmune) .... ▣**768**
None cited in PDR database.

IMMUNOCAL POWDER SACHETS

(Whey Protein Isolate) **1642**
None cited in PDR database.

IMODIUM CAPSULES

(Loperamide Hydrochloride) **1834**
None cited in PDR database.

IMODIUM A-D LIQUID AND CAPLETS

(Loperamide Hydrochloride) **1835**
None cited in PDR database.

IMODIUM ADVANCED CAPLETS AND CHEWABLE TABLETS

(Loperamide Hydrochloride, Simethicone) **1835**
None cited in PDR database.

INCRELEX INJECTION

(Mecasermin [rDNA origin]) **3290**
None cited in PDR database.

INDAPAMIDE TABLETS

(Indapamide) **2119**
May interact with antihypertensives, barbiturates, corticosteroids, cardiac glycosides, insulin, lithium preparations, narcotic analgesics, and certain other agents. Compounds in these categories include:

Acebutolol Hydrochloride (Indapamide may add to or potentiate the therapeutic effect of other antihypertensive drugs).
No products indexed under this heading.

ACTH (Co-administration with ACTH may increase the risk of hypokalemia).
No products indexed under this heading.

Alfentanil Hydrochloride (Aggravates orthostatic hypotension).
No products indexed under this heading.

Amlodipine Besylate (Indapamide may add to or potentiate the therapeutic effect of other antihypertensive drugs). Products include:
Caduet Tablets **2507**
Lotrel Capsules **2238**
Norvasc Tablets **2529**

Aprobarbital (Aggravates orthostatic hypotension).
No products indexed under this heading.

Atenolol (Indapamide may add to or potentiate the therapeutic effect of other antihypertensive drugs). Products include:
Tenormin I.V. Injection **698**
Tenormin Tablets **695**

Benazepril Hydrochloride (Indapamide may add to or potentiate the therapeutic effect of other antihypertensive drugs). Products include:
Lotensin Tablets **2232**
Lotensin HCT Tablets **2235**
Lotrel Capsules **2238**

Bendroflumethiazide (Indapamide may add to or potentiate the therapeutic effect of other antihypertensive drugs).
No products indexed under this heading.

Betamethasone Acetate (Co-administration with corticosteroids may increase the risk of hypokalemia).
No products indexed under this heading.

Betamethasone Sodium Phosphate (Co-administration with corticosteroids may increase the risk of hypokalemia).
No products indexed under this heading.

Betaxolol Hydrochloride (Indapamide may add to or potentiate the therapeutic effect of other antihypertensive drugs). Products include:
Betoptic S Ophthalmic Suspension........ **554**

Bisoprolol Fumarate (Indapamide may add to or potentiate the therapeutic effect of other antihypertensive drugs).
No products indexed under this heading.

Buprenorphine Hydrochloride (Aggravates orthostatic hypotension). Products include:
Buprenex Injectable **2718**
Suboxone Tablets **2719**

Subutex Tablets 2719

Butabarbital (Aggravates orthostatic hypotension).
No products indexed under this heading.

Butalbital (Aggravates orthostatic hypotension). Products include:
Sedapap Tablets 50 mg/650 mg 2098

Candesartan Cilexetil (Indapamide may add to or potentiate the therapeutic effect of other antihypertensive drugs). Products include:
Atacand Tablets 634
Atacand HCT 637

Captopril (Indapamide may add to or potentiate the therapeutic effect of other antihypertensive drugs). Products include:
Captopril Tablets 2114

Carteolol Hydrochloride (Indapamide may add to or potentiate the therapeutic effect of other antihypertensive drugs). Products include:
Carteolol Hydrochloride Ophthalmic Solution USP, 1%....... ⊙246

Chlorothiazide (Indapamide may add to or potentiate the therapeutic effect of other antihypertensive drugs). Products include:
Aldoclor Tablets 1881
Diuril Oral 1936

Chlorothiazide Sodium (Indapamide may add to or potentiate the therapeutic effect of other antihypertensive drugs). Products include:
Diuril Sodium Intravenous 1934

Chlorthalidone (Indapamide may add to or potentiate the therapeutic effect of other antihypertensive drugs). Products include:
Clorpres Tablets 2139

Clonidine (Indapamide may add to or potentiate the therapeutic effect of other antihypertensive drugs). Products include:
Catapres-TTS 875

Clonidine Hydrochloride (Indapamide may add to or potentiate the therapeutic effect of other antihypertensive drugs). Products include:
Catapres Tablets 874
Clorpres Tablets 2139

Codeine Phosphate (Aggravates orthostatic hypotension). Products include:
Tylenol with Codeine 2461

Cortisone Acetate (Co-administration with corticosteroids may increase the risk of hypokalemia).
No products indexed under this heading.

Deserpidine (Indapamide may add to or potentiate the therapeutic effect of other antihypertensive drugs).
No products indexed under this heading.

Deslanoside (Concurrent digitalis therapy may exaggerate metabolic effects of hypokalemia; especially myocardial effects such as increase ventricular irritability).
No products indexed under this heading.

Dexamethasone (Co-administration with corticosteroids may increase the risk of hypokalemia). Products include:
Ciprodex Otic Suspension 555
Decadron Tablets 1929
TobraDex Ophthalmic Ointment 558
TobraDex Ophthalmic Suspension ... 558

Dexamethasone Acetate (Co-administration with corticosteroids may increase the risk of hypokalemia).
No products indexed under this heading.

Dexamethasone Sodium Phosphate (Co-administration with corticosteroids may increase the risk of hypokalemia). Products include:
Decadron Phosphate Injection 1931

Dezocine (Aggravates orthostatic hypotension).
No products indexed under this heading.

Diazoxide (Indapamide may add to or potentiate the therapeutic effect of other antihypertensive drugs). Products include:
Hyperstat I.V. Injection 3031

Digitalis Glycoside Preparations (Concurrent digitalis therapy may exaggerate metabolic effects of hypokalemia; especially myocardial effects such as increase ventricular irritability).
No products indexed under this heading.

Digitoxin (Concurrent digitalis therapy may exaggerate metabolic effects of hypokalemia; especially myocardial effects such as increase ventricular irritability).
No products indexed under this heading.

Digoxin (Concurrent digitalis therapy may exaggerate metabolic effects of hypokalemia; especially myocardial effects such as increase ventricular irritability). Products include:
Digitek Tablets 2146
Lanoxicaps Capsules 1458
Lanoxin Injection 1462
Lanoxin Tablets 1468
Lanoxin Injection Pediatric 1465

Diltiazem Hydrochloride (Indapamide may add to or potentiate the therapeutic effect of other antihypertensive drugs). Products include:
Cardizem LA Extended Release Tablets 1699
Tiazac Capsules 1204

Doxazosin Mesylate (Indapamide may add to or potentiate the therapeutic effect of other antihypertensive drugs).
No products indexed under this heading.

Enalapril Maleate (Indapamide may add to or potentiate the therapeutic effect of other antihypertensive drugs). Products include:
Vaseretic Tablets 2073
Vasotec I.V. Injection 2076

Enalaprilat (Indapamide may add to or potentiate the therapeutic effect of other antihypertensive drugs).
No products indexed under this heading.

Eprosartan Mesylate (Indapamide may add to or potentiate the therapeutic effect of other antihypertensive drugs). Products include:
Teveten Tablets 1707
Teveten HCT Tablets 1710

Esmolol Hydrochloride (Indapamide may add to or potentiate the therapeutic effect of other antihypertensive drugs). Products include:
Brevibloc Concentrate 766
Brevibloc Injection 766
Brevibloc Double Strength Injection.. 766
Brevibloc Premixed Injection 766
Brevibloc Double Strength Premixed Injection 766

Felodipine (Indapamide may add to or potentiate the therapeutic effect of other antihypertensive drugs). Products include:
Plendil Extended-Release Tablets 651

Fentanyl (Aggravates orthostatic hypotension). Products include:
Duragesic Transdermal System 2448

Fentanyl Citrate (Aggravates orthostatic hypotension). Products include:
Actiq 993

Fludrocortisone Acetate (Co-administration with corticosteroids may increase the risk of hypokalemia).
No products indexed under this heading.

Fosinopril Sodium (Indapamide may add to or potentiate the therapeutic effect of other antihypertensive drugs).
No products indexed under this heading.

Furosemide (Indapamide may add to or potentiate the therapeutic effect of other antihypertensive drugs). Products include:
Furosemide Tablets 2117

Guanabenz Acetate (Indapamide may add to or potentiate the therapeutic effect of other antihypertensive drugs).
No products indexed under this heading.

Guanethidine Monosulfate (Indapamide may add to or potentiate the therapeutic effect of other antihypertensive drugs).
No products indexed under this heading.

Hydralazine Hydrochloride (Indapamide may add to or potentiate the therapeutic effect of other antihypertensive drugs). Products include:
BiDil Tablets 2161

Hydrochlorothiazide (Indapamide may add to or potentiate the therapeutic effect of other antihypertensive drugs). Products include:
Aldoril Tablets 1884
Atacand HCT 637
Avalide Tablets 2889
Avalide Tablets 922
Benicar HCT Tablets 2852
Diovan HCT Tablets 2195
Dyazide Capsules 1389
Hyzaar 1964
Lotensin HCT Tablets 2235
Maxzide 2150
Micardis HCT Tablets 886
Moduretic Tablets 2003
Prinzide Tablets 2033
Teveten HCT Tablets 1710
Timolide Tablets 2056
Uniretic Tablets 3114
Vaseretic Tablets 2073
Zestoretic Tablets 701

Hydrocodone Bitartrate (Aggravates orthostatic hypotension). Products include:
Hycodan 1104
Hycomine Compound Tablets 1105
Hycotuss Expectorant Syrup 1106
Lortab 3315
Lortab Elixir 3312
Vicodin Tablets 530
Vicodin ES Tablets 531
Vicodin HP Tablets 532
Vicoprofen Tablets 533
Zydone Tablets 1118

Hydrocodone Polistirex (Aggravates orthostatic hypotension). Products include:
Tussionex Pennkinetic Extended-Release Suspension 3322

Hydrocortisone (Co-administration with corticosteroids may increase the risk of hypokalemia). Products include:
Cortizone•5 Ointment .... ▣699
Cortizone•10 Creme .... ▣699
Cortizone•10 Ointment .... ▣699
Cortizone•10 Plus Creme .... ▣700
Cortizone•10 Maximum Strength Quick Shot Spray .... ▣700
Hydrocortone Tablets 1963
Preparation H Hydrocortisone Cream .... ▣748

Hydrocortisone Acetate (Co-administration with corticosteroids may increase the risk of hypokalemia). Products include:
Analpram-HC 1136
Pramosone 1139
ProctoFoam-HC 3113
Tucks Anti-Itch Ointment .... ▣712
U-cort 1% Cream 3289

Hydrocortisone Sodium Phosphate (Co-administration with corticosteroids may increase the risk of hypokalemia).
No products indexed under this heading.

Hydrocortisone Sodium Succinate (Co-administration with corticosteroids may increase the risk of hypokalemia).
No products indexed under this heading.

Hydroflumethiazide (Indapamide may add to or potentiate the therapeutic effect of other antihypertensive drugs).
No products indexed under this heading.

Hydromorphone Hydrochloride (Aggravates orthostatic hypotension). Products include:
Dilaudid 439
Dilaudid Oral Liquid 443
Dilaudid Non-Sterile Powder 439
Dilaudid Rectal Suppositories 439
Dilaudid Tablets 439
Dilaudid Tablets - 8 mg 443
Dilaudid-HP 441

Insulin, Human, Zinc Suspension (Hyperglycemia has been reported with the use of indapamide; co-administration may require adjustment in insulin dosage in diabetic patients). Products include:
Humulin L, 100 Units 1763
Humulin U, 100 Units 1770

Insulin, Human NPH (Hyperglycemia has been reported with the use of indapamide; co-administration may require adjustment in insulin dosage in diabetic patients). Products include:
Humulin N, 100 Units 1764
Humulin N Pen 1765
Novolin N Human Insulin 10 ml Vials 2322
Novolin N InnoLet 2322
Novolin N PenFill 3 ml Cartridges 2325
Novolin R InnoLet 2322

Insulin, Human Regular (Hyperglycemia has been reported with the use of indapamide; co-administration may require adjustment in insulin dosage in diabetic patients). Products include:
Humulin R (U-500) 1768
Humulin R, 100 Units 1767
Novolin R Human Insulin 10 ml Vials 2322
Novolin R PenFill 2325

Insulin, Human Regular and Human NPH Mixture (Hyperglycemia has been reported with the use of indapamide; co-administration may require adjustment in insulin dosage in diabetic patients). Products include:

Humulin 50/50, 100 Units 1760
Humulin 70/30 Pen 1761
Novolin 70/30 Human Insulin
10 ml Vials 2321
Novolin 70/30 InnoLet 2322
Novolin 70/30 PenFill 3 ml
Cartridges 2325

Insulin, NPH (Hyperglycemia has been reported with the use of indapamide; co-administration may require adjustment in insulin dosage in diabetic patients).
No products indexed under this heading.

Insulin, Regular (Hyperglycemia has been reported with the use of indapamide; co-administration may require adjustment in insulin dosage in diabetic patients).
No products indexed under this heading.

Insulin, Zinc Crystals (Hyperglycemia has been reported with the use of indapamide; co-administration may require adjustment in insulin dosage in diabetic patients).
No products indexed under this heading.

Insulin, Zinc Suspension (Hyperglycemia has been reported with the use of indapamide; co-administration may require adjustment in insulin dosage in diabetic patients).
No products indexed under this heading.

Insulin Aspart, Human Regular (Hyperglycemia has been reported with the use of indapamide; co-administration may require adjustment in insulin dosage in diabetic patients). Products include:
NovoLog Injection 2326

Insulin glargine (Hyperglycemia has been reported with the use of indapamide; co-administration may require adjustment in insulin dosage in diabetic patients). Products include:
Lantus Injection 2925

Insulin Lispro, Human (Hyperglycemia has been reported with the use of indapamide; co-administration may require adjustment in insulin dosage in diabetic patients). Products include:
Humalog-Pen 1751
Humalog Mix 75/25-Pen 1754

Insulin Lispro Protamine, Human (Hyperglycemia has been reported with the use of indapamide; co-administration may require adjustment in insulin dosage in diabetic patients). Products include:
Humalog Mix 75/25-Pen 1754

Irbesartan (Indapamide may add to or potentiate the therapeutic effect of other antihypertensive drugs). Products include:
Avalide Tablets 922
Avalide Tablets 2889
Avapro Tablets 925
Avapro Tablets 2886

Isradipine (Indapamide may add to or potentiate the therapeutic effect of other antihypertensive drugs). Products include:
DynaCirc CR Tablets 2726

Labetalol Hydrochloride (Indapamide may add to or potentiate the therapeutic effect of other antihypertensive drugs).
No products indexed under this heading.

Levorphanol Tartrate (Aggravates orthostatic hypotension).
No products indexed under this heading.

Lisinopril (Indapamide may add to or potentiate the therapeutic effect of other antihypertensive drugs). Products include:
Prinivil Tablets 2029
Prinzide Tablets 2033
Zestoretic Tablets 701
Zestril Tablets 704

Lithium (Diuretics reduce lithium's renal clearance and add a high risk of lithium toxicity).
No products indexed under this heading.

Lithium Carbonate (Diuretics reduce lithium's renal clearance and add a high risk of lithium toxicity). Products include:
Eskalith 1406
Lithobid Tablets 1670

Lithium Citrate (Diuretics reduce lithium's renal clearance and add a high risk of lithium toxicity).
No products indexed under this heading.

Losartan Potassium (Indapamide may add to or potentiate the therapeutic effect of other antihypertensive drugs). Products include:
Cozaar Tablets 1913
Hyzaar 1964

Mecamylamine Hydrochloride (Indapamide may add to or potentiate the therapeutic effect of other antihypertensive drugs). Products include:
Inversine Tablets 3286

Meperidine Hydrochloride (Aggravates orthostatic hypotension).
No products indexed under this heading.

Mephobarbital (Aggravates orthostatic hypotension). Products include:
Mebaral Tablets, USP 2483

Methadone Hydrochloride (Aggravates orthostatic hypotension).
No products indexed under this heading.

Methyclothiazide (Indapamide may add to or potentiate the therapeutic effect of other antihypertensive drugs).
No products indexed under this heading.

Methyldopa (Indapamide may add to or potentiate the therapeutic effect of other antihypertensive drugs). Products include:
Aldoclor Tablets 1881
Aldoril Tablets 1884

Methyldopate Hydrochloride (Indapamide may add to or potentiate the therapeutic effect of other antihypertensive drugs).
No products indexed under this heading.

Methylprednisolone Acetate (Co-administration with corticosteroids may increase the risk of hypokalemia). Products include:
Depo-Medrol Injectable
Suspension 2615
Depo-Medrol Single-Dose Vial 2617

Methylprednisolone Sodium Succinate (Co-administration with corticosteroids may increase the risk of hypokalemia).
No products indexed under this heading.

Metolazone (Indapamide may add to or potentiate the therapeutic effect of other antihypertensive drugs).
No products indexed under this heading.

Metoprolol Succinate (Indapamide may add to or potentiate the therapeutic effect of other antihypertensive drugs). Products include:
Toprol-XL Tablets 660

Metoprolol Tartrate (Indapamide may add to or potentiate the therapeutic effect of other antihypertensive drugs).
No products indexed under this heading.

Metyrosine (Indapamide may add to or potentiate the therapeutic effect of other antihypertensive drugs). Products include:
Demser Capsules 1933

Mibefradil Dihydrochloride (Indapamide may add to or potentiate the therapeutic effect of other antihypertensive drugs).
No products indexed under this heading.

Minoxidil (Indapamide may add to or potentiate the therapeutic effect of other antihypertensive drugs). Products include:
Men's Rogaine Extra Strength
Topical Solution, Ocean Rush
Scent and Original Unscented ..... ■ 706
Women's Rogaine Topical
Solution, Spring Bloom Scent
and Original Unscented .... ■ 707

Moexipril Hydrochloride (Indapamide may add to or potentiate the therapeutic effect of other antihypertensive drugs). Products include:
Uniretic Tablets 3114
Univasc Tablets 3118

Morphine Sulfate (Aggravates orthostatic hypotension). Products include:
Avinza Capsules 1714
Kadian Capsules 572
MS Contin Tablets 2703

Nadolol (Indapamide may add to or potentiate the therapeutic effect of other antihypertensive drugs). Products include:
Nadolol Tablets 2121

Nicardipine Hydrochloride (Indapamide may add to or potentiate the therapeutic effect of other antihypertensive drugs). Products include:
Cardene I.V. 1129

Nifedipine (Indapamide may add to or potentiate the therapeutic effect of other antihypertensive drugs). Products include:
Adalat CC Tablets 2978

Nisoldipine (Indapamide may add to or potentiate the therapeutic effect of other antihypertensive drugs). Products include:
Sular Tablets 1163

Nitroglycerin (Indapamide may add to or potentiate the therapeutic effect of other antihypertensive drugs). Products include:
Nitro-Dur Transdermal Infusion
System 3060
Nitrolingual Pumpspray 1161

Norepinephrine Bitartrate (Indapamide may decrease arterial responsiveness to norepinephrine).
No products indexed under this heading.

Oxycodone Hydrochloride (Aggravates orthostatic hypotension). Products include:
Combunox Tablets 1183
OxyContin Tablets 2699
OxyFast Oral Concentrate
Solution 2704
OxyIR Capsules 2704
Percocet Tablets 1114
Percodan Tablets 1115

Penbutolol Sulfate (Indapamide may add to or potentiate the therapeutic effect of other antihypertensive drugs).
No products indexed under this heading.

Pentobarbital Sodium (Aggravates orthostatic hypotension). Products include:
Nembutal Sodium Solution, USP 2484

Perindopril Erbumine (Indapamide may add to or potentiate the therapeutic effect of other antihypertensive drugs). Products include:
Aceon Tablets (2 mg, 4 mg,
8 mg) 3191

Phenobarbital (Aggravates orthostatic hypotension).
No products indexed under this heading.

Phenoxybenzamine Hydrochloride (Indapamide may add to or potentiate the therapeutic effect of other antihypertensive drugs). Products include:
Dibenzyline Capsules 3390

Phentolamine Mesylate (Indapamide may add to or potentiate the therapeutic effect of other antihypertensive drugs).
No products indexed under this heading.

Pindolol (Indapamide may add to or potentiate the therapeutic effect of other antihypertensive drugs).
No products indexed under this heading.

Polythiazide (Indapamide may add to or potentiate the therapeutic effect of other antihypertensive drugs).
No products indexed under this heading.

Prazosin Hydrochloride (Indapamide may add to or potentiate the therapeutic effect of other antihypertensive drugs).
No products indexed under this heading.

Prednisolone Acetate (Co-administration with corticosteroids may increase the risk of hypokalemia). Products include:
Blephamide Ophthalmic Ointment 563
Blephamide Ophthalmic
Suspension 564
Poly-Pred Liquifilm Ophthalmic
Suspension .... ⊙ 231
Pred Forte Ophthalmic
Suspension .... ⊙ 233
Pred Mild Sterile Ophthalmic
Suspension .... ⊙ 236
Pred-G Ophthalmic Suspension ...... ⊙ 234
Pred-G Sterile Ophthalmic
Ointment .... ⊙ 235

Prednisolone Sodium Phosphate (Co-administration with corticosteroids may increase the risk of hypokalemia). Products include:
Pediapred Oral Solution 3319

Prednisolone Tebutate (Co-administration with corticosteroids may increase the risk of hypokalemia).
No products indexed under this heading.

Prednisone (Co-administration with corticosteroids may increase the risk of hypokalemia).
No products indexed under this heading.

Propoxyphene Hydrochloride (Aggravates orthostatic hypotension).
No products indexed under this heading.

Propoxyphene Napsylate (Aggravates orthostatic hypotension). Products include:
Darvocet A 500 Tablets 3497

Propranolol Hydrochloride (Indapamide may add to or potentiate the therapeutic effect of other antihypertensive drugs). Products include:
Inderal LA Long-Acting Capsules 3421
InnoPran XL Capsules 2728

Quinapril Hydrochloride (Indapamide may add to or potentiate the therapeutic effect of other antihypertensive drugs).
No products indexed under this heading.

Ramipril (Indapamide may add to or potentiate the therapeutic effect of other antihypertensive drugs). Products include:
Altace Capsules 1673

Rauwolfia Serpentina (Indapamide may add to or potentiate the therapeutic effect of other antihypertensive drugs).
No products indexed under this heading.

Remifentanil Hydrochloride (Aggravates orthostatic hypotension).
No products indexed under this heading.

Rescinnamine (Indapamide may add to or potentiate the therapeutic effect of other antihypertensive drugs).
No products indexed under this heading.

Reserpine (Indapamide may add to or potentiate the therapeutic effect of other antihypertensive drugs).
No products indexed under this heading.

Secobarbital Sodium (Aggravates orthostatic hypotension).
No products indexed under this heading.

Sodium Nitroprusside (Indapamide may add to or potentiate the therapeutic effect of other antihypertensive drugs).
No products indexed under this heading.

Sotalol Hydrochloride (Indapamide may add to or potentiate the therapeutic effect of other antihypertensive drugs).
No products indexed under this heading.

Spirapril Hydrochloride (Indapamide may add to or potentiate the therapeutic effect of other antihypertensive drugs).
No products indexed under this heading.

Sufentanil Citrate (Aggravates orthostatic hypotension).
No products indexed under this heading.

Telmisartan (Indapamide may add to or potentiate the therapeutic effect of other antihypertensive drugs). Products include:
Micardis Tablets 884
Micardis HCT Tablets 886

Terazosin Hydrochloride (Indapamide may add to or potentiate the therapeutic effect of other antihypertensive drugs). Products include:
Hytrin Capsules 469

Thiamylal Sodium (Aggravates orthostatic hypotension).
No products indexed under this heading.

Timolol Maleate (Indapamide may add to or potentiate the therapeutic effect of other antihypertensive drugs). Products include:
Blocadren Tablets 1891
Cosopt Sterile Ophthalmic Solution 1910
Timolide Tablets 2056
Timoptic in Ocudose 2061
Timoptic Sterile Ophthalmic Solution 2058
Timoptic-XE Sterile Ophthalmic Gel Forming Solution 2062

Torsemide (Indapamide may add to or potentiate the therapeutic effect of other antihypertensive drugs).
No products indexed under this heading.

Trandolapril (Indapamide may add to or potentiate the therapeutic effect of other antihypertensive drugs). Products include:
Mavik Tablets 482
Tarka Tablets 519

Triamcinolone (Co-administration with corticosteroids may increase the risk of hypokalemia).
No products indexed under this heading.

Triamcinolone Acetonide (Co-administration with corticosteroids may increase the risk of hypokalemia). Products include:
Azmacort Inhalation Aerosol 1701
Nasacort HFA Inhalation Aerosol 2939
Nasacort AQ Nasal Spray 2937

Triamcinolone Diacetate (Co-administration with corticosteroids may increase the risk of hypokalemia).
No products indexed under this heading.

Triamcinolone Hexacetonide (Co-administration with corticosteroids may increase the risk of hypokalemia).
No products indexed under this heading.

Trimethaphan Camsylate (Indapamide may add to or potentiate the therapeutic effect of other antihypertensive drugs).
No products indexed under this heading.

Valsartan (Indapamide may add to or potentiate the therapeutic effect of other antihypertensive drugs). Products include:
Diovan HCT Tablets 2195
Diovan Tablets 2191

Verapamil Hydrochloride (Indapamide may add to or potentiate the therapeutic effect of other antihypertensive drugs). Products include:
Covera-HS Tablets 3135
Tarka Tablets 519
Verelan PM Capsules 3120

Food Interactions

Alcohol (Aggravates orthostatic hypotension).

INDERAL LA LONG-ACTING CAPSULES

(Propranolol Hydrochloride) 3421
May interact with beta-adrenergic stimulating agents, calcium channel blockers, oral hypoglycemic agents, insulin, non-steroidal anti-inflammatory agents, phenytoin, xanthines, and certain other agents. Compounds in these categories include:

Acarbose (Beta-adrenergic blockade may prevent the appearance of certain premonitory signs and symptoms of acute hypoglycemia in labile insulin-dependent diabetes). Products include:
Precose Tablets 776

Albuterol (Propranolol may block bronchodilation produced by exogenous catecholamine stimulation of beta receptors). Products include:
Proventil Inhalation Aerosol 3067

Albuterol Sulfate (Propranolol may block bronchodilation produced by exogenous catecholamine stimulation of beta receptors). Products include:
AccuNeb Inhalation Solution 1055
Combivent Inhalation Aerosol 878
DuoNeb Inhalation Solution 1058
Proventil Inhalation Solution 0.083%...................................... 3069
Proventil HFA Inhalation Aerosol 3071
Ventolin HFA Inhalation Aerosol 1576
VoSpire Extended-Release Tablets ... 2352

Aluminum Hydroxide (Greatly reduces intestinal absorption of propranolol). Products include:
Gaviscon Regular Strength Liquid .. 620
Gaviscon Regular Strength Tablets... 619
Gaviscon Extra Strength Liquid 620
Gaviscon Extra Strength Tablets 619
Maalox Max Maximum Strength Antacid/Anti-Gas Liquid................ 2165
Maalox Regular Strength Antacid/Antigas Liquid................. 2164

Aminophylline (Co-administration of theophylline with propranolol results in reduced theophylline clearance).
No products indexed under this heading.

Amlodipine Besylate (Both agents may depress myocardial contractility or AV conduction resulting in increased adverse reactions). Products include:
Caduet Tablets 2507
Lotrel Capsules 2238
Norvasc Tablets 2529

Antipyrine (Reduced clearance of antipyrine).
No products indexed under this heading.

Bepridil Hydrochloride (Both agents may depress myocardial contractility or AV conduction resulting in increased adverse reactions).
No products indexed under this heading.

Bitolterol Mesylate (Propranolol may block bronchodilation produced by exogenous catecholamine stimulation of beta receptors).
No products indexed under this heading.

Celecoxib (Blunts antihypertensive effect of beta-blocker). Products include:
Celebrex Capsules 3130

Chlorpromazine (Increased plasma levels of both drugs).
No products indexed under this heading.

Chlorpromazine Hydrochloride (Increased plasma levels of both drugs).
No products indexed under this heading.

Chlorpropamide (Beta-adrenergic blockade may prevent the appearance of certain premonitory signs and symptoms of acute hypoglycemia in labile insulin-dependent diabetes).
No products indexed under this heading.

Cimetidine (Decreases hepatic metabolism of propranolol resulting in increased blood levels). Products include:
Tagamet HB 200 Tablets 637
Tagamet Tablets 1547

Cimetidine Hydrochloride (Decreases hepatic metabolism of propranolol resulting in increased blood levels).
No products indexed under this heading.

Diclofenac Potassium (Blunts antihypertensive effect of beta-blocker). Products include:
Cataflam Tablets 2173

Diclofenac Sodium (Blunts antihypertensive effect of beta-blocker). Products include:
Arthrotec Tablets 3126
Voltaren Ophthalmic Solution 2300
Voltaren Tablets 2298
Voltaren-XR Tablets 2301

Diltiazem Hydrochloride (Both agents may depress myocardial contractility or AV conduction resulting in increased adverse reactions). Products include:
Cardizem LA Extended Release Tablets... 1699
Tiazac Capsules 1204

Dobutamine (Propranolol may block bronchodilation produced by exogenous catecholamine stimulation of beta receptors).
No products indexed under this heading.

Dobutamine Hydrochloride (Reversed effects of propranolol).
No products indexed under this heading.

Dyphylline (Co-administration of theophylline with propranolol results in reduced theophylline clearance).
No products indexed under this heading.

Ephedrine Hydrochloride (Propranolol may block bronchodilation produced by exogenous catecholamine stimulation of beta receptors). Products include:
Primatene Tablets 749

Ephedrine Sulfate (Propranolol may block bronchodilation produced by exogenous catecholamine stimulation of beta receptors).
No products indexed under this heading.

Ephedrine Tannate (Propranolol may block bronchodilation produced by exogenous catecholamine stimulation of beta receptors).
No products indexed under this heading.

Epinephrine (Potential for unresponsiveness to the usual dose of epinephrine to treat allergic reaction). Products include:
EpiPen 1061
Primatene Mist 749

Epinephrine Hydrochloride (Potential for unresponsiveness to the usual dose of epinephrine to treat allergic reaction).
No products indexed under this heading.

Etodolac (Blunts antihypertensive effect of beta-blocker).
No products indexed under this heading.

Felodipine (Both agents may depress myocardial contractility or AV conduction resulting in increased adverse reactions). Products include:
Plendil Extended-Release Tablets 651

Fenoprofen Calcium (Blunts antihypertensive effect of beta-blocker). Products include:
Nalfon Capsules 2504

IMPORTANT NOTE: Always consult each drug listing in the patient's regimen for possible interactions.

Flurbiprofen (Blunts antihypertensive effect of beta-blocker).
No products indexed under this heading.

Fosphenytoin Sodium (Accelerates propranolol clearance).
No products indexed under this heading.

Glimepiride (Beta-adrenergic blockade may prevent the appearance of certain premonitory signs and symptoms of acute hypoglycemia in labile insulin-dependent diabetes).
Products include:
Amaryl Tablets ... 2864

Glipizide (Beta-adrenergic blockade may prevent the appearance of certain premonitory signs and symptoms of acute hypoglycemia in labile insulin-dependent diabetes).
No products indexed under this heading.

Glyburide (Beta-adrenergic blockade may prevent the appearance of certain premonitory signs and symptoms of acute hypoglycemia in labile insulin-dependent diabetes).
No products indexed under this heading.

Haloperidol (Hypotension and cardiac arrest have been reported with the concomitant use of propranolol and haloperidol).
No products indexed under this heading.

Haloperidol Decanoate (Hypotension and cardiac arrest have been reported with the concomitant use of propranolol and haloperidol).
No products indexed under this heading.

Ibuprofen (Blunts antihypertensive effect of beta-blocker). Products include:
Advil Allergy Sinus Caplets ... ▣737
Advil ... ▣737
Children's Advil Suspension ... ▣742
Children's Advil Chewable Tablets ... ▣741
Advil Cold & Sinus ... ▣739
Advil Flu & Body Ache Caplets ... ▣739
Children's Advil Cold Suspension ... ▣741
Infants' Advil Concentrated Drops ... ▣743
Junior Strength Advil Swallow Tablets ... ▣740
Advil Migraine Liquigels ... ▣740
Advil Multi-Symptom Cold Caplets ... ▣738
Combunox Tablets ... 1183
Children's Motrin Oral Suspension and Chewable Tablets ... 1837
Children's Motrin Cold Non-Staining Dye-Free Oral Suspension ... 1838
Children's Motrin Cold Oral Suspension ... 1838
Children's Motrin Non-Staining Dye-Free Oral Suspension ... 1837
Motrin Cold & Sinus Caplets ... 1836
Motrin IB Tablets and Caplets ... 1836
Infants' Motrin Concentrated Drops ... 1837
Infants' Motrin Non-Staining Dye-Free Drops ... 1837
Junior Strength Motrin Caplets and Chewable Tablets ... 1837
Vicoprofen Tablets ... 533

Indomethacin (Blunts antihypertensive effect of beta-blocker). Products include:
Indocin ... 1968

Indomethacin Sodium Trihydrate (Blunts antihypertensive effect of beta-blocker). Products include:
Indocin I.V. ... 1973

Insulin, Human, Zinc Suspension (Beta-adrenergic blockade may prevent the appearance of certain premonitory signs and symptoms of acute hypoglycemia in labile insulin-dependent diabetes; acute increases in blood pressure occurred after insulin-induced hypoglycemia in patients on propranolol). Products include:
Humulin L, 100 Units ... 1763
Humulin U, 100 Units ... 1770

Insulin, Human NPH (Beta-adrenergic blockade may prevent the appearance of certain premonitory signs and symptoms of acute hypoglycemia in labile insulin-dependent diabetes; acute increases in blood pressure occurred after insulin-induced hypoglycemia in patients on propranolol). Products include:
Humulin N, 100 Units ... 1764
Humulin N Pen ... 1765
Novolin N Human Insulin 10 ml Vials ... 2322
Novolin N InnoLet ... 2322
Novolin N PenFill 3 ml Cartridges ... 2325
Novolin R InnoLet ... 2322

Insulin, Human Regular (Beta-adrenergic blockade may prevent the appearance of certain premonitory signs and symptoms of acute hypoglycemia in labile insulin-dependent diabetes; acute increases in blood pressure occurred after insulin-induced hypoglycemia in patients on propranolol). Products include:
Humulin R (U-500) ... 1768
Humulin R, 100 Units ... 1767
Novolin R Human Insulin 10 ml Vials ... 2322
Novolin R PenFill ... 2325

Insulin, Human Regular and Human NPH Mixture (Beta-adrenergic blockade may prevent the appearance of certain premonitory signs and symptoms of acute hypoglycemia in labile insulin-dependent diabetes; acute increases in blood pressure occurred after insulin-induced hypoglycemia in patients on propranolol). Products include:
Humulin 50/50, 100 Units ... 1760
Humulin 70/30 Pen ... 1761
Novolin 70/30 Human Insulin 10 ml Vials ... 2321
Novolin 70/30 InnoLet ... 2322
Novolin 70/30 PenFill 3 ml Cartridges ... 2325

Insulin, NPH (Beta-adrenergic blockade may prevent the appearance of certain premonitory signs and symptoms of acute hypoglycemia in labile insulin-dependent diabetes; acute increases in blood pressure occurred after insulin-induced hypoglycemia in patients on propranolol).
No products indexed under this heading.

Insulin, Regular (Beta-adrenergic blockade may prevent the appearance of certain premonitory signs and symptoms of acute hypoglycemia in labile insulin-dependent diabetes; acute increases in blood pressure occurred after insulin-induced hypoglycemia in patients on propranolol).
No products indexed under this heading.

Insulin, Zinc Crystals (Beta-adrenergic blockade may prevent the appearance of certain premonitory signs and symptoms of acute hypoglycemia in labile insulin-dependent diabetes; acute increases in blood pressure occurred after insulin-induced hypoglycemia in patients on propranolol).
No products indexed under this heading.

Insulin, Zinc Suspension (Beta-adrenergic blockade may prevent the appearance of certain premonitory signs and symptoms of acute hypoglycemia in labile insulin-dependent diabetes; acute increases in blood pressure occurred after insulin-induced hypoglycemia in patients on propranolol).
No products indexed under this heading.

Insulin Aspart, Human Regular (Beta-adrenergic blockade may prevent the appearance of certain premonitory signs and symptoms of acute hypoglycemia in labile insulin-dependent diabetes; acute increases in blood pressure occurred after insulin-induced hypoglycemia in patients on propranolol). Products include:
NovoLog Injection ... 2326

Insulin glargine (Beta-adrenergic blockade may prevent the appearance of certain premonitory signs and symptoms of acute hypoglycemia in labile insulin-dependent diabetes; acute increases in blood pressure occurred after insulin-induced hypoglycemia in patients on propranolol). Products include:
Lantus Injection ... 2925

Insulin Lispro, Human (Beta-adrenergic blockade may prevent the appearance of certain premonitory signs and symptoms of acute hypoglycemia in labile insulin-dependent diabetes; acute increases in blood pressure occurred after insulin-induced hypoglycemia in patients on propranolol). Products include:
Humalog-Pen ... 1751
Humalog Mix 75/25-Pen ... 1754

Insulin Lispro Protamine, Human (Beta-adrenergic blockade may prevent the appearance of certain premonitory signs and symptoms of acute hypoglycemia in labile insulin-dependent diabetes; acute increases in blood pressure occurred after insulin-induced hypoglycemia in patients on propranolol). Products include:
Humalog Mix 75/25-Pen ... 1754

Isoetharine (Propranolol may block bronchodilation produced by exogenous catecholamine stimulation of beta receptors).
No products indexed under this heading.

Isoproterenol Hydrochloride (Propranolol may block bronchodilation produced by exogenous catecholamine stimulation of beta receptors).
No products indexed under this heading.

Isoproterenol Sulfate (Propranolol may block bronchodilation produced by exogenous catecholamine stimulation of beta receptors).
No products indexed under this heading.

Isradipine (Both agents may depress myocardial contractility or AV conduction resulting in increased adverse reactions). Products include:
DynaCirc CR Tablets ... 2726

Ketoprofen (Blunts antihypertensive effect of beta-blocker).
No products indexed under this heading.

Ketorolac Tromethamine (Blunts antihypertensive effect of beta-blocker). Products include:
Acular Ophthalmic Solution ... 561
Acular LS Ophthalmic Solution ... 562

Levalbuterol Hydrochloride (Propranolol may block bronchodilation produced by exogenous catecholamine stimulation of beta receptors). Products include:
Xopenex Inhalation Solution ... 3143
Xopenex Inhalation Solution Concentrate ... 3147

Levothyroxine Sodium (Concurrent use may result in lower than expected T_3 concentration). Products include:
Levothroid Tablets ... 1189
Levoxyl Tablets ... 1680
Synthroid Tablets ... 515
Unithroid Tablets ... 3521

Lidocaine Hydrochloride (Reduced clearance of lidocaine).
No products indexed under this heading.

Meclofenamate Sodium (Blunts antihypertensive effect of beta-blocker).
No products indexed under this heading.

Mefenamic Acid (Blunts antihypertensive effect of beta-blocker).
No products indexed under this heading.

Meloxicam (Blunts antihypertensive effect of beta-blocker). Products include:
Mobic Oral Suspension ... 893
Mobic Tablets ... 893

Metaproterenol Sulfate (Propranolol may block bronchodilation produced by exogenous catecholamine stimulation of beta receptors). Products include:
Alupent Inhalation Aerosol ... 858

Metformin Hydrochloride (Beta-adrenergic blockade may prevent the appearance of certain premonitory signs and symptoms of acute hypoglycemia in labile insulin-dependent diabetes). Products include:
ActoPlus Met Tablets ... 3219
Avandamet Tablets ... 1343
Fortamet Extended-Release Tablets ... 1156

Mibefradil Dihydrochloride (Both agents may depress myocardial contractility or AV conduction resulting in increased adverse reactions).
No products indexed under this heading.

Miglitol (Beta-adrenergic blockade may prevent the appearance of certain premonitory signs and symptoms of acute hypoglycemia in labile insulin-dependent diabetes).
No products indexed under this heading.

Nabumetone (Blunts antihypertensive effect of beta-blocker). Products include:
Relafen Tablets ... 1523

Naproxen (Blunts antihypertensive effect of beta-blocker). Products include:
EC-Naprosyn Delayed-Release Tablets ... 2769
Naprosyn Suspension ... 2769
Naprosyn Tablets ... 2769
Prevacid NapraPAC ... 3277

Naproxen Sodium (Blunts antihypertensive effect of beta-blocker). Products include:
Aleve Tablets, Caplets and Gelcaps ... ▣605
Anaprox Tablets ... 2769
Anaprox DS Tablets ... 2769

Nicardipine Hydrochloride (Both agents may depress myocardial con-

tractility or AV conduction resulting in increased adverse reactions). Products include:
- Cardene I.V. 1129

Nifedipine (Both agents may depress myocardial contractility or AV conduction resulting in increased adverse reactions). Products include:
- Adalat CC Tablets 2978

Nimodipine (Both agents may depress myocardial contractility or AV conduction resulting in increased adverse reactions). Products include:
- Nimotop Capsules 774

Nisoldipine (Both agents may depress myocardial contractility or AV conduction resulting in increased adverse reactions). Products include:
- Sular Tablets 1163

Oxaprozin (Blunts antihypertensive effect of beta-blocker).
- No products indexed under this heading.

Phenobarbital (Accelerates propranolol clearance).
- No products indexed under this heading.

Phenylbutazone (Blunts antihypertensive effect of beta-blocker).
- No products indexed under this heading.

Phenytoin (Accelerates propranolol clearance).
- No products indexed under this heading.

Phenytoin Sodium (Accelerates propranolol clearance). Products include:
- Phenytek Capsules 2153

Pioglitazone Hydrochloride (Beta-adrenergic blockade may prevent the appearance of certain premonitory signs and symptoms of acute hypoglycemia in labile insulin-dependent diabetes). Products include:
- ActoPlus Met Tablets 3219
- Actos Tablets 3224

Pirbuterol Acetate (Propranolol may block bronchodilation produced by exogenous catecholamine stimulation of beta receptors). Products include:
- Maxair Autohaler 1820

Piroxicam (Blunts antihypertensive effect of beta-blocker).
- No products indexed under this heading.

Repaglinide (Beta-adrenergic blockade may prevent the appearance of certain premonitory signs and symptoms of acute hypoglycemia in labile insulin-dependent diabetes). Products include:
- Prandin Tablets (0.5, 1, and 2 mg) 2337

Reserpine (Co-administration of catecholamine-depleting drugs, such as reserpine, may produce an excessive reduction of resting sympathetic nervous activity, which may result in hypotension, vertigo, marked bradycardia, syncopal attacks or orthostatic hypotension).
- No products indexed under this heading.

Rifampin (Accelerates propranolol clearance).
- No products indexed under this heading.

Rofecoxib (Blunts antihypertensive effect of beta-blocker).
- No products indexed under this heading.

Rosiglitazone Maleate (Beta-adrenergic blockade may prevent the appearance of certain premonitory signs and symptoms of acute hypoglycemia in labile insulin-dependent diabetes). Products include:
- Avandamet Tablets 1343
- Avandia Tablets 1348

Salmeterol Xinafoate (Propranolol may block bronchodilation produced by exogenous catecholamine stimulation of beta receptors). Products include:
- Advair Diskus 100/50 1291
- Advair Diskus 250/50 1291
- Advair Diskus 500/50 1291
- Serevent Diskus 1540

Sulindac (Blunts antihypertensive effect of beta-blocker). Products include:
- Clinoril Tablets 1899

Terbutaline Sulfate (Propranolol may block bronchodilation produced by exogenous catecholamine stimulation of beta receptors).
- No products indexed under this heading.

Theophylline (Co-administration of theophylline with propranolol results in reduced theophylline clearance).
- No products indexed under this heading.

Theophylline Anhydrous (Co-administration of theophylline with propranolol results in reduced theophylline clearance). Products include:
- Uniphyl Tablets 2708

Theophylline Calcium Salicylate (Co-administration of theophylline with propranolol results in reduced theophylline clearance).
- No products indexed under this heading.

Theophylline Dihydroxypropyl (Glyceryl) (Co-administration of theophylline with propranolol results in reduced theophylline clearance).
- No products indexed under this heading.

Theophylline Ethylenediamine (Co-administration of theophylline with propranolol results in reduced theophylline clearance).
- No products indexed under this heading.

Theophylline Sodium Glycinate (Co-administration of theophylline with propranolol results in reduced theophylline clearance).
- No products indexed under this heading.

Tolazamide (Beta-adrenergic blockade may prevent the appearance of certain premonitory signs and symptoms of acute hypoglycemia in labile insulin-dependent diabetes).
- No products indexed under this heading.

Tolbutamide (Beta-adrenergic blockade may prevent the appearance of certain premonitory signs and symptoms of acute hypoglycemia in labile insulin-dependent diabetes).
- No products indexed under this heading.

Tolmetin Sodium (Blunts antihypertensive effect of beta-blocker).
- No products indexed under this heading.

Troglitazone (Beta-adrenergic blockade may prevent the appearance of certain premonitory signs and symptoms of acute hypoglycemia in labile insulin-dependent diabetes).
- No products indexed under this heading.

Valdecoxib (Blunts antihypertensive effect of beta-blocker).
- No products indexed under this heading.

Verapamil Hydrochloride (On rare occasion, co-administration of intravenous beta-blocker and verapamil, has resulted in serious adverse reactions, especially in patients with severe cardiomyopathy, congestive heart failure or recent myocardial infarction; calcium channel blockers and beta-blockers may depress myocardial contractility or AV conduction). Products include:
- Covera-HS Tablets 3135
- Tarka Tablets 519
- Verelan PM Capsules 3120

Food Interactions

Alcohol (Slows the rate of absorption of propranolol).

INDOCIN CAPSULES

(Indomethacin) 1968

May interact with ACE inhibitors, angiotensin-II receptor antagonists, beta blockers, anticoagulants, lithium preparations, loop diuretics, non-steroidal anti-inflammatory agents, potassium sparing diuretics, thiazides, and certain other agents. Compounds in these categories include:

Acebutolol Hydrochloride (Blunting of antihypertensive effect of beta blockers).
- No products indexed under this heading.

Amiloride Hydrochloride (Reduced diuretic, natriuretic and antihypertensive effects of increased serum potassium levels). Products include:
- Midamor Tablets 2000
- Moduretic Tablets 2003

Anisindione (Bleeding has been reported in patients on concomitant treatment with anticoagulants and indomethacin. Caution should be exercised when indomethacin and anticoagulants are administered concomitantly). Products include:
- Miradon Tablets 3056

Ardeparin Sodium (Bleeding has been reported in patients on concomitant treatment with anticoagulants and indomethacin. Caution should be exercised when indomethacin and anticoagulants are administered concomitantly).
- No products indexed under this heading.

Aspirin (When indomethacin is administered with aspirin, its protein binding is reduced, although the clearance of free indomethacin is not altered. The clinical significance of this interaction is not known; however, as with other NSAIDs, concomitant administration of indomethacin and aspirin is not generally recommended because of the potential of increased adverse effects). Products include:
- Aggrenox Capsules 855
- Bayer, Aspirin Regimen .... ▣606
- Bayer Aspirin Tablets 3515
- BC Powder .... ▣612
- BC Allergy Sinus Cold Powder .... ▣612
- Arthritis Strength BC Powder .... ▣612
- BC Sinus Cold Powder .... ▣612
- Ecotrin Enteric Coated Aspirin Low, Regular and Maximum Strength Tablets 1627
- Goody's Body Pain Formula Powder .... ▣621
- Goody's Extra Strength Headache Powder .... ▣621
- Goody's Extra Strength Pain Relief Tablets .... ▣621
- Percodan Tablets 1115
- St. Joseph 81 mg Aspirin Chewable and Enteric Coated Tablets 1841

Atenolol (Blunting of antihypertensive effect of beta blockers). Products include:
- Tenormin I.V. Injection 698
- Tenormin Tablets 695

Benazepril Hydrochloride (Reports suggest that NSAIDs may diminish the antihypertensive effect of ACE-inhibitors and angiotensin II antagonists. These interactions should be given consideration in patients taking NSAIDs concomitantly with ACE-inhibitors or angiotensin II antagonists. In some patients with compromised renal function, the co-administration of an NSAID and an ACE-inhibitor or an angiotensin II antagonist may result in further deterioration of renal funchtion, including possible acute renal failure, which is usually reversible). Products include:
- Lotensin Tablets 2232
- Lotensin HCT Tablets 2235
- Lotrel Capsules 2238

Bendroflumethiazide (Reduced diuretic, natriuretic, and antihypertensive effects of thiazide diuretics).
- No products indexed under this heading.

Betaxolol Hydrochloride (Blunting of antihypertensive effect of beta blockers). Products include:
- Betoptic S Ophthalmic Suspension 554

Bisoprolol Fumarate (Blunting of antihypertensive effect of beta blockers).
- No products indexed under this heading.

Bumetanide (Reduced diuretic, natriuretic, and antihypertensive effects of loop diuretics).
- No products indexed under this heading.

Candesartan Cilexetil (Reports suggest that NSAIDs may diminish the antihypertensive effect of ACE-inhibitors and angiotensin II antagonists. These interactions should be given consideration in patients taking NSAIDs concomitantly with ACE-inhibitors or angiotensin II antagonists. In some patients with compromised renal function, the co-administration of an NSAID and an ACE-inhibitor or an angiotensin II antagonist may result in further deterioration of renal funchtion, including possible acute renal failure, which is usually reversible). Products include:
- Atacand Tablets 634
- Atacand HCT 637

Captopril (Reduced antihypertensive effect of captopril). Products include:
- Captopril Tablets 2114

Carteolol Hydrochloride (Blunting of antihypertensive effect of beta blockers). Products include:
- Carteolol Hydrochloride Ophthalmic Solution USP, 1% .... ⊙246

Celecoxib (Concomitant use is not recommended due to the increased

possibility of gastrointestinal toxicity, with little or no increase in efficacy). Products include:
Celebrex Capsules 3130

Chlorothiazide (Reduced diuretic, natriuretic, and antihypertensive effects of thiazide diuretics). Products include:
Aldoclor Tablets 1881
Diuril Oral 1936

Chlorothiazide Sodium (Reduced diuretic, natriuretic, and antihypertensive effects of thiazide diuretics). Products include:
Diuril Sodium Intravenous 1934

Cyclosporine (Increase in cyclosporine-induced toxicity). Products include:
Gengraf Capsules 458
Neoral Soft Gelatin Capsules 2247
Neoral Oral Solution 2247
Restasis Ophthalmic Emulsion 570
Sandimmune 2259

Dalteparin Sodium (Bleeding has been reported in patients on concomitant treatment with anticoagulants and indomethacin. Caution should be exercised when indomethacin and anticoagulants are administered concomitantly). Products include:
Fragmin Injection 2638

Danaparoid Sodium (Bleeding has been reported in patients on concomitant treatment with anticoagulants and indomethacin. Caution should be exercised when indomethacin and anticoagulants are administered concomitantly).
No products indexed under this heading.

Dexamethasone (False-negative results in dexamethasone suppression test). Products include:
Ciprodex Otic Suspension 555
Decadron Tablets 1929
TobraDex Ophthalmic Ointment 558
TobraDex Ophthalmic Suspension 558

Dexamethasone Acetate (False-negative results in dexamethasone suppression test).
No products indexed under this heading.

Dexamethasone Sodium Phosphate (False-negative results in dexamethasone suppression test). Products include:
Decadron Phosphate Injection 1931

Diclofenac Potassium (Concomitant use is not recommended due to the increased possibility of gastrointestinal toxicity, with little or no increase in efficacy). Products include:
Cataflam Tablets 2173

Diclofenac Sodium (Concomitant use is not recommended due to the increased possibility of gastrointestinal toxicity, with little or no increase in efficacy). Products include:
Arthrotec Tablets 3126
Voltaren Ophthalmic Solution 2300
Voltaren Tablets 2298
Voltaren-XR Tablets 2301

Dicumarol (Bleeding has been reported in patients on concomitant treatment with anticoagulants and indomethacin. Caution should be exercised when indomethacin and anticoagulants are administered concomitantly).
No products indexed under this heading.

Diflunisal (Co-administration results in decreased renal clearance and significant increase in the plasma levels of indomethacin; in some patients combined therapy has been associated with fatal gastrointestinal hemorrhage; concurrent use is not recommended). Products include:
Dolobid Tablets 1937

Digoxin (Increased serum digoxin concentration and prolonged half-life). Products include:
Digitek Tablets 2146
Lanoxicaps Capsules 1458
Lanoxin Injection 1462
Lanoxin Tablets 1468
Lanoxin Injection Pediatric 1465

Enalapril Maleate (Reports suggest that NSAIDs may diminish the antihypertensive effect of ACE-inhibitors and angiotensin II antagonists. These interactions should be given consideration in patients taking NSAIDs concomitantly with ACE-inhibitors or angiotensin II antagonists. In some patients with compromised renal function, the co-administration of an NSAID and an ACE-inhibitor or an angiotensin II antagonist may result in further deterioration of renal funchtion, including possible acute renal failure, which is usually reversible). Products include:
Vaseretic Tablets 2073
Vasotec I.V. Injection 2076

Enalaprilat (Reports suggest that NSAIDs may diminish the antihypertensive effect of ACE-inhibitors and angiotensin II antagonists. These interactions should be given consideration in patients taking NSAIDs concomitantly with ACE-inhibitors or angiotensin II antagonists. In some patients with compromised renal function, the co-administration of an NSAID and an ACE-inhibitor or an angiotensin II antagonist may result in further deterioration of renal funchtion, including possible acute renal failure, which is usually reversible).
No products indexed under this heading.

Enoxaparin Sodium (Bleeding has been reported in patients on concomitant treatment with anticoagulants and indomethacin. Caution should be exercised when indomethacin and anticoagulants are administered concomitantly). Products include:
Lovenox Injection 2931

Eprosartan Mesylate (Reports suggest that NSAIDs may diminish the antihypertensive effect of ACE-inhibitors and angiotensin II antagonists. These interactions should be given consideration in patients taking NSAIDs concomitantly with ACE-inhibitors or angiotensin II antagonists. In some patients with compromised renal function, the co-administration of an NSAID and an ACE-inhibitor or an angiotensin II antagonist may result in further deterioration of renal funchtion, including possible acute renal failure, which is usually reversible). Products include:
Teveten Tablets 1707
Teveten HCT Tablets 1710

Esmolol Hydrochloride (Blunting of antihypertensive effect of beta blockers). Products include:
Brevibloc Concentrate 766
Brevibloc Injection 766
Brevibloc Double Strength Injection 766
Brevibloc Premixed Injection 766
Brevibloc Double Strength Premixed Injection 766

Ethacrynic Acid (Reduced diuretic, natriuretic, and antihypertensive effects of loop diuretics). Products include:
Edecrin Tablets 1941

Etodolac (Concomitant use is not recommended due to the increased possibility of gastrointestinal toxicity, with little or no increase in efficacy).
No products indexed under this heading.

Fenoprofen Calcium (Concomitant use is not recommended due to the increased possibility of gastrointestinal toxicity, with little or no increase in efficacy). Products include:
Nalfon Capsules 2504

Flurbiprofen (Concomitant use is not recommended due to the increased possibility of gastrointestinal toxicity, with little or no increase in efficacy).
No products indexed under this heading.

Fondaparinux Sodium (Bleeding has been reported in patients on concomitant treatment with anticoagulants and indomethacin. Caution should be exercised when indomethacin and anticoagulants are administered concomitantly). Products include:
Arixtra Injection 1325

Fosinopril Sodium (Reports suggest that NSAIDs may diminish the antihypertensive effect of ACE-inhibitors and angiotensin II antagonists. These interactions should be given consideration in patients taking NSAIDs concomitantly with ACE-inhibitors or angiotensin II antagonists. In some patients with compromised renal function, the co-administration of an NSAID and an ACE-inhibitor or an angiotensin II antagonist may result in further deterioration of renal funchtion, including possible acute renal failure, which is usually reversible).
No products indexed under this heading.

Furosemide (Indomethacin reduces basal plasma renin activity (PRA) induced by furosemide; reduced diuretic, natriuretic, and antihypertensive effects of loop diuretics). Products include:
Furosemide Tablets 2117

Heparin Calcium (Bleeding has been reported in patients on concomitant treatment with anticoagulants and indomethacin. Caution should be exercised when indomethacin and anticoagulants are administered concomitantly).
No products indexed under this heading.

Heparin Sodium (Bleeding has been reported in patients on concomitant treatment with anticoagulants and indomethacin. Caution should be exercised when indomethacin and anticoagulants are administered concomitantly).
No products indexed under this heading.

Hydrochlorothiazide (Reduced diuretic, natriuretic, and antihypertensive effects of thiazide diuretics). Products include:
Aldoril Tablets 1884
Atacand HCT 637
Avalide Tablets 2889
Avalide Tablets 922
Benicar HCT Tablets 2852
Diovan HCT Tablets 2195
Dyazide Capsules 1389
Hyzaar 1964
Lotensin HCT Tablets 2235
Maxzide 2150
Micardis HCT Tablets 886
Moduretic Tablets 2003
Prinzide Tablets 2033
Teveten HCT Tablets 1710
Timolide Tablets 2056
Uniretic Tablets 3114
Vaseretic Tablets 2073
Zestoretic Tablets 701

Hydroflumethiazide (Reduced diuretic, natriuretic, and antihypertensive effects of thiazide diuretics).
No products indexed under this heading.

Ibuprofen (Concomitant use is not recommended due to the increased possibility of gastrointestinal toxicity, with little or no increase in efficacy). Products include:
Advil Allergy Sinus Caplets .... ■737
Advil .... ■737
Children's Advil Suspension .... ■742
Children's Advil Chewable Tablets .... ■741
Advil Cold & Sinus .... ■739
Advil Flu & Body Ache Caplets .... ■739
Children's Advil Cold Suspension .... ■741
Infants' Advil Concentrated Drops .... ■743
Junior Strength Advil Swallow Tablets .... ■740
Advil Migraine Liquigels .... ■740
Advil Multi-Symptom Cold Caplets .... ■738
Combunox Tablets 1183
Children's Motrin Oral Suspension and Chewable Tablets 1837
Children's Motrin Cold Non-Staining Dye-Free Oral Suspension 1838
Children's Motrin Cold Oral Suspension 1838
Children's Motrin Non-Staining Dye-Free Oral Suspension 1837
Motrin Cold & Sinus Caplets 1836
Motrin IB Tablets and Caplets 1836
Infants' Motrin Concentrated Drops 1837
Infants' Motrin Non-Staining Dye-Free Drops 1837
Junior Strength Motrin Caplets and Chewable Tablets 1837
Vicoprofen Tablets 533

Indomethacin Sodium Trihydrate (Concomitant use is not recommended due to the increased possibility of gastrointestinal toxicity, with little or no increase in efficacy). Products include:
Indocin I.V. 1973

Irbesartan (Reports suggest that NSAIDs may diminish the antihypertensive effect of ACE-inhibitors and angiotensin II antagonists. These interactions should be given consideration in patients taking NSAIDs concomitantly with ACE-inhibitors or angiotensin II antagonists. In some patients with compromised renal function, the co-administration of an NSAID and an ACE-inhibitor or an angiotensin II antagonist may result in further deterioration of renal funchtion, including possible acute renal failure, which is usually reversible). Products include:
Avalide Tablets 922
Avalide Tablets 2889
Avapro Tablets 925
Avapro Tablets 2886

Ketoprofen (Concomitant use is not recommended due to the increased possibility of gastrointestinal toxicity, with little or no increase in efficacy).
No products indexed under this heading.

Ketorolac Tromethamine (Concomitant use is not recommended due to the increased possibility of

gastrointestinal toxicity, with little or no increase in efficacy). Products include:
Acular Ophthalmic Solution 561
Acular LS Ophthalmic Solution 562

Labetalol Hydrochloride (Blunting of antihypertensive effect of beta blockers).
No products indexed under this heading.

Levobunolol Hydrochloride (Blunting of antihypertensive effect of beta blockers). Products include:
Betagan Ophthalmic Solution, USP.. ⊙217

Lisinopril (Reports suggest that NSAIDs may diminish the antihypertensive effect of ACE-inhibitors and angiotensin II antagonists. These interactions should be given consideration in patients taking NSAIDs concomitantly with ACE-inhibitors or angiotensin II antagonists. In some patients with compromised renal function, the co-administration of an NSAID and an ACE-inhibitor or an angiotensin II antagonist may result in further deterioration of renal funchtion, including possible acute renal failure, which is usually reversible). Products include:
Prinivil Tablets 2029
Prinzide Tablets 2033
Zestoretic Tablets 701
Zestril Tablets 704

Lithium (Co-administration produces a clinically relevant elevation of plasma lithium and reduction in renal lithium clearance with a potential for lithium toxicity).
No products indexed under this heading.

Lithium Carbonate (Co-administration produces a clinically relevant elevation of plasma lithium and reduction in renal lithium clearance with a potential for lithium toxicity). Products include:
Eskalith 1406
Lithobid Tablets 1670

Lithium Citrate (Co-administration produces a clinically relevant elevation of plasma lithium and reduction in renal lithium clearance with a potential for lithium toxicity).
No products indexed under this heading.

Losartan Potassium (Reports suggest that NSAIDs may diminish the antihypertensive effect of ACE-inhibitors and angiotensin II antagonists. These interactions should be given consideration in patients taking NSAIDs concomitantly with ACE-inhibitors or angiotensin II antagonists. In some patients with compromised renal function, the co-administration of an NSAID and an ACE-inhibitor or an angiotensin II antagonist may result in further deterioration of renal funchtion, including possible acute renal failure, which is usually reversible). Products include:
Cozaar Tablets 1913
Hyzaar 1964

Low Molecular Weight Heparins (Bleeding has been reported in patients on concomitant treatment with anticoagulants and indomethacin. Caution should be exercised when indomethacin and anticoagulants are administered concomitantly).
No products indexed under this heading.

Meclofenamate Sodium (Concomitant use is not recommended due to the increased possibility of gastrointestinal toxicity, with little or no increase in efficacy).
No products indexed under this heading.

Mefenamic Acid (Concomitant use is not recommended due to the increased possibility of gastrointestinal toxicity, with little or no increase in efficacy).
No products indexed under this heading.

Meloxicam (Concomitant use is not recommended due to the increased possibility of gastrointestinal toxicity, with little or no increase in efficacy). Products include:
Mobic Oral Suspension 893
Mobic Tablets 893

Methotrexate Sodium (Potentiation of methotrexate toxicity).
No products indexed under this heading.

Methyclothiazide (Reduced diuretic, natriuretic, and antihypertensive effects of thiazide diuretics).
No products indexed under this heading.

Metipranolol Hydrochloride (Blunting of antihypertensive effect of beta blockers).
No products indexed under this heading.

Metoprolol Succinate (Blunting of antihypertensive effect of beta blockers). Products include:
Toprol-XL Tablets 660

Metoprolol Tartrate (Blunting of antihypertensive effect of beta blockers).
No products indexed under this heading.

Moexipril Hydrochloride (Reports suggest that NSAIDs may diminish the antihypertensive effect of ACE-inhibitors and angiotensin II antagonists. These interactions should be given consideration in patients taking NSAIDs concomitantly with ACE-inhibitors or angiotensin II antagonists. In some patients with compromised renal function, the co-administration of an NSAID and an ACE-inhibitor or an angiotensin II antagonist may result in further deterioration of renal funchtion, including possible acute renal failure, which is usually reversible). Products include:
Uniretic Tablets 3114
Univasc Tablets 3118

Nabumetone (Concomitant use is not recommended due to the increased possibility of gastrointestinal toxicity, with little or no increase in efficacy). Products include:
Relafen Tablets 1523

Nadolol (Blunting of antihypertensive effect of beta blockers). Products include:
Nadolol Tablets 2121

Naproxen (Concomitant use is not recommended due to the increased possibility of gastrointestinal toxicity, with little or no increase in efficacy). Products include:
EC-Naprosyn Delayed-Release Tablets 2769
Naprosyn Suspension 2769
Naprosyn Tablets 2769
Prevacid NapraPAC 3277

Naproxen Sodium (Concomitant use is not recommended due to the increased possibility of gastrointestinal toxicity, with little or no increase in efficacy). Products include:
Aleve Tablets, Caplets and Gelcaps 605
Anaprox Tablets 2769
Anaprox DS Tablets 2769

Nephrotoxic Drugs (Overt renal decompensation).
No products indexed under this heading.

Oxaprozin (Concomitant use is not recommended due to the increased possibility of gastrointestinal toxicity, with little or no increase in efficacy).
No products indexed under this heading.

Penbutolol Sulfate (Blunting of antihypertensive effect of beta blockers).
No products indexed under this heading.

Perindopril Erbumine (Reports suggest that NSAIDs may diminish the antihypertensive effect of ACE-inhibitors and angiotensin II antagonists. These interactions should be given consideration in patients taking NSAIDs concomitantly with ACE-inhibitors or angiotensin II antagonists. In some patients with compromised renal function, the co-administration of an NSAID and an ACE-inhibitor or an angiotensin II antagonist may result in further deterioration of renal funchtion, including possible acute renal failure, which is usually reversible). Products include:
Aceon Tablets (2 mg, 4 mg, 8 mg)... 3191

Phenylbutazone (Concomitant use is not recommended due to the increased possibility of gastrointestinal toxicity, with little or no increase in efficacy).
No products indexed under this heading.

Pindolol (Blunting of antihypertensive effect of beta blockers).
No products indexed under this heading.

Piroxicam (Concomitant use is not recommended due to the increased possibility of gastrointestinal toxicity, with little or no increase in efficacy).
No products indexed under this heading.

Polythiazide (Reduced diuretic, natriuretic, and antihypertensive effects of thiazide diuretics).
No products indexed under this heading.

Probenecid (Increased plasma levels of indomethacin).
No products indexed under this heading.

Propranolol Hydrochloride (Blunting of antihypertensive effect of beta blockers). Products include:
Inderal LA Long-Acting Capsules 3421
InnoPran XL Capsules 2728

Quinapril Hydrochloride (Reports suggest that NSAIDs may diminish the antihypertensive effect of ACE-inhibitors and angiotensin II antagonists. These interactions should be given consideration in patients taking NSAIDs concomitantly with ACE-inhibitors or angiotensin II antagonists. In some patients with compromised renal function, the co-administration of an NSAID and an ACE-inhibitor or an angiotensin II antagonist may result in further deterioration of renal funchtion, including possible acute renal failure, which is usually reversible).
No products indexed under this heading.

Ramipril (Reports suggest that NSAIDs may diminish the antihypertensive effect of ACE-inhibitors and angiotensin II antagonists. These interactions should be given consideration in patients taking NSAIDs concomitantly with ACE-inhibitors or angiotensin II antagonists. In some patients with compromised renal function, the co-administration of an NSAID and an ACE-inhibitor or an angiotensin II antagonist may result in further deterioration of renal funchtion, including possible acute renal failure, which is usually reversible). Products include:
Altace Capsules 1673

Rofecoxib (Concomitant use is not recommended due to the increased possibility of gastrointestinal toxicity, with little or no increase in efficacy).
No products indexed under this heading.

Sotalol Hydrochloride (Blunting of antihypertensive effect of beta blockers).
No products indexed under this heading.

Spirapril Hydrochloride (Reports suggest that NSAIDs may diminish the antihypertensive effect of ACE-inhibitors and angiotensin II antagonists. These interactions should be given consideration in patients taking NSAIDs concomitantly with ACE-inhibitors or angiotensin II antagonists. In some patients with compromised renal function, the co-administration of an NSAID and an ACE-inhibitor or an angiotensin II antagonist may result in further deterioration of renal funchtion, including possible acute renal failure, which is usually reversible).
No products indexed under this heading.

Spironolactone (Reduced diuretic, natriuretic and antihypertensive effects of increased serum potassium levels).
No products indexed under this heading.

Sulindac (Concomitant use is not recommended due to the increased possibility of gastrointestinal toxicity, with little or no increase in efficacy). Products include:
Clinoril Tablets 1899

Telmisartan (Reports suggest that NSAIDs may diminish the antihypertensive effect of ACE-inhibitors and angiotensin II antagonists. These interactions should be given consideration in patients taking NSAIDs concomitantly with ACE-inhibitors or angiotensin II antagonists. In some patients with compromised renal function, the co-administration of an NSAID and an ACE-inhibitor or an angiotensin II antagonist may result in further deterioration of renal funchtion, including possible acute renal failure, which is usually reversible). Products include:
Micardis Tablets 884
Micardis HCT Tablets 886

Timolol Hemihydrate (Blunting of antihypertensive effect of beta blockers). Products include:
Betimol Ophthalmic Solution 3371
Betimol Ophthalmic Solution .... ⊙283

Timolol Maleate (Blunting of antihypertensive effect of beta blockers). Products include:
Blocadren Tablets 1891
Cosopt Sterile Ophthalmic Solution.. 1910

Timolide Tablets 2056
Timoptic in Ocudose 2061
Timoptic Sterile Ophthalmic Solution 2058
Timoptic-XE Sterile Ophthalmic Gel Forming Solution 2062

Tinzaparin Sodium (Bleeding has been reported in patients on concomitant treatment with anticoagulants and indomethacin. Caution should be exercised when indomethacin and anticoagulants are administered concomitantly).
No products indexed under this heading.

Tolmetin Sodium (Concomitant use is not recommended due to the increased possibility of gastrointestinal toxicity, with little or no increase in efficacy).
No products indexed under this heading.

Torsemide (Reduced diuretic, natriuretic, and antihypertensive effects of loop diuretics).
No products indexed under this heading.

Trandolapril (Reports suggest that NSAIDs may diminish the antihypertensive effect of ACE-inhibitors and angiotensin II antagonists. These interactions should be given consideration in patients taking NSAIDs concomitantly with ACE-inhibitors or angiotensin II antagonists. In some patients with compromised renal function, the co-administration of an NSAID and an ACE-inhibitor or an angiotensin II antagonist may result in further deterioration of renal funchtion, including possible acute renal failure, which is usually reversible). Products include:
Mavik Tablets 482
Tarka Tablets 519

Triamterene (The addition of triamterene to maintenance schedule of indomethacin has resulted in reversible acute renal failure; potential for increased hyperkalemia; concurrent therapy should be avoided).
Products include:
Dyazide Capsules 1389
Dyrenium Capsules 3390
Maxzide 2150

Valdecoxib (Concomitant use is not recommended due to the increased possibility of gastrointestinal toxicity, with little or no increase in efficacy).
No products indexed under this heading.

Valsartan (Reports suggest that NSAIDs may diminish the antihypertensive effect of ACE-inhibitors and angiotensin II antagonists. These interactions should be given consideration in patients taking NSAIDs concomitantly with ACE-inhibitors or angiotensin II antagonists. In some patients with compromised renal function, the co-administration of an NSAID and an ACE-inhibitor or an angiotensin II antagonist may result in further deterioration of renal funchtion, including possible acute renal failure, which is usually reversible). Products include:
Diovan HCT Tablets 2195
Diovan Tablets 2191

Warfarin Sodium (Bleeding has been reported in patients on concomitant treatment with anticoagulants and indomethacin. Caution should be exercised when indomethacin and anticoagulants are administered concomitantly). Products include:
Coumadin for Injection 932
Coumadin Tablets 932

INDOCIN I.V.

(Indomethacin Sodium Trihydrate) 1973
May interact with cardiac glycosides and certain other agents. Compounds in these categories include:

Amikacin Sulfate (Serum levels of amikacin significantly elevated).
No products indexed under this heading.

Deslanoside (Half-life of digitalis may be prolonged when given concomitantly).
No products indexed under this heading.

Digitalis Glycoside Preparations (Half-life of digitalis may be prolonged when given concomitantly).
No products indexed under this heading.

Digitoxin (Half-life of digitalis may be prolonged when given concomitantly).
No products indexed under this heading.

Digoxin (Half-life of digitalis may be prolonged when given concomitantly). Products include:
Digitek Tablets 2146
Lanoxicaps Capsules 1458
Lanoxin Injection 1462
Lanoxin Tablets 1468
Lanoxin Injection Pediatric 1465

Furosemide (Blunted natriuretic effect of furosemide). Products include:
Furosemide Tablets 2117

Gentamicin Sulfate (Serum levels of gentamicin significantly elevated).
Products include:
Garamycin Injectable 3028
Genoptic Sterile Ophthalmic Solution .... ⊙227
Pred-G Ophthalmic Suspension ...... ⊙234
Pred-G Sterile Ophthalmic Ointment .... ⊙235

INDOCIN ORAL SUSPENSION

(Indomethacin) 1968
See Indocin Capsules

INDOCIN SUPPOSITORIES

(Indomethacin) 1968
See Indocin Capsules

INFANRIX VACCINE

(Diphtheria & Tetanus Toxoids and Acellular Pertussis Vaccine Adsorbed) 1444
May interact with alkylating agents, antimetabolites, corticosteroids, cytotoxic drugs, and immunosuppressive agents. Compounds in these categories include:

Azathioprine (Concurrent immunosuppressive therapy may reduce the immune response to vaccine).
Products include:
Azasan Tablets 2844

Basiliximab (Concurrent immunosuppressive therapy may reduce the immune response to vaccine).
Products include:
Simulect for Injection 2268

Betamethasone Acetate (Concurrent immunosuppressive therapy with greater than physiologic doses of corticosteroids may reduce the immune response to vaccine).
No products indexed under this heading.

Betamethasone Sodium Phosphate (Concurrent immunosuppressive therapy with greater than physiologic doses of corticosteroids may reduce the immune response to vaccine).
No products indexed under this heading.

Bleomycin Sulfate (Cytotoxic drugs may reduce the immune response to vaccine).
No products indexed under this heading.

Busulfan (Alkylating drugs may reduce the immune response to vaccine). Products include:
I.V. Busulfex 1125
Myleran Tablets 1492

Capecitabine (Immunosuppressive therapies may reduce the immune response to vaccines). Products include:
Xeloda Tablets 2825

Carmustine (BCNU) (Alkylating drugs may reduce the immune response to vaccine).
No products indexed under this heading.

Chlorambucil (Alkylating drugs may reduce the immune response to vaccine). Products include:
Leukeran Tablets 1472

Cladribine (Immunosuppressive therapies may reduce the immune response to vaccines). Products include:
Leustatin Injection 2368

Cortisone Acetate (Concurrent immunosuppressive therapy with greater than physiologic doses of corticosteroids may reduce the immune response to vaccine).
No products indexed under this heading.

Cyclophosphamide (Alkylating drugs may reduce the immune response to vaccine).
No products indexed under this heading.

Cyclosporine (Concurrent immunosuppressive therapy may reduce the immune response to vaccine).
Products include:
Gengraf Capsules 458
Neoral Soft Gelatin Capsules 2247
Neoral Oral Solution 2247
Restasis Ophthalmic Emulsion 570
Sandimmune 2259

Cytarabine (Immunosuppressive therapies may reduce the immune response to vaccines).
No products indexed under this heading.

Dacarbazine (Alkylating drugs may reduce the immune response to vaccine).
No products indexed under this heading.

Daunorubicin Hydrochloride (Cytotoxic drugs may reduce the immune response to vaccine).
Products include:
Cerubidine for Injection 788

Dexamethasone (Concurrent immunosuppressive therapy with greater than physiologic doses of corticosteroids may reduce the immune response to vaccine).
Products include:
Ciprodex Otic Suspension 555
Decadron Tablets 1929
TobraDex Ophthalmic Ointment 558
TobraDex Ophthalmic Suspension 558

Dexamethasone Acetate (Concurrent immunosuppressive therapy with greater than physiologic doses of corticosteroids may reduce the immune response to vaccine).
No products indexed under this heading.

Dexamethasone Sodium Phosphate (Concurrent immunosuppressive therapy with greater than physiologic doses of corticosteroids may reduce the immune response to vaccine). Products include:
Decadron Phosphate Injection 1931

Doxorubicin Hydrochloride (Cytotoxic drugs may reduce the immune response to vaccine). Products, include:
Adriamycin for Injection, USP 786
Adriamycin Injection, USP 786

Epirubicin Hydrochloride (Cytotoxic drugs may reduce the immune response to vaccine). Products include:
Ellence Injection 2632

Floxuridine (Immunosuppressive therapies may reduce the immune response to vaccines).
No products indexed under this heading.

Fludarabine Phosphate (Immunosuppressive therapies may reduce the immune response to vaccines).
No products indexed under this heading.

Fludrocortisone Acetate (Concurrent immunosuppressive therapy with greater than physiologic doses of corticosteroids may reduce the immune response to vaccine).
No products indexed under this heading.

Fluorouracil (Immunosuppressive therapies may reduce the immune response to vaccines). Products include:
Carac Cream, 0.5% 1048
Efudex 3348

Gemcitabine Hydrochloride (Immunosuppressive therapies may reduce the immune response to vaccines). Products include:
Gemzar for Injection 1743

Hydrocortisone (Concurrent immunosuppressive therapy with greater than physiologic doses of corticosteroids may reduce the immune response to vaccine). Products include:
Cortizone•5 Ointment .... ▣699
Cortizone•10 Creme .... ▣699
Cortizone•10 Ointment .... ▣699
Cortizone•10 Plus Creme .... ▣700
Cortizone•10 Maximum Strength Quick Shot Spray .... ▣700
Hydrocortone Tablets 1963
Preparation H Hydrocortisone Cream .... ▣748

Hydrocortisone Acetate (Concurrent immunosuppressive therapy with greater than physiologic doses of corticosteroids may reduce the immune response to vaccine).
Products include:
Analpram-HC 1136
Pramosone 1139
ProctoFoam-HC 3113
Tucks Anti-Itch Ointment .... ▣712
U-cort 1% Cream 3289

Hydrocortisone Sodium Phosphate (Concurrent immunosuppressive therapy with greater than physiologic doses of corticosteroids may reduce the immune response to vaccine).
No products indexed under this heading.

Hydrocortisone Sodium Succinate (Concurrent immunosuppressive therapy with greater than physiologic doses of corticosteroids may reduce the immune response to vaccine).
No products indexed under this heading.

Hydroxyurea (Cytotoxic drugs may reduce the immune response to vaccine).
No products indexed under this heading.

Lomustine (CCNU) (Alkylating drugs may reduce the immune response to vaccine).
No products indexed under this heading.

Mechlorethamine Hydrochloride (Alkylating drugs may reduce the immune response to vaccine).
Products include:
- Mustargen for Injection 2007

Melphalan (Alkylating drugs may reduce the immune response to vaccine). Products include:
- Alkeran Tablets 977

Mercaptopurine (Immunosuppressive therapies may reduce the immune response to vaccines).
Products include:
- Purinethol Tablets 1222

Methotrexate (Immunosuppressive therapies may reduce the immune response to vaccines).
No products indexed under this heading.

Methotrexate Sodium (Cytotoxic drugs may reduce the immune response to vaccine).
No products indexed under this heading.

Methylprednisolone Acetate (Concurrent immunosuppressive therapy with greater than physiologic doses of corticosteroids may reduce the immune response to vaccine).
Products include:
- Depo-Medrol Injectable Suspension 2615
- Depo-Medrol Single-Dose Vial 2617

Methylprednisolone Sodium Succinate (Concurrent immunosuppressive therapy with greater than physiologic doses of corticosteroids may reduce the immune response to vaccine).
No products indexed under this heading.

Mitotane (Cytotoxic drugs may reduce the immune response to vaccine).
No products indexed under this heading.

Mitoxantrone Hydrochloride (Cytotoxic drugs may reduce the immune response to vaccine).
Products include:
- Novantrone for Injection Concentrate 3158

Muromonab-CD3 (Concurrent immunosuppressive therapy may reduce the immune response to vaccine). Products include:
- Orthoclone OKT3 Sterile Solution 2370

Mycophenolate Mofetil (Concurrent immunosuppressive therapy may reduce the immune response to vaccine). Products include:
- CellCept Capsules 2751
- CellCept Oral Suspension 2751
- CellCept Tablets 2751

Pentostatin (Immunosuppressive therapies may reduce the immune response to vaccines). Products include:
- Nipent for Injection 3216

Prednisolone Acetate (Concurrent immunosuppressive therapy with greater than physiologic doses of corticosteroids may reduce the immune response to vaccine).
Products include:
- Blephamide Ophthalmic Ointment 563
- Blephamide Ophthalmic Suspension 564
- Poly-Pred Liquifilm Ophthalmic Suspension .... ⊙231
- Pred Forte Ophthalmic Suspension .... ⊙233
- Pred Mild Sterile Ophthalmic Suspension .... ⊙236
- Pred-G Ophthalmic Suspension .... ⊙234
- Pred-G Sterile Ophthalmic Ointment .... ⊙235

Prednisolone Sodium Phosphate (Concurrent immunosuppressive therapy with greater than physiologic doses of corticosteroids may reduce the immune response to vaccine).
Products include:
- Pediapred Oral Solution 3319

Prednisolone Tebutate (Concurrent immunosuppressive therapy with greater than physiologic doses of corticosteroids may reduce the immune response to vaccine).
No products indexed under this heading.

Prednisone (Concurrent immunosuppressive therapy with greater than physiologic doses of corticosteroids may reduce the immune response to vaccine).
No products indexed under this heading.

Procarbazine Hydrochloride (Cytotoxic drugs may reduce the immune response to vaccine).
Products include:
- Matulane Capsules 3188

Sirolimus (Concurrent immunosuppressive therapy may reduce the immune response to vaccine).
Products include:
- Rapamune Oral Solution and Tablets 3472

Tacrolimus (Concurrent immunosuppressive therapy may reduce the immune response to vaccine).
Products include:
- Prograf Capsules and Injection 624
- Protopic Ointment 629

Tamoxifen Citrate (Cytotoxic drugs may reduce the immune response to vaccine).
No products indexed under this heading.

Thioguanine (Immunosuppressive therapies may reduce the immune response to vaccines). Products include:
- Tabloid Tablets 1545

Thiotepa (Alkylating drugs may reduce the immune response to vaccine).
No products indexed under this heading.

Triamcinolone (Concurrent immunosuppressive therapy with greater than physiologic doses of corticosteroids may reduce the immune response to vaccine).
No products indexed under this heading.

Triamcinolone Acetonide (Concurrent immunosuppressive therapy with greater than physiologic doses of corticosteroids may reduce the immune response to vaccine).
Products include:
- Azmacort Inhalation Aerosol 1701
- Nasacort HFA Inhalation Aerosol 2939
- Nasacort AQ Nasal Spray 2937

Triamcinolone Diacetate (Concurrent immunosuppressive therapy with greater than physiologic doses of corticosteroids may reduce the immune response to vaccine).
No products indexed under this heading.

Triamcinolone Hexacetonide (Concurrent immunosuppressive therapy with greater than physiologic doses of corticosteroids may reduce the immune response to vaccine).
No products indexed under this heading.

Vincristine Sulfate (Cytotoxic drugs may reduce the immune response to vaccine).
No products indexed under this heading.

INFASURF INTRATRACHEAL SUSPENSION

(Calfactant) 1188
None cited in PDR database.

INFED INJECTION

(Iron Dextran) 3381
None cited in PDR database.

INFERGEN

(Interferon Alfacon-1) 1647
May interact with drugs which undergo biotransformation by cytochrome p-450 mixed function oxidase and certain other agents. Compounds in these categories include:

Acarbose (Concurrent use with agents known to be metabolized via cytochrome P450 pathway requires caution). Products include:
- Precose Tablets 776

Acetaminophen (Concurrent use with agents known to be metabolized via cytochrome P450 pathway requires caution). Products include:
- Benadryl Allergy & Cold Tablets .... ◘692
- Benadryl Allergy & Sinus Headache Caplets & Gelcaps .... ◘693
- Benadryl Maximum Strength Severe Allergy & Sinus Headache Caplets .... ◘694
- Contac Severe Cold and Flu Caplets Maximum Strength .... ◘615
- Contac Severe Cold and Flu Caplets Non-Drowsy .... ◘615
- Darvocet A 500 Tablets 3497
- Goody's Body Pain Formula Powder .... ◘621
- Goody's Extra Strength Headache Powder .... ◘621
- Goody's Extra Strength Pain Relief Tablets .... ◘621
- Goody's PM Powder .... ◘622
- Hycomine Compound Tablets 1105
- Lortab 3315
- Lortab Elixir 3312
- Percocet Tablets 1114
- Robitussin Cough, Cold & Flu Liquid-filled Capsules .... ◘750
- Robitussin Flu Liquid .... ◘752
- Sedapap Tablets 50 mg/650 mg 2098
- Singlet Caplets .... ◘636
- Sudafed Severe Cold .... ◘710
- Sudafed Sinus Headache .... ◘711
- TheraFlu Cold & Cough Hot Liquid .... ◘680
- TheraFlu Cold & Sore Throat Hot Liquid .... ◘680
- TheraFlu Flu & Chest Congestion Non-Drowsy Hot Liquid .... ◘681
- TheraFlu Flu & Sore Throat Hot Liquid .... ◘681
- TheraFlu Severe Cold Non-Drowsy Hot Liquid .... ◘683
- TheraFlu Severe Cold & Cough Hot Liquid .... ◘683
- TheraFlu Severe Cold Caplets .... ◘679
- TheraFlu Severe Cold Hot Liquid .... ◘682
- TheraFlu Severe Cold Non-Drowsy Caplets .... ◘679
- Triaminic Cough & Sore Throat Liquid .... ◘687
- Triaminic Flu, Cough & Fever Liquid .... ◘685
- Triaminic Cough & Sore Throat Softchews .... ◘689
- Tylenol 8 Hour Extended Release Geltabs and Caplets 1843
- Tylenol Sinus NightTime Caplets .... ◘663
- Children's Tylenol Suspension Liquid and Meltaways 1850
- Children's Tylenol Plus Cold & Allergy Suspension Liquid 1850
- Children's Tylenol Plus Cold NightTime Suspension Liquid 1851
- Children's Tylenol Plus Cold & Cough Suspension Liquid and Chewable Tablets 1851
- Children's Tylenol Plus Cold Chewable Tablets 1851
- Children's Tylenol Plus Cold Daytime Non-Drowsy Suspension Liquid 1851
- Children's Tylenol Plus Flu Suspension Liquid 1853
- Concentrated Tylenol Infants' Drops Plus Cold 1851
- Concentrated Tylenol Infants' Drops Plus Cold and Cough 1851
- Concentrated Tylenol Infants' Drops 1850
- Junior Tylenol Meltaways 1850
- Tylenol Cold & Flu Severe Daytime Liquid with Cool Bust 1846
- Tylenol Cold & Flu Severe NightTime Liquid with Cool Burst 1846
- Tylenol Cold Severe Congestion Non-Drowsy Caplets with Cool Burst 1846
- Tylenol Cough & Sore Throat Daytime Liquid with Cool Burst 1849
- Tylenol Cough & Sore Throat NightTime Liquid with Cool Burst 1849
- Tylenol 1843
- Extra Strength Tylenol Rapid Release Gels 1843
- Tylenol 1843
- Tylenol Allergy Complete Night Time Caplets 1844
- Tylenol Allergy Complete Multi-Symptom Caplets and Gelcaps with Cool Burst 1844
- Tylenol Severe Allergy Caplets 1844
- Tylenol Flu NightTime Gelcaps 1846
- Tylenol Flu Day Non-Drowsy Gelcaps 1846
- Concentrated Tylenol Infants' Drops Plus Cold Nasal Congestant, Fever Reducer & Pain Reliever .... ◘668
- Concentrated Tylenol Infants' Drops Plus Cold & Cough Nasal Decongestant, Fever Reducer & Pain Reliever .... ◘668
- Multi-Symptom Tylenol Cold Night Time Caplets 1845
- Multi-Symptom Tylenol Cold Day Non-Drowsy Caplets and Gelcaps 1845
- Extra Strength Tylenol PM Caplets, Geltabs, Gelcaps and Liquid 1847
- Tylenol Sinus Day Non-Drowsy 1848
- Tylenol Sinus Night Time Caplets 1848
- Tylenol Sinus Severe Congestion Caplets with Cool Burst 1848
- Tylenol Sore Throat Daytime Liquid with Cool Burst 1849
- Tylenol Sore Throat NightTime Liquid with Cool Burst 1849
- Tylenol with Codeine 2461
- Women's Tylenol Menstrual Relief Caplets 1849
- Ultracet Tablets 2462
- Vicks 44M Cough, Cold & Flu Relief 2676
- Vicks DayQuil LiquiCaps/Liquid Multi-Symptom Cold/Flu Relief .... ◘723
- Vicks DayQuil Multi-Symptom Cold/Flu Relief LiquiCaps 2675
- Vicks DayQuil Multi-Symptom Cold/Flu Relief Liquid 2675
- Vicks NyQuil LiquiCaps 2677

Vicks NyQuil LiquiCaps/Liquid Multi-Symptom Cold/Flu Relief ..... ■ 725
Vicks NyQuil Liquid 2677
Vicodin Tablets 530
Vicodin ES Tablets 531
Vicodin HP Tablets 532
Zydone Tablets 1118

Alatrofloxacin Mesylate (Concurrent use with agents known to be metabolized via cytochrome P450 pathway requires caution).
No products indexed under this heading.

Alfentanil Hydrochloride (Concurrent use with agents known to be metabolized via cytochrome P450 pathway requires caution).
No products indexed under this heading.

Alprazolam (Concurrent use with agents known to be metabolized via cytochrome P450 pathway requires caution). Products include:
Niravam Orally Disintegrating Tablets 3106
Xanax XR Tablets 2655

Aminophylline (Concurrent use with agents known to be metabolized via cytochrome P450 pathway requires caution).
No products indexed under this heading.

Amiodarone Hydrochloride (Concurrent use with agents known to be metabolized via cytochrome P450 pathway requires caution). Products include:
Pacerone Tablets 3337

Amitriptyline Hydrochloride (Concurrent use with agents known to be metabolized via cytochrome P450 pathway requires caution).
No products indexed under this heading.

Amlodipine Besylate (Concurrent use with agents known to be metabolized via cytochrome P450 pathway requires caution). Products include:
Caduet Tablets 2507
Lotrel Capsules 2238
Norvasc Tablets 2529

Amoxapine (Concurrent use with agents known to be metabolized via cytochrome P450 pathway requires caution).
No products indexed under this heading.

Amphetamine Aspartate (Concurrent use with agents known to be metabolized via cytochrome P450 pathway requires caution). Products include:
Adderall Tablets 3168
Adderall XR Capsules 3169

Amphetamine Aspartate Monohydrate (Concurrent use with agents known to be metabolized via cytochrome P450 pathway requires caution).
No products indexed under this heading.

Amphetamine Sulfate (Concurrent use with agents known to be metabolized via cytochrome P450 pathway requires caution). Products include:
Adderall Tablets 3168
Adderall XR Capsules 3169

Aprepitant (Concurrent use with agents known to be metabolized via cytochrome P450 pathway requires caution). Products include:
Emend Capsules 1944

Astemizole (Concurrent use with agents known to be metabolized via cytochrome P450 pathway requires caution).
No products indexed under this heading.

Atomoxetine Hydrochloride (Concurrent use with agents known to be metabolized via cytochrome P450 pathway requires caution). Products include:
Strattera Capsules 1784

Atorvastatin Calcium (Concurrent use with agents known to be metabolized via cytochrome P450 pathway requires caution). Products include:
Caduet Tablets 2507
Lipitor Tablets 2495

Belladonna Ergotamine (Concurrent use with agents known to be metabolized via cytochrome P450 pathway requires caution).
No products indexed under this heading.

Benzphetamine Hydrochloride (Concurrent use with agents known to be metabolized via cytochrome P450 pathway requires caution).
No products indexed under this heading.

Bisoprolol Fumarate (Concurrent use with agents known to be metabolized via cytochrome P450 pathway requires caution).
No products indexed under this heading.

Bone Marrow Depressants, unspecified (Concurrent use with agents known to cause myelosuppression requires caution).
No products indexed under this heading.

Buspirone Hydrochloride (Concurrent use with agents known to be metabolized via cytochrome P450 pathway requires caution).
No products indexed under this heading.

Busulfan (Concurrent use with agents known to be metabolized via cytochrome P450 pathway requires caution). Products include:
I.V. Busulfex 1125
Myleran Tablets 1492

Caffeine (Concurrent use with agents known to be metabolized via cytochrome P450 pathway requires caution). Products include:
Athena Hair System Shampoo ..... ■ 767
BC Powder ..... ■ 612
Arthritis Strength BC Powder ..... ■ 612
Goody's Extra Strength Headache Powder ..... ■ 621
Goody's Extra Strength Pain Relief Tablets ..... ■ 621
Hycomine Compound Tablets 1105
Spartan Hair System Shampoo ..... ■ 767
Vivarin ..... ■ 639

Caffeine Anhydrous (Concurrent use with agents known to be metabolized via cytochrome P450 pathway requires caution).
No products indexed under this heading.

Caffeine Citrate (Concurrent use with agents known to be metabolized via cytochrome P450 pathway requires caution). Products include:
Cafcit 1854

Candesartan Cilexetil (Concurrent use with agents known to be metabolized via cytochrome P450 pathway requires caution). Products include:
Atacand Tablets 634
Atacand HCT 637

Captopril (Concurrent use with agents known to be metabolized via cytochrome P450 pathway requires caution). Products include:
Captopril Tablets 2114

Carbamazepine (Concurrent use with agents known to be metabolized via cytochrome P450 pathway requires caution). Products include:
Carbatrol Capsules 3174
Equetro Extended-Release Capsules 3178
Tegretol/Tegretol-XR 2278

Carisoprodol (Concurrent use with agents known to be metabolized via cytochrome P450 pathway requires caution).
No products indexed under this heading.

Carvedilol (Concurrent use with agents known to be metabolized via cytochrome P450 pathway requires caution). Products include:
Coreg Tablets 1376

Celecoxib (Concurrent use with agents known to be metabolized via cytochrome P450 pathway requires caution). Products include:
Celebrex Capsules 3130

Cerivastatin Sodium (Concurrent use with agents known to be metabolized via cytochrome P450 pathway requires caution).
No products indexed under this heading.

Cevimeline Hydrochloride (Concurrent use with agents known to be metabolized via cytochrome P450 pathway requires caution). Products include:
Evoxac Capsules 1042

Chlordiazepoxide (Concurrent use with agents known to be metabolized via cytochrome P450 pathway requires caution).
No products indexed under this heading.

Chlordiazepoxide Hydrochloride (Concurrent use with agents known to be metabolized via cytochrome P450 pathway requires caution). Products include:
Librium Capsules 3349

Chlorpheniramine (Concurrent use with agents known to be metabolized via cytochrome P450 pathway requires caution).
No products indexed under this heading.

Chlorpheniramine Maleate (Concurrent use with agents known to be metabolized via cytochrome P450 pathway requires caution). Products include:
Advil Allergy Sinus Caplets ..... ■ 737
Advil Multi-Symptom Cold Caplets ..... ■ 738
BC Allergy Sinus Cold Powder ..... ■ 612
Contac Severe Cold and Flu Caplets Maximum Strength ..... ■ 615
Hycomine Compound Tablets 1105
PediaCare Multi-Symptom Cold Liquid ..... ■ 704
PediaCare NightRest Cough & Cold Liquid ..... ■ 704
Robitussin Flu Liquid ..... ■ 752
Robitussin PM Cough & Cold Liquid ..... ■ 752
Singlet Caplets ..... ■ 636
Sudafed Sinus & Allergy Tablets ..... ■ 710
TheraFlu Cold & Cough Hot Liquid ..... ■ 680
TheraFlu Cold & Sore Throat Hot Liquid ..... ■ 680
TheraFlu Flu & Sore Throat Hot Liquid ..... ■ 681
TheraFlu Severe Cold & Cough Hot Liquid ..... ■ 683
TheraFlu Severe Cold Caplets ..... ■ 679
TheraFlu Severe Cold Hot Liquid ..... ■ 682
Triaminic Cold & Allergy Liquid ..... ■ 685
Triaminic Cold & Cough Liquid ..... ■ 685
Triaminic Flu, Cough & Fever Liquid ..... ■ 685
Triaminic Night Time Cough & Cold Liquid ..... ■ 685
Triaminic Allergy Runny Nose & Congestion Softchews ..... ■ 688
Triaminic Cold & Cough Softchews ..... ■ 688
Children's Tylenol Plus Cold NightTime Suspension Liquid 1851
Children's Tylenol Plus Cold & Cough Suspension Liquid and Chewable Tablets 1851
Children's Tylenol Plus Cold Chewable Tablets 1851
Children's Tylenol Plus Flu Suspension Liquid 1853
Tylenol Allergy Complete Multi-Symptom Caplets and Gelcaps with Cool Burst 1844
Multi-Symptom Tylenol Cold Night Time Caplets 1845
Vicks 44M Cough, Cold & Flu Relief 2676
Pediatric Vicks 44m Cough & Cold Relief 2673
Children's Vicks NyQuil Cold/Cough Relief 2671

Chlorpheniramine Polistirex (Concurrent use with agents known to be metabolized via cytochrome P450 pathway requires caution). Products include:
Tussionex Pennkinetic Extended-Release Suspension 3322

Chlorpheniramine Tannate (Concurrent use with agents known to be metabolized via cytochrome P450 pathway requires caution).
No products indexed under this heading.

Chlorpromazine (Concurrent use with agents known to be metabolized via cytochrome P450 pathway requires caution).
No products indexed under this heading.

Chlorpromazine Hydrochloride (Concurrent use with agents known to be metabolized via cytochrome P450 pathway requires caution).
No products indexed under this heading.

Chlorpropamide (Concurrent use with agents known to be metabolized via cytochrome P450 pathway requires caution).
No products indexed under this heading.

Cilostazol (Concurrent use with agents known to be metabolized via cytochrome P450 pathway requires caution). Products include:
Pletal Tablets 2478

Cimetidine Hydrochloride (Concurrent use with agents known to be metabolized via cytochrome P450 pathway requires caution).
No products indexed under this heading.

Ciprofloxacin (Concurrent use with agents known to be metabolized via cytochrome P450 pathway requires caution). Products include:
Cipro I.V. 2998
Cipro I.V. Pharmacy Bulk Package 3509
Cipro Oral Suspension 2991
Cipro XR Tablets 3004
Ciprodex Otic Suspension 555

Ciprofloxacin Hydrochloride (Concurrent use with agents known to be metabolized via cytochrome P450 pathway requires caution). Products include:
Ciloxan Ophthalmic Ointment 554
Cipro Tablets 2991

Cisapride (Concurrent use with agents known to be metabolized via cytochrome P450 pathway requires caution).
No products indexed under this heading.

Citalopram Hydrobromide (Concurrent use with agents known to be metabolized via cytochrome P450 pathway requires caution). Products include:
Celexa ... 1177

Clarithromycin (Concurrent use with agents known to be metabolized via cytochrome P450 pathway requires caution). Products include:
Biaxin/Biaxin XL ... 402
PREVPAC ... 3281

Clomipramine Hydrochloride (Concurrent use with agents known to be metabolized via cytochrome P450 pathway requires caution).
No products indexed under this heading.

Clopidogrel Hydrogen Sulfate (Concurrent use with agents known to be metabolized via cytochrome P450 pathway requires caution).
No products indexed under this heading.

Clozapine (Concurrent use with agents known to be metabolized via cytochrome P450 pathway requires caution). Products include:
Clozapine Tablets ... 2141
Clozaril Tablets ... 2174
FazaClo Orally Disintegrating Tablets ... 547

Codeine Phosphate (Concurrent use with agents known to be metabolized via cytochrome P450 pathway requires caution). Products include:
Tylenol with Codeine ... 2461

Codeine Sulfate (Concurrent use with agents known to be metabolized via cytochrome P450 pathway requires caution).
No products indexed under this heading.

Cyclobenzaprine (Concurrent use with agents known to be metabolized via cytochrome P450 pathway requires caution).
No products indexed under this heading.

Cyclobenzaprine Hydrochloride (Concurrent use with agents known to be metabolized via cytochrome P450 pathway requires caution). Products include:
Flexeril Tablets ... 1832

Cyclophosphamide (Concurrent use with agents known to be metabolized via cytochrome P450 pathway requires caution).
No products indexed under this heading.

Cyclosporine (Concurrent use with agents known to be metabolized via cytochrome P450 pathway requires caution). Products include:
Gengraf Capsules ... 458
Neoral Soft Gelatin Capsules ... 2247
Neoral Oral Solution ... 2247
Restasis Ophthalmic Emulsion ... 570
Sandimmune ... 2259

Desipramine Hydrochloride (Concurrent use with agents known to be metabolized via cytochrome P450 pathway requires caution).
No products indexed under this heading.

Desogestrel (Concurrent use with agents known to be metabolized via cytochrome P450 pathway requires caution). Products include:
Ortho-Cept Tablets ... 2395

Dexamethasone (Concurrent use with agents known to be metabolized via cytochrome P450 pathway requires caution). Products include:
Ciprodex Otic Suspension ... 555
Decadron Tablets ... 1929
TobraDex Ophthalmic Ointment ... 558
TobraDex Ophthalmic Suspension ... 558

Dexamethasone Acetate (Concurrent use with agents known to be metabolized via cytochrome P450 pathway requires caution).
No products indexed under this heading.

Dexamethasone Phosphate (Concurrent use with agents known to be metabolized via cytochrome P450 pathway requires caution).
No products indexed under this heading.

Dexamethasone Sodium (Concurrent use with agents known to be metabolized via cytochrome P450 pathway requires caution).
No products indexed under this heading.

Dexamethasone Sodium Phosphate (Concurrent use with agents known to be metabolized via cytochrome P450 pathway requires caution). Products include:
Decadron Phosphate Injection ... 1931

Dexfenfluramine Hydrochloride (Concurrent use with agents known to be metabolized via cytochrome P450 pathway requires caution).
No products indexed under this heading.

Dextromethorphan (Concurrent use with agents known to be metabolized via cytochrome P450 pathway requires caution).
No products indexed under this heading.

Dextromethorphan Hydrobromide (Concurrent use with agents known to be metabolized via cytochrome P450 pathway requires caution). Products include:
Alacol DM Syrup ... 739
Balamine DM ... 739
Contac Severe Cold and Flu Caplets Maximum Strength ... 615
Contac Severe Cold and Flu Caplets Non-Drowsy ... 615
Children's Dimetapp DM Cold & Cough Elixir ... 745
Children's Dimetapp Long Acting Cough Plus Cold Syrup ... 746
Dimetapp Infant Drops Decongestant Plus Cough ... 746
Mucinex DM Tablets ... 602
PediaCare Decongestant & Cough Infant Drops ... 705
PediaCare Freezer Pops Long-Acting Cough-Glacier Grape and Polar Berry Blue ... 706
PediaCare Long-Acting Cough Infant Drops ... 705
PediaCare Long-Acting Cough Plus Cold Liquid ... 704
PediaCare Multi-Symptom Cold Liquid ... 704
PediaCare NightRest Cough & Cold Liquid ... 704
Robitussin Allergy & Cough Syrup ... 750
Robitussin CF Liquid ... 755
Robitussin Cough & Cold Liquid-filled Capsules ... 750
Robitussin Cough, Cold & Flu Liquid-filled Capsules ... 750
Robitussin Cough & Cold Infant Drops ... 755
Robitussin DM Infant Drops ... 753
Robitussin DM Liquid ... 753
Robitussin Flu Liquid ... 752
Robitussin Maximum Strength Cough Liquid ... 754
Robitussin Maximum Strength Cough & Cold Liquid ... 754
Robitussin Pediatric Cough Liquid ... 754
Robitussin Pediatric Cough & Cold Liquid ... 754
Robitussin PM Cough & Cold Liquid ... 752
Robitussin Sugar Free Cough Liquid ... 753
Simply Cough Liquid ... 1840
Sudafed Severe Cold ... 710
TheraFlu Cold & Cough Hot Liquid ... 680
TheraFlu Flu & Chest Congestion Non-Drowsy Hot Liquid ... 681
TheraFlu Severe Cold Non-Drowsy Hot Liquid ... 683
TheraFlu Severe Cold & Cough Hot Liquid ... 683
TheraFlu Severe Cold Caplets ... 679
TheraFlu Severe Cold Hot Liquid ... 682
TheraFlu Severe Cold Non-Drowsy Caplets ... 679
TheraFlu Thin Strips Long Acting Cough ... 684
Triaminic Cold & Cough Liquid ... 685
Triaminic Cough Liquid ... 687
Triaminic Cough & Nasal Congestion Liquid ... 687
Triaminic Cough & Sore Throat Liquid ... 687
Triaminic Flu, Cough & Fever Liquid ... 685
Triaminic Night Time Cough & Cold Liquid ... 685
Triaminic Cold & Cough Softchews ... 688
Triaminic Cough & Sore Throat Softchews ... 689
Triaminic Thin Strips Long Acting Cough ... 689
Children's Tylenol Plus Cold & Cough Suspension Liquid and Chewable Tablets ... 1851
Children's Tylenol Plus Flu Suspension Liquid ... 1853
Concentrated Tylenol Infants' Drops Plus Cold and Cough ... 1851
Tylenol Cold & Flu Severe Daytime Liquid with Cool Burst ... 1846
Tylenol Cold & Flu Severe NightTime Liquid with Cool Burst ... 1846
Tylenol Cold Severe Congestion Non-Drowsy Caplets with Cool Burst ... 1846
Tylenol Cough & Sore Throat Daytime Liquid with Cool Burst ... 1849
Tylenol Cough & Sore Throat NightTime Liquid with Cool Burst ... 1849
Tylenol Flu Day Non-Drowsy Gelcaps ... 1846
Concentrated Tylenol Infants' Drops Plus Cold & Cough Nasal Decongestant, Fever Reducer & Pain Reliever ... 668
Multi-Symptom Tylenol Cold Night Time Caplets ... 1845
Multi-Symptom Tylenol Cold Day Non-Drowsy Caplets and Gelcaps ... 1845
Vicks 44 Cough Relief ... 2675
Vicks 44D Cough & Head Congestion Relief ... 2676
Vicks 44D Cough & Head Congestion Relief Liquid ... 721
Vicks 44E Cough & Chest Congestion Relief ... 2676
Pediatric Vicks 44e Cough & Chest Congestion Relief Liquid ... 2673
Vicks 44M Cough, Cold & Flu Relief ... 2676
Pediatric Vicks 44m Cough & Cold Relief ... 2673
Vicks DayQuil LiquiCaps/Liquid Multi-Symptom Cold/Flu Relief ... 723
Vicks DayQuil Multi-Symptom Cold/Flu Relief LiquiCaps ... 2675
Vicks DayQuil Multi-Symptom Cold/Flu Relief Liquid ... 2675
Children's Vicks NyQuil Cold/Cough Relief ... 2671
Vicks NyQuil Cough Liquid ... 2677
Vicks NyQuil LiquiCaps ... 2677
Vicks NyQuil LiquiCaps/Liquid Multi-Symptom Cold/Flu Relief ... 725
Vicks NyQuil Liquid ... 2677
Zicam Concentrated Cough Mist for Kids Cool Cherry ... 643
Zicam Concentrated Cough Mist for Kids Plus D Cool Cherry ... 643
Zicam Concentrated Cough Mist Nite-Cool Cherry ... 642
Zicam Concentrated Cough Mist Plus D Cool Cherry ... 642
Zicam Concentrated Cough Mist-Honey Lemon & Cool Cherry ... 642

Dextromethorphan Polistirex (Concurrent use with agents known to be metabolized via cytochrome P450 pathway requires caution). Products include:
Delsym Extended-Release Suspension ... 611
Delsym 12 Hour Cough Suppressant for Children ... 611

Diazepam (Concurrent use with agents known to be metabolized via cytochrome P450 pathway requires caution). Products include:
Diastat Rectal Delivery System ... 3344
Valium Tablets ... 2822

Diclofenac Potassium (Concurrent use with agents known to be metabolized via cytochrome P450 pathway requires caution). Products include:
Cataflam Tablets ... 2173

Diclofenac Sodium (Concurrent use with agents known to be metabolized via cytochrome P450 pathway requires caution). Products include:
Arthrotec Tablets ... 3126
Voltaren Ophthalmic Solution ... 2300
Voltaren Tablets ... 2298
Voltaren-XR Tablets ... 2301

Dihydroergotamine Mesylate (Concurrent use with agents known to be metabolized via cytochrome P450 pathway requires caution). Products include:
Migranal Nasal Spray ... 3350

Diltiazem Hydrochloride (Concurrent use with agents known to be metabolized via cytochrome P450 pathway requires caution). Products include:
Cardizem LA Extended Release Tablets ... 1699
Tiazac Capsules ... 1204

Diltiazem Maleate (Concurrent use with agents known to be metabolized via cytochrome P450 pathway requires caution).
No products indexed under this heading.

Disopyramide (Concurrent use with agents known to be metabolized via cytochrome P450 pathway requires caution).
No products indexed under this heading.

Disopyramide Phosphate (Concurrent use with agents known to be metabolized via cytochrome P450 pathway requires caution).
No products indexed under this heading.

Divalproex Sodium (Concurrent use with agents known to be metabolized via cytochrome P450 pathway requires caution). Products include:
Depakote Sprinkle Capsules ... 422
Depakote Tablets ... 427
Depakote ER Tablets ... 433

Docetaxel (Concurrent use with agents known to be metabolized via cytochrome P450 pathway requires caution). Products include:
Taxotere Injection Concentrate ... 2947

Dolasetron Mesylate (Concurrent use with agents known to be metabolized via cytochrome P450 pathway requires caution). Products include:
Anzemet Injection ... 2871

Anzemet Tablets 2874

Donepezil Hydrochloride (Concurrent use with agents known to be metabolized via cytochrome P450 pathway requires caution). Products include:
Aricept Tablets 1086
Aricept ODT Tablets 1086

Doxepin Hydrochloride (Concurrent use with agents known to be metabolized via cytochrome P450 pathway requires caution).
No products indexed under this heading.

Doxorubicin Hydrochloride (Concurrent use with agents known to be metabolized via cytochrome P450 pathway requires caution). Products include:
Adriamycin for Injection, USP 786
Adriamycin Injection, USP 786

Dronabinol (Concurrent use with agents known to be metabolized via cytochrome P450 pathway requires caution). Products include:
Marinol Capsules 3334

Drugs that Undergo Biotransformation by Cytochrome P-450 Mixed Function Oxidase (Concurrent use with agents known to be metabolized via cytochrome P450 pathway requires caution).
No products indexed under this heading.

Dyphylline (Concurrent use with agents known to be metabolized via cytochrome P450 pathway requires caution).
No products indexed under this heading.

Encainide Hydrochloride (Concurrent use with agents known to be metabolized via cytochrome P450 pathway requires caution).
No products indexed under this heading.

Enoxacin (Concurrent use with agents known to be metabolized via cytochrome P450 pathway requires caution).
No products indexed under this heading.

Eprosartan Mesylate (Concurrent use with agents known to be metabolized via cytochrome P450 pathway requires caution). Products include:
Teveten Tablets 1707
Teveten HCT Tablets 1710

Ergotamine Tartrate (Concurrent use with agents known to be metabolized via cytochrome P450 pathway requires caution).
No products indexed under this heading.

Erythromycin (Concurrent use with agents known to be metabolized via cytochrome P450 pathway requires caution). Products include:
Erygel Topical Gel 2096
Ery-Tab Tablets 447
Erythromycin Base Filmtab Tablets 454
Erythromycin Delayed-Release Capsules, USP............................... 456
PCE Dispertab Tablets 510

Erythromycin Estolate (Concurrent use with agents known to be metabolized via cytochrome P450 pathway requires caution).
No products indexed under this heading.

Erythromycin Ethylsuccinate (Concurrent use with agents known to be metabolized via cytochrome P450 pathway requires caution). Products include:
E.E.S. 449
EryPed 445

Erythromycin Gluceptate (Concurrent use with agents known to be metabolized via cytochrome P450 pathway requires caution).
No products indexed under this heading.

Erythromycin Lactobionate (Concurrent use with agents known to be metabolized via cytochrome P450 pathway requires caution).
No products indexed under this heading.

Erythromycin Stearate (Concurrent use with agents known to be metabolized via cytochrome P450 pathway requires caution). Products include:
Erythrocin Stearate Filmtab Tablets 452

Esomeprazole Magnesium (Concurrent use with agents known to be metabolized via cytochrome P450 pathway requires caution). Products include:
Nexium Delayed-Release Capsules 645

Estradiol (Concurrent use with agents known to be metabolized via cytochrome P450 pathway requires caution). Products include:
Activella Tablets 2311
Climara Transdermal System 795
Climara Pro Transdermal System 800
CombiPatch Transdermal System 2180
Estrogel 0.06% 3200
Menostar Transdermal System 805
Prefest Tablets 1069
Vagifem Tablets 2340
Vivelle Transdermal System 2288
Vivelle-Dot Transdermal System 2293

Estradiol Benzoate (Concurrent use with agents known to be metabolized via cytochrome P450 pathway requires caution).
No products indexed under this heading.

Estradiol Cypionate (Concurrent use with agents known to be metabolized via cytochrome P450 pathway requires caution).
No products indexed under this heading.

Estradiol Valerate (Concurrent use with agents known to be metabolized via cytochrome P450 pathway requires caution).
No products indexed under this heading.

Estrogen (Concurrent use with agents known to be metabolized via cytochrome P450 pathway requires caution).
No products indexed under this heading.

Estrogens, Conjugated (Concurrent use with agents known to be metabolized via cytochrome P450 pathway requires caution). Products include:
Premarin Intravenous 3440
Premarin Tablets 3443
Premarin Vaginal Cream 3449
Premphase Tablets 3452
Prempro Tablets 3452

Estrogens, Conjugated, Synthetic A (Concurrent use with agents known to be metabolized via cytochrome P450 pathway requires caution). Products include:
Cenestin Tablets, 0.45mg, 0.625mg, 0.9mg, 1.25mg........... 1063
Cenestin Tablets, 0.3mg 1063

Estrogens, Esterified (Concurrent use with agents known to be metabolized via cytochrome P450 pathway requires caution). Products include:
Estratest Tablets 3196
Estratest H.S. Tablets 3196

Ethinyl Estradiol (Concurrent use with agents known to be metabolized via cytochrome P450 pathway requires caution). Products include:
Alesse-28 Tablets 3392
Lo/Ovral-28 Tablets 3423
NuvaRing 2357
Ortho-Cept Tablets 2395
Ortho-Cyclen/Ortho Tri-Cyclen 2414
Ortho Evra Transdermal System 2402
Ortho Tri-Cyclen Lo Tablets 2421
Seasonale Tablets 1073
Triphasil-28 Tablets 3483
Yasmin 28 Tablets 818

Ethosuximide (Concurrent use with agents known to be metabolized via cytochrome P450 pathway requires caution).
No products indexed under this heading.

Ethotoin (Concurrent use with agents known to be metabolized via cytochrome P450 pathway requires caution). Products include:
Peganone Tablets, USP 2487

Ethynodiol Diacetate (Concurrent use with agents known to be metabolized via cytochrome P450 pathway requires caution).
No products indexed under this heading.

Etodolac (Concurrent use with agents known to be metabolized via cytochrome P450 pathway requires caution).
No products indexed under this heading.

Etoposide (Concurrent use with agents known to be metabolized via cytochrome P450 pathway requires caution).
No products indexed under this heading.

Etoposide Phosphate (Concurrent use with agents known to be metabolized via cytochrome P450 pathway requires caution).
No products indexed under this heading.

Felbamate (Concurrent use with agents known to be metabolized via cytochrome P450 pathway requires caution).
No products indexed under this heading.

Felodipine (Concurrent use with agents known to be metabolized via cytochrome P450 pathway requires caution). Products include:
Plendil Extended-Release Tablets 651

Fenoprofen Calcium (Concurrent use with agents known to be metabolized via cytochrome P450 pathway requires caution). Products include:
Nalfon Capsules 2504

Fentanyl (Concurrent use with agents known to be metabolized via cytochrome P450 pathway requires caution). Products include:
Duragesic Transdermal System 2448

Fentanyl Citrate (Concurrent use with agents known to be metabolized via cytochrome P450 pathway requires caution). Products include:
Actiq 993

Flecainide Acetate (Concurrent use with agents known to be metabolized via cytochrome P450 pathway requires caution). Products include:
Tambocor Tablets 1824

Fluoxetine (Concurrent use with agents known to be metabolized via cytochrome P450 pathway requires caution).
No products indexed under this heading.

Fluoxetine Hydrochloride (Concurrent use with agents known to be metabolized via cytochrome P450 pathway requires caution). Products include:
Prozac Pulvules and Liquid 1771
Symbyax Capsules 1788

Fluphenazine Decanoate (Concurrent use with agents known to be metabolized via cytochrome P450 pathway requires caution).
No products indexed under this heading.

Fluphenazine Enanthate (Concurrent use with agents known to be metabolized via cytochrome P450 pathway requires caution).
No products indexed under this heading.

Fluphenazine Hydrochloride (Concurrent use with agents known to be metabolized via cytochrome P450 pathway requires caution).
No products indexed under this heading.

Flurbiprofen (Concurrent use with agents known to be metabolized via cytochrome P450 pathway requires caution).
No products indexed under this heading.

Flurbiprofen Sodium (Concurrent use with agents known to be metabolized via cytochrome P450 pathway requires caution). Products include:
Ocufen Ophthalmic Solution .... ⊙ 230

Flutamide (Concurrent use with agents known to be metabolized via cytochrome P450 pathway requires caution). Products include:
Eulexin Capsules 3023

Fluticasone Propionate (Concurrent use with agents known to be metabolized via cytochrome P450 pathway requires caution). Products include:
Advair Diskus 100/50 1291
Advair Diskus 250/50 1291
Advair Diskus 500/50 1291
Cutivate Cream 1381
Cutivate Lotion 0.05% 1383
Cutivate Ointment 1384
Flonase Nasal Spray 1412
Flovent Diskus 100 mcg 1418
Flovent Diskus 50 mcg 1415

Fluvastatin Sodium (Concurrent use with agents known to be metabolized via cytochrome P450 pathway requires caution). Products include:
Lescol Capsules 2227
Lescol 2730
Lescol XL Tablets 2227

Fluvoxamine Maleate (Concurrent use with agents known to be metabolized via cytochrome P450 pathway requires caution).
No products indexed under this heading.

Formoterol Fumarate (Concurrent use with agents known to be metabolized via cytochrome P450 pathway requires caution). Products include:
Foradil Aerolizer 3024

Fosphenytoin (Concurrent use with agents known to be metabolized via cytochrome P450 pathway requires caution).
No products indexed under this heading.

Fosphenytoin Sodium (Concurrent use with agents known to be metabolized via cytochrome P450 pathway requires caution).
No products indexed under this heading.

Gabapentin (Concurrent use with agents known to be metabolized via cytochrome P450 pathway requires caution). Products include:
Neurontin Capsules 2498
Neurontin Oral Solution 2498
Neurontin Tablets 2498

Galantamine Hydrobromide (Concurrent use with agents known to be metabolized via cytochrome P450 pathway requires caution). Products include:
Razadyne ER Extended-Release Capsules 2434
Razadyne 2434

Glimepiride (Concurrent use with agents known to be metabolized via cytochrome P450 pathway requires caution). Products include:
Amaryl Tablets 2864

Glipizide (Concurrent use with agents known to be metabolized via cytochrome P450 pathway requires caution).
No products indexed under this heading.

Glyburide (Concurrent use with agents known to be metabolized via cytochrome P450 pathway requires caution).
No products indexed under this heading.

Grepafloxacin Hydrochloride (Concurrent use with agents known to be metabolized via cytochrome P450 pathway requires caution).
No products indexed under this heading.

Haloperidol (Concurrent use with agents known to be metabolized via cytochrome P450 pathway requires caution).
No products indexed under this heading.

Haloperidol Decanoate (Concurrent use with agents known to be metabolized via cytochrome P450 pathway requires caution).
No products indexed under this heading.

Haloperidol Lactate (Concurrent use with agents known to be metabolized via cytochrome P450 pathway requires caution).
No products indexed under this heading.

Hydrocodone Bitartrate (Concurrent use with agents known to be metabolized via cytochrome P450 pathway requires caution). Products include:
Hycodan 1104
Hycomine Compound Tablets 1105
Hycotuss Expectorant Syrup 1106
Lortab 3315
Lortab Elixir 3312
Vicodin Tablets 530
Vicodin ES Tablets 531
Vicodin HP Tablets 532
Vicoprofen Tablets 533
Zydone Tablets 1118

Ibuprofen (Concurrent use with agents known to be metabolized via cytochrome P450 pathway requires caution). Products include:
Advil Allergy Sinus Caplets 737
Advil 737
Children's Advil Suspension 742
Children's Advil Chewable Tablets 741
Advil Cold & Sinus 739
Advil Flu & Body Ache Caplets 739
Children's Advil Cold Suspension 741
Infants' Advil Concentrated Drops 743
Junior Strength Advil Swallow Tablets 740
Advil Migraine Liquigels 740
Advil Multi-Symptom Cold Caplets 738
Combunox Tablets 1183
Children's Motrin Oral Suspension and Chewable Tablets 1837
Children's Motrin Cold Non-Staining Dye-Free Oral Suspension 1838
Children's Motrin Cold Oral Suspension 1838
Children's Motrin Non-Staining Dye-Free Oral Suspension 1837
Motrin Cold & Sinus Caplets 1836
Motrin IB Tablets and Caplets 1836
Infants' Motrin Concentrated Drops 1837
Infants' Motrin Non-Staining Dye-Free Drops 1837
Junior Strength Motrin Caplets and Chewable Tablets 1837
Vicoprofen Tablets 533

Imipramine Hydrochloride (Concurrent use with agents known to be metabolized via cytochrome P450 pathway requires caution).
No products indexed under this heading.

Imipramine Pamoate (Concurrent use with agents known to be metabolized via cytochrome P450 pathway requires caution).
No products indexed under this heading.

Indinavir Sulfate (Concurrent use with agents known to be metabolized via cytochrome P450 pathway requires caution). Products include:
Crixivan Capsules 1918

Indomethacin (Concurrent use with agents known to be metabolized via cytochrome P450 pathway requires caution). Products include:
Indocin 1968

Indomethacin Sodium Trihydrate (Concurrent use with agents known to be metabolized via cytochrome P450 pathway requires caution). Products include:
Indocin I.V. 1973

Indoramin Hydrochloride (Concurrent use with agents known to be metabolized via cytochrome P450 pathway requires caution).
No products indexed under this heading.

Irbesartan (Concurrent use with agents known to be metabolized via cytochrome P450 pathway requires caution). Products include:
Avalide Tablets 922
Avalide Tablets 2889
Avapro Tablets 925
Avapro Tablets 2886

Isotretinoin (Concurrent use with agents known to be metabolized via cytochrome P450 pathway requires caution). Products include:
Accutane Capsules 2740
Amnesteem Capsules 2126

Isradipine (Concurrent use with agents known to be metabolized via cytochrome P450 pathway requires caution). Products include:
DynaCirc CR Tablets 2726

Itraconazole (Concurrent use with agents known to be metabolized via cytochrome P450 pathway requires caution).
No products indexed under this heading.

Ketoconazole (Concurrent use with agents known to be metabolized via cytochrome P450 pathway requires caution). Products include:
Nizoral A-D Shampoo, 1% 1839
Nizoral 2% Shampoo 1838

Ketoprofen (Concurrent use with agents known to be metabolized via cytochrome P450 pathway requires caution).
No products indexed under this heading.

Ketorolac Tromethamine (Concurrent use with agents known to be metabolized via cytochrome P450 pathway requires caution). Products include:
Acular Ophthalmic Solution 561
Acular LS Ophthalmic Solution 562

Labetalol Hydrochloride (Concurrent use with agents known to be metabolized via cytochrome P450 pathway requires caution).
No products indexed under this heading.

Lamotrigine (Concurrent use with agents known to be metabolized via cytochrome P450 pathway requires caution). Products include:
Lamictal 1449

Lansoprazole (Concurrent use with agents known to be metabolized via cytochrome P450 pathway requires caution). Products include:
Prevacid Delayed-Release Capsules 3268
Prevacid for Delayed-Release Oral Suspension 3268
Prevacid I.V. for Injection 3274
Prevacid NapraPAC 3277
Prevacid SoluTab Delayed-Release Orally Disintegrating Tablets 3268
PREVPAC 3281

Levetiracetam (Concurrent use with agents known to be metabolized via cytochrome P450 pathway requires caution). Products include:
Keppra Oral Solution 3307
Keppra Tablets 3307

Levobupivacaine Hydrochloride (Concurrent use with agents known to be metabolized via cytochrome P450 pathway requires caution).
No products indexed under this heading.

Levonorgestrel (Concurrent use with agents known to be metabolized via cytochrome P450 pathway requires caution). Products include:
Alesse-28 Tablets 3392
Climara Pro Transdermal System 800
Mirena Intrauterine System 810
Plan B Tablets 1068
Seasonale Tablets 1073
Triphasil-28 Tablets 3483

Lidocaine (Concurrent use with agents known to be metabolized via cytochrome P450 pathway requires caution). Products include:
Lidoderm Patch 1107

Lidocaine Base (Concurrent use with agents known to be metabolized via cytochrome P450 pathway requires caution).
No products indexed under this heading.

Lidocaine Hydrochloride (Concurrent use with agents known to be metabolized via cytochrome P450 pathway requires caution).
No products indexed under this heading.

Lomefloxacin Hydrochloride (Concurrent use with agents known to be metabolized via cytochrome P450 pathway requires caution).
No products indexed under this heading.

Losartan Potassium (Concurrent use with agents known to be metabolized via cytochrome P450 pathway requires caution). Products include:
Cozaar Tablets 1913
Hyzaar 1964

Lovastatin (Concurrent use with agents known to be metabolized via cytochrome P450 pathway requires caution). Products include:
Advicor Tablets 1694
Altoprev Extended-Release Tablets 1151
Mevacor Tablets 1996

Maprotiline Hydrochloride (Concurrent use with agents known to be metabolized via cytochrome P450 pathway requires caution).
No products indexed under this heading.

Meclofenamate Sodium (Concurrent use with agents known to be metabolized via cytochrome P450 pathway requires caution).
No products indexed under this heading.

Mefenamic Acid (Concurrent use with agents known to be metabolized via cytochrome P450 pathway requires caution).
No products indexed under this heading.

Meloxicam (Concurrent use with agents known to be metabolized via cytochrome P450 pathway requires caution). Products include:
Mobic Oral Suspension 893
Mobic Tablets 893

Meperidine Hydrochloride (Concurrent use with agents known to be metabolized via cytochrome P450 pathway requires caution).
No products indexed under this heading.

Mephenytoin (Concurrent use with agents known to be metabolized via cytochrome P450 pathway requires caution).
No products indexed under this heading.

Mephobarbital (Concurrent use with agents known to be metabolized via cytochrome P450 pathway requires caution). Products include:
Mebaral Tablets, USP 2483

Meprobamate (Concurrent use with agents known to be metabolized via cytochrome P450 pathway requires caution).
No products indexed under this heading.

Mestranol (Concurrent use with agents known to be metabolized via cytochrome P450 pathway requires caution).
No products indexed under this heading.

Metformin Hydrochloride (Concurrent use with agents known to be metabolized via cytochrome P450 pathway requires caution). Products include:
ActoPlus Met Tablets 3219
Avandamet Tablets 1343
Fortamet Extended-Release Tablets 1156

Methadone Hydrochloride (Concurrent use with agents known to be metabolized via cytochrome P450 pathway requires caution).
No products indexed under this heading.

Methamphetamine Hydrochloride (Concurrent use with agents known to be metabolized via cytochrome P450 pathway requires caution). Products include:
Desoxyn Tablets, USP 2482

Methsuximide (Concurrent use with agents known to be metabolized via cytochrome P450 pathway requires caution).
No products indexed under this heading.

Metoprolol Succinate (Concurrent use with agents known to be metabolized via cytochrome P450 pathway requires caution). Products include:
Toprol-XL Tablets 660

Metoprolol Tartrate (Concurrent use with agents known to be metabolized via cytochrome P450 pathway requires caution).
No products indexed under this heading.

Mexiletine Hydrochloride (Concurrent use with agents known to be metabolized via cytochrome P450 pathway requires caution).
No products indexed under this heading.

Midazolam Hydrochloride (Concurrent use with agents known to be metabolized via cytochrome P450 pathway requires caution).
No products indexed under this heading.

Miglitol (Concurrent use with agents known to be metabolized via cytochrome P450 pathway requires caution).
No products indexed under this heading.

Mirtazapine (Concurrent use with agents known to be metabolized via cytochrome P450 pathway requires caution).
No products indexed under this heading.

Montelukast Sodium (Concurrent use with agents known to be metabolized via cytochrome P450 pathway requires caution). Products include:
Singulair 2047

Morphine Sulfate (Concurrent use with agents known to be metabolized via cytochrome P450 pathway requires caution). Products include:
Avinza Capsules 1714
Kadian Capsules 572
MS Contin Tablets 2703

Moxifloxacin Hydrochloride (Concurrent use with agents known to be metabolized via cytochrome P450 pathway requires caution). Products include:
Avelox 2984
Vigamox Ophthalmic Solution 560

Nabumetone (Concurrent use with agents known to be metabolized via cytochrome P450 pathway requires caution). Products include:
Relafen Tablets 1523

Nafcillin Sodium (Concurrent use with agents known to be metabolized via cytochrome P450 pathway requires caution).
No products indexed under this heading.

Naproxen (Concurrent use with agents known to be metabolized via cytochrome P450 pathway requires caution). Products include:
EC-Naprosyn Delayed-Release Tablets 2769
Naprosyn Suspension 2769
Naprosyn Tablets 2769
Prevacid NapraPAC 3277

Naproxen Sodium (Concurrent use with agents known to be metabolized via cytochrome P450 pathway requires caution). Products include:
Aleve Tablets, Caplets and Gelcaps .... ▣ 605
Anaprox Tablets 2769
Anaprox DS Tablets 2769

Nateglinide (Concurrent use with agents known to be metabolized via cytochrome P450 pathway requires caution). Products include:
Starlix Tablets 2276

Nefazodone Hydrochloride (Concurrent use with agents known to be metabolized via cytochrome P450 pathway requires caution).
No products indexed under this heading.

Nelfinavir Mesylate (Concurrent use with agents known to be metabolized via cytochrome P450 pathway requires caution). Products include:
Viracept 2556

Nicardipine (Concurrent use with agents known to be metabolized via cytochrome P450 pathway requires caution).
No products indexed under this heading.

Nicardipine Hydrochloride (Concurrent use with agents known to be metabolized via cytochrome P450 pathway requires caution). Products include:
Cardene I.V. 1129

Nicotine Polacrilex (Concurrent use with agents known to be metabolized via cytochrome P450 pathway requires caution). Products include:
Commit Lozenges 1625
Nicorette Gum 1632

Nicotine Salicylate (Concurrent use with agents known to be metabolized via cytochrome P450 pathway requires caution).
No products indexed under this heading.

Nicotine Sulfate (Concurrent use with agents known to be metabolized via cytochrome P450 pathway requires caution).
No products indexed under this heading.

Nifedipine (Concurrent use with agents known to be metabolized via cytochrome P450 pathway requires caution). Products include:
Adalat CC Tablets 2978

Nilutamide (Concurrent use with agents known to be metabolized via cytochrome P450 pathway requires caution).
No products indexed under this heading.

Nimodipine (Concurrent use with agents known to be metabolized via cytochrome P450 pathway requires caution). Products include:
Nimotop Capsules 774

Nisoldipine (Concurrent use with agents known to be metabolized via cytochrome P450 pathway requires caution). Products include:
Sular Tablets 1163

Nitrendipine (Concurrent use with agents known to be metabolized via cytochrome P450 pathway requires caution).
No products indexed under this heading.

Norethindrone (Concurrent use with agents known to be metabolized via cytochrome P450 pathway requires caution). Products include:
Ortho Micronor Tablets 2411

Norethindrone Acetate (Concurrent use with agents known to be metabolized via cytochrome P450 pathway requires caution). Products include:
Activella Tablets 2311
Aygestin Tablets 1062
CombiPatch Transdermal System 2180

Norfloxacin (Concurrent use with agents known to be metabolized via cytochrome P450 pathway requires caution). Products include:
Noroxin Tablets 2009

Norgestrel (Concurrent use with agents known to be metabolized via cytochrome P450 pathway requires caution). Products include:
Lo/Ovral-28 Tablets 3423

Nortriptyline Hydrochloride (Concurrent use with agents known to be metabolized via cytochrome P450 pathway requires caution).
No products indexed under this heading.

Ofloxacin (Concurrent use with agents known to be metabolized via cytochrome P450 pathway requires caution). Products include:
Floxin Otic Singles 1045
Floxin Otic Solution 1043

Olanzapine (Concurrent use with agents known to be metabolized via cytochrome P450 pathway requires caution). Products include:
Symbyax Capsules 1788
Zyprexa Tablets 1798
Zyprexa IntraMuscular 1798
Zyprexa ZYDIS Orally Disintegrating Tablets 1798

Omeprazole (Concurrent use with agents known to be metabolized via cytochrome P450 pathway requires caution). Products include:
Zegerid Powder for Oral Solution 2972

Ondansetron (Concurrent use with agents known to be metabolized via cytochrome P450 pathway requires caution). Products include:
Zofran ODT Orally Disintegrating Tablets 1613

Ondansetron Hydrochloride (Concurrent use with agents known to be metabolized via cytochrome P450 pathway requires caution). Products include:
Zofran Injection 1607
Zofran 1613

Oxaprozin (Concurrent use with agents known to be metabolized via cytochrome P450 pathway requires caution).
No products indexed under this heading.

Oxcarbazepine (Concurrent use with agents known to be metabolized via cytochrome P450 pathway requires caution). Products include:
Trileptal Oral Suspension 2281
Trileptal Tablets 2281

Oxycodone Hydrochloride (Concurrent use with agents known to be metabolized via cytochrome P450 pathway requires caution). Products include:
Combunox Tablets 1183
OxyContin Tablets 2699
OxyFast Oral Concentrate Solution 2704
OxyIR Capsules 2704
Percocet Tablets 1114
Percodan Tablets 1115

Paclitaxel (Concurrent use with agents known to be metabolized via cytochrome P450 pathway requires caution).
No products indexed under this heading.

Pantoprazole Sodium (Concurrent use with agents known to be metabolized via cytochrome P450 pathway requires caution). Products include:
Protonix I.V. 3468
Protonix Tablets 3465

Paramethadione (Concurrent use with agents known to be metabolized via cytochrome P450 pathway requires caution).
No products indexed under this heading.

Paroxetine Hydrochloride (Concurrent use with agents known to be metabolized via cytochrome P450 pathway requires caution). Products include:
Paxil CR Controlled-Release Tablets 1509
Paxil 1501

Pentamidine Isethionate (Concurrent use with agents known to be metabolized via cytochrome P450 pathway requires caution).
No products indexed under this heading.

Phenacemide (Concurrent use with agents known to be metabolized via cytochrome P450 pathway requires caution).
No products indexed under this heading.

Phenobarbital (Concurrent use with agents known to be metabolized via cytochrome P450 pathway requires caution).
No products indexed under this heading.

Phenobarbital Sodium (Concurrent use with agents known to be metabolized via cytochrome P450 pathway requires caution).
No products indexed under this heading.

Phensuximide (Concurrent use with agents known to be metabolized via cytochrome P450 pathway requires caution).
No products indexed under this heading.

Phenylbutazone (Concurrent use with agents known to be metabolized via cytochrome P450 pathway requires caution).
No products indexed under this heading.

Phenytoin (Concurrent use with agents known to be metabolized via cytochrome P450 pathway requires caution).
No products indexed under this heading.

Phenytoin Sodium (Concurrent use with agents known to be metabolized via cytochrome P450 pathway requires caution). Products include:
Phenytek Capsules 2153

Pimozide (Concurrent use with agents known to be metabolized via cytochrome P450 pathway requires caution). Products include:
Orap Tablets 1220

Pindolol (Concurrent use with agents known to be metabolized via cytochrome P450 pathway requires caution).
No products indexed under this heading.

Pioglitazone Hydrochloride (Concurrent use with agents known to be metabolized via cytochrome P450 pathway requires caution). Products include:
ActoPlus Met Tablets 3219
Actos Tablets 3224

Piroxicam (Concurrent use with agents known to be metabolized via cytochrome P450 pathway requires caution).
No products indexed under this heading.

Polyestradiol Phosphate (Concurrent use with agents known to be metabolized via cytochrome P450 pathway requires caution).
No products indexed under this heading.

Primidone (Concurrent use with agents known to be metabolized via cytochrome P450 pathway requires caution).
No products indexed under this heading.

Progesterone (Concurrent use with agents known to be metabolized via cytochrome P450 pathway requires caution). Products include:
Prochieve 4% Gel 1018
Prochieve 8% Gel 1018
Prometrium Capsules (100 mg, 200 mg) 3205

Proguanil Hydrochloride (Concurrent use with agents known to be metabolized via cytochrome P450 pathway requires caution). Products include:
Malarone Tablets 1484
Malarone Pediatric Tablets 1484

Propafenone Hydrochloride (Concurrent use with agents known to be metabolized via cytochrome P450 pathway requires caution). Products include:
Rythmol SR Capsules 2736

Propoxyphene Hydrochloride (Concurrent use with agents known to be metabolized via cytochrome P450 pathway requires caution).
No products indexed under this heading.

Propoxyphene Napsylate (Concurrent use with agents known to be metabolized via cytochrome P450 pathway requires caution). Products include:
Darvocet A 500 Tablets 3497

Propranolol Hydrochloride (Concurrent use with agents known to be metabolized via cytochrome P450 pathway requires caution). Products include:
Inderal LA Long-Acting Capsules 3421
InnoPran XL Capsules 2728

Protriptyline Hydrochloride (Concurrent use with agents known to be metabolized via cytochrome P450 pathway requires caution). Products include:
Vivactil Tablets 2350

Quetiapine Fumarate (Concurrent use with agents known to be metabolized via cytochrome P450 pathway requires caution). Products include:
Seroquel Tablets 691

Quinidine Gluconate (Concurrent use with agents known to be metabolized via cytochrome P450 pathway requires caution).
No products indexed under this heading.

Quinidine Hydrochloride (Concurrent use with agents known to be metabolized via cytochrome P450 pathway requires caution).
No products indexed under this heading.

Quinidine Polygalacturonate (Concurrent use with agents known to be metabolized via cytochrome P450 pathway requires caution).
No products indexed under this heading.

Quinidine Sulfate (Concurrent use with agents known to be metabolized via cytochrome P450 pathway requires caution).
No products indexed under this heading.

Quinine (Concurrent use with agents known to be metabolized via cytochrome P450 pathway requires caution).
No products indexed under this heading.

Quinine Sulfate (Concurrent use with agents known to be metabolized via cytochrome P450 pathway requires caution).
No products indexed under this heading.

Rabeprazole Sodium (Concurrent use with agents known to be metabolized via cytochrome P450 pathway requires caution). Products include:
Aciphex Tablets 1081

Repaglinide (Concurrent use with agents known to be metabolized via cytochrome P450 pathway requires caution). Products include:
Prandin Tablets (0.5, 1, and 2 mg) 2337

Rifabutin (Concurrent use with agents known to be metabolized via cytochrome P450 pathway requires caution).
No products indexed under this heading.

Riluzole (Concurrent use with agents known to be metabolized via cytochrome P450 pathway requires caution). Products include:
Rilutek Tablets 2945

Risperidone (Concurrent use with agents known to be metabolized via cytochrome P450 pathway requires caution). Products include:
Risperdal Consta Long-Acting Injection 1664
Risperdal M-Tab Orally Disintegrating Tablets 1658
Risperdal 1658

Ritonavir (Concurrent use with agents known to be metabolized via cytochrome P450 pathway requires caution). Products include:
Kaletra 474
Norvir 499

Rofecoxib (Concurrent use with agents known to be metabolized via cytochrome P450 pathway requires caution).
No products indexed under this heading.

Ropinirole Hydrochloride (Concurrent use with agents known to be metabolized via cytochrome P450 pathway requires caution). Products include:
Requip Tablets 1528

Ropivacaine Hydrochloride (Concurrent use with agents known to be metabolized via cytochrome P450 pathway requires caution). Products include:
Naropin Injection 640

Rosiglitazone Maleate (Concurrent use with agents known to be metabolized via cytochrome P450 pathway requires caution). Products include:
Avandamet Tablets 1343
Avandia Tablets 1348

Saquinavir (Concurrent use with agents known to be metabolized via cytochrome P450 pathway requires caution).
No products indexed under this heading.

Saquinavir Mesylate (Concurrent use with agents known to be metabolized via cytochrome P450 pathway requires caution). Products include:
Invirase 2776

Sertraline Hydrochloride (Concurrent use with agents known to be metabolized via cytochrome P450 pathway requires caution). Products include:
Zoloft 2581

Sildenafil Citrate (Concurrent use with agents known to be metabolized via cytochrome P450 pathway requires caution). Products include:
Revatio Tablets 2541
Viagra Tablets 2552

Simvastatin (Concurrent use with agents known to be metabolized via cytochrome P450 pathway requires caution). Products include:
Vytorin 10/10 Tablets 2084
Vytorin 10/10 Tablets 3092
Vytorin 10/20 Tablets 2084
Vytorin 10/20 Tablets 3092
Vytorin 10/40 Tablets 3092
Vytorin 10/40 Tablets 2084
Vytorin 10/80 Tablets 2084
Vytorin 10/80 Tablets 3092
Zocor Tablets 2078

Sirolimus (Concurrent use with agents known to be metabolized via cytochrome P450 pathway requires caution). Products include:
Rapamune Oral Solution and Tablets 3472

Sulfamethoxazole (Concurrent use with agents known to be metabolized via cytochrome P450 pathway requires caution).
No products indexed under this heading.

Sulindac (Concurrent use with agents known to be metabolized via cytochrome P450 pathway requires caution). Products include:
Clinoril Tablets 1899

Suprofen (Concurrent use with agents known to be metabolized via cytochrome P450 pathway requires caution).
No products indexed under this heading.

Tacrine Hydrochloride (Concurrent use with agents known to be metabolized via cytochrome P450 pathway requires caution).
No products indexed under this heading.

Tacrolimus (Concurrent use with agents known to be metabolized via cytochrome P450 pathway requires caution). Products include:
Prograf Capsules and Injection 624
Protopic Ointment 629

Tamoxifen Citrate (Concurrent use with agents known to be metabolized via cytochrome P450 pathway requires caution).
No products indexed under this heading.

Telmisartan (Concurrent use with agents known to be metabolized via cytochrome P450 pathway requires caution). Products include:
Micardis Tablets 884
Micardis HCT Tablets 886

Teniposide (Concurrent use with agents known to be metabolized via cytochrome P450 pathway requires caution).
No products indexed under this heading.

Terfenadine (Concurrent use with agents known to be metabolized via cytochrome P450 pathway requires caution).
No products indexed under this heading.

Testosterone (Concurrent use with agents known to be metabolized via cytochrome P450 pathway requires caution). Products include:
AndroGel 3330
Striant Mucoadhesive 1022
Testim 1% Gel 722

Testosterone Cypionate (Concurrent use with agents known to be metabolized via cytochrome P450 pathway requires caution).
No products indexed under this heading.

Testosterone Enanthate (Concurrent use with agents known to be metabolized via cytochrome P450 pathway requires caution). Products include:
Delatestryl Injection 2976

Testosterone Propionate (Concurrent use with agents known to be metabolized via cytochrome P450 pathway requires caution).
No products indexed under this heading.

Theophylline (Concurrent use with agents known to be metabolized via cytochrome P450 pathway requires caution).
No products indexed under this heading.

Theophylline Anhydrous (Concurrent use with agents known to be metabolized via cytochrome P450 pathway requires caution). Products include:
Uniphyl Tablets 2708

Theophylline Sodium Glycinate (Concurrent use with agents known to be metabolized via cytochrome P450 pathway requires caution).
No products indexed under this heading.

Thioridazine (Concurrent use with agents known to be metabolized via cytochrome P450 pathway requires caution).
No products indexed under this heading.

Thioridazine Hydrochloride (Concurrent use with agents known to be metabolized via cytochrome P450 pathway requires caution). Products include:
Thioridazine Hydrochloride Tablets 2122

Tiagabine Hydrochloride (Concurrent use with agents known to be metabolized via cytochrome P450 pathway requires caution). Products include:
Gabitril Tablets 998

Timolol Maleate (Concurrent use with agents known to be metabolized via cytochrome P450 pathway requires caution). Products include:
Blocadren Tablets 1891
Cosopt Sterile Ophthalmic Solution 1910
Timolide Tablets 2056
Timoptic in Ocudose 2061
Timoptic Sterile Ophthalmic Solution 2058
Timoptic-XE Sterile Ophthalmic Gel Forming Solution 2062

Tolazamide (Concurrent use with agents known to be metabolized via cytochrome P450 pathway requires caution).
No products indexed under this heading.

Tolbutamide (Concurrent use with agents known to be metabolized via cytochrome P450 pathway requires caution).
No products indexed under this heading.

Tolbutamide Sodium (Concurrent use with agents known to be metabolized via cytochrome P450 pathway requires caution).
No products indexed under this heading.

Tolmetin Sodium (Concurrent use with agents known to be metabolized via cytochrome P450 pathway requires caution).
No products indexed under this heading.

Tolterodine Tartrate (Concurrent use with agents known to be metabolized via cytochrome P450 pathway requires caution). Products include:
Detrol Tablets 2626
Detrol LA Capsules 2629

Topiramate (Concurrent use with agents known to be metabolized via cytochrome P450 pathway requires caution). Products include:
Topamax Sprinkle Capsules 2438
Topamax Tablets 2438

Torsemide (Concurrent use with agents known to be metabolized via cytochrome P450 pathway requires caution).
No products indexed under this heading.

Tramadol Hydrochloride (Concurrent use with agents known to be metabolized via cytochrome P450 pathway requires caution). Products include:
Ultracet Tablets 2462

Trazodone Hydrochloride (Concurrent use with agents known to be metabolized via cytochrome P450 pathway requires caution).
No products indexed under this heading.

Tretinoin (Concurrent use with agents known to be metabolized via cytochrome P450 pathway requires caution). Products include:
Avita Cream 2136
Avita Gel 2138
Renova 0.02% Cream 2384
Renova 0.05% Cream 2387
Retin-A Micro 0.1%/0.04% 2388
Solage Topical Solution 740
Tri-Luma Cream 1213
Vesanoid Capsules 2823

Triazolam (Concurrent use with agents known to be metabolized via cytochrome P450 pathway requires caution).
No products indexed under this heading.

Trimethadione (Concurrent use with agents known to be metabolized via cytochrome P450 pathway requires caution).
No products indexed under this heading.

Trimethaphan Camsylate (Concurrent use with agents known to be metabolized via cytochrome P450 pathway requires caution).
No products indexed under this heading.

Trimipramine Maleate (Concurrent use with agents known to be metabolized via cytochrome P450 pathway requires caution). Products include:
Surmontil Capsules 2347

Troglitazone (Concurrent use with agents known to be metabolized via cytochrome P450 pathway requires caution).
No products indexed under this heading.

Trovafloxacin Mesylate (Concurrent use with agents known to be metabolized via cytochrome P450 pathway requires caution).
No products indexed under this heading.

Valdecoxib (Concurrent use with agents known to be metabolized via cytochrome P450 pathway requires caution).
No products indexed under this heading.

Valproate Sodium (Concurrent use with agents known to be metabolized via cytochrome P450 pathway requires caution). Products include:
Depacon Injection 412

Valproic Acid (Concurrent use with agents known to be metabolized via cytochrome P450 pathway requires caution). Products include:
Depakene 417

Valsartan (Concurrent use with agents known to be metabolized via cytochrome P450 pathway requires caution). Products include:
Diovan HCT Tablets 2195
Diovan Tablets 2191

Venlafaxine Hydrochloride (Concurrent use with agents known to be metabolized via cytochrome P450 pathway requires caution). Products include:
Effexor Tablets 3405
Effexor XR Capsules 3411

Verapamil Hydrochloride (Concurrent use with agents known to be metabolized via cytochrome P450 pathway requires caution). Products include:
Covera-HS Tablets 3135
Tarka Tablets 519
Verelan PM Capsules 3120

Vinblastine Sulfate (Concurrent use with agents known to be metabolized via cytochrome P450 pathway requires caution).
No products indexed under this heading.

Vincristine Sulfate (Concurrent use with agents known to be metabolized via cytochrome P450 pathway requires caution).
No products indexed under this heading.

Vitamin A (Concurrent use with agents known to be metabolized via cytochrome P450 pathway requires caution). Products include:
Visutein Capsules 3328

Vitamin A Acetate (Concurrent use with agents known to be metabolized via cytochrome P450 pathway requires caution).
No products indexed under this heading.

Voriconazole (Concurrent use with agents known to be metabolized via cytochrome P450 pathway requires caution). Products include:
VFEND I.V. 2543
VFEND Oral Suspension 2543
VFEND Tablets 2543

Warfarin Sodium (Concurrent use with agents known to be metabolized via cytochrome P450 pathway requires caution). Products include:
Coumadin for Injection 932
Coumadin Tablets 932

Zafirlukast (Concurrent use with agents known to be metabolized via cytochrome P450 pathway requires caution). Products include:
Accolate Tablets 663

Zileuton (Concurrent use with agents known to be metabolized via cytochrome P450 pathway requires caution).
No products indexed under this heading.

Zolmitriptan (Concurrent use with agents known to be metabolized via cytochrome P450 pathway requires caution). Products include:
Zomig Nasal Spray 718
Zomig Tablets 714
Zomig-ZMT Tablets 714

Zonisamide (Concurrent use with agents known to be metabolized via cytochrome P450 pathway requires caution). Products include:
Zonegran Capsules 1089

Zopiclone (Concurrent use with agents known to be metabolized via cytochrome P450 pathway requires caution).
No products indexed under this heading.

INNOPRAN XL CAPSULES

(Propranolol Hydrochloride) 2728
May interact with ACE inhibitors, beta-adrenergic stimulating agents, catecholamine depleting drugs, calcium channel blockers, cytochrome p450 1a2 inhibitors (selected), cytochrome p450 1a2 substrates (selected), cytochrome p450 2c19 inhibitors (selected), cytochrome p450 2c19 substrates (selected), cytochrome p450 2d6 inhibitors (selected), cytochrome p450 2d6 substrates (selected), cardiac glycosides, hepatic microsomal enzyme inducers, monoamine oxidase inhibitors, non-steroidal anti-inflammatory agents, tricyclic antidepressants, and certain other agents. Compounds in these categories include:

Acetaminophen (Blood levels and/or toxicity of propranolol may be increased by administration of propranolol hydrochloride extended-release capsules with substrates of CYP1A2). Products include:
Benadryl Allergy & Cold Tablets .... ■692
Benadryl Allergy & Sinus Headache Caplets & Gelcaps .... ■693
Benadryl Maximum Strength Severe Allergy & Sinus Headache Caplets .... ■694
Contac Severe Cold and Flu Caplets Maximum Strength .... ■615
Contac Severe Cold and Flu Caplets Non-Drowsy .... ■615
Darvocet A 500 Tablets 3497
Goody's Body Pain Formula Powder .... ■621
Goody's Extra Strength Headache Powder .... ■621
Goody's Extra Strength Pain Relief Tablets .... ■621
Goody's PM Powder .... ■622
Hycomine Compound Tablets 1105
Lortab 3315
Lortab Elixir 3312
Percocet Tablets 1114
Robitussin Cough, Cold & Flu Liquid-filled Capsules .... ■750
Robitussin Flu Liquid .... ■752
Sedapap Tablets 50 mg/650 mg 2098
Singlet Caplets .... ■636
Sudafed Severe Cold .... ■710
Sudafed Sinus Headache .... ■711
TheraFlu Cold & Cough Hot Liquid .... ■680
TheraFlu Cold & Sore Throat Hot Liquid .... ■680
TheraFlu Flu & Chest Congestion Non-Drowsy Hot Liquid .... ■681
TheraFlu Flu & Sore Throat Hot Liquid .... ■681
TheraFlu Severe Cold Non-Drowsy Hot Liquid .... ■683
TheraFlu Severe Cold & Cough Hot Liquid .... ■683
TheraFlu Severe Cold Caplets .... ■679
TheraFlu Severe Cold Hot Liquid .... ■682
TheraFlu Severe Cold Non-Drowsy Caplets .... ■679
Triaminic Cough & Sore Throat Liquid .... ■687
Triaminic Flu, Cough & Fever Liquid .... ■685
Triaminic Cough & Sore Throat Softchews .... ■689
Tylenol 8 Hour Extended Release Geltabs and Caplets 1843
Tylenol Sinus NightTime Caplets .... ■663
Children's Tylenol Suspension Liquid and Meltaways 1850
Children's Tylenol Plus Cold & Allergy Suspension Liquid 1850
Children's Tylenol Plus Cold NightTime Suspension Liquid 1851
Children's Tylenol Plus Cold & Cough Suspension Liquid and Chewable Tablets 1851
Children's Tylenol Plus Cold Chewable Tablets 1851
Children's Tylenol Plus Cold Daytime Non-Drowsy Suspension Liquid 1851
Children's Tylenol Plus Flu Suspension Liquid 1853
Concentrated Tylenol Infants' Drops Plus Cold 1851
Concentrated Tylenol Infants' Drops Plus Cold and Cough 1851
Concentrated Tylenol Infants' Drops 1850
Junior Tylenol Meltaways 1850
Tylenol Cold & Flu Severe Daytime Liquid with Cool Bust 1846
Tylenol Cold & Flu Severe NightTime Liquid with Cool Burst 1846
Tylenol Cold Severe Congestion Non-Drowsy Caplets with Cool Burst 1846
Tylenol Cough & Sore Throat Daytime Liquid with Cool Burst 1849
Tylenol Cough & Sore Throat NightTime Liquid with Cool Burst 1849
Tylenol 1843
Extra Strength Tylenol Rapid Release Gels 1843
Tylenol 1843
Tylenol Allergy Complete Night Time Caplets 1844
Tylenol Allergy Complete Multi-Symptom Caplets and Gelcaps with Cool Burst 1844
Tylenol Severe Allergy Caplets 1844
Tylenol Flu NightTime Gelcaps 1846
Tylenol Flu Day Non-Drowsy Gelcaps 1846
Concentrated Tylenol Infants' Drops Plus Cold Nasal Congestant, Fever Reducer & Pain Reliever .... ■668
Concentrated Tylenol Infants' Drops Plus Cold & Cough Nasal Decongestant, Fever Reducer & Pain Reliever .... ■668
Multi-Symptom Tylenol Cold Night Time Caplets 1845
Multi-Symptom Tylenol Cold Day Non-Drowsy Caplets and Gelcaps 1845
Extra Strength Tylenol PM Caplets, Geltabs, Gelcaps and Liquid 1847
Tylenol Sinus Day Non-Drowsy 1848
Tylenol Sinus Night Time Caplets 1848
Tylenol Sinus Severe Congestion Caplets with Cool Burst 1848
Tylenol Sore Throat Daytime Liquid with Cool Burst 1849
Tylenol Sore Throat NightTime Liquid with Cool Burst 1849
Tylenol with Codeine 2461
Women's Tylenol Menstrual Relief Caplets 1849
Ultracet Tablets 2462
Vicks 44M Cough, Cold & Flu Relief 2676
Vicks DayQuil LiquiCaps/Liquid Multi-Symptom Cold/Flu Relief .... ■723
Vicks DayQuil Multi-Symptom Cold/Flu Relief LiquiCaps 2675
Vicks DayQuil Multi-Symptom Cold/Flu Relief Liquid 2675
Vicks NyQuil LiquiCaps 2677
Vicks NyQuil LiquiCaps/Liquid Multi-Symptom Cold/Flu Relief .... ■725
Vicks NyQuil Liquid 2677
Vicodin Tablets 530
Vicodin ES Tablets 531
Vicodin HP Tablets 532
Zydone Tablets 1118

Alatrofloxacin Mesylate (Blood levels and/or toxicity of propranolol may be increased by administration of propranolol hydrochloride extended-release capsules with substrates of CYP1A2).
No products indexed under this heading.

Albuterol (Propranolol is a competitive inhibitor of beta-receptor agonists and its effects can be reversed by administration of such agents (e.g., isoproterenol)). Products include:
Proventil Inhalation Aerosol 3067

Albuterol Sulfate (Propranolol is a competitive inhibitor of beta-receptor agonists and its effects can be reversed by administration of such agents (e.g., isoproterenol)).
Products include:
AccuNeb Inhalation Solution 1055
Combivent Inhalation Aerosol 878
DuoNeb Inhalation Solution 1058
Proventil Inhalation Solution 0.083% 3069
Proventil HFA Inhalation Aerosol 3071
Ventolin HFA Inhalation Aerosol 1576
VoSpire Extended-Release Tablets ... 2352

Aluminum Hydroxide (Co-administration of propranolol with aluminum hydroxide gel (1200 mg) resulted in a 50% decrease in propranolol concentrations). Products include:
Gaviscon Regular Strength Liquid .. 620
Gaviscon Regular Strength Tablets.. 619
Gaviscon Extra Strength Liquid 620
Gaviscon Extra Strength Tablets 619
Maalox Max Maximum Strength Antacid/Anti-Gas Liquid................ 2165
Maalox Regular Strength Antacid/Antigas Liquid.................. 2164

Aluminum Hydroxide Preparations (Co-administration of propranolol with aluminum hydroxide gel (1200 mg) resulted in a 50% decrease in propranolol concentrations).
No products indexed under this heading.

Amiodarone Hydrochloride (Amiodarone is an antiarrhythmic agent with negative chronotropic properties that may be additive to those seen with propranolol).
Products include:
Pacerone Tablets 3337

Amitriptyline Hydrochloride (Blood levels and/or toxicity of propranolol may be increased by administration of propranolol hydrochloride extended-release capsules with substrates of CYP2D6).
No products indexed under this heading.

Amlodipine Besylate (Caution should be exercised when patients receiving a beta-blocker are administered a calcium channel blocking drug with negative inotropic and/or chronotropic effects. Both agents may depress cardiac contractility or atrioventricular conduction).
Products include:
Caduet Tablets 2507
Lotrel Capsules 2238
Norvasc Tablets 2529

Amoxapine (Blood levels and/or toxicity of propranolol may be increased by administration of propranolol hydrochloride extended-release capsules with inhibitors of CYP2D6).
No products indexed under this heading.

Amphetamine Aspartate (Blood levels and/or toxicity of propranolol may be increased by administration of propranolol hydrochloride extended-release capsules with substrates of CYP2D6). Products include:
Adderall Tablets 3168
Adderall XR Capsules 3169

Amphetamine Aspartate Monohydrate (Blood levels and/or toxicity of propranolol may be increased by administration of propranolol hydrochloride extended-release capsules with substrates of CYP2D6).
No products indexed under this heading.

Amphetamine Sulfate (Blood levels and/or toxicity of propranolol may be increased by administration of propranolol hydrochloride extended-release capsules with substrates of CYP2D6). Products include:
Adderall Tablets 3168
Adderall XR Capsules 3169

Anagrelide Hydrochloride (Blood levels and/or toxicity of propranolol may be increased by administration of propranolol hydrochloride extended-release capsules with substrates of CYP1A2). Products include:
Agrylin Capsules 3172

Anastrozole (Blood levels and/or toxicity of propranolol may be increased by administration of propranolol hydrochloride extended-release capsules with inhibitors of CYP1A2). Products include:
Arimidex Tablets 665

Atomoxetine Hydrochloride (Blood levels and/or toxicity of propranolol may be increased by administration of propranolol hydrochloride extended-release capsules with substrates of CYP2D6). Products include:
Strattera Capsules 1784

Benazepril Hydrochloride (When combined with beta-blockers, ACE inhibitors can cause hypotension, particularly in the setting of acute myocardial infarction. Certain ACE inhibitors have been reported to increase bronchial hyper-reactivity when administered with propranolol).
Products include:
Lotensin Tablets 2232
Lotensin HCT Tablets 2235
Lotrel Capsules 2238

Bepridil Hydrochloride (Caution should be exercised when patients receiving a beta-blocker are administered a calcium channel blocking drug with negative inotropic and/or chronotropic effects. Both agents may depress cardiac contractility or atrioventricular conduction).
No products indexed under this heading.

Bisoprolol Fumarate (Blood levels and/or toxicity of propranolol may be increased by administration of propranolol hydrochloride extended-release capsules with substrates of CYP2D6).
No products indexed under this heading.

Bitolterol Mesylate (Propranolol is a competitive inhibitor of beta-receptor agonists and its effects can be reversed by administration of such agents (e.g., isoproterenol)).
No products indexed under this heading.

Bupropion Hydrochloride (Blood levels and/or toxicity of propranolol may be increased by administration of propranolol hydrochloride extended-release capsules with inhibitors of CYP2D6). Products include:
Wellbutrin Tablets 1579
Wellbutrin SR Sustained-Release Tablets 1583
Wellbutrin XL Extended-Release Tablets 1588
Zyban Sustained-Release Tablets 1620

Caffeine (Blood levels and/or toxicity of propranolol may be increased by administration of propranolol hydrochloride extended-release capsules with substrates of CYP1A2).
Products include:
Athena Hair System Shampoo 767
BC Powder 612
Arthritis Strength BC Powder 612
Goody's Extra Strength Headache Powder....................... 621
Goody's Extra Strength Pain Relief Tablets 621
Hycomine Compound Tablets 1105
Spartan Hair System Shampoo 767
Vivarin 639

Caffeine Anhydrous (Blood levels and/or toxicity of propranolol may be increased by administration of propranolol hydrochloride extended-release capsules with substrates of CYP1A2).
No products indexed under this heading.

Captopril (Blood levels and/or toxicity of propranolol may be increased by administration of propranolol hydrochloride extended-release capsules with substrates of CYP2D6).
Products include:
Captopril Tablets 2114

Carbamazepine (Blood levels of propranolol may be decreased by co-administration of propranolol hydrochloride extended-release capsules with inducers of hepatic drug metabolism). Products include:
Carbatrol Capsules 3174
Equetro Extended-Release Capsules 3178
Tegretol/Tegretol-XR 2278

Carisoprodol (Blood levels and/or toxicity of propranolol may be increased by administration of propranolol hydrochloride extended-release capsules with substrates of CYP2C19).
No products indexed under this heading.

Carvedilol (Blood levels and/or toxicity of propranolol may be increased by administration of propranolol hydrochloride extended-release capsules with substrates of CYP2D6). Products include:
Coreg Tablets 1376

Celecoxib (Blood levels and/or toxicity of propranolol may be increased by administration of propranolol hydrochloride extended-release capsules with inhibitors of CYP2D6).
Products include:
Celebrex Capsules 3130

Cevimeline Hydrochloride (Blood levels and/or toxicity of propranolol may be increased by administration of propranolol hydrochloride extended-release capsules with substrates of CYP2D6). Products include:
Evoxac Capsules 1042

Chlordiazepoxide (Blood levels and/or toxicity of propranolol may be increased by administration of propranolol hydrochloride extended-release capsules with substrates of CYP1A2).
No products indexed under this heading.

Chlordiazepoxide Hydrochloride (Blood levels and/or toxicity of propranolol may be increased by administration of propranolol hydrochloride extended-release capsules with substrates of CYP1A2). Products include:
Librium Capsules 3349

Chloroquine Hydrochloride (Blood levels and/or toxicity of propranolol may be increased by administration of propranolol hydrochloride extended-release capsules with inhibitors of CYP2D6).
No products indexed under this heading.

Chloroquine Phosphate (Blood levels and/or toxicity of propranolol may be increased by administration of propranolol hydrochloride extended-release capsules with inhibitors of CYP2D6).
No products indexed under this heading.

Chlorpheniramine (Blood levels and/or toxicity of propranolol may be increased by administration of propranolol hydrochloride extended-release capsules with inhibitors of CYP2D6).
No products indexed under this heading.

Chlorpheniramine Maleate (Blood levels and/or toxicity of propranolol may be increased by administration of propranolol hydrochloride extended-release capsules with inhibitors of CYP2D6). Products include:
Advil Allergy Sinus Caplets 737
Advil Multi-Symptom Cold Caplets 738
BC Allergy Sinus Cold Powder 612
Contac Severe Cold and Flu Caplets Maximum Strength......... 615
Hycomine Compound Tablets 1105
PediaCare Multi-Symptom Cold Liquid 704
PediaCare NightRest Cough & Cold Liquid..................................... 704
Robitussin Flu Liquid 752
Robitussin PM Cough & Cold Liquid 752
Singlet Caplets 636
Sudafed Sinus & Allergy Tablets 710
TheraFlu Cold & Cough Hot Liquid 680
TheraFlu Cold & Sore Throat Hot Liquid 680
TheraFlu Flu & Sore Throat Hot Liquid 681
TheraFlu Severe Cold & Cough Hot Liquid 683
TheraFlu Severe Cold Caplets 679
TheraFlu Severe Cold Hot Liquid 682
Triaminic Cold & Allergy Liquid 685
Triaminic Cold & Cough Liquid 685
Triaminic Flu, Cough & Fever Liquid 685
Triaminic Night Time Cough & Cold Liquid..................................... 685
Triaminic Allergy Runny Nose & Congestion Softchews................ 688
Triaminic Cold & Cough Softchews 688
Children's Tylenol Plus Cold NightTime Suspension Liquid........ 1851
Children's Tylenol Plus Cold & Cough Suspension Liquid and Chewable Tablets 1851
Children's Tylenol Plus Cold Chewable Tablets 1851

Children's Tylenol Plus Flu Suspension Liquid 1853
Tylenol Allergy Complete Multi-Symptom Caplets and Gelcaps with Cool Burst........ 1844
Multi-Symptom Tylenol Cold Night Time Caplets........ 1845
Vicks 44M Cough, Cold & Flu Relief........ 2676
Pediatric Vicks 44m Cough & Cold Relief........ 2673
Children's Vicks NyQuil Cold/Cough Relief........ 2671

Chlorpheniramine Polistirex (Blood levels and/or toxicity of propranolol may be increased by administration of propranolol hydrochloride extended-release capsules with inhibitors of CYP2D6). Products include:
Tussionex Pennkinetic Extended-Release Suspension........ 3322

Chlorpheniramine Tannate (Blood levels and/or toxicity of propranolol may be increased by administration of propranolol hydrochloride extended-release capsules with inhibitors of CYP2D6).
No products indexed under this heading.

Chlorpromazine (Co-administration of chlorpromazine with propranolol resulted in increased plasma levels of both drugs (70% increase in propranolol concentrations)).
No products indexed under this heading.

Chlorpromazine Hydrochloride (Co-administration of chlorpromazine with propranolol resulted in increased plasma levels of both drugs (70% increase in propranolol concentrations)).
No products indexed under this heading.

Chlorpropamide (Blood levels and/or toxicity of propranolol may be increased by administration of propranolol hydrochloride extended-release capsules with substrates of CYP2D6).
No products indexed under this heading.

Cholestyramine (Co-administration of cholestyramine with propranolol decreased propranolol concentrations by up to 50%).
No products indexed under this heading.

Cilostazol (Blood levels and/or toxicity of propranolol may be increased by administration of propranolol hydrochloride extended-release capsules with substrates of CYP2C19). Products include:
Pletal Tablets........ 2478

Cimetidine (Co-administration of propranolol with cimetidine, a non-specific CYP450 inhibitor, increased propranolol concentrations by about 40%). Products include:
Tagamet HB 200 Tablets........ ■ 637
Tagamet Tablets........ 1547

Cimetidine Hydrochloride (Co-administration of propranolol with cimetidine, a non-specific CYP450 inhibitor, increased propranolol concentrations by about 40%).
No products indexed under this heading.

Ciprofloxacin (Blood levels and/or toxicity of propranolol may be increased by administration of propranolol hydrochloride extended-release capsules with substrates of CYP1A2). Products include:
Cipro I.V. 2998
Cipro I.V. Pharmacy Bulk Package........ 3509
Cipro Oral Suspension........ 2991
Cipro XR Tablets........ 3004
Ciprodex Otic Suspension........ 555

Ciprofloxacin Hydrochloride (Blood levels and/or toxicity of propranolol may be increased by administration of propranolol hydrochloride extended-release capsules with substrates of CYP1A2). Products include:
Ciloxan Ophthalmic Ointment........ 554
Cipro Tablets........ 2991

Citalopram Hydrobromide (Blood levels and/or toxicity of propranolol may be increased by administration of propranolol hydrochloride extended-release capsules with inhibitors of CYP2D6). Products include:
Celexa........ 1177

Clarithromycin (Blood levels and/or toxicity of propranolol may be increased by administration of propranolol hydrochloride extended-release capsules with inhibitors of CYP1A2). Products include:
Biaxin/Biaxin XL........ 402
PREVPAC........ 3281

Clomipramine Hydrochloride (Blood levels and/or toxicity of propranolol may be increased by administration of propranolol hydrochloride extended-release capsules with substrates of CYP2D6).
No products indexed under this heading.

Clonidine (The antihypertensive effects of clonidine may be antagonized by beta-blockers. Propranolol extended-release capsules should be administered cautiously to patients withdrawing from clonidine). Products include:
Catapres-TTS........ 875

Clonidine Hydrochloride (The antihypertensive effects of clonidine may be antagonized by beta-blockers. Propranolol extended-release capsules should be administered cautiously to patients withdrawing from clonidine). Products include:
Catapres Tablets........ 874
Clorpres Tablets........ 2139

Clopidogrel Bisulfate (Blood levels and/or toxicity of propranolol may be increased by administration of propranolol hydrochloride extended-release capsules with substrates of CYP1A2). Products include:
Plavix Tablets........ 940
Plavix Tablets........ 2942

Clozapine (Blood levels and/or toxicity of propranolol may be increased by administration of propranolol hydrochloride extended-release capsules with substrates of CYP2D6). Products include:
Clozapine Tablets........ 2141
Clozaril Tablets........ 2174
FazaClo Orally Disintegrating Tablets........ 547

Cocaine Hydrochloride (Blood levels and/or toxicity of propranolol may be increased by administration of propranolol hydrochloride extended-release capsules with inhibitors of CYP2D6).
No products indexed under this heading.

Codeine Phosphate (Blood levels and/or toxicity of propranolol may be increased by administration of propranolol hydrochloride extended-release capsules with substrates of CYP2D6). Products include:
Tylenol with Codeine........ 2461

Codeine Sulfate (Blood levels and/or toxicity of propranolol may be increased by administration of propranolol hydrochloride extended-release capsules with substrates of CYP2D6).
No products indexed under this heading.

Colestipol (Co-administration of colestipol with propranolol decreased propranolol concentrations by up to 50%).
No products indexed under this heading.

Colestipol Hydrochloride (Co-administration of colestipol with propranolol decreased propranolol concentrations by up to 50%).
No products indexed under this heading.

Cyclobenzaprine (Blood levels and/or toxicity of propranolol may be increased by administration of propranolol hydrochloride extended-release capsules with substrates of CYP1A2).
No products indexed under this heading.

Cyclobenzaprine Hydrochloride (Blood levels and/or toxicity of propranolol may be increased by administration of propranolol hydrochloride extended-release capsules with substrates of CYP2D6). Products include:
Flexeril Tablets........ 1832

Cyclophosphamide (Blood levels and/or toxicity of propranolol may be increased by administration of propranolol hydrochloride extended-release capsules with substrates of CYP2C19).
No products indexed under this heading.

Delavirdine Mesylate (Blood levels and/or toxicity of propranolol may be increased by administration of propranolol hydrochloride extended-release capsules with inhibitors of CYP2C19). Products include:
Rescriptor Tablets........ 2535

Deserpidine (Patients receiving catecholamine-depleting drugs (e.g., reserpine) and propranolol hydrochloride extended-release capsules should be observed closely for excessive reduction of resting sympathetic nervous activity, which may result in hypotension, marked bradycardia, vertigo, syncopal attacks, or orthostatic hypotension).
No products indexed under this heading.

Desipramine Hydrochloride (Blood levels and/or toxicity of propranolol may be increased by administration of propranolol hydrochloride extended-release capsules with substrates of CYP2D6).
No products indexed under this heading.

Deslanoside (Use caution when administering propranolol hydrochloride extended-release tablets with drugs that slow AV nodal conduction (e.g., digitalis)).
No products indexed under this heading.

Desogestrel (Blood levels and/or toxicity of propranolol may be increased by administration of propranolol hydrochloride extended-release capsules with inhibitors of CYP1A2). Products include:
Ortho-Cept Tablets........ 2395

Dexfenfluramine Hydrochloride (Blood levels and/or toxicity of propranolol may be increased by administration of propranolol hydrochloride extended-release capsules with substrates of CYP2D6).
No products indexed under this heading.

Dextromethorphan (Blood levels and/or toxicity of propranolol may be increased by administration of propranolol hydrochloride extended-release capsules with substrates of CYP2C19).
No products indexed under this heading.

Dextromethorphan Hydrobromide (Blood levels and/or toxicity of propranolol may be increased by administration of propranolol hydrochloride extended-release capsules with substrates of CYP2D6). Products include:
Alacol DM Syrup........ 739
Balamine DM........ 739
Contac Severe Cold and Flu Caplets Maximum Strength........ ■ 615
Contac Severe Cold and Flu Caplets Non-Drowsy........ ■ 615
Children's Dimetapp DM Cold & Cough Elixir........ ■ 745
Children's Dimetapp Long Acting Cough Plus Cold Syrup........ ■ 746
Dimetapp Infant Drops Decongestant Plus Cough........ ■ 746
Mucinex DM Tablets........ ■ 602
PediaCare Decongestant & Cough Infant Drops........ ■ 705
PediaCare Freezer Pops Long-Acting Cough-Glacier Grape and Polar Berry Blue........ ■ 706
PediaCare Long-Acting Cough Infant Drops........ ■ 705
PediaCare Long-Acting Cough Plus Cold Liquid........ ■ 704
PediaCare Multi-Symptom Cold Liquid........ ■ 704
PediaCare NightRest Cough & Cold Liquid........ ■ 704
Robitussin Allergy & Cough Syrup........ ■ 750
Robitussin CF Liquid........ ■ 755
Robitussin Cough & Cold Liquid-filled Capsules........ ■ 750
Robitussin Cough, Cold & Flu Liquid-filled Capsules........ ■ 750
Robitussin Cough & Cold Infant Drops........ ■ 755
Robitussin DM Infant Drops........ ■ 753
Robitussin DM Liquid........ ■ 753
Robitussin Flu Liquid........ ■ 752
Robitussin Maximum Strength Cough Liquid........ ■ 754
Robitussin Maximum Strength Cough & Cold Liquid........ ■ 754
Robitussin Pediatric Cough Liquid........ ■ 754
Robitussin Pediatric Cough & Cold Liquid........ ■ 754
Robitussin PM Cough & Cold Liquid........ ■ 752
Robitussin Sugar Free Cough Liquid........ ■ 753
Simply Cough Liquid........ 1840
Sudafed Severe Cold........ ■ 710
TheraFlu Cold & Cough Hot Liquid........ ■ 680
TheraFlu Flu & Chest Congestion Non-Drowsy Hot Liquid........ ■ 681
TheraFlu Severe Cold Non-Drowsy Hot Liquid........ ■ 683
TheraFlu Severe Cold & Cough Hot Liquid........ ■ 683
TheraFlu Severe Cold Caplets........ ■ 679
TheraFlu Severe Cold Hot Liquid........ ■ 682
TheraFlu Severe Cold Non-Drowsy Caplets........ ■ 679
TheraFlu Thin Strips Long Acting Cough........ ■ 684
Triaminic Cold & Cough Liquid........ ■ 685
Triaminic Cough Liquid........ ■ 687
Triaminic Cough & Nasal Congestion Liquid........ ■ 687

Triaminic Cough & Sore Throat Liquid 687
Triaminic Flu, Cough & Fever Liquid 685
Triaminic Night Time Cough & Cold Liquid 685
Triaminic Cold & Cough Softchews 688
Triaminic Cough & Sore Throat Softchews 689
Triaminic Thin Strips Long Acting Cough 689
Children's Tylenol Plus Cold & Cough Suspension Liquid and Chewable Tablets 1851
Children's Tylenol Plus Flu Suspension Liquid 1853
Concentrated Tylenol Infants' Drops Plus Cold and Cough 1851
Tylenol Cold & Flu Severe Daytime Liquid with Cool Burst 1846
Tylenol Cold & Flu Severe NightTime Liquid with Cool Burst 1846
Tylenol Cold Severe Congestion Non-Drowsy Caplets with Cool Burst 1846
Tylenol Cough & Sore Throat Daytime Liquid with Cool Burst 1849
Tylenol Cough & Sore Throat NightTime Liquid with Cool Burst 1849
Tylenol Flu Day Non-Drowsy Gelcaps 1846
Concentrated Tylenol Infants' Drops Plus Cold & Cough Nasal Decongestant, Fever Reducer & Pain Reliever 668
Multi-Symptom Tylenol Cold Night Time Caplets 1845
Multi-Symptom Tylenol Cold Day Non-Drowsy Caplets and Gelcaps 1845
Vicks 44 Cough Relief 2675
Vicks 44D Cough & Head Congestion Relief 2676
Vicks 44D Cough & Head Congestion Relief Liquid 721
Vicks 44E Cough & Chest Congestion Relief 2676
Pediatric Vicks 44e Cough & Chest Congestion Relief Liquid 2673
Vicks 44M Cough, Cold & Flu Relief 2676
Pediatric Vicks 44m Cough & Cold Relief 2673
Vicks DayQuil LiquiCaps/Liquid Multi-Symptom Cold/Flu Relief 723
Vicks DayQuil Multi-Symptom Cold/Flu Relief LiquiCaps 2675
Vicks DayQuil Multi-Symptom Cold/Flu Relief Liquid 2675
Children's Vicks NyQuil Cold/Cough Relief 2671
Vicks NyQuil Cough Liquid 2677
Vicks NyQuil LiquiCaps 2677
Vicks NyQuil LiquiCaps/Liquid Multi-Symptom Cold/Flu Relief 725
Vicks NyQuil Liquid 2677
Zicam Concentrated Cough Mist for Kids Cool Cherry 643
Zicam Concentrated Cough Mist for Kids Plus D Cool Cherry 643
Zicam Concentrated Cough Mist Nite-Cool Cherry 642
Zicam Concentrated Cough Mist Plus D Cool Cherry 642
Zicam Concentrated Cough Mist-Honey Lemon & Cool Cherry 642

Dextromethorphan Polistirex (Blood levels and/or toxicity of propranolol may be increased by administration of propranolol hydrochloride extended-release capsules with substrates of CYP2D6). Products include:
Delsym Extended-Release Suspension 611
Delsym 12 Hour Cough Suppressant for Children 611

Diazepam (Propranolol can inhibit the metabolism of diazepam, resulting in increased concentrations of diazepam and its metabolites. Diazepam does not alter the pharmacokinetics of propranolol). Products include:
Diastat Rectal Delivery System 3344
Valium Tablets 2822

Diclofenac Potassium (Non-steroidal anti-inflammatory drugs have been reported to blunt the antihypertensive effects of beta-adrenoreceptor blocking agents). Products include:
Cataflam Tablets 2173

Diclofenac Sodium (Non-steroidal anti-inflammatory drugs have been reported to blunt the antihypertensive effects of beta-adrenoreceptor blocking agents). Products include:
Arthrotec Tablets 3126
Voltaren Ophthalmic Solution 2300
Voltaren Tablets 2298
Voltaren-XR Tablets 2301

Digitalis Glycoside Preparations (Use caution when administering propranolol hydrochloride extended-release tablets with drugs that slow AV nodal conduction (e.g., digitalis)).
No products indexed under this heading.

Digitoxin (Use caution when administering propranolol hydrochloride extended-release tablets with drugs that slow AV nodal conduction (e.g., digitalis)).
No products indexed under this heading.

Digoxin (Use caution when administering propranolol hydrochloride extended-release tablets with drugs that slow AV nodal conduction (e.g., digitalis)). Products include:
Digitek Tablets 2146
Lanoxicaps Capsules 1458
Lanoxin Injection 1462
Lanoxin Tablets 1468
Lanoxin Injection Pediatric 1465

Diltiazem Hydrochloride (Co-administration of propranolol and diltiazem in patients with cardiac disease has been associated with bradycardia, hypotension, high degree heart block, and heart failure). Products include:
Cardizem LA Extended Release Tablets 1699
Tiazac Capsules 1204

Diltiazem Maleate (Co-administration of propranolol and diltiazem in patients with cardiac disease has been associated with bradycardia, hypotension, high degree heart block, and heart failure).
No products indexed under this heading.

Diphenhydramine (Blood levels and/or toxicity of propranolol may be increased by administration of propranolol hydrochloride extended-release capsules with inhibitors of CYP2D6). Products include:
Tylenol Sore Throat NightTime Liquid with Cool Burst 1849

Diphenhydramine Hydrochloride (Blood levels and/or toxicity of propranolol may be increased by administration of propranolol hydrochloride extended-release capsules with inhibitors of CYP2D6). Products include:
Benadryl Allergy & Cold Tablets 692
Benadryl Allergy 691
Benadryl Allergy & Sinus Headache Caplets & Gelcaps 693
Children's Benadryl Allergy Liquid 695
Children's Benadryl Dye-Free Allergy Liquid 695
Benadryl Dye-Free Allergy Liqui-Gels Softgels 692
Benadryl Itch Relief Stick Extra Strength 696
Benadryl Itch Stopping Cream Extra Strength 697
Benadryl Itch Stopping Gel Extra Strength 697
Benadryl Itch Stopping Spray Extra Strength 697
Benadryl Maximum Strength Severe Allergy & Sinus Headache Caplets 694
Children's Benadryl D Liquid Medication 693
Benadryl D Tablets 694
Nytol QuickCaps Caplets 635
Maximum Strength Nytol QuickGels Softgels 635
Simply Sleep Caplets 1841
Sominex Original Formula Tablets 637
TheraFlu Thin Strips Multi Symptom 684
Triaminic Thin Strips Cough & Runny Nose 690
Children's Tylenol Plus Cold & Allergy Suspension Liquid 1850
Tylenol Allergy Complete Night Time Caplets 1844
Tylenol Severe Allergy Caplets 1844
Tylenol Flu NightTime Gelcaps 1846
Extra Strength Tylenol PM Caplets, Geltabs, Gelcaps and Liquid 1847
Unisom Maximum Strength SleepGels 712

Disopyramide (Disopyramide, a Type I antiarrhythmic drug with potent negative inotropic and chronotropic effects, has been associated with severe bradycardia, asystole, and heart failure when administered with propranolol).
No products indexed under this heading.

Disopyramide Phosphate (Disopyramide, a Type I antiarrhythmic drug with potent negative inotropic and chronotropic effects, has been associated with severe bradycardia, asystole, and heart failure when administered with propranolol).
No products indexed under this heading.

Divalproex Sodium (Blood levels and/or toxicity of propranolol may be increased by administration of propranolol hydrochloride extended-release capsules with substrates of CYP2C19). Products include:
Depakote Sprinkle Capsules 422
Depakote Tablets 427
Depakote ER Tablets 433

Dobutamine (Propranolol is a competitive inhibitor of beta-receptor agonists and its effects can be reversed by administration of such agents (e.g., dobutamine)).
No products indexed under this heading.

Dobutamine Hydrochloride (Propranolol is a competitive inhibitor of beta-receptor agonists and its effects can be reversed by administration of such agents (e.g., dobutamine)).
No products indexed under this heading.

Dolasetron Mesylate (Blood levels and/or toxicity of propranolol may be increased by administration of propranolol hydrochloride extended-release capsules with substrates of CYP2D6). Products include:
Anzemet Injection 2871
Anzemet Tablets 2874

Donepezil Hydrochloride (Blood levels and/or toxicity of propranolol may be increased by administration of propranolol hydrochloride extended-release capsules with substrates of CYP2D6). Products include:
Aricept Tablets 1086
Aricept ODT Tablets 1086

Doxazosin Mesylate (Postural hypotension has been reported in patients taking both beta-blockers and doxazosin).
No products indexed under this heading.

Doxepin Hydrochloride (Blood levels and/or toxicity of propranolol may be increased by administration of propranolol hydrochloride extended-release capsules with substrates of CYP2D6).
No products indexed under this heading.

Efavirenz (Blood levels and/or toxicity of propranolol may be increased by administration of propranolol hydrochloride extended-release capsules with inhibitors of CYP2C19). Products include:
Sustiva Capsules 957

Enalapril Maleate (When combined with beta-blockers, ACE inhibitors can cause hypotension, particularly in the setting of acute myocardial infarction. Certain ACE inhibitors have been reported to increase bronchial hyper-reactivity when administered with propranolol). Products include:
Vaseretic Tablets 2073
Vasotec I.V. Injection 2076

Enalaprilat (When combined with beta-blockers, ACE inhibitors can cause hypotension, particularly in the setting of acute myocardial infarction. Certain ACE inhibitors have been reported to increase bronchial hyper-reactivity when administered with propranolol).
No products indexed under this heading.

Encainide Hydrochloride (Blood levels and/or toxicity of propranolol may be increased by administration of propranolol hydrochloride extended-release capsules with substrates of CYP2D6).
No products indexed under this heading.

Enoxacin (Blood levels and/or toxicity of propranolol may be increased by administration of propranolol hydrochloride extended-release capsules with substrates of CYP1A2).
No products indexed under this heading.

Ephedrine Hydrochloride (Propranolol is a competitive inhibitor of beta-receptor agonists and its effects can be reversed by administration of such agents (e.g., isoproterenol)). Products include:
Primatene Tablets 749

Ephedrine Sulfate (Propranolol is a competitive inhibitor of beta-receptor agonists and its effects can be reversed by administration of such agents (e.g., isoproterenol)).
No products indexed under this heading.

Ephedrine Tannate (Propranolol is a competitive inhibitor of beta-receptor agonists and its effects can be reversed by administration of such agents (e.g., isoproterenol)).
No products indexed under this heading.

Epinephrine (Patients on long-term therapy with propranolol may experience uncontrolled hypertension if they are administered epinephrine as a consequence of unopposed alpha-receptor stimulation. Epineph-

rine is, therefore, not indicated in the treatment of propranolol overdose). Products include:

- EpiPen ... 1061
- Primatene Mist ... ▣ 749

Epinephrine, Racemic (Patients on long-term therapy with propranolol may experience uncontrolled hypertension if they are administered epinephrine as a consequence of unopposed alpha-receptor stimulation. Epinephrine is, therefore, not indicated in the treatment of propranolol overdose).

No products indexed under this heading.

Epinephrine Bitartrate (Patients on long-term therapy with propranolol may experience uncontrolled hypertension if they are administered epinephrine as a consequence of unopposed alpha-receptor stimulation. Epinephrine is, therefore, not indicated in the treatment of propranolol overdose).

No products indexed under this heading.

Epinephrine Hydrochloride (Patients on long-term therapy with propranolol may experience uncontrolled hypertension if they are administered epinephrine as a consequence of unopposed alpha-receptor stimulation. Epinephrine is, therefore, not indicated in the treatment of propranolol overdose).

No products indexed under this heading.

Erythromycin (Blood levels and/or toxicity of propranolol may be increased by administration of propranolol hydrochloride extended-release capsules with substrates of CYP1A2). Products include:

- Erygel Topical Gel ... 2096
- Ery-Tab Tablets ... 447
- Erythromycin Base Filmtab Tablets ... 454
- Erythromycin Delayed-Release Capsules, USP ... 456
- PCE Dispertab Tablets ... 510

Erythromycin Estolate (Blood levels and/or toxicity of propranolol may be increased by administration of propranolol hydrochloride extended-release capsules with substrates of CYP1A2).

No products indexed under this heading.

Erythromycin Ethylsuccinate (Blood levels and/or toxicity of propranolol may be increased by administration of propranolol hydrochloride extended-release capsules with substrates of CYP1A2). Products include:

- E.E.S. ... 449
- EryPed ... 445

Erythromycin Gluceptate (Blood levels and/or toxicity of propranolol may be increased by administration of propranolol hydrochloride extended-release capsules with substrates of CYP1A2).

No products indexed under this heading.

Erythromycin Lactobionate (Blood levels and/or toxicity of propranolol may be increased by administration of propranolol hydrochloride extended-release capsules with substrates of CYP1A2).

No products indexed under this heading.

Erythromycin Stearate (Blood levels and/or toxicity of propranolol may be increased by administration of propranolol hydrochloride extended-release capsules with substrates of CYP1A2). Products include:

- Erythrocin Stearate Filmtab Tablets ... 452

Escitalopram Oxalate (Blood levels and/or toxicity of propranolol may be increased by administration of propranolol hydrochloride extended-release capsules with inhibitors of CYP2D6). Products include:

- Lexapro Oral Solution ... 1193
- Lexapro Tablets ... 1193

Esomeprazole Magnesium (Blood levels and/or toxicity of propranolol may be increased by administration of propranolol hydrochloride extended-release capsules with substrates of CYP2C19). Products include:

- Nexium Delayed-Release Capsules ... 645

Estradiol (Blood levels and/or toxicity of propranolol may be increased by administration of propranolol hydrochloride extended-release capsules with substrates of CYP1A2). Products include:

- Activella Tablets ... 2311
- Climara Transdermal System ... 795
- Climara Pro Transdermal System ... 800
- CombiPatch Transdermal System ... 2180
- Estrogel 0.06% ... 3200
- Menostar Transdermal System ... 805
- Prefest Tablets ... 1069
- Vagifem Tablets ... 2340
- Vivelle Transdermal System ... 2288
- Vivelle-Dot Transdermal System ... 2293

Estradiol Benzoate (Blood levels and/or toxicity of propranolol may be increased by administration of propranolol hydrochloride extended-release capsules with substrates of CYP1A2).

No products indexed under this heading.

Estradiol Cypionate (Blood levels and/or toxicity of propranolol may be increased by administration of propranolol hydrochloride extended-release capsules with substrates of CYP1A2).

No products indexed under this heading.

Ethanol (Blood levels of propranolol may be decreased by co-administration of propranolol hydrochloride extended-release capsules with inducers of hepatic drug metabolism (e.g., ethanol)).

No products indexed under this heading.

Ethinyl Estradiol (Blood levels and/or toxicity of propranolol may be increased by administration of propranolol hydrochloride extended-release capsules with inhibitors of CYP1A2). Products include:

- Alesse-28 Tablets ... 3392
- Lo/Ovral-28 Tablets ... 3423
- NuvaRing ... 2357
- Ortho-Cept Tablets ... 2395
- Ortho-Cyclen/Ortho Tri-Cyclen ... 2414
- Ortho Evra Transdermal System ... 2402
- Ortho Tri-Cyclen Lo Tablets ... 2421
- Seasonale Tablets ... 1073
- Triphasil-28 Tablets ... 3483
- Yasmin 28 Tablets ... 818

Ethosuximide (Blood levels and/or toxicity of propranolol may be increased by administration of propranolol hydrochloride extended-release capsules with substrates of CYP2C19).

No products indexed under this heading.

Ethotoin (Blood levels and/or toxicity of propranolol may be increased by administration of propranolol hydrochloride extended-release capsules with substrates of CYP2C19). Products include:

- Peganone Tablets, USP ... 2487

Ethynodiol Diacetate (Blood levels and/or toxicity of propranolol may be increased by administration of propranolol hydrochloride extended-release capsules with inhibitors of CYP2C19).

No products indexed under this heading.

Etodolac (Non-steroidal anti-inflammatory drugs have been reported to blunt the antihypertensive effects of beta-adrenoreceptor blocking agents).

No products indexed under this heading.

Felbamate (Blood levels and/or toxicity of propranolol may be increased by administration of propranolol hydrochloride extended-release capsules with inhibitors of CYP2C19).

No products indexed under this heading.

Felodipine (Caution should be exercised when patients receiving a beta-blocker are administered a calcium channel blocking drug with negative inotropic and/or chronotropic effects. Both agents may depress cardiac contractility or atrioventricular conduction). Products include:

- Plendil Extended-Release Tablets ... 651

Fenoprofen Calcium (Non-steroidal anti-inflammatory drugs have been reported to blunt the antihypertensive effects of beta-adrenoreceptor blocking agents). Products include:

- Nalfon Capsules ... 2504

Fentanyl (Blood levels and/or toxicity of propranolol may be increased by administration of propranolol hydrochloride extended-release capsules with substrates of CYP2D6). Products include:

- Duragesic Transdermal System ... 2448

Fentanyl Citrate (Blood levels and/or toxicity of propranolol may be increased by administration of propranolol hydrochloride extended-release capsules with substrates of CYP2D6). Products include:

- Actiq ... 993

Flecainide Acetate (Blood levels and/or toxicity of propranolol may be increased by administration of propranolol hydrochloride extended-release capsules with substrates of CYP2D6). Products include:

- Tambocor Tablets ... 1824

Fluoxetine (Blood levels and/or toxicity of propranolol may be increased by administration of propranolol hydrochloride extended-release capsules with substrates of CYP2D6).

No products indexed under this heading.

Fluoxetine Hydrochloride (Blood levels and/or toxicity of propranolol may be increased by administration of propranolol hydrochloride extended-release capsules with substrates of CYP2D6). Products include:

- Prozac Pulvules and Liquid ... 1771
- Symbyax Capsules ... 1788

Fluphenazine Decanoate (Blood levels and/or toxicity of propranolol may be increased by administration of propranolol hydrochloride extended-release capsules with substrates of CYP2D6).

No products indexed under this heading.

Fluphenazine Enanthate (Blood levels and/or toxicity of propranolol may be increased by administration of propranolol hydrochloride extended-release capsules with substrates of CYP2D6).

No products indexed under this heading.

Fluphenazine Hydrochloride (Blood levels and/or toxicity of propranolol may be increased by administration of propranolol hydrochloride extended-release capsules with substrates of CYP2D6).

No products indexed under this heading.

Flurbiprofen (Non-steroidal anti-inflammatory drugs have been reported to blunt the antihypertensive effects of beta-adrenoreceptor blocking agents).

No products indexed under this heading.

Flutamide (Blood levels and/or toxicity of propranolol may be increased by administration of propranolol hydrochloride extended-release capsules with substrates of CYP1A2). Products include:

- Eulexin Capsules ... 3023

Fluticasone Propionate (Blood levels and/or toxicity of propranolol may be increased by administration of propranolol hydrochloride extended-release capsules with substrates of CYP1A2). Products include:

- Advair Diskus 100/50 ... 1291
- Advair Diskus 250/50 ... 1291
- Advair Diskus 500/50 ... 1291
- Cutivate Cream ... 1381
- Cutivate Lotion 0.05% ... 1383
- Cutivate Ointment ... 1384
- Flonase Nasal Spray ... 1412
- Flovent Diskus 100 mcg ... 1418
- Flovent Diskus 50 mcg ... 1415

Fluvastatin Sodium (Blood levels and/or toxicity of propranolol may be increased by administration of propranolol hydrochloride extended-release capsules with inhibitors of CYP2C19). Products include:

- Lescol Capsules ... 2227
- Lescol ... 2730
- Lescol XL Tablets ... 2227

Fluvoxamine (Blood levels and/or toxicity of propranolol may be increased by administration of propranolol hydrochloride extended-release capsules with inhibitors of CYP1A2).

No products indexed under this heading.

Fluvoxamine Maleate (Blood levels and/or toxicity of propranolol may be increased by administration of propranolol hydrochloride extended-release capsules with substrates of CYP2D6).

No products indexed under this heading.

Formoterol Fumarate (Blood levels and/or toxicity of propranolol may be increased by administration of propranolol hydrochloride extended-release capsules with substrates of CYP2D6). Products include:

- Foradil Aerolizer ... 3024

Fosinopril Sodium (When combined with beta-blockers, ACE inhibitors can cause hypotension, particularly in the setting of acute myocardial infarction. Certain ACE inhibitors have been reported to increase bronchial hyper-reactivity when administered with propranolol).
No products indexed under this heading.

Fosphenytoin (Blood levels and/or toxicity of propranolol may be increased by administration of propranolol hydrochloride extended-release capsules with substrates of CYP2C19).
No products indexed under this heading.

Fosphenytoin Sodium (Blood levels and/or toxicity of propranolol may be increased by administration of propranolol hydrochloride extended-release capsules with substrates of CYP2C19).
No products indexed under this heading.

Gabapentin (Blood levels and/or toxicity of propranolol may be increased by administration of propranolol hydrochloride extended-release capsules with substrates of CYP2C19). Products include:
Neurontin Capsules **2498**
Neurontin Oral Solution **2498**
Neurontin Tablets **2498**

Galantamine Hydrobromide (Blood levels and/or toxicity of propranolol may be increased by administration of propranolol hydrochloride extended-release capsules with substrates of CYP2D6). Products include:
Razadyne ER Extended-Release Capsules **2434**
Razadyne **2434**

Gatifloxacin (Blood levels and/or toxicity of propranolol may be increased by administration of propranolol hydrochloride extended-release capsules with inhibitors of CYP1A2). Products include:
Tequin Injection **964**
Tequin Tablets **964**
Zymar Ophthalmic Solution **571**

Gemifloxacin Mesylate (Blood levels and/or toxicity of propranolol may be increased by administration of propranolol hydrochloride extended-release capsules with inhibitors of CYP1A2). Products include:
Factive Tablets **2464**

Glipizide (Blood levels of propranolol may be decreased by co-administration of propranolol hydrochloride extended-release capsules with inducers of hepatic drug metabolism).
No products indexed under this heading.

Glyburide (Blood levels of propranolol may be decreased by co-administration of propranolol hydrochloride extended-release capsules with inducers of hepatic drug metabolism).
No products indexed under this heading.

Grepafloxacin Hydrochloride (Blood levels and/or toxicity of propranolol may be increased by administration of propranolol hydrochloride extended-release capsules with substrates of CYP1A2).
No products indexed under this heading.

Guanethidine Monosulfate (Patients receiving catecholamine-depleting drugs (e.g., reserpine) and propranolol hydrochloride extended-release capsules should be observed closely for excessive reduction of resting sympathetic nervous activity, which may result in hypotension, marked bradycardia, vertigo, syncopal attacks, or orthostatic hypotension).
No products indexed under this heading.

Halofantrine Hydrochloride (Blood levels and/or toxicity of propranolol may be increased by administration of propranolol hydrochloride extended-release capsules with inhibitors of CYP2D6).
No products indexed under this heading.

Haloperidol (Hypotension and cardiac arrest have been reported with the concomitant use of propranolol and haloperidol).
No products indexed under this heading.

Haloperidol Decanoate (Hypotension and cardiac arrest have been reported with the concomitant use of propranolol and haloperidol).
No products indexed under this heading.

Haloperidol Lactate (Hypotension and cardiac arrest have been reported with the concomitant use of propranolol and haloperidol).
No products indexed under this heading.

Hydrocodone Bitartrate (Blood levels and/or toxicity of propranolol may be increased by administration of propranolol hydrochloride extended-release capsules with substrates of CYP2D6). Products include:
Hycodan **1104**
Hycomine Compound Tablets **1105**
Hycotuss Expectorant Syrup **1106**
Lortab **3315**
Lortab Elixir **3312**
Vicodin Tablets **530**
Vicodin ES Tablets **531**
Vicodin HP Tablets **532**
Vicoprofen Tablets **533**
Zydone Tablets **1118**

Hydroxychloroquine Sulfate (Blood levels and/or toxicity of propranolol may be increased by administration of propranolol hydrochloride extended-release capsules with inhibitors of CYP2D6).
No products indexed under this heading.

Ibuprofen (Non-steroidal anti-inflammatory drugs have been reported to blunt the antihypertensive effects of beta-adrenoreceptor blocking agents). Products include:
Advil Allergy Sinus Caplets **737**
Advil **737**
Children's Advil Suspension **742**
Children's Advil Chewable Tablets **741**
Advil Cold & Sinus **739**
Advil Flu & Body Ache Caplets **739**
Children's Advil Cold Suspension **741**
Infants' Advil Concentrated Drops **743**
Junior Strength Advil Swallow Tablets **740**
Advil Migraine Liquigels **740**
Advil Multi-Symptom Cold Caplets **738**
Combunox Tablets **1183**
Children's Motrin Oral Suspension and Chewable Tablets **1837**
Children's Motrin Cold Non-Staining Dye-Free Oral Suspension **1838**
Children's Motrin Cold Oral Suspension **1838**
Children's Motrin Non-Staining Dye-Free Oral Suspension **1837**
Motrin Cold & Sinus Caplets **1836**
Motrin IB Tablets and Caplets **1836**
Infants' Motrin Concentrated Drops **1837**
Infants' Motrin Non-Staining Dye-Free Drops **1837**
Junior Strength Motrin Caplets and Chewable Tablets **1837**
Vicoprofen Tablets **533**

Imatinib Mesylate (Blood levels and/or toxicity of propranolol may be increased by administration of propranolol hydrochloride extended-release capsules with inhibitors of CYP2D6). Products include:
Gleevec Tablets **2221**

Imipramine Hydrochloride (Blood levels and/or toxicity of propranolol may be increased by administration of propranolol hydrochloride extended-release capsules with substrates of CYP2D6).
No products indexed under this heading.

Imipramine Pamoate (Blood levels and/or toxicity of propranolol may be increased by administration of propranolol hydrochloride extended-release capsules with substrates of CYP2D6).
No products indexed under this heading.

Indomethacin (Administration of indomethacin with propranolol may reduce the efficacy of propranolol in reducing blood pressure and heart rate). Products include:
Indocin **1968**

Indomethacin Sodium Trihydrate (Administration of indomethacin with propranolol may reduce the efficacy of propranolol in reducing blood pressure and heart rate). Products include:
Indocin I.V. **1973**

Indoramin Hydrochloride (Blood levels and/or toxicity of propranolol may be increased by administration of propranolol hydrochloride extended-release capsules with substrates of CYP2D6).
No products indexed under this heading.

Isocarboxazid (The hypotensive effects of MAO inhibitors may be exacerbated when administered with beta-blockers by interfering with the beta-blocking activity of propranolol).
No products indexed under this heading.

Isoetharine (Propranolol is a competitive inhibitor of beta-receptor agonists and its effects can be reversed by administration of such agents (e.g., isoproterenol)).
No products indexed under this heading.

Isoniazid (Blood levels and/or toxicity of propranolol may be increased by administration of propranolol hydrochloride extended-release capsules with inhibitors of CYP1A2).
No products indexed under this heading.

Isoproterenol Hydrochloride (Propranolol is a competitive inhibitor of beta-receptor agonists and its effects can be reversed by administration of such agents (e.g., isoproterenol)).
No products indexed under this heading.

Isoproterenol Sulfate (Propranolol is a competitive inhibitor of beta-receptor agonists and its effects can be reversed by administration of such agents (e.g., isoproterenol)).
No products indexed under this heading.

Isradipine (Caution should be exercised when patients receiving a beta-blocker are administered a calcium channel blocking drug with negative inotropic and/or chronotropic effects. Both agents may depress cardiac contractility or atrioventricular conduction). Products include:
DynaCirc CR Tablets **2726**

Ketoconazole (Blood levels and/or toxicity of propranolol may be increased by administration of propranolol hydrochloride extended-release capsules with inhibitors of CYP1A2). Products include:
Nizoral A-D Shampoo, 1% **1839**
Nizoral 2% Shampoo **1838**

Ketoprofen (Non-steroidal anti-inflammatory drugs have been reported to blunt the antihypertensive effects of beta-adrenoreceptor blocking agents).
No products indexed under this heading.

Ketorolac Tromethamine (Non-steroidal anti-inflammatory drugs have been reported to blunt the antihypertensive effects of beta-adrenoreceptor blocking agents). Products include:
Acular Ophthalmic Solution **561**
Acular LS Ophthalmic Solution **562**

Labetalol Hydrochloride (Blood levels and/or toxicity of propranolol may be increased by administration of propranolol hydrochloride extended-release capsules with substrates of CYP2D6).
No products indexed under this heading.

Lamotrigine (Blood levels and/or toxicity of propranolol may be increased by administration of propranolol hydrochloride extended-release capsules with substrates of CYP2C19). Products include:
Lamictal **1449**

Lansoprazole (Although blood levels and/or toxicity of propranolol may be increased by administration of propranolol hydrochloride extended-release capsules with substrates or inhibitors of CYP2D6, no interaction was observed with lansoprazole). Products include:
Prevacid Delayed-Release Capsules **3268**
Prevacid for Delayed-Release Oral Suspension **3268**
Prevacid I.V. for Injection **3274**
Prevacid NapraPAC **3277**
Prevacid SoluTab Delayed-Release Orally Disintegrating Tablets **3268**
PREVPAC **3281**

Letrozole (Blood levels and/or toxicity of propranolol may be increased by administration of propranolol hydrochloride extended-release capsules with inhibitors of CYP2C19). Products include:
Femara Tablets **2210**

Levalbuterol Hydrochloride (Propranolol is a competitive inhibitor of beta-receptor agonists and its effects can be reversed by administration of such agents (e.g., isoproterenol)). Products include:
Xopenex Inhalation Solution **3143**
Xopenex Inhalation Solution Concentrate **3147**

IMPORTANT NOTE: Always consult each drug listing in the patient's regimen for possible interactions.

Levetiracetam (Blood levels and/or toxicity of propranolol may be increased by administration of propranolol hydrochloride extended-release capsules with substrates of CYP2C19). Products include:
Keppra Oral Solution 3307
Keppra Tablets 3307

Levobupivacaine Hydrochloride (Blood levels and/or toxicity of propranolol may be increased by administration of propranolol hydrochloride extended-release capsules with substrates of CYP1A2).
No products indexed under this heading.

Levofloxacin (Blood levels and/or toxicity of propranolol may be increased by administration of propranolol hydrochloride extended-release capsules with inhibitors of CYP1A2). Products include:
Levaquin in 5% Dextrose Injection 2453
Levaquin 2453
Quixin Ophthalmic Solution 3373

Levonorgestrel (Blood levels and/or toxicity of propranolol may be increased by administration of propranolol hydrochloride extended-release capsules with inhibitors of CYP1A2). Products include:
Alesse-28 Tablets 3392
Climara Pro Transdermal System 800
Mirena Intrauterine System 810
Plan B Tablets 1068
Seasonale Tablets 1073
Triphasil-28 Tablets 3483

Lidocaine (The clearance of lidocaine is reduced with administration of propranolol. Lidocaine toxicity has been reported following co-administration with propranolol. Use caution when administering propranolol hydrochloride extended-release capsules with drugs that slow AV nodal conduction (e.g., lidocaine)). Products include:
Lidoderm Patch 1107

Lidocaine Base (The clearance of lidocaine is reduced with administration of propranolol. Lidocaine toxicity has been reported following co-administration with propranolol. Use caution when administering propranolol hydrochloride extended-release capsules with drugs that slow AV nodal conduction (e.g., lidocaine)).
No products indexed under this heading.

Lidocaine Hydrochloride (The clearance of lidocaine is reduced with administration of propranolol. Lidocaine toxicity has been reported following co-administration with propranolol. Use caution when administering propranolol hydrochloride extended-release capsules with drugs that slow AV nodal conduction (e.g., lidocaine)).
No products indexed under this heading.

Lisinopril (When combined with beta-blockers, ACE inhibitors can cause hypotension, particularly in the setting of acute myocardial infarction. Certain ACE inhibitors have been reported to increase bronchial hyper-reactivity when administered with propranolol). Products include:
Prinivil Tablets 2029
Prinzide Tablets 2033
Zestoretic Tablets 701
Zestril Tablets 704

Lomefloxacin Hydrochloride (Blood levels and/or toxicity of propranolol may be increased by administration of propranolol hydrochloride extended-release capsules with substrates of CYP1A2).
No products indexed under this heading.

Lovastatin (Co-administration of propranolol with lovastatin decreased the AUC of lovastatin but did not alter its pharmacodynamics). Products include:
Advicor Tablets 1694
Altoprev Extended-Release Tablets 1151
Mevacor Tablets 1996

Maprotiline Hydrochloride (Blood levels and/or toxicity of propranolol may be increased by administration of propranolol hydrochloride extended-release capsules with substrates of CYP2D6).
No products indexed under this heading.

Meclofenamate Sodium (Non-steroidal anti-inflammatory drugs have been reported to blunt the antihypertensive effects of beta-adrenoreceptor blocking agents).
No products indexed under this heading.

Mefenamic Acid (Non-steroidal anti-inflammatory drugs have been reported to blunt the antihypertensive effects of beta-adrenoreceptor blocking agents).
No products indexed under this heading.

Meloxicam (Non-steroidal anti-inflammatory drugs have been reported to blunt the antihypertensive effects of beta-adrenoreceptor blocking agents). Products include:
Mobic Oral Suspension 893
Mobic Tablets 893

Meperidine Hydrochloride (Blood levels and/or toxicity of propranolol may be increased by administration of propranolol hydrochloride extended-release capsules with substrates of CYP2D6).
No products indexed under this heading.

Mephenytoin (Blood levels and/or toxicity of propranolol may be increased by administration of propranolol hydrochloride extended-release capsules with substrates of CYP2C19).
No products indexed under this heading.

Mephobarbital (Blood levels and/or toxicity of propranolol may be increased by administration of propranolol hydrochloride extended-release capsules with substrates of CYP2C19). Products include:
Mebaral Tablets, USP 2483

Meprobamate (Blood levels and/or toxicity of propranolol may be increased by administration of propranolol hydrochloride extended-release capsules with substrates of CYP2C19).
No products indexed under this heading.

Mestranol (Blood levels and/or toxicity of propranolol may be increased by administration of propranolol hydrochloride extended-release capsules with inhibitors of CYP1A2).
No products indexed under this heading.

Metaproterenol Sulfate (Propranolol is a competitive inhibitor of beta-receptor agonists and its effects can be reversed by administration of such agents (e.g., isoproterenol)). Products include:
Alupent Inhalation Aerosol 858

Methadone Hydrochloride (Blood levels and/or toxicity of propranolol may be increased by administration of propranolol hydrochloride extended-release capsules with substrates of CYP2D6).
No products indexed under this heading.

Methamphetamine Hydrochloride (Blood levels and/or toxicity of propranolol may be increased by administration of propranolol hydrochloride extended-release capsules with substrates of CYP2D6). Products include:
Desoxyn Tablets, USP 2482

Methoxsalen (Blood levels and/or toxicity of propranolol may be increased by administration of propranolol hydrochloride extended-release capsules with inhibitors of CYP1A2). Products include:
Oxsoralen Lotion 1% 3354
Oxsoralen-Ultra Capsules 3354

Methoxyflurane (May depress myocardial contractility when administered with propranolol).
No products indexed under this heading.

Methsuximide (Blood levels and/or toxicity of propranolol may be increased by administration of propranolol hydrochloride extended-release capsules with substrates of CYP2C19).
No products indexed under this heading.

Metoprolol Succinate (Blood levels and/or toxicity of propranolol may be increased by administration of propranolol hydrochloride extended-release capsules with substrates of CYP2D6). Products include:
Toprol-XL Tablets 660

Metoprolol Tartrate (Blood levels and/or toxicity of propranolol may be increased by administration of propranolol hydrochloride extended-release capsules with substrates of CYP2D6).
No products indexed under this heading.

Mexiletine Hydrochloride (Blood levels and/or toxicity of propranolol may be increased by administration of propranolol hydrochloride extended-release capsules with substrates of CYP2D6).
No products indexed under this heading.

Mibefradil Dihydrochloride (Blood levels and/or toxicity of propranolol may be increased by administration of propranolol hydrochloride extended-release capsules with inhibitors of CYP2D6).
No products indexed under this heading.

Midazolam Hydrochloride (Blood levels and/or toxicity of propranolol may be increased by administration of propranolol hydrochloride extended-release capsules with substrates of CYP2C19).
No products indexed under this heading.

Mirtazapine (Blood levels and/or toxicity of propranolol may be increased by administration of propranolol hydrochloride extended-release capsules with substrates of CYP2D6).
No products indexed under this heading.

Moclobemide (Blood levels and/or toxicity of propranolol may be increased by administration of propranolol hydrochloride extended-release capsules with inhibitors of CYP2D6).
No products indexed under this heading.

Modafinil (Blood levels and/or toxicity of propranolol may be increased by administration of propranolol hydrochloride extended-release capsules with inhibitors of CYP2C19). Products include:
Provigil Tablets 1002

Moexipril Hydrochloride (When combined with beta-blockers, ACE inhibitors can cause hypotension, particularly in the setting of acute myocardial infarction. Certain ACE inhibitors have been reported to increase bronchial hyper-reactivity when administered with propranolol). Products include:
Uniretic Tablets 3114
Univasc Tablets 3118

Morphine Sulfate (Blood levels and/or toxicity of propranolol may be increased by administration of propranolol hydrochloride extended-release capsules with substrates of CYP2D6). Products include:
Avinza Capsules 1714
Kadian Capsules 572
MS Contin Tablets 2703

Moxifloxacin Hydrochloride (Blood levels and/or toxicity of propranolol may be increased by administration of propranolol hydrochloride extended-release capsules with substrates of CYP1A2). Products include:
Avelox 2984
Vigamox Ophthalmic Solution 560

Nabumetone (Non-steroidal anti-inflammatory drugs have been reported to blunt the antihypertensive effects of beta-adrenoreceptor blocking agents). Products include:
Relafen Tablets 1523

Nafcillin Sodium (Blood levels and/or toxicity of propranolol may be increased by administration of propranolol hydrochloride extended-release capsules with substrates of CYP1A2).
No products indexed under this heading.

Nalidixic Acid (Blood levels and/or toxicity of propranolol may be increased by administration of propranolol hydrochloride extended-release capsules with inhibitors of CYP1A2).
No products indexed under this heading.

Naproxen (Blood levels and/or toxicity of propranolol may be increased by administration of propranolol hydrochloride extended-release capsules with substrates of CYP1A2). Products include:
EC-Naprosyn Delayed-Release Tablets 2769
Naprosyn Suspension 2769
Naprosyn Tablets 2769
Prevacid NapraPAC 3277

Naproxen Sodium (Blood levels and/or toxicity of propranolol may

be increased by administration of propranolol hydrochloride extended-release capsules with substrates of CYP1A2). Products include:
Aleve Tablets, Caplets and Gelcaps 605
Anaprox Tablets 2769
Anaprox DS Tablets 2769

Nelfinavir Mesylate (Blood levels and/or toxicity of propranolol may be increased by administration of propranolol hydrochloride extended-release capsules with substrates of CYP2D6). Products include:
Viracept 2556

Nicardipine (The mean Cmax and AUC of propranolol are increased by 80% and 47%, respectively, by co-administration with nicardipine).
No products indexed under this heading.

Nicardipine Hydrochloride (The mean Cmax and AUC of propranolol are increased by 80% and 47%, respectively, by co-administration with nicardipine). Products include:
Cardene I.V. 1129

Nicotine Polacrilex (Blood levels and/or toxicity of propranolol may be increased by administration of propranolol hydrochloride extended-release capsules with substrates of CYP1A2). Products include:
Commit Lozenges 1625
Nicorette Gum 1632

Nicotine Salicylate (Blood levels and/or toxicity of propranolol may be increased by administration of propranolol hydrochloride extended-release capsules with substrates of CYP1A2).
No products indexed under this heading.

Nicotine Sulfate (Blood levels and/or toxicity of propranolol may be increased by administration of propranolol hydrochloride extended-release capsules with substrates of CYP1A2).
No products indexed under this heading.

Nifedipine (The mean Cmax and AUC of nifedipine are increased by 64% and 79%, respectively, by co-administration with propranolol). Products include:
Adalat CC Tablets 2978

Nilutamide (Blood levels and/or toxicity of propranolol may be increased by administration of propranolol hydrochloride extended-release capsules with substrates of CYP2C19).
No products indexed under this heading.

Nimodipine (Caution should be exercised when patients receiving a beta-blocker are administered a calcium channel blocking drug with negative inotropic and/or chronotropic effects. Both agents may depress cardiac contractility or atrioventricular conduction). Products include:
Nimotop Capsules 774

Nisoldipine (The mean Cmax and AUC of propranolol are increased by 50% and 30%, respectively, by co-administration with nisoldipine). Products include:
Sular Tablets 1163

Norethindrone (Blood levels and/or toxicity of propranolol may be increased by administration of propranolol hydrochloride extended-release capsules with inhibitors of CYP1A2). Products include:
Ortho Micronor Tablets 2411

Norethindrone Acetate (Blood levels and/or toxicity of propranolol may be increased by administration of propranolol hydrochloride extended-release capsules with substrates of CYP1A2). Products include:
Activella Tablets 2311
Aygestin Tablets 1062
CombiPatch Transdermal System 2180

Norethynodrel (Blood levels and/or toxicity of propranolol may be increased by administration of propranolol hydrochloride extended-release capsules with inhibitors of CYP2C19).
No products indexed under this heading.

Norfloxacin (Blood levels and/or toxicity of propranolol may be increased by administration of propranolol hydrochloride extended-release capsules with substrates of CYP1A2). Products include:
Noroxin Tablets 2009

Norgestimate (Blood levels and/or toxicity of propranolol may be increased by administration of propranolol hydrochloride extended-release capsules with inhibitors of CYP2C19). Products include:
Ortho-Cyclen/Ortho Tri-Cyclen 2414
Ortho Tri-Cyclen Lo Tablets 2421
Prefest Tablets 1069

Norgestrel (Blood levels and/or toxicity of propranolol may be increased by administration of propranolol hydrochloride extended-release capsules with inhibitors of CYP1A2). Products include:
Lo/Ovral-28 Tablets 3423

Nortriptyline Hydrochloride (Blood levels and/or toxicity of propranolol may be increased by administration of propranolol hydrochloride extended-release capsules with substrates of CYP2D6).
No products indexed under this heading.

Ofloxacin (Blood levels and/or toxicity of propranolol may be increased by administration of propranolol hydrochloride extended-release capsules with substrates of CYP1A2). Products include:
Floxin Otic Singles 1045
Floxin Otic Solution 1043

Olanzapine (Blood levels and/or toxicity of propranolol may be increased by administration of propranolol hydrochloride extended-release capsules with substrates of CYP2D6). Products include:
Symbyax Capsules 1788
Zyprexa Tablets 1798
Zyprexa IntraMuscular 1798
Zyprexa ZYDIS Orally Disintegrating Tablets 1798

Omeprazole (Although blood levels and/or toxicity of propranolol may be increased by administration of propranolol hydrochloride extended-release capsules with substrates or inhibitors of CYP2C19, no interaction was observed with omeprazole). Products include:
Zegerid Powder for Oral Solution 2972

Omeprazole magnesium (Although blood levels and/or toxicity of propranolol may be increased by administration of propranolol hydrochloride extended-release capsules with substrates or inhibitors of CYP2C19, no interaction was observed with omeprazole). Products include:
Prilosec OTC Tablets 2674

Ondansetron (Blood levels and/or toxicity of propranolol may be increased by administration of propranolol hydrochloride extended-release capsules with substrates of CYP2D6). Products include:
Zofran ODT Orally Disintegrating Tablets 1613

Ondansetron Hydrochloride (Blood levels and/or toxicity of propranolol may be increased by administration of propranolol hydrochloride extended-release capsules with substrates of CYP2D6). Products include:
Zofran Injection 1607
Zofran 1613

Oxaprozin (Non-steroidal anti-inflammatory drugs have been reported to blunt the antihypertensive effects of beta-adrenoreceptor blocking agents).
No products indexed under this heading.

Oxcarbazepine (Blood levels and/or toxicity of propranolol may be increased by administration of propranolol hydrochloride extended-release capsules with inhibitors of CYP2C19). Products include:
Trileptal Oral Suspension 2281
Trileptal Tablets 2281

Oxycodone Hydrochloride (Blood levels and/or toxicity of propranolol may be increased by administration of propranolol hydrochloride extended-release capsules with substrates of CYP2D6). Products include:
Combunox Tablets 1183
OxyContin Tablets 2699
OxyFast Oral Concentrate Solution 2704
OxyIR Capsules 2704
Percocet Tablets 1114
Percodan Tablets 1115

Paclitaxel (Blood levels and/or toxicity of propranolol may be increased by administration of propranolol hydrochloride extended-release capsules with substrates of CYP2D6).
No products indexed under this heading.

Pantoprazole Sodium (Blood levels and/or toxicity of propranolol may be increased by administration of propranolol hydrochloride extended-release capsules with substrates of CYP2C19). Products include:
Protonix I.V. 3468
Protonix Tablets 3465

Paramethadione (Blood levels and/or toxicity of propranolol may be increased by administration of propranolol hydrochloride extended-release capsules with substrates of CYP2C19).
No products indexed under this heading.

Pargyline Hydrochloride (The hypotensive effects of MAO inhibitors may be exacerbated when administered with beta-blockers by interfering with the beta-blocking activity of propranolol).
No products indexed under this heading.

Paroxetine Hydrochloride (Blood levels and/or toxicity of propranolol may be increased by administration of propranolol hydrochloride extended-release capsules with substrates of CYP2D6). Products include:
Paxil CR Controlled-Release Tablets 1509
Paxil 1501

Pentamidine Isethionate (Blood levels and/or toxicity of propranolol may be increased by administration of propranolol hydrochloride extended-release capsules with substrates of CYP2C19).
No products indexed under this heading.

Perindopril Erbumine (When combined with beta-blockers, ACE inhibitors can cause hypotension, particularly in the setting of acute myocardial infarction. Certain ACE inhibitors have been reported to increase bronchial hyper-reactivity when administered with propranolol). Products include:
Aceon Tablets (2 mg, 4 mg, 8 mg) 3191

Perphenazine (Blood levels and/or toxicity of propranolol may be increased by administration of propranolol hydrochloride extended-release capsules with inhibitors of CYP2D6).
No products indexed under this heading.

Phenacemide (Blood levels and/or toxicity of propranolol may be increased by administration of propranolol hydrochloride extended-release capsules with substrates of CYP2C19).
No products indexed under this heading.

Phenelzine Sulfate (The hypotensive effects of MAO inhibitors may be exacerbated when administered with beta-blockers by interfering with the beta-blocking activity of propranolol).
No products indexed under this heading.

Phenobarbital (Blood levels and/or toxicity of propranolol may be increased by administration of propranolol hydrochloride extended-release capsules with substrates of CYP2C19).
No products indexed under this heading.

Phenobarbital Sodium (Blood levels and/or toxicity of propranolol may be increased by administration of propranolol hydrochloride extended-release capsules with substrates of CYP1A2).
No products indexed under this heading.

Phensuximide (Blood levels and/or toxicity of propranolol may be increased by administration of propranolol hydrochloride extended-release capsules with substrates of CYP2C19).
No products indexed under this heading.

Phenylbutazone (Non-steroidal anti-inflammatory drugs have been reported to blunt the antihypertensive effects of beta-adrenoreceptor blocking agents).
No products indexed under this heading.

Phenytoin (Blood levels and/or toxicity of propranolol may be increased by administration of propranolol hydrochloride extended-release capsules with substrates of CYP2C19).
No products indexed under this heading.

Phenytoin Sodium (Blood levels and/or toxicity of propranolol may be increased by administration of propranolol hydrochloride extended-release capsules with substrates of CYP1A2). Products include:

Phenytek Capsules 2153

Pindolol (Blood levels and/or toxicity of propranolol may be increased by administration of propranolol hydrochloride extended-release capsules with substrates of CYP2D6).
No products indexed under this heading.

Pirbuterol Acetate (Propranolol is a competitive inhibitor of beta-receptor agonists and its effects can be reversed by administration of such agents (e.g., isoproterenol)). Products include:
Maxair Autohaler 1820

Piroxicam (Non-steroidal anti-inflammatory drugs have been reported to blunt the antihypertensive effects of beta-adrenoreceptor blocking agents).
No products indexed under this heading.

Pravastatin Sodium (Co-administration of propranolol with pravastatin decreased the AUC of pravastatin but did not alter its pharmacodynamics). Products include:
Pravachol Tablets 943

Prazosin Hydrochloride (Prazosin has been associated with prolongation of first dose hypotension in the presence of beta-blockers).
No products indexed under this heading.

Primidone (Blood levels and/or toxicity of propranolol may be increased by administration of propranolol hydrochloride extended-release capsules with substrates of CYP2C19).
No products indexed under this heading.

Procarbazine Hydrochloride (The hypotensive effects of MAO inhibitors may be exacerbated when administered with beta-blockers by interfering with the beta-blocking activity of propranolol). Products include:
Matulane Capsules 3188

Progesterone (Blood levels and/or toxicity of propranolol may be increased by administration of propranolol hydrochloride extended-release capsules with substrates of CYP2C19). Products include:
Prochieve 4% Gel 1018
Prochieve 8% Gel 1018
Prometrium Capsules (100 mg, 200 mg).. 3205

Proguanil Hydrochloride (Blood levels and/or toxicity of propranolol may be increased by administration of propranolol hydrochloride extended-release capsules with substrates of CYP2C19). Products include:
Malarone Tablets 1484
Malarone Pediatric Tablets 1484

Propafenone Hydrochloride (Propafenone has negative inotropic and beta-blocking properties that can be additive to those of propranolol. The AUC of propafenone is increased by more than 200% by co-administration with propranolol). Products include:
Rythmol SR Capsules 2736

Propoxyphene Hydrochloride (Blood levels and/or toxicity of propranolol may be increased by administration of propranolol hydrochloride extended-release capsules with substrates of CYP2D6).
No products indexed under this heading.

Propoxyphene Napsylate (Blood levels and/or toxicity of propranolol may be increased by administration of propranolol hydrochloride extended-release capsules with substrates of CYP2D6). Products include:
Darvocet A 500 Tablets 3497

Protriptyline Hydrochloride (Blood levels and/or toxicity of propranolol may be increased by administration of propranolol hydrochloride extended-release capsules with inhibitors of CYP2D6). Products include:
Vivactil Tablets 2350

Quetiapine Fumarate (Blood levels and/or toxicity of propranolol may be increased by administration of propranolol hydrochloride extended-release capsules with substrates of CYP2D6). Products include:
Seroquel Tablets 691

Quinacrine Hydrochloride (Blood levels and/or toxicity of propranolol may be increased by administration of propranolol hydrochloride extended-release capsules with inhibitors of CYP2D6).
No products indexed under this heading.

Quinapril Hydrochloride (When combined with beta-blockers, ACE inhibitors can cause hypotension, particularly in the setting of acute myocardial infarction. Certain ACE inhibitors have been reported to increase bronchial hyper-reactivity when administered with propranolol).
No products indexed under this heading.

Quinidine (Quinidine increases the concentration of propranolol and produces greater degrees of clinical beta-blockade and may cause postural hypotension).
No products indexed under this heading.

Quinidine Gluconate (Quinidine increases the concentration of propranolol and produces greater degrees of clinical beta-blockade and may cause postural hypotension).
No products indexed under this heading.

Quinidine Hydrochloride (Quinidine increases the concentration of propranolol and produces greater degrees of clinical beta-blockade and may cause postural hypotension).
No products indexed under this heading.

Quinidine Polygalacturonate (Quinidine increases the concentration of propranolol and produces greater degrees of clinical beta-blockade and may cause postural hypotension).
No products indexed under this heading.

Quinidine Sulfate (Quinidine increases the concentration of propranolol and produces greater degrees of clinical beta-blockade and may cause postural hypotension).
No products indexed under this heading.

Rabeprazole Sodium (Blood levels and/or toxicity of propranolol may be increased by administration of propranolol hydrochloride extended-release capsules with substrates of CYP2C19). Products include:
Aciphex Tablets 1081

Ramipril (When combined with beta-blockers, ACE inhibitors can cause hypotension, particularly in the setting of acute myocardial infarction. Certain ACE inhibitors have been reported to increase bronchial hyper-reactivity when administered with propranolol). Products include:
Altace Capsules 1673

Ranitidine Bismuth Citrate (Although blood levels and/or toxicity of propranolol may be increased by administration of propranolol hydrochloride extended-release capsules with substrates or inhibitors of CYP2D6, no interaction was observed with ranitidine).
No products indexed under this heading.

Ranitidine Hydrochloride (Although blood levels and/or toxicity of propranolol may be increased by administration of propranolol hydrochloride extended-release capsules with substrates or inhibitors of CYP2D6, no interaction was observed with ranitidine). Products include:
Zantac 1597
Zantac Injection 1593
Zantac 75 Tablets .... ▣715
Zantac 150 Maximum Strength Tablets.. ▣715
Zantac Injection Pharmacy Bulk Package.. 1595

Rauwolfia Serpentina (Patients receiving catecholamine-depleting drugs (e.g., reserpine) and propranolol hydrochloride extended-release capsules should be observed closely for excessive reduction of resting sympathetic nervous activity, which may result in hypotension, marked bradycardia, vertigo, syncopal attacks, or orthostatic hypotension).
No products indexed under this heading.

Rescinnamine (Patients receiving catecholamine-depleting drugs (e.g., reserpine) and propranolol hydrochloride extended-release capsules should be observed closely for excessive reduction of resting sympathetic nervous activity, which may result in hypotension, marked bradycardia, vertigo, syncopal attacks, or orthostatic hypotension).
No products indexed under this heading.

Reserpine (Patients receiving catecholamine-depleting drugs (e.g., reserpine) and propranolol hydrochloride extended-release capsules should be observed closely for excessive reduction of resting sympathetic nervous activity, which may result in hypotension, marked bradycardia, vertigo, syncopal attacks, or orthostatic hypotension. Administration of reserpine with propranolol may also potentiate depression).
No products indexed under this heading.

Rifampin (Blood levels of propranolol may be decreased by administration of propranolol hydrochloride extended-release capsules with inducers of hepatic drug metabolism, such as rifampin).
No products indexed under this heading.

Rifapentine (Blood levels of propranolol may be decreased by co-administration of propranolol hydrochloride extended-release capsules with inducers of hepatic drug metabolism).
No products indexed under this heading.

Riluzole (Blood levels and/or toxicity of propranolol may be increased by administration of propranolol hydrochloride extended-release capsules with substrates of CYP1A2). Products include:
Rilutek Tablets 2945

Risperidone (Blood levels and/or toxicity of propranolol may be increased by administration of propranolol hydrochloride extended-release capsules with substrates of CYP2D6). Products include:
Risperdal Consta Long-Acting Injection 1664
Risperdal M-Tab Orally Disintegrating Tablets................. 1658
Risperdal 1658

Ritonavir (Blood levels and/or toxicity of propranolol may be increased by administration of propranolol hydrochloride extended-release capsules with substrates of CYP2D6). Products include:
Kaletra 474
Norvir 499

Rizatriptan Benzoate (Co-administration of rizatriptan with propranolol resulted in increased concentrations of rizatriptan (AUC increased by 67% and Cmax by 75%)). Products include:
Maxalt Tablets 1983
Maxalt-MLT Orally Disintegrating Tablets 1983

Rofecoxib (Non-steroidal anti-inflammatory drugs have been reported to blunt the antihypertensive effects of beta-adrenoreceptor blocking agents).
No products indexed under this heading.

Ropinirole Hydrochloride (Blood levels and/or toxicity of propranolol may be increased by administration of propranolol hydrochloride extended-release capsules with substrates of CYP1A2). Products include:
Requip Tablets 1528

Ropivacaine Hydrochloride (Blood levels and/or toxicity of propranolol may be increased by administration of propranolol hydrochloride extended-release capsules with substrates of CYP1A2). Products include:
Naropin Injection 640

Salmeterol Xinafoate (Propranolol is a competitive inhibitor of beta-receptor agonists and its effects can be reversed by administration of such agents (e.g., isoproterenol)). Products include:
Advair Diskus 100/50 1291
Advair Diskus 250/50 1291
Advair Diskus 500/50 1291
Serevent Diskus 1540

Selegiline Hydrochloride (The hypotensive effects of MAO inhibitors may be exacerbated when administered with beta-blockers by interfering with the beta-blocking activity of propranolol). Products include:
Eldepryl Capsules 3209

Sertraline Hydrochloride (Blood levels and/or toxicity of propranolol may be increased by administration of propranolol hydrochloride

extended-release capsules with inhibitors of CYP2D6). Products include:

Zoloft 2581

Sparfloxacin (Blood levels and/or toxicity of propranolol may be increased by administration of propranolol hydrochloride extended-release capsules with inhibitors of CYP1A2).

No products indexed under this heading.

Spirapril Hydrochloride (When combined with beta-blockers, ACE inhibitors can cause hypotension, particularly in the setting of acute myocardial infarction. Certain ACE inhibitors have been reported to increase bronchial hyper-reactivity when administered with propranolol).

No products indexed under this heading.

Sulfaphenazole (Blood levels and/or toxicity of propranolol may be increased by administration of propranolol hydrochloride extended-release capsules with inhibitors of CYP2C19).

No products indexed under this heading.

Sulindac (Non-steroidal anti-inflammatory drugs have been reported to blunt the antihypertensive effects of beta-adrenoreceptor blocking agents). Products include:

Clinoril Tablets 1899

Tacrine Hydrochloride (Blood levels and/or toxicity of propranolol may be increased by administration of propranolol hydrochloride extended-release capsules with substrates of CYP1A2).

No products indexed under this heading.

Tamoxifen Citrate (Blood levels and/or toxicity of propranolol may be increased by administration of propranolol hydrochloride extended-release capsules with substrates of CYP2D6).

No products indexed under this heading.

Telmisartan (Blood levels and/or toxicity of propranolol may be increased by administration of propranolol hydrochloride extended-release capsules with inhibitors of CYP2C19). Products include:

Micardis Tablets 884
Micardis HCT Tablets 886

Teniposide (Blood levels and/or toxicity of propranolol may be increased by administration of propranolol hydrochloride extended-release capsules with substrates of CYP2D6).

No products indexed under this heading.

Terazosin Hydrochloride (Postural hypotension has been reported in patients taking both beta-blockers and terazosin). Products include:

Hytrin Capsules 469

Terbinafine Hydrochloride (Blood levels and/or toxicity of propranolol may be increased by administration of propranolol hydrochloride extended-release capsules with inhibitors of CYP2D6). Products include:

Lamisil AT Creams (Athlete's Foot & Jock Itch) 676
Lamisil Tablets 2226

Terbutaline Sulfate (Propranolol is a competitive inhibitor of beta-receptor agonists and its effects can be reversed by administration of such agents (e.g., isoproterenol)).

No products indexed under this heading.

Testosterone (Blood levels and/or toxicity of propranolol may be increased by administration of propranolol hydrochloride extended-release capsules with substrates of CYP2D6). Products include:

AndroGel 3330
Striant Mucoadhesive 1022
Testim 1% Gel 722

Testosterone Cypionate (Blood levels and/or toxicity of propranolol may be increased by administration of propranolol hydrochloride extended-release capsules with substrates of CYP2D6).

No products indexed under this heading.

Testosterone Enanthate (Blood levels and/or toxicity of propranolol may be increased by administration of propranolol hydrochloride extended-release capsules with substrates of CYP2D6). Products include:

Delatestryl Injection 2976

Testosterone Propionate (Blood levels and/or toxicity of propranolol may be increased by administration of propranolol hydrochloride extended-release capsules with substrates of CYP2D6).

No products indexed under this heading.

Theophylline (Co-administration of theophylline with propranolol decreases theophylline oral clearance by 33% to 52%).

No products indexed under this heading.

Theophylline Anhydrous (Co-administration of theophylline with propranolol decreases theophylline oral clearance by 33% to 52%). Products include:

Uniphyl Tablets 2708

Theophylline Calcium Salicylate (Co-administration of theophylline with propranolol decreases theophylline oral clearance by 33% to 52%).

No products indexed under this heading.

Theophylline Dihydroxypropyl (Glyceryl) (Co-administration of theophylline with propranolol decreases theophylline oral clearance by 33% to 52%).

No products indexed under this heading.

Theophylline Ethylenediamine (Co-administration of theophylline with propranolol decreases theophylline oral clearance by 33% to 52%).

No products indexed under this heading.

Theophylline Sodium Glycinate (Co-administration of theophylline with propranolol decreases theophylline oral clearance by 33% to 52%).

No products indexed under this heading.

Thioridazine (Co-administration of propranolol at doses greater than or equal to 160 mg/day resulted in increased thioridazine plasma concentrations, ranging from 50% to 370%, and increased thioridazine metabolites concentrations, ranging from 33% to 210%).

No products indexed under this heading.

Thioridazine Hydrochloride (Co-administration of propranolol at doses greater than or equal to 160 mg/day resulted in increased thioridazine plasma concentrations, ranging from 50% to 370%, and increased thioridazine metabolites concentrations, ranging from 33% to 210%). Products include:

Thioridazine Hydrochloride Tablets 2122

Thyroxine (Thyroxine may result in a lower than expected T3 concentration when used concomitantly with propranolol).

No products indexed under this heading.

Thyroxine Sodium (Thyroxine may result in a lower than expected T3 concentration when used concomitantly with propranolol).

No products indexed under this heading.

Tiagabine Hydrochloride (Blood levels and/or toxicity of propranolol may be increased by administration of propranolol hydrochloride extended-release capsules with substrates of CYP2C19). Products include:

Gabitril Tablets 998

Ticlopidine Hydrochloride (Blood levels and/or toxicity of propranolol may be increased by administration of propranolol hydrochloride extended-release capsules with inhibitors of CYP1A2). Products include:

Ticlid Tablets 2813

Timolol Maleate (Blood levels and/or toxicity of propranolol may be increased by administration of propranolol hydrochloride extended-release capsules with substrates of CYP2D6). Products include:

Blocadren Tablets 1891
Cosopt Sterile Ophthalmic Solution 1910
Timolide Tablets 2056
Timoptic in Ocudose 2061
Timoptic Sterile Ophthalmic Solution 2058
Timoptic-XE Sterile Ophthalmic Gel Forming Solution 2062

Tolazamide (Blood levels of propranolol may be decreased by co-administration of propranolol hydrochloride extended-release capsules with inducers of hepatic drug metabolism).

No products indexed under this heading.

Tolbutamide (Blood levels and/or toxicity of propranolol may be increased by administration of propranolol hydrochloride extended-release capsules with inhibitors of CYP2C19).

No products indexed under this heading.

Tolbutamide Sodium (Blood levels and/or toxicity of propranolol may be increased by administration of propranolol hydrochloride extended-release capsules with inhibitors of CYP2C19).

No products indexed under this heading.

Tolmetin Sodium (Non-steroidal anti-inflammatory drugs have been reported to blunt the antihypertensive effects of beta-adrenoreceptor blocking agents).

No products indexed under this heading.

Tolterodine Tartrate (Blood levels and/or toxicity of propranolol may be increased by administration of propranolol hydrochloride extended-release capsules with substrates of CYP2D6). Products include:

Detrol Tablets 2626
Detrol LA Capsules 2629

Topiramate (Blood levels and/or toxicity of propranolol may be increased by administration of propranolol hydrochloride extended-release capsules with inhibitors of CYP2C19). Products include:

Topamax Sprinkle Capsules 2438
Topamax Tablets 2438

Tramadol Hydrochloride (Blood levels and/or toxicity of propranolol may be increased by administration of propranolol hydrochloride extended-release capsules with substrates of CYP2D6). Products include:

Ultracet Tablets 2462

Trandolapril (When combined with beta-blockers, ACE inhibitors can cause hypotension, particularly in the setting of acute myocardial infarction. Certain ACE inhibitors have been reported to increase bronchial hyper-reactivity when administered with propranolol). Products include:

Mavik Tablets 482
Tarka Tablets 519

Tranylcypromine Sulfate (The hypotensive effects of MAO inhibitors may be exacerbated when administered with beta-blockers by interfering with the beta-blocking activity of propranolol). Products include:

Parnate Tablets 1499

Trazodone Hydrochloride (Blood levels and/or toxicity of propranolol may be increased by administration of propranolol hydrochloride extended-release capsules with substrates of CYP2D6).

No products indexed under this heading.

Triazolam (Blood levels and/or toxicity of propranolol may be increased by administration of propranolol hydrochloride extended-release capsules with substrates of CYP2D6).

No products indexed under this heading.

Trichloroethylene (May depress myocardial contractility when administered with propranolol).

No products indexed under this heading.

Trimethadione (Blood levels and/or toxicity of propranolol may be increased by administration of propranolol hydrochloride extended-release capsules with substrates of CYP2C19).

No products indexed under this heading.

Trimethaphan Camsylate (Blood levels and/or toxicity of propranolol may be increased by administration of propranolol hydrochloride extended-release capsules with substrates of CYP1A2).

No products indexed under this heading.

Trimipramine Maleate (Blood levels and/or toxicity of propranolol may be increased by administration of propranolol hydrochloride extended-release capsules with substrates of CYP2D6). Products include:

Surmontil Capsules 2347

IMPORTANT NOTE: Always consult each drug listing in the patient's regimen for possible interactions.

Troleandomycin (Blood levels and/or toxicity of propranolol may be increased by administration of propranolol hydrochloride extended-release capsules with inhibitors of CYP1A2).
No products indexed under this heading.

Trovafloxacin Mesylate (Blood levels and/or toxicity of propranolol may be increased by administration of propranolol hydrochloride extended-release capsules with substrates of CYP1A2).
No products indexed under this heading.

Valdecoxib (Non-steroidal anti-inflammatory drugs have been reported to blunt the antihypertensive effects of beta-adrenoreceptor blocking agents).
No products indexed under this heading.

Valproate Sodium (Blood levels and/or toxicity of propranolol may be increased by administration of propranolol hydrochloride extended-release capsules with substrates of CYP2C19). Products include:
Depacon Injection **412**

Valproic Acid (Blood levels and/or toxicity of propranolol may be increased by administration of propranolol hydrochloride extended-release capsules with substrates of CYP2C19). Products include:
Depakene **417**

Venlafaxine Hydrochloride (Blood levels and/or toxicity of propranolol may be increased by administration of propranolol hydrochloride extended-release capsules with substrates of CYP2D6). Products include:
Effexor Tablets **3405**
Effexor XR Capsules **3411**

Verapamil Hydrochloride (There have been reports of significant bradycardia, heart failure, and cardiovascular collapse with concurrent use of verapamil and beta-blockers). Products include:
Covera-HS Tablets **3135**
Tarka Tablets **519**
Verelan PM Capsules **3120**

Vinblastine Sulfate (Blood levels and/or toxicity of propranolol may be increased by administration of propranolol hydrochloride extended-release capsules with substrates of CYP2D6).
No products indexed under this heading.

Voriconazole (Blood levels and/or toxicity of propranolol may be increased by administration of propranolol hydrochloride extended-release capsules with inhibitors of CYP2C19). Products include:
VFEND I.V. **2543**
VFEND Oral Suspension **2543**
VFEND Tablets **2543**

Warfarin Sodium (Concomitant administration of propranolol and warfarin has been shown to increase warfarin bioavailability and concentration, as well as increasing prothrombin time; therefore, prothrombin time should be monitored). Products include:
Coumadin for Injection **932**
Coumadin Tablets **932**

Zileuton (Blood levels and/or toxicity of propranolol may be increased by administration of propranolol hydrochloride extended-release capsules with substrates of CYP1A2).
No products indexed under this heading.

Zolmitriptan (Co-administration of zolmitriptan with propranolol resulted in increased concentrations of zolmitriptan (AUC increased by 56% and Cmax by 37%)). Products include:
Zomig Nasal Spray **718**
Zomig Tablets **714**
Zomig-ZMT Tablets **714**

Zonisamide (Blood levels and/or toxicity of propranolol may be increased by administration of propranolol hydrochloride extended-release capsules with substrates of CYP2D6). Products include:
Zonegran Capsules **1089**

Food Interactions

Grapefruit Juice (Blood levels and/or toxicity of propranolol may be increased by administration of propranolol hydrochloride extended-release capsules with inhibitors of CYP1A2).

INNOVO

(Device) **2314**
None cited in PDR database.

INSPRA TABLETS

(Eplerenone) **2520**
May interact with ACE inhibitors, angiotensin-II receptor antagonists, cytochrome p450 3a4 inhibitors (selected), non-steroidal anti-inflammatory agents, potassium preparations, potassium sparing diuretics, and certain other agents. Compounds in these categories include:

Acetazolamide (Eplerenone should not be used with strong inhibitors of CYP450 3A4. Potent inhibitors of CYP3A4 caused increased exposure of about 5-fold, while less potent CYP3A4 inhibitors (e.g., erythromycin, saquinavir, verapamil, fluconazole) gave approximately 2-fold increases in exposure. Grapefruit juice caused only a small increase (about 25%) in exposure).
No products indexed under this heading.

Amiloride Hydrochloride (Eplerenone is contraindicated in patients treated concomitantly with potassium-sparing diuretics). Products include:
Midamor Tablets **2000**
Moduretic Tablets **2003**

Amiodarone Hydrochloride (Eplerenone should not be used with strong inhibitors of CYP450 3A4. Potent inhibitors of CYP3A4 caused increased exposure of about 5-fold, while less potent CYP3A4 inhibitors (e.g., erythromycin, saquinavir, verapamil, fluconazole) gave approximately 2-fold increases in exposure. Grapefruit juice caused only a small increase (about 25%) in exposure). Products include:
Pacerone Tablets **3337**

Amprenavir (Eplerenone should not be used with strong inhibitors of CYP450 3A4. Potent inhibitors of CYP3A4 caused increased exposure of about 5-fold, while less potent CYP3A4 inhibitors (e.g., erythromycin, saquinavir, verapamil, fluconazole) gave approximately 2-fold increases in exposure. Grapefruit juice caused only a small increase (about 25%) in exposure). Products include:
Agenerase Capsules **1299**
Agenerase Oral Solution **1304**

Anastrozole (Eplerenone should not be used with strong inhibitors of CYP450 3A4. Potent inhibitors of CYP3A4 caused increased exposure of about 5-fold, while less potent CYP3A4 inhibitors (e.g., erythromycin, saquinavir, verapamil, fluconazole) gave approximately 2-fold increases in exposure. Grapefruit juice caused only a small increase (about 25%) in exposure). Products include:
Arimidex Tablets **665**

Aprepitant (Eplerenone should not be used with strong inhibitors of CYP450 3A4. Potent inhibitors of CYP3A4 caused increased exposure of about 5-fold, while less potent CYP3A4 inhibitors (e.g., erythromycin, saquinavir, verapamil, fluconazole) gave approximately 2-fold increases in exposure. Grapefruit juice caused only a small increase (about 25%) in exposure). Products include:
Emend Capsules **1944**

Benazepril Hydrochloride (Because the concomitant use of another mineralocorticoid receptor blocker and ACE inhibitors has led to clinically relevant hyperkalemia; caution should be used). Products include:
Lotensin Tablets **2232**
Lotensin HCT Tablets **2235**
Lotrel Capsules **2238**

Candesartan Cilexetil (Because the concomitant use of another mineralocorticoid receptor blocker and angiotensin II receptor antagonists has led to clinically relevant hyperkalemia; caution should be used). Products include:
Atacand Tablets **634**
Atacand HCT **637**

Captopril (Because the concomitant use of another mineralocorticoid receptor blocker and ACE inhibitors has led to clinically relevant hyperkalemia; caution should be used). Products include:
Captopril Tablets **2114**

Celecoxib (When eplerenone and NSAIDs are used concomitantly, patients should be observed to determine whether the desired effect on blood pressure is obtained). Products include:
Celebrex Capsules **3130**

Cimetidine (Eplerenone should not be used with strong inhibitors of CYP450 3A4. Potent inhibitors of CYP3A4 caused increased exposure of about 5-fold, while less potent CYP3A4 inhibitors (e.g., erythromycin, saquinavir, verapamil, fluconazole) gave approximately 2-fold increases in exposure. Grapefruit juice caused only a small increase (about 25%) in exposure). Products include:
Tagamet HB 200 Tablets .... ▣ **637**
Tagamet Tablets **1547**

Cimetidine Hydrochloride (Eplerenone should not be used with strong inhibitors of CYP450 3A4. Potent inhibitors of CYP3A4 caused increased exposure of about 5-fold, while less potent CYP3A4 inhibitors (e.g., erythromycin, saquinavir, verapamil, fluconazole) gave approximately 2-fold increases in exposure. Grapefruit juice caused only a small increase (about 25%) in exposure).
No products indexed under this heading.

Ciprofloxacin (Eplerenone should not be used with strong inhibitors of CYP450 3A4. Potent inhibitors of CYP3A4 caused increased exposure of about 5-fold, while less potent CYP3A4 inhibitors (e.g., erythromycin, saquinavir, verapamil, fluconazole) gave approximately 2-fold increases in exposure. Grapefruit juice caused only a small increase (about 25%) in exposure). Products include:
Cipro I.V. **2998**
Cipro I.V. Pharmacy Bulk Package **3509**
Cipro Oral Suspension **2991**
Cipro XR Tablets **3004**
Ciprodex Otic Suspension **555**

Clarithromycin (Concomitant use with the potent CYP3A4 inhibitor clarithromycin is contraindicated). Products include:
Biaxin/Biaxin XL **402**
PREVPAC **3281**

Clotrimazole (Eplerenone should not be used with strong inhibitors of CYP450 3A4. Potent inhibitors of CYP3A4 caused increased exposure of about 5-fold, while less potent CYP3A4 inhibitors (e.g., erythromycin, saquinavir, verapamil, fluconazole) gave approximately 2-fold increases in exposure. Grapefruit juice caused only a small increase (about 25%) in exposure). Products include:
Lotrimin **3053**
Lotrisone **3054**

Cyclosporine (Eplerenone should not be used with strong inhibitors of CYP450 3A4. Potent inhibitors of CYP3A4 caused increased exposure of about 5-fold, while less potent CYP3A4 inhibitors (e.g., erythromycin, saquinavir, verapamil, fluconazole) gave approximately 2-fold increases in exposure. Grapefruit juice caused only a small increase (about 25%) in exposure). Products include:
Gengraf Capsules **458**
Neoral Soft Gelatin Capsules **2247**
Neoral Oral Solution **2247**
Restasis Ophthalmic Emulsion **570**
Sandimmune **2259**

Dalfopristin (Eplerenone should not be used with strong inhibitors of CYP450 3A4. Potent inhibitors of CYP3A4 caused increased exposure of about 5-fold, while less potent CYP3A4 inhibitors (e.g., erythromycin, saquinavir, verapamil, fluconazole) gave approximately 2-fold increases in exposure. Grapefruit juice caused only a small increase (about 25%) in exposure). Products include:
Synercid I.V. **1690**

Danazol (Eplerenone should not be used with strong inhibitors of CYP450 3A4. Potent inhibitors of CYP3A4 caused increased exposure of about 5-fold, while less potent CYP3A4 inhibitors (e.g., erythromycin, saquinavir, verapamil, fluconazole) gave approximately 2-fold increases in exposure. Grapefruit juice caused only a small increase (about 25%) in exposure).
No products indexed under this heading.

Delavirdine Mesylate (Eplerenone should not be used with strong inhibitors of CYP450 3A4. Potent inhibitors of CYP3A4 caused increased exposure of about 5-fold, while less potent CYP3A4 inhibitors (e.g., erythromycin, saquinavir, verapamil, fluconazole) gave approximately 2-fold increases in exposure. Grapefruit juice caused only a small increase (about 25%) in exposure). Products include:
Rescriptor Tablets 2535

Diclofenac Potassium (When eplerenone and NSAIDs are used concomitantly, patients should be observed to determine whether the desired effect on blood pressure is obtained). Products include:
Cataflam Tablets 2173

Diclofenac Sodium (When eplerenone and NSAIDs are used concomitantly, patients should be observed to determine whether the desired effect on blood pressure is obtained). Products include:
Arthrotec Tablets 3126
Voltaren Ophthalmic Solution 2300
Voltaren Tablets 2298
Voltaren-XR Tablets 2301

Diltiazem Hydrochloride (Eplerenone should not be used with strong inhibitors of CYP450 3A4. Potent inhibitors of CYP3A4 caused increased exposure of about 5-fold, while less potent CYP3A4 inhibitors (e.g., erythromycin, saquinavir, verapamil, fluconazole) gave approximately 2-fold increases in exposure. Grapefruit juice caused only a small increase (about 25%) in exposure). Products include:
Cardizem LA Extended Release Tablets 1699
Tiazac Capsules 1204

Diltiazem Maleate (Eplerenone should not be used with strong inhibitors of CYP450 3A4. Potent inhibitors of CYP3A4 caused increased exposure of about 5-fold, while less potent CYP3A4 inhibitors (e.g., erythromycin, saquinavir, verapamil, fluconazole) gave approximately 2-fold increases in exposure. Grapefruit juice caused only a small increase (about 25%) in exposure).
No products indexed under this heading.

Efavirenz (Eplerenone should not be used with strong inhibitors of CYP450 3A4. Potent inhibitors of CYP3A4 caused increased exposure of about 5-fold, while less potent CYP3A4 inhibitors (e.g., erythromycin, saquinavir, verapamil, fluconazole) gave approximately 2-fold increases in exposure. Grapefruit juice caused only a small increase (about 25%) in exposure). Products include:
Sustiva Capsules 957

Enalapril Maleate (Because the concomitant use of another mineralocorticoid receptor blocker and ACE inhibitors has led to clinically relevant hyperkalemia; caution should be used). Products include:
Vaseretic Tablets 2073
Vasotec I.V. Injection 2076

Enalaprilat (Because the concomitant use of another mineralocorticoid receptor blocker and ACE inhibitors has led to clinically relevant hyperkalemia; caution should be used).
No products indexed under this heading.

Eprosartan Mesylate (Because the concomitant use of another mineralocorticoid receptor blocker and angiotensin II receptor antagonists has led to clinically relevant hyperkalemia; caution should be used). Products include:
Teveten Tablets 1707
Teveten HCT Tablets 1710

Erythromycin (Eplerenone should not be used with strong inhibitors of CYP450 3A4. Potent inhibitors of CYP3A4 caused increased exposure of about 5-fold, while less potent CYP3A4 inhibitors (e.g., erythromycin, saquinavir, verapamil, fluconazole) gave approximately 2-fold increases in exposure. Grapefruit juice caused only a small increase (about 25%) in exposure). Products include:
Erygel Topical Gel 2096
Ery-Tab Tablets 447
Erythromycin Base Filmtab Tablets 454
Erythromycin Delayed-Release Capsules, USP 456
PCE Dispertab Tablets 510

Erythromycin Estolate (Eplerenone should not be used with strong inhibitors of CYP450 3A4. Potent inhibitors of CYP3A4 caused increased exposure of about 5-fold, while less potent CYP3A4 inhibitors (e.g., erythromycin, saquinavir, verapamil, fluconazole) gave approximately 2-fold increases in exposure. Grapefruit juice caused only a small increase (about 25%) in exposure).
No products indexed under this heading.

Erythromycin Ethylsuccinate (Eplerenone should not be used with strong inhibitors of CYP450 3A4. Potent inhibitors of CYP3A4 caused increased exposure of about 5-fold, while less potent CYP3A4 inhibitors (e.g., erythromycin, saquinavir, verapamil, fluconazole) gave approximately 2-fold increases in exposure. Grapefruit juice caused only a small increase (about 25%) in exposure). Products include:
E.E.S. 449
EryPed 445

Erythromycin Gluceptate (Eplerenone should not be used with strong inhibitors of CYP450 3A4. Potent inhibitors of CYP3A4 caused increased exposure of about 5-fold, while less potent CYP3A4 inhibitors (e.g., erythromycin, saquinavir, verapamil, fluconazole) gave approximately 2-fold increases in exposure. Grapefruit juice caused only a small increase (about 25%) in exposure).
No products indexed under this heading.

Erythromycin Lactobionate (Eplerenone should not be used with strong inhibitors of CYP450 3A4. Potent inhibitors of CYP3A4 caused increased exposure of about 5-fold, while less potent CYP3A4 inhibitors (e.g., erythromycin, saquinavir, verapamil, fluconazole) gave approximately 2-fold increases in exposure. Grapefruit juice caused only a small increase (about 25%) in exposure).
No products indexed under this heading.

Erythromycin Stearate (Eplerenone should not be used with strong inhibitors of CYP450 3A4. Potent inhibitors of CYP3A4 caused increased exposure of about 5-fold, while less potent CYP3A4 inhibitors (e.g., erythromycin, saquinavir, verapamil, fluconazole) gave approximately 2-fold increases in exposure. Grapefruit juice caused only a small increase (about 25%) in exposure). Products include:
Erythrocin Stearate Filmtab Tablets 452

Esomeprazole Magnesium (Eplerenone should not be used with strong inhibitors of CYP450 3A4. Potent inhibitors of CYP3A4 caused increased exposure of about 5-fold, while less potent CYP3A4 inhibitors (e.g., erythromycin, saquinavir, verapamil, fluconazole) gave approximately 2-fold increases in exposure. Grapefruit juice caused only a small increase (about 25%) in exposure). Products include:
Nexium Delayed-Release Capsules 645

Etodolac (When eplerenone and NSAIDs are used concomitantly, patients should be observed to determine whether the desired effect on blood pressure is obtained).
No products indexed under this heading.

Fenoprofen Calcium (When eplerenone and NSAIDs are used concomitantly, patients should be observed to determine whether the desired effect on blood pressure is obtained). Products include:
Nalfon Capsules 2504

Fluconazole (Eplerenone should not be used with strong inhibitors of CYP450 3A4. Potent inhibitors of CYP3A4 caused increased exposure of about 5-fold, while less potent CYP3A4 inhibitors (e.g., erythromycin, saquinavir, verapamil, fluconazole) gave approximately 2-fold increases in exposure. Grapefruit juice caused only a small increase (about 25%) in exposure).
No products indexed under this heading.

Fluoxetine Hydrochloride (Eplerenone should not be used with strong inhibitors of CYP450 3A4. Potent inhibitors of CYP3A4 caused increased exposure of about 5-fold, while less potent CYP3A4 inhibitors (e.g., erythromycin, saquinavir, verapamil, fluconazole) gave approximately 2-fold increases in exposure. Grapefruit juice caused only a small increase (about 25%) in exposure). Products include:
Prozac Pulvules and Liquid 1771
Symbyax Capsules 1788

Flurbiprofen (When eplerenone and NSAIDs are used concomitantly, patients should be observed to determine whether the desired effect on blood pressure is obtained).
No products indexed under this heading.

Fluvoxamine Maleate (Eplerenone should not be used with strong inhibitors of CYP450 3A4. Potent inhibitors of CYP3A4 caused increased exposure of about 5-fold, while less potent CYP3A4 inhibitors (e.g., erythromycin, saquinavir, verapamil, fluconazole) gave approximately 2-fold increases in exposure. Grapefruit juice caused only a small increase (about 25%) in exposure).
No products indexed under this heading.

Fosamprenavir Calcium (Eplerenone should not be used with strong inhibitors of CYP450 3A4. Potent inhibitors of CYP3A4 caused increased exposure of about 5-fold, while less potent CYP3A4 inhibitors (e.g., erythromycin, saquinavir, verapamil, fluconazole) gave approximately 2-fold increases in exposure. Grapefruit juice caused only a small increase (about 25%) in exposure). Products include:
Lexiva Tablets 1473

Fosinopril Sodium (Because the concomitant use of another mineralocorticoid receptor blocker and ACE inhibitors has led to clinically relevant hyperkalemia; caution should be used).
No products indexed under this heading.

Ibuprofen (When eplerenone and NSAIDs are used concomitantly, patients should be observed to determine whether the desired effect on blood pressure is obtained). Products include:
Advil Allergy Sinus Caplets 737
Advil 737
Children's Advil Suspension 742
Children's Advil Chewable Tablets 741
Advil Cold & Sinus 739
Advil Flu & Body Ache Caplets 739
Children's Advil Cold Suspension 741
Infants' Advil Concentrated Drops 743
Junior Strength Advil Swallow Tablets 740
Advil Migraine Liquigels 740
Advil Multi-Symptom Cold Caplets 738
Combunox Tablets 1183
Children's Motrin Oral Suspension and Chewable Tablets 1837
Children's Motrin Cold Non-Staining Dye-Free Oral Suspension 1838
Children's Motrin Cold Oral Suspension 1838
Children's Motrin Non-Staining Dye-Free Oral Suspension 1837
Motrin Cold & Sinus Caplets 1836
Motrin IB Tablets and Caplets 1836
Infants' Motrin Concentrated Drops 1837
Infants' Motrin Non-Staining Dye-Free Drops 1837
Junior Strength Motrin Caplets and Chewable Tablets 1837
Vicoprofen Tablets 533

Indinavir Sulfate (Eplerenone should not be used with strong inhibitors of CYP450 3A4. Potent inhibitors of CYP3A4 caused increased exposure of about 5-fold, while less potent CYP3A4 inhibitors (e.g., erythromycin, saquinavir, verapamil, fluconazole) gave approximately 2-fold increases in exposure. Grape-

fruit juice caused only a small increase (about 25%) in exposure). Products include:
- Crixivan Capsules ... 1918

Indomethacin (When eplerenone and NSAIDs are used concomitantly, patients should be observed to determine whether the desired effect on blood pressure is obtained). Products include:
- Indocin ... 1968

Indomethacin Sodium Trihydrate (When eplerenone and NSAIDs are used concomitantly, patients should be observed to determine whether the desired effect on blood pressure is obtained). Products include:
- Indocin I.V. ... 1973

Irbesartan (Because the concomitant use of another mineralocorticoid receptor blocker and angiotensin II receptor antagonists has led to clinically relevant hyperkalemia; caution should be used). Products include:
- Avalide Tablets ... 922
- Avalide Tablets ... 2889
- Avapro Tablets ... 925
- Avapro Tablets ... 2886

Isoniazid (Eplerenone should not be used with strong inhibitors of CYP450 3A4. Potent inhibitors of CYP3A4 caused increased exposure of about 5-fold, while less potent CYP3A4 inhibitors (e.g., erythromycin, saquinavir, verapamil, fluconazole) gave approximately 2-fold increases in exposure. Grapefruit juice caused only a small increase (about 25%) in exposure).

No products indexed under this heading.

Itraconazole (Concomitant use with the potent CYP3A4 inhibitor itraconazole is contraindicated).

No products indexed under this heading.

Ketoconazole (Concomitant use with the potent CYP3A4 inhibitor ketoconazole is contraindicated). Products include:
- Nizoral A-D Shampoo, 1% ... 1839
- Nizoral 2% Shampoo ... 1838

Ketoprofen (When eplerenone and NSAIDs are used concomitantly, patients should be observed to determine whether the desired effect on blood pressure is obtained).

No products indexed under this heading.

Ketorolac Tromethamine (When eplerenone and NSAIDs are used concomitantly, patients should be observed to determine whether the desired effect on blood pressure is obtained). Products include:
- Acular Ophthalmic Solution ... 561
- Acular LS Ophthalmic Solution ... 562

Lisinopril (Because the concomitant use of another mineralocorticoid receptor blocker and ACE inhibitors has led to clinically relevant hyperkalemia; caution should be used). Products include:
- Prinivil Tablets ... 2029
- Prinzide Tablets ... 2033
- Zestoretic Tablets ... 701
- Zestril Tablets ... 704

Lithium (Serum lithium levels should be monitored frequently if eplerenone is administered concomitantly with lithium).

No products indexed under this heading.

Lithium Carbonate (Serum lithium levels should be monitored frequently if eplerenone is administered concomitantly with lithium). Products include:
- Eskalith ... 1406
- Lithobid Tablets ... 1670

Lithium Citrate (Serum lithium levels should be monitored frequently if eplerenone is administered concomitantly with lithium).

No products indexed under this heading.

Lopinavir (Eplerenone should not be used with strong inhibitors of CYP450 3A4. Potent inhibitors of CYP3A4 caused increased exposure of about 5-fold, while less potent CYP3A4 inhibitors (e.g., erythromycin, saquinavir, verapamil, fluconazole) gave approximately 2-fold increases in exposure. Grapefruit juice caused only a small increase (about 25%) in exposure). Products include:
- Kaletra ... 474

Loratadine (Eplerenone should not be used with strong inhibitors of CYP450 3A4. Potent inhibitors of CYP3A4 caused increased exposure of about 5-fold, while less potent CYP3A4 inhibitors (e.g., erythromycin, saquinavir, verapamil, fluconazole) gave approximately 2-fold increases in exposure. Grapefruit juice caused only a small increase (about 25%) in exposure). Products include:
- Alavert Allergy & Sinus D-12 Hour Tablets ... ▣ 743
- Alavert ... ▣ 743
- Children's Claritin 24 Hour Non-Drowsy Allergy Syrup ... ▣ 732
- Claritin Non-Drowsy 24 Hour Tablets ... ▣ 731
- Non-Drowsy Claritin Hives Relief Tablets ... ▣ 733
- Claritin Reditabs 24 Hour Non-Drowsy Tablets ... ▣ 732
- Claritin-D Non-Drowsy 12 Hour Tablets ... ▣ 731
- Claritin-D Non-Drowsy 24 Hour Tablets ... ▣ 731
- Children's Dimetapp ND Non-Drowsy Allergy Syrup ... ▣ 746
- Triaminic Allerchews ... ▣ 684

Losartan Potassium (Because the concomitant use of another mineralocorticoid receptor blocker and angiotensin II receptor antagonists has led to clinically relevant hyperkalemia; caution should be used). Products include:
- Cozaar Tablets ... 1913
- Hyzaar ... 1964

Meclofenamate Sodium (When eplerenone and NSAIDs are used concomitantly, patients should be observed to determine whether the desired effect on blood pressure is obtained).

No products indexed under this heading.

Mefenamic Acid (When eplerenone and NSAIDs are used concomitantly, patients should be observed to determine whether the desired effect on blood pressure is obtained).

No products indexed under this heading.

Meloxicam (When eplerenone and NSAIDs are used concomitantly, patients should be observed to determine whether the desired effect on blood pressure is obtained). Products include:
- Mobic Oral Suspension ... 893
- Mobic Tablets ... 893

Metronidazole (Eplerenone should not be used with strong inhibitors of CYP450 3A4. Potent inhibitors of CYP3A4 caused increased exposure of about 5-fold, while less potent CYP3A4 inhibitors (e.g., erythromycin, saquinavir, verapamil, fluconazole) gave approximately 2-fold increases in exposure. Grapefruit juice caused only a small increase (about 25%) in exposure). Products include:
- Metrogel 1% ... 1212
- MetroGel-Vaginal Gel ... 1822
- Noritate Cream, 1% ... 1051

Metronidazole Benzoate (Eplerenone should not be used with strong inhibitors of CYP450 3A4. Potent inhibitors of CYP3A4 caused increased exposure of about 5-fold, while less potent CYP3A4 inhibitors (e.g., erythromycin, saquinavir, verapamil, fluconazole) gave approximately 2-fold increases in exposure. Grapefruit juice caused only a small increase (about 25%) in exposure).

No products indexed under this heading.

Metronidazole Hydrochloride (Eplerenone should not be used with strong inhibitors of CYP450 3A4. Potent inhibitors of CYP3A4 caused increased exposure of about 5-fold, while less potent CYP3A4 inhibitors (e.g., erythromycin, saquinavir, verapamil, fluconazole) gave approximately 2-fold increases in exposure. Grapefruit juice caused only a small increase (about 25%) in exposure).

No products indexed under this heading.

Miconazole (Eplerenone should not be used with strong inhibitors of CYP450 3A4. Potent inhibitors of CYP3A4 caused increased exposure of about 5-fold, while less potent CYP3A4 inhibitors (e.g., erythromycin, saquinavir, verapamil, fluconazole) gave approximately 2-fold increases in exposure. Grapefruit juice caused only a small increase (about 25%) in exposure).

No products indexed under this heading.

Miconazole Nitrate (Eplerenone should not be used with strong inhibitors of CYP450 3A4. Potent inhibitors of CYP3A4 caused increased exposure of about 5-fold, while less potent CYP3A4 inhibitors (e.g., erythromycin, saquinavir, verapamil, fluconazole) gave approximately 2-fold increases in exposure. Grapefruit juice caused only a small increase (about 25%) in exposure). Products include:
- Desenex ... ▣ 674
- Desenex Jock Itch Spray Powder ... ▣ 674

Moexipril Hydrochloride (Because the concomitant use of another mineralocorticoid receptor blocker and ACE inhibitors has led to clinically relevant hyperkalemia; caution should be used). Products include:
- Uniretic Tablets ... 3114
- Univasc Tablets ... 3118

Nabumetone (When eplerenone and NSAIDs are used concomitantly, patients should be observed to determine whether the desired effect on blood pressure is obtained). Products include:
- Relafen Tablets ... 1523

Naproxen (When eplerenone and NSAIDs are used concomitantly, patients should be observed to determine whether the desired effect on blood pressure is obtained). Products include:
- EC-Naprosyn Delayed-Release Tablets ... 2769
- Naprosyn Suspension ... 2769
- Naprosyn Tablets ... 2769
- Prevacid NapraPAC ... 3277

Naproxen Sodium (When eplerenone and NSAIDs are used concomitantly, patients should be observed to determine whether the desired effect on blood pressure is obtained). Products include:
- Aleve Tablets, Caplets and Gelcaps ... ▣ 605
- Anaprox Tablets ... 2769
- Anaprox DS Tablets ... 2769

Nefazodone Hydrochloride (Concomitant use with the potent CYP3A4 inhibitor nefazodone is contraindicated).

No products indexed under this heading.

Nelfinavir Mesylate (Concomitant use with the potent CYP3A4 inhibitor nelfinavir is contraindicated). Products include:
- Viracept ... 2556

Nevirapine (Eplerenone should not be used with strong inhibitors of CYP450 3A4. Potent inhibitors of CYP3A4 caused increased exposure of about 5-fold, while less potent CYP3A4 inhibitors (e.g., erythromycin, saquinavir, verapamil, fluconazole) gave approximately 2-fold increases in exposure. Grapefruit juice caused only a small increase (about 25%) in exposure). Products include:
- Viramune Oral Suspension ... 903
- Viramune Tablets ... 903

Niacinamide (Eplerenone should not be used with strong inhibitors of CYP450 3A4. Potent inhibitors of CYP3A4 caused increased exposure of about 5-fold, while less potent CYP3A4 inhibitors (e.g., erythromycin, saquinavir, verapamil, fluconazole) gave approximately 2-fold increases in exposure. Grapefruit juice caused only a small increase (about 25%) in exposure).

No products indexed under this heading.

Nicotinamide (Eplerenone should not be used with strong inhibitors of CYP450 3A4. Potent inhibitors of CYP3A4 caused increased exposure of about 5-fold, while less potent CYP3A4 inhibitors (e.g., erythromycin, saquinavir, verapamil, fluconazole) gave approximately 2-fold increases in exposure. Grapefruit juice caused only a small increase (about 25%) in exposure). Products include:
- Nicomide Tablets ... 3190

Nifedipine (Eplerenone should not be used with strong inhibitors of CYP450 3A4. Potent inhibitors of CYP3A4 caused increased exposure of about 5-fold, while less potent CYP3A4 inhibitors (e.g., erythromycin, saquinavir, verapamil, fluconazole) gave approximately 2-fold increases in exposure. Grapefruit juice caused only a small increase (about 25%) in exposure). Products include:
- Adalat CC Tablets ... 2978

Norfloxacin (Eplerenone should not be used with strong inhibitors of CYP450 3A4. Potent inhibitors of CYP3A4 caused increased exposure of about 5-fold, while less potent CYP3A4 inhibitors (e.g., erythromycin, saquinavir, verapamil, fluconazole) gave approximately 2-fold increases in exposure. Grapefruit

juice caused only a small increase (about 25%) in exposure). Products include:

Noroxin Tablets 2009

Omeprazole (Eplerenone should not be used with strong inhibitors of CYP450 3A4. Potent inhibitors of CYP3A4 caused increased exposure of about 5-fold, while less potent CYP3A4 inhibitors (e.g., erythromycin, saquinavir, verapamil, fluconazole) gave approximately 2-fold increases in exposure. Grapefruit juice caused only a small increase (about 25%) in exposure). Products include:

Zegerid Powder for Oral Solution 2972

Oxaprozin (When eplerenone and NSAIDs are used concomitantly, patients should be observed to determine whether the desired effect on blood pressure is obtained).

No products indexed under this heading.

Paroxetine Hydrochloride (Eplerenone should not be used with strong inhibitors of CYP450 3A4. Potent inhibitors of CYP3A4 caused increased exposure of about 5-fold, while less potent CYP3A4 inhibitors (e.g., erythromycin, saquinavir, verapamil, fluconazole) gave approximately 2-fold increases in exposure. Grapefruit juice caused only a small increase (about 25%) in exposure). Products include:

Paxil CR Controlled-Release Tablets 1509
Paxil 1501

Perindopril Erbumine (Because the concomitant use of another mineralocorticoid receptor blocker and ACE inhibitors has led to clinically relevant hyperkalemia; caution should be used). Products include:

Aceon Tablets (2 mg, 4 mg, 8 mg) 3191

Phenylbutazone (When eplerenone and NSAIDs are used concomitantly, patients should be observed to determine whether the desired effect on blood pressure is obtained).

No products indexed under this heading.

Piroxicam (When eplerenone and NSAIDs are used concomitantly, patients should be observed to determine whether the desired effect on blood pressure is obtained).

No products indexed under this heading.

Potassium Acid Phosphate (Eplerenone is contraindicated in patients treated concomitantly with potassium supplements). Products include:

K-Phos Original (Sodium Free) Tablets 785

Potassium Bicarbonate (Eplerenone is contraindicated in patients treated concomitantly with potassium supplements).

No products indexed under this heading.

Potassium Chloride (Eplerenone is contraindicated in patients treated concomitantly with potassium supplements). Products include:

Colyte with Flavor Packs for Oral Solution 3102
HalfLytely and Bisacodyl Tablets Bowel Prep Kit with Flavors Packs 915
K-Dur Extended-Relase Tablets 3047
K-Lor Powder Packets 472
K-Tab Filmtab Tablets 473
TriLyte with Flavor Packs for Oral Solution 3114

Potassium Citrate (Eplerenone is contraindicated in patients treated concomitantly with potassium supplements). Products include:

Urocit-K Tablets 2109

Potassium Gluconate (Eplerenone is contraindicated in patients treated concomitantly with potassium supplements).

No products indexed under this heading.

Potassium Phosphate (Eplerenone is contraindicated in patients treated concomitantly with potassium supplements). Products include:

K-Phos Neutral Tablets 785

Propoxyphene Hydrochloride (Eplerenone should not be used with strong inhibitors of CYP450 3A4. Potent inhibitors of CYP3A4 caused increased exposure of about 5-fold, while less potent CYP3A4 inhibitors (e.g., erythromycin, saquinavir, verapamil, fluconazole) gave approximately 2-fold increases in exposure. Grapefruit juice caused only a small increase (about 25%) in exposure).

No products indexed under this heading.

Propoxyphene Napsylate (Eplerenone should not be used with strong inhibitors of CYP450 3A4. Potent inhibitors of CYP3A4 caused increased exposure of about 5-fold, while less potent CYP3A4 inhibitors (e.g., erythromycin, saquinavir, verapamil, fluconazole) gave approximately 2-fold increases in exposure. Grapefruit juice caused only a small increase (about 25%) in exposure). Products include:

Darvocet A 500 Tablets 3497

Quinapril Hydrochloride (Because the concomitant use of another mineralocorticoid receptor blocker and ACE inhibitors has led to clinically relevant hyperkalemia; caution should be used).

No products indexed under this heading.

Quinidine (Eplerenone should not be used with strong inhibitors of CYP450 3A4. Potent inhibitors of CYP3A4 caused increased exposure of about 5-fold, while less potent CYP3A4 inhibitors (e.g., erythromycin, saquinavir, verapamil, fluconazole) gave approximately 2-fold increases in exposure. Grapefruit juice caused only a small increase (about 25%) in exposure).

No products indexed under this heading.

Quinidine Hydrochloride (Eplerenone should not be used with strong inhibitors of CYP450 3A4. Potent inhibitors of CYP3A4 caused increased exposure of about 5-fold, while less potent CYP3A4 inhibitors (e.g., erythromycin, saquinavir, verapamil, fluconazole) gave approximately 2-fold increases in exposure. Grapefruit juice caused only a small increase (about 25%) in exposure).

No products indexed under this heading.

Quinidine Polygalacturonate (Eplerenone should not be used with strong inhibitors of CYP450 3A4. Potent inhibitors of CYP3A4 caused increased exposure of about 5-fold, while less potent CYP3A4 inhibitors (e.g., erythromycin, saquinavir, verapamil, fluconazole) gave approximately 2-fold increases in exposure. Grapefruit juice caused only a small increase (about 25%) in exposure).

No products indexed under this heading.

Quinidine Sulfate (Eplerenone should not be used with strong inhibitors of CYP450 3A4. Potent inhibitors of CYP3A4 caused increased exposure of about 5-fold, while less potent CYP3A4 inhibitors (e.g., erythromycin, saquinavir, verapamil, fluconazole) gave approximately 2-fold increases in exposure. Grapefruit juice caused only a small increase (about 25%) in exposure).

No products indexed under this heading.

Quinine (Eplerenone should not be used with strong inhibitors of CYP450 3A4. Potent inhibitors of CYP3A4 caused increased exposure of about 5-fold, while less potent CYP3A4 inhibitors (e.g., erythromycin, saquinavir, verapamil, fluconazole) gave approximately 2-fold increases in exposure. Grapefruit juice caused only a small increase (about 25%) in exposure).

No products indexed under this heading.

Quinine Sulfate (Eplerenone should not be used with strong inhibitors of CYP450 3A4. Potent inhibitors of CYP3A4 caused increased exposure of about 5-fold, while less potent CYP3A4 inhibitors (e.g., erythromycin, saquinavir, verapamil, fluconazole) gave approximately 2-fold increases in exposure. Grapefruit juice caused only a small increase (about 25%) in exposure).

No products indexed under this heading.

Quinupristin (Eplerenone should not be used with strong inhibitors of CYP450 3A4. Potent inhibitors of CYP3A4 caused increased exposure of about 5-fold, while less potent CYP3A4 inhibitors (e.g., erythromycin, saquinavir, verapamil, fluconazole) gave approximately 2-fold increases in exposure. Grapefruit juice caused only a small increase (about 25%) in exposure). Products include:

Synercid I.V. 1690

Ramipril (Because the concomitant use of another mineralocorticoid receptor blocker and ACE inhibitors has led to clinically relevant hyperkalemia; caution should be used). Products include:

Altace Capsules 1673

Ranitidine Bismuth Citrate (Eplerenone should not be used with strong inhibitors of CYP450 3A4. Potent inhibitors of CYP3A4 caused increased exposure of about 5-fold, while less potent CYP3A4 inhibitors (e.g., erythromycin, saquinavir, verapamil, fluconazole) gave approximately 2-fold increases in exposure. Grapefruit juice caused only a small increase (about 25%) in exposure).

No products indexed under this heading.

Ranitidine Hydrochloride (Eplerenone should not be used with strong inhibitors of CYP450 3A4. Potent inhibitors of CYP3A4 caused increased exposure of about 5-fold, while less potent CYP3A4 inhibitors (e.g., erythromycin, saquinavir, verapamil, fluconazole) gave approximately 2-fold increases in exposure. Grapefruit juice caused only a small increase (about 25%) in exposure). Products include:

Zantac 1597
Zantac Injection 1593
Zantac 75 Tablets 715
Zantac 150 Maximum Strength Tablets 715
Zantac Injection Pharmacy Bulk Package 1595

Ritonavir (Concomitant use with the potent CYP3A4 inhibitor ritonavir is contraindicated). Products include:

Kaletra 474
Norvir 499

Rofecoxib (When eplerenone and NSAIDs are used concomitantly, patients should be observed to determine whether the desired effect on blood pressure is obtained).

No products indexed under this heading.

Saquinavir (Eplerenone should not be used with strong inhibitors of CYP450 3A4. Potent inhibitors of CYP3A4 caused increased exposure of about 5-fold, while less potent CYP3A4 inhibitors (e.g., erythromycin, saquinavir, verapamil, fluconazole) gave approximately 2-fold increases in exposure. Grapefruit juice caused only a small increase (about 25%) in exposure).

No products indexed under this heading.

Saquinavir Mesylate (Eplerenone should not be used with strong inhibitors of CYP450 3A4. Potent inhibitors of CYP3A4 caused increased exposure of about 5-fold, while less potent CYP3A4 inhibitors (e.g., erythromycin, saquinavir, verapamil, fluconazole) gave approximately 2-fold increases in exposure. Grapefruit juice caused only a small increase (about 25%) in exposure). Products include:

Invirase 2776

Sertraline Hydrochloride (Eplerenone should not be used with strong inhibitors of CYP450 3A4. Potent inhibitors of CYP3A4 caused increased exposure of about 5-fold, while less potent CYP3A4 inhibitors (e.g., erythromycin, saquinavir, verapamil, fluconazole) gave approximately 2-fold increases in exposure. Grapefruit juice caused only a small increase (about 25%) in exposure). Products include:

Zoloft 2581

Spirapril Hydrochloride (Because the concomitant use of another mineralocorticoid receptor blocker and ACE inhibitors has led to clinically relevant hyperkalemia; caution should be used).

No products indexed under this heading.

Spironolactone (Eplerenone is contraindicated in patients treated concomitantly with potassium-sparing diuretics).

No products indexed under this heading.

Sulindac (When eplerenone and NSAIDs are used concomitantly, patients should be observed to determine whether the desired effect on blood pressure is obtained). Products include:

Clinoril Tablets 1899

Telithromycin (Eplerenone should not be used with strong inhibitors of CYP450 3A4. Potent inhibitors of CYP3A4 caused increased exposure of about 5-fold, while less potent CYP3A4 inhibitors (e.g., erythromycin, saquinavir, verapamil, fluconazole) gave approximately 2-fold increases in exposure. Grapefruit juice caused only a small increase (about 25%) in exposure). Products include:

Ketek Tablets 2920

Telmisartan (Because the concomitant use of another mineralocorticoid receptor blocker and angiotensin II receptor antagonists has led to clinically relevant hyperkalemia; caution should be used). Products include:

Micardis Tablets 884
Micardis HCT Tablets 886

Tolmetin Sodium (When eplerenone and NSAIDs are used concomitantly, patients should be observed to determine whether the desired effect on blood pressure is obtained).

No products indexed under this heading.

Trandolapril (Because the concomitant use of another mineralocorticoid receptor blocker and ACE inhibitors has led to clinically relevant hyperkalemia; caution should be used). Products include:

Mavik Tablets 482
Tarka Tablets 519

Triamterene (Eplerenone is contraindicated in patients treated concomitantly with potassium-sparing diuretics). Products include:

Dyazide Capsules 1389
Dyrenium Capsules 3390
Maxzide 2150

Troglitazone (Eplerenone should not be used with strong inhibitors of CYP450 3A4. Potent inhibitors of CYP3A4 caused increased exposure of about 5-fold, while less potent CYP3A4 inhibitors (e.g., erythromycin, saquinavir, verapamil, fluconazole) gave approximately 2-fold increases in exposure. Grapefruit juice caused only a small increase (about 25%) in exposure).

No products indexed under this heading.

Troleandomycin (Concomitant use with the potent CYP3A4 inhibitor troleandomycin is contraindicated).

No products indexed under this heading.

Valdecoxib (When eplerenone and NSAIDs are used concomitantly, patients should be observed to determine whether the desired effect on blood pressure is obtained).

No products indexed under this heading.

Valproate Sodium (Eplerenone should not be used with strong inhibitors of CYP450 3A4. Potent inhibitors of CYP3A4 caused increased exposure of about 5-fold, while less potent CYP3A4 inhibitors (e.g., erythromycin, saquinavir, verapamil, fluconazole) gave approximately 2-fold increases in exposure. Grapefruit juice caused only a small increase (about 25%) in exposure). Products include:

Depacon Injection 412

Valsartan (Because the concomitant use of another mineralocorticoid receptor blocker and angiotensin II receptor antagonists has led to clinically relevant hyperkalemia; caution should be used). Products include:

Diovan HCT Tablets 2195
Diovan Tablets 2191

Verapamil Hydrochloride (Eplerenone should not be used with strong inhibitors of CYP450 3A4. Potent inhibitors of CYP3A4 caused increased exposure of about 5-fold, while less potent CYP3A4 inhibitors (e.g., erythromycin, saquinavir, verapamil, fluconazole) gave approximately 2-fold increases in exposure. Grapefruit juice caused only a small increase (about 25%) in exposure). Products include:

Covera-HS Tablets 3135
Tarka Tablets 519
Verelan PM Capsules 3120

Voriconazole (Eplerenone should not be used with strong inhibitors of CYP450 3A4. Potent inhibitors of CYP3A4 caused increased exposure of about 5-fold, while less potent CYP3A4 inhibitors (e.g., erythromycin, saquinavir, verapamil, fluconazole) gave approximately 2-fold increases in exposure. Grapefruit juice caused only a small increase (about 25%) in exposure). Products include:

VFEND I.V. 2543
VFEND Oral Suspension 2543
VFEND Tablets 2543

Zafirlukast (Eplerenone should not be used with strong inhibitors of CYP450 3A4. Potent inhibitors of CYP3A4 caused increased exposure of about 5-fold, while less potent CYP3A4 inhibitors (e.g., erythromycin, saquinavir, verapamil, fluconazole) gave approximately 2-fold increases in exposure. Grapefruit juice caused only a small increase (about 25%) in exposure). Products include:

Accolate Tablets 663

Zileuton (Eplerenone should not be used with strong inhibitors of CYP450 3A4. Potent inhibitors of CYP3A4 caused increased exposure of about 5-fold, while less potent CYP3A4 inhibitors (e.g., erythromycin, saquinavir, verapamil, fluconazole) gave approximately 2-fold increases in exposure. Grapefruit juice caused only a small increase (about 25%) in exposure).

No products indexed under this heading.

Food Interactions

Grapefruit (Eplerenone should not be used with strong inhibitors of CYP450 3A4. Potent inhibitors of CYP3A4 caused increased exposure of about 5-fold, while less potent CYP3A4 inhibitors (e.g., erythromycin, saquinavir, verapamil, fluconazole) gave approximately 2-fold increases in exposure. Grapefruit juice caused only a small increase (about 25%) in exposure).

Grapefruit Juice (Eplerenone should not be used with strong inhibitors of CYP450 3A4. Potent inhibitors of CYP3A4 caused increased exposure of about 5-fold, while less potent CYP3A4 inhibitors (e.g., erythromycin, saquinavir, verapamil, fluconazole) gave approximately 2-fold increases in exposure. Grapefruit juice caused only a small increase (about 25%) in exposure).

Salt Substitutes, Potassium-Containing (Eplerenone is contraindicated in patients treated concomitantly with salt substitutes containing potassium).

INTEGRILIN INJECTION

(Eptifibatide) 3034

May interact with oral anticoagulants, glycoprotein (GP) IIb/IIIa inhibitors, non-steroidal anti-inflammatory agents, and certain other agents. Compounds in these categories include:

Abciximab (Current or planned administration of another parenteral GP IIb/IIIa inhibitor is contraindicated). Products include:

ReoPro Vials 1779

Anisindione (Potential for additive pharmacologic effects because eptifibatide inhibits platelet aggregation; concurrent use requires caution). Products include:

Miradon Tablets 3056

Aspirin (Co-administration of eptifibatide with heparin and aspirin has resulted in cerebral, GI and pulmonary hemorrhage). Products include:

Aggrenox Capsules 855
Bayer, Aspirin Regimen .... ■606
Bayer Aspirin Tablets 3515
BC Powder .... ■612
BC Allergy Sinus Cold Powder .... ■612
Arthritis Strength BC Powder .... ■612
BC Sinus Cold Powder .... ■612
Ecotrin Enteric Coated Aspirin Low, Regular and Maximum Strength Tablets 1627
Goody's Body Pain Formula Powder .... ■621
Goody's Extra Strength Headache Powder .... ■621
Goody's Extra Strength Pain Relief Tablets .... ■621
Percodan Tablets 1115
St. Joseph 81 mg Aspirin Chewable and Enteric Coated Tablets 1841

Celecoxib (Potential for additive pharmacologic effects because eptifibatide inhibits platelet aggregation; concurrent use requires caution). Products include:

Celebrex Capsules 3130

Clopidogrel Bisulfate (Potential for additive pharmacologic effects because eptifibatide inhibits platelet aggregation; concurrent use requires caution). Products include:

Plavix Tablets 940
Plavix Tablets 2942

Diclofenac Potassium (Potential for additive pharmacologic effects because eptifibatide inhibits platelet aggregation; concurrent use requires caution). Products include:

Cataflam Tablets 2173

Diclofenac Sodium (Potential for additive pharmacologic effects because eptifibatide inhibits platelet aggregation; concurrent use requires caution). Products include:

Arthrotec Tablets 3126
Voltaren Ophthalmic Solution 2300
Voltaren Tablets 2298
Voltaren-XR Tablets 2301

Dicumarol (Potential for additive pharmacologic effects because eptifibatide inhibits platelet aggregation; concurrent use requires caution).

No products indexed under this heading.

Dipyridamole (Potential for additive pharmacologic effects because eptifibatide inhibits platelet aggregation; concurrent use requires caution). Products include:

Aggrenox Capsules 855
Persantine Tablets 898

Etodolac (Potential for additive pharmacologic effects because eptifibatide inhibits platelet aggregation; concurrent use requires caution).

No products indexed under this heading.

Fenoprofen Calcium (Potential for additive pharmacologic effects because eptifibatide inhibits platelet aggregation; concurrent use requires caution). Products include:

Nalfon Capsules 2504

Flurbiprofen (Potential for additive pharmacologic effects because eptifibatide inhibits platelet aggregation; concurrent use requires caution).

No products indexed under this heading.

Heparin Sodium (Co-administration of eptifibatide with heparin and aspirin has resulted in cerebral, GI and pulmonary hemorrhage).

No products indexed under this heading.

Ibuprofen (Potential for additive pharmacologic effects because eptifibatide inhibits platelet aggregation; concurrent use requires caution). Products include:

Advil Allergy Sinus Caplets .... ■737
Advil .... ■737
Children's Advil Suspension .... ■742
Children's Advil Chewable Tablets .... ■741
Advil Cold & Sinus .... ■739
Advil Flu & Body Ache Caplets .... ■739
Children's Advil Cold Suspension .... ■741
Infants' Advil Concentrated Drops .... ■743
Junior Strength Advil Swallow Tablets .... ■740
Advil Migraine Liquigels .... ■740
Advil Multi-Symptom Cold Caplets .... ■738
Combunox Tablets 1183
Children's Motrin Oral Suspension and Chewable Tablets 1837
Children's Motrin Cold Non-Staining Dye-Free Oral Suspension 1838
Children's Motrin Cold Oral Suspension 1838
Children's Motrin Non-Staining Dye-Free Oral Suspension 1837
Motrin Cold & Sinus Caplets 1836
Motrin IB Tablets and Caplets 1836
Infants' Motrin Concentrated Drops 1837
Infants' Motrin Non-Staining Dye-Free Drops 1837
Junior Strength Motrin Caplets and Chewable Tablets 1837
Vicoprofen Tablets 533

Indomethacin (Potential for additive pharmacologic effects because eptifibatide inhibits platelet aggregation; concurrent use requires caution). Products include:

Indocin 1968

Indomethacin Sodium Trihydrate (Potential for additive pharmacologic effects because eptifibatide inhibits platelet aggregation; concurrent use requires caution). Products include:

Indocin I.V. 1973

Ketoprofen (Potential for additive pharmacologic effects because eptifibatide inhibits platelet aggregation; concurrent use requires caution).

No products indexed under this heading.

Ketorolac Tromethamine (Potential for additive pharmacologic effects because eptifibatide inhibits platelet aggregation; concurrent use requires caution). Products include:

Acular Ophthalmic Solution 561
Acular LS Ophthalmic Solution 562

Meclofenamate Sodium (Potential for additive pharmacologic effects because eptifibatide inhibits platelet aggregation; concurrent use requires caution).

No products indexed under this heading.

Mefenamic Acid (Potential for additive pharmacologic effects because eptifibatide inhibits platelet aggregation; concurrent use requires caution).

No products indexed under this heading.

Meloxicam (Potential for additive pharmacologic effects because eptifibatide inhibits platelet aggregation; concurrent use requires caution). Products include:
Mobic Oral Suspension 893
Mobic Tablets 893

Nabumetone (Potential for additive pharmacologic effects because eptifibatide inhibits platelet aggregation; concurrent use requires caution). Products include:
Relafen Tablets 1523

Naproxen (Potential for additive pharmacologic effects because eptifibatide inhibits platelet aggregation; concurrent use requires caution). Products include:
EC-Naprosyn Delayed-Release Tablets 2769
Naprosyn Suspension 2769
Naprosyn Tablets 2769
Prevacid NapraPAC 3277

Naproxen Sodium (Potential for additive pharmacologic effects because eptifibatide inhibits platelet aggregation; concurrent use requires caution). Products include:
Aleve Tablets, Caplets and Gelcaps 605
Anaprox Tablets 2769
Anaprox DS Tablets 2769

Oxaprozin (Potential for additive pharmacologic effects because eptifibatide inhibits platelet aggregation; concurrent use requires caution).
No products indexed under this heading.

Phenylbutazone (Potential for additive pharmacologic effects because eptifibatide inhibits platelet aggregation; concurrent use requires caution).
No products indexed under this heading.

Piroxicam (Potential for additive pharmacologic effects because eptifibatide inhibits platelet aggregation; concurrent use requires caution).
No products indexed under this heading.

Rofecoxib (Potential for additive pharmacologic effects because eptifibatide inhibits platelet aggregation; concurrent use requires caution).
No products indexed under this heading.

Sulindac (Potential for additive pharmacologic effects because eptifibatide inhibits platelet aggregation; concurrent use requires caution). Products include:
Clinoril Tablets 1899

Ticlopidine Hydrochloride (Potential for additive pharmacologic effects because eptifibatide inhibits platelet aggregation; concurrent use requires caution). Products include:
Ticlid Tablets 2813

Tirofiban Hydrochloride (Current or planned administration of another parenteral GP IIb/IIIa inhibitor is contraindicated). Products include:
Aggrastat 1878

Tolmetin Sodium (Potential for additive pharmacologic effects because eptifibatide inhibits platelet aggregation; concurrent use requires caution).
No products indexed under this heading.

Valdecoxib (Potential for additive pharmacologic effects because eptifibatide inhibits platelet aggregation; concurrent use requires caution).
No products indexed under this heading.

Warfarin Sodium (Potential for additive pharmacologic effects because eptifibatide inhibits platelet aggregation; concurrent use requires caution). Products include:
Coumadin for Injection 932
Coumadin Tablets 932

INTELECTOL TABLETS

(Vinpocetine) 770
None cited in PDR database.

INTRON A FOR INJECTION

(Interferon alfa-2b, Recombinant) 3038
May interact with xanthines and certain other agents. Compounds in these categories include:

Aminophylline (Co-administration results in decreased theophylline clearance resulting in a 100% increase in serum theophylline levels).
No products indexed under this heading.

Bone Marrow Depressants, unspecified (Careful monitoring of the WBC count is indicated).
No products indexed under this heading.

Dyphylline (Co-administration results in decreased theophylline clearance resulting in a 100% increase in serum theophylline levels).
No products indexed under this heading.

Theophylline (Co-administration results in decreased theophylline clearance resulting in a 100% increase in serum theophylline levels).
No products indexed under this heading.

Theophylline Anhydrous (Co-administration results in decreased theophylline clearance resulting in a 100% increase in serum theophylline levels). Products include:
Uniphyl Tablets 2708

Theophylline Calcium Salicylate (Co-administration results in decreased theophylline clearance resulting in a 100% increase in serum theophylline levels).
No products indexed under this heading.

Theophylline Dihydroxypropyl (Glyceryl) (Co-administration results in decreased theophylline clearance resulting in a 100% increase in serum theophylline levels).
No products indexed under this heading.

Theophylline Ethylenediamine (Co-administration results in decreased theophylline clearance resulting in a 100% increase in serum theophylline levels).
No products indexed under this heading.

Theophylline Sodium Glycinate (Co-administration results in decreased theophylline clearance resulting in a 100% increase in serum theophylline levels).
No products indexed under this heading.

Zidovudine (Concomitant administration may result in a higher incidence of neutropenia). Products include:
Combivir Tablets 1373
Retrovir 1533
Retrovir IV Infusion 1537
Trizivir Tablets 1565

INVANZ FOR INJECTION

(Ertapenem) 1974
May interact with:

Probenecid (Competes for active tubular secretion and reduces the renal clearance of ertapenem).
No products indexed under this heading.

INVERSINE TABLETS

(Mecamylamine Hydrochloride) 3286
May interact with anesthetics, antihypertensives, and certain other agents. Compounds in these categories include:

Acebutolol Hydrochloride (The action of mecamylamine may be potentiated by other antihypertensives).
No products indexed under this heading.

Alfentanil Hydrochloride (The action of mecamylamine may be potentiated by anesthetics).
No products indexed under this heading.

Amlodipine Besylate (The action of mecamylamine may be potentiated by other antihypertensives). Products include:
Caduet Tablets 2507
Lotrel Capsules 2238
Norvasc Tablets 2529

Antibiotics, unspecified (Concurrent use of ganglionic blockers in patients receiving antibiotics should be avoided).
No products indexed under this heading.

Atenolol (The action of mecamylamine may be potentiated by other antihypertensives). Products include:
Tenormin I.V. Injection 698
Tenormin Tablets 695

Benazepril Hydrochloride (The action of mecamylamine may be potentiated by other antihypertensives). Products include:
Lotensin Tablets 2232
Lotensin HCT Tablets 2235
Lotrel Capsules 2238

Bendroflumethiazide (The action of mecamylamine may be potentiated by other antihypertensives).
No products indexed under this heading.

Betaxolol Hydrochloride (The action of mecamylamine may be potentiated by other antihypertensives). Products include:
Betoptic S Ophthalmic Suspension 554

Bisoprolol Fumarate (The action of mecamylamine may be potentiated by other antihypertensives).
No products indexed under this heading.

Candesartan Cilexetil (The action of mecamylamine may be potentiated by other antihypertensives). Products include:
Atacand Tablets 634
Atacand HCT 637

Captopril (The action of mecamylamine may be potentiated by other antihypertensives). Products include:
Captopril Tablets 2114

Carteolol Hydrochloride (The action of mecamylamine may be potentiated by other antihypertensives). Products include:
Carteolol Hydrochloride Ophthalmic Solution USP, 1% .... ⊙246

Chlorothiazide (The action of mecamylamine may be potentiated by other antihypertensives). Products include:
Aldoclor Tablets 1881
Diuril Oral 1936

Chlorothiazide Sodium (The action of mecamylamine may be potentiated by other antihypertensives). Products include:
Diuril Sodium Intravenous 1934

Chlorthalidone (The action of mecamylamine may be potentiated by other antihypertensives). Products include:
Clorpres Tablets 2139

Clonidine (The action of mecamylamine may be potentiated by other antihypertensives). Products include:
Catapres-TTS 875

Clonidine Hydrochloride (The action of mecamylamine may be potentiated by other antihypertensives). Products include:
Catapres Tablets 874
Clorpres Tablets 2139

Deserpidine (The action of mecamylamine may be potentiated by other antihypertensives).
No products indexed under this heading.

Diazoxide (The action of mecamylamine may be potentiated by other antihypertensives). Products include:
Hyperstat I.V. Injection 3031

Diltiazem Hydrochloride (The action of mecamylamine may be potentiated by other antihypertensives). Products include:
Cardizem LA Extended Release Tablets 1699
Tiazac Capsules 1204

Doxazosin Mesylate (The action of mecamylamine may be potentiated by other antihypertensives).
No products indexed under this heading.

Enalapril Maleate (The action of mecamylamine may be potentiated by other antihypertensives). Products include:
Vaseretic Tablets 2073
Vasotec I.V. Injection 2076

Enalaprilat (The action of mecamylamine may be potentiated by other antihypertensives).
No products indexed under this heading.

Enflurane (The action of mecamylamine may be potentiated by anesthetics).
No products indexed under this heading.

Eprosartan Mesylate (The action of mecamylamine may be potentiated by other antihypertensives). Products include:
Teveten Tablets 1707
Teveten HCT Tablets 1710

Esmolol Hydrochloride (The action of mecamylamine may be potentiated by other antihypertensives). Products include:
Brevibloc Concentrate 766
Brevibloc Injection 766
Brevibloc Double Strength Injection 766
Brevibloc Premixed Injection 766
Brevibloc Double Strength Premixed Injection 766

Felodipine (The action of mecamylamine may be potentiated by other antihypertensives). Products include:
Plendil Extended-Release Tablets 651

Fentanyl Citrate (The action of mecamylamine may be potentiated by anesthetics). Products include:

Actiq 993

Fosinopril Sodium (The action of mecamylamine may be potentiated by other antihypertensives).
No products indexed under this heading.

Furosemide (The action of mecamylamine may be potentiated by other antihypertensives). Products include:
Furosemide Tablets 2117

Guanabenz Acetate (The action of mecamylamine may be potentiated by other antihypertensives).
No products indexed under this heading.

Guanethidine Monosulfate (The action of mecamylamine may be potentiated by other antihypertensives).
No products indexed under this heading.

Halothane (The action of mecamylamine may be potentiated by anesthetics).
No products indexed under this heading.

Hydralazine Hydrochloride (The action of mecamylamine may be potentiated by other antihypertensives). Products include:
BiDil Tablets 2161

Hydrochlorothiazide (The action of mecamylamine may be potentiated by other antihypertensives). Products include:
Aldoril Tablets 1884
Atacand HCT 637
Avalide Tablets 2889
Avalide Tablets 922
Benicar HCT Tablets 2852
Diovan HCT Tablets 2195
Dyazide Capsules 1389
Hyzaar 1964
Lotensin HCT Tablets 2235
Maxzide 2150
Micardis HCT Tablets 886
Moduretic Tablets 2003
Prinzide Tablets 2033
Teveten HCT Tablets 1710
Timolide Tablets 2056
Uniretic Tablets 3114
Vaseretic Tablets 2073
Zestoretic Tablets 701

Hydroflumethiazide (The action of mecamylamine may be potentiated by other antihypertensives).
No products indexed under this heading.

Indapamide (The action of mecamylamine may be potentiated by other antihypertensives). Products include:
Indapamide Tablets 2119

Irbesartan (The action of mecamylamine may be potentiated by other antihypertensives). Products include:
Avalide Tablets 922
Avalide Tablets 2889
Avapro Tablets 925
Avapro Tablets 2886

Isoflurane (The action of mecamylamine may be potentiated by anesthetics).
No products indexed under this heading.

Isradipine (The action of mecamylamine may be potentiated by other antihypertensives). Products include:
DynaCirc CR Tablets 2726

Ketamine Hydrochloride (The action of mecamylamine may be potentiated by anesthetics).
No products indexed under this heading.

Labetalol Hydrochloride (The action of mecamylamine may be potentiated by other antihypertensives).
No products indexed under this heading.

Lisinopril (The action of mecamylamine may be potentiated by other antihypertensives). Products include:
Prinivil Tablets 2029
Prinzide Tablets 2033
Zestoretic Tablets 701
Zestril Tablets 704

Losartan Potassium (The action of mecamylamine may be potentiated by other antihypertensives). Products include:
Cozaar Tablets 1913
Hyzaar 1964

Methohexital Sodium (The action of mecamylamine may be potentiated by anesthetics).
No products indexed under this heading.

Methyclothiazide (The action of mecamylamine may be potentiated by other antihypertensives).
No products indexed under this heading.

Methyldopa (The action of mecamylamine may be potentiated by other antihypertensives). Products include:
Aldoclor Tablets 1881
Aldoril Tablets 1884

Methyldopate Hydrochloride (The action of mecamylamine may be potentiated by other antihypertensives).
No products indexed under this heading.

Metolazone (The action of mecamylamine may be potentiated by other antihypertensives).
No products indexed under this heading.

Metoprolol Succinate (The action of mecamylamine may be potentiated by other antihypertensives). Products include:
Toprol-XL Tablets 660

Metoprolol Tartrate (The action of mecamylamine may be potentiated by other antihypertensives).
No products indexed under this heading.

Metyrosine (The action of mecamylamine may be potentiated by other antihypertensives). Products include:
Demser Capsules 1933

Mibefradil Dihydrochloride (The action of mecamylamine may be potentiated by other antihypertensives).
No products indexed under this heading.

Midazolam Hydrochloride (The action of mecamylamine may be potentiated by anesthetics).
No products indexed under this heading.

Minoxidil (The action of mecamylamine may be potentiated by other antihypertensives). Products include:
Men's Rogaine Extra Strength Topical Solution, Ocean Rush Scent and Original Unscented .... ▣706
Women's Rogaine Topical Solution, Spring Bloom Scent and Original Unscented .... ▣707

Moexipril Hydrochloride (The action of mecamylamine may be potentiated by other antihypertensives). Products include:
Uniretic Tablets 3114

Univasc Tablets 3118

Nadolol (The action of mecamylamine may be potentiated by other antihypertensives). Products include:
Nadolol Tablets 2121

Nicardipine Hydrochloride (The action of mecamylamine may be potentiated by other antihypertensives). Products include:
Cardene I.V. 1129

Nifedipine (The action of mecamylamine may be potentiated by other antihypertensives). Products include:
Adalat CC Tablets 2978

Nisoldipine (The action of mecamylamine may be potentiated by other antihypertensives). Products include:
Sular Tablets 1163

Nitroglycerin (The action of mecamylamine may be potentiated by other antihypertensives). Products include:
Nitro-Dur Transdermal Infusion System 3060
Nitrolingual Pumpspray 1161

Penbutolol Sulfate (The action of mecamylamine may be potentiated by other antihypertensives).
No products indexed under this heading.

Perindopril Erbumine (The action of mecamylamine may be potentiated by other antihypertensives). Products include:
Aceon Tablets (2 mg, 4 mg, 8 mg) 3191

Phenoxybenzamine Hydrochloride (The action of mecamylamine may be potentiated by other antihypertensives). Products include:
Dibenzyline Capsules 3390

Phentolamine Mesylate (The action of mecamylamine may be potentiated by other antihypertensives).
No products indexed under this heading.

Pindolol (The action of mecamylamine may be potentiated by other antihypertensives).
No products indexed under this heading.

Polythiazide (The action of mecamylamine may be potentiated by other antihypertensives).
No products indexed under this heading.

Prazosin Hydrochloride (The action of mecamylamine may be potentiated by other antihypertensives).
No products indexed under this heading.

Propofol (The action of mecamylamine may be potentiated by anesthetics). Products include:
Diprivan Injectable Emulsion 676

Propranolol Hydrochloride (The action of mecamylamine may be potentiated by other antihypertensives). Products include:
Inderal LA Long-Acting Capsules 3421
InnoPran XL Capsules 2728

Quinapril Hydrochloride (The action of mecamylamine may be potentiated by other antihypertensives).
No products indexed under this heading.

Ramipril (The action of mecamylamine may be potentiated by other antihypertensives). Products include:
Altace Capsules 1673

Rauwolfia Serpentina (The action of mecamylamine may be potentiated by other antihypertensives).
No products indexed under this heading.

Remifentanil Hydrochloride (The action of mecamylamine may be potentiated by anesthetics).
No products indexed under this heading.

Rescinnamine (The action of mecamylamine may be potentiated by other antihypertensives).
No products indexed under this heading.

Reserpine (The action of mecamylamine may be potentiated by other antihypertensives).
No products indexed under this heading.

Sodium Nitroprusside (The action of mecamylamine may be potentiated by other antihypertensives).
No products indexed under this heading.

Sotalol Hydrochloride (The action of mecamylamine may be potentiated by other antihypertensives).
No products indexed under this heading.

Spirapril Hydrochloride (The action of mecamylamine may be potentiated by other antihypertensives).
No products indexed under this heading.

Sufentanil Citrate (The action of mecamylamine may be potentiated by anesthetics).
No products indexed under this heading.

Sulfamethoxazole (Concurrent use of ganglionic blockers in patients receiving sulfonamides should be avoided).
No products indexed under this heading.

Sulfisoxazole Acetyl (Concurrent use of ganglionic blockers in patients receiving sulfonamides should be avoided).
No products indexed under this heading.

Telmisartan (The action of mecamylamine may be potentiated by other antihypertensives). Products include:
Micardis Tablets 884
Micardis HCT Tablets 886

Terazosin Hydrochloride (The action of mecamylamine may be potentiated by other antihypertensives). Products include:
Hytrin Capsules 469

Thiamylal Sodium (The action of mecamylamine may be potentiated by anesthetics).
No products indexed under this heading.

Timolol Maleate (The action of mecamylamine may be potentiated by other antihypertensives). Products include:
Blocadren Tablets 1891
Cosopt Sterile Ophthalmic Solution 1910
Timolide Tablets 2056
Timoptic in Ocudose 2061
Timoptic Sterile Ophthalmic Solution 2058
Timoptic-XE Sterile Ophthalmic Gel Forming Solution 2062

Torsemide (The action of mecamylamine may be potentiated by other antihypertensives).
No products indexed under this heading.

Trandolapril (The action of mecamylamine may be potentiated by other antihypertensives). Products include:
Mavik Tablets 482
Tarka Tablets 519

Trimethaphan Camsylate (The action of mecamylamine may be potentiated by other antihypertensives).
No products indexed under this heading.

Valsartan (The action of mecamylamine may be potentiated by other antihypertensives). Products include:
Diovan HCT Tablets 2195
Diovan Tablets 2191

Verapamil Hydrochloride (The action of mecamylamine may be potentiated by other antihypertensives). Products include:
Covera-HS Tablets 3135
Tarka Tablets 519
Verelan PM Capsules 3120

Food Interactions

Alcohol (The action of mecamylamine may be potentiated by alcohol).

INVIRASE CAPSULES

(Saquinavir Mesylate) 2776

May interact with calcium channel blockers, cytochrome p450 3a4 inducers (selected), cytochrome p450 3a4 substrates (selected), dexamethasone, ergot-containing drugs, oral contraceptives, phenytoin, and certain other agents. Compounds in these categories include:

Alfentanil Hydrochloride (Co-administration with drugs that are mainly metabolized by CYP3A4 may have elevated plasma concentrations when co-administered with saquinavir; these combinations should be used with caution).
No products indexed under this heading.

Allium sativum (Co-administration with compounds that are potent inducers of CYP3A4 may result in decreased plasma levels of saquinavir).
No products indexed under this heading.

Alprazolam (Concomitant administration with saquinavir may lead to increased alprazolam levels; a decrease in alprazolam dose may be needed). Products include:
Niravam Orally Disintegrating Tablets 3106
Xanax XR Tablets 2655

Amiodarone Hydrochloride (Inhibition of CYP3A4 by saquinavir could result in elevated plasma concentrations of amiodarone, potentially causing serious or life-threatening reactions; concurrent use is contraindicated). Products include:
Pacerone Tablets 3337

Amitriptyline Hydrochloride (Concomitant administration with saquinavir may cause increased levels of amitriptyline; therapeutic concentration monitoring is recommended for tricyclic antidepressants when co-administered with saquinavir).
No products indexed under this heading.

Amlodipine Besylate (Concomitant administration with saquinavir may lead to increased amlodipine levels; caution is warranted and clinical monitoring of patient is recommended). Products include:
Caduet Tablets 2507
Lotrel Capsules 2238
Norvasc Tablets 2529

Aprepitant (Co-administration with drugs that are mainly metabolized by CYP3A4 may have elevated plasma concentrations when co-administered with saquinavir; these combinations should be used with caution). Products include:
Emend Capsules 1944

Astemizole (Inhibition of CYP3A4 by saquinavir could result in increased astemizole plasma levels and create the potential for serious and/or life-threatening reactions, such as rare cases of serious cardiovascular adverse events; concurrent use is contraindicated).
No products indexed under this heading.

Atorvastatin Calcium (Concomitant administration with saquinavir may cause increased atorvastatin levels. Use lowest possible dose of atorvastatin and with careful monitoring or consider other HMG-CoA reductase inhibitors, such as pravastatin, fluvastatin, and rosuvastatin). Products include:
Caduet Tablets 2507
Lipitor Tablets 2495

Belladonna Ergotamine (Co-administration with drugs that are mainly metabolized by CYP3A4 may have elevated plasma concentrations when co-administered with saquinavir; these combinations should be used with caution).

Bepridil Hydrochloride (Inhibition of CYP3A4 by saquinavir could result in elevated plasma concentrations of bepridil, potentially causing serious or life-threatening reactions; concurrent use is contraindicated).
No products indexed under this heading.

Betamethasone Acetate (Co-administration with compounds that are potent inducers of CYP3A4 may result in decreased plasma levels of saquinavir).
No products indexed under this heading.

Betamethasone Sodium Phosphate (Co-administration with compounds that are potent inducers of CYP3A4 may result in decreased plasma levels of saquinavir).
No products indexed under this heading.

Buspirone Hydrochloride (Co-administration with drugs that are mainly metabolized by CYP3A4 may have elevated plasma concentrations when co-administered with saquinavir; these combinations should be used with caution).
No products indexed under this heading.

Busulfan (Co-administration with drugs that are mainly metabolized by CYP3A4 may have elevated plasma concentrations when co-administered with saquinavir; these combinations should be used with caution). Products include:
I.V. Busulfex 1125
Myleran Tablets 1492

Carbamazepine (Concomitant administration with saquinavir may decrease saquinavir levels. Use with caution since saquinavir may be less effective due to decreased saquinavir plasma concentrations). Products include:
Carbatrol Capsules 3174
Equetro Extended-Release Capsules 3178
Tegretol/Tegretol-XR 2278

Cerivastatin Sodium (Co-administration of Invirase and other HMG-CoA reductase inhibitors that are metabolized by the CYP3A4 pathway, such as cerivastatin, may result in increased concentrations of statins; potential for, in rare cases, severe adverse events, such as myopathy, including rhabdomyolysis).
No products indexed under this heading.

Chlorpheniramine (Co-administration with drugs that are mainly metabolized by CYP3A4 may have elevated plasma concentrations when co-administered with saquinavir; these combinations should be used with caution).
No products indexed under this heading.

Chlorpheniramine Maleate (Co-administration with drugs that are mainly metabolized by CYP3A4 may have elevated plasma concentrations when co-administered with saquinavir; these combinations should be used with caution). Products include:
Advil Allergy Sinus Caplets 737
Advil Multi-Symptom Cold Caplets 738
BC Allergy Sinus Cold Powder 612
Contac Severe Cold and Flu Caplets Maximum Strength 615
Hycomine Compound Tablets 1105
PediaCare Multi-Symptom Cold Liquid 704
PediaCare NightRest Cough & Cold Liquid 704
Robitussin Flu Liquid 752
Robitussin PM Cough & Cold Liquid 752
Singlet Caplets 636
Sudafed Sinus & Allergy Tablets 710
TheraFlu Cold & Cough Hot Liquid 680
TheraFlu Cold & Sore Throat Hot Liquid 680
TheraFlu Flu & Sore Throat Hot Liquid 681
TheraFlu Severe Cold & Cough Hot Liquid 683
TheraFlu Severe Cold Caplets 679
TheraFlu Severe Cold Hot Liquid 682
Triaminic Cold & Allergy Liquid 685
Triaminic Cold & Cough Liquid 685
Triaminic Flu, Cough & Fever Liquid 685
Triaminic Night Time Cough & Cold Liquid 685
Triaminic Allergy Runny Nose & Congestion Softchews 688
Triaminic Cold & Cough Softchews 688
Children's Tylenol Plus Cold NightTime Suspension Liquid 1851
Children's Tylenol Plus Cold & Cough Suspension Liquid and Chewable Tablets 1851
Children's Tylenol Plus Cold Chewable Tablets 1851
Children's Tylenol Plus Flu Suspension Liquid 1853
Tylenol Allergy Complete Multi-Symptom Caplets and Gelcaps with Cool Burst 1844
Multi-Symptom Tylenol Cold Night Time Caplets 1845
Vicks 44M Cough, Cold & Flu Relief 2676
Pediatric Vicks 44m Cough & Cold Relief 2673
Children's Vicks NyQuil Cold/Cough Relief 2671

Chlorpheniramine Polistirex (Co-administration with drugs that are mainly metabolized by CYP3A4 may have elevated plasma concentrations when co-administered with saquinavir; these combinations should be used with caution). Products include:
Tussionex Pennkinetic Extended-Release Suspension 3322

Chlorpheniramine Tannate (Co-administration with drugs that are mainly metabolized by CYP3A4 may have elevated plasma concentrations when co-administered with saquinavir; these combinations should be used with caution).
No products indexed under this heading.

Ciprofloxacin Hydrochloride (Co-administration with compounds that are potent inducers of CYP3A4 may result in decreased plasma levels of saquinavir). Products include:
Ciloxan Ophthalmic Ointment 554
Cipro Tablets 2991

Cisapride (Inhibition of CYP3A4 by saquinavir could result in increased cisapride plasma levels and create the potential for serious and/or life-threatening reactions, such as rare cases of serious cardiovascular adverse events; concurrent use is contraindicated).
No products indexed under this heading.

Cisplatin (Co-administration with compounds that are potent inducers of CYP3A4 may result in decreased plasma levels of saquinavir).
No products indexed under this heading.

Clarithromycin (Concomitant administration with saquinavir may cause increased levels of clarithromycin and/or saquinavir). Products include:
Biaxin/Biaxin XL 402
PREVPAC 3281

Clindamycin Hydrochloride (Potential for elevated plasma concentrations of compounds that are substrate of CYP3A4, such as clindamycin). Products include:
Cleocin Vaginal Ovules 2613

Clindamycin Palmitate Hydrochloride (Potential for elevated plasma concentrations of compounds that are substrate of CYP3A4, such as clindamycin).
No products indexed under this heading.

Clindamycin Phosphate (Potential for elevated plasma concentrations of compounds that are substrate of CYP3A4, such as clindamycin). Products include:
Benzaclin Topical Gel 1046
Clindagel 1207
Clindesse Vaginal Cream 3296
Clindets Pledgets 3212
Evoclin Foam, 1% 1025

Clorazepate Dipotassium (Concomitant administration with saquinavir may lead to increased clorazepate levels; a decrease in clorazepate dose may be needed). Products include:
Tranxene 2488

Cortisone Acetate (Co-administration with compounds that are potent inducers of CYP3A4 may result in decreased plasma levels of saquinavir).
No products indexed under this heading.

IMPORTANT NOTE: Always consult each drug listing in the patient's regimen for possible interactions.

Cyclosporine (Concomitant administration with saquinavir may lead to increased levels of cyclosporine. Therapeutic concentration monitoring is recommended for all immunosuppressant agents when co-administered with saquinavir). Products include:
Gengraf Capsules 458
Neoral Soft Gelatin Capsules 2247
Neoral Oral Solution 2247
Restasis Ophthalmic Emulsion 570
Sandimmune 2259

Dapsone (Potential for elevated plasma concentrations of compounds that are substrate of CYP3A4, such as dapsone). Products include:
Dapsone Tablets USP 1656

Delavirdine Mesylate (Co-administration has resulted in a 5-fold increase in saquinavir plasma AUC; currently, there are no safety and efficacy data available from use of this combination; hepatocellular enzyme elevations have occurred in some patients). Products include:
Rescriptor Tablets 2535

Desogestrel (Concomitant administration with saquinavir/ritonavir may lead to decreased ethinyl estradiol levels. Alternative or additional contraceptive measures should be used when estrogen-based oral contraceptives and saquinavir/ritonavir are co-administered). Products include:
Ortho-Cept Tablets 2395

Dexamethasone (Concomitant administration with saquinavir may cause decreased saquinavir levels. Use with caution since saquinavir may be less effective due to decreased saquinavir plasma concentrations). Products include:
Ciprodex Otic Suspension 555
Decadron Tablets 1929
TobraDex Ophthalmic Ointment 558
TobraDex Ophthalmic Suspension 558

Dexamethasone Acetate (Concomitant administration with saquinavir may cause decreased saquinavir levels. Use with caution since saquinavir may be less effective due to decreased saquinavir plasma concentrations).
No products indexed under this heading.

Dexamethasone Sodium Phosphate (Concomitant administration with saquinavir may cause decreased saquinavir levels. Use with caution since saquinavir may be less effective due to decreased saquinavir plasma concentrations). Products include:
Decadron Phosphate Injection 1931

Diazepam (Concomitant administration with saquinavir may lead to increased diazepam levels; a decrease in diazepam dose may be needed). Products include:
Diastat Rectal Delivery System 3344
Valium Tablets 2822

Dihydroergotamine Mesylate (Inhibition of CYP3A4 by saquinavir could result in increased ergot derivatives plasma levels and create the potential for serious and/or life-threatening reactions; concurrent use is contraindicated). Products include:
Migranal Nasal Spray 3350

Diltiazem Hydrochloride (Concomitant administration with saquinavir may lead to increased diltiazem levels; caution is warranted and clinical monitoring of patient is recommended). Products include:
Cardizem LA Extended Release Tablets 1699
Tiazac Capsules 1204

Diltiazem Maleate (Concomitant administration with saquinavir may lead to increased diltiazem levels; caution is warranted and clinical monitoring of patient is recommended).
No products indexed under this heading.

Disopyramide (Co-administration with drugs that are mainly metabolized by CYP3A4 may have elevated plasma concentrations when co-administered with saquinavir; these combinations should be used with caution).
No products indexed under this heading.

Disopyramide Phosphate (Co-administration with drugs that are mainly metabolized by CYP3A4 may have elevated plasma concentrations when co-administered with saquinavir; these combinations should be used with caution).
No products indexed under this heading.

Disulfiram (Co-administration with drugs that are mainly metabolized by CYP3A4 may have elevated plasma concentrations when co-administered with saquinavir; these combinations should be used with caution). Products include:
Antabuse Tablets 2343

Doxorubicin Hydrochloride (Co-administration with drugs that are mainly metabolized by CYP3A4 may have elevated plasma concentrations when co-administered with saquinavir; these combinations should be used with caution). Products include:
Adriamycin for Injection, USP 786
Adriamycin Injection, USP 786

Dronabinol (Co-administration with drugs that are mainly metabolized by CYP3A4 may have elevated plasma concentrations when co-administered with saquinavir; these combinations should be used with caution). Products include:
Marinol Capsules 3334

Efavirenz (Concomitant administration with saquinavir may lead to decreased levels of saquinavir and efavirenz. Saquinavir should not be given as the sole protease inhibitor to patients taking efavirenz). Products include:
Sustiva Capsules 957

Ergonovine Maleate (Inhibition of CYP3A4 by saquinavir could result in increased ergot derivatives plasma levels and create the potential for serious and/or life-threatening reactions; concurrent use is contraindicated).
No products indexed under this heading.

Ergotamine Tartrate (Inhibition of CYP3A4 by saquinavir could result in increased ergot derivatives plasma levels and create the potential for serious and/or life-threatening reactions; concurrent use is contraindicated).
No products indexed under this heading.

Erythromycin (Co-administration with drugs that are mainly metabolized by CYP3A4 may have elevated plasma concentrations when co-administered with saquinavir; these combinations should be used with caution). Products include:
Erygel Topical Gel 2096
Ery-Tab Tablets 447
Erythromycin Base Filmtab Tablets 454
Erythromycin Delayed-Release Capsules, USP 456
PCE Dispertab Tablets 510

Erythromycin Estolate (Co-administration with drugs that are mainly metabolized by CYP3A4 may have elevated plasma concentrations when co-administered with saquinavir; these combinations should be used with caution).
No products indexed under this heading.

Erythromycin Ethylsuccinate (Co-administration with drugs that are mainly metabolized by CYP3A4 may have elevated plasma concentrations when co-administered with saquinavir; these combinations should be used with caution). Products include:
E.E.S. 449
EryPed 445

Erythromycin Gluceptate (Co-administration with drugs that are mainly metabolized by CYP3A4 may have elevated plasma concentrations when co-administered with saquinavir; these combinations should be used with caution).
No products indexed under this heading.

Erythromycin Lactobionate (Co-administration with drugs that are mainly metabolized by CYP3A4 may have elevated plasma concentrations when co-administered with saquinavir; these combinations should be used with caution).
No products indexed under this heading.

Erythromycin Stearate (Co-administration with drugs that are mainly metabolized by CYP3A4 may have elevated plasma concentrations when co-administered with saquinavir; these combinations should be used with caution). Products include:
Erythrocin Stearate Filmtab Tablets 452

Estradiol (Co-administration with drugs that are mainly metabolized by CYP3A4 may have elevated plasma concentrations when co-administered with saquinavir; these combinations should be used with caution). Products include:
Activella Tablets 2311
Climara Transdermal System 795
Climara Pro Transdermal System 800
CombiPatch Transdermal System 2180
Estrogel 0.06% 3200
Menostar Transdermal System 805
Prefest Tablets 1069
Vagifem Tablets 2340
Vivelle Transdermal System 2288
Vivelle-Dot Transdermal System 2293

Estradiol Benzoate (Co-administration with drugs that are mainly metabolized by CYP3A4 may have elevated plasma concentrations when co-administered with saquinavir; these combinations should be used with caution).
No products indexed under this heading.

Estradiol Cypionate (Co-administration with drugs that are mainly metabolized by CYP3A4 may have elevated plasma concentrations when co-administered with saquinavir; these combinations should be used with caution).
No products indexed under this heading.

Estradiol Valerate (Co-administration with drugs that are mainly metabolized by CYP3A4 may have elevated plasma concentrations when co-administered with saquinavir; these combinations should be used with caution).
No products indexed under this heading.

Ethinyl Estradiol (Concomitant administration with saquinavir/ritonavir may lead to decreased ethinyl estradiol levels. Alternative or additional contraceptive measures should be used when estrogen-based oral contraceptives and saquinavir/ritonavir are co-administered). Products include:
Alesse-28 Tablets 3392
Lo/Ovral-28 Tablets 3423
NuvaRing 2357
Ortho-Cept Tablets 2395
Ortho-Cyclen/Ortho Tri-Cyclen 2414
Ortho Evra Transdermal System 2402
Ortho Tri-Cyclen Lo Tablets 2421
Seasonale Tablets 1073
Triphasil-28 Tablets 3483
Yasmin 28 Tablets 818

Ethosuximide (Co-administration with drugs that are mainly metabolized by CYP3A4 may have elevated plasma concentrations when co-administered with saquinavir; these combinations should be used with caution).
No products indexed under this heading.

Ethynodiol Diacetate (Concomitant administration with saquinavir/ritonavir may lead to decreased ethinyl estradiol levels. Alternative or additional contraceptive measures should be used when estrogen-based oral contraceptives and saquinavir/ritonavir are co-administered).
No products indexed under this heading.

Etoposide (Co-administration with drugs that are mainly metabolized by CYP3A4 may have elevated plasma concentrations when co-administered with saquinavir; these combinations should be used with caution).
No products indexed under this heading.

Etoposide Phosphate (Co-administration with drugs that are mainly metabolized by CYP3A4 may have elevated plasma concentrations when co-administered with saquinavir; these combinations should be used with caution).
No products indexed under this heading.

Felbamate (Co-administration with compounds that are potent inducers of CYP3A4 may result in decreased plasma levels of saquinavir).
No products indexed under this heading.

Felodipine (Concomitant administration with saquinavir may lead to increased felodipine levels; caution is warranted and clinical monitoring of patient is recommended). Products include:

Plendil Extended-Release Tablets 651

Fentanyl (Co-administration with drugs that are mainly metabolized by CYP3A4 may have elevated plasma concentrations when co-administered with saquinavir; these combinations should be used with caution). Products include:

Duragesic Transdermal System 2448

Fentanyl Citrate (Co-administration with drugs that are mainly metabolized by CYP3A4 may have elevated plasma concentrations when co-administered with saquinavir; these combinations should be used with caution). Products include:

Actiq 993

Flecainide Acetate (Inhibition of CYP3A4 by saquinavir could result in elevated plasma concentrations of flecainide, potentially causing serious or life-threatening reactions; concurrent use is contraindicated). Products include:

Tambocor Tablets 1824

Fludrocortisone Acetate (Co-administration with compounds that are potent inducers of CYP3A4 may result in decreased plasma levels of saquinavir).

No products indexed under this heading.

Flurazepam Hydrochloride (Concomitant administration with saquinavir may lead to increased flurazepam levels; a decrease in flurazepam dose may be needed). Products include:

Dalmane Capsules 3343

Fosphenytoin Sodium (Concomitant administration with saquinavir may decrease saquinavir levels. Use with caution since saquinavir may be less effective due to decreased saquinavir plasma concentrations).

No products indexed under this heading.

Garlic Extract (Garlic capsules should not be used while taking saquinavir as the sole protease inhibitor due to the increased risk of decreased saquinavir plasma concentrations).

No products indexed under this heading.

Garlic Oil (Garlic capsules should not be used while taking saquinavir as the sole protease inhibitor due to the increased risk of decreased saquinavir plasma concentrations).

No products indexed under this heading.

Haloperidol (Co-administration with drugs that are mainly metabolized by CYP3A4 may have elevated plasma concentrations when co-administered with saquinavir; these combinations should be used with caution).

No products indexed under this heading.

Haloperidol Decanoate (Co-administration with drugs that are mainly metabolized by CYP3A4 may have elevated plasma concentrations when co-administered with saquinavir; these combinations should be used with caution).

No products indexed under this heading.

Haloperidol Lactate (Co-administration with drugs that are mainly metabolized by CYP3A4 may have elevated plasma concentrations when co-administered with saquinavir; these combinations should be used with caution).

No products indexed under this heading.

Hydrocortisone (Co-administration with compounds that are potent inducers of CYP3A4 may result in decreased plasma levels of saquinavir). Products include:

Cortizone•5 Ointment 699
Cortizone•10 Creme 699
Cortizone•10 Ointment 699
Cortizone•10 Plus Creme 700
Cortizone•10 Maximum Strength Quick Shot Spray 700
Hydrocortone Tablets 1963
Preparation H Hydrocortisone Cream 748

Hydrocortisone Acetate (Co-administration with compounds that are potent inducers of CYP3A4 may result in decreased plasma levels of saquinavir). Products include:

Analpram-HC 1136
Pramosone 1139
ProctoFoam-HC 3113
Tucks Anti-Itch Ointment 712
U-cort 1% Cream 3289

Hydrocortisone Butyrate (Co-administration with compounds that are potent inducers of CYP3A4 may result in decreased plasma levels of saquinavir). Products include:

Locoid 1138
Locoid Lipocream Cream 1138

Hydrocortisone Cypionate (Co-administration with compounds that are potent inducers of CYP3A4 may result in decreased plasma levels of saquinavir).

No products indexed under this heading.

Hydrocortisone Hemisuccinate (Co-administration with compounds that are potent inducers of CYP3A4 may result in decreased plasma levels of saquinavir).

No products indexed under this heading.

Hydrocortisone Probutate (Co-administration with compounds that are potent inducers of CYP3A4 may result in decreased plasma levels of saquinavir). Products include:

Pandel Cream, 0.1% 1017

Hydrocortisone Sodium Phosphate (Co-administration with compounds that are potent inducers of CYP3A4 may result in decreased plasma levels of saquinavir).

No products indexed under this heading.

Hydrocortisone Sodium Succinate (Co-administration with compounds that are potent inducers of CYP3A4 may result in decreased plasma levels of saquinavir).

No products indexed under this heading.

Hydrocortisone Valerate (Co-administration with compounds that are potent inducers of CYP3A4 may result in decreased plasma levels of saquinavir).

No products indexed under this heading.

Hypericum (Co-administration of protease inhibitors with St. John's Wort is expected to substantially decrease protease inhibitor concentrations and may result in suboptimal levels of protease inhibitor and loss of virologic response and possible resistance to protease inhibitors; concurrent use is not recommended).

No products indexed under this heading.

Hypericum Perforatum (Co-administration with compounds that are potent inducers of CYP3A4 may result in decreased plasma levels of saquinavir).

No products indexed under this heading.

Imipramine Hydrochloride (Concomitant administration with saquinavir may cause increased levels of imipramine; therapeutic concentration monitoring is recommended for tricyclic antidepressants when co-administered with saquinavir).

No products indexed under this heading.

Imipramine Pamoate (Concomitant administration with saquinavir may cause increased levels of imipramine; therapeutic concentration monitoring is recommended for tricyclic antidepressants when co-administered with saquinavir).

No products indexed under this heading.

Indinavir Sulfate (Co-administration with drugs that are mainly metabolized by CYP3A4 may have elevated plasma concentrations when co-administered with saquinavir; these combinations should be used with caution). Products include:

Crixivan Capsules 1918

Isradipine (Concomitant administration with saquinavir may lead to increased isradipine levels; caution is warranted and clinical monitoring of patient is recommended). Products include:

DynaCirc CR Tablets 2726

Itraconazole (Concomitant administration with saquinavir may lead to increased saquinavir levels).

No products indexed under this heading.

Ketoconazole (Concomitant administration with saquinavir may lead to increased saquinavir levels). Products include:

Nizoral A-D Shampoo, 1% 1839
Nizoral 2% Shampoo 1838

Levonorgestrel (Concomitant administration with saquinavir/ritonavir may lead to decreased ethinyl estradiol levels. Alternative or additional contraceptive measures should be used when estrogen-based oral contraceptives and saquinavir/ritonavir are co-administered). Products include:

Alesse-28 Tablets 3392
Climara Pro Transdermal System 800
Mirena Intrauterine System 810
Plan B Tablets 1068
Seasonale Tablets 1073
Triphasil-28 Tablets 3483

Lidocaine (Caution is warranted and therapeutic concentration monitoring is recommended for antiarrhythmics given with saquinavir). Products include:

Lidoderm Patch 1107

Lidocaine Hydrochloride (Caution is warranted and therapeutic concentration monitoring is recommended for antiarrhythmics given with saquinavir).

No products indexed under this heading.

Lovastatin (Co-administration of Invirase and lovastatin may result in increased concentrations of statins; potential for, in rare cases, severe adverse events, such as myopathy including rhabdomyolysis; concomitant use is not recommended). Products include:

Advicor Tablets 1694
Altoprev Extended-Release Tablets 1151
Mevacor Tablets 1996

Mephenytoin (Co-administration with compounds that are potent inducers of CYP3A4 may result in decreased plasma levels of saquinavir).

No products indexed under this heading.

Mestranol (Concomitant administration with saquinavir/ritonavir may lead to decreased ethinyl estradiol levels. Alternative or additional contraceptive measures should be used when estrogen-based oral contraceptives and saquinavir/ritonavir are co-administered).

No products indexed under this heading.

Methadone Hydrochloride (Concomitant administration with saquinavir/ritonavir may lead to decreased methadone levels. Dosage of methadone may need to be increased when co-administered with saquinavir/ritonavir).

No products indexed under this heading.

Methsuximide (Co-administration with compounds that are potent inducers of CYP3A4 may result in decreased plasma levels of saquinavir).

No products indexed under this heading.

Methylergonovine Maleate (Inhibition of CYP3A4 by saquinavir could result in increased ergot derivatives plasma levels and create the potential for serious and/or life-threatening reactions; concurrent use is contraindicated).

No products indexed under this heading.

Methylprednisolone (Co-administration with compounds that are potent inducers of CYP3A4 may result in decreased plasma levels of saquinavir).

No products indexed under this heading.

Methylprednisolone Acetate (Co-administration with compounds that are potent inducers of CYP3A4 may result in decreased plasma levels of saquinavir). Products include:

Depo-Medrol Injectable Suspension 2615
Depo-Medrol Single-Dose Vial 2617

Methylprednisolone Sodium Succinate (Co-administration with compounds that are potent inducers of CYP3A4 may result in decreased plasma levels of saquinavir).

No products indexed under this heading.

Methysergide Maleate (Inhibition of CYP3A4 by saquinavir could result in increased ergot derivatives plasma levels and create the potential for serious and/or life-threatening reactions; concurrent use is contraindicated).

No products indexed under this heading.

Mibefradil Dihydrochloride (Potential for elevated plasma concentrations of compounds that are substrate of CYP3A4, such as calcium channel blockers).

No products indexed under this heading.

Midazolam Hydrochloride (Inhibition of CYP3A4 by saquinavir could result in increased midazolam plasma levels and create the potential for serious and/or life-threatening reactions; concurrent use is contraindicated).

No products indexed under this heading.

Modafinil (Co-administration with compounds that are potent inducers of CYP3A4 may result in decreased plasma levels of saquinavir). Products include:

Provigil Tablets 1002

Nefazodone Hydrochloride (Co-administration with drugs that are mainly metabolized by CYP3A4 may have elevated plasma concentrations when co-administered with saquinavir; these combinations should be used with caution).

No products indexed under this heading.

Nelfinavir Mesylate (Co-administration has resulted in an 18% increase in nelfinavir plasma AUC and a 392% increase in saquinavir plasma AUC; currently, there are no safety and efficacy data available from use of this combination). Products include:

Viracept 2556

Nevirapine (Co-administration has resulted in a 24% decrease in saquinavir plasma AUC; currently, there are no safety and efficacy data available from use of this combination). Products include:

Viramune Oral Suspension 903
Viramune Tablets 903

Nicardipine (Concomitant administration with saquinavir may lead to increased nicardipine levels; caution is warranted and clinical monitoring of patient is recommended).

No products indexed under this heading.

Nicardipine Hydrochloride (Concomitant administration with saquinavir may lead to increased nicardipine levels; caution is warranted and clinical monitoring of patient is recommended). Products include:

Cardene I.V. 1129

Nifedipine (Concomitant administration with saquinavir may lead to increased nifedipine levels; caution is warranted and clinical monitoring of patient is recommended). Products include:

Adalat CC Tablets 2978

Nimodipine (Concomitant administration with saquinavir may lead to increased nimodipine levels; caution is warranted and clinical monitoring of patient is recommended). Products include:

Nimotop Capsules 774

Nisoldipine (Concomitant administration with saquinavir may lead to increased nisoldipine levels; caution is warranted and clinical monitoring of patient is recommended). Products include:

Sular Tablets 1163

Nitrendipine (Co-administration with drugs that are mainly metabolized by CYP3A4 may have elevated plasma concentrations when co-administered with saquinavir; these combinations should be used with caution).

No products indexed under this heading.

Norethindrone (Concomitant administration with saquinavir/ritonavir may lead to decreased ethinyl estradiol levels. Alternative or additional contraceptive measures should be used when estrogen-based oral contraceptives and saquinavir/ritonavir are co-administered). Products include:

Ortho Micronor Tablets 2411

Norethindrone Acetate (Co-administration with drugs that are mainly metabolized by CYP3A4 may have elevated plasma concentrations when co-administered with saquinavir; these combinations should be used with caution). Products include:

Activella Tablets 2311
Aygestin Tablets 1062
CombiPatch Transdermal System 2180

Norethynodrel (Concomitant administration with saquinavir/ritonavir may lead to decreased ethinyl estradiol levels. Alternative or additional contraceptive measures should be used when estrogen-based oral contraceptives and saquinavir/ritonavir are co-administered).

No products indexed under this heading.

Norgestimate (Concomitant administration with saquinavir/ritonavir may lead to decreased ethinyl estradiol levels. Alternative or additional contraceptive measures should be used when estrogen-based oral contraceptives and saquinavir/ritonavir are co-administered). Products include:

Ortho-Cyclen/Ortho Tri-Cyclen 2414
Ortho Tri-Cyclen Lo Tablets 2421
Prefest Tablets 1069

Norgestrel (Concomitant administration with saquinavir/ritonavir may lead to decreased ethinyl estradiol levels. Alternative or additional contraceptive measures should be used when estrogen-based oral contraceptives and saquinavir/ritonavir are co-administered). Products include:

Lo/Ovral-28 Tablets 3423

Ondansetron (Co-administration with drugs that are mainly metabolized by CYP3A4 may have elevated plasma concentrations when co-administered with saquinavir; these combinations should be used with caution). Products include:

Zofran ODT Orally Disintegrating Tablets 1613

Ondansetron Hydrochloride (Co-administration with drugs that are mainly metabolized by CYP3A4 may have elevated plasma concentrations when co-administered with saquinavir; these combinations should be used with caution). Products include:

Zofran Injection 1607
Zofran 1613

Oxcarbazepine (Co-administration with compounds that are potent inducers of CYP3A4 may result in decreased plasma levels of saquinavir). Products include:

Trileptal Oral Suspension 2281
Trileptal Tablets 2281

Paclitaxel (Co-administration with drugs that are mainly metabolized by CYP3A4 may have elevated plasma concentrations when co-administered with saquinavir; these combinations should be used with caution).

No products indexed under this heading.

Phenobarbital (Anticonvulsants, such as phenobarbital, may decrease saquinavir plasma concentrations).

No products indexed under this heading.

Phenobarbital Sodium (Co-administration with compounds that are potent inducers of CYP3A4 may result in decreased plasma levels of saquinavir).

No products indexed under this heading.

Phenytoin (Concomitant administration with saquinavir may decrease saquinavir levels. Use with caution since saquinavir may be less effective due to decreased saquinavir plasma concentrations).

No products indexed under this heading.

Phenytoin Sodium (Concomitant administration with saquinavir may decrease saquinavir levels. Use with caution since saquinavir may be less effective due to decreased saquinavir plasma concentrations). Products include:

Phenytek Capsules 2153

Pimozide (Inhibition of CYP3A4 by saquinavir could result in elevated plasma concentrations of pimozide, potentially causing serious or life-threatening reactions; concurrent use is contraindicated). Products include:

Orap Tablets 1220

Polyestradiol Phosphate (Co-administration with drugs that are mainly metabolized by CYP3A4 may have elevated plasma concentrations when co-administered with saquinavir; these combinations should be used with caution).

No products indexed under this heading.

Prednisolone Acetate (Co-administration with compounds that are potent inducers of CYP3A4 may result in decreased plasma levels of saquinavir). Products include:

Blephamide Ophthalmic Ointment 563
Blephamide Ophthalmic Suspension.............................. 564
Poly-Pred Liquifilm Ophthalmic Suspension .... ⊙231
Pred Forte Ophthalmic Suspension .... ⊙233
Pred Mild Sterile Ophthalmic Suspension .... ⊙236
Pred-G Ophthalmic Suspension ..... ⊙234
Pred-G Sterile Ophthalmic Ointment .... ⊙235

Prednisolone Sodium Phosphate (Co-administration with compounds that are potent inducers of CYP3A4 may result in decreased plasma levels of saquinavir). Products include:

Pediapred Oral Solution 3319

Prednisolone Tebutate (Co-administration with compounds that are potent inducers of CYP3A4 may result in decreased plasma levels of saquinavir).

No products indexed under this heading.

Prednisone (Co-administration with compounds that are potent inducers of CYP3A4 may result in decreased plasma levels of saquinavir).

No products indexed under this heading.

Primidone (Co-administration with compounds that are potent inducers of CYP3A4 may result in decreased plasma levels of saquinavir).

No products indexed under this heading.

Propafenone Hydrochloride (Inhibition of CYP3A4 by saquinavir could result in elevated plasma concentrations of propafenone, potentially causing serious or life-threatening reactions; concurrent use is contraindicated). Products include:

Rythmol SR Capsules 2736

Quinidine (Inhibition of CYP3A4 by saquinavir could result in elevated plasma concentrations of quinidine, potentially causing serious or life-threatening reactions; concurrent use is contraindicated).

No products indexed under this heading.

Quinidine Gluconate (Inhibition of CYP3A4 by saquinavir could result in elevated plasma concentrations of quinidine, potentially causing serious or life-threatening reactions; concurrent use is contraindicated).

No products indexed under this heading.

Quinidine Hydrochloride (Inhibition of CYP3A4 by saquinavir could result in elevated plasma concentrations of quinidine, potentially causing serious or life-threatening reactions; concurrent use is contraindicated).

No products indexed under this heading.

Quinidine Polygalacturonate (Inhibition of CYP3A4 by saquinavir could result in elevated plasma concentrations of quinidine, potentially causing serious or life-threatening reactions; concurrent use is contraindicated).

No products indexed under this heading.

Quinidine Sulfate (Inhibition of CYP3A4 by saquinavir could result in elevated plasma concentrations of quinidine, potentially causing serious or life-threatening reactions; concurrent use is contraindicated).

No products indexed under this heading.

Ranitidine Hydrochloride (Concomitant administration may cause increased saquinavir levels; no dosage adjustment of saquinavir is recommended). Products include:

Zantac 1597
Zantac Injection 1593
Zantac 75 Tablets .... ▣715
Zantac 150 Maximum Strength Tablets.............................. ▣715
Zantac Injection Pharmacy Bulk Package.............................. 1595

(▣ Described in PDR For Nonprescription Drugs)

(⊙ Described in PDR For Ophthalmic Medicines™)

Rapamycin (Concomitant administration with saquinavir may lead to increased levels of rapamycin. Therapeutic concentration monitoring is recommended for all immunosuppressant agents when co-administered with saquinavir).
No products indexed under this heading.

Rifabutin (Concomitant administration with saquinavir may lead to decreased saquinavir and/or increased rifabutin levels. Saquinavir should not be given as the sole protease inhibitor to patients taking rifabutin).
No products indexed under this heading.

Rifampicin (Co-administration with compounds that are potent inducers of CYP3A4 may result in decreased plasma levels of saquinavir).
No products indexed under this heading.

Rifampin (Inhibition of CYP3A4 by saquinavir could result in elevated plasma concentrations of rifampin, potentially causing serious or life-threatening reactions; concurrent use is contraindicated).
No products indexed under this heading.

Rifapentine (Co-administration with compounds that are potent inducers of CYP3A4 may result in decreased plasma levels of saquinavir).
No products indexed under this heading.

Ritonavir (Combination therapy in HIV-infected patients has resulted in AUC values which were at least 17-fold greater than historical AUC values from patients who received saquinavir without ritonavir).
Products include:
Kaletra 474
Norvir 499

Saquinavir (Co-administration with drugs that are mainly metabolized by CYP3A4 may have elevated plasma concentrations when co-administered with saquinavir; these combinations should be used with caution).
No products indexed under this heading.

Sertraline Hydrochloride (Co-administration with drugs that are mainly metabolized by CYP3A4 may have elevated plasma concentrations when co-administered with saquinavir; these combinations should be used with caution).
Products include:
Zoloft 2581

Sildenafil Citrate (Concomitant administration may lead to increased sildenafil levels; use sildenafil with caution at reduced doses of 25mg every 48 hours with increased monitoring of adverse events when co-administered with saquinavir).
Products include:
Revatio Tablets 2541
Viagra Tablets 2552

Simvastatin (Co-administration of Invirase and simvastatin may result in increased concentrations of statins; potential for, in rare cases, severe adverse events, such as myopathy including rhabdomyolysis; concomitant use is not recommended). Products include:
Vytorin 10/10 Tablets 2084
Vytorin 10/10 Tablets 3092
Vytorin 10/20 Tablets 2084
Vytorin 10/20 Tablets 3092
Vytorin 10/40 Tablets 3092
Vytorin 10/40 Tablets 2084
Vytorin 10/80 Tablets 2084
Vytorin 10/80 Tablets 3092
Zocor Tablets 2078

Sirolimus (Co-administration with drugs that are mainly metabolized by CYP3A4 may have elevated plasma concentrations when co-administered with saquinavir; these combinations should be used with caution). Products include:
Rapamune Oral Solution and Tablets 3472

Sulfinpyrazone (Co-administration with compounds that are potent inducers of CYP3A4 may result in decreased plasma levels of saquinavir).
No products indexed under this heading.

Tacrolimus (Concomitant administration with saquinavir may lead to increased levels of tacrolimus. Therapeutic concentration monitoring is recommended for all immunosuppressant agents when co-administered with saquinavir).
Products include:
Prograf Capsules and Injection 624
Protopic Ointment 629

Tadalafil (Concomitant administration may lead to increased tadalafil levels; use tadalafil with caution at reduced doses of no more than 10mg every 72 hours with increased monitoring of adverse events when co-administered with saquinavir).
Products include:
Cialis Tablets 1806

Tamoxifen Citrate (Co-administration with drugs that are mainly metabolized by CYP3A4 may have elevated plasma concentrations when co-administered with saquinavir; these combinations should be used with caution).
No products indexed under this heading.

Terfenadine (Inhibition of CYP3A4 by saquinavir could result in increased terfenadine plasma levels and create the potential for serious and/or life-threatening reactions, such as rare cases of serious cardiovascular adverse events; concurrent use is contraindicated).
No products indexed under this heading.

Theophylline (Co-administration with compounds that are potent inducers of CYP3A4 may result in decreased plasma levels of saquinavir).
No products indexed under this heading.

Tiagabine Hydrochloride (Co-administration with drugs that are mainly metabolized by CYP3A4 may have elevated plasma concentrations when co-administered with saquinavir; these combinations should be used with caution).
Products include:
Gabitril Tablets 998

Tolterodine Tartrate (Co-administration with drugs that are mainly metabolized by CYP3A4 may have elevated plasma concentrations when co-administered with saquinavir; these combinations should be used with caution).
Products include:
Detrol Tablets 2626
Detrol LA Capsules 2629

Trazodone Hydrochloride (Co-administration with drugs that are mainly metabolized by CYP3A4 may have elevated plasma concentrations when co-administered with saquinavir; these combinations should be used with caution).
No products indexed under this heading.

Triamcinolone (Co-administration with compounds that are potent inducers of CYP3A4 may result in decreased plasma levels of saquinavir).
No products indexed under this heading.

Triamcinolone Acetonide (Co-administration with compounds that are potent inducers of CYP3A4 may result in decreased plasma levels of saquinavir). Products include:
Azmacort Inhalation Aerosol 1701
Nasacort HFA Inhalation Aerosol 2939
Nasacort AQ Nasal Spray 2937

Triamcinolone Diacetate (Co-administration with compounds that are potent inducers of CYP3A4 may result in decreased plasma levels of saquinavir).
No products indexed under this heading.

Triamcinolone Hexacetonide (Co-administration with compounds that are potent inducers of CYP3A4 may result in decreased plasma levels of saquinavir).
No products indexed under this heading.

Triazolam (Inhibition of CYP3A4 by saquinavir could result in increased triazolam plasma levels and create the potential for serious and/or life-threatening reactions; concurrent use is contraindicated).
No products indexed under this heading.

Troglitazone (Co-administration with compounds that are potent inducers of CYP3A4 may result in decreased plasma levels of saquinavir).
No products indexed under this heading.

Vardenafil Hydrochloride (Concomitant administration may lead to increased vardenafil levels; use vardenafil with caution at reduced doses of no more than 2.5mg every 72 hours with increased monitoring of adverse events when co-administered with saquinavir).
Products include:
Levitra Tablets 3048

Verapamil Hydrochloride (Concomitant administration with saquinavir may lead to increased verapamil levels; caution is warranted and clinical monitoring of patient is recommended). Products include:
Covera-HS Tablets 3135
Tarka Tablets 519
Verelan PM Capsules 3120

Vinblastine Sulfate (Co-administration with drugs that are mainly metabolized by CYP3A4 may have elevated plasma concentrations when co-administered with saquinavir; these combinations should be used with caution).
No products indexed under this heading.

Vincristine Sulfate (Co-administration with drugs that are mainly metabolized by CYP3A4 may have elevated plasma concentrations when co-administered with saquinavir; these combinations should be used with caution).
No products indexed under this heading.

Warfarin Sodium (Concentrations of warfarin may be affected. It is recommended that INR be monitored). Products include:
Coumadin for Injection 932
Coumadin Tablets 932

Food Interactions

Food, unspecified (Saquinavir 24-hour AUC and Cmax following the administration of a high calorie meal were an average two times higher than after a lower calorie, lower fat meal; the effect of food has been shown to persist for up to 2 hours).

INVIRASE TABLETS

(Saquinavir Mesylate) 2776
See Invirase Capsules

IRESSA TABLETS

(Gefitinib) 684
May interact with cytochrome p450 3a4 inducers (selected), histamine H_2-receptor antagonists, and certain other agents. Compounds in these categories include:

Allium sativum (Substances that are inducers of CYP3A4 activity increase the metabolism of gefitinib and decrease its plasma concentrations).
No products indexed under this heading.

Aprepitant (Substances that are inducers of CYP3A4 activity increase the metabolism of gefitinib and decrease its plasma concentrations).
Products include:
Emend Capsules 1944

Betamethasone Acetate (Substances that are inducers of CYP3A4 activity increase the metabolism of gefitinib and decrease its plasma concentrations).
No products indexed under this heading.

Betamethasone Sodium Phosphate (Substances that are inducers of CYP3A4 activity increase the metabolism of gefitinib and decrease its plasma concentrations).
No products indexed under this heading.

Carbamazepine (Substances that are inducers of CYP3A4 activity increase the metabolism of gefitinib and decrease its plasma concentrations). Products include:
Carbatrol Capsules 3174
Equetro Extended-Release Capsules 3178
Tegretol/Tegretol-XR 2278

Cimetidine (Drugs that cause significant sustained elevation in gastric pH may reduce plasma concentrations of IRESSA and therefore potentially may reduce efficacy). Products include:
Tagamet HB 200 Tablets 637
Tagamet Tablets 1547

IMPORTANT NOTE: Always consult each drug listing in the patient's regimen for possible interactions.

Cimetidine Hydrochloride (Drugs that cause significant sustained elevation in gastric pH may reduce plasma concentrations of IRESSA and therefore potentially may reduce efficacy).
No products indexed under this heading.

Ciprofloxacin Hydrochloride (Substances that are inducers of CYP3A4 activity increase the metabolism of gefitinib and decrease its plasma concentrations). Products include:
Ciloxan Ophthalmic Ointment 554
Cipro Tablets 2991

Cisplatin (Substances that are inducers of CYP3A4 activity increase the metabolism of gefitinib and decrease its plasma concentrations).
No products indexed under this heading.

Cortisone Acetate (Substances that are inducers of CYP3A4 activity increase the metabolism of gefitinib and decrease its plasma concentrations).
No products indexed under this heading.

Dexamethasone (Substances that are inducers of CYP3A4 activity increase the metabolism of gefitinib and decrease its plasma concentrations). Products include:
Ciprodex Otic Suspension 555
Decadron Tablets 1929
TobraDex Ophthalmic Ointment 558
TobraDex Ophthalmic Suspension ... 558

Dexamethasone Acetate (Substances that are inducers of CYP3A4 activity increase the metabolism of gefitinib and decrease its plasma concentrations).
No products indexed under this heading.

Dexamethasone Sodium Phosphate (Substances that are inducers of CYP3A4 activity increase the metabolism of gefitinib and decrease its plasma concentrations). Products include:
Decadron Phosphate Injection 1931

Doxorubicin Hydrochloride (Substances that are inducers of CYP3A4 activity increase the metabolism of gefitinib and decrease its plasma concentrations). Products include:
Adriamycin for Injection, USP 786
Adriamycin Injection, USP 786

Efavirenz (Substances that are inducers of CYP3A4 activity increase the metabolism of gefitinib and decrease its plasma concentrations). Products include:
Sustiva Capsules 957

Ethosuximide (Substances that are inducers of CYP3A4 activity increase the metabolism of gefitinib and decrease its plasma concentrations).
No products indexed under this heading.

Famotidine (Drugs that cause significant sustained elevation in gastric pH may reduce plasma concentrations of IRESSA and therefore potentially may reduce efficacy). Products include:
Pepcid AC Chewable Tablets 1672
Pepcid AC Gelcaps 1672
Pepcid AC Tablets 1672
Maximum Strength Pepcid AC Tablets 1672
Pepcid Complete Chewable Tablets 1672
Pepcid Injection 2017
Pepcid 2014

Felbamate (Substances that are inducers of CYP3A4 activity increase the metabolism of gefitinib and decrease its plasma concentrations).
No products indexed under this heading.

Fludrocortisone Acetate (Substances that are inducers of CYP3A4 activity increase the metabolism of gefitinib and decrease its plasma concentrations).
No products indexed under this heading.

Fosphenytoin Sodium (Substances that are inducers of CYP3A4 activity increase the metabolism of gefitinib and decrease its plasma concentrations).
No products indexed under this heading.

Garlic Extract (Substances that are inducers of CYP3A4 activity increase the metabolism of gefitinib and decrease its plasma concentrations).
No products indexed under this heading.

Garlic Oil (Substances that are inducers of CYP3A4 activity increase the metabolism of gefitinib and decrease its plasma concentrations).
No products indexed under this heading.

Hydrocortisone (Substances that are inducers of CYP3A4 activity increase the metabolism of gefitinib and decrease its plasma concentrations). Products include:
Cortizone•5 Ointment .... ■ 699
Cortizone•10 Creme .... ■ 699
Cortizone•10 Ointment .... ■ 699
Cortizone•10 Plus Creme .... ■ 700
Cortizone•10 Maximum Strength Quick Shot Spray .... ■ 700
Hydrocortone Tablets 1963
Preparation H Hydrocortisone Cream .... ■ 748

Hydrocortisone Acetate (Substances that are inducers of CYP3A4 activity increase the metabolism of gefitinib and decrease its plasma concentrations). Products include:
Analpram-HC 1136
Pramosone 1139
ProctoFoam-HC 3113
Tucks Anti-Itch Ointment .... ■ 712
U-cort 1% Cream 3289

Hydrocortisone Butyrate (Substances that are inducers of CYP3A4 activity increase the metabolism of gefitinib and decrease its plasma concentrations). Products include:
Locoid 1138
Locoid Lipocream Cream 1138

Hydrocortisone Cypionate (Substances that are inducers of CYP3A4 activity increase the metabolism of gefitinib and decrease its plasma concentrations).
No products indexed under this heading.

Hydrocortisone Hemisuccinate (Substances that are inducers of CYP3A4 activity increase the metabolism of gefitinib and decrease its plasma concentrations).
No products indexed under this heading.

Hydrocortisone Probutate (Substances that are inducers of CYP3A4 activity increase the metabolism of gefitinib and decrease its plasma concentrations). Products include:
Pandel Cream, 0.1% 1017

Hydrocortisone Sodium Phosphate (Substances that are inducers of CYP3A4 activity increase the metabolism of gefitinib and decrease its plasma concentrations).
No products indexed under this heading.

Hydrocortisone Sodium Succinate (Substances that are inducers of CYP3A4 activity increase the metabolism of gefitinib and decrease its plasma concentrations).
No products indexed under this heading.

Hydrocortisone Valerate (Substances that are inducers of CYP3A4 activity increase the metabolism of gefitinib and decrease its plasma concentrations).
No products indexed under this heading.

Hypericum (Substances that are inducers of CYP3A4 activity increase the metabolism of gefitinib and decrease its plasma concentrations).
No products indexed under this heading.

Hypericum Perforatum (Substances that are inducers of CYP3A4 activity increase the metabolism of gefitinib and decrease its plasma concentrations).
No products indexed under this heading.

Itraconazole (Concomitant administration of itraconazole with gefitinib to healthy male volunteers increased mean gefitinib AUC by 88%).
No products indexed under this heading.

Mephenytoin (Substances that are inducers of CYP3A4 activity increase the metabolism of gefitinib and decrease its plasma concentrations).
No products indexed under this heading.

Methsuximide (Substances that are inducers of CYP3A4 activity increase the metabolism of gefitinib and decrease its plasma concentrations).
No products indexed under this heading.

Methylprednisolone (Substances that are inducers of CYP3A4 activity increase the metabolism of gefitinib and decrease its plasma concentrations).
No products indexed under this heading.

Methylprednisolone Acetate (Substances that are inducers of CYP3A4 activity increase the metabolism of gefitinib and decrease its plasma concentrations). Products include:
Depo-Medrol Injectable Suspension 2615
Depo-Medrol Single-Dose Vial 2617

Methylprednisolone Sodium Succinate (Substances that are inducers of CYP3A4 activity increase the metabolism of gefitinib and decrease its plasma concentrations).
No products indexed under this heading.

Metoprolol Succinate (Exposure to metoprolol was increased by 30% when it was given in combination with gefitinib in patients with solid tumors). Products include:
Toprol-XL Tablets 660

Metoprolol Tartrate (Exposure to metoprolol was increased by 30% when it was given in combination with gefitinib in patients with solid tumors).
No products indexed under this heading.

Modafinil (Substances that are inducers of CYP3A4 activity increase the metabolism of gefitinib and decrease its plasma concentrations). Products include:
Provigil Tablets 1002

Nevirapine (Substances that are inducers of CYP3A4 activity increase the metabolism of gefitinib and decrease its plasma concentrations). Products include:
Viramune Oral Suspension 903
Viramune Tablets 903

Nizatidine (Drugs that cause significant sustained elevation in gastric pH may reduce plasma concentrations of IRESSA and therefore potentially may reduce efficacy). Products include:
Axid Oral Solution 913

Oxcarbazepine (Substances that are inducers of CYP3A4 activity increase the metabolism of gefitinib and decrease its plasma concentrations). Products include:
Trileptal Oral Suspension 2281
Trileptal Tablets 2281

Phenobarbital (Substances that are inducers of CYP3A4 activity increase the metabolism of gefitinib and decrease its plasma concentrations).
No products indexed under this heading.

Phenobarbital Sodium (Substances that are inducers of CYP3A4 activity increase the metabolism of gefitinib and decrease its plasma concentrations).
No products indexed under this heading.

Phenytoin (Substances that are inducers of CYP3A4 activity increase the metabolism of gefitinib and decrease its plasma concentrations).
No products indexed under this heading.

Phenytoin Sodium (Substances that are inducers of CYP3A4 activity increase the metabolism of gefitinib and decrease its plasma concentrations). Products include:
Phenytek Capsules 2153

Prednisolone Acetate (Substances that are inducers of CYP3A4 activity increase the metabolism of gefitinib and decrease its plasma concentrations). Products include:
Blephamide Ophthalmic Ointment 563
Blephamide Ophthalmic Suspension 564
Poly-Pred Liquifilm Ophthalmic Suspension .... ⊙ 231
Pred Forte Ophthalmic Suspension .... ⊙ 233
Pred Mild Sterile Ophthalmic Suspension .... ⊙ 236
Pred-G Ophthalmic Suspension .... ⊙ 234
Pred-G Sterile Ophthalmic Ointment .... ⊙ 235

Prednisolone Sodium Phosphate (Substances that are inducers of CYP3A4 activity increase the metabolism of gefitinib and decrease its plasma concentrations). Products include:
Pediapred Oral Solution 3319

Prednisolone Tebutate (Substances that are inducers of CYP3A4 activity increase the metabolism of gefitinib and decrease its plasma concentrations).
No products indexed under this heading.

Prednisone (Substances that are inducers of CYP3A4 activity increase the metabolism of gefitinib and decrease its plasma concentrations).
No products indexed under this heading.

Primidone (Substances that are inducers of CYP3A4 activity increase the metabolism of gefitinib and decrease its plasma concentrations).
No products indexed under this heading.

Ranitidine Bismuth Citrate (Co-administration of high doses of ranitidine with sodium bicarbonate reduced mean gefitinib AUC by 44%).
No products indexed under this heading.

Ranitidine Hydrochloride (Co-administration of high doses of ranitidine with sodium bicarbonate reduced mean gefitinib AUC by 44%). Products include:
Zantac ... **1597**
Zantac Injection ... **1593**
Zantac 75 Tablets ... ■ **715**
Zantac 150 Maximum Strength Tablets ... ■ **715**
Zantac Injection Pharmacy Bulk Package ... **1595**

Rifabutin (Substances that are inducers of CYP3A4 activity increase the metabolism of gefitinib and decrease its plasma concentrations).
No products indexed under this heading.

Rifampicin (Rifampicin reduced mean AUC of gefitinib by 85% in healthy male volunteers).
No products indexed under this heading.

Rifampin (Substances that are inducers of CYP3A4 activity increase the metabolism of gefitinib and decrease its plasma concentrations).
No products indexed under this heading.

Rifapentine (Substances that are inducers of CYP3A4 activity increase the metabolism of gefitinib and decrease its plasma concentrations).
No products indexed under this heading.

Sulfinpyrazone (Substances that are inducers of CYP3A4 activity increase the metabolism of gefitinib and decrease its plasma concentrations).
No products indexed under this heading.

Theophylline (Substances that are inducers of CYP3A4 activity increase the metabolism of gefitinib and decrease its plasma concentrations).
No products indexed under this heading.

Triamcinolone (Substances that are inducers of CYP3A4 activity increase the metabolism of gefitinib and decrease its plasma concentrations).
No products indexed under this heading.

Triamcinolone Acetonide (Substances that are inducers of CYP3A4 activity increase the metabolism of gefitinib and decrease its plasma concentrations). Products include:
Azmacort Inhalation Aerosol ... **1701**
Nasacort HFA Inhalation Aerosol ... **2939**
Nasacort AQ Nasal Spray ... **2937**

Triamcinolone Diacetate (Substances that are inducers of CYP3A4 activity increase the metabolism of gefitinib and decrease its plasma concentrations).
No products indexed under this heading.

Triamcinolone Hexacetonide (Substances that are inducers of CYP3A4 activity increase the metabolism of gefitinib and decrease its plasma concentrations).
No products indexed under this heading.

Troglitazone (Substances that are inducers of CYP3A4 activity increase the metabolism of gefitinib and decrease its plasma concentrations).
No products indexed under this heading.

Vinorelbine Tartrate (Phase II clinical trial data indicates that gefitinib may exacerbate the neutropenic effect of vinorelbine). Products include:
Navelbine Injection ... **1494**

Warfarin Sodium (International Normalized Ratio elevations and/or bleeding events have been reported in some patients taking warfarin while on gefitinib therapy). Products include:
Coumadin for Injection ... **932**
Coumadin Tablets ... **932**

I.V. BUSULFEX

(Busulfan) ... **1125**
May interact with phenytoin and certain other agents. Compounds in these categories include:

Acetaminophen (Use of acetaminophen prior to (less than 72 hours) or concurrent with Busulfex may result in reduced busulfan clearance since acetaminophen decreases glutathione levels in the blood and tissues). Products include:
Benadryl Allergy & Cold Tablets ... ■ **692**
Benadryl Allergy & Sinus Headache Caplets & Gelcaps ... ■ **693**
Benadryl Maximum Strength Severe Allergy & Sinus Headache Caplets ... ■ **694**
Contac Severe Cold and Flu Caplets Maximum Strength ... ■ **615**
Contac Severe Cold and Flu Caplets Non-Drowsy ... ■ **615**
Darvocet A 500 Tablets ... **3497**
Goody's Body Pain Formula Powder ... ■ **621**
Goody's Extra Strength Headache Powder ... ■ **621**
Goody's Extra Strength Pain Relief Tablets ... ■ **621**
Goody's PM Powder ... ■ **622**
Hycomine Compound Tablets ... **1105**
Lortab ... **3315**
Lortab Elixir ... **3312**
Percocet Tablets ... **1114**
Robitussin Cough, Cold & Flu Liquid-filled Capsules ... ■ **750**
Robitussin Flu Liquid ... ■ **752**
Sedapap Tablets 50 mg/650 mg ... **2098**
Singlet Caplets ... ■ **636**
Sudafed Severe Cold ... ■ **710**
Sudafed Sinus Headache ... ■ **711**
TheraFlu Cold & Cough Hot Liquid ... ■ **680**
TheraFlu Cold & Sore Throat Hot Liquid ... ■ **680**
TheraFlu Flu & Chest Congestion Non-Drowsy Hot Liquid ... ■ **681**
TheraFlu Flu & Sore Throat Hot Liquid ... ■ **681**
TheraFlu Severe Cold Non-Drowsy Hot Liquid ... ■ **683**
TheraFlu Severe Cold & Cough Hot Liquid ... ■ **683**
TheraFlu Severe Cold Caplets ... ■ **679**
TheraFlu Severe Cold Hot Liquid ... ■ **682**
TheraFlu Severe Cold Non-Drowsy Caplets ... ■ **679**
Triaminic Cough & Sore Throat Liquid ... ■ **687**
Triaminic Flu, Cough & Fever Liquid ... ■ **685**
Triaminic Cough & Sore Throat Softchews ... ■ **689**
Tylenol 8 Hour Extended Release Geltabs and Caplets ... **1843**
Tylenol Sinus NightTime Caplets ... ■ **663**
Children's Tylenol Suspension Liquid and Meltaways ... **1850**
Children's Tylenol Plus Cold & Allergy Suspension Liquid ... **1850**
Children's Tylenol Plus Cold NightTime Suspension Liquid ... **1851**
Children's Tylenol Plus Cold & Cough Suspension Liquid and Chewable Tablets ... **1851**
Children's Tylenol Plus Cold Chewable Tablets ... **1851**
Children's Tylenol Plus Cold Daytime Non-Drowsy Suspension Liquid ... **1851**
Children's Tylenol Plus Flu Suspension Liquid ... **1853**
Concentrated Tylenol Infants' Drops Plus Cold ... **1851**
Concentrated Tylenol Infants' Drops Plus Cold and Cough ... **1851**
Concentrated Tylenol Infants' Drops ... **1850**
Junior Tylenol Meltaways ... **1850**
Tylenol Cold & Flu Severe Daytime Liquid with Cool Bust ... **1846**
Tylenol Cold & Flu Severe NightTime Liquid with Cool Burst ... **1846**
Tylenol Cold Severe Congestion Non-Drowsy Caplets with Cool Burst ... **1846**
Tylenol Cough & Sore Throat Daytime Liquid with Cool Burst ... **1849**
Tylenol Cough & Sore Throat NightTime Liquid with Cool Burst ... **1849**
Tylenol ... **1843**
Extra Strength Tylenol Rapid Release Gels ... **1843**
Tylenol ... **1843**
Tylenol Allergy Complete Night Time Caplets ... **1844**
Tylenol Allergy Complete Multi-Symptom Caplets and Gelcaps with Cool Burst ... **1844**
Tylenol Severe Allergy Caplets ... **1844**
Tylenol Flu NightTime Gelcaps ... **1846**
Tylenol Flu Day Non-Drowsy Gelcaps ... **1846**
Concentrated Tylenol Infants' Drops Plus Cold Nasal Congestant, Fever Reducer & Pain Reliever ... ■ **668**
Concentrated Tylenol Infants' Drops Plus Cold & Cough Nasal Decongestant, Fever Reducer & Pain Reliever ... ■ **668**
Multi-Symptom Tylenol Cold Night Time Caplets ... **1845**
Multi-Symptom Tylenol Cold Day Non-Drowsy Caplets and Gelcaps ... **1845**
Extra Strength Tylenol PM Caplets, Geltabs, Gelcaps and Liquid ... **1847**
Tylenol Sinus Day Non-Drowsy ... **1848**
Tylenol Sinus Night Time Caplets ... **1848**
Tylenol Sinus Severe Congestion Caplets with Cool Burst ... **1848**
Tylenol Sore Throat Daytime Liquid with Cool Burst ... **1849**
Tylenol Sore Throat NightTime Liquid with Cool Burst ... **1849**
Tylenol with Codeine ... **2461**
Women's Tylenol Menstrual Relief Caplets ... **1849**
Ultracet Tablets ... **2462**
Vicks 44M Cough, Cold & Flu Relief ... **2676**
Vicks DayQuil LiquiCaps/Liquid Multi-Symptom Cold/Flu Relief ... ■ **723**
Vicks DayQuil Multi-Symptom Cold/Flu Relief LiquiCaps ... **2675**
Vicks DayQuil Multi-Symptom Cold/Flu Relief Liquid ... **2675**
Vicks NyQuil LiquiCaps ... **2677**
Vicks NyQuil LiquiCaps/Liquid Multi-Symptom Cold/Flu Relief ... ■ **725**
Vicks NyQuil Liquid ... **2677**
Vicodin Tablets ... **530**
Vicodin ES Tablets ... **531**
Vicodin HP Tablets ... **532**
Zydone Tablets ... **1118**

Fosphenytoin Sodium (Phenytoin increases the clearance of busulfan by 15% or more, possibly due to the induction of glutathione-S-transferase).
No products indexed under this heading.

Itraconazole (Itraconazole decreases busulfan clearance by up to 25%).
No products indexed under this heading.

Phenytoin (Phenytoin increases the clearance of busulfan by 15% or more, possibly due to the induction of glutathione-S-transferase).
No products indexed under this heading.

Phenytoin Sodium (Phenytoin increases the clearance of busulfan by 15% or more, possibly due to the induction of glutathione-S-transferase). Products include:
Phenytek Capsules ... **2153**

IVEEGAM EN

(Immune Globulin Intravenous (Human)) ... **759**
May interact with vaccines, live and certain other agents. Compounds in these categories include:

BCG Vaccine (It is reported that antibodies in immune globulin preparations may interfere with the responses by patients to live viral vaccines).
No products indexed under this heading.

Measles, Mumps & Rubella Virus Vaccine, Live (It is reported that antibodies in immune globulin preparations may interfere with the responses by patients to live viral vaccines). Products include:
M-M-R II ... **1980**

Measles & Rubella Virus Vaccine Live (It is reported that antibodies in immune globulin preparations may interfere with the responses by patients to live viral vaccines).
No products indexed under this heading.

Measles Virus Vaccine Live (It is reported that antibodies in immune globulin preparations may interfere with the responses by patients to live viral vaccines). Products include:
Attenuvax ... **1889**

Mumps Skin Test Antigen (It is reported that antibodies in immune globulin preparations may interfere with the responses by patients to live viral vaccines).
No products indexed under this heading.

Mumps Virus Vaccine, Live (It is reported that antibodies in immune globulin preparations may interfere with the responses by patients to live viral vaccines). Products include:
Mumpsvax ... **2005**

Poliovirus Vaccine, Live, Oral, Trivalent, Types 1,2,3 (Sabin) (It is reported that antibodies in immune globulin preparations may interfere with the responses by patients to live viral vaccines).
No products indexed under this heading.

Rotavirus Vaccine, Live, Oral, Tetravalent (It is reported that antibodies in immune globulin preparations may interfere with the responses by patients to live viral vaccines).
No products indexed under this heading.

Rubella & Mumps Virus Vaccine Live (It is reported that antibodies in immune globulin preparations may interfere with the responses by patients to live viral vaccines).
No products indexed under this heading.

Rubella Virus Vaccine Live (It is reported that antibodies in immune globulin preparations may interfere with the responses by patients to live viral vaccines). Products include:
Meruvax II 1994

Smallpox Vaccine (It is reported that antibodies in immune globulin preparations may interfere with the responses by patients to live viral vaccines).
No products indexed under this heading.

Typhoid Vaccine (It is reported that antibodies in immune globulin preparations may interfere with the responses by patients to live viral vaccines).
No products indexed under this heading.

Varicella Virus Vaccine Live (It is reported that antibodies in immune globulin preparations may interfere with the responses by patients to live viral vaccines). Products include:
Varivax 2070

Yellow Fever Vaccine (It is reported that antibodies in immune globulin preparations may interfere with the responses by patients to live viral vaccines).
No products indexed under this heading.

KADIAN CAPSULES

(Morphine Sulfate) 572

May interact with central nervous system depressants, diuretics, general anesthetics, hypnotics and sedatives, monoamine oxidase inhibitors, mixed agonist/antagonist opioid analgesics, neuromuscular blocking agents, phenothiazines, and tranquilizers. Compounds in these categories include:

Alfentanil Hydrochloride (Co-administration may increase the risk of respiratory depression, hypotension and profound sedation and coma; when such combined therapy is contemplated, the initial dose of one or both agents should be reduced by at least 50%).
No products indexed under this heading.

Alprazolam (Co-administration may increase the risk of respiratory depression, hypotension and profound sedation and coma; when such combined therapy is contemplated, the initial dose of one or both agents should be reduced by at least 50%). Products include:
Niravam Orally Disintegrating Tablets 3106
Xanax XR Tablets 2655

Amiloride Hydrochloride (Morphine can reduce the efficacy of diuretics by inducing the release of antidiuretic hormone and by causing spasm of the sphincter of the bladder leading to acute retention of urine). Products include:
Midamor Tablets 2000
Moduretic Tablets 2003

Aprobarbital (Co-administration may increase the risk of respiratory depression, hypotension and profound sedation and coma; when such combined therapy is contemplated, the initial dose of one or both agents should be reduced by at least 50%).
No products indexed under this heading.

Atracurium Besylate (Morphine may enhance the neuromuscular blocking action of skeletal relaxants and produce an increased degree of respiratory depression).
No products indexed under this heading.

Bendroflumethiazide (Morphine can reduce the efficacy of diuretics by inducing the release of antidiuretic hormone and by causing spasm of the sphincter of the bladder leading to acute retention of urine).
No products indexed under this heading.

Bumetanide (Morphine can reduce the efficacy of diuretics by inducing the release of antidiuretic hormone and by causing spasm of the sphincter of the bladder leading to acute retention of urine).
No products indexed under this heading.

Buprenorphine Hydrochloride (May reduce the analgesic effect and/or precipitate withdrawal symptoms). Products include:
Buprenex Injectable 2718
Suboxone Tablets 2719
Subutex Tablets 2719

Buspirone Hydrochloride (Co-administration may increase the risk of respiratory depression, hypotension and profound sedation and coma; when such combined therapy is contemplated, the initial dose of one or both agents should be reduced by at least 50%).
No products indexed under this heading.

Butabarbital (Co-administration may increase the risk of respiratory depression, hypotension and profound sedation and coma; when such combined therapy is contemplated, the initial dose of one or both agents should be reduced by at least 50%).
No products indexed under this heading.

Butalbital (Co-administration may increase the risk of respiratory depression, hypotension and profound sedation and coma; when such combined therapy is contemplated, the initial dose of one or both agents should be reduced by at least 50%). Products include:
Sedapap Tablets 50 mg/650 mg 2098

Butorphanol Tartrate (May reduce the analgesic effect and/or precipitate withdrawal symptoms).
No products indexed under this heading.

Chlordiazepoxide (Co-administration may increase the risk of respiratory depression, hypotension and profound sedation and coma; when such combined therapy is contemplated, the initial dose of one or both agents should be reduced by at least 50%).
No products indexed under this heading.

Chlordiazepoxide Hydrochloride (Co-administration may increase the risk of respiratory depression, hypotension and profound sedation and coma; when such combined therapy is contemplated, the initial dose of one or both agents should be reduced by at least 50%). Products include:
Librium Capsules 3349

Chlorothiazide (Morphine can reduce the efficacy of diuretics by inducing the release of antidiuretic hormone and by causing spasm of the sphincter of the bladder leading to acute retention of urine). Products include:
Aldoclor Tablets 1881
Diuril Oral 1936

Chlorothiazide Sodium (Morphine can reduce the efficacy of diuretics by inducing the release of antidiuretic hormone and by causing spasm of the sphincter of the bladder leading to acute retention of urine). Products include:
Diuril Sodium Intravenous 1934

Chlorpromazine (Co-administration may increase the risk of respiratory depression, hypotension and profound sedation and coma; when such combined therapy is contemplated, the initial dose of one or both agents should be reduced by at least 50%).
No products indexed under this heading.

Chlorpromazine Hydrochloride (Co-administration may increase the risk of respiratory depression, hypotension and profound sedation and coma; when such combined therapy is contemplated, the initial dose of one or both agents should be reduced by at least 50%).
No products indexed under this heading.

Chlorprothixene (Co-administration may increase the risk of respiratory depression, hypotension and profound sedation and coma; when such combined therapy is contemplated, the initial dose of one or both agents should be reduced by at least 50%).
No products indexed under this heading.

Chlorprothixene Hydrochloride (Co-administration may increase the risk of respiratory depression, hypotension and profound sedation and coma; when such combined therapy is contemplated, the initial dose of one or both agents should be reduced by at least 50%).
No products indexed under this heading.

Chlorprothixene Lactate (Co-administration may increase the risk of respiratory depression, hypotension and profound sedation and coma; when such combined therapy is contemplated, the initial dose of one or both agents should be reduced by at least 50%).
No products indexed under this heading.

Chlorthalidone (Morphine can reduce the efficacy of diuretics by inducing the release of antidiuretic hormone and by causing spasm of the sphincter of the bladder leading to acute retention of urine). Products include:
Clorpres Tablets 2139

Cimetidine (Co-administration has resulted in an isolated report of confusion and severe respiratory depression). Products include:
Tagamet HB 200 Tablets 637
Tagamet Tablets 1547

Cimetidine Hydrochloride (Co-administration has resulted in an isolated report of confusion and severe respiratory depression).
No products indexed under this heading.

Cisatracurium Besylate (Morphine may enhance the neuromuscular blocking action of skeletal relaxants and produce an increased degree of respiratory depression). Products include:
Nimbex Injection 494

Clorazepate Dipotassium (Co-administration may increase the risk of respiratory depression, hypotension and profound sedation and coma; when such combined therapy is contemplated, the initial dose of one or both agents should be reduced by at least 50%). Products include:
Tranxene 2488

Clozapine (Co-administration may increase the risk of respiratory depression, hypotension and profound sedation and coma; when such combined therapy is contemplated, the initial dose of one or both agents should be reduced by at least 50%). Products include:
Clozapine Tablets 2141
Clozaril Tablets 2174
FazaClo Orally Disintegrating Tablets 547

Codeine Phosphate (Co-administration may increase the risk of respiratory depression, hypotension and profound sedation and coma; when such combined therapy is contemplated, the initial dose of one or both agents should be reduced by at least 50%). Products include:
Tylenol with Codeine 2461

Desflurane (Co-administration may increase the risk of respiratory depression, hypotension and profound sedation and coma; when such combined therapy is contemplated, the initial dose of one or both agents should be reduced by at least 50%). Products include:
Suprane Liquid for Inhalation 770

Dezocine (Co-administration may increase the risk of respiratory depression, hypotension and profound sedation and coma; when such combined therapy is contemplated, the initial dose of one or both agents should be reduced by at least 50%).
No products indexed under this heading.

Diazepam (Co-administration may increase the risk of respiratory depression, hypotension and profound sedation and coma; when such combined therapy is contemplated, the initial dose of one or both agents should be reduced by at least 50%). Products include:
Diastat Rectal Delivery System 3344

Valium Tablets 2822

Doxacurium Chloride (Morphine may enhance the neuromuscular blocking action of skeletal relaxants and produce an increased degree of respiratory depression).
No products indexed under this heading.

Droperidol (Co-administration may increase the risk of respiratory depression, hypotension and profound sedation and coma; when such combined therapy is contemplated, the initial dose of one or both agents should be reduced by at least 50%).
No products indexed under this heading.

Enflurane (Co-administration may increase the risk of respiratory depression, hypotension and profound sedation and coma; when such combined therapy is contemplated, the initial dose of one or both agents should be reduced by at least 50%).
No products indexed under this heading.

Estazolam (Co-administration may increase the risk of respiratory depression, hypotension and profound sedation and coma; when such combined therapy is contemplated, the initial dose of one or both agents should be reduced by at least 50%). Products include:
ProSom Tablets 512

Ethacrynic Acid (Morphine can reduce the efficacy of diuretics by inducing the release of antidiuretic hormone and by causing spasm of the sphincter of the bladder leading to acute retention of urine). Products include:
Edecrin Tablets 1941

Ethanol (Co-administration may increase the risk of respiratory depression, hypotension and profound sedation and coma; when such combined therapy is contemplated, the initial dose of one or both agents should be reduced by at least 50%).
No products indexed under this heading.

Ethchlorvynol (Co-administration may increase the risk of respiratory depression, hypotension and profound sedation and coma; when such combined therapy is contemplated, the initial dose of one or both agents should be reduced by at least 50%).
No products indexed under this heading.

Ethinamate (Co-administration may increase the risk of respiratory depression, hypotension and profound sedation and coma; when such combined therapy is contemplated, the initial dose of one or both agents should be reduced by at least 50%).
No products indexed under this heading.

Ethyl Alcohol (Co-administration may increase the risk of respiratory depression, hypotension and profound sedation and coma; when such combined therapy is contemplated, the initial dose of one or both agents should be reduced by at least 50%).
No products indexed under this heading.

Fentanyl (Co-administration may increase the risk of respiratory depression, hypotension and profound sedation and coma; when such combined therapy is contemplated, the initial dose of one or both agents should be reduced by at least 50%). Products include:
Duragesic Transdermal System 2448

Fentanyl Citrate (Co-administration may increase the risk of respiratory depression, hypotension and profound sedation and coma; when such combined therapy is contemplated, the initial dose of one or both agents should be reduced by at least 50%). Products include:
Actiq 993

Fluphenazine Decanoate (Co-administration may increase the risk of respiratory depression, hypotension and profound sedation and coma; when such combined therapy is contemplated, the initial dose of one or both agents should be reduced by at least 50%).
No products indexed under this heading.

Fluphenazine Enanthate (Co-administration may increase the risk of respiratory depression, hypotension and profound sedation and coma; when such combined therapy is contemplated, the initial dose of one or both agents should be reduced by at least 50%).
No products indexed under this heading.

Fluphenazine Hydrochloride (Co-administration may increase the risk of respiratory depression, hypotension and profound sedation and coma; when such combined therapy is contemplated, the initial dose of one or both agents should be reduced by at least 50%).
No products indexed under this heading.

Flurazepam Hydrochloride (Co-administration may increase the risk of respiratory depression, hypotension and profound sedation and coma; when such combined therapy is contemplated, the initial dose of one or both agents should be reduced by at least 50%). Products include:
Dalmane Capsules 3343

Furosemide (Morphine can reduce the efficacy of diuretics by inducing the release of antidiuretic hormone and by causing spasm of the sphincter of the bladder leading to acute retention of urine). Products include:
Furosemide Tablets 2117

Glutethimide (Co-administration may increase the risk of respiratory depression, hypotension and profound sedation and coma; when such combined therapy is contemplated, the initial dose of one or both agents should be reduced by at least 50%).
No products indexed under this heading.

Haloperidol (Co-administration may increase the risk of respiratory depression, hypotension and profound sedation and coma; when such combined therapy is contemplated, the initial dose of one or both agents should be reduced by at least 50%).
No products indexed under this heading.

Haloperidol Decanoate (Co-administration may increase the risk of respiratory depression, hypotension and profound sedation and coma; when such combined therapy is contemplated, the initial dose of one or both agents should be reduced by at least 50%).
No products indexed under this heading.

Hydrochlorothiazide (Morphine can reduce the efficacy of diuretics by inducing the release of antidiuretic hormone and by causing spasm of the sphincter of the bladder leading to acute retention of urine). Products include:
Aldoril Tablets 1884
Atacand HCT 637
Avalide Tablets 2889
Avalide Tablets 922
Benicar HCT Tablets 2852
Diovan HCT Tablets 2195
Dyazide Capsules 1389
Hyzaar 1964
Lotensin HCT Tablets 2235
Maxzide 2150
Micardis HCT Tablets 886
Moduretic Tablets 2003
Prinzide Tablets 2033
Teveten HCT Tablets 1710
Timolide Tablets 2056
Uniretic Tablets 3114
Vaseretic Tablets 2073
Zestoretic Tablets 701

Hydrocodone Bitartrate (Co-administration may increase the risk of respiratory depression, hypotension and profound sedation and coma; when such combined therapy is contemplated, the initial dose of one or both agents should be reduced by at least 50%). Products include:
Hycodan 1104
Hycomine Compound Tablets 1105
Hycotuss Expectorant Syrup 1106
Lortab 3315
Lortab Elixir 3312
Vicodin Tablets 530
Vicodin ES Tablets 531
Vicodin HP Tablets 532
Vicoprofen Tablets 533
Zydone Tablets 1118

Hydrocodone Polistirex (Co-administration may increase the risk of respiratory depression, hypotension and profound sedation and coma; when such combined therapy is contemplated, the initial dose of one or both agents should be reduced by at least 50%). Products include:
Tussionex Pennkinetic Extended-Release Suspension 3322

Hydroflumethiazide (Morphine can reduce the efficacy of diuretics by inducing the release of antidiuretic hormone and by causing spasm of the sphincter of the bladder leading to acute retention of urine).
No products indexed under this heading.

Hydromorphone Hydrochloride (Co-administration may increase the risk of respiratory depression, hypotension and profound sedation and coma; when such combined therapy is contemplated, the initial dose of one or both agents should be reduced by at least 50%). Products include:
Dilaudid 439
Dilaudid Oral Liquid 443
Dilaudid Non-Sterile Powder 439
Dilaudid Rectal Suppositories 439
Dilaudid Tablets 439
Dilaudid Tablets - 8 mg 443
Dilaudid-HP 441

Hydroxyzine Hydrochloride (Co-administration may increase the risk of respiratory depression, hypotension and profound sedation and coma; when such combined therapy is contemplated, the initial dose of one or both agents should be reduced by at least 50%).
No products indexed under this heading.

Indapamide (Morphine can reduce the efficacy of diuretics by inducing the release of antidiuretic hormone and by causing spasm of the sphincter of the bladder leading to acute retention of urine). Products include:
Indapamide Tablets 2119

Isocarboxazid (MAO inhibitors have been reported to intensify the effects of opioids causing anxiety, confusion and significant depression of respiration or coma; concurrent and/or sequential use is not recommended).
No products indexed under this heading.

Isoflurane (Co-administration may increase the risk of respiratory depression, hypotension and profound sedation and coma; when such combined therapy is contemplated, the initial dose of one or both agents should be reduced by at least 50%).
No products indexed under this heading.

Ketamine Hydrochloride (Co-administration may increase the risk of respiratory depression, hypotension and profound sedation and coma; when such combined therapy is contemplated, the initial dose of one or both agents should be reduced by at least 50%).
No products indexed under this heading.

Levomethadyl Acetate Hydrochloride (Co-administration may increase the risk of respiratory depression, hypotension and profound sedation and coma; when such combined therapy is contemplated, the initial dose of one or both agents should be reduced by at least 50%).
No products indexed under this heading.

Levorphanol Tartrate (Co-administration may increase the risk of respiratory depression, hypotension and profound sedation and coma; when such combined therapy is contemplated, the initial dose of one or both agents should be reduced by at least 50%).
No products indexed under this heading.

Lorazepam (Co-administration may increase the risk of respiratory depression, hypotension and profound sedation and coma; when such combined therapy is contemplated, the initial dose of one or both agents should be reduced by at least 50%).
No products indexed under this heading.

Loxapine Hydrochloride (Co-administration may increase the risk of respiratory depression, hypotension and profound sedation and coma; when such combined therapy is contemplated, the initial dose of one or both agents should be reduced by at least 50%).
No products indexed under this heading.

Loxapine Succinate (Co-administration may increase the risk of respiratory depression, hypotension and profound sedation and coma; when such combined therapy is contemplated, the initial dose of one or both agents should be reduced by at least 50%).
No products indexed under this heading.

Meperidine Hydrochloride (Co-administration may increase the risk of respiratory depression, hypotension and profound sedation and coma; when such combined therapy is contemplated, the initial dose of one or both agents should be reduced by at least 50%).
No products indexed under this heading.

Mephobarbital (Co-administration may increase the risk of respiratory depression, hypotension and profound sedation and coma; when such combined therapy is contemplated, the initial dose of one or both agents should be reduced by at least 50%). Products include:
Mebaral Tablets, USP 2483

Meprobamate (Co-administration may increase the risk of respiratory depression, hypotension and profound sedation and coma; when such combined therapy is contemplated, the initial dose of one or both agents should be reduced by at least 50%).
No products indexed under this heading.

Mesoridazine Besylate (Co-administration may increase the risk of respiratory depression, hypotension and profound sedation and coma; when such combined therapy is contemplated, the initial dose of one or both agents should be reduced by at least 50%).
No products indexed under this heading.

Methadone Hydrochloride (Co-administration may increase the risk of respiratory depression, hypotension and profound sedation and coma; when such combined therapy is contemplated, the initial dose of one or both agents should be reduced by at least 50%).
No products indexed under this heading.

Methohexital Sodium (Co-administration may increase the risk of respiratory depression, hypotension and profound sedation and coma; when such combined therapy is contemplated, the initial dose of one or both agents should be reduced by at least 50%).
No products indexed under this heading.

Methotrimeprazine (Co-administration may increase the risk of respiratory depression, hypotension and profound sedation and coma; when such combined therapy is contemplated, the initial dose of one or both agents should be reduced by at least 50%).
No products indexed under this heading.

Methoxyflurane (Co-administration may increase the risk of respiratory depression, hypotension and profound sedation and coma; when such combined therapy is contemplated, the initial dose of one or both agents should be reduced by at least 50%).
No products indexed under this heading.

Methyclothiazide (Morphine can reduce the efficacy of diuretics by inducing the release of antidiuretic hormone and by causing spasm of the sphincter of the bladder leading to acute retention of urine).
No products indexed under this heading.

Metocurine Iodide (Morphine may enhance the neuromuscular blocking action of skeletal relaxants and produce an increased degree of respiratory depression).
No products indexed under this heading.

Metolazone (Morphine can reduce the efficacy of diuretics by inducing the release of antidiuretic hormone and by causing spasm of the sphincter of the bladder leading to acute retention of urine).
No products indexed under this heading.

Midazolam Hydrochloride (Co-administration may increase the risk of respiratory depression, hypotension and profound sedation and coma; when such combined therapy is contemplated, the initial dose of one or both agents should be reduced by at least 50%).
No products indexed under this heading.

Mivacurium Chloride (Morphine may enhance the neuromuscular blocking action of skeletal relaxants and produce an increased degree of respiratory depression). Products include:
Mivacron Injection 489

Moclobemide (MAO inhibitors have been reported to intensify the effects of opioids causing anxiety, confusion and significant depression of respiration or coma; concurrent and/or sequential use is not recommended).
No products indexed under this heading.

Molindone Hydrochloride (Co-administration may increase the risk of respiratory depression, hypotension and profound sedation and coma; when such combined therapy is contemplated, the initial dose of one or both agents should be reduced by at least 50%). Products include:
Moban Tablets 1108

Nalbuphine Hydrochloride (May reduce the analgesic effect and/or precipitate withdrawal symptoms). Products include:
Nubain Injection 1111

Olanzapine (Co-administration may increase the risk of respiratory depression, hypotension and profound sedation and coma; when such combined therapy is contemplated, the initial dose of one or both agents should be reduced by at least 50%). Products include:
Symbyax Capsules 1788
Zyprexa Tablets 1798
Zyprexa IntraMuscular 1798
Zyprexa ZYDIS Orally Disintegrating Tablets 1798

Oxazepam (Co-administration may increase the risk of respiratory depression, hypotension and profound sedation and coma; when such combined therapy is contemplated, the initial dose of one or both agents should be reduced by at least 50%).
No products indexed under this heading.

Oxycodone Hydrochloride (Co-administration may increase the risk of respiratory depression, hypotension and profound sedation and coma; when such combined therapy is contemplated, the initial dose of one or both agents should be reduced by at least 50%). Products include:
Combunox Tablets 1183
OxyContin Tablets 2699
OxyFast Oral Concentrate Solution 2704
OxyIR Capsules 2704
Percocet Tablets 1114
Percodan Tablets 1115

Pancuronium Bromide (Morphine may enhance the neuromuscular blocking action of skeletal relaxants and produce an increased degree of respiratory depression).
No products indexed under this heading.

Pargyline Hydrochloride (MAO inhibitors have been reported to intensify the effects of opioids causing anxiety, confusion and significant depression of respiration or coma; concurrent and/or sequential use is not recommended).
No products indexed under this heading.

Pentazocine Hydrochloride (May reduce the analgesic effect and/or precipitate withdrawal symptoms).
No products indexed under this heading.

Pentazocine Lactate (May reduce the analgesic effect and/or precipitate withdrawal symptoms).
No products indexed under this heading.

Pentobarbital Sodium (Co-administration may increase the risk of respiratory depression, hypotension and profound sedation and coma; when such combined therapy is contemplated, the initial dose of one or both agents should be reduced by at least 50%). Products include:
Nembutal Sodium Solution, USP 2484

Perphenazine (Co-administration may increase the risk of respiratory depression, hypotension and profound sedation and coma; when such combined therapy is contemplated, the initial dose of one or both agents should be reduced by at least 50%).
No products indexed under this heading.

Phenelzine Sulfate (MAO inhibitors have been reported to intensify the effects of opioids causing anxiety, confusion and significant depression of respiration or coma; concurrent and/or sequential use is not recommended).
No products indexed under this heading.

Phenobarbital (Co-administration may increase the risk of respiratory depression, hypotension and profound sedation and coma; when such combined therapy is contemplated, the initial dose of one or both agents should be reduced by at least 50%).
No products indexed under this heading.

Polythiazide (Morphine can reduce the efficacy of diuretics by inducing the release of antidiuretic hormone and by causing spasm of the sphincter of the bladder leading to acute retention of urine).
No products indexed under this heading.

Prazepam (Co-administration may increase the risk of respiratory depression, hypotension and profound sedation and coma; when such combined therapy is contemplated, the initial dose of one or both agents should be reduced by at least 50%).
No products indexed under this heading.

Procarbazine Hydrochloride (MAO inhibitors have been reported to intensify the effects of opioids causing anxiety, confusion and significant depression of respiration or coma; concurrent and/or sequential use is not recommended). Products include:
Matulane Capsules 3188

Prochlorperazine (Co-administration may increase the risk of respiratory depression, hypotension and profound sedation and coma; when such combined therapy is contemplated, the initial dose of one or both agents should be reduced by at least 50%).
No products indexed under this heading.

Promethazine Hydrochloride (Co-administration may increase the risk of respiratory depression, hypotension and profound sedation and coma; when such combined therapy is contemplated, the initial dose of one or both agents should be reduced by at least 50%). Products include:
Phenergan 3438

Propofol (Co-administration may increase the risk of respiratory depression, hypotension and profound sedation and coma; when such combined therapy is contemplated, the initial dose of one or both agents should be reduced by at least 50%). Products include:
Diprivan Injectable Emulsion 676

Propoxyphene Hydrochloride (Co-administration may increase the risk of respiratory depression, hypotension and profound sedation and coma; when such combined therapy is contemplated, the initial dose of one or both agents should be reduced by at least 50%).
No products indexed under this heading.

Propoxyphene Napsylate (Co-administration may increase the risk of respiratory depression, hypotension and profound sedation and coma; when such combined therapy is contemplated, the initial dose of one or both agents should be reduced by at least 50%). Products include:
Darvocet A 500 Tablets 3497

Quazepam (Co-administration may increase the risk of respiratory depression, hypotension and profound sedation and coma; when such combined therapy is contemplated, the initial dose of one or both agents should be reduced by at least 50%).
No products indexed under this heading.

Quetiapine Fumarate (Co-administration may increase the risk of respiratory depression, hypotension and profound sedation and coma; when such combined therapy is contemplated, the initial dose of one or both agents should be reduced by at least 50%). Products include:

Seroquel Tablets 691

Rapacuronium Bromide (Morphine may enhance the neuromuscular blocking action of skeletal relaxants and produce an increased degree of respiratory depression).
No products indexed under this heading.

Remifentanil Hydrochloride (Co-administration may increase the risk of respiratory depression, hypotension and profound sedation and coma; when such combined therapy is contemplated, the initial dose of one or both agents should be reduced by at least 50%).
No products indexed under this heading.

Risperidone (Co-administration may increase the risk of respiratory depression, hypotension and profound sedation and coma; when such combined therapy is contemplated, the initial dose of one or both agents should be reduced by at least 50%). Products include:

Risperdal Consta Long-Acting Injection 1664
Risperdal M-Tab Orally Disintegrating Tablets 1658
Risperdal 1658

Rocuronium Bromide (Morphine may enhance the neuromuscular blocking action of skeletal relaxants and produce an increased degree of respiratory depression). Products include:

Zemuron Injection 2363

Secobarbital Sodium (Co-administration may increase the risk of respiratory depression, hypotension and profound sedation and coma; when such combined therapy is contemplated, the initial dose of one or both agents should be reduced by at least 50%).
No products indexed under this heading.

Selegiline Hydrochloride (MAO inhibitors have been reported to intensify the effects of opioids causing anxiety, confusion and significant depression of respiration or coma; concurrent and/or sequential use is not recommended). Products include:

Eldepryl Capsules 3209

Sevoflurane (Co-administration may increase the risk of respiratory depression, hypotension and profound sedation and coma; when such combined therapy is contemplated, the initial dose of one or both agents should be reduced by at least 50%). Products include:

Ultane Liquid for Inhalation 526

Spironolactone (Morphine can reduce the efficacy of diuretics by inducing the release of antidiuretic hormone and by causing spasm of the sphincter of the bladder leading to acute retention of urine).
No products indexed under this heading.

Succinylcholine Chloride (Morphine may enhance the neuromuscular blocking action of skeletal relaxants and produce an increased degree of respiratory depression).
No products indexed under this heading.

Sufentanil Citrate (Co-administration may increase the risk of respiratory depression, hypotension and profound sedation and coma; when such combined therapy is contemplated, the initial dose of one or both agents should be reduced by at least 50%).
No products indexed under this heading.

Temazepam (Co-administration may increase the risk of respiratory depression, hypotension and profound sedation and coma; when such combined therapy is contemplated, the initial dose of one or both agents should be reduced by at least 50%).
No products indexed under this heading.

Thiamylal Sodium (Co-administration may increase the risk of respiratory depression, hypotension and profound sedation and coma; when such combined therapy is contemplated, the initial dose of one or both agents should be reduced by at least 50%).
No products indexed under this heading.

Thioridazine Hydrochloride (Co-administration may increase the risk of respiratory depression, hypotension and profound sedation and coma; when such combined therapy is contemplated, the initial dose of one or both agents should be reduced by at least 50%). Products include:

Thioridazine Hydrochloride Tablets 2122

Thiothixene (Co-administration may increase the risk of respiratory depression, hypotension and profound sedation and coma; when such combined therapy is contemplated, the initial dose of one or both agents should be reduced by at least 50%). Products include:

Thiothixene Capsules 2124

Torsemide (Morphine can reduce the efficacy of diuretics by inducing the release of antidiuretic hormone and by causing spasm of the sphincter of the bladder leading to acute retention of urine).
No products indexed under this heading.

Tranylcypromine Sulfate (MAO inhibitors have been reported to intensify the effects of opioids causing anxiety, confusion and significant depression of respiration or coma; concurrent and/or sequential use is not recommended). Products include:

Parnate Tablets 1499

Triamterene (Morphine can reduce the efficacy of diuretics by inducing the release of antidiuretic hormone and by causing spasm of the sphincter of the bladder leading to acute retention of urine). Products include:

Dyazide Capsules 1389
Dyrenium Capsules 3390
Maxzide 2150

Triazolam (Co-administration may increase the risk of respiratory depression, hypotension and profound sedation and coma; when such combined therapy is contemplated, the initial dose of one or both agents should be reduced by at least 50%).
No products indexed under this heading.

Trifluoperazine Hydrochloride (Co-administration may increase the risk of respiratory depression, hypotension and profound sedation and coma; when such combined therapy is contemplated, the initial dose of one or both agents should be reduced by at least 50%).
No products indexed under this heading.

Vecuronium Bromide (Morphine may enhance the neuromuscular blocking action of skeletal relaxants and produce an increased degree of respiratory depression).
No products indexed under this heading.

Zaleplon (Co-administration may increase the risk of respiratory depression, hypotension and profound sedation and coma; when such combined therapy is contemplated, the initial dose of one or both agents should be reduced by at least 50%). Products include:

Sonata Capsules 1686

Ziprasidone Hydrochloride (Co-administration may increase the risk of respiratory depression, hypotension and profound sedation and coma; when such combined therapy is contemplated, the initial dose of one or both agents should be reduced by at least 50%). Products include:

Geodon Capsules 2514

Zolpidem Tartrate (Co-administration may increase the risk of respiratory depression, hypotension and profound sedation and coma; when such combined therapy is contemplated, the initial dose of one or both agents should be reduced by at least 50%). Products include:

Ambien Tablets 2867

Food Interactions

Alcohol (Co-administration may increase the risk of respiratory depression, hypotension and profound sedation and coma).

Food, unspecified (Slows the rate of absorption of Kadian, the extent of absorption is not affected and Kadian can be administered without regard to meals; the pellets in Kadian should not be dissolved).

KALETRA CAPSULES

(Lopinavir, Ritonavir) 474

May interact with dexamethasone, dihydropyridine calcium channel blockers, ergot-containing drugs, phenytoin, quinidine, and certain other agents. Compounds in these categories include:

Abacavir Sulfate (Kaletra induces glucuronidation; therefore, Kaletra has the potential to reduce abacavir plasma concentrations; the clinical significance is unknown). Products include:

Epzicom Tablets 1402
Trizivir Tablets 1565
Ziagen 1600

Amiodarone Hydrochloride (Co-administration can result in increased amiodarone plasma concentrations; caution and monitoring is recommended). Products include:

Pacerone Tablets 3337

Amlodipine Besylate (Increased plasma concentrations of dihydropyridine calcium channel blockers; caution is warranted and clinical monitoring of patients is recommended). Products include:

Caduet Tablets 2507
Lotrel Capsules 2238
Norvasc Tablets 2529

Amprenavir (Co-administration results in increased amprenavir plasma concentrations, decreased Cmax and increased Cmin; dosage adjustments may be needed). Products include:

Agenerase Capsules 1299
Agenerase Oral Solution 1304

Astemizole (Kaletra is an inhibitor of the CYP450 3A. Co-administration with drugs that are highly dependent on CYP450 3A for clearance and for which elevated plasma concentrations are associated with serious and/or life threatening events, such as astemizole, is contraindicated).
No products indexed under this heading.

Atorvastatin Calcium (Co-administration with HMG-CoA reductase inhibitors that are metabolized by the CYP3A pathway, such as atorvastatin, increases the risk of myopathy including rhabdomyolysis; caution is recommended). Products include:

Caduet Tablets 2507
Lipitor Tablets 2495

Atovaquone (Co-administration can result in decreased atovaquone plasma concentrations; clinical significance is unknown; however, increase in atovaquone doses may be needed). Products include:

Malarone Tablets 1484
Malarone Pediatric Tablets 1484
Mepron Suspension 1487

Bepridil Hydrochloride (Co-administration can result in increased bepridil plasma concentrations; caution and monitoring is recommended).
No products indexed under this heading.

Carbamazepine (Co-administration can result in decreased lopinavir plasma concentrations; Kaletra may be less effective due to decreased lopinavir plasma concentrations; use with caution). Products include:

Carbatrol Capsules 3174
Equetro Extended-Release Capsules 3178
Tegretol/Tegretol-XR 2278

Cisapride (Kaletra is an inhibitor of the CYP450 3A. Co-administration with drugs that are highly dependent on CYP450 3A for clearance and for which elevated plasma concentrations are associated with serious and/or life threatening events, such as cisapride, is contraindicated).
No products indexed under this heading.

Clarithromycin (Co-administration can result in increased clarithromycin plasma concentrations; for patients with renal impairment, the dosage may need to be adjusted). Products include:

Biaxin/Biaxin XL 402
PREVPAC 3281

Cyclosporine (Co-administration results in increased plasma concen-

trations of immunosuppressants; monitoring is recommended). Products include:
Gengraf Capsules 458
Neoral Soft Gelatin Capsules 2247
Neoral Oral Solution 2247
Restasis Ophthalmic Emulsion 570
Sandimmune 2259

Delavirdine Mesylate (Co-administration has a potential to increase lopinavir plasma concentrations). Products include:
Rescriptor Tablets 2535

Dexamethasone (Co-administration can result in decreased lopinavir plasma concentrations; Kaletra may be less effective due to decreased lopinavir plasma concentrations in patients taking these agents concomitantly. Co-administer with caution). Products include:
Ciprodex Otic Suspension 555
Decadron Tablets 1929
TobraDex Ophthalmic Ointment 558
TobraDex Ophthalmic Suspension 558

Dexamethasone Acetate (Co-administration can result in decreased lopinavir plasma concentrations; Kaletra may be less effective due to decreased lopinavir plasma concentrations in patients taking these agents concomitantly. Co-administer with caution).
No products indexed under this heading.

Dexamethasone Sodium Phosphate (Co-administration can result in decreased lopinavir plasma concentrations; Kaletra may be less effective due to decreased lopinavir plasma concentrations in patients taking these agents concomitantly. Co-administer with caution). Products include:
Decadron Phosphate Injection 1931

Didanosine (Simultaneous administration is not recommended; it is recommended that didanosine be administered on an empty stomach; therefore, didanosine should be given one hour before or two hours after Kaletra).
No products indexed under this heading.

Dihydroergotamine Mesylate (Kaletra is an inhibitor of CYP450 3A. Co-administration is contraindicated due to potential for serious and/or life threatening reactions such as acute ergot toxicity). Products include:
Migranal Nasal Spray 3350

Disulfiram (Kaletra oral solution contains alcohol which can produce disulfiram-like reactions when co-administered with disulfiram). Products include:
Antabuse Tablets 2343

Efavirenz (Co-administration with efavirenz has a potential to decrease plasma concentrations of protease inhibitors by inducing the activity of CYP3A; dosage adjustments may be needed). Products include:
Sustiva Capsules 957

Ergonovine Maleate (Kaletra is an inhibitor of CYP450 3A. Co-administration is contraindicated due to potential for serious and/or life threatening reactions such as acute ergot toxicity).
No products indexed under this heading.

Ergotamine Tartrate (Kaletra is an inhibitor of CYP450 3A. Co-administration is contraindicated due to potential for serious and/or life threatening reactions such as acute ergot toxicity).
No products indexed under this heading.

Ethinyl Estradiol (Co-administration results in decreased plasma concentrations of ethinyl estradiol; alternative methods of non-hormonal contraception should be used when estrogen-based oral contraceptives and Kaletra are co-administered). Products include:
Alesse-28 Tablets 3392
Lo/Ovral-28 Tablets 3423
NuvaRing 2357
Ortho-Cept Tablets 2395
Ortho-Cyclen/Ortho Tri-Cyclen 2414
Ortho Evra Transdermal System 2402
Ortho Tri-Cyclen Lo Tablets 2421
Seasonale Tablets 1073
Triphasil-28 Tablets 3483
Yasmin 28 Tablets 818

Felodipine (Increased plasma concentrations of dihydropyridine calcium channel blockers; caution is warranted and clinical monitoring of patients is recommended). Products include:
Plendil Extended-Release Tablets 651

Flecainide Acetate (Kaletra is an in vitro inhibitor of the CYP450 3A and inhibits CYP2D6 to a lesser extent; co-administration with drugs that are highly dependent on these isoforms for clearance and for which elevated plasma concentrations are associated with serious and/or life threatening events, such as flecainide, is contraindicated). Products include:
Tambocor Tablets 1824

Fosamprenavir Calcium (Co-administration may result in decreased levels of amprenavir and/or lopinavir. An increased rate of adverse effects has also been observed with co-administration of these medications). Products include:
Lexiva Tablets 1473

Fosphenytoin Sodium (Co-administration can result in decreased lopinavir plasma concentrations; Kaletra may be less effective due to decreased lopinavir plasma concentrations. Co-administer with caution).
No products indexed under this heading.

Hypericum (Co-administration is expected to substantially decrease protease inhibitor concentrations and may result in sub-optimal levels of lopinavir and lead to loss of virologic response and possible resistance to lopinavir or to the class of protease inhibitors; concomitant use is not recommended).
No products indexed under this heading.

Indinavir Sulfate (Co-administration results in increased indinavir plasma concentrations, decreased Cmax and increased Cmin; dosage adjustment may be needed). Products include:
Crixivan Capsules 1918

Isradipine (Increased plasma concentrations of dihydropyridine calcium channel blockers; caution is warranted and clinical monitoring of patients is recommended). Products include:
DynaCirc CR Tablets 2726

Itraconazole (Co-administration can result in increased itraconazole plasma concentrations; high doses of itraconazole (>200 mg/day) are not recommended).
No products indexed under this heading.

Ketoconazole (Co-administration can result in increased ketoconazole plasma concentrations; high doses of ketoconazole (>200 mg/day) are not recommended). Products include:
Nizoral A-D Shampoo, 1% 1839
Nizoral 2% Shampoo 1838

Lidocaine Hydrochloride (Co-administration with systemic lidocaine can result in increased lidocaine plasma concentrations; caution and monitoring is recommended).
No products indexed under this heading.

Lovastatin (Co-administration of Kaletra and lovastatin may increase the risk of myopathy, including rhabdomyolysis; concomitant use is not recommended). Products include:
Advicor Tablets 1694
Altoprev Extended-Release Tablets 1151
Mevacor Tablets 1996

Methadone Hydrochloride (Co-administration results in decreased plasma concentrations of methadone; dosage of methadone may need to be increased when co-administered).
No products indexed under this heading.

Methylergonovine Maleate (Kaletra is an inhibitor of CYP450 3A. Co-administration is contraindicated due to potential for serious and/or life threatening reactions such as acute ergot toxicity).
No products indexed under this heading.

Methysergide Maleate (Kaletra is an inhibitor of CYP450 3A. Co-administration is contraindicated due to potential for serious and/or life threatening reactions such as acute ergot toxicity).
No products indexed under this heading.

Metronidazole (Kaletra oral solution contains alcohol, which can produce disulfiram-like reactions when co-administered with disulfiram or other drugs that produce this reaction, such as metronidazole). Products include:
Metrogel 1% 1212
MetroGel-Vaginal Gel 1822
Noritate Cream, 1% 1051

Metronidazole Hydrochloride (Kaletra oral solution contains alcohol, which can produce disulfiram-like reactions when co-administered with disulfiram or other drugs that produce this reaction, such as metronidazole).
No products indexed under this heading.

Midazolam Hydrochloride (Kaletra is an in vitro inhibitor of the CYP450 3A and inhibits CYP2D6 to a lesser extent; co-administration with drugs that are highly dependent on these isoforms for clearance and for which elevated plasma concentrations are associated with serious and/or life threatening events, such as midazolam, is contraindicated).
No products indexed under this heading.

Nelfinavir Mesylate (Co-administration may require dosage adjustment). Products include:
Viracept 2556

Nevirapine (Co-administration with nevirapine has a potential to decrease plasma concentrations of protease inhibitors by inducing the activity of CYP3A; dosage adjustment may be needed). Products include:
Viramune Oral Suspension 903
Viramune Tablets 903

Nicardipine Hydrochloride (Increased plasma concentrations of dihydropyridine calcium channel blockers; caution is warranted and clinical monitoring of patients is recommended). Products include:
Cardene I.V. 1129

Nifedipine (Increased plasma concentrations of dihydropyridine calcium channel blockers; caution is warranted and clinical monitoring of patients is recommended). Products include:
Adalat CC Tablets 2978

Nimodipine (Increased plasma concentrations of dihydropyridine calcium channel blockers; caution is warranted and clinical monitoring of patients is recommended). Products include:
Nimotop Capsules 774

Phenobarbital (Co-administration can result in decreased lopinavir plasma concentrations; Kaletra may be less effective due to decreased lopinavir plasma concentrations. Co-administer with caution).
No products indexed under this heading.

Phenytoin (Co-administration can result in decreased lopinavir plasma concentrations; Kaletra may be less effective due to decreased lopinavir plasma concentrations. Co-administer with caution).
No products indexed under this heading.

Phenytoin Sodium (Co-administration can result in decreased lopinavir plasma concentrations; Kaletra may be less effective due to decreased lopinavir plasma concentrations. Co-administer with caution). Products include:
Phenytek Capsules 2153

Pimozide (Kaletra is an inhibitor of CYP450 3A. Co-administration with drugs that are highly dependent on CYP450 3A for clearance and for which elevated plasma concentrations are associated with serious and/or life threatening events, such as pimozide, is contraindicated). Products include:
Orap Tablets 1220

Propafenone Hydrochloride (Kaletra is an inhibitor of CYP450 3A. Co-administration with drugs that are highly dependent on CYP450 3A for clearance and for which elevated plasma concentrations are associated with serious and/or life threatening events, such as propafenone, is contraindicated). Products include:
Rythmol SR Capsules 2736

Quinidine (Co-administration can result in increased quinidine plasma concentrations; caution and monitoring is recommended).
No products indexed under this heading.

Quinidine Gluconate (Co-administration can result in increased quinidine plasma concentrations; caution and monitoring is recommended).
No products indexed under this heading.

Quinidine Hydrochloride (Co-administration can result in increased quinidine plasma concentrations; caution and monitoring is recommended).
No products indexed under this heading.

Quinidine Polygalacturonate (Co-administration can result in increased quinidine plasma concentrations; caution and monitoring is recommended).
No products indexed under this heading.

Quinidine Sulfate (Co-administration can result in increased quinidine plasma concentrations; caution and monitoring is recommended).
No products indexed under this heading.

Rapamycin (Co-administration results in increased plasma concentrations of immunosuppressants; monitoring is recommended).
No products indexed under this heading.

Rifabutin (Co-administration can result in increased rifabutin and rifabutin metabolite plasma concentrations; dosage reduction of rifabutin by at least 75% of the usual dose of 300 mg/day is recommended; increased monitoring for adverse reactions is warranted).
No products indexed under this heading.

Rifampin (Co-administration may lead to loss of virologic response and possible resistance to Kaletra; concomitant use should be avoided).
No products indexed under this heading.

Saquinavir (Co-administration results in increased saquinavir plasma concentrations, decreased Cmax and increased Cmin).
No products indexed under this heading.

Saquinavir Mesylate (Co-administration results in increased saquinavir plasma concentrations, increased in Cmax and increased in Cmin; dosage adjustments may be needed). Products include:
Invirase 2776

Sildenafil Citrate (Co-administration is expected to substantially increase sildenafil concentrations and may result in an increase in sildenafil-associated adverse events including hypotension, syncope, visual changes and prolonged erection; Dosage reductions of 25 mg every 48 hours with increased monitoring for adverse events). Products include:
Revatio Tablets 2541
Viagra Tablets 2552

Simvastatin (Co-administration of Kaletra and simvastatin may increase the risk of myopathy, including rhabdomyolysis; concomitant use is not recommended).
Products include:
Vytorin 10/10 Tablets 2084
Vytorin 10/10 Tablets 3092
Vytorin 10/20 Tablets 2084
Vytorin 10/20 Tablets 3092
Vytorin 10/40 Tablets 3092
Vytorin 10/40 Tablets 2084
Vytorin 10/80 Tablets 2084
Vytorin 10/80 Tablets 3092
Zocor Tablets 2078

Tacrolimus (Co-administration results in increased plasma concentrations of immunosuppressants; monitoring is recommended).
Products include:
Prograf Capsules and Injection 624
Protopic Ointment 629

Tadalafil (Co-administration is expected to substantially increase tadalafil concentrations and may result in an increase in tadalafil associated adverse drug events including hypotension, syncope, visual changes and prolonged erection; Dosage reduction recommended10 mg every 72 hours with increased monitoring for adverse events). Products include:
Cialis Tablets 1806

Tenofovir Disoproxil Fumarate (Co-administration results in increased plasma concentrations of nucleoside reverse transcriptase inhibitors; Co-administer with caution). Products include:
Truvada Tablets 1279
Viread Tablets 1284

Terfenadine (Kaletra is an inhibitor of CYP450 3A. Co-administration with drugs that are highly dependent on CYP450 3A for clearance and for which elevated plasma concentrations are associated with serious and/or life threatening events, such as terfenadine, is contraindicated).
No products indexed under this heading.

Triazolam (Kaletra is an inhibitor of CYP450 3A. Co-administration with drugs that are highly dependent on CYP450 3A for clearance and for which elevated plasma concentrations are associated with serious and/or life threatening events, such as triazolam, is contraindicated).
No products indexed under this heading.

Vardenafil Hydrochloride (Co-administration is expected to substantially increase vardenafil concentrations and may result in an increase in vardenafil associated adverse drug events including hypotension, syncope, visual changes and prolonged erection; Dosage reduction of 2.5 mg every 72 hours with increased monitoring for adverse effects). Products include:
Levitra Tablets 3048

Voriconazole (Co-administration of voriconazole with Kaletra has not been studied. However, administration of voriconazole with ritonavir 400 mg every 12 hours decreased voriconazole steady-state AUC by an average of 82%. The effect of lower ritonavir doses on voriconazole is not known at this time. Until data is available, voriconazole should not be administered to patients receiving Kaletra). Products include:
VFEND I.V. 2543
VFEND Oral Suspension 2543
VFEND Tablets 2543

Warfarin Sodium (Co-administration can affect concentrations of warfarin; it is recommended that INR be monitored). Products include:
Coumadin for Injection 932
Coumadin Tablets 932

Zidovudine (Kaletra induces glucuronidation; therefore, Kaletra has the potential to reduce zidovudine plasma concentrations; the clinical significance is unknown). Products include:
Combivir Tablets 1373
Retrovir 1533
Retrovir IV Infusion 1537
Trizivir Tablets 1565

Food Interactions

Food, unspecified (Co-administration with moderate fat meal was associated with a mean increase in AUC and Cmax; to enhance bioavailability Kaletra should be taken with food).

KALETRA ORAL SOLUTION

(Lopinavir, Ritonavir) 474
See Kaletra Capsules

KAOPECTATE ANTI-DIARRHEAL/UPSET STOMACH RELIEVER LIQUID

(Bismuth Subsalicylate) 701
None cited in PDR database.

EXTRA STRENGTH KAOPECTATE ANTI-DIARRHEAL LIQUID

(Bismuth Subsalicylate) 701
None cited in PDR database.

KAOPECTATE STOOL SOFTENER

(Docusate Calcium) 702
None cited in PDR database.

K-DUR EXTENDED-RELEASE TABLETS

(Potassium Chloride) 3047
May interact with ACE inhibitors, potassium sparing diuretics, and certain other agents. Compounds in these categories include:

Amiloride Hydrochloride (Co-administration of these agents can produce severe hyperkalemia; concurrent use is not recommended).
Products include:
Midamor Tablets 2000
Moduretic Tablets 2003

Benazepril Hydrochloride (Potential for increased potassium retention). Products include:
Lotensin Tablets 2232
Lotensin HCT Tablets 2235
Lotrel Capsules 2238

Captopril (Potential for increased potassium retention). Products include:
Captopril Tablets 2114

Enalapril Maleate (Potential for increased potassium retention).
Products include:
Vaseretic Tablets 2073
Vasotec I.V. Injection 2076

Enalaprilat (Potential for increased potassium retention).
No products indexed under this heading.

Fosinopril Sodium (Potential for increased potassium retention).
No products indexed under this heading.

Lisinopril (Potential for increased potassium retention). Products include:
Prinivil Tablets 2029
Prinzide Tablets 2033
Zestoretic Tablets 701
Zestril Tablets 704

Moexipril Hydrochloride (Potential for increased potassium retention). Products include:
Uniretic Tablets 3114
Univasc Tablets 3118

Perindopril Erbumine (Potential for increased potassium retention).
Products include:
Aceon Tablets (2 mg, 4 mg, 8 mg) 3191

Quinapril Hydrochloride (Potential for increased potassium retention).
No products indexed under this heading.

Ramipril (Potential for increased potassium retention). Products include:
Altace Capsules 1673

Spirapril Hydrochloride (Potential for increased potassium retention).
No products indexed under this heading.

Spironolactone (Co-administration of these agents can produce severe hyperkalemia; concurrent use is not recommended).
No products indexed under this heading.

Trandolapril (Potential for increased potassium retention).
Products include:
Mavik Tablets 482
Tarka Tablets 519

Triamterene (Co-administration of these agents can produce severe hyperkalemia; concurrent use is not recommended). Products include:
Dyazide Capsules 1389
Dyrenium Capsules 3390
Maxzide 2150

KEPIVANCE

(Palifermin) 592
May interact with:

Heparin Calcium (Palifermin has been shown to bind to heparin in vitro. Therefore, if heparin is used to maintain an IV line, saline should be used to rinse the line prior to and after palifermin administration).
No products indexed under this heading.

Heparin Sodium (Palifermin has been shown to bind to heparin in vitro. Therefore, if heparin is used to maintain an IV line, saline should be used to rinse the line prior to and after palifermin administration).
No products indexed under this heading.

KEPPRA ORAL SOLUTION

(Levetiracetam) 3307
See Keppra Tablets

KEPPRA TABLETS

(Levetiracetam) 3307
May interact with:

Probenecid (Co-administration has resulted in double Cmax of the metabolite, ucb L057, while the fraction of the drug excreted remained unchanged in the urine; renal clearance of ucb L057 in the presence of probenecid decreased 60%).
No products indexed under this heading.

Food Interactions

Food, unspecified (Decreases Cmax by 20% and delays Tmax by 1.5 hours; does not affect the extent of absorption).

KETEK TABLETS

(Telithromycin) 2920

May interact with benzodiazepine that are metabolized by CYP3A4, cytochrome p450 3a4 inducers (selected), cytochrome p450 3a4 substrates (selected), ergot-containing drugs, and drugs which undergo biotransformation by cytochrome p-450 mixed function oxidase. Compounds in these categories include:

Acarbose (Elevated levels of drugs metabolized by the CYP450 system may be observed when co-administered with telithromycin; therefore, increases or prolongation of the therapeutic and/or adverse effects of the concomitant drug may be observed). Products include:

- Precose Tablets 776

Acetaminophen (Elevated levels of drugs metabolized by the CYP450 system may be observed when co-administered with telithromycin; therefore, increases or prolongation of the therapeutic and/or adverse effects of the concomitant drug may be observed). Products include:

- Benadryl Allergy & Cold Tablets .... ▣692
- Benadryl Allergy & Sinus Headache Caplets & Gelcaps .... ▣693
- Benadryl Maximum Strength Severe Allergy & Sinus Headache Caplets .... ▣694
- Contac Severe Cold and Flu Caplets Maximum Strength .... ▣615
- Contac Severe Cold and Flu Caplets Non-Drowsy .... ▣615
- Darvocet A 500 Tablets 3497
- Goody's Body Pain Formula Powder .... ▣621
- Goody's Extra Strength Headache Powder .... ▣621
- Goody's Extra Strength Pain Relief Tablets .... ▣621
- Goody's PM Powder .... ▣622
- Hycomine Compound Tablets 1105
- Lortab 3315
- Lortab Elixir 3312
- Percocet Tablets 1114
- Robitussin Cough, Cold & Flu Liquid-filled Capsules .... ▣750
- Robitussin Flu Liquid .... ▣752
- Sedapap Tablets 50 mg/650 mg 2098
- Singlet Caplets .... ▣636
- Sudafed Severe Cold .... ▣710
- Sudafed Sinus Headache .... ▣711
- TheraFlu Cold & Cough Hot Liquid .... ▣680
- TheraFlu Cold & Sore Throat Hot Liquid .... ▣680
- TheraFlu Flu & Chest Congestion Non-Drowsy Hot Liquid .... ▣681
- TheraFlu Flu & Sore Throat Hot Liquid .... ▣681
- TheraFlu Severe Cold Non-Drowsy Hot Liquid .... ▣683
- TheraFlu Severe Cold & Cough Hot Liquid .... ▣683
- TheraFlu Severe Cold Caplets .... ▣679
- TheraFlu Severe Cold Hot Liquid .... ▣682
- TheraFlu Severe Cold Non-Drowsy Caplets .... ▣679
- Triaminic Cough & Sore Throat Liquid .... ▣687
- Triaminic Flu, Cough & Fever Liquid .... ▣685
- Triaminic Cough & Sore Throat Softchews .... ▣689
- Tylenol 8 Hour Extended Release Geltabs and Caplets 1843
- Tylenol Sinus NightTime Caplets .... ▣663
- Children's Tylenol Suspension Liquid and Meltaways 1850
- Children's Tylenol Plus Cold & Allergy Suspension Liquid 1850
- Children's Tylenol Plus Cold NightTime Suspension Liquid 1851
- Children's Tylenol Plus Cold & Cough Suspension Liquid and Chewable Tablets 1851
- Children's Tylenol Plus Cold Chewable Tablets 1851
- Children's Tylenol Plus Cold Daytime Non-Drowsy Suspension Liquid 1851
- Children's Tylenol Plus Flu Suspension Liquid 1853
- Concentrated Tylenol Infants' Drops Plus Cold 1851
- Concentrated Tylenol Infants' Drops Plus Cold and Cough 1851
- Concentrated Tylenol Infants' Drops 1850
- Junior Tylenol Meltaways 1850
- Tylenol Cold & Flu Severe Daytime Liquid with Cool Bust 1846
- Tylenol Cold & Flu Severe NightTime Liquid with Cool Burst 1846
- Tylenol Cold Severe Congestion Non-Drowsy Caplets with Cool Burst 1846
- Tylenol Cough & Sore Throat Daytime Liquid with Cool Burst 1849
- Tylenol Cough & Sore Throat NightTime Liquid with Cool Burst 1849
- Tylenol 1843
- Extra Strength Tylenol Rapid Release Gels 1843
- Tylenol 1843
- Tylenol Allergy Complete Night Time Caplets 1844
- Tylenol Allergy Complete Multi-Symptom Caplets and Gelcaps with Cool Burst 1844
- Tylenol Severe Allergy Caplets 1844
- Tylenol Flu NightTime Gelcaps 1846
- Tylenol Flu Day Non-Drowsy Gelcaps 1846
- Concentrated Tylenol Infants' Drops Plus Cold Nasal Congestant, Fever Reducer & Pain Reliever .... ▣668
- Concentrated Tylenol Infants' Drops Plus Cold & Cough Nasal Decongestant, Fever Reducer & Pain Reliever .... ▣668
- Multi-Symptom Tylenol Cold Night Time Caplets 1845
- Multi-Symptom Tylenol Cold Day Non-Drowsy Caplets and Gelcaps 1845
- Extra Strength Tylenol PM Caplets, Geltabs, Gelcaps and Liquid 1847
- Tylenol Sinus Day Non-Drowsy 1848
- Tylenol Sinus Night Time Caplets 1848
- Tylenol Sinus Severe Congestion Caplets with Cool Burst 1848
- Tylenol Sore Throat Daytime Liquid with Cool Burst 1849
- Tylenol Sore Throat NightTime Liquid with Cool Burst 1849
- Tylenol with Codeine 2461
- Women's Tylenol Menstrual Relief Caplets 1849
- Ultracet Tablets 2462
- Vicks 44M Cough, Cold & Flu Relief 2676
- Vicks DayQuil LiquiCaps/Liquid Multi-Symptom Cold/Flu Relief .... ▣723
- Vicks DayQuil Multi-Symptom Cold/Flu Relief LiquiCaps 2675
- Vicks DayQuil Multi-Symptom Cold/Flu Relief Liquid 2675
- Vicks NyQuil LiquiCaps 2677
- Vicks NyQuil LiquiCaps/Liquid Multi-Symptom Cold/Flu Relief .... ▣725
- Vicks NyQuil Liquid 2677
- Vicodin Tablets 530
- Vicodin ES Tablets 531
- Vicodin HP Tablets 532
- Zydone Tablets 1118

Alatrofloxacin Mesylate (Elevated levels of drugs metabolized by the CYP450 system may be observed when co-administered with telithromycin; therefore, increases or prolongation of the therapeutic and/or adverse effects of the concomitant drug may be observed).

No products indexed under this heading.

Alfentanil Hydrochloride (Co-administration of telithromycin with a drug primarily metabolized by the CYP 3A4 enzyme system may result in increased plasma concentrations of the drug co-administered with telithromycin that could increase or prolong both the therapeutic and adverse effects).

No products indexed under this heading.

Allium sativum (Concomitant administration of CYP 3A4 inducers is likely to result in subtherapeutic levels of telithromycin and loss of effect).

No products indexed under this heading.

Alprazolam (Co-administration of telithromycin with a drug primarily metabolized by the CYP 3A4 enzyme system may result in increased plasma concentrations of the drug co-administered with telithromycin that could increase or prolong both the therapeutic and adverse effects). Products include:

- Niravam Orally Disintegrating Tablets 3106
- Xanax XR Tablets 2655

Aminophylline (Elevated levels of drugs metabolized by the CYP450 system may be observed when co-administered with telithromycin; therefore, increases or prolongation of the therapeutic and/or adverse effects of the concomitant drug may be observed).

No products indexed under this heading.

Amiodarone Hydrochloride (Elevated levels of drugs metabolized by the CYP450 system may be observed when co-administered with telithromycin; therefore, increases or prolongation of the therapeutic and/or adverse effects of the concomitant drug may be observed). Products include:

- Pacerone Tablets 3337

Amitriptyline Hydrochloride (Co-administration of telithromycin with a drug primarily metabolized by the CYP 3A4 enzyme system may result in increased plasma concentrations of the drug co-administered with telithromycin that could increase or prolong both the therapeutic and adverse effects).

No products indexed under this heading.

Amlodipine Besylate (Co-administration of telithromycin with a drug primarily metabolized by the CYP 3A4 enzyme system may result in increased plasma concentrations of the drug co-administered with telithromycin that could increase or prolong both the therapeutic and adverse effects). Products include:

- Caduet Tablets 2507
- Lotrel Capsules 2238
- Norvasc Tablets 2529

Amoxapine (Elevated levels of drugs metabolized by the CYP450 system may be observed when co-administered with telithromycin; therefore, increases or prolongation of the therapeutic and/or adverse effects of the concomitant drug may be observed).

No products indexed under this heading.

Amphetamine Aspartate (Elevated levels of drugs metabolized by the CYP450 system may be observed when co-administered with telithromycin; therefore, increases or prolongation of the therapeutic and/or adverse effects of the concomitant drug may be observed). Products include:

- Adderall Tablets 3168
- Adderall XR Capsules 3169

Amphetamine Aspartate Monohydrate (Elevated levels of drugs metabolized by the CYP450 system may be observed when co-administered with telithromycin; therefore, increases or prolongation of the therapeutic and/or adverse effects of the concomitant drug may be observed).

No products indexed under this heading.

Amphetamine Sulfate (Elevated levels of drugs metabolized by the CYP450 system may be observed when co-administered with telithromycin; therefore, increases or prolongation of the therapeutic and/or adverse effects of the concomitant drug may be observed). Products include:

- Adderall Tablets 3168
- Adderall XR Capsules 3169

Aprepitant (Co-administration of telithromycin with a drug primarily metabolized by the CYP 3A4 enzyme system may result in increased plasma concentrations of the drug co-administered with telithromycin that could increase or prolong both the therapeutic and adverse effects). Products include:

- Emend Capsules 1944

Astemizole (Co-administration of telithromycin with a drug primarily metabolized by the CYP 3A4 enzyme system may result in increased plasma concentrations of the drug co-administered with telithromycin that could increase or prolong both the therapeutic and adverse effects).

No products indexed under this heading.

Atomoxetine Hydrochloride (Elevated levels of drugs metabolized by the CYP450 system may be observed when co-administered with telithromycin; therefore, increases or prolongation of the therapeutic and/or adverse effects of the concomitant drug may be observed). Products include:

- Strattera Capsules 1784

Atorvastatin Calcium (Atorvastatin levels were increased due to CYP 3A4 inhibition by telithromycin, thereby increasing the risk of myopathy. Co-administration should be avoided). Products include:

- Caduet Tablets 2507
- Lipitor Tablets 2495

Belladonna Ergotamine (Co-administration of telithromycin with a drug primarily metabolized by the CYP 3A4 enzyme system may result in increased plasma concentrations of the drug co-administered with telithromycin that could increase or prolong both the therapeutic and adverse effects).

No products indexed under this heading.

Benzphetamine Hydrochloride (Elevated levels of drugs metabolized by the CYP450 system may be observed when co-administered with telithromycin; therefore, increases or prolongation of the therapeutic and/or adverse effects of the concomitant drug may be observed).

No products indexed under this heading.

Betamethasone Acetate (Concomitant administration of CYP 3A4 inducers is likely to result in subtherapeutic levels of telithromycin and loss of effect).
No products indexed under this heading.

Betamethasone Sodium Phosphate (Concomitant administration of CYP 3A4 inducers is likely to result in subtherapeutic levels of telithromycin and loss of effect).
No products indexed under this heading.

Bisoprolol Fumarate (Elevated levels of drugs metabolized by the CYP450 system may be observed when co-administered with telithromycin; therefore, increases or prolongation of the therapeutic and/or adverse effects of the concomitant drug may be observed).
No products indexed under this heading.

Buspirone Hydrochloride (Co-administration of telithromycin with a drug primarily metabolized by the CYP 3A4 enzyme system may result in increased plasma concentrations of the drug co-administered with telithromycin that could increase or prolong both the therapeutic and adverse effects).
No products indexed under this heading.

Busulfan (Co-administration of telithromycin with a drug primarily metabolized by the CYP 3A4 enzyme system may result in increased plasma concentrations of the drug co-administered with telithromycin that could increase or prolong both the therapeutic and adverse effects). Products include:
I.V. Busulfex 1125
Myleran Tablets 1492

Caffeine (Elevated levels of drugs metabolized by the CYP450 system may be observed when co-administered with telithromycin; therefore, increases or prolongation of the therapeutic and/or adverse effects of the concomitant drug may be observed). Products include:
Athena Hair System Shampoo 767
BC Powder 612
Arthritis Strength BC Powder 612
Goody's Extra Strength Headache Powder 621
Goody's Extra Strength Pain Relief Tablets 621
Hycomine Compound Tablets 1105
Spartan Hair System Shampoo 767
Vivarin 639

Caffeine Anhydrous (Elevated levels of drugs metabolized by the CYP450 system may be observed when co-administered with telithromycin; therefore, increases or prolongation of the therapeutic and/or adverse effects of the concomitant drug may be observed).
No products indexed under this heading.

Caffeine Citrate (Elevated levels of drugs metabolized by the CYP450 system may be observed when co-administered with telithromycin; therefore, increases or prolongation of the therapeutic and/or adverse effects of the concomitant drug may be observed). Products include:
Cafcit 1854

Candesartan Cilexetil (Elevated levels of drugs metabolized by the CYP450 system may be observed when co-administered with telithromycin; therefore, increases or prolongation of the therapeutic and/or adverse effects of the concomitant drug may be observed). Products include:
Atacand Tablets 634
Atacand HCT 637

Captopril (Elevated levels of drugs metabolized by the CYP450 system may be observed when co-administered with telithromycin; therefore, increases or prolongation of the therapeutic and/or adverse effects of the concomitant drug may be observed). Products include:
Captopril Tablets 2114

Carbamazepine (Co-administration of telithromycin with a drug primarily metabolized by the CYP 3A4 enzyme system may result in increased plasma concentrations of the drug co-administered with telithromycin that could increase or prolong both the therapeutic and adverse effects). Products include:
Carbatrol Capsules 3174
Equetro Extended-Release Capsules 3178
Tegretol/Tegretol-XR 2278

Carisoprodol (Elevated levels of drugs metabolized by the CYP450 system may be observed when co-administered with telithromycin; therefore, increases or prolongation of the therapeutic and/or adverse effects of the concomitant drug may be observed).
No products indexed under this heading.

Carvedilol (Elevated levels of drugs metabolized by the CYP450 system may be observed when co-administered with telithromycin; therefore, increases or prolongation of the therapeutic and/or adverse effects of the concomitant drug may be observed). Products include:
Coreg Tablets 1376

Celecoxib (Elevated levels of drugs metabolized by the CYP450 system may be observed when co-administered with telithromycin; therefore, increases or prolongation of the therapeutic and/or adverse effects of the concomitant drug may be observed). Products include:
Celebrex Capsules 3130

Cerivastatin Sodium (Co-administration of telithromycin with a drug primarily metabolized by the CYP 3A4 enzyme system may result in increased plasma concentrations of the drug co-administered with telithromycin that could increase or prolong both the therapeutic and adverse effects).
No products indexed under this heading.

Cevimeline Hydrochloride (Elevated levels of drugs metabolized by the CYP450 system may be observed when co-administered with telithromycin; therefore, increases or prolongation of the therapeutic and/or adverse effects of the concomitant drug may be observed). Products include:
Evoxac Capsules 1042

Chlordiazepoxide (Elevated levels of drugs metabolized by the CYP450 system may be observed when co-administered with telithromycin; therefore, increases or prolongation of the therapeutic and/or adverse effects of the concomitant drug may be observed).
No products indexed under this heading.

Chlordiazepoxide Hydrochloride (Elevated levels of drugs metabolized by the CYP450 system may be observed when co-administered with telithromycin; therefore, increases or prolongation of the therapeutic and/or adverse effects of the concomitant drug may be observed). Products include:
Librium Capsules 3349

Chlorpheniramine (Co-administration of telithromycin with a drug primarily metabolized by the CYP 3A4 enzyme system may result in increased plasma concentrations of the drug co-administered with telithromycin that could increase or prolong both the therapeutic and adverse effects).
No products indexed under this heading.

Chlorpheniramine Maleate (Co-administration of telithromycin with a drug primarily metabolized by the CYP 3A4 enzyme system may result in increased plasma concentrations of the drug co-administered with telithromycin that could increase or prolong both the therapeutic and adverse effects). Products include:
Advil Allergy Sinus Caplets 737
Advil Multi-Symptom Cold Caplets 738
BC Allergy Sinus Cold Powder 612
Contac Severe Cold and Flu Caplets Maximum Strength 615
Hycomine Compound Tablets 1105
PediaCare Multi-Symptom Cold Liquid 704
PediaCare NightRest Cough & Cold Liquid 704
Robitussin Flu Liquid 752
Robitussin PM Cough & Cold Liquid 752
Singlet Caplets 636
Sudafed Sinus & Allergy Tablets 710
TheraFlu Cold & Cough Hot Liquid 680
TheraFlu Cold & Sore Throat Hot Liquid 680
TheraFlu Flu & Sore Throat Hot Liquid 681
TheraFlu Severe Cold & Cough Hot Liquid 683
TheraFlu Severe Cold Caplets 679
TheraFlu Severe Cold Hot Liquid 682
Triaminic Cold & Allergy Liquid 685
Triaminic Cold & Cough Liquid 685
Triaminic Flu, Cough & Fever Liquid 685
Triaminic Night Time Cough & Cold Liquid 685
Triaminic Allergy Runny Nose & Congestion Softchews 688
Triaminic Cold & Cough Softchews 688
Children's Tylenol Plus Cold NightTime Suspension Liquid 1851
Children's Tylenol Plus Cold & Cough Suspension Liquid and Chewable Tablets 1851
Children's Tylenol Plus Cold Chewable Tablets 1851
Children's Tylenol Plus Flu Suspension Liquid 1853
Tylenol Allergy Complete Multi-Symptom Caplets and Gelcaps with Cool Burst 1844
Multi-Symptom Tylenol Cold Night Time Caplets 1845
Vicks 44M Cough, Cold & Flu Relief 2676
Pediatric Vicks 44m Cough & Cold Relief 2673
Children's Vicks NyQuil Cold/Cough Relief 2671

Chlorpheniramine Polistirex (Co-administration of telithromycin with a drug primarily metabolized by the CYP 3A4 enzyme system may result in increased plasma concentrations of the drug co-administered with telithromycin that could increase or prolong both the therapeutic and adverse effects). Products include:
Tussionex Pennkinetic Extended-Release Suspension 3322

Chlorpheniramine Tannate (Co-administration of telithromycin with a drug primarily metabolized by the CYP 3A4 enzyme system may result in increased plasma concentrations of the drug co-administered with telithromycin that could increase or prolong both the therapeutic and adverse effects).
No products indexed under this heading.

Chlorpromazine (Elevated levels of drugs metabolized by the CYP450 system may be observed when co-administered with telithromycin; therefore, increases or prolongation of the therapeutic and/or adverse effects of the concomitant drug may be observed).
No products indexed under this heading.

Chlorpromazine Hydrochloride (Elevated levels of drugs metabolized by the CYP450 system may be observed when co-administered with telithromycin; therefore, increases or prolongation of the therapeutic and/or adverse effects of the concomitant drug may be observed).
No products indexed under this heading.

Chlorpropamide (Elevated levels of drugs metabolized by the CYP450 system may be observed when co-administered with telithromycin; therefore, increases or prolongation of the therapeutic and/or adverse effects of the concomitant drug may be observed).
No products indexed under this heading.

Cilostazol (Elevated levels of drugs metabolized by the CYP450 system may be observed when co-administered with telithromycin; therefore, increases or prolongation of the therapeutic and/or adverse effects of the concomitant drug may be observed). Products include:
Pletal Tablets 2478

Cimetidine Hydrochloride (Elevated levels of drugs metabolized by the CYP450 system may be observed when co-administered with telithromycin; therefore, increases or prolongation of the therapeutic and/or adverse effects of the concomitant drug may be observed).
No products indexed under this heading.

Ciprofloxacin (Elevated levels of drugs metabolized by the CYP450 system may be observed when co-administered with telithromycin; therefore, increases or prolongation of the therapeutic and/or adverse effects of the concomitant drug may be observed). Products include:
Cipro I.V. 2998
Cipro I.V. Pharmacy Bulk Package 3509
Cipro Oral Suspension 2991
Cipro XR Tablets 3004
Ciprodex Otic Suspension 555

Ciprofloxacin Hydrochloride (Concomitant administration of CYP 3A4 inducers is likely to result in subtherapeutic levels of telithromycin and loss of effect). Products include:
Ciloxan Ophthalmic Ointment 554
Cipro Tablets 2991

Cisapride (Steady-state peak plasma concentrations of cisapride were increased when co-administered with repeated doses of telithromycin, resulting in significant increases in QTc. Co-administration is contraindicated).
No products indexed under this heading.

Cisplatin (Concomitant administration of CYP 3A4 inducers is likely to result in subtherapeutic levels of telithromycin and loss of effect).
No products indexed under this heading.

Citalopram Hydrobromide (Elevated levels of drugs metabolized by the CYP450 system may be observed when co-administered with telithromycin; therefore, increases or prolongation of the therapeutic and/or adverse effects of the concomitant drug may be observed).
Products include:
Celexa 1177

Clarithromycin (Co-administration of telithromycin with a drug primarily metabolized by the CYP 3A4 enzyme system may result in increased plasma concentrations of the drug co-administered with telithromycin that could increase or prolong both the therapeutic and adverse effects).
Products include:
Biaxin/Biaxin XL 402
PREVPAC 3281

Clomipramine Hydrochloride (Elevated levels of drugs metabolized by the CYP450 system may be observed when co-administered with telithromycin; therefore, increases or prolongation of the therapeutic and/or adverse effects of the concomitant drug may be observed).
No products indexed under this heading.

Clopidogrel Hydrogen Sulfate (Elevated levels of drugs metabolized by the CYP450 system may be observed when co-administered with telithromycin; therefore, increases or prolongation of the therapeutic and/or adverse effects of the concomitant drug may be observed).
No products indexed under this heading.

Clozapine (Elevated levels of drugs metabolized by the CYP450 system may be observed when co-administered with telithromycin; therefore, increases or prolongation of the therapeutic and/or adverse effects of the concomitant drug may be observed). Products include:
Clozapine Tablets 2141
Clozaril Tablets 2174
FazaClo Orally Disintegrating Tablets 547

Codeine Phosphate (Elevated levels of drugs metabolized by the CYP450 system may be observed when co-administered with telithromycin; therefore, increases or prolongation of the therapeutic and/or adverse effects of the concomitant drug may be observed). Products include:
Tylenol with Codeine 2461

Codeine Sulfate (Elevated levels of drugs metabolized by the CYP450 system may be observed when co-administered with telithromycin; therefore, increases or prolongation of the therapeutic and/or adverse effects of the concomitant drug may be observed).
No products indexed under this heading.

Cortisone Acetate (Concomitant administration of CYP 3A4 inducers is likely to result in subtherapeutic levels of telithromycin and loss of effect).
No products indexed under this heading.

Cyclobenzaprine (Elevated levels of drugs metabolized by the CYP450 system may be observed when co-administered with telithromycin; therefore, increases or prolongation of the therapeutic and/or adverse effects of the concomitant drug may be observed).
No products indexed under this heading.

Cyclobenzaprine Hydrochloride (Elevated levels of drugs metabolized by the CYP450 system may be observed when co-administered with telithromycin; therefore, increases or prolongation of the therapeutic and/or adverse effects of the concomitant drug may be observed).
Products include:
Flexeril Tablets 1832

Cyclophosphamide (Elevated levels of drugs metabolized by the CYP450 system may be observed when co-administered with telithromycin; therefore, increases or prolongation of the therapeutic and/or adverse effects of the concomitant drug may be observed).
No products indexed under this heading.

Cyclosporine (Co-administration of telithromycin with a drug primarily metabolized by the CYP 3A4 enzyme system may result in increased plasma concentrations of the drug co-administered with telithromycin that could increase or prolong both the therapeutic and adverse effects).
Products include:
Gengraf Capsules 458
Neoral Soft Gelatin Capsules 2247
Neoral Oral Solution 2247
Restasis Ophthalmic Emulsion 570
Sandimmune 2259

Desipramine Hydrochloride (Elevated levels of drugs metabolized by the CYP450 system may be observed when co-administered with telithromycin; therefore, increases or prolongation of the therapeutic and/or adverse effects of the concomitant drug may be observed).
No products indexed under this heading.

Desogestrel (Co-administration of telithromycin with a drug primarily metabolized by the CYP 3A4 enzyme system may result in increased plasma concentrations of the drug co-administered with telithromycin that could increase or prolong both the therapeutic and adverse effects).
Products include:
Ortho-Cept Tablets 2395

Dexamethasone (Concomitant administration of CYP 3A4 inducers is likely to result in subtherapeutic levels of telithromycin and loss of effect). Products include:
Ciprodex Otic Suspension 555
Decadron Tablets 1929
TobraDex Ophthalmic Ointment 558
TobraDex Ophthalmic Suspension 558

Dexamethasone Acetate (Concomitant administration of CYP 3A4 inducers is likely to result in subtherapeutic levels of telithromycin and loss of effect).
No products indexed under this heading.

Dexamethasone Phosphate (Elevated levels of drugs metabolized by the CYP450 system may be observed when co-administered with telithromycin; therefore, increases or prolongation of the therapeutic and/or adverse effects of the concomitant drug may be observed).
No products indexed under this heading.

Dexamethasone Sodium (Elevated levels of drugs metabolized by the CYP450 system may be observed when co-administered with telithromycin; therefore, increases or prolongation of the therapeutic and/or adverse effects of the concomitant drug may be observed).
No products indexed under this heading.

Dexamethasone Sodium Phosphate (Concomitant administration of CYP 3A4 inducers is likely to result in subtherapeutic levels of telithromycin and loss of effect).
Products include:
Decadron Phosphate Injection 1931

Dexfenfluramine Hydrochloride (Elevated levels of drugs metabolized by the CYP450 system may be observed when co-administered with telithromycin; therefore, increases or prolongation of the therapeutic and/or adverse effects of the concomitant drug may be observed).
No products indexed under this heading.

Dextromethorphan (Elevated levels of drugs metabolized by the CYP450 system may be observed when co-administered with telithromycin; therefore, increases or prolongation of the therapeutic and/or adverse effects of the concomitant drug may be observed).
No products indexed under this heading.

Dextromethorphan Hydrobromide (Elevated levels of drugs metabolized by the CYP450 system may be observed when co-administered with telithromycin; therefore, increases or prolongation of the therapeutic and/or adverse effects of the concomitant drug may be observed). Products include:
Alacol DM Syrup 739
Balamine DM 739
Contac Severe Cold and Flu Caplets Maximum Strength .... ▣ 615
Contac Severe Cold and Flu Caplets Non-Drowsy .... ▣ 615
Children's Dimetapp DM Cold & Cough Elixir .... ▣ 745
Children's Dimetapp Long Acting Cough Plus Cold Syrup .... ▣ 746
Dimetapp Infant Drops Decongestant Plus Cough .... ▣ 746
Mucinex DM Tablets .... ▣ 602
PediaCare Decongestant & Cough Infant Drops .... ▣ 705
PediaCare Freezer Pops Long-Acting Cough-Glacier Grape and Polar Berry Blue .... ▣ 706
PediaCare Long-Acting Cough Infant Drops .... ▣ 705
PediaCare Long-Acting Cough Plus Cold Liquid .... ▣ 704
PediaCare Multi-Symptom Cold Liquid .... ▣ 704
PediaCare NightRest Cough & Cold Liquid .... ▣ 704
Robitussin Allergy & Cough Syrup .... ▣ 750
Robitussin CF Liquid .... ▣ 755
Robitussin Cough & Cold Liquid-filled Capsules .... ▣ 750
Robitussin Cough, Cold & Flu Liquid-filled Capsules .... ▣ 750
Robitussin Cough & Cold Infant Drops .... ▣ 755
Robitussin DM Infant Drops .... ▣ 753
Robitussin DM Liquid .... ▣ 753
Robitussin Flu Liquid .... ▣ 752
Robitussin Maximum Strength Cough Liquid .... ▣ 754
Robitussin Maximum Strength Cough & Cold Liquid .... ▣ 754
Robitussin Pediatric Cough Liquid .... ▣ 754
Robitussin Pediatric Cough & Cold Liquid .... ▣ 754
Robitussin PM Cough & Cold Liquid .... ▣ 752
Robitussin Sugar Free Cough Liquid .... ▣ 753
Simply Cough Liquid 1840
Sudafed Severe Cold .... ▣ 710
TheraFlu Cold & Cough Hot Liquid .... ▣ 680
TheraFlu Flu & Chest Congestion Non-Drowsy Hot Liquid .... ▣ 681
TheraFlu Severe Cold Non-Drowsy Hot Liquid .... ▣ 683
TheraFlu Severe Cold & Cough Hot Liquid .... ▣ 683
TheraFlu Severe Cold Caplets .... ▣ 679
TheraFlu Severe Cold Hot Liquid .... ▣ 682
TheraFlu Severe Cold Non-Drowsy Caplets .... ▣ 679
TheraFlu Thin Strips Long Acting Cough .... ▣ 684
Triaminic Cold & Cough Liquid .... ▣ 685
Triaminic Cough Liquid .... ▣ 687
Triaminic Cough & Nasal Congestion Liquid .... ▣ 687
Triaminic Cough & Sore Throat Liquid .... ▣ 687
Triaminic Flu, Cough & Fever Liquid .... ▣ 685
Triaminic Night Time Cough & Cold Liquid .... ▣ 685
Triaminic Cold & Cough Softchews .... ▣ 688
Triaminic Cough & Sore Throat Softchews .... ▣ 689
Triaminic Thin Strips Long Acting Cough .... ▣ 689
Children's Tylenol Plus Cold & Cough Suspension Liquid and Chewable Tablets 1851
Children's Tylenol Plus Flu Suspension Liquid 1853
Concentrated Tylenol Infants' Drops Plus Cold and Cough 1851
Tylenol Cold & Flu Severe Daytime Liquid with Cool Bust 1846
Tylenol Cold & Flu Severe NightTime Liquid with Cool Burst 1846
Tylenol Cold Severe Congestion Non-Drowsy Caplets with Cool Burst 1846
Tylenol Cough & Sore Throat Daytime Liquid with Cool Burst 1849
Tylenol Cough & Sore Throat NightTime Liquid with Cool Burst 1849
Tylenol Flu Day Non-Drowsy Gelcaps 1846
Concentrated Tylenol Infants' Drops Plus Cold & Cough Nasal Decongestant, Fever Reducer & Pain Reliever .... ▣ 668
Multi-Symptom Tylenol Cold Night Time Caplets 1845
Multi-Symptom Tylenol Cold Day Non-Drowsy Caplets and Gelcaps 1845
Vicks 44 Cough Relief 2675
Vicks 44D Cough & Head Congestion Relief 2676
Vicks 44D Cough & Head Congestion Relief Liquid .... ▣ 721
Vicks 44E Cough & Chest Congestion Relief 2676
Pediatric Vicks 44e Cough & Chest Congestion Relief Liquid 2673
Vicks 44M Cough, Cold & Flu Relief 2676
Pediatric Vicks 44m Cough & Cold Relief 2673
Vicks DayQuil LiquiCaps/Liquid Multi-Symptom Cold/Flu Relief .... ▣ 723
Vicks DayQuil Multi-Symptom Cold/Flu Relief LiquiCaps 2675
Vicks DayQuil Multi-Symptom Cold/Flu Relief Liquid 2675

(▣ Described in PDR For Nonprescription Drugs)

(⊙ Described in PDR For Ophthalmic Medicines™)

Children's Vicks NyQuil Cold/Cough Relief 2671
Vicks NyQuil Cough Liquid 2677
Vicks NyQuil LiquiCaps 2677
Vicks NyQuil LiquiCaps/Liquid Multi-Symptom Cold/Flu Relief 725
Vicks NyQuil Liquid 2677
Zicam Concentrated Cough Mist for Kids Cool Cherry 643
Zicam Concentrated Cough Mist for Kids Plus D Cool Cherry 643
Zicam Concentrated Cough Mist Nite-Cool Cherry 642
Zicam Concentrated Cough Mist Plus D Cool Cherry 642
Zicam Concentrated Cough Mist-Honey Lemon & Cool Cherry 642

Dextromethorphan Polistirex (Elevated levels of drugs metabolized by the CYP450 system may be observed when co-administered with telithromycin; therefore, increases or prolongation of the therapeutic and/or adverse effects of the concomitant drug may be observed). Products include:
Delsym Extended-Release Suspension 611
Delsym 12 Hour Cough Suppressant for Children 611

Diazepam (Co-administration of telithromycin with a drug primarily metabolized by the CYP 3A4 enzyme system may result in increased plasma concentrations of the drug co-administered with telithromycin that could increase or prolong both the therapeutic and adverse effects). Products include:
Diastat Rectal Delivery System 3344
Valium Tablets 2822

Diclofenac Potassium (Elevated levels of drugs metabolized by the CYP450 system may be observed when co-administered with telithromycin; therefore, increases or prolongation of the therapeutic and/or adverse effects of the concomitant drug may be observed). Products include:
Cataflam Tablets 2173

Diclofenac Sodium (Elevated levels of drugs metabolized by the CYP450 system may be observed when co-administered with telithromycin; therefore, increases or prolongation of the therapeutic and/or adverse effects of the concomitant drug may be observed). Products include:
Arthrotec Tablets 3126
Voltaren Ophthalmic Solution 2300
Voltaren Tablets 2298
Voltaren-XR Tablets 2301

Digoxin (Plasma peak and trough levels of digoxin were increased when co-adminstered with telithromycin; however, trough concentrations of digoxin ranged from 0.74 to 2.17 ng/mL). Products include:
Digitek Tablets 2146
Lanoxicaps Capsules 1458
Lanoxin Injection 1462
Lanoxin Tablets 1468
Lanoxin Injection Pediatric 1465

Dihydroergotamine Mesylate (Co-administration is not recommended because acute ergot toxicity characterized by severe peripheral vasospasm and dyesthesia have been reported with macrolide antibiotics). Products include:
Migranal Nasal Spray 3350

Diltiazem Hydrochloride (Co-administration of telithromycin with a drug primarily metabolized by the CYP 3A4 enzyme system may result in increased plasma concentrations of the drug co-administered with telithromycin that could increase or prolong both the therapeutic and adverse effects). Products include:
Cardizem LA Extended Release Tablets 1699
Tiazac Capsules 1204

Diltiazem Maleate (Co-administration of telithromycin with a drug primarily metabolized by the CYP 3A4 enzyme system may result in increased plasma concentrations of the drug co-administered with telithromycin that could increase or prolong both the therapeutic and adverse effects).
No products indexed under this heading.

Disopyramide (Co-administration of telithromycin with a drug primarily metabolized by the CYP 3A4 enzyme system may result in increased plasma concentrations of the drug co-administered with telithromycin that could increase or prolong both the therapeutic and adverse effects).
No products indexed under this heading.

Disopyramide Phosphate (Co-administration of telithromycin with a drug primarily metabolized by the CYP 3A4 enzyme system may result in increased plasma concentrations of the drug co-administered with telithromycin that could increase or prolong both the therapeutic and adverse effects).
No products indexed under this heading.

Disulfiram (Co-administration of telithromycin with a drug primarily metabolized by the CYP 3A4 enzyme system may result in increased plasma concentrations of the drug co-administered with telithromycin that could increase or prolong both the therapeutic and adverse effects). Products include:
Antabuse Tablets 2343

Divalproex Sodium (Elevated levels of drugs metabolized by the CYP450 system may be observed when co-administered with telithromycin; therefore, increases or prolongation of the therapeutic and/or adverse effects of the concomitant drug may be observed). Products include:
Depakote Sprinkle Capsules 422
Depakote Tablets 427
Depakote ER Tablets 433

Docetaxel (Elevated levels of drugs metabolized by the CYP450 system may be observed when co-administered with telithromycin; therefore, increases or prolongation of the therapeutic and/or adverse effects of the concomitant drug may be observed). Products include:
Taxotere Injection Concentrate 2947

Dolasetron Mesylate (Elevated levels of drugs metabolized by the CYP450 system may be observed when co-administered with telithromycin; therefore, increases or prolongation of the therapeutic and/or adverse effects of the concomitant drug may be observed). Products include:
Anzemet Injection 2871
Anzemet Tablets 2874

Donepezil Hydrochloride (Elevated levels of drugs metabolized by the CYP450 system may be observed when co-administered with telithromycin; therefore, increases or prolongation of the therapeutic and/or adverse effects of the concomitant drug may be observed). Products include:
Aricept Tablets 1086
Aricept ODT Tablets 1086

Doxepin Hydrochloride (Elevated levels of drugs metabolized by the CYP450 system may be observed when co-administered with telithromycin; therefore, increases or prolongation of the therapeutic and/or adverse effects of the concomitant drug may be observed).
No products indexed under this heading.

Doxorubicin Hydrochloride (Co-administration of telithromycin with a drug primarily metabolized by the CYP 3A4 enzyme system may result in increased plasma concentrations of the drug co-administered with telithromycin that could increase or prolong both the therapeutic and adverse effects). Products include:
Adriamycin for Injection, USP 786
Adriamycin Injection, USP 786

Dronabinol (Co-administration of telithromycin with a drug primarily metabolized by the CYP 3A4 enzyme system may result in increased plasma concentrations of the drug co-administered with telithromycin that could increase or prolong both the therapeutic and adverse effects). Products include:
Marinol Capsules 3334

Drugs that Undergo Biotransformation by Cytochrome P-450 Mixed Function Oxidase (Elevated levels of drugs metabolized by the CYP450 system may be observed when co-administered with telithromycin; therefore, increases or prolongation of the therapeutic and/or adverse effects of the concomitant drug may be observed).
No products indexed under this heading.

Dyphylline (Elevated levels of drugs metabolized by the CYP450 system may be observed when co-administered with telithromycin; therefore, increases or prolongation of the therapeutic and/or adverse effects of the concomitant drug may be observed).
No products indexed under this heading.

Efavirenz (Concomitant administration of CYP 3A4 inducers is likely to result in subtherapeutic levels of telithromycin and loss of effect). Products include:
Sustiva Capsules 957

Encainide Hydrochloride (Elevated levels of drugs metabolized by the CYP450 system may be observed when co-administered with telithromycin; therefore, increases or prolongation of the therapeutic and/or adverse effects of the concomitant drug may be observed).
No products indexed under this heading.

Enoxacin (Elevated levels of drugs metabolized by the CYP450 system may be observed when co-administered with telithromycin; therefore, increases or prolongation of the therapeutic and/or adverse effects of the concomitant drug may be observed).
No products indexed under this heading.

Eprosartan Mesylate (Elevated levels of drugs metabolized by the CYP450 system may be observed when co-administered with telithromycin; therefore, increases or prolongation of the therapeutic and/or adverse effects of the concomitant drug may be observed). Products include:
Teveten Tablets 1707
Teveten HCT Tablets 1710

Ergonovine Maleate (Co-administration is not recommended because acute ergot toxicity characterized by severe peripheral vasospasm and dyesthesia have been reported with macrolide antibiotics).
No products indexed under this heading.

Ergotamine Tartrate (Co-administration is not recommended because acute ergot toxicity characterized by severe peripheral vasospasm and dyesthesia have been reported with macrolide antibiotics).
No products indexed under this heading.

Erythromycin (Co-administration of telithromycin with a drug primarily metabolized by the CYP 3A4 enzyme system may result in increased plasma concentrations of the drug co-administered with telithromycin that could increase or prolong both the therapeutic and adverse effects). Products include:
Erygel Topical Gel 2096
Ery-Tab Tablets 447
Erythromycin Base Filmtab Tablets 454
Erythromycin Delayed-Release Capsules, USP 456
PCE Dispertab Tablets 510

Erythromycin Estolate (Co-administration of telithromycin with a drug primarily metabolized by the CYP 3A4 enzyme system may result in increased plasma concentrations of the drug co-administered with telithromycin that could increase or prolong both the therapeutic and adverse effects).
No products indexed under this heading.

Erythromycin Ethylsuccinate (Co-administration of telithromycin with a drug primarily metabolized by the CYP 3A4 enzyme system may result in increased plasma concentrations of the drug co-administered with telithromycin that could increase or prolong both the therapeutic and adverse effects). Products include:
E.E.S. 449
EryPed 445

Erythromycin Gluceptate (Co-administration of telithromycin with a drug primarily metabolized by the CYP 3A4 enzyme system may result in increased plasma concentrations of the drug co-administered with telithromycin that could increase or prolong both the therapeutic and adverse effects).
No products indexed under this heading.

Erythromycin Lactobionate (Co-administration of telithromycin with a drug primarily metabolized by the CYP 3A4 enzyme system may result in increased plasma concentrations of the drug co-administered with telithromycin that could increase or prolong both the therapeutic and adverse effects).
No products indexed under this heading.

Erythromycin Stearate (Co-administration of telithromycin with a drug primarily metabolized by the

CYP 3A4 enzyme system may result in increased plasma concentrations of the drug co-administered with telithromycin that could increase or prolong both the therapeutic and adverse effects). Products include:
Erythrocin Stearate Filmtab Tablets 452

Esomeprazole Magnesium (Elevated levels of drugs metabolized by the CYP450 system may be observed when co-administered with telithromycin; therefore, increases or prolongation of the therapeutic and/or adverse effects of the concomitant drug may be observed). Products include:
Nexium Delayed-Release Capsules 645

Estradiol (Co-administration of telithromycin with a drug primarily metabolized by the CYP 3A4 enzyme system may result in increased plasma concentrations of the drug co-administered with telithromycin that could increase or prolong both the therapeutic and adverse effects). Products include:
Activella Tablets 2311
Climara Transdermal System 795
Climara Pro Transdermal System 800
CombiPatch Transdermal System 2180
Estrogel 0.06% 3200
Menostar Transdermal System 805
Prefest Tablets 1069
Vagifem Tablets 2340
Vivelle Transdermal System 2288
Vivelle-Dot Transdermal System 2293

Estradiol Benzoate (Co-administration of telithromycin with a drug primarily metabolized by the CYP 3A4 enzyme system may result in increased plasma concentrations of the drug co-administered with telithromycin that could increase or prolong both the therapeutic and adverse effects).
No products indexed under this heading.

Estradiol Cypionate (Co-administration of telithromycin with a drug primarily metabolized by the CYP 3A4 enzyme system may result in increased plasma concentrations of the drug co-administered with telithromycin that could increase or prolong both the therapeutic and adverse effects).
No products indexed under this heading.

Estradiol Valerate (Co-administration of telithromycin with a drug primarily metabolized by the CYP 3A4 enzyme system may result in increased plasma concentrations of the drug co-administered with telithromycin that could increase or prolong both the therapeutic and adverse effects).
No products indexed under this heading.

Estrogen (Elevated levels of drugs metabolized by the CYP450 system may be observed when co-administered with telithromycin; therefore, increases or prolongation of the therapeutic and/or adverse effects of the concomitant drug may be observed).
No products indexed under this heading.

Estrogens, Conjugated (Elevated levels of drugs metabolized by the CYP450 system may be observed when co-administered with telithromycin; therefore, increases or prolongation of the therapeutic and/or adverse effects of the concomitant drug may be observed). Products include:
Premarin Intravenous 3440
Premarin Tablets 3443
Premarin Vaginal Cream 3449
Premphase Tablets 3452
Prempro Tablets 3452

Estrogens, Conjugated, Synthetic A (Elevated levels of drugs metabolized by the CYP450 system may be observed when co-administered with telithromycin; therefore, increases or prolongation of the therapeutic and/or adverse effects of the concomitant drug may be observed). Products include:
Cenestin Tablets, 0.45mg, 0.625mg, 0.9mg, 1.25mg 1063
Cenestin Tablets, 0.3mg 1063

Estrogens, Esterified (Elevated levels of drugs metabolized by the CYP450 system may be observed when co-administered with telithromycin; therefore, increases or prolongation of the therapeutic and/or adverse effects of the concomitant drug may be observed). Products include:
Estratest Tablets 3196
Estratest H.S. Tablets 3196

Ethinyl Estradiol (Co-administration of telithromycin with a drug primarily metabolized by the CYP 3A4 enzyme system may result in increased plasma concentrations of the drug co-administered with telithromycin that could increase or prolong both the therapeutic and adverse effects). Products include:
Alesse-28 Tablets 3392
Lo/Ovral-28 Tablets 3423
NuvaRing 2357
Ortho-Cept Tablets 2395
Ortho-Cyclen/Ortho Tri-Cyclen 2414
Ortho Evra Transdermal System 2402
Ortho Tri-Cyclen Lo Tablets 2421
Seasonale Tablets 1073
Triphasil-28 Tablets 3483
Yasmin 28 Tablets 818

Ethosuximide (Co-administration of telithromycin with a drug primarily metabolized by the CYP 3A4 enzyme system may result in increased plasma concentrations of the drug co-administered with telithromycin that could increase or prolong both the therapeutic and adverse effects).
No products indexed under this heading.

Ethotoin (Elevated levels of drugs metabolized by the CYP450 system may be observed when co-administered with telithromycin; therefore, increases or prolongation of the therapeutic and/or adverse effects of the concomitant drug may be observed). Products include:
Peganone Tablets, USP 2487

Ethynodiol Diacetate (Co-administration of telithromycin with a drug primarily metabolized by the CYP 3A4 enzyme system may result in increased plasma concentrations of the drug co-administered with telithromycin that could increase or prolong both the therapeutic and adverse effects).
No products indexed under this heading.

Etodolac (Elevated levels of drugs metabolized by the CYP450 system may be observed when co-administered with telithromycin; therefore, increases or prolongation of the therapeutic and/or adverse effects of the concomitant drug may be observed).
No products indexed under this heading.

Etoposide (Co-administration of telithromycin with a drug primarily metabolized by the CYP 3A4 enzyme system may result in increased plasma concentrations of the drug co-administered with telithromycin that could increase or prolong both the therapeutic and adverse effects).
No products indexed under this heading.

Etoposide Phosphate (Co-administration of telithromycin with a drug primarily metabolized by the CYP 3A4 enzyme system may result in increased plasma concentrations of the drug co-administered with telithromycin that could increase or prolong both the therapeutic and adverse effects).
No products indexed under this heading.

Felbamate (Concomitant administration of CYP 3A4 inducers is likely to result in subtherapeutic levels of telithromycin and loss of effect).
No products indexed under this heading.

Felodipine (Co-administration of telithromycin with a drug primarily metabolized by the CYP 3A4 enzyme system may result in increased plasma concentrations of the drug co-administered with telithromycin that could increase or prolong both the therapeutic and adverse effects). Products include:
Plendil Extended-Release Tablets 651

Fenoprofen Calcium (Elevated levels of drugs metabolized by the CYP450 system may be observed when co-administered with telithromycin; therefore, increases or prolongation of the therapeutic and/or adverse effects of the concomitant drug may be observed). Products include:
Nalfon Capsules 2504

Fentanyl (Co-administration of telithromycin with a drug primarily metabolized by the CYP 3A4 enzyme system may result in increased plasma concentrations of the drug co-administered with telithromycin that could increase or prolong both the therapeutic and adverse effects). Products include:
Duragesic Transdermal System 2448

Fentanyl Citrate (Co-administration of telithromycin with a drug primarily metabolized by the CYP 3A4 enzyme system may result in increased plasma concentrations of the drug co-administered with telithromycin that could increase or prolong both the therapeutic and adverse effects). Products include:
Actiq 993

Flecainide Acetate (Elevated levels of drugs metabolized by the CYP450 system may be observed when co-administered with telithromycin; therefore, increases or prolongation of the therapeutic and/or adverse effects of the concomitant drug may be observed). Products include:
Tambocor Tablets 1824

Fludrocortisone Acetate (Concomitant administration of CYP 3A4 inducers is likely to result in subtherapeutic levels of telithromycin and loss of effect).
No products indexed under this heading.

Fluoxetine (Elevated levels of drugs metabolized by the CYP450 system may be observed when co-administered with telithromycin; therefore, increases or prolongation of the therapeutic and/or adverse effects of the concomitant drug may be observed).
No products indexed under this heading.

Fluoxetine Hydrochloride (Elevated levels of drugs metabolized by the CYP450 system may be observed when co-administered with telithromycin; therefore, increases or prolongation of the therapeutic and/or adverse effects of the concomitant drug may be observed). Products include:
Prozac Pulvules and Liquid 1771
Symbyax Capsules 1788

Fluphenazine Decanoate (Elevated levels of drugs metabolized by the CYP450 system may be observed when co-administered with telithromycin; therefore, increases or prolongation of the therapeutic and/or adverse effects of the concomitant drug may be observed).
No products indexed under this heading.

Fluphenazine Enanthate (Elevated levels of drugs metabolized by the CYP450 system may be observed when co-administered with telithromycin; therefore, increases or prolongation of the therapeutic and/or adverse effects of the concomitant drug may be observed).
No products indexed under this heading.

Fluphenazine Hydrochloride (Elevated levels of drugs metabolized by the CYP450 system may be observed when co-administered with telithromycin; therefore, increases or prolongation of the therapeutic and/or adverse effects of the concomitant drug may be observed).
No products indexed under this heading.

Flurbiprofen (Elevated levels of drugs metabolized by the CYP450 system may be observed when co-administered with telithromycin; therefore, increases or prolongation of the therapeutic and/or adverse effects of the concomitant drug may be observed).
No products indexed under this heading.

Flurbiprofen Sodium (Elevated levels of drugs metabolized by the CYP450 system may be observed when co-administered with telithromycin; therefore, increases or prolongation of the therapeutic and/or adverse effects of the concomitant drug may be observed). Products include:
Ocufen Ophthalmic Solution .... ⊙230

Flutamide (Elevated levels of drugs metabolized by the CYP450 system may be observed when co-administered with telithromycin; therefore, increases or prolongation of the therapeutic and/or adverse effects of the concomitant drug may be observed). Products include:
Eulexin Capsules 3023

Fluticasone Propionate (Elevated levels of drugs metabolized by the CYP450 system may be observed when co-administered with telithromycin; therefore, increases or prolongation of the therapeutic and/or

adverse effects of the concomitant drug may be observed). Products include:

- Advair Diskus 100/50 .... **1291**
- Advair Diskus 250/50 .... **1291**
- Advair Diskus 500/50 .... **1291**
- Cutivate Cream **1381**
- Cutivate Lotion 0.05% **1383**
- Cutivate Ointment **1384**
- Flonase Nasal Spray **1412**
- Flovent Diskus 100 mcg **1418**
- Flovent Diskus 50 mcg **1415**

Fluvastatin Sodium (Elevated levels of drugs metabolized by the CYP450 system may be observed when co-administered with telithromycin; therefore, increases or prolongation of the therapeutic and/or adverse effects of the concomitant drug may be observed). Products include:

- Lescol Capsules **2227**
- Lescol **2730**
- Lescol XL Tablets **2227**

Fluvoxamine Maleate (Elevated levels of drugs metabolized by the CYP450 system may be observed when co-administered with telithromycin; therefore, increases or prolongation of the therapeutic and/or adverse effects of the concomitant drug may be observed).

No products indexed under this heading.

Formoterol Fumarate (Elevated levels of drugs metabolized by the CYP450 system may be observed when co-administered with telithromycin; therefore, increases or prolongation of the therapeutic and/or adverse effects of the concomitant drug may be observed). Products include:

- Foradil Aerolizer **3024**

Fosphenytoin (Elevated levels of drugs metabolized by the CYP450 system may be observed when co-administered with telithromycin; therefore, increases or prolongation of the therapeutic and/or adverse effects of the concomitant drug may be observed).

No products indexed under this heading.

Fosphenytoin Sodium (Concomitant administration of CYP 3A4 inducers is likely to result in subtherapeutic levels of telithromycin and loss of effect).

No products indexed under this heading.

Gabapentin (Elevated levels of drugs metabolized by the CYP450 system may be observed when co-administered with telithromycin; therefore, increases or prolongation of the therapeutic and/or adverse effects of the concomitant drug may be observed). Products include:

- Neurontin Capsules **2498**
- Neurontin Oral Solution **2498**
- Neurontin Tablets **2498**

Galantamine Hydrobromide (Elevated levels of drugs metabolized by the CYP450 system may be observed when co-administered with telithromycin; therefore, increases or prolongation of the therapeutic and/or adverse effects of the concomitant drug may be observed). Products include:

- Razadyne ER Extended-Release Capsules **2434**
- Razadyne **2434**

Garlic Extract (Concomitant administration of CYP 3A4 inducers is likely to result in subtherapeutic levels of telithromycin and loss of effect).

No products indexed under this heading.

Garlic Oil (Concomitant administration of CYP 3A4 inducers is likely to result in subtherapeutic levels of telithromycin and loss of effect).

No products indexed under this heading.

Glimepiride (Elevated levels of drugs metabolized by the CYP450 system may be observed when co-administered with telithromycin; therefore, increases or prolongation of the therapeutic and/or adverse effects of the concomitant drug may be observed). Products include:

- Amaryl Tablets **2864**

Glipizide (Elevated levels of drugs metabolized by the CYP450 system may be observed when co-administered with telithromycin; therefore, increases or prolongation of the therapeutic and/or adverse effects of the concomitant drug may be observed).

No products indexed under this heading.

Glyburide (Elevated levels of drugs metabolized by the CYP450 system may be observed when co-administered with telithromycin; therefore, increases or prolongation of the therapeutic and/or adverse effects of the concomitant drug may be observed).

No products indexed under this heading.

Grepafloxacin Hydrochloride (Elevated levels of drugs metabolized by the CYP450 system may be observed when co-administered with telithromycin; therefore, increases or prolongation of the therapeutic and/or adverse effects of the concomitant drug may be observed).

No products indexed under this heading.

Haloperidol (Co-administration of telithromycin with a drug primarily metabolized by the CYP 3A4 enzyme system may result in increased plasma concentrations of the drug co-administered with telithromycin that could increase or prolong both the therapeutic and adverse effects).

No products indexed under this heading.

Haloperidol Decanoate (Co-administration of telithromycin with a drug primarily metabolized by the CYP 3A4 enzyme system may result in increased plasma concentrations of the drug co-administered with telithromycin that could increase or prolong both the therapeutic and adverse effects).

No products indexed under this heading.

Haloperidol Lactate (Co-administration of telithromycin with a drug primarily metabolized by the CYP 3A4 enzyme system may result in increased plasma concentrations of the drug co-administered with telithromycin that could increase or prolong both the therapeutic and adverse effects).

No products indexed under this heading.

Hydrocodone Bitartrate (Elevated levels of drugs metabolized by the CYP450 system may be observed when co-administered with telithromycin; therefore, increases or prolongation of the therapeutic and/or adverse effects of the concomitant drug may be observed). Products include:

- Hycodan **1104**
- Hycomine Compound Tablets **1105**
- Hycotuss Expectorant Syrup **1106**
- Lortab **3315**
- Lortab Elixir **3312**
- Vicodin Tablets **530**
- Vicodin ES Tablets **531**
- Vicodin HP Tablets **532**
- Vicoprofen Tablets **533**
- Zydone Tablets **1118**

Hydrocortisone (Concomitant administration of CYP 3A4 inducers is likely to result in subtherapeutic levels of telithromycin and loss of effect). Products include:

- Cortizone•5 Ointment **699**
- Cortizone•10 Creme **699**
- Cortizone•10 Ointment **699**
- Cortizone•10 Plus Creme **700**
- Cortizone•10 Maximum Strength Quick Shot Spray **700**
- Hydrocortone Tablets **1963**
- Preparation H Hydrocortisone Cream **748**

Hydrocortisone Acetate (Concomitant administration of CYP 3A4 inducers is likely to result in subtherapeutic levels of telithromycin and loss of effect). Products include:

- Analpram-HC **1136**
- Pramosone **1139**
- ProctoFoam-HC **3113**
- Tucks Anti-Itch Ointment **712**
- U-cort 1% Cream **3289**

Hydrocortisone Butyrate (Concomitant administration of CYP 3A4 inducers is likely to result in subtherapeutic levels of telithromycin and loss of effect). Products include:

- Locoid **1138**
- Locoid Lipocream Cream **1138**

Hydrocortisone Cypionate (Concomitant administration of CYP 3A4 inducers is likely to result in subtherapeutic levels of telithromycin and loss of effect).

No products indexed under this heading.

Hydrocortisone Hemisuccinate (Concomitant administration of CYP 3A4 inducers is likely to result in subtherapeutic levels of telithromycin and loss of effect).

No products indexed under this heading.

Hydrocortisone Probutate (Concomitant administration of CYP 3A4 inducers is likely to result in subtherapeutic levels of telithromycin and loss of effect). Products include:

- Pandel Cream, 0.1% **1017**

Hydrocortisone Sodium Phosphate (Concomitant administration of CYP 3A4 inducers is likely to result in subtherapeutic levels of telithromycin and loss of effect).

No products indexed under this heading.

Hydrocortisone Sodium Succinate (Concomitant administration of CYP 3A4 inducers is likely to result in subtherapeutic levels of telithromycin and loss of effect).

No products indexed under this heading.

Hydrocortisone Valerate (Concomitant administration of CYP 3A4 inducers is likely to result in subtherapeutic levels of telithromycin and loss of effect).

No products indexed under this heading.

Hypericum (Concomitant administration of CYP 3A4 inducers is likely to result in subtherapeutic levels of telithromycin and loss of effect).

No products indexed under this heading.

Hypericum Perforatum (Concomitant administration of CYP 3A4 inducers is likely to result in subtherapeutic levels of telithromycin and loss of effect).

No products indexed under this heading.

Ibuprofen (Elevated levels of drugs metabolized by the CYP450 system may be observed when co-administered with telithromycin; therefore, increases or prolongation of the therapeutic and/or adverse effects of the concomitant drug may be observed). Products include:

- Advil Allergy Sinus Caplets **737**
- Advil **737**
- Children's Advil Suspension **742**
- Children's Advil Chewable Tablets **741**
- Advil Cold & Sinus **739**
- Advil Flu & Body Ache Caplets **739**
- Children's Advil Cold Suspension **741**
- Infants' Advil Concentrated Drops **743**
- Junior Strength Advil Swallow Tablets **740**
- Advil Migraine Liquigels **740**
- Advil Multi-Symptom Cold Caplets **738**
- Combunox Tablets **1183**
- Children's Motrin Oral Suspension and Chewable Tablets **1837**
- Children's Motrin Cold Non-Staining Dye-Free Oral Suspension **1838**
- Children's Motrin Cold Oral Suspension **1838**
- Children's Motrin Non-Staining Dye-Free Oral Suspension **1837**
- Motrin Cold & Sinus Caplets **1836**
- Motrin IB Tablets and Caplets **1836**
- Infants' Motrin Concentrated Drops **1837**
- Infants' Motrin Non-Staining Dye-Free Drops **1837**
- Junior Strength Motrin Caplets and Chewable Tablets **1837**
- Vicoprofen Tablets **533**

Imipramine Hydrochloride (Elevated levels of drugs metabolized by the CYP450 system may be observed when co-administered with telithromycin; therefore, increases or prolongation of the therapeutic and/or adverse effects of the concomitant drug may be observed).

No products indexed under this heading.

Imipramine Pamoate (Elevated levels of drugs metabolized by the CYP450 system may be observed when co-administered with telithromycin; therefore, increases or prolongation of the therapeutic and/or adverse effects of the concomitant drug may be observed).

No products indexed under this heading.

Indinavir Sulfate (Co-administration of telithromycin with a drug primarily metabolized by the CYP 3A4 enzyme system may result in increased plasma concentrations of the drug co-administered with telithromycin that could increase or prolong both the therapeutic and adverse effects). Products include:

- Crixivan Capsules **1918**

Indomethacin (Elevated levels of drugs metabolized by the CYP450 system may be observed when co-administered with telithromycin; therefore, increases or prolongation

of the therapeutic and/or adverse effects of the concomitant drug may be observed). Products include:

Indocin ... 1968

Indomethacin Sodium Trihydrate (Elevated levels of drugs metabolized by the CYP450 system may be observed when co-administered with telithromycin; therefore, increases or prolongation of the therapeutic and/or adverse effects of the concomitant drug may be observed). Products include:

Indocin I.V. ... 1973

Indoramin Hydrochloride (Elevated levels of drugs metabolized by the CYP450 system may be observed when co-administered with telithromycin; therefore, increases or prolongation of the therapeutic and/or adverse effects of the concomitant drug may be observed).

No products indexed under this heading.

Irbesartan (Elevated levels of drugs metabolized by the CYP450 system may be observed when co-administered with telithromycin; therefore, increases or prolongation of the therapeutic and/or adverse effects of the concomitant drug may be observed). Products include:

Avalide Tablets ... 922
Avalide Tablets ... 2889
Avapro Tablets ... 925
Avapro Tablets ... 2886

Isotretinoin (Elevated levels of drugs metabolized by the CYP450 system may be observed when co-administered with telithromycin; therefore, increases or prolongation of the therapeutic and/or adverse effects of the concomitant drug may be observed). Products include:

Accutane Capsules ... 2740
Amnesteem Capsules ... 2126

Isradipine (Co-administration of telithromycin with a drug primarily metabolized by the CYP 3A4 enzyme system may result in increased plasma concentrations of the drug co-administered with telithromycin that could increase or prolong both the therapeutic and adverse effects). Products include:

DynaCirc CR Tablets ... 2726

Itraconazole (A study with itraconazole showed the Cmax and AUC of telithromycin were increased).

No products indexed under this heading.

Ketoconazole (A study with ketoconazole showed the Cmax and AUC of telithromycin were increased). Products include:

Nizoral A-D Shampoo, 1% ... 1839
Nizoral 2% Shampoo ... 1838

Ketoprofen (Elevated levels of drugs metabolized by the CYP450 system may be observed when co-administered with telithromycin; therefore, increases or prolongation of the therapeutic and/or adverse effects of the concomitant drug may be observed).

No products indexed under this heading.

Ketorolac Tromethamine (Elevated levels of drugs metabolized by the CYP450 system may be observed when co-administered with telithromycin; therefore, increases or prolongation of the therapeutic and/or adverse effects of the concomitant drug may be observed). Products include:

Acular Ophthalmic Solution ... 561
Acular LS Ophthalmic Solution ... 562

Labetalol Hydrochloride (Elevated levels of drugs metabolized by the CYP450 system may be observed when co-administered with telithromycin; therefore, increases or prolongation of the therapeutic and/or adverse effects of the concomitant drug may be observed).

No products indexed under this heading.

Lamotrigine (Elevated levels of drugs metabolized by the CYP450 system may be observed when co-administered with telithromycin; therefore, increases or prolongation of the therapeutic and/or adverse effects of the concomitant drug may be observed). Products include:

Lamictal ... 1449

Lansoprazole (Elevated levels of drugs metabolized by the CYP450 system may be observed when co-administered with telithromycin; therefore, increases or prolongation of the therapeutic and/or adverse effects of the concomitant drug may be observed). Products include:

Prevacid Delayed-Release Capsules ... 3268
Prevacid for Delayed-Release Oral Suspension ... 3268
Prevacid I.V. for Injection ... 3274
Prevacid NapraPAC ... 3277
Prevacid SoluTab Delayed-Release Orally Disintegrating Tablets ... 3268
PREVPAC ... 3281

Levetiracetam (Elevated levels of drugs metabolized by the CYP450 system may be observed when co-administered with telithromycin; therefore, increases or prolongation of the therapeutic and/or adverse effects of the concomitant drug may be observed). Products include:

Keppra Oral Solution ... 3307
Keppra Tablets ... 3307

Levobupivacaine Hydrochloride (Elevated levels of drugs metabolized by the CYP450 system may be observed when co-administered with telithromycin; therefore, increases or prolongation of the therapeutic and/or adverse effects of the concomitant drug may be observed).

No products indexed under this heading.

Levonorgestrel (When oral contraceptives containing ethinyl estradiol and levonorgestrel were co-administered with telithromycin, the steady-state AUC of ethinyl estradiol did not change but the AUC of levonorgestrel increased. However, telithromycin did not interfere with the antiovulatory effect of the oral contraceptives). Products include:

Alesse-28 Tablets ... 3392
Climara Pro Transdermal System ... 800
Mirena Intrauterine System ... 810
Plan B Tablets ... 1068
Seasonale Tablets ... 1073
Triphasil-28 Tablets ... 3483

Lidocaine (Co-administration of telithromycin with a drug primarily metabolized by the CYP 3A4 enzyme system may result in increased plasma concentrations of the drug co-administered with telithromycin that could increase or prolong both the therapeutic and adverse effects). Products include:

Lidoderm Patch ... 1107

Lidocaine Base (Elevated levels of drugs metabolized by the CYP450 system may be observed when co-administered with telithromycin; therefore, increases or prolongation of the therapeutic and/or adverse effects of the concomitant drug may be observed).

No products indexed under this heading.

Lidocaine Hydrochloride (Co-administration of telithromycin with a drug primarily metabolized by the CYP 3A4 enzyme system may result in increased plasma concentrations of the drug co-administered with telithromycin that could increase or prolong both the therapeutic and adverse effects).

No products indexed under this heading.

Lomefloxacin Hydrochloride (Elevated levels of drugs metabolized by the CYP450 system may be observed when co-administered with telithromycin; therefore, increases or prolongation of the therapeutic and/or adverse effects of the concomitant drug may be observed).

No products indexed under this heading.

Losartan Potassium (Elevated levels of drugs metabolized by the CYP450 system may be observed when co-administered with telithromycin; therefore, increases or prolongation of the therapeutic and/or adverse effects of the concomitant drug may be observed). Products include:

Cozaar Tablets ... 1913
Hyzaar ... 1964

Lovastatin (Lovastatin levels were increased due to CYP 3A4 inhibition by telithromycin, thereby increasing the risk of myopathy. Co-administration should be avoided). Products include:

Advicor Tablets ... 1694
Altoprev Extended-Release Tablets ... 1151
Mevacor Tablets ... 1996

Maprotiline Hydrochloride (Elevated levels of drugs metabolized by the CYP450 system may be observed when co-administered with telithromycin; therefore, increases or prolongation of the therapeutic and/or adverse effects of the concomitant drug may be observed).

No products indexed under this heading.

Meclofenamate Sodium (Elevated levels of drugs metabolized by the CYP450 system may be observed when co-administered with telithromycin; therefore, increases or prolongation of the therapeutic and/or adverse effects of the concomitant drug may be observed).

No products indexed under this heading.

Mefenamic Acid (Elevated levels of drugs metabolized by the CYP450 system may be observed when co-administered with telithromycin; therefore, increases or prolongation of the therapeutic and/or adverse effects of the concomitant drug may be observed).

No products indexed under this heading.

Meloxicam (Elevated levels of drugs metabolized by the CYP450 system may be observed when co-administered with telithromycin; therefore, increases or prolongation of the therapeutic and/or adverse effects of the concomitant drug may be observed). Products include:

Mobic Oral Suspension ... 893
Mobic Tablets ... 893

Meperidine Hydrochloride (Elevated levels of drugs metabolized by the CYP450 system may be observed when co-administered with telithromycin; therefore, increases or prolongation of the therapeutic and/or adverse effects of the concomitant drug may be observed).

No products indexed under this heading.

Mephenytoin (Concomitant administration of CYP 3A4 inducers is likely to result in subtherapeutic levels of telithromycin and loss of effect).

No products indexed under this heading.

Mephobarbital (Elevated levels of drugs metabolized by the CYP450 system may be observed when co-administered with telithromycin; therefore, increases or prolongation of the therapeutic and/or adverse effects of the concomitant drug may be observed). Products include:

Mebaral Tablets, USP ... 2483

Meprobamate (Elevated levels of drugs metabolized by the CYP450 system may be observed when co-administered with telithromycin; therefore, increases or prolongation of the therapeutic and/or adverse effects of the concomitant drug may be observed).

No products indexed under this heading.

Mestranol (Co-administration of telithromycin with a drug primarily metabolized by the CYP 3A4 enzyme system may result in increased plasma concentrations of the drug co-administered with telithromycin that could increase or prolong both the therapeutic and adverse effects).

No products indexed under this heading.

Metformin Hydrochloride (Elevated levels of drugs metabolized by the CYP450 system may be observed when co-administered with telithromycin; therefore, increases or prolongation of the therapeutic and/or adverse effects of the concomitant drug may be observed). Products include:

ActoPlus Met Tablets ... 3219
Avandamet Tablets ... 1343
Fortamet Extended-Release Tablets ... 1156

Methadone Hydrochloride (Co-administration of telithromycin with a drug primarily metabolized by the CYP 3A4 enzyme system may result in increased plasma concentrations of the drug co-administered with telithromycin that could increase or prolong both the therapeutic and adverse effects).

No products indexed under this heading.

Methamphetamine Hydrochloride (Elevated levels of drugs metabolized by the CYP450 system may be observed when co-administered with telithromycin; therefore, increases or prolongation of the therapeutic and/or adverse effects of the concomitant drug may be observed). Products include:

Desoxyn Tablets, USP ... 2482

Methsuximide (Concomitant administration of CYP 3A4 inducers is likely to result in subtherapeutic levels of telithromycin and loss of effect).
No products indexed under this heading.

Methylergonovine Maleate (Co-administration is not recommended because acute ergot toxicity characterized by severe peripheral vasospasm and dyesthesia have been reported with macrolide antibiotics).
No products indexed under this heading.

Methylprednisolone (Concomitant administration of CYP 3A4 inducers is likely to result in subtherapeutic levels of telithromycin and loss of effect).
No products indexed under this heading.

Methylprednisolone Acetate (Concomitant administration of CYP 3A4 inducers is likely to result in subtherapeutic levels of telithromycin and loss of effect). Products include:
Depo-Medrol Injectable Suspension **2615**
Depo-Medrol Single-Dose Vial **2617**

Methylprednisolone Sodium Succinate (Concomitant administration of CYP 3A4 inducers is likely to result in subtherapeutic levels of telithromycin and loss of effect).
No products indexed under this heading.

Methysergide Maleate (Co-administration is not recommended because acute ergot toxicity characterized by severe peripheral vasospasm and dyesthesia have been reported with macrolide antibiotics).
No products indexed under this heading.

Metoprolol Succinate (Co-administration increased the Cmax and AUC of metoprolol; however, there was no effect on the elimination half-life. The increased exposure to metoprolol may be of clinical importance). Products include:
Toprol-XL Tablets **660**

Metoprolol Tartrate (Co-administration increased the Cmax and AUC of metoprolol; however, there was no effect on the elimination half-life. The increased exposure to metoprolol may be of clinical importance).
No products indexed under this heading.

Mexiletine Hydrochloride (Elevated levels of drugs metabolized by the CYP450 system may be observed when co-administered with telithromycin; therefore, increases or prolongation of the therapeutic and/or adverse effects of the concomitant drug may be observed).
No products indexed under this heading.

Midazolam Hydrochloride (Concomitant administration of telithromycin with midazolam increased the AUC of midazolam. Dosage adjustment of midazolam should be considered if necessary).
No products indexed under this heading.

Miglitol (Elevated levels of drugs metabolized by the CYP450 system may be observed when co-administered with telithromycin; therefore, increases or prolongation of the therapeutic and/or adverse effects of the concomitant drug may be observed).
No products indexed under this heading.

Mirtazapine (Elevated levels of drugs metabolized by the CYP450 system may be observed when co-administered with telithromycin; therefore, increases or prolongation of the therapeutic and/or adverse effects of the concomitant drug may be observed).
No products indexed under this heading.

Modafinil (Concomitant administration of CYP 3A4 inducers is likely to result in subtherapeutic levels of telithromycin and loss of effect). Products include:
Provigil Tablets **1002**

Montelukast Sodium (Elevated levels of drugs metabolized by the CYP450 system may be observed when co-administered with telithromycin; therefore, increases or prolongation of the therapeutic and/or adverse effects of the concomitant drug may be observed). Products include:
Singulair **2047**

Morphine Sulfate (Elevated levels of drugs metabolized by the CYP450 system may be observed when co-administered with telithromycin; therefore, increases or prolongation of the therapeutic and/or adverse effects of the concomitant drug may be observed). Products include:
Avinza Capsules **1714**
Kadian Capsules **572**
MS Contin Tablets **2703**

Moxifloxacin Hydrochloride (Elevated levels of drugs metabolized by the CYP450 system may be observed when co-administered with telithromycin; therefore, increases or prolongation of the therapeutic and/or adverse effects of the concomitant drug may be observed). Products include:
Avelox **2984**
Vigamox Ophthalmic Solution **560**

Nabumetone (Elevated levels of drugs metabolized by the CYP450 system may be observed when co-administered with telithromycin; therefore, increases or prolongation of the therapeutic and/or adverse effects of the concomitant drug may be observed). Products include:
Relafen Tablets **1523**

Nafcillin Sodium (Elevated levels of drugs metabolized by the CYP450 system may be observed when co-administered with telithromycin; therefore, increases or prolongation of the therapeutic and/or adverse effects of the concomitant drug may be observed).
No products indexed under this heading.

Naproxen (Elevated levels of drugs metabolized by the CYP450 system may be observed when co-administered with telithromycin; therefore, increases or prolongation of the therapeutic and/or adverse effects of the concomitant drug may be observed). Products include:
EC-Naprosyn Delayed-Release Tablets **2769**
Naprosyn Suspension **2769**
Naprosyn Tablets **2769**
Prevacid NapraPAC **3277**

Naproxen Sodium (Elevated levels of drugs metabolized by the CYP450 system may be observed when co-administered with telithromycin; therefore, increases or prolongation of the therapeutic and/or adverse effects of the concomitant drug may be observed). Products include:
Aleve Tablets, Caplets and Gelcaps **605**
Anaprox Tablets **2769**
Anaprox DS Tablets **2769**

Nateglinide (Elevated levels of drugs metabolized by the CYP450 system may be observed when co-administered with telithromycin; therefore, increases or prolongation of the therapeutic and/or adverse effects of the concomitant drug may be observed). Products include:
Starlix Tablets **2276**

Nefazodone Hydrochloride (Co-administration of telithromycin with a drug primarily metabolized by the CYP 3A4 enzyme system may result in increased plasma concentrations of the drug co-administered with telithromycin that could increase or prolong both the therapeutic and adverse effects).
No products indexed under this heading.

Nelfinavir Mesylate (Co-administration of telithromycin with a drug primarily metabolized by the CYP 3A4 enzyme system may result in increased plasma concentrations of the drug co-administered with telithromycin that could increase or prolong both the therapeutic and adverse effects). Products include:
Viracept **2556**

Nevirapine (Concomitant administration of CYP 3A4 inducers is likely to result in subtherapeutic levels of telithromycin and loss of effect). Products include:
Viramune Oral Suspension **903**
Viramune Tablets **903**

Nicardipine (Elevated levels of drugs metabolized by the CYP450 system may be observed when co-administered with telithromycin; therefore, increases or prolongation of the therapeutic and/or adverse effects of the concomitant drug may be observed).
No products indexed under this heading.

Nicardipine Hydrochloride (Co-administration of telithromycin with a drug primarily metabolized by the CYP 3A4 enzyme system may result in increased plasma concentrations of the drug co-administered with telithromycin that could increase or prolong both the therapeutic and adverse effects). Products include:
Cardene I.V. **1129**

Nicotine Polacrilex (Elevated levels of drugs metabolized by the CYP450 system may be observed when co-administered with telithromycin; therefore, increases or prolongation of the therapeutic and/or adverse effects of the concomitant drug may be observed). Products include:
Commit Lozenges **1625**
Nicorette Gum **1632**

Nicotine Salicylate (Elevated levels of drugs metabolized by the CYP450 system may be observed when co-administered with telithromycin; therefore, increases or prolongation of the therapeutic and/or adverse effects of the concomitant drug may be observed).
No products indexed under this heading.

Nicotine Sulfate (Elevated levels of drugs metabolized by the CYP450 system may be observed when co-administered with telithromycin; therefore, increases or prolongation of the therapeutic and/or adverse effects of the concomitant drug may be observed).
No products indexed under this heading.

Nifedipine (Co-administration of telithromycin with a drug primarily metabolized by the CYP 3A4 enzyme system may result in increased plasma concentrations of the drug co-administered with telithromycin that could increase or prolong both the therapeutic and adverse effects). Products include:
Adalat CC Tablets **2978**

Nilutamide (Elevated levels of drugs metabolized by the CYP450 system may be observed when co-administered with telithromycin; therefore, increases or prolongation of the therapeutic and/or adverse effects of the concomitant drug may be observed).
No products indexed under this heading.

Nimodipine (Co-administration of telithromycin with a drug primarily metabolized by the CYP 3A4 enzyme system may result in increased plasma concentrations of the drug co-administered with telithromycin that could increase or prolong both the therapeutic and adverse effects). Products include:
Nimotop Capsules **774**

Nisoldipine (Co-administration of telithromycin with a drug primarily metabolized by the CYP 3A4 enzyme system may result in increased plasma concentrations of the drug co-administered with telithromycin that could increase or prolong both the therapeutic and adverse effects). Products include:
Sular Tablets **1163**

Nitrendipine (Co-administration of telithromycin with a drug primarily metabolized by the CYP 3A4 enzyme system may result in increased plasma concentrations of the drug co-administered with telithromycin that could increase or prolong both the therapeutic and adverse effects).
No products indexed under this heading.

Norethindrone (Co-administration of telithromycin with a drug primarily metabolized by the CYP 3A4 enzyme system may result in increased plasma concentrations of the drug co-administered with telithromycin that could increase or prolong both the therapeutic and adverse effects). Products include:
Ortho Micronor Tablets **2411**

Norethindrone Acetate (Co-administration of telithromycin with a drug primarily metabolized by the CYP 3A4 enzyme system may result in increased plasma concentrations of the drug co-administered with

telithromycin that could increase or prolong both the therapeutic and adverse effects). Products include:
- Activella Tablets 2311
- Aygestin Tablets 1062
- CombiPatch Transdermal System 2180

Norfloxacin (Elevated levels of drugs metabolized by the CYP450 system may be observed when co-administered with telithromycin; therefore, increases or prolongation of the therapeutic and/or adverse effects of the concomitant drug may be observed). Products include:
- Noroxin Tablets 2009

Norgestrel (Co-administration of telithromycin with a drug primarily metabolized by the CYP 3A4 enzyme system may result in increased plasma concentrations of the drug co-administered with telithromycin that could increase or prolong both the therapeutic and adverse effects). Products include:
- Lo/Ovral-28 Tablets 3423

Nortriptyline Hydrochloride (Elevated levels of drugs metabolized by the CYP450 system may be observed when co-administered with telithromycin; therefore, increases or prolongation of the therapeutic and/or adverse effects of the concomitant drug may be observed).
No products indexed under this heading.

Ofloxacin (Elevated levels of drugs metabolized by the CYP450 system may be observed when co-administered with telithromycin; therefore, increases or prolongation of the therapeutic and/or adverse effects of the concomitant drug may be observed). Products include:
- Floxin Otic Singles 1045
- Floxin Otic Solution 1043

Olanzapine (Elevated levels of drugs metabolized by the CYP450 system may be observed when co-administered with telithromycin; therefore, increases or prolongation of the therapeutic and/or adverse effects of the concomitant drug may be observed). Products include:
- Symbyax Capsules 1788
- Zyprexa Tablets 1798
- Zyprexa IntraMuscular 1798
- Zyprexa ZYDIS Orally Disintegrating Tablets 1798

Omeprazole (Elevated levels of drugs metabolized by the CYP450 system may be observed when co-administered with telithromycin; therefore, increases or prolongation of the therapeutic and/or adverse effects of the concomitant drug may be observed). Products include:
- Zegerid Powder for Oral Solution 2972

Ondansetron (Co-administration of telithromycin with a drug primarily metabolized by the CYP 3A4 enzyme system may result in increased plasma concentrations of the drug co-administered with telithromycin that could increase or prolong both the therapeutic and adverse effects). Products include:
- Zofran ODT Orally Disintegrating Tablets 1613

Ondansetron Hydrochloride (Co-administration of telithromycin with a drug primarily metabolized by the CYP 3A4 enzyme system may result in increased plasma concentrations of the drug co-administered with telithromycin that could increase or prolong both the therapeutic and adverse effects). Products include:
- Zofran Injection 1607
- Zofran 1613

Oxaprozin (Elevated levels of drugs metabolized by the CYP450 system may be observed when co-administered with telithromycin; therefore, increases or prolongation of the therapeutic and/or adverse effects of the concomitant drug may be observed).
No products indexed under this heading.

Oxcarbazepine (Concomitant administration of CYP 3A4 inducers is likely to result in subtherapeutic levels of telithromycin and loss of effect). Products include:
- Trileptal Oral Suspension 2281
- Trileptal Tablets 2281

Oxycodone Hydrochloride (Elevated levels of drugs metabolized by the CYP450 system may be observed when co-administered with telithromycin; therefore, increases or prolongation of the therapeutic and/or adverse effects of the concomitant drug may be observed). Products include:
- Combunox Tablets 1183
- OxyContin Tablets 2699
- OxyFast Oral Concentrate Solution 2704
- OxyIR Capsules 2704
- Percocet Tablets 1114
- Percodan Tablets 1115

Paclitaxel (Co-administration of telithromycin with a drug primarily metabolized by the CYP 3A4 enzyme system may result in increased plasma concentrations of the drug co-administered with telithromycin that could increase or prolong both the therapeutic and adverse effects).
No products indexed under this heading.

Pantoprazole Sodium (Elevated levels of drugs metabolized by the CYP450 system may be observed when co-administered with telithromycin; therefore, increases or prolongation of the therapeutic and/or adverse effects of the concomitant drug may be observed). Products include:
- Protonix I.V. 3468
- Protonix Tablets 3465

Paramethadione (Elevated levels of drugs metabolized by the CYP450 system may be observed when co-administered with telithromycin; therefore, increases or prolongation of the therapeutic and/or adverse effects of the concomitant drug may be observed).
No products indexed under this heading.

Paroxetine Hydrochloride (Elevated levels of drugs metabolized by the CYP450 system may be observed when co-administered with telithromycin; therefore, increases or prolongation of the therapeutic and/or adverse effects of the concomitant drug may be observed). Products include:
- Paxil CR Controlled-Release Tablets 1509
- Paxil 1501

Pentamidine Isethionate (Elevated levels of drugs metabolized by the CYP450 system may be observed when co-administered with telithromycin; therefore, increases or prolongation of the therapeutic and/or adverse effects of the concomitant drug may be observed).
No products indexed under this heading.

Phenacemide (Elevated levels of drugs metabolized by the CYP450 system may be observed when co-administered with telithromycin; therefore, increases or prolongation of the therapeutic and/or adverse effects of the concomitant drug may be observed).
No products indexed under this heading.

Phenobarbital (Concomitant administration of CYP 3A4 inducers is likely to result in subtherapeutic levels of telithromycin and loss of effect).
No products indexed under this heading.

Phenobarbital Sodium (Concomitant administration of CYP 3A4 inducers is likely to result in subtherapeutic levels of telithromycin and loss of effect).
No products indexed under this heading.

Phensuximide (Elevated levels of drugs metabolized by the CYP450 system may be observed when co-administered with telithromycin; therefore, increases or prolongation of the therapeutic and/or adverse effects of the concomitant drug may be observed).
No products indexed under this heading.

Phenylbutazone (Elevated levels of drugs metabolized by the CYP450 system may be observed when co-administered with telithromycin; therefore, increases or prolongation of the therapeutic and/or adverse effects of the concomitant drug may be observed).
No products indexed under this heading.

Phenytoin (Concomitant administration of CYP 3A4 inducers is likely to result in subtherapeutic levels of telithromycin and loss of effect).
No products indexed under this heading.

Phenytoin Sodium (Concomitant administration of CYP 3A4 inducers is likely to result in subtherapeutic levels of telithromycin and loss of effect). Products include:
- Phenytek Capsules 2153

Pimozide (There is a potential risk of increased pimozide plasma levels by inhibition of CYP 3A4 pathways by telithromycin. Coadministration is contraindicated). Products include:
- Orap Tablets 1220

Pindolol (Elevated levels of drugs metabolized by the CYP450 system may be observed when co-administered with telithromycin; therefore, increases or prolongation of the therapeutic and/or adverse effects of the concomitant drug may be observed).
No products indexed under this heading.

Pioglitazone Hydrochloride (Elevated levels of drugs metabolized by the CYP450 system may be observed when co-administered with telithromycin; therefore, increases or prolongation of the therapeutic and/or adverse effects of the concomitant drug may be observed). Products include:
- ActoPlus Met Tablets 3219
- Actos Tablets 3224

Piroxicam (Elevated levels of drugs metabolized by the CYP450 system may be observed when co-administered with telithromycin; therefore, increases or prolongation of the therapeutic and/or adverse effects of the concomitant drug may be observed).
No products indexed under this heading.

Polyestradiol Phosphate (Co-administration of telithromycin with a drug primarily metabolized by the CYP 3A4 enzyme system may result in increased plasma concentrations of the drug co-administered with telithromycin that could increase or prolong both the therapeutic and adverse effects).
No products indexed under this heading.

Prednisolone Acetate (Concomitant administration of CYP 3A4 inducers is likely to result in subtherapeutic levels of telithromycin and loss of effect). Products include:
- Blephamide Ophthalmic Ointment 563
- Blephamide Ophthalmic Suspension 564
- Poly-Pred Liquifilm Ophthalmic Suspension .... ⊙231
- Pred Forte Ophthalmic Suspension .... ⊙233
- Pred Mild Sterile Ophthalmic Suspension .... ⊙236
- Pred-G Ophthalmic Suspension .... ⊙234
- Pred-G Sterile Ophthalmic Ointment .... ⊙235

Prednisolone Sodium Phosphate (Concomitant administration of CYP 3A4 inducers is likely to result in subtherapeutic levels of telithromycin and loss of effect). Products include:
- Pediapred Oral Solution 3319

Prednisolone Tebutate (Concomitant administration of CYP 3A4 inducers is likely to result in subtherapeutic levels of telithromycin and loss of effect).
No products indexed under this heading.

Prednisone (Concomitant administration of CYP 3A4 inducers is likely to result in subtherapeutic levels of telithromycin and loss of effect).
No products indexed under this heading.

Primidone (Concomitant administration of CYP 3A4 inducers is likely to result in subtherapeutic levels of telithromycin and loss of effect).
No products indexed under this heading.

Progesterone (Elevated levels of drugs metabolized by the CYP450 system may be observed when co-administered with telithromycin; therefore, increases or prolongation of the therapeutic and/or adverse effects of the concomitant drug may be observed). Products include:
- Prochieve 4% Gel 1018
- Prochieve 8% Gel 1018
- Prometrium Capsules (100 mg, 200 mg) 3205

Proguanil Hydrochloride (Elevated levels of drugs metabolized by the CYP450 system may be observed when co-administered with telithromycin; therefore, increases or prolongation of the therapeutic and/or adverse effects of the concomitant drug may be observed). Products include:
- Malarone Tablets 1484
- Malarone Pediatric Tablets 1484

Propafenone Hydrochloride (Elevated levels of drugs metabolized by the CYP450 system may be observed when co-administered with telithromycin; therefore, increases or prolongation of the therapeutic and/ or adverse effects of the concomitant drug may be observed). Products include:
Rythmol SR Capsules 2736

Propoxyphene Hydrochloride (Elevated levels of drugs metabolized by the CYP450 system may be observed when co-administered with telithromycin; therefore, increases or prolongation of the therapeutic and/ or adverse effects of the concomitant drug may be observed).
No products indexed under this heading.

Propoxyphene Napsylate (Elevated levels of drugs metabolized by the CYP450 system may be observed when co-administered with telithromycin; therefore, increases or prolongation of the therapeutic and/ or adverse effects of the concomitant drug may be observed). Products include:
Darvocet A 500 Tablets 3497

Propranolol Hydrochloride (Elevated levels of drugs metabolized by the CYP450 system may be observed when co-administered with telithromycin; therefore, increases or prolongation of the therapeutic and/ or adverse effects of the concomitant drug may be observed). Products include:
Inderal LA Long-Acting Capsules 3421
InnoPran XL Capsules 2728

Protriptyline Hydrochloride (Elevated levels of drugs metabolized by the CYP450 system may be observed when co-administered with telithromycin; therefore, increases or prolongation of the therapeutic and/ or adverse effects of the concomitant drug may be observed). Products include:
Vivactil Tablets 2350

Quetiapine Fumarate (Elevated levels of drugs metabolized by the CYP450 system may be observed when co-administered with telithromycin; therefore, increases or prolongation of the therapeutic and/or adverse effects of the concomitant drug may be observed). Products include:
Seroquel Tablets 691

Quinidine Gluconate (Co-administration of telithromycin with a drug primarily metabolized by the CYP 3A4 enzyme system may result in increased plasma concentrations of the drug co-administered with telithromycin that could increase or prolong both the therapeutic and adverse effects).
No products indexed under this heading.

Quinidine Hydrochloride (Elevated levels of drugs metabolized by the CYP450 system may be observed when co-administered with telithromycin; therefore, increases or prolongation of the therapeutic and/ or adverse effects of the concomitant drug may be observed).
No products indexed under this heading.

Quinidine Polygalacturonate (Co-administration of telithromycin with a drug primarily metabolized by the CYP 3A4 enzyme system may result in increased plasma concentrations of the drug co-administered with telithromycin that could increase or prolong both the therapeutic and adverse effects).
No products indexed under this heading.

Quinidine Sulfate (Co-administration of telithromycin with a drug primarily metabolized by the CYP 3A4 enzyme system may result in increased plasma concentrations of the drug co-administered with telithromycin that could increase or prolong both the therapeutic and adverse effects).
No products indexed under this heading.

Quinine (Elevated levels of drugs metabolized by the CYP450 system may be observed when co-administered with telithromycin; therefore, increases or prolongation of the therapeutic and/or adverse effects of the concomitant drug may be observed).
No products indexed under this heading.

Quinine Sulfate (Elevated levels of drugs metabolized by the CYP450 system may be observed when co-administered with telithromycin; therefore, increases or prolongation of the therapeutic and/or adverse effects of the concomitant drug may be observed).
No products indexed under this heading.

Rabeprazole Sodium (Elevated levels of drugs metabolized by the CYP450 system may be observed when co-administered with telithromycin; therefore, increases or prolongation of the therapeutic and/or adverse effects of the concomitant drug may be observed). Products include:
Aciphex Tablets 1081

Repaglinide (Elevated levels of drugs metabolized by the CYP450 system may be observed when co-administered with telithromycin; therefore, increases or prolongation of the therapeutic and/or adverse effects of the concomitant drug may be observed). Products include:
Prandin Tablets (0.5, 1, and 2 mg)... 2337

Rifabutin (Co-administration of telithromycin with a drug primarily metabolized by the CYP 3A4 enzyme system may result in increased plasma concentrations of the drug co-administered with telithromycin that could increase or prolong both the therapeutic and adverse effects).
No products indexed under this heading.

Rifampicin (Concomitant administration of CYP 3A4 inducers is likely to result in subtherapeutic levels of telithromycin and loss of effect).
No products indexed under this heading.

Rifampin (Co-administration of rifampin, a CYP 3A4 inducer, with telithromycin in repeated doses decreased the Cmax and AUC of telithromycin. Avoid concomitant treatment).
No products indexed under this heading.

Rifapentine (Concomitant administration of CYP 3A4 inducers is likely to result in subtherapeutic levels of telithromycin and loss of effect).
No products indexed under this heading.

Riluzole (Elevated levels of drugs metabolized by the CYP450 system may be observed when co-administered with telithromycin; therefore, increases or prolongation of the therapeutic and/or adverse effects of the concomitant drug may be observed). Products include:
Rilutek Tablets 2945

Risperidone (Elevated levels of drugs metabolized by the CYP450 system may be observed when co-administered with telithromycin; therefore, increases or prolongation of the therapeutic and/or adverse effects of the concomitant drug may be observed). Products include:
Risperdal Consta Long-Acting Injection 1664
Risperdal M-Tab Orally Disintegrating Tablets.................. 1658
Risperdal 1658

Ritonavir (Co-administration of telithromycin with a drug primarily metabolized by the CYP 3A4 enzyme system may result in increased plasma concentrations of the drug co-administered with telithromycin that could increase or prolong both the therapeutic and adverse effects). Products include:
Kaletra 474
Norvir 499

Rofecoxib (Elevated levels of drugs metabolized by the CYP450 system may be observed when co-administered with telithromycin; therefore, increases or prolongation of the therapeutic and/or adverse effects of the concomitant drug may be observed).
No products indexed under this heading.

Ropinirole Hydrochloride (Elevated levels of drugs metabolized by the CYP450 system may be observed when co-administered with telithromycin; therefore, increases or prolongation of the therapeutic and/ or adverse effects of the concomitant drug may be observed). Products include:
Requip Tablets 1528

Ropivacaine Hydrochloride (Elevated levels of drugs metabolized by the CYP450 system may be observed when co-administered with telithromycin; therefore, increases or prolongation of the therapeutic and/ or adverse effects of the concomitant drug may be observed). Products include:
Naropin Injection 640

Rosiglitazone Maleate (Elevated levels of drugs metabolized by the CYP450 system may be observed when co-administered with telithromycin; therefore, increases or prolongation of the therapeutic and/or adverse effects of the concomitant drug may be observed). Products include:
Avandamet Tablets 1343
Avandia Tablets 1348

Saquinavir (Co-administration of telithromycin with a drug primarily metabolized by the CYP 3A4 enzyme system may result in increased plasma concentrations of the drug co-administered with telithromycin that could increase or prolong both the therapeutic and adverse effects).
No products indexed under this heading.

Saquinavir Mesylate (Co-administration of telithromycin with a drug primarily metabolized by the CYP 3A4 enzyme system may result in increased plasma concentrations of the drug co-administered with telithromycin that could increase or prolong both the therapeutic and adverse effects). Products include:
Invirase 2776

Sertraline Hydrochloride (Co-administration of telithromycin with a drug primarily metabolized by the CYP 3A4 enzyme system may result in increased plasma concentrations of the drug co-administered with telithromycin that could increase or prolong both the therapeutic and adverse effects). Products include:
Zoloft 2581

Sildenafil Citrate (Co-administration of telithromycin with a drug primarily metabolized by the CYP 3A4 enzyme system may result in increased plasma concentrations of the drug co-administered with telithromycin that could increase or prolong both the therapeutic and adverse effects). Products include:
Revatio Tablets 2541
Viagra Tablets 2552

Simvastatin (Simvastatin levels were increased due to CYP 3A4 inhibition by telithromycin, thereby increasing the risk of myopathy. Co-administration should be avoided). Products include:
Vytorin 10/10 Tablets 2084
Vytorin 10/10 Tablets 3092
Vytorin 10/20 Tablets 2084
Vytorin 10/20 Tablets 3092
Vytorin 10/40 Tablets 3092
Vytorin 10/40 Tablets 2084
Vytorin 10/80 Tablets 2084
Vytorin 10/80 Tablets 3092
Zocor Tablets 2078

Sirolimus (Co-administration of telithromycin with a drug primarily metabolized by the CYP 3A4 enzyme system may result in increased plasma concentrations of the drug co-administered with telithromycin that could increase or prolong both the therapeutic and adverse effects). Products include:
Rapamune Oral Solution and Tablets 3472

Sotalol Hydrochloride (Telithromycin has been shown to decrease the Cmax and AUC of sotalol due to decreased absorption).
No products indexed under this heading.

Sulfamethoxazole (Elevated levels of drugs metabolized by the CYP450 system may be observed when co-administered with telithromycin; therefore, increases or prolongation of the therapeutic and/or adverse effects of the concomitant drug may be observed).
No products indexed under this heading.

Sulfinpyrazone (Concomitant administration of CYP 3A4 inducers is likely to result in subtherapeutic levels of telithromycin and loss of effect).
No products indexed under this heading.

Sulindac (Elevated levels of drugs metabolized by the CYP450 system may be observed when co-administered with telithromycin; therefore, increases or prolongation of the therapeutic and/or adverse effects of the concomitant drug may be observed). Products include:
Clinoril Tablets 1899

Suprofen (Elevated levels of drugs metabolized by the CYP450 system may be observed when co-administered with telithromycin; therefore, increases or prolongation of the therapeutic and/or adverse effects of the concomitant drug may be observed).
No products indexed under this heading.

Tacrine Hydrochloride (Elevated levels of drugs metabolized by the CYP450 system may be observed when co-administered with telithromycin; therefore, increases or prolongation of the therapeutic and/or adverse effects of the concomitant drug may be observed).
No products indexed under this heading.

Tacrolimus (Co-administration of telithromycin with a drug primarily metabolized by the CYP 3A4 enzyme system may result in increased plasma concentrations of the drug co-administered with telithromycin that could increase or prolong both the therapeutic and adverse effects). Products include:
Prograf Capsules and Injection 624
Protopic Ointment 629

Tamoxifen Citrate (Co-administration of telithromycin with a drug primarily metabolized by the CYP 3A4 enzyme system may result in increased plasma concentrations of the drug co-administered with telithromycin that could increase or prolong both the therapeutic and adverse effects).
No products indexed under this heading.

Telmisartan (Elevated levels of drugs metabolized by the CYP450 system may be observed when co-administered with telithromycin; therefore, increases or prolongation of the therapeutic and/or adverse effects of the concomitant drug may be observed). Products include:
Micardis Tablets 884
Micardis HCT Tablets 886

Teniposide (Elevated levels of drugs metabolized by the CYP450 system may be observed when co-administered with telithromycin; therefore, increases or prolongation of the therapeutic and/or adverse effects of the concomitant drug may be observed).
No products indexed under this heading.

Terfenadine (Elevated levels of drugs metabolized by the CYP450 system may be observed when co-administered with telithromycin; therefore, increases or prolongation of the therapeutic and/or adverse effects of the concomitant drug may be observed).
No products indexed under this heading.

Testosterone (Elevated levels of drugs metabolized by the CYP450 system may be observed when co-administered with telithromycin; therefore, increases or prolongation of the therapeutic and/or adverse effects of the concomitant drug may be observed). Products include:
AndroGel 3330
Striant Mucoadhesive 1022
Testim 1% Gel 722

Testosterone Cypionate (Elevated levels of drugs metabolized by the CYP450 system may be observed when co-administered with telithromycin; therefore, increases or prolongation of the therapeutic and/or adverse effects of the concomitant drug may be observed).
No products indexed under this heading.

Testosterone Enanthate (Elevated levels of drugs metabolized by the CYP450 system may be observed when co-administered with telithromycin; therefore, increases or prolongation of the therapeutic and/or adverse effects of the concomitant drug may be observed). Products include:
Delatestryl Injection 2976

Testosterone Propionate (Elevated levels of drugs metabolized by the CYP450 system may be observed when co-administered with telithromycin; therefore, increases or prolongation of the therapeutic and/or adverse effects of the concomitant drug may be observed).
No products indexed under this heading.

Theophylline (Co-administration increased steady state Cmax and AUC of theophylline and may worsen GI side effects, especially in female patients. Theophylline and telithromycin should be taken 1 hour apart).
No products indexed under this heading.

Theophylline Anhydrous (Co-administration increased steady state Cmax and AUC of theophylline and may worsen GI side effects, especially in female patients. Theophylline and telithromycin should be taken 1 hour apart). Products include:
Uniphyl Tablets 2708

Theophylline Calcium Salicylate (Co-administration increased steady state Cmax and AUC of theophylline and may worsen GI side effects, especially in female patients. Theophylline and telithromycin should be taken 1 hour apart).
No products indexed under this heading.

Theophylline Dihydroxypropyl (Glyceryl) (Co-administration increased steady state Cmax and AUC of theophylline and may worsen GI side effects, especially in female patients. Theophylline and telithromycin should be taken 1 hour apart).
No products indexed under this heading.

Theophylline Ethylenediamine (Co-administration increased steady state Cmax and AUC of theophylline and may worsen GI side effects, especially in female patients. Theophylline and telithromycin should be taken 1 hour apart).
No products indexed under this heading.

Theophylline Sodium Glycinate (Co-administration increased steady state Cmax and AUC of theophylline and may worsen GI side effects, especially in female patients. Theophylline and telithromycin should be taken 1 hour apart).
No products indexed under this heading.

Thioridazine (Elevated levels of drugs metabolized by the CYP450 system may be observed when co-administered with telithromycin; therefore, increases or prolongation of the therapeutic and/or adverse effects of the concomitant drug may be observed).
No products indexed under this heading.

Thioridazine Hydrochloride (Elevated levels of drugs metabolized by the CYP450 system may be observed when co-administered with telithromycin; therefore, increases or prolongation of the therapeutic and/or adverse effects of the concomitant drug may be observed). Products include:
Thioridazine Hydrochloride Tablets 2122

Tiagabine Hydrochloride (Co-administration of telithromycin with a drug primarily metabolized by the CYP 3A4 enzyme system may result in increased plasma concentrations of the drug co-administered with telithromycin that could increase or prolong both the therapeutic and adverse effects). Products include:
Gabitril Tablets 998

Timolol Maleate (Elevated levels of drugs metabolized by the CYP450 system may be observed when co-administered with telithromycin; therefore, increases or prolongation of the therapeutic and/or adverse effects of the concomitant drug may be observed). Products include:
Blocadren Tablets 1891
Cosopt Sterile Ophthalmic Solution 1910
Timolide Tablets 2056
Timoptic in Ocudose 2061
Timoptic Sterile Ophthalmic Solution 2058
Timoptic-XE Sterile Ophthalmic Gel Forming Solution 2062

Tolazamide (Elevated levels of drugs metabolized by the CYP450 system may be observed when co-administered with telithromycin; therefore, increases or prolongation of the therapeutic and/or adverse effects of the concomitant drug may be observed).
No products indexed under this heading.

Tolbutamide (Elevated levels of drugs metabolized by the CYP450 system may be observed when co-administered with telithromycin; therefore, increases or prolongation of the therapeutic and/or adverse effects of the concomitant drug may be observed).
No products indexed under this heading.

Tolbutamide Sodium (Elevated levels of drugs metabolized by the CYP450 system may be observed when co-administered with telithromycin; therefore, increases or prolongation of the therapeutic and/or adverse effects of the concomitant drug may be observed).
No products indexed under this heading.

Tolmetin Sodium (Elevated levels of drugs metabolized by the CYP450 system may be observed when co-administered with telithromycin; therefore, increases or prolongation of the therapeutic and/or adverse effects of the concomitant drug may be observed).
No products indexed under this heading.

Tolterodine Tartrate (Co-administration of telithromycin with a drug primarily metabolized by the CYP 3A4 enzyme system may result in increased plasma concentrations of the drug co-administered with telithromycin that could increase or prolong both the therapeutic and adverse effects). Products include:
Detrol Tablets 2626
Detrol LA Capsules 2629

Topiramate (Elevated levels of drugs metabolized by the CYP450 system may be observed when co-administered with telithromycin; therefore, increases or prolongation of the therapeutic and/or adverse effects of the concomitant drug may be observed). Products include:
Topamax Sprinkle Capsules 2438
Topamax Tablets 2438

Torsemide (Elevated levels of drugs metabolized by the CYP450 system may be observed when co-administered with telithromycin; therefore, increases or prolongation of the therapeutic and/or adverse effects of the concomitant drug may be observed).
No products indexed under this heading.

Tramadol Hydrochloride (Elevated levels of drugs metabolized by the CYP450 system may be observed when co-administered with telithromycin; therefore, increases or prolongation of the therapeutic and/or adverse effects of the concomitant drug may be observed). Products include:
Ultracet Tablets 2462

Trazodone Hydrochloride (Co-administration of telithromycin with a drug primarily metabolized by the CYP 3A4 enzyme system may result in increased plasma concentrations of the drug co-administered with telithromycin that could increase or prolong both the therapeutic and adverse effects).
No products indexed under this heading.

Tretinoin (Elevated levels of drugs metabolized by the CYP450 system may be observed when co-administered with telithromycin; therefore, increases or prolongation of the therapeutic and/or adverse effects of the concomitant drug may be observed). Products include:
Avita Cream 2136
Avita Gel 2138
Renova 0.02% Cream 2384
Renova 0.05% Cream 2387
Retin-A Micro 0.1%/0.04% 2388
Solage Topical Solution 740
Tri-Luma Cream 1213
Vesanoid Capsules 2823

Triamcinolone (Concomitant administration of CYP 3A4 inducers is likely to result in subtherapeutic levels of telithromycin and loss of effect).
No products indexed under this heading.

Triamcinolone Acetonide (Concomitant administration of CYP 3A4 inducers is likely to result in sub-

therapeutic levels of telithromycin and loss of effect). Products include:
Azmacort Inhalation Aerosol 1701
Nasacort HFA Inhalation Aerosol 2939
Nasacort AQ Nasal Spray 2937

Triamcinolone Diacetate (Concomitant administration of CYP 3A4 inducers is likely to result in subtherapeutic levels of telithromycin and loss of effect).
No products indexed under this heading.

Triamcinolone Hexacetonide (Concomitant administration of CYP 3A4 inducers is likely to result in subtherapeutic levels of telithromycin and loss of effect).
No products indexed under this heading.

Triazolam (Co-administration of telithromycin with a drug primarily metabolized by the CYP 3A4 enzyme system may result in increased plasma concentrations of the drug co-administered with telithromycin that could increase or prolong both the therapeutic and adverse effects).
No products indexed under this heading.

Trimethadione (Elevated levels of drugs metabolized by the CYP450 system may be observed when co-administered with telithromycin; therefore, increases or prolongation of the therapeutic and/or adverse effects of the concomitant drug may be observed).
No products indexed under this heading.

Trimethaphan Camsylate (Elevated levels of drugs metabolized by the CYP450 system may be observed when co-administered with telithromycin; therefore, increases or prolongation of the therapeutic and/or adverse effects of the concomitant drug may be observed).
No products indexed under this heading.

Trimipramine Maleate (Elevated levels of drugs metabolized by the CYP450 system may be observed when co-administered with telithromycin; therefore, increases or prolongation of the therapeutic and/or adverse effects of the concomitant drug may be observed). Products include:
Surmontil Capsules 2347

Troglitazone (Concomitant administration of CYP 3A4 inducers is likely to result in subtherapeutic levels of telithromycin and loss of effect).
No products indexed under this heading.

Trovafloxacin Mesylate (Elevated levels of drugs metabolized by the CYP450 system may be observed when co-administered with telithromycin; therefore, increases or prolongation of the therapeutic and/or adverse effects of the concomitant drug may be observed).
No products indexed under this heading.

Valdecoxib (Elevated levels of drugs metabolized by the CYP450 system may be observed when co-administered with telithromycin; therefore, increases or prolongation of the therapeutic and/or adverse effects of the concomitant drug may be observed).
No products indexed under this heading.

Valproate Sodium (Elevated levels of drugs metabolized by the CYP450 system may be observed when co-administered with telithromycin; therefore, increases or prolongation of the therapeutic and/or adverse effects of the concomitant drug may be observed). Products include:
Depacon Injection 412

Valproic Acid (Elevated levels of drugs metabolized by the CYP450 system may be observed when co-administered with telithromycin; therefore, increases or prolongation of the therapeutic and/or adverse effects of the concomitant drug may be observed). Products include:
Depakene 417

Valsartan (Elevated levels of drugs metabolized by the CYP450 system may be observed when co-administered with telithromycin; therefore, increases or prolongation of the therapeutic and/or adverse effects of the concomitant drug may be observed). Products include:
Diovan HCT Tablets 2195
Diovan Tablets 2191

Venlafaxine Hydrochloride (Elevated levels of drugs metabolized by the CYP450 system may be observed when co-administered with telithromycin; therefore, increases or prolongation of the therapeutic and/or adverse effects of the concomitant drug may be observed). Products include:
Effexor Tablets 3405
Effexor XR Capsules 3411

Verapamil Hydrochloride (Co-administration of telithromycin with a drug primarily metabolized by the CYP 3A4 enzyme system may result in increased plasma concentrations of the drug co-administered with telithromycin that could increase or prolong both the therapeutic and adverse effects). Products include:
Covera-HS Tablets 3135
Tarka Tablets 519
Verelan PM Capsules 3120

Vinblastine Sulfate (Co-administration of telithromycin with a drug primarily metabolized by the CYP 3A4 enzyme system may result in increased plasma concentrations of the drug co-administered with telithromycin that could increase or prolong both the therapeutic and adverse effects).
No products indexed under this heading.

Vincristine Sulfate (Co-administration of telithromycin with a drug primarily metabolized by the CYP 3A4 enzyme system may result in increased plasma concentrations of the drug co-administered with telithromycin that could increase or prolong both the therapeutic and adverse effects).
No products indexed under this heading.

Vitamin A (Elevated levels of drugs metabolized by the CYP450 system may be observed when co-administered with telithromycin; therefore, increases or prolongation of the therapeutic and/or adverse effects of the concomitant drug may be observed). Products include:
Visutein Capsules 3328

Vitamin A Acetate (Elevated levels of drugs metabolized by the CYP450 system may be observed when co-administered with telithromycin; therefore, increases or prolongation of the therapeutic and/or adverse effects of the concomitant drug may be observed).
No products indexed under this heading.

Voriconazole (Elevated levels of drugs metabolized by the CYP450 system may be observed when co-administered with telithromycin; therefore, increases or prolongation of the therapeutic and/or adverse effects of the concomitant drug may be observed). Products include:
VFEND I.V. 2543
VFEND Oral Suspension 2543
VFEND Tablets 2543

Warfarin Sodium (Co-administration of telithromycin with a drug primarily metabolized by the CYP 3A4 enzyme system may result in increased plasma concentrations of the drug co-administered with telithromycin that could increase or prolong both the therapeutic and adverse effects). Products include:
Coumadin for Injection 932
Coumadin Tablets 932

Zafirlukast (Elevated levels of drugs metabolized by the CYP450 system may be observed when co-administered with telithromycin; therefore, increases or prolongation of the therapeutic and/or adverse effects of the concomitant drug may be observed). Products include:
Accolate Tablets 663

Zileuton (Elevated levels of drugs metabolized by the CYP450 system may be observed when co-administered with telithromycin; therefore, increases or prolongation of the therapeutic and/or adverse effects of the concomitant drug may be observed).
No products indexed under this heading.

Zolmitriptan (Elevated levels of drugs metabolized by the CYP450 system may be observed when co-administered with telithromycin; therefore, increases or prolongation of the therapeutic and/or adverse effects of the concomitant drug may be observed). Products include:
Zomig Nasal Spray 718
Zomig Tablets 714
Zomig-ZMT Tablets 714

Zonisamide (Elevated levels of drugs metabolized by the CYP450 system may be observed when co-administered with telithromycin; therefore, increases or prolongation of the therapeutic and/or adverse effects of the concomitant drug may be observed). Products include:
Zonegran Capsules 1089

Zopiclone (Elevated levels of drugs metabolized by the CYP450 system may be observed when co-administered with telithromycin; therefore, increases or prolongation of the therapeutic and/or adverse effects of the concomitant drug may be observed).
No products indexed under this heading.

KINERET INJECTION

(Anakinra) 594
May interact with killed/inactivated vaccines and certain other agents. Compounds in these categories include:

Adalimumab (Use of anakinra in combination with TNF-blocking agents is not recommended). Products include:
Humira Injection 464

Diphtheria & Tetanus Toxoids and Acellular Pertussis Vaccine Adsorbed, Hepatitis B (recombinant) and Inactivated Poliovirus Vaccine Combined (Vaccination may not be effective in patients receiving anakinra).
No products indexed under this heading.

Etanercept (In a study in which patients with active RA were treated for up to 24 weeks with concurrent anakinra and etanercept therapy, a 7% rate of serious infections was observed, which was higher than that observed with etanercept alone (0%). Two percent of patients treated concurrently with anakinra and etanercept developed neutropenia. Use of anakinra in combination with TNF-blocking agents is not recommended). Products include:
Enbrel for Injection 580

Hepatitis A Vaccine, Inactivated (Vaccination may not be effective in patients receiving anakinra). Products include:
Havrix Vaccine 1425
Twinrix Vaccine 1571
Vaqta 2067

Infliximab (Use of anakinra in combination with TNF-blocking agents is not recommended). Products include:
Remicade for IV Injection 987

Influenza Virus Vaccine (Vaccination may not be effective in patients receiving anakinra). Products include:
Flumist Vaccine 1872

Japanese Encephalitis Vaccine Inactivated (Vaccination may not be effective in patients receiving anakinra).
No products indexed under this heading.

Poliovirus Vaccine Inactivated, Trivalent Types 1,2,3 (Vaccination may not be effective in patients receiving anakinra). Products include:
Pediarix Vaccine 1518

Vaccines (Live) (Vaccination may not be effective in patients receiving anakinra. Live vaccines should not be given concurrently with anakinra).
No products indexed under this heading.

KLARON LOTION 10%

(Sulfacetamide Sodium) 1050
None cited in PDR database.

KLONOPIN TABLETS

(Clonazepam) 2782
May interact with central nervous system depressants, anticonvulsants, monoamine oxidase inhibitors, phenytoin, tricyclic antidepressants, and certain other agents. Compounds in these categories include:

Alfentanil Hydrochloride (Potentiates CNS-depressant action).
No products indexed under this heading.

Alprazolam (Potentiates CNS-depressant action). Products include:

Niravam Orally Disintegrating Tablets 3106
Xanax XR Tablets 2655

Amitriptyline Hydrochloride (Potentiates CNS-depressant action).
No products indexed under this heading.

Amoxapine (Potentiates CNS-depressant action).
No products indexed under this heading.

Aprobarbital (Potentiates CNS-depressant action).
No products indexed under this heading.

Buprenorphine Hydrochloride (Potentiates CNS-depressant action). Products include:
Buprenex Injectable 2718
Suboxone Tablets 2719
Subutex Tablets 2719

Buspirone Hydrochloride (Potentiates CNS-depressant action).
No products indexed under this heading.

Butabarbital (Potentiates CNS-depressant action).
No products indexed under this heading.

Butalbital (Potentiates CNS-depressant action). Products include:
Sedapap Tablets 50 mg/650 mg 2098

Carbamazepine (Induces clonazepam metabolism causing an approximately 30% decrease in plasma clonazepam levels). Products include:
Carbatrol Capsules 3174
Equetro Extended-Release Capsules 3178
Tegretol/Tegretol-XR 2278

Chlordiazepoxide (Potentiates CNS-depressant action).
No products indexed under this heading.

Chlordiazepoxide Hydrochloride (Potentiates CNS-depressant action). Products include:
Librium Capsules 3349

Chlorpromazine (Potentiates CNS-depressant action).
No products indexed under this heading.

Chlorpromazine Hydrochloride (Potentiates CNS-depressant action).
No products indexed under this heading.

Chlorprothixene (Potentiates CNS-depressant action).
No products indexed under this heading.

Chlorprothixene Hydrochloride (Potentiates CNS-depressant action).
No products indexed under this heading.

Chlorprothixene Lactate (Potentiates CNS-depressant action).
No products indexed under this heading.

Clomipramine Hydrochloride (Potentiates CNS-depressant action).
No products indexed under this heading.

Clorazepate Dipotassium (Potentiates CNS-depressant action). Products include:
Tranxene 2488

Clozapine (Potentiates CNS-depressant action). Products include:
Clozapine Tablets 2141
Clozaril Tablets 2174
FazaClo Orally Disintegrating Tablets 547

Codeine Phosphate (Potentiates CNS-depressant action). Products include:
Tylenol with Codeine 2461

Desflurane (Potentiates CNS-depressant action). Products include:
Suprane Liquid for Inhalation 770

Desipramine Hydrochloride (Potentiates CNS-depressant action).
No products indexed under this heading.

Dezocine (Potentiates CNS-depressant action).
No products indexed under this heading.

Diazepam (Potentiates CNS-depressant action). Products include:
Diastat Rectal Delivery System 3344
Valium Tablets 2822

Divalproex Sodium (Potentiates CNS-depressant action). Products include:
Depakote Sprinkle Capsules 422
Depakote Tablets 427
Depakote ER Tablets 433

Doxepin Hydrochloride (Potentiates CNS-depressant action).
No products indexed under this heading.

Droperidol (Potentiates CNS-depressant action).
No products indexed under this heading.

Enflurane (Potentiates CNS-depressant action).
No products indexed under this heading.

Estazolam (Potentiates CNS-depressant action). Products include:
ProSom Tablets 512

Ethanol (Potentiates CNS-depressant action).
No products indexed under this heading.

Ethchlorvynol (Potentiates CNS-depressant action).
No products indexed under this heading.

Ethinamate (Potentiates CNS-depressant action).
No products indexed under this heading.

Ethosuximide (Potentiates CNS-depressant action).
No products indexed under this heading.

Ethotoin (Potentiates CNS-depressant action). Products include:
Peganone Tablets, USP 2487

Ethyl Alcohol (Potentiates CNS-depressant action).
No products indexed under this heading.

Felbamate (Potentiates CNS-depressant action).
No products indexed under this heading.

Fentanyl (Potentiates CNS-depressant action). Products include:
Duragesic Transdermal System 2448

Fentanyl Citrate (Potentiates CNS-depressant action). Products include:
Actiq 993

Fluphenazine Decanoate (Potentiates CNS-depressant action).
No products indexed under this heading.

Fluphenazine Enanthate (Potentiates CNS-depressant action).
No products indexed under this heading.

Fluphenazine Hydrochloride (Potentiates CNS-depressant action).
No products indexed under this heading.

Flurazepam Hydrochloride (Potentiates CNS-depressant action). Products include:
Dalmane Capsules 3343

Fosphenytoin (Potentiates CNS-depressant action).
No products indexed under this heading.

Fosphenytoin Sodium (Induces clonazepam metabolism causing an approximately 30% decrease in plasma clonazepam levels).
No products indexed under this heading.

Gabapentin (Potentiates CNS-depressant action). Products include:
Neurontin Capsules 2498
Neurontin Oral Solution 2498
Neurontin Tablets 2498

Glutethimide (Potentiates CNS-depressant action).
No products indexed under this heading.

Haloperidol (Potentiates CNS-depressant action).
No products indexed under this heading.

Haloperidol Decanoate (Potentiates CNS-depressant action).
No products indexed under this heading.

Hydrocodone Bitartrate (Potentiates CNS-depressant action). Products include:
Hycodan 1104
Hycomine Compound Tablets 1105
Hycotuss Expectorant Syrup 1106
Lortab 3315
Lortab Elixir 3312
Vicodin Tablets 530
Vicodin ES Tablets 531
Vicodin HP Tablets 532
Vicoprofen Tablets 533
Zydone Tablets 1118

Hydrocodone Polistirex (Potentiates CNS-depressant action). Products include:
Tussionex Pennkinetic Extended-Release Suspension 3322

Hydromorphone Hydrochloride (Potentiates CNS-depressant action). Products include:
Dilaudid 439
Dilaudid Oral Liquid 443
Dilaudid Non-Sterile Powder 439
Dilaudid Rectal Suppositories 439
Dilaudid Tablets 439
Dilaudid Tablets - 8 mg 443
Dilaudid-HP 441

Hydroxyzine Hydrochloride (Potentiates CNS-depressant action).
No products indexed under this heading.

Imipramine Hydrochloride (Potentiates CNS-depressant action).
No products indexed under this heading.

Imipramine Pamoate (Potentiates CNS-depressant action).
No products indexed under this heading.

Isocarboxazid (Potentiates CNS-depressant action).
No products indexed under this heading.

Isoflurane (Potentiates CNS-depressant action).
No products indexed under this heading.

Itraconazole (Co-administration with CYP450 3A inhibitors should be undertaken with caution).
No products indexed under this heading.

Ketamine Hydrochloride (Potentiates CNS-depressant action).
No products indexed under this heading.

Ketoconazole (Co-administration with CYP450 3A inhibitors should be undertaken with caution). Products include:
Nizoral A-D Shampoo, 1% 1839
Nizoral 2% Shampoo 1838

Lamotrigine (Potentiates CNS-depressant action). Products include:
Lamictal 1449

Levetiracetam (Potentiates CNS-depressant action). Products include:
Keppra Oral Solution 3307
Keppra Tablets 3307

Levomethadyl Acetate Hydrochloride (Potentiates CNS-depressant action).
No products indexed under this heading.

Levorphanol Tartrate (Potentiates CNS-depressant action).
No products indexed under this heading.

Lorazepam (Potentiates CNS-depressant action).
No products indexed under this heading.

Loxapine Hydrochloride (Potentiates CNS-depressant action).
No products indexed under this heading.

Loxapine Succinate (Potentiates CNS-depressant action).
No products indexed under this heading.

Maprotiline Hydrochloride (Potentiates CNS-depressant action).
No products indexed under this heading.

Meperidine Hydrochloride (Potentiates CNS-depressant action).
No products indexed under this heading.

Mephenytoin (Potentiates CNS-depressant action).
No products indexed under this heading.

Mephobarbital (Potentiates CNS-depressant action). Products include:
Mebaral Tablets, USP 2483

Meprobamate (Potentiates CNS-depressant action).
No products indexed under this heading.

Mesoridazine Besylate (Potentiates CNS-depressant action).
No products indexed under this heading.

Methadone Hydrochloride (Potentiates CNS-depressant action).
No products indexed under this heading.

Methohexital Sodium (Potentiates CNS-depressant action).
No products indexed under this heading.

Methotrimeprazine (Potentiates CNS-depressant action).
No products indexed under this heading.

Methoxyflurane (Potentiates CNS-depressant action).
No products indexed under this heading.

Methsuximide (Potentiates CNS-depressant action).
No products indexed under this heading.

Midazolam Hydrochloride (Potentiates CNS-depressant action).
No products indexed under this heading.

Moclobemide (Potentiates CNS-depressant action).
No products indexed under this heading.

Molindone Hydrochloride (Potentiates CNS-depressant action). Products include:
Moban Tablets ... 1108

Morphine Sulfate (Potentiates CNS-depressant action). Products include:
Avinza Capsules ... 1714
Kadian Capsules ... 572
MS Contin Tablets ... 2703

Nortriptyline Hydrochloride (Potentiates CNS-depressant action).
No products indexed under this heading.

Olanzapine (Potentiates CNS-depressant action). Products include:
Symbyax Capsules ... 1788
Zyprexa Tablets ... 1798
Zyprexa IntraMuscular ... 1798
Zyprexa ZYDIS Orally Disintegrating Tablets ... 1798

Oxazepam (Potentiates CNS-depressant action).
No products indexed under this heading.

Oxcarbazepine (Potentiates CNS-depressant action). Products include:
Trileptal Oral Suspension ... 2281
Trileptal Tablets ... 2281

Oxycodone Hydrochloride (Potentiates CNS-depressant action). Products include:
Combunox Tablets ... 1183
OxyContin Tablets ... 2699
OxyFast Oral Concentrate Solution ... 2704
OxyIR Capsules ... 2704
Percocet Tablets ... 1114
Percodan Tablets ... 1115

Paramethadione (Potentiates CNS-depressant action).
No products indexed under this heading.

Pargyline Hydrochloride (Potentiates CNS-depressant action).
No products indexed under this heading.

Pentobarbital Sodium (Potentiates CNS-depressant action). Products include:
Nembutal Sodium Solution, USP ... 2484

Perphenazine (Potentiates CNS-depressant action).
No products indexed under this heading.

Phenacemide (Potentiates CNS-depressant action).
No products indexed under this heading.

Phenelzine Sulfate (Potentiates CNS-depressant action).
No products indexed under this heading.

Phenobarbital (Induces clonazepam metabolism causing an approximately 30% decrease in plasma clonazepam levels; CNS depressant action may be potentiated).
No products indexed under this heading.

Phensuximide (Potentiates CNS-depressant action).
No products indexed under this heading.

Phenytoin (Induces clonazepam metabolism causing an approximately 30% decrease in plasma clonazepam levels).
No products indexed under this heading.

Phenytoin Sodium (Induces clonazepam metabolism causing an approximately 30% decrease in plasma clonazepam levels). Products include:
Phenytek Capsules ... 2153

Prazepam (Potentiates CNS-depressant action).
No products indexed under this heading.

Primidone (Potentiates CNS-depressant action).
No products indexed under this heading.

Procarbazine Hydrochloride (Potentiates CNS-depressant action). Products include:
Matulane Capsules ... 3188

Prochlorperazine (Potentiates CNS-depressant action).
No products indexed under this heading.

Promethazine Hydrochloride (Potentiates CNS-depressant action). Products include:
Phenergan ... 3438

Propofol (Potentiates CNS-depressant action). Products include:
Diprivan Injectable Emulsion ... 676

Propoxyphene Hydrochloride (Potentiates CNS-depressant action).
No products indexed under this heading.

Propoxyphene Napsylate (Potentiates CNS-depressant action). Products include:
Darvocet A 500 Tablets ... 3497

Protriptyline Hydrochloride (Potentiates CNS-depressant action). Products include:
Vivactil Tablets ... 2350

Quazepam (Potentiates CNS-depressant action).
No products indexed under this heading.

Quetiapine Fumarate (Potentiates CNS-depressant action). Products include:
Seroquel Tablets ... 691

Remifentanil Hydrochloride (Potentiates CNS-depressant action).
No products indexed under this heading.

Risperidone (Potentiates CNS-depressant action). Products include:
Risperdal Consta Long-Acting Injection ... 1664
Risperdal M-Tab Orally Disintegrating Tablets ... 1658
Risperdal ... 1658

Secobarbital Sodium (Potentiates CNS-depressant action).
No products indexed under this heading.

Selegiline Hydrochloride (Potentiates CNS-depressant action). Products include:
Eldepryl Capsules ... 3209

Sevoflurane (Potentiates CNS-depressant action). Products include:
Ultane Liquid for Inhalation ... 526

Sufentanil Citrate (Potentiates CNS-depressant action).
No products indexed under this heading.

Temazepam (Potentiates CNS-depressant action).
No products indexed under this heading.

Thiamylal Sodium (Potentiates CNS-depressant action).
No products indexed under this heading.

Thioridazine Hydrochloride (Potentiates CNS-depressant action). Products include:
Thioridazine Hydrochloride Tablets ... 2122

Thiothixene (Potentiates CNS-depressant action). Products include:
Thiothixene Capsules ... 2124

Tiagabine Hydrochloride (Potentiates CNS-depressant action). Products include:
Gabitril Tablets ... 998

Topiramate (Potentiates CNS-depressant action). Products include:
Topamax Sprinkle Capsules ... 2438
Topamax Tablets ... 2438

Tranylcypromine Sulfate (Potentiates CNS-depressant action). Products include:
Parnate Tablets ... 1499

Triazolam (Potentiates CNS-depressant action).
No products indexed under this heading.

Trifluoperazine Hydrochloride (Potentiates CNS-depressant action).
No products indexed under this heading.

Trimethadione (Potentiates CNS-depressant action).
No products indexed under this heading.

Trimipramine Maleate (Potentiates CNS-depressant action). Products include:
Surmontil Capsules ... 2347

Valproate Sodium (Potentiates CNS-depressant action). Products include:
Depacon Injection ... 412

Valproic Acid (Potentiates CNS-depressant action). Products include:
Depakene ... 417

Zaleplon (Potentiates CNS-depressant action). Products include:
Sonata Capsules ... 1686

Ziprasidone Hydrochloride (Potentiates CNS-depressant action). Products include:
Geodon Capsules ... 2514

Zolpidem Tartrate (Potentiates CNS-depressant action). Products include:
Ambien Tablets ... 2867

Zonisamide (Potentiates CNS-depressant action). Products include:
Zonegran Capsules ... 1089

Food Interactions

Alcohol (Potentiates CNS-depressant action).

KLONOPIN WAFERS

(Clonazepam) ... 2782
See Klonopin Tablets

K-LOR POWDER PACKETS

(Potassium Chloride) ... 472
May interact with ACE inhibitors and potassium sparing diuretics. Compounds in these categories include:

Amiloride Hydrochloride (Co-administration of these agents can produce severe hyperkalemia; concurrent use is not recommended). Products include:
Midamor Tablets ... 2000
Moduretic Tablets ... 2003

Benazepril Hydrochloride (Potential for hyperkalemia). Products include:
Lotensin Tablets ... 2232
Lotensin HCT Tablets ... 2235
Lotrel Capsules ... 2238

Captopril (Potential for hyperkalemia). Products include:
Captopril Tablets ... 2114

Enalapril Maleate (Potential for hyperkalemia). Products include:
Vaseretic Tablets ... 2073
Vasotec I.V. Injection ... 2076

Enalaprilat (Potential for hyperkalemia).
No products indexed under this heading.

Fosinopril Sodium (Potential for hyperkalemia).
No products indexed under this heading.

Lisinopril (Potential for hyperkalemia). Products include:
Prinivil Tablets ... 2029
Prinzide Tablets ... 2033
Zestoretic Tablets ... 701
Zestril Tablets ... 704

Moexipril Hydrochloride (Potential for hyperkalemia). Products include:
Uniretic Tablets ... 3114
Univasc Tablets ... 3118

Perindopril Erbumine (Potential for hyperkalemia). Products include:
Aceon Tablets (2 mg, 4 mg, 8 mg) ... 3191

Quinapril Hydrochloride (Potential for hyperkalemia).
No products indexed under this heading.

Ramipril (Potential for hyperkalemia). Products include:
Altace Capsules ... 1673

Spirapril Hydrochloride (Potential for hyperkalemia).
No products indexed under this heading.

Spironolactone (Co-administration of these agents can produce severe hyperkalemia; concurrent use is not recommended).
No products indexed under this heading.

Trandolapril (Potential for hyperkalemia). Products include:
Mavik Tablets ... 482
Tarka Tablets ... 519

Triamterene (Co-administration of these agents can produce severe hyperkalemia; concurrent use is not recommended). Products include:
Dyazide Capsules ... 1389
Dyrenium Capsules ... 3390
Maxzide ... 2150

KOĀTE-DVI

(Antihemophilic Factor (Human)) ... 3247
None cited in PDR database.

IMPORTANT NOTE: Always consult each drug listing in the patient's regimen for possible interactions.

KOGENATE FS
(Antihemophilic Factor (Recombinant)) ... 3517
None cited in PDR database.

K-PHOS NEUTRAL TABLETS
(Potassium Phosphate, Sodium Phosphate) ... 785
May interact with antacids containing aluminum, calcium and magnesium, calcium preparations, potassium sparing diuretics, and certain other agents. Compounds in these categories include:

ACTH (Concurrent use with corticotropin may result in hypernatremia).
No products indexed under this heading.

Aluminum Carbonate (Co-administration with antacids may bind the phosphate and prevent its absorption).
No products indexed under this heading.

Aluminum Hydroxide (Co-administration with antacids may bind the phosphate and prevent its absorption). Products include:
Gaviscon Regular Strength Liquid .. ▣620
Gaviscon Regular Strength Tablets ... ▣619
Gaviscon Extra Strength Liquid ... ▣620
Gaviscon Extra Strength Tablets ... ▣619
Maalox Max Maximum Strength Antacid/Anti-Gas Liquid ... 2165
Maalox Regular Strength Antacid/Antigas Liquid ... 2164

Amiloride Hydrochloride (Concurrent use with potassium-sparing diuretics may cause hyperkalemia). Products include:
Midamor Tablets ... 2000
Moduretic Tablets ... 2003

Calcium Carbonate (Concurrent use with calcium-containing preparations may antagonize the effects of phosphates in the treatment of hypercalcemia). Products include:
Actonel with Calcium Tablets ... 2684
Caltrate 600 PLUS Chewables ... ▣779
Caltrate 600 PLUS Tablets ... ▣779
Caltrate 600 + D Tablets ... ▣779
Encora Capsules ... 3298
Encora AM Tablets ... 3298
Encora PM Tablets ... 3298
Gas-X with Maalox ... ▣675
Maalox Regular Strength Antacid Tablets ... 2166
Quick Dissolve Maalox Max Maximum Strength Antacid/Antigas Tablets ... 2165
Maalox Max Quick Dissolve Maximum Strength Chewable Tablets ... ▣678
Os-Cal Chewable Tablets ... ▣765
Pepcid Complete Chewable Tablets ... 1672
PremCal Light, Regular, and Extra Strength Tablets ... ▣762
Rolaids Tablets ... ▣707
Extra Strength Rolaids Softchews ... ▣708
Extra Strength Rolaids Tablets ... ▣707
Rolaids Multi-Symptom Antacid & Antigas Tablets ... ▣708
Tums ... ▣639

Calcium Chloride (Concurrent use with calcium-containing preparations may antagonize the effects of phosphates in the treatment of hypercalcemia).
No products indexed under this heading.

Calcium Citrate (Concurrent use with calcium-containing preparations may antagonize the effects of phosphates in the treatment of hypercalcemia). Products include:
Active Calcium Tablets ... 3342
Citracal Tablets ... 2108

Calcium Glubionate (Concurrent use with calcium-containing preparations may antagonize the effects of phosphates in the treatment of hypercalcemia).
No products indexed under this heading.

Deserpidine (Concurrent use with antihypertensives, such as rauwolfia alkaloids, may result in hypernatremia).
No products indexed under this heading.

Diazoxide (Concurrent use with antihypertensives, such as diazoxide, may result in hypernatremia). Products include:
Hyperstat I.V. Injection ... 3031

Fludrocortisone Acetate (Concurrent use with mineralocorticoids may result in hypernatremia).
No products indexed under this heading.

Guanethidine Monosulfate (Concurrent use with antihypertensives, such as guanethidine, may result in hypernatremia).
No products indexed under this heading.

Hydralazine Hydrochloride (Concurrent use with antihypertensives, such as hydralazine, may result in hypernatremia). Products include:
BiDil Tablets ... 2161

Magaldrate (Co-administration with antacids may bind the phosphate and prevent its absorption).
No products indexed under this heading.

Magnesium Hydroxide (Co-administration with antacids may bind the phosphate and prevent its absorption). Products include:
Maalox Max Maximum Strength Antacid/Anti-Gas Liquid ... 2165
Maalox Regular Strength Antacid/Antigas Liquid ... 2164
Pepcid Complete Chewable Tablets ... 1672
Rolaids Tablets ... ▣707
Extra Strength Rolaids Tablets ... ▣707
Rolaids Multi-Symptom Antacid & Antigas Tablets ... ▣708

Magnesium Oxide (Co-administration with antacids may bind the phosphate and prevent its absorption). Products include:
Beelith Tablets ... 784
PremCal Light, Regular, and Extra Strength Tablets ... ▣762

Methyldopa (Concurrent use with antihypertensives, such as methyldopa, may result in hypernatremia). Products include:
Aldoclor Tablets ... 1881
Aldoril Tablets ... 1884

Potassium Acid Phosphate (Concurrent use with potassium-containing medications may cause hyperkalemia). Products include:
K-Phos Original (Sodium Free) Tablets ... 785

Potassium Bicarbonate (Concurrent use with potassium-containing medications may cause hyperkalemia).
No products indexed under this heading.

Potassium Chloride (Concurrent use with potassium-containing medications may cause hyperkalemia). Products include:
Colyte with Flavor Packs for Oral Solution ... 3102
HalfLytely and Bisacodyl Tablets Bowel Prep Kit with Flavors Packs ... 915
K-Dur Extended-Relase Tablets ... 3047
K-Lor Powder Packets ... 472
K-Tab Filmtab Tablets ... 473
TriLyte with Flavor Packs for Oral Solution ... 3114

Potassium Citrate (Concurrent use with potassium-containing medications may cause hyperkalemia). Products include:
Urocit-K Tablets ... 2109

Potassium Gluconate (Concurrent use with potassium-containing medications may cause hyperkalemia).
No products indexed under this heading.

Rauwolfia Serpentina (Concurrent use with antihypertensives, such as rauwolfia alkaloids, may result in hypernatremia).
No products indexed under this heading.

Rescinnamine (Concurrent use with antihypertensives, such as rauwolfia alkaloids, may result in hypernatremia).
No products indexed under this heading.

Reserpine (Concurrent use with antihypertensives, such as rauwolfia alkaloids, may result in hypernatremia).
No products indexed under this heading.

Spironolactone (Concurrent use with potassium-sparing diuretics may cause hyperkalemia).
No products indexed under this heading.

Triamterene (Concurrent use with potassium-sparing diuretics may cause hyperkalemia). Products include:
Dyazide Capsules ... 1389
Dyrenium Capsules ... 3390
Maxzide ... 2150

Vitamin D (Concurrent use with vitamin D may antagonize the effects of phosphates in the treatment of hypercalcemia). Products include:
Active Calcium Tablets ... 3342
Caltrate 600 PLUS Chewables ... ▣779
Caltrate 600 PLUS Tablets ... ▣779
Caltrate 600 + D Tablets ... ▣779
Os-Cal 250 + D Tablets ... ▣765
Os-Cal 500 + D Tablets ... ▣766

K-PHOS ORIGINAL (SODIUM FREE) TABLETS
(Potassium Acid Phosphate) ... 785
May interact with antacids, potassium preparations, potassium sparing diuretics, salicylates, and certain other agents. Compounds in these categories include:

Aluminum Carbonate (May bind phosphate and prevent its absorption).
No products indexed under this heading.

Aluminum Hydroxide (May bind phosphate and prevent its absorption). Products include:
Gaviscon Regular Strength Liquid .. ▣620
Gaviscon Regular Strength Tablets ... ▣619
Gaviscon Extra Strength Liquid ... ▣620
Gaviscon Extra Strength Tablets ... ▣619
Maalox Max Maximum Strength Antacid/Anti-Gas Liquid ... 2165
Maalox Regular Strength Antacid/Antigas Liquid ... 2164

Amiloride Hydrochloride (Hyperkalemia). Products include:
Midamor Tablets ... 2000
Moduretic Tablets ... 2003

Aspirin (Increased serum salicylate levels; possible toxicity). Products include:
Aggrenox Capsules ... 855
Bayer, Aspirin Regimen ... ▣606
Bayer Aspirin Tablets ... 3515
BC Powder ... ▣612
BC Allergy Sinus Cold Powder ... ▣612
Arthritis Strength BC Powder ... ▣612
BC Sinus Cold Powder ... ▣612
Ecotrin Enteric Coated Aspirin Low, Regular and Maximum Strength Tablets ... 1627
Goody's Body Pain Formula Powder ... ▣621
Goody's Extra Strength Headache Powder ... ▣621
Goody's Extra Strength Pain Relief Tablets ... ▣621
Percodan Tablets ... 1115
St. Joseph 81 mg Aspirin Chewable and Enteric Coated Tablets ... 1841

Aspirin, Enteric Coated (Increased serum salicylate levels; possible toxicity).
No products indexed under this heading.

Aspirin Buffered (Increased serum salicylate levels; possible toxicity).
No products indexed under this heading.

Choline Magnesium Trisalicylate (Increased serum salicylate levels; possible toxicity).
No products indexed under this heading.

Diflunisal (Increased serum salicylate levels; possible toxicity). Products include:
Dolobid Tablets ... 1937

Magaldrate (May bind phosphate and prevent its absorption).
No products indexed under this heading.

Magnesium Hydroxide (May bind phosphate and prevent its absorption). Products include:
Maalox Max Maximum Strength Antacid/Anti-Gas Liquid ... 2165
Maalox Regular Strength Antacid/Antigas Liquid ... 2164
Pepcid Complete Chewable Tablets ... 1672
Rolaids Tablets ... ▣707
Extra Strength Rolaids Tablets ... ▣707
Rolaids Multi-Symptom Antacid & Antigas Tablets ... ▣708

Magnesium Oxide (May bind phosphate and prevent its absorption). Products include:
Beelith Tablets ... 784
PremCal Light, Regular, and Extra Strength Tablets ... ▣762

Magnesium Salicylate (Increased serum salicylate levels; possible toxicity).
No products indexed under this heading.

Potassium Bicarbonate (Potential for hyperkalemia).
No products indexed under this heading.

Potassium Chloride (Potential for hyperkalemia). Products include:
Colyte with Flavor Packs for Oral Solution ... 3102
HalfLytely and Bisacodyl Tablets Bowel Prep Kit with Flavors Packs ... 915
K-Dur Extended-Relase Tablets ... 3047
K-Lor Powder Packets ... 472
K-Tab Filmtab Tablets ... 473
TriLyte with Flavor Packs for Oral Solution ... 3114

Potassium Citrate (Potential for hyperkalemia). Products include:
Urocit-K Tablets ... 2109

Potassium Gluconate (Potential for hyperkalemia).
No products indexed under this heading.

Potassium Phosphate (Potential for hyperkalemia). Products include:
K-Phos Neutral Tablets 785

Salsalate (Increased serum salicylate levels; possible toxicity).
No products indexed under this heading.

Sodium Bicarbonate (May bind phosphate and prevent its absorption). Products include:
Ceo-Two Evacuant Suppository 607
Colyte with Flavor Packs for Oral Solution 3102
HalfLytely and Bisacodyl Tablets Bowel Prep Kit with Flavors Packs 915
TriLyte with Flavor Packs for Oral Solution 3114

Spironolactone (Hyperkalemia).
No products indexed under this heading.

Triamterene (Hyperkalemia). Products include:
Dyazide Capsules 1389
Dyrenium Capsules 3390
Maxzide 2150

KRISTALOSE FOR ORAL SOLUTION

(Lactulose) 2149
May interact with nonabsorbable antacids. Compounds in these categories include:

Aluminum Carbonate (Results of preliminary studies suggests that nonabsorbable antacids given concurrently with lactulose may inhibit the desired lactulose-induced drop in colonic pH).
No products indexed under this heading.

Aluminum Hydroxide (Results of preliminary studies suggests that nonabsorbable antacids given concurrently with lactulose may inhibit the desired lactulose-induced drop in colonic pH). Products include:
Gaviscon Regular Strength Liquid .. 620
Gaviscon Regular Strength Tablets 619
Gaviscon Extra Strength Liquid 620
Gaviscon Extra Strength Tablets 619
Maalox Max Maximum Strength Antacid/Anti-Gas Liquid................. 2165
Maalox Regular Strength Antacid/Antigas Liquid.................. 2164

Calcium Carbonate (Results of preliminary studies suggests that nonabsorbable antacids given concurrently with lactulose may inhibit the desired lactulose-induced drop in colonic pH). Products include:
Actonel with Calcium Tablets 2684
Caltrate 600 PLUS Chewables 779
Caltrate 600 PLUS Tablets 779
Caltrate 600 + D Tablets 779
Encora Capsules 3298
Encora AM Tablets 3298
Encora PM Tablets 3298
Gas-X with Maalox 675
Maalox Regular Strength Antacid Tablets 2166
Quick Dissolve Maalox Max Maximum Strength Antacid/Antigas Tablets................ 2165
Maalox Max Quick Dissolve Maximum Strength Chewable Tablets.. 678
Os-Cal Chewable Tablets 765
Pepcid Complete Chewable Tablets 1672
PremCal Light, Regular, and Extra Strength Tablets................. 762
Rolaids Tablets 707
Extra Strength Rolaids Softchews 708
Extra Strength Rolaids Tablets 707
Rolaids Multi-Symptom Antacid & Antigas Tablets 708
Tums 639

Magnesium Carbonate (Results of preliminary studies suggests that nonabsorbable antacids given concurrently with lactulose may inhibit the desired lactulose-induced drop in colonic pH). Products include:
Gaviscon Regular Strength Liquid .. 620
Gaviscon Extra Strength Liquid 620
Gaviscon Extra Strength Tablets 619

Magnesium Hydroxide (Results of preliminary studies suggests that nonabsorbable antacids given concurrently with lactulose may inhibit the desired lactulose-induced drop in colonic pH). Products include:
Maalox Max Maximum Strength Antacid/Anti-Gas Liquid................ 2165
Maalox Regular Strength Antacid/Antigas Liquid................. 2164
Pepcid Complete Chewable Tablets 1672
Rolaids Tablets 707
Extra Strength Rolaids Tablets 707
Rolaids Multi-Symptom Antacid & Antigas Tablets 708

K-TAB FILMTAB TABLETS

(Potassium Chloride) 473
May interact with ACE inhibitors, anticholinergics, and potassium sparing diuretics. Compounds in these categories include:

Amiloride Hydrochloride (Potential for severe hyperkalemia). Products include:
Midamor Tablets 2000
Moduretic Tablets 2003

Atropine Sulfate (Anticholinergic drugs can be cause for delay or arrest in tablet passage through the gastrointestinal tract; concomitant administration of drugs capable of decreasing GI motility should be avoided).
No products indexed under this heading.

Belladonna Alkaloids (Anticholinergic drugs can be cause for delay or arrest in tablet passage through the gastrointestinal tract; concomitant administration of drugs capable of decreasing GI motility should be avoided). Products include:
Hyland's Teething Tablets 736

Benazepril Hydrochloride (Concomitant therapy may result in hyperkalemia; close monitoring is advised). Products include:
Lotensin Tablets 2232
Lotensin HCT Tablets 2235
Lotrel Capsules 2238

Benztropine Mesylate (Anticholinergic drugs can be cause for delay or arrest in tablet passage through the gastrointestinal tract; concomitant administration of drugs capable of decreasing GI motility should be avoided). Products include:
Cogentin Injection 1903

Biperiden Hydrochloride (Anticholinergic drugs can be cause for delay or arrest in tablet passage through the gastrointestinal tract; concomitant administration of drugs capable of decreasing GI motility should be avoided).
No products indexed under this heading.

Captopril (Concomitant therapy may result in hyperkalemia; close monitoring is advised). Products include:
Captopril Tablets 2114

Clidinium Bromide (Anticholinergic drugs can be cause for delay or arrest in tablet passage through the gastrointestinal tract; concomitant administration of drugs capable of decreasing GI motility should be avoided).
No products indexed under this heading.

Dicyclomine Hydrochloride (Anticholinergic drugs can be cause for delay or arrest in tablet passage through the gastrointestinal tract; concomitant administration of drugs capable of decreasing GI motility should be avoided). Products include:
Bentyl Capsules 724
Bentyl Injection 724
Bentyl Syrup 724
Bentyl Tablets 724

Enalapril Maleate (Concomitant therapy may result in hyperkalemia; close monitoring is advised). Products include:
Vaseretic Tablets 2073
Vasotec I.V. Injection 2076

Enalaprilat (Concomitant therapy may result in hyperkalemia; close monitoring is advised).
No products indexed under this heading.

Fosinopril Sodium (Concomitant therapy may result in hyperkalemia; close monitoring is advised).
No products indexed under this heading.

Glycopyrrolate (Anticholinergic drugs can be cause for delay or arrest in tablet passage through the gastrointestinal tract; concomitant administration of drugs capable of decreasing GI motility should be avoided).
No products indexed under this heading.

Hyoscyamine (Anticholinergic drugs can be cause for delay or arrest in tablet passage through the gastrointestinal tract; concomitant administration of drugs capable of decreasing GI motility should be avoided).
No products indexed under this heading.

Hyoscyamine Sulfate (Anticholinergic drugs can be cause for delay or arrest in tablet passage through the gastrointestinal tract; concomitant administration of drugs capable of decreasing GI motility should be avoided).
No products indexed under this heading.

Ipratropium Bromide (Anticholinergic drugs can be cause for delay or arrest in tablet passage through the gastrointestinal tract; concomitant administration of drugs capable of decreasing GI motility should be avoided). Products include:
Atrovent HFA Inhalation Aerosol 872
Atrovent Inhalation Solution 868
Atrovent Nasal Spray 0.03% 869
Atrovent Nasal Spray 0.06% 870
Combivent Inhalation Aerosol 878
DuoNeb Inhalation Solution 1058

Lisinopril (Concomitant therapy may result in hyperkalemia; close monitoring is advised). Products include:
Prinivil Tablets 2029
Prinzide Tablets 2033
Zestoretic Tablets 701
Zestril Tablets 704

Mepenzolate Bromide (Anticholinergic drugs can be cause for delay or arrest in tablet passage through the gastrointestinal tract; concomitant administration of drugs capable of decreasing GI motility should be avoided).
No products indexed under this heading.

Moexipril Hydrochloride (Concomitant therapy may result in hyperkalemia; close monitoring is advised). Products include:
Uniretic Tablets 3114
Univasc Tablets 3118

Oxybutynin Chloride (Anticholinergic drugs can be cause for delay or arrest in tablet passage through the gastrointestinal tract; concomitant administration of drugs capable of decreasing GI motility should be avoided). Products include:
Ditropan XL Extended Release Tablets 2391

Perindopril Erbumine (Concomitant therapy may result in hyperkalemia; close monitoring is advised). Products include:
Aceon Tablets (2 mg, 4 mg, 8 mg)... 3191

Procyclidine Hydrochloride (Anticholinergic drugs can be cause for delay or arrest in tablet passage through the gastrointestinal tract; concomitant administration of drugs capable of decreasing GI motility should be avoided).
No products indexed under this heading.

Propantheline Bromide (Anticholinergic drugs can be cause for delay or arrest in tablet passage through the gastrointestinal tract; concomitant administration of drugs capable of decreasing GI motility should be avoided).
No products indexed under this heading.

Quinapril Hydrochloride (Concomitant therapy may result in hyperkalemia; close monitoring is advised).
No products indexed under this heading.

Ramipril (Concomitant therapy may result in hyperkalemia; close monitoring is advised). Products include:
Altace Capsules 1673

Scopolamine (Anticholinergic drugs can be cause for delay or arrest in tablet passage through the gastrointestinal tract; concomitant administration of drugs capable of decreasing GI motility should be avoided). Products include:
Transderm Scōp Transdermal Therapeutic System 2166

Scopolamine Hydrobromide (Anticholinergic drugs can be cause for delay or arrest in tablet passage through the gastrointestinal tract; concomitant administration of drugs capable of decreasing GI motility should be avoided).
No products indexed under this heading.

Spirapril Hydrochloride (Concomitant therapy may result in hyperkalemia; close monitoring is advised).
No products indexed under this heading.

Spironolactone (Potential for severe hyperkalemia).
No products indexed under this heading.

Tolterodine Tartrate (Anticholinergic drugs can be cause for delay

or arrest in tablet passage through the gastrointestinal tract; concomitant administration of drugs capable of decreasing GI motility should be avoided). Products include:

Detrol Tablets 2626
Detrol LA Capsules 2629

Trandolapril (Concomitant therapy may result in hyperkalemia; close monitoring is advised). Products include:

Mavik Tablets 482
Tarka Tablets 519

Triamterene (Potential for severe hyperkalemia). Products include:

Dyazide Capsules 1389
Dyrenium Capsules 3390
Maxzide 2150

Tridihexethyl Chloride (Anticholinergic drugs can be cause for delay or arrest in tablet passage through the gastrointestinal tract; concomitant administration of drugs capable of decreasing GI motility should be avoided).

No products indexed under this heading.

Trihexyphenidyl Hydrochloride (Anticholinergic drugs can be cause for delay or arrest in tablet passage through the gastrointestinal tract; concomitant administration of drugs capable of decreasing GI motility should be avoided).

No products indexed under this heading.

KYTRIL INJECTION

(Granisetron Hydrochloride) 2785
See Kytril Tablets

KYTRIL ORAL SOLUTION

(Granisetron Hydrochloride) 2788
See Kytril Tablets

KYTRIL TABLETS

(Granisetron Hydrochloride) 2788
May interact with drugs affecting hepatic drug metabolizing enzyme systems and certain other agents. Compounds in these categories include:

Carbamazepine (May change the clearance and, hence the half-life of granisetron). Products include:

Carbatrol Capsules 3174
Equetro Extended-Release Capsules 3178
Tegretol/Tegretol-XR 2278

Cimetidine (May change the clearance and, hence the half-life of granisetron). Products include:

Tagamet HB 200 Tablets .... ▣637
Tagamet Tablets 1547

Cimetidine Hydrochloride (May change the clearance and, hence the half-life of granisetron).

No products indexed under this heading.

Fosphenytoin Sodium (May change the clearance and, hence the half-life of granisetron).

No products indexed under this heading.

Phenobarbital (May change the clearance and, hence the half-life of granisetron).

No products indexed under this heading.

Phenytoin (May change the clearance and, hence the half-life of granisetron).

No products indexed under this heading.

Phenytoin Sodium (May change the clearance and, hence the half-life of granisetron). Products include:

Phenytek Capsules 2153

Food Interactions

Food, unspecified (When oral granisetron was administered with food, AUC was decreased by 5% and Cmax increased by 30% in non-fasted individuals).

LACRISERT STERILE OPHTHALMIC INSERT

(Hydroxypropyl Cellulose) 1979
None cited in PDR database.

LACTAID ORIGINAL STRENGTH CAPLETS

(Lactase (beta-d-Galactosidase)) 1836
None cited in PDR database.

LACTAID FAST ACT CAPLETS AND CHEWABLE TABLETS

(Lactase (beta-d-Galactosidase)) 1836
None cited in PDR database.

LAMICTAL TABLETS

(Lamotrigine) 1449
May interact with dihydrofolate reductase inhibitors, oral contraceptives, phenytoin, valproate, and certain other agents. Compounds in these categories include:

Carbamazepine (Potential for higher incidence of dizziness, diplopia, ataxia, and blurred vision; decreases lamotrigine steady-state concentrations by approximately 40%; lamotrigine has no appreciable effect on steady-state carbamazepine plasma concentration). Products include:

Carbatrol Capsules 3174
Equetro Extended-Release Capsules 3178
Tegretol/Tegretol-XR 2278

Desogestrel (Oral contraceptive have been shown to increase the apparent clearance of lamotrigine. There have been reports of decreased lamotrigine concentrations following introduction of oral contraceptives and reports of increased lamotrigine concentrations following withdrawal of oral contraceptives). Products include:

Ortho-Cept Tablets 2395

Divalproex Sodium (Co-administration in healthy volunteers resulted in decreased trough steady-state VPA concentrations; the addition of VPA increases lamotrigine steady-state concentrations in normal volunteers by slightly more than two-fold). Products include:

Depakote Sprinkle Capsules 422
Depakote Tablets 427
Depakote ER Tablets 433

Ethinyl Estradiol (Oral contraceptive have been shown to increase the apparent clearance of lamotrigine. There have been reports of decreased lamotrigine concentrations following introduction of oral contraceptives and reports of increased lamotrigine concentrations following withdrawal of oral contraceptives). Products include:

Alesse-28 Tablets 3392
Lo/Ovral-28 Tablets 3423
NuvaRing 2357
Ortho-Cept Tablets 2395
Ortho-Cyclen/Ortho Tri-Cyclen 2414
Ortho Evra Transdermal System 2402
Ortho Tri-Cyclen Lo Tablets 2421
Seasonale Tablets 1073
Triphasil-28 Tablets 3483
Yasmin 28 Tablets 818

Ethynodiol Diacetate (Oral contraceptive have been shown to increase the apparent clearance of lamotrigine. There have been reports of decreased lamotrigine concentrations following introduction of oral contraceptives and reports of increased lamotrigine concentrations following withdrawal of oral contraceptives).

No products indexed under this heading.

Fosphenytoin Sodium (Decreases lamotrigine steady-state concentrations by approximately 40%).

No products indexed under this heading.

Levonorgestrel (Oral contraceptive have been shown to increase the apparent clearance of lamotrigine. There have been reports of decreased lamotrigine concentrations following introduction of oral contraceptives and reports of increased lamotrigine concentrations following withdrawal of oral contraceptives). Products include:

Alesse-28 Tablets 3392
Climara Pro Transdermal System 800
Mirena Intrauterine System 810
Plan B Tablets 1068
Seasonale Tablets 1073
Triphasil-28 Tablets 3483

Mestranol (Oral contraceptive have been shown to increase the apparent clearance of lamotrigine. There have been reports of decreased lamotrigine concentrations following introduction of oral contraceptives and reports of increased lamotrigine concentrations following withdrawal of oral contraceptives).

No products indexed under this heading.

Methotrexate Sodium (Lamotrigine is an inhibitor of dihydrofolate reductase; use caution when prescribing other medications that inhibit folate metabolism).

No products indexed under this heading.

Norethindrone (Oral contraceptive have been shown to increase the apparent clearance of lamotrigine. There have been reports of decreased lamotrigine concentrations following introduction of oral contraceptives and reports of increased lamotrigine concentrations following withdrawal of oral contraceptives). Products include:

Ortho Micronor Tablets 2411

Norethynodrel (Oral contraceptive have been shown to increase the apparent clearance of lamotrigine. There have been reports of decreased lamotrigine concentrations following introduction of oral contraceptives and reports of increased lamotrigine concentrations following withdrawal of oral contraceptives).

No products indexed under this heading.

Norgestimate (Oral contraceptive have been shown to increase the apparent clearance of lamotrigine. There have been reports of decreased lamotrigine concentrations following introduction of oral contraceptives and reports of increased lamotrigine concentrations following withdrawal of oral contraceptives). Products include:

Ortho-Cyclen/Ortho Tri-Cyclen 2414
Ortho Tri-Cyclen Lo Tablets 2421
Prefest Tablets 1069

Norgestrel (Oral contraceptive have been shown to increase the apparent clearance of lamotrigine. There have been reports of decreased lamotrigine concentrations following introduction of oral contraceptives and reports of increased lamotrigine concentrations following withdrawal of oral contraceptives). Products include:

Lo/Ovral-28 Tablets 3423

Olanzapine (The AUC and Cmax of lamotrigine was reduced on average by 24% and 20%, respectively, following the addition of olanzapine (15 mg once daily) to lamotrigine (200 mg once daily) in healthy male volunteers (n=16) compared to healthy male volunteers receiving lamotrigine alone (n=12). This reduction in lamotrigine plasma concentration is not expected to be clinically relevant). Products include:

Symbyax Capsules 1788
Zyprexa Tablets 1798
Zyprexa IntraMuscular 1798
Zyprexa ZYDIS Orally Disintegrating Tablets 1798

Oral Contraceptives (There have been reports of decreased lamotrigine concentrations following introduction of oral contraceptives and reports of increased lamotrigine concentrations following withdrawal of oral contraceptives).

No products indexed under this heading.

Phenobarbital (Decreases lamotrigine steady-state concentrations by approximately 40%).

No products indexed under this heading.

Phenytoin (Decreases lamotrigine steady-state concentrations by approximately 40%).

No products indexed under this heading.

Phenytoin Sodium (Decreases lamotrigine steady-state concentrations by approximately 40%). Products include:

Phenytek Capsules 2153

Primidone (Decreases lamotrigine steady-state concentrations by approximately 40%).

No products indexed under this heading.

Rifampin (Co-administration of rifampin has been shown to increase the apparent clearance of lamotrigine).

No products indexed under this heading.

Trimethoprim (Lamotrigine is an inhibitor of dihydrofolate reductase; use caution when prescribing other medications that inhibit folate metabolism).

No products indexed under this heading.

Trimetrexate Glucuronate (Lamotrigine is an inhibitor of dihydrofolate reductase; use caution when prescribing other medications that inhibit folate metabolism).

No products indexed under this heading.

Valproate Sodium (Co-administration in healthy volunteers resulted in decreased trough steady-state VPA concentrations; the addition of VPA increases lamotrigine steady-state concentrations in normal volunteers by slightly more than two-fold). Products include:

Depacon Injection 412

Valproic Acid (Co-administration in healthy volunteers resulted in decreased trough steady-state VPA concentrations; the addition of VPA increases lamotrigine steady-state concentrations in normal volunteers by slightly more than two-fold). Products include:

Depakene 417

LAMICTAL CHEWABLE DISPERSIBLE TABLETS

(Lamotrigine) 1449

See Lamictal Tablets

LAMISIL AT CREAMS (ATHLETE'S FOOT & JOCK ITCH)

(Terbinafine Hydrochloride) 676

None cited in PDR database.

LAMISIL TABLETS

(Terbinafine Hydrochloride) 2226

May interact with beta blockers, cytochrome p450 2d6 substrates (selected), monoamine oxidase inhibitors, selective serotonin reuptake inhibitors, tricyclic antidepressants, and certain other agents. Compounds in these categories include:

Acebutolol Hydrochloride (Studies have shown that terbinafine is an inhibitor of the CYP450 2D6 isoenzyme. Co-administration of terbinafine with drugs predominantly metabolized by the CYP450 2D6 isoenzyme should be done with careful monitoring and may require a reduction in dose of the 2D6-metabolized drug).

No products indexed under this heading.

Amitriptyline Hydrochloride (Studies have shown that terbinafine is an inhibitor of the CYP450 2D6 isoenzyme. Co-administration of terbinafine with drugs predominantly metabolized by the CYP450 2D6 isoenzyme should be done with careful monitoring and may require a reduction in dose of the 2D6-metabolized drug).

No products indexed under this heading.

Amoxapine (Studies have shown that terbinafine is an inhibitor of the CYP450 2D6 isoenzyme. Co-administration of terbinafine with drugs predominantly metabolized by the CYP450 2D6 isoenzyme should be done with careful monitoring and may require a reduction in dose of the 2D6-metabolized drug).

No products indexed under this heading.

Amphetamine Aspartate (Studies have shown that terbinafine is an inhibitor of the CYP450 2D6 isoenzyme. Co-administration of terbinafine with drugs predominantly metabolized by the CYP450 2D6 isoenzyme should be done with careful monitoring and may require a reduction in dose of the 2D6-metabolized drug). Products include:

Adderall Tablets 3168
Adderall XR Capsules 3169

Amphetamine Aspartate Monohydrate (Studies have shown that terbinafine is an inhibitor of the CYP450 2D6 isoenzyme. Co-administration of terbinafine with drugs predominantly metabolized by the CYP450 2D6 isoenzyme should be done with careful monitoring and may require a reduction in dose of the 2D6-metabolized drug).

No products indexed under this heading.

Amphetamine Sulfate (Studies have shown that terbinafine is an inhibitor of the CYP450 2D6 isoenzyme. Co-administration of terbinafine with drugs predominantly metabolized by the CYP450 2D6 isoenzyme should be done with careful monitoring and may require a reduction in dose of the 2D6-metabolized drug). Products include:

Adderall Tablets 3168
Adderall XR Capsules 3169

Atenolol (Studies have shown that terbinafine is an inhibitor of the CYP450 2D6 isoenzyme. Co-administration of terbinafine with drugs predominantly metabolized by the CYP450 2D6 isoenzyme should be done with careful monitoring and may require a reduction in dose of the 2D6-metabolized drug). Products include:

Tenormin I.V. Injection 698
Tenormin Tablets 695

Atomoxetine Hydrochloride (Studies have shown that terbinafine is an inhibitor of the CYP450 2D6 isoenzyme. Co-administration of terbinafine with drugs predominantly metabolized by the CYP450 2D6 isoenzyme should be done with careful monitoring and may require a reduction in dose of the 2D6-metabolized drug). Products include:

Strattera Capsules 1784

Betaxolol Hydrochloride (Studies have shown that terbinafine is an inhibitor of the CYP450 2D6 isoenzyme. Co-administration of terbinafine with drugs predominantly metabolized by the CYP450 2D6 isoenzyme should be done with careful monitoring and may require a reduction in dose of the 2D6-metabolized drug). Products include:

Betoptic S Ophthalmic Suspension.................................. 554

Bisoprolol Fumarate (Studies have shown that terbinafine is an inhibitor of the CYP450 2D6 isoenzyme. Co-administration of terbinafine with drugs predominantly metabolized by the CYP450 2D6 isoenzyme should be done with careful monitoring and may require a reduction in dose of the 2D6-metabolized drug).

No products indexed under this heading.

Caffeine (Terbinafine decreases the clearance of intravenously administered caffeine by 19%). Products include:

Athena Hair System Shampoo 767
BC Powder 612
Arthritis Strength BC Powder 612
Goody's Extra Strength Headache Powder....................... 621
Goody's Extra Strength Pain Relief Tablets............................. 621
Hycomine Compound Tablets 1105
Spartan Hair System Shampoo 767
Vivarin 639

Caffeine Citrate (Terbinafine decreases the clearance of intravenously administered caffeine by 19%). Products include:

Cafcit 1854

Captopril (Studies have shown that terbinafine is an inhibitor of the CYP450 2D6 isoenzyme. Co-administration of terbinafine with drugs predominantly metabolized by the CYP450 2D6 isoenzyme should be done with careful monitoring and may require a reduction in dose of the 2D6-metabolized drug). Products include:

Captopril Tablets 2114

Carteolol Hydrochloride (Studies have shown that terbinafine is an inhibitor of the CYP450 2D6 isoenzyme. Co-administration of terbinafine with drugs predominantly metabolized by the CYP450 2D6 isoenzyme should be done with careful monitoring and may require a reduction in dose of the 2D6-metabolized drug). Products include:

Carteolol Hydrochloride Ophthalmic Solution USP, 1%....... ⊙246

Carvedilol (Studies have shown that terbinafine is an inhibitor of the CYP450 2D6 isoenzyme. Co-administration of terbinafine with drugs predominantly metabolized by the CYP450 2D6 isoenzyme should be done with careful monitoring and may require a reduction in dose of the 2D6-metabolized drug). Products include:

Coreg Tablets 1376

Cevimeline Hydrochloride (Studies have shown that terbinafine is an inhibitor of the CYP450 2D6 isoenzyme. Co-administration of terbinafine with drugs predominantly metabolized by the CYP450 2D6 isoenzyme should be done with careful monitoring and may require a reduction in dose of the 2D6-metabolized drug). Products include:

Evoxac Capsules 1042

Chlorpromazine (Studies have shown that terbinafine is an inhibitor of the CYP450 2D6 isoenzyme. Co-administration of terbinafine with drugs predominantly metabolized by the CYP450 2D6 isoenzyme should be done with careful monitoring and may require a reduction in dose of the 2D6-metabolized drug).

No products indexed under this heading.

Chlorpromazine Hydrochloride (Studies have shown that terbinafine is an inhibitor of the CYP450 2D6 isoenzyme. Co-administration of terbinafine with drugs predominantly metabolized by the CYP450 2D6 isoenzyme should be done with careful monitoring and may require a reduction in dose of the 2D6-metabolized drug).

No products indexed under this heading.

Chlorpropamide (Studies have shown that terbinafine is an inhibitor of the CYP450 2D6 isoenzyme. Co-administration of terbinafine with drugs predominantly metabolized by the CYP450 2D6 isoenzyme should be done with careful monitoring and may require a reduction in dose of the 2D6-metabolized drug).

No products indexed under this heading.

Cimetidine (Terbinafine clearance is decreased 33% by cimetidine, a CYP450 enzyme inhibitor). Products include:

Tagamet HB 200 Tablets 637
Tagamet Tablets 1547

Cimetidine Hydrochloride (Terbinafine clearance is decreased 33% by cimetidine, a CYP450 enzyme inhibitor).

No products indexed under this heading.

Citalopram Hydrobromide (Studies have shown that terbinafine is an inhibitor of the CYP450 2D6 isoenzyme. Co-administration of terbinafine with drugs predominantly metabolized by the CYP450 2D6 isoenzyme should be done with careful monitoring and may require a reduction in dose of the 2D6-metabolized drug). Products include:

Celexa 1177

Clomipramine Hydrochloride (Studies have shown that terbinafine is an inhibitor of the CYP450 2D6 isoenzyme. Co-administration of terbinafine with drugs predominantly metabolized by the CYP450 2D6 isoenzyme should be done with careful monitoring and may require a reduction in dose of the 2D6-metabolized drug).

No products indexed under this heading.

Clozapine (Studies have shown that terbinafine is an inhibitor of the CYP450 2D6 isoenzyme. Co-administration of terbinafine with drugs predominantly metabolized by the CYP450 2D6 isoenzyme should be done with careful monitoring and may require a reduction in dose of the 2D6-metabolized drug). Products include:

Clozapine Tablets 2141
Clozaril Tablets 2174
FazaClo Orally Disintegrating Tablets.. 547

Codeine Phosphate (Studies have shown that terbinafine is an inhibitor of the CYP450 2D6 isoenzyme. Co-administration of terbinafine with drugs predominantly metabolized by the CYP450 2D6 isoenzyme should be done with careful monitoring and may require a reduction in dose of the 2D6-metabolized drug). Products include:

Tylenol with Codeine 2461

Codeine Sulfate (Studies have shown that terbinafine is an inhibitor of the CYP450 2D6 isoenzyme. Co-administration of terbinafine with drugs predominantly metabolized by the CYP450 2D6 isoenzyme should be done with careful monitoring and may require a reduction in dose of the 2D6-metabolized drug).

No products indexed under this heading.

Cyclobenzaprine Hydrochloride (Studies have shown that terbinafine is an inhibitor of the CYP450 2D6 isoenzyme. Co-administration of terbinafine with drugs predominantly metabolized by the CYP450 2D6 isoenzyme should be done with careful monitoring and may require a reduction in dose of the 2D6-metabolized drug). Products include:

Flexeril Tablets 1832

Cyclosporine (Terbinafine increases the clearance of cyclospo-

rine by 15%; terbinafine clearance is unaffected by cyclosporine). Products include:

- Gengraf Capsules 458
- Neoral Soft Gelatin Capsules 2247
- Neoral Oral Solution 2247
- Restasis Ophthalmic Emulsion 570
- Sandimmune 2259

Desipramine Hydrochloride (Studies have shown that terbinafine is an inhibitor of the CYP450 2D6 isoenzyme. Co-administration of terbinafine with drugs predominantly metabolized by the CYP450 2D6 isoenzyme should be done with careful monitoring and may require a reduction in dose of the 2D6-metabolized drug).

No products indexed under this heading.

Dexfenfluramine Hydrochloride (Studies have shown that terbinafine is an inhibitor of the CYP450 2D6 isoenzyme. Co-administration of terbinafine with drugs predominantly metabolized by the CYP450 2D6 isoenzyme should be done with careful monitoring and may require a reduction in dose of the 2D6-metabolized drug).

No products indexed under this heading.

Dextromethorphan Hydrobromide (Studies have shown that terbinafine is an inhibitor of the CYP450 2D6 isoenzyme. Co-administration of terbinafine with drugs predominantly metabolized by the CYP450 2D6 isoenzyme should be done with careful monitoring and may require a reduction in dose of the 2D6-metabolized drug). Products include:

- Alacol DM Syrup 739
- Balamine DM 739
- Contac Severe Cold and Flu Caplets Maximum Strength .... ■615
- Contac Severe Cold and Flu Caplets Non-Drowsy .... ■615
- Children's Dimetapp DM Cold & Cough Elixir .... ■745
- Children's Dimetapp Long Acting Cough Plus Cold Syrup .... ■746
- Dimetapp Infant Drops Decongestant Plus Cough .... ■746
- Mucinex DM Tablets .... ■602
- PediaCare Decongestant & Cough Infant Drops .... ■705
- PediaCare Freezer Pops Long-Acting Cough-Glacier Grape and Polar Berry Blue .... ■706
- PediaCare Long-Acting Cough Infant Drops .... ■705
- PediaCare Long-Acting Cough Plus Cold Liquid .... ■704
- PediaCare Multi-Symptom Cold Liquid .... ■704
- PediaCare NightRest Cough & Cold Liquid .... ■704
- Robitussin Allergy & Cough Syrup .... ■750
- Robitussin CF Liquid .... ■755
- Robitussin Cough & Cold Liquid-filled Capsules .... ■750
- Robitussin Cough, Cold & Flu Liquid-filled Capsules .... ■750
- Robitussin Cough & Cold Infant Drops .... ■755
- Robitussin DM Infant Drops .... ■753
- Robitussin DM Liquid .... ■753
- Robitussin Flu Liquid .... ■752
- Robitussin Maximum Strength Cough Liquid .... ■754
- Robitussin Maximum Strength Cough & Cold Liquid .... ■754
- Robitussin Pediatric Cough Liquid .... ■754
- Robitussin Pediatric Cough & Cold Liquid .... ■754
- Robitussin PM Cough & Cold Liquid .... ■752
- Robitussin Sugar Free Cough Liquid .... ■753
- Simply Cough Liquid 1840
- Sudafed Severe Cold .... ■710
- TheraFlu Cold & Cough Hot Liquid .... ■680
- TheraFlu Flu & Chest Congestion Non-Drowsy Hot Liquid .... ■681
- TheraFlu Severe Cold Non-Drowsy Hot Liquid .... ■683
- TheraFlu Severe Cold & Cough Hot Liquid .... ■683
- TheraFlu Severe Cold Caplets .... ■679
- TheraFlu Severe Cold Hot Liquid .... ■682
- TheraFlu Severe Cold Non-Drowsy Caplets .... ■679
- TheraFlu Thin Strips Long Acting Cough .... ■684
- Triaminic Cold & Cough Liquid .... ■685
- Triaminic Cough Liquid .... ■687
- Triaminic Cough & Nasal Congestion Liquid .... ■687
- Triaminic Cough & Sore Throat Liquid .... ■687
- Triaminic Flu, Cough & Fever Liquid .... ■685
- Triaminic Night Time Cough & Cold Liquid .... ■685
- Triaminic Cold & Cough Softchews .... ■688
- Triaminic Cough & Sore Throat Softchews .... ■689
- Triaminic Thin Strips Long Acting Cough .... ■689
- Children's Tylenol Plus Cold & Cough Suspension Liquid and Chewable Tablets 1851
- Children's Tylenol Plus Flu Suspension Liquid 1853
- Concentrated Tylenol Infants' Drops Plus Cold and Cough 1851
- Tylenol Cold & Flu Severe Daytime Liquid with Cool Bust 1846
- Tylenol Cold & Flu Severe NightTime Liquid with Cool Burst 1846
- Tylenol Cold Severe Congestion Non-Drowsy Caplets with Cool Burst 1846
- Tylenol Cough & Sore Throat Daytime Liquid with Cool Burst 1849
- Tylenol Cough & Sore Throat NightTime Liquid with Cool Burst 1849
- Tylenol Flu Day Non-Drowsy Gelcaps 1846
- Concentrated Tylenol Infants' Drops Plus Cold & Cough Nasal Decongestant, Fever Reducer & Pain Reliever .... ■668
- Multi-Symptom Tylenol Cold Night Time Caplets 1845
- Multi-Symptom Tylenol Cold Day Non-Drowsy Caplets and Gelcaps 1845
- Vicks 44 Cough Relief 2675
- Vicks 44D Cough & Head Congestion Relief 2676
- Vicks 44D Cough & Head Congestion Relief Liquid .... ■721
- Vicks 44E Cough & Chest Congestion Relief 2676
- Pediatric Vicks 44e Cough & Chest Congestion Relief Liquid 2673
- Vicks 44M Cough, Cold & Flu Relief 2676
- Pediatric Vicks 44m Cough & Cold Relief 2673
- Vicks DayQuil LiquiCaps/Liquid Multi-Symptom Cold/Flu Relief .... ■723
- Vicks DayQuil Multi-Symptom Cold/Flu Relief LiquiCaps 2675
- Vicks DayQuil Multi-Symptom Cold/Flu Relief Liquid 2675
- Children's Vicks NyQuil Cold/Cough Relief 2671
- Vicks NyQuil Cough Liquid 2677
- Vicks NyQuil LiquiCaps 2677
- Vicks NyQuil LiquiCaps/Liquid Multi-Symptom Cold/Flu Relief .... ■725
- Vicks NyQuil Liquid 2677
- Zicam Concentrated Cough Mist for Kids Cool Cherry .... ■643
- Zicam Concentrated Cough Mist for Kids Plus D Cool Cherry .... ■643
- Zicam Concentrated Cough Mist Nite-Cool Cherry .... ■642
- Zicam Concentrated Cough Mist Plus D Cool Cherry .... ■642
- Zicam Concentrated Cough Mist-Honey Lemon & Cool Cherry .... ■642

Dextromethorphan Polistirex (Studies have shown that terbinafine is an inhibitor of the CYP450 2D6 isoenzyme. Co-administration of terbinafine with drugs predominantly metabolized by the CYP450 2D6 isoenzyme should be done with careful monitoring and may require a reduction in dose of the 2D6-metabolized drug). Products include:

- Delsym Extended-Release Suspension .... ■611
- Delsym 12 Hour Cough Suppressant for Children .... ■611

Dolasetron Mesylate (Studies have shown that terbinafine is an inhibitor of the CYP450 2D6 isoenzyme. Co-administration of terbinafine with drugs predominantly metabolized by the CYP450 2D6 isoenzyme should be done with careful monitoring and may require a reduction in dose of the 2D6-metabolized drug). Products include:

- Anzemet Injection 2871
- Anzemet Tablets 2874

Donepezil Hydrochloride (Studies have shown that terbinafine is an inhibitor of the CYP450 2D6 isoenzyme. Co-administration of terbinafine with drugs predominantly metabolized by the CYP450 2D6 isoenzyme should be done with careful monitoring and may require a reduction in dose of the 2D6-metabolized drug). Products include:

- Aricept Tablets 1086
- Aricept ODT Tablets 1086

Doxepin Hydrochloride (Studies have shown that terbinafine is an inhibitor of the CYP450 2D6 isoenzyme. Co-administration of terbinafine with drugs predominantly metabolized by the CYP450 2D6 isoenzyme should be done with careful monitoring and may require a reduction in dose of the 2D6-metabolized drug).

No products indexed under this heading.

Encainide Hydrochloride (Studies have shown that terbinafine is an inhibitor of the CYP450 2D6 isoenzyme. Co-administration of terbinafine with drugs predominantly metabolized by the CYP450 2D6 isoenzyme should be done with careful monitoring and may require a reduction in dose of the 2D6-metabolized drug).

No products indexed under this heading.

Escitalopram Oxalate (Studies have shown that terbinafine is an inhibitor of the CYP450 2D6 isoenzyme. Co-administration of terbinafine with drugs predominantly metabolized by the CYP450 2D6 isoenzyme should be done with careful monitoring and may require a reduction in dose of the 2D6-metabolized drug). Products include:

- Lexapro Oral Solution 1193
- Lexapro Tablets 1193

Esmolol Hydrochloride (Studies have shown that terbinafine is an inhibitor of the CYP450 2D6 isoenzyme. Co-administration of terbinafine with drugs predominantly metabolized by the CYP450 2D6 isoenzyme should be done with careful monitoring and may require a reduction in dose of the 2D6-metabolized drug). Products include:

- Brevibloc Concentrate 766
- Brevibloc Injection 766
- Brevibloc Double Strength Injection 766
- Brevibloc Premixed Injection 766
- Brevibloc Double Strength Premixed Injection 766

Fentanyl (Studies have shown that terbinafine is an inhibitor of the CYP450 2D6 isoenzyme. Co-administration of terbinafine with drugs predominantly metabolized by the CYP450 2D6 isoenzyme should be done with careful monitoring and may require a reduction in dose of the 2D6-metabolized drug). Products include:

- Duragesic Transdermal System 2448

Fentanyl Citrate (Studies have shown that terbinafine is an inhibitor of the CYP450 2D6 isoenzyme. Co-administration of terbinafine with drugs predominantly metabolized by the CYP450 2D6 isoenzyme should be done with careful monitoring and may require a reduction in dose of the 2D6-metabolized drug). Products include:

- Actiq 993

Flecainide Acetate (Studies have shown that terbinafine is an inhibitor of the CYP450 2D6 isoenzyme. Co-administration of terbinafine with drugs predominantly metabolized by the CYP450 2D6 isoenzyme should be done with careful monitoring and may require a reduction in dose of the 2D6-metabolized drug). Products include:

- Tambocor Tablets 1824

Fluoxetine (Studies have shown that terbinafine is an inhibitor of the CYP450 2D6 isoenzyme. Co-administration of terbinafine with drugs predominantly metabolized by the CYP450 2D6 isoenzyme should be done with careful monitoring and may require a reduction in dose of the 2D6-metabolized drug).

No products indexed under this heading.

Fluoxetine Hydrochloride (Studies have shown that terbinafine is an inhibitor of the CYP450 2D6 isoenzyme. Co-administration of terbinafine with drugs predominantly metabolized by the CYP450 2D6 isoenzyme should be done with careful monitoring and may require a reduction in dose of the 2D6-metabolized drug). Products include:

- Prozac Pulvules and Liquid 1771
- Symbyax Capsules 1788

Fluphenazine Decanoate (Studies have shown that terbinafine is an inhibitor of the CYP450 2D6 isoenzyme. Co-administration of terbinafine with drugs predominantly metabolized by the CYP450 2D6 isoenzyme should be done with careful monitoring and may require a reduction in dose of the 2D6-metabolized drug).

No products indexed under this heading.

Fluphenazine Enanthate (Studies have shown that terbinafine is an inhibitor of the CYP450 2D6 isoenzyme. Co-administration of terbinafine with drugs predominantly metabolized by the CYP450 2D6 isoenzyme should be done with careful monitoring and may require a reduction in dose of the 2D6-metabolized drug).
No products indexed under this heading.

Fluphenazine Hydrochloride (Studies have shown that terbinafine is an inhibitor of the CYP450 2D6 isoenzyme. Co-administration of terbinafine with drugs predominantly metabolized by the CYP450 2D6 isoenzyme should be done with careful monitoring and may require a reduction in dose of the 2D6-metabolized drug).
No products indexed under this heading.

Fluvoxamine Maleate (Studies have shown that terbinafine is an inhibitor of the CYP450 2D6 isoenzyme. Co-administration of terbinafine with drugs predominantly metabolized by the CYP450 2D6 isoenzyme should be done with careful monitoring and may require a reduction in dose of the 2D6-metabolized drug).
No products indexed under this heading.

Formoterol Fumarate (Studies have shown that terbinafine is an inhibitor of the CYP450 2D6 isoenzyme. Co-administration of terbinafine with drugs predominantly metabolized by the CYP450 2D6 isoenzyme should be done with careful monitoring and may require a reduction in dose of the 2D6-metabolized drug). Products include:
Foradil Aerolizer **3024**

Galantamine Hydrobromide (Studies have shown that terbinafine is an inhibitor of the CYP450 2D6 isoenzyme. Co-administration of terbinafine with drugs predominantly metabolized by the CYP450 2D6 isoenzyme should be done with careful monitoring and may require a reduction in dose of the 2D6-metabolized drug). Products include:
Razadyne ER Extended-Release Capsules **2434**
Razadyne **2434**

Haloperidol (Studies have shown that terbinafine is an inhibitor of the CYP450 2D6 isoenzyme. Co-administration of terbinafine with drugs predominantly metabolized by the CYP450 2D6 isoenzyme should be done with careful monitoring and may require a reduction in dose of the 2D6-metabolized drug).
No products indexed under this heading.

Haloperidol Decanoate (Studies have shown that terbinafine is an inhibitor of the CYP450 2D6 isoenzyme. Co-administration of terbinafine with drugs predominantly metabolized by the CYP450 2D6 isoenzyme should be done with careful monitoring and may require a reduction in dose of the 2D6-metabolized drug).
No products indexed under this heading.

Hydrocodone Bitartrate (Studies have shown that terbinafine is an inhibitor of the CYP450 2D6 isoenzyme. Co-administration of terbinafine with drugs predominantly metabolized by the CYP450 2D6 isoenzyme should be done with careful monitoring and may require a reduction in dose of the 2D6-metabolized drug). Products include:
Hycodan **1104**
Hycomine Compound Tablets **1105**
Hycotuss Expectorant Syrup **1106**
Lortab **3315**
Lortab Elixir **3312**
Vicodin Tablets **530**
Vicodin ES Tablets **531**
Vicodin HP Tablets **532**
Vicoprofen Tablets **533**
Zydone Tablets **1118**

Imipramine Hydrochloride (Studies have shown that terbinafine is an inhibitor of the CYP450 2D6 isoenzyme. Co-administration of terbinafine with drugs predominantly metabolized by the CYP450 2D6 isoenzyme should be done with careful monitoring and may require a reduction in dose of the 2D6-metabolized drug).
No products indexed under this heading.

Imipramine Pamoate (Studies have shown that terbinafine is an inhibitor of the CYP450 2D6 isoenzyme. Co-administration of terbinafine with drugs predominantly metabolized by the CYP450 2D6 isoenzyme should be done with careful monitoring and may require a reduction in dose of the 2D6-metabolized drug).
No products indexed under this heading.

Indoramin Hydrochloride (Studies have shown that terbinafine is an inhibitor of the CYP450 2D6 isoenzyme. Co-administration of terbinafine with drugs predominantly metabolized by the CYP450 2D6 isoenzyme should be done with careful monitoring and may require a reduction in dose of the 2D6-metabolized drug).
No products indexed under this heading.

Isocarboxazid (Studies have shown that terbinafine is an inhibitor of the CYP450 2D6 isoenzyme. Co-administration of terbinafine with drugs predominantly metabolized by the CYP450 2D6 isoenzyme should be done with careful monitoring and may require a reduction in dose of the 2D6-metabolized drug).
No products indexed under this heading.

Labetalol Hydrochloride (Studies have shown that terbinafine is an inhibitor of the CYP450 2D6 isoenzyme. Co-administration of terbinafine with drugs predominantly metabolized by the CYP450 2D6 isoenzyme should be done with careful monitoring and may require a reduction in dose of the 2D6-metabolized drug).
No products indexed under this heading.

Levobunolol Hydrochloride (Studies have shown that terbinafine is an inhibitor of the CYP450 2D6 isoenzyme. Co-administration of terbinafine with drugs predominantly metabolized by the CYP450 2D6 isoenzyme should be done with careful monitoring and may require a reduction in dose of the 2D6-metabolized drug). Products include:
Betagan Ophthalmic Solution, USP .... ⊙**217**

Lidocaine (Studies have shown that terbinafine is an inhibitor of the CYP450 2D6 isoenzyme. Co-administration of terbinafine with drugs predominantly metabolized by the CYP450 2D6 isoenzyme should be done with careful monitoring and may require a reduction in dose of the 2D6-metabolized drug). Products include:
Lidoderm Patch **1107**

Lidocaine Hydrochloride (Studies have shown that terbinafine is an inhibitor of the CYP450 2D6 isoenzyme. Co-administration of terbinafine with drugs predominantly metabolized by the CYP450 2D6 isoenzyme should be done with careful monitoring and may require a reduction in dose of the 2D6-metabolized drug).
No products indexed under this heading.

Maprotiline Hydrochloride (Studies have shown that terbinafine is an inhibitor of the CYP450 2D6 isoenzyme. Co-administration of terbinafine with drugs predominantly metabolized by the CYP450 2D6 isoenzyme should be done with careful monitoring and may require a reduction in dose of the 2D6-metabolized drug).
No products indexed under this heading.

Meperidine Hydrochloride (Studies have shown that terbinafine is an inhibitor of the CYP450 2D6 isoenzyme. Co-administration of terbinafine with drugs predominantly metabolized by the CYP450 2D6 isoenzyme should be done with careful monitoring and may require a reduction in dose of the 2D6-metabolized drug).
No products indexed under this heading.

Methadone Hydrochloride (Studies have shown that terbinafine is an inhibitor of the CYP450 2D6 isoenzyme. Co-administration of terbinafine with drugs predominantly metabolized by the CYP450 2D6 isoenzyme should be done with careful monitoring and may require a reduction in dose of the 2D6-metabolized drug).
No products indexed under this heading.

Methamphetamine Hydrochloride (Studies have shown that terbinafine is an inhibitor of the CYP450 2D6 isoenzyme. Co-administration of terbinafine with drugs predominantly metabolized by the CYP450 2D6 isoenzyme should be done with careful monitoring and may require a reduction in dose of the 2D6-metabolized drug). Products include:
Desoxyn Tablets, USP **2482**

Metipranolol Hydrochloride (Studies have shown that terbinafine is an inhibitor of the CYP450 2D6 isoenzyme. Co-administration of terbinafine with drugs predominantly metabolized by the CYP450 2D6 isoenzyme should be done with careful monitoring and may require a reduction in dose of the 2D6-metabolized drug).
No products indexed under this heading.

Metoprolol Succinate (Studies have shown that terbinafine is an inhibitor of the CYP450 2D6 isoenzyme. Co-administration of terbinafine with drugs predominantly metabolized by the CYP450 2D6 isoenzyme should be done with careful monitoring and may require a reduction in dose of the 2D6-metabolized drug). Products include:
Toprol-XL Tablets **660**

Metoprolol Tartrate (Studies have shown that terbinafine is an inhibitor of the CYP450 2D6 isoenzyme. Co-administration of terbinafine with drugs predominantly metabolized by the CYP450 2D6 isoenzyme should be done with careful monitoring and may require a reduction in dose of the 2D6-metabolized drug).
No products indexed under this heading.

Mexiletine Hydrochloride (Studies have shown that terbinafine is an inhibitor of the CYP450 2D6 isoenzyme. Co-administration of terbinafine with drugs predominantly metabolized by the CYP450 2D6 isoenzyme should be done with careful monitoring and may require a reduction in dose of the 2D6-metabolized drug).
No products indexed under this heading.

Mirtazapine (Studies have shown that terbinafine is an inhibitor of the CYP450 2D6 isoenzyme. Co-administration of terbinafine with drugs predominantly metabolized by the CYP450 2D6 isoenzyme should be done with careful monitoring and may require a reduction in dose of the 2D6-metabolized drug).
No products indexed under this heading.

Moclobemide (Studies have shown that terbinafine is an inhibitor of the CYP450 2D6 isoenzyme. Co-administration of terbinafine with drugs predominantly metabolized by the CYP450 2D6 isoenzyme should be done with careful monitoring and may require a reduction in dose of the 2D6-metabolized drug).
No products indexed under this heading.

Morphine Sulfate (Studies have shown that terbinafine is an inhibitor of the CYP450 2D6 isoenzyme. Co-administration of terbinafine with drugs predominantly metabolized by the CYP450 2D6 isoenzyme should be done with careful monitoring and may require a reduction in dose of the 2D6-metabolized drug). Products include:
Avinza Capsules **1714**
Kadian Capsules **572**
MS Contin Tablets **2703**

Nadolol (Studies have shown that terbinafine is an inhibitor of the CYP450 2D6 isoenzyme. Co-administration of terbinafine with drugs predominantly metabolized by the CYP450 2D6 isoenzyme should be done with careful monitoring and may require a reduction in dose of the 2D6-metabolized drug). Products include:
Nadolol Tablets **2121**

Nelfinavir Mesylate (Studies have shown that terbinafine is an inhibitor of the CYP450 2D6 isoenzyme. Co-administration of terbinafine with drugs predominantly metabolized by the CYP450 2D6 isoenzyme should be done with careful monitoring and may require a reduction in dose of the 2D6-metabolized drug). Products include:

Viracept 2556

Nortriptyline Hydrochloride (Studies have shown that terbinafine is an inhibitor of the CYP450 2D6 isoenzyme. Co-administration of terbinafine with drugs predominantly metabolized by the CYP450 2D6 isoenzyme should be done with careful monitoring and may require a reduction in dose of the 2D6-metabolized drug).

No products indexed under this heading.

Olanzapine (Studies have shown that terbinafine is an inhibitor of the CYP450 2D6 isoenzyme. Co-administration of terbinafine with drugs predominantly metabolized by the CYP450 2D6 isoenzyme should be done with careful monitoring and may require a reduction in dose of the 2D6-metabolized drug). Products include:

Symbyax Capsules 1788
Zyprexa Tablets 1798
Zyprexa IntraMuscular 1798
Zyprexa ZYDIS Orally Disintegrating Tablets 1798

Omeprazole (Studies have shown that terbinafine is an inhibitor of the CYP450 2D6 isoenzyme. Co-administration of terbinafine with drugs predominantly metabolized by the CYP450 2D6 isoenzyme should be done with careful monitoring and may require a reduction in dose of the 2D6-metabolized drug). Products include:

Zegerid Powder for Oral Solution 2972

Ondansetron (Studies have shown that terbinafine is an inhibitor of the CYP450 2D6 isoenzyme. Co-administration of terbinafine with drugs predominantly metabolized by the CYP450 2D6 isoenzyme should be done with careful monitoring and may require a reduction in dose of the 2D6-metabolized drug). Products include:

Zofran ODT Orally Disintegrating Tablets 1613

Ondansetron Hydrochloride (Studies have shown that terbinafine is an inhibitor of the CYP450 2D6 isoenzyme. Co-administration of terbinafine with drugs predominantly metabolized by the CYP450 2D6 isoenzyme should be done with careful monitoring and may require a reduction in dose of the 2D6-metabolized drug). Products include:

Zofran Injection 1607
Zofran 1613

Oxycodone Hydrochloride (Studies have shown that terbinafine is an inhibitor of the CYP450 2D6 isoenzyme. Co-administration of terbinafine with drugs predominantly metabolized by the CYP450 2D6 isoenzyme should be done with careful monitoring and may require a reduction in dose of the 2D6-metabolized drug). Products include:

Combunox Tablets 1183
OxyContin Tablets 2699
OxyFast Oral Concentrate Solution 2704
OxyIR Capsules 2704
Percocet Tablets 1114
Percodan Tablets 1115

Paclitaxel (Studies have shown that terbinafine is an inhibitor of the CYP450 2D6 isoenzyme. Co-administration of terbinafine with drugs predominantly metabolized by the CYP450 2D6 isoenzyme should be done with careful monitoring and may require a reduction in dose of the 2D6-metabolized drug).

No products indexed under this heading.

Pargyline Hydrochloride (Studies have shown that terbinafine is an inhibitor of the CYP450 2D6 isoenzyme. Co-administration of terbinafine with drugs predominantly metabolized by the CYP450 2D6 isoenzyme should be done with careful monitoring and may require a reduction in dose of the 2D6-metabolized drug).

No products indexed under this heading.

Paroxetine Hydrochloride (Studies have shown that terbinafine is an inhibitor of the CYP450 2D6 isoenzyme. Co-administration of terbinafine with drugs predominantly metabolized by the CYP450 2D6 isoenzyme should be done with careful monitoring and may require a reduction in dose of the 2D6-metabolized drug). Products include:

Paxil CR Controlled-Release Tablets 1509
Paxil 1501

Penbutolol Sulfate (Studies have shown that terbinafine is an inhibitor of the CYP450 2D6 isoenzyme. Co-administration of terbinafine with drugs predominantly metabolized by the CYP450 2D6 isoenzyme should be done with careful monitoring and may require a reduction in dose of the 2D6-metabolized drug).

No products indexed under this heading.

Phenelzine Sulfate (Studies have shown that terbinafine is an inhibitor of the CYP450 2D6 isoenzyme. Co-administration of terbinafine with drugs predominantly metabolized by the CYP450 2D6 isoenzyme should be done with careful monitoring and may require a reduction in dose of the 2D6-metabolized drug).

No products indexed under this heading.

Pindolol (Studies have shown that terbinafine is an inhibitor of the CYP450 2D6 isoenzyme. Co-administration of terbinafine with drugs predominantly metabolized by the CYP450 2D6 isoenzyme should be done with careful monitoring and may require a reduction in dose of the 2D6-metabolized drug).

No products indexed under this heading.

Procarbazine Hydrochloride (Studies have shown that terbinafine is an inhibitor of the CYP450 2D6 isoenzyme. Co-administration of terbinafine with drugs predominantly metabolized by the CYP450 2D6 isoenzyme should be done with careful monitoring and may require a reduction in dose of the 2D6-metabolized drug). Products include:

Matulane Capsules 3188

Propafenone Hydrochloride (Studies have shown that terbinafine is an inhibitor of the CYP450 2D6 isoenzyme. Co-administration of terbinafine with drugs predominantly metabolized by the CYP450 2D6 isoenzyme should be done with careful monitoring and may require a reduction in dose of the 2D6-metabolized drug). Products include:

Rythmol SR Capsules 2736

Propoxyphene Hydrochloride (Studies have shown that terbinafine is an inhibitor of the CYP450 2D6 isoenzyme. Co-administration of terbinafine with drugs predominantly metabolized by the CYP450 2D6 isoenzyme should be done with careful monitoring and may require a reduction in dose of the 2D6-metabolized drug).

No products indexed under this heading.

Propoxyphene Napsylate (Studies have shown that terbinafine is an inhibitor of the CYP450 2D6 isoenzyme. Co-administration of terbinafine with drugs predominantly metabolized by the CYP450 2D6 isoenzyme should be done with careful monitoring and may require a reduction in dose of the 2D6-metabolized drug). Products include:

Darvocet A 500 Tablets 3497

Propranolol Hydrochloride (Studies have shown that terbinafine is an inhibitor of the CYP450 2D6 isoenzyme. Co-administration of terbinafine with drugs predominantly metabolized by the CYP450 2D6 isoenzyme should be done with careful monitoring and may require a reduction in dose of the 2D6-metabolized drug). Products include:

Inderal LA Long-Acting Capsules 3421
InnoPran XL Capsules 2728

Protriptyline Hydrochloride (Studies have shown that terbinafine is an inhibitor of the CYP450 2D6 isoenzyme. Co-administration of terbinafine with drugs predominantly metabolized by the CYP450 2D6 isoenzyme should be done with careful monitoring and may require a reduction in dose of the 2D6-metabolized drug). Products include:

Vivactil Tablets 2350

Quetiapine Fumarate (Studies have shown that terbinafine is an inhibitor of the CYP450 2D6 isoenzyme. Co-administration of terbinafine with drugs predominantly metabolized by the CYP450 2D6 isoenzyme should be done with careful monitoring and may require a reduction in dose of the 2D6-metabolized drug). Products include:

Seroquel Tablets 691

Quinidine Gluconate (Studies have shown that terbinafine is an inhibitor of the CYP450 2D6 isoenzyme. Co-administration of terbinafine with drugs predominantly metabolized by the CYP450 2D6 isoenzyme should be done with careful monitoring and may require a reduction in dose of the 2D6-metabolized drug).

No products indexed under this heading.

Quinidine Hydrochloride (Studies have shown that terbinafine is an inhibitor of the CYP450 2D6 isoenzyme. Co-administration of terbinafine with drugs predominantly metabolized by the CYP450 2D6 isoenzyme should be done with careful monitoring and may require a reduction in dose of the 2D6-metabolized drug).

No products indexed under this heading.

Quinidine Polygalacturonate (Studies have shown that terbinafine is an inhibitor of the CYP450 2D6 isoenzyme. Co-administration of terbinafine with drugs predominantly metabolized by the CYP450 2D6 isoenzyme should be done with careful monitoring and may require a reduction in dose of the 2D6-metabolized drug).

No products indexed under this heading.

Quinidine Sulfate (Studies have shown that terbinafine is an inhibitor of the CYP450 2D6 isoenzyme. Co-administration of terbinafine with drugs predominantly metabolized by the CYP450 2D6 isoenzyme should be done with careful monitoring and may require a reduction in dose of the 2D6-metabolized drug).

No products indexed under this heading.

Rifampin (Terbinafine clearance is increased 100% by rifampin, a CYP450 enzyme inducer).

No products indexed under this heading.

Risperidone (Studies have shown that terbinafine is an inhibitor of the CYP450 2D6 isoenzyme. Co-administration of terbinafine with drugs predominantly metabolized by the CYP450 2D6 isoenzyme should be done with careful monitoring and may require a reduction in dose of the 2D6-metabolized drug). Products include:

Risperdal Consta Long-Acting Injection 1664
Risperdal M-Tab Orally Disintegrating Tablets 1658
Risperdal 1658

Ritonavir (Studies have shown that terbinafine is an inhibitor of the CYP450 2D6 isoenzyme. Co-administration of terbinafine with drugs predominantly metabolized by the CYP450 2D6 isoenzyme should be done with careful monitoring and may require a reduction in dose of the 2D6-metabolized drug). Products include:

Kaletra 474
Norvir 499

Selegiline Hydrochloride (In vitro studies show that terbinafine inhibits CYP2D6 mediated metabolism; this may be of clinical relevance for compounds predominantly metabolized by this enzyme, such as type B MAO inhibitor, if they have a narrow therapeutic window). Products include:

Eldepryl Capsules 3209

Sertraline Hydrochloride (Studies have shown that terbinafine is an inhibitor of the CYP450 2D6 isoenzyme. Co-administration of terbinafine with drugs predominantly metabolized by the CYP450 2D6 isoenzyme should be done with careful monitoring and may require a reduction in dose of the 2D6-metabolized drug). Products include:

Zoloft 2581

Sotalol Hydrochloride (Studies have shown that terbinafine is an inhibitor of the CYP450 2D6 isoenzyme. Co-administration of terbinafine with drugs predominantly metabolized by the CYP450 2D6 isoenzyme should be done with careful monitoring and may require a reduction in dose of the 2D6-metabolized drug).
No products indexed under this heading.

Tamoxifen Citrate (Studies have shown that terbinafine is an inhibitor of the CYP450 2D6 isoenzyme. Co-administration of terbinafine with drugs predominantly metabolized by the CYP450 2D6 isoenzyme should be done with careful monitoring and may require a reduction in dose of the 2D6-metabolized drug).
No products indexed under this heading.

Teniposide (Studies have shown that terbinafine is an inhibitor of the CYP450 2D6 isoenzyme. Co-administration of terbinafine with drugs predominantly metabolized by the CYP450 2D6 isoenzyme should be done with careful monitoring and may require a reduction in dose of the 2D6-metabolized drug).
No products indexed under this heading.

Terfenadine (Terbinafine clearance is decreased 16% by terfenadine).
No products indexed under this heading.

Testosterone (Studies have shown that terbinafine is an inhibitor of the CYP450 2D6 isoenzyme. Co-administration of terbinafine with drugs predominantly metabolized by the CYP450 2D6 isoenzyme should be done with careful monitoring and may require a reduction in dose of the 2D6-metabolized drug). Products include:
AndroGel 3330
Striant Mucoadhesive 1022
Testim 1% Gel 722

Testosterone Cypionate (Studies have shown that terbinafine is an inhibitor of the CYP450 2D6 isoenzyme. Co-administration of terbinafine with drugs predominantly metabolized by the CYP450 2D6 isoenzyme should be done with careful monitoring and may require a reduction in dose of the 2D6-metabolized drug).
No products indexed under this heading.

Testosterone Enanthate (Studies have shown that terbinafine is an inhibitor of the CYP450 2D6 isoenzyme. Co-administration of terbinafine with drugs predominantly metabolized by the CYP450 2D6 isoenzyme should be done with careful monitoring and may require a reduction in dose of the 2D6-metabolized drug). Products include:
Delatestryl Injection 2976

Testosterone Propionate (Studies have shown that terbinafine is an inhibitor of the CYP450 2D6 isoenzyme. Co-administration of terbinafine with drugs predominantly metabolized by the CYP450 2D6 isoenzyme should be done with careful monitoring and may require a reduction in dose of the 2D6-metabolized drug).
No products indexed under this heading.

Thioridazine (Studies have shown that terbinafine is an inhibitor of the CYP450 2D6 isoenzyme. Co-administration of terbinafine with drugs predominantly metabolized by the CYP450 2D6 isoenzyme should be done with careful monitoring and may require a reduction in dose of the 2D6-metabolized drug).
No products indexed under this heading.

Thioridazine Hydrochloride (Studies have shown that terbinafine is an inhibitor of the CYP450 2D6 isoenzyme. Co-administration of terbinafine with drugs predominantly metabolized by the CYP450 2D6 isoenzyme should be done with careful monitoring and may require a reduction in dose of the 2D6-metabolized drug). Products include:
Thioridazine Hydrochloride Tablets 2122

Timolol Hemihydrate (Studies have shown that terbinafine is an inhibitor of the CYP450 2D6 isoenzyme. Co-administration of terbinafine with drugs predominantly metabolized by the CYP450 2D6 isoenzyme should be done with careful monitoring and may require a reduction in dose of the 2D6-metabolized drug). Products include:
Betimol Ophthalmic Solution 3371
Betimol Ophthalmic Solution .... ⊙283

Timolol Maleate (Studies have shown that terbinafine is an inhibitor of the CYP450 2D6 isoenzyme. Co-administration of terbinafine with drugs predominantly metabolized by the CYP450 2D6 isoenzyme should be done with careful monitoring and may require a reduction in dose of the 2D6-metabolized drug). Products include:
Blocadren Tablets 1891
Cosopt Sterile Ophthalmic Solution 1910
Timolide Tablets 2056
Timoptic in Ocudose 2061
Timoptic Sterile Ophthalmic Solution 2058
Timoptic-XE Sterile Ophthalmic Gel Forming Solution 2062

Tolterodine Tartrate (Studies have shown that terbinafine is an inhibitor of the CYP450 2D6 isoenzyme. Co-administration of terbinafine with drugs predominantly metabolized by the CYP450 2D6 isoenzyme should be done with careful monitoring and may require a reduction in dose of the 2D6-metabolized drug). Products include:
Detrol Tablets 2626
Detrol LA Capsules 2629

Tramadol Hydrochloride (Studies have shown that terbinafine is an inhibitor of the CYP450 2D6 isoenzyme. Co-administration of terbinafine with drugs predominantly metabolized by the CYP450 2D6 isoenzyme should be done with careful monitoring and may require a reduction in dose of the 2D6-metabolized drug). Products include:
Ultracet Tablets 2462

Tranylcypromine Sulfate (Studies have shown that terbinafine is an inhibitor of the CYP450 2D6 isoenzyme. Co-administration of terbinafine with drugs predominantly metabolized by the CYP450 2D6 isoenzyme should be done with careful monitoring and may require a reduction in dose of the 2D6-metabolized drug). Products include:
Parnate Tablets 1499

Trazodone Hydrochloride (Studies have shown that terbinafine is an inhibitor of the CYP450 2D6 isoenzyme. Co-administration of terbinafine with drugs predominantly metabolized by the CYP450 2D6 isoenzyme should be done with careful monitoring and may require a reduction in dose of the 2D6-metabolized drug).
No products indexed under this heading.

Triazolam (Studies have shown that terbinafine is an inhibitor of the CYP450 2D6 isoenzyme. Co-administration of terbinafine with drugs predominantly metabolized by the CYP450 2D6 isoenzyme should be done with careful monitoring and may require a reduction in dose of the 2D6-metabolized drug).
No products indexed under this heading.

Trimipramine Maleate (Studies have shown that terbinafine is an inhibitor of the CYP450 2D6 isoenzyme. Co-administration of terbinafine with drugs predominantly metabolized by the CYP450 2D6 isoenzyme should be done with careful monitoring and may require a reduction in dose of the 2D6-metabolized drug). Products include:
Surmontil Capsules 2347

Venlafaxine Hydrochloride (Studies have shown that terbinafine is an inhibitor of the CYP450 2D6 isoenzyme. Co-administration of terbinafine with drugs predominantly metabolized by the CYP450 2D6 isoenzyme should be done with careful monitoring and may require a reduction in dose of the 2D6-metabolized drug). Products include:
Effexor Tablets 3405
Effexor XR Capsules 3411

Vinblastine Sulfate (Studies have shown that terbinafine is an inhibitor of the CYP450 2D6 isoenzyme. Co-administration of terbinafine with drugs predominantly metabolized by the CYP450 2D6 isoenzyme should be done with careful monitoring and may require a reduction in dose of the 2D6-metabolized drug).
No products indexed under this heading.

Warfarin Sodium (Co-administration has resulted in altered prothrombin time (prolongation and reduction)). Products include:
Coumadin for Injection 932
Coumadin Tablets 932

Zonisamide (Studies have shown that terbinafine is an inhibitor of the CYP450 2D6 isoenzyme. Co-administration of terbinafine with drugs predominantly metabolized by the CYP450 2D6 isoenzyme should be done with careful monitoring and may require a reduction in dose of the 2D6-metabolized drug). Products include:
Zonegran Capsules 1089

Food Interactions

Food, unspecified (Co-administration has resulted in an increase in the AUC of terbinafine of less than 20%).

LANOXICAPS CAPSULES

(Digoxin) 1458
See Lanoxin Tablets

LANOXIN INJECTION

(Digoxin) 1462
See Lanoxin Tablets

LANOXIN TABLETS

(Digoxin) 1468
May interact with antacids, beta blockers, calcium channel blockers, corticosteroids, erythromycin, macrolide antibiotics, potassium-depleting diuretics, quinidine, sympathomimetics, tetracyclines, thyroid preparations, and certain other agents. Compounds in these categories include:

Acebutolol Hydrochloride (Concomitant use of digoxin and beta-andrenergic blockers may result in the additive effects on AV node conduction).
No products indexed under this heading.

Albuterol (Concomitant use of digoxin and sympathomimetics increases the risk of cardiac arrhythmias). Products include:
Proventil Inhalation Aerosol 3067

Albuterol Sulfate (Concomitant use of digoxin and sympathomimetics increases the risk of cardiac arrhythmias). Products include:
AccuNeb Inhalation Solution 1055
Combivent Inhalation Aerosol 878
DuoNeb Inhalation Solution 1058
Proventil Inhalation Solution 0.083% 3069
Proventil HFA Inhalation Aerosol 3071
Ventolin HFA Inhalation Aerosol 1576
VoSpire Extended-Release Tablets 2352

Alprazolam (Raises the serum digoxin concentration due to reduction in clearance and/or volume of distribution of the drug, with the implication that digitalis intoxication may result). Products include:
Niravam Orally Disintegrating Tablets 3106
Xanax XR Tablets 2655

Aluminum Carbonate (Antacids may interfere with intestinal digoxin absorption, resulting in unexpectedly low serum concentrations; antacids may cause hypokalemia or hypomagnesemia and co-administration can cause digitalis toxicity).
No products indexed under this heading.

Aluminum Hydroxide (Antacids may interfere with intestinal digoxin absorption, resulting in unexpectedly low serum concentrations; antacids may cause hypokalemia or hypomagnesemia and co-administration can cause digitalis toxicity). Products include:
Gaviscon Regular Strength Liquid 620
Gaviscon Regular Strength Tablets 619
Gaviscon Extra Strength Liquid 620
Gaviscon Extra Strength Tablets 619
Maalox Max Maximum Strength Antacid/Anti-Gas Liquid 2165
Maalox Regular Strength Antacid/Antigas Liquid 2164

Amiodarone Hydrochloride (Raises the serum digoxin concentration due to reduction in clearance and/or volume of distribution of the drug, with the implication that digitalis intoxication may result). Products include:
Pacerone Tablets 3337

Amlodipine Besylate (Concomitant use of digoxin and calcium chan-

nel blockers may result in the additive effects on AV node conduction). Products include:

Caduet Tablets 2507
Lotrel Capsules 2238
Norvasc Tablets 2529

Amphotericin B (Can cause hypokalemia or hypomagnesemia and potassium or magnesium depletion can sensitize the myocardium to digoxin resulting in digitails toxicity).
No products indexed under this heading.

Anticancer Drugs, unspecified (May interfere with intestinal digoxin absorption, resulting in unexpectedly low serum concentrations).
No products indexed under this heading.

Atenolol (Concomitant use of digoxin and beta-andrenergic blockers may result in the additive effects on AV node conduction). Products include:

Tenormin I.V. Injection 698
Tenormin Tablets 695

Azithromycin Dihydrate (Macrolide antibiotics may possibly increase digoxin absorption in patients who inactivate digoxin by bacterial metabolism in the lower intestine, so that digitalis intoxication may result). Products include:

Zithromax 2568
Zithromax for IV Infusion 2573
Zithromax for Oral Suspension, 300 mg, 600 mg, 900 mg, 1200 mg 2561
Zithromax Tablets, 250 mg, 500 mg 2561
Zithromax Tri-Pak 2561
Zithromax Z-Pak 2568

Bendroflumethiazide (Potassium-depleting diuretics can cause hypokalemia and co-administration can result in digitalis toxicity).
No products indexed under this heading.

Bepridil Hydrochloride (Concomitant use of digoxin and calcium channel blockers may result in the additive effects on AV node conduction).
No products indexed under this heading.

Betamethasone Acetate (Corticosteroids can cause hypokalemia or hypomagnesemia and potassium or magnesium depletion can sensitize the myocardium to digoxin resulting in digitalis toxicity).
No products indexed under this heading.

Betamethasone Sodium Phosphate (Corticosteroids can cause hypokalemia or hypomagnesemia and potassium or magnesium depletion can sensitize the myocardium to digoxin resulting in digitalis toxicity).
No products indexed under this heading.

Betaxolol Hydrochloride (Concomitant use of digoxin and beta-andrenergic blockers may result in the additive effects on AV node conduction). Products include:

Betoptic S Ophthalmic Suspension 554

Bisoprolol Fumarate (Concomitant use of digoxin and beta-andrenergic blockers may result in the additive effects on AV node conduction).
No products indexed under this heading.

Bumetanide (Potassium-depleting diuretics can cause hypokalemia and co-administration can result in digitalis toxicity).
No products indexed under this heading.

Calcium, intravenous (Co-administration with calcium, particularly if administered rapidly by the intravenous route may produce serious arrhythmias in digitalized patients).
No products indexed under this heading.

Carteolol Hydrochloride (Concomitant use of digoxin and beta-andrenergic blockers may result in the additive effects on AV node conduction). Products include:

Carteolol Hydrochloride Ophthalmic Solution USP, 1% .... ⊙246

Chlorothiazide (Potassium-depleting diuretics can cause hypokalemia and co-administration can result in digitalis toxicity). Products include:

Aldoclor Tablets 1881
Diuril Oral 1936

Chlorothiazide Sodium (Potassium-depleting diuretics can cause hypokalemia and co-administration can result in digitalis toxicity). Products include:

Diuril Sodium Intravenous 1934

Cholestyramine (May interfere with intestinal digoxin absorption, resulting in unexpectedly low serum concentrations).
No products indexed under this heading.

Clarithromycin (May increase digoxin absorption in patients who inactivate digoxin by bacterial metabolism in the lower intestine, so that digitalis intoxication may result). Products include:

Biaxin/Biaxin XL 402
PREVPAC 3281

Cortisone Acetate (Corticosteroids can cause hypokalemia or hypomagnesemia and potassium or magnesium depletion can sensitize the myocardium to digoxin resulting in digitalis toxicity).
No products indexed under this heading.

Demeclocycline Hydrochloride (May increase digoxin absorption in patients who inactivate digoxin by bacterial metabolism in the lower intestine, so that digitalis intoxication may result).
No products indexed under this heading.

Dexamethasone (Corticosteroids can cause hypokalemia or hypomagnesemia and potassium or magnesium depletion can sensitize the myocardium to digoxin resulting in digitalis toxicity). Products include:

Ciprodex Otic Suspension 555
Decadron Tablets 1929
TobraDex Ophthalmic Ointment 558
TobraDex Ophthalmic Suspension 558

Dexamethasone Acetate (Corticosteroids can cause hypokalemia or hypomagnesemia and potassium or magnesium depletion can sensitize the myocardium to digoxin resulting in digitalis toxicity).
No products indexed under this heading.

Dexamethasone Sodium Phosphate (Corticosteroids can cause hypokalemia or hypomagnesemia and potassium or magnesium depletion can sensitize the myocardium to digoxin resulting in digitalis toxicity). Products include:

Decadron Phosphate Injection 1931

Diltiazem Hydrochloride (Concomitant use of digoxin and calcium channel blockers may result in the additive effects on AV node conduction). Products include:

Cardizem LA Extended Release Tablets 1699
Tiazac Capsules 1204

Diphenoxylate Hydrochloride (Decreases gut motility and may increase digoxin absorption).
No products indexed under this heading.

Dirithromycin (Macrolide antibiotics may possibly increase digoxin absorption in patients who inactivate digoxin by bacterial metabolism in the lower intestine, so that digitalis intoxication may result).
No products indexed under this heading.

Dobutamine Hydrochloride (Concomitant use of digoxin and sympathomimetics increases the risk of cardiac arrhythmias).
No products indexed under this heading.

Dopamine Hydrochloride (Concomitant use of digoxin and sympathomimetics increases the risk of cardiac arrhythmias).
No products indexed under this heading.

Doxycycline Calcium (May increase digoxin absorption in patients who inactivate digoxin by bacterial metabolism in the lower intestine, so that digitalis intoxication may result).
No products indexed under this heading.

Doxycycline Hyclate (May increase digoxin absorption in patients who inactivate digoxin by bacterial metabolism in the lower intestine, so that digitalis intoxication may result).
No products indexed under this heading.

Doxycycline Monohydrate (May increase digoxin absorption in patients who inactivate digoxin by bacterial metabolism in the lower intestine, so that digitalis intoxication may result).
No products indexed under this heading.

Ephedrine Hydrochloride (Concomitant use of digoxin and sympathomimetics increases the risk of cardiac arrhythmias). Products include:

Primatene Tablets .... ■749

Ephedrine Sulfate (Concomitant use of digoxin and sympathomimetics increases the risk of cardiac arrhythmias).
No products indexed under this heading.

Ephedrine Tannate (Concomitant use of digoxin and sympathomimetics increases the risk of cardiac arrhythmias).
No products indexed under this heading.

Epinephrine (Concomitant use of digoxin and sympathomimetics increases the risk of cardiac arrhythmias). Products include:

EpiPen 1061
Primatene Mist .... ■749

Epinephrine Bitartrate (Concomitant use of digoxin and sympathomimetics increases the risk of cardiac arrhythmias).
No products indexed under this heading.

Epinephrine Hydrochloride (Concomitant use of digoxin and sympathomimetics increases the risk of cardiac arrhythmias).
No products indexed under this heading.

Erythromycin (May increase digoxin absorption in patients who inactivate digoxin by bacterial metabolism in the lower intestine, so that digitalis intoxication may result). Products include:

Erygel Topical Gel 2096
Ery-Tab Tablets 447
Erythromycin Base Filmtab Tablets 454
Erythromycin Delayed-Release Capsules, USP 456
PCE Dispertab Tablets 510

Erythromycin Estolate (May increase digoxin absorption in patients who inactivate digoxin by bacterial metabolism in the lower intestine, so that digitalis intoxication may result).
No products indexed under this heading.

Erythromycin Ethylsuccinate (May increase digoxin absorption in patients who inactivate digoxin by bacterial metabolism in the lower intestine, so that digitalis intoxication may result). Products include:

E.E.S. 449
EryPed 445

Erythromycin Gluceptate (May increase digoxin absorption in patients who inactivate digoxin by bacterial metabolism in the lower intestine, so that digitalis intoxication may result).
No products indexed under this heading.

Erythromycin Lactobionate (May increase digoxin absorption in patients who inactivate digoxin by bacterial metabolism in the lower intestine, so that digitalis intoxication may result).
No products indexed under this heading.

Erythromycin Stearate (May increase digoxin absorption in patients who inactivate digoxin by bacterial metabolism in the lower intestine, so that digitalis intoxication may result). Products include:

Erythrocin Stearate Filmtab Tablets 452

Esmolol Hydrochloride (Concomitant use of digoxin and beta-andrenergic blockers may result in the additive effects on AV node conduction). Products include:

Brevibloc Concentrate 766
Brevibloc Injection 766
Brevibloc Double Strength Injection 766
Brevibloc Premixed Injection 766
Brevibloc Double Strength Premixed Injection 766

Ethacrynic Acid (Potassium-depleting diuretics can cause hypokalemia and co-administration can result in digitalis toxicity). Products include:

Edecrin Tablets 1941

Felodipine (Concomitant use of digoxin and calcium channel blockers may result in the additive effects on AV node conduction). Products include:

Plendil Extended-Release Tablets 651

Fludrocortisone Acetate (Corticosteroids can cause hypokalemia or hypomagnesemia and potassium or magnesium depletion can sensitize the myocardium to digoxin resulting in digitalis toxicity).
No products indexed under this heading.

Furosemide (Potassium-depleting diuretics can cause hypokalemia and co-administration can result in digitalis toxicity). Products include:
Furosemide Tablets 2117

Hydrochlorothiazide (Potassium-depleting diuretics can cause hypokalemia and co-administration can result in digitalis toxicity). Products include:
Aldoril Tablets 1884
Atacand HCT 637
Avalide Tablets 2889
Avalide Tablets 922
Benicar HCT Tablets 2852
Diovan HCT Tablets 2195
Dyazide Capsules 1389
Hyzaar 1964
Lotensin HCT Tablets 2235
Maxzide 2150
Micardis HCT Tablets 886
Moduretic Tablets 2003
Prinzide Tablets 2033
Teveten HCT Tablets 1710
Timolide Tablets 2056
Uniretic Tablets 3114
Vaseretic Tablets 2073
Zestoretic Tablets 701

Hydrocortisone (Corticosteroids can cause hypokalemia or hypomagnesemia and potassium or magnesium depletion can sensitize the myocardium to digoxin resulting in digitalis toxicity). Products include:
Cortizone•5 Ointment .... ⊡ 699
Cortizone•10 Creme .... ⊡ 699
Cortizone•10 Ointment .... ⊡ 699
Cortizone•10 Plus Creme .... ⊡ 700
Cortizone•10 Maximum Strength Quick Shot Spray .... ⊡ 700
Hydrocortone Tablets 1963
Preparation H Hydrocortisone Cream .... ⊡ 748

Hydrocortisone Acetate (Corticosteroids can cause hypokalemia or hypomagnesemia and potassium or magnesium depletion can sensitize the myocardium to digoxin resulting in digitalis toxicity). Products include:
Analpram-HC 1136
Pramosone 1139
ProctoFoam-HC 3113
Tucks Anti-Itch Ointment .... ⊡ 712
U-cort 1% Cream 3289

Hydrocortisone Sodium Phosphate (Corticosteroids can cause hypokalemia or hypomagnesemia and potassium or magnesium depletion can sensitize the myocardium to digoxin resulting in digitalis toxicity).
No products indexed under this heading.

Hydrocortisone Sodium Succinate (Corticosteroids can cause hypokalemia or hypomagnesemia and potassium or magnesium depletion can sensitize the myocardium to digoxin resulting in digitalis toxicity).
No products indexed under this heading.

Hydroflumethiazide (Potassium-depleting diuretics can cause hypokalemia and co-administration can result in digitalis toxicity).
No products indexed under this heading.

Indomethacin (Raises the serum digoxin concentration due to reduction in clearance and/or volume of distribution of the drug, with the implication that digitalis intoxication may result). Products include:
Indocin 1968

Indomethacin Sodium Trihydrate (Raises the serum digoxin concentration due to reduction in clearance and/or volume of distribution of the drug, with the implication that digitalis intoxication may result). Products include:
Indocin I.V. 1973

Isoproterenol Hydrochloride (Concomitant use of digoxin and sympathomimetics increases the risk of cardiac arrhythmias).
No products indexed under this heading.

Isoproterenol Sulfate (Concomitant use of digoxin and sympathomimetics increases the risk of cardiac arrhythmias).
No products indexed under this heading.

Isradipine (Concomitant use of digoxin and calcium channel blockers may result in the additive effects on AV node conduction). Products include:
DynaCirc CR Tablets 2726

Itraconazole (Raises the serum digoxin concentration due to reduction in clearance and/or volume of distribution of the drug, with the implication that digitalis intoxication may result).
No products indexed under this heading.

Kaolin (May interfere with intestinal digoxin absorption, resulting in unexpectedly low serum concentrations).
No products indexed under this heading.

Labetalol Hydrochloride (Concomitant use of digoxin and beta-andrenergic blockers may result in the additive effects on AV node conduction).
No products indexed under this heading.

Levalbuterol Hydrochloride (Concomitant use of digoxin and sympathomimetics increases the risk of cardiac arrhythmias). Products include:
Xopenex Inhalation Solution 3143
Xopenex Inhalation Solution Concentrate 3147

Levobunolol Hydrochloride (Concomitant use of digoxin and beta-andrenergic blockers may result in the additive effects on AV node conduction). Products include:
Betagan Ophthalmic Solution, USP .... ⊙ 217

Levothyroxine Sodium (Thyroid administration to a digitalized, hypothyroid patient may increase the dose requirement of digoxin). Products include:
Levothroid Tablets 1189
Levoxyl Tablets 1680
Synthroid Tablets 515
Unithroid Tablets 3521

Liothyronine Sodium (Thyroid administration to a digitalized, hypothyroid patient may increase the dose requirement of digoxin). Products include:
Cytomel Tablets 1678

Liotrix (Thyroid administration to a digitalized, hypothyroid patient may increase the dose requirement of digoxin). Products include:
Thyrolar 1203

Magaldrate (Antacids may interfere with intestinal digoxin absorption, resulting in unexpectedly low serum concentrations; antacids may cause hypokalemia or hypomagnesemia and co-administration can cause digitalis toxicity).
No products indexed under this heading.

Magnesium Hydroxide (Antacids may interfere with intestinal digoxin absorption, resulting in unexpectedly low serum concentrations; antacids may cause hypokalemia or hypomagnesemia and co-administration can cause digitalis toxicity). Products include:
Maalox Max Maximum Strength Antacid/Anti-Gas Liquid 2165
Maalox Regular Strength Antacid/Antigas Liquid 2164
Pepcid Complete Chewable Tablets 1672
Rolaids Tablets .... ⊡ 707
Extra Strength Rolaids Tablets .... ⊡ 707
Rolaids Multi-Symptom Antacid & Antigas Tablets .... ⊡ 708

Magnesium Oxide (Antacids may interfere with intestinal digoxin absorption, resulting in unexpectedly low serum concentrations; antacids may cause hypokalemia or hypomagnesemia and co-administration can cause digitalis toxicity). Products include:
Beelith Tablets 784
PremCal Light, Regular, and Extra Strength Tablets .... ⊡ 762

Metaproterenol Sulfate (Concomitant use of digoxin and sympathomimetics increases the risk of cardiac arrhythmias). Products include:
Alupent Inhalation Aerosol 858

Metaraminol Bitartrate (Concomitant use of digoxin and sympathomimetics increases the risk of cardiac arrhythmias). Products include:
Aramine Injection 1889

Methacycline Hydrochloride (May increase digoxin absorption in patients who inactivate digoxin by bacterial metabolism in the lower intestine, so that digitalis intoxication may result).
No products indexed under this heading.

Methoxamine Hydrochloride (Concomitant use of digoxin and sympathomimetics increases the risk of cardiac arrhythmias).
No products indexed under this heading.

Methyclothiazide (Potassium-depleting diuretics can cause hypokalemia and co-administration can result in digitalis toxicity).
No products indexed under this heading.

Methylprednisolone Acetate (Corticosteroids can cause hypokalemia or hypomagnesemia and potassium or magnesium depletion can sensitize the myocardium to digoxin resulting in digitalis toxicity). Products include:
Depo-Medrol Injectable Suspension 2615
Depo-Medrol Single-Dose Vial 2617

Methylprednisolone Sodium Succinate (Corticosteroids can cause hypokalemia or hypomagnesemia and potassium or magnesium depletion can sensitize the myocardium to digoxin resulting in digitalis toxicity).
No products indexed under this heading.

Metipranolol Hydrochloride (Concomitant use of digoxin and beta-andrenergic blockers may result in the additive effects on AV node conduction).
No products indexed under this heading.

Metoclopramide Hydrochloride (May interfere with intestinal digoxin absorption, resulting in unexpectedly low serum concentrations).
No products indexed under this heading.

Metoprolol Succinate (Concomitant use of digoxin and beta-andrenergic blockers may result in the additive effects on AV node conduction). Products include:
Toprol-XL Tablets 660

Metoprolol Tartrate (Concomitant use of digoxin and beta-andrenergic blockers may result in the additive effects on AV node conduction).
No products indexed under this heading.

Mibefradil Dihydrochloride (Concomitant use of digoxin and calcium channel blockers may result in the additive effects on AV node conduction).
No products indexed under this heading.

Minocycline Hydrochloride (May increase digoxin absorption in patients who inactivate digoxin by bacterial metabolism in the lower intestine, so that digitalis intoxication may result). Products include:
Dynacin Tablets 1859

Nadolol (Concomitant use of digoxin and beta-andrenergic blockers may result in the additive effects on AV node conduction). Products include:
Nadolol Tablets 2121

Neomycin, oral (May interfere with intestinal digoxin absorption, resulting in unexpectedly low serum concentrations).
No products indexed under this heading.

Nicardipine Hydrochloride (Concomitant use of digoxin and calcium channel blockers may result in the additive effects on AV node conduction). Products include:
Cardene I.V. 1129

Nifedipine (Concomitant use of digoxin and calcium channel blockers may result in the additive effects on AV node conduction). Products include:
Adalat CC Tablets 2978

Nimodipine (Concomitant use of digoxin and calcium channel blockers may result in the additive effects on AV node conduction). Products include:
Nimotop Capsules 774

Nisoldipine (Concomitant use of digoxin and calcium channel blockers may result in the additive effects on AV node conduction). Products include:
Sular Tablets 1163

Norepinephrine Bitartrate (Concomitant use of digoxin and sympathomimetics increases the risk of cardiac arrhythmias).
No products indexed under this heading.

Oxytetracycline Hydrochloride (May increase digoxin absorption in patients who inactivate digoxin by bacterial metabolism in the lower intestine, so that digitalis intoxication may result).

No products indexed under this heading.

Pectin (May interfere with intestinal digoxin absorption, resulting in unexpectedly low serum concentrations). Products include:

- Halls Fruit Breezers Pectin Throat Drops .... ▣ 609
- Halls Plus Cough Drops .... ▣ 609

Penbutolol Sulfate (Concomitant use of digoxin and beta-andrenergic blockers may result in the additive effects on AV node conduction).

No products indexed under this heading.

Penicillamine (Co-administration has resulted in inconsistent reports regarding the effects of penicillamine on serum digoxin concentration). Products include:

- Cuprimine Capsules 1925

Phenylephrine Bitartrate (Concomitant use of digoxin and sympathomimetics increases the risk of cardiac arrhythmias).

No products indexed under this heading.

Phenylephrine Hydrochloride (Concomitant use of digoxin and sympathomimetics increases the risk of cardiac arrhythmias). Products include:

- Alacol DM Syrup 739
- Hycomine Compound Tablets 1105
- Preparation H Maximum Strength Cream .... ▣ 747
- Preparation H Cooling Gel .... ▣ 747
- Preparation H .... ▣ 747
- Sudafed PE Tablets .... ▣ 711
- Vicks Sinex Nasal Spray and Ultra Fine Mist for Sinus Relief 2677
- Zicam Concentrated Cough Mist for Kids Plus D Cool Cherry .... ▣ 643
- Zicam Concentrated Cough Mist Plus D Cool Cherry .... ▣ 642

Phenylephrine Tannate (Concomitant use of digoxin and sympathomimetics increases the risk of cardiac arrhythmias).

No products indexed under this heading.

Phenylpropanolamine Hydrochloride (Concomitant use of digoxin and sympathomimetics increases the risk of cardiac arrhythmias).

No products indexed under this heading.

Pindolol (Concomitant use of digoxin and beta-andrenergic blockers may result in the additive effects on AV node conduction).

No products indexed under this heading.

Pirbuterol Acetate (Concomitant use of digoxin and sympathomimetics increases the risk of cardiac arrhythmias). Products include:

- Maxair Autohaler 1820

Polythiazide (Potassium-depleting diuretics can cause hypokalemia and co-administration can result in digitalis toxicity).

No products indexed under this heading.

Prednisolone Acetate (Corticosteroids can cause hypokalemia or hypomagnesemia and potassium or magnesium depletion can sensitize the myocardium to digoxin resulting in digitalis toxicity). Products include:

- Blephamide Ophthalmic Ointment 563
- Blephamide Ophthalmic Suspension 564
- Poly-Pred Liquifilm Ophthalmic Suspension .... ⊙ 231
- Pred Forte Ophthalmic Suspension .... ⊙ 233
- Pred Mild Sterile Ophthalmic Suspension .... ⊙ 236
- Pred-G Ophthalmic Suspension .... ⊙ 234
- Pred-G Sterile Ophthalmic Ointment .... ⊙ 235

Prednisolone Sodium Phosphate (Corticosteroids can cause hypokalemia or hypomagnesemia and potassium or magnesium depletion can sensitize the myocardium to digoxin resulting in digitalis toxicity). Products include:

- Pediapred Oral Solution 3319

Prednisolone Tebutate (Corticosteroids can cause hypokalemia or hypomagnesemia and potassium or magnesium depletion can sensitize the myocardium to digoxin resulting in digitalis toxicity).

No products indexed under this heading.

Prednisone (Corticosteroids can cause hypokalemia or hypomagnesemia and potassium or magnesium depletion can sensitize the myocardium to digoxin resulting in digitalis toxicity).

No products indexed under this heading.

Propafenone Hydrochloride (Raises the serum digoxin concentration due to reduction in clearance and/or volume of distribution of the drug, with the implication that digitalis intoxication may result). Products include:

- Rythmol SR Capsules 2736

Propantheline Bromide (Decreases gut motility and may increase digoxin absorption).

No products indexed under this heading.

Propranolol Hydrochloride (Concomitant use of digoxin and beta-andrenergic blockers may result in the additive effects on AV node conduction). Products include:

- Inderal LA Long-Acting Capsules 3421
- InnoPran XL Capsules 2728

Pseudoephedrine Hydrochloride (Concomitant use of digoxin and sympathomimetics increases the risk of cardiac arrhythmias). Products include:

- Advil Allergy Sinus Caplets .... ▣ 737
- Advil Cold & Sinus .... ▣ 739
- Advil Flu & Body Ache Caplets .... ▣ 739
- Children's Advil Cold Suspension .... ▣ 741
- Advil Multi-Symptom Cold Caplets .... ▣ 738
- Allegra-D 12 Hour Extended-Release Tablets 2860
- Allegra-D 24 Hour Extended-Release Tablets 2862
- Balamine DM 739
- BC Cold Powder .... ▣ 612
- Benadryl Allergy & Cold Tablets .... ▣ 692
- Benadryl Allergy & Sinus Headache Caplets & Gelcaps .... ▣ 693
- Children's Benadryl Allergy & Cold Fastmelt Tablets .... ▣ 695
- Benadryl Maximum Strength Severe Allergy & Sinus Headache Caplets .... ▣ 694
- Children's Benadryl D Allergy & Sinus Fastmelt Tablets .... ▣ 694
- Children's Benadryl D Liquid Medication .... ▣ 693
- Benadryl D Tablets .... ▣ 694
- Contac Non-Drowsy 12 Hour Cold Caplets .... ▣ 614
- Contac Non-Drowsy Timed Release 12 Hour Cold Caplets .... ▣ 615
- Contac Severe Cold and Flu Caplets Maximum Strength .... ▣ 615
- Contac Severe Cold and Flu Caplets Non-Drowsy .... ▣ 615
- Children's Dimetapp Cold & Allergy Elixir .... ▣ 745
- Children's Dimetapp DM Cold & Cough Elixir .... ▣ 745
- Children's Dimetapp Long Acting Cough Plus Cold Syrup .... ▣ 746
- Dimetapp Infant Drops Decongestant Plus Cough .... ▣ 746
- Children's Motrin Cold Non-Staining Dye-Free Oral Suspension 1838
- Children's Motrin Cold Oral Suspension 1838
- Motrin Cold & Sinus Caplets 1836
- PediaCare Decongestant & Cough Infant Drops .... ▣ 705
- PediaCare Decongestant Infants' Drops .... ▣ 705
- PediaCare Long-Acting Cough Plus Cold Liquid .... ▣ 704
- PediaCare Multi-Symptom Cold Liquid .... ▣ 704
- PediaCare NightRest Cough & Cold Liquid .... ▣ 704
- Robitussin Allergy & Cough Syrup .... ▣ 750
- Robitussin CF Liquid .... ▣ 755
- Robitussin Cough & Cold Liquid-filled Capsules .... ▣ 750
- Robitussin Cough, Cold & Flu Liquid-filled Capsules .... ▣ 750
- Robitussin Cough & Cold Infant Drops .... ▣ 755
- Robitussin Flu Liquid .... ▣ 752
- Robitussin Maximum Strength Cough & Cold Liquid .... ▣ 754
- Robitussin PE Syrup .... ▣ 753
- Robitussin Pediatric Cough & Cold Liquid .... ▣ 754
- Robitussin PM Cough & Cold Liquid .... ▣ 752
- Robitussin Severe Congestion Liquid-filled Capsules .... ▣ 751
- Simply Stuffy Liquid 1841
- Singlet Caplets .... ▣ 636
- Sudafed 12 Hour Caplets .... ▣ 708
- Sudafed 24 Hour Tablets .... ▣ 709
- Sudafed Nasal Decongestant Tablets .... ▣ 709
- Sudafed Severe Cold .... ▣ 710
- Sudafed Non-Drying Sinus Liquid Caps .... ▣ 709
- Sudafed Sinus & Allergy Tablets .... ▣ 710
- Sudafed Sinus Headache .... ▣ 711
- TheraFlu Cold & Cough Hot Liquid .... ▣ 680
- TheraFlu Cold & Sore Throat Hot Liquid .... ▣ 680
- TheraFlu Flu & Chest Congestion Non-Drowsy Hot Liquid .... ▣ 681
- TheraFlu Flu & Sore Throat Hot Liquid .... ▣ 681
- TheraFlu Severe Cold Non-Drowsy Hot Liquid .... ▣ 683
- TheraFlu Severe Cold & Cough Hot Liquid .... ▣ 683
- TheraFlu Severe Cold Caplets .... ▣ 679
- TheraFlu Severe Cold Hot Liquid .... ▣ 682
- TheraFlu Severe Cold Non-Drowsy Caplets .... ▣ 679
- Triaminic Chest & Nasal Congestion Liquid .... ▣ 685
- Triaminic Cold & Allergy Liquid .... ▣ 685
- Triaminic Cold & Cough Liquid .... ▣ 685
- Triaminic Cough Liquid .... ▣ 687
- Triaminic Cough & Nasal Congestion Liquid .... ▣ 687
- Triaminic Cough & Sore Throat Liquid .... ▣ 687
- Triaminic Flu, Cough & Fever Liquid .... ▣ 685
- Triaminic Night Time Cough & Cold Liquid .... ▣ 685
- Triaminic Allergy Runny Nose & Congestion Softchews .... ▣ 688
- Triaminic Cold & Cough Softchews .... ▣ 688
- Triaminic Cough & Sore Throat Softchews .... ▣ 689
- Tylenol Sinus NightTime Caplets .... ▣ 663
- Children's Tylenol Plus Cold & Allergy Suspension Liquid 1850
- Children's Tylenol Plus Cold NightTime Suspension Liquid 1851
- Children's Tylenol Plus Cold & Cough Suspension Liquid and Chewable Tablets 1851
- Children's Tylenol Plus Cold Chewable Tablets 1851
- Children's Tylenol Plus Cold Daytime Non-Drowsy Suspension Liquid 1851
- Children's Tylenol Plus Flu Suspension Liquid 1853
- Concentrated Tylenol Infants' Drops Plus Cold 1851
- Concentrated Tylenol Infants' Drops Plus Cold and Cough 1851
- Tylenol Cold & Flu Severe Daytime Liquid with Cool Bust 1846
- Tylenol Cold & Flu Severe NightTime Liquid with Cool Burst 1846
- Tylenol Cold Severe Congestion Non-Drowsy Caplets with Cool Burst 1846
- Tylenol Allergy Complete Night Time Caplets 1844
- Tylenol Allergy Complete Multi-Symptom Caplets and Gelcaps with Cool Burst 1844
- Tylenol Flu NightTime Gelcaps 1846
- Tylenol Flu Day Non-Drowsy Gelcaps 1846
- Concentrated Tylenol Infants' Drops Plus Cold Nasal Congestant, Fever Reducer & Pain Reliever .... ▣ 668
- Concentrated Tylenol Infants' Drops Plus Cold & Cough Nasal Decongestant, Fever Reducer & Pain Reliever .... ▣ 668
- Multi-Symptom Tylenol Cold Night Time Caplets 1845
- Multi-Symptom Tylenol Cold Day Non-Drowsy Caplets and Gelcaps 1845
- Tylenol Sinus Day Non-Drowsy 1848
- Tylenol Sinus Night Time Caplets 1848
- Tylenol Sinus Severe Congestion Caplets with Cool Burst 1848
- Vicks 44D Cough & Head Congestion Relief 2676
- Vicks 44D Cough & Head Congestion Relief Liquid .... ▣ 721
- Vicks 44M Cough, Cold & Flu Relief 2676
- Pediatric Vicks 44m Cough & Cold Relief 2673
- Vicks DayQuil LiquiCaps/Liquid Multi-Symptom Cold/Flu Relief .... ▣ 723
- Vicks DayQuil Multi-Symptom Cold/Flu Relief LiquiCaps 2675
- Vicks DayQuil Multi-Symptom Cold/Flu Relief Liquid 2675
- Children's Vicks NyQuil Cold/Cough Relief 2671
- Vicks NyQuil LiquiCaps 2677
- Vicks NyQuil LiquiCaps/Liquid Multi-Symptom Cold/Flu Relief .... ▣ 725
- Vicks NyQuil Liquid 2677
- Zyrtec-D 12 Hour Extended Release Tablets 2591

Pseudoephedrine Sulfate (Concomitant use of digoxin and sympathomimetics increases the risk of cardiac arrhythmias). Products include:

- Alavert Allergy & Sinus D-12 Hour Tablets .... ▣ 743
- Clarinex-D 24-Hour Extended-Release Tablets 3012
- Claritin-D Non-Drowsy 12 Hour Tablets .... ▣ 731
- Claritin-D Non-Drowsy 24 Hour Tablets .... ▣ 731

Quinidine (Raises the serum digoxin concentration due to reduction in clearance and/or volume of distribution of the drug, with the implication that digitalis intoxication may result).

No products indexed under this heading.

Quinidine Gluconate (Raises the serum digoxin concentration due to reduction in clearance and/or volume of distribution of the drug, with the implication that digitalis intoxication may result).

No products indexed under this heading.

Quinidine Hydrochloride (Raises the serum digoxin concentration due to reduction in clearance and/or volume of distribution of the drug, with the implication that digitalis intoxication may result).
No products indexed under this heading.

Quinidine Polygalacturonate (Raises the serum digoxin concentration due to reduction in clearance and/or volume of distribution of the drug, with the implication that digitalis intoxication may result).
No products indexed under this heading.

Quinidine Sulfate (Raises the serum digoxin concentration due to reduction in clearance and/or volume of distribution of the drug, with the implication that digitalis intoxication may result).
No products indexed under this heading.

Quinine (Co-administration has resulted in inconsistent reports regarding the effects of quinine on serum digoxin concentration).
No products indexed under this heading.

Rifampin (May decrease serum digoxin concentration, especially in patients with renal dysfunction, by increasing the non-renal clearance of digoxin).
No products indexed under this heading.

Salmeterol Xinafoate (Concomitant use of digoxin and sympathomimetics increases the risk of cardiac arrhythmias). Products include:
- Advair Diskus 100/50 .... **1291**
- Advair Diskus 250/50 .... **1291**
- Advair Diskus 500/50 .... **1291**
- Serevent Diskus **1540**

Sodium Bicarbonate (Antacids may interfere with intestinal digoxin absorption, resulting in unexpectedly low serum concentrations; antacids may cause hypokalemia or hypomagnesemia and co-administration can cause digitalis toxicity). Products include:
- Ceo-Two Evacuant Suppository **607**
- Colyte with Flavor Packs for Oral Solution **3102**
- HalfLytely and Bisacodyl Tablets Bowel Prep Kit with Flavors Packs **915**
- TriLyte with Flavor Packs for Oral Solution **3114**

Sotalol Hydrochloride (Concomitant use of digoxin and beta-andrenergic blockers may result in the additive effects on AV node conduction).
No products indexed under this heading.

Spironolactone (Raises the serum digoxin concentration due to reduction in clearance and/or volume of distribution of the drug, with the implication that digitalis intoxication may result).
No products indexed under this heading.

Succinylcholine Chloride (May cause a sudden extrusion of potassium from muscle cells, and may thereby cause arrhythmias in digitalized patients).
No products indexed under this heading.

Sulfasalazine (May interfere with intestinal digoxin absorption, resulting in unexpectedly low serum concentrations).
No products indexed under this heading.

Terbutaline Sulfate (Concomitant use of digoxin and sympathomimetics increases the risk of cardiac arrhythmias).
No products indexed under this heading.

Tetracycline Hydrochloride (May increase digoxin absorption in patients who inactivate digoxin by bacterial metabolism in the lower intestine, so that digitalis intoxication may result).
No products indexed under this heading.

Thyroglobulin (Thyroid administration to a digitalized, hypothyroid patient may increase the dose requirement of digoxin).
No products indexed under this heading.

Thyroid (Thyroid administration to a digitalized, hypothyroid patient may increase the dose requirement of digoxin).
No products indexed under this heading.

Thyroxine (Thyroid administration to a digitalized, hypothyroid patient may increase the dose requirement of digoxin).
No products indexed under this heading.

Thyroxine Sodium (Thyroid administration to a digitalized, hypothyroid patient may increase the dose requirement of digoxin).
No products indexed under this heading.

Timolol Hemihydrate (Concomitant use of digoxin and beta-andrenergic blockers may result in the additive effects on AV node conduction). Products include:
- Betimol Ophthalmic Solution **3371**
- Betimol Ophthalmic Solution .... ⊙ **283**

Timolol Maleate (Concomitant use of digoxin and beta-andrenergic blockers may result in the additive effects on AV node conduction). Products include:
- Blocadren Tablets **1891**
- Cosopt Sterile Ophthalmic Solution **1910**
- Timolide Tablets **2056**
- Timoptic in Ocudose **2061**
- Timoptic Sterile Ophthalmic Solution **2058**
- Timoptic-XE Sterile Ophthalmic Gel Forming Solution **2062**

Torsemide (Potassium-depleting diuretics can cause hypokalemia and co-administration can result in digitalis toxicity).
No products indexed under this heading.

Triamcinolone (Corticosteroids can cause hypokalemia or hypomagnesemia and potassium or magnesium depletion can sensitize the myocardium to digoxin resulting in digitalis toxicity).
No products indexed under this heading.

Triamcinolone Acetonide (Corticosteroids can cause hypokalemia or hypomagnesemia and potassium or magnesium depletion can sensitize the myocardium to digoxin resulting in digitalis toxicity). Products include:
- Azmacort Inhalation Aerosol **1701**
- Nasacort HFA Inhalation Aerosol **2939**
- Nasacort AQ Nasal Spray **2937**

Triamcinolone Diacetate (Corticosteroids can cause hypokalemia or hypomagnesemia and potassium or magnesium depletion can sensitize the myocardium to digoxin resulting in digitalis toxicity).
No products indexed under this heading.

Triamcinolone Hexacetonide (Corticosteroids can cause hypokalemia or hypomagnesemia and potassium or magnesium depletion can sensitize the myocardium to digoxin resulting in digitalis toxicity).
No products indexed under this heading.

Troleandomycin (Macrolide antibiotics may possibly increase digoxin absorption in patients who inactivate digoxin by bacterial metabolism in the lower intestine, so that digitalis intoxication may result).
No products indexed under this heading.

Verapamil Hydrochloride (Raises the serum digoxin concentration due to reduction in clearance and/or volume of distribution of the drug, with the implication that digitalis intoxication may result). Products include:
- Covera-HS Tablets **3135**
- Tarka Tablets **519**
- Verelan PM Capsules **3120**

Food Interactions

Meal, high in bran fiber (The amount of digoxin from an oral dose may be reduced).

Meal, unspecified (Slows the rate of absorption).

LANOXIN INJECTION PEDIATRIC

(Digoxin) **1465**
See Lanoxin Tablets

LANTUS INJECTION

(Insulin glargine) **2925**
May interact with ACE inhibitors, beta blockers, corticosteroids, diuretics, fibrates, oral hypoglycemic agents, lithium preparations, monoamine oxidase inhibitors, oral contraceptives, phenothiazines, salicylates, sympathomimetics, thyroid preparations, and certain other agents. Compounds in these categories include:

Acarbose (May increase the blood-glucose-lowering effect and susceptibility to hypoglycemia). Products include:
- Precose Tablets **776**

Acebutolol Hydrochloride (Beta-blockers may either potentiate or weaken the blood-glucose-lowering effect of insulin; signs of hypoglycemia may be reduced or absent with co-administration).
No products indexed under this heading.

Albuterol (Sympathomimetic agents may reduce the blood-glucose-lowering effect of insulin). Products include:
- Proventil Inhalation Aerosol **3067**

Albuterol Sulfate (Sympathomimetic agents may reduce the blood-glucose-lowering effect of insulin). Products include:
- AccuNeb Inhalation Solution **1055**
- Combivent Inhalation Aerosol **878**
- DuoNeb Inhalation Solution **1058**
- Proventil Inhalation Solution 0.083% **3069**
- Proventil HFA Inhalation Aerosol **3071**
- Ventolin HFA Inhalation Aerosol **1576**
- VoSpire Extended-Release Tablets ... **2352**

Amiloride Hydrochloride (Diuretics may reduce the blood-glucose-lowering effect of insulin). Products include:
- Midamor Tablets **2000**
- Moduretic Tablets **2003**

Aspirin (May increase the blood-glucose-lowering effect and susceptibility to hypoglycemia). Products include:
- Aggrenox Capsules **855**
- Bayer, Aspirin Regimen **606**
- Bayer Aspirin Tablets **3515**
- BC Powder **612**
- BC Allergy Sinus Cold Powder **612**
- Arthritis Strength BC Powder **612**
- BC Sinus Cold Powder **612**
- Ecotrin Enteric Coated Aspirin Low, Regular and Maximum Strength Tablets **1627**
- Goody's Body Pain Formula Powder **621**
- Goody's Extra Strength Headache Powder **621**
- Goody's Extra Strength Pain Relief Tablets **621**
- Percodan Tablets **1115**
- St. Joseph 81 mg Aspirin Chewable and Enteric Coated Tablets **1841**

Aspirin, Enteric Coated (May increase the blood-glucose-lowering effect and susceptibility to hypoglycemia).
No products indexed under this heading.

Aspirin Buffered (May increase the blood-glucose-lowering effect and susceptibility to hypoglycemia).
No products indexed under this heading.

Atenolol (Beta-blockers may either potentiate or weaken the blood-glucose-lowering effect of insulin; signs of hypoglycemia may be reduced or absent with co-administration). Products include:
- Tenormin I.V. Injection **698**
- Tenormin Tablets **695**

Benazepril Hydrochloride (May increase the blood-glucose-lowering effect and susceptibility to hypoglycemia). Products include:
- Lotensin Tablets **2232**
- Lotensin HCT Tablets **2235**
- Lotrel Capsules **2238**

Bendroflumethiazide (Diuretics may reduce the blood-glucose-lowering effect of insulin).
No products indexed under this heading.

Betamethasone Acetate (Co-administration with corticosteroids may reduce the blood-glucose-lowering effect of insulin).
No products indexed under this heading.

Betamethasone Sodium Phosphate (Co-administration with corticosteroids may reduce the blood-glucose-lowering effect of insulin).
No products indexed under this heading.

Betaxolol Hydrochloride (Beta-blockers may either potentiate or weaken the blood-glucose-lowering effect of insulin; signs of hypoglycemia may be reduced or absent with co-administration). Products include:
- Betoptic S Ophthalmic Suspension.................................. **554**

IMPORTANT NOTE: Always consult each drug listing in the patient's regimen for possible interactions.

Bisoprolol Fumarate (Beta-blockers may either potentiate or weaken the blood-glucose-lowering effect of insulin; signs of hypoglycemia may be reduced or absent with co-administration).
No products indexed under this heading.

Bumetanide (Diuretics may reduce the blood-glucose-lowering effect of insulin).
No products indexed under this heading.

Captopril (May increase the blood-glucose-lowering effect and susceptibility to hypoglycemia). Products include:
Captopril Tablets 2114

Carteolol Hydrochloride (Beta-blockers may either potentiate or weaken the blood-glucose-lowering effect of insulin; signs of hypoglycemia may be reduced or absent with co-administration). Products include:
Carteolol Hydrochloride Ophthalmic Solution USP, 1% .... ⊙ 246

Chlorothiazide (Diuretics may reduce the blood-glucose-lowering effect of insulin). Products include:
Aldoclor Tablets 1881
Diuril Oral 1936

Chlorothiazide Sodium (Diuretics may reduce the blood-glucose-lowering effect of insulin). Products include:
Diuril Sodium Intravenous 1934

Chlorpromazine (Phenothiazine derivatives may reduce the blood-glucose-lowering effect of insulin).
No products indexed under this heading.

Chlorpromazine Hydrochloride (Phenothiazine derivatives may reduce the blood-glucose-lowering effect of insulin).
No products indexed under this heading.

Chlorpropamide (May increase the blood-glucose-lowering effect and susceptibility to hypoglycemia).
No products indexed under this heading.

Chlorthalidone (Diuretics may reduce the blood-glucose-lowering effect of insulin). Products include:
Clorpres Tablets 2139

Choline Magnesium Trisalicylate (May increase the blood-glucose-lowering effect and susceptibility to hypoglycemia).
No products indexed under this heading.

Clofibrate (May increase the blood-glucose-lowering effect and susceptibility to hypoglycemia).
No products indexed under this heading.

Clonidine (Signs of hypoglycemia may be reduced or absent with co-administration). Products include:
Catapres-TTS 875

Clonidine Hydrochloride (Signs of hypoglycemia may be reduced or absent with co-administration). Products include:
Catapres Tablets 874
Clorpres Tablets 2139

Cortisone Acetate (Co-administration with corticosteroids may reduce the blood-glucose-lowering effect of insulin).
No products indexed under this heading.

Danazol (May reduce the blood-glucose-lowering effect of insulin).
No products indexed under this heading.

Desogestrel (Oral contraceptives may reduce the blood-glucose-lowering effect of insulin). Products include:
Ortho-Cept Tablets 2395

Dexamethasone (Co-administration with corticosteroids may reduce the blood-glucose-lowering effect of insulin). Products include:
Ciprodex Otic Suspension 555
Decadron Tablets 1929
TobraDex Ophthalmic Ointment 558
TobraDex Ophthalmic Suspension 558

Dexamethasone Acetate (Co-administration with corticosteroids may reduce the blood-glucose-lowering effect of insulin).
No products indexed under this heading.

Dexamethasone Sodium Phosphate (Co-administration with corticosteroids may reduce the blood-glucose-lowering effect of insulin). Products include:
Decadron Phosphate Injection 1931

Diflunisal (May increase the blood-glucose-lowering effect and susceptibility to hypoglycemia). Products include:
Dolobid Tablets 1937

Disopyramide Phosphate (May increase the blood-glucose-lowering effect and susceptibility to hypoglycemia).
No products indexed under this heading.

Dobutamine Hydrochloride (Sympathomimetic agents may reduce the blood-glucose-lowering effect of insulin).
No products indexed under this heading.

Dopamine Hydrochloride (Sympathomimetic agents may reduce the blood-glucose-lowering effect of insulin).
No products indexed under this heading.

Enalapril Maleate (May increase the blood-glucose-lowering effect and susceptibility to hypoglycemia). Products include:
Vaseretic Tablets 2073
Vasotec I.V. Injection 2076

Enalaprilat (May increase the blood-glucose-lowering effect and susceptibility to hypoglycemia).
No products indexed under this heading.

Ephedrine Hydrochloride (Sympathomimetic agents may reduce the blood-glucose-lowering effect of insulin). Products include:
Primatene Tablets .... ▣ 749

Ephedrine Sulfate (Sympathomimetic agents may reduce the blood-glucose-lowering effect of insulin).
No products indexed under this heading.

Ephedrine Tannate (Sympathomimetic agents may reduce the blood-glucose-lowering effect of insulin).
No products indexed under this heading.

Epinephrine (Sympathomimetic agents may reduce the blood-glucose-lowering effect of insulin). Products include:
EpiPen 1061
Primatene Mist .... ▣ 749

Epinephrine Bitartrate (Sympathomimetic agents may reduce the blood-glucose-lowering effect of insulin).
No products indexed under this heading.

Epinephrine Hydrochloride (Sympathomimetic agents may reduce the blood-glucose-lowering effect of insulin).
No products indexed under this heading.

Esmolol Hydrochloride (Beta-blockers may either potentiate or weaken the blood-glucose-lowering effect of insulin; signs of hypoglycemia may be reduced or absent with co-administration). Products include:
Brevibloc Concentrate 766
Brevibloc Injection 766
Brevibloc Double Strength Injection 766
Brevibloc Premixed Injection 766
Brevibloc Double Strength Premixed Injection 766

Ethacrynic Acid (Diuretics may reduce the blood-glucose-lowering effect of insulin). Products include:
Edecrin Tablets 1941

Ethinyl Estradiol (Oral contraceptives may reduce the blood-glucose-lowering effect of insulin). Products include:
Alesse-28 Tablets 3392
Lo/Ovral-28 Tablets 3423
NuvaRing 2357
Ortho-Cept Tablets 2395
Ortho-Cyclen/Ortho Tri-Cyclen 2414
Ortho Evra Transdermal System 2402
Ortho Tri-Cyclen Lo Tablets 2421
Seasonale Tablets 1073
Triphasil-28 Tablets 3483
Yasmin 28 Tablets 818

Ethynodiol Diacetate (Oral contraceptives may reduce the blood-glucose-lowering effect of insulin).
No products indexed under this heading.

Fenofibrate (May increase the blood-glucose-lowering effect and susceptibility to hypoglycemia). Products include:
Antara Capsules 2723
Lofibra Capsules 1217
Tricor Tablets 523
Triglide Tablets 1165

Fludrocortisone Acetate (Co-administration with corticosteroids may reduce the blood-glucose-lowering effect of insulin).
No products indexed under this heading.

Fluoxetine Hydrochloride (May increase the blood-glucose-lowering effect and susceptibility to hypoglycemia). Products include:
Prozac Pulvules and Liquid 1771
Symbyax Capsules 1788

Fluphenazine Decanoate (Phenothiazine derivatives may reduce the blood-glucose-lowering effect of insulin).
No products indexed under this heading.

Fluphenazine Enanthate (Phenothiazine derivatives may reduce the blood-glucose-lowering effect of insulin).
No products indexed under this heading.

Fluphenazine Hydrochloride (Phenothiazine derivatives may reduce the blood-glucose-lowering effect of insulin).
No products indexed under this heading.

Fosinopril Sodium (May increase the blood-glucose-lowering effect and susceptibility to hypoglycemia).
No products indexed under this heading.

Furosemide (Diuretics may reduce the blood-glucose-lowering effect of insulin). Products include:
Furosemide Tablets 2117

Gemfibrozil (May increase the blood-glucose-lowering effect and susceptibility to hypoglycemia).
No products indexed under this heading.

Glimepiride (May increase the blood-glucose-lowering effect and susceptibility to hypoglycemia). Products include:
Amaryl Tablets 2864

Glipizide (May increase the blood-glucose-lowering effect and susceptibility to hypoglycemia).
No products indexed under this heading.

Glyburide (May increase the blood-glucose-lowering effect and susceptibility to hypoglycemia).
No products indexed under this heading.

Guanethidine Monosulfate (Signs of hypoglycemia may be reduced or absent with co-administration).
No products indexed under this heading.

Hydrochlorothiazide (Diuretics may reduce the blood-glucose-lowering effect of insulin). Products include:
Aldoril Tablets 1884
Atacand HCT 637
Avalide Tablets 2889
Avalide Tablets 922
Benicar HCT Tablets 2852
Diovan HCT Tablets 2195
Dyazide Capsules 1389
Hyzaar 1964
Lotensin HCT Tablets 2235
Maxzide 2150
Micardis HCT Tablets 886
Moduretic Tablets 2003
Prinzide Tablets 2033
Teveten HCT Tablets 1710
Timolide Tablets 2056
Uniretic Tablets 3114
Vaseretic Tablets 2073
Zestoretic Tablets 701

Hydrocortisone (Co-administration with corticosteroids may reduce the blood-glucose-lowering effect of insulin). Products include:
Cortizone•5 Ointment .... ▣ 699
Cortizone•10 Creme .... ▣ 699
Cortizone•10 Ointment .... ▣ 699
Cortizone•10 Plus Creme .... ▣ 700
Cortizone•10 Maximum Strength Quick Shot Spray .... ▣ 700
Hydrocortone Tablets 1963
Preparation H Hydrocortisone Cream .... ▣ 748

Hydrocortisone Acetate (Co-administration with corticosteroids may reduce the blood-glucose-lowering effect of insulin). Products include:
Analpram-HC 1136
Pramosone 1139
ProctoFoam-HC 3113
Tucks Anti-Itch Ointment .... ▣ 712
U-cort 1% Cream 3289

Hydrocortisone Sodium Phosphate (Co-administration with corticosteroids may reduce the blood-glucose-lowering effect of insulin).
No products indexed under this heading.

Hydrocortisone Sodium Succinate (Co-administration with corticosteroids may reduce the blood-glucose-lowering effect of insulin).
No products indexed under this heading.

Hydroflumethiazide (Diuretics may reduce the blood-glucose-lowering effect of insulin).
No products indexed under this heading.

Indapamide (Diuretics may reduce the blood-glucose-lowering effect of insulin). Products include:
Indapamide Tablets 2119

Isocarboxazid (May increase the blood-glucose-lowering effect and susceptibility to hypoglycemia).
No products indexed under this heading.

Isoniazid (May reduce the blood-glucose-lowering effect of insulin).
No products indexed under this heading.

Isoproterenol Hydrochloride (Sympathomimetic agents may reduce the blood-glucose-lowering effect of insulin).
No products indexed under this heading.

Isoproterenol Sulfate (Sympathomimetic agents may reduce the blood-glucose-lowering effect of insulin).
No products indexed under this heading.

Labetalol Hydrochloride (Beta-blockers may either potentiate or weaken the blood-glucose-lowering effect of insulin; signs of hypoglycemia may be reduced or absent with co-administration).
No products indexed under this heading.

Levalbuterol Hydrochloride (Sympathomimetic agents may reduce the blood-glucose-lowering effect of insulin). Products include:
Xopenex Inhalation Solution 3143
Xopenex Inhalation Solution Concentrate 3147

Levobunolol Hydrochloride (Beta-blockers may either potentiate or weaken the blood-glucose-lowering effect of insulin; signs of hypoglycemia may be reduced or absent with co-administration). Products include:
Betagan Ophthalmic Solution, USP.. ⊙217

Levonorgestrel (Oral contraceptives may reduce the blood-glucose-lowering effect of insulin). Products include:
Alesse-28 Tablets 3392
Climara Pro Transdermal System 800
Mirena Intrauterine System 810
Plan B Tablets 1068
Seasonale Tablets 1073
Triphasil-28 Tablets 3483

Levothyroxine Sodium (May reduce the blood-glucose-lowering effect of insulin). Products include:
Levothroid Tablets 1189
Levoxyl Tablets 1680
Synthroid Tablets 515
Unithroid Tablets 3521

Liothyronine Sodium (May reduce the blood-glucose-lowering effect of insulin). Products include:
Cytomel Tablets 1678

Liotrix (May reduce the blood-glucose-lowering effect of insulin). Products include:
Thyrolar 1203

Lisinopril (May increase the blood-glucose-lowering effect and susceptibility to hypoglycemia). Products include:
Prinivil Tablets 2029
Prinzide Tablets 2033
Zestoretic Tablets 701
Zestril Tablets 704

Lithium (May either potentiate or weaken the blood-glucose-lowering effect of insulin).
No products indexed under this heading.

Lithium Carbonate (May either potentiate or weaken the blood-glucose-lowering effect of insulin). Products include:
Eskalith 1406
Lithobid Tablets 1670

Lithium Citrate (May either potentiate or weaken the blood-glucose-lowering effect of insulin).
No products indexed under this heading.

Magnesium Salicylate (May increase the blood-glucose-lowering effect and susceptibility to hypoglycemia).
No products indexed under this heading.

Mesoridazine Besylate (Phenothiazine derivatives may reduce the blood-glucose-lowering effect of insulin).
No products indexed under this heading.

Mestranol (Oral contraceptives may reduce the blood-glucose-lowering effect of insulin).
No products indexed under this heading.

Metaproterenol Sulfate (Sympathomimetic agents may reduce the blood-glucose-lowering effect of insulin). Products include:
Alupent Inhalation Aerosol 858

Metaraminol Bitartrate (Sympathomimetic agents may reduce the blood-glucose-lowering effect of insulin). Products include:
Aramine Injection 1889

Metformin Hydrochloride (May increase the blood-glucose-lowering effect and susceptibility to hypoglycemia). Products include:
ActoPlus Met Tablets 3219
Avandamet Tablets 1343
Fortamet Extended-Release Tablets 1156

Methotrimeprazine (Phenothiazine derivatives may reduce the blood-glucose-lowering effect of insulin).
No products indexed under this heading.

Methoxamine Hydrochloride (Sympathomimetic agents may reduce the blood-glucose-lowering effect of insulin).
No products indexed under this heading.

Methyclothiazide (Diuretics may reduce the blood-glucose-lowering effect of insulin).
No products indexed under this heading.

Methylprednisolone Acetate (Co-administration with corticosteroids may reduce the blood-glucose-lowering effect of insulin). Products include:
Depo-Medrol Injectable Suspension 2615
Depo-Medrol Single-Dose Vial 2617

Methylprednisolone Sodium Succinate (Co-administration with corticosteroids may reduce the blood-glucose-lowering effect of insulin).
No products indexed under this heading.

Metipranolol Hydrochloride (Beta-blockers may either potentiate or weaken the blood-glucose-lowering effect of insulin; signs of hypoglycemia may be reduced or absent with co-administration).
No products indexed under this heading.

Metolazone (Diuretics may reduce the blood-glucose-lowering effect of insulin).
No products indexed under this heading.

Metoprolol Succinate (Beta-blockers may either potentiate or weaken the blood-glucose-lowering effect of insulin; signs of hypoglycemia may be reduced or absent with co-administration). Products include:
Toprol-XL Tablets 660

Metoprolol Tartrate (Beta-blockers may either potentiate or weaken the blood-glucose-lowering effect of insulin; signs of hypoglycemia may be reduced or absent with co-administration).
No products indexed under this heading.

Miglitol (May increase the blood-glucose-lowering effect and susceptibility to hypoglycemia).
No products indexed under this heading.

Moclobemide (May increase the blood-glucose-lowering effect and susceptibility to hypoglycemia).
No products indexed under this heading.

Moexipril Hydrochloride (May increase the blood-glucose-lowering effect and susceptibility to hypoglycemia). Products include:
Uniretic Tablets 3114
Univasc Tablets 3118

Nadolol (Beta-blockers may either potentiate or weaken the blood-glucose-lowering effect of insulin; signs of hypoglycemia may be reduced or absent with co-administration). Products include:
Nadolol Tablets 2121

Norepinephrine Bitartrate (Sympathomimetic agents may reduce the blood-glucose-lowering effect of insulin).
No products indexed under this heading.

Norethindrone (Oral contraceptives may reduce the blood-glucose-lowering effect of insulin). Products include:
Ortho Micronor Tablets 2411

Norethynodrel (Oral contraceptives may reduce the blood-glucose-lowering effect of insulin).
No products indexed under this heading.

Norgestimate (Oral contraceptives may reduce the blood-glucose-lowering effect of insulin). Products include:
Ortho-Cyclen/Ortho Tri-Cyclen 2414
Ortho Tri-Cyclen Lo Tablets 2421
Prefest Tablets 1069

Norgestrel (Oral contraceptives may reduce the blood-glucose-lowering effect of insulin). Products include:
Lo/Ovral-28 Tablets 3423

Octreotide Acetate (May increase the blood-glucose-lowering effect and susceptibility to hypoglycemia). Products include:
Sandostatin Injection 2263
Sandostatin LAR Depot 2264

Pargyline Hydrochloride (May increase the blood-glucose-lowering effect and susceptibility to hypoglycemia).
No products indexed under this heading.

Penbutolol Sulfate (Beta-blockers may either potentiate or weaken the blood-glucose-lowering effect of insulin; signs of hypoglycemia may be reduced or absent with co-administration).
No products indexed under this heading.

Pentamidine Isethionate (May cause hypoglycemia, which may sometimes be followed by hyperglycemia).
No products indexed under this heading.

Perindopril Erbumine (May increase the blood-glucose-lowering effect and susceptibility to hypoglycemia). Products include:
Aceon Tablets (2 mg, 4 mg, 8 mg).. 3191

Perphenazine (Phenothiazine derivatives may reduce the blood-glucose-lowering effect of insulin).
No products indexed under this heading.

Phenelzine Sulfate (May increase the blood-glucose-lowering effect and susceptibility to hypoglycemia).
No products indexed under this heading.

Phenylephrine Bitartrate (Sympathomimetic agents may reduce the blood-glucose-lowering effect of insulin).
No products indexed under this heading.

Phenylephrine Hydrochloride (Sympathomimetic agents may reduce the blood-glucose-lowering effect of insulin). Products include:
Alacol DM Syrup 739
Hycomine Compound Tablets 1105
Preparation H Maximum Strength Cream 747
Preparation H Cooling Gel 747
Preparation H 747
Sudafed PE Tablets 711
Vicks Sinex Nasal Spray and Ultra Fine Mist for Sinus Relief.............. 2677
Zicam Concentrated Cough Mist for Kids Plus D Cool Cherry........ 643
Zicam Concentrated Cough Mist Plus D Cool Cherry...................... 642

Phenylephrine Tannate (Sympathomimetic agents may reduce the blood-glucose-lowering effect of insulin).
No products indexed under this heading.

Phenylpropanolamine Hydrochloride (Sympathomimetic agents may reduce the blood-glucose-lowering effect of insulin).
No products indexed under this heading.

Pindolol (Beta-blockers may either potentiate or weaken the blood-glucose-lowering effect of insulin; signs of hypoglycemia may be reduced or absent with co-administration).
No products indexed under this heading.

Pioglitazone Hydrochloride (May increase the blood-glucose-lowering effect and susceptibility to hypoglycemia). Products include:

ActoPlus Met Tablets 3219
Actos Tablets 3224

Pirbuterol Acetate (Sympathomimetic agents may reduce the blood-glucose-lowering effect of insulin). Products include:

Maxair Autohaler 1820

Polythiazide (Diuretics may reduce the blood-glucose-lowering effect of insulin).

No products indexed under this heading.

Prednisolone Acetate (Co-administration with corticosteroids may reduce the blood-glucose-lowering effect of insulin). Products include:

Blephamide Ophthalmic Ointment 563
Blephamide Ophthalmic Suspension 564
Poly-Pred Liquifilm Ophthalmic Suspension .... ⊙231
Pred Forte Ophthalmic Suspension .... ⊙233
Pred Mild Sterile Ophthalmic Suspension .... ⊙236
Pred-G Ophthalmic Suspension .... ⊙234
Pred-G Sterile Ophthalmic Ointment .... ⊙235

Prednisolone Sodium Phosphate (Co-administration with corticosteroids may reduce the blood-glucose-lowering effect of insulin). Products include:

Pediapred Oral Solution 3319

Prednisolone Tebutate (Co-administration with corticosteroids may reduce the blood-glucose-lowering effect of insulin).

No products indexed under this heading.

Prednisone (Co-administration with corticosteroids may reduce the blood-glucose-lowering effect of insulin).

No products indexed under this heading.

Procarbazine Hydrochloride (May increase the blood-glucose-lowering effect and susceptibility to hypoglycemia). Products include:

Matulane Capsules 3188

Prochlorperazine (Phenothiazine derivatives may reduce the blood-glucose-lowering effect of insulin).

No products indexed under this heading.

Promethazine Hydrochloride (Phenothiazine derivatives may reduce the blood-glucose-lowering effect of insulin). Products include:

Phenergan 3438

Propoxyphene Hydrochloride (May increase the blood-glucose-lowering effect and susceptibility to hypoglycemia).

No products indexed under this heading.

Propoxyphene Napsylate (May increase the blood-glucose-lowering effect and susceptibility to hypoglycemia). Products include:

Darvocet A 500 Tablets 3497

Propranolol Hydrochloride (Beta-blockers may either potentiate or weaken the blood-glucose-lowering effect of insulin; signs of hypoglycemia may be reduced or absent with co-administration). Products include:

Inderal LA Long-Acting Capsules 3421
InnoPran XL Capsules 2728

Pseudoephedrine Hydrochloride (Sympathomimetic agents may reduce the blood-glucose-lowering effect of insulin). Products include:

Advil Allergy Sinus Caplets .... ◙737
Advil Cold & Sinus .... ◙739
Advil Flu & Body Ache Caplets .... ◙739
Children's Advil Cold Suspension .... ◙741
Advil Multi-Symptom Cold Caplets .... ◙738
Allegra-D 12 Hour Extended-Release Tablets 2860
Allegra-D 24 Hour Extended-Release Tablets 2862
Balamine DM 739
BC Cold Powder .... ◙612
Benadryl Allergy & Cold Tablets .... ◙692
Benadryl Allergy & Sinus Headache Caplets & Gelcaps .... ◙693
Children's Benadryl Allergy & Cold Fastmelt Tablets .... ◙695
Benadryl Maximum Strength Severe Allergy & Sinus Headache Caplets .... ◙694
Children's Benadryl D Allergy & Sinus Fastmelt Tablets .... ◙694
Children's Benadryl D Liquid Medication .... ◙693
Benadryl D Tablets .... ◙694
Contac Non-Drowsy 12 Hour Cold Caplets .... ◙614
Contac Non-Drowsy Timed Release 12 Hour Cold Caplets .... ◙615
Contac Severe Cold and Flu Caplets Maximum Strength .... ◙615
Contac Severe Cold and Flu Caplets Non-Drowsy .... ◙615
Children's Dimetapp Cold & Allergy Elixir .... ◙745
Children's Dimetapp DM Cold & Cough Elixir .... ◙745
Children's Dimetapp Long Acting Cough Plus Cold Syrup .... ◙746
Dimetapp Infant Drops Decongestant Plus Cough .... ◙746
Children's Motrin Cold Non-Staining Dye-Free Oral Suspension 1838
Children's Motrin Cold Oral Suspension 1838
Motrin Cold & Sinus Caplets 1836
PediaCare Decongestant & Cough Infant Drops .... ◙705
PediaCare Decongestant Infants' Drops .... ◙705
PediaCare Long-Acting Cough Plus Cold Liquid .... ◙704
PediaCare Multi-Symptom Cold Liquid .... ◙704
PediaCare NightRest Cough & Cold Liquid .... ◙704
Robitussin Allergy & Cough Syrup .... ◙750
Robitussin CF Liquid .... ◙755
Robitussin Cough & Cold Liquid-filled Capsules .... ◙750
Robitussin Cough, Cold & Flu Liquid-filled Capsules .... ◙750
Robitussin Cough & Cold Infant Drops .... ◙755
Robitussin Flu Liquid .... ◙752
Robitussin Maximum Strength Cough & Cold Liquid .... ◙754
Robitussin PE Syrup .... ◙753
Robitussin Pediatric Cough & Cold Liquid .... ◙754
Robitussin PM Cough & Cold Liquid .... ◙752
Robitussin Severe Congestion Liquid-filled Capsules .... ◙751
Simply Stuffy Liquid 1841
Singlet Caplets .... ◙636
Sudafed 12 Hour Caplets .... ◙708
Sudafed 24 Hour Tablets .... ◙709
Sudafed Nasal Decongestant Tablets .... ◙709
Sudafed Severe Cold .... ◙710
Sudafed Non-Drying Sinus Liquid Caps .... ◙709
Sudafed Sinus & Allergy Tablets .... ◙710
Sudafed Sinus Headache .... ◙711
TheraFlu Cold & Cough Hot Liquid .... ◙680
TheraFlu Cold & Sore Throat Hot Liquid .... ◙680
TheraFlu Flu & Chest Congestion Non-Drowsy Hot Liquid .... ◙681
TheraFlu Flu & Sore Throat Hot Liquid .... ◙681
TheraFlu Severe Cold Non-Drowsy Hot Liquid .... ◙683
TheraFlu Severe Cold & Cough Hot Liquid .... ◙683
TheraFlu Severe Cold Caplets .... ◙679
TheraFlu Severe Cold Hot Liquid .... ◙682
TheraFlu Severe Cold Non-Drowsy Caplets .... ◙679
Triaminic Chest & Nasal Congestion Liquid .... ◙685
Triaminic Cold & Allergy Liquid .... ◙685
Triaminic Cold & Cough Liquid .... ◙685
Triaminic Cough Liquid .... ◙687
Triaminic Cough & Nasal Congestion Liquid .... ◙687
Triaminic Cough & Sore Throat Liquid .... ◙687
Triaminic Flu, Cough & Fever Liquid .... ◙685
Triaminic Night Time Cough & Cold Liquid .... ◙685
Triaminic Allergy Runny Nose & Congestion Softchews .... ◙688
Triaminic Cold & Cough Softchews .... ◙688
Triaminic Cough & Sore Throat Softchews .... ◙689
Tylenol Sinus NightTime Caplets .... ◙663
Children's Tylenol Plus Cold & Allergy Suspension Liquid 1850
Children's Tylenol Plus Cold NightTime Suspension Liquid 1851
Children's Tylenol Plus Cold & Cough Suspension Liquid and Chewable Tablets 1851
Children's Tylenol Plus Cold Chewable Tablets 1851
Children's Tylenol Plus Cold Daytime Non-Drowsy Suspension Liquid 1851
Children's Tylenol Plus Flu Suspension Liquid 1853
Concentrated Tylenol Infants' Drops Plus Cold 1851
Concentrated Tylenol Infants' Drops Plus Cold and Cough 1851
Tylenol Cold & Flu Severe Daytime Liquid with Cool Bust 1846
Tylenol Cold & Flu Severe NightTime Liquid with Cool Burst 1846
Tylenol Cold Severe Congestion Non-Drowsy Caplets with Cool Burst 1846
Tylenol Allergy Complete Night Time Caplets 1844
Tylenol Allergy Complete Multi-Symptom Caplets and Gelcaps with Cool Burst 1844
Tylenol Flu NightTime Gelcaps 1846
Tylenol Flu Day Non-Drowsy Gelcaps 1846
Concentrated Tylenol Infants' Drops Plus Cold Nasal Congestant, Fever Reducer & Pain Reliever .... ◙668
Concentrated Tylenol Infants' Drops Plus Cold & Cough Nasal Decongestant, Fever Reducer & Pain Reliever .... ◙668
Multi-Symptom Tylenol Cold Night Time Caplets 1845
Multi-Symptom Tylenol Cold Day Non-Drowsy Caplets and Gelcaps 1845
Tylenol Sinus Day Non-Drowsy 1848
Tylenol Sinus Night Time Caplets 1848
Tylenol Sinus Severe Congestion Caplets with Cool Burst 1848
Vicks 44D Cough & Head Congestion Relief 2676
Vicks 44D Cough & Head Congestion Relief Liquid .... ◙721
Vicks 44M Cough, Cold & Flu Relief 2676
Pediatric Vicks 44m Cough & Cold Relief 2673
Vicks DayQuil LiquiCaps/Liquid Multi-Symptom Cold/Flu Relief .... ◙723
Vicks DayQuil Multi-Symptom Cold/Flu Relief LiquiCaps 2675
Vicks DayQuil Multi-Symptom Cold/Flu Relief Liquid 2675
Children's Vicks NyQuil Cold/Cough Relief 2671
Vicks NyQuil LiquiCaps 2677
Vicks NyQuil LiquiCaps/Liquid Multi-Symptom Cold/Flu Relief .... ◙725
Vicks NyQuil Liquid 2677
Zyrtec-D 12 Hour Extended Release Tablets 2591

Pseudoephedrine Sulfate (Sympathomimetic agents may reduce the blood-glucose-lowering effect of insulin). Products include:

Alavert Allergy & Sinus D-12 Hour Tablets .... ◙743
Clarinex-D 24-Hour Extended-Release Tablets 3012
Claritin-D Non-Drowsy 12 Hour Tablets .... ◙731
Claritin-D Non-Drowsy 24 Hour Tablets .... ◙731

Quinapril Hydrochloride (May increase the blood-glucose-lowering effect and susceptibility to hypoglycemia).

No products indexed under this heading.

Ramipril (May increase the blood-glucose-lowering effect and susceptibility to hypoglycemia). Products include:

Altace Capsules 1673

Repaglinide (May increase the blood-glucose-lowering effect and susceptibility to hypoglycemia). Products include:

Prandin Tablets (0.5, 1, and 2 mg) 2337

Reserpine (Signs of hypoglycemia may be reduced or absent with co-administration).

No products indexed under this heading.

Rosiglitazone Maleate (May increase the blood-glucose-lowering effect and susceptibility to hypoglycemia). Products include:

Avandamet Tablets 1343
Avandia Tablets 1348

Salmeterol Xinafoate (Sympathomimetic agents may reduce the blood-glucose-lowering effect of insulin). Products include:

Advair Diskus 100/50 1291
Advair Diskus 250/50 1291
Advair Diskus 500/50 1291
Serevent Diskus 1540

Salsalate (May increase the blood-glucose-lowering effect and susceptibility to hypoglycemia).

No products indexed under this heading.

Selegiline Hydrochloride (May increase the blood-glucose-lowering effect and susceptibility to hypoglycemia). Products include:

Eldepryl Capsules 3209

Somatropin (May reduce the blood-glucose-lowering effect of insulin). Products include:

Genotropin Lyophilized Powder 2642
Humatrope Vials and Cartridges 1756
Norditropin Cartridges 2318
Nutropin for Injection 1238
Nutropin AQ Injection 1241
Nutropin AQ Pen 1241
Nutropin AQ Pen Cartridge 1241

Sotalol Hydrochloride (Beta-blockers may either potentiate or weaken the blood-glucose-lowering effect of insulin; signs of hypoglycemia may be reduced or absent with co-administration).

No products indexed under this heading.

Spirapril Hydrochloride (May increase the blood-glucose-lowering effect and susceptibility to hypoglycemia).

No products indexed under this heading.

(◙ Described in PDR For Nonprescription Drugs)

(⊙ Described in PDR For Ophthalmic Medicines™)

Spironolactone (Diuretics may reduce the blood-glucose-lowering effect of insulin).
No products indexed under this heading.

Sulfamethoxazole (Co-administration with sulfonamide antibiotics may increase the blood-glucose-lowering effect and susceptibility to hypoglycemia).
No products indexed under this heading.

Sulfisoxazole Acetyl (Co-administration with sulfonamide antibiotics may increase the blood-glucose-lowering effect and susceptibility to hypoglycemia).
No products indexed under this heading.

Terbutaline Sulfate (Sympathomimetic agents may reduce the blood-glucose-lowering effect of insulin).
No products indexed under this heading.

Thioridazine Hydrochloride (Phenothiazine derivatives may reduce the blood-glucose-lowering effect of insulin). Products include:
Thioridazine Hydrochloride Tablets 2122

Thyroglobulin (May reduce the blood-glucose-lowering effect of insulin).
No products indexed under this heading.

Thyroid (May reduce the blood-glucose-lowering effect of insulin).
No products indexed under this heading.

Thyroxine (May reduce the blood-glucose-lowering effect of insulin).
No products indexed under this heading.

Thyroxine Sodium (May reduce the blood-glucose-lowering effect of insulin).
No products indexed under this heading.

Timolol Hemihydrate (Beta-blockers may either potentiate or weaken the blood-glucose-lowering effect of insulin; signs of hypoglycemia may be reduced or absent with co-administration). Products include:
Betimol Ophthalmic Solution 3371
Betimol Ophthalmic Solution .... ⊙ 283

Timolol Maleate (Beta-blockers may either potentiate or weaken the blood-glucose-lowering effect of insulin; signs of hypoglycemia may be reduced or absent with co-administration). Products include:
Blocadren Tablets 1891
Cosopt Sterile Ophthalmic Solution 1910
Timolide Tablets 2056
Timoptic in Ocudose 2061
Timoptic Sterile Ophthalmic Solution 2058
Timoptic-XE Sterile Ophthalmic Gel Forming Solution 2062

Tolazamide (May increase the blood-glucose-lowering effect and susceptibility to hypoglycemia).
No products indexed under this heading.

Tolbutamide (May increase the blood-glucose-lowering effect and susceptibility to hypoglycemia).
No products indexed under this heading.

Torsemide (Diuretics may reduce the blood-glucose-lowering effect of insulin).
No products indexed under this heading.

Trandolapril (May increase the blood-glucose-lowering effect and susceptibility to hypoglycemia). Products include:
Mavik Tablets 482
Tarka Tablets 519

Tranylcypromine Sulfate (May increase the blood-glucose-lowering effect and susceptibility to hypoglycemia). Products include:
Parnate Tablets 1499

Triamcinolone (Co-administration with corticosteroids may reduce the blood-glucose-lowering effect of insulin).
No products indexed under this heading.

Triamcinolone Acetonide (Co-administration with corticosteroids may reduce the blood-glucose-lowering effect of insulin). Products include:
Azmacort Inhalation Aerosol 1701
Nasacort HFA Inhalation Aerosol 2939
Nasacort AQ Nasal Spray 2937

Triamcinolone Diacetate (Co-administration with corticosteroids may reduce the blood-glucose-lowering effect of insulin).
No products indexed under this heading.

Triamcinolone Hexacetonide (Co-administration with corticosteroids may reduce the blood-glucose-lowering effect of insulin).
No products indexed under this heading.

Triamterene (Diuretics may reduce the blood-glucose-lowering effect of insulin). Products include:
Dyazide Capsules 1389
Dyrenium Capsules 3390
Maxzide 2150

Trifluoperazine Hydrochloride (Phenothiazine derivatives may reduce the blood-glucose-lowering effect of insulin).
No products indexed under this heading.

Troglitazone (May increase the blood-glucose-lowering effect and susceptibility to hypoglycemia).
No products indexed under this heading.

Food Interactions

Alcohol (May either potentiate or weaken the blood-glucose-lowering effect of insulin).

LARIAM TABLETS

(Mefloquine Hydrochloride) 2790

May interact with antiarrhythmics, beta blockers, calcium channel blockers, anticonvulsants, phenothiazines, quinidine, tricyclic antidepressants, and certain other agents. Compounds in these categories include:

Acebutolol Hydrochloride (There is a theoretical possibility that co-administration of other drugs known to alter cardiac conduction, such as beta blockers, might also contribute to a prolongation of the QTc interval).
No products indexed under this heading.

Adenosine (There is a theoretical possibility that co-administration of other drugs known to alter cardiac conduction, such as antiarrhythmic agents, might also contribute to a prolongation of the QTc interval). Products include:
Adenocard Injection 612
Adenoscan 613

Amiodarone Hydrochloride (There is a theoretical possibility that co-administration of other drugs known to alter cardiac conduction, such as antiarrhythmic agents, might also contribute to a prolongation of the QTc interval). Products include:
Pacerone Tablets 3337

Amitriptyline Hydrochloride (There is a theoretical possibility that co-administration of other drugs known to alter cardiac conduction, such as tricyclic antidepressants, might also contribute to a prolongation of the QTc interval).
No products indexed under this heading.

Amlodipine Besylate (There is a theoretical possibility that co-administration of other drugs known to alter cardiac conduction, such as calcium channel blockers, might also contribute to a prolongation of the QTc interval). Products include:
Caduet Tablets 2507
Lotrel Capsules 2238
Norvasc Tablets 2529

Amoxapine (There is a theoretical possibility that co-administration of other drugs known to alter cardiac conduction, such as tricyclic antidepressants, might also contribute to a prolongation of the QTc interval).
No products indexed under this heading.

Astemizole (There is a theoretical possibility that co-administration of other drugs known to alter cardiac conduction, such as antihistamine astemizole, might also contribute to a prolongation of the QTc interval).
No products indexed under this heading.

Atenolol (There is a theoretical possibility that co-administration of other drugs known to alter cardiac conduction, such as beta blockers, might also contribute to a prolongation of the QTc interval). Products include:
Tenormin I.V. Injection 698
Tenormin Tablets 695

Bepridil Hydrochloride (There is a theoretical possibility that co-administration of other drugs known to alter cardiac conduction, such as calcium channel blockers, might also contribute to a prolongation of the QTc interval).
No products indexed under this heading.

Betaxolol Hydrochloride (There is a theoretical possibility that co-administration of other drugs known to alter cardiac conduction, such as beta blockers, might also contribute to a prolongation of the QTc interval). Products include:
Betoptic S Ophthalmic Suspension 554

Bisoprolol Fumarate (There is a theoretical possibility that co-administration of other drugs known to alter cardiac conduction, such as beta blockers, might also contribute to a prolongation of the QTc interval).
No products indexed under this heading.

Bretylium Tosylate (There is a theoretical possibility that co-administration of other drugs known to alter cardiac conduction, such as antiarrhythmic agents, might also contribute to a prolongation of the QTc interval).
No products indexed under this heading.

Carbamazepine (Co-administration may reduce seizure control by lowering the plasma levels of anticonvulsant; dosage of anticonvulsant may need to be adjusted). Products include:
Carbatrol Capsules 3174
Equetro Extended-Release Capsules 3178
Tegretol/Tegretol-XR 2278

Carteolol Hydrochloride (There is a theoretical possibility that co-administration of other drugs known to alter cardiac conduction, such as beta blockers, might also contribute to a prolongation of the QTc interval). Products include:
Carteolol Hydrochloride Ophthalmic Solution USP, 1% .... ⊙ 246

Chloroquine Hydrochloride (Co-administration may produce electrocardiographic abnormalities and increase the risk of convulsions; if these drugs are to be used in the initial treatment of severe malaria, mefloquine administration should be delayed at least 12 hours after the last dose).
No products indexed under this heading.

Chloroquine Phosphate (Co-administration may produce electrocardiographic abnormalities and increase the risk of convulsions; if these drugs are to be used in the initial treatment of severe malaria, mefloquine administration should be delayed at least 12 hours after the last dose).
No products indexed under this heading.

Chlorpromazine (There is a theoretical possibility that co-administration of other drugs known to alter cardiac conduction, such as phenothiazines, might also contribute to a prolongation of the QTc interval).
No products indexed under this heading.

Chlorpromazine Hydrochloride (There is a theoretical possibility that co-administration of other drugs known to alter cardiac conduction, such as phenothiazines, might also contribute to a prolongation of the QTc interval).
No products indexed under this heading.

Clomipramine Hydrochloride (There is a theoretical possibility that co-administration of other drugs known to alter cardiac conduction, such as tricyclic antidepressants, might also contribute to a prolongation of the QTc interval).
No products indexed under this heading.

Desipramine Hydrochloride (There is a theoretical possibility that co-administration of other drugs known to alter cardiac conduction, such as tricyclic antidepressants, might also contribute to a prolongation of the QTc interval).
No products indexed under this heading.

Diltiazem Hydrochloride (There is a theoretical possibility that co-administration of other drugs known to alter cardiac conduction, such as calcium channel blockers, might also contribute to a prolongation of the QTc interval). Products include:
Cardizem LA Extended Release Tablets 1699
Tiazac Capsules 1204

Disopyramide Phosphate (There is a theoretical possibility that co-administration of other drugs known to alter cardiac conduction, such as antiarrhythmic agents, might also contribute to a prolongation of the QTc interval).
No products indexed under this heading.

Divalproex Sodium (Co-administration may reduce seizure control by lowering the plasma levels of anticonvulsant; dosage of anticonvulsant may need to be adjusted). Products include:
Depakote Sprinkle Capsules 422
Depakote Tablets 427
Depakote ER Tablets 433

Dofetilide (There is a theoretical possibility that co-administration of other drugs known to alter cardiac conduction, such as antiarrhythmic agents, might also contribute to a prolongation of the QTc interval).
No products indexed under this heading.

Doxepin Hydrochloride (There is a theoretical possibility that co-administration of other drugs known to alter cardiac conduction, such as tricyclic antidepressants, might also contribute to a prolongation of the QTc interval).
No products indexed under this heading.

Esmolol Hydrochloride (There is a theoretical possibility that co-administration of other drugs known to alter cardiac conduction, such as beta blockers, might also contribute to a prolongation of the QTc interval). Products include:
Brevibloc Concentrate 766
Brevibloc Injection 766
Brevibloc Double Strength Injection..................................... 766
Brevibloc Premixed Injection 766
Brevibloc Double Strength Premixed Injection....................... 766

Ethosuximide (Co-administration may reduce seizure control by lowering the plasma levels of anticonvulsant; dosage of anticonvulsant may need to be adjusted).
No products indexed under this heading.

Ethotoin (Co-administration may reduce seizure control by lowering the plasma levels of anticonvulsant; dosage of anticonvulsant may need to be adjusted). Products include:
Peganone Tablets, USP 2487

Felbamate (Co-administration may reduce seizure control by lowering the plasma levels of anticonvulsant; dosage of anticonvulsant may need to be adjusted).
No products indexed under this heading.

Felodipine (There is a theoretical possibility that co-administration of other drugs known to alter cardiac conduction, such as calcium channel blockers, might also contribute to a prolongation of the QTc interval).
Products include:
Plendil Extended-Release Tablets 651

Flecainide Acetate (There is a theoretical possibility that co-administration of other drugs known to alter cardiac conduction, such as antiarrhythmic agents, might also contribute to a prolongation of the QTc interval). Products include:
Tambocor Tablets 1824

Fluphenazine Decanoate (There is a theoretical possibility that co-administration of other drugs known to alter cardiac conduction, such as phenothiazines, might also contribute to a prolongation of the QTc interval).
No products indexed under this heading.

Fluphenazine Enanthate (There is a theoretical possibility that co-administration of other drugs known to alter cardiac conduction, such as phenothiazines, might also contribute to a prolongation of the QTc interval).
No products indexed under this heading.

Fluphenazine Hydrochloride (There is a theoretical possibility that co-administration of other drugs known to alter cardiac conduction, such as phenothiazines, might also contribute to a prolongation of the QTc interval).
No products indexed under this heading.

Fosphenytoin (Co-administration may reduce seizure control by lowering the plasma levels of anticonvulsant; dosage of anticonvulsant may need to be adjusted).
No products indexed under this heading.

Fosphenytoin Sodium (Co-administration may reduce seizure control by lowering the plasma levels of anticonvulsant; dosage of anticonvulsant may need to be adjusted).
No products indexed under this heading.

Gabapentin (Co-administration may reduce seizure control by lowering the plasma levels of anticonvulsant; dosage of anticonvulsant may need to be adjusted). Products include:
Neurontin Capsules 2498
Neurontin Oral Solution 2498
Neurontin Tablets 2498

Halofantrine (Administration of halofantrine subsequent to mefloquine suggests a significant, potentially fatal, prolongation of the QTc interval of ECG; halofantrine must not be given simultaneously with or subsequent to mefloquine).
No products indexed under this heading.

Imipramine Hydrochloride (There is a theoretical possibility that co-administration of other drugs known to alter cardiac conduction, such as tricyclic antidepressants, might also contribute to a prolongation of the QTc interval).
No products indexed under this heading.

Imipramine Pamoate (There is a theoretical possibility that co-administration of other drugs known to alter cardiac conduction, such as tricyclic antidepressants, might also contribute to a prolongation of the QTc interval).
No products indexed under this heading.

Isradipine (There is a theoretical possibility that co-administration of other drugs known to alter cardiac conduction, such as calcium channel blockers, might also contribute to a prolongation of the QTc interval).
Products include:
DynaCirc CR Tablets 2726

Labetalol Hydrochloride (There is a theoretical possibility that co-administration of other drugs known to alter cardiac conduction, such as beta blockers, might also contribute to a prolongation of the QTc interval).
No products indexed under this heading.

Lamotrigine (Co-administration may reduce seizure control by lowering the plasma levels of anticonvulsant; dosage of anticonvulsant may need to be adjusted). Products include:
Lamictal 1449

Levetiracetam (Co-administration may reduce seizure control by lowering the plasma levels of anticonvulsant; dosage of anticonvulsant may need to be adjusted). Products include:
Keppra Oral Solution 3307
Keppra Tablets 3307

Levobunolol Hydrochloride (There is a theoretical possibility that co-administration of other drugs known to alter cardiac conduction, such as beta blockers, might also contribute to a prolongation of the QTc interval). Products include:
Betagan Ophthalmic Solution, USP.. ⊙ 217

Lidocaine Hydrochloride (There is a theoretical possibility that co-administration of other drugs known to alter cardiac conduction, such as antiarrhythmic agents, might also contribute to a prolongation of the QTc interval).
No products indexed under this heading.

Maprotiline Hydrochloride (There is a theoretical possibility that co-administration of other drugs known to alter cardiac conduction, such as tricyclic antidepressants, might also contribute to a prolongation of the QTc interval).
No products indexed under this heading.

Mephenytoin (Co-administration may reduce seizure control by lowering the plasma levels of anticonvulsant; dosage of anticonvulsant may need to be adjusted).
No products indexed under this heading.

Mesoridazine Besylate (There is a theoretical possibility that co-administration of other drugs known to alter cardiac conduction, such as phenothiazines, might also contribute to a prolongation of the QTc interval).
No products indexed under this heading.

Methotrimeprazine (There is a theoretical possibility that co-administration of other drugs known to alter cardiac conduction, such as phenothiazines, might also contribute to a prolongation of the QTc interval).
No products indexed under this heading.

Methsuximide (Co-administration may reduce seizure control by lowering the plasma levels of anticonvulsant; dosage of anticonvulsant may need to be adjusted).
No products indexed under this heading.

Metipranolol Hydrochloride (There is a theoretical possibility that co-administration of other drugs known to alter cardiac conduction, such as beta blockers, might also contribute to a prolongation of the QTc interval).
No products indexed under this heading.

Metoprolol Succinate (There is a theoretical possibility that co-administration of other drugs known to alter cardiac conduction, such as beta blockers, might also contribute to a prolongation of the QTc interval). Products include:
Toprol-XL Tablets 660

Metoprolol Tartrate (There is a theoretical possibility that co-administration of other drugs known to alter cardiac conduction, such as beta blockers, might also contribute to a prolongation of the QTc interval).
No products indexed under this heading.

Mexiletine Hydrochloride (There is a theoretical possibility that co-administration of other drugs known to alter cardiac conduction, such as antiarrhythmic agents, might also contribute to a prolongation of the QTc interval).
No products indexed under this heading.

Mibefradil Dihydrochloride (There is a theoretical possibility that co-administration of other drugs known to alter cardiac conduction, such as calcium channel blockers, might also contribute to a prolongation of the QTc interval).
No products indexed under this heading.

Moricizine Hydrochloride (There is a theoretical possibility that co-administration of other drugs known to alter cardiac conduction, such as antiarrhythmic agents, might also contribute to a prolongation of the QTc interval).
No products indexed under this heading.

Nadolol (There is a theoretical possibility that co-administration of other drugs known to alter cardiac conduction, such as beta blockers, might also contribute to a prolongation of the QTc interval). Products include:
Nadolol Tablets 2121

Nicardipine Hydrochloride (There is a theoretical possibility that co-administration of other drugs known to alter cardiac conduction, such as calcium channel blockers, might also contribute to a prolongation of the QTc interval). Products include:
Cardene I.V. 1129

Nifedipine (There is a theoretical possibility that co-administration of other drugs known to alter cardiac conduction, such as calcium channel blockers, might also contribute to a prolongation of the QTc interval).
Products include:
Adalat CC Tablets 2978

Nimodipine (There is a theoretical possibility that co-administration of other drugs known to alter cardiac conduction, such as calcium channel blockers, might also contribute to a prolongation of the QTc interval).
Products include:
Nimotop Capsules 774

Nisoldipine (There is a theoretical possibility that co-administration of other drugs known to alter cardiac

conduction, such as calcium channel blockers, might also contribute to a prolongation of the QTc interval). Products include:

Sular Tablets **1163**

Nortriptyline Hydrochloride (There is a theoretical possibility that co-administration of other drugs known to alter cardiac conduction, such as tricyclic antidepressants, might also contribute to a prolongation of the QTc interval).

No products indexed under this heading.

Oxcarbazepine (Co-administration may reduce seizure control by lowering the plasma levels of anticonvulsant; dosage of anticonvulsant may need to be adjusted). Products include:

Trileptal Oral Suspension **2281**
Trileptal Tablets **2281**

Paramethadione (Co-administration may reduce seizure control by lowering the plasma levels of anticonvulsant; dosage of anticonvulsant may need to be adjusted).

No products indexed under this heading.

Penbutolol Sulfate (There is a theoretical possibility that co-administration of other drugs known to alter cardiac conduction, such as beta blockers, might also contribute to a prolongation of the QTc interval).

No products indexed under this heading.

Perphenazine (There is a theoretical possibility that co-administration of other drugs known to alter cardiac conduction, such as phenothiazines, might also contribute to a prolongation of the QTc interval).

No products indexed under this heading.

Phenacemide (Co-administration may reduce seizure control by lowering the plasma levels of anticonvulsant; dosage of anticonvulsant may need to be adjusted).

No products indexed under this heading.

Phenobarbital (Co-administration may reduce seizure control by lowering the plasma levels of anticonvulsant; dosage of anticonvulsant may need to be adjusted).

No products indexed under this heading.

Phensuximide (Co-administration may reduce seizure control by lowering the plasma levels of anticonvulsant; dosage of anticonvulsant may need to be adjusted).

No products indexed under this heading.

Phenytoin (Co-administration may reduce seizure control by lowering the plasma levels of anticonvulsant; dosage of anticonvulsant may need to be adjusted).

No products indexed under this heading.

Phenytoin Sodium (Co-administration may reduce seizure control by lowering the plasma levels of anticonvulsant; dosage of anticonvulsant may need to be adjusted). Products include:

Phenytek Capsules **2153**

Pindolol (There is a theoretical possibility that co-administration of other drugs known to alter cardiac conduction, such as beta blockers, might also contribute to a prolongation of the QTc interval).

No products indexed under this heading.

Primidone (Co-administration may reduce seizure control by lowering the plasma levels of anticonvulsant; dosage of anticonvulsant may need to be adjusted).

No products indexed under this heading.

Procainamide Hydrochloride (There is a theoretical possibility that co-administration of other drugs known to alter cardiac conduction, such as antiarrhythmic agents, might also contribute to a prolongation of the QTc interval).

No products indexed under this heading.

Prochlorperazine (There is a theoretical possibility that co-administration of other drugs known to alter cardiac conduction, such as phenothiazines, might also contribute to a prolongation of the QTc interval).

No products indexed under this heading.

Promethazine Hydrochloride (There is a theoretical possibility that co-administration of other drugs known to alter cardiac conduction, such as phenothiazines, might also contribute to a prolongation of the QTc interval). Products include:

Phenergan **3438**

Propafenone Hydrochloride (There is a theoretical possibility that co-administration of other drugs known to alter cardiac conduction, such as antiarrhythmic agents, might also contribute to a prolongation of the QTc interval). Products include:

Rythmol SR Capsules **2736**

Propranolol Hydrochloride (Co-administration has resulted in one report of cardiopulmonary arrest, with full recovery, in a patient; there is a theoretical possibility that co-administration of other drugs known to alter cardiac conduction, such as beta blockers, might also contribute to a prolongation of the QTc interval). Products include:

Inderal LA Long-Acting Capsules **3421**
InnoPran XL Capsules **2728**

Protriptyline Hydrochloride (There is a theoretical possibility that co-administration of other drugs known to alter cardiac conduction, such as tricyclic antidepressants, might also contribute to a prolongation of the QTc interval). Products include:

Vivactil Tablets **2350**

Quinidine (Co-administration may produce electrocardiographic abnormalities and increase the risk of convulsions; if these drugs are to be used in the initial treatment of severe malaria, mefloquine administration should be delayed at least 12 hours after the last dose).

No products indexed under this heading.

Quinidine Gluconate (Co-administration may produce electrocardiographic abnormalities and increase the risk of convulsions; if these drugs are to be used in the initial treatment of severe malaria, mefloquine administration should be delayed at least 12 hours after the last dose).

No products indexed under this heading.

Quinidine Hydrochloride (Co-administration may produce electrocardiographic abnormalities and increase the risk of convulsions; if these drugs are to be used in the initial treatment of severe malaria, mefloquine administration should be delayed at least 12 hours after the last dose).

No products indexed under this heading.

Quinidine Polygalacturonate (Co-administration may produce electrocardiographic abnormalities and increase the risk of convulsions; if these drugs are to be used in the initial treatment of severe malaria, mefloquine administration should be delayed at least 12 hours after the last dose).

No products indexed under this heading.

Quinidine Sulfate (Co-administration may produce electrocardiographic abnormalities and increase the risk of convulsions; if these drugs are to be used in the initial treatment of severe malaria, mefloquine administration should be delayed at least 12 hours after the last dose).

No products indexed under this heading.

Quinine Sulfate (Co-administration may produce electrocardiographic abnormalities and increase the risk of convulsions; if these drugs are to be used in the initial treatment of severe malaria, mefloquine administration should be delayed at least 12 hours after the last dose).

No products indexed under this heading.

Sotalol Hydrochloride (There is a theoretical possibility that co-administration of other drugs known to alter cardiac conduction, such as beta blockers, might also contribute to a prolongation of the QTc interval).

No products indexed under this heading.

Terfenadine (There is a theoretical possibility that the co-administration of other drugs known to alter cardiac conduction, such as antihistamine terfenadine, might also contribute to a prolongation of the QTc interval).

No products indexed under this heading.

Thioridazine Hydrochloride (There is a theoretical possibility that co-administration of other drugs known to alter cardiac conduction, such as phenothiazines, might also contribute to a prolongation of the QTc interval). Products include:

Thioridazine Hydrochloride Tablets **2122**

Tiagabine Hydrochloride (Co-administration may reduce seizure control by lowering the plasma levels of anticonvulsant; dosage of anticonvulsant may need to be adjusted). Products include:

Gabitril Tablets **998**

Timolol Hemihydrate (There is a theoretical possibility that co-administration of other drugs known to alter cardiac conduction, such as beta blockers, might also contribute to a prolongation of the QTc interval). Products include:

Betimol Ophthalmic Solution **3371**
Betimol Ophthalmic Solution .... ⊙**283**

Timolol Maleate (There is a theoretical possibility that co-administration of other drugs known to alter cardiac conduction, such as beta blockers, might also contribute to a prolongation of the QTc interval). Products include:

Blocadren Tablets **1891**
Cosopt Sterile Ophthalmic Solution **1910**
Timolide Tablets **2056**
Timoptic in Ocudose **2061**
Timoptic Sterile Ophthalmic Solution **2058**
Timoptic-XE Sterile Ophthalmic Gel Forming Solution **2062**

Tocainide Hydrochloride (There is a theoretical possibility that co-administration of other drugs known to alter cardiac conduction, such as antiarrhythmic agents, might also contribute to a prolongation of the QTc interval).

No products indexed under this heading.

Topiramate (Co-administration may reduce seizure control by lowering the plasma levels of anticonvulsant; dosage of anticonvulsant may need to be adjusted). Products include:

Topamax Sprinkle Capsules **2438**
Topamax Tablets **2438**

Trifluoperazine Hydrochloride (There is a theoretical possibility that co-administration of other drugs known to alter cardiac conduction, such as phenothiazines, might also contribute to a prolongation of the QTc interval).

No products indexed under this heading.

Trimethadione (Co-administration may reduce seizure control by lowering the plasma levels of anticonvulsant; dosage of anticonvulsant may need to be adjusted).

No products indexed under this heading.

Trimipramine Maleate (There is a theoretical possibility that co-administration of other drugs known to alter cardiac conduction, such as tricyclic antidepressants, might also contribute to a prolongation of the QTc interval). Products include:

Surmontil Capsules **2347**

Typhoid Vaccine Live Oral TY21a (Attenuation of immunization cannot be excluded when co-administered). Products include:

Vivotif **834**

Valproate Sodium (Co-administration may reduce seizure control by lowering the plasma levels of anticonvulsant; dosage of anticonvulsant may need to be adjusted). Products include:

Depacon Injection **412**

Valproic Acid (Co-administration may reduce seizure control by lowering the plasma levels of anticonvulsant; dosage of anticonvulsant may need to be adjusted). Products include:

Depakene **417**

Verapamil Hydrochloride (There is a theoretical possibility that co-administration of other drugs known to alter cardiac conduction, such as

calcium channel blockers, might also contribute to a prolongation of the QTc interval). Products include:

Covera-HS Tablets ... 3135
Tarka Tablets ... 519
Verelan PM Capsules ... 3120

Zonisamide (Co-administration may reduce seizure control by lowering the plasma levels of anticonvulsant; dosage of anticonvulsant may need to be adjusted). Products include:

Zonegran Capsules ... 1089

LESCOL CAPSULES

(Fluvastatin Sodium) ... 2730

May interact with erythromycin, fibrates, and certain other agents. Compounds in these categories include:

Cholestyramine (Administration of fluvastatin with, or up to 4 hours, after cholestyramine results in significant reductions in AUC and Cmax of fluvastatin; however, use of fluvastatin 4 hours after resin results in clinically significant additive effect).

No products indexed under this heading.

Cimetidine (Co-administration results in a significant increase in the fluvastatin Cmax and AUC and a decrease in plasma clearance). Products include:

Tagamet HB 200 Tablets ... ▣637
Tagamet Tablets ... 1547

Cimetidine Hydrochloride (Co-administration results in a significant increase in the fluvastatin Cmax and AUC and a decrease in plasma clearance).

No products indexed under this heading.

Clofibrate (Myopathy has occasionally been associated with fibrates; combined use should generally be avoided).

No products indexed under this heading.

Cyclosporine (The risk of myopathy and/or rhabdomyolysis during treatment with HMG-CoA reductase inhibitors has been reported to be increased with concurrent cyclosporine; caution should be exercised). Products include:

Gengraf Capsules ... 458
Neoral Soft Gelatin Capsules ... 2247
Neoral Oral Solution ... 2247
Restasis Ophthalmic Emulsion ... 570
Sandimmune ... 2259

Diclofenac Potassium (Co-administration increases the mean Cmax and AUC of diclofenac by 60% and 25% respectively). Products include:

Cataflam Tablets ... 2173

Diclofenac Sodium (Co-administration increases the mean Cmax and AUC of diclofenac by 60% and 25% respectively). Products include:

Arthrotec Tablets ... 3126
Voltaren Ophthalmic Solution ... 2300
Voltaren Tablets ... 2298
Voltaren-XR Tablets ... 2301

Digoxin (Co-administration in patients on chronic digoxin may result in a small increase in digoxin Cmax (11%) and urinary clearance). Products include:

Digitek Tablets ... 2146
Lanoxicaps Capsules ... 1458
Lanoxin Injection ... 1462
Lanoxin Tablets ... 1468
Lanoxin Injection Pediatric ... 1465

Erythromycin (The risk of myopathy and/or rhabdomyolysis during treatment with HMG-CoA reductase inhibitors has been reported to be increased with concurrent erythromycin; caution should be exercised). Products include:

Erygel Topical Gel ... 2096
Ery-Tab Tablets ... 447
Erythromycin Base Filmtab Tablets ... 454
Erythromycin Delayed-Release Capsules, USP ... 456
PCE Dispertab Tablets ... 510

Erythromycin Estolate (The risk of myopathy and/or rhabdomyolysis during treatment with HMG-CoA reductase inhibitors has been reported to be increased with concurrent erythromycin; caution should be exercised).

No products indexed under this heading.

Erythromycin Ethylsuccinate (The risk of myopathy and/or rhabdomyolysis during treatment with HMG-CoA reductase inhibitors has been reported to be increased with concurrent erythromycin; caution should be exercised). Products include:

E.E.S. ... 449
EryPed ... 445

Erythromycin Gluceptate (The risk of myopathy and/or rhabdomyolysis during treatment with HMG-CoA reductase inhibitors has been reported to be increased with concurrent erythromycin; caution should be exercised).

No products indexed under this heading.

Erythromycin Lactobionate (The risk of myopathy and/or rhabdomyolysis during treatment with HMG-CoA reductase inhibitors has been reported to be increased with concurrent erythromycin; caution should be exercised).

No products indexed under this heading.

Erythromycin Stearate (The risk of myopathy and/or rhabdomyolysis during treatment with HMG-CoA reductase inhibitors has been reported to be increased with concurrent erythromycin; caution should be exercised). Products include:

Erythrocin Stearate Filmtab Tablets ... 452

Fenofibrate (Myopathy has occasionally been associated with fibrates; combined use should generally be avoided). Products include:

Antara Capsules ... 2723
Lofibra Capsules ... 1217
Tricor Tablets ... 523
Triglide Tablets ... 1165

Gemfibrozil (The risk of myopathy and/or rhabdomyolysis during treatment with HMG-CoA reductase inhibitors has been reported to be increased with concurrent gemfibrozil; combined use should generally be avoided).

No products indexed under this heading.

Glyburide (Co-administration results in increased mean Cmax, AUC, and t1/2 of glyburide approximately 50%, 69% and 121% respectively; glyburide increased the mean Cmax and AUC of fluvastatin by 44% and 51% respectively).

No products indexed under this heading.

Ketoconazole (Caution should be exercised if used concurrently with drugs that may decrease the levels of endogenous steroid hormones; increased potential for endocrine dysfunction). Products include:

Nizoral A-D Shampoo, 1% ... 1839
Nizoral 2% Shampoo ... 1838

Nicotinic Acid (The risk of myopathy and/or rhabdomyolysis during treatment with HMG-CoA reductase inhibitors has been reported to be increased with concurrent niacin; caution should be exercised).

No products indexed under this heading.

Omeprazole (Co-administration results in a significant increase in the fluvastatin Cmax and AUC and a decrease in plasma clearance). Products include:

Zegerid Powder for Oral Solution ... 2972

Ranitidine Hydrochloride (Co-administration results in a significant increase in the fluvastatin Cmax and AUC and a decrease in plasma clearance). Products include:

Zantac ... 1597
Zantac Injection ... 1593
Zantac 75 Tablets ... ▣715
Zantac 150 Maximum Strength Tablets ... ▣715
Zantac Injection Pharmacy Bulk Package ... 1595

Rifampin (Co-administration in patients pretreated with rifampin results in significant reduction in Cmax (59%) and AUC (51%) with a large increase (95%) in plasma clearance).

No products indexed under this heading.

Spironolactone (Caution should be exercised if used concurrently with drugs that may decrease the levels of endogenous steroid hormones; increased potential for endocrine dysfunction).

No products indexed under this heading.

Warfarin Sodium (Bleeding and/or increased prothrombin time has been reported with other HMG-CoA reductase inhibitors when used concurrently; no interactions at therapeutic concentrations have been demonstrated with fluvastatin and warfarin). Products include:

Coumadin for Injection ... 932
Coumadin Tablets ... 932

Food Interactions

Food, unspecified (Administration of regular formulation of fluvastatin with food reduces the rate but not the extent of absorption; administration with evening meal results in a two-fold decrease in Cmax and more than a two-fold increase in tmax as compared to administration 4 hours after the evening meal; administration of Lescol XL with a high fat meal delayed the absorption and increased the bioavailability by 50%).

LESCOL CAPSULES

(Fluvastatin Sodium) ... 2227

May interact with erythromycin, fibrates, and certain other agents. Compounds in these categories include:

Cholestyramine (Administration of fluvastatin with, or up to 4 hours after cholestyramine results in significant reductions in AUC and Cmax of fluvastatin; however, use of fluvastatin 4 hours after resin results in clinically significant additive effect).

No products indexed under this heading.

Cimetidine (Co-administration results in a significant increase in the fluvastatin Cmax and AUC and a decrease in plasma clearance). Products include:

Tagamet HB 200 Tablets ... ▣637
Tagamet Tablets ... 1547

Cimetidine Hydrochloride (Co-administration results in a significant increase in the fluvastatin Cmax and AUC and a decrease in plasma clearance).

No products indexed under this heading.

Clofibrate (Myopathy has occasionally been associated with fibrates; combined use should generally be avoided).

No products indexed under this heading.

Cyclosporine (The risk of myopathy and/or rhabdomyolysis during treatment with HMG-CoA reductase inhibitor has been reported to be increased with concurrent cyclosporine; caution should be exercised). Products include:

Gengraf Capsules ... 458
Neoral Soft Gelatin Capsules ... 2247
Neoral Oral Solution ... 2247
Restasis Ophthalmic Emulsion ... 570
Sandimmune ... 2259

Diclofenac Potassium (Co-administration increases the mean Cmax and AUC of diclofenac by 60% and 25% respectively). Products include:

Cataflam Tablets ... 2173

Diclofenac Sodium (Co-administration increases the mean Cmax and AUC of diclofenac by 60% and 25% respectively). Products include:

Arthrotec Tablets ... 3126
Voltaren Ophthalmic Solution ... 2300
Voltaren Tablets ... 2298
Voltaren-XR Tablets ... 2301

Digoxin (Co-administration in patients on chronic digoxin may result in a small increase in digoxin Cmax (11%) and urinary clearance). Products include:

Digitek Tablets ... 2146
Lanoxicaps Capsules ... 1458
Lanoxin Injection ... 1462
Lanoxin Tablets ... 1468
Lanoxin Injection Pediatric ... 1465

Erythromycin (The risk of myopathy and/or rhabdomyolysis during treatment with HMG-CoA reductase inhibitor has been reported to be increased with concurrent erythromycin; caution should be exercised). Products include:

Erygel Topical Gel ... 2096
Ery-Tab Tablets ... 447
Erythromycin Base Filmtab Tablets ... 454
Erythromycin Delayed-Release Capsules, USP ... 456
PCE Dispertab Tablets ... 510

Erythromycin Estolate (The risk of myopathy and/or rhabdomyolysis during treatment with HMG-CoA reductase inhibitor has been reported to be increased with concurrent erythromycin; caution should be exercised).

No products indexed under this heading.

Erythromycin Ethylsuccinate (The risk of myopathy and/or rhabdomyolysis during treatment with HMG-CoA reductase inhibitor has been reported to be increased with concurrent erythromycin; caution should be exercised). Products include:

E.E.S. ... 449
EryPed ... 445

Erythromycin Gluceptate (The risk of myopathy and/or rhabdomyolysis during treatment with HMG-CoA reductase inhibitor has been reported to be increased with concurrent erythromycin; caution should be exercised).
No products indexed under this heading.

Erythromycin Lactobionate (The risk of myopathy and/or rhabdomyolysis during treatment with HMG-CoA reductase inhibitor has been reported to be increased with concurrent erythromycin; caution should be exercised).
No products indexed under this heading.

Erythromycin Stearate (The risk of myopathy and/or rhabdomyolysis during treatment with HMG-CoA reductase inhibitor has been reported to be increased with concurrent erythromycin; caution should be exercised). Products include:
Erythrocin Stearate Filmtab Tablets **452**

Fenofibrate (Myopathy has occasionally been associated with fibrates; combined use should generally be avoided). Products include:
Antara Capsules **2723**
Lofibra Capsules **1217**
Tricor Tablets **523**
Triglide Tablets **1165**

Gemfibrozil (The risk of myopathy and/or rhabdomyolysis during treatment with HMG-CoA reductase inhibitor has been reported to be increased with concurrent gemfibrozil; combined use should generally be avoided).
No products indexed under this heading.

Glyburide (Co-administration results in increased mean Cmax, AUC, and t1/2 of glyburide approximately 50%, 69% and 121% respectively; glyburide increased the mean Cmax and AUC of fluvastatin by 44% and 51% respectively).
No products indexed under this heading.

Ketoconazole (Caution should be exercised if used concurrently with drugs that may decrease the levels of endogenous steroid hormones; increased potential for endocrine dysfunction). Products include:
Nizoral A-D Shampoo, 1% **1839**
Nizoral 2% Shampoo **1838**

Nicotinic Acid (The risk of myopathy and/or rhabdomyolysis during treatment with HMG-CoA reductase inhibitor has been reported to be increased with concurrent niacin; caution should be exercised).
No products indexed under this heading.

Omeprazole (Co-administration results in a significant increase in the fluvastatin Cmax and AUC and a decrease in plasma clearance). Products include:
Zegerid Powder for Oral Solution **2972**

Ranitidine Hydrochloride (Co-administration results in a significant increase in the fluvastatin Cmax and AUC and a decrease in plasma clearance). Products include:
Zantac **1597**
Zantac Injection **1593**
Zantac 75 Tablets **715**
Zantac 150 Maximum Strength Tablets **715**
Zantac Injection Pharmacy Bulk Package **1595**

Rifampin (Co-administration in patients pretreated with rifampin results in significant reduction in Cmax (59%) and AUC (51%) with a large increase (95%) in plasma clearance).
No products indexed under this heading.

Spironolactone (Caution should be exercised if used concurrently with drugs that may decrease the levels of endogenous steroid hormones; increased potential for endocrine dysfunction).
No products indexed under this heading.

Warfarin Sodium (Bleeding and/or increased prothrombin time has been reported with other HMG-CoA reductase inhibitors when used concurrently; no interactions at therapeutic concentrations have been demonstrated with fluvastatin and warfarin). Products include:
Coumadin for Injection **932**
Coumadin Tablets **932**

Food Interactions

Food, unspecified (Administration of regular formulation of fluvastatin with food reduces the rate but not the extent of absorption; administration with evening meal results in a two-fold decrease in Cmax and more than a two-fold increase in tmax as compared to administration 4 hours after the evening meal; administration of Lescol XL with a high fat meal delayed the absorption and increased the bioavailability by 50%).

LESCOL XL TABLETS

(Fluvastatin Sodium) **2730**
See Lescol Capsules

LESCOL XL TABLETS

(Fluvastatin Sodium) **2227**
See Lescol Capsules

LEUKERAN TABLETS

(Chlorambucil) **1472**
May interact with vaccines, live. Compounds in these categories include:

BCG Vaccine (Administration of live vaccines to immunocompromised patients should be avoided).
No products indexed under this heading.

Measles, Mumps & Rubella Virus Vaccine, Live (Administration of live vaccines to immunocompromised patients should be avoided). Products include:
M-M-R II **1980**

Measles & Rubella Virus Vaccine Live (Administration of live vaccines to immunocompromised patients should be avoided).
No products indexed under this heading.

Measles Virus Vaccine Live (Administration of live vaccines to immunocompromised patients should be avoided). Products include:
Attenuvax **1889**

Mumps Virus Vaccine, Live (Administration of live vaccines to immunocompromised patients should be avoided). Products include:
Mumpsvax **2005**

Poliovirus Vaccine, Live, Oral, Trivalent, Types 1,2,3 (Sabin) (Administration of live vaccines to immunocompromised patients should be avoided).
No products indexed under this heading.

Rotavirus Vaccine, Live, Oral, Tetravalent (Administration of live vaccines to immunocompromised patients should be avoided).
No products indexed under this heading.

Rubella & Mumps Virus Vaccine Live (Administration of live vaccines to immunocompromised patients should be avoided).
No products indexed under this heading.

Rubella Virus Vaccine Live (Administration of live vaccines to immunocompromised patients should be avoided). Products include:
Meruvax II **1994**

Smallpox Vaccine (Administration of live vaccines to immunocompromised patients should be avoided).
No products indexed under this heading.

Typhoid Vaccine (Administration of live vaccines to immunocompromised patients should be avoided).
No products indexed under this heading.

Varicella Virus Vaccine Live (Administration of live vaccines to immunocompromised patients should be avoided). Products include:
Varivax **2070**

Yellow Fever Vaccine (Administration of live vaccines to immunocompromised patients should be avoided).
No products indexed under this heading.

LEUKINE

(Sargramostim) **829**
May interact with antimetabolites, cytotoxic drugs, drugs with myeloproliferative effects, and certain other agents. Compounds in these categories include:

Betamethasone Acetate (May potentiate the myeloproliferative effect).
No products indexed under this heading.

Betamethasone Sodium Phosphate (May potentiate the myeloproliferative effect).
No products indexed under this heading.

Bleomycin Sulfate (Coadministration within 24 hours preceding or following chemotherapy is not recommended because of potential sensitivity of rapidly dividing hematopoietic progenitor cells to cytotoxic therapy).
No products indexed under this heading.

Capecitabine (In patients who have been exposed to multiple myelotoxic agents, the effect of Leukine on myeloid reconstitution may be limited). Products include:
Xeloda Tablets **2825**

Cladribine (In patients who have been exposed to multiple myelotoxic agents, the effect of Leukine on myeloid reconstitution may be limited). Products include:
Leustatin Injection **2368**

Cortisone Acetate (May potentiate the myeloproliferative effect).
No products indexed under this heading.

Cyclophosphamide (Coadministration within 24 hours preceding or following chemotherapy is not recommended because of potential sensitivity of rapidly dividing hematopoietic progenitor cells to cytotoxic therapy).
No products indexed under this heading.

Cytarabine (In patients who have been exposed to multiple myelotoxic agents, the effect of Leukine on myeloid reconstitution may be limited).
No products indexed under this heading.

Daunorubicin Hydrochloride (Coadministration within 24 hours preceding or following chemotherapy is not recommended because of potential sensitivity of rapidly dividing hematopoietic progenitor cells to cytotoxic therapy). Products include:
Cerubidine for Injection **788**

Dexamethasone (May potentiate the myeloproliferative effect). Products include:
Ciprodex Otic Suspension **555**
Decadron Tablets **1929**
TobraDex Ophthalmic Ointment **558**
TobraDex Ophthalmic Suspension ... **558**

Dexamethasone Acetate (May potentiate the myeloproliferative effect).
No products indexed under this heading.

Dexamethasone Sodium Phosphate (May potentiate the myeloproliferative effect). Products include:
Decadron Phosphate Injection **1931**

Doxorubicin Hydrochloride (Coadministration within 24 hours preceding or following chemotherapy is not recommended because of potential sensitivity of rapidly dividing hematopoietic progenitor cells to cytotoxic therapy). Products include:
Adriamycin for Injection, USP **786**
Adriamycin Injection, USP **786**

Epirubicin Hydrochloride (Coadministration within 24 hours preceding or following chemotherapy is not recommended because of potential sensitivity of rapidly dividing hematopoietic progenitor cells to cytotoxic therapy). Products include:
Ellence Injection **2632**

Floxuridine (In patients who have been exposed to multiple myelotoxic agents, the effect of Leukine on myeloid reconstitution may be limited).
No products indexed under this heading.

Fludarabine Phosphate (In patients who have been exposed to multiple myelotoxic agents, the effect of Leukine on myeloid reconstitution may be limited).
No products indexed under this heading.

Fluorouracil (Coadministration within 24 hours preceding or following chemotherapy is not recommended because of potential sensitivity of rapidly dividing hematopoietic progenitor cells to cytotoxic therapy). Products include:
Carac Cream, 0.5% **1048**
Efudex **3348**

Gemcitabine Hydrochloride (In patients who have been exposed to multiple myelotoxic agents, the effect of Leukine on myeloid reconstitution may be limited). Products include:

Gemzar for Injection 1743

Hydrocortisone (May potentiate the myeloproliferative effect). Products include:

Cortizone•5 Ointment .... ▣ 699
Cortizone•10 Creme .... ▣ 699
Cortizone•10 Ointment .... ▣ 699
Cortizone•10 Plus Creme .... ▣ 700
Cortizone•10 Maximum Strength Quick Shot Spray .... ▣ 700
Hydrocortone Tablets 1963
Preparation H Hydrocortisone Cream .... ▣ 748

Hydrocortisone Acetate (May potentiate the myeloproliferative effect). Products include:

Analpram-HC 1136
Pramosone 1139
ProctoFoam-HC 3113
Tucks Anti-Itch Ointment .... ▣ 712
U-cort 1% Cream 3289

Hydrocortisone Sodium Phosphate (May potentiate the myeloproliferative effect).

No products indexed under this heading.

Hydrocortisone Sodium Succinate (May potentiate the myeloproliferative effect).

No products indexed under this heading.

Hydroxyurea (Coadministration within 24 hours preceding or following chemotherapy is not recommended because of potential sensitivity of rapidly dividing hematopoietic progenitor cells to cytotoxic therapy).

No products indexed under this heading.

Lithium Carbonate (May potentiate the myeloproliferative effect). Products include:

Eskalith 1406
Lithobid Tablets 1670

Lithium Citrate (May potentiate the myeloproliferative effect).

No products indexed under this heading.

Mercaptopurine (In patients who have been exposed to multiple myelotoxic agents, the effect of Leukine on myeloid reconstitution may be limited). Products include:

Purinethol Tablets 1222

Methotrexate (In patients who have been exposed to multiple myelotoxic agents, the effect of Leukine on myeloid reconstitution may be limited).

No products indexed under this heading.

Methotrexate Sodium (Coadministration within 24 hours preceding or following chemotherapy is not recommended because of potential sensitivity of rapidly dividing hematopoietic progenitor cells to cytotoxic therapy).

No products indexed under this heading.

Methylprednisolone Acetate (May potentiate the myeloproliferative effect). Products include:

Depo-Medrol Injectable Suspension 2615
Depo-Medrol Single-Dose Vial 2617

Methylprednisolone Sodium Succinate (May potentiate the myeloproliferative effect).

No products indexed under this heading.

Mitotane (Coadministration within 24 hours preceding or following chemotherapy is not recommended because of potential sensitivity of rapidly dividing hematopoietic progenitor cells to cytotoxic therapy).

No products indexed under this heading.

Mitoxantrone Hydrochloride (Coadministration within 24 hours preceding or following chemotherapy is not recommended because of potential sensitivity of rapidly dividing hematopoietic progenitor cells to cytotoxic therapy). Products include:

Novantrone for Injection Concentrate 3158

Pentostatin (In patients who have been exposed to multiple myelotoxic agents, the effect of Leukine on myeloid reconstitution may be limited). Products include:

Nipent for Injection 3216

Prednisolone Acetate (May potentiate the myeloproliferative effect). Products include:

Blephamide Ophthalmic Ointment 563
Blephamide Ophthalmic Suspension.................................. 564
Poly-Pred Liquifilm Ophthalmic Suspension .... ⊙ 231
Pred Forte Ophthalmic Suspension .... ⊙ 233
Pred Mild Sterile Ophthalmic Suspension .... ⊙ 236
Pred-G Ophthalmic Suspension ...... ⊙ 234
Pred-G Sterile Ophthalmic Ointment .... ⊙ 235

Prednisolone Sodium Phosphate (May potentiate the myeloproliferative effect). Products include:

Pediapred Oral Solution 3319

Prednisolone Tebutate (May potentiate the myeloproliferative effect).

No products indexed under this heading.

Prednisone (May potentiate the myeloproliferative effect).

No products indexed under this heading.

Procarbazine Hydrochloride (Coadministration within 24 hours preceding or following chemotherapy is not recommended because of potential sensitivity of rapidly dividing hematopoietic progenitor cells to cytotoxic therapy). Products include:

Matulane Capsules 3188

Tamoxifen Citrate (Coadministration within 24 hours preceding or following chemotherapy is not recommended because of potential sensitivity of rapidly dividing hematopoietic progenitor cells to cytotoxic therapy).

No products indexed under this heading.

Thioguanine (In patients who have been exposed to multiple myelotoxic agents, the effect of Leukine on myeloid reconstitution may be limited). Products include:

Tabloid Tablets 1545

Triamcinolone (May potentiate the myeloproliferative effect).

No products indexed under this heading.

Triamcinolone Acetonide (May potentiate the myeloproliferative effect). Products include:

Azmacort Inhalation Aerosol 1701
Nasacort HFA Inhalation Aerosol 2939
Nasacort AQ Nasal Spray 2937

Triamcinolone Diacetate (May potentiate the myeloproliferative effect).

No products indexed under this heading.

Triamcinolone Hexacetonide (May potentiate the myeloproliferative effect).

No products indexed under this heading.

Vincristine Sulfate (Coadministration within 24 hours preceding or following chemotherapy is not recommended because of potential sensitivity of rapidly dividing hematopoietic progenitor cells to cytotoxic therapy).

No products indexed under this heading.

LEUSTATIN INJECTION

(Cladribine) 2368
May interact with:

Bone Marrow Depressants, unspecified (Caution should be exercised if co-administered with other drugs known to cause myelosuppression).

No products indexed under this heading.

LEVAQUIN IN 5% DEXTROSE INJECTION

(Levofloxacin) 2453
See Levaquin Tablets

LEVAQUIN INJECTION

(Levofloxacin) 2453
See Levaquin Tablets

LEVAQUIN ORAL SOLUTION

(Levofloxacin) 2453
See Levaquin Tablets

LEVAQUIN TABLETS

(Levofloxacin) 2453
May interact with antacids containing aluminum, calcium and magnesium, class 1A antiarrhythmics, class III antiarrhythmics, cations, corticosteroids, erythromycin, oral hypoglycemic agents, iron containing oral preparations, non-steroidal anti-inflammatory agents, psychotropics, quinidine, tricyclic antidepressants, xanthines, and certain other agents. Compounds in these categories include:

Acarbose (Disturbances of blood glucose, including hyper- and hypoglycemia, have been reported in patients treated concomitantly with quinolones and an antidiabetic agent; careful monitoring of blood glucose levels is recommended). Products include:

Precose Tablets 776

Alprazolam (Levofloxacin has been associated with prolongation of the QTc interval; co-administration with drugs known to prolong QT interval should be avoided). Products include:

Niravam Orally Disintegrating Tablets 3106
Xanax XR Tablets 2655

Aluminum Carbonate (Antacids containing aluminum or magnesium may interfere with the gastrointestinal absorption of levofloxacin resulting in systemic levels considerably lower than desired; these agents should be taken at least 2 hours before or after levofloxacin administration).

No products indexed under this heading.

Aluminum-containing Compounds, unspecified (Concurrent administration of levofloxacin with metal cations may interfere with the GI absorption of levofloxacin, resulting in systemic levels considerably lower than desired; these agents containing metal cations should be taken at least 2 hours before or 2 hours after levofloxacin administration).

No products indexed under this heading.

Aluminum Hydroxide (Antacids containing aluminum or magnesium may interfere with the gastrointestinal absorption of levofloxacin resulting in systemic levels considerably lower than desired; these agents should be taken at least 2 hours before or after levofloxacin administration). Products include:

Gaviscon Regular Strength Liquid .. ▣ 620
Gaviscon Regular Strength Tablets .... ▣ 619
Gaviscon Extra Strength Liquid ...... ▣ 620
Gaviscon Extra Strength Tablets .... ▣ 619
Maalox Max Maximum Strength Antacid/Anti-Gas Liquid 2165
Maalox Regular Strength Antacid/Antigas Liquid 2164

Aminophylline (Co-administration of other quinolones with theophylline has resulted in prolonged elimination half-life, elevated serum theophylline levels, and increased risk of theophylline related toxicity; no significant effect of levofloxacin on theophylline pharmacokinetic parameters has been detected, however, caution should be exercised).

No products indexed under this heading.

Amiodarone Hydrochloride (Levofloxacin has been associated with prolongation of the QTc interval; co-administration with drugs known to prolong QT interval should be avoided). Products include:

Pacerone Tablets 3337

Amitriptyline Hydrochloride (Levofloxacin has been associated with prolongation of the QTc interval; co-administration with drugs known to prolong QT interval should be avoided).

No products indexed under this heading.

Amoxapine (Levofloxacin has been associated with prolongation of the QTc interval; co-administration with drugs known to prolong QT interval should be avoided).

No products indexed under this heading.

Arsenic Trioxide (Levofloxacin has been associated with prolongation of the QTc interval; co-administration with drugs known to prolong QT interval should be avoided). Products include:

Trisenox Injection 983

Betamethasone Acetate (Achilles and other tendon ruptures have been reported with quinolones, post-market surveillance reports indicate that the risk may be increased in patients on concomitant corticosteroids).

No products indexed under this heading.

Betamethasone Sodium Phosphate (Achilles and other tendon ruptures have been reported with quinolones, post-market surveillance reports indicate that the risk may be increased in patients on concomitant corticosteroids).
No products indexed under this heading.

Bretylium Tosylate (Levofloxacin has been associated with prolongation of the QT interval and infrequent cases of arrhythmia. Rare cases of torsades de pointes have been spontaneously reported during post-marketing surveillance in patients receiving levofloxacin. Levofloxacin should be avoided in patients receiving class III antiarrhythmic agents).
No products indexed under this heading.

Buspirone Hydrochloride (Levofloxacin has been associated with prolongation of the QTc interval; co-administration with drugs known to prolong QT interval should be avoided).
No products indexed under this heading.

Calcium (Concurrent administration of levofloxacin with metal cations may interfere with the GI absorption of levofloxacin, resulting in systemic levels considerably lower than desired; these agents containing metal cations should be taken at least 2 hours before or 2 hours after levofloxacin administration).
Products include:
Os-Cal 250 + D Tablets 765
Os-Cal 500 Tablets 765
Os-Cal 500 + D Tablets 766
Perdiem Overnight Relief Pills 2166
Slow-Mag Tablets 2717

Celecoxib (Co-administration may increase the risk of CNS stimulation and convulsive seizures). Products include:
Celebrex Capsules 3130

Chlordiazepoxide (Levofloxacin has been associated with prolongation of the QTc interval; co-administration with drugs known to prolong QT interval should be avoided).
No products indexed under this heading.

Chlordiazepoxide Hydrochloride (Levofloxacin has been associated with prolongation of the QTc interval; co-administration with drugs known to prolong QT interval should be avoided). Products include:
Librium Capsules 3349

Chlorpromazine (Levofloxacin has been associated with prolongation of the QTc interval; co-administration with drugs known to prolong QT interval should be avoided).
No products indexed under this heading.

Chlorpromazine Hydrochloride (Levofloxacin has been associated with prolongation of the QTc interval; co-administration with drugs known to prolong QT interval should be avoided).
No products indexed under this heading.

Chlorpropamide (Disturbances of blood glucose, including hyper- and hypoglycemia, have been reported in patients treated concomitantly with quinolones and an antidiabetic agent; careful monitoring of blood glucose levels is recommended).
No products indexed under this heading.

Chlorprothixene (Levofloxacin has been associated with prolongation of the QTc interval; co-administration with drugs known to prolong QT interval should be avoided).
No products indexed under this heading.

Chlorprothixene Hydrochloride (Levofloxacin has been associated with prolongation of the QTc interval; co-administration with drugs known to prolong QT interval should be avoided).
No products indexed under this heading.

Cimetidine (Co-administration has resulted in higher levofloxacin AUC and t1/2, while CL/F and CLr were lower during concomitant treatment with cimetidine). Products include:
Tagamet HB 200 Tablets 637
Tagamet Tablets 1547

Cimetidine Hydrochloride (Co-administration has resulted in higher levofloxacin AUC and t1/2, while CL/F and CLr were lower during concomitant treatment with cimetidine).
No products indexed under this heading.

Cisapride (Levofloxacin has been associated with prolongation of the QTc interval; co-administration with drugs known to prolong QT interval should be avoided).
No products indexed under this heading.

Clomipramine Hydrochloride (Levofloxacin has been associated with prolongation of the QTc interval; co-administration with drugs known to prolong QT interval should be avoided).
No products indexed under this heading.

Clorazepate Dipotassium (Levofloxacin has been associated with prolongation of the QTc interval; co-administration with drugs known to prolong QT interval should be avoided). Products include:
Tranxene 2488

Clozapine (Levofloxacin has been associated with prolongation of the QTc interval; co-administration with drugs known to prolong QT interval should be avoided). Products include:
Clozapine Tablets 2141
Clozaril Tablets 2174
FazaClo Orally Disintegrating Tablets 547

Cortisone Acetate (Achilles and other tendon ruptures have been reported with quinolones, post-market surveillance reports indicate that the risk may be increased in patients on concomitant corticosteroids).
No products indexed under this heading.

Cyclosporine (Levofloxacin Cmax and Ke were slightly lower while Tmax and t1/2 were slightly longer in the presence of cyclosporine; these differences, however, are not clinically significant, therefore, no dosage adjustment is required). Products include:
Gengraf Capsules 458
Neoral Soft Gelatin Capsules 2247
Neoral Oral Solution 2247
Restasis Ophthalmic Emulsion 570
Sandimmune 2259

Desipramine Hydrochloride (Levofloxacin has been associated with prolongation of the QTc interval; co-administration with drugs known to prolong QT interval should be avoided).
No products indexed under this heading.

Dexamethasone (Achilles and other tendon ruptures have been reported with quinolones, post-market surveillance reports indicate that the risk may be increased in patients on concomitant corticosteroids).
Products include:
Ciprodex Otic Suspension 555
Decadron Tablets 1929
TobraDex Ophthalmic Ointment 558
TobraDex Ophthalmic Suspension ... 558

Dexamethasone Acetate (Achilles and other tendon ruptures have been reported with quinolones, post-market surveillance reports indicate that the risk may be increased in patients on concomitant corticosteroids).
No products indexed under this heading.

Dexamethasone Sodium Phosphate (Achilles and other tendon ruptures have been reported with quinolones, post-market surveillance reports indicate that the risk may be increased in patients on concomitant corticosteroids). Products include:
Decadron Phosphate Injection 1931

Diazepam (Levofloxacin has been associated with prolongation of the QTc interval; co-administration with drugs known to prolong QT interval should be avoided). Products include:
Diastat Rectal Delivery System 3344
Valium Tablets 2822

Diclofenac Potassium (Co-administration may increase the risk of CNS stimulation and convulsive seizures). Products include:
Cataflam Tablets 2173

Diclofenac Sodium (Co-administration may increase the risk of CNS stimulation and convulsive seizures). Products include:
Arthrotec Tablets 3126
Voltaren Ophthalmic Solution 2300
Voltaren Tablets 2298
Voltaren-XR Tablets 2301

Didanosine (Antacids contained in Videx chewable/buffered tablets or pediatric powder for oral solution may substantially interfere with the gastrointestinal absorption of levofloxacin, resulting in systemic levels considerably lower than desired).
No products indexed under this heading.

Disopyramide (Levofloxacin has been associated with prolongation of the QT interval and infrequent cases of arrhythmia. Rare cases of torsades de pointes have been spontaneously reported during post-marketing surveillance in patients receiving levofloxacin. Levofloxacin should be avoided in patients receiving class IA antiarrhythmic agents).
No products indexed under this heading.

Doxepin Hydrochloride (Levofloxacin has been associated with prolongation of the QTc interval; co-administration with drugs known to prolong QT interval should be avoided).
No products indexed under this heading.

Droperidol (Levofloxacin has been associated with prolongation of the QTc interval; co-administration with drugs known to prolong QT interval should be avoided).
No products indexed under this heading.

Dyphylline (Co-administration of other quinolones with theophylline has resulted in prolonged elimination half-life, elevated serum theophylline levels, and increased risk of theophylline related toxicity; no significant effect of levofloxacin on theophylline pharmacokinetic parameters has been detected, however, caution should be exercised).
No products indexed under this heading.

Erythromycin (Levofloxacin has been associated with prolongation of the QTc interval; co-administration with drugs known to prolong QT interval should be avoided). Products include:
Erygel Topical Gel 2096
Ery-Tab Tablets 447
Erythromycin Base Filmtab Tablets 454
Erythromycin Delayed-Release Capsules, USP 456
PCE Dispertab Tablets 510

Erythromycin Estolate (Levofloxacin has been associated with prolongation of the QTc interval; co-administration with drugs known to prolong QT interval should be avoided).
No products indexed under this heading.

Erythromycin Ethylsuccinate (Levofloxacin has been associated with prolongation of the QTc interval; co-administration with drugs known to prolong QT interval should be avoided). Products include:
E.E.S. 449
EryPed 445

Erythromycin Gluceptate (Levofloxacin has been associated with prolongation of the QTc interval; co-administration with drugs known to prolong QT interval should be avoided).
No products indexed under this heading.

Erythromycin Lactobionate (Levofloxacin has been associated with prolongation of the QTc interval; co-administration with drugs known to prolong QT interval should be avoided).
No products indexed under this heading.

Erythromycin Stearate (Levofloxacin has been associated with prolongation of the QTc interval; co-administration with drugs known to prolong QT interval should be avoided). Products include:
Erythrocin Stearate Filmtab Tablets 452

Etodolac (Co-administration may increase the risk of CNS stimulation and convulsive seizures).
No products indexed under this heading.

IMPORTANT NOTE: Always consult each drug listing in the patient's regimen for possible interactions.

Fenoprofen Calcium (Co-administration may increase the risk of CNS stimulation and convulsive seizures). Products include:

Nalfon Capsules **2504**

Ferrous Fumarate (Iron-containing preparations may interfere with the gastrointestinal absorption of levofloxacin resulting in systemic levels considerably lower than desired; these agents should be taken at least 2 hours before or after levofloxacin administration). Products include:

Chromagen Forte Soft Gelatin Capsules **3296**
Ferretts Tablets .... ▣ **773**
Repliva 21/7 Tablets **3301**

Ferrous Gluconate (Iron-containing preparations may interfere with the gastrointestinal absorption of levofloxacin resulting in systemic levels considerably lower than desired; these agents should be taken at least 2 hours before or after levofloxacin administration).

No products indexed under this heading.

Ferrous Sulfate (Iron-containing preparations may interfere with the gastrointestinal absorption of levofloxacin resulting in systemic levels considerably lower than desired; these agents should be taken at least 2 hours before or after levofloxacin administration). Products include:

Feosol Tablets **1629**
Slow Fe Iron Tablets .... ▣ **772**
Slow Fe with Folic Acid Tablets .... ▣ **773**

Fludrocortisone Acetate (Achilles and other tendon ruptures have been reported with quinolones, post-market surveillance reports indicate that the risk may be increased in patients on concomitant corticosteroids).

No products indexed under this heading.

Fluphenazine Decanoate (Levofloxacin has been associated with prolongation of the QTc interval; co-administration with drugs known to prolong QT interval should be avoided).

No products indexed under this heading.

Fluphenazine Enanthate (Levofloxacin has been associated with prolongation of the QTc interval; co-administration with drugs known to prolong QT interval should be avoided).

No products indexed under this heading.

Fluphenazine Hydrochloride (Levofloxacin has been associated with prolongation of the QTc interval; co-administration with drugs known to prolong QT interval should be avoided).

No products indexed under this heading.

Flurbiprofen (Co-administration may increase the risk of CNS stimulation and convulsive seizures).

No products indexed under this heading.

Glimepiride (Disturbances of blood glucose, including hyper- and hypoglycemia, have been reported in patients treated concomitantly with quinolones and an antidiabetic agent; careful monitoring of blood glucose levels is recommended). Products include:

Amaryl Tablets **2864**

Glipizide (Disturbances of blood glucose, including hyper- and hypoglycemia, have been reported in patients treated concomitantly with quinolones and an antidiabetic agent; careful monitoring of blood glucose levels is recommended).

No products indexed under this heading.

Glyburide (Disturbances of blood glucose, including hyper- and hypoglycemia, have been reported in patients treated concomitantly with quinolones and an antidiabetic agent; careful monitoring of blood glucose levels is recommended).

No products indexed under this heading.

Haloperidol (Levofloxacin has been associated with prolongation of the QTc interval; co-administration with drugs known to prolong QT interval should be avoided).

No products indexed under this heading.

Haloperidol Decanoate (Levofloxacin has been associated with prolongation of the QTc interval; co-administration with drugs known to prolong QT interval should be avoided).

No products indexed under this heading.

Hydrocortisone (Achilles and other tendon ruptures have been reported with quinolones, post-market surveillance reports indicate that the risk may be increased in patients on concomitant corticosteroids). Products include:

Cortizone•5 Ointment .... ▣ **699**
Cortizone•10 Creme .... ▣ **699**
Cortizone•10 Ointment .... ▣ **699**
Cortizone•10 Plus Creme .... ▣ **700**
Cortizone•10 Maximum Strength Quick Shot Spray .... ▣ **700**
Hydrocortone Tablets **1963**
Preparation H Hydrocortisone Cream .... ▣ **748**

Hydrocortisone Acetate (Achilles and other tendon ruptures have been reported with quinolones, post-market surveillance reports indicate that the risk may be increased in patients on concomitant corticosteroids). Products include:

Analpram-HC **1136**
Pramosone **1139**
ProctoFoam-HC **3113**
Tucks Anti-Itch Ointment .... ▣ **712**
U-cort 1% Cream **3289**

Hydrocortisone Sodium Phosphate (Achilles and other tendon ruptures have been reported with quinolones, post-market surveillance reports indicate that the risk may be increased in patients on concomitant corticosteroids).

No products indexed under this heading.

Hydrocortisone Sodium Succinate (Achilles and other tendon ruptures have been reported with quinolones, post-market surveillance reports indicate that the risk may be increased in patients on concomitant corticosteroids).

No products indexed under this heading.

Hydroxyzine Hydrochloride (Levofloxacin has been associated with prolongation of the QTc interval; co-administration with drugs known to prolong QT interval should be avoided).

No products indexed under this heading.

Ibuprofen (Co-administration may increase the risk of CNS stimulation and convulsive seizures). Products include:

Advil Allergy Sinus Caplets .... ▣ **737**
Advil .... ▣ **737**
Children's Advil Suspension .... ▣ **742**
Children's Advil Chewable Tablets .... ▣ **741**
Advil Cold & Sinus .... ▣ **739**
Advil Flu & Body Ache Caplets .... ▣ **739**
Children's Advil Cold Suspension .... ▣ **741**
Infants' Advil Concentrated Drops .... ▣ **743**
Junior Strength Advil Swallow Tablets .... ▣ **740**
Advil Migraine Liquigels .... ▣ **740**
Advil Multi-Symptom Cold Caplets .... ▣ **738**
Combunox Tablets **1183**
Children's Motrin Oral Suspension and Chewable Tablets **1837**
Children's Motrin Cold Non-Staining Dye-Free Oral Suspension **1838**
Children's Motrin Cold Oral Suspension **1838**
Children's Motrin Non-Staining Dye-Free Oral Suspension **1837**
Motrin Cold & Sinus Caplets **1836**
Motrin IB Tablets and Caplets **1836**
Infants' Motrin Concentrated Drops **1837**
Infants' Motrin Non-Staining Dye-Free Drops **1837**
Junior Strength Motrin Caplets and Chewable Tablets **1837**
Vicoprofen Tablets **533**

Imipramine Hydrochloride (Levofloxacin has been associated with prolongation of the QTc interval; co-administration with drugs known to prolong QT interval should be avoided).

No products indexed under this heading.

Imipramine Pamoate (Levofloxacin has been associated with prolongation of the QTc interval; co-administration with drugs known to prolong QT interval should be avoided).

No products indexed under this heading.

Indomethacin (Co-administration may increase the risk of CNS stimulation and convulsive seizures). Products include:

Indocin **1968**

Indomethacin Sodium Trihydrate (Co-administration may increase the risk of CNS stimulation and convulsive seizures). Products include:

Indocin I.V. **1973**

Iron (Iron-containing preparations may interfere with the gastrointestinal absorption of levofloxacin resulting in systemic levels considerably lower than desired; these agents should be taken at least 2 hours before or after levofloxacin administration). Products include:

Chromagen Forte Soft Gelatin Capsules **3296**
Ferretts IPS Liquid .... ▣ **773**
OptiNate **1162**
Repliva 21/7 Tablets **3301**

Isocarboxazid (Levofloxacin has been associated with prolongation of the QTc interval; co-administration with drugs known to prolong QT interval should be avoided).

No products indexed under this heading.

Ketoprofen (Co-administration may increase the risk of CNS stimulation and convulsive seizures).

No products indexed under this heading.

Ketorolac Tromethamine (Co-administration may increase the risk of CNS stimulation and convulsive seizures). Products include:

Acular Ophthalmic Solution **561**
Acular LS Ophthalmic Solution **562**

Lithium Carbonate (Levofloxacin has been associated with prolongation of the QTc interval; co-administration with drugs known to prolong QT interval should be avoided). Products include:

Eskalith **1406**
Lithobid Tablets **1670**

Lithium Citrate (Levofloxacin has been associated with prolongation of the QTc interval; co-administration with drugs known to prolong QT interval should be avoided).

No products indexed under this heading.

Lorazepam (Levofloxacin has been associated with prolongation of the QTc interval; co-administration with drugs known to prolong QT interval should be avoided).

No products indexed under this heading.

Loxapine Hydrochloride (Levofloxacin has been associated with prolongation of the QTc interval; co-administration with drugs known to prolong QT interval should be avoided).

No products indexed under this heading.

Loxapine Succinate (Levofloxacin has been associated with prolongation of the QTc interval; co-administration with drugs known to prolong QT interval should be avoided).

No products indexed under this heading.

Magaldrate (Antacids containing aluminum or magnesium may interfere with the gastrointestinal absorption of levofloxacin resulting in systemic levels considerably lower than desired; these agents should be taken at least 2 hours before or after levofloxacin administration).

No products indexed under this heading.

Magnesium (Concurrent administration of levofloxacin with metal cations may interfere with the GI absorption of levofloxacin, resulting in systemic levels considerably lower than desired; these agents containing metal cations should be taken at least 2 hours before or 2 hours after levofloxacin administration).

No products indexed under this heading.

Magnesium Hydroxide (Antacids containing aluminum or magnesium may interfere with the gastrointestinal absorption of levofloxacin resulting in systemic levels considerably lower than desired; these agents should be taken at least 2 hours before or after levofloxacin administration). Products include:

Maalox Max Maximum Strength Antacid/Anti-Gas Liquid **2165**
Maalox Regular Strength Antacid/Antigas Liquid **2164**
Pepcid Complete Chewable Tablets **1672**
Rolaids Tablets .... ▣ **707**
Extra Strength Rolaids Tablets .... ▣ **707**
Rolaids Multi-Symptom Antacid & Antigas Tablets .... ▣ **708**

Magnesium Oxide (Antacids containing aluminum or magnesium may interfere with the gastrointestinal absorption of levofloxacin resulting

in systemic levels considerably lower than desired; these agents should be taken at least 2 hours before or after levofloxacin administration).
Products include:
- Beelith Tablets ... **784**
- PremCal Light, Regular, and Extra Strength Tablets ... **762**

Maprotiline Hydrochloride (Levofloxacin has been associated with prolongation of the QTc interval; co-administration with drugs known to prolong QT interval should be avoided).
No products indexed under this heading.

Meclofenamate Sodium (Co-administration may increase the risk of CNS stimulation and convulsive seizures).
No products indexed under this heading.

Mefenamic Acid (Co-administration may increase the risk of CNS stimulation and convulsive seizures).
No products indexed under this heading.

Meloxicam (Co-administration may increase the risk of CNS stimulation and convulsive seizures). Products include:
- Mobic Oral Suspension ... **893**
- Mobic Tablets ... **893**

Meprobamate (Levofloxacin has been associated with prolongation of the QTc interval; co-administration with drugs known to prolong QT interval should be avoided).
No products indexed under this heading.

Mesoridazine Besylate (Levofloxacin has been associated with prolongation of the QTc interval; co-administration with drugs known to prolong QT interval should be avoided).
No products indexed under this heading.

Metformin Hydrochloride (Disturbances of blood glucose, including hyper- and hypoglycemia, have been reported in patients treated concomitantly with quinolones and an antidiabetic agent; careful monitoring of blood glucose levels is recommended). Products include:
- ActoPlus Met Tablets ... **3219**
- Avandamet Tablets ... **1343**
- Fortamet Extended-Release Tablets ... **1156**

Methylprednisolone Acetate (Achilles and other tendon ruptures have been reported with quinolones, post-market surveillance reports indicate that the risk may be increased in patients on concomitant corticosteroids). Products include:
- Depo-Medrol Injectable Suspension ... **2615**
- Depo-Medrol Single-Dose Vial ... **2617**

Methylprednisolone Sodium Succinate (Achilles and other tendon ruptures have been reported with quinolones, post-market surveillance reports indicate that the risk may be increased in patients on concomitant corticosteroids).
No products indexed under this heading.

Midazolam Hydrochloride (Levofloxacin has been associated with prolongation of the QTc interval; co-administration with drugs known to prolong QT interval should be avoided).
No products indexed under this heading.

Miglitol (Disturbances of blood glucose, including hyper- and hypoglycemia, have been reported in patients treated concomitantly with quinolones and an antidiabetic agent; careful monitoring of blood glucose levels is recommended).
No products indexed under this heading.

Molindone Hydrochloride (Levofloxacin has been associated with prolongation of the QTc interval; co-administration with drugs known to prolong QT interval should be avoided). Products include:
- Moban Tablets ... **1108**

Moricizine Hydrochloride (Levofloxacin has been associated with prolongation of the QT interval and infrequent cases of arrhythmia. Rare cases of torsades de pointes have been spontaneously reported during post-marketing surveillance in patients receiving levofloxacin. Levofloxacin should be avoided in patients receiving class IA antiarrhythmic agents).
No products indexed under this heading.

Nabumetone (Co-administration may increase the risk of CNS stimulation and convulsive seizures).
Products include:
- Relafen Tablets ... **1523**

Naproxen (Co-administration may increase the risk of CNS stimulation and convulsive seizures). Products include:
- EC-Naprosyn Delayed-Release Tablets ... **2769**
- Naprosyn Suspension ... **2769**
- Naprosyn Tablets ... **2769**
- Prevacid NapraPAC ... **3277**

Naproxen Sodium (Co-administration may increase the risk of CNS stimulation and convulsive seizures). Products include:
- Aleve Tablets, Caplets and Gelcaps ... **605**
- Anaprox Tablets ... **2769**
- Anaprox DS Tablets ... **2769**

Nortriptyline Hydrochloride (Levofloxacin has been associated with prolongation of the QTc interval; co-administration with drugs known to prolong QT interval should be avoided).
No products indexed under this heading.

Olanzapine (Levofloxacin has been associated with prolongation of the QTc interval; co-administration with drugs known to prolong QT interval should be avoided). Products include:
- Symbyax Capsules ... **1788**
- Zyprexa Tablets ... **1798**
- Zyprexa IntraMuscular ... **1798**
- Zyprexa ZYDIS Orally Disintegrating Tablets ... **1798**

Oxaprozin (Co-administration may increase the risk of CNS stimulation and convulsive seizures).
No products indexed under this heading.

Oxazepam (Levofloxacin has been associated with prolongation of the QTc interval; co-administration with drugs known to prolong QT interval should be avoided).
No products indexed under this heading.

Perphenazine (Levofloxacin has been associated with prolongation of the QTc interval; co-administration with drugs known to prolong QT interval should be avoided).
No products indexed under this heading.

Phenelzine Sulfate (Levofloxacin has been associated with prolongation of the QTc interval; co-administration with drugs known to prolong QT interval should be avoided).
No products indexed under this heading.

Phenylbutazone (Co-administration may increase the risk of CNS stimulation and convulsive seizures).
No products indexed under this heading.

Pimozide (Levofloxacin has been associated with prolongation of the QTc interval; co-administration with drugs known to prolong QT interval should be avoided). Products include:
- Orap Tablets ... **1220**

Pioglitazone Hydrochloride (Disturbances of blood glucose, including hyper- and hypoglycemia, have been reported in patients treated concomitantly with quinolones and an antidiabetic agent; careful monitoring of blood glucose levels is recommended). Products include:
- ActoPlus Met Tablets ... **3219**
- Actos Tablets ... **3224**

Piroxicam (Co-administration may increase the risk of CNS stimulation and convulsive seizures).
No products indexed under this heading.

Polysaccharide Iron Complex (Iron-containing preparations may interfere with the gastrointestinal absorption of levofloxacin resulting in systemic levels considerably lower than desired; these agents should be taken at least 2 hours before or after levofloxacin administration).
Products include:
- Niferex-150 Forte Capsules ... **3299**
- Nu-Iron 150 Capsules ... **2098**

Prazepam (Levofloxacin has been associated with prolongation of the QTc interval; co-administration with drugs known to prolong QT interval should be avoided).
No products indexed under this heading.

Prednisolone Acetate (Achilles and other tendon ruptures have been reported with quinolones, post-market surveillance reports indicate that the risk may be increased in patients on concomitant corticosteroids). Products include:
- Blephamide Ophthalmic Ointment ... **563**
- Blephamide Ophthalmic Suspension ... **564**
- Poly-Pred Liquifilm Ophthalmic Suspension ... ⊙**231**
- Pred Forte Ophthalmic Suspension ... ⊙**233**
- Pred Mild Sterile Ophthalmic Suspension ... ⊙**236**
- Pred-G Ophthalmic Suspension ... ⊙**234**
- Pred-G Sterile Ophthalmic Ointment ... ⊙**235**

Prednisolone Sodium Phosphate (Achilles and other tendon ruptures have been reported with quinolones, post-market surveillance reports indicate that the risk may be increased in patients on concomitant corticosteroids). Products include:
- Pediapred Oral Solution ... **3319**

Prednisolone Tebutate (Achilles and other tendon ruptures have been reported with quinolones, post-market surveillance reports indicate that the risk may be increased in patients on concomitant corticosteroids).
No products indexed under this heading.

Prednisone (Achilles and other tendon ruptures have been reported with quinolones, post-market surveillance reports indicate that the risk may be increased in patients on concomitant corticosteroids).
No products indexed under this heading.

Probenecid (Co-administration has resulted in higher levofloxacin AUC and t1/2, while CL/F and CLr were lower during concomitant treatment with probenecid).
No products indexed under this heading.

Procainamide (Levofloxacin has been associated with prolongation of the QT interval and infrequent cases of arrhythmia. Rare cases of torsades de pointes have been spontaneously reported during post-marketing surveillance in patients receiving levofloxacin. Levofloxacin should be avoided in patients receiving class IA antiarrhythmic agents).
No products indexed under this heading.

Procainamide Hydrochloride (Levofloxacin has been associated with prolongation of the QTc interval; co-administration with drugs known to prolong QT interval should be avoided).
No products indexed under this heading.

Prochlorperazine (Levofloxacin has been associated with prolongation of the QTc interval; co-administration with drugs known to prolong QT interval should be avoided).
No products indexed under this heading.

Promethazine Hydrochloride (Levofloxacin has been associated with prolongation of the QTc interval; co-administration with drugs known to prolong QT interval should be avoided). Products include:
- Phenergan ... **3438**

Protriptyline Hydrochloride (Levofloxacin has been associated with prolongation of the QTc interval; co-administration with drugs known to prolong QT interval should be avoided). Products include:
- Vivactil Tablets ... **2350**

Quetiapine Fumarate (Levofloxacin has been associated with prolongation of the QTc interval; co-administration with drugs known to prolong QT interval should be avoided). Products include:
- Seroquel Tablets ... **691**

Quinidine (Levofloxacin has been associated with prolongation of the QTc interval; co-administration with drugs known to prolong QT interval should be avoided).
No products indexed under this heading.

Quinidine Gluconate (Levofloxacin has been associated with prolongation of the QTc interval; co-administration with drugs known to prolong QT interval should be avoided).
No products indexed under this heading.

Quinidine Hydrochloride (Levofloxacin has been associated with prolongation of the QTc interval; co-administration with drugs known to prolong QT interval should be avoided).
No products indexed under this heading.

Quinidine Polygalacturonate (Levofloxacin has been associated with prolongation of the QTc interval; co-administration with drugs known to prolong QT interval should be avoided).
No products indexed under this heading.

Quinidine Sulfate (Levofloxacin has been associated with prolongation of the QTc interval; co-administration with drugs known to prolong QT interval should be avoided).
No products indexed under this heading.

Repaglinide (Disturbances of blood glucose, including hyper- and hypoglycemia, have been reported in patients treated concomitantly with quinolones and an antidiabetic agent; careful monitoring of blood glucose levels is recommended). Products include:
Prandin Tablets (0.5, 1, and 2 mg) **2337**

Risperidone (Levofloxacin has been associated with prolongation of the QTc interval; co-administration with drugs known to prolong QT interval should be avoided). Products include:
Risperdal Consta Long-Acting Injection **1664**
Risperdal M-Tab Orally Disintegrating Tablets **1658**
Risperdal **1658**

Rofecoxib (Co-administration may increase the risk of CNS stimulation and convulsive seizures).
No products indexed under this heading.

Rosiglitazone Maleate (Disturbances of blood glucose, including hyper- and hypoglycemia, have been reported in patients treated concomitantly with quinolones and an antidiabetic agent; careful monitoring of blood glucose levels is recommended). Products include:
Avandamet Tablets **1343**
Avandia Tablets **1348**

Sotalol Hydrochloride (Levofloxacin has been associated with prolongation of the QTc interval; co-administration with drugs known to prolong QT interval should be avoided).
No products indexed under this heading.

Sucralfate (May interfere with the gastrointestinal absorption of levofloxacin resulting in systemic levels considerably lower than desired; sucralfate should be taken at least 2 hours before or after levofloxacin administration). Products include:
Carafate Suspension **727**
Carafate Tablets **728**

Sulindac (Co-administration may increase the risk of CNS stimulation and convulsive seizures). Products include:
Clinoril Tablets **1899**

Theophylline (Co-administration of other quinolones with theophylline has resulted in prolonged elimination half-life, elevated serum theophylline levels, and increased risk of theophylline related toxicity; no significant effect of levofloxacin on theophylline pharmacokinetic parameters has been detected, however, caution should be exercised).
No products indexed under this heading.

Theophylline Anhydrous (Co-administration of other quinolones with theophylline has resulted in prolonged elimination half-life, elevated serum theophylline levels, and increased risk of theophylline related toxicity; no significant effect of levofloxacin on theophylline pharmacokinetic parameters has been detected, however, caution should be exercised). Products include:
Uniphyl Tablets **2708**

Theophylline Calcium Salicylate (Co-administration of other quinolones with theophylline has resulted in prolonged elimination half-life, elevated serum theophylline levels, and increased risk of theophylline related toxicity; no significant effect of levofloxacin on theophylline pharmacokinetic parameters has been detected, however, caution should be exercised).
No products indexed under this heading.

Theophylline Dihydroxypropyl (Glyceryl) (Co-administration of other quinolones with theophylline has resulted in prolonged elimination half-life, elevated serum theophylline levels, and increased risk of theophylline related toxicity; no significant effect of levofloxacin on theophylline pharmacokinetic parameters has been detected, however, caution should be exercised).
No products indexed under this heading.

Theophylline Ethylenediamine (Co-administration of other quinolones with theophylline has resulted in prolonged elimination half-life, elevated serum theophylline levels, and increased risk of theophylline related toxicity; no significant effect of levofloxacin on theophylline pharmacokinetic parameters has been detected, however, caution should be exercised).
No products indexed under this heading.

Theophylline Sodium Glycinate (Co-administration of other quinolones with theophylline has resulted in prolonged elimination half-life, elevated serum theophylline levels, and increased risk of theophylline related toxicity; no significant effect of levofloxacin on theophylline pharmacokinetic parameters has been detected, however, caution should be exercised).
No products indexed under this heading.

Thioridazine Hydrochloride (Levofloxacin has been associated with prolongation of the QTc interval; co-administration with drugs known to prolong QT interval should be avoided). Products include:
Thioridazine Hydrochloride Tablets **2122**

Thiothixene (Levofloxacin has been associated with prolongation of the QTc interval; co-administration with drugs known to prolong QT interval should be avoided). Products include:
Thiothixene Capsules **2124**

Tolazamide (Disturbances of blood glucose, including hyper- and hypoglycemia, have been reported in patients treated concomitantly with quinolones and an antidiabetic agent; careful monitoring of blood glucose levels is recommended).
No products indexed under this heading.

Tolbutamide (Disturbances of blood glucose, including hyper- and hypoglycemia, have been reported in patients treated concomitantly with quinolones and an antidiabetic agent; careful monitoring of blood glucose levels is recommended).
No products indexed under this heading.

Tolmetin Sodium (Co-administration may increase the risk of CNS stimulation and convulsive seizures).
No products indexed under this heading.

Tranylcypromine Sulfate (Levofloxacin has been associated with prolongation of the QTc interval; co-administration with drugs known to prolong QT interval should be avoided). Products include:
Parnate Tablets **1499**

Triamcinolone (Achilles and other tendon ruptures have been reported with quinolones, post-market surveillance reports indicate that the risk may be increased in patients on concomitant corticosteroids).
No products indexed under this heading.

Triamcinolone Acetonide (Achilles and other tendon ruptures have been reported with quinolones, post-market surveillance reports indicate that the risk may be increased in patients on concomitant corticosteroids). Products include:
Azmacort Inhalation Aerosol **1701**
Nasacort HFA Inhalation Aerosol **2939**
Nasacort AQ Nasal Spray **2937**

Triamcinolone Diacetate (Achilles and other tendon ruptures have been reported with quinolones, post-market surveillance reports indicate that the risk may be increased in patients on concomitant corticosteroids).
No products indexed under this heading.

Triamcinolone Hexacetonide (Achilles and other tendon ruptures have been reported with quinolones, post-market surveillance reports indicate that the risk may be increased in patients on concomitant corticosteroids).
No products indexed under this heading.

Trifluoperazine Hydrochloride (Levofloxacin has been associated with prolongation of the QTc interval; co-administration with drugs known to prolong QT interval should be avoided).
No products indexed under this heading.

Trimipramine Maleate (Levofloxacin has been associated with prolongation of the QTc interval; co-administration with drugs known to prolong QT interval should be avoided). Products include:
Surmontil Capsules **2347**

Troglitazone (Disturbances of blood glucose, including hyper- and hypoglycemia, have been reported in patients treated concomitantly with quinolones and an antidiabetic agent; careful monitoring of blood glucose levels is recommended).
No products indexed under this heading.

Valdecoxib (Co-administration may increase the risk of CNS stimulation and convulsive seizures).
No products indexed under this heading.

Warfarin Sodium (Co-administration of other quinolones with warfarin has resulted in enhanced effects of warfarin; no significant effect of levofloxacin on warfarin pharmacokinetic parameters has been detected in clinical studies, however, caution should be exercised and coagulation test should be closely monitored). Products include:
Coumadin for Injection **932**
Coumadin Tablets **932**

Zinc (Concurrent administration of levofloxacin with metal cations may interfere with the GI absorption of levofloxacin, resulting in systemic levels considerably lower than desired; these agents containing metal cations should be taken at least 2 hours before or 2 hours after levofloxacin administration). Products include:
Visutein Capsules **3328**

Ziprasidone Hydrochloride (Levofloxacin has been associated with prolongation of the QTc interval; co-administration with drugs known to prolong QT interval should be avoided). Products include:
Geodon Capsules **2514**

Food Interactions

Food, unspecified (Co-administration slightly prolongs the time to peak concentration by approximately 1 hour and slightly decreases the peak concentration by approximately 14%; levofloxacin can be administered without regard to food).

LEVITRA TABLETS

(Vardenafil Hydrochloride) **3048**
May interact with alpha adrenergic blockers, class 1A antiarrhythmics, class III antiarrhythmics, cytochrome p450 3a4 inhibitors (selected), erythromycin, nitrates and nitrites, and certain other agents. Compounds in these categories include:

Acetazolamide (Concomitant use with moderate/strong CYP 3A4 inhibitors results in significant increases in plasma levels of vardenafil).
No products indexed under this heading.

Amiodarone Hydrochloride (Vardenafil hydrochloride may increase the QTc interval. Patients with congenital QT prolongation and those taking Class III antiarrhythmic medications should avoid using vardenafil hydrochloride). Products include:
Pacerone Tablets **3337**

Amprenavir (Concomitant use with moderate/strong CYP 3A4 inhibitors results in significant increases in plasma levels of vardenafil). Products include:

Agenerase Capsules 1299
Agenerase Oral Solution 1304

Amyl Nitrite (The blood pressure lowering effects of sublingual nitrates taken 1 and 4 hours after vardenafil and increases in heart rate when taken at 1, 4 and 8 hours, were potentiated by vardenafil hydrochloride. These effects were not observed when vardenafil hydrochloride was taken 24 hours before the nitroglycerin. Concomitant use of vardenafil and nitrates is contraindicated).
No products indexed under this heading.

Anastrozole (Concomitant use with moderate/strong CYP 3A4 inhibitors results in significant increases in plasma levels of vardenafil). Products include:
Arimidex Tablets 665

Aprepitant (Concomitant use with moderate/strong CYP 3A4 inhibitors results in significant increases in plasma levels of vardenafil). Products include:
Emend Capsules 1944

Bretylium Tosylate (Vardenafil hydrochloride may increase the QTc interval. Patients with congenital QT prolongation and those taking Class III antiarrhythmic medications should avoid using vardenafil hydrochloride).
No products indexed under this heading.

Cimetidine (Concomitant use with moderate/strong CYP 3A4 inhibitors results in significant increases in plasma levels of vardenafil). Products include:
Tagamet HB 200 Tablets 637
Tagamet Tablets 1547

Cimetidine Hydrochloride (Concomitant use with moderate/strong CYP 3A4 inhibitors results in significant increases in plasma levels of vardenafil).
No products indexed under this heading.

Ciprofloxacin (Concomitant use with moderate/strong CYP 3A4 inhibitors results in significant increases in plasma levels of vardenafil). Products include:
Cipro I.V. 2998
Cipro I.V. Pharmacy Bulk Package ... 3509
Cipro Oral Suspension 2991
Cipro XR Tablets 3004
Ciprodex Otic Suspension 555

Clarithromycin (Concomitant use with moderate/strong CYP 3A4 inhibitors results in significant increases in plasma levels of vardenafil). Products include:
Biaxin/Biaxin XL 402
PREVPAC 3281

Clotrimazole (Concomitant use with moderate/strong CYP 3A4 inhibitors results in significant increases in plasma levels of vardenafil). Products include:
Lotrimin 3053
Lotrisone 3054

Cyclosporine (Concomitant use with moderate/strong CYP 3A4 inhibitors results in significant increases in plasma levels of vardenafil). Products include:
Gengraf Capsules 458
Neoral Soft Gelatin Capsules 2247
Neoral Oral Solution 2247
Restasis Ophthalmic Emulsion 570
Sandimmune 2259

Dalfopristin (Concomitant use with moderate/strong CYP 3A4 inhibitors results in significant increases in plasma levels of vardenafil). Products include:
Synercid I.V. 1690

Danazol (Concomitant use with moderate/strong CYP 3A4 inhibitors results in significant increases in plasma levels of vardenafil).
No products indexed under this heading.

Delavirdine Mesylate (Concomitant use with moderate/strong CYP 3A4 inhibitors results in significant increases in plasma levels of vardenafil). Products include:
Rescriptor Tablets 2535

Diltiazem Hydrochloride (Concomitant use with moderate/strong CYP 3A4 inhibitors results in significant increases in plasma levels of vardenafil). Products include:
Cardizem LA Extended Release Tablets 1699
Tiazac Capsules 1204

Diltiazem Maleate (Concomitant use with moderate/strong CYP 3A4 inhibitors results in significant increases in plasma levels of vardenafil).
No products indexed under this heading.

Disopyramide (Vardenafil hydrochloride may increase the QTc interval. Patients with congenital QT prolongation and those taking Class IA antiarrhythmic medications should avoid using vardenafil hydrochloride).
No products indexed under this heading.

Doxazosin Mesylate (Caution is advised when Phosphodiesterase Type 5 (PDE5) inhibitors are co-administered with alpha-blockers. Concomitant use of these two drug classes may lower blood pressure significantly leading to symptomatic hypotension. Patients should be stable on alpha-blocker therapy prior to initiating a PDE5 inhibitor. Patients who demonstrate hemodynamic instability on alpha-blocker therapy alone are at an increased risk of symptomatic hypotention with concomitant use of PDE5 inhibitors. In those patients who are stable on alpha-blocker therapy, PDE5 inhibitors should be initiated at the lowest recommended starting dose. In those patients already taking an optimized dose of PDE5 inhibitor, alpha-blocker therapy should be initiated at the lowest dose).
No products indexed under this heading.

Efavirenz (Concomitant use with moderate/strong CYP 3A4 inhibitors results in significant increases in plasma levels of vardenafil). Products include:
Sustiva Capsules 957

Erythrityl Tetranitrate (The blood pressure lowering effects of sublingual nitrates taken 1 and 4 hours after vardenafil and increases in heart rate when taken at 1, 4 and 8 hours, were potentiated by vardenafil hydrochloride. These effects were not observed when vardenafil hydrochloride was taken 24 hours before the nitroglycerin. Concomitant use of vardenafil and nitrates is contraindicated).
No products indexed under this heading.

Erythromycin (Erythromycin produced a 4-fold increase in vardenafil AUC and a 3-fold increase in Cmax when co-administered with vardenafil hydrochloride in healthy volunteers. It is not recommended to exceed a single 5mg dose of vardenafil hydrochloride in a 24-hour period when used in combination with erythromycin). Products include:
Erygel Topical Gel 2096
Ery-Tab Tablets 447
Erythromycin Base Filmtab Tablets 454
Erythromycin Delayed-Release Capsules, USP 456
PCE Dispertab Tablets 510

Erythromycin Estolate (Erythromycin produced a 4-fold increase in vardenafil AUC and a 3-fold increase in Cmax when co-administered with vardenafil hydrochloride in healthy volunteers. It is not recommended to exceed a single 5mg dose of vardenafil hydrochloride in a 24-hour period when used in combination with erythromycin).
No products indexed under this heading.

Erythromycin Ethylsuccinate (Erythromycin produced a 4-fold increase in vardenafil AUC and a 3-fold increase in Cmax when co-administered with vardenafil hydrochloride in healthy volunteers. It is not recommended to exceed a single 5mg dose of vardenafil hydrochloride in a 24-hour period when used in combination with erythromycin). Products include:
E.E.S. 449
EryPed 445

Erythromycin Gluceptate (Erythromycin produced a 4-fold increase in vardenafil AUC and a 3-fold increase in Cmax when co-administered with vardenafil hydrochloride in healthy volunteers. It is not recommended to exceed a single 5mg dose of vardenafil hydrochloride in a 24-hour period when used in combination with erythromycin).
No products indexed under this heading.

Erythromycin Lactobionate (Erythromycin produced a 4-fold increase in vardenafil AUC and a 3-fold increase in Cmax when co-administered with vardenafil hydrochloride in healthy volunteers. It is not recommended to exceed a single 5mg dose of vardenafil hydrochloride in a 24-hour period when used in combination with erythromycin).
No products indexed under this heading.

Erythromycin Stearate (Erythromycin produced a 4-fold increase in vardenafil AUC and a 3-fold increase in Cmax when co-administered with vardenafil hydrochloride in healthy volunteers. It is not recommended to exceed a single 5mg dose of vardenafil hydrochloride in a 24-hour period when used in combination with erythromycin). Products include:
Erythrocin Stearate Filmtab Tablets 452

Esomeprazole Magnesium (Concomitant use with moderate/strong CYP 3A4 inhibitors results in significant increases in plasma levels of vardenafil). Products include:
Nexium Delayed-Release Capsules 645

Fluconazole (Concomitant use with moderate/strong CYP 3A4 inhibitors results in significant increases in plasma levels of vardenafil).
No products indexed under this heading.

Fluoxetine Hydrochloride (Concomitant use with moderate/strong CYP 3A4 inhibitors results in significant increases in plasma levels of vardenafil). Products include:
Prozac Pulvules and Liquid 1771
Symbyax Capsules 1788

Fluvoxamine Maleate (Concomitant use with moderate/strong CYP 3A4 inhibitors results in significant increases in plasma levels of vardenafil).
No products indexed under this heading.

Fosamprenavir Calcium (Concomitant use with moderate/strong CYP 3A4 inhibitors results in significant increases in plasma levels of vardenafil). Products include:
Lexiva Tablets 1473

Indinavir Sulfate (Indinavir, co-administered with vardenafil hydrochloride, resulted in a 16-fold increase in vardenafil AUC, a 7-fold increase in vardenafil Cmax and a 2-fold increase in vardenafil half-life. It is recommended not to exceed a single 2.5mg vardenafil hydrochloride dose in a 24-hour period when used in combination with indinavir). Products include:
Crixivan Capsules 1918

Isoniazid (Concomitant use with moderate/strong CYP 3A4 inhibitors results in significant increases in plasma levels of vardenafil).
No products indexed under this heading.

Isosorbide Dinitrate (The blood pressure lowering effects of sublingual nitrates taken 1 and 4 hours after vardenafil and increases in heart rate when taken at 1, 4 and 8 hours, were potentiated by vardenafil hydrochloride. These effects were not observed when vardenafil hydrochloride was taken 24 hours before the nitroglycerin. Concomitant use of vardenafil and nitrates is contraindicated). Products include:
BiDil Tablets 2161

Isosorbide Mononitrate (The blood pressure lowering effects of sublingual nitrates taken 1 and 4 hours after vardenafil and increases in heart rate when taken at 1, 4 and 8 hours, were potentiated by vardenafil hydrochloride. These effects were not observed when vardenafil hydrochloride was taken 24 hours before the nitroglycerin. Concomitant use of vardenafil and nitrates is contraindicated). Products include:
Imdur Tablets 3032

Itraconazole (Patients taking itraconazole 400mg daily should not exceed vardenafil hydrochloride 2.5mg once daily. For patients taking itraconazole 200mg daily, a single dose of 5mg vardenafil hydrochloride should not be exceeded in a 24-hour period).
No products indexed under this heading.

Ketoconazole (Ketoconazole may produce an increase in vardenafil AUC and Cmax when co-administered. Patients taking ketoconazole 400mg daily should not exceed vardenafil hydrochloride 2.5mg once daily. For patients tak-

ing ketoconazole 200mg daily, a single dose of 5mg vardenafil hydrochloride should not be exceeded in a 24-hour period). Products include:

Nizoral A-D Shampoo, 1% ... 1839
Nizoral 2% Shampoo ... 1838

Lopinavir (Concomitant use with moderate/strong CYP 3A4 inhibitors results in significant increases in plasma levels of vardenafil). Products include:

Kaletra ... 474

Loratadine (Concomitant use with moderate/strong CYP 3A4 inhibitors results in significant increases in plasma levels of vardenafil). Products include:

Alavert Allergy & Sinus D-12 Hour Tablets ... ▣743
Alavert ... ▣743
Children's Claritin 24 Hour Non-Drowsy Allergy Syrup ... ▣732
Claritin Non-Drowsy 24 Hour Tablets ... ▣731
Non-Drowsy Claritin Hives Relief Tablets ... ▣733
Claritin Reditabs 24 Hour Non-Drowsy Tablets ... ▣732
Claritin-D Non-Drowsy 12 Hour Tablets ... ▣731
Claritin-D Non-Drowsy 24 Hour Tablets ... ▣731
Children's Dimetapp ND Non-Drowsy Allergy Syrup ... ▣746
Triaminic Allerchews ... ▣684

Metronidazole (Concomitant use with moderate/strong CYP 3A4 inhibitors results in significant increases in plasma levels of vardenafil). Products include:

Metrogel 1% ... 1212
MetroGel-Vaginal Gel ... 1822
Noritate Cream, 1% ... 1051

Metronidazole Benzoate (Concomitant use with moderate/strong CYP 3A4 inhibitors results in significant increases in plasma levels of vardenafil).

No products indexed under this heading.

Metronidazole Hydrochloride (Concomitant use with moderate/strong CYP 3A4 inhibitors results in significant increases in plasma levels of vardenafil).

No products indexed under this heading.

Miconazole (Concomitant use with moderate/strong CYP 3A4 inhibitors results in significant increases in plasma levels of vardenafil).

No products indexed under this heading.

Miconazole Nitrate (Concomitant use with moderate/strong CYP 3A4 inhibitors results in significant increases in plasma levels of vardenafil). Products include:

Desenex ... ▣674
Desenex Jock Itch Spray Powder ... ▣674

Moricizine Hydrochloride (Vardenafil hydrochloride may increase the QTc interval. Patients with congenital QT prolongation and those taking Class IA antiarrhythmic medications should avoid using vardenafil hydrochloride).

No products indexed under this heading.

Nefazodone Hydrochloride (Concomitant use with moderate/strong CYP 3A4 inhibitors results in significant increases in plasma levels of vardenafil).

No products indexed under this heading.

Nelfinavir Mesylate (Concomitant use with moderate/strong CYP 3A4 inhibitors results in significant increases in plasma levels of vardenafil). Products include:

Viracept ... 2556

Nevirapine (Concomitant use with moderate/strong CYP 3A4 inhibitors results in significant increases in plasma levels of vardenafil). Products include:

Viramune Oral Suspension ... 903
Viramune Tablets ... 903

Niacinamide (Concomitant use with moderate/strong CYP 3A4 inhibitors results in significant increases in plasma levels of vardenafil).

No products indexed under this heading.

Nicotinamide (Concomitant use with moderate/strong CYP 3A4 inhibitors results in significant increases in plasma levels of vardenafil). Products include:

Nicomide Tablets ... 3190

Nifedipine (In patients whose hypertension was controlled with nifedipine, vardenafil hydrochloride produced mean additional supine systolic/diastolic blood pressure reductions of 6/5mm Hg compared to placebo). Products include:

Adalat CC Tablets ... 2978

Nitroglycerin (The blood pressure lowering effects of sublingual nitrates taken 1 and 4 hours after vardenafil and increases in heart rate when taken at 1, 4 and 8 hours, were potentiated by vardenafil hydrochloride. These effects were not observed when vardenafil hydrochloride was taken 24 hours before the nitroglycerin. Concomitant use of vardenafil and nitrates is contraindicated). Products include:

Nitro-Dur Transdermal Infusion System ... 3060
Nitrolingual Pumpspray ... 1161

Norfloxacin (Concomitant use with moderate/strong CYP 3A4 inhibitors results in significant increases in plasma levels of vardenafil). Products include:

Noroxin Tablets ... 2009

Omeprazole (Concomitant use with moderate/strong CYP 3A4 inhibitors results in significant increases in plasma levels of vardenafil). Products include:

Zegerid Powder for Oral Solution ... 2972

Paroxetine Hydrochloride (Concomitant use with moderate/strong CYP 3A4 inhibitors results in significant increases in plasma levels of vardenafil). Products include:

Paxil CR Controlled-Release Tablets ... 1509
Paxil ... 1501

Pentaerythritol Tetranitrate (The blood pressure lowering effects of sublingual nitrates taken 1 and 4 hours after vardenafil and increases in heart rate when taken at 1, 4 and 8 hours, were potentiated by vardenafil hydrochloride. These effects were not observed when vardenafil hydrochloride was taken 24 hours before the nitroglycerin. Concomitant use of vardenafil and nitrates is contraindicated).

No products indexed under this heading.

Prazosin Hydrochloride (Caution is advised when Phosphodiesterase Type 5 (PDE5) inhibitors are co-administered with alpha-blockers. Concomitant use of these two drug classes may lower blood pressure significantly leading to symptomatic hypotention. Patients should be stable on alpha-blocker therapy prior to initiating a PDE5 inhibitor. Patients who demonstrate hemodynamic instability on alpha-blocker therapy alone are at an increased risk of symptomatic hypotention with concomitant use of PDE5 inhibitors. In those patients who are stable on alpha-blocker therapy, PDE5 inhibitors should be initiated at the lowest recommended starting dose. In those patients already taking an optimized dose of PDE5 inhibitor, alpha-blocker therapy should be initiated at the lowest dose).

No products indexed under this heading.

Procainamide (Vardenafil hydrochloride may increase the QTc interval. Patients with congenital QT prolongation and those taking Class IA antiarrhythmic medications should avoid using vardenafil hydrochloride).

No products indexed under this heading.

Propoxyphene Hydrochloride (Concomitant use with moderate/strong CYP 3A4 inhibitors results in significant increases in plasma levels of vardenafil).

No products indexed under this heading.

Propoxyphene Napsylate (Concomitant use with moderate/strong CYP 3A4 inhibitors results in significant increases in plasma levels of vardenafil). Products include:

Darvocet A 500 Tablets ... 3497

Quinidine (Vardenafil hydrochloride may increase the QTc interval. Patients with congenital QT prolongation and those taking Class IA antiarrhythmic medications should avoid using vardenafil hydrochloride).

No products indexed under this heading.

Quinidine Gluconate (Vardenafil hydrochloride may increase the QTc interval. Patients with congenital QT prolongation and those taking Class IA antiarrhythmic medications should avoid using vardenafil hydrochloride).

No products indexed under this heading.

Quinidine Hydrochloride (Concomitant use with moderate/strong CYP 3A4 inhibitors results in significant increases in plasma levels of vardenafil).

No products indexed under this heading.

Quinidine Polygalacturonate (Concomitant use with moderate/strong CYP 3A4 inhibitors results in significant increases in plasma levels of vardenafil).

No products indexed under this heading.

Quinidine Sulfate (Concomitant use with moderate/strong CYP 3A4 inhibitors results in significant increases in plasma levels of vardenafil).

No products indexed under this heading.

Quinine (Concomitant use with moderate/strong CYP 3A4 inhibitors results in significant increases in plasma levels of vardenafil).

No products indexed under this heading.

Quinine Sulfate (Concomitant use with moderate/strong CYP 3A4 inhibitors results in significant increases in plasma levels of vardenafil).

No products indexed under this heading.

Quinupristin (Concomitant use with moderate/strong CYP 3A4 inhibitors results in significant increases in plasma levels of vardenafil). Products include:

Synercid I.V. ... 1690

Ranitidine Bismuth Citrate (Concomitant use with moderate/strong CYP 3A4 inhibitors results in significant increases in plasma levels of vardenafil).

No products indexed under this heading.

Ranitidine Hydrochloride (Concomitant use with moderate/strong CYP 3A4 inhibitors results in significant increases in plasma levels of vardenafil). Products include:

Zantac ... 1597
Zantac Injection ... 1593
Zantac 75 Tablets ... ▣715
Zantac 150 Maximum Strength Tablets ... ▣715
Zantac Injection Pharmacy Bulk Package ... 1595

Ritonavir (Ritonavir co-administered with vardenafil hydrochloride resulted in a 49-fold increase in vardenafil AUC, a 13-fold increase in vardenafil Cmax, and significantly prolonged the half-life of vardenafil to 26 hours. The interaction is a consequence of blocking the hepatic metabolism of vardenafil by ritonavir, a highly potent CYP3A4 inhibitor. It is recommended not to exceed a single 2.5mg dose of vardenafil hydrochloride in a 72-hour period when used in combination with ritonavir). Products include:

Kaletra ... 474
Norvir ... 499

Saquinavir (Concomitant use with moderate/strong CYP 3A4 inhibitors results in significant increases in plasma levels of vardenafil).

No products indexed under this heading.

Saquinavir Mesylate (Concomitant use with moderate/strong CYP 3A4 inhibitors results in significant increases in plasma levels of vardenafil). Products include:

Invirase ... 2776

Sertraline Hydrochloride (Concomitant use with moderate/strong CYP 3A4 inhibitors results in significant increases in plasma levels of vardenafil). Products include:

Zoloft ... 2581

Sildenafil Citrate (The safety and efficacy of vardenafil hydrochloride used in combination with other treatments for erectile dysfunction have not been studied. Therefore, the use of such combinations is not recommended). Products include:

Revatio Tablets ... 2541
Viagra Tablets ... 2552

Sotalol Hydrochloride (Vardenafil hydrochloride may increase the QTc interval. Patients with congenital QT prolongation and those taking Class III antiarrhythmic medications should avoid using vardenafil hydrochloride).

No products indexed under this heading.

Tamsulosin Hydrochloride (Caution is advised when Phosphodiesterase Type 5 (PDE5) inhibitors are co-administered with alpha-blockers.

Concomitant use of these two drug classes may lower blood pressure significantly leading to symptomatic hypotention. Patients should be stable on alpha-blocker therapy prior to initiating a PDE5 inhibitor. Patients who demonstrate hemodynamic instability on alpha-blocker therapy alone are at an increased risk of symptomatic hypotention with concomitant use of PDE5 inhibitors. In those patients who are stable on alpha-blocker therapy, PDE5 inhibitors should be initiated at the lowest recommended starting dose. In those patients already taking an optimized dose of PDE5 inhibitor, alpha-blocker therapy should be initiated at the lowest dose). Products include:

Flomax Capsules 881

Telithromycin (Concomitant use with moderate/strong CYP 3A4 inhibitors results in significant increases in plasma levels of vardenafil). Products include:

Ketek Tablets 2920

Terazosin Hydrochloride (Caution is advised when Phosphodiesterase Type 5 (PDE5) inhibitors are co-administered with alpha-blockers. Concomitant use of these two drug classes may lower blood pressure significantly leading to symptomatic hypotention. Patients should be stable on alpha-blocker therapy prior to initiating a PDE5 inhibitor. Patients who demonstrate hemodynamic instability on alpha-blocker therapy alone are at an increased risk of symptomatic hypotention with concomitant use of PDE5 inhibitors. In those patients who are stable on alpha-blocker therapy, PDE5 inhibitors should be initiated at the lowest recommended starting dose. In those patients already taking an optimized dose of PDE5 inhibitor, alpha-blocker therapy should be initiated at the lowest dose). Products include:

Hytrin Capsules 469

Troglitazone (Concomitant use with moderate/strong CYP 3A4 inhibitors results in significant increases in plasma levels of vardenafil).

No products indexed under this heading.

Troleandomycin (Concomitant use with moderate/strong CYP 3A4 inhibitors results in significant increases in plasma levels of vardenafil).

No products indexed under this heading.

Valproate Sodium (Concomitant use with moderate/strong CYP 3A4 inhibitors results in significant increases in plasma levels of vardenafil). Products include:

Depacon Injection 412

Verapamil Hydrochloride (Concomitant use with moderate/strong CYP 3A4 inhibitors results in significant increases in plasma levels of vardenafil). Products include:

Covera-HS Tablets 3135
Tarka Tablets 519
Verelan PM Capsules 3120

Voriconazole (Concomitant use with moderate/strong CYP 3A4 inhibitors results in significant increases in plasma levels of vardenafil). Products include:

VFEND I.V. 2543
VFEND Oral Suspension 2543
VFEND Tablets 2543

Zafirlukast (Concomitant use with moderate/strong CYP 3A4 inhibitors results in significant increases in plasma levels of vardenafil). Products include:

Accolate Tablets 663

Zileuton (Concomitant use with moderate/strong CYP 3A4 inhibitors results in significant increases in plasma levels of vardenafil).

No products indexed under this heading.

Food Interactions

Grapefruit (Concomitant use with moderate/strong CYP 3A4 inhibitors results in significant increases in plasma levels of vardenafil).

Grapefruit Juice (Concomitant use with moderate/strong CYP 3A4 inhibitors results in significant increases in plasma levels of vardenafil).

LEVOTHROID TABLETS

(Levothyroxine Sodium) 1189

May interact with androgens, antacids, beta blockers, oral anticoagulants, dopamine agonists, estrogens, glucocorticoids, cardiac glycosides, hydantoin anticonvulsants, oral hypoglycemic agents, insulin, oral contraceptives, radiographic iodinated contrast media, salicylates, sympathomimetics, thiazides, tricyclic antidepressants, xanthines, and certain other agents. Compounds in these categories include:

Acarbose (Addition of levothyroxine to antidiabetic therapy may result in increased antidiabetic agent requirements. Careful monitoring of diabetic control is recommended, especially when thyroid therapy is started, changed, or discontinued). Products include:

Precose Tablets 776

Acebutolol Hydrochloride (Actions of particular beta-adrenergic antagonists may be impaired when the hypothyroid patient is converted to the euthroid state).

No products indexed under this heading.

Albuterol (Concurrent use may increase the effects of sympathomimetics or thyroid hormone. Thyroid hormones may increase the risk of coronary insufficiency when sympathomimetic agents are administered to patients with coronary artery disease). Products include:

Proventil Inhalation Aerosol 3067

Albuterol Sulfate (Concurrent use may increase the effects of sympathomimetics or thyroid hormone. Thyroid hormones may increase the risk of coronary insufficiency when sympathomimetic agents are administered to patients with coronary artery disease). Products include:

AccuNeb Inhalation Solution 1055
Combivent Inhalation Aerosol 878
DuoNeb Inhalation Solution 1058
Proventil Inhalation Solution 0.083% 3069
Proventil HFA Inhalation Aerosol 3071
Ventolin HFA Inhalation Aerosol 1576
VoSpire Extended-Release Tablets ... 2352

Aluminum Carbonate (Concurrent use with antacids may reduce the efficacy of levothyroxine by binding and delaying or preventing the absorption, potentially resulting in hypothyroidism. Administer levothyroxine at least four hours apart from these agents).

No products indexed under this heading.

Aluminum Hydroxide (Concurrent use with antacids may reduce the efficacy of levothyroxine by binding and delaying or preventing the absorption, potentially resulting in hypothyroidism. Administer levothyroxine at least four hours apart from these agents). Products include:

Gaviscon Regular Strength Liquid .. 620
Gaviscon Regular Strength Tablets 619
Gaviscon Extra Strength Liquid 620
Gaviscon Extra Strength Tablets 619
Maalox Max Maximum Strength Antacid/Anti-Gas Liquid 2165
Maalox Regular Strength Antacid/Antigas Liquid 2164

Aminoglutethimide (Long-term aminoglutethimide therapy may minimally decrease T4 and T3 levels and increase TSH, although all values remain within normal limits in most patients).

No products indexed under this heading.

Aminophylline (Decreased theophylline clearance may occur in hypothyroid patients; clearance returns to normal when the euthroid state is achieved).

No products indexed under this heading.

Amiodarone Hydrochloride (Administration may decrease the peripheral conversion of T4 to T3, leading to decreased T3 levels. However, serum T4 levels are usually normal but may occasionally be slightly increased. Amiodarone may also induce hyperthyroidism by causing thyroiditis). Products include:

Pacerone Tablets 3337

Amitriptyline Hydrochloride (Concurrent use of tricyclic antidepressants and levothyroxine may increase the therapeutic and toxic effects of both drugs, possibly due to increased receptor sensitivity to catecholamines. Onset of action of tricyclics may be accelerated).

No products indexed under this heading.

Amoxapine (Concurrent use of tricyclic antidepressants and levothyroxine may increase the therapeutic and toxic effects of both drugs, possibly due to increased receptor sensitivity to catecholamines. Onset of action of tricyclics may be accelerated).

No products indexed under this heading.

Anisindione (Thyroid hormones appear to increase the catabolism of vitamin-K dependent clotting factors, thereby increasing the anticoagulant activity of oral anticoagulants. Concomitant use of these agents impairs the compensatory increases in clotting factor synthesis. Prothrombin time should be carefully monitored in patients taking levothyroxine and oral anticoagulants and the dose of anticoagulant therapy adjusted accordingly). Products include:

Miradon Tablets 3056

Asparaginase (Asparaginase may decrease serum TBG concentration). Products include:

Elspar for Injection 1943

Aspirin (Salicylates inhibit binding of T4 and T3 to TBG and transthyretin. An initial increase in FT4 is followed by return of FT4 to normal levels with sustained therapeutic serum salicylate concentrations, although total T4 levels may decrease by as much as 30%). Products include:

Aggrenox Capsules 855
Bayer, Aspirin Regimen 606
Bayer Aspirin Tablets 3515
BC Powder 612
BC Allergy Sinus Cold Powder 612
Arthritis Strength BC Powder 612
BC Sinus Cold Powder 612
Ecotrin Enteric Coated Aspirin Low, Regular and Maximum Strength Tablets 1627
Goody's Body Pain Formula Powder 621
Goody's Extra Strength Headache Powder 621
Goody's Extra Strength Pain Relief Tablets 621
Percodan Tablets 1115
St. Joseph 81 mg Aspirin Chewable and Enteric Coated Tablets 1841

Aspirin, Enteric Coated (Salicylates inhibit binding of T4 and T3 to TBG and transthyretin. An initial increase in FT4 is followed by return of FT4 to normal levels with sustained therapeutic serum salicylate concentrations, although total T4 levels may decrease by as much as 30%).

No products indexed under this heading.

Aspirin Buffered (Salicylates inhibit binding of T4 and T3 to TBG and transthyretin. An initial increase in FT4 is followed by return of FT4 to normal levels with sustained therapeutic serum salicylate concentrations, although total T4 levels may decrease by as much as 30%).

No products indexed under this heading.

Atenolol (Actions of particular beta-adrenergic antagonists may be impaired when the hypothyroid patient is converted to the euthroid state). Products include:

Tenormin I.V. Injection 698
Tenormin Tablets 695

Bendroflumethiazide (Thiazide diuretics are associated with thyroid hormone and/or TSH level alterations).

No products indexed under this heading.

Betamethasone Acetate (Glucocorticoids may result in a transient reduction in TSH secretion when administered at doses greater than 100mg/day of hydrocortisone or equivalent. Short-term administration of large doses of glucocorticoids may decrease serum T3 concentrations by 30% with minimal change in serum T4 levels. However, long-term glucocorticoid therapy may result in slightly decreased T3 and T4 levels due to decreased TBG production).

No products indexed under this heading.

Betamethasone Sodium Phosphate (Glucocorticoids may result in a transient reduction in TSH secretion when administered at doses greater than 100mg/day of hydrocortisone or equivalent. Short-term administration of large doses of glucocorticoids may decrease serum T3 concentrations by 30% with minimal change in serum T4 levels. However, long-term glucocorticoid therapy may result in slightly decreased T3 and T4 levels due to decreased TBG production).

No products indexed under this heading.

Betaxolol Hydrochloride (Actions of particular beta-adrenergic antagonists may be impaired when the hypothyroid patient is converted to the euthroid state). Products include:

Betoptic S Ophthalmic Suspension.................................. 554

Bisoprolol Fumarate (Actions of particular beta-adrenergic antagonists may be impaired when the hypothyroid patient is converted to the euthroid state).
No products indexed under this heading.

Bromocriptine Mesylate (Dopamine and dopamine agonists may result in a transient reduction in TSH secretion when administered at dopamine doses greater than or equal to 1 mcg/kg/min).
No products indexed under this heading.

Calcium Carbonate (Calcium carbonate may form an insoluble chelate with levothyroxine. Concurrent use may reduce the efficacy of levothyroxine by binding and delaying or preventing the absorption, potentially resulting in hypothyroidism. Administer levothyroxine at least four hours apart from calcium carbonate-containing products). Products include:

Actonel with Calcium Tablets........... 2684
Caltrate 600 PLUS Chewables....... ▣779
Caltrate 600 PLUS Tablets............ ▣779
Caltrate 600 + D Tablets.............. ▣779
Encora Capsules............................ 3298
Encora AM Tablets......................... 3298
Encora PM Tablets......................... 3298
Gas-X with Maalox......................... ▣675
Maalox Regular Strength Antacid Tablets... 2166
Quick Dissolve Maalox Max Maximum Strength Antacid/Antigas Tablets................ 2165
Maalox Max Quick Dissolve Maximum Strength Chewable Tablets.. ▣678
Os-Cal Chewable Tablets................ ▣765
Pepcid Complete Chewable Tablets... 1672
PremCal Light, Regular, and Extra Strength Tablets................ ▣762
Rolaids Tablets.............................. ▣707
Extra Strength Rolaids Softchews................................. ▣708
Extra Strength Rolaids Tablets....... ▣707
Rolaids Multi-Symptom Antacid & Antigas Tablets.......................... ▣708
Tums... ▣639

Carbamazepine (Stimulation of hepatic microsomal drug-metabolizing activity may cause increased hepatic degradation of levothyroxine, resulting in increased levothyroxine requirements).
Products include:

Carbatrol Capsules........................ 3174
Equetro Extended-Release Capsules.. 3178
Tegretol/Tegretol-XR...................... 2278

Carteolol Hydrochloride (Actions of particular beta-adrenergic antagonists may be impaired when the hypothyroid patient is converted to the euthroid state). Products include:

Carteolol Hydrochloride Ophthalmic Solution USP, 1%....... ⊙246

Chloral Hydrate (Chloral Hydrate has been associated with thyroid hormone and/or TSH level alterations).
No products indexed under this heading.

Chlorothiazide (Thiazide diuretics are associated with thyroid hormone and/or TSH level alterations).
Products include:

Aldoclor Tablets............................. 1881
Diuril Oral....................................... 1936

Chlorothiazide Sodium (Thiazide diuretics are associated with thyroid hormone and/or TSH level alterations). Products include:

Diuril Sodium Intravenous................ 1934

Chlorotrianisene (Estrogen may increase serum TBG concentration).
No products indexed under this heading.

Chlorpropamide (Addition of levothyroxine to antidiabetic therapy may result in increased antidiabetic agent requirements. Careful monitoring of diabetic control is recommended, especially when thyroid therapy is started, changed, or discontinued).
No products indexed under this heading.

Cholestyramine (Concurrent use with cholestyramine may reduce the efficacy of levothyroxine by binding and delaying or preventing the absorption, potentially resulting in hypothyroidism. Administer levothyroxine at least four hours apart from cholestyramine).
No products indexed under this heading.

Choline Magnesium Trisalicylate (Salicylates inhibit binding of T4 and T3 to TBG and transthyretin. An initial increase in FT4 is followed by return of FT4 to normal levels with sustained therapeutic serum salicylate concentrations, although total T4 levels may decrease by as much as 30%).
No products indexed under this heading.

Clofibrate (Clofibrate may increase serum TBG concentration).
No products indexed under this heading.

Clomipramine Hydrochloride (Concurrent use of tricyclic antidepressants and levothyroxine may increase the therapeutic and toxic effects of both drugs, possibly due to increased receptor sensitivity to catecholamines. Onset of action of tricyclics may be accelerated).
No products indexed under this heading.

Colestipol (Concurrent use with colestipol may reduce the efficacy of levothyroxine by binding and delaying or preventing the absorption, potentially resulting in hypothyroidism. Administer levothyroxine at least four hours apart from colestipol).
No products indexed under this heading.

Colestipol Hydrochloride (Concurrent use with colestipol may reduce the efficacy of levothyroxine by binding and delaying or preventing the absorption, potentially resulting in hypothyroidism. Administer levothyroxine at least four hours apart from colestipol).
No products indexed under this heading.

Cortisone Acetate (Glucocorticoids may result in a transient reduction in TSH secretion when administered at doses greater than 100mg/day of hydrocortisone or equivalent. Short-term administration of large doses of glucocorticoids may decrease serum T3 concentrations by 30% with minimal change in serum T4 levels. However, long-term glucocorticoid therapy may result in slightly decreased T3 and T4 levels due to decreased TBG production).
No products indexed under this heading.

Desipramine Hydrochloride (Concurrent use of tricyclic antidepressants and levothyroxine may increase the therapeutic and toxic effects of both drugs, possibly due to increased receptor sensitivity to catecholamines. Onset of action of tricyclics may be accelerated).
No products indexed under this heading.

Deslanoside (Serum digitalis glycoside levels may be reduced in hyperthyroidism or when the hypothyroid patient is converted to the euthroid state. Therapeutic effect of digitalis glycosides may be reduced).
No products indexed under this heading.

Desogestrel (Estrogen-containing oral contraceptives may increase serum TBG concentration). Products include:

Ortho-Cept Tablets.......................... 2395

Dexamethasone (Glucocorticoids may result in a transient reduction in TSH secretion when administered at doses greater than 100mg/day of hydrocortisone or equivalent. Short-term administration of large doses of glucocorticoids may decrease serum T3 concentrations by 30% with minimal change in serum T4 levels. However, long-term glucocorticoid therapy may result in slightly decreased T3 and T4 levels due to decreased TBG production).
Products include:

Ciprodex Otic Suspension.............. 555
Decadron Tablets.......................... 1929
TobraDex Ophthalmic Ointment....... 558
TobraDex Ophthalmic Suspension... 558

Dexamethasone Acetate (Glucocorticoids may result in a transient reduction in TSH secretion when administered at doses greater than 100mg/day of hydrocortisone or equivalent. Short-term administration of large doses of glucocorticoids may decrease serum T3 concentrations by 30% with minimal change in serum T4 levels. However, long-term glucocorticoid therapy may result in slightly decreased T3 and T4 levels due to decreased TBG production).
No products indexed under this heading.

Dexamethasone Sodium Phosphate (Glucocorticoids may result in a transient reduction in TSH secretion when administered at doses greater than 100mg/day of hydrocortisone or equivalent. Short-term administration of large doses of glucocorticoids may decrease serum T3 concentrations by 30% with minimal change in serum T4 levels. However, long-term glucocorticoid therapy may result in slightly decreased T3 and T4 levels due to decreased TBG production). Products include:

Decadron Phosphate Injection......... 1931

Diatrizoate Meglumine (Iodide and drugs that contain pharmacologic amounts of iodide may cause hyperthyroidism in euthroid patients with Grave's disease previously treated with antithyroid drugs or in euthroid patients with thyroid autonomy. Hyperthyroidism may develop over several weeks and may persist for several months after therapy discontinuation. Thyroid hormones may also reduce the uptake of I-123 and I-131).
No products indexed under this heading.

Diatrizoate Sodium (Iodide and drugs that contain pharmacologic amounts of iodide may cause hyperthyroidism in euthroid patients with Grave's disease previously treated with antithyroid drugs or in euthroid patients with thyroid autonomy. Hyperthyroidism may develop over several weeks and may persist for several months after therapy discontinuation. Thyroid hormones may also reduce the uptake of I-123 and I-131).
No products indexed under this heading.

Diazepam (Diazepam is associated with thyroid hormone and/or TSH level alterations). Products include:

Diastat Rectal Delivery System........ 3344
Valium Tablets................................ 2822

Dicumarol (Thyroid hormones appear to increase the catabolism of vitamin-K dependent clotting factors, thereby increasing the anticoagulant activity of oral anticoagulants. Concomitant use of these agents impairs the compensatory increases in clotting factor synthesis. Prothrombin time should be carefully monitored in patients taking levothyroxine and oral anticoagulants and the dose of anticoagulant therapy adjusted accordingly).
No products indexed under this heading.

Dienestrol (Estrogen may increase serum TBG concentration).
No products indexed under this heading.

Diethylstilbestrol (Estrogen may increase serum TBG concentration).
No products indexed under this heading.

Diflunisal (Salicylates inhibit binding of T4 and T3 to TBG and transthyretin. An initial increase in FT4 is followed by return of FT4 to normal levels with sustained therapeutic serum salicylate concentrations, although total T4 levels may decrease by as much as 30%).
Products include:

Dolobid Tablets.............................. 1937

Digitalis Glycoside Preparations (Serum digitalis glycoside levels may be reduced in hyperthyroidism or when the hypothyroid patient is converted to the euthroid state. Therapeutic effect of digitalis glycosides may be reduced).
No products indexed under this heading.

Digitoxin (Serum digitalis glycoside levels may be reduced in hyperthyroidism or when the hypothyroid patient is converted to the euthroid state. Therapeutic effect of digitalis glycosides may be reduced).
No products indexed under this heading.

Digoxin (Serum digitalis glycoside levels may be reduced in hyperthyroidism or when the hypothyroid patient is converted to the euthroid state. Therapeutic effect of digitalis glycosides may be reduced).
Products include:

Digitek Tablets................................ 2146
Lanoxicaps Capsules...................... 1458
Lanoxin Injection............................ 1462
Lanoxin Tablets.............................. 1468
Lanoxin Injection Pediatric.............. 1465

Dobutamine Hydrochloride (Concurrent use may increase the effects of sympathomimetics or thyroid hormone. Thyroid hormones may increase the risk of coronary insufficiency when sympathomimetic agents are administered to patients with coronary artery disease).
No products indexed under this heading.

Dopamine Hydrochloride (Concurrent use may increase the effects of sympathomimetics or thyroid hormone. Thyroid hormones may increase the risk of coronary insufficiency when sympathomimetic agents are administered to patients with coronary artery disease).
No products indexed under this heading.

Doxepin Hydrochloride (Concurrent use of tricyclic antidepressants and levothyroxine may increase the therapeutic and toxic effects of both drugs, possibly due to increased receptor sensitivity to catecholamines. Onset of action of tricyclics may be accelerated).
No products indexed under this heading.

Dyphylline (Decreased theophylline clearance may occur in hypothyroid patients; clearance returns to normal when the euthroid state is achieved).
No products indexed under this heading.

Ephedrine Hydrochloride (Concurrent use may increase the effects of sympathomimetics or thyroid hormone. Thyroid hormones may increase the risk of coronary insufficiency when sympathomimetic agents are administered to patients with coronary artery disease). Products include:
Primatene Tablets 749

Ephedrine Sulfate (Concurrent use may increase the effects of sympathomimetics or thyroid hormone. Thyroid hormones may increase the risk of coronary insufficiency when sympathomimetic agents are administered to patients with coronary artery disease).
No products indexed under this heading.

Ephedrine Tannate (Concurrent use may increase the effects of sympathomimetics or thyroid hormone. Thyroid hormones may increase the risk of coronary insufficiency when sympathomimetic agents are administered to patients with coronary artery disease).
No products indexed under this heading.

Epinephrine (Concurrent use may increase the effects of sympathomimetics or thyroid hormone. Thyroid hormones may increase the risk of coronary insufficiency when sympathomimetic agents are administered to patients with coronary artery disease). Products include:
EpiPen 1061
Primatene Mist 749

Epinephrine Bitartrate (Concurrent use may increase the effects of sympathomimetics or thyroid hormone. Thyroid hormones may increase the risk of coronary insufficiency when sympathomimetic agents are administered to patients with coronary artery disease).
No products indexed under this heading.

Epinephrine Hydrochloride (Concurrent use may increase the effects of sympathomimetics or thyroid hormone. Thyroid hormones may increase the risk of coronary insufficiency when sympathomimetic agents are administered to patients with coronary artery disease).
No products indexed under this heading.

Esmolol Hydrochloride (Actions of particular beta-adrenergic antagonists may be impaired when the hypothyroid patient is converted to the euthroid state). Products include:
Brevibloc Concentrate 766
Brevibloc Injection 766
Brevibloc Double Strength Injection 766
Brevibloc Premixed Injection 766
Brevibloc Double Strength Premixed Injection 766

Estradiol (Estrogen may increase serum TBG concentration). Products include:
Activella Tablets 2311
Climara Transdermal System 795
Climara Pro Transdermal System 800
CombiPatch Transdermal System 2180
Estrogel 0.06% 3200
Menostar Transdermal System 805
Prefest Tablets 1069
Vagifem Tablets 2340
Vivelle Transdermal System 2288
Vivelle-Dot Transdermal System 2293

Estrogens, Conjugated (Estrogen may increase serum TBG concentration). Products include:
Premarin Intravenous 3440
Premarin Tablets 3443
Premarin Vaginal Cream 3449
Premphase Tablets 3452
Prempro Tablets 3452

Estrogens, Esterified (Estrogen may increase serum TBG concentration). Products include:
Estratest Tablets 3196
Estratest H.S. Tablets 3196

Estropipate (Estrogen may increase serum TBG concentration).
No products indexed under this heading.

Ethinyl Estradiol (Estrogen-containing oral contraceptives may increase serum TBG concentration). Products include:
Alesse-28 Tablets 3392
Lo/Ovral-28 Tablets 3423
NuvaRing 2357
Ortho-Cept Tablets 2395
Ortho-Cyclen/Ortho Tri-Cyclen 2414
Ortho Evra Transdermal System 2402
Ortho Tri-Cyclen Lo Tablets 2421
Seasonale Tablets 1073
Triphasil-28 Tablets 3483
Yasmin 28 Tablets 818

Ethiodized Oil (Iodide and drugs that contain pharmacologic amounts of iodide may cause hyperthyroidism in euthroid patients with Grave's disease previously treated with antithyroid drugs or in euthroid patients with thyroid autonomy. Hyperthyroidism may develop over several weeks and may persist for several months after therapy discontinuation. Thyroid hormones may also reduce the uptake of I-123 and I-131).
No products indexed under this heading.

Ethionamide (Ethionamide is associated with thyroid hormone and/or TSH level alterations). Products include:
Trecator Tablets 3482

Ethotoin (Stimulation of hepatic microsomal drug-metabolizing activity may cause increased hepatic degradation of levothyroxine, resulting in increased levothyroxine requirements). Products include:
Peganone Tablets, USP 2487

Ethynodiol Diacetate (Estrogen-containing oral contraceptives may increase serum TBG concentration).
No products indexed under this heading.

Ferrous Sulfate (Ferrous sulfate likely forms a ferric-thyroxine complex. Concurrent use may reduce the efficacy of levothyroxine by binding and delaying or preventing the absorption, potentially resulting in hypothyroidism. Administer levothyroxine at least four hours apart from ferrous sulfate-containing products). Products include:
Feosol Tablets 1629
Slow Fe Iron Tablets 772
Slow Fe with Folic Acid Tablets 773

Fludrocortisone Acetate (Glucocorticoids may result in a transient reduction in TSH secretion when administered at doses greater than 100mg/day of hydrocortisone or equivalent. Short-term administration of large doses of glucocorticoids may decrease serum T3 concentrations by 30% with minimal change in serum T4 levels. However, long-term glucocorticoid therapy may result in slightly decreased T3 and T4 levels due to decreased TBG production).
No products indexed under this heading.

Fluorouracil (Fluorouracil may increase serum TBG concentration). Products include:
Carac Cream, 0.5% 1048
Efudex 3348

Fluoxymesterone (Androgens/anabolic steroids may decrease serum TBG concentration).
No products indexed under this heading.

Fosphenytoin Sodium (Stimulation of hepatic microsomal drug-metabolizing activity may cause increased hepatic degradation of levothyroxine, resulting in increased levothyroxine requirements).
No products indexed under this heading.

Furosemide (Co-administration of furosemide (greater than 80mg IV) with levothyroxine results in an initial transient increase in FT4. Continued administration results in a decrease in serum T4 and normal FT4 and TSH concentrations and, therefore, patients are clinically euthroid). Products include:
Furosemide Tablets 2117

Gadopentetate Dimeglumine (Iodide and drugs that contain pharmacologic amounts of iodide may cause hyperthyroidism in euthroid patients with Grave's disease previously treated with antithyroid drugs or in euthroid patients with thyroid autonomy. Hyperthyroidism may develop over several weeks and may persist for several months after therapy discontinuation. Thyroid hormones may also reduce the uptake of I-123 and I-131).
No products indexed under this heading.

Glimepiride (Addition of levothyroxine to antidiabetic therapy may result in increased antidiabetic agent requirements. Careful monitoring of diabetic control is recommended, especially when thyroid therapy is started, changed, or discontinued). Products include:
Amaryl Tablets 2864

Glipizide (Addition of levothyroxine to antidiabetic therapy may result in increased antidiabetic agent requirements. Careful monitoring of diabetic control is recommended, especially when thyroid therapy is started, changed, or discontinued).
No products indexed under this heading.

Glyburide (Addition of levothyroxine to antidiabetic therapy may result in increased antidiabetic agent requirements. Careful monitoring of diabetic control is recommended, especially when thyroid therapy is started, changed, or discontinued).
No products indexed under this heading.

Heparin Calcium (Co-administration of heparin with levothyroxine results in an initial transient increase in FT4. Continued administration results in a decrease in serum T4 and normal FT4 and TSH concentrations and, therefore, patients are clinically euthroid).
No products indexed under this heading.

Heparin Sodium (Co-administration of heparin with levothyroxine results in an initial transient increase in FT4. Continued administration results in a decrease in serum T4 and normal FT4 and TSH concentrations and, therefore, patients are clinically euthroid).
No products indexed under this heading.

Heroin (Heroin may increase serum TBG concentration).
No products indexed under this heading.

Hydrochlorothiazide (Thiazide diuretics are associated with thyroid hormone and/or TSH level alterations). Products include:
Aldoril Tablets 1884
Atacand HCT 637
Avalide Tablets 2889
Avalide Tablets 922
Benicar HCT Tablets 2852
Diovan HCT Tablets 2195
Dyazide Capsules 1389
Hyzaar 1964
Lotensin HCT Tablets 2235
Maxzide 2150
Micardis HCT Tablets 886
Moduretic Tablets 2003
Prinzide Tablets 2033
Teveten HCT Tablets 1710
Timolide Tablets 2056
Uniretic Tablets 3114
Vaseretic Tablets 2073
Zestoretic Tablets 701

Hydrocortisone (Glucocorticoids may result in a transient reduction in TSH secretion when administered at doses greater than 100mg/day of hydrocortisone or equivalent. Short-term administration of large doses of glucocorticoids may decrease serum T3 concentrations by 30% with minimal change in serum T4 levels. However, long-term glucocorticoid therapy may result in slightly decreased T3 and T4 levels due to decreased TBG production). Products include:
Cortizone•5 Ointment 699
Cortizone•10 Creme 699
Cortizone•10 Ointment 699
Cortizone•10 Plus Creme 700
Cortizone•10 Maximum Strength Quick Shot Spray 700

Hydrocortone Tablets 1963
Preparation H Hydrocortisone Cream .... ▣ 748

Hydrocortisone Acetate (Glucocorticoids may result in a transient reduction in TSH secretion when administered at doses greater than 100mg/day of hydrocortisone or equivalent. Short-term administration of large doses of glucocorticoids may decrease serum T3 concentrations by 30% with minimal change in serum T4 levels. However, long-term glucocorticoid therapy may result in slightly decreased T3 and T4 levels due to decreased TBG production). Products include:
Analpram-HC 1136
Pramosone 1139
ProctoFoam-HC 3113
Tucks Anti-Itch Ointment .... ▣ 712
U-cort 1% Cream 3289

Hydrocortisone Sodium Phosphate (Glucocorticoids may result in a transient reduction in TSH secretion when administered at doses greater than 100mg/day of hydrocortisone or equivalent. Short-term administration of large doses of glucocorticoids may decrease serum T3 concentrations by 30% with minimal change in serum T4 levels. However, long-term glucocorticoid therapy may result in slightly decreased T3 and T4 levels due to decreased TBG production).
No products indexed under this heading.

Hydrocortisone Sodium Succinate (Glucocorticoids may result in a transient reduction in TSH secretion when administered at doses greater than 100mg/day of hydrocortisone or equivalent. Short-term administration of large doses of glucocorticoids may decrease serum T3 concentrations by 30% with minimal change in serum T4 levels. However, long-term glucocorticoid therapy may result in slightly decreased T3 and T4 levels due to decreased TBG production).
No products indexed under this heading.

Hydroflumethiazide (Thiazide diuretics are associated with thyroid hormone and/or TSH level alterations).
No products indexed under this heading.

Imipramine Hydrochloride (Concurrent use of tricyclic antidepressants and levothyroxine may increase the therapeutic and toxic effects of both drugs, possibly due to increased receptor sensitivity to catecholamines. Onset of action of tricyclics may be accelerated).
No products indexed under this heading.

Imipramine Pamoate (Concurrent use of tricyclic antidepressants and levothyroxine may increase the therapeutic and toxic effects of both drugs, possibly due to increased receptor sensitivity to catecholamines. Onset of action of tricyclics may be accelerated).
No products indexed under this heading.

Insulin, Human, Zinc Suspension (Addition of levothyroxine to insulin therapy may result in increased insulin requirements. Careful monitoring of diabetic control is recommended, especially when thyroid therapy is started, changed, or discontinued). Products include:
Humulin L, 100 Units 1763
Humulin U, 100 Units 1770

Insulin, Human NPH (Addition of levothyroxine to insulin therapy may result in increased insulin requirements. Careful monitoring of diabetic control is recommended, especially when thyroid therapy is started, changed, or discontinued). Products include:
Humulin N, 100 Units 1764
Humulin N Pen 1765
Novolin N Human Insulin 10 ml Vials 2322
Novolin N InnoLet 2322
Novolin N PenFill 3 ml Cartridges 2325
Novolin R InnoLet 2322

Insulin, Human Regular (Addition of levothyroxine to insulin therapy may result in increased insulin requirements. Careful monitoring of diabetic control is recommended, especially when thyroid therapy is started, changed, or discontinued). Products include:
Humulin R (U-500) 1768
Humulin R, 100 Units 1767
Novolin R Human Insulin 10 ml Vials 2322
Novolin R PenFill 2325

Insulin, Human Regular and Human NPH Mixture (Addition of levothyroxine to insulin therapy may result in increased insulin requirements. Careful monitoring of diabetic control is recommended, especially when thyroid therapy is started, changed, or discontinued). Products include:
Humulin 50/50, 100 Units 1760
Humulin 70/30 Pen 1761
Novolin 70/30 Human Insulin 10 ml Vials 2321
Novolin 70/30 InnoLet 2322
Novolin 70/30 PenFill 3 ml Cartridges 2325

Insulin, NPH (Addition of levothyroxine to insulin therapy may result in increased insulin requirements. Careful monitoring of diabetic control is recommended, especially when thyroid therapy is started, changed, or discontinued).
No products indexed under this heading.

Insulin, Regular (Addition of levothyroxine to insulin therapy may result in increased insulin requirements. Careful monitoring of diabetic control is recommended, especially when thyroid therapy is started, changed, or discontinued).
No products indexed under this heading.

Insulin, Zinc Crystals (Addition of levothyroxine to insulin therapy may result in increased insulin requirements. Careful monitoring of diabetic control is recommended, especially when thyroid therapy is started, changed, or discontinued).
No products indexed under this heading.

Insulin, Zinc Suspension (Addition of levothyroxine to insulin therapy may result in increased insulin requirements. Careful monitoring of diabetic control is recommended, especially when thyroid therapy is started, changed, or discontinued).
No products indexed under this heading.

Insulin Aspart, Human Regular (Addition of levothyroxine to insulin therapy may result in increased insulin requirements. Careful monitoring of diabetic control is recommended, especially when thyroid therapy is started, changed, or discontinued). Products include:
NovoLog Injection 2326

Insulin glargine (Addition of levothyroxine to insulin therapy may result in increased insulin requirements. Careful monitoring of diabetic control is recommended, especially when thyroid therapy is started, changed, or discontinued). Products include:
Lantus Injection 2925

Insulin Lispro, Human (Addition of levothyroxine to insulin therapy may result in increased insulin requirements. Careful monitoring of diabetic control is recommended, especially when thyroid therapy is started, changed, or discontinued). Products include:
Humalog-Pen 1751
Humalog Mix 75/25-Pen 1754

Insulin Lispro Protamine, Human (Addition of levothyroxine to insulin therapy may result in increased insulin requirements. Careful monitoring of diabetic control is recommended, especially when thyroid therapy is started, changed, or discontinued). Products include:
Humalog Mix 75/25-Pen 1754

Interferon alfa-2a, Recombinant (Therapy with interferon-alpha has been associated with the development of antithyroid microsomal antibodies in 20% of patients and some have transient hypothyroidism, hyperthyroidism, or both). Products include:
Roferon-A Injection 2805

Interferon alfa-2b, Recombinant (Therapy with interferon-alpha has been associated with the development of antithyroid microsomal antibodies in 20% of patients and some have transient hypothyroidism, hyperthyroidism, or both). Products include:
Intron A for Injection 3038
Rebetron Combination Therapy 3078

Iodamide Meglumine (Iodide and drugs that contain pharmacologic amounts of iodide may cause hyperthyroidism in euthroid patients with Grave's disease previously treated with antithyroid drugs or in euthroid patients with thyroid autonomy. Hyperthyroidism may develop over several weeks and may persist for several months after therapy discontinuation. Thyroid hormones may also reduce the uptake of I-123 and I-131).
No products indexed under this heading.

Iohexol (Iodide and drugs that contain pharmacologic amounts of iodide may cause hyperthyroidism in euthroid patients with Grave's disease previously treated with antithyroid drugs or in euthroid patients with thyroid autonomy. Hyperthyroidism may develop over several weeks and may persist for several months after therapy discontinuation. Thyroid hormones may also reduce the uptake of I-123 and I-131).
No products indexed under this heading.

Iopamidol (Iodide and drugs that contain pharmacologic amounts of iodide may cause hyperthyroidism in euthroid patients with Grave's disease previously treated with antithyroid drugs or in euthroid patients with thyroid autonomy. Hyperthyroidism may develop over several weeks and may persist for several months after therapy discontinuation. Thyroid hormones may also reduce the uptake of I-123 and I-131).
No products indexed under this heading.

Iopanoic Acid (Iodide and drugs that contain pharmacologic amounts of iodide may cause hyperthyroidism in euthroid patients with Grave's disease previously treated with antithyroid drugs or in euthroid patients with thyroid autonomy. Hyperthyroidism may develop over several weeks and may persist for several months after therapy discontinuation. Thyroid hormones may also reduce the uptake of I-123 and I-131).
No products indexed under this heading.

Iothalamate Meglumine (Iodide and drugs that contain pharmacologic amounts of iodide may cause hyperthyroidism in euthroid patients with Grave's disease previously treated with antithyroid drugs or in euthroid patients with thyroid autonomy. Hyperthyroidism may develop over several weeks and may persist for several months after therapy discontinuation. Thyroid hormones may also reduce the uptake of I-123 and I-131).
No products indexed under this heading.

Ioxaglate Meglumine (Iodide and drugs that contain pharmacologic amounts of iodide may cause hyperthyroidism in euthroid patients with Grave's disease previously treated with antithyroid drugs or in euthroid patients with thyroid autonomy. Hyperthyroidism may develop over several weeks and may persist for several months after therapy discontinuation. Thyroid hormones may also reduce the uptake of I-123 and I-131).
No products indexed under this heading.

Ioxaglate Sodium (Iodide and drugs that contain pharmacologic amounts of iodide may cause hyperthyroidism in euthroid patients with Grave's disease previously treated with antithyroid drugs or in euthroid patients with thyroid autonomy. Hyperthyroidism may develop over several weeks and may persist for several months after therapy discontinuation. Thyroid hormones may also reduce the uptake of I-123 and I-131).
No products indexed under this heading.

Isoproterenol Hydrochloride (Concurrent use may increase the effects of sympathomimetics or thyroid hormone. Thyroid hormones may increase the risk of coronary insufficiency when sympathomimetic agents are administered to patients with coronary artery disease).
No products indexed under this heading.

Isoproterenol Sulfate (Concurrent use may increase the effects of sympathomimetics or thyroid hormone. Thyroid hormones may increase the risk of coronary insufficiency when sympathomimetic agents are administered to patients with coronary artery disease).
No products indexed under this heading.

Ketamine (Concurrent use may produce marked hypertension and tachycardia; cautious administration to patients receiving thyroid therapy is recommended).
No products indexed under this heading.

Ketamine Hydrochloride (Concurrent use may produce marked hypertension and tachycardia; cautious administration to patients receiving thyroid therapy is recommended).
No products indexed under this heading.

Labetalol Hydrochloride (Actions of particular beta-adrenergic antagonists may be impaired when the hypothyroid patient is converted to the euthroid state).
No products indexed under this heading.

Levalbuterol Hydrochloride (Concurrent use may increase the effects of sympathomimetics or thyroid hormone. Thyroid hormones may increase the risk of coronary insufficiency when sympathomimetic agents are administered to patients with coronary artery disease). Products include:
Xopenex Inhalation Solution 3143
Xopenex Inhalation Solution Concentrate 3147

Levobunolol Hydrochloride (Actions of particular beta-adrenergic antagonists may be impaired when the hypothyroid patient is converted to the euthroid state). Products include:
Betagan Ophthalmic Solution, USP .... ⊙ 217

Levonorgestrel (Estrogen-containing oral contraceptives may increase serum TBG concentration). Products include:
Alesse-28 Tablets 3392
Climara Pro Transdermal System 800
Mirena Intrauterine System 810
Plan B Tablets 1068
Seasonale Tablets 1073
Triphasil-28 Tablets 3483

Lithium (Long-term lithium therapy can result in goiter in up to 50% of patients, and either subclinical or overt hypothyroidism, each in up to 20% of patients).
No products indexed under this heading.

Lithium Carbonate (Long-term lithium therapy can result in goiter in up to 50% of patients, and either subclinical or overt hypothyroidism, each in up to 20% of patients). Products include:
Eskalith 1406
Lithobid Tablets 1670

Lithium Citrate (Long-term lithium therapy can result in goiter in up to 50% of patients, and either subclinical or overt hypothyroidism, each in up to 20% of patients).
No products indexed under this heading.

Lovastatin (Lovastatin is associated with thyroid hormone and/or TSH level alterations). Products include:
Advicor Tablets 1694
Altoprev Extended-Release Tablets 1151
Mevacor Tablets 1996

Magaldrate (Concurrent use with antacids may reduce the efficacy of levothyroxine by binding and delaying or preventing the absorption, potentially resulting in hypothyroidism. Administer levothyroxine at least four hours apart from these agents).
No products indexed under this heading.

Magnesium Hydroxide (Concurrent use with antacids may reduce the efficacy of levothyroxine by binding and delaying or preventing the absorption, potentially resulting in hypothyroidism. Administer levothyroxine at least four hours apart from these agents). Products include:
Maalox Max Maximum Strength Antacid/Anti-Gas Liquid 2165
Maalox Regular Strength Antacid/Antigas Liquid 2164
Pepcid Complete Chewable Tablets 1672
Rolaids Tablets 707
Extra Strength Rolaids Tablets 707
Rolaids Multi-Symptom Antacid & Antigas Tablets 708

Magnesium Oxide (Concurrent use with antacids may reduce the efficacy of levothyroxine by binding and delaying or preventing the absorption, potentially resulting in hypothyroidism. Administer levothyroxine at least four hours apart from these agents). Products include:
Beelith Tablets 784
PremCal Light, Regular, and Extra Strength Tablets 762

Magnesium Salicylate (Salicylates inhibit binding of T4 and T3 to TBG and transthyretin. An initial increase in FT4 is followed by return of FT4 to normal levels with sustained therapeutic serum salicylate concentrations, although total T4 levels may decrease by as much as 30%).
No products indexed under this heading.

Maprotiline Hydrochloride (Concurrent use of tetracyclic antidepressants and levothyroxine may increase the therapeutic and toxic effects of both drugs, possibly due to increased receptor sensitivity to catecholamines).
No products indexed under this heading.

Meclofenamate Sodium (Co-administration of fenamates with levothyroxine results in an initial transient increase in FT4. Continued administration results in a decrease in serum T4 and normal FT4 and TSH concentrations and, therefore, patients are clinically euthroid).
No products indexed under this heading.

Mephenytoin (Stimulation of hepatic microsomal drug-metabolizing activity may cause increased hepatic degradation of levothyroxine, resulting in increased levothyroxine requirements).
No products indexed under this heading.

Mercaptopurine (Mercaptopurine is associated with thyroid hormone and/or TSH level alterations). Products include:
Purinethol Tablets 1222

Mestranol (Estrogen-containing oral contraceptives may increase serum TBG concentration).
No products indexed under this heading.

Metaproterenol Sulfate (Concurrent use may increase the effects of sympathomimetics or thyroid hormone. Thyroid hormones may increase the risk of coronary insufficiency when sympathomimetic agents are administered to patients with coronary artery disease). Products include:
Alupent Inhalation Aerosol 858

Metaraminol Bitartrate (Concurrent use may increase the effects of sympathomimetics or thyroid hormone. Thyroid hormones may increase the risk of coronary insufficiency when sympathomimetic agents are administered to patients with coronary artery disease). Products include:
Aramine Injection 1889

Metformin Hydrochloride (Addition of levothyroxine to antidiabetic therapy may result in increased antidiabetic agent requirements. Careful monitoring of diabetic control is recommended, especially when thyroid therapy is started, changed, or discontinued). Products include:
ActoPlus Met Tablets 3219
Avandamet Tablets 1343
Fortamet Extended-Release Tablets 1156

Methadone Hydrochloride (Methadone may increase serum TBG concentration).
No products indexed under this heading.

Methoxamine Hydrochloride (Concurrent use may increase the effects of sympathomimetics or thyroid hormone. Thyroid hormones may increase the risk of coronary insufficiency when sympathomimetic agents are administered to patients with coronary artery disease).
No products indexed under this heading.

Methyclothiazide (Thiazide diuretics are associated with thyroid hormone and/or TSH level alterations).
No products indexed under this heading.

Methylprednisolone Acetate (Glucocorticoids may result in a transient reduction in TSH secretion when administered at doses greater than 100mg/day of hydrocortisone or equivalent. Short-term administration of large doses of glucocorticoids may decrease serum T3 concentrations by 30% with minimal change in serum T4 levels. However, long-term glucocorticoid therapy may result in slightly decreased T3 and T4 levels due to decreased TBG production). Products include:
Depo-Medrol Injectable Suspension 2615
Depo-Medrol Single-Dose Vial 2617

Methylprednisolone Sodium Succinate (Glucocorticoids may result in a transient reduction in TSH secretion when administered at doses greater than 100mg/day of hydrocortisone or equivalent. Short-term administration of large doses of glucocorticoids may decrease serum T3 concentrations by 30% with minimal change in serum T4 levels. However, long-term glucocorticoid therapy may result in slightly decreased T3 and T4 levels due to decreased TBG production).
No products indexed under this heading.

Methyltestosterone (Androgens/anabolic steroids may decrease serum TBG concentration). Products include:
Estratest Tablets 3196
Estratest H.S. Tablets 3196

Metipranolol Hydrochloride (Actions of particular beta-adrenergic antagonists may be impaired when the hypothyroid patient is converted to the euthroid state).
No products indexed under this heading.

Metoclopramide Hydrochloride (Metoclopramide is associated with thyroid hormone and/or TSH level alterations).
No products indexed under this heading.

Metoprolol Succinate (Actions of particular beta-adrenergic antagonists may be impaired when the hypothyroid patient is converted to the euthroid state). Products include:
Toprol-XL Tablets 660

Metoprolol Tartrate (Actions of particular beta-adrenergic antagonists may be impaired when the hypothyroid patient is converted to the euthroid state).
No products indexed under this heading.

Miglitol (Addition of levothyroxine to antidiabetic therapy may result in increased antidiabetic agent requirements. Careful monitoring of diabetic control is recommended, especially when thyroid therapy is started, changed, or discontinued).
No products indexed under this heading.

Mirtazapine (Concurrent use of tetracyclic antidepressants and levothyroxine may increase the therapeutic and toxic effects of both drugs, possibly due to increased receptor sensitivity to catecholamines).
No products indexed under this heading.

Mitotane (Mitotane may increase serum TBG concentration).
No products indexed under this heading.

Nadolol (Actions of particular beta-adrenergic antagonists may be impaired when the hypothyroid patient is converted to the euthroid state). Products include:
Nadolol Tablets 2121

Nicotinic Acid (Slow-release nicotinic acid may decrease TBG concentration).
No products indexed under this heading.

Norepinephrine Bitartrate (Concurrent use may increase the effects of sympathomimetics or thyroid hormone. Thyroid hormones may increase the risk of coronary insufficiency when sympathomimetic agents are administered to patients with coronary artery disease).
No products indexed under this heading.

Norethindrone (Estrogen-containing oral contraceptives may increase serum TBG concentration). Products include:
Ortho Micronor Tablets 2411

Norethynodrel (Estrogen-containing oral contraceptives may increase serum TBG concentration).
No products indexed under this heading.

Norgestimate (Estrogen-containing oral contraceptives may increase serum TBG concentration). Products include:
Ortho-Cyclen/Ortho Tri-Cyclen 2414
Ortho Tri-Cyclen Lo Tablets 2421

Prefest Tablets ... 1069

Norgestrel (Estrogen-containing oral contraceptives may increase serum TBG concentration). Products include:

Lo/Ovral-28 Tablets ... 3423

Nortriptyline Hydrochloride (Concurrent use of tricyclic antidepressants and levothyroxine may increase the therapeutic and toxic effects of both drugs, possibly due to increased receptor sensitivity to catecholamines. Onset of action of tricyclics may be accelerated).

No products indexed under this heading.

Octreotide Acetate (Octreotide may result in a transient reduction in TSH secretion when administered at doses greater than 100 mcg/day). Products include:

Sandostatin Injection ... 2263
Sandostatin LAR Depot ... 2264

Oxandrolone (Androgens/anabolic steroids may decrease serum TBG concentration). Products include:

Oxandrin Tablets ... 2977

Oxymetholone (Androgens/anabolic steroids may decrease serum TBG concentration). Products include:

Anadrol-50 Tablets ... 3329

Para-Aminosalicylate Sodium (Para-aminosalicylate sodium is associated with thyroid hormone and/or TSH level alterations).

No products indexed under this heading.

Penbutolol Sulfate (Actions of particular beta-adrenergic antagonists may be impaired when the hypothyroid patient is converted to the euthroid state).

No products indexed under this heading.

Pergolide Mesylate (Dopamine and dopamine agonists may result in a transient reduction in TSH secretion when administered at dopamine doses greater than or equal to 1 mcg/kg/min). Products include:

Permax Tablets ... 3357

Perphenazine (Perphenazine is associated with thyroid hormone and/or TSH level alterations).

No products indexed under this heading.

Phenobarbital (Stimulation of hepatic microsomal drug-metabolizing activity may cause increased hepatic degradation of levothyroxine, resulting in increased levothyroxine requirements).

No products indexed under this heading.

Phenobarbital Sodium (Stimulation of hepatic microsomal drug-metabolizing activity may cause increased hepatic degradation of levothyroxine, resulting in increased levothyroxine requirements).

No products indexed under this heading.

Phenylbutazone (Co-administration of phenylbutazone with levothyroxine results in an initial transient increase in FT4. Continued administration results in a decrease in serum T4 and normal FT4 and TSH concentrations and, therefore, patients are clinically euthroid).

No products indexed under this heading.

Phenylephrine Bitartrate (Concurrent use may increase the effects of sympathomimetics or thyroid hormone. Thyroid hormones may increase the risk of coronary insufficiency when sympathomimetic agents are administered to patients with coronary artery disease).

No products indexed under this heading.

Phenylephrine Hydrochloride (Concurrent use may increase the effects of sympathomimetics or thyroid hormone. Thyroid hormones may increase the risk of coronary insufficiency when sympathomimetic agents are administered to patients with coronary artery disease). Products include:

Alacol DM Syrup ... 739
Hycomine Compound Tablets ... 1105
Preparation H Maximum Strength Cream ... ■□ 747
Preparation H Cooling Gel ... ■□ 747
Preparation H ... ■□ 747
Sudafed PE Tablets ... ■□ 711
Vicks Sinex Nasal Spray and Ultra Fine Mist for Sinus Relief ... 2677
Zicam Concentrated Cough Mist for Kids Plus D Cool Cherry ... ■□ 643
Zicam Concentrated Cough Mist Plus D Cool Cherry ... ■□ 642

Phenylephrine Tannate (Concurrent use may increase the effects of sympathomimetics or thyroid hormone. Thyroid hormones may increase the risk of coronary insufficiency when sympathomimetic agents are administered to patients with coronary artery disease).

No products indexed under this heading.

Phenylpropanolamine Hydrochloride (Concurrent use may increase the effects of sympathomimetics or thyroid hormone. Thyroid hormones may increase the risk of coronary insufficiency when sympathomimetic agents are administered to patients with coronary artery disease).

No products indexed under this heading.

Phenytoin (Stimulation of hepatic microsomal drug-metabolizing activity may cause increased hepatic degradation of levothyroxine, resulting in increased levothyroxine requirements).

No products indexed under this heading.

Phenytoin Sodium (Stimulation of hepatic microsomal drug-metabolizing activity may cause increased hepatic degradation of levothyroxine, resulting in increased levothyroxine requirements). Products include:

Phenytek Capsules ... 2153

Pindolol (Actions of particular beta-adrenergic antagonists may be impaired when the hypothyroid patient is converted to the euthroid state).

No products indexed under this heading.

Pioglitazone Hydrochloride (Addition of levothyroxine to antidiabetic therapy may result in increased antidiabetic agent requirements. Careful monitoring of diabetic control is recommended, especially when thyroid therapy is started, changed, or discontinued). Products include:

ActoPlus Met Tablets ... 3219
Actos Tablets ... 3224

Pirbuterol Acetate (Concurrent use may increase the effects of sympathomimetics or thyroid hormone. Thyroid hormones may increase the risk of coronary insufficiency when sympathomimetic agents are administered to patients with coronary artery disease). Products include:

Maxair Autohaler ... 1820

Polyestradiol Phosphate (Estrogen may increase serum TBG concentration).

No products indexed under this heading.

Polythiazide (Thiazide diuretics are associated with thyroid hormone and/or TSH level alterations).

No products indexed under this heading.

Pramipexole Dihydrochloride (Dopamine and dopamine agonists may result in a transient reduction in TSH secretion when administered at dopamine doses greater than or equal to 1 mcg/kg/min). Products include:

Mirapex Tablets ... 889

Prednisolone Acetate (Glucocorticoids may result in a transient reduction in TSH secretion when administered at doses greater than 100mg/day of hydrocortisone or equivalent. Short-term administration of large doses of glucocorticoids may decrease serum T3 concentrations by 30% with minimal change in serum T4 levels. However, long-term glucocorticoid therapy may result in slightly decreased T3 and T4 levels due to decreased TBG production). Products include:

Blephamide Ophthalmic Ointment ... 563
Blephamide Ophthalmic Suspension ... 564
Poly-Pred Liquifilm Ophthalmic Suspension ... ⊙ 231
Pred Forte Ophthalmic Suspension ... ⊙ 233
Pred Mild Sterile Ophthalmic Suspension ... ⊙ 236
Pred-G Ophthalmic Suspension ... ⊙ 234
Pred-G Sterile Ophthalmic Ointment ... ⊙ 235

Prednisolone Sodium Phosphate (Glucocorticoids may result in a transient reduction in TSH secretion when administered at doses greater than 100mg/day of hydrocortisone or equivalent. Short-term administration of large doses of glucocorticoids may decrease serum T3 concentrations by 30% with minimal change in serum T4 levels. However, long-term glucocorticoid therapy may result in slightly decreased T3 and T4 levels due to decreased TBG production). Products include:

Pediapred Oral Solution ... 3319

Prednisolone Tebutate (Glucocorticoids may result in a transient reduction in TSH secretion when administered at doses greater than 100mg/day of hydrocortisone or equivalent. Short-term administration of large doses of glucocorticoids may decrease serum T3 concentrations by 30% with minimal change in serum T4 levels. However, long-term glucocorticoid therapy may result in slightly decreased T3 and T4 levels due to decreased TBG production).

No products indexed under this heading.

Prednisone (Glucocorticoids may result in a transient reduction in TSH secretion when administered at doses greater than 100mg/day of hydrocortisone or equivalent. Short-term administration of large doses of glucocorticoids may decrease serum T3 concentrations by 30% with minimal change in serum T4 levels. However, long-term glucocorticoid therapy may result in slightly decreased T3 and T4 levels due to decreased TBG production).

No products indexed under this heading.

Propranolol Hydrochloride (In patients treated with large doses of propranolol (greater than 160mg/day), T3 and T4 levels change slightly, TSH levels remain normal, and patients are clinically euthroid). Products include:

Inderal LA Long-Acting Capsules ... 3421
InnoPran XL Capsules ... 2728

Protriptyline Hydrochloride (Concurrent use of tricyclic antidepressants and levothyroxine may increase the therapeutic and toxic effects of both drugs, possibly due to increased receptor sensitivity to catecholamines. Onset of action of tricyclics may be accelerated). Products include:

Vivactil Tablets ... 2350

Pseudoephedrine Hydrochloride (Concurrent use may increase the effects of sympathomimetics or thyroid hormone. Thyroid hormones may increase the risk of coronary insufficiency when sympathomimetic agents are administered to patients with coronary artery disease). Products include:

Advil Allergy Sinus Caplets ... ■□ 737
Advil Cold & Sinus ... ■□ 739
Advil Flu & Body Ache Caplets ... ■□ 739
Children's Advil Cold Suspension ... ■□ 741
Advil Multi-Symptom Cold Caplets ... ■□ 738
Allegra-D 12 Hour Extended-Release Tablets ... 2860
Allegra-D 24 Hour Extended-Release Tablets ... 2862
Balamine DM ... 739
BC Cold Powder ... ■□ 612
Benadryl Allergy & Cold Tablets ... ■□ 692
Benadryl Allergy & Sinus Headache Caplets & Gelcaps ... ■□ 693
Children's Benadryl Allergy & Cold Fastmelt Tablets ... ■□ 695
Benadryl Maximum Strength Severe Allergy & Sinus Headache Caplets ... ■□ 694
Children's Benadryl D Allergy & Sinus Fastmelt Tablets ... ■□ 694
Children's Benadryl D Liquid Medication ... ■□ 693
Benadryl D Tablets ... ■□ 694
Contac Non-Drowsy 12 Hour Cold Caplets ... ■□ 614
Contac Non-Drowsy Timed Release 12 Hour Cold Caplets ... ■□ 615
Contac Severe Cold and Flu Caplets Maximum Strength ... ■□ 615
Contac Severe Cold and Flu Caplets Non-Drowsy ... ■□ 615
Children's Dimetapp Cold & Allergy Elixir ... ■□ 745
Children's Dimetapp DM Cold & Cough Elixir ... ■□ 745
Children's Dimetapp Long Acting Cough Plus Cold Syrup ... ■□ 746
Dimetapp Infant Drops Decongestant Plus Cough ... ■□ 746
Children's Motrin Cold Non-Staining Dye-Free Oral Suspension ... 1838
Children's Motrin Cold Oral Suspension ... 1838
Motrin Cold & Sinus Caplets ... 1836
PediaCare Decongestant & Cough Infant Drops ... ■□ 705
PediaCare Decongestant Infants' Drops ... ■□ 705
PediaCare Long-Acting Cough Plus Cold Liquid ... ■□ 704
PediaCare Multi-Symptom Cold Liquid ... ■□ 704
PediaCare NightRest Cough & Cold Liquid ... ■□ 704

Robitussin Allergy & Cough Syrup .. 750
Robitussin CF Liquid 755
Robitussin Cough & Cold Liquid-filled Capsules 750
Robitussin Cough, Cold & Flu Liquid-filled Capsules 750
Robitussin Cough & Cold Infant Drops 755
Robitussin Flu Liquid 752
Robitussin Maximum Strength Cough & Cold Liquid 754
Robitussin PE Syrup 753
Robitussin Pediatric Cough & Cold Liquid 754
Robitussin PM Cough & Cold Liquid 752
Robitussin Severe Congestion Liquid-filled Capsules 751
Simply Stuffy Liquid 1841
Singlet Caplets 636
Sudafed 12 Hour Caplets 708
Sudafed 24 Hour Tablets 709
Sudafed Nasal Decongestant Tablets 709
Sudafed Severe Cold 710
Sudafed Non-Drying Sinus Liquid Caps 709
Sudafed Sinus & Allergy Tablets 710
Sudafed Sinus Headache 711
TheraFlu Cold & Cough Hot Liquid 680
TheraFlu Cold & Sore Throat Hot Liquid 680
TheraFlu Flu & Chest Congestion Non-Drowsy Hot Liquid 681
TheraFlu Flu & Sore Throat Hot Liquid 681
TheraFlu Severe Cold Non-Drowsy Hot Liquid 683
TheraFlu Severe Cold & Cough Hot Liquid 683
TheraFlu Severe Cold Caplets 679
TheraFlu Severe Cold Hot Liquid 682
TheraFlu Severe Cold Non-Drowsy Caplets 679
Triaminic Chest & Nasal Congestion Liquid 685
Triaminic Cold & Allergy Liquid 685
Triaminic Cold & Cough Liquid 685
Triaminic Cough Liquid 687
Triaminic Cough & Nasal Congestion Liquid 687
Triaminic Cough & Sore Throat Liquid 687
Triaminic Flu, Cough & Fever Liquid 685
Triaminic Night Time Cough & Cold Liquid 685
Triaminic Allergy Runny Nose & Congestion Softchews 688
Triaminic Cold & Cough Softchews 688
Triaminic Cough & Sore Throat Softchews 689
Tylenol Sinus NightTime Caplets 663
Children's Tylenol Plus Cold & Allergy Suspension Liquid 1850
Children's Tylenol Plus Cold NightTime Suspension Liquid 1851
Children's Tylenol Plus Cold & Cough Suspension Liquid and Chewable Tablets 1851
Children's Tylenol Plus Cold Chewable Tablets 1851
Children's Tylenol Plus Cold Daytime Non-Drowsy Suspension Liquid 1851
Children's Tylenol Plus Flu Suspension Liquid 1853
Concentrated Tylenol Infants' Drops Plus Cold 1851
Concentrated Tylenol Infants' Drops Plus Cold and Cough 1851
Tylenol Cold & Flu Severe Daytime Liquid with Cool Bust 1846
Tylenol Cold & Flu Severe NightTime Liquid with Cool Burst 1846
Tylenol Cold Severe Congestion Non-Drowsy Caplets with Cool Burst 1846
Tylenol Allergy Complete Night Time Caplets 1844
Tylenol Allergy Complete Multi-Symptom Caplets and Gelcaps with Cool Burst 1844
Tylenol Flu NightTime Gelcaps 1846
Tylenol Flu Day Non-Drowsy Gelcaps 1846
Concentrated Tylenol Infants' Drops Plus Cold Nasal Congestant, Fever Reducer & Pain Reliever 668
Concentrated Tylenol Infants' Drops Plus Cold & Cough Nasal Decongestant, Fever Reducer & Pain Reliever 668
Multi-Symptom Tylenol Cold Night Time Caplets 1845
Multi-Symptom Tylenol Cold Day Non-Drowsy Caplets and Gelcaps 1845
Tylenol Sinus Day Non-Drowsy 1848
Tylenol Sinus Night Time Caplets 1848
Tylenol Sinus Severe Congestion Caplets with Cool Burst 1848
Vicks 44D Cough & Head Congestion Relief 2676
Vicks 44D Cough & Head Congestion Relief Liquid 721
Vicks 44M Cough, Cold & Flu Relief 2676
Pediatric Vicks 44m Cough & Cold Relief 2673
Vicks DayQuil LiquiCaps/Liquid Multi-Symptom Cold/Flu Relief 723
Vicks DayQuil Multi-Symptom Cold/Flu Relief LiquiCaps 2675
Vicks DayQuil Multi-Symptom Cold/Flu Relief Liquid 2675
Children's Vicks NyQuil Cold/Cough Relief 2671
Vicks NyQuil LiquiCaps 2677
Vicks NyQuil LiquiCaps/Liquid Multi-Symptom Cold/Flu Relief 725
Vicks NyQuil Liquid 2677
Zyrtec-D 12 Hour Extended Release Tablets 2591

Pseudoephedrine Sulfate (Concurrent use may increase the effects of sympathomimetics or thyroid hormone. Thyroid hormones may increase the risk of coronary insufficiency when sympathomimetic agents are administered to patients with coronary artery disease). Products include:
Alavert Allergy & Sinus D-12 Hour Tablets 743
Clarinex-D 24-Hour Extended-Release Tablets 3012
Claritin-D Non-Drowsy 12 Hour Tablets 731
Claritin-D Non-Drowsy 24 Hour Tablets 731

Quinestrol (Estrogen may increase serum TBG concentration).
No products indexed under this heading.

Repaglinide (Addition of levothyroxine to antidiabetic therapy may result in increased antidiabetic agent requirements. Careful monitoring of diabetic control is recommended, especially when thyroid therapy is started, changed, or discontinued). Products include:
Prandin Tablets (0.5, 1, and 2 mg) 2337

Resorcinol (Excessive topical use of resorcinol has been associated with thyroid hormone and/or TSH level alterations).
No products indexed under this heading.

Rifampin (Stimulation of hepatic microsomal drug-metabolizing activity may cause increased hepatic degradation of levothyroxine, resulting in increased levothyroxine requirements).
No products indexed under this heading.

Ropinirole Hydrochloride (Dopamine and dopamine agonists may result in a transient reduction in TSH secretion when administered at dopamine doses greater than or equal to 1 mcg/kg/min). Products include:
Requip Tablets 1528

Rosiglitazone Maleate (Addition of levothyroxine to antidiabetic therapy may result in increased antidiabetic agent requirements. Careful monitoring of diabetic control is recommended, especially when thyroid therapy is started, changed, or discontinued). Products include:
Avandamet Tablets 1343
Avandia Tablets 1348

Salmeterol Xinafoate (Concurrent use may increase the effects of sympathomimetics or thyroid hormone. Thyroid hormones may increase the risk of coronary insufficiency when sympathomimetic agents are administered to patients with coronary artery disease). Products include:
Advair Diskus 100/50 1291
Advair Diskus 250/50 1291
Advair Diskus 500/50 1291
Serevent Diskus 1540

Salsalate (Salicylates inhibit binding of T4 and T3 to TBG and transthyretin. An initial increase in FT4 is followed by return of FT4 to normal levels with sustained therapeutic serum salicylate concentrations, although total T4 levels may decrease by as much as 30%).
No products indexed under this heading.

Sertraline Hydrochloride (Administration of sertraline in patients stabilized on levothyroxine may result in increased levothyroxine requirements). Products include:
Zoloft 2581

Simethicone (Concurrent use with simethicone may reduce the efficacy of levothyroxine by binding and delaying or preventing the absorption, potentially resulting in hypothyroidism. Administer levothyroxine at least 4 hours apart from simethicone). Products include:
Gas-X Regular Strength Chewable Tablets 675
Gas-X Extra Strength 675
Gas-X Maximum Strength Softgels 675
Gas-X with Maalox 675
Imodium Advanced Caplets and Chewable Tablets 1835
Maalox Max Maximum Strength Antacid/Anti-Gas Liquid 2165
Maalox Regular Strength Antacid/Antigas Liquid 2164
Maalox Max Quick Dissolve Maximum Strength Chewable Tablets 678
Phazyme-125 mg Quick Dissolve Chewable Tablets 635
Phazyme-180 mg Ultra Strength Softgels 635
Rolaids Multi-Symptom Antacid & Antigas Tablets 708

Sodium Bicarbonate (Concurrent use with antacids may reduce the efficacy of levothyroxine by binding and delaying or preventing the absorption, potentially resulting in hypothyroidism. Administer levothyroxine at least four hours apart from these agents). Products include:
Ceo-Two Evacuant Suppository 607
Colyte with Flavor Packs for Oral Solution 3102
HalfLytely and Bisacodyl Tablets Bowel Prep Kit with Flavors Packs 915
TriLyte with Flavor Packs for Oral Solution 3114

Sodium Nitroprusside (Nitroprusside is associated with thyroid hormone and/or TSH level alterations).
No products indexed under this heading.

Sodium Polystyrene Sulfonate (Concurrent use with sodium polystyrene sulfonate may reduce the efficacy of levothyroxine by binding and delaying or preventing the absorption, potentially resulting in hypothyroidism. Administer levothyroxine at least 4 hours apart from sodium polystyrene sodium).
No products indexed under this heading.

Somatrem (Excessive use of thyroid hormones with growth hormones may accelerate epiphyseal closure. However, untreated hypothyroidism may interfere with growth response to growth hormone).
No products indexed under this heading.

Somatropin (Excessive use of thyroid hormones with growth hormones may accelerate epiphyseal closure. However, untreated hypothyroidism may interfere with growth response to growth hormone). Products include:
Genotropin Lyophilized Powder 2642
Humatrope Vials and Cartridges 1756
Norditropin Cartridges 2318
Nutropin for Injection 1238
Nutropin AQ Injection 1241
Nutropin AQ Pen 1241
Nutropin AQ Pen Cartridge 1241

Sotalol Hydrochloride (Actions of particular beta-adrenergic antagonists may be impaired when the hypothyroid patient is converted to the euthroid state).
No products indexed under this heading.

Stanozolol (Androgens/anabolic steroids may decrease serum TBG concentration).
No products indexed under this heading.

Sucralfate (Concurrent use with sucralfate may reduce the efficacy of levothyroxine by binding and delaying or preventing the absorption, potentially resulting in hypothyroidism. Administer levothyroxine at least four hours apart from sucralfate). Products include:
Carafate Suspension 727
Carafate Tablets 728

Tamoxifen Citrate (Tamoxifen may increase serum TBG concentration).
No products indexed under this heading.

Terbutaline Sulfate (Concurrent use may increase the effects of sympathomimetics or thyroid hormone. Thyroid hormones may increase the risk of coronary insufficiency when sympathomimetic agents are administered to patients with coronary artery disease).
No products indexed under this heading.

Theophylline (Decreased theophylline clearance may occur in hypothyroid patients; clearance returns to normal when the euthroid state is achieved).
No products indexed under this heading.

Theophylline Anhydrous (Decreased theophylline clearance may occur in hypothyroid patients; clearance returns to normal when the euthroid state is achieved). Products include:

Uniphyl Tablets 2708

Theophylline Calcium Salicylate (Decreased theophylline clearance may occur in hypothyroid patients; clearance returns to normal when the euthroid state is achieved).
No products indexed under this heading.

Theophylline Dihydroxypropyl (Glyceryl) (Decreased theophylline clearance may occur in hypothyroid patients; clearance returns to normal when the euthroid state is achieved).
No products indexed under this heading.

Theophylline Ethylenediamine (Decreased theophylline clearance may occur in hypothyroid patients; clearance returns to normal when the euthroid state is achieved).
No products indexed under this heading.

Theophylline Sodium Glycinate (Decreased theophylline clearance may occur in hypothyroid patients; clearance returns to normal when the euthroid state is achieved).
No products indexed under this heading.

Timolol Hemihydrate (Actions of particular beta-adrenergic antagonists may be impaired when the hypothyroid patient is converted to the euthroid state). Products include:
Betimol Ophthalmic Solution 3371
Betimol Ophthalmic Solution .... ⊙283

Timolol Maleate (Actions of particular beta-adrenergic antagonists may be impaired when the hypothyroid patient is converted to the euthroid state). Products include:
Blocadren Tablets 1891
Cosopt Sterile Ophthalmic Solution 1910
Timolide Tablets 2056
Timoptic in Ocudose 2061
Timoptic Sterile Ophthalmic Solution 2058
Timoptic-XE Sterile Ophthalmic Gel Forming Solution 2062

Tolazamide (Addition of levothyroxine to antidiabetic therapy may result in increased antidiabetic agent requirements. Careful monitoring of diabetic control is recommended, especially when thyroid therapy is started, changed, or discontinued).
No products indexed under this heading.

Tolbutamide (Addition of levothyroxine to antidiabetic therapy may result in increased antidiabetic agent requirements. Careful monitoring of diabetic control is recommended, especially when thyroid therapy is started, changed, or discontinued).
No products indexed under this heading.

Triamcinolone (Glucocorticoids may result in a transient reduction in TSH secretion when administered at doses greater than 100mg/day of hydrocortisone or equivalent. Short-term administration of large doses of glucocorticoids may decrease serum T3 concentrations by 30% with minimal change in serum T4 levels. However, long-term glucocorticoid therapy may result in slightly decreased T3 and T4 levels due to decreased TBG production).
No products indexed under this heading.

Triamcinolone Acetonide (Glucocorticoids may result in a transient reduction in TSH secretion when administered at doses greater than 100mg/day of hydrocortisone or equivalent. Short-term administration of large doses of glucocorticoids may decrease serum T3 concentrations by 30% with minimal change in serum T4 levels. However, long-term glucocorticoid therapy may result in slightly decreased T3 and T4 levels due to decreased TBG production). Products include:
Azmacort Inhalation Aerosol 1701
Nasacort HFA Inhalation Aerosol 2939
Nasacort AQ Nasal Spray 2937

Triamcinolone Diacetate (Glucocorticoids may result in a transient reduction in TSH secretion when administered at doses greater than 100mg/day of hydrocortisone or equivalent. Short-term administration of large doses of glucocorticoids may decrease serum T3 concentrations by 30% with minimal change in serum T4 levels. However, long-term glucocorticoid therapy may result in slightly decreased T3 and T4 levels due to decreased TBG production).
No products indexed under this heading.

Triamcinolone Hexacetonide (Glucocorticoids may result in a transient reduction in TSH secretion when administered at doses greater than 100mg/day of hydrocortisone or equivalent. Short-term administration of large doses of glucocorticoids may decrease serum T3 concentrations by 30% with minimal change in serum T4 levels. However, long-term glucocorticoid therapy may result in slightly decreased T3 and T4 levels due to decreased TBG production).
No products indexed under this heading.

Trimipramine Maleate (Concurrent use of tricyclic antidepressants and levothyroxine may increase the therapeutic and toxic effects of both drugs, possibly due to increased receptor sensitivity to catecholamines. Onset of action of tricyclics may be accelerated). Products include:
Surmontil Capsules 2347

Troglitazone (Addition of levothyroxine to antidiabetic therapy may result in increased antidiabetic agent requirements. Careful monitoring of diabetic control is recommended, especially when thyroid therapy is started, changed, or discontinued).
No products indexed under this heading.

Tyropanoate Sodium (Iodide and drugs that contain pharmacologic amounts of iodide may cause hyperthyroidism in euthroid patients with Grave's disease previously treated with antithyroid drugs or in euthroid patients with thyroid autonomy. Hyperthyroidism may develop over several weeks and may persist for several months after therapy discontinuation. Thyroid hormones may also reduce the uptake of I-123 and I-131).
No products indexed under this heading.

Warfarin Sodium (Thyroid hormones appear to increase the catabolism of vitamin-K dependent clotting factors, thereby increasing the anticoagulant activity of oral anticoagulants. Concomitant use of these agents impairs the compensatory increases in clotting factor synthesis. Prothrombin time should be carefully monitored in patients taking levothyroxine and oral anticoagulants and the dose of anticoagulant therapy adjusted accordingly). Products include:
Coumadin for Injection 932
Coumadin Tablets 932

LEVOXYL TABLETS

(Levothyroxine Sodium) 1680

May interact with androgens, antacids containing aluminum, calcium and magnesium, beta blockers, oral anticoagulants, dopamine agonists, estrogens, glucocorticoids, cardiac glycosides, hydantoin anticonvulsants, oral hypoglycemic agents, insulin, lithium preparations, phenytoin, radiographic iodinated contrast media, salicylates, sympathomimetics, thiazides, tricyclic antidepressants, and xanthines. Compounds in these categories include:

Acarbose (Addition of levothyroxine to antidiabetic therapy may result in increased antidiabetic agent requirements). Products include:
Precose Tablets 776

Acebutolol Hydrochloride (Co-administration with beta-blockers may decrease T_4 5'-deiodinase activity; action of beta-blocker may be impaired when the hypothyroid patient is converted to euthyroid).
No products indexed under this heading.

Albuterol (Co-administration of sympathomimetic agents may increase the effects of sympathomimetics or thyroid hormone; thyroid hormones may increase risk of coronary insufficiency when sympathomimetic agents are administered to patients with coronary disease). Products include:
Proventil Inhalation Aerosol 3067

Albuterol Sulfate (Co-administration of sympathomimetic agents may increase the effects of sympathomimetics or thyroid hormone; thyroid hormones may increase risk of coronary insufficiency when sympathomimetic agents are administered to patients with coronary disease). Products include:
AccuNeb Inhalation Solution 1055
Combivent Inhalation Aerosol 878
DuoNeb Inhalation Solution 1058
Proventil Inhalation Solution 0.083% 3069
Proventil HFA Inhalation Aerosol 3071
Ventolin HFA Inhalation Aerosol 1576
VoSpire Extended-Release Tablets 2352

Aldesleukin (Co-administration has been associated with transient painless thyroiditis in 20% of patients). Products include:
Proleukin for Injection 1007

Aluminum Carbonate (Co-administration with antacids may reduce the efficacy of levothyroxine by binding and delaying or preventing absorption, potentially resulting in hypothyroidism; administer levothyroxine at least 4 hours apart from these agents).
No products indexed under this heading.

Aluminum Hydroxide (Co-administration with antacids may reduce the efficacy of levothyroxine by binding and delaying or preventing absorption, potentially resulting in hypothyroidism; administer levothyroxine at least 4 hours apart from these agents). Products include:
Gaviscon Regular Strength Liquid .... ▣620
Gaviscon Regular Strength Tablets .... ▣619
Gaviscon Extra Strength Liquid .... ▣620
Gaviscon Extra Strength Tablets .... ▣619
Maalox Max Maximum Strength Antacid/Anti-Gas Liquid 2165
Maalox Regular Strength Antacid/Antigas Liquid 2164

Aminoglutethimide (May decrease thyroid hormone secretion, which may result in hypothyrodism).
No products indexed under this heading.

Aminophylline (Decreased theophylline clearance may occur in hypothyroid patients; clearance returns to normal when euthyroid state is achieved).
No products indexed under this heading.

p-Aminosalicylic Acid (Co-administration has been associated with thyroid hormone and/or TSH level alterations by various mechanisms).
No products indexed under this heading.

Amiodarone Hydrochloride (May decrease thyroid hormone secretion, which may result in hypothyrodism; amiodarone is slowly excreted, producing more prolonged hypothyroidism; amiodarone may induce hyperthyroidism by causing thyroiditis). Products include:
Pacerone Tablets 3337

Amitriptyline Hydrochloride (Co-administration may increase the therapeutic and toxic effects of both drugs possibly due to increased receptor sensitivity to catecholamines; toxic effects may include increased risk of arrhythmias and CNS stimulation; onset of tricyclics may be accelerated).
No products indexed under this heading.

Amoxapine (Co-administration may increase the therapeutic and toxic effects of both drugs possibly due to increased receptor sensitivity to catecholamines; toxic effects may include increased risk of arrhythmias and CNS stimulation; onset of tricyclics may be accelerated).
No products indexed under this heading.

Anisindione (Thyroid hormones appear to increase the catabolism of vitamin K-dependent clotting factors, thereby increasing the anticoagulant activity of oral anticoagulants). Products include:
Miradon Tablets 3056

Asparaginase (Co-administration may result in decreased serum TBG concentration). Products include:
Elspar for Injection 1943

Aspirin (Co-administration with salicylates at greater than 2 gm inhibit binding of T_4 and T_3 to TBG and transthyrelin; an initial increase in serum FT_4 is followed by return of FT_4 to normal levels with sustained therapeutic salicylate concentrations, although total T_4 levels may decrease by as much as 30%). Products include:
Aggrenox Capsules 855
Bayer, Aspirin Regimen .... ▣606
Bayer Aspirin Tablets 3515
BC Powder .... ▣612
BC Allergy Sinus Cold Powder .... ▣612
Arthritis Strength BC Powder .... ▣612
BC Sinus Cold Powder .... ▣612
Ecotrin Enteric Coated Aspirin Low, Regular and Maximum Strength Tablets 1627
Goody's Body Pain Formula Powder .... ▣621

(▣ Described in PDR For Nonprescription Drugs)

(⊙ Described in PDR For Ophthalmic Medicines™)

Goody's Extra Strength Headache Powder 621
Goody's Extra Strength Pain Relief Tablets 621
Percodan Tablets 1115
St. Joseph 81 mg Aspirin Chewable and Enteric Coated Tablets 1841

Aspirin, Enteric Coated (Co-administration with salicylates at greater than 2 gm inhibit binding of T_4 and T_3 to TBG and transthyrelin; an initial increase in serum FT_4 is followed by return of FT_4 to normal levels with sustained therapeutic salicylate concentrations, although total T_4 levels may decrease by as much as 30%).
No products indexed under this heading.

Aspirin Buffered (Co-administration with salicylates at greater than 2 gm inhibit binding of T_4 and T_3 to TBG and transthyrelin; an initial increase in serum FT_4 is followed by return of FT_4 to normal levels with sustained therapeutic salicylate concentrations, although total T_4 levels may decrease by as much as 30%).
No products indexed under this heading.

Atenolol (Co-administration with beta-blockers may decrease T_4 5'-deiodinase activity; action of beta-blocker may be impaired when the hypothyroid patient is converted to euthyroid). Products include:
Tenormin I.V. Injection 698
Tenormin Tablets 695

Bendroflumethiazide (Co-administration has been associated with thyroid hormone and/or TSH level alterations by various mechanisms).
No products indexed under this heading.

Betamethasone Acetate (Co-administration with glucocorticoids may result in a transient reduction in TSH secretion; the reduction is not sustained, therefore, hypothyroidism does not occur; glucocorticoids may decrease serum TBG concentration).
No products indexed under this heading.

Betamethasone Sodium Phosphate (Co-administration with glucocorticoids may result in a transient reduction in TSH secretion; the reduction is not sustained, therefore, hypothyroidism does not occur; glucocorticoids may decrease serum TBG concentration).
No products indexed under this heading.

Betaxolol Hydrochloride (Co-administration with beta-blockers may decrease T_4 5'-deiodinase activity; action of beta-blocker may be impaired when the hypothyroid patient is converted to euthyroid). Products include:
Betoptic S Ophthalmic Suspension 554

Bisoprolol Fumarate (Co-administration with beta-blockers may decrease T_4 5'-deiodinase activity; action of beta-blocker may be impaired when the hypothyroid patient is converted to euthyroid).
No products indexed under this heading.

Bromocriptine Mesylate (Co-administration with dopamine agonists may result in a transient reduction in TSH secretion; the reduction is not sustained, therefore, hypothyroidism does not occur).
No products indexed under this heading.

Calcium Carbonate (Co-administration with calcium carbonate may form insoluble chelate with levothyroxine, which may result in hypothyroidism; administer levothyroxine at least 4 hours apart from these agents). Products include:
Actonel with Calcium Tablets 2684
Caltrate 600 PLUS Chewables 779
Caltrate 600 PLUS Tablets 779
Caltrate 600 + D Tablets 779
Encora Capsules 3298
Encora AM Tablets 3298
Encora PM Tablets 3298
Gas-X with Maalox 675
Maalox Regular Strength Antacid Tablets 2166
Quick Dissolve Maalox Max Maximum Strength Antacid/Antigas Tablets 2165
Maalox Max Quick Dissolve Maximum Strength Chewable Tablets 678
Os-Cal Chewable Tablets 765
Pepcid Complete Chewable Tablets 1672
PremCal Light, Regular, and Extra Strength Tablets 762
Rolaids Tablets 707
Extra Strength Rolaids Softchews 708
Extra Strength Rolaids Tablets 707
Rolaids Multi-Symptom Antacid & Antigas Tablets 708
Tums 639

Carbamazepine (Co-administration may increase hepatic metabolism, which may result in hypothyroidism, resulting in increased levothyroxine requirements; carbamazepine reduces serum protein binding of levothyroxine, and total- and free-T_4 may be reduced by 20% to 40%, but most patients have normal serum TSH levels and are clinically euthyroid). Products include:
Carbatrol Capsules 3174
Equetro Extended-Release Capsules 3178
Tegretol/Tegretol-XR 2278

Carteolol Hydrochloride (Co-administration with beta-blockers may decrease T_4 5'-deiodinase activity; action of beta-blocker may be impaired when the hypothyroid patient is converted to euthyroid). Products include:
Carteolol Hydrochloride Ophthalmic Solution USP, 1% .... ⊙246

Chloral Hydrate (Co-administration has been associated with thyroid hormone and/or TSH level alterations by various mechanisms).
No products indexed under this heading.

Chlorothiazide (Co-administration has been associated with thyroid hormone and/or TSH level alterations by various mechanisms). Products include:
Aldoclor Tablets 1881
Diuril Oral 1936

Chlorothiazide Sodium (Co-administration has been associated with thyroid hormone and/or TSH level alterations by various mechanisms). Products include:
Diuril Sodium Intravenous 1934

Chlorotrianisene (Co-administration with oral estrogens may result in increased serum TBG concentrations).
No products indexed under this heading.

Chlorpropamide (Addition of levothyroxine to antidiabetic therapy may result in increased antidiabetic agent requirements).
No products indexed under this heading.

Cholestyramine (Co-administration may result in decreased T_4 absorption, which may result in hypothyroidism; administer levothyroxine at least 4 hours apart from these agents).
No products indexed under this heading.

Choline Magnesium Trisalicylate (Co-administration with salicylates at greater than 2 gm inhibit binding of T_4 and T_3 to TBG and transthyrelin; an initial increase in serum FT_4 is followed by return of FT_4 to normal levels with sustained therapeutic salicylate concentrations, although total T_4 levels may decrease by as much as 30%).
No products indexed under this heading.

Clofibrate (Co-administration may result in increased serum TBG concentrations).
No products indexed under this heading.

Clomipramine Hydrochloride (Co-administration may increase the therapeutic and toxic effects of both drugs possibly due to increased receptor sensitivity to catecholamines; toxic effects may include increased risk of arrhythmias and CNS stimulation; onset of tricyclics may be accelerated).
No products indexed under this heading.

Colestipol Hydrochloride (Co-administration may result in decreased T_4 absorption, which may result in hypothyroidism; administer levothyroxine at least 4 hours apart from these agents).
No products indexed under this heading.

Cortisone Acetate (Co-administration with glucocorticoids may result in a transient reduction in TSH secretion; the reduction is not sustained, therefore, hypothyroidism does not occur; glucocorticoids may decrease serum TBG concentration).
No products indexed under this heading.

Desipramine Hydrochloride (Co-administration may increase the therapeutic and toxic effects of both drugs possibly due to increased receptor sensitivity to catecholamines; toxic effects may include increased risk of arrhythmias and CNS stimulation; onset of tricyclics may be accelerated).
No products indexed under this heading.

Deslanoside (Co-administration may result in reduced serum digitalis glycosides in hyperthyroidism or when the hypothyroid patient is converted to euthyroid state; therapeutic effect of digitalis glycoside may be reduced).
No products indexed under this heading.

Dexamethasone (Co-administration with glucocorticoids may result in a transient reduction in TSH secretion; the reduction is not sustained, therefore, hypothyroidism does not occur; glucocorticoids may decrease serum TBG concentration). Products include:
Ciprodex Otic Suspension 555
Decadron Tablets 1929
TobraDex Ophthalmic Ointment 558
TobraDex Ophthalmic Suspension 558

Dexamethasone Acetate (Co-administration with glucocorticoids may result in a transient reduction in TSH secretion; the reduction is not sustained, therefore, hypothyroidism does not occur; glucocorticoids may decrease serum TBG concentration).
No products indexed under this heading.

Dexamethasone Sodium Phosphate (Co-administration with glucocorticoids may result in a transient reduction in TSH secretion; the reduction is not sustained, therefore, hypothyroidism does not occur; glucocorticoids may decrease serum TBG concentration). Products include:
Decadron Phosphate Injection 1931

Diatrizoate Meglumine (May decrease thyroid hormone secretion, which may result in hypothyrodism; the fetus, elderly, and euthyroid patients with underlying thyroid disease are among those individuals who are susceptible to iodine-induced hypothyroidism; oral cholecytographic agents slowly excreted, producing more prolonged hypothyroidism; iodide drugs that contain pharmacologic amounts of iodide may cause hypothyroidism in euthyroid patients with Grave's disease previously treated with thyroid autonomy; hyperthyroidism may develop over several weeks and may persist for several months after therapy discontinuation).
No products indexed under this heading.

Diatrizoate Sodium (May decrease thyroid hormone secretion, which may result in hypothyrodism; the fetus, elderly, and euthyroid patients with underlying thyroid disease are among those individuals who are susceptible to iodine-induced hypothyroidism; oral cholecytographic agents slowly excreted, producing more prolonged hypothyroidism; iodide drugs that contain pharmacologic amounts of iodide may cause hypothyroidism in euthyroid patients with Grave's disease previously treated with thyroid autonomy; hyperthyroidism may develop over several weeks and may persist for several months after therapy discontinuation).
No products indexed under this heading.

Diazepam (Co-administration has been associated with thyroid hormone and/or TSH level alterations by various mechanisms). Products include:
Diastat Rectal Delivery System 3344
Valium Tablets 2822

Dicumarol (Thyroid hormones appear to increase the catabolism of vitamin K-dependent clotting factors, thereby increasing the anticoagulant activity of oral anticoagulants).
No products indexed under this heading.

Dienestrol (Co-administration with oral estrogens may result in increased serum TBG concentrations).
No products indexed under this heading.

Diethylstilbestrol (Co-administration with oral estrogens may result in increased serum TBG concentrations).
No products indexed under this heading.

Diflunisal (Co-administration with salicylates at greater than 2 gm inhibit binding of T_4 and T_3 to TBG and transthyrelin; an initial increase in serum FT_4 is followed by return of FT_4 to normal levels with sustained therapeutic salicylate concentrations, although total T_4 levels may decrease by as much as 30%). Products include:
Dolobid Tablets 1937

Digitalis Glycoside Preparations (Co-administration may result in reduced serum digitalis glycosides in hyperthyroidism or when the hypothyroid patient is converted to euthyroid state; therapeutic effect of digitalis glycoside may be reduced).
No products indexed under this heading.

Digitoxin (Co-administration may result in reduced serum digitalis glycosides in hyperthyroidism or when the hypothyroid patient is converted to euthyroid state; therapeutic effect of digitalis glycoside may be reduced).
No products indexed under this heading.

Digoxin (Co-administration may result in reduced serum digitalis glycosides in hyperthyroidism or when the hypothyroid patient is converted to euthyroid state; therapeutic effect of digitalis glycoside may be reduced). Products include:
Digitek Tablets 2146
Lanoxicaps Capsules 1458
Lanoxin Injection 1462
Lanoxin Tablets 1468
Lanoxin Injection Pediatric 1465

Dobutamine Hydrochloride (Co-administration of sympathomimetic agents may increase the effects of sympathomimetics or thyroid hormone; thyroid hormones may increase risk of coronary insufficiency when sympathomimetic agents are administered to patients with coronary disease).
No products indexed under this heading.

Dopamine Hydrochloride (Co-administration with dopamine may result in a transient reduction in TSH secretion; the reduction is not sustained, therefore, hypothyroidism does not occur).
No products indexed under this heading.

Doxepin Hydrochloride (Co-administration may increase the therapeutic and toxic effects of both drugs possibly due to increased receptor sensitivity to catecholamines; toxic effects may include increased risk of arrhythmias and CNS stimulation; onset of tricyclics may be accelerated).
No products indexed under this heading.

Dyphylline (Decreased theophylline clearance may occur in hypothyroid patients; clearance returns to normal when euthyroid state is achieved).
No products indexed under this heading.

Ephedrine Hydrochloride (Co-administration of sympathomimetic agents may increase the effects of sympathomimetics or thyroid hormone; thyroid hormones may increase risk of coronary insufficiency when sympathomimetic agents are administered to patients with coronary disease). Products include:
Primatene Tablets .... ▣ 749

Ephedrine Sulfate (Co-administration of sympathomimetic agents may increase the effects of sympathomimetics or thyroid hormone; thyroid hormones may increase risk of coronary insufficiency when sympathomimetic agents are administered to patients with coronary disease).
No products indexed under this heading.

Ephedrine Tannate (Co-administration of sympathomimetic agents may increase the effects of sympathomimetics or thyroid hormone; thyroid hormones may increase risk of coronary insufficiency when sympathomimetic agents are administered to patients with coronary disease).
No products indexed under this heading.

Epinephrine (Co-administration of sympathomimetic agents may increase the effects of sympathomimetics or thyroid hormone; thyroid hormones may increase risk of coronary insufficiency when sympathomimetic agents are administered to patients with coronary disease). Products include:
EpiPen 1061
Primatene Mist .... ▣ 749

Epinephrine Bitartrate (Co-administration of sympathomimetic agents may increase the effects of sympathomimetics or thyroid hormone; thyroid hormones may increase risk of coronary insufficiency when sympathomimetic agents are administered to patients with coronary disease).
No products indexed under this heading.

Epinephrine Hydrochloride (Co-administration of sympathomimetic agents may increase the effects of sympathomimetics or thyroid hormone; thyroid hormones may increase risk of coronary insufficiency when sympathomimetic agents are administered to patients with coronary disease).
No products indexed under this heading.

Esmolol Hydrochloride (Co-administration with beta-blockers may decrease T_4 5'-deiodinase activity; action of beta-blocker may be impaired when the hypothyroid patient is converted to euthyroid). Products include:
Brevibloc Concentrate 766
Brevibloc Injection 766
Brevibloc Double Strength Injection 766
Brevibloc Premixed Injection 766
Brevibloc Double Strength Premixed Injection 766

Estradiol (Co-administration with oral estrogens may result in increased serum TBG concentrations). Products include:
Activella Tablets 2311
Climara Transdermal System 795
Climara Pro Transdermal System 800
CombiPatch Transdermal System 2180
Estrogel 0.06% 3200
Menostar Transdermal System 805
Prefest Tablets 1069
Vagifem Tablets 2340
Vivelle Transdermal System 2288
Vivelle-Dot Transdermal System 2293

Estrogens, Conjugated (Co-administration with oral estrogens may result in increased serum TBG concentrations). Products include:
Premarin Intravenous 3440
Premarin Tablets 3443
Premarin Vaginal Cream 3449
Premphase Tablets 3452
Prempro Tablets 3452

Estrogens, Esterified (Co-administration with oral estrogens may result in increased serum TBG concentrations). Products include:
Estratest Tablets 3196
Estratest H.S. Tablets 3196

Estropipate (Co-administration with oral estrogens may result in increased serum TBG concentrations).
No products indexed under this heading.

Ethinyl Estradiol (Co-administration with estrogen containing oral contraceptives may result in increased serum TBG concentrations). Products include:
Alesse-28 Tablets 3392
Lo/Ovral-28 Tablets 3423
NuvaRing 2357
Ortho-Cept Tablets 2395
Ortho-Cyclen/Ortho Tri-Cyclen 2414
Ortho Evra Transdermal System 2402
Ortho Tri-Cyclen Lo Tablets 2421
Seasonale Tablets 1073
Triphasil-28 Tablets 3483
Yasmin 28 Tablets 818

Ethiodized Oil (May decrease thyroid hormone secretion, which may result in hypothyrodism; the fetus, elderly, and euthyroid patients with underlying thyroid disease are among those individuals who are susceptible to iodine-induced hypothyroidism; oral cholecytographic agents slowly excreted, producing more prolonged hypothyroidism; iodide drugs that contain pharmacologic amounts of iodide may cause hypothyroidism in euthyroid patients with Grave's disease previously treated with thyroid autonomy; hyperthyroidism may develop over several weeks and may persist for several months after therapy discontinuation).
No products indexed under this heading.

Ethionamide (Co-administration has been associated with thyroid hormone and/or TSH level alterations by various mechanisms). Products include:
Trecator Tablets 3482

Ethotoin (Hydantoins may cause protein-binding site displacement; co-administration results in an initial transient increase in FT_4; continued administration results in a decrease in serum T_4 and normal FT_4 and TSH concentrations and, therefore, patients are clinically euthyroid). Products include:
Peganone Tablets, USP 2487

Ferrous Sulfate (Co-administration may result in decreased T_4 absorption, which may result in hypothyroidism; ferrous sulfate may form a ferric-thyroxine complex; administer levothyroxine at least 4 hours apart from these agents). Products include:
Feosol Tablets 1629
Slow Fe Iron Tablets .... ▣ 772
Slow Fe with Folic Acid Tablets .... ▣ 773

Fiber Supplement (Concurrent use of dietary fiber may bind and decrease the absorption of levothyroxine sodium from GI tract).
No products indexed under this heading.

Fludrocortisone Acetate (Co-administration with glucocorticoids may result in a transient reduction in TSH secretion; the reduction is not sustained, therefore, hypothyroidism does not occur; glucocorticoids may decrease serum TBG concentration).
No products indexed under this heading.

Fluorouracil (Co-administration with 5-FU may result in increased serum TBG concentrations). Products include:
Carac Cream, 0.5% 1048
Efudex 3348

Fluoxymesterone (Co-administration with androgens/anabolic steroids may result in decreased serum TBG concentration).
No products indexed under this heading.

Fosphenytoin Sodium (Hydantoins may cause protein-binding site displacement; co-administration results in an initial transient increase in FT_4; co-administration may increase hepatic metabolism, which may result in hypothyroidism, resulting in increased levothyroxine requirements; phenytoin reduces serum protein binding of levothyroxine, and total- and free-T_4 may be reduced by 20% to 40%, but most patients have normal serum TSH levels and are clinicly euthyroid).
No products indexed under this heading.

Furosemide (May cause protein-binding site displacement at greater than 80 mg IV; co-administration results in an initial transient increase in FT_4; continued administration results in a decrease in serum T_4 and normal FT_4 and TSH concentrations and, therefore, patients are clinically euthyroid). Products include:
Furosemide Tablets 2117

Gadopentetate Dimeglumine (May decrease thyroid hormone secretion, which may result in hypothyrodism; the fetus, elderly, and euthyroid patients with underlying thyroid disease are among those individuals who are susceptible to iodine-induced hypothyroidism; oral cholecytographic agents slowly excreted, producing more prolonged hypothyroidism; iodide drugs that contain pharmacologic amounts of iodide may cause hypothyroidism in euthyroid patients with Grave's disease previously treated with thyroid autonomy; hyperthyroidism may develop over several weeks and may persist for several months after therapy discontinuation).
No products indexed under this heading.

Glimepiride (Addition of levothyroxine to antidiabetic therapy may result in increased antidiabetic agent requirements). Products include:
- Amaryl Tablets 2864

Glipizide (Addition of levothyroxine to antidiabetic therapy may result in increased antidiabetic agent requirements).
No products indexed under this heading.

Glyburide (Addition of levothyroxine to antidiabetic therapy may result in increased antidiabetic agent requirements).
No products indexed under this heading.

Heparin Sodium (May cause protein-binding site displacement; co-administration results in an initial transient increase in FT_4; continued administration results in a decrease in serum T_4 and normal FT_4 and TSH concentrations and, therefore, patients are clinically euthyroid).
No products indexed under this heading.

Heroin (Co-administration may result in increased serum TBG concentrations).
No products indexed under this heading.

Hydrochlorothiazide (Co-administration has been associated with thyroid hormone and/or TSH level alterations by various mechanisms). Products include:
- Aldoril Tablets 1884
- Atacand HCT 637
- Avalide Tablets 2889
- Avalide Tablets 922
- Benicar HCT Tablets 2852
- Diovan HCT Tablets 2195
- Dyazide Capsules 1389
- Hyzaar 1964
- Lotensin HCT Tablets 2235
- Maxzide 2150
- Micardis HCT Tablets 886
- Moduretic Tablets 2003
- Prinzide Tablets 2033
- Teveten HCT Tablets 1710
- Timolide Tablets 2056
- Uniretic Tablets 3114
- Vaseretic Tablets 2073
- Zestoretic Tablets 701

Hydrocortisone (Co-administration with glucocorticoids may result in a transient reduction in TSH secretion; the reduction is not sustained, therefore, hypothyroidism does not occur; glucocorticoids may decrease serum TBG concentration). Products include:
- Cortizone•5 Ointment 699
- Cortizone•10 Creme 699
- Cortizone•10 Ointment 699
- Cortizone•10 Plus Creme 700
- Cortizone•10 Maximum Strength Quick Shot Spray 700
- Hydrocortone Tablets 1963
- Preparation H Hydrocortisone Cream 748

Hydrocortisone Acetate (Co-administration with glucocorticoids may result in a transient reduction in TSH secretion; the reduction is not sustained, therefore, hypothyroidism does not occur; glucocorticoids may decrease serum TBG concentration). Products include:
- Analpram-HC 1136
- Pramosone 1139
- ProctoFoam-HC 3113
- Tucks Anti-Itch Ointment 712
- U-cort 1% Cream 3289

Hydrocortisone Sodium Phosphate (Co-administration with glucocorticoids may result in a transient reduction in TSH secretion; the reduction is not sustained, therefore, hypothyroidism does not occur; glucocorticoids may decrease serum TBG concentration).
No products indexed under this heading.

Hydrocortisone Sodium Succinate (Co-administration with glucocorticoids may result in a transient reduction in TSH secretion; the reduction is not sustained, therefore, hypothyroidism does not occur; glucocorticoids may decrease serum TBG concentration).
No products indexed under this heading.

Hydroflumethiazide (Co-administration has been associated with thyroid hormone and/or TSH level alterations by various mechanisms).
No products indexed under this heading.

Imipramine Hydrochloride (Co-administration may increase the therapeutic and toxic effects of both drugs possibly due to increased receptor sensitivity to catecholamines; toxic effects may include increased risk of arrhythmias and CNS stimulation; onset of tricyclics may be accelerated).
No products indexed under this heading.

Imipramine Pamoate (Co-administration may increase the therapeutic and toxic effects of both drugs possibly due to increased receptor sensitivity to catecholamines; toxic effects may include increased risk of arrhythmias and CNS stimulation; onset of tricyclics may be accelerated).
No products indexed under this heading.

Infant Formula (Concurrent use of soybean flour may bind and decrease the absorption of levothyroxine sodium from GI tract).
No products indexed under this heading.

Insulin, Human, Zinc Suspension (Addition of levothyroxine to insulin therapy may result in increased insulin requirements). Products include:
- Humulin L, 100 Units 1763
- Humulin U, 100 Units 1770

Insulin, Human NPH (Addition of levothyroxine to insulin therapy may result in increased insulin requirements). Products include:
- Humulin N, 100 Units 1764
- Humulin N Pen 1765
- Novolin N Human Insulin 10 ml Vials 2322
- Novolin N InnoLet 2322
- Novolin N PenFill 3 ml Cartridges 2325
- Novolin R InnoLet 2322

Insulin, Human Regular (Addition of levothyroxine to insulin therapy may result in increased insulin requirements). Products include:
- Humulin R (U-500) 1768
- Humulin R, 100 Units 1767
- Novolin R Human Insulin 10 ml Vials 2322
- Novolin R PenFill 2325

Insulin, Human Regular and Human NPH Mixture (Addition of levothyroxine to insulin therapy may result in increased insulin requirements). Products include:
- Humulin 50/50, 100 Units 1760
- Humulin 70/30 Pen 1761
- Novolin 70/30 Human Insulin 10 ml Vials 2321
- Novolin 70/30 InnoLet 2322
- Novolin 70/30 PenFill 3 ml Cartridges 2325

Insulin, NPH (Addition of levothyroxine to insulin therapy may result in increased insulin requirements).
No products indexed under this heading.

Insulin, Regular (Addition of levothyroxine to insulin therapy may result in increased insulin requirements).
No products indexed under this heading.

Insulin, Zinc Crystals (Addition of levothyroxine to insulin therapy may result in increased insulin requirements).
No products indexed under this heading.

Insulin, Zinc Suspension (Addition of levothyroxine to insulin therapy may result in increased insulin requirements).
No products indexed under this heading.

Insulin Aspart, Human Regular (Addition of levothyroxine to insulin therapy may result in increased insulin requirements). Products include:
- NovoLog Injection 2326

Insulin glargine (Addition of levothyroxine to insulin therapy may result in increased insulin requirements). Products include:
- Lantus Injection 2925

Insulin Lispro, Human (Addition of levothyroxine to insulin therapy may result in increased insulin requirements). Products include:
- Humalog-Pen 1751
- Humalog Mix 75/25-Pen 1754

Insulin Lispro Protamine, Human (Addition of levothyroxine to insulin therapy may result in increased insulin requirements). Products include:
- Humalog Mix 75/25-Pen 1754

Interferon alfa-2a, Recombinant (Co-administration with interferon alpha has been associated with the development of antithyroid microsomal antibodies in 20% of patients and some have transient hypothyroidism, hyperthyroidism, or both; patients who have antithyroid antibodies before treatment are at higher risk for thyroid dysfunction). Products include:
- Roferon-A Injection 2805

Interferon alfa-2b, Recombinant (Co-administration with interferon alpha has been associated with the development of antithyroid microsomal antibodies in 20% of patients and some have transient hypothyroidism, hyperthyroidism, or both; patients who have antithyroid antibodies before treatment are at higher risk for thyroid dysfunction). Products include:
- Intron A for Injection 3038
- Rebetron Combination Therapy 3078

Interferon alfa-N3 (Human Leukocyte Derived) (Co-administration with interferon alpha has been associated with the development of antithyroid microsomal antibodies in 20% of patients and some have transient hypothyroidism, hyperthyroidism, or both; patients who have antithyroid antibodies before treatment are at higher risk for thyroid dysfunction). Products include:
- Alferon N Injection 1640

Iodamide Meglumine (May decrease thyroid hormone secretion, which may result in hypothyrodism; the fetus, elderly, and euthyroid patients with underlying thyroid disease are among those individuals who are susceptible to iodine-induced hypothyroidism; oral cholecytographic agents slowly excreted, producing more prolonged hypothyroidism; iodide drugs that contain pharmacologic amounts of iodide may cause hypothyroidism in euthyroid patients with Grave's disease previously treated with thyroid autonomy; hyperthyroidism may develop over several weeks and may persist for several months after therapy discontinuation).
No products indexed under this heading.

Iohexol (May decrease thyroid hormone secretion, which may result in hypothyrodism; the fetus, elderly, and euthyroid patients with underlying thyroid disease are among those individuals who are susceptible to iodine-induced hypothyroidism; oral cholecytographic agents slowly excreted, producing more prolonged hypothyroidism; iodide drugs that contain pharmacologic amounts of iodide may cause hypothyroidism in euthyroid patients with Grave's disease previously treated with thyroid autonomy; hyperthyroidism may develop over several weeks and may persist for several months after therapy discontinuation).
No products indexed under this heading.

Iopamidol (May decrease thyroid hormone secretion, which may result in hypothyrodism; the fetus, elderly, and euthyroid patients with underlying thyroid disease are among those individuals who are susceptible to iodine-induced hypothyroidism; oral cholecytographic agents slowly excreted, producing more prolonged hypothyroidism; iodide drugs that contain pharmacologic amounts of iodide may cause hypothyroidism in euthyroid patients with Grave's disease previously treated with thyroid autonomy; hyperthyroidism may develop over several weeks and may persist for several months after therapy discontinuation).
No products indexed under this heading.

Iopanoic Acid (May decrease thyroid hormone secretion, which may result in hypothyrodism; the fetus, elderly, and euthyroid patients with underlying thyroid disease are among those individuals who are susceptible to iodine-induced hypothyroidism; oral cholecytographic agents slowly excreted, producing more prolonged hypothyroidism; iodide drugs that contain pharmacologic amounts of iodide may cause hypothyroidism in euthyroid patients with Grave's disease previously treated with thyroid autonomy; hyperthyroidism may develop over several weeks and may persist for several months after therapy discontinuation).
No products indexed under this heading.

Iothalamate Meglumine (May decrease thyroid hormone secretion, which may result in hypothyrodism; the fetus, elderly, and euthyroid patients with underlying thyroid disease are among those individuals

IMPORTANT NOTE: Always consult each drug listing in the patient's regimen for possible interactions.

who are susceptible to iodine-induced hypothyroidism; oral cholecytographic agents slowly excreted, producing more prolonged hypothyroidism; iodide drugs that contain pharmacologic amounts of iodide may cause hypothyroidism in euthyroid patients with Grave's disease previously treated with thyroid autonomy; hyperthyroidism may develop over several weeks and may persist for several months after therapy discontinuation).

No products indexed under this heading.

Ioxaglate Meglumine (May decrease thyroid hormone secretion, which may result in hypothyrodism; the fetus, elderly, and euthyroid patients with underlying thyroid disease are among those individuals who are susceptible to iodine-induced hypothyroidism; oral cholecytographic agents slowly excreted, producing more prolonged hypothyroidism; iodide drugs that contain pharmacologic amounts of iodide may cause hypothyroidism in euthyroid patients with Grave's disease previously treated with thyroid autonomy; hyperthyroidism may develop over several weeks and may persist for several months after therapy discontinuation).

No products indexed under this heading.

Ioxaglate Sodium (May decrease thyroid hormone secretion, which may result in hypothyrodism; the fetus, elderly, and euthyroid patients with underlying thyroid disease are among those individuals who are susceptible to iodine-induced hypothyroidism; oral cholecytographic agents slowly excreted, producing more prolonged hypothyroidism; iodide drugs that contain pharmacologic amounts of iodide may cause hypothyroidism in euthyroid patients with Grave's disease previously treated with thyroid autonomy; hyperthyroidism may develop over several weeks and may persist for several months after therapy discontinuation).

No products indexed under this heading.

Isoproterenol Hydrochloride (Co-administration of sympathomimetic agents may increase the effects of sympathomimetics or thyroid hormone; thyroid hormones may increase risk of coronary insufficiency when sympathomimetic agents are administered to patients with coronary disease).

No products indexed under this heading.

Isoproterenol Sulfate (Co-administration of sympathomimetic agents may increase the effects of sympathomimetics or thyroid hormone; thyroid hormones may increase risk of coronary insufficiency when sympathomimetic agents are administered to patients with coronary disease).

No products indexed under this heading.

Ketamine Hydrochloride (Co-administration may produce marked hypertension and tachycardia).

No products indexed under this heading.

Labetalol Hydrochloride (Co-administration with beta-blockers may decrease T_4 5'-deiodinase activity; action of beta-blocker may be impaired when the hypothyroid patient is converted to euthyroid).

No products indexed under this heading.

Levalbuterol Hydrochloride (Co-administration of sympathomimetic agents may increase the effects of sympathomimetics or thyroid hormone; thyroid hormones may increase risk of coronary insufficiency when sympathomimetic agents are administered to patients with coronary disease). Products include:

Xopenex Inhalation Solution 3143
Xopenex Inhalation Solution Concentrate 3147

Levobunolol Hydrochloride (Co-administration with beta-blockers may decrease T_4 5'-deiodinase activity; action of beta-blocker may be impaired when the hypothyroid patient is converted to euthyroid). Products include:

Betagan Ophthalmic Solution, USP............ ⊙217

Lithium (May decrease thyroid hormone secretion, which may result in hypothyrodism; long-term lithium therapy can result in goiter in up to 50% of patients, and either subclinical or overt hypothyroidism, each in up to 20% of patients).

No products indexed under this heading.

Lithium Carbonate (May decrease thyroid hormone secretion, which may result in hypothyrodism; long-term lithium therapy can result in goiter in up to 50% of patients, and either subclinical or overt hypothyroidism, each in up to 20% of patients). Products include:

Eskalith 1406
Lithobid Tablets 1670

Lithium Citrate (May decrease thyroid hormone secretion, which may result in hypothyrodism; long-term lithium therapy can result in goiter in up to 50% of patients, and either subclinical or overt hypothyroidism, each in up to 20% of patients).

No products indexed under this heading.

Lovastatin (Co-administration has been associated with thyroid hormone and/or TSH level alterations by various mechanisms). Products include:

Advicor Tablets 1694
Altoprev Extended-Release Tablets 1151
Mevacor Tablets 1996

Magaldrate (Co-administration with antacids may reduce the efficacy of levothyroxine by binding and delaying or preventing absorption, potentially resulting in hypothyroidism; administer levothyroxine at least 4 hours apart from these agents).

No products indexed under this heading.

Magnesium Hydroxide (Co-administration with antacids may reduce the efficacy of levothyroxine by binding and delaying or preventing absorption, potentially resulting in hypothyroidism; administer levothyroxine at least 4 hours apart from these agents). Products include:

Maalox Max Maximum Strength Antacid/Anti-Gas Liquid............ 2165
Maalox Regular Strength Antacid/Antigas Liquid............ 2164
Pepcid Complete Chewable Tablets............ 1672
Rolaids Tablets .... ▣707
Extra Strength Rolaids Tablets .... ▣707
Rolaids Multi-Symptom Antacid & Antigas Tablets .... ▣708

Magnesium Oxide (Co-administration with antacids may reduce the efficacy of levothyroxine by binding and delaying or preventing absorption, potentially resulting in hypothyroidism; administer levothyroxine at least 4 hours apart from these agents). Products include:

Beelith Tablets 784
PremCal Light, Regular, and Extra Strength Tablets............ ▣762

Magnesium Salicylate (Co-administration with salicylates at greater than 2 gm inhibit binding of T_4 and T_3 to TBG and transthyrelin; an initial increase in serum FT_4 is followed by return of FT_4 to normal levels with sustained therapeutic salicylate concentrations, although total T_4 levels may decrease by as much as 30%).

No products indexed under this heading.

Maprotiline Hydrochloride (Co-administration may increase the therapeutic and toxic effects of both drugs possibly due to increased receptor sensitivity to catecholamines; toxic effects may include increased risk of arrhythmias and CNS stimulation; onset of tricyclics may be accelerated).

No products indexed under this heading.

Meclofenamate Sodium (Co-administration with fenamate NSAID may result in decreased serum TBG concentration).

No products indexed under this heading.

Mefenamic Acid (Co-administration with fenamate NSAID may result in decreased serum TBG concentration).

No products indexed under this heading.

Mephenytoin (Hydantoins may cause protein-binding site displacement; co-administration results in an initial transient increase in FT_4; continued administration results in a decrease in serum T_4 and normal FT_4 and TSH concentrations and, therefore, patients are clinically euthyroid).

No products indexed under this heading.

Mercaptopurine (Co-administration has been associated with thyroid hormone and/or TSH level alterations by various mechanisms). Products include:

Purinethol Tablets 1222

Mestranol (Co-administration with estrogen containing oral contraceptives may result in increased serum TBG concentrations).

No products indexed under this heading.

Metaproterenol Sulfate (Co-administration of sympathomimetic agents may increase the effects of sympathomimetics or thyroid hormone; thyroid hormones may increase risk of coronary insufficiency when sympathomimetic agents are administered to patients with coronary disease). Products include:

Alupent Inhalation Aerosol 858

Metaraminol Bitartrate (Co-administration of sympathomimetic agents may increase the effects of sympathomimetics or thyroid hormone; thyroid hormones may increase risk of coronary insufficiency when sympathomimetic agents are administered to patients with coronary disease). Products include:

Aramine Injection 1889

Metformin Hydrochloride (Addition of levothyroxine to antidiabetic therapy may result in increased antidiabetic agent requirements). Products include:

ActoPlus Met Tablets 3219
Avandamet Tablets 1343
Fortamet Extended-Release Tablets 1156

Methadone Hydrochloride (Co-administration may result in increased serum TBG concentrations).

No products indexed under this heading.

Methimazole (May decrease thyroid hormone secretion, which may result in hypothyrodism).

No products indexed under this heading.

Methoxamine Hydrochloride (Co-administration of sympathomimetic agents may increase the effects of sympathomimetics or thyroid hormone; thyroid hormones may increase risk of coronary insufficiency when sympathomimetic agents are administered to patients with coronary disease).

No products indexed under this heading.

Methyclothiazide (Co-administration has been associated with thyroid hormone and/or TSH level alterations by various mechanisms).

No products indexed under this heading.

Methylprednisolone Acetate (Co-administration with glucocorticoids may result in a transient reduction in TSH secretion; the reduction is not sustained, therefore, hypothyroidism does not occur; glucocorticoids may decrease serum TBG concentration). Products include:

Depo-Medrol Injectable Suspension 2615
Depo-Medrol Single-Dose Vial 2617

Methylprednisolone Sodium Succinate (Co-administration with glucocorticoids may result in a transient reduction in TSH secretion; the reduction is not sustained, therefore, hypothyroidism does not occur; glucocorticoids may decrease serum TBG concentration).

No products indexed under this heading.

Methyltestosterone (Co-administration with androgens/anabolic steroids may result in decreased serum TBG concentration). Products include:

Estratest Tablets 3196
Estratest H.S. Tablets 3196

Metipranolol Hydrochloride (Co-administration with beta-blockers may decrease T_4 5'-deiodinase activity; action of beta-blocker may be impaired when the hypothyroid patient is converted to euthyroid).

No products indexed under this heading.

Metoclopramide Hydrochloride (Co-administration has been associated with thyroid hormone and/or TSH level alterations by various mechanisms).
No products indexed under this heading.

Metoprolol Succinate (Co-administration with beta-blockers may decrease T_4 5'-deiodinase activity; action of beta-blocker may be impaired when the hypothyroid patient is converted to euthyroid). Products include:
Toprol-XL Tablets 660

Metoprolol Tartrate (Co-administration with beta-blockers may decrease T_4 5'-deiodinase activity; action of beta-blocker may be impaired when the hypothyroid patient is converted to euthyroid).
No products indexed under this heading.

Miglitol (Addition of levothyroxine to antidiabetic therapy may result in increased antidiabetic agent requirements).
No products indexed under this heading.

Mitotane (Co-administration may result in increased serum TBG concentrations).
No products indexed under this heading.

Nadolol (Co-administration with beta-blockers may decrease T_4 5'-deiodinase activity; action of beta-blocker may be impaired when the hypothyroid patient is converted to euthyroid). Products include:
Nadolol Tablets 2121

Niacin (Co-administration with slow-release nicotinic acid may result in decreased serum TBG concentration). Products include:
Advicor Tablets 1694
Niaspan Extended-Release Tablets 1703

Norepinephrine Bitartrate (Co-administration of sympathomimetic agents may increase the effects of sympathomimetics or thyroid hormone; thyroid hormones may increase risk of coronary insufficiency when sympathomimetic agents are administered to patients with coronary disease).
No products indexed under this heading.

Nortriptyline Hydrochloride (Co-administration may increase the therapeutic and toxic effects of both drugs possibly due to increased receptor sensitivity to catecholamines; toxic effects may include increased risk of arrhythmias and CNS stimulation; onset of tricyclics may be accelerated).
No products indexed under this heading.

Octreotide Acetate (Co-administration with octreotide may result in a transient reduction in TSH secretion; the reduction is not sustained, therefore, hypothyroidism does not occur). Products include:
Sandostatin Injection 2263
Sandostatin LAR Depot 2264

Oxandrolone (Co-administration with androgens/anabolic steroids may result in decreased serum TBG concentration). Products include:
Oxandrin Tablets 2977

Oxymetholone (Co-administration with androgens/anabolic steroids may result in decreased serum TBG concentration). Products include:
Anadrol-50 Tablets 3329

Penbutolol Sulfate (Co-administration with beta-blockers may decrease T_4 5'-deiodinase activity; action of beta-blocker may be impaired when the hypothyroid patient is converted to euthyroid).
No products indexed under this heading.

Pergolide Mesylate (Co-administration with dopamine agonists may result in a transient reduction in TSH secretion; the reduction is not sustained, therefore, hypothyroidism does not occur). Products include:
Permax Tablets 3357

Perphenazine (Co-administration has been associated with thyroid hormone and/or TSH level alterations by various mechanisms).
No products indexed under this heading.

Phenobarbital (Co-administration may increase hepatic metabolism, which may result in hypothyroidism, resulting in increased levothyroxine requirements).
No products indexed under this heading.

Phenylbutazone (Co-administration may cause protein-binding site displacement).
No products indexed under this heading.

Phenylephrine Bitartrate (Co-administration of sympathomimetic agents may increase the effects of sympathomimetics or thyroid hormone; thyroid hormones may increase risk of coronary insufficiency when sympathomimetic agents are administered to patients with coronary disease).
No products indexed under this heading.

Phenylephrine Hydrochloride (Co-administration of sympathomimetic agents may increase the effects of sympathomimetics or thyroid hormone; thyroid hormones may increase risk of coronary insufficiency when sympathomimetic agents are administered to patients with coronary disease). Products include:
Alacol DM Syrup 739
Hycomine Compound Tablets 1105
Preparation H Maximum Strength Cream 747
Preparation H Cooling Gel 747
Preparation H 747
Sudafed PE Tablets 711
Vicks Sinex Nasal Spray and Ultra Fine Mist for Sinus Relief 2677
Zicam Concentrated Cough Mist for Kids Plus D Cool Cherry 643
Zicam Concentrated Cough Mist Plus D Cool Cherry 642

Phenylephrine Tannate (Co-administration of sympathomimetic agents may increase the effects of sympathomimetics or thyroid hormone; thyroid hormones may increase risk of coronary insufficiency when sympathomimetic agents are administered to patients with coronary disease).
No products indexed under this heading.

Phenylpropanolamine Hydrochloride (Co-administration of sympathomimetic agents may increase the effects of sympathomimetics or thyroid hormone; thyroid hormones may increase risk of coronary insufficiency when sympathomimetic agents are administered to patients with coronary disease).
No products indexed under this heading.

Phenytoin (Hydantoins may cause protein-binding site displacement; co-administration results in an initial transient increase in FT_4; co-administration may increase hepatic metabolism, which may result in hypothyroidism, resulting in increased levothyroxine requirements; phenytoin reduces serum protein binding of levothyroxine, and total- and free-T_4 may be reduced by 20% to 40%, but most patients have normal serum TSH levels and are clinicly euthyroid).
No products indexed under this heading.

Phenytoin Sodium (Hydantoins may cause protein-binding site displacement; co-administration results in an initial transient increase in FT_4; co-administration may increase hepatic metabolism, which may result in hypothyroidism, resulting in increased levothyroxine requirements; phenytoin reduces serum protein binding of levothyroxine, and total- and free-T_4 may be reduced by 20% to 40%, but most patients have normal serum TSH levels and are clinicly euthyroid). Products include:
Phenytek Capsules 2153

Pindolol (Co-administration with beta-blockers may decrease T_4 5'-deiodinase activity; action of beta-blocker may be impaired when the hypothyroid patient is converted to euthyroid).
No products indexed under this heading.

Pioglitazone Hydrochloride (Addition of levothyroxine to antidiabetic therapy may result in increased antidiabetic agent requirements). Products include:
ActoPlus Met Tablets 3219
Actos Tablets 3224

Pirbuterol Acetate (Co-administration of sympathomimetic agents may increase the effects of sympathomimetics or thyroid hormone; thyroid hormones may increase risk of coronary insufficiency when sympathomimetic agents are administered to patients with coronary disease). Products include:
Maxair Autohaler 1820

Polyestradiol Phosphate (Co-administration with oral estrogens may result in increased serum TBG concentrations).
No products indexed under this heading.

Polythiazide (Co-administration has been associated with thyroid hormone and/or TSH level alterations by various mechanisms).
No products indexed under this heading.

Potassium Iodide (May decrease thyroid hormone secretion, which may result in hypothyroidism; iodide drugs that contain pharmacologic amounts of iodide may cause hypothyroidism in euthyroid patients with Grave's disease previously treated with thyroid autonomy; hyperthyroidism may develop over several weeks and may persist for several months after therapy discontinuation).
No products indexed under this heading.

Pramipexole Dihydrochloride (Co-administration with dopamine agonists may result in a transient reduction in TSH secretion; the reduction is not sustained, therefore, hypothyroidism does not occur). Products include:
Mirapex Tablets 889

Prednisolone Acetate (Co-administration with glucocorticoids may result in a transient reduction in TSH secretion; the reduction is not sustained, therefore, hypothyroidism does not occur; glucocorticoids may decrease serum TBG concentration). Products include:
Blephamide Ophthalmic Ointment 563
Blephamide Ophthalmic Suspension 564
Poly-Pred Liquifilm Ophthalmic Suspension .... ⊙231
Pred Forte Ophthalmic Suspension .... ⊙233
Pred Mild Sterile Ophthalmic Suspension .... ⊙236
Pred-G Ophthalmic Suspension .... ⊙234
Pred-G Sterile Ophthalmic Ointment .... ⊙235

Prednisolone Sodium Phosphate (Co-administration with glucocorticoids may result in a transient reduction in TSH secretion; the reduction is not sustained, therefore, hypothyroidism does not occur; glucocorticoids may decrease serum TBG concentration). Products include:
Pediapred Oral Solution 3319

Prednisolone Tebutate (Co-administration with glucocorticoids may result in a transient reduction in TSH secretion; the reduction is not sustained, therefore, hypothyroidism does not occur; glucocorticoids may decrease serum TBG concentration).
No products indexed under this heading.

Prednisone (Co-administration with glucocorticoids may result in a transient reduction in TSH secretion; the reduction is not sustained, therefore, hypothyroidism does not occur; glucocorticoids may decrease serum TBG concentration).
No products indexed under this heading.

Propranolol Hydrochloride (Co-administration with beta-blockers may decrease T_4 5'-deiodinase activity; in patients treated with large doses of propranolol, greater than 160 mg/day, T_3 and T_4 levels change slightly, TSH levels remain normal, and patients are clinically euthyroid; action of beta-blocker may be impaired when the hypothyroid patient is converted to euthyroid). Products include:
Inderal LA Long-Acting Capsules 3421
InnoPran XL Capsules 2728

Propylthiouracil (May decrease thyroid hormone secretion, which may result in hypothyrodism).
No products indexed under this heading.

Protriptyline Hydrochloride (Co-administration may increase the therapeutic and toxic effects of both drugs possibly due to increased receptor sensitivity to catecholamines; toxic effects may include increased risk of arrhythmias and CNS stimulation; onset of tricyclics may be accelerated). Products include:

Vivactil Tablets 2350

Pseudoephedrine Hydrochloride (Co-administration of sympathomimetic agents may increase the effects of sympathomimetics or thyroid hormone; thyroid hormones may increase risk of coronary insufficiency when sympathomimetic agents are administered to patients with coronary disease). Products include:

Advil Allergy Sinus Caplets .... ■ 737
Advil Cold & Sinus .... ■ 739
Advil Flu & Body Ache Caplets .... ■ 739
Children's Advil Cold Suspension .... ■ 741
Advil Multi-Symptom Cold Caplets .... ■ 738
Allegra-D 12 Hour Extended-Release Tablets 2860
Allegra-D 24 Hour Extended-Release Tablets 2862
Balamine DM 739
BC Cold Powder .... ■ 612
Benadryl Allergy & Cold Tablets .... ■ 692
Benadryl Allergy & Sinus Headache Caplets & Gelcaps .... ■ 693
Children's Benadryl Allergy & Cold Fastmelt Tablets .... ■ 695
Benadryl Maximum Strength Severe Allergy & Sinus Headache Caplets .... ■ 694
Children's Benadryl D Allergy & Sinus Fastmelt Tablets .... ■ 694
Children's Benadryl D Liquid Medication .... ■ 693
Benadryl D Tablets .... ■ 694
Contac Non-Drowsy 12 Hour Cold Caplets .... ■ 614
Contac Non-Drowsy Timed Release 12 Hour Cold Caplets .... ■ 615
Contac Severe Cold and Flu Caplets Maximum Strength .... ■ 615
Contac Severe Cold and Flu Caplets Non-Drowsy .... ■ 615
Children's Dimetapp Cold & Allergy Elixir .... ■ 745
Children's Dimetapp DM Cold & Cough Elixir .... ■ 745
Children's Dimetapp Long Acting Cough Plus Cold Syrup .... ■ 746
Dimetapp Infant Drops Decongestant Plus Cough .... ■ 746
Children's Motrin Cold Non-Staining Dye-Free Oral Suspension 1838
Children's Motrin Cold Oral Suspension 1838
Motrin Cold & Sinus Caplets 1836
PediaCare Decongestant & Cough Infant Drops .... ■ 705
PediaCare Decongestant Infants' Drops .... ■ 705
PediaCare Long-Acting Cough Plus Cold Liquid .... ■ 704
PediaCare Multi-Symptom Cold Liquid .... ■ 704
PediaCare NightRest Cough & Cold Liquid .... ■ 704
Robitussin Allergy & Cough Syrup .... ■ 750
Robitussin CF Liquid .... ■ 755
Robitussin Cough & Cold Liquid-filled Capsules .... ■ 750
Robitussin Cough, Cold & Flu Liquid-filled Capsules .... ■ 750
Robitussin Cough & Cold Infant Drops .... ■ 755
Robitussin Flu Liquid .... ■ 752
Robitussin Maximum Strength Cough & Cold Liquid .... ■ 754
Robitussin PE Syrup .... ■ 753
Robitussin Pediatric Cough & Cold Liquid .... ■ 754
Robitussin PM Cough & Cold Liquid .... ■ 752
Robitussin Severe Congestion Liquid-filled Capsules .... ■ 751
Simply Stuffy Liquid 1841
Singlet Caplets .... ■ 636
Sudafed 12 Hour Caplets .... ■ 708
Sudafed 24 Hour Tablets .... ■ 709
Sudafed Nasal Decongestant Tablets .... ■ 709
Sudafed Severe Cold .... ■ 710
Sudafed Non-Drying Sinus Liquid Caps .... ■ 709
Sudafed Sinus & Allergy Tablets .... ■ 710
Sudafed Sinus Headache .... ■ 711
TheraFlu Cold & Cough Hot Liquid .... ■ 680
TheraFlu Cold & Sore Throat Hot Liquid .... ■ 680
TheraFlu Flu & Chest Congestion Non-Drowsy Hot Liquid .... ■ 681
TheraFlu Flu & Sore Throat Hot Liquid .... ■ 681
TheraFlu Severe Cold Non-Drowsy Hot Liquid .... ■ 683
TheraFlu Severe Cold & Cough Hot Liquid .... ■ 683
TheraFlu Severe Cold Caplets .... ■ 679
TheraFlu Severe Cold Hot Liquid .... ■ 682
TheraFlu Severe Cold Non-Drowsy Caplets .... ■ 679
Triaminic Chest & Nasal Congestion Liquid .... ■ 685
Triaminic Cold & Allergy Liquid .... ■ 685
Triaminic Cold & Cough Liquid .... ■ 685
Triaminic Cough Liquid .... ■ 687
Triaminic Cough & Nasal Congestion Liquid .... ■ 687
Triaminic Cough & Sore Throat Liquid .... ■ 687
Triaminic Flu, Cough & Fever Liquid .... ■ 685
Triaminic Night Time Cough & Cold Liquid .... ■ 685
Triaminic Allergy Runny Nose & Congestion Softchews .... ■ 688
Triaminic Cold & Cough Softchews .... ■ 688
Triaminic Cough & Sore Throat Softchews .... ■ 689
Tylenol Sinus NightTime Caplets .... ■ 663
Children's Tylenol Plus Cold & Allergy Suspension Liquid 1850
Children's Tylenol Plus Cold NightTime Suspension Liquid 1851
Children's Tylenol Plus Cold & Cough Suspension Liquid and Chewable Tablets 1851
Children's Tylenol Plus Cold Chewable Tablets 1851
Children's Tylenol Plus Cold Daytime Non-Drowsy Suspension Liquid 1851
Children's Tylenol Plus Flu Suspension Liquid 1853
Concentrated Tylenol Infants' Drops Plus Cold 1851
Concentrated Tylenol Infants' Drops Plus Cold and Cough 1851
Tylenol Cold & Flu Severe Daytime Liquid with Cool Bust 1846
Tylenol Cold & Flu Severe NightTime Liquid with Cool Burst 1846
Tylenol Cold Severe Congestion Non-Drowsy Caplets with Cool Burst 1846
Tylenol Allergy Complete Night Time Caplets 1844
Tylenol Allergy Complete Multi-Symptom Caplets and Gelcaps with Cool Burst 1844
Tylenol Flu NightTime Gelcaps 1846
Tylenol Flu Day Non-Drowsy Gelcaps 1846
Concentrated Tylenol Infants' Drops Plus Cold Nasal Congestant, Fever Reducer & Pain Reliever .... ■ 668
Concentrated Tylenol Infants' Drops Plus Cold & Cough Nasal Decongestant, Fever Reducer & Pain Reliever .... ■ 668
Multi-Symptom Tylenol Cold Night Time Caplets 1845
Multi-Symptom Tylenol Cold Day Non-Drowsy Caplets and Gelcaps 1845
Tylenol Sinus Day Non-Drowsy 1848
Tylenol Sinus Night Time Caplets 1848
Tylenol Sinus Severe Congestion Caplets with Cool Burst 1848
Vicks 44D Cough & Head Congestion Relief 2676
Vicks 44D Cough & Head Congestion Relief Liquid .... ■ 721
Vicks 44M Cough, Cold & Flu Relief 2676
Pediatric Vicks 44m Cough & Cold Relief 2673
Vicks DayQuil LiquiCaps/Liquid Multi-Symptom Cold/Flu Relief .... ■ 723
Vicks DayQuil Multi-Symptom Cold/Flu Relief LiquiCaps 2675
Vicks DayQuil Multi-Symptom Cold/Flu Relief Liquid 2675
Children's Vicks NyQuil Cold/Cough Relief 2671
Vicks NyQuil LiquiCaps 2677
Vicks NyQuil LiquiCaps/Liquid Multi-Symptom Cold/Flu Relief .... ■ 725
Vicks NyQuil Liquid 2677
Zyrtec-D 12 Hour Extended Release Tablets 2591

Pseudoephedrine Sulfate (Co-administration of sympathomimetic agents may increase the effects of sympathomimetics or thyroid hormone; thyroid hormones may increase risk of coronary insufficiency when sympathomimetic agents are administered to patients with coronary disease). Products include:

Alavert Allergy & Sinus D-12 Hour Tablets .... ■ 743
Clarinex-D 24-Hour Extended-Release Tablets 3012
Claritin-D Non-Drowsy 12 Hour Tablets .... ■ 731
Claritin-D Non-Drowsy 24 Hour Tablets .... ■ 731

Quinestrol (Co-administration with oral estrogens may result in increased serum TBG concentrations).

No products indexed under this heading.

Repaglinide (Addition of levothyroxine to antidiabetic therapy may result in increased antidiabetic agent requirements). Products include:

Prandin Tablets (0.5, 1, and 2 mg) 2337

Resorcinol (Co-administration of excessive topical use of resorcinol has been associated with thyroid hormone and/or TSH level alterations by various mechanisms).

No products indexed under this heading.

Rifampin (Co-administration may increase hepatic metabolism, which may result in hypothyroidism, resulting in increased levothyroxine requirements).

No products indexed under this heading.

Ropinirole Hydrochloride (Co-administration with dopamine agonists may result in a transient reduction in TSH secretion; the reduction is not sustained, therefore, hypothyroidism does not occur). Products include:

Requip Tablets 1528

Rosiglitazone Maleate (Addition of levothyroxine to antidiabetic therapy may result in increased antidiabetic agent requirements). Products include:

Avandamet Tablets 1343
Avandia Tablets 1348

Salmeterol Xinafoate (Co-administration of sympathomimetic agents may increase the effects of sympathomimetics or thyroid hormone; thyroid hormones may increase risk of coronary insufficiency when sympathomimetic agents are administered to patients with coronary disease). Products include:

Advair Diskus 100/50 1291
Advair Diskus 250/50 1291
Advair Diskus 500/50 1291
Serevent Diskus 1540

Salsalate (Co-administration with salicylates at greater than 2 gm inhibit binding of T_4 and T_3 to TBG and transthyrelin; an initial increase in serum FT_4 is followed by return of FT_4 to normal levels with sustained therapeutic salicylate concentrations, although total T_4 levels may decrease by as much as 30%).

No products indexed under this heading.

Sertraline Hydrochloride (Co-administration of sertraline in patients stabilized on levothyroxine may result in increased levothyroxine requirements). Products include:

Zoloft 2581

Sodium Nitroprusside (Co-administration has been associated with thyroid hormone and/or TSH level alterations by various mechanisms).

No products indexed under this heading.

Sodium Polystyrene Sulfonate (Co-administration may result in decreased T_4 absorption, which may result in hypothyroidism; administer levothyroxine at least 4 hours apart from these agents).

No products indexed under this heading.

Somatrem (Excessive use of thyroid hormone with growth hormones may accelerate epiphyseal closure; however, untreated hypothyroidism may interfere with growth response to growth hormone).

No products indexed under this heading.

Somatropin (Excessive use of thyroid hormone with growth hormones may accelerate epiphyseal closure; however, untreated hypothyroidism may interfere with growth response to growth hormone). Products include:

Genotropin Lyophilized Powder 2642
Humatrope Vials and Cartridges 1756
Norditropin Cartridges 2318
Nutropin for Injection 1238
Nutropin AQ Injection 1241
Nutropin AQ Pen 1241
Nutropin AQ Pen Cartridge 1241

Sotalol Hydrochloride (Co-administration with beta-blockers may decrease T_4 5'-deiodinase activity; action of beta-blocker may be impaired when the hypothyroid patient is converted to euthyroid).

No products indexed under this heading.

Soybean Preparations (Concurrent use of soybean flour may bind and decrease the absorption of levothyroxine sodium from GI tract).

No products indexed under this heading.

Stanozolol (Co-administration with androgens/anabolic steroids may result in decreased serum TBG concentration).

No products indexed under this heading.

Sucralfate (Co-administration may result in decreased T_4 absorption, which may result in hypothyroidism; administer levothyroxine at least 4 hours apart from these agents). Products include:

Carafate Suspension 727
Carafate Tablets 728

Sulfamethoxazole (May decrease thyroid hormone secretion, which may result in hypothyrodism).
No products indexed under this heading.

Sulfisoxazole Acetyl (May decrease thyroid hormone secretion, which may result in hypothyrodism).
No products indexed under this heading.

Tamoxifen Citrate (Co-administration may result in increased serum TBG concentrations).
No products indexed under this heading.

Terbutaline Sulfate (Co-administration of sympathomimetic agents may increase the effects of sympathomimetics or thyroid hormone; thyroid hormones may increase risk of coronary insufficiency when sympathomimetic agents are administered to patients with coronary disease).
No products indexed under this heading.

Theophylline (Decreased theophylline clearance may occur in hypothyroid patients; clearance returns to normal when euthyroid state is achieved).
No products indexed under this heading.

Theophylline Anhydrous (Decreased theophylline clearance may occur in hypothyroid patients; clearance returns to normal when euthyroid state is achieved). Products include:
Uniphyl Tablets 2708

Theophylline Calcium Salicylate (Decreased theophylline clearance may occur in hypothyroid patients; clearance returns to normal when euthyroid state is achieved).
No products indexed under this heading.

Theophylline Dihydroxypropyl (Glyceryl) (Decreased theophylline clearance may occur in hypothyroid patients; clearance returns to normal when euthyroid state is achieved).
No products indexed under this heading.

Theophylline Ethylenediamine (Decreased theophylline clearance may occur in hypothyroid patients; clearance returns to normal when euthyroid state is achieved).
No products indexed under this heading.

Theophylline Sodium Glycinate (Decreased theophylline clearance may occur in hypothyroid patients; clearance returns to normal when euthyroid state is achieved).
No products indexed under this heading.

Timolol Hemihydrate (Co-administration with beta-blockers may decrease T_4 5'-deiodinase activity; action of beta-blocker may be impaired when the hypothyroid patient is converted to euthyroid). Products include:
Betimol Ophthalmic Solution 3371
Betimol Ophthalmic Solution .... ⊙283

Timolol Maleate (Co-administration with beta-blockers may decrease T_4 5'-deiodinase activity; action of beta-blocker may be impaired when the hypothyroid patient is converted to euthyroid). Products include:
Blocadren Tablets 1891
Cosopt Sterile Ophthalmic Solution 1910
Timolide Tablets 2056
Timoptic in Ocudose 2061
Timoptic Sterile Ophthalmic Solution 2058
Timoptic-XE Sterile Ophthalmic Gel Forming Solution 2062

Tolazamide (Addition of levothyroxine to antidiabetic therapy may result in increased antidiabetic agent requirements).
No products indexed under this heading.

Tolbutamide (May decrease thyroid hormone secretion, which may result in hypothyrodism).
No products indexed under this heading.

Triamcinolone (Co-administration with glucocorticoids may result in a transient reduction in TSH secretion; the reduction is not sustained, therefore, hypothyroidism does not occur; glucocorticoids may decrease serum TBG concentration).
No products indexed under this heading.

Triamcinolone Acetonide (Co-administration with glucocorticoids may result in a transient reduction in TSH secretion; the reduction is not sustained, therefore, hypothyroidism does not occur; glucocorticoids may decrease serum TBG concentration). Products include:
Azmacort Inhalation Aerosol 1701
Nasacort HFA Inhalation Aerosol 2939
Nasacort AQ Nasal Spray 2937

Triamcinolone Diacetate (Co-administration with glucocorticoids may result in a transient reduction in TSH secretion; the reduction is not sustained, therefore, hypothyroidism does not occur; glucocorticoids may decrease serum TBG concentration).
No products indexed under this heading.

Triamcinolone Hexacetonide (Co-administration with glucocorticoids may result in a transient reduction in TSH secretion; the reduction is not sustained, therefore, hypothyroidism does not occur; glucocorticoids may decrease serum TBG concentration).
No products indexed under this heading.

Trimipramine Maleate (Co-administration may increase the therapeutic and toxic effects of both drugs possibly due to increased receptor sensitivity to catecholamines; toxic effects may include increased risk of arrhythmias and CNS stimulation; onset of tricyclics may be accelerated). Products include:
Surmontil Capsules 2347

Troglitazone (Addition of levothyroxine to antidiabetic therapy may result in increased antidiabetic agent requirements).
No products indexed under this heading.

Tyropanoate Sodium (May decrease thyroid hormone secretion, which may result in hypothyrodism; the fetus, elderly, and euthyroid patients with underlying thyroid disease are among those individuals who are susceptible to iodine-induced hypothyroidism; oral cholecytographic agents slowly excreted, producing more prolonged hypothyroidism; iodide drugs that contain pharmacologic amounts of iodide may cause hypothyroidism in euthyroid patients with Grave's disease previously treated with thyroid autonomy; hyperthyroidism may develop over several weeks and may persist for several months after therapy discontinuation).
No products indexed under this heading.

Warfarin Sodium (Thyroid hormones appear to increase the catabolism of vitamin K-dependent clotting factors, thereby increasing the anticoagulant activity of oral anticoagulants). Products include:
Coumadin for Injection 932
Coumadin Tablets 932

Food Interactions

Cotton seed meal (Concurrent use of cotton seed meal may bind and decrease the absorption of levothyroxine sodium from GI tract).

Dietary Fiber (Concurrent use of dietary fiber may bind and decrease the absorption of levothyroxine sodium from GI tract).

Soybean Formula, Children's (Concurrent use of soybean flour may bind and decrease the absorption of levothyroxine sodium from GI tract).

Walnuts (Concurrent use of walnuts may bind and decrease the absorption of levothyroxine sodium from GI tract).

LEXAPRO ORAL SOLUTION

(Escitalopram Oxalate) 1193
See Lexapro Tablets

LEXAPRO TABLETS

(Escitalopram Oxalate) 1193
May interact with anticoagulants, cytochrome p450 2d6 substrates (selected), lithium preparations, monoamine oxidase inhibitors, non-steroidal anti-inflammatory agents, and certain other agents. Compounds in these categories include:

Amitriptyline Hydrochloride (Caution is indicated in the co-administration of escitalopram and drugs metabolized by CYP2D6).
No products indexed under this heading.

Amphetamine Aspartate (Caution is indicated in the co-administration of escitalopram and drugs metabolized by CYP2D6). Products include:
Adderall Tablets 3168
Adderall XR Capsules 3169

Amphetamine Aspartate Monohydrate (Caution is indicated in the co-administration of escitalopram and drugs metabolized by CYP2D6).
No products indexed under this heading.

Amphetamine Sulfate (Caution is indicated in the co-administration of escitalopram and drugs metabolized by CYP2D6). Products include:
Adderall Tablets 3168
Adderall XR Capsules 3169

Anisindione (The combined use of psychotropic drugs that interfere with serotonin reuptake and drugs that affect coagulation has been associated with an increased risk of bleeding). Products include:
Miradon Tablets 3056

Ardeparin Sodium (The combined use of psychotropic drugs that interfere with serotonin reuptake and drugs that affect coagulation has been associated with an increased risk of bleeding).
No products indexed under this heading.

Aspirin (The combined use of psychotropic drugs that interfere with serotonin reuptake and drugs that affect coagulation has been associated with an increased risk of bleeding. Use caution when co-administering). Products include:
Aggrenox Capsules 855
Bayer, Aspirin Regimen 606
Bayer Aspirin Tablets 3515
BC Powder 612
BC Allergy Sinus Cold Powder 612
Arthritis Strength BC Powder 612
BC Sinus Cold Powder 612
Ecotrin Enteric Coated Aspirin Low, Regular and Maximum Strength Tablets 1627
Goody's Body Pain Formula Powder 621
Goody's Extra Strength Headache Powder 621
Goody's Extra Strength Pain Relief Tablets 621
Percodan Tablets 1115
St. Joseph 81 mg Aspirin Chewable and Enteric Coated Tablets 1841

Aspirin, Enteric Coated (The combined use of psychotropic drugs that interfere with serotonin reuptake and drugs that affect coagulation has been associated with an increased risk of bleeding. Use caution when co-administering).
No products indexed under this heading.

Aspirin Buffered (The combined use of psychotropic drugs that interfere with serotonin reuptake and drugs that affect coagulation has been associated with an increased risk of bleeding. Use caution when co-administering).
No products indexed under this heading.

Atomoxetine Hydrochloride (Caution is indicated in the co-administration of escitalopram and drugs metabolized by CYP2D6). Products include:
Strattera Capsules 1784

Bisoprolol Fumarate (Caution is indicated in the co-administration of escitalopram and drugs metabolized by CYP2D6).
No products indexed under this heading.

Captopril (Caution is indicated in the co-administration of escitalopram and drugs metabolized by CYP2D6). Products include:
Captopril Tablets 2114

Carbamazepine (Potential for increased clearance of escitalopram, although trough citalopram plasma levels were unaffected during co-administration. The possibility that carbamazepine might increase the clearance of escitalopram should be considered if the two drugs are co-administered). Products include:
Carbatrol Capsules 3174
Equetro Extended-Release Capsules 3178
Tegretol/Tegretol-XR 2278

Carvedilol (Caution is indicated in the co-administration of escitalopram and drugs metabolized by CYP2D6). Products include:
Coreg Tablets 1376

Celecoxib (The combined use of psychotropic drugs that interfere with serotonin reuptake and drugs that affect coagulation has been associated with an increased risk of bleeding; use caution when co-administering). Products include:
Celebrex Capsules 3130

Cevimeline Hydrochloride (Caution is indicated in the co-administration of escitalopram and drugs metabolized by CYP2D6). Products include:
Evoxac Capsules 1042

Chlorpromazine (Caution is indicated in the co-administration of escitalopram and drugs metabolized by CYP2D6).
No products indexed under this heading.

Chlorpromazine Hydrochloride (Caution is indicated in the co-administration of escitalopram and drugs metabolized by CYP2D6).
No products indexed under this heading.

Chlorpropamide (Caution is indicated in the co-administration of escitalopram and drugs metabolized by CYP2D6).
No products indexed under this heading.

Cimetidine (Co-administration of racemic citalopram with cimetidine has resulted in an increase in citalopram AUC and Cmax). Products include:
Tagamet HB 200 Tablets .... ■ 637
Tagamet Tablets 1547

Cimetidine Hydrochloride (Co-administration of racemic citalopram with cimetidine has resulted in an increase in citalopram AUC and Cmax).
No products indexed under this heading.

Citalopram Hydrobromide (Since escitalopram is the active isomer of racemic citalopram, the two agents should not be co-administered). Products include:
Celexa 1177

Clomipramine Hydrochloride (Caution is indicated in the co-administration of escitalopram and drugs metabolized by CYP2D6).
No products indexed under this heading.

Clozapine (Caution is indicated in the co-administration of escitalopram and drugs metabolized by CYP2D6). Products include:
Clozapine Tablets 2141
Clozaril Tablets 2174
FazaClo Orally Disintegrating Tablets 547

Codeine Phosphate (Caution is indicated in the co-administration of escitalopram and drugs metabolized by CYP2D6). Products include:
Tylenol with Codeine 2461

Codeine Sulfate (Caution is indicated in the co-administration of escitalopram and drugs metabolized by CYP2D6).
No products indexed under this heading.

Cyclobenzaprine Hydrochloride (Caution is indicated in the co-administration of escitalopram and drugs metabolized by CYP2D6). Products include:
Flexeril Tablets 1832

Dalteparin Sodium (The combined use of psychotropic drugs that interfere with serotonin reuptake and drugs that affect coagulation has been associated with an increased risk of bleeding). Products include:
Fragmin Injection 2638

Danaparoid Sodium (The combined use of psychotropic drugs that interfere with serotonin reuptake and drugs that affect coagulation has been associated with an increased risk of bleeding).
No products indexed under this heading.

Desipramine Hydrochloride (Co-administration has resulted in an increase in Cmax and AUC of desipramine; the clinical significance of this finding is unknown).
No products indexed under this heading.

Dexfenfluramine Hydrochloride (Caution is indicated in the co-administration of escitalopram and drugs metabolized by CYP2D6).
No products indexed under this heading.

Dextromethorphan Hydrobromide (Caution is indicated in the co-administration of escitalopram and drugs metabolized by CYP2D6). Products include:
Alacol DM Syrup 739
Balamine DM 739
Contac Severe Cold and Flu Caplets Maximum Strength .... ■ 615
Contac Severe Cold and Flu Caplets Non-Drowsy .... ■ 615
Children's Dimetapp DM Cold & Cough Elixir .... ■ 745
Children's Dimetapp Long Acting Cough Plus Cold Syrup .... ■ 746
Dimetapp Infant Drops Decongestant Plus Cough .... ■ 746
Mucinex DM Tablets .... ■ 602
PediaCare Decongestant & Cough Infant Drops .... ■ 705
PediaCare Freezer Pops Long-Acting Cough-Glacier Grape and Polar Berry Blue .... ■ 706
PediaCare Long-Acting Cough Infant Drops .... ■ 705
PediaCare Long-Acting Cough Plus Cold Liquid .... ■ 704
PediaCare Multi-Symptom Cold Liquid .... ■ 704
PediaCare NightRest Cough & Cold Liquid .... ■ 704
Robitussin Allergy & Cough Syrup .... ■ 750
Robitussin CF Liquid .... ■ 755
Robitussin Cough & Cold Liquid-filled Capsules .... ■ 750
Robitussin Cough, Cold & Flu Liquid-filled Capsules .... ■ 750
Robitussin Cough & Cold Infant Drops .... ■ 755
Robitussin DM Infant Drops .... ■ 753
Robitussin DM Liquid .... ■ 753
Robitussin Flu Liquid .... ■ 752
Robitussin Maximum Strength Cough Liquid .... ■ 754
Robitussin Maximum Strength Cough & Cold Liquid .... ■ 754
Robitussin Pediatric Cough Liquid .... ■ 754
Robitussin Pediatric Cough & Cold Liquid .... ■ 754
Robitussin PM Cough & Cold Liquid .... ■ 752
Robitussin Sugar Free Cough Liquid .... ■ 753
Simply Cough Liquid 1840
Sudafed Severe Cold .... ■ 710
TheraFlu Cold & Cough Hot Liquid .... ■ 680
TheraFlu Flu & Chest Congestion Non-Drowsy Hot Liquid .... ■ 681
TheraFlu Severe Cold Non-Drowsy Hot Liquid .... ■ 683
TheraFlu Severe Cold & Cough Hot Liquid .... ■ 683
TheraFlu Severe Cold Caplets .... ■ 679
TheraFlu Severe Cold Hot Liquid .... ■ 682
TheraFlu Severe Cold Non-Drowsy Caplets .... ■ 679
TheraFlu Thin Strips Long Acting Cough .... ■ 684
Triaminic Cold & Cough Liquid .... ■ 685
Triaminic Cough Liquid .... ■ 687
Triaminic Cough & Nasal Congestion Liquid .... ■ 687
Triaminic Cough & Sore Throat Liquid .... ■ 687
Triaminic Flu, Cough & Fever Liquid .... ■ 685
Triaminic Night Time Cough & Cold Liquid .... ■ 685
Triaminic Cold & Cough Softchews .... ■ 688
Triaminic Cough & Sore Throat Softchews .... ■ 689
Triaminic Thin Strips Long Acting Cough .... ■ 689
Children's Tylenol Plus Cold & Cough Suspension Liquid and Chewable Tablets 1851
Children's Tylenol Plus Flu Suspension Liquid 1853
Concentrated Tylenol Infants' Drops Plus Cold and Cough 1851
Tylenol Cold & Flu Severe Daytime Liquid with Cool Bust 1846
Tylenol Cold & Flu Severe NightTime Liquid with Cool Burst 1846
Tylenol Cold Severe Congestion Non-Drowsy Caplets with Cool Burst 1846
Tylenol Cough & Sore Throat Daytime Liquid with Cool Burst 1849
Tylenol Cough & Sore Throat NightTime Liquid with Cool Burst 1849
Tylenol Flu Day Non-Drowsy Gelcaps 1846
Concentrated Tylenol Infants' Drops Plus Cold & Cough Nasal Decongestant, Fever Reducer & Pain Reliever .... ■ 668
Multi-Symptom Tylenol Cold Night Time Caplets 1845
Multi-Symptom Tylenol Cold Day Non-Drowsy Caplets and Gelcaps 1845
Vicks 44 Cough Relief 2675
Vicks 44D Cough & Head Congestion Relief 2676
Vicks 44D Cough & Head Congestion Relief Liquid .... ■ 721
Vicks 44E Cough & Chest Congestion Relief 2676
Pediatric Vicks 44e Cough & Chest Congestion Relief Liquid 2673
Vicks 44M Cough, Cold & Flu Relief 2676
Pediatric Vicks 44m Cough & Cold Relief 2673
Vicks DayQuil LiquiCaps/Liquid Multi-Symptom Cold/Flu Relief .... ■ 723
Vicks DayQuil Multi-Symptom Cold/Flu Relief LiquiCaps 2675
Vicks DayQuil Multi-Symptom Cold/Flu Relief Liquid 2675
Children's Vicks NyQuil Cold/Cough Relief 2671
Vicks NyQuil Cough Liquid 2677
Vicks NyQuil LiquiCaps 2677
Vicks NyQuil LiquiCaps/Liquid Multi-Symptom Cold/Flu Relief .... ■ 725
Vicks NyQuil Liquid 2677
Zicam Concentrated Cough Mist for Kids Cool Cherry .... ■ 643
Zicam Concentrated Cough Mist for Kids Plus D Cool Cherry .... ■ 643
Zicam Concentrated Cough Mist Nite-Cool Cherry .... ■ 642
Zicam Concentrated Cough Mist Plus D Cool Cherry .... ■ 642
Zicam Concentrated Cough Mist-Honey Lemon & Cool Cherry .... ■ 642

Dextromethorphan Polistirex (Caution is indicated in the co-administration of escitalopram and drugs metabolized by CYP2D6). Products include:
Delsym Extended-Release Suspension .... ■ 611
Delsym 12 Hour Cough Suppressant for Children .... ■ 611

Diclofenac Potassium (The combined use of psychotropic drugs that interfere with serotonin reuptake and drugs that affect coagulation has been associated with an increased risk of bleeding; use caution when co-administering). Products include:
Cataflam Tablets 2173

Diclofenac Sodium (The combined use of psychotropic drugs that interfere with serotonin reuptake and drugs that affect coagulation has been associated with an increased risk of bleeding; use caution when co-administering). Products include:
Arthrotec Tablets 3126
Voltaren Ophthalmic Solution 2300
Voltaren Tablets 2298
Voltaren-XR Tablets 2301

Dicumarol (The combined use of psychotropic drugs that interfere with serotonin reuptake and drugs that affect coagulation has been associated with an increased risk of bleeding).
No products indexed under this heading.

Dolasetron Mesylate (Caution is indicated in the co-administration of escitalopram and drugs metabolized by CYP2D6). Products include:
Anzemet Injection 2871
Anzemet Tablets 2874

Donepezil Hydrochloride (Caution is indicated in the co-administration of escitalopram and drugs metabolized by CYP2D6). Products include:
Aricept Tablets 1086
Aricept ODT Tablets 1086

Doxepin Hydrochloride (Caution is indicated in the co-administration of escitalopram and drugs metabolized by CYP2D6).
No products indexed under this heading.

Encainide Hydrochloride (Caution is indicated in the co-administration of escitalopram and drugs metabolized by CYP2D6).
No products indexed under this heading.

Enoxaparin Sodium (The combined use of psychotropic drugs that interfere with serotonin reuptake and drugs that affect coagulation has been associated with an increased risk of bleeding). Products include:
Lovenox Injection 2931

Etodolac (The combined use of psychotropic drugs that interfere with serotonin reuptake and drugs that affect coagulation has been associated with an increased risk of bleeding; use caution when co-administering).
No products indexed under this heading.

Fenoprofen Calcium (The combined use of psychotropic drugs that interfere with serotonin reuptake and drugs that affect coagulation has been associated with an increased risk of bleeding; use caution when co-administering). Products include:
Nalfon Capsules 2504

Fentanyl (Caution is indicated in the co-administration of escitalopram and drugs metabolized by CYP2D6). Products include:
Duragesic Transdermal System 2448

Fentanyl Citrate (Caution is indicated in the co-administration of escitalopram and drugs metabolized by CYP2D6). Products include:
Actiq 993

Flecainide Acetate (Caution is indicated in the co-administration of escitalopram and drugs metabolized by CYP2D6). Products include:

Tambocor Tablets 1824

Fluoxetine (Caution is indicated in the co-administration of escitalopram and drugs metabolized by CYP2D6).
No products indexed under this heading.

Fluoxetine Hydrochloride (Caution is indicated in the co-administration of escitalopram and drugs metabolized by CYP2D6). Products include:
Prozac Pulvules and Liquid 1771
Symbyax Capsules 1788

Fluphenazine Decanoate (Caution is indicated in the co-administration of escitalopram and drugs metabolized by CYP2D6).
No products indexed under this heading.

Fluphenazine Enanthate (Caution is indicated in the co-administration of escitalopram and drugs metabolized by CYP2D6).
No products indexed under this heading.

Fluphenazine Hydrochloride (Caution is indicated in the co-administration of escitalopram and drugs metabolized by CYP2D6).
No products indexed under this heading.

Flurbiprofen (The combined use of psychotropic drugs that interfere with serotonin reuptake and drugs that affect coagulation has been associated with an increased risk of bleeding; use caution when co-administering).
No products indexed under this heading.

Fluvoxamine Maleate (Caution is indicated in the co-administration of escitalopram and drugs metabolized by CYP2D6).
No products indexed under this heading.

Fondaparinux Sodium (The combined use of psychotropic drugs that interfere with serotonin reuptake and drugs that affect coagulation has been associated with an increased risk of bleeding). Products include:
Arixtra Injection 1325

Formoterol Fumarate (Caution is indicated in the co-administration of escitalopram and drugs metabolized by CYP2D6). Products include:
Foradil Aerolizer 3024

Galantamine Hydrobromide (Caution is indicated in the co-administration of escitalopram and drugs metabolized by CYP2D6). Products include:
Razadyne ER Extended-Release Capsules 2434
Razadyne 2434

Haloperidol (Caution is indicated in the co-administration of escitalopram and drugs metabolized by CYP2D6).
No products indexed under this heading.

Haloperidol Decanoate (Caution is indicated in the co-administration of escitalopram and drugs metabolized by CYP2D6).
No products indexed under this heading.

Heparin Calcium (The combined use of psychotropic drugs that interfere with serotonin reuptake and drugs that affect coagulation has been associated with an increased risk of bleeding).
No products indexed under this heading.

Heparin Sodium (The combined use of psychotropic drugs that interfere with serotonin reuptake and drugs that affect coagulation has been associated with an increased risk of bleeding).
No products indexed under this heading.

Hydrocodone Bitartrate (Caution is indicated in the co-administration of escitalopram and drugs metabolized by CYP2D6). Products include:
Hycodan 1104
Hycomine Compound Tablets 1105
Hycotuss Expectorant Syrup 1106
Lortab 3315
Lortab Elixir 3312
Vicodin Tablets 530
Vicodin ES Tablets 531
Vicodin HP Tablets 532
Vicoprofen Tablets 533
Zydone Tablets 1118

Ibuprofen (The combined use of psychotropic drugs that interfere with serotonin reuptake and drugs that affect coagulation has been associated with an increased risk of bleeding; use caution when co-administering). Products include:
Advil Allergy Sinus Caplets ..... ▣737
Advil ..... ▣737
Children's Advil Suspension ..... ▣742
Children's Advil Chewable Tablets ..... ▣741
Advil Cold & Sinus ..... ▣739
Advil Flu & Body Ache Caplets ..... ▣739
Children's Advil Cold Suspension ..... ▣741
Infants' Advil Concentrated Drops ..... ▣743
Junior Strength Advil Swallow Tablets ..... ▣740
Advil Migraine Liquigels ..... ▣740
Advil Multi-Symptom Cold Caplets ..... ▣738
Combunox Tablets 1183
Children's Motrin Oral Suspension and Chewable Tablets 1837
Children's Motrin Cold Non-Staining Dye-Free Oral Suspension 1838
Children's Motrin Cold Oral Suspension 1838
Children's Motrin Non-Staining Dye-Free Oral Suspension 1837
Motrin Cold & Sinus Caplets 1836
Motrin IB Tablets and Caplets 1836
Infants' Motrin Concentrated Drops 1837
Infants' Motrin Non-Staining Dye-Free Drops 1837
Junior Strength Motrin Caplets and Chewable Tablets 1837
Vicoprofen Tablets 533

Imipramine Hydrochloride (Caution is indicated in the co-administration of escitalopram and drugs metabolized by CYP2D6).
No products indexed under this heading.

Imipramine Pamoate (Caution is indicated in the co-administration of escitalopram and drugs metabolized by CYP2D6).
No products indexed under this heading.

Indomethacin (The combined use of psychotropic drugs that interfere with serotonin reuptake and drugs that affect coagulation has been associated with an increased risk of bleeding; use caution when co-administering). Products include:
Indocin 1968

Indomethacin Sodium Trihydrate (The combined use of psychotropic drugs that interfere with serotonin reuptake and drugs that affect coagulation has been associated with an increased risk of bleeding; use caution when co-administering). Products include:
Indocin I.V. 1973

Indoramin Hydrochloride (Caution is indicated in the co-administration of escitalopram and drugs metabolized by CYP2D6).
No products indexed under this heading.

Isocarboxazid (Co-administration of SSRIs and MAO inhibitors has resulted in serious, sometimes fatal, reactions including hyperthermia, rigidity, myoclonus, autonomic instability, agitation progressing to delirium and coma; concurrent and/or sequential use is contraindicated).
No products indexed under this heading.

Ketoconazole (Co-administration of racemic citalopram and ketoconazole resulted in decrease in Cmax and AUC of ketoconazole). Products include:
Nizoral A-D Shampoo, 1% 1839
Nizoral 2% Shampoo 1838

Ketoprofen (The combined use of psychotropic drugs that interfere with serotonin reuptake and drugs that affect coagulation has been associated with an increased risk of bleeding; use caution when co-administering).
No products indexed under this heading.

Ketorolac Tromethamine (The combined use of psychotropic drugs that interfere with serotonin reuptake and drugs that affect coagulation has been associated with an increased risk of bleeding; use caution when co-administering). Products include:
Acular Ophthalmic Solution 561
Acular LS Ophthalmic Solution 562

Labetalol Hydrochloride (Caution is indicated in the co-administration of escitalopram and drugs metabolized by CYP2D6).
No products indexed under this heading.

Lidocaine (Caution is indicated in the co-administration of escitalopram and drugs metabolized by CYP2D6). Products include:
Lidoderm Patch 1107

Lidocaine Hydrochloride (Caution is indicated in the co-administration of escitalopram and drugs metabolized by CYP2D6).
No products indexed under this heading.

Lithium (Serotonergic effects of escitalopram may be enhanced by lithium; co-administration had no significant effect on the pharmacokinetics of citalopram or lithium. Use caution when co-administering).
No products indexed under this heading.

Lithium Carbonate (Serotonergic effects of escitalopram may be enhanced by lithium; co-administration had no significant effect on the pharmacokinetics of citalopram or lithium. Use caution when co-administering). Products include:
Eskalith 1406
Lithobid Tablets 1670

Lithium Citrate (Serotonergic effects of escitalopram may be enhanced by lithium; co-administration had no significant effect on the pharmacokinetics of citalopram or lithium. Use caution when co-administering).
No products indexed under this heading.

Low Molecular Weight Heparins (The combined use of psychotropic drugs that interfere with serotonin reuptake and drugs that affect coagulation has been associated with an increased risk of bleeding).
No products indexed under this heading.

Maprotiline Hydrochloride (Caution is indicated in the co-administration of escitalopram and drugs metabolized by CYP2D6).
No products indexed under this heading.

Meclofenamate Sodium (The combined use of psychotropic drugs that interfere with serotonin reuptake and drugs that affect coagulation has been associated with an increased risk of bleeding; use caution when co-administering).
No products indexed under this heading.

Mefenamic Acid (The combined use of psychotropic drugs that interfere with serotonin reuptake and drugs that affect coagulation has been associated with an increased risk of bleeding; use caution when co-administering).
No products indexed under this heading.

Meloxicam (The combined use of psychotropic drugs that interfere with serotonin reuptake and drugs that affect coagulation has been associated with an increased risk of bleeding; use caution when co-administering). Products include:
Mobic Oral Suspension 893
Mobic Tablets 893

Meperidine Hydrochloride (Caution is indicated in the co-administration of escitalopram and drugs metabolized by CYP2D6).
No products indexed under this heading.

Methadone Hydrochloride (Caution is indicated in the co-administration of escitalopram and drugs metabolized by CYP2D6).
No products indexed under this heading.

Methamphetamine Hydrochloride (Caution is indicated in the co-administration of escitalopram and drugs metabolized by CYP2D6). Products include:
Desoxyn Tablets, USP 2482

Metoprolol Succinate (Co-administration has resulted in an increase in Cmax and AUC of metoprolol; increased metoprolol plasma levels have been associated with decreased cardioselectivity). Products include:
Toprol-XL Tablets 660

Metoprolol Tartrate (Co-administration has resulted in an increase in Cmax and AUC of metoprolol; increased metoprolol plasma levels have been associated with decreased cardioselectivity).
No products indexed under this heading.

Mexiletine Hydrochloride (Caution is indicated in the co-administration of escitalopram and drugs metabolized by CYP2D6).
No products indexed under this heading.

Mirtazapine (Caution is indicated in the co-administration of escitalopram and drugs metabolized by CYP2D6).
No products indexed under this heading.

IMPORTANT NOTE: Always consult each drug listing in the patient's regimen for possible interactions.

Moclobemide (Co-administration of SSRIs and MAO inhibitors has resulted in serious, sometimes fatal, reactions including hyperthermia, rigidity, myoclonus, autonomic instability, agitation progressing to delirium and coma; concurrent and/or sequential use is contraindicated).
No products indexed under this heading.

Morphine Sulfate (Caution is indicated in the co-administration of escitalopram and drugs metabolized by CYP2D6). Products include:
Avinza Capsules 1714
Kadian Capsules 572
MS Contin Tablets 2703

Nabumetone (The combined use of psychotropic drugs that interfere with serotonin reuptake and drugs that affect coagulation has been associated with an increased risk of bleeding; use caution when co-administering). Products include:
Relafen Tablets 1523

Naproxen (The combined use of psychotropic drugs that interfere with serotonin reuptake and drugs that affect coagulation has been associated with an increased risk of bleeding; use caution when co-administering). Products include:
EC-Naprosyn Delayed-Release Tablets 2769
Naprosyn Suspension 2769
Naprosyn Tablets 2769
Prevacid NapraPAC 3277

Naproxen Sodium (The combined use of psychotropic drugs that interfere with serotonin reuptake and drugs that affect coagulation has been associated with an increased risk of bleeding; use caution when co-administering). Products include:
Aleve Tablets, Caplets and Gelcaps .... ▣605
Anaprox Tablets 2769
Anaprox DS Tablets 2769

Nelfinavir Mesylate (Caution is indicated in the co-administration of escitalopram and drugs metabolized by CYP2D6). Products include:
Viracept 2556

Nortriptyline Hydrochloride (Caution is indicated in the co-administration of escitalopram and drugs metabolized by CYP2D6).
No products indexed under this heading.

Olanzapine (Caution is indicated in the co-administration of escitalopram and drugs metabolized by CYP2D6). Products include:
Symbyax Capsules 1788
Zyprexa Tablets 1798
Zyprexa IntraMuscular 1798
Zyprexa ZYDIS Orally Disintegrating Tablets 1798

Omeprazole (Caution is indicated in the co-administration of escitalopram and drugs metabolized by CYP2D6). Products include:
Zegerid Powder for Oral Solution 2972

Ondansetron (Caution is indicated in the co-administration of escitalopram and drugs metabolized by CYP2D6). Products include:
Zofran ODT Orally Disintegrating Tablets 1613

Ondansetron Hydrochloride (Caution is indicated in the co-administration of escitalopram and drugs metabolized by CYP2D6). Products include:
Zofran Injection 1607
Zofran 1613

Oxaprozin (The combined use of psychotropic drugs that interfere with serotonin reuptake and drugs that affect coagulation has been associated with an increased risk of bleeding; use caution when co-administering).
No products indexed under this heading.

Oxycodone Hydrochloride (Caution is indicated in the co-administration of escitalopram and drugs metabolized by CYP2D6). Products include:
Combunox Tablets 1183
OxyContin Tablets 2699
OxyFast Oral Concentrate Solution 2704
OxyIR Capsules 2704
Percocet Tablets 1114
Percodan Tablets 1115

Paclitaxel (Caution is indicated in the co-administration of escitalopram and drugs metabolized by CYP2D6).
No products indexed under this heading.

Pargyline Hydrochloride (Co-administration of SSRIs and MAO inhibitors has resulted in serious, sometimes fatal, reactions including hyperthermia, rigidity, myoclonus, autonomic instability, agitation progressing to delirium and coma; concurrent and/or sequential use is contraindicated).
No products indexed under this heading.

Paroxetine Hydrochloride (Caution is indicated in the co-administration of escitalopram and drugs metabolized by CYP2D6). Products include:
Paxil CR Controlled-Release Tablets 1509
Paxil 1501

Phenelzine Sulfate (Co-administration of SSRIs and MAO inhibitors has resulted in serious, sometimes fatal, reactions including hyperthermia, rigidity, myoclonus, autonomic instability, agitation progressing to delirium and coma; concurrent and/or sequential use is contraindicated).
No products indexed under this heading.

Phenylbutazone (The combined use of psychotropic drugs that interfere with serotonin reuptake and drugs that affect coagulation has been associated with an increased risk of bleeding; use caution when co-administering).
No products indexed under this heading.

Pimozide (In a controlled study, a single dose of pimozide 2 mg co-administered with citalopram 40 mg given once daily for 11 days was associated with a mean increase in QTc values of approximately 10 msec. compared to pimozide given alone). Products include:
Orap Tablets 1220

Pindolol (Caution is indicated in the co-administration of escitalopram and drugs metabolized by CYP2D6).
No products indexed under this heading.

Piroxicam (The combined use of psychotropic drugs that interfere with serotonin reuptake and drugs that affect coagulation has been associated with an increased risk of bleeding; use caution when co-administering).
No products indexed under this heading.

Procarbazine Hydrochloride (Co-administration of SSRIs and MAO inhibitors has resulted in serious, sometimes fatal, reactions including hyperthermia, rigidity, myoclonus, autonomic instability, agitation progressing to delirium and coma; concurrent and/or sequential use is contraindicated). Products include:
Matulane Capsules 3188

Propafenone Hydrochloride (Caution is indicated in the co-administration of escitalopram and drugs metabolized by CYP2D6). Products include:
Rythmol SR Capsules 2736

Propoxyphene Hydrochloride (Caution is indicated in the co-administration of escitalopram and drugs metabolized by CYP2D6).
No products indexed under this heading.

Propoxyphene Napsylate (Caution is indicated in the co-administration of escitalopram and drugs metabolized by CYP2D6). Products include:
Darvocet A 500 Tablets 3497

Propranolol Hydrochloride (Caution is indicated in the co-administration of escitalopram and drugs metabolized by CYP2D6). Products include:
Inderal LA Long-Acting Capsules 3421
InnoPran XL Capsules 2728

Quetiapine Fumarate (Caution is indicated in the co-administration of escitalopram and drugs metabolized by CYP2D6). Products include:
Seroquel Tablets 691

Quinidine Gluconate (Caution is indicated in the co-administration of escitalopram and drugs metabolized by CYP2D6).
No products indexed under this heading.

Quinidine Hydrochloride (Caution is indicated in the co-administration of escitalopram and drugs metabolized by CYP2D6).
No products indexed under this heading.

Quinidine Polygalacturonate (Caution is indicated in the co-administration of escitalopram and drugs metabolized by CYP2D6).
No products indexed under this heading.

Quinidine Sulfate (Caution is indicated in the co-administration of escitalopram and drugs metabolized by CYP2D6).
No products indexed under this heading.

Risperidone (Caution is indicated in the co-administration of escitalopram and drugs metabolized by CYP2D6). Products include:
Risperdal Consta Long-Acting Injection 1664
Risperdal M-Tab Orally Disintegrating Tablets 1658
Risperdal 1658

Ritonavir (Caution is indicated in the co-administration of escitalopram and drugs metabolized by CYP2D6). Products include:
Kaletra 474
Norvir 499

Rofecoxib (The combined use of psychotropic drugs that interfere with serotonin reuptake and drugs that affect coagulation has been associated with an increased risk of bleeding; use caution when co-administering).
No products indexed under this heading.

Selegiline Hydrochloride (Co-administration of SSRIs and MAO inhibitors has resulted in serious, sometimes fatal, reactions including hyperthermia, rigidity, myoclonus, autonomic instability, agitation progressing to delirium and coma; concurrent and/or sequential use is contraindicated). Products include:
Eldepryl Capsules 3209

Sulindac (The combined use of psychotropic drugs that interfere with serotonin reuptake and drugs that affect coagulation has been associated with an increased risk of bleeding; use caution when co-administering). Products include:
Clinoril Tablets 1899

Sumatriptan (Co-administration of SSRIs and sumatriptan has resulted in weakness, hyperreflexia, and incoordination). Products include:
Imitrex Nasal Spray 1435

Sumatriptan Succinate (Co-administration of SSRIs and sumatriptan has resulted in weakness, hyperreflexia, and incoordination). Products include:
Imitrex Injection 1431
Imitrex Tablets 1440

Tamoxifen Citrate (Caution is indicated in the co-administration of escitalopram and drugs metabolized by CYP2D6).
No products indexed under this heading.

Teniposide (Caution is indicated in the co-administration of escitalopram and drugs metabolized by CYP2D6).
No products indexed under this heading.

Testosterone (Caution is indicated in the co-administration of escitalopram and drugs metabolized by CYP2D6). Products include:
AndroGel 3330
Striant Mucoadhesive 1022
Testim 1% Gel 722

Testosterone Cypionate (Caution is indicated in the co-administration of escitalopram and drugs metabolized by CYP2D6).
No products indexed under this heading.

Testosterone Enanthate (Caution is indicated in the co-administration of escitalopram and drugs metabolized by CYP2D6). Products include:
Delatestryl Injection 2976

Testosterone Propionate (Caution is indicated in the co-administration of escitalopram and drugs metabolized by CYP2D6).
No products indexed under this heading.

Thioridazine (Caution is indicated in the co-administration of escitalopram and drugs metabolized by CYP2D6).
No products indexed under this heading.

Thioridazine Hydrochloride (Caution is indicated in the co-

administration of escitalopram and drugs metabolized by CYP2D6). Products include:
Thioridazine Hydrochloride Tablets 2122

Timolol Maleate (Caution is indicated in the co-administration of escitalopram and drugs metabolized by CYP2D6). Products include:
Blocadren Tablets 1891
Cosopt Sterile Ophthalmic Solution 1910
Timolide Tablets 2056
Timoptic in Ocudose 2061
Timoptic Sterile Ophthalmic Solution 2058
Timoptic-XE Sterile Ophthalmic Gel Forming Solution 2062

Tinzaparin Sodium (The combined use of psychotropic drugs that interfere with serotonin reuptake and drugs that affect coagulation has been associated with an increased risk of bleeding).
No products indexed under this heading.

Tolmetin Sodium (The combined use of psychotropic drugs that interfere with serotonin reuptake and drugs that affect coagulation has been associated with an increased risk of bleeding; use caution when co-administering).
No products indexed under this heading.

Tolterodine Tartrate (Caution is indicated in the co-administration of escitalopram and drugs metabolized by CYP2D6). Products include:
Detrol Tablets 2626
Detrol LA Capsules 2629

Tramadol Hydrochloride (Caution is indicated in the co-administration of escitalopram and drugs metabolized by CYP2D6). Products include:
Ultracet Tablets 2462

Tranylcypromine Sulfate (Co-administration of SSRIs and MAO inhibitors has resulted in serious, sometimes fatal, reactions including hyperthermia, rigidity, myoclonus, autonomic instability, agitation progressing to delirium and coma; concurrent and/or sequential use is contraindicated). Products include:
Parnate Tablets 1499

Trazodone Hydrochloride (Caution is indicated in the co-administration of escitalopram and drugs metabolized by CYP2D6).
No products indexed under this heading.

Triazolam (Caution is indicated in the co-administration of escitalopram and drugs metabolized by CYP2D6).
No products indexed under this heading.

Trimipramine Maleate (Caution is indicated in the co-administration of escitalopram and drugs metabolized by CYP2D6). Products include:
Surmontil Capsules 2347

Valdecoxib (The combined use of psychotropic drugs that interfere with serotonin reuptake and drugs that affect coagulation has been associated with an increased risk of bleeding; use caution when co-administering).
No products indexed under this heading.

Venlafaxine Hydrochloride (Caution is indicated in the co-administration of escitalopram and drugs metabolized by CYP2D6). Products include:
Effexor Tablets 3405
Effexor XR Capsules 3411

Vinblastine Sulfate (Caution is indicated in the co-administration of escitalopram and drugs metabolized by CYP2D6).
No products indexed under this heading.

Warfarin Sodium (The combined use of psychotropic drugs that interfere with serotonin reuptake and drugs that affect coagulation has been associated with an increased risk of bleeding). Products include:
Coumadin for Injection 932
Coumadin Tablets 932

Zonisamide (Caution is indicated in the co-administration of escitalopram and drugs metabolized by CYP2D6). Products include:
Zonegran Capsules 1089

Food Interactions

Alcohol (Given the primary CNS effects of escitalopram, concurrent use is not recommended).

LEXIVA TABLETS

(Fosamprenavir Calcium) 1473

May interact with cytochrome p450 3a4 inducers (selected), cytochrome p450 3a4 inhibitors (selected), cytochrome p450 3a4 substrates (selected), histamine H_2-receptor antagonists, phenytoin, proton pump inhibitor, and certain other agents. Compounds in these categories include:

Acetazolamide (Amprenavir, the active metabolite of fosamprenavir, is metabolized in the liver by the cytochrome P450 enzyme system. Amprenavir may inhibit or induce CYP3A4. Caution should be used when co-administering medications that are substrates, inhibitors, or inducers of CYP3A4, or potentially toxic medications that are metabolized by CYP3A4).
No products indexed under this heading.

Alfentanil Hydrochloride (Amprenavir, the active metabolite of fosamprenavir, is metabolized in the liver by the cytochrome P450 enzyme system. Amprenavir may inhibit or induce CYP3A4. Caution should be used when co-administering medications that are substrates, inhibitors, or inducers of CYP3A4, or potentially toxic medications that are metabolized by CYP3A4).
No products indexed under this heading.

Allium sativum (Amprenavir, the active metabolite of fosamprenavir, is metabolized in the liver by the cytochrome P450 enzyme system. Amprenavir may inhibit or induce CYP3A4. Caution should be used when co-administering medications that are substrates, inhibitors, or inducers of CYP3A4, or potentially toxic medications that are metabolized by CYP3A4).
No products indexed under this heading.

Alprazolam (Co-administration may increase alprazolam levels; may need to decrease alprazolam dose). Products include:
Niravam Orally Disintegrating Tablets 3106
Xanax XR Tablets 2655

Amiodarone Hydrochloride (Co-administration may lead to increased levels of amiodarone. Caution is warranted and therapeutic concentration monitoring is recommended for antiarrhythmics when co-administered with fosamprenavir). Products include:
Pacerone Tablets 3337

Amitriptyline Hydrochloride (Co-administration may lead to increased levels of amitriptyline. Therapeutic concentration monitoring is recommended for tricyclic antidepressants when co-administered with fosamprenavir).
No products indexed under this heading.

Amlodipine Besylate (Co-administration may increase levels of amlodipine; caution is warranted and clinical monitoring is recommended). Products include:
Caduet Tablets 2507
Lotrel Capsules 2238
Norvasc Tablets 2529

Amprenavir (Amprenavir, the active metabolite of fosamprenavir, is metabolized in the liver by the cytochrome P450 enzyme system. Amprenavir may inhibit or induce CYP3A4. Caution should be used when co-administering medications that are substrates, inhibitors, or inducers of CYP3A4, or potentially toxic medications that are metabolized by CYP3A4). Products include:
Agenerase Capsules 1299
Agenerase Oral Solution 1304

Anastrozole (Amprenavir, the active metabolite of fosamprenavir, is metabolized in the liver by the cytochrome P450 enzyme system. Amprenavir may inhibit or induce CYP3A4. Caution should be used when co-administering medications that are substrates, inhibitors, or inducers of CYP3A4, or potentially toxic medications that are metabolized by CYP3A4). Products include:
Arimidex Tablets 665

Aprepitant (Amprenavir, the active metabolite of fosamprenavir, is metabolized in the liver by the cytochrome P450 enzyme system. Amprenavir may inhibit or induce CYP3A4. Caution should be used when co-administering medications that are substrates, inhibitors, or inducers of CYP3A4, or potentially toxic medications that are metabolized by CYP3A4). Products include:
Emend Capsules 1944

Astemizole (Amprenavir, the active metabolite of fosamprenavir, is metabolized in the liver by the cytochrome P450 enzyme system. Amprenavir may inhibit or induce CYP3A4. Caution should be used when co-administering medications that are substrates, inhibitors, or inducers of CYP3A4, or potentially toxic medications that are metabolized by CYP3A4).
No products indexed under this heading.

Atorvastatin Calcium (Co-administration may lead to increased atorvastatin levels. Use ≤20mg/day of atorvastatin with careful monitoring or consider other HMG-CoA reductase inhibitors in combination with fosamprenavir). Products include:
Caduet Tablets 2507
Lipitor Tablets 2495

Belladonna Ergotamine (Amprenavir, the active metabolite of fosamprenavir, is metabolized in the liver by the cytochrome P450 enzyme system. Amprenavir may inhibit or induce CYP3A4. Caution should be used when co-administering medications that are substrates, inhibitors, or inducers of CYP3A4, or potentially toxic medications that are metabolized by CYP3A4).
No products indexed under this heading.

Bepridil Hydrochloride (Co-administration may lead to increased levels of bepridil. Use with caution; increased levels of bepridil may be associated with life-threatening reactions such as cardiac arrhythmias).
No products indexed under this heading.

Betamethasone Acetate (Amprenavir, the active metabolite of fosamprenavir, is metabolized in the liver by the cytochrome P450 enzyme system. Amprenavir may inhibit or induce CYP3A4. Caution should be used when co-administering medications that are substrates, inhibitors, or inducers of CYP3A4, or potentially toxic medications that are metabolized by CYP3A4).
No products indexed under this heading.

Betamethasone Sodium Phosphate (Amprenavir, the active metabolite of fosamprenavir, is metabolized in the liver by the cytochrome P450 enzyme system. Amprenavir may inhibit or induce CYP3A4. Caution should be used when co-administering medications that are substrates, inhibitors, or inducers of CYP3A4, or potentially toxic medications that are metabolized by CYP3A4).
No products indexed under this heading.

Buspirone Hydrochloride (Amprenavir, the active metabolite of fosamprenavir, is metabolized in the liver by the cytochrome P450 enzyme system. Amprenavir may inhibit or induce CYP3A4. Caution should be used when co-administering medications that are substrates, inhibitors, or inducers of CYP3A4, or potentially toxic medications that are metabolized by CYP3A4).
No products indexed under this heading.

Busulfan (Amprenavir, the active metabolite of fosamprenavir, is metabolized in the liver by the cytochrome P450 enzyme system. Amprenavir may inhibit or induce CYP3A4. Caution should be used when co-administering medications that are substrates, inhibitors, or inducers of CYP3A4, or potentially toxic medications that are metabolized by CYP3A4). Products include:
I.V. Busulfex 1125
Myleran Tablets 1492

Carbamazepine (Co-administration may lead to decreased amprenavir levels. Use with caution; fosamprenavir may be less effective due to decreased plasma concentrations in patients taking these agents concomitantly). Products include:
Carbatrol Capsules 3174
Equetro Extended-Release Capsules 3178

Tegretol/Tegretol-XR **2278**

Cerivastatin Sodium (Amprenavir, the active metabolite of fosamprenavir, is metabolized in the liver by the cytochrome P450 enzyme system. Amprenavir may inhibit or induce CYP3A4. Caution should be used when co-administering medications that are substrates, inhibitors, or inducers of CYP3A4, or potentially toxic medications that are metabolized by CYP3A4).

No products indexed under this heading.

Chlorpheniramine (Amprenavir, the active metabolite of fosamprenavir, is metabolized in the liver by the cytochrome P450 enzyme system. Amprenavir may inhibit or induce CYP3A4. Caution should be used when co-administering medications that are substrates, inhibitors, or inducers of CYP3A4, or potentially toxic medications that are metabolized by CYP3A4).

No products indexed under this heading.

Chlorpheniramine Maleate (Amprenavir, the active metabolite of fosamprenavir, is metabolized in the liver by the cytochrome P450 enzyme system. Amprenavir may inhibit or induce CYP3A4. Caution should be used when co-administering medications that are substrates, inhibitors, or inducers of CYP3A4, or potentially toxic medications that are metabolized by CYP3A4). Products include:

Advil Allergy Sinus Caplets .... ▣ **737**
Advil Multi-Symptom Cold Caplets .... ▣ **738**
BC Allergy Sinus Cold Powder .... ▣ **612**
Contac Severe Cold and Flu Caplets Maximum Strength .... ▣ **615**
Hycomine Compound Tablets **1105**
PediaCare Multi-Symptom Cold Liquid .... ▣ **704**
PediaCare NightRest Cough & Cold Liquid .... ▣ **704**
Robitussin Flu Liquid .... ▣ **752**
Robitussin PM Cough & Cold Liquid .... ▣ **752**
Singlet Caplets .... ▣ **636**
Sudafed Sinus & Allergy Tablets ..... ▣ **710**
TheraFlu Cold & Cough Hot Liquid .... ▣ **680**
TheraFlu Cold & Sore Throat Hot Liquid .... ▣ **680**
TheraFlu Flu & Sore Throat Hot Liquid .... ▣ **681**
TheraFlu Severe Cold & Cough Hot Liquid .... ▣ **683**
TheraFlu Severe Cold Caplets .... ▣ **679**
TheraFlu Severe Cold Hot Liquid ..... ▣ **682**
Triaminic Cold & Allergy Liquid ..... ▣ **685**
Triaminic Cold & Cough Liquid .... ▣ **685**
Triaminic Flu, Cough & Fever Liquid .... ▣ **685**
Triaminic Night Time Cough & Cold Liquid .... ▣ **685**
Triaminic Allergy Runny Nose & Congestion Softchews .... ▣ **688**
Triaminic Cold & Cough Softchews .... ▣ **688**
Children's Tylenol Plus Cold NightTime Suspension Liquid **1851**
Children's Tylenol Plus Cold & Cough Suspension Liquid and Chewable Tablets **1851**
Children's Tylenol Plus Cold Chewable Tablets **1851**
Children's Tylenol Plus Flu Suspension Liquid **1853**
Tylenol Allergy Complete Multi-Symptom Caplets and Gelcaps with Cool Burst............ **1844**
Multi-Symptom Tylenol Cold Night Time Caplets **1845**
Vicks 44M Cough, Cold & Flu Relief............ **2676**
Pediatric Vicks 44m Cough & Cold Relief **2673**
Children's Vicks NyQuil Cold/Cough Relief **2671**

Chlorpheniramine Polistirex (Amprenavir, the active metabolite of fosamprenavir, is metabolized in the liver by the cytochrome P450 enzyme system. Amprenavir may inhibit or induce CYP3A4. Caution should be used when co-administering medications that are substrates, inhibitors, or inducers of CYP3A4, or potentially toxic medications that are metabolized by CYP3A4). Products include:

Tussionex Pennkinetic Extended-Release Suspension **3322**

Chlorpheniramine Tannate (Amprenavir, the active metabolite of fosamprenavir, is metabolized in the liver by the cytochrome P450 enzyme system. Amprenavir may inhibit or induce CYP3A4. Caution should be used when co-administering medications that are substrates, inhibitors, or inducers of CYP3A4, or potentially toxic medications that are metabolized by CYP3A4).

No products indexed under this heading.

Cimetidine (Amprenavir, the active metabolite of fosamprenavir, is metabolized in the liver by the cytochrome P450 enzyme system. Amprenavir may inhibit or induce CYP3A4. Caution should be used when co-administering medications that are substrates, inhibitors, or inducers of CYP3A4, or potentially toxic medications that are metabolized by CYP3A4). Products include:

Tagamet HB 200 Tablets .... ▣ **637**
Tagamet Tablets **1547**

Cimetidine Hydrochloride (Amprenavir, the active metabolite of fosamprenavir, is metabolized in the liver by the cytochrome P450 enzyme system. Amprenavir may inhibit or induce CYP3A4. Caution should be used when co-administering medications that are substrates, inhibitors, or inducers of CYP3A4, or potentially toxic medications that are metabolized by CYP3A4).

No products indexed under this heading.

Ciprofloxacin (Amprenavir, the active metabolite of fosamprenavir, is metabolized in the liver by the cytochrome P450 enzyme system. Amprenavir may inhibit or induce CYP3A4. Caution should be used when co-administering medications that are substrates, inhibitors, or inducers of CYP3A4, or potentially toxic medications that are metabolized by CYP3A4). Products include:

Cipro I.V. **2998**
Cipro I.V. Pharmacy Bulk Package ... **3509**
Cipro Oral Suspension **2991**
Cipro XR Tablets **3004**
Ciprodex Otic Suspension **555**

Ciprofloxacin Hydrochloride (Amprenavir, the active metabolite of fosamprenavir, is metabolized in the liver by the cytochrome P450 enzyme system. Amprenavir may inhibit or induce CYP3A4. Caution should be used when co-administering medications that are substrates, inhibitors, or inducers of CYP3A4, or potentially toxic medications that are metabolized by CYP3A4). Products include:

Ciloxan Ophthalmic Ointment **554**
Cipro Tablets **2991**

Cisapride (Co-administration with cisapride is contraindicated due to the potential for serious and/or life-threatening reactions such as cardiac arrhythmias).

No products indexed under this heading.

Cisplatin (Amprenavir, the active metabolite of fosamprenavir, is metabolized in the liver by the cytochrome P450 enzyme system. Amprenavir may inhibit or induce CYP3A4. Caution should be used when co-administering medications that are substrates, inhibitors, or inducers of CYP3A4, or potentially toxic medications that are metabolized by CYP3A4).

No products indexed under this heading.

Clarithromycin (Amprenavir, the active metabolite of fosamprenavir, is metabolized in the liver by the cytochrome P450 enzyme system. Amprenavir may inhibit or induce CYP3A4. Caution should be used when co-administering medications that are substrates, inhibitors, or inducers of CYP3A4, or potentially toxic medications that are metabolized by CYP3A4). Products include:

Biaxin/Biaxin XL **402**
PREVPAC **3281**

Clorazepate Dipotassium (Co-administration may increase clorazepate levels; may need to decrease clorazepate dose). Products include:

Tranxene **2488**

Clotrimazole (Amprenavir, the active metabolite of fosamprenavir, is metabolized in the liver by the cytochrome P450 enzyme system. Amprenavir may inhibit or induce CYP3A4. Caution should be used when co-administering medications that are substrates, inhibitors, or inducers of CYP3A4, or potentially toxic medications that are metabolized by CYP3A4). Products include:

Lotrimin **3053**
Lotrisone **3054**

Cortisone Acetate (Amprenavir, the active metabolite of fosamprenavir, is metabolized in the liver by the cytochrome P450 enzyme system. Amprenavir may inhibit or induce CYP3A4. Caution should be used when co-administering medications that are substrates, inhibitors, or inducers of CYP3A4, or potentially toxic medications that are metabolized by CYP3A4).

No products indexed under this heading.

Cyclosporine (Co-administration may lead to increased levels of cyclosporine. Therapeutic concentration monitoring is recommended for immunosuppressant agents when co-administered with fosamprenavir). Products include:

Gengraf Capsules **458**
Neoral Soft Gelatin Capsules **2247**
Neoral Oral Solution **2247**
Restasis Ophthalmic Emulsion **570**
Sandimmune **2259**

Dalfopristin (Amprenavir, the active metabolite of fosamprenavir, is metabolized in the liver by the cytochrome P450 enzyme system. Amprenavir may inhibit or induce CYP3A4. Caution should be used when co-administering medications that are substrates, inhibitors, or inducers of CYP3A4, or potentially toxic medications that are metabolized by CYP3A4). Products include:

Synercid I.V. **1690**

Danazol (Amprenavir, the active metabolite of fosamprenavir, is metabolized in the liver by the cytochrome P450 enzyme system. Amprenavir may inhibit or induce CYP3A4. Caution should be used when co-administering medications that are substrates, inhibitors, or inducers of CYP3A4, or potentially toxic medications that are metabolized by CYP3A4).

No products indexed under this heading.

Delavirdine Mesylate (Co-administration may lead to loss of virologic response and possible resistance to delavirdine). Products include:

Rescriptor Tablets **2535**

Desogestrel (Amprenavir, the active metabolite of fosamprenavir, is metabolized in the liver by the cytochrome P450 enzyme system. Amprenavir may inhibit or induce CYP3A4. Caution should be used when co-administering medications that are substrates, inhibitors, or inducers of CYP3A4, or potentially toxic medications that are metabolized by CYP3A4). Products include:

Ortho-Cept Tablets **2395**

Dexamethasone (Co-administration may decrease amprenavir levels. Use with caution since fosamprenavir may be less effective due to decreased amprenavir plasma concentrations in patients taking these agents concomitantly). Products include:

Ciprodex Otic Suspension **555**
Decadron Tablets **1929**
TobraDex Ophthalmic Ointment **558**
TobraDex Ophthalmic Suspension ... **558**

Dexamethasone Acetate (Co-administration may decrease amprenavir levels. Use with caution since fosamprenavir may be less effective due to decreased amprenavir plasma concentrations in patients taking these agents concomitantly).

No products indexed under this heading.

Dexamethasone Phosphate (Co-administration may decrease amprenavir levels. Use with caution since fosamprenavir may be less effective due to decreased amprenavir plasma concentrations in patients taking these agents concomitantly).

No products indexed under this heading.

Dexamethasone Sodium (Co-administration may decrease amprenavir levels. Use with caution since fosamprenavir may be less effective due to decreased amprenavir plasma concentrations in patients taking these agents concomitantly).

No products indexed under this heading.

Dexamethasone Sodium Phosphate (Co-administration may decrease amprenavir levels. Use with caution since fosamprenavir may be less effective due to decreased amprenavir plasma concentrations in patients taking these agents concomitantly). Products include:

Decadron Phosphate Injection **1931**

Dexamethasone Sodium Phosphate Injection (Co-administration may decrease amprenavir levels. Use with caution since fosamprenavir may be less effective due to decreased amprenavir plasma concentrations in patients taking these agents concomitantly).
No products indexed under this heading.

Diazepam (Co-administration may increase diazepam levels; may need to decrease diazepam dose). Products include:
Diastat Rectal Delivery System **3344**
Valium Tablets **2822**

Dihydroergotamine Mesylate (Co-administration with dihydroergotamine is contraindicated due to the potential for serious and/or life-threatening reactions such as acute ergot toxicity characterized by peripheral vasospasm and ischemia of the extremities and other tissues). Products include:
Migranal Nasal Spray **3350**

Diltiazem Hydrochloride (Co-administration may increase levels of diltiazem; caution is warranted and clinical monitoring is recommended). Products include:
Cardizem LA Extended Release Tablets **1699**
Tiazac Capsules **1204**

Diltiazem Maleate (Co-administration may increase levels of diltiazem; caution is warranted and clinical monitoring is recommended).
No products indexed under this heading.

Disopyramide (Amprenavir, the active metabolite of fosamprenavir, is metabolized in the liver by the cytochrome P450 enzyme system. Amprenavir may inhibit or induce CYP3A4. Caution should be used when co-administering medications that are substrates, inhibitors, or inducers of CYP3A4, or potentially toxic medications that are metabolized by CYP3A4).
No products indexed under this heading.

Disopyramide Phosphate (Amprenavir, the active metabolite of fosamprenavir, is metabolized in the liver by the cytochrome P450 enzyme system. Amprenavir may inhibit or induce CYP3A4. Caution should be used when co-administering medications that are substrates, inhibitors, or inducers of CYP3A4, or potentially toxic medications that are metabolized by CYP3A4).
No products indexed under this heading.

Disulfiram (Amprenavir, the active metabolite of fosamprenavir, is metabolized in the liver by the cytochrome P450 enzyme system. Amprenavir may inhibit or induce CYP3A4. Caution should be used when co-administering medications that are substrates, inhibitors, or inducers of CYP3A4, or potentially toxic medications that are metabolized by CYP3A4). Products include:
Antabuse Tablets **2343**

Doxorubicin Hydrochloride (Amprenavir, the active metabolite of fosamprenavir, is metabolized in the liver by the cytochrome P450 enzyme system. Amprenavir may inhibit or induce CYP3A4. Caution should be used when co-administering medications that are substrates, inhibitors, or inducers of CYP3A4, or potentially toxic medications that are metabolized by CYP3A4). Products include:
Adriamycin for Injection, USP **786**
Adriamycin Injection, USP **786**

Dronabinol (Amprenavir, the active metabolite of fosamprenavir, is metabolized in the liver by the cytochrome P450 enzyme system. Amprenavir may inhibit or induce CYP3A4. Caution should be used when co-administering medications that are substrates, inhibitors, or inducers of CYP3A4, or potentially toxic medications that are metabolized by CYP3A4). Products include:
Marinol Capsules **3334**

Efavirenz (Co-administration may lead to decreased amprenavir levels. An additional 100mg/day (300mg total) of ritonavir is recommended when efavirenz is administered with fosamprenavir/ritonavir once daily. No change in the ritonavir dose is required when efavirenz is administered with fosamprenavir plus ritonavir twice daily). Products include:
Sustiva Capsules **957**

Ergonovine Maleate (Co-administration with ergonovine is contraindicated due to the potential for serious and/or life-threatening reactions such as acute ergot toxicity characterized by peripheral vasospasm and ischemia of the extremities and other tissues).
No products indexed under this heading.

Ergotamine Tartrate (Co-administration with ergotamine is contraindicated due to the potential for serious and/or life-threatening reactions such as acute ergot toxicity characterized by peripheral vasospasm and ischemia of the extremities and other tissues).
No products indexed under this heading.

Erythromycin (Amprenavir, the active metabolite of fosamprenavir, is metabolized in the liver by the cytochrome P450 enzyme system. Amprenavir may inhibit or induce CYP3A4. Caution should be used when co-administering medications that are substrates, inhibitors, or inducers of CYP3A4, or potentially toxic medications that are metabolized by CYP3A4). Products include:
Erygel Topical Gel **2096**
Ery-Tab Tablets **447**
Erythromycin Base Filmtab Tablets **454**
Erythromycin Delayed-Release Capsules, USP **456**
PCE Dispertab Tablets **510**

Erythromycin Estolate (Amprenavir, the active metabolite of fosamprenavir, is metabolized in the liver by the cytochrome P450 enzyme system. Amprenavir may inhibit or induce CYP3A4. Caution should be used when co-administering medications that are substrates, inhibitors, or inducers of CYP3A4, or potentially toxic medications that are metabolized by CYP3A4).
No products indexed under this heading.

Erythromycin Ethylsuccinate (Amprenavir, the active metabolite of fosamprenavir, is metabolized in the liver by the cytochrome P450 enzyme system. Amprenavir may inhibit or induce CYP3A4. Caution should be used when co-administering medications that are substrates, inhibitors, or inducers of CYP3A4, or potentially toxic medications that are metabolized by CYP3A4). Products include:
E.E.S. **449**
EryPed **445**

Erythromycin Gluceptate (Amprenavir, the active metabolite of fosamprenavir, is metabolized in the liver by the cytochrome P450 enzyme system. Amprenavir may inhibit or induce CYP3A4. Caution should be used when co-administering medications that are substrates, inhibitors, or inducers of CYP3A4, or potentially toxic medications that are metabolized by CYP3A4).
No products indexed under this heading.

Erythromycin Lactobionate (Amprenavir, the active metabolite of fosamprenavir, is metabolized in the liver by the cytochrome P450 enzyme system. Amprenavir may inhibit or induce CYP3A4. Caution should be used when co-administering medications that are substrates, inhibitors, or inducers of CYP3A4, or potentially toxic medications that are metabolized by CYP3A4).
No products indexed under this heading.

Erythromycin Stearate (Amprenavir, the active metabolite of fosamprenavir, is metabolized in the liver by the cytochrome P450 enzyme system. Amprenavir may inhibit or induce CYP3A4. Caution should be used when co-administering medications that are substrates, inhibitors, or inducers of CYP3A4, or potentially toxic medications that are metabolized by CYP3A4). Products include:
Erythrocin Stearate Filmtab Tablets **452**

Esomeprazole Magnesium (Amprenavir, the active metabolite of fosamprenavir, is metabolized in the liver by the cytochrome P450 enzyme system. Amprenavir may inhibit or induce CYP3A4. Caution should be used when co-administering medications that are substrates, inhibitors, or inducers of CYP3A4, or potentially toxic medications that are metabolized by CYP3A4). Products include:
Nexium Delayed-Release Capsules **645**

Estradiol (Amprenavir, the active metabolite of fosamprenavir, is metabolized in the liver by the cytochrome P450 enzyme system. Amprenavir may inhibit or induce CYP3A4. Caution should be used when co-administering medications that are substrates, inhibitors, or inducers of CYP3A4, or potentially toxic medications that are metabolized by CYP3A4). Products include:
Activella Tablets **2311**
Climara Transdermal System **795**
Climara Pro Transdermal System **800**
CombiPatch Transdermal System **2180**
Estrogel 0.06% **3200**
Menostar Transdermal System **805**
Prefest Tablets **1069**
Vagifem Tablets **2340**
Vivelle Transdermal System **2288**
Vivelle-Dot Transdermal System **2293**

Estradiol Benzoate (Amprenavir, the active metabolite of fosamprenavir, is metabolized in the liver by the cytochrome P450 enzyme system. Amprenavir may inhibit or induce CYP3A4. Caution should be used when co-administering medications that are substrates, inhibitors, or inducers of CYP3A4, or potentially toxic medications that are metabolized by CYP3A4).
No products indexed under this heading.

Estradiol Cypionate (Amprenavir, the active metabolite of fosamprenavir, is metabolized in the liver by the cytochrome P450 enzyme system. Amprenavir may inhibit or induce CYP3A4. Caution should be used when co-administering medications that are substrates, inhibitors, or inducers of CYP3A4, or potentially toxic medications that are metabolized by CYP3A4).
No products indexed under this heading.

Estradiol Valerate (Amprenavir, the active metabolite of fosamprenavir, is metabolized in the liver by the cytochrome P450 enzyme system. Amprenavir may inhibit or induce CYP3A4. Caution should be used when co-administering medications that are substrates, inhibitors, or inducers of CYP3A4, or potentially toxic medications that are metabolized by CYP3A4).
No products indexed under this heading.

Ethinyl Estradiol (Co-administration of fosamprenavir alone with oral contraceptives containing the combination ethinyl estradiol/norethindrone may lead to increased levels of ethinyl estradiol/norethindrone. Because these hormonal levels may be altered, alternative methods of non-hormonal contraception are recommended). Products include:
Alesse-28 Tablets **3392**
Lo/Ovral-28 Tablets **3423**
NuvaRing **2357**
Ortho-Cept Tablets **2395**
Ortho-Cyclen/Ortho Tri-Cyclen **2414**
Ortho Evra Transdermal System **2402**
Ortho Tri-Cyclen Lo Tablets **2421**
Seasonale Tablets **1073**
Triphasil-28 Tablets **3483**
Yasmin 28 Tablets **818**

Ethosuximide (Amprenavir, the active metabolite of fosamprenavir, is metabolized in the liver by the cytochrome P450 enzyme system. Amprenavir may inhibit or induce CYP3A4. Caution should be used when co-administering medications that are substrates, inhibitors, or inducers of CYP3A4, or potentially toxic medications that are metabolized by CYP3A4).
No products indexed under this heading.

Ethynodiol Diacetate (Amprenavir, the active metabolite of fosamprenavir, is metabolized in the liver by the cytochrome P450 enzyme system. Amprenavir may inhibit or induce CYP3A4. Caution should be used when co-administering medications that are substrates, inhibitors, or inducers of CYP3A4, or potentially toxic medications that are metabolized by CYP3A4).
No products indexed under this heading.

Etoposide (Amprenavir, the active metabolite of fosamprenavir, is metabolized in the liver by the cytochrome P450 enzyme system. Amprenavir may inhibit or induce CYP3A4. Caution should be used when co-administering medications that are substrates, inhibitors, or inducers of CYP3A4, or potentially toxic medications that are metabolized by CYP3A4).
No products indexed under this heading.

Etoposide Phosphate (Amprenavir, the active metabolite of fosamprenavir, is metabolized in the liver by the cytochrome P450 enzyme system. Amprenavir may inhibit or induce CYP3A4. Caution should be used when co-administering medications that are substrates, inhibitors, or inducers of CYP3A4, or potentially toxic medications that are metabolized by CYP3A4).
No products indexed under this heading.

Famotidine (Co-administration of fosamprenavir alone and histamine H2-receptor antagonists may lead to decreased levels of fosamprenavir. Use with caution since fosamprenavir may be less effective due to decreased amprenavir plasma concentrations in patients takingthese agents concomitantly). Products include:
Pepcid AC Chewable Tablets **1672**
Pepcid AC Gelcaps **1672**
Pepcid AC Tablets **1672**
Maximum Strength Pepcid AC Tablets **1672**
Pepcid Complete Chewable Tablets **1672**
Pepcid Injection **2017**
Pepcid **2014**

Felbamate (Amprenavir, the active metabolite of fosamprenavir, is metabolized in the liver by the cytochrome P450 enzyme system. Amprenavir may inhibit or induce CYP3A4. Caution should be used when co-administering medications that are substrates, inhibitors, or inducers of CYP3A4, or potentially toxic medications that are metabolized by CYP3A4).
No products indexed under this heading.

Felodipine (Co-administration may increase levels of felodipine; caution is warranted and clinical monitoring is recommended). Products include:
Plendil Extended-Release Tablets **651**

Fentanyl (Amprenavir, the active metabolite of fosamprenavir, is metabolized in the liver by the cytochrome P450 enzyme system. Amprenavir may inhibit or induce CYP3A4. Caution should be used when co-administering medications that are substrates, inhibitors, or inducers of CYP3A4, or potentially toxic medications that are metabolized by CYP3A4). Products include:
Duragesic Transdermal System **2448**

Fentanyl Citrate (Amprenavir, the active metabolite of fosamprenavir, is metabolized in the liver by the cytochrome P450 enzyme system. Amprenavir may inhibit or induce CYP3A4. Caution should be used when co-administering medications that are substrates, inhibitors, or inducers of CYP3A4, or potentially toxic medications that are metabolized by CYP3A4). Products include:
Actiq **993**

Flecainide Acetate (If fosamprenavir is co-administered with ritonavir, the antiarrhythmic agent flecainide is contraindicated due to the potential for serious and/or life-threatening reactions such as cardiac arrhythmias secondary to increases in plasma concentrations of flecainide). Products include:
Tambocor Tablets **1824**

Fluconazole (Amprenavir, the active metabolite of fosamprenavir, is metabolized in the liver by the cytochrome P450 enzyme system. Amprenavir may inhibit or induce CYP3A4. Caution should be used when co-administering medications that are substrates, inhibitors, or inducers of CYP3A4, or potentially toxic medications that are metabolized by CYP3A4).
No products indexed under this heading.

Fludrocortisone Acetate (Amprenavir, the active metabolite of fosamprenavir, is metabolized in the liver by the cytochrome P450 enzyme system. Amprenavir may inhibit or induce CYP3A4. Caution should be used when co-administering medications that are substrates, inhibitors, or inducers of CYP3A4, or potentially toxic medications that are metabolized by CYP3A4).
No products indexed under this heading.

Fluoxetine Hydrochloride (Amprenavir, the active metabolite of fosamprenavir, is metabolized in the liver by the cytochrome P450 enzyme system. Amprenavir may inhibit or induce CYP3A4. Caution should be used when co-administering medications that are substrates, inhibitors, or inducers of CYP3A4, or potentially toxic medications that are metabolized by CYP3A4). Products include:
Prozac Pulvules and Liquid **1771**
Symbyax Capsules **1788**

Flurazepam Hydrochloride (Co-administration may increase flurazepam levels; may need to decrease flurazepam dose). Products include:
Dalmane Capsules **3343**

Fluvoxamine Maleate (Amprenavir, the active metabolite of fosamprenavir, is metabolized in the liver by the cytochrome P450 enzyme system. Amprenavir may inhibit or induce CYP3A4. Caution should be used when co-administering medications that are substrates, inhibitors, or inducers of CYP3A4, or potentially toxic medications that are metabolized by CYP3A4).
No products indexed under this heading.

Fosphenytoin Sodium (Amprenavir, the active metabolite of fosamprenavir, is metabolized in the liver by the cytochrome P450 enzyme system. Amprenavir may inhibit or induce CYP3A4. Caution should be used when co-administering medications that are substrates, inhibitors, or inducers of CYP3A4, or potentially toxic medications that are metabolized by CYP3A4).
No products indexed under this heading.

Garlic Extract (Amprenavir, the active metabolite of fosamprenavir, is metabolized in the liver by the cytochrome P450 enzyme system. Amprenavir may inhibit or induce CYP3A4. Caution should be used when co-administering medications that are substrates, inhibitors, or inducers of CYP3A4, or potentially toxic medications that are metabolized by CYP3A4).
No products indexed under this heading.

Garlic Oil (Amprenavir, the active metabolite of fosamprenavir, is metabolized in the liver by the cytochrome P450 enzyme system. Amprenavir may inhibit or induce CYP3A4. Caution should be used when co-administering medications that are substrates, inhibitors, or inducers of CYP3A4, or potentially toxic medications that are metabolized by CYP3A4).
No products indexed under this heading.

Haloperidol (Amprenavir, the active metabolite of fosamprenavir, is metabolized in the liver by the cytochrome P450 enzyme system. Amprenavir may inhibit or induce CYP3A4. Caution should be used when co-administering medications that are substrates, inhibitors, or inducers of CYP3A4, or potentially toxic medications that are metabolized by CYP3A4).
No products indexed under this heading.

Haloperidol Decanoate (Amprenavir, the active metabolite of fosamprenavir, is metabolized in the liver by the cytochrome P450 enzyme system. Amprenavir may inhibit or induce CYP3A4. Caution should be used when co-administering medications that are substrates, inhibitors, or inducers of CYP3A4, or potentially toxic medications that are metabolized by CYP3A4).
No products indexed under this heading.

Haloperidol Lactate (Amprenavir, the active metabolite of fosamprenavir, is metabolized in the liver by the cytochrome P450 enzyme system. Amprenavir may inhibit or induce CYP3A4. Caution should be used when co-administering medications that are substrates, inhibitors, or inducers of CYP3A4, or potentially toxic medications that are metabolized by CYP3A4).
No products indexed under this heading.

Hydrocortisone (Amprenavir, the active metabolite of fosamprenavir, is metabolized in the liver by the cytochrome P450 enzyme system. Amprenavir may inhibit or induce CYP3A4. Caution should be used when co-administering medications that are substrates, inhibitors, or inducers of CYP3A4, or potentially toxic medications that are metabolized by CYP3A4). Products include:
Cortizone•5 Ointment .... ▣ **699**
Cortizone•10 Creme .... ▣ **699**
Cortizone•10 Ointment .... ▣ **699**
Cortizone•10 Plus Creme .... ▣ **700**
Cortizone•10 Maximum Strength Quick Shot Spray .... ▣ **700**
Hydrocortone Tablets **1963**
Preparation H Hydrocortisone Cream .... ▣ **748**

Hydrocortisone Acetate (Amprenavir, the active metabolite of fosamprenavir, is metabolized in the liver by the cytochrome P450 enzyme system. Amprenavir may inhibit or induce CYP3A4. Caution should be used when co-administering medications that are substrates, inhibitors, or inducers of CYP3A4, or potentially toxic medications that are metabolized by CYP3A4). Products include:
Analpram-HC **1136**
Pramosone **1139**
ProctoFoam-HC **3113**
Tucks Anti-Itch Ointment .... ▣ **712**
U-cort 1% Cream **3289**

Hydrocortisone Butyrate (Amprenavir, the active metabolite of fosamprenavir, is metabolized in the liver by the cytochrome P450 enzyme system. Amprenavir may inhibit or induce CYP3A4. Caution should be used when co-administering medications that are substrates, inhibitors, or inducers of CYP3A4, or potentially toxic medications that are metabolized by CYP3A4). Products include:
Locoid **1138**
Locoid Lipocream Cream **1138**

Hydrocortisone Cypionate (Amprenavir, the active metabolite of fosamprenavir, is metabolized in the liver by the cytochrome P450 enzyme system. Amprenavir may inhibit or induce CYP3A4. Caution should be used when co-administering medications that are substrates, inhibitors, or inducers of CYP3A4, or potentially toxic medications that are metabolized by CYP3A4).
No products indexed under this heading.

Hydrocortisone Hemisuccinate (Amprenavir, the active metabolite of fosamprenavir, is metabolized in the liver by the cytochrome P450 enzyme system. Amprenavir may inhibit or induce CYP3A4. Caution should be used when co-administering medications that are substrates, inhibitors, or inducers of CYP3A4, or potentially toxic medications that are metabolized by CYP3A4).
No products indexed under this heading.

Hydrocortisone Probutate (Amprenavir, the active metabolite of fosamprenavir, is metabolized in the liver by the cytochrome P450 enzyme system. Amprenavir may inhibit or induce CYP3A4. Caution should be used when co-administering medications that are substrates, inhibitors, or inducers of CYP3A4, or potentially toxic medications that are metabolized by CYP3A4). Products include:
Pandel Cream, 0.1% **1017**

Hydrocortisone Sodium Phosphate (Amprenavir, the active metabolite of fosamprenavir, is metabolized in the liver by the cytochrome P450 enzyme system. Amprenavir may inhibit or induce CYP3A4. Caution should be used when co-administering medications that are substrates, inhibitors, or inducers of CYP3A4, or potentially toxic medications that are metabolized by CYP3A4).
No products indexed under this heading.

Hydrocortisone Sodium Succinate (Amprenavir, the active metabolite of fosamprenavir, is metabolized in the liver by the cytochrome P450 enzyme system. Amprenavir may inhibit or induce CYP3A4. Caution should be used when co-administering medications that are substrates, inhibitors, or inducers of CYP3A4, or potentially toxic medications that are metabolized by CYP3A4).
No products indexed under this heading.

Hydrocortisone Valerate (Amprenavir, the active metabolite of fosamprenavir, is metabolized in the liver by the cytochrome P450 enzyme system. Amprenavir may inhibit or induce CYP3A4. Caution should be used when co-administering medications that are substrates, inhibitors, or inducers of CYP3A4, or potentially toxic medications that are metabolized by CYP3A4).
No products indexed under this heading.

Hypericum (Co-administration may lead to loss of virologic response and possible resistance to fosamprenavir or other protease inhibitors).
No products indexed under this heading.

Hypericum Perforatum (Co-administration may lead to loss of virologic response and possible resistance to fosamprenavir or other protease inhibitors).
No products indexed under this heading.

Imipramine Hydrochloride (Co-administration may lead to increased levels of imipramine. Therapeutic concentration monitoring is recommended for tricyclic antidepressants when co-administered with fosamprenavir).
No products indexed under this heading.

Imipramine Pamoate (Co-administration may lead to increased levels of imipramine. Therapeutic concentration monitoring is recommended for tricyclic antidepressants when co-administered with fosamprenavir).
No products indexed under this heading.

Indinavir Sulfate (Co-administration with fosamprenavir alone may lead to increased amprenavir levels). Products include:
Crixivan Capsules 1918

Isoniazid (Amprenavir, the active metabolite of fosamprenavir, is metabolized in the liver by the cytochrome P450 enzyme system. Amprenavir may inhibit or induce CYP3A4. Caution should be used when co-administering medications that are substrates, inhibitors, or inducers of CYP3A4, or potentially toxic medications that are metabolized by CYP3A4).
No products indexed under this heading.

Isradipine (Co-administration may increase levels of isradipine; caution is warranted and clinical monitoring is recommended). Products include:
DynaCirc CR Tablets 2726

Itraconazole (Co-administration may increase itraconazole levels; increase monitoring for adverse events due to itraconazole. When co-administered with fosamprenavir alone; itraconazole dose reduction may be needed for patients receiving more than 400mg of itraconazole per day. If patient is receiving fosamprenavir/ritonavir combination, co-administration of high doses of itraconazole (>200mg/day) is not recommended).
No products indexed under this heading.

Ketoconazole (Co-administration may increase ketoconazole levels; increase monitoring for adverse events due to ketoconazole. When co-administered with fosamprenavir alone; ketoconazole dose reduction may be needed for patients receiving more than 400mg of ketoconazole per day. If patient is receiving fosamprenavir/ritonavir combination, co-administration of high doses of ketoconazole (>200mg/day) is not recommended). Products include:
Nizoral A-D Shampoo, 1% 1839
Nizoral 2% Shampoo 1838

Lansoprazole (Co-administration of fosamprenavir alone and proton-pump inhibitors may lead to decreased levels of fosamprenavir. Use with caution since fosamprenavir may be less effective due to decreased amprenavir plasma concentrations in patients taking these agents concomitantly). Products include:
Prevacid Delayed-Release Capsules 3268
Prevacid for Delayed-Release Oral Suspension 3268
Prevacid I.V. for Injection 3274
Prevacid NapraPAC 3277
Prevacid SoluTab Delayed-Release Orally Disintegrating Tablets 3268
PREVPAC 3281

Levonorgestrel (Amprenavir, the active metabolite of fosamprenavir, is metabolized in the liver by the cytochrome P450 enzyme system. Amprenavir may inhibit or induce CYP3A4. Caution should be used when co-administering medications that are substrates, inhibitors, or inducers of CYP3A4, or potentially toxic medications that are metabolized by CYP3A4). Products include:
Alesse-28 Tablets 3392
Climara Pro Transdermal System 800
Mirena Intrauterine System 810
Plan B Tablets 1068
Seasonale Tablets 1073
Triphasil-28 Tablets 3483

Lidocaine (Co-administration may lead to increased levels of lidocaine. Caution is warranted and therapeutic concentration monitoring is recommended for antiarrhythmics when co-administered with fosamprenavir). Products include:
Lidoderm Patch 1107

Lidocaine Hydrochloride (Co-administration may lead to increased levels of lidocaine. Caution is warranted and therapeutic concentration monitoring is recommended for antiarrhythmics when co-administered with fosamprenavir).
No products indexed under this heading.

Lopinavir (Co-administration of lopinavir/ritonavir and fosamprenavir may lead to decreased levels of amprenavir and lopinavir. An increased rate of adverse events has also been observed with co-administration of these medications). Products include:
Kaletra 474

Loratadine (Amprenavir, the active metabolite of fosamprenavir, is metabolized in the liver by the cytochrome P450 enzyme system. Amprenavir may inhibit or induce CYP3A4. Caution should be used when co-administering medications that are substrates, inhibitors, or inducers of CYP3A4, or potentially toxic medications that are metabolized by CYP3A4). Products include:
Alavert Allergy & Sinus D-12 Hour Tablets 743
Alavert 743
Children's Claritin 24 Hour Non-Drowsy Allergy Syrup 732
Claritin Non-Drowsy 24 Hour Tablets 731
Non-Drowsy Claritin Hives Relief Tablets 733
Claritin Reditabs 24 Hour Non-Drowsy Tablets 732
Claritin-D Non-Drowsy 12 Hour Tablets 731
Claritin-D Non-Drowsy 24 Hour Tablets 731
Children's Dimetapp ND Non-Drowsy Allergy Syrup 746
Triaminic Allerchews 684

Lovastatin (Co-administration may lead to the potential for serious reactions such as risk of myopathy including rhabdomyolysis). Products include:
Advicor Tablets 1694
Altoprev Extended-Release Tablets 1151
Mevacor Tablets 1996

Mephenytoin (Amprenavir, the active metabolite of fosamprenavir, is metabolized in the liver by the cytochrome P450 enzyme system. Amprenavir may inhibit or induce CYP3A4. Caution should be used when co-administering medications that are substrates, inhibitors, or inducers of CYP3A4, or potentially toxic medications that are metabolized by CYP3A4).
No products indexed under this heading.

Mestranol (Amprenavir, the active metabolite of fosamprenavir, is metabolized in the liver by the cytochrome P450 enzyme system. Amprenavir may inhibit or induce CYP3A4. Caution should be used when co-administering medications that are substrates, inhibitors, or inducers of CYP3A4, or potentially toxic medications that are metabolized by CYP3A4).
No products indexed under this heading.

Methadone Hydrochloride (Co-administration may lead to decreased levels of methadone; dosage of methadone may need to be increased when co-administered with fosamprenavir).
No products indexed under this heading.

Methsuximide (Amprenavir, the active metabolite of fosamprenavir, is metabolized in the liver by the cytochrome P450 enzyme system. Amprenavir may inhibit or induce CYP3A4. Caution should be used when co-administering medications that are substrates, inhibitors, or inducers of CYP3A4, or potentially toxic medications that are metabolized by CYP3A4).
No products indexed under this heading.

Methylergonovine Maleate (Co-administration with methylergonovine is contraindicated due to the potential for serious and/or life-threatening reactions such as acute ergot toxicity characterized by peripheral vasospasm and ischemia of the extremities and other tissues).
No products indexed under this heading.

Methylprednisolone (Amprenavir, the active metabolite of fosamprenavir, is metabolized in the liver by the cytochrome P450 enzyme system. Amprenavir may inhibit or induce CYP3A4. Caution should be used when co-administering medications that are substrates, inhibitors, or inducers of CYP3A4, or potentially toxic medications that are metabolized by CYP3A4).
No products indexed under this heading.

Methylprednisolone Acetate (Amprenavir, the active metabolite of fosamprenavir, is metabolized in the liver by the cytochrome P450 enzyme system. Amprenavir may inhibit or induce CYP3A4. Caution should be used when co-administering medications that are substrates, inhibitors, or inducers of CYP3A4, or potentially toxic medications that are metabolized by CYP3A4). Products include:
Depo-Medrol Injectable Suspension 2615
Depo-Medrol Single-Dose Vial 2617

Methylprednisolone Sodium Succinate (Amprenavir, the active metabolite of fosamprenavir, is metabolized in the liver by the cytochrome P450 enzyme system. Amprenavir may inhibit or induce CYP3A4. Caution should be used when co-administering medications that are substrates, inhibitors, or inducers of CYP3A4, or potentially toxic medications that are metabolized by CYP3A4).
No products indexed under this heading.

Metronidazole (Amprenavir, the active metabolite of fosamprenavir, is metabolized in the liver by the cytochrome P450 enzyme system. Amprenavir may inhibit or induce CYP3A4. Caution should be used when co-administering medications that are substrates, inhibitors, or inducers of CYP3A4, or potentially toxic medications that are metabolized by CYP3A4). Products include:
Metrogel 1% 1212
MetroGel-Vaginal Gel 1822
Noritate Cream, 1% 1051

Metronidazole Benzoate (Amprenavir, the active metabolite of fosamprenavir, is metabolized in the liver by the cytochrome P450 enzyme system. Amprenavir may inhibit or induce CYP3A4. Caution should be used when co-administering medications that are substrates, inhibitors, or inducers of CYP3A4, or potentially toxic medications that are metabolized by CYP3A4).
No products indexed under this heading.

Metronidazole Hydrochloride (Amprenavir, the active metabolite of fosamprenavir, is metabolized in the liver by the cytochrome P450 enzyme system. Amprenavir may inhibit or induce CYP3A4. Caution should be used when co-administering medications that are substrates, inhibitors, or inducers of CYP3A4, or potentially toxic medications that are metabolized by CYP3A4).
No products indexed under this heading.

Miconazole (Amprenavir, the active metabolite of fosamprenavir, is metabolized in the liver by the cytochrome P450 enzyme system. Amprenavir may inhibit or induce CYP3A4. Caution should be used when co-administering medications that are substrates, inhibitors, or inducers of CYP3A4, or potentially toxic medications that are metabolized by CYP3A4).
No products indexed under this heading.

Miconazole Nitrate (Amprenavir, the active metabolite of fosamprenavir, is metabolized in the liver by the cytochrome P450 enzyme system. Amprenavir may inhibit or induce CYP3A4. Caution should be used when co-administering medications that are substrates, inhibitors, or inducers of CYP3A4, or potentially toxic medications that are metabolized by CYP3A4). Products include:
Desenex .... ▣ 674
Desenex Jock Itch Spray Powder .... ▣ 674

Midazolam Hydrochloride (Co-administration with midazolam is contraindicated due to potential for serious and/or life-threatening reactions such as prolonged or increased sedation or respiratory depression).
No products indexed under this heading.

Modafinil (Amprenavir, the active metabolite of fosamprenavir, is metabolized in the liver by the cytochrome P450 enzyme system. Amprenavir may inhibit or induce CYP3A4. Caution should be used when co-administering medications that are substrates, inhibitors, or inducers of CYP3A4, or potentially toxic medications that are metabolized by CYP3A4). Products include:
Provigil Tablets 1002

Nefazodone Hydrochloride (Amprenavir, the active metabolite of fosamprenavir, is metabolized in the liver by the cytochrome P450 enzyme system. Amprenavir may inhibit or induce CYP3A4. Caution should be used when co-administering medications that are substrates, inhibitors, or inducers of CYP3A4, or potentially toxic medications that are metabolized by CYP3A4).
No products indexed under this heading.

Nelfinavir Mesylate (Co-administration with fosamprenavir alone may lead to increased amprenavir levels). Products include:
Viracept 2556

Nevirapine (Co-administration may lead to decreased amprenavir levels and increased nevirapine levels. Co-administration of nevirapine and fosamprenavir calcium is not recommended). Products include:
Viramune Oral Suspension 903
Viramune Tablets 903

Niacinamide (Amprenavir, the active metabolite of fosamprenavir, is metabolized in the liver by the cytochrome P450 enzyme system. Amprenavir may inhibit or induce CYP3A4. Caution should be used when co-administering medications that are substrates, inhibitors, or inducers of CYP3A4, or potentially toxic medications that are metabolized by CYP3A4).
No products indexed under this heading.

Nicardipine (Co-administration may increase levels of nicardipine; caution is warranted and clinical monitoring is recommended).
No products indexed under this heading.

Nicardipine Hydrochloride (Co-administration may increase levels of nicardipine; caution is warranted and clinical monitoring is recommended). Products include:
Cardene I.V. 1129

Nicotinamide (Amprenavir, the active metabolite of fosamprenavir, is metabolized in the liver by the cytochrome P450 enzyme system. Amprenavir may inhibit or induce CYP3A4. Caution should be used when co-administering medications that are substrates, inhibitors, or inducers of CYP3A4, or potentially toxic medications that are metabolized by CYP3A4). Products include:
Nicomide Tablets 3190

Nifedipine (Co-administration may increase levels of nifedipine, caution is warranted and clinical monitoring is recommended). Products include:
Adalat CC Tablets 2978

Nimodipine (Co-administration may increase levels of nimodipine; caution is warranted and clinical monitoring is recommended). Products include:
Nimotop Capsules 774

Nisoldipine (Co-administration may increase levels of nisoldipine; caution is warranted and clinical monitoring is recommended). Products include:
Sular Tablets 1163

Nitrendipine (Amprenavir, the active metabolite of fosamprenavir, is metabolized in the liver by the cytochrome P450 enzyme system. Amprenavir may inhibit or induce CYP3A4. Caution should be used when co-administering medications that are substrates, inhibitors, or inducers of CYP3A4, or potentially toxic medications that are metabolized by CYP3A4).
No products indexed under this heading.

Nizatidine (Co-administration of fosamprenavir alone and histamine H2-receptor antagonists may lead to decreased levels of fosamprenavir. Use with caution since fosamprenavir may be less effective due to decreased amprenavir plasma concentrations in patients takingthese agents concomitantly). Products include:
Axid Oral Solution 913

Norethindrone (Co-administration of fosamprenavir alone with oral contraceptives containing the combination ethinyl estradiol/norethindrone may lead to increased levels of ethinyl estradiol/norethindrone. Because these hormonal levels may be altered, alternative methods of non-hormonal contraception are recommended). Products include:
Ortho Micronor Tablets 2411

Norethindrone Acetate (Amprenavir, the active metabolite of fosamprenavir, is metabolized in the liver by the cytochrome P450 enzyme system. Amprenavir may inhibit or induce CYP3A4. Caution should be used when co-administering medications that are substrates, inhibitors, or inducers of CYP3A4, or potentially toxic medications that are metabolized by CYP3A4). Products include:
Activella Tablets 2311
Aygestin Tablets 1062
CombiPatch Transdermal System 2180

Norfloxacin (Amprenavir, the active metabolite of fosamprenavir, is metabolized in the liver by the cytochrome P450 enzyme system. Amprenavir may inhibit or induce CYP3A4. Caution should be used when co-administering medications that are substrates, inhibitors, or inducers of CYP3A4, or potentially toxic medications that are metabolized by CYP3A4). Products include:
Noroxin Tablets 2009

Norgestrel (Amprenavir, the active metabolite of fosamprenavir, is metabolized in the liver by the cytochrome P450 enzyme system. Amprenavir may inhibit or induce CYP3A4. Caution should be used when co-administering medications that are substrates, inhibitors, or inducers of CYP3A4, or potentially toxic medications that are metabolized by CYP3A4). Products include:
Lo/Ovral-28 Tablets 3423

Omeprazole (Amprenavir, the active metabolite of fosamprenavir, is metabolized in the liver by the cytochrome P450 enzyme system. Amprenavir may inhibit or induce CYP3A4. Caution should be used when co-administering medications that are substrates, inhibitors, or inducers of CYP3A4, or potentially toxic medications that are metabolized by CYP3A4). Products include:
Zegerid Powder for Oral Solution 2972

Ondansetron (Amprenavir, the active metabolite of fosamprenavir, is metabolized in the liver by the cytochrome P450 enzyme system. Amprenavir may inhibit or induce CYP3A4. Caution should be used when co-administering medications that are substrates, inhibitors, or inducers of CYP3A4, or potentially toxic medications that are metabolized by CYP3A4). Products include:
Zofran ODT Orally Disintegrating Tablets 1613

Ondansetron Hydrochloride (Amprenavir, the active metabolite of fosamprenavir, is metabolized in the liver by the cytochrome P450 enzyme system. Amprenavir may inhibit or induce CYP3A4. Caution should be used when co-administering medications that are substrates, inhibitors, or inducers of CYP3A4, or potentially toxic medications that are metabolized by CYP3A4). Products include:
Zofran Injection 1607
Zofran 1613

Oxcarbazepine (Amprenavir, the active metabolite of fosamprenavir, is metabolized in the liver by the cytochrome P450 enzyme system. Amprenavir may inhibit or induce CYP3A4. Caution should be used when co-administering medications that are substrates, inhibitors, or inducers of CYP3A4, or potentially toxic medications that are metabolized by CYP3A4). Products include:
Trileptal Oral Suspension 2281
Trileptal Tablets 2281

Paclitaxel (Amprenavir, the active metabolite of fosamprenavir, is metabolized in the liver by the cytochrome P450 enzyme system. Amprenavir may inhibit or induce CYP3A4. Caution should be used when co-administering medications that are substrates, inhibitors, or inducers of CYP3A4, or potentially toxic medications that are metabolized by CYP3A4).
No products indexed under this heading.

Pantoprazole Sodium (Co-administration of fosamprenavir alone and proton-pump inhibitors may lead to decreased levels of fosamprenavir. Use with caution since fosamprenavir may be less effective due to decreased amprenavir plasma concentrations in patients taking these agents concomitantly). Products include:
Protonix I.V. 3468
Protonix Tablets 3465

Paroxetine Hydrochloride (Amprenavir, the active metabolite of fosamprenavir, is metabolized in the liver by the cytochrome P450 enzyme system. Amprenavir may inhibit or induce CYP3A4. Caution should be used when co-administering medications that are substrates, inhibitors, or inducers of CYP3A4, or potentially toxic medications that are metabolized by CYP3A4). Products include:
Paxil CR Controlled-Release Tablets 1509
Paxil 1501

Phenobarbital (Co-administration may lead to decreased amprenavir levels. Use with caution; fosamprenavir may be less effective due to decreased plasma concentrations in patients taking these agents concomitantly).
No products indexed under this heading.

Phenobarbital Sodium (Co-administration may lead to decreased amprenavir levels. Use with caution; fosamprenavir may be less effective due to decreased plasma concentrations in patients taking these agents concomitantly).
No products indexed under this heading.

Phenytoin (Amprenavir, the active metabolite of fosamprenavir, is metabolized in the liver by the cytochrome P450 enzyme system. Amprenavir may inhibit or induce CYP3A4. Caution should be used when co-administering medications that are substrates, inhibitors, or inducers of CYP3A4, or potentially toxic medications that are metabolized by CYP3A4).
No products indexed under this heading.

Phenytoin Sodium (Amprenavir, the active metabolite of fosamprenavir, is metabolized in the liver by the cytochrome P450 enzyme system. Amprenavir may inhibit or induce CYP3A4. Caution should be used when co-administering medications that are substrates, inhibitors, or inducers of CYP3A4, or potential-

ly toxic medications that are metabolized by CYP3A4). Products include:
Phenytek Capsules 2153

Pimozide (Co-administration with pimozide is contraindicated due to potential for serious and/or life-threatening reactions such as cardiac arrhythmias). Products include:
Orap Tablets 1220

Polyestradiol Phosphate (Amprenavir, the active metabolite of fosamprenavir, is metabolized in the liver by the cytochrome P450 enzyme system. Amprenavir may inhibit or induce CYP3A4. Caution should be used when co-administering medications that are substrates, inhibitors, or inducers of CYP3A4, or potentially toxic medications that are metabolized by CYP3A4).
No products indexed under this heading.

Prednisolone Acetate (Amprenavir, the active metabolite of fosamprenavir, is metabolized in the liver by the cytochrome P450 enzyme system. Amprenavir may inhibit or induce CYP3A4. Caution should be used when co-administering medications that are substrates, inhibitors, or inducers of CYP3A4, or potentially toxic medications that are metabolized by CYP3A4). Products include:
Blephamide Ophthalmic Ointment 563
Blephamide Ophthalmic Suspension.................................. 564
Poly-Pred Liquifilm Ophthalmic Suspension .... ⊙ 231
Pred Forte Ophthalmic Suspension .... ⊙ 233
Pred Mild Sterile Ophthalmic Suspension .... ⊙ 236
Pred-G Ophthalmic Suspension ...... ⊙ 234
Pred-G Sterile Ophthalmic Ointment.................................... ⊙ 235

Prednisolone Sodium Phosphate (Amprenavir, the active metabolite of fosamprenavir, is metabolized in the liver by the cytochrome P450 enzyme system. Amprenavir may inhibit or induce CYP3A4. Caution should be used when co-administering medications that are substrates, inhibitors, or inducers of CYP3A4, or potentially toxic medications that are metabolized by CYP3A4). Products include:
Pediapred Oral Solution 3319

Prednisolone Tebutate (Amprenavir, the active metabolite of fosamprenavir, is metabolized in the liver by the cytochrome P450 enzyme system. Amprenavir may inhibit or induce CYP3A4. Caution should be used when co-administering medications that are substrates, inhibitors, or inducers of CYP3A4, or potentially toxic medications that are metabolized by CYP3A4).
No products indexed under this heading.

Prednisone (Amprenavir, the active metabolite of fosamprenavir, is metabolized in the liver by the cytochrome P450 enzyme system. Amprenavir may inhibit or induce CYP3A4. Caution should be used when co-administering medications that are substrates, inhibitors, or inducers of CYP3A4, or potentially toxic medications that are metabolized by CYP3A4).
No products indexed under this heading.

Primidone (Amprenavir, the active metabolite of fosamprenavir, is metabolized in the liver by the cytochrome P450 enzyme system. Amprenavir may inhibit or induce CYP3A4. Caution should be used when co-administering medications that are substrates, inhibitors, or inducers of CYP3A4, or potentially toxic medications that are metabolized by CYP3A4).
No products indexed under this heading.

Propafenone Hydrochloride (If fosamprenavir is co-administered with ritonavir, the antiarrhythmic agent propafenone is contraindicated due to the potential for serious and/or life-threatening reactions such as cardiac arrhythmias secondary to increases in plasma concentrations of propafenone). Products include:
Rythmol SR Capsules 2736

Propoxyphene Hydrochloride (Amprenavir, the active metabolite of fosamprenavir, is metabolized in the liver by the cytochrome P450 enzyme system. Amprenavir may inhibit or induce CYP3A4. Caution should be used when co-administering medications that are substrates, inhibitors, or inducers of CYP3A4, or potentially toxic medications that are metabolized by CYP3A4).
No products indexed under this heading.

Propoxyphene Napsylate (Amprenavir, the active metabolite of fosamprenavir, is metabolized in the liver by the cytochrome P450 enzyme system. Amprenavir may inhibit or induce CYP3A4. Caution should be used when co-administering medications that are substrates, inhibitors, or inducers of CYP3A4, or potentially toxic medications that are metabolized by CYP3A4). Products include:
Darvocet A 500 Tablets 3497

Quinidine (Co-administration may lead to increased levels of quinidine. Caution is warranted and therapeutic concentration monitoring is recommended for antiarrhythmics when co-administered with fosamprenavir).
No products indexed under this heading.

Quinidine Gluconate (Co-administration may lead to increased levels of quinidine. Caution is warranted and therapeutic concentration monitoring is recommended for antiarrhythmics when co-administered with fosamprenavir).
No products indexed under this heading.

Quinidine Hydrochloride (Co-administration may lead to increased levels of quinidine. Caution is warranted and therapeutic concentration monitoring is recommended for antiarrhythmics when co-administered with fosamprenavir).
No products indexed under this heading.

Quinidine Polygalacturonate (Co-administration may lead to increased levels of quinidine. Caution is warranted and therapeutic concentration monitoring is recommended for antiarrhythmics when co-administered with fosamprenavir).
No products indexed under this heading.

Quinidine Sulfate (Co-administration may lead to increased levels of quinidine. Caution is warranted and therapeutic concentration monitoring is recommended for antiarrhythmics when co-administered with fosamprenavir).
No products indexed under this heading.

Quinine (Amprenavir, the active metabolite of fosamprenavir, is metabolized in the liver by the cytochrome P450 enzyme system. Amprenavir may inhibit or induce CYP3A4. Caution should be used when co-administering medications that are substrates, inhibitors, or inducers of CYP3A4, or potentially toxic medications that are metabolized by CYP3A4).
No products indexed under this heading.

Quinine Sulfate (Amprenavir, the active metabolite of fosamprenavir, is metabolized in the liver by the cytochrome P450 enzyme system. Amprenavir may inhibit or induce CYP3A4. Caution should be used when co-administering medications that are substrates, inhibitors, or inducers of CYP3A4, or potentially toxic medications that are metabolized by CYP3A4).
No products indexed under this heading.

Quinupristin (Amprenavir, the active metabolite of fosamprenavir, is metabolized in the liver by the cytochrome P450 enzyme system. Amprenavir may inhibit or induce CYP3A4. Caution should be used when co-administering medications that are substrates, inhibitors, or inducers of CYP3A4, or potentially toxic medications that are metabolized by CYP3A4). Products include:
Synercid I.V. 1690

Rabeprazole Sodium (Co-administration of fosamprenavir alone and proton-pump inhibitors may lead to decreased levels of fosamprenavir. Use with caution since fosamprenavir may be less effective due to decreased amprenavir plasma concentrations in patients taking these agents concomitantly). Products include:
Aciphex Tablets 1081

Ranitidine Bismuth Citrate (Amprenavir, the active metabolite of fosamprenavir, is metabolized in the liver by the cytochrome P450 enzyme system. Amprenavir may inhibit or induce CYP3A4. Caution should be used when co-administering medications that are substrates, inhibitors, or inducers of CYP3A4, or potentially toxic medications that are metabolized by CYP3A4).
No products indexed under this heading.

Ranitidine Hydrochloride (Amprenavir, the active metabolite of fosamprenavir, is metabolized in the liver by the cytochrome P450 enzyme system. Amprenavir may inhibit or induce CYP3A4. Caution should be used when co-administering medications that are substrates, inhibitors, or inducers of CYP3A4, or potentially toxic medications that are metabolized by CYP3A4). Products include:
Zantac 1597
Zantac Injection 1593
Zantac 75 Tablets 715
Zantac 150 Maximum Strength Tablets.. 715
Zantac Injection Pharmacy Bulk Package 1595

Rapamycin (Co-administration may lead to increased levels of rapamycin. Therapeutic concentration monitoring is recommended for immunosuppressant agents when co-administered with fosamprenavir).
No products indexed under this heading.

Rifabutin (Co-administration may cause increased levels of rifabutin and its metabolite; perform CBC weekly and as clinically indicated in order to monitor for neutropenia in patients receiving concurrent administration. In patients receiving fosamprenavir alone, a dosage reduction of rifabutin by at least half the recommended dose is required. In patients receiving fosamprenavir/ritonavir combination, dosage reduction of rifabutin by at least 75% of the usual dose of 300mg/day is recommended (maximum dose of 150mg every other day or three times weekly)).
No products indexed under this heading.

Rifampicin (Amprenavir, the active metabolite of fosamprenavir, is metabolized in the liver by the cytochrome P450 enzyme system. Amprenavir may inhibit or induce CYP3A4. Caution should be used when co-administering medications that are substrates, inhibitors, or inducers of CYP3A4, or potentially toxic medications that are metabolized by CYP3A4).
No products indexed under this heading.

Rifampin (Co-administration may lead to loss of virologic response and possible resistance to fosamprenavir or other protease inhibitors).
No products indexed under this heading.

Rifapentine (Amprenavir, the active metabolite of fosamprenavir, is metabolized in the liver by the cytochrome P450 enzyme system. Amprenavir may inhibit or induce CYP3A4. Caution should be used when co-administering medications that are substrates, inhibitors, or inducers of CYP3A4, or potentially toxic medications that are metabolized by CYP3A4).
No products indexed under this heading.

Ritonavir (Co-administration of lopinavir/ritonavir and fosamprenavir may lead to decreased levels of amprenavir and lopinavir (when given in combination with ritonavir). An increased rate of adverse events has also been observed with co-administration of these medications). Products include:
Kaletra 474
Norvir 499

Saquinavir (Co-administration with fosamprenavir alone may lead to decreased levels of amprenavir).
No products indexed under this heading.

Saquinavir Mesylate (Amprenavir, the active metabolite of fosamprenavir, is metabolized in the liver by the cytochrome P450 enzyme system. Amprenavir may inhibit or induce CYP3A4. Caution should be used when co-administering medications that are substrates, inhibitors,

or inducers of CYP3A4, or potentially toxic medications that are metabolized by CYP3A4). Products include:
Invirase 2776

Sertraline Hydrochloride (Amprenavir, the active metabolite of fosamprenavir, is metabolized in the liver by the cytochrome P450 enzyme system. Amprenavir may inhibit or induce CYP3A4. Caution should be used when co-administering medications that are substrates, inhibitors, or inducers of CYP3A4, or potentially toxic medications that are metabolized by CYP3A4). Products include:
Zoloft 2581

Sildenafil Citrate (Co-administration may lead to increased levels of sildenafil; use sildenafil with caution at reduced doses of 25mg every 48 hours with increased monitoring for adverse events). Products include:
Revatio Tablets 2541
Viagra Tablets 2552

Simvastatin (Co-administration may lead to the potential for serious reactions such as risk of myopathy including rhabdomyolysis). Products include:
Vytorin 10/10 Tablets 2084
Vytorin 10/10 Tablets 3092
Vytorin 10/20 Tablets 2084
Vytorin 10/20 Tablets 3092
Vytorin 10/40 Tablets 3092
Vytorin 10/40 Tablets 2084
Vytorin 10/80 Tablets 2084
Vytorin 10/80 Tablets 3092
Zocor Tablets 2078

Sirolimus (Amprenavir, the active metabolite of fosamprenavir, is metabolized in the liver by the cytochrome P450 enzyme system. Amprenavir may inhibit or induce CYP3A4. Caution should be used when co-administering medications that are substrates, inhibitors, or inducers of CYP3A4, or potentially toxic medications that are metabolized by CYP3A4). Products include:
Rapamune Oral Solution and Tablets 3472

Sulfinpyrazone (Amprenavir, the active metabolite of fosamprenavir, is metabolized in the liver by the cytochrome P450 enzyme system. Amprenavir may inhibit or induce CYP3A4. Caution should be used when co-administering medications that are substrates, inhibitors, or inducers of CYP3A4, or potentially toxic medications that are metabolized by CYP3A4).
No products indexed under this heading.

Tacrolimus (Co-administration may lead to increased levels of tacrolimus. Therapeutic concentration monitoring is recommended for immunosuppressant agents when co-administered with fosamprenavir). Products include:
Prograf Capsules and Injection 624
Protopic Ointment 629

Tamoxifen Citrate (Amprenavir, the active metabolite of fosamprenavir, is metabolized in the liver by the cytochrome P450 enzyme system. Amprenavir may inhibit or induce CYP3A4. Caution should be used when co-administering medications that are substrates, inhibitors, or inducers of CYP3A4, or potentially toxic medications that are metabolized by CYP3A4).
No products indexed under this heading.

Telithromycin (Amprenavir, the active metabolite of fosamprenavir, is metabolized in the liver by the cytochrome P450 enzyme system. Amprenavir may inhibit or induce CYP3A4. Caution should be used when co-administering medications that are substrates, inhibitors, or inducers of CYP3A4, or potentially toxic medications that are metabolized by CYP3A4). Products include:
Ketek Tablets 2920

Theophylline (Amprenavir, the active metabolite of fosamprenavir, is metabolized in the liver by the cytochrome P450 enzyme system. Amprenavir may inhibit or induce CYP3A4. Caution should be used when co-administering medications that are substrates, inhibitors, or inducers of CYP3A4, or potentially toxic medications that are metabolized by CYP3A4).
No products indexed under this heading.

Tiagabine Hydrochloride (Amprenavir, the active metabolite of fosamprenavir, is metabolized in the liver by the cytochrome P450 enzyme system. Amprenavir may inhibit or induce CYP3A4. Caution should be used when co-administering medications that are substrates, inhibitors, or inducers of CYP3A4, or potentially toxic medications that are metabolized by CYP3A4). Products include:
Gabitril Tablets 998

Tolterodine Tartrate (Amprenavir, the active metabolite of fosamprenavir, is metabolized in the liver by the cytochrome P450 enzyme system. Amprenavir may inhibit or induce CYP3A4. Caution should be used when co-administering medications that are substrates, inhibitors, or inducers of CYP3A4, or potentially toxic medications that are metabolized by CYP3A4). Products include:
Detrol Tablets 2626
Detrol LA Capsules 2629

Trazodone Hydrochloride (Amprenavir, the active metabolite of fosamprenavir, is metabolized in the liver by the cytochrome P450 enzyme system. Amprenavir may inhibit or induce CYP3A4. Caution should be used when co-administering medications that are substrates, inhibitors, or inducers of CYP3A4, or potentially toxic medications that are metabolized by CYP3A4).
No products indexed under this heading.

Triamcinolone (Amprenavir, the active metabolite of fosamprenavir, is metabolized in the liver by the cytochrome P450 enzyme system. Amprenavir may inhibit or induce CYP3A4. Caution should be used when co-administering medications that are substrates, inhibitors, or inducers of CYP3A4, or potentially toxic medications that are metabolized by CYP3A4).
No products indexed under this heading.

Triamcinolone Acetonide (Amprenavir, the active metabolite of fosamprenavir, is metabolized in the liver by the cytochrome P450 enzyme system. Amprenavir may inhibit or induce CYP3A4. Caution should be used when co-administering medications that are substrates, inhibitors, or inducers of CYP3A4, or potentially toxic medications that are metabolized by CYP3A4). Products include:
Azmacort Inhalation Aerosol 1701
Nasacort HFA Inhalation Aerosol 2939
Nasacort AQ Nasal Spray 2937

Triamcinolone Diacetate (Amprenavir, the active metabolite of fosamprenavir, is metabolized in the liver by the cytochrome P450 enzyme system. Amprenavir may inhibit or induce CYP3A4. Caution should be used when co-administering medications that are substrates, inhibitors, or inducers of CYP3A4, or potentially toxic medications that are metabolized by CYP3A4).
No products indexed under this heading.

Triamcinolone Hexacetonide (Amprenavir, the active metabolite of fosamprenavir, is metabolized in the liver by the cytochrome P450 enzyme system. Amprenavir may inhibit or induce CYP3A4. Caution should be used when co-administering medications that are substrates, inhibitors, or inducers of CYP3A4, or potentially toxic medications that are metabolized by CYP3A4).
No products indexed under this heading.

Triazolam (Co-administration with triazolam is contraindicated due to potential for serious and/or life-threatening reactions such as prolonged or increased sedation or respiratory depression).
No products indexed under this heading.

Troglitazone (Amprenavir, the active metabolite of fosamprenavir, is metabolized in the liver by the cytochrome P450 enzyme system. Amprenavir may inhibit or induce CYP3A4. Caution should be used when co-administering medications that are substrates, inhibitors, or inducers of CYP3A4, or potentially toxic medications that are metabolized by CYP3A4).
No products indexed under this heading.

Troleandomycin (Amprenavir, the active metabolite of fosamprenavir, is metabolized in the liver by the cytochrome P450 enzyme system. Amprenavir may inhibit or induce CYP3A4. Caution should be used when co-administering medications that are substrates, inhibitors, or inducers of CYP3A4, or potentially toxic medications that are metabolized by CYP3A4).
No products indexed under this heading.

Valproate Sodium (Amprenavir, the active metabolite of fosamprenavir, is metabolized in the liver by the cytochrome P450 enzyme system. Amprenavir may inhibit or induce CYP3A4. Caution should be used when co-administering medications that are substrates, inhibitors, or inducers of CYP3A4, or potentially toxic medications that are metabolized by CYP3A4). Products include:
Depacon Injection 412

Vardenafil Hydrochloride (Co-administration may lead to increased levels of vardenafil. When co-administered with fosamprenavir alone, use vardenafil with caution at reduced doses of no more than 2.5mg every 24 hours with increased monitoring for adverse events. When co-administered with fosamprenavir/ritonavir combination, use vardenafil with caution at reduced doses of no more than 2.5mg every 72 hours with increased monitoring for adverse events). Products include:
Levitra Tablets 3048

Verapamil Hydrochloride (Co-administration may increase levels of verapamil; caution is warranted and clinical monitoring is recommended). Products include:
Covera-HS Tablets 3135
Tarka Tablets 519
Verelan PM Capsules 3120

Vinblastine Sulfate (Amprenavir, the active metabolite of fosamprenavir, is metabolized in the liver by the cytochrome P450 enzyme system. Amprenavir may inhibit or induce CYP3A4. Caution should be used when co-administering medications that are substrates, inhibitors, or inducers of CYP3A4, or potentially toxic medications that are metabolized by CYP3A4).
No products indexed under this heading.

Vincristine Sulfate (Amprenavir, the active metabolite of fosamprenavir, is metabolized in the liver by the cytochrome P450 enzyme system. Amprenavir may inhibit or induce CYP3A4. Caution should be used when co-administering medications that are substrates, inhibitors, or inducers of CYP3A4, or potentially toxic medications that are metabolized by CYP3A4).
No products indexed under this heading.

Voriconazole (Amprenavir, the active metabolite of fosamprenavir, is metabolized in the liver by the cytochrome P450 enzyme system. Amprenavir may inhibit or induce CYP3A4. Caution should be used when co-administering medications that are substrates, inhibitors, or inducers of CYP3A4, or potentially toxic medications that are metabolized by CYP3A4). Products include:
VFEND I.V. 2543
VFEND Oral Suspension 2543
VFEND Tablets 2543

Warfarin Sodium (Concentrations of warfarin may be affected. It is recommended that INR be monitored). Products include:
Coumadin for Injection 932
Coumadin Tablets 932

Zafirlukast (Amprenavir, the active metabolite of fosamprenavir, is metabolized in the liver by the cytochrome P450 enzyme system. Amprenavir may inhibit or induce CYP3A4. Caution should be used when co-administering medications that are substrates, inhibitors, or inducers of CYP3A4, or potentially toxic medications that are metabolized by CYP3A4). Products include:
Accolate Tablets 663

Zileuton (Amprenavir, the active metabolite of fosamprenavir, is metabolized in the liver by the cytochrome P450 enzyme system. Amprenavir may inhibit or induce CYP3A4. Caution should be used when co-administering medications that are substrates, inhibitors, or inducers of CYP3A4, or potentially toxic medications that are metabolized by CYP3A4).
No products indexed under this heading.

Food Interactions

Grapefruit (Amprenavir, the active metabolite of fosamprenavir, is metabolized in the liver by the cytochrome P450 enzyme system. Amprenavir may inhibit or induce CYP3A4. Caution should be used when co-administering medications that are substrates, inhibitors, or inducers of CYP3A4, or potentially toxic medications that are metabolized by CYP3A4).

Grapefruit Juice (Amprenavir, the active metabolite of fosamprenavir, is metabolized in the liver by the cytochrome P450 enzyme system. Amprenavir may inhibit or induce CYP3A4. Caution should be used when co-administering medications that are substrates, inhibitors, or inducers of CYP3A4, or potentially toxic medications that are metabolized by CYP3A4).

LIBRIUM CAPSULES

(Chlordiazepoxide Hydrochloride) 3349
None cited in PDR database.

LIDODERM PATCH

(Lidocaine) 1107
May interact with:

Mexiletine Hydrochloride (Co-administration in patients receiving Class-1 antiarrhythmic drugs, such as mexiletine, may result in additive toxic effects).
No products indexed under this heading.

Tocainide Hydrochloride (Co-administration in patients receiving Class-1 antiarrhythmic drugs, such as tocainide, may result in additive toxic effects).
No products indexed under this heading.

LIFEPAK CAPSULES

(Vitamins with Minerals) 2669
None cited in PDR database.

LIPITOR TABLETS

(Atorvastatin Calcium) 2495
May interact with azole antifungals, erythromycin, fibrates, and certain other agents. Compounds in these categories include:

Aluminum Hydroxide (Co-administration with aluminum hydroxide/magnesium hydroxide antacid has resulted in decreased atorvastatin plasma concentrations by 35%; LDL-C reduction was unaltered). Products include:

- Gaviscon Regular Strength Liquid .. 620
- Gaviscon Regular Strength Tablets 619
- Gaviscon Extra Strength Liquid 620
- Gaviscon Extra Strength Tablets 619
- Maalox Max Maximum Strength Antacid/Anti-Gas Liquid 2165
- Maalox Regular Strength Antacid/Antigas Liquid 2164

Clofibrate (Co-administration with fibric acid derivatives increases the risk of myopathy).
No products indexed under this heading.

Clotrimazole (Co-administration with azole antifungals increases the risk of myopathy). Products include:

- Lotrimin 3053
- Lotrisone 3054

Colestipol Hydrochloride (Co-administration has resulted in decreased atorvastatin plasma concentrations by 25%; however, LDL-C reduction was greater when these drugs were given together than when either drug was given alone).
No products indexed under this heading.

Cyclosporine (Co-administration increases the risk of myopathy). Products include:

- Gengraf Capsules 458
- Neoral Soft Gelatin Capsules 2247
- Neoral Oral Solution 2247
- Restasis Ophthalmic Emulsion 570
- Sandimmune 2259

Digoxin (Co-administration has resulted in increased steady-state digoxin plasma concentrations by 20%). Products include:

- Digitek Tablets 2146
- Lanoxicaps Capsules 1458
- Lanoxin Injection 1462
- Lanoxin Tablets 1468
- Lanoxin Injection Pediatric 1465

Erythromycin (Co-administration increases the risk of myopathy; plasma concentrations of atorvastatin has increased by 40% when co-administered with erythromycin, a known inhibitor of cytochrome P4503A4). Products include:

- Erygel Topical Gel 2096
- Ery-Tab Tablets 447
- Erythromycin Base Filmtab Tablets 454
- Erythromycin Delayed-Release Capsules, USP 456
- PCE Dispertab Tablets 510

Erythromycin Estolate (Co-administration increases the risk of myopathy; plasma concentrations of atorvastatin has increased by 40% when co-administered with erythromycin, a known inhibitor of cytochrome P4503A4).
No products indexed under this heading.

Erythromycin Ethylsuccinate (Co-administration increases the risk of myopathy; plasma concentrations of atorvastatin has increased by 40% when co-administered with erythromycin, a known inhibitor of cytochrome P4503A4). Products include:

- E.E.S. 449
- EryPed 445

Erythromycin Gluceptate (Co-administration increases the risk of myopathy; plasma concentrations of atorvastatin has increased by 40% when co-administered with erythromycin, a known inhibitor of cytochrome P4503A4).
No products indexed under this heading.

Erythromycin Lactobionate (Co-administration increases the risk of myopathy; plasma concentrations of atorvastatin has increased by 40% when co-administered with erythromycin, a known inhibitor of cytochrome P4503A4).
No products indexed under this heading.

Erythromycin Stearate (Co-administration increases the risk of myopathy; plasma concentrations of atorvastatin has increased by 40% when co-administered with erythromycin, a known inhibitor of cytochrome P4503A4). Products include:

- Erythrocin Stearate Filmtab Tablets 452

Ethinyl Estradiol (Co-administration with an oral contraceptive has increased AUC values for norethindrone and ethinyl estradiol by 30% and 20%, respectively). Products include:

- Alesse-28 Tablets 3392
- Lo/Ovral-28 Tablets 3423
- NuvaRing 2357
- Ortho-Cept Tablets 2395
- Ortho-Cyclen/Ortho Tri-Cyclen 2414
- Ortho Evra Transdermal System 2402
- Ortho Tri-Cyclen Lo Tablets 2421
- Seasonale Tablets 1073
- Triphasil-28 Tablets 3483
- Yasmin 28 Tablets 818

Fenofibrate (Co-administration with fibric acid derivatives increases the risk of myopathy). Products include:

- Antara Capsules 2723
- Lofibra Capsules 1217
- Tricor Tablets 523
- Triglide Tablets 1165

Fluconazole (Co-administration with azole antifungals increases the risk of myopathy).
No products indexed under this heading.

Gemfibrozil (Co-administration with fibric acid derivatives increases the risk of myopathy).
No products indexed under this heading.

Itraconazole (Co-administration with azole antifungals increases the risk of myopathy).
No products indexed under this heading.

Ketoconazole (Co-administration with azole antifungals increases the risk of myopathy). Products include:

- Nizoral A-D Shampoo, 1% 1839
- Nizoral 2% Shampoo 1838

Miconazole (Co-administration with azole antifungals increases the risk of myopathy).
No products indexed under this heading.

Niacin (Co-administration increases the risk of myopathy). Products include:

- Advicor Tablets 1694
- Niaspan Extended-Release Tablets 1703

Norethindrone (Co-administration with an oral contraceptive has increased AUC values for norethindrone and ethinyl estradiol by 30% and 20%, respectively). Products include:

- Ortho Micronor Tablets 2411

Oxiconazole Nitrate (Co-administration with azole antifungals increases the risk of myopathy). Products include:

- Oxistat 1498

Terconazole (Co-administration with azole antifungals increases the risk of myopathy).
No products indexed under this heading.

LITHOBID TABLETS

(Lithium Carbonate) 1670
May interact with ACE inhibitors, calcium channel blockers, diuretics, nondepolarizing neuromuscular blocking agents, antipsychotic agents, non-steroidal anti-inflammatory agents, urinary alkalinizing agents, xanthines, and certain other agents. Compounds in these categories include:

Acetazolamide (Concurrent use of acetazolamide with lithium may lower serum lithium concentrations by increasing urinary lithium excretion).
No products indexed under this heading.

Acetazolamide Sodium (Concurrent use of acetazolamide with lithium may lower serum lithium concentrations by increasing urinary lithium excretion).
No products indexed under this heading.

Amiloride Hydrochloride (Concurrent use of lithium with diuretics is not recommended since the risk of lithium toxicity is very high. If psychiatric indication is life threatening, and if such a patient fails to respond to other measures, lithium treatment may be undertaken withextreme caution including daily serum lithium determinations and adjustment to the usually low doses ordinarily tolerated by these individuals. In such instances, hospitilization is a necessity). Products include:

- Midamor Tablets 2000
- Moduretic Tablets 2003

Aminophylline (Concurrent use of xanthine preparations with lithium may lower serum lithium concentrations by increasing urinary lithium excretion).
No products indexed under this heading.

Amlodipine Besylate (Concurrent use of calcium channel blocking agents with lithium may increase the risk of neurotoxicity in the form of ataxia, tremors, nausea, vomiting, diarrhea and/or tinnitus). Products include:

- Caduet Tablets 2507
- Lotrel Capsules 2238
- Norvasc Tablets 2529

Aripiprazole (An encephalopathic syndrome (characterized by weakness, lethargy, fever, tremulousness and confusion, extrapyramidal symptoms, leukocytois, elevated serum enzymes, BUN and FBS) has occurred in a few patients treated with lithium plus a neuroleptic, most notably haloperidol. In some instance, the syndrome was followed by irreversible brain damage. Monitor these patients closely for early evidence of neurologic toxicity and discontinue treatment promptly if such signs appear). Products include:

- Abilify Tablets 2472
- Abilify Tablets 916

Atracurium Besylate (Concurrent use of lithium with neuromuscular blocking agents may prolong the effect of neuromuscular blocking agents. Neuromuscular blocking agents should be given with caution to patients receiving lithium).
No products indexed under this heading.

Benazepril Hydrochloride (Concurrent use of lithium with ACE inhibitors is not recommended since the risk of lithium toxicity is very high. If psychiatric indication is life threatening, and if such a patient fails to respond to other measures, lithium treatment may be undertakenwith extreme caution including daily serum lithium determinations and adjustment to the usually low doses ordinarily tolerated by these individuals. In such instances, hospitilization is a necessity). Products include:

- Lotensin Tablets 2232
- Lotensin HCT Tablets 2235
- Lotrel Capsules 2238

Bendroflumethiazide (Concurrent use of lithium with diuretics is not recommended since the risk of lithium toxicity is very high. If psychiatric

indication is life threatening, and if such a patient fails to respond to other measures, lithium treatment may be undertaken withextreme caution including daily serum lithium determinations and adjustment to the usually low doses ordinarily tolerated by these individuals. In such instances, hospitilization is a necessity).
No products indexed under this heading.

Bepridil Hydrochloride (Concurrent use of calcium channel blocking agents with lithium may increase the risk of neurotoxicity in the form of ataxia, tremors, nausea, vomiting, diarrhea and/or tinnitus).
No products indexed under this heading.

Bismuth Oxyiodide (Concomitant use of iodide preparations with lithium may produce hypothyroidism).
No products indexed under this heading.

Bumetanide (Concurrent use of lithium with diuretics is not recommended since the risk of lithium toxicity is very high. If psychiatric indication is life threatening, and if such a patient fails to respond to other measures, lithium treatment may be undertaken withextreme caution including daily serum lithium determinations and adjustment to the usually low doses ordinarily tolerated by these individuals. In such instances, hospitilization is a necessity).
No products indexed under this heading.

Calcium Iodide (Concomitant use of iodide preparations with lithium may produce hypothyroidism).
No products indexed under this heading.

Captopril (Concurrent use of lithium with ACE inhibitors is not recommended since the risk of lithium toxicity is very high. If psychiatric indication is life threatening, and if such a patient fails to respond to other measures, lithium treatment may be undertakenwith extreme caution including daily serum lithium determinations and adjustment to the usually low doses ordinarily tolerated by these individuals. In such instances, hospitilization is a necessity). Products include:
Captopril Tablets 2114

Carbamazepine (Concomitant administration of carbamazepine and lithium may increase the risk of neurotoxic side effects). Products include:
Carbatrol Capsules 3174
Equetro Extended-Release Capsules 3178
Tegretol/Tegretol-XR 2278

Celecoxib (Lithium levels should be closely monitored when patients initiate or discontinue NSAID use. In some cases, lithium toxicity has resulted from interactions between an NSAID and lithium. Significantly increased steady-state plasma lithium concentrations are reported with concurrent use of lithium with NSAIDs and selective COX-2 inhibitors). Products include:
Celebrex Capsules 3130

Chlorothiazide (Concurrent use of lithium with diuretics is not recommended since the risk of lithium toxicity is very high. If psychiatric indication is life threatening, and if such a patient fails to respond to other measures, lithium treatment may be undertaken withextreme caution including daily serum lithium determinations and adjustment to the usually low doses ordinarily tolerated by these individuals. In such instances, hospitilization is a necessity).
Products include:
Aldoclor Tablets 1881
Diuril Oral 1936

Chlorothiazide Sodium (Concurrent use of lithium with diuretics is not recommended since the risk of lithium toxicity is very high. If psychiatric indication is life threatening, and if such a patient fails to respond to other measures, lithium treatment may be undertaken withextreme caution including daily serum lithium determinations and adjustment to the usually low doses ordinarily tolerated by these individuals. In such instances, hospitilization is a necessity). Products include:
Diuril Sodium Intravenous 1934

Chlorpromazine (An encephalopathic syndrome (characterized by weakness, lethargy, fever, tremulousness and confusion, extrapyramidal symptoms, leukocytois, elevated serum enzymes, BUN and FBS) has occurred in a few patients treated with lithium plus a neuroleptic, most notably haloperidol. In some instance, the syndrome was followed by irreversible brain damage. Monitor these patients closely for early evidence of neurologic toxicity and discontinue treatment promptly if such signs appear).
No products indexed under this heading.

Chlorpromazine Hydrochloride (An encephalopathic syndrome (characterized by weakness, lethargy, fever, tremulousness and confusion, extrapyramidal symptoms, leukocytois, elevated serum enzymes, BUN and FBS) has occurred in a few patients treated with lithium plus a neuroleptic, most notably haloperidol. In some instance, the syndrome was followed by irreversible brain damage. Monitor these patients closely for early evidence of neurologic toxicity and discontinue treatment promptly if such signs appear).
No products indexed under this heading.

Chlorprothixene (An encephalopathic syndrome (characterized by weakness, lethargy, fever, tremulousness and confusion, extrapyramidal symptoms, leukocytois, elevated serum enzymes, BUN and FBS) has occurred in a few patients treated with lithium plus a neuroleptic, most notably haloperidol. In some instance, the syndrome was followed by irreversible brain damage. Monitor these patients closely for early evidence of neurologic toxicity and discontinue treatment promptly if such signs appear).
No products indexed under this heading.

Chlorprothixene Hydrochloride (An encephalopathic syndrome (characterized by weakness, lethargy, fever, tremulousness and confusion, extrapyramidal symptoms, leukocytois, elevated serum enzymes, BUN and FBS) has occurred in a few patients treated with lithium plus a neuroleptic, most notably haloperidol. In some instance, the syndrome was followed by irreversible brain damage. Monitor these patients closely for early evidence of neurologic toxicity and discontinue treatment promptly if such signs appear).
No products indexed under this heading.

Chlorthalidone (Concurrent use of lithium with diuretics is not recommended since the risk of lithium toxicity is very high. If psychiatric indication is life threatening, and if such a patient fails to respond to other measures, lithium treatment may be undertaken withextreme caution including daily serum lithium determinations and adjustment to the usually low doses ordinarily tolerated by these individuals. In such instances, hospitilization is a necessity).
Products include:
Clorpres Tablets 2139

Cisatracurium Besylate (Concurrent use of lithium with neuromuscular blocking agents may prolong the effect of neuromuscular blocking agents. Neuromuscular blocking agents should be given with caution to patients receiving lithium).
Products include:
Nimbex Injection 494

Clozapine (An encephalopathic syndrome (characterized by weakness, lethargy, fever, tremulousness and confusion, extrapyramidal symptoms, leukocytois, elevated serum enzymes, BUN and FBS) has occurred in a few patients treated with lithium plus a neuroleptic, most notably haloperidol. In some instance, the syndrome was followed by irreversible brain damage. Monitor these patients closely for early evidence of neurologic toxicity and discontinue treatment promptly if such signs appear). Products include:
Clozapine Tablets 2141
Clozaril Tablets 2174
FazaClo Orally Disintegrating Tablets 547

Diclofenac Potassium (Lithium levels should be closely monitored when patients initiate or discontinue NSAID use. In some cases, lithium toxicity has resulted from interactions between an NSAID and lithium. Significantly increased steady-state plasma lithium concentrations are reported with concurrent use of lithium with NSAIDs and selective COX-2 inhibitors). Products include:
Cataflam Tablets 2173

Diclofenac Sodium (Lithium levels should be closely monitored when patients initiate or discontinue NSAID use. In some cases, lithium toxicity has resulted from interactions between an NSAID and lithium. Significantly increased steady-state plasma lithium concentrations are reported with concurrent use of lithium with NSAIDs and selective COX-2 inhibitors). Products include:
Arthrotec Tablets 3126
Voltaren Ophthalmic Solution 2300
Voltaren Tablets 2298
Voltaren-XR Tablets 2301

Diltiazem Hydrochloride (Concurrent use of calcium channel blocking agents with lithium may increase the risk of neurotoxicity in the form of ataxia, tremors, nausea, vomiting, diarrhea and/or tinnitus). Products include:
Cardizem LA Extended Release Tablets 1699
Tiazac Capsules 1204

Dyphylline (Concurrent use of xanthine preparations with lithium may lower serum lithium concentrations by increasing urinary lithium excretion).
No products indexed under this heading.

Echothiophate Iodide (Concomitant use of iodide preparations with lithium may produce hypothyroidism).
No products indexed under this heading.

Enalapril Maleate (Concurrent use of lithium with ACE inhibitors is not recommended since the risk of lithium toxicity is very high. If psychiatric indication is life threatening, and if such a patient fails to respond to other measures, lithium treatment may be undertakenwith extreme caution including daily serum lithium determinations and adjustment to the usually low doses ordinarily tolerated by these individuals. In such instances, hospitilization is a necessity). Products include:
Vaseretic Tablets 2073
Vasotec I.V. Injection 2076

Enalaprilat (Concurrent use of lithium with ACE inhibitors is not recommended since the risk of lithium toxicity is very high. If psychiatric indication is life threatening, and if such a patient fails to respond to other measures, lithium treatment may be undertakenwith extreme caution including daily serum lithium determinations and adjustment to the usually low doses ordinarily tolerated by these individuals. In such instances, hospitilization is a necessity).
No products indexed under this heading.

Ethacrynic Acid (Concurrent use of lithium with diuretics is not recommended since the risk of lithium toxicity is very high. If psychiatric indication is life threatening, and if such a patient fails to respond to other measures, lithium treatment may be undertaken withextreme caution including daily serum lithium determinations and adjustment to the usually low doses ordinarily tolerated by these individuals. In such instances, hospitilization is a necessity).
Products include:
Edecrin Tablets 1941

Etodolac (Lithium levels should be closely monitored when patients initiate or discontinue NSAID use. In some cases, lithium toxicity has resulted from interactions between an NSAID and lithium. Significantly increased steady-state plasma lithium concentrations are reported with concurrent use of lithium with NSAIDs and selective COX-2 inhibitors).
No products indexed under this heading.

Felodipine (Concurrent use of calcium channel blocking agents with lithium may increase the risk of neurotoxicity in the form of ataxia, tremors, nausea, vomiting, diarrhea and/or tinnitus). Products include:
Plendil Extended-Release Tablets 651

Fenoprofen Calcium (Lithium levels should be closely monitored when patients initiate or discontinue NSAID use. In some cases, lithium toxicity has resulted from interactions between an NSAID and lithium. Significantly increased steady-state plasma lithium concentrations are

reported with concurrent use of lithium with NSAIDs and selective COX-2 inhibitors). Products include:

Nalfon Capsules **2504**

Fluoxetine (Concurrent use of fluoxetine with lithium has resulted in both increased and decreased serum lithium concentration. Patients receiving such combined therapy should be monitored closely).

No products indexed under this heading.

Fluoxetine Hydrochloride (Concurrent use of fluoxetine with lithium has resulted in both increased and decreased serum lithium concentration. Patients receiving such combined therapy should be monitored closely). Products include:

Prozac Pulvules and Liquid **1771**
Symbyax Capsules **1788**

Fluphenazine Decanoate (An encephalopathic syndrome (characterized by weakness, lethargy, fever, tremulousness and confusion, extrapyramidal symptoms, leukocytois, elevated serum enzymes, BUN and FBS) has occurred in a few patients treated with lithium plus a neuroleptic, most notably haloperidol. In some instance, the syndrome was followed by irreversible brain damage. Monitor these patients closely for early evidence of neurologic toxicity and discontinue treatment promptly if such signs appear).

No products indexed under this heading.

Fluphenazine Enanthate (An encephalopathic syndrome (characterized by weakness, lethargy, fever, tremulousness and confusion, extrapyramidal symptoms, leukocytois, elevated serum enzymes, BUN and FBS) has occurred in a few patients treated with lithium plus a neuroleptic, most notably haloperidol. In some instance, the syndrome was followed by irreversible brain damage. Monitor these patients closely for early evidence of neurologic toxicity and discontinue treatment promptly if such signs appear).

No products indexed under this heading.

Fluphenazine Hydrochloride (An encephalopathic syndrome (characterized by weakness, lethargy, fever, tremulousness and confusion, extrapyramidal symptoms, leukocytois, elevated serum enzymes, BUN and FBS) has occurred in a few patients treated with lithium plus a neuroleptic, most notably haloperidol. In some instance, the syndrome was followed by irreversible brain damage. Monitor these patients closely for early evidence of neurologic toxicity and discontinue treatment promptly if such signs appear).

No products indexed under this heading.

Flurbiprofen (Lithium levels should be closely monitored when patients initiate or discontinue NSAID use. In some cases, lithium toxicity has resulted from interactions between an NSAID and lithium. Significantly increased steady-state plasma lithium concentrations are reported with concurrent use of lithium with NSAIDs and selective COX-2 inhibitors).

No products indexed under this heading.

Fosinopril Sodium (Concurrent use of lithium with ACE inhibitors is not recommended since the risk of lithium toxicity is very high. If psychiatric indication is life threatening, and if such a patient fails to respond to other measures, lithium treatment may be undertakenwith extreme caution including daily serum lithium determinations and adjustment to the usually low doses ordinarily tolerated by these individuals. In such instances, hospitilization is a necessity).

No products indexed under this heading.

Furosemide (Concurrent use of lithium with diuretics is not recommended since the risk of lithium toxicity is very high. If psychiatric indication is life threatening, and if such a patient fails to respond to other measures, lithium treatment may be undertaken withextreme caution including daily serum lithium determinations and adjustment to the usually low doses ordinarily tolerated by these individuals. In such instances, hospitilization is a necessity). Products include:

Furosemide Tablets **2117**

Gallamine Triethiodide (Concomitant use of iodide preparations with lithium may produce hypothyroidism).

No products indexed under this heading.

Haloperidol (An encephalopathic syndrome (characterized by weakness, lethargy, fever, tremulousness and confusion, extrapyramidal symptoms, leukocytois, elevated serum enzymes, BUN and FBS) has occurred in a few patients treated with lithium plus a neuroleptic, most notably haloperidol. In some instance, the syndrome was followed by irreversible brain damage. Monitor these patients closely for early evidence of neurologic toxicity and discontinue treatment promptly if such signs appear).

No products indexed under this heading.

Haloperidol Decanoate (An encephalopathic syndrome (characterized by weakness, lethargy, fever, tremulousness and confusion, extrapyramidal symptoms, leukocytois, elevated serum enzymes, BUN and FBS) has occurred in a few patients treated with lithium plus a neuroleptic, most notably haloperidol. In some instance, the syndrome was followed by irreversible brain damage. Monitor these patients closely for early evidence of neurologic toxicity and discontinue treatment promptly if such signs appear).

No products indexed under this heading.

Hydrochlorothiazide (Concurrent use of lithium with diuretics is not recommended since the risk of lithium toxicity is very high. If psychiatric indication is life threatening, and if such a patient fails to respond to other measures, lithium treatment may be undertaken withextreme caution including daily serum lithium determinations and adjustment to the usually low doses ordinarily tolerated by these individuals. In such instances, hospitilization is a necessity). Products include:

Aldoril Tablets **1884**
Atacand HCT **637**
Avalide Tablets **2889**
Avalide Tablets **922**
Benicar HCT Tablets **2852**
Diovan HCT Tablets **2195**
Dyazide Capsules **1389**
Hyzaar **1964**
Lotensin HCT Tablets **2235**
Maxzide **2150**
Micardis HCT Tablets **886**
Moduretic Tablets **2003**
Prinzide Tablets **2033**
Teveten HCT Tablets **1710**
Timolide Tablets **2056**
Uniretic Tablets **3114**
Vaseretic Tablets **2073**
Zestoretic Tablets **701**

Hydroflumethiazide (Concurrent use of lithium with diuretics is not recommended since the risk of lithium toxicity is very high. If psychiatric indication is life threatening, and if such a patient fails to respond to other measures, lithium treatment may be undertaken withextreme caution including daily serum lithium determinations and adjustment to the usually low doses ordinarily tolerated by these individuals. In such instances, hospitilization is a necessity).

No products indexed under this heading.

Ibuprofen (Lithium levels should be closely monitored when patients initiate or discontinue NSAID use. In some cases, lithium toxicity has resulted from interactions between an NSAID and lithium. Significantly increased steady-state plasma lithium concentrations are reported with concurrent use of lithium with NSAIDs and selective COX-2 inhibitors). Products include:

Advil Allergy Sinus Caplets **737**
Advil **737**
Children's Advil Suspension **742**
Children's Advil Chewable Tablets .. **741**
Advil Cold & Sinus **739**
Advil Flu & Body Ache Caplets **739**
Children's Advil Cold Suspension ... **741**
Infants' Advil Concentrated Drops .. **743**
Junior Strength Advil Swallow Tablets **740**
Advil Migraine Liquigels **740**
Advil Multi-Symptom Cold Caplets **738**
Combunox Tablets **1183**
Children's Motrin Oral Suspension and Chewable Tablets **1837**
Children's Motrin Cold Non-Staining Dye-Free Oral Suspension **1838**
Children's Motrin Cold Oral Suspension **1838**
Children's Motrin Non-Staining Dye-Free Oral Suspension **1837**
Motrin Cold & Sinus Caplets **1836**
Motrin IB Tablets and Caplets **1836**
Infants' Motrin Concentrated Drops **1837**
Infants' Motrin Non-Staining Dye-Free Drops **1837**
Junior Strength Motrin Caplets and Chewable Tablets **1837**
Vicoprofen Tablets **533**

Indapamide (Concurrent use of lithium with diuretics is not recommended since the risk of lithium toxicity is very high. If psychiatric indication is life threatening, and if such a patient fails to respond to other measures, lithium treatment may be undertaken withextreme caution including daily serum lithium determinations and adjustment to the usually low doses ordinarily tolerated by these individuals. In such instances, hospitilization is a necessity). Products include:

Indapamide Tablets **2119**

Indomethacin (Lithium levels should be closely monitored when patients initiate or discontinue NSAID use. In some cases, lithium toxicity has resulted from interactions between an NSAID and lithium. Significantly increased steady-state plasma lithium concentrations are reported with concurrent use of lithium with NSAIDs and selective COX-2 inhibitors). Products include:

Indocin **1968**

Indomethacin Sodium Trihydrate (Lithium levels should be closely monitored when patients initiate or discontinue NSAID use. In some cases, lithium toxicity has resulted from interactions between an NSAID and lithium. Significantly increased steady-state plasma lithium concentrations are reported with concurrent use of lithium with NSAIDs and selective COX-2 inhibitors). Products include:

Indocin I.V. **1973**

Isopropamide Iodide (Concomitant use of iodide preparations with lithium may produce hypothyroidism).

No products indexed under this heading.

Isradipine (Concurrent use of calcium channel blocking agents with lithium may increase the risk of neurotoxicity in the form of ataxia, tremors, nausea, vomiting, diarrhea and/or tinnitus). Products include:

DynaCirc CR Tablets **2726**

Ketoprofen (Lithium levels should be closely monitored when patients initiate or discontinue NSAID use. In some cases, lithium toxicity has resulted from interactions between an NSAID and lithium. Significantly increased steady-state plasma lithium concentrations are reported with concurrent use of lithium with NSAIDs and selective COX-2 inhibitors).

No products indexed under this heading.

Ketorolac Tromethamine (Lithium levels should be closely monitored when patients initiate or discontinue NSAID use. In some cases, lithium toxicity has resulted from interactions between an NSAID and lithium. Significantly increased steady-state plasma lithium concentrations are reported with concurrent use of lithium with NSAIDs and selective COX-2 inhibitors). Products include:

Acular Ophthalmic Solution **561**
Acular LS Ophthalmic Solution **562**

Lisinopril (Concurrent use of lithium with ACE inhibitors is not recommended since the risk of lithium toxicity is very high. If psychiatric indication is life threatening, and if such a patient fails to respond to other measures, lithium treatment may be undertakenwith extreme caution including daily serum lithium determinations and adjustment to the usually low doses ordinarily tolerated by these individuals. In such instances, hospitilization is a necessity). Products include:

Prinivil Tablets **2029**
Prinzide Tablets **2033**
Zestoretic Tablets **701**
Zestril Tablets **704**

Lithium Citrate (An encephalopathic syndrome (characterized by weakness, lethargy, fever, tremulousness and confusion, extrapyramidal symptoms, leukocytois, elevated serum enzymes, BUN and FBS) has occurred in a few patients treated with lithium plus a neuroleptic, most notably haloperidol. In some instance, the syndrome was followed by irreversible brain damage. Moni-

tor these patients closely for early evidence of neurologic toxicity and discontinue treatment promptly if such signs appear).
No products indexed under this heading.

Loxapine Hydrochloride (An encephalopathic syndrome (characterized by weakness, lethargy, fever, tremulousness and confusion, extrapyramidal symptoms, leukocytois, elevated serum enzymes, BUN and FBS) has occurred in a few patients treated with lithium plus a neuroleptic, most notably haloperidol. In some instance, the syndrome was followed by irreversible brain damage. Monitor these patients closely for early evidence of neurologic toxicity and discontinue treatment promptly if such signs appear).
No products indexed under this heading.

Loxapine Succinate (An encephalopathic syndrome (characterized by weakness, lethargy, fever, tremulousness and confusion, extrapyramidal symptoms, leukocytois, elevated serum enzymes, BUN and FBS) has occurred in a few patients treated with lithium plus a neuroleptic, most notably haloperidol. In some instance, the syndrome was followed by irreversible brain damage. Monitor these patients closely for early evidence of neurologic toxicity and discontinue treatment promptly if such signs appear).
No products indexed under this heading.

Meclofenamate Sodium (Lithium levels should be closely monitored when patients initiate or discontinue NSAID use. In some cases, lithium toxicity has resulted from interactions between an NSAID and lithium. Significantly increased steady-state plasma lithium concentrations are reported with concurrent use of lithium with NSAIDs and selective COX-2 inhibitors).
No products indexed under this heading.

Mefenamic Acid (Lithium levels should be closely monitored when patients initiate or discontinue NSAID use. In some cases, lithium toxicity has resulted from interactions between an NSAID and lithium. Significantly increased steady-state plasma lithium concentrations are reported with concurrent use of lithium with NSAIDs and selective COX-2 inhibitors).
No products indexed under this heading.

Meloxicam (Lithium levels should be closely monitored when patients initiate or discontinue NSAID use. In some cases, lithium toxicity has resulted from interactions between an NSAID and lithium. Significantly increased steady-state plasma lithium concentrations are reported with concurrent use of lithium with NSAIDs and selective COX-2 inhibitors). Products include:

Mobic Oral Suspension 893
Mobic Tablets 893

Mesoridazine Besylate (An encephalopathic syndrome (characterized by weakness, lethargy, fever, tremulousness and confusion, extrapyramidal symptoms, leukocytois, elevated serum enzymes, BUN and FBS) has occurred in a few patients treated with lithium plus a neuroleptic, most notably haloperidol. In some instance, the syndrome was followed by irreversible brain damage. Monitor these patients closely for early evidence of neurologic toxicity and discontinue treatment promptly if such signs appear).
No products indexed under this heading.

Methotrimeprazine (An encephalopathic syndrome (characterized by weakness, lethargy, fever, tremulousness and confusion, extrapyramidal symptoms, leukocytois, elevated serum enzymes, BUN and FBS) has occurred in a few patients treated with lithium plus a neuroleptic, most notably haloperidol. In some instance, the syndrome was followed by irreversible brain damage. Monitor these patients closely for early evidence of neurologic toxicity and discontinue treatment promptly if such signs appear).
No products indexed under this heading.

Methyclothiazide (Concurrent use of lithium with diuretics is not recommended since the risk of lithium toxicity is very high. If psychiatric indication is life threatening, and if such a patient fails to respond to other measures, lithium treatment may be undertaken withextreme caution including daily serum lithium determinations and adjustment to the usually low doses ordinarily tolerated by these individuals. In such instances, hospitilization is a necessity).
No products indexed under this heading.

Metocurine Iodide (Concomitant use of iodide preparations with lithium may produce hypothyroidism).
No products indexed under this heading.

Metolazone (Concurrent use of lithium with diuretics is not recommended since the risk of lithium toxicity is very high. If psychiatric indication is life threatening, and if such a patient fails to respond to other measures, lithium treatment may be undertaken withextreme caution including daily serum lithium determinations and adjustment to the usually low doses ordinarily tolerated by these individuals. In such instances, hospitilization is a necessity).
No products indexed under this heading.

Metronidazole (Concurrent use of metronidazole with lithium may provoke lithium toxicity due to reduced renal clearance. Patients receiving such combined therapy should be monitored closely). Products include:

Metrogel 1% 1212
MetroGel-Vaginal Gel 1822
Noritate Cream, 1% 1051

Metronidazole Benzoate (Concurrent use of metronidazole with lithium may provoke lithium toxicity due to reduced renal clearance. Patients receiving such combined therapy should be monitored closely).
No products indexed under this heading.

Metronidazole Hydrochloride (Concurrent use of metronidazole with lithium may provoke lithium toxicity due to reduced renal clearance. Patients receiving such combined therapy should be monitored closely).
No products indexed under this heading.

Metronidazole Sodium (Concurrent use of metronidazole with lithium may provoke lithium toxicity due to reduced renal clearance. Patients receiving such combined therapy should be monitored closely).
No products indexed under this heading.

Mibefradil Dihydrochloride (Concurrent use of calcium channel blocking agents with lithium may increase the risk of neurotoxicity in the form of ataxia, tremors, nausea, vomiting, diarrhea and/or tinnitus).
No products indexed under this heading.

Mivacurium Chloride (Concurrent use of lithium with neuromuscular blocking agents may prolong the effect of neuromuscular blocking agents. Neuromuscular blocking agents should be given with caution to patients receiving lithium). Products include:

Mivacron Injection 489

Moexipril Hydrochloride (Concurrent use of lithium with ACE inhibitors is not recommended since the risk of lithium toxicity is very high. If psychiatric indication is life threatening, and if such a patient fails to respond to other measures, lithium treatment may be undertakenwith extreme caution including daily serum lithium determinations and adjustment to the usually low doses ordinarily tolerated by these individuals. In such instances, hospitilization is a necessity). Products include:

Uniretic Tablets 3114
Univasc Tablets 3118

Molindone Hydrochloride (An encephalopathic syndrome (characterized by weakness, lethargy, fever, tremulousness and confusion, extrapyramidal symptoms, leukocytois, elevated serum enzymes, BUN and FBS) has occurred in a few patients treated with lithium plus a neuroleptic, most notably haloperidol. In some instance, the syndrome was followed by irreversible brain damage. Monitor these patients closely for early evidence of neurologic toxicity and discontinue treatment promptly if such signs appear). Products include:

Moban Tablets 1108

Nabumetone (Lithium levels should be closely monitored when patients initiate or discontinue NSAID use. In some cases, lithium toxicity has resulted from interactions between an NSAID and lithium. Significantly increased steady-state plasma lithium concentrations are reported with concurrent use of lithium with NSAIDs and selective COX-2 inhibitors). Products include:

Relafen Tablets 1523

Naproxen (Lithium levels should be closely monitored when patients initiate or discontinue NSAID use. In some cases, lithium toxicity has resulted from interactions between an NSAID and lithium. Significantly increased steady-state plasma lithium concentrations are reported with concurrent use of lithium with NSAIDs and selective COX-2 inhibitors). Products include:

EC-Naprosyn Delayed-Release Tablets 2769
Naprosyn Suspension 2769
Naprosyn Tablets 2769
Prevacid NapraPAC 3277

Naproxen Sodium (Lithium levels should be closely monitored when patients initiate or discontinue NSAID use. In some cases, lithium toxicity has resulted from interactions between an NSAID and lithium. Significantly increased steady-state plasma lithium concentrations are reported with concurrent use of lithium with NSAIDs and selective COX-2 inhibitors). Products include:

Aleve Tablets, Caplets and Gelcaps .... ⊡605
Anaprox Tablets 2769
Anaprox DS Tablets 2769

Niacinamide Hydroiodide (Concomitant use of iodide preparations with lithium may produce hypothyroidism).
No products indexed under this heading.

Nicardipine Hydrochloride (Concurrent use of calcium channel blocking agents with lithium may increase the risk of neurotoxicity in the form of ataxia, tremors, nausea, vomiting, diarrhea and/or tinnitus). Products include:

Cardene I.V. 1129

Nifedipine (Concurrent use of calcium channel blocking agents with lithium may increase the risk of neurotoxicity in the form of ataxia, tremors, nausea, vomiting, diarrhea and/or tinnitus). Products include:

Adalat CC Tablets 2978

Nimodipine (Concurrent use of calcium channel blocking agents with lithium may increase the risk of neurotoxicity in the form of ataxia, tremors, nausea, vomiting, diarrhea and/or tinnitus). Products include:

Nimotop Capsules 774

Nisoldipine (Concurrent use of calcium channel blocking agents with lithium may increase the risk of neurotoxicity in the form of ataxia, tremors, nausea, vomiting, diarrhea and/or tinnitus). Products include:

Sular Tablets 1163

Olanzapine (An encephalopathic syndrome (characterized by weakness, lethargy, fever, tremulousness and confusion, extrapyramidal symptoms, leukocytois, elevated serum enzymes, BUN and FBS) has occurred in a few patients treated with lithium plus a neuroleptic, most notably haloperidol. In some instance, the syndrome was followed by irreversible brain damage. Monitor these patients closely for early evidence of neurologic toxicity and discontinue treatment promptly if such signs appear). Products include:

Symbyax Capsules 1788
Zyprexa Tablets 1798
Zyprexa IntraMuscular 1798
Zyprexa ZYDIS Orally Disintegrating Tablets 1798

Oxaprozin (Lithium levels should be closely monitored when patients initiate or discontinue NSAID use. In some cases, lithium toxicity has resulted from interactions between an NSAID and lithium. Significantly increased steady-state plasma lithium concentrations are reported with concurrent use of lithium with NSAIDs and selective COX-2 inhibitors).
No products indexed under this heading.

Pancuronium Bromide (Concurrent use of lithium with neuromuscular blocking agents may prolong the effect of neuromuscular blocking agents. Neuromuscular blocking agents should be given with caution to patients receiving lithium).
No products indexed under this heading.

Perindopril Erbumine (Concurrent use of lithium with ACE inhibitors is not recommended since the risk of lithium toxicity is very high. If psychiatric indication is life threatening, and if such a patient fails to respond to other measures, lithium treatment may be undertakenwith extreme caution including daily serum lithium determinations and adjustment to the usually low doses ordinarily tolerated by these individuals. In such instances, hospitilization is a necessity). Products include:
Aceon Tablets (2 mg, 4 mg, 8 mg) 3191

Perphenazine (An encephalopathic syndrome (characterized by weakness, lethargy, fever, tremulousness and confusion, extrapyramidal symptoms, leukocytois, elevated serum enzymes, BUN and FBS) has occurred in a few patients treated with lithium plus a neuroleptic, most notably haloperidol. In some instance, the syndrome was followed by irreversible brain damage. Monitor these patients closely for early evidence of neurologic toxicity and discontinue treatment promptly if such signs appear).
No products indexed under this heading.

Phenylbutazone (Lithium levels should be closely monitored when patients initiate or discontinue NSAID use. In some cases, lithium toxicity has resulted from interactions between an NSAID and lithium. Significantly increased steady-state plasma lithium concentrations are reported with concurrent use of lithium with NSAIDs and selective COX-2 inhibitors).
No products indexed under this heading.

Pimozide (An encephalopathic syndrome (characterized by weakness, lethargy, fever, tremulousness and confusion, extrapyramidal symptoms, leukocytois, elevated serum enzymes, BUN and FBS) has occurred in a few patients treated with lithium plus a neuroleptic, most notably haloperidol. In some instance, the syndrome was followed by irreversible brain damage. Monitor these patients closely for early evidence of neurologic toxicity and discontinue treatment promptly if such signs appear). Products include:
Orap Tablets 1220

Piroxicam (Lithium levels should be closely monitored when patients initiate or discontinue NSAID use. In some cases, lithium toxicity has resulted from interactions between an NSAID and lithium. Significantly increased steady-state plasma lithium concentrations are reported with concurrent use of lithium with NSAIDs and selective COX-2 inhibitors).
No products indexed under this heading.

Polythiazide (Concurrent use of lithium with diuretics is not recommended since the risk of lithium toxicity is very high. If psychiatric indication is life threatening, and if such a patient fails to respond to other measures, lithium treatment may be undertaken withextreme caution including daily serum lithium determinations and adjustment to the usually low doses ordinarily tolerated by these individuals. In such instances, hospitilization is a necessity).
No products indexed under this heading.

Potassium Citrate (Concurrent use of alkalinizing agents, such as sodium bicarbonate, with lithium may lower the serum lithium concentration by increasing urinary lithium excretion). Products include:
Urocit-K Tablets 2109

Potassium Iodide (Concomitant use of iodide preparations, especially potassium iodide, with lithium may produce hypothyroidism).
No products indexed under this heading.

Prochlorperazine (An encephalopathic syndrome (characterized by weakness, lethargy, fever, tremulousness and confusion, extrapyramidal symptoms, leukocytois, elevated serum enzymes, BUN and FBS) has occurred in a few patients treated with lithium plus a neuroleptic, most notably haloperidol. In some instance, the syndrome was followed by irreversible brain damage. Monitor these patients closely for early evidence of neurologic toxicity and discontinue treatment promptly if such signs appear).
No products indexed under this heading.

Promethazine Hydrochloride (An encephalopathic syndrome (characterized by weakness, lethargy, fever, tremulousness and confusion, extrapyramidal symptoms, leukocytois, elevated serum enzymes, BUN and FBS) has occurred in a few patients treated with lithium plus a neuroleptic, most notably haloperidol. In some instance, the syndrome was followed by irreversible brain damage. Monitor these patients closely for early evidence of neurologic toxicity and discontinue treatment promptly if such signs appear). Products include:
Phenergan 3438

Quetiapine Fumarate (An encephalopathic syndrome (characterized by weakness, lethargy, fever, tremulousness and confusion, extrapyramidal symptoms, leukocytois, elevated serum enzymes, BUN and FBS) has occurred in a few patients treated with lithium plus a neuroleptic, most notably haloperidol. In some instance, the syndrome was followed by irreversible brain damage. Monitor these patients closely for early evidence of neurologic toxicity and discontinue treatment promptly if such signs appear). Products include:
Seroquel Tablets 691

Quinapril Hydrochloride (Concurrent use of lithium with ACE inhibitors is not recommended since the risk of lithium toxicity is very high. If psychiatric indication is life threatening, and if such a patient fails to respond to other measures, lithium treatment may be undertakenwith extreme caution including daily serum lithium determinations and adjustment to the usually low doses ordinarily tolerated by these individuals. In such instances, hospitilization is a necessity).
No products indexed under this heading.

Ramipril (Concurrent use of lithium with ACE inhibitors is not recommended since the risk of lithium toxicity is very high. If psychiatric indication is life threatening, and if such a patient fails to respond to other measures, lithium treatment may be undertakenwith extreme caution including daily serum lithium determinations and adjustment to the usually low doses ordinarily tolerated by these individuals. In such instances, hospitilization is a necessity). Products include:
Altace Capsules 1673

Rapacuronium Bromide (Concurrent use of lithium with neuromuscular blocking agents may prolong the effect of neuromuscular blocking agents. Neuromuscular blocking agents should be given with caution to patients receiving lithium).
No products indexed under this heading.

Risperidone (An encephalopathic syndrome (characterized by weakness, lethargy, fever, tremulousness and confusion, extrapyramidal symptoms, leukocytois, elevated serum enzymes, BUN and FBS) has occurred in a few patients treated with lithium plus a neuroleptic, most notably haloperidol. In some instance, the syndrome was followed by irreversible brain damage. Monitor these patients closely for early evidence of neurologic toxicity and discontinue treatment promptly if such signs appear). Products include:
Risperdal Consta Long-Acting Injection 1664
Risperdal M-Tab Orally Disintegrating Tablets 1658
Risperdal 1658

Rocuronium Bromide (Concurrent use of lithium with neuromuscular blocking agents may prolong the effect of neuromuscular blocking agents. Neuromuscular blocking agents should be given with caution to patients receiving lithium). Products include:
Zemuron Injection 2363

Rofecoxib (Lithium levels should be closely monitored when patients initiate or discontinue NSAID use. In some cases, lithium toxicity has resulted from interactions between an NSAID and lithium. Significantly increased steady-state plasma lithium concentrations are reported with concurrent use of lithium with NSAIDs and selective COX-2 inhibitors).
No products indexed under this heading.

Sodium Bicarbonate (Concurrent use of alkalinizing agents, such as sodium bicarbonate, with lithium may lower the serum lithium concentration by increasing urinary lithium excretion). Products include:
Ceo-Two Evacuant Suppository 607
Colyte with Flavor Packs for Oral Solution 3102
HalfLytely and Bisacodyl Tablets Bowel Prep Kit with Flavors Packs 915
TriLyte with Flavor Packs for Oral Solution 3114

Sodium Citrate (Concurrent use of alkalinizing agents, such as sodium bicarbonate, with lithium may lower the serum lithium concentration by increasing urinary lithium excretion).
No products indexed under this heading.

Sodium Iodide I 123 (Concomitant use of iodide preparations with lithium may produce hypothyroidism).
No products indexed under this heading.

Sodium Iodide I 131 (Concomitant use of iodide preparations with lithium may produce hypothyroidism).
No products indexed under this heading.

Spirapril Hydrochloride (Concurrent use of lithium with ACE inhibitors is not recommended since the risk of lithium toxicity is very high. If psychiatric indication is life threatening, and if such a patient fails to respond to other measures, lithium treatment may be undertakenwith extreme caution including daily serum lithium determinations and adjustment to the usually low doses ordinarily tolerated by these individuals. In such instances, hospitilization is a necessity).
No products indexed under this heading.

Spironolactone (Concurrent use of lithium with diuretics is not recommended since the risk of lithium toxicity is very high. If psychiatric indication is life threatening, and if such a patient fails to respond to other measures, lithium treatment may be undertaken withextreme caution including daily serum lithium determinations and adjustment to the usually low doses ordinarily tolerated by these individuals. In such instances, hospitilization is a necessity).
No products indexed under this heading.

Sulindac (Lithium levels should be closely monitored when patients initiate or discontinue NSAID use. In some cases, lithium toxicity has resulted from interactions between an NSAID and lithium. Significantly increased steady-state plasma lithium concentrations are reported with concurrent use of lithium with NSAIDs and selective COX-2 inhibitors). Products include:
Clinoril Tablets 1899

Theophylline (Concurrent use of xanthine preparations with lithium may lower serum lithium concentrations by increasing urinary lithium excretion).
No products indexed under this heading.

Theophylline Anhydrous (Concurrent use of xanthine preparations with lithium may lower serum lithium concentrations by increasing urinary lithium excretion). Products include:
Uniphyl Tablets 2708

Theophylline Calcium Salicylate (Concurrent use of xanthine preparations with lithium may lower serum lithium concentrations by increasing urinary lithium excretion).
No products indexed under this heading.

Theophylline Dihydroxypropyl (Glyceryl) (Concurrent use of xanthine preparations with lithium may lower serum lithium concentrations by increasing urinary lithium excretion).
No products indexed under this heading.

Theophylline Ethylenediamine (Concurrent use of xanthine preparations with lithium may lower serum lithium concentrations by increasing urinary lithium excretion).
No products indexed under this heading.

Theophylline Sodium Glycinate (Concurrent use of xanthine preparations with lithium may lower serum lithium concentrations by increasing urinary lithium excretion).
No products indexed under this heading.

Thioridazine Hydrochloride (An encephalopathic syndrome (characterized by weakness, lethargy, fever, tremulousness and confusion, extrapyramidal symptoms, leukocytosis, elevated serum enzymes, BUN and FBS) has occurred in a few patients treated with lithium plus a neuroleptic, most notably haloperidol. In some instance, the syndrome was followed by irreversible brain damage. Monitor these patients closely for early evidence of neurologic toxicity and discontinue treatment promptly if such signs appear). Products include:
- Thioridazine Hydrochloride Tablets **2122**

Thiothixene (An encephalopathic syndrome (characterized by weakness, lethargy, fever, tremulousness and confusion, extrapyramidal symptoms, leukocytosis, elevated serum enzymes, BUN and FBS) has occurred in a few patients treated with lithium plus a neuroleptic, most notably haloperidol. In some instance, the syndrome was followed by irreversible brain damage. Monitor these patients closely for early evidence of neurologic toxicity and discontinue treatment promptly if such signs appear). Products include:
- Thiothixene Capsules **2124**

Tolmetin Sodium (Lithium levels should be closely monitored when patients initiate or discontinue NSAID use. In some cases, lithium toxicity has resulted from interactions between an NSAID and lithium. Significantly increased steady-state plasma lithium concentrations are reported with concurrent use of lithium with NSAIDs and selective COX-2 inhibitors).
No products indexed under this heading.

Torsemide (Concurrent use of lithium with diuretics is not recommended since the risk of lithium toxicity is very high. If psychiatric indication is life threatening, and if such a patient fails to respond to other measures, lithium treatment may be undertaken withextreme caution including daily serum lithium determinations and adjustment to the usually low doses ordinarily tolerated by these individuals. In such instances, hospitilization is a necessity).
No products indexed under this heading.

Trandolapril (Concurrent use of lithium with ACE inhibitors is not recommended since the risk of lithium toxicity is very high. If psychiatric indication is life threatening, and if such a patient fails to respond to other measures, lithium treatment may be undertakenwith extreme caution including daily serum lithium determinations and adjustment to the usually low doses ordinarily tolerated by these individuals. In such instances, hospitilization is a necessity). Products include:
- Mavik Tablets **482**
- Tarka Tablets **519**

Triamterene (Concurrent use of lithium with diuretics is not recommended since the risk of lithium toxicity is very high. If psychiatric indication is life threatening, and if such a patient fails to respond to other measures, lithium treatment may be undertaken withextreme caution including daily serum lithium determinations and adjustment to the usually low doses ordinarily tolerated by these individuals. In such instances, hospitilization is a necessity). Products include:
- Dyazide Capsules **1389**
- Dyrenium Capsules **3390**
- Maxzide **2150**

Trifluoperazine Hydrochloride (An encephalopathic syndrome (characterized by weakness, lethargy, fever, tremulousness and confusion, extrapyramidal symptoms, leukocytosis, elevated serum enzymes, BUN and FBS) has occurred in a few patients treated with lithium plus a neuroleptic, most notably haloperidol. In some instance, the syndrome was followed by irreversible brain damage. Monitor these patients closely for early evidence of neurologic toxicity and discontinue treatment promptly if such signs appear).
No products indexed under this heading.

Urea (Concurrent use of urea with lithium may lower serum lithium concentrations by increasing urinary lithium excretion). Products include:
- Accuzyme Debriding Ointment **1636**
- Accuzyme Spray **1637**
- Panafil Ointment **1637**
- Panafil Spray **1637**
- U-Kera Cream **3290**
- Ultralytic 2 Cream 20% **1651**
- Ultralytic 2 Foam 20% **1652**

Valdecoxib (Lithium levels should be closely monitored when patients initiate or discontinue NSAID use. In some cases, lithium toxicity has resulted from interactions between an NSAID and lithium. Significantly increased steady-state plasma lithium concentrations are reported with concurrent use of lithium with NSAIDs and selective COX-2 inhibitors).
No products indexed under this heading.

Vecuronium Bromide (Concurrent use of lithium with neuromuscular blocking agents may prolong the effect of neuromuscular blocking agents. Neuromuscular blocking agents should be given with caution to patients receiving lithium).
No products indexed under this heading.

Verapamil Hydrochloride (Concurrent use of calcium channel blocking agents with lithium may increase the risk of neurotoxicity in the form of ataxia, tremors, nausea, vomiting, diarrhea and/or tinnitus). Products include:
- Covera-HS Tablets **3135**
- Tarka Tablets **519**
- Verelan PM Capsules **3120**

Ziprasidone Hydrochloride (An encephalopathic syndrome (characterized by weakness, lethargy, fever, tremulousness and confusion, extrapyramidal symptoms, leukocytosis, elevated serum enzymes, BUN and FBS) has occurred in a few patients treated with lithium plus a neuroleptic, most notably haloperidol. In some instance, the syndrome was followed by irreversible brain damage. Monitor these patients closely for early evidence of neurologic toxicity and discontinue treatment promptly if such signs appear). Products include:
- Geodon Capsules **2514**

LOCOID CREAM

(Hydrocortisone Butyrate) **1138**
None cited in PDR database.

LOCOID LIPOCREAM CREAM

(Hydrocortisone Butyrate) **1138**
None cited in PDR database.

LOCOID OINTMENT

(Hydrocortisone Butyrate) **1138**
None cited in PDR database.

LOCOID TOPICAL SOLUTION

(Hydrocortisone Butyrate) **1138**
None cited in PDR database.

LOFIBRA CAPSULES

(Fenofibrate) **1217**
May interact with bile acid sequestering agents, oral anticoagulants, HMG-CoA reductase inhibitors, and certain other agents. Compounds in these categories include:

Anisindione (Co-administration with coumarin-type anticoagulants has resulted in potentiation of oral anticoagulants resulting in prolonged prothrombin time; the dosage of the anticoaguant should be reduced to maintain the PT at the desired level). Products include:
- Miradon Tablets **3056**

Atorvastatin Calcium (Co-administration of fibric acid derivatives and HMG-CoA reductase inhibitors has been associated, in numerous case reports, with rhabdomyolysis, markedly elevated creatine kinase (CK) levels and myoglobulinuria, leading in a high proportion of cases to acute renal failure; the combined use should be avoided unless the benefit of further alterations in lipid levels is likely to outweigh the increased risk of this combination). Products include:
- Caduet Tablets **2507**
- Lipitor Tablets **2495**

Cerivastatin Sodium (Co-administration of fibric acid derivatives and HMG-CoA reductase inhibitors has been associated, in numerous case reports, with rhabdomyolysis, markedly elevated creatine kinase (CK) levels and myoglobulinuria, leading in a high proportion of cases to acute renal failure; the combined use should be avoided unless the benefit of further alterations in lipid levels is likely to outweigh the increased risk of this combination).
No products indexed under this heading.

Cholestyramine (Bile acid sequestrants may bind fenofibrate; Lofibra should be taken at least 1 hour before or 4-6 hours after a bile acid binding resin to avoid impeding its absorption).
No products indexed under this heading.

Colesevelam Hydrochloride (Bile acid sequestrants may bind fenofibrate; Lofibra should be taken at least 1 hour before or 4-6 hours after a bile acid binding resin to avoid impeding its absorption). Products include:
- WelChol Tablets **2855**

Colestipol Hydrochloride (Bile acid sequestrants may bind fenofibrate; Lofibra should be taken at least 1 hour before or 4-6 hours after a bile acid binding resin to avoid impeding its absorption).
No products indexed under this heading.

Cyclosporine (Renal excretion is the primary elimination route for fibrates and because cyclosporine can produce nephrotoxicity with decrease in creatinine clearance and rise in serum clearance, there is a risk that an interaction will lead to deterioration). Products include:
- Gengraf Capsules **458**
- Neoral Soft Gelatin Capsules **2247**
- Neoral Oral Solution **2247**
- Restasis Ophthalmic Emulsion **570**
- Sandimmune **2259**

Dicumarol (Co-administration with coumarin-type anticoagulants has resulted in potentiation of oral anticoagulants resulting in prolonged prothrombin time; the dosage of the anticoaguant should be reduced to maintain the PT at the desired level).
No products indexed under this heading.

Fluvastatin Sodium (Co-administration of fibric acid derivatives and HMG-CoA reductase inhibitors has been associated, in numerous case reports, with rhabdomyolysis, markedly elevated creatine kinase (CK) levels and myoglobulinuria, leading in a high proportion of cases to acute renal failure; the combined use should be avoided unless the benefit of further alterations in lipid levels is likely to outweigh the increased risk of this combination). Products include:
- Lescol Capsules **2227**
- Lescol **2730**
- Lescol XL Tablets **2227**

Lovastatin (Co-administration of fibric acid derivatives and HMG-CoA reductase inhibitors has been associated, in numerous case reports, with rhabdomyolysis, markedly elevated creatine kinase (CK) levels and myoglobulinuria, leading in a high proportion of cases to acute renal failure; the combined use should be avoided unless the benefit of further alterations in lipid levels is likely to outweigh the increased risk of this combination). Products include:
- Advicor Tablets **1694**
- Altoprev Extended-Release Tablets **1151**
- Mevacor Tablets **1996**

Pravastatin Sodium (Co-administration of fibric acid derivatives and HMG-CoA reductase inhibitors has been associated, in numerous case reports, with rhabdomyolysis, markedly elevated creatine kinase (CK) levels and myoglobulinuria, leading in a high proportion of

cases to acute renal failure; the combined use should be avoided unless the benefit of further alterations in lipid levels is likely to outweigh the increased risk of this combination). Products include:

Pravachol Tablets 943

Simvastatin (Co-administration of fibric acid derivatives and HMG-CoA reductase inhibitors has been associated, in numerous case reports, with rhabdomyolysis, markedly elevated creatine kinase (CK) levels and myoglobulinuria, leading in a high proportion of cases to acute renal failure; the combined use should be avoided unless the benefit of further alterations in lipid levels is likely to outweigh the increased risk of this combination). Products include:

Vytorin 10/10 Tablets 2084
Vytorin 10/10 Tablets 3092
Vytorin 10/20 Tablets 2084
Vytorin 10/20 Tablets 3092
Vytorin 10/40 Tablets 3092
Vytorin 10/40 Tablets 2084
Vytorin 10/80 Tablets 2084
Vytorin 10/80 Tablets 3092
Zocor Tablets 2078

Warfarin Sodium (Co-administration with coumarin-type anticoagulants has resulted in potentiation of oral anticoagulants resulting in prolonged prothrombin time; the dosage of the anticoaguant should be reduced to maintain the PT at the desired level). Products include:

Coumadin for Injection 932
Coumadin Tablets 932

Food Interactions

Food, unspecified (The absorption of fenofibrate is increased when administered with food; Lofibra should be given with meals).

LO/OVRAL-28 TABLETS

(Ethinyl Estradiol, Norgestrel) 3423

May interact with barbiturates, corticosteroids, penicillins, phenytoin, protease inhibitors, tetracyclines, xanthines, and certain other agents. Compounds in these categories include:

Acetaminophen (May increase plasma ethinyl estradiol concentrations). Products include:

Benadryl Allergy & Cold Tablets 692
Benadryl Allergy & Sinus Headache Caplets & Gelcaps...... 693
Benadryl Maximum Strength Severe Allergy & Sinus Headache Caplets....................... 694
Contac Severe Cold and Flu Caplets Maximum Strength......... 615
Contac Severe Cold and Flu Caplets Non-Drowsy.................... 615
Darvocet A 500 Tablets 3497
Goody's Body Pain Formula Powder.. 621
Goody's Extra Strength Headache Powder........................ 621
Goody's Extra Strength Pain Relief Tablets 621
Goody's PM Powder 622
Hycomine Compound Tablets 1105
Lortab 3315
Lortab Elixir 3312
Percocet Tablets 1114
Robitussin Cough, Cold & Flu Liquid-filled Capsules.................. 750
Robitussin Flu Liquid 752
Sedapap Tablets 50 mg/650 mg 2098
Singlet Caplets 636
Sudafed Severe Cold 710
Sudafed Sinus Headache 711
TheraFlu Cold & Cough Hot Liquid 680
TheraFlu Cold & Sore Throat Hot Liquid 680
TheraFlu Flu & Chest Congestion Non-Drowsy Hot Liquid............... 681
TheraFlu Flu & Sore Throat Hot Liquid 681
TheraFlu Severe Cold Non-Drowsy Hot Liquid................ 683
TheraFlu Severe Cold & Cough Hot Liquid...................................... 683
TheraFlu Severe Cold Caplets 679
TheraFlu Severe Cold Hot Liquid 682
TheraFlu Severe Cold Non-Drowsy Caplets.................... 679
Triaminic Cough & Sore Throat Liquid 687
Triaminic Flu, Cough & Fever Liquid 685
Triaminic Cough & Sore Throat Softchews 689
Tylenol 8 Hour Extended Release Geltabs and Caplets 1843
Tylenol Sinus NightTime Caplets 663
Children's Tylenol Suspension Liquid and Meltaways.................... 1850
Children's Tylenol Plus Cold & Allergy Suspension Liquid............ 1850
Children's Tylenol Plus Cold NightTime Suspension Liquid........ 1851
Children's Tylenol Plus Cold & Cough Suspension Liquid and Chewable Tablets 1851
Children's Tylenol Plus Cold Chewable Tablets 1851
Children's Tylenol Plus Cold Daytime Non-Drowsy Suspension Liquid 1851
Children's Tylenol Plus Flu Suspension Liquid 1853
Concentrated Tylenol Infants' Drops Plus Cold........................ 1851
Concentrated Tylenol Infants' Drops Plus Cold and Cough 1851
Concentrated Tylenol Infants' Drops.. 1850
Junior Tylenol Meltaways 1850
Tylenol Cold & Flu Severe Daytime Liquid with Cool Bust....... 1846
Tylenol Cold & Flu Severe NightTime Liquid with Cool Burst.. 1846
Tylenol Cold Severe Congestion Non-Drowsy Caplets with Cool Burst.. 1846
Tylenol Cough & Sore Throat Daytime Liquid with Cool Burst...... 1849
Tylenol Cough & Sore Throat NightTime Liquid with Cool Burst.. 1849
Tylenol 1843
Extra Strength Tylenol Rapid Release Gels 1843
Tylenol 1843
Tylenol Allergy Complete Night Time Caplets 1844
Tylenol Allergy Complete Multi-Symptom Caplets and Gelcaps with Cool Burst............... 1844
Tylenol Severe Allergy Caplets 1844
Tylenol Flu NightTime Gelcaps 1846
Tylenol Flu Day Non-Drowsy Gelcaps.. 1846
Concentrated Tylenol Infants' Drops Plus Cold Nasal Congestant, Fever Reducer & Pain Reliever 668
Concentrated Tylenol Infants' Drops Plus Cold & Cough Nasal Decongestant, Fever Reducer & Pain Reliever............. 668
Multi-Symptom Tylenol Cold Night Time Caplets 1845
Multi-Symptom Tylenol Cold Day Non-Drowsy Caplets and Gelcaps.. 1845
Extra Strength Tylenol PM Caplets, Geltabs, Gelcaps and Liquid 1847
Tylenol Sinus Day Non-Drowsy 1848
Tylenol Sinus Night Time Caplets 1848
Tylenol Sinus Severe Congestion Caplets with Cool Burst 1848
Tylenol Sore Throat Daytime Liquid with Cool Burst.................. 1849
Tylenol Sore Throat NightTime Liquid with Cool Burst.................. 1849
Tylenol with Codeine 2461
Women's Tylenol Menstrual Relief Caplets... 1849
Ultracet Tablets 2462
Vicks 44M Cough, Cold & Flu Relief... 2676
Vicks DayQuil LiquiCaps/Liquid Multi-Symptom Cold/Flu Relief..... 723
Vicks DayQuil Multi-Symptom Cold/Flu Relief LiquiCaps............. 2675
Vicks DayQuil Multi-Symptom Cold/Flu Relief Liquid.................... 2675
Vicks NyQuil LiquiCaps 2677
Vicks NyQuil LiquiCaps/Liquid Multi-Symptom Cold/Flu Relief..... 725
Vicks NyQuil Liquid 2677
Vicodin Tablets 530
Vicodin ES Tablets 531
Vicodin HP Tablets 532
Zydone Tablets 1118

Aminophylline (Co-administration increases the plasma concentrations of theophylline).

No products indexed under this heading.

Amoxicillin (Penicillins may decrease ethinyl estradiol plasma concentrations that may cause an increased incidence of breakthrough bleeding and menstrual irregularities and may possibly reduce efficacy of combination contraceptives). Products include:

Amoxil Capsules 1315
Amoxil Chewable Tablets 1315
Amoxil Pediatric Drops for Oral Suspension 1315
Amoxil Powder for Oral Suspension 1315
Amoxil Tablets 1315
Augmentin 1331
Augmentin Tablets 1334
Augmentin XR Extended-Release Tablets 1340
Augmentin ES-600 Powder for Oral Suspension 1337
PREVPAC 3281

Amoxicillin Trihydrate (Penicillins may decrease ethinyl estradiol plasma concentrations that may cause an increased incidence of breakthrough bleeding and menstrual irregularities and may possibly reduce efficacy of combination contraceptives).

No products indexed under this heading.

Ampicillin (May decrease ethinyl estradiol plasma concentrations that may cause an increased incidence of breakthrough bleeding and menstrual irregularities and may possibly reduce efficacy of combination contraceptives).

No products indexed under this heading.

Ampicillin Sodium (May decrease ethinyl estradiol plasma concentrations that may cause an increased incidence of breakthrough bleeding and menstrual irregularities and may possibly reduce efficacy of combination contraceptives).

No products indexed under this heading.

Ampicillin Trihydrate (Penicillins may decrease ethinyl estradiol plasma concentrations that may cause an increased incidence of breakthrough bleeding and menstrual irregularities and may possibly reduce efficacy of combination contraceptives).

No products indexed under this heading.

Amprenavir (Some protease inhibitors increase the metabolism of ethinyl estradiol leading to decreased ethinyl estradiol plasma concentrations which may cause an increased incidence of breakthrough bleeding and menstrual irregularities and may possibly reduce efficacy of combination contraceptives). Products include:

Agenerase Capsules 1299
Agenerase Oral Solution 1304

Aprobarbital (Barbiturates increase the metabolism of ethinyl estradiol leading to decreased ethinyl estradiol plasma concentrations which may cause an increased incidence of breakthrough bleeding and menstrual irregularities and may possibly reduce efficacy of combination contraceptives).

No products indexed under this heading.

Atorvastatin Calcium (May increase plasma ethinyl estradiol concentrations). Products include:

Caduet Tablets 2507
Lipitor Tablets 2495

Azlocillin Sodium (Penicillins may decrease ethinyl estradiol plasma concentrations that may cause an increased incidence of breakthrough bleeding and menstrual irregularities and may possibly reduce efficacy of combination contraceptives).

No products indexed under this heading.

Bacampicillin Hydrochloride (Penicillins may decrease ethinyl estradiol plasma concentrations that may cause an increased incidence of breakthrough bleeding and menstrual irregularities and may possibly reduce efficacy of combination contraceptives).

No products indexed under this heading.

Betamethasone Acetate (Co-administration with corticosteroids may increase the plasma concentrations of corticosteroids).

No products indexed under this heading.

Betamethasone Sodium Phosphate (Co-administration with corticosteroids may increase the plasma concentrations of corticosteroids).

No products indexed under this heading.

Butabarbital (Barbiturates increase the metabolism of ethinyl estradiol leading to decreased ethinyl estradiol plasma concentrations which may cause an increased incidence of breakthrough bleeding and menstrual irregularities and may possibly reduce efficacy of combination contraceptives).

No products indexed under this heading.

Butalbital (Barbiturates increase the metabolism of ethinyl estradiol leading to decreased ethinyl estradiol plasma concentrations which may cause an increased incidence of breakthrough bleeding and menstrual irregularities and may possibly reduce efficacy of combination contraceptives). Products include:

Sedapap Tablets 50 mg/650 mg 2098

Carbenicillin Disodium (Penicillins may decrease ethinyl estradiol plasma concentrations that may cause an increased incidence of breakthrough bleeding and menstrual irregularities and may possibly reduce efficacy of combination contraceptives).

No products indexed under this heading.

Carbenicillin Indanyl Sodium (Penicillins may decrease ethinyl estradiol plasma concentrations that may cause an increased incidence of breakthrough bleeding and menstrual irregularities and may possibly reduce efficacy of combination contraceptives).
No products indexed under this heading.

Cortisone Acetate (Co-administration with corticosteroids may increase the plasma concentrations of corticosteroids).
No products indexed under this heading.

Cyclosporine (Co-administration increases the plasma concentrations of cyclosporine). Products include:
Gengraf Capsules 458
Neoral Soft Gelatin Capsules 2247
Neoral Oral Solution 2247
Restasis Ophthalmic Emulsion 570
Sandimmune 2259

Demeclocycline Hydrochloride (Tetracyclines may decrease ethinyl estradiol plasma concentrations that may cause an increased incidence of breakthrough bleeding and menstrual irregularities and may possibly reduce efficacy of combination contraceptives).
No products indexed under this heading.

Dexamethasone (Co-administration with corticosteroids may increase the plasma concentrations of corticosteroids). Products include:
Ciprodex Otic Suspension 555
Decadron Tablets 1929
TobraDex Ophthalmic Ointment 558
TobraDex Ophthalmic Suspension ... 558

Dexamethasone Acetate (Co-administration with corticosteroids may increase the plasma concentrations of corticosteroids).
No products indexed under this heading.

Dexamethasone Sodium Phosphate (Co-administration with corticosteroids may increase the plasma concentrations of corticosteroids). Products include:
Decadron Phosphate Injection 1931

Dicloxacillin Sodium (Penicillins may decrease ethinyl estradiol plasma concentrations that may cause an increased incidence of breakthrough bleeding and menstrual irregularities and may possibly reduce efficacy of combination contraceptives).
No products indexed under this heading.

Doxycycline Calcium (Tetracyclines may decrease ethinyl estradiol plasma concentrations that may cause an increased incidence of breakthrough bleeding and menstrual irregularities and may possibly reduce efficacy of combination contraceptives).
No products indexed under this heading.

Doxycycline Hyclate (Tetracyclines may decrease ethinyl estradiol plasma concentrations that may cause an increased incidence of breakthrough bleeding and menstrual irregularities and may possibly reduce efficacy of combination contraceptives).
No products indexed under this heading.

Doxycycline Monohydrate (Tetracyclines may decrease ethinyl estradiol plasma concentrations that may cause an increased incidence of breakthrough bleeding and menstrual irregularities and may possibly reduce efficacy of combination contraceptives).
No products indexed under this heading.

Dyphylline (Co-administration increases the plasma concentrations of theophylline).
No products indexed under this heading.

Fluconazole (Co-administration with CYP3A4 inhibitors may increase plasma ethinyl estradiol concentrations).
No products indexed under this heading.

Fludrocortisone Acetate (Co-administration with corticosteroids may increase the plasma concentrations of corticosteroids).
No products indexed under this heading.

Fosphenytoin Sodium (Increases the metabolism of ethinyl estradiol leading to decreased ethinyl estradiol plasma concentrations that may cause an increased incidence of breakthrough bleeding and menstrual irregularities and may possibly reduce efficacy of combination contraceptives).
No products indexed under this heading.

Griseofulvin (Increases the metabolism of ethinyl estradiol leading to decreased ethinyl estradiol plasma concentrations that may cause an increased incidence of breakthrough bleeding and menstrual irregularities and may possibly reduce efficacy of combination contraceptives). Products include:
Grifulvin V Tablets Microsize and Oral Suspension Microsize........... 2384
Gris-PEG Tablets 2504

Hydrocortisone (Co-administration with corticosteroids may increase the plasma concentrations of corticosteroids). Products include:
Cortizone•5 Ointment .... ▣699
Cortizone•10 Creme .... ▣699
Cortizone•10 Ointment .... ▣699
Cortizone•10 Plus Creme .... ▣700
Cortizone•10 Maximum Strength Quick Shot Spray........................ ▣700
Hydrocortone Tablets 1963
Preparation H Hydrocortisone Cream .... ▣748

Hydrocortisone Acetate (Co-administration with corticosteroids may increase the plasma concentrations of corticosteroids). Products include:
Analpram-HC 1136
Pramosone 1139
ProctoFoam-HC 3113
Tucks Anti-Itch Ointment .... ▣712
U-cort 1% Cream 3289

Hydrocortisone Sodium Phosphate (Co-administration with corticosteroids may increase the plasma concentrations of corticosteroids).
No products indexed under this heading.

Hydrocortisone Sodium Succinate (Co-administration with corticosteroids may increase the plasma concentrations of corticosteroids).
No products indexed under this heading.

Hypericum (Increases the metabolism of ethinyl estradiol leading to decreased ethinyl estradiol plasma concentrations that may cause an increased incidence of breakthrough bleeding and menstrual irregularities and may possibly reduce efficacy of combination contraceptives).
No products indexed under this heading.

Indinavir Sulfate (May increase plasma ethinyl estradiol concentrations; some protease inhibitors increase the metabolism of ethinyl estradiol leading to decreased ethinyl estradiol plasma concentrations which may cause an increased incidence of breakthrough bleeding and menstrual irregularities and may possibly reduce efficacy of combination contraceptives). Products include:
Crixivan Capsules 1918

Lopinavir (Some protease inhibitors increase the metabolism of ethinyl estradiol leading to decreased ethinyl estradiol plasma concentrations which may cause an increased incidence of breakthrough bleeding and menstrual irregularities and may possibly reduce efficacy of combination contraceptives). Products include:
Kaletra 474

Mephobarbital (Barbiturates increase the metabolism of ethinyl estradiol leading to decreased ethinyl estradiol plasma concentrations which may cause an increased incidence of breakthrough bleeding and menstrual irregularities and may possibly reduce efficacy of combination contraceptives). Products include:
Mebaral Tablets, USP 2483

Methacycline Hydrochloride (Tetracyclines may decrease ethinyl estradiol plasma concentrations that may cause an increased incidence of breakthrough bleeding and menstrual irregularities and may possibly reduce efficacy of combination contraceptives).
No products indexed under this heading.

Methylprednisolone Acetate (Co-administration with corticosteroids may increase the plasma concentrations of corticosteroids). Products include:
Depo-Medrol Injectable Suspension.................................. 2615
Depo-Medrol Single-Dose Vial 2617

Methylprednisolone Sodium Succinate (Co-administration with corticosteroids may increase the plasma concentrations of corticosteroids).
No products indexed under this heading.

Mezlocillin Sodium (Penicillins may decrease ethinyl estradiol plasma concentrations that may cause an increased incidence of breakthrough bleeding and menstrual irregularities and may possibly reduce efficacy of combination contraceptives).
No products indexed under this heading.

Minocycline Hydrochloride (Tetracyclines may decrease ethinyl estradiol plasma concentrations that may cause an increased incidence of breakthrough bleeding and menstrual irregularities and may possibly reduce efficacy of combination contraceptives). Products include:
Dynacin Tablets 1859

Modafinil (Increases the metabolism of ethinyl estradiol leading to decreased ethinyl estradiol plasma concentrations that may cause an increased incidence of breakthrough bleeding and menstrual irregularities and may possibly reduce efficacy of combination contraceptives). Products include:
Provigil Tablets 1002

Nafcillin Sodium (Penicillins may decrease ethinyl estradiol plasma concentrations that may cause an increased incidence of breakthrough bleeding and menstrual irregularities and may possibly reduce efficacy of combination contraceptives).
No products indexed under this heading.

Nelfinavir Mesylate (Some protease inhibitors increase the metabolism of ethinyl estradiol leading to decreased ethinyl estradiol plasma concentrations which may cause an increased incidence of breakthrough bleeding and menstrual irregularities and may possibly reduce efficacy of combination contraceptives). Products include:
Viracept 2556

Oxytetracycline Hydrochloride (Tetracyclines may decrease ethinyl estradiol plasma concentrations that may cause an increased incidence of breakthrough bleeding and menstrual irregularities and may possibly reduce efficacy of combination contraceptives).
No products indexed under this heading.

Penicillin G Benzathine (Penicillins may decrease ethinyl estradiol plasma concentrations that may cause an increased incidence of breakthrough bleeding and menstrual irregularities and may possibly reduce efficacy of combination contraceptives).
No products indexed under this heading.

Penicillin G Potassium (Penicillins may decrease ethinyl estradiol plasma concentrations that may cause an increased incidence of breakthrough bleeding and menstrual irregularities and may possibly reduce efficacy of combination contraceptives).
No products indexed under this heading.

Penicillin G Procaine (Penicillins may decrease ethinyl estradiol plasma concentrations that may cause an increased incidence of breakthrough bleeding and menstrual irregularities and may possibly reduce efficacy of combination contraceptives).
No products indexed under this heading.

Penicillin G Sodium (Penicillins may decrease ethinyl estradiol plasma concentrations that may cause an increased incidence of breakthrough bleeding and menstrual irregularities and may possibly reduce efficacy of combination contraceptives).
No products indexed under this heading.

Penicillin V Potassium (Penicillins may decrease ethinyl estradiol plasma concentrations that may cause an increased incidence of breakthrough bleeding and menstrual irregularities and may possibly reduce efficacy of combination contraceptives).
No products indexed under this heading.

Pentobarbital Sodium (Barbiturates increase the metabolism of ethinyl estradiol leading to decreased ethinyl estradiol plasma concentrations which may cause an increased incidence of breakthrough bleeding and menstrual irregularities and may possibly reduce efficacy of combination contraceptives).
Products include:
Nembutal Sodium Solution, USP **2484**

Phenobarbital (Barbiturates increase the metabolism of ethinyl estradiol leading to decreased ethinyl estradiol plasma concentrations which may cause an increased incidence of breakthrough bleeding and menstrual irregularities and may possibly reduce efficacy of combination contraceptives).
No products indexed under this heading.

Phenylbutazone (Increases the metabolism of ethinyl estradiol leading to decreased ethinyl estradiol plasma concentrations that may cause an increased incidence of breakthrough bleeding and menstrual irregularities and may possibly reduce efficacy of combination contraceptives).
No products indexed under this heading.

Phenytoin (Increases the metabolism of ethinyl estradiol leading to decreased ethinyl estradiol plasma concentrations that may cause an increased incidence of breakthrough bleeding and menstrual irregularities and may possibly reduce efficacy of combination contraceptives).
No products indexed under this heading.

Phenytoin Sodium (Increases the metabolism of ethinyl estradiol leading to decreased ethinyl estradiol plasma concentrations that may cause an increased incidence of breakthrough bleeding and menstrual irregularities and may possibly reduce efficacy of combination contraceptives). Products include:
Phenytek Capsules **2153**

Prednisolone Acetate (Co-administration with corticosteroids may increase the plasma concentrations of corticosteroids). Products include:
Blephamide Ophthalmic Ointment **563**
Blephamide Ophthalmic Suspension.................................. **564**
Poly-Pred Liquifilm Ophthalmic Suspension .... **⊙231**
Pred Forte Ophthalmic Suspension .... **⊙233**
Pred Mild Sterile Ophthalmic Suspension .... **⊙236**
Pred-G Ophthalmic Suspension ...... **⊙234**
Pred-G Sterile Ophthalmic Ointment.................................... **⊙235**

Prednisolone Sodium Phosphate (Co-administration with corticosteroids may increase the plasma concentrations of corticosteroids).
Products include:
Pediapred Oral Solution **3319**

Prednisolone Tebutate (Co-administration with corticosteroids may increase the plasma concentrations of corticosteroids).
No products indexed under this heading.

Prednisone (Co-administration with corticosteroids may increase the plasma concentrations of corticosteroids).
No products indexed under this heading.

Rifabutin (Increases the metabolism of ethinyl estradiol leading to decreased ethinyl estradiol plasma concentrations that may cause an increased incidence of breakthrough bleeding and menstrual irregularities and may possibly reduce efficacy of combination contraceptives).
No products indexed under this heading.

Rifampin (Increases the metabolism of ethinyl estradiol leading to decreased ethinyl estradiol plasma concentrations that may cause an increased incidence of breakthrough bleeding and menstrual irregularities and may possibly reduce efficacy of combination contraceptives).
No products indexed under this heading.

Ritonavir (Some protease inhibitors increase the metabolism of ethinyl estradiol leading to decreased ethinyl estradiol plasma concentrations which may cause an increased incidence of breakthrough bleeding and menstrual irregularities and may possibly reduce efficacy of combination contraceptives). Products include:
Kaletra **474**
Norvir **499**

Saquinavir (Some protease inhibitors increase the metabolism of ethinyl estradiol leading to decreased ethinyl estradiol plasma concentrations which may cause an increased incidence of breakthrough bleeding and menstrual irregularities and may possibly reduce efficacy of combination contraceptives).
No products indexed under this heading.

Saquinavir Mesylate (Some protease inhibitors increase the metabolism of ethinyl estradiol leading to decreased ethinyl estradiol plasma concentrations which may cause an increased incidence of breakthrough bleeding and menstrual irregularities and may possibly reduce efficacy of combination contraceptives).
Products include:
Invirase **2776**

Secobarbital Sodium (Barbiturates increase the metabolism of ethinyl estradiol leading to decreased ethinyl estradiol plasma concentrations which may cause an increased incidence of breakthrough bleeding and menstrual irregularities and may possibly reduce efficacy of combination contraceptives).
No products indexed under this heading.

Tetracycline Hydrochloride (Tetracyclines may decrease ethinyl estradiol plasma concentrations that may cause an increased incidence of breakthrough bleeding and menstrual irregularities and may possibly reduce efficacy of combination contraceptives).
No products indexed under this heading.

Theophylline (Co-administration increases the plasma concentrations of theophylline).
No products indexed under this heading.

Theophylline Anhydrous (Co-administration increases the plasma concentrations of theophylline).
Products include:
Uniphyl Tablets **2708**

Theophylline Calcium Salicylate (Co-administration increases the plasma concentrations of theophylline).
No products indexed under this heading.

Theophylline Dihydroxypropyl (Glyceryl) (Co-administration increases the plasma concentrations of theophylline).
No products indexed under this heading.

Theophylline Ethylenediamine (Co-administration increases the plasma concentrations of theophylline).
No products indexed under this heading.

Theophylline Sodium Glycinate (Co-administration increases the plasma concentrations of theophylline).
No products indexed under this heading.

Thiamylal Sodium (Barbiturates increase the metabolism of ethinyl estradiol leading to decreased ethinyl estradiol plasma concentrations which may cause an increased incidence of breakthrough bleeding and menstrual irregularities and may possibly reduce efficacy of combination contraceptives).
No products indexed under this heading.

Ticarcillin Disodium (Penicillins may decrease ethinyl estradiol plasma concentrations that may cause an increased incidence of breakthrough bleeding and menstrual irregularities and may possibly reduce efficacy of combination contraceptives). Products include:
Timentin ADD-Vantage **1556**
Timentin Injection Galaxy Container **1559**
Timentin IV Infusion **1553**
Timentin Pharmacy Bulk Package **1562**

Topiramate (Increases the metabolism of ethinyl estradiol leading to decreased ethinyl estradiol plasma concentrations that may cause an increased incidence of breakthrough bleeding and menstrual irregularities and may possibly reduce efficacy of combination contraceptives).
Products include:
Topamax Sprinkle Capsules **2438**
Topamax Tablets **2438**

Triamcinolone (Co-administration with corticosteroids may increase the plasma concentrations of corticosteroids).
No products indexed under this heading.

Triamcinolone Acetonide (Co-administration with corticosteroids may increase the plasma concentrations of corticosteroids). Products include:
Azmacort Inhalation Aerosol **1701**
Nasacort HFA Inhalation Aerosol **2939**
Nasacort AQ Nasal Spray **2937**

Triamcinolone Diacetate (Co-administration with corticosteroids may increase the plasma concentrations of corticosteroids).
No products indexed under this heading.

Triamcinolone Hexacetonide (Co-administration with corticosteroids may increase the plasma concentrations of corticosteroids).
No products indexed under this heading.

Troleandomycin (May increase plasma ethinyl estradiol concentrations; may increase the risk of intrahepatic cholestasis).
No products indexed under this heading.

Vitamin C (May increase plasma ethinyl estradiol concentrations).
Products include:
Chromagen Forte Soft Gelatin Capsules **3296**
Halls Defense Sugarfree Vitamin C Drops .... **▣611**
Niferex-150 Forte Capsules **3299**
Peridin-C Tablets .... **▣761**
Repliva 21/7 Tablets **3301**

LOPROX GEL
(Ciclopirox) **1861**
None cited in PDR database.

LOPROX SHAMPOO
(Ciclopirox) **1862**
None cited in PDR database.

LORTAB 2.5/500 TABLETS
(Acetaminophen, Hydrocodone Bitartrate)... **3315**
See Lortab 10/500 Tablets

LORTAB 5/500 TABLETS
(Acetaminophen, Hydrocodone Bitartrate)... **3315**
See Lortab 10/500 Tablets

LORTAB 7.5/500 TABLETS
(Acetaminophen, Hydrocodone Bitartrate)... **3315**
See Lortab 10/500 Tablets

LORTAB 10/500 TABLETS
(Acetaminophen, Hydrocodone Bitartrate)... **3315**
May interact with antihistamines, central nervous system depressants, monoamine oxidase inhibitors, narcotic analgesics, tranquilizers, tricyclic antidepressants, and certain other agents. Compounds in these categories include:

Acrivastine (Co-administration may exhibit additive CNS-depression).
No products indexed under this heading.

Alfentanil Hydrochloride (Co-administration may exhibit additive CNS-depression).
No products indexed under this heading.

Alprazolam (Co-administration may exhibit additive CNS-depression).
Products include:
Niravam Orally Disintegrating Tablets **3106**
Xanax XR Tablets **2655**

Amitriptyline Hydrochloride (Co-administration may increase the effect of either the antidepressant or hydrocodone).
No products indexed under this heading.

Amoxapine (Co-administration may increase the effect of either the antidepressant or hydrocodone).
No products indexed under this heading.

Aprobarbital (Co-administration may exhibit additive CNS-depression).
No products indexed under this heading.

Astemizole (Co-administration may exhibit additive CNS-depression).
No products indexed under this heading.

Azatadine Maleate (Co-administration may exhibit additive CNS-depression).
No products indexed under this heading.

Bromodiphenhydramine Hydrochloride (Co-administration may exhibit additive CNS-depression).
No products indexed under this heading.

Brompheniramine Maleate (Co-administration may exhibit additive CNS-depression). Products include:
Alacol DM Syrup ... 739
Children's Dimetapp Cold & Allergy Elixir ... ▣745
Children's Dimetapp DM Cold & Cough Elixir ... ▣745
Robitussin Allergy & Cough Syrup ... ▣750

Buprenorphine Hydrochloride (Co-administration may exhibit additive CNS-depression). Products include:
Buprenex Injectable ... 2718
Suboxone Tablets ... 2719
Subutex Tablets ... 2719

Buspirone Hydrochloride (Co-administration may exhibit additive CNS-depression).
No products indexed under this heading.

Butabarbital (Co-administration may exhibit additive CNS-depression).
No products indexed under this heading.

Butalbital (Co-administration may exhibit additive CNS-depression). Products include:
Sedapap Tablets 50 mg/650 mg ... 2098

Cetirizine Hydrochloride (Co-administration may exhibit additive CNS-depression). Products include:
Zyrtec Chewable Tablets ... 2589
Zyrtec ... 2589
Zyrtec-D 12 Hour Extended Release Tablets ... 2591

Chlordiazepoxide (Co-administration may exhibit additive CNS-depression).
No products indexed under this heading.

Chlordiazepoxide Hydrochloride (Co-administration may exhibit additive CNS-depression). Products include:
Librium Capsules ... 3349

Chlorpheniramine Maleate (Co-administration may exhibit additive CNS-depression). Products include:
Advil Allergy Sinus Caplets ... ▣737
Advil Multi-Symptom Cold Caplets ... ▣738
BC Allergy Sinus Cold Powder ... ▣612
Contac Severe Cold and Flu Caplets Maximum Strength ... ▣615
Hycomine Compound Tablets ... 1105
PediaCare Multi-Symptom Cold Liquid ... ▣704
PediaCare NightRest Cough & Cold Liquid ... ▣704
Robitussin Flu Liquid ... ▣752
Robitussin PM Cough & Cold Liquid ... ▣752
Singlet Caplets ... ▣636
Sudafed Sinus & Allergy Tablets ... ▣710
TheraFlu Cold & Cough Hot Liquid ... ▣680
TheraFlu Cold & Sore Throat Hot Liquid ... ▣680
TheraFlu Flu & Sore Throat Hot Liquid ... ▣681
TheraFlu Severe Cold & Cough Hot Liquid ... ▣683
TheraFlu Severe Cold Caplets ... ▣679
TheraFlu Severe Cold Hot Liquid ... ▣682
Triaminic Cold & Allergy Liquid ... ▣685
Triaminic Cold & Cough Liquid ... ▣685
Triaminic Flu, Cough & Fever Liquid ... ▣685
Triaminic Night Time Cough & Cold Liquid ... ▣685
Triaminic Allergy Runny Nose & Congestion Softchews ... ▣688
Triaminic Cold & Cough Softchews ... ▣688
Children's Tylenol Plus Cold NightTime Suspension Liquid ... 1851
Children's Tylenol Plus Cold & Cough Suspension Liquid and Chewable Tablets ... 1851
Children's Tylenol Plus Cold Chewable Tablets ... 1851
Children's Tylenol Plus Flu Suspension Liquid ... 1853
Tylenol Allergy Complete Multi-Symptom Caplets and Gelcaps with Cool Burst ... 1844
Multi-Symptom Tylenol Cold Night Time Caplets ... 1845
Vicks 44M Cough, Cold & Flu Relief ... 2676
Pediatric Vicks 44m Cough & Cold Relief ... 2673
Children's Vicks NyQuil Cold/Cough Relief ... 2671

Chlorpheniramine Polistirex (Co-administration may exhibit additive CNS-depression). Products include:
Tussionex Pennkinetic Extended-Release Suspension ... 3322

Chlorpheniramine Tannate (Co-administration may exhibit additive CNS-depression).
No products indexed under this heading.

Chlorpromazine (Co-administration may exhibit additive CNS-depression).
No products indexed under this heading.

Chlorpromazine Hydrochloride (Co-administration may exhibit additive CNS-depression).
No products indexed under this heading.

Chlorprothixene (Co-administration may exhibit additive CNS-depression).
No products indexed under this heading.

Chlorprothixene Hydrochloride (Co-administration may exhibit additive CNS-depression).
No products indexed under this heading.

Chlorprothixene Lactate (Co-administration may exhibit additive CNS-depression).
No products indexed under this heading.

Clemastine Fumarate (Co-administration may exhibit additive CNS-depression).
No products indexed under this heading.

Clomipramine Hydrochloride (Co-administration may increase the effect of either the antidepressant or hydrocodone).
No products indexed under this heading.

Clorazepate Dipotassium (Co-administration may exhibit additive CNS-depression). Products include:
Tranxene ... 2488

Clozapine (Co-administration may exhibit additive CNS-depression). Products include:
Clozapine Tablets ... 2141
Clozaril Tablets ... 2174
FazaClo Orally Disintegrating Tablets ... 547

Codeine Phosphate (Co-administration may exhibit additive CNS-depression). Products include:
Tylenol with Codeine ... 2461

Cyproheptadine Hydrochloride (Co-administration may exhibit additive CNS-depression).
No products indexed under this heading.

Desflurane (Co-administration may exhibit additive CNS-depression). Products include:
Suprane Liquid for Inhalation ... 770

Desipramine Hydrochloride (Co-administration may increase the effect of either the antidepressant or hydrocodone).
No products indexed under this heading.

Dexchlorpheniramine Maleate (Co-administration may exhibit additive CNS-depression).
No products indexed under this heading.

Dezocine (Co-administration may exhibit additive CNS-depression).
No products indexed under this heading.

Diazepam (Co-administration may exhibit additive CNS-depression). Products include:
Diastat Rectal Delivery System ... 3344
Valium Tablets ... 2822

Diphenhydramine Citrate (Co-administration may exhibit additive CNS-depression). Products include:
Children's Benadryl Allergy & Cold Fastmelt Tablets ... ▣695
Children's Benadryl D Allergy & Sinus Fastmelt Tablets ... ▣694
Children's Benadryl Allergy Fastmelt Tablets ... ▣696
Goody's PM Powder ... ▣622

Diphenhydramine Hydrochloride (Co-administration may exhibit additive CNS-depression). Products include:
Benadryl Allergy & Cold Tablets ... ▣692
Benadryl Allergy ... ▣691
Benadryl Allergy & Sinus Headache Caplets & Gelcaps ... ▣693
Children's Benadryl Allergy Liquid ... ▣695
Children's Benadryl Dye-Free Allergy Liquid ... ▣695
Benadryl Dye-Free Allergy Liqui-Gels Softgels ... ▣692
Benadryl Itch Relief Stick Extra Strength ... ▣696
Benadryl Itch Stopping Cream Extra Strength ... ▣697
Benadryl Itch Stopping Gel Extra Strength ... ▣697
Benadryl Itch Stopping Spray Extra Strength ... ▣697
Benadryl Maximum Strength Severe Allergy & Sinus Headache Caplets ... ▣694
Children's Benadryl D Liquid Medication ... ▣693
Benadryl D Tablets ... ▣694
Nytol QuickCaps Caplets ... ▣635
Maximum Strength Nytol QuickGels Softgels ... ▣635
Simply Sleep Caplets ... 1841
Sominex Original Formula Tablets ... ▣637
TheraFlu Thin Strips Multi Symptom ... ▣684
Triaminic Thin Strips Cough & Runny Nose ... ▣690
Children's Tylenol Plus Cold & Allergy Suspension Liquid ... 1850
Tylenol Allergy Complete Night Time Caplets ... 1844
Tylenol Severe Allergy Caplets ... 1844
Tylenol Flu NightTime Gelcaps ... 1846
Extra Strength Tylenol PM Caplets, Geltabs, Gelcaps and Liquid ... 1847
Unisom Maximum Strength SleepGels ... ▣712

Diphenylpyraline Hydrochloride (Co-administration may exhibit additive CNS-depression).
No products indexed under this heading.

Doxepin Hydrochloride (Co-administration may increase the effect of either the antidepressant or hydrocodone).
No products indexed under this heading.

Droperidol (Co-administration may exhibit additive CNS-depression).
No products indexed under this heading.

Enflurane (Co-administration may exhibit additive CNS-depression).
No products indexed under this heading.

Estazolam (Co-administration may exhibit additive CNS-depression). Products include:
ProSom Tablets ... 512

Ethanol (Co-administration may exhibit additive CNS-depression).
No products indexed under this heading.

Ethchlorvynol (Co-administration may exhibit additive CNS-depression).
No products indexed under this heading.

Ethinamate (Co-administration may exhibit additive CNS-depression).
No products indexed under this heading.

Ethyl Alcohol (Co-administration may exhibit additive CNS-depression).
No products indexed under this heading.

Fentanyl (Co-administration may exhibit additive CNS-depression). Products include:
Duragesic Transdermal System ... 2448

Fentanyl Citrate (Co-administration may exhibit additive CNS-depression). Products include:
Actiq ... 993

Fexofenadine Hydrochloride (Co-administration may exhibit additive CNS-depression). Products include:
Allegra ... 2857
Allegra-D 12 Hour Extended-Release Tablets ... 2860
Allegra-D 24 Hour Extended-Release Tablets ... 2862

Fluphenazine Decanoate (Co-administration may exhibit additive CNS-depression).
No products indexed under this heading.

Fluphenazine Enanthate (Co-administration may exhibit additive CNS-depression).
No products indexed under this heading.

Fluphenazine Hydrochloride (Co-administration may exhibit additive CNS-depression).
No products indexed under this heading.

Flurazepam Hydrochloride (Co-administration may exhibit additive CNS-depression). Products include:
Dalmane Capsules ... 3343

Glutethimide (Co-administration may exhibit additive CNS-depression).
No products indexed under this heading.

Haloperidol (Co-administration may exhibit additive CNS-depression).
No products indexed under this heading.

Haloperidol Decanoate (Co-administration may exhibit additive CNS-depression).
No products indexed under this heading.

Hydrocodone Polistirex (Co-administration may exhibit additive CNS-depression). Products include:
Tussionex Pennkinetic Extended-Release Suspension 3322

Hydromorphone Hydrochloride (Co-administration may exhibit additive CNS depression). Products include:
Dilaudid 439
Dilaudid Oral Liquid 443
Dilaudid Non-Sterile Powder 439
Dilaudid Rectal Suppositories 439
Dilaudid Tablets 439
Dilaudid Tablets - 8 mg 443
Dilaudid-HP 441

Hydroxyzine Hydrochloride (Co-administration may exhibit additive CNS-depression).
No products indexed under this heading.

Imipramine Hydrochloride (Co-administration may increase the effect of either the antidepressant or hydrocodone).
No products indexed under this heading.

Imipramine Pamoate (Co-administration may increase the effect of either the antidepressant or hydrocodone).
No products indexed under this heading.

Isocarboxazid (Co-administration may increase the effect of either the MAO inhibitor or hydrocodone).
No products indexed under this heading.

Isoflurane (Co-administration may exhibit additive CNS-depression).
No products indexed under this heading.

Ketamine Hydrochloride (Co-administration may exhibit additive CNS-depression).
No products indexed under this heading.

Levomethadyl Acetate Hydrochloride (Co-administration may exhibit additive CNS-depression).
No products indexed under this heading.

Levorphanol Tartrate (Co-administration may exhibit additive CNS-depression).
No products indexed under this heading.

Loratadine (Co-administration may exhibit additive CNS-depression). Products include:
Alavert Allergy & Sinus D-12 Hour Tablets 743
Alavert 743
Children's Claritin 24 Hour Non-Drowsy Allergy Syrup 732
Claritin Non-Drowsy 24 Hour Tablets 731
Non-Drowsy Claritin Hives Relief Tablets 733
Claritin Reditabs 24 Hour Non-Drowsy Tablets 732
Claritin-D Non-Drowsy 12 Hour Tablets 731
Claritin-D Non-Drowsy 24 Hour Tablets 731
Children's Dimetapp ND Non-Drowsy Allergy Syrup 746
Triaminic Allerchews 684

Lorazepam (Co-administration may exhibit additive CNS-depression).
No products indexed under this heading.

Loxapine Hydrochloride (Co-administration may exhibit additive CNS-depression).
No products indexed under this heading.

Loxapine Succinate (Co-administration may exhibit additive CNS-depression).
No products indexed under this heading.

Maprotiline Hydrochloride (Co-administration may increase the effect of either the antidepressant or hydrocodone).
No products indexed under this heading.

Meperidine Hydrochloride (Co-administration may exhibit additive CNS-depression).
No products indexed under this heading.

Mephobarbital (Co-administration may exhibit additive CNS-depression). Products include:
Mebaral Tablets, USP 2483

Meprobamate (Co-administration may exhibit additive CNS-depression).
No products indexed under this heading.

Mesoridazine Besylate (Co-administration may exhibit additive CNS-depression).
No products indexed under this heading.

Methadone Hydrochloride (Co-administration may exhibit additive CNS-depression).
No products indexed under this heading.

Methdilazine Hydrochloride (Co-administration may exhibit additive CNS-depression).
No products indexed under this heading.

Methohexital Sodium (Co-administration may exhibit additive CNS-depression).
No products indexed under this heading.

Methotrimeprazine (Co-administration may exhibit additive CNS-depression).
No products indexed under this heading.

Methoxyflurane (Co-administration may exhibit additive CNS-depression).
No products indexed under this heading.

Midazolam Hydrochloride (Co-administration may exhibit additive CNS-depression).
No products indexed under this heading.

Moclobemide (Co-administration may increase the effect of either the MAO inhibitor or hydrocodone).
No products indexed under this heading.

Molindone Hydrochloride (Co-administration may exhibit additive CNS-depression). Products include:
Moban Tablets 1108

Morphine Sulfate (Co-administration may exhibit additive CNS-depression). Products include:
Avinza Capsules 1714
Kadian Capsules 572
MS Contin Tablets 2703

Nortriptyline Hydrochloride (Co-administration may increase the effect of either the antidepressant or hydrocodone).
No products indexed under this heading.

Olanzapine (Co-administration may exhibit additive CNS-depression). Products include:
Symbyax Capsules 1788
Zyprexa Tablets 1798
Zyprexa IntraMuscular 1798
Zyprexa ZYDIS Orally Disintegrating Tablets 1798

Oxazepam (Co-administration may exhibit additive CNS-depression).
No products indexed under this heading.

Oxycodone Hydrochloride (Co-administration may exhibit additive CNS-depression). Products include:
Combunox Tablets 1183
OxyContin Tablets 2699
OxyFast Oral Concentrate Solution 2704
OxyIR Capsules 2704
Percocet Tablets 1114
Percodan Tablets 1115

Pargyline Hydrochloride (Co-administration may increase the effect of either the MAO inhibitor or hydrocodone).
No products indexed under this heading.

Pentobarbital Sodium (Co-administration may exhibit additive CNS-depression). Products include:
Nembutal Sodium Solution, USP 2484

Perphenazine (Co-administration may exhibit additive CNS-depression).
No products indexed under this heading.

Phenelzine Sulfate (Co-administration may increase the effect of either the MAO inhibitor or hydrocodone).
No products indexed under this heading.

Phenobarbital (Co-administration may exhibit additive CNS-depression).
No products indexed under this heading.

Prazepam (Co-administration may exhibit additive CNS-depression).
No products indexed under this heading.

Procarbazine Hydrochloride (Co-administration may increase the effect of either the MAO inhibitor or hydrocodone). Products include:
Matulane Capsules 3188

Prochlorperazine (Co-administration may exhibit additive CNS-depression).
No products indexed under this heading.

Promethazine Hydrochloride (Co-administration may exhibit additive CNS-depression). Products include:
Phenergan 3438

Propofol (Co-administration may exhibit additive CNS-depression). Products include:
Diprivan Injectable Emulsion 676

Propoxyphene Hydrochloride (Co-administration may exhibit additive CNS-depression).
No products indexed under this heading.

Propoxyphene Napsylate (Co-administration may exhibit additive CNS-depression). Products include:
Darvocet A 500 Tablets 3497

Protriptyline Hydrochloride (Co-administration may increase the effect of either the antidepressant or hydrocodone). Products include:
Vivactil Tablets 2350

Pyrilamine Maleate (Co-administration may exhibit additive CNS-depression).
No products indexed under this heading.

Pyrilamine Tannate (Co-administration may exhibit additive CNS-depression).
No products indexed under this heading.

Quazepam (Co-administration may exhibit additive CNS-depression).
No products indexed under this heading.

Quetiapine Fumarate (Co-administration may exhibit additive CNS-depression). Products include:
Seroquel Tablets 691

Remifentanil Hydrochloride (Co-administration may exhibit additive CNS-depression).
No products indexed under this heading.

Risperidone (Co-administration may exhibit additive CNS-depression). Products include:
Risperdal Consta Long-Acting Injection 1664
Risperdal M-Tab Orally Disintegrating Tablets 1658
Risperdal 1658

Secobarbital Sodium (Co-administration may exhibit additive CNS-depression).
No products indexed under this heading.

Selegiline Hydrochloride (Co-administration may increase the effect of either the MAO inhibitor or hydrocodone). Products include:
Eldepryl Capsules 3209

Sevoflurane (Co-administration may exhibit additive CNS-depression). Products include:
Ultane Liquid for Inhalation 526

Sufentanil Citrate (Co-administration may exhibit additive CNS-depression).
No products indexed under this heading.

Temazepam (Co-administration may exhibit additive CNS-depression).
No products indexed under this heading.

Terfenadine (Co-administration may exhibit additive CNS-depression).
No products indexed under this heading.

Thiamylal Sodium (Co-administration may exhibit additive CNS-depression).
No products indexed under this heading.

Thioridazine Hydrochloride (Co-administration may exhibit additive CNS-depression). Products include:
Thioridazine Hydrochloride Tablets 2122

Thiothixene (Co-administration may exhibit additive CNS-depression). Products include:
Thiothixene Capsules 2124

IMPORTANT NOTE: Always consult each drug listing in the patient's regimen for possible interactions.

Tranylcypromine Sulfate (Co-administration may increase the effect of either the MAO inhibitor or hydrocodone). Products include:
Parnate Tablets 1499

Triazolam (Co-administration may exhibit additive CNS-depression).
No products indexed under this heading.

Trifluoperazine Hydrochloride (Co-administration may exhibit additive CNS-depression).
No products indexed under this heading.

Trimeprazine Tartrate (Co-administration may exhibit additive CNS-depression).
No products indexed under this heading.

Trimipramine Maleate (Co-administration may increase the effect of either the antidepressant or hydrocodone). Products include:
Surmontil Capsules 2347

Tripelennamine Hydrochloride (Co-administration may exhibit additive CNS-depression).
No products indexed under this heading.

Triprolidine Hydrochloride (Co-administration may exhibit additive CNS-depression).
No products indexed under this heading.

Zaleplon (Co-administration may exhibit additive CNS-depression). Products include:
Sonata Capsules 1686

Ziprasidone Hydrochloride (Co-administration may exhibit additive CNS-depression). Products include:
Geodon Capsules 2514

Zolpidem Tartrate (Co-administration may exhibit additive CNS-depression). Products include:
Ambien Tablets 2867

Food Interactions

Alcohol (Co-administration may exhibit additive CNS-depression; concurrent use should be avoided).

LORTAB ELIXIR
(Acetaminophen, Hydrocodone Bitartrate) 3312
See Lortab 10/500 Tablets

LOTEMAX OPHTHALMIC SUSPENSION 0.5%
(Loteprednol Etabonate) .... ⊙249
None cited in PDR database.

LOTENSIN TABLETS
(Benazepril Hydrochloride) 2232
May interact with diuretics, lithium preparations, potassium preparations, and potassium sparing diuretics. Compounds in these categories include:

Amiloride Hydrochloride (Co-administration with potassium-sparing diuretics can increase the risk of hyperkalemia). Products include:
Midamor Tablets 2000
Moduretic Tablets 2003

Bendroflumethiazide (Patients on diuretics, especially those in whom diuretic therapy was recently instituted, may occasionally experience an excessive reduction in blood pressure).
No products indexed under this heading.

Bumetanide (Patients on diuretics, especially those in whom diuretic therapy was recently instituted, may occasionally experience an excessive reduction in blood pressure).
No products indexed under this heading.

Chlorothiazide (Patients on diuretics, especially those in whom diuretic therapy was recently instituted, may occasionally experience an excessive reduction in blood pressure). Products include:
Aldoclor Tablets 1881
Diuril Oral 1936

Chlorothiazide Sodium (Patients on diuretics, especially those in whom diuretic therapy was recently instituted, may occasionally experience an excessive reduction in blood pressure). Products include:
Diuril Sodium Intravenous 1934

Chlorthalidone (Patients on diuretics, especially those in whom diuretic therapy was recently instituted, may occasionally experience an excessive reduction in blood pressure). Products include:
Clorpres Tablets 2139

Ethacrynic Acid (Patients on diuretics, especially those in whom diuretic therapy was recently instituted, may occasionally experience an excessive reduction in blood pressure). Products include:
Edecrin Tablets 1941

Furosemide (Patients on diuretics, especially those in whom diuretic therapy was recently instituted, may occasionally experience an excessive reduction in blood pressure). Products include:
Furosemide Tablets 2117

Hydrochlorothiazide (Patients on diuretics, especially those in whom diuretic therapy was recently instituted, may occasionally experience an excessive reduction in blood pressure). Products include:
Aldoril Tablets 1884
Atacand HCT 637
Avalide Tablets 2889
Avalide Tablets 922
Benicar HCT Tablets 2852
Diovan HCT Tablets 2195
Dyazide Capsules 1389
Hyzaar 1964
Lotensin HCT Tablets 2235
Maxzide 2150
Micardis HCT Tablets 886
Moduretic Tablets 2003
Prinzide Tablets 2033
Teveten HCT Tablets 1710
Timolide Tablets 2056
Uniretic Tablets 3114
Vaseretic Tablets 2073
Zestoretic Tablets 701

Hydroflumethiazide (Patients on diuretics, especially those in whom diuretic therapy was recently instituted, may occasionally experience an excessive reduction in blood pressure).
No products indexed under this heading.

Indapamide (Patients on diuretics, especially those in whom diuretic therapy was recently instituted, may occasionally experience an excessive reduction in blood pressure). Products include:
Indapamide Tablets 2119

Lithium (Co-administration with lithium results in increased serum lithium levels and symptoms of lithium toxicity).
No products indexed under this heading.

Lithium Carbonate (Co-administration with lithium results in increased serum lithium levels and symptoms of lithium toxicity). Products include:
Eskalith 1406
Lithobid Tablets 1670

Lithium Citrate (Co-administration with lithium results in increased serum lithium levels and symptoms of lithium toxicity).
No products indexed under this heading.

Methyclothiazide (Patients on diuretics, especially those in whom diuretic therapy was recently instituted, may occasionally experience an excessive reduction in blood pressure).
No products indexed under this heading.

Metolazone (Patients on diuretics, especially those in whom diuretic therapy was recently instituted, may occasionally experience an excessive reduction in blood pressure).
No products indexed under this heading.

Polythiazide (Patients on diuretics, especially those in whom diuretic therapy was recently instituted, may occasionally experience an excessive reduction in blood pressure).
No products indexed under this heading.

Potassium Acid Phosphate (Co-administration with potassium supplements can increase the risk of hyperkalemia). Products include:
K-Phos Original (Sodium Free) Tablets 785

Potassium Bicarbonate (Co-administration with potassium supplements can increase the risk of hyperkalemia).
No products indexed under this heading.

Potassium Chloride (Co-administration with potassium supplements can increase the risk of hyperkalemia). Products include:
Colyte with Flavor Packs for Oral Solution 3102
HalfLytely and Bisacodyl Tablets Bowel Prep Kit with Flavors Packs 915
K-Dur Extended-Relase Tablets 3047
K-Lor Powder Packets 472
K-Tab Filmtab Tablets 473
TriLyte with Flavor Packs for Oral Solution 3114

Potassium Citrate (Co-administration with potassium supplements can increase the risk of hyperkalemia). Products include:
Urocit-K Tablets 2109

Potassium Gluconate (Co-administration with potassium supplements can increase the risk of hyperkalemia).
No products indexed under this heading.

Potassium Phosphate (Co-administration with potassium supplements can increase the risk of hyperkalemia). Products include:
K-Phos Neutral Tablets 785

Spironolactone (Co-administration with potassium-sparing diuretics can increase the risk of hyperkalemia).
No products indexed under this heading.

Torsemide (Patients on diuretics, especially those in whom diuretic therapy was recently instituted, may occasionally experience an excessive reduction in blood pressure).
No products indexed under this heading.

Triamterene (Co-administration with potassium-sparing diuretics can increase the risk of hyperkalemia). Products include:
Dyazide Capsules 1389
Dyrenium Capsules 3390
Maxzide 2150

LOTENSIN HCT TABLETS
(Benazepril Hydrochloride, Hydrochlorothiazide) 2235
May interact with barbiturates, insulin, lithium preparations, narcotic analgesics, non-steroidal anti-inflammatory agents, potassium preparations, potassium sparing diuretics, and certain other agents. Compounds in these categories include:

Alfentanil Hydrochloride (Orthostatic hypotension produced by thiazides may be potentiated by narcotics).
No products indexed under this heading.

Amiloride Hydrochloride (Co-administration with potassium-sparing diuretics can increase the risk of hyperkalemia). Products include:
Midamor Tablets 2000
Moduretic Tablets 2003

Aprobarbital (Orthostatic hypotension produced by thiazides may be potentiated by barbiturates).
No products indexed under this heading.

Buprenorphine Hydrochloride (Orthostatic hypotension produced by thiazides may be potentiated by narcotics). Products include:
Buprenex Injectable 2718
Suboxone Tablets 2719
Subutex Tablets 2719

Butabarbital (Orthostatic hypotension produced by thiazides may be potentiated by barbiturates).
No products indexed under this heading.

Butalbital (Orthostatic hypotension produced by thiazides may be potentiated by barbiturates). Products include:
Sedapap Tablets 50 mg/650 mg 2098

Celecoxib (The diuretic, natriuretic, and antihypertensive effects of thiazide diuretics may be reduced by concurrent administration of non-steroidal anti-inflammatory agents). Products include:
Celebrex Capsules 3130

Cholestyramine (Absorption of hydrochlorothiazide is impaired in the presence of anionic exchange resins; cholestyramine resins bind the hydrochlorothiazide and reduce its absorption from GI tract by up to 85%).
No products indexed under this heading.

Codeine Phosphate (Orthostatic hypotension produced by thiazides may be potentiated by narcotics). Products include:
Tylenol with Codeine 2461

Colestipol Hydrochloride (Absorption of hydrochlorothiazide is impaired in the presence of anionic exchange resins; colestipol resins bind the hydrochlorothiazide and reduce its absorption from GI tract by up to 43%).
No products indexed under this heading.

Dezocine (Orthostatic hypotension produced by thiazides may be potentiated by narcotics).
No products indexed under this heading.

Diclofenac Potassium (The diuretic, natriuretic, and antihypertensive effects of thiazide diuretics may be reduced by concurrent administration of non-steroidal anti-inflammatory agents). Products include:
Cataflam Tablets **2173**

Diclofenac Sodium (The diuretic, natriuretic, and antihypertensive effects of thiazide diuretics may be reduced by concurrent administration of non-steroidal anti-inflammatory agents). Products include:
Arthrotec Tablets **3126**
Voltaren Ophthalmic Solution **2300**
Voltaren Tablets **2298**
Voltaren-XR Tablets **2301**

Etodolac (The diuretic, natriuretic, and antihypertensive effects of thiazide diuretics may be reduced by concurrent administration of non-steroidal anti-inflammatory agents).
No products indexed under this heading.

Fenoprofen Calcium (The diuretic, natriuretic, and antihypertensive effects of thiazide diuretics may be reduced by concurrent administration of non-steroidal anti-inflammatory agents). Products include:
Nalfon Capsules **2504**

Fentanyl (Orthostatic hypotension produced by thiazides may be potentiated by narcotics). Products include:
Duragesic Transdermal System **2448**

Fentanyl Citrate (Orthostatic hypotension produced by thiazides may be potentiated by narcotics). Products include:
Actiq **993**

Flurbiprofen (The diuretic, natriuretic, and antihypertensive effects of thiazide diuretics may be reduced by concurrent administration of non-steroidal anti-inflammatory agents).
No products indexed under this heading.

Hydrocodone Bitartrate (Orthostatic hypotension produced by thiazides may be potentiated by narcotics). Products include:
Hycodan **1104**
Hycomine Compound Tablets **1105**
Hycotuss Expectorant Syrup **1106**
Lortab **3315**
Lortab Elixir **3312**
Vicodin Tablets **530**
Vicodin ES Tablets **531**
Vicodin HP Tablets **532**
Vicoprofen Tablets **533**
Zydone Tablets **1118**

Hydrocodone Polistirex (Orthostatic hypotension produced by thiazides may be potentiated by narcotics). Products include:
Tussionex Pennkinetic Extended-Release Suspension **3322**

Hydromorphone Hydrochloride (Orthostatic hypotension produced by thiazides may be potentiated by narcotics). Products include:
Dilaudid **439**
Dilaudid Oral Liquid **443**
Dilaudid Non-Sterile Powder **439**
Dilaudid Rectal Suppositories **439**
Dilaudid Tablets **439**
Dilaudid Tablets - 8 mg **443**
Dilaudid-HP **441**

Ibuprofen (The diuretic, natriuretic, and antihypertensive effects of thiazide diuretics may be reduced by concurrent administration of non-steroidal anti-inflammatory agents). Products include:
Advil Allergy Sinus Caplets **737**
Advil **737**
Children's Advil Suspension **742**
Children's Advil Chewable Tablets **741**
Advil Cold & Sinus **739**
Advil Flu & Body Ache Caplets **739**
Children's Advil Cold Suspension **741**
Infants' Advil Concentrated Drops **743**
Junior Strength Advil Swallow Tablets **740**
Advil Migraine Liquigels **740**
Advil Multi-Symptom Cold Caplets **738**
Combunox Tablets **1183**
Children's Motrin Oral Suspension and Chewable Tablets **1837**
Children's Motrin Cold Non-Staining Dye-Free Oral Suspension **1838**
Children's Motrin Cold Oral Suspension **1838**
Children's Motrin Non-Staining Dye-Free Oral Suspension **1837**
Motrin Cold & Sinus Caplets **1836**
Motrin IB Tablets and Caplets **1836**
Infants' Motrin Concentrated Drops **1837**
Infants' Motrin Non-Staining Dye-Free Drops **1837**
Junior Strength Motrin Caplets and Chewable Tablets **1837**
Vicoprofen Tablets **533**

Indomethacin (The diuretic, natriuretic, and antihypertensive effects of thiazide diuretics may be reduced by concurrent administration of non-steroidal anti-inflammatory agents). Products include:
Indocin **1968**

Indomethacin Sodium Trihydrate (The diuretic, natriuretic, and antihypertensive effects of thiazide diuretics may be reduced by concurrent administration of non-steroidal anti-inflammatory agents). Products include:
Indocin I.V. **1973**

Insulin, Human, Zinc Suspension (Hydrochlorothiazide causes hyperglycemia and tends to reduce glucose tolerance; insulin requirements may be increased, decreased, or unchanged). Products include:
Humulin L, 100 Units **1763**
Humulin U, 100 Units **1770**

Insulin, Human NPH (Hydrochlorothiazide causes hyperglycemia and tends to reduce glucose tolerance; insulin requirements may be increased, decreased, or unchanged). Products include:
Humulin N, 100 Units **1764**
Humulin N Pen **1765**
Novolin N Human Insulin 10 ml Vials **2322**
Novolin N InnoLet **2322**
Novolin N PenFill 3 ml Cartridges **2325**
Novolin R InnoLet **2322**

Insulin, Human Regular (Hydrochlorothiazide causes hyperglycemia and tends to reduce glucose tolerance; insulin requirements may be increased, decreased, or unchanged). Products include:
Humulin R (U-500) **1768**
Humulin R, 100 Units **1767**
Novolin R Human Insulin 10 ml Vials **2322**
Novolin R PenFill **2325**

Insulin, Human Regular and Human NPH Mixture (Hydrochlorothiazide causes hyperglycemia and tends to reduce glucose tolerance; insulin requirements may be increased, decreased, or unchanged). Products include:
Humulin 50/50, 100 Units **1760**
Humulin 70/30 Pen **1761**
Novolin 70/30 Human Insulin 10 ml Vials **2321**
Novolin 70/30 InnoLet **2322**
Novolin 70/30 PenFill 3 ml Cartridges **2325**

Insulin, NPH (Hydrochlorothiazide causes hyperglycemia and tends to reduce glucose tolerance; insulin requirements may be increased, decreased, or unchanged).
No products indexed under this heading.

Insulin, Regular (Hydrochlorothiazide causes hyperglycemia and tends to reduce glucose tolerance; insulin requirements may be increased, decreased, or unchanged).
No products indexed under this heading.

Insulin, Zinc Crystals (Hydrochlorothiazide causes hyperglycemia and tends to reduce glucose tolerance; insulin requirements may be increased, decreased, or unchanged).
No products indexed under this heading.

Insulin, Zinc Suspension (Hydrochlorothiazide causes hyperglycemia and tends to reduce glucose tolerance; insulin requirements may be increased, decreased, or unchanged).
No products indexed under this heading.

Insulin Aspart, Human Regular (Hydrochlorothiazide causes hyperglycemia and tends to reduce glucose tolerance; insulin requirements may be increased, decreased, or unchanged). Products include:
NovoLog Injection **2326**

Insulin glargine (Hydrochlorothiazide causes hyperglycemia and tends to reduce glucose tolerance; insulin requirements may be increased, decreased, or unchanged). Products include:
Lantus Injection **2925**

Insulin Lispro, Human (Hydrochlorothiazide causes hyperglycemia and tends to reduce glucose tolerance; insulin requirements may be increased, decreased, or unchanged). Products include:
Humalog-Pen **1751**
Humalog Mix 75/25-Pen **1754**

Insulin Lispro Protamine, Human (Hydrochlorothiazide causes hyperglycemia and tends to reduce glucose tolerance; insulin requirements may be increased, decreased, or unchanged). Products include:
Humalog Mix 75/25-Pen **1754**

Ketoprofen (The diuretic, natriuretic, and antihypertensive effects of thiazide diuretics may be reduced by concurrent administration of non-steroidal anti-inflammatory agents).
No products indexed under this heading.

Ketorolac Tromethamine (The diuretic, natriuretic, and antihypertensive effects of thiazide diuretics may be reduced by concurrent administration of non-steroidal anti-inflammatory agents). Products include:
Acular Ophthalmic Solution **561**
Acular LS Ophthalmic Solution **562**

Levorphanol Tartrate (Orthostatic hypotension produced by thiazides may be potentiated by narcotics).
No products indexed under this heading.

Lithium (Co-administration with lithium results in increased serum lithium levels; renal clearance of lithium is reduced by thiazides; increased risk of lithium toxicity).
No products indexed under this heading.

Lithium Carbonate (Co-administration with lithium results in increased serum lithium levels; renal clearance of lithium is reduced by thiazides; increased risk of lithium toxicity). Products include:
Eskalith **1406**
Lithobid Tablets **1670**

Lithium Citrate (Co-administration with lithium results in increased serum lithium levels; renal clearance of lithium is reduced by thiazides; increased risk of lithium toxicity).
No products indexed under this heading.

Meclofenamate Sodium (The diuretic, natriuretic, and antihypertensive effects of thiazide diuretics may be reduced by concurrent administration of non-steroidal anti-inflammatory agents).
No products indexed under this heading.

Mefenamic Acid (The diuretic, natriuretic, and antihypertensive effects of thiazide diuretics may be reduced by concurrent administration of non-steroidal anti-inflammatory agents).
No products indexed under this heading.

Meloxicam (The diuretic, natriuretic, and antihypertensive effects of thiazide diuretics may be reduced by concurrent administration of non-steroidal anti-inflammatory agents). Products include:
Mobic Oral Suspension **893**
Mobic Tablets **893**

Meperidine Hydrochloride (Orthostatic hypotension produced by thiazides may be potentiated by narcotics).
No products indexed under this heading.

Mephobarbital (Orthostatic hypotension produced by thiazides may be potentiated by barbiturates). Products include:
Mebaral Tablets, USP **2483**

Methadone Hydrochloride (Orthostatic hypotension produced by thiazides may be potentiated by narcotics).
No products indexed under this heading.

Morphine Sulfate (Orthostatic hypotension produced by thiazides may be potentiated by narcotics). Products include:
Avinza Capsules **1714**
Kadian Capsules **572**
MS Contin Tablets **2703**

Nabumetone (The diuretic, natriuretic, and antihypertensive effects of thiazide diuretics may be reduced by concurrent administration of non-steroidal anti-inflammatory agents). Products include:
Relafen Tablets **1523**

Naproxen (The diuretic, natriuretic, and antihypertensive effects of thia-

zide diuretics may be reduced by concurrent administration of non-steroidal anti-inflammatory agents). Products include:
EC-Naprosyn Delayed-Release Tablets 2769
Naprosyn Suspension 2769
Naprosyn Tablets 2769
Prevacid NapraPAC 3277

Naproxen Sodium (The diuretic, natriuretic, and antihypertensive effects of thiazide diuretics may be reduced by concurrent administration of non-steroidal anti-inflammatory agents). Products include:
Aleve Tablets, Caplets and Gelcaps 605
Anaprox Tablets 2769
Anaprox DS Tablets 2769

Norepinephrine Hydrochloride (Thiazides may decrease arterial responsiveness to norepinephrine).
No products indexed under this heading.

Oxaprozin (The diuretic, natriuretic, and antihypertensive effects of thiazide diuretics may be reduced by concurrent administration of non-steroidal anti-inflammatory agents).
No products indexed under this heading.

Oxycodone Hydrochloride (Orthostatic hypotension produced by thiazides may be potentiated by narcotics). Products include:
Combunox Tablets 1183
OxyContin Tablets 2699
OxyFast Oral Concentrate Solution 2704
OxyIR Capsules 2704
Percocet Tablets 1114
Percodan Tablets 1115

Pentobarbital Sodium (Orthostatic hypotension produced by thiazides may be potentiated by barbiturates). Products include:
Nembutal Sodium Solution, USP 2484

Phenobarbital (Orthostatic hypotension produced by thiazides may be potentiated by barbiturates).
No products indexed under this heading.

Phenylbutazone (The diuretic, natriuretic, and antihypertensive effects of thiazide diuretics may be reduced by concurrent administration of non-steroidal anti-inflammatory agents).
No products indexed under this heading.

Piroxicam (The diuretic, natriuretic, and antihypertensive effects of thiazide diuretics may be reduced by concurrent administration of non-steroidal anti-inflammatory agents).
No products indexed under this heading.

Potassium Acid Phosphate (Co-administration with potassium supplements can increase the risk of hyperkalemia). Products include:
K-Phos Original (Sodium Free) Tablets 785

Potassium Bicarbonate (Co-administration with potassium supplements can increase the risk of hyperkalemia).
No products indexed under this heading.

Potassium Chloride (Co-administration with potassium supplements can increase the risk of hyperkalemia). Products include:
Colyte with Flavor Packs for Oral Solution 3102
HalfLytely and Bisacodyl Tablets Bowel Prep Kit with Flavors Packs 915
K-Dur Extended-Relase Tablets 3047
K-Lor Powder Packets 472
K-Tab Filmtab Tablets 473
TriLyte with Flavor Packs for Oral Solution 3114

Potassium Citrate (Co-administration with potassium supplements can increase the risk of hyperkalemia). Products include:
Urocit-K Tablets 2109

Potassium Gluconate (Co-administration with potassium supplements can increase the risk of hyperkalemia).
No products indexed under this heading.

Potassium Phosphate (Co-administration with potassium supplements can increase the risk of hyperkalemia). Products include:
K-Phos Neutral Tablets 785

Propoxyphene Hydrochloride (Orthostatic hypotension produced by thiazides may be potentiated by narcotics).
No products indexed under this heading.

Propoxyphene Napsylate (Orthostatic hypotension produced by thiazides may be potentiated by narcotics). Products include:
Darvocet A 500 Tablets 3497

Remifentanil Hydrochloride (Orthostatic hypotension produced by thiazides may be potentiated by narcotics).
No products indexed under this heading.

Rofecoxib (The diuretic, natriuretic, and antihypertensive effects of thiazide diuretics may be reduced by concurrent administration of non-steroidal anti-inflammatory agents).
No products indexed under this heading.

Secobarbital Sodium (Orthostatic hypotension produced by thiazides may be potentiated by barbiturates).
No products indexed under this heading.

Spironolactone (Co-administration with potassium-sparing diuretics can increase the risk of hyperkalemia).
No products indexed under this heading.

Sufentanil Citrate (Orthostatic hypotension produced by thiazides may be potentiated by narcotics).
No products indexed under this heading.

Sulindac (The diuretic, natriuretic, and antihypertensive effects of thiazide diuretics may be reduced by concurrent administration of non-steroidal anti-inflammatory agents). Products include:
Clinoril Tablets 1899

Thiamylal Sodium (Orthostatic hypotension produced by thiazides may be potentiated by barbiturates).
No products indexed under this heading.

Tolmetin Sodium (The diuretic, natriuretic, and antihypertensive effects of thiazide diuretics may be reduced by concurrent administration of non-steroidal anti-inflammatory agents).
No products indexed under this heading.

Triamterene (Co-administration with potassium-sparing diuretics can increase the risk of hyperkalemia). Products include:
Dyazide Capsules 1389
Dyrenium Capsules 3390
Maxzide 2150

Tubocurarine Chloride (Thiazides may increase the responsiveness to tubocurarine).
No products indexed under this heading.

Valdecoxib (The diuretic, natriuretic, and antihypertensive effects of thiazide diuretics may be reduced by concurrent administration of non-steroidal anti-inflammatory agents).
No products indexed under this heading.

Food Interactions

Alcohol (Orthostatic hypotension produced by thiazides may be potentiated by alcohol).

LOTREL CAPSULES

(Amlodipine Besylate, Benazepril Hydrochloride) 2238
May interact with diuretics, lithium preparations, potassium preparations, and potassium sparing diuretics. Compounds in these categories include:

Amiloride Hydrochloride (Potential for the increased risk of hyperkalemia; patients on diuretics, especially those in whom diuretic therapy was recently instituted, may experience an excessive reduction in blood pressure). Products include:
Midamor Tablets 2000
Moduretic Tablets 2003

Bendroflumethiazide (Patients on diuretics, especially those in whom diuretic therapy was recently instituted, may experience an excessive reduction in blood pressure).
No products indexed under this heading.

Bumetanide (Patients on diuretics, especially those in whom diuretic therapy was recently instituted, may experience an excessive reduction in blood pressure).
No products indexed under this heading.

Chlorothiazide (Patients on diuretics, especially those in whom diuretic therapy was recently instituted, may experience an excessive reduction in blood pressure). Products include:
Aldoclor Tablets 1881
Diuril Oral 1936

Chlorothiazide Sodium (Patients on diuretics, especially those in whom diuretic therapy was recently instituted, may experience an excessive reduction in blood pressure). Products include:
Diuril Sodium Intravenous 1934

Chlorthalidone (Patients on diuretics, especially those in whom diuretic therapy was recently instituted, may experience an excessive reduction in blood pressure). Products include:
Clorpres Tablets 2139

Ethacrynic Acid (Patients on diuretics, especially those in whom diuretic therapy was recently instituted, may experience an excessive reduction in blood pressure). Products include:
Edecrin Tablets 1941

Furosemide (Patients on diuretics, especially those in whom diuretic therapy was recently instituted, may experience an excessive reduction in blood pressure). Products include:
Furosemide Tablets 2117

Hydrochlorothiazide (Patients on diuretics, especially those in whom diuretic therapy was recently instituted, may experience an excessive reduction in blood pressure). Products include:
Aldoril Tablets 1884
Atacand HCT 637
Avalide Tablets 2889
Avalide Tablets 922
Benicar HCT Tablets 2852
Diovan HCT Tablets 2195
Dyazide Capsules 1389
Hyzaar 1964
Lotensin HCT Tablets 2235
Maxzide 2150
Micardis HCT Tablets 886
Moduretic Tablets 2003
Prinzide Tablets 2033
Teveten HCT Tablets 1710
Timolide Tablets 2056
Uniretic Tablets 3114
Vaseretic Tablets 2073
Zestoretic Tablets 701

Hydroflumethiazide (Patients on diuretics, especially those in whom diuretic therapy was recently instituted, may experience an excessive reduction in blood pressure).
No products indexed under this heading.

Indapamide (Patients on diuretics, especially those in whom diuretic therapy was recently instituted, may experience an excessive reduction in blood pressure). Products include:
Indapamide Tablets 2119

Lithium (Potential for increased serum lithium levels and symptoms of lithium toxicity).
No products indexed under this heading.

Lithium Carbonate (Potential for increased serum lithium levels and symptoms of lithium toxicity). Products include:
Eskalith 1406
Lithobid Tablets 1670

Lithium Citrate (Potential for increased serum lithium levels and symptoms of lithium toxicity).
No products indexed under this heading.

Methyclothiazide (Patients on diuretics, especially those in whom diuretic therapy was recently instituted, may experience an excessive reduction in blood pressure).
No products indexed under this heading.

Metolazone (Patients on diuretics, especially those in whom diuretic therapy was recently instituted, may experience an excessive reduction in blood pressure).
No products indexed under this heading.

Polythiazide (Patients on diuretics, especially those in whom diuretic therapy was recently instituted, may experience an excessive reduction in blood pressure).
No products indexed under this heading.

Potassium Acid Phosphate (Potential for the increased risk of hyperkalemia). Products include:
K-Phos Original (Sodium Free) Tablets 785

Potassium Bicarbonate (Potential for the increased risk of hyperkalemia).
No products indexed under this heading.

Potassium Chloride (Potential for the increased risk of hyperkalemia). Products include:
Colyte with Flavor Packs for Oral Solution 3102

HalfLytely and Bisacodyl Tablets Bowel Prep Kit with Flavors Packs ... 915
K-Dur Extended-Relase Tablets ... 3047
K-Lor Powder Packets ... 472
K-Tab Filmtab Tablets ... 473
TriLyte with Flavor Packs for Oral Solution ... 3114

Potassium Citrate (Potential for the increased risk of hyperkalemia). Products include:
Urocit-K Tablets ... 2109

Potassium Gluconate (Potential for the increased risk of hyperkalemia).
No products indexed under this heading.

Potassium Phosphate (Potential for the increased risk of hyperkalemia). Products include:
K-Phos Neutral Tablets ... 785

Spironolactone (Potential for the increased risk of hyperkalemia; patients on diuretics, especially those in whom diuretic therapy was recently instituted, may experience an excessive reduction in blood pressure).
No products indexed under this heading.

Torsemide (Patients on diuretics, especially those in whom diuretic therapy was recently instituted, may experience an excessive reduction in blood pressure).
No products indexed under this heading.

Triamterene (Potential for the increased risk of hyperkalemia; patients on diuretics, especially those in whom diuretic therapy was recently instituted, may experience an excessive reduction in blood pressure). Products include:
Dyazide Capsules ... 1389
Dyrenium Capsules ... 3390
Maxzide ... 2150

LOTRIMIN CREAM
(Clotrimazole) ... 3053
None cited in PDR database.

LOTRIMIN LOTION 1%
(Clotrimazole) ... 3053
None cited in PDR database.

LOTRIMIN TOPICAL SOLUTION 1%
(Clotrimazole) ... 3053
None cited in PDR database.

LOTRIMIN ULTRA CREAM 1%
(Butenafine Hydrochloride) ... 733
None cited in PDR database.

LOTRISONE CREAM
(Betamethasone Dipropionate, Clotrimazole) ... 3054
None cited in PDR database.

LOTRISONE LOTION
(Betamethasone Dipropionate, Clotrimazole) ... 3054
None cited in PDR database.

LOTRONEX TABLETS
(Alosetron Hydrochloride) ... 1479
May interact with cytochrome p450 1a2 inhibitors (selected), cytochrome p450 3a4 inhibitors, potent, and certain other agents. Compounds in these categories include:

Alatrofloxacin Mesylate (Concomitant administration of alosetron and moderate CYP1A2 inhibitors, including quinolone antibiotics and cimetidine, has not been evaluated, but should be avoided unless clinically necessary because of potential drug interactions).
No products indexed under this heading.

Amiodarone Hydrochloride (Concomitant administration of alosetron and moderate CYP1A2 inhibitors, including quinolone antibiotics and cimetidine, has not been evaluated, but should be avoided unless clinically necessary because of potential drug interactions). Products include:
Pacerone Tablets ... 3337

Amprenavir (Ketoconazole is a known strong inhibitor of CYP3A4. In a pharmacokinetic study, 38 healthy female subjects received ketoconazole 200 mg twice daily for 7 days, with co-administration of alosetron 1 mg on the last day. Ketoconazole increased mean alosetron plasma concentrations (AUC) by 29%. Caution should be used when alosetron and ketoconazole are administered concomitantly. Co-administration of alosetron and strong SYP3A4 inhibitors has not been evaluated but should be undertaken with caution because of similar potential drug interactions). Products include:
Agenerase Capsules ... 1299
Agenerase Oral Solution ... 1304

Anastrozole (Concomitant administration of alosetron and moderate CYP1A2 inhibitors, including quinolone antibiotics and cimetidine, has not been evaluated, but should be avoided unless clinically necessary because of potential drug interactions). Products include:
Arimidex Tablets ... 665

Atazanavir (Ketoconazole is a known strong inhibitor of CYP3A4. In a pharmacokinetic study, 38 healthy female subjects received ketoconazole 200 mg twice daily for 7 days, with co-administration of alosetron 1 mg on the last day. Ketoconazole increased mean alosetron plasma concentrations (AUC) by 29%. Caution should be used when alosetron and ketoconazole are administered concomitantly. Co-administration of alosetron and strong SYP3A4 inhibitors has not been evaluated but should be undertaken with caution because of similar potential drug interactions).
No products indexed under this heading.

Atazanavir sulfate (Ketoconazole is a known strong inhibitor of CYP3A4. In a pharmacokinetic study, 38 healthy female subjects received ketoconazole 200 mg twice daily for 7 days, with co-administration of alosetron 1 mg on the last day. Ketoconazole increased mean alosetron plasma concentrations (AUC) by 29%. Caution should be used when alosetron and ketoconazole are administered concomitantly. Co-administration of alosetron and strong SYP3A4 inhibitors has not been evaluated but should be undertaken with caution because of similar potential drug interactions). Products include:
Reyataz Capsules ... 948

Cimetidine (Concomitant administration of alosetron and moderate CYP1A2 inhibitors, including quinolone antibiotics and cimetidine, has not been evaluated, but should be avoided unless clinically necessary because of potential drug interactions). Products include:
Tagamet HB 200 Tablets ... 637
Tagamet Tablets ... 1547

Cimetidine Hydrochloride (Concomitant administration of alosetron and moderate CYP1A2 inhibitors, including quinolone antibiotics and cimetidine, has not been evaluated, but should be avoided unless clinically necessary because of potential drug interactions).
No products indexed under this heading.

Ciprofloxacin (Concomitant administration of alosetron and moderate CYP1A2 inhibitors, including quinolone antibiotics and cimetidine, has not been evaluated, but should be avoided unless clinically necessary because of potential drug interactions). Products include:
Cipro I.V. ... 2998
Cipro I.V. Pharmacy Bulk Package ... 3509
Cipro Oral Suspension ... 2991
Cipro XR Tablets ... 3004
Ciprodex Otic Suspension ... 555

Ciprofloxacin Hydrochloride (Concomitant administration of alosetron and moderate CYP1A2 inhibitors, including quinolone antibiotics and cimetidine, has not been evaluated, but should be avoided unless clinically necessary because of potential drug interactions). Products include:
Ciloxan Ophthalmic Ointment ... 554
Cipro Tablets ... 2991

Clarithromycin (Ketoconazole is a known strong inhibitor of CYP3A4. In a pharmacokinetic study, 38 healthy female subjects received ketoconazole 200 mg twice daily for 7 days, with co-administration of alosetron 1 mg on the last day. Ketoconazole increased mean alosetron plasma concentrations (AUC) by 29%. Caution should be used when alosetron and ketoconazole are administered concomitantly. Co-administration of alosetron and strong SYP3A4 inhibitors has not been evaluated but should be undertaken with caution because of similar potential drug interactions). Products include:
Biaxin/Biaxin XL ... 402
PREVPAC ... 3281

Desogestrel (Concomitant administration of alosetron and moderate CYP1A2 inhibitors, including quinolone antibiotics and cimetidine, has not been evaluated, but should be avoided unless clinically necessary because of potential drug interactions). Products include:
Ortho-Cept Tablets ... 2395

Enoxacin (Concomitant administration of alosetron and moderate CYP1A2 inhibitors, including quinolone antibiotics and cimetidine, has not been evaluated, but should be avoided unless clinically necessary because of potential drug interactions).
No products indexed under this heading.

Ethinyl Estradiol (Concomitant administration of alosetron and moderate CYP1A2 inhibitors, including quinolone antibiotics and cimetidine, has not been evaluated, but should be avoided unless clinically necessary because of potential drug interactions). Products include:
Alesse-28 Tablets ... 3392
Lo/Ovral-28 Tablets ... 3423
NuvaRing ... 2357
Ortho-Cept Tablets ... 2395
Ortho-Cyclen/Ortho Tri-Cyclen ... 2414
Ortho Evra Transdermal System ... 2402
Ortho Tri-Cyclen Lo Tablets ... 2421
Seasonale Tablets ... 1073
Triphasil-28 Tablets ... 3483
Yasmin 28 Tablets ... 818

Fluvoxamine (Concomitant administration of alosetron with fluvoxamine is contraindicated. Fluvoxamine, a known strong inhibitor of CYP1A2, has been shown to increase mean alosetron plasma concentrations (AUC) approximately 6 fold and prolong the half-life by approximately 3 fold).
No products indexed under this heading.

Fluvoxamine Maleate (Concomitant administration of alosetron and moderate CYP1A2 inhibitors, including quinolone antibiotics and cimetidine, has not been evaluated, but should be avoided unless clinically necessary because of potential drug interactions).
No products indexed under this heading.

Fosamprenavir Calcium (Ketoconazole is a known strong inhibitor of CYP3A4. In a pharmacokinetic study, 38 healthy female subjects received ketoconazole 200 mg twice daily for 7 days, with co-administration of alosetron 1 mg on the last day. Ketoconazole increased mean alosetron plasma concentrations (AUC) by 29%. Caution should be used when alosetron and ketoconazole are administered concomitantly. Co-administration of alosetron and strong SYP3A4 inhibitors has not been evaluated but should be undertaken with caution because of similar potential drug interactions). Products include:
Lexiva Tablets ... 1473

Gatifloxacin (Concomitant administration of alosetron and moderate CYP1A2 inhibitors, including quinolone antibiotics and cimetidine, has not been evaluated, but should be avoided unless clinically necessary because of potential drug interactions). Products include:
Tequin Injection ... 964
Tequin Tablets ... 964
Zymar Ophthalmic Solution ... 571

Gemifloxacin Mesylate (Concomitant administration of alosetron and moderate CYP1A2 inhibitors, including quinolone antibiotics and cimetidine, has not been evaluated, but should be avoided unless clinically necessary because of potential drug interactions). Products include:
Factive Tablets ... 2464

Grepafloxacin Hydrochloride (Concomitant administration of alosetron and moderate CYP1A2 inhibitors, including quinolone antibiotics and cimetidine, has not been evaluated, but should be avoided unless clinically necessary because of potential drug interactions).
No products indexed under this heading.

Hydralazine Hydrochloride (Although not studied with alosetron,

inhibition of N-acetyltransferase may have clinically relevant consequences for drugs such as hydralazine). Products include:
- BiDil Tablets **2161**

Indinavir Sulfate (Ketoconazole is a known strong inhibitor of CYP3A4. In a pharmacokinetic study, 38 healthy female subjects received ketoconazole 200 mg twice daily for 7 days, with co-administration of alosetron 1 mg on the last day. Ketoconazole increased mean alosetron plasma concentrations (AUC) by 29%. Caution should be used when alosetron and ketoconazole are administered concomitantly. Co-administration of alosetron and strong SYP3A4 inhibitors has not been evaluated but should be undertaken with caution because of similar potential drug interactions). Products include:
- Crixivan Capsules **1918**

Isoniazid (Although not studied with alosetron, inhibition of N-acetyltransferase may have clinically relevant consequences for drugs such as isoniazid).
- No products indexed under this heading.

Itraconazole (Ketoconazole is a known strong inhibitor of CYP3A4. In a pharmacokinetic study, 38 healthy female subjects received ketoconazole 200 mg twice daily for 7 days, with co-administration of alosetron 1 mg on the last day. Ketoconazole increased mean alosetron plasma concentrations (AUC) by 29%. Caution should be used when alosetron and ketoconazole are administered concomitantly. Co-administration of alosetron and strong SYP3A4 inhibitors has not been evaluated but should be undertaken with caution because of similar potential drug interactions).
- No products indexed under this heading.

Ketoconazole (Ketoconazole is a known strong inhibitor of CYP3A4. In a pharmacokinetic study, 38 healthy female subjects recieved ketoconazole 200 mg twice daily for 7 days, with co-administration of alosetron 1 mg on the last day. Ketoconazole increased mean alosetron plasma concentrations (AUC) by 29%. Caution should be used when alosetron and ketoconazole are administered concomitantly). Products include:
- Nizoral A-D Shampoo, 1% **1839**
- Nizoral 2% Shampoo **1838**

Levofloxacin (Concomitant administration of alosetron and moderate CYP1A2 inhibitors, including quinolone antibiotics and cimetidine, has not been evaluated, but should be avoided unless clinically necessary because of potential drug interactions). Products include:
- Levaquin in 5% Dextrose Injection **2453**
- Levaquin **2453**
- Quixin Ophthalmic Solution **3373**

Levonorgestrel (Concomitant administration of alosetron and moderate CYP1A2 inhibitors, including quinolone antibiotics and cimetidine, has not been evaluated, but should be avoided unless clinically necessary because of potential drug interactions). Products include:
- Alesse-28 Tablets **3392**
- Climara Pro Transdermal System **800**
- Mirena Intrauterine System **810**
- Plan B Tablets **1068**
- Seasonale Tablets **1073**
- Triphasil-28 Tablets **3483**

Lomefloxacin Hydrochloride (Concomitant administration of alosetron and moderate CYP1A2 inhibitors, including quinolone antibiotics and cimetidine, has not been evaluated, but should be avoided unless clinically necessary because of potential drug interactions).
- No products indexed under this heading.

Lopinavir (Ketoconazole is a known strong inhibitor of CYP3A4. In a pharmacokinetic study, 38 healthy female subjects received ketoconazole 200 mg twice daily for 7 days, with co-administration of alosetron 1 mg on the last day. Ketoconazole increased mean alosetron plasma concentrations (AUC) by 29%. Caution should be used when alosetron and ketoconazole are administered concomitantly. Co-administration of alosetron and strong SYP3A4 inhibitors has not been evaluated but should be undertaken with caution because of similar potential drug interactions). Products include:
- Kaletra **474**

Mestranol (Concomitant administration of alosetron and moderate CYP1A2 inhibitors, including quinolone antibiotics and cimetidine, has not been evaluated, but should be avoided unless clinically necessary because of potential drug interactions).
- No products indexed under this heading.

Methoxsalen (Concomitant administration of alosetron and moderate CYP1A2 inhibitors, including quinolone antibiotics and cimetidine, has not been evaluated, but should be avoided unless clinically necessary because of potential drug interactions). Products include:
- Oxsoralen Lotion 1% **3354**
- Oxsoralen-Ultra Capsules **3354**

Mexiletine Hydrochloride (Concomitant administration of alosetron and moderate CYP1A2 inhibitors, including quinolone antibiotics and cimetidine, has not been evaluated, but should be avoided unless clinically necessary because of potential drug interactions).
- No products indexed under this heading.

Mibefradil Dihydrochloride (Concomitant administration of alosetron and moderate CYP1A2 inhibitors, including quinolone antibiotics and cimetidine, has not been evaluated, but should be avoided unless clinically necessary because of potential drug interactions).
- No products indexed under this heading.

Moxifloxacin Hydrochloride (Concomitant administration of alosetron and moderate CYP1A2 inhibitors, including quinolone antibiotics and cimetidine, has not been evaluated, but should be avoided unless clinically necessary because of potential drug interactions). Products include:
- Avelox **2984**
- Vigamox Ophthalmic Solution **560**

Nalidixic Acid (Concomitant administration of alosetron and moderate CYP1A2 inhibitors, including quinolone antibiotics and cimetidine, has not been evaluated, but should be avoided unless clinically necessary because of potential drug interactions).
- No products indexed under this heading.

Nefazodone Hydrochloride (Ketoconazole is a known strong inhibitor of CYP3A4. In a pharmacokinetic study, 38 healthy female subjects received ketoconazole 200 mg twice daily for 7 days, with co-administration of alosetron 1 mg on the last day. Ketoconazole increased mean alosetron plasma concentrations (AUC) by 29%. Caution should be used when alosetron and ketoconazole are administered concomitantly. Co-administration of alosetron and strong SYP3A4 inhibitors has not been evaluated but should be undertaken with caution because of similar potential drug interactions).
- No products indexed under this heading.

Nelfinavir Mesylate (Ketoconazole is a known strong inhibitor of CYP3A4. In a pharmacokinetic study, 38 healthy female subjects received ketoconazole 200 mg twice daily for 7 days, with co-administration of alosetron 1 mg on the last day. Ketoconazole increased mean alosetron plasma concentrations (AUC) by 29%. Caution should be used when alosetron and ketoconazole are administered concomitantly. Co-administration of alosetron and strong SYP3A4 inhibitors has not been evaluated but should be undertaken with caution because of similar potential drug interactions). Products include:
- Viracept **2556**

Norethindrone (Concomitant administration of alosetron and moderate CYP1A2 inhibitors, including quinolone antibiotics and cimetidine, has not been evaluated, but should be avoided unless clinically necessary because of potential drug interactions). Products include:
- Ortho Micronor Tablets **2411**

Norfloxacin (Concomitant administration of alosetron and moderate CYP1A2 inhibitors, including quinolone antibiotics and cimetidine, has not been evaluated, but should be avoided unless clinically necessary because of potential drug interactions). Products include:
- Noroxin Tablets **2009**

Norgestrel (Concomitant administration of alosetron and moderate CYP1A2 inhibitors, including quinolone antibiotics and cimetidine, has not been evaluated, but should be avoided unless clinically necessary because of potential drug interactions). Products include:
- Lo/Ovral-28 Tablets **3423**

Ofloxacin (Concomitant administration of alosetron and moderate CYP1A2 inhibitors, including quinolone antibiotics and cimetidine, has not been evaluated, but should be avoided unless clinically necessary because of potential drug interactions). Products include:
- Floxin Otic Singles **1045**
- Floxin Otic Solution **1043**

Omeprazole (Concomitant administration of alosetron and moderate CYP1A2 inhibitors, including quinolone antibiotics and cimetidine, has not been evaluated, but should be avoided unless clinically necessary because of potential drug interactions). Products include:
- Zegerid Powder for Oral Solution **2972**

Paroxetine Hydrochloride (Concomitant administration of alosetron and moderate CYP1A2 inhibitors, including quinolone antibiotics and cimetidine, has not been evaluated, but should be avoided unless clinically necessary because of potential drug interactions). Products include:
- Paxil CR Controlled-Release Tablets **1509**
- Paxil **1501**

Procainamide Hydrochloride (Although not studied with alosetron, inhibition of N-acetyltransferase may have clinically relevant consequences for drugs such as procainamide).
- No products indexed under this heading.

Ranitidine Hydrochloride (Concomitant administration of alosetron and moderate CYP1A2 inhibitors, including quinolone antibiotics and cimetidine, has not been evaluated, but should be avoided unless clinically necessary because of potential drug interactions). Products include:
- Zantac **1597**
- Zantac Injection **1593**
- Zantac 75 Tablets .... ▣**715**
- Zantac 150 Maximum Strength Tablets .... ▣**715**
- Zantac Injection Pharmacy Bulk Package **1595**

Ritonavir (Ketoconazole is a known strong inhibitor of CYP3A4. In a pharmacokinetic study, 38 healthy female subjects received ketoconazole 200 mg twice daily for 7 days, with co-administration of alosetron 1 mg on the last day. Ketoconazole increased mean alosetron plasma concentrations (AUC) by 29%. Caution should be used when alosetron and ketoconazole are administered concomitantly. Co-administration of alosetron and strong SYP3A4 inhibitors has not been evaluated but should be undertaken with caution because of similar potential drug interactions). Products include:
- Kaletra **474**
- Norvir **499**

Saquinavir (Ketoconazole is a known strong inhibitor of CYP3A4. In a pharmacokinetic study, 38 healthy female subjects received ketoconazole 200 mg twice daily for 7 days, with co-administration of alosetron 1 mg on the last day. Ketoconazole increased mean alosetron plasma concentrations (AUC) by 29%. Caution should be used when alosetron and ketoconazole are administered concomitantly. Co-administration of alosetron and strong SYP3A4 inhibitors has not been evaluated but should be undertaken with caution because of similar potential drug interactions).
- No products indexed under this heading.

Saquinavir Mesylate (Ketoconazole is a known strong inhibitor of CYP3A4. In a pharmacokinetic study, 38 healthy female subjects received ketoconazole 200 mg twice daily for 7 days, with co-administration of alosetron 1 mg on the last day. Ketoconazole increased mean alosetron plasma concentrations (AUC) by 29%. Caution should be used when alosetron and ketoconazole are administered concomitantly. Co-administration of alosetron and strong SYP3A4 inhibitors has not been evaluated but should be undertaken with caution because of similar potential drug interactions). Products include:
- Invirase **2776**

Sparfloxacin (Concomitant administration of alosetron and moderate CYP1A2 inhibitors, including quinolone antibiotics and cimetidine, has not been evaluated, but should be avoided unless clinically necessary because of potential drug interactions).
No products indexed under this heading.

Tacrine Hydrochloride (Concomitant administration of alosetron and moderate CYP1A2 inhibitors, including quinolone antibiotics and cimetidine, has not been evaluated, but should be avoided unless clinically necessary because of potential drug interactions).
No products indexed under this heading.

Telithromycin (Ketoconazole is a known strong inhibitor of CYP3A4. In a pharmacokinetic study, 38 healthy female subjects received ketoconazole 200 mg twice daily for 7 days, with co-administration of alosetron 1 mg on the last day. Ketoconazole increased mean alosetron plasma concentrations (AUC) by 29%. Caution should be used when alosetron and ketoconazole are administered concomitantly. Co-administration of alosetron and strong SYP3A4 inhibitors has not been evaluated but should be undertaken with caution because of similar potential drug interactions). Products include:
Ketek Tablets 2920

Ticlopidine Hydrochloride (Concomitant administration of alosetron and moderate CYP1A2 inhibitors, including quinolone antibiotics and cimetidine, has not been evaluated, but should be avoided unless clinically necessary because of potential drug interactions). Products include:
Ticlid Tablets 2813

Troleandomycin (Ketoconazole is a known strong inhibitor of CYP3A4. In a pharmacokinetic study, 38 healthy female subjects received ketoconazole 200 mg twice daily for 7 days, with co-administration of alosetron 1 mg on the last day. Ketoconazole increased mean alosetron plasma concentrations (AUC) by 29%. Caution should be used when alosetron and ketoconazole are administered concomitantly. Co-administration of alosetron and strong SYP3A4 inhibitors has not been evaluated but should be undertaken with caution because of similar potential drug interactions).
No products indexed under this heading.

Trovafloxacin Mesylate (Concomitant administration of alosetron and moderate CYP1A2 inhibitors, including quinolone antibiotics and cimetidine, has not been evaluated, but should be avoided unless clinically necessary because of potential drug interactions).
No products indexed under this heading.

Voriconazole (Ketoconazole is a known strong inhibitor of CYP3A4. In a pharmacokinetic study, 38 healthy female subjects received ketoconazole 200 mg twice daily for 7 days, with co-administration of alosetron 1 mg on the last day. Ketoconazole increased mean alosetron plasma concentrations (AUC) by 29%. Caution should be used when alosetron and ketoconazole are administered concomitantly. Co-administration of alosetron and strong SYP3A4 inhibitors has not been evaluated but should be undertaken with caution because of similar potential drug interactions). Products include:
VFEND I.V. 2543
VFEND Oral Suspension 2543
VFEND Tablets 2543

Zileuton (Concomitant administration of alosetron and moderate CYP1A2 inhibitors, including quinolone antibiotics and cimetidine, has not been evaluated, but should be avoided unless clinically necessary because of potential drug interactions).
No products indexed under this heading.

Food Interactions

Food, unspecified (Alosetron absorption is decreased by approximately 25% by co-administration with food with a mean delay in time to peak concentration of 15 minutes; Lotronex can be taken with or without food).

Grapefruit Juice (Concomitant administration of alosetron and moderate CYP1A2 inhibitors, including quinolone antibiotics and cimetidine, has not been evaluated, but should be avoided unless clinically necessary because of potential drug interactions).

LOVENOX INJECTION

(Enoxaparin Sodium) 2931

May interact with anticoagulants, non-steroidal anti-inflammatory agents, salicylates, and certain other agents. Compounds in these categories include:

Anisindione (Agents which may enhance the risk of hemorrhage, such as other anticoagulants, should be discontinued prior to initiation of Lovenox therapy; the risk of developing epidural or spinal hematoma which can result in long-term or permanent paralysis is increased by the concomitant use of drugs affecting hemostasis). Products include:
Miradon Tablets 3056

Ardeparin Sodium (Agents which may enhance the risk of hemorrhage, such as other anticoagulants, should be discontinued prior to initiation of Lovenox therapy; the risk of developing epidural or spinal hematoma which can result in long-term or permanent paralysis is increased by the concomitant use of drugs affecting hemostasis).
No products indexed under this heading.

Aspirin (Agents which may enhance the risk of hemorrhage, such as platelet inhibitors, should be discontinued prior to initiation of Lovenox therapy; the risk of developing epidural or spinal hematoma which can result in long-term or permanent paralysis is increased by the concomitant use of drugs affecting hemostasis). Products include:
Aggrenox Capsules 855
Bayer, Aspirin Regimen 606
Bayer Aspirin Tablets 3515
BC Powder 612
BC Allergy Sinus Cold Powder 612
Arthritis Strength BC Powder 612
BC Sinus Cold Powder 612
Ecotrin Enteric Coated Aspirin Low, Regular and Maximum Strength Tablets 1627
Goody's Body Pain Formula Powder 621
Goody's Extra Strength Headache Powder 621
Goody's Extra Strength Pain Relief Tablets 621
Percodan Tablets 1115
St. Joseph 81 mg Aspirin Chewable and Enteric Coated Tablets 1841

Aspirin, Enteric Coated (Agents which may enhance the risk of hemorrhage, such as platelet inhibitors, should be discontinued prior to initiation of Lovenox therapy; the risk of developing epidural or spinal hematoma which can result in long-term or permanent paralysis is increased by the concomitant use of drugs affecting hemostasis).
No products indexed under this heading.

Aspirin Buffered (Agents which may enhance the risk of hemorrhage, such as platelet inhibitors, should be discontinued prior to initiation of Lovenox therapy; the risk of developing epidural or spinal hematoma which can result in long-term or permanent paralysis is increased by the concomitant use of drugs affecting hemostasis).
No products indexed under this heading.

Celecoxib (Agents which may enhance the risk of hemorrhage, such as platelet inhibitors, should be discontinued prior to initiation of Lovenox therapy; the risk of developing epidural or spinal hematoma which can result in long-term or permanent paralysis is increased by the concomitant use of drugs affecting hemostasis). Products include:
Celebrex Capsules 3130

Choline Magnesium Trisalicylate (Agents which may enhance the risk of hemorrhage, such as platelet inhibitors, should be discontinued prior to initiation of Lovenox therapy; the risk of developing epidural or spinal hematoma which can result in long-term or permanent paralysis is increased by the concomitant use of drugs affecting hemostasis).
No products indexed under this heading.

Clopidogrel Bisulfate (Agents which may enhance the risk of hemorrhage, such as platelet aggregation inhibitors, should be discontinued prior to initiation of Lovenox therapy; the risk of developing epidural or spinal hematoma which can result in long-term or permanent paralysis is increased by the concomitant use of drugs affecting hemostasis). Products include:
Plavix Tablets 940
Plavix Tablets 2942

Dalteparin Sodium (Agents which may enhance the risk of hemorrhage, such as other anticoagulants, should be discontinued prior to initiation of Lovenox therapy; the risk of developing epidural or spinal hematoma which can result in long-term or permanent paralysis is increased by the concomitant use of drugs affecting hemostasis). Products include:
Fragmin Injection 2638

Danaparoid Sodium (Agents which may enhance the risk of hemorrhage, such as other anticoagulants, should be discontinued prior to initiation of Lovenox therapy; the risk of developing epidural or spinal hematoma which can result in long-term or permanent paralysis is increased by the concomitant use of drugs affecting hemostasis).
No products indexed under this heading.

Diclofenac Potassium (Agents which may enhance the risk of hemorrhage, such as platelet inhibitors, should be discontinued prior to initiation of Lovenox therapy; the risk of developing epidural or spinal hematoma which can result in long-term or permanent paralysis is increased by the concomitant use of drugs affecting hemostasis). Products include:
Cataflam Tablets 2173

Diclofenac Sodium (Agents which may enhance the risk of hemorrhage, such as platelet inhibitors, should be discontinued prior to initiation of Lovenox therapy; the risk of developing epidural or spinal hematoma which can result in long-term or permanent paralysis is increased by the concomitant use of drugs affecting hemostasis). Products include:
Arthrotec Tablets 3126
Voltaren Ophthalmic Solution 2300
Voltaren Tablets 2298
Voltaren-XR Tablets 2301

Dicumarol (Agents which may enhance the risk of hemorrhage, such as other anticoagulants, should be discontinued prior to initiation of Lovenox therapy; the risk of developing epidural or spinal hematoma which can result in long-term or permanent paralysis is increased by the concomitant use of drugs affecting hemostasis).
No products indexed under this heading.

Diflunisal (Agents which may enhance the risk of hemorrhage, such as platelet inhibitors, should be discontinued prior to initiation of Lovenox therapy; the risk of developing epidural or spinal hematoma which can result in long-term or permanent paralysis is increased by the concomitant use of drugs affecting hemostasis). Products include:
Dolobid Tablets 1937

Dipyridamole (Agents which may enhance the risk of hemorrhage, such as dipyridamole, should be discontinued prior to initiation of Lovenox therapy). Products include:
Aggrenox Capsules 855
Persantine Tablets 898

Eptifibatide (Agents which may enhance the risk of hemorrhage, such as platelet aggregation inhibitors, should be discontinued prior to initiation of Lovenox therapy; the risk of developing epidural or spinal hematoma which can result in long-term or permanent paralysis is increased by the concomitant use of drugs affecting hemostasis). Products include:
Integrilin Injection 3034

Etodolac (Agents which may enhance the risk of hemorrhage, such as platelet inhibitors, should be discontinued prior to initiation of Lovenox therapy; the risk of developing epidural or spinal hematoma which can result in long-term or permanent paralysis is increased by the concomitant use of drugs affecting hemostasis).
No products indexed under this heading.

Fenoprofen Calcium (Agents which may enhance the risk of hemorrhage, such as platelet inhibitors, should be discontinued prior to initiation of Lovenox therapy; the risk of developing epidural or spinal hematoma which can result in long-term or

permanent paralysis is increased by the concomitant use of drugs affecting hemostasis). Products include:
Nalfon Capsules **2504**

Flurbiprofen (Agents which may enhance the risk of hemorrhage, such as platelet inhibitors, should be discontinued prior to initiation of Lovenox therapy; the risk of developing epidural or spinal hematoma which can result in long-term or permanent paralysis is increased by the concomitant use of drugs affecting hemostasis).
No products indexed under this heading.

Fondaparinux Sodium (Agents which may enhance the risk of hemorrhage, such as other anticoagulants, should be discontinued prior to initiation of Lovenox therapy; the risk of developing epidural or spinal hematoma which can result in long-term or permanent paralysis is increased by the concomitant use of drugs affecting hemostasis).
Products include:
Arixtra Injection **1325**

Heparin Calcium (Agents which may enhance the risk of hemorrhage, such as other anticoagulants, should be discontinued prior to initiation of Lovenox therapy; the risk of developing epidural or spinal hematoma which can result in long-term or permanent paralysis is increased by the concomitant use of drugs affecting hemostasis).
No products indexed under this heading.

Heparin Sodium (Agents which may enhance the risk of hemorrhage, such as other anticoagulants, should be discontinued prior to initiation of Lovenox therapy; the risk of developing epidural or spinal hematoma which can result in long-term or permanent paralysis is increased by the concomitant use of drugs affecting hemostasis).
No products indexed under this heading.

Ibuprofen (Agents which may enhance the risk of hemorrhage, such as platelet inhibitors, should be discontinued prior to initiation of Lovenox therapy; the risk of developing epidural or spinal hematoma which can result in long-term or permanent paralysis is increased by the concomitant use of drugs affecting hemostasis). Products include:
Advil Allergy Sinus Caplets .... ▣ **737**
Advil .... ▣ **737**
Children's Advil Suspension .... ▣ **742**
Children's Advil Chewable Tablets .. ▣ **741**
Advil Cold & Sinus .... ▣ **739**
Advil Flu & Body Ache Caplets .... ▣ **739**
Children's Advil Cold Suspension .... ▣ **741**
Infants' Advil Concentrated Drops .. ▣ **743**
Junior Strength Advil Swallow Tablets .... ▣ **740**
Advil Migraine Liquigels .... ▣ **740**
Advil Multi-Symptom Cold Caplets .... ▣ **738**
Combunox Tablets **1183**
Children's Motrin Oral Suspension and Chewable Tablets **1837**
Children's Motrin Cold Non-Staining Dye-Free Oral Suspension **1838**
Children's Motrin Cold Oral Suspension **1838**
Children's Motrin Non-Staining Dye-Free Oral Suspension **1837**
Motrin Cold & Sinus Caplets **1836**
Motrin IB Tablets and Caplets **1836**
Infants' Motrin Concentrated Drops **1837**
Infants' Motrin Non-Staining Dye-Free Drops **1837**
Junior Strength Motrin Caplets and Chewable Tablets **1837**
Vicoprofen Tablets **533**

Indomethacin (Agents which may enhance the risk of hemorrhage, such as platelet inhibitors, should be discontinued prior to initiation of Lovenox therapy; the risk of developing epidural or spinal hematoma which can result in long-term or permanent paralysis is increased by the concomitant use of drugs affecting hemostasis). Products include:
Indocin **1968**

Indomethacin Sodium Trihydrate (Agents which may enhance the risk of hemorrhage, such as platelet inhibitors, should be discontinued prior to initiation of Lovenox therapy; the risk of developing epidural or spinal hematoma which can result in long-term or permanent paralysis is increased by the concomitant use of drugs affecting hemostasis). Products include:
Indocin I.V. **1973**

Ketoprofen (Agents which may enhance the risk of hemorrhage, such as platelet inhibitors, should be discontinued prior to initiation of Lovenox therapy; the risk of developing epidural or spinal hematoma which can result in long-term or permanent paralysis is increased by the concomitant use of drugs affecting hemostasis).
No products indexed under this heading.

Ketorolac Tromethamine (Agents which may enhance the risk of hemorrhage, such as platelet inhibitors, should be discontinued prior to initiation of Lovenox therapy; the risk of developing epidural or spinal hematoma which can result in long-term or permanent paralysis is increased by the concomitant use of drugs affecting hemostasis). Products include:
Acular Ophthalmic Solution **561**
Acular LS Ophthalmic Solution **562**

Low Molecular Weight Heparins (Agents which may enhance the risk of hemorrhage, such as other anticoagulants, should be discontinued prior to initiation of Lovenox therapy; the risk of developing epidural or spinal hematoma which can result in long-term or permanent paralysis is increased by the concomitant use of drugs affecting hemostasis).
No products indexed under this heading.

Magnesium Salicylate (Agents which may enhance the risk of hemorrhage, such as platelet inhibitors, should be discontinued prior to initiation of Lovenox therapy; the risk of developing epidural or spinal hematoma which can result in long-term or permanent paralysis is increased by the concomitant use of drugs affecting hemostasis).
No products indexed under this heading.

Meclofenamate Sodium (Agents which may enhance the risk of hemorrhage, such as platelet inhibitors, should be discontinued prior to initiation of Lovenox therapy; the risk of developing epidural or spinal hematoma which can result in long-term or permanent paralysis is increased by the concomitant use of drugs affecting hemostasis).
No products indexed under this heading.

Mefenamic Acid (Agents which may enhance the risk of hemorrhage, such as platelet inhibitors, should be discontinued prior to initiation of Lovenox therapy; the risk of developing epidural or spinal hematoma which can result in long-term or permanent paralysis is increased by the concomitant use of drugs affecting hemostasis).
No products indexed under this heading.

Meloxicam (Agents which may enhance the risk of hemorrhage, such as platelet inhibitors, should be discontinued prior to initiation of Lovenox therapy; the risk of developing epidural or spinal hematoma which can result in long-term or permanent paralysis is increased by the concomitant use of drugs affecting hemostasis). Products include:
Mobic Oral Suspension **893**
Mobic Tablets **893**

Nabumetone (Agents which may enhance the risk of hemorrhage, such as platelet inhibitors, should be discontinued prior to initiation of Lovenox therapy; the risk of developing epidural or spinal hematoma which can result in long-term or permanent paralysis is increased by the concomitant use of drugs affecting hemostasis). Products include:
Relafen Tablets **1523**

Naproxen (Agents which may enhance the risk of hemorrhage, such as platelet inhibitors, should be discontinued prior to initiation of Lovenox therapy; the risk of developing epidural or spinal hematoma which can result in long-term or permanent paralysis is increased by the concomitant use of drugs affecting hemostasis). Products include:
EC-Naprosyn Delayed-Release Tablets **2769**
Naprosyn Suspension **2769**
Naprosyn Tablets **2769**
Prevacid NapraPAC **3277**

Naproxen Sodium (Agents which may enhance the risk of hemorrhage, such as platelet inhibitors, should be discontinued prior to initiation of Lovenox therapy; the risk of developing epidural or spinal hematoma which can result in long-term or permanent paralysis is increased by the concomitant use of drugs affecting hemostasis). Products include:
Aleve Tablets, Caplets and Gelcaps .... ▣ **605**
Anaprox Tablets **2769**
Anaprox DS Tablets **2769**

Oxaprozin (Agents which may enhance the risk of hemorrhage, such as platelet inhibitors, should be discontinued prior to initiation of Lovenox therapy; the risk of developing epidural or spinal hematoma which can result in long-term or permanent paralysis is increased by the concomitant use of drugs affecting hemostasis).
No products indexed under this heading.

Phenylbutazone (Agents which may enhance the risk of hemorrhage, such as platelet inhibitors, should be discontinued prior to initiation of Lovenox therapy; the risk of developing epidural or spinal hematoma which can result in long-term or permanent paralysis is increased by the concomitant use of drugs affecting hemostasis).
No products indexed under this heading.

Piroxicam (Agents which may enhance the risk of hemorrhage, such as platelet inhibitors, should be discontinued prior to initiation of Lovenox therapy; the risk of developing epidural or spinal hematoma which can result in long-term or permanent paralysis is increased by the concomitant use of drugs affecting hemostasis).
No products indexed under this heading.

Rofecoxib (Agents which may enhance the risk of hemorrhage, such as platelet inhibitors, should be discontinued prior to initiation of Lovenox therapy; the risk of developing epidural or spinal hematoma which can result in long-term or permanent paralysis is increased by the concomitant use of drugs affecting hemostasis).
No products indexed under this heading.

Salsalate (Agents which may enhance the risk of hemorrhage, such as platelet inhibitors, should be discontinued prior to initiation of Lovenox therapy; the risk of developing epidural or spinal hematoma which can result in long-term or permanent paralysis is increased by the concomitant use of drugs affecting hemostasis).
No products indexed under this heading.

Sulfinpyrazone (Agents which may enhance the risk of hemorrhage, such as sulfinpyrazone, should be discontinued prior to initiation of Lovenox therapy).
No products indexed under this heading.

Sulindac (Agents which may enhance the risk of hemorrhage, such as platelet inhibitors, should be discontinued prior to initiation of Lovenox therapy; the risk of developing epidural or spinal hematoma which can result in long-term or permanent paralysis is increased by the concomitant use of drugs affecting hemostasis). Products include:
Clinoril Tablets **1899**

Tinzaparin Sodium (Agents which may enhance the risk of hemorrhage, such as other anticoagulants, should be discontinued prior to initiation of Lovenox therapy; the risk of developing epidural or spinal hematoma which can result in long-term or permanent paralysis is increased by the concomitant use of drugs affecting hemostasis).
No products indexed under this heading.

Tirofiban Hydrochloride (Agents which may enhance the risk of hemorrhage, such as platelet aggregation inhibitors, should be discontinued prior to initiation of Lovenox therapy; the risk of developing epidural or spinal hematoma which can result in long-term or permanent paralysis is increased by the concomitant use of drugs affecting hemostasis). Products include:
Aggrastat **1878**

Tolmetin Sodium (Agents which may enhance the risk of hemorrhage, such as platelet inhibitors, should be discontinued prior to initiation of Lovenox therapy; the risk of developing epidural or spinal hematoma which can result in long-term or permanent paralysis is increased by the concomitant use of drugs affecting hemostasis).
No products indexed under this heading.

Valdecoxib (Agents which may enhance the risk of hemorrhage, such as platelet inhibitors, should be discontinued prior to initiation of Lovenox therapy; the risk of developing epidural or spinal hematoma which can result in long-term or permanent paralysis is increased by the concomitant use of drugs affecting hemostasis).
No products indexed under this heading.

Warfarin Sodium (Agents which may enhance the risk of hemorrhage, such as other anticoagulants, should be discontinued prior to initiation of Lovenox therapy; the risk of developing epidural or spinal hematoma which can result in long-term or permanent paralysis is increased by the concomitant use of drugs affecting hemostasis). Products include:
Coumadin for Injection 932
Coumadin Tablets 932

LUBRIDERM ADVANCED THERAPY MOISTURIZING LOTION

(Cetyl Alcohol, Glycerin, Mineral Oil) 702
None cited in PDR database.

LUMIGAN OPHTHALMIC SOLUTION

(Bimatoprost) 569
None cited in PDR database.

LUNESTA TABLETS

(Eszopiclone) 3139
May interact with cytochrome p450 3a4 inhibitors, potent and certain other agents. Compounds in these categories include:

Amprenavir (CYP3A4 is a major metabolic pathway for elimination of eszopiclone. The AUC of eszopiclone was increased 2.2-fold by co-administration of ketoconazole, a potent inhibitor of CYP3A4, 400 mg daily for 5 days. Cmax and T1/2 were increased 1.4-fold and 1.3-fold, respectively. Other strong inhibitors of CYP3A4 (e.g., itraconazole, clarithromycin, nefazodone, troleandomycin, ritonavir, nelfinavir) would be expected to behave similarly). Products include:
Agenerase Capsules 1299
Agenerase Oral Solution 1304

Atazanavir (CYP3A4 is a major metabolic pathway for elimination of eszopiclone. The AUC of eszopiclone was increased 2.2-fold by co-administration of ketoconazole, a potent inhibitor of CYP3A4, 400 mg daily for 5 days. Cmax and T1/2 were increased 1.4-fold and 1.3-fold, respectively. Other strong inhibitors of CYP3A4 (e.g., itraconazole, clarithromycin, nefazodone, troleandomycin, ritonavir, nelfinavir) would be expected to behave similarly).
No products indexed under this heading.

Atazanavir sulfate (CYP3A4 is a major metabolic pathway for elimination of eszopiclone. The AUC of eszopiclone was increased 2.2-fold by co-administration of ketoconazole, a potent inhibitor of CYP3A4, 400 mg daily for 5 days. Cmax and T1/2 were increased 1.4-fold and 1.3-fold, respectively. Other strong inhibitors of CYP3A4 (e.g., itraconazole, clarithromycin, nefazodone, troleandomycin, ritonavir, nelfinavir) would be expected to behave similarly). Products include:
Reyataz Capsules 948

Clarithromycin (CYP3A4 is a major metabolic pathway for elimination of eszopiclone. The AUC of eszopiclone was increased 2.2-fold by co-administration of ketoconazole, a potent inhibitor of CYP3A4, 400 mg daily for 5 days. Cmax and T1/2 were increased 1.4-fold and 1.3-fold, respectively. Other strong inhibitors of CYP3A4 (e.g., itraconazole, clarithromycin, nefazodone, troleandomycin, ritonavir, nelfinavir) would be expected to behave similarly). Products include:
Biaxin/Biaxin XL 402
PREVPAC 3281

Ethanol (An additive effect on psychomotor performance was seen with co-administration of eszopiclone and ethanol 0.70 g/kg for up to 4 hours after ethanol administration).
No products indexed under this heading.

Fosamprenavir Calcium (CYP3A4 is a major metabolic pathway for elimination of eszopiclone. The AUC of eszopiclone was increased 2.2-fold by co-administration of ketoconazole, a potent inhibitor of CYP3A4, 400 mg daily for 5 days. Cmax and T1/2 were increased 1.4-fold and 1.3-fold, respectively. Other strong inhibitors of CYP3A4 (e.g., itraconazole, clarithromycin, nefazodone, troleandomycin, ritonavir, nelfinavir) would be expected to behave similarly). Products include:
Lexiva Tablets 1473

Indinavir Sulfate (CYP3A4 is a major metabolic pathway for elimination of eszopiclone. The AUC of eszopiclone was increased 2.2-fold by co-administration of ketoconazole, a potent inhibitor of CYP3A4, 400 mg daily for 5 days. Cmax and T1/2 were increased 1.4-fold and 1.3-fold, respectively. Other strong inhibitors of CYP3A4 (e.g., itraconazole, clarithromycin, nefazodone, troleandomycin, ritonavir, nelfinavir) would be expected to behave similarly). Products include:
Crixivan Capsules 1918

Itraconazole (CYP3A4 is a major metabolic pathway for elimination of eszopiclone. The AUC of eszopiclone was increased 2.2-fold by co-administration of ketoconazole, a potent inhibitor of CYP3A4, 400 mg daily for 5 days. Cmax and T1/2 were increased 1.4-fold and 1.3-fold, respectively. Other strong inhibitors of CYP3A4 (e.g., itraconazole, clarithromycin, nefazodone, troleandomycin, ritonavir, nelfinavir) would be expected to behave similarly).
No products indexed under this heading.

Ketoconazole (CYP3A4 is a major metabolic pathway for elimination of eszopiclone. The AUC of eszopiclone was increased 2.2-fold by co-administration of ketoconazole, a potent inhibitor of CYP3A4, 400 mg daily for 5 days. Cmax and T1/2 were increased 1.4-fold and 1.3-fold, respectively. Other strong inhibitors of CYP3A4 (e.g., itraconazole, clarithromycin, nefazodone, troleandomycin, ritonavir, nelfinavir) would be expected to behave similarly). Products include:
Nizoral A-D Shampoo, 1% 1839
Nizoral 2% Shampoo 1838

Lopinavir (CYP3A4 is a major metabolic pathway for elimination of eszopiclone. The AUC of eszopiclone was increased 2.2-fold by co-administration of ketoconazole, a potent inhibitor of CYP3A4, 400 mg daily for 5 days. Cmax and T1/2 were increased 1.4-fold and 1.3-fold, respectively. Other strong inhibitors of CYP3A4 (e.g., itraconazole, clarithromycin, nefazodone, troleandomycin, ritonavir, nelfinavir) would be expected to behave similarly). Products include:
Kaletra 474

Nefazodone Hydrochloride (CYP3A4 is a major metabolic pathway for elimination of eszopiclone. The AUC of eszopiclone was increased 2.2-fold by co-administration of ketoconazole, a potent inhibitor of CYP3A4, 400 mg daily for 5 days. Cmax and T1/2 were increased 1.4-fold and 1.3-fold, respectively. Other strong inhibitors of CYP3A4 (e.g., itraconazole, clarithromycin, nefazodone, troleandomycin, ritonavir, nelfinavir) would be expected to behave similarly).
No products indexed under this heading.

Nelfinavir Mesylate (CYP3A4 is a major metabolic pathway for elimination of eszopiclone. The AUC of eszopiclone was increased 2.2-fold by co-administration of ketoconazole, a potent inhibitor of CYP3A4, 400 mg daily for 5 days. Cmax and T1/2 were increased 1.4-fold and 1.3-fold, respectively. Other strong inhibitors of CYP3A4 (e.g., itraconazole, clarithromycin, nefazodone, troleandomycin, ritonavir, nelfinavir) would be expected to behave similarly). Products include:
Viracept 2556

Olanzapine (Co-administration of eszopiclone 3 mg and olanzapine 10 mg produced a decrease in DSST scores. The interaction was pharmacodynamic; there was no alteration in the pharmacokinetics of either drug). Products include:
Symbyax Capsules 1788
Zyprexa Tablets 1798
Zyprexa IntraMuscular 1798
Zyprexa ZYDIS Orally Disintegrating Tablets 1798

Rifampicin (Racemic zopiclone exposure was decreased 80% by concomitant use of rifampicin, a potent inducer of CYP3A4. A similar effect would be expected with eszopiclone).
No products indexed under this heading.

Ritonavir (CYP3A4 is a major metabolic pathway for elimination of eszopiclone. The AUC of eszopiclone was increased 2.2-fold by co-administration of ketoconazole, a potent inhibitor of CYP3A4, 400 mg daily for 5 days. Cmax and T1/2 were increased 1.4-fold and 1.3-fold, respectively. Other strong inhibitors of CYP3A4 (e.g., itraconazole, clarithromycin, nefazodone, troleandomycin, ritonavir, nelfinavir) would be expected to behave similarly). Products include:
Kaletra 474
Norvir 499

Saquinavir (CYP3A4 is a major metabolic pathway for elimination of eszopiclone. The AUC of eszopiclone was increased 2.2-fold by co-administration of ketoconazole, a potent inhibitor of CYP3A4, 400 mg daily for 5 days. Cmax and T1/2 were increased 1.4-fold and 1.3-fold, respectively. Other strong inhibitors of CYP3A4 (e.g., itraconazole, clarithromycin, nefazodone, troleandomycin, ritonavir, nelfinavir) would be expected to behave similarly).
No products indexed under this heading.

Saquinavir Mesylate (CYP3A4 is a major metabolic pathway for elimination of eszopiclone. The AUC of eszopiclone was increased 2.2-fold by co-administration of ketoconazole, a potent inhibitor of CYP3A4, 400 mg daily for 5 days. Cmax and T1/2 were increased 1.4-fold and 1.3-fold, respectively. Other strong inhibitors of CYP3A4 (e.g., itraconazole, clarithromycin, nefazodone, troleandomycin, ritonavir, nelfinavir) would be expected to behave similarly). Products include:
Invirase 2776

Telithromycin (CYP3A4 is a major metabolic pathway for elimination of eszopiclone. The AUC of eszopiclone was increased 2.2-fold by co-administration of ketoconazole, a potent inhibitor of CYP3A4, 400 mg daily for 5 days. Cmax and T1/2 were increased 1.4-fold and 1.3-fold, respectively. Other strong inhibitors of CYP3A4 (e.g., itraconazole, clarithromycin, nefazodone, troleandomycin, ritonavir, nelfinavir) would be expected to behave similarly). Products include:
Ketek Tablets 2920

Troleandomycin (CYP3A4 is a major metabolic pathway for elimination of eszopiclone. The AUC of eszopiclone was increased 2.2-fold by co-administration of ketoconazole, a potent inhibitor of CYP3A4, 400 mg daily for 5 days. Cmax and T1/2 were increased 1.4-fold and 1.3-fold, respectively. Other strong inhibitors of CYP3A4 (e.g., itraconazole, clarithromycin, nefazodone, troleandomycin, ritonavir, nelfinavir) would be expected to behave similarly).
No products indexed under this heading.

Voriconazole (CYP3A4 is a major metabolic pathway for elimination of eszopiclone. The AUC of eszopiclone was increased 2.2-fold by co-administration of ketoconazole, a potent inhibitor of CYP3A4, 400 mg daily for 5 days. Cmax and T1/2 were increased 1.4-fold and 1.3-fold, respectively. Other strong inhibitors of CYP3A4 (e.g., itraconazole, clarithromycin, nefazodone, troleandomycin, ritonavir, nelfinavir) would be expected to behave similarly). Products include:
VFEND I.V. 2543
VFEND Oral Suspension 2543
VFEND Tablets 2543

Food Interactions

Alcohol (An additive effect on psychomotor performance was seen with co-administration of eszopiclone and alcohol 0.70 g/kg for up to 4 hours after alcohol consumption).

LUPRON DEPOT 3.75 MG
(Leuprolide Acetate) 3257
None cited in PDR database.

LUPRON DEPOT 7.5 MG
(Leuprolide Acetate) 3261
None cited in PDR database.

LUPRON DEPOT--3 MONTH 11.25 MG
(Leuprolide Acetate) 3262
None cited in PDR database.

LUPRON DEPOT-PED 7.5 MG, 11.25 MG AND 15 MG
(Leuprolide Acetate) 3266
None cited in PDR database.

LUPRON INJECTION PEDIATRIC
(Leuprolide Acetate) 3256
None cited in PDR database.

LUSTRA CREAM
(Hydroquinone) 3287
None cited in PDR database.

LUSTRA-AF CREAM
(Hydroquinone) 3287
None cited in PDR database.

LUSTRA-ULTRA CREAM
(Hydroquinone) 3287
None cited in PDR database.

LUXIQ FOAM
(Betamethasone Valerate) 1026
None cited in PDR database.

LYRICA CAPSULES
(Pregabalin) 2524
None cited in PDR database.

MAALOX REGULAR STRENGTH ANTACID/ ANTI-GAS LIQUID
(Aluminum Hydroxide, Magnesium Hydroxide, Simethicone).................. ▣677
May interact with:

Prescription Drugs, unspecified
(Antacids may interact with certain unspecified prescription drugs).
No products indexed under this heading.

MAALOX REGULAR STRENGTH ANTACID TABLETS
(Calcium Carbonate) 2166
May interact with:

Drugs, Oral, unspecified (Antacids may interact with certain unspecified prescription drugs).
No products indexed under this heading.

MAALOX MAX MAXIMUM STRENGTH ANTACID/ ANTI-GAS LIQUID
(Aluminum Hydroxide, Magnesium Hydroxide, Simethicone).................... 2165
May interact with:

Prescription Drugs, unspecified
(Antacids may interfere with certain unspecified prescription drugs; resulting effect not specified).
No products indexed under this heading.

MAALOX REGULAR STRENGTH ANTACID/ ANTIGAS LIQUID
(Aluminum Hydroxide, Magnesium Hydroxide, Simethicone).................... 2164
May interact with:

Prescription Drugs, unspecified
(Antacids may interact with certain unspecified prescription drugs).
No products indexed under this heading.

MAALOX MAXIMUM STRENGTH TOTAL STOMACH RELIEF PEPPERMINT LIQUID
(Bismuth Subsalicylate) .... ▣677
None cited in PDR database.

MAALOX MAXIMUM STRENGTH TOTAL STOMACH RELIEF STRAWBERRY LIQUID
(Bismuth Subsalicylate) .... ▣678
None cited in PDR database.

MALARONE TABLETS
(Atovaquone, Proguanil Hydrochloride)................................ 1484
May interact with tetracyclines and certain other agents. Compounds in these categories include:

Demeclocycline Hydrochloride
(Co-administration with tetracyclines has been associated with approximately a 40% reduction in plasma concentrations of atovaquone).
No products indexed under this heading.

Doxycycline Calcium (Co-administration with tetracyclines has been associated with approximately a 40% reduction in plasma concentrations of atovaquone).
No products indexed under this heading.

Doxycycline Hyclate (Co-administration with tetracyclines has been associated with approximately a 40% reduction in plasma concentrations of atovaquone).
No products indexed under this heading.

Doxycycline Monohydrate (Co-administration with tetracyclines has been associated with approximately a 40% reduction in plasma concentrations of atovaquone).
No products indexed under this heading.

Methacycline Hydrochloride (Co-administration with tetracyclines has been associated with approximately a 40% reduction in plasma concentrations of atovaquone).
No products indexed under this heading.

Metoclopramide Hydrochloride
(May reduce the bioavailability of atovaquone and should be used only if other antiemetics are not available).
No products indexed under this heading.

Minocycline Hydrochloride (Co-administration with tetracyclines has been associated with approximately a 40% reduction in plasma concentrations of atovaquone). Products include:
Dynacin Tablets 1859

Oxytetracycline Hydrochloride
(Co-administration with tetracyclines has been associated with approximately a 40% reduction in plasma concentrations of atovaquone).
No products indexed under this heading.

Rifabutin (Co-administration of rifabutin is known to reduce atovaquone levels by approximately 34%; concomitant therapy is not recommended).
No products indexed under this heading.

Rifampin (Co-administration of rifampin is known to reduce atovaquone levels by approximately 50%; concomitant therapy is not recommended).
No products indexed under this heading.

Tetracycline Hydrochloride (Co-administration with tetracyclines has been associated with approximately a 40% reduction in plasma concentrations of atovaquone).
No products indexed under this heading.

Food Interactions

Food, unspecified (Dietary fat intake with atovaquone increases the rate and extent of absorption; Malarone should be taken with food or milky drink).

MALARONE PEDIATRIC TABLETS
(Atovaquone, Proguanil Hydrochloride).................................. 1484
See Malarone Tablets

MARINEOMEGA SOFTGEL CAPSULES
(Fatty Acids, Vitamin E) 2669
None cited in PDR database.

MARINOL CAPSULES
(Dronabinol) 3334
May interact with anticholinergics, antihistamines, barbiturates, benzodiazepines, central nervous system depressants, lithium preparations, narcotic analgesics, sympathomimetics, tricyclic antidepressants, xanthines, and certain other agents. Compounds in these categories include:

Acrivastine (Co-administration results in additive CNS depression or super-additive tachycardia and drowsiness).
No products indexed under this heading.

Albuterol (Co-administration with sympathomimetics may result in additive hypertension, tachycardia, and possibly cardiotoxicity). Products include:
Proventil Inhalation Aerosol 3067

Albuterol Sulfate (Co-administration with sympathomimetics may result in additive hypertension, tachycardia, and possibly cardiotoxicity). Products include:
AccuNeb Inhalation Solution 1055
Combivent Inhalation Aerosol 878
DuoNeb Inhalation Solution 1058
Proventil Inhalation Solution 0.083%.................................... 3069
Proventil HFA Inhalation Aerosol 3071
Ventolin HFA Inhalation Aerosol 1576
VoSpire Extended-Release Tablets ... 2352

Alfentanil Hydrochloride (Co-administration results in additive drowsiness and CNS depression).
No products indexed under this heading.

Alprazolam (Co-administration results in additive drowsiness and CNS depression). Products include:
Niravam Orally Disintegrating Tablets 3106
Xanax XR Tablets 2655

Aminophylline (Increased theophylline metabolism has resulted with smoking marijuana).
No products indexed under this heading.

Amitriptyline Hydrochloride (Co-administration results in additive tachycardia, hypertension, and drowsiness).
No products indexed under this heading.

Amoxapine (Co-administration results in additive tachycardia, hypertension, and drowsiness).
No products indexed under this heading.

Amphetamine Sulfate (Co-administration with amphetamine may result in additive hypertension, tachycardia, and possibly cardiotoxicity). Products include:
Adderall Tablets 3168
Adderall XR Capsules 3169

Aprobarbital (Co-administration results in decreased clearance of barbiturates via competitive inhibition of metabolism; additive drowsiness and CNS depression).
No products indexed under this heading.

Astemizole (Co-administration results in additive CNS depression or super-additive tachycardia and drowsiness).
No products indexed under this heading.

Atropine Sulfate (Co-administration with anticholinergic agents may result in additive or super-additive tachycardia and drowsiness).
No products indexed under this heading.

Azatadine Maleate (Co-administration results in additive CNS depression or super-additive tachycardia and drowsiness).
No products indexed under this heading.

Belladonna Alkaloids (Co-administration with anticholinergic agents may result in additive or super-additive tachycardia and drowsiness). Products include:
Hyland's Teething Tablets .... ▣736

Benztropine Mesylate (Co-administration with anticholinergic agents may result in additive or super-additive tachycardia and drowsiness). Products include:
Cogentin Injection 1903

Biperiden Hydrochloride (Co-administration with anticholinergic agents may result in additive or super-additive tachycardia and drowsiness).
No products indexed under this heading.

Bromodiphenhydramine Hydrochloride (Co-administration results in additive CNS depression or super-additive tachycardia and drowsiness).
No products indexed under this heading.

Brompheniramine Maleate (Co-administration results in additive CNS depression or super-additive tachycardia and drowsiness). Products include:
Alacol DM Syrup 739
Children's Dimetapp Cold & Allergy Elixir 745
Children's Dimetapp DM Cold & Cough Elixir 745
Robitussin Allergy & Cough Syrup 750
Sudafed Sinus & Allergy Tablets 710
TheraFlu Cold & Cough Hot Liquid 680
TheraFlu Cold & Sore Throat Hot Liquid 680
TheraFlu Flu & Sore Throat Hot Liquid 681
TheraFlu Severe Cold & Cough Hot Liquid 683
TheraFlu Severe Cold Caplets 679
TheraFlu Severe Cold Hot Liquid 682
Triaminic Cold & Allergy Liquid 685
Triaminic Cold & Cough Liquid 685
Triaminic Flu, Cough & Fever Liquid 685
Triaminic Night Time Cough & Cold Liquid 685
Triaminic Allergy Runny Nose & Congestion Softchews 688
Triaminic Cold & Cough Softchews 688
Children's Tylenol Plus Cold NightTime Suspension Liquid 1851
Children's Tylenol Plus Cold & Cough Suspension Liquid and Chewable Tablets 1851
Children's Tylenol Plus Cold Chewable Tablets 1851
Children's Tylenol Plus Flu Suspension Liquid 1853
Tylenol Allergy Complete Multi-Symptom Caplets and Gelcaps with Cool Burst 1844
Multi-Symptom Tylenol Cold Night Time Caplets 1845
Vicks 44M Cough, Cold & Flu Relief 2676
Pediatric Vicks 44m Cough & Cold Relief 2673
Children's Vicks NyQuil Cold/Cough Relief 2671

Buprenorphine Hydrochloride (Co-administration results in additive drowsiness and CNS depression). Products include:
Buprenex Injectable 2718
Suboxone Tablets 2719
Subutex Tablets 2719

Buspirone Hydrochloride (Co-administration results in additive drowsiness and CNS depression).
No products indexed under this heading.

Butabarbital (Co-administration results in decreased clearance of barbiturates via competitive inhibition of metabolism; additive drowsiness and CNS depression).
No products indexed under this heading.

Butalbital (Co-administration results in decreased clearance of barbiturates via competitive inhibition of metabolism; additive drowsiness and CNS depression). Products include:
Sedapap Tablets 50 mg/650 mg 2098

Carisoprodol (Co-administration with muscle relaxants may result in additive drowsiness and CNS depression).
No products indexed under this heading.

Cetirizine Hydrochloride (Co-administration results in additive CNS depression or super-additive tachycardia and drowsiness). Products include:
Zyrtec Chewable Tablets 2589
Zyrtec 2589
Zyrtec-D 12 Hour Extended Release Tablets 2591

Chlordiazepoxide (Co-administration results in additive drowsiness and CNS depression).
No products indexed under this heading.

Chlordiazepoxide Hydrochloride (Co-administration results in additive drowsiness and CNS depression). Products include:
Librium Capsules 3349

Chlorpheniramine Maleate (Co-administration results in additive CNS depression or super-additive tachycardia and drowsiness). Products include:
Advil Allergy Sinus Caplets 737
Advil Multi-Symptom Cold Caplets 738
BC Allergy Sinus Cold Powder 612
Contac Severe Cold and Flu Caplets Maximum Strength 615
Hycomine Compound Tablets 1105
PediaCare Multi-Symptom Cold Liquid 704
PediaCare NightRest Cough & Cold Liquid 704
Robitussin Flu Liquid 752
Robitussin PM Cough & Cold Liquid 752
Singlet Caplets 636

Chlorpheniramine Polistirex (Co-administration results in additive CNS depression or super-additive tachycardia and drowsiness). Products include:
Tussionex Pennkinetic Extended-Release Suspension 3322

Chlorpheniramine Tannate (Co-administration results in additive CNS depression or super-additive tachycardia and drowsiness).
No products indexed under this heading.

Chlorpromazine (Co-administration results in additive drowsiness and CNS depression).
No products indexed under this heading.

Chlorpromazine Hydrochloride (Co-administration results in additive drowsiness and CNS depression).
No products indexed under this heading.

Chlorprothixene (Co-administration results in additive drowsiness and CNS depression).
No products indexed under this heading.

Chlorprothixene Hydrochloride (Co-administration results in additive drowsiness and CNS depression).
No products indexed under this heading.

Chlorprothixene Lactate (Co-administration results in additive drowsiness and CNS depression).
No products indexed under this heading.

Chlorzoxazone (Co-administration with muscle relaxants may result in additive drowsiness and CNS depression).
No products indexed under this heading.

Clemastine Fumarate (Co-administration results in additive CNS depression or super-additive tachycardia and drowsiness).
No products indexed under this heading.

Clidinium Bromide (Co-administration with anticholinergic agents may result in additive or super-additive tachycardia and drowsiness).
No products indexed under this heading.

Clomipramine Hydrochloride (Co-administration results in additive tachycardia, hypertension, and drowsiness).
No products indexed under this heading.

Clorazepate Dipotassium (Co-administration results in additive drowsiness and CNS depression). Products include:
Tranxene 2488

Clozapine (Co-administration results in additive drowsiness and CNS depression). Products include:
Clozapine Tablets 2141
Clozaril Tablets 2174
FazaClo Orally Disintegrating Tablets 547

Cocaine Hydrochloride (Co-administration with cocaine may result in additive hypertension, tachycardia, and possibly cardiotoxicity).
No products indexed under this heading.

Codeine Phosphate (Co-administration results in additive drowsiness and CNS depression). Products include:
Tylenol with Codeine 2461

Cyclobenzaprine Hydrochloride (Co-administration with muscle relaxants may result in additive drowsiness and CNS depression). Products include:
Flexeril Tablets 1832

Cyproheptadine Hydrochloride (Co-administration results in additive CNS depression or super-additive tachycardia and drowsiness).
No products indexed under this heading.

Desflurane (Co-administration results in additive drowsiness and CNS depression). Products include:
Suprane Liquid for Inhalation 770

Desipramine Hydrochloride (Co-administration results in additive tachycardia, hypertension, and drowsiness).
No products indexed under this heading.

Dexchlorpheniramine Maleate (Co-administration results in additive CNS depression or super-additive tachycardia and drowsiness).
No products indexed under this heading.

Dextroamphetamine Sulfate (Co-administration with amphetamine may result in additive hypertension, tachycardia, and possibly cardiotoxicity). Products include:
Adderall Tablets 3168
Adderall XR Capsules 3169
Dexedrine 1386
DextroStat Tablets 3177

Dezocine (Co-administration results in additive drowsiness and CNS depression).
No products indexed under this heading.

Diazepam (Co-administration results in additive drowsiness and CNS depression). Products include:
Diastat Rectal Delivery System 3344
Valium Tablets 2822

Dicyclomine Hydrochloride (Co-administration with anticholinergic agents may result in additive or super-additive tachycardia and drowsiness). Products include:
Bentyl Capsules 724
Bentyl Injection 724
Bentyl Syrup 724
Bentyl Tablets 724

Diphenhydramine Citrate (Co-administration results in additive CNS depression or super-additive tachycardia and drowsiness). Products include:
Children's Benadryl Allergy & Cold Fastmelt Tablets 695
Children's Benadryl D Allergy & Sinus Fastmelt Tablets 694
Children's Benadryl Allergy Fastmelt Tablets 696
Goody's PM Powder 622

Diphenhydramine Hydrochloride (Co-administration results in additive CNS depression or super-additive tachycardia and drowsiness). Products include:
Benadryl Allergy & Cold Tablets 692
Benadryl Allergy 691
Benadryl Allergy & Sinus Headache Caplets & Gelcaps 693
Children's Benadryl Allergy Liquid 695
Children's Benadryl Dye-Free Allergy Liquid 695
Benadryl Dye-Free Allergy Liqui-Gels Softgels 692
Benadryl Itch Relief Stick Extra Strength 696
Benadryl Itch Stopping Cream Extra Strength 697
Benadryl Itch Stopping Gel Extra Strength 697
Benadryl Itch Stopping Spray Extra Strength 697
Benadryl Maximum Strength Severe Allergy & Sinus Headache Caplets 694
Children's Benadryl D Liquid Medication 693
Benadryl D Tablets 694
Nytol QuickCaps Caplets 635
Maximum Strength Nytol QuickGels Softgels 635
Simply Sleep Caplets 1841
Sominex Original Formula Tablets 637
TheraFlu Thin Strips Multi Symptom 684
Triaminic Thin Strips Cough & Runny Nose 690
Children's Tylenol Plus Cold & Allergy Suspension Liquid 1850
Tylenol Allergy Complete Night Time Caplets 1844
Tylenol Severe Allergy Caplets 1844
Tylenol Flu NightTime Gelcaps 1846
Extra Strength Tylenol PM Caplets, Geltabs, Gelcaps and Liquid 1847
Unisom Maximum Strength SleepGels 712

Diphenylpyraline Hydrochloride (Co-administration results in additive CNS depression or super-additive tachycardia and drowsiness).
No products indexed under this heading.

Disulfiram (Co-administration of disulfiram in a patient who smoked marijuana has resulted in a reversible hypomanic reaction). Products include:
Antabuse Tablets 2343

Dobutamine Hydrochloride (Co-administration with sympathomimetics may result in additive hypertension, tachycardia, and possibly cardiotoxicity).
No products indexed under this heading.

Dopamine Hydrochloride (Co-administration with sympathomimetics may result in additive hypertension, tachycardia, and possibly cardiotoxicity).
No products indexed under this heading.

Doxepin Hydrochloride (Co-administration results in additive tachycardia, hypertension, and drowsiness).
No products indexed under this heading.

Droperidol (Co-administration results in additive drowsiness and CNS depression).
No products indexed under this heading.

Dyphylline (Increased theophylline metabolism has resulted with smoking marijuana).
No products indexed under this heading.

Enflurane (Co-administration results in additive drowsiness and CNS depression).
No products indexed under this heading.

Ephedrine Hydrochloride (Co-administration with sympathomimetics may result in additive hypertension, tachycardia, and possibly cardiotoxicity). Products include:
Primatene Tablets .... ◘ 749

Ephedrine Sulfate (Co-administration with sympathomimetics may result in additive hypertension, tachycardia, and possibly cardiotoxicity).
No products indexed under this heading.

Ephedrine Tannate (Co-administration with sympathomimetics may result in additive hypertension, tachycardia, and possibly cardiotoxicity).
No products indexed under this heading.

Epinephrine (Co-administration with sympathomimetics may result in additive hypertension, tachycardia, and possibly cardiotoxicity).
Products include:
EpiPen 1061
Primatene Mist .... ◘ 749

Epinephrine Bitartrate (Co-administration with sympathomimetics may result in additive hypertension, tachycardia, and possibly cardiotoxicity).
No products indexed under this heading.

Epinephrine Hydrochloride (Co-administration with sympathomimetics may result in additive hypertension, tachycardia, and possibly cardiotoxicity).
No products indexed under this heading.

Estazolam (Co-administration results in additive drowsiness and CNS depression). Products include:
ProSom Tablets 512

Ethanol (Co-administration results in additive drowsiness and CNS depression).
No products indexed under this heading.

Ethchlorvynol (Co-administration results in additive drowsiness and CNS depression).
No products indexed under this heading.

Ethinamate (Co-administration results in additive drowsiness and CNS depression).
No products indexed under this heading.

Ethyl Alcohol (Co-administration results in additive drowsiness and CNS depression).
No products indexed under this heading.

Fentanyl (Co-administration results in additive drowsiness and CNS depression). Products include:
Duragesic Transdermal System 2448

Fentanyl Citrate (Co-administration results in additive drowsiness and CNS depression). Products include:
Actiq 993

Fexofenadine Hydrochloride (Co-administration results in additive CNS depression or super-additive tachycardia and drowsiness).
Products include:
Allegra 2857
Allegra-D 12 Hour Extended-Release Tablets 2860
Allegra-D 24 Hour Extended-Release Tablets 2862

Fluoxetine Hydrochloride (Co-administration of fluoxetine in a patient who smoked marijuana has resulted in a hypomanic reaction).
Products include:
Prozac Pulvules and Liquid 1771
Symbyax Capsules 1788

Fluphenazine Decanoate (Co-administration results in additive drowsiness and CNS depression).
No products indexed under this heading.

Fluphenazine Enanthate (Co-administration results in additive drowsiness and CNS depression).
No products indexed under this heading.

Fluphenazine Hydrochloride (Co-administration results in additive drowsiness and CNS depression).
No products indexed under this heading.

Flurazepam Hydrochloride (Co-administration results in additive drowsiness and CNS depression).
Products include:
Dalmane Capsules 3343

Glutethimide (Co-administration results in additive drowsiness and CNS depression).
No products indexed under this heading.

Glycopyrrolate (Co-administration with anticholinergic agents may result in additive or super-additive tachycardia and drowsiness).
No products indexed under this heading.

Halazepam (Co-administration results in additive drowsiness and CNS depression).
No products indexed under this heading.

Haloperidol (Co-administration results in additive drowsiness and CNS depression).
No products indexed under this heading.

Haloperidol Decanoate (Co-administration results in additive drowsiness and CNS depression).
No products indexed under this heading.

Hydrocodone Bitartrate (Co-administration results in additive drowsiness and CNS depression).
Products include:
Hycodan 1104
Hycomine Compound Tablets 1105
Hycotuss Expectorant Syrup 1106
Lortab 3315
Lortab Elixir 3312
Vicodin Tablets 530
Vicodin ES Tablets 531
Vicodin HP Tablets 532
Vicoprofen Tablets 533
Zydone Tablets 1118

Hydrocodone Polistirex (Co-administration results in additive drowsiness and CNS depression).
Products include:
Tussionex Pennkinetic Extended-Release Suspension 3322

Hydromorphone Hydrochloride (Co-administration results in additive drowsiness and CNS depression).
Products include:
Dilaudid 439
Dilaudid Oral Liquid 443
Dilaudid Non-Sterile Powder 439
Dilaudid Rectal Suppositories 439
Dilaudid Tablets 439
Dilaudid Tablets - 8 mg 443
Dilaudid-HP 441

Hydroxyzine Hydrochloride (Co-administration results in additive drowsiness and CNS depression).
No products indexed under this heading.

Hyoscyamine (Co-administration with anticholinergic agents may result in additive or super-additive tachycardia and drowsiness).
No products indexed under this heading.

Hyoscyamine Sulfate (Co-administration with anticholinergic agents may result in additive or super-additive tachycardia and drowsiness).
No products indexed under this heading.

Imipramine Hydrochloride (Co-administration results in additive tachycardia, hypertension, and drowsiness).
No products indexed under this heading.

Imipramine Pamoate (Co-administration results in additive tachycardia, hypertension, and drowsiness).
No products indexed under this heading.

Ipratropium Bromide (Co-administration with anticholinergic agents may result in additive or super-additive tachycardia and drowsiness). Products include:
Atrovent HFA Inhalation Aerosol 872
Atrovent Inhalation Solution 868
Atrovent Nasal Spray 0.03% 869
Atrovent Nasal Spray 0.06% 870
Combivent Inhalation Aerosol 878
DuoNeb Inhalation Solution 1058

Isoflurane (Co-administration results in additive drowsiness and CNS depression).
No products indexed under this heading.

Isoproterenol Hydrochloride (Co-administration with sympathomimetics may result in additive hypertension, tachycardia, and possibly cardiotoxicity).
No products indexed under this heading.

Isoproterenol Sulfate (Co-administration with sympathomimetics may result in additive hypertension, tachycardia, and possibly cardiotoxicity).
No products indexed under this heading.

Ketamine Hydrochloride (Co-administration results in additive drowsiness and CNS depression).
No products indexed under this heading.

Levalbuterol Hydrochloride (Co-administration with sympathomimetics may result in additive hypertension, tachycardia, and possibly cardiotoxicity). Products include:
Xopenex Inhalation Solution 3143
Xopenex Inhalation Solution Concentrate 3147

Levomethadyl Acetate Hydrochloride (Co-administration results in additive drowsiness and CNS depression).
No products indexed under this heading.

Levorphanol Tartrate (Co-administration results in additive drowsiness and CNS depression).
No products indexed under this heading.

Lithium (Co-administration results in additive drowsiness and CNS depression).
No products indexed under this heading.

Lithium Carbonate (Co-administration results in additive drowsiness and CNS depression).
Products include:
Eskalith 1406
Lithobid Tablets 1670

Lithium Citrate (Co-administration results in additive drowsiness and CNS depression).
No products indexed under this heading.

Loratadine (Co-administration results in additive CNS depression or super-additive tachycardia and drowsiness). Products include:
Alavert Allergy & Sinus D-12 Hour Tablets .... ◘ 743
Alavert .... ◘ 743
Children's Claritin 24 Hour Non-Drowsy Allergy Syrup .... ◘ 732
Claritin Non-Drowsy 24 Hour Tablets .... ◘ 731
Non-Drowsy Claritin Hives Relief Tablets .... ◘ 733
Claritin Reditabs 24 Hour Non-Drowsy Tablets .... ◘ 732
Claritin-D Non-Drowsy 12 Hour Tablets .... ◘ 731
Claritin-D Non-Drowsy 24 Hour Tablets .... ◘ 731
Children's Dimetapp ND Non-Drowsy Allergy Syrup .... ◘ 746
Triaminic Allerchews .... ◘ 684

Lorazepam (Co-administration results in additive drowsiness and CNS depression).
No products indexed under this heading.

Loxapine Hydrochloride (Co-administration results in additive drowsiness and CNS depression).
No products indexed under this heading.

Loxapine Succinate (Co-administration results in additive drowsiness and CNS depression).
No products indexed under this heading.

Maprotiline Hydrochloride (Co-administration results in additive tachycardia, hypertension, and drowsiness).
No products indexed under this heading.

Mepenzolate Bromide (Co-administration with anticholinergic agents may result in additive or super-additive tachycardia and drowsiness).
No products indexed under this heading.

Meperidine Hydrochloride (Co-administration results in additive drowsiness and CNS depression).
No products indexed under this heading.

Mephobarbital (Co-administration results in decreased clearance of barbiturates via competitive inhibition of metabolism; additive drowsiness and CNS depression). Products include:
Mebaral Tablets, USP 2483

Meprobamate (Co-administration results in additive drowsiness and CNS depression).
No products indexed under this heading.

Mesoridazine Besylate (Co-administration results in additive drowsiness and CNS depression).
No products indexed under this heading.

Metaproterenol Sulfate (Co-administration with sympathomimetics may result in additive hypertension, tachycardia, and possibly cardiotoxicity). Products include:
Alupent Inhalation Aerosol 858

Metaraminol Bitartrate (Co-administration with sympathomimetics may result in additive hypertension, tachycardia, and possibly cardiotoxicity). Products include:
Aramine Injection 1889

Methadone Hydrochloride (Co-administration results in additive drowsiness and CNS depression).
No products indexed under this heading.

Methamphetamine Hydrochloride (Co-administration with amphetamine may result in additive hypertension, tachycardia, and possibly cardiotoxicity). Products include:
Desoxyn Tablets, USP 2482

Methdilazine Hydrochloride (Co-administration results in additive CNS depression or super-additive tachycardia and drowsiness).
No products indexed under this heading.

Methocarbamol (Co-administration with muscle relaxants may result in additive drowsiness and CNS depression).
No products indexed under this heading.

Methohexital Sodium (Co-administration results in additive drowsiness and CNS depression).
No products indexed under this heading.

Methotrimeprazine (Co-administration results in additive drowsiness and CNS depression).
No products indexed under this heading.

Methoxamine Hydrochloride (Co-administration with sympathomimetics may result in additive hypertension, tachycardia, and possibly cardiotoxicity).
No products indexed under this heading.

Methoxyflurane (Co-administration results in additive drowsiness and CNS depression).
No products indexed under this heading.

Midazolam Hydrochloride (Co-administration results in additive drowsiness and CNS depression).
No products indexed under this heading.

Molindone Hydrochloride (Co-administration results in additive drowsiness and CNS depression). Products include:
Moban Tablets 1108

Morphine Sulfate (Co-administration results in additive drowsiness and CNS depression). Products include:
Avinza Capsules 1714
Kadian Capsules 572
MS Contin Tablets 2703

Norepinephrine Bitartrate (Co-administration with sympathomimetics may result in additive hypertension, tachycardia, and possibly cardiotoxicity).
No products indexed under this heading.

Nortriptyline Hydrochloride (Co-administration results in additive tachycardia, hypertension, and drowsiness).
No products indexed under this heading.

Olanzapine (Co-administration results in additive drowsiness and CNS depression). Products include:
Symbyax Capsules 1788
Zyprexa Tablets 1798
Zyprexa IntraMuscular 1798
Zyprexa ZYDIS Orally Disintegrating Tablets 1798

Orphenadrine Citrate (Co-administration with muscle relaxants may result in additive drowsiness and CNS depression). Products include:
Norflex Injection 1824

Oxazepam (Co-administration results in additive drowsiness and CNS depression).
No products indexed under this heading.

Oxybutynin Chloride (Co-administration with anticholinergic agents may result in additive or super-additive tachycardia and drowsiness). Products include:
Ditropan XL Extended Release Tablets 2391

Oxycodone Hydrochloride (Co-administration results in additive drowsiness and CNS depression). Products include:
Combunox Tablets 1183
OxyContin Tablets 2699
OxyFast Oral Concentrate Solution 2704
OxyIR Capsules 2704
Percocet Tablets 1114
Percodan Tablets 1115

Pentobarbital Sodium (Co-administration results in decreased clearance of barbiturates via competitive inhibition of metabolism; additive drowsiness and CNS depression). Products include:
Nembutal Sodium Solution, USP 2484

Perphenazine (Co-administration results in additive drowsiness and CNS depression).
No products indexed under this heading.

Phenobarbital (Co-administration results in decreased clearance of barbiturates via competitive inhibition of metabolism; additive drowsiness and CNS depression).
No products indexed under this heading.

Phenylephrine Bitartrate (Co-administration with sympathomimetics may result in additive hypertension, tachycardia, and possibly cardiotoxicity).
No products indexed under this heading.

Phenylephrine Hydrochloride (Co-administration with sympathomimetics may result in additive hypertension, tachycardia, and possibly cardiotoxicity). Products include:
Alacol DM Syrup 739
Hycomine Compound Tablets 1105
Preparation H Maximum Strength Cream 747
Preparation H Cooling Gel 747
Preparation H 747
Sudafed PE Tablets 711
Vicks Sinex Nasal Spray and Ultra Fine Mist for Sinus Relief.............. 2677
Zicam Concentrated Cough Mist for Kids Plus D Cool Cherry......... 643
Zicam Concentrated Cough Mist Plus D Cool Cherry..................... 642

Phenylephrine Tannate (Co-administration with sympathomimetics may result in additive hypertension, tachycardia, and possibly cardiotoxicity).
No products indexed under this heading.

Phenylpropanolamine Hydrochloride (Co-administration with sympathomimetics may result in additive hypertension, tachycardia, and possibly cardiotoxicity).
No products indexed under this heading.

Pirbuterol Acetate (Co-administration with sympathomimetics may result in additive hypertension, tachycardia, and possibly cardiotoxicity). Products include:
Maxair Autohaler 1820

Prazepam (Co-administration results in additive drowsiness and CNS depression).
No products indexed under this heading.

Prochlorperazine (Co-administration results in additive drowsiness and CNS depression).
No products indexed under this heading.

Procyclidine Hydrochloride (Co-administration with anticholinergic agents may result in additive or super-additive tachycardia and drowsiness).
No products indexed under this heading.

Promethazine Hydrochloride (Co-administration results in additive drowsiness and CNS depression). Products include:
Phenergan 3438

Propantheline Bromide (Co-administration with anticholinergic agents may result in additive or super-additive tachycardia and drowsiness).
No products indexed under this heading.

Propofol (Co-administration results in additive drowsiness and CNS depression). Products include:
Diprivan Injectable Emulsion 676

Propoxyphene Hydrochloride (Co-administration results in additive drowsiness and CNS depression).
No products indexed under this heading.

Propoxyphene Napsylate (Co-administration results in additive drowsiness and CNS depression). Products include:
Darvocet A 500 Tablets 3497

Protriptyline Hydrochloride (Co-administration results in additive tachycardia, hypertension, and drowsiness). Products include:
Vivactil Tablets 2350

Pseudoephedrine Hydrochloride (Co-administration with sympathomimetics may result in additive hypertension, tachycardia, and possibly cardiotoxicity). Products include:
Advil Allergy Sinus Caplets 737
Advil Cold & Sinus 739
Advil Flu & Body Ache Caplets 739
Children's Advil Cold Suspension ... 741
Advil Multi-Symptom Cold Caplets....................................... 738
Allegra-D 12 Hour Extended-Release Tablets............ 2860
Allegra-D 24 Hour Extended-Release Tablets............ 2862
Balamine DM 739
BC Cold Powder 612
Benadryl Allergy & Cold Tablets 692
Benadryl Allergy & Sinus Headache Caplets & Gelcaps...... 693
Children's Benadryl Allergy & Cold Fastmelt Tablets.................. 695
Benadryl Maximum Strength Severe Allergy & Sinus Headache Caplets........................ 694
Children's Benadryl D Allergy & Sinus Fastmelt Tablets............... 694
Children's Benadryl D Liquid Medication...................................... 693
Benadryl D Tablets 694
Contac Non-Drowsy 12 Hour Cold Caplets.............................. 614
Contac Non-Drowsy Timed Release 12 Hour Cold Caplets.... 615
Contac Severe Cold and Flu Caplets Maximum Strength......... 615
Contac Severe Cold and Flu Caplets Non-Drowsy.................... 615
Children's Dimetapp Cold & Allergy Elixir................................ 745
Children's Dimetapp DM Cold & Cough Elixir................................ 745
Children's Dimetapp Long Acting Cough Plus Cold Syrup............... 746
Dimetapp Infant Drops Decongestant Plus Cough.......... 746
Children's Motrin Cold Non-Staining Dye-Free Oral Suspension................................ 1838
Children's Motrin Cold Oral Suspension................................ 1838
Motrin Cold & Sinus Caplets 1836
PediaCare Decongestant & Cough Infant Drops..................... 705
PediaCare Decongestant Infants' Drops.. 705
PediaCare Long-Acting Cough Plus Cold Liquid......................... 704
PediaCare Multi-Symptom Cold Liquid.. 704
PediaCare NightRest Cough & Cold Liquid................................. 704
Robitussin Allergy & Cough Syrup .. 750
Robitussin CF Liquid 755
Robitussin Cough & Cold Liquid-filled Capsules.................. 750
Robitussin Cough, Cold & Flu Liquid-filled Capsules.................. 750
Robitussin Cough & Cold Infant Drops.. 755
Robitussin Flu Liquid 752
Robitussin Maximum Strength Cough & Cold Liquid................. 754
Robitussin PE Syrup 753
Robitussin Pediatric Cough & Cold Liquid................................. 754
Robitussin PM Cough & Cold Liquid.. 752
Robitussin Severe Congestion Liquid-filled Capsules................. 751
Simply Stuffy Liquid 1841
Singlet Caplets 636
Sudafed 12 Hour Caplets 708
Sudafed 24 Hour Tablets 709
Sudafed Nasal Decongestant Tablets....................................... 709
Sudafed Severe Cold 710
Sudafed Non-Drying Sinus Liquid Caps.. 709
Sudafed Sinus & Allergy Tablets 710

IMPORTANT NOTE: Always consult each drug listing in the patient's regimen for possible interactions.

Sudafed Sinus Headache .... ▣711
TheraFlu Cold & Cough Hot Liquid .... ▣680
TheraFlu Cold & Sore Throat Hot Liquid .... ▣680
TheraFlu Flu & Chest Congestion Non-Drowsy Hot Liquid .... ▣681
TheraFlu Flu & Sore Throat Hot Liquid .... ▣681
TheraFlu Severe Cold Non-Drowsy Hot Liquid .... ▣683
TheraFlu Severe Cold & Cough Hot Liquid .... ▣683
TheraFlu Severe Cold Caplets .... ▣679
TheraFlu Severe Cold Hot Liquid .... ▣682
TheraFlu Severe Cold Non-Drowsy Caplets .... ▣679
Triaminic Chest & Nasal Congestion Liquid .... ▣685
Triaminic Cold & Allergy Liquid .... ▣685
Triaminic Cold & Cough Liquid .... ▣685
Triaminic Cough Liquid .... ▣687
Triaminic Cough & Nasal Congestion Liquid .... ▣687
Triaminic Cough & Sore Throat Liquid .... ▣687
Triaminic Flu, Cough & Fever Liquid .... ▣685
Triaminic Night Time Cough & Cold Liquid .... ▣685
Triaminic Allergy Runny Nose & Congestion Softchews .... ▣688
Triaminic Cold & Cough Softchews .... ▣688
Triaminic Cough & Sore Throat Softchews .... ▣689
Tylenol Sinus NightTime Caplets .... ▣663
Children's Tylenol Plus Cold & Allergy Suspension Liquid 1850
Children's Tylenol Plus Cold NightTime Suspension Liquid 1851
Children's Tylenol Plus Cold & Cough Suspension Liquid and Chewable Tablets 1851
Children's Tylenol Plus Cold Chewable Tablets 1851
Children's Tylenol Plus Cold Daytime Non-Drowsy Suspension Liquid 1851
Children's Tylenol Plus Flu Suspension Liquid 1853
Concentrated Tylenol Infants' Drops Plus Cold 1851
Concentrated Tylenol Infants' Drops Plus Cold and Cough 1851
Tylenol Cold & Flu Severe Daytime Liquid with Cool Burst 1846
Tylenol Cold & Flu Severe NightTime Liquid with Cool Burst 1846
Tylenol Cold Severe Congestion Non-Drowsy Caplets with Cool Burst 1846
Tylenol Allergy Complete Night Time Caplets 1844
Tylenol Allergy Complete Multi-Symptom Caplets and Gelcaps with Cool Burst 1844
Tylenol Flu NightTime Gelcaps 1846
Tylenol Flu Day Non-Drowsy Gelcaps 1846
Concentrated Tylenol Infants' Drops Plus Cold Nasal Congestant, Fever Reducer & Pain Reliever .... ▣668
Concentrated Tylenol Infants' Drops Plus Cold & Cough Nasal Decongestant, Fever Reducer & Pain Reliever .... ▣668
Multi-Symptom Tylenol Cold Night Time Caplets 1845
Multi-Symptom Tylenol Cold Day Non-Drowsy Caplets and Gelcaps 1845
Tylenol Sinus Day Non-Drowsy 1848
Tylenol Sinus Night Time Caplets 1848
Tylenol Sinus Severe Congestion Caplets with Cool Burst 1848
Vicks 44D Cough & Head Congestion Relief 2676
Vicks 44D Cough & Head Congestion Relief Liquid .... ▣721
Vicks 44M Cough, Cold & Flu Relief 2676
Pediatric Vicks 44m Cough & Cold Relief 2673
Vicks DayQuil LiquiCaps/Liquid Multi-Symptom Cold/Flu Relief .... ▣723
Vicks DayQuil Multi-Symptom Cold/Flu Relief LiquiCaps 2675
Vicks DayQuil Multi-Symptom Cold/Flu Relief Liquid 2675
Children's Vicks NyQuil Cold/Cough Relief 2671
Vicks NyQuil LiquiCaps 2677
Vicks NyQuil LiquiCaps/Liquid Multi-Symptom Cold/Flu Relief .... ▣725
Vicks NyQuil Liquid 2677
Zyrtec-D 12 Hour Extended Release Tablets 2591

Pseudoephedrine Sulfate (Co-administration with sympathomimetics may result in additive hypertension, tachycardia, and possibly cardiotoxicity). Products include:

Alavert Allergy & Sinus D-12 Hour Tablets .... ▣743
Clarinex-D 24-Hour Extended-Release Tablets 3012
Claritin-D Non-Drowsy 12 Hour Tablets .... ▣731
Claritin-D Non-Drowsy 24 Hour Tablets .... ▣731

Pyrilamine Maleate (Co-administration results in additive CNS depression or super-additive tachycardia and drowsiness).
No products indexed under this heading.

Pyrilamine Tannate (Co-administration results in additive CNS depression or super-additive tachycardia and drowsiness).
No products indexed under this heading.

Quazepam (Co-administration results in additive drowsiness and CNS depression).
No products indexed under this heading.

Quetiapine Fumarate (Co-administration results in additive drowsiness and CNS depression). Products include:

Seroquel Tablets 691

Remifentanil Hydrochloride (Co-administration results in additive drowsiness and CNS depression).
No products indexed under this heading.

Risperidone (Co-administration results in additive drowsiness and CNS depression). Products include:

Risperdal Consta Long-Acting Injection 1664
Risperdal M-Tab Orally Disintegrating Tablets 1658
Risperdal 1658

Salmeterol Xinafoate (Co-administration with sympathomimetics may result in additive hypertension, tachycardia, and possibly cardiotoxicity). Products include:

Advair Diskus 100/50 1291
Advair Diskus 250/50 1291
Advair Diskus 500/50 1291
Serevent Diskus 1540

Scopolamine (Co-administration with anticholinergic agents may result in additive or super-additive tachycardia and drowsiness). Products include:

Transderm Scōp Transdermal Therapeutic System 2166

Scopolamine Hydrobromide (Co-administration with anticholinergic agents may result in additive or super-additive tachycardia and drowsiness).
No products indexed under this heading.

Secobarbital Sodium (Co-administration results in decreased clearance of barbiturates via competitive inhibition of metabolism; additive drowsiness and CNS depression).
No products indexed under this heading.

Sevoflurane (Co-administration results in additive drowsiness and CNS depression). Products include:

Ultane Liquid for Inhalation 526

Sodium Oxybate (Co-administration results in additive drowsiness and CNS depression).
No products indexed under this heading.

Sufentanil Citrate (Co-administration results in additive drowsiness and CNS depression).
No products indexed under this heading.

Temazepam (Co-administration results in additive drowsiness and CNS depression).
No products indexed under this heading.

Terbutaline Sulfate (Co-administration with sympathomimetics may result in additive hypertension, tachycardia, and possibly cardiotoxicity).
No products indexed under this heading.

Terfenadine (Co-administration results in additive CNS depression or super-additive tachycardia and drowsiness).
No products indexed under this heading.

Theophylline (Increased theophylline metabolism has resulted with smoking marijuana).
No products indexed under this heading.

Theophylline Anhydrous (Increased theophylline metabolism has resulted with smoking marijuana). Products include:

Uniphyl Tablets 2708

Theophylline Calcium Salicylate (Increased theophylline metabolism has resulted with smoking marijuana).
No products indexed under this heading.

Theophylline Dihydroxypropyl (Glyceryl) (Increased theophylline metabolism has resulted with smoking marijuana).
No products indexed under this heading.

Theophylline Ethylenediamine (Increased theophylline metabolism has resulted with smoking marijuana).
No products indexed under this heading.

Theophylline Sodium Glycinate (Increased theophylline metabolism has resulted with smoking marijuana).
No products indexed under this heading.

Thiamylal Sodium (Co-administration results in decreased clearance of barbiturates via competitive inhibition of metabolism; additive drowsiness and CNS depression).
No products indexed under this heading.

Thioridazine Hydrochloride (Co-administration results in additive drowsiness and CNS depression). Products include:

Thioridazine Hydrochloride Tablets 2122

Thiothixene (Co-administration results in additive drowsiness and CNS depression). Products include:

Thiothixene Capsules 2124

Tolterodine Tartrate (Co-administration with anticholinergic agents may result in additive or super-additive tachycardia and drowsiness). Products include:

Detrol Tablets 2626
Detrol LA Capsules 2629

Triazolam (Co-administration results in additive drowsiness and CNS depression).
No products indexed under this heading.

Tridihexethyl Chloride (Co-administration with anticholinergic agents may result in additive or super-additive tachycardia and drowsiness).
No products indexed under this heading.

Trifluoperazine Hydrochloride (Co-administration results in additive drowsiness and CNS depression).
No products indexed under this heading.

Trihexyphenidyl Hydrochloride (Co-administration with anticholinergic agents may result in additive or super-additive tachycardia and drowsiness).
No products indexed under this heading.

Trimeprazine Tartrate (Co-administration results in additive CNS depression or super-additive tachycardia and drowsiness).
No products indexed under this heading.

Trimipramine Maleate (Co-administration results in additive tachycardia, hypertension, and drowsiness). Products include:

Surmontil Capsules 2347

Tripelennamine Hydrochloride (Co-administration results in additive CNS depression or super-additive tachycardia and drowsiness).
No products indexed under this heading.

Triprolidine Hydrochloride (Co-administration results in additive CNS depression or super-additive tachycardia and drowsiness).
No products indexed under this heading.

Zaleplon (Co-administration results in additive drowsiness and CNS depression). Products include:

Sonata Capsules 1686

Ziprasidone Hydrochloride (Co-administration results in additive drowsiness and CNS depression). Products include:

Geodon Capsules 2514

Zolpidem Tartrate (Co-administration results in additive drowsiness and CNS depression). Products include:

Ambien Tablets 2867

Food Interactions

Alcohol (Co-administration results in additive drowsiness and CNS depression).

MARLYN FORMULA 50 CAPSULES

(Amino Acid Preparations, Vitamin B_6) 3525
None cited in PDR database.

MASSENGILL FEMININE CLEANSING WASH
(Cleanser) 622
None cited in PDR database.

MASSENGILL BABY POWDER SCENT SOFT CLOTH TOWELETTE
(Lactic Acid, Potassium Sorbate, Sodium Lactate).............................. 622
None cited in PDR database.

MATULANE CAPSULES
(Procarbazine Hydrochloride) **3188**
May interact with antihistamines, antihypertensives, barbiturates, narcotic analgesics, phenothiazines, sympathomimetics, tricyclic antidepressants, and certain other agents. Compounds in these categories include:

Acebutolol Hydrochloride (To minimize CNS depression and possible potentiation, hypotensive agents should be used with caution).
No products indexed under this heading.

Acrivastine (Potential for increased CNS depression and possible potentiation).
No products indexed under this heading.

Albuterol (Procarbazine exhibits some MAO inhibitory activity; concurrent use should be avoided). Products include:
Proventil Inhalation Aerosol **3067**

Albuterol Sulfate (Procarbazine exhibits some MAO inhibitory activity; concurrent use should be avoided). Products include:
AccuNeb Inhalation Solution **1055**
Combivent Inhalation Aerosol **878**
DuoNeb Inhalation Solution **1058**
Proventil Inhalation Solution 0.083%.. **3069**
Proventil HFA Inhalation Aerosol **3071**
Ventolin HFA Inhalation Aerosol **1576**
VoSpire Extended-Release Tablets ... **2352**

Alfentanil Hydrochloride (Potential for increased CNS depression and possible potentiation).
No products indexed under this heading.

Amitriptyline Hydrochloride (Procarbazine exhibits some MAO inhibitory activity; concurrent use should be avoided).
No products indexed under this heading.

Amlodipine Besylate (To minimize CNS depression and possible potentiation, hypotensive agents should be used with caution). Products include:
Caduet Tablets **2507**
Lotrel Capsules **2238**
Norvasc Tablets **2529**

Amoxapine (Procarbazine exhibits some MAO inhibitory activity; concurrent use should be avoided).
No products indexed under this heading.

Aprobarbital (Potential for increased CNS depression and possible potentiation).
No products indexed under this heading.

Astemizole (Potential for increased CNS depression and possible potentiation).
No products indexed under this heading.

Atenolol (To minimize CNS depression and possible potentiation, hypotensive agents should be used with caution). Products include:
Tenormin I.V. Injection **698**
Tenormin Tablets **695**

Azatadine Maleate (Potential for increased CNS depression and possible potentiation).
No products indexed under this heading.

Benazepril Hydrochloride (To minimize CNS depression and possible potentiation, hypotensive agents should be used with caution). Products include:
Lotensin Tablets **2232**
Lotensin HCT Tablets **2235**
Lotrel Capsules **2238**

Bendroflumethiazide (To minimize CNS depression and possible potentiation, hypotensive agents should be used with caution).
No products indexed under this heading.

Betaxolol Hydrochloride (To minimize CNS depression and possible potentiation, hypotensive agents should be used with caution). Products include:
Betoptic S Ophthalmic Suspension.................................. **554**

Bisoprolol Fumarate (To minimize CNS depression and possible potentiation, hypotensive agents should be used with caution).
No products indexed under this heading.

Bromodiphenhydramine Hydrochloride (Potential for increased CNS depression and possible potentiation).
No products indexed under this heading.

Brompheniramine Maleate (Potential for increased CNS depression and possible potentiation). Products include:
Alacol DM Syrup **739**
Children's Dimetapp Cold & Allergy Elixir **745**
Children's Dimetapp DM Cold & Cough Elixir **745**
Robitussin Allergy & Cough Syrup .. **750**

Buprenorphine Hydrochloride (Potential for increased CNS depression and possible potentiation). Products include:
Buprenex Injectable **2718**
Suboxone Tablets **2719**
Subutex Tablets **2719**

Butabarbital (Potential for increased CNS depression and possible potentiation).
No products indexed under this heading.

Butalbital (Potential for increased CNS depression and possible potentiation). Products include:
Sedapap Tablets 50 mg/650 mg **2098**

Candesartan Cilexetil (To minimize CNS depression and possible potentiation, hypotensive agents should be used with caution). Products include:
Atacand Tablets **634**
Atacand HCT **637**

Captopril (To minimize CNS depression and possible potentiation, hypotensive agents should be used with caution). Products include:
Captopril Tablets **2114**

Carteolol Hydrochloride (To minimize CNS depression and possible potentiation, hypotensive agents should be used with caution). Products include:
Carteolol Hydrochloride Ophthalmic Solution USP, 1%....... ⊙**246**

Cetirizine Hydrochloride (Potential for increased CNS depression and possible potentiation). Products include:
Zyrtec Chewable Tablets **2589**
Zyrtec **2589**
Zyrtec-D 12 Hour Extended Release Tablets.......................... **2591**

Chlorothiazide (To minimize CNS depression and possible potentiation, hypotensive agents should be used with caution). Products include:
Aldoclor Tablets **1881**
Diuril Oral **1936**

Chlorothiazide Sodium (To minimize CNS depression and possible potentiation, hypotensive agents should be used with caution). Products include:
Diuril Sodium Intravenous **1934**

Chlorpheniramine Maleate (Potential for increased CNS depression and possible potentiation). Products include:
Advil Allergy Sinus Caplets **737**
Advil Multi-Symptom Cold Caplets.. **738**
BC Allergy Sinus Cold Powder **612**
Contac Severe Cold and Flu Caplets Maximum Strength......... **615**
Hycomine Compound Tablets **1105**
PediaCare Multi-Symptom Cold Liquid **704**
PediaCare NightRest Cough & Cold Liquid.................................. **704**
Robitussin Flu Liquid **752**
Robitussin PM Cough & Cold Liquid **752**
Singlet Caplets **636**
Sudafed Sinus & Allergy Tablets **710**
TheraFlu Cold & Cough Hot Liquid **680**
TheraFlu Cold & Sore Throat Hot Liquid **680**
TheraFlu Flu & Sore Throat Hot Liquid **681**
TheraFlu Severe Cold & Cough Hot Liquid...................................... **683**
TheraFlu Severe Cold Caplets **679**
TheraFlu Severe Cold Hot Liquid **682**
Triaminic Cold & Allergy Liquid **685**
Triaminic Cold & Cough Liquid **685**
Triaminic Flu, Cough & Fever Liquid **685**
Triaminic Night Time Cough & Cold Liquid.................................. **685**
Triaminic Allergy Runny Nose & Congestion Softchews.............. **688**
Triaminic Cold & Cough Softchews **688**
Children's Tylenol Plus Cold NightTime Suspension Liquid........ **1851**
Children's Tylenol Plus Cold & Cough Suspension Liquid and Chewable Tablets **1851**
Children's Tylenol Plus Cold Chewable Tablets **1851**
Children's Tylenol Plus Flu Suspension Liquid **1853**
Tylenol Allergy Complete Multi-Symptom Caplets and Gelcaps with Cool Burst............... **1844**
Multi-Symptom Tylenol Cold Night Time Caplets **1845**
Vicks 44M Cough, Cold & Flu Relief.. **2676**
Pediatric Vicks 44m Cough & Cold Relief...................................... **2673**
Children's Vicks NyQuil Cold/Cough Relief **2671**

Chlorpheniramine Polistirex (Potential for increased CNS depression and possible potentiation). Products include:
Tussionex Pennkinetic Extended-Release Suspension...... **3322**

Chlorpheniramine Tannate (Potential for increased CNS depression and possible potentiation).
No products indexed under this heading.

Chlorpromazine (Potential for increased CNS depression and possible potentiation).
No products indexed under this heading.

Chlorpromazine Hydrochloride (Potential for increased CNS depression and possible potentiation).
No products indexed under this heading.

Chlorthalidone (To minimize CNS depression and possible potentiation, hypotensive agents should be used with caution). Products include:
Clorpres Tablets **2139**

Clemastine Fumarate (Potential for increased CNS depression and possible potentiation).
No products indexed under this heading.

Clomipramine Hydrochloride (Procarbazine exhibits some MAO inhibitory activity; concurrent use should be avoided).
No products indexed under this heading.

Clonidine (To minimize CNS depression and possible potentiation, hypotensive agents should be used with caution). Products include:
Catapres-TTS **875**

Clonidine Hydrochloride (To minimize CNS depression and possible potentiation, hypotensive agents should be used with caution). Products include:
Catapres Tablets **874**
Clorpres Tablets **2139**

Codeine Phosphate (Potential for increased CNS depression and possible potentiation). Products include:
Tylenol with Codeine **2461**

Cyproheptadine Hydrochloride (Potential for increased CNS depression and possible potentiation).
No products indexed under this heading.

Deserpidine (To minimize CNS depression and possible potentiation, hypotensive agents should be used with caution).
No products indexed under this heading.

Desipramine Hydrochloride (Procarbazine exhibits some MAO inhibitory activity; concurrent use should be avoided).
No products indexed under this heading.

Dexchlorpheniramine Maleate (Potential for increased CNS depression and possible potentiation).
No products indexed under this heading.

Dezocine (Potential for increased CNS depression and possible potentiation).
No products indexed under this heading.

Diazoxide (To minimize CNS depression and possible potentiation, hypotensive agents should be used with caution). Products include:
Hyperstat I.V. Injection **3031**

Diltiazem Hydrochloride (To minimize CNS depression and possible potentiation, hypotensive agents should be used with caution). Products include:
Cardizem LA Extended Release Tablets **1699**
Tiazac Capsules **1204**

Diphenhydramine Citrate (Potential for increased CNS depression and possible potentiation). Products include:

IMPORTANT NOTE: Always consult each drug listing in the patient's regimen for possible interactions.

Children's Benadryl Allergy & Cold Fastmelt Tablets .... ▣695
Children's Benadryl D Allergy & Sinus Fastmelt Tablets .... ▣694
Children's Benadryl Allergy Fastmelt Tablets .... ▣696
Goody's PM Powder .... ▣622

Diphenhydramine Hydrochloride (Potential for increased CNS depression and possible potentiation). Products include:
Benadryl Allergy & Cold Tablets .... ▣692
Benadryl Allergy .... ▣691
Benadryl Allergy & Sinus Headache Caplets & Gelcaps .... ▣693
Children's Benadryl Allergy Liquid .... ▣695
Children's Benadryl Dye-Free Allergy Liquid .... ▣695
Benadryl Dye-Free Allergy Liqui-Gels Softgels .... ▣692
Benadryl Itch Relief Stick Extra Strength .... ▣696
Benadryl Itch Stopping Cream Extra Strength .... ▣697
Benadryl Itch Stopping Gel Extra Strength .... ▣697
Benadryl Itch Stopping Spray Extra Strength .... ▣697
Benadryl Maximum Strength Severe Allergy & Sinus Headache Caplets .... ▣694
Children's Benadryl D Liquid Medication .... ▣693
Benadryl D Tablets .... ▣694
Nytol QuickCaps Caplets .... ▣635
Maximum Strength Nytol QuickGels Softgels .... ▣635
Simply Sleep Caplets 1841
Sominex Original Formula Tablets .... ▣637
TheraFlu Thin Strips Multi Symptom .... ▣684
Triaminic Thin Strips Cough & Runny Nose .... ▣690
Children's Tylenol Plus Cold & Allergy Suspension Liquid 1850
Tylenol Allergy Complete Night Time Caplets 1844
Tylenol Severe Allergy Caplets 1844
Tylenol Flu NightTime Gelcaps 1846
Extra Strength Tylenol PM Caplets, Geltabs, Gelcaps and Liquid 1847
Unisom Maximum Strength SleepGels .... ▣712

Diphenylpyraline Hydrochloride (Potential for increased CNS depression and possible potentiation).
No products indexed under this heading.

Dobutamine Hydrochloride (Procarbazine exhibits some MAO inhibitory activity; concurrent use should be avoided).
No products indexed under this heading.

Dopamine Hydrochloride (Procarbazine exhibits some MAO inhibitory activity; concurrent use should be avoided).
No products indexed under this heading.

Doxazosin Mesylate (To minimize CNS depression and possible potentiation, hypotensive agents should be used with caution).
No products indexed under this heading.

Doxepin Hydrochloride (Procarbazine exhibits some MAO inhibitory activity; concurrent use should be avoided).
No products indexed under this heading.

Enalapril Maleate (To minimize CNS depression and possible potentiation, hypotensive agents should be used with caution). Products include:
Vaseretic Tablets 2073
Vasotec I.V. Injection 2076

Enalaprilat (To minimize CNS depression and possible potentiation, hypotensive agents should be used with caution).
No products indexed under this heading.

Ephedrine Hydrochloride (Procarbazine exhibits some MAO inhibitory activity; concurrent use should be avoided). Products include:
Primatene Tablets .... ▣749

Ephedrine Sulfate (Procarbazine exhibits some MAO inhibitory activity; concurrent use should be avoided).
No products indexed under this heading.

Ephedrine Tannate (Procarbazine exhibits some MAO inhibitory activity; concurrent use should be avoided).
No products indexed under this heading.

Epinephrine (Procarbazine exhibits some MAO inhibitory activity; concurrent use should be avoided). Products include:
EpiPen 1061
Primatene Mist .... ▣749

Epinephrine Bitartrate (Procarbazine exhibits some MAO inhibitory activity; concurrent use should be avoided).
No products indexed under this heading.

Epinephrine Hydrochloride (Procarbazine exhibits some MAO inhibitory activity; concurrent use should be avoided).
No products indexed under this heading.

Eprosartan Mesylate (To minimize CNS depression and possible potentiation, hypotensive agents should be used with caution). Products include:
Teveten Tablets 1707
Teveten HCT Tablets 1710

Esmolol Hydrochloride (To minimize CNS depression and possible potentiation, hypotensive agents should be used with caution). Products include:
Brevibloc Concentrate 766
Brevibloc Injection 766
Brevibloc Double Strength Injection 766
Brevibloc Premixed Injection 766
Brevibloc Double Strength Premixed Injection 766

Felodipine (To minimize CNS depression and possible potentiation, hypotensive agents should be used with caution). Products include:
Plendil Extended-Release Tablets 651

Fentanyl (Potential for increased CNS depression and possible potentiation). Products include:
Duragesic Transdermal System 2448

Fentanyl Citrate (Potential for increased CNS depression and possible potentiation). Products include:
Actiq 993

Fexofenadine Hydrochloride (Potential for increased CNS depression and possible potentiation). Products include:
Allegra 2857
Allegra-D 12 Hour Extended-Release Tablets 2860
Allegra-D 24 Hour Extended-Release Tablets 2862

Fluphenazine Decanoate (Potential for increased CNS depression and possible potentiation).
No products indexed under this heading.

Fluphenazine Enanthate (Potential for increased CNS depression and possible potentiation).
No products indexed under this heading.

Fluphenazine Hydrochloride (Potential for increased CNS depression and possible potentiation).
No products indexed under this heading.

Fosinopril Sodium (To minimize CNS depression and possible potentiation, hypotensive agents should be used with caution).
No products indexed under this heading.

Furosemide (To minimize CNS depression and possible potentiation, hypotensive agents should be used with caution). Products include:
Furosemide Tablets 2117

Guanabenz Acetate (To minimize CNS depression and possible potentiation, hypotensive agents should be used with caution).
No products indexed under this heading.

Guanethidine Monosulfate (To minimize CNS depression and possible potentiation, hypotensive agents should be used with caution).
No products indexed under this heading.

Hydralazine Hydrochloride (To minimize CNS depression and possible potentiation, hypotensive agents should be used with caution). Products include:
BiDil Tablets 2161

Hydrochlorothiazide (To minimize CNS depression and possible potentiation, hypotensive agents should be used with caution). Products include:
Aldoril Tablets 1884
Atacand HCT 637
Avalide Tablets 2889
Avalide Tablets 922
Benicar HCT Tablets 2852
Diovan HCT Tablets 2195
Dyazide Capsules 1389
Hyzaar 1964
Lotensin HCT Tablets 2235
Maxzide 2150
Micardis HCT Tablets 886
Moduretic Tablets 2003
Prinzide Tablets 2033
Teveten HCT Tablets 1710
Timolide Tablets 2056
Uniretic Tablets 3114
Vaseretic Tablets 2073
Zestoretic Tablets 701

Hydrocodone Bitartrate (Potential for increased CNS depression and possible potentiation). Products include:
Hycodan 1104
Hycomine Compound Tablets 1105
Hycotuss Expectorant Syrup 1106
Lortab 3315
Lortab Elixir 3312
Vicodin Tablets 530
Vicodin ES Tablets 531
Vicodin HP Tablets 532
Vicoprofen Tablets 533
Zydone Tablets 1118

Hydrocodone Polistirex (Potential for increased CNS depression and possible potentiation). Products include:
Tussionex Pennkinetic Extended-Release Suspension 3322

Hydroflumethiazide (To minimize CNS depression and possible potentiation, hypotensive agents should be used with caution).
No products indexed under this heading.

Hydromorphone Hydrochloride (Potential for increased CNS depression and possible potentiation). Products include:
Dilaudid 439
Dilaudid Oral Liquid 443
Dilaudid Non-Sterile Powder 439
Dilaudid Rectal Suppositories 439
Dilaudid Tablets 439
Dilaudid Tablets - 8 mg 443
Dilaudid-HP 441

Imipramine Hydrochloride (Procarbazine exhibits some MAO inhibitory activity; concurrent use should be avoided).
No products indexed under this heading.

Imipramine Pamoate (Procarbazine exhibits some MAO inhibitory activity; concurrent use should be avoided).
No products indexed under this heading.

Indapamide (To minimize CNS depression and possible potentiation, hypotensive agents should be used with caution). Products include:
Indapamide Tablets 2119

Irbesartan (To minimize CNS depression and possible potentiation, hypotensive agents should be used with caution). Products include:
Avalide Tablets 922
Avalide Tablets 2889
Avapro Tablets 925
Avapro Tablets 2886

Isoproterenol Hydrochloride (Procarbazine exhibits some MAO inhibitory activity; concurrent use should be avoided).
No products indexed under this heading.

Isoproterenol Sulfate (Procarbazine exhibits some MAO inhibitory activity; concurrent use should be avoided).
No products indexed under this heading.

Isradipine (To minimize CNS depression and possible potentiation, hypotensive agents should be used with caution). Products include:
DynaCirc CR Tablets 2726

Labetalol Hydrochloride (To minimize CNS depression and possible potentiation, hypotensive agents should be used with caution).
No products indexed under this heading.

Levalbuterol Hydrochloride (Procarbazine exhibits some MAO inhibitory activity; concurrent use should be avoided). Products include:
Xopenex Inhalation Solution 3143
Xopenex Inhalation Solution Concentrate 3147

Levorphanol Tartrate (Potential for increased CNS depression and possible potentiation).
No products indexed under this heading.

Lisinopril (To minimize CNS depression and possible potentiation, hypotensive agents should be used with caution). Products include:
Prinivil Tablets 2029
Prinzide Tablets 2033
Zestoretic Tablets 701
Zestril Tablets 704

Loratadine (Potential for increased CNS depression and possible potentiation). Products include:
Alavert Allergy & Sinus D-12 Hour Tablets .... ▣743
Alavert .... ▣743
Children's Claritin 24 Hour Non-Drowsy Allergy Syrup .... ▣732

Claritin Non-Drowsy 24 Hour Tablets ... 731
Non-Drowsy Claritin Hives Relief Tablets ... 733
Claritin Reditabs 24 Hour Non-Drowsy Tablets ... 732
Claritin-D Non-Drowsy 12 Hour Tablets ... 731
Claritin-D Non-Drowsy 24 Hour Tablets ... 731
Children's Dimetapp ND Non-Drowsy Allergy Syrup ... 746
Triaminic Allerchews ... 684

Losartan Potassium (To minimize CNS depression and possible potentiation, hypotensive agents should be used with caution). Products include:
Cozaar Tablets ... 1913
Hyzaar ... 1964

Maprotiline Hydrochloride (Procarbazine exhibits some MAO inhibitory activity; concurrent use should be avoided).
No products indexed under this heading.

Mecamylamine Hydrochloride (To minimize CNS depression and possible potentiation, hypotensive agents should be used with caution). Products include:
Inversine Tablets ... 3286

Meperidine Hydrochloride (Potential for increased CNS depression and possible potentiation).
No products indexed under this heading.

Mephobarbital (Potential for increased CNS depression and possible potentiation). Products include:
Mebaral Tablets, USP ... 2483

Mesoridazine Besylate (Potential for increased CNS depression and possible potentiation).
No products indexed under this heading.

Metaproterenol Sulfate (Procarbazine exhibits some MAO inhibitory activity; concurrent use should be avoided). Products include:
Alupent Inhalation Aerosol ... 858

Metaraminol Bitartrate (Procarbazine exhibits some MAO inhibitory activity; concurrent use should be avoided). Products include:
Aramine Injection ... 1889

Methadone Hydrochloride (Potential for increased CNS depression and possible potentiation).
No products indexed under this heading.

Methdilazine Hydrochloride (Potential for increased CNS depression and possible potentiation).
No products indexed under this heading.

Methotrimeprazine (Potential for increased CNS depression and possible potentiation).
No products indexed under this heading.

Methoxamine Hydrochloride (Procarbazine exhibits some MAO inhibitory activity; concurrent use should be avoided).
No products indexed under this heading.

Methyclothiazide (To minimize CNS depression and possible potentiation, hypotensive agents should be used with caution).
No products indexed under this heading.

Methyldopa (To minimize CNS depression and possible potentiation, hypotensive agents should be used with caution). Products include:
Aldoclor Tablets ... 1881
Aldoril Tablets ... 1884

Methyldopate Hydrochloride (To minimize CNS depression and possible potentiation, hypotensive agents should be used with caution).
No products indexed under this heading.

Metolazone (To minimize CNS depression and possible potentiation, hypotensive agents should be used with caution).
No products indexed under this heading.

Metoprolol Succinate (To minimize CNS depression and possible potentiation, hypotensive agents should be used with caution). Products include:
Toprol-XL Tablets ... 660

Metoprolol Tartrate (To minimize CNS depression and possible potentiation, hypotensive agents should be used with caution).
No products indexed under this heading.

Metyrosine (To minimize CNS depression and possible potentiation, hypotensive agents should be used with caution). Products include:
Demser Capsules ... 1933

Mibefradil Dihydrochloride (To minimize CNS depression and possible potentiation, hypotensive agents should be used with caution).
No products indexed under this heading.

Minoxidil (To minimize CNS depression and possible potentiation, hypotensive agents should be used with caution). Products include:
Men's Rogaine Extra Strength Topical Solution, Ocean Rush Scent and Original Unscented ... 706
Women's Rogaine Topical Solution, Spring Bloom Scent and Original Unscented ... 707

Moexipril Hydrochloride (To minimize CNS depression and possible potentiation, hypotensive agents should be used with caution). Products include:
Uniretic Tablets ... 3114
Univasc Tablets ... 3118

Morphine Sulfate (Potential for increased CNS depression and possible potentiation). Products include:
Avinza Capsules ... 1714
Kadian Capsules ... 572
MS Contin Tablets ... 2703

Nadolol (To minimize CNS depression and possible potentiation, hypotensive agents should be used with caution). Products include:
Nadolol Tablets ... 2121

Nicardipine Hydrochloride (To minimize CNS depression and possible potentiation, hypotensive agents should be used with caution). Products include:
Cardene I.V. ... 1129

Nifedipine (To minimize CNS depression and possible potentiation, hypotensive agents should be used with caution). Products include:
Adalat CC Tablets ... 2978

Nisoldipine (To minimize CNS depression and possible potentiation, hypotensive agents should be used with caution). Products include:
Sular Tablets ... 1163

Nitroglycerin (To minimize CNS depression and possible potentiation, hypotensive agents should be used with caution). Products include:
Nitro-Dur Transdermal Infusion System ... 3060
Nitrolingual Pumpspray ... 1161

Norepinephrine Bitartrate (Procarbazine exhibits some MAO inhibitory activity; concurrent use should be avoided).
No products indexed under this heading.

Nortriptyline Hydrochloride (Procarbazine exhibits some MAO inhibitory activity; concurrent use should be avoided).
No products indexed under this heading.

Oxycodone Hydrochloride (Potential for increased CNS depression and possible potentiation). Products include:
Combunox Tablets ... 1183
OxyContin Tablets ... 2699
OxyFast Oral Concentrate Solution ... 2704
OxyIR Capsules ... 2704
Percocet Tablets ... 1114
Percodan Tablets ... 1115

Penbutolol Sulfate (To minimize CNS depression and possible potentiation, hypotensive agents should be used with caution).
No products indexed under this heading.

Pentobarbital Sodium (Potential for increased CNS depression and possible potentiation). Products include:
Nembutal Sodium Solution, USP ... 2484

Perindopril Erbumine (To minimize CNS depression and possible potentiation, hypotensive agents should be used with caution). Products include:
Aceon Tablets (2 mg, 4 mg, 8 mg) ... 3191

Perphenazine (Potential for increased CNS depression and possible potentiation).
No products indexed under this heading.

Phenobarbital (Potential for increased CNS depression and possible potentiation).
No products indexed under this heading.

Phenoxybenzamine Hydrochloride (To minimize CNS depression and possible potentiation, hypotensive agents should be used with caution). Products include:
Dibenzyline Capsules ... 3390

Phentolamine Mesylate (To minimize CNS depression and possible potentiation, hypotensive agents should be used with caution).
No products indexed under this heading.

Phenylephrine Bitartrate (Procarbazine exhibits some MAO inhibitory activity; concurrent use should be avoided).
No products indexed under this heading.

Phenylephrine Hydrochloride (Procarbazine exhibits some MAO inhibitory activity; concurrent use should be avoided). Products include:
Alacol DM Syrup ... 739
Hycomine Compound Tablets ... 1105
Preparation H Maximum Strength Cream ... 747
Preparation H Cooling Gel ... 747
Preparation H ... 747
Sudafed PE Tablets ... 711
Vicks Sinex Nasal Spray and Ultra Fine Mist for Sinus Relief ... 2677
Zicam Concentrated Cough Mist for Kids Plus D Cool Cherry ... 643
Zicam Concentrated Cough Mist Plus D Cool Cherry ... 642

Phenylephrine Tannate (Procarbazine exhibits some MAO inhibitory activity; concurrent use should be avoided).
No products indexed under this heading.

Phenylpropanolamine Hydrochloride (Procarbazine exhibits some MAO inhibitory activity; concurrent use should be avoided).
No products indexed under this heading.

Pindolol (To minimize CNS depression and possible potentiation, hypotensive agents should be used with caution).
No products indexed under this heading.

Pirbuterol Acetate (Procarbazine exhibits some MAO inhibitory activity; concurrent use should be avoided). Products include:
Maxair Autohaler ... 1820

Polythiazide (To minimize CNS depression and possible potentiation, hypotensive agents should be used with caution).
No products indexed under this heading.

Prazosin Hydrochloride (To minimize CNS depression and possible potentiation, hypotensive agents should be used with caution).
No products indexed under this heading.

Prochlorperazine (Potential for increased CNS depression and possible potentiation).
No products indexed under this heading.

Promethazine Hydrochloride (Potential for increased CNS depression and possible potentiation). Products include:
Phenergan ... 3438

Propoxyphene Hydrochloride (Potential for increased CNS depression and possible potentiation).
No products indexed under this heading.

Propoxyphene Napsylate (Potential for increased CNS depression and possible potentiation). Products include:
Darvocet A 500 Tablets ... 3497

Propranolol Hydrochloride (To minimize CNS depression and possible potentiation, hypotensive agents should be used with caution). Products include:
Inderal LA Long-Acting Capsules ... 3421
InnoPran XL Capsules ... 2728

Protriptyline Hydrochloride (Procarbazine exhibits some MAO inhibitory activity; concurrent use should be avoided). Products include:
Vivactil Tablets ... 2350

Pseudoephedrine Hydrochloride (Procarbazine exhibits some MAO inhibitory activity; concurrent use should be avoided). Products include:
Advil Allergy Sinus Caplets ... 737
Advil Cold & Sinus ... 739
Advil Flu & Body Ache Caplets ... 739
Children's Advil Cold Suspension ... 741
Advil Multi-Symptom Cold Caplets ... 738
Allegra-D 12 Hour Extended-Release Tablets ... 2860
Allegra-D 24 Hour Extended-Release Tablets ... 2862
Balamine DM ... 739
BC Cold Powder ... 612
Benadryl Allergy & Cold Tablets ... 692
Benadryl Allergy & Sinus Headache Caplets & Gelcaps ... 693

Children's Benadryl Allergy & Cold Fastmelt Tablets ■ 695
Benadryl Maximum Strength Severe Allergy & Sinus Headache Caplets ■ 694
Children's Benadryl D Allergy & Sinus Fastmelt Tablets ■ 694
Children's Benadryl D Liquid Medication ■ 693
Benadryl D Tablets ■ 694
Contac Non-Drowsy 12 Hour Cold Caplets ■ 614
Contac Non-Drowsy Timed Release 12 Hour Cold Caplets ■ 615
Contac Severe Cold and Flu Caplets Maximum Strength ■ 615
Contac Severe Cold and Flu Caplets Non-Drowsy ■ 615
Children's Dimetapp Cold & Allergy Elixir ■ 745
Children's Dimetapp DM Cold & Cough Elixir ■ 745
Children's Dimetapp Long Acting Cough Plus Cold Syrup ■ 746
Dimetapp Infant Drops Decongestant Plus Cough ■ 746
Children's Motrin Cold Non-Staining Dye-Free Oral Suspension 1838
Children's Motrin Cold Oral Suspension 1838
Motrin Cold & Sinus Caplets 1836
PediaCare Decongestant & Cough Infant Drops ■ 705
PediaCare Decongestant Infants' Drops ■ 705
PediaCare Long-Acting Cough Plus Cold Liquid ■ 704
PediaCare Multi-Symptom Cold Liquid ■ 704
PediaCare NightRest Cough & Cold Liquid ■ 704
Robitussin Allergy & Cough Syrup ■ 750
Robitussin CF Liquid ■ 755
Robitussin Cough & Cold Liquid-filled Capsules ■ 750
Robitussin Cough, Cold & Flu Liquid-filled Capsules ■ 750
Robitussin Cough & Cold Infant Drops ■ 755
Robitussin Flu Liquid ■ 752
Robitussin Maximum Strength Cough & Cold Liquid ■ 754
Robitussin PE Syrup ■ 753
Robitussin Pediatric Cough & Cold Liquid ■ 754
Robitussin PM Cough & Cold Liquid ■ 752
Robitussin Severe Congestion Liquid-filled Capsules ■ 751
Simply Stuffy Liquid 1841
Singlet Caplets ■ 636
Sudafed 12 Hour Caplets ■ 708
Sudafed 24 Hour Tablets ■ 709
Sudafed Nasal Decongestant Tablets ■ 709
Sudafed Severe Cold ■ 710
Sudafed Non-Drying Sinus Liquid Caps ■ 709
Sudafed Sinus & Allergy Tablets ■ 710
Sudafed Sinus Headache ■ 711
TheraFlu Cold & Cough Hot Liquid ■ 680
TheraFlu Cold & Sore Throat Hot Liquid ■ 680
TheraFlu Flu & Chest Congestion Non-Drowsy Hot Liquid ■ 681
TheraFlu Flu & Sore Throat Hot Liquid ■ 681
TheraFlu Severe Cold Non-Drowsy Hot Liquid ■ 683
TheraFlu Severe Cold & Cough Hot Liquid ■ 683
TheraFlu Severe Cold Caplets ■ 679
TheraFlu Severe Cold Hot Liquid ■ 682
TheraFlu Severe Cold Non-Drowsy Caplets ■ 679
Triaminic Chest & Nasal Congestion Liquid ■ 685
Triaminic Cold & Allergy Liquid ■ 685
Triaminic Cold & Cough Liquid ■ 685
Triaminic Cough Liquid ■ 687
Triaminic Cough & Nasal Congestion Liquid ■ 687
Triaminic Cough & Sore Throat Liquid ■ 687
Triaminic Flu, Cough & Fever Liquid ■ 685
Triaminic Night Time Cough & Cold Liquid ■ 685
Triaminic Allergy Runny Nose & Congestion Softchews ■ 688
Triaminic Cold & Cough Softchews ■ 688
Triaminic Cough & Sore Throat Softchews ■ 689
Tylenol Sinus NightTime Caplets ■ 663
Children's Tylenol Plus Cold & Allergy Suspension Liquid 1850
Children's Tylenol Plus Cold NightTime Suspension Liquid 1851
Children's Tylenol Plus Cold & Cough Suspension Liquid and Chewable Tablets 1851
Children's Tylenol Plus Cold Chewable Tablets 1851
Children's Tylenol Plus Cold Daytime Non-Drowsy Suspension Liquid 1851
Children's Tylenol Plus Flu Suspension Liquid 1853
Concentrated Tylenol Infants' Drops Plus Cold 1851
Concentrated Tylenol Infants' Drops Plus Cold and Cough 1851
Tylenol Cold & Flu Severe Daytime Liquid with Cool Burst 1846
Tylenol Cold & Flu Severe NightTime Liquid with Cool Burst 1846
Tylenol Cold Severe Congestion Non-Drowsy Caplets with Cool Burst 1846
Tylenol Allergy Complete Night Time Caplets 1844
Tylenol Allergy Complete Multi-Symptom Caplets and Gelcaps with Cool Burst 1844
Tylenol Flu NightTime Gelcaps 1846
Tylenol Flu Day Non-Drowsy Gelcaps 1846
Concentrated Tylenol Infants' Drops Plus Cold Nasal Congestant, Fever Reducer & Pain Reliever ■ 668
Concentrated Tylenol Infants' Drops Plus Cold & Cough Nasal Decongestant, Fever Reducer & Pain Reliever ■ 668
Multi-Symptom Tylenol Cold Night Time Caplets 1845
Multi-Symptom Tylenol Cold Day Non-Drowsy Caplets and Gelcaps 1845
Tylenol Sinus Day Non-Drowsy 1848
Tylenol Sinus Night Time Caplets 1848
Tylenol Sinus Severe Congestion Caplets with Cool Burst 1848
Vicks 44D Cough & Head Congestion Relief 2676
Vicks 44D Cough & Head Congestion Relief Liquid ■ 721
Vicks 44M Cough, Cold & Flu Relief 2676
Pediatric Vicks 44m Cough & Cold Relief 2673
Vicks DayQuil LiquiCaps/Liquid Multi-Symptom Cold/Flu Relief ■ 723
Vicks DayQuil Multi-Symptom Cold/Flu Relief LiquiCaps 2675
Vicks DayQuil Multi-Symptom Cold/Flu Relief Liquid 2675
Children's Vicks NyQuil Cold/Cough Relief 2671
Vicks NyQuil LiquiCaps 2677
Vicks NyQuil LiquiCaps/Liquid Multi-Symptom Cold/Flu Relief ■ 725
Vicks NyQuil Liquid 2677
Zyrtec-D 12 Hour Extended Release Tablets 2591

Pseudoephedrine Sulfate (Procarbazine exhibits some MAO inhibitory activity; concurrent use should be avoided). Products include:
Alavert Allergy & Sinus D-12 Hour Tablets ■ 743
Clarinex-D 24-Hour Extended-Release Tablets 3012
Claritin-D Non-Drowsy 12 Hour Tablets ■ 731
Claritin-D Non-Drowsy 24 Hour Tablets ■ 731

Pyrilamine Maleate (Potential for increased CNS depression and possible potentiation).
No products indexed under this heading.

Pyrilamine Tannate (Potential for increased CNS depression and possible potentiation).
No products indexed under this heading.

Quinapril Hydrochloride (To minimize CNS depression and possible potentiation, hypotensive agents should be used with caution).
No products indexed under this heading.

Ramipril (To minimize CNS depression and possible potentiation, hypotensive agents should be used with caution). Products include:
Altace Capsules 1673

Rauwolfia Serpentina (To minimize CNS depression and possible potentiation, hypotensive agents should be used with caution).
No products indexed under this heading.

Remifentanil Hydrochloride (Potential for increased CNS depression and possible potentiation).
No products indexed under this heading.

Rescinnamine (To minimize CNS depression and possible potentiation, hypotensive agents should be used with caution).
No products indexed under this heading.

Reserpine (To minimize CNS depression and possible potentiation, hypotensive agents should be used with caution).
No products indexed under this heading.

Salmeterol Xinafoate (Procarbazine exhibits some MAO inhibitory activity; concurrent use should be avoided). Products include:
Advair Diskus 100/50 1291
Advair Diskus 250/50 1291
Advair Diskus 500/50 1291
Serevent Diskus 1540

Secobarbital Sodium (Potential for increased CNS depression and possible potentiation).
No products indexed under this heading.

Sodium Nitroprusside (To minimize CNS depression and possible potentiation, hypotensive agents should be used with caution).
No products indexed under this heading.

Sotalol Hydrochloride (To minimize CNS depression and possible potentiation, hypotensive agents should be used with caution).
No products indexed under this heading.

Spirapril Hydrochloride (To minimize CNS depression and possible potentiation, hypotensive agents should be used with caution).
No products indexed under this heading.

Sufentanil Citrate (Potential for increased CNS depression and possible potentiation).
No products indexed under this heading.

Telmisartan (To minimize CNS depression and possible potentiation, hypotensive agents should be used with caution). Products include:
Micardis Tablets 884
Micardis HCT Tablets 886

Terazosin Hydrochloride (To minimize CNS depression and possible potentiation, hypotensive agents should be used with caution).
Products include:
Hytrin Capsules 469

Terbutaline Sulfate (Procarbazine exhibits some MAO inhibitory activity; concurrent use should be avoided).
No products indexed under this heading.

Terfenadine (Potential for increased CNS depression and possible potentiation).
No products indexed under this heading.

Thiamylal Sodium (Potential for increased CNS depression and possible potentiation).
No products indexed under this heading.

Thioridazine Hydrochloride (Potential for increased CNS depression and possible potentiation).
Products include:
Thioridazine Hydrochloride Tablets 2122

Timolol Maleate (To minimize CNS depression and possible potentiation, hypotensive agents should be used with caution). Products include:
Blocadren Tablets 1891
Cosopt Sterile Ophthalmic Solution 1910
Timolide Tablets 2056
Timoptic in Ocudose 2061
Timoptic Sterile Ophthalmic Solution 2058
Timoptic-XE Sterile Ophthalmic Gel Forming Solution 2062

Torsemide (To minimize CNS depression and possible potentiation, hypotensive agents should be used with caution).
No products indexed under this heading.

Trandolapril (To minimize CNS depression and possible potentiation, hypotensive agents should be used with caution). Products include:
Mavik Tablets 482
Tarka Tablets 519

Trifluoperazine Hydrochloride (Potential for increased CNS depression and possible potentiation).
No products indexed under this heading.

Trimeprazine Tartrate (Potential for increased CNS depression and possible potentiation).
No products indexed under this heading.

Trimethaphan Camsylate (To minimize CNS depression and possible potentiation, hypotensive agents should be used with caution).
No products indexed under this heading.

Trimipramine Maleate (Procarbazine exhibits some MAO inhibitory activity; concurrent use should be avoided). Products include:
Surmontil Capsules 2347

Tripelennamine Hydrochloride (Potential for increased CNS depression and possible potentiation).
No products indexed under this heading.

Triprolidine Hydrochloride (Potential for increased CNS depression and possible potentiation).
No products indexed under this heading.

Valsartan (To minimize CNS depression and possible potentiation, hypotensive agents should be used with caution). Products include:

- Diovan HCT Tablets ... 2195
- Diovan Tablets ... 2191

Verapamil Hydrochloride (To minimize CNS depression and possible potentiation, hypotensive agents should be used with caution). Products include:

- Covera-HS Tablets ... 3135
- Tarka Tablets ... 519
- Verelan PM Capsules ... 3120

Food Interactions

Alcohol (Concurrent use may produce an Antabuse-like reaction; concomitant use should be avoided).

Bananas (Procarbazine exhibits some MAO inhibitory activity: concurrent use should be avoided).

Cheese, aged (Procarbazine exhibits some MAO inhibitory activity: concurrent use should be avoided).

Food with high concentration of tyramine (Procarbazine exhibits some MAO inhibitory activity: concurrent use should be avoided).

Wine, unspecified (Procarbazine exhibits some MAO inhibitory activity: concurrent use should be avoided).

Yogurt (Procarbazine exhibits some MAO inhibitory activity: concurrent use should be avoided).

MAVIK TABLETS

(Trandolapril) ... 482

May interact with diuretics, lithium preparations, potassium preparations, potassium sparing diuretics, and certain other agents. Compounds in these categories include:

Amiloride Hydrochloride (Co-administration increases the risk of hyperkalemia; patients on diuretics, especially those on recently instituted diuretic therapy, may experience an excessive reduction in blood pressure after initiation of therapy with trandolapril). Products include:

- Midamor Tablets ... 2000
- Moduretic Tablets ... 2003

Bendroflumethiazide (Patients on diuretics, especially those on recently instituted diuretic therapy, may experience an excessive reduction in blood pressure after initiation of therapy with trandolapril).

No products indexed under this heading.

Bumetanide (Patients on diuretics, especially those on recently instituted diuretic therapy, may experience an excessive reduction in blood pressure after initiation of therapy with trandolapril).

No products indexed under this heading.

Chlorothiazide (Patients on diuretics, especially those on recently instituted diuretic therapy, may experience an excessive reduction in blood pressure after initiation of therapy with trandolapril). Products include:

- Aldoclor Tablets ... 1881
- Diuril Oral ... 1936

Chlorothiazide Sodium (Patients on diuretics, especially those on recently instituted diuretic therapy, may experience an excessive reduction in blood pressure after initiation of therapy with trandolapril). Products include:

- Diuril Sodium Intravenous ... 1934

Chlorthalidone (Patients on diuretics, especially those on recently instituted diuretic therapy, may experience an excessive reduction in blood pressure after initiation of therapy with trandolapril). Products include:

- Clorpres Tablets ... 2139

Cimetidine (Co-administration has led to an increase of about 44% in Cmax for trandolapril with no effect on ACE inhibition). Products include:

- Tagamet HB 200 Tablets ... 637
- Tagamet Tablets ... 1547

Cimetidine Hydrochloride (Co-administration has led to an increase of about 44% in Cmax for trandolapril with no effect on ACE inhibition).

No products indexed under this heading.

Ethacrynic Acid (Patients on diuretics, especially those on recently instituted diuretic therapy, may experience an excessive reduction in blood pressure after initiation of therapy with trandolapril). Products include:

- Edecrin Tablets ... 1941

Furosemide (Co-administration has led to an increase of about 25% in the renal clearance of trandolapril with no effect on ACE inhibition; patients on diuretics, especially those on recently instituted diuretic therapy, may experience an excessive reduction in blood pressure after initiation of therapy with trandolapril). Products include:

- Furosemide Tablets ... 2117

Hydrochlorothiazide (Patients on diuretics, especially those on recently instituted diuretic therapy, may experience an excessive reduction in blood pressure after initiation of therapy with trandolapril). Products include:

- Aldoril Tablets ... 1884
- Atacand HCT ... 637
- Avalide Tablets ... 2889
- Avalide Tablets ... 922
- Benicar HCT Tablets ... 2852
- Diovan HCT Tablets ... 2195
- Dyazide Capsules ... 1389
- Hyzaar ... 1964
- Lotensin HCT Tablets ... 2235
- Maxzide ... 2150
- Micardis HCT Tablets ... 886
- Moduretic Tablets ... 2003
- Prinzide Tablets ... 2033
- Teveten HCT Tablets ... 1710
- Timolide Tablets ... 2056
- Uniretic Tablets ... 3114
- Vaseretic Tablets ... 2073
- Zestoretic Tablets ... 701

Hydroflumethiazide (Patients on diuretics, especially those on recently instituted diuretic therapy, may experience an excessive reduction in blood pressure after initiation of therapy with trandolapril).

No products indexed under this heading.

Indapamide (Patients on diuretics, especially those on recently instituted diuretic therapy, may experience an excessive reduction in blood pressure after initiation of therapy with trandolapril). Products include:

- Indapamide Tablets ... 2119

Lithium (Co-administration of ACE inhibitors and lithium has resulted in increased serum lithium levels and symptoms of lithium toxicity).

No products indexed under this heading.

Lithium Carbonate (Co-administration of ACE inhibitors and lithium has resulted in increased serum lithium levels and symptoms of lithium toxicity). Products include:

- Eskalith ... 1406
- Lithobid Tablets ... 1670

Lithium Citrate (Co-administration of ACE inhibitors and lithium has resulted in increased serum lithium levels and symptoms of lithium toxicity).

No products indexed under this heading.

Methyclothiazide (Patients on diuretics, especially those on recently instituted diuretic therapy, may experience an excessive reduction in blood pressure after initiation of therapy with trandolapril).

No products indexed under this heading.

Metolazone (Patients on diuretics, especially those on recently instituted diuretic therapy, may experience an excessive reduction in blood pressure after initiation of therapy with trandolapril).

No products indexed under this heading.

Polythiazide (Patients on diuretics, especially those on recently instituted diuretic therapy, may experience an excessive reduction in blood pressure after initiation of therapy with trandolapril).

No products indexed under this heading.

Potassium Acid Phosphate (Co-administration increases the risk of hyperkalemia). Products include:

- K-Phos Original (Sodium Free) Tablets ... 785

Potassium Bicarbonate (Co-administration increases the risk of hyperkalemia).

No products indexed under this heading.

Potassium Chloride (Co-administration increases the risk of hyperkalemia). Products include:

- Colyte with Flavor Packs for Oral Solution ... 3102
- HalfLytely and Bisacodyl Tablets Bowel Prep Kit with Flavors Packs ... 915
- K-Dur Extended-Relase Tablets ... 3047
- K-Lor Powder Packets ... 472
- K-Tab Filmtab Tablets ... 473
- TriLyte with Flavor Packs for Oral Solution ... 3114

Potassium Citrate (Co-administration increases the risk of hyperkalemia). Products include:

- Urocit-K Tablets ... 2109

Potassium Gluconate (Co-administration increases the risk of hyperkalemia).

No products indexed under this heading.

Potassium Phosphate (Co-administration increases the risk of hyperkalemia). Products include:

- K-Phos Neutral Tablets ... 785

Spironolactone (Co-administration increases the risk of hyperkalemia; patients on diuretics, especially those on recently instituted diuretic therapy, may experience an excessive reduction in blood pressure after initiation of therapy with trandolapril).

No products indexed under this heading.

Torsemide (Patients on diuretics, especially those on recently instituted diuretic therapy, may experience an excessive reduction in blood pressure after initiation of therapy with trandolapril).

No products indexed under this heading.

Triamterene (Co-administration increases the risk of hyperkalemia; patients on diuretics, especially those on recently instituted diuretic therapy, may experience an excessive reduction in blood pressure after initiation of therapy with trandolapril). Products include:

- Dyazide Capsules ... 1389
- Dyrenium Capsules ... 3390
- Maxzide ... 2150

Food Interactions

Food, unspecified (Slows absorption of trandolapril but does not affect AUC or Cmax).

MAXAIR AUTOHALER

(Pirbuterol Acetate) ... 1820

May interact with beta blockers, monoamine oxidase inhibitors, potassium-depleting diuretics, sympathomimetic aerosol bronchodilators, and tricyclic antidepressants. Compounds in these categories include:

Acebutolol Hydrochloride (Co-administration with beta adrenergic receptor blocking agents blocks the pulmonary effect of pirbuterol and may produce severe bronchospasm in asthmatic patients).

No products indexed under this heading.

Albuterol (Potential for additive effects). Products include:

- Proventil Inhalation Aerosol ... 3067

Amitriptyline Hydrochloride (Concurrent and/or sequential use with tricyclic antidepressants can result in the potentiation of pirbuterol's action on the vascular system).

No products indexed under this heading.

Amoxapine (Concurrent and/or sequential use with tricyclic antidepressants can result in the potentiation of pirbuterol's action on the vascular system).

No products indexed under this heading.

Atenolol (Co-administration with beta adrenergic receptor blocking agents blocks the pulmonary effect of pirbuterol and may produce severe bronchospasm in asthmatic patients). Products include:

- Tenormin I.V. Injection ... 698
- Tenormin Tablets ... 695

Bendroflumethiazide (The ECG changes and/or hypokalemia that may result from administration of non-potassium sparing diuretics can be acutely worsened by beta-agonists; clinical significance is not known).

No products indexed under this heading.

Betaxolol Hydrochloride (Co-administration with beta adrenergic receptor blocking agents blocks the pulmonary effect of pirbuterol and may produce severe bronchospasm in asthmatic patients). Products include:

- Betoptic S Ophthalmic Suspension ... 554

IMPORTANT NOTE: Always consult each drug listing in the patient's regimen for possible interactions.

Bisoprolol Fumarate (Co-administration with beta adrenergic receptor blocking agents blocks the pulmonary effect of pirbuterol and may produce severe bronchospasm in asthmatic patients).
No products indexed under this heading.

Bitolterol Mesylate (Potential for additive effects).
No products indexed under this heading.

Bumetanide (The ECG changes and/or hypokalemia that may result from administration of non-potassium sparing diuretics can be acutely worsened by beta-agonists; clinical significance is not known).
No products indexed under this heading.

Carteolol Hydrochloride (Co-administration with beta adrenergic receptor blocking agents blocks the pulmonary effect of pirbuterol and may produce severe bronchospasm in asthmatic patients). Products include:
Carteolol Hydrochloride Ophthalmic Solution USP, 1%....... ⊙246

Chlorothiazide (The ECG changes and/or hypokalemia that may result from administration of non-potassium sparing diuretics can be acutely worsened by beta-agonists; clinical significance is not known). Products include:
Aldoclor Tablets 1881
Diuril Oral 1936

Chlorothiazide Sodium (The ECG changes and/or hypokalemia that may result from administration of non-potassium sparing diuretics can be acutely worsened by beta-agonists; clinical significance is not known). Products include:
Diuril Sodium Intravenous 1934

Clomipramine Hydrochloride (Concurrent and/or sequential use with tricyclic antidepressants can result in the potentiation of pirbuterol's action on the vascular system).
No products indexed under this heading.

Desipramine Hydrochloride (Concurrent and/or sequential use with tricyclic antidepressants can result in the potentiation of pirbuterol's action on the vascular system).
No products indexed under this heading.

Doxepin Hydrochloride (Concurrent and/or sequential use with tricyclic antidepressants can result in the potentiation of pirbuterol's action on the vascular system).
No products indexed under this heading.

Esmolol Hydrochloride (Co-administration with beta adrenergic receptor blocking agents blocks the pulmonary effect of pirbuterol and may produce severe bronchospasm in asthmatic patients). Products include:
Brevibloc Concentrate 766
Brevibloc Injection 766
Brevibloc Double Strength Injection..................... 766
Brevibloc Premixed Injection 766
Brevibloc Double Strength Premixed Injection 766

Ethacrynic Acid (The ECG changes and/or hypokalemia that may result from administration of non-potassium sparing diuretics can be acutely worsened by beta-agonists; clinical significance is not known). Products include:
Edecrin Tablets 1941

Furosemide (The ECG changes and/or hypokalemia that may result from administration of non-potassium sparing diuretics can be acutely worsened by beta-agonists; clinical significance is not known). Products include:
Furosemide Tablets 2117

Hydrochlorothiazide (The ECG changes and/or hypokalemia that may result from administration of non-potassium sparing diuretics can be acutely worsened by beta-agonists; clinical significance is not known). Products include:
Aldoril Tablets 1884
Atacand HCT 637
Avalide Tablets 2889
Avalide Tablets 922
Benicar HCT Tablets 2852
Diovan HCT Tablets 2195
Dyazide Capsules 1389
Hyzaar 1964
Lotensin HCT Tablets 2235
Maxzide 2150
Micardis HCT Tablets 886
Moduretic Tablets 2003
Prinzide Tablets 2033
Teveten HCT Tablets 1710
Timolide Tablets 2056
Uniretic Tablets 3114
Vaseretic Tablets 2073
Zestoretic Tablets 701

Hydroflumethiazide (The ECG changes and/or hypokalemia that may result from administration of non-potassium sparing diuretics can be acutely worsened by beta-agonists; clinical significance is not known).
No products indexed under this heading.

Imipramine Hydrochloride (Concurrent and/or sequential use with tricyclic antidepressants can result in the potentiation of pirbuterol's action on the vascular system).
No products indexed under this heading.

Imipramine Pamoate (Concurrent and/or sequential use with tricyclic antidepressants can result in the potentiation of pirbuterol's action on the vascular system).
No products indexed under this heading.

Isocarboxazid (Concurrent and/or sequential use with MAO inhibitors can result in the potentiation of pirbuterol's action on the vascular system).
No products indexed under this heading.

Isoetharine (Potential for additive effects).
No products indexed under this heading.

Isoproterenol Hydrochloride (Potential for additive effects).
No products indexed under this heading.

Labetalol Hydrochloride (Co-administration with beta adrenergic receptor blocking agents blocks the pulmonary effect of pirbuterol and may produce severe bronchospasm in asthmatic patients).
No products indexed under this heading.

Levalbuterol Hydrochloride (Potential for additive effects). Products include:
Xopenex Inhalation Solution 3143
Xopenex Inhalation Solution Concentrate 3147

Levobunolol Hydrochloride (Co-administration with beta adrenergic receptor blocking agents blocks the pulmonary effect of pirbuterol and may produce severe bronchospasm in asthmatic patients). Products include:
Betagan Ophthalmic Solution, USP..................... ⊙217

Maprotiline Hydrochloride (Concurrent and/or sequential use with tricyclic antidepressants can result in the potentiation of pirbuterol's action on the vascular system).
No products indexed under this heading.

Metaproterenol Sulfate (Potential for additive effects). Products include:
Alupent Inhalation Aerosol 858

Methyclothiazide (The ECG changes and/or hypokalemia that may result from administration of non-potassium sparing diuretics can be acutely worsened by beta-agonists; clinical significance is not known).
No products indexed under this heading.

Metipranolol Hydrochloride (Co-administration with beta adrenergic receptor blocking agents blocks the pulmonary effect of pirbuterol and may produce severe bronchospasm in asthmatic patients).
No products indexed under this heading.

Metoprolol Succinate (Co-administration with beta adrenergic receptor blocking agents blocks the pulmonary effect of pirbuterol and may produce severe bronchospasm in asthmatic patients). Products include:
Toprol-XL Tablets 660

Metoprolol Tartrate (Co-administration with beta adrenergic receptor blocking agents blocks the pulmonary effect of pirbuterol and may produce severe bronchospasm in asthmatic patients).
No products indexed under this heading.

Moclobemide (Concurrent and/or sequential use with MAO inhibitors can result in the potentiation of pirbuterol's action on the vascular system).
No products indexed under this heading.

Nadolol (Co-administration with beta adrenergic receptor blocking agents blocks the pulmonary effect of pirbuterol and may produce severe bronchospasm in asthmatic patients). Products include:
Nadolol Tablets 2121

Nortriptyline Hydrochloride (Concurrent and/or sequential use with tricyclic antidepressants can result in the potentiation of pirbuterol's action on the vascular system).
No products indexed under this heading.

Pargyline Hydrochloride (Concurrent and/or sequential use with MAO inhibitors can result in the potentiation of pirbuterol's action on the vascular system).
No products indexed under this heading.

Penbutolol Sulfate (Co-administration with beta adrenergic receptor blocking agents blocks the pulmonary effect of pirbuterol and may produce severe bronchospasm in asthmatic patients).
No products indexed under this heading.

Phenelzine Sulfate (Concurrent and/or sequential use with MAO inhibitors can result in the potentiation of pirbuterol's action on the vascular system).
No products indexed under this heading.

Pindolol (Co-administration with beta adrenergic receptor blocking agents blocks the pulmonary effect of pirbuterol and may produce severe bronchospasm in asthmatic patients).
No products indexed under this heading.

Polythiazide (The ECG changes and/or hypokalemia that may result from administration of non-potassium sparing diuretics can be acutely worsened by beta-agonists; clinical significance is not known).
No products indexed under this heading.

Procarbazine Hydrochloride (Concurrent and/or sequential use with MAO inhibitors can result in the potentiation of pirbuterol's action on the vascular system). Products include:
Matulane Capsules 3188

Propranolol Hydrochloride (Co-administration with beta adrenergic receptor blocking agents blocks the pulmonary effect of pirbuterol and may produce severe bronchospasm in asthmatic patients). Products include:
Inderal LA Long-Acting Capsules 3421
InnoPran XL Capsules 2728

Protriptyline Hydrochloride (Concurrent and/or sequential use with tricyclic antidepressants can result in the potentiation of pirbuterol's action on the vascular system). Products include:
Vivactil Tablets 2350

Salmeterol Xinafoate (Potential for additive effects). Products include:
Advair Diskus 100/50 1291
Advair Diskus 250/50 1291
Advair Diskus 500/50 1291
Serevent Diskus 1540

Selegiline Hydrochloride (Concurrent and/or sequential use with MAO inhibitors can result in the potentiation of pirbuterol's action on the vascular system). Products include:
Eldepryl Capsules 3209

Sotalol Hydrochloride (Co-administration with beta adrenergic receptor blocking agents blocks the pulmonary effect of pirbuterol and may produce severe bronchospasm in asthmatic patients).
No products indexed under this heading.

Terbutaline Sulfate (Potential for additive effects).
No products indexed under this heading.

Timolol Hemihydrate (Co-administration with beta adrenergic receptor blocking agents blocks the pulmonary effect of pirbuterol and may produce severe bronchospasm in asthmatic patients). Products include:

Betimol Ophthalmic Solution 3371
Betimol Ophthalmic Solution .... ⊙283

Timolol Maleate (Co-administration with beta adrenergic receptor blocking agents blocks the pulmonary effect of pirbuterol and may produce severe bronchospasm in asthmatic patients). Products include:
Blocadren Tablets 1891
Cosopt Sterile Ophthalmic Solution 1910
Timolide Tablets 2056
Timoptic in Ocudose 2061
Timoptic Sterile Ophthalmic Solution 2058
Timoptic-XE Sterile Ophthalmic Gel Forming Solution 2062

Torsemide (The ECG changes and/or hypokalemia that may result from administration of non-potassium sparing diuretics can be acutely worsened by beta-agonists; clinical significance is not known).
No products indexed under this heading.

Tranylcypromine Sulfate (Concurrent and/or sequential use with MAO inhibitors can result in the potentiation of pirbuterol's action on the vascular system). Products include:
Parnate Tablets 1499

Trimipramine Maleate (Concurrent and/or sequential use with tricyclic antidepressants can result in the potentiation of pirbuterol's action on the vascular system). Products include:
Surmontil Capsules 2347

MAXALT TABLETS

(Rizatriptan Benzoate) 1983

May interact with 5HT1-receptor agonists, ergot-containing drugs, monoamine oxidase inhibitors, selective serotonin reuptake inhibitors, and certain other agents. Compounds in these categories include:

Citalopram Hydrobromide (Co-administration of 5-HT1 agonists with selective serotonin reuptake inhibitors (SSRIs) has resulted, rarely, in hyperreflexia, weakness, and incoordination). Products include:
Celexa 1177

Dihydroergotamine Mesylate (Ergot-containing drugs have been reported to cause prolonged vasospastic reactions; because there is a theoretical basis that these effects may be additive, use of ergot-type agents and rizatriptan within 24 hours is contraindicated). Products include:
Migranal Nasal Spray 3350

Ergonovine Maleate (Ergot-containing drugs have been reported to cause prolonged vasospastic reactions; because there is a theoretical basis that these effects may be additive, use of ergot-type agents and rizatriptan within 24 hours is contraindicated).
No products indexed under this heading.

Ergotamine Tartrate (Ergot-containing drugs have been reported to cause prolonged vasospastic reactions; because there is a theoretical basis that these effects may be additive, use of ergot-type agents and rizatriptan within 24 hours is contraindicated).
No products indexed under this heading.

Fluoxetine Hydrochloride (Co-administration of 5-HT1 agonists with selective serotonin reuptake inhibitors (SSRIs) has resulted, rarely, in hyperreflexia, weakness, and incoordination). Products include:
Prozac Pulvules and Liquid 1771
Symbyax Capsules 1788

Fluvoxamine Maleate (Co-administration of 5-HT1 agonists with selective serotonin reuptake inhibitors (SSRIs) has resulted, rarely, in hyperreflexia, weakness, and incoordination).
No products indexed under this heading.

Isocarboxazid (Plasma concentrations of rizatriptan may be increased by MAO inhibitors; concurrent and/or sequential use is contraindicated).
No products indexed under this heading.

Methylergonovine Maleate (Ergot-containing drugs have been reported to cause prolonged vasospastic reactions; because there is a theoretical basis that these effects may be additive, use of ergot-type agents and rizatriptan within 24 hours is contraindicated).
No products indexed under this heading.

Methysergide Maleate (Ergot-containing drugs have been reported to cause prolonged vasospastic reactions; because there is a theoretical basis that these effects may be additive, use of ergot-type agents and rizatriptan within 24 hours is contraindicated).
No products indexed under this heading.

Moclobemide (Concomitant therapy with the selective, reversible MAO-A inhibitor, moclobemide, has resulted in increased systemic exposure of rizatriptan and its metabolite; concurrent and/or sequential use is contraindicated).
No products indexed under this heading.

Naratriptan Hydrochloride (Co-administration with other 5-HT1 agonists within 24 hours of each other is contraindicated because the vasospastic effects may be additive). Products include:
Amerge Tablets 1312

Pargyline Hydrochloride (Plasma concentrations of rizatriptan may be increased by MAO inhibitors; concurrent and/or sequential use is contraindicated).
No products indexed under this heading.

Paroxetine Hydrochloride (Co-administration of 5-HT1 agonists with selective serotonin reuptake inhibitors (SSRIs) has resulted, rarely, in hyperreflexia, weakness, and incoordination; no pharmacokinetic interaction was observed with a single dose study). Products include:
Paxil CR Controlled-Release Tablets 1509
Paxil 1501

Phenelzine Sulfate (Plasma concentrations of rizatriptan may be increased by MAO inhibitors; concurrent and/or sequential use is contraindicated).
No products indexed under this heading.

Procarbazine Hydrochloride (Plasma concentrations of rizatriptan may be increased by MAO inhibitors; concurrent and/or sequential use is contraindicated). Products include:
Matulane Capsules 3188

Propranolol Hydrochloride (Co-administration has resulted in an increase in mean plasma AUC for rizatriptan by 70%). Products include:
Inderal LA Long-Acting Capsules 3421
InnoPran XL Capsules 2728

Selegiline Hydrochloride (Plasma concentrations of rizatriptan may be increased by MAO inhibitors; concurrent and/or sequential use is contraindicated). Products include:
Eldepryl Capsules 3209

Sertraline Hydrochloride (Co-administration of 5-HT1 agonists with selective serotonin reuptake inhibitors (SSRIs) has resulted, rarely, in hyperreflexia, weakness, and incoordination). Products include:
Zoloft 2581

Sumatriptan (Co-administration with other 5-HT1 agonists within 24 hours of each other is contraindicated because the vasospastic effects may be additive). Products include:
Imitrex Nasal Spray 1435

Sumatriptan Succinate (Co-administration with other 5-HT1 agonists within 24 hours of each other is contraindicated because the vasospastic effects may be additive). Products include:
Imitrex Injection 1431
Imitrex Tablets 1440

Tranylcypromine Sulfate (Plasma concentrations of rizatriptan may be increased by MAO inhibitors; concurrent and/or sequential use is contraindicated). Products include:
Parnate Tablets 1499

Zolmitriptan (Co-administration with other 5-HT1 agonists within 24 hours of each other is contraindicated because the vasospastic effects may be additive). Products include:
Zomig Nasal Spray 718
Zomig Tablets 714
Zomig-ZMT Tablets 714

Food Interactions

Food, unspecified (Delays the time to reach peak concentration by an hour; no significant effect on the bioavailability).

MAXALT-MLT ORALLY DISINTEGRATING TABLETS

(Rizatriptan Benzoate) 1983
See Maxalt Tablets

MAXIPIME FOR INJECTION

(Cefepime Hydrochloride) 1093

May interact with aminoglycosides and certain other agents. Compounds in these categories include:

Amikacin Sulfate (Co-administration increases the potential for nephrotoxicity and ototoxicity of aminoglycoside antibiotics).
No products indexed under this heading.

Furosemide (Co-administration with furosemide and other cephalosporins has resulted in nephrotoxicity). Products include:
Furosemide Tablets 2117

Gentamicin Sulfate (Co-administration increases the potential for nephrotoxicity and ototoxicity of aminoglycoside antibiotics). Products include:
Garamycin Injectable 3028
Genoptic Sterile Ophthalmic Solution .... ⊙227
Pred-G Ophthalmic Suspension .... ⊙234
Pred-G Sterile Ophthalmic Ointment .... ⊙235

Kanamycin Sulfate (Co-administration increases the potential for nephrotoxicity and ototoxicity of aminoglycoside antibiotics).
No products indexed under this heading.

Streptomycin Sulfate (Co-administration increases the potential for nephrotoxicity and ototoxicity of aminoglycoside antibiotics).
No products indexed under this heading.

Tobramycin (Co-administration increases the potential for nephrotoxicity and ototoxicity of aminoglycoside antibiotics). Products include:
TOBI Solution for Inhalation 1015
TobraDex Ophthalmic Ointment 558
TobraDex Ophthalmic Suspension 558
Zylet Ophthalmic Suspension 3508

Tobramycin Sulfate (Co-administration increases the potential for nephrotoxicity and ototoxicity of aminoglycoside antibiotics).
No products indexed under this heading.

MAXZIDE TABLETS

(Hydrochlorothiazide, Triamterene) 2150

May interact with ACE inhibitors, antihypertensives, barbiturates, cardiac glycosides, insulin, lithium preparations, narcotic analgesics, non-steroidal anti-inflammatory agents, potassium preparations, potassium sparing diuretics, and certain other agents. Compounds in these categories include:

Acebutolol Hydrochloride (Potential for additive or augmentative effect).
No products indexed under this heading.

Alfentanil Hydrochloride (May aggravate orthostatic hypotension).
No products indexed under this heading.

Amiloride Hydrochloride (Increased risk of hyperkalemia; co-administration with other potassium-conserving agents is contraindicated). Products include:
Midamor Tablets 2000
Moduretic Tablets 2003

Amlodipine Besylate (Potential for additive or augmentative effect). Products include:
Caduet Tablets 2507
Lotrel Capsules 2238
Norvasc Tablets 2529

Aprobarbital (May aggravate orthostatic hypotension).
No products indexed under this heading.

Atenolol (Potential for additive or augmentative effect). Products include:
Tenormin I.V. Injection 698
Tenormin Tablets 695

Benazepril Hydrochloride (Co-administration of potassium-sparing agents with ACE inhibitors greatly increases the risk of hyperkalemia; concurrent use should be undertaken with extreme caution). Products include:
Lotensin Tablets 2232
Lotensin HCT Tablets 2235
Lotrel Capsules 2238

Bendroflumethiazide (Potential for additive or augmentative effect).
No products indexed under this heading.

Betaxolol Hydrochloride (Potential for additive or augmentative effect). Products include:
Betoptic S Ophthalmic Suspension 554

Bisoprolol Fumarate (Potential for additive or augmentative effect).
No products indexed under this heading.

Buprenorphine Hydrochloride (May aggravate orthostatic hypotension). Products include:
Buprenex Injectable 2718
Suboxone Tablets 2719
Subutex Tablets 2719

Butabarbital (May aggravate orthostatic hypotension).
No products indexed under this heading.

Butalbital (May aggravate orthostatic hypotension). Products include:
Sedapap Tablets 50 mg/650 mg 2098

Candesartan Cilexetil (Potential for additive or augmentative effect). Products include:
Atacand Tablets 634
Atacand HCT 637

Captopril (Co-administration of potassium-sparing agents with ACE inhibitors greatly increases the risk of hyperkalemia; concurrent use should be undertaken with extreme caution). Products include:
Captopril Tablets 2114

Carteolol Hydrochloride (Potential for additive or augmentative effect). Products include:
Carteolol Hydrochloride Ophthalmic Solution USP, 1% .... ⊙246

Celecoxib (Potential for acute renal failure). Products include:
Celebrex Capsules 3130

Chlorothiazide (Potential for additive or augmentative effect). Products include:
Aldoclor Tablets 1881
Diuril Oral 1936

Chlorothiazide Sodium (Potential for additive or augmentative effect). Products include:
Diuril Sodium Intravenous 1934

Chlorthalidone (Potential for additive or augmentative effect). Products include:
Clorpres Tablets 2139

Clonidine (Potential for additive or augmentative effect). Products include:
Catapres-TTS 875

Clonidine Hydrochloride (Potential for additive or augmentative effect). Products include:
Catapres Tablets 874
Clorpres Tablets 2139

Codeine Phosphate (May aggravate orthostatic hypotension). Products include:
Tylenol with Codeine 2461

Deserpidine (Potential for additive or augmentative effect).
No products indexed under this heading.

Deslanoside (Potential for digitalis toxicity due to hypokalemia).
No products indexed under this heading.

Dezocine (May aggravate orthostatic hypotension).
No products indexed under this heading.

Diazoxide (Potential for additive or augmentative effect). Products include:
Hyperstat I.V. Injection 3031

Diclofenac Potassium (Potential for acute renal failure). Products include:
Cataflam Tablets 2173

Diclofenac Sodium (Potential for acute renal failure). Products include:
Arthrotec Tablets 3126
Voltaren Ophthalmic Solution 2300
Voltaren Tablets 2298
Voltaren-XR Tablets 2301

Digitalis Glycoside Preparations (Potential for digitalis toxicity due to hypokalemia).
No products indexed under this heading.

Digitoxin (Potential for digitalis toxicity due to hypokalemia).
No products indexed under this heading.

Digoxin (Potential for digitalis toxicity due to hypokalemia). Products include:
Digitek Tablets 2146
Lanoxicaps Capsules 1458
Lanoxin Injection 1462
Lanoxin Tablets 1468
Lanoxin Injection Pediatric 1465

Diltiazem Hydrochloride (Potential for additive or augmentative effect). Products include:
Cardizem LA Extended Release Tablets 1699
Tiazac Capsules 1204

Doxazosin Mesylate (Potential for additive or augmentative effect).
No products indexed under this heading.

Enalapril Maleate (Co-administration of potassium-sparing agents with ACE inhibitors greatly increases the risk of hyperkalemia; concurrent use should be undertaken with extreme caution). Products include:
Vaseretic Tablets 2073
Vasotec I.V. Injection 2076

Enalaprilat (Co-administration of potassium-sparing agents with ACE inhibitors greatly increases the risk of hyperkalemia; concurrent use should be undertaken with extreme caution).
No products indexed under this heading.

Eprosartan Mesylate (Potential for additive or augmentative effect). Products include:
Teveten Tablets 1707
Teveten HCT Tablets 1710

Esmolol Hydrochloride (Potential for additive or augmentative effect). Products include:
Brevibloc Concentrate 766
Brevibloc Injection 766
Brevibloc Double Strength Injection 766
Brevibloc Premixed Injection 766
Brevibloc Double Strength Premixed Injection 766

Etodolac (Potential for acute renal failure).
No products indexed under this heading.

Felodipine (Potential for additive or augmentative effect). Products include:
Plendil Extended-Release Tablets 651

Fenoprofen Calcium (Potential for acute renal failure). Products include:
Nalfon Capsules 2504

Fentanyl (May aggravate orthostatic hypotension). Products include:
Duragesic Transdermal System 2448

Fentanyl Citrate (May aggravate orthostatic hypotension). Products include:
Actiq 993

Flurbiprofen (Potential for acute renal failure).
No products indexed under this heading.

Fosinopril Sodium (Co-administration of potassium-sparing agents with ACE inhibitors greatly increases the risk of hyperkalemia; concurrent use should be undertaken with extreme caution).
No products indexed under this heading.

Furosemide (Potential for additive or augmentative effect). Products include:
Furosemide Tablets 2117

Guanabenz Acetate (Potential for additive or augmentative effect).
No products indexed under this heading.

Guanethidine Monosulfate (Potential for additive or augmentative effect).
No products indexed under this heading.

Hydralazine Hydrochloride (Potential for additive or augmentative effect). Products include:
BiDil Tablets 2161

Hydrocodone Bitartrate (May aggravate orthostatic hypotension). Products include:
Hycodan 1104
Hycomine Compound Tablets 1105
Hycotuss Expectorant Syrup 1106
Lortab 3315
Lortab Elixir 3312
Vicodin Tablets 530
Vicodin ES Tablets 531
Vicodin HP Tablets 532
Vicoprofen Tablets 533
Zydone Tablets 1118

Hydrocodone Polistirex (May aggravate orthostatic hypotension). Products include:
Tussionex Pennkinetic Extended-Release Suspension 3322

Hydroflumethiazide (Potential for additive or augmentative effect).
No products indexed under this heading.

Hydromorphone Hydrochloride (May aggravate orthostatic hypotension). Products include:
Dilaudid 439
Dilaudid Oral Liquid 443
Dilaudid Non-Sterile Powder 439
Dilaudid Rectal Suppositories 439
Dilaudid Tablets 439
Dilaudid Tablets - 8 mg 443
Dilaudid-HP 441

Ibuprofen (Potential for acute renal failure). Products include:
Advil Allergy Sinus Caplets .... ▣737
Advil .... ▣737
Children's Advil Suspension .... ▣742
Children's Advil Chewable Tablets .... ▣741
Advil Cold & Sinus .... ▣739
Advil Flu & Body Ache Caplets .... ▣739
Children's Advil Cold Suspension .... ▣741
Infants' Advil Concentrated Drops .... ▣743
Junior Strength Advil Swallow Tablets .... ▣740
Advil Migraine Liquigels .... ▣740
Advil Multi-Symptom Cold Caplets .... ▣738
Combunox Tablets 1183
Children's Motrin Oral Suspension and Chewable Tablets 1837
Children's Motrin Cold Non-Staining Dye-Free Oral Suspension 1838
Children's Motrin Cold Oral Suspension 1838
Children's Motrin Non-Staining Dye-Free Oral Suspension 1837
Motrin Cold & Sinus Caplets 1836
Motrin IB Tablets and Caplets 1836
Infants' Motrin Concentrated Drops 1837
Infants' Motrin Non-Staining Dye-Free Drops 1837
Junior Strength Motrin Caplets and Chewable Tablets 1837
Vicoprofen Tablets 533

Indapamide (Potential for additive or augmentative effect). Products include:
Indapamide Tablets 2119

Indomethacin (Potential for acute renal failure). Products include:
Indocin 1968

Indomethacin Sodium Trihydrate (Potential for acute renal failure). Products include:
Indocin I.V. 1973

Insulin, Human, Zinc Suspension (Insulin requirements in diabetics may be altered). Products include:
Humulin L, 100 Units 1763
Humulin U, 100 Units 1770

Insulin, Human NPH (Insulin requirements in diabetics may be altered). Products include:
Humulin N, 100 Units 1764
Humulin N Pen 1765
Novolin N Human Insulin 10 ml Vials 2322
Novolin N InnoLet 2322
Novolin N PenFill 3 ml Cartridges 2325
Novolin R InnoLet 2322

Insulin, Human Regular (Insulin requirements in diabetics may be altered). Products include:
Humulin R (U-500) 1768
Humulin R, 100 Units 1767
Novolin R Human Insulin 10 ml Vials 2322
Novolin R PenFill 2325

Insulin, Human Regular and Human NPH Mixture (Insulin requirements in diabetics may be altered). Products include:
Humulin 50/50, 100 Units 1760
Humulin 70/30 Pen 1761
Novolin 70/30 Human Insulin 10 ml Vials 2321
Novolin 70/30 InnoLet 2322
Novolin 70/30 PenFill 3 ml Cartridges 2325

Insulin, NPH (Insulin requirements in diabetics may be altered).
No products indexed under this heading.

Insulin, Regular (Insulin requirements in diabetics may be altered).
No products indexed under this heading.

Insulin, Zinc Crystals (Insulin requirements in diabetics may be altered).
No products indexed under this heading.

Insulin, Zinc Suspension (Insulin requirements in diabetics may be altered).
No products indexed under this heading.

Insulin Aspart, Human Regular (Insulin requirements in diabetics may be altered). Products include:
NovoLog Injection 2326

Insulin glargine (Insulin requirements in diabetics may be altered). Products include:
Lantus Injection 2925

Insulin Lispro, Human (Insulin requirements in diabetics may be altered). Products include:
Humalog-Pen 1751
Humalog Mix 75/25-Pen 1754

Insulin Lispro Protamine, Human (Insulin requirements in diabetics may be altered). Products include:
Humalog Mix 75/25-Pen 1754

Irbesartan (Potential for additive or augmentative effect). Products include:
Avalide Tablets 922
Avalide Tablets 2889
Avapro Tablets 925
Avapro Tablets 2886

Isradipine (Potential for additive or augmentative effect). Products include:
DynaCirc CR Tablets 2726

Ketoprofen (Potential for acute renal failure).
No products indexed under this heading.

Ketorolac Tromethamine (Potential for acute renal failure). Products include:
Acular Ophthalmic Solution 561
Acular LS Ophthalmic Solution 562

Labetalol Hydrochloride (Potential for additive or augmentative effect).
No products indexed under this heading.

Levorphanol Tartrate (May aggravate orthostatic hypotension).
No products indexed under this heading.

Lisinopril (Co-administration of potassium-sparing agents with ACE inhibitors greatly increases the risk of hyperkalemia; concurrent use should be undertaken with extreme caution). Products include:
Prinivil Tablets 2029
Prinzide Tablets 2033
Zestoretic Tablets 701
Zestril Tablets 704

Lithium (Diuretics tend to reduce lithium renal clearance and add a high risk of lithium toxicity).
No products indexed under this heading.

Lithium Carbonate (Diuretics tend to reduce lithium renal clearance and add a high risk of lithium toxicity). Products include:
Eskalith 1406
Lithobid Tablets 1670

Lithium Citrate (Diuretics tend to reduce lithium renal clearance and add a high risk of lithium toxicity).
No products indexed under this heading.

Losartan Potassium (Potential for additive or augmentative effect). Products include:
Cozaar Tablets 1913
Hyzaar 1964

Mecamylamine Hydrochloride (Potential for additive or augmentative effect). Products include:
Inversine Tablets 3286

Meclofenamate Sodium (Potential for acute renal failure).
No products indexed under this heading.

Mefenamic Acid (Potential for acute renal failure).
No products indexed under this heading.

Meloxicam (Potential for acute renal failure). Products include:
Mobic Oral Suspension 893
Mobic Tablets 893

Meperidine Hydrochloride (May aggravate orthostatic hypotension).
No products indexed under this heading.

Mephobarbital (May aggravate orthostatic hypotension). Products include:
Mebaral Tablets, USP 2483

Methadone Hydrochloride (May aggravate orthostatic hypotension).
No products indexed under this heading.

Methyclothiazide (Potential for additive or augmentative effect).
No products indexed under this heading.

Methyldopa (Potential for additive or augmentative effect). Products include:
Aldoclor Tablets 1881
Aldoril Tablets 1884

Methyldopate Hydrochloride (Potential for additive or augmentative effect).
No products indexed under this heading.

Metolazone (Potential for additive or augmentative effect).
No products indexed under this heading.

Metoprolol Succinate (Potential for additive or augmentative effect). Products include:
Toprol-XL Tablets 660

Metoprolol Tartrate (Potential for additive or augmentative effect).
No products indexed under this heading.

Metyrosine (Potential for additive or augmentative effect). Products include:
Demser Capsules 1933

Mibefradil Dihydrochloride (Potential for additive or augmentative effect).
No products indexed under this heading.

Minoxidil (Potential for additive or augmentative effect). Products include:
Men's Rogaine Extra Strength Topical Solution, Ocean Rush Scent and Original Unscented 706
Women's Rogaine Topical Solution, Spring Bloom Scent and Original Unscented 707

Moexipril Hydrochloride (Co-administration of potassium-sparing agents with ACE inhibitors greatly increases the risk of hyperkalemia; concurrent use should be undertaken with extreme caution). Products include:
Uniretic Tablets 3114
Univasc Tablets 3118

Morphine Sulfate (May aggravate orthostatic hypotension). Products include:
Avinza Capsules 1714
Kadian Capsules 572
MS Contin Tablets 2703

Nabumetone (Potential for acute renal failure). Products include:
Relafen Tablets 1523

Nadolol (Potential for additive or augmentative effect). Products include:
Nadolol Tablets 2121

Naproxen (Potential for acute renal failure). Products include:
EC-Naprosyn Delayed-Release Tablets 2769
Naprosyn Suspension 2769
Naprosyn Tablets 2769
Prevacid NapraPAC 3277

Naproxen Sodium (Potential for acute renal failure). Products include:
Aleve Tablets, Caplets and Gelcaps 605
Anaprox Tablets 2769
Anaprox DS Tablets 2769

Nicardipine Hydrochloride (Potential for additive or augmentative effect). Products include:
Cardene I.V. 1129

Nifedipine (Potential for additive or augmentative effect). Products include:
Adalat CC Tablets 2978

Nisoldipine (Potential for additive or augmentative effect). Products include:
Sular Tablets 1163

Nitroglycerin (Potential for additive or augmentative effect). Products include:
Nitro-Dur Transdermal Infusion System 3060
Nitrolingual Pumpspray 1161

Oxaprozin (Potential for acute renal failure).
No products indexed under this heading.

Oxycodone Hydrochloride (May aggravate orthostatic hypotension). Products include:
Combunox Tablets 1183
OxyContin Tablets 2699
OxyFast Oral Concentrate Solution 2704
OxyIR Capsules 2704
Percocet Tablets 1114
Percodan Tablets 1115

Penbutolol Sulfate (Potential for additive or augmentative effect).
No products indexed under this heading.

Pentobarbital Sodium (May aggravate orthostatic hypotension). Products include:
Nembutal Sodium Solution, USP 2484

Perindopril Erbumine (Co-administration of potassium-sparing agents with ACE inhibitors greatly increases the risk of hyperkalemia; concurrent use should be undertaken with extreme caution). Products include:
Aceon Tablets (2 mg, 4 mg, 8 mg) 3191

Phenobarbital (May aggravate orthostatic hypotension).
No products indexed under this heading.

Phenoxybenzamine Hydrochloride (Potential for additive or augmentative effect). Products include:
Dibenzyline Capsules 3390

Phentolamine Mesylate (Potential for additive or augmentative effect).
No products indexed under this heading.

Phenylbutazone (Potential for acute renal failure).
No products indexed under this heading.

Pindolol (Potential for additive or augmentative effect).
No products indexed under this heading.

Piroxicam (Potential for acute renal failure).
No products indexed under this heading.

Polythiazide (Potential for additive or augmentative effect).
No products indexed under this heading.

Potassium Acid Phosphate (Concomitant administration is contraindicated). Products include:
K-Phos Original (Sodium Free) Tablets 785

Potassium Bicarbonate (Concomitant administration is contraindicated).
No products indexed under this heading.

Potassium Chloride (Concomitant administration is contraindicated). Products include:
Colyte with Flavor Packs for Oral Solution 3102
HalfLytely and Bisacodyl Tablets Bowel Prep Kit with Flavors Packs 915
K-Dur Extended-Relase Tablets 3047
K-Lor Powder Packets 472
K-Tab Filmtab Tablets 473
TriLyte with Flavor Packs for Oral Solution 3114

Potassium Citrate (Concomitant administration is contraindicated). Products include:
Urocit-K Tablets 2109

Potassium Gluconate (Concomitant administration is contraindicated).
No products indexed under this heading.

Potassium Phosphate (Concomitant administration is contraindicated). Products include:
K-Phos Neutral Tablets 785

Prazosin Hydrochloride (Potential for additive or augmentative effect).
No products indexed under this heading.

Propoxyphene Hydrochloride (May aggravate orthostatic hypotension).
No products indexed under this heading.

Propoxyphene Napsylate (May aggravate orthostatic hypotension). Products include:
Darvocet A 500 Tablets 3497

Propranolol Hydrochloride (Potential for additive or augmentative effect). Products include:
Inderal LA Long-Acting Capsules 3421
InnoPran XL Capsules 2728

Quinapril Hydrochloride (Co-administration of potassium-sparing agents with ACE inhibitors greatly increases the risk of hyperkalemia; concurrent use should be undertaken with extreme caution).
No products indexed under this heading.

Ramipril (Co-administration of potassium-sparing agents with ACE inhibitors greatly increases the risk of hyperkalemia; concurrent use should be undertaken with extreme caution). Products include:
Altace Capsules 1673

Rauwolfia Serpentina (Potential for additive or augmentative effect).
No products indexed under this heading.

Remifentanil Hydrochloride (May aggravate orthostatic hypotension).
No products indexed under this heading.

Rescinnamine (Potential for additive or augmentative effect).
No products indexed under this heading.

Reserpine (Potential for additive or augmentative effect).
No products indexed under this heading.

Rofecoxib (Potential for acute renal failure).
No products indexed under this heading.

Secobarbital Sodium (May aggravate orthostatic hypotension).
No products indexed under this heading.

Sodium Nitroprusside (Potential for additive or augmentative effect).
No products indexed under this heading.

Sotalol Hydrochloride (Potential for additive or augmentative effect).
No products indexed under this heading.

Spirapril Hydrochloride (Co-administration of potassium-sparing agents with ACE inhibitors greatly increases the risk of hyperkalemia; concurrent use should be undertaken with extreme caution).
No products indexed under this heading.

Spironolactone (Increased risk of hyperkalemia; co-administration with other potassium-conserving agents is contraindicated).
No products indexed under this heading.

Sufentanil Citrate (May aggravate orthostatic hypotension).
No products indexed under this heading.

Sulindac (Potential for acute renal failure). Products include:
Clinoril Tablets **1899**

Telmisartan (Potential for additive or augmentative effect). Products include:
Micardis Tablets **884**
Micardis HCT Tablets **886**

Terazosin Hydrochloride (Potential for additive or augmentative effect). Products include:
Hytrin Capsules **469**

Thiamylal Sodium (May aggravate orthostatic hypotension).
No products indexed under this heading.

Timolol Maleate (Potential for additive or augmentative effect). Products include:
Blocadren Tablets **1891**
Cosopt Sterile Ophthalmic Solution **1910**
Timolide Tablets **2056**
Timoptic in Ocudose **2061**
Timoptic Sterile Ophthalmic Solution **2058**
Timoptic-XE Sterile Ophthalmic Gel Forming Solution **2062**

Tolmetin Sodium (Potential for acute renal failure).
No products indexed under this heading.

Torsemide (Potential for additive or augmentative effect).
No products indexed under this heading.

Trandolapril (Co-administration of potassium-sparing agents with ACE inhibitors greatly increases the risk of hyperkalemia; concurrent use should be undertaken with extreme caution). Products include:
Mavik Tablets **482**
Tarka Tablets **519**

Trimethaphan Camsylate (Potential for additive or augmentative effect).
No products indexed under this heading.

Valdecoxib (Potential for acute renal failure).
No products indexed under this heading.

Valsartan (Potential for additive or augmentative effect). Products include:
Diovan HCT Tablets **2195**
Diovan Tablets **2191**

Verapamil Hydrochloride (Potential for additive or augmentative effect). Products include:
Covera-HS Tablets **3135**
Tarka Tablets **519**
Verelan PM Capsules **3120**

Food Interactions

Alcohol (May aggravate orthostatic hypotension).

Diet, potassium-rich (Concurrent use is contraindicated).

MAXZIDE-25 MG TABLETS

(Hydrochlorothiazide, Triamterene) **2150**
See Maxzide Tablets

MDR FITNESS TABS FOR MEN AND WOMEN

(Vitamins with Minerals) **1854**
None cited in PDR database.

MDR VITAL FACTORS

(Vitamins with Minerals) **1854**
None cited in PDR database.

MEBARAL TABLETS, USP

(Mephobarbital) **2483**
May interact with central nervous system depressants, corticosteroids, oral anticoagulants, monoamine oxidase inhibitors, oral contraceptives, and certain other agents. Compounds in these categories include:

Alfentanil Hydrochloride (The concomitant use of other central nervous system depressants, including other sedatives or hypnotics, antihistamines, tranquilizers, or alcohol, may produce additive depressant effects).
No products indexed under this heading.

Alprazolam (The concomitant use of other central nervous system depressants, including other sedatives or hypnotics, antihistamines, tranquilizers, or alcohol, may produce additive depressant effects). Products include:
Niravam Orally Disintegrating Tablets **3106**
Xanax XR Tablets **2655**

Anisindione (Barbiturates can induce hepatic microsomal enzymes resulting in increased metabolism and decreased anticoagulant response of oral anticoagulants. Patients stabilized on anticoagulant therapy may require dosage adjustments if barbiturates are added to or withdrawn from their dosage regimen). Products include:
Miradon Tablets **3056**

Aprobarbital (The concomitant use of other central nervous system depressants, including other sedatives or hypnotics, antihistamines, tranquilizers, or alcohol, may produce additive depressant effects).
No products indexed under this heading.

Betamethasone Acetate (Barbiturates appear to enhance the metabolism of exogenous corticosteroids probably through the induction of hepatic microsomal enzymes. Patients stabilized on corticosteroid therapy may require dosage adjustments if barbiturates are added to or withdrawn from their dosage regimen).
No products indexed under this heading.

Betamethasone Sodium Phosphate (Barbiturates appear to enhance the metabolism of exogenous corticosteroids probably through the induction of hepatic microsomal enzymes. Patients stabilized on corticosteroid therapy may require dosage adjustments if barbiturates are added to or withdrawn from their dosage regimen).
No products indexed under this heading.

Buprenorphine Hydrochloride (The concomitant use of other central nervous system depressants, including other sedatives or hypnotics, antihistamines, tranquilizers, or alcohol, may produce additive depressant effects). Products include:
Buprenex Injectable **2718**
Suboxone Tablets **2719**
Subutex Tablets **2719**

Buspirone Hydrochloride (The concomitant use of other central nervous system depressants, including other sedatives or hypnotics, antihistamines, tranquilizers, or alcohol, may produce additive depressant effects).
No products indexed under this heading.

Butabarbital (The concomitant use of other central nervous system depressants, including other sedatives or hypnotics, antihistamines, tranquilizers, or alcohol, may produce additive depressant effects).
No products indexed under this heading.

Butalbital (The concomitant use of other central nervous system depressants, including other sedatives or hypnotics, antihistamines, tranquilizers, or alcohol, may produce additive depressant effects). Products include:
Sedapap Tablets 50 mg/650 mg **2098**

Chlordiazepoxide (The concomitant use of other central nervous system depressants, including other sedatives or hypnotics, antihistamines, tranquilizers, or alcohol, may produce additive depressant effects).
No products indexed under this heading.

Chlordiazepoxide Hydrochloride (The concomitant use of other central nervous system depressants, including other sedatives or hypnotics, antihistamines, tranquilizers, or alcohol, may produce additive depressant effects). Products include:
Librium Capsules **3349**

Chlorpromazine (The concomitant use of other central nervous system depressants, including other sedatives or hypnotics, antihistamines, tranquilizers, or alcohol, may produce additive depressant effects).
No products indexed under this heading.

Chlorpromazine Hydrochloride (The concomitant use of other central nervous system depressants, including other sedatives or hypnotics, antihistamines, tranquilizers, or alcohol, may produce additive depressant effects).
No products indexed under this heading.

Chlorprothixene (The concomitant use of other central nervous system depressants, including other sedatives or hypnotics, antihistamines, tranquilizers, or alcohol, may produce additive depressant effects).
No products indexed under this heading.

Chlorprothixene Hydrochloride (The concomitant use of other central nervous system depressants, including other sedatives or hypnotics, antihistamines, tranquilizers, or alcohol, may produce additive depressant effects).
No products indexed under this heading.

Chlorprothixene Lactate (The concomitant use of other central nervous system depressants, including other sedatives or hypnotics, antihistamines, tranquilizers, or alcohol, may produce additive depressant effects).
No products indexed under this heading.

Clorazepate Dipotassium (The concomitant use of other central nervous system depressants, including other sedatives or hypnotics, antihistamines, tranquilizers, or alcohol, may produce additive depressant effects). Products include:
Tranxene **2488**

Clozapine (The concomitant use of other central nervous system depressants, including other sedatives or hypnotics, antihistamines, tranquilizers, or alcohol, may produce additive depressant effects). Products include:
Clozapine Tablets **2141**
Clozaril Tablets **2174**
FazaClo Orally Disintegrating Tablets **547**

Codeine Phosphate (The concomitant use of other central nervous system depressants, including other sedatives or hypnotics, antihistamines, tranquilizers, or alcohol, may produce additive depressant effects). Products include:
Tylenol with Codeine **2461**

Cortisone Acetate (Barbiturates appear to enhance the metabolism of exogenous corticosteroids probably through the induction of hepatic microsomal enzymes. Patients stabilized on corticosteroid therapy may require dosage adjustments if barbiturates are added to or withdrawn from their dosage regimen).
No products indexed under this heading.

Desflurane (The concomitant use of other central nervous system depressants, including other sedatives or hypnotics, antihistamines, tranquilizers, or alcohol, may produce additive depressant effects). Products include:
Suprane Liquid for Inhalation **770**

Desogestrel (There have been reports of patients treated with antiepileptic drugs who become pregnant while taking oral contraceptives. An alternate contraceptive method might be suggested to women taking phenobarbital). Products include:
Ortho-Cept Tablets **2395**

Dexamethasone (Barbiturates appear to enhance the metabolism of exogenous corticosteroids probably through the induction of hepatic microsomal enzymes. Patients stabilized on corticosteroid therapy may

require dosage adjustments if barbiturates are added to or withdrawn from their dosage regimen). Products include:

Ciprodex Otic Suspension 555
Decadron Tablets 1929
TobraDex Ophthalmic Ointment 558
TobraDex Ophthalmic Suspension ... 558

Dexamethasone Acetate (Barbiturates appear to enhance the metabolism of exogenous corticosteroids probably through the induction of hepatic microsomal enzymes. Patients stabilized on corticosteroid therapy may require dosage adjustments if barbiturates are added to or withdrawn from their dosage regimen).

No products indexed under this heading.

Dexamethasone Sodium Phosphate (Barbiturates appear to enhance the metabolism of exogenous corticosteroids probably through the induction of hepatic microsomal enzymes. Patients stabilized on corticosteroid therapy may require dosage adjustments if barbiturates are added to or withdrawn from their dosage regimen). Products include:

Decadron Phosphate Injection 1931

Dezocine (The concomitant use of other central nervous system depressants, including other sedatives or hypnotics, antihistamines, tranquilizers, or alcohol, may produce additive depressant effects).

No products indexed under this heading.

Diazepam (The concomitant use of other central nervous system depressants, including other sedatives or hypnotics, antihistamines, tranquilizers, or alcohol, may produce additive depressant effects). Products include:

Diastat Rectal Delivery System 3344
Valium Tablets 2822

Dicumarol (Barbiturates can induce hepatic microsomal enzymes resulting in increased metabolism and decreased anticoagulant response of oral anticoagulants. Patients stabilized on anticoagulant therapy may require dosage adjustments if barbiturates are added to or withdrawn from their dosage regimen).

No products indexed under this heading.

Doxycycline Calcium (Phenobarbital has been shown to shorten the half-life of doxycycline for as long as two weeks after barbiturate therapy is discontinued).

No products indexed under this heading.

Doxycycline Hyclate (Phenobarbital has been shown to shorten the half-life of doxycycline for as long as two weeks after barbiturate therapy is discontinued).

No products indexed under this heading.

Droperidol (The concomitant use of other central nervous system depressants, including other sedatives or hypnotics, antihistamines, tranquilizers, or alcohol, may produce additive depressant effects).

No products indexed under this heading.

Enflurane (The concomitant use of other central nervous system depressants, including other sedatives or hypnotics, antihistamines, tranquilizers, or alcohol, may produce additive depressant effects).

No products indexed under this heading.

Estazolam (The concomitant use of other central nervous system depressants, including other sedatives or hypnotics, antihistamines, tranquilizers, or alcohol, may produce additive depressant effects). Products include:

ProSom Tablets 512

Ethanol (The concomitant use of other central nervous system depressants, including other sedatives or hypnotics, antihistamines, tranquilizers, or alcohol, may produce additive depressant effects).

No products indexed under this heading.

Ethchlorvynol (The concomitant use of other central nervous system depressants, including other sedatives or hypnotics, antihistamines, tranquilizers, or alcohol, may produce additive depressant effects).

No products indexed under this heading.

Ethinamate (The concomitant use of other central nervous system depressants, including other sedatives or hypnotics, antihistamines, tranquilizers, or alcohol, may produce additive depressant effects).

No products indexed under this heading.

Ethinyl Estradiol (There have been reports of patients treated with antiepileptic drugs who become pregnant while taking oral contraceptives. An alternate contraceptive method might be suggested to women taking phenobarbital). Products include:

Alesse-28 Tablets 3392
Lo/Ovral-28 Tablets 3423
NuvaRing 2357
Ortho-Cept Tablets 2395
Ortho-Cyclen/Ortho Tri-Cyclen 2414
Ortho Evra Transdermal System 2402
Ortho Tri-Cyclen Lo Tablets 2421
Seasonale Tablets 1073
Triphasil-28 Tablets 3483
Yasmin 28 Tablets 818

Ethyl Alcohol (The concomitant use of other central nervous system depressants, including other sedatives or hypnotics, antihistamines, tranquilizers, or alcohol, may produce additive depressant effects).

No products indexed under this heading.

Ethynodiol Diacetate (There have been reports of patients treated with antiepileptic drugs who become pregnant while taking oral contraceptives. An alternate contraceptive method might be suggested to women taking phenobarbital).

No products indexed under this heading.

Fentanyl (The concomitant use of other central nervous system depressants, including other sedatives or hypnotics, antihistamines, tranquilizers, or alcohol, may produce additive depressant effects). Products include:

Duragesic Transdermal System 2448

Fentanyl Citrate (The concomitant use of other central nervous system depressants, including other sedatives or hypnotics, antihistamines, tranquilizers, or alcohol, may produce additive depressant effects). Products include:

Actiq 993

Fludrocortisone Acetate (Barbiturates appear to enhance the metabolism of exogenous corticosteroids probably through the induction of hepatic microsomal enzymes. Patients stabilized on corticosteroid therapy may require dosage adjustments if barbiturates are added to or withdrawn from their dosage regimen).

No products indexed under this heading.

Fluphenazine Decanoate (The concomitant use of other central nervous system depressants, including other sedatives or hypnotics, antihistamines, tranquilizers, or alcohol, may produce additive depressant effects).

No products indexed under this heading.

Fluphenazine Enanthate (The concomitant use of other central nervous system depressants, including other sedatives or hypnotics, antihistamines, tranquilizers, or alcohol, may produce additive depressant effects).

No products indexed under this heading.

Fluphenazine Hydrochloride (The concomitant use of other central nervous system depressants, including other sedatives or hypnotics, antihistamines, tranquilizers, or alcohol, may produce additive depressant effects).

No products indexed under this heading.

Flurazepam Hydrochloride (The concomitant use of other central nervous system depressants, including other sedatives or hypnotics, antihistamines, tranquilizers, or alcohol, may produce additive depressant effects). Products include:

Dalmane Capsules 3343

Glutethimide (The concomitant use of other central nervous system depressants, including other sedatives or hypnotics, antihistamines, tranquilizers, or alcohol, may produce additive depressant effects).

No products indexed under this heading.

Griseofulvin (Phenobarbital appears to interfere with the absorption of orally administered griseofulvin, thus decreasing its blood level. The effect of the resultant decreased blood levels of griseofulvin on therapeutic response has not been established. However, it would be preferable to avoid concomitant administration of these drugs). Products include:

Grifulvin V Tablets Microsize and Oral Suspension Microsize........... 2384
Gris-PEG Tablets 2504

Haloperidol (The concomitant use of other central nervous system depressants, including other sedatives or hypnotics, antihistamines, tranquilizers, or alcohol, may produce additive depressant effects).

No products indexed under this heading.

Haloperidol Decanoate (The concomitant use of other central nervous system depressants, including other sedatives or hypnotics, antihistamines, tranquilizers, or alcohol, may produce additive depressant effects).

No products indexed under this heading.

Hydrocodone Bitartrate (The concomitant use of other central nervous system depressants, including other sedatives or hypnotics, antihistamines, tranquilizers, or alcohol, may produce additive depressant effects). Products include:

Hycodan 1104
Hycomine Compound Tablets 1105
Hycotuss Expectorant Syrup 1106
Lortab 3315
Lortab Elixir 3312
Vicodin Tablets 530
Vicodin ES Tablets 531
Vicodin HP Tablets 532
Vicoprofen Tablets 533
Zydone Tablets 1118

Hydrocodone Polistirex (The concomitant use of other central nervous system depressants, including other sedatives or hypnotics, antihistamines, tranquilizers, or alcohol, may produce additive depressant effects). Products include:

Tussionex Pennkinetic Extended-Release Suspension 3322

Hydrocortisone (Barbiturates appear to enhance the metabolism of exogenous corticosteroids probably through the induction of hepatic microsomal enzymes. Patients stabilized on corticosteroid therapy may require dosage adjustments if barbiturates are added to or withdrawn from their dosage regimen). Products include:

Cortizone•5 Ointment 699
Cortizone•10 Creme 699
Cortizone•10 Ointment 699
Cortizone•10 Plus Creme 700
Cortizone•10 Maximum Strength Quick Shot Spray 700
Hydrocortone Tablets 1963
Preparation H Hydrocortisone Cream 748

Hydrocortisone Acetate (Barbiturates appear to enhance the metabolism of exogenous corticosteroids probably through the induction of hepatic microsomal enzymes. Patients stabilized on corticosteroid therapy may require dosage adjustments if barbiturates are added to or withdrawn from their dosage regimen). Products include:

Analpram-HC 1136
Pramosone 1139
ProctoFoam-HC 3113
Tucks Anti-Itch Ointment 712
U-cort 1% Cream 3289

Hydrocortisone Sodium Phosphate (Barbiturates appear to enhance the metabolism of exogenous corticosteroids probably through the induction of hepatic microsomal enzymes. Patients stabilized on corticosteroid therapy may require dosage adjustments if barbiturates are added to or withdrawn from their dosage regimen).

No products indexed under this heading.

Hydrocortisone Sodium Succinate (Barbiturates appear to enhance the metabolism of exogenous corticosteroids probably through the induction of hepatic microsomal enzymes. Patients stabilized on corticosteroid therapy may require dosage adjustments if barbiturates are added to or withdrawn from their dosage regimen).
No products indexed under this heading.

Hydromorphone Hydrochloride (The concomitant use of other central nervous system depressants, including other sedatives or hypnotics, antihistamines, tranquilizers, or alcohol, may produce additive depressant effects). Products include:
Dilaudid 439
Dilaudid Oral Liquid 443
Dilaudid Non-Sterile Powder 439
Dilaudid Rectal Suppositories 439
Dilaudid Tablets 439
Dilaudid Tablets - 8 mg 443
Dilaudid-HP 441

Hydroxyzine Hydrochloride (The concomitant use of other central nervous system depressants, including other sedatives or hypnotics, antihistamines, tranquilizers, or alcohol, may produce additive depressant effects).
No products indexed under this heading.

Isocarboxazid (MAO inhibitors prolong the effects of barbiturates probably because metabolism of the barbiturate is inhibited).
No products indexed under this heading.

Isoflurane (The concomitant use of other central nervous system depressants, including other sedatives or hypnotics, antihistamines, tranquilizers, or alcohol, may produce additive depressant effects).
No products indexed under this heading.

Ketamine Hydrochloride (The concomitant use of other central nervous system depressants, including other sedatives or hypnotics, antihistamines, tranquilizers, or alcohol, may produce additive depressant effects).
No products indexed under this heading.

Levomethadyl Acetate Hydrochloride (The concomitant use of other central nervous system depressants, including other sedatives or hypnotics, antihistamines, tranquilizers, or alcohol, may produce additive depressant effects).
No products indexed under this heading.

Levonorgestrel (There have been reports of patients treated with antiepileptic drugs who become pregnant while taking oral contraceptives. An alternate contraceptive method might be suggested to women taking phenobarbital). Products include:
Alesse-28 Tablets 3392
Climara Pro Transdermal System 800
Mirena Intrauterine System 810
Plan B Tablets 1068
Seasonale Tablets 1073
Triphasil-28 Tablets 3483

Levorphanol Tartrate (The concomitant use of other central nervous system depressants, including other sedatives or hypnotics, antihistamines, tranquilizers, or alcohol, may produce additive depressant effects).
No products indexed under this heading.

Lorazepam (The concomitant use of other central nervous system depressants, including other sedatives or hypnotics, antihistamines, tranquilizers, or alcohol, may produce additive depressant effects).
No products indexed under this heading.

Loxapine Hydrochloride (The concomitant use of other central nervous system depressants, including other sedatives or hypnotics, antihistamines, tranquilizers, or alcohol, may produce additive depressant effects).
No products indexed under this heading.

Loxapine Succinate (The concomitant use of other central nervous system depressants, including other sedatives or hypnotics, antihistamines, tranquilizers, or alcohol, may produce additive depressant effects).
No products indexed under this heading.

Meperidine Hydrochloride (The concomitant use of other central nervous system depressants, including other sedatives or hypnotics, antihistamines, tranquilizers, or alcohol, may produce additive depressant effects).
No products indexed under this heading.

Meprobamate (The concomitant use of other central nervous system depressants, including other sedatives or hypnotics, antihistamines, tranquilizers, or alcohol, may produce additive depressant effects).
No products indexed under this heading.

Mesoridazine Besylate (The concomitant use of other central nervous system depressants, including other sedatives or hypnotics, antihistamines, tranquilizers, or alcohol, may produce additive depressant effects).
No products indexed under this heading.

Mestranol (There have been reports of patients treated with antiepileptic drugs who become pregnant while taking oral contraceptives. An alternate contraceptive method might be suggested to women taking phenobarbital).
No products indexed under this heading.

Methadone Hydrochloride (The concomitant use of other central nervous system depressants, including other sedatives or hypnotics, antihistamines, tranquilizers, or alcohol, may produce additive depressant effects).
No products indexed under this heading.

Methohexital Sodium (The concomitant use of other central nervous system depressants, including other sedatives or hypnotics, antihistamines, tranquilizers, or alcohol, may produce additive depressant effects).
No products indexed under this heading.

Methotrimeprazine (The concomitant use of other central nervous system depressants, including other sedatives or hypnotics, antihistamines, tranquilizers, or alcohol, may produce additive depressant effects).
No products indexed under this heading.

Methoxyflurane (The concomitant use of other central nervous system depressants, including other sedatives or hypnotics, antihistamines, tranquilizers, or alcohol, may produce additive depressant effects).
No products indexed under this heading.

Methylprednisolone Acetate (Barbiturates appear to enhance the metabolism of exogenous corticosteroids probably through the induction of hepatic microsomal enzymes. Patients stabilized on corticosteroid therapy may require dosage adjustments if barbiturates are added to or withdrawn from their dosage regimen). Products include:
Depo-Medrol Injectable Suspension 2615
Depo-Medrol Single-Dose Vial 2617

Methylprednisolone Sodium Succinate (Barbiturates appear to enhance the metabolism of exogenous corticosteroids probably through the induction of hepatic microsomal enzymes. Patients stabilized on corticosteroid therapy may require dosage adjustments if barbiturates are added to or withdrawn from their dosage regimen).
No products indexed under this heading.

Midazolam Hydrochloride (The concomitant use of other central nervous system depressants, including other sedatives or hypnotics, antihistamines, tranquilizers, or alcohol, may produce additive depressant effects).
No products indexed under this heading.

Moclobemide (MAO inhibitors prolong the effects of barbiturates probably because metabolism of the barbiturate is inhibited).
No products indexed under this heading.

Molindone Hydrochloride (The concomitant use of other central nervous system depressants, including other sedatives or hypnotics, antihistamines, tranquilizers, or alcohol, may produce additive depressant effects). Products include:
Moban Tablets 1108

Morphine Sulfate (The concomitant use of other central nervous system depressants, including other sedatives or hypnotics, antihistamines, tranquilizers, or alcohol, may produce additive depressant effects). Products include:
Avinza Capsules 1714
Kadian Capsules 572
MS Contin Tablets 2703

Norethindrone (There have been reports of patients treated with antiepileptic drugs who become pregnant while taking oral contraceptives. An alternate contraceptive method might be suggested to women taking phenobarbital). Products include:
Ortho Micronor Tablets 2411

Norethynodrel (There have been reports of patients treated with antiepileptic drugs who become pregnant while taking oral contraceptives. An alternate contraceptive method might be suggested to women taking phenobarbital).
No products indexed under this heading.

Norgestimate (There have been reports of patients treated with antiepileptic drugs who become pregnant while taking oral contraceptives. An alternate contraceptive method might be suggested to women taking phenobarbital). Products include:
Ortho-Cyclen/Ortho Tri-Cyclen 2414
Ortho Tri-Cyclen Lo Tablets 2421
Prefest Tablets 1069

Norgestrel (There have been reports of patients treated with antiepileptic drugs who become pregnant while taking oral contraceptives. An alternate contraceptive method might be suggested to women taking phenobarbital). Products include:
Lo/Ovral-28 Tablets 3423

Olanzapine (The concomitant use of other central nervous system depressants, including other sedatives or hypnotics, antihistamines, tranquilizers, or alcohol, may produce additive depressant effects). Products include:
Symbyax Capsules 1788
Zyprexa Tablets 1798
Zyprexa IntraMuscular 1798
Zyprexa ZYDIS Orally Disintegrating Tablets 1798

Oxazepam (The concomitant use of other central nervous system depressants, including other sedatives or hypnotics, antihistamines, tranquilizers, or alcohol, may produce additive depressant effects).
No products indexed under this heading.

Oxycodone Hydrochloride (The concomitant use of other central nervous system depressants, including other sedatives or hypnotics, antihistamines, tranquilizers, or alcohol, may produce additive depressant effects). Products include:
Combunox Tablets 1183
OxyContin Tablets 2699
OxyFast Oral Concentrate Solution 2704
OxyIR Capsules 2704
Percocet Tablets 1114
Percodan Tablets 1115

Pargyline Hydrochloride (MAO inhibitors prolong the effects of barbiturates probably because metabolism of the barbiturate is inhibited).
No products indexed under this heading.

Pentobarbital Sodium (The concomitant use of other central nervous system depressants, including other sedatives or hypnotics, antihistamines, tranquilizers, or alcohol, may produce additive depressant effects). Products include:
Nembutal Sodium Solution, USP 2484

Perphenazine (The concomitant use of other central nervous system depressants, including other sedatives or hypnotics, antihistamines, tranquilizers, or alcohol, may produce additive depressant effects).
No products indexed under this heading.

Phenelzine Sulfate (MAO inhibitors prolong the effects of barbiturates probably because metabolism of the barbiturate is inhibited).
No products indexed under this heading.

Phenobarbital (The concomitant use of other central nervous system depressants, including other sedatives or hypnotics, antihistamines, tranquilizers, or alcohol, may produce additive depressant effects).
No products indexed under this heading.

Phenytoin (The effect of barbiturates on the metabolism of phenytoin appears to be variable. Some investigators report an accelerating effect, while others report no effect. Because this is unpredictable, phenytoin and barbiturate blood levels should be monitored more frequently if these drugs are given concurrently).
No products indexed under this heading.

Prazepam (The concomitant use of other central nervous system depressants, including other sedatives or hypnotics, antihistamines, tranquilizers, or alcohol, may produce additive depressant effects).
No products indexed under this heading.

Prednisolone Acetate (Barbiturates appear to enhance the metabolism of exogenous corticosteroids probably through the induction of hepatic microsomal enzymes. Patients stabilized on corticosteroid therapy may require dosage adjustments if barbiturates are added to or withdrawn from their dosage regimen). Products include:
Blephamide Ophthalmic Ointment 563
Blephamide Ophthalmic Suspension.................................. 564
Poly-Pred Liquifilm Ophthalmic Suspension .... ⊙ 231
Pred Forte Ophthalmic Suspension .... ⊙ 233
Pred Mild Sterile Ophthalmic Suspension .... ⊙ 236
Pred-G Ophthalmic Suspension ...... ⊙ 234
Pred-G Sterile Ophthalmic Ointment.................................. ⊙ 235

Prednisolone Sodium Phosphate (Barbiturates appear to enhance the metabolism of exogenous corticosteroids probably through the induction of hepatic microsomal enzymes. Patients stabilized on corticosteroid therapy may require dosage adjustments if barbiturates are added to or withdrawn from their dosage regimen). Products include:
Pediapred Oral Solution 3319

Prednisolone Tebutate (Barbiturates appear to enhance the metabolism of exogenous corticosteroids probably through the induction of hepatic microsomal enzymes. Patients stabilized on corticosteroid therapy may require dosage adjustments if barbiturates are added to or withdrawn from their dosage regimen).
No products indexed under this heading.

Prednisone (Barbiturates appear to enhance the metabolism of exogenous corticosteroids probably through the induction of hepatic microsomal enzymes. Patients stabilized on corticosteroid therapy may require dosage adjustments if barbiturates are added to or withdrawn from their dosage regimen).
No products indexed under this heading.

Procarbazine Hydrochloride (MAO inhibitors prolong the effects of barbiturates probably because metabolism of the barbiturate is inhibited). Products include:
Matulane Capsules 3188

Prochlorperazine (The concomitant use of other central nervous system depressants, including other sedatives or hypnotics, antihistamines, tranquilizers, or alcohol, may produce additive depressant effects).
No products indexed under this heading.

Promethazine Hydrochloride (The concomitant use of other central nervous system depressants, including other sedatives or hypnotics, antihistamines, tranquilizers, or alcohol, may produce additive depressant effects). Products include:
Phenergan 3438

Propofol (The concomitant use of other central nervous system depressants, including other sedatives or hypnotics, antihistamines, tranquilizers, or alcohol, may produce additive depressant effects). Products include:
Diprivan Injectable Emulsion 676

Propoxyphene Hydrochloride (The concomitant use of other central nervous system depressants, including other sedatives or hypnotics, antihistamines, tranquilizers, or alcohol, may produce additive depressant effects).
No products indexed under this heading.

Propoxyphene Napsylate (The concomitant use of other central nervous system depressants, including other sedatives or hypnotics, antihistamines, tranquilizers, or alcohol, may produce additive depressant effects). Products include:
Darvocet A 500 Tablets 3497

Quazepam (The concomitant use of other central nervous system depressants, including other sedatives or hypnotics, antihistamines, tranquilizers, or alcohol, may produce additive depressant effects).
No products indexed under this heading.

Quetiapine Fumarate (The concomitant use of other central nervous system depressants, including other sedatives or hypnotics, antihistamines, tranquilizers, or alcohol, may produce additive depressant effects). Products include:
Seroquel Tablets 691

Remifentanil Hydrochloride (The concomitant use of other central nervous system depressants, including other sedatives or hypnotics, antihistamines, tranquilizers, or alcohol, may produce additive depressant effects).
No products indexed under this heading.

Risperidone (The concomitant use of other central nervous system depressants, including other sedatives or hypnotics, antihistamines, tranquilizers, or alcohol, may produce additive depressant effects). Products include:
Risperdal Consta Long-Acting Injection 1664
Risperdal M-Tab Orally Disintegrating Tablets.................. 1658
Risperdal 1658

Secobarbital Sodium (The concomitant use of other central nervous system depressants, including other sedatives or hypnotics, antihistamines, tranquilizers, or alcohol, may produce additive depressant effects).
No products indexed under this heading.

Selegiline Hydrochloride (MAO inhibitors prolong the effects of barbiturates probably because metabolism of the barbiturate is inhibited). Products include:
Eldepryl Capsules 3209

Sevoflurane (The concomitant use of other central nervous system depressants, including other sedatives or hypnotics, antihistamines, tranquilizers, or alcohol, may produce additive depressant effects). Products include:
Ultane Liquid for Inhalation 526

Sodium Oxybate (The concomitant use of other central nervous system depressants, including other sedatives or hypnotics, antihistamines, tranquilizers, or alcohol, may produce additive depressant effects).
No products indexed under this heading.

Sufentanil Citrate (The concomitant use of other central nervous system depressants, including other sedatives or hypnotics, antihistamines, tranquilizers, or alcohol, may produce additive depressant effects).
No products indexed under this heading.

Temazepam (The concomitant use of other central nervous system depressants, including other sedatives or hypnotics, antihistamines, tranquilizers, or alcohol, may produce additive depressant effects).
No products indexed under this heading.

Thiamylal Sodium (The concomitant use of other central nervous system depressants, including other sedatives or hypnotics, antihistamines, tranquilizers, or alcohol, may produce additive depressant effects).
No products indexed under this heading.

Thioridazine Hydrochloride (The concomitant use of other central nervous system depressants, including other sedatives or hypnotics, antihistamines, tranquilizers, or alcohol, may produce additive depressant effects). Products include:
Thioridazine Hydrochloride Tablets.. 2122

Thiothixene (The concomitant use of other central nervous system depressants, including other sedatives or hypnotics, antihistamines, tranquilizers, or alcohol, may produce additive depressant effects). Products include:
Thiothixene Capsules 2124

Tranylcypromine Sulfate (MAO inhibitors prolong the effects of barbiturates probably because metabolism of the barbiturate is inhibited). Products include:
Parnate Tablets 1499

Triamcinolone (Barbiturates appear to enhance the metabolism of exogenous corticosteroids probably through the induction of hepatic microsomal enzymes. Patients stabilized on corticosteroid therapy may require dosage adjustments if barbiturates are added to or withdrawn from their dosage regimen).
No products indexed under this heading.

Triamcinolone Acetonide (Barbiturates appear to enhance the metabolism of exogenous corticosteroids probably through the induction of hepatic microsomal enzymes. Patients stabilized on corticosteroid therapy may require dosage adjustments if barbiturates are added to or withdrawn from their dosage regimen). Products include:
Azmacort Inhalation Aerosol 1701
Nasacort HFA Inhalation Aerosol 2939
Nasacort AQ Nasal Spray 2937

Triamcinolone Diacetate (Barbiturates appear to enhance the metabolism of exogenous corticosteroids probably through the induction of hepatic microsomal enzymes. Patients stabilized on corticosteroid therapy may require dosage adjustments if barbiturates are added to or withdrawn from their dosage regimen).
No products indexed under this heading.

Triamcinolone Hexacetonide (Barbiturates appear to enhance the metabolism of exogenous corticosteroids probably through the induction of hepatic microsomal enzymes. Patients stabilized on corticosteroid therapy may require dosage adjustments if barbiturates are added to or withdrawn from their dosage regimen).
No products indexed under this heading.

Triazolam (The concomitant use of other central nervous system depressants, including other sedatives or hypnotics, antihistamines, tranquilizers, or alcohol, may produce additive depressant effects).
No products indexed under this heading.

Trifluoperazine Hydrochloride (The concomitant use of other central nervous system depressants, including other sedatives or hypnotics, antihistamines, tranquilizers, or alcohol, may produce additive depressant effects).
No products indexed under this heading.

Valproate Sodium (Sodium valproate and valproic acid appear to decrease barbiturate metabolism, therefore barbiturate blood levels should be monitored and appropriate dosage adjustments made as indicated). Products include:
Depacon Injection 412

Valproic Acid (Sodium valproate and valproic acid appear to decrease barbiturate metabolism; therefore, barbiturate blood levels should be monitored and appropriate dosage adjustments made as indicated). Products include:
Depakene 417

Warfarin Sodium (Barbiturates can induce hepatic microsomal enzymes

resulting in increased metabolism and decreased anticoagulant response of oral anticoagulants. Patients stabilized on anticoagulant therapy may require dosage adjustments if barbiturates are added to or withdrawn from their dosage regimen). Products include:
Coumadin for Injection 932
Coumadin Tablets 932

Zaleplon (The concomitant use of other central nervous system depressants, including other sedatives or hypnotics, antihistamines, tranquilizers, or alcohol, may produce additive depressant effects). Products include:
Sonata Capsules 1686

Ziprasidone Hydrochloride (The concomitant use of other central nervous system depressants, including other sedatives or hypnotics, antihistamines, tranquilizers, or alcohol, may produce additive depressant effects). Products include:
Geodon Capsules 2514

Zolpidem Tartrate (The concomitant use of other central nervous system depressants, including other sedatives or hypnotics, antihistamines, tranquilizers, or alcohol, may produce additive depressant effects). Products include:
Ambien Tablets 2867

MEDERMA FOR KIDS TOPICAL GEL
(Allantoin, Allium cepa) 2097
None cited in PDR database.

MEDERMA TOPICAL GEL
(Allantoin, Allium cepa) 2096
None cited in PDR database.

MEFOXIN FOR INJECTION
(Cefoxitin Sodium) 1987
May interact with aminoglycosides and certain other agents. Compounds in these categories include:

Amikacin Sulfate (Increased nephrotoxicity).
No products indexed under this heading.

Gentamicin Sulfate (Increased nephrotoxicity). Products include:
Garamycin Injectable 3028
Genoptic Sterile Ophthalmic Solution.. ⊙ 227
Pred-G Ophthalmic Suspension ...... ⊙ 234
Pred-G Sterile Ophthalmic Ointment.. ⊙ 235

Kanamycin Sulfate (Increased nephrotoxicity).
No products indexed under this heading.

Probenecid (Higher serum levels of cefoxitin).
No products indexed under this heading.

Streptomycin Sulfate (Increased nephrotoxicity).
No products indexed under this heading.

Tobramycin (Increased nephrotoxicity). Products include:
TOBI Solution for Inhalation 1015
TobraDex Ophthalmic Ointment 558
TobraDex Ophthalmic Suspension ... 558
Zylet Ophthalmic Suspension 3508

Tobramycin Sulfate (Increased nephrotoxicity).
No products indexed under this heading.

MEFOXIN PREMIXED INTRAVENOUS SOLUTION
(Cefoxitin Sodium) 1990
May interact with aminoglycosides and certain other agents. Compounds in these categories include:

Amikacin Sulfate (Increased nephrotoxicity).
No products indexed under this heading.

Gentamicin Sulfate (Increased nephrotoxicity). Products include:
Garamycin Injectable 3028
Genoptic Sterile Ophthalmic Solution.. ⊙ 227
Pred-G Ophthalmic Suspension ...... ⊙ 234
Pred-G Sterile Ophthalmic Ointment.. ⊙ 235

Kanamycin Sulfate (Increased nephrotoxicity).
No products indexed under this heading.

Probenecid (Higher serum levels of cefoxitin).
No products indexed under this heading.

Streptomycin Sulfate (Increased nephrotoxicity).
No products indexed under this heading.

Tobramycin (Increased nephrotoxicity). Products include:
TOBI Solution for Inhalation 1015
TobraDex Ophthalmic Ointment 558
TobraDex Ophthalmic Suspension ... 558
Zylet Ophthalmic Suspension 3508

Tobramycin Sulfate (Increased nephrotoxicity).
No products indexed under this heading.

MEGA ANTIOXIDANT TABLETS
(Vitamins, Multiple) 3343
None cited in PDR database.

MEGA-B TABLETS
(Vitamin B Complex) 612
None cited in PDR database.

MEGACE ES ORAL SUSPENSION
(Megestrol Acetate) 2492
May interact with insulin and certain other agents. Compounds in these categories include:

Indinavir Sulfate (A pharmacokinetic study demonstrated that co-administration of megestrol acetate and indinavir results in a significant decrease in the pharmacokinetic parameters (approximately 36% for Cmax and approximately 28% for AUC) of indinavir. Administration of a higher dose of indinavir should be considered when co-administering with megestrol acetate). Products include:
Crixivan Capsules 1918

Insulin, Human, Zinc Suspension (Exacerbation of pre-existing diabetes with increased insulin requirements has been reported in association with concomitant use of megestrol acetate). Products include:
Humulin L, 100 Units 1763
Humulin U, 100 Units 1770

Insulin, Human NPH (Exacerbation of pre-existing diabetes with increased insulin requirements has been reported in association with concomitant use of megestrol acetate). Products include:
Humulin N, 100 Units 1764
Humulin N Pen 1765
Novolin N Human Insulin 10 ml Vials 2322
Novolin N InnoLet 2322
Novolin N PenFill 3 ml Cartridges 2325
Novolin R InnoLet 2322

Insulin, Human Regular (Exacerbation of pre-existing diabetes with increased insulin requirements has been reported in association with concomitant use of megestrol acetate). Products include:
Humulin R (U-500) 1768
Humulin R, 100 Units 1767
Novolin R Human Insulin 10 ml Vials 2322
Novolin R PenFill 2325

Insulin, Human Regular and Human NPH Mixture (Exacerbation of pre-existing diabetes with increased insulin requirements has been reported in association with concomitant use of megestrol acetate). Products include:
Humulin 50/50, 100 Units 1760
Humulin 70/30 Pen 1761
Novolin 70/30 Human Insulin 10 ml Vials 2321
Novolin 70/30 InnoLet 2322
Novolin 70/30 PenFill 3 ml Cartridges.................................... 2325

Insulin, NPH (Exacerbation of pre-existing diabetes with increased insulin requirements has been reported in association with concomitant use of megestrol acetate).
No products indexed under this heading.

Insulin, Regular (Exacerbation of pre-existing diabetes with increased insulin requirements has been reported in association with concomitant use of megestrol acetate).
No products indexed under this heading.

Insulin, Zinc Crystals (Exacerbation of pre-existing diabetes with increased insulin requirements has been reported in association with concomitant use of megestrol acetate).
No products indexed under this heading.

Insulin, Zinc Suspension (Exacerbation of pre-existing diabetes with increased insulin requirements has been reported in association with concomitant use of megestrol acetate).
No products indexed under this heading.

Insulin Aspart, Human Regular (Exacerbation of pre-existing diabetes with increased insulin requirements has been reported in association with concomitant use of megestrol acetate). Products include:
NovoLog Injection 2326

Insulin glargine (Exacerbation of pre-existing diabetes with increased insulin requirements has been reported in association with concomitant use of megestrol acetate). Products include:
Lantus Injection 2925

Insulin Lispro, Human (Exacerbation of pre-existing diabetes with increased insulin requirements has been reported in association with concomitant use of megestrol acetate). Products include:
Humalog-Pen 1751
Humalog Mix 75/25-Pen 1754

Insulin Lispro Protamine, Human (Exacerbation of pre-existing diabetes with increased insulin requirements has been reported in association with concomitant use of megestrol acetate). Products include:
Humalog Mix 75/25-Pen 1754

MENACTRA VACCINE
(Meningococcal Polysaccharide Diphtheria Toxoid Conjugate Vaccine).. 2968
May interact with alkylating agents, antimetabolites, anticoagulants, corticosteroids, oral anticoagulants, cytotoxic drugs, immunosuppressive agents, and nitrogen-mustard-type alkylating agents. Compounds in these categories include:

Anisindione (Because of the risk of hemorrhage, avoid use with concomitant anticoagulant therapy unless the potential benefit clearly outweighs the risk of administration). Products include:
Miradon Tablets 3056

Ardeparin Sodium (Because of the risk of hemorrhage, avoid use with concomitant anticoagulant therapy unless the potential benefit clearly outweighs the risk of administration).
No products indexed under this heading.

Azathioprine (Immunosuppressive therapies, including irradiation, antimetabolites, alkylating agents, cytotoxic drugs, and corticosteroids (used in greater than physiologic doses) may reduce the immune response to vaccines). Products include:
Azasan Tablets 2844

Basiliximab (Immunosuppressive therapies, including irradiation, antimetabolites, alkylating agents, cytotoxic drugs, and corticosteroids (used in greater than physiologic doses) may reduce the immune response to vaccines). Products include:
Simulect for Injection 2268

Betamethasone Acetate (Immunosuppressive therapies, including irradiation, antimetabolites, alkylating agents, cytotoxic drugs, and corticosteroids (used in greater than physiologic doses) may reduce the immune response to vaccines).
No products indexed under this heading.

Betamethasone Sodium Phosphate (Immunosuppressive therapies, including irradiation, antimetabolites, alkylating agents, cytotoxic drugs, and corticosteroids (used in greater than physiologic doses) may reduce the immune response to vaccines).
No products indexed under this heading.

Bleomycin Sulfate (Immunosuppressive therapies, including irradiation, antimetabolites, alkylating agents, cytotoxic drugs, and corticosteroids (used in greater than physiologic doses) may reduce the immune response to vaccines).
No products indexed under this heading.

Busulfan (Immunosuppressive therapies, including irradiation, antimetabolites, alkylating agents, cytotoxic drugs, and corticosteroids (used in greater than physiologic doses) may reduce the immune response to vaccines). Products include:
I.V. Busulfex 1125
Myleran Tablets 1492

Capecitabine (Immunosuppressive therapies, including irradiation, anti-

metabolites, alkylating agents, cytotoxic drugs, and corticosteroids (used in greater than physiologic doses) may reduce the immune response to vaccines). Products include:

Xeloda Tablets 2825

Carmustine (BCNU) (Immunosuppressive therapies, including irradiation, antimetabolites, alkylating agents, cytotoxic drugs, and corticosteroids (used in greater than physiologic doses) may reduce the immune response to vaccines).

No products indexed under this heading.

Chlorambucil (Immunosuppressive therapies, including irradiation, antimetabolites, alkylating agents, cytotoxic drugs, and corticosteroids (used in greater than physiologic doses) may reduce the immune response to vaccines). Products include:

Leukeran Tablets 1472

Cladribine (Immunosuppressive therapies, including irradiation, antimetabolites, alkylating agents, cytotoxic drugs, and corticosteroids (used in greater than physiologic doses) may reduce the immune response to vaccines). Products include:

Leustatin Injection 2368

Cortisone Acetate (Immunosuppressive therapies, including irradiation, antimetabolites, alkylating agents, cytotoxic drugs, and corticosteroids (used in greater than physiologic doses) may reduce the immune response to vaccines).

No products indexed under this heading.

Cyclophosphamide (Immunosuppressive therapies, including irradiation, antimetabolites, alkylating agents, cytotoxic drugs, and corticosteroids (used in greater than physiologic doses) may reduce the immune response to vaccines).

No products indexed under this heading.

Cyclosporine (Immunosuppressive therapies, including irradiation, antimetabolites, alkylating agents, cytotoxic drugs, and corticosteroids (used in greater than physiologic doses) may reduce the immune response to vaccines). Products include:

Gengraf Capsules 458
Neoral Soft Gelatin Capsules 2247
Neoral Oral Solution 2247
Restasis Ophthalmic Emulsion 570
Sandimmune 2259

Cytarabine (Immunosuppressive therapies, including irradiation, antimetabolites, alkylating agents, cytotoxic drugs, and corticosteroids (used in greater than physiologic doses) may reduce the immune response to vaccines).

No products indexed under this heading.

Dacarbazine (Immunosuppressive therapies, including irradiation, antimetabolites, alkylating agents, cytotoxic drugs, and corticosteroids (used in greater than physiologic doses) may reduce the immune response to vaccines).

No products indexed under this heading.

Dalteparin Sodium (Because of the risk of hemorrhage, avoid use with concomitant anticoagulant therapy unless the potential benefit clearly outweighs the risk of administration). Products include:

Fragmin Injection 2638

Danaparoid Sodium (Because of the risk of hemorrhage, avoid use with concomitant anticoagulant therapy unless the potential benefit clearly outweighs the risk of administration).

No products indexed under this heading.

Daunorubicin Hydrochloride (Immunosuppressive therapies, including irradiation, antimetabolites, alkylating agents, cytotoxic drugs, and corticosteroids (used in greater than physiologic doses) may reduce the immune response to vaccines). Products include:

Cerubidine for Injection 788

Dexamethasone (Immunosuppressive therapies, including irradiation, antimetabolites, alkylating agents, cytotoxic drugs, and corticosteroids (used in greater than physiologic doses) may reduce the immune response to vaccines). Products include:

Ciprodex Otic Suspension 555
Decadron Tablets 1929
TobraDex Ophthalmic Ointment 558
TobraDex Ophthalmic Suspension 558

Dexamethasone Acetate (Immunosuppressive therapies, including irradiation, antimetabolites, alkylating agents, cytotoxic drugs, and corticosteroids (used in greater than physiologic doses) may reduce the immune response to vaccines).

No products indexed under this heading.

Dexamethasone Sodium Phosphate (Immunosuppressive therapies, including irradiation, antimetabolites, alkylating agents, cytotoxic drugs, and corticosteroids (used in greater than physiologic doses) may reduce the immune response to vaccines). Products include:

Decadron Phosphate Injection 1931

Dicumarol (Because of the risk of hemorrhage, avoid use with concomitant anticoagulant therapy unless the potential benefit clearly outweighs the risk of administration).

No products indexed under this heading.

Doxorubicin Hydrochloride (Immunosuppressive therapies, including irradiation, antimetabolites, alkylating agents, cytotoxic drugs, and corticosteroids (used in greater than physiologic doses) may reduce the immune response to vaccines). Products include:

Adriamycin for Injection, USP 786
Adriamycin Injection, USP 786

Enoxaparin Sodium (Because of the risk of hemorrhage, avoid use with concomitant anticoagulant therapy unless the potential benefit clearly outweighs the risk of administration). Products include:

Lovenox Injection 2931

Epirubicin Hydrochloride (Immunosuppressive therapies, including irradiation, antimetabolites, alkylating agents, cytotoxic drugs, and corticosteroids (used in greater than physiologic doses) may reduce the immune response to vaccines). Products include:

Ellence Injection 2632

Estramustine Phosphate Sodium (Immunosuppressive therapies, including irradiation, antimetabolites, alkylating agents, cytotoxic drugs, and corticosteroids (used in greater than physiologic doses) may reduce the immune response to vaccines). Products include:

Emcyt Capsules 3137

Floxuridine (Immunosuppressive therapies, including irradiation, antimetabolites, alkylating agents, cytotoxic drugs, and corticosteroids (used in greater than physiologic doses) may reduce the immune response to vaccines).

No products indexed under this heading.

Fludarabine Phosphate (Immunosuppressive therapies, including irradiation, antimetabolites, alkylating agents, cytotoxic drugs, and corticosteroids (used in greater than physiologic doses) may reduce the immune response to vaccines).

No products indexed under this heading.

Fludrocortisone Acetate (Immunosuppressive therapies, including irradiation, antimetabolites, alkylating agents, cytotoxic drugs, and corticosteroids (used in greater than physiologic doses) may reduce the immune response to vaccines).

No products indexed under this heading.

Fluorouracil (Immunosuppressive therapies, including irradiation, antimetabolites, alkylating agents, cytotoxic drugs, and corticosteroids (used in greater than physiologic doses) may reduce the immune response to vaccines). Products include:

Carac Cream, 0.5% 1048
Efudex 3348

Fondaparinux Sodium (Because of the risk of hemorrhage, avoid use with concomitant anticoagulant therapy unless the potential benefit clearly outweighs the risk of administration). Products include:

Arixtra Injection 1325

Gemcitabine Hydrochloride (Immunosuppressive therapies, including irradiation, antimetabolites, alkylating agents, cytotoxic drugs, and corticosteroids (used in greater than physiologic doses) may reduce the immune response to vaccines). Products include:

Gemzar for Injection 1743

Heparin Calcium (Because of the risk of hemorrhage, avoid use with concomitant anticoagulant therapy unless the potential benefit clearly outweighs the risk of administration).

No products indexed under this heading.

Heparin Sodium (Because of the risk of hemorrhage, avoid use with concomitant anticoagulant therapy unless the potential benefit clearly outweighs the risk of administration).

No products indexed under this heading.

Hydrocortisone (Immunosuppressive therapies, including irradiation, antimetabolites, alkylating agents, cytotoxic drugs, and corticosteroids (used in greater than physiologic doses) may reduce the immune response to vaccines). Products include:

Cortizone•5 Ointment 699
Cortizone•10 Creme 699
Cortizone•10 Ointment 699
Cortizone•10 Plus Creme 700
Cortizone•10 Maximum Strength Quick Shot Spray 700
Hydrocortone Tablets 1963
Preparation H Hydrocortisone Cream 748

Hydrocortisone Acetate (Immunosuppressive therapies, including irradiation, antimetabolites, alkylating agents, cytotoxic drugs, and corticosteroids (used in greater than physiologic doses) may reduce the immune response to vaccines). Products include:

Analpram-HC 1136
Pramosone 1139
ProctoFoam-HC 3113
Tucks Anti-Itch Ointment 712
U-cort 1% Cream 3289

Hydrocortisone Sodium Phosphate (Immunosuppressive therapies, including irradiation, antimetabolites, alkylating agents, cytotoxic drugs, and corticosteroids (used in greater than physiologic doses) may reduce the immune response to vaccines).

No products indexed under this heading.

Hydrocortisone Sodium Succinate (Immunosuppressive therapies, including irradiation, antimetabolites, alkylating agents, cytotoxic drugs, and corticosteroids (used in greater than physiologic doses) may reduce the immune response to vaccines).

No products indexed under this heading.

Hydroxyurea (Immunosuppressive therapies, including irradiation, antimetabolites, alkylating agents, cytotoxic drugs, and corticosteroids (used in greater than physiologic doses) may reduce the immune response to vaccines).

No products indexed under this heading.

Lomustine (CCNU) (Immunosuppressive therapies, including irradiation, antimetabolites, alkylating agents, cytotoxic drugs, and corticosteroids (used in greater than physiologic doses) may reduce the immune response to vaccines).

No products indexed under this heading.

Low Molecular Weight Heparins (Because of the risk of hemorrhage, avoid use with concomitant anticoagulant therapy unless the potential benefit clearly outweighs the risk of administration).

No products indexed under this heading.

Mechlorethamine Hydrochloride (Immunosuppressive therapies, including irradiation, antimetabolites, alkylating agents, cytotoxic drugs, and corticosteroids (used in greater than physiologic doses) may reduce the immune response to vaccines). Products include:

Mustargen for Injection 2007

Melphalan (Immunosuppressive therapies, including irradiation, antimetabolites, alkylating agents, cytotoxic drugs, and corticosteroids (used in greater than physiologic doses) may reduce the immune response to vaccines). Products include:

Alkeran Tablets 977

Mercaptopurine (Immunosuppressive therapies, including irradiation, antimetabolites, alkylating agents, cytotoxic drugs, and corticosteroids (used in greater than physiologic

doses) may reduce the immune response to vaccines). Products include:

Purinethol Tablets 1222

Methotrexate (Immunosuppressive therapies, including irradiation, antimetabolites, alkylating agents, cytotoxic drugs, and corticosteroids (used in greater than physiologic doses) may reduce the immune response to vaccines).

No products indexed under this heading.

Methotrexate Sodium (Immunosuppressive therapies, including irradiation, antimetabolites, alkylating agents, cytotoxic drugs, and corticosteroids (used in greater than physiologic doses) may reduce the immune response to vaccines).

No products indexed under this heading.

Methylprednisolone Acetate (Immunosuppressive therapies, including irradiation, antimetabolites, alkylating agents, cytotoxic drugs, and corticosteroids (used in greater than physiologic doses) may reduce the immune response to vaccines). Products include:

Depo-Medrol Injectable Suspension 2615
Depo-Medrol Single-Dose Vial 2617

Methylprednisolone Sodium Succinate (Immunosuppressive therapies, including irradiation, antimetabolites, alkylating agents, cytotoxic drugs, and corticosteroids (used in greater than physiologic doses) may reduce the immune response to vaccines).

No products indexed under this heading.

Mitotane (Immunosuppressive therapies, including irradiation, antimetabolites, alkylating agents, cytotoxic drugs, and corticosteroids (used in greater than physiologic doses) may reduce the immune response to vaccines).

No products indexed under this heading.

Mitoxantrone Hydrochloride (Immunosuppressive therapies, including irradiation, antimetabolites, alkylating agents, cytotoxic drugs, and corticosteroids (used in greater than physiologic doses) may reduce the immune response to vaccines). Products include:

Novantrone for Injection Concentrate 3158

Muromonab-CD3 (Immunosuppressive therapies, including irradiation, antimetabolites, alkylating agents, cytotoxic drugs, and corticosteroids (used in greater than physiologic doses) may reduce the immune response to vaccines). Products include:

Orthoclone OKT3 Sterile Solution 2370

Mycophenolate Mofetil (Immunosuppressive therapies, including irradiation, antimetabolites, alkylating agents, cytotoxic drugs, and corticosteroids (used in greater than physiologic doses) may reduce the immune response to vaccines). Products include:

CellCept Capsules 2751
CellCept Oral Suspension 2751
CellCept Tablets 2751

Pentostatin (Immunosuppressive therapies, including irradiation, antimetabolites, alkylating agents, cytotoxic drugs, and corticosteroids (used in greater than physiologic doses) may reduce the immune response to vaccines). Products include:

Nipent for Injection 3216

Prednisolone Acetate (Immunosuppressive therapies, including irradiation, antimetabolites, alkylating agents, cytotoxic drugs, and corticosteroids (used in greater than physiologic doses) may reduce the immune response to vaccines). Products include:

Blephamide Ophthalmic Ointment 563
Blephamide Ophthalmic Suspension 564
Poly-Pred Liquifilm Ophthalmic Suspension .... ⊙231
Pred Forte Ophthalmic Suspension .... ⊙233
Pred Mild Sterile Ophthalmic Suspension .... ⊙236
Pred-G Ophthalmic Suspension .... ⊙234
Pred-G Sterile Ophthalmic Ointment .... ⊙235

Prednisolone Sodium Phosphate (Immunosuppressive therapies, including irradiation, antimetabolites, alkylating agents, cytotoxic drugs, and corticosteroids (used in greater than physiologic doses) may reduce the immune response to vaccines). Products include:

Pediapred Oral Solution 3319

Prednisolone Tebutate (Immunosuppressive therapies, including irradiation, antimetabolites, alkylating agents, cytotoxic drugs, and corticosteroids (used in greater than physiologic doses) may reduce the immune response to vaccines).

No products indexed under this heading.

Prednisone (Immunosuppressive therapies, including irradiation, antimetabolites, alkylating agents, cytotoxic drugs, and corticosteroids (used in greater than physiologic doses) may reduce the immune response to vaccines).

No products indexed under this heading.

Procarbazine Hydrochloride (Immunosuppressive therapies, including irradiation, antimetabolites, alkylating agents, cytotoxic drugs, and corticosteroids (used in greater than physiologic doses) may reduce the immune response to vaccines). Products include:

Matulane Capsules 3188

Sirolimus (Immunosuppressive therapies, including irradiation, antimetabolites, alkylating agents, cytotoxic drugs, and corticosteroids (used in greater than physiologic doses) may reduce the immune response to vaccines). Products include:

Rapamune Oral Solution and Tablets 3472

Tacrolimus (Immunosuppressive therapies, including irradiation, antimetabolites, alkylating agents, cytotoxic drugs, and corticosteroids (used in greater than physiologic doses) may reduce the immune response to vaccines). Products include:

Prograf Capsules and Injection 624
Protopic Ointment 629

Tamoxifen Citrate (Immunosuppressive therapies, including irradiation, antimetabolites, alkylating agents, cytotoxic drugs, and corticosteroids (used in greater than physiologic doses) may reduce the immune response to vaccines).

No products indexed under this heading.

Thioguanine (Immunosuppressive therapies, including irradiation, antimetabolites, alkylating agents, cytotoxic drugs, and corticosteroids (used in greater than physiologic doses) may reduce the immune response to vaccines). Products include:

Tabloid Tablets 1545

Thiotepa (Immunosuppressive therapies, including irradiation, antimetabolites, alkylating agents, cytotoxic drugs, and corticosteroids (used in greater than physiologic doses) may reduce the immune response to vaccines).

No products indexed under this heading.

Tinzaparin Sodium (Because of the risk of hemorrhage, avoid use with concomitant anticoagulant therapy unless the potential benefit clearly outweighs the risk of administration).

No products indexed under this heading.

Triamcinolone (Immunosuppressive therapies, including irradiation, antimetabolites, alkylating agents, cytotoxic drugs, and corticosteroids (used in greater than physiologic doses) may reduce the immune response to vaccines).

No products indexed under this heading.

Triamcinolone Acetonide (Immunosuppressive therapies, including irradiation, antimetabolites, alkylating agents, cytotoxic drugs, and corticosteroids (used in greater than physiologic doses) may reduce the immune response to vaccines). Products include:

Azmacort Inhalation Aerosol 1701
Nasacort HFA Inhalation Aerosol 2939
Nasacort AQ Nasal Spray 2937

Triamcinolone Diacetate (Immunosuppressive therapies, including irradiation, antimetabolites, alkylating agents, cytotoxic drugs, and corticosteroids (used in greater than physiologic doses) may reduce the immune response to vaccines).

No products indexed under this heading.

Triamcinolone Hexacetonide (Immunosuppressive therapies, including irradiation, antimetabolites, alkylating agents, cytotoxic drugs, and corticosteroids (used in greater than physiologic doses) may reduce the immune response to vaccines).

No products indexed under this heading.

Vincristine Sulfate (Immunosuppressive therapies, including irradiation, antimetabolites, alkylating agents, cytotoxic drugs, and corticosteroids (used in greater than physiologic doses) may reduce the immune response to vaccines).

No products indexed under this heading.

Warfarin Sodium (Because of the risk of hemorrhage, avoid use with concomitant anticoagulant therapy unless the potential benefit clearly outweighs the risk of administration). Products include:

Coumadin for Injection 932
Coumadin Tablets 932

MENOPUR FOR SUBCUTANEOUS INJECTION

(Menotropins) 1145
None cited in PDR database.

MENOSTAR TRANSDERMAL SYSTEM

(Estradiol) 805
May interact with erythromycin. Compounds in these categories include:

Carbamazepine (Inducers of CYP3A4, such as carbamazepine, may reduce plasma concentrations of estrogens, possibly resulting in a decrease in therapeutic effects and/or changes in uterine bleeding profile). Products include:

Carbatrol Capsules 3174
Equetro Extended-Release Capsules 3178
Tegretol/Tegretol-XR 2278

Clarithromycin (Inhibitors of CYP3A4, such as clarithromycin, may increase plasma concentrations of estrogens and may result in side effects). Products include:

Biaxin/Biaxin XL 402
PREVPAC 3281

Erythromycin (Inhibitors of CYP3A4, such as erythromycin, may increase plasma concentrations of estrogens and may result in side effects). Products include:

Erygel Topical Gel 2096
Ery-Tab Tablets 447
Erythromycin Base Filmtab Tablets 454
Erythromycin Delayed-Release Capsules, USP 456
PCE Dispertab Tablets 510

Erythromycin Estolate (Inhibitors of CYP3A4, such as erythromycin, may increase plasma concentrations of estrogens and may result in side effects).

No products indexed under this heading.

Erythromycin Ethylsuccinate (Inhibitors of CYP3A4, such as erythromycin, may increase plasma concentrations of estrogens and may result in side effects). Products include:

E.E.S. 449
EryPed 445

Erythromycin Gluceptate (Inhibitors of CYP3A4, such as erythromycin, may increase plasma concentrations of estrogens and may result in side effects).

No products indexed under this heading.

Erythromycin Lactobionate (Inhibitors of CYP3A4, such as erythromycin, may increase plasma concentrations of estrogens and may result in side effects).

No products indexed under this heading.

Erythromycin Stearate (Inhibitors of CYP3A4, such as erythromycin, may increase plasma concentrations of estrogens and may result in side effects). Products include:

Erythrocin Stearate Filmtab Tablets 452

Hypericum Perforatum (Inducers of CYP3A4, such as St. John's Wort preparations (Hypericum perforatum), may reduce plasma concentrations of estrogens, possibly resulting in a decrease in therapeutic effects and/or changes in uterine bleeding profile).

No products indexed under this heading.

Itraconazole (Inhibitors of CYP3A4, such as itraconazole, may increase plasma concentrations of estrogens and may result in side effects).
No products indexed under this heading.

Ketoconazole (Inhibitors of CYP3A4, such as ketoconazole, may increase plasma concentrations of estrogens and may result in side effects). Products include:
Nizoral A-D Shampoo, 1% 1839
Nizoral 2% Shampoo 1838

Phenobarbital (Inducers of CYP3A4, such as phenobarbital, may reduce plasma concentrations of estrogens, possibly resulting in a decrease in therapeutic effects and/or changes in uterine bleeding profile).
No products indexed under this heading.

Phenobarbital Sodium (Inducers of CYP3A4, such as phenobarbital, may reduce plasma concentrations of estrogens, possibly resulting in a decrease in therapeutic effects and/or changes in uterine bleeding profile).
No products indexed under this heading.

Rifampin (Inducers of CYP3A4, such as rifampin, may reduce plasma concentrations of estrogens, possibly resulting in a decrease in therapeutic effects and/or changes in uterine bleeding profile).
No products indexed under this heading.

Ritonavir (Inhibitors of CYP3A4, such as ritonavir, may increase plasma concentrations of estrogens and may result in side effects). Products include:
Kaletra 474
Norvir 499

Food Interactions

Grapefruit Juice (Inhibitors of CYP3A4, such as grapefruit juice, may increase plasma concentrations of estrogens and may result in side effects).

MENTAX CREAM

(Butenafine Hydrochloride) 2152
None cited in PDR database.

MEPHYTON TABLETS

(Vitamin K_1) 1993
None cited in PDR database.

MEPRON SUSPENSION

(Atovaquone) 1487
May interact with highly protein bound drugs (selected) and certain other agents. Compounds in these categories include:

Amiodarone Hydrochloride (Atovaquone is highly bound to plasma protein (greater than 99.9%); caution is advised when co-administered with other highly protein bound drugs with narrow therapeutic indices). Products include:
Pacerone Tablets 3337

Amitriptyline Hydrochloride (Atovaquone is highly bound to plasma protein (greater than 99.9%); caution is advised when co-administered with other highly protein bound drugs with narrow therapeutic indices).
No products indexed under this heading.

Cefonicid Sodium (Atovaquone is highly bound to plasma protein (greater than 99.9%); caution is advised when co-administered with other highly protein bound drugs with narrow therapeutic indices).
No products indexed under this heading.

Celecoxib (Atovaquone is highly bound to plasma protein (greater than 99.9%); caution is advised when co-administered with other highly protein bound drugs with narrow therapeutic indices). Products include:
Celebrex Capsules 3130

Chlordiazepoxide (Atovaquone is highly bound to plasma protein (greater than 99.9%); caution is advised when co-administered with other highly protein bound drugs with narrow therapeutic indices).
No products indexed under this heading.

Chlordiazepoxide Hydrochloride (Atovaquone is highly bound to plasma protein (greater than 99.9%); caution is advised when co-administered with other highly protein bound drugs with narrow therapeutic indices). Products include:
Librium Capsules 3349

Chlorpromazine (Atovaquone is highly bound to plasma protein (greater than 99.9%); caution is advised when co-administered with other highly protein bound drugs with narrow therapeutic indices).
No products indexed under this heading.

Chlorpromazine Hydrochloride (Atovaquone is highly bound to plasma protein (greater than 99.9%); caution is advised when co-administered with other highly protein bound drugs with narrow therapeutic indices).
No products indexed under this heading.

Clomipramine Hydrochloride (Atovaquone is highly bound to plasma protein (greater than 99.9%); caution is advised when co-administered with other highly protein bound drugs with narrow therapeutic indices).
No products indexed under this heading.

Clozapine (Atovaquone is highly bound to plasma protein (greater than 99.9%); caution is advised when co-administered with other highly protein bound drugs with narrow therapeutic indices). Products include:
Clozapine Tablets 2141
Clozaril Tablets 2174
FazaClo Orally Disintegrating Tablets 547

Cyclosporine (Atovaquone is highly bound to plasma protein (greater than 99.9%); caution is advised when co-administered with other highly protein bound drugs with narrow therapeutic indices). Products include:
Gengraf Capsules 458
Neoral Soft Gelatin Capsules 2247
Neoral Oral Solution 2247
Restasis Ophthalmic Emulsion 570
Sandimmune 2259

Diazepam (Atovaquone is highly bound to plasma protein (greater than 99.9%); caution is advised when co-administered with other highly protein bound drugs with narrow therapeutic indices). Products include:
Diastat Rectal Delivery System 3344
Valium Tablets 2822

Diclofenac Potassium (Atovaquone is highly bound to plasma protein (greater than 99.9%); caution is advised when co-administered with other highly protein bound drugs with narrow therapeutic indices). Products include:
Cataflam Tablets 2173

Diclofenac Sodium (Atovaquone is highly bound to plasma protein (greater than 99.9%); caution is advised when co-administered with other highly protein bound drugs with narrow therapeutic indices). Products include:
Arthrotec Tablets 3126
Voltaren Ophthalmic Solution 2300
Voltaren Tablets 2298
Voltaren-XR Tablets 2301

Dipyridamole (Atovaquone is highly bound to plasma protein (greater than 99.9%); caution is advised when co-administered with other highly protein bound drugs with narrow therapeutic indices). Products include:
Aggrenox Capsules 855
Persantine Tablets 898

Fenoprofen Calcium (Atovaquone is highly bound to plasma protein (greater than 99.9%); caution is advised when co-administered with other highly protein bound drugs with narrow therapeutic indices). Products include:
Nalfon Capsules 2504

Flurazepam Hydrochloride (Atovaquone is highly bound to plasma protein (greater than 99.9%); caution is advised when co-administered with other highly protein bound drugs with narrow therapeutic indices). Products include:
Dalmane Capsules 3343

Flurbiprofen (Atovaquone is highly bound to plasma protein (greater than 99.9%); caution is advised when co-administered with other highly protein bound drugs with narrow therapeutic indices).
No products indexed under this heading.

Glipizide (Atovaquone is highly bound to plasma protein (greater than 99.9%); caution is advised when co-administered with other highly protein bound drugs with narrow therapeutic indices).
No products indexed under this heading.

Ibuprofen (Atovaquone is highly bound to plasma protein (greater than 99.9%); caution is advised when co-administered with other highly protein bound drugs with narrow therapeutic indices). Products include:
Advil Allergy Sinus Caplets 737
Advil 737
Children's Advil Suspension 742
Children's Advil Chewable Tablets .. 741
Advil Cold & Sinus 739
Advil Flu & Body Ache Caplets 739
Children's Advil Cold Suspension ... 741
Infants' Advil Concentrated Drops .. 743
Junior Strength Advil Swallow Tablets 740
Advil Migraine Liquigels 740
Advil Multi-Symptom Cold Caplets 738
Combunox Tablets 1183
Children's Motrin Oral Suspension and Chewable Tablets 1837
Children's Motrin Cold Non-Staining Dye-Free Oral Suspension 1838
Children's Motrin Cold Oral Suspension 1838
Children's Motrin Non-Staining Dye-Free Oral Suspension 1837
Motrin Cold & Sinus Caplets 1836
Motrin IB Tablets and Caplets 1836
Infants' Motrin Concentrated Drops 1837
Infants' Motrin Non-Staining Dye-Free Drops 1837
Junior Strength Motrin Caplets and Chewable Tablets 1837
Vicoprofen Tablets 533

Imipramine Hydrochloride (Atovaquone is highly bound to plasma protein (greater than 99.9%); caution is advised when co-administered with other highly protein bound drugs with narrow therapeutic indices).
No products indexed under this heading.

Imipramine Pamoate (Atovaquone is highly bound to plasma protein (greater than 99.9%); caution is advised when co-administered with other highly protein bound drugs with narrow therapeutic indices).
No products indexed under this heading.

Indomethacin (Atovaquone is highly bound to plasma protein (greater than 99.9%); caution is advised when co-administered with other highly protein bound drugs with narrow therapeutic indices). Products include:
Indocin 1968

Indomethacin Sodium Trihydrate (Atovaquone is highly bound to plasma protein (greater than 99.9%); caution is advised when co-administered with other highly protein bound drugs with narrow therapeutic indices). Products include:
Indocin I.V. 1973

Ketoprofen (Atovaquone is highly bound to plasma protein (greater than 99.9%); caution is advised when co-administered with other highly protein bound drugs with narrow therapeutic indices).
No products indexed under this heading.

Ketorolac Tromethamine (Atovaquone is highly bound to plasma protein (greater than 99.9%); caution is advised when co-administered with other highly protein bound drugs with narrow therapeutic indices). Products include:
Acular Ophthalmic Solution 561
Acular LS Ophthalmic Solution 562

Meclofenamate Sodium (Atovaquone is highly bound to plasma protein (greater than 99.9%); caution is advised when co-administered with other highly protein bound drugs with narrow therapeutic indices).
No products indexed under this heading.

Mefenamic Acid (Atovaquone is highly bound to plasma protein (greater than 99.9%); caution is advised when co-administered with other highly protein bound drugs with narrow therapeutic indices).
No products indexed under this heading.

Midazolam Hydrochloride (Atovaquone is highly bound to plasma protein (greater than 99.9%); caution is advised when co-administered with other highly protein bound drugs with narrow therapeutic indices).
No products indexed under this heading.

Naproxen (Atovaquone is highly bound to plasma protein (greater than 99.9%); caution is advised when co-administered with other highly protein bound drugs with narrow therapeutic indices). Products include:
EC-Naprosyn Delayed-Release Tablets 2769
Naprosyn Suspension 2769
Naprosyn Tablets 2769
Prevacid NapraPAC 3277

Naproxen Sodium (Atovaquone is highly bound to plasma protein (greater than 99.9%); caution is advised when co-administered with other highly protein bound drugs with narrow therapeutic indices). Products include:
Aleve Tablets, Caplets and Gelcaps .... ▣605
Anaprox Tablets 2769
Anaprox DS Tablets 2769

Nortriptyline Hydrochloride (Atovaquone is highly bound to plasma protein (greater than 99.9%); caution is advised when co-administered with other highly protein bound drugs with narrow therapeutic indices).
No products indexed under this heading.

Oxaprozin (Atovaquone is highly bound to plasma protein (greater than 99.9%); caution is advised when co-administered with other highly protein bound drugs with narrow therapeutic indices).
No products indexed under this heading.

Oxazepam (Atovaquone is highly bound to plasma protein (greater than 99.9%); caution is advised when co-administered with other highly protein bound drugs with narrow therapeutic indices).
No products indexed under this heading.

Phenylbutazone (Atovaquone is highly bound to plasma protein (greater than 99.9%); caution is advised when co-administered with other highly protein bound drugs with narrow therapeutic indices).
No products indexed under this heading.

Piroxicam (Atovaquone is highly bound to plasma protein (greater than 99.9%); caution is advised when co-administered with other highly protein bound drugs with narrow therapeutic indices).
No products indexed under this heading.

Propranolol Hydrochloride (Atovaquone is highly bound to plasma protein (greater than 99.9%); caution is advised when co-administered with other highly protein bound drugs with narrow therapeutic indices). Products include:
Inderal LA Long-Acting Capsules 3421
InnoPran XL Capsules 2728

Rifabutin (Due to structural similarity to rifampin, rifabutin may decrease average steady-state plasma atovaquone concentration).
No products indexed under this heading.

Rifampin (Co-administration with oral rifampin in HIV-infected individuals may result in a 52% ± 13% decrease in the average steady-state plasma atovaquone concentration and a 37% ± 42% increase in the average steady-state plasma rifampin concentration).
No products indexed under this heading.

Sulfamethoxazole (Co-administration with TMP-SMX may result in slight decrease in average steady-state concentrations of TMP-SMX; this effect is minor and would not expect to produce clinically significant events).
No products indexed under this heading.

Sulindac (Atovaquone is highly bound to plasma protein (greater than 99.9%); caution is advised when co-administered with other highly protein bound drugs with narrow therapeutic indices). Products include:
Clinoril Tablets 1899

Temazepam (Atovaquone is highly bound to plasma protein (greater than 99.9%); caution is advised when co-administered with other highly protein bound drugs with narrow therapeutic indices).
No products indexed under this heading.

Tolbutamide (Atovaquone is highly bound to plasma protein (greater than 99.9%); caution is advised when co-administered with other highly protein bound drugs with narrow therapeutic indices).
No products indexed under this heading.

Tolmetin Sodium (Atovaquone is highly bound to plasma protein (greater than 99.9%); caution is advised when co-administered with other highly protein bound drugs with narrow therapeutic indices).
No products indexed under this heading.

Trimethoprim (Co-administration with TMP-SMX may result in slight decrease in average steady-state concentrations of TMP-SMX; this effect is minor and would not expect to produce clinically significant events).
No products indexed under this heading.

Trimipramine Maleate (Atovaquone is highly bound to plasma protein (greater than 99.9%); caution is advised when co-administered with other highly protein bound drugs with narrow therapeutic indices). Products include:
Surmontil Capsules 2347

Warfarin Sodium (Atovaquone is highly bound to plasma protein (greater than 99.9%); caution is advised when co-administered with other highly protein bound drugs with narrow therapeutic indices). Products include:
Coumadin for Injection 932
Coumadin Tablets 932

Zidovudine (Atovaquone tablets have shown to decrease zidovudine apparent oral clearance leading to an increase in plasma zidovudine AUC; this effect is minor and would not expect to produce clinically significant events). Products include:
Combivir Tablets 1373
Retrovir 1533
Retrovir IV Infusion 1537
Trizivir Tablets 1565

Food Interactions

Food, unspecified (Food enhances absorption by approximately two-fold).

MERIDIA CAPSULES

(Sibutramine Hydrochloride Monohydrate) 485
May interact with anorexiants, erythromycin, lithium preparations, monoamine oxidase inhibitors, serotonergic agents, and certain other agents. Compounds in these categories include:

Amphetamine Resins (Concurrent use with other centrally acting appetite suppressant drugs is contraindicated).
No products indexed under this heading.

Benzphetamine Hydrochloride (Concurrent use with other centrally acting appetite suppressant drugs is contraindicated).
No products indexed under this heading.

Cimetidine (Co-administration has resulted in small increases in combined (M1 and M2 metabolites) plasma Cmax and AUC; these differences are unlikely to be of clinical significance). Products include:
Tagamet HB 200 Tablets .... ▣637
Tagamet Tablets 1547

Cimetidine Hydrochloride (Co-administration has resulted in small increases in combined (M1 and M2 metabolites) plasma Cmax and AUC; these differences are unlikely to be of clinical significance).
No products indexed under this heading.

Citalopram Hydrobromide (Sibutramine inhibits serotonin reuptake and serotonin syndrome, a rare, but serious constellation of symptoms, has been reported with the concomitant use of two SSRIs; concurrent use should be avoided). Products include:
Celexa 1177

Dexfenfluramine Hydrochloride (Concurrent use with other centrally acting appetite suppressant drugs is contraindicated).
No products indexed under this heading.

Dextroamphetamine Sulfate (Concurrent use with other centrally acting appetite suppressant drugs is contraindicated). Products include:
Adderall Tablets 3168
Adderall XR Capsules 3169
Dexedrine 1386
DextroStat Tablets 3177

Dextromethorphan Hydrobromide (Sibutramine inhibits serotonin reuptake and combination of SSRIs and dextromethorphan has resulted in serious, sometimes fatal, reactions, serotonin syndrome). Products include:
Alacol DM Syrup 739
Balamine DM 739
Contac Severe Cold and Flu Caplets Maximum Strength .... ▣615
Contac Severe Cold and Flu Caplets Non-Drowsy .... ▣615
Children's Dimetapp DM Cold & Cough Elixir .... ▣745
Children's Dimetapp Long Acting Cough Plus Cold Syrup .... ▣746
Dimetapp Infant Drops Decongestant Plus Cough .... ▣746
Mucinex DM Tablets .... ▣602
PediaCare Decongestant & Cough Infant Drops .... ▣705
PediaCare Freezer Pops Long-Acting Cough-Glacier Grape and Polar Berry Blue .... ▣706
PediaCare Long-Acting Cough Infant Drops .... ▣705
PediaCare Long-Acting Cough Plus Cold Liquid .... ▣704
PediaCare Multi-Symptom Cold Liquid .... ▣704
PediaCare NightRest Cough & Cold Liquid .... ▣704
Robitussin Allergy & Cough Syrup .. ▣750
Robitussin CF Liquid .... ▣755
Robitussin Cough & Cold Liquid-filled Capsules .... ▣750
Robitussin Cough, Cold & Flu Liquid-filled Capsules .... ▣750
Robitussin Cough & Cold Infant Drops .... ▣755
Robitussin DM Infant Drops .... ▣753
Robitussin DM Liquid .... ▣753
Robitussin Flu Liquid .... ▣752
Robitussin Maximum Strength Cough Liquid .... ▣754
Robitussin Maximum Strength Cough & Cold Liquid .... ▣754
Robitussin Pediatric Cough Liquid .... ▣754
Robitussin Pediatric Cough & Cold Liquid .... ▣754
Robitussin PM Cough & Cold Liquid .... ▣752
Robitussin Sugar Free Cough Liquid .... ▣753
Simply Cough Liquid 1840
Sudafed Severe Cold .... ▣710
TheraFlu Cold & Cough Hot Liquid .... ▣680
TheraFlu Flu & Chest Congestion Non-Drowsy Hot Liquid .... ▣681
TheraFlu Severe Cold Non-Drowsy Hot Liquid .... ▣683
TheraFlu Severe Cold & Cough Hot Liquid .... ▣683
TheraFlu Severe Cold Caplets .... ▣679
TheraFlu Severe Cold Hot Liquid .... ▣682
TheraFlu Severe Cold Non-Drowsy Caplets .... ▣679
TheraFlu Thin Strips Long Acting Cough .... ▣684
Triaminic Cold & Cough Liquid .... ▣685
Triaminic Cough Liquid .... ▣687
Triaminic Cough & Nasal Congestion Liquid .... ▣687
Triaminic Cough & Sore Throat Liquid .... ▣687
Triaminic Flu, Cough & Fever Liquid .... ▣685
Triaminic Night Time Cough & Cold Liquid .... ▣685
Triaminic Cold & Cough Softchews .... ▣688
Triaminic Cough & Sore Throat Softchews .... ▣689
Triaminic Thin Strips Long Acting Cough .... ▣689
Children's Tylenol Plus Cold & Cough Suspension Liquid and Chewable Tablets 1851
Children's Tylenol Plus Flu Suspension Liquid 1853
Concentrated Tylenol Infants' Drops Plus Cold and Cough 1851
Tylenol Cold & Flu Severe Daytime Liquid with Cool Burst 1846
Tylenol Cold & Flu Severe NightTime Liquid with Cool Burst 1846
Tylenol Cold Severe Congestion Non-Drowsy Caplets with Cool Burst 1846
Tylenol Cough & Sore Throat Daytime Liquid with Cool Burst 1849
Tylenol Cough & Sore Throat NightTime Liquid with Cool Burst 1849
Tylenol Flu Day Non-Drowsy Gelcaps 1846
Concentrated Tylenol Infants' Drops Plus Cold & Cough Nasal Decongestant, Fever Reducer & Pain Reliever .... ▣668
Multi-Symptom Tylenol Cold Night Time Caplets 1845
Multi-Symptom Tylenol Cold Day Non-Drowsy Caplets and Gelcaps 1845
Vicks 44 Cough Relief 2675

Vicks 44D Cough & Head Congestion Relief 2676
Vicks 44D Cough & Head Congestion Relief Liquid 721
Vicks 44E Cough & Chest Congestion Relief 2676
Pediatric Vicks 44e Cough & Chest Congestion Relief Liquid 2673
Vicks 44M Cough, Cold & Flu Relief 2676
Pediatric Vicks 44m Cough & Cold Relief 2673
Vicks DayQuil LiquiCaps/Liquid Multi-Symptom Cold/Flu Relief 723
Vicks DayQuil Multi-Symptom Cold/Flu Relief LiquiCaps 2675
Vicks DayQuil Multi-Symptom Cold/Flu Relief Liquid 2675
Children's Vicks NyQuil Cold/Cough Relief 2671
Vicks NyQuil Cough Liquid 2677
Vicks NyQuil LiquiCaps 2677
Vicks NyQuil LiquiCaps/Liquid Multi-Symptom Cold/Flu Relief 725
Vicks NyQuil Liquid 2677
Zicam Concentrated Cough Mist for Kids Cool Cherry 643
Zicam Concentrated Cough Mist for Kids Plus D Cool Cherry 643
Zicam Concentrated Cough Mist Nite-Cool Cherry 642
Zicam Concentrated Cough Mist Plus D Cool Cherry 642
Zicam Concentrated Cough Mist-Honey Lemon & Cool Cherry 642

Dextromethorphan Polistirex (Sibutramine inhibits serotonin reuptake and combination of SSRIs and dextromethorphan has resulted in serious, sometimes fatal, reactions, serotonin syndrome). Products include:
Delsym Extended-Release Suspension 611
Delsym 12 Hour Cough Suppressant for Children 611

Diethylpropion Hydrochloride (Concurrent use with other centrally acting appetite suppressant drugs is contraindicated).
No products indexed under this heading.

Dihydroergotamine Mesylate (Sibutramine inhibits serotonin reuptake and combination of SSRIs and agents for migraine, such as dihydroergotamine, has resulted in serious, sometimes fatal, reactions, serotonin syndrome). Products include:
Migranal Nasal Spray 3350

Erythromycin (Co-administration has resulted in a small increase in the AUC and a small reduction in Cmax of sibutramine metabolites). Products include:
Erygel Topical Gel 2096
Ery-Tab Tablets 447
Erythromycin Base Filmtab Tablets 454
Erythromycin Delayed-Release Capsules, USP 456
PCE Dispertab Tablets 510

Erythromycin Estolate (Co-administration has resulted in a small increase in the AUC and a small reduction in Cmax of sibutramine metabolites).
No products indexed under this heading.

Erythromycin Ethylsuccinate (Co-administration has resulted in a small increase in the AUC and a small reduction in Cmax of sibutramine metabolites). Products include:
E.E.S. 449
EryPed 445

Erythromycin Gluceptate (Co-administration has resulted in a small increase in the AUC and a small reduction in Cmax of sibutramine metabolites).
No products indexed under this heading.

Erythromycin Lactobionate (Co-administration has resulted in a small increase in the AUC and a small reduction in Cmax of sibutramine metabolites).
No products indexed under this heading.

Erythromycin Stearate (Co-administration has resulted in a small increase in the AUC and a small reduction in Cmax of sibutramine metabolites). Products include:
Erythrocin Stearate Filmtab Tablets 452

Escitalopram Oxalate (Sibutramine inhibits serotonin reuptake and serotonin syndrome, a rare, but serious constellation of symptoms, has been reported with the concomitant use of two SSRIs; concurrent use should be avoided). Products include:
Lexapro Oral Solution 1193
Lexapro Tablets 1193

Fenfluramine Hydrochloride (Concurrent use with other centrally acting appetite suppressant drugs is contraindicated).
No products indexed under this heading.

Fentanyl (Sibutramine inhibits serotonin reuptake and combination of SSRIs and certain opioids, such as fentanyl, has resulted in serious, sometimes fatal, reactions, serotonin syndrome). Products include:
Duragesic Transdermal System 2448

Fentanyl Citrate (Sibutramine inhibits serotonin reuptake and combination of SSRIs and certain opioids, such as fentanyl, has resulted in serious, sometimes fatal, reactions, serotonin syndrome). Products include:
Actiq 993

Fluoxetine Hydrochloride (Sibutramine inhibits serotonin reuptake and serotonin syndrome, a rare, but serious constellation of symptoms, has been reported with the concomitant use of two SSRIs; concurrent use should be avoided). Products include:
Prozac Pulvules and Liquid 1771
Symbyax Capsules 1788

Fluvoxamine Maleate (Sibutramine inhibits serotonin reuptake and serotonin syndrome, a rare, but serious constellation of symptoms, has been reported with the concomitant use of two SSRIs; concurrent use should be avoided).
No products indexed under this heading.

Isocarboxazid (Concurrent and/or sequential use with MAO inhibitors is contraindicated; sibutramine inhibits serotonin reuptake and combination of MAO inhibitor and serotonergic agents has resulted in serious, sometimes fatal, reactions, serotonin syndrome).
No products indexed under this heading.

Ketoconazole (Co-administration has resulted in a moderate increase in AUC and Cmax of sibutramine). Products include:
Nizoral A-D Shampoo, 1% 1839
Nizoral 2% Shampoo 1838

Lithium (Sibutramine inhibits serotonin reuptake and combination of SSRIs and lithium has resulted in serious, sometimes fatal, reactions, serotonin syndrome).
No products indexed under this heading.

Lithium Carbonate (Sibutramine inhibits serotonin reuptake and combination of SSRIs and lithium has resulted in serious, sometimes fatal, reactions, serotonin syndrome). Products include:
Eskalith 1406
Lithobid Tablets 1670

Lithium Citrate (Sibutramine inhibits serotonin reuptake and combination of SSRIs and lithium has resulted in serious, sometimes fatal, reactions, serotonin syndrome).
No products indexed under this heading.

Mazindol (Concurrent use with other centrally acting appetite suppressant drugs is contraindicated).
No products indexed under this heading.

Meperidine Hydrochloride (Sibutramine inhibits serotonin reuptake and combination of SSRIs and certain opioids, such as meperidine, has resulted in serious, sometimes fatal, reactions, serotonin syndrome).
No products indexed under this heading.

Methamphetamine Hydrochloride (Concurrent use with other centrally acting appetite suppressant drugs is contraindicated). Products include:
Desoxyn Tablets, USP 2482

Moclobemide (Concurrent and/or sequential use with MAO inhibitors is contraindicated; sibutramine inhibits serotonin reuptake and combination of MAO inhibitor and serotonergic agents has resulted in serious, sometimes fatal, reactions, serotonin syndrome).
No products indexed under this heading.

Pargyline Hydrochloride (Concurrent and/or sequential use with MAO inhibitors is contraindicated; sibutramine inhibits serotonin reuptake and combination of MAO inhibitor and serotonergic agents has resulted in serious, sometimes fatal, reactions, serotonin syndrome).
No products indexed under this heading.

Paroxetine Hydrochloride (Sibutramine inhibits serotonin reuptake and serotonin syndrome, a rare, but serious constellation of symptoms, has been reported with the concomitant use of two SSRIs; concurrent use should be avoided). Products include:
Paxil CR Controlled-Release Tablets 1509
Paxil 1501

Pentazocine Hydrochloride (Sibutramine inhibits serotonin reuptake and combination of SSRIs and pentazocine has resulted in serious, sometimes fatal, reactions, serotonin syndrome).
No products indexed under this heading.

Phendimetrazine Tartrate (Concurrent use with other centrally acting appetite suppressant drugs is contraindicated).
No products indexed under this heading.

Phenelzine Sulfate (Concurrent and/or sequential use with MAO inhibitors is contraindicated; sibutramine inhibits serotonin reuptake and combination of MAO inhibitor and serotonergic agents has resulted in serious, sometimes fatal, reactions, serotonin syndrome).
No products indexed under this heading.

Phenmetrazine Hydrochloride (Concurrent use with other centrally acting appetite suppressant drugs is contraindicated).
No products indexed under this heading.

Phentermine Hydrochloride (Concurrent use with other centrally acting appetite suppressant drugs is contraindicated). Products include:
Adipex-P 1216

Phentermine Resin (Concurrent use with other centrally acting appetite suppressant drugs is contraindicated).
No products indexed under this heading.

Phenylephrine Hydrochloride (Sibutramine substantially raises blood in some patients and concomitant use of sibutramine and drugs that raise blood pressure and/or heart rate, such as decongestants, requires caution). Products include:
Alacol DM Syrup 739
Hycomine Compound Tablets 1105
Preparation H Maximum Strength Cream 747
Preparation H Cooling Gel 747
Preparation H 747
Sudafed PE Tablets 711
Vicks Sinex Nasal Spray and Ultra Fine Mist for Sinus Relief 2677
Zicam Concentrated Cough Mist for Kids Plus D Cool Cherry 643
Zicam Concentrated Cough Mist Plus D Cool Cherry 642

Phenylephrine Tannate (Sibutramine substantially raises blood in some patients and concomitant use of sibutramine and drugs that raise blood pressure and/or heart rate, such as decongestants, requires caution).
No products indexed under this heading.

Phenylpropanolamine Hydrochloride (Sibutramine substantially raises blood in some patients and concomitant use of sibutramine and drugs that raise blood pressure and/or heart rate, such as decongestants, requires caution).
No products indexed under this heading.

Procarbazine Hydrochloride (Concurrent and/or sequential use with MAO inhibitors is contraindicated; sibutramine inhibits serotonin reuptake and combination of MAO inhibitor and serotonergic agents has resulted in serious, sometimes fatal, reactions, serotonin syndrome). Products include:
Matulane Capsules 3188

Pseudoephedrine Hydrochloride (Sibutramine substantially raises blood in some patients and concomitant use of sibutramine and drugs that raise blood pressure and/or heart rate, such as decongestants, requires caution). Products include:
Advil Allergy Sinus Caplets 737
Advil Cold & Sinus 739
Advil Flu & Body Ache Caplets 739
Children's Advil Cold Suspension 741
Advil Multi-Symptom Cold Caplets 738

Allegra-D 12 Hour Extended-Release Tablets............ 2860
Allegra-D 24 Hour Extended-Release Tablets............ 2862
Balamine DM.............................. 739
BC Cold Powder .... ■ 612
Benadryl Allergy & Cold Tablets ..... ■ 692
Benadryl Allergy & Sinus Headache Caplets & Gelcaps...... ■ 693
Children's Benadryl Allergy & Cold Fastmelt Tablets.................... ■ 695
Benadryl Maximum Strength Severe Allergy & Sinus Headache Caplets.................... ■ 694
Children's Benadryl D Allergy & Sinus Fastmelt Tablets.............. ■ 694
Children's Benadryl D Liquid Medication................................ ■ 693
Benadryl D Tablets .... ■ 694
Contac Non-Drowsy 12 Hour Cold Caplets................................. ■ 614
Contac Non-Drowsy Timed Release 12 Hour Cold Caplets....... ■ 615
Contac Severe Cold and Flu Caplets Maximum Strength........ ■ 615
Contac Severe Cold and Flu Caplets Non-Drowsy..................... ■ 615
Children's Dimetapp Cold & Allergy Elixir............................. ■ 745
Children's Dimetapp DM Cold & Cough Elixir.......................... ■ 745
Children's Dimetapp Long Acting Cough Plus Cold Syrup............. ■ 746
Dimetapp Infant Drops Decongestant Plus Cough.......... ■ 746
Children's Motrin Cold Non-Staining Dye-Free Oral Suspension............................. 1838
Children's Motrin Cold Oral Suspension............................. 1838
Motrin Cold & Sinus Caplets 1836
PediaCare Decongestant & Cough Infant Drops.................... ■ 705
PediaCare Decongestant Infants' Drops....................................... ■ 705
PediaCare Long-Acting Cough Plus Cold Liquid......................... ■ 704
PediaCare Multi-Symptom Cold Liquid.. ■ 704
PediaCare NightRest Cough & Cold Liquid.................................. ■ 704
Robitussin Allergy & Cough Syrup .. ■ 750
Robitussin CF Liquid .... ■ 755
Robitussin Cough & Cold Liquid-filled Capsules................. ■ 750
Robitussin Cough, Cold & Flu Liquid-filled Capsules................. ■ 750
Robitussin Cough & Cold Infant Drops... ■ 755
Robitussin Flu Liquid .... ■ 752
Robitussin Maximum Strength Cough & Cold Liquid .... ■ 754
Robitussin PE Syrup .... ■ 753
Robitussin Pediatric Cough & Cold Liquid.................................. ■ 754
Robitussin PM Cough & Cold Liquid .... ■ 752
Robitussin Severe Congestion Liquid-filled Capsules................. ■ 751
Simply Stuffy Liquid 1841
Singlet Caplets .... ■ 636
Sudafed 12 Hour Caplets .... ■ 708
Sudafed 24 Hour Tablets .... ■ 709
Sudafed Nasal Decongestant Tablets...................................... ■ 709
Sudafed Severe Cold .... ■ 710
Sudafed Non-Drying Sinus Liquid Caps.. ■ 709
Sudafed Sinus & Allergy Tablets ..... ■ 710
Sudafed Sinus Headache .... ■ 711
TheraFlu Cold & Cough Hot Liquid.. ■ 680
TheraFlu Cold & Sore Throat Hot Liquid.. ■ 680
TheraFlu Flu & Chest Congestion Non-Drowsy Hot Liquid............... ■ 681
TheraFlu Flu & Sore Throat Hot Liquid.. ■ 681
TheraFlu Severe Cold Non-Drowsy Hot Liquid............... ■ 683
TheraFlu Severe Cold & Cough Hot Liquid.................................. ■ 683
TheraFlu Severe Cold Caplets .... ■ 679
TheraFlu Severe Cold Hot Liquid .... ■ 682
TheraFlu Severe Cold Non-Drowsy Caplets.................. ■ 679
Triaminic Chest & Nasal Congestion Liquid.................... ■ 685
Triaminic Cold & Allergy Liquid .... ■ 685
Triaminic Cold & Cough Liquid .... ■ 685
Triaminic Cough Liquid .... ■ 687
Triaminic Cough & Nasal Congestion Liquid.................... ■ 687
Triaminic Cough & Sore Throat Liquid.. ■ 687
Triaminic Flu, Cough & Fever Liquid.. ■ 685
Triaminic Night Time Cough & Cold Liquid.................................. ■ 685
Triaminic Allergy Runny Nose & Congestion Softchews.................. ■ 688
Triaminic Cold & Cough Softchews.. ■ 688
Triaminic Cough & Sore Throat Softchews.. ■ 689
Tylenol Sinus NightTime Caplets .... ■ 663
Children's Tylenol Plus Cold & Allergy Suspension Liquid............ 1850
Children's Tylenol Plus Cold NightTime Suspension Liquid....... 1851
Children's Tylenol Plus Cold & Cough Suspension Liquid and Chewable Tablets....................... 1851
Children's Tylenol Plus Cold Chewable Tablets.......................... 1851
Children's Tylenol Plus Cold Daytime Non-Drowsy Suspension Liquid........................ 1851
Children's Tylenol Plus Flu Suspension Liquid........................ 1853
Concentrated Tylenol Infants' Drops Plus Cold........................... 1851
Concentrated Tylenol Infants' Drops Plus Cold and Cough.......... 1851
Tylenol Cold & Flu Severe Daytime Liquid with Cool Burst....... 1846
Tylenol Cold & Flu Severe NightTime Liquid with Cool Burst.. 1846
Tylenol Cold Severe Congestion Non-Drowsy Caplets with Cool Burst.. 1846
Tylenol Allergy Complete Night Time Caplets.............................. 1844
Tylenol Allergy Complete Multi-Symptom Caplets and Gelcaps with Cool Burst............... 1844
Tylenol Flu NightTime Gelcaps 1846
Tylenol Flu Day Non-Drowsy Gelcaps...................................... 1846
Concentrated Tylenol Infants' Drops Plus Cold Nasal Congestant, Fever Reducer & Pain Reliever....................... ■ 668
Concentrated Tylenol Infants' Drops Plus Cold & Cough Nasal Decongestant, Fever Reducer & Pain Reliever............... ■ 668
Multi-Symptom Tylenol Cold Night Time Caplets.............................. 1845
Multi-Symptom Tylenol Cold Day Non-Drowsy Caplets and Gelcaps...................................... 1845
Tylenol Sinus Day Non-Drowsy.......... 1848
Tylenol Sinus Night Time Caplets 1848
Tylenol Sinus Severe Congestion Caplets with Cool Burst............ 1848
Vicks 44D Cough & Head Congestion Relief......................... 2676
Vicks 44D Cough & Head Congestion Relief Liquid............. ■ 721
Vicks 44M Cough, Cold & Flu Relief.. 2676
Pediatric Vicks 44m Cough & Cold Relief.................................. 2673
Vicks DayQuil LiquiCaps/Liquid Multi-Symptom Cold/Flu Relief..... ■ 723
Vicks DayQuil Multi-Symptom Cold/Flu Relief LiquiCaps............. 2675
Vicks DayQuil Multi-Symptom Cold/Flu Relief Liquid.................. 2675
Children's Vicks NyQuil Cold/Cough Relief........................ 2671
Vicks NyQuil LiquiCaps 2677
Vicks NyQuil LiquiCaps/Liquid Multi-Symptom Cold/Flu Relief..... ■ 725
Vicks NyQuil Liquid 2677
Zyrtec-D 12 Hour Extended Release Tablets............................. 2591

Pseudoephedrine Sulfate (Sibutramine substantially raises blood in some patients and concomitant use of sibutramine and drugs that raise blood pressure and/or heart rate, such as decongestants, requires caution). Products include:

Alavert Allergy & Sinus D-12 Hour Tablets.. ■ 743
Clarinex-D 24-Hour Extended-Release Tablets............ 3012
Claritin-D Non-Drowsy 12 Hour Tablets.. ■ 731
Claritin-D Non-Drowsy 24 Hour Tablets.. ■ 731

Selegiline Hydrochloride (Concurrent and/or sequential use with MAO inhibitors is contraindicated; sibutramine inhibits serotonin reuptake and combination of MAO inhibitor and serotonergic agents has resulted in serious, sometimes fatal, reactions, serotonin syndrome). Products include:

Eldepryl Capsules 3209

Sertraline Hydrochloride (Sibutramine inhibits serotonin reuptake and serotonin syndrome, a rare, but serious constellation of symptoms, has been reported with the concomitant use of two SSRIs; concurrent use should be avoided). Products include:

Zoloft 2581

Sumatriptan (Sibutramine inhibits serotonin reuptake and combination of SSRIs and agents for migraine, such as sumatriptan, has resulted in serious, sometimes fatal, reactions, serotonin syndrome). Products include:

Imitrex Nasal Spray 1435

Sumatriptan Succinate (Sibutramine inhibits serotonin reuptake and combination of SSRIs and agents for migraine, such as sumatriptan, has resulted in serious, sometimes fatal, reactions, serotonin syndrome). Products include:

Imitrex Injection 1431
Imitrex Tablets 1440

Tranylcypromine Sulfate (Concurrent and/or sequential use with MAO inhibitors is contraindicated; sibutramine inhibits serotonin reuptake and combination of MAO inhibitor and serotonergic agents has resulted in serious, sometimes fatal, reactions, serotonin syndrome). Products include:

Parnate Tablets 1499

L-Tryptophan (Sibutramine inhibits serotonin reuptake and combination of SSRIs and tryptophan has resulted in serious, sometimes fatal, reactions, serotonin syndrome).

No products indexed under this heading.

Venlafaxine Hydrochloride (Sibutramine inhibits serotonin reuptake and serotonin syndrome, a rare, but serious constellation of symptoms, has been reported with the concomitant use of two SSRIs; concurrent use should be avoided). Products include:

Effexor Tablets 3405
Effexor XR Capsules 3411

Food Interactions

Alcohol (Concurrent use has not resulted in psychomotor reactions of clinical significance, however, concomitant use with excessive alcohol is not recommended).

Food, unspecified (Co-administration with a standard breakfast has resulted in reduced peak M1 and M2 amine concentrations and delayed the time to peak by approximately three hours; the AUCs of M1 and M2 were not significantly altered).

MERREM I.V.

(Meropenem) 687
May interact with:

Probenecid (Competes with meropenem for active tubular secretion and, thus, inhibits the renal excretion of meropenem. Statistically significant increases in the elimination half-life and the extent of systemic exposure have been reported; co-administration is not recommended).

No products indexed under this heading.

MERUVAX II

(Rubella Virus Vaccine Live) 1994
May interact with immunosuppressive agents. Compounds in these categories include:

Azathioprine (Concurrent immunosuppressive therapy is contraindicated). Products include:

Azasan Tablets 2844

Basiliximab (Concurrent immunosuppressive therapy is contraindicated). Products include:

Simulect for Injection 2268

Cyclosporine (Concurrent immunosuppressive therapy is contraindicated). Products include:

Gengraf Capsules 458
Neoral Soft Gelatin Capsules 2247
Neoral Oral Solution 2247
Restasis Ophthalmic Emulsion 570
Sandimmune 2259

Muromonab-CD3 (Concurrent immunosuppressive therapy is contraindicated). Products include:

Orthoclone OKT3 Sterile Solution 2370

Mycophenolate Mofetil (Concurrent immunosuppressive therapy is contraindicated). Products include:

CellCept Capsules 2751
CellCept Oral Suspension 2751
CellCept Tablets 2751

Sirolimus (Concurrent immunosuppressive therapy is contraindicated). Products include:

Rapamune Oral Solution and Tablets.. 3472

Tacrolimus (Concurrent immunosuppressive therapy is contraindicated). Products include:

Prograf Capsules and Injection 624
Protopic Ointment 629

METADATE CD CAPSULES

(Methylphenidate Hydrochloride) 3316
May interact with oral anticoagulants, monoamine oxidase inhibitors, phenytoin, selective serotonin reuptake inhibitors, tricyclic antidepressants, vasopressors, and certain other agents. Compounds in these categories include:

Amitriptyline Hydrochloride (Methylphenidate may inhibit the metabolism of tricyclic antidepressants; downward dosage adjustment of tricyclic antidepressants may be required).

No products indexed under this heading.

Amoxapine (Methylphenidate may inhibit the metabolism of tricyclic antidepressants; downward dosage adjustment of tricyclic antidepressants may be required).

No products indexed under this heading.

Anisindione (Methylphenidate may inhibit the metabolism of coumarin anticoagulants; downward dosage adjustment of anticoagulants may be required). Products include:

Miradon Tablets 3056

Citalopram Hydrobromide (Methylphenidate may inhibit the metabolism of selective serotonin reuptake inhibitors; downward dosage adjustment of SSRI may be required). Products include:

Celexa 1177

Clomipramine Hydrochloride (Methylphenidate may inhibit the metabolism of tricyclic antidepressants; downward dosage adjustment of tricyclic antidepressants may be required).

No products indexed under this heading.

Clonidine (Co-administration has resulted in serious adverse events; the safety of this combination has not been systemically established). Products include:

Catapres-TTS 875

Clonidine Hydrochloride (Co-administration has resulted in serious adverse events; the safety of this combination has not been systemically established). Products include:

Catapres Tablets 874
Clorpres Tablets 2139

Desipramine Hydrochloride (Methylphenidate may inhibit the metabolism of tricyclic antidepressants; downward dosage adjustment of tricyclic antidepressants may be required).

No products indexed under this heading.

Dicumarol (Methylphenidate may inhibit the metabolism of coumarin anticoagulants; downward dosage adjustment of anticoagulants may be required).

No products indexed under this heading.

Dobutamine (Methylphenidate causes rise in blood pressure; co-administration with other pressor agents should be undertaken with caution).

No products indexed under this heading.

Dobutamine Hydrochloride (Methylphenidate causes rise in blood pressure; co-administration with other pressor agents should be undertaken with caution).

No products indexed under this heading.

Dopamine Hydrochloride (Methylphenidate causes rise in blood pressure; co-administration with other pressor agents should be undertaken with caution).

No products indexed under this heading.

Doxepin Hydrochloride (Methylphenidate may inhibit the metabolism of tricyclic antidepressants; downward dosage adjustment of tricyclic antidepressants may be required).

No products indexed under this heading.

Ephedrine Sulfate (Methylphenidate causes rise in blood pressure; co-administration with other pressor agents should be undertaken with caution).

No products indexed under this heading.

Epinephrine Bitartrate (Methylphenidate causes rise in blood pressure; co-administration with other pressor agents should be undertaken with caution).

No products indexed under this heading.

Epinephrine Hydrochloride (Methylphenidate causes rise in blood pressure; co-administration with other pressor agents should be undertaken with caution).

No products indexed under this heading.

Escitalopram Oxalate (Methylphenidate may inhibit the metabolism of selective serotonin reuptake inhibitors; downward dosage adjustment of SSRI may be required). Products include:

Lexapro Oral Solution 1193
Lexapro Tablets 1193

Fluoxetine Hydrochloride (Methylphenidate may inhibit the metabolism of selective serotonin reuptake inhibitors; downward dosage adjustment of SSRI may be required). Products include:

Prozac Pulvules and Liquid 1771
Symbyax Capsules 1788

Fluvoxamine Maleate (Methylphenidate may inhibit the metabolism of selective serotonin reuptake inhibitors; downward dosage adjustment of SSRI may be required).

No products indexed under this heading.

Fosphenytoin Sodium (Methylphenidate may inhibit the metabolism of anticonvulsants, such as phenytoin; additionally methylphenidate may lower the convulsive threshold in patients with prior history of seizures).

No products indexed under this heading.

Guanethidine Monosulfate (Methylphenidate may decrease the hypotensive effect of guanethidine).

No products indexed under this heading.

Imipramine Hydrochloride (Methylphenidate may inhibit the metabolism of tricyclic antidepressants; downward dosage adjustment of tricyclic antidepressants may be required).

No products indexed under this heading.

Imipramine Pamoate (Methylphenidate may inhibit the metabolism of tricyclic antidepressants; downward dosage adjustment of tricyclic antidepressants may be required).

No products indexed under this heading.

Isocarboxazid (Co-administration is contraindicated during treatment with monoamine oxidase inhibitors, and also within a minimum of 14 days following discontinuation of a monoamine oxidase inhibitor (hypertensive crises may result)).

No products indexed under this heading.

Isoproterenol Hydrochloride (Methylphenidate causes rise in blood pressure; co-administration with other pressor agents should be undertaken with caution).

No products indexed under this heading.

Isoproterenol Sulfate (Methylphenidate causes rise in blood pressure; co-administration with other pressor agents should be undertaken with caution).

No products indexed under this heading.

Maprotiline Hydrochloride (Methylphenidate may inhibit the metabolism of tricyclic antidepressants; downward dosage adjustment of tricyclic antidepressants may be required).

No products indexed under this heading.

Mephentermine Sulfate (Methylphenidate causes rise in blood pressure; co-administration with other pressor agents should be undertaken with caution).

No products indexed under this heading.

Metaraminol Bitartrate (Methylphenidate causes rise in blood pressure; co-administration with other pressor agents should be undertaken with caution). Products include:

Aramine Injection 1889

Methoxamine Hydrochloride (Methylphenidate causes rise in blood pressure; co-administration with other pressor agents should be undertaken with caution).

No products indexed under this heading.

Moclobemide (Co-administration is contraindicated during treatment with monoamine oxidase inhibitors, and also within a minimum of 14 days following discontinuation of a monoamine oxidase inhibitor (hypertensive crises may result)).

No products indexed under this heading.

Norepinephrine Bitartrate (Methylphenidate causes rise in blood pressure; co-administration with other pressor agents should be undertaken with caution).

No products indexed under this heading.

Nortriptyline Hydrochloride (Methylphenidate may inhibit the metabolism of tricyclic antidepressants; downward dosage adjustment of tricyclic antidepressants may be required).

No products indexed under this heading.

Pargyline Hydrochloride (Co-administration is contraindicated during treatment with monoamine oxidase inhibitors, and also within a minimum of 14 days following discontinuation of a monoamine oxidase inhibitor (hypertensive crises may result)).

No products indexed under this heading.

Paroxetine Hydrochloride (Methylphenidate may inhibit the metabolism of selective serotonin reuptake inhibitors; downward dosage adjustment of SSRI may be required). Products include:

Paxil CR Controlled-Release Tablets 1509
Paxil 1501

Phenelzine Sulfate (Co-administration is contraindicated during treatment with monoamine oxidase inhibitors, and also within a minimum of 14 days following discontinuation of a monoamine oxidase inhibitor (hypertensive crises may result)).

No products indexed under this heading.

Phenobarbital (Methylphenidate may inhibit the metabolism of anticonvulsants, such as phenobarbital; additionally methylphenidate may lower the convulsive threshold in patients with prior history of seizures).

No products indexed under this heading.

Phenylephrine Hydrochloride (Methylphenidate causes rise in blood pressure; co-administration with other pressor agents should be undertaken with caution). Products include:

Alacol DM Syrup 739
Hycomine Compound Tablets 1105
Preparation H Maximum Strength Cream 747
Preparation H Cooling Gel 747
Preparation H 747
Sudafed PE Tablets 711
Vicks Sinex Nasal Spray and Ultra Fine Mist for Sinus Relief 2677
Zicam Concentrated Cough Mist for Kids Plus D Cool Cherry 643
Zicam Concentrated Cough Mist Plus D Cool Cherry 642

Phenytoin (Methylphenidate may inhibit the metabolism of anticonvulsants, such as phenytoin; additionally methylphenidate may lower the convulsive threshold in patients with prior history of seizures).

No products indexed under this heading.

Phenytoin Sodium (Methylphenidate may inhibit the metabolism of anticonvulsants, such as phenytoin; additionally methylphenidate may lower the convulsive threshold in patients with prior history of seizures). Products include:

Phenytek Capsules 2153

Primidone (Methylphenidate may inhibit the metabolism of anticonvulsants, such as primidone; additionally methylphenidate may lower the convulsive threshold in patients with prior history of seizures).

No products indexed under this heading.

Procarbazine Hydrochloride (Co-administration is contraindicated during treatment with monoamine oxidase inhibitors, and also within a minimum of 14 days following discontinuation of a monoamine oxidase inhibitor (hypertensive crises may result)). Products include:

Matulane Capsules 3188

Protriptyline Hydrochloride (Methylphenidate may inhibit the metabolism of tricyclic antidepressants; downward dosage adjustment of tricyclic antidepressants may be required). Products include:

Vivactil Tablets 2350

Selegiline Hydrochloride (Co-administration is contraindicated during treatment with monoamine oxidase inhibitors, and also within a minimum of 14 days following discontinuation of a monoamine oxidase inhibitor (hypertensive crises may result)). Products include:

Eldepryl Capsules 3209

Sertraline Hydrochloride (Methylphenidate may inhibit the metabolism of selective serotonin reuptake inhibitors; downward dosage adjustment of SSRI may be required). Products include:
Zoloft ... 2581

Tranylcypromine Sulfate (Co-administration is contraindicated during treatment with monoamine oxidase inhibitors, and also within a minimum of 14 days following discontinuation of a monoamine oxidase inhibitor (hypertensive crises may result)). Products include:
Parnate Tablets ... 1499

Trimipramine Maleate (Methylphenidate may inhibit the metabolism of tricyclic antidepressants; downward dosage adjustment of tricyclic antidepressants may be required). Products include:
Surmontil Capsules ... 2347

Venlafaxine Hydrochloride (Co-administration in a patient on methylphenidate for 18 months has resulted in neuroleptic malignant syndrome within 45 minutes of ingesting his first dose of venlafaxine). Products include:
Effexor Tablets ... 3405
Effexor XR Capsules ... 3411

Warfarin Sodium (Methylphenidate may inhibit the metabolism of coumarin anticoagulants; downward dosage adjustment of anticoagulants may be required). Products include:
Coumadin for Injection ... 932
Coumadin Tablets ... 932

METAMUCIL CAPSULES
(Psyllium Preparations) ... 2672
None cited in PDR database.

METAMUCIL COARSE MILLED ORANGE FLAVOR POWDER
(Psyllium Preparations) ... 2672
None cited in PDR database.

METAMUCIL COARSE MILLED UNFLAVORED POWDER
(Psyllium Preparations) ... 2672
None cited in PDR database.

METAMUCIL DIETARY FIBER SUPPLEMENT
(Psyllium Preparations) ... ▣774
None cited in PDR database.

METAMUCIL SMOOTH TEXTURE ORANGE FLAVOR POWDER
(Psyllium Preparations) ... 2672
None cited in PDR database.

METAMUCIL SMOOTH TEXTURE SUGAR-FREE ORANGE FLAVOR POWDER
(Psyllium Preparations) ... 2672
None cited in PDR database.

METAMUCIL SMOOTH TEXTURE SUGAR-FREE UNFLAVORED POWDER
(Psyllium Preparations) ... 2672
None cited in PDR database.

METAMUCIL WAFERS, APPLE CRISP AND CINNAMON SPICE FLAVORS
(Psyllium Preparations) ... 2672
None cited in PDR database.

METROGEL 1%
(Metronidazole) ... 1212
May interact with oral anticoagulants. Compounds in these categories include:

Anisindione (Prolonged prothrombin time and potentiation of oral anticoagulant with oral metronidazole; the effect of topical metronidazole on prothrombin time is unknown). Products include:
Miradon Tablets ... 3056

Dicumarol (Prolonged prothrombin time and potentiation of oral anticoagulant with oral metronidazole; the effect of topical metronidazole on prothrombin time is unknown).
No products indexed under this heading.

Warfarin Sodium (Prolonged prothrombin time and potentiation of oral anticoagulant with oral metronidazole; the effect of topical metronidazole on prothrombin time is unknown). Products include:
Coumadin for Injection ... 932
Coumadin Tablets ... 932

METROGEL-VAGINAL GEL
(Metronidazole) ... 1822
May interact with oral anticoagulants and certain other agents. Compounds in these categories include:

Anisindione (Oral metronidazole potentiates the anticoagulant effect of warfarin). Products include:
Miradon Tablets ... 3056

Dicumarol (Oral metronidazole potentiates the anticoagulant effect of warfarin).
No products indexed under this heading.

Disulfiram (Psychotic reactions to oral metronidazole have been reported in alcoholics who are using metronidazole and disulfiram concurrently). Products include:
Antabuse Tablets ... 2343

Warfarin Sodium (Oral metronidazole potentiates the anticoagulant effect of warfarin). Products include:
Coumadin for Injection ... 932
Coumadin Tablets ... 932

Food Interactions

Alcohol (Possibility of a disulfiram-like reaction).

MEVACOR TABLETS
(Lovastatin) ... 1996
May interact with azole antifungals, oral anticoagulants, cytochrome p450 3a4 inhibitors (selected), erythromycin, fibrates, protease inhibitors, and certain other agents. Compounds in these categories include:

Acetazolamide (The risk of myopathy/rhabdomyolysis is increased by concomitant use of lovastatin with potent inhibitors of CYP3A4, particularly with higher doses of lovastatin; concomitant use should be avoided unless the benefits of combined therapy outweigh the increased risk).
No products indexed under this heading.

Amiodarone Hydrochloride (The combined use of lovastatin at doses higher than 40 mg daily with amiodarone should be avoided unless the clinical benefit is likely to outweigh the increased risk of myopathy). Products include:
Pacerone Tablets ... 3337

Amprenavir (The risk of myopathy/rhabdomyolysis is increased by concomitant use of lovastatin with potent inhibitors of CYP3A4, particularly with higher doses of lovastatin; concomitant use should be avoided unless the benefits of combined therapy outweigh the increased risk). Products include:
Agenerase Capsules ... 1299
Agenerase Oral Solution ... 1304

Anastrozole (The risk of myopathy/rhabdomyolysis is increased by concomitant use of lovastatin with potent inhibitors of CYP3A4, particularly with higher doses of lovastatin; concomitant use should be avoided unless the benefits of combined therapy outweigh the increased risk). Products include:
Arimidex Tablets ... 665

Anisindione (Co-administration has resulted in bleeding and/or increased prothrombin time in few patients). Products include:
Miradon Tablets ... 3056

Aprepitant (The risk of myopathy/rhabdomyolysis is increased by concomitant use of lovastatin with potent inhibitors of CYP3A4, particularly with higher doses of lovastatin; concomitant use should be avoided unless the benefits of combined therapy outweigh the increased risk). Products include:
Emend Capsules ... 1944

Cimetidine (The risk of myopathy/rhabdomyolysis is increased by concomitant use of lovastatin with potent inhibitors of CYP3A4, particularly with higher doses of lovastatin; concomitant use should be avoided unless the benefits of combined therapy outweigh the increased risk). Products include:
Tagamet HB 200 Tablets ... ▣637
Tagamet Tablets ... 1547

Cimetidine Hydrochloride (The risk of myopathy/rhabdomyolysis is increased by concomitant use of lovastatin with potent inhibitors of CYP3A4, particularly with higher doses of lovastatin; concomitant use should be avoided unless the benefits of combined therapy outweigh the increased risk).
No products indexed under this heading.

Ciprofloxacin (The risk of myopathy/rhabdomyolysis is increased by concomitant use of lovastatin with potent inhibitors of CYP3A4, particularly with higher doses of lovastatin; concomitant use should be avoided unless the benefits of combined therapy outweigh the increased risk). Products include:
Cipro I.V. ... 2998
Cipro I.V. Pharmacy Bulk Package ... 3509
Cipro Oral Suspension ... 2991
Cipro XR Tablets ... 3004
Ciprodex Otic Suspension ... 555

Clarithromycin (The risk of myopathy appears to be increased by high levels of HMG-CoA reductase inhibitory activity in plasma; lovastatin is metabolized by CYP3A4 isoenzyme, certain agents, such as macrolide antibiotics clarithromycin, share this metabolic pathway and can raise the plasma levels of lovastatin and may increase the risk of myopathy). Products include:
Biaxin/Biaxin XL ... 402
PREVPAC ... 3281

Clofibrate (The incidence and severity of myopathy are increased by co-administration of HMG-CoA reductase inhibitors with drugs that cause myopathy when given alone, such as fibrates; combined use should be avoided; if used concurrently, the dose of lovastatin should generally not exceed 20 mg).
No products indexed under this heading.

Clotrimazole (The risk of myopathy appears to be increased by high levels of HMG-CoA reductase inhibitory activity in plasma; lovastatin is metabolized by CYP3A4 isoenzyme, certain agents, such as azole antifungals, share this metabolic pathway and can raise the plasma levels of lovastatin and may increase the risk of myopathy). Products include:
Lotrimin ... 3053
Lotrisone ... 3054

Cyclosporine (The risk of myopathy appears to be increased by high levels of HMG-CoA reductase inhibitory activity in plasma; lovastatin is metabolized by CYP3A4 isoenzyme, certain agents, such as cyclosporine, share this metabolic pathway and can raise the plasma levels of lovastatin and may increase the risk of myopathy; the dose of lovastatin should generally not exceed 20 mg if used concomitantly). Products include:
Gengraf Capsules ... 458
Neoral Soft Gelatin Capsules ... 2247
Neoral Oral Solution ... 2247
Restasis Ophthalmic Emulsion ... ⊙570
Sandimmune ... 2259

Dalfopristin (The risk of myopathy/rhabdomyolysis is increased by concomitant use of lovastatin with potent inhibitors of CYP3A4, particularly with higher doses of lovastatin; concomitant use should be avoided unless the benefits of combined therapy outweigh the increased risk). Products include:
Synercid I.V. ... 1690

Danazol (The risk of rhabdomyolysis/myopathy is increased by concomitant administration of danazol, particularly with higher doses of lovastatin. The dose of lovastatin should not exceed 20 mg daily in patients receiving concomitant medication with danazol).
No products indexed under this heading.

Delavirdine Mesylate (The risk of myopathy/rhabdomyolysis is increased by concomitant use of lovastatin with potent inhibitors of CYP3A4, particularly with higher doses of lovastatin; concomitant use should be avoided unless the benefits of combined therapy outweigh the increased risk). Products include:
Rescriptor Tablets ... 2535

Dicumarol (Co-administration has resulted in bleeding and/or increased prothrombin time in few patients).
No products indexed under this heading.

Diltiazem Hydrochloride (The risk of myopathy/rhabdomyolysis is increased by concomitant use of lovastatin with potent inhibitors of CYP3A4, particularly with higher doses of lovastatin; concomitant use should be avoided unless the ben-

efits of combined therapy outweigh the increased risk). Products include:

- Cardizem LA Extended Release Tablets **1699**
- Tiazac Capsules **1204**

Diltiazem Maleate (The risk of myopathy/rhabdomyolysis is increased by concomitant use of lovastatin with potent inhibitors of CYP3A4, particularly with higher doses of lovastatin; concomitant use should be avoided unless the benefits of combined therapy outweigh the increased risk).

No products indexed under this heading.

Efavirenz (The risk of myopathy/rhabdomyolysis is increased by concomitant use of lovastatin with potent inhibitors of CYP3A4, particularly with higher doses of lovastatin; concomitant use should be avoided unless the benefits of combined therapy outweigh the increased risk). Products include:

- Sustiva Capsules **957**

Erythromycin (The risk of myopathy/rhabdomyolysis is increased by concomitant use of lovastatin with potent inhibitors of CYP3A4, particularly with higher doses of lovastatin; concomitant use should be avoided unless the benefits of combined therapy outweigh the increased risk). Products include:

- Erygel Topical Gel **2096**
- Ery-Tab Tablets **447**
- Erythromycin Base Filmtab Tablets **454**
- Erythromycin Delayed-Release Capsules, USP **456**
- PCE Dispertab Tablets **510**

Erythromycin Estolate (The risk of myopathy/rhabdomyolysis is increased by concomitant use of lovastatin with potent inhibitors of CYP3A4, particularly with higher doses of lovastatin; concomitant use should be avoided unless the benefits of combined therapy outweigh the increased risk).

No products indexed under this heading.

Erythromycin Ethylsuccinate (The risk of myopathy/rhabdomyolysis is increased by concomitant use of lovastatin with potent inhibitors of CYP3A4, particularly with higher doses of lovastatin; concomitant use should be avoided unless the benefits of combined therapy outweigh the increased risk). Products include:

- E.E.S. **449**
- EryPed **445**

Erythromycin Gluceptate (The risk of myopathy/rhabdomyolysis is increased by concomitant use of lovastatin with potent inhibitors of CYP3A4, particularly with higher doses of lovastatin; concomitant use should be avoided unless the benefits of combined therapy outweigh the increased risk).

No products indexed under this heading.

Erythromycin Lactobionate (The risk of myopathy/rhabdomyolysis is increased by concomitant use of lovastatin with potent inhibitors of CYP3A4, particularly with higher doses of lovastatin; concomitant use should be avoided unless the benefits of combined therapy outweigh the increased risk).

No products indexed under this heading.

Erythromycin Stearate (The risk of myopathy/rhabdomyolysis is increased by concomitant use of lovastatin with potent inhibitors of CYP3A4, particularly with higher doses of lovastatin; concomitant use should be avoided unless the benefits of combined therapy outweigh the increased risk). Products include:

- Erythrocin Stearate Filmtab Tablets **452**

Esomeprazole Magnesium (The risk of myopathy/rhabdomyolysis is increased by concomitant use of lovastatin with potent inhibitors of CYP3A4, particularly with higher doses of lovastatin; concomitant use should be avoided unless the benefits of combined therapy outweigh the increased risk). Products include:

- Nexium Delayed-Release Capsules **645**

Fenofibrate (The incidence and severity of myopathy are increased by co-administration of HMG-CoA reductase inhibitors with drugs that cause myopathy when given alone, such as fibrates; combined use should be avoided; if used concurrently, the dose of lovastatin should generally not exceed 20 mg). Products include:

- Antara Capsules **2723**
- Lofibra Capsules **1217**
- Tricor Tablets **523**
- Triglide Tablets **1165**

Fluconazole (The risk of myopathy appears to be increased by high levels of HMG-CoA reductase inhibitory activity in plasma; lovastatin is metabolized by CYP3A4 isoenzyme, certain agents, such as azole antifungals, share this metabolic pathway and can raise the plasma levels of lovastatin and may increase the risk of myopathy).

No products indexed under this heading.

Fluoxetine Hydrochloride (The risk of myopathy/rhabdomyolysis is increased by concomitant use of lovastatin with potent inhibitors of CYP3A4, particularly with higher doses of lovastatin; concomitant use should be avoided unless the benefits of combined therapy outweigh the increased risk). Products include:

- Prozac Pulvules and Liquid **1771**
- Symbyax Capsules **1788**

Fluvoxamine Maleate (The risk of myopathy/rhabdomyolysis is increased by concomitant use of lovastatin with potent inhibitors of CYP3A4, particularly with higher doses of lovastatin; concomitant use should be avoided unless the benefits of combined therapy outweigh the increased risk).

No products indexed under this heading.

Fosamprenavir Calcium (The risk of myopathy/rhabdomyolysis is increased by concomitant use of lovastatin with potent inhibitors of CYP3A4, particularly with higher doses of lovastatin; concomitant use should be avoided unless the benefits of combined therapy outweigh the increased risk). Products include:

- Lexiva Tablets **1473**

Gemfibrozil (The incidence and severity of myopathy are increased by co-administration of HMG-CoA reductase inhibitors with drugs that cause myopathy when given alone, such as fibrates; combined use should be avoided; if used concurrently, the dose of lovastatin should generally not exceed 20 mg).

No products indexed under this heading.

Indinavir Sulfate (The risk of myopathy/rhabdomyolysis is increased by concomitant use of lovastatin with potent inhibitors of CYP3A4, particularly with higher doses of lovastatin; concomitant use should be avoided unless the benefits of combined therapy outweigh the increased risk). Products include:

- Crixivan Capsules **1918**

Isoniazid (The risk of myopathy/rhabdomyolysis is increased by concomitant use of lovastatin with potent inhibitors of CYP3A4, particularly with higher doses of lovastatin; concomitant use should be avoided unless the benefits of combined therapy outweigh the increased risk).

No products indexed under this heading.

Itraconazole (The risk of myopathy appears to be increased by high levels of HMG-CoA reductase inhibitory activity in plasma; lovastatin is metabolized by CYP3A4 isoenzyme, certain agents, such as itraconazole, share this metabolic pathway and can raise the plasma levels of lovastatin and may increase the risk of myopathy).

No products indexed under this heading.

Ketoconazole (The risk of myopathy appears to be increased by high levels of HMG-CoA reductase inhibitory activity in plasma; lovastatin is metabolized by CYP3A4 isoenzyme, certain agents, such as ketoconazole, share this metabolic pathway and can raise the plasma levels of lovastatin and may increase the risk of myopathy). Products include:

- Nizoral A-D Shampoo, 1% **1839**
- Nizoral 2% Shampoo **1838**

Lopinavir (The risk of myopathy/rhabdomyolysis is increased by concomitant use of lovastatin with potent inhibitors of CYP3A4, particularly with higher doses of lovastatin; concomitant use should be avoided unless the benefits of combined therapy outweigh the increased risk). Products include:

- Kaletra **474**

Loratadine (The risk of myopathy/rhabdomyolysis is increased by concomitant use of lovastatin with potent inhibitors of CYP3A4, particularly with higher doses of lovastatin; concomitant use should be avoided unless the benefits of combined therapy outweigh the increased risk). Products include:

- Alavert Allergy & Sinus D-12 Hour Tablets **743**
- Alavert **743**
- Children's Claritin 24 Hour Non-Drowsy Allergy Syrup **732**
- Claritin Non-Drowsy 24 Hour Tablets **731**
- Non-Drowsy Claritin Hives Relief Tablets **733**
- Claritin Reditabs 24 Hour Non-Drowsy Tablets **732**
- Claritin-D Non-Drowsy 12 Hour Tablets **731**
- Claritin-D Non-Drowsy 24 Hour Tablets **731**
- Children's Dimetapp ND Non-Drowsy Allergy Syrup **746**
- Triaminic Allerchews **684**

Metronidazole (The risk of myopathy/rhabdomyolysis is increased by concomitant use of lovastatin with potent inhibitors of CYP3A4, particularly with higher doses of lovastatin; concomitant use should be avoided unless the benefits of combined therapy outweigh the increased risk). Products include:

- Metrogel 1% **1212**
- MetroGel-Vaginal Gel **1822**
- Noritate Cream, 1% **1051**

Metronidazole Benzoate (The risk of myopathy/rhabdomyolysis is increased by concomitant use of lovastatin with potent inhibitors of CYP3A4, particularly with higher doses of lovastatin; concomitant use should be avoided unless the benefits of combined therapy outweigh the increased risk).

No products indexed under this heading.

Metronidazole Hydrochloride (The risk of myopathy/rhabdomyolysis is increased by concomitant use of lovastatin with potent inhibitors of CYP3A4, particularly with higher doses of lovastatin; concomitant use should be avoided unless the benefits of combined therapy outweigh the increased risk).

No products indexed under this heading.

Miconazole (The risk of myopathy appears to be increased by high levels of HMG-CoA reductase inhibitory activity in plasma; lovastatin is metabolized by CYP3A4 isoenzyme, certain agents, such as azole antifungals, share this metabolic pathway and can raise the plasma levels of lovastatin and may increase the risk of myopathy).

No products indexed under this heading.

Miconazole Nitrate (The risk of myopathy/rhabdomyolysis is increased by concomitant use of lovastatin with potent inhibitors of CYP3A4, particularly with higher doses of lovastatin; concomitant use should be avoided unless the benefits of combined therapy outweigh the increased risk). Products include:

- Desenex **674**
- Desenex Jock Itch Spray Powder **674**

Nefazodone Hydrochloride (The risk of myopathy appears to be increased by high levels of HMG-CoA reductase inhibitory activity in plasma; lovastatin is metabolized by CYP3A4 isoenzyme, certain agents, such as antidepressant nefazodone, share this metabolic pathway and can raise the plasma levels of lovastatin and may increase the risk of myopathy).

No products indexed under this heading.

Nelfinavir Mesylate (The risk of myopathy/rhabdomyolysis is increased by concomitant use of lovastatin with potent inhibitors of CYP3A4, particularly with higher doses of lovastatin; concomitant use should be avoided unless the benefits of combined therapy outweigh the increased risk). Products include:

- Viracept **2556**

Nevirapine (The risk of myopathy/ rhabdomyolysis is increased by concomitant use of lovastatin with potent inhibitors of CYP3A4, particularly with higher doses of lovastatin; concomitant use should be avoided unless the benefits of combined therapy outweigh the increased risk). Products include:
- Viramune Oral Suspension **903**
- Viramune Tablets **903**

Niacin (The incidence and severity of myopathy are increased by coadministration of HMG-CoA reductase inhibitors with drugs that cause myopathy when given alone, such as lipid-lowering doses of niacin; combined use should be avoided; if used concurrently, the dose of lovastatin should generally not exceed 20 mg). Products include:
- Advicor Tablets **1694**
- Niaspan Extended-Release Tablets **1703**

Niacinamide (The risk of myopathy/rhabdomyolysis is increased by concomitant use of lovastatin with potent inhibitors of CYP3A4, particularly with higher doses of lovastatin; concomitant use should be avoided unless the benefits of combined therapy outweigh the increased risk).
No products indexed under this heading.

Nicotinamide (The risk of myopathy/rhabdomyolysis is increased by concomitant use of lovastatin with potent inhibitors of CYP3A4, particularly with higher doses of lovastatin; concomitant use should be avoided unless the benefits of combined therapy outweigh the increased risk). Products include:
- Nicomide Tablets **3190**

Nifedipine (The risk of myopathy/ rhabdomyolysis is increased by concomitant use of lovastatin with potent inhibitors of CYP3A4, particularly with higher doses of lovastatin; concomitant use should be avoided unless the benefits of combined therapy outweigh the increased risk). Products include:
- Adalat CC Tablets **2978**

Norfloxacin (The risk of myopathy/ rhabdomyolysis is increased by concomitant use of lovastatin with potent inhibitors of CYP3A4, particularly with higher doses of lovastatin; concomitant use should be avoided unless the benefits of combined therapy outweigh the increased risk). Products include:
- Noroxin Tablets **2009**

Omeprazole (The risk of myopathy/rhabdomyolysis is increased by concomitant use of lovastatin with potent inhibitors of CYP3A4, particularly with higher doses of lovastatin; concomitant use should be avoided unless the benefits of combined therapy outweigh the increased risk). Products include:
- Zegerid Powder for Oral Solution **2972**

Oxiconazole Nitrate (The risk of myopathy appears to be increased by high levels of HMG-CoA reductase inhibitory activity in plasma; lovastatin is metabolized by CYP3A4 isoenzyme, certain agents, such as azole antifungals, share this metabolic pathway and can raise the plasma levels of lovastatin and may increase the risk of myopathy). Products include:
- Oxistat **1498**

Paroxetine Hydrochloride (The risk of myopathy/rhabdomyolysis is increased by concomitant use of lovastatin with potent inhibitors of CYP3A4, particularly with higher doses of lovastatin; concomitant use should be avoided unless the benefits of combined therapy outweigh the increased risk). Products include:
- Paxil CR Controlled-Release Tablets **1509**
- Paxil **1501**

Propoxyphene Hydrochloride (The risk of myopathy/ rhabdomyolysis is increased by concomitant use of lovastatin with potent inhibitors of CYP3A4, particularly with higher doses of lovastatin; concomitant use should be avoided unless the benefits of combined therapy outweigh the increased risk).
No products indexed under this heading.

Propoxyphene Napsylate (The risk of myopathy/rhabdomyolysis is increased by concomitant use of lovastatin with potent inhibitors of CYP3A4, particularly with higher doses of lovastatin; concomitant use should be avoided unless the benefits of combined therapy outweigh the increased risk). Products include:
- Darvocet A 500 Tablets **3497**

Quinidine (The risk of myopathy/ rhabdomyolysis is increased by concomitant use of lovastatin with potent inhibitors of CYP3A4, particularly with higher doses of lovastatin; concomitant use should be avoided unless the benefits of combined therapy outweigh the increased risk).
No products indexed under this heading.

Quinidine Hydrochloride (The risk of myopathy/rhabdomyolysis is increased by concomitant use of lovastatin with potent inhibitors of CYP3A4, particularly with higher doses of lovastatin; concomitant use should be avoided unless the benefits of combined therapy outweigh the increased risk).
No products indexed under this heading.

Quinidine Polygalacturonate (The risk of myopathy/ rhabdomyolysis is increased by concomitant use of lovastatin with potent inhibitors of CYP3A4, particularly with higher doses of lovastatin; concomitant use should be avoided unless the benefits of combined therapy outweigh the increased risk).
No products indexed under this heading.

Quinidine Sulfate (The risk of myopathy/rhabdomyolysis is increased by concomitant use of lovastatin with potent inhibitors of CYP3A4, particularly with higher doses of lovastatin; concomitant use should be avoided unless the benefits of combined therapy outweigh the increased risk).
No products indexed under this heading.

Quinine (The risk of myopathy/ rhabdomyolysis is increased by concomitant use of lovastatin with potent inhibitors of CYP3A4, particularly with higher doses of lovastatin; concomitant use should be avoided unless the benefits of combined therapy outweigh the increased risk).
No products indexed under this heading.

Quinine Sulfate (The risk of myopathy/rhabdomyolysis is increased by concomitant use of lovastatin with potent inhibitors of CYP3A4, particularly with higher doses of lovastatin; concomitant use should be avoided unless the benefits of combined therapy outweigh the increased risk).
No products indexed under this heading.

Quinupristin (The risk of myopathy/rhabdomyolysis is increased by concomitant use of lovastatin with potent inhibitors of CYP3A4, particularly with higher doses of lovastatin; concomitant use should be avoided unless the benefits of combined therapy outweigh the increased risk). Products include:
- Synercid I.V. **1690**

Ranitidine Bismuth Citrate (The risk of myopathy/rhabdomyolysis is increased by concomitant use of lovastatin with potent inhibitors of CYP3A4, particularly with higher doses of lovastatin; concomitant use should be avoided unless the benefits of combined therapy outweigh the increased risk).
No products indexed under this heading.

Ranitidine Hydrochloride (The risk of myopathy/rhabdomyolysis is increased by concomitant use of lovastatin with potent inhibitors of CYP3A4, particularly with higher doses of lovastatin; concomitant use should be avoided unless the benefits of combined therapy outweigh the increased risk). Products include:
- Zantac **1597**
- Zantac Injection **1593**
- Zantac 75 Tablets .... ▣ **715**
- Zantac 150 Maximum Strength Tablets.. ▣ **715**
- Zantac Injection Pharmacy Bulk Package.. **1595**

Ritonavir (The risk of myopathy/ rhabdomyolysis is increased by concomitant use of lovastatin with potent inhibitors of CYP3A4, particularly with higher doses of lovastatin; concomitant use should be avoided unless the benefits of combined therapy outweigh the increased risk). Products include:
- Kaletra **474**
- Norvir **499**

Saquinavir (The risk of myopathy/ rhabdomyolysis is increased by concomitant use of lovastatin with potent inhibitors of CYP3A4, particularly with higher doses of lovastatin; concomitant use should be avoided unless the benefits of combined therapy outweigh the increased risk).
No products indexed under this heading.

Saquinavir Mesylate (The risk of myopathy/rhabdomyolysis is increased by concomitant use of lovastatin with potent inhibitors of CYP3A4, particularly with higher doses of lovastatin; concomitant use should be avoided unless the benefits of combined therapy outweigh the increased risk). Products include:
- Invirase **2776**

Sertraline Hydrochloride (The risk of myopathy/rhabdomyolysis is increased by concomitant use of lovastatin with potent inhibitors of CYP3A4, particularly with higher doses of lovastatin; concomitant use should be avoided unless the benefits of combined therapy outweigh the increased risk). Products include:
- Zoloft **2581**

Telithromycin (The risk of myopathy appears to be increased by high levels of HMG-CoA reductase inhibitory activity in plasma; lovastatin is metabolized by CYP3A4 isoenzyme, certain agents, such as macrolide antibiotics telithromycin, share this metabolic pathway and can raise the plasma levels of lovastatin and may increase the risk of myopathy). Products include:
- Ketek Tablets **2920**

Terconazole (The risk of myopathy appears to be increased by high levels of HMG-CoA reductase inhibitory activity in plasma; lovastatin is metabolized by CYP3A4 isoenzyme, certain agents, such as azole antifungals, share this metabolic pathway and can raise the plasma levels of lovastatin and may increase the risk of myopathy).
No products indexed under this heading.

Troglitazone (The risk of myopathy/rhabdomyolysis is increased by concomitant use of lovastatin with potent inhibitors of CYP3A4, particularly with higher doses of lovastatin; concomitant use should be avoided unless the benefits of combined therapy outweigh the increased risk).
No products indexed under this heading.

Troleandomycin (The risk of myopathy/rhabdomyolysis is increased by concomitant use of lovastatin with potent inhibitors of CYP3A4, particularly with higher doses of lovastatin; concomitant use should be avoided unless the benefits of combined therapy outweigh the increased risk).
No products indexed under this heading.

Valproate Sodium (The risk of myopathy/rhabdomyolysis is increased by concomitant use of lovastatin with potent inhibitors of CYP3A4, particularly with higher doses of lovastatin; concomitant use should be avoided unless the benefits of combined therapy outweigh the increased risk). Products include:
- Depacon Injection **412**

Verapamil Hydrochloride (The combined use of lovastatin at doses higher than 40 mg daily with verapamil should be avoided unless the clinical benefit is likely to outweigh the increased risk of myopathy). Products include:
- Covera-HS Tablets **3135**
- Tarka Tablets **519**
- Verelan PM Capsules **3120**

Voriconazole (The risk of myopathy/rhabdomyolysis is increased by concomitant use of lovastatin with potent inhibitors of CYP3A4, particularly with higher doses of lovastatin; concomitant use should be avoided unless the benefits of combined therapy outweigh the increased risk). Products include:
- VFEND I.V. **2543**
- VFEND Oral Suspension **2543**
- VFEND Tablets **2543**

Warfarin Sodium (Co-administration has resulted in bleed-

ing and/or increased prothrombin time in few patients). Products include:
Coumadin for Injection 932
Coumadin Tablets 932
Zafirlukast (The risk of myopathy/rhabdomyolysis is increased by concomitant use of lovastatin with potent inhibitors of CYP3A4, particularly with higher doses of lovastatin; concomitant use should be avoided unless the benefits of combined therapy outweigh the increased risk). Products include:
Accolate Tablets 663
Zileuton (The risk of myopathy/rhabdomyolysis is increased by concomitant use of lovastatin with potent inhibitors of CYP3A4, particularly with higher doses of lovastatin; concomitant use should be avoided unless the benefits of combined therapy outweigh the increased risk).
No products indexed under this heading.

Food Interactions

Alcohol (Lovastatin should be used with caution in patients who have consumed substantial quantity of alcohol and have a past history of liver disease; active liver disease and unexplained elevation in transaminase are contraindications to the use of lovastatin).
Grapefruit (The risk of myopathy/rhabdomyolysis is increased by concomitant use of lovastatin with potent inhibitors of CYP3A4, particularly with higher doses of lovastatin; concomitant use should be avoided unless the benefits of combined therapy outweigh the increased risk).
Grapefruit Juice (The risk of myopathy/rhabdomyolysis is increased by concomitant use of lovastatin with potent inhibitors of CYP3A4, particularly with higher doses of lovastatin; concomitant use should be avoided unless the benefits of combined therapy outweigh the increased risk).
Meal, unspecified (When lovastatin was given under fasting conditions, plasma concentrations of total inhibitors were on average about two-thirds those found when lovastatin was administered immediately after a standard meal).

MIACALCIN INJECTION

(Calcitonin-Salmon) 2241
None cited in PDR database.

MIACALCIN NASAL SPRAY

(Calcitonin-Salmon) 2242
May interact with:

Etidronate Disodium (Diphosphonate) (Prior diphosphonate use may reduce the anti-resorptive response to calcitonin-salmon nasal spray).
No products indexed under this heading.
Pamidronate Disodium (Prior diphosphonate use may reduce the anti-resorptive response to calcitonin-salmon nasal spray). Products include:
Aredia for Injection 2168

MICARDIS TABLETS

(Telmisartan) 884
May interact with:

Digoxin (Co-administration has resulted in median increases in digoxin peak plasma concentration (49%) and in trough concentration (20%); digoxin levels should be monitored when initiating, adjusting, and discontinuing telmisartan to avoid possible over- or under- digitalization). Products include:
Digitek Tablets 2146
Lanoxicaps Capsules 1458
Lanoxin Injection 1462
Lanoxin Tablets 1468
Lanoxin Injection Pediatric 1465
Warfarin Sodium (Co-administration has resulted in slight decrease in the mean warfarin trough plasma concentration; this decrease did not result in a change in INR). Products include:
Coumadin for Injection 932
Coumadin Tablets 932

Food Interactions

Food, unspecified (Slightly reduces the bioavailability of telmisartan; Micardis tablets may be administered with or without food).

MICARDIS HCT TABLETS

(Hydrochlorothiazide, Telmisartan) 886
May interact with antihypertensives, barbiturates, corticosteroids, oral hypoglycemic agents, insulin, lithium preparations, narcotic analgesics, nondepolarizing neuromuscular blocking agents, and non-steroidal anti-inflammatory agents. Compounds in these categories include:

Acarbose (Thiazide diuretics may cause hyperglycemia; dosage adjustment of oral hypoglycemia agents may be required). Products include:
Precose Tablets 776
Acebutolol Hydrochloride (Co-administration with other antihypertensive agents may result in additive effect or potentiation).
No products indexed under this heading.
ACTH (Intensifies electrolyte depletion, particularly hypokalemia).
No products indexed under this heading.
Alfentanil Hydrochloride (Potentiation of orthostatic hypotension).
No products indexed under this heading.
Amlodipine Besylate (Co-administration with other antihypertensive agents may result in additive effect or potentiation). Products include:
Caduet Tablets 2507
Lotrel Capsules 2238
Norvasc Tablets 2529
Aprobarbital (Potentiation of orthostatic hypotension).
No products indexed under this heading.
Atenolol (Co-administration with other antihypertensive agents may result in additive effect or potentiation). Products include:
Tenormin I.V. Injection 698
Tenormin Tablets 695
Atracurium Besylate (Possible increased responsiveness to the muscle relaxants).
No products indexed under this heading.
Benazepril Hydrochloride (Co-administration with other antihypertensive agents may result in additive effect or potentiation). Products include:
Lotensin Tablets 2232
Lotensin HCT Tablets 2235
Lotrel Capsules 2238
Bendroflumethiazide (Co-administration with other antihypertensive agents may result in additive effect or potentiation).
No products indexed under this heading.
Betamethasone Acetate (Corticosteroids intensify electrolyte depletion, particularly hypokalemia).
No products indexed under this heading.
Betamethasone Sodium Phosphate (Corticosteroids intensify electrolyte depletion, particularly hypokalemia).
No products indexed under this heading.
Betaxolol Hydrochloride (Co-administration with other antihypertensive agents may result in additive effect or potentiation). Products include:
Betoptic S Ophthalmic Suspension................................. 554
Bisoprolol Fumarate (Co-administration with other antihypertensive agents may result in additive effect or potentiation).
No products indexed under this heading.
Buprenorphine Hydrochloride (Potentiation of orthostatic hypotension). Products include:
Buprenex Injectable 2718
Suboxone Tablets 2719
Subutex Tablets 2719
Butabarbital (Potentiation of orthostatic hypotension).
No products indexed under this heading.
Butalbital (Potentiation of orthostatic hypotension). Products include:
Sedapap Tablets 50 mg/650 mg 2098
Candesartan Cilexetil (Co-administration with other antihypertensive agents may result in additive effect or potentiation). Products include:
Atacand Tablets 634
Atacand HCT 637
Captopril (Co-administration with other antihypertensive agents may result in additive effect or potentiation). Products include:
Captopril Tablets 2114
Carteolol Hydrochloride (Co-administration with other antihypertensive agents may result in additive effect or potentiation). Products include:
Carteolol Hydrochloride Ophthalmic Solution USP, 1%....... ⊙246
Celecoxib (Co-administration in some patients can result in reduced diuretic, natriuretic, and antihypertensive effects). Products include:
Celebrex Capsules 3130
Chlorothiazide (Co-administration with other antihypertensive agents may result in additive effect or potentiation). Products include:
Aldoclor Tablets 1881
Diuril Oral 1936
Chlorothiazide Sodium (Co-administration with other antihypertensive agents may result in additive effect or potentiation). Products include:
Diuril Sodium Intravenous 1934
Chlorpropamide (Thiazide diuretics may cause hyperglycemia; dosage adjustment of oral hypoglycemia agents may be required).
No products indexed under this heading.
Chlorthalidone (Co-administration with other antihypertensive agents may result in additive effect or potentiation). Products include:
Clorpres Tablets 2139
Cholestyramine (Absorption of hydrochlorothiazide is impaired in the presence of anionic exchange resins; cholestyramine binds the hydrochlorothiazide from the GI tract by up to 85%).
No products indexed under this heading.
Cisatracurium Besylate (Possible increased responsiveness to the muscle relaxants). Products include:
Nimbex Injection 494
Clonidine (Co-administration with other antihypertensive agents may result in additive effect or potentiation). Products include:
Catapres-TTS 875
Clonidine Hydrochloride (Co-administration with other antihypertensive agents may result in additive effect or potentiation). Products include:
Catapres Tablets 874
Clorpres Tablets 2139
Codeine Phosphate (Potentiation of orthostatic hypotension). Products include:
Tylenol with Codeine 2461
Colestipol Hydrochloride (Absorption of hydrochlorothiazide is impaired in the presence of anionic exchange resins; colestipol binds the hydroclorothiazide from the GI tract by up to 43%).
No products indexed under this heading.
Cortisone Acetate (Corticosteroids intensify electrolyte depletion, particularly hypokalemia).
No products indexed under this heading.
Deserpidine (Co-administration with other antihypertensive agents may result in additive effect or potentiation).
No products indexed under this heading.
Dexamethasone (Corticosteroids intensify electrolyte depletion, particularly hypokalemia). Products include:
Ciprodex Otic Suspension 555
Decadron Tablets 1929
TobraDex Ophthalmic Ointment 558
TobraDex Ophthalmic Suspension ... 558
Dexamethasone Acetate (Corticosteroids intensify electrolyte depletion, particularly hypokalemia).
No products indexed under this heading.
Dexamethasone Sodium Phosphate (Corticosteroids intensify electrolyte depletion, particularly hypokalemia). Products include:
Decadron Phosphate Injection 1931
Dezocine (Potentiation of orthostatic hypotension).
No products indexed under this heading.
Diazoxide (Co-administration with other antihypertensive agents may result in additive effect or potentiation). Products include:
Hyperstat I.V. Injection 3031
Diclofenac Potassium (Co-administration in some patients can result in reduced diuretic, natriuretic, and antihypertensive effects). Products include:
Cataflam Tablets 2173

Diclofenac Sodium (Co-administration in some patients can result in reduced diuretic, natriuretic, and antihypertensive effects). Products include:
Arthrotec Tablets 3126
Voltaren Ophthalmic Solution 2300
Voltaren Tablets 2298
Voltaren-XR Tablets 2301

Digoxin (Co-administration has resulted in median increases in digoxin peak plasma concentration (49%) and in trough concentration (20%); digoxin levels should be monitored when initiating, adjusting, and discontinuing telmisartan to avoid possible over- or under-digitalization; thiazide-induced hypokalemia exaggerates or sensitizes the response of the heart to the toxic effects of digitalis, i.e., increased ventricular irritability). Products include:
Digitek Tablets 2146
Lanoxicaps Capsules 1458
Lanoxin Injection 1462
Lanoxin Tablets 1468
Lanoxin Injection Pediatric 1465

Diltiazem Hydrochloride (Co-administration with other antihypertensive agents may result in additive effect or potentiation). Products include:
Cardizem LA Extended Release Tablets 1699
Tiazac Capsules 1204

Doxazosin Mesylate (Co-administration with other antihypertensive agents may result in additive effect or potentiation).
No products indexed under this heading.

Enalapril Maleate (Co-administration with other antihypertensive agents may result in additive effect or potentiation). Products include:
Vaseretic Tablets 2073
Vasotec I.V. Injection 2076

Enalaprilat (Co-administration with other antihypertensive agents may result in additive effect or potentiation).
No products indexed under this heading.

Eprosartan Mesylate (Co-administration with other antihypertensive agents may result in additive effect or potentiation). Products include:
Teveten Tablets 1707
Teveten HCT Tablets 1710

Esmolol Hydrochloride (Co-administration with other antihypertensive agents may result in additive effect or potentiation). Products include:
Brevibloc Concentrate 766
Brevibloc Injection 766
Brevibloc Double Strength Injection 766
Brevibloc Premixed Injection 766
Brevibloc Double Strength Premixed Injection 766

Etodolac (Co-administration in some patients can result in reduced diuretic, natriuretic, and antihypertensive effects).
No products indexed under this heading.

Felodipine (Co-administration with other antihypertensive agents may result in additive effect or potentiation). Products include:
Plendil Extended-Release Tablets 651

Fenoprofen Calcium (Co-administration in some patients can result in reduced diuretic, natriuretic, and antihypertensive effects). Products include:
Nalfon Capsules 2504

Fentanyl (Potentiation of orthostatic hypotension). Products include:
Duragesic Transdermal System 2448

Fentanyl Citrate (Potentiation of orthostatic hypotension). Products include:
Actiq 993

Fludrocortisone Acetate (Corticosteroids intensify electrolyte depletion, particularly hypokalemia).
No products indexed under this heading.

Flurbiprofen (Co-administration in some patients can result in reduced diuretic, natriuretic, and antihypertensive effects).
No products indexed under this heading.

Fosinopril Sodium (Co-administration with other antihypertensive agents may result in additive effect or potentiation).
No products indexed under this heading.

Furosemide (Co-administration with other antihypertensive agents may result in additive effect or potentiation). Products include:
Furosemide Tablets 2117

Glimepiride (Thiazide diuretics may cause hyperglycemia; dosage adjustment of oral hypoglycemia agents may be required). Products include:
Amaryl Tablets 2864

Glipizide (Thiazide diuretics may cause hyperglycemia; dosage adjustment of oral hypoglycemia agents may be required).
No products indexed under this heading.

Glyburide (Thiazide diuretics may cause hyperglycemia; dosage adjustment of oral hypoglycemia agents may be required).
No products indexed under this heading.

Guanabenz Acetate (Co-administration with other antihypertensive agents may result in additive effect or potentiation).
No products indexed under this heading.

Guanethidine Monosulfate (Co-administration with other antihypertensive agents may result in additive effect or potentiation).
No products indexed under this heading.

Hydralazine Hydrochloride (Co-administration with other antihypertensive agents may result in additive effect or potentiation). Products include:
BiDil Tablets 2161

Hydrocodone Bitartrate (Potentiation of orthostatic hypotension). Products include:
Hycodan 1104
Hycomine Compound Tablets 1105
Hycotuss Expectorant Syrup 1106
Lortab 3315
Lortab Elixir 3312
Vicodin Tablets 530
Vicodin ES Tablets 531
Vicodin HP Tablets 532
Vicoprofen Tablets 533
Zydone Tablets 1118

Hydrocodone Polistirex (Potentiation of orthostatic hypotension). Products include:
Tussionex Pennkinetic Extended-Release Suspension 3322

Hydrocortisone (Corticosteroids intensify electrolyte depletion, particularly hypokalemia). Products include:
Cortizone•5 Ointment .... ■ 699
Cortizone•10 Creme .... ■ 699
Cortizone•10 Ointment .... ■ 699
Cortizone•10 Plus Creme .... ■ 700
Cortizone•10 Maximum Strength Quick Shot Spray .... ■ 700
Hydrocortone Tablets 1963
Preparation H Hydrocortisone Cream .... ■ 748

Hydrocortisone Acetate (Corticosteroids intensify electrolyte depletion, particularly hypokalemia). Products include:
Analpram-HC 1136
Pramosone 1139
ProctoFoam-HC 3113
Tucks Anti-Itch Ointment .... ■ 712
U-cort 1% Cream 3289

Hydrocortisone Sodium Phosphate (Corticosteroids intensify electrolyte depletion, particularly hypokalemia).
No products indexed under this heading.

Hydrocortisone Sodium Succinate (Corticosteroids intensify electrolyte depletion, particularly hypokalemia).
No products indexed under this heading.

Hydroflumethiazide (Co-administration with other antihypertensive agents may result in additive effect or potentiation).
No products indexed under this heading.

Hydromorphone Hydrochloride (Potentiation of orthostatic hypotension). Products include:
Dilaudid 439
Dilaudid Oral Liquid 443
Dilaudid Non-Sterile Powder 439
Dilaudid Rectal Suppositories 439
Dilaudid Tablets 439
Dilaudid Tablets - 8 mg 443
Dilaudid-HP 441

Ibuprofen (Co-administration in some patients can result in reduced diuretic, natriuretic, and antihypertensive effects). Products include:
Advil Allergy Sinus Caplets .... ■ 737
Advil .... ■ 737
Children's Advil Suspension .... ■ 742
Children's Advil Chewable Tablets .. ■ 741
Advil Cold & Sinus .... ■ 739
Advil Flu & Body Ache Caplets .... ■ 739
Children's Advil Cold Suspension ... ■ 741
Infants' Advil Concentrated Drops .. ■ 743
Junior Strength Advil Swallow Tablets .... ■ 740
Advil Migraine Liquigels .... ■ 740
Advil Multi-Symptom Cold Caplets .... ■ 738
Combunox Tablets 1183
Children's Motrin Oral Suspension and Chewable Tablets 1837
Children's Motrin Cold Non-Staining Dye-Free Oral Suspension 1838
Children's Motrin Cold Oral Suspension 1838
Children's Motrin Non-Staining Dye-Free Oral Suspension 1837
Motrin Cold & Sinus Caplets 1836
Motrin IB Tablets and Caplets 1836
Infants' Motrin Concentrated Drops 1837
Infants' Motrin Non-Staining Dye-Free Drops 1837
Junior Strength Motrin Caplets and Chewable Tablets 1837
Vicoprofen Tablets 533

Indapamide (Co-administration with other antihypertensive agents may result in additive effect or potentiation). Products include:
Indapamide Tablets 2119

Indomethacin (Co-administration in some patients can result in reduced diuretic, natriuretic, and antihypertensive effects). Products include:
Indocin 1968

Indomethacin Sodium Trihydrate (Co-administration in some patients can result in reduced diuretic, natriuretic, and antihypertensive effects). Products include:
Indocin I.V. 1973

Insulin, Human, Zinc Suspension (Thiazide diuretics may cause hyperglycemia; dosage adjustment of insulin may be required). Products include:
Humulin L, 100 Units 1763
Humulin U, 100 Units 1770

Insulin, Human NPH (Thiazide diuretics may cause hyperglycemia; dosage adjustment of insulin may be required). Products include:
Humulin N, 100 Units 1764
Humulin N Pen 1765
Novolin N Human Insulin 10 ml Vials 2322
Novolin N InnoLet 2322
Novolin N PenFill 3 ml Cartridges 2325
Novolin R InnoLet 2322

Insulin, Human Regular (Thiazide diuretics may cause hyperglycemia; dosage adjustment of insulin may be required). Products include:
Humulin R (U-500) 1768
Humulin R, 100 Units 1767
Novolin R Human Insulin 10 ml Vials 2322
Novolin R PenFill 2325

Insulin, Human Regular and Human NPH Mixture (Thiazide diuretics may cause hyperglycemia; dosage adjustment of insulin may be required). Products include:
Humulin 50/50, 100 Units 1760
Humulin 70/30 Pen 1761
Novolin 70/30 Human Insulin 10 ml Vials 2321
Novolin 70/30 InnoLet 2322
Novolin 70/30 PenFill 3 ml Cartridges 2325

Insulin, NPH (Thiazide diuretics may cause hyperglycemia; dosage adjustment of insulin may be required).
No products indexed under this heading.

Insulin, Regular (Thiazide diuretics may cause hyperglycemia; dosage adjustment of insulin may be required).
No products indexed under this heading.

Insulin, Zinc Crystals (Thiazide diuretics may cause hyperglycemia; dosage adjustment of insulin may be required).
No products indexed under this heading.

Insulin, Zinc Suspension (Thiazide diuretics may cause hyperglycemia; dosage adjustment of insulin may be required).
No products indexed under this heading.

Insulin Aspart, Human Regular (Thiazide diuretics may cause hyperglycemia; dosage adjustment of insulin may be required). Products include:
NovoLog Injection 2326

Insulin glargine (Thiazide diuretics may cause hyperglycemia; dosage adjustment of insulin may be required). Products include:
Lantus Injection 2925

Insulin Lispro, Human (Thiazide diuretics may cause hyperglycemia; dosage adjustment of insulin may be required). Products include:
- Humalog-Pen 1751
- Humalog Mix 75/25-Pen 1754

Insulin Lispro Protamine, Human (Thiazide diuretics may cause hyperglycemia; dosage adjustment of insulin may be required). Products include:
- Humalog Mix 75/25-Pen 1754

Irbesartan (Co-administration with other antihypertensive agents may result in additive effect or potentiation). Products include:
- Avalide Tablets 922
- Avalide Tablets 2889
- Avapro Tablets 925
- Avapro Tablets 2886

Isradipine (Co-administration with other antihypertensive agents may result in additive effect or potentiation). Products include:
- DynaCirc CR Tablets 2726

Ketoprofen (Co-administration in some patients can result in reduced diuretic, natriuretic, and antihypertensive effects).
No products indexed under this heading.

Ketorolac Tromethamine (Co-administration in some patients can result in reduced diuretic, natriuretic, and antihypertensive effects). Products include:
- Acular Ophthalmic Solution 561
- Acular LS Ophthalmic Solution 562

Labetalol Hydrochloride (Co-administration with other antihypertensive agents may result in additive effect or potentiation).
No products indexed under this heading.

Levorphanol Tartrate (Potentiation of orthostatic hypotension).
No products indexed under this heading.

Lisinopril (Co-administration with other antihypertensive agents may result in additive effect or potentiation). Products include:
- Prinivil Tablets 2029
- Prinzide Tablets 2033
- Zestoretic Tablets 701
- Zestril Tablets 704

Lithium (Diuretics reduce the renal clearance of lithium and add a high risk of lithium toxicity; concurrent use should be avoided).
No products indexed under this heading.

Lithium Carbonate (Diuretics reduce the renal clearance of lithium and add a high risk of lithium toxicity; concurrent use should be avoided). Products include:
- Eskalith 1406
- Lithobid Tablets 1670

Lithium Citrate (Diuretics reduce the renal clearance of lithium and add a high risk of lithium toxicity; concurrent use should be avoided).
No products indexed under this heading.

Losartan Potassium (Co-administration with other antihypertensive agents may result in additive effect or potentiation). Products include:
- Cozaar Tablets 1913
- Hyzaar 1964

Mecamylamine Hydrochloride (Co-administration with other antihypertensive agents may result in additive effect or potentiation). Products include:
- Inversine Tablets 3286

Meclofenamate Sodium (Co-administration in some patients can result in reduced diuretic, natriuretic, and antihypertensive effects).
No products indexed under this heading.

Mefenamic Acid (Co-administration in some patients can result in reduced diuretic, natriuretic, and antihypertensive effects).
No products indexed under this heading.

Meloxicam (Co-administration in some patients can result in reduced diuretic, natriuretic, and antihypertensive effects). Products include:
- Mobic Oral Suspension 893
- Mobic Tablets 893

Meperidine Hydrochloride (Potentiation of orthostatic hypotension).
No products indexed under this heading.

Mephobarbital (Potentiation of orthostatic hypotension). Products include:
- Mebaral Tablets, USP 2483

Metformin Hydrochloride (Thiazide diuretics may cause hyperglycemia; dosage adjustment of oral hypoglycemia agents may be required). Products include:
- ActoPlus Met Tablets 3219
- Avandamet Tablets 1343
- Fortamet Extended-Release Tablets 1156

Methadone Hydrochloride (Potentiation of orthostatic hypotension).
No products indexed under this heading.

Methyclothiazide (Co-administration with other antihypertensive agents may result in additive effect or potentiation).
No products indexed under this heading.

Methyldopa (Co-administration with other antihypertensive agents may result in additive effect or potentiation). Products include:
- Aldoclor Tablets 1881
- Aldoril Tablets 1884

Methyldopate Hydrochloride (Co-administration with other antihypertensive agents may result in additive effect or potentiation).
No products indexed under this heading.

Methylprednisolone Acetate (Corticosteroids intensify electrolyte depletion, particularly hypokalemia). Products include:
- Depo-Medrol Injectable Suspension 2615
- Depo-Medrol Single-Dose Vial 2617

Methylprednisolone Sodium Succinate (Corticosteroids intensify electrolyte depletion, particularly hypokalemia).
No products indexed under this heading.

Metocurine Iodide (Possible increased responsiveness to the muscle relaxants).
No products indexed under this heading.

Metolazone (Co-administration with other antihypertensive agents may result in additive effect or potentiation).
No products indexed under this heading.

Metoprolol Succinate (Co-administration with other antihypertensive agents may result in additive effect or potentiation). Products include:
- Toprol-XL Tablets 660

Metoprolol Tartrate (Co-administration with other antihypertensive agents may result in additive effect or potentiation).
No products indexed under this heading.

Metyrosine (Co-administration with other antihypertensive agents may result in additive effect or potentiation). Products include:
- Demser Capsules 1933

Mibefradil Dihydrochloride (Co-administration with other antihypertensive agents may result in additive effect or potentiation).
No products indexed under this heading.

Miglitol (Thiazide diuretics may cause hyperglycemia; dosage adjustment of oral hypoglycemia agents may be required).
No products indexed under this heading.

Minoxidil (Co-administration with other antihypertensive agents may result in additive effect or potentiation). Products include:
- Men's Rogaine Extra Strength Topical Solution, Ocean Rush Scent and Original Unscented 706
- Women's Rogaine Topical Solution, Spring Bloom Scent and Original Unscented 707

Mivacurium Chloride (Possible increased responsiveness to the muscle relaxants). Products include:
- Mivacron Injection 489

Moexipril Hydrochloride (Co-administration with other antihypertensive agents may result in additive effect or potentiation). Products include:
- Uniretic Tablets 3114
- Univasc Tablets 3118

Morphine Sulfate (Potentiation of orthostatic hypotension). Products include:
- Avinza Capsules 1714
- Kadian Capsules 572
- MS Contin Tablets 2703

Nabumetone (Co-administration in some patients can result in reduced diuretic, natriuretic, and antihypertensive effects). Products include:
- Relafen Tablets 1523

Nadolol (Co-administration with other antihypertensive agents may result in additive effect or potentiation). Products include:
- Nadolol Tablets 2121

Naproxen (Co-administration in some patients can result in reduced diuretic, natriuretic, and antihypertensive effects). Products include:
- EC-Naprosyn Delayed-Release Tablets 2769
- Naprosyn Suspension 2769
- Naprosyn Tablets 2769
- Prevacid NapraPAC 3277

Naproxen Sodium (Co-administration in some patients can result in reduced diuretic, natriuretic, and antihypertensive effects). Products include:
- Aleve Tablets, Caplets and Gelcaps 605
- Anaprox Tablets 2769
- Anaprox DS Tablets 2769

Nicardipine Hydrochloride (Co-administration with other antihypertensive agents may result in additive effect or potentiation). Products include:
- Cardene I.V. 1129

Nifedipine (Co-administration with other antihypertensive agents may result in additive effect or potentiation). Products include:
- Adalat CC Tablets 2978

Nisoldipine (Co-administration with other antihypertensive agents may result in additive effect or potentiation). Products include:
- Sular Tablets 1163

Nitroglycerin (Co-administration with other antihypertensive agents may result in additive effect or potentiation). Products include:
- Nitro-Dur Transdermal Infusion System 3060
- Nitrolingual Pumpspray 1161

Norepinephrine Bitartrate (Possible decreased response to pressor amines).
No products indexed under this heading.

Oxaprozin (Co-administration in some patients can result in reduced diuretic, natriuretic, and antihypertensive effects).
No products indexed under this heading.

Oxycodone Hydrochloride (Potentiation of orthostatic hypotension). Products include:
- Combunox Tablets 1183
- OxyContin Tablets 2699
- OxyFast Oral Concentrate Solution 2704
- OxyIR Capsules 2704
- Percocet Tablets 1114
- Percodan Tablets 1115

Pancuronium Bromide (Possible increased responsiveness to the muscle relaxants).
No products indexed under this heading.

Penbutolol Sulfate (Co-administration with other antihypertensive agents may result in additive effect or potentiation).
No products indexed under this heading.

Pentobarbital Sodium (Potentiation of orthostatic hypotension). Products include:
- Nembutal Sodium Solution, USP 2484

Perindopril Erbumine (Co-administration with other antihypertensive agents may result in additive effect or potentiation). Products include:
- Aceon Tablets (2 mg, 4 mg, 8 mg) 3191

Phenobarbital (Potentiation of orthostatic hypotension).
No products indexed under this heading.

Phenoxybenzamine Hydrochloride (Co-administration with other antihypertensive agents may result in additive effect or potentiation). Products include:
- Dibenzyline Capsules 3390

Phentolamine Mesylate (Co-administration with other antihypertensive agents may result in additive effect or potentiation).
No products indexed under this heading.

Phenylbutazone (Co-administration in some patients can result in reduced diuretic, natriuretic, and antihypertensive effects).
No products indexed under this heading.

Pindolol (Co-administration with other antihypertensive agents may result in additive effect or potentiation).
No products indexed under this heading.

Pioglitazone Hydrochloride (Thiazide diuretics may cause hyperglycemia; dosage adjustment of oral hypoglycemia agents may be required). Products include:
ActoPlus Met Tablets 3219
Actos Tablets 3224

Piroxicam (Co-administration in some patients can result in reduced diuretic, natriuretic, and antihypertensive effects).
No products indexed under this heading.

Polythiazide (Co-administration with other antihypertensive agents may result in additive effect or potentiation).
No products indexed under this heading.

Potassium Acid Phosphate (Concurrent use of potassium supplements or salt substitute is not recommended). Products include:
K-Phos Original (Sodium Free) Tablets 785

Potassium Bicarbonate (Concurrent use of potassium supplements or salt substitute is not recommended).
No products indexed under this heading.

Potassium Chloride (Concurrent use of potassium supplements or salt substitute is not recommended). Products include:
Colyte with Flavor Packs for Oral Solution 3102
HalfLytely and Bisacodyl Tablets Bowel Prep Kit with Flavors Packs 915
K-Dur Extended-Relase Tablets 3047
K-Lor Powder Packets 472
K-Tab Filmtab Tablets 473
TriLyte with Flavor Packs for Oral Solution 3114

Potassium Citrate (Concurrent use of potassium supplements or salt substitute is not recommended). Products include:
Urocit-K Tablets 2109

Potassium Gluconate (Concurrent use of potassium supplements or salt substitute is not recommended).
No products indexed under this heading.

Potassium Phosphate (Concurrent use of potassium supplements or salt substitute is not recommended). Products include:
K-Phos Neutral Tablets 785

Prazosin Hydrochloride (Co-administration with other antihypertensive agents may result in additive effect or potentiation).
No products indexed under this heading.

Prednisolone Acetate (Corticosteroids intensify electrolyte depletion, particularly hypokalemia). Products include:
Blephamide Ophthalmic Ointment 563
Blephamide Ophthalmic Suspension 564
Poly-Pred Liquifilm Ophthalmic Suspension .... ⊙231
Pred Forte Ophthalmic Suspension .... ⊙233
Pred Mild Sterile Ophthalmic Suspension .... ⊙236
Pred-G Ophthalmic Suspension .... ⊙234
Pred-G Sterile Ophthalmic Ointment .... ⊙235

Prednisolone Sodium Phosphate (Corticosteroids intensify electrolyte depletion, particularly hypokalemia). Products include:
Pediapred Oral Solution 3319

Prednisolone Tebutate (Corticosteroids intensify electrolyte depletion, particularly hypokalemia).
No products indexed under this heading.

Prednisone (Corticosteroids intensify electrolyte depletion, particularly hypokalemia).
No products indexed under this heading.

Propoxyphene Hydrochloride (Potentiation of orthostatic hypotension).
No products indexed under this heading.

Propoxyphene Napsylate (Potentiation of orthostatic hypotension). Products include:
Darvocet A 500 Tablets 3497

Propranolol Hydrochloride (Co-administration with other antihypertensive agents may result in additive effect or potentiation). Products include:
Inderal LA Long-Acting Capsules 3421
InnoPran XL Capsules 2728

Quinapril Hydrochloride (Co-administration with other antihypertensive agents may result in additive effect or potentiation).
No products indexed under this heading.

Ramipril (Co-administration with other antihypertensive agents may result in additive effect or potentiation). Products include:
Altace Capsules 1673

Rapacuronium Bromide (Possible increased responsiveness to the muscle relaxants).
No products indexed under this heading.

Rauwolfia Serpentina (Co-administration with other antihypertensive agents may result in additive effect or potentiation).
No products indexed under this heading.

Remifentanil Hydrochloride (Potentiation of orthostatic hypotension).
No products indexed under this heading.

Repaglinide (Thiazide diuretics may cause hyperglycemia; dosage adjustment of oral hypoglycemia agents may be required). Products include:
Prandin Tablets (0.5, 1, and 2 mg) 2337

Rescinnamine (Co-administration with other antihypertensive agents may result in additive effect or potentiation).
No products indexed under this heading.

Reserpine (Co-administration with other antihypertensive agents may result in additive effect or potentiation).
No products indexed under this heading.

Rocuronium Bromide (Possible increased responsiveness to the muscle relaxants). Products include:
Zemuron Injection 2363

Rofecoxib (Co-administration in some patients can result in reduced diuretic, natriuretic, and antihypertensive effects).
No products indexed under this heading.

Rosiglitazone Maleate (Thiazide diuretics may cause hyperglycemia; dosage adjustment of oral hypoglycemia agents may be required). Products include:
Avandamet Tablets 1343
Avandia Tablets 1348

Secobarbital Sodium (Potentiation of orthostatic hypotension).
No products indexed under this heading.

Sodium Nitroprusside (Co-administration with other antihypertensive agents may result in additive effect or potentiation).
No products indexed under this heading.

Sotalol Hydrochloride (Co-administration with other antihypertensive agents may result in additive effect or potentiation).
No products indexed under this heading.

Spirapril Hydrochloride (Co-administration with other antihypertensive agents may result in additive effect or potentiation).
No products indexed under this heading.

Sufentanil Citrate (Potentiation of orthostatic hypotension).
No products indexed under this heading.

Sulindac (Co-administration in some patients can result in reduced diuretic, natriuretic, and antihypertensive effects). Products include:
Clinoril Tablets 1899

Terazosin Hydrochloride (Co-administration with other antihypertensive agents may result in additive effect or potentiation). Products include:
Hytrin Capsules 469

Thiamylal Sodium (Potentiation of orthostatic hypotension).
No products indexed under this heading.

Timolol Maleate (Co-administration with other antihypertensive agents may result in additive effect or potentiation). Products include:
Blocadren Tablets 1891
Cosopt Sterile Ophthalmic Solution 1910
Timolide Tablets 2056
Timoptic in Ocudose 2061
Timoptic Sterile Ophthalmic Solution 2058
Timoptic-XE Sterile Ophthalmic Gel Forming Solution 2062

Tolazamide (Thiazide diuretics may cause hyperglycemia; dosage adjustment of oral hypoglycemia agents may be required).
No products indexed under this heading.

Tolbutamide (Thiazide diuretics may cause hyperglycemia; dosage adjustment of oral hypoglycemia agents may be required).
No products indexed under this heading.

Tolmetin Sodium (Co-administration in some patients can result in reduced diuretic, natriuretic, and antihypertensive effects).
No products indexed under this heading.

Torsemide (Co-administration with other antihypertensive agents may result in additive effect or potentiation).
No products indexed under this heading.

Trandolapril (Co-administration with other antihypertensive agents may result in additive effect or potentiation). Products include:
Mavik Tablets 482
Tarka Tablets 519

Triamcinolone (Corticosteroids intensify electrolyte depletion, particularly hypokalemia).
No products indexed under this heading.

Triamcinolone Acetonide (Corticosteroids intensify electrolyte depletion, particularly hypokalemia). Products include:
Azmacort Inhalation Aerosol 1701
Nasacort HFA Inhalation Aerosol 2939
Nasacort AQ Nasal Spray 2937

Triamcinolone Diacetate (Corticosteroids intensify electrolyte depletion, particularly hypokalemia).
No products indexed under this heading.

Triamcinolone Hexacetonide (Corticosteroids intensify electrolyte depletion, particularly hypokalemia).
No products indexed under this heading.

Trimethaphan Camsylate (Co-administration with other antihypertensive agents may result in additive effect or potentiation).
No products indexed under this heading.

Troglitazone (Thiazide diuretics may cause hyperglycemia; dosage adjustment of oral hypoglycemia agents may be required).
No products indexed under this heading.

Valdecoxib (Co-administration in some patients can result in reduced diuretic, natriuretic, and antihypertensive effects).
No products indexed under this heading.

Valsartan (Co-administration with other antihypertensive agents may result in additive effect or potentiation). Products include:
Diovan HCT Tablets 2195
Diovan Tablets 2191

Vecuronium Bromide (Possible increased responsiveness to the muscle relaxants).
No products indexed under this heading.

Verapamil Hydrochloride (Co-administration with other antihypertensive agents may result in additive effect or potentiation). Products include:
Covera-HS Tablets 3135
Tarka Tablets 519
Verelan PM Capsules 3120

Warfarin Sodium (Co-administration has resulted in slight decrease in the mean warfarin trough plasma concentration; this decrease did not result in a change in INR). Products include:
Coumadin for Injection 932
Coumadin Tablets 932

Food Interactions

Alcohol (Potentiation of orthostatic hypotension).

Food, unspecified (Slightly reduces the bioavailability of telmisartan with reduction in AUC of about 6%).

MICRHOGAM ULTRA-FILTERED
(Rh_o (D) Immune Globulin (Human)) 2429
None cited in PDR database.

MICRODIET DIETARY SUPPLEMENT
(Multivitamins with Minerals) 775
None cited in PDR database.

MIDAMOR TABLETS
(Amiloride Hydrochloride) 2000
May interact with ACE inhibitors, angiotensin-II receptor antagonists, diuretics, lithium preparations, nonsteroidal anti-inflammatory agents, potassium preparations, potassium sparing diuretics, and certain other agents. Compounds in these categories include:

Benazepril Hydrochloride (Co-administration increases the risk of hyperkalemia). Products include:
Lotensin Tablets 2232
Lotensin HCT Tablets 2235
Lotrel Capsules 2238

Bendroflumethiazide (Co-administration with other diuretics may result in hypochloremia, hyponatremia, and increases in BUN).
No products indexed under this heading.

Bumetanide (Co-administration with other diuretics may result in hypochloremia, hyponatremia, and increases in BUN).
No products indexed under this heading.

Candesartan Cilexetil (Co-administration increases the risk of hyperkalemia). Products include:
Atacand Tablets 634
Atacand HCT 637

Captopril (Co-administration increases the risk of hyperkalemia). Products include:
Captopril Tablets 2114

Celecoxib (Co-administration of non-steroidal anti-inflammatory agents can reduce the diuretic, natriuretic, and antihypertensive effects). Products include:
Celebrex Capsules 3130

Chlorothiazide (Co-administration with other diuretics may result in hypochloremia, hyponatremia, and increases in BUN). Products include:
Aldoclor Tablets 1881
Diuril Oral 1936

Chlorothiazide Sodium (Co-administration with other diuretics may result in hypochloremia, hyponatremia, and increases in BUN). Products include:
Diuril Sodium Intravenous 1934

Chlorthalidone (Co-administration with other diuretics may result in hypochloremia, hyponatremia, and increases in BUN). Products include:
Clorpres Tablets 2139

Cyclosporine (Co-administration increases the risk of hyperkalemia). Products include:
Gengraf Capsules 458
Neoral Soft Gelatin Capsules 2247
Neoral Oral Solution 2247
Restasis Ophthalmic Emulsion 570
Sandimmune 2259

Diclofenac Potassium (Co-administration of non-steroidal anti-inflammatory agents can reduce the diuretic, natriuretic, and antihypertensive effects). Products include:
Cataflam Tablets 2173

Diclofenac Sodium (Co-administration of non-steroidal anti-inflammatory agents can reduce the diuretic, natriuretic, and antihypertensive effects). Products include:
Arthrotec Tablets 3126
Voltaren Ophthalmic Solution 2300
Voltaren Tablets 2298
Voltaren-XR Tablets 2301

Enalapril Maleate (Co-administration increases the risk of hyperkalemia). Products include:
Vaseretic Tablets 2073
Vasotec I.V. Injection 2076

Enalaprilat (Co-administration increases the risk of hyperkalemia).
No products indexed under this heading.

Eprosartan Mesylate (Co-administration increases the risk of hyperkalemia). Products include:
Teveten Tablets 1707
Teveten HCT Tablets 1710

Ethacrynic Acid (Co-administration with other diuretics may result in hypochloremia, hyponatremia, and increases in BUN). Products include:
Edecrin Tablets 1941

Etodolac (Co-administration of non-steroidal anti-inflammatory agents can reduce the diuretic, natriuretic, and antihypertensive effects).
No products indexed under this heading.

Fenoprofen Calcium (Co-administration of non-steroidal anti-inflammatory agents can reduce the diuretic, natriuretic, and antihypertensive effects). Products include:
Nalfon Capsules 2504

Flurbiprofen (Co-administration of non-steroidal anti-inflammatory agents can reduce the diuretic, natriuretic, and antihypertensive effects).
No products indexed under this heading.

Fosinopril Sodium (Co-administration increases the risk of hyperkalemia).
No products indexed under this heading.

Furosemide (Co-administration with other diuretics may result in hypochloremia, hyponatremia, and increases in BUN). Products include:
Furosemide Tablets 2117

Hydrochlorothiazide (Co-administration with other diuretics may result in hypochloremia, hyponatremia, and increases in BUN). Products include:
Aldoril Tablets 1884
Atacand HCT 637
Avalide Tablets 2889
Avalide Tablets 922
Benicar HCT Tablets 2852
Diovan HCT Tablets 2195
Dyazide Capsules 1389
Hyzaar 1964
Lotensin HCT Tablets 2235
Maxzide 2150
Micardis HCT Tablets 886
Moduretic Tablets 2003
Prinzide Tablets 2033
Teveten HCT Tablets 1710
Timolide Tablets 2056
Uniretic Tablets 3114
Vaseretic Tablets 2073
Zestoretic Tablets 701

Hydroflumethiazide (Co-administration with other diuretics may result in hypochloremia, hyponatremia, and increases in BUN).
No products indexed under this heading.

Ibuprofen (Co-administration of non-steroidal anti-inflammatory agents can reduce the diuretic, natriuretic, and antihypertensive effects). Products include:
Advil Allergy Sinus Caplets 737
Advil 737
Children's Advil Suspension 742
Children's Advil Chewable Tablets .. 741
Advil Cold & Sinus 739
Advil Flu & Body Ache Caplets 739
Children's Advil Cold Suspension 741
Infants' Advil Concentrated Drops .. 743
Junior Strength Advil Swallow Tablets 740
Advil Migraine Liquigels 740
Advil Multi-Symptom Cold Caplets 738
Combunox Tablets 1183
Children's Motrin Oral Suspension and Chewable Tablets 1837
Children's Motrin Cold Non-Staining Dye-Free Oral Suspension 1838
Children's Motrin Cold Oral Suspension 1838
Children's Motrin Non-Staining Dye-Free Oral Suspension 1837
Motrin Cold & Sinus Caplets 1836
Motrin IB Tablets and Caplets 1836
Infants' Motrin Concentrated Drops 1837
Infants' Motrin Non-Staining Dye-Free Drops 1837
Junior Strength Motrin Caplets and Chewable Tablets 1837
Vicoprofen Tablets 533

Indapamide (Co-administration with other diuretics may result in hypochloremia, hyponatremia, and increases in BUN). Products include:
Indapamide Tablets 2119

Indomethacin (Co-administration of non-steroidal anti-inflammatory agents can reduce the diuretic, natriuretic, and antihypertensive effects; both indomethacin and amiloride are associated with hyperkalemia, the potential effect on potassium kinetic and renal function should be considered if used concurrently). Products include:
Indocin 1968

Indomethacin Sodium Trihydrate (Co-administration of non-steroidal anti-inflammatory agents can reduce the diuretic, natriuretic, and antihypertensive effects; both indomethacin and amiloride are associated with hyperkalemia, the potential effect on potassium kinetic and renal function should be considered if used concurrently). Products include:
Indocin I.V. 1973

Irbesartan (Co-administration increases the risk of hyperkalemia). Products include:
Avalide Tablets 922
Avalide Tablets 2889
Avapro Tablets 925
Avapro Tablets 2886

Ketoprofen (Co-administration of non-steroidal anti-inflammatory agents can reduce the diuretic, natriuretic, and antihypertensive effects).
No products indexed under this heading.

Ketorolac Tromethamine (Co-administration of non-steroidal anti-inflammatory agents can reduce the diuretic, natriuretic, and antihypertensive effects). Products include:
Acular Ophthalmic Solution 561
Acular LS Ophthalmic Solution 562

Lisinopril (Co-administration increases the risk of hyperkalemia). Products include:
Prinivil Tablets 2029
Prinzide Tablets 2033
Zestoretic Tablets 701
Zestril Tablets 704

Lithium (Diuretics reduce the renal clearance and add a high risk of lithium toxicity).
No products indexed under this heading.

Lithium Carbonate (Diuretics reduce the renal clearance and add a high risk of lithium toxicity). Products include:
Eskalith 1406
Lithobid Tablets 1670

Lithium Citrate (Diuretics reduce the renal clearance and add a high risk of lithium toxicity).
No products indexed under this heading.

Losartan Potassium (Co-administration increases the risk of hyperkalemia). Products include:
Cozaar Tablets 1913
Hyzaar 1964

Meclofenamate Sodium (Co-administration of non-steroidal anti-inflammatory agents can reduce the diuretic, natriuretic, and antihypertensive effects).
No products indexed under this heading.

Mefenamic Acid (Co-administration of non-steroidal anti-inflammatory agents can reduce the diuretic, natriuretic, and antihypertensive effects).
No products indexed under this heading.

Meloxicam (Co-administration of non-steroidal anti-inflammatory agents can reduce the diuretic, natriuretic, and antihypertensive effects). Products include:
Mobic Oral Suspension 893
Mobic Tablets 893

Methyclothiazide (Co-administration with other diuretics may result in hypochloremia, hyponatremia, and increases in BUN).
No products indexed under this heading.

Metolazone (Co-administration with other diuretics may result in hypochloremia, hyponatremia, and increases in BUN).
No products indexed under this heading.

Moexipril Hydrochloride (Co-administration increases the risk of hyperkalemia). Products include:
Uniretic Tablets 3114
Univasc Tablets 3118

Nabumetone (Co-administration of non-steroidal anti-inflammatory agents can reduce the diuretic, natriuretic, and antihypertensive effects). Products include:
Relafen Tablets 1523

Naproxen (Co-administration of non-steroidal anti-inflammatory agents can reduce the diuretic, natriuretic, and antihypertensive effects). Products include:
EC-Naprosyn Delayed-Release Tablets 2769
Naprosyn Suspension 2769
Naprosyn Tablets 2769
Prevacid NapraPAC 3277

Naproxen Sodium (Co-administration of non-steroidal anti-inflammatory agents can reduce the diuretic, natriuretic, and antihypertensive effects). Products include:
Aleve Tablets, Caplets and Gelcaps 605
Anaprox Tablets 2769
Anaprox DS Tablets 2769

IMPORTANT NOTE: Always consult each drug listing in the patient's regimen for possible interactions.

Oxaprozin (Co-administration of non-steroidal anti-inflammatory agents can reduce the diuretic, natriuretic, and antihypertensive effects).
No products indexed under this heading.

Perindopril Erbumine (Co-administration increases the risk of hyperkalemia). Products include:
Aceon Tablets (2 mg, 4 mg, 8 mg) **3191**

Phenylbutazone (Co-administration of non-steroidal anti-inflammatory agents can reduce the diuretic, natriuretic, and antihypertensive effects).
No products indexed under this heading.

Piroxicam (Co-administration of non-steroidal anti-inflammatory agents can reduce the diuretic, natriuretic, and antihypertensive effects).
No products indexed under this heading.

Polythiazide (Co-administration with other diuretics may result in hypochloremia, hyponatremia, and increases in BUN).
No products indexed under this heading.

Potassium Acid Phosphate (Amiloride is associated with hyperkalemia; concurrent use with potassium supplements is contraindicated). Products include:
K-Phos Original (Sodium Free) Tablets **785**

Potassium Bicarbonate (Amiloride is associated with hyperkalemia; concurrent use with potassium supplements is contraindicated).
No products indexed under this heading.

Potassium Chloride (Amiloride is associated with hyperkalemia; concurrent use with potassium supplements is contraindicated). Products include:
Colyte with Flavor Packs for Oral Solution **3102**
HalfLytely and Bisacodyl Tablets Bowel Prep Kit with Flavors Packs **915**
K-Dur Extended-Relase Tablets **3047**
K-Lor Powder Packets **472**
K-Tab Filmtab Tablets **473**
TriLyte with Flavor Packs for Oral Solution **3114**

Potassium Citrate (Amiloride is associated with hyperkalemia; concurrent use with potassium supplements is contraindicated). Products include:
Urocit-K Tablets **2109**

Potassium Gluconate (Amiloride is associated with hyperkalemia; concurrent use with potassium supplements is contraindicated).
No products indexed under this heading.

Potassium Phosphate (Amiloride is associated with hyperkalemia; concurrent use with potassium supplements is contraindicated). Products include:
K-Phos Neutral Tablets **785**

Quinapril Hydrochloride (Co-administration increases the risk of hyperkalemia).
No products indexed under this heading.

Ramipril (Co-administration increases the risk of hyperkalemia). Products include:
Altace Capsules **1673**

Rofecoxib (Co-administration of non-steroidal anti-inflammatory agents can reduce the diuretic, natriuretic, and antihypertensive effects).
No products indexed under this heading.

Spirapril Hydrochloride (Co-administration increases the risk of hyperkalemia).
No products indexed under this heading.

Spironolactone (Amiloride is associated with hyperkalemia; concurrent use with potassium sparing diuretics is contraindicated).
No products indexed under this heading.

Sulindac (Co-administration of non-steroidal anti-inflammatory agents can reduce the diuretic, natriuretic, and antihypertensive effects). Products include:
Clinoril Tablets **1899**

Tacrolimus (Co-administration increases the risk of hyperkalemia). Products include:
Prograf Capsules and Injection **624**
Protopic Ointment **629**

Telmisartan (Co-administration increases the risk of hyperkalemia). Products include:
Micardis Tablets **884**
Micardis HCT Tablets **886**

Tolmetin Sodium (Co-administration of non-steroidal anti-inflammatory agents can reduce the diuretic, natriuretic, and antihypertensive effects).
No products indexed under this heading.

Torsemide (Co-administration with other diuretics may result in hypochloremia, hyponatremia, and increases in BUN).
No products indexed under this heading.

Trandolapril (Co-administration increases the risk of hyperkalemia). Products include:
Mavik Tablets **482**
Tarka Tablets **519**

Triamterene (Amiloride is associated with hyperkalemia; concurrent use with potassium sparing diuretics is contraindicated). Products include:
Dyazide Capsules **1389**
Dyrenium Capsules **3390**
Maxzide **2150**

Valdecoxib (Co-administration of non-steroidal anti-inflammatory agents can reduce the diuretic, natriuretic, and antihypertensive effects).
No products indexed under this heading.

Valsartan (Co-administration increases the risk of hyperkalemia). Products include:
Diovan HCT Tablets **2195**
Diovan Tablets **2191**

Food Interactions

Diet, potassium-rich (Potential for rapid increases in serum potassium levels).

MIGRANAL NASAL SPRAY

(Dihydroergotamine Mesylate) **3350**
May interact with 5HT1-receptor agonists, cytochrome p450 3a4 inhibitors (selected), cytochrome p450 3a4 inhibitors, potent, macrolide antibiotics, vasopressors, and certain other agents. Compounds in these categories include:

Acetazolamide (Co-administration of dihydroergotamin with potent CYP3A4 inhibitors results in vasospasm that can lead to cerebral ischemia and/or ischemia of the extremities, therefore it is contraindicated).
No products indexed under this heading.

Amiodarone Hydrochloride (Co-administration of dihydroergotamin with potent CYP3A4 inhibitors results in vasospasm that can lead to cerebral ischemia and/or ischemia of the extremities, therefore it is contraindicated). Products include:
Pacerone Tablets **3337**

Amprenavir (Co-administration of dihydroergotamin and potent CYP3A4 inhibitors results in vasospasm that can lead to cerebral ischemia and/or ischemia of the extremities, therefore it is contraindicated). Products include:
Agenerase Capsules **1299**
Agenerase Oral Solution **1304**

Anastrozole (Co-administration of dihydroergotamin with potent CYP3A4 inhibitors results in vasospasm that can lead to cerebral ischemia and/or ischemia of the extremities, therefore it is contraindicated). Products include:
Arimidex Tablets **665**

Aprepitant (Co-administration of dihydroergotamin with potent CYP3A4 inhibitors results in vasospasm that can lead to cerebral ischemia and/or ischemia of the extremities, therefore it is contraindicated). Products include:
Emend Capsules **1944**

Atazanavir (Co-administration of dihydroergotamin and potent CYP3A4 inhibitors results in vasospasm that can lead to cerebral ischemia and/or ischemia of the extremities, therefore it is contraindicated).
No products indexed under this heading.

Atazanavir sulfate (Co-administration of dihydroergotamin and potent CYP3A4 inhibitors results in vasospasm that can lead to cerebral ischemia and/or ischemia of the extremities, therefore it is contraindicated). Products include:
Reyataz Capsules **948**

Azithromycin Dihydrate (Co-administration of ergot alkaloids with macrolide antibiotics has resulted in increased plasma levels of unchanged alkaloids and peripheral vasoconstriction; vasospastic reactions have been reported with concurrent use at therapeutic doses). Products include:
Zithromax **2568**
Zithromax for IV Infusion **2573**
Zithromax for Oral Suspension, 300 mg, 600 mg, 900 mg, 1200 mg **2561**
Zithromax Tablets, 250 mg, 500 mg **2561**
Zithromax Tri-Pak **2561**
Zithromax Z-Pak **2568**

Cimetidine (Co-administration of dihydroergotamin with potent CYP3A4 inhibitors results in vasospasm that can lead to cerebral ischemia and/or ischemia of the extremities, therefore it is contraindicated). Products include:
Tagamet HB 200 Tablets .... ▣ **637**
Tagamet Tablets **1547**

Cimetidine Hydrochloride (Co-administration of dihydroergotamin with potent CYP3A4 inhibitors results in vasospasm that can lead to cerebral ischemia and/or ischemia of the extremities, therefore it is contraindicated).
No products indexed under this heading.

Ciprofloxacin (Co-administration of dihydroergotamin with potent CYP3A4 inhibitors results in vasospasm that can lead to cerebral ischemia and/or ischemia of the extremities, therefore it is contraindicated). Products include:
Cipro I.V. **2998**
Cipro I.V. Pharmacy Bulk Package **3509**
Cipro Oral Suspension **2991**
Cipro XR Tablets **3004**
Ciprodex Otic Suspension **555**

Clarithromycin (Co-administration of dihydroergotamin and potent CYP3A4 inhibitors results in vasospasm that can lead to cerebral ischemia and/or ischemia of the extremities, therefore it is contraindicated). Products include:
Biaxin/Biaxin XL **402**
PREVPAC **3281**

Clotrimazole (Co-administration of dihydroergotamin with potent CYP3A4 inhibitors results in vasospasm that can lead to cerebral ischemia and/or ischemia of the extremities, therefore it is contraindicated). Products include:
Lotrimin **3053**
Lotrisone **3054**

Cyclosporine (Co-administration of dihydroergotamin with potent CYP3A4 inhibitors results in vasospasm that can lead to cerebral ischemia and/or ischemia of the extremities, therefore it is contraindicated). Products include:
Gengraf Capsules **458**
Neoral Soft Gelatin Capsules **2247**
Neoral Oral Solution **2247**
Restasis Ophthalmic Emulsion **570**
Sandimmune **2259**

Dalfopristin (Co-administration of dihydroergotamin with potent CYP3A4 inhibitors results in vasospasm that can lead to cerebral ischemia and/or ischemia of the extremities, therefore it is contraindicated). Products include:
Synercid I.V. **1690**

Danazol (Co-administration of dihydroergotamin with potent CYP3A4 inhibitors results in vasospasm that can lead to cerebral ischemia and/or ischemia of the extremities, therefore it is contraindicated).
No products indexed under this heading.

Delavirdine Mesylate (Co-administration of dihydroergotamin with potent CYP3A4 inhibitors results in vasospasm that can lead to cerebral ischemia and/or ischemia of the extremities, therefore it is contraindicated). Products include:
Rescriptor Tablets **2535**

Diltiazem Hydrochloride (Co-administration of dihydroergotamin with potent CYP3A4 inhibitors results in vasospasm that can lead to cere-

bral ischemia and/or ischemia of the extremities, therefore it is contraindicated). Products include:

Cardizem LA Extended Release Tablets 1699
Tiazac Capsules 1204

Diltiazem Maleate (Co-administration of dihydroergotamin with potent CYP3A4 inhibitors results in vasospasm that can lead to cerebral ischemia and/or ischemia of the extremities, therefore it is contraindicated).

No products indexed under this heading.

3-Diphenylacrylate (Concurrent use of 5-HT1 agonists and ergot-containing or ergot-type medications should not be undertaken within 24 hours of each other).

No products indexed under this heading.

Dirithromycin (Co-administration of ergot alkaloids with macrolide antibiotics has resulted in increased plasma levels of unchanged alkaloids and peripheral vasoconstriction; vasospastic reactions have been reported with concurrent use at therapeutic doses).

No products indexed under this heading.

Dobutamine (Concurrent use with peripheral and central vasoconstrictors is not recommended because the combination may result in additive or synergistic elevation of blood pressure).

No products indexed under this heading.

Dobutamine Hydrochloride (Concurrent use with peripheral and central vasoconstrictors is not recommended because the combination may result in additive or synergistic elevation of blood pressure).

No products indexed under this heading.

Dopamine Hydrochloride (Concurrent use with peripheral and central vasoconstrictors is not recommended because the combination may result in additive or synergistic elevation of blood pressure).

No products indexed under this heading.

Efavirenz (Co-administration of dihydroergotamin with potent CYP3A4 inhibitors results in vasospasm that can lead to cerebral ischemia and/or ischemia of the extremities, therefore it is contraindicated). Products include:

Sustiva Capsules 957

Ephedrine Sulfate (Concurrent use with peripheral and central vasoconstrictors is not recommended because the combination may result in additive or synergistic elevation of blood pressure).

No products indexed under this heading.

Epinephrine Bitartrate (Concurrent use with peripheral and central vasoconstrictors is not recommended because the combination may result in additive or synergistic elevation of blood pressure).

No products indexed under this heading.

Epinephrine Hydrochloride (Concurrent use with peripheral and central vasoconstrictors is not recommended because the combination may result in additive or synergistic elevation of blood pressure).

No products indexed under this heading.

Erythromycin (Co-administration of dihydroergotamin with potent CYP3A4 inhibitors results in vasospasm that can lead to cerebral ischemia and/or ischemia of the extremities, therefore it is contraindicated). Products include:

Erygel Topical Gel 2096
Ery-Tab Tablets 447
Erythromycin Base Filmtab Tablets 454
Erythromycin Delayed-Release Capsules, USP 456
PCE Dispertab Tablets 510

Erythromycin Estolate (Co-administration of dihydroergotamin with potent CYP3A4 inhibitors results in vasospasm that can lead to cerebral ischemia and/or ischemia of the extremities, therefore it is contraindicated).

No products indexed under this heading.

Erythromycin Ethylsuccinate (Co-administration of dihydroergotamin with potent CYP3A4 inhibitors results in vasospasm that can lead to cerebral ischemia and/or ischemia of the extremities, therefore it is contraindicated). Products include:

E.E.S. 449
EryPed 445

Erythromycin Gluceptate (Co-administration of dihydroergotamin with potent CYP3A4 inhibitors results in vasospasm that can lead to cerebral ischemia and/or ischemia of the extremities, therefore it is contraindicated).

No products indexed under this heading.

Erythromycin Lactobionate (Co-administration of dihydroergotamin with potent CYP3A4 inhibitors results in vasospasm that can lead to cerebral ischemia and/or ischemia of the extremities, therefore it is contraindicated).

No products indexed under this heading.

Erythromycin Stearate (Co-administration of dihydroergotamin with potent CYP3A4 inhibitors results in vasospasm that can lead to cerebral ischemia and/or ischemia of the extremities, therefore it is contraindicated). Products include:

Erythrocin Stearate Filmtab Tablets 452

Esomeprazole Magnesium (Co-administration of dihydroergotamin with potent CYP3A4 inhibitors results in vasospasm that can lead to cerebral ischemia and/or ischemia of the extremities, therefore it is contraindicated). Products include:

Nexium Delayed-Release Capsules 645

Fluconazole (Co-administration of dihydroergotamin with potent CYP3A4 inhibitors results in vasospasm that can lead to cerebral ischemia and/or ischemia of the extremities, therefore it is contraindicated).

No products indexed under this heading.

Fluoxetine Hydrochloride (Co-administration of dihydroergotamin with potent CYP3A4 inhibitors results in vasospasm that can lead to cerebral ischemia and/or ischemia of the extremities, therefore it is contraindicated). Products include:

Prozac Pulvules and Liquid 1771
Symbyax Capsules 1788

Fluvoxamine Maleate (Co-administration of dihydroergotamin with potent CYP3A4 inhibitors results in vasospasm that can lead to cerebral ischemia and/or ischemia of the extremities, therefore it is contraindicated).

No products indexed under this heading.

Fosamprenavir Calcium (Co-administration of dihydroergotamin and potent CYP3A4 inhibitors results in vasospasm that can lead to cerebral ischemia and/or ischemia of the extremities, therefore it is contraindicated). Products include:

Lexiva Tablets 1473

Indinavir Sulfate (Co-administration of dihydroergotamin and potent CYP3A4 inhibitors results in vasospasm that can lead to cerebral ischemia and/or ischemia of the extremities, therefore it is contraindicated). Products include:

Crixivan Capsules 1918

Isoniazid (Co-administration of dihydroergotamin with potent CYP3A4 inhibitors results in vasospasm that can lead to cerebral ischemia and/or ischemia of the extremities, therefore it is contraindicated).

No products indexed under this heading.

Isoproterenol Hydrochloride (Concurrent use with peripheral and central vasoconstrictors is not recommended because the combination may result in additive or synergistic elevation of blood pressure).

No products indexed under this heading.

Isoproterenol Sulfate (Concurrent use with peripheral and central vasoconstrictors is not recommended because the combination may result in additive or synergistic elevation of blood pressure).

No products indexed under this heading.

Itraconazole (Co-administration of dihydroergotamin and potent CYP3A4 inhibitors results in vasospasm that can lead to cerebral ischemia and/or ischemia of the extremities, therefore it is contraindicated).

No products indexed under this heading.

Ketoconazole (Co-administration of dihydroergotamin and potent CYP3A4 inhibitors results in vasospasm that can lead to cerebral ischemia and/or ischemia of the extremities, therefore it is contraindicated). Products include:

Nizoral A-D Shampoo, 1% 1839
Nizoral 2% Shampoo 1838

Lopinavir (Co-administration of dihydroergotamin and potent CYP3A4 inhibitors results in vasospasm that can lead to cerebral ischemia and/or ischemia of the extremities, therefore it is contraindicated). Products include:

Kaletra 474

Loratadine (Co-administration of dihydroergotamin with potent CYP3A4 inhibitors results in vasospasm that can lead to cerebral ischemia and/or ischemia of the extremities, therefore it is contraindicated). Products include:

Alavert Allergy & Sinus D-12 Hour Tablets 743
Alavert 743
Children's Claritin 24 Hour Non-Drowsy Allergy Syrup 732
Claritin Non-Drowsy 24 Hour Tablets 731
Non-Drowsy Claritin Hives Relief Tablets 733
Claritin Reditabs 24 Hour Non-Drowsy Tablets 732
Claritin-D Non-Drowsy 12 Hour Tablets 731
Claritin-D Non-Drowsy 24 Hour Tablets 731
Children's Dimetapp ND Non-Drowsy Allergy Syrup 746
Triaminic Allerchews 684

Mephentermine Sulfate (Concurrent use with peripheral and central vasoconstrictors is not recommended because the combination may result in additive or synergistic elevation of blood pressure).

No products indexed under this heading.

Metaraminol Bitartrate (Concurrent use with peripheral and central vasoconstrictors is not recommended because the combination may result in additive or synergistic elevation of blood pressure). Products include:

Aramine Injection 1889

Methoxamine Hydrochloride (Concurrent use with peripheral and central vasoconstrictors is not recommended because the combination may result in additive or synergistic elevation of blood pressure).

No products indexed under this heading.

Metronidazole (Co-administration of dihydroergotamin with potent CYP3A4 inhibitors results in vasospasm that can lead to cerebral ischemia and/or ischemia of the extremities, therefore it is contraindicated). Products include:

Metrogel 1% 1212
MetroGel-Vaginal Gel 1822
Noritate Cream, 1% 1051

Metronidazole Benzoate (Co-administration of dihydroergotamin with potent CYP3A4 inhibitors results in vasospasm that can lead to cerebral ischemia and/or ischemia of the extremities, therefore it is contraindicated).

No products indexed under this heading.

Metronidazole Hydrochloride (Co-administration of dihydroergotamin with potent CYP3A4 inhibitors results in vasospasm that can lead to cerebral ischemia and/or ischemia of the extremities, therefore it is contraindicated).

No products indexed under this heading.

Miconazole (Co-administration of dihydroergotamin with potent CYP3A4 inhibitors results in vasospasm that can lead to cerebral ischemia and/or ischemia of the extremities, therefore it is contraindicated).

No products indexed under this heading.

Miconazole Nitrate (Co-administration of dihydroergotamin with potent CYP3A4 inhibitors results in vasospasm that can lead to cerebral ischemia and/or ischemia of the extremities, therefore it is contraindicated). Products include:

Desenex ■674
Desenex Jock Itch Spray Powder ■674

Naratriptan Hydrochloride (Concurrent use of 5-HT1 agonists and ergot-containing or ergot-type medications should not be undertaken within 24 hours of each other). Products include:
Amerge Tablets 1312

Nefazodone Hydrochloride (Co-administration of dihydroergotamin and potent CYP3A4 inhibitors results in vasospasm that can lead to cerebral ischemia and/or ischemia of the extremities, therefore it is contraindicated).
No products indexed under this heading.

Nelfinavir Mesylate (Co-administration of dihydroergotamin and potent CYP3A4 inhibitors results in vasospasm that can lead to cerebral ischemia and/or ischemia of the extremities, therefore it is contraindicated). Products include:
Viracept 2556

Nevirapine (Co-administration of dihydroergotamin with potent CYP3A4 inhibitors results in vasospasm that can lead to cerebral ischemia and/or ischemia of the extremities, therefore it is contraindicated). Products include:
Viramune Oral Suspension 903
Viramune Tablets 903

Niacinamide (Co-administration of dihydroergotamin with potent CYP3A4 inhibitors results in vasospasm that can lead to cerebral ischemia and/or ischemia of the extremities, therefore it is contraindicated).
No products indexed under this heading.

Nicotinamide (Co-administration of dihydroergotamin with potent CYP3A4 inhibitors results in vasospasm that can lead to cerebral ischemia and/or ischemia of the extremities, therefore it is contraindicated). Products include:
Nicomide Tablets 3190

Nicotine (May provoke vasoconstriction in some patients, predisposing to a greater ischemic response to ergot). Products include:
Nicoderm CQ Patch 1629
NicoDerm CQ Clear Patch ■627
Nicotrol Inhaler 2594
Nicotrol NS 2596

Nicotine Polacrilex (May provoke vasoconstriction in some patients, predisposing to a greater ischemic response to ergot). Products include:
Commit Lozenges 1625
Nicorette Gum 1632

Nifedipine (Co-administration of dihydroergotamin with potent CYP3A4 inhibitors results in vasospasm that can lead to cerebral ischemia and/or ischemia of the extremities, therefore it is contraindicated). Products include:
Adalat CC Tablets 2978

Norepinephrine Bitartrate (Concurrent use with peripheral and central vasoconstrictors is not recommended because the combination may result in additive or synergistic elevation of blood pressure).
No products indexed under this heading.

Norfloxacin (Co-administration of dihydroergotamin with potent CYP3A4 inhibitors results in vasospasm that can lead to cerebral ischemia and/or ischemia of the extremities, therefore it is contraindicated). Products include:
Noroxin Tablets 2009

Omeprazole (Co-administration of dihydroergotamin with potent CYP3A4 inhibitors results in vasospasm that can lead to cerebral ischemia and/or ischemia of the extremities, therefore it is contraindicated). Products include:
Zegerid Powder for Oral Solution 2972

Paroxetine Hydrochloride (Co-administration of dihydroergotamin with potent CYP3A4 inhibitors results in vasospasm that can lead to cerebral ischemia and/or ischemia of the extremities, therefore it is contraindicated). Products include:
Paxil CR Controlled-Release Tablets 1509
Paxil 1501

Phenylephrine Hydrochloride (Concurrent use with peripheral and central vasoconstrictors is not recommended because the combination may result in additive or synergistic elevation of blood pressure). Products include:
Alacol DM Syrup 739
Hycomine Compound Tablets 1105
Preparation H Maximum Strength Cream ■747
Preparation H Cooling Gel ■747
Preparation H ■747
Sudafed PE Tablets ■711
Vicks Sinex Nasal Spray and Ultra Fine Mist for Sinus Relief 2677
Zicam Concentrated Cough Mist for Kids Plus D Cool Cherry ■643
Zicam Concentrated Cough Mist Plus D Cool Cherry ■642

Propoxyphene Hydrochloride (Co-administration of dihydroergotamin with potent CYP3A4 inhibitors results in vasospasm that can lead to cerebral ischemia and/or ischemia of the extremities, therefore it is contraindicated).
No products indexed under this heading.

Propoxyphene Napsylate (Co-administration of dihydroergotamin with potent CYP3A4 inhibitors results in vasospasm that can lead to cerebral ischemia and/or ischemia of the extremities, therefore it is contraindicated). Products include:
Darvocet A 500 Tablets 3497

Propranolol Hydrochloride (May potentiate the vasoconstrictive action of ergotamine by blocking the vasodilating property of epinephrine). Products include:
Inderal LA Long-Acting Capsules 3421
InnoPran XL Capsules 2728

Quinidine (Co-administration of dihydroergotamin with potent CYP3A4 inhibitors results in vasospasm that can lead to cerebral ischemia and/or ischemia of the extremities, therefore it is contraindicated).
No products indexed under this heading.

Quinidine Hydrochloride (Co-administration of dihydroergotamin with potent CYP3A4 inhibitors results in vasospasm that can lead to cerebral ischemia and/or ischemia of the extremities, therefore it is contraindicated).
No products indexed under this heading.

Quinidine Polygalacturonate (Co-administration of dihydroergotamin with potent CYP3A4 inhibitors results in vasospasm that can lead to cerebral ischemia and/or ischemia of the extremities, therefore it is contraindicated).
No products indexed under this heading.

Quinidine Sulfate (Co-administration of dihydroergotamin with potent CYP3A4 inhibitors results in vasospasm that can lead to cerebral ischemia and/or ischemia of the extremities, therefore it is contraindicated).
No products indexed under this heading.

Quinine (Co-administration of dihydroergotamin with potent CYP3A4 inhibitors results in vasospasm that can lead to cerebral ischemia and/or ischemia of the extremities, therefore it is contraindicated).
No products indexed under this heading.

Quinine Sulfate (Co-administration of dihydroergotamin with potent CYP3A4 inhibitors results in vasospasm that can lead to cerebral ischemia and/or ischemia of the extremities, therefore it is contraindicated).
No products indexed under this heading.

Quinupristin (Co-administration of dihydroergotamin with potent CYP3A4 inhibitors results in vasospasm that can lead to cerebral ischemia and/or ischemia of the extremities, therefore it is contraindicated). Products include:
Synercid I.V. 1690

Ranitidine Bismuth Citrate (Co-administration of dihydroergotamin with potent CYP3A4 inhibitors results in vasospasm that can lead to cerebral ischemia and/or ischemia of the extremities, therefore it is contraindicated).
No products indexed under this heading.

Ranitidine Hydrochloride (Co-administration of dihydroergotamin with potent CYP3A4 inhibitors results in vasospasm that can lead to cerebral ischemia and/or ischemia of the extremities, therefore it is contraindicated). Products include:
Zantac 1597
Zantac Injection 1593
Zantac 75 Tablets ■715
Zantac 150 Maximum Strength Tablets ■715
Zantac Injection Pharmacy Bulk Package 1595

Ritonavir (Co-administration of dihydroergotamin and potent CYP3A4 inhibitors results in vasospasm that can lead to cerebral ischemia and/or ischemia of the extremities, therefore it is contraindicated). Products include:
Kaletra 474
Norvir 499

Rizatriptan Benzoate (Concurrent use of 5-HT1 agonists and ergot-containing or ergot-type medications should not be undertaken within 24 hours of each other). Products include:
Maxalt Tablets 1983
Maxalt-MLT Orally Disintegrating Tablets 1983

Saquinavir (Co-administration of dihydroergotamin and potent CYP3A4 inhibitors results in vasospasm that can lead to cerebral ischemia and/or ischemia of the extremities, therefore it is contraindicated).
No products indexed under this heading.

Saquinavir Mesylate (Co-administration of dihydroergotamin and potent CYP3A4 inhibitors results in vasospasm that can lead to cerebral ischemia and/or ischemia of the extremities, therefore it is contraindicated). Products include:
Invirase 2776

Sertraline Hydrochloride (Co-administration of dihydroergotamin with potent CYP3A4 inhibitors results in vasospasm that can lead to cerebral ischemia and/or ischemia of the extremities, therefore it is contraindicated). Products include:
Zoloft 2581

Sumatriptan (Co-administration could lead to additive coronary artery vasospasm effect; concurrent use should not be undertaken within 24 hours of each other). Products include:
Imitrex Nasal Spray 1435

Sumatriptan Succinate (Co-administration could lead to additive coronary artery vasospasm effect; concurrent use should not be undertaken within 24 hours of each other). Products include:
Imitrex Injection 1431
Imitrex Tablets 1440

Telithromycin (Co-administration of dihydroergotamin and potent CYP3A4 inhibitors results in vasospasm that can lead to cerebral ischemia and/or ischemia of the extremities, therefore it is contraindicated). Products include:
Ketek Tablets 2920

Troglitazone (Co-administration of dihydroergotamin with potent CYP3A4 inhibitors results in vasospasm that can lead to cerebral ischemia and/or ischemia of the extremities, therefore it is contraindicated).
No products indexed under this heading.

Troleandomycin (Co-administration of dihydroergotamin and potent CYP3A4 inhibitors results in vasospasm that can lead to cerebral ischemia and/or ischemia of the extremities, therefore it is contraindicated).
No products indexed under this heading.

Valproate Sodium (Co-administration of dihydroergotamin with potent CYP3A4 inhibitors results in vasospasm that can lead to cerebral ischemia and/or ischemia of the extremities, therefore it is contraindicated). Products include:
Depacon Injection 412

Verapamil Hydrochloride (Co-administration of dihydroergotamin with potent CYP3A4 inhibitors results in vasospasm that can lead to cerebral ischemia and/or ischemia of the extremities, therefore it is contraindicated). Products include:
Covera-HS Tablets 3135
Tarka Tablets 519
Verelan PM Capsules 3120

Voriconazole (Co-administration of dihydroergotamin and potent CYP3A4 inhibitors results in vaso-

spasm that can lead to cerebral ischemia and/or ischemia of the extremities, therefore it is contraindicated). Products include:
- VFEND I.V. 2543
- VFEND Oral Suspension 2543
- VFEND Tablets 2543

Zafirlukast (Co-administration of dihydroergotamin with potent CYP3A4 inhibitors results in vasospasm that can lead to cerebral ischemia and/or ischemia of the extremities, therefore it is contraindicated). Products include:
- Accolate Tablets 663

Zileuton (Co-administration of dihydroergotamin with potent CYP3A4 inhibitors results in vasospasm that can lead to cerebral ischemia and/or ischemia of the extremities, therefore it is contraindicated).
No products indexed under this heading.

Zolmitriptan (Concurrent use of 5-HT1 agonists and ergot-containing or ergot-type medications should not be undertaken within 24 hours of each other). Products include:
- Zomig Nasal Spray 718
- Zomig Tablets 714
- Zomig-ZMT Tablets 714

Food Interactions

Grapefruit (Co-administration of dihydroergotamin with potent CYP3A4 inhibitors results in vasospasm that can lead to cerebral ischemia and/or ischemia of the extremities, therefore it is contraindicated).

Grapefruit Juice (Co-administration of dihydroergotamin with potent CYP3A4 inhibitors results in vasospasm that can lead to cerebral ischemia and/or ischemia of the extremities, therefore it is contraindicated).

MINERAL OIL

(Mineral Oil) 2716

May interact with stool softener laxatives. Compounds in these categories include:

Docusate Calcium (Do not use mineral oil if you are presently taking a stool softener laxative). Products include:
- Kaopectate Stool Softener 702

Docusate Potassium (Do not use mineral oil if you are presently taking a stool softener laxative).
No products indexed under this heading.

Docusate Sodium (Do not use mineral oil if you are presently taking a stool softener laxative). Products include:
- Colace Capsules 729
- Colace Capsules 50 mg 2715
- Colace Capsules 100 mg 2715
- Colace Liquid 1% Solution 2716
- Colace Syrup 2716
- Dulcolax Stool Softener 608
- Peri-Colace Tablets 2716
- Senokot-S Tablets 2717

MINTEZOL SUSPENSION

(Thiabendazole) 2002

See Mintezol Chewable Tablets

MINTEZOL CHEWABLE TABLETS

(Thiabendazole) 2002

May interact with xanthines. Compounds in these categories include:

Aminophylline (Thiabendazole may compete with theophylline for sites of metabolism in the liver, thus elevating the serum levels of theophylline to toxic levels; monitor theophylline blood levels).
No products indexed under this heading.

Dyphylline (Thiabendazole may compete with theophylline for sites of metabolism in the liver, thus elevating the serum levels of theophylline to toxic levels; monitor theophylline blood levels).
No products indexed under this heading.

Theophylline (Thiabendazole may compete with theophylline for sites of metabolism in the liver, thus elevating the serum levels of theophylline to toxic levels; monitor theophylline blood levels).
No products indexed under this heading.

Theophylline Anhydrous (Thiabendazole may compete with theophylline for sites of metabolism in the liver, thus elevating the serum levels of theophylline to toxic levels; monitor theophylline blood levels). Products include:
- Uniphyl Tablets 2708

Theophylline Calcium Salicylate (Thiabendazole may compete with theophylline for sites of metabolism in the liver, thus elevating the serum levels of theophylline to toxic levels; monitor theophylline blood levels).
No products indexed under this heading.

Theophylline Dihydroxypropyl (Glyceryl) (Thiabendazole may compete with theophylline for sites of metabolism in the liver, thus elevating the serum levels of theophylline to toxic levels; monitor theophylline blood levels).
No products indexed under this heading.

Theophylline Ethylenediamine (Thiabendazole may compete with theophylline for sites of metabolism in the liver, thus elevating the serum levels of theophylline to toxic levels; monitor theophylline blood levels).
No products indexed under this heading.

Theophylline Sodium Glycinate (Thiabendazole may compete with theophylline for sites of metabolism in the liver, thus elevating the serum levels of theophylline to toxic levels; monitor theophylline blood levels).
No products indexed under this heading.

MIRADON TABLETS

(Anisindione) 3056

May interact with androgens, antacids, antihistamines, barbiturates, corticosteroids, diuretics, inhalant anesthetics, monoamine oxidase inhibitors, narcotic analgesics, non-steroidal anti-inflammatory agents, oral contraceptives, phenytoin, pyrazolon derivatives, quinidine, salicylates, thrombolytics, thyroid preparations, and certain other agents. Compounds in these categories include:

Acrivastine (Antihistamines have been reported to diminish oral anticoagulant response, i.e., decreased prothrombin time response significantly).
No products indexed under this heading.

Alfentanil Hydrochloride (Prolonged use of narcotics may increase oral anticoagulant response, i.e., increased prothrombin time response).
No products indexed under this heading.

Allopurinol (May increase oral anticoagulant response, i.e., increased prothrombin time response).
No products indexed under this heading.

Alteplase (Co-administration with thrombolytics is not recommended and may be hazardous). Products include:
- Activase I.V. 1225
- Cathflo Activase 1232

Aluminum Carbonate (Antacids have been reported to diminish oral anticoagulant response, i.e., decreased prothrombin time response significantly).
No products indexed under this heading.

Aluminum Hydroxide (Antacids have been reported to diminish oral anticoagulant response, i.e., decreased prothrombin time response significantly). Products include:
- Gaviscon Regular Strength Liquid 620
- Gaviscon Regular Strength Tablets 619
- Gaviscon Extra Strength Liquid 620
- Gaviscon Extra Strength Tablets 619
- Maalox Max Maximum Strength Antacid/Anti-Gas Liquid 2165
- Maalox Regular Strength Antacid/Antigas Liquid 2164

Amiloride Hydrochloride (Diuretics have been reported to diminish or increase oral anticoagulant response, i.e., decreased or increased prothrombin time response significantly). Products include:
- Midamor Tablets 2000
- Moduretic Tablets 2003

p-Aminosalicylic Acid (May increase oral anticoagulant response, i.e., increased prothrombin time response).
No products indexed under this heading.

Amiodarone Hydrochloride (May increase oral anticoagulant response, i.e., increased prothrombin time response). Products include:
- Pacerone Tablets 3337

Anistreplase (Co-administration with thrombolytics is not recommended and may be hazardous).
No products indexed under this heading.

Antipyrine (May increase oral anticoagulant response, i.e., increased prothrombin time response).
No products indexed under this heading.

Aprobarbital (Barbiturates have been reported to diminish oral anticoagulant response, i.e., decreased prothrombin time response significantly).
No products indexed under this heading.

Aspirin (May increase oral anticoagulant response, i.e., increased prothrombin time response; aspirin may increase the bleeding tendency produced by anticoagulants without altering prothrombin time determination). Products include:
- Aggrenox Capsules 855
- Bayer, Aspirin Regimen 606
- Bayer Aspirin Tablets 3515
- BC Powder 612
- BC Allergy Sinus Cold Powder 612
- Arthritis Strength BC Powder 612
- BC Sinus Cold Powder 612
- Ecotrin Enteric Coated Aspirin Low, Regular and Maximum Strength Tablets 1627
- Goody's Body Pain Formula Powder 621
- Goody's Extra Strength Headache Powder 621
- Goody's Extra Strength Pain Relief Tablets 621
- Percodan Tablets 1115
- St. Joseph 81 mg Aspirin Chewable and Enteric Coated Tablets 1841

Astemizole (Antihistamines have been reported to diminish oral anticoagulant response, i.e., decreased prothrombin time response significantly).
No products indexed under this heading.

Azatadine Maleate (Antihistamines have been reported to diminish oral anticoagulant response, i.e., decreased prothrombin time response significantly).
No products indexed under this heading.

Bendroflumethiazide (Diuretics have been reported to diminish or increase oral anticoagulant response, i.e., decreased or increased prothrombin time response significantly).
No products indexed under this heading.

Betamethasone Acetate (Adrenocorticosteroids have been reported to diminish oral anticoagulant response, i.e., decreased prothrombin time response significantly).
No products indexed under this heading.

Betamethasone Sodium Phosphate (Adrenocorticosteroids have been reported to diminish oral anticoagulant response, i.e., decreased prothrombin time response significantly).
No products indexed under this heading.

Bromelains (May increase oral anticoagulant response, i.e., increased prothrombin time response).
No products indexed under this heading.

Bromodiphenhydramine Hydrochloride (Antihistamines have been reported to diminish oral anticoagulant response, i.e., decreased prothrombin time response significantly).
No products indexed under this heading.

Brompheniramine Maleate (Antihistamines have been reported to diminish oral anticoagulant response, i.e., decreased prothrombin time response significantly). Products include:
- Alacol DM Syrup 739
- Children's Dimetapp Cold & Allergy Elixir 745
- Children's Dimetapp DM Cold & Cough Elixir 745
- Robitussin Allergy & Cough Syrup 750

Bumetanide (Diuretics have been reported to diminish or increase oral anticoagulant response, i.e., decreased or increased prothrombin time response significantly).
No products indexed under this heading.

Buprenorphine Hydrochloride (Prolonged use of narcotics may increase oral anticoagulant response, i.e., increased prothrombin time response). Products include:
- Buprenex Injectable 2718
- Suboxone Tablets 2719
- Subutex Tablets 2719

Butabarbital (Barbiturates have been reported to diminish oral anticoagulant response, i.e., decreased prothrombin time response significantly).
No products indexed under this heading.

Butalbital (Barbiturates have been reported to diminish oral anticoagulant response, i.e., decreased prothrombin time response significantly). Products include:
Sedapap Tablets 50 mg/650 mg 2098

Carbamazepine (Has been reported to diminish oral anticoagulant response, i.e., decreased prothrombin time response significantly). Products include:
Carbatrol Capsules 3174
Equetro Extended-Release Capsules 3178
Tegretol/Tegretol-XR 2278

Celecoxib (Drugs that reduce the number of blood platelets by causing bone marrow depression, such as non-steroidal anti-inflammatory agents, may increase the bleeding tendency produced by anticoagulants without altering prothrombin time determination). Products include:
Celebrex Capsules 3130

Cetirizine Hydrochloride (Antihistamines have been reported to diminish oral anticoagulant response, i.e., decreased prothrombin time response significantly). Products include:
Zyrtec Chewable Tablets 2589
Zyrtec 2589
Zyrtec-D 12 Hour Extended Release Tablets 2591

Chloral Hydrate (May cause an increased prothrombin response by displacing the anticoagulant from protein binding sites or an increased metabolism of the unbound drug by hepatic enzyme induction).
No products indexed under this heading.

Chlorothiazide (Diuretics have been reported to diminish or increase oral anticoagulant response, i.e., decreased or increased prothrombin time response significantly). Products include:
Aldoclor Tablets 1881
Diuril Oral 1936

Chlorothiazide Sodium (Diuretics have been reported to diminish or increase oral anticoagulant response, i.e., decreased or increased prothrombin time response significantly). Products include:
Diuril Sodium Intravenous 1934

Chlorpheniramine Maleate (Antihistamines have been reported to diminish oral anticoagulant response, i.e., decreased prothrombin time response significantly). Products include:
Advil Allergy Sinus Caplets .... ■737
Advil Multi-Symptom Cold Caplets .... ■738
BC Allergy Sinus Cold Powder .... ■612
Contac Severe Cold and Flu Caplets Maximum Strength .... ■615
Hycomine Compound Tablets 1105
PediaCare Multi-Symptom Cold Liquid .... ■704
PediaCare NightRest Cough & Cold Liquid .... ■704
Robitussin Flu Liquid .... ■752
Robitussin PM Cough & Cold Liquid .... ■752
Singlet Caplets .... ■636
Sudafed Sinus & Allergy Tablets .... ■710
TheraFlu Cold & Cough Hot Liquid .... ■680
TheraFlu Cold & Sore Throat Hot Liquid .... ■680
TheraFlu Flu & Sore Throat Hot Liquid .... ■681
TheraFlu Severe Cold & Cough Hot Liquid .... ■683
TheraFlu Severe Cold Caplets .... ■679
TheraFlu Severe Cold Hot Liquid .... ■682
Triaminic Cold & Allergy Liquid .... ■685
Triaminic Cold & Cough Liquid .... ■685
Triaminic Flu, Cough & Fever Liquid .... ■685
Triaminic Night Time Cough & Cold Liquid .... ■685
Triaminic Allergy Runny Nose & Congestion Softchews .... ■688
Triaminic Cold & Cough Softchews .... ■688
Children's Tylenol Plus Cold NightTime Suspension Liquid 1851
Children's Tylenol Plus Cold & Cough Suspension Liquid and Chewable Tablets 1851
Children's Tylenol Plus Cold Chewable Tablets 1851
Children's Tylenol Plus Flu Suspension Liquid 1853
Tylenol Allergy Complete Multi-Symptom Caplets and Gelcaps with Cool Burst 1844
Multi-Symptom Tylenol Cold Night Time Caplets 1845
Vicks 44M Cough, Cold & Flu Relief 2676
Pediatric Vicks 44m Cough & Cold Relief 2673
Children's Vicks NyQuil Cold/Cough Relief 2671

Chlorpheniramine Polistirex (Antihistamines have been reported to diminish oral anticoagulant response, i.e., decreased prothrombin time response significantly). Products include:
Tussionex Pennkinetic Extended-Release Suspension 3322

Chlorpheniramine Tannate (Antihistamines have been reported to diminish oral anticoagulant response, i.e., decreased prothrombin time response significantly).
No products indexed under this heading.

Chlorpropamide (May increase oral anticoagulant response, i.e., increased prothrombin time response; oral anticoagulants may potentiate the hypoglycemic agents; such as chlorpropamide by inhibiting their metabolism in the liver).
No products indexed under this heading.

Chlorthalidone (Diuretics have been reported to diminish or increase oral anticoagulant response, i.e., decreased or increased prothrombin time response significantly). Products include:
Clorpres Tablets 2139

Cholestyramine (May reduce the gastrointestinal absorption of both the anticoagulants and Vitamin K; net effect is unpredictable).
No products indexed under this heading.

Choline Magnesium Trisalicylate (May increase oral anticoagulant response, i.e., increased prothrombin time response).
No products indexed under this heading.

Chymotrypsin (May increase oral anticoagulant response, i.e., increased prothrombin time response).
No products indexed under this heading.

Cimetidine (May increase oral anticoagulant response, i.e., increased prothrombin time response). Products include:
Tagamet HB 200 Tablets .... ■637
Tagamet Tablets 1547

Cimetidine Hydrochloride (May increase oral anticoagulant response, i.e., increased prothrombin time response).
No products indexed under this heading.

Cinchophen (May increase oral anticoagulant response, i.e., increased prothrombin time response).
No products indexed under this heading.

Clemastine Fumarate (Antihistamines have been reported to diminish oral anticoagulant response, i.e., decreased prothrombin time response significantly).
No products indexed under this heading.

Clofibrate (Drugs that reduce the number of blood platelets by causing bone marrow depression, such as clofibrate, may increase the bleeding tendency produced by anticoagulants without altering prothrombin time determination; may increase oral anticoagulant response, i.e. increased prothrombin time response).
No products indexed under this heading.

Clopidogrel Bisulfate (Drugs that reduce the number of blood platelets by causing bone marrow depression, such as clopidogrel, may increase the bleeding tendency produced by anticoagulants without altering prothrombin time determination). Products include:
Plavix Tablets 940
Plavix Tablets 2942

Codeine Phosphate (Prolonged use of narcotics may increase oral anticoagulant response, i.e., increased prothrombin time response). Products include:
Tylenol with Codeine 2461

Cortisone Acetate (Adrenocorticosteroids have been reported to diminish oral anticoagulant response, i.e., decreased prothrombin time response significantly).
No products indexed under this heading.

Cyproheptadine Hydrochloride (Antihistamines have been reported to diminish oral anticoagulant response, i.e., decreased prothrombin time response significantly).
No products indexed under this heading.

Desflurane (May increase oral anticoagulant response, i.e., increased prothrombin time response). Products include:
Suprane Liquid for Inhalation 770

Desogestrel (Oral contraceptives have been reported to diminish oral anticoagulant response, i.e., decreased prothrombin time response significantly). Products include:
Ortho-Cept Tablets 2395

Dexamethasone (Adrenocorticosteroids have been reported to diminish oral anticoagulant response, i.e., decreased prothrombin time response significantly). Products include:
Ciprodex Otic Suspension 555
Decadron Tablets 1929
TobraDex Ophthalmic Ointment 558
TobraDex Ophthalmic Suspension 558

Dexamethasone Acetate (Adrenocorticosteroids have been reported to diminish oral anticoagulant response, i.e., decreased prothrombin time response significantly).
No products indexed under this heading.

Dexamethasone Sodium Phosphate (Adrenocorticosteroids have been reported to diminish oral anticoagulant response, i.e., decreased prothrombin time response significantly). Products include:
Decadron Phosphate Injection 1931

Dexchlorpheniramine Maleate (Antihistamines have been reported to diminish oral anticoagulant response, i.e., decreased prothrombin time response significantly).
No products indexed under this heading.

Dextrans (Low Molecular Weight) (May increase oral anticoagulant response, i.e., increased prothrombin time response; drugs that reduce the number of blood platelets by causing bone marrow depression, such as dextran, may increase the bleeding tendency produced by anticoagulants withoutaltering prothrombin time determination).
No products indexed under this heading.

Dextrothyroxine Sodium (May increase oral anticoagulant response, i.e., increased prothrombin time response).
No products indexed under this heading.

Dezocine (Prolonged use of narcotics may increase oral anticoagulant response, i.e., increased prothrombin time response).
No products indexed under this heading.

Diazoxide (May increase oral anticoagulant response, i.e., increased prothrombin time response). Products include:
Hyperstat I.V. Injection 3031

Diclofenac Potassium (Drugs that reduce the number of blood platelets by causing bone marrow depression, such as non-steroidal anti-inflammatory agents, may increase the bleeding tendency produced by anticoagulants without altering prothrombin time determination). Products include:
Cataflam Tablets 2173

Diclofenac Sodium (Drugs that reduce the number of blood platelets by causing bone marrow depression, such as non-steroidal anti-inflammatory agents, may increase the bleeding tendency produced by anticoagulants without altering prothrombin time determination). Products include:
Arthrotec Tablets 3126
Voltaren Ophthalmic Solution 2300
Voltaren Tablets 2298
Voltaren-XR Tablets 2301

Diflunisal (May increase oral anticoagulant response, i.e., increased prothrombin time response; drugs that reduce the number of platelets by causing bone marrow depression, such as non-steroidal anti-inflammatory agents, may increase the bleeding tendency produced by anticoagu-

lants without altering prothrombin time determination). Products include:

- Dolobid Tablets 1937

Diphenhydramine Citrate (Antihistamines have been reported to diminish oral anticoagulant response, i.e., decreased prothrombin time response significantly). Products include:

- Children's Benadryl Allergy & Cold Fastmelt Tablets 695
- Children's Benadryl D Allergy & Sinus Fastmelt Tablets 694
- Children's Benadryl Allergy Fastmelt Tablets 696
- Goody's PM Powder 622

Diphenhydramine Hydrochloride (Antihistamines have been reported to diminish oral anticoagulant response, i.e., decreased prothrombin time response significantly). Products include:

- Benadryl Allergy & Cold Tablets 692
- Benadryl Allergy 691
- Benadryl Allergy & Sinus Headache Caplets & Gelcaps 693
- Children's Benadryl Allergy Liquid 695
- Children's Benadryl Dye-Free Allergy Liquid 695
- Benadryl Dye-Free Allergy Liqui-Gels Softgels 692
- Benadryl Itch Relief Stick Extra Strength 696
- Benadryl Itch Stopping Cream Extra Strength 697
- Benadryl Itch Stopping Gel Extra Strength 697
- Benadryl Itch Stopping Spray Extra Strength 697
- Benadryl Maximum Strength Severe Allergy & Sinus Headache Caplets 694
- Children's Benadryl D Liquid Medication 693
- Benadryl D Tablets 694
- Nytol QuickCaps Caplets 635
- Maximum Strength Nytol QuickGels Softgels 635
- Simply Sleep Caplets 1841
- Sominex Original Formula Tablets 637
- TheraFlu Thin Strips Multi Symptom 684
- Triaminic Thin Strips Cough & Runny Nose 690
- Children's Tylenol Plus Cold & Allergy Suspension Liquid 1850
- Tylenol Allergy Complete Night Time Caplets 1844
- Tylenol Severe Allergy Caplets 1844
- Tylenol Flu NightTime Gelcaps 1846
- Extra Strength Tylenol PM Caplets, Geltabs, Gelcaps and Liquid 1847
- Unisom Maximum Strength SleepGels 712

Diphenylpyraline Hydrochloride (Antihistamines have been reported to diminish oral anticoagulant response, i.e., decreased prothrombin time response significantly).
No products indexed under this heading.

Dipyridamole (Drugs that reduce the number of blood platelets by causing bone marrow depression, such as dipyridamole, may increase the bleeding tendency produced by anticoagulants without altering prothrombin time determination). Products include:

- Aggrenox Capsules 855
- Persantine Tablets 898

Disulfiram (May increase oral anticoagulant response, i.e., increased prothrombin time response). Products include:

- Antabuse Tablets 2343

Enflurane (May increase oral anticoagulant response, i.e., increased prothrombin time response).
No products indexed under this heading.

Ethacrynic Acid (Diuretics have been reported to diminish or increase oral anticoagulant response, i.e., decreased or increased prothrombin time response significantly). Products include:

- Edecrin Tablets 1941

Ethchlorvynol (Has been reported to diminish oral anticoagulant response, i.e., decreased prothrombin time response significantly).
No products indexed under this heading.

Ethinyl Estradiol (Oral contraceptives have been reported to diminish oral anticoagulant response, i.e., decreased prothrombin time response significantly). Products include:

- Alesse-28 Tablets 3392
- Lo/Ovral-28 Tablets 3423
- NuvaRing 2357
- Ortho-Cept Tablets 2395
- Ortho-Cyclen/Ortho Tri-Cyclen 2414
- Ortho Evra Transdermal System 2402
- Ortho Tri-Cyclen Lo Tablets 2421
- Seasonale Tablets 1073
- Triphasil-28 Tablets 3483
- Yasmin 28 Tablets 818

Ethynodiol Diacetate (Oral contraceptives have been reported to diminish oral anticoagulant response, i.e., decreased prothrombin time response significantly).
No products indexed under this heading.

Etodolac (Drugs that reduce the number of blood platelets by causing bone marrow depression, such as non-steroidal anti-inflammatory agents, may increase the bleeding tendency produced by anticoagulants without altering prothrombin time determination).
No products indexed under this heading.

Fenoprofen Calcium (May increase oral anticoagulant response, i.e., increased prothrombin time response; drugs that reduce the number of blood platelets by causing bone marrow depression, such as non-steroidal anti-inflammatory agents, may increase the bleeding tendency produced by anticoagulants without altering prothrombin time determination). Products include:

- Nalfon Capsules 2504

Fentanyl (Prolonged use of narcotics may increase oral anticoagulant response, i.e., increased prothrombin time response). Products include:

- Duragesic Transdermal System 2448

Fentanyl Citrate (Prolonged use of narcotics may increase oral anticoagulant response, i.e., increased prothrombin time response). Products include:

- Actiq 993

Fexofenadine Hydrochloride (Antihistamines have been reported to diminish oral anticoagulant response, i.e., decreased prothrombin time response significantly). Products include:

- Allegra 2857
- Allegra-D 12 Hour Extended-Release Tablets 2860
- Allegra-D 24 Hour Extended-Release Tablets 2862

Fludrocortisone Acetate (Adrenocorticosteroids have been reported to diminish oral anticoagulant response, i.e., decreased prothrombin time response significantly).
No products indexed under this heading.

Fluoxymesterone (Anabolic steroids may increase oral anticoagulant response, i.e., increased prothrombin time response).
No products indexed under this heading.

Flurbiprofen (Drugs that reduce the number of blood platelets by causing bone marrow depression, such as non-steroidal anti-inflammatory agents, may increase the bleeding tendency produced by anticoagulants without altering prothrombin time determination).
No products indexed under this heading.

Fosphenytoin Sodium (May increase oral anticoagulant response, i.e., increased prothrombin time response; oral anticoagulants may interfere with the hepatic metabolism of phenytoin, toxic levels of phenytoin may occur).
No products indexed under this heading.

Furosemide (Diuretics have been reported to diminish or increase oral anticoagulant response, i.e., decreased or increased prothrombin time response significantly). Products include:

- Furosemide Tablets 2117

Glucagon (May increase oral anticoagulant response, i.e., increased prothrombin time response). Products include:

- GlucaGen for Injection 790
- Glucagon for Injection Vials and Emergency Kit 1749

Glutethimide (Has been reported to diminish oral anticoagulant response, i.e., decreased prothrombin time response significantly).
No products indexed under this heading.

Griseofulvin (Has been reported to diminish oral anticoagulant response, i.e., decreased prothrombin time response significantly). Products include:

- Grifulvin V Tablets Microsize and Oral Suspension Microsize 2384
- Gris-PEG Tablets 2504

Haloperidol (Has been reported to diminish oral anticoagulant response, i.e., decreased prothrombin time response significantly).
No products indexed under this heading.

Haloperidol Decanoate (Has been reported to diminish oral anticoagulant response, i.e., decreased prothrombin time response significantly).
No products indexed under this heading.

Halothane (May increase oral anticoagulant response, i.e., increased prothrombin time response).
No products indexed under this heading.

Hepatotoxic Drugs, unspecified (May increase oral anticoagulant response, i.e., increased prothrombin time response).
No products indexed under this heading.

Hydrochloroquine (Drugs that reduce the number of blood platelets by causing bone marrow depression, such as hydrochloroquine, may increase the bleeding tendency produced by anticoagulants without altering prothrombin time determination).
No products indexed under this heading.

Hydrochlorothiazide (Diuretics have been reported to diminish or increase oral anticoagulant response, i.e., decreased or increased prothrombin time response significantly). Products include:

- Aldoril Tablets 1884
- Atacand HCT 637
- Avalide Tablets 2889
- Avalide Tablets 922
- Benicar HCT Tablets 2852
- Diovan HCT Tablets 2195
- Dyazide Capsules 1389
- Hyzaar 1964
- Lotensin HCT Tablets 2235
- Maxzide 2150
- Micardis HCT Tablets 886
- Moduretic Tablets 2003
- Prinzide Tablets 2033
- Teveten HCT Tablets 1710
- Timolide Tablets 2056
- Uniretic Tablets 3114
- Vaseretic Tablets 2073
- Zestoretic Tablets 701

Hydrocodone Bitartrate (Prolonged use of narcotics may increase oral anticoagulant response, i.e., increased prothrombin time response). Products include:

- Hycodan 1104
- Hycomine Compound Tablets 1105
- Hycotuss Expectorant Syrup 1106
- Lortab 3315
- Lortab Elixir 3312
- Vicodin Tablets 530
- Vicodin ES Tablets 531
- Vicodin HP Tablets 532
- Vicoprofen Tablets 533
- Zydone Tablets 1118

Hydrocodone Polistirex (Prolonged use of narcotics may increase oral anticoagulant response, i.e., increased prothrombin time response). Products include:

- Tussionex Pennkinetic Extended-Release Suspension 3322

Hydrocortisone (Adrenocorticosteroids have been reported to diminish oral anticoagulant response, i.e., decreased prothrombin time response significantly). Products include:

- Cortizone•5 Ointment 699
- Cortizone•10 Creme 699
- Cortizone•10 Ointment 699
- Cortizone•10 Plus Creme 700
- Cortizone•10 Maximum Strength Quick Shot Spray 700
- Hydrocortone Tablets 1963
- Preparation H Hydrocortisone Cream 748

Hydrocortisone Acetate (Adrenocorticosteroids have been reported to diminish oral anticoagulant response, i.e., decreased prothrombin time response significantly). Products include:

- Analpram-HC 1136
- Pramosone 1139
- ProctoFoam-HC 3113
- Tucks Anti-Itch Ointment 712
- U-cort 1% Cream 3289

IMPORTANT NOTE: Always consult each drug listing in the patient's regimen for possible interactions.

Hydrocortisone Sodium Phosphate (Adrenocorticosteroids have been reported to diminish oral anticoagulant response, i.e., decreased prothrombin time response significantly).
No products indexed under this heading.

Hydrocortisone Sodium Succinate (Adrenocorticosteroids have been reported to diminish oral anticoagulant response, i.e., decreased prothrombin time response significantly).
No products indexed under this heading.

Hydroflumethiazide (Diuretics have been reported to diminish or increase oral anticoagulant response, i.e., decreased or increased prothrombin time response significantly).
No products indexed under this heading.

Hydromorphone Hydrochloride (Prolonged use of narcotics may increase oral anticoagulant response, i.e., increased prothrombin time response). Products include:
Dilaudid 439
Dilaudid Oral Liquid 443
Dilaudid Non-Sterile Powder 439
Dilaudid Rectal Suppositories 439
Dilaudid Tablets 439
Dilaudid Tablets - 8 mg 443
Dilaudid-HP 441

Ibuprofen (May increase oral anticoagulant response, i.e., increased prothrombin time response; drugs that reduce the number of blood platelets by causing bone marrow depression, such as non-steroidal anti-inflammatory agents, may increase the bleeding tendency produced by anticoagulants without altering prothrombin time determination). Products include:
Advil Allergy Sinus Caplets 737
Advil 737
Children's Advil Suspension 742
Children's Advil Chewable Tablets 741
Advil Cold & Sinus 739
Advil Flu & Body Ache Caplets 739
Children's Advil Cold Suspension 741
Infants' Advil Concentrated Drops 743
Junior Strength Advil Swallow Tablets 740
Advil Migraine Liquigels 740
Advil Multi-Symptom Cold Caplets 738
Combunox Tablets 1183
Children's Motrin Oral Suspension and Chewable Tablets 1837
Children's Motrin Cold Non-Staining Dye-Free Oral Suspension 1838
Children's Motrin Cold Oral Suspension 1838
Children's Motrin Non-Staining Dye-Free Oral Suspension 1837
Motrin Cold & Sinus Caplets 1836
Motrin IB Tablets and Caplets 1836
Infants' Motrin Concentrated Drops 1837
Infants' Motrin Non-Staining Dye-Free Drops 1837
Junior Strength Motrin Caplets and Chewable Tablets 1837
Vicoprofen Tablets 533

Indapamide (Diuretics have been reported to diminish or increase oral anticoagulant response, i.e., decreased or increased prothrombin time response significantly). Products include:
Indapamide Tablets 2119

Indomethacin (May increase oral anticoagulant response, i.e., increased prothrombin time response; drugs that reduce the number of blood platelets by causing bone marrow depression, such as non-steroidal anti-inflammatory agents, may increase the bleeding tendency produced by anticoagulants without altering prothrombin time determination). Products include:
Indocin 1968

Indomethacin Sodium Trihydrate (Drugs that reduce the number of blood platelets by causing bone marrow depression, such as non-steroidal anti-inflammatory agents, may increase the bleeding tendency produced by anticoagulants without altering prothrombin time determination). Products include:
Indocin I.V. 1973

Influenza Virus Vaccine (May increase oral anticoagulant response, i.e., increased prothrombin time response). Products include:
Flumist Vaccine 1872

Isocarboxazid (May increase oral anticoagulant response, i.e., increased prothrombin time response).
No products indexed under this heading.

Isoflurane (May increase oral anticoagulant response, i.e., increased prothrombin time response).
No products indexed under this heading.

Ketoprofen (Drugs that reduce the number of blood platelets by causing bone marrow depression, such as non-steroidal anti-inflammatory agents, may increase the bleeding tendency produced by anticoagulants without altering prothrombin time determination).
No products indexed under this heading.

Ketorolac Tromethamine (Drugs that reduce the number of blood platelets by causing bone marrow depression, such as non-steroidal anti-inflammatory agents, may increase the bleeding tendency produced by anticoagulants without altering prothrombin time determination). Products include:
Acular Ophthalmic Solution 561
Acular LS Ophthalmic Solution 562

Levonorgestrel (Oral contraceptives have been reported to diminish oral anticoagulant response, i.e., decreased prothrombin time response significantly). Products include:
Alesse-28 Tablets 3392
Climara Pro Transdermal System 800
Mirena Intrauterine System 810
Plan B Tablets 1068
Seasonale Tablets 1073
Triphasil-28 Tablets 3483

Levorphanol Tartrate (Prolonged use of narcotics may increase oral anticoagulant response, i.e., increased prothrombin time response).
No products indexed under this heading.

Levothyroxine Sodium (May increase oral anticoagulant response, i.e., increased prothrombin time response). Products include:
Levothroid Tablets 1189
Levoxyl Tablets 1680
Synthroid Tablets 515
Unithroid Tablets 3521

Liothyronine Sodium (May increase oral anticoagulant response, i.e., increased prothrombin time response). Products include:
Cytomel Tablets 1678

Liotrix (May increase oral anticoagulant response, i.e., increased prothrombin time response). Products include:
Thyrolar 1203

Loratadine (Antihistamines have been reported to diminish oral anticoagulant response, i.e., decreased prothrombin time response significantly). Products include:
Alavert Allergy & Sinus D-12 Hour Tablets 743
Alavert 743
Children's Claritin 24 Hour Non-Drowsy Allergy Syrup 732
Claritin Non-Drowsy 24 Hour Tablets 731
Non-Drowsy Claritin Hives Relief Tablets 733
Claritin Reditabs 24 Hour Non-Drowsy Tablets 732
Claritin-D Non-Drowsy 12 Hour Tablets 731
Claritin-D Non-Drowsy 24 Hour Tablets 731
Children's Dimetapp ND Non-Drowsy Allergy Syrup 746
Triaminic Allerchews 684

Magaldrate (Antacids have been reported to diminish oral anticoagulant response, i.e., decreased prothrombin time response significantly).
No products indexed under this heading.

Magnesium Hydroxide (Antacids have been reported to diminish oral anticoagulant response, i.e., decreased prothrombin time response significantly). Products include:
Maalox Max Maximum Strength Antacid/Anti-Gas Liquid 2165
Maalox Regular Strength Antacid/Antigas Liquid 2164
Pepcid Complete Chewable Tablets 1672
Rolaids Tablets 707
Extra Strength Rolaids Tablets 707
Rolaids Multi-Symptom Antacid & Antigas Tablets 708

Magnesium Oxide (Antacids have been reported to diminish oral anticoagulant response, i.e., decreased prothrombin time response significantly). Products include:
Beelith Tablets 784
PremCal Light, Regular, and Extra Strength Tablets 762

Magnesium Salicylate (May increase oral anticoagulant response, i.e., increased prothrombin time response).
No products indexed under this heading.

Meclofenamate Sodium (Drugs that reduce the number of blood platelets by causing bone marrow depression, such as non-steroidal anti-inflammatory agents, may increase the bleeding tendency produced by anticoagulants without altering prothrombin time determination).
No products indexed under this heading.

Mefenamic Acid (May increase oral anticoagulant response, i.e., increased prothrombin time response; drugs that reduce the number of blood platelets by causing bone marrow depression, such as non-steroidal anti-inflammatory agents, may increase the bleeding tendency produced by anticoagulants without altering prothrombin time determination).
No products indexed under this heading.

Meloxicam (Drugs that reduce the number of blood platelets by causing bone marrow depression, such as non-steroidal anti-inflammatory agents, may increase the bleeding tendency produced by anticoagulants without altering prothrombin time determination). Products include:
Mobic Oral Suspension 893
Mobic Tablets 893

Meperidine Hydrochloride (Prolonged use of narcotics may increase oral anticoagulant response, i.e., increased prothrombin time response).
No products indexed under this heading.

Mephobarbital (Barbiturates have been reported to diminish oral anticoagulant response, i.e., decreased prothrombin time response significantly). Products include:
Mebaral Tablets, USP 2483

Meprobamate (Has been reported to diminish oral anticoagulant response, i.e., decreased prothrombin time response significantly).
No products indexed under this heading.

Mestranol (Oral contraceptives have been reported to diminish oral anticoagulant response, i.e., decreased prothrombin time response significantly).
No products indexed under this heading.

Methadone Hydrochloride (Prolonged use of narcotics may increase oral anticoagulant response, i.e., increased prothrombin time response).
No products indexed under this heading.

Methdilazine Hydrochloride (Antihistamines have been reported to diminish oral anticoagulant response, i.e., decreased prothrombin time response significantly).
No products indexed under this heading.

Methoxyflurane (May increase oral anticoagulant response, i.e., increased prothrombin time response).
No products indexed under this heading.

Methyclothiazide (Diuretics have been reported to diminish or increase oral anticoagulant response, i.e., decreased or increased prothrombin time response significantly).
No products indexed under this heading.

Methyldopa (May increase oral anticoagulant response, i.e., increased prothrombin time response). Products include:
Aldoclor Tablets 1881
Aldoril Tablets 1884

Methylphenidate Hydrochloride (May increase oral anticoagulant

response, i.e., increased prothrombin time response). Products include:
Concerta Extended-Release Tablets ... 1828
Metadate CD Capsules ... 3316
Ritalin ... 2254
Ritalin LA Capsules ... 2255

Methylprednisolone Acetate (Adrenocorticosteroids have been reported to diminish oral anticoagulant response, i.e., decreased prothrombin time response significantly). Products include:
Depo-Medrol Injectable Suspension ... 2615
Depo-Medrol Single-Dose Vial ... 2617

Methylprednisolone Sodium Succinate (Adrenocorticosteroids have been reported to diminish oral anticoagulant response, i.e., decreased prothrombin time response significantly).
No products indexed under this heading.

Methyltestosterone (Anabolic steroids may increase oral anticoagulant response, i.e., increased prothrombin time response). Products include:
Estratest Tablets ... 3196
Estratest H.S. Tablets ... 3196

Metolazone (Diuretics have been reported to diminish or increase oral anticoagulant response, i.e., decreased or increased prothrombin time response significantly).
No products indexed under this heading.

Metronidazole (May increase oral anticoagulant response, i.e., increased prothrombin time response). Products include:
Metrogel 1% ... 1212
MetroGel-Vaginal Gel ... 1822
Noritate Cream, 1% ... 1051

Metronidazole Hydrochloride (May increase oral anticoagulant response, i.e., increased prothrombin time response).
No products indexed under this heading.

Miconazole (May increase oral anticoagulant response, i.e., increased prothrombin time response).
No products indexed under this heading.

Moclobemide (May increase oral anticoagulant response, i.e., increased prothrombin time response).
No products indexed under this heading.

Morphine Sulfate (Prolonged use of narcotics may increase oral anticoagulant response, i.e., increased prothrombin time response). Products include:
Avinza Capsules ... 1714
Kadian Capsules ... 572
MS Contin Tablets ... 2703

Nabumetone (Drugs that reduce the number of blood platelets by causing bone marrow depression, such as non-steroidal anti-inflammatory agents, may increase the bleeding tendency produced by anticoagulants without altering prothrombin time determination). Products include:
Relafen Tablets ... 1523

Nalidixic Acid (May increase oral anticoagulant response, i.e., increased prothrombin time response).
No products indexed under this heading.

Naproxen (May increase oral anticoagulant response, i.e., increased prothrombin time response; drugs that reduce the number of blood platelets by causing bone marrow depression, such as non-steroidal anti-inflammatory agents, may increase the bleeding tendency produced by anticoagulants without altering prothrombin time determination). Products include:
EC-Naprosyn Delayed-Release Tablets ... 2769
Naprosyn Suspension ... 2769
Naprosyn Tablets ... 2769
Prevacid NapraPAC ... 3277

Naproxen Sodium (May increase oral anticoagulant response, i.e., increased prothrombin time response; drugs that reduce the number of blood platelets by causing bone marrow depression, such as non-steroidal anti-inflammatory agents, may increase the bleeding tendency produced by anticoagulants without altering prothrombin time determination). Products include:
Aleve Tablets, Caplets and Gelcaps ... 605
Anaprox Tablets ... 2769
Anaprox DS Tablets ... 2769

Norethindrone (Oral contraceptives have been reported to diminish oral anticoagulant response, i.e., decreased prothrombin time response significantly). Products include:
Ortho Micronor Tablets ... 2411

Norethynodrel (Oral contraceptives have been reported to diminish oral anticoagulant response, i.e., decreased prothrombin time response significantly).
No products indexed under this heading.

Norgestimate (Oral contraceptives have been reported to diminish oral anticoagulant response, i.e., decreased prothrombin time response significantly). Products include:
Ortho-Cyclen/Ortho Tri-Cyclen ... 2414
Ortho Tri-Cyclen Lo Tablets ... 2421
Prefest Tablets ... 1069

Norgestrel (Oral contraceptives have been reported to diminish oral anticoagulant response, i.e., decreased prothrombin time response significantly). Products include:
Lo/Ovral-28 Tablets ... 3423

Oxandrolone (Anabolic steroids may increase oral anticoagulant response, i.e., increased prothrombin time response). Products include:
Oxandrin Tablets ... 2977

Oxaprozin (Drugs that reduce the number of blood platelets by causing bone marrow depression, such as non-steroidal anti-inflammatory agents, may increase the bleeding tendency produced by anticoagulants without altering prothrombin time determination).
No products indexed under this heading.

Oxolinic Acid (May increase oral anticoagulant response, i.e., increased prothrombin time response).
No products indexed under this heading.

Oxycodone Hydrochloride (Prolonged use of narcotics may increase oral anticoagulant response, i.e., increased prothrombin time response). Products include:
Combunox Tablets ... 1183
OxyContin Tablets ... 2699
OxyFast Oral Concentrate Solution ... 2704
OxyIR Capsules ... 2704
Percocet Tablets ... 1114
Percodan Tablets ... 1115

Oxymetholone (Anabolic steroids may increase oral anticoagulant response, i.e., increased prothrombin time response). Products include:
Anadrol-50 Tablets ... 3329

Oxyphenbutazone (May increase oral anticoagulant response, i.e., increased prothrombin time response).
No products indexed under this heading.

Paraldehyde (Has been reported to diminish oral anticoagulant response, i.e., decreased prothrombin time response significantly).
No products indexed under this heading.

Pargyline Hydrochloride (May increase oral anticoagulant response, i.e., increased prothrombin time response).
No products indexed under this heading.

Pentobarbital Sodium (Barbiturates have been reported to diminish oral anticoagulant response, i.e., decreased prothrombin time response significantly). Products include:
Nembutal Sodium Solution, USP ... 2484

Phenelzine Sulfate (May increase oral anticoagulant response, i.e., increased prothrombin time response).
No products indexed under this heading.

Phenobarbital (Barbiturates have been reported to diminish oral anticoagulant response, i.e., decreased prothrombin time response significantly).
No products indexed under this heading.

Phenylbutazone (May increase oral anticoagulant response, i.e., increased prothrombin time response).
No products indexed under this heading.

Phenyramidol (May increase oral anticoagulant response, i.e., increased prothrombin time response).
No products indexed under this heading.

Phenytoin (May increase oral anticoagulant response, i.e., increased prothrombin time response; oral anticoagulants may interfere with the hepatic metabolism of phenytoin, toxic levels of phenytoin may occur).
No products indexed under this heading.

Phenytoin Sodium (May increase oral anticoagulant response, i.e., increased prothrombin time response; oral anticoagulants may interfere with the hepatic metabolism of phenytoin, toxic levels of phenytoin may occur). Products include:
Phenytek Capsules ... 2153

Piroxicam (Drugs that reduce the number of blood platelets by causing bone marrow depression, such as non-steroidal anti-inflammatory agents, may increase the bleeding tendency produced by anticoagulants without altering prothrombin time determination).
No products indexed under this heading.

Polythiazide (Diuretics have been reported to diminish or increase oral anticoagulant response, i.e., decreased or increased prothrombin time response significantly).
No products indexed under this heading.

Prednisolone Acetate (Adrenocorticosteroids have been reported to diminish oral anticoagulant response, i.e., decreased prothrombin time response significantly). Products include:
Blephamide Ophthalmic Ointment ... 563
Blephamide Ophthalmic Suspension ... 564
Poly-Pred Liquifilm Ophthalmic Suspension ... ⊙231
Pred Forte Ophthalmic Suspension ... ⊙233
Pred Mild Sterile Ophthalmic Suspension ... ⊙236
Pred-G Ophthalmic Suspension ... ⊙234
Pred-G Sterile Ophthalmic Ointment ... ⊙235

Prednisolone Sodium Phosphate (Adrenocorticosteroids have been reported to diminish oral anticoagulant response, i.e., decreased prothrombin time response significantly). Products include:
Pediapred Oral Solution ... 3319

Prednisolone Tebutate (Adrenocorticosteroids have been reported to diminish oral anticoagulant response, i.e., decreased prothrombin time response significantly).
No products indexed under this heading.

Prednisone (Adrenocorticosteroids have been reported to diminish oral anticoagulant response, i.e., decreased prothrombin time response significantly).
No products indexed under this heading.

Primidone (Has been reported to diminish oral anticoagulant response, i.e., decreased prothrombin time response significantly).
No products indexed under this heading.

Procarbazine Hydrochloride (May increase oral anticoagulant response, i.e., increased prothrombin time response). Products include:
Matulane Capsules ... 3188

Promethazine Hydrochloride (Antihistamines have been reported to diminish oral anticoagulant response, i.e., decreased prothrombin time response significantly). Products include:
Phenergan ... 3438

Propoxyphene Hydrochloride (Prolonged use of narcotics may increase oral anticoagulant response, i.e., increased prothrombin time response).
No products indexed under this heading.

Propoxyphene Napsylate (Prolonged use of narcotics may increase oral anticoagulant response, i.e., increased prothrombin time response). Products include:

Darvocet A 500 Tablets 3497

Pyrilamine Maleate (Antihistamines have been reported to diminish oral anticoagulant response, i.e., decreased prothrombin time response significantly).
No products indexed under this heading.

Pyrilamine Tannate (Antihistamines have been reported to diminish oral anticoagulant response, i.e., decreased prothrombin time response significantly).
No products indexed under this heading.

Quinidine Gluconate (May increase oral anticoagulant response, i.e., increased prothrombin time response).
No products indexed under this heading.

Quinidine Polygalacturonate (May increase oral anticoagulant response, i.e., increased prothrombin time response).
No products indexed under this heading.

Quinidine Sulfate (May increase oral anticoagulant response, i.e., increased prothrombin time response).
No products indexed under this heading.

Quinine Sulfate (May increase oral anticoagulant response, i.e., increased prothrombin time response).
No products indexed under this heading.

Ranitidine Hydrochloride (Has been reported to diminish or increase oral anticoagulant response, i.e., decreased or increased prothrombin time response significantly). Products include:
Zantac 1597
Zantac Injection 1593
Zantac 75 Tablets .... ▣715
Zantac 150 Maximum Strength Tablets .... ▣715
Zantac Injection Pharmacy Bulk Package 1595

Remifentanil Hydrochloride (Prolonged use of narcotics may increase oral anticoagulant response, i.e., increased prothrombin time response).
No products indexed under this heading.

Reteplase (Co-administration with thrombolytics is not recommended and may be hazardous). Products include:
Retavase 1131

Rifampin (Has been reported to diminish oral anticoagulant response, i.e., decreased prothrombin time response significantly).
No products indexed under this heading.

Rofecoxib (Drugs that reduce the number of blood platelets by causing bone marrow depression, such as non-steroidal anti-inflammatory agents, may increase the bleeding tendency produced by anticoagulants without altering prothrombin time determination).
No products indexed under this heading.

Salsalate (May increase oral anticoagulant response, i.e., increased prothrombin time response).
No products indexed under this heading.

Secobarbital Sodium (Barbiturates have been reported to diminish oral anticoagulant response, i.e., decreased prothrombin time response significantly).
No products indexed under this heading.

Selegiline Hydrochloride (May increase oral anticoagulant response, i.e., increased prothrombin time response). Products include:
Eldepryl Capsules 3209

Sodium Bicarbonate (Antacids have been reported to diminish oral anticoagulant response, i.e., decreased prothrombin time response significantly). Products include:
Ceo-Two Evacuant Suppository ...... ▣607
Colyte with Flavor Packs for Oral Solution 3102
HalfLytely and Bisacodyl Tablets Bowel Prep Kit with Flavors Packs 915
TriLyte with Flavor Packs for Oral Solution 3114

Spironolactone (Diuretics have been reported to diminish or increase oral anticoagulant response, i.e., decreased or increased prothrombin time response significantly).
No products indexed under this heading.

Stanozolol (Anabolic steroids may increase oral anticoagulant response, i.e., increased prothrombin time response).
No products indexed under this heading.

Streptokinase (Co-administration with thrombolytics is not recommended and may be hazardous).
No products indexed under this heading.

Sufentanil Citrate (Prolonged use of narcotics may increase oral anticoagulant response, i.e., increased prothrombin time response).
No products indexed under this heading.

Sulfamethizole (May increase oral anticoagulant response, i.e., increased prothrombin time response).
No products indexed under this heading.

Sulfamethoxazole (May increase oral anticoagulant response, i.e., increased prothrombin time response).
No products indexed under this heading.

Sulfinpyrazone (May increase oral anticoagulant response, i.e., increased prothrombin time response).
No products indexed under this heading.

Sulfisoxazole Acetyl (May increase oral anticoagulant response, i.e., increased prothrombin time response).
No products indexed under this heading.

Sulindac (Long acting sulindac may increase oral anticoagulant response, i.e., increased prothrombin time response; drugs that reduce the number of blood platelets by causing bone marrow depression, such as non-steroidal anti-inflammatory agents, may increase the bleeding tendency produced by anticoagulants without altering prothrombin time determination). Products include:
Clinoril Tablets 1899

Terfenadine (Antihistamines have been reported to diminish oral anticoagulant response, i.e., decreased prothrombin time response significantly).
No products indexed under this heading.

Thiamylal Sodium (Barbiturates have been reported to diminish oral anticoagulant response, i.e., decreased prothrombin time response significantly).
No products indexed under this heading.

Thyroglobulin (May increase oral anticoagulant response, i.e., increased prothrombin time response).
No products indexed under this heading.

Thyroid (May increase oral anticoagulant response, i.e., increased prothrombin time response).
No products indexed under this heading.

Thyroxine (May increase oral anticoagulant response, i.e., increased prothrombin time response).
No products indexed under this heading.

Thyroxine Sodium (May increase oral anticoagulant response, i.e., increased prothrombin time response).
No products indexed under this heading.

Tolbutamide (May increase oral anticoagulant response, i.e., increased prothrombin time response; oral anticoagulants may potentiate the hypoglycemic agents; such as tolbutamide by inhibiting their metabolism in the liver).
No products indexed under this heading.

Tolmetin Sodium (Drugs that reduce the number of blood platelets by causing bone marrow depression, such as non-steroidal anti-inflammatory agents, may increase the bleeding tendency produced by anticoagulants without altering prothrombin time determination).
No products indexed under this heading.

Torsemide (Diuretics have been reported to diminish or increase oral anticoagulant response, i.e., decreased or increased prothrombin time response significantly).
No products indexed under this heading.

Tranylcypromine Sulfate (May increase oral anticoagulant response, i.e., increased prothrombin time response). Products include:
Parnate Tablets 1499

Triamcinolone (Adrenocorticosteroids have been reported to diminish oral anticoagulant response, i.e., decreased prothrombin time response significantly).
No products indexed under this heading.

Triamcinolone Acetonide (Adrenocorticosteroids have been reported to diminish oral anticoagulant response, i.e., decreased prothrombin time response significantly). Products include:
Azmacort Inhalation Aerosol 1701
Nasacort HFA Inhalation Aerosol 2939
Nasacort AQ Nasal Spray 2937

Triamcinolone Diacetate (Adrenocorticosteroids have been reported to diminish oral anticoagulant response, i.e., decreased prothrombin time response significantly).
No products indexed under this heading.

Triamcinolone Hexacetonide (Adrenocorticosteroids have been reported to diminish oral anticoagulant response, i.e., decreased prothrombin time response significantly).
No products indexed under this heading.

Triamterene (Diuretics have been reported to diminish or increase oral anticoagulant response, i.e., decreased or increased prothrombin time response significantly). Products include:
Dyazide Capsules 1389
Dyrenium Capsules 3390
Maxzide 2150

Trimeprazine Tartrate (Antihistamines have been reported to diminish oral anticoagulant response, i.e., decreased prothrombin time response significantly).
No products indexed under this heading.

Trimethoprim (Sulfamethoxazole/trimethoprim may increase oral anticoagulant response, i.e., increased prothrombin time response).
No products indexed under this heading.

Tripelennamine Hydrochloride (Antihistamines have been reported to diminish oral anticoagulant response, i.e., decreased prothrombin time response significantly).
No products indexed under this heading.

Triprolidine Hydrochloride (Antihistamines have been reported to diminish oral anticoagulant response, i.e., decreased prothrombin time response significantly).
No products indexed under this heading.

Urokinase (Co-administration with thrombolytics is not recommended and may be hazardous).
No products indexed under this heading.

Valdecoxib (Drugs that reduce the number of blood platelets by causing bone marrow depression, such as non-steroidal anti-inflammatory agents, may increase the bleeding tendency produced by anticoagulants without altering prothrombin time determination).
No products indexed under this heading.

Vitamin C (Has been reported to diminish oral anticoagulant response, i.e., decreased prothrombin time response significantly). Products include:
Chromagen Forte Soft Gelatin Capsules 3296
Halls Defense Sugarfree Vitamin C Drops .... ▣611
Niferex-150 Forte Capsules 3299
Peridin-C Tablets .... ▣761
Repliva 21/7 Tablets 3301

Warfarin Sodium (Under dosage of warfarin sodium has been reported to diminish oral anticoagulant response, i.e., decreased prothrombin time response significantly; overdosage of warfarin may increase oral anticoagulant response, i.e., increased prothrombin time response). Products include:

Coumadin for Injection 932
Coumadin Tablets 932

Food Interactions

Alcohol (Has been reported to diminish and/or increase oral anticoagulant response, i.e., decreased prothrombin time response significantly).

Diet high in vitamin K (Has been reported to diminish oral anticoagulant response, i.e., decreased prothrombin time response significantly).

MIRAPEX TABLETS

(Pramipexole Dihydrochloride) 889

May interact with dopamine D2 antagonists, quinidine, and certain other agents. Compounds in these categories include:

Chlorpromazine (Co-administration with dopamine antagonists may diminish the effectiveness of pramipexole).
No products indexed under this heading.

Chlorpromazine Hydrochloride (Co-administration with dopamine antagonists may diminish the effectiveness of pramipexole).
No products indexed under this heading.

Chlorprothixene (Co-administration with dopamine antagonists may diminish the effectiveness of pramipexole).
No products indexed under this heading.

Chlorprothixene Hydrochloride (Co-administration with dopamine antagonists may diminish the effectiveness of pramipexole).
No products indexed under this heading.

Cimetidine (Co-administration with cimetidine, a known inhibitor of renal tubular secretion of organic acids via anionic transport, has caused a 50% increase in pramipexole AUC and a 40% increase in half-life). Products include:
Tagamet HB 200 Tablets 637
Tagamet Tablets 1547

Cimetidine Hydrochloride (Co-administration with cimetidine, a known inhibitor of renal tubular secretion of organic acids via anionic transport, has caused a 50% increase in pramipexole AUC and a 40% increase in half-life).
No products indexed under this heading.

Diltiazem Hydrochloride (Co-administration of drugs that are secreted by the cationic transport system, e.g., diltiazem, decrease the oral clearance of pramipexole by about 20%). Products include:
Cardizem LA Extended Release Tablets 1699
Tiazac Capsules 1204

Fluphenazine Decanoate (Co-administration with dopamine antagonists may diminish the effectiveness of pramipexole).
No products indexed under this heading.

Fluphenazine Enanthate (Co-administration with dopamine antagonists may diminish the effectiveness of pramipexole).
No products indexed under this heading.

Fluphenazine Hydrochloride (Co-administration with dopamine antagonists may diminish the effectiveness of pramipexole).
No products indexed under this heading.

Haloperidol (Co-administration with dopamine antagonists may diminish the effectiveness of pramipexole).
No products indexed under this heading.

Haloperidol Decanoate (Co-administration with dopamine antagonists may diminish the effectiveness of pramipexole).
No products indexed under this heading.

Levodopa (Pramipexole may potentiate the dopaminergic side effects of levodopa and may cause or exacerbate pre-existing dyskinesia; pramipexole may cause an increase in levodopa Cmax by about 40% and a decrease in Tmax from 2.5 to 0.6 hours). Products include:
Parcopa Orally Disintegrating Tablets 3111
Stalevo Tablets 2270

Loxapine Hydrochloride (Co-administration with dopamine antagonists may diminish the effectiveness of pramipexole).
No products indexed under this heading.

Loxapine Succinate (Co-administration with dopamine antagonists may diminish the effectiveness of pramipexole).
No products indexed under this heading.

Mesoridazine Besylate (Co-administration with dopamine antagonists may diminish the effectiveness of pramipexole).
No products indexed under this heading.

Methotrimeprazine (Co-administration with dopamine antagonists may diminish the effectiveness of pramipexole).
No products indexed under this heading.

Metoclopramide Hydrochloride (Co-administration with dopamine antagonists may diminish the effectiveness of pramipexole).
No products indexed under this heading.

Molindone Hydrochloride (Co-administration with dopamine antagonists may diminish the effectiveness of pramipexole). Products include:
Moban Tablets 1108

Perphenazine (Co-administration with dopamine antagonists may diminish the effectiveness of pramipexole).
No products indexed under this heading.

Prochlorperazine (Co-administration with dopamine antagonists may diminish the effectiveness of pramipexole).
No products indexed under this heading.

Promethazine Hydrochloride (Co-administration with dopamine antagonists may diminish the effectiveness of pramipexole). Products include:
Phenergan 3438

Quetiapine Fumarate (Co-administration with dopamine antagonists may diminish the effectiveness of pramipexole). Products include:
Seroquel Tablets 691

Quinidine (Co-administration of drugs that are secreted by the cationic transport system, e.g., quinidine, decrease the oral clearance of pramipexole by about 20%).
No products indexed under this heading.

Quinidine Gluconate (Co-administration of drugs that are secreted by the cationic transport system, e.g., quinidine, decrease the oral clearance of pramipexole by about 20%).
No products indexed under this heading.

Quinidine Hydrochloride (Co-administration of drugs that are secreted by the cationic transport system, e.g., quinidine, decrease the oral clearance of pramipexole by about 20%).
No products indexed under this heading.

Quinidine Polygalacturonate (Co-administration of drugs that are secreted by the cationic transport system, e.g., quinidine, decrease the oral clearance of pramipexole by about 20%).
No products indexed under this heading.

Quinidine Sulfate (Co-administration of drugs that are secreted by the cationic transport system, e.g., quinidine, decrease the oral clearance of pramipexole by about 20%).
No products indexed under this heading.

Quinine Sulfate (Co-administration of drugs that are secreted by the cationic transport system, e.g., quinine, decrease the oral clearance of pramipexole by about 20%).
No products indexed under this heading.

Ranitidine Hydrochloride (Co-administration of drugs that are secreted by the cationic transport system, e.g., ranitidine, decrease the oral clearance of pramipexole by about 20%). Products include:
Zantac 1597
Zantac Injection 1593
Zantac 75 Tablets 715
Zantac 150 Maximum Strength Tablets 715
Zantac Injection Pharmacy Bulk Package 1595

Risperidone (Co-administration with dopamine antagonists may diminish the effectiveness of pramipexole). Products include:
Risperdal Consta Long-Acting Injection 1664
Risperdal M-Tab Orally Disintegrating Tablets 1658
Risperdal 1658

Thioridazine Hydrochloride (Co-administration with dopamine antagonists may diminish the effectiveness of pramipexole). Products include:
Thioridazine Hydrochloride Tablets 2122

Thiothixene (Co-administration with dopamine antagonists may diminish the effectiveness of pramipexole). Products include:
Thiothixene Capsules 2124

Triamterene (Co-administration of drugs that are secreted by the cationic transport system, e.g., triamterene, decrease the oral clearance of pramipexole by about 20%). Products include:
Dyazide Capsules 1389
Dyrenium Capsules 3390
Maxzide 2150

Trifluoperazine Hydrochloride (Co-administration with dopamine antagonists may diminish the effectiveness of pramipexole).
No products indexed under this heading.

Verapamil Hydrochloride (Co-administration of drugs that are secreted by the cationic transport system, e.g., verapamil, decrease the oral clearance of pramipexole by about 20%). Products include:
Covera-HS Tablets 3135
Tarka Tablets 519
Verelan PM Capsules 3120

Food Interactions

Food, unspecified (Food does not affect the extent of pramipexole absorption, although the time of maximum plasma concentration is increased by about 1 hour when the drug is taken with a meal).

MIRENA INTRAUTERINE SYSTEM

(Levonorgestrel) 810

May interact with phenytoin and certain other agents. Compounds in these categories include:

Carbamazepine (Co-administration with drugs that induce liver enzymes may impair the effect of hormonal contraceptives). Products include:
Carbatrol Capsules 3174
Equetro Extended-Release Capsules 3178
Tegretol/Tegretol-XR 2278

Fosphenytoin Sodium (Co-administration with drugs that induce liver enzymes may impair the effect of hormonal contraceptives).
No products indexed under this heading.

Phenytoin (Co-administration with drugs that induce liver enzymes may impair the effect of hormonal contraceptives).
No products indexed under this heading.

Phenytoin Sodium (Co-administration with drugs that induce liver enzymes may impair the effect of hormonal contraceptives). Products include:
Phenytek Capsules 2153

Rifampin (Co-administration with drugs that induce liver enzymes may impair the effect of hormonal contraceptives).
No products indexed under this heading.

MIVACRON INJECTION

(Mivacurium Chloride) 489

May interact with aminoglycosides, antineoplastics, glucocorticoids, lithium preparations, local anesthetics, monoamine oxidase inhibitors, oral contraceptives, phenytoin, quinidine, tetracyclines, and certain other agents. Compounds in these categories include:

Altretamine (Irreversible inhibition of plasma cholinesterase by certain unspecified antineoplastic drugs resulting in possible prolonged neuromuscular block). Products include:
Hexalen Capsules 2101

Amikacin Sulfate (Enhances the neuromuscular blocking action).
No products indexed under this heading.

Anastrozole (Irreversible inhibition of plasma cholinesterase by certain

unspecified antineoplastic drugs resulting in possible prolonged neuromuscular block). Products include:

Arimidex Tablets 665

Asparaginase (Irreversible inhibition of plasma cholinesterase by certain unspecified antineoplastic drugs resulting in possible prolonged neuromuscular block). Products include:

Elspar for Injection 1943

Bacitracin (Enhances neuromuscular blocking action). Products include:

Neosporin Ointment .... ▣702
Neosporin + Pain Relief Maximum Strength Ointment .... ▣703
Polysporin Ointment .... ▣706

Betamethasone Acetate (Enhances the neuromuscular blocking effects by a reduction in plasma cholinesterase activity induced by chronic administration of glucocorticoids).

No products indexed under this heading.

Betamethasone Sodium Phosphate (Enhances the neuromuscular blocking effects by a reduction in plasma cholinesterase activity induced by chronic administration of glucocorticoids).

No products indexed under this heading.

Bicalutamide (Irreversible inhibition of plasma cholinesterase by certain unspecified antineoplastic drugs resulting in possible prolonged neuromuscular block). Products include:

Casodex Tablets 670

Bleomycin Sulfate (Irreversible inhibition of plasma cholinesterase by certain unspecified antineoplastic drugs resulting in possible prolonged neuromuscular block).

No products indexed under this heading.

Bupivacaine Hydrochloride (Enhances neuromuscular blocking action).

No products indexed under this heading.

Busulfan (Irreversible inhibition of plasma cholinesterase by certain unspecified antineoplastic drugs resulting in possible prolonged neuromuscular block). Products include:

I.V. Busulfex 1125
Myleran Tablets 1492

Carbamazepine (Potential for resistance to the neuromuscular blocking action in patients on chronic carbamazepine therapy). Products include:

Carbatrol Capsules 3174
Equetro Extended-Release Capsules 3178
Tegretol/Tegretol-XR 2278

Carboplatin (Irreversible inhibition of plasma cholinesterase by certain unspecified antineoplastic drugs resulting in possible prolonged neuromuscular block).

No products indexed under this heading.

Carmustine (BCNU) (Irreversible inhibition of plasma cholinesterase by certain unspecified antineoplastic drugs resulting in possible prolonged neuromuscular block).

No products indexed under this heading.

Chlorambucil (Irreversible inhibition of plasma cholinesterase by certain unspecified antineoplastic drugs resulting in possible prolonged neuromuscular block). Products include:

Leukeran Tablets 1472

Chloroprocaine Hydrochloride (Enhances neuromuscular blocking action).

No products indexed under this heading.

Cisplatin (Irreversible inhibition of plasma cholinesterase by certain unspecified antineoplastic drugs resulting in possible prolonged neuromuscular block).

No products indexed under this heading.

Clindamycin Hydrochloride (Enhances neuromuscular blocking action). Products include:

Cleocin Vaginal Ovules 2613

Clindamycin Palmitate Hydrochloride (Enhances neuromuscular blocking action).

No products indexed under this heading.

Clindamycin Phosphate (Enhances neuromuscular blocking action). Products include:

Benzaclin Topical Gel 1046
Clindagel 1207
Clindesse Vaginal Cream 3296
Clindets Pledgets 3212
Evoclin Foam, 1% 1025

Colistimethate Sodium (Enhances neuromuscular blocking action).

No products indexed under this heading.

Colistin Sulfate (Enhances neuromuscular blocking action).

No products indexed under this heading.

Cortisone Acetate (Enhances the neuromuscular blocking effects by a reduction in plasma cholinesterase activity induced by chronic administration of glucocorticoids).

No products indexed under this heading.

Cyclophosphamide (Irreversible inhibition of plasma cholinesterase by certain unspecified antineoplastic drugs resulting in possible prolonged neuromuscular block).

No products indexed under this heading.

Dacarbazine (Irreversible inhibition of plasma cholinesterase by certain unspecified antineoplastic drugs resulting in possible prolonged neuromuscular block).

No products indexed under this heading.

Daunorubicin Citrate (Irreversible inhibition of plasma cholinesterase by certain unspecified antineoplastic drugs resulting in possible prolonged neuromuscular block).

No products indexed under this heading.

Daunorubicin Hydrochloride (Irreversible inhibition of plasma cholinesterase by certain unspecified antineoplastic drugs resulting in possible prolonged neuromuscular block). Products include:

Cerubidine for Injection 788

Demeclocycline Hydrochloride (Enhances neuromuscular blocking action).

No products indexed under this heading.

Denileukin Diftitox (Irreversible inhibition of plasma cholinesterase by certain unspecified antineoplastic drugs resulting in possible prolonged neuromuscular block). Products include:

Ontak Vials 1717

Desogestrel (Enhances the neuromuscular blocking effects by a reduction in plasma cholinesterase activity induced by chronic administration of oral contraceptives). Products include:

Ortho-Cept Tablets 2395

Dexamethasone (Enhances the neuromuscular blocking effects by a reduction in plasma cholinesterase activity induced by chronic administration of glucocorticoids). Products include:

Ciprodex Otic Suspension 555
Decadron Tablets 1929
TobraDex Ophthalmic Ointment 558
TobraDex Ophthalmic Suspension ... 558

Dexamethasone Acetate (Enhances the neuromuscular blocking effects by a reduction in plasma cholinesterase activity induced by chronic administration of glucocorticoids).

No products indexed under this heading.

Dexamethasone Sodium Phosphate (Enhances the neuromuscular blocking effects by a reduction in plasma cholinesterase activity induced by chronic administration of glucocorticoids). Products include:

Decadron Phosphate Injection 1931

Docetaxel (Irreversible inhibition of plasma cholinesterase by certain unspecified antineoplastic drugs resulting in possible prolonged neuromuscular block). Products include:

Taxotere Injection Concentrate 2947

Doxorubicin Hydrochloride (Irreversible inhibition of plasma cholinesterase by certain unspecified antineoplastic drugs resulting in possible prolonged neuromuscular block). Products include:

Adriamycin for Injection, USP 786
Adriamycin Injection, USP 786

Doxycycline Calcium (Enhances neuromuscular blocking action).

No products indexed under this heading.

Doxycycline Hyclate (Enhances neuromuscular blocking action).

No products indexed under this heading.

Doxycycline Monohydrate (Enhances neuromuscular blocking action).

No products indexed under this heading.

Echothiophate Iodide (Irreversible inhibition of plasma cholinesterase by echothiophate resulting in possible prolonged neuromuscular block).

No products indexed under this heading.

Enflurane (Decreases ED_{50} of Mivacron by as much as 35% to 40%; prolongs the clinically effective duration of action).

No products indexed under this heading.

Epirubicin Hydrochloride (Irreversible inhibition of plasma cholinesterase by certain unspecified antineoplastic drugs resulting in possible prolonged neuromuscular block). Products include:

Ellence Injection 2632

Estramustine Phosphate Sodium (Irreversible inhibition of plasma cholinesterase by certain unspecified antineoplastic drugs resulting in possible prolonged neuromuscular block). Products include:

Emcyt Capsules 3137

Ethinyl Estradiol (Enhances the neuromuscular blocking effects by a reduction in plasma cholinesterase activity induced by chronic administration of oral contraceptives). Products include:

Alesse-28 Tablets 3392
Lo/Ovral-28 Tablets 3423
NuvaRing 2357
Ortho-Cept Tablets 2395
Ortho-Cyclen/Ortho Tri-Cyclen 2414
Ortho Evra Transdermal System 2402
Ortho Tri-Cyclen Lo Tablets 2421
Seasonale Tablets 1073
Triphasil-28 Tablets 3483
Yasmin 28 Tablets 818

Ethynodiol Diacetate (Enhances the neuromuscular blocking effects by a reduction in plasma cholinesterase activity induced by chronic administration of oral contraceptives).

No products indexed under this heading.

Etidocaine Hydrochloride (Enhances neuromuscular blocking action).

No products indexed under this heading.

Etoposide (Irreversible inhibition of plasma cholinesterase by certain unspecified antineoplastic drugs resulting in possible prolonged neuromuscular block).

No products indexed under this heading.

Exemestane (Irreversible inhibition of plasma cholinesterase by certain unspecified antineoplastic drugs resulting in possible prolonged neuromuscular block). Products include:

Aromasin Tablets 2600

Floxuridine (Irreversible inhibition of plasma cholinesterase by certain unspecified antineoplastic drugs resulting in possible prolonged neuromuscular block).

No products indexed under this heading.

Fludrocortisone Acetate (Enhances the neuromuscular blocking effects by a reduction in plasma cholinesterase activity induced by chronic administration of glucocorticoids).

No products indexed under this heading.

Fluorouracil (Irreversible inhibition of plasma cholinesterase by certain unspecified antineoplastic drugs resulting in possible prolonged neuromuscular block). Products include:

Carac Cream, 0.5% 1048
Efudex 3348

Flutamide (Irreversible inhibition of plasma cholinesterase by certain unspecified antineoplastic drugs resulting in possible prolonged neuromuscular block). Products include:

Eulexin Capsules 3023

Fosphenytoin Sodium (Potential for resistance to the neuromuscular blocking action in patients on chronic phenytoin therapy).

No products indexed under this heading.

Gemcitabine Hydrochloride (Irreversible inhibition of plasma cholinesterase by certain unspecified antineoplastic drugs resulting in possible prolonged neuromuscular block). Products include:

Gemzar for Injection 1743

Gentamicin Sulfate (Enhances the neuromuscular blocking action). Products include:

Garamycin Injectable 3028

Genoptic Sterile Ophthalmic Solution .... ⊙ 227
Pred-G Ophthalmic Suspension .... ⊙ 234
Pred-G Sterile Ophthalmic Ointment .... ⊙ 235

Halothane (Prolongs the duration of action).
No products indexed under this heading.

Hydrocortisone (Enhances the neuromuscular blocking effects by a reduction in plasma cholinesterase activity induced by chronic administration of glucocorticoids). Products include:
Cortizone•5 Ointment 699
Cortizone•10 Creme 699
Cortizone•10 Ointment 699
Cortizone•10 Plus Creme 700
Cortizone•10 Maximum Strength Quick Shot Spray 700
Hydrocortone Tablets 1963
Preparation H Hydrocortisone Cream 748

Hydrocortisone Acetate (Enhances the neuromuscular blocking effects by a reduction in plasma cholinesterase activity induced by chronic administration of glucocorticoids). Products include:
Analpram-HC 1136
Pramosone 1139
ProctoFoam-HC 3113
Tucks Anti-Itch Ointment 712
U-cort 1% Cream 3289

Hydrocortisone Sodium Phosphate (Enhances the neuromuscular blocking effects by a reduction in plasma cholinesterase activity induced by chronic administration of glucocorticoids).
No products indexed under this heading.

Hydrocortisone Sodium Succinate (Enhances the neuromuscular blocking effects by a reduction in plasma cholinesterase activity induced by chronic administration of glucocorticoids).
No products indexed under this heading.

Hydroxyurea (Irreversible inhibition of plasma cholinesterase by certain unspecified antineoplastic drugs resulting in possible prolonged neuromuscular block).
No products indexed under this heading.

Idarubicin Hydrochloride (Irreversible inhibition of plasma cholinesterase by certain unspecified antineoplastic drugs resulting in possible prolonged neuromuscular block). Products include:
Idamycin PFS Injection 2645

Ifosfamide (Irreversible inhibition of plasma cholinesterase by certain unspecified antineoplastic drugs resulting in possible prolonged neuromuscular block).
No products indexed under this heading.

Interferon alfa-2a, Recombinant (Irreversible inhibition of plasma cholinesterase by certain unspecified antineoplastic drugs resulting in possible prolonged neuromuscular block). Products include:
Roferon-A Injection 2805

Interferon alfa-2b, Recombinant (Irreversible inhibition of plasma cholinesterase by certain unspecified antineoplastic drugs resulting in possible prolonged neuromuscular block). Products include:
Intron A for Injection 3038
Rebetron Combination Therapy 3078

Irinotecan Hydrochloride (Irreversible inhibition of plasma cholinesterase by certain unspecified antineoplastic drugs resulting in possible prolonged neuromuscular block). Products include:
Camptosar Injection 2602

Isocarboxazid (Enhances the neuromuscular blocking effects by a reduction in plasma cholinesterase activity induced by chronic administration of certain unspecified monoamine oxidase inhibitors).
No products indexed under this heading.

Isoflurane (Decreases ED_{50} of Mivacron by as much as 35% to 40%; prolongs the clinically effective duration of action).
No products indexed under this heading.

Kanamycin Sulfate (Enhances the neuromuscular blocking action).
No products indexed under this heading.

Levamisole Hydrochloride (Irreversible inhibition of plasma cholinesterase by certain unspecified antineoplastic drugs resulting in possible prolonged neuromuscular block).
No products indexed under this heading.

Levobupivacaine Hydrochloride (Enhances neuromuscular blocking action).
No products indexed under this heading.

Levonorgestrel (Enhances the neuromuscular blocking effects by a reduction in plasma cholinesterase activity induced by chronic administration of oral contraceptives). Products include:
Alesse-28 Tablets 3392
Climara Pro Transdermal System 800
Mirena Intrauterine System 810
Plan B Tablets 1068
Seasonale Tablets 1073
Triphasil-28 Tablets 3483

Lidocaine Hydrochloride (Enhances neuromuscular blocking action).
No products indexed under this heading.

Lincomycin Hydrochloride (Enhances neuromuscular blocking action).
No products indexed under this heading.

Lithium (Enhances neuromuscular blocking action).
No products indexed under this heading.

Lithium Carbonate (Enhances neuromuscular blocking action). Products include:
Eskalith 1406
Lithobid Tablets 1670

Lithium Citrate (Enhances neuromuscular blocking action).
No products indexed under this heading.

Lomustine (CCNU) (Irreversible inhibition of plasma cholinesterase by certain unspecified antineoplastic drugs resulting in possible prolonged neuromuscular block).
No products indexed under this heading.

Magnesium Salts (Enhances neuromuscular blocking action).
No products indexed under this heading.

Mechlorethamine Hydrochloride (Irreversible inhibition of plasma cholinesterase by certain unspecified antineoplastic drugs resulting in possible prolonged neuromuscular block). Products include:
Mustargen for Injection 2007

Megestrol Acetate (Irreversible inhibition of plasma cholinesterase by certain unspecified antineoplastic drugs resulting in possible prolonged neuromuscular block). Products include:
Megace ES Oral Suspension 2492

Melphalan (Irreversible inhibition of plasma cholinesterase by certain unspecified antineoplastic drugs resulting in possible prolonged neuromuscular block). Products include:
Alkeran Tablets 977

Mepivacaine Hydrochloride (Enhances neuromuscular blocking action).
No products indexed under this heading.

Mercaptopurine (Irreversible inhibition of plasma cholinesterase by certain unspecified antineoplastic drugs resulting in possible prolonged neuromuscular block). Products include:
Purinethol Tablets 1222

Mestranol (Enhances the neuromuscular blocking effects by a reduction in plasma cholinesterase activity induced by chronic administration of oral contraceptives).
No products indexed under this heading.

Methacycline Hydrochloride (Enhances neuromuscular blocking action).
No products indexed under this heading.

Methotrexate Sodium (Irreversible inhibition of plasma cholinesterase by certain unspecified antineoplastic drugs resulting in possible prolonged neuromuscular block).
No products indexed under this heading.

Methylprednisolone Acetate (Enhances the neuromuscular blocking effects by a reduction in plasma cholinesterase activity induced by chronic administration of glucocorticoids). Products include:
Depo-Medrol Injectable Suspension 2615
Depo-Medrol Single-Dose Vial 2617

Methylprednisolone Sodium Succinate (Enhances the neuromuscular blocking effects by a reduction in plasma cholinesterase activity induced by chronic administration of glucocorticoids).
No products indexed under this heading.

Minocycline Hydrochloride (Enhances neuromuscular blocking action). Products include:
Dynacin Tablets 1859

Mitomycin (Mitomycin-C) (Irreversible inhibition of plasma cholinesterase by certain unspecified antineoplastic drugs resulting in possible prolonged neuromuscular block).
No products indexed under this heading.

Mitotane (Irreversible inhibition of plasma cholinesterase by certain unspecified antineoplastic drugs resulting in possible prolonged neuromuscular block).
No products indexed under this heading.

Mitoxantrone Hydrochloride (Irreversible inhibition of plasma cholinesterase by certain unspecified antineoplastic drugs resulting in possible prolonged neuromuscular block). Products include:
Novantrone for Injection Concentrate 3158

Moclobemide (Enhances the neuromuscular blocking effects by a reduction in plasma cholinesterase activity induced by chronic administration of certain unspecified monoamine oxidase inhibitors).
No products indexed under this heading.

Norethindrone (Enhances the neuromuscular blocking effects by a reduction in plasma cholinesterase activity induced by chronic administration of oral contraceptives). Products include:
Ortho Micronor Tablets 2411

Norethynodrel (Enhances the neuromuscular blocking effects by a reduction in plasma cholinesterase activity induced by chronic administration of oral contraceptives).
No products indexed under this heading.

Norgestimate (Enhances the neuromuscular blocking effects by a reduction in plasma cholinesterase activity induced by chronic administration of oral contraceptives). Products include:
Ortho-Cyclen/Ortho Tri-Cyclen 2414
Ortho Tri-Cyclen Lo Tablets 2421
Prefest Tablets 1069

Norgestrel (Enhances the neuromuscular blocking effects by a reduction in plasma cholinesterase activity induced by chronic administration of oral contraceptives). Products include:
Lo/Ovral-28 Tablets 3423

Oxaliplatin (Irreversible inhibition of plasma cholinesterase by certain unspecified antineoplastic drugs resulting in possible prolonged neuromuscular block). Products include:
Eloxatin for Injection 2908

Oxytetracycline Hydrochloride (Enhances neuromuscular blocking action).
No products indexed under this heading.

Paclitaxel (Irreversible inhibition of plasma cholinesterase by certain unspecified antineoplastic drugs resulting in possible prolonged neuromuscular block).
No products indexed under this heading.

Pargyline Hydrochloride (Enhances the neuromuscular blocking effects by a reduction in plasma cholinesterase activity induced by chronic administration of certain unspecified monoamine oxidase inhibitors).
No products indexed under this heading.

Phenelzine Sulfate (Enhances the neuromuscular blocking effects by a reduction in plasma cholinesterase activity induced by chronic administration of certain unspecified monoamine oxidase inhibitors).
No products indexed under this heading.

Phenytoin (Potential for resistance to the neuromuscular blocking action in patients on chronic phenytoin therapy).
No products indexed under this heading.

Phenytoin Sodium (Potential for resistance to the neuromuscular

blocking action in patients on chronic phenytoin therapy). Products include:
Phenytek Capsules 2153

Polymyxin Preparations (Enhances neuromuscular blocking action).
No products indexed under this heading.

Prednisolone Acetate (Enhances the neuromuscular blocking effects by a reduction in plasma cholinesterase activity induced by chronic administration of glucocorticoids). Products include:
Blephamide Ophthalmic Ointment 563
Blephamide Ophthalmic Suspension 564
Poly-Pred Liquifilm Ophthalmic Suspension .... ⊙ 231
Pred Forte Ophthalmic Suspension .... ⊙ 233
Pred Mild Sterile Ophthalmic Suspension .... ⊙ 236
Pred-G Ophthalmic Suspension ...... ⊙ 234
Pred-G Sterile Ophthalmic Ointment .... ⊙ 235

Prednisolone Sodium Phosphate (Enhances the neuromuscular blocking effects by a reduction in plasma cholinesterase activity induced by chronic administration of glucocorticoids). Products include:
Pediapred Oral Solution 3319

Prednisolone Tebutate (Enhances the neuromuscular blocking effects by a reduction in plasma cholinesterase activity induced by chronic administration of glucocorticoids).
No products indexed under this heading.

Prednisone (Enhances the neuromuscular blocking effects by a reduction in plasma cholinesterase activity induced by chronic administration of glucocorticoids).
No products indexed under this heading.

Procainamide Hydrochloride (Enhances neuromuscular blocking action).
No products indexed under this heading.

Procaine Hydrochloride (Enhances neuromuscular blocking action).
No products indexed under this heading.

Procarbazine Hydrochloride (Irreversible inhibition of plasma cholinesterase by certain unspecified antineoplastic drugs resulting in possible prolonged neuromuscular block). Products include:
Matulane Capsules 3188

Quinidine (Enhances neuromuscular blocking action).
No products indexed under this heading.

Quinidine Gluconate (Enhances neuromuscular blocking action).
No products indexed under this heading.

Quinidine Hydrochloride (Enhances neuromuscular blocking action).
No products indexed under this heading.

Quinidine Polygalacturonate (Enhances neuromuscular blocking action).
No products indexed under this heading.

Quinidine Sulfate (Enhances neuromuscular blocking action).
No products indexed under this heading.

Selegiline Hydrochloride (Enhances the neuromuscular blocking effects by a reduction in plasma cholinesterase activity induced by chronic administration of certain unspecified monoamine oxidase inhibitors). Products include:
Eldepryl Capsules 3209

Streptomycin Sulfate (Enhances the neuromuscular blocking action).
No products indexed under this heading.

Streptozocin (Irreversible inhibition of plasma cholinesterase by certain unspecified antineoplastic drugs resulting in possible prolonged neuromuscular block).
No products indexed under this heading.

Succinylcholine Chloride (Prior administration of succinylcholine can potentiate neuromuscular blockade).
No products indexed under this heading.

Tamoxifen Citrate (Irreversible inhibition of plasma cholinesterase by certain unspecified antineoplastic drugs resulting in possible prolonged neuromuscular block).
No products indexed under this heading.

Teniposide (Irreversible inhibition of plasma cholinesterase by certain unspecified antineoplastic drugs resulting in possible prolonged neuromuscular block).
No products indexed under this heading.

Tetracaine Hydrochloride (Enhances neuromuscular blocking action). Products include:
Cetacaine Topical Anesthetic 1007

Tetracycline Hydrochloride (Enhances neuromuscular blocking action).
No products indexed under this heading.

Thioguanine (Irreversible inhibition of plasma cholinesterase by certain unspecified antineoplastic drugs resulting in possible prolonged neuromuscular block). Products include:
Tabloid Tablets 1545

Thiotepa (Irreversible inhibition of plasma cholinesterase by certain unspecified antineoplastic drugs resulting in possible prolonged neuromuscular block).
No products indexed under this heading.

Tobramycin (Enhances the neuromuscular blocking action). Products include:
TOBI Solution for Inhalation 1015
TobraDex Ophthalmic Ointment 558
TobraDex Ophthalmic Suspension ... 558
Zylet Ophthalmic Suspension 3508

Tobramycin Sulfate (Enhances the neuromuscular blocking action).
No products indexed under this heading.

Topotecan Hydrochloride (Irreversible inhibition of plasma cholinesterase by certain unspecified antineoplastic drugs resulting in possible prolonged neuromuscular block). Products include:
Hycamtin for Injection 1427

Toremifene Citrate (Irreversible inhibition of plasma cholinesterase by certain unspecified antineoplastic drugs resulting in possible prolonged neuromuscular block).
No products indexed under this heading.

Tranylcypromine Sulfate (Enhances the neuromuscular blocking effects by a reduction in plasma cholinesterase activity induced by chronic administration of certain unspecified monoamine oxidase inhibitors). Products include:
Parnate Tablets 1499

Triamcinolone (Enhances the neuromuscular blocking effects by a reduction in plasma cholinesterase activity induced by chronic administration of glucocorticoids).
No products indexed under this heading.

Triamcinolone Acetonide (Enhances the neuromuscular blocking effects by a reduction in plasma cholinesterase activity induced by chronic administration of glucocorticoids). Products include:
Azmacort Inhalation Aerosol 1701
Nasacort HFA Inhalation Aerosol 2939
Nasacort AQ Nasal Spray 2937

Triamcinolone Diacetate (Enhances the neuromuscular blocking effects by a reduction in plasma cholinesterase activity induced by chronic administration of glucocorticoids).
No products indexed under this heading.

Triamcinolone Hexacetonide (Enhances the neuromuscular blocking effects by a reduction in plasma cholinesterase activity induced by chronic administration of glucocorticoids).
No products indexed under this heading.

Valrubicin (Irreversible inhibition of plasma cholinesterase by certain unspecified antineoplastic drugs resulting in possible prolonged neuromuscular block).
No products indexed under this heading.

Vincristine Sulfate (Irreversible inhibition of plasma cholinesterase by certain unspecified antineoplastic drugs resulting in possible prolonged neuromuscular block).
No products indexed under this heading.

Vinorelbine Tartrate (Irreversible inhibition of plasma cholinesterase by certain unspecified antineoplastic drugs resulting in possible prolonged neuromuscular block). Products include:
Navelbine Injection 1494

M-M-R II

(Measles, Mumps & Rubella Virus Vaccine, Live) 1980
May interact with immunosuppressive agents. Compounds in these categories include:

Azathioprine (Concurrent administration with immunosuppressant is contraindicated). Products include:
Azasan Tablets 2844

Basiliximab (Concurrent administration with immunosuppressant is contraindicated). Products include:
Simulect for Injection 2268

Cyclosporine (Concurrent administration with immunosuppressant is contraindicated). Products include:
Gengraf Capsules 458
Neoral Soft Gelatin Capsules 2247
Neoral Oral Solution 2247
Restasis Ophthalmic Emulsion 570
Sandimmune 2259

Muromonab-CD3 (Concurrent administration with immunosuppressant is contraindicated). Products include:
Orthoclone OKT3 Sterile Solution 2370

Mycophenolate Mofetil (Concurrent administration with immunosuppressant is contraindicated). Products include:
CellCept Capsules 2751
CellCept Oral Suspension 2751
CellCept Tablets 2751

Sirolimus (Concurrent administration with immunosuppressant is contraindicated). Products include:
Rapamune Oral Solution and Tablets 3472

Tacrolimus (Concurrent administration with immunosuppressant is contraindicated). Products include:
Prograf Capsules and Injection 624
Protopic Ointment 629

MOBAN TABLETS

(Molindone Hydrochloride) 1108
May interact with tetracyclines and certain other agents. Compounds in these categories include:

Demeclocycline Hydrochloride (Calcium sulfate present as an excipient may interfere with the absorption of oral tetracyclines).
No products indexed under this heading.

Doxycycline Calcium (Calcium sulfate present as an excipient may interfere with the absorption of oral tetracyclines).
No products indexed under this heading.

Doxycycline Hyclate (Calcium sulfate present as an excipient may interfere with the absorption of oral tetracyclines).
No products indexed under this heading.

Doxycycline Monohydrate (Calcium sulfate present as an excipient may interfere with the absorption of oral tetracyclines).
No products indexed under this heading.

Methacycline Hydrochloride (Calcium sulfate present as an excipient may interfere with the absorption of oral tetracyclines).
No products indexed under this heading.

Minocycline Hydrochloride (Calcium sulfate present as an excipient may interfere with the absorption of oral tetracyclines). Products include:
Dynacin Tablets 1859

Oxytetracycline Hydrochloride (Calcium sulfate present as an excipient may interfere with the absorption of oral tetracyclines).
No products indexed under this heading.

Phenytoin Sodium (Calcium sulfate present as an excipient may interfere with the absorption of oral phenytoin sodium). Products include:
Phenytek Capsules 2153

Tetracycline Hydrochloride (Calcium sulfate present as an excipient may interfere with the absorption of oral tetracyclines).
No products indexed under this heading.

MOBIC ORAL SUSPENSION

(Meloxicam) 893
See Mobic Tablets

MOBIC TABLETS

(Meloxicam) 893

May interact with ACE inhibitors, lithium preparations, loop diuretics, thiazides, and certain other agents. Compounds in these categories include:

Aspirin (Co-administration of aspirin to healthy volunteers tended to increase the AUC and Cmax of meloxicam; the clinical significance of this interaction is not known; concurrent use may result in an increased rate of GI ulceration or other complications). Products include:

Aggrenox Capsules 855
Bayer, Aspirin Regimen 606
Bayer Aspirin Tablets 3515
BC Powder 612
BC Allergy Sinus Cold Powder 612
Arthritis Strength BC Powder 612
BC Sinus Cold Powder 612
Ecotrin Enteric Coated Aspirin Low, Regular and Maximum Strength Tablets 1627
Goody's Body Pain Formula Powder 621
Goody's Extra Strength Headache Powder 621
Goody's Extra Strength Pain Relief Tablets 621
Percodan Tablets 1115
St. Joseph 81 mg Aspirin Chewable and Enteric Coated Tablets 1841

Benazepril Hydrochloride (Co-administration of NSAIDs with ACE inhibitors may diminish the antihypertensive effects of ACE inhibitors). Products include:

Lotensin Tablets 2232
Lotensin HCT Tablets 2235
Lotrel Capsules 2238

Bendroflumethiazide (NSAIDs can reduce the natriuretic effect of thiazide diuretics in some patients. Patients taking thiazides may have impaired response when taking NSAIDs).

No products indexed under this heading.

Bumetanide (Patients taking loop diuretics may have impaired response when taking NSAIDs).

No products indexed under this heading.

Captopril (Co-administration of NSAIDs with ACE inhibitors may diminish the antihypertensive effects of ACE inhibitors). Products include:

Captopril Tablets 2114

Chlorothiazide (NSAIDs can reduce the natriuretic effect of thiazide diuretics in some patients. Patients taking thiazides may have impaired response when taking NSAIDs). Products include:

Aldoclor Tablets 1881
Diuril Oral 1936

Chlorothiazide Sodium (NSAIDs can reduce the natriuretic effect of thiazide diuretics in some patients. Patients taking thiazides may have impaired response when taking NSAIDs). Products include:

Diuril Sodium Intravenous 1934

Cholestyramine (Pretreatment for four days with cholestyramine significantly increased clearance of meloxicam by 50% resulting in a decrease in t1/2 from 19.2 hours to 12.5 hours and a 35% reduction in AUC; the clinical significance of this interaction is not known).

No products indexed under this heading.

Enalapril Maleate (Co-administration of NSAIDs with ACE inhibitors may diminish the antihypertensive effects of ACE inhibitors). Products include:

Vaseretic Tablets 2073
Vasotec I.V. Injection 2076

Enalaprilat (Co-administration of NSAIDs with ACE inhibitors may diminish the antihypertensive effects of ACE inhibitors).

No products indexed under this heading.

Ethacrynic Acid (Patients taking loop diuretics may have impaired response when taking NSAIDs). Products include:

Edecrin Tablets 1941

Fosinopril Sodium (Co-administration of NSAIDs with ACE inhibitors may diminish the antihypertensive effects of ACE inhibitors).

No products indexed under this heading.

Furosemide (NSAIDs can reduce the natriuretic effect of furosemide in some patients; in clinical studies, pharmacokinetics and pharmacodynamics of furosemide were not affected by multiple doses of meloxicam). Products include:

Furosemide Tablets 2117

Hydrochlorothiazide (NSAIDs can reduce the natriuretic effect of thiazide diuretics in some patients. Patients taking thiazides may have impaired response when taking NSAIDs). Products include:

Aldoril Tablets 1884
Atacand HCT 637
Avalide Tablets 2889
Avalide Tablets 922
Benicar HCT Tablets 2852
Diovan HCT Tablets 2195
Dyazide Capsules 1389
Hyzaar 1964
Lotensin HCT Tablets 2235
Maxzide 2150
Micardis HCT Tablets 886
Moduretic Tablets 2003
Prinzide Tablets 2033
Teveten HCT Tablets 1710
Timolide Tablets 2056
Uniretic Tablets 3114
Vaseretic Tablets 2073
Zestoretic Tablets 701

Hydroflumethiazide (NSAIDs can reduce the natriuretic effect of thiazide diuretics in some patients. Patients taking thiazides may have impaired response when taking NSAIDs).

No products indexed under this heading.

Lisinopril (Co-administration of NSAIDs with ACE inhibitors may diminish the antihypertensive effects of ACE inhibitors). Products include:

Prinivil Tablets 2029
Prinzide Tablets 2033
Zestoretic Tablets 701
Zestril Tablets 704

Lithium (NSAIDs can produce an elevation of plasma lithium levels and a reduction in renal lithium clearance; co-administration in healthy subjects has resulted in increased lithium concentration and AUC).

No products indexed under this heading.

Lithium Carbonate (NSAIDs can produce an elevation of plasma lithium levels and a reduction in renal lithium clearance; co-administration in healthy subjects has resulted in increased lithium concentration and AUC). Products include:

Eskalith 1406
Lithobid Tablets 1670

Lithium Citrate (NSAIDs can produce an elevation of plasma lithium levels and a reduction in renal lithium clearance; co-administration in healthy subjects has resulted in increased lithium concentration and AUC).

No products indexed under this heading.

Methotrexate (Caution should be used when NSAIDs are administered concomitantly with methotrexate).

No products indexed under this heading.

Methotrexate Sodium (Caution should be used when NSAIDs are administered concomitantly with methotrexate).

No products indexed under this heading.

Methyclothiazide (NSAIDs can reduce the natriuretic effect of thiazide diuretics in some patients. Patients taking thiazides may have impaired response when taking NSAIDs).

No products indexed under this heading.

Moexipril Hydrochloride (Co-administration of NSAIDs with ACE inhibitors may diminish the antihypertensive effects of ACE inhibitors). Products include:

Uniretic Tablets 3114
Univasc Tablets 3118

Perindopril Erbumine (Co-administration of NSAIDs with ACE inhibitors may diminish the antihypertensive effects of ACE inhibitors). Products include:

Aceon Tablets (2 mg, 4 mg, 8 mg) 3191

Polythiazide (NSAIDs can reduce the natriuretic effect of thiazide diuretics in some patients. Patients taking thiazides may have impaired response when taking NSAIDs).

No products indexed under this heading.

Quinapril Hydrochloride (Co-administration of NSAIDs with ACE inhibitors may diminish the antihypertensive effects of ACE inhibitors).

No products indexed under this heading.

Ramipril (Co-administration of NSAIDs with ACE inhibitors may diminish the antihypertensive effects of ACE inhibitors). Products include:

Altace Capsules 1673

Spirapril Hydrochloride (Co-administration of NSAIDs with ACE inhibitors may diminish the antihypertensive effects of ACE inhibitors).

No products indexed under this heading.

Torsemide (Patients taking loop diuretics may have impaired response when taking NSAIDs).

No products indexed under this heading.

Trandolapril (Co-administration of NSAIDs with ACE inhibitors may diminish the antihypertensive effects of ACE inhibitors). Products include:

Mavik Tablets 482
Tarka Tablets 519

Warfarin Sodium (Potential for increased risk of bleeding). Products include:

Coumadin for Injection 932
Coumadin Tablets 932

Food Interactions

Food, unspecified (Co-administration with a high-fat breakfast did not affect extent of absorption of meloxicam capsules but led to 22% higher Cmax values; mean Cmax values were achieved between 5 to 6 hours; Mobic tablets can be administered without regard to timing of meals).

MODURETIC TABLETS

(Amiloride Hydrochloride, Hydrochlorothiazide)......................... 2003

May interact with ACE inhibitors, angiotensin-II receptor antagonists, antihypertensives, barbiturates, corticosteroids, cardiac glycosides, oral hypoglycemic agents, insulin, lithium preparations, narcotic analgesics, nondepolarizing neuromuscular blocking agents, non-steroidal anti-inflammatory agents, potassium preparations, potassium sparing diuretics, and certain other agents. Compounds in these categories include:

Acarbose (Hydrochlorothiazide produces hyperglycemia; dosage adjustment of the antidiabetic agent may be required). Products include:

Precose Tablets 776

Acebutolol Hydrochloride (Co-administration with other antihypertensive drugs may result in additive effect or potentiation).

No products indexed under this heading.

ACTH (Intensifies electrolyte depletion particularly hypokalemia).

No products indexed under this heading.

Alfentanil Hydrochloride (Potentiation of orthostatic hypotension).

No products indexed under this heading.

Amlodipine Besylate (Co-administration with other antihypertensive drugs may result in additive effect or potentiation). Products include:

Caduet Tablets 2507
Lotrel Capsules 2238
Norvasc Tablets 2529

Aprobarbital (Potentiation of orthostatic hypotension).

No products indexed under this heading.

Atenolol (Co-administration with other antihypertensive drugs may result in additive effect or potentiation). Products include:

Tenormin I.V. Injection 698
Tenormin Tablets 695

Atracurium Besylate (Possible increased responsiveness to muscle relaxant).

No products indexed under this heading.

Benazepril Hydrochloride (Co-administration increases the risk of hyperkalemia; potential for additive antihypertensive effect). Products include:

Lotensin Tablets 2232
Lotensin HCT Tablets 2235
Lotrel Capsules 2238

Bendroflumethiazide (Co-administration with other antihypertensive drugs may result in additive effect or potentiation).

No products indexed under this heading.

Betamethasone Acetate (Corticosteroids intensify electrolyte depletion particularly hypokalemia).

No products indexed under this heading.

Betamethasone Sodium Phosphate (Corticosteroids intensify electrolyte depletion particularly hypokalemia).
No products indexed under this heading.

Betaxolol Hydrochloride (Co-administration with other antihypertensive drugs may result in additive effect or potentiation). Products include:
Betoptic S Ophthalmic Suspension 554

Bisoprolol Fumarate (Co-administration with other antihypertensive drugs may result in additive effect or potentiation).
No products indexed under this heading.

Buprenorphine Hydrochloride (Potentiation of orthostatic hypotension). Products include:
Buprenex Injectable 2718
Suboxone Tablets 2719
Subutex Tablets 2719

Butabarbital (Potentiation of orthostatic hypotension).
No products indexed under this heading.

Butalbital (Potentiation of orthostatic hypotension). Products include:
Sedapap Tablets 50 mg/650 mg 2098

Candesartan Cilexetil (Co-administration increases the risk of hyperkalemia; potential for additive antihypertensive effect). Products include:
Atacand Tablets 634
Atacand HCT 637

Captopril (Co-administration increases the risk of hyperkalemia; potential for additive antihypertensive effect). Products include:
Captopril Tablets 2114

Carteolol Hydrochloride (Co-administration with other antihypertensive drugs may result in additive effect or potentiation). Products include:
Carteolol Hydrochloride Ophthalmic Solution USP, 1% .... ⊙ 246

Celecoxib (Co-administration of non-steroidal anti-inflammatory agents can reduce the diuretic, natriuretic, and antihypertensive effects). Products include:
Celebrex Capsules 3130

Chlorothiazide (Co-administration with other antihypertensive drugs may result in additive effect or potentiation). Products include:
Aldoclor Tablets 1881
Diuril Oral 1936

Chlorothiazide Sodium (Co-administration with other antihypertensive drugs may result in additive effect or potentiation). Products include:
Diuril Sodium Intravenous 1934

Chlorpropamide (Hydrochlorothiazide produces hyperglycemia; dosage adjustment of the antidiabetic agent may be required).
No products indexed under this heading.

Chlorthalidone (Co-administration with other antihypertensive drugs may result in additive effect or potentiation). Products include:
Clorpres Tablets 2139

Cholestyramine (Impairs the absorption of hydrochlorothiazide by binding in the GI tract and reducing the absorption by 85%).
No products indexed under this heading.

Cisatracurium Besylate (Possible increased responsiveness to muscle relaxant). Products include:
Nimbex Injection 494

Clonidine (Co-administration with other antihypertensive drugs may result in additive effect or potentiation). Products include:
Catapres-TTS 875

Clonidine Hydrochloride (Co-administration with other antihypertensive drugs may result in additive effect or potentiation). Products include:
Catapres Tablets 874
Clorpres Tablets 2139

Codeine Phosphate (Potentiation of orthostatic hypotension). Products include:
Tylenol with Codeine 2461

Colestipol Hydrochloride (Impairs the absorption of hydrochlorothiazide by binding in the GI tract and reducing the absorption by 43%).
No products indexed under this heading.

Cortisone Acetate (Corticosteroids intensify electrolyte depletion particularly hypokalemia).
No products indexed under this heading.

Cyclosporine (Co-administration increases the risk of hyperkalemia). Products include:
Gengraf Capsules 458
Neoral Soft Gelatin Capsules 2247
Neoral Oral Solution 2247
Restasis Ophthalmic Emulsion 570
Sandimmune 2259

Deserpidine (Co-administration with other antihypertensive drugs may result in additive effect or potentiation).
No products indexed under this heading.

Deslanoside (Hypokalemia may develop during thiazide therapy and may sensitize or exaggerate the response of the heart to the toxic effects of digitalis, such as increased ventricular irritability).
No products indexed under this heading.

Dexamethasone (Corticosteroids intensify electrolyte depletion particularly hypokalemia). Products include:
Ciprodex Otic Suspension 555
Decadron Tablets 1929
TobraDex Ophthalmic Ointment 558
TobraDex Ophthalmic Suspension 558

Dexamethasone Acetate (Corticosteroids intensify electrolyte depletion particularly hypokalemia).
No products indexed under this heading.

Dexamethasone Sodium Phosphate (Corticosteroids intensify electrolyte depletion particularly hypokalemia). Products include:
Decadron Phosphate Injection 1931

Dezocine (Potentiation of orthostatic hypotension).
No products indexed under this heading.

Diazoxide (Co-administration with other antihypertensive drugs may result in additive effect or potentiation). Products include:
Hyperstat I.V. Injection 3031

Diclofenac Potassium (Co-administration of non-steroidal anti-inflammatory agents can reduce the diuretic, natriuretic, and antihypertensive effects). Products include:
Cataflam Tablets 2173

Diclofenac Sodium (Co-administration of non-steroidal anti-inflammatory agents can reduce the diuretic, natriuretic, and antihypertensive effects). Products include:
Arthrotec Tablets 3126
Voltaren Ophthalmic Solution 2300
Voltaren Tablets 2298
Voltaren-XR Tablets 2301

Digitalis Glycoside Preparations (Hypokalemia may develop during thiazide therapy and may sensitize or exaggerate the response of the heart to the toxic effects of digitalis, such as increased ventricular irritability).
No products indexed under this heading.

Digitoxin (Hypokalemia may develop during thiazide therapy and may sensitize or exaggerate the response of the heart to the toxic effects of digitalis, such as increased ventricular irritability).
No products indexed under this heading.

Digoxin (Hypokalemia may develop during thiazide therapy and may sensitize or exaggerate the response of the heart to the toxic effects of digitalis, such as increased ventricular irritability). Products include:
Digitek Tablets 2146
Lanoxicaps Capsules 1458
Lanoxin Injection 1462
Lanoxin Tablets 1468
Lanoxin Injection Pediatric 1465

Diltiazem Hydrochloride (Co-administration with other antihypertensive drugs may result in additive effect or potentiation). Products include:
Cardizem LA Extended Release Tablets 1699
Tiazac Capsules 1204

Doxazosin Mesylate (Co-administration with other antihypertensive drugs may result in additive effect or potentiation).
No products indexed under this heading.

Enalapril Maleate (Co-administration increases the risk of hyperkalemia; potential for additive antihypertensive effect). Products include:
Vaseretic Tablets 2073
Vasotec I.V. Injection 2076

Enalaprilat (Co-administration increases the risk of hyperkalemia; potential for additive antihypertensive effect).
No products indexed under this heading.

Eprosartan Mesylate (Co-administration increases the risk of hyperkalemia; potential for additive antihypertensive effect). Products include:
Teveten Tablets 1707
Teveten HCT Tablets 1710

Esmolol Hydrochloride (Co-administration with other antihypertensive drugs may result in additive effect or potentiation). Products include:
Brevibloc Concentrate 766
Brevibloc Injection 766
Brevibloc Double Strength Injection 766
Brevibloc Premixed Injection 766
Brevibloc Double Strength Premixed Injection 766

Etodolac (Co-administration of non-steroidal anti-inflammatory agents can reduce the diuretic, natriuretic, and antihypertensive effects).
No products indexed under this heading.

Felodipine (Co-administration with other antihypertensive drugs may result in additive effect or potentiation). Products include:
Plendil Extended-Release Tablets 651

Fenoprofen Calcium (Co-administration of non-steroidal anti-inflammatory agents can reduce the diuretic, natriuretic, and antihypertensive effects). Products include:
Nalfon Capsules 2504

Fentanyl (Potentiation of orthostatic hypotension). Products include:
Duragesic Transdermal System 2448

Fentanyl Citrate (Potentiation of orthostatic hypotension). Products include:
Actiq 993

Fludrocortisone Acetate (Corticosteroids intensify electrolyte depletion particularly hypokalemia).
No products indexed under this heading.

Flurbiprofen (Co-administration of non-steroidal anti-inflammatory agents can reduce the diuretic, natriuretic, and antihypertensive effects).
No products indexed under this heading.

Fosinopril Sodium (Co-administration increases the risk of hyperkalemia; potential for additive antihypertensive effect).
No products indexed under this heading.

Furosemide (Co-administration with other antihypertensive drugs may result in additive effect or potentiation). Products include:
Furosemide Tablets 2117

Glimepiride (Hydrochlorothiazide produces hyperglycemia; dosage adjustment of the antidiabetic agent may be required). Products include:
Amaryl Tablets 2864

Glipizide (Hydrochlorothiazide produces hyperglycemia; dosage adjustment of the antidiabetic agent may be required).
No products indexed under this heading.

Glyburide (Hydrochlorothiazide produces hyperglycemia; dosage adjustment of the antidiabetic agent may be required).
No products indexed under this heading.

Guanabenz Acetate (Co-administration with other antihypertensive drugs may result in additive effect or potentiation).
No products indexed under this heading.

Guanethidine Monosulfate (Co-administration with other antihypertensive drugs may result in additive effect or potentiation).
No products indexed under this heading.

Hydralazine Hydrochloride (Co-administration with other antihypertensive drugs may result in additive effect or potentiation). Products include:
BiDil Tablets 2161

Hydrocodone Bitartrate (Potentiation of orthostatic hypotension). Products include:
Hycodan 1104

Hycomine Compound Tablets 1105
Hycotuss Expectorant Syrup 1106
Lortab 3315
Lortab Elixir 3312
Vicodin Tablets 530
Vicodin ES Tablets 531
Vicodin HP Tablets 532
Vicoprofen Tablets 533
Zydone Tablets 1118

Hydrocodone Polistirex (Potentiation of orthostatic hypotension). Products include:
Tussionex Pennkinetic Extended-Release Suspension 3322

Hydrocortisone (Corticosteroids intensify electrolyte depletion particularly hypokalemia). Products include:
Cortizone•5 Ointment 699
Cortizone•10 Creme 699
Cortizone•10 Ointment 699
Cortizone•10 Plus Creme 700
Cortizone•10 Maximum Strength Quick Shot Spray 700
Hydrocortone Tablets 1963
Preparation H Hydrocortisone Cream 748

Hydrocortisone Acetate (Corticosteroids intensify electrolyte depletion particularly hypokalemia). Products include:
Analpram-HC 1136
Pramosone 1139
ProctoFoam-HC 3113
Tucks Anti-Itch Ointment 712
U-cort 1% Cream 3289

Hydrocortisone Sodium Phosphate (Corticosteroids intensify electrolyte depletion particularly hypokalemia).
No products indexed under this heading.

Hydrocortisone Sodium Succinate (Corticosteroids intensify electrolyte depletion particularly hypokalemia).
No products indexed under this heading.

Hydroflumethiazide (Co-administration with other antihypertensive drugs may result in additive effect or potentiation).
No products indexed under this heading.

Hydromorphone Hydrochloride (Potentiation of orthostatic hypotension). Products include:
Dilaudid 439
Dilaudid Oral Liquid 443
Dilaudid Non-Sterile Powder 439
Dilaudid Rectal Suppositories 439
Dilaudid Tablets 439
Dilaudid Tablets - 8 mg 443
Dilaudid-HP 441

Ibuprofen (Co-administration of non-steroidal anti-inflammatory agents can reduce the diuretic, natriuretic, and antihypertensive effects). Products include:
Advil Allergy Sinus Caplets 737
Advil 737
Children's Advil Suspension 742
Children's Advil Chewable Tablets 741
Advil Cold & Sinus 739
Advil Flu & Body Ache Caplets 739
Children's Advil Cold Suspension 741
Infants' Advil Concentrated Drops 743
Junior Strength Advil Swallow Tablets 740
Advil Migraine Liquigels 740
Advil Multi-Symptom Cold Caplets 738
Combunox Tablets 1183
Children's Motrin Oral Suspension and Chewable Tablets 1837
Children's Motrin Cold Non-Staining Dye-Free Oral Suspension 1838
Children's Motrin Cold Oral Suspension 1838
Children's Motrin Non-Staining Dye-Free Oral Suspension 1837
Motrin Cold & Sinus Caplets 1836
Motrin IB Tablets and Caplets 1836
Infants' Motrin Concentrated Drops 1837
Infants' Motrin Non-Staining Dye-Free Drops 1837
Junior Strength Motrin Caplets and Chewable Tablets 1837
Vicoprofen Tablets 533

Indapamide (Co-administration with other antihypertensive drugs may result in additive effect or potentiation). Products include:
Indapamide Tablets 2119

Indomethacin (Co-administration of non-steroidal anti-inflammatory agents can reduce the diuretic, natriuretic, and antihypertensive effects; both indomethacin and amiloride are associated with hyperkalemia, the potential effect on potassium kinetic and renal function should be considered if used concurrently). Products include:
Indocin 1968

Indomethacin Sodium Trihydrate (Co-administration of non-steroidal anti-inflammatory agents can reduce the diuretic, natriuretic, and antihypertensive effects; both indomethacin and amiloride are associated with hyperkalemia, the potential effect on potassium kinetic and renal function should be considered if used concurrently). Products include:
Indocin I.V. 1973

Insulin, Human, Zinc Suspension (Hydrochlorothiazide produces hyperglycemia; dosage adjustment of the insulin agent may be required). Products include:
Humulin L, 100 Units 1763
Humulin U, 100 Units 1770

Insulin, Human NPH (Hydrochlorothiazide produces hyperglycemia; dosage adjustment of the insulin agent may be required). Products include:
Humulin N, 100 Units 1764
Humulin N Pen 1765
Novolin N Human Insulin 10 ml Vials 2322
Novolin N InnoLet 2322
Novolin N PenFill 3 ml Cartridges 2325
Novolin R InnoLet 2322

Insulin, Human Regular (Hydrochlorothiazide produces hyperglycemia; dosage adjustment of the insulin agent may be required). Products include:
Humulin R (U-500) 1768
Humulin R, 100 Units 1767
Novolin R Human Insulin 10 ml Vials 2322
Novolin R PenFill 2325

Insulin, Human Regular and Human NPH Mixture (Hydrochlorothiazide produces hyperglycemia; dosage adjustment of the insulin agent may be required). Products include:
Humulin 50/50, 100 Units 1760
Humulin 70/30 Pen 1761
Novolin 70/30 Human Insulin 10 ml Vials 2321
Novolin 70/30 InnoLet 2322
Novolin 70/30 PenFill 3 ml Cartridges 2325

Insulin, NPH (Hydrochlorothiazide produces hyperglycemia; dosage adjustment of the insulin agent may be required).
No products indexed under this heading.

Insulin, Regular (Hydrochlorothiazide produces hyperglycemia; dosage adjustment of the insulin agent may be required).
No products indexed under this heading.

Insulin, Zinc Crystals (Hydrochlorothiazide produces hyperglycemia; dosage adjustment of the insulin agent may be required).
No products indexed under this heading.

Insulin, Zinc Suspension (Hydrochlorothiazide produces hyperglycemia; dosage adjustment of the insulin agent may be required).
No products indexed under this heading.

Insulin Aspart, Human Regular (Hydrochlorothiazide produces hyperglycemia; dosage adjustment of the insulin agent may be required). Products include:
NovoLog Injection 2326

Insulin glargine (Hydrochlorothiazide produces hyperglycemia; dosage adjustment of the insulin agent may be required). Products include:
Lantus Injection 2925

Insulin Lispro, Human (Hydrochlorothiazide produces hyperglycemia; dosage adjustment of the insulin agent may be required). Products include:
Humalog-Pen 1751
Humalog Mix 75/25-Pen 1754

Insulin Lispro Protamine, Human (Hydrochlorothiazide produces hyperglycemia; dosage adjustment of the insulin agent may be required). Products include:
Humalog Mix 75/25-Pen 1754

Irbesartan (Co-administration increases the risk of hyperkalemia; potential for additive antihypertensive effect). Products include:
Avalide Tablets 922
Avalide Tablets 2889
Avapro Tablets 925
Avapro Tablets 2886

Isradipine (Co-administration with other antihypertensive drugs may result in additive effect or potentiation). Products include:
DynaCirc CR Tablets 2726

Ketoprofen (Co-administration of non-steroidal anti-inflammatory agents can reduce the diuretic, natriuretic, and antihypertensive effects).
No products indexed under this heading.

Ketorolac Tromethamine (Co-administration of non-steroidal anti-inflammatory agents can reduce the diuretic, natriuretic, and antihypertensive effects). Products include:
Acular Ophthalmic Solution 561
Acular LS Ophthalmic Solution 562

Labetalol Hydrochloride (Co-administration with other antihypertensive drugs may result in additive effect or potentiation).
No products indexed under this heading.

Levorphanol Tartrate (Potentiation of orthostatic hypotension).
No products indexed under this heading.

Lisinopril (Co-administration increases the risk of hyperkalemia; potential for additive antihypertensive effect). Products include:
Prinivil Tablets 2029
Prinzide Tablets 2033
Zestoretic Tablets 701
Zestril Tablets 704

Lithium (Diuretics reduce the renal clearance and add a high risk of lithium toxicity).
No products indexed under this heading.

Lithium Carbonate (Diuretics reduce the renal clearance and add a high risk of lithium toxicity). Products include:
Eskalith 1406
Lithobid Tablets 1670

Lithium Citrate (Diuretics reduce the renal clearance and add a high risk of lithium toxicity).
No products indexed under this heading.

Losartan Potassium (Co-administration increases the risk of hyperkalemia; potential for additive antihypertensive effect). Products include:
Cozaar Tablets 1913
Hyzaar 1964

Mecamylamine Hydrochloride (Co-administration with other antihypertensive drugs may result in additive effect or potentiation). Products include:
Inversine Tablets 3286

Meclofenamate Sodium (Co-administration of non-steroidal anti-inflammatory agents can reduce the diuretic, natriuretic, and antihypertensive effects).
No products indexed under this heading.

Mefenamic Acid (Co-administration of non-steroidal anti-inflammatory agents can reduce the diuretic, natriuretic, and antihypertensive effects).
No products indexed under this heading.

Meloxicam (Co-administration of non-steroidal anti-inflammatory agents can reduce the diuretic, natriuretic, and antihypertensive effects). Products include:
Mobic Oral Suspension 893
Mobic Tablets 893

Meperidine Hydrochloride (Potentiation of orthostatic hypotension).
No products indexed under this heading.

Mephobarbital (Potentiation of orthostatic hypotension). Products include:
Mebaral Tablets, USP 2483

Metformin Hydrochloride (Hydrochlorothiazide produces hyperglycemia; dosage adjustment of the antidiabetic agent may be required). Products include:
ActoPlus Met Tablets 3219
Avandamet Tablets 1343
Fortamet Extended-Release Tablets 1156

Methadone Hydrochloride (Potentiation of orthostatic hypotension).
No products indexed under this heading.

Methyclothiazide (Co-administration with other antihypertensive drugs may result in additive effect or potentiation).
No products indexed under this heading.

Methyldopa (Co-administration with other antihypertensive drugs may result in additive effect or potentiation). Products include:
Aldoclor Tablets 1881
Aldoril Tablets 1884

Methyldopate Hydrochloride (Co-administration with other antihypertensive drugs may result in additive effect or potentiation).
No products indexed under this heading.

Methylprednisolone Acetate (Corticosteroids intensify electrolyte depletion particularly hypokalemia). Products include:
Depo-Medrol Injectable Suspension 2615
Depo-Medrol Single-Dose Vial 2617

Methylprednisolone Sodium Succinate (Corticosteroids intensify electrolyte depletion particularly hypokalemia).
No products indexed under this heading.

Metocurine Iodide (Possible increased responsiveness to muscle relaxant).
No products indexed under this heading.

Metolazone (Co-administration with other antihypertensive drugs may result in additive effect or potentiation).
No products indexed under this heading.

Metoprolol Succinate (Co-administration with other antihypertensive drugs may result in additive effect or potentiation). Products include:
Toprol-XL Tablets 660

Metoprolol Tartrate (Co-administration with other antihypertensive drugs may result in additive effect or potentiation).
No products indexed under this heading.

Metyrosine (Co-administration with other antihypertensive drugs may result in additive effect or potentiation). Products include:
Demser Capsules 1933

Mibefradil Dihydrochloride (Co-administration with other antihypertensive drugs may result in additive effect or potentiation).
No products indexed under this heading.

Miglitol (Hydrochlorothiazide produces hyperglycemia; dosage adjustment of the antidiabetic agent may be required).
No products indexed under this heading.

Minoxidil (Co-administration with other antihypertensive drugs may result in additive effect or potentiation). Products include:
Men's Rogaine Extra Strength Topical Solution, Ocean Rush Scent and Original Unscented .... ▣ 706
Women's Rogaine Topical Solution, Spring Bloom Scent and Original Unscented .... ▣ 707

Mivacurium Chloride (Possible increased responsiveness to muscle relaxant). Products include:
Mivacron Injection 489

Moexipril Hydrochloride (Co-administration increases the risk of hyperkalemia; potential for additive antihypertensive effect). Products include:
Uniretic Tablets 3114
Univasc Tablets 3118

Morphine Sulfate (Potentiation of orthostatic hypotension). Products include:
Avinza Capsules 1714
Kadian Capsules 572
MS Contin Tablets 2703

Nabumetone (Co-administration of non-steroidal anti-inflammatory agents can reduce the diuretic, natriuretic, and antihypertensive effects). Products include:
Relafen Tablets 1523

Nadolol (Co-administration with other antihypertensive drugs may result in additive effect or potentiation). Products include:
Nadolol Tablets 2121

Naproxen (Co-administration of non-steroidal anti-inflammatory agents can reduce the diuretic, natriuretic, and antihypertensive effects). Products include:
EC-Naprosyn Delayed-Release Tablets 2769
Naprosyn Suspension 2769
Naprosyn Tablets 2769
Prevacid NapraPAC 3277

Naproxen Sodium (Co-administration of non-steroidal anti-inflammatory agents can reduce the diuretic, natriuretic, and antihypertensive effects). Products include:
Aleve Tablets, Caplets and Gelcaps .... ▣ 605
Anaprox Tablets 2769
Anaprox DS Tablets 2769

Nicardipine Hydrochloride (Co-administration with other antihypertensive drugs may result in additive effect or potentiation). Products include:
Cardene I.V. 1129

Nifedipine (Co-administration with other antihypertensive drugs may result in additive effect or potentiation). Products include:
Adalat CC Tablets 2978

Nisoldipine (Co-administration with other antihypertensive drugs may result in additive effect or potentiation). Products include:
Sular Tablets 1163

Nitroglycerin (Co-administration with other antihypertensive drugs may result in additive effect or potentiation). Products include:
Nitro-Dur Transdermal Infusion System 3060
Nitrolingual Pumpspray 1161

Norepinephrine Bitartrate (Possible decreased response to pressor amines).
No products indexed under this heading.

Oxaprozin (Co-administration of non-steroidal anti-inflammatory agents can reduce the diuretic, natriuretic, and antihypertensive effects).
No products indexed under this heading.

Oxycodone Hydrochloride (Potentiation of orthostatic hypotension). Products include:
Combunox Tablets 1183
OxyContin Tablets 2699
OxyFast Oral Concentrate Solution 2704
OxyIR Capsules 2704
Percocet Tablets 1114
Percodan Tablets 1115

Pancuronium Bromide (Possible increased responsiveness to muscle relaxant).
No products indexed under this heading.

Penbutolol Sulfate (Co-administration with other antihypertensive drugs may result in additive effect or potentiation).
No products indexed under this heading.

Pentobarbital Sodium (Potentiation of orthostatic hypotension). Products include:
Nembutal Sodium Solution, USP 2484

Perindopril Erbumine (Co-administration increases the risk of hyperkalemia; potential for additive antihypertensive effect). Products include:
Aceon Tablets (2 mg, 4 mg, 8 mg) 3191

Phenobarbital (Potentiation of orthostatic hypotension).
No products indexed under this heading.

Phenoxybenzamine Hydrochloride (Co-administration with other antihypertensive drugs may result in additive effect or potentiation). Products include:
Dibenzyline Capsules 3390

Phentolamine Mesylate (Co-administration with other antihypertensive drugs may result in additive effect or potentiation).
No products indexed under this heading.

Phenylbutazone (Co-administration of non-steroidal anti-inflammatory agents can reduce the diuretic, natriuretic, and antihypertensive effects).
No products indexed under this heading.

Pindolol (Co-administration with other antihypertensive drugs may result in additive effect or potentiation).
No products indexed under this heading.

Pioglitazone Hydrochloride (Hydrochlorothiazide produces hyperglycemia; dosage adjustment of the antidiabetic agent may be required). Products include:
ActoPlus Met Tablets 3219
Actos Tablets 3224

Piroxicam (Co-administration of non-steroidal anti-inflammatory agents can reduce the diuretic, natriuretic, and antihypertensive effects).
No products indexed under this heading.

Polythiazide (Co-administration with other antihypertensive drugs may result in additive effect or potentiation).
No products indexed under this heading.

Potassium Acid Phosphate (Amiloride is associated with hyperkalemia; concurrent use with potassium supplements is contraindicated). Products include:
K-Phos Original (Sodium Free) Tablets 785

Potassium Bicarbonate (Amiloride is associated with hyperkalemia; concurrent use with potassium supplements is contraindicated).
No products indexed under this heading.

Potassium Chloride (Amiloride is associated with hyperkalemia; concurrent use with potassium supplements is contraindicated). Products include:
Colyte with Flavor Packs for Oral Solution 3102
HalfLytely and Bisacodyl Tablets Bowel Prep Kit with Flavors Packs 915
K-Dur Extended-Relase Tablets 3047
K-Lor Powder Packets 472
K-Tab Filmtab Tablets 473
TriLyte with Flavor Packs for Oral Solution 3114

Potassium Citrate (Amiloride is associated with hyperkalemia; concurrent use with potassium supplements is contraindicated). Products include:
Urocit-K Tablets 2109

Potassium Gluconate (Amiloride is associated with hyperkalemia; concurrent use with potassium supplements is contraindicated).
No products indexed under this heading.

Potassium Phosphate (Amiloride is associated with hyperkalemia; concurrent use with potassium supplements is contraindicated). Products include:
K-Phos Neutral Tablets 785

Prazosin Hydrochloride (Co-administration with other antihypertensive drugs may result in additive effect or potentiation).
No products indexed under this heading.

Prednisolone Acetate (Corticosteroids intensify electrolyte depletion particularly hypokalemia). Products include:
Blephamide Ophthalmic Ointment 563
Blephamide Ophthalmic Suspension 564
Poly-Pred Liquifilm Ophthalmic Suspension .... ⊙ 231
Pred Forte Ophthalmic Suspension .... ⊙ 233
Pred Mild Sterile Ophthalmic Suspension .... ⊙ 236
Pred-G Ophthalmic Suspension .... ⊙ 234
Pred-G Sterile Ophthalmic Ointment .... ⊙ 235

Prednisolone Sodium Phosphate (Corticosteroids intensify electrolyte depletion particularly hypokalemia). Products include:
Pediapred Oral Solution 3319

Prednisolone Tebutate (Corticosteroids intensify electrolyte depletion particularly hypokalemia).
No products indexed under this heading.

Prednisone (Corticosteroids intensify electrolyte depletion particularly hypokalemia).
No products indexed under this heading.

Propoxyphene Hydrochloride (Potentiation of orthostatic hypotension).
No products indexed under this heading.

Propoxyphene Napsylate (Potentiation of orthostatic hypotension). Products include:
Darvocet A 500 Tablets 3497

Propranolol Hydrochloride (Co-administration with other antihypertensive drugs may result in additive effect or potentiation). Products include:
Inderal LA Long-Acting Capsules 3421
InnoPran XL Capsules 2728

Quinapril Hydrochloride (Co-administration increases the risk of hyperkalemia; potential for additive antihypertensive effect).
No products indexed under this heading.

Ramipril (Co-administration increases the risk of hyperkalemia; potential for additive antihypertensive effect). Products include:
Altace Capsules 1673

Rapacuronium Bromide (Possible increased responsiveness to muscle relaxant).
No products indexed under this heading.

Rauwolfia Serpentina (Co-administration with other antihypertensive drugs may result in additive effect or potentiation).
No products indexed under this heading.

Remifentanil Hydrochloride (Potentiation of orthostatic hypotension).
No products indexed under this heading.

Repaglinide (Hydrochlorothiazide produces hyperglycemia; dosage adjustment of the antidiabetic agent may be required). Products include:
Prandin Tablets (0.5, 1, and 2 mg) 2337

Rescinnamine (Co-administration with other antihypertensive drugs may result in additive effect or potentiation).
No products indexed under this heading.

Reserpine (Co-administration with other antihypertensive drugs may result in additive effect or potentiation).
No products indexed under this heading.

Rocuronium Bromide (Possible increased responsiveness to muscle relaxant). Products include:
Zemuron Injection 2363

Rofecoxib (Co-administration of non-steroidal anti-inflammatory agents can reduce the diuretic, natriuretic, and antihypertensive effects).
No products indexed under this heading.

Rosiglitazone Maleate (Hydrochlorothiazide produces hyperglycemia; dosage adjustment of the antidiabetic agent may be required). Products include:
Avandamet Tablets 1343
Avandia Tablets 1348

Secobarbital Sodium (Potentiation of orthostatic hypotension).
No products indexed under this heading.

Sodium Nitroprusside (Co-administration with other antihypertensive drugs may result in additive effect or potentiation).
No products indexed under this heading.

Sotalol Hydrochloride (Co-administration with other antihypertensive drugs may result in additive effect or potentiation).
No products indexed under this heading.

Spirapril Hydrochloride (Co-administration increases the risk of hyperkalemia; potential for additive antihypertensive effect).
No products indexed under this heading.

Spironolactone (Amiloride is associated with hyperkalemia; concurrent use with potassium sparing diuretics is contraindicated).
No products indexed under this heading.

Sufentanil Citrate (Potentiation of orthostatic hypotension).
No products indexed under this heading.

Sulindac (Co-administration of non-steroidal anti-inflammatory agents can reduce the diuretic, natriuretic, and antihypertensive effects). Products include:
Clinoril Tablets 1899

Tacrolimus (Co-administration increases the risk of hyperkalemia). Products include:
Prograf Capsules and Injection 624
Protopic Ointment 629

Telmisartan (Co-administration increases the risk of hyperkalemia; potential for additive antihypertensive effect). Products include:
Micardis Tablets 884
Micardis HCT Tablets 886

Terazosin Hydrochloride (Co-administration with other antihypertensive drugs may result in additive effect or potentiation). Products include:
Hytrin Capsules 469

Thiamylal Sodium (Potentiation of orthostatic hypotension).
No products indexed under this heading.

Timolol Maleate (Co-administration with other antihypertensive drugs may result in additive effect or potentiation). Products include:
Blocadren Tablets 1891
Cosopt Sterile Ophthalmic Solution 1910
Timolide Tablets 2056
Timoptic in Ocudose 2061
Timoptic Sterile Ophthalmic Solution 2058
Timoptic-XE Sterile Ophthalmic Gel Forming Solution 2062

Tolazamide (Hydrochlorothiazide produces hyperglycemia; dosage adjustment of the antidiabetic agent may be required).
No products indexed under this heading.

Tolbutamide (Hydrochlorothiazide produces hyperglycemia; dosage adjustment of the antidiabetic agent may be required).
No products indexed under this heading.

Tolmetin Sodium (Co-administration of non-steroidal anti-inflammatory agents can reduce the diuretic, natriuretic, and antihypertensive effects).
No products indexed under this heading.

Torsemide (Co-administration with other antihypertensive drugs may result in additive effect or potentiation).
No products indexed under this heading.

Trandolapril (Co-administration increases the risk of hyperkalemia; potential for additive antihypertensive effect). Products include:
Mavik Tablets 482
Tarka Tablets 519

Triamcinolone (Corticosteroids intensify electrolyte depletion particularly hypokalemia).
No products indexed under this heading.

Triamcinolone Acetonide (Corticosteroids intensify electrolyte depletion particularly hypokalemia). Products include:
Azmacort Inhalation Aerosol 1701
Nasacort HFA Inhalation Aerosol 2939
Nasacort AQ Nasal Spray 2937

Triamcinolone Diacetate (Corticosteroids intensify electrolyte depletion particularly hypokalemia).
No products indexed under this heading.

Triamcinolone Hexacetonide (Corticosteroids intensify electrolyte depletion particularly hypokalemia).
No products indexed under this heading.

Triamterene (Amiloride is associated with hyperkalemia; concurrent use with potassium sparing diuretics is contraindicated). Products include:
Dyazide Capsules 1389
Dyrenium Capsules 3390
Maxzide 2150

Trimethaphan Camsylate (Co-administration with other antihypertensive drugs may result in additive effect or potentiation).
No products indexed under this heading.

Troglitazone (Hydrochlorothiazide produces hyperglycemia; dosage adjustment of the antidiabetic agent may be required).
No products indexed under this heading.

Tubocurarine Chloride (Possible increased responsiveness to the muscle relaxant).
No products indexed under this heading.

Valdecoxib (Co-administration of non-steroidal anti-inflammatory agents can reduce the diuretic, natriuretic, and antihypertensive effects).
No products indexed under this heading.

Valsartan (Co-administration increases the risk of hyperkalemia; potential for additive antihypertensive effect). Products include:
Diovan HCT Tablets 2195
Diovan Tablets 2191

Vecuronium Bromide (Possible increased responsiveness to muscle relaxant).
No products indexed under this heading.

Verapamil Hydrochloride (Co-administration with other antihypertensive drugs may result in additive effect or potentiation). Products include:
Covera-HS Tablets 3135
Tarka Tablets 519
Verelan PM Capsules 3120

Food Interactions

Alcohol (Potentiation of orthostatic hypotension).

Diet, potassium-rich (Potential for rapid increases in serum potassium levels).

CHILDREN'S MOTRIN ORAL SUSPENSION AND CHEWABLE TABLETS

(Ibuprofen) 1837
None cited in PDR database.

CHILDREN'S MOTRIN COLD NON-STAINING DYE-FREE ORAL SUSPENSION

(Ibuprofen, Pseudoephedrine Hydrochloride) 1838
None cited in PDR database.

CHILDREN'S MOTRIN COLD ORAL SUSPENSION

(Ibuprofen, Pseudoephedrine Hydrochloride) 648
May interact with monoamine oxidase inhibitors. Compounds in these categories include:

Isocarboxazid (Concurrent and/or sequential use with MAO inhibitors is not recommended).
No products indexed under this heading.

Moclobemide (Concurrent and/or sequential use with MAO inhibitors is not recommended).
No products indexed under this heading.

Pargyline Hydrochloride (Concurrent and/or sequential use with MAO inhibitors is not recommended).
No products indexed under this heading.

Phenelzine Sulfate (Concurrent and/or sequential use with MAO inhibitors is not recommended).
No products indexed under this heading.

Procarbazine Hydrochloride (Concurrent and/or sequential use with MAO inhibitors is not recommended). Products include:
Matulane Capsules 3188

Selegiline Hydrochloride (Concurrent and/or sequential use with MAO inhibitors is not recommended). Products include:
Eldepryl Capsules 3209

Tranylcypromine Sulfate (Concurrent and/or sequential use with MAO inhibitors is not recommended). Products include:
Parnate Tablets 1499

CHILDREN'S MOTRIN COLD NON-STAINING DYE-FREE ORAL SUSPENSION

(Ibuprofen, Pseudoephedrine Hydrochloride) 648
See Children's Motrin Cold Oral Suspension

CHILDREN'S MOTRIN COLD ORAL SUSPENSION

(Ibuprofen, Pseudoephedrine Hydrochloride) 1838
See Motrin Cold & Sinus Caplets

CHILDREN'S MOTRIN NON-STAINING DYE-FREE ORAL SUSPENSION

(Ibuprofen) 1837
See Children's Motrin Oral Suspension and Chewable Tablets

MOTRIN COLD & SINUS CAPLETS

(Ibuprofen, Pseudoephedrine Hydrochloride) 1836
May interact with monoamine oxidase inhibitors and certain other agents. Compounds in these categories include:

Isocarboxazid (Concurrent and/or sequential use with MAO inhibitors is not recommended).
No products indexed under this heading.

Moclobemide (Concurrent and/or sequential use with MAO inhibitors is not recommended).
No products indexed under this heading.

Pargyline Hydrochloride (Concurrent and/or sequential use with MAO inhibitors is not recommended).
No products indexed under this heading.

Phenelzine Sulfate (Concurrent and/or sequential use with MAO inhibitors is not recommended).
No products indexed under this heading.

Procarbazine Hydrochloride (Concurrent and/or sequential use with MAO inhibitors is not recommended). Products include:
Matulane Capsules 3188

Selegiline Hydrochloride (Concurrent and/or sequential use with MAO inhibitors is not recommended). Products include:
Eldepryl Capsules 3209

Tranylcypromine Sulfate (Concurrent and/or sequential use with MAO inhibitors is not recommended). Products include:
Parnate Tablets 1499

Food Interactions

Alcohol (Chronic heavy alcohol users, three or more drinks per day, should consult their physicians for advice on when and how they should take pain relievers/fever reducers including ibuprofen).

MOTRIN IB TABLETS AND CAPLETS

(Ibuprofen) 1836

May interact with aspirin-acetylsalicylic acid, anticoagulants, corticosteroids, non-steroidal anti-inflammatory agents, and certain other agents. Compounds in these categories include:

Anisindione (Increased risk of stomach bleeding if co-administered with anticoagulants). Products include:
Miradon Tablets 3056

Ardeparin Sodium (Increased risk of stomach bleeding if co-administered with anticoagulants).
No products indexed under this heading.

Aspirin (Increased risk of stomach bleeding if co-administered with non-steroidal anti-inflammatory drugs). Products include:
Aggrenox Capsules 855
Bayer, Aspirin Regimen .... ▣ 606
Bayer Aspirin Tablets 3515
BC Powder .... ▣ 612
BC Allergy Sinus Cold Powder .... ▣ 612
Arthritis Strength BC Powder .... ▣ 612
BC Sinus Cold Powder .... ▣ 612
Ecotrin Enteric Coated Aspirin Low, Regular and Maximum Strength Tablets 1627
Goody's Body Pain Formula Powder .... ▣ 621
Goody's Extra Strength Headache Powder .... ▣ 621
Goody's Extra Strength Pain Relief Tablets .... ▣ 621
Percodan Tablets 1115
St. Joseph 81 mg Aspirin Chewable and Enteric Coated Tablets 1841

Aspirin, Enteric Coated (Increased risk of stomach bleeding if co-administered with non-steroidal anti-inflammatory drugs).
No products indexed under this heading.

Aspirin Buffered (Increased risk of stomach bleeding if co-administered with non-steroidal anti-inflammatory drugs).
No products indexed under this heading.

Betamethasone Acetate (Increased risk of stomach bleeding if co-administered with steroidal drugs).
No products indexed under this heading.

Betamethasone Sodium Phosphate (Increased risk of stomach bleeding if co-administered with steroidal drugs).
No products indexed under this heading.

Celecoxib (Increased risk of stomach bleeding if co-administered with non-steroidal anti-inflammatory drugs). Products include:
Celebrex Capsules 3130

Cortisone Acetate (Increased risk of stomach bleeding if co-administered with steroidal drugs).
No products indexed under this heading.

Dalteparin Sodium (Increased risk of stomach bleeding if co-administered with anticoagulants). Products include:
Fragmin Injection 2638

Danaparoid Sodium (Increased risk of stomach bleeding if co-administered with anticoagulants).
No products indexed under this heading.

Dexamethasone (Increased risk of stomach bleeding if co-administered with steroidal drugs). Products include:
Ciprodex Otic Suspension 555
Decadron Tablets 1929
TobraDex Ophthalmic Ointment 558
TobraDex Ophthalmic Suspension 558

Dexamethasone Acetate (Increased risk of stomach bleeding if co-administered with steroidal drugs).
No products indexed under this heading.

Dexamethasone Sodium Phosphate (Increased risk of stomach bleeding if co-administered with steroidal drugs). Products include:
Decadron Phosphate Injection 1931

Diclofenac Potassium (Increased risk of stomach bleeding if co-administered with non-steroidal anti-inflammatory drugs). Products include:
Cataflam Tablets 2173

Diclofenac Sodium (Increased risk of stomach bleeding if co-administered with non-steroidal anti-inflammatory drugs). Products include:
Arthrotec Tablets 3126
Voltaren Ophthalmic Solution 2300
Voltaren Tablets 2298
Voltaren-XR Tablets 2301

Dicumarol (Increased risk of stomach bleeding if co-administered with anticoagulants).
No products indexed under this heading.

Enoxaparin Sodium (Increased risk of stomach bleeding if co-administered with anticoagulants). Products include:
Lovenox Injection 2931

Etodolac (Increased risk of stomach bleeding if co-administered with non-steroidal anti-inflammatory drugs).
No products indexed under this heading.

Fenoprofen Calcium (Increased risk of stomach bleeding if co-administered with non-steroidal anti-inflammatory drugs). Products include:
Nalfon Capsules 2504

Fludrocortisone Acetate (Increased risk of stomach bleeding if co-administered with steroidal drugs).
No products indexed under this heading.

Flurbiprofen (Increased risk of stomach bleeding if co-administered with non-steroidal anti-inflammatory drugs).
No products indexed under this heading.

Fondaparinux Sodium (Increased risk of stomach bleeding if co-administered with anticoagulants). Products include:
Arixtra Injection 1325

Heparin Calcium (Increased risk of stomach bleeding if co-administered with anticoagulants).
No products indexed under this heading.

Heparin Sodium (Increased risk of stomach bleeding if co-administered with anticoagulants).
No products indexed under this heading.

Hydrocortisone (Increased risk of stomach bleeding if co-administered with steroidal drugs). Products include:
Cortizone•5 Ointment .... ▣ 699
Cortizone•10 Creme .... ▣ 699
Cortizone•10 Ointment .... ▣ 699
Cortizone•10 Plus Creme .... ▣ 700
Cortizone•10 Maximum Strength Quick Shot Spray .... ▣ 700
Hydrocortone Tablets 1963
Preparation H Hydrocortisone Cream .... ▣ 748

Hydrocortisone Acetate (Increased risk of stomach bleeding if co-administered with steroidal drugs). Products include:
Analpram-HC 1136
Pramosone 1139
ProctoFoam-HC 3113
Tucks Anti-Itch Ointment .... ▣ 712
U-cort 1% Cream 3289

Hydrocortisone Sodium Phosphate (Increased risk of stomach bleeding if co-administered with steroidal drugs).
No products indexed under this heading.

Hydrocortisone Sodium Succinate (Increased risk of stomach bleeding if co-administered with steroidal drugs).
No products indexed under this heading.

Indomethacin (Increased risk of stomach bleeding if co-administered with non-steroidal anti-inflammatory drugs). Products include:
Indocin 1968

Indomethacin Sodium Trihydrate (Increased risk of stomach bleeding if co-administered with non-steroidal anti-inflammatory drugs). Products include:
Indocin I.V. 1973

Ketoprofen (Increased risk of stomach bleeding if co-administered with non-steroidal anti-inflammatory drugs).
No products indexed under this heading.

Ketorolac Tromethamine (Increased risk of stomach bleeding if co-administered with non-steroidal anti-inflammatory drugs). Products include:
Acular Ophthalmic Solution 561
Acular LS Ophthalmic Solution 562

Low Molecular Weight Heparins (Increased risk of stomach bleeding if co-administered with anticoagulants).
No products indexed under this heading.

Meclofenamate Sodium (Increased risk of stomach bleeding if co-administered with non-steroidal anti-inflammatory drugs).
No products indexed under this heading.

Mefenamic Acid (Increased risk of stomach bleeding if co-administered with non-steroidal anti-inflammatory drugs).
No products indexed under this heading.

Meloxicam (Increased risk of stomach bleeding if co-administered with non-steroidal anti-inflammatory drugs). Products include:
Mobic Oral Suspension 893
Mobic Tablets 893

Methylprednisolone Acetate (Increased risk of stomach bleeding if co-administered with steroidal drugs). Products include:
Depo-Medrol Injectable Suspension 2615
Depo-Medrol Single-Dose Vial 2617

Methylprednisolone Sodium Succinate (Increased risk of stomach bleeding if co-administered with steroidal drugs).
No products indexed under this heading.

Nabumetone (Increased risk of stomach bleeding if co-administered with non-steroidal anti-inflammatory drugs). Products include:
Relafen Tablets 1523

Naproxen (Increased risk of stomach bleeding if co-administered with non-steroidal anti-inflammatory drugs). Products include:
EC-Naprosyn Delayed-Release Tablets 2769
Naprosyn Suspension 2769
Naprosyn Tablets 2769
Prevacid NapraPAC 3277

Naproxen Sodium (Increased risk of stomach bleeding if co-administered with non-steroidal anti-inflammatory drugs). Products include:
Aleve Tablets, Caplets and Gelcaps .... ▣ 605
Anaprox Tablets 2769
Anaprox DS Tablets 2769

Oxaprozin (Increased risk of stomach bleeding if co-administered with non-steroidal anti-inflammatory drugs).
No products indexed under this heading.

Phenylbutazone (Increased risk of stomach bleeding if co-administered with non-steroidal anti-inflammatory drugs).
No products indexed under this heading.

Piroxicam (Increased risk of stomach bleeding if co-administered with non-steroidal anti-inflammatory drugs).
No products indexed under this heading.

Prednisolone Acetate (Increased risk of stomach bleeding if co-administered with steroidal drugs). Products include:
Blephamide Ophthalmic Ointment 563
Blephamide Ophthalmic Suspension 564

Poly-Pred Liquifilm Ophthalmic Suspension ⊙231
Pred Forte Ophthalmic Suspension ⊙233
Pred Mild Sterile Ophthalmic Suspension ⊙236
Pred-G Ophthalmic Suspension ⊙234
Pred-G Sterile Ophthalmic Ointment ⊙235

Prednisolone Sodium Phosphate (Increased risk of stomach bleeding if co-administered with steroidal drugs). Products include:
Pediapred Oral Solution 3319

Prednisolone Tebutate (Increased risk of stomach bleeding if co-administered with steroidal drugs).
No products indexed under this heading.

Prednisone (Increased risk of stomach bleeding if co-administered with steroidal drugs).
No products indexed under this heading.

Rofecoxib (Increased risk of stomach bleeding if co-administered with non-steroidal anti-inflammatory drugs).
No products indexed under this heading.

Sulindac (Increased risk of stomach bleeding if co-administered with non-steroidal anti-inflammatory drugs). Products include:
Clinoril Tablets 1899

Tinzaparin Sodium (Increased risk of stomach bleeding if co-administered with anticoagulants).
No products indexed under this heading.

Tolmetin Sodium (Increased risk of stomach bleeding if co-administered with non-steroidal anti-inflammatory drugs).
No products indexed under this heading.

Triamcinolone (Increased risk of stomach bleeding if co-administered with steroidal drugs).
No products indexed under this heading.

Triamcinolone Acetonide (Increased risk of stomach bleeding if co-administered with steroidal drugs). Products include:
Azmacort Inhalation Aerosol 1701
Nasacort HFA Inhalation Aerosol 2939
Nasacort AQ Nasal Spray 2937

Triamcinolone Diacetate (Increased risk of stomach bleeding if co-administered with steroidal drugs).
No products indexed under this heading.

Triamcinolone Hexacetonide (Increased risk of stomach bleeding if co-administered with steroidal drugs).
No products indexed under this heading.

Valdecoxib (Increased risk of stomach bleeding if co-administered with non-steroidal anti-inflammatory drugs).
No products indexed under this heading.

Warfarin Sodium (Increased risk of stomach bleeding if co-administered with anticoagulants). Products include:
Coumadin for Injection 932
Coumadin Tablets 932

INFANTS' MOTRIN CONCENTRATED DROPS

(Ibuprofen) 1837
None cited in PDR database.

INFANTS' MOTRIN NON-STAINING DYE-FREE DROPS

(Ibuprofen) 1837
None cited in PDR database.

JUNIOR STRENGTH MOTRIN CAPLETS AND CHEWABLE TABLETS

(Ibuprofen) 1837
None cited in PDR database.

MS CONTIN TABLETS

(Morphine Sulfate) 2703
May interact with central nervous system depressants, general anesthetics, hypnotics and sedatives, mixed agonist/antagonist opioid analgesics, neuromuscular blocking agents, phenothiazines, tranquilizers, and certain other agents. Compounds in these categories include:

Alfentanil Hydrochloride (Profound sedation, coma, severe hypotension, respiratory depression).
No products indexed under this heading.

Alprazolam (Profound sedation, coma, severe hypotension, respiratory depression). Products include:
Niravam Orally Disintegrating Tablets 3106
Xanax XR Tablets 2655

Aprobarbital (Profound sedation, coma, severe hypotension, respiratory depression).
No products indexed under this heading.

Atracurium Besylate (Increased respiratory depression).
No products indexed under this heading.

Buprenorphine Hydrochloride (Mixed agonist/antagonist analgesics may reduce the analgesic effect or may precipitate withdrawal symptoms). Products include:
Buprenex Injectable 2718
Suboxone Tablets 2719
Subutex Tablets 2719

Buspirone Hydrochloride (Profound sedation, coma, severe hypotension, respiratory depression).
No products indexed under this heading.

Butabarbital (Profound sedation, coma, severe hypotension, respiratory depression).
No products indexed under this heading.

Butalbital (Profound sedation, coma, severe hypotension, respiratory depression). Products include:
Sedapap Tablets 50 mg/650 mg 2098

Butorphanol Tartrate (Mixed agonist/antagonist analgesics may reduce the analgesic effect or may precipitate withdrawal symptoms).
No products indexed under this heading.

Chlordiazepoxide (Profound sedation, coma, severe hypotension, respiratory depression).
No products indexed under this heading.

Chlordiazepoxide Hydrochloride (Profound sedation, coma, severe hypotension, respiratory depression). Products include:
Librium Capsules 3349

Chlorpromazine (Profound sedation, coma, severe hypotension, respiratory depression).
No products indexed under this heading.

Chlorpromazine Hydrochloride (Profound sedation, coma, severe hypotension, respiratory depression).
No products indexed under this heading.

Chlorprothixene (Profound sedation, coma, severe hypotension, respiratory depression).
No products indexed under this heading.

Chlorprothixene Hydrochloride (Profound sedation, coma, severe hypotension, respiratory depression).
No products indexed under this heading.

Chlorprothixene Lactate (Profound sedation, coma, severe hypotension, respiratory depression).
No products indexed under this heading.

Cisatracurium Besylate (Increased respiratory depression). Products include:
Nimbex Injection 494

Clorazepate Dipotassium (Profound sedation, coma, severe hypotension, respiratory depression). Products include:
Tranxene 2488

Clozapine (Profound sedation, coma, severe hypotension, respiratory depression). Products include:
Clozapine Tablets 2141
Clozaril Tablets 2174
FazaClo Orally Disintegrating Tablets 547

Codeine Phosphate (Profound sedation, coma, severe hypotension, respiratory depression). Products include:
Tylenol with Codeine 2461

Desflurane (Profound sedation, coma, severe hypotension, respiratory depression). Products include:
Suprane Liquid for Inhalation 770

Dezocine (Profound sedation, coma, severe hypotension, respiratory depression).
No products indexed under this heading.

Diazepam (Profound sedation, coma, severe hypotension, respiratory depression). Products include:
Diastat Rectal Delivery System 3344
Valium Tablets 2822

Doxacurium Chloride (Increased respiratory depression).
No products indexed under this heading.

Droperidol (Profound sedation, coma, severe hypotension, respiratory depression).
No products indexed under this heading.

Enflurane (Profound sedation, coma, severe hypotension, respiratory depression).
No products indexed under this heading.

Estazolam (Profound sedation, coma, severe hypotension, respiratory depression). Products include:
ProSom Tablets 512

Ethanol (Profound sedation, coma, severe hypotension, respiratory depression).
No products indexed under this heading.

Ethchlorvynol (Profound sedation, coma, severe hypotension, respiratory depression).
No products indexed under this heading.

Ethinamate (Profound sedation, coma, severe hypotension, respiratory depression).
No products indexed under this heading.

Ethyl Alcohol (Profound sedation, coma, severe hypotension, respiratory depression).
No products indexed under this heading.

Fentanyl (Profound sedation, coma, severe hypotension, respiratory depression). Products include:
Duragesic Transdermal System 2448

Fentanyl Citrate (Profound sedation, coma, severe hypotension, respiratory depression). Products include:
Actiq 993

Fluphenazine Decanoate (Profound sedation, coma, severe hypotension, respiratory depression).
No products indexed under this heading.

Fluphenazine Enanthate (Profound sedation, coma, severe hypotension, respiratory depression).
No products indexed under this heading.

Fluphenazine Hydrochloride (Profound sedation, coma, severe hypotension, respiratory depression).
No products indexed under this heading.

Flurazepam Hydrochloride (Profound sedation, coma, severe hypotension, respiratory depression). Products include:
Dalmane Capsules 3343

Glutethimide (Profound sedation, coma, severe hypotension, respiratory depression).
No products indexed under this heading.

Haloperidol (Profound sedation, coma, severe hypotension, respiratory depression).
No products indexed under this heading.

Haloperidol Decanoate (Profound sedation, coma, severe hypotension, respiratory depression).
No products indexed under this heading.

Hydrocodone Bitartrate (Profound sedation, coma, severe hypotension, respiratory depression). Products include:
Hycodan 1104
Hycomine Compound Tablets 1105
Hycotuss Expectorant Syrup 1106
Lortab 3315
Lortab Elixir 3312
Vicodin Tablets 530
Vicodin ES Tablets 531
Vicodin HP Tablets 532
Vicoprofen Tablets 533
Zydone Tablets 1118

Hydrocodone Polistirex (Profound sedation, coma, severe hypotension, respiratory depression). Products include:
Tussionex Pennkinetic Extended-Release Suspension 3322

Hydromorphone Hydrochloride (Profound sedation, coma, severe hypotension, respiratory depression). Products include:
Dilaudid 439
Dilaudid Oral Liquid 443
Dilaudid Non-Sterile Powder 439
Dilaudid Rectal Suppositories 439
Dilaudid Tablets 439
Dilaudid Tablets - 8 mg 443
Dilaudid-HP 441

Hydroxyzine Hydrochloride (Profound sedation, coma, severe hypotension, respiratory depression).
No products indexed under this heading.

Isoflurane (Profound sedation, coma, severe hypotension, respiratory depression).
No products indexed under this heading.

Ketamine Hydrochloride (Profound sedation, coma, severe hypotension, respiratory depression).
No products indexed under this heading.

Levomethadyl Acetate Hydrochloride (Profound sedation, coma, severe hypotension, respiratory depression).
No products indexed under this heading.

Levorphanol Tartrate (Profound sedation, coma, severe hypotension, respiratory depression).
No products indexed under this heading.

Lorazepam (Profound sedation, coma, severe hypotension, respiratory depression).
No products indexed under this heading.

Loxapine Hydrochloride (Profound sedation, coma, severe hypotension, respiratory depression).
No products indexed under this heading.

Loxapine Succinate (Profound sedation, coma, severe hypotension, respiratory depression).
No products indexed under this heading.

Meperidine Hydrochloride (Profound sedation, coma, severe hypotension, respiratory depression).
No products indexed under this heading.

Mephobarbital (Profound sedation, coma, severe hypotension, respiratory depression). Products include:
Mebaral Tablets, USP 2483

Meprobamate (Profound sedation, coma, severe hypotension, respiratory depression).
No products indexed under this heading.

Mesoridazine Besylate (Profound sedation, coma, severe hypotension, respiratory depression).
No products indexed under this heading.

Methadone Hydrochloride (Profound sedation, coma, severe hypotension, respiratory depression).
No products indexed under this heading.

Methohexital Sodium (Profound sedation, coma, severe hypotension, respiratory depression).
No products indexed under this heading.

Methotrimeprazine (Profound sedation, coma, severe hypotension, respiratory depression).
No products indexed under this heading.

Methoxyflurane (Profound sedation, coma, severe hypotension, respiratory depression).
No products indexed under this heading.

Metocurine Iodide (Increased respiratory depression).
No products indexed under this heading.

Midazolam Hydrochloride (Profound sedation, coma, severe hypotension, respiratory depression).
No products indexed under this heading.

Mivacurium Chloride (Increased respiratory depression). Products include:
Mivacron Injection 489

Molindone Hydrochloride (Profound sedation, coma, severe hypotension, respiratory depression). Products include:
Moban Tablets 1108

Nalbuphine Hydrochloride (Mixed agonist/antagonist analgesics may reduce the analgesic effect or may precipitate withdrawal symptoms). Products include:
Nubain Injection 1111

Olanzapine (Profound sedation, coma, severe hypotension, respiratory depression). Products include:
Symbyax Capsules 1788
Zyprexa Tablets 1798
Zyprexa IntraMuscular 1798
Zyprexa ZYDIS Orally Disintegrating Tablets.................. 1798

Oxazepam (Profound sedation, coma, severe hypotension, respiratory depression).
No products indexed under this heading.

Oxycodone Hydrochloride (Profound sedation, coma, severe hypotension, respiratory depression). Products include:
Combunox Tablets 1183
OxyContin Tablets 2699
OxyFast Oral Concentrate Solution 2704
OxyIR Capsules 2704
Percocet Tablets 1114
Percodan Tablets 1115

Pancuronium Bromide (Increased respiratory depression).
No products indexed under this heading.

Pentazocine Hydrochloride (Mixed agonist/antagonist analgesics may reduce the analgesic effect or may precipitate withdrawal symptoms).
No products indexed under this heading.

Pentazocine Lactate (Mixed agonist/antagonist analgesics may reduce the analgesic effect or may precipitate withdrawal symptoms).
No products indexed under this heading.

Pentobarbital Sodium (Profound sedation, coma, severe hypotension, respiratory depression). Products include:
Nembutal Sodium Solution, USP 2484

Perphenazine (Profound sedation, coma, severe hypotension, respiratory depression).
No products indexed under this heading.

Phenobarbital (Profound sedation, coma, severe hypotension, respiratory depression).
No products indexed under this heading.

Prazepam (Profound sedation, coma, severe hypotension, respiratory depression).
No products indexed under this heading.

Prochlorperazine (Profound sedation, coma, severe hypotension, respiratory depression).
No products indexed under this heading.

Promethazine Hydrochloride (Profound sedation, coma, severe hypotension, respiratory depression). Products include:
Phenergan 3438

Propofol (Profound sedation, coma, severe hypotension, respiratory depression). Products include:
Diprivan Injectable Emulsion 676

Propoxyphene Hydrochloride (Profound sedation, coma, severe hypotension, respiratory depression).
No products indexed under this heading.

Propoxyphene Napsylate (Profound sedation, coma, severe hypotension, respiratory depression). Products include:
Darvocet A 500 Tablets 3497

Quazepam (Profound sedation, coma, severe hypotension, respiratory depression).
No products indexed under this heading.

Quetiapine Fumarate (Profound sedation, coma, severe hypotension, respiratory depression). Products include:
Seroquel Tablets 691

Rapacuronium Bromide (Increased respiratory depression).
No products indexed under this heading.

Remifentanil Hydrochloride (Profound sedation, coma, severe hypotension, respiratory depression).
No products indexed under this heading.

Risperidone (Profound sedation, coma, severe hypotension, respiratory depression). Products include:
Risperdal Consta Long-Acting Injection 1664
Risperdal M-Tab Orally Disintegrating Tablets..................... 1658
Risperdal 1658

Rocuronium Bromide (Increased respiratory depression). Products include:
Zemuron Injection 2363

Secobarbital Sodium (Profound sedation, coma, severe hypotension, respiratory depression).
No products indexed under this heading.

Sevoflurane (Profound sedation, coma, severe hypotension, respiratory depression). Products include:
Ultane Liquid for Inhalation 526

Sodium Oxybate (Profound sedation, coma, severe hypotension, respiratory depression).
No products indexed under this heading.

Succinylcholine Chloride (Increased respiratory depression).
No products indexed under this heading.

Sufentanil Citrate (Profound sedation, coma, severe hypotension, respiratory depression).
No products indexed under this heading.

Temazepam (Profound sedation, coma, severe hypotension, respiratory depression).
No products indexed under this heading.

Thiamylal Sodium (Profound sedation, coma, severe hypotension, respiratory depression).
No products indexed under this heading.

Thioridazine Hydrochloride (Profound sedation, coma, severe hypotension, respiratory depression). Products include:
Thioridazine Hydrochloride Tablets 2122

Thiothixene (Profound sedation, coma, severe hypotension, respiratory depression). Products include:
Thiothixene Capsules 2124

Triazolam (Profound sedation, coma, severe hypotension, respiratory depression).
No products indexed under this heading.

Trifluoperazine Hydrochloride (Profound sedation, coma, severe hypotension, respiratory depression).
No products indexed under this heading.

Vecuronium Bromide (Increased respiratory depression).
No products indexed under this heading.

Zaleplon (Profound sedation, coma, severe hypotension, respiratory depression). Products include:
Sonata Capsules 1686

Ziprasidone Hydrochloride (Profound sedation, coma, severe hypotension, respiratory depression). Products include:
Geodon Capsules 2514

Zolpidem Tartrate (Profound sedation, coma, severe hypotension, respiratory depression). Products include:
Ambien Tablets 2867

Food Interactions

Alcohol (Respiratory depression, hypotension and profound sedation or coma may result).

MUCINEX 600MG EXTENDED-RELEASE TABLETS

(Guaifenesin) .... ▣602
None cited in PDR database.

MUCINEX DM TABLETS

(Dextromethorphan Hydrobromide, Guaifenesin)............... ▣602
May interact with monoamine oxidase inhibitors. Compounds in these categories include:

Isocarboxazid (Avoid use with, or for two weeks after stopping, MAOI drugs).
No products indexed under this heading.

Moclobemide (Avoid use with, or for two weeks after stopping, MAOI drugs).
No products indexed under this heading.

Pargyline Hydrochloride (Avoid use with, or for two weeks after stopping, MAOI drugs).
No products indexed under this heading.

Phenelzine Sulfate (Avoid use with, or for two weeks after stopping, MAOI drugs).
No products indexed under this heading.

Procarbazine Hydrochloride (Avoid use with, or for two weeks after stopping, MAOI drugs). Products include:
Matulane Capsules 3188

Selegiline Hydrochloride (Avoid use with, or for two weeks after stopping, MAOI drugs). Products include:

Eldepryl Capsules 3209

Tranylcypromine Sulfate (Avoid use with, or for two weeks after stopping, MAOI drugs). Products include:
Parnate Tablets 1499

MUMPSVAX
(Mumps Virus Vaccine, Live) 2005
May interact with immunosuppressive agents. Compounds in these categories include:

Azathioprine (Concurrent immunosuppressive therapy is contraindicated). Products include:
Azasan Tablets 2844

Basiliximab (Concurrent immunosuppressive therapy is contraindicated). Products include:
Simulect for Injection 2268

Cyclosporine (Concurrent immunosuppressive therapy is contraindicated). Products include:
Gengraf Capsules 458
Neoral Soft Gelatin Capsules 2247
Neoral Oral Solution 2247
Restasis Ophthalmic Emulsion 570
Sandimmune 2259

Muromonab-CD3 (Concurrent immunosuppressive therapy is contraindicated). Products include:
Orthoclone OKT3 Sterile Solution 2370

Mycophenolate Mofetil (Concurrent immunosuppressive therapy is contraindicated). Products include:
CellCept Capsules 2751
CellCept Oral Suspension 2751
CellCept Tablets 2751

Sirolimus (Concurrent immunosuppressive therapy is contraindicated). Products include:
Rapamune Oral Solution and Tablets 3472

Tacrolimus (Concurrent immunosuppressive therapy is contraindicated). Products include:
Prograf Capsules and Injection 624
Protopic Ointment 629

MURO 128 OPHTHALMIC OINTMENT
(Sodium Chloride) .... ⊙251
None cited in PDR database.

MURO 128 OPHTHALMIC SOLUTION 2% AND 5%
(Sodium Chloride) .... ⊙251
None cited in PDR database.

MUSTARGEN FOR INJECTION
(Mechlorethamine Hydrochloride) 2007
May interact with antineoplastics. Compounds in these categories include:

Altretamine (Hematopoiesis may be further compromised in patients who have been previously treated with chemotherapeutic agents). Products include:
Hexalen Capsules 2101

Anastrozole (Hematopoiesis may be further compromised in patients who have been previously treated with chemotherapeutic agents). Products include:
Arimidex Tablets 665

Asparaginase (Hematopoiesis may be further compromised in patients who have been previously treated with chemotherapeutic agents). Products include:
Elspar for Injection 1943

Bicalutamide (Hematopoiesis may be further compromised in patients who have been previously treated with chemotherapeutic agents). Products include:
Casodex Tablets 670

Bleomycin Sulfate (Hematopoiesis may be further compromised in patients who have been previously treated with chemotherapeutic agents).
No products indexed under this heading.

Busulfan (Hematopoiesis may be further compromised in patients who have been previously treated with chemotherapeutic agents). Products include:
I.V. Busulfex 1125
Myleran Tablets 1492

Carboplatin (Hematopoiesis may be further compromised in patients who have been previously treated with chemotherapeutic agents).
No products indexed under this heading.

Carmustine (BCNU) (Hematopoiesis may be further compromised in patients who have been previously treated with chemotherapeutic agents).
No products indexed under this heading.

Chlorambucil (Hematopoiesis may be further compromised in patients who have been previously treated with chemotherapeutic agents). Products include:
Leukeran Tablets 1472

Cisplatin (Hematopoiesis may be further compromised in patients who have been previously treated with chemotherapeutic agents).
No products indexed under this heading.

Cyclophosphamide (Hematopoiesis may be further compromised in patients who have been previously treated with chemotherapeutic agents).
No products indexed under this heading.

Dacarbazine (Hematopoiesis may be further compromised in patients who have been previously treated with chemotherapeutic agents).
No products indexed under this heading.

Daunorubicin Citrate (Hematopoiesis may be further compromised in patients who have been previously treated with chemotherapeutic agents).
No products indexed under this heading.

Daunorubicin Hydrochloride (Hematopoiesis may be further compromised in patients who have been previously treated with chemotherapeutic agents). Products include:
Cerubidine for Injection 788

Denileukin Diftitox (Hematopoiesis may be further compromised in patients who have been previously treated with chemotherapeutic agents). Products include:
Ontak Vials 1717

Docetaxel (Hematopoiesis may be further compromised in patients who have been previously treated with chemotherapeutic agents). Products include:
Taxotere Injection Concentrate 2947

Doxorubicin Hydrochloride (Hematopoiesis may be further compromised in patients who have been previously treated with chemotherapeutic agents). Products include:
Adriamycin for Injection, USP 786
Adriamycin Injection, USP 786

Epirubicin Hydrochloride (Hematopoiesis may be further compromised in patients who have been previously treated with chemotherapeutic agents). Products include:
Ellence Injection 2632

Estramustine Phosphate Sodium (Hematopoiesis may be further compromised in patients who have been previously treated with chemotherapeutic agents). Products include:
Emcyt Capsules 3137

Etoposide (Hematopoiesis may be further compromised in patients who have been previously treated with chemotherapeutic agents).
No products indexed under this heading.

Exemestane (Hematopoiesis may be further compromised in patients who have been previously treated with chemotherapeutic agents). Products include:
Aromasin Tablets 2600

Floxuridine (Hematopoiesis may be further compromised in patients who have been previously treated with chemotherapeutic agents).
No products indexed under this heading.

Fluorouracil (Hematopoiesis may be further compromised in patients who have been previously treated with chemotherapeutic agents). Products include:
Carac Cream, 0.5% 1048
Efudex 3348

Flutamide (Hematopoiesis may be further compromised in patients who have been previously treated with chemotherapeutic agents). Products include:
Eulexin Capsules 3023

Gemcitabine Hydrochloride (Hematopoiesis may be further compromised in patients who have been previously treated with chemotherapeutic agents). Products include:
Gemzar for Injection 1743

Hydroxyurea (Hematopoiesis may be further compromised in patients who have been previously treated with chemotherapeutic agents).
No products indexed under this heading.

Idarubicin Hydrochloride (Hematopoiesis may be further compromised in patients who have been previously treated with chemotherapeutic agents). Products include:
Idamycin PFS Injection 2645

Ifosfamide (Hematopoiesis may be further compromised in patients who have been previously treated with chemotherapeutic agents).
No products indexed under this heading.

Interferon alfa-2a, Recombinant (Hematopoiesis may be further compromised in patients who have been previously treated with chemotherapeutic agents). Products include:
Roferon-A Injection 2805

Interferon alfa-2b, Recombinant (Hematopoiesis may be further compromised in patients who have been previously treated with chemotherapeutic agents). Products include:
Intron A for Injection 3038
Rebetron Combination Therapy 3078

Irinotecan Hydrochloride (Hematopoiesis may be further compromised in patients who have been previously treated with chemotherapeutic agents). Products include:
Camptosar Injection 2602

Levamisole Hydrochloride (Hematopoiesis may be further compromised in patients who have been previously treated with chemotherapeutic agents).
No products indexed under this heading.

Lomustine (CCNU) (Hematopoiesis may be further compromised in patients who have been previously treated with chemotherapeutic agents).
No products indexed under this heading.

Megestrol Acetate (Hematopoiesis may be further compromised in patients who have been previously treated with chemotherapeutic agents). Products include:
Megace ES Oral Suspension 2492

Melphalan (Hematopoiesis may be further compromised in patients who have been previously treated with chemotherapeutic agents). Products include:
Alkeran Tablets 977

Mercaptopurine (Hematopoiesis may be further compromised in patients who have been previously treated with chemotherapeutic agents). Products include:
Purinethol Tablets 1222

Methotrexate Sodium (Hematopoiesis may be further compromised in patients who have been previously treated with chemotherapeutic agents).
No products indexed under this heading.

Mitomycin (Mitomycin-C) (Hematopoiesis may be further compromised in patients who have been previously treated with chemotherapeutic agents).
No products indexed under this heading.

Mitotane (Hematopoiesis may be further compromised in patients who have been previously treated with chemotherapeutic agents).
No products indexed under this heading.

Mitoxantrone Hydrochloride (Hematopoiesis may be further compromised in patients who have been previously treated with chemotherapeutic agents). Products include:
Novantrone for Injection Concentrate 3158

Paclitaxel (Hematopoiesis may be further compromised in patients who have been previously treated with chemotherapeutic agents).
No products indexed under this heading.

Procarbazine Hydrochloride (Hematopoiesis may be further compromised in patients who have been previously treated with chemotherapeutic agents). Products include:
Matulane Capsules 3188

Streptozocin (Hematopoiesis may be further compromised in patients who have been previously treated with chemotherapeutic agents).
No products indexed under this heading.

Tamoxifen Citrate (Hematopoiesis may be further compromised in patients who have been previously treated with chemotherapeutic agents).
No products indexed under this heading.

Teniposide (Hematopoiesis may be further compromised in patients who have been previously treated with chemotherapeutic agents).
No products indexed under this heading.

Thioguanine (Hematopoiesis may be further compromised in patients who have been previously treated with chemotherapeutic agents). Products include:
Tabloid Tablets 1545

Thiotepa (Hematopoiesis may be further compromised in patients who have been previously treated with chemotherapeutic agents).
No products indexed under this heading.

Topotecan Hydrochloride (Hematopoiesis may be further compromised in patients who have been previously treated with chemotherapeutic agents). Products include:
Hycamtin for Injection 1427

Toremifene Citrate (Hematopoiesis may be further compromised in patients who have been previously treated with chemotherapeutic agents).
No products indexed under this heading.

Valrubicin (Hematopoiesis may be further compromised in patients who have been previously treated with chemotherapeutic agents).
No products indexed under this heading.

Vincristine Sulfate (Hematopoiesis may be further compromised in patients who have been previously treated with chemotherapeutic agents).
No products indexed under this heading.

Vinorelbine Tartrate (Hematopoiesis may be further compromised in patients who have been previously treated with chemotherapeutic agents). Products include:
Navelbine Injection 1494

MYCAMINE FOR INJECTION

(Micafungin Sodium) 620
May interact with:

Nifedipine (Nifedipine AUC and Cmax were increased by 18% and 42% respectively, in the presence of steady state micafungin sodium compared with nifedipine alone. Patients receiving nifedipine in combination with micafungin sodium should be monitored for nifedipine toxicity and nifedipine dosage should be reduced if necessary). Products include:
Adalat CC Tablets 2978

Sirolimus (Sirolimus AUC and Cmax were increased by 18% and 42% respectively, in the presence of steady state micafungin sodium compared with Sirolimus alone. Patients receiving Sirolimus in combination with micafungin sodium should be monitored for Sirolimus toxicity and Sirolimus dosage should be reduced if necessary). Products include:
Rapamune Oral Solution and Tablets 3472

MYFORTIC TABLETS

(Mycophenolic Acid) 2244
May interact with antacids, bacteriostatic antibiotics, bile acid sequestering agents, oral contraceptives, vaccines, live, and certain other agents. Compounds in these categories include:

Acyclovir (May be taken with mycophenolic acid; however, during the period of treatment, physicians should monitor blood cell counts. Both acyclovir and MPAG concentrations are increased in the presence of renal impairment; their coexistence may compete for tubular secretion and further increase in the concentrations of the two). Products include:
Zovirax 1616
Zovirax Cream 853
Zovirax Ointment 854

Acyclovir Sodium (May be taken with mycophenolic acid; however, during the period of treatment, physicians should monitor blood cell counts. Both acyclovir and MPAG concentrations are increased in the presence of renal impairment; their coexistence may compete for tubular secretion and further increase in the concentrations of the two). Products include:
Zovirax for Injection 1618

Aluminum Carbonate (Absorption of a single dose of mycophenolic acid was decreased when administered to stable renal transplant patients also taking magnesium-aluminum containing antacids. Concurrent use with antacids is not recommended).
No products indexed under this heading.

Aluminum Hydroxide (Absorption of a single dose of mycophenolic acid was decreased when administered to stable renal transplant patients also taking magnesium-aluminum containing antacids. Concurrent use with antacids is not recommended). Products include:
Gaviscon Regular Strength Liquid .. ▣ 620
Gaviscon Regular Strength Tablets .... ▣ 619
Gaviscon Extra Strength Liquid ...... ▣ 620
Gaviscon Extra Strength Tablets .... ▣ 619
Maalox Max Maximum Strength Antacid/Anti-Gas Liquid 2165
Maalox Regular Strength Antacid/Antigas Liquid 2164

Azathioprine (Given that azathioprine inhibits purine metabolism, it is recommended that mycophenolic acid not be administered concomitantly with azathioprine). Products include:
Azasan Tablets 2844

Azathioprine Sodium (Given that azathioprine inhibits purine metabolism, it is recommended that mycophenolic acid not be administered concomitantly with azathioprine).
No products indexed under this heading.

BCG Vaccine (During treatment with mycophenolic acid, the use of live attenuated vaccines should be avoided and patients should be advised that vaccinations may be less effective. Influenza vaccination may be of value).
No products indexed under this heading.

Charcoal, Activated (Do not administer mycophenolic acid with agents that may interfere with enterohepatic recirculation, or drugs that may bind bile acids, for example, oral activated charcoal, because of the potential to reduce the efficacy of mycophenolic acid).
No products indexed under this heading.

Chloramphenicol (Drugs that alter the gastrointestinal flora may interact with mycophenolic acid by disrupting enterohepatic recirculation. Interference of MPAG hydrolysis may lead to less mycophenolic acid available for absorption).
No products indexed under this heading.

Chloramphenicol Palmitate (Drugs that alter the gastrointestinal flora may interact with mycophenolic acid by disrupting enterohepatic recirculation. Interference of MPAG hydrolysis may lead to less mycophenolic acid available for absorption).
No products indexed under this heading.

Chloramphenicol Sodium Succinate (Drugs that alter the gastrointestinal flora may interact with mycophenolic acid by disrupting enterohepatic recirculation. Interference of MPAG hydrolysis may lead to less mycophenolic acid available for absorption).
No products indexed under this heading.

Cholestyramine (Do not administer mycophenolic acid with agents that may interfere with enterohepatic recirculation, or drugs that may bind bile acids, for example, bile acid sequestrates, because of the potential to reduce the efficacy of mycophenolic acid).
No products indexed under this heading.

Colesevelam Hydrochloride (Do not administer mycophenolic acid with agents that may interfere with enterohepatic recirculation, or drugs that may bind bile acids, for example, bile acid sequestrates, because of the potential to reduce the efficacy of mycophenolic acid). Products include:
WelChol Tablets 2855

Colestipol Hydrochloride (Do not administer mycophenolic acid with agents that may interfere with enterohepatic recirculation, or drugs that may bind bile acids, for example, bile acid sequestrates, because of the potential to reduce the efficacy of mycophenolic acid).
No products indexed under this heading.

Demeclocycline Hydrochloride (Drugs that alter the gastrointestinal flora may interact with mycophenolic acid by disrupting enterohepatic recirculation. Interference of MPAG hydrolysis may lead to less mycophenolic acid available for absorption).
No products indexed under this heading.

Desogestrel (In a drug-drug interaction study, mean levonorgesterol AUC was decreased by 15% when co-administered with mycophenolate mofetil; therefore, it is recommended that oral contraceptives are co-administered with mycophenolic acid with caution, and additional birth control methods be considered). Products include:
Ortho-Cept Tablets 2395

Doxycycline Calcium (Drugs that alter the gastrointestinal flora may interact with mycophenolic acid by disrupting enterohepatic recirculation. Interference of MPAG hydrolysis may lead to less mycophenolic acid available for absorption).
No products indexed under this heading.

Doxycycline Hyclate (Drugs that alter the gastrointestinal flora may interact with mycophenolic acid by disrupting enterohepatic recirculation. Interference of MPAG hydrolysis may lead to less mycophenolic acid available for absorption).
No products indexed under this heading.

Doxycycline Monohydrate (Drugs that alter the gastrointestinal flora may interact with mycophenolic acid by disrupting enterohepatic recirculation. Interference of MPAG hydrolysis may lead to less mycophenolic acid available for absorption).
No products indexed under this heading.

Erythromycin (Drugs that alter the gastrointestinal flora may interact with mycophenolic acid by disrupting enterohepatic recirculation. Interference of MPAG hydrolysis may lead to less mycophenolic acid available for absorption). Products include:
Erygel Topical Gel 2096
Ery-Tab Tablets 447
Erythromycin Base Filmtab Tablets 454
Erythromycin Delayed-Release Capsules, USP 456
PCE Dispertab Tablets 510

Erythromycin Estolate (Drugs that alter the gastrointestinal flora may interact with mycophenolic acid by disrupting enterohepatic recirculation. Interference of MPAG hydrolysis may lead to less mycophenolic acid available for absorption).
No products indexed under this heading.

Erythromycin Ethylsuccinate (Drugs that alter the gastrointestinal flora may interact with mycophenolic acid by disrupting enterohepatic recirculation. Interference of MPAG hydrolysis may lead to less mycophenolic acid available for absorption). Products include:
E.E.S. 449
EryPed 445

Erythromycin Gluceptate (Drugs that alter the gastrointestinal flora may interact with mycophenolic acid by disrupting enterohepatic recirculation. Interference of MPAG hydrolysis may lead to less mycophenolic acid available for absorption).
No products indexed under this heading.

Erythromycin Stearate (Drugs that alter the gastrointestinal flora may interact with mycophenolic acid by disrupting enterohepatic recirculation. Interference of MPAG hydrolysis may lead to less mycophenolic acid available for absorption). Products include:
Erythrocin Stearate Filmtab Tablets 452

Ethinyl Estradiol (In a drug-drug interaction study, mean levonorgesterol AUC was decreased by 15% when co-administered with mycophenolate mofetil; therefore, it is recom-

mended that oral contraceptives are co-administered with mycophenolic acid with caution, and additional birth control methods be considered). Products include:

- Alesse-28 Tablets 3392
- Lo/Ovral-28 Tablets 3423
- NuvaRing 2357
- Ortho-Cept Tablets 2395
- Ortho-Cyclen/Ortho Tri-Cyclen 2414
- Ortho Evra Transdermal System 2402
- Ortho Tri-Cyclen Lo Tablets 2421
- Seasonale Tablets 1073
- Triphasil-28 Tablets 3483
- Yasmin 28 Tablets 818

Ethynodiol Diacetate (In a drug-drug interaction study, mean levonorgesterol AUC was decreased by 15% when co-administered with mycophenolate mofetil; therefore, it is recommended that oral contraceptives are co-administered with mycophenolic acid with caution, and additional birth control methods be considered).

No products indexed under this heading.

Ganciclovir (May be taken with mycophenolic acid; however, during the period of treatment, physicians should monitor blood cell counts. Both ganciclovir and MPAG concentrations are increased in the presence of renal impairment; their coexistence may compete for tubular secretion and further increase in the concentrations of the two). Products include:

- Cytovene Capsules 2763

Ganciclovir Sodium (May be taken with mycophenolic acid; however, during the period of treatment, physicians should monitor blood cell counts. Both ganciclovir and MPAG concentrations are increased in the presence of renal impairment; their coexistence may compete for tubular secretion and further increase in the concentrations of the two). Products include:

- Cytovene-IV 2763

Levonorgestrel (In a drug-drug interaction study, mean levonorgesterol AUC was decreased by 15% when co-administered with mycophenolate mofetil; therefore, it is recommended that oral contraceptives are co-administered with mycophenolic acid with caution, and additional birth control methods be considered). Products include:

- Alesse-28 Tablets 3392
- Climara Pro Transdermal System 800
- Mirena Intrauterine System 810
- Plan B Tablets 1068
- Seasonale Tablets 1073
- Triphasil-28 Tablets 3483

Magaldrate (Absorption of a single dose of mycophenolic acid was decreased when administered to stable renal transplant patients also taking magnesium-aluminum containing antacids. Concurrent use with antacids is not recommended).

No products indexed under this heading.

Magnesium Hydroxide (Absorption of a single dose of mycophenolic acid was decreased when administered to stable renal transplant patients also taking magnesium-aluminum containing antacids. Concurrent use with antacids is not recommended). Products include:

- Maalox Max Maximum Strength Antacid/Anti-Gas Liquid 2165
- Maalox Regular Strength Antacid/Antigas Liquid 2164
- Pepcid Complete Chewable Tablets 1672
- Rolaids Tablets 707
- Extra Strength Rolaids Tablets 707
- Rolaids Multi-Symptom Antacid & Antigas Tablets 708

Magnesium Oxide (Absorption of a single dose of mycophenolic acid was decreased when administered to stable renal transplant patients also taking magnesium-aluminum containing antacids. Concurrent use with antacids is not recommended). Products include:

- Beelith Tablets 784
- PremCal Light, Regular, and Extra Strength Tablets 762

Measles, Mumps & Rubella Virus Vaccine, Live (During treatment with mycophenolic acid, the use of live attenuated vaccines should be avoided and patients should be advised that vaccinations may be less effective. Influenza vaccination may be of value). Products include:

- M-M-R II 1980

Measles & Rubella Virus Vaccine Live (During treatment with mycophenolic acid, the use of live attenuated vaccines should be avoided and patients should be advised that vaccinations may be less effective. Influenza vaccination may be of value).

No products indexed under this heading.

Measles Virus Vaccine Live (During treatment with mycophenolic acid, the use of live attenuated vaccines should be avoided and patients should be advised that vaccinations may be less effective. Influenza vaccination may be of value). Products include:

- Attenuvax 1889

Mestranol (In a drug-drug interaction study, mean levonorgesterol AUC was decreased by 15% when co-administered with mycophenolate mofetil; therefore, it is recommended that oral contraceptives are co-administered with mycophenolic acid with caution, and additional birth control methods be considered).

No products indexed under this heading.

Methacycline Hydrochloride (Drugs that alter the gastrointestinal flora may interact with mycophenolic acid by disrupting enterohepatic recirculation. Interference of MPAG hydrolysis may lead to less mycophenolic acid available for absorption).

No products indexed under this heading.

Minocycline Hydrochloride (Drugs that alter the gastrointestinal flora may interact with mycophenolic acid by disrupting enterohepatic recirculation. Interference of MPAG hydrolysis may lead to less mycophenolic acid available for absorption). Products include:

- Dynacin Tablets 1859

Mumps Virus Vaccine, Live (During treatment with mycophenolic acid, the use of live attenuated vaccines should be avoided and patients should be advised that vaccinations may be less effective. Influenza vaccination may be of value). Products include:

- Mumpsvax 2005

Mycophenolate Mofetil (Given that mycophenolate mofetil inhibits purine metabolism, it is recommended that mycophenolic acid not be administered concomitantly with mycophenolate mofetil). Products include:

- CellCept Capsules 2751
- CellCept Oral Suspension 2751
- CellCept Tablets 2751

Mycophenolate Mofetil Hydrochloride (Given that mycophenolate mofetil inhibits purine metabolism, it is recommended that mycophenolic acid not be administered concomitantly with mycophenolate mofetil). Products include:

- CellCept Intravenous 2751

Norethindrone (In a drug-drug interaction study, mean levonorgesterol AUC was decreased by 15% when co-administered with mycophenolate mofetil; therefore, it is recommended that oral contraceptives are co-administered with mycophenolic acid with caution, and additional birth control methods be considered). Products include:

- Ortho Micronor Tablets 2411

Norethynodrel (In a drug-drug interaction study, mean levonorgesterol AUC was decreased by 15% when co-administered with mycophenolate mofetil; therefore, it is recommended that oral contraceptives are co-administered with mycophenolic acid with caution, and additional birth control methods be considered).

No products indexed under this heading.

Norgestimate (In a drug-drug interaction study, mean levonorgesterol AUC was decreased by 15% when co-administered with mycophenolate mofetil; therefore, it is recommended that oral contraceptives are co-administered with mycophenolic acid with caution, and additional birth control methods be considered). Products include:

- Ortho-Cyclen/Ortho Tri-Cyclen 2414
- Ortho Tri-Cyclen Lo Tablets 2421
- Prefest Tablets 1069

Norgestrel (In a drug-drug interaction study, mean levonorgesterol AUC was decreased by 15% when co-administered with mycophenolate mofetil; therefore, it is recommended that oral contraceptives are co-administered with mycophenolic acid with caution, and additional birth control methods be considered). Products include:

- Lo/Ovral-28 Tablets 3423

Oxytetracycline Hydrochloride (Drugs that alter the gastrointestinal flora may interact with mycophenolic acid by disrupting enterohepatic recirculation. Interference of MPAG hydrolysis may lead to less mycophenolic acid available for absorption).

No products indexed under this heading.

Poliovirus Vaccine, Live, Oral, Trivalent, Types 1,2,3 (Sabin) (During treatment with mycophenolic acid, the use of live attenuated vaccines should be avoided and patients should be advised that vaccinations may be less effective. Influenza vaccination may be of value).

No products indexed under this heading.

Rotavirus Vaccine, Live, Oral, Tetravalent (During treatment with mycophenolic acid, the use of live attenuated vaccines should be avoided and patients should be advised that vaccinations may be less effective. Influenza vaccination may be of value).

No products indexed under this heading.

Rubella & Mumps Virus Vaccine Live (During treatment with mycophenolic acid, the use of live attenuated vaccines should be avoided and patients should be advised that vaccinations may be less effective. Influenza vaccination may be of value).

No products indexed under this heading.

Rubella Virus Vaccine Live (During treatment with mycophenolic acid, the use of live attenuated vaccines should be avoided and patients should be advised that vaccinations may be less effective. Influenza vaccination may be of value). Products include:

- Meruvax II 1994

Smallpox Vaccine (During treatment with mycophenolic acid, the use of live attenuated vaccines should be avoided and patients should be advised that vaccinations may be less effective. Influenza vaccination may be of value).

No products indexed under this heading.

Sodium Bicarbonate (Absorption of a single dose of mycophenolic acid was decreased when administered to stable renal transplant patients also taking magnesium-aluminum containing antacids. Concurrent use with antacids is not recommended). Products include:

- Ceo-Two Evacuant Suppository 607
- Colyte with Flavor Packs for Oral Solution 3102
- HalfLytely and Bisacodyl Tablets Bowel Prep Kit with Flavors Packs 915
- TriLyte with Flavor Packs for Oral Solution 3114

Sulfamethizole (Drugs that alter the gastrointestinal flora may interact with mycophenolic acid by disrupting enterohepatic recirculation. Interference of MPAG hydrolysis may lead to less mycophenolic acid available for absorption).

No products indexed under this heading.

Sulfamethoxazole (Drugs that alter the gastrointestinal flora may interact with mycophenolic acid by disrupting enterohepatic recirculation. Interference of MPAG hydrolysis may lead to less mycophenolic acid available for absorption).

No products indexed under this heading.

Sulfisoxazole (Drugs that alter the gastrointestinal flora may interact with mycophenolic acid by disrupting enterohepatic recirculation. Interference of MPAG hydrolysis may lead to less mycophenolic acid available for absorption).

No products indexed under this heading.

Sulfisoxazole Acetyl (Drugs that alter the gastrointestinal flora may interact with mycophenolic acid by disrupting enterohepatic recirculation. Interference of MPAG hydrolysis may lead to less mycophenolic acid available for absorption).

No products indexed under this heading.

Tetracycline Hydrochloride (Drugs that alter the gastrointestinal flora may interact with mycophenolic acid by disrupting enterohepatic recirculation. Interference of MPAG hydrolysis may lead to less mycophenolic acid available for absorption).
No products indexed under this heading.

Typhoid Vaccine (During treatment with mycophenolic acid, the use of live attenuated vaccines should be avoided and patients should be advised that vaccinations may be less effective. Influenza vaccination may be of value).
No products indexed under this heading.

Varicella Virus Vaccine Live (During treatment with mycophenolic acid, the use of live attenuated vaccines should be avoided and patients should be advised that vaccinations may be less effective. Influenza vaccination may be of value). Products include:
Varivax 2070

Yellow Fever Vaccine (During treatment with mycophenolic acid, the use of live attenuated vaccines should be avoided and patients should be advised that vaccinations may be less effective. Influenza vaccination may be of value).
No products indexed under this heading.

MYLERAN TABLETS

(Busulfan) 1492
May interact with antineoplastics, cytotoxic drugs, agents associated with myelosuppression, and certain other agents. Compounds in these categories include:

Altretamine (Potential for rare life-threatening hepatic veno-occlusive disease). Products include:
Hexalen Capsules 2101

Anastrozole (Potential for rare life-threatening hepatic veno-occlusive disease). Products include:
Arimidex Tablets 665

Asparaginase (Potential for rare life-threatening hepatic veno-occlusive disease). Products include:
Elspar for Injection 1943

Bicalutamide (Potential for rare life-threatening hepatic veno-occlusive disease). Products include:
Casodex Tablets 670

Bleomycin Sulfate (Busulfan-induced pulmonary toxicity may be additive to the effects produced by other cytotoxic agents).
No products indexed under this heading.

Bone Marrow Depressants, unspecified (Additive myelosuppression).
No products indexed under this heading.

Carboplatin (Potential for rare life-threatening hepatic veno-occlusive disease).
No products indexed under this heading.

Carmustine (BCNU) (Potential for rare life-threatening hepatic veno-occlusive disease).
No products indexed under this heading.

Chlorambucil (Potential for rare life-threatening hepatic veno-occlusive disease). Products include:
Leukeran Tablets 1472

Cisplatin (Potential for rare life-threatening hepatic veno-occlusive disease).
No products indexed under this heading.

Cladribine (Busulfan may cause additive myelosuppression when used with other myelosuppressive drugs). Products include:
Leustatin Injection 2368

Cyclophosphamide (Potential for rare life-threatening hepatic veno-occlusive disease; potential for cardiac temponade; co-administration may result in reduced busulfan clearance).
No products indexed under this heading.

Dacarbazine (Potential for rare life-threatening hepatic veno-occlusive disease).
No products indexed under this heading.

Daunorubicin Citrate (Potential for rare life-threatening hepatic veno-occlusive disease).
No products indexed under this heading.

Daunorubicin Citrate Liposome (Busulfan may cause additive myelosuppression when used with other myelosuppressive drugs).
No products indexed under this heading.

Daunorubicin Hydrochloride (Busulfan-induced pulmonary toxicity may be additive to the effects produced by other cytotoxic agents). Products include:
Cerubidine for Injection 788

Denileukin Diftitox (Potential for rare life-threatening hepatic veno-occlusive disease). Products include:
Ontak Vials 1717

Dexrazoxane (Busulfan may cause additive myelosuppression when used with other myelosuppressive drugs). Products include:
Zinecard for Injection 2659

Docetaxel (Potential for rare life-threatening hepatic veno-occlusive disease). Products include:
Taxotere Injection Concentrate 2947

Doxorubicin Hydrochloride (Busulfan-induced pulmonary toxicity may be additive to the effects produced by other cytotoxic agents). Products include:
Adriamycin for Injection, USP 786
Adriamycin Injection, USP 786

Doxorubicin Hydrochloride Liposome (Busulfan may cause additive myelosuppression when used with other myelosuppressive drugs). Products include:
Doxil Injection 3302

Epirubicin Hydrochloride (Busulfan-induced pulmonary toxicity may be additive to the effects produced by other cytotoxic agents). Products include:
Ellence Injection 2632

Estramustine Phosphate Sodium (Potential for rare life-threatening hepatic veno-occlusive disease). Products include:
Emcyt Capsules 3137

Etoposide (Potential for rare life-threatening hepatic veno-occlusive disease).
No products indexed under this heading.

Exemestane (Potential for rare life-threatening hepatic veno-occlusive disease). Products include:
Aromasin Tablets 2600

Floxuridine (Potential for rare life-threatening hepatic veno-occlusive disease).
No products indexed under this heading.

Fludarabine Phosphate (Busulfan may cause additive myelosuppression when used with other myelosuppressive drugs).
No products indexed under this heading.

Fluorouracil (Busulfan-induced pulmonary toxicity may be additive to the effects produced by other cytotoxic agents). Products include:
Carac Cream, 0.5% 1048
Efudex 3348

Flutamide (Potential for rare life-threatening hepatic veno-occlusive disease). Products include:
Eulexin Capsules 3023

Gemcitabine Hydrochloride (Potential for rare life-threatening hepatic veno-occlusive disease). Products include:
Gemzar for Injection 1743

Gemtuzumab Ozogamicin (Busulfan may cause additive myelosuppression when used with other myelosuppressive drugs). Products include:
Mylotarg for Injection 3429

Hydroxyurea (Busulfan-induced pulmonary toxicity may be additive to the effects produced by other cytotoxic agents).
No products indexed under this heading.

Idarubicin Hydrochloride (Potential for rare life-threatening hepatic veno-occlusive disease). Products include:
Idamycin PFS Injection 2645

Ifosfamide (Potential for rare life-threatening hepatic veno-occlusive disease).
No products indexed under this heading.

Interferon alfa-2a, Recombinant (Potential for rare life-threatening hepatic veno-occlusive disease). Products include:
Roferon-A Injection 2805

Interferon alfa-2b, Recombinant (Potential for rare life-threatening hepatic veno-occlusive disease). Products include:
Intron A for Injection 3038
Rebetron Combination Therapy 3078

Irinotecan Hydrochloride (Potential for rare life-threatening hepatic veno-occlusive disease). Products include:
Camptosar Injection 2602

Itraconazole (The concomitant systemic administration of itraconazole to patients receiving high-dose busulfan may result in reduced busulfan clearance. Patients should be monitored for signs of busulfan toxicity when itraconazole is used concomitantly with busulfan).
No products indexed under this heading.

Levamisole Hydrochloride (Potential for rare life-threatening hepatic veno-occlusive disease).
No products indexed under this heading.

Lomustine (CCNU) (Potential for rare life-threatening hepatic veno-occlusive disease).
No products indexed under this heading.

Mechlorethamine Hydrochloride (Potential for rare life-threatening hepatic veno-occlusive disease). Products include:
Mustargen for Injection 2007

Megestrol Acetate (Potential for rare life-threatening hepatic veno-occlusive disease). Products include:
Megace ES Oral Suspension 2492

Melphalan (Potential for rare life-threatening hepatic veno-occlusive disease). Products include:
Alkeran Tablets 977

Melphalan Hydrochloride (Busulfan may cause additive myelosuppression when used with other myelosuppressive drugs). Products include:
Alkeran for Injection 976

Mercaptopurine (Potential for rare life-threatening hepatic veno-occlusive disease). Products include:
Purinethol Tablets 1222

Methotrexate Sodium (Busulfan-induced pulmonary toxicity may be additive to the effects produced by other cytotoxic agents).
No products indexed under this heading.

Metronidazole (The concomitant administration of metronidazole and high-dose busulfan may result in increased trough levels of busulfan and, therefore, it is not recommended). Products include:
Metrogel 1% 1212
MetroGel-Vaginal Gel 1822
Noritate Cream, 1% 1051

Metronidazole Benzoate (The concomitant administration of metronidazole and high-dose busulfan may result in increased trough levels of busulfan and, therefore, it is not recommended).
No products indexed under this heading.

Metronidazole Hydrochloride (The concomitant administration of metronidazole and high-dose busulfan may result in increased trough levels of busulfan and, therefore, it is not recommended).
No products indexed under this heading.

Metronidazole Sodium (The concomitant administration of metronidazole and high-dose busulfan may result in increased trough levels of busulfan and, therefore, it is not recommended).
No products indexed under this heading.

Mitomycin (Mitomycin-C) (Potential for rare life-threatening hepatic veno-occlusive disease).
No products indexed under this heading.

Mitotane (Busulfan-induced pulmonary toxicity may be additive to the effects produced by other cytotoxic agents).
No products indexed under this heading.

Mitoxantrone Hydrochloride (Busulfan-induced pulmonary toxicity may be additive to the effects produced by other cytotoxic agents). Products include:
Novantrone for Injection Concentrate 3158

Oxaliplatin (Potential for rare life-threatening hepatic veno-occlusive disease). Products include:
Eloxatin for Injection 2908

Paclitaxel (Potential for rare life-threatening hepatic veno-occlusive disease).
No products indexed under this heading.

Procarbazine Hydrochloride (Busulfan-induced pulmonary toxicity may be additive to the effects produced by other cytotoxic agents). Products include:
Matulane Capsules 3188

Streptozocin (Potential for rare life-threatening hepatic veno-occlusive disease).
No products indexed under this heading.

Tamoxifen Citrate (Busulfan-induced pulmonary toxicity may be additive to the effects produced by other cytotoxic agents).
No products indexed under this heading.

Temozolomide (Busulfan may cause additive myelosuppression when used with other myelosuppressive drugs). Products include:
Temodar Capsules 3088

Teniposide (Potential for rare life-threatening hepatic veno-occlusive disease).
No products indexed under this heading.

Thioguanine (Potential for portal hypertension and esophageal varices associated with abnormal liver function tests; potential for rare life-threatening hepatic veno-occlusive disease). Products include:
Tabloid Tablets 1545

Thiotepa (Potential for rare life-threatening hepatic veno-occlusive disease).
No products indexed under this heading.

Topotecan Hydrochloride (Potential for rare life-threatening hepatic veno-occlusive disease). Products include:
Hycamtin for Injection 1427

Toremifene Citrate (Potential for rare life-threatening hepatic veno-occlusive disease).
No products indexed under this heading.

Valrubicin (Potential for rare life-threatening hepatic veno-occlusive disease).
No products indexed under this heading.

Vincristine Sulfate (Busulfan-induced pulmonary toxicity may be additive to the effects produced by other cytotoxic agents).
No products indexed under this heading.

Vinorelbine Tartrate (Potential for rare life-threatening hepatic veno-occlusive disease). Products include:
Navelbine Injection 1494

MYLOTARG FOR INJECTION

(Gemtuzumab Ozogamicin) 3429
May interact with drugs which undergo biotransformation by cytochrome p-450 mixed function oxidase. Compounds in these categories include:

Acarbose (Potential for drug-drug interaction with drugs affected by CYP450 enzymes). Products include:
Precose Tablets 776

Acetaminophen (Potential for drug-drug interaction with drugs affected by CYP450 enzymes). Products include:
Benadryl Allergy & Cold Tablets 692
Benadryl Allergy & Sinus Headache Caplets & Gelcaps 693
Benadryl Maximum Strength Severe Allergy & Sinus Headache Caplets 694
Contac Severe Cold and Flu Caplets Maximum Strength 615
Contac Severe Cold and Flu Caplets Non-Drowsy 615
Darvocet A 500 Tablets 3497
Goody's Body Pain Formula Powder 621
Goody's Extra Strength Headache Powder 621
Goody's Extra Strength Pain Relief Tablets 621
Goody's PM Powder 622
Hycomine Compound Tablets 1105
Lortab 3315
Lortab Elixir 3312
Percocet Tablets 1114
Robitussin Cough, Cold & Flu Liquid-filled Capsules 750
Robitussin Flu Liquid 752
Sedapap Tablets 50 mg/650 mg 2098
Singlet Caplets 636
Sudafed Severe Cold 710
Sudafed Sinus Headache 711
TheraFlu Cold & Cough Hot Liquid 680
TheraFlu Cold & Sore Throat Hot Liquid 680
TheraFlu Flu & Chest Congestion Non-Drowsy Hot Liquid 681
TheraFlu Flu & Sore Throat Hot Liquid 681
TheraFlu Severe Cold Non-Drowsy Hot Liquid 683
TheraFlu Severe Cold & Cough Hot Liquid 683
TheraFlu Severe Cold Caplets 679
TheraFlu Severe Cold Hot Liquid 682
TheraFlu Severe Cold Non-Drowsy Caplets 679
Triaminic Cough & Sore Throat Liquid 687
Triaminic Flu, Cough & Fever Liquid 685
Triaminic Cough & Sore Throat Softchews 689
Tylenol 8 Hour Extended Release Geltabs and Caplets 1843
Tylenol Sinus NightTime Caplets 663
Children's Tylenol Suspension Liquid and Meltaways 1850
Children's Tylenol Plus Cold & Allergy Suspension Liquid 1850
Children's Tylenol Plus Cold NightTime Suspension Liquid 1851
Children's Tylenol Plus Cold & Cough Suspension Liquid and Chewable Tablets 1851
Children's Tylenol Plus Cold Chewable Tablets 1851
Children's Tylenol Plus Cold Daytime Non-Drowsy Suspension Liquid 1851
Children's Tylenol Plus Flu Suspension Liquid 1853
Concentrated Tylenol Infants' Drops Plus Cold 1851
Concentrated Tylenol Infants' Drops Plus Cold and Cough 1851
Concentrated Tylenol Infants' Drops 1850
Junior Tylenol Meltaways 1850
Tylenol Cold & Flu Severe Daytime Liquid with Cool Bust 1846
Tylenol Cold & Flu Severe NightTime Liquid with Cool Burst 1846
Tylenol Cold Severe Congestion Non-Drowsy Caplets with Cool Burst 1846
Tylenol Cough & Sore Throat Daytime Liquid with Cool Burst 1849
Tylenol Cough & Sore Throat NightTime Liquid with Cool Burst 1849
Tylenol 1843
Extra Strength Tylenol Rapid Release Gels 1843
Tylenol 1843
Tylenol Allergy Complete Night Time Caplets 1844
Tylenol Allergy Complete Multi-Symptom Caplets and Gelcaps with Cool Burst 1844
Tylenol Severe Allergy Caplets 1844
Tylenol Flu NightTime Gelcaps 1846
Tylenol Flu Day Non-Drowsy Gelcaps 1846
Concentrated Tylenol Infants' Drops Plus Cold Nasal Congestant, Fever Reducer & Pain Reliever 668
Concentrated Tylenol Infants' Drops Plus Cold & Cough Nasal Decongestant, Fever Reducer & Pain Reliever 668
Multi-Symptom Tylenol Cold Night Time Caplets 1845
Multi-Symptom Tylenol Cold Day Non-Drowsy Caplets and Gelcaps 1845
Extra Strength Tylenol PM Caplets, Geltabs, Gelcaps and Liquid 1847
Tylenol Sinus Day Non-Drowsy 1848
Tylenol Sinus Night Time Caplets 1848
Tylenol Sinus Severe Congestion Caplets with Cool Burst 1848
Tylenol Sore Throat Daytime Liquid with Cool Burst 1849
Tylenol Sore Throat NightTime Liquid with Cool Burst 1849
Tylenol with Codeine 2461
Women's Tylenol Menstrual Relief Caplets 1849
Ultracet Tablets 2462
Vicks 44M Cough, Cold & Flu Relief 2676
Vicks DayQuil LiquiCaps/Liquid Multi-Symptom Cold/Flu Relief 723
Vicks DayQuil Multi-Symptom Cold/Flu Relief LiquiCaps 2675
Vicks DayQuil Multi-Symptom Cold/Flu Relief Liquid 2675
Vicks NyQuil LiquiCaps 2677
Vicks NyQuil LiquiCaps/Liquid Multi-Symptom Cold/Flu Relief 725
Vicks NyQuil Liquid 2677
Vicodin Tablets 530
Vicodin ES Tablets 531
Vicodin HP Tablets 532
Zydone Tablets 1118

Alatrofloxacin Mesylate (Potential for drug-drug interaction with drugs affected by CYP450 enzymes).
No products indexed under this heading.

Alfentanil Hydrochloride (Potential for drug-drug interaction with drugs affected by CYP450 enzymes).
No products indexed under this heading.

Alprazolam (Potential for drug-drug interaction with drugs affected by CYP450 enzymes). Products include:
Niravam Orally Disintegrating Tablets 3106
Xanax XR Tablets 2655

Aminophylline (Potential for drug-drug interaction with drugs affected by CYP450 enzymes).
No products indexed under this heading.

Amiodarone Hydrochloride (Potential for drug-drug interaction with drugs affected by CYP450 enzymes). Products include:
Pacerone Tablets 3337

Amitriptyline Hydrochloride (Potential for drug-drug interaction with drugs affected by CYP450 enzymes).
No products indexed under this heading.

Amlodipine Besylate (Potential for drug-drug interaction with drugs affected by CYP450 enzymes). Products include:
Caduet Tablets 2507
Lotrel Capsules 2238
Norvasc Tablets 2529

Amoxapine (Potential for drug-drug interaction with drugs affected by CYP450 enzymes).
No products indexed under this heading.

Amphetamine Aspartate (Potential for drug-drug interaction with drugs affected by CYP450 enzymes). Products include:
Adderall Tablets 3168
Adderall XR Capsules 3169

Amphetamine Aspartate Monohydrate (Potential for drug-drug interaction with drugs affected by CYP450 enzymes).
No products indexed under this heading.

Amphetamine Sulfate (Potential for drug-drug interaction with drugs affected by CYP450 enzymes). Products include:
Adderall Tablets 3168
Adderall XR Capsules 3169

Aprepitant (Potential for drug-drug interaction with drugs affected by CYP450 enzymes). Products include:
Emend Capsules 1944

Astemizole (Potential for drug-drug interaction with drugs affected by CYP450 enzymes).
No products indexed under this heading.

Atomoxetine Hydrochloride (Potential for drug-drug interaction with drugs affected by CYP450 enzymes). Products include:
Strattera Capsules 1784

Atorvastatin Calcium (Potential for drug-drug interaction with drugs affected by CYP450 enzymes). Products include:
Caduet Tablets 2507
Lipitor Tablets 2495

Belladonna Ergotamine (Potential for drug-drug interaction with drugs affected by CYP450 enzymes).
No products indexed under this heading.

Benzphetamine Hydrochloride (Potential for drug-drug interaction with drugs affected by CYP450 enzymes).
No products indexed under this heading.

Bisoprolol Fumarate (Potential for drug-drug interaction with drugs affected by CYP450 enzymes).
No products indexed under this heading.

Buspirone Hydrochloride (Potential for drug-drug interaction with drugs affected by CYP450 enzymes).
No products indexed under this heading.

Busulfan (Potential for drug-drug interaction with drugs affected by CYP450 enzymes). Products include:
I.V. Busulfex 1125
Myleran Tablets 1492

Caffeine (Potential for drug-drug interaction with drugs affected by CYP450 enzymes). Products include:
Athena Hair System Shampoo 767
BC Powder 612
Arthritis Strength BC Powder 612
Goody's Extra Strength Headache Powder 621
Goody's Extra Strength Pain Relief Tablets 621
Hycomine Compound Tablets 1105

IMPORTANT NOTE: Always consult each drug listing in the patient's regimen for possible interactions.

Spartan Hair System Shampoo ...... ▣767
Vivarin .... ▣639

Caffeine Anhydrous (Potential for drug-drug interaction with drugs affected by CYP450 enzymes).
No products indexed under this heading.

Caffeine Citrate (Potential for drug-drug interaction with drugs affected by CYP450 enzymes). Products include:
Cafcit 1854

Candesartan Cilexetil (Potential for drug-drug interaction with drugs affected by CYP450 enzymes). Products include:
Atacand Tablets 634
Atacand HCT 637

Captopril (Potential for drug-drug interaction with drugs affected by CYP450 enzymes). Products include:
Captopril Tablets 2114

Carbamazepine (Potential for drug-drug interaction with drugs affected by CYP450 enzymes). Products include:
Carbatrol Capsules 3174
Equetro Extended-Release Capsules 3178
Tegretol/Tegretol-XR 2278

Carisoprodol (Potential for drug-drug interaction with drugs affected by CYP450 enzymes).
No products indexed under this heading.

Carvedilol (Potential for drug-drug interaction with drugs affected by CYP450 enzymes). Products include:
Coreg Tablets 1376

Celecoxib (Potential for drug-drug interaction with drugs affected by CYP450 enzymes). Products include:
Celebrex Capsules 3130

Cerivastatin Sodium (Potential for drug-drug interaction with drugs affected by CYP450 enzymes).
No products indexed under this heading.

Cevimeline Hydrochloride (Potential for drug-drug interaction with drugs affected by CYP450 enzymes). Products include:
Evoxac Capsules 1042

Chlordiazepoxide (Potential for drug-drug interaction with drugs affected by CYP450 enzymes).
No products indexed under this heading.

Chlordiazepoxide Hydrochloride (Potential for drug-drug interaction with drugs affected by CYP450 enzymes). Products include:
Librium Capsules 3349

Chlorpheniramine (Potential for drug-drug interaction with drugs affected by CYP450 enzymes).
No products indexed under this heading.

Chlorpheniramine Maleate (Potential for drug-drug interaction with drugs affected by CYP450 enzymes). Products include:
Advil Allergy Sinus Caplets .... ▣737
Advil Multi-Symptom Cold Caplets .... ▣738
BC Allergy Sinus Cold Powder .... ▣612
Contac Severe Cold and Flu Caplets Maximum Strength .... ▣615
Hycomine Compound Tablets 1105
PediaCare Multi-Symptom Cold Liquid .... ▣704
PediaCare NightRest Cough & Cold Liquid .... ▣704
Robitussin Flu Liquid .... ▣752
Robitussin PM Cough & Cold Liquid .... ▣752
Singlet Caplets .... ▣636
Sudafed Sinus & Allergy Tablets ..... ▣710
TheraFlu Cold & Cough Hot Liquid .... ▣680
TheraFlu Cold & Sore Throat Hot Liquid .... ▣680
TheraFlu Flu & Sore Throat Hot Liquid .... ▣681
TheraFlu Severe Cold & Cough Hot Liquid .... ▣683
TheraFlu Severe Cold Caplets .... ▣679
TheraFlu Severe Cold Hot Liquid ..... ▣682
Triaminic Cold & Allergy Liquid ...... ▣685
Triaminic Cold & Cough Liquid .... ▣685
Triaminic Flu, Cough & Fever Liquid .... ▣685
Triaminic Night Time Cough & Cold Liquid .... ▣685
Triaminic Allergy Runny Nose & Congestion Softchews .... ▣688
Triaminic Cold & Cough Softchews .... ▣688
Children's Tylenol Plus Cold NightTime Suspension Liquid 1851
Children's Tylenol Plus Cold & Cough Suspension Liquid and Chewable Tablets 1851
Children's Tylenol Plus Cold Chewable Tablets 1851
Children's Tylenol Plus Flu Suspension Liquid 1853
Tylenol Allergy Complete Multi-Symptom Caplets and Gelcaps with Cool Burst 1844
Multi-Symptom Tylenol Cold Night Time Caplets 1845
Vicks 44M Cough, Cold & Flu Relief 2676
Pediatric Vicks 44m Cough & Cold Relief 2673
Children's Vicks NyQuil Cold/Cough Relief 2671

Chlorpheniramine Polistirex (Potential for drug-drug interaction with drugs affected by CYP450 enzymes). Products include:
Tussionex Pennkinetic Extended-Release Suspension 3322

Chlorpheniramine Tannate (Potential for drug-drug interaction with drugs affected by CYP450 enzymes).
No products indexed under this heading.

Chlorpromazine (Potential for drug-drug interaction with drugs affected by CYP450 enzymes).
No products indexed under this heading.

Chlorpromazine Hydrochloride (Potential for drug-drug interaction with drugs affected by CYP450 enzymes).
No products indexed under this heading.

Chlorpropamide (Potential for drug-drug interaction with drugs affected by CYP450 enzymes).
No products indexed under this heading.

Cilostazol (Potential for drug-drug interaction with drugs affected by CYP450 enzymes). Products include:
Pletal Tablets 2478

Cimetidine Hydrochloride (Potential for drug-drug interaction with drugs affected by CYP450 enzymes).
No products indexed under this heading.

Ciprofloxacin (Potential for drug-drug interaction with drugs affected by CYP450 enzymes). Products include:
Cipro I.V. 2998
Cipro I.V. Pharmacy Bulk Package ... 3509
Cipro Oral Suspension 2991
Cipro XR Tablets 3004
Ciprodex Otic Suspension 555

Ciprofloxacin Hydrochloride (Potential for drug-drug interaction with drugs affected by CYP450 enzymes). Products include:
Ciloxan Ophthalmic Ointment 554
Cipro Tablets 2991

Cisapride (Potential for drug-drug interaction with drugs affected by CYP450 enzymes).
No products indexed under this heading.

Citalopram Hydrobromide (Potential for drug-drug interaction with drugs affected by CYP450 enzymes). Products include:
Celexa 1177

Clarithromycin (Potential for drug-drug interaction with drugs affected by CYP450 enzymes). Products include:
Biaxin/Biaxin XL 402
PREVPAC 3281

Clomipramine Hydrochloride (Potential for drug-drug interaction with drugs affected by CYP450 enzymes).
No products indexed under this heading.

Clopidogrel Hydrogen Sulfate (Potential for drug-drug interaction with drugs affected by CYP450 enzymes).
No products indexed under this heading.

Clozapine (Potential for drug-drug interaction with drugs affected by CYP450 enzymes). Products include:
Clozapine Tablets 2141
Clozaril Tablets 2174
FazaClo Orally Disintegrating Tablets 547

Codeine Phosphate (Potential for drug-drug interaction with drugs affected by CYP450 enzymes). Products include:
Tylenol with Codeine 2461

Codeine Sulfate (Potential for drug-drug interaction with drugs affected by CYP450 enzymes).
No products indexed under this heading.

Cyclobenzaprine (Potential for drug-drug interaction with drugs affected by CYP450 enzymes).
No products indexed under this heading.

Cyclobenzaprine Hydrochloride (Potential for drug-drug interaction with drugs affected by CYP450 enzymes). Products include:
Flexeril Tablets 1832

Cyclophosphamide (Potential for drug-drug interaction with drugs affected by CYP450 enzymes).
No products indexed under this heading.

Cyclosporine (Potential for drug-drug interaction with drugs affected by CYP450 enzymes). Products include:
Gengraf Capsules 458
Neoral Soft Gelatin Capsules 2247
Neoral Oral Solution 2247
Restasis Ophthalmic Emulsion 570
Sandimmune 2259

Desipramine Hydrochloride (Potential for drug-drug interaction with drugs affected by CYP450 enzymes).
No products indexed under this heading.

Desogestrel (Potential for drug-drug interaction with drugs affected by CYP450 enzymes). Products include:
Ortho-Cept Tablets 2395

Dexamethasone (Potential for drug-drug interaction with drugs affected by CYP450 enzymes). Products include:
Ciprodex Otic Suspension 555
Decadron Tablets 1929
TobraDex Ophthalmic Ointment 558
TobraDex Ophthalmic Suspension ... 558

Dexamethasone Acetate (Potential for drug-drug interaction with drugs affected by CYP450 enzymes).
No products indexed under this heading.

Dexamethasone Phosphate (Potential for drug-drug interaction with drugs affected by CYP450 enzymes).
No products indexed under this heading.

Dexamethasone Sodium (Potential for drug-drug interaction with drugs affected by CYP450 enzymes).
No products indexed under this heading.

Dexamethasone Sodium Phosphate (Potential for drug-drug interaction with drugs affected by CYP450 enzymes). Products include:
Decadron Phosphate Injection 1931

Dexfenfluramine Hydrochloride (Potential for drug-drug interaction with drugs affected by CYP450 enzymes).
No products indexed under this heading.

Dextromethorphan (Potential for drug-drug interaction with drugs affected by CYP450 enzymes).
No products indexed under this heading.

Dextromethorphan Hydrobromide (Potential for drug-drug interaction with drugs affected by CYP450 enzymes). Products include:
Alacol DM Syrup 739
Balamine DM 739
Contac Severe Cold and Flu Caplets Maximum Strength .... ▣615
Contac Severe Cold and Flu Caplets Non-Drowsy .... ▣615
Children's Dimetapp DM Cold & Cough Elixir .... ▣745
Children's Dimetapp Long Acting Cough Plus Cold Syrup .... ▣746
Dimetapp Infant Drops Decongestant Plus Cough .... ▣746
Mucinex DM Tablets .... ▣602
PediaCare Decongestant & Cough Infant Drops .... ▣705
PediaCare Freezer Pops Long-Acting Cough-Glacier Grape and Polar Berry Blue .... ▣706
PediaCare Long-Acting Cough Infant Drops .... ▣705
PediaCare Long-Acting Cough Plus Cold Liquid .... ▣704
PediaCare Multi-Symptom Cold Liquid .... ▣704
PediaCare NightRest Cough & Cold Liquid .... ▣704
Robitussin Allergy & Cough Syrup .. ▣750
Robitussin CF Liquid .... ▣755
Robitussin Cough & Cold Liquid-filled Capsules .... ▣750
Robitussin Cough, Cold & Flu Liquid-filled Capsules .... ▣750
Robitussin Cough & Cold Infant Drops .... ▣755
Robitussin DM Infant Drops .... ▣753
Robitussin DM Liquid .... ▣753
Robitussin Flu Liquid .... ▣752
Robitussin Maximum Strength Cough Liquid .... ▣754
Robitussin Maximum Strength Cough & Cold Liquid .... ▣754

Robitussin Pediatric Cough Liquid ... 754
Robitussin Pediatric Cough & Cold Liquid ... 754
Robitussin PM Cough & Cold Liquid ... 752
Robitussin Sugar Free Cough Liquid ... 753
Simply Cough Liquid ... 1840
Sudafed Severe Cold ... 710
TheraFlu Cold & Cough Hot Liquid ... 680
TheraFlu Flu & Chest Congestion Non-Drowsy Hot Liquid ... 681
TheraFlu Severe Cold Non-Drowsy Hot Liquid ... 683
TheraFlu Severe Cold & Cough Hot Liquid ... 683
TheraFlu Severe Cold Caplets ... 679
TheraFlu Severe Cold Hot Liquid ... 682
TheraFlu Severe Cold Non-Drowsy Caplets ... 679
TheraFlu Thin Strips Long Acting Cough ... 684
Triaminic Cold & Cough Liquid ... 685
Triaminic Cough Liquid ... 687
Triaminic Cough & Nasal Congestion Liquid ... 687
Triaminic Cough & Sore Throat Liquid ... 687
Triaminic Flu, Cough & Fever Liquid ... 685
Triaminic Night Time Cough & Cold Liquid ... 685
Triaminic Cold & Cough Softchews ... 688
Triaminic Cough & Sore Throat Softchews ... 689
Triaminic Thin Strips Long Acting Cough ... 689
Children's Tylenol Plus Cold & Cough Suspension Liquid and Chewable Tablets ... 1851
Children's Tylenol Plus Flu Suspension Liquid ... 1853
Concentrated Tylenol Infants' Drops Plus Cold and Cough ... 1851
Tylenol Cold & Flu Severe Daytime Liquid with Cool Bust ... 1846
Tylenol Cold & Flu Severe NightTime Liquid with Cool Burst ... 1846
Tylenol Cold Severe Congestion Non-Drowsy Caplets with Cool Burst ... 1846
Tylenol Cough & Sore Throat Daytime Liquid with Cool Burst ... 1849
Tylenol Cough & Sore Throat NightTime Liquid with Cool Burst ... 1849
Tylenol Flu Day Non-Drowsy Gelcaps ... 1846
Concentrated Tylenol Infants' Drops Plus Cold & Cough Nasal Decongestant, Fever Reducer & Pain Reliever ... 668
Multi-Symptom Tylenol Cold Night Time Caplets ... 1845
Multi-Symptom Tylenol Cold Day Non-Drowsy Caplets and Gelcaps ... 1845
Vicks 44 Cough Relief ... 2675
Vicks 44D Cough & Head Congestion Relief ... 2676
Vicks 44D Cough & Head Congestion Relief Liquid ... 721
Vicks 44E Cough & Chest Congestion Relief ... 2676
Pediatric Vicks 44e Cough & Chest Congestion Relief Liquid ... 2673
Vicks 44M Cough, Cold & Flu Relief ... 2676
Pediatric Vicks 44m Cough & Cold Relief ... 2673
Vicks DayQuil LiquiCaps/Liquid Multi-Symptom Cold/Flu Relief ... 723
Vicks DayQuil Multi-Symptom Cold/Flu Relief LiquiCaps ... 2675
Vicks DayQuil Multi-Symptom Cold/Flu Relief Liquid ... 2675
Children's Vicks NyQuil Cold/Cough Relief ... 2671
Vicks NyQuil Cough Liquid ... 2677
Vicks NyQuil LiquiCaps ... 2677
Vicks NyQuil LiquiCaps/Liquid Multi-Symptom Cold/Flu Relief ... 725
Vicks NyQuil Liquid ... 2677
Zicam Concentrated Cough Mist for Kids Cool Cherry ... 643
Zicam Concentrated Cough Mist for Kids Plus D Cool Cherry ... 643
Zicam Concentrated Cough Mist Nite-Cool Cherry ... 642
Zicam Concentrated Cough Mist Plus D Cool Cherry ... 642
Zicam Concentrated Cough Mist-Honey Lemon & Cool Cherry ... 642

Dextromethorphan Polistirex (Potential for drug-drug interaction with drugs affected by CYP450 enzymes). Products include:
Delsym Extended-Release Suspension ... 611
Delsym 12 Hour Cough Suppressant for Children ... 611

Diazepam (Potential for drug-drug interaction with drugs affected by CYP450 enzymes). Products include:
Diastat Rectal Delivery System ... 3344
Valium Tablets ... 2822

Diclofenac Potassium (Potential for drug-drug interaction with drugs affected by CYP450 enzymes). Products include:
Cataflam Tablets ... 2173

Diclofenac Sodium (Potential for drug-drug interaction with drugs affected by CYP450 enzymes). Products include:
Arthrotec Tablets ... 3126
Voltaren Ophthalmic Solution ... 2300
Voltaren Tablets ... 2298
Voltaren-XR Tablets ... 2301

Dihydroergotamine Mesylate (Potential for drug-drug interaction with drugs affected by CYP450 enzymes). Products include:
Migranal Nasal Spray ... 3350

Diltiazem Hydrochloride (Potential for drug-drug interaction with drugs affected by CYP450 enzymes). Products include:
Cardizem LA Extended Release Tablets ... 1699
Tiazac Capsules ... 1204

Diltiazem Maleate (Potential for drug-drug interaction with drugs affected by CYP450 enzymes).
No products indexed under this heading.

Disopyramide (Potential for drug-drug interaction with drugs affected by CYP450 enzymes).
No products indexed under this heading.

Disopyramide Phosphate (Potential for drug-drug interaction with drugs affected by CYP450 enzymes).
No products indexed under this heading.

Divalproex Sodium (Potential for drug-drug interaction with drugs affected by CYP450 enzymes). Products include:
Depakote Sprinkle Capsules ... 422
Depakote Tablets ... 427
Depakote ER Tablets ... 433

Docetaxel (Potential for drug-drug interaction with drugs affected by CYP450 enzymes). Products include:
Taxotere Injection Concentrate ... 2947

Dolasetron Mesylate (Potential for drug-drug interaction with drugs affected by CYP450 enzymes). Products include:
Anzemet Injection ... 2871
Anzemet Tablets ... 2874

Donepezil Hydrochloride (Potential for drug-drug interaction with drugs affected by CYP450 enzymes). Products include:
Aricept Tablets ... 1086
Aricept ODT Tablets ... 1086

Doxepin Hydrochloride (Potential for drug-drug interaction with drugs affected by CYP450 enzymes).
No products indexed under this heading.

Doxorubicin Hydrochloride (Potential for drug-drug interaction with drugs affected by CYP450 enzymes). Products include:
Adriamycin for Injection, USP ... 786
Adriamycin Injection, USP ... 786

Dronabinol (Potential for drug-drug interaction with drugs affected by CYP450 enzymes). Products include:
Marinol Capsules ... 3334

Drugs that Undergo Biotransformation by Cytochrome P-450 Mixed Function Oxidase (Potential for drug-drug interaction with drugs affected by CYP450 enzymes).
No products indexed under this heading.

Dyphylline (Potential for drug-drug interaction with drugs affected by CYP450 enzymes).
No products indexed under this heading.

Encainide Hydrochloride (Potential for drug-drug interaction with drugs affected by CYP450 enzymes).
No products indexed under this heading.

Enoxacin (Potential for drug-drug interaction with drugs affected by CYP450 enzymes).
No products indexed under this heading.

Eprosartan Mesylate (Potential for drug-drug interaction with drugs affected by CYP450 enzymes). Products include:
Teveten Tablets ... 1707
Teveten HCT Tablets ... 1710

Ergotamine Tartrate (Potential for drug-drug interaction with drugs affected by CYP450 enzymes).
No products indexed under this heading.

Erythromycin (Potential for drug-drug interaction with drugs affected by CYP450 enzymes). Products include:
Erygel Topical Gel ... 2096
Ery-Tab Tablets ... 447
Erythromycin Base Filmtab Tablets ... 454
Erythromycin Delayed-Release Capsules, USP ... 456
PCE Dispertab Tablets ... 510

Erythromycin Estolate (Potential for drug-drug interaction with drugs affected by CYP450 enzymes).
No products indexed under this heading.

Erythromycin Ethylsuccinate (Potential for drug-drug interaction with drugs affected by CYP450 enzymes). Products include:
E.E.S. ... 449
EryPed ... 445

Erythromycin Gluceptate (Potential for drug-drug interaction with drugs affected by CYP450 enzymes).
No products indexed under this heading.

Erythromycin Lactobionate (Potential for drug-drug interaction with drugs affected by CYP450 enzymes).
No products indexed under this heading.

Erythromycin Stearate (Potential for drug-drug interaction with drugs affected by CYP450 enzymes). Products include:
Erythrocin Stearate Filmtab Tablets ... 452

Esomeprazole Magnesium (Potential for drug-drug interaction with drugs affected by CYP450 enzymes). Products include:
Nexium Delayed-Release Capsules ... 645

Estradiol (Potential for drug-drug interaction with drugs affected by CYP450 enzymes). Products include:
Activella Tablets ... 2311
Climara Transdermal System ... 795
Climara Pro Transdermal System ... 800
CombiPatch Transdermal System ... 2180
Estrogel 0.06% ... 3200
Menostar Transdermal System ... 805
Prefest Tablets ... 1069
Vagifem Tablets ... 2340
Vivelle Transdermal System ... 2288
Vivelle-Dot Transdermal System ... 2293

Estradiol Benzoate (Potential for drug-drug interaction with drugs affected by CYP450 enzymes).
No products indexed under this heading.

Estradiol Cypionate (Potential for drug-drug interaction with drugs affected by CYP450 enzymes).
No products indexed under this heading.

Estradiol Valerate (Potential for drug-drug interaction with drugs affected by CYP450 enzymes).
No products indexed under this heading.

Estrogen (Potential for drug-drug interaction with drugs affected by CYP450 enzymes).
No products indexed under this heading.

Estrogens, Conjugated (Potential for drug-drug interaction with drugs affected by CYP450 enzymes). Products include:
Premarin Intravenous ... 3440
Premarin Tablets ... 3443
Premarin Vaginal Cream ... 3449
Premphase Tablets ... 3452
Prempro Tablets ... 3452

Estrogens, Conjugated, Synthetic A (Potential for drug-drug interaction with drugs affected by CYP450 enzymes). Products include:
Cenestin Tablets, 0.45mg, 0.625mg, 0.9mg, 1.25mg ... 1063
Cenestin Tablets, 0.3mg ... 1063

Estrogens, Esterified (Potential for drug-drug interaction with drugs affected by CYP450 enzymes). Products include:
Estratest Tablets ... 3196
Estratest H.S. Tablets ... 3196

Ethinyl Estradiol (Potential for drug-drug interaction with drugs affected by CYP450 enzymes). Products include:
Alesse-28 Tablets ... 3392
Lo/Ovral-28 Tablets ... 3423
NuvaRing ... 2357
Ortho-Cept Tablets ... 2395
Ortho-Cyclen/Ortho Tri-Cyclen ... 2414
Ortho Evra Transdermal System ... 2402
Ortho Tri-Cyclen Lo Tablets ... 2421
Seasonale Tablets ... 1073
Triphasil-28 Tablets ... 3483
Yasmin 28 Tablets ... 818

Ethosuximide (Potential for drug-drug interaction with drugs affected by CYP450 enzymes).
No products indexed under this heading.

Ethotoin (Potential for drug-drug interaction with drugs affected by CYP450 enzymes). Products include:
Peganone Tablets, USP 2487

Ethynodiol Diacetate (Potential for drug-drug interaction with drugs affected by CYP450 enzymes).
No products indexed under this heading.

Etodolac (Potential for drug-drug interaction with drugs affected by CYP450 enzymes).
No products indexed under this heading.

Etoposide (Potential for drug-drug interaction with drugs affected by CYP450 enzymes).
No products indexed under this heading.

Etoposide Phosphate (Potential for drug-drug interaction with drugs affected by CYP450 enzymes).
No products indexed under this heading.

Felbamate (Potential for drug-drug interaction with drugs affected by CYP450 enzymes).
No products indexed under this heading.

Felodipine (Potential for drug-drug interaction with drugs affected by CYP450 enzymes). Products include:
Plendil Extended-Release Tablets 651

Fenoprofen Calcium (Potential for drug-drug interaction with drugs affected by CYP450 enzymes). Products include:
Nalfon Capsules 2504

Fentanyl (Potential for drug-drug interaction with drugs affected by CYP450 enzymes). Products include:
Duragesic Transdermal System 2448

Fentanyl Citrate (Potential for drug-drug interaction with drugs affected by CYP450 enzymes). Products include:
Actiq 993

Flecainide Acetate (Potential for drug-drug interaction with drugs affected by CYP450 enzymes). Products include:
Tambocor Tablets 1824

Fluoxetine (Potential for drug-drug interaction with drugs affected by CYP450 enzymes).
No products indexed under this heading.

Fluoxetine Hydrochloride (Potential for drug-drug interaction with drugs affected by CYP450 enzymes). Products include:
Prozac Pulvules and Liquid 1771
Symbyax Capsules 1788

Fluphenazine Decanoate (Potential for drug-drug interaction with drugs affected by CYP450 enzymes).
No products indexed under this heading.

Fluphenazine Enanthate (Potential for drug-drug interaction with drugs affected by CYP450 enzymes).
No products indexed under this heading.

Fluphenazine Hydrochloride (Potential for drug-drug interaction with drugs affected by CYP450 enzymes).
No products indexed under this heading.

Flurbiprofen (Potential for drug-drug interaction with drugs affected by CYP450 enzymes).
No products indexed under this heading.

Flurbiprofen Sodium (Potential for drug-drug interaction with drugs affected by CYP450 enzymes). Products include:
Ocufen Ophthalmic Solution .... ⊙230

Flutamide (Potential for drug-drug interaction with drugs affected by CYP450 enzymes). Products include:
Eulexin Capsules 3023

Fluticasone Propionate (Potential for drug-drug interaction with drugs affected by CYP450 enzymes). Products include:
Advair Diskus 100/50 1291
Advair Diskus 250/50 1291
Advair Diskus 500/50 1291
Cutivate Cream 1381
Cutivate Lotion 0.05% 1383
Cutivate Ointment 1384
Flonase Nasal Spray 1412
Flovent Diskus 100 mcg 1418
Flovent Diskus 50 mcg 1415

Fluvastatin Sodium (Potential for drug-drug interaction with drugs affected by CYP450 enzymes). Products include:
Lescol Capsules 2227
Lescol 2730
Lescol XL Tablets 2227

Fluvoxamine Maleate (Potential for drug-drug interaction with drugs affected by CYP450 enzymes).
No products indexed under this heading.

Formoterol Fumarate (Potential for drug-drug interaction with drugs affected by CYP450 enzymes). Products include:
Foradil Aerolizer 3024

Fosphenytoin (Potential for drug-drug interaction with drugs affected by CYP450 enzymes).
No products indexed under this heading.

Fosphenytoin Sodium (Potential for drug-drug interaction with drugs affected by CYP450 enzymes).
No products indexed under this heading.

Gabapentin (Potential for drug-drug interaction with drugs affected by CYP450 enzymes). Products include:
Neurontin Capsules 2498
Neurontin Oral Solution 2498
Neurontin Tablets 2498

Galantamine Hydrobromide (Potential for drug-drug interaction with drugs affected by CYP450 enzymes). Products include:
Razadyne ER Extended-Release Capsules 2434
Razadyne 2434

Glimepiride (Potential for drug-drug interaction with drugs affected by CYP450 enzymes). Products include:
Amaryl Tablets 2864

Glipizide (Potential for drug-drug interaction with drugs affected by CYP450 enzymes).
No products indexed under this heading.

Glyburide (Potential for drug-drug interaction with drugs affected by CYP450 enzymes).
No products indexed under this heading.

Grepafloxacin Hydrochloride (Potential for drug-drug interaction with drugs affected by CYP450 enzymes).
No products indexed under this heading.

Haloperidol (Potential for drug-drug interaction with drugs affected by CYP450 enzymes).
No products indexed under this heading.

Haloperidol Decanoate (Potential for drug-drug interaction with drugs affected by CYP450 enzymes).
No products indexed under this heading.

Haloperidol Lactate (Potential for drug-drug interaction with drugs affected by CYP450 enzymes).
No products indexed under this heading.

Hydrocodone Bitartrate (Potential for drug-drug interaction with drugs affected by CYP450 enzymes). Products include:
Hycodan 1104
Hycomine Compound Tablets 1105
Hycotuss Expectorant Syrup 1106
Lortab 3315
Lortab Elixir 3312
Vicodin Tablets 530
Vicodin ES Tablets 531
Vicodin HP Tablets 532
Vicoprofen Tablets 533
Zydone Tablets 1118

Ibuprofen (Potential for drug-drug interaction with drugs affected by CYP450 enzymes). Products include:
Advil Allergy Sinus Caplets .... ▣737
Advil .... ▣737
Children's Advil Suspension .... ▣742
Children's Advil Chewable Tablets .. ▣741
Advil Cold & Sinus .... ▣739
Advil Flu & Body Ache Caplets .... ▣739
Children's Advil Cold Suspension ... ▣741
Infants' Advil Concentrated Drops .. ▣743
Junior Strength Advil Swallow Tablets .... ▣740
Advil Migraine Liquigels .... ▣740
Advil Multi-Symptom Cold Caplets .... ▣738
Combunox Tablets 1183
Children's Motrin Oral Suspension and Chewable Tablets 1837
Children's Motrin Cold Non-Staining Dye-Free Oral Suspension 1838
Children's Motrin Cold Oral Suspension 1838
Children's Motrin Non-Staining Dye-Free Oral Suspension 1837
Motrin Cold & Sinus Caplets 1836
Motrin IB Tablets and Caplets 1836
Infants' Motrin Concentrated Drops 1837
Infants' Motrin Non-Staining Dye-Free Drops 1837
Junior Strength Motrin Caplets and Chewable Tablets 1837
Vicoprofen Tablets 533

Imipramine Hydrochloride (Potential for drug-drug interaction with drugs affected by CYP450 enzymes).
No products indexed under this heading.

Imipramine Pamoate (Potential for drug-drug interaction with drugs affected by CYP450 enzymes).
No products indexed under this heading.

Indinavir Sulfate (Potential for drug-drug interaction with drugs affected by CYP450 enzymes). Products include:
Crixivan Capsules 1918

Indomethacin (Potential for drug-drug interaction with drugs affected by CYP450 enzymes). Products include:
Indocin 1968

Indomethacin Sodium Trihydrate (Potential for drug-drug interaction with drugs affected by CYP450 enzymes). Products include:
Indocin I.V. 1973

Indoramin Hydrochloride (Potential for drug-drug interaction with drugs affected by CYP450 enzymes).
No products indexed under this heading.

Irbesartan (Potential for drug-drug interaction with drugs affected by CYP450 enzymes). Products include:
Avalide Tablets 922
Avalide Tablets 2889
Avapro Tablets 925
Avapro Tablets 2886

Isotretinoin (Potential for drug-drug interaction with drugs affected by CYP450 enzymes). Products include:
Accutane Capsules 2740
Amnesteem Capsules 2126

Isradipine (Potential for drug-drug interaction with drugs affected by CYP450 enzymes). Products include:
DynaCirc CR Tablets 2726

Itraconazole (Potential for drug-drug interaction with drugs affected by CYP450 enzymes).
No products indexed under this heading.

Ketoconazole (Potential for drug-drug interaction with drugs affected by CYP450 enzymes). Products include:
Nizoral A-D Shampoo, 1% 1839
Nizoral 2% Shampoo 1838

Ketoprofen (Potential for drug-drug interaction with drugs affected by CYP450 enzymes).
No products indexed under this heading.

Ketorolac Tromethamine (Potential for drug-drug interaction with drugs affected by CYP450 enzymes). Products include:
Acular Ophthalmic Solution 561
Acular LS Ophthalmic Solution 562

Labetalol Hydrochloride (Potential for drug-drug interaction with drugs affected by CYP450 enzymes).
No products indexed under this heading.

Lamotrigine (Potential for drug-drug interaction with drugs affected by CYP450 enzymes). Products include:
Lamictal 1449

Lansoprazole (Potential for drug-drug interaction with drugs affected by CYP450 enzymes). Products include:
Prevacid Delayed-Release Capsules 3268
Prevacid for Delayed-Release Oral Suspension 3268
Prevacid I.V. for Injection 3274
Prevacid NapraPAC 3277
Prevacid SoluTab Delayed-Release Orally Disintegrating Tablets 3268
PREVPAC 3281

Levetiracetam (Potential for drug-drug interaction with drugs affected by CYP450 enzymes). Products include:

(▣ Described in PDR For Nonprescription Drugs)

(⊙ Described in PDR For Ophthalmic Medicines™)

Keppra Oral Solution 3307
Keppra Tablets 3307

Levobupivacaine Hydrochloride (Potential for drug-drug interaction with drugs affected by CYP450 enzymes).
No products indexed under this heading.

Levonorgestrel (Potential for drug-drug interaction with drugs affected by CYP450 enzymes). Products include:
Alesse-28 Tablets 3392
Climara Pro Transdermal System 800
Mirena Intrauterine System 810
Plan B Tablets 1068
Seasonale Tablets 1073
Triphasil-28 Tablets 3483

Lidocaine (Potential for drug-drug interaction with drugs affected by CYP450 enzymes). Products include:
Lidoderm Patch 1107

Lidocaine Base (Potential for drug-drug interaction with drugs affected by CYP450 enzymes).
No products indexed under this heading.

Lidocaine Hydrochloride (Potential for drug-drug interaction with drugs affected by CYP450 enzymes).
No products indexed under this heading.

Lomefloxacin Hydrochloride (Potential for drug-drug interaction with drugs affected by CYP450 enzymes).
No products indexed under this heading.

Losartan Potassium (Potential for drug-drug interaction with drugs affected by CYP450 enzymes). Products include:
Cozaar Tablets 1913
Hyzaar 1964

Lovastatin (Potential for drug-drug interaction with drugs affected by CYP450 enzymes). Products include:
Advicor Tablets 1694
Altoprev Extended-Release Tablets 1151
Mevacor Tablets 1996

Maprotiline Hydrochloride (Potential for drug-drug interaction with drugs affected by CYP450 enzymes).
No products indexed under this heading.

Meclofenamate Sodium (Potential for drug-drug interaction with drugs affected by CYP450 enzymes).
No products indexed under this heading.

Mefenamic Acid (Potential for drug-drug interaction with drugs affected by CYP450 enzymes).
No products indexed under this heading.

Meloxicam (Potential for drug-drug interaction with drugs affected by CYP450 enzymes). Products include:
Mobic Oral Suspension 893
Mobic Tablets 893

Meperidine Hydrochloride (Potential for drug-drug interaction with drugs affected by CYP450 enzymes).
No products indexed under this heading.

Mephenytoin (Potential for drug-drug interaction with drugs affected by CYP450 enzymes).
No products indexed under this heading.

Mephobarbital (Potential for drug-drug interaction with drugs affected by CYP450 enzymes). Products include:
Mebaral Tablets, USP 2483

Meprobamate (Potential for drug-drug interaction with drugs affected by CYP450 enzymes).
No products indexed under this heading.

Mestranol (Potential for drug-drug interaction with drugs affected by CYP450 enzymes).
No products indexed under this heading.

Metformin Hydrochloride (Potential for drug-drug interaction with drugs affected by CYP450 enzymes). Products include:
ActoPlus Met Tablets 3219
Avandamet Tablets 1343
Fortamet Extended-Release Tablets 1156

Methadone Hydrochloride (Potential for drug-drug interaction with drugs affected by CYP450 enzymes).
No products indexed under this heading.

Methamphetamine Hydrochloride (Potential for drug-drug interaction with drugs affected by CYP450 enzymes). Products include:
Desoxyn Tablets, USP 2482

Methsuximide (Potential for drug-drug interaction with drugs affected by CYP450 enzymes).
No products indexed under this heading.

Metoprolol Succinate (Potential for drug-drug interaction with drugs affected by CYP450 enzymes). Products include:
Toprol-XL Tablets 660

Metoprolol Tartrate (Potential for drug-drug interaction with drugs affected by CYP450 enzymes).
No products indexed under this heading.

Mexiletine Hydrochloride (Potential for drug-drug interaction with drugs affected by CYP450 enzymes).
No products indexed under this heading.

Midazolam Hydrochloride (Potential for drug-drug interaction with drugs affected by CYP450 enzymes).
No products indexed under this heading.

Miglitol (Potential for drug-drug interaction with drugs affected by CYP450 enzymes).
No products indexed under this heading.

Mirtazapine (Potential for drug-drug interaction with drugs affected by CYP450 enzymes).
No products indexed under this heading.

Montelukast Sodium (Potential for drug-drug interaction with drugs affected by CYP450 enzymes). Products include:
Singulair 2047

Morphine Sulfate (Potential for drug-drug interaction with drugs affected by CYP450 enzymes). Products include:
Avinza Capsules 1714
Kadian Capsules 572
MS Contin Tablets 2703

Moxifloxacin Hydrochloride (Potential for drug-drug interaction with drugs affected by CYP450 enzymes). Products include:
Avelox 2984
Vigamox Ophthalmic Solution 560

Nabumetone (Potential for drug-drug interaction with drugs affected by CYP450 enzymes). Products include:
Relafen Tablets 1523

Nafcillin Sodium (Potential for drug-drug interaction with drugs affected by CYP450 enzymes).
No products indexed under this heading.

Naproxen (Potential for drug-drug interaction with drugs affected by CYP450 enzymes). Products include:
EC-Naprosyn Delayed-Release Tablets 2769
Naprosyn Suspension 2769
Naprosyn Tablets 2769
Prevacid NapraPAC 3277

Naproxen Sodium (Potential for drug-drug interaction with drugs affected by CYP450 enzymes). Products include:
Aleve Tablets, Caplets and Gelcaps 605
Anaprox Tablets 2769
Anaprox DS Tablets 2769

Nateglinide (Potential for drug-drug interaction with drugs affected by CYP450 enzymes). Products include:
Starlix Tablets 2276

Nefazodone Hydrochloride (Potential for drug-drug interaction with drugs affected by CYP450 enzymes).
No products indexed under this heading.

Nelfinavir Mesylate (Potential for drug-drug interaction with drugs affected by CYP450 enzymes). Products include:
Viracept 2556

Nicardipine (Potential for drug-drug interaction with drugs affected by CYP450 enzymes).
No products indexed under this heading.

Nicardipine Hydrochloride (Potential for drug-drug interaction with drugs affected by CYP450 enzymes). Products include:
Cardene I.V. 1129

Nicotine Polacrilex (Potential for drug-drug interaction with drugs affected by CYP450 enzymes). Products include:
Commit Lozenges 1625
Nicorette Gum 1632

Nicotine Salicylate (Potential for drug-drug interaction with drugs affected by CYP450 enzymes).
No products indexed under this heading.

Nicotine Sulfate (Potential for drug-drug interaction with drugs affected by CYP450 enzymes).
No products indexed under this heading.

Nifedipine (Potential for drug-drug interaction with drugs affected by CYP450 enzymes). Products include:
Adalat CC Tablets 2978

Nilutamide (Potential for drug-drug interaction with drugs affected by CYP450 enzymes).
No products indexed under this heading.

Nimodipine (Potential for drug-drug interaction with drugs affected by CYP450 enzymes). Products include:
Nimotop Capsules 774

Nisoldipine (Potential for drug-drug interaction with drugs affected by CYP450 enzymes). Products include:
Sular Tablets 1163

Nitrendipine (Potential for drug-drug interaction with drugs affected by CYP450 enzymes).
No products indexed under this heading.

Norethindrone (Potential for drug-drug interaction with drugs affected by CYP450 enzymes). Products include:
Ortho Micronor Tablets 2411

Norethindrone Acetate (Potential for drug-drug interaction with drugs affected by CYP450 enzymes). Products include:
Activella Tablets 2311
Aygestin Tablets 1062
CombiPatch Transdermal System 2180

Norfloxacin (Potential for drug-drug interaction with drugs affected by CYP450 enzymes). Products include:
Noroxin Tablets 2009

Norgestrel (Potential for drug-drug interaction with drugs affected by CYP450 enzymes). Products include:
Lo/Ovral-28 Tablets 3423

Nortriptyline Hydrochloride (Potential for drug-drug interaction with drugs affected by CYP450 enzymes).
No products indexed under this heading.

Ofloxacin (Potential for drug-drug interaction with drugs affected by CYP450 enzymes). Products include:
Floxin Otic Singles 1045
Floxin Otic Solution 1043

Olanzapine (Potential for drug-drug interaction with drugs affected by CYP450 enzymes). Products include:
Symbyax Capsules 1788
Zyprexa Tablets 1798
Zyprexa IntraMuscular 1798
Zyprexa ZYDIS Orally Disintegrating Tablets 1798

Omeprazole (Potential for drug-drug interaction with drugs affected by CYP450 enzymes). Products include:
Zegerid Powder for Oral Solution 2972

Ondansetron (Potential for drug-drug interaction with drugs affected by CYP450 enzymes). Products include:
Zofran ODT Orally Disintegrating Tablets 1613

Ondansetron Hydrochloride (Potential for drug-drug interaction with drugs affected by CYP450 enzymes). Products include:
Zofran Injection 1607
Zofran 1613

Oxaprozin (Potential for drug-drug interaction with drugs affected by CYP450 enzymes).
No products indexed under this heading.

Oxcarbazepine (Potential for drug-drug interaction with drugs affected by CYP450 enzymes). Products include:
Trileptal Oral Suspension 2281
Trileptal Tablets 2281

Oxycodone Hydrochloride (Potential for drug-drug interaction with drugs affected by CYP450 enzymes). Products include:
- Combunox Tablets ... **1183**
- OxyContin Tablets ... **2699**
- OxyFast Oral Concentrate Solution ... **2704**
- OxyIR Capsules ... **2704**
- Percocet Tablets ... **1114**
- Percodan Tablets ... **1115**

Paclitaxel (Potential for drug-drug interaction with drugs affected by CYP450 enzymes).
No products indexed under this heading.

Pantoprazole Sodium (Potential for drug-drug interaction with drugs affected by CYP450 enzymes). Products include:
- Protonix I.V. ... **3468**
- Protonix Tablets ... **3465**

Paramethadione (Potential for drug-drug interaction with drugs affected by CYP450 enzymes).
No products indexed under this heading.

Paroxetine Hydrochloride (Potential for drug-drug interaction with drugs affected by CYP450 enzymes). Products include:
- Paxil CR Controlled-Release Tablets ... **1509**
- Paxil ... **1501**

Pentamidine Isethionate (Potential for drug-drug interaction with drugs affected by CYP450 enzymes).
No products indexed under this heading.

Phenacemide (Potential for drug-drug interaction with drugs affected by CYP450 enzymes).
No products indexed under this heading.

Phenobarbital (Potential for drug-drug interaction with drugs affected by CYP450 enzymes).
No products indexed under this heading.

Phenobarbital Sodium (Potential for drug-drug interaction with drugs affected by CYP450 enzymes).
No products indexed under this heading.

Phensuximide (Potential for drug-drug interaction with drugs affected by CYP450 enzymes).
No products indexed under this heading.

Phenylbutazone (Potential for drug-drug interaction with drugs affected by CYP450 enzymes).
No products indexed under this heading.

Phenytoin (Potential for drug-drug interaction with drugs affected by CYP450 enzymes).
No products indexed under this heading.

Phenytoin Sodium (Potential for drug-drug interaction with drugs affected by CYP450 enzymes). Products include:
- Phenytek Capsules ... **2153**

Pimozide (Potential for drug-drug interaction with drugs affected by CYP450 enzymes). Products include:
- Orap Tablets ... **1220**

Pindolol (Potential for drug-drug interaction with drugs affected by CYP450 enzymes).
No products indexed under this heading.

Pioglitazone Hydrochloride (Potential for drug-drug interaction with drugs affected by CYP450 enzymes). Products include:
- ActoPlus Met Tablets ... **3219**
- Actos Tablets ... **3224**

Piroxicam (Potential for drug-drug interaction with drugs affected by CYP450 enzymes).
No products indexed under this heading.

Polyestradiol Phosphate (Potential for drug-drug interaction with drugs affected by CYP450 enzymes).
No products indexed under this heading.

Primidone (Potential for drug-drug interaction with drugs affected by CYP450 enzymes).
No products indexed under this heading.

Progesterone (Potential for drug-drug interaction with drugs affected by CYP450 enzymes). Products include:
- Prochieve 4% Gel ... **1018**
- Prochieve 8% Gel ... **1018**
- Prometrium Capsules (100 mg, 200 mg) ... **3205**

Proguanil Hydrochloride (Potential for drug-drug interaction with drugs affected by CYP450 enzymes). Products include:
- Malarone Tablets ... **1484**
- Malarone Pediatric Tablets ... **1484**

Propafenone Hydrochloride (Potential for drug-drug interaction with drugs affected by CYP450 enzymes). Products include:
- Rythmol SR Capsules ... **2736**

Propoxyphene Hydrochloride (Potential for drug-drug interaction with drugs affected by CYP450 enzymes).
No products indexed under this heading.

Propoxyphene Napsylate (Potential for drug-drug interaction with drugs affected by CYP450 enzymes). Products include:
- Darvocet A 500 Tablets ... **3497**

Propranolol Hydrochloride (Potential for drug-drug interaction with drugs affected by CYP450 enzymes). Products include:
- Inderal LA Long-Acting Capsules ... **3421**
- InnoPran XL Capsules ... **2728**

Protriptyline Hydrochloride (Potential for drug-drug interaction with drugs affected by CYP450 enzymes). Products include:
- Vivactil Tablets ... **2350**

Quetiapine Fumarate (Potential for drug-drug interaction with drugs affected by CYP450 enzymes). Products include:
- Seroquel Tablets ... **691**

Quinidine Gluconate (Potential for drug-drug interaction with drugs affected by CYP450 enzymes).
No products indexed under this heading.

Quinidine Hydrochloride (Potential for drug-drug interaction with drugs affected by CYP450 enzymes).
No products indexed under this heading.

Quinidine Polygalacturonate (Potential for drug-drug interaction with drugs affected by CYP450 enzymes).
No products indexed under this heading.

Quinidine Sulfate (Potential for drug-drug interaction with drugs affected by CYP450 enzymes).
No products indexed under this heading.

Quinine (Potential for drug-drug interaction with drugs affected by CYP450 enzymes).
No products indexed under this heading.

Quinine Sulfate (Potential for drug-drug interaction with drugs affected by CYP450 enzymes).
No products indexed under this heading.

Rabeprazole Sodium (Potential for drug-drug interaction with drugs affected by CYP450 enzymes). Products include:
- Aciphex Tablets ... **1081**

Repaglinide (Potential for drug-drug interaction with drugs affected by CYP450 enzymes). Products include:
- Prandin Tablets (0.5, 1, and 2 mg) ... **2337**

Rifabutin (Potential for drug-drug interaction with drugs affected by CYP450 enzymes).
No products indexed under this heading.

Riluzole (Potential for drug-drug interaction with drugs affected by CYP450 enzymes). Products include:
- Rilutek Tablets ... **2945**

Risperidone (Potential for drug-drug interaction with drugs affected by CYP450 enzymes). Products include:
- Risperdal Consta Long-Acting Injection ... **1664**
- Risperdal M-Tab Orally Disintegrating Tablets ... **1658**
- Risperdal ... **1658**

Ritonavir (Potential for drug-drug interaction with drugs affected by CYP450 enzymes). Products include:
- Kaletra ... **474**
- Norvir ... **499**

Rofecoxib (Potential for drug-drug interaction with drugs affected by CYP450 enzymes).
No products indexed under this heading.

Ropinirole Hydrochloride (Potential for drug-drug interaction with drugs affected by CYP450 enzymes). Products include:
- Requip Tablets ... **1528**

Ropivacaine Hydrochloride (Potential for drug-drug interaction with drugs affected by CYP450 enzymes). Products include:
- Naropin Injection ... **640**

Rosiglitazone Maleate (Potential for drug-drug interaction with drugs affected by CYP450 enzymes). Products include:
- Avandamet Tablets ... **1343**
- Avandia Tablets ... **1348**

Saquinavir (Potential for drug-drug interaction with drugs affected by CYP450 enzymes).
No products indexed under this heading.

Saquinavir Mesylate (Potential for drug-drug interaction with drugs affected by CYP450 enzymes). Products include:
- Invirase ... **2776**

Sertraline Hydrochloride (Potential for drug-drug interaction with drugs affected by CYP450 enzymes). Products include:
- Zoloft ... **2581**

Sildenafil Citrate (Potential for drug-drug interaction with drugs affected by CYP450 enzymes). Products include:
- Revatio Tablets ... **2541**
- Viagra Tablets ... **2552**

Simvastatin (Potential for drug-drug interaction with drugs affected by CYP450 enzymes). Products include:
- Vytorin 10/10 Tablets ... **2084**
- Vytorin 10/10 Tablets ... **3092**
- Vytorin 10/20 Tablets ... **2084**
- Vytorin 10/20 Tablets ... **3092**
- Vytorin 10/40 Tablets ... **3092**
- Vytorin 10/40 Tablets ... **2084**
- Vytorin 10/80 Tablets ... **2084**
- Vytorin 10/80 Tablets ... **3092**
- Zocor Tablets ... **2078**

Sirolimus (Potential for drug-drug interaction with drugs affected by CYP450 enzymes). Products include:
- Rapamune Oral Solution and Tablets ... **3472**

Sulfamethoxazole (Potential for drug-drug interaction with drugs affected by CYP450 enzymes).
No products indexed under this heading.

Sulindac (Potential for drug-drug interaction with drugs affected by CYP450 enzymes). Products include:
- Clinoril Tablets ... **1899**

Suprofen (Potential for drug-drug interaction with drugs affected by CYP450 enzymes).
No products indexed under this heading.

Tacrine Hydrochloride (Potential for drug-drug interaction with drugs affected by CYP450 enzymes).
No products indexed under this heading.

Tacrolimus (Potential for drug-drug interaction with drugs affected by CYP450 enzymes). Products include:
- Prograf Capsules and Injection ... **624**
- Protopic Ointment ... **629**

Tamoxifen Citrate (Potential for drug-drug interaction with drugs affected by CYP450 enzymes).
No products indexed under this heading.

Telmisartan (Potential for drug-drug interaction with drugs affected by CYP450 enzymes). Products include:
- Micardis Tablets ... **884**
- Micardis HCT Tablets ... **886**

Teniposide (Potential for drug-drug interaction with drugs affected by CYP450 enzymes).
No products indexed under this heading.

Terfenadine (Potential for drug-drug interaction with drugs affected by CYP450 enzymes).
No products indexed under this heading.

Testosterone (Potential for drug-drug interaction with drugs affected by CYP450 enzymes). Products include:
- AndroGel ... **3330**
- Striant Mucoadhesive ... **1022**
- Testim 1% Gel ... **722**

Testosterone Cypionate (Potential for drug-drug interaction with drugs affected by CYP450 enzymes).
No products indexed under this heading.

Testosterone Enanthate (Potential for drug-drug interaction with drugs affected by CYP450 enzymes). Products include:
Delatestryl Injection 2976

Testosterone Propionate (Potential for drug-drug interaction with drugs affected by CYP450 enzymes).
No products indexed under this heading.

Theophylline (Potential for drug-drug interaction with drugs affected by CYP450 enzymes).
No products indexed under this heading.

Theophylline Anhydrous (Potential for drug-drug interaction with drugs affected by CYP450 enzymes). Products include:
Uniphyl Tablets 2708

Theophylline Sodium Glycinate (Potential for drug-drug interaction with drugs affected by CYP450 enzymes).
No products indexed under this heading.

Thioridazine (Potential for drug-drug interaction with drugs affected by CYP450 enzymes).
No products indexed under this heading.

Thioridazine Hydrochloride (Potential for drug-drug interaction with drugs affected by CYP450 enzymes). Products include:
Thioridazine Hydrochloride Tablets 2122

Tiagabine Hydrochloride (Potential for drug-drug interaction with drugs affected by CYP450 enzymes). Products include:
Gabitril Tablets 998

Timolol Maleate (Potential for drug-drug interaction with drugs affected by CYP450 enzymes). Products include:
Blocadren Tablets 1891
Cosopt Sterile Ophthalmic Solution 1910
Timolide Tablets 2056
Timoptic in Ocudose 2061
Timoptic Sterile Ophthalmic Solution 2058
Timoptic-XE Sterile Ophthalmic Gel Forming Solution 2062

Tolazamide (Potential for drug-drug interaction with drugs affected by CYP450 enzymes).
No products indexed under this heading.

Tolbutamide (Potential for drug-drug interaction with drugs affected by CYP450 enzymes).
No products indexed under this heading.

Tolbutamide Sodium (Potential for drug-drug interaction with drugs affected by CYP450 enzymes).
No products indexed under this heading.

Tolmetin Sodium (Potential for drug-drug interaction with drugs affected by CYP450 enzymes).
No products indexed under this heading.

Tolterodine Tartrate (Potential for drug-drug interaction with drugs affected by CYP450 enzymes). Products include:
Detrol Tablets 2626
Detrol LA Capsules 2629

Topiramate (Potential for drug-drug interaction with drugs affected by CYP450 enzymes). Products include:
Topamax Sprinkle Capsules 2438
Topamax Tablets 2438

Torsemide (Potential for drug-drug interaction with drugs affected by CYP450 enzymes).
No products indexed under this heading.

Tramadol Hydrochloride (Potential for drug-drug interaction with drugs affected by CYP450 enzymes). Products include:
Ultracet Tablets 2462

Trazodone Hydrochloride (Potential for drug-drug interaction with drugs affected by CYP450 enzymes).
No products indexed under this heading.

Tretinoin (Potential for drug-drug interaction with drugs affected by CYP450 enzymes). Products include:
Avita Cream 2136
Avita Gel 2138
Renova 0.02% Cream 2384
Renova 0.05% Cream 2387
Retin-A Micro 0.1%/0.04% 2388
Solage Topical Solution 740
Tri-Luma Cream 1213
Vesanoid Capsules 2823

Triazolam (Potential for drug-drug interaction with drugs affected by CYP450 enzymes).
No products indexed under this heading.

Trimethadione (Potential for drug-drug interaction with drugs affected by CYP450 enzymes).
No products indexed under this heading.

Trimethaphan Camsylate (Potential for drug-drug interaction with drugs affected by CYP450 enzymes).
No products indexed under this heading.

Trimipramine Maleate (Potential for drug-drug interaction with drugs affected by CYP450 enzymes). Products include:
Surmontil Capsules 2347

Troglitazone (Potential for drug-drug interaction with drugs affected by CYP450 enzymes).
No products indexed under this heading.

Trovafloxacin Mesylate (Potential for drug-drug interaction with drugs affected by CYP450 enzymes).
No products indexed under this heading.

Valdecoxib (Potential for drug-drug interaction with drugs affected by CYP450 enzymes).
No products indexed under this heading.

Valproate Sodium (Potential for drug-drug interaction with drugs affected by CYP450 enzymes). Products include:
Depacon Injection 412

Valproic Acid (Potential for drug-drug interaction with drugs affected by CYP450 enzymes). Products include:
Depakene 417

Valsartan (Potential for drug-drug interaction with drugs affected by CYP450 enzymes). Products include:
Diovan HCT Tablets 2195
Diovan Tablets 2191

Venlafaxine Hydrochloride (Potential for drug-drug interaction with drugs affected by CYP450 enzymes). Products include:
Effexor Tablets 3405
Effexor XR Capsules 3411

Verapamil Hydrochloride (Potential for drug-drug interaction with drugs affected by CYP450 enzymes). Products include:
Covera-HS Tablets 3135
Tarka Tablets 519
Verelan PM Capsules 3120

Vinblastine Sulfate (Potential for drug-drug interaction with drugs affected by CYP450 enzymes).
No products indexed under this heading.

Vincristine Sulfate (Potential for drug-drug interaction with drugs affected by CYP450 enzymes).
No products indexed under this heading.

Vitamin A (Potential for drug-drug interaction with drugs affected by CYP450 enzymes). Products include:
Visutein Capsules 3328

Vitamin A Acetate (Potential for drug-drug interaction with drugs affected by CYP450 enzymes).
No products indexed under this heading.

Voriconazole (Potential for drug-drug interaction with drugs affected by CYP450 enzymes). Products include:
VFEND I.V. 2543
VFEND Oral Suspension 2543
VFEND Tablets 2543

Warfarin Sodium (Potential for drug-drug interaction with drugs affected by CYP450 enzymes). Products include:
Coumadin for Injection 932
Coumadin Tablets 932

Zafirlukast (Potential for drug-drug interaction with drugs affected by CYP450 enzymes). Products include:
Accolate Tablets 663

Zileuton (Potential for drug-drug interaction with drugs affected by CYP450 enzymes).
No products indexed under this heading.

Zolmitriptan (Potential for drug-drug interaction with drugs affected by CYP450 enzymes). Products include:
Zomig Nasal Spray 718
Zomig Tablets 714
Zomig-ZMT Tablets 714

Zonisamide (Potential for drug-drug interaction with drugs affected by CYP450 enzymes). Products include:
Zonegran Capsules 1089

Zopiclone (Potential for drug-drug interaction with drugs affected by CYP450 enzymes).
No products indexed under this heading.

NABI-HB

(Hepatitis B Immune Globulin (Human)) 2159
May interact with:

Mumps Virus Vaccine, Live (H-BIG may interfere with the immune response to vaccination, therefore, vaccination with live virus vaccine should be deferred until approximately 3 months). Products include:
Mumpsvax 2005

Rubella & Mumps Virus Vaccine Live (H-BIG may interfere with the immune response to vaccination, therefore, vaccination with live virus vaccine should be deferred until approximately 3 months).
No products indexed under this heading.

Rubella Virus Vaccine Live (H-BIG may interfere with the immune response to vaccination, therefore, vaccination with live virus vaccine should be deferred until approximately 3 months). Products include:
Meruvax II 1994

NADOLOL TABLETS

(Nadolol) 2121
May interact with general anesthetics, oral hypoglycemic agents, insulin, and certain other agents. Compounds in these categories include:

Acarbose (Beta-adrenergic blockade may prevent the appearance of premonitory signs and symptoms, such as tachycardia and blood pressure changes, of acute hypoglycemia; beta-blockade also reduces the release of insulin in response to hyperglycemia; adjust dosage of oral antidiabetic drugs). Products include:
Precose Tablets 776

Chlorpropamide (Beta-adrenergic blockade may prevent the appearance of premonitory signs and symptoms, such as tachycardia and blood pressure changes, of acute hypoglycemia; beta-blockade also reduces the release of insulin in response to hyperglycemia; adjust dosage of oral antidiabetic drugs).
No products indexed under this heading.

Enflurane (Co-administration may result in exaggeration of the hypotension induced by general anesthetics).
No products indexed under this heading.

Epinephrine (Patients with a history of severe anaphylactic reaction to variety of allergens may be more reactive to repeated challenge; potential for unresponsiveness to the usual dose of epinephrine). Products include:
EpiPen 1061
Primatene Mist 749

Epinephrine Hydrochloride (Patients with a history of severe anaphylactic reaction to variety of allergens may be more reactive to repeated challenge; potential for unresponsiveness to the usual dose of epinephrine).
No products indexed under this heading.

Glimepiride (Beta-adrenergic blockade may prevent the appearance of premonitory signs and symptoms, such as tachycardia and blood pressure changes, of acute hypoglycemia; beta-blockade also reduces the release of insulin in response to hyperglycemia; adjust dosage of oral antidiabetic drugs). Products include:
Amaryl Tablets 2864

Glipizide (Beta-adrenergic blockade may prevent the appearance of premonitory signs and symptoms, such as tachycardia and blood pressure changes, of acute hypoglycemia; beta-blockade also reduces the release of insulin in response to hyperglycemia; adjust dosage of oral antidiabetic drugs).
No products indexed under this heading.

Glyburide (Beta-adrenergic blockade may prevent the appearance of premonitory signs and symptoms, such as tachycardia and blood pressure changes, of acute hypoglycemia; beta-blockade also reduces the release of insulin in response to hyperglycemia; adjust dosage of oral antidiabetic drugs).
No products indexed under this heading.

Insulin, Human, Zinc Suspension (Beta-adrenergic blockade may prevent the appearance of premonitory signs and symptoms, such as tachycardia and blood pressure changes, of acute hypoglycemia; beta-blockade also reduces the release of insulin in response to hyperglycemia; adjust dosage of insulin). Products include:
Humulin L, 100 Units 1763
Humulin U, 100 Units 1770

Insulin, Human NPH (Beta-adrenergic blockade may prevent the appearance of premonitory signs and symptoms, such as tachycardia and blood pressure changes, of acute hypoglycemia; beta-blockade also reduces the release of insulin in response to hyperglycemia; adjust dosage of insulin). Products include:
Humulin N, 100 Units 1764
Humulin N Pen 1765
Novolin N Human Insulin 10 ml Vials 2322
Novolin N InnoLet 2322
Novolin N PenFill 3 ml Cartridges 2325
Novolin R InnoLet 2322

Insulin, Human Regular (Beta-adrenergic blockade may prevent the appearance of premonitory signs and symptoms, such as tachycardia and blood pressure changes, of acute hypoglycemia; beta-blockade also reduces the release of insulin in response to hyperglycemia; adjust dosage of insulin). Products include:
Humulin R (U-500) 1768
Humulin R, 100 Units 1767
Novolin R Human Insulin 10 ml Vials 2322
Novolin R PenFill 2325

Insulin, Human Regular and Human NPH Mixture (Beta-adrenergic blockade may prevent the appearance of premonitory signs and symptoms, such as tachycardia and blood pressure changes, of acute hypoglycemia; beta-blockade also reduces the release of insulin in response to hyperglycemia; adjust dosage of insulin). Products include:
Humulin 50/50, 100 Units 1760
Humulin 70/30 Pen 1761
Novolin 70/30 Human Insulin 10 ml Vials 2321
Novolin 70/30 InnoLet 2322
Novolin 70/30 PenFill 3 ml Cartridges 2325

Insulin, NPH (Beta-adrenergic blockade may prevent the appearance of premonitory signs and symptoms, such as tachycardia and blood pressure changes, of acute hypoglycemia; beta-blockade also reduces the release of insulin in response to hyperglycemia; adjust dosage of insulin).
No products indexed under this heading.

Insulin, Regular (Beta-adrenergic blockade may prevent the appearance of premonitory signs and symptoms, such as tachycardia and blood pressure changes, of acute hypoglycemia; beta-blockade also reduces the release of insulin in response to hyperglycemia; adjust dosage of insulin).
No products indexed under this heading.

Insulin, Zinc Crystals (Beta-adrenergic blockade may prevent the appearance of premonitory signs and symptoms, such as tachycardia and blood pressure changes, of acute hypoglycemia; beta-blockade also reduces the release of insulin in response to hyperglycemia; adjust dosage of insulin).
No products indexed under this heading.

Insulin, Zinc Suspension (Beta-adrenergic blockade may prevent the appearance of premonitory signs and symptoms, such as tachycardia and blood pressure changes, of acute hypoglycemia; beta-blockade also reduces the release of insulin in response to hyperglycemia; adjust dosage of insulin).
No products indexed under this heading.

Insulin Aspart, Human Regular (Beta-adrenergic blockade may prevent the appearance of premonitory signs and symptoms, such as tachycardia and blood pressure changes, of acute hypoglycemia; beta-blockade also reduces the release of insulin in response to hyperglycemia; adjust dosage of insulin). Products include:
NovoLog Injection 2326

Insulin glargine (Beta-adrenergic blockade may prevent the appearance of premonitory signs and symptoms, such as tachycardia and blood pressure changes, of acute hypoglycemia; beta-blockade also reduces the release of insulin in response to hyperglycemia; adjust dosage of insulin). Products include:
Lantus Injection 2925

Insulin Lispro, Human (Beta-adrenergic blockade may prevent the appearance of premonitory signs and symptoms, such as tachycardia and blood pressure changes, of acute hypoglycemia; beta-blockade also reduces the release of insulin in response to hyperglycemia; adjust dosage of insulin). Products include:
Humalog-Pen 1751
Humalog Mix 75/25-Pen 1754

Insulin Lispro Protamine, Human (Beta-adrenergic blockade may prevent the appearance of premonitory signs and symptoms, such as tachycardia and blood pressure changes, of acute hypoglycemia; beta-blockade also reduces the release of insulin in response to hyperglycemia; adjust dosage of insulin). Products include:
Humalog Mix 75/25-Pen 1754

Isoflurane (Co-administration may result in exaggeration of the hypotension induced by general anesthetics).
No products indexed under this heading.

Ketamine Hydrochloride (Co-administration may result in exaggeration of the hypotension induced by general anesthetics).
No products indexed under this heading.

Metformin Hydrochloride (Beta-adrenergic blockade may prevent the appearance of premonitory signs and symptoms, such as tachycardia and blood pressure changes, of acute hypoglycemia; beta-blockade also reduces the release of insulin in response to hyperglycemia; adjust dosage of oral antidiabetic drugs). Products include:
ActoPlus Met Tablets 3219
Avandamet Tablets 1343
Fortamet Extended-Release Tablets 1156

Methohexital Sodium (Co-administration may result in exaggeration of the hypotension induced by general anesthetics).
No products indexed under this heading.

Methoxyflurane (Co-administration may result in exaggeration of the hypotension induced by general anesthetics).
No products indexed under this heading.

Miglitol (Beta-adrenergic blockade may prevent the appearance of premonitory signs and symptoms, such as tachycardia and blood pressure changes, of acute hypoglycemia; beta-blockade also reduces the release of insulin in response to hyperglycemia; adjust dosage of oral antidiabetic drugs).
No products indexed under this heading.

Pioglitazone Hydrochloride (Beta-adrenergic blockade may prevent the appearance of premonitory signs and symptoms, such as tachycardia and blood pressure changes, of acute hypoglycemia; beta-blockade also reduces the release of insulin in response to hyperglycemia; adjust dosage of oral antidiabetic drugs). Products include:
ActoPlus Met Tablets 3219
Actos Tablets 3224

Propofol (Co-administration may result in exaggeration of the hypotension induced by general anesthetics). Products include:
Diprivan Injectable Emulsion 676

Repaglinide (Beta-adrenergic blockade may prevent the appearance of premonitory signs and symptoms, such as tachycardia and blood pressure changes, of acute hypoglycemia; beta-blockade also reduces the release of insulin in response to hyperglycemia; adjust dosage of oral antidiabetic drugs). Products include:
Prandin Tablets (0.5, 1, and 2 mg) 2337

Reserpine (Potential for additive effects resulting in hypotension and/or excessive bradycardia (vertigo, syncope, postural hypotension)).
No products indexed under this heading.

Rosiglitazone Maleate (Beta-adrenergic blockade may prevent the appearance of premonitory signs and symptoms, such as tachycardia and blood pressure changes, of acute hypoglycemia; beta-blockade also reduces the release of insulin in response to hyperglycemia; adjust dosage of oral antidiabetic drugs). Products include:
Avandamet Tablets 1343
Avandia Tablets 1348

Sevoflurane (Co-administration may result in exaggeration of the hypotension induced by general anesthetics). Products include:
Ultane Liquid for Inhalation 526

Tolazamide (Beta-adrenergic blockade may prevent the appearance of premonitory signs and symptoms, such as tachycardia and blood pressure changes, of acute hypoglycemia; beta-blockade also reduces the release of insulin in response to hyperglycemia; adjust dosage of oral antidiabetic drugs).
No products indexed under this heading.

Tolbutamide (Beta-adrenergic blockade may prevent the appearance of premonitory signs and symptoms, such as tachycardia and blood pressure changes, of acute hypoglycemia; beta-blockade also reduces the release of insulin in response to hyperglycemia; adjust dosage of oral antidiabetic drugs).
No products indexed under this heading.

Troglitazone (Beta-adrenergic blockade may prevent the appearance of premonitory signs and symptoms, such as tachycardia and blood pressure changes, of acute hypoglycemia; beta-blockade also reduces the release of insulin in response to hyperglycemia; adjust dosage of oral antidiabetic drugs).
No products indexed under this heading.

NAFTIN CREAM

(Naftifine Hydrochloride) 2097
None cited in PDR database.

NAFTIN GEL

(Naftifine Hydrochloride) 2097
None cited in PDR database.

NALFON CAPSULES

(Fenoprofen Calcium) 2504
May interact with oral anticoagulants, hydantoin anticonvulsants, loop diuretics, salicylates, sulfonamides, sulfonylureas, and certain other agents. Compounds in these categories include:

Anisindione (In patients receiving coumarin-type anticoagulants, the addition of fenoprofen calcium to therapy could prolong the prothrombin time. Patients receiving both drugs should be under careful observation). Products include:
Miradon Tablets 3056

Aspirin (The co-administration of aspirin decreases the biologic half-life of fenoprofen because of an increase in metabolic clearance that results in a greater amount of hydroxylated fenoprofen in the urine. Although the mechanism of interaction between fenoprofen and aspirin is not totally known, enzyme induction and displacement of fenoprofen from plasma albumin binding sites are possibilities. Because fenoprofen

calcium has not been shown to produce any additional effect beyond that obtained with aspirin alone and because aspirin increases the rate of excretion of fenoprofen calcium, concomitant use of fenoprofen calcium and salicylates is not recommended). Products include:

- Aggrenox Capsules 855
- Bayer, Aspirin Regimen 606
- Bayer Aspirin Tablets 3515
- BC Powder 612
- BC Allergy Sinus Cold Powder 612
- Arthritis Strength BC Powder 612
- BC Sinus Cold Powder 612
- Ecotrin Enteric Coated Aspirin Low, Regular and Maximum Strength Tablets 1627
- Goody's Body Pain Formula Powder 621
- Goody's Extra Strength Headache Powder 621
- Goody's Extra Strength Pain Relief Tablets 621
- Percodan Tablets 1115
- St. Joseph 81 mg Aspirin Chewable and Enteric Coated Tablets 1841

Aspirin, Enteric Coated (The co-administration of aspirin decreases the biologic half-life of fenoprofen because of an increase in metabolic clearance that results in a greater amount of hydroxylated fenoprofen in the urine. Although the mechanism of interaction between fenoprofen and aspirin is not totally known, enzyme induction and displacement of fenoprofen from plasma albumin binding sites are possibilities. Because fenoprofen calcium has not been shown to produce any additional effect beyond that obtained with aspirin alone and because aspirin increases the rate of excretion of fenoprofen calcium, concomitant use of fenoprofen calcium and salicylates is not recommended).

No products indexed under this heading.

Aspirin Buffered (The co-administration of aspirin decreases the biologic half-life of fenoprofen because of an increase in metabolic clearance that results in a greater amount of hydroxylated fenoprofen in the urine. Although the mechanism of interaction between fenoprofen and aspirin is not totally known, enzyme induction and displacement of fenoprofen from plasma albumin binding sites are possibilities. Because fenoprofen calcium has not been shown to produce any additional effect beyond that obtained with aspirin alone and because aspirin increases the rate of excretion of fenoprofen calcium, concomitant use of fenoprofen calcium and salicylates is not recommended).

No products indexed under this heading.

Bendroflumethiazide (In vitro studies have shown that fenoprofen, because of its affinity for albumin, may displace from their bindings sites other drugs that are also albumin bound, and this may lead to drug interaction. Theoretically, fenoprofen could likewise be displayed. Patients receiving sulfonamides should be observed for increased activity of these drugs and, therefore, signs of toxicity from these drugs).

No products indexed under this heading.

Bumetanide (Patients treated with fenoprofen calcium may be resistant to the effects of loop diuretics).

No products indexed under this heading.

Chlorothiazide (In vitro studies have shown that fenoprofen, because of its affinity for albumin, may displace from their bindings sites other drugs that are also albumin bound, and this may lead to drug interaction. Theoretically, fenoprofen could likewise be displayed. Patients receiving sulfonamides should be observed for increased activity of these drugs and, therefore, signs of toxicity from these drugs). Products include:

- Aldoclor Tablets 1881
- Diuril Oral 1936

Chlorothiazide Sodium (In vitro studies have shown that fenoprofen, because of its affinity for albumin, may displace from their bindings sites other drugs that are also albumin bound, and this may lead to drug interaction. Theoretically, fenoprofen could likewise be displayed. Patients receiving sulfonamides should be observed for increased activity of these drugs and, therefore, signs of toxicity from these drugs). Products include:

- Diuril Sodium Intravenous 1934

Chlorpropamide (In vitro studies have shown that fenoprofen, because of its affinity for albumin, may displace from their bindings sites other drugs that are also albumin bound, and this may lead to drug interaction. Theoretically, fenoprofen could likewise be displayed. Patients receiving sulfonamides should be observed for increased activity of these drugs and, therefore, signs of toxicity from these drugs).

No products indexed under this heading.

Choline Magnesium Trisalicylate (The co-administration of aspirin decreases the biologic half-life of fenoprofen because of an increase in metabolic clearance that results in a greater amount of hydroxylated fenoprofen in the urine. Although the mechanism of interaction between fenoprofen and aspirin is not totally known, enzyme induction and displacement of fenoprofen from plasma albumin binding sites are possibilities. Because fenoprofen calcium has not been shown to produce any additional effect beyond that obtained with aspirin alone and because aspirin increases the rate of excretion of fenoprofen calcium, concomitant use of fenoprofen calcium and salicylates is not recommended).

No products indexed under this heading.

Dicumarol (In patients receiving coumarin-type anticoagulants, the addition of fenoprofen calcium to therapy could prolong the prothrombin time. Patients receiving both drugs should be under careful observation).

No products indexed under this heading.

Diflunisal (The co-administration of aspirin decreases the biologic half-life of fenoprofen because of an increase in metabolic clearance that results in a greater amount of hydroxylated fenoprofen in the urine. Although the mechanism of interaction between fenoprofen and aspirin is not totally known, enzyme induction and displacement of fenoprofen from plasma albumin binding sites are possibilities. Because fenoprofen calcium has not been shown to produce any additional effect beyond that obtained with aspirin alone and because aspirin increases the rate of excretion of fenoprofen calcium, concomitant use of fenoprofen calcium and salicylates is not recommended). Products include:

- Dolobid Tablets 1937

Ethacrynic Acid (Patients treated with fenoprofen calcium may be resistant to the effects of loop diuretics). Products include:

- Edecrin Tablets 1941

Ethotoin (In vitro studies have shown that fenoprofen, because of its affinity for albumin, may displace from their binding sites other drugs that are also albumin bound, and this may lead to drug interaction. Theoretically, fenoprofen could likewise be displayed.Patients receiving hydantins should be observed for increased activity drugs and, therefore, signs of toxicity from these drugs). Products include:

- Peganone Tablets, USP 2487

Fosphenytoin Sodium (In vitro studies have shown that fenoprofen, because of its affinity for albumin, may displace from their binding sites other drugs that are also albumin bound, and this may lead to drug interaction. Theoretically, fenoprofen could likewise be displayed.Patients receiving hydantins should be observed for increased activity drugs and, therefore, signs of toxicity from these drugs).

No products indexed under this heading.

Furosemide (Patients treated with fenoprofen calcium may be resistant to the effects of loop diuretics). Products include:

- Furosemide Tablets 2117

Glimepiride (In vitro studies have shown that fenoprofen, because of its affinity for albumin, may displace from their bindings sites other drugs that are also albumin bound, and this may lead to drug interaction. Theoretically, fenoprofen could likewise be displayed. Patients receiving sulfonylureas should be observed for increased activity of these drugs and, therefore, signs of toxicity from these drugs). Products include:

- Amaryl Tablets 2864

Glipizide (In vitro studies have shown that fenoprofen, because of its affinity for albumin, may displace from their bindings sites other drugs that are also albumin bound, and this may lead to drug interaction. Theoretically, fenoprofen could likewise be displayed. Patients receiving sulfonamides should be observed for increased activity of these drugs and, therefore, signs of toxicity from these drugs).

No products indexed under this heading.

Glyburide (In vitro studies have shown that fenoprofen, because of its affinity for albumin, may displace from their bindings sites other drugs that are also albumin bound, and this may lead to drug interaction. Theoretically, fenoprofen could likewise be displayed. Patients receiving sulfonamides should be observed for increased activity of these drugs and, therefore, signs of toxicity from these drugs).

No products indexed under this heading.

Hydrochlorothiazide (In vitro studies have shown that fenoprofen, because of its affinity for albumin, may displace from their bindings sites other drugs that are also albumin bound, and this may lead to drug interaction. Theoretically, fenoprofen could likewise be displayed. Patients receiving sulfonamides should be observed for increased activity of these drugs and, therefore, signs of toxicity from these drugs). Products include:

- Aldoril Tablets 1884
- Atacand HCT 637
- Avalide Tablets 2889
- Avalide Tablets 922
- Benicar HCT Tablets 2852
- Diovan HCT Tablets 2195
- Dyazide Capsules 1389
- Hyzaar 1964
- Lotensin HCT Tablets 2235
- Maxzide 2150
- Micardis HCT Tablets 886
- Moduretic Tablets 2003
- Prinzide Tablets 2033
- Teveten HCT Tablets 1710
- Timolide Tablets 2056
- Uniretic Tablets 3114
- Vaseretic Tablets 2073
- Zestoretic Tablets 701

Hydroflumethiazide (In vitro studies have shown that fenoprofen, because of its affinity for albumin, may displace from their bindings sites other drugs that are also albumin bound, and this may lead to drug interaction. Theoretically, fenoprofen could likewise be displayed. Patients receiving sulfonamides should be observed for increased activity of these drugs and, therefore, signs of toxicity from these drugs).

No products indexed under this heading.

Magnesium Salicylate (The co-administration of aspirin decreases the biologic half-life of fenoprofen because of an increase in metabolic clearance that results in a greater amount of hydroxylated fenoprofen in the urine. Although the mechanism of interaction between fenoprofen and aspirin is not totally known, enzyme induction and displacement of fenoprofen from plasma albumin binding sites are possibilities. Because fenoprofen calcium has not been shown to produce any additional effect beyond that obtained with aspirin alone and because aspirin increases the rate of excretion of fenoprofen calcium, concomitant use of fenoprofen calcium and salicylates is not recommended).

No products indexed under this heading.

Mephenytoin (In vitro studies have shown that fenoprofen, because of its affinity for albumin, may displace from their binding sites other drugs that are also albumin bound, and this may lead to drug interaction. Theoretically, fenoprofen could likewise be displayed.Patients receiving hydantins should be observed for increased activity drugs and, therefore, signs of toxicity from these drugs).

No products indexed under this heading.

Methyclothiazide (In vitro studies have shown that fenoprofen, because of its affinity for albumin,

may displace from their bindings sites other drugs that are also albumin bound, and this may lead to drug interaction. Theoretically, fenoprofen could likewise be displayed. Patients receiving sulfonamides should be observed for increased activity of these drugs and, therefore, signs of toxicity from these drugs).
No products indexed under this heading.

Phenobarbital (Chronic administration of phenobarbital, a known enzyme inducer, may be associated with a decrease in the plasma half-life of fenoprofen. When phenobarbital is added to or withdrawn from treatment, dosage adjustment of fenoprofen calcium may be required).
No products indexed under this heading.

Phenobarbital Sodium (Chronic administration of phenobarbital, a known enzyme inducer, may be associated with a decrease in the plasma half-life of fenoprofen. When phenobarbital is added to or withdrawn from treatment, dosage adjustment of fenoprofen calcium may be required).
No products indexed under this heading.

Phenytoin (In vitro studies have shown that fenoprofen, because of its affinity for albumin, may displace from their binding sites other drugs that are also albumin bound, and this may lead to drug interaction. Theoretically, fenoprofen could likewise be displayed.Patients receiving hydantins should be observed for increased activity drugs and, therefore, signs of toxicity from these drugs).
No products indexed under this heading.

Phenytoin Sodium (In vitro studies have shown that fenoprofen, because of its affinity for albumin, may displace from their binding sites other drugs that are also albumin bound, and this may lead to drug interaction. Theoretically, fenoprofen could likewise be displayed.Patients receiving hydantins should be observed for increased activity drugs and, therefore, signs of toxicity from these drugs). Products include:
Phenytek Capsules 2153

Polythiazide (In vitro studies have shown that fenoprofen, because of its affinity for albumin, may displace from their bindings sites other drugs that are also albumin bound, and this may lead to drug interaction. Theoretically, fenoprofen could likewise be displayed. Patients receiving sulfonamides should be observed for increased activity of these drugs and, therefore, signs of toxicity from these drugs).
No products indexed under this heading.

Salsalate (The co-administration of aspirin decreases the biologic half-life of fenoprofen because of an increase in metabolic clearance that results in a greater amount of hydroxylated fenoprofen in the urine. Although the mechanism of interaction between fenoprofen and aspirin is not totally known, enzyme induction and displacement of fenoprofen from plasma albumin binding sites are possibilities. Because fenoprofen calcium has not been shown to produce any additional effect beyond that obtained with aspirin alone and because aspirin increases the rate of excretion of fenoprofen calcium, concomitant use of fenoprofen calcium and salicylates is not recommended).
No products indexed under this heading.

Sulfacytine (In vitro studies have shown that fenoprofen, because of its affinity for albumin, may displace from their bindings sites other drugs that are also albumin bound, and this may lead to drug interaction. Theoretically, fenoprofen could likewise be displayed. Patients receiving sulfonamides should be observed for increased activity of these drugs and, therefore, signs of toxicity from these drugs).
No products indexed under this heading.

Sulfamethizole (In vitro studies have shown that fenoprofen, because of its affinity for albumin, may displace from their bindings sites other drugs that are also albumin bound, and this may lead to drug interaction. Theoretically, fenoprofen could likewise be displayed. Patients receiving sulfonamides should be observed for increased activity of these drugs and, therefore, signs of toxicity from these drugs).
No products indexed under this heading.

Sulfamethoxazole (In vitro studies have shown that fenoprofen, because of its affinity for albumin, may displace from their bindings sites other drugs that are also albumin bound, and this may lead to drug interaction. Theoretically, fenoprofen could likewise be displayed. Patients receiving sulfonamides should be observed for increased activity of these drugs and, therefore, signs of toxicity from these drugs).
No products indexed under this heading.

Sulfasalazine (In vitro studies have shown that fenoprofen, because of its affinity for albumin, may displace from their bindings sites other drugs that are also albumin bound, and this may lead to drug interaction. Theoretically, fenoprofen could likewise be displayed. Patients receiving sulfonamides should be observed for increased activity of these drugs and, therefore, signs of toxicity from these drugs).
No products indexed under this heading.

Sulfinpyrazone (In vitro studies have shown that fenoprofen, because of its affinity for albumin, may displace from their bindings sites other drugs that are also albumin bound, and this may lead to drug interaction. Theoretically, fenoprofen could likewise be displayed. Patients receiving sulfonamides should be observed for increased activity of these drugs and, therefore, signs of toxicity from these drugs).
No products indexed under this heading.

Sulfisoxazole (In vitro studies have shown that fenoprofen, because of its affinity for albumin, may displace from their bindings sites other drugs that are also albumin bound, and this may lead to drug interaction. Theoretically, fenoprofen could likewise be displayed. Patients receiving sulfonamides should be observed for increased activity of these drugs and, therefore, signs of toxicity from these drugs).
No products indexed under this heading.

Sulfisoxazole Acetyl (In vitro studies have shown that fenoprofen, because of its affinity for albumin, may displace from their bindings sites other drugs that are also albumin bound, and this may lead to drug interaction. Theoretically, fenoprofen could likewise be displayed. Patients receiving sulfonamides should be observed for increased activity of these drugs and, therefore, signs of toxicity from these drugs).
No products indexed under this heading.

Sulfisoxazole Diolamine (In vitro studies have shown that fenoprofen, because of its affinity for albumin, may displace from their bindings sites other drugs that are also albumin bound, and this may lead to drug interaction. Theoretically, fenoprofen could likewise be displayed. Patients receiving sulfonamides should be observed for increased activity of these drugs and, therefore, signs of toxicity from these drugs).
No products indexed under this heading.

Tolazamide (In vitro studies have shown that fenoprofen, because of its affinity for albumin, may displace from their bindings sites other drugs that are also albumin bound, and this may lead to drug interaction. Theoretically, fenoprofen could likewise be displayed. Patients receiving sulfonamides should be observed for increased activity of these drugs and, therefore, signs of toxicity from these drugs).
No products indexed under this heading.

Tolbutamide (In vitro studies have shown that fenoprofen, because of its affinity for albumin, may displace from their bindings sites other drugs that are also albumin bound, and this may lead to drug interaction. Theoretically, fenoprofen could likewise be displayed. Patients receiving sulfonamides should be observed for increased activity of these drugs and, therefore, signs of toxicity from these drugs).
No products indexed under this heading.

Torsemide (Patients treated with fenoprofen calcium may be resistant to the effects of loop diuretics).
No products indexed under this heading.

Warfarin Sodium (In patients receiving coumarin-type anticoagulants, the addition of fenoprofen calcium to therapy could prolong the prothrombin time. Patients receiving both drugs should be under careful observation). Products include:
Coumadin for Injection 932
Coumadin Tablets 932

NAMENDA ORAL SOLUTION

(Memantine Hydrochloride) 1199
See Namenda Tablets

NAMENDA TABLETS

(Memantine Hydrochloride) 1199
May interact with carbonic anhydrase inhibitors, quinidine, urinary alkalinizing agents, and certain other agents. Compounds in these categories include:

Acetazolamide (Alterations of urine pH towards the alkaline condition by drugs that make the urine alkaline (e.g., carbonic anhydrase inhibitors) may lead to an accumulation of memantine with a possible increase in adverse effects; use with caution).
No products indexed under this heading.

Amantadine Hydrochloride (The combined use of memantine with other NMDA antagonists, like amantadine, has not been systemically evaluated and such use should be approached with caution). Products include:
Symmetrel 1115

Cimetidine (Co-administration with drugs that use the same renal cationic system, including cimetidine, could potentially result in altered plasma levels of both drugs). Products include:
Tagamet HB 200 Tablets .... ▣637
Tagamet Tablets 1547

Cimetidine Hydrochloride (Co-administration with drugs that use the same renal cationic system, including cimetidine, could potentially result in altered plasma levels of both drugs).
No products indexed under this heading.

Dextromethorphan (The combined use of memantine with other NMDA antagonists, like dextromethorphan, has not been systemically evaluated and such use should be approached with caution).
No products indexed under this heading.

Dextromethorphan Hydrobromide (The combined use of memantine with other NMDA antagonists, like dextromethorphan, has not been systemically evaluated and such use should be approached with caution). Products include:
Alacol DM Syrup 739
Balamine DM 739
Contac Severe Cold and Flu Caplets Maximum Strength .... ▣615
Contac Severe Cold and Flu Caplets Non-Drowsy .... ▣615
Children's Dimetapp DM Cold & Cough Elixir .... ▣745
Children's Dimetapp Long Acting Cough Plus Cold Syrup .... ▣746
Dimetapp Infant Drops Decongestant Plus Cough .... ▣746
Mucinex DM Tablets .... ▣602
PediaCare Decongestant & Cough Infant Drops .... ▣705
PediaCare Freezer Pops Long-Acting Cough-Glacier Grape and Polar Berry Blue .... ▣706
PediaCare Long-Acting Cough Infant Drops .... ▣705
PediaCare Long-Acting Cough Plus Cold Liquid .... ▣704
PediaCare Multi-Symptom Cold Liquid .... ▣704
PediaCare NightRest Cough & Cold Liquid .... ▣704
Robitussin Allergy & Cough Syrup .. ▣750
Robitussin CF Liquid .... ▣755
Robitussin Cough & Cold Liquid-filled Capsules .... ▣750
Robitussin Cough, Cold & Flu Liquid-filled Capsules .... ▣750
Robitussin Cough & Cold Infant Drops .... ▣755

Robitussin DM Infant Drops .... ▣753
Robitussin DM Liquid .... ▣753
Robitussin Flu Liquid .... ▣752
Robitussin Maximum Strength Cough Liquid.............................. ▣754
Robitussin Maximum Strength Cough & Cold Liquid .... ▣754
Robitussin Pediatric Cough Liquid .... ▣754
Robitussin Pediatric Cough & Cold Liquid.................................. ▣754
Robitussin PM Cough & Cold Liquid .... ▣752
Robitussin Sugar Free Cough Liquid .... ▣753
Simply Cough Liquid 1840
Sudafed Severe Cold .... ▣710
TheraFlu Cold & Cough Hot Liquid .... ▣680
TheraFlu Flu & Chest Congestion Non-Drowsy Hot Liquid............... ▣681
TheraFlu Severe Cold Non-Drowsy Hot Liquid............... ▣683
TheraFlu Severe Cold & Cough Hot Liquid................................. ▣683
TheraFlu Severe Cold Caplets .... ▣679
TheraFlu Severe Cold Hot Liquid .... ▣682
TheraFlu Severe Cold Non-Drowsy Caplets................... ▣679
TheraFlu Thin Strips Long Acting Cough.. ▣684
Triaminic Cold & Cough Liquid .... ▣685
Triaminic Cough Liquid .... ▣687
Triaminic Cough & Nasal Congestion Liquid....................... ▣687
Triaminic Cough & Sore Throat Liquid .... ▣687
Triaminic Flu, Cough & Fever Liquid .... ▣685
Triaminic Night Time Cough & Cold Liquid.................................. ▣685
Triaminic Cold & Cough Softchews .... ▣688
Triaminic Cough & Sore Throat Softchews .... ▣689
Triaminic Thin Strips Long Acting Cough.. ▣689
Children's Tylenol Plus Cold & Cough Suspension Liquid and Chewable Tablets 1851
Children's Tylenol Plus Flu Suspension Liquid 1853
Concentrated Tylenol Infants' Drops Plus Cold and Cough.......... 1851
Tylenol Cold & Flu Severe Daytime Liquid with Cool Bust....... 1846
Tylenol Cold & Flu Severe NightTime Liquid with Cool Burst.. 1846
Tylenol Cold Severe Congestion Non-Drowsy Caplets with Cool Burst.. 1846
Tylenol Cough & Sore Throat Daytime Liquid with Cool Burst...... 1849
Tylenol Cough & Sore Throat NightTime Liquid with Cool Burst.. 1849
Tylenol Flu Day Non-Drowsy Gelcaps.. 1846
Concentrated Tylenol Infants' Drops Plus Cold & Cough Nasal Decongestant, Fever Reducer & Pain Reliever.................. ▣668
Multi-Symptom Tylenol Cold Night Time Caplets............................... 1845
Multi-Symptom Tylenol Cold Day Non-Drowsy Caplets and Gelcaps.. 1845
Vicks 44 Cough Relief 2675
Vicks 44D Cough & Head Congestion Relief......................... 2676
Vicks 44D Cough & Head Congestion Relief Liquid............. ▣721
Vicks 44E Cough & Chest Congestion Relief......................... 2676
Pediatric Vicks 44e Cough & Chest Congestion Relief Liquid...... 2673
Vicks 44M Cough, Cold & Flu Relief.. 2676
Pediatric Vicks 44m Cough & Cold Relief..................................... 2673
Vicks DayQuil LiquiCaps/Liquid Multi-Symptom Cold/Flu Relief..... ▣723
Vicks DayQuil Multi-Symptom Cold/Flu Relief LiquiCaps............. 2675
Vicks DayQuil Multi-Symptom Cold/Flu Relief Liquid................... 2675
Children's Vicks NyQuil Cold/Cough Relief........................ 2671
Vicks NyQuil Cough Liquid 2677
Vicks NyQuil LiquiCaps 2677
Vicks NyQuil LiquiCaps/Liquid Multi-Symptom Cold/Flu Relief..... ▣725
Vicks NyQuil Liquid 2677
Zicam Concentrated Cough Mist for Kids Cool Cherry................... ▣643
Zicam Concentrated Cough Mist for Kids Plus D Cool Cherry......... ▣643
Zicam Concentrated Cough Mist Nite-Cool Cherry .... ▣642
Zicam Concentrated Cough Mist Plus D Cool Cherry...................... ▣642
Zicam Concentrated Cough Mist-Honey Lemon & Cool Cherry .... ▣642

Dextromethorphan Polistirex (The combined use of memantine with other NMDA antagonists, like dextromethorphan, has not been systemically evaluated and such use should be approached with caution). Products include:

Delsym Extended-Release Suspension................................ ▣611
Delsym 12 Hour Cough Suppressant for Children............ ▣611

Dextromethorphan tannate (The combined use of memantine with other NMDA antagonists, like dextromethorphan, has not been systemically evaluated and such use should be approached with caution).

No products indexed under this heading.

Dichlorphenamide (Alterations of urine pH towards the alkaline condition by drugs that make the urine alkaline (e.g., carbonic anhydrase inhibitors) may lead to an accumulation of memantine with a possible increase in adverse effects; use with caution). Products include:

Daranide Tablets 1928

Dorzolamide Hydrochloride (Alterations of urine pH towards the alkaline condition by drugs that make the urine alkaline (e.g., carbonic anhydrase inhibitors) may lead to an accumulation of memantine with a possible increase in adverse effects; use with caution). Products include:

Cosopt Sterile Ophthalmic Solution.. 1910
Trusopt Sterile Ophthalmic Solution.. 2065

Hydrochlorothiazide (Co-administration with drugs that use the same renal cationic system, including hydrochlorothiazide, could potentially result in altered plasma levels of both drugs. The co-administration of memantine and hydrochlorothiazide/triamterene decreased the bioavailability of hydrochlorothiazide by 20%). Products include:

Aldoril Tablets 1884
Atacand HCT 637
Avalide Tablets 2889
Avalide Tablets 922
Benicar HCT Tablets 2852
Diovan HCT Tablets 2195
Dyazide Capsules 1389
Hyzaar 1964
Lotensin HCT Tablets 2235
Maxzide 2150
Micardis HCT Tablets 886
Moduretic Tablets 2003
Prinzide Tablets 2033
Teveten HCT Tablets 1710
Timolide Tablets 2056
Uniretic Tablets 3114
Vaseretic Tablets 2073
Zestoretic Tablets 701

Hydrochlorothiazide Hydrochloride (Co-administration with drugs that use the same renal cationic system, including hydrochlorothiazide, could potentially result in altered plasma levels of both drugs. The co-administration of memantine and hydrochlorothiazide/triamterene decreased the bioavailability of hydrochlorothiazide by 20%).

No products indexed under this heading.

Ketamine (The combined use of memantine with other NMDA antagonists, like ketamine, has not been systemically evaluated and such use should be approached with caution).

No products indexed under this heading.

Ketamine Hydrochloride (The combined use of memantine with other NMDA antagonists, like ketamine, has not been systemically evaluated and such use should be approached with caution).

No products indexed under this heading.

Methazolamide (Alterations of urine pH towards the alkaline condition by drugs that make the urine alkaline (e.g., carbonic anhydrase inhibitors) may lead to an accumulation of memantine with a possible increase in adverse effects; use with caution).

No products indexed under this heading.

Nicotine (Co-administration with drugs that use the same renal cationic system, including nicotine, could potentially result in altered plasma levels of both drugs). Products include:

Nicoderm CQ Patch 1629
NicoDerm CQ Clear Patch .... ▣627
Nicotrol Inhaler 2594
Nicotrol NS 2596

Nicotine Polacrilex (Co-administration with drugs that use the same renal cationic system, including nicotine, could potentially result in altered plasma levels of both drugs). Products include:

Commit Lozenges 1625
Nicorette Gum 1632

Nicotine Salicylate (Co-administration with drugs that use the same renal cationic system, including nicotine, could potentially result in altered plasma levels of both drugs).

No products indexed under this heading.

Nicotine Sulfate (Co-administration with drugs that use the same renal cationic system, including nicotine, could potentially result in altered plasma levels of both drugs).

No products indexed under this heading.

Potassium Citrate (Alterations of urine pH towards the alkaline condition by drugs that make the urine alkaline may lead to an accumulation of memantine with a possible increase in adverse effects; use with caution). Products include:

Urocit-K Tablets 2109

Quinidine (Co-administration with drugs that use the same renal cationic system, including quinidine, could potentially result in altered plasma levels of both drugs).

No products indexed under this heading.

Quinidine Gluconate (Co-administration with drugs that use the same renal cationic system, including quinidine, could potentially result in altered plasma levels of both drugs).

No products indexed under this heading.

Quinidine Hydrochloride (Co-administration with drugs that use the same renal cationic system, including quinidine, could potentially result in altered plasma levels of both drugs).

No products indexed under this heading.

Quinidine Polygalacturonate (Co-administration with drugs that use the same renal cationic system, including quinidine, could potentially result in altered plasma levels of both drugs).

No products indexed under this heading.

Quinidine Sulfate (Co-administration with drugs that use the same renal cationic system, including quinidine, could potentially result in altered plasma levels of both drugs).

No products indexed under this heading.

Ranitidine Bismuth Citrate (Co-administration with drugs that use the same renal cationic system, including ranitidine, could potentially result in altered plasma levels of both drugs).

No products indexed under this heading.

Ranitidine Hydrochloride (Co-administration with drugs that use the same renal cationic system, including ranitidine, could potentially result in altered plasma levels of both drugs). Products include:

Zantac 1597
Zantac Injection 1593
Zantac 75 Tablets .... ▣715
Zantac 150 Maximum Strength Tablets.. ▣715
Zantac Injection Pharmacy Bulk Package.. 1595

Sodium Bicarbonate (Alterations of urine pH towards the alkaline condition by drugs that make the urine alkaline (e.g., sodium bicarbonate) may lead to an accumulation of memantine with a possible increase in adverse effects; hence, use with caution). Products include:

Ceo-Two Evacuant Suppository ...... ▣607
Colyte with Flavor Packs for Oral Solution.. 3102
HalfLytely and Bisacodyl Tablets Bowel Prep Kit with Flavors Packs... 915
TriLyte with Flavor Packs for Oral Solution.. 3114

Sodium Citrate (Alterations of urine pH towards the alkaline condition by drugs that make the urine alkaline may lead to an accumulation of memantine with a possible increase in adverse effects; use with caution).

No products indexed under this heading.

Triamterene (Co-administration with drugs that use the same renal cationic system, including triamterene, could potentially result in altered plasma levels of both drugs. However, co-administration of memantine and hydrochlorothiazide/triamterene did not affect the bioavailability of either memantine or triamterene). Products include:

Dyazide Capsules **1389**
Dyrenium Capsules **3390**
Maxzide **2150**

NAPROSYN SUSPENSION

(Naproxen) **2769**
See EC-Naprosyn Delayed-Release Tablets

NAPROSYN TABLETS

(Naproxen) **2769**
See EC-Naprosyn Delayed-Release Tablets

NARCAN INJECTION

(Naloxone Hydrochloride) **1109**
May interact with:

Cardiotoxic drugs, unspecified (Narcan should be used with caution in patients who have received potentially cardiotoxic drugs).
No products indexed under this heading.

NAROPIN INJECTION

(Ropivacaine Hydrochloride) **640**
May interact with class III antiarrhythmics, local anesthetics, xanthines, and certain other agents. Compounds in these categories include:

Aminophylline (Co-administration with drugs known to be metabolized by CYP1A2 via competitive inhibition, such as theophylline, may result in an interaction; caution is advised if used concurrently).
No products indexed under this heading.

Amiodarone Hydrochloride (Patients treated with class III antiarrhythmic drugs should be under close surveillance and ECG monitoring considered, since cardiac effects may be additive. Caution is advised). Products include:
Pacerone Tablets **3337**

Bretylium Tosylate (Patients treated with class III antiarrhythmic drugs should be under close surveillance and ECG monitoring considered, since cardiac effects may be additive. Caution is advised).
No products indexed under this heading.

Bupivacaine Hydrochloride (Co-administration with other local anesthetics or agents structurally related to amide-type local anesthetics may result in additive toxic effects).
No products indexed under this heading.

Chloroprocaine Hydrochloride (Co-administration with other local anesthetics or agents structurally related to amide-type local anesthetics may result in additive toxic effects).
No products indexed under this heading.

Dyphylline (Co-administration with drugs known to be metabolized by CYP1A2 via competitive inhibition, such as theophylline, may result in an interaction; caution is advised if used concurrently).
No products indexed under this heading.

Etidocaine Hydrochloride (Co-administration with other local anesthetics or agents structurally related to amide-type local anesthetics may result in additive toxic effects).
No products indexed under this heading.

Fluvoxamine Maleate (Co-administration with fluvoxamine, a selective and potent inhibitor of CYP1A2, has resulted in reduced plasma clearance by 70% leading to increased ropivacaine plasma levels).
No products indexed under this heading.

Imipramine Hydrochloride (Co-administration with drugs known to be metabolized by CYP1A2 via competitive inhibition, such as imipramine, may result in an interaction; caution is advised if used concurrently).
No products indexed under this heading.

Imipramine Pamoate (Co-administration with drugs known to be metabolized by CYP1A2 via competitive inhibition, such as imipramine, may result in an interaction; caution is advised if used concurrently).
No products indexed under this heading.

Ketoconazole (Co-administration has resulted in a 15% reduction in in vivo plasma clearance of ropivacaine). Products include:
Nizoral A-D Shampoo, 1% **1839**
Nizoral 2% Shampoo **1838**

Levobupivacaine Hydrochloride (Co-administration with other local anesthetics or agents structurally related to amide-type local anesthetics may result in additive toxic effects).
No products indexed under this heading.

Lidocaine Hydrochloride (Co-administration with other local anesthetics or agents structurally related to amide-type local anesthetics may result in additive toxic effects).
No products indexed under this heading.

Mepivacaine Hydrochloride (Co-administration with other local anesthetics or agents structurally related to amide-type local anesthetics may result in additive toxic effects).
No products indexed under this heading.

Procaine Hydrochloride (Co-administration with other local anesthetics or agents structurally related to amide-type local anesthetics may result in additive toxic effects).
No products indexed under this heading.

Sotalol Hydrochloride (Patients treated with class III antiarrhythmic drugs should be under close surveillance and ECG monitoring considered, since cardiac effects may be additive. Caution is advised).
No products indexed under this heading.

Tetracaine Hydrochloride (Co-administration with other local anesthetics or agents structurally related to amide-type local anesthetics may result in additive toxic effects). Products include:
Cetacaine Topical Anesthetic **1007**

Theophylline (Co-administration with drugs known to be metabolized by CYP1A2 via competitive inhibition, such as theophylline, may result in an interaction; caution is advised if used concurrently).
No products indexed under this heading.

Theophylline Anhydrous (Co-administration with drugs known to be metabolized by CYP1A2 via competitive inhibition, such as theophylline, may result in an interaction; caution is advised if used concurrently). Products include:
Uniphyl Tablets **2708**

Theophylline Calcium Salicylate (Co-administration with drugs known to be metabolized by CYP1A2 via competitive inhibition, such as theophylline, may result in an interaction; caution is advised if used concurrently).
No products indexed under this heading.

Theophylline Dihydroxypropyl (Glyceryl) (Co-administration with drugs known to be metabolized by CYP1A2 via competitive inhibition, such as theophylline, may result in an interaction; caution is advised if used concurrently).
No products indexed under this heading.

Theophylline Ethylenediamine (Co-administration with drugs known to be metabolized by CYP1A2 via competitive inhibition, such as theophylline, may result in an interaction; caution is advised if used concurrently).
No products indexed under this heading.

Theophylline Sodium Glycinate (Co-administration with drugs known to be metabolized by CYP1A2 via competitive inhibition, such as theophylline, may result in an interaction; caution is advised if used concurrently).
No products indexed under this heading.

Verapamil Hydrochloride (*In vitro* studies indicate that cytochrome P450 IA is involved in the formation of 3-hydroxy ropivacaine, the major metabolite; co-administration with other agents which are potent inhibitors of this enzyme, such as verapamil, may potentially interact with Naropin). Products include:
Covera-HS Tablets **3135**
Tarka Tablets **519**
Verelan PM Capsules **3120**

NASACORT HFA INHALATION AEROSOL

(Triamcinolone Acetonide) **2939**
None cited in PDR database.

NASACORT AQ NASAL SPRAY

(Triamcinolone Acetonide) **2937**
None cited in PDR database.

NASAREL NASAL SPRAY

(Flunisolide) **1652**
None cited in PDR database.

NASONEX NASAL SPRAY

(Mometasone Furoate Monohydrate) **3058**
None cited in PDR database.

NATACYN ANTIFUNGAL OPHTHALMIC SUSPENSION

(Natamycin) .... ⊙**207**
None cited in PDR database.

NATRECOR FOR INJECTION

(Nesiritide) **3123**
None cited in PDR database.

NAVELBINE INJECTION

(Vinorelbine Tartrate) **1494**
May interact with cytochrome p450 3a4 inhibitors (selected) and certain other agents. Compounds in these categories include:

Acetazolamide (Co-administration of vinorelbine with an inhibitor of CYP3A metabolic pathway may cause an earlier onset and/or an increased severity of side effects).
No products indexed under this heading.

Amiodarone Hydrochloride (Co-administration of vinorelbine with an inhibitor of CYP3A metabolic pathway may cause an earlier onset and/or an increased severity of side effects). Products include:
Pacerone Tablets **3337**

Amprenavir (Co-administration of vinorelbine with an inhibitor of CYP3A metabolic pathway may cause an earlier onset and/or an increased severity of side effects). Products include:
Agenerase Capsules **1299**
Agenerase Oral Solution **1304**

Anastrozole (Co-administration of vinorelbine with an inhibitor of CYP3A metabolic pathway may cause an earlier onset and/or an increased severity of side effects). Products include:
Arimidex Tablets **665**

Aprepitant (Co-administration of vinorelbine with an inhibitor of CYP3A metabolic pathway may cause an earlier onset and/or an increased severity of side effects). Products include:
Emend Capsules **1944**

Cimetidine (Co-administration of vinorelbine with an inhibitor of CYP3A metabolic pathway may cause an earlier onset and/or an increased severity of side effects). Products include:
Tagamet HB 200 Tablets .... ▣**637**
Tagamet Tablets **1547**

Cimetidine Hydrochloride (Co-administration of vinorelbine with an inhibitor of CYP3A metabolic pathway may cause an earlier onset and/or an increased severity of side effects).
No products indexed under this heading.

Ciprofloxacin (Co-administration of vinorelbine with an inhibitor of CYP3A metabolic pathway may cause an earlier onset and/or an increased severity of side effects). Products include:
Cipro I.V. **2998**
Cipro I.V. Pharmacy Bulk Package ... **3509**
Cipro Oral Suspension **2991**
Cipro XR Tablets **3004**
Ciprodex Otic Suspension **555**

Cisplatin (Potential for higher incidence of granulocytopenia with vinorelbine used in combination with cisplatin; vestibular and auditory deficits have been observed with combination therapy).
No products indexed under this heading.

Clarithromycin (Co-administration of vinorelbine with an inhibitor of CYP3A metabolic pathway may cause an earlier onset and/or an increased severity of side effects). Products include:
Biaxin/Biaxin XL **402**
PREVPAC **3281**

Clotrimazole (Co-administration of vinorelbine with an inhibitor of CYP3A

metabolic pathway may cause an earlier onset and/or an increased severity of side effects). Products include:

Lotrimin 3053
Lotrisone 3054

Cyclosporine (Co-administration of vinorelbine with an inhibitor of CYP3A metabolic pathway may cause an earlier onset and/or an increased severity of side effects). Products include:

Gengraf Capsules 458
Neoral Soft Gelatin Capsules 2247
Neoral Oral Solution 2247
Restasis Ophthalmic Emulsion 570
Sandimmune 2259

Dalfopristin (Co-administration of vinorelbine with an inhibitor of CYP3A metabolic pathway may cause an earlier onset and/or an increased severity of side effects). Products include:

Synercid I.V. 1690

Danazol (Co-administration of vinorelbine with an inhibitor of CYP3A metabolic pathway may cause an earlier onset and/or an increased severity of side effects).

No products indexed under this heading.

Delavirdine Mesylate (Co-administration of vinorelbine with an inhibitor of CYP3A metabolic pathway may cause an earlier onset and/or an increased severity of side effects). Products include:

Rescriptor Tablets 2535

Diltiazem Hydrochloride (Co-administration of vinorelbine with an inhibitor of CYP3A metabolic pathway may cause an earlier onset and/or an increased severity of side effects). Products include:

Cardizem LA Extended Release Tablets 1699
Tiazac Capsules 1204

Diltiazem Maleate (Co-administration of vinorelbine with an inhibitor of CYP3A metabolic pathway may cause an earlier onset and/or an increased severity of side effects).

No products indexed under this heading.

Efavirenz (Co-administration of vinorelbine with an inhibitor of CYP3A metabolic pathway may cause an earlier onset and/or an increased severity of side effects). Products include:

Sustiva Capsules 957

Erythromycin (Co-administration of vinorelbine with an inhibitor of CYP3A metabolic pathway may cause an earlier onset and/or an increased severity of side effects). Products include:

Erygel Topical Gel 2096
Ery-Tab Tablets 447
Erythromycin Base Filmtab Tablets 454
Erythromycin Delayed-Release Capsules, USP 456
PCE Dispertab Tablets 510

Erythromycin Estolate (Co-administration of vinorelbine with an inhibitor of CYP3A metabolic pathway may cause an earlier onset and/or an increased severity of side effects).

No products indexed under this heading.

Erythromycin Ethylsuccinate (Co-administration of vinorelbine with an inhibitor of CYP3A metabolic pathway may cause an earlier onset and/or an increased severity of side effects). Products include:

E.E.S. 449
EryPed 445

Erythromycin Gluceptate (Co-administration of vinorelbine with an inhibitor of CYP3A metabolic pathway may cause an earlier onset and/or an increased severity of side effects).

No products indexed under this heading.

Erythromycin Lactobionate (Co-administration of vinorelbine with an inhibitor of CYP3A metabolic pathway may cause an earlier onset and/or an increased severity of side effects).

No products indexed under this heading.

Erythromycin Stearate (Co-administration of vinorelbine with an inhibitor of CYP3A metabolic pathway may cause an earlier onset and/or an increased severity of side effects). Products include:

Erythrocin Stearate Filmtab Tablets 452

Esomeprazole Magnesium (Co-administration of vinorelbine with an inhibitor of CYP3A metabolic pathway may cause an earlier onset and/or an increased severity of side effects). Products include:

Nexium Delayed-Release Capsules 645

Fluconazole (Co-administration of vinorelbine with an inhibitor of CYP3A metabolic pathway may cause an earlier onset and/or an increased severity of side effects).

No products indexed under this heading.

Fluoxetine Hydrochloride (Co-administration of vinorelbine with an inhibitor of CYP3A metabolic pathway may cause an earlier onset and/or an increased severity of side effects). Products include:

Prozac Pulvules and Liquid 1771
Symbyax Capsules 1788

Fluvoxamine Maleate (Co-administration of vinorelbine with an inhibitor of CYP3A metabolic pathway may cause an earlier onset and/or an increased severity of side effects).

No products indexed under this heading.

Fosamprenavir Calcium (Co-administration of vinorelbine with an inhibitor of CYP3A metabolic pathway may cause an earlier onset and/or an increased severity of side effects). Products include:

Lexiva Tablets 1473

Indinavir Sulfate (Co-administration of vinorelbine with an inhibitor of CYP3A metabolic pathway may cause an earlier onset and/or an increased severity of side effects). Products include:

Crixivan Capsules 1918

Isoniazid (Co-administration of vinorelbine with an inhibitor of CYP3A metabolic pathway may cause an earlier onset and/or an increased severity of side effects).

No products indexed under this heading.

Itraconazole (Co-administration of vinorelbine with an inhibitor of CYP3A metabolic pathway may cause an earlier onset and/or an increased severity of side effects).

No products indexed under this heading.

Ketoconazole (Co-administration of vinorelbine with an inhibitor of CYP3A metabolic pathway may cause an earlier onset and/or an increased severity of side effects). Products include:

Nizoral A-D Shampoo, 1% 1839
Nizoral 2% Shampoo 1838

Lopinavir (Co-administration of vinorelbine with an inhibitor of CYP3A metabolic pathway may cause an earlier onset and/or an increased severity of side effects). Products include:

Kaletra 474

Loratadine (Co-administration of vinorelbine with an inhibitor of CYP3A metabolic pathway may cause an earlier onset and/or an increased severity of side effects). Products include:

Alavert Allergy & Sinus D-12 Hour Tablets 743
Alavert 743
Children's Claritin 24 Hour Non-Drowsy Allergy Syrup 732
Claritin Non-Drowsy 24 Hour Tablets 731
Non-Drowsy Claritin Hives Relief Tablets 733
Claritin Reditabs 24 Hour Non-Drowsy Tablets 732
Claritin-D Non-Drowsy 12 Hour Tablets 731
Claritin-D Non-Drowsy 24 Hour Tablets 731
Children's Dimetapp ND Non-Drowsy Allergy Syrup 746
Triaminic Allerchews 684

Metronidazole (Co-administration of vinorelbine with an inhibitor of CYP3A metabolic pathway may cause an earlier onset and/or an increased severity of side effects). Products include:

Metrogel 1% 1212
MetroGel-Vaginal Gel 1822
Noritate Cream, 1% 1051

Metronidazole Benzoate (Co-administration of vinorelbine with an inhibitor of CYP3A metabolic pathway may cause an earlier onset and/or an increased severity of side effects).

No products indexed under this heading.

Metronidazole Hydrochloride (Co-administration of vinorelbine with an inhibitor of CYP3A metabolic pathway may cause an earlier onset and/or an increased severity of side effects).

No products indexed under this heading.

Miconazole (Co-administration of vinorelbine with an inhibitor of CYP3A metabolic pathway may cause an earlier onset and/or an increased severity of side effects).

No products indexed under this heading.

Miconazole Nitrate (Co-administration of vinorelbine with an inhibitor of CYP3A metabolic pathway may cause an earlier onset and/or an increased severity of side effects). Products include:

Desenex 674
Desenex Jock Itch Spray Powder 674

Mitomycin (Mitomycin-C) (Acute pulmonary reactions have been reported with vinorelbine and other vinca alkaloids used in conjunction with mitomycin).

No products indexed under this heading.

Nefazodone Hydrochloride (Co-administration of vinorelbine with an inhibitor of CYP3A metabolic pathway may cause an earlier onset and/or an increased severity of side effects).

No products indexed under this heading.

Nelfinavir Mesylate (Co-administration of vinorelbine with an inhibitor of CYP3A metabolic pathway may cause an earlier onset and/or an increased severity of side effects). Products include:

Viracept 2556

Nevirapine (Co-administration of vinorelbine with an inhibitor of CYP3A metabolic pathway may cause an earlier onset and/or an increased severity of side effects). Products include:

Viramune Oral Suspension 903
Viramune Tablets 903

Niacinamide (Co-administration of vinorelbine with an inhibitor of CYP3A metabolic pathway may cause an earlier onset and/or an increased severity of side effects).

No products indexed under this heading.

Nicotinamide (Co-administration of vinorelbine with an inhibitor of CYP3A metabolic pathway may cause an earlier onset and/or an increased severity of side effects). Products include:

Nicomide Tablets 3190

Nifedipine (Co-administration of vinorelbine with an inhibitor of CYP3A metabolic pathway may cause an earlier onset and/or an increased severity of side effects). Products include:

Adalat CC Tablets 2978

Norfloxacin (Co-administration of vinorelbine with an inhibitor of CYP3A metabolic pathway may cause an earlier onset and/or an increased severity of side effects). Products include:

Noroxin Tablets 2009

Omeprazole (Co-administration of vinorelbine with an inhibitor of CYP3A metabolic pathway may cause an earlier onset and/or an increased severity of side effects). Products include:

Zegerid Powder for Oral Solution 2972

Paclitaxel (Patients on concomitant and/or sequential administration should be monitored for signs and symptoms of neuropathy).

No products indexed under this heading.

Paroxetine Hydrochloride (Co-administration of vinorelbine with an inhibitor of CYP3A metabolic pathway may cause an earlier onset and/or an increased severity of side effects). Products include:

Paxil CR Controlled-Release Tablets 1509
Paxil 1501

Propoxyphene Hydrochloride (Co-administration of vinorelbine with an inhibitor of CYP3A metabolic pathway may cause an earlier onset and/or an increased severity of side effects).
No products indexed under this heading.

Propoxyphene Napsylate (Co-administration of vinorelbine with an inhibitor of CYP3A metabolic pathway may cause an earlier onset and/or an increased severity of side effects). Products include:
Darvocet A 500 Tablets ... **3497**

Quinidine (Co-administration of vinorelbine with an inhibitor of CYP3A metabolic pathway may cause an earlier onset and/or an increased severity of side effects).
No products indexed under this heading.

Quinidine Hydrochloride (Co-administration of vinorelbine with an inhibitor of CYP3A metabolic pathway may cause an earlier onset and/or an increased severity of side effects).
No products indexed under this heading.

Quinidine Polygalacturonate (Co-administration of vinorelbine with an inhibitor of CYP3A metabolic pathway may cause an earlier onset and/or an increased severity of side effects).
No products indexed under this heading.

Quinidine Sulfate (Co-administration of vinorelbine with an inhibitor of CYP3A metabolic pathway may cause an earlier onset and/or an increased severity of side effects).
No products indexed under this heading.

Quinine (Co-administration of vinorelbine with an inhibitor of CYP3A metabolic pathway may cause an earlier onset and/or an increased severity of side effects).
No products indexed under this heading.

Quinine Sulfate (Co-administration of vinorelbine with an inhibitor of CYP3A metabolic pathway may cause an earlier onset and/or an increased severity of side effects).
No products indexed under this heading.

Quinupristin (Co-administration of vinorelbine with an inhibitor of CYP3A metabolic pathway may cause an earlier onset and/or an increased severity of side effects). Products include:
Synercid I.V. ... **1690**

Ranitidine Bismuth Citrate (Co-administration of vinorelbine with an inhibitor of CYP3A metabolic pathway may cause an earlier onset and/or an increased severity of side effects).
No products indexed under this heading.

Ranitidine Hydrochloride (Co-administration of vinorelbine with an inhibitor of CYP3A metabolic pathway may cause an earlier onset and/or an increased severity of side effects). Products include:
Zantac ... **1597**
Zantac Injection ... **1593**
Zantac 75 Tablets ... ▣ **715**
Zantac 150 Maximum Strength Tablets ... ▣ **715**
Zantac Injection Pharmacy Bulk Package ... **1595**

Ritonavir (Co-administration of vinorelbine with an inhibitor of CYP3A metabolic pathway may cause an earlier onset and/or an increased severity of side effects). Products include:
Kaletra ... **474**
Norvir ... **499**

Saquinavir (Co-administration of vinorelbine with an inhibitor of CYP3A metabolic pathway may cause an earlier onset and/or an increased severity of side effects).
No products indexed under this heading.

Saquinavir Mesylate (Co-administration of vinorelbine with an inhibitor of CYP3A metabolic pathway may cause an earlier onset and/or an increased severity of side effects). Products include:
Invirase ... **2776**

Sertraline Hydrochloride (Co-administration of vinorelbine with an inhibitor of CYP3A metabolic pathway may cause an earlier onset and/or an increased severity of side effects). Products include:
Zoloft ... **2581**

Telithromycin (Co-administration of vinorelbine with an inhibitor of CYP3A metabolic pathway may cause an earlier onset and/or an increased severity of side effects). Products include:
Ketek Tablets ... **2920**

Troglitazone (Co-administration of vinorelbine with an inhibitor of CYP3A metabolic pathway may cause an earlier onset and/or an increased severity of side effects).
No products indexed under this heading.

Troleandomycin (Co-administration of vinorelbine with an inhibitor of CYP3A metabolic pathway may cause an earlier onset and/or an increased severity of side effects).
No products indexed under this heading.

Valproate Sodium (Co-administration of vinorelbine with an inhibitor of CYP3A metabolic pathway may cause an earlier onset and/or an increased severity of side effects). Products include:
Depacon Injection ... **412**

Verapamil Hydrochloride (Co-administration of vinorelbine with an inhibitor of CYP3A metabolic pathway may cause an earlier onset and/or an increased severity of side effects). Products include:
Covera-HS Tablets ... **3135**
Tarka Tablets ... **519**
Verelan PM Capsules ... **3120**

Voriconazole (Co-administration of vinorelbine with an inhibitor of CYP3A metabolic pathway may cause an earlier onset and/or an increased severity of side effects). Products include:
VFEND I.V. ... **2543**
VFEND Oral Suspension ... **2543**
VFEND Tablets ... **2543**

Zafirlukast (Co-administration of vinorelbine with an inhibitor of CYP3A metabolic pathway may cause an earlier onset and/or an increased severity of side effects). Products include:
Accolate Tablets ... **663**

Zileuton (Co-administration of vinorelbine with an inhibitor of CYP3A metabolic pathway may cause an earlier onset and/or an increased severity of side effects).
No products indexed under this heading.

Food Interactions

Grapefruit (Co-administration of vinorelbine with an inhibitor of CYP3A metabolic pathway may cause an earlier onset and/or an increased severity of side effects).

Grapefruit Juice (Co-administration of vinorelbine with an inhibitor of CYP3A metabolic pathway may cause an earlier onset and/or an increased severity of side effects).

NEMBUTAL SODIUM SOLUTION, USP

(Pentobarbital Sodium) ... **2484**

May interact with central nervous system depressants, corticosteroids, oral anticoagulants, doxycycline, estrogens, monoamine oxidase inhibitors, oral contraceptives, phenytoin, and certain other agents. Compounds in these categories include:

Alfentanil Hydrochloride (Concomitant use of other CNS depressants may produce additive depressant effects).
No products indexed under this heading.

Alprazolam (Concomitant use of other CNS depressants may produce additive depressant effects). Products include:
Niravam Orally Disintegrating Tablets ... **3106**
Xanax XR Tablets ... **2655**

Anisindione (Barbiturates can induce hepatic microsomal enzymes resulting in increased metabolism and decreased anticoagulant response of oral anticoagulants). Products include:
Miradon Tablets ... **3056**

Aprobarbital (Concomitant use of other CNS depressants may produce additive depressant effects).
No products indexed under this heading.

Betamethasone Acetate (Barbiturates appear to enhance the metabolism of exogenous corticosteroids probably through the induction of hepatic microsomal enzymes).
No products indexed under this heading.

Betamethasone Sodium Phosphate (Barbiturates appear to enhance the metabolism of exogenous corticosteroids probably through the induction of hepatic microsomal enzymes).
No products indexed under this heading.

Buprenorphine Hydrochloride (Concomitant use of other CNS depressants may produce additive depressant effects). Products include:
Buprenex Injectable ... **2718**
Suboxone Tablets ... **2719**
Subutex Tablets ... **2719**

Buspirone Hydrochloride (Concomitant use of other CNS depressants may produce additive depressant effects).
No products indexed under this heading.

Butabarbital (Concomitant use of other CNS depressants may produce additive depressant effects).
No products indexed under this heading.

Butalbital (Concomitant use of other CNS depressants may produce additive depressant effects). Products include:
Sedapap Tablets 50 mg/650 mg ... **2098**

Chlordiazepoxide (Concomitant use of other CNS depressants may produce additive depressant effects).
No products indexed under this heading.

Chlordiazepoxide Hydrochloride (Concomitant use of other CNS depressants may produce additive depressant effects). Products include:
Librium Capsules ... **3349**

Chlorotrianisene (Pretreatment with or co-administration of phenobarbital may decrease the effect of estrogen by increasing its metabolism; application of this data to other barbiturates appears valid).
No products indexed under this heading.

Chlorpromazine (Concomitant use of other CNS depressants may produce additive depressant effects).
No products indexed under this heading.

Chlorpromazine Hydrochloride (Concomitant use of other CNS depressants may produce additive depressant effects).
No products indexed under this heading.

Chlorprothixene (Concomitant use of other CNS depressants may produce additive depressant effects).
No products indexed under this heading.

Chlorprothixene Hydrochloride (Concomitant use of other CNS depressants may produce additive depressant effects).
No products indexed under this heading.

Chlorprothixene Lactate (Concomitant use of other CNS depressants may produce additive depressant effects).
No products indexed under this heading.

Clorazepate Dipotassium (Concomitant use of other CNS depressants may produce additive depressant effects). Products include:
Tranxene ... **2488**

Clozapine (Concomitant use of other CNS depressants may produce additive depressant effects). Products include:
Clozapine Tablets ... **2141**
Clozaril Tablets ... **2174**
FazaClo Orally Disintegrating Tablets ... **547**

Codeine Phosphate (Concomitant use of other CNS depressants may produce additive depressant effects). Products include:
Tylenol with Codeine ... **2461**

Cortisone Acetate (Barbiturates appear to enhance the metabolism of exogenous corticosteroids probably through the induction of hepatic microsomal enzymes).
No products indexed under this heading.

Desflurane (Concomitant use of other CNS depressants may produce additive depressant effects). Products include:

Suprane Liquid for Inhalation 770

Desogestrel (Pretreatment with or co-administration of phenobarbital may decrease the effect of estrogen by increasing its metabolism; application of this data to other barbiturates appears valid; higher incidence of pregnancy in patients on co-administration). Products include:
Ortho-Cept Tablets 2395

Dexamethasone (Barbiturates appear to enhance the metabolism of exogenous corticosteroids probably through the induction of hepatic microsomal enzymes). Products include:
Ciprodex Otic Suspension 555
Decadron Tablets 1929
TobraDex Ophthalmic Ointment 558
TobraDex Ophthalmic Suspension ... 558

Dexamethasone Acetate (Barbiturates appear to enhance the metabolism of exogenous corticosteroids probably through the induction of hepatic microsomal enzymes).
No products indexed under this heading.

Dexamethasone Sodium Phosphate (Barbiturates appear to enhance the metabolism of exogenous corticosteroids probably through the induction of hepatic microsomal enzymes). Products include:
Decadron Phosphate Injection 1931

Dezocine (Concomitant use of other CNS depressants may produce additive depressant effects).
No products indexed under this heading.

Diazepam (Concomitant use of other CNS depressants may produce additive depressant effects). Products include:
Diastat Rectal Delivery System 3344
Valium Tablets 2822

Dicumarol (Barbiturates can induce hepatic microsomal enzymes resulting in increased metabolism and decreased anticoagulant response of oral anticoagulants).
No products indexed under this heading.

Dienestrol (Pretreatment with or co-administration of phenobarbital may decrease the effect of estrogen by increasing its metabolism; application of this data to other barbiturates appears valid).
No products indexed under this heading.

Diethylstilbestrol (Pretreatment with or co-administration of phenobarbital may decrease the effect of estrogen by increasing its metabolism; application of this data to other barbiturates appears valid).
No products indexed under this heading.

Divalproex Sodium (Valproate appears to decrease barbiturate metabolism). Products include:
Depakote Sprinkle Capsules 422
Depakote Tablets 427
Depakote ER Tablets 433

Doxycycline Calcium (Phenobarbital has been shown to shorten the half-life of doxycycline for as long as 2 weeks after barbiturate therapy is discontinued; application of this data to other barbiturates appears valid).
No products indexed under this heading.

Doxycycline Hyclate (Phenobarbital has been shown to shorten the half-life of doxycycline for as long as 2 weeks after barbiturate therapy is discontinued; application of this data to other barbiturates appears valid).
No products indexed under this heading.

Doxycycline Monohydrate (Phenobarbital has been shown to shorten the half-life of doxycycline for as long as 2 weeks after barbiturate therapy is discontinued; application of this data to other barbiturates appears valid).
No products indexed under this heading.

Droperidol (Concomitant use of other CNS depressants may produce additive depressant effects).
No products indexed under this heading.

Enflurane (Concomitant use of other CNS depressants may produce additive depressant effects).
No products indexed under this heading.

Estazolam (Concomitant use of other CNS depressants may produce additive depressant effects). Products include:
ProSom Tablets 512

Estradiol (Pretreatment with or co-administration of phenobarbital may decrease the effect of estrogen by increasing its metabolism; application of this data to other barbiturates appears valid). Products include:
Activella Tablets 2311
Climara Transdermal System 795
Climara Pro Transdermal System 800
CombiPatch Transdermal System 2180
Estrogel 0.06% 3200
Menostar Transdermal System 805
Prefest Tablets 1069
Vagifem Tablets 2340
Vivelle Transdermal System 2288
Vivelle-Dot Transdermal System 2293

Estrogens, Conjugated (Pretreatment with or co-administration of phenobarbital may decrease the effect of estrogen by increasing its metabolism; application of this data to other barbiturates appears valid). Products include:
Premarin Intravenous 3440
Premarin Tablets 3443
Premarin Vaginal Cream 3449
Premphase Tablets 3452
Prempro Tablets 3452

Estrogens, Esterified (Pretreatment with or co-administration of phenobarbital may decrease the effect of estrogen by increasing its metabolism; application of this data to other barbiturates appears valid). Products include:
Estratest Tablets 3196
Estratest H.S. Tablets 3196

Estropipate (Pretreatment with or co-administration of phenobarbital may decrease the effect of estrogen by increasing its metabolism; application of this data to other barbiturates appears valid).
No products indexed under this heading.

Ethanol (Concomitant use of other CNS depressants may produce additive depressant effects).
No products indexed under this heading.

Ethchlorvynol (Concomitant use of other CNS depressants may produce additive depressant effects).
No products indexed under this heading.

Ethinamate (Concomitant use of other CNS depressants may produce additive depressant effects).
No products indexed under this heading.

Ethinyl Estradiol (Pretreatment with or co-administration of phenobarbital may decrease the effect of estrogen by increasing its metabolism; application of this data to other barbiturates appears valid; higher incidence of pregnancy in patients on co-administration). Products include:
Alesse-28 Tablets 3392
Lo/Ovral-28 Tablets 3423
NuvaRing 2357
Ortho-Cept Tablets 2395
Ortho-Cyclen/Ortho Tri-Cyclen 2414
Ortho Evra Transdermal System 2402
Ortho Tri-Cyclen Lo Tablets 2421
Seasonale Tablets 1073
Triphasil-28 Tablets 3483
Yasmin 28 Tablets 818

Ethyl Alcohol (Concomitant use of other CNS depressants may produce additive depressant effects).
No products indexed under this heading.

Ethynodiol Diacetate (Pretreatment with or co-administration of phenobarbital may decrease the effect of estrogen by increasing its metabolism; application of this data to other barbiturates appears valid; higher incidence of pregnancy in patients on co-administration).
No products indexed under this heading.

Fentanyl (Concomitant use of other CNS depressants may produce additive depressant effects). Products include:
Duragesic Transdermal System 2448

Fentanyl Citrate (Concomitant use of other CNS depressants may produce additive depressant effects). Products include:
Actiq 993

Fludrocortisone Acetate (Barbiturates appear to enhance the metabolism of exogenous corticosteroids probably through the induction of hepatic microsomal enzymes).
No products indexed under this heading.

Fluphenazine Decanoate (Concomitant use of other CNS depressants may produce additive depressant effects).
No products indexed under this heading.

Fluphenazine Enanthate (Concomitant use of other CNS depressants may produce additive depressant effects).
No products indexed under this heading.

Fluphenazine Hydrochloride (Concomitant use of other CNS depressants may produce additive depressant effects).
No products indexed under this heading.

Flurazepam Hydrochloride (Concomitant use of other CNS depressants may produce additive depressant effects). Products include:
Dalmane Capsules 3343

Fosphenytoin Sodium (The effect of barbiturates on the metabolism of phenytoin appears to be variable).
No products indexed under this heading.

Furazolidone (Co-administration with MAO inhibitors prolongs the effects of barbiturates probably because the metabolism of the barbiturate is inhibited).
No products indexed under this heading.

Glutethimide (Concomitant use of other CNS depressants may produce additive depressant effects).
No products indexed under this heading.

Griseofulvin (Phenobarbital appears to interfere with the absorption of orally administered griseofulvin, thus decreasing its blood level; application of this data to other barbiturates appears valid). Products include:
Grifulvin V Tablets Microsize and Oral Suspension Microsize............ 2384
Gris-PEG Tablets 2504

Haloperidol (Concomitant use of other CNS depressants may produce additive depressant effects).
No products indexed under this heading.

Haloperidol Decanoate (Concomitant use of other CNS depressants may produce additive depressant effects).
No products indexed under this heading.

Hydrocodone Bitartrate (Concomitant use of other CNS depressants may produce additive depressant effects). Products include:
Hycodan 1104
Hycomine Compound Tablets 1105
Hycotuss Expectorant Syrup 1106
Lortab 3315
Lortab Elixir 3312
Vicodin Tablets 530
Vicodin ES Tablets 531
Vicodin HP Tablets 532
Vicoprofen Tablets 533
Zydone Tablets 1118

Hydrocodone Polistirex (Concomitant use of other CNS depressants may produce additive depressant effects). Products include:
Tussionex Pennkinetic Extended-Release Suspension 3322

Hydrocortisone (Barbiturates appear to enhance the metabolism of exogenous corticosteroids probably through the induction of hepatic microsomal enzymes). Products include:
Cortizone•5 Ointment 699
Cortizone•10 Creme 699
Cortizone•10 Ointment 699
Cortizone•10 Plus Creme 700
Cortizone•10 Maximum Strength Quick Shot Spray 700
Hydrocortone Tablets 1963
Preparation H Hydrocortisone Cream 748

Hydrocortisone Acetate (Barbiturates appear to enhance the metabolism of exogenous corticosteroids probably through the induction of hepatic microsomal enzymes). Products include:
Analpram-HC 1136
Pramosone 1139
ProctoFoam-HC 3113
Tucks Anti-Itch Ointment 712
U-cort 1% Cream 3289

Hydrocortisone Sodium Phosphate (Barbiturates appear to enhance the metabolism of exogenous corticosteroids probably through the induction of hepatic microsomal enzymes).
No products indexed under this heading.

IMPORTANT NOTE: Always consult each drug listing in the patient's regimen for possible interactions.

Hydrocortisone Sodium Succinate (Barbiturates appear to enhance the metabolism of exogenous corticosteroids probably through the induction of hepatic microsomal enzymes).
No products indexed under this heading.

Hydromorphone Hydrochloride (Concomitant use of other CNS depressants may produce additive depressant effects). Products include:
- Dilaudid ... 439
- Dilaudid Oral Liquid ... 443
- Dilaudid Non-Sterile Powder ... 439
- Dilaudid Rectal Suppositories ... 439
- Dilaudid Tablets ... 439
- Dilaudid Tablets - 8 mg ... 443
- Dilaudid-HP ... 441

Hydroxyzine Hydrochloride (Concomitant use of other CNS depressants may produce additive depressant effects).
No products indexed under this heading.

Isocarboxazid (Co-administration with MAO inhibitors prolongs the effects of barbiturates probably because the metabolism of the barbiturate is inhibited).
No products indexed under this heading.

Isoflurane (Concomitant use of other CNS depressants may produce additive depressant effects).
No products indexed under this heading.

Ketamine Hydrochloride (Concomitant use of other CNS depressants may produce additive depressant effects).
No products indexed under this heading.

Levomethadyl Acetate Hydrochloride (Concomitant use of other CNS depressants may produce additive depressant effects).
No products indexed under this heading.

Levonorgestrel (Pretreatment with or co-administration of phenobarbital may decrease the effect of estrogen by increasing its metabolism; application of this data to other barbiturates appears valid; higher incidence of pregnancy in patients on co-administration). Products include:
- Alesse-28 Tablets ... 3392
- Climara Pro Transdermal System ... 800
- Mirena Intrauterine System ... 810
- Plan B Tablets ... 1068
- Seasonale Tablets ... 1073
- Triphasil-28 Tablets ... 3483

Levorphanol Tartrate (Concomitant use of other CNS depressants may produce additive depressant effects).
No products indexed under this heading.

Lorazepam (Concomitant use of other CNS depressants may produce additive depressant effects).
No products indexed under this heading.

Loxapine Hydrochloride (Concomitant use of other CNS depressants may produce additive depressant effects).
No products indexed under this heading.

Loxapine Succinate (Concomitant use of other CNS depressants may produce additive depressant effects).
No products indexed under this heading.

Meperidine Hydrochloride (Concomitant use of other CNS depressants may produce additive depressant effects).
No products indexed under this heading.

Mephobarbital (Concomitant use of other CNS depressants may produce additive depressant effects). Products include:
- Mebaral Tablets, USP ... 2483

Meprobamate (Concomitant use of other CNS depressants may produce additive depressant effects).
No products indexed under this heading.

Mesoridazine Besylate (Concomitant use of other CNS depressants may produce additive depressant effects).
No products indexed under this heading.

Mestranol (Pretreatment with or co-administration of phenobarbital may decrease the effect of estrogen by increasing its metabolism; application of this data to other barbiturates appears valid; higher incidence of pregnancy in patients on co-administration).
No products indexed under this heading.

Methadone Hydrochloride (Concomitant use of other CNS depressants may produce additive depressant effects).
No products indexed under this heading.

Methohexital Sodium (Concomitant use of other CNS depressants may produce additive depressant effects).
No products indexed under this heading.

Methotrimeprazine (Concomitant use of other CNS depressants may produce additive depressant effects).
No products indexed under this heading.

Methoxyflurane (Concomitant use of other CNS depressants may produce additive depressant effects).
No products indexed under this heading.

Methylprednisolone Acetate (Barbiturates appear to enhance the metabolism of exogenous corticosteroids probably through the induction of hepatic microsomal enzymes). Products include:
- Depo-Medrol Injectable Suspension ... 2615
- Depo-Medrol Single-Dose Vial ... 2617

Methylprednisolone Sodium Succinate (Barbiturates appear to enhance the metabolism of exogenous corticosteroids probably through the induction of hepatic microsomal enzymes).
No products indexed under this heading.

Midazolam Hydrochloride (Concomitant use of other CNS depressants may produce additive depressant effects).
No products indexed under this heading.

Moclobemide (Co-administration with MAO inhibitors prolongs the effects of barbiturates probably because the metabolism of the barbiturate is inhibited).
No products indexed under this heading.

Molindone Hydrochloride (Concomitant use of other CNS depressants may produce additive depressant effects). Products include:
- Moban Tablets ... 1108

Morphine Sulfate (Concomitant use of other CNS depressants may produce additive depressant effects). Products include:
- Avinza Capsules ... 1714
- Kadian Capsules ... 572
- MS Contin Tablets ... 2703

Norethindrone (Pretreatment with or co-administration of phenobarbital may decrease the effect of estrogen by increasing its metabolism; application of this data to other barbiturates appears valid; higher incidence of pregnancy in patients on co-administration). Products include:
- Ortho Micronor Tablets ... 2411

Norethynodrel (Pretreatment with or co-administration of phenobarbital may decrease the effect of estrogen by increasing its metabolism; application of this data to other barbiturates appears valid; higher incidence of pregnancy in patients on co-administration).
No products indexed under this heading.

Norgestimate (Pretreatment with or co-administration of phenobarbital may decrease the effect of estrogen by increasing its metabolism; application of this data to other barbiturates appears valid; higher incidence of pregnancy in patients on co-administration). Products include:
- Ortho-Cyclen/Ortho Tri-Cyclen ... 2414
- Ortho Tri-Cyclen Lo Tablets ... 2421
- Prefest Tablets ... 1069

Norgestrel (Pretreatment with or co-administration of phenobarbital may decrease the effect of estrogen by increasing its metabolism; application of this data to other barbiturates appears valid; higher incidence of pregnancy in patients on co-administration). Products include:
- Lo/Ovral-28 Tablets ... 3423

Olanzapine (Concomitant use of other CNS depressants may produce additive depressant effects). Products include:
- Symbyax Capsules ... 1788
- Zyprexa Tablets ... 1798
- Zyprexa IntraMuscular ... 1798
- Zyprexa ZYDIS Orally Disintegrating Tablets ... 1798

Oxazepam (Concomitant use of other CNS depressants may produce additive depressant effects).
No products indexed under this heading.

Oxycodone Hydrochloride (Concomitant use of other CNS depressants may produce additive depressant effects). Products include:
- Combunox Tablets ... 1183
- OxyContin Tablets ... 2699
- OxyFast Oral Concentrate Solution ... 2704
- OxyIR Capsules ... 2704
- Percocet Tablets ... 1114
- Percodan Tablets ... 1115

Pargyline Hydrochloride (Co-administration with MAO inhibitors prolongs the effects of barbiturates probably because the metabolism of the barbiturate is inhibited).
No products indexed under this heading.

Perphenazine (Concomitant use of other CNS depressants may produce additive depressant effects).
No products indexed under this heading.

Phenelzine Sulfate (Co-administration with MAO inhibitors prolongs the effects of barbiturates probably because the metabolism of the barbiturate is inhibited).
No products indexed under this heading.

Phenobarbital (Concomitant use of other CNS depressants may produce additive depressant effects).
No products indexed under this heading.

Phenytoin (The effect of barbiturates on the metabolism of phenytoin appears to be variable).
No products indexed under this heading.

Phenytoin Sodium (The effect of barbiturates on the metabolism of phenytoin appears to be variable). Products include:
- Phenytek Capsules ... 2153

Polyestradiol Phosphate (Pretreatment with or co-administration of phenobarbital may decrease the effect of estrogen by increasing its metabolism; application of this data to other barbiturates appears valid).
No products indexed under this heading.

Prazepam (Concomitant use of other CNS depressants may produce additive depressant effects).
No products indexed under this heading.

Prednisolone Acetate (Barbiturates appear to enhance the metabolism of exogenous corticosteroids probably through the induction of hepatic microsomal enzymes). Products include:
- Blephamide Ophthalmic Ointment ... 563
- Blephamide Ophthalmic Suspension ... 564
- Poly-Pred Liquifilm Ophthalmic Suspension ... ⊙231
- Pred Forte Ophthalmic Suspension ... ⊙233
- Pred Mild Sterile Ophthalmic Suspension ... ⊙236
- Pred-G Ophthalmic Suspension ... ⊙234
- Pred-G Sterile Ophthalmic Ointment ... ⊙235

Prednisolone Sodium Phosphate (Barbiturates appear to enhance the metabolism of exogenous corticosteroids probably through the induction of hepatic microsomal enzymes). Products include:
- Pediapred Oral Solution ... 3319

Prednisolone Tebutate (Barbiturates appear to enhance the metabolism of exogenous corticosteroids probably through the induction of hepatic microsomal enzymes).
No products indexed under this heading.

Prednisone (Barbiturates appear to enhance the metabolism of exogenous corticosteroids probably through the induction of hepatic microsomal enzymes).
No products indexed under this heading.

Procarbazine Hydrochloride (Co-administration with MAO inhibitors prolongs the effects of barbiturates probably because the metabolism of the barbiturate is inhibited). Products include:
- Matulane Capsules ... 3188

Prochlorperazine (Concomitant use of other CNS depressants may produce additive depressant effects).
No products indexed under this heading.

Promethazine Hydrochloride (Concomitant use of other CNS depressants may produce additive depressant effects). Products include:
- Phenergan 3438

Propofol (Concomitant use of other CNS depressants may produce additive depressant effects). Products include:
- Diprivan Injectable Emulsion 676

Propoxyphene Hydrochloride (Concomitant use of other CNS depressants may produce additive depressant effects).
- No products indexed under this heading.

Propoxyphene Napsylate (Concomitant use of other CNS depressants may produce additive depressant effects). Products include:
- Darvocet A 500 Tablets 3497

Quazepam (Concomitant use of other CNS depressants may produce additive depressant effects).
- No products indexed under this heading.

Quetiapine Fumarate (Concomitant use of other CNS depressants may produce additive depressant effects). Products include:
- Seroquel Tablets 691

Quinestrol (Pretreatment with or co-administration of phenobarbital may decrease the effect of estrogen by increasing its metabolism; application of this data to other barbiturates appears valid).
- No products indexed under this heading.

Remifentanil Hydrochloride (Concomitant use of other CNS depressants may produce additive depressant effects).
- No products indexed under this heading.

Risperidone (Concomitant use of other CNS depressants may produce additive depressant effects). Products include:
- Risperdal Consta Long-Acting Injection 1664
- Risperdal M-Tab Orally Disintegrating Tablets.................. 1658
- Risperdal 1658

Secobarbital Sodium (Concomitant use of other CNS depressants may produce additive depressant effects).
- No products indexed under this heading.

Selegiline Hydrochloride (Co-administration with MAO inhibitors prolongs the effects of barbiturates probably because the metabolism of the barbiturate is inhibited). Products include:
- Eldepryl Capsules 3209

Sevoflurane (Concomitant use of other CNS depressants may produce additive depressant effects). Products include:
- Ultane Liquid for Inhalation 526

Sufentanil Citrate (Concomitant use of other CNS depressants may produce additive depressant effects).
- No products indexed under this heading.

Temazepam (Concomitant use of other CNS depressants may produce additive depressant effects).
- No products indexed under this heading.

Thiamylal Sodium (Concomitant use of other CNS depressants may produce additive depressant effects).
- No products indexed under this heading.

Thioridazine Hydrochloride (Concomitant use of other CNS depressants may produce additive depressant effects). Products include:
- Thioridazine Hydrochloride Tablets 2122

Thiothixene (Concomitant use of other CNS depressants may produce additive depressant effects). Products include:
- Thiothixene Capsules 2124

Tranylcypromine Sulfate (Co-administration with MAO inhibitors prolongs the effects of barbiturates probably because the metabolism of the barbiturate is inhibited). Products include:
- Parnate Tablets 1499

Triamcinolone (Barbiturates appear to enhance the metabolism of exogenous corticosteroids probably through the induction of hepatic microsomal enzymes).
- No products indexed under this heading.

Triamcinolone Acetonide (Barbiturates appear to enhance the metabolism of exogenous corticosteroids probably through the induction of hepatic microsomal enzymes). Products include:
- Azmacort Inhalation Aerosol 1701
- Nasacort HFA Inhalation Aerosol 2939
- Nasacort AQ Nasal Spray 2937

Triamcinolone Diacetate (Barbiturates appear to enhance the metabolism of exogenous corticosteroids probably through the induction of hepatic microsomal enzymes).
- No products indexed under this heading.

Triamcinolone Hexacetonide (Barbiturates appear to enhance the metabolism of exogenous corticosteroids probably through the induction of hepatic microsomal enzymes).
- No products indexed under this heading.

Triazolam (Concomitant use of other CNS depressants may produce additive depressant effects).
- No products indexed under this heading.

Trifluoperazine Hydrochloride (Concomitant use of other CNS depressants may produce additive depressant effects).
- No products indexed under this heading.

Valproate Sodium (Valproate appears to decrease barbiturate metabolism). Products include:
- Depacon Injection 412

Valproic Acid (Appears to decrease barbiturate metabolism). Products include:
- Depakene 417

Warfarin Sodium (Barbiturates can induce hepatic microsomal enzymes resulting in increased metabolism and decreased anticoagulant response of oral anticoagulants). Products include:
- Coumadin for Injection 932
- Coumadin Tablets 932

Zaleplon (Concomitant use of other CNS depressants may produce additive depressant effects). Products include:
- Sonata Capsules 1686

Ziprasidone Hydrochloride (Concomitant use of other CNS depressants may produce additive depressant effects). Products include:
- Geodon Capsules 2514

Zolpidem Tartrate (Concomitant use of other CNS depressants may produce additive depressant effects). Products include:
- Ambien Tablets 2867

Food Interactions

Alcohol (Concomitant use of other CNS depressants may produce additive depressant effects).

NEORAL SOFT GELATIN CAPSULES

(Cyclosporine) 2247

May interact with erythromycin, nonsteroidal anti-inflammatory agents, protease inhibitors, potassium sparing diuretics, vaccines, live, and certain other agents. Compounds in these categories include:

Allopurinol (Increases cyclosporine concentrations).
- No products indexed under this heading.

Amiloride Hydrochloride (Cyclosporine may cause hyperkalemia; concurrent use should be avoided). Products include:
- Midamor Tablets 2000
- Moduretic Tablets 2003

Amiodarone Hydrochloride (Increases cyclosporine concentrations). Products include:
- Pacerone Tablets 3337

Amphotericin B (May potentiate renal dysfunction).
- No products indexed under this heading.

Amprenavir (The HIV protease inhibitors are known to inhibit cytochrome P450IIIA and increase the concentration of drugs metabolized by this enzyme system; agents that inhibit this enzyme could decrease metabolism and increase cyclosporine concentrations; this interaction has not been studied; however, care should be exercised). Products include:
- Agenerase Capsules 1299
- Agenerase Oral Solution 1304

Atorvastatin Calcium (Co-administration may result in myotoxicity; atorvastatin dosage should be reduced according to label recommendations. Atorvastatin needs to be temporarily withheld or discontinued in patients with signs and symptoms of myopathy or those with risk factors predisposing to severe renal injury secondary to rhabdomyolysis). Products include:
- Caduet Tablets 2507
- Lipitor Tablets 2495

Azapropazon (May potentiate renal dysfunction).
- No products indexed under this heading.

Azathioprine (May potentiate renal dysfunction). Products include:
- Azasan Tablets 2844

BCG Vaccine (The use of live vaccines should be avoided).
- No products indexed under this heading.

Bromocriptine Mesylate (Increases cyclosporine concentrations).
- No products indexed under this heading.

Carbamazepine (Decreases cyclosporine concentrations). Products include:
- Carbatrol Capsules 3174
- Equetro Extended-Release Capsules.. 3178
- Tegretol/Tegretol-XR 2278

Celecoxib (Co-administration with NSAID's particularly in the setting of dehydration, may potentiate renal dysfunction). Products include:
- Celebrex Capsules 3130

Cimetidine (May potentiate renal dysfunction). Products include:
- Tagamet HB 200 Tablets 637
- Tagamet Tablets 1547

Cimetidine Hydrochloride (May potentiate renal dysfunction).
- No products indexed under this heading.

Clarithromycin (Increases cyclosporine concentrations). Products include:
- Biaxin/Biaxin XL 402
- PREVPAC 3281

Colchicine (Cyclosporine may reduce the clearance of colchicine and enhance the toxic effects of colchicine, such as myopathy and neuropathy, especially in patients with renal dysfunction. Close clinical observation is required during concurrent therapy to enable early detection of colchicine toxicity, followed by reduction of dosage or its withdrawal).
- No products indexed under this heading.

Dalfopristin (Co-administration with substrates that inhibit CYP450 3A, such as dalfopristin, could decrease metabolism and increase cyclosporine concentrations). Products include:
- Synercid I.V. 1690

Danazol (Increases cyclosporine concentrations).
- No products indexed under this heading.

Diclofenac Potassium (Co-administration has been associated with approximate doubling of diclofenac blood levels and occasional reports of reversible decreases in renal function; possible potentiation of renal dysfunction; the dose of diclofenac should be in the lower end of the therapeutic range). Products include:
- Cataflam Tablets 2173

Diclofenac Sodium (Co-administration has been associated with approximate doubling of diclofenac blood levels and occasional reports of reversible decreases in renal function; possible potentiation of renal dysfunction; the dose of diclofenac should be in the lower end of the therapeutic range). Products include:
- Arthrotec Tablets 3126
- Voltaren Ophthalmic Solution 2300
- Voltaren Tablets 2298
- Voltaren-XR Tablets 2301

Digoxin (Cyclosporine may reduce the clearance of digoxin; severe digitalis toxicity may result. Closed clinical observation is required during concurrent therapy to enable early detection of digitalis toxicity, followed by reduction of dosage or its withdrawal). Products include:
- Digitek Tablets 2146
- Lanoxicaps Capsules 1458
- Lanoxin Injection 1462
- Lanoxin Tablets 1468
- Lanoxin Injection Pediatric 1465

IMPORTANT NOTE: Always consult each drug listing in the patient's regimen for possible interactions.

Diltiazem Hydrochloride (Increases cyclosporine concentrations). Products include:
- Cardizem LA Extended Release Tablets 1699
- Tiazac Capsules 1204

Erythromycin (Co-administration with substrates that inhibit CYP450 3A, such as erythromycin, could decrease metabolism and increase cyclosporine concentrations). Products include:
- Erygel Topical Gel 2096
- Ery-Tab Tablets 447
- Erythromycin Base Filmtab Tablets 454
- Erythromycin Delayed-Release Capsules, USP 456
- PCE Dispertab Tablets 510

Erythromycin Estolate (Co-administration with substrates that inhibit CYP450 3A, such as erythromycin, could decrease metabolism and increase cyclosporine concentrations).
- No products indexed under this heading.

Erythromycin Ethylsuccinate (Co-administration with substrates that inhibit CYP450 3A, such as erythromycin, could decrease metabolism and increase cyclosporine concentrations). Products include:
- E.E.S. 449
- EryPed 445

Erythromycin Gluceptate (Co-administration with substrates that inhibit CYP450 3A, such as erythromycin, could decrease metabolism and increase cyclosporine concentrations).
- No products indexed under this heading.

Erythromycin Lactobionate (Co-administration with substrates that inhibit CYP450 3A, such as erythromycin, could decrease metabolism and increase cyclosporine concentrations).
- No products indexed under this heading.

Erythromycin Stearate (Co-administration with substrates that inhibit CYP450 3A, such as erythromycin, could decrease metabolism and increase cyclosporine concentrations). Products include:
- Erythrocin Stearate Filmtab Tablets 452

Etodolac (Co-administration with NSAID's particularly in the setting of dehydration, may potentiate renal dysfunction).
- No products indexed under this heading.

Fenoprofen Calcium (Co-administration with NSAID's particularly in the setting of dehydration, may potentiate renal dysfunction). Products include:
- Nalfon Capsules 2504

Fluconazole (Increases cyclosporine concentrations).
- No products indexed under this heading.

Flurbiprofen (Co-administration with NSAID's particularly in the setting of dehydration, may potentiate renal dysfunction).
- No products indexed under this heading.

Fluvastatin Sodium (Co-administration may rarely result in myotoxicity; fluvastatin dosage should be reduced according to label recommendations. Fluvastatin needs to be temporarily withheld or discontinued in patients with signs and symptons of myopathy or those with risk factors predisposing to severe renal injury secondary to rhabdomyolysis). Products include:
- Lescol Capsules 2227
- Lescol 2730
- Lescol XL Tablets 2227

Gentamicin Sulfate (May potentiate renal dysfunction). Products include:
- Garamycin Injectable 3028
- Genoptic Sterile Ophthalmic Solution ⊙227
- Pred-G Ophthalmic Suspension ⊙234
- Pred-G Sterile Ophthalmic Ointment ⊙235

Hypericum (Co-administration has been reported to produce a marked reduction in blood cyclosporine concentrations, resulting in subtherapeutic levels, rejection of transplanted organs, and graft loss).
- No products indexed under this heading.

Ibuprofen (Co-administration with NSAID's particularly in the setting of dehydration, may potentiate renal dysfunction). Products include:
- Advil Allergy Sinus Caplets ▣737
- Advil ▣737
- Children's Advil Suspension ▣742
- Children's Advil Chewable Tablets ▣741
- Advil Cold & Sinus ▣739
- Advil Flu & Body Ache Caplets ▣739
- Children's Advil Cold Suspension ▣741
- Infants' Advil Concentrated Drops ▣743
- Junior Strength Advil Swallow Tablets ▣740
- Advil Migraine Liquigels ▣740
- Advil Multi-Symptom Cold Caplets ▣738
- Combunox Tablets 1183
- Children's Motrin Oral Suspension and Chewable Tablets 1837
- Children's Motrin Cold Non-Staining Dye-Free Oral Suspension 1838
- Children's Motrin Cold Oral Suspension 1838
- Children's Motrin Non-Staining Dye-Free Oral Suspension 1837
- Motrin Cold & Sinus Caplets 1836
- Motrin IB Tablets and Caplets 1836
- Infants' Motrin Concentrated Drops 1837
- Infants' Motrin Non-Staining Dye-Free Drops 1837
- Junior Strength Motrin Caplets and Chewable Tablets 1837
- Vicoprofen Tablets 533

Indinavir Sulfate (The HIV protease inhibitors are known to inhibit cytochrome P450IIIA and increase the concentration of drugs metabolized by this enzyme system; agents that inhibit this enzyme could decrease metabolism and increase cyclosporine concentrations; this interaction has not been studied; however, care should be exercised). Products include:
- Crixivan Capsules 1918

Indomethacin (Co-administration with NSAID's particularly in the setting of dehydration, may potentiate renal dysfunction). Products include:
- Indocin 1968

Indomethacin Sodium Trihydrate (Co-administration with NSAID's particularly in the setting of dehydration, may potentiate renal dysfunction). Products include:
- Indocin I.V. 1973

Itraconazole (Increases cyclosporine concentrations).
- No products indexed under this heading.

Ketoconazole (May potentiate renal dysfunction; co-administration with substrates that inhibit CYP450 3A, such as ketoconazole, could decrease metabolism and increase cyclosporine concentrations). Products include:
- Nizoral A-D Shampoo, 1% 1839
- Nizoral 2% Shampoo 1838

Ketoprofen (Co-administration with NSAID's particularly in the setting of dehydration, may potentiate renal dysfunction).
- No products indexed under this heading.

Ketorolac Tromethamine (Co-administration with NSAID's particularly in the setting of dehydration, may potentiate renal dysfunction). Products include:
- Acular Ophthalmic Solution 561
- Acular LS Ophthalmic Solution 562

Lopinavir (The HIV protease inhibitors are known to inhibit cytochrome P450IIIA and increase the concentration of drugs metabolized by this enzyme system; agents that inhibit this enzyme could decrease metabolism and increase cyclosporine concentrations; this interaction has not been studied; however, care should be exercised). Products include:
- Kaletra 474

Lovastatin (Co-administration may results in myotoxicity; lovastatin dosage should be reduced according to label recommendations. Lovastatin needs to be temporarily withheld or discontinued in patients with signs and symptoms of myopathy or those with risk factors predisposing to severe renal injury secondary to rhabdomyolysis). Products include:
- Advicor Tablets 1694
- Altoprev Extended-Release Tablets 1151
- Mevacor Tablets 1996

Measles, Mumps & Rubella Virus Vaccine, Live (The use of live vaccines should be avoided). Products include:
- M-M-R II 1980

Measles & Rubella Virus Vaccine Live (The use of live vaccines should be avoided).
- No products indexed under this heading.

Measles Virus Vaccine Live (The use of live vaccines should be avoided). Products include:
- Attenuvax 1889

Meclofenamate Sodium (Co-administration with NSAID's particularly in the setting of dehydration, may potentiate renal dysfunction).
- No products indexed under this heading.

Mefenamic Acid (Co-administration with NSAID's particularly in the setting of dehydration, may potentiate renal dysfunction).
- No products indexed under this heading.

Meloxicam (Co-administration with NSAID's particularly in the setting of dehydration, may potentiate renal dysfunction). Products include:
- Mobic Oral Suspension 893
- Mobic Tablets 893

Melphalan (May potentiate renal dysfunction). Products include:
- Alkeran Tablets 977

Methotrexate Sodium (Increased risk of developing skin malignancies in psoriasis patients with concurrent use; in rheumatoid arthritis patients, methotrexate concentrations (AUCs) were increased approximately 30% and concentrations (AUCs) of its metabolites were decreased approximately 80%; the clinical significance is unknown).
- No products indexed under this heading.

Methylprednisolone (Convulsions have been reported with high doses of methylprednisolone).
- No products indexed under this heading.

Methylprednisolone Acetate (Convulsions have been reported with high doses of methylprednisolone). Products include:
- Depo-Medrol Injectable Suspension 2615
- Depo-Medrol Single-Dose Vial 2617

Methylprednisolone Sodium Succinate (Convulsions have been reported with high doses of methylprednisolone).
- No products indexed under this heading.

Metoclopramide Hydrochloride (Increases cyclosporine concentrations).
- No products indexed under this heading.

Mumps Virus Vaccine, Live (The use of live vaccines should be avoided). Products include:
- Mumpsvax 2005

Muromonab-CD3 (Psoriasis patients receiving other immunosuppressive agents, such as muromonab-CD3, should not receive concurrent cyclosporine because of the possibility of excessive immunosuppression). Products include:
- Orthoclone OKT3 Sterile Solution 2370

Mycophenolate Mofetil (Psoriasis patients receiving other immunosuppressive agents, such as mycophenolate mofetil, should not receive concurrent cyclosporine because of the possibility of excessive immunosuppression). Products include:
- CellCept Capsules 2751
- CellCept Oral Suspension 2751
- CellCept Tablets 2751

Nabumetone (Co-administration with NSAID's particularly in the setting of dehydration, may potentiate renal dysfunction). Products include:
- Relafen Tablets 1523

Nafcillin Sodium (Decreases cyclosporine concentrations).
- No products indexed under this heading.

Naproxen (Concomitant use is associated with additive decreases in renal function with possible potentiation of renal dysfunction). Products include:
- EC-Naprosyn Delayed-Release Tablets 2769
- Naprosyn Suspension 2769
- Naprosyn Tablets 2769
- Prevacid NapraPAC 3277

Naproxen Sodium (Concomitant use is associated with additive decreases in renal function with possible potentiation of renal dysfunction). Products include:
- Aleve Tablets, Caplets and Gelcaps ▣605
- Anaprox Tablets 2769
- Anaprox DS Tablets 2769

Nelfinavir Mesylate (The HIV protease inhibitors are known to inhibit

cytochrome P450IIIA and increase the concentration of drugs metabolized by this enzyme system; agents that inhibit this enzyme could decrease metabolism and increase cyclosporine concentrations; this interaction has not been studied; however, care should be exercised). Products include:

Viracept 2556

Nephrotoxic Drugs (Potential for increased nephrotoxicity; careful monitoring of renal function is required).

No products indexed under this heading.

Nicardipine Hydrochloride (Increases cyclosporine concentrations). Products include:

Cardene I.V. 1129

Nifedipine (Potential for frequent gingival hyperplasia). Products include:

Adalat CC Tablets 2978

Octreotide Acetate (Decreases cyclosporine concentrations). Products include:

Sandostatin Injection 2263
Sandostatin LAR Depot 2264

Orlistat (Co-administration can result in decreased absorption of cyclosporine; concomitant use should be avoided). Products include:

Xenical Capsules 2834

Oxaprozin (Co-administration with NSAID's particularly in the setting of dehydration, may potentiate renal dysfunction).

No products indexed under this heading.

Phenobarbital (Decreases cyclosporine concentrations).

No products indexed under this heading.

Phenylbutazone (Co-administration with NSAID's particularly in the setting of dehydration, may potentiate renal dysfunction).

No products indexed under this heading.

Piroxicam (Co-administration with NSAID's particularly in the setting of dehydration, may potentiate renal dysfunction).

No products indexed under this heading.

Poliovirus Vaccine, Live, Oral, Trivalent, Types 1,2,3 (Sabin) (The use of live vaccines should be avoided).

No products indexed under this heading.

Pravastatin Sodium (Co-administration may result in myotoxicity; pravastatin dosage should be reduced according to label recommendations. Pravastatin needs to be temporarily withheld or discontinued in patients with signs and symptoms of myopathy or those with risk factors predisposing to severe renal injury secondary to rhabdomyolysis). Products include:

Pravachol Tablets 943

Prednisolone (Cyclosporine may reduce the clearance of prednisolone).

No products indexed under this heading.

Prednisolone Acetate (Cyclosporine may reduce the clearance of prednisolone). Products include:

Blephamide Ophthalmic Ointment 563
Blephamide Ophthalmic Suspension 564
Poly-Pred Liquifilm Ophthalmic Suspension .... ⊙231
Pred Forte Ophthalmic Suspension .... ⊙233
Pred Mild Sterile Ophthalmic Suspension .... ⊙236
Pred-G Ophthalmic Suspension .... ⊙234
Pred-G Sterile Ophthalmic Ointment .... ⊙235

Prednisolone Sodium Phosphate (Cyclosporine may reduce the clearance of prednisolone). Products include:

Pediapred Oral Solution 3319

Quinupristin (Co-administration with substrates that inhibit CYP450 3A, such as quinupristin, could decrease metabolism and increase cyclosporine concentrations). Products include:

Synercid I.V. 1690

Ranitidine Hydrochloride (May potentiate renal dysfunction). Products include:

Zantac 1597
Zantac Injection 1593
Zantac 75 Tablets .... ▣715
Zantac 150 Maximum Strength Tablets .... ▣715
Zantac Injection Pharmacy Bulk Package 1595

Rifabutin (Substances that are inducers of cyctochrome P450 activity could increase metabolism and decrease cyclosporine concentrations; rifabutin is known to increase the metabolism of other drugs metabolized by the cytochrome P450; this interaction has not been studied, however, care should be exercised).

No products indexed under this heading.

Rifampin (Decreases cyclosporine concentrations).

No products indexed under this heading.

Ritonavir (The HIV protease inhibitors are known to inhibit cytochrome P450IIIA and increase the concentration of drugs metabolized by this enzyme system; agents that inhibit this enzyme could decrease metabolism and increase cyclosporine concentrations; this interaction has not been studied; however, care should be exercised). Products include:

Kaletra 474
Norvir 499

Rofecoxib (Co-administration with NSAID's particularly in the setting of dehydration, may potentiate renal dysfunction).

No products indexed under this heading.

Rotavirus Vaccine, Live, Oral, Tetravalent (The use of live vaccines should be avoided).

No products indexed under this heading.

Rubella & Mumps Virus Vaccine Live (The use of live vaccines should be avoided).

No products indexed under this heading.

Rubella Virus Vaccine Live (The use of live vaccines should be avoided). Products include:

Meruvax II 1994

Saquinavir (The HIV protease inhibitors are known to inhibit cytochrome P450IIIA and increase the concentration of drugs metabolized by this enzyme system; agents that inhibit this enzyme could decrease metabolism and increase cyclosporine concentrations; this interaction has not been studied; however, care should be exercised).

No products indexed under this heading.

Saquinavir Mesylate (The HIV protease inhibitors are known to inhibit cytochrome P450IIIA and increase the concentration of drugs metabolized by this enzyme system; agents that inhibit this enzyme could decrease metabolism and increase cyclosporine concentrations; this interaction has not been studied; however, care should be exercised). Products include:

Invirase 2776

Simvastatin (Co-administration may result in myotoxicity; simvastation dosage should be reduced according to label recommendations. Simvastatin needs to be temporarily withheld or discontinued in patients with signs and symptoms of myopathy or those with risk factors predisposing to severe renal injury secondary to rhabdomyolysis). Products include:

Vytorin 10/10 Tablets 2084
Vytorin 10/10 Tablets 3092
Vytorin 10/20 Tablets 2084
Vytorin 10/20 Tablets 3092
Vytorin 10/40 Tablets 3092
Vytorin 10/40 Tablets 2084
Vytorin 10/80 Tablets 2084
Vytorin 10/80 Tablets 3092
Zocor Tablets 2078

Smallpox Vaccine (The use of live vaccines should be avoided).

No products indexed under this heading.

Spironolactone (Cyclosporine may cause hyperkalemia; concurrent use should be avoided).

No products indexed under this heading.

Sulfamethoxazole (Co-administration with trimethoprim/sulfamethoxazole may potentiate renal dysfunction).

No products indexed under this heading.

Sulindac (Concomitant use is associated with additive decreases in renal function with possible potentiation of renal dysfunction). Products include:

Clinoril Tablets 1899

Tacrolimus (May potentiate renal dysfunction). Products include:

Prograf Capsules and Injection 624
Protopic Ointment 629

Ticlopidine Hydrochloride (Decreases cyclosporine concentrations). Products include:

Ticlid Tablets 2813

Tobramycin (May potentiate renal dysfunction). Products include:

TOBI Solution for Inhalation 1015
TobraDex Ophthalmic Ointment 558
TobraDex Ophthalmic Suspension 558
Zylet Ophthalmic Suspension 3508

Tobramycin Sulfate (May potentiate renal dysfunction).

No products indexed under this heading.

Tolmetin Sodium (Co-administration with NSAID's particularly in the setting of dehydration, may potentiate renal dysfunction).

No products indexed under this heading.

Triamterene (Cyclosporine may cause hyperkalemia; concurrent use should be avoided). Products include:

Dyazide Capsules 1389
Dyrenium Capsules 3390
Maxzide 2150

Trimethoprim (Co-administration with trimethoprim/sulfamethoxazole may potentiate renal dysfunction).

No products indexed under this heading.

Typhoid Vaccine (The use of live vaccines should be avoided).

No products indexed under this heading.

Vaccines (Live) (Vaccination may be less effective).

No products indexed under this heading.

Valdecoxib (Co-administration with NSAID's particularly in the setting of dehydration, may potentiate renal dysfunction).

No products indexed under this heading.

Vancomycin Hydrochloride (May potentiate renal dysfunction). Products include:

Vancocin HCl Capsules, USP 3370

Varicella Virus Vaccine Live (The use of live vaccines should be avoided). Products include:

Varivax 2070

Verapamil Hydrochloride (Increases cyclosporine concentrations). Products include:

Covera-HS Tablets 3135
Tarka Tablets 519
Verelan PM Capsules 3120

Yellow Fever Vaccine (The use of live vaccines should be avoided).

No products indexed under this heading.

Food Interactions

Diet, high-lipid (A high-fat meal consumed within one-half hour before Neoral administration decreased the AUC by 13% and Cmax by 33%).

Food, unspecified (Administration of food with Neoral decreases the AUC and Cmax).

Grapefruit (Affects the metabolism of cyclosporine and should be avoided).

Grapefruit Juice (Affects the metabolism of cyclosporine and should be avoided).

NEORAL ORAL SOLUTION

(Cyclosporine) 2247
See Neoral Soft Gelatin Capsules

NEOSPORIN OINTMENT

(Bacitracin, Neomycin, Polymyxin B Sulfate) .... ▣702
None cited in PDR database.

NEOSPORIN + PAIN RELIEF MAXIMUM STRENGTH CREAM

(Neomycin, Polymyxin B Sulfate, Pramoxine Hydrochloride) .... ▣703
None cited in PDR database.

NEOSPORIN + PAIN RELIEF MAXIMUM STRENGTH OINTMENT

(Bacitracin, Neomycin, Polymyxin B Sulfate, Pramoxine Hydrochloride) .... ▣703
None cited in PDR database.

NEOSPORIN SCAR SOLUTION

(Silicone) .... ▣702
None cited in PDR database.

NEULASTA INJECTION
(Pegfilgrastim) 596
May interact with drugs which potentiate the release of neutrophils. Compounds in these categories include:

Lithium Carbonate (Concurrent use should be undertaken with caution since lithium potentiates the release of neutrophils). Products include:
- Eskalith 1406
- Lithobid Tablets 1670

Lithium Citrate (Concurrent use should be undertaken with caution since lithium potentiates the release of neutrophils).
No products indexed under this heading.

NEUMEGA FOR INJECTION
(Oprelvekin) 3433
None cited in PDR database.

NEUPOGEN FOR INJECTION
(Filgrastim) 598
May interact with drugs which potentiate the release of neutrophils. Compounds in these categories include:

Lithium Carbonate (Concurrent use should be undertaken with caution since lithium potentiates the release of neutrophils). Products include:
- Eskalith 1406
- Lithobid Tablets 1670

Lithium Citrate (Concurrent use should be undertaken with caution since lithium potentiates the release of neutrophils).
No products indexed under this heading.

NEURONTIN CAPSULES
(Gabapentin) 2498
May interact with:

Aluminum Hydroxide (Coadministration reduces bioavailability of gabapentin by 20%; gabapentin should be taken at least 2 hours following antacid containing aluminum hydroxide and magnesium hydroxide). Products include:
- Gaviscon Regular Strength Liquid .. ▣620
- Gaviscon Regular Strength Tablets .... ▣619
- Gaviscon Extra Strength Liquid ...... ▣620
- Gaviscon Extra Strength Tablets .... ▣619
- Maalox Max Maximum Strength Antacid/Anti-Gas Liquid................ 2165
- Maalox Regular Strength Antacid/Antigas Liquid................ 2164

Cimetidine (Alters renal clearance of gabapentin and creatinine; this small decrease in excretion of gabapentin is not expected to be of clinical importance). Products include:
- Tagamet HB 200 Tablets .... ▣637
- Tagamet Tablets 1547

Cimetidine Hydrochloride (Alters renal clearance of gabapentin and creatinine; this small decrease in excretion of gabapentin is not expected to be of clinical importance).
No products indexed under this heading.

Hydrocodone Bitartrate (Co-administration decreases hydrocodone CMax and AUC values in a dose-dependent manner relative to administration of hydrocodone alone; hydrocodone increases gabapentin AUC values by 14%). Products include:
- Hycodan 1104
- Hycomine Compound Tablets 1105
- Hycotuss Expectorant Syrup 1106
- Lortab 3315
- Lortab Elixir 3312
- Vicodin Tablets 530
- Vicodin ES Tablets 531
- Vicodin HP Tablets 532
- Vicoprofen Tablets 533
- Zydone Tablets 1118

Magnesium Hydroxide (Coadministration reduces bioavailability of gabapentin by 20%; gabapentin should be taken at least 2 hours following antacid containing aluminum hydroxide and magnesium hydroxide). Products include:
- Maalox Max Maximum Strength Antacid/Anti-Gas Liquid................ 2165
- Maalox Regular Strength Antacid/Antigas Liquid................ 2164
- Pepcid Complete Chewable Tablets 1672
- Rolaids Tablets .... ▣707
- Extra Strength Rolaids Tablets .... ▣707
- Rolaids Multi-Symptom Antacid & Antigas Tablets .... ▣708

Morphine Sulfate (Co-administration results in increased gabapentin concentrations; patients should be observed for signs of CNS depression, such as somnolence). Products include:
- Avinza Capsules 1714
- Kadian Capsules 572
- MS Contin Tablets 2703

Naproxen (Co-administration appears to increase the amount of gabapentin absorbed by 12% to 15%; the doses for both drugs were lower than the therapeutic doses; magnitude of interaction within the recommended dose ranges for either drug is not known). Products include:
- EC-Naprosyn Delayed-Release Tablets 2769
- Naprosyn Suspension 2769
- Naprosyn Tablets 2769
- Prevacid NapraPAC 3277

Naproxen Sodium (Co-administration appears to increase the amount of gabapentin absorbed by 12% to 15%; the doses for both drugs were lower than the therapeutic doses; magnitude of interaction within the recommended dose ranges for either drug is not known). Products include:
- Aleve Tablets, Caplets and Gelcaps .... ▣605
- Anaprox Tablets 2769
- Anaprox DS Tablets 2769

Norethindrone (The Cmax of norethindrone was 13% higher when it was coadministered with gabapentin; this interaction is not expected to be of clinical importance). Products include:
- Ortho Micronor Tablets 2411

Norethindrone Acetate (The Cmax of norethindrone was 13% higher when it was coadministered with gabapentin; this interaction is not expected to be of clinical importance). Products include:
- Activella Tablets 2311
- Aygestin Tablets 1062
- CombiPatch Transdermal System 2180

NEURONTIN ORAL SOLUTION
(Gabapentin) 2498
See Neurontin Capsules

NEURONTIN TABLETS
(Gabapentin) 2498
See Neurontin Capsules

NEXIUM DELAYED-RELEASE CAPSULES
(Esomeprazole Magnesium) 645
May interact with iron containing oral preparations and certain other agents. Compounds in these categories include:

Amoxicillin (Co-administration of esomeprazole, clarithromycin, and amoxicillin has resulted in an increase in the plasma levels of esomeprazole and 14-hydroxyclarithromycin; the observed increase in esomeprazole exposure during co-administration with clarithromycin and amoxicillin is not expected to produce safety concerns). Products include:
- Amoxil Capsules 1315
- Amoxil Chewable Tablets 1315
- Amoxil Pediatric Drops for Oral Suspension 1315
- Amoxil Powder for Oral Suspension 1315
- Amoxil Tablets 1315
- Augmentin 1331
- Augmentin Tablets 1334
- Augmentin XR Extended-Release Tablets 1340
- Augmentin ES-600 Powder for Oral Suspension 1337
- PREVPAC 3281

Amoxicillin Trihydrate (Co-administration of esomeprazole, clarithromycin, and amoxicillin has resulted in an increase in the plasma levels of esomeprazole and 14-hydroxyclarithromycin; the observed increase in esomeprazole exposure during co-administration with clarithromycin and amoxicillin is not expected to produce safety concerns).
No products indexed under this heading.

Clarithromycin (Co-administration of esomeprazole, clarithromycin, and amoxicillin has resulted in an increase in the plasma levels of esomeprazole and 14-hydroxyclarithromycin; the observed increase in esomeprazole exposure during co-administration with clarithromycin and amoxicillin is not expected to produce safety concerns). Products include:
- Biaxin/Biaxin XL 402
- PREVPAC 3281

Diazepam (Esomeprazole may interfere with CYP2C19, the major metabolizing enzyme; co-administration of esomeprazole and diazepam, a CYP2C19 substrate, resulted in a 45% decrease in clearance of diazepam; increased plasma levels of diazepam were observed 12 hours after dosing and onwards; however, at that time the plasma levels of diazepam were below the therapeutic interval, and this interaction is unlikely to be of clinical relevance). Products include:
- Diastat Rectal Delivery System 3344
- Valium Tablets 2822

Digoxin (Esomeprazole inhibits gastric acid secretion; therefore, esomeprazole may interfere with the absorption of drugs where gastric pH is an important determinant of bioavailability, such as digoxin). Products include:
- Digitek Tablets 2146
- Lanoxicaps Capsules 1458
- Lanoxin Injection 1462
- Lanoxin Tablets 1468
- Lanoxin Injection Pediatric 1465

Ferrous Fumarate (Esomeprazole inhibits gastric acid secretion; therefore, esomeprazole may interfere with the absorption of drugs where gastric pH is an important determinant of bioavailability, such as oral iron salts). Products include:
- Chromagen Forte Soft Gelatin Capsules 3296
- Ferretts Tablets .... ▣773
- Repliva 21/7 Tablets 3301

Ferrous Gluconate (Esomeprazole inhibits gastric acid secretion; therefore, esomeprazole may interfere with the absorption of drugs where gastric pH is an important determinant of bioavailability, such as oral iron salts).
No products indexed under this heading.

Ferrous Sulfate (Esomeprazole inhibits gastric acid secretion; therefore, esomeprazole may interfere with the absorption of drugs where gastric pH is an important determinant of bioavailability, such as oral iron salts). Products include:
- Feosol Tablets 1629
- Slow Fe Iron Tablets .... ▣772
- Slow Fe with Folic Acid Tablets .... ▣773

Iron (Esomeprazole inhibits gastric acid secretion; therefore, esomeprazole may interfere with the absorption of drugs where gastric pH is an important determinant of bioavailability, such as oral iron salts). Products include:
- Chromagen Forte Soft Gelatin Capsules 3296
- Ferretts IPS Liquid .... ▣773
- OptiNate 1162
- Repliva 21/7 Tablets 3301

Ketoconazole (Esomeprazole inhibits gastric acid secretion; therefore, esomeprazole may interfere with the absorption of drugs where gastric pH is an important determinant of bioavailability, such as ketoconazole). Products include:
- Nizoral A-D Shampoo, 1% 1839
- Nizoral 2% Shampoo 1838

Pimozide (Co-administration of clarithromycin-esomeprazole combination with pimozide is contraindicated; concurrent use of clarithromycin and/or erythromycin with pimozide has resulted in cardiac arrhythmias including QT prolongation, ventricular tachycardia, ventricular fibrillations and torsade de pointes). Products include:
- Orap Tablets 1220

Polysaccharide Iron Complex (Esomeprazole inhibits gastric acid secretion; therefore, esomeprazole may interfere with the absorption of drugs where gastric pH is an important determinant of bioavailability, such as oral iron salts). Products include:
- Niferex-150 Forte Capsules 3299
- Nu-Iron 150 Capsules 2098

Warfarin Sodium (Changes in prothrombin measures have been reported among patients on concomitant warfarin and esomeprazole therapy. Increases in INR and prothrombin time may lead to abnormal bleeding and even death. Patients treated with proton pump inhibitors and warfarin concomitantly may need to be monitored for increases in INR and prothrombin time). Products include:
- Coumadin for Injection 932

Coumadin Tablets 932

NEXIUM I.V.
(Esomeprazole Sodium) 649
May interact with iron containing oral preparations and certain other agents. Compounds in these categories include:

Diazepam (Esomeprazole may interfere with CYP2C19, the major metabolizing enzyme; co-administration of esomeprazole and diazepam, a CYP2C19 substrate, resulted in a 45% decrease in clearance of diazepam; increased plasma levels of diazepam were observed 12 hours after dosing and onwards; however, at that time the plasma levels of diazepam were below the therapeutic interval, and this interaction is unlikely to be of clinical relevance). Products include:
Diastat Rectal Delivery System 3344
Valium Tablets 2822

Digoxin (Esomeprazole inhibits gastric acid secretion; therefore, esomeprazole may interfere with the absorption of drugs where gastric pH is an important determinant of bioavailability, such as digoxin). Products include:
Digitek Tablets 2146
Lanoxicaps Capsules 1458
Lanoxin Injection 1462
Lanoxin Tablets 1468
Lanoxin Injection Pediatric 1465

Ferrous Fumarate (Esomeprazole inhibits gastric acid secretion; therefore, esomeprazole may interfere with the absorption of drugs where gastric pH is an important determinant of bioavailability, such as oral iron salts). Products include:
Chromagen Forte Soft Gelatin Capsules 3296
Ferretts Tablets 773
Repliva 21/7 Tablets 3301

Ferrous Gluconate (Esomeprazole inhibits gastric acid secretion; therefore, esomeprazole may interfere with the absorption of drugs where gastric pH is an important determinant of bioavailability, such as oral iron salts).
No products indexed under this heading.

Ferrous Sulfate (Esomeprazole inhibits gastric acid secretion; therefore, esomeprazole may interfere with the absorption of drugs where gastric pH is an important determinant of bioavailability, such as oral iron salts). Products include:
Feosol Tablets 1629
Slow Fe Iron Tablets 772
Slow Fe with Folic Acid Tablets 773

Iron (Esomeprazole inhibits gastric acid secretion; therefore, esomeprazole may interfere with the absorption of drugs where gastric pH is an important determinant of bioavailability, such as oral iron salts). Products include:
Chromagen Forte Soft Gelatin Capsules 3296
Ferretts IPS Liquid 773
OptiNate 1162
Repliva 21/7 Tablets 3301

Ketoconazole (Esomeprazole inhibits gastric acid secretion; therefore, esomeprazole may interfere with the absorption of drugs where gastric pH is an important determinant of bioavailability, such as ketoconazole). Products include:
Nizoral A-D Shampoo, 1% 1839
Nizoral 2% Shampoo 1838

Pimozide (Co-administration of clarithromycin-esomeprazole combination with pimozide is contraindicated; concurrent use of clarithromycin and/or erythromycin with pimozide has resulted in cardiac arrhythmias including QT prolongation, ventricular tachycardia, ventricular fibrillations and torsade de pointes). Products include:
Orap Tablets 1220

Polysaccharide Iron Complex (Esomeprazole inhibits gastric acid secretion; therefore, esomeprazole may interfere with the absorption of drugs where gastric pH is an important determinant of bioavailability, such as oral iron salts). Products include:
Niferex-150 Forte Capsules 3299
Nu-Iron 150 Capsules 2098

Warfarin Sodium (Changes in prothrombin measures have been reported among patients on concomitant warfarin and esomeprazole therapy. Increases in INR and prothrombin time may lead to abnormal bleeding and even death. Patients treated with proton pump inhibitors and warfarin concomitantly may need to be monitored for increases in INR and prothrombin time). Products include:
Coumadin for Injection 932
Coumadin Tablets 932

NIASPAN EXTENDED-RELEASE TABLETS
(Niacin) 1703
May interact with beta blockers, calcium channel blockers, oral anticoagulants, HMG-CoA reductase inhibitors, nitrates and nitrites, and certain other agents. Compounds in these categories include:

Acebutolol Hydrochloride (Co-administration with vasoactive drugs, such as adrenergic blocking agents, may result in postural hypotension, particularly in patients with unstable angina or acute phase of myocardial infarction).
No products indexed under this heading.

Amlodipine Besylate (Co-administration with vasoactive drugs, such as calcium channel blockers, may result in postural hypotension, particularly in patients with unstable angina or acute phase of myocardial infarction). Products include:
Caduet Tablets 2507
Lotrel Capsules 2238
Norvasc Tablets 2529

Amyl Nitrite (Co-administration with vasoactive drugs, such as nitrates, may result in postural hypotension, particularly in patients with unstable angina or acute phase of myocardial infarction).
No products indexed under this heading.

Anisindione (Niacin prolongs prothrombin time; caution should be exercised when used concurrently). Products include:
Miradon Tablets 3056

Aspirin (Concomitant aspirin may decrease the metabolic clearance of nicotinic acid; the clinical relevance of this finding is unclear). Products include:
Aggrenox Capsules 855
Bayer, Aspirin Regimen 606
Bayer Aspirin Tablets 3515
BC Powder 612
BC Allergy Sinus Cold Powder 612
Arthritis Strength BC Powder 612
BC Sinus Cold Powder 612
Ecotrin Enteric Coated Aspirin Low, Regular and Maximum Strength Tablets 1627
Goody's Body Pain Formula Powder 621
Goody's Extra Strength Headache Powder 621
Goody's Extra Strength Pain Relief Tablets 621
Percodan Tablets 1115
St. Joseph 81 mg Aspirin Chewable and Enteric Coated Tablets 1841

Atenolol (Co-administration with vasoactive drugs, such as adrenergic blocking agents, may result in postural hypotension, particularly in patients with unstable angina or acute phase of myocardial infarction). Products include:
Tenormin I.V. Injection 698
Tenormin Tablets 695

Atorvastatin Calcium (Co-administration of lipid-altering doses ($\geq$ 1 g/day) of niacin and HMG-CoA reductase inhibitors has resulted in rare cases of rhabdomyolysis). Products include:
Caduet Tablets 2507
Lipitor Tablets 2495

Bepridil Hydrochloride (Co-administration with vasoactive drugs, such as calcium channel blockers, may result in postural hypotension, particularly in patients with unstable angina or acute phase of myocardial infarction).
No products indexed under this heading.

Betaxolol Hydrochloride (Co-administration with vasoactive drugs, such as adrenergic blocking agents, may result in postural hypotension, particularly in patients with unstable angina or acute phase of myocardial infarction). Products include:
Betoptic S Ophthalmic Suspension 554

Bisoprolol Fumarate (Co-administration with vasoactive drugs, such as adrenergic blocking agents, may result in postural hypotension, particularly in patients with unstable angina or acute phase of myocardial infarction).
No products indexed under this heading.

Carteolol Hydrochloride (Co-administration with vasoactive drugs, such as adrenergic blocking agents, may result in postural hypotension, particularly in patients with unstable angina or acute phase of myocardial infarction). Products include:
Carteolol Hydrochloride Ophthalmic Solution USP, 1% .... ⊙246

Cerivastatin Sodium (Co-administration of lipid-altering doses ($\geq$ 1 g/day) of niacin and HMG-CoA reductase inhibitors has resulted in rare cases of rhabdomyolysis).
No products indexed under this heading.

Cholestyramine (*In vitro* study resulted in approximately 10% to 30% of available niacin bound to cholestyramine; 4 to 6 hours or greater should elapse between ingestion of bile acid-binding resins and the administration of Niaspan).
No products indexed under this heading.

Colestipol Hydrochloride (*In vitro* study resulted in approximately 90% of available niacin bound to colestipol; 4 to 6 hours or greater should elapse between ingestion of bile acid-binding resins and the administration of Niaspan).
No products indexed under this heading.

Dicumarol (Niacin prolongs prothrombin time; caution should be exercised when used concurrently).
No products indexed under this heading.

Diltiazem Hydrochloride (Co-administration with vasoactive drugs, such as calcium channel blockers, may result in postural hypotension, particularly in patients with unstable angina or acute phase of myocardial infarction). Products include:
Cardizem LA Extended Release Tablets 1699
Tiazac Capsules 1204

Erythrityl Tetranitrate (Co-administration with vasoactive drugs, such as nitrates, may result in postural hypotension, particularly in patients with unstable angina or acute phase of myocardial infarction).
No products indexed under this heading.

Esmolol Hydrochloride (Co-administration with vasoactive drugs, such as adrenergic blocking agents, may result in postural hypotension, particularly in patients with unstable angina or acute phase of myocardial infarction). Products include:
Brevibloc Concentrate 766
Brevibloc Injection 766
Brevibloc Double Strength Injection 766
Brevibloc Premixed Injection 766
Brevibloc Double Strength Premixed Injection 766

Felodipine (Co-administration with vasoactive drugs, such as calcium channel blockers, may result in postural hypotension, particularly in patients with unstable angina or acute phase of myocardial infarction). Products include:
Plendil Extended-Release Tablets 651

Fluvastatin Sodium (Co-administration of lipid-altering doses ($\geq$ 1 g/day) of niacin and HMG-CoA reductase inhibitors has resulted in rare cases of rhabdomyolysis). Products include:
Lescol Capsules 2227
Lescol 2730
Lescol XL Tablets 2227

Isosorbide Dinitrate (Co-administration with vasoactive drugs, such as nitrates, may result in postural hypotension, particularly in patients with unstable angina or acute phase of myocardial infarction). Products include:
BiDil Tablets 2161

Isosorbide Mononitrate (Co-administration with vasoactive drugs, such as nitrates, may result in postural hypotension, particularly in patients with unstable angina or acute phase of myocardial infarction). Products include:
Imdur Tablets 3032

Isradipine (Co-administration with vasoactive drugs, such as calcium channel blockers, may result in postural hypotension, particularly in

patients with unstable angina or acute phase of myocardial infarction). Products include:
DynaCirc CR Tablets 2726

Labetalol Hydrochloride (Co-administration with vasoactive drugs, such as adrenergic blocking agents, may result in postural hypotension, particularly in patients with unstable angina or acute phase of myocardial infarction).
No products indexed under this heading.

Levobunolol Hydrochloride (Co-administration with vasoactive drugs, such as adrenergic blocking agents, may result in postural hypotension, particularly in patients with unstable angina or acute phase of myocardial infarction). Products include:
Betagan Ophthalmic Solution, USP .... ⊙217

Lovastatin (Co-administration of lipid-altering doses (≥ 1 g/day) of niacin and HMG-CoA reductase inhibitors has resulted in rare cases of rhabdomyolysis). Products include:
Advicor Tablets 1694
Altoprev Extended-Release Tablets 1151
Mevacor Tablets 1996

Mecamylamine Hydrochloride (Niacin may potentiate the effects of ganglionic blocking agents, such as mecamylamine, resulting in postural hypotension). Products include:
Inversine Tablets 3286

Metipranolol Hydrochloride (Co-administration with vasoactive drugs, such as adrenergic blocking agents, may result in postural hypotension, particularly in patients with unstable angina or acute phase of myocardial infarction).
No products indexed under this heading.

Metoprolol Succinate (Co-administration with vasoactive drugs, such as adrenergic blocking agents, may result in postural hypotension, particularly in patients with unstable angina or acute phase of myocardial infarction). Products include:
Toprol-XL Tablets 660

Metoprolol Tartrate (Co-administration with vasoactive drugs, such as adrenergic blocking agents, may result in postural hypotension, particularly in patients with unstable angina or acute phase of myocardial infarction).
No products indexed under this heading.

Mibefradil Dihydrochloride (Co-administration with vasoactive drugs, such as calcium channel blockers, may result in postural hypotension, particularly in patients with unstable angina or acute phase of myocardial infarction).
No products indexed under this heading.

Nadolol (Co-administration with vasoactive drugs, such as adrenergic blocking agents, may result in postural hypotension, particularly in patients with unstable angina or acute phase of myocardial infarction). Products include:
Nadolol Tablets 2121

Nicardipine Hydrochloride (Co-administration with vasoactive drugs, such as calcium channel blockers, may result in postural hypotension, particularly in patients with unstable angina or acute phase of myocardial infarction). Products include:
Cardene I.V. 1129

Nicotinamide (May potentiate the adverse effects of Niaspan). Products include:
Nicomide Tablets 3190

Nifedipine (Co-administration with vasoactive drugs, such as calcium channel blockers, may result in postural hypotension, particularly in patients with unstable angina or acute phase of myocardial infarction). Products include:
Adalat CC Tablets 2978

Nimodipine (Co-administration with vasoactive drugs, such as calcium channel blockers, may result in postural hypotension, particularly in patients with unstable angina or acute phase of myocardial infarction). Products include:
Nimotop Capsules 774

Nisoldipine (Co-administration with vasoactive drugs, such as calcium channel blockers, may result in postural hypotension, particularly in patients with unstable angina or acute phase of myocardial infarction). Products include:
Sular Tablets 1163

Nitroglycerin (Co-administration with vasoactive drugs, such as nitrates, may result in postural hypotension, particularly in patients with unstable angina or acute phase of myocardial infarction). Products include:
Nitro-Dur Transdermal Infusion System 3060
Nitrolingual Pumpspray 1161

Penbutolol Sulfate (Co-administration with vasoactive drugs, such as adrenergic blocking agents, may result in postural hypotension, particularly in patients with unstable angina or acute phase of myocardial infarction).
No products indexed under this heading.

Pentaerythritol Tetranitrate (Co-administration with vasoactive drugs, such as nitrates, may result in postural hypotension, particularly in patients with unstable angina or acute phase of myocardial infarction).
No products indexed under this heading.

Pindolol (Co-administration with vasoactive drugs, such as adrenergic blocking agents, may result in postural hypotension, particularly in patients with unstable angina or acute phase of myocardial infarction).
No products indexed under this heading.

Pravastatin Sodium (Co-administration of lipid-altering doses (≥ 1 g/day) of niacin and HMG-CoA reductase inhibitors has resulted in rare cases of rhabdomyolysis). Products include:
Pravachol Tablets 943

Propranolol Hydrochloride (Co-administration with vasoactive drugs, such as adrenergic blocking agents, may result in postural hypotension, particularly in patients with unstable angina or acute phase of myocardial infarction). Products include:
Inderal LA Long-Acting Capsules 3421
InnoPran XL Capsules 2728

Simvastatin (Co-administration of lipid-altering doses (≥ 1 g/day) of niacin and HMG-CoA reductase inhibitors has resulted in rare cases of rhabdomyolysis). Products include:
Vytorin 10/10 Tablets 2084
Vytorin 10/10 Tablets 3092
Vytorin 10/20 Tablets 2084
Vytorin 10/20 Tablets 3092
Vytorin 10/40 Tablets 3092
Vytorin 10/40 Tablets 2084
Vytorin 10/80 Tablets 2084
Vytorin 10/80 Tablets 3092
Zocor Tablets 2078

Sotalol Hydrochloride (Co-administration with vasoactive drugs, such as adrenergic blocking agents, may result in postural hypotension, particularly in patients with unstable angina or acute phase of myocardial infarction).
No products indexed under this heading.

Timolol Hemihydrate (Co-administration with vasoactive drugs, such as adrenergic blocking agents, may result in postural hypotension, particularly in patients with unstable angina or acute phase of myocardial infarction). Products include:
Betimol Ophthalmic Solution 3371
Betimol Ophthalmic Solution .... ⊙283

Timolol Maleate (Co-administration with vasoactive drugs, such as adrenergic blocking agents, may result in postural hypotension, particularly in patients with unstable angina or acute phase of myocardial infarction). Products include:
Blocadren Tablets 1891
Cosopt Sterile Ophthalmic Solution 1910
Timolide Tablets 2056
Timoptic in Ocudose 2061
Timoptic Sterile Ophthalmic Solution 2058
Timoptic-XE Sterile Ophthalmic Gel Forming Solution 2062

Verapamil Hydrochloride (Co-administration with vasoactive drugs, such as calcium channel blockers, may result in postural hypotension, particularly in patients with unstable angina or acute phase of myocardial infarction). Products include:
Covera-HS Tablets 3135
Tarka Tablets 519
Verelan PM Capsules 3120

Warfarin Sodium (Niacin prolongs prothrombin time; caution should be exercised when used concurrently). Products include:
Coumadin for Injection 932
Coumadin Tablets 932

Food Interactions

Alcohol (Concomitant alcohol may increase the side effects of flushing and pruritus and should be avoided around the time of Niaspan ingestion).

Drinks, hot, unspecified (Concomitant hot drinks may increase the side effects of flushing and pruritus and should be avoided around the time of Niaspan ingestion).

NICODERM CQ PATCH

(Nicotine) 1629
See Nicorette Gum

NICODERM CQ CLEAR PATCH

(Nicotine) .... ▣627
See Nicorette Gum

NICOMIDE TABLETS

(Folic Acid, Nicotinamide, Zinc Oxide)... 3190

May interact with fluoroquinolone antibiotics, tetracyclines, and certain other agents. Compounds in these categories include:

Alatrofloxacin Mesylate (Decreased absorption of oral quinolones).
No products indexed under this heading.

Carbamazepine (Reduced clearance of carbamazepine). Products include:
Carbatrol Capsules 3174
Equetro Extended-Release Capsules 3178
Tegretol/Tegretol-XR 2278

Ciprofloxacin (Decreased absorption of oral quinolones). Products include:
Cipro I.V. 2998
Cipro I.V. Pharmacy Bulk Package ... 3509
Cipro Oral Suspension 2991
Cipro XR Tablets 3004
Ciprodex Otic Suspension 555

Ciprofloxacin Hydrochloride (Decreased absorption of oral quinolones). Products include:
Ciloxan Ophthalmic Ointment 554
Cipro Tablets 2991

Demeclocycline Hydrochloride (Decreased absorption of oral tetracyclines).
No products indexed under this heading.

Doxycycline Calcium (Decreased absorption of oral tetracyclines).
No products indexed under this heading.

Doxycycline Hyclate (Decreased absorption of oral tetracyclines).
No products indexed under this heading.

Doxycycline Monohydrate (Decreased absorption of oral tetracyclines).
No products indexed under this heading.

Enoxacin (Decreased absorption of oral quinolones).
No products indexed under this heading.

Grepafloxacin Hydrochloride (Decreased absorption of oral quinolones).
No products indexed under this heading.

Lomefloxacin Hydrochloride (Decreased absorption of oral quinolones).
No products indexed under this heading.

Methacycline Hydrochloride (Decreased absorption of oral tetracyclines).
No products indexed under this heading.

Minocycline Hydrochloride (Decreased absorption of oral tetracyclines). Products include:
Dynacin Tablets 1859

Moxifloxacin Hydrochloride (Decreased absorption of oral quinolones). Products include:
Avelox 2984
Vigamox Ophthalmic Solution 560

Norfloxacin (Decreased absorption of oral quinolones). Products include:
Noroxin Tablets 2009

Ofloxacin (Decreased absorption of oral quinolones). Products include:
Floxin Otic Singles 1045

Floxin Otic Solution 1043

Oxytetracycline Hydrochloride (Decreased absorption of oral tetracyclines).
No products indexed under this heading.

Primidone (Reduced clearance of primidone).
No products indexed under this heading.

Tetracycline Hydrochloride (Decreased absorption of oral tetracyclines).
No products indexed under this heading.

Trovafloxacin Mesylate (Decreased absorption of oral quinolones).
No products indexed under this heading.

NICORETTE GUM

(Nicotine Polacrilex) 1632
May interact with asthma medications and antidepressant drugs. Compounds in these categories include:

Albuterol (Concurrent use with asthma medications should be undertaken under physician's supervision). Products include:
Proventil Inhalation Aerosol 3067

Albuterol Sulfate (Concurrent use with asthma medications should be undertaken under physician's supervision). Products include:
AccuNeb Inhalation Solution 1055
Combivent Inhalation Aerosol 878
DuoNeb Inhalation Solution 1058
Proventil Inhalation Solution 0.083% 3069
Proventil HFA Inhalation Aerosol 3071
Ventolin HFA Inhalation Aerosol 1576
VoSpire Extended-Release Tablets ... 2352

Amitriptyline Hydrochloride (Concurrent use with antidepressant should be undertaken under physician's supervision).
No products indexed under this heading.

Amoxapine (Concurrent use with antidepressant should be undertaken under physician's supervision).
No products indexed under this heading.

Bitolterol Mesylate (Concurrent use with asthma medications should be undertaken under physician's supervision).
No products indexed under this heading.

Bupropion Hydrochloride (Concurrent use with antidepressant should be undertaken under physician's supervision). Products include:
Wellbutrin Tablets 1579
Wellbutrin SR Sustained-Release Tablets 1583
Wellbutrin XL Extended-Release Tablets 1588
Zyban Sustained-Release Tablets 1620

Citalopram Hydrobromide (Concurrent use with antidepressant should be undertaken under physician's supervision). Products include:
Celexa 1177

Desipramine Hydrochloride (Concurrent use with antidepressant should be undertaken under physician's supervision).
No products indexed under this heading.

Doxepin Hydrochloride (Concurrent use with antidepressant should be undertaken under physician's supervision).
No products indexed under this heading.

Ephedrine Hydrochloride (Concurrent use with asthma medications should be undertaken under physician's supervision). Products include:
Primatene Tablets 749

Ephedrine Sulfate (Concurrent use with asthma medications should be undertaken under physician's supervision).
No products indexed under this heading.

Ephedrine Tannate (Concurrent use with asthma medications should be undertaken under physician's supervision).
No products indexed under this heading.

Epinephrine (Concurrent use with asthma medications should be undertaken under physician's supervision). Products include:
EpiPen 1061
Primatene Mist 749

Epinephrine Bitartrate (Concurrent use with asthma medications should be undertaken under physician's supervision).
No products indexed under this heading.

Epinephrine Hydrochloride (Concurrent use with asthma medications should be undertaken under physician's supervision).
No products indexed under this heading.

Fluoxetine Hydrochloride (Concurrent use with antidepressant should be undertaken under physician's supervision). Products include:
Prozac Pulvules and Liquid 1771
Symbyax Capsules 1788

Imipramine Hydrochloride (Concurrent use with antidepressant should be undertaken under physician's supervision).
No products indexed under this heading.

Imipramine Pamoate (Concurrent use with antidepressant should be undertaken under physician's supervision).
No products indexed under this heading.

Isocarboxazid (Concurrent use with antidepressant should be undertaken under physician's supervision).
No products indexed under this heading.

Isoetharine (Concurrent use with asthma medications should be undertaken under physician's supervision).
No products indexed under this heading.

Isoproterenol Hydrochloride (Concurrent use with asthma medications should be undertaken under physician's supervision).
No products indexed under this heading.

Isoproterenol Sulfate (Concurrent use with asthma medications should be undertaken under physician's supervision).
No products indexed under this heading.

Levalbuterol Hydrochloride (Concurrent use with asthma medications should be undertaken under physician's supervision). Products include:
Xopenex Inhalation Solution 3143
Xopenex Inhalation Solution Concentrate 3147

Maprotiline Hydrochloride (Concurrent use with antidepressant should be undertaken under physician's supervision).
No products indexed under this heading.

Metaproterenol Sulfate (Concurrent use with asthma medications should be undertaken under physician's supervision). Products include:
Alupent Inhalation Aerosol 858

Mirtazapine (Concurrent use with antidepressant should be undertaken under physician's supervision).
No products indexed under this heading.

Nefazodone Hydrochloride (Concurrent use with antidepressant should be undertaken under physician's supervision).
No products indexed under this heading.

Nortriptyline Hydrochloride (Concurrent use with antidepressant should be undertaken under physician's supervision).
No products indexed under this heading.

Paroxetine Hydrochloride (Concurrent use with antidepressant should be undertaken under physician's supervision). Products include:
Paxil CR Controlled-Release Tablets 1509
Paxil 1501

Phenelzine Sulfate (Concurrent use with antidepressant should be undertaken under physician's supervision).
No products indexed under this heading.

Pirbuterol Acetate (Concurrent use with asthma medications should be undertaken under physician's supervision). Products include:
Maxair Autohaler 1820

Protriptyline Hydrochloride (Concurrent use with antidepressant should be undertaken under physician's supervision). Products include:
Vivactil Tablets 2350

Salmeterol Xinafoate (Concurrent use with asthma medications should be undertaken under physician's supervision). Products include:
Advair Diskus 100/50 1291
Advair Diskus 250/50 1291
Advair Diskus 500/50 1291
Serevent Diskus 1540

Sertraline Hydrochloride (Concurrent use with antidepressant should be undertaken under physician's supervision). Products include:
Zoloft 2581

Terbutaline Sulfate (Concurrent use with asthma medications should be undertaken under physician's supervision).
No products indexed under this heading.

Tranylcypromine Sulfate (Concurrent use with antidepressant should be undertaken under physician's supervision). Products include:
Parnate Tablets 1499

Trazodone Hydrochloride (Concurrent use with antidepressant should be undertaken under physician's supervision).
No products indexed under this heading.

Trimipramine Maleate (Concurrent use with antidepressant should be undertaken under physician's supervision). Products include:
Surmontil Capsules 2347

Venlafaxine Hydrochloride (Concurrent use with antidepressant should be undertaken under physician's supervision). Products include:
Effexor Tablets 3405
Effexor XR Capsules 3411

NICOTROL INHALER

(Nicotine) 2594
May interact with theophyllines and tricyclic antidepressants. Compounds in these categories include:

Amitriptyline Hydrochloride (Physiological changes resulting from smoking cessation, with or without nicotine replacement, may alter the pharmacokinetics of certain concomitant medications, such as tricyclic antidepressants. Doses of tricyclic antidepressants, and perhaps other medications, may need to be adjusted in patients who successfully quit smoking).
No products indexed under this heading.

Amoxapine (Physiological changes resulting from smoking cessation, with or without nicotine replacement, may alter the pharmacokinetics of certain concomitant medications, such as tricyclic antidepressants. Doses of tricyclic antidepressants, and perhaps other medications, may need to be adjusted in patients who successfully quit smoking).
No products indexed under this heading.

Clomipramine Hydrochloride (Physiological changes resulting from smoking cessation, with or without nicotine replacement, may alter the pharmacokinetics of certain concomitant medications, such as tricyclic antidepressants. Doses of tricyclic antidepressants, and perhaps other medications, may need to be adjusted in patients who successfully quit smoking).
No products indexed under this heading.

Desipramine Hydrochloride (Physiological changes resulting from smoking cessation, with or without nicotine replacement, may alter the pharmacokinetics of certain concomitant medications, such as tricyclic antidepressants. Doses of tricyclic antidepressants, and perhaps other medications, may need to be adjusted in patients who successfully quit smoking).
No products indexed under this heading.

Doxepin Hydrochloride (Physiological changes resulting from smoking cessation, with or without nicotine replacement, may alter the pharmacokinetics of certain concomitant medications, such as tricyclic antidepressants. Doses of tricyclic antidepressants, and perhaps other medications, may need to be adjusted in patients who successfully quit smoking).
No products indexed under this heading.

Imipramine Hydrochloride (Physiological changes resulting from smoking cessation, with or without nicotine replacement, may alter the pharmacokinetics of certain concomitant medications, such as tricyclic antidepressants. Doses of tricyclic antidepressants, and perhaps other medications, may need to be adjusted in patients who successfully quit smoking).

No products indexed under this heading.

Imipramine Pamoate (Physiological changes resulting from smoking cessation, with or without nicotine replacement, may alter the pharmacokinetics of certain concomitant medications, such as tricyclic antidepressants. Doses of tricyclic antidepressants, and perhaps other medications, may need to be adjusted in patients who successfully quit smoking).

No products indexed under this heading.

Maprotiline Hydrochloride (Physiological changes resulting from smoking cessation, with or without nicotine replacement, may alter the pharmacokinetics of certain concomitant medications, such as tricyclic antidepressants. Doses of tricyclic antidepressants, and perhaps other medications, may need to be adjusted in patients who successfully quit smoking).

No products indexed under this heading.

Nortriptyline Hydrochloride (Physiological changes resulting from smoking cessation, with or without nicotine replacement, may alter the pharmacokinetics of certain concomitant medications, such as tricyclic antidepressants. Doses of tricyclic antidepressants, and perhaps other medications, may need to be adjusted in patients who successfully quit smoking).

No products indexed under this heading.

Protriptyline Hydrochloride (Physiological changes resulting from smoking cessation, with or without nicotine replacement, may alter the pharmacokinetics of certain concomitant medications, such as tricyclic antidepressants. Doses of tricyclic antidepressants, and perhaps other medications, may need to be adjusted in patients who successfully quit smoking). Products include:

Vivactil Tablets ... 2350

Theophylline (Physiological changes resulting from smoking cessation, with or without nicotine replacement, may alter the pharmacokinetics of certain concomitant medications, such as theophylline. Doses of theophylline, and perhaps other medications, may need to be adjusted in patients who successfully quit smoking).

No products indexed under this heading.

Theophylline Anhydrous (Physiological changes resulting from smoking cessation, with or without nicotine replacement, may alter the pharmacokinetics of certain concomitant medications, such as theophylline. Doses of theophylline, and perhaps other medications, may need to be adjusted in patients who successfully quit smoking). Products include:

Uniphyl Tablets ... 2708

Theophylline Calcium Salicylate (Physiological changes resulting from smoking cessation, with or without nicotine replacement, may alter the pharmacokinetics of certain concomitant medications, such as theophylline. Doses of theophylline, and perhaps other medications, may need to be adjusted in patients who successfully quit smoking).

No products indexed under this heading.

Theophylline Dihydroxypropyl (Glyceryl) (Physiological changes resulting from smoking cessation, with or without nicotine replacement, may alter the pharmacokinetics of certain concomitant medications, such as theophylline. Doses of theophylline, and perhaps other medications, may need to be adjusted in patients who successfully quit smoking).

No products indexed under this heading.

Theophylline Ethylenediamine (Physiological changes resulting from smoking cessation, with or without nicotine replacement, may alter the pharmacokinetics of certain concomitant medications, such as theophylline. Doses of theophylline, and perhaps other medications, may need to be adjusted in patients who successfully quit smoking).

No products indexed under this heading.

Theophylline Sodium Glycinate (Physiological changes resulting from smoking cessation, with or without nicotine replacement, may alter the pharmacokinetics of certain concomitant medications, such as theophylline. Doses of theophylline, and perhaps other medications, may need to be adjusted in patients who successfully quit smoking).

No products indexed under this heading.

Trimipramine Maleate (Physiological changes resulting from smoking cessation, with or without nicotine replacement, may alter the pharmacokinetics of certain concomitant medications, such as tricyclic antidepressants. Doses of tricyclic antidepressants, and perhaps other medications, may need to be adjusted in patients who successfully quit smoking). Products include:

Surmontil Capsules ... 2347

NICOTROL NS

(Nicotine) ... 2596

May interact with alpha adrenergic stimulants, alpha adrenergic blockers, beta blockers, beta-adrenergic stimulating agents, insulin, sympathomimetics, xanthines, and certain other agents. Compounds in these categories include:

Acebutolol Hydrochloride (Deinduction of hepatic enzyme on smoking cessation; may require a decrease in dose at cessation of smoking).

No products indexed under this heading.

Acetaminophen (Deinduction of hepatic enzyme on smoking cessation; may require a decrease in dose at cessation of smoking). Products include:

Benadryl Allergy & Cold Tablets ... ▣692
Benadryl Allergy & Sinus Headache Caplets & Gelcaps ... ▣693
Benadryl Maximum Strength Severe Allergy & Sinus Headache Caplets ... ▣694
Contac Severe Cold and Flu Caplets Maximum Strength ... ▣615
Contac Severe Cold and Flu Caplets Non-Drowsy ... ▣615
Darvocet A 500 Tablets ... 3497
Goody's Body Pain Formula Powder ... ▣621
Goody's Extra Strength Headache Powder ... ▣621
Goody's Extra Strength Pain Relief Tablets ... ▣621
Goody's PM Powder ... ▣622
Hycomine Compound Tablets ... 1105
Lortab ... 3315
Lortab Elixir ... 3312
Percocet Tablets ... 1114
Robitussin Cough, Cold & Flu Liquid-filled Capsules ... ▣750
Robitussin Flu Liquid ... ▣752
Sedapap Tablets 50 mg/650 mg ... 2098
Singlet Caplets ... ▣636
Sudafed Severe Cold ... ▣710
Sudafed Sinus Headache ... ▣711
TheraFlu Cold & Cough Hot Liquid ... ▣680
TheraFlu Cold & Sore Throat Hot Liquid ... ▣680
TheraFlu Flu & Chest Congestion Non-Drowsy Hot Liquid ... ▣681
TheraFlu Flu & Sore Throat Hot Liquid ... ▣681
TheraFlu Severe Cold Non-Drowsy Hot Liquid ... ▣683
TheraFlu Severe Cold & Cough Hot Liquid ... ▣683
TheraFlu Severe Cold Caplets ... ▣679
TheraFlu Severe Cold Hot Liquid ... ▣682
TheraFlu Severe Cold Non-Drowsy Caplets ... ▣679
Triaminic Cough & Sore Throat Liquid ... ▣687
Triaminic Flu, Cough & Fever Liquid ... ▣685
Triaminic Cough & Sore Throat Softchews ... ▣689
Tylenol 8 Hour Extended Release Geltabs and Caplets ... 1843
Tylenol Sinus NightTime Caplets ... ▣663
Children's Tylenol Suspension Liquid and Meltaways ... 1850
Children's Tylenol Plus Cold & Allergy Suspension Liquid ... 1850
Children's Tylenol Plus Cold NightTime Suspension Liquid ... 1851
Children's Tylenol Plus Cold & Cough Suspension Liquid and Chewable Tablets ... 1851
Children's Tylenol Plus Cold Chewable Tablets ... 1851
Children's Tylenol Plus Cold Daytime Non-Drowsy Suspension Liquid ... 1851
Children's Tylenol Plus Flu Suspension Liquid ... 1853
Concentrated Tylenol Infants' Drops Plus Cold ... 1851
Concentrated Tylenol Infants' Drops Plus Cold and Cough ... 1851
Concentrated Tylenol Infants' Drops ... 1850
Junior Tylenol Meltaways ... 1850
Tylenol Cold & Flu Severe Daytime Liquid with Cool Bust ... 1846
Tylenol Cold & Flu Severe NightTime Liquid with Cool Burst ... 1846
Tylenol Cold Severe Congestion Non-Drowsy Caplets with Cool Burst ... 1846
Tylenol Cough & Sore Throat Daytime Liquid with Cool Burst ... 1849
Tylenol Cough & Sore Throat NightTime Liquid with Cool Burst ... 1849
Tylenol ... 1843
Extra Strength Tylenol Rapid Release Gels ... 1843
Tylenol ... 1843
Tylenol Allergy Complete Night Time Caplets ... 1844
Tylenol Allergy Complete Multi-Symptom Caplets and Gelcaps with Cool Burst ... 1844
Tylenol Severe Allergy Caplets ... 1844
Tylenol Flu NightTime Gelcaps ... 1846
Tylenol Flu Day Non-Drowsy Gelcaps ... 1846
Concentrated Tylenol Infants' Drops Plus Cold Nasal Congestant, Fever Reducer & Pain Reliever ... ▣668
Concentrated Tylenol Infants' Drops Plus Cold & Cough Nasal Decongestant, Fever Reducer & Pain Reliever ... ▣668
Multi-Symptom Tylenol Cold Night Time Caplets ... 1845
Multi-Symptom Tylenol Cold Day Non-Drowsy Caplets and Gelcaps ... 1845
Extra Strength Tylenol PM Caplets, Geltabs, Gelcaps and Liquid ... 1847
Tylenol Sinus Day Non-Drowsy ... 1848
Tylenol Sinus Night Time Caplets ... 1848
Tylenol Sinus Severe Congestion Caplets with Cool Burst ... 1848
Tylenol Sore Throat Daytime Liquid with Cool Burst ... 1849
Tylenol Sore Throat NightTime Liquid with Cool Burst ... 1849
Tylenol with Codeine ... 2461
Women's Tylenol Menstrual Relief Caplets ... 1849
Ultracet Tablets ... 2462
Vicks 44M Cough, Cold & Flu Relief ... 2676
Vicks DayQuil LiquiCaps/Liquid Multi-Symptom Cold/Flu Relief ... ▣723
Vicks DayQuil Multi-Symptom Cold/Flu Relief LiquiCaps ... 2675
Vicks DayQuil Multi-Symptom Cold/Flu Relief Liquid ... 2675
Vicks NyQuil LiquiCaps ... 2677
Vicks NyQuil LiquiCaps/Liquid Multi-Symptom Cold/Flu Relief ... ▣725
Vicks NyQuil Liquid ... 2677
Vicodin Tablets ... 530
Vicodin ES Tablets ... 531
Vicodin HP Tablets ... 532
Zydone Tablets ... 1118

Albuterol (Decrease in circulating catecholamines with smoking cessation; may require an increase in dose at cessation of smoking). Products include:

Proventil Inhalation Aerosol ... 3067

Albuterol Sulfate (Decrease in circulating catecholamines with smoking cessation; may require an increase in dose at cessation of smoking). Products include:

AccuNeb Inhalation Solution ... 1055
Combivent Inhalation Aerosol ... 878
DuoNeb Inhalation Solution ... 1058
Proventil Inhalation Solution 0.083% ... 3069
Proventil HFA Inhalation Aerosol ... 3071
Ventolin HFA Inhalation Aerosol ... 1576
VoSpire Extended-Release Tablets ... 2352

Aminophylline (Deinduction of hepatic enzyme on smoking cessation; may require a decrease in dose at cessation of smoking).

No products indexed under this heading.

Atenolol (Deinduction of hepatic enzyme on smoking cessation; may require a decrease in dose at cessation of smoking). Products include:

Tenormin I.V. Injection ... 698
Tenormin Tablets ... 695

Betaxolol Hydrochloride (Deinduction of hepatic enzyme on smoking cessation; may require a decrease in dose at cessation of smoking). Products include:

Betoptic S Ophthalmic Suspension ... 554

Bisoprolol Fumarate (Deinduction of hepatic enzyme on smoking cessation; may require a decrease in dose at cessation of smoking).

No products indexed under this heading.

Bitolterol Mesylate (Decrease in circulating catecholamines with smoking cessation; may require an increase in dose at cessation of smoking).
No products indexed under this heading.

Caffeine (Deinduction of hepatic enzyme on smoking cessation; may require a decrease in dose at cessation of smoking). Products include:
Athena Hair System Shampoo .... ■ 767
BC Powder .... ■ 612
Arthritis Strength BC Powder .... ■ 612
Goody's Extra Strength Headache Powder....... ■ 621
Goody's Extra Strength Pain Relief Tablets....... ■ 621
Hycomine Compound Tablets 1105
Spartan Hair System Shampoo .... ■ 767
Vivarin .... ■ 639

Carteolol Hydrochloride (Deinduction of hepatic enzyme on smoking cessation; may require a decrease in dose at cessation of smoking). Products include:
Carteolol Hydrochloride Ophthalmic Solution USP, 1%....... ⊙ 246

Dobutamine (Decrease in circulating catecholamines with smoking cessation; may require an increase in dose at cessation of smoking).
No products indexed under this heading.

Dobutamine Hydrochloride (Decrease in circulating catecholamines with smoking cessation; may require an increase in dose at cessation of smoking).
No products indexed under this heading.

Dopamine Hydrochloride (Decrease in circulating catecholamines with smoking cessation; may require an increase in dose at cessation of smoking).
No products indexed under this heading.

Doxazosin Mesylate (Decrease in circulating catecholamines with smoking cessation; may require a decrease in dose at cessation of smoking).
No products indexed under this heading.

Dyphylline (Deinduction of hepatic enzyme on smoking cessation; may require a decrease in dose at cessation of smoking).
No products indexed under this heading.

Ephedrine Hydrochloride (Decrease in circulating catecholamines with smoking cessation; may require an increase in dose at cessation of smoking). Products include:
Primatene Tablets .... ■ 749

Ephedrine Sulfate (Decrease in circulating catecholamines with smoking cessation; may require an increase in dose at cessation of smoking).
No products indexed under this heading.

Ephedrine Tannate (Decrease in circulating catecholamines with smoking cessation; may require an increase in dose at cessation of smoking).
No products indexed under this heading.

Epinephrine (Decrease in circulating catecholamines with smoking cessation; may require an increase in dose at cessation of smoking). Products include:
EpiPen 1061
Primatene Mist .... ■ 749

Epinephrine Bitartrate (Decrease in circulating catecholamines with smoking cessation; may require an increase in dose at cessation of smoking).
No products indexed under this heading.

Epinephrine Hydrochloride (Decrease in circulating catecholamines with smoking cessation; may require an increase in dose at cessation of smoking).
No products indexed under this heading.

Esmolol Hydrochloride (Deinduction of hepatic enzyme on smoking cessation; may require a decrease in dose at cessation of smoking). Products include:
Brevibloc Concentrate 766
Brevibloc Injection 766
Brevibloc Double Strength Injection....... 766
Brevibloc Premixed Injection 766
Brevibloc Double Strength Premixed Injection 766

Imipramine Hydrochloride (Deinduction of hepatic enzyme on smoking cessation; may require a decrease in dose at cessation of smoking).
No products indexed under this heading.

Imipramine Pamoate (Deinduction of hepatic enzyme on smoking cessation; may require a decrease in dose at cessation of smoking).
No products indexed under this heading.

Insulin, Human, Zinc Suspension (Increase of subcutaneous insulin absorption with smoking cessation; may require a decrease in dose at cessation of smoking). Products include:
Humulin L, 100 Units 1763
Humulin U, 100 Units 1770

Insulin, Human NPH (Increase of subcutaneous insulin absorption with smoking cessation; may require a decrease in dose at cessation of smoking). Products include:
Humulin N, 100 Units 1764
Humulin N Pen 1765
Novolin N Human Insulin 10 ml Vials 2322
Novolin N InnoLet 2322
Novolin N PenFill 3 ml Cartridges 2325
Novolin R InnoLet 2322

Insulin, Human Regular (Increase of subcutaneous insulin absorption with smoking cessation; may require a decrease in dose at cessation of smoking). Products include:
Humulin R (U-500) 1768
Humulin R, 100 Units 1767
Novolin R Human Insulin 10 ml Vials 2322
Novolin R PenFill 2325

Insulin, Human Regular and Human NPH Mixture (Increase of subcutaneous insulin absorption with smoking cessation; may require a decrease in dose at cessation of smoking). Products include:
Humulin 50/50, 100 Units 1760
Humulin 70/30 Pen 1761
Novolin 70/30 Human Insulin 10 ml Vials 2321
Novolin 70/30 InnoLet 2322
Novolin 70/30 PenFill 3 ml Cartridges 2325

Insulin, NPH (Increase of subcutaneous insulin absorption with smoking cessation; may require a decrease in dose at cessation of smoking).
No products indexed under this heading.

Insulin, Regular (Increase of subcutaneous insulin absorption with smoking cessation; may require a decrease in dose at cessation of smoking).
No products indexed under this heading.

Insulin, Zinc Crystals (Increase of subcutaneous insulin absorption with smoking cessation; may require a decrease in dose at cessation of smoking).
No products indexed under this heading.

Insulin, Zinc Suspension (Increase of subcutaneous insulin absorption with smoking cessation; may require a decrease in dose at cessation of smoking).
No products indexed under this heading.

Insulin Aspart, Human Regular (Increase of subcutaneous insulin absorption with smoking cessation; may require a decrease in dose at cessation of smoking). Products include:
NovoLog Injection 2326

Insulin glargine (Increase of subcutaneous insulin absorption with smoking cessation; may require a decrease in dose at cessation of smoking). Products include:
Lantus Injection 2925

Insulin Lispro, Human (Increase of subcutaneous insulin absorption with smoking cessation; may require a decrease in dose at cessation of smoking). Products include:
Humalog-Pen 1751
Humalog Mix 75/25-Pen 1754

Insulin Lispro Protamine, Human (Increase of subcutaneous insulin absorption with smoking cessation; may require a decrease in dose at cessation of smoking). Products include:
Humalog Mix 75/25-Pen 1754

Isoetharine (Decrease in circulating catecholamines with smoking cessation; may require an increase in dose at cessation of smoking).
No products indexed under this heading.

Isoproterenol Hydrochloride (Decrease in circulating catecholamines with smoking cessation; may require an increase in dose at cessation of smoking).
No products indexed under this heading.

Isoproterenol Sulfate (Decrease in circulating catecholamines with smoking cessation; may require an increase in dose at cessation of smoking).
No products indexed under this heading.

Labetalol Hydrochloride (Decrease in circulating catecholamines with smoking cessation; may require a decrease in dose at cessation of smoking).
No products indexed under this heading.

Levalbuterol Hydrochloride (Decrease in circulating catecholamines with smoking cessation; may require an increase in dose at cessation of smoking). Products include:
Xopenex Inhalation Solution 3143
Xopenex Inhalation Solution Concentrate 3147

Levobunolol Hydrochloride (Deinduction of hepatic enzyme on smoking cessation; may require a decrease in dose at cessation of smoking). Products include:
Betagan Ophthalmic Solution, USP....... ⊙ 217

Metaproterenol Sulfate (Decrease in circulating catecholamines with smoking cessation; may require an increase in dose at cessation of smoking). Products include:
Alupent Inhalation Aerosol 858

Metaraminol Bitartrate (Decrease in circulating catecholamines with smoking cessation; may require an increase in dose at cessation of smoking). Products include:
Aramine Injection 1889

Methoxamine Hydrochloride (Decrease in circulating catecholamines with smoking cessation; may require an increase in dose at cessation of smoking).
No products indexed under this heading.

Metipranolol Hydrochloride (Deinduction of hepatic enzyme on smoking cessation; may require a decrease in dose at cessation of smoking).
No products indexed under this heading.

Metoprolol Succinate (Deinduction of hepatic enzyme on smoking cessation; may require a decrease in dose at cessation of smoking). Products include:
Toprol-XL Tablets 660

Metoprolol Tartrate (Deinduction of hepatic enzyme on smoking cessation; may require a decrease in dose at cessation of smoking).
No products indexed under this heading.

Nadolol (Deinduction of hepatic enzyme on smoking cessation; may require a decrease in dose at cessation of smoking). Products include:
Nadolol Tablets 2121

Naphazoline Hydrochloride (Decrease in circulating catecholamines with smoking cessation; may require an increase in dose at cessation of smoking). Products include:
Albalon Ophthalmic Solution .... ⊙ 216
Visine-A Eye Drops .... ■ 713

Norepinephrine Bitartrate (Decrease in circulating catecholamines with smoking cessation; may require an increase in dose at cessation of smoking).
No products indexed under this heading.

Oxazepam (Deinduction of hepatic enzyme on smoking cessation; may require a decrease in dose at cessation of smoking).
No products indexed under this heading.

Oxymetazoline Hydrochloride (Decrease in circulating catecholamines with smoking cessation; may require an increase in dose at cessation of smoking). Products include:
Vicks Sinex 12-Hour Nasal Spray and Ultra Fine Mist for Sinus Relief....... 2678
Visine L.R. Long Lasting Eye Drops....... ⊙ 279
Zicam Extreme Congestion Relief Nasal Pump .... ■
Zicam Sinus Relief Nasal Pump .... ■

Penbutolol Sulfate (Deinduction of hepatic enzyme on smoking cessation; may require a decrease in dose at cessation of smoking).
No products indexed under this heading.

Pentazocine Hydrochloride (Deinduction of hepatic enzyme on smoking cessation; may require a decrease in dose at cessation of smoking).
No products indexed under this heading.

Pentazocine Lactate (Deinduction of hepatic enzyme on smoking cessation; may require a decrease in dose at cessation of smoking).
No products indexed under this heading.

Phenylephrine Bitartrate (Decrease in circulating catecholamines with smoking cessation; may require an increase in dose at cessation of smoking).
No products indexed under this heading.

Phenylephrine Hydrochloride (Decrease in circulating catecholamines with smoking cessation; may require an increase in dose at cessation of smoking). Products include:
Alacol DM Syrup ... 739
Hycomine Compound Tablets ... 1105
Preparation H Maximum Strength Cream ... ▣ 747
Preparation H Cooling Gel ... ▣ 747
Preparation H ... ▣ 747
Sudafed PE Tablets ... ▣ 711
Vicks Sinex Nasal Spray and Ultra Fine Mist for Sinus Relief ... 2677
Zicam Concentrated Cough Mist for Kids Plus D Cool Cherry ... ▣ 643
Zicam Concentrated Cough Mist Plus D Cool Cherry ... ▣ 642

Phenylephrine Tannate (Decrease in circulating catecholamines with smoking cessation; may require an increase in dose at cessation of smoking).
No products indexed under this heading.

Phenylpropanolamine Hydrochloride (Decrease in circulating catecholamines with smoking cessation; may require an increase in dose at cessation of smoking).
No products indexed under this heading.

Pindolol (Deinduction of hepatic enzyme on smoking cessation; may require a decrease in dose at cessation of smoking).
No products indexed under this heading.

Pirbuterol Acetate (Decrease in circulating catecholamines with smoking cessation; may require an increase in dose at cessation of smoking). Products include:
Maxair Autohaler ... 1820

Prazosin Hydrochloride (Decrease in circulating catecholamines with smoking cessation; may require a decrease in dose at cessation of smoking).
No products indexed under this heading.

Propranolol Hydrochloride (Deinduction of hepatic enzyme on smoking cessation; may require a decrease in dose at cessation of smoking). Products include:
Inderal LA Long-Acting Capsules ... 3421
InnoPran XL Capsules ... 2728

Pseudoephedrine Hydrochloride (Decrease in circulating catecholamines with smoking cessation; may require an increase in dose at cessation of smoking). Products include:
Advil Allergy Sinus Caplets ... ▣ 737
Advil Cold & Sinus ... ▣ 739
Advil Flu & Body Ache Caplets ... ▣ 739
Children's Advil Cold Suspension ... ▣ 741
Advil Multi-Symptom Cold Caplets ... ▣ 738
Allegra-D 12 Hour Extended-Release Tablets ... 2860
Allegra-D 24 Hour Extended-Release Tablets ... 2862
Balamine DM ... 739
BC Cold Powder ... ▣ 612
Benadryl Allergy & Cold Tablets ... ▣ 692
Benadryl Allergy & Sinus Headache Caplets & Gelcaps ... ▣ 693
Children's Benadryl Allergy & Cold Fastmelt Tablets ... ▣ 695
Benadryl Maximum Strength Severe Allergy & Sinus Headache Caplets ... ▣ 694
Children's Benadryl D Allergy & Sinus Fastmelt Tablets ... ▣ 694
Children's Benadryl D Liquid Medication ... ▣ 693
Benadryl D Tablets ... ▣ 694
Contac Non-Drowsy 12 Hour Cold Caplets ... ▣ 614
Contac Non-Drowsy Timed Release 12 Hour Cold Caplets ... ▣ 615
Contac Severe Cold and Flu Caplets Maximum Strength ... ▣ 615
Contac Severe Cold and Flu Caplets Non-Drowsy ... ▣ 615
Children's Dimetapp Cold & Allergy Elixir ... ▣ 745
Children's Dimetapp DM Cold & Cough Elixir ... ▣ 745
Children's Dimetapp Long Acting Cough Plus Cold Syrup ... ▣ 746
Dimetapp Infant Drops Decongestant Plus Cough ... ▣ 746
Children's Motrin Cold Non-Staining Dye-Free Oral Suspension ... 1838
Children's Motrin Cold Oral Suspension ... 1838
Motrin Cold & Sinus Caplets ... 1836
PediaCare Decongestant & Cough Infant Drops ... ▣ 705
PediaCare Decongestant Infants' Drops ... ▣ 705
PediaCare Long-Acting Cough Plus Cold Liquid ... ▣ 704
PediaCare Multi-Symptom Cold Liquid ... ▣ 704
PediaCare NightRest Cough & Cold Liquid ... ▣ 704
Robitussin Allergy & Cough Syrup ... ▣ 750
Robitussin CF Liquid ... ▣ 755
Robitussin Cough & Cold Liquid-filled Capsules ... ▣ 750
Robitussin Cough, Cold & Flu Liquid-filled Capsules ... ▣ 750
Robitussin Cough & Cold Infant Drops ... ▣ 755
Robitussin Flu Liquid ... ▣ 752
Robitussin Maximum Strength Cough & Cold Liquid ... ▣ 754
Robitussin PE Syrup ... ▣ 753
Robitussin Pediatric Cough & Cold Liquid ... ▣ 754
Robitussin PM Cough & Cold Liquid ... ▣ 752
Robitussin Severe Congestion Liquid-filled Capsules ... ▣ 751
Simply Stuffy Liquid ... 1841
Singlet Caplets ... ▣ 636
Sudafed 12 Hour Caplets ... ▣ 708
Sudafed 24 Hour Tablets ... ▣ 709
Sudafed Nasal Decongestant Tablets ... ▣ 709
Sudafed Severe Cold ... ▣ 710
Sudafed Non-Drying Sinus Liquid Caps ... ▣ 709
Sudafed Sinus & Allergy Tablets ... ▣ 710
Sudafed Sinus Headache ... ▣ 711
TheraFlu Cold & Cough Hot Liquid ... ▣ 680
TheraFlu Cold & Sore Throat Hot Liquid ... ▣ 680
TheraFlu Flu & Chest Congestion Non-Drowsy Hot Liquid ... ▣ 681
TheraFlu Flu & Sore Throat Hot Liquid ... ▣ 681
TheraFlu Severe Cold Non-Drowsy Hot Liquid ... ▣ 683
TheraFlu Severe Cold & Cough Hot Liquid ... ▣ 683
TheraFlu Severe Cold Caplets ... ▣ 679
TheraFlu Severe Cold Hot Liquid ... ▣ 682
TheraFlu Severe Cold Non-Drowsy Caplets ... ▣ 679
Triaminic Chest & Nasal Congestion Liquid ... ▣ 685
Triaminic Cold & Allergy Liquid ... ▣ 685
Triaminic Cold & Cough Liquid ... ▣ 685
Triaminic Cough Liquid ... ▣ 687
Triaminic Cough & Nasal Congestion Liquid ... ▣ 687
Triaminic Cough & Sore Throat Liquid ... ▣ 687
Triaminic Flu, Cough & Fever Liquid ... ▣ 685
Triaminic Night Time Cough & Cold Liquid ... ▣ 685
Triaminic Allergy Runny Nose & Congestion Softchews ... ▣ 688
Triaminic Cold & Cough Softchews ... ▣ 688
Triaminic Cough & Sore Throat Softchews ... ▣ 689
Tylenol Sinus NightTime Caplets ... ▣ 663
Children's Tylenol Plus Cold & Allergy Suspension Liquid ... 1850
Children's Tylenol Plus Cold NightTime Suspension Liquid ... 1851
Children's Tylenol Plus Cold & Cough Suspension Liquid and Chewable Tablets ... 1851
Children's Tylenol Plus Cold Chewable Tablets ... 1851
Children's Tylenol Plus Cold Daytime Non-Drowsy Suspension Liquid ... 1851
Children's Tylenol Plus Flu Suspension Liquid ... 1853
Concentrated Tylenol Infants' Drops Plus Cold ... 1851
Concentrated Tylenol Infants' Drops Plus Cold and Cough ... 1851
Tylenol Cold & Flu Severe Daytime Liquid with Cool Burst ... 1846
Tylenol Cold & Flu Severe NightTime Liquid with Cool Burst ... 1846
Tylenol Cold Severe Congestion Non-Drowsy Caplets with Cool Burst ... 1846
Tylenol Allergy Complete Night Time Caplets ... 1844
Tylenol Allergy Complete Multi-Symptom Caplets and Gelcaps with Cool Burst ... 1844
Tylenol Flu NightTime Gelcaps ... 1846
Tylenol Flu Day Non-Drowsy Gelcaps ... 1846
Concentrated Tylenol Infants' Drops Plus Cold Nasal Congestant, Fever Reducer & Pain Reliever ... ▣ 668
Concentrated Tylenol Infants' Drops Plus Cold & Cough Nasal Decongestant, Fever Reducer & Pain Reliever ... ▣ 668
Multi-Symptom Tylenol Cold Night Time Caplets ... 1845
Multi-Symptom Tylenol Cold Day Non-Drowsy Caplets and Gelcaps ... 1845
Tylenol Sinus Day Non-Drowsy ... 1848
Tylenol Sinus Night Time Caplets ... 1848
Tylenol Sinus Severe Congestion Caplets with Cool Burst ... 1848
Vicks 44D Cough & Head Congestion Relief ... 2676
Vicks 44D Cough & Head Congestion Relief Liquid ... ▣ 721
Vicks 44M Cough, Cold & Flu Relief ... 2676
Pediatric Vicks 44m Cough & Cold Relief ... 2673
Vicks DayQuil LiquiCaps/Liquid Multi-Symptom Cold/Flu Relief ... ▣ 723
Vicks DayQuil Multi-Symptom Cold/Flu Relief LiquiCaps ... 2675
Vicks DayQuil Multi-Symptom Cold/Flu Relief Liquid ... 2675
Children's Vicks NyQuil Cold/Cough Relief ... 2671
Vicks NyQuil LiquiCaps ... 2677
Vicks NyQuil LiquiCaps/Liquid Multi-Symptom Cold/Flu Relief ... ▣ 725
Vicks NyQuil Liquid ... 2677
Zyrtec-D 12 Hour Extended Release Tablets ... 2591

Pseudoephedrine Sulfate (Decrease in circulating catecholamines with smoking cessation; may require an increase in dose at cessation of smoking). Products include:
Alavert Allergy & Sinus D-12 Hour Tablets ... ▣ 743
Clarinex-D 24-Hour Extended-Release Tablets ... 3012
Claritin-D Non-Drowsy 12 Hour Tablets ... ▣ 731
Claritin-D Non-Drowsy 24 Hour Tablets ... ▣ 731

Salmeterol Xinafoate (Decrease in circulating catecholamines with smoking cessation; may require an increase in dose at cessation of smoking). Products include:
Advair Diskus 100/50 ... 1291
Advair Diskus 250/50 ... 1291
Advair Diskus 500/50 ... 1291
Serevent Diskus ... 1540

Sotalol Hydrochloride (Deinduction of hepatic enzyme on smoking cessation; may require a decrease in dose at cessation of smoking).
No products indexed under this heading.

Tamsulosin Hydrochloride (Decrease in circulating catecholamines with smoking cessation; may require a decrease in dose at cessation of smoking). Products include:
Flomax Capsules ... 881

Terazosin Hydrochloride (Decrease in circulating catecholamines with smoking cessation; may require a decrease in dose at cessation of smoking). Products include:
Hytrin Capsules ... 469

Terbutaline Sulfate (Decrease in circulating catecholamines with smoking cessation; may require an increase in dose at cessation of smoking).
No products indexed under this heading.

Tetrahydrozoline Hydrochloride (Decrease in circulating catecholamines with smoking cessation; may require an increase in dose at cessation of smoking). Products include:
Visine A.C. Seasonal Itching and Redness Relief Drops ... ⊙ 278
Advanced Relief Visine Eye Drops ... ⊙ 278

Theophylline (Deinduction of hepatic enzyme on smoking cessation; may require a decrease in dose at cessation of smoking).
No products indexed under this heading.

Theophylline Anhydrous (Deinduction of hepatic enzyme on smoking cessation; may require a decrease in dose at cessation of smoking). Products include:
Uniphyl Tablets ... 2708

Theophylline Calcium Salicylate (Deinduction of hepatic enzyme on smoking cessation; may require a decrease in dose at cessation of smoking).
No products indexed under this heading.

Theophylline Dihydroxypropyl (Glyceryl) (Deinduction of hepatic enzyme on smoking cessation; may require a decrease in dose at cessation of smoking).
No products indexed under this heading.

Theophylline Ethylenediamine (Deinduction of hepatic enzyme on smoking cessation; may require a decrease in dose at cessation of smoking).
No products indexed under this heading.

Theophylline Sodium Glycinate (Deinduction of hepatic enzyme on smoking cessation; may require a decrease in dose at cessation of smoking).
No products indexed under this heading.

Timolol Hemihydrate (Deinduction of hepatic enzyme on smoking cessation; may require a decrease in dose at cessation of smoking). Products include:
Betimol Ophthalmic Solution 3371
Betimol Ophthalmic Solution .... ⊙ 283

Timolol Maleate (Deinduction of hepatic enzyme on smoking cessation; may require a decrease in dose at cessation of smoking). Products include:
Blocadren Tablets 1891
Cosopt Sterile Ophthalmic Solution.. 1910
Timolide Tablets 2056
Timoptic in Ocudose 2061
Timoptic Sterile Ophthalmic Solution.. 2058
Timoptic-XE Sterile Ophthalmic Gel Forming Solution 2062

Xylometazoline Hydrochloride (The extent of absorption and peak plasma concentration is slightly reduced in patients with common cold/rhinitis; time to peak concentration is prolonged with the use of xylometazoline).
No products indexed under this heading.

NIFEREX-150 FORTE CAPSULES
(Folic Acid, Polysaccharide Iron Complex, Vitamin B_{12}, Vitamin C)........ 3299
None cited in PDR database.

NIMBEX INJECTION
(Cisatracurium Besylate) 494
May interact with aminoglycosides, lithium preparations, local anesthetics, phenytoin, tetracyclines, and certain other agents. Compounds in these categories include:

Amikacin Sulfate (Enhances neuromuscular blocking action).
No products indexed under this heading.

Bacitracin (Enhances neuromuscular blocking action). Products include:
Neosporin Ointment .... 🅾 702
Neosporin + Pain Relief Maximum Strength Ointment....... 🅾 703
Polysporin Ointment .... 🅾 706

Bupivacaine Hydrochloride (Enhances neuromuscular blocking action).
No products indexed under this heading.

Carbamazepine (Chronic administration of carbamazepine may produce resistance to the neuromuscular blocking action; slightly shorter durations of neuromuscular block may be anticipated). Products include:
Carbatrol Capsules 3174
Equetro Extended-Release Capsules.. 3178
Tegretol/Tegretol-XR 2278

Chloroprocaine Hydrochloride (Enhances neuromuscular blocking action).
No products indexed under this heading.

Clindamycin Hydrochloride (Enhances neuromuscular blocking action). Products include:
Cleocin Vaginal Ovules 2613

Clindamycin Palmitate Hydrochloride (Enhances neuromuscular blocking action).
No products indexed under this heading.

Clindamycin Phosphate (Enhances neuromuscular blocking action). Products include:
Benzaclin Topical Gel 1046
Clindagel 1207
Clindesse Vaginal Cream 3296
Clindets Pledgets 3212
Evoclin Foam, 1% 1025

Colistimethate Sodium (Enhances neuromuscular blocking action).
No products indexed under this heading.

Colistin Sulfate (Enhances neuromuscular blocking action).
No products indexed under this heading.

Demeclocycline Hydrochloride (Enhances neuromuscular blocking action).
No products indexed under this heading.

Doxycycline Calcium (Enhances neuromuscular blocking action).
No products indexed under this heading.

Doxycycline Hyclate (Enhances neuromuscular blocking action).
No products indexed under this heading.

Doxycycline Monohydrate (Enhances neuromuscular blocking action).
No products indexed under this heading.

Enflurane (Enflurane administered with nitrous oxide/oxygen may prolong the clinically effective duration of action of initial and maintenance doses of cisatracurium and decrease the required infusion rate of cisatracurium).
No products indexed under this heading.

Etidocaine Hydrochloride (Enhances neuromuscular blocking action).
No products indexed under this heading.

Fosphenytoin Sodium (Chronic administration of phenytoin may produce resistance to the neuromuscular blocking action; slightly shorter durations of neuromuscular block may be anticipated).
No products indexed under this heading.

Gentamicin Sulfate (Enhances neuromuscular blocking action). Products include:
Garamycin Injectable 3028
Genoptic Sterile Ophthalmic Solution.. ⊙ 227
Pred-G Ophthalmic Suspension ...... ⊙ 234
Pred-G Sterile Ophthalmic Ointment.. ⊙ 235

Isoflurane (Isoflurane administered with nitrous oxide/oxygen may prolong the clinically effective duration of action of initial and maintenance doses of cisatracurium and decrease the required infusion rate of cisatracurium).
No products indexed under this heading.

Kanamycin Sulfate (Enhances neuromuscular blocking action).
No products indexed under this heading.

Levobupivacaine Hydrochloride (Enhances neuromuscular blocking action).
No products indexed under this heading.

Lidocaine Hydrochloride (Enhances neuromuscular blocking action).
No products indexed under this heading.

Lincomycin Hydrochloride (Enhances neuromuscular blocking action).
No products indexed under this heading.

Lithium (Enhances neuromuscular blocking action).
No products indexed under this heading.

Lithium Carbonate (Enhances neuromuscular blocking action). Products include:
Eskalith 1406
Lithobid Tablets 1670

Lithium Citrate (Enhances neuromuscular blocking action).
No products indexed under this heading.

Magnesium Salts (Enhances neuromuscular blocking action).
No products indexed under this heading.

Mepivacaine Hydrochloride (Enhances neuromuscular blocking action).
No products indexed under this heading.

Methacycline Hydrochloride (Enhances neuromuscular blocking action).
No products indexed under this heading.

Minocycline Hydrochloride (Enhances neuromuscular blocking action). Products include:
Dynacin Tablets 1859

Oxytetracycline Hydrochloride (Enhances neuromuscular blocking action).
No products indexed under this heading.

Phenytoin (Chronic administration of phenytoin may produce resistance to the neuromuscular blocking action; slightly shorter durations of neuromuscular block may be anticipated).
No products indexed under this heading.

Phenytoin Sodium (Chronic administration of phenytoin may produce resistance to the neuromuscular blocking action; slightly shorter durations of neuromuscular block may be anticipated). Products include:
Phenytek Capsules 2153

Polymyxin Preparations (Enhances neuromuscular blocking action).
No products indexed under this heading.

Procainamide Hydrochloride (Enhances neuromuscular blocking action).
No products indexed under this heading.

Procaine Hydrochloride (Enhances neuromuscular blocking action).
No products indexed under this heading.

Quinidine Gluconate (Enhances neuromuscular blocking action).
No products indexed under this heading.

Quinidine Polygalacturonate (Enhances neuromuscular blocking action).
No products indexed under this heading.

Quinidine Sulfate (Enhances neuromuscular blocking action).
No products indexed under this heading.

Streptomycin Sulfate (Enhances neuromuscular blocking action).
No products indexed under this heading.

Tetracaine Hydrochloride (Enhances neuromuscular blocking action). Products include:
Cetacaine Topical Anesthetic 1007

Tetracycline Hydrochloride (Enhances neuromuscular blocking action).
No products indexed under this heading.

Tobramycin (Enhances neuromuscular blocking action). Products include:
TOBI Solution for Inhalation 1015
TobraDex Ophthalmic Ointment 558
TobraDex Ophthalmic Suspension ... 558
Zylet Ophthalmic Suspension 3508

Tobramycin Sulfate (Enhances neuromuscular blocking action).
No products indexed under this heading.

NIMOTOP CAPSULES
(Nimodipine) 774
May interact with antihypertensives, calcium channel blockers, and certain other agents. Compounds in these categories include:

Acebutolol Hydrochloride (Concomitant administration results in intensified effect).
No products indexed under this heading.

Amlodipine Besylate (Possibility of enhanced cardiovascular action). Products include:
Caduet Tablets 2507
Lotrel Capsules 2238
Norvasc Tablets 2529

Atenolol (Concomitant administration results in intensified effect). Products include:
Tenormin I.V. Injection 698
Tenormin Tablets 695

Benazepril Hydrochloride (Concomitant administration results in intensified effect). Products include:
Lotensin Tablets 2232
Lotensin HCT Tablets 2235
Lotrel Capsules 2238

Bendroflumethiazide (Concomitant administration results in intensified effect).
No products indexed under this heading.

Bepridil Hydrochloride (Possibility of enhanced cardiovascular action).
No products indexed under this heading.

IMPORTANT NOTE: Always consult each drug listing in the patient's regimen for possible interactions.

Betaxolol Hydrochloride (Concomitant administration results in intensified effect). Products include:
Betoptic S Ophthalmic Suspension 554

Bisoprolol Fumarate (Concomitant administration results in intensified effect).
No products indexed under this heading.

Candesartan Cilexetil (Concomitant administration results in intensified effect). Products include:
Atacand Tablets 634
Atacand HCT 637

Captopril (Concomitant administration results in intensified effect). Products include:
Captopril Tablets 2114

Carteolol Hydrochloride (Concomitant administration results in intensified effect). Products include:
Carteolol Hydrochloride Ophthalmic Solution USP, 1% .... ⊙246

Chlorothiazide (Concomitant administration results in intensified effect). Products include:
Aldoclor Tablets 1881
Diuril Oral 1936

Chlorothiazide Sodium (Concomitant administration results in intensified effect). Products include:
Diuril Sodium Intravenous 1934

Chlorthalidone (Concomitant administration results in intensified effect). Products include:
Clorpres Tablets 2139

Cimetidine (May increase peak nimodipine plasma concentrations and AUC). Products include:
Tagamet HB 200 Tablets .... ▣637
Tagamet Tablets 1547

Cimetidine Hydrochloride (May increase peak nimodipine plasma concentrations and AUC).
No products indexed under this heading.

Clonidine (Concomitant administration results in intensified effect). Products include:
Catapres-TTS 875

Clonidine Hydrochloride (Concomitant administration results in intensified effect). Products include:
Catapres Tablets 874
Clorpres Tablets 2139

Deserpidine (Concomitant administration results in intensified effect).
No products indexed under this heading.

Diazoxide (Concomitant administration results in intensified effect). Products include:
Hyperstat I.V. Injection 3031

Diltiazem Hydrochloride (Possibility of enhanced cardiovascular action). Products include:
Cardizem LA Extended Release Tablets 1699
Tiazac Capsules 1204

Doxazosin Mesylate (Concomitant administration results in intensified effect).
No products indexed under this heading.

Enalapril Maleate (Concomitant administration results in intensified effect). Products include:
Vaseretic Tablets 2073
Vasotec I.V. Injection 2076

Enalaprilat (Concomitant administration results in intensified effect).
No products indexed under this heading.

Eprosartan Mesylate (Concomitant administration results in intensified effect). Products include:
Teveten Tablets 1707
Teveten HCT Tablets 1710

Esmolol Hydrochloride (Concomitant administration results in intensified effect). Products include:
Brevibloc Concentrate 766
Brevibloc Injection 766
Brevibloc Double Strength Injection 766
Brevibloc Premixed Injection 766
Brevibloc Double Strength Premixed Injection 766

Felodipine (Possibility of enhanced cardiovascular action). Products include:
Plendil Extended-Release Tablets 651

Fosinopril Sodium (Concomitant administration results in intensified effect).
No products indexed under this heading.

Furosemide (Concomitant administration results in intensified effect). Products include:
Furosemide Tablets 2117

Guanabenz Acetate (Concomitant administration results in intensified effect).
No products indexed under this heading.

Guanethidine Monosulfate (Concomitant administration results in intensified effect).
No products indexed under this heading.

Hydralazine Hydrochloride (Concomitant administration results in intensified effect). Products include:
BiDil Tablets 2161

Hydrochlorothiazide (Concomitant administration results in intensified effect). Products include:
Aldoril Tablets 1884
Atacand HCT 637
Avalide Tablets 2889
Avalide Tablets 922
Benicar HCT Tablets 2852
Diovan HCT Tablets 2195
Dyazide Capsules 1389
Hyzaar 1964
Lotensin HCT Tablets 2235
Maxzide 2150
Micardis HCT Tablets 886
Moduretic Tablets 2003
Prinzide Tablets 2033
Teveten HCT Tablets 1710
Timolide Tablets 2056
Uniretic Tablets 3114
Vaseretic Tablets 2073
Zestoretic Tablets 701

Hydroflumethiazide (Concomitant administration results in intensified effect).
No products indexed under this heading.

Indapamide (Concomitant administration results in intensified effect). Products include:
Indapamide Tablets 2119

Irbesartan (Concomitant administration results in intensified effect). Products include:
Avalide Tablets 922
Avalide Tablets 2889
Avapro Tablets 925
Avapro Tablets 2886

Isradipine (Possibility of enhanced cardiovascular action). Products include:
DynaCirc CR Tablets 2726

Labetalol Hydrochloride (Concomitant administration results in intensified effect).
No products indexed under this heading.

Lisinopril (Concomitant administration results in intensified effect). Products include:
Prinivil Tablets 2029
Prinzide Tablets 2033
Zestoretic Tablets 701
Zestril Tablets 704

Losartan Potassium (Concomitant administration results in intensified effect). Products include:
Cozaar Tablets 1913
Hyzaar 1964

Mecamylamine Hydrochloride (Concomitant administration results in intensified effect). Products include:
Inversine Tablets 3286

Methyclothiazide (Concomitant administration results in intensified effect).
No products indexed under this heading.

Methyldopa (Concomitant administration results in intensified effect). Products include:
Aldoclor Tablets 1881
Aldoril Tablets 1884

Methyldopate Hydrochloride (Concomitant administration results in intensified effect).
No products indexed under this heading.

Metolazone (Concomitant administration results in intensified effect).
No products indexed under this heading.

Metoprolol Succinate (Concomitant administration results in intensified effect). Products include:
Toprol-XL Tablets 660

Metoprolol Tartrate (Concomitant administration results in intensified effect).
No products indexed under this heading.

Metyrosine (Concomitant administration results in intensified effect). Products include:
Demser Capsules 1933

Mibefradil Dihydrochloride (Possibility of enhanced cardiovascular action).
No products indexed under this heading.

Minoxidil (Concomitant administration results in intensified effect). Products include:
Men's Rogaine Extra Strength Topical Solution, Ocean Rush Scent and Original Unscented .... ▣706
Women's Rogaine Topical Solution, Spring Bloom Scent and Original Unscented .... ▣707

Moexipril Hydrochloride (Concomitant administration results in intensified effect). Products include:
Uniretic Tablets 3114
Univasc Tablets 3118

Nadolol (Concomitant administration results in intensified effect). Products include:
Nadolol Tablets 2121

Nicardipine Hydrochloride (Possibility of enhanced cardiovascular action). Products include:
Cardene I.V. 1129

Nifedipine (Possibility of enhanced cardiovascular action). Products include:
Adalat CC Tablets 2978

Nisoldipine (Possibility of enhanced cardiovascular action). Products include:
Sular Tablets 1163

Nitroglycerin (Concomitant administration results in intensified effect). Products include:
Nitro-Dur Transdermal Infusion System 3060
Nitrolingual Pumpspray 1161

Penbutolol Sulfate (Concomitant administration results in intensified effect).
No products indexed under this heading.

Perindopril Erbumine (Concomitant administration results in intensified effect). Products include:
Aceon Tablets (2 mg, 4 mg, 8 mg) 3191

Phenoxybenzamine Hydrochloride (Concomitant administration results in intensified effect). Products include:
Dibenzyline Capsules 3390

Phentolamine Mesylate (Concomitant administration results in intensified effect).
No products indexed under this heading.

Phenytoin (Potential for phenytoin toxicity).
No products indexed under this heading.

Phenytoin Sodium (Potential for phenytoin toxicity). Products include:
Phenytek Capsules 2153

Pindolol (Concomitant administration results in intensified effect).
No products indexed under this heading.

Polythiazide (Concomitant administration results in intensified effect).
No products indexed under this heading.

Prazosin Hydrochloride (Concomitant administration results in intensified effect).
No products indexed under this heading.

Propranolol Hydrochloride (Concomitant administration results in intensified effect). Products include:
Inderal LA Long-Acting Capsules 3421
InnoPran XL Capsules 2728

Quinapril Hydrochloride (Concomitant administration results in intensified effect).
No products indexed under this heading.

Ramipril (Concomitant administration results in intensified effect). Products include:
Altace Capsules 1673

Rauwolfia Serpentina (Concomitant administration results in intensified effect).
No products indexed under this heading.

Rescinnamine (Concomitant administration results in intensified effect).
No products indexed under this heading.

Reserpine (Concomitant administration results in intensified effect).
No products indexed under this heading.

Sodium Nitroprusside (Concomitant administration results in intensified effect).
No products indexed under this heading.

Sotalol Hydrochloride (Concomitant administration results in intensified effect).
No products indexed under this heading.

Spirapril Hydrochloride (Concomitant administration results in intensified effect).
No products indexed under this heading.

Telmisartan (Concomitant administration results in intensified effect). Products include:
Micardis Tablets 884
Micardis HCT Tablets 886

Terazosin Hydrochloride (Concomitant administration results in intensified effect). Products include:
Hytrin Capsules 469

Timolol Maleate (Concomitant administration results in intensified effect). Products include:
Blocadren Tablets 1891
Cosopt Sterile Ophthalmic Solution 1910
Timolide Tablets 2056
Timoptic in Ocudose 2061
Timoptic Sterile Ophthalmic Solution 2058
Timoptic-XE Sterile Ophthalmic Gel Forming Solution 2062

Torsemide (Concomitant administration results in intensified effect).
No products indexed under this heading.

Trandolapril (Concomitant administration results in intensified effect). Products include:
Mavik Tablets 482
Tarka Tablets 519

Trimethaphan Camsylate (Concomitant administration results in intensified effect).
No products indexed under this heading.

Valsartan (Concomitant administration results in intensified effect). Products include:
Diovan HCT Tablets 2195
Diovan Tablets 2191

Verapamil Hydrochloride (Possibility of enhanced cardiovascular action). Products include:
Covera-HS Tablets 3135
Tarka Tablets 519
Verelan PM Capsules 3120

Food Interactions

Meal, unspecified (Administration of nimodipine capsules following a standard breakfast resulted in 68% lower peak plasma concentration and 38% lower bioavailability).

NIPENT FOR INJECTION

(Pentostatin) 3216
May interact with:

Allopurinol (Both drugs are associated with skin rashes; concomitant therapy in one patient has resulted in a fatal hypersensitivity vasculitis).
No products indexed under this heading.

Carmustine (BCNU) (Co-administration with high dose cyclophosphamide, carmustine, and etoposide has resulted in a report of acute pulmonary edema, hypotension, and death).
No products indexed under this heading.

Cyclophosphamide (Co-administration with high dose cyclophosphamide, carmustine, and etoposide has resulted in a report of acute pulmonary edema, hypotension, and death).
No products indexed under this heading.

Etoposide (Co-administration with high dose cyclophosphamide, carmustine, and etoposide has resulted in a report of acute pulmonary edema, hypotension, and death).
No products indexed under this heading.

Fludarabine Phosphate (Increased risk of fatal pulmonary toxicity; combined use is not recommended).
No products indexed under this heading.

Vidarabine (Enhanced effects of vidarabine and may result in increased adverse reactions associated with each drug).
No products indexed under this heading.

NIRAVAM ORALLY DISINTEGRATING TABLETS

(Alprazolam) 3106
May interact with antacids, antihistamines, central nervous system depressants, cytochrome p450 3a inhibitors (selected), anticonvulsants, histamine H_2-receptor antagonists, macrolide antibiotics, oral contraceptives, proton pump inhibitor, psychotropics, and certain other agents. Compounds in these categories include:

Acrivastine (The benzodiazepines, including alprazolam, produce additive CNS depressant effects when co-administered with antihistamines).
No products indexed under this heading.

Alfentanil Hydrochloride (The benzodiazepines, including alprazolam, produce additive CNS depressant effects when co-administered with other drugs which themselves produce CNS depression).
No products indexed under this heading.

Aluminum Carbonate (Because Niravam disintegrates in the presence of saliva and the formulation requires an acidic environment to dissolve, concomitant drugs or diseases that raise stomach pH might slow disintegration or dissolution, resulting in slowed or decreased absorption).
No products indexed under this heading.

Aluminum Hydroxide (Because Niravam disintegrates in the presence of saliva and the formulation requires an acidic environment to dissolve, concomitant drugs or diseases that raise stomach pH might slow disintegration or dissolution, resulting in slowed or decreased absorption). Products include:
Gaviscon Regular Strength Liquid 620
Gaviscon Regular Strength Tablets 619
Gaviscon Extra Strength Liquid 620
Gaviscon Extra Strength Tablets 619
Maalox Max Maximum Strength Antacid/Anti-Gas Liquid 2165
Maalox Regular Strength Antacid/Antigas Liquid 2164

Amiodarone Hydrochloride (Data from in vitro studies of benzodiazepines, other than alprazolam, suggest a possible drug interaction with amiodarone; caution is recommended during co-administration). Products include:
Pacerone Tablets 3337

Amitriptyline Hydrochloride (The benzodiazepines, including alprazolam, produce additive CNS depressant effects when co-administered with other psychotropic medications. If alprazolam is to be combined with other psychotropic agents, careful consideration should be given to the pharmacology of the agents to be employed, particularly with compounds which might potentiate the action of benzodiazepines).
No products indexed under this heading.

Amoxapine (The benzodiazepines, including alprazolam, produce additive CNS depressant effects when co-administered with other psychotropic medications. If alprazolam is to be combined with other psychotropic agents, careful consideration should be given to the pharmacology of the agents to be employed, particularly with compounds which might potentiate the action of benzodiazepines).
No products indexed under this heading.

Amprenavir (The initial step in alprazolam metabolism is hydroxylation catalyzed by cytochrome P450 3A (CYP3A). Drugs which inhibit this metabolic pathway may have a profound effect on the clearance of alprazolam). Products include:
Agenerase Capsules 1299
Agenerase Oral Solution 1304

Aprepitant (The initial step in alprazolam metabolism is hydroxylation catalyzed by cytochrome P450 3A (CYP3A). Drugs which inhibit this metabolic pathway may have a profound effect on the clearance of alprazolam). Products include:
Emend Capsules 1944

Aprobarbital (The benzodiazepines, including alprazolam, produce additive CNS depressant effects when co-administered with other drugs which themselves produce CNS depression).
No products indexed under this heading.

Azatadine Maleate (The benzodiazepines, including alprazolam, produce additive CNS depressant effects when co-administered with antihistamines).
No products indexed under this heading.

Azithromycin Dihydrate (Available data from clinical studies of benzodiazepines, other than alprazolam, suggest a possible drug interaction with alprazolam and macrolide antibiotics; caution is recommended during co-administration). Products include:
Zithromax 2568
Zithromax for IV Infusion 2573
Zithromax for Oral Suspension, 300 mg, 600 mg, 900 mg, 1200 mg 2561
Zithromax Tablets, 250 mg, 500 mg 2561
Zithromax Tri-Pak 2561
Zithromax Z-Pak 2568

Belladonna Ergotamine (Data from in vitro studies of benzodiazepines, other than alprazolam, suggest a possible drug interaction with ergotamine; caution is recommended during co-administration).
No products indexed under this heading.

Bromodiphenhydramine Hydrochloride (The benzodiazepines, including alprazolam, produce additive CNS depressant effects when co-administered with antihistamines).
No products indexed under this heading.

Brompheniramine Maleate (The benzodiazepines, including alprazolam, produce additive CNS depressant effects when co-administered with antihistamines). Products include:
Alacol DM Syrup 739
Children's Dimetapp Cold & Allergy Elixir 745
Children's Dimetapp DM Cold & Cough Elixir 745
Robitussin Allergy & Cough Syrup 750

Buprenorphine Hydrochloride (The benzodiazepines, including alprazolam, produce additive CNS depressant effects when co-administered with other drugs which themselves produce CNS depression). Products include:
Buprenex Injectable 2718
Suboxone Tablets 2719
Subutex Tablets 2719

Buspirone Hydrochloride (The benzodiazepines, including alprazolam, produce additive CNS depressant effects when co-administered with other psychotropic medications. If alprazolam is to be combined with other psychotropic agents, careful consideration should be given to the pharmacology of the agents to be employed, particularly with compounds which might potentiate the action of benzodiazepines).
No products indexed under this heading.

Butabarbital (The benzodiazepines, including alprazolam, produce additive CNS depressant effects when co-administered with other drugs which themselves produce CNS depression).
No products indexed under this heading.

Butalbital (The benzodiazepines, including alprazolam, produce additive CNS depressant effects when co-administered with other drugs which themselves produce CNS depression). Products include:
Sedapap Tablets 50 mg/650 mg 2098

Carbamazepine (Carbamazepine can increase alprazolam metabolism and therefore can decrease plasma levels of alprazolam). Products include:
Carbatrol Capsules 3174
Equetro Extended-Release Capsules 3178
Tegretol/Tegretol-XR 2278

Cetirizine Hydrochloride (The benzodiazepines, including alprazolam, produce additive CNS depressant effects when co-administered with antihistamines). Products include:
Zyrtec Chewable Tablets 2589
Zyrtec 2589
Zyrtec-D 12 Hour Extended Release Tablets 2591

Chlordiazepoxide (The benzodiazepines, including alprazolam, produce additive CNS depressant effects when co-administered with other psychotropic medications. If alprazolam is to be combined with other psychotropic agents, careful consideration should be given to the pharmacology of the agents to be employed, particularly with compounds which might potentiate the

action of benzodiazepines).
No products indexed under this heading.

Chlordiazepoxide Hydrochloride (The benzodiazepines, including alprazolam, produce additive CNS depressant effects when co-administered with other psychotropic medications. If alprazolam is to be combined with other psychotropic agents, careful consideration should be given to the pharmacology of the agents to be employed, particularly with compounds which might potentiate the action of benzodiazepines). Products include:
- Librium Capsules 3349

Chlorpheniramine Maleate (The benzodiazepines, including alprazolam, produce additive CNS depressant effects when co-administered with antihistamines). Products include:
- Advil Allergy Sinus Caplets .... ▣ 737
- Advil Multi-Symptom Cold Caplets .... ▣ 738
- BC Allergy Sinus Cold Powder .... ▣ 612
- Contac Severe Cold and Flu Caplets Maximum Strength .... ▣ 615
- Hycomine Compound Tablets 1105
- PediaCare Multi-Symptom Cold Liquid .... ▣ 704
- PediaCare NightRest Cough & Cold Liquid .... ▣ 704
- Robitussin Flu Liquid .... ▣ 752
- Robitussin PM Cough & Cold Liquid .... ▣ 752
- Singlet Caplets .... ▣ 636
- Sudafed Sinus & Allergy Tablets .... ▣ 710
- TheraFlu Cold & Cough Hot Liquid .... ▣ 680
- TheraFlu Cold & Sore Throat Hot Liquid .... ▣ 680
- TheraFlu Flu & Sore Throat Hot Liquid .... ▣ 681
- TheraFlu Severe Cold & Cough Hot Liquid .... ▣ 683
- TheraFlu Severe Cold Caplets .... ▣ 679
- TheraFlu Severe Cold Hot Liquid .... ▣ 682
- Triaminic Cold & Allergy Liquid .... ▣ 685
- Triaminic Cold & Cough Liquid .... ▣ 685
- Triaminic Flu, Cough & Fever Liquid .... ▣ 685
- Triaminic Night Time Cough & Cold Liquid .... ▣ 685
- Triaminic Allergy Runny Nose & Congestion Softchews .... ▣ 688
- Triaminic Cold & Cough Softchews .... ▣ 688
- Children's Tylenol Plus Cold NightTime Suspension Liquid 1851
- Children's Tylenol Plus Cold & Cough Suspension Liquid and Chewable Tablets 1851
- Children's Tylenol Plus Cold Chewable Tablets 1851
- Children's Tylenol Plus Flu Suspension Liquid 1853
- Tylenol Allergy Complete Multi-Symptom Caplets and Gelcaps with Cool Burst 1844
- Multi-Symptom Tylenol Cold Night Time Caplets 1845
- Vicks 44M Cough, Cold & Flu Relief 2676
- Pediatric Vicks 44m Cough & Cold Relief 2673
- Children's Vicks NyQuil Cold/Cough Relief 2671

Chlorpheniramine Polistirex (The benzodiazepines, including alprazolam, produce additive CNS depressant effects when co-administered with antihistamines). Products include:
- Tussionex Pennkinetic Extended-Release Suspension 3322

Chlorpheniramine Tannate (The benzodiazepines, including alprazolam, produce additive CNS depressant effects when co-administered with antihistamines).
No products indexed under this heading.

Chlorpromazine (The benzodiazepines, including alprazolam, produce additive CNS depressant effects when co-administered with other psychotropic medications. If alprazolam is to be combined with other psychotropic agents, careful consideration should be given to the pharmacology of the agents to be employed, particularly with compounds which might potentiate the action of benzodiazepines).
No products indexed under this heading.

Chlorpromazine Hydrochloride (The benzodiazepines, including alprazolam, produce additive CNS depressant effects when co-administered with other psychotropic medications. If alprazolam is to be combined with other psychotropic agents, careful consideration should be given to the pharmacology of the agents to be employed, particularly with compounds which might potentiate the action of benzodiazepines).
No products indexed under this heading.

Chlorprothixene (The benzodiazepines, including alprazolam, produce additive CNS depressant effects when co-administered with other psychotropic medications. If alprazolam is to be combined with other psychotropic agents, careful consideration should be given to the pharmacology of the agents to be employed, particularly with compounds which might potentiate the action of benzodiazepines).
No products indexed under this heading.

Chlorprothixene Hydrochloride (The benzodiazepines, including alprazolam, produce additive CNS depressant effects when co-administered with other psychotropic medications. If alprazolam is to be combined with other psychotropic agents, careful consideration should be given to the pharmacology of the agents to be employed, particularly with compounds which might potentiate the action of benzodiazepines).
No products indexed under this heading.

Chlorprothixene Lactate (The benzodiazepines, including alprazolam, produce additive CNS depressant effects when co-administered with other drugs which themselves produce CNS depression).
No products indexed under this heading.

Cimetidine (Because Niravam disintegrates in the presence of saliva and the formulation requires an acidic environment to dissolve, concomitant drugs or diseases that raise stomach pH might slow disintegration or dissolution, resulting in slowed or decreased absorption). Products include:
- Tagamet HB 200 Tablets .... ▣ 637
- Tagamet Tablets 1547

Cimetidine Hydrochloride (Because Niravam disintegrates in the presence of saliva and the formulation requires an acidic environment to dissolve, concomitant drugs or diseases that raise stomach pH might slow disintegration or dissolution, resulting in slowed or decreased absorption).
No products indexed under this heading.

Ciprofloxacin (The initial step in alprazolam metabolism is hydroxylation catalyzed by cytochrome P450 3A (CYP3A). Drugs which inhibit this metabolic pathway may have a profound effect on the clearance of alprazolam). Products include:
- Cipro I.V. 2998
- Cipro I.V. Pharmacy Bulk Package 3509
- Cipro Oral Suspension 2991
- Cipro XR Tablets 3004
- Ciprodex Otic Suspension 555

Ciprofloxacin Hydrochloride (The initial step in alprazolam metabolism is hydroxylation catalyzed by cytochrome P450 3A (CYP3A). Drugs which inhibit this metabolic pathway may have a profound effect on the clearance of alprazolam). Products include:
- Ciloxan Ophthalmic Ointment 554
- Cipro Tablets 2991

Clarithromycin (The initial step in alprazolam metabolism is hydroxylation catalyzed by cytochrome P450 3A (CYP3A). Drugs which inhibit this metabolic pathway may have a profound effect on the clearance of alprazolam). Products include:
- Biaxin/Biaxin XL 402
- PREVPAC 3281

Clemastine Fumarate (The benzodiazepines, including alprazolam, produce additive CNS depressant effects when co-administered with antihistamines).
No products indexed under this heading.

Clorazepate Dipotassium (The benzodiazepines, including alprazolam, produce additive CNS depressant effects when co-administered with other psychotropic medications. If alprazolam is to be combined with other psychotropic agents, careful consideration should be given to the pharmacology of the agents to be employed, particularly with compounds which might potentiate the action of benzodiazepines). Products include:
- Tranxene 2488

Clozapine (The benzodiazepines, including alprazolam, produce additive CNS depressant effects when co-administered with other psychotropic medications. If alprazolam is to be combined with other psychotropic agents, careful consideration should be given to the pharmacology of the agents to be employed, particularly with compounds which might potentiate the action of benzodiazepines). Products include:
- Clozapine Tablets 2141
- Clozaril Tablets 2174
- FazaClo Orally Disintegrating Tablets 547

Codeine Phosphate (The benzodiazepines, including alprazolam, produce additive CNS depressant effects when co-administered with other drugs which themselves produce CNS depression). Products include:
- Tylenol with Codeine 2461

Cyclosporine (Data from in vitro studies of benzodiazepines, other than alprazolam, suggest a possible drug interaction with cyclosporine; caution is recommended during co-administration). Products include:
- Gengraf Capsules 458
- Neoral Soft Gelatin Capsules 2247
- Neoral Oral Solution 2247
- Restasis Ophthalmic Emulsion 570
- Sandimmune 2259

Cyproheptadine Hydrochloride (The benzodiazepines, including alprazolam, produce additive CNS depressant effects when co-administered with antihistamines).
No products indexed under this heading.

Delavirdine Mesylate (The initial step in alprazolam metabolism is hydroxylation catalyzed by cytochrome P450 3A (CYP3A). Drugs which inhibit this metabolic pathway may have a profound effect on the clearance of alprazolam). Products include:
- Rescriptor Tablets 2535

Desflurane (The benzodiazepines, including alprazolam, produce additive CNS depressant effects when co-administered with other drugs which themselves produce CNS depression). Products include:
- Suprane Liquid for Inhalation 770

Desipramine Hydrochloride (The steady state plasma concentration of desipramine has been reported to be increased an average of 20% by the concomitant administration of alprazolam in doses up to 4 mg/day. The clinical significance of these changes is unknown).
No products indexed under this heading.

Desogestrel (Co-administration of oral contraceptives increased the maximum plasma concentration of alprazolam by 18%, decreased clearance by 22%, and increased half-life by 29%). Products include:
- Ortho-Cept Tablets 2395

Dexchlorpheniramine Maleate (The benzodiazepines, including alprazolam, produce additive CNS depressant effects when co-administered with antihistamines).
No products indexed under this heading.

Dezocine (The benzodiazepines, including alprazolam, produce additive CNS depressant effects when co-administered with other drugs which themselves produce CNS depression).
No products indexed under this heading.

Diazepam (The benzodiazepines, including alprazolam, produce additive CNS depressant effects when co-administered with other psychotropic medications. If alprazolam is to be combined with other psychotropic agents, careful consideration should be given to the pharmacology of the agents to be employed, particularly with compounds which might potentiate the action of benzodiazepines). Products include:
- Diastat Rectal Delivery System 3344
- Valium Tablets 2822

Dihydroergotamine Mesylate (Data from in vitro studies of benzodiazepines other than alprazolam suggest a possible drug interaction with ergotamine; caution is recommended during co-administration). Products include:

Migranal Nasal Spray 3350

Diltiazem Hydrochloride (Available data from clinical studies of benzodiazepines other than alprazolam suggest a possible drug interaction with alprazolam and diltiazem; caution is recommended during co-administration). Products include:

Cardizem LA Extended Release Tablets 1699
Tiazac Capsules 1204

Diltiazem Maleate (Available data from clinical studies of benzodiazepines other than alprazolam suggest a possible drug interaction with alprazolam and diltiazem; caution is recommended during co-administration).

No products indexed under this heading.

Diphenhydramine Citrate (The benzodiazepines, including alprazolam, produce additive CNS depressant effects when co-administered with antihistamines). Products include:

Children's Benadryl Allergy & Cold Fastmelt Tablets.................. 695
Children's Benadryl D Allergy & Sinus Fastmelt Tablets 694
Children's Benadryl Allergy Fastmelt Tablets 696
Goody's PM Powder 622

Diphenhydramine Hydrochloride (The benzodiazepines, including alprazolam, produce additive CNS depressant effects when co-administered with antihistamines). Products include:

Benadryl Allergy & Cold Tablets 692
Benadryl Allergy 691
Benadryl Allergy & Sinus Headache Caplets & Gelcaps...... 693
Children's Benadryl Allergy Liquid ... 695
Children's Benadryl Dye-Free Allergy Liquid 695
Benadryl Dye-Free Allergy Liqui-Gels Softgels 692
Benadryl Itch Relief Stick Extra Strength 696
Benadryl Itch Stopping Cream Extra Strength 697
Benadryl Itch Stopping Gel Extra Strength 697
Benadryl Itch Stopping Spray Extra Strength 697
Benadryl Maximum Strength Severe Allergy & Sinus Headache Caplets....................... 694
Children's Benadryl D Liquid Medication.................................. 693
Benadryl D Tablets 694
Nytol QuickCaps Caplets 635
Maximum Strength Nytol QuickGels Softgels 635
Simply Sleep Caplets 1841
Sominex Original Formula Tablets .. 637
TheraFlu Thin Strips Multi Symptom.................................. 684
Triaminic Thin Strips Cough & Runny Nose 690
Children's Tylenol Plus Cold & Allergy Suspension Liquid............ 1850
Tylenol Allergy Complete Night Time Caplets 1844
Tylenol Severe Allergy Caplets 1844
Tylenol Flu NightTime Gelcaps 1846
Extra Strength Tylenol PM Caplets, Geltabs, Gelcaps and Liquid 1847
Unisom Maximum Strength SleepGels................................... 712

Diphenylpyraline Hydrochloride (The benzodiazepines, including alprazolam, produce additive CNS depressant effects when co-administered with antihistamines).

No products indexed under this heading.

Dirithromycin (Available data from clinical studies of benzodiazepines, other than alprazolam, suggest a possible drug interaction with alprazolam and macrolide antibiotics; caution is recommended during co-administration).

No products indexed under this heading.

Divalproex Sodium (If alprazolam is to be combined with anticonvulsant drugs, careful consideration should be given to the pharmacology of the agents to be employed, particularly with compounds which might potentiate the action of benzodiazepines. The benzodiazepines, including alprazolam, produce additive CNS depressant effects when co-administered with anticonvulsants). Products include:

Depakote Sprinkle Capsules 422
Depakote Tablets 427
Depakote ER Tablets 433

Doxepin Hydrochloride (The benzodiazepines, including alprazolam, produce additive CNS depressant effects when co-administered with other psychotropic medications. If alprazolam is to be combined with other psychotropic agents, careful consideration should be given to the pharmacology of the agents to be employed, particularly with compounds which might potentiate the action of benzodiazepines).

No products indexed under this heading.

Droperidol (The benzodiazepines, including alprazolam, produce additive CNS depressant effects when co-administered with other psychotropic medications. If alprazolam is to be combined with other psychotropic agents, careful consideration should be given to the pharmacology of the agents to be employed, particularly with compounds which might potentiate the action of benzodiazepines).

No products indexed under this heading.

Efavirenz (The initial step in alprazolam metabolism is hydroxylation catalyzed by cytochrome P450 3A (CYP3A). Drugs which inhibit this metabolic pathway may have a profound effect on the clearance of alprazolam). Products include:

Sustiva Capsules 957

Enflurane (The benzodiazepines, including alprazolam, produce additive CNS depressant effects when co-administered with other drugs which themselves produce CNS depression).

No products indexed under this heading.

Ergotamine Tartrate (Data from in vitro studies of benzodiazepines, other than alprazolam, suggest a possible drug interaction with ergotamine; caution is recommended during co-administration).

No products indexed under this heading.

Erythromycin (The initial step in alprazolam metabolism is hydroxylation catalyzed by cytochrome P450 3A (CYP3A). Drugs which inhibit this metabolic pathway may have a profound effect on the clearance of alprazolam). Products include:

Erygel Topical Gel 2096
Ery-Tab Tablets 447
Erythromycin Base Filmtab Tablets 454
Erythromycin Delayed-Release Capsules, USP............................. 456
PCE Dispertab Tablets 510

Erythromycin Estolate (Available data from clinical studies of benzodiazepines, other than alprazolam, suggest a possible drug interaction with alprazolam and macrolide antibiotics; caution is recommended during co-administration).

No products indexed under this heading.

Erythromycin Ethylsuccinate (Available data from clinical studies of benzodiazepines, other than alprazolam, suggest a possible drug interaction with alprazolam and macrolide antibiotics; caution is recommended during co-administration). Products include:

E.E.S. 449
EryPed 445

Erythromycin Gluceptate (Available data from clinical studies of benzodiazepines, other than alprazolam, suggest a possible drug interaction with alprazolam and macrolide antibiotics; caution is recommended during co-administration).

No products indexed under this heading.

Erythromycin Stearate (Available data from clinical studies of benzodiazepines, other than alprazolam, suggest a possible drug interaction with alprazolam and macrolide antibiotics; caution is recommended during co-administration). Products include:

Erythrocin Stearate Filmtab Tablets 452

Esomeprazole Magnesium (Because Niravam disintegrates in the presence of saliva and the formulation requires an acidic environment to dissolve, concomitant drugs or diseases that raise stomach pH might slow disintegration or dissolution, resulting in slowed or decreased absorption). Products include:

Nexium Delayed-Release Capsules 645

Estazolam (The benzodiazepines, including alprazolam, produce additive CNS depressant effects when co-administered with other drugs which themselves produce CNS depression). Products include:

ProSom Tablets 512

Ethanol (The benzodiazepines, including alprazolam, produce additive CNS depressant effects when co-administered with ethanol).

No products indexed under this heading.

Ethchlorvynol (The benzodiazepines, including alprazolam, produce additive CNS depressant effects when co-administered with other drugs which themselves produce CNS depression).

No products indexed under this heading.

Ethinamate (The benzodiazepines, including alprazolam, produce additive CNS depressant effects when co-administered with other drugs which themselves produce CNS depression).

No products indexed under this heading.

Ethinyl Estradiol (Co-administration of oral contraceptives increased the maximum plasma concentration of alprazolam by 18%, decreased clearance by 22%, and increased half-life by 29%). Products include:

Alesse-28 Tablets 3392
Lo/Ovral-28 Tablets 3423
NuvaRing 2357
Ortho-Cept Tablets 2395
Ortho-Cyclen/Ortho Tri-Cyclen 2414
Ortho Evra Transdermal System 2402
Ortho Tri-Cyclen Lo Tablets 2421
Seasonale Tablets 1073
Triphasil-28 Tablets 3483
Yasmin 28 Tablets 818

Ethosuximide (If alprazolam is to be combined with anticonvulsant drugs, careful consideration should be given to the pharmacology of the agents to be employed, particularly with compounds which might potentiate the action of benzodiazepines. The benzodiazepines, including alprazolam, produce additive CNS depressant effects when co-administered with anticonvulsants).

No products indexed under this heading.

Ethotoin (If alprazolam is to be combined with anticonvulsant drugs, careful consideration should be given to the pharmacology of the agents to be employed, particularly with compounds which might potentiate the action of benzodiazepines. The benzodiazepines, including alprazolam, produce additive CNS depressant effects when co-administered with anticonvulsants). Products include:

Peganone Tablets, USP 2487

Ethyl Alcohol (The benzodiazepines, including alprazolam, produce additive CNS depressant effects when co-administered with other drugs which themselves produce CNS depression).

No products indexed under this heading.

Ethynodiol Diacetate (Co-administration of oral contraceptives increased the maximum plasma concentration of alprazolam by 18%, decreased clearance by 22%, and increased half-life by 29%).

No products indexed under this heading.

Famotidine (Because Niravam disintegrates in the presence of saliva and the formulation requires an acidic environment to dissolve, concomitant drugs or diseases that raise stomach pH might slow disintegration or dissolution, resulting in slowed or decreased absorption). Products include:

Pepcid AC Chewable Tablets 1672
Pepcid AC Gelcaps 1672
Pepcid AC Tablets 1672
Maximum Strength Pepcid AC Tablets 1672
Pepcid Complete Chewable Tablets 1672
Pepcid Injection 2017
Pepcid 2014

Felbamate (If alprazolam is to be combined with anticonvulsant drugs, careful consideration should be given to the pharmacology of the agents to be employed, particularly with compounds which might potentiate the action of benzodiazepines. The benzodiazepines, including alprazolam, produce additive CNS depressant effects when co-administered with anticonvulsants).

No products indexed under this heading.

Fentanyl (The benzodiazepines, including alprazolam, produce additive CNS depressant effects when

co-administered with other drugs which themselves produce CNS depression). Products include:
Duragesic Transdermal System 2448

Fentanyl Citrate (The benzodiazepines, including alprazolam, produce additive CNS depressant effects when co-administered with other drugs which themselves produce CNS depression). Products include:
Actiq 993

Fexofenadine Hydrochloride (The benzodiazepines, including alprazolam, produce additive CNS depressant effects when co-administered with antihistamines). Products include:
Allegra 2857
Allegra-D 12 Hour Extended-Release Tablets............ 2860
Allegra-D 24 Hour Extended-Release Tablets............ 2862

Fluconazole (The initial step in alprazolam metabolism is hydroxylation catalyzed by cytochrome P450 3A (CYP3A). Drugs which inhibit this metabolic pathway may have a profound effect on the clearance of alprazolam).
No products indexed under this heading.

Fluoxetine (Co-administration of fluoxetine with alprazolam increased the maximum plasma concentration of alprazolam by 46%, decreased clearance by 21%, increased half-life by 17%, and decreased measured psychomotor performance).
No products indexed under this heading.

Fluoxetine Hydrochloride (Co-administration of fluoxetine with alprazolam increased the maximum plasma concentration of alprazolam by 46%, decreased clearance by 21%, increased half-life by 17%, and decreased measured psychomotor performance). Products include:
Prozac Pulvules and Liquid 1771
Symbyax Capsules 1788

Fluphenazine Decanoate (The benzodiazepines, including alprazolam, produce additive CNS depressant effects when co-administered with other psychotropic medications. If alprazolam is to be combined with other psychotropic agents, careful consideration should be given to the pharmacology of the agents to be employed, particularly with compounds which might potentiate the action of benzodiazepines).
No products indexed under this heading.

Fluphenazine Enanthate (The benzodiazepines, including alprazolam, produce additive CNS depressant effects when co-administered with other psychotropic medications. If alprazolam is to be combined with other psychotropic agents, careful consideration should be given to the pharmacology of the agents to be employed, particularly with compounds which might potentiate the action of benzodiazepines).
No products indexed under this heading.

Fluphenazine Hydrochloride (The benzodiazepines, including alprazolam, produce additive CNS depressant effects when co-administered with other psychotropic medications. If alprazolam is to be combined with other psychotropic agents, careful consideration should be given to the pharmacology of the agents to be employed, particularly with compounds which might potentiate the action of benzodiazepines).
No products indexed under this heading.

Flurazepam Hydrochloride (The benzodiazepines, including alprazolam, produce additive CNS depressant effects when co-administered with other drugs which themselves produce CNS depression). Products include:
Dalmane Capsules 3343

Fluvoxamine Maleate (The initial step in alprazolam metabolism is hydroxylation catalyzed by cytochrome P450 3A (CYP3A). Drugs which inhibit this metabolic pathway may have a profound effect on the clearance of alprazolam).
No products indexed under this heading.

Fosphenytoin (If alprazolam is to be combined with anticonvulsant drugs, careful consideration should be given to the pharmacology of the agents to be employed, particularly with compounds which might potentiate the action of benzodiazepines. The benzodiazepines, including alprazolam, produce additive CNS depressant effects when co-administered with anticonvulsants).
No products indexed under this heading.

Fosphenytoin Sodium (If alprazolam is to be combined with anticonvulsant drugs, careful consideration should be given to the pharmacology of the agents to be employed, particularly with compounds which might potentiate the action of benzodiazepines. The benzodiazepines, including alprazolam, produce additive CNS depressant effects when co-administered with anticonvulsants).
No products indexed under this heading.

Gabapentin (If alprazolam is to be combined with anticonvulsant drugs, careful consideration should be given to the pharmacology of the agents to be employed, particularly with compounds which might potentiate the action of benzodiazepines. The benzodiazepines, including alprazolam, produce additive CNS depressant effects when co-administered with anticonvulsants). Products include:
Neurontin Capsules 2498
Neurontin Oral Solution 2498
Neurontin Tablets 2498

Glutethimide (The benzodiazepines, including alprazolam, produce additive CNS depressant effects when co-administered with other drugs which themselves produce CNS depression).
No products indexed under this heading.

Haloperidol (The benzodiazepines, including alprazolam, produce additive CNS depressant effects when co-administered with other psychotropic medications. If alprazolam is to be combined with other psychotropic agents, careful consideration should be given to the pharmacology of the agents to be employed, particularly with compounds which might potentiate the action of benzodiazepines).
No products indexed under this heading.

Haloperidol Decanoate (The benzodiazepines, including alprazolam, produce additive CNS depressant effects when co-administered with other psychotropic medications. If alprazolam is to be combined with other psychotropic agents, careful consideration should be given to the pharmacology of the agents to be employed, particularly with compounds which might potentiate the action of benzodiazepines).
No products indexed under this heading.

Hydrocodone Bitartrate (The benzodiazepines, including alprazolam, produce additive CNS depressant effects when co-administered with other drugs which themselves produce CNS depression). Products include:
Hycodan 1104
Hycomine Compound Tablets 1105
Hycotuss Expectorant Syrup 1106
Lortab 3315
Lortab Elixir 3312
Vicodin Tablets 530
Vicodin ES Tablets 531
Vicodin HP Tablets 532
Vicoprofen Tablets 533
Zydone Tablets 1118

Hydrocodone Polistirex (The benzodiazepines, including alprazolam, produce additive CNS depressant effects when co-administered with other drugs which themselves produce CNS depression). Products include:
Tussionex Pennkinetic Extended-Release Suspension...... 3322

Hydromorphone Hydrochloride (The benzodiazepines, including alprazolam, produce additive CNS depressant effects when co-administered with other drugs which themselves produce CNS depression). Products include:
Dilaudid 439
Dilaudid Oral Liquid 443
Dilaudid Non-Sterile Powder 439
Dilaudid Rectal Suppositories 439
Dilaudid Tablets 439
Dilaudid Tablets - 8 mg 443
Dilaudid-HP 441

Hydroxyzine Hydrochloride (The benzodiazepines, including alprazolam, produce additive CNS depressant effects when co-administered with other psychotropic medications. If alprazolam is to be combined with other psychotropic agents, careful consideration should be given to the pharmacology of the agents to be employed, particularly with compounds which might potentiate the action of benzodiazepines).
No products indexed under this heading.

Imipramine Hydrochloride (The steady state plasma concentration of imipramine has been reported to be increased an average of 31% by the concomitant administration of alprazolam in doses up to 4 mg/day. The clinical significance of these changes is unknown).
No products indexed under this heading.

Imipramine Pamoate (The steady state plasma concentration of imipramine has been reported to be increased an average of 31% by the concomitant administration of alprazolam in doses up to 4 mg/day. The clinical significance of these changes is unknown).
No products indexed under this heading.

Indinavir Sulfate (The initial step in alprazolam metabolism is hydroxylation catalyzed by cytochrome P450 3A (CYP3A). Drugs which inhibit this metabolic pathway may have a profound effect on the clearance of alprazolam). Products include:
Crixivan Capsules 1918

Isocarboxazid (The benzodiazepines, including alprazolam, produce additive CNS depressant effects when co-administered with other psychotropic medications. If alprazolam is to be combined with other psychotropic agents, careful consideration should be given to the pharmacology of the agents to be employed, particularly with compounds which might potentiate the action of benzodiazepines).
No products indexed under this heading.

Isoflurane (The benzodiazepines, including alprazolam, produce additive CNS depressant effects when co-administered with other drugs which themselves produce CNS depression).
No products indexed under this heading.

Isoniazid (Available data from clinical studies of benzodiazepines other than alprazolam suggest a possible drug interaction with alprazolam and isoniazid; caution is recommended during co-administration).
No products indexed under this heading.

Itraconazole (Alprazolam is contraindicated with itraconazole since this medication significantly impairs the oxidative metabolism mediated by cytochrome P450 3A (CYP3A)).
No products indexed under this heading.

Ketamine Hydrochloride (The benzodiazepines, including alprazolam, produce additive CNS depressant effects when co-administered with other drugs which themselves produce CNS depression).
No products indexed under this heading.

Ketoconazole (Alprazolam is contraindicated with ketoconazole since this medication significantly impairs the oxidative metabolism mediated by cytochrome P450 3A (CYP3A)). Products include:
Nizoral A-D Shampoo, 1% 1839
Nizoral 2% Shampoo 1838

Lamotrigine (If alprazolam is to be combined with anticonvulsant drugs, careful consideration should be given to the pharmacology of the agents to be employed, particularly with compounds which might potentiate the action of benzodiazepines. The benzodiazepines, including alprazolam, produce additive CNS depressant effects when co-administered with anticonvulsants). Products include:
Lamictal 1449

Lansoprazole (Because Niravam disintegrates in the presence of saliva and the formulation requires an acidic environment to dissolve, concomitant drugs or diseases that raise stomach pH might slow disintegration or dissolution, resulting in slowed or decreased absorption). Products include:
Prevacid Delayed-Release Capsules 3268

Prevacid for Delayed-Release Oral Suspension 3268
Prevacid I.V. for Injection 3274
Prevacid NapraPAC 3277
Prevacid SoluTab Delayed-Release Orally Disintegrating Tablets 3268
PREVPAC 3281

Levetiracetam (If alprazolam is to be combined with anticonvulsant drugs, careful consideration should be given to the pharmacology of the agents to be employed, particularly with compounds which might potentiate the action of benzodiazepines. The benzodiazepines, including alprazolam, produce additive CNS depressant effects when co-administered with anticonvulsants). Products include:
Keppra Oral Solution 3307
Keppra Tablets 3307

Levomethadyl Acetate Hydrochloride (The benzodiazepines, including alprazolam, produce additive CNS depressant effects when co-administered with other drugs which themselves produce CNS depression).
No products indexed under this heading.

Levonorgestrel (Co-administration of oral contraceptives increased the maximum plasma concentration of alprazolam by 18%, decreased clearance by 22%, and increased half-life by 29%). Products include:
Alesse-28 Tablets 3392
Climara Pro Transdermal System 800
Mirena Intrauterine System 810
Plan B Tablets 1068
Seasonale Tablets 1073
Triphasil-28 Tablets 3483

Levorphanol Tartrate (The benzodiazepines, including alprazolam, produce additive CNS depressant effects when co-administered with other drugs which themselves produce CNS depression).
No products indexed under this heading.

Lithium Carbonate (The benzodiazepines, including alprazolam, produce additive CNS depressant effects when co-administered with other psychotropic medications. If alprazolam is to be combined with other psychotropic agents, careful consideration should be given to the pharmacology of the agents to be employed, particularly with compounds which might potentiate the action of benzodiazepines). Products include:
Eskalith 1406
Lithobid Tablets 1670

Lithium Citrate (The benzodiazepines, including alprazolam, produce additive CNS depressant effects when co-administered with other psychotropic medications. If alprazolam is to be combined with other psychotropic agents, careful consideration should be given to the pharmacology of the agents to be employed, particularly with compounds which might potentiate the action of benzodiazepines).
No products indexed under this heading.

Lopinavir (The initial step in alprazolam metabolism is hydroxylation catalyzed by cytochrome P450 3A (CYP3A). Drugs which inhibit this metabolic pathway may have a profound effect on the clearance of alprazolam). Products include:
Kaletra 474

Loratadine (The benzodiazepines, including alprazolam, produce additive CNS depressant effects when co-administered with antihistamines). Products include:
Alavert Allergy & Sinus D-12 Hour Tablets 743
Alavert 743
Children's Claritin 24 Hour Non-Drowsy Allergy Syrup 732
Claritin Non-Drowsy 24 Hour Tablets 731
Non-Drowsy Claritin Hives Relief Tablets 733
Claritin Reditabs 24 Hour Non-Drowsy Tablets 732
Claritin-D Non-Drowsy 12 Hour Tablets 731
Claritin-D Non-Drowsy 24 Hour Tablets 731
Children's Dimetapp ND Non-Drowsy Allergy Syrup 746
Triaminic Allerchews 684

Lorazepam (The benzodiazepines, including alprazolam, produce additive CNS depressant effects when co-administered with other psychotropic medications. If alprazolam is to be combined with other psychotropic agents, careful consideration should be given to the pharmacology of the agents to be employed, particularly with compounds which might potentiate the action of benzodiazepines).
No products indexed under this heading.

Loxapine Hydrochloride (The benzodiazepines, including alprazolam, produce additive CNS depressant effects when co-administered with other psychotropic medications. If alprazolam is to be combined with other psychotropic agents, careful consideration should be given to the pharmacology of the agents to be employed, particularly with compounds which might potentiate the action of benzodiazepines).
No products indexed under this heading.

Loxapine Succinate (The benzodiazepines, including alprazolam, produce additive CNS depressant effects when co-administered with other psychotropic medications. If alprazolam is to be combined with other psychotropic agents, careful consideration should be given to the pharmacology of the agents to be employed, particularly with compounds which might potentiate the action of benzodiazepines).
No products indexed under this heading.

Magaldrate (Because Niravam disintegrates in the presence of saliva and the formulation requires an acidic environment to dissolve, concomitant drugs or diseases that raise stomach pH might slow disintegration or dissolution, resulting in slowed or decreased absorption).
No products indexed under this heading.

Magnesium Hydroxide (Because Niravam disintegrates in the presence of saliva and the formulation requires an acidic environment to dissolve, concomitant drugs or diseases that raise stomach pH might slow disintegration or dissolution, resulting in slowed or decreased absorption). Products include:
Maalox Max Maximum Strength Antacid/Anti-Gas Liquid 2165
Maalox Regular Strength Antacid/Antigas Liquid 2164
Pepcid Complete Chewable Tablets 1672
Rolaids Tablets 707
Extra Strength Rolaids Tablets 707
Rolaids Multi-Symptom Antacid & Antigas Tablets 708

Magnesium Oxide (Because Niravam disintegrates in the presence of saliva and the formulation requires an acidic environment to dissolve, concomitant drugs or diseases that raise stomach pH might slow disintegration or dissolution, resulting in slowed or decreased absorption). Products include:
Beelith Tablets 784
PremCal Light, Regular, and Extra Strength Tablets 762

Maprotiline Hydrochloride (The benzodiazepines, including alprazolam, produce additive CNS depressant effects when co-administered with other psychotropic medications. If alprazolam is to be combined with other psychotropic agents, careful consideration should be given to the pharmacology of the agents to be employed, particularly with compounds which might potentiate the action of benzodiazepines).
No products indexed under this heading.

Meperidine Hydrochloride (The benzodiazepines, including alprazolam, produce additive CNS depressant effects when co-administered with other drugs which themselves produce CNS depression).
No products indexed under this heading.

Mephenytoin (If alprazolam is to be combined with anticonvulsant drugs, careful consideration should be given to the pharmacology of the agents to be employed, particularly with compounds which might potentiate the action of benzodiazepines. The benzodiazepines, including alprazolam, produce additive CNS depressant effects when co-administered with anticonvulsants).
No products indexed under this heading.

Mephobarbital (The benzodiazepines, including alprazolam, produce additive CNS depressant effects when co-administered with other drugs which themselves produce CNS depression). Products include:
Mebaral Tablets, USP 2483

Meprobamate (The benzodiazepines, including alprazolam, produce additive CNS depressant effects when co-administered with other psychotropic medications. If alprazolam is to be combined with other psychotropic agents, careful consideration should be given to the pharmacology of the agents to be employed, particularly with compounds which might potentiate the action of benzodiazepines).
No products indexed under this heading.

Mesoridazine Besylate (The benzodiazepines, including alprazolam, produce additive CNS depressant effects when co-administered with other psychotropic medications. If alprazolam is to be combined with other psychotropic agents, careful consideration should be given to the pharmacology of the agents to be employed, particularly with compounds which might potentiate the action of benzodiazepines).
No products indexed under this heading.

Mestranol (Co-administration of oral contraceptives increased the maximum plasma concentration of alprazolam by 18%, decreased clearance by 22%, and increased half-life by 29%).
No products indexed under this heading.

Methadone Hydrochloride (The benzodiazepines, including alprazolam, produce additive CNS depressant effects when co-administered with other drugs which themselves produce CNS depression).
No products indexed under this heading.

Methdilazine Hydrochloride (The benzodiazepines, including alprazolam, produce additive CNS depressant effects when co-administered with antihistamines).
No products indexed under this heading.

Methohexital Sodium (The benzodiazepines, including alprazolam, produce additive CNS depressant effects when co-administered with other drugs which themselves produce CNS depression).
No products indexed under this heading.

Methotrimeprazine (The benzodiazepines, including alprazolam, produce additive CNS depressant effects when co-administered with other drugs which themselves produce CNS depression).
No products indexed under this heading.

Methoxyflurane (The benzodiazepines, including alprazolam, produce additive CNS depressant effects when co-administered with other drugs which themselves produce CNS depression).
No products indexed under this heading.

Methsuximide (If alprazolam is to be combined with anticonvulsant drugs, careful consideration should be given to the pharmacology of the agents to be employed, particularly with compounds which might potentiate the action of benzodiazepines. The benzodiazepines, including alprazolam, produce additive CNS depressant effects when co-administered with anticonvulsants).
No products indexed under this heading.

Metronidazole (The initial step in alprazolam metabolism is hydroxylation catalyzed by cytochrome P450 3A (CYP3A). Drugs which inhibit this metabolic pathway may have a profound effect on the clearance of alprazolam). Products include:
Metrogel 1% 1212
MetroGel-Vaginal Gel 1822
Noritate Cream, 1% 1051

Metronidazole Benzoate (The initial step in alprazolam metabolism is hydroxylation catalyzed by cytochrome P450 3A (CYP3A). Drugs which inhibit this metabolic pathway may have a profound effect on the clearance of alprazolam).
No products indexed under this heading.

Metronidazole Hydrochloride (The initial step in alprazolam metabolism is hydroxylation catalyzed by cytochrome P450 3A (CYP3A). Drugs which inhibit this metabolic pathway may have a profound effect on the clearance of alprazolam).
No products indexed under this heading.

Miconazole (The initial step in alprazolam metabolism is hydroxylation catalyzed by cytochrome P450 3A (CYP3A). Drugs which inhibit this metabolic pathway may have a profound effect on the clearance of alprazolam).
No products indexed under this heading.

Midazolam Hydrochloride (The benzodiazepines, including alprazolam, produce additive CNS depressant effects when co-administered with other psychotropic medications. If alprazolam is to be combined with other psychotropic agents, careful consideration should be given to the pharmacology of the agents to be employed, particularly with compounds which might potentiate the action of benzodiazepines).
No products indexed under this heading.

Molindone Hydrochloride (The benzodiazepines, including alprazolam, produce additive CNS depressant effects when co-administered with other psychotropic medications. If alprazolam is to be combined with other psychotropic agents, careful consideration should be given to the pharmacology of the agents to be employed, particularly with compounds which might potentiate the action of benzodiazepines). Products include:
Moban Tablets 1108

Morphine Sulfate (The benzodiazepines, including alprazolam, produce additive CNS depressant effects when co-administered with other drugs which themselves produce CNS depression). Products include:
Avinza Capsules 1714
Kadian Capsules 572
MS Contin Tablets 2703

Nefazodone Hydrochloride (The initial step in alprazolam metabolism is hydroxylation catalyzed by cytochrome P450 3A (CYP3A). Drugs which inhibit this metabolic pathway may have a profound effect on the clearance of alprazolam).
No products indexed under this heading.

Nelfinavir Mesylate (The initial step in alprazolam metabolism is hydroxylation catalyzed by cytochrome P450 3A (CYP3A). Drugs which inhibit this metabolic pathway may have a profound effect on the clearance of alprazolam). Products include:
Viracept 2556

Nicardipine (Data from in vitro studies of benzodiazepines, other than alprazolam, suggest a possible drug interaction with nicardipine; caution is recommended during co-administration).
No products indexed under this heading.

Nicardipine Hydrochloride (Data from in vitro studies of benzodiazepines, other than alprazolam, suggest a possible drug interaction with nicardipine; caution is recommended during co-administration). Products include:
Cardene I.V. 1129

Nifedipine (Data from in vitro studies of benzodiazepines, other than alprazolam, suggest a possible drug interaction with nifedipine; caution is recommended during co-administration). Products include:
Adalat CC Tablets 2978

Nizatidine (Because Niravam disintegrates in the presence of saliva and the formulation requires an acidic environment to dissolve, concomitant drugs or diseases that raise stomach pH might slow disintegration or dissolution, resulting in slowed or decreased absorption). Products include:
Axid Oral Solution 913

Norethindrone (Co-administration of oral contraceptives increased the maximum plasma concentration of alprazolam by 18%, decreased clearance by 22%, and increased half-life by 29%). Products include:
Ortho Micronor Tablets 2411

Norethynodrel (Co-administration of oral contraceptives increased the maximum plasma concentration of alprazolam by 18%, decreased clearance by 22%, and increased half-life by 29%).
No products indexed under this heading.

Norfloxacin (The initial step in alprazolam metabolism is hydroxylation catalyzed by cytochrome P450 3A (CYP3A). Drugs which inhibit this metabolic pathway may have a profound effect on the clearance of alprazolam). Products include:
Noroxin Tablets 2009

Norgestimate (Co-administration of oral contraceptives increased the maximum plasma concentration of alprazolam by 18%, decreased clearance by 22%, and increased half-life by 29%). Products include:
Ortho-Cyclen/Ortho Tri-Cyclen 2414
Ortho Tri-Cyclen Lo Tablets 2421
Prefest Tablets 1069

Norgestrel (Co-administration of oral contraceptives increased the maximum plasma concentration of alprazolam by 18%, decreased clearance by 22%, and increased half-life by 29%). Products include:
Lo/Ovral-28 Tablets 3423

Nortriptyline Hydrochloride (The benzodiazepines, including alprazolam, produce additive CNS depressant effects when co-administered with other psychotropic medications. If alprazolam is to be combined with other psychotropic agents, careful consideration should be given to the pharmacology of the agents to be employed, particularly with compounds which might potentiate the action of benzodiazepines).
No products indexed under this heading.

Olanzapine (The benzodiazepines, including alprazolam, produce additive CNS depressant effects when co-administered with other psychotropic medications. If alprazolam is to be combined with other psychotropic agents, careful consideration should be given to the pharmacology of the agents to be employed, particularly with compounds which might potentiate the action of benzodiazepines). Products include:
Symbyax Capsules 1788
Zyprexa Tablets 1798
Zyprexa IntraMuscular 1798
Zyprexa ZYDIS Orally Disintegrating Tablets 1798

Omeprazole (Because Niravam disintegrates in the presence of saliva and the formulation requires an acidic environment to dissolve, concomitant drugs or diseases that raise stomach pH might slow disintegration or dissolution, resulting in slowed or decreased absorption). Products include:
Zegerid Powder for Oral Solution 2972

Oxazepam (The benzodiazepines, including alprazolam, produce additive CNS depressant effects when co-administered with other psychotropic medications. If alprazolam is to be combined with other psychotropic agents, careful consideration should be given to the pharmacology of the agents to be employed, particularly with compounds which might potentiate the action of benzodiazepines).
No products indexed under this heading.

Oxcarbazepine (If alprazolam is to be combined with anticonvulsant drugs, careful consideration should be given to the pharmacology of the agents to be employed, particularly with compounds which might potentiate the action of benzodiazepines. The benzodiazepines, including alprazolam, produce additive CNS depressant effects when co-administered with anticonvulsants). Products include:
Trileptal Oral Suspension 2281
Trileptal Tablets 2281

Oxycodone Hydrochloride (The benzodiazepines, including alprazolam, produce additive CNS depressant effects when co-administered with other drugs which themselves produce CNS depression). Products include:
Combunox Tablets 1183
OxyContin Tablets 2699
OxyFast Oral Concentrate Solution 2704
OxyIR Capsules 2704
Percocet Tablets 1114
Percodan Tablets 1115

Pantoprazole Sodium (Because Niravam disintegrates in the presence of saliva and the formulation requires an acidic environment to dissolve, concomitant drugs or diseases that raise stomach pH might slow disintegration or dissolution, resulting in slowed or decreased absorption). Products include:
Protonix I.V. 3468
Protonix Tablets 3465

Paramethadione (If alprazolam is to be combined with anticonvulsant drugs, careful consideration should be given to the pharmacology of the agents to be employed, particularly with compounds which might potentiate the action of benzodiazepines. The benzodiazepines, including alprazolam, produce additive CNS depressant effects when co-administered with anticonvulsants).
No products indexed under this heading.

Paroxetine Hydrochloride (Data from in vitro studies of alprazolam suggest a possible drug interaction with alprazolam and sertraline. However, data from an in vivo drug interaction study involving a single dose of alprazolam 1 mg and steady state doses of sertraline (50 to 150 mg/day) did not reveal any clinically significant changes in the pharmacokinetics of alprazolam; caution is recommended during co-administration). Products include:
Paxil CR Controlled-Release Tablets 1509
Paxil 1501

Paroxetine Mesylate (Data from in vitro studies of alprazolam suggest a possible drug interaction with alprazolam and sertraline. However, data from an in vivo drug interaction study involving a single dose of alprazolam 1 mg and steady state doses of sertraline (50 to 150 mg/day) did not reveal any clinically significant changes in the pharmacokinetics of alprazolam; caution is recommended during co-administration).
No products indexed under this heading.

Pentobarbital Sodium (The benzodiazepines, including alprazolam, produce additive CNS depressant effects when co-administered with other drugs which themselves produce CNS depression). Products include:
Nembutal Sodium Solution, USP 2484

Perphenazine (The benzodiazepines, including alprazolam, produce additive CNS depressant effects when co-administered with other psychotropic medications. If alprazolam is to be combined with other psychotropic agents, careful consideration should be given to the pharmacology of the agents to be employed, particularly with compounds which might potentiate the action of benzodiazepines).
No products indexed under this heading.

Phenacemide (If alprazolam is to be combined with anticonvulsant drugs, careful consideration should be given to the pharmacology of the agents to be employed, particularly with compounds which might potentiate the action of benzodiazepines. The benzodiazepines, including alprazolam, produce additive CNS depressant effects when co-administered with anticonvulsants).
No products indexed under this heading.

Phenelzine Sulfate (The benzodiazepines, including alprazolam, produce additive CNS depressant effects when co-administered with other psychotropic medications. If alprazolam is to be combined with other psychotropic agents, careful consideration should be given to the pharmacology of the agents to be employed, particularly with compounds which might potentiate the action of benzodiazepines).
No products indexed under this heading.

Phenobarbital (If alprazolam is to be combined with anticonvulsant drugs, careful consideration should be given to the pharmacology of the agents to be employed, particularly with compounds which might potentiate the action of benzodiazepines. The benzodiazepines, including alprazolam, produce additive CNS depressant effects when co-administered with anticonvulsants).
No products indexed under this heading.

Phensuximide (If alprazolam is to be combined with anticonvulsant drugs, careful consideration should be given to the pharmacology of the agents to be employed, particularly with compounds which might potentiate the action of benzodiazepines. The benzodiazepines, including alprazolam, produce additive CNS depressant effects when co-administered with anticonvulsants).
No products indexed under this heading.

Phenytoin (If alprazolam is to be combined with anticonvulsant drugs, careful consideration should be given to the pharmacology of the agents to be employed, particularly with compounds which might potentiate the action of benzodiazepines. The benzodiazepines, including alprazolam, produce additive CNS depressant effects when co-administered with anticonvulsants).
No products indexed under this heading.

Phenytoin Sodium (If alprazolam is to be combined with anticonvulsant drugs, careful consideration should be given to the pharmacology of the agents to be employed, particularly with compounds which might potentiate the action of benzodiazepines. The benzodiazepines, including alprazolam, produce additive CNS depressant effects when co-administered with anticonvulsants). Products include:
Phenytek Capsules 2153

Prazepam (The benzodiazepines, including alprazolam, produce additive CNS depressant effects when co-administered with other psychotropic medications. If alprazolam is to be combined with other psychotropic agents, careful consideration should be given to the pharmacology of the agents to be employed, particularly with compounds which might potentiate the action of benzodiazepines).
No products indexed under this heading.

Primidone (If alprazolam is to be combined with anticonvulsant drugs, careful consideration should be given to the pharmacology of the agents to be employed, particularly with compounds which might potentiate the action of benzodiazepines. The benzodiazepines, including alprazolam, produce additive CNS depressant effects when co-administered with anticonvulsants).
No products indexed under this heading.

Prochlorperazine (The benzodiazepines, including alprazolam, produce additive CNS depressant effects when co-administered with other psychotropic medications. If alprazolam is to be combined with other psychotropic agents, careful consideration should be given to the pharmacology of the agents to be employed, particularly with compounds which might potentiate the action of benzodiazepines).
No products indexed under this heading.

Promethazine Hydrochloride (The benzodiazepines, including alprazolam, produce additive CNS depressant effects when co-administered with other psychotropic medications. If alprazolam is to be combined with other psychotropic agents, careful consideration should be given to the pharmacology of the agents to be employed, particularly with compounds which might potentiate the action of benzodiazepines). Products include:
Phenergan 3438

Propofol (The benzodiazepines, including alprazolam, produce additive CNS depressant effects when co-administered with other drugs which themselves produce CNS depression). Products include:
Diprivan Injectable Emulsion 676

Propoxyphene Hydrochloride (Co-administration of propoxyphene decreased the maximum plasma concentration of alprazolam by 6%, decreased clearance by 38%, and increased half-life by 58%).
No products indexed under this heading.

Propoxyphene Napsylate (Co-administration of propoxyphene decreased the maximum plasma concentration of alprazolam by 6%, decreased clearance by 38%, and increased half-life by 58%). Products include:
Darvocet A 500 Tablets 3497

Protriptyline Hydrochloride (The benzodiazepines, including alprazolam, produce additive CNS depressant effects when co-administered with other psychotropic medications. If alprazolam is to be combined with other psychotropic agents, careful consideration should be given to the pharmacology of the agents to be employed, particularly with compounds which might potentiate the action of benzodiazepines). Products include:
Vivactil Tablets 2350

Pyrilamine Maleate (The benzodiazepines, including alprazolam, produce additive CNS depressant effects when co-administered with antihistamines).
No products indexed under this heading.

Pyrilamine Tannate (The benzodiazepines, including alprazolam, produce additive CNS depressant effects when co-administered with antihistamines).
No products indexed under this heading.

Quazepam (The benzodiazepines, including alprazolam, produce additive CNS depressant effects when co-administered with other drugs which themselves produce CNS depression).
No products indexed under this heading.

Quetiapine Fumarate (The benzodiazepines, including alprazolam, produce additive CNS depressant effects when co-administered with other psychotropic medications. If alprazolam is to be combined with other psychotropic agents, careful consideration should be given to the pharmacology of the agents to be employed, particularly with compounds which might potentiate the action of benzodiazepines). Products include:
Seroquel Tablets 691

Quinine (The initial step in alprazolam metabolism is hydroxylation catalyzed by cytochrome P450 3A (CYP3A). Drugs which inhibit this metabolic pathway may have a profound effect on the clearance of alprazolam).
No products indexed under this heading.

Quinine Sulfate (The initial step in alprazolam metabolism is hydroxylation catalyzed by cytochrome P450 3A (CYP3A). Drugs which inhibit this metabolic pathway may have a profound effect on the clearance of alprazolam).
No products indexed under this heading.

Rabeprazole Sodium (Because Niravam disintegrates in the presence of saliva and the formulation requires an acidic environment to dissolve, concomitant drugs or diseases that raise stomach pH might slow disintegration or dissolution, resulting in slowed or decreased absorption). Products include:
Aciphex Tablets 1081

Ranitidine Bismuth Citrate (Because Niravam disintegrates in the presence of saliva and the formulation requires an acidic environment to dissolve, concomitant drugs or diseases that raise stomach pH might slow disintegration or dissolution, resulting in slowed or decreased absorption).
No products indexed under this heading.

Ranitidine Hydrochloride (Because Niravam disintegrates in the presence of saliva and the formulation requires an acidic environment to dissolve, concomitant drugs or diseases that raise stomach pH might slow disintegration or dissolution, resulting in slowed or decreased absorption). Products include:
Zantac 1597
Zantac Injection 1593
Zantac 75 Tablets .... ▣715
Zantac 150 Maximum Strength Tablets .... ▣715
Zantac Injection Pharmacy Bulk Package 1595

Remifentanil Hydrochloride (The benzodiazepines, including alprazolam, produce additive CNS depressant effects when co-administered with other drugs which themselves produce CNS depression).
No products indexed under this heading.

Risperidone (The benzodiazepines, including alprazolam, produce additive CNS depressant effects when co-administered with other psychotropic medications. If alprazolam is to be combined with other psychotropic agents, careful consideration should be given to the pharmacology of the agents to be employed, particularly with compounds which might potentiate the action of benzodiazepines). Products include:
Risperdal Consta Long-Acting Injection 1664
Risperdal M-Tab Orally Disintegrating Tablets 1658
Risperdal 1658

Ritonavir (The initial step in alprazolam metabolism is hydroxylation catalyzed by cytochrome P450 3A (CYP3A). Drugs which inhibit this metabolic pathway may have a profound effect on the clearance of alprazolam). Products include:
Kaletra 474
Norvir 499

Saquinavir (The initial step in alprazolam metabolism is hydroxylation catalyzed by cytochrome P450 3A (CYP3A). Drugs which inhibit this metabolic pathway may have a profound effect on the clearance of alprazolam).
No products indexed under this heading.

Saquinavir Mesylate (The initial step in alprazolam metabolism is hydroxylation catalyzed by cytochrome P450 3A (CYP3A). Drugs which inhibit this metabolic pathway may have a profound effect on the clearance of alprazolam). Products include:
Invirase 2776

Secobarbital Sodium (The benzodiazepines, including alprazolam, produce additive CNS depressant effects when co-administered with other drugs which themselves produce CNS depression).
No products indexed under this heading.

Sertraline Hydrochloride (Data from in vitro studies of alprazolam suggest a possible drug interaction with alprazolam and sertraline. However, data from an in vivo drug interaction study involving a single dose of alprazolam 1 mg and steady state doses of sertraline (50 to 150 mg/day) did not reveal any clinically significant changes in the pharmacokinetics of alprazolam; caution is recommended during co-administration). Products include:
Zoloft 2581

Sevoflurane (The benzodiazepines, including alprazolam, produce additive CNS depressant effects when co-administered with other drugs which themselves produce CNS depression). Products include:
Ultane Liquid for Inhalation 526

Sodium Bicarbonate (Because Niravam disintegrates in the presence of saliva and the formulation requires an acidic environment to dissolve, concomitant drugs or diseases that raise stomach pH might slow disintegration or dissolution, resulting in slowed or decreased absorption). Products include:
Ceo-Two Evacuant Suppository ...... ▣607
Colyte with Flavor Packs for Oral Solution 3102
HalfLytely and Bisacodyl Tablets Bowel Prep Kit with Flavors Packs 915
TriLyte with Flavor Packs for Oral Solution 3114

Sodium Oxybate (The benzodiazepines, including alprazolam, produce additive CNS depressant effects when co-administered with other drugs which themselves produce CNS depression).
No products indexed under this heading.

Sufentanil Citrate (The benzodiazepines, including alprazolam, produce additive CNS depressant effects when co-administered with other drugs which themselves produce CNS depression).
No products indexed under this heading.

Temazepam (The benzodiazepines, including alprazolam, produce additive CNS depressant effects when co-administered with other drugs which themselves produce CNS depression).
No products indexed under this heading.

Terfenadine (The benzodiazepines, including alprazolam, produce additive CNS depressant effects when co-administered with antihistamines).
No products indexed under this heading.

Thiamylal Sodium (The benzodiazepines, including alprazolam, produce additive CNS depressant effects when co-administered with other drugs which themselves produce CNS depression).
No products indexed under this heading.

Thioridazine Hydrochloride (The benzodiazepines, including alprazolam, produce additive CNS depressant effects when co-administered with other psychotropic medications. If alprazolam is to be combined with other psychotropic agents, careful consideration should be given to the pharmacology of the agents to be employed, particularly with compounds which might potentiate the action of benzodiazepines). Products include:
Thioridazine Hydrochloride Tablets 2122

Thiothixene (The benzodiazepines, including alprazolam, produce additive CNS depressant effects when co-administered with other psychotropic medications. If alprazolam is to be combined with other psychotropic agents, careful consideration should be given to the pharmacology of the agents to be employed, particularly with compounds which might potentiate the action of benzodiazepines). Products include:
Thiothixene Capsules 2124

Tiagabine Hydrochloride (If alprazolam is to be combined with anticonvulsant drugs, careful consideration should be given to the pharmacology of the agents to be employed, particularly with compounds which might potentiate the action of benzodiazepines. The benzodiazepines, including alprazolam, produce additive CNS depressant effects when co-administered with anticonvulsants). Products include:
Gabitril Tablets 998

Topiramate (If alprazolam is to be combined with anticonvulsant drugs, careful consideration should be given to the pharmacology of the agents to be employed, particularly with compounds which might potentiate the action of benzodiazepines. The benzodiazepines, including alprazolam, produce additive CNS depressant effects when co-administered with anticonvulsants). Products include:
Topamax Sprinkle Capsules 2438
Topamax Tablets 2438

Tranylcypromine Sulfate (The benzodiazepines, including alprazolam, produce additive CNS depressant effects when co-administered with other psychotropic medications. If alprazolam is to be combined with other psychotropic agents, careful consideration should be given to the pharmacology of the agents to be employed, particularly with compounds which might potentiate the action of benzodiazepines). Products include:
Parnate Tablets 1499

Triazolam (The benzodiazepines, including alprazolam, produce additive CNS depressant effects when co-administered with other drugs which themselves produce CNS depression).
No products indexed under this heading.

Trifluoperazine Hydrochloride (The benzodiazepines, including alprazolam, produce additive CNS depressant effects when co-administered with other psychotropic medications. If alprazolam is to be combined with other psychotropic agents, careful consideration should be given to the pharmacology of the agents to be employed, particularly with compounds which might potentiate the action of benzodiazepines).
No products indexed under this heading.

Trimeprazine Tartrate (The benzodiazepines, including alprazolam, produce additive CNS depressant effects when co-administered with antihistamines).
No products indexed under this heading.

Trimethadione (If alprazolam is to be combined with anticonvulsant drugs, careful consideration should be given to the pharmacology of the agents to be employed, particularly with compounds which might potentiate the action of benzodiazepines. The benzodiazepines, including alprazolam, produce additive CNS depressant effects when co-administered with anticonvulsants).
No products indexed under this heading.

Trimipramine Maleate (The benzodiazepines, including alprazolam, produce additive CNS depressant effects when co-administered with other psychotropic medications. If alprazolam is to be combined with other psychotropic agents, careful consideration should be given to the pharmacology of the agents to be employed, particularly with compounds which might potentiate the action of benzodiazepines). Products include:
Surmontil Capsules 2347

Tripelennamine Hydrochloride (The benzodiazepines, including alprazolam, produce additive CNS depressant effects when co-administered with antihistamines).
No products indexed under this heading.

Triprolidine Hydrochloride (The benzodiazepines, including alprazolam, produce additive CNS depressant effects when co-administered with antihistamines).
No products indexed under this heading.

Troleandomycin (The initial step in alprazolam metabolism is hydroxylation catalyzed by cytochrome P450 3A (CYP3A). Drugs which inhibit this metabolic pathway may have a profound effect on the clearance of alprazolam).
No products indexed under this heading.

Valproate Sodium (If alprazolam is to be combined with anticonvulsant drugs, careful consideration should be given to the pharmacology of the agents to be employed, particularly with compounds which might potentiate the action of benzodiazepines. The benzodiazepines, including alprazolam, produce additive CNS depressant effects when co-administered with anticonvulsants). Products include:
Depacon Injection 412

Valproic Acid (If alprazolam is to be combined with anticonvulsant drugs, careful consideration should be given to the pharmacology of the agents to be employed, particularly with compounds which might potentiate the action of benzodiazepines. The benzodiazepines, including alprazolam, produce additive CNS depressant effects when co-administered with anticonvulsants). Products include:
Depakene 417

Venlafaxine Hydrochloride (The initial step in alprazolam metabolism is hydroxylation catalyzed by cytochrome P450 3A (CYP3A). Drugs which inhibit this metabolic pathway may have a profound effect on the clearance of alprazolam). Products include:
Effexor Tablets 3405
Effexor XR Capsules 3411

Verapamil Hydrochloride (The initial step in alprazolam metabolism is hydroxylation catalyzed by cytochrome P450 3A (CYP3A). Drugs which inhibit this metabolic pathway may have a profound effect on the clearance of alprazolam). Products include:
Covera-HS Tablets 3135
Tarka Tablets 519
Verelan PM Capsules 3120

Voriconazole (The initial step in alprazolam metabolism is hydroxylation catalyzed by cytochrome P450 3A (CYP3A). Drugs which inhibit this metabolic pathway may have a profound effect on the clearance of alprazolam). Products include:
VFEND I.V. 2543
VFEND Oral Suspension 2543
VFEND Tablets 2543

Zafirlukast (The initial step in alprazolam metabolism is hydroxylation catalyzed by cytochrome P450 3A (CYP3A). Drugs which inhibit this metabolic pathway may have a profound effect on the clearance of alprazolam). Products include:
Accolate Tablets 663

Zaleplon (The benzodiazepines, including alprazolam, produce additive CNS depressant effects when co-administered with other drugs which themselves produce CNS depression). Products include:
Sonata Capsules 1686

Zileuton (The initial step in alprazolam metabolism is hydroxylation catalyzed by cytochrome P450 3A (CYP3A). Drugs which inhibit this metabolic pathway may have a profound effect on the clearance of alprazolam).
No products indexed under this heading.

Ziprasidone Hydrochloride (The benzodiazepines, including alprazolam, produce additive CNS depressant effects when co-administered with other psychotropic medications. If alprazolam is to be combined with other psychotropic agents, careful consideration should be given to the pharmacology of the agents to be employed, particularly with compounds which might potentiate the action of benzodiazepines). Products include:
Geodon Capsules 2514

Zolpidem Tartrate (The benzodiazepines, including alprazolam, produce additive CNS depressant effects when co-administered with other drugs which themselves produce CNS depression). Products include:
Ambien Tablets 2867

Zonisamide (If alprazolam is to be combined with anticonvulsant drugs, careful consideration should be given to the pharmacology of the agents to be employed, particularly with compounds which might potentiate the action of benzodiazepines. The benzodiazepines, including alprazolam, produce additive CNS depressant effects when co-administered with anticonvulsants). Products include:
Zonegran Capsules 1089

Food Interactions

Grapefruit (Available data from clinical studies of benzodiazepines, other than alprazolam, suggest a possible drug interaction with alprazolam and grapefruit juice; caution is recommended during co-administration).

Grapefruit Juice (Available data from clinical studies of benzodiazepines, other than alprazolam, suggest a possible drug interaction with alprazolam and grapefruit juice; caution is recommended during co-administration).

NITRO-DUR TRANSDERMAL INFUSION SYSTEM

(Nitroglycerin) 3060
May interact with calcium channel blockers, vasodilators, and certain other agents. Compounds in these categories include:

Amlodipine Besylate (Vasodilating effects of nitroglycerin may be additive with those of other vasodilators). Products include:
Caduet Tablets 2507
Lotrel Capsules 2238
Norvasc Tablets 2529

Amyl Nitrite (Vasodilating effects of nitroglycerin may be additive with those of other vasodilators).
No products indexed under this heading.

Bepridil Hydrochloride (Vasodilating effects of nitroglycerin may be additive with those of other vasodilators).
No products indexed under this heading.

Diazoxide (Vasodilating effects of nitroglycerin may be additive with those of other vasodilators). Products include:
Hyperstat I.V. Injection 3031

Diltiazem Hydrochloride (Vasodilating effects of nitroglycerin may be additive with those of other vasodilators). Products include:
Cardizem LA Extended Release Tablets 1699
Tiazac Capsules 1204

Epoprostenol Sodium (Vasodilating effects of nitroglycerin may be additive with those of other vasodilators). Products include:
Flolan for Injection 1408

Ethaverine Hydrochloride (Vasodilating effects of nitroglycerin may be additive with those of other vasodilators).
No products indexed under this heading.

Felodipine (Vasodilating effects of nitroglycerin may be additive with those of other vasodilators).
Products include:
Plendil Extended-Release Tablets 651

Hydralazine Hydrochloride (Vasodilating effects of nitroglycerin may be additive with those of other vasodilators). Products include:
BiDil Tablets 2161

Isosorbide Dinitrate (Vasodilating effects of nitroglycerin may be additive with those of other vasodilators).
Products include:
BiDil Tablets 2161

Isosorbide Mononitrate (Vasodilating effects of nitroglycerin may be additive with those of other vasodilators). Products include:
Imdur Tablets 3032

Isoxsuprine Hydrochloride (Vasodilating effects of nitroglycerin may be additive with those of other vasodilators).
No products indexed under this heading.

Isradipine (Vasodilating effects of nitroglycerin may be additive with those of other vasodilators).
Products include:
DynaCirc CR Tablets 2726

Mibefradil Dihydrochloride (Vasodilating effects of nitroglycerin may be additive with those of other vasodilators).
No products indexed under this heading.

Minoxidil (Vasodilating effects of nitroglycerin may be additive with those of other vasodilators).
Products include:
Men's Rogaine Extra Strength Topical Solution, Ocean Rush Scent and Original Unscented..... 706
Women's Rogaine Topical Solution, Spring Bloom Scent and Original Unscented.............. 707

Nicardipine Hydrochloride (Vasodilating effects of nitroglycerin may be additive with those of other vasodilators). Products include:
Cardene I.V. 1129

Nifedipine (Vasodilating effects of nitroglycerin may be additive with those of other vasodilators).
Products include:
Adalat CC Tablets 2978

Nimodipine (Vasodilating effects of nitroglycerin may be additive with those of other vasodilators).
Products include:
Nimotop Capsules 774

Nisoldipine (Vasodilating effects of nitroglycerin may be additive with those of other vasodilators).
Products include:
Sular Tablets 1163

Nitroglycerin, long-acting formulations (Vasodilating effects of nitroglycerin may be additive with those of other vasodilators).
No products indexed under this heading.

Nitroglycerin Intravenous (Vasodilating effects of nitroglycerin may be additive with those of other vasodilators).
No products indexed under this heading.

Papaverine (Vasodilating effects of nitroglycerin may be additive with those of other vasodilators).
No products indexed under this heading.

Papaverine Hydrochloride (Vasodilating effects of nitroglycerin may be additive with those of other vasodilators).
No products indexed under this heading.

Sildenafil Citrate (Amplification of the vasodilatory effects of the nitroglycerin patch by sildenafil can result in severe hypotension). Products include:
Revatio Tablets 2541
Viagra Tablets 2552

Tolazoline Hydrochloride (Vasodilating effects of nitroglycerin may be additive with those of other vasodilators).
No products indexed under this heading.

Verapamil Hydrochloride (Vasodilating effects of nitroglycerin may be additive with those of other vasodilators). Products include:
Covera-HS Tablets 3135
Tarka Tablets 519
Verelan PM Capsules 3120

Food Interactions

Alcohol (Enhances sensitivity to the hypotensive effects).

NITROLINGUAL PUMPSPRAY

(Nitroglycerin) 1161
May interact with calcium channel blockers and certain other agents. Compounds in these categories include:

Amlodipine Besylate (Marked symptomatic orthostatic hypotension). Products include:
Caduet Tablets 2507
Lotrel Capsules 2238
Norvasc Tablets 2529

Bepridil Hydrochloride (Marked symptomatic orthostatic hypotension).
No products indexed under this heading.

Diltiazem Hydrochloride (Marked symptomatic orthostatic hypotension). Products include:
Cardizem LA Extended Release Tablets 1699
Tiazac Capsules 1204

Drugs Depending On Vascular Smooth Muscle (Decreased or increased effect).
No products indexed under this heading.

Felodipine (Marked symptomatic orthostatic hypotension). Products include:
Plendil Extended-Release Tablets 651

Isradipine (Marked symptomatic orthostatic hypotension). Products include:
DynaCirc CR Tablets 2726

Mibefradil Dihydrochloride (Marked symptomatic orthostatic hypotension).
No products indexed under this heading.

Nicardipine Hydrochloride (Marked symptomatic orthostatic hypotension). Products include:
Cardene I.V. 1129

Nifedipine (Marked symptomatic orthostatic hypotension). Products include:
Adalat CC Tablets 2978

Nimodipine (Marked symptomatic orthostatic hypotension). Products include:
Nimotop Capsules 774

Nisoldipine (Marked symptomatic orthostatic hypotension). Products include:
Sular Tablets 1163

Sildenafil Citrate (Concomitant administration with phosphodiesterase inhibitors can cause severe hypotension. The time, course and dose dependency of this interaction are not known. Concurrent use is contraindicated). Products include:
Revatio Tablets 2541
Viagra Tablets 2552

Tadalafil (Concomitant administration with phosphodiesterase inhibitors can cause severe hypotension. The time, course and dose dependency of this interaction are not known. Concurrent use is contraindicated). Products include:
Cialis Tablets 1806

Vardenafil Hydrochloride (Concomitant administration with phosphodiesterase inhibitors can cause severe hypotension. The time, course and dose dependency of this interaction are not known. Concurrent use is contraindicated).
Products include:
Levitra Tablets 3048

Verapamil Hydrochloride (Marked symptomatic orthostatic hypotension). Products include:
Covera-HS Tablets 3135
Tarka Tablets 519
Verelan PM Capsules 3120

Food Interactions

Alcohol (Enhanced sensitivity to hypotensive effects).

NIZORAL A-D SHAMPOO, 1%

(Ketoconazole) 1839
None cited in PDR database.

NIZORAL 2% SHAMPOO

(Ketoconazole) 1838
None cited in PDR database.

NONI PLUS PLUS LIQUID

(Multivitamins with Minerals) 759
None cited in PDR database.

NORDITROPIN CARTRIDGES

(Somatropin) 2318
May interact with corticosteroids, cytochrome p450 3a4 substrates (selected), oral hypoglycemic agents, and insulin. Compounds in these categories include:

Acarbose (In patients with diabetes mellitus requiring drug therapy, the dose of insulin and/or oral agents may require adjustment when somatropin therapy is initiated). Products include:
Precose Tablets 776

Alfentanil Hydrochloride (Data indicates that growth hormone may be an inducer of cytochrome p450 3A4. When growth hormone is administered in combination with drugs known to be metabolized by cytochrome P450 3A4 hepatic enzymes, it is advisable to monitor the clinical effectiveness of such drugs).
No products indexed under this heading.

Alprazolam (Data indicates that growth hormone may be an inducer of cytochrome p450 3A4. When growth hormone is administered in combination with drugs known to be metabolized by cytochrome P450 3A4 hepatic enzymes, it is advisable to monitor the clinical effectiveness of such drugs). Products include:
Niravam Orally Disintegrating Tablets 3106
Xanax XR Tablets 2655

Amitriptyline Hydrochloride (Data indicates that growth hormone may be an inducer of cytochrome p450 3A4. When growth hormone is administered in combination with drugs known to be metabolized by cytochrome P450 3A4 hepatic enzymes, it is advisable to monitor the clinical effectiveness of such drugs).
No products indexed under this heading.

Amlodipine Besylate (Data indicates that growth hormone may be an inducer of cytochrome p450 3A4. When growth hormone is administered in combination with drugs known to be metabolized by cytochrome P450 3A4 hepatic enzymes, it is advisable to monitor the clinical effectiveness of such drugs). Products include:
Caduet Tablets 2507
Lotrel Capsules 2238
Norvasc Tablets 2529

Aprepitant (Data indicates that growth hormone may be an inducer of cytochrome p450 3A4. When growth hormone is administered in combination with drugs known to be metabolized by cytochrome P450 3A4 hepatic enzymes, it is advisable to monitor the clinical effectiveness of such drugs). Products include:
Emend Capsules 1944

Astemizole (Data indicates that growth hormone may be an inducer of cytochrome p450 3A4. When growth hormone is administered in combination with drugs known to be metabolized by cytochrome P450 3A4 hepatic enzymes, it is advisable to monitor the clinical effectiveness of such drugs).
No products indexed under this heading.

Atorvastatin Calcium (Data indicates that growth hormone may be an inducer of cytochrome p450 3A4. When growth hormone is administered in combination with drugs known to be metabolized by cytochrome P450 3A4 hepatic enzymes, it is advisable to monitor the clinical effectiveness of such drugs). Products include:
Caduet Tablets 2507
Lipitor Tablets 2495

Belladonna Ergotamine (Data indicates that growth hormone may be an inducer of cytochrome p450 3A4. When growth hormone is administered in combination with drugs known to be metabolized by cytochrome P450 3A4 hepatic enzymes, it is advisable to monitor the clinical effectiveness of such drugs).
No products indexed under this heading.

Betamethasone Acetate (Concomitant glucocorticoid therapy may inhibit the growth promoting effect of somatropin).
No products indexed under this heading.

Betamethasone Sodium Phosphate (Concomitant glucocorticoid therapy may inhibit the growth promoting effect of somatropin).
No products indexed under this heading.

Buspirone Hydrochloride (Data indicates that growth hormone may be an inducer of cytochrome p450 3A4. When growth hormone is administered in combination with drugs known to be metabolized by cytochrome P450 3A4 hepatic enzymes, it is advisable to monitor the clinical effectiveness of such drugs).
No products indexed under this heading.

Busulfan (Data indicates that growth hormone may be an inducer of cytochrome p450 3A4. When growth hormone is administered in combination with drugs known to be metabolized by cytochrome P450 3A4 hepatic enzymes, it is advisable to monitor the clinical effectiveness of such drugs). Products include:
I.V. Busulfex 1125
Myleran Tablets 1492

Carbamazepine (Data indicates that growth hormone may be an inducer of cytochrome p450 3A4. When growth hormone is administered in combination with drugs known to be metabolized by cytochrome P450 3A4 hepatic enzymes, it is advisable to monitor the clinical effectiveness of such drugs). Products include:
Carbatrol Capsules 3174
Equetro Extended-Release Capsules 3178
Tegretol/Tegretol-XR 2278

Cerivastatin Sodium (Data indicates that growth hormone may be an inducer of cytochrome p450 3A4. When growth hormone is administered in combination with drugs known to be metabolized by cytochrome P450 3A4 hepatic enzymes, it is advisable to monitor the clinical effectiveness of such drugs).
No products indexed under this heading.

Chlorpheniramine (Data indicates that growth hormone may be an inducer of cytochrome p450 3A4. When growth hormone is administered in combination with drugs known to be metabolized by cytochrome P450 3A4 hepatic enzymes, it is advisable to monitor the clinical effectiveness of such drugs).
No products indexed under this heading.

Chlorpheniramine Maleate (Data indicates that growth hormone may be an inducer of cytochrome p450 3A4. When growth hormone is administered in combination with drugs known to be metabolized by cytochrome P450 3A4 hepatic enzymes, it is advisable to monitor the clinical effectiveness of such drugs). Products include:
Advil Allergy Sinus Caplets .... ▣ 737
Advil Multi-Symptom Cold Caplets .... ▣ 738
BC Allergy Sinus Cold Powder .... ▣ 612
Contac Severe Cold and Flu Caplets Maximum Strength .... ▣ 615
Hycomine Compound Tablets 1105
PediaCare Multi-Symptom Cold Liquid .... ▣ 704
PediaCare NightRest Cough & Cold Liquid .... ▣ 704
Robitussin Flu Liquid .... ▣ 752
Robitussin PM Cough & Cold Liquid .... ▣ 752
Singlet Caplets .... ▣ 636
Sudafed Sinus & Allergy Tablets ..... ▣ 710
TheraFlu Cold & Cough Hot Liquid .... ▣ 680
TheraFlu Cold & Sore Throat Hot Liquid .... ▣ 680
TheraFlu Flu & Sore Throat Hot Liquid .... ▣ 681
TheraFlu Severe Cold & Cough Hot Liquid .... ▣ 683
TheraFlu Severe Cold Caplets .... ▣ 679
TheraFlu Severe Cold Hot Liquid .... ▣ 682
Triaminic Cold & Allergy Liquid .... ▣ 685
Triaminic Cold & Cough Liquid .... ▣ 685
Triaminic Flu, Cough & Fever Liquid .... ▣ 685
Triaminic Night Time Cough & Cold Liquid .... ▣ 685
Triaminic Allergy Runny Nose & Congestion Softchews .... ▣ 688
Triaminic Cold & Cough Softchews .... ▣ 688
Children's Tylenol Plus Cold NightTime Suspension Liquid 1851
Children's Tylenol Plus Cold & Cough Suspension Liquid and Chewable Tablets 1851
Children's Tylenol Plus Cold Chewable Tablets 1851
Children's Tylenol Plus Flu Suspension Liquid 1853
Tylenol Allergy Complete Multi-Symptom Caplets and Gelcaps with Cool Burst 1844
Multi-Symptom Tylenol Cold Night Time Caplets 1845
Vicks 44M Cough, Cold & Flu Relief 2676
Pediatric Vicks 44m Cough & Cold Relief 2673
Children's Vicks NyQuil Cold/Cough Relief 2671

Chlorpheniramine Polistirex (Data indicates that growth hormone may be an inducer of cytochrome p450 3A4. When growth hormone is administered in combination with drugs known to be metabolized by cytochrome P450 3A4 hepatic enzymes, it is advisable to monitor the clinical effectiveness of such drugs). Products include:
Tussionex Pennkinetic Extended-Release Suspension 3322

Chlorpheniramine Tannate (Data indicates that growth hormone may be an inducer of cytochrome p450 3A4. When growth hormone is administered in combination with drugs known to be metabolized by cytochrome P450 3A4 hepatic enzymes, it is advisable to monitor the clinical effectiveness of such drugs).
No products indexed under this heading.

Chlorpropamide (In patients with diabetes mellitus requiring drug therapy, the dose of insulin and/or oral agents may require adjustment when somatropin therapy is initiated).
No products indexed under this heading.

Cisapride (Data indicates that growth hormone may be an inducer of cytochrome p450 3A4. When growth hormone is administered in combination with drugs known to be metabolized by cytochrome P450 3A4 hepatic enzymes, it is advisable to monitor the clinical effectiveness of such drugs).
No products indexed under this heading.

Clarithromycin (Data indicates that growth hormone may be an inducer of cytochrome p450 3A4. When growth hormone is administered in combination with drugs known to be metabolized by cytochrome P450 3A4 hepatic enzymes, it is advisable to monitor the clinical effectiveness of such drugs). Products include:
Biaxin/Biaxin XL 402
PREVPAC 3281

Cortisone Acetate (Concomitant glucocorticoid therapy may inhibit the growth promoting effect of somatropin).
No products indexed under this heading.

Cyclosporine (Data indicates that growth hormone may be an inducer of cytochrome p450 3A4. When growth hormone is administered in combination with drugs known to be metabolized by cytochrome P450 3A4 hepatic enzymes, it is advisable to monitor the clinical effectiveness of such drugs). Products include:
Gengraf Capsules 458
Neoral Soft Gelatin Capsules 2247
Neoral Oral Solution 2247
Restasis Ophthalmic Emulsion 570
Sandimmune 2259

Desogestrel (Data indicates that growth hormone may be an inducer of cytochrome p450 3A4. When growth hormone is administered in combination with drugs known to be metabolized by cytochrome P450 3A4 hepatic enzymes, it is advisable to monitor the clinical effectiveness of such drugs). Products include:
Ortho-Cept Tablets 2395

Dexamethasone (Concomitant glucocorticoid therapy may inhibit the growth promoting effect of somatropin). Products include:
Ciprodex Otic Suspension 555
Decadron Tablets 1929
TobraDex Ophthalmic Ointment 558
TobraDex Ophthalmic Suspension ... 558

Dexamethasone Acetate (Concomitant glucocorticoid therapy may inhibit the growth promoting effect of somatropin).
No products indexed under this heading.

Dexamethasone Sodium Phosphate (Concomitant glucocorticoid therapy may inhibit the growth promoting effect of somatropin). Products include:
Decadron Phosphate Injection 1931

Diazepam (Data indicates that growth hormone may be an inducer of cytochrome p450 3A4. When growth hormone is administered in combination with drugs known to be metabolized by cytochrome P450 3A4 hepatic enzymes, it is advisable to monitor the clinical effectiveness of such drugs). Products include:
Diastat Rectal Delivery System 3344
Valium Tablets 2822

Dihydroergotamine Mesylate (Data indicates that growth hormone may be an inducer of cytochrome p450 3A4. When growth hormone is administered in combination with drugs known to be metabolized by cytochrome P450 3A4 hepatic enzymes, it is advisable to monitor the clinical effectiveness of such drugs). Products include:
Migranal Nasal Spray 3350

Diltiazem Hydrochloride (Data indicates that growth hormone may be an inducer of cytochrome p450 3A4. When growth hormone is administered in combination with drugs known to be metabolized by cytochrome P450 3A4 hepatic enzymes, it is advisable to monitor the clinical effectiveness of such drugs). Products include:
Cardizem LA Extended Release Tablets 1699
Tiazac Capsules 1204

Diltiazem Maleate (Data indicates that growth hormone may be an inducer of cytochrome p450 3A4. When growth hormone is administered in combination with drugs known to be metabolized by cytochrome P450 3A4 hepatic enzymes, it is advisable to monitor the clinical effectiveness of such drugs).
No products indexed under this heading.

Disopyramide (Data indicates that growth hormone may be an inducer of cytochrome p450 3A4. When growth hormone is administered in combination with drugs known to be metabolized by cytochrome P450 3A4 hepatic enzymes, it is advisable to monitor the clinical effectiveness of such drugs).
No products indexed under this heading.

Disopyramide Phosphate (Data indicates that growth hormone may be an inducer of cytochrome p450 3A4. When growth hormone is administered in combination with drugs known to be metabolized by cytochrome P450 3A4 hepatic enzymes, it is advisable to monitor the clinical effectiveness of such drugs).
No products indexed under this heading.

Disulfiram (Data indicates that growth hormone may be an inducer of cytochrome p450 3A4. When growth hormone is administered in combination with drugs known to be metabolized by cytochrome P450 3A4 hepatic enzymes, it is advisable to monitor the clinical effectiveness of such drugs). Products include:
Antabuse Tablets 2343

Doxorubicin Hydrochloride (Data indicates that growth hormone may be an inducer of cytochrome p450 3A4. When growth hormone is administered in combination with drugs known to be metabolized by cytochrome P450 3A4 hepatic enzymes, it is advisable to monitor the clinical effectiveness of such drugs). Products include:
Adriamycin for Injection, USP 786
Adriamycin Injection, USP 786

Dronabinol (Data indicates that growth hormone may be an inducer of cytochrome p450 3A4. When growth hormone is administered in combination with drugs known to be metabolized by cytochrome P450 3A4 hepatic enzymes, it is advisable to monitor the clinical effectiveness of such drugs). Products include:
Marinol Capsules 3334

Ergotamine Tartrate (Data indicates that growth hormone may be an inducer of cytochrome p450 3A4. When growth hormone is administered in combination with drugs known to be metabolized by cytochrome P450 3A4 hepatic enzymes, it is advisable to monitor the clinical effectiveness of such drugs).
No products indexed under this heading.

Erythromycin (Data indicates that growth hormone may be an inducer of cytochrome p450 3A4. When growth hormone is administered in combination with drugs known to be metabolized by cytochrome P450

3A4 hepatic enzymes, it is advisable to monitor the clinical effectiveness of such drugs). Products include:

- Erygel Topical Gel 2096
- Ery-Tab Tablets 447
- Erythromycin Base Filmtab Tablets 454
- Erythromycin Delayed-Release Capsules, USP 456
- PCE Dispertab Tablets 510

Erythromycin Estolate (Data indicates that growth hormone may be an inducer of cytochrome p450 3A4. When growth hormone is administered in combination with drugs known to be metabolized by cytochrome P450 3A4 hepatic enzymes, it is advisable to monitor the clinical effectiveness of such drugs).

No products indexed under this heading.

Erythromycin Ethylsuccinate (Data indicates that growth hormone may be an inducer of cytochrome p450 3A4. When growth hormone is administered in combination with drugs known to be metabolized by cytochrome P450 3A4 hepatic enzymes, it is advisable to monitor the clinical effectiveness of such drugs). Products include:

- E.E.S. 449
- EryPed 445

Erythromycin Gluceptate (Data indicates that growth hormone may be an inducer of cytochrome p450 3A4. When growth hormone is administered in combination with drugs known to be metabolized by cytochrome P450 3A4 hepatic enzymes, it is advisable to monitor the clinical effectiveness of such drugs).

No products indexed under this heading.

Erythromycin Lactobionate (Data indicates that growth hormone may be an inducer of cytochrome p450 3A4. When growth hormone is administered in combination with drugs known to be metabolized by cytochrome P450 3A4 hepatic enzymes, it is advisable to monitor the clinical effectiveness of such drugs).

No products indexed under this heading.

Erythromycin Stearate (Data indicates that growth hormone may be an inducer of cytochrome p450 3A4. When growth hormone is administered in combination with drugs known to be metabolized by cytochrome P450 3A4 hepatic enzymes, it is advisable to monitor the clinical effectiveness of such drugs). Products include:

- Erythrocin Stearate Filmtab Tablets 452

Estradiol (Data indicates that growth hormone may be an inducer of cytochrome p450 3A4. When growth hormone is administered in combination with drugs known to be metabolized by cytochrome P450 3A4 hepatic enzymes, it is advisable to monitor the clinical effectiveness of such drugs). Products include:

- Activella Tablets 2311
- Climara Transdermal System 795
- Climara Pro Transdermal System 800
- CombiPatch Transdermal System 2180
- Estrogel 0.06% 3200
- Menostar Transdermal System 805
- Prefest Tablets 1069
- Vagifem Tablets 2340
- Vivelle Transdermal System 2288
- Vivelle-Dot Transdermal System 2293

Estradiol Benzoate (Data indicates that growth hormone may be an inducer of cytochrome p450 3A4. When growth hormone is administered in combination with drugs known to be metabolized by cytochrome P450 3A4 hepatic enzymes, it is advisable to monitor the clinical effectiveness of such drugs).

No products indexed under this heading.

Estradiol Cypionate (Data indicates that growth hormone may be an inducer of cytochrome p450 3A4. When growth hormone is administered in combination with drugs known to be metabolized by cytochrome P450 3A4 hepatic enzymes, it is advisable to monitor the clinical effectiveness of such drugs).

No products indexed under this heading.

Estradiol Valerate (Data indicates that growth hormone may be an inducer of cytochrome p450 3A4. When growth hormone is administered in combination with drugs known to be metabolized by cytochrome P450 3A4 hepatic enzymes, it is advisable to monitor the clinical effectiveness of such drugs).

No products indexed under this heading.

Ethinyl Estradiol (Data indicates that growth hormone may be an inducer of cytochrome p450 3A4. When growth hormone is administered in combination with drugs known to be metabolized by cytochrome P450 3A4 hepatic enzymes, it is advisable to monitor the clinical effectiveness of such drugs). Products include:

- Alesse-28 Tablets 3392
- Lo/Ovral-28 Tablets 3423
- NuvaRing 2357
- Ortho-Cept Tablets 2395
- Ortho-Cyclen/Ortho Tri-Cyclen 2414
- Ortho Evra Transdermal System 2402
- Ortho Tri-Cyclen Lo Tablets 2421
- Seasonale Tablets 1073
- Triphasil-28 Tablets 3483
- Yasmin 28 Tablets 818

Ethosuximide (Data indicates that growth hormone may be an inducer of cytochrome p450 3A4. When growth hormone is administered in combination with drugs known to be metabolized by cytochrome P450 3A4 hepatic enzymes, it is advisable to monitor the clinical effectiveness of such drugs).

No products indexed under this heading.

Ethynodiol Diacetate (Data indicates that growth hormone may be an inducer of cytochrome p450 3A4. When growth hormone is administered in combination with drugs known to be metabolized by cytochrome P450 3A4 hepatic enzymes, it is advisable to monitor the clinical effectiveness of such drugs).

No products indexed under this heading.

Etoposide (Data indicates that growth hormone may be an inducer of cytochrome p450 3A4. When growth hormone is administered in combination with drugs known to be metabolized by cytochrome P450 3A4 hepatic enzymes, it is advisable to monitor the clinical effectiveness of such drugs).

No products indexed under this heading.

Etoposide Phosphate (Data indicates that growth hormone may be an inducer of cytochrome p450 3A4. When growth hormone is administered in combination with drugs known to be metabolized by cytochrome P450 3A4 hepatic enzymes, it is advisable to monitor the clinical effectiveness of such drugs).

No products indexed under this heading.

Felodipine (Data indicates that growth hormone may be an inducer of cytochrome p450 3A4. When growth hormone is administered in combination with drugs known to be metabolized by cytochrome P450 3A4 hepatic enzymes, it is advisable to monitor the clinical effectiveness of such drugs). Products include:

- Plendil Extended-Release Tablets 651

Fentanyl (Data indicates that growth hormone may be an inducer of cytochrome p450 3A4. When growth hormone is administered in combination with drugs known to be metabolized by cytochrome P450 3A4 hepatic enzymes, it is advisable to monitor the clinical effectiveness of such drugs). Products include:

- Duragesic Transdermal System 2448

Fentanyl Citrate (Data indicates that growth hormone may be an inducer of cytochrome p450 3A4. When growth hormone is administered in combination with drugs known to be metabolized by cytochrome P450 3A4 hepatic enzymes, it is advisable to monitor the clinical effectiveness of such drugs). Products include:

- Actiq 993

Fludrocortisone Acetate (Concomitant glucocorticoid therapy may inhibit the growth promoting effect of somatropin).

No products indexed under this heading.

Glimepiride (In patients with diabetes mellitus requiring drug therapy, the dose of insulin and/or oral agents may require adjustment when somatropin therapy is initiated). Products include:

- Amaryl Tablets 2864

Glipizide (In patients with diabetes mellitus requiring drug therapy, the dose of insulin and/or oral agents may require adjustment when somatropin therapy is initiated).

No products indexed under this heading.

Glyburide (In patients with diabetes mellitus requiring drug therapy, the dose of insulin and/or oral agents may require adjustment when somatropin therapy is initiated).

No products indexed under this heading.

Haloperidol (Data indicates that growth hormone may be an inducer of cytochrome p450 3A4. When growth hormone is administered in combination with drugs known to be metabolized by cytochrome P450 3A4 hepatic enzymes, it is advisable to monitor the clinical effectiveness of such drugs).

No products indexed under this heading.

Haloperidol Decanoate (Data indicates that growth hormone may be an inducer of cytochrome p450 3A4. When growth hormone is administered in combination with drugs known to be metabolized by cytochrome P450 3A4 hepatic enzymes, it is advisable to monitor the clinical effectiveness of such drugs).

No products indexed under this heading.

Haloperidol Lactate (Data indicates that growth hormone may be an inducer of cytochrome p450 3A4. When growth hormone is administered in combination with drugs known to be metabolized by cytochrome P450 3A4 hepatic enzymes, it is advisable to monitor the clinical effectiveness of such drugs).

No products indexed under this heading.

Hydrocortisone (Concomitant glucocorticoid therapy may inhibit the growth promoting effect of somatropin). Products include:

- Cortizone•5 Ointment 699
- Cortizone•10 Creme 699
- Cortizone•10 Ointment 699
- Cortizone•10 Plus Creme 700
- Cortizone•10 Maximum Strength Quick Shot Spray 700
- Hydrocortone Tablets 1963
- Preparation H Hydrocortisone Cream 748

Hydrocortisone Acetate (Concomitant glucocorticoid therapy may inhibit the growth promoting effect of somatropin). Products include:

- Analpram-HC 1136
- Pramosone 1139
- ProctoFoam-HC 3113
- Tucks Anti-Itch Ointment 712
- U-cort 1% Cream 3289

Hydrocortisone Sodium Phosphate (Concomitant glucocorticoid therapy may inhibit the growth promoting effect of somatropin).

No products indexed under this heading.

Hydrocortisone Sodium Succinate (Concomitant glucocorticoid therapy may inhibit the growth promoting effect of somatropin).

No products indexed under this heading.

Indinavir Sulfate (Data indicates that growth hormone may be an inducer of cytochrome p450 3A4. When growth hormone is administered in combination with drugs known to be metabolized by cytochrome P450 3A4 hepatic enzymes, it is advisable to monitor the clinical effectiveness of such drugs). Products include:

- Crixivan Capsules 1918

Insulin, Human, Zinc Suspension (In patients with diabetes mellitus requiring drug therapy, the dose of insulin and/or oral agents may require adjustment when somatropin therapy is initiated). Products include:

- Humulin L, 100 Units 1763
- Humulin U, 100 Units 1770

Insulin, Human NPH (In patients with diabetes mellitus requiring drug therapy, the dose of insulin and/or oral agents may require adjustment when somatropin therapy is initiated). Products include:

- Humulin N, 100 Units 1764
- Humulin N Pen 1765
- Novolin N Human Insulin 10 ml Vials 2322

Novolin N InnoLet 2322
Novolin N PenFill 3 ml Cartridges 2325
Novolin R InnoLet 2322

Insulin, Human Regular (In patients with diabetes mellitus requiring drug therapy, the dose of insulin and/or oral agents may require adjustment when somatropin therapy is initiated). Products include:
Humulin R (U-500) 1768
Humulin R, 100 Units 1767
Novolin R Human Insulin 10 ml Vials 2322
Novolin R PenFill 2325

Insulin, Human Regular and Human NPH Mixture (In patients with diabetes mellitus requiring drug therapy, the dose of insulin and/or oral agents may require adjustment when somatropin therapy is initiated). Products include:
Humulin 50/50, 100 Units 1760
Humulin 70/30 Pen 1761
Novolin 70/30 Human Insulin 10 ml Vials 2321
Novolin 70/30 InnoLet 2322
Novolin 70/30 PenFill 3 ml Cartridges 2325

Insulin, NPH (In patients with diabetes mellitus requiring drug therapy, the dose of insulin and/or oral agents may require adjustment when somatropin therapy is initiated).
No products indexed under this heading.

Insulin, Regular (In patients with diabetes mellitus requiring drug therapy, the dose of insulin and/or oral agents may require adjustment when somatropin therapy is initiated).
No products indexed under this heading.

Insulin, Zinc Crystals (In patients with diabetes mellitus requiring drug therapy, the dose of insulin and/or oral agents may require adjustment when somatropin therapy is initiated).
No products indexed under this heading.

Insulin, Zinc Suspension (In patients with diabetes mellitus requiring drug therapy, the dose of insulin and/or oral agents may require adjustment when somatropin therapy is initiated).
No products indexed under this heading.

Insulin Aspart, Human Regular (In patients with diabetes mellitus requiring drug therapy, the dose of insulin and/or oral agents may require adjustment when somatropin therapy is initiated). Products include:
NovoLog Injection 2326

Insulin glargine (In patients with diabetes mellitus requiring drug therapy, the dose of insulin and/or oral agents may require adjustment when somatropin therapy is initiated). Products include:
Lantus Injection 2925

Insulin Lispro, Human (In patients with diabetes mellitus requiring drug therapy, the dose of insulin and/or oral agents may require adjustment when somatropin therapy is initiated). Products include:
Humalog-Pen 1751
Humalog Mix 75/25-Pen 1754

Insulin Lispro Protamine, Human (In patients with diabetes mellitus requiring drug therapy, the dose of insulin and/or oral agents may require adjustment when somatropin therapy is initiated). Products include:
Humalog Mix 75/25-Pen 1754

Isradipine (Data indicates that growth hormone may be an inducer of cytochrome p450 3A4. When growth hormone is administered in combination with drugs known to be metabolized by cytochrome P450 3A4 hepatic enzymes, it is advisable to monitor the clinical effectiveness of such drugs). Products include:
DynaCirc CR Tablets 2726

Itraconazole (Data indicates that growth hormone may be an inducer of cytochrome p450 3A4. When growth hormone is administered in combination with drugs known to be metabolized by cytochrome P450 3A4 hepatic enzymes, it is advisable to monitor the clinical effectiveness of such drugs).
No products indexed under this heading.

Ketoconazole (Data indicates that growth hormone may be an inducer of cytochrome p450 3A4. When growth hormone is administered in combination with drugs known to be metabolized by cytochrome P450 3A4 hepatic enzymes, it is advisable to monitor the clinical effectiveness of such drugs). Products include:
Nizoral A-D Shampoo, 1% 1839
Nizoral 2% Shampoo 1838

Levonorgestrel (Data indicates that growth hormone may be an inducer of cytochrome p450 3A4. When growth hormone is administered in combination with drugs known to be metabolized by cytochrome P450 3A4 hepatic enzymes, it is advisable to monitor the clinical effectiveness of such drugs). Products include:
Alesse-28 Tablets 3392
Climara Pro Transdermal System 800
Mirena Intrauterine System 810
Plan B Tablets 1068
Seasonale Tablets 1073
Triphasil-28 Tablets 3483

Lidocaine (Data indicates that growth hormone may be an inducer of cytochrome p450 3A4. When growth hormone is administered in combination with drugs known to be metabolized by cytochrome P450 3A4 hepatic enzymes, it is advisable to monitor the clinical effectiveness of such drugs). Products include:
Lidoderm Patch 1107

Lidocaine Hydrochloride (Data indicates that growth hormone may be an inducer of cytochrome p450 3A4. When growth hormone is administered in combination with drugs known to be metabolized by cytochrome P450 3A4 hepatic enzymes, it is advisable to monitor the clinical effectiveness of such drugs).
No products indexed under this heading.

Lovastatin (Data indicates that growth hormone may be an inducer of cytochrome p450 3A4. When growth hormone is administered in combination with drugs known to be metabolized by cytochrome P450 3A4 hepatic enzymes, it is advisable to monitor the clinical effectiveness of such drugs). Products include:
Advicor Tablets 1694
Altoprev Extended-Release Tablets 1151
Mevacor Tablets 1996

Mestranol (Data indicates that growth hormone may be an inducer of cytochrome p450 3A4. When growth hormone is administered in combination with drugs known to be metabolized by cytochrome P450 3A4 hepatic enzymes, it is advisable to monitor the clinical effectiveness of such drugs).
No products indexed under this heading.

Metformin Hydrochloride (In patients with diabetes mellitus requiring drug therapy, the dose of insulin and/or oral agents may require adjustment when somatropin therapy is initiated). Products include:
ActoPlus Met Tablets 3219
Avandamet Tablets 1343
Fortamet Extended-Release Tablets 1156

Methadone Hydrochloride (Data indicates that growth hormone may be an inducer of cytochrome p450 3A4. When growth hormone is administered in combination with drugs known to be metabolized by cytochrome P450 3A4 hepatic enzymes, it is advisable to monitor the clinical effectiveness of such drugs).
No products indexed under this heading.

Methylprednisolone Acetate (Concomitant glucocorticoid therapy may inhibit the growth promoting effect of somatropin). Products include:
Depo-Medrol Injectable Suspension 2615
Depo-Medrol Single-Dose Vial 2617

Methylprednisolone Sodium Succinate (Concomitant glucocorticoid therapy may inhibit the growth promoting effect of somatropin).
No products indexed under this heading.

Midazolam Hydrochloride (Data indicates that growth hormone may be an inducer of cytochrome p450 3A4. When growth hormone is administered in combination with drugs known to be metabolized by cytochrome P450 3A4 hepatic enzymes, it is advisable to monitor the clinical effectiveness of such drugs).
No products indexed under this heading.

Miglitol (In patients with diabetes mellitus requiring drug therapy, the dose of insulin and/or oral agents may require adjustment when somatropin therapy is initiated).
No products indexed under this heading.

Nefazodone Hydrochloride (Data indicates that growth hormone may be an inducer of cytochrome p450 3A4. When growth hormone is administered in combination with drugs known to be metabolized by cytochrome P450 3A4 hepatic enzymes, it is advisable to monitor the clinical effectiveness of such drugs).
No products indexed under this heading.

Nelfinavir Mesylate (Data indicates that growth hormone may be an inducer of cytochrome p450 3A4. When growth hormone is administered in combination with drugs known to be metabolized by cytochrome P450 3A4 hepatic enzymes, it is advisable to monitor the clinical effectiveness of such drugs). Products include:
Viracept 2556

Nicardipine Hydrochloride (Data indicates that growth hormone may be an inducer of cytochrome p450 3A4. When growth hormone is administered in combination with drugs known to be metabolized by cytochrome P450 3A4 hepatic enzymes, it is advisable to monitor the clinical effectiveness of such drugs). Products include:
Cardene I.V. 1129

Nifedipine (Data indicates that growth hormone may be an inducer of cytochrome p450 3A4. When growth hormone is administered in combination with drugs known to be metabolized by cytochrome P450 3A4 hepatic enzymes, it is advisable to monitor the clinical effectiveness of such drugs). Products include:
Adalat CC Tablets 2978

Nimodipine (Data indicates that growth hormone may be an inducer of cytochrome p450 3A4. When growth hormone is administered in combination with drugs known to be metabolized by cytochrome P450 3A4 hepatic enzymes, it is advisable to monitor the clinical effectiveness of such drugs). Products include:
Nimotop Capsules 774

Nisoldipine (Data indicates that growth hormone may be an inducer of cytochrome p450 3A4. When growth hormone is administered in combination with drugs known to be metabolized by cytochrome P450 3A4 hepatic enzymes, it is advisable to monitor the clinical effectiveness of such drugs). Products include:
Sular Tablets 1163

Nitrendipine (Data indicates that growth hormone may be an inducer of cytochrome p450 3A4. When growth hormone is administered in combination with drugs known to be metabolized by cytochrome P450 3A4 hepatic enzymes, it is advisable to monitor the clinical effectiveness of such drugs).
No products indexed under this heading.

Norethindrone (Data indicates that growth hormone may be an inducer of cytochrome p450 3A4. When growth hormone is administered in combination with drugs known to be metabolized by cytochrome P450 3A4 hepatic enzymes, it is advisable to monitor the clinical effectiveness of such drugs). Products include:
Ortho Micronor Tablets 2411

Norethindrone Acetate (Data indicates that growth hormone may be an inducer of cytochrome p450 3A4. When growth hormone is administered in combination with drugs known to be metabolized by cytochrome P450 3A4 hepatic enzymes, it is advisable to monitor the clinical effectiveness of such drugs). Products include:
Activella Tablets 2311
Aygestin Tablets 1062
CombiPatch Transdermal System 2180

Norgestrel (Data indicates that growth hormone may be an inducer of cytochrome p450 3A4. When growth hormone is administered in combination with drugs known to be metabolized by cytochrome P450 3A4 hepatic enzymes, it is advisable to monitor the clinical effectiveness of such drugs). Products include:
Lo/Ovral-28 Tablets 3423

Ondansetron (Data indicates that growth hormone may be an inducer of cytochrome p450 3A4. When growth hormone is administered in combination with drugs known to be metabolized by cytochrome P450 3A4 hepatic enzymes, it is advisable to monitor the clinical effectiveness of such drugs). Products include:

Zofran ODT Orally Disintegrating Tablets **1613**

Ondansetron Hydrochloride (Data indicates that growth hormone may be an inducer of cytochrome p450 3A4. When growth hormone is administered in combination with drugs known to be metabolized by cytochrome P450 3A4 hepatic enzymes, it is advisable to monitor the clinical effectiveness of such drugs). Products include:

Zofran Injection **1607**
Zofran **1613**

Paclitaxel (Data indicates that growth hormone may be an inducer of cytochrome p450 3A4. When growth hormone is administered in combination with drugs known to be metabolized by cytochrome P450 3A4 hepatic enzymes, it is advisable to monitor the clinical effectiveness of such drugs).

No products indexed under this heading.

Pimozide (Data indicates that growth hormone may be an inducer of cytochrome p450 3A4. When growth hormone is administered in combination with drugs known to be metabolized by cytochrome P450 3A4 hepatic enzymes, it is advisable to monitor the clinical effectiveness of such drugs). Products include:

Orap Tablets **1220**

Pioglitazone Hydrochloride (In patients with diabetes mellitus requiring drug therapy, the dose of insulin and/or oral agents may require adjustment when somatropin therapy is initiated). Products include:

ActoPlus Met Tablets **3219**
Actos Tablets **3224**

Polyestradiol Phosphate (Data indicates that growth hormone may be an inducer of cytochrome p450 3A4. When growth hormone is administered in combination with drugs known to be metabolized by cytochrome P450 3A4 hepatic enzymes, it is advisable to monitor the clinical effectiveness of such drugs).

No products indexed under this heading.

Prednisolone Acetate (Concomitant glucocorticoid therapy may inhibit the growth promoting effect of somatropin). Products include:

Blephamide Ophthalmic Ointment **563**
Blephamide Ophthalmic Suspension **564**
Poly-Pred Liquifilm Ophthalmic Suspension .... **⊙231**
Pred Forte Ophthalmic Suspension .... **⊙233**
Pred Mild Sterile Ophthalmic Suspension .... **⊙236**
Pred-G Ophthalmic Suspension .... **⊙234**
Pred-G Sterile Ophthalmic Ointment .... **⊙235**

Prednisolone Sodium Phosphate (Concomitant glucocorticoid therapy may inhibit the growth promoting effect of somatropin). Products include:

Pediapred Oral Solution **3319**

Prednisolone Tebutate (Concomitant glucocorticoid therapy may inhibit the growth promoting effect of somatropin).

No products indexed under this heading.

Prednisone (Concomitant glucocorticoid therapy may inhibit the growth promoting effect of somatropin).

No products indexed under this heading.

Quinidine Gluconate (Data indicates that growth hormone may be an inducer of cytochrome p450 3A4. When growth hormone is administered in combination with drugs known to be metabolized by cytochrome P450 3A4 hepatic enzymes, it is advisable to monitor the clinical effectiveness of such drugs).

No products indexed under this heading.

Quinidine Polygalacturonate (Data indicates that growth hormone may be an inducer of cytochrome p450 3A4. When growth hormone is administered in combination with drugs known to be metabolized by cytochrome P450 3A4 hepatic enzymes, it is advisable to monitor the clinical effectiveness of such drugs).

No products indexed under this heading.

Quinidine Sulfate (Data indicates that growth hormone may be an inducer of cytochrome p450 3A4. When growth hormone is administered in combination with drugs known to be metabolized by cytochrome P450 3A4 hepatic enzymes, it is advisable to monitor the clinical effectiveness of such drugs).

No products indexed under this heading.

Repaglinide (In patients with diabetes mellitus requiring drug therapy, the dose of insulin and/or oral agents may require adjustment when somatropin therapy is initiated). Products include:

Prandin Tablets (0.5, 1, and 2 mg) **2337**

Rifabutin (Data indicates that growth hormone may be an inducer of cytochrome p450 3A4. When growth hormone is administered in combination with drugs known to be metabolized by cytochrome P450 3A4 hepatic enzymes, it is advisable to monitor the clinical effectiveness of such drugs).

No products indexed under this heading.

Ritonavir (Data indicates that growth hormone may be an inducer of cytochrome p450 3A4. When growth hormone is administered in combination with drugs known to be metabolized by cytochrome P450 3A4 hepatic enzymes, it is advisable to monitor the clinical effectiveness of such drugs). Products include:

Kaletra **474**
Norvir **499**

Rosiglitazone Maleate (In patients with diabetes mellitus requiring drug therapy, the dose of insulin and/or oral agents may require adjustment when somatropin therapy is initiated). Products include:

Avandamet Tablets **1343**
Avandia Tablets **1348**

Saquinavir (Data indicates that growth hormone may be an inducer of cytochrome p450 3A4. When growth hormone is administered in combination with drugs known to be metabolized by cytochrome P450 3A4 hepatic enzymes, it is advisable to monitor the clinical effectiveness of such drugs).

No products indexed under this heading.

Saquinavir Mesylate (Data indicates that growth hormone may be an inducer of cytochrome p450 3A4. When growth hormone is administered in combination with drugs known to be metabolized by cytochrome P450 3A4 hepatic enzymes, it is advisable to monitor the clinical effectiveness of such drugs). Products include:

Invirase **2776**

Sertraline Hydrochloride (Data indicates that growth hormone may be an inducer of cytochrome p450 3A4. When growth hormone is administered in combination with drugs known to be metabolized by cytochrome P450 3A4 hepatic enzymes, it is advisable to monitor the clinical effectiveness of such drugs). Products include:

Zoloft **2581**

Sildenafil Citrate (Data indicates that growth hormone may be an inducer of cytochrome p450 3A4. When growth hormone is administered in combination with drugs known to be metabolized by cytochrome P450 3A4 hepatic enzymes, it is advisable to monitor the clinical effectiveness of such drugs). Products include:

Revatio Tablets **2541**
Viagra Tablets **2552**

Simvastatin (Data indicates that growth hormone may be an inducer of cytochrome p450 3A4. When growth hormone is administered in combination with drugs known to be metabolized by cytochrome P450 3A4 hepatic enzymes, it is advisable to monitor the clinical effectiveness of such drugs). Products include:

Vytorin 10/10 Tablets **2084**
Vytorin 10/10 Tablets **3092**
Vytorin 10/20 Tablets **2084**
Vytorin 10/20 Tablets **3092**
Vytorin 10/40 Tablets **3092**
Vytorin 10/40 Tablets **2084**
Vytorin 10/80 Tablets **2084**
Vytorin 10/80 Tablets **3092**
Zocor Tablets **2078**

Sirolimus (Data indicates that growth hormone may be an inducer of cytochrome p450 3A4. When growth hormone is administered in combination with drugs known to be metabolized by cytochrome P450 3A4 hepatic enzymes, it is advisable to monitor the clinical effectiveness of such drugs). Products include:

Rapamune Oral Solution and Tablets **3472**

Tacrolimus (Data indicates that growth hormone may be an inducer of cytochrome p450 3A4. When growth hormone is administered in combination with drugs known to be metabolized by cytochrome P450 3A4 hepatic enzymes, it is advisable to monitor the clinical effectiveness of such drugs). Products include:

Prograf Capsules and Injection **624**
Protopic Ointment **629**

Tamoxifen Citrate (Data indicates that growth hormone may be an inducer of cytochrome p450 3A4. When growth hormone is administered in combination with drugs known to be metabolized by cytochrome P450 3A4 hepatic enzymes, it is advisable to monitor the clinical effectiveness of such drugs).

No products indexed under this heading.

Tiagabine Hydrochloride (Data indicates that growth hormone may be an inducer of cytochrome p450 3A4. When growth hormone is administered in combination with drugs known to be metabolized by cytochrome P450 3A4 hepatic enzymes, it is advisable to monitor the clinical effectiveness of such drugs). Products include:

Gabitril Tablets **998**

Tolazamide (In patients with diabetes mellitus requiring drug therapy, the dose of insulin and/or oral agents may require adjustment when somatropin therapy is initiated).

No products indexed under this heading.

Tolbutamide (In patients with diabetes mellitus requiring drug therapy, the dose of insulin and/or oral agents may require adjustment when somatropin therapy is initiated).

No products indexed under this heading.

Tolterodine Tartrate (Data indicates that growth hormone may be an inducer of cytochrome p450 3A4. When growth hormone is administered in combination with drugs known to be metabolized by cytochrome P450 3A4 hepatic enzymes, it is advisable to monitor the clinical effectiveness of such drugs). Products include:

Detrol Tablets **2626**
Detrol LA Capsules **2629**

Trazodone Hydrochloride (Data indicates that growth hormone may be an inducer of cytochrome p450 3A4. When growth hormone is administered in combination with drugs known to be metabolized by cytochrome P450 3A4 hepatic enzymes, it is advisable to monitor the clinical effectiveness of such drugs).

No products indexed under this heading.

Triamcinolone (Concomitant glucocorticoid therapy may inhibit the growth promoting effect of somatropin).

No products indexed under this heading.

Triamcinolone Acetonide (Concomitant glucocorticoid therapy may inhibit the growth promoting effect of somatropin). Products include:

Azmacort Inhalation Aerosol **1701**
Nasacort HFA Inhalation Aerosol **2939**
Nasacort AQ Nasal Spray **2937**

Triamcinolone Diacetate (Concomitant glucocorticoid therapy may inhibit the growth promoting effect of somatropin).

No products indexed under this heading.

Triamcinolone Hexacetonide (Concomitant glucocorticoid therapy may inhibit the growth promoting effect of somatropin).

No products indexed under this heading.

Triazolam (Data indicates that growth hormone may be an inducer of cytochrome p450 3A4. When growth hormone is administered in combination with drugs known to be metabolized by cytochrome P450 3A4 hepatic enzymes, it is advisable to monitor the clinical effectiveness of such drugs).
No products indexed under this heading.

Troglitazone (In patients with diabetes mellitus requiring drug therapy, the dose of insulin and/or oral agents may require adjustment when somatropin therapy is initiated).
No products indexed under this heading.

Verapamil Hydrochloride (Data indicates that growth hormone may be an inducer of cytochrome p450 3A4. When growth hormone is administered in combination with drugs known to be metabolized by cytochrome P450 3A4 hepatic enzymes, it is advisable to monitor the clinical effectiveness of such drugs). Products include:
Covera-HS Tablets **3135**
Tarka Tablets **519**
Verelan PM Capsules **3120**

Vinblastine Sulfate (Data indicates that growth hormone may be an inducer of cytochrome p450 3A4. When growth hormone is administered in combination with drugs known to be metabolized by cytochrome P450 3A4 hepatic enzymes, it is advisable to monitor the clinical effectiveness of such drugs).
No products indexed under this heading.

Vincristine Sulfate (Data indicates that growth hormone may be an inducer of cytochrome p450 3A4. When growth hormone is administered in combination with drugs known to be metabolized by cytochrome P450 3A4 hepatic enzymes, it is advisable to monitor the clinical effectiveness of such drugs).
No products indexed under this heading.

Warfarin Sodium (Data indicates that growth hormone may be an inducer of cytochrome p450 3A4. When growth hormone is administered in combination with drugs known to be metabolized by cytochrome P450 3A4 hepatic enzymes, it is advisable to monitor the clinical effectiveness of such drugs). Products include:
Coumadin for Injection **932**
Coumadin Tablets **932**

NORFLEX INJECTION

(Orphenadrine Citrate) **1824**
May interact with:

Propoxyphene Hydrochloride (Concomitant use results in confusion, anxiety and tremors).
No products indexed under this heading.

Propoxyphene Napsylate (Concomitant use results in confusion, anxiety and tremors). Products include:
Darvocet A 500 Tablets **3497**

NORITATE CREAM, 1%

(Metronidazole) **1051**
May interact with oral anticoagulants. Compounds in these categories include:

Anisindione (Oral metronidazole has been reported to potentiate the anticoagulant effect of coumarin and warfarin resulting in a prolongation of prothrombin time; this interaction should be kept in mind if Noritate is used concurrently with oral coagulants). Products include:
Miradon Tablets **3056**

Dicumarol (Oral metronidazole has been reported to potentiate the anticoagulant effect of coumarin and warfarin resulting in a prolongation of prothrombin time; this interaction should be kept in mind if Noritate is used concurrently with oral coagulants).
No products indexed under this heading.

Warfarin Sodium (Oral metronidazole has been reported to potentiate the anticoagulant effect of coumarin and warfarin resulting in a prolongation of prothrombin time; this interaction should be kept in mind if Noritate is used concurrently with oral coagulants). Products include:
Coumadin for Injection **932**
Coumadin Tablets **932**

NOROXIN TABLETS

(Norfloxacin) **2009**
May interact with antacids containing aluminum, calcium and magnesium, class 1A antiarrhythmics, class III antiarrhythmics, corticosteroids, oral anticoagulants, erythromycin, iron containing oral preparations, antipsychotic agents, tricyclic antidepressants, xanthines, and certain other agents. Compounds in these categories include:

Aluminum Carbonate (May interfere with absorption resulting in lower serum and urine levels of norfloxacin; antacids should not be administered concomitantly with, or within 2 hours of, the administration of norfloxacin).
No products indexed under this heading.

Aluminum Hydroxide (May interfere with absorption resulting in lower serum and urine levels of norfloxacin; antacids should not be administered concomitantly with, or within 2 hours of, the administration of norfloxacin). Products include:
Gaviscon Regular Strength Liquid .. ▣**620**
Gaviscon Regular Strength Tablets .... ▣**619**
Gaviscon Extra Strength Liquid .... ▣**620**
Gaviscon Extra Strength Tablets .... ▣**619**
Maalox Max Maximum Strength Antacid/Anti-Gas Liquid **2165**
Maalox Regular Strength Antacid/Antigas Liquid **2164**

Aminophylline (Co-administration of quinolone with theophylline has resulted in elevated plasma levels of theophylline resulting in theophylline-related side effects).
No products indexed under this heading.

Amiodarone Hydrochloride (Risk of developing arrhythmias with norfloxacin may be reduced by avoiding concurrent treatment with class III antiarrhythmic agents). Products include:
Pacerone Tablets **3337**

Amitriptyline Hydrochloride (Norfloxacin should be used with caution in subjects receiving drugs that affect the QTc interval, such as tricyclic antidepressants).
No products indexed under this heading.

Amoxapine (Norfloxacin should be used with caution in subjects receiving drugs that affect the QTc interval, such as tricyclic antidepressants).
No products indexed under this heading.

Anisindione (Co-administration may enhance the effects of oral anticoagulants). Products include:
Miradon Tablets **3056**

Aripiprazole (Norfloxacin should be used with caution in subjects receiving drugs that affect the QTc interval, such as antipsychotics). Products include:
Abilify Tablets **2472**
Abilify Tablets **916**

Betamethasone Acetate (The risk of ruptures of the shoulder, hand or Achilles tendons may be increased in patients receiving concomitant corticosteroids, especially in the elderly).
No products indexed under this heading.

Betamethasone Sodium Phosphate (The risk of ruptures of the shoulder, hand or Achilles tendons may be increased in patients receiving concomitant corticosteroids, especially in the elderly).
No products indexed under this heading.

Bretylium Tosylate (Risk of developing arrhythmias with norfloxacin may be reduced by avoiding concurrent treatment with class III antiarrhythmic agents).
No products indexed under this heading.

Caffeine (Some quinolones have been shown to interfere with the metabolism of caffeine leading to reduced clearance of caffeine and a prolongation of its plasma half-life). Products include:
Athena Hair System Shampoo .... ▣**767**
BC Powder .... ▣**612**
Arthritis Strength BC Powder .... ▣**612**
Goody's Extra Strength Headache Powder .... ▣**621**
Goody's Extra Strength Pain Relief Tablets .... ▣**621**
Hycomine Compound Tablets **1105**
Spartan Hair System Shampoo .... ▣**767**
Vivarin .... ▣**639**

Chlorpromazine (Norfloxacin should be used with caution in subjects receiving drugs that affect the QTc interval, such as antipsychotics).
No products indexed under this heading.

Chlorpromazine Hydrochloride (Norfloxacin should be used with caution in subjects receiving drugs that affect the QTc interval, such as antipsychotics).
No products indexed under this heading.

Chlorprothixene (Norfloxacin should be used with caution in subjects receiving drugs that affect the QTc interval, such as antipsychotics).
No products indexed under this heading.

Chlorprothixene Hydrochloride (Norfloxacin should be used with caution in subjects receiving drugs that affect the QTc interval, such as antipsychotics).
No products indexed under this heading.

Cisapride (Norfloxacin should be used with caution in subjects receiving drugs that affect the QTc interval, such as cispride).
No products indexed under this heading.

Clomipramine Hydrochloride (Norfloxacin should be used with caution in subjects receiving drugs that affect the QTc interval, such as tricyclic antidepressants).
No products indexed under this heading.

Clozapine (Norfloxacin should be used with caution in subjects receiving drugs that affect the QTc interval, such as antipsychotics). Products include:
Clozapine Tablets **2141**
Clozaril Tablets **2174**
FazaClo Orally Disintegrating Tablets **547**

Cortisone Acetate (The risk of ruptures of the shoulder, hand or Achilles tendons may be increased in patients receiving concomitant corticosteroids, especially in the elderly).
No products indexed under this heading.

Cyclosporine (Co-administration has resulted in elevated serum levels of cyclosporine). Products include:
Gengraf Capsules **458**
Neoral Soft Gelatin Capsules **2247**
Neoral Oral Solution **2247**
Restasis Ophthalmic Emulsion **570**
Sandimmune **2259**

Desipramine Hydrochloride (Norfloxacin should be used with caution in subjects receiving drugs that affect the QTc interval, such as tricyclic antidepressants).
No products indexed under this heading.

Dexamethasone (The risk of ruptures of the shoulder, hand or Achilles tendons may be increased in patients receiving concomitant corticosteroids, especially in the elderly). Products include:
Ciprodex Otic Suspension **555**
Decadron Tablets **1929**
TobraDex Ophthalmic Ointment **558**
TobraDex Ophthalmic Suspension ... **558**

Dexamethasone Acetate (The risk of ruptures of the shoulder, hand or Achilles tendons may be increased in patients receiving concomitant corticosteroids, especially in the elderly).
No products indexed under this heading.

Dexamethasone Sodium Phosphate (The risk of ruptures of the shoulder, hand or Achilles tendons may be increased in patients receiving concomitant corticosteroids, especially in the elderly). Products include:
Decadron Phosphate Injection **1931**

Dicumarol (Co-administration may enhance the effects of oral anticoagulants).
No products indexed under this heading.

Didanosine (Co-administration with Videx, didanosine chewable/buffered tablets or the pediatric powder for oral solution may interfere with absorption resulting in lower serum and urine levels of norfloxacin; this combination should not be administered concomitantlyor within 2 hours of administration of norfloxacin).
No products indexed under this heading.

Disopyramide (Risk of developing arrhythmias with norfloxacin may be reduced by avoiding concurrent treatment with class IA antiarrhythmic agents).
No products indexed under this heading.

Doxepin Hydrochloride (Norfloxacin should be used with caution in subjects receiving drugs that affect the QTc interval, such as tricyclic antidepressants).
No products indexed under this heading.

Dyphylline (Co-administration of quinolone with theophylline has resulted in elevated plasma levels of theophylline resulting in theophylline-related side effects).
No products indexed under this heading.

Erythromycin (Norfloxacin should be used with caution in subjects receiving drugs that affect the QTc interval, such as erythromycin). Products include:
Erygel Topical Gel **2096**
Ery-Tab Tablets **447**
Erythromycin Base Filmtab Tablets **454**
Erythromycin Delayed-Release Capsules, USP **456**
PCE Dispertab Tablets **510**

Erythromycin Estolate (Norfloxacin should be used with caution in subjects receiving drugs that affect the QTc interval, such as erythromycin).
No products indexed under this heading.

Erythromycin Ethylsuccinate (Norfloxacin should be used with caution in subjects receiving drugs that affect the QTc interval, such as erythromycin). Products include:
E.E.S. **449**
EryPed **445**

Erythromycin Gluceptate (Norfloxacin should be used with caution in subjects receiving drugs that affect the QTc interval, such as erythromycin).
No products indexed under this heading.

Erythromycin Lactobionate (Norfloxacin should be used with caution in subjects receiving drugs that affect the QTc interval, such as erythromycin).
No products indexed under this heading.

Erythromycin Stearate (Norfloxacin should be used with caution in subjects receiving drugs that affect the QTc interval, such as erythromycin). Products include:
Erythrocin Stearate Filmtab Tablets **452**

Ferrous Fumarate (May interfere with absorption resulting in lower serum and urine levels of norfloxacin; iron-containing products should not be administered concomitantly with, or within 2 hours of, the administration of norfloxacin). Products include:
Chromagen Forte Soft Gelatin Capsules **3296**
Ferretts Tablets .... ▣ **773**
Repliva 21/7 Tablets **3301**

Ferrous Gluconate (May interfere with absorption resulting in lower serum and urine levels of norfloxacin; iron-containing products should not be administered concomitantly with, or within 2 hours of, the administration of norfloxacin).
No products indexed under this heading.

Ferrous Sulfate (May interfere with absorption resulting in lower serum and urine levels of norfloxacin; iron-containing products should not be administered concomitantly with, or within 2 hours of, the administration of norfloxacin). Products include:
Feosol Tablets **1629**
Slow Fe Iron Tablets .... ▣ **772**
Slow Fe with Folic Acid Tablets .... ▣ **773**

Fludrocortisone Acetate (The risk of ruptures of the shoulder, hand or Achilles tendons may be increased in patients receiving concomitant corticosteroids, especially in the elderly).
No products indexed under this heading.

Fluphenazine Decanoate (Norfloxacin should be used with caution in subjects receiving drugs that affect the QTc interval, such as antipsychotics).
No products indexed under this heading.

Fluphenazine Enanthate (Norfloxacin should be used with caution in subjects receiving drugs that affect the QTc interval, such as antipsychotics).
No products indexed under this heading.

Fluphenazine Hydrochloride (Norfloxacin should be used with caution in subjects receiving drugs that affect the QTc interval, such as antipsychotics).
No products indexed under this heading.

Glyburide (Concomitant administration of norfloxacin with glyburide has rarely resulted in severe hypoglycemia; monitoring of blood glucose is recommended when these agents are co-administered).
No products indexed under this heading.

Haloperidol (Norfloxacin should be used with caution in subjects receiving drugs that affect the QTc interval, such as antipsychotics).
No products indexed under this heading.

Haloperidol Decanoate (Norfloxacin should be used with caution in subjects receiving drugs that affect the QTc interval, such as antipsychotics).
No products indexed under this heading.

Hydrocortisone (The risk of ruptures of the shoulder, hand or Achilles tendons may be increased in patients receiving concomitant corticosteroids, especially in the elderly). Products include:
Cortizone•5 Ointment .... ▣ **699**
Cortizone•10 Creme .... ▣ **699**
Cortizone•10 Ointment .... ▣ **699**
Cortizone•10 Plus Creme .... ▣ **700**
Cortizone•10 Maximum Strength Quick Shot Spray .... ▣ **700**
Hydrocortone Tablets **1963**
Preparation H Hydrocortisone Cream .... ▣ **748**

Hydrocortisone Acetate (The risk of ruptures of the shoulder, hand or Achilles tendons may be increased in patients receiving concomitant corticosteroids, especially in the elderly). Products include:
Analpram-HC **1136**
Pramosone **1139**
ProctoFoam-HC **3113**
Tucks Anti-Itch Ointment .... ▣ **712**
U-cort 1% Cream **3289**

Hydrocortisone Sodium Phosphate (The risk of ruptures of the shoulder, hand or Achilles tendons may be increased in patients receiving concomitant corticosteroids, especially in the elderly).
No products indexed under this heading.

Hydrocortisone Sodium Succinate (The risk of ruptures of the shoulder, hand or Achilles tendons may be increased in patients receiving concomitant corticosteroids, especially in the elderly).
No products indexed under this heading.

Imipramine Hydrochloride (Norfloxacin should be used with caution in subjects receiving drugs that affect the QTc interval, such as tricyclic antidepressants).
No products indexed under this heading.

Imipramine Pamoate (Norfloxacin should be used with caution in subjects receiving drugs that affect the QTc interval, such as tricyclic antidepressants).
No products indexed under this heading.

Iron (May interfere with absorption resulting in lower serum and urine levels of norfloxacin; iron-containing products should not be administered concomitantly with, or within 2 hours of, the administration of norfloxacin). Products include:
Chromagen Forte Soft Gelatin Capsules **3296**
Ferretts IPS Liquid .... ▣ **773**
OptiNate **1162**
Repliva 21/7 Tablets **3301**

Lithium Carbonate (Norfloxacin should be used with caution in subjects receiving drugs that affect the QTc interval, such as antipsychotics). Products include:
Eskalith **1406**
Lithobid Tablets **1670**

Lithium Citrate (Norfloxacin should be used with caution in subjects receiving drugs that affect the QTc interval, such as antipsychotics).
No products indexed under this heading.

Loxapine Hydrochloride (Norfloxacin should be used with caution in subjects receiving drugs that affect the QTc interval, such as antipsychotics).
No products indexed under this heading.

Loxapine Succinate (Norfloxacin should be used with caution in subjects receiving drugs that affect the QTc interval, such as antipsychotics).
No products indexed under this heading.

Magaldrate (May interfere with absorption resulting in lower serum and urine levels of norfloxacin; antacids should not be administered concomitantly with, or within 2 hours of, the administration of norfloxacin).
No products indexed under this heading.

Magnesium Hydroxide (May interfere with absorption resulting in lower serum and urine levels of norfloxacin; antacids should not be administered concomitantly with, or within 2 hours of, the administration of norfloxacin). Products include:
Maalox Max Maximum Strength Antacid/Anti-Gas Liquid **2165**
Maalox Regular Strength Antacid/Antigas Liquid **2164**
Pepcid Complete Chewable Tablets **1672**
Rolaids Tablets .... ▣ **707**
Extra Strength Rolaids Tablets .... ▣ **707**
Rolaids Multi-Symptom Antacid & Antigas Tablets .... ▣ **708**

Magnesium Oxide (May interfere with absorption resulting in lower serum and urine levels of norfloxacin; antacids should not be administered concomitantly with, or within 2 hours of, the administration of norfloxacin). Products include:
Beelith Tablets **784**
PremCal Light, Regular, and Extra Strength Tablets .... ▣ **762**

Maprotiline Hydrochloride (Norfloxacin should be used with caution in subjects receiving drugs that affect the QTc interval, such as tricyclic antidepressants).
No products indexed under this heading.

Mesoridazine Besylate (Norfloxacin should be used with caution in subjects receiving drugs that affect the QTc interval, such as antipsychotics).
No products indexed under this heading.

Methotrimeprazine (Norfloxacin should be used with caution in subjects receiving drugs that affect the QTc interval, such as antipsychotics).
No products indexed under this heading.

Methylprednisolone Acetate (The risk of ruptures of the shoulder, hand or Achilles tendons may be increased in patients receiving concomitant corticosteroids, especially in the elderly). Products include:
Depo-Medrol Injectable Suspension **2615**
Depo-Medrol Single-Dose Vial **2617**

Methylprednisolone Sodium Succinate (The risk of ruptures of the shoulder, hand or Achilles tendons may be increased in patients receiving concomitant corticosteroids, especially in the elderly).
No products indexed under this heading.

Molindone Hydrochloride (Norfloxacin should be used with caution in subjects receiving drugs that affect the QTc interval, such as antipsychotics). Products include:
Moban Tablets **1108**

Moricizine Hydrochloride (Risk of developing arrhythmias with norfloxacin may be reduced by avoiding concurrent treatment with class IA antiarrhythmic agents).
No products indexed under this heading.

Nitrofurantoin (Nitrofurantoin may antagonize the antibacterial effect of norfloxacin in the urinary tract; concurrent use is not recommended).
No products indexed under this heading.

Nortriptyline Hydrochloride (Norfloxacin should be used with caution in subjects receiving drugs that affect the QTc interval, such as tricyclic antidepressants).
No products indexed under this heading.

Olanzapine (Norfloxacin should be used with caution in subjects receiving drugs that affect the QTc interval, such as antipsychotics).
Products include:
- Symbyax Capsules 1788
- Zyprexa Tablets 1798
- Zyprexa IntraMuscular 1798
- Zyprexa ZYDIS Orally Disintegrating Tablets 1798

Perphenazine (Norfloxacin should be used with caution in subjects receiving drugs that affect the QTc interval, such as antipsychotics).
No products indexed under this heading.

Pimozide (Norfloxacin should be used with caution in subjects receiving drugs that affect the QTc interval, such as antipsychotics).
Products include:
- Orap Tablets 1220

Polysaccharide Iron Complex (May interfere with absorption resulting in lower serum and urine levels of norfloxacin; iron-containing products should not be administered concomitantly with, or within 2 hours of, the administration of norfloxacin).
Products include:
- Niferex-150 Forte Capsules 3299
- Nu-Iron 150 Capsules 2098

Prednisolone Acetate (The risk of ruptures of the shoulder, hand or Achilles tendons may be increased in patients receiving concomitant corticosteroids, especially in the elderly).
Products include:
- Blephamide Ophthalmic Ointment 563
- Blephamide Ophthalmic Suspension 564
- Poly-Pred Liquifilm Ophthalmic Suspension .... ⊙231
- Pred Forte Ophthalmic Suspension .... ⊙233
- Pred Mild Sterile Ophthalmic Suspension .... ⊙236
- Pred-G Ophthalmic Suspension .... ⊙234
- Pred-G Sterile Ophthalmic Ointment .... ⊙235

Prednisolone Sodium Phosphate (The risk of ruptures of the shoulder, hand or Achilles tendons may be increased in patients receiving concomitant corticosteroids, especially in the elderly). Products include:
- Pediapred Oral Solution 3319

Prednisolone Tebutate (The risk of ruptures of the shoulder, hand or Achilles tendons may be increased in patients receiving concomitant corticosteroids, especially in the elderly).
No products indexed under this heading.

Prednisone (The risk of ruptures of the shoulder, hand or Achilles tendons may be increased in patients receiving concomitant corticosteroids, especially in the elderly).
No products indexed under this heading.

Probenecid (Co-administration with probenecid has resulted in diminished urinary excretion).
No products indexed under this heading.

Procainamide (Risk of developing arrhythmias with norfloxacin may be reduced by avoiding concurrent treatment with class IA antiarrhythmic agents).
No products indexed under this heading.

Prochlorperazine (Norfloxacin should be used with caution in subjects receiving drugs that affect the QTc interval, such as antipsychotics).
No products indexed under this heading.

Promethazine Hydrochloride (Norfloxacin should be used with caution in subjects receiving drugs that affect the QTc interval, such as antipsychotics). Products include:
- Phenergan 3438

Protriptyline Hydrochloride (Norfloxacin should be used with caution in subjects receiving drugs that affect the QTc interval, such as tricyclic antidepressants). Products include:
- Vivactil Tablets 2350

Quetiapine Fumarate (Norfloxacin should be used with caution in subjects receiving drugs that affect the QTc interval, such as antipsychotics). Products include:
- Seroquel Tablets 691

Quinidine (Risk of developing arrhythmias with norfloxacin may be reduced by avoiding concurrent treatment with class IA antiarrhythmic agents).
No products indexed under this heading.

Quinidine Gluconate (Risk of developing arrhythmias with norfloxacin may be reduced by avoiding concurrent treatment with class IA antiarrhythmic agents).
No products indexed under this heading.

Risperidone (Norfloxacin should be used with caution in subjects receiving drugs that affect the QTc interval, such as antipsychotics).
Products include:
- Risperdal Consta Long-Acting Injection 1664
- Risperdal M-Tab Orally Disintegrating Tablets 1658
- Risperdal 1658

Sotalol Hydrochloride (Risk of developing arrhythmias with norfloxacin may be reduced by avoiding concurrent treatment with class III antiarrhythmic agents).
No products indexed under this heading.

Sucralfate (May interfere with absorption resulting in lower serum and urine levels of norfloxacin; sucralfate should not be administered concomitantly with, or within 2 hours of, the administration of norfloxacin). Products include:
- Carafate Suspension 727
- Carafate Tablets 728

Theophylline (Co-administration of quinolone with theophylline has resulted in elevated plasma levels of theophylline resulting in theophylline-related side effects).
No products indexed under this heading.

Theophylline Calcium Salicylate (Co-administration of quinolone with theophylline has resulted in elevated plasma levels of theophylline resulting in theophylline-related side effects).
No products indexed under this heading.

Theophylline Dihydroxypropyl (Glyceryl) (Co-administration of quinolone with theophylline has resulted in elevated plasma levels of theophylline resulting in theophylline-related side effects).
No products indexed under this heading.

Theophylline Ethylenediamine (Co-administration of quinolone with theophylline has resulted in elevated plasma levels of theophylline resulting in theophylline-related side effects).
No products indexed under this heading.

Theophylline Sodium Glycinate (Co-administration of quinolone with theophylline has resulted in elevated plasma levels of theophylline resulting in theophylline-related side effects).
No products indexed under this heading.

Thioridazine Hydrochloride (Norfloxacin should be used with caution in subjects receiving drugs that affect the QTc interval, such as antipsychotics). Products include:
- Thioridazine Hydrochloride Tablets 2122

Thiothixene (Norfloxacin should be used with caution in subjects receiving drugs that affect the QTc interval, such as antipsychotics).
Products include:
- Thiothixene Capsules 2124

Triamcinolone (The risk of ruptures of the shoulder, hand or Achilles tendons may be increased in patients receiving concomitant corticosteroids, especially in the elderly).
No products indexed under this heading.

Triamcinolone Acetonide (The risk of ruptures of the shoulder, hand or Achilles tendons may be increased in patients receiving concomitant corticosteroids, especially in the elderly). Products include:
- Azmacort Inhalation Aerosol 1701
- Nasacort HFA Inhalation Aerosol 2939
- Nasacort AQ Nasal Spray 2937

Triamcinolone Diacetate (The risk of ruptures of the shoulder, hand or Achilles tendons may be increased in patients receiving concomitant corticosteroids, especially in the elderly).
No products indexed under this heading.

Triamcinolone Hexacetonide (The risk of ruptures of the shoulder, hand or Achilles tendons may be increased in patients receiving concomitant corticosteroids, especially in the elderly).
No products indexed under this heading.

Trifluoperazine Hydrochloride (Norfloxacin should be used with caution in subjects receiving drugs that affect the QTc interval, such as antipsychotics).
No products indexed under this heading.

Trimipramine Maleate (Norfloxacin should be used with caution in subjects receiving drugs that affect the QTc interval, such as tricyclic antidepressants). Products include:
- Surmontil Capsules 2347

Warfarin Sodium (Co-administration may enhance the effects of oral anticoagulants).
Products include:
- Coumadin for Injection 932
- Coumadin Tablets 932

Zinc Sulfate (May interfere with absorption resulting in lower serum and urine levels of norfloxacin; zinc-containing oral products should not be administered concomitantly with, or within 2 hours of, the administration of norfloxacin). Products include:
- Athena Hair System Shampoo .... ▣767
- Spartan Hair System Shampoo .... ▣767
- Visine A.C. Seasonal Itching and Redness Relief Drops .... ⊙278
- Zinc-220 Capsules 576

Ziprasidone Hydrochloride (Norfloxacin should be used with caution in subjects receiving drugs that affect the QTc interval, such as antipsychotics). Products include:
- Geodon Capsules 2514

Food Interactions

Dairy products (Avoid simultaneous ingestion; administer norfloxacin at least one hour before or two hours after ingestion of milk and/or other dairy products).

Food, unspecified (Co-administration may decrease the absorption of norfloxacin; administer at least one hour before or two hours after a meal).

NORVASC TABLETS

(Amlodipine Besylate) 2529
None cited in PDR database.

NORVIR SOFT GELATIN CAPSULES

(Ritonavir) 499
May interact with beta blockers, cytochrome p450 3a inducers (selected), dexamethasone, ergot-containing drugs, erythromycin, oral hypoglycemic agents, highly metabolized sedatives and hypnotics, insulin, phenytoin, quinidine, selective serotonin reuptake inhibitors, tricyclic antidepressants, valproate, xanthines, and certain other agents. Compounds in these categories include:

Acarbose (New onset diabetes mellitus, exacerbation of pre-existing diabetes, and hyperglycemia have been reported with protease inhibitors; dosage adjustment of oral hypoglycemic agents may be required). Products include:
- Precose Tablets 776

Acebutolol Hydrochloride (Co-administration with beta-blockers has resulted in cardiac and neurologic events).
No products indexed under this heading.

Albendazole (Co-administration results in a possible increase in AUC of albendazole; dosage adjustments may be required). Products include:
- Albenza Tablets 1310

Alfentanil Hydrochloride (Co-administration results in a large increase (> 3x) in AUC of alfentanil; dosage adjustments may be required).
No products indexed under this heading.

(▣ Described in PDR For Nonprescription Drugs) (⊙ Described in PDR For Ophthalmic Medicines™)

Allium sativum (Potential for increase in the clearance of ritonavir resulting in decreased ritonavir plasma concentrations).
No products indexed under this heading.

Alprazolam (Co-administration is likely to produce large increases in highly metabolized sedatives and hypnotics resulting in extreme sedation and respiratory depression; concurrent use is contraindicated). Products include:
Niravam Orally Disintegrating Tablets 3106
Xanax XR Tablets 2655

Aminophylline (Co-administration results in the reduction of the average AUC of theophylline; increased dosage of theophylline may be required and therapeutic monitoring should be considered).
No products indexed under this heading.

Amiodarone Hydrochloride (Co-administration is contraindicated due to potential for serious and/or life-threatening reactions, such as cardiac arrhythmias). Products include:
Pacerone Tablets 3337

Amitriptyline Hydrochloride (Co-administration may result in increased tricyclic antidepressants' plasma concentrations; dose decrease of tricyclics may be needed. Use with caution).
No products indexed under this heading.

Amoxapine (Co-administration may result in increased tricyclic antidepressants' plasma concentrations; dose decrease of tricyclics may be needed. Use with caution).
No products indexed under this heading.

Aprepitant (Potential for increase in the clearance of ritonavir resulting in decreased ritonavir plasma concentrations). Products include:
Emend Capsules 1944

Astemizole (Co-administration is contraindicated due to potential for serious and/or life-threatening reactions, such as cardiac arrhythmias).
No products indexed under this heading.

Atenolol (Co-administration with beta-blockers has resulted in cardiac and neurologic events). Products include:
Tenormin I.V. Injection 698
Tenormin Tablets 695

Atorvastatin Calcium (Co-administration may result in increased plasma concentrations of atorvastatin calcium; the risk of myopathy, including rhabdomyolysis, may be increased. Dosage adjustment may be needed. Use with caution). Products include:
Caduet Tablets 2507
Lipitor Tablets 2495

Atovaquone (Co-administration may result in decreased atovaquone plasma concentrations; dose increase of atovaquone may be needed. Use with caution). Products include:
Malarone Tablets 1484
Malarone Pediatric Tablets 1484
Mepron Suspension 1487

Bepridil Hydrochloride (Co-administration is contraindicated due to potential for serious and/or life-threatening reactions, such as cardiac arrhythmias).
No products indexed under this heading.

Betaxolol Hydrochloride (Co-administration results in a possible increase in AUC of betaxolol; dosage adjustments may be required). Products include:
Betoptic S Ophthalmic Suspension 554

Bisoprolol Fumarate (Co-administration with beta-blockers has resulted in cardiac and neurologic events).
No products indexed under this heading.

Bromocriptine Mesylate (Co-administration results in a large increase (> 3x) in AUC of bromocriptine; dosage adjustments may be required).
No products indexed under this heading.

Bupropion Hydrochloride (Co-administration may result in increased bupropion plasma concentrations; dose decrease of bupropion may be needed. Use with caution). Products include:
Wellbutrin Tablets 1579
Wellbutrin SR Sustained-Release Tablets 1583
Wellbutrin XL Extended-Release Tablets 1588
Zyban Sustained-Release Tablets 1620

Carbamazepine (Co-administration may result in increased carbamazepine plasma concentrations; dose decrease of carbamazepine may be needed. Use with caution). Products include:
Carbatrol Capsules 3174
Equetro Extended-Release Capsules 3178
Tegretol/Tegretol-XR 2278

Carteolol Hydrochloride (Co-administration with beta-blockers has resulted in cardiac and neurologic events). Products include:
Carteolol Hydrochloride Ophthalmic Solution USP, 1% .... ⊙246

Chloroquine Hydrochloride (Co-administration results in a possible increase in AUC of chloroquine; dosage adjustments may be required).
No products indexed under this heading.

Chloroquine Phosphate (Co-administration results in a possible increase in AUC of chloroquine; dosage adjustments may be required).
No products indexed under this heading.

Chlorpromazine (Co-administration results in a moderate increase (1.5 to 3x) in AUC of chlorpromazine; dosage adjustments may be required).
No products indexed under this heading.

Chlorpromazine Hydrochloride (Co-administration results in a moderate increase (1.5 to 3x) in AUC of chlorpromazine; dosage adjustments may be required).
No products indexed under this heading.

Chlorpropamide (New onset diabetes mellitus, exacerbation of pre-existing diabetes, and hyperglycemia have been reported with protease inhibitors; dosage adjustment of oral hypoglycemic agents may be required).
No products indexed under this heading.

Cisapride (Co-administration is contraindicated due to potential for serious and/or life-threatening reactions, such as cardiac arrhythmias).
No products indexed under this heading.

Citalopram Hydrobromide (Co-administration may result in increased selective serotonin reuptake inhibitors' plasma concentrations; dose decrease of SSRIs may be needed. Use with caution). Products include:
Celexa 1177

Clarithromycin (Co-administration may result in increased clarithromycin concentration; for patients with renal impairment, dosage adjustments should be considered). Products include:
Biaxin/Biaxin XL 402
PREVPAC 3281

Clofibrate (Ritonavir may increase the activity of glucuronosyltransferase; co-administration results in a decrease in AUC of clofibrate; dosage adjustments may be required).
No products indexed under this heading.

Clomipramine Hydrochloride (Co-administration may result in increased tricyclic antidepressants' plasma concentrations; dose decrease of tricyclics may be needed. Use with caution).
No products indexed under this heading.

Clonazepam (Co-administration may result in increased clonazepam plasma concentrations; dose decrease of clonazepam may be needed. Use with caution). Products include:
Klonopin 2782

Clorazepate Dipotassium (Co-administration may result in increased clorazepate plasma concentrations; dose decrease of clorazepate may be needed. Use with caution). Products include:
Tranxene 2488

Clozapine (Ritonavir is expected to produce a large increase in the plasma clozapine concentrations; clozapine has recognized risk to induce hematologic abnormalities; co-administration is contraindicated). Products include:
Clozapine Tablets 2141
Clozaril Tablets 2174
FazaClo Orally Disintegrating Tablets 547

Codeine Phosphate (Ritonavir may increase the activity of glucuronosyltransferase; co-administration results in possible decrease in AUC of codeine; possible need for dosage alterations of codeine). Products include:
Tylenol with Codeine 2461

Cyclophosphamide (An increase in the AUC of cyclophosphamide, activated by CYP, may correspond to a decrease in the AUC of the active metabolite(s) and a possible decrease in efficacy of cyclophosphamide).
No products indexed under this heading.

Cyclosporine (Co-administration may result in increased cyclosporine plasma concentrations; dose decrease of cyclosporine may be needed. Use with caution). Products include:
Gengraf Capsules 458
Neoral Soft Gelatin Capsules 2247
Neoral Oral Solution 2247
Restasis Ophthalmic Emulsion 570
Sandimmune 2259

Daunorubicin Hydrochloride (Co-administration results in a possible increase in AUC of daunorubicin; dosage adjustments may be required). Products include:
Cerubidine for Injection 788

Desipramine Hydrochloride (Co-administration may lead to increased desipramine levels. Dosage reduction and concentration monitoring of desipramine is recommended).
No products indexed under this heading.

Dexamethasone (Co-administration may result in increased dexamethasone plasma concentrations; dose decrease of dexamethasone may be needed. Use with caution). Products include:
Ciprodex Otic Suspension 555
Decadron Tablets 1929
TobraDex Ophthalmic Ointment 558
TobraDex Ophthalmic Suspension 558

Dexamethasone Acetate (Co-administration may result in increased dexamethasone plasma concentrations; dose decrease of dexamethasone may be needed. Use with caution).
No products indexed under this heading.

Dexamethasone Sodium Phosphate (Co-administration may result in increased dexamethasone plasma concentrations; dose decrease of dexamethasone may be needed. Use with caution). Products include:
Decadron Phosphate Injection 1931

Dexfenfluramine Hydrochloride (Co-administration may lead to increased desipramine levels. Dosage reduction and concentration monitoring of desipramine is recommended).
No products indexed under this heading.

Diazepam (Co-administration may result in increased diazepam plasma concentrations; dose decrease of diazepam may be needed. Use with caution). Products include:
Diastat Rectal Delivery System 3344
Valium Tablets 2822

Diclofenac Potassium (Co-administration results in a moderate (1.5 to 3x) increase or decrease in AUC of diclofenac). Products include:
Cataflam Tablets 2173

Diclofenac Sodium (Co-administration results in a moderate (1.5 to 3x) increase or decrease in AUC of diclofenac). Products include:
Arthrotec Tablets 3126
Voltaren Ophthalmic Solution 2300
Voltaren Tablets 2298
Voltaren-XR Tablets 2301

Didanosine (Dosing of these two drugs should be separated by 2.5 hours to avoid formulation incompatability).
No products indexed under this heading.

Dihydroergotamine Mesylate (Co-administration is contraindicated due to potential for serious and/or life-threatening reactions, such as acute ergot toxicity characterized by vasospasm and ischemia of the extremities and other tissues including the CNS). Products include:
Migranal Nasal Spray 3350

IMPORTANT NOTE: Always consult each drug listing in the patient's regimen for possible interactions.

Diltiazem Hydrochloride (Co-administration may result in increased diltiazem plasma concentrations; dose decrease of diltiazem may be needed. Use with caution). Products include:
- Cardizem LA Extended Release Tablets ... 1699
- Tiazac Capsules ... 1204

Diphenoxylate Hydrochloride (Ritonavir may increase the activity of glucuronosyltransferase; co-administration results in a decrease in AUC of diphenoxylate; dosage adjustments may be required).
No products indexed under this heading.

Disopyramide Phosphate (Co-administration may result in increased disopyramide plasma concentrations; cardiac and neurologic events have been reported with co-administration. Dosage adjustment may be needed. Use with caution).
No products indexed under this heading.

Disulfiram (Potential for disulfiram-like reactions due to the presence of ethanol in the ritonavir formulations). Products include:
- Antabuse Tablets ... 2343

Divalproex Sodium (Co-administration may result in decreased valproate plasma concentrations; dose increase of valproate may be needed. Use with caution). Products include:
- Depakote Sprinkle Capsules ... 422
- Depakote Tablets ... 427
- Depakote ER Tablets ... 433

Doxazosin Mesylate (Co-administration results in a possible increase in AUC of doxazosin; dosage adjustments may be required).
No products indexed under this heading.

Doxepin Hydrochloride (Co-administration results in a possible increase in the AUC of doxepin; dosage adjustment of doxepin may be required).
No products indexed under this heading.

Doxorubicin Hydrochloride (Co-administration results in a possible increase in AUC of doxorubicin; dosage adjustments may be required). Products include:
- Adriamycin for Injection, USP ... 786
- Adriamycin Injection, USP ... 786

Dronabinol (Co-administration may result in increased dronabinol plasma concentrations; dose decrease of dronabinol may be needed. Use with caution). Products include:
- Marinol Capsules ... 3334

Dyphylline (Co-administration results in the reduction of the average AUC of theophylline; increased dosage of theophylline may be required and therapeutic monitoring should be considered).
No products indexed under this heading.

Efavirenz (Potential for increase in the clearance of ritonavir resulting in decreased ritonavir plasma concentrations). Products include:
- Sustiva Capsules ... 957

Encainide Hydrochloride (Ritonavir is expected to produce a large increase in the plasma concentrations of encainide; concurrent use is contraindicated).
No products indexed under this heading.

Ergonovine Maleate (Co-administration may result in a possible increase in concentrations of ergonovine; in general, concurrent use with ergot alkaloid preparations is contraindicated).
No products indexed under this heading.

Ergotamine Tartrate (Co-administration is contraindicated due to potential for serious and/or life-threatening reactions, such as acute ergot toxicity characterized by vasospasm and ischemia of the extremities and other tissues including the CNS).
No products indexed under this heading.

Erythromycin (Co-administration results in a large increase (> 3x) in AUC of erythromycin; dosage adjustments may be required). Products include:
- Erygel Topical Gel ... 2096
- Ery-Tab Tablets ... 447
- Erythromycin Base Filmtab Tablets ... 454
- Erythromycin Delayed-Release Capsules, USP ... 456
- PCE Dispertab Tablets ... 510

Erythromycin Estolate (Co-administration results in a large increase (> 3x) in AUC of erythromycin; dosage adjustments may be required).
No products indexed under this heading.

Erythromycin Ethylsuccinate (Co-administration results in a large increase (> 3x) in AUC of erythromycin; dosage adjustments may be required). Products include:
- E.E.S. ... 449
- EryPed ... 445

Erythromycin Gluceptate (Co-administration results in a large increase (> 3x) in AUC of erythromycin; dosage adjustments may be required).
No products indexed under this heading.

Erythromycin Lactobionate (Co-administration results in a large increase (> 3x) in AUC of erythromycin; dosage adjustments may be required).
No products indexed under this heading.

Erythromycin Stearate (Co-administration results in a large increase (> 3x) in AUC of erythromycin; dosage adjustments may be required). Products include:
- Erythrocin Stearate Filmtab Tablets ... 452

Escitalopram Oxalate (Co-administration may result in increased selective serotonin reuptake inhibitors' plasma concentrations; dose decrease of SSRIs may be needed. Use with caution). Products include:
- Lexapro Oral Solution ... 1193
- Lexapro Tablets ... 1193

Esmolol Hydrochloride (Co-administration with beta-blockers has resulted in cardiac and neurologic events). Products include:
- Brevibloc Concentrate ... 766
- Brevibloc Injection ... 766
- Brevibloc Double Strength Injection ... 766
- Brevibloc Premixed Injection ... 766
- Brevibloc Double Strength Premixed Injection ... 766

Estazolam (Co-administration may result in increased estazolam plasma concentrations; dose decrease of estazolam may be needed. Use with caution). Products include:
- ProSom Tablets ... 512

Ethinyl Estradiol (Co-administration may result in the reduction of ethinyl estradiol levels; dosage increase or alternate contraceptive measures should be considered). Products include:
- Alesse-28 Tablets ... 3392
- Lo/Ovral-28 Tablets ... 3423
- NuvaRing ... 2357
- Ortho-Cept Tablets ... 2395
- Ortho-Cyclen/Ortho Tri-Cyclen ... 2414
- Ortho Evra Transdermal System ... 2402
- Ortho Tri-Cyclen Lo Tablets ... 2421
- Seasonale Tablets ... 1073
- Triphasil-28 Tablets ... 3483
- Yasmin 28 Tablets ... 818

Ethosuximide (Co-administration may result in increased ethosuximide plasma concentrations; dose decrease of ethosuximide may be needed. Use with caution).
No products indexed under this heading.

Etoposide (Co-administration results in a large increase (> 3x) in AUC of etoposide; dosage adjustments may be required).
No products indexed under this heading.

Fentanyl (Co-administration results in a large increase (> 3x) in AUC of fentanyl; dosage adjustments may be required). Products include:
- Duragesic Transdermal System ... 2448

Fentanyl Citrate (Co-administration results in a large increase (> 3x) in AUC of fentanyl; dosage adjustments may be required). Products include:
- Actiq ... 993

Flecainide Acetate (Co-administration is contraindicated due to potential for serious and/or life-threatening reactions, such as cardiac arrhythmias). Products include:
- Tambocor Tablets ... 1824

Fluconazole (Co-administration has resulted in an increase in AUC and Cmax of ritonavir by 12% and 15%, respectively).
No products indexed under this heading.

Fluoxetine Hydrochloride (Cardiac and neurologic events have been reported when ritonavir has been co-administered with fluoxetine, Co-administration may result in increased selective serotonin reuptake inhibitors' plasma concentrations; dose decrease of SSRIs may be needed. Use with caution). Products include:
- Prozac Pulvules and Liquid ... 1771
- Symbyax Capsules ... 1788

Flurazepam Hydrochloride (Co-administration may result in increased flurazepam plasma concentrations; dose decrease of flurazepam may be needed. Use with caution). Products include:
- Dalmane Capsules ... 3343

Flurbiprofen (Co-administration results in a moderate (1.5 to 3x) increase or decrease in AUC of flurbiprofen).
No products indexed under this heading.

Fluticasone Propionate (Co-administration may result in increased fluticasone plasma concentrations; dose decrease of fluticasone may be needed. Use with caution). Products include:
- Advair Diskus 100/50 ... 1291
- Advair Diskus 250/50 ... 1291
- Advair Diskus 500/50 ... 1291
- Cutivate Cream ... 1381
- Cutivate Lotion 0.05% ... 1383
- Cutivate Ointment ... 1384
- Flonase Nasal Spray ... 1412
- Flovent Diskus 100 mcg ... 1418
- Flovent Diskus 50 mcg ... 1415

Fluvastatin Sodium (Co-administration results in a possible increase in AUC of fluvastatin; dosage adjustments may be required). Products include:
- Lescol Capsules ... 2227
- Lescol ... 2730
- Lescol XL Tablets ... 2227

Fluvoxamine Maleate (Co-administration may result in increased selective serotonin reuptake inhibitors' plasma concentrations; dose decrease of SSRIs may be needed. Use with caution).
No products indexed under this heading.

Fosphenytoin Sodium (Co-administration results in a moderate increase or decrease in AUC of phenytoin; dosage adjustments may be required; potential for increase in the clearance of ritonavir resulting in decreased ritonavir plasma concentrations).
No products indexed under this heading.

Gemfibrozil (Co-administration results in a possible increase in AUC of gemfibrozil; dosage adjustments may be required).
No products indexed under this heading.

Glimepiride (Co-administration results in a moderate increase or decrease in AUC of glimepiride; dosage adjustments may be required). Products include:
- Amaryl Tablets ... 2864

Glipizide (Co-administration results in a moderate increase or decrease in AUC of glipizide; dosage adjustments may be required).
No products indexed under this heading.

Glyburide (Co-administration results in a moderate increase or decrease in AUC of glyburide; dosage adjustments may be required).
No products indexed under this heading.

Haloperidol (Co-administration results in a moderate increase (1.5 to 3x) in AUC of haloperidol; dosage adjustments may be required).
No products indexed under this heading.

Haloperidol Decanoate (Co-administration results in a moderate increase (1.5 to 3x) in AUC of haloperidol; dosage adjustments may be required).
No products indexed under this heading.

Hydrocodone Bitartrate (Co-administration results in a moderate increase (1.5 to 3x) in AUC of hydrocodone; dosage adjustments may be required). Products include:
- Hycodan ... 1104
- Hycomine Compound Tablets ... 1105
- Hycotuss Expectorant Syrup ... 1106
- Lortab ... 3315
- Lortab Elixir ... 3312
- Vicodin Tablets ... 530
- Vicodin ES Tablets ... 531
- Vicodin HP Tablets ... 532
- Vicoprofen Tablets ... 533
- Zydone Tablets ... 1118

Hydromorphone Hydrochloride (Ritonavir may increase the activity of glucuronosyltransferase; co-administration results in possible decrease in AUC of hydromorphone; possible need for dosage alterations of hydromorphone). Products include:
- Dilaudid ... 439
- Dilaudid Oral Liquid ... 443
- Dilaudid Non-Sterile Powder ... 439
- Dilaudid Rectal Suppositories ... 439
- Dilaudid Tablets ... 439
- Dilaudid Tablets - 8 mg ... 443
- Dilaudid-HP ... 441

Hypericum (May lead to loss of virologic response and possible resistance to ritonavir or to the class of protease inhibitors).
No products indexed under this heading.

Ibuprofen (Co-administration results in a moderate (1.5 to 3x) increase or decrease in AUC of ibuprofen). Products include:
- Advil Allergy Sinus Caplets ... 737
- Advil ... 737
- Children's Advil Suspension ... 742
- Children's Advil Chewable Tablets ... 741
- Advil Cold & Sinus ... 739
- Advil Flu & Body Ache Caplets ... 739
- Children's Advil Cold Suspension ... 741
- Infants' Advil Concentrated Drops ... 743
- Junior Strength Advil Swallow Tablets ... 740
- Advil Migraine Liquigels ... 740
- Advil Multi-Symptom Cold Caplets ... 738
- Combunox Tablets ... 1183
- Children's Motrin Oral Suspension and Chewable Tablets ... 1837
- Children's Motrin Cold Non-Staining Dye-Free Oral Suspension ... 1838
- Children's Motrin Cold Oral Suspension ... 1838
- Children's Motrin Non-Staining Dye-Free Oral Suspension ... 1837
- Motrin Cold & Sinus Caplets ... 1836
- Motrin IB Tablets and Caplets ... 1836
- Infants' Motrin Concentrated Drops ... 1837
- Infants' Motrin Non-Staining Dye-Free Drops ... 1837
- Junior Strength Motrin Caplets and Chewable Tablets ... 1837
- Vicoprofen Tablets ... 533

Ifosfamide (An increase in the AUC of ifosfamide, activated by CYP, may correspond to a decrease in the AUC of the active metabolite(s) and a possible decrease in efficacy of ifosfamide).
No products indexed under this heading.

Imipramine Hydrochloride (Co-administration may result in increased tricyclic antidepressants' plasma concentrations; dose decrease of tricyclics may be needed. Use with caution).
No products indexed under this heading.

Imipramine Pamoate (Co-administration may result in increased tricyclic antidepressants' plasma concentrations; dose decrease of tricyclics may be needed. Use with caution).
No products indexed under this heading.

Indinavir Sulfate (When co-administered with reduced doses of indinavir, ritonavir increased indinavir concentration, decreased Cmax, and increased Cmin; appropriate doses for this combination with respect to efficacy and safety have not been established). Products include:
- Crixivan Capsules ... 1918

Indomethacin (Co-administration results in a moderate (1.5 to 3x) increase or decrease in AUC of indomethacin). Products include:
- Indocin ... 1968

Insulin, Human, Zinc Suspension (New onset diabetes mellitus, exacerbation of pre-existing diabetes, and hyperglycemia have been reported with protease inhibitors; dosage adjustment of insulin may be required). Products include:
- Humulin L, 100 Units ... 1763
- Humulin U, 100 Units ... 1770

Insulin, Human NPH (New onset diabetes mellitus, exacerbation of pre-existing diabetes, and hyperglycemia have been reported with protease inhibitors; dosage adjustment of insulin may be required). Products include:
- Humulin N, 100 Units ... 1764
- Humulin N Pen ... 1765
- Novolin N Human Insulin 10 ml Vials ... 2322
- Novolin N InnoLet ... 2322
- Novolin N PenFill 3 ml Cartridges ... 2325
- Novolin R InnoLet ... 2322

Insulin, Human Regular (New onset diabetes mellitus, exacerbation of pre-existing diabetes, and hyperglycemia have been reported with protease inhibitors; dosage adjustment of insulin may be required). Products include:
- Humulin R (U-500) ... 1768
- Humulin R, 100 Units ... 1767
- Novolin R Human Insulin 10 ml Vials ... 2322
- Novolin R PenFill ... 2325

Insulin, Human Regular and Human NPH Mixture (New onset diabetes mellitus, exacerbation of pre-existing diabetes, and hyperglycemia have been reported with protease inhibitors; dosage adjustment of insulin may be required). Products include:
- Humulin 50/50, 100 Units ... 1760
- Humulin 70/30 Pen ... 1761
- Novolin 70/30 Human Insulin 10 ml Vials ... 2321
- Novolin 70/30 InnoLet ... 2322
- Novolin 70/30 PenFill 3 ml Cartridges ... 2325

Insulin, NPH (New onset diabetes mellitus, exacerbation of pre-existing diabetes, and hyperglycemia have been reported with protease inhibitors; dosage adjustment of insulin may be required).
No products indexed under this heading.

Insulin, Regular (New onset diabetes mellitus, exacerbation of pre-existing diabetes, and hyperglycemia have been reported with protease inhibitors; dosage adjustment of insulin may be required).
No products indexed under this heading.

Insulin, Zinc Crystals (New onset diabetes mellitus, exacerbation of pre-existing diabetes, and hyperglycemia have been reported with protease inhibitors; dosage adjustment of insulin may be required).
No products indexed under this heading.

Insulin, Zinc Suspension (New onset diabetes mellitus, exacerbation of pre-existing diabetes, and hyperglycemia have been reported with protease inhibitors; dosage adjustment of insulin may be required).
No products indexed under this heading.

Insulin Aspart, Human Regular (New onset diabetes mellitus, exacerbation of pre-existing diabetes, and hyperglycemia have been reported with protease inhibitors; dosage adjustment of insulin may be required). Products include:
- NovoLog Injection ... 2326

Insulin glargine (New onset diabetes mellitus, exacerbation of pre-existing diabetes, and hyperglycemia have been reported with protease inhibitors; dosage adjustment of insulin may be required). Products include:
- Lantus Injection ... 2925

Insulin Lispro, Human (New onset diabetes mellitus, exacerbation of pre-existing diabetes, and hyperglycemia have been reported with protease inhibitors; dosage adjustment of insulin may be required). Products include:
- Humalog-Pen ... 1751
- Humalog Mix 75/25-Pen ... 1754

Insulin Lispro Protamine, Human (New onset diabetes mellitus, exacerbation of pre-existing diabetes, and hyperglycemia have been reported with protease inhibitors; dosage adjustment of insulin may be required). Products include:
- Humalog Mix 75/25-Pen ... 1754

Itraconazole (Co-administration may result in a possible increase in plasma concentrations of itraconazole; dosage adjustment may be required. Use with caution).
No products indexed under this heading.

Ketoconazole (Co-administration may result in increased ketoconazole concentration; high doses of ketoconazole (>200 mg/day) are not recommended). Products include:
- Nizoral A-D Shampoo, 1% ... 1839
- Nizoral 2% Shampoo ... 1838

Ketoprofen (Ritonavir may increase the activity of glucuronosyltransferase; co-administration results in possible decrease in AUC of ketoprofen; possible need for dosage alterations of ketoprofen).
No products indexed under this heading.

Ketorolac Tromethamine (Ritonavir may increase the activity of glucuronosyltransferase; co-administration results in possible decrease in AUC of ketorolac; possible need for dosage alterations of ketorolac). Products include:
- Acular Ophthalmic Solution ... 561
- Acular LS Ophthalmic Solution ... 562

Labetalol Hydrochloride (Co-administration with beta-blockers has resulted in cardiac and neurologic events).
No products indexed under this heading.

Lamotrigine (Co-administration may result in decreased lamotrigine plasma concentrations; dose increase of lamotrigine may be needed. Use with caution). Products include:
- Lamictal ... 1449

Lansoprazole (Co-administration results in a moderate increase or decrease in AUC of lansoprazole; dosage adjustments may be required). Products include:
- Prevacid Delayed-Release Capsules ... 3268
- Prevacid for Delayed-Release Oral Suspension ... 3268
- Prevacid I.V. for Injection ... 3274
- Prevacid NapraPAC ... 3277
- Prevacid SoluTab Delayed-Release Orally Disintegrating Tablets ... 3268
- PREVPAC ... 3281

Levobunolol Hydrochloride (Co-administration with beta-blockers has resulted in cardiac and neurologic events). Products include:
- Betagan Ophthalmic Solution, USP ... ⊙217

Lidocaine Hydrochloride (Co-administration may result in an increase in plasma concentrations of lidocaine; dosage adjustments may be required. Use with caution).
No products indexed under this heading.

Loperamide Hydrochloride (Co-administration results in a decrease in AUC of loperamide). Products include:
- Imodium Capsules ... 1834
- Imodium A-D Liquid and Caplets ... 1835
- Imodium Advanced Caplets and Chewable Tablets ... 1835

Loratadine (Ritonavir is expected to produce a large increase (> 3x) in the plasma concentrations of loratadine; dosage adjustments may be required). Products include:
- Alavert Allergy & Sinus D-12 Hour Tablets ... 743
- Alavert ... 743
- Children's Claritin 24 Hour Non-Drowsy Allergy Syrup ... 732
- Claritin Non-Drowsy 24 Hour Tablets ... 731
- Non-Drowsy Claritin Hives Relief Tablets ... 733
- Claritin Reditabs 24 Hour Non-Drowsy Tablets ... 732
- Claritin-D Non-Drowsy 12 Hour Tablets ... 731
- Claritin-D Non-Drowsy 24 Hour Tablets ... 731
- Children's Dimetapp ND Non-Drowsy Allergy Syrup ... 746
- Triaminic Allerchews ... 684

Lorazepam (Ritonavir may increase the activity of glucuronosyltransferase; co-administration results in a decrease in AUC of lorazepam; dosage adjustments may be required).
No products indexed under this heading.

Losartan Potassium (Co-administration results in a moderate increase or decrease in AUC of losartan; dosage adjustments may be required). Products include:
- Cozaar Tablets ... 1913
- Hyzaar ... 1964

Lovastatin (Co-administration results in increased plasma concentrations of lovastatin; the risk of myopathy, including rhabdomyolysis, may be increased). Products include:
- Advicor Tablets ... 1694
- Altoprev Extended-Release Tablets ... 1151
- Mevacor Tablets ... 1996

Maprotiline Hydrochloride (Co-administration may result in increased tricyclic antidepressants' plasma concentrations; dose decrease of tricyclics may be needed. Use with caution).
No products indexed under this heading.

IMPORTANT NOTE: Always consult each drug listing in the patient's regimen for possible interactions.

Meperidine Hydrochloride (Co-administration results in decreased meperidine concentration and increased normeperidine concentration; dosage increase and long-term use of meperidine with ritonavir are not recommended due to the increased concentrations of the metabolite normeperidine which has both analgesic activity and CNS stimulant activity, such as seizures).
No products indexed under this heading.

Metformin Hydrochloride (New onset diabetes mellitus, exacerbation of pre-existing diabetes, and hyperglycemia have been reported with protease inhibitors; dosage adjustment of oral hypoglycemic agents may be required). Products include:
- ActoPlus Met Tablets 3219
- Avandamet Tablets 1343
- Fortamet Extended-Release Tablets 1156

Methadone Hydrochloride (Co-administration may result may result in decreased methadone concentration; dosage increase of methadone may be considered).
No products indexed under this heading.

Methamphetamine Hydrochloride (Co-administration may result in increased methamphetamine plasma concentrations; dose decrease of methamphetamine may be needed. Use with caution). Products include:
- Desoxyn Tablets, USP 2482

Methylergonovine Maleate (Co-administration is contraindicated due to potential for serious and/or life-threatening reactions, such as acute ergot toxicity characterized by vasospasm and ischemia of the extremities and other tissues including the CNS).
No products indexed under this heading.

Methylphenidate Hydrochloride (Co-administration results in a possible increase in AUC of methylphenidate; dosage adjustments may be required). Products include:
- Concerta Extended-Release Tablets 1828
- Metadate CD Capsules 3316
- Ritalin 2254
- Ritalin LA Capsules 2255

Methysergide Maleate (Co-administration is contraindicated due to potential for serious and/or life-threatening reactions, such as acute ergot toxicity characterized by vasospasm and ischemia of the extremities and other tissues including the CNS).
No products indexed under this heading.

Metipranolol Hydrochloride (Co-administration with beta-blockers has resulted in cardiac and neurologic events).
No products indexed under this heading.

Metoclopramide Hydrochloride (Ritonavir may increase the activity of glucuronosyltransferase; co-administration results in a decrease in AUC of metoclopramide; dosage adjustments may be required).
No products indexed under this heading.

Metoprolol Succinate (Co-administration may result in increased metoprolol plasma concentrations; cardiac and neurologic events have been reported with co-administration. Dosage adjustment may be needed. Use with caution). Products include:
- Toprol-XL Tablets 660

Metoprolol Tartrate (Co-administration may result in increased metoprolol plasma concentrations; cardiac and neurologic events have been reported with co-administration. Dosage adjustment may be needed. Use with caution).
No products indexed under this heading.

Metronidazole (Potential for disulfiram-like reactions due to the presence of ethanol in the ritonavir formulations). Products include:
- Metrogel 1% 1212
- MetroGel-Vaginal Gel 1822
- Noritate Cream, 1% 1051

Metronidazole Hydrochloride (Potential for disulfiram-like reactions due to the presence of ethanol in the ritonavir formulations).
No products indexed under this heading.

Mexiletine Hydrochloride (Co-administration may result in increased mexiletine plasma concentrations; cardiac and neurologic events have been reported with co-administration. Dosage adjustment may be needed. Use with caution).
No products indexed under this heading.

Miconazole (Co-administration results in a possible increase in AUC of miconazole; dosage adjustments may be required).
No products indexed under this heading.

Miconazole Nitrate (Co-administration results in a possible increase in AUC of miconazole; dosage adjustments may be required). Products include:
- Desenex .... ■674
- Desenex Jock Itch Spray Powder .... ■674

Midazolam Hydrochloride (Co-administration is contraindicated due to potential for prolonged or increased sedation and/or respiratory depression).
No products indexed under this heading.

Miglitol (New onset diabetes mellitus, exacerbation of pre-existing diabetes, and hyperglycemia have been reported with protease inhibitors; dosage adjustment of oral hypoglycemic agents may be required).
No products indexed under this heading.

Modafinil (Potential for increase in the clearance of ritonavir resulting in decreased ritonavir plasma concentrations). Products include:
- Provigil Tablets 1002

Morphine Sulfate (Ritonavir may increase the activity of glucuronosyltransferase; co-administration results in possible decrease in AUC of morphine; possible need for dosage alterations of morphine). Products include:
- Avinza Capsules 1714
- Kadian Capsules 572
- MS Contin Tablets 2703

Nadolol (Co-administration with beta-blockers has resulted in cardiac and neurologic events). Products include:
- Nadolol Tablets 2121

Naproxen (Ritonavir may increase the activity of glucuronosyltransferase; co-administration results in possible decrease in AUC of naproxen; possible need for dosage alterations of naproxen). Products include:
- EC-Naprosyn Delayed-Release Tablets 2769
- Naprosyn Suspension 2769
- Naprosyn Tablets 2769
- Prevacid NapraPAC 3277

Naproxen Sodium (Ritonavir may increase the activity of glucuronosyltransferase; co-administration results in possible decrease in AUC of naproxen; possible need for dosage alterations of naproxen). Products include:
- Aleve Tablets, Caplets and Gelcaps .... ■605
- Anaprox Tablets 2769
- Anaprox DS Tablets 2769

Nefazodone Hydrochloride (Co-administration may result in increased nefazodone plasma concentrations; cardiac and neurologic events have been reported with co-administration. Dosage adjustment may be needed. Use with caution).
No products indexed under this heading.

Nevirapine (Co-administration may result in a possible increase in concentrations of nevirapine). Products include:
- Viramune Oral Suspension 903
- Viramune Tablets 903

Nifedipine (Co-administration may result in increased nifedipine plasma concentrations; dose decrease of nifedipine may be needed. Use with caution). Products include:
- Adalat CC Tablets 2978

Nitrendipine (Co-administration results in a large increase (> 3x) in AUC of nitrendipine; dosage adjustments may be required).
No products indexed under this heading.

Nortriptyline Hydrochloride (Co-administration may result in increased tricyclic antidepressants' plasma concentrations; dose decrease of tricyclics may be needed. Use with caution).
No products indexed under this heading.

Omeprazole (Co-administration results in a moderate increase or decrease in AUC of omeprazole; dosage adjustments may be required). Products include:
- Zegerid Powder for Oral Solution 2972

Ondansetron Hydrochloride (Co-administration results in a large increase (> 3x) in AUC of ondansetron; dosage adjustments may be required). Products include:
- Zofran Injection 1607
- Zofran 1613

Oxazepam (Ritonavir may increase the activity of glucuronosyltransferase; co-administration results in a decrease in AUC of oxazepam; dosage adjustments may be required).
No products indexed under this heading.

Oxycodone Hydrochloride (Co-administration results in a moderate increase (1.5 to 3x) in AUC of oxycodone; dosage adjustments may be required). Products include:
- Combunox Tablets 1183
- OxyContin Tablets 2699
- OxyFast Oral Concentrate Solution 2704
- OxyIR Capsules 2704
- Percocet Tablets 1114
- Percodan Tablets 1115

Paclitaxel (Co-administration results in a large increase (> 3x) in AUC of paclitaxel; dosage adjustments may be required).
No products indexed under this heading.

Paroxetine Hydrochloride (Co-administration results in a moderate increase (1.5 to 3x) in AUC of paroxetine; dosage adjustments may be required). Products include:
- Paxil CR Controlled-Release Tablets 1509
- Paxil 1501

Penbutolol Sulfate (Co-administration results in a possible increase in AUC of penbutolol; dosage adjustments may be required).
No products indexed under this heading.

Pentoxifylline (Co-administration results in a possible increase in AUC of pentoxifylline; dosage adjustments may be required).
No products indexed under this heading.

Perphenazine (Co-administration may result in increased perphenazine plasma concentrations; dose decrease of perphenazine may be needed).
No products indexed under this heading.

Phenobarbital (Co-administration results in a possible increase in AUC of phenobarbital; dosage adjustments may be required; potential for increase in the clearance of ritonavir resulting in decreased ritonavir plasma concentrations).
No products indexed under this heading.

Phenytoin (Co-administration may result in decreased phenytoin plasma concentrations; dose increase of phenytoin may be needed. Use with caution).
No products indexed under this heading.

Phenytoin Sodium (Co-administration may result in decreased phenytoin plasma concentrations; dose increase of phenytoin may be needed. Use with caution). Products include:
- Phenytek Capsules 2153

Pimozide (Co-administration is contraindicated due to potential for serious and/or life-threatening reactions, such as cardiac arrhythmias). Products include:
- Orap Tablets 1220

Pindolol (Co-administration results in a possible increase in AUC of pindolol; dosage adjustments may be required).
No products indexed under this heading.

Pioglitazone Hydrochloride (New onset diabetes mellitus, exacerbation of pre-existing diabetes, and hyperglycemia have been reported with protease inhibitors; dosage adjustment of oral hypoglycemic agents may be required). Products include:
- ActoPlus Met Tablets 3219
- Actos Tablets 3224

Piroxicam (Ritonavir is expected to produce a large increase in the plasma concentrations of piroxicam; concurrent use is contraindicated).
No products indexed under this heading.

Pravastatin Sodium (Co-administration results in a large

increase (> 3x) in AUC of pravastatin; dosage adjustments may be required). Products include:
Pravachol Tablets 943

Prazosin Hydrochloride (Co-administration results in a possible increase in AUC of prazosin; dosage adjustments may be required).
No products indexed under this heading.

Prednisone (Co-administration may result in increased prednisone plasma concentrations; dose decrease of prednisone may be needed. Use with caution).
No products indexed under this heading.

Primaquine Phosphate (Co-administration results in a possible increase in AUC of primaquine; dosage adjustments may be required).
No products indexed under this heading.

Prochlorperazine (Co-administration results in a possible increase in AUC of prochlorperazine; dosage adjustments may be required).
No products indexed under this heading.

Proguanil (Co-administration results in a moderate increase or decrease in AUC of proguanil; dosage adjustments may be required).
No products indexed under this heading.

Promethazine Hydrochloride (Co-administration results in a possible increase in AUC of promethazine; dosage adjustments may be required). Products include:
Phenergan 3438

Propafenone Hydrochloride (Co-administration is contraindicated due to potential for serious and/or life-threatening reactions, such as cardiac arrhythmias). Products include:
Rythmol SR Capsules 2736

Propofol (Ritonavir may increase the activity of glucuronosyltransferase; co-administration results in a decrease in AUC of propofol; dosage adjustments may be required). Products include:
Diprivan Injectable Emulsion 676

Propoxyphene Hydrochloride (Ritonavir may produce an increase in the plasma concentrations of propoxyphene. Dosage adjustment may be needed. Use with caution).
No products indexed under this heading.

Propoxyphene Napsylate (Ritonavir may produce an increase in the plasma concentrations of propoxyphene. Dosage adjustment may be needed. Use with caution). Products include:
Darvocet A 500 Tablets 3497

Propranolol Hydrochloride (Co-administration results in a moderate increase (1.5 to 3x) in AUC of propranolol; dosage adjustments may be required). Products include:
Inderal LA Long-Acting Capsules 3421
InnoPran XL Capsules 2728

Protriptyline Hydrochloride (Co-administration may result in increased tricyclic antidepressants' plasma concentrations; dose decrease of tricyclics may be needed. Use with caution). Products include:
Vivactil Tablets 2350

Pyrimethamine (Co-administration results in a possible increase in AUC of pyrimethamine; dosage adjustments may be required). Products include:
Daraprim Tablets 1385

Quinidine (Co-administration is contraindicated due to potential for serious and/or life-threatening reactions, such as cardiac arrhythmias).
No products indexed under this heading.

Quinidine Gluconate (Co-administration is contraindicated due to potential for serious and/or life-threatening reactions, such as cardiac arrhythmias).
No products indexed under this heading.

Quinidine Hydrochloride (Co-administration is contraindicated due to potential for serious and/or life-threatening reactions, such as cardiac arrhythmias).
No products indexed under this heading.

Quinidine Polygalacturonate (Co-administration is contraindicated due to potential for serious and/or life-threatening reactions, such as cardiac arrhythmias).
No products indexed under this heading.

Quinidine Sulfate (Co-administration is contraindicated due to potential for serious and/or life-threatening reactions, such as cardiac arrhythmias).
No products indexed under this heading.

Quinine Sulfate (Co-administration may result in increased quinine plasma concentrations; dose decrease of quinine may be needed. Use with caution).
No products indexed under this heading.

Repaglinide (New onset diabetes mellitus, exacerbation of pre-existing diabetes, and hyperglycemia have been reported with protease inhibitors; dosage adjustment of oral hypoglycemic agents may be required). Products include:
Prandin Tablets (0.5, 1, and 2 mg) 2337

Rifabutin (Co-administration results in increased rifabutin and rifabutin metabolite concentration; dosage reduction of rifabutin by at least three-quarters of the usual dose of 300 mg/day is recommended).
No products indexed under this heading.

Rifampicin (Potential for increase in the clearance of ritonavir resulting in decreased ritonavir plasma concentrations).
No products indexed under this heading.

Rifampin (Co-administration has resulted in decreased ritonavir concentration leading to loss of virologic response. Consider alternate antimyobacterial agents).
No products indexed under this heading.

Rifapentine (Potential for increase in the clearance of ritonavir resulting in decreased ritonavir plasma concentrations).
No products indexed under this heading.

Risperidone (Co-administration may result in increased risperidone plasma concentrations; dose decrease of risperidone may be needed. Use with caution). Products include:
Risperdal Consta Long-Acting Injection 1664
Risperdal M-Tab Orally Disintegrating Tablets 1658
Risperdal 1658

Rosiglitazone Maleate (New onset diabetes mellitus, exacerbation of pre-existing diabetes, and hyperglycemia have been reported with protease inhibitors; dosage adjustment of oral hypoglycemic agents may be required). Products include:
Avandamet Tablets 1343
Avandia Tablets 1348

Saquinavir (When co-administered with reduced doses of saquinavir and ritonavir increased saquinavir concentration, increased AUC, Cmax, and Cmin have resulted).
No products indexed under this heading.

Saquinavir Mesylate (When co-administered with reduced doses of saquinavir and ritonavir, increased saquinavir concentration, increased AUC, Cmax, and Cmin have resulted). Products include:
Invirase 2776

Sertraline Hydrochloride (Co-administration results in a large increase (> 3x) in AUC of sertraline; dosage adjustments may be required). Products include:
Zoloft 2581

Sildenafil Citrate (Co-administration is expected to substantially increase sildenafil concentrations, 11-fold increase in AUC, and may result in an increase in sildenafil-associated adverse events, including hypotension, syncope, visual changes, and prolonged erection; sildenafil should not exceed a maximum dose of 25 mg in a 48-hour period in patients receiving concomitant therapy). Products include:
Revatio Tablets 2541
Viagra Tablets 2552

Simvastatin (Co-administration results in increased plasma concentrations of simvastatin; the risk of myopathy, including rhabdomyolysis, may be increased). Products include:
Vytorin 10/10 Tablets 2084
Vytorin 10/10 Tablets 3092
Vytorin 10/20 Tablets 2084
Vytorin 10/20 Tablets 3092
Vytorin 10/40 Tablets 3092
Vytorin 10/40 Tablets 2084
Vytorin 10/80 Tablets 2084
Vytorin 10/80 Tablets 3092
Zocor Tablets 2078

Sirolimus (Co-administration may result in increased sirolimus plasma concentrations; dose decrease of sirolimus may be needed. Use with caution). Products include:
Rapamune Oral Solution and Tablets 3472

Sotalol Hydrochloride (Co-administration with beta-blockers has resulted in cardiac and neurologic events).
No products indexed under this heading.

Sulfamethoxazole (Co-administration with a combination tablet containing sulfamethoxazole and trimethoprim has resulted in decreased AUC of sulfamethoxazole by 20% and no change in AUC).
No products indexed under this heading.

Tacrolimus (Co-administration may result in increased tacrolimus plasma concentrations; dose decrease of tacrolimus may be needed. Use with caution). Products include:
Prograf Capsules and Injection 624
Protopic Ointment 629

Tamoxifen Citrate (Co-administration results in a large increase (> 3x) in AUC of tamoxifen; dosage adjustments may be required).
No products indexed under this heading.

Temazepam (Ritonavir may increase the activity of glucuronosyltransferase; co-administration results in a decrease in AUC of temazepam; dosage adjustments may be required).
No products indexed under this heading.

Terazosin Hydrochloride (Co-administration results in a possible increase in AUC of terazosin; dosage adjustments may be required). Products include:
Hytrin Capsules 469

Terfenadine (Co-administration is contraindicated due to potential for serious and/or life-threatening reactions, such as cardiac arrhythmias).
No products indexed under this heading.

Theophylline (Co-administration results in the reduction of the average AUC of theophylline; increased dosage of theophylline may be required and therapeutic monitoring should be considered).
No products indexed under this heading.

Theophylline Anhydrous (Co-administration results in the reduction of the average AUC of theophylline; increased dosage of theophylline may be required and therapeutic monitoring should be considered). Products include:
Uniphyl Tablets 2708

Theophylline Calcium Salicylate (Co-administration results in the reduction of the average AUC of theophylline; increased dosage of theophylline may be required and therapeutic monitoring should be considered).
No products indexed under this heading.

Theophylline Dihydroxypropyl (Glyceryl) (Co-administration results in the reduction of the average AUC of theophylline; increased dosage of theophylline may be required and therapeutic monitoring should be considered).
No products indexed under this heading.

Theophylline Ethylenediamine (Co-administration results in the reduction of the average AUC of theophylline; increased dosage of theophylline may be required and therapeutic monitoring should be considered).
No products indexed under this heading.

Theophylline Sodium Glycinate (Co-administration results in the reduction of the average AUC of theophylline; increased dosage of theophylline may be required and therapeutic monitoring should be considered).
No products indexed under this heading.

Thioridazine Hydrochloride (Co-administration may result in increased thioridazine plasma con-

centrations; dose decrease of thioridazine may be needed. Use with caution). Products include:
Thioridazine Hydrochloride Tablets 2122

Timolol Hemihydrate (Co-administration may result in increased timolol plasma concentrations; cardiac and neurologic events have been reported with co-administration. Dosage adjustment may be needed. Use with caution). Products include:
Betimol Ophthalmic Solution 3371
Betimol Ophthalmic Solution .... ⊙283

Timolol Maleate (Co-administration may result in increased timolol plasma concentrations; dosage adjustment may be needed). Products include:
Blocadren Tablets 1891
Cosopt Sterile Ophthalmic Solution 1910
Timolide Tablets 2056
Timoptic in Ocudose 2061
Timoptic Sterile Ophthalmic Solution 2058
Timoptic-XE Sterile Ophthalmic Gel Forming Solution 2062

Tocainide Hydrochloride (Co-administration results in a possible increase in AUC of tocainide; dosage adjustments may be required).
No products indexed under this heading.

Tolazamide (New onset diabetes mellitus, exacerbation of pre-existing diabetes, and hyperglycemia have been reported with protease inhibitors; dosage adjustment of oral hypoglycemic agents may be required).
No products indexed under this heading.

Tolbutamide (Co-administration results in a moderate increase or decrease in AUC of tolbutamide; dosage adjustments may be required).
No products indexed under this heading.

Tramadol Hydrochloride (Co-administration may result in an increase in AUC of tramadol; dosage adjustments may be required. Use with caution). Products include:
Ultracet Tablets 2462

Trazodone Hydrochloride (Co-administration results in a large increase (> 3x) in AUC of trazodone; dosage adjustments may be required).
No products indexed under this heading.

Triazolam (Co-administration is contraindicated due to potential for prolonged or increased sedation and/or respiratory depression).
No products indexed under this heading.

Trimethoprim (Co-administration with a combination tablet containing sulfamethoxazole and trimethoprim has resulted in increased AUC of trimethoprim by 20% and no change in AUC of ritonavir).
No products indexed under this heading.

Trimipramine Maleate (Co-administration may result in increased tricyclic antidepressants' plasma concentrations; dose decrease of tricyclics may be needed. Use with caution). Products include:
Surmontil Capsules 2347

Troglitazone (New onset diabetes mellitus, exacerbation of pre-existing diabetes, and hyperglycemia have been reported with protease inhibitors; dosage adjustment of oral hypoglycemic agents may be required).
No products indexed under this heading.

Valproate Sodium (Co-administration may result in decreased valproate plasma concentrations; dose increase of valproate may be needed. Use with caution). Products include:
Depacon Injection 412

Valproic Acid (Co-administration may result in decreased valproate plasma concentrations; dose increase of valproate may be needed. Use with caution). Products include:
Depakene 417

Venlafaxine Hydrochloride (Co-administration results in a moderate increase (1.5 to 3x) in AUC of venlafaxine; dosage adjustments may be required). Products include:
Effexor Tablets 3405
Effexor XR Capsules 3411

Verapamil Hydrochloride (Co-administration may result in increased verapamil plasma concentrations; dose decrease of verapamil may be needed. Use with caution). Products include:
Covera-HS Tablets 3135
Tarka Tablets 519
Verelan PM Capsules 3120

Vinblastine Sulfate (Co-administration results in a large increase (> 3x) in AUC of vinblastine; dosage adjustments may be required).
No products indexed under this heading.

Vincristine Sulfate (Co-administration results in a large increase (> 3x) in AUC of vincristine; dosage adjustments may be required).
No products indexed under this heading.

Warfarin Sodium (Co-administration may result in decreased warfarin plasma concentrations; initial frequent monitoring of the INR during ritonavir and nartarin co-administration is indicated). Products include:
Coumadin for Injection 932
Coumadin Tablets 932

Zidovudine (Co-administration has resulted in decreased AUC and Cmax of zidovudine by 25% and 27%, respectively, and no change in ritonavir AUC and/or Cmax). Products include:
Combivir Tablets 1373
Retrovir 1533
Retrovir IV Infusion 1537
Trizivir Tablets 1565

Zolpidem Tartrate (Co-administration may result in increased zolpidem plasma concentrations; dose decrease of zolpidem may be needed. Use with caution). Products include:
Ambien Tablets 2867

Food Interactions

Meal, unspecified (Relative to fasting conditions, the extent of absorption of ritonavir from capsule formulation was 15% higher when administered with a meal; decreased peak ritonavir concentrations when oral solution was given under non-fasting condition).

NORVIR ORAL SOLUTION
(Ritonavir) 499
See Norvir Soft Gelatin Capsules

NOVANTRONE FOR INJECTION CONCENTRATE
(Mitoxantrone Hydrochloride) 3158
None cited in PDR database.

NOVAREL FOR INJECTION
(Chorionic Gonadotropin) 1147
None cited in PDR database.

NOVOLIN 70/30 HUMAN INSULIN 10 ML VIALS
(Insulin, Human Regular and Human NPH Mixture) 2321
None cited in PDR database.

NOVOLIN 70/30 INNOLET
(Insulin, Human Regular and Human NPH Mixture) 2322
None cited in PDR database.

NOVOLIN 70/30 PENFILL 3 ML CARTRIDGES
(Insulin, Human Regular and Human NPH Mixture) 2325
None cited in PDR database.

NOVOLIN N HUMAN INSULIN 10 ML VIALS
(Insulin, Human NPH) 2322
None cited in PDR database.

NOVOLIN N INNOLET
(Insulin, Human NPH) 2322
None cited in PDR database.

NOVOLIN N PENFILL 3 ML CARTRIDGES
(Insulin, Human NPH) 2325
None cited in PDR database.

NOVOLIN R HUMAN INSULIN 10 ML VIALS
(Insulin, Human Regular) 2322
None cited in PDR database.

NOVOLIN R INNOLET
(Insulin, Human NPH) 2322
None cited in PDR database.

NOVOLIN R PENFILL 1.5 ML CARTRIDGES
(Insulin, Human Regular) 2325
None cited in PDR database.

NOVOLIN R PENFILL 3 ML CARTRIDGES
(Insulin, Human Regular) 2325
None cited in PDR database.

NOVOLOG INJECTION
(Insulin Aspart, Human Regular) 2326
May interact with ACE inhibitors, beta blockers, corticosteroids, diuretics, fibrates, oral hypoglycemic agents, lithium preparations, monoamine oxidase inhibitors, oral contraceptives, phenothiazines, salicylates, sympathomimetics, thyroid preparations, and certain other agents. Compounds in these categories include:

Acarbose (May increase the blood-glucose-lowering effect and susceptibility to hypoglycemia). Products include:
Precose Tablets 776

Acebutolol Hydrochloride (Beta-blockers may either potentiate or weaken the blood-glucose-lowering effect of insulin; signs of hypoglycemia may be reduced or absent with co-administration).
No products indexed under this heading.

Albuterol (Sympathomimetic agents may reduce the blood-glucose-lowering effect of insulin). Products include:
Proventil Inhalation Aerosol 3067

Albuterol Sulfate (Sympathomimetic agents may reduce the blood-glucose-lowering effect of insulin). Products include:
AccuNeb Inhalation Solution 1055
Combivent Inhalation Aerosol 878
DuoNeb Inhalation Solution 1058
Proventil Inhalation Solution 0.083% 3069
Proventil HFA Inhalation Aerosol 3071
Ventolin HFA Inhalation Aerosol 1576
VoSpire Extended-Release Tablets 2352

Amiloride Hydrochloride (Diuretics may reduce the blood-glucose-lowering effect of insulin). Products include:
Midamor Tablets 2000
Moduretic Tablets 2003

Aspirin (May increase the blood-glucose-lowering effect and susceptibility to hypoglycemia). Products include:
Aggrenox Capsules 855
Bayer, Aspirin Regimen .... ▣606
Bayer Aspirin Tablets 3515
BC Powder .... ▣612
BC Allergy Sinus Cold Powder .... ▣612
Arthritis Strength BC Powder .... ▣612
BC Sinus Cold Powder .... ▣612
Ecotrin Enteric Coated Aspirin Low, Regular and Maximum Strength Tablets 1627
Goody's Body Pain Formula Powder .... ▣621
Goody's Extra Strength Headache Powder .... ▣621
Goody's Extra Strength Pain Relief Tablets .... ▣621
Percodan Tablets 1115
St. Joseph 81 mg Aspirin Chewable and Enteric Coated Tablets 1841

Aspirin, Enteric Coated (May increase the blood-glucose-lowering effect and susceptibility to hypoglycemia).
No products indexed under this heading.

Aspirin Buffered (May increase the blood-glucose-lowering effect and susceptibility to hypoglycemia).
No products indexed under this heading.

Atenolol (Beta-blockers may either potentiate or weaken the blood-glucose-lowering effect of insulin; signs of hypoglycemia may be reduced or absent with co-administration). Products include:
Tenormin I.V. Injection 698
Tenormin Tablets 695

Benazepril Hydrochloride (May increase the blood-glucose-lowering effect and susceptibility to hypoglycemia). Products include:
Lotensin Tablets 2232
Lotensin HCT Tablets 2235
Lotrel Capsules 2238

Bendroflumethiazide (Diuretics may reduce the blood-glucose-lowering effect of insulin).
No products indexed under this heading.

Betamethasone Acetate (Co-administration with corticosteroids may reduce the blood-glucose-lowering effect of insulin).
No products indexed under this heading.

Betamethasone Sodium Phosphate (Co-administration with corticosteroids may reduce the blood-glucose-lowering effect of insulin).
No products indexed under this heading.

Betaxolol Hydrochloride (Beta-blockers may either potentiate or weaken the blood-glucose-lowering effect of insulin; signs of hypoglycemia may be reduced or absent with co-administration). Products include:
Betoptic S Ophthalmic Suspension 554

Bisoprolol Fumarate (Beta-blockers may either potentiate or weaken the blood-glucose-lowering effect of insulin; signs of hypoglycemia may be reduced or absent with co-administration).
No products indexed under this heading.

Bumetanide (Diuretics may reduce the blood-glucose-lowering effect of insulin).
No products indexed under this heading.

Captopril (May increase the blood-glucose-lowering effect and susceptibility to hypoglycemia). Products include:
Captopril Tablets 2114

Carteolol Hydrochloride (Beta-blockers may either potentiate or weaken the blood-glucose-lowering effect of insulin; signs of hypoglycemia may be reduced or absent with co-administration). Products include:
Carteolol Hydrochloride Ophthalmic Solution USP, 1% .... ⊙246

Chlorothiazide (Diuretics may reduce the blood-glucose-lowering effect of insulin). Products include:
Aldoclor Tablets 1881
Diuril Oral 1936

Chlorothiazide Sodium (Diuretics may reduce the blood-glucose-lowering effect of insulin). Products include:
Diuril Sodium Intravenous 1934

Chlorpromazine (Phenothiazine derivatives may reduce the blood-glucose-lowering effect of insulin).
No products indexed under this heading.

Chlorpromazine Hydrochloride (Phenothiazine derivatives may reduce the blood-glucose-lowering effect of insulin).
No products indexed under this heading.

Chlorpropamide (May increase the blood-glucose-lowering effect and susceptibility to hypoglycemia).
No products indexed under this heading.

Chlorthalidone (Diuretics may reduce the blood-glucose-lowering effect of insulin). Products include:
Clorpres Tablets 2139

Choline Magnesium Trisalicylate (May increase the blood-glucose-lowering effect and susceptibility to hypoglycemia).
No products indexed under this heading.

Clofibrate (May increase the blood-glucose-lowering effect and susceptibility to hypoglycemia).
No products indexed under this heading.

Clonidine (Signs of hypoglycemia may be reduced or absent with co-administration). Products include:
Catapres-TTS 875

Clonidine Hydrochloride (Signs of hypoglycemia may be reduced or absent with co-administration). Products include:
Catapres Tablets 874
Clorpres Tablets 2139

Cortisone Acetate (Co-administration with corticosteroids may reduce the blood-glucose-lowering effect of insulin).
No products indexed under this heading.

Danazol (May reduce the blood-glucose-lowering effect of insulin).
No products indexed under this heading.

Desogestrel (Oral contraceptives may reduce the blood-glucose-lowering effect of insulin). Products include:
Ortho-Cept Tablets 2395

Dexamethasone (Co-administration with corticosteroids may reduce the blood-glucose-lowering effect of insulin). Products include:
Ciprodex Otic Suspension 555
Decadron Tablets 1929
TobraDex Ophthalmic Ointment 558
TobraDex Ophthalmic Suspension ... 558

Dexamethasone Acetate (Co-administration with corticosteroids may reduce the blood-glucose-lowering effect of insulin).
No products indexed under this heading.

Dexamethasone Sodium Phosphate (Co-administration with corticosteroids may reduce the blood-glucose-lowering effect of insulin). Products include:
Decadron Phosphate Injection 1931

Diflunisal (May increase the blood-glucose-lowering effect and susceptibility to hypoglycemia). Products include:
Dolobid Tablets 1937

Disopyramide Phosphate (May increase the blood-glucose-lowering effect and susceptibility to hypoglycemia).
No products indexed under this heading.

Dobutamine Hydrochloride (Sympathomimetic agents may reduce the blood-glucose-lowering effect of insulin).
No products indexed under this heading.

Dopamine Hydrochloride (Sympathomimetic agents may reduce the blood-glucose-lowering effect of insulin).
No products indexed under this heading.

Enalapril Maleate (May increase the blood-glucose-lowering effect and susceptibility to hypoglycemia). Products include:
Vaseretic Tablets 2073
Vasotec I.V. Injection 2076

Enalaprilat (May increase the blood-glucose-lowering effect and susceptibility to hypoglycemia).
No products indexed under this heading.

Ephedrine Hydrochloride (Sympathomimetic agents may reduce the blood-glucose-lowering effect of insulin). Products include:
Primatene Tablets .... ▣749

Ephedrine Sulfate (Sympathomimetic agents may reduce the blood-glucose-lowering effect of insulin).
No products indexed under this heading.

Ephedrine Tannate (Sympathomimetic agents may reduce the blood-glucose-lowering effect of insulin).
No products indexed under this heading.

Epinephrine (Sympathomimetic agents may reduce the blood-glucose-lowering effect of insulin). Products include:
EpiPen 1061
Primatene Mist .... ▣749

Epinephrine Bitartrate (Sympathomimetic agents may reduce the blood-glucose-lowering effect of insulin).
No products indexed under this heading.

Epinephrine Hydrochloride (Sympathomimetic agents may reduce the blood-glucose-lowering effect of insulin).
No products indexed under this heading.

Esmolol Hydrochloride (Beta-blockers may either potentiate or weaken the blood-glucose-lowering effect of insulin; signs of hypoglycemia may be reduced or absent with co-administration). Products include:
Brevibloc Concentrate 766
Brevibloc Injection 766
Brevibloc Double Strength Injection 766
Brevibloc Premixed Injection 766
Brevibloc Double Strength Premixed Injection 766

Ethacrynic Acid (Diuretics may reduce the blood-glucose-lowering effect of insulin). Products include:
Edecrin Tablets 1941

Ethinyl Estradiol (Oral contraceptives may reduce the blood-glucose-lowering effect of insulin). Products include:
Alesse-28 Tablets 3392
Lo/Ovral-28 Tablets 3423
NuvaRing 2357
Ortho-Cept Tablets 2395
Ortho-Cyclen/Ortho Tri-Cyclen 2414
Ortho Evra Transdermal System 2402
Ortho Tri-Cyclen Lo Tablets 2421
Seasonale Tablets 1073
Triphasil-28 Tablets 3483
Yasmin 28 Tablets 818

Ethynodiol Diacetate (Oral contraceptives may reduce the blood-glucose-lowering effect of insulin).
No products indexed under this heading.

Fenofibrate (May increase the blood-glucose-lowering effect and susceptibility to hypoglycemia). Products include:
Antara Capsules 2723
Lofibra Capsules 1217
Tricor Tablets 523
Triglide Tablets 1165

Fludrocortisone Acetate (Co-administration with corticosteroids may reduce the blood-glucose-lowering effect of insulin).
No products indexed under this heading.

Fluoxetine Hydrochloride (May increase the blood-glucose-lowering effect and susceptibility to hypoglycemia). Products include:
Prozac Pulvules and Liquid 1771
Symbyax Capsules 1788

Fluphenazine Decanoate (Phenothiazine derivatives may reduce the blood-glucose-lowering effect of insulin).
No products indexed under this heading.

Fluphenazine Enanthate (Phenothiazine derivatives may reduce the blood-glucose-lowering effect of insulin).
No products indexed under this heading.

Fluphenazine Hydrochloride (Phenothiazine derivatives may reduce the blood-glucose-lowering effect of insulin).
No products indexed under this heading.

Fosinopril Sodium (May increase the blood-glucose-lowering effect and susceptibility to hypoglycemia).
No products indexed under this heading.

Furosemide (Diuretics may reduce the blood-glucose-lowering effect of insulin). Products include:
Furosemide Tablets 2117

Gemfibrozil (May increase the blood-glucose-lowering effect and susceptibility to hypoglycemia).
No products indexed under this heading.

Glimepiride (May increase the blood-glucose-lowering effect and susceptibility to hypoglycemia). Products include:
Amaryl Tablets 2864

Glipizide (May increase the blood-glucose-lowering effect and susceptibility to hypoglycemia).
No products indexed under this heading.

Glyburide (May increase the blood-glucose-lowering effect and susceptibility to hypoglycemia).
No products indexed under this heading.

Guanethidine Monosulfate (Signs of hypoglycemia may be reduced or absent with co-administration).
No products indexed under this heading.

Hydrochlorothiazide (Diuretics may reduce the blood-glucose-lowering effect of insulin). Products include:
Aldoril Tablets 1884
Atacand HCT 637
Avalide Tablets 2889
Avalide Tablets 922
Benicar HCT Tablets 2852
Diovan HCT Tablets 2195
Dyazide Capsules 1389
Hyzaar 1964
Lotensin HCT Tablets 2235
Maxzide 2150
Micardis HCT Tablets 886
Moduretic Tablets 2003
Prinzide Tablets 2033
Teveten HCT Tablets 1710
Timolide Tablets 2056
Uniretic Tablets 3114
Vaseretic Tablets 2073
Zestoretic Tablets 701

Hydrocortisone (Co-administration with corticosteroids may reduce the blood-glucose-lowering effect of insulin). Products include:
Cortizone•5 Ointment .... ▣699
Cortizone•10 Creme .... ▣699
Cortizone•10 Ointment .... ▣699
Cortizone•10 Plus Creme .... ▣700
Cortizone•10 Maximum Strength Quick Shot Spray .... ▣700
Hydrocortone Tablets 1963
Preparation H Hydrocortisone Cream .... ▣748

IMPORTANT NOTE: Always consult each drug listing in the patient's regimen for possible interactions.

Hydrocortisone Acetate (Co-administration with corticosteroids may reduce the blood-glucose-lowering effect of insulin). Products include:
- Analpram-HC 1136
- Pramosone 1139
- ProctoFoam-HC 3113
- Tucks Anti-Itch Ointment .... ▣712
- U-cort 1% Cream 3289

Hydrocortisone Sodium Phosphate (Co-administration with corticosteroids may reduce the blood-glucose-lowering effect of insulin).
No products indexed under this heading.

Hydrocortisone Sodium Succinate (Co-administration with corticosteroids may reduce the blood-glucose-lowering effect of insulin).
No products indexed under this heading.

Hydroflumethiazide (Diuretics may reduce the blood-glucose-lowering effect of insulin).
No products indexed under this heading.

Indapamide (Diuretics may reduce the blood-glucose-lowering effect of insulin). Products include:
- Indapamide Tablets 2119

Isocarboxazid (May increase the blood-glucose-lowering effect and susceptibility to hypoglycemia).
No products indexed under this heading.

Isoniazid (May reduce the blood-glucose-lowering effect of insulin).
No products indexed under this heading.

Isoproterenol Hydrochloride (Sympathomimetic agents may reduce the blood-glucose-lowering effect of insulin).
No products indexed under this heading.

Isoproterenol Sulfate (Sympathomimetic agents may reduce the blood-glucose-lowering effect of insulin).
No products indexed under this heading.

Labetalol Hydrochloride (Beta-blockers may either potentiate or weaken the blood-glucose-lowering effect of insulin; signs of hypoglycemia may be reduced or absent with co-administration).
No products indexed under this heading.

Levalbuterol Hydrochloride (Sympathomimetic agents may reduce the blood-glucose-lowering effect of insulin). Products include:
- Xopenex Inhalation Solution 3143
- Xopenex Inhalation Solution Concentrate 3147

Levobunolol Hydrochloride (Beta-blockers may either potentiate or weaken the blood-glucose-lowering effect of insulin; signs of hypoglycemia may be reduced or absent with co-administration). Products include:
- Betagan Ophthalmic Solution, USP .... ⊙217

Levonorgestrel (Oral contraceptives may reduce the blood-glucose-lowering effect of insulin). Products include:
- Alesse-28 Tablets 3392
- Climara Pro Transdermal System 800
- Mirena Intrauterine System 810
- Plan B Tablets 1068
- Seasonale Tablets 1073
- Triphasil-28 Tablets 3483

Levothyroxine Sodium (May reduce the blood-glucose-lowering effect of insulin). Products include:
- Levothroid Tablets 1189
- Levoxyl Tablets 1680
- Synthroid Tablets 515
- Unithroid Tablets 3521

Liothyronine Sodium (May reduce the blood-glucose-lowering effect of insulin). Products include:
- Cytomel Tablets 1678

Liotrix (May reduce the blood-glucose-lowering effect of insulin). Products include:
- Thyrolar 1203

Lisinopril (May increase the blood-glucose-lowering effect and susceptibility to hypoglycemia). Products include:
- Prinivil Tablets 2029
- Prinzide Tablets 2033
- Zestoretic Tablets 701
- Zestril Tablets 704

Lithium (May either potentiate or weaken the blood-glucose-lowering effect of insulin).
No products indexed under this heading.

Lithium Carbonate (May either potentiate or weaken the blood-glucose-lowering effect of insulin). Products include:
- Eskalith 1406
- Lithobid Tablets 1670

Lithium Citrate (May either potentiate or weaken the blood-glucose-lowering effect of insulin).
No products indexed under this heading.

Magnesium Salicylate (May increase the blood-glucose-lowering effect and susceptibility to hypoglycemia).
No products indexed under this heading.

Mesoridazine Besylate (Phenothiazine derivatives may reduce the blood-glucose-lowering effect of insulin).
No products indexed under this heading.

Mestranol (Oral contraceptives may reduce the blood-glucose-lowering effect of insulin).
No products indexed under this heading.

Metaproterenol Sulfate (Sympathomimetic agents may reduce the blood-glucose-lowering effect of insulin). Products include:
- Alupent Inhalation Aerosol 858

Metaraminol Bitartrate (Sympathomimetic agents may reduce the blood-glucose-lowering effect of insulin). Products include:
- Aramine Injection 1889

Metformin Hydrochloride (May increase the blood-glucose-lowering effect and susceptibility to hypoglycemia). Products include:
- ActoPlus Met Tablets 3219
- Avandamet Tablets 1343
- Fortamet Extended-Release Tablets 1156

Methotrimeprazine (Phenothiazine derivatives may reduce the blood-glucose-lowering effect of insulin).
No products indexed under this heading.

Methoxamine Hydrochloride (Sympathomimetic agents may reduce the blood-glucose-lowering effect of insulin).
No products indexed under this heading.

Methyclothiazide (Diuretics may reduce the blood-glucose-lowering effect of insulin).
No products indexed under this heading.

Methylprednisolone Acetate (Co-administration with corticosteroids may reduce the blood-glucose-lowering effect of insulin). Products include:
- Depo-Medrol Injectable Suspension 2615
- Depo-Medrol Single-Dose Vial 2617

Methylprednisolone Sodium Succinate (Co-administration with corticosteroids may reduce the blood-glucose-lowering effect of insulin).
No products indexed under this heading.

Metipranolol Hydrochloride (Beta-blockers may either potentiate or weaken the blood-glucose-lowering effect of insulin; signs of hypoglycemia may be reduced or absent with co-administration).
No products indexed under this heading.

Metolazone (Diuretics may reduce the blood-glucose-lowering effect of insulin).
No products indexed under this heading.

Metoprolol Succinate (Beta-blockers may either potentiate or weaken the blood-glucose-lowering effect of insulin; signs of hypoglycemia may be reduced or absent with co-administration). Products include:
- Toprol-XL Tablets 660

Metoprolol Tartrate (Beta-blockers may either potentiate or weaken the blood-glucose-lowering effect of insulin; signs of hypoglycemia may be reduced or absent with co-administration).
No products indexed under this heading.

Miglitol (May increase the blood-glucose-lowering effect and susceptibility to hypoglycemia).
No products indexed under this heading.

Moclobemide (May increase the blood-glucose-lowering effect and susceptibility to hypoglycemia).
No products indexed under this heading.

Moexipril Hydrochloride (May increase the blood-glucose-lowering effect and susceptibility to hypoglycemia). Products include:
- Uniretic Tablets 3114
- Univasc Tablets 3118

Nadolol (Beta-blockers may either potentiate or weaken the blood-glucose-lowering effect of insulin; signs of hypoglycemia may be reduced or absent with co-administration). Products include:
- Nadolol Tablets 2121

Niacin (May reduce the blood-glucose-lowering effect of insulin). Products include:
- Advicor Tablets 1694
- Niaspan Extended-Release Tablets 1703

Norepinephrine Bitartrate (Sympathomimetic agents may reduce the blood-glucose-lowering effect of insulin).
No products indexed under this heading.

Norethindrone (Oral contraceptives may reduce the blood-glucose-lowering effect of insulin). Products include:
- Ortho Micronor Tablets 2411

Norethynodrel (Oral contraceptives may reduce the blood-glucose-lowering effect of insulin).
No products indexed under this heading.

Norgestimate (Oral contraceptives may reduce the blood-glucose-lowering effect of insulin). Products include:
- Ortho-Cyclen/Ortho Tri-Cyclen 2414
- Ortho Tri-Cyclen Lo Tablets 2421
- Prefest Tablets 1069

Norgestrel (Oral contraceptives may reduce the blood-glucose-lowering effect of insulin). Products include:
- Lo/Ovral-28 Tablets 3423

Octreotide Acetate (May increase the blood-glucose-lowering effect and susceptibility to hypoglycemia). Products include:
- Sandostatin Injection 2263
- Sandostatin LAR Depot 2264

Pargyline Hydrochloride (May increase the blood-glucose-lowering effect and susceptibility to hypoglycemia).
No products indexed under this heading.

Penbutolol Sulfate (Beta-blockers may either potentiate or weaken the blood-glucose-lowering effect of insulin; signs of hypoglycemia may be reduced or absent with co-administration).
No products indexed under this heading.

Pentamidine Isethionate (May cause hypoglycemia, which may sometimes be followed by hyperglycemia).
No products indexed under this heading.

Perindopril Erbumine (May increase the blood-glucose-lowering effect and susceptibility to hypoglycemia). Products include:
- Aceon Tablets (2 mg, 4 mg, 8 mg) 3191

Perphenazine (Phenothiazine derivatives may reduce the blood-glucose-lowering effect of insulin).
No products indexed under this heading.

Phenelzine Sulfate (May increase the blood-glucose-lowering effect and susceptibility to hypoglycemia).
No products indexed under this heading.

Phenylephrine Bitartrate (Sympathomimetic agents may reduce the blood-glucose-lowering effect of insulin).
No products indexed under this heading.

Phenylephrine Hydrochloride (Sympathomimetic agents may reduce the blood-glucose-lowering effect of insulin). Products include:
- Alacol DM Syrup 739
- Hycomine Compound Tablets 1105
- Preparation H Maximum Strength Cream .... ▣747
- Preparation H Cooling Gel .... ▣747
- Preparation H .... ▣747
- Sudafed PE Tablets .... ▣711
- Vicks Sinex Nasal Spray and Ultra Fine Mist for Sinus Relief 2677
- Zicam Concentrated Cough Mist for Kids Plus D Cool Cherry .... ▣643
- Zicam Concentrated Cough Mist Plus D Cool Cherry .... ▣642

Phenylephrine Tannate (Sympathomimetic agents may reduce the blood-glucose-lowering effect of insulin).
No products indexed under this heading.

Phenylpropanolamine Hydrochloride (Sympathomimetic agents may reduce the blood-glucose-lowering effect of insulin).
No products indexed under this heading.

Pindolol (Beta-blockers may either potentiate or weaken the blood-glucose-lowering effect of insulin; signs of hypoglycemia may be reduced or absent with co-administration).
No products indexed under this heading.

Pioglitazone Hydrochloride (May increase the blood-glucose-lowering effect and susceptibility to hypoglycemia). Products include:
ActoPlus Met Tablets ... 3219
Actos Tablets ... 3224

Pirbuterol Acetate (Sympathomimetic agents may reduce the blood-glucose-lowering effect of insulin). Products include:
Maxair Autohaler ... 1820

Polythiazide (Diuretics may reduce the blood-glucose-lowering effect of insulin).
No products indexed under this heading.

Prednisolone Acetate (Co-administration with corticosteroids may reduce the blood-glucose-lowering effect of insulin). Products include:
Blephamide Ophthalmic Ointment ... 563
Blephamide Ophthalmic Suspension ... 564
Poly-Pred Liquifilm Ophthalmic Suspension ... ⊙ 231
Pred Forte Ophthalmic Suspension ... ⊙ 233
Pred Mild Sterile Ophthalmic Suspension ... ⊙ 236
Pred-G Ophthalmic Suspension ... ⊙ 234
Pred-G Sterile Ophthalmic Ointment ... ⊙ 235

Prednisolone Sodium Phosphate (Co-administration with corticosteroids may reduce the blood-glucose-lowering effect of insulin). Products include:
Pediapred Oral Solution ... 3319

Prednisolone Tebutate (Co-administration with corticosteroids may reduce the blood-glucose-lowering effect of insulin).
No products indexed under this heading.

Prednisone (Co-administration with corticosteroids may reduce the blood-glucose-lowering effect of insulin).
No products indexed under this heading.

Procarbazine Hydrochloride (May increase the blood-glucose-lowering effect and susceptibility to hypoglycemia). Products include:
Matulane Capsules ... 3188

Prochlorperazine (Phenothiazine derivatives may reduce the blood-glucose-lowering effect of insulin).
No products indexed under this heading.

Promethazine Hydrochloride (Phenothiazine derivatives may reduce the blood-glucose-lowering effect of insulin). Products include:
Phenergan ... 3438

Propoxyphene Hydrochloride (May increase the blood-glucose-lowering effect and susceptibility to hypoglycemia).
No products indexed under this heading.

Propoxyphene Napsylate (May increase the blood-glucose-lowering effect and susceptibility to hypoglycemia). Products include:
Darvocet A 500 Tablets ... 3497

Propranolol Hydrochloride (Beta-blockers may either potentiate or weaken the blood-glucose-lowering effect of insulin; signs of hypoglycemia may be reduced or absent with co-administration). Products include:
Inderal LA Long-Acting Capsules ... 3421
InnoPran XL Capsules ... 2728

Pseudoephedrine Hydrochloride (Sympathomimetic agents may reduce the blood-glucose-lowering effect of insulin). Products include:
Advil Allergy Sinus Caplets ... 737
Advil Cold & Sinus ... 739
Advil Flu & Body Ache Caplets ... 739
Children's Advil Cold Suspension ... 741
Advil Multi-Symptom Cold Caplets ... 738
Allegra-D 12 Hour Extended-Release Tablets ... 2860
Allegra-D 24 Hour Extended-Release Tablets ... 2862
Balamine DM ... 739
BC Cold Powder ... 612
Benadryl Allergy & Cold Tablets ... 692
Benadryl Allergy & Sinus Headache Caplets & Gelcaps ... 693
Children's Benadryl Allergy & Cold Fastmelt Tablets ... 695
Benadryl Maximum Strength Severe Allergy & Sinus Headache Caplets ... 694
Children's Benadryl D Allergy & Sinus Fastmelt Tablets ... 694
Children's Benadryl D Liquid Medication ... 693
Benadryl D Tablets ... 694
Contac Non-Drowsy 12 Hour Cold Caplets ... 614
Contac Non-Drowsy Timed Release 12 Hour Cold Caplets ... 615
Contac Severe Cold and Flu Caplets Maximum Strength ... 615
Contac Severe Cold and Flu Caplets Non-Drowsy ... 615
Children's Dimetapp Cold & Allergy Elixir ... 745
Children's Dimetapp DM Cold & Cough Elixir ... 745
Children's Dimetapp Long Acting Cough Plus Cold Syrup ... 746
Dimetapp Infant Drops Decongestant Plus Cough ... 746
Children's Motrin Cold Non-Staining Dye-Free Oral Suspension ... 1838
Children's Motrin Cold Oral Suspension ... 1838
Motrin Cold & Sinus Caplets ... 1836
PediaCare Decongestant & Cough Infant Drops ... 705
PediaCare Decongestant Infants' Drops ... 705
PediaCare Long-Acting Cough Plus Cold Liquid ... 704
PediaCare Multi-Symptom Cold Liquid ... 704
PediaCare NightRest Cough & Cold Liquid ... 704
Robitussin Allergy & Cough Syrup ... 750
Robitussin CF Liquid ... 755
Robitussin Cough & Cold Liquid-filled Capsules ... 750
Robitussin Cough, Cold & Flu Liquid-filled Capsules ... 750
Robitussin Cough & Cold Infant Drops ... 755
Robitussin Flu Liquid ... 752
Robitussin Maximum Strength Cough & Cold Liquid ... 754
Robitussin PE Syrup ... 753
Robitussin Pediatric Cough & Cold Liquid ... 754
Robitussin PM Cough & Cold Liquid ... 752
Robitussin Severe Congestion Liquid-filled Capsules ... 751
Simply Stuffy Liquid ... 1841
Singlet Caplets ... 636
Sudafed 12 Hour Caplets ... 708
Sudafed 24 Hour Tablets ... 709
Sudafed Nasal Decongestant Tablets ... 709
Sudafed Severe Cold ... 710
Sudafed Non-Drying Sinus Liquid Caps ... 709
Sudafed Sinus & Allergy Tablets ... 710
Sudafed Sinus Headache ... 711
TheraFlu Cold & Cough Hot Liquid ... 680
TheraFlu Cold & Sore Throat Hot Liquid ... 680
TheraFlu Flu & Chest Congestion Non-Drowsy Hot Liquid ... 681
TheraFlu Flu & Sore Throat Hot Liquid ... 681
TheraFlu Severe Cold Non-Drowsy Hot Liquid ... 683
TheraFlu Severe Cold & Cough Hot Liquid ... 683
TheraFlu Severe Cold Caplets ... 679
TheraFlu Severe Cold Hot Liquid ... 682
TheraFlu Severe Cold Non-Drowsy Caplets ... 679
Triaminic Chest & Nasal Congestion Liquid ... 685
Triaminic Cold & Allergy Liquid ... 685
Triaminic Cold & Cough Liquid ... 685
Triaminic Cough Liquid ... 687
Triaminic Cough & Nasal Congestion Liquid ... 687
Triaminic Cough & Sore Throat Liquid ... 687
Triaminic Flu, Cough & Fever Liquid ... 685
Triaminic Night Time Cough & Cold Liquid ... 685
Triaminic Allergy Runny Nose & Congestion Softchews ... 688
Triaminic Cold & Cough Softchews ... 688
Triaminic Cough & Sore Throat Softchews ... 689
Tylenol Sinus NightTime Caplets ... 663
Children's Tylenol Plus Cold & Allergy Suspension Liquid ... 1850
Children's Tylenol Plus Cold NightTime Suspension Liquid ... 1851
Children's Tylenol Plus Cold & Cough Suspension Liquid and Chewable Tablets ... 1851
Children's Tylenol Plus Cold Chewable Tablets ... 1851
Children's Tylenol Plus Cold Daytime Non-Drowsy Suspension Liquid ... 1851
Children's Tylenol Plus Flu Suspension Liquid ... 1853
Concentrated Tylenol Infants' Drops Plus Cold ... 1851
Concentrated Tylenol Infants' Drops Plus Cold and Cough ... 1851
Tylenol Cold & Flu Severe Daytime Liquid with Cool Bust ... 1846
Tylenol Cold & Flu Severe NightTime Liquid with Cool Burst ... 1846
Tylenol Cold Severe Congestion Non-Drowsy Caplets with Cool Burst ... 1846
Tylenol Allergy Complete Night Time Caplets ... 1844
Tylenol Allergy Complete Multi-Symptom Caplets and Gelcaps with Cool Burst ... 1844
Tylenol Flu NightTime Gelcaps ... 1846
Tylenol Flu Day Non-Drowsy Gelcaps ... 1846
Concentrated Tylenol Infants' Drops Plus Cold Nasal Congestant, Fever Reducer & Pain Reliever ... 668
Concentrated Tylenol Infants' Drops Plus Cold & Cough Nasal Decongestant, Fever Reducer & Pain Reliever ... 668
Multi-Symptom Tylenol Cold Night Time Caplets ... 1845
Multi-Symptom Tylenol Cold Day Non-Drowsy Caplets and Gelcaps ... 1845
Tylenol Sinus Day Non-Drowsy ... 1848
Tylenol Sinus Night Time Caplets ... 1848
Tylenol Sinus Severe Congestion Caplets with Cool Burst ... 1848
Vicks 44D Cough & Head Congestion Relief ... 2676
Vicks 44D Cough & Head Congestion Relief Liquid ... 721
Vicks 44M Cough, Cold & Flu Relief ... 2676
Pediatric Vicks 44m Cough & Cold Relief ... 2673
Vicks DayQuil LiquiCaps/Liquid Multi-Symptom Cold/Flu Relief ... 723
Vicks DayQuil Multi-Symptom Cold/Flu Relief LiquiCaps ... 2675
Vicks DayQuil Multi-Symptom Cold/Flu Relief Liquid ... 2675
Children's Vicks NyQuil Cold/Cough Relief ... 2671
Vicks NyQuil LiquiCaps ... 2677
Vicks NyQuil LiquiCaps/Liquid Multi-Symptom Cold/Flu Relief ... 725
Vicks NyQuil Liquid ... 2677
Zyrtec-D 12 Hour Extended Release Tablets ... 2591

Pseudoephedrine Sulfate (Sympathomimetic agents may reduce the blood-glucose-lowering effect of insulin). Products include:
Alavert Allergy & Sinus D-12 Hour Tablets ... 743
Clarinex-D 24-Hour Extended-Release Tablets ... 3012
Claritin-D Non-Drowsy 12 Hour Tablets ... 731
Claritin-D Non-Drowsy 24 Hour Tablets ... 731

Quinapril Hydrochloride (May increase the blood-glucose-lowering effect and susceptibility to hypoglycemia).
No products indexed under this heading.

Ramipril (May increase the blood-glucose-lowering effect and susceptibility to hypoglycemia). Products include:
Altace Capsules ... 1673

Repaglinide (May increase the blood-glucose-lowering effect and susceptibility to hypoglycemia). Products include:
Prandin Tablets (0.5, 1, and 2 mg) ... 2337

Reserpine (Signs of hypoglycemia may be reduced or absent with co-administration).
No products indexed under this heading.

Rosiglitazone Maleate (May increase the blood-glucose-lowering effect and susceptibility to hypoglycemia). Products include:
Avandamet Tablets ... 1343
Avandia Tablets ... 1348

Salmeterol Xinafoate (Sympathomimetic agents may reduce the blood-glucose-lowering effect of insulin). Products include:
Advair Diskus 100/50 ... 1291
Advair Diskus 250/50 ... 1291
Advair Diskus 500/50 ... 1291
Serevent Diskus ... 1540

Salsalate (May increase the blood-glucose-lowering effect and susceptibility to hypoglycemia).
No products indexed under this heading.

Selegiline Hydrochloride (May increase the blood-glucose-lowering effect and susceptibility to hypoglycemia). Products include:
Eldepryl Capsules ... 3209

Somatropin (May reduce the blood-glucose-lowering effect of insulin). Products include:
Genotropin Lyophilized Powder ... 2642
Humatrope Vials and Cartridges ... 1756
Norditropin Cartridges ... 2318

IMPORTANT NOTE: Always consult each drug listing in the patient's regimen for possible interactions.

Nutropin for Injection 1238
Nutropin AQ Injection 1241
Nutropin AQ Pen 1241
Nutropin AQ Pen Cartridge 1241

Sotalol Hydrochloride (Beta-blockers may either potentiate or weaken the blood-glucose-lowering effect of insulin; signs of hypoglycemia may be reduced or absent with co-administration).
No products indexed under this heading.

Spirapril Hydrochloride (May increase the blood-glucose-lowering effect and susceptibility to hypoglycemia).
No products indexed under this heading.

Spironolactone (Diuretics may reduce the blood-glucose-lowering effect of insulin).
No products indexed under this heading.

Sulfamethoxazole (Co-administration with sulfonamide antibiotics may increase the blood-glucose-lowering effect and susceptibility to hypoglycemia).
No products indexed under this heading.

Sulfisoxazole Acetyl (Co-administration with sulfonamide antibiotics may increase the blood-glucose-lowering effect and susceptibility to hypoglycemia).
No products indexed under this heading.

Terbutaline Sulfate (Sympathomimetic agents may reduce the blood-glucose-lowering effect of insulin).
No products indexed under this heading.

Thioridazine Hydrochloride (Phenothiazine derivatives may reduce the blood-glucose-lowering effect of insulin). Products include:
Thioridazine Hydrochloride Tablets 2122

Thyroglobulin (May reduce the blood-glucose-lowering effect of insulin).
No products indexed under this heading.

Thyroid (May reduce the blood-glucose-lowering effect of insulin).
No products indexed under this heading.

Thyroxine (May reduce the blood-glucose-lowering effect of insulin).
No products indexed under this heading.

Thyroxine Sodium (May reduce the blood-glucose-lowering effect of insulin).
No products indexed under this heading.

Timolol Hemihydrate (Beta-blockers may either potentiate or weaken the blood-glucose-lowering effect of insulin; signs of hypoglycemia may be reduced or absent with co-administration). Products include:
Betimol Ophthalmic Solution 3371
Betimol Ophthalmic Solution .... ⊙283

Timolol Maleate (Beta-blockers may either potentiate or weaken the blood-glucose-lowering effect of insulin; signs of hypoglycemia may be reduced or absent with co-administration). Products include:
Blocadren Tablets 1891
Cosopt Sterile Ophthalmic Solution 1910
Timolide Tablets 2056
Timoptic in Ocudose 2061
Timoptic Sterile Ophthalmic Solution 2058
Timoptic-XE Sterile Ophthalmic Gel Forming Solution 2062

Tolazamide (May increase the blood-glucose-lowering effect and susceptibility to hypoglycemia).
No products indexed under this heading.

Tolbutamide (May increase the blood-glucose-lowering effect and susceptibility to hypoglycemia).
No products indexed under this heading.

Torsemide (Diuretics may reduce the blood-glucose-lowering effect of insulin).
No products indexed under this heading.

Trandolapril (May increase the blood-glucose-lowering effect and susceptibility to hypoglycemia). Products include:
Mavik Tablets 482
Tarka Tablets 519

Tranylcypromine Sulfate (May increase the blood-glucose-lowering effect and susceptibility to hypoglycemia). Products include:
Parnate Tablets 1499

Triamcinolone (Co-administration with corticosteroids may reduce the blood-glucose-lowering effect of insulin).
No products indexed under this heading.

Triamcinolone Acetonide (Co-administration with corticosteroids may reduce the blood-glucose-lowering effect of insulin). Products include:
Azmacort Inhalation Aerosol 1701
Nasacort HFA Inhalation Aerosol 2939
Nasacort AQ Nasal Spray 2937

Triamcinolone Diacetate (Co-administration with corticosteroids may reduce the blood-glucose-lowering effect of insulin).
No products indexed under this heading.

Triamcinolone Hexacetonide (Co-administration with corticosteroids may reduce the blood-glucose-lowering effect of insulin).
No products indexed under this heading.

Triamterene (Diuretics may reduce the blood-glucose-lowering effect of insulin). Products include:
Dyazide Capsules 1389
Dyrenium Capsules 3390
Maxzide 2150

Trifluoperazine Hydrochloride (Phenothiazine derivatives may reduce the blood-glucose-lowering effect of insulin).
No products indexed under this heading.

Troglitazone (May increase the blood-glucose-lowering effect and susceptibility to hypoglycemia).
No products indexed under this heading.

Food Interactions

Alcohol (May either potentiate or weaken the blood-glucose-lowering effect of insulin).

NOVOLOG MIX 70/30

(Insulin Aspart, Human, Insulin Aspart Protamine, Human) 2331
May interact with ACE inhibitors, beta blockers, corticosteroids, diuretics, estrogens, fibrates, monoamine oxidase inhibitors, oral contraceptives, phenothiazines, progestins, sulfonamides, sympathomimetics, thyroid preparations, and certain other agents. Compounds in these categories include:

Acebutolol Hydrochloride (May potentiate or weaken the blood-glucose-lowering effect of insulin. The signs of hypoglycemia may be reduced or absent).
No products indexed under this heading.

Albuterol (Substances that may reduce the blood-glucose-lowering effect). Products include:
Proventil Inhalation Aerosol 3067

Albuterol Sulfate (Substances that may reduce the blood-glucose-lowering effect). Products include:
AccuNeb Inhalation Solution 1055
Combivent Inhalation Aerosol 878
DuoNeb Inhalation Solution 1058
Proventil Inhalation Solution 0.083% 3069
Proventil HFA Inhalation Aerosol 3071
Ventolin HFA Inhalation Aerosol 1576
VoSpire Extended-Release Tablets 2352

Amiloride Hydrochloride (Substances that may reduce the blood-glucose-lowering effect). Products include:
Midamor Tablets 2000
Moduretic Tablets 2003

Atenolol (May potentiate or weaken the blood-glucose-lowering effect of insulin. The signs of hypoglycemia may be reduced or absent). Products include:
Tenormin I.V. Injection 698
Tenormin Tablets 695

Benazepril Hydrochloride (Substances that may increase the blood-glucose-lowering effect and susceptibility to hypoglycemia). Products include:
Lotensin Tablets 2232
Lotensin HCT Tablets 2235
Lotrel Capsules 2238

Bendroflumethiazide (Substances that may increase the blood-glucose-lowering effect and susceptibility to hypoglycemia).
No products indexed under this heading.

Betamethasone Acetate (Substances that may reduce the blood-glucose-lowering effect).
No products indexed under this heading.

Betamethasone Sodium Phosphate (Substances that may reduce the blood-glucose-lowering effect).
No products indexed under this heading.

Betaxolol Hydrochloride (May potentiate or weaken the blood-glucose-lowering effect of insulin. The signs of hypoglycemia may be reduced or absent). Products include:
Betoptic S Ophthalmic Suspension 554

Bisoprolol Fumarate (May potentiate or weaken the blood-glucose-lowering effect of insulin. The signs of hypoglycemia may be reduced or absent).
No products indexed under this heading.

Bumetanide (Substances that may reduce the blood-glucose-lowering effect).
No products indexed under this heading.

Captopril (Substances that may increase the blood-glucose-lowering effect and susceptibility to hypoglycemia). Products include:
Captopril Tablets 2114

Carteolol Hydrochloride (May potentiate or weaken the blood-glucose-lowering effect of insulin. The signs of hypoglycemia may be reduced or absent). Products include:
Carteolol Hydrochloride Ophthalmic Solution USP, 1% .... ⊙246

Chlorothiazide (Substances that may increase the blood-glucose-lowering effect and susceptibility to hypoglycemia). Products include:
Aldoclor Tablets 1881
Diuril Oral 1936

Chlorothiazide Sodium (Substances that may increase the blood-glucose-lowering effect and susceptibility to hypoglycemia). Products include:
Diuril Sodium Intravenous 1934

Chlorotrianisene (Substances that may reduce the blood-glucose-lowering effect).
No products indexed under this heading.

Chlorpromazine (Substances that may reduce the blood-glucose-lowering effect).
No products indexed under this heading.

Chlorpromazine Hydrochloride (Substances that may reduce the blood-glucose-lowering effect).
No products indexed under this heading.

Chlorpropamide (Substances that may increase the blood-glucose-lowering effect and susceptibility to hypoglycemia).
No products indexed under this heading.

Chlorthalidone (Substances that may reduce the blood-glucose-lowering effect). Products include:
Clorpres Tablets 2139

Clofibrate (Substances that may increase the blood-glucose-lowering effect and susceptibility to hypoglycemia).
No products indexed under this heading.

Clonidine Hydrochloride (May potentiate or weaken the blood-glucose-lowering effect of insulin. The signs of hypoglycemia may be reduced or absent). Products include:
Catapres Tablets 874
Clorpres Tablets 2139

Cortisone Acetate (Substances that may reduce the blood-glucose-lowering effect).
No products indexed under this heading.

Danazol (Substances that may reduce the blood-glucose-lowering effect).
No products indexed under this heading.

Desogestrel (Substances that may reduce the blood-glucose-lowering effect). Products include:
Ortho-Cept Tablets 2395

Dexamethasone (Substances that may reduce the blood-glucose-lowering effect). Products include:

Ciprodex Otic Suspension **555**
Decadron Tablets **1929**
TobraDex Ophthalmic Ointment **558**
TobraDex Ophthalmic Suspension ... **558**

Dexamethasone Acetate (Substances that may reduce the blood-glucose-lowering effect).
No products indexed under this heading.

Dexamethasone Sodium Phosphate (Substances that may reduce the blood-glucose-lowering effect). Products include:
Decadron Phosphate Injection **1931**

Dienestrol (Substances that may reduce the blood-glucose-lowering effect).
No products indexed under this heading.

Diethylstilbestrol (Substances that may reduce the blood-glucose-lowering effect).
No products indexed under this heading.

Disopyramide Phosphate (Substances that may increase the blood-glucose-lowering effect and susceptibility to hypoglycemia).
No products indexed under this heading.

Dobutamine Hydrochloride (Substances that may reduce the blood-glucose-lowering effect).
No products indexed under this heading.

Dopamine Hydrochloride (Substances that may reduce the blood-glucose-lowering effect).
No products indexed under this heading.

Enalapril Maleate (Substances that may increase the blood-glucose-lowering effect and susceptibility to hypoglycemia). Products include:
Vaseretic Tablets **2073**
Vasotec I.V. Injection **2076**

Enalaprilat (Substances that may increase the blood-glucose-lowering effect and susceptibility to hypoglycemia).
No products indexed under this heading.

Ephedrine Hydrochloride (Substances that may reduce the blood-glucose-lowering effect). Products include:
Primatene Tablets **749**

Ephedrine Sulfate (Substances that may reduce the blood-glucose-lowering effect).
No products indexed under this heading.

Ephedrine Tannate (Substances that may reduce the blood-glucose-lowering effect).
No products indexed under this heading.

Epinephrine (Substances that may reduce the blood-glucose-lowering effect). Products include:
EpiPen **1061**
Primatene Mist **749**

Epinephrine Bitartrate (Substances that may reduce the blood-glucose-lowering effect).
No products indexed under this heading.

Epinephrine Hydrochloride (Substances that may reduce the blood-glucose-lowering effect).
No products indexed under this heading.

Esmolol Hydrochloride (May potentiate or weaken the blood-glucose-lowering effect of insulin. The signs of hypoglycemia may be reduced or absent). Products include:
Brevibloc Concentrate **766**
Brevibloc Injection **766**
Brevibloc Double Strength Injection... **766**
Brevibloc Premixed Injection **766**
Brevibloc Double Strength Premixed Injection **766**

Estradiol (Substances that may reduce the blood-glucose-lowering effect). Products include:
Activella Tablets **2311**
Climara Transdermal System **795**
Climara Pro Transdermal System **800**
CombiPatch Transdermal System **2180**
Estrogel 0.06% **3200**
Menostar Transdermal System **805**
Prefest Tablets **1069**
Vagifem Tablets **2340**
Vivelle Transdermal System **2288**
Vivelle-Dot Transdermal System **2293**

Estrogens, Conjugated (Substances that may reduce the blood-glucose-lowering effect). Products include:
Premarin Intravenous **3440**
Premarin Tablets **3443**
Premarin Vaginal Cream **3449**
Premphase Tablets **3452**
Prempro Tablets **3452**

Estrogens, Esterified (Substances that may reduce the blood-glucose-lowering effect). Products include:
Estratest Tablets **3196**
Estratest H.S. Tablets **3196**

Estropipate (Substances that may reduce the blood-glucose-lowering effect).
No products indexed under this heading.

Ethacrynic Acid (Substances that may reduce the blood-glucose-lowering effect). Products include:
Edecrin Tablets **1941**

Ethinyl Estradiol (Substances that may reduce the blood-glucose-lowering effect). Products include:
Alesse-28 Tablets **3392**
Lo/Ovral-28 Tablets **3423**
NuvaRing **2357**
Ortho-Cept Tablets **2395**
Ortho-Cyclen/Ortho Tri-Cyclen **2414**
Ortho Evra Transdermal System **2402**
Ortho Tri-Cyclen Lo Tablets **2421**
Seasonale Tablets **1073**
Triphasil-28 Tablets **3483**
Yasmin 28 Tablets **818**

Ethynodiol Diacetate (Substances that may reduce the blood-glucose-lowering effect).
No products indexed under this heading.

Fenofibrate (Substances that may increase the blood-glucose-lowering effect and susceptibility to hypoglycemia). Products include:
Antara Capsules **2723**
Lofibra Capsules **1217**
Tricor Tablets **523**
Triglide Tablets **1165**

Fludrocortisone Acetate (Substances that may reduce the blood-glucose-lowering effect).
No products indexed under this heading.

Fluoxetine Hydrochloride (Substances that may increase the blood-glucose-lowering effect and susceptibility to hypoglycemia). Products include:
Prozac Pulvules and Liquid **1771**
Symbyax Capsules **1788**

Fluphenazine Decanoate (Substances that may reduce the blood-glucose-lowering effect).
No products indexed under this heading.

Fluphenazine Enanthate (Substances that may reduce the blood-glucose-lowering effect).
No products indexed under this heading.

Fluphenazine Hydrochloride (Substances that may reduce the blood-glucose-lowering effect).
No products indexed under this heading.

Fosinopril Sodium (Substances that may increase the blood-glucose-lowering effect and susceptibility to hypoglycemia).
No products indexed under this heading.

Furosemide (Substances that may reduce the blood-glucose-lowering effect). Products include:
Furosemide Tablets **2117**

Gemfibrozil (Substances that may increase the blood-glucose-lowering effect and susceptibility to hypoglycemia).
No products indexed under this heading.

Glipizide (Substances that may increase the blood-glucose-lowering effect and susceptibility to hypoglycemia).
No products indexed under this heading.

Glyburide (Substances that may increase the blood-glucose-lowering effect and susceptibility to hypoglycemia).
No products indexed under this heading.

Guanethidine Monosulfate (The signs of hypoglycemia may be reduced or absent when under the influence of guanethidine).
No products indexed under this heading.

Hydrochlorothiazide (Substances that may increase the blood-glucose-lowering effect and susceptibility to hypoglycemia). Products include:
Aldoril Tablets **1884**
Atacand HCT **637**
Avalide Tablets **2889**
Avalide Tablets **922**
Benicar HCT Tablets **2852**
Diovan HCT Tablets **2195**
Dyazide Capsules **1389**
Hyzaar **1964**
Lotensin HCT Tablets **2235**
Maxzide **2150**
Micardis HCT Tablets **886**
Moduretic Tablets **2003**
Prinzide Tablets **2033**
Teveten HCT Tablets **1710**
Timolide Tablets **2056**
Uniretic Tablets **3114**
Vaseretic Tablets **2073**
Zestoretic Tablets **701**

Hydrocortisone (Substances that may reduce the blood-glucose-lowering effect). Products include:
Cortizone•5 Ointment **699**
Cortizone•10 Creme **699**
Cortizone•10 Ointment **699**
Cortizone•10 Plus Creme **700**
Cortizone•10 Maximum Strength Quick Shot Spray **700**
Hydrocortone Tablets **1963**
Preparation H Hydrocortisone Cream **748**

Hydrocortisone Acetate (Substances that may reduce the blood-glucose-lowering effect). Products include:
Analpram-HC **1136**
Pramosone **1139**
ProctoFoam-HC **3113**
Tucks Anti-Itch Ointment **712**
U-cort 1% Cream **3289**

Hydrocortisone Sodium Phosphate (Substances that may reduce the blood-glucose-lowering effect).
No products indexed under this heading.

Hydrocortisone Sodium Succinate (Substances that may reduce the blood-glucose-lowering effect).
No products indexed under this heading.

Hydroflumethiazide (Substances that may increase the blood-glucose-lowering effect and susceptibility to hypoglycemia).
No products indexed under this heading.

Indapamide (Substances that may reduce the blood-glucose-lowering effect). Products include:
Indapamide Tablets **2119**

Isocarboxazid (Substances that may increase the blood-glucose-lowering effect and susceptibility to hypoglycemia).
No products indexed under this heading.

Isoniazid (Substances that may reduce the blood-glucose-lowering effect).
No products indexed under this heading.

Isoproterenol Hydrochloride (Substances that may reduce the blood-glucose-lowering effect).
No products indexed under this heading.

Isoproterenol Sulfate (Substances that may reduce the blood-glucose-lowering effect).
No products indexed under this heading.

Labetalol Hydrochloride (May potentiate or weaken the blood-glucose-lowering effect of insulin. The signs of hypoglycemia may be reduced or absent).
No products indexed under this heading.

Levalbuterol Hydrochloride (Substances that may reduce the blood-glucose-lowering effect). Products include:
Xopenex Inhalation Solution **3143**
Xopenex Inhalation Solution Concentrate **3147**

Levobunolol Hydrochloride (May potentiate or weaken the blood-glucose-lowering effect of insulin. The signs of hypoglycemia may be reduced or absent). Products include:
Betagan Ophthalmic Solution, USP .... ⊙**217**

Levonorgestrel (Substances that may reduce the blood-glucose-lowering effect). Products include:
Alesse-28 Tablets **3392**
Climara Pro Transdermal System **800**
Mirena Intrauterine System **810**
Plan B Tablets **1068**
Seasonale Tablets **1073**
Triphasil-28 Tablets **3483**

Levothyroxine Sodium (Substances that may reduce the blood-glucose-lowering effect). Products include:
Levothroid Tablets **1189**
Levoxyl Tablets **1680**
Synthroid Tablets **515**
Unithroid Tablets **3521**

Liothyronine Sodium (Substances that may reduce the blood-glucose-lowering effect). Products include:
Cytomel Tablets **1678**

Liotrix (Substances that may reduce the blood-glucose-lowering effect). Products include:
- Thyrolar 1203

Lisinopril (Substances that may increase the blood-glucose-lowering effect and susceptibility to hypoglycemia). Products include:
- Prinivil Tablets 2029
- Prinzide Tablets 2033
- Zestoretic Tablets 701
- Zestril Tablets 704

Lithium Carbonate (May potentiate or weaken the blood-glucose-lowering effect of insulin). Products include:
- Eskalith 1406
- Lithobid Tablets 1670

Lithium Citrate (May potentiate or weaken the blood-glucose-lowering effect of insulin).
No products indexed under this heading.

Medroxyprogesterone Acetate (Substances that may reduce the blood-glucose-lowering effect). Products include:
- Depo-Provera Contraceptive Injection 2619
- depo-subQ provera 104 Injectable Suspension 2622
- Premphase Tablets 3452
- Prempro Tablets 3452

Megestrol Acetate (Substances that may reduce the blood-glucose-lowering effect). Products include:
- Megace ES Oral Suspension 2492

Mesoridazine Besylate (Substances that may reduce the blood-glucose-lowering effect).
No products indexed under this heading.

Mestranol (Substances that may reduce the blood-glucose-lowering effect).
No products indexed under this heading.

Metaproterenol Sulfate (Substances that may reduce the blood-glucose-lowering effect). Products include:
- Alupent Inhalation Aerosol 858

Metaraminol Bitartrate (Substances that may reduce the blood-glucose-lowering effect). Products include:
- Aramine Injection 1889

Methotrimeprazine (Substances that may reduce the blood-glucose-lowering effect).
No products indexed under this heading.

Methoxamine Hydrochloride (Substances that may reduce the blood-glucose-lowering effect).
No products indexed under this heading.

Methyclothiazide (Substances that may increase the blood-glucose-lowering effect and susceptibility to hypoglycemia).
No products indexed under this heading.

Methylprednisolone Acetate (Substances that may reduce the blood-glucose-lowering effect). Products include:
- Depo-Medrol Injectable Suspension 2615
- Depo-Medrol Single-Dose Vial 2617

Methylprednisolone Sodium Succinate (Substances that may reduce the blood-glucose-lowering effect).
No products indexed under this heading.

Metipranolol Hydrochloride (May potentiate or weaken the blood-glucose-lowering effect of insulin. The signs of hypoglycemia may be reduced or absent).
No products indexed under this heading.

Metolazone (Substances that may reduce the blood-glucose-lowering effect).
No products indexed under this heading.

Metoprolol Succinate (May potentiate or weaken the blood-glucose-lowering effect of insulin. The signs of hypoglycemia may be reduced or absent). Products include:
- Toprol-XL Tablets 660

Metoprolol Tartrate (May potentiate or weaken the blood-glucose-lowering effect of insulin. The signs of hypoglycemia may be reduced or absent).
No products indexed under this heading.

Moclobemide (Substances that may increase the blood-glucose-lowering effect and susceptibility to hypoglycemia).
No products indexed under this heading.

Moexipril Hydrochloride (Substances that may increase the blood-glucose-lowering effect and susceptibility to hypoglycemia). Products include:
- Uniretic Tablets 3114
- Univasc Tablets 3118

Nadolol (May potentiate or weaken the blood-glucose-lowering effect of insulin. The signs of hypoglycemia may be reduced or absent). Products include:
- Nadolol Tablets 2121

Niacin (Substances that may reduce the blood-glucose-lowering effect). Products include:
- Advicor Tablets 1694
- Niaspan Extended-Release Tablets 1703

Norepinephrine Bitartrate (Substances that may reduce the blood-glucose-lowering effect).
No products indexed under this heading.

Norethindrone (Substances that may reduce the blood-glucose-lowering effect). Products include:
- Ortho Micronor Tablets 2411

Norethynodrel (Substances that may reduce the blood-glucose-lowering effect).
No products indexed under this heading.

Norgestimate (Substances that may reduce the blood-glucose-lowering effect). Products include:
- Ortho-Cyclen/Ortho Tri-Cyclen 2414
- Ortho Tri-Cyclen Lo Tablets 2421
- Prefest Tablets 1069

Norgestrel (Substances that may reduce the blood-glucose-lowering effect). Products include:
- Lo/Ovral-28 Tablets 3423

Octreotide Acetate (Substances that may increase the blood-glucose-lowering effect and susceptibility to hypoglycemia). Products include:
- Sandostatin Injection 2263
- Sandostatin LAR Depot 2264

Pargyline Hydrochloride (Substances that may increase the blood-glucose-lowering effect and susceptibility to hypoglycemia).
No products indexed under this heading.

Penbutolol Sulfate (May potentiate or weaken the blood-glucose-lowering effect of insulin. The signs of hypoglycemia may be reduced or absent).
No products indexed under this heading.

Pentamidine Isethionate (May cause hypoglycemia, which may sometimes be followed by hyperglycemia).
No products indexed under this heading.

Perindopril Erbumine (Substances that may increase the blood-glucose-lowering effect and susceptibility to hypoglycemia). Products include:
- Aceon Tablets (2 mg, 4 mg, 8 mg) 3191

Perphenazine (Substances that may reduce the blood-glucose-lowering effect).
No products indexed under this heading.

Phenelzine Sulfate (Substances that may increase the blood-glucose-lowering effect and susceptibility to hypoglycemia).
No products indexed under this heading.

Phenylephrine Bitartrate (Substances that may reduce the blood-glucose-lowering effect).
No products indexed under this heading.

Phenylephrine Hydrochloride (Substances that may reduce the blood-glucose-lowering effect). Products include:
- Alacol DM Syrup 739
- Hycomine Compound Tablets 1105
- Preparation H Maximum Strength Cream .... ▣747
- Preparation H Cooling Gel .... ▣747
- Preparation H .... ▣747
- Sudafed PE Tablets .... ▣711
- Vicks Sinex Nasal Spray and Ultra Fine Mist for Sinus Relief 2677
- Zicam Concentrated Cough Mist for Kids Plus D Cool Cherry .... ▣643
- Zicam Concentrated Cough Mist Plus D Cool Cherry .... ▣642

Phenylephrine Tannate (Substances that may reduce the blood-glucose-lowering effect).
No products indexed under this heading.

Phenylpropanolamine Hydrochloride (Substances that may reduce the blood-glucose-lowering effect).
No products indexed under this heading.

Pindolol (May potentiate or weaken the blood-glucose-lowering effect of insulin. The signs of hypoglycemia may be reduced or absent).
No products indexed under this heading.

Pirbuterol Acetate (Substances that may reduce the blood-glucose-lowering effect). Products include:
- Maxair Autohaler 1820

Polyestradiol Phosphate (Substances that may reduce the blood-glucose-lowering effect).
No products indexed under this heading.

Polythiazide (Substances that may increase the blood-glucose-lowering effect and susceptibility to hypoglycemia).
No products indexed under this heading.

Prednisolone Acetate (Substances that may reduce the blood-glucose-lowering effect). Products include:
- Blephamide Ophthalmic Ointment 563
- Blephamide Ophthalmic Suspension 564
- Poly-Pred Liquifilm Ophthalmic Suspension .... ⊙231
- Pred Forte Ophthalmic Suspension .... ⊙233
- Pred Mild Sterile Ophthalmic Suspension .... ⊙236
- Pred-G Ophthalmic Suspension .... ⊙234
- Pred-G Sterile Ophthalmic Ointment .... ⊙235

Prednisolone Sodium Phosphate (Substances that may reduce the blood-glucose-lowering effect). Products include:
- Pediapred Oral Solution 3319

Prednisolone Tebutate (Substances that may reduce the blood-glucose-lowering effect).
No products indexed under this heading.

Prednisone (Substances that may reduce the blood-glucose-lowering effect).
No products indexed under this heading.

Procarbazine Hydrochloride (Substances that may increase the blood-glucose-lowering effect and susceptibility to hypoglycemia). Products include:
- Matulane Capsules 3188

Prochlorperazine (Substances that may reduce the blood-glucose-lowering effect).
No products indexed under this heading.

Promethazine Hydrochloride (Substances that may reduce the blood-glucose-lowering effect). Products include:
- Phenergan 3438

Propoxyphene Hydrochloride (Substances that may increase the blood-glucose-lowering effect and susceptibility to hypoglycemia).
No products indexed under this heading.

Propoxyphene Napsylate (Substances that may increase the blood-glucose-lowering effect and susceptibility to hypoglycemia). Products include:
- Darvocet A 500 Tablets 3497

Propranolol Hydrochloride (May potentiate or weaken the blood-glucose-lowering effect of insulin. The signs of hypoglycemia may be reduced or absent). Products include:
- Inderal LA Long-Acting Capsules 3421
- InnoPran XL Capsules 2728

Pseudoephedrine Hydrochloride (Substances that may reduce the blood-glucose-lowering effect). Products include:
- Advil Allergy Sinus Caplets .... ▣737
- Advil Cold & Sinus .... ▣739
- Advil Flu & Body Ache Caplets .... ▣739
- Children's Advil Cold Suspension .... ▣741
- Advil Multi-Symptom Cold Caplets .... ▣738
- Allegra-D 12 Hour Extended-Release Tablets 2860
- Allegra-D 24 Hour Extended-Release Tablets 2862
- Balamine DM 739
- BC Cold Powder .... ▣612
- Benadryl Allergy & Cold Tablets .... ▣692
- Benadryl Allergy & Sinus Headache Caplets & Gelcaps .... ▣693
- Children's Benadryl Allergy & Cold Fastmelt Tablets .... ▣695

Benadryl Maximum Strength Severe Allergy & Sinus Headache Caplets 694
Children's Benadryl D Allergy & Sinus Fastmelt Tablets 694
Children's Benadryl D Liquid Medication 693
Benadryl D Tablets 694
Contac Non-Drowsy 12 Hour Cold Caplets 614
Contac Non-Drowsy Timed Release 12 Hour Cold Caplets 615
Contac Severe Cold and Flu Caplets Maximum Strength 615
Contac Severe Cold and Flu Caplets Non-Drowsy 615
Children's Dimetapp Cold & Allergy Elixir 745
Children's Dimetapp DM Cold & Cough Elixir 745
Children's Dimetapp Long Acting Cough Plus Cold Syrup 746
Dimetapp Infant Drops Decongestant Plus Cough 746
Children's Motrin Cold Non-Staining Dye-Free Oral Suspension 1838
Children's Motrin Cold Oral Suspension 1838
Motrin Cold & Sinus Caplets 1836
PediaCare Decongestant & Cough Infant Drops 705
PediaCare Decongestant Infants' Drops 705
PediaCare Long-Acting Cough Plus Cold Liquid 704
PediaCare Multi-Symptom Cold Liquid 704
PediaCare NightRest Cough & Cold Liquid 704
Robitussin Allergy & Cough Syrup 750
Robitussin CF Liquid 755
Robitussin Cough & Cold Liquid-filled Capsules 750
Robitussin Cough, Cold & Flu Liquid-filled Capsules 750
Robitussin Cough & Cold Infant Drops 755
Robitussin Flu Liquid 752
Robitussin Maximum Strength Cough & Cold Liquid 754
Robitussin PE Syrup 753
Robitussin Pediatric Cough & Cold Liquid 754
Robitussin PM Cough & Cold Liquid 752
Robitussin Severe Congestion Liquid-filled Capsules 751
Simply Stuffy Liquid 1841
Singlet Caplets 636
Sudafed 12 Hour Caplets 708
Sudafed 24 Hour Tablets 709
Sudafed Nasal Decongestant Tablets 709
Sudafed Severe Cold 710
Sudafed Non-Drying Sinus Liquid Caps 709
Sudafed Sinus & Allergy Tablets 710
Sudafed Sinus Headache 711
TheraFlu Cold & Cough Hot Liquid 680
TheraFlu Cold & Sore Throat Hot Liquid 680
TheraFlu Flu & Chest Congestion Non-Drowsy Hot Liquid 681
TheraFlu Flu & Sore Throat Hot Liquid 681
TheraFlu Severe Cold Non-Drowsy Hot Liquid 683
TheraFlu Severe Cold & Cough Hot Liquid 683
TheraFlu Severe Cold Caplets 679
TheraFlu Severe Cold Hot Liquid 682
TheraFlu Severe Cold Non-Drowsy Caplets 679
Triaminic Chest & Nasal Congestion Liquid 685
Triaminic Cold & Allergy Liquid 685
Triaminic Cold & Cough Liquid 685
Triaminic Cough Liquid 687
Triaminic Cough & Nasal Congestion Liquid 687
Triaminic Cough & Sore Throat Liquid 687
Triaminic Flu, Cough & Fever Liquid 685
Triaminic Night Time Cough & Cold Liquid 685
Triaminic Allergy Runny Nose & Congestion Softchews 688
Triaminic Cold & Cough Softchews 688
Triaminic Cough & Sore Throat Softchews 689
Tylenol Sinus NightTime Caplets 663
Children's Tylenol Plus Cold & Allergy Suspension Liquid 1850
Children's Tylenol Plus Cold NightTime Suspension Liquid 1851
Children's Tylenol Plus Cold & Cough Suspension Liquid and Chewable Tablets 1851
Children's Tylenol Plus Cold Chewable Tablets 1851
Children's Tylenol Plus Cold Daytime Non-Drowsy Suspension Liquid 1851
Children's Tylenol Plus Flu Suspension Liquid 1853
Concentrated Tylenol Infants' Drops Plus Cold 1851
Concentrated Tylenol Infants' Drops Plus Cold and Cough 1851
Tylenol Cold & Flu Severe Daytime Liquid with Cool Bust 1846
Tylenol Cold & Flu Severe NightTime Liquid with Cool Burst 1846
Tylenol Cold Severe Congestion Non-Drowsy Caplets with Cool Burst 1846
Tylenol Allergy Complete Night Time Caplets 1844
Tylenol Allergy Complete Multi-Symptom Caplets and Gelcaps with Cool Burst 1844
Tylenol Flu NightTime Gelcaps 1846
Tylenol Flu Day Non-Drowsy Gelcaps 1846
Concentrated Tylenol Infants' Drops Plus Cold Nasal Congestant, Fever Reducer & Pain Reliever 668
Concentrated Tylenol Infants' Drops Plus Cold & Cough Nasal Decongestant, Fever Reducer & Pain Reliever 668
Multi-Symptom Tylenol Cold Night Time Caplets 1845
Multi-Symptom Tylenol Cold Day Non-Drowsy Caplets and Gelcaps 1845
Tylenol Sinus Day Non-Drowsy 1848
Tylenol Sinus Night Time Caplets 1848
Tylenol Sinus Severe Congestion Caplets with Cool Burst 1848
Vicks 44D Cough & Head Congestion Relief 2676
Vicks 44D Cough & Head Congestion Relief Liquid 721
Vicks 44M Cough, Cold & Flu Relief 2676
Pediatric Vicks 44m Cough & Cold Relief 2673
Vicks DayQuil LiquiCaps/Liquid Multi-Symptom Cold/Flu Relief 723
Vicks DayQuil Multi-Symptom Cold/Flu Relief LiquiCaps 2675
Vicks DayQuil Multi-Symptom Cold/Flu Relief Liquid 2675
Children's Vicks NyQuil Cold/Cough Relief 2671
Vicks NyQuil LiquiCaps 2677
Vicks NyQuil LiquiCaps/Liquid Multi-Symptom Cold/Flu Relief 725
Vicks NyQuil Liquid 2677
Zyrtec-D 12 Hour Extended Release Tablets 2591

Pseudoephedrine Sulfate (Substances that may reduce the blood-glucose-lowering effect). Products include:
Alavert Allergy & Sinus D-12 Hour Tablets 743
Clarinex-D 24-Hour Extended-Release Tablets 3012
Claritin-D Non-Drowsy 12 Hour Tablets 731
Claritin-D Non-Drowsy 24 Hour Tablets 731

Quinapril Hydrochloride (Substances that may increase the blood-glucose-lowering effect and susceptibility to hypoglycemia).
No products indexed under this heading.

Quinestrol (Substances that may reduce the blood-glucose-lowering effect).
No products indexed under this heading.

Ramipril (Substances that may increase the blood-glucose-lowering effect and susceptibility to hypoglycemia). Products include:
Altace Capsules 1673

Reserpine (The signs of hypoglycemia may be reduced or absent when under the influence of reserpine).
No products indexed under this heading.

Salmeterol Xinafoate (Substances that may reduce the blood-glucose-lowering effect). Products include:
Advair Diskus 100/50 1291
Advair Diskus 250/50 1291
Advair Diskus 500/50 1291
Serevent Diskus 1540

Selegiline Hydrochloride (Substances that may increase the blood-glucose-lowering effect and susceptibility to hypoglycemia). Products include:
Eldepryl Capsules 3209

Somatropin (Substances that may reduce the blood-glucose-lowering effect). Products include:
Genotropin Lyophilized Powder 2642
Humatrope Vials and Cartridges 1756
Norditropin Cartridges 2318
Nutropin for Injection 1238
Nutropin AQ Injection 1241
Nutropin AQ Pen 1241
Nutropin AQ Pen Cartridge 1241

Sotalol Hydrochloride (May potentiate or weaken the blood-glucose-lowering effect of insulin. The signs of hypoglycemia may be reduced or absent).
No products indexed under this heading.

Spirapril Hydrochloride (Substances that may increase the blood-glucose-lowering effect and susceptibility to hypoglycemia).
No products indexed under this heading.

Spironolactone (Substances that may reduce the blood-glucose-lowering effect).
No products indexed under this heading.

Sulfacytine (Substances that may increase the blood-glucose-lowering effect and susceptibility to hypoglycemia).
No products indexed under this heading.

Sulfamethizole (Substances that may increase the blood-glucose-lowering effect and susceptibility to hypoglycemia).
No products indexed under this heading.

Sulfamethoxazole (Substances that may increase the blood-glucose-lowering effect and susceptibility to hypoglycemia).
No products indexed under this heading.

Sulfasalazine (Substances that may increase the blood-glucose-lowering effect and susceptibility to hypoglycemia).
No products indexed under this heading.

Sulfinpyrazone (Substances that may increase the blood-glucose-lowering effect and susceptibility to hypoglycemia).
No products indexed under this heading.

Sulfisoxazole (Substances that may increase the blood-glucose-lowering effect and susceptibility to hypoglycemia).
No products indexed under this heading.

Sulfisoxazole Acetyl (Substances that may increase the blood-glucose-lowering effect and susceptibility to hypoglycemia).
No products indexed under this heading.

Sulfisoxazole Diolamine (Substances that may increase the blood-glucose-lowering effect and susceptibility to hypoglycemia).
No products indexed under this heading.

Terbutaline Sulfate (Substances that may reduce the blood-glucose-lowering effect).
No products indexed under this heading.

Thioridazine Hydrochloride (Substances that may reduce the blood-glucose-lowering effect). Products include:
Thioridazine Hydrochloride Tablets 2122

Thyroglobulin (Substances that may reduce the blood-glucose-lowering effect).
No products indexed under this heading.

Thyroid (Substances that may reduce the blood-glucose-lowering effect).
No products indexed under this heading.

Thyroxine (Substances that may reduce the blood-glucose-lowering effect).
No products indexed under this heading.

Thyroxine Sodium (Substances that may reduce the blood-glucose-lowering effect).
No products indexed under this heading.

Timolol Hemihydrate (May potentiate or weaken the blood-glucose-lowering effect of insulin. The signs of hypoglycemia may be reduced or absent). Products include:
Betimol Ophthalmic Solution 3371
Betimol Ophthalmic Solution ...... ⊙283

Timolol Maleate (May potentiate or weaken the blood-glucose-lowering effect of insulin. The signs of hypoglycemia may be reduced or absent). Products include:
Blocadren Tablets 1891
Cosopt Sterile Ophthalmic Solution 1910
Timolide Tablets 2056
Timoptic in Ocudose 2061
Timoptic Sterile Ophthalmic Solution 2058
Timoptic-XE Sterile Ophthalmic Gel Forming Solution 2062

Tolazamide (Substances that may increase the blood-glucose-lowering effect and susceptibility to hypoglycemia).
No products indexed under this heading.

IMPORTANT NOTE: Always consult each drug listing in the patient's regimen for possible interactions.

Tolbutamide (Substances that may increase the blood-glucose-lowering effect and susceptibility to hypoglycemia).
No products indexed under this heading.

Torsemide (Substances that may reduce the blood-glucose-lowering effect).
No products indexed under this heading.

Trandolapril (Substances that may increase the blood-glucose-lowering effect and susceptibility to hypoglycemia). Products include:
Mavik Tablets 482
Tarka Tablets 519

Tranylcypromine Sulfate (Substances that may increase the blood-glucose-lowering effect and susceptibility to hypoglycemia). Products include:
Parnate Tablets 1499

Triamcinolone (Substances that may reduce the blood-glucose-lowering effect).
No products indexed under this heading.

Triamcinolone Acetonide (Substances that may reduce the blood-glucose-lowering effect). Products include:
Azmacort Inhalation Aerosol 1701
Nasacort HFA Inhalation Aerosol 2939
Nasacort AQ Nasal Spray 2937

Triamcinolone Diacetate (Substances that may reduce the blood-glucose-lowering effect).
No products indexed under this heading.

Triamcinolone Hexacetonide (Substances that may reduce the blood-glucose-lowering effect).
No products indexed under this heading.

Triamterene (Substances that may reduce the blood-glucose-lowering effect). Products include:
Dyazide Capsules 1389
Dyrenium Capsules 3390
Maxzide 2150

Trifluoperazine Hydrochloride (Substances that may reduce the blood-glucose-lowering effect).
No products indexed under this heading.

NOVOSEVEN

(Antihemophilic Factor (Recombinant)) 2335
None cited in PDR database.

NUBAIN INJECTION

(Nalbuphine Hydrochloride) 1111
May interact with anesthetics, central nervous system depressants, general anesthetics, hypnotics and sedatives, narcotic analgesics, phenothiazines, tranquilizers, and certain other agents. Compounds in these categories include:

Alfentanil Hydrochloride (Additive CNS depression).
No products indexed under this heading.

Alprazolam (Additive CNS depression). Products include:
Niravam Orally Disintegrating Tablets 3106
Xanax XR Tablets 2655

Aprobarbital (Additive CNS depression).
No products indexed under this heading.

Buprenorphine Hydrochloride (Additive CNS depression). Products include:
Buprenex Injectable 2718
Suboxone Tablets 2719
Subutex Tablets 2719

Buspirone Hydrochloride (Additive CNS depression).
No products indexed under this heading.

Butabarbital (Additive CNS depression).
No products indexed under this heading.

Butalbital (Additive CNS depression). Products include:
Sedapap Tablets 50 mg/650 mg 2098

Chlordiazepoxide (Additive CNS depression).
No products indexed under this heading.

Chlordiazepoxide Hydrochloride (Additive CNS depression). Products include:
Librium Capsules 3349

Chlorpromazine (Additive CNS depression).
No products indexed under this heading.

Chlorpromazine Hydrochloride (Additive CNS depression).
No products indexed under this heading.

Chlorprothixene (Additive CNS depression).
No products indexed under this heading.

Chlorprothixene Hydrochloride (Additive CNS depression).
No products indexed under this heading.

Chlorprothixene Lactate (Additive CNS depression).
No products indexed under this heading.

Clorazepate Dipotassium (Additive CNS depression). Products include:
Tranxene 2488

Clozapine (Additive CNS depression). Products include:
Clozapine Tablets 2141
Clozaril Tablets 2174
FazaClo Orally Disintegrating Tablets 547

Codeine Phosphate (Additive CNS depression). Products include:
Tylenol with Codeine 2461

Desflurane (Additive CNS depression). Products include:
Suprane Liquid for Inhalation 770

Dezocine (Additive CNS depression).
No products indexed under this heading.

Diazepam (Additive CNS depression). Products include:
Diastat Rectal Delivery System 3344
Valium Tablets 2822

Droperidol (Additive CNS depression).
No products indexed under this heading.

Enflurane (Additive CNS depression).
No products indexed under this heading.

Estazolam (Additive CNS depression). Products include:
ProSom Tablets 512

Ethanol (Additive CNS depression).
No products indexed under this heading.

Ethchlorvynol (Additive CNS depression).
No products indexed under this heading.

Ethinamate (Additive CNS depression).
No products indexed under this heading.

Ethyl Alcohol (Additive CNS depression).
No products indexed under this heading.

Fentanyl (Additive CNS depression). Products include:
Duragesic Transdermal System 2448

Fentanyl Citrate (Additive CNS depression). Products include:
Actiq 993

Fluphenazine Decanoate (Additive CNS depression).
No products indexed under this heading.

Fluphenazine Enanthate (Additive CNS depression).
No products indexed under this heading.

Fluphenazine Hydrochloride (Additive CNS depression).
No products indexed under this heading.

Flurazepam Hydrochloride (Additive CNS depression). Products include:
Dalmane Capsules 3343

Glutethimide (Additive CNS depression).
No products indexed under this heading.

Haloperidol (Additive CNS depression).
No products indexed under this heading.

Haloperidol Decanoate (Additive CNS depression).
No products indexed under this heading.

Halothane (Additive CNS depression).
No products indexed under this heading.

Hydrocodone Bitartrate (Additive CNS depression). Products include:
Hycodan 1104
Hycomine Compound Tablets 1105
Hycotuss Expectorant Syrup 1106
Lortab 3315
Lortab Elixir 3312
Vicodin Tablets 530
Vicodin ES Tablets 531
Vicodin HP Tablets 532
Vicoprofen Tablets 533
Zydone Tablets 1118

Hydrocodone Polistirex (Additive CNS depression). Products include:
Tussionex Pennkinetic Extended-Release Suspension 3322

Hydromorphone Hydrochloride (Additive CNS depression). Products include:
Dilaudid 439
Dilaudid Oral Liquid 443
Dilaudid Non-Sterile Powder 439
Dilaudid Rectal Suppositories 439
Dilaudid Tablets 439
Dilaudid Tablets - 8 mg 443
Dilaudid-HP 441

Hydroxyzine Hydrochloride (Additive CNS depression).
No products indexed under this heading.

Isoflurane (Additive CNS depression).
No products indexed under this heading.

Ketamine Hydrochloride (Additive CNS depression).
No products indexed under this heading.

Levomethadyl Acetate Hydrochloride (Additive CNS depression).
No products indexed under this heading.

Levorphanol Tartrate (Additive CNS depression).
No products indexed under this heading.

Lorazepam (Additive CNS depression).
No products indexed under this heading.

Loxapine Hydrochloride (Additive CNS depression).
No products indexed under this heading.

Loxapine Succinate (Additive CNS depression).
No products indexed under this heading.

Meperidine Hydrochloride (Additive CNS depression).
No products indexed under this heading.

Mephobarbital (Additive CNS depression). Products include:
Mebaral Tablets, USP 2483

Meprobamate (Additive CNS depression).
No products indexed under this heading.

Mesoridazine Besylate (Additive CNS depression).
No products indexed under this heading.

Methadone Hydrochloride (Additive CNS depression).
No products indexed under this heading.

Methohexital Sodium (Additive CNS depression).
No products indexed under this heading.

Methotrimeprazine (Additive CNS depression).
No products indexed under this heading.

Methoxyflurane (Additive CNS depression).
No products indexed under this heading.

Midazolam Hydrochloride (Additive CNS depression).
No products indexed under this heading.

Molindone Hydrochloride (Additive CNS depression). Products include:
Moban Tablets 1108

Morphine Sulfate (Additive CNS depression). Products include:
Avinza Capsules 1714
Kadian Capsules 572
MS Contin Tablets 2703

Olanzapine (Additive CNS depression). Products include:
Symbyax Capsules 1788
Zyprexa Tablets 1798
Zyprexa IntraMuscular 1798
Zyprexa ZYDIS Orally Disintegrating Tablets 1798

Oxazepam (Additive CNS depression).
No products indexed under this heading.

Oxycodone Hydrochloride (Additive CNS depression). Products include:
Combunox Tablets 1183
OxyContin Tablets 2699
OxyFast Oral Concentrate Solution 2704
OxyIR Capsules 2704
Percocet Tablets 1114
Percodan Tablets 1115

Pentobarbital Sodium (Additive CNS depression). Products include:
Nembutal Sodium Solution, USP 2484

Perphenazine (Additive CNS depression).
No products indexed under this heading.

Phenobarbital (Additive CNS depression).
No products indexed under this heading.

Prazepam (Additive CNS depression).
No products indexed under this heading.

Prochlorperazine (Additive CNS depression).
No products indexed under this heading.

Promethazine Hydrochloride (Additive CNS depression). Products include:
Phenergan 3438

Propofol (Additive CNS depression). Products include:
Diprivan Injectable Emulsion 676

Propoxyphene Hydrochloride (Additive CNS depression).
No products indexed under this heading.

Propoxyphene Napsylate (Additive CNS depression). Products include:
Darvocet A 500 Tablets 3497

Quazepam (Additive CNS depression).
No products indexed under this heading.

Quetiapine Fumarate (Additive CNS depression). Products include:
Seroquel Tablets 691

Remifentanil Hydrochloride (Additive CNS depression).
No products indexed under this heading.

Risperidone (Additive CNS depression). Products include:
Risperdal Consta Long-Acting Injection 1664
Risperdal M-Tab Orally Disintegrating Tablets 1658
Risperdal 1658

Secobarbital Sodium (Additive CNS depression).
No products indexed under this heading.

Sevoflurane (Additive CNS depression). Products include:
Ultane Liquid for Inhalation 526

Sodium Oxybate (Additive CNS depression).
No products indexed under this heading.

Sufentanil Citrate (Additive CNS depression).
No products indexed under this heading.

Temazepam (Additive CNS depression).
No products indexed under this heading.

Thiamylal Sodium (Additive CNS depression).
No products indexed under this heading.

Thioridazine Hydrochloride (Additive CNS depression). Products include:
Thioridazine Hydrochloride Tablets 2122

Thiothixene (Additive CNS depression). Products include:
Thiothixene Capsules 2124

Triazolam (Additive CNS depression).
No products indexed under this heading.

Trifluoperazine Hydrochloride (Additive CNS depression).
No products indexed under this heading.

Zaleplon (Additive CNS depression). Products include:
Sonata Capsules 1686

Ziprasidone Hydrochloride (Additive CNS depression). Products include:
Geodon Capsules 2514

Zolpidem Tartrate (Additive CNS depression). Products include:
Ambien Tablets 2867

Food Interactions

Alcohol (Additive CNS depression).

NU-IRON 150 CAPSULES

(Polysaccharide Iron Complex) 2098
None cited in PDR database.

NUMORPHAN INJECTION

(Oxymorphone Hydrochloride) 1112
May interact with anticholinergics, central nervous system depressants, general anesthetics, hypnotics and sedatives, monoamine oxidase inhibitors, narcotic analgesics, phenothiazines, tranquilizers, tricyclic antidepressants, and certain other agents. Compounds in these categories include:

Alfentanil Hydrochloride (Concomitant use may produce additive CNS depressant effects).
No products indexed under this heading.

Alprazolam (Concomitant use may produce additive CNS depressant effects). Products include:
Niravam Orally Disintegrating Tablets 3106
Xanax XR Tablets 2655

Amitriptyline Hydrochloride (Concomitant use may produce additive CNS depressant effects).
No products indexed under this heading.

Amoxapine (Concomitant use may produce additive CNS depressant effects).
No products indexed under this heading.

Aprobarbital (Concomitant use may produce additive CNS depressant effects).
No products indexed under this heading.

Atropine Sulfate (Co-administration of anticholinergics and opiod analgesics may result in increased risk of urinary retention and/or severe constipation and paralytic ileus).
No products indexed under this heading.

Belladonna Alkaloids (Co-administration of anticholinergics and opiod analgesics may result in increased risk of urinary retention and/or severe constipation and paralytic ileus). Products include:
Hyland's Teething Tablets 736

Benztropine Mesylate (Co-administration of anticholinergics and opiod analgesics may result in increased risk of urinary retention and/or severe constipation and paralytic ileus). Products include:
Cogentin Injection 1903

Biperiden Hydrochloride (Co-administration of anticholinergics and opiod analgesics may result in increased risk of urinary retention and/or severe constipation and paralytic ileus).
No products indexed under this heading.

Buprenorphine Hydrochloride (Concomitant use may produce additive CNS depressant effects). Products include:
Buprenex Injectable 2718
Suboxone Tablets 2719
Subutex Tablets 2719

Buspirone Hydrochloride (Concomitant use may produce additive CNS depressant effects).
No products indexed under this heading.

Butabarbital (Concomitant use may produce additive CNS depressant effects).
No products indexed under this heading.

Butalbital (Concomitant use may produce additive CNS depressant effects). Products include:
Sedapap Tablets 50 mg/650 mg 2098

Chlordiazepoxide (Concomitant use may produce additive CNS depressant effects).
No products indexed under this heading.

Chlordiazepoxide Hydrochloride (Concomitant use may produce additive CNS depressant effects). Products include:
Librium Capsules 3349

Chlorpromazine (Concomitant use may produce additive CNS depressant effects).
No products indexed under this heading.

Chlorpromazine Hydrochloride (Concomitant use may produce additive CNS depressant effects).
No products indexed under this heading.

Chlorprothixene (Concomitant use may produce additive CNS depressant effects).
No products indexed under this heading.

Chlorprothixene Hydrochloride (Concomitant use may produce additive CNS depressant effects).
No products indexed under this heading.

Chlorprothixene Lactate (Concomitant use may produce additive CNS depressant effects).
No products indexed under this heading.

Cimetidine (Co-administration of cimetidine and opioid analgesics has resulted in confusion, disorientation, respiratory depression, apnea, and seizures; no clear-cut cause and effect relationship was established). Products include:
Tagamet HB 200 Tablets 637
Tagamet Tablets 1547

Cimetidine Hydrochloride (Co-administration of cimetidine and opioid analgesics has resulted in confusion, disorientation, respiratory depression, apnea, and seizures; no clear-cut cause and effect relationship was established).
No products indexed under this heading.

Clidinium Bromide (Co-administration of anticholinergics and opiod analgesics may result in increased risk of urinary retention and/or severe constipation and paralytic ileus).
No products indexed under this heading.

Clomipramine Hydrochloride (Concomitant use may produce additive CNS depressant effects).
No products indexed under this heading.

Clorazepate Dipotassium (Concomitant use may produce additive CNS depressant effects). Products include:
Tranxene 2488

Clozapine (Concomitant use may produce additive CNS depressant effects). Products include:
Clozapine Tablets 2141
Clozaril Tablets 2174
FazaClo Orally Disintegrating Tablets 547

Codeine Phosphate (Concomitant use may produce additive CNS depressant effects). Products include:
Tylenol with Codeine 2461

Desflurane (Concomitant use may produce additive CNS depressant effects). Products include:
Suprane Liquid for Inhalation 770

Desipramine Hydrochloride (Concomitant use may produce additive CNS depressant effects).
No products indexed under this heading.

Dezocine (Concomitant use may produce additive CNS depressant effects).
No products indexed under this heading.

Diazepam (Concomitant use may produce additive CNS depressant effects). Products include:
Diastat Rectal Delivery System 3344
Valium Tablets 2822

Dicyclomine Hydrochloride (Co-administration of anticholinergics and opiod analgesics may result in increased risk of urinary retention and/or severe constipation and paralytic ileus). Products include:
Bentyl Capsules 724
Bentyl Injection 724
Bentyl Syrup 724
Bentyl Tablets 724

Doxepin Hydrochloride (Concomitant use may produce additive CNS depressant effects).
No products indexed under this heading.

Droperidol (Concomitant use may produce additive CNS depressant effects).
No products indexed under this heading.

Enflurane (Concomitant use may produce additive CNS depressant effects).
No products indexed under this heading.

Estazolam (Concomitant use may produce additive CNS depressant effects). Products include:
ProSom Tablets 512

Ethanol (Concomitant use may produce additive CNS depressant effects).
No products indexed under this heading.

IMPORTANT NOTE: Always consult each drug listing in the patient's regimen for possible interactions.

Ethchlorvynol (Concomitant use may produce additive CNS depressant effects).
No products indexed under this heading.

Ethinamate (Concomitant use may produce additive CNS depressant effects).
No products indexed under this heading.

Ethyl Alcohol (Concomitant use may produce additive CNS depressant effects).
No products indexed under this heading.

Fentanyl (Concomitant use may produce additive CNS depressant effects). Products include:
Duragesic Transdermal System **2448**

Fentanyl Citrate (Concomitant use may produce additive CNS depressant effects). Products include:
Actiq **993**

Fluphenazine Decanoate (Concomitant use may produce additive CNS depressant effects).
No products indexed under this heading.

Fluphenazine Enanthate (Concomitant use may produce additive CNS depressant effects).
No products indexed under this heading.

Fluphenazine Hydrochloride (Concomitant use may produce additive CNS depressant effects).
No products indexed under this heading.

Flurazepam Hydrochloride (Concomitant use may produce additive CNS depressant effects). Products include:
Dalmane Capsules **3343**

Glutethimide (Concomitant use may produce additive CNS depressant effects).
No products indexed under this heading.

Glycopyrrolate (Co-administration of anticholinergics and opiod analgesics may result in increased risk of urinary retention and/or severe constipation and paralytic ileus).
No products indexed under this heading.

Haloperidol (Concomitant use may produce additive CNS depressant effects).
No products indexed under this heading.

Haloperidol Decanoate (Concomitant use may produce additive CNS depressant effects).
No products indexed under this heading.

Hydrocodone Bitartrate (Concomitant use may produce additive CNS depressant effects). Products include:
Hycodan **1104**
Hycomine Compound Tablets **1105**
Hycotuss Expectorant Syrup **1106**
Lortab **3315**
Lortab Elixir **3312**
Vicodin Tablets **530**
Vicodin ES Tablets **531**
Vicodin HP Tablets **532**
Vicoprofen Tablets **533**
Zydone Tablets **1118**

Hydrocodone Polistirex (Concomitant use may produce additive CNS depressant effects). Products include:
Tussionex Pennkinetic Extended-Release Suspension **3322**

Hydromorphone Hydrochloride (Concomitant use may produce additive CNS depressant effects). Products include:
Dilaudid **439**
Dilaudid Oral Liquid **443**
Dilaudid Non-Sterile Powder **439**
Dilaudid Rectal Suppositories **439**
Dilaudid Tablets **439**
Dilaudid Tablets - 8 mg **443**
Dilaudid-HP **441**

Hydroxyzine Hydrochloride (Concomitant use may produce additive CNS depressant effects).
No products indexed under this heading.

Hyoscyamine (Co-administration of anticholinergics and opiod analgesics may result in increased risk of urinary retention and/or severe constipation and paralytic ileus).
No products indexed under this heading.

Hyoscyamine Sulfate (Co-administration of anticholinergics and opiod analgesics may result in increased risk of urinary retention and/or severe constipation and paralytic ileus).
No products indexed under this heading.

Imipramine Hydrochloride (Concomitant use may produce additive CNS depressant effects).
No products indexed under this heading.

Imipramine Pamoate (Concomitant use may produce additive CNS depressant effects).
No products indexed under this heading.

Ipratropium Bromide (Co-administration of anticholinergics and opiod analgesics may result in increased risk of urinary retention and/or severe constipation and paralytic ileus). Products include:
Atrovent HFA Inhalation Aerosol **872**
Atrovent Inhalation Solution **868**
Atrovent Nasal Spray 0.03% **869**
Atrovent Nasal Spray 0.06% **870**
Combivent Inhalation Aerosol **878**
DuoNeb Inhalation Solution **1058**

Isocarboxazid (Concomitant use may produce additive CNS depressant effects).
No products indexed under this heading.

Isoflurane (Concomitant use may produce additive CNS depressant effects).
No products indexed under this heading.

Ketamine Hydrochloride (Concomitant use may produce additive CNS depressant effects).
No products indexed under this heading.

Levomethadyl Acetate Hydrochloride (Concomitant use may produce additive CNS depressant effects).
No products indexed under this heading.

Levorphanol Tartrate (Concomitant use may produce additive CNS depressant effects).
No products indexed under this heading.

Lorazepam (Concomitant use may produce additive CNS depressant effects).
No products indexed under this heading.

Loxapine Hydrochloride (Concomitant use may produce additive CNS depressant effects).
No products indexed under this heading.

Loxapine Succinate (Concomitant use may produce additive CNS depressant effects).
No products indexed under this heading.

Maprotiline Hydrochloride (Concomitant use may produce additive CNS depressant effects).
No products indexed under this heading.

Mepenzolate Bromide (Co-administration of anticholinergics and opiod analgesics may result in increased risk of urinary retention and/or severe constipation and paralytic ileus).
No products indexed under this heading.

Meperidine Hydrochloride (Concomitant use may produce additive CNS depressant effects).
No products indexed under this heading.

Mephobarbital (Concomitant use may produce additive CNS depressant effects). Products include:
Mebaral Tablets, USP **2483**

Meprobamate (Concomitant use may produce additive CNS depressant effects).
No products indexed under this heading.

Mesoridazine Besylate (Concomitant use may produce additive CNS depressant effects).
No products indexed under this heading.

Methadone Hydrochloride (Concomitant use may produce additive CNS depressant effects).
No products indexed under this heading.

Methohexital Sodium (Concomitant use may produce additive CNS depressant effects).
No products indexed under this heading.

Methotrimeprazine (Concomitant use may produce additive CNS depressant effects).
No products indexed under this heading.

Methoxyflurane (Concomitant use may produce additive CNS depressant effects).
No products indexed under this heading.

Midazolam Hydrochloride (Concomitant use may produce additive CNS depressant effects).
No products indexed under this heading.

Moclobemide (Concomitant use may produce additive CNS depressant effects).
No products indexed under this heading.

Molindone Hydrochloride (Concomitant use may produce additive CNS depressant effects). Products include:
Moban Tablets **1108**

Morphine Sulfate (Concomitant use may produce additive CNS depressant effects). Products include:
Avinza Capsules **1714**
Kadian Capsules **572**
MS Contin Tablets **2703**

Nortriptyline Hydrochloride (Concomitant use may produce additive CNS depressant effects).
No products indexed under this heading.

Olanzapine (Concomitant use may produce additive CNS depressant effects). Products include:
Symbyax Capsules **1788**
Zyprexa Tablets **1798**
Zyprexa IntraMuscular **1798**
Zyprexa ZYDIS Orally Disintegrating Tablets **1798**

Oxazepam (Concomitant use may produce additive CNS depressant effects).
No products indexed under this heading.

Oxybutynin Chloride (Co-administration of anticholinergics and opiod analgesics may result in increased risk of urinary retention and/or severe constipation and paralytic ileus). Products include:
Ditropan XL Extended Release Tablets **2391**

Oxycodone Hydrochloride (Concomitant use may produce additive CNS depressant effects). Products include:
Combunox Tablets **1183**
OxyContin Tablets **2699**
OxyFast Oral Concentrate Solution **2704**
OxyIR Capsules **2704**
Percocet Tablets **1114**
Percodan Tablets **1115**

Pargyline Hydrochloride (Concomitant use may produce additive CNS depressant effects).
No products indexed under this heading.

Pentobarbital Sodium (Concomitant use may produce additive CNS depressant effects). Products include:
Nembutal Sodium Solution, USP **2484**

Perphenazine (Concomitant use may produce additive CNS depressant effects).
No products indexed under this heading.

Phenelzine Sulfate (Concomitant use may produce additive CNS depressant effects).
No products indexed under this heading.

Phenobarbital (Concomitant use may produce additive CNS depressant effects).
No products indexed under this heading.

Prazepam (Concomitant use may produce additive CNS depressant effects).
No products indexed under this heading.

Procarbazine Hydrochloride (Concomitant use may produce additive CNS depressant effects). Products include:
Matulane Capsules **3188**

Prochlorperazine (Concomitant use may produce additive CNS depressant effects).
No products indexed under this heading.

Procyclidine Hydrochloride (Co-administration of anticholinergics and opiod analgesics may result in increased risk of urinary retention and/or severe constipation and paralytic ileus).
No products indexed under this heading.

Promethazine Hydrochloride (Concomitant use may produce additive CNS depressant effects). Products include:
Phenergan 3438

Propantheline Bromide (Co-administration of anticholinergics and opioid analgesics may result in increased risk of urinary retention and/or severe constipation and paralytic ileus).
No products indexed under this heading.

Propofol (Co-administration has resulted in increased incidence of bradycardia; concomitant use may produce additive CNS depressant effects). Products include:
Diprivan Injectable Emulsion 676

Propoxyphene Hydrochloride (Concomitant use may produce additive CNS depressant effects).
No products indexed under this heading.

Propoxyphene Napsylate (Concomitant use may produce additive CNS depressant effects). Products include:
Darvocet A 500 Tablets 3497

Protriptyline Hydrochloride (Concomitant use may produce additive CNS depressant effects). Products include:
Vivactil Tablets 2350

Quazepam (Concomitant use may produce additive CNS depressant effects).
No products indexed under this heading.

Quetiapine Fumarate (Concomitant use may produce additive CNS depressant effects). Products include:
Seroquel Tablets 691

Remifentanil Hydrochloride (Concomitant use may produce additive CNS depressant effects).
No products indexed under this heading.

Risperidone (Concomitant use may produce additive CNS depressant effects). Products include:
Risperdal Consta Long-Acting Injection 1664
Risperdal M-Tab Orally Disintegrating Tablets.................. 1658
Risperdal 1658

Scopolamine (Co-administration of anticholinergics and opiod analgesics may result in increased risk of urinary retention and/or severe constipation and paralytic ileus).
Products include:
Transderm Scōp Transdermal Therapeutic System 2166

Scopolamine Hydrobromide (Co-administration of anticholinergics and opioid analgesics may result in increased risk of urinary retention and/or severe constipation and paralytic ileus).
No products indexed under this heading.

Secobarbital Sodium (Concomitant use may produce additive CNS depressant effects).
No products indexed under this heading.

Selegiline Hydrochloride (Concomitant use may produce additive CNS depressant effects). Products include:
Eldepryl Capsules 3209

Sevoflurane (Concomitant use may produce additive CNS depressant effects). Products include:
Ultane Liquid for Inhalation 526

Sodium Oxybate (Concomitant use may produce additive CNS depressant effects).
No products indexed under this heading.

Sufentanil Citrate (Concomitant use may produce additive CNS depressant effects).
No products indexed under this heading.

Temazepam (Concomitant use may produce additive CNS depressant effects).
No products indexed under this heading.

Thiamylal Sodium (Concomitant use may produce additive CNS depressant effects).
No products indexed under this heading.

Thioridazine Hydrochloride (Concomitant use may produce additive CNS depressant effects). Products include:
Thioridazine Hydrochloride Tablets 2122

Thiothixene (Concomitant use may produce additive CNS depressant effects). Products include:
Thiothixene Capsules 2124

Tolterodine Tartrate (Co-administration of anticholinergics and opioid analgesics may result in increased risk of urinary retention and/or severe constipation and paralytic ileus). Products include:
Detrol Tablets 2626
Detrol LA Capsules 2629

Tranylcypromine Sulfate (Concomitant use may produce additive CNS depressant effects). Products include:
Parnate Tablets 1499

Triazolam (Concomitant use may produce additive CNS depressant effects).
No products indexed under this heading.

Tridihexethyl Chloride (Co-administration of anticholinergics and opioid analgesics may result in increased risk of urinary retention and/or severe constipation and paralytic ileus).
No products indexed under this heading.

Trifluoperazine Hydrochloride (Concomitant use may produce additive CNS depressant effects).
No products indexed under this heading.

Trihexyphenidyl Hydrochloride (Co-administration of anticholinergics and opioid analgesics may result in increased risk of urinary retention and/or severe constipation and paralytic ileus).
No products indexed under this heading.

Trimipramine Maleate (Concomitant use may produce additive CNS depressant effects). Products include:
Surmontil Capsules 2347

Zaleplon (Concomitant use may produce additive CNS depressant effects). Products include:
Sonata Capsules 1686

Ziprasidone Hydrochloride (Concomitant use may produce additive CNS depressant effects). Products include:
Geodon Capsules 2514

Zolpidem Tartrate (Concomitant use may produce additive CNS depressant effects). Products include:
Ambien Tablets 2867

Food Interactions

Alcohol (Concomitant use may produce additive CNS depressant effects).

NUMORPHAN SUPPOSITORIES
(Oxymorphone Hydrochloride) 1112
See Numorphan Injection

NUTRISURE OTC TABLETS
(Folic Acid, Herbals, Multiple, Vitamins with Minerals)...................... 3392
None cited in PDR database.

NUTROPIN FOR INJECTION
(Somatropin) 1238
May interact with corticosteroids, phenytoin, and certain other agents. Compounds in these categories include:

Betamethasone Acetate (Excessive glucocorticoid therapy will inhibit the growth-promoting effect of human growth hormone).
No products indexed under this heading.

Betamethasone Sodium Phosphate (Excessive glucocorticoid therapy will inhibit the growth-promoting effect of human growth hormone).
No products indexed under this heading.

Carbamazepine (Limited published data suggests that growth hormone treatment increased CYP450 mediated antipyrine clearance in man; therefore, growth hormone administration may alter the clearance of compounds known to be metabolized by CYP450 liver enzymes, such as anticonvulsants including carbamazepine). Products include:
Carbatrol Capsules 3174
Equetro Extended-Release Capsules 3178
Tegretol/Tegretol-XR 2278

Cortisone Acetate (Excessive glucocorticoid therapy will inhibit the growth-promoting effect of human growth hormone).
No products indexed under this heading.

Cyclosporine (Limited published data suggests that growth hormone treatment increases CYP450 mediated antipyrine clearance in man, therefore, growth hormone administration may alter the clearance of compounds known to be metabolized by CYP450 liver enzymes, such as cyclosporine). Products include:
Gengraf Capsules 458
Neoral Soft Gelatin Capsules 2247
Neoral Oral Solution 2247
Restasis Ophthalmic Emulsion 570
Sandimmune 2259

Dexamethasone (Excessive glucocorticoid therapy will inhibit the growth-promoting effect of human growth hormone). Products include:
Ciprodex Otic Suspension 555
Decadron Tablets 1929
TobraDex Ophthalmic Ointment 558
TobraDex Ophthalmic Suspension ... 558

Dexamethasone Acetate (Excessive glucocorticoid therapy will inhibit the growth-promoting effect of human growth hormone).
No products indexed under this heading.

Dexamethasone Sodium Phosphate (Excessive glucocorticoid therapy will inhibit the growth-promoting effect of human growth hormone). Products include:
Decadron Phosphate Injection 1931

Fludrocortisone Acetate (Excessive glucocorticoid therapy will inhibit the growth-promoting effect of human growth hormone).
No products indexed under this heading.

Fosphenytoin Sodium (Limited published data suggests that growth hormone treatment increases CYP450 mediated antipyrine clearance in man; therefore, growth hormone administration may alter the clearance of compounds known to be metabolized by CYP450 liver enzymes, such as anticonvulsants, including phenytoin).
No products indexed under this heading.

Hydrocortisone (Excessive glucocorticoid therapy will inhibit the growth-promoting effect of human growth hormone). Products include:
Cortizone•5 Ointment 699
Cortizone•10 Creme 699
Cortizone•10 Ointment 699
Cortizone•10 Plus Creme 700
Cortizone•10 Maximum Strength Quick Shot Spray........................ 700
Hydrocortone Tablets 1963
Preparation H Hydrocortisone Cream 748

Hydrocortisone Acetate (Excessive glucocorticoid therapy will inhibit the growth-promoting effect of human growth hormone). Products include:
Analpram-HC 1136
Pramosone 1139
ProctoFoam-HC 3113
Tucks Anti-Itch Ointment 712
U-cort 1% Cream 3289

Hydrocortisone Sodium Phosphate (Excessive glucocorticoid therapy will inhibit the growth-promoting effect of human growth hormone).
No products indexed under this heading.

Hydrocortisone Sodium Succinate (Excessive glucocorticoid therapy will inhibit the growth-promoting effect of human growth hormone).
No products indexed under this heading.

Methylprednisolone Acetate (Excessive glucocorticoid therapy will inhibit the growth-promoting effect of human growth hormone).
Products include:
Depo-Medrol Injectable Suspension 2615
Depo-Medrol Single-Dose Vial 2617

Methylprednisolone Sodium Succinate (Excessive glucocorticoid therapy will inhibit the growth-promoting effect of human growth hormone).
No products indexed under this heading.

IMPORTANT NOTE: Always consult each drug listing in the patient's regimen for possible interactions.

Phenytoin (Limited published data suggests that growth hormone treatment increases CYP450 mediated antipyrine clearance in man; therefore, growth hormone administration may alter the clearance of compounds known to be metabolized by CYP450 liver enzymes, such as anticonvulsants, including phenytoin).
No products indexed under this heading.

Phenytoin Sodium (Limited published data suggests that growth hormone treatment increases CYP450 mediated antipyrine clearance in man; therefore, growth hormone administration may alter the clearance of compounds known to be metabolized by CYP450 liver enzymes, such as anticonvulsants, including phenytoin). Products include:
Phenytek Capsules 2153

Prednisolone Acetate (Excessive glucocorticoid therapy will inhibit the growth-promoting effect of human growth hormone). Products include:
Blephamide Ophthalmic Ointment 563
Blephamide Ophthalmic Suspension 564
Poly-Pred Liquifilm Ophthalmic Suspension .... ⊙231
Pred Forte Ophthalmic Suspension .... ⊙233
Pred Mild Sterile Ophthalmic Suspension .... ⊙236
Pred-G Ophthalmic Suspension ..... ⊙234
Pred-G Sterile Ophthalmic Ointment .... ⊙235

Prednisolone Sodium Phosphate (Excessive glucocorticoid therapy will inhibit the growth-promoting effect of human growth hormone). Products include:
Pediapred Oral Solution 3319

Prednisolone Tebutate (Excessive glucocorticoid therapy will inhibit the growth-promoting effect of human growth hormone).
No products indexed under this heading.

Prednisone (Excessive glucocorticoid therapy will inhibit the growth-promoting effect of human growth hormone).
No products indexed under this heading.

Triamcinolone (Excessive glucocorticoid therapy will inhibit the growth-promoting effect of human growth hormone).
No products indexed under this heading.

Triamcinolone Acetonide (Excessive glucocorticoid therapy will inhibit the growth-promoting effect of human growth hormone). Products include:
Azmacort Inhalation Aerosol 1701
Nasacort HFA Inhalation Aerosol 2939
Nasacort AQ Nasal Spray 2937

Triamcinolone Diacetate (Excessive glucocorticoid therapy will inhibit the growth-promoting effect of human growth hormone).
No products indexed under this heading.

Triamcinolone Hexacetonide (Excessive glucocorticoid therapy will inhibit the growth-promoting effect of human growth hormone).
No products indexed under this heading.

NUTROPIN AQ INJECTION
(Somatropin) 1241
See Nutropin for Injection

NUTROPIN AQ PEN
(Somatropin) 1241
See Nutropin for Injection

NUTROPIN AQ PEN CARTRIDGE
(Somatropin) 1241
See Nutropin for Injection

NUVARING
(Ethinyl Estradiol, Etonogestrel) 2357
None cited in PDR database.

NYSTATIN VAGINAL TABLETS, USP
(Nystatin) 2347
None cited in PDR database.

NYSTOP TOPICAL POWDER USP
(Nystatin) 2490
None cited in PDR database.

NYTOL QUICKCAPS CAPLETS
(Diphenhydramine Hydrochloride) ..... ▣635
See Maximum Strength Nytol QuickGels Softgels

MAXIMUM STRENGTH NYTOL QUICKGELS SOFTGELS
(Diphenhydramine Hydrochloride) ..... ▣635
May interact with central nervous system depressants, monoamine oxidase inhibitors, and certain other agents. Compounds in these categories include:

Alfentanil Hydrochloride (Concurrent use with CNS depressant will heighten the depressant effect of Nytol).
No products indexed under this heading.

Alprazolam (Concurrent use with CNS depressant will heighten the depressant effect of Nytol). Products include:
Niravam Orally Disintegrating Tablets 3106
Xanax XR Tablets 2655

Aprobarbital (Concurrent use with CNS depressant will heighten the depressant effect of Nytol).
No products indexed under this heading.

Buprenorphine Hydrochloride (Concurrent use with CNS depressant will heighten the depressant effect of Nytol). Products include:
Buprenex Injectable 2718
Suboxone Tablets 2719
Subutex Tablets 2719

Buspirone Hydrochloride (Concurrent use with CNS depressant will heighten the depressant effect of Nytol).
No products indexed under this heading.

Butabarbital (Concurrent use with CNS depressant will heighten the depressant effect of Nytol).
No products indexed under this heading.

Butalbital (Concurrent use with CNS depressant will heighten the depressant effect of Nytol). Products include:
Sedapap Tablets 50 mg/650 mg 2098

Chlordiazepoxide (Concurrent use with CNS depressant will heighten the depressant effect of Nytol).
No products indexed under this heading.

Chlordiazepoxide Hydrochloride (Concurrent use with CNS depressant will heighten the depressant effect of Nytol). Products include:
Librium Capsules 3349

Chlorpromazine (Concurrent use with CNS depressant will heighten the depressant effect of Nytol).
No products indexed under this heading.

Chlorpromazine Hydrochloride (Concurrent use with CNS depressant will heighten the depressant effect of Nytol).
No products indexed under this heading.

Chlorprothixene (Concurrent use with CNS depressant will heighten the depressant effect of Nytol).
No products indexed under this heading.

Chlorprothixene Hydrochloride (Concurrent use with CNS depressant will heighten the depressant effect of Nytol).
No products indexed under this heading.

Chlorprothixene Lactate (Concurrent use with CNS depressant will heighten the depressant effect of Nytol).
No products indexed under this heading.

Clorazepate Dipotassium (Concurrent use with CNS depressant will heighten the depressant effect of Nytol). Products include:
Tranxene 2488

Clozapine (Concurrent use with CNS depressant will heighten the depressant effect of Nytol). Products include:
Clozapine Tablets 2141
Clozaril Tablets 2174
FazaClo Orally Disintegrating Tablets 547

Codeine Phosphate (Concurrent use with CNS depressant will heighten the depressant effect of Nytol). Products include:
Tylenol with Codeine 2461

Desflurane (Concurrent use with CNS depressant will heighten the depressant effect of Nytol). Products include:
Suprane Liquid for Inhalation 770

Dezocine (Concurrent use with CNS depressant will heighten the depressant effect of Nytol).
No products indexed under this heading.

Diazepam (Concurrent use with CNS depressant will heighten the depressant effect of Nytol). Products include:
Diastat Rectal Delivery System 3344
Valium Tablets 2822

Droperidol (Concurrent use with CNS depressant will heighten the depressant effect of Nytol).
No products indexed under this heading.

Enflurane (Concurrent use with CNS depressant will heighten the depressant effect of Nytol).
No products indexed under this heading.

Estazolam (Concurrent use with CNS depressant will heighten the depressant effect of Nytol). Products include:
ProSom Tablets 512

Ethanol (Concurrent use with CNS depressant will heighten the depressant effect of Nytol).
No products indexed under this heading.

Ethchlorvynol (Concurrent use with CNS depressant will heighten the depressant effect of Nytol).
No products indexed under this heading.

Ethinamate (Concurrent use with CNS depressant will heighten the depressant effect of Nytol).
No products indexed under this heading.

Ethyl Alcohol (Concurrent use with CNS depressant will heighten the depressant effect of Nytol).
No products indexed under this heading.

Fentanyl (Concurrent use with CNS depressant will heighten the depressant effect of Nytol). Products include:
Duragesic Transdermal System 2448

Fentanyl Citrate (Concurrent use with CNS depressant will heighten the depressant effect of Nytol). Products include:
Actiq 993

Fluphenazine Decanoate (Concurrent use with CNS depressant will heighten the depressant effect of Nytol).
No products indexed under this heading.

Fluphenazine Enanthate (Concurrent use with CNS depressant will heighten the depressant effect of Nytol).
No products indexed under this heading.

Fluphenazine Hydrochloride (Concurrent use with CNS depressant will heighten the depressant effect of Nytol).
No products indexed under this heading.

Flurazepam Hydrochloride (Concurrent use with CNS depressant will heighten the depressant effect of Nytol). Products include:
Dalmane Capsules 3343

Glutethimide (Concurrent use with CNS depressant will heighten the depressant effect of Nytol).
No products indexed under this heading.

Haloperidol (Concurrent use with CNS depressant will heighten the depressant effect of Nytol).
No products indexed under this heading.

Haloperidol Decanoate (Concurrent use with CNS depressant will heighten the depressant effect of Nytol).
No products indexed under this heading.

Hydrocodone Bitartrate (Concurrent use with CNS depressant will heighten the depressant effect of Nytol). Products include:
Hycodan 1104
Hycomine Compound Tablets 1105
Hycotuss Expectorant Syrup 1106
Lortab 3315
Lortab Elixir 3312
Vicodin Tablets 530
Vicodin ES Tablets 531
Vicodin HP Tablets 532
Vicoprofen Tablets 533
Zydone Tablets 1118

Hydrocodone Polistirex (Concurrent use with CNS depressant will heighten the depressant effect of Nytol). Products include:
Tussionex Pennkinetic Extended-Release Suspension 3322

Hydromorphone Hydrochloride (Concurrent use with CNS depressant will heighten the depressant effect of Nytol). Products include:
Dilaudid ... 439
Dilaudid Oral Liquid ... 443
Dilaudid Non-Sterile Powder ... 439
Dilaudid Rectal Suppositories ... 439
Dilaudid Tablets ... 439
Dilaudid Tablets - 8 mg ... 443
Dilaudid-HP ... 441

Hydroxyzine Hydrochloride (Concurrent use with CNS depressant will heighten the depressant effect of Nytol).
No products indexed under this heading.

Isocarboxazid (Concurrent use with MAO inhibitor will prolong and intensify the anticholinergic effects of antihistamines).
No products indexed under this heading.

Isoflurane (Concurrent use with CNS depressant will heighten the depressant effect of Nytol).
No products indexed under this heading.

Ketamine Hydrochloride (Concurrent use with CNS depressant will heighten the depressant effect of Nytol).
No products indexed under this heading.

Levomethadyl Acetate Hydrochloride (Concurrent use with CNS depressant will heighten the depressant effect of Nytol).
No products indexed under this heading.

Levorphanol Tartrate (Concurrent use with CNS depressant will heighten the depressant effect of Nytol).
No products indexed under this heading.

Lorazepam (Concurrent use with CNS depressant will heighten the depressant effect of Nytol).
No products indexed under this heading.

Loxapine Hydrochloride (Concurrent use with CNS depressant will heighten the depressant effect of Nytol).
No products indexed under this heading.

Loxapine Succinate (Concurrent use with CNS depressant will heighten the depressant effect of Nytol).
No products indexed under this heading.

Meperidine Hydrochloride (Concurrent use with CNS depressant will heighten the depressant effect of Nytol).
No products indexed under this heading.

Mephobarbital (Concurrent use with CNS depressant will heighten the depressant effect of Nytol). Products include:
Mebaral Tablets, USP ... 2483

Meprobamate (Concurrent use with CNS depressant will heighten the depressant effect of Nytol).
No products indexed under this heading.

Mesoridazine Besylate (Concurrent use with CNS depressant will heighten the depressant effect of Nytol).
No products indexed under this heading.

Methadone Hydrochloride (Concurrent use with CNS depressant will heighten the depressant effect of Nytol).
No products indexed under this heading.

Methohexital Sodium (Concurrent use with CNS depressant will heighten the depressant effect of Nytol).
No products indexed under this heading.

Methotrimeprazine (Concurrent use with CNS depressant will heighten the depressant effect of Nytol).
No products indexed under this heading.

Methoxyflurane (Concurrent use with CNS depressant will heighten the depressant effect of Nytol).
No products indexed under this heading.

Midazolam Hydrochloride (Concurrent use with CNS depressant will heighten the depressant effect of Nytol).
No products indexed under this heading.

Moclobemide (Concurrent use with MAO inhibitor will prolong and intensify the anticholinergic effects of antihistamines).
No products indexed under this heading.

Molindone Hydrochloride (Concurrent use with CNS depressant will heighten the depressant effect of Nytol). Products include:
Moban Tablets ... 1108

Morphine Sulfate (Concurrent use with CNS depressant will heighten the depressant effect of Nytol). Products include:
Avinza Capsules ... 1714
Kadian Capsules ... 572
MS Contin Tablets ... 2703

Olanzapine (Concurrent use with CNS depressant will heighten the depressant effect of Nytol). Products include:
Symbyax Capsules ... 1788
Zyprexa Tablets ... 1798
Zyprexa IntraMuscular ... 1798
Zyprexa ZYDIS Orally Disintegrating Tablets ... 1798

Oxazepam (Concurrent use with CNS depressant will heighten the depressant effect of Nytol).
No products indexed under this heading.

Oxycodone Hydrochloride (Concurrent use with CNS depressant will heighten the depressant effect of Nytol). Products include:
Combunox Tablets ... 1183
OxyContin Tablets ... 2699
OxyFast Oral Concentrate Solution ... 2704
OxyIR Capsules ... 2704
Percocet Tablets ... 1114
Percodan Tablets ... 1115

Pargyline Hydrochloride (Concurrent use with MAO inhibitor will prolong and intensify the anticholinergic effects of antihistamines).
No products indexed under this heading.

Pentobarbital Sodium (Concurrent use with CNS depressant will heighten the depressant effect of Nytol). Products include:
Nembutal Sodium Solution, USP ... 2484

Perphenazine (Concurrent use with CNS depressant will heighten the depressant effect of Nytol).
No products indexed under this heading.

Phenelzine Sulfate (Concurrent use with MAO inhibitor will prolong and intensify the anticholinergic effects of antihistamines).
No products indexed under this heading.

Phenobarbital (Concurrent use with CNS depressant will heighten the depressant effect of Nytol).
No products indexed under this heading.

Prazepam (Concurrent use with CNS depressant will heighten the depressant effect of Nytol).
No products indexed under this heading.

Procarbazine Hydrochloride (Concurrent use with MAO inhibitor will prolong and intensify the anticholinergic effects of antihistamines). Products include:
Matulane Capsules ... 3188

Prochlorperazine (Concurrent use with CNS depressant will heighten the depressant effect of Nytol).
No products indexed under this heading.

Promethazine Hydrochloride (Concurrent use with CNS depressant will heighten the depressant effect of Nytol). Products include:
Phenergan ... 3438

Propofol (Concurrent use with CNS depressant will heighten the depressant effect of Nytol). Products include:
Diprivan Injectable Emulsion ... 676

Propoxyphene Hydrochloride (Concurrent use with CNS depressant will heighten the depressant effect of Nytol).
No products indexed under this heading.

Propoxyphene Napsylate (Concurrent use with CNS depressant will heighten the depressant effect of Nytol). Products include:
Darvocet A 500 Tablets ... 3497

Quazepam (Concurrent use with CNS depressant will heighten the depressant effect of Nytol).
No products indexed under this heading.

Quetiapine Fumarate (Concurrent use with CNS depressant will heighten the depressant effect of Nytol). Products include:
Seroquel Tablets ... 691

Remifentanil Hydrochloride (Concurrent use with CNS depressant will heighten the depressant effect of Nytol).
No products indexed under this heading.

Risperidone (Concurrent use with CNS depressant will heighten the depressant effect of Nytol). Products include:
Risperdal Consta Long-Acting Injection ... 1664
Risperdal M-Tab Orally Disintegrating Tablets ... 1658
Risperdal ... 1658

Secobarbital Sodium (Concurrent use with CNS depressant will heighten the depressant effect of Nytol).
No products indexed under this heading.

Selegiline Hydrochloride (Concurrent use with MAO inhibitor will prolong and intensify the anticholinergic effects of antihistamines). Products include:
Eldepryl Capsules ... 3209

Sevoflurane (Concurrent use with CNS depressant will heighten the depressant effect of Nytol). Products include:
Ultane Liquid for Inhalation ... 526

Sufentanil Citrate (Concurrent use with CNS depressant will heighten the depressant effect of Nytol).
No products indexed under this heading.

Temazepam (Concurrent use with CNS depressant will heighten the depressant effect of Nytol).
No products indexed under this heading.

Thiamylal Sodium (Concurrent use with CNS depressant will heighten the depressant effect of Nytol).
No products indexed under this heading.

Thioridazine Hydrochloride (Concurrent use with CNS depressant will heighten the depressant effect of Nytol). Products include:
Thioridazine Hydrochloride Tablets ... 2122

Thiothixene (Concurrent use with CNS depressant will heighten the depressant effect of Nytol). Products include:
Thiothixene Capsules ... 2124

Tranylcypromine Sulfate (Concurrent use with MAO inhibitor will prolong and intensify the anticholinergic effects of antihistamines). Products include:
Parnate Tablets ... 1499

Triazolam (Concurrent use with CNS depressant will heighten the depressant effect of Nytol).
No products indexed under this heading.

Trifluoperazine Hydrochloride (Concurrent use with CNS depressant will heighten the depressant effect of Nytol).
No products indexed under this heading.

Zaleplon (Concurrent use with CNS depressant will heighten the depressant effect of Nytol). Products include:
Sonata Capsules ... 1686

Ziprasidone Hydrochloride (Concurrent use with CNS depressant will heighten the depressant effect of Nytol). Products include:
Geodon Capsules ... 2514

Zolpidem Tartrate (Concurrent use with CNS depressant will heighten the depressant effect of Nytol). Products include:
Ambien Tablets ... 2867

Food Interactions

Alcohol (Concurrent use will heighten the depressant effect of Nytol; avoid alcoholic beverages while taking this product).

OCUCOAT

(Hydroxypropyl Methylcellulose) ... ⊙290
None cited in PDR database.

OCUFEN OPHTHALMIC SOLUTION
(Flurbiprofen Sodium) .... ⊙230
May interact with:

Acetylcholine Chloride (There have been reports that acetylcholine chloride is ineffective when used in patients treated with ophthalmic flurbiprofen).
No products indexed under this heading.

Carbachol (There have been reports that carbachol is ineffective when used in patients treated with ophthalmic flurbiprofen).
No products indexed under this heading.

OCUVITE LUTEIN VITAMIN AND MINERAL SUPPLEMENT
(Vitamins with Minerals) .... ⊙252
None cited in PDR database.

OCUVITE VITAMIN AND MINERAL SUPPLEMENT
(Vitamins with Minerals) .... ⊙251
None cited in PDR database.

OCUVITE EXTRA VITAMIN AND MINERAL SUPPLEMENT
(Vitamins with Minerals) .... ⊙252
None cited in PDR database.

OLUX FOAM
(Clobetasol Propionate) 1027
None cited in PDR database.

OMACOR CAPSULES
(Omega-3-acid ethyl esters) 2735
May interact with anticoagulants and oral anticoagulants. Compounds in these categories include:

Anisindione (Some studies with omega-3-acids demonstrated prolongation of bleeding time. Patients receiving treatment with omega-3-acid ethyl esters and anticoagulants should be monitored periodically). Products include:
Miradon Tablets 3056

Ardeparin Sodium (Some studies with omega-3-acids demonstrated prolongation of bleeding time. Patients receiving treatment with omega-3-acid ethyl esters and anticoagulants should be monitored periodically).
No products indexed under this heading.

Dalteparin Sodium (Some studies with omega-3-acids demonstrated prolongation of bleeding time. Patients receiving treatment with omega-3-acid ethyl esters and anticoagulants should be monitored periodically). Products include:
Fragmin Injection 2638

Danaparoid Sodium (Some studies with omega-3-acids demonstrated prolongation of bleeding time. Patients receiving treatment with omega-3-acid ethyl esters and anticoagulants should be monitored periodically).
No products indexed under this heading.

Dicumarol (Some studies with omega-3-acids demonstrated prolongation of bleeding time. Patients receiving treatment with omega-3-acid ethyl esters and anticoagulants should be monitored periodically).
No products indexed under this heading.

Enoxaparin Sodium (Some studies with omega-3-acids demonstrated prolongation of bleeding time. Patients receiving treatment with omega-3-acid ethyl esters and anticoagulants should be monitored periodically). Products include:
Lovenox Injection 2931

Fondaparinux Sodium (Some studies with omega-3-acids demonstrated prolongation of bleeding time. Patients receiving treatment with omega-3-acid ethyl esters and anticoagulants should be monitored periodically). Products include:
Arixtra Injection 1325

Heparin Calcium (Some studies with omega-3-acids demonstrated prolongation of bleeding time. Patients receiving treatment with omega-3-acid ethyl esters and anticoagulants should be monitored periodically).
No products indexed under this heading.

Heparin Sodium (Some studies with omega-3-acids demonstrated prolongation of bleeding time. Patients receiving treatment with omega-3-acid ethyl esters and anticoagulants should be monitored periodically).
No products indexed under this heading.

Low Molecular Weight Heparins (Some studies with omega-3-acids demonstrated prolongation of bleeding time. Patients receiving treatment with omega-3-acid ethyl esters and anticoagulants should be monitored periodically).
No products indexed under this heading.

Tinzaparin Sodium (Some studies with omega-3-acids demonstrated prolongation of bleeding time. Patients receiving treatment with omega-3-acid ethyl esters and anticoagulants should be monitored periodically).
No products indexed under this heading.

Warfarin Sodium (Some studies with omega-3-acids demonstrated prolongation of bleeding time. Patients receiving treatment with omega-3-acid ethyl esters and anticoagulants should be monitored periodically). Products include:
Coumadin for Injection 932
Coumadin Tablets 932

OMNICEF CAPSULES
(Cefdinir) 506
May interact with antacids containing aluminum, calcium and magnesium, iron containing oral preparations, and certain other agents. Compounds in these categories include:

Aluminum Carbonate (Antacids (aluminum- or magnesium-containing) interfere with the absorption of cefdinir; Omnicef should be taken at least 2 hours before or after the antacids).
No products indexed under this heading.

Aluminum Hydroxide (Antacids (aluminum- or magnesium-containing) interfere with the absorption of cefdinir; Omnicef should be taken at least 2 hours before or after the antacids). Products include:
Gaviscon Regular Strength Liquid .. ▣620
Gaviscon Regular Strength Tablets .... ▣619
Gaviscon Extra Strength Liquid ...... ▣620
Gaviscon Extra Strength Tablets .... ▣619
Maalox Max Maximum Strength Antacid/Anti-Gas Liquid 2165
Maalox Regular Strength Antacid/Antigas Liquid 2164

Ferrous Fumarate (Iron supplements, including multivitamins that contain iron, interfere with the absorption of cefdinir; Omnicef should be taken at least 2 hours before or after the administration of iron-containing products). Products include:
Chromagen Forte Soft Gelatin Capsules 3296
Ferretts Tablets .... ▣773
Repliva 21/7 Tablets 3301

Ferrous Gluconate (Iron supplements, including multivitamins that contain iron, interfere with the absorption of cefdinir; Omnicef should be taken at least 2 hours before or after the administration of iron-containing products).
No products indexed under this heading.

Ferrous Sulfate (Iron supplements, including multivitamins that contain iron, interfere with the absorption of cefdinir; Omnicef should be taken at least 2 hours before or after the administration of iron-containing products). Products include:
Feosol Tablets 1629
Slow Fe Iron Tablets .... ▣772
Slow Fe with Folic Acid Tablets .... ▣773

Iron (Iron supplements, including multivitamins that contain iron, interfere with the absorption of cefdinir; Omnicef should be taken at least 2 hours before or after the administration of iron-containing products). Products include:
Chromagen Forte Soft Gelatin Capsules 3296
Ferretts IPS Liquid .... ▣773
OptiNate 1162
Repliva 21/7 Tablets 3301

Magaldrate (Antacids (aluminum- or magnesium-containing) interfere with the absorption of cefdinir; Omnicef should be taken at least 2 hours before or after the antacids).
No products indexed under this heading.

Magnesium Hydroxide (Antacids (aluminum- or magnesium-containing) interfere with the absorption of cefdinir; Omnicef should be taken at least 2 hours before or after the antacids). Products include:
Maalox Max Maximum Strength Antacid/Anti-Gas Liquid 2165
Maalox Regular Strength Antacid/Antigas Liquid 2164
Pepcid Complete Chewable Tablets 1672
Rolaids Tablets .... ▣707
Extra Strength Rolaids Tablets .... ▣707
Rolaids Multi-Symptom Antacid & Antigas Tablets .... ▣708

Magnesium Oxide (Antacids (aluminum- or magnesium-containing) interfere with the absorption of cefdinir; Omnicef should be taken at least 2 hours before or after the antacids). Products include:
Beelith Tablets 784
PremCal Light, Regular, and Extra Strength Tablets .... ▣762

Polysaccharide Iron Complex (Iron supplements, including multivitamins that contain iron, interfere with the absorption of cefdinir; Omnicef should be taken at least 2 hours before or after the administration of iron-containing products). Products include:
Niferex-150 Forte Capsules 3299
Nu-Iron 150 Capsules 2098

Probenecid (Inhibits renal excretion of cefdinir, resulting in an approximate doubling in AUC, a 54% increase in peak cefdinir plasma levels, and a 50% prolongation in the apparent elimination).
No products indexed under this heading.

Food Interactions

Food, unspecified (Although Cmax and AUC of cefdinir absorption from capsules are reduced by 44% and 33%, respectively, when given with a high-fat meal, the magnitude of these reductions is not likely to be clinically significant; therefore, cefdinir may be taken without regard to food).

OMNICEF FOR ORAL SUSPENSION
(Cefdinir) 506
See Omnicef Capsules

ONCASPAR
(Pegaspargase) 1123
May interact with antineoplastics, anticoagulants, non-steroidal anti-inflammatory agents, highly protein bound drugs (selected), and certain other agents. Compounds in these categories include:

Altretamine (Potential for unspecified unfavorable interactions). Products include:
Hexalen Capsules 2101

Amiodarone Hydrochloride (Depletion of serum proteins by pegaspargase may increase the toxicity of other drugs which are protein bound). Products include:
Pacerone Tablets 3337

Amitriptyline Hydrochloride (Depletion of serum proteins by pegaspargase may increase the toxicity of other drugs which are protein bound).
No products indexed under this heading.

Anastrozole (Potential for unspecified unfavorable interactions). Products include:
Arimidex Tablets 665

Anisindione (Increased risk of bleeding and/or thrombosis). Products include:
Miradon Tablets 3056

Ardeparin Sodium (Increased risk of bleeding and/or thrombosis).
No products indexed under this heading.

Asparaginase (Potential for unspecified unfavorable interactions). Products include:
Elspar for Injection 1943

Aspirin (Increased risk of bleeding and/or thrombosis). Products include:
Aggrenox Capsules 855
Bayer, Aspirin Regimen .... ▣606
Bayer Aspirin Tablets 3515
BC Powder .... ▣612
BC Allergy Sinus Cold Powder .... ▣612
Arthritis Strength BC Powder .... ▣612
BC Sinus Cold Powder .... ▣612

Ecotrin Enteric Coated Aspirin Low, Regular and Maximum Strength Tablets 1627
Goody's Body Pain Formula Powder 621
Goody's Extra Strength Headache Powder 621
Goody's Extra Strength Pain Relief Tablets 621
Percodan Tablets 1115
St. Joseph 81 mg Aspirin Chewable and Enteric Coated Tablets 1841

Atovaquone (Depletion of serum proteins by pegaspargase may increase the toxicity of other drugs which are protein bound). Products include:
Malarone Tablets 1484
Malarone Pediatric Tablets 1484
Mepron Suspension 1487

Bicalutamide (Potential for unspecified unfavorable interactions). Products include:
Casodex Tablets 670

Bleomycin Sulfate (Potential for unspecified unfavorable interactions).
No products indexed under this heading.

Busulfan (Potential for unspecified unfavorable interactions). Products include:
I.V. Busulfex 1125
Myleran Tablets 1492

Carboplatin (Potential for unspecified unfavorable interactions).
No products indexed under this heading.

Carmustine (BCNU) (Potential for unspecified unfavorable interactions).
No products indexed under this heading.

Cefonicid Sodium (Depletion of serum proteins by pegaspargase may increase the toxicity of other drugs which are protein bound).
No products indexed under this heading.

Celecoxib (Increased risk of bleeding and/or thrombosis). Products include:
Celebrex Capsules 3130

Chlorambucil (Potential for unspecified unfavorable interactions). Products include:
Leukeran Tablets 1472

Chlordiazepoxide (Depletion of serum proteins by pegaspargase may increase the toxicity of other drugs which are protein bound).
No products indexed under this heading.

Chlordiazepoxide Hydrochloride (Depletion of serum proteins by pegaspargase may increase the toxicity of other drugs which are protein bound). Products include:
Librium Capsules 3349

Chlorpromazine (Depletion of serum proteins by pegaspargase may increase the toxicity of other drugs which are protein bound).
No products indexed under this heading.

Chlorpromazine Hydrochloride (Depletion of serum proteins by pegaspargase may increase the toxicity of other drugs which are protein bound).
No products indexed under this heading.

Cisplatin (Potential for unspecified unfavorable interactions).
No products indexed under this heading.

Clomipramine Hydrochloride (Depletion of serum proteins by pegaspargase may increase the toxicity of other drugs which are protein bound).
No products indexed under this heading.

Clozapine (Depletion of serum proteins by pegaspargase may increase the toxicity of other drugs which are protein bound). Products include:
Clozapine Tablets 2141
Clozaril Tablets 2174
FazaClo Orally Disintegrating Tablets 547

Cyclophosphamide (Potential for unspecified unfavorable interactions).
No products indexed under this heading.

Cyclosporine (Depletion of serum proteins by pegaspargase may increase the toxicity of other drugs which are protein bound). Products include:
Gengraf Capsules 458
Neoral Soft Gelatin Capsules 2247
Neoral Oral Solution 2247
Restasis Ophthalmic Emulsion 570
Sandimmune 2259

Dacarbazine (Potential for unspecified unfavorable interactions).
No products indexed under this heading.

Dalteparin Sodium (Increased risk of bleeding and/or thrombosis). Products include:
Fragmin Injection 2638

Danaparoid Sodium (Increased risk of bleeding and/or thrombosis).
No products indexed under this heading.

Daunorubicin Citrate (Potential for unspecified unfavorable interactions).
No products indexed under this heading.

Daunorubicin Hydrochloride (Potential for unspecified unfavorable interactions). Products include:
Cerubidine for Injection 788

Denileukin Diftitox (Potential for unspecified unfavorable interactions). Products include:
Ontak Vials 1717

Diazepam (Depletion of serum proteins by pegaspargase may increase the toxicity of other drugs which are protein bound). Products include:
Diastat Rectal Delivery System 3344
Valium Tablets 2822

Diclofenac Potassium (Depletion of serum proteins by pegaspargase may increase the toxicity of other drugs which are protein bound; increased risk of bleeding and/or thrombosis). Products include:
Cataflam Tablets 2173

Diclofenac Sodium (Depletion of serum proteins by pegaspargase may increase the toxicity of other drugs which are protein bound; increased risk of bleeding and/or thrombosis). Products include:
Arthrotec Tablets 3126
Voltaren Ophthalmic Solution 2300
Voltaren Tablets 2298
Voltaren-XR Tablets 2301

Dicumarol (Increased risk of bleeding and/or thrombosis).
No products indexed under this heading.

Dipyridamole (Depletion of serum proteins by pegaspargase may increase the toxicity of other drugs which are protein bound). Products include:
Aggrenox Capsules 855
Persantine Tablets 898

Docetaxel (Potential for unspecified unfavorable interactions). Products include:
Taxotere Injection Concentrate 2947

Doxorubicin Hydrochloride (Potential for unspecified unfavorable interactions). Products include:
Adriamycin for Injection, USP 786
Adriamycin Injection, USP 786

Enoxaparin Sodium (Increased risk of bleeding and/or thrombosis). Products include:
Lovenox Injection 2931

Epirubicin Hydrochloride (Potential for unspecified unfavorable interactions). Products include:
Ellence Injection 2632

Estramustine Phosphate Sodium (Potential for unspecified unfavorable interactions). Products include:
Emcyt Capsules 3137

Etodolac (Increased risk of bleeding and/or thrombosis).
No products indexed under this heading.

Etoposide (Potential for unspecified unfavorable interactions).
No products indexed under this heading.

Exemestane (Potential for unspecified unfavorable interactions). Products include:
Aromasin Tablets 2600

Fenoprofen Calcium (Depletion of serum proteins by pegaspargase may increase the toxicity of other drugs which are protein bound; increased risk of bleeding and/or thrombosis). Products include:
Nalfon Capsules 2504

Floxuridine (Potential for unspecified unfavorable interactions).
No products indexed under this heading.

Fluorouracil (Potential for unspecified unfavorable interactions). Products include:
Carac Cream, 0.5% 1048
Efudex 3348

Flurazepam Hydrochloride (Depletion of serum proteins by pegaspargase may increase the toxicity of other drugs which are protein bound). Products include:
Dalmane Capsules 3343

Flurbiprofen (Depletion of serum proteins by pegaspargase may increase the toxicity of other drugs which are protein bound; increased risk of bleeding and/or thrombosis).
No products indexed under this heading.

Flutamide (Potential for unspecified unfavorable interactions). Products include:
Eulexin Capsules 3023

Fondaparinux Sodium (Increased risk of bleeding and/or thrombosis). Products include:
Arixtra Injection 1325

Gemcitabine Hydrochloride (Potential for unspecified unfavorable interactions). Products include:
Gemzar for Injection 1743

Glipizide (Depletion of serum proteins by pegaspargase may increase the toxicity of other drugs which are protein bound).
No products indexed under this heading.

Heparin Calcium (Increased risk of bleeding and/or thrombosis).
No products indexed under this heading.

Heparin Sodium (Increased risk of bleeding and/or thrombosis).
No products indexed under this heading.

Hydroxyurea (Potential for unspecified unfavorable interactions).
No products indexed under this heading.

Ibuprofen (Depletion of serum proteins by pegaspargase may increase the toxicity of other drugs which are protein bound; increased risk of bleeding and/or thrombosis). Products include:
Advil Allergy Sinus Caplets 737
Advil 737
Children's Advil Suspension 742
Children's Advil Chewable Tablets 741
Advil Cold & Sinus 739
Advil Flu & Body Ache Caplets 739
Children's Advil Cold Suspension 741
Infants' Advil Concentrated Drops 743
Junior Strength Advil Swallow Tablets 740
Advil Migraine Liquigels 740
Advil Multi-Symptom Cold Caplets 738
Combunox Tablets 1183
Children's Motrin Oral Suspension and Chewable Tablets 1837
Children's Motrin Cold Non-Staining Dye-Free Oral Suspension 1838
Children's Motrin Cold Oral Suspension 1838
Children's Motrin Non-Staining Dye-Free Oral Suspension 1837
Motrin Cold & Sinus Caplets 1836
Motrin IB Tablets and Caplets 1836
Infants' Motrin Concentrated Drops 1837
Infants' Motrin Non-Staining Dye-Free Drops 1837
Junior Strength Motrin Caplets and Chewable Tablets 1837
Vicoprofen Tablets 533

Idarubicin Hydrochloride (Potential for unspecified unfavorable interactions). Products include:
Idamycin PFS Injection 2645

Ifosfamide (Potential for unspecified unfavorable interactions).
No products indexed under this heading.

Imipramine Hydrochloride (Depletion of serum proteins by pegaspargase may increase the toxicity of other drugs which are protein bound).
No products indexed under this heading.

Imipramine Pamoate (Depletion of serum proteins by pegaspargase may increase the toxicity of other drugs which are protein bound).
No products indexed under this heading.

Indomethacin (Depletion of serum proteins by pegaspargase may increase the toxicity of other drugs which are protein bound; increased risk of bleeding and/or thrombosis). Products include:
Indocin 1968

Indomethacin Sodium Trihydrate (Depletion of serum proteins by pegaspargase may increase the toxicity of other drugs which are protein bound; increased risk of bleeding and/or thrombosis). Products include:
Indocin I.V. 1973

Interferon alfa-2a, Recombinant (Potential for unspecified unfavorable interactions). Products include:
Roferon-A Injection 2805

Interferon alfa-2b, Recombinant (Potential for unspecified unfavorable interactions). Products include:

IMPORTANT NOTE: Always consult each drug listing in the patient's regimen for possible interactions.

Intron A for Injection 3038
Rebetron Combination Therapy 3078

Irinotecan Hydrochloride (Potential for unspecified unfavorable interactions). Products include:
Camptosar Injection 2602

Ketoprofen (Depletion of serum proteins by pegaspargase may increase the toxicity of other drugs which are protein bound; increased risk of bleeding and/or thrombosis).
No products indexed under this heading.

Ketorolac Tromethamine (Depletion of serum proteins by pegaspargase may increase the toxicity of other drugs which are protein bound; increased risk of bleeding and/or thrombosis). Products include:
Acular Ophthalmic Solution 561
Acular LS Ophthalmic Solution 562

Levamisole Hydrochloride (Potential for unspecified unfavorable interactions).
No products indexed under this heading.

Lomustine (CCNU) (Potential for unspecified unfavorable interactions).
No products indexed under this heading.

Low Molecular Weight Heparins (Increased risk of bleeding and/or thrombosis).
No products indexed under this heading.

Mechlorethamine Hydrochloride (Potential for unspecified unfavorable interactions). Products include:
Mustargen for Injection 2007

Meclofenamate Sodium (Depletion of serum proteins by pegaspargase may increase the toxicity of other drugs which are protein bound; increased risk of bleeding and/or thrombosis).
No products indexed under this heading.

Mefenamic Acid (Depletion of serum proteins by pegaspargase may increase the toxicity of other drugs which are protein bound; increased risk of bleeding and/or thrombosis).
No products indexed under this heading.

Megestrol Acetate (Potential for unspecified unfavorable interactions). Products include:
Megace ES Oral Suspension 2492

Meloxicam (Increased risk of bleeding and/or thrombosis). Products include:
Mobic Oral Suspension 893
Mobic Tablets 893

Melphalan (Potential for unspecified unfavorable interactions). Products include:
Alkeran Tablets 977

Mercaptopurine (Potential for unspecified unfavorable interactions). Products include:
Purinethol Tablets 1222

Methotrexate Sodium (Pegaspargase inhibits protein synthesis and cell replication and thus interferes with the action of methotrexate which requires cell replication for its lethal effect; potential for unspecified unfavorable interactions).
No products indexed under this heading.

Midazolam Hydrochloride (Depletion of serum proteins by pegaspargase may increase the toxicity of other drugs which are protein bound).
No products indexed under this heading.

Mitomycin (Mitomycin-C) (Potential for unspecified unfavorable interactions).
No products indexed under this heading.

Mitotane (Potential for unspecified unfavorable interactions).
No products indexed under this heading.

Mitoxantrone Hydrochloride (Potential for unspecified unfavorable interactions). Products include:
Novantrone for Injection Concentrate 3158

Nabumetone (Increased risk of bleeding and/or thrombosis). Products include:
Relafen Tablets 1523

Naproxen (Depletion of serum proteins by pegaspargase may increase the toxicity of other drugs which are protein bound; increased risk of bleeding and/or thrombosis). Products include:
EC-Naprosyn Delayed-Release Tablets 2769
Naprosyn Suspension 2769
Naprosyn Tablets 2769
Prevacid NapraPAC 3277

Naproxen Sodium (Depletion of serum proteins by pegaspargase may increase the toxicity of other drugs which are protein bound; increased risk of bleeding and/or thrombosis). Products include:
Aleve Tablets, Caplets and Gelcaps .... ▣605
Anaprox Tablets 2769
Anaprox DS Tablets 2769

Nortriptyline Hydrochloride (Depletion of serum proteins by pegaspargase may increase the toxicity of other drugs which are protein bound).
No products indexed under this heading.

Oxaliplatin (Potential for unspecified unfavorable interactions). Products include:
Eloxatin for Injection 2908

Oxaprozin (Depletion of serum proteins by pegaspargase may increase the toxicity of other drugs which are protein bound; increased risk of bleeding and/or thrombosis).
No products indexed under this heading.

Oxazepam (Depletion of serum proteins by pegaspargase may increase the toxicity of other drugs which are protein bound).
No products indexed under this heading.

Paclitaxel (Potential for unspecified unfavorable interactions).
No products indexed under this heading.

Phenylbutazone (Depletion of serum proteins by pegaspargase may increase the toxicity of other drugs which are protein bound; increased risk of bleeding and/or thrombosis).
No products indexed under this heading.

Piroxicam (Depletion of serum proteins by pegaspargase may increase the toxicity of other drugs which are protein bound; increased risk of bleeding and/or thrombosis).
No products indexed under this heading.

Procarbazine Hydrochloride (Potential for unspecified unfavorable interactions). Products include:
Matulane Capsules 3188

Propranolol Hydrochloride (Depletion of serum proteins by pegaspargase may increase the toxicity of other drugs which are protein bound). Products include:
Inderal LA Long-Acting Capsules 3421
InnoPran XL Capsules 2728

Rofecoxib (Increased risk of bleeding and/or thrombosis).
No products indexed under this heading.

Streptozocin (Potential for unspecified unfavorable interactions).
No products indexed under this heading.

Sulindac (Depletion of serum proteins by pegaspargase may increase the toxicity of other drugs which are protein bound; increased risk of bleeding and/or thrombosis). Products include:
Clinoril Tablets 1899

Tamoxifen Citrate (Potential for unspecified unfavorable interactions).
No products indexed under this heading.

Temazepam (Depletion of serum proteins by pegaspargase may increase the toxicity of other drugs which are protein bound).
No products indexed under this heading.

Teniposide (Potential for unspecified unfavorable interactions).
No products indexed under this heading.

Thioguanine (Potential for unspecified unfavorable interactions). Products include:
Tabloid Tablets 1545

Thiotepa (Potential for unspecified unfavorable interactions).
No products indexed under this heading.

Tinzaparin Sodium (Increased risk of bleeding and/or thrombosis).
No products indexed under this heading.

Tolbutamide (Depletion of serum proteins by pegaspargase may increase the toxicity of other drugs which are protein bound).
No products indexed under this heading.

Tolmetin Sodium (Depletion of serum proteins by pegaspargase may increase the toxicity of other drugs which are protein bound; increased risk of bleeding and/or thrombosis).
No products indexed under this heading.

Topotecan Hydrochloride (Potential for unspecified unfavorable interactions). Products include:
Hycamtin for Injection 1427

Toremifene Citrate (Potential for unspecified unfavorable interactions).
No products indexed under this heading.

Trimipramine Maleate (Depletion of serum proteins by pegaspargase may increase the toxicity of other drugs which are protein bound). Products include:
Surmontil Capsules 2347

Valdecoxib (Increased risk of bleeding and/or thrombosis).
No products indexed under this heading.

Valrubicin (Potential for unspecified unfavorable interactions).
No products indexed under this heading.

Vincristine Sulfate (Potential for unspecified unfavorable interactions).
No products indexed under this heading.

Vinorelbine Tartrate (Potential for unspecified unfavorable interactions). Products include:
Navelbine Injection 1494

Warfarin Sodium (Depletion of serum proteins by pegaspargase may increase the toxicity of other drugs which are protein bound; increased risk of bleeding and/or thrombosis). Products include:
Coumadin for Injection 932
Coumadin Tablets 932

ONTAK VIALS

(Denileukin Diftitox) 1717
None cited in PDR database.

OPHTHETIC OPHTHALMIC SOLUTION

(Proparacaine Hydrochloride) .... ⊙230
None cited in PDR database.

OPTINATE OMEGA-3 L-VCAPS

(Docosahexaenoic Acid (DHA), Folic Acid, Iron, Multivitamins with Minerals) 1162
May interact with anticoagulants. Compounds in these categories include:

Anisindione (Ingestion of more than 3 grams of omega-3 fatty acids per day has been shown to have potential antithrombotic effects, including an increased bleeding time and INR. Administration of omega-3 fatty acids should be avoided in patients on anticoagulants and in those known to have an inherited or acquired bleeding diathesis). Products include:
Miradon Tablets 3056

Ardeparin Sodium (Ingestion of more than 3 grams of omega-3 fatty acids per day has been shown to have potential antithrombotic effects, including an increased bleeding time and INR. Administration of omega-3 fatty acids should be avoided in patients on anticoagulants and in those known to have an inherited or acquired bleeding diathesis).
No products indexed under this heading.

Dalteparin Sodium (Ingestion of more than 3 grams of omega-3 fatty acids per day has been shown to have potential antithrombotic effects, including an increased bleeding time and INR. Administration of omega-3 fatty acids should be avoided in patients on anticoagulants and in those known to have an inherited or acquired bleeding diathesis). Products include:
Fragmin Injection 2638

Danaparoid Sodium (Ingestion of more than 3 grams of omega-3 fatty acids per day has been shown to have potential antithrombotic effects, including an increased bleeding time and INR. Administration of omega-3 fatty acids should be avoided in patients on anticoagulants and in those known to have an inherited or acquired bleeding diathesis).
No products indexed under this heading.

Dicumarol (Ingestion of more than 3 grams of omega-3 fatty acids per day has been shown to have potential antithrombotic effects, including an increased bleeding time and INR. Administration of omega-3 fatty acids should be avoided in patients on anticoagulants and in those known to have an inherited or acquired bleeding diathesis).
No products indexed under this heading.

Enoxaparin Sodium (Ingestion of more than 3 grams of omega-3 fatty acids per day has been shown to have potential antithrombotic effects, including an increased bleeding time and INR. Administration of omega-3 fatty acids should be avoided in patients on anticoagulants and in those known to have an inherited or acquired bleeding diathesis). Products include:
Lovenox Injection **2931**

Fondaparinux Sodium (Ingestion of more than 3 grams of omega-3 fatty acids per day has been shown to have potential antithrombotic effects, including an increased bleeding time and INR. Administration of omega-3 fatty acids should be avoided in patients on anticoagulants and in those known to have an inherited or acquired bleeding diathesis). Products include:
Arixtra Injection **1325**

Heparin Calcium (Ingestion of more than 3 grams of omega-3 fatty acids per day has been shown to have potential antithrombotic effects, including an increased bleeding time and INR. Administration of omega-3 fatty acids should be avoided in patients on anticoagulants and in those known to have an inherited or acquired bleeding diathesis).
No products indexed under this heading.

Heparin Sodium (Ingestion of more than 3 grams of omega-3 fatty acids per day has been shown to have potential antithrombotic effects, including an increased bleeding time and INR. Administration of omega-3 fatty acids should be avoided in patients on anticoagulants and in those known to have an inherited or acquired bleeding diathesis).
No products indexed under this heading.

Low Molecular Weight Heparins (Ingestion of more than 3 grams of omega-3 fatty acids per day has been shown to have potential antithrombotic effects, including an increased bleeding time and INR. Administration of omega-3 fatty acids should be avoided in patients on anticoagulants and in those known to have an inherited or acquired bleeding diathesis).
No products indexed under this heading.

Tinzaparin Sodium (Ingestion of more than 3 grams of omega-3 fatty acids per day has been shown to have potential antithrombotic effects, including an increased bleeding time and INR. Administration of omega-3 fatty acids should be avoided in patients on anticoagulants and in those known to have an inherited or acquired bleeding diathesis).
No products indexed under this heading.

Warfarin Sodium (Ingestion of more than 3 grams of omega-3 fatty acids per day has been shown to have potential antithrombotic effects, including an increased bleeding time and INR. Administration of omega-3 fatty acids should be avoided in patients on anticoagulants and in those known to have an inherited or acquired bleeding diathesis). Products include:
Coumadin for Injection **932**
Coumadin Tablets **932**

OPTINATE TABLETS

(Docosahexaenoic Acid (DHA), Folic Acid, Iron, Multivitamins with Minerals) **1162**
May interact with anticoagulants. Compounds in these categories include:

Anisindione (Ingestion of more than 3 grams of omega-3 fatty acids per day has been shown to have potential antithrombotic effects, including an increased bleeding time and INR. Administration of omega-3 fatty acids should be avoided in patients on anticoagulants and in those known to have an inherited or acquired bleeding diathesis). Products include:
Miradon Tablets **3056**

Ardeparin Sodium (Ingestion of more than 3 grams of omega-3 fatty acids per day has been shown to have potential antithrombotic effects, including an increased bleeding time and INR. Administration of omega-3 fatty acids should be avoided in patients on anticoagulants and in those known to have an inherited or acquired bleeding diathesis).
No products indexed under this heading.

Dalteparin Sodium (Ingestion of more than 3 grams of omega-3 fatty acids per day has been shown to have potential antithrombotic effects, including an increased bleeding time and INR. Administration of omega-3 fatty acids should be avoided in patients on anticoagulants and in those known to have an inherited or acquired bleeding diathesis). Products include:
Fragmin Injection **2638**

Danaparoid Sodium (Ingestion of more than 3 grams of omega-3 fatty acids per day has been shown to have potential antithrombotic effects, including an increased bleeding time and INR. Administration of omega-3 fatty acids should be avoided in patients on anticoagulants and in those known to have an inherited or acquired bleeding diathesis).
No products indexed under this heading.

Dicumarol (Ingestion of more than 3 grams of omega-3 fatty acids per day has been shown to have potential antithrombotic effects, including an increased bleeding time and INR. Administration of omega-3 fatty acids should be avoided in patients on anticoagulants and in those known to have an inherited or acquired bleeding diathesis).
No products indexed under this heading.

Enoxaparin Sodium (Ingestion of more than 3 grams of omega-3 fatty acids per day has been shown to have potential antithrombotic effects, including an increased bleeding time and INR. Administration of omega-3 fatty acids should be avoided in patients on anticoagulants and in those known to have an inherited or acquired bleeding diathesis). Products include:
Lovenox Injection **2931**

Fondaparinux Sodium (Ingestion of more than 3 grams of omega-3 fatty acids per day has been shown to have potential antithrombotic effects, including an increased bleeding time and INR. Administration of omega-3 fatty acids should be avoided in patients on anticoagulants and in those known to have an inherited or acquired bleeding diathesis). Products include:
Arixtra Injection **1325**

Heparin Calcium (Ingestion of more than 3 grams of omega-3 fatty acids per day has been shown to have potential antithrombotic effects, including an increased bleeding time and INR. Administration of omega-3 fatty acids should be avoided in patients on anticoagulants and in those known to have an inherited or acquired bleeding diathesis).
No products indexed under this heading.

Heparin Sodium (Ingestion of more than 3 grams of omega-3 fatty acids per day has been shown to have potential antithrombotic effects, including an increased bleeding time and INR. Administration of omega-3 fatty acids should be avoided in patients on anticoagulants and in those known to have an inherited or acquired bleeding diathesis).
No products indexed under this heading.

Low Molecular Weight Heparins (Ingestion of more than 3 grams of omega-3 fatty acids per day has been shown to have potential antithrombotic effects, including an increased bleeding time and INR. Administration of omega-3 fatty acids should be avoided in patients on anticoagulants and in those known to have an inherited or acquired bleeding diathesis).
No products indexed under this heading.

Tinzaparin Sodium (Ingestion of more than 3 grams of omega-3 fatty acids per day has been shown to have potential antithrombotic effects, including an increased bleeding time and INR. Administration of omega-3 fatty acids should be avoided in patients on anticoagulants and in those known to have an inherited or acquired bleeding diathesis).
No products indexed under this heading.

Warfarin Sodium (Ingestion of more than 3 grams of omega-3 fatty acids per day has been shown to have potential antithrombotic effects, including an increased bleeding time and INR. Administration of omega-3 fatty acids should be avoided in patients on anticoagulants and in those known to have an inherited or acquired bleeding diathesis). Products include:
Coumadin for Injection **932**
Coumadin Tablets **932**

OPTIPRANOLOL METIPRANOLOL OPHTHALMIC SOLUTION 0.3%

(Metipranolol) .... **⊙254**
May interact with adrenergic augmenting psychotropics, beta blockers, calcium channel blockers, cardiac glycosides, and certain other agents. Compounds in these categories include:

Acebutolol Hydrochloride (Co-administration with oral beta blockers may result in additive effects or systemic beta blockade).
No products indexed under this heading.

Amlodipine Besylate (Co-administration with oral or intravenous calcium channel antagonists may result in possible precipitation of left ventricular failure and hypotension). Products include:
Caduet Tablets **2507**
Lotrel Capsules **2238**
Norvasc Tablets **2529**

Atenolol (Co-administration with oral beta blockers may result in additive effects or systemic beta blockade). Products include:
Tenormin I.V. Injection **698**
Tenormin Tablets **695**

Bepridil Hydrochloride (Co-administration with oral or intravenous calcium channel antagonists may result in possible precipitation of left ventricular failure and hypotension).
No products indexed under this heading.

Betaxolol Hydrochloride (Co-administration with oral beta blockers may result in additive effects or systemic beta blockade). Products include:
Betoptic S Ophthalmic Suspension **554**

Bisoprolol Fumarate (Co-administration with oral beta blockers may result in additive effects or systemic beta blockade).
No products indexed under this heading.

Carteolol Hydrochloride (Co-administration with oral beta blockers may result in additive effects or systemic beta blockade). Products include:
Carteolol Hydrochloride Ophthalmic Solution USP, 1% .... **⊙246**

Deserpidine (Possible additive effects and production of hypotension and/or bradycardia when beta blocker is concurrently used with catecholamine-depleting drugs).
No products indexed under this heading.

IMPORTANT NOTE: Always consult each drug listing in the patient's regimen for possible interactions.

Deslanoside (Concomitant use of beta blockers with digitalis and calcium channel blockers may result in additive effects in prolonging atrioventricular conduction time).
No products indexed under this heading.

Digitalis Glycoside Preparations (Concomitant use of beta blockers with digitalis and calcium channel blockers may result in additive effects in prolonging atrioventricular conduction time).
No products indexed under this heading.

Digitoxin (Concomitant use of beta blockers with digitalis and calcium channel blockers may result in additive effects in prolonging atrioventricular conduction time).
No products indexed under this heading.

Digoxin (Concomitant use of beta blockers with digitalis and calcium channel blockers may result in additive effects in prolonging atrioventricular conduction time). Products include:
Digitek Tablets **2146**
Lanoxicaps Capsules **1458**
Lanoxin Injection **1462**
Lanoxin Tablets **1468**
Lanoxin Injection Pediatric **1465**

Diltiazem Hydrochloride (Co-administration with oral or intravenous calcium channel antagonists may result in possible precipitation of left ventricular failure and hypotension). Products include:
Cardizem LA Extended Release Tablets **1699**
Tiazac Capsules **1204**

Epinephrine (Concurrent use in patients with history of atopy or severe anaphylactic reaction to allergens may be unresponsive to the usual doses of epinephrine used to treat anaphylactic reaction). Products include:
EpiPen **1061**
Primatene Mist .... ▣ **749**

Epinephrine Hydrochloride (Concurrent use in patients with history of atopy or severe anaphylactic reaction to allergens may be unresponsive to the usual doses of epinephrine used to treat anaphylactic reaction).
No products indexed under this heading.

Esmolol Hydrochloride (Co-administration with oral beta blockers may result in additive effects or systemic beta blockade). Products include:
Brevibloc Concentrate **766**
Brevibloc Injection **766**
Brevibloc Double Strength Injection.. **766**
Brevibloc Premixed Injection **766**
Brevibloc Double Strength Premixed Injection....................... **766**

Felodipine (Co-administration with oral or intravenous calcium channel antagonists may result in possible precipitation of left ventricular failure and hypotension). Products include:
Plendil Extended-Release Tablets **651**

Isocarboxazid (Exercise caution when used concurrently with adrenergic psychotropic drugs).
No products indexed under this heading.

Isradipine (Co-administration with oral or intravenous calcium channel antagonists may result in possible precipitation of left ventricular failure and hypotension). Products include:
DynaCirc CR Tablets **2726**

Labetalol Hydrochloride (Co-administration with oral beta blockers may result in additive effects or systemic beta blockade).
No products indexed under this heading.

Levobunolol Hydrochloride (Co-administration with oral beta blockers may result in additive effects or systemic beta blockade). Products include:
Betagan Ophthalmic Solution, USP.. ⊙ **217**

Metoprolol Succinate (Co-administration with oral beta blockers may result in additive effects or systemic beta blockade). Products include:
Toprol-XL Tablets **660**

Metoprolol Tartrate (Co-administration with oral beta blockers may result in additive effects or systemic beta blockade).
No products indexed under this heading.

Mibefradil Dihydrochloride (Co-administration with oral or intravenous calcium channel antagonists may result in possible precipitation of left ventricular failure and hypotension).
No products indexed under this heading.

Nadolol (Co-administration with oral beta blockers may result in additive effects or systemic beta blockade). Products include:
Nadolol Tablets **2121**

Nicardipine Hydrochloride (Co-administration with oral or intravenous calcium channel antagonists may result in possible precipitation of left ventricular failure and hypotension). Products include:
Cardene I.V. **1129**

Nifedipine (Co-administration with oral or intravenous calcium channel antagonists may result in possible precipitation of left ventricular failure and hypotension). Products include:
Adalat CC Tablets **2978**

Nimodipine (Co-administration with oral or intravenous calcium channel antagonists may result in possible precipitation of left ventricular failure and hypotension). Products include:
Nimotop Capsules **774**

Nisoldipine (Co-administration with oral or intravenous calcium channel antagonists may result in possible precipitation of left ventricular failure and hypotension). Products include:
Sular Tablets **1163**

Pargyline Hydrochloride (Exercise caution when used concurrently with adrenergic psychotropic drugs).
No products indexed under this heading.

Penbutolol Sulfate (Co-administration with oral beta blockers may result in additive effects or systemic beta blockade).
No products indexed under this heading.

Phenelzine Sulfate (Exercise caution when used concurrently with adrenergic psychotropic drugs).
No products indexed under this heading.

Pindolol (Co-administration with oral beta blockers may result in additive effects or systemic beta blockade).
No products indexed under this heading.

Propranolol Hydrochloride (Co-administration with oral beta blockers may result in additive effects or systemic beta blockade). Products include:
Inderal LA Long-Acting Capsules **3421**
InnoPran XL Capsules **2728**

Rauwolfia Serpentina (Possible additive effects and production of hypotension and/or bradycardia when beta blocker is concurrently used with catecholamine-depleting drugs).
No products indexed under this heading.

Rescinnamine (Possible additive effects and production of hypotension and/or bradycardia when beta blocker is concurrently used with catecholamine-depleting drugs).
No products indexed under this heading.

Reserpine (Possible additive effects and production of hypotension and/or bradycardia when beta blocker is concurrently used with catecholamine-depleting drugs).
No products indexed under this heading.

Sotalol Hydrochloride (Co-administration with oral beta blockers may result in additive effects or systemic beta blockade).
No products indexed under this heading.

Timolol Hemihydrate (Co-administration with oral beta blockers may result in additive effects or systemic beta blockade). Products include:
Betimol Ophthalmic Solution **3371**
Betimol Ophthalmic Solution .... ⊙ **283**

Timolol Maleate (Co-administration with oral beta blockers may result in additive effects or systemic beta blockade). Products include:
Blocadren Tablets **1891**
Cosopt Sterile Ophthalmic Solution... **1910**
Timolide Tablets **2056**
Timoptic in Ocudose **2061**
Timoptic Sterile Ophthalmic Solution... **2058**
Timoptic-XE Sterile Ophthalmic Gel Forming Solution **2062**

Tranylcypromine Sulfate (Exercise caution when used concurrently with adrenergic psychotropic drugs). Products include:
Parnate Tablets **1499**

Verapamil Hydrochloride (Co-administration with oral or intravenous calcium channel antagonists may result in possible precipitation of left ventricular failure and hypotension). Products include:
Covera-HS Tablets **3135**
Tarka Tablets **519**
Verelan PM Capsules **3120**

OPTIVAR OPHTHALMIC SOLUTION

(Azelastine Hydrochloride) **1877**
None cited in PDR database.

ORAP TABLETS

(Pimozide) **1220**
May interact with central nervous system depressants, macrolide antibiotics, protease inhibitors, drugs that prolong the QT interval, and certain other agents. Compounds in these categories include:

Alfentanil Hydrochloride (Pimozide may be capable of potentiating CNS depressants).
No products indexed under this heading.

Alprazolam (Pimozide may be capable of potentiating CNS depressants). Products include:
Niravam Orally Disintegrating Tablets **3106**
Xanax XR Tablets **2655**

Amiodarone Hydrochloride (Co-administration with other drugs which prolong the QT interval may result in additive effect on the QT interval). Products include:
Pacerone Tablets **3337**

Amitriptyline Hydrochloride (Co-administration with other drugs which prolong the QT interval may result in additive effect on the QT interval).
No products indexed under this heading.

Amoxapine (Co-administration with other drugs which prolong the QT interval may result in additive effect on the QT interval).
No products indexed under this heading.

Amphetamine Sulfate (Pimozide should not be used in patients taking drugs that themselves cause motor and phonic tics; such as amphetamine). Products include:
Adderall Tablets **3168**
Adderall XR Capsules **3169**

Amprenavir (Protease inhibitor drugs are inhibitors of CYP3A and thus could potentially impede pimozide metabolism; co-administration is contraindicated). Products include:
Agenerase Capsules **1299**
Agenerase Oral Solution **1304**

Aprobarbital (Pimozide may be capable of potentiating CNS depressants).
No products indexed under this heading.

Astemizole (Co-administration with other drugs which prolong the QT interval may result in additive effect on the QT interval).
No products indexed under this heading.

Azithromycin Dihydrate (Macrolide antibiotics are inhibitors of CYP3A and thus could potentially impede pimozide metabolism; ventricular arrhythmias have been rarely associated with the use of macrolide antibiotics in patients with prolonged QT intervals, as might be produced by pimozide; co-administration is contraindicated). Products include:
Zithromax **2568**
Zithromax for IV Infusion **2573**
Zithromax for Oral Suspension, 300 mg, 600 mg, 900 mg, 1200 mg.. **2561**
Zithromax Tablets, 250 mg, 500 mg.. **2561**
Zithromax Tri-Pak **2561**
Zithromax Z-Pak **2568**

Bretylium Tosylate (Co-administration with other drugs which prolong the QT interval may result in additive effect on the QT interval).
No products indexed under this heading.

Buprenorphine Hydrochloride (Pimozide may be capable of potentiating CNS depressants). Products include:
Buprenex Injectable **2718**
Suboxone Tablets **2719**
Subutex Tablets **2719**

Buspirone Hydrochloride (Pimozide may be capable of potentiating CNS depressants).
No products indexed under this heading.

Butabarbital (Pimozide may be capable of potentiating CNS depressants).
No products indexed under this heading.

Butalbital (Pimozide may be capable of potentiating CNS depressants). Products include:
Sedapap Tablets 50 mg/650 mg 2098

Chlordiazepoxide (Pimozide may be capable of potentiating CNS depressants).
No products indexed under this heading.

Chlordiazepoxide Hydrochloride (Pimozide may be capable of potentiating CNS depressants). Products include:
Librium Capsules 3349

Chlorpromazine (Co-administration with other drugs which prolong the QT interval may result in additive effect on the QT interval).
No products indexed under this heading.

Chlorpromazine Hydrochloride (Co-administration with other drugs which prolong the QT interval may result in additive effect on the QT interval).
No products indexed under this heading.

Chlorprothixene (Pimozide may be capable of potentiating CNS depressants).
No products indexed under this heading.

Chlorprothixene Hydrochloride (Pimozide may be capable of potentiating CNS depressants).
No products indexed under this heading.

Chlorprothixene Lactate (Pimozide may be capable of potentiating CNS depressants).
No products indexed under this heading.

Clarithromycin (Marcolide antibiotics are inhibitors of CYP3A and thus could potentially impede pimozide metabolism; ventricular arrhythmias have been rarely associated with the use of macrolide antibiotics in patients with prolonged QT intervals, as might be produced by pimozide; two sudden deaths have been reported when clarithromycin was added to ongoing pimozide therapy; co-administration is contraindicated). Products include:
Biaxin/Biaxin XL 402
PREVPAC 3281

Clomipramine Hydrochloride (Co-administration with other drugs which prolong the QT interval may result in additive effect on the QT interval).
No products indexed under this heading.

Clorazepate Dipotassium (Pimozide may be capable of potentiating CNS depressants). Products include:
Tranxene 2488

Clozapine (Pimozide may be capable of potentiating CNS depressants). Products include:
Clozapine Tablets 2141
Clozaril Tablets 2174
FazaClo Orally Disintegrating Tablets 547

Codeine Phosphate (Pimozide may be capable of potentiating CNS depressants). Products include:
Tylenol with Codeine 2461

Desflurane (Pimozide may be capable of potentiating CNS depressants). Products include:
Suprane Liquid for Inhalation 770

Desipramine Hydrochloride (Co-administration with other drugs which prolong the QT interval may result in additive effect on the QT interval).
No products indexed under this heading.

Dextroamphetamine Sulfate (Pimozide should not be used in patients taking drugs that themselves cause motor and phonic tics; such as amphetamine). Products include:
Adderall Tablets 3168
Adderall XR Capsules 3169
Dexedrine 1386
DextroStat Tablets 3177

Dezocine (Pimozide may be capable of potentiating CNS depressants).
No products indexed under this heading.

Diazepam (Pimozide may be capable of potentiating CNS depressants). Products include:
Diastat Rectal Delivery System 3344
Valium Tablets 2822

Dirithromycin (Macrolide antibiotics are inhibitors of CYP3A and thus could potentially impede pimozide metabolism; ventricular arrhythmias have been rarely associated with the use of macrolide antibiotics in patients with prolonged QT intervals, as might be produced by pimozide; co-administration is contraindicated).
No products indexed under this heading.

Disopyramide Phosphate (Co-administration with other drugs which prolong the QT interval may result in additive effect on the QT interval).
No products indexed under this heading.

Dofetilide (Co-administration with other drugs which prolong the QT interval may result in additive effect on the QT interval).
No products indexed under this heading.

Doxepin Hydrochloride (Co-administration with other drugs which prolong the QT interval may result in additive effect on the QT interval).
No products indexed under this heading.

Droperidol (Pimozide may be capable of potentiating CNS depressants).
No products indexed under this heading.

Enflurane (Pimozide may be capable of potentiating CNS depressants).
No products indexed under this heading.

Erythromycin (Macrolide antibiotics are inhibitors of CYP3A and thus could potentially impede pimozide metabolism; ventricular arrhythmias have been rarely associated with the use of macrolide antibiotics in patients with prolonged QT intervals, as might be produced by pimozide; co-administration is contraindicated). Products include:
Erygel Topical Gel 2096
Ery-Tab Tablets 447
Erythromycin Base Filmtab Tablets 454
Erythromycin Delayed-Release Capsules, USP 456
PCE Dispertab Tablets 510

Erythromycin Estolate (Macrolide antibiotics are inhibitors of CYP3A and thus could potentially impede pimozide metabolism; ventricular arrhythmias have been rarely associated with the use of macrolide antibiotics in patients with prolonged QT intervals, as might be produced by pimozide; co-administration is contraindicated).
No products indexed under this heading.

Erythromycin Ethylsuccinate (Macrolide antibiotics are inhibitors of CYP3A and thus could potentially impede pimozide metabolism; ventricular arrhythmias have been rarely associated with the use of macrolide antibiotics in patients with prolonged QT intervals, as might be produced by pimozide; co-administration is contraindicated). Products include:
E.E.S. 449
EryPed 445

Erythromycin Gluceptate (Macrolide antibiotics are inhibitors of CYP3A and thus could potentially impede pimozide metabolism; ventricular arrhythmias have been rarely associated with the use of macrolide antibiotics in patients with prolonged QT intervals, as might be produced by pimozide; co-administration is contraindicated).
No products indexed under this heading.

Erythromycin Stearate (Macrolide antibiotics are inhibitors of CYP3A and thus could potentially impede pimozide metabolism; ventricular arrhythmias have been rarely associated with the use of macrolide antibiotics in patients with prolonged QT intervals, as might be produced by pimozide; co-administration is contraindicated). Products include:
Erythrocin Stearate Filmtab Tablets 452

Estazolam (Pimozide may be capable of potentiating CNS depressants). Products include:
ProSom Tablets 512

Ethanol (Pimozide may be capable of potentiating CNS depressants).
No products indexed under this heading.

Ethchlorvynol (Pimozide may be capable of potentiating CNS depressants).
No products indexed under this heading.

Ethinamate (Pimozide may be capable of potentiating CNS depressants).
No products indexed under this heading.

Ethyl Alcohol (Pimozide may be capable of potentiating CNS depressants).
No products indexed under this heading.

Fentanyl (Pimozide may be capable of potentiating CNS depressants). Products include:
Duragesic Transdermal System 2448

Fentanyl Citrate (Pimozide may be capable of potentiating CNS depressants). Products include:
Actiq 993

Flecainide Acetate (Co-administration with other drugs which prolong the QT interval may result in additive effect on the QT interval). Products include:
Tambocor Tablets 1824

Fluoxetine Hydrochloride (Co-administration has resulted in a single case report of possible additive effects of pimozide and fluoxetine leading to bradycardia). Products include:
Prozac Pulvules and Liquid 1771
Symbyax Capsules 1788

Fluphenazine Decanoate (Co-administration with other drugs which prolong the QT interval may result in additive effect on the QT interval).
No products indexed under this heading.

Fluphenazine Enanthate (Co-administration with other drugs which prolong the QT interval may result in additive effect on the QT interval).
No products indexed under this heading.

Fluphenazine Hydrochloride (Co-administration with other drugs which prolong the QT interval may result in additive effect on the QT interval).
No products indexed under this heading.

Flurazepam Hydrochloride (Pimozide may be capable of potentiating CNS depressants). Products include:
Dalmane Capsules 3343

Glutethimide (Pimozide may be capable of potentiating CNS depressants).
No products indexed under this heading.

Haloperidol (Pimozide may be capable of potentiating CNS depressants).
No products indexed under this heading.

Haloperidol Decanoate (Pimozide may be capable of potentiating CNS depressants).
No products indexed under this heading.

Hydrocodone Bitartrate (Pimozide may be capable of potentiating CNS depressants). Products include:
Hycodan 1104
Hycomine Compound Tablets 1105
Hycotuss Expectorant Syrup 1106
Lortab 3315
Lortab Elixir 3312
Vicodin Tablets 530
Vicodin ES Tablets 531
Vicodin HP Tablets 532
Vicoprofen Tablets 533
Zydone Tablets 1118

Hydrocodone Polistirex (Pimozide may be capable of potentiating CNS depressants). Products include:
Tussionex Pennkinetic Extended-Release Suspension 3322

Hydromorphone Hydrochloride (Pimozide may be capable of potentiating CNS depressants). Products include:
Dilaudid 439
Dilaudid Oral Liquid 443
Dilaudid Non-Sterile Powder 439
Dilaudid Rectal Suppositories 439
Dilaudid Tablets 439
Dilaudid Tablets - 8 mg 443
Dilaudid-HP 441

Hydroxyzine Hydrochloride (Pimozide may be capable of potentiating CNS depressants).
No products indexed under this heading.

Imipramine Hydrochloride (Co-administration with other drugs which prolong the QT interval may result in additive effect on the QT interval).
No products indexed under this heading.

Imipramine Pamoate (Co-administration with other drugs which prolong the QT interval may result in additive effect on the QT interval).
No products indexed under this heading.

Indinavir Sulfate (Protease inhibitor drugs are inhibitors of CYP3A and thus could potentially impede pimozide metabolism; co-administration is contraindicated). Products include:
Crixivan Capsules **1918**

Isoflurane (Pimozide may be capable of potentiating CNS depressants).
No products indexed under this heading.

Itraconazole (Azole antifungals are inhibitors of CYP3A and thus could potentially impede pimozide metabolism; co-administration is contraindicated).
No products indexed under this heading.

Ketamine Hydrochloride (Pimozide may be capable of potentiating CNS depressants).
No products indexed under this heading.

Ketoconazole (Azole antifungals are inhibitors of CYP3A and thus could potentially impede pimozide metabolism; co-administration is contraindicated). Products include:
Nizoral A-D Shampoo, 1% **1839**
Nizoral 2% Shampoo **1838**

Levomethadyl Acetate Hydrochloride (Pimozide may be capable of potentiating CNS depressants).
No products indexed under this heading.

Levorphanol Tartrate (Pimozide may be capable of potentiating CNS depressants).
No products indexed under this heading.

Lidocaine Hydrochloride (Co-administration with other drugs which prolong the QT interval may result in additive effect on the QT interval).
No products indexed under this heading.

Lopinavir (Protease inhibitor drugs are inhibitors of CYP3A and thus could potentially impede pimozide metabolism; co-administration is contraindicated). Products include:
Kaletra **474**

Lorazepam (Pimozide may be capable of potentiating CNS depressants).
No products indexed under this heading.

Loxapine Hydrochloride (Pimozide may be capable of potentiating CNS depressants).
No products indexed under this heading.

Loxapine Succinate (Pimozide may be capable of potentiating CNS depressants).
No products indexed under this heading.

Maprotiline Hydrochloride (Co-administration with other drugs which prolong the QT interval may result in additive effect on the QT interval).
No products indexed under this heading.

Meperidine Hydrochloride (Pimozide may be capable of potentiating CNS depressants).
No products indexed under this heading.

Mephobarbital (Pimozide may be capable of potentiating CNS depressants). Products include:
Mebaral Tablets, USP **2483**

Meprobamate (Pimozide may be capable of potentiating CNS depressants).
No products indexed under this heading.

Mesoridazine Besylate (Co-administration with other drugs which prolong the QT interval may result in additive effect on the QT interval).
No products indexed under this heading.

Methadone Hydrochloride (Pimozide may be capable of potentiating CNS depressants).
No products indexed under this heading.

Methamphetamine Hydrochloride (Pimozide should not be used in patients taking drugs that themselves cause motor and phonic tics; such as amphetamine). Products include:
Desoxyn Tablets, USP **2482**

Methohexital Sodium (Pimozide may be capable of potentiating CNS depressants).
No products indexed under this heading.

Methotrimeprazine (Pimozide may be capable of potentiating CNS depressants).
No products indexed under this heading.

Methoxyflurane (Pimozide may be capable of potentiating CNS depressants).
No products indexed under this heading.

Methylphenidate Hydrochloride (Pimozide should not be used in patients taking drugs that themselves cause motor and phonic tics; such as methylphenidate). Products include:
Concerta Extended-Release Tablets **1828**
Metadate CD Capsules **3316**
Ritalin **2254**
Ritalin LA Capsules **2255**

Mexiletine Hydrochloride (Co-administration with other drugs which prolong the QT interval may result in additive effect on the QT interval).
No products indexed under this heading.

Midazolam Hydrochloride (Pimozide may be capable of potentiating CNS depressants).
No products indexed under this heading.

Molindone Hydrochloride (Pimozide may be capable of potentiating CNS depressants). Products include:
Moban Tablets **1108**

Morphine Sulfate (Pimozide may be capable of potentiating CNS depressants). Products include:
Avinza Capsules **1714**
Kadian Capsules **572**
MS Contin Tablets **2703**

Nefazodone Hydrochloride (Pimozide is metabolized by CYP3A; co-administration with potent inhibitors of this enzyme system, such as nefazodone, could potentially impede pimozide metabolism; concurrent use is contraindicated).
No products indexed under this heading.

Nelfinavir Mesylate (Protease inhibitor drugs are inhibitors of CYP3A and thus could potentially impede pimozide metabolism; co-administration is contraindicated). Products include:
Viracept **2556**

Nortriptyline Hydrochloride (Co-administration with other drugs which prolong the QT interval may result in additive effect on the QT interval).
No products indexed under this heading.

Olanzapine (Pimozide may be capable of potentiating CNS depressants). Products include:
Symbyax Capsules **1788**
Zyprexa Tablets **1798**
Zyprexa IntraMuscular **1798**
Zyprexa ZYDIS Orally Disintegrating Tablets **1798**

Oxazepam (Pimozide may be capable of potentiating CNS depressants).
No products indexed under this heading.

Oxycodone Hydrochloride (Pimozide may be capable of potentiating CNS depressants). Products include:
Combunox Tablets **1183**
OxyContin Tablets **2699**
OxyFast Oral Concentrate Solution **2704**
OxyIR Capsules **2704**
Percocet Tablets **1114**
Percodan Tablets **1115**

Pemoline (Pimozide should not be used in patients taking drugs that themselves cause motor and phonic tics; such as pemoline).
No products indexed under this heading.

Pentobarbital Sodium (Pimozide may be capable of potentiating CNS depressants). Products include:
Nembutal Sodium Solution, USP **2484**

Perphenazine (Co-administration with other drugs which prolong the QT interval may result in additive effect on the QT interval).
No products indexed under this heading.

Phenobarbital (Pimozide may be capable of potentiating CNS depressants).
No products indexed under this heading.

Prazepam (Pimozide may be capable of potentiating CNS depressants).
No products indexed under this heading.

Procainamide Hydrochloride (Co-administration with other drugs which prolong the QT interval may result in additive effect on the QT interval).
No products indexed under this heading.

Prochlorperazine (Co-administration with other drugs which prolong the QT interval may result in additive effect on the QT interval).
No products indexed under this heading.

Promethazine Hydrochloride (Co-administration with other drugs which prolong the QT interval may result in additive effect on the QT interval). Products include:
Phenergan **3438**

Propafenone Hydrochloride (Co-administration with other drugs which prolong the QT interval may result in additive effect on the QT interval). Products include:
Rythmol SR Capsules **2736**

Propofol (Pimozide may be capable of potentiating CNS depressants). Products include:
Diprivan Injectable Emulsion **676**

Propoxyphene Hydrochloride (Pimozide may be capable of potentiating CNS depressants).
No products indexed under this heading.

Propoxyphene Napsylate (Pimozide may be capable of potentiating CNS depressants). Products include:
Darvocet A 500 Tablets **3497**

Protriptyline Hydrochloride (Co-administration with other drugs which prolong the QT interval may result in additive effect on the QT interval). Products include:
Vivactil Tablets **2350**

Quazepam (Pimozide may be capable of potentiating CNS depressants).
No products indexed under this heading.

Quetiapine Fumarate (Pimozide may be capable of potentiating CNS depressants). Products include:
Seroquel Tablets **691**

Quinidine Gluconate (Co-administration with other drugs which prolong the QT interval may result in additive effect on the QT interval).
No products indexed under this heading.

Quinidine Polygalacturonate (Co-administration with other drugs which prolong the QT interval may result in additive effect on the QT interval).
No products indexed under this heading.

Quinidine Sulfate (Co-administration with other drugs which prolong the QT interval may result in additive effect on the QT interval).
No products indexed under this heading.

Remifentanil Hydrochloride (Pimozide may be capable of potentiating CNS depressants).
No products indexed under this heading.

Risperidone (Pimozide may be capable of potentiating CNS depressants). Products include:
Risperdal Consta Long-Acting Injection **1664**
Risperdal M-Tab Orally Disintegrating Tablets **1658**
Risperdal **1658**

Ritonavir (Protease inhibitor drugs are inhibitors of CYP3A and thus

could potentially impede pimozide metabolism; co-administration is contraindicated). Products include:
Kaletra ... 474
Norvir ... 499

Saquinavir (Protease inhibitor drugs are inhibitors of CYP3A and thus could potentially impede pimozide metabolism; co-administration is contraindicated).
No products indexed under this heading.

Saquinavir Mesylate (Protease inhibitor drugs are inhibitors of CYP3A and thus could potentially impede pimozide metabolism; co-administration is contraindicated). Products include:
Invirase ... 2776

Secobarbital Sodium (Pimozide may be capable of potentiating CNS depressants).
No products indexed under this heading.

Sevoflurane (Pimozide may be capable of potentiating CNS depressants). Products include:
Ultane Liquid for Inhalation ... 526

Sodium Oxybate (Pimozide may be capable of potentiating CNS depressants).
No products indexed under this heading.

Sufentanil Citrate (Pimozide may be capable of potentiating CNS depressants).
No products indexed under this heading.

Temazepam (Pimozide may be capable of potentiating CNS depressants).
No products indexed under this heading.

Thiamylal Sodium (Pimozide may be capable of potentiating CNS depressants).
No products indexed under this heading.

Thioridazine Hydrochloride (Co-administration with other drugs which prolong the QT interval may result in additive effect on the QT interval). Products include:
Thioridazine Hydrochloride Tablets ... 2122

Thiothixene (Pimozide may be capable of potentiating CNS depressants). Products include:
Thiothixene Capsules ... 2124

Tocainide Hydrochloride (Co-administration with other drugs which prolong the QT interval may result in additive effect on the QT interval).
No products indexed under this heading.

Triazolam (Pimozide may be capable of potentiating CNS depressants).
No products indexed under this heading.

Trifluoperazine Hydrochloride (Co-administration with other drugs which prolong the QT interval may result in additive effect on the QT interval).
No products indexed under this heading.

Trimipramine Maleate (Co-administration with other drugs which prolong the QT interval may result in additive effect on the QT interval). Products include:
Surmontil Capsules ... 2347

Troleandomycin (Macrolide antibiotics are inhibitors of CYP3A and thus could potentially impede pimozide metabolism; ventricular arrhythmias have been rarely associated with the use of macrolide antibiotics in patients with prolonged QT intervals, as might be produced by pimozide; co-administration is contraindicated).
No products indexed under this heading.

Zaleplon (Pimozide may be capable of potentiating CNS depressants). Products include:
Sonata Capsules ... 1686

Zileuton (Pimozide is metabolized by CYP3A; co-administration with inhibitors of this enzyme system, such as zileuton, could potentially impede pimozide metabolism; concurrent use should be avoided).
No products indexed under this heading.

Ziprasidone Hydrochloride (Co-administration with other drugs which prolong the QT interval may result in additive effect on the QT interval). Products include:
Geodon Capsules ... 2514

Zolpidem Tartrate (Pimozide may be capable of potentiating CNS depressants). Products include:
Ambien Tablets ... 2867

Food Interactions

Alcohol (Pimozide may be capable of potentiating CNS depressants, including alcohol).

ORTHO-CEPT TABLETS

(Desogestrel, Ethinyl Estradiol) ... 2395
May interact with barbiturates, protease inhibitors, tetracyclines, and certain other agents. Compounds in these categories include:

Acetaminophen (Increased plasma ethinyl estradiol levels and decreased acetaminophen plasma concentrations with concomitant use). Products include:
Benadryl Allergy & Cold Tablets ... 692
Benadryl Allergy & Sinus Headache Caplets & Gelcaps ... 693
Benadryl Maximum Strength Severe Allergy & Sinus Headache Caplets ... 694
Contac Severe Cold and Flu Caplets Maximum Strength ... 615
Contac Severe Cold and Flu Caplets Non-Drowsy ... 615
Darvocet A 500 Tablets ... 3497
Goody's Body Pain Formula Powder ... 621
Goody's Extra Strength Headache Powder ... 621
Goody's Extra Strength Pain Relief Tablets ... 621
Goody's PM Powder ... 622
Hycomine Compound Tablets ... 1105
Lortab ... 3315
Lortab Elixir ... 3312
Percocet Tablets ... 1114
Robitussin Cough, Cold & Flu Liquid-filled Capsules ... 750
Robitussin Flu Liquid ... 752
Sedapap Tablets 50 mg/650 mg ... 2098
Singlet Caplets ... 636
Sudafed Severe Cold ... 710
Sudafed Sinus Headache ... 711
TheraFlu Cold & Cough Hot Liquid ... 680
TheraFlu Cold & Sore Throat Hot Liquid ... 680
TheraFlu Flu & Chest Congestion Non-Drowsy Hot Liquid ... 681
TheraFlu Flu & Sore Throat Hot Liquid ... 681
TheraFlu Severe Cold Non-Drowsy Hot Liquid ... 683
TheraFlu Severe Cold & Cough Hot Liquid ... 683
TheraFlu Severe Cold Caplets ... 679
TheraFlu Severe Cold Hot Liquid ... 682
TheraFlu Severe Cold Non-Drowsy Caplets ... 679
Triaminic Cough & Sore Throat Liquid ... 687
Triaminic Flu, Cough & Fever Liquid ... 685
Triaminic Cough & Sore Throat Softchews ... 689
Tylenol 8 Hour Extended Release Geltabs and Caplets ... 1843
Tylenol Sinus NightTime Caplets ... 663
Children's Tylenol Suspension Liquid and Meltaways ... 1850
Children's Tylenol Plus Cold & Allergy Suspension Liquid ... 1850
Children's Tylenol Plus Cold NightTime Suspension Liquid ... 1851
Children's Tylenol Plus Cold & Cough Suspension Liquid and Chewable Tablets ... 1851
Children's Tylenol Plus Cold Chewable Tablets ... 1851
Children's Tylenol Plus Cold Daytime Non-Drowsy Suspension Liquid ... 1851
Children's Tylenol Plus Flu Suspension Liquid ... 1853
Concentrated Tylenol Infants' Drops Plus Cold ... 1851
Concentrated Tylenol Infants' Drops Plus Cold and Cough ... 1851
Concentrated Tylenol Infants' Drops ... 1850
Junior Tylenol Meltaways ... 1850
Tylenol Cold & Flu Severe Daytime Liquid with Cool Burst ... 1846
Tylenol Cold & Flu Severe NightTime Liquid with Cool Burst ... 1846
Tylenol Cold Severe Congestion Non-Drowsy Caplets with Cool Burst ... 1846
Tylenol Cough & Sore Throat Daytime Liquid with Cool Burst ... 1849
Tylenol Cough & Sore Throat NightTime Liquid with Cool Burst ... 1849
Tylenol ... 1843
Extra Strength Tylenol Rapid Release Gels ... 1843
Tylenol ... 1843
Tylenol Allergy Complete Night Time Caplets ... 1844
Tylenol Allergy Complete Multi-Symptom Caplets and Gelcaps with Cool Burst ... 1844
Tylenol Severe Allergy Caplets ... 1844
Tylenol Flu NightTime Gelcaps ... 1846
Tylenol Flu Day Non-Drowsy Gelcaps ... 1846
Concentrated Tylenol Infants' Drops Plus Cold Nasal Congestant, Fever Reducer & Pain Reliever ... 668
Concentrated Tylenol Infants' Drops Plus Cold & Cough Nasal Decongestant, Fever Reducer & Pain Reliever ... 668
Multi-Symptom Tylenol Cold Night Time Caplets ... 1845
Multi-Symptom Tylenol Cold Day Non-Drowsy Caplets and Gelcaps ... 1845
Extra Strength Tylenol PM Caplets, Geltabs, Gelcaps and Liquid ... 1847
Tylenol Sinus Day Non-Drowsy ... 1848
Tylenol Sinus Night Time Caplets ... 1848
Tylenol Sinus Severe Congestion Caplets with Cool Burst ... 1848
Tylenol Sore Throat Daytime Liquid with Cool Burst ... 1849
Tylenol Sore Throat NightTime Liquid with Cool Burst ... 1849
Tylenol with Codeine ... 2461
Women's Tylenol Menstrual Relief Caplets ... 1849
Ultracet Tablets ... 2462
Vicks 44M Cough, Cold & Flu Relief ... 2676
Vicks DayQuil LiquiCaps/Liquid Multi-Symptom Cold/Flu Relief ... 723
Vicks DayQuil Multi-Symptom Cold/Flu Relief LiquiCaps ... 2675
Vicks DayQuil Multi-Symptom Cold/Flu Relief Liquid ... 2675
Vicks NyQuil LiquiCaps ... 2677
Vicks NyQuil LiquiCaps/Liquid Multi-Symptom Cold/Flu Relief ... 725
Vicks NyQuil Liquid ... 2677
Vicodin Tablets ... 530
Vicodin ES Tablets ... 531
Vicodin HP Tablets ... 532
Zydone Tablets ... 1118

Ampicillin (Potential for reduced efficacy and increased incidence of breakthrough bleeding and unintended pregnancy with concomitant use).
No products indexed under this heading.

Ampicillin Sodium (Potential for reduced efficacy and increased incidence of breakthrough bleeding and unintended pregnancy with concomitant use).
No products indexed under this heading.

Amprenavir (Safety and efficacy of oral contraceptive products may be affected by anti-HIV protease inhibitors. Refer to the label of the individual anti-HIV protease inhibitors for further information). Products include:
Agenerase Capsules ... 1299
Agenerase Oral Solution ... 1304

Aprobarbital (Potential for reduced efficacy and increased incidence of breakthrough bleeding and unintended pregnancy with concomitant use).
No products indexed under this heading.

Ascorbic Acid (May increase plasma ethinyl estradiol levels).
No products indexed under this heading.

Atorvastatin Calcium (Co-administration of atorvastatin and certain oral contraceptives containing ethinyl estradiol increase AUC values for ethinyl estradiol by 20%). Products include:
Caduet Tablets ... 2507
Lipitor Tablets ... 2495

Butabarbital (Potential for reduced efficacy and increased incidence of breakthrough bleeding and unintended pregnancy with concomitant use).
No products indexed under this heading.

Butalbital (Potential for reduced efficacy and increased incidence of breakthrough bleeding and unintended pregnancy with concomitant use). Products include:
Sedapap Tablets 50 mg/650 mg ... 2098

Carbamazepine (Potential for reduced efficacy and increased incidence of breakthrough bleeding and unintended pregnancy with concomitant use). Products include:
Carbatrol Capsules ... 3174
Equetro Extended-Release Capsules ... 3178
Tegretol/Tegretol-XR ... 2278

Clofibrate (Increased clearance of clofibrate concomitant use).
No products indexed under this heading.

Cyclosporine (Increased concentration of cyclosporine has been reported with concomitant use). Products include:
Gengraf Capsules ... 458
Neoral Soft Gelatin Capsules ... 2247
Neoral Oral Solution ... 2247
Restasis Ophthalmic Emulsion ... 570
Sandimmune ... 2259

IMPORTANT NOTE: Always consult each drug listing in the patient's regimen for possible interactions.

Demeclocycline Hydrochloride (Potential for reduced efficacy and increased incidence of breakthrough bleeding and unintended pregnancy with concomitant use).
No products indexed under this heading.

Doxycycline Calcium (Potential for reduced efficacy and increased incidence of breakthrough bleeding and unintended pregnancy with concomitant use).
No products indexed under this heading.

Doxycycline Hyclate (Potential for reduced efficacy and increased incidence of breakthrough bleeding and unintended pregnancy with concomitant use).
No products indexed under this heading.

Doxycycline Monohydrate (Potential for reduced efficacy and increased incidence of breakthrough bleeding and unintended pregnancy with concomitant use).
No products indexed under this heading.

Felbamate (Potential for reduced efficacy and increased incidence of breakthrough bleeding and unintended pregnancy with concomitant use).
No products indexed under this heading.

Fosphenytoin Sodium (Potential for reduced efficacy and increased incidence of breakthrough bleeding and unintended pregnancy with concomitant use).
No products indexed under this heading.

Griseofulvin (Potential for reduced efficacy and increased incidence of breakthrough bleeding and unintended pregnancy with concomitant use). Products include:
Grifulvin V Tablets Microsize and Oral Suspension Microsize 2384
Gris-PEG Tablets 2504

Hypericum (Co-administration of hormonal contraceptives and St. John's Wort may reduce effectiveness and result in beakthrough bleeding).
No products indexed under this heading.

Indinavir Sulfate (Safety and efficacy of oral contraceptive products may be affected by anti-HIV protease inhibitors. Refer to the label of the individual anti-HIV protease inhibitors for further information). Products include:
Crixivan Capsules 1918

Itraconazole (CYP3A4 inhibitors, such as itraconazole, may increase plasma hormone levels).
No products indexed under this heading.

Ketoconazole (CYP3A4 inhibitors, such as ketoconazole, may increase plasma hormone levels). Products include:
Nizoral A-D Shampoo, 1% 1839
Nizoral 2% Shampoo 1838

Lopinavir (Safety and efficacy of oral contraceptive products may be affected by anti-HIV protease inhibitors. Refer to the label of the individual anti-HIV protease inhibitors for further information). Products include:
Kaletra 474

Mephobarbital (Potential for reduced efficacy and increased incidence of breakthrough bleeding and unintended pregnancy with concomitant use). Products include:
Mebaral Tablets, USP 2483

Methacycline Hydrochloride (Potential for reduced efficacy and increased incidence of breakthrough bleeding and unintended pregnancy with concomitant use).
No products indexed under this heading.

Minocycline Hydrochloride (Potential for reduced efficacy and increased incidence of breakthrough bleeding and unintended pregnancy with concomitant use). Products include:
Dynacin Tablets 1859

Morphine Sulfate (Increased clearance of morphine sulfate with concomitant use). Products include:
Avinza Capsules 1714
Kadian Capsules 572
MS Contin Tablets 2703

Nelfinavir Mesylate (Safety and efficacy of oral contraceptive products may be affected by anti-HIV protease inhibitors. Refer to the label of the individual anti-HIV protease inhibitors for further information). Products include:
Viracept 2556

Oxcarbazepine (Potential for reduced efficacy and increased incidence of breakthrough bleeding and unintended pregnancy with concomitant use). Products include:
Trileptal Oral Suspension 2281
Trileptal Tablets 2281

Oxytetracycline Hydrochloride (Potential for reduced efficacy and increased incidence of breakthrough bleeding and unintended pregnancy with concomitant use).
No products indexed under this heading.

Pentobarbital Sodium (Potential for reduced efficacy and increased incidence of breakthrough bleeding and unintended pregnancy with concomitant use). Products include:
Nembutal Sodium Solution, USP 2484

Phenobarbital (Potential for reduced efficacy and increased incidence of breakthrough bleeding and unintended pregnancy with concomitant use).
No products indexed under this heading.

Phenylbutazone (Potential for reduced efficacy and increased incidence of breakthrough bleeding and unintended pregnancy with concomitant use).
No products indexed under this heading.

Phenytoin (Potential for reduced efficacy and increased incidence of breakthrough bleeding and unintended pregnancy with concomitant use).
No products indexed under this heading.

Phenytoin Sodium (Potential for reduced efficacy and increased incidence of breakthrough bleeding and unintended pregnancy with concomitant use). Products include:
Phenytek Capsules 2153

Prednisolone (Increased concentration of prenisolone has been reported with concomitant use).
No products indexed under this heading.

Prednisolone Acetate (Increased concentration of prednisolone has been reported with concomitant use). Products include:
Blephamide Ophthalmic Ointment 563
Blephamide Ophthalmic Suspension 564
Poly-Pred Liquifilm Ophthalmic Suspension .... ⊙231
Pred Forte Ophthalmic Suspension .... ⊙233
Pred Mild Sterile Ophthalmic Suspension .... ⊙236
Pred-G Ophthalmic Suspension .... ⊙234
Pred-G Sterile Ophthalmic Ointment .... ⊙235

Prednisolone Sodium Phosphate (Increased concentration of prednisolone has been reported with concomitant use). Products include:
Pediapred Oral Solution 3319

Prednisolone Tebutate (Increased concentration of prednisolone has been reported with concomitant use).
No products indexed under this heading.

Rifampin (Co-administration has been associated with reduced efficacy and increased incidence of breakthrough bleeding and unintended pregnancy).
No products indexed under this heading.

Ritonavir (Safety and efficacy of oral contraceptive products may be affected by anti-HIV protease inhibitors. Refer to the label of the individual anti-HIV protease inhibitors for further information). Products include:
Kaletra 474
Norvir 499

Salicylic Acid (Increased clearance of salicylic acid with concomitant use).
No products indexed under this heading.

Saquinavir (Safety and efficacy of oral contraceptive products may be affected by anti-HIV protease inhibitors. Refer to the label of the individual anti-HIV protease inhibitors for further information).
No products indexed under this heading.

Saquinavir Mesylate (Safety and efficacy of oral contraceptive products may be affected by anti-HIV protease inhibitors. Refer to the label of the individual anti-HIV protease inhibitors for further information). Products include:
Invirase 2776

Secobarbital Sodium (Potential for reduced efficacy and increased incidence of breakthrough bleeding and unintended pregnancy with concomitant use).
No products indexed under this heading.

Temazepam (Increased clearance of temazepam with concomitant use).
No products indexed under this heading.

Tetracycline Hydrochloride (Potential for reduced efficacy and increased incidence of breakthrough bleeding and unintended pregnancy with concomitant use).
No products indexed under this heading.

Theophylline (Increased concentration of theophylline has been reported with concomitant use).
No products indexed under this heading.

Theophylline Anhydrous (Increased concentration of theophylline has been reported with concomitant use). Products include:
Uniphyl Tablets 2708

Theophylline Calcium Salicylate (Increased concentration of theophylline has been reported with concomitant use).
No products indexed under this heading.

Theophylline Dihydroxypropyl (Glyceryl) (Increased concentration of theophylline has been reported with concomitant use).
No products indexed under this heading.

Theophylline Ethylenediamine (Increased concentration of theophylline has been reported with concomitant use).
No products indexed under this heading.

Theophylline Sodium Glycinate (Increased concentration of theophylline has been reported with concomitant use).
No products indexed under this heading.

Thiamylal Sodium (Potential for reduced efficacy and increased incidence of breakthrough bleeding and unintended pregnancy with concomitant use).
No products indexed under this heading.

Topiramate (Potential for reduced efficacy and increased incidence of breakthrough bleeding and unintended pregnancy with concomitant use). Products include:
Topamax Sprinkle Capsules 2438
Topamax Tablets 2438

ORTHO-CYCLEN TABLETS

(Ethinyl Estradiol, Norgestimate) 2414
May interact with barbiturates, phenytoin, tetracyclines, and certain other agents. Compounds in these categories include:

Ampicillin (Potential for reduced efficacy and increased incidence of breakthrough bleeding and menstrual irregularities with concomitant use).
No products indexed under this heading.

Ampicillin Sodium (Potential for reduced efficacy and increased incidence of breakthrough bleeding and menstrual irregularities with concomitant use).
No products indexed under this heading.

Aprobarbital (Potential for reduced efficacy and increased incidence of breakthrough bleeding and menstrual irregularities with concomitant use).
No products indexed under this heading.

Butabarbital (Potential for reduced efficacy and increased incidence of breakthrough bleeding and menstrual irregularities with concomitant use).
No products indexed under this heading.

Butalbital (Potential for reduced efficacy and increased incidence of breakthrough bleeding and menstrual irregularities with concomitant use). Products include:
Sedapap Tablets 50 mg/650 mg 2098

Carbamazepine (Potential for reduced efficacy and increased inci-

dence of breakthrough bleeding and menstrual irregularities with concomitant use). Products include:

Carbatrol Capsules 3174
Equetro Extended-Release Capsules 3178
Tegretol/Tegretol-XR 2278

Demeclocycline Hydrochloride (Potential for reduced efficacy and increased incidence of breakthrough bleeding and menstrual irregularities with concomitant use).
No products indexed under this heading.

Doxycycline Calcium (Potential for reduced efficacy and increased incidence of breakthrough bleeding and menstrual irregularities with concomitant use).
No products indexed under this heading.

Doxycycline Hyclate (Potential for reduced efficacy and increased incidence of breakthrough bleeding and menstrual irregularities with concomitant use).
No products indexed under this heading.

Doxycycline Monohydrate (Potential for reduced efficacy and increased incidence of breakthrough bleeding and menstrual irregularities with concomitant use).
No products indexed under this heading.

Fosphenytoin Sodium (Potential for reduced efficacy and increased incidence of breakthrough bleeding and menstrual irregularities with concomitant use).
No products indexed under this heading.

Griseofulvin (Potential for reduced efficacy and increased incidence of breakthrough bleeding and menstrual irregularities with concomitant use). Products include:

Grifulvin V Tablets Microsize and Oral Suspension Microsize........... 2384
Gris-PEG Tablets 2504

Hypericum (Co-administration of hormonal contraceptives and St. John's Wort containing herbal supplements has resulted in breakthrough bleeding shortly after starting St. John's Wort and pregnancies have been reported with concomitant therapy in some patients).
No products indexed under this heading.

Mephobarbital (Potential for reduced efficacy and increased incidence of breakthrough bleeding and menstrual irregularities with concomitant use). Products include:

Mebaral Tablets, USP 2483

Methacycline Hydrochloride (Potential for reduced efficacy and increased incidence of breakthrough bleeding and menstrual irregularities with concomitant use).
No products indexed under this heading.

Minocycline Hydrochloride (Potential for reduced efficacy and increased incidence of breakthrough bleeding and menstrual irregularities with concomitant use). Products include:

Dynacin Tablets 1859

Oxytetracycline Hydrochloride (Potential for reduced efficacy and increased incidence of breakthrough bleeding and menstrual irregularities with concomitant use).
No products indexed under this heading.

Pentobarbital Sodium (Potential for reduced efficacy and increased incidence of breakthrough bleeding and menstrual irregularities with concomitant use). Products include:

Nembutal Sodium Solution, USP 2484

Phenobarbital (Potential for reduced efficacy and increased incidence of breakthrough bleeding and menstrual irregularities with concomitant use).
No products indexed under this heading.

Phenylbutazone (Potential for reduced efficacy and increased incidence of breakthrough bleeding and menstrual irregularities with concomitant use).
No products indexed under this heading.

Phenytoin (Potential for reduced efficacy and increased incidence of breakthrough bleeding and menstrual irregularities with concomitant use).
No products indexed under this heading.

Phenytoin Sodium (Potential for reduced efficacy and increased incidence of breakthrough bleeding and menstrual irregularities with concomitant use). Products include:

Phenytek Capsules 2153

Rifampin (Co-administration has been associated with reduced efficacy and increased incidence of breakthrough bleeding and menstrual irregularities).
No products indexed under this heading.

Secobarbital Sodium (Potential for reduced efficacy and increased incidence of breakthrough bleeding and menstrual irregularities with concomitant use).
No products indexed under this heading.

Tetracycline Hydrochloride (Potential for reduced efficacy and increased incidence of breakthrough bleeding and menstrual irregularities with concomitant use).
No products indexed under this heading.

Thiamylal Sodium (Potential for reduced efficacy and increased incidence of breakthrough bleeding and menstrual irregularities with concomitant use).
No products indexed under this heading.

Topiramate (Co-administration may result in reduced efficacy and increased incidence of breakthrough bleeding and menstrual irregularities). Products include:

Topamax Sprinkle Capsules 2438
Topamax Tablets 2438

ORTHO EVRA TRANSDERMAL SYSTEM

(Ethinyl Estradiol, Norelgestromin) 2402
May interact with barbiturates, phenytoin, prednisolone, protease inhibitors, xanthines, and certain other agents. Compounds in these categories include:

Acetaminophen (Co-administration with certain oral contraceptives containing ethinyl estradiol increases plasma ethinyl estradiol levels possibly by inhibition of conjugation; decreased plasma levels of acetaminophen). Products include:

Benadryl Allergy & Cold Tablets 692
Benadryl Allergy & Sinus Headache Caplets & Gelcaps...... 693
Benadryl Maximum Strength Severe Allergy & Sinus Headache Caplets........................ 694
Contac Severe Cold and Flu Caplets Maximum Strength......... 615
Contac Severe Cold and Flu Caplets Non-Drowsy.................. 615
Darvocet A 500 Tablets 3497
Goody's Body Pain Formula Powder........................ 621
Goody's Extra Strength Headache Powder.................. 621
Goody's Extra Strength Pain Relief Tablets 621
Goody's PM Powder 622
Hycomine Compound Tablets 1105
Lortab 3315
Lortab Elixir 3312
Percocet Tablets 1114
Robitussin Cough, Cold & Flu Liquid-filled Capsules.................. 750
Robitussin Flu Liquid 752
Sedapap Tablets 50 mg/650 mg 2098
Singlet Caplets 636
Sudafed Severe Cold 710
Sudafed Sinus Headache 711
TheraFlu Cold & Cough Hot Liquid 680
TheraFlu Cold & Sore Throat Hot Liquid 680
TheraFlu Flu & Chest Congestion Non-Drowsy Hot Liquid............... 681
TheraFlu Flu & Sore Throat Hot Liquid 681
TheraFlu Severe Cold Non-Drowsy Hot Liquid............... 683
TheraFlu Severe Cold & Cough Hot Liquid 683
TheraFlu Severe Cold Caplets 679
TheraFlu Severe Cold Hot Liquid 682
TheraFlu Severe Cold Non-Drowsy Caplets.................. 679
Triaminic Cough & Sore Throat Liquid 687
Triaminic Flu, Cough & Fever Liquid 685
Triaminic Cough & Sore Throat Softchews 689
Tylenol 8 Hour Extended Release Geltabs and Caplets 1843
Tylenol Sinus NightTime Caplets 663
Children's Tylenol Suspension Liquid and Meltaways.................. 1850
Children's Tylenol Plus Cold & Allergy Suspension Liquid............ 1850
Children's Tylenol Plus Cold NightTime Suspension Liquid........ 1851
Children's Tylenol Plus Cold & Cough Suspension Liquid and Chewable Tablets 1851
Children's Tylenol Plus Cold Chewable Tablets 1851
Children's Tylenol Plus Cold Daytime Non-Drowsy Suspension Liquid 1851
Children's Tylenol Plus Flu Suspension Liquid 1853
Concentrated Tylenol Infants' Drops Plus Cold........................ 1851
Concentrated Tylenol Infants' Drops Plus Cold and Cough 1851
Concentrated Tylenol Infants' Drops........................ 1850
Junior Tylenol Meltaways 1850
Tylenol Cold & Flu Severe Daytime Liquid with Cool Bust....... 1846
Tylenol Cold & Flu Severe NightTime Liquid with Cool Burst........................ 1846
Tylenol Cold Severe Congestion Non-Drowsy Caplets with Cool Burst........................ 1846
Tylenol Cough & Sore Throat Daytime Liquid with Cool Burst...... 1849
Tylenol Cough & Sore Throat NightTime Liquid with Cool Burst........................ 1849
Tylenol 1843
Extra Strength Tylenol Rapid Release Gels........................ 1843
Tylenol 1843
Tylenol Allergy Complete Night Time Caplets........................ 1844
Tylenol Allergy Complete Multi-Symptom Caplets and Gelcaps with Cool Burst............... 1844
Tylenol Severe Allergy Caplets 1844
Tylenol Flu NightTime Gelcaps 1846
Tylenol Flu Day Non-Drowsy Gelcaps........................ 1846
Concentrated Tylenol Infants' Drops Plus Cold Nasal Congestant, Fever Reducer & Pain Reliever........................ 668
Concentrated Tylenol Infants' Drops Plus Cold & Cough Nasal Decongestant, Fever Reducer & Pain Reliever 668
Multi-Symptom Tylenol Cold Night Time Caplets 1845
Multi-Symptom Tylenol Cold Day Non-Drowsy Caplets and Gelcaps........................ 1845
Extra Strength Tylenol PM Caplets, Geltabs, Gelcaps and Liquid 1847
Tylenol Sinus Day Non-Drowsy 1848
Tylenol Sinus Night Time Caplets 1848
Tylenol Sinus Severe Congestion Caplets with Cool Burst............... 1848
Tylenol Sore Throat Daytime Liquid with Cool Burst................. 1849
Tylenol Sore Throat NightTime Liquid with Cool Burst................. 1849
Tylenol with Codeine 2461
Women's Tylenol Menstrual Relief Caplets........................ 1849
Ultracet Tablets 2462
Vicks 44M Cough, Cold & Flu Relief........................ 2676
Vicks DayQuil LiquiCaps/Liquid Multi-Symptom Cold/Flu Relief..... 723
Vicks DayQuil Multi-Symptom Cold/Flu Relief LiquiCaps............. 2675
Vicks DayQuil Multi-Symptom Cold/Flu Relief Liquid.................. 2675
Vicks NyQuil LiquiCaps 2677
Vicks NyQuil LiquiCaps/Liquid Multi-Symptom Cold/Flu Relief..... 725
Vicks NyQuil Liquid 2677
Vicodin Tablets 530
Vicodin ES Tablets 531
Vicodin HP Tablets 532
Zydone Tablets 1118

Aminophylline (Co-administration increases the plasma concentrations of theophylline).
No products indexed under this heading.

Ampicillin (Increases the metabolism of contraceptive steroids resulting in reduced contraceptive effectiveness which could precipitate unintended pregnancy).
No products indexed under this heading.

Ampicillin Sodium (Increases the metabolism of contraceptive steroids resulting in reduced contraceptive effectiveness which could precipitate unintended pregnancy).
No products indexed under this heading.

Amprenavir (Several of the protease inhibitors have induced significant changes in the AUC of the estrogen and progestins in some cases; it is not known if this applies to Ortho Evra). Products include:

Agenerase Capsules 1299
Agenerase Oral Solution 1304

Aprobarbital (Barbiturates increase the metabolism of contraceptive steroids resulting in reduced contraceptive effectiveness which could precipitate unintended pregnancy).
No products indexed under this heading.

Atorvastatin Calcium (Co-administration with certain oral contraceptives containing ethinyl estradiol increases AUC values for ethinyl estradiol by approximately 20%). Products include:

Caduet Tablets 2507

Lipitor Tablets 2495

Butabarbital (Barbiturates increase the metabolism of contraceptive steroids resulting in reduced contraceptive effectiveness which could precipitate unintended pregnancy).
No products indexed under this heading.

Butalbital (Barbiturates increase the metabolism of contraceptive steroids resulting in reduced contraceptive effectiveness which could precipitate unintended pregnancy). Products include:
Sedapap Tablets 50 mg/650 mg 2098

Carbamazepine (Increases the metabolism of contraceptive steroids resulting in reduced contraceptive effectiveness which could precipitate unintended pregnancy). Products include:
Carbatrol Capsules 3174
Equetro Extended-Release Capsules 3178
Tegretol/Tegretol-XR 2278

Clofibrate (Increased clearance of clofibric acid).
No products indexed under this heading.

Cyclosporine (Co-administration increases the plasma concentrations of cyclosporine). Products include:
Gengraf Capsules 458
Neoral Soft Gelatin Capsules 2247
Neoral Oral Solution 2247
Restasis Ophthalmic Emulsion 570
Sandimmune 2259

Dyphylline (Co-administration increases the plasma concentrations of theophylline).
No products indexed under this heading.

Fosphenytoin Sodium (Increases the metabolism of contraceptive steroids resulting in reduced contraceptive effectiveness which could precipitate unintended pregnancy).
No products indexed under this heading.

Griseofulvin (Increases the metabolism of contraceptive steroids resulting in reduced contraceptive effectiveness which could precipitate unintended pregnancy). Products include:
Grifulvin V Tablets Microsize and Oral Suspension Microsize........ 2384
Gris-PEG Tablets 2504

Hypericum (May induce hepatic enzymes and p-glycoprotein transporter and may reduce the effectiveness of contraceptive steroids which may result in breakthrough bleeding).
No products indexed under this heading.

Indinavir Sulfate (Several of the protease inhibitors have induced significant changes in the AUC of the estrogen and progestins in some cases; it is not known if this applies to Ortho Evra). Products include:
Crixivan Capsules 1918

Itraconazole (Co-administration with CYP 3A4 inhibitors may increase plasma hormone levels).
No products indexed under this heading.

Ketoconazole (Co-administration with CYP 3A4 inhibitors may increase plasma hormone levels). Products include:
Nizoral A-D Shampoo, 1% 1839
Nizoral 2% Shampoo 1838

Lopinavir (Several of the protease inhibitors have induced significant changes in the AUC of the estrogen and progestins in some cases; it is not known if this applies to Ortho Evra). Products include:
Kaletra 474

Mephobarbital (Barbiturates increase the metabolism of contraceptive steroids resulting in reduced contraceptive effectiveness which could precipitate unintended pregnancy). Products include:
Mebaral Tablets, USP 2483

Morphine Sulfate (Increased clearance of morphine). Products include:
Avinza Capsules 1714
Kadian Capsules 572
MS Contin Tablets 2703

Nelfinavir Mesylate (Several of the protease inhibitors have induced significant changes in the AUC of the estrogen and progestins in some cases; it is not known if this applies to Ortho Evra). Products include:
Viracept 2556

Pentobarbital Sodium (Barbiturates increase the metabolism of contraceptive steroids resulting in reduced contraceptive effectiveness which could precipitate unintended pregnancy). Products include:
Nembutal Sodium Solution, USP 2484

Phenobarbital (Barbiturates increase the metabolism of contraceptive steroids resulting in reduced contraceptive effectiveness which could precipitate unintended pregnancy).
No products indexed under this heading.

Phenylbutazone (Increases the metabolism of contraceptive steroids resulting in reduced contraceptive effectiveness which could precipitate unintended pregnancy).
No products indexed under this heading.

Phenytoin (Increases the metabolism of contraceptive steroids resulting in reduced contraceptive effectiveness which could precipitate unintended pregnancy).
No products indexed under this heading.

Phenytoin Sodium (Increases the metabolism of contraceptive steroids resulting in reduced contraceptive effectiveness which could precipitate unintended pregnancy). Products include:
Phenytek Capsules 2153

Prednisolone (Co-administration increases the plasma concentrations of prednisolone).
No products indexed under this heading.

Prednisolone Acetate (Co-administration increases the plasma concentrations of prednisolone). Products include:
Blephamide Ophthalmic Ointment 563
Blephamide Ophthalmic Suspension........ 564
Poly-Pred Liquifilm Ophthalmic Suspension .... ⊙231
Pred Forte Ophthalmic Suspension .... ⊙233
Pred Mild Sterile Ophthalmic Suspension .... ⊙236
Pred-G Ophthalmic Suspension ...... ⊙234
Pred-G Sterile Ophthalmic Ointment .... ⊙235

Prednisolone Sodium Phosphate (Co-administration increases the plasma concentrations of prednisolone). Products include:
Pediapred Oral Solution 3319

Prednisolone Tebutate (Co-administration increases the plasma concentrations of prednisolone).
No products indexed under this heading.

Rifampin (Increases the metabolism of contraceptive steroids resulting in reduced contraceptive effectiveness which could precipitate unintended pregnancy).
No products indexed under this heading.

Ritonavir (Several of the protease inhibitors have induced significant changes in the AUC of the estrogen and progestins in some cases; it is not known if this applies to Ortho Evra). Products include:
Kaletra 474
Norvir 499

Salicylic Acid (Increased clearance of salicylic acid).
No products indexed under this heading.

Saquinavir (Several of the protease inhibitors have induced significant changes in the AUC of the estrogen and progestins in some cases; it is not known if this applies to Ortho Evra).
No products indexed under this heading.

Saquinavir Mesylate (Several of the protease inhibitors have induced significant changes in the AUC of the estrogen and progestins in some cases; it is not known if this applies to Ortho Evra). Products include:
Invirase 2776

Secobarbital Sodium (Barbiturates increase the metabolism of contraceptive steroids resulting in reduced contraceptive effectiveness which could precipitate unintended pregnancy).
No products indexed under this heading.

Temazepam (Increased clearance of temazepam).
No products indexed under this heading.

Theophylline (Co-administration increases the plasma concentrations of theophylline).
No products indexed under this heading.

Theophylline Anhydrous (Co-administration increases the plasma concentrations of theophylline). Products include:
Uniphyl Tablets 2708

Theophylline Calcium Salicylate (Co-administration increases the plasma concentrations of theophylline).
No products indexed under this heading.

Theophylline Dihydroxypropyl (Glyceryl) (Co-administration increases the plasma concentrations of theophylline).
No products indexed under this heading.

Theophylline Ethylenediamine (Co-administration increases the plasma concentrations of theophylline).
No products indexed under this heading.

Theophylline Sodium Glycinate (Co-administration increases the plasma concentrations of theophylline).
No products indexed under this heading.

Thiamylal Sodium (Barbiturates increase the metabolism of contraceptive steroids resulting in reduced contraceptive effectiveness which could precipitate unintended pregnancy).
No products indexed under this heading.

Topiramate (Increases the metabolism of contraceptive steroids resulting in reduced contraceptive effectiveness which could precipitate unintended pregnancy). Products include:
Topamax Sprinkle Capsules 2438
Topamax Tablets 2438

Vitamin C (Co-administration with certain oral contraceptives containing ethinyl estradiol increases plasma ethinyl estradiol levels possibly by inhibition of conjugation). Products include:
Chromagen Forte Soft Gelatin Capsules 3296
Halls Defense Sugarfree Vitamin C Drops .... ⊡611
Niferex-150 Forte Capsules 3299
Peridin-C Tablets .... ⊡761
Repliva 21/7 Tablets 3301

ORTHO MICRONOR TABLETS

(Norethindrone) 2411
May interact with barbiturates, phenytoin, and certain other agents. Compounds in these categories include:

Aprobarbital (The effectiveness of progestin-only oral contraceptives is reduced by hepatic enzyme-inducing agents such as barbiturates).
No products indexed under this heading.

Butabarbital (The effectiveness of progestin-only oral contraceptives is reduced by hepatic enzyme-inducing agents such as barbiturates).
No products indexed under this heading.

Butalbital (The effectiveness of progestin-only oral contraceptives is reduced by hepatic enzyme-inducing agents such as barbiturates). Products include:
Sedapap Tablets 50 mg/650 mg 2098

Carbamazepine (The effectiveness of progestin-only oral contraceptives is reduced by hepatic enzyme-inducing agents such as carbamazepine). Products include:
Carbatrol Capsules 3174
Equetro Extended-Release Capsules 3178
Tegretol/Tegretol-XR 2278

Fosphenytoin Sodium (The effectiveness of progestin-only oral contraceptives is reduced by hepatic enzyme-inducing agents such as phenytoin).
No products indexed under this heading.

Mephobarbital (The effectiveness of progestin-only oral contraceptives is reduced by hepatic enzyme-inducing agents such as barbiturates). Products include:
Mebaral Tablets, USP 2483

Pentobarbital Sodium (The effectiveness of progestin-only oral contraceptives is reduced by hepatic enzyme-inducing agents such as barbiturates). Products include:
Nembutal Sodium Solution, USP 2484

Phenobarbital (The effectiveness of progestin-only oral contraceptives is reduced by hepatic enzyme-inducing agents such as barbiturates).
No products indexed under this heading.

Phenytoin (The effectiveness of progestin-only oral contraceptives is reduced by hepatic enzyme-inducing agents such as phenytoin).
No products indexed under this heading.

Phenytoin Sodium (The effectiveness of progestin-only oral contraceptives is reduced by hepatic enzyme-inducing agents such as phenytoin). Products include:
- Phenytek Capsules **2153**

Rifampin (The effectiveness of progestin-only oral contraceptives is reduced by hepatic enzyme-inducing agents such as rifampin).
No products indexed under this heading.

Secobarbital Sodium (The effectiveness of progestin-only oral contraceptives is reduced by hepatic enzyme-inducing agents such as barbiturates).
No products indexed under this heading.

Thiamylal Sodium (The effectiveness of progestin-only oral contraceptives is reduced by hepatic enzyme-inducing agents such as barbiturates).
No products indexed under this heading.

ORTHO TRI-CYCLEN TABLETS
(Ethinyl Estradiol, Norgestimate) **2414**
See Ortho Tri-Cyclen Lo Tablets

ORTHO TRI-CYCLEN LO TABLETS
(Ethinyl Estradiol, Norgestimate) **2421**
May interact with barbiturates, phenytoin, prednisolone, protease inhibitors, tetracyclines, xanthines, and certain other agents. Compounds in these categories include:

Acetaminophen (Co-administration with certain oral contraceptives containing ethinyl estradiol increases plasma ethinyl estradiol levels possibly by inhibition of conjugation; decreased plasma levels of acetaminophen). Products include:
- Benadryl Allergy & Cold Tablets .... ■**692**
- Benadryl Allergy & Sinus Headache Caplets & Gelcaps .... ■**693**
- Benadryl Maximum Strength Severe Allergy & Sinus Headache Caplets .... ■**694**
- Contac Severe Cold and Flu Caplets Maximum Strength .... ■**615**
- Contac Severe Cold and Flu Caplets Non-Drowsy .... ■**615**
- Darvocet A 500 Tablets **3497**
- Goody's Body Pain Formula Powder .... ■**621**
- Goody's Extra Strength Headache Powder .... ■**621**
- Goody's Extra Strength Pain Relief Tablets .... ■**621**
- Goody's PM Powder .... ■**622**
- Hycomine Compound Tablets **1105**
- Lortab **3315**
- Lortab Elixir **3312**
- Percocet Tablets **1114**
- Robitussin Cough, Cold & Flu Liquid-filled Capsules .... ■**750**
- Robitussin Flu Liquid .... ■**752**
- Sedapap Tablets 50 mg/650 mg **2098**
- Singlet Caplets .... ■**636**
- Sudafed Severe Cold .... ■**710**
- Sudafed Sinus Headache .... ■**711**
- TheraFlu Cold & Cough Hot Liquid .... ■**680**
- TheraFlu Cold & Sore Throat Hot Liquid .... ■**680**
- TheraFlu Flu & Chest Congestion Non-Drowsy Hot Liquid .... ■**681**
- TheraFlu Flu & Sore Throat Hot Liquid .... ■**681**
- TheraFlu Severe Cold Non-Drowsy Hot Liquid .... ■**683**
- TheraFlu Severe Cold & Cough Hot Liquid .... ■**683**
- TheraFlu Severe Cold Caplets .... ■**679**
- TheraFlu Severe Cold Hot Liquid .... ■**682**
- TheraFlu Severe Cold Non-Drowsy Caplets .... ■**679**
- Triaminic Cough & Sore Throat Liquid .... ■**687**
- Triaminic Flu, Cough & Fever Liquid .... ■**685**
- Triaminic Cough & Sore Throat Softchews .... ■**689**
- Tylenol 8 Hour Extended Release Geltabs and Caplets **1843**
- Tylenol Sinus NightTime Caplets .... ■**663**
- Children's Tylenol Suspension Liquid and Meltaways **1850**
- Children's Tylenol Plus Cold & Allergy Suspension Liquid **1850**
- Children's Tylenol Plus Cold NightTime Suspension Liquid **1851**
- Children's Tylenol Plus Cold & Cough Suspension Liquid and Chewable Tablets **1851**
- Children's Tylenol Plus Cold Chewable Tablets **1851**
- Children's Tylenol Plus Cold Daytime Non-Drowsy Suspension Liquid **1851**
- Children's Tylenol Plus Flu Suspension Liquid **1853**
- Concentrated Tylenol Infants' Drops Plus Cold **1851**
- Concentrated Tylenol Infants' Drops Plus Cold and Cough **1851**
- Concentrated Tylenol Infants' Drops **1850**
- Junior Tylenol Meltaways **1850**
- Tylenol Cold & Flu Severe Daytime Liquid with Cool Bust **1846**
- Tylenol Cold & Flu Severe NightTime Liquid with Cool Burst **1846**
- Tylenol Cold Severe Congestion Non-Drowsy Caplets with Cool Burst **1846**
- Tylenol Cough & Sore Throat Daytime Liquid with Cool Burst **1849**
- Tylenol Cough & Sore Throat NightTime Liquid with Cool Burst **1849**
- Tylenol **1843**
- Extra Strength Tylenol Rapid Release Gels **1843**
- Tylenol **1843**
- Tylenol Allergy Complete Night Time Caplets **1844**
- Tylenol Allergy Complete Multi-Symptom Caplets and Gelcaps with Cool Burst **1844**
- Tylenol Severe Allergy Caplets **1844**
- Tylenol Flu NightTime Gelcaps **1846**
- Tylenol Flu Day Non-Drowsy Gelcaps **1846**
- Concentrated Tylenol Infants' Drops Plus Cold Nasal Congestant, Fever Reducer & Pain Reliever .... ■**668**
- Concentrated Tylenol Infants' Drops Plus Cold & Cough Nasal Decongestant, Fever Reducer & Pain Reliever .... ■**668**
- Multi-Symptom Tylenol Cold Night Time Caplets **1845**
- Multi-Symptom Tylenol Cold Day Non-Drowsy Caplets and Gelcaps **1845**
- Extra Strength Tylenol PM Caplets, Geltabs, Gelcaps and Liquid **1847**
- Tylenol Sinus Day Non-Drowsy **1848**
- Tylenol Sinus Night Time Caplets **1848**
- Tylenol Sinus Severe Congestion Caplets with Cool Burst **1848**
- Tylenol Sore Throat Daytime Liquid with Cool Burst **1849**
- Tylenol Sore Throat NightTime Liquid with Cool Burst **1849**
- Tylenol with Codeine **2461**
- Women's Tylenol Menstrual Relief Caplets **1849**
- Ultracet Tablets **2462**
- Vicks 44M Cough, Cold & Flu Relief **2676**
- Vicks DayQuil LiquiCaps/Liquid Multi-Symptom Cold/Flu Relief .... ■**723**
- Vicks DayQuil Multi-Symptom Cold/Flu Relief LiquiCaps **2675**
- Vicks DayQuil Multi-Symptom Cold/Flu Relief Liquid **2675**
- Vicks NyQuil LiquiCaps **2677**
- Vicks NyQuil LiquiCaps/Liquid Multi-Symptom Cold/Flu Relief .... ■**725**
- Vicks NyQuil Liquid **2677**
- Vicodin Tablets **530**
- Vicodin ES Tablets **531**
- Vicodin HP Tablets **532**
- Zydone Tablets **1118**

Aminophylline (Co-administration increases the plasma concentrations of theophylline).
No products indexed under this heading.

Ampicillin (Several cases of contraceptive failure and breakthrough bleeding have been reported in the literature with concomitant administration of antibiotics, such as tetracyclines. However, clinical pharmacology studies investigating drug interaction between combined oral contraceptives and tetracyclines have reported inconsistent results).
No products indexed under this heading.

Ampicillin Sodium (Several cases of contraceptive failure and breakthrough bleeding have been reported in the literature with concomitant administration of antibiotics, such as tetracyclines. However, clinical pharmacology studies investigating drug interaction between combined oral contraceptives and tetracyclines have reported inconsistent results).
No products indexed under this heading.

Amprenavir (Several of the protease inhibitors have induced significant changes in the AUC of the estrogen and progestins in some cases; co-administration may affect safety and efficacy of oral contraceptives). Products include:
- Agenerase Capsules **1299**
- Agenerase Oral Solution **1304**

Aprobarbital (Barbiturates increase the metabolism of contraceptive steroids resulting in reduced contraceptive effectiveness and this could precipitate unintended pregnancy or breakthrough bleeding).
No products indexed under this heading.

Atorvastatin Calcium (Co-administration with certain oral contraceptives containing ethinyl estradiol increases AUC values for ethinyl estradiol by approximately 20%). Products include:
- Caduet Tablets **2507**
- Lipitor Tablets **2495**

Butabarbital (Barbiturates increase the metabolism of contraceptive steroids resulting in reduced contraceptive effectiveness and this could precipitate unintended pregnancy or breakthrough bleeding).
No products indexed under this heading.

Butalbital (Barbiturates increase the metabolism of contraceptive steroids resulting in reduced contraceptive effectiveness and this could precipitate unintended pregnancy or breakthrough bleeding). Products include:
- Sedapap Tablets 50 mg/650 mg **2098**

Carbamazepine (Increases the metabolism of contraceptive steroids resulting in reduced contraceptive effectiveness and this could precipitate unintended pregnancy or breakthrough bleeding). Products include:
- Carbatrol Capsules **3174**
- Equetro Extended-Release Capsules **3178**
- Tegretol/Tegretol-XR **2278**

Clofibrate (Increased clearance of clofibric acid).
No products indexed under this heading.

Cyclosporine (Co-administration increases the plasma concentrations of cyclosporine). Products include:
- Gengraf Capsules **458**
- Neoral Soft Gelatin Capsules **2247**
- Neoral Oral Solution **2247**
- Restasis Ophthalmic Emulsion **570**
- Sandimmune **2259**

Demeclocycline Hydrochloride (Several cases of contraceptive failure and breakthrough bleeding have been reported in the literature with concomitant administration of antibiotics, such as tetracyclines. However, clinical pharmacology studies investigating drug interaction between combined oral contraceptives and tetracyclines have reported inconsistent results).
No products indexed under this heading.

Doxycycline Calcium (Several cases of contraceptive failure and breakthrough bleeding have been reported in the literature with concomitant administration of antibiotics, such as tetracyclines. However, clinical pharmacology studies investigating drug interaction between combined oral contraceptives and tetracyclines have reported inconsistent results).
No products indexed under this heading.

Doxycycline Hyclate (Several cases of contraceptive failure and breakthrough bleeding have been reported in the literature with concomitant administration of antibiotics, such as tetracyclines. However, clinical pharmacology studies investigating drug interaction between combined oral contraceptives and tetracyclines have reported inconsistent results).
No products indexed under this heading.

Doxycycline Monohydrate (Several cases of contraceptive failure and breakthrough bleeding have been reported in the literature with concomitant administration of antibiotics, such as tetracyclines. However, clinical pharmacology studies investigating drug interaction between combined oral contraceptives and tetracyclines have reported inconsistent results).
No products indexed under this heading.

Dyphylline (Co-administration increases the plasma concentrations of theophylline).
No products indexed under this heading.

Felbamate (Increases the metabolism of contraceptive steroids resulting in reduced contraceptive effectiveness and this could precipitate unintended pregnancy or breakthrough bleeding).
No products indexed under this heading.

Fosphenytoin Sodium (Increases the metabolism of contraceptive steroids resulting in reduced contraceptive effectiveness and this could precipitate unintended pregnancy or breakthrough bleeding).
No products indexed under this heading.

Griseofulvin (Increases the metabolism of contraceptive steroids resulting in reduced contraceptive effectiveness and this could precipitate unintended pregnancy or breakthrough bleeding). Products include:
Grifulvin V Tablets Microsize and Oral Suspension Microsize **2384**
Gris-PEG Tablets **2504**

Hypericum (May induce hepatic enzymes and p-glycoprotein transporter and may reduce the effectiveness of contraceptive steroids and this may result in breakthrough bleeding).
No products indexed under this heading.

Indinavir Sulfate (Several of the protease inhibitors have induced significant changes in the AUC of the estrogen and progestins in some cases; co-administration may affect safety and efficacy of oral contraceptives). Products include:
Crixivan Capsules **1918**

Itraconazole (Co-administration with CYP 3A4 inhibitors may increase plasma hormone levels).
No products indexed under this heading.

Ketoconazole (Co-administration with CYP 3A4 inhibitors may increase plasma hormone levels).
Products include:
Nizoral A-D Shampoo, 1% **1839**
Nizoral 2% Shampoo **1838**

Lopinavir (Several of the protease inhibitors have induced significant changes in the AUC of the estrogen and progestins in some cases; co-administration may affect safety and efficacy of oral contraceptives).
Products include:
Kaletra **474**

Mephobarbital (Barbiturates increase the metabolism of contraceptive steroids resulting in reduced contraceptive effectiveness and this could precipitate unintended pregnancy or breakthrough bleeding).
Products include:
Mebaral Tablets, USP **2483**

Methacycline Hydrochloride (Several cases of contraceptive failure and breakthrough bleeding have been reported in the literature with concomitant administration of antibiotics, such as tetracyclines. However, clinical pharmacology studies investigating drug interaction between combined oral contraceptives and tetracyclines have reported inconsistent results).
No products indexed under this heading.

Minocycline Hydrochloride (Several cases of contraceptive failure and breakthrough bleeding have been reported in the literature with concomitant administration of antibiotics, such as tetracyclines. However, clinical pharmacology studies investigating drug interaction between combined oral contraceptives and tetracyclines have reported inconsistent results). Products include:
Dynacin Tablets **1859**

Morphine Sulfate (Increased clearance of morphine). Products include:
Avinza Capsules **1714**
Kadian Capsules **572**
MS Contin Tablets **2703**

Nelfinavir Mesylate (Several of the protease inhibitors have induced significant changes in the AUC of the estrogen and progestins in some cases; co-administration may affect safety and efficacy of oral contraceptives). Products include:
Viracept **2556**

Oxcarbazepine (Increases the metabolism of contraceptive steroids resulting in reduced contraceptive effectiveness and this could precipitate unintended pregnancy or breakthrough bleeding). Products include:
Trileptal Oral Suspension **2281**
Trileptal Tablets **2281**

Oxytetracycline Hydrochloride (Several cases of contraceptive failure and breakthrough bleeding have been reported in the literature with concomitant administration of antibiotics, such as tetracyclines. However, clinical pharmacology studies investigating drug interaction between combined oral contraceptives and tetracyclines have reported inconsistent results).
No products indexed under this heading.

Pentobarbital Sodium (Barbiturates increase the metabolism of contraceptive steroids resulting in reduced contraceptive effectiveness and this could precipitate unintended pregnancy or breakthrough bleeding). Products include:
Nembutal Sodium Solution, USP **2484**

Phenobarbital (Barbiturates increase the metabolism of contraceptive steroids resulting in reduced contraceptive effectiveness and this could precipitate unintended pregnancy or breakthrough bleeding).
No products indexed under this heading.

Phenylbutazone (Increases the metabolism of contraceptive steroids resulting in reduced contraceptive effectiveness and this could precipitate unintended pregnancy or breakthrough bleeding).
No products indexed under this heading.

Phenytoin (Increases the metabolism of contraceptive steroids resulting in reduced contraceptive effectiveness and this could precipitate unintended pregnancy or breakthrough bleeding).
No products indexed under this heading.

Phenytoin Sodium (Increases the metabolism of contraceptive steroids resulting in reduced contraceptive effectiveness and this could precipitate unintended pregnancy or breakthrough bleeding). Products include:
Phenytek Capsules **2153**

Prednisolone (Co-administration increases the plasma concentrations of prednisolone).
No products indexed under this heading.

Prednisolone Acetate (Co-administration increases the plasma concentrations of prednisolone).
Products include:
Blephamide Ophthalmic Ointment **563**
Blephamide Ophthalmic Suspension **564**
Poly-Pred Liquifilm Ophthalmic Suspension .... ⊙**231**
Pred Forte Ophthalmic Suspension .... ⊙**233**
Pred Mild Sterile Ophthalmic Suspension .... ⊙**236**
Pred-G Ophthalmic Suspension .... ⊙**234**
Pred-G Sterile Ophthalmic Ointment .... ⊙**235**

Prednisolone Sodium Phosphate (Co-administration increases the plasma concentrations of prednisolone). Products include:
Pediapred Oral Solution **3319**

Prednisolone Tebutate (Co-administration increases the plasma concentrations of prednisolone).
No products indexed under this heading.

Rifampin (Increases the metabolism of contraceptive steroids resulting in reduced contraceptive effectiveness and this could precipitate unintended pregnancy or breakthrough bleeding).
No products indexed under this heading.

Ritonavir (Several of the protease inhibitors have induced significant changes in the AUC of the estrogen and progestins in some cases; co-administration may affect safety and efficacy of oral contraceptives).
Products include:
Kaletra **474**
Norvir **499**

Salicylic Acid (Increased clearance of salicylic acid).
No products indexed under this heading.

Saquinavir (Several of the protease inhibitors have induced significant changes in the AUC of the estrogen and progestins in some cases; co-administration may affect safety and efficacy of oral contraceptives).
No products indexed under this heading.

Saquinavir Mesylate (Several of the protease inhibitors have induced significant changes in the AUC of the estrogen and progestins in some cases; co-administration may affect safety and efficacy of oral contraceptives). Products include:
Invirase **2776**

Secobarbital Sodium (Barbiturates increase the metabolism of contraceptive steroids resulting in reduced contraceptive effectiveness and this could precipitate unintended pregnancy or breakthrough bleeding).
No products indexed under this heading.

Temazepam (Increased clearance of temazepam).
No products indexed under this heading.

Tetracycline Hydrochloride (Several cases of contraceptive failure and breakthrough bleeding have been reported in the literature with concomitant administration of antibiotics, such as tetracyclines. However, clinical pharmacology studies investigating drug interaction between combined oral contraceptives and tetracyclines have reported inconsistent results).
No products indexed under this heading.

Theophylline (Co-administration increases the plasma concentrations of theophylline).
No products indexed under this heading.

Theophylline Anhydrous (Co-administration increases the plasma concentrations of theophylline).
Products include:
Uniphyl Tablets **2708**

Theophylline Calcium Salicylate (Co-administration increases the plasma concentrations of theophylline).
No products indexed under this heading.

Theophylline Dihydroxypropyl (Glyceryl) (Co-administration increases the plasma concentrations of theophylline).
No products indexed under this heading.

Theophylline Ethylenediamine (Co-administration increases the plasma concentrations of theophylline).
No products indexed under this heading.

Theophylline Sodium Glycinate (Co-administration increases the plasma concentrations of theophylline).
No products indexed under this heading.

Thiamylal Sodium (Barbiturates increase the metabolism of contraceptive steroids resulting in reduced contraceptive effectiveness and this could precipitate unintended pregnancy or breakthrough bleeding).
No products indexed under this heading.

Topiramate (Increases the metabolism of contraceptive steroids resulting in reduced contraceptive effectiveness and this could precipitate unintended pregnancy or breakthrough bleeding). Products include:
Topamax Sprinkle Capsules **2438**
Topamax Tablets **2438**

Vitamin C (Co-administration with certain oral contraceptives containing ethinyl estradiol increases plasma ethinyl estradiol levels possibly by inhibition of conjugation).
Products include:
Chromagen Forte Soft Gelatin Capsules **3296**
Halls Defense Sugarfree Vitamin C Drops .... ▣**611**
Niferex-150 Forte Capsules **3299**
Peridin-C Tablets .... ▣**761**
Repliva 21/7 Tablets **3301**

ORTHOCLONE OKT3 STERILE SOLUTION

(Muromonab-CD3) **2370**

May interact with corticosteroids and certain other agents. Compounds in these categories include:

Azathioprine (Infection or malignancies have been reported with azathioprine alone and in conjunction with muromonab-CD3). Products include:
Azasan Tablets **2844**

Betamethasone Acetate (Psychosis and infection have been reported in patients treated with corticosteroids alone and in conjunction with muromonab-CD3).
No products indexed under this heading.

Betamethasone Sodium Phosphate (Psychosis and infection have been reported in patients treated with corticosteroids alone and in conjunction with muromonab-CD3).
No products indexed under this heading.

Cortisone Acetate (Psychosis and infection have been reported in patients treated with corticosteroids alone and in conjunction with muromonab-CD3).
No products indexed under this heading.

Cyclosporine (Seizures, encephalopathy, infections, malignancies, and thrombotic events have been reported in patients receiving cyclosporine alone and in conjunction with muromonab-CD3). Products include:
Gengraf Capsules 458
Neoral Soft Gelatin Capsules 2247
Neoral Oral Solution 2247
Restasis Ophthalmic Emulsion 570
Sandimmune 2259

Dexamethasone (Psychosis and infection have been reported in patients treated with corticosteroids alone and in conjunction with muromonab-CD3). Products include:
Ciprodex Otic Suspension 555
Decadron Tablets 1929
TobraDex Ophthalmic Ointment 558
TobraDex Ophthalmic Suspension ... 558

Dexamethasone Acetate (Psychosis and infection have been reported in patients treated with corticosteroids alone and in conjunction with muromonab-CD3).
No products indexed under this heading.

Dexamethasone Sodium Phosphate (Psychosis and infection have been reported in patients treated with corticosteroids alone and in conjunction with muromonab-CD3). Products include:
Decadron Phosphate Injection 1931

Fludrocortisone Acetate (Psychosis and infection have been reported in patients treated with corticosteroids alone and in conjunction with muromonab-CD3).
No products indexed under this heading.

Hydrocortisone (Psychosis and infection have been reported in patients treated with corticosteroids alone and in conjunction with muromonab-CD3). Products include:
Cortizone•5 Ointment .... ⊡699
Cortizone•10 Creme .... ⊡699
Cortizone•10 Ointment .... ⊡699
Cortizone•10 Plus Creme .... ⊡700
Cortizone•10 Maximum Strength Quick Shot Spray .... ⊡700
Hydrocortone Tablets 1963
Preparation H Hydrocortisone Cream .... ⊡748

Hydrocortisone Acetate (Psychosis and infection have been reported in patients treated with corticosteroids alone and in conjunction with muromonab-CD3). Products include:
Analpram-HC 1136
Pramosone 1139
ProctoFoam-HC 3113
Tucks Anti-Itch Ointment .... ⊡712
U-cort 1% Cream 3289

Hydrocortisone Sodium Phosphate (Psychosis and infection have been reported in patients treated with corticosteroids alone and in conjunction with muromonab-CD3).
No products indexed under this heading.

Hydrocortisone Sodium Succinate (Psychosis and infection have been reported in patients treated with corticosteroids alone and in conjunction with muromonab-CD3).
No products indexed under this heading.

Indomethacin (Encephalopathy and other CNS effects have been reported in patients treated with indomethacin alone and in conjunction with muromonab-CD3). Products include:
Indocin 1968

Indomethacin Sodium Trihydrate (Encephalopathy and other CNS effects have been reported in patients treated with indomethacin alone and in conjunction with muromonab-CD3). Products include:
Indocin I.V. 1973

Methylprednisolone Acetate (Psychosis and infection have been reported in patients treated with corticosteroids alone and in conjunction with muromonab-CD3). Products include:
Depo-Medrol Injectable Suspension 2615
Depo-Medrol Single-Dose Vial 2617

Methylprednisolone Sodium Succinate (Psychosis and infection have been reported in patients treated with corticosteroids alone and in conjunction with muromonab-CD3).
No products indexed under this heading.

Prednisolone Acetate (Psychosis and infection have been reported in patients treated with corticosteroids alone and in conjunction with muromonab-CD3). Products include:
Blephamide Ophthalmic Ointment 563
Blephamide Ophthalmic Suspension.................................. 564
Poly-Pred Liquifilm Ophthalmic Suspension .... ⊙231
Pred Forte Ophthalmic Suspension .... ⊙233
Pred Mild Sterile Ophthalmic Suspension .... ⊙236
Pred-G Ophthalmic Suspension ...... ⊙234
Pred-G Sterile Ophthalmic Ointment .... ⊙235

Prednisolone Sodium Phosphate (Psychosis and infection have been reported in patients treated with corticosteroids alone and in conjunction with muromonab-CD3). Products include:
Pediapred Oral Solution 3319

Prednisolone Tebutate (Psychosis and infection have been reported in patients treated with corticosteroids alone and in conjunction with muromonab-CD3).
No products indexed under this heading.

Prednisone (Psychosis and infection have been reported in patients treated with corticosteroids alone and in conjunction with muromonab-CD3).
No products indexed under this heading.

Triamcinolone (Psychosis and infection have been reported in patients treated with corticosteroids alone and in conjunction with muromonab-CD3).
No products indexed under this heading.

Triamcinolone Acetonide (Psychosis and infection have been reported in patients treated with corticosteroids alone and in conjunction with muromonab-CD3). Products include:
Azmacort Inhalation Aerosol 1701
Nasacort HFA Inhalation Aerosol 2939
Nasacort AQ Nasal Spray 2937

Triamcinolone Diacetate (Psychosis and infection have been reported in patients treated with corticosteroids alone and in conjunction with muromonab-CD3).
No products indexed under this heading.

Triamcinolone Hexacetonide (Psychosis and infection have been reported in patients treated with corticosteroids alone and in conjunction with muromonab-CD3).
No products indexed under this heading.

ORTHOVISC INJECTION

(Hyaluronan) 3518
May interact with quarternary ammonium compounds. Compounds in these categories include:

Benzalkonium Chloride (Avoid concomitant use of disinfectants containing quarternary ammonium salts for skin preparation as hyaluronic acid can precipitate in their presence).
No products indexed under this heading.

Benzethonium Chloride (Avoid concomitant use of disinfectants containing quarternary ammonium salts for skin preparation as hyaluronic acid can precipitate in their presence).
No products indexed under this heading.

Cetylpyridinium Chloride (Avoid concomitant use of disinfectants containing quarternary ammonium salts for skin preparation as hyaluronic acid can precipitate in their presence).
No products indexed under this heading.

OS-CAL CHEWABLE TABLETS

(Calcium Carbonate) .... ⊡765
None cited in PDR database.

OS-CAL 250 + D TABLETS

(Calcium, Vitamin D) .... ⊡765
None cited in PDR database.

OS-CAL 500 TABLETS

(Calcium) .... ⊡765
None cited in PDR database.

OS-CAL 500 + D TABLETS

(Calcium, Vitamin D) .... ⊡766
None cited in PDR database.

OVIDE .5% LOTION

(Malathion) 3287
None cited in PDR database.

OXANDRIN TABLETS

(Oxandrolone) 2977
May interact with corticosteroids, oral anticoagulants, oral hypoglycemic agents, and certain other agents. Compounds in these categories include:

Acarbose (Oxandrolone may inhibit the metabolism of oral hypoglycemic agents). Products include:
Precose Tablets 776

ACTH (In patients with edema, co-administration with ACTH may increase the edema).
No products indexed under this heading.

Anisindione (Concurrent dosing of oxandrolone and warfarin may result in unexpectedly large increases in the INR or prothrombin time (PT). When oxandrolone is prescribed to patients being treated with warfarin, doses of warfarin may need to be decreased significantlyto maintain the desirable INR level and diminish the risk of potentially serious bleeding. Furthermore, in patients receiving both drugs, careful monitoring of the PT or INR and adjustment of the warfarin dosage if indicated are recommended when the oxandrolone dose is changed or discontinued. Patients should be closely monitored for signs and symptoms of occult bleeding). Products include:
Miradon Tablets 3056

Betamethasone Acetate (In patients with edema, co-administration with adrenal cortical steroids may increase the edema).
No products indexed under this heading.

Betamethasone Sodium Phosphate (In patients with edema, co-administration with adrenal cortical steroids may increase the edema).
No products indexed under this heading.

Chlorpropamide (Oxandrolone may inhibit the metabolism of oral hypoglycemic agents).
No products indexed under this heading.

Cortisone Acetate (In patients with edema, co-administration with adrenal cortical steroids may increase the edema).
No products indexed under this heading.

Dexamethasone (In patients with edema, co-administration with adrenal cortical steroids may increase the edema). Products include:
Ciprodex Otic Suspension 555
Decadron Tablets 1929
TobraDex Ophthalmic Ointment 558
TobraDex Ophthalmic Suspension ... 558

Dexamethasone Acetate (In patients with edema, co-administration with adrenal cortical steroids may increase the edema).
No products indexed under this heading.

Dexamethasone Sodium Phosphate (In patients with edema, co-administration with adrenal cortical steroids may increase the edema). Products include:
Decadron Phosphate Injection 1931

Dicumarol (Concurrent dosing of oxandrolone and warfarin may result in unexpectedly large increases in the INR or prothrombin time (PT). When oxandrolone is prescribed to patients being treated with warfarin, doses of warfarin may need to be decreased significantlyto maintain the desirable INR level and diminish the risk of potentially serious bleeding. Furthermore, in patients receiving both drugs, careful monitoring of the PT or INR and adjustment of the warfarin dosage if indicated are recommended when the oxandrolone dose is changed or discontinued. Patients should be closely monitored for signs and symptoms of occult bleeding).
No products indexed under this heading.

Fludrocortisone Acetate (In patients with edema, co-administration with adrenal cortical steroids may increase the edema).
No products indexed under this heading.

Glimepiride (Oxandrolone may inhibit the metabolism of oral hypoglycemic agents). Products include:
Amaryl Tablets 2864

Glipizide (Oxandrolone may inhibit the metabolism of oral hypoglycemic agents).
No products indexed under this heading.

Glyburide (Oxandrolone may inhibit the metabolism of oral hypoglycemic agents).
No products indexed under this heading.

Hydrocortisone (In patients with edema, co-administration with adrenal cortical steroids may increase the edema). Products include:
Cortizone•5 Ointment .... ▣699
Cortizone•10 Creme .... ▣699
Cortizone•10 Ointment .... ▣699
Cortizone•10 Plus Creme .... ▣700
Cortizone•10 Maximum Strength Quick Shot Spray .... ▣700
Hydrocortone Tablets 1963
Preparation H Hydrocortisone Cream .... ▣748

Hydrocortisone Acetate (In patients with edema, co-administration with adrenal cortical steroids may increase the edema). Products include:
Analpram-HC 1136
Pramosone 1139
ProctoFoam-HC 3113
Tucks Anti-Itch Ointment .... ▣712
U-cort 1% Cream 3289

Hydrocortisone Sodium Phosphate (In patients with edema, co-administration with adrenal cortical steroids may increase the edema).
No products indexed under this heading.

Hydrocortisone Sodium Succinate (In patients with edema, co-administration with adrenal cortical steroids may increase the edema).
No products indexed under this heading.

Metformin Hydrochloride (Oxandrolone may inhibit the metabolism of oral hypoglycemic agents). Products include:
ActoPlus Met Tablets 3219
Avandamet Tablets 1343
Fortamet Extended-Release Tablets 1156

Methylprednisolone Acetate (In patients with edema, co-administration with adrenal cortical steroids may increase the edema). Products include:
Depo-Medrol Injectable Suspension 2615
Depo-Medrol Single-Dose Vial 2617

Methylprednisolone Sodium Succinate (In patients with edema, co-administration with adrenal cortical steroids may increase the edema).
No products indexed under this heading.

Miglitol (Oxandrolone may inhibit the metabolism of oral hypoglycemic agents).
No products indexed under this heading.

Pioglitazone Hydrochloride (Oxandrolone may inhibit the metabolism of oral hypoglycemic agents). Products include:
ActoPlus Met Tablets 3219
Actos Tablets 3224

Prednisolone Acetate (In patients with edema, co-administration with adrenal cortical steroids may increase the edema). Products include:
Blephamide Ophthalmic Ointment 563
Blephamide Ophthalmic Suspension............................... 564
Poly-Pred Liquifilm Ophthalmic Suspension .... ⊙231
Pred Forte Ophthalmic Suspension .... ⊙233
Pred Mild Sterile Ophthalmic Suspension .... ⊙236
Pred-G Ophthalmic Suspension ...... ⊙234
Pred-G Sterile Ophthalmic Ointment.................................. ⊙235

Prednisolone Sodium Phosphate (In patients with edema, co-administration with adrenal cortical steroids may increase the edema). Products include:
Pediapred Oral Solution 3319

Prednisolone Tebutate (In patients with edema, co-administration with adrenal cortical steroids may increase the edema).
No products indexed under this heading.

Prednisone (In patients with edema, co-administration with adrenal cortical steroids may increase the edema).
No products indexed under this heading.

Repaglinide (Oxandrolone may inhibit the metabolism of oral hypoglycemic agents). Products include:
Prandin Tablets (0.5, 1, and 2 mg).. 2337

Rosiglitazone Maleate (Oxandrolone may inhibit the metabolism of oral hypoglycemic agents). Products include:
Avandamet Tablets 1343
Avandia Tablets 1348

Tolazamide (Oxandrolone may inhibit the metabolism of oral hypoglycemic agents).
No products indexed under this heading.

Tolbutamide (Oxandrolone may inhibit the metabolism of oral hypoglycemic agents).
No products indexed under this heading.

Triamcinolone (In patients with edema, co-administration with adrenal cortical steroids may increase the edema).
No products indexed under this heading.

Triamcinolone Acetonide (In patients with edema, co-administration with adrenal cortical steroids may increase the edema). Products include:
Azmacort Inhalation Aerosol 1701
Nasacort HFA Inhalation Aerosol 2939
Nasacort AQ Nasal Spray 2937

Triamcinolone Diacetate (In patients with edema, co-administration with adrenal cortical steroids may increase the edema).
No products indexed under this heading.

Triamcinolone Hexacetonide (In patients with edema, co-administration with adrenal cortical steroids may increase the edema).
No products indexed under this heading.

Troglitazone (Oxandrolone may inhibit the metabolism of oral hypoglycemic agents).
No products indexed under this heading.

Warfarin Sodium (Concurrent dosing of oxandrolone and warfarin may result in unexpectedly large increases in the INR or prothrombin time (PT). When oxandrolone is prescribed to patients being treated with warfarin, doses of warfarin may need to be decreased significantlyto maintain the desirable INR level and diminish the risk of potentially serious bleeding. Furthermore, in patients receiving both drugs, careful monitoring of the PT or INR and adjustment of the warfarin dosage if indicated are recommended when the oxandrolone dose is changed or discontinued. Patients should be closely monitored for signs and symptoms of occult bleeding). Products include:
Coumadin for Injection 932
Coumadin Tablets 932

OXISTAT CREAM
(Oxiconazole Nitrate) 1498
None cited in PDR database.

OXISTAT LOTION
(Oxiconazole Nitrate) 1498
None cited in PDR database.

OXSORALEN LOTION 1%
(Methoxsalen) 3354
May interact with phenothiazines, sulfonamides, tetracyclines, thiazides, and certain other agents. Compounds in these categories include:

Anthralin (Possible photosensitivity effects). Products include:
Psoriatec Cream 3191

Bendroflumethiazide (Possible photosensitivity effects).
No products indexed under this heading.

Chlorothiazide (Possible photosensitivity effects). Products include:
Aldoclor Tablets 1881
Diuril Oral 1936

Chlorothiazide Sodium (Possible photosensitivity effects). Products include:
Diuril Sodium Intravenous 1934

Chlorpromazine (Possible photosensitivity effects).
No products indexed under this heading.

Chlorpromazine Hydrochloride (Possible photosensitivity effects).
No products indexed under this heading.

Chlorpropamide (Possible photosensitivity effects).
No products indexed under this heading.

Coal Tar (Possible photosensitivity effects). Products include:
Tegrin Dandruff Shampoo - Extra Conditioning.................................. ▣637
Tegrin Dandruff Shampoo - Fresh Herbal.. ▣638
Tegrin Skin Cream .... ▣638

Demeclocycline Hydrochloride (Possible photosensitivity effects).
No products indexed under this heading.

Doxycycline Calcium (Possible photosensitivity effects).
No products indexed under this heading.

Doxycycline Hyclate (Possible photosensitivity effects).
No products indexed under this heading.

Doxycycline Monohydrate (Possible photosensitivity effects).
No products indexed under this heading.

Fluphenazine Decanoate (Possible photosensitivity effects).
No products indexed under this heading.

Fluphenazine Enanthate (Possible photosensitivity effects).
No products indexed under this heading.

Fluphenazine Hydrochloride (Possible photosensitivity effects).
No products indexed under this heading.

Glipizide (Possible photosensitivity effects).
No products indexed under this heading.

Glyburide (Possible photosensitivity effects).
No products indexed under this heading.

Griseofulvin (Possible photosensitivity effects). Products include:
Grifulvin V Tablets Microsize and Oral Suspension Microsize........... 2384
Gris-PEG Tablets 2504

Hydrochlorothiazide (Possible photosensitivity effects). Products include:
Aldoril Tablets 1884
Atacand HCT 637
Avalide Tablets 2889
Avalide Tablets 922
Benicar HCT Tablets 2852
Diovan HCT Tablets 2195
Dyazide Capsules 1389
Hyzaar 1964
Lotensin HCT Tablets 2235
Maxzide 2150
Micardis HCT Tablets 886
Moduretic Tablets 2003
Prinzide Tablets 2033
Teveten HCT Tablets 1710
Timolide Tablets 2056
Uniretic Tablets 3114
Vaseretic Tablets 2073
Zestoretic Tablets 701

Hydroflumethiazide (Possible photosensitivity effects).
No products indexed under this heading.

Mesoridazine Besylate (Possible photosensitivity effects).
No products indexed under this heading.

Methacycline Hydrochloride (Possible photosensitivity effects).
No products indexed under this heading.

Methotrimeprazine (Possible photosensitivity effects).
No products indexed under this heading.

Methyclothiazide (Possible photosensitivity effects).
No products indexed under this heading.

Methylene Blue (Possible photosensitivity effects).
No products indexed under this heading.

Minocycline Hydrochloride (Possible photosensitivity effects). Products include:
Dynacin Tablets 1859

Nalidixic Acid (Possible photosensitivity effects).
No products indexed under this heading.

Oxytetracycline (Possible photosensitivity effects).
No products indexed under this heading.

Oxytetracycline Hydrochloride (Possible photosensitivity effects).
No products indexed under this heading.

Perphenazine (Possible photosensitivity effects).
No products indexed under this heading.

Polythiazide (Possible photosensitivity effects).
No products indexed under this heading.

Prochlorperazine (Possible photosensitivity effects).
No products indexed under this heading.

Promethazine Hydrochloride (Possible photosensitivity effects). Products include:
Phenergan 3438

Sulfacytine (Possible photosensitivity effects).
No products indexed under this heading.

Sulfamethizole (Possible photosensitivity effects).
No products indexed under this heading.

Sulfamethoxazole (Possible photosensitivity effects).
No products indexed under this heading.

Sulfasalazine (Possible photosensitivity effects).
No products indexed under this heading.

Sulfinpyrazone (Possible photosensitivity effects).
No products indexed under this heading.

Sulfisoxazole (Possible photosensitivity effects).
No products indexed under this heading.

Sulfisoxazole Acetyl (Possible photosensitivity effects).
No products indexed under this heading.

Sulfisoxazole Diolamine (Possible photosensitivity effects).
No products indexed under this heading.

Tetracycline Hydrochloride (Possible photosensitivity effects).
No products indexed under this heading.

Thioridazine Hydrochloride (Possible photosensitivity effects). Products include:
Thioridazine Hydrochloride Tablets 2122

Tolazamide (Possible photosensitivity effects).
No products indexed under this heading.

Tolbutamide (Possible photosensitivity effects).
No products indexed under this heading.

Trifluoperazine Hydrochloride (Possible photosensitivity effects).
No products indexed under this heading.

OXSORALEN-ULTRA CAPSULES

(Methoxsalen) 3354

May interact with phenothiazines, sulfonamides, tetracyclines, thiazides, and certain other agents. Compounds in these categories include:

Anthralin (Possible photosensitivity effects). Products include:
Psoriatec Cream 3191

Bendroflumethiazide (Possible photosensitivity effects).
No products indexed under this heading.

Chlorothiazide (Possible photosensitivity effects). Products include:
Aldoclor Tablets 1881
Diuril Oral 1936

Chlorothiazide Sodium (Possible photosensitivity effects). Products include:
Diuril Sodium Intravenous 1934

Chlorpromazine (Possible photosensitivity effects).
No products indexed under this heading.

Chlorpromazine Hydrochloride (Possible photosensitivity effects).
No products indexed under this heading.

Chlorpropamide (Possible photosensitivity effects).
No products indexed under this heading.

Coal Tar (Possible photosensitivity effects). Products include:
Tegrin Dandruff Shampoo - Extra Conditioning 637
Tegrin Dandruff Shampoo - Fresh Herbal 638
Tegrin Skin Cream 638

Demeclocycline Hydrochloride (Possible photosensitivity effects).
No products indexed under this heading.

Doxycycline Calcium (Possible photosensitivity effects).
No products indexed under this heading.

Doxycycline Hyclate (Possible photosensitivity effects).
No products indexed under this heading.

Doxycycline Monohydrate (Possible photosensitivity effects).
No products indexed under this heading.

Fluphenazine Decanoate (Possible photosensitivity effects).
No products indexed under this heading.

Fluphenazine Enanthate (Possible photosensitivity effects).
No products indexed under this heading.

Fluphenazine Hydrochloride (Possible photosensitivity effects).
No products indexed under this heading.

Glipizide (Possible photosensitivity effects).
No products indexed under this heading.

Glyburide (Possible photosensitivity effects).
No products indexed under this heading.

Griseofulvin (Possible photosensitivity effects). Products include:
Grifulvin V Tablets Microsize and Oral Suspension Microsize............ 2384
Gris-PEG Tablets 2504

Hydrochlorothiazide (Possible photosensitivity effects). Products include:
Aldoril Tablets 1884
Atacand HCT 637
Avalide Tablets 2889
Avalide Tablets 922
Benicar HCT Tablets 2852
Diovan HCT Tablets 2195
Dyazide Capsules 1389
Hyzaar 1964
Lotensin HCT Tablets 2235
Maxzide 2150
Micardis HCT Tablets 886
Moduretic Tablets 2003
Prinzide Tablets 2033
Teveten HCT Tablets 1710
Timolide Tablets 2056
Uniretic Tablets 3114
Vaseretic Tablets 2073
Zestoretic Tablets 701

Hydroflumethiazide (Possible photosensitivity effects).
No products indexed under this heading.

Mesoridazine Besylate (Possible photosensitivity effects).
No products indexed under this heading.

Methacycline Hydrochloride (Possible photosensitivity effects).
No products indexed under this heading.

Methotrimeprazine (Possible photosensitivity effects).
No products indexed under this heading.

Methyclothiazide (Possible photosensitivity effects).
No products indexed under this heading.

Methylene Blue (Possible photosensitivity effects).
No products indexed under this heading.

Minocycline Hydrochloride (Possible photosensitivity effects). Products include:
Dynacin Tablets 1859

Nalidixic Acid (Possible photosensitivity effects).
No products indexed under this heading.

Oxytetracycline (Possible photosensitivity effects).
No products indexed under this heading.

Oxytetracycline Hydrochloride (Possible photosensitivity effects).
No products indexed under this heading.

Perphenazine (Possible photosensitivity effects).
No products indexed under this heading.

Polythiazide (Possible photosensitivity effects).
No products indexed under this heading.

Prochlorperazine (Possible photosensitivity effects).
No products indexed under this heading.

Promethazine Hydrochloride (Possible photosensitivity effects). Products include:
Phenergan 3438

Sulfacytine (Possible photosensitivity effects).
No products indexed under this heading.

Sulfamethizole (Possible photosensitivity effects).
No products indexed under this heading.

Sulfamethoxazole (Possible photosensitivity effects).
No products indexed under this heading.

Sulfasalazine (Possible photosensitivity effects).
No products indexed under this heading.

Sulfinpyrazone (Possible photosensitivity effects).
No products indexed under this heading.

Sulfisoxazole (Possible photosensitivity effects).
No products indexed under this heading.

Sulfisoxazole Acetyl (Possible photosensitivity effects).
No products indexed under this heading.

Sulfisoxazole Diolamine (Possible photosensitivity effects).
No products indexed under this heading.

Tetracycline Hydrochloride (Possible photosensitivity effects).
No products indexed under this heading.

Thioridazine Hydrochloride (Possible photosensitivity effects). Products include:
Thioridazine Hydrochloride Tablets 2122

Tolazamide (Possible photosensitivity effects).
No products indexed under this heading.

Tolbutamide (Possible photosensitivity effects).
No products indexed under this heading.

Trifluoperazine Hydrochloride (Possible photosensitivity effects).
No products indexed under this heading.

OXYCONTIN TABLETS

(Oxycodone Hydrochloride) 2699

May interact with central nervous system depressants, general anesthetics, hypnotics and sedatives, mixed agonist/antagonist opioid analgesics, phenothiazines, tranquilizers, and certain other agents. Compounds in these categories include:

Alfentanil Hydrochloride (Concurrent use with the usual dose of OxyContin may result in respiratory depression, profound sedation or coma; reduced dosage (1/3 to 1/2 of the usual dosage) may be necessary).
No products indexed under this heading.

Alprazolam (Concurrent use with the usual dose of OxyContin may result in respiratory depression, profound sedation or coma; reduced dosage (1/3 to 1/2 of the usual dosage) may be necessary). Products include:
Niravam Orally Disintegrating Tablets 3106
Xanax XR Tablets 2655

Aprobarbital (Concurrent use with the usual dose of OxyContin may result in respiratory depression, profound sedation or coma; reduced dosage (1/3 to 1/2 of the usual dosage) may be necessary).
No products indexed under this heading.

Buprenorphine Hydrochloride (Mixed agonist/antagonist analgesics may reduce the analgesic effect of oxycodone and/or may precipitate withdrawal symptoms). Products include:
Buprenex Injectable 2718
Suboxone Tablets 2719
Subutex Tablets 2719

Buspirone Hydrochloride (Concurrent use with the usual dose of OxyContin may result in respiratory depression, profound sedation or coma; reduced dosage (1/3 to 1/2 of the usual dosage) may be necessary).
No products indexed under this heading.

Butabarbital (Concurrent use with the usual dose of OxyContin may result in respiratory depression, profound sedation or coma; reduced dosage (1/3 to 1/2 of the usual dosage) may be necessary).
No products indexed under this heading.

Butalbital (Concurrent use with the usual dose of OxyContin may result in respiratory depression, profound sedation or coma; reduced dosage (1/3 to 1/2 of the usual dosage) may be necessary). Products include:
Sedapap Tablets 50 mg/650 mg 2098

Butorphanol Tartrate (Mixed agonist/antagonist analgesics may reduce the analgesic effect of oxycodone and/or may precipitate withdrawal symptoms).
No products indexed under this heading.

Chlordiazepoxide (Concurrent use with the usual dose of OxyContin may result in respiratory depression, profound sedation or coma; reduced dosage (1/3 to 1/2 of the usual dosage) may be necessary).
No products indexed under this heading.

Chlordiazepoxide Hydrochloride (Concurrent use with the usual dose of OxyContin may result in respiratory depression, profound sedation or coma; reduced dosage (1/3 to 1/2 of the usual dosage) may be necessary). Products include:
Librium Capsules 3349

Chlorpromazine (Concurrent use with the usual dose of OxyContin may result in respiratory depression, profound sedation or coma; reduced dosage (1/3 to 1/2 of the usual dosage) may be necessary).
No products indexed under this heading.

Chlorpromazine Hydrochloride (Concurrent use with the usual dose of OxyContin may result in respiratory depression, profound sedation or coma; reduced dosage (1/3 to 1/2 of the usual dosage) may be necessary).
No products indexed under this heading.

Chlorprothixene (Concurrent use with the usual dose of OxyContin may result in respiratory depression, profound sedation or coma; reduced dosage (1/3 to 1/2 of the usual dosage) may be necessary).
No products indexed under this heading.

Chlorprothixene Hydrochloride (Concurrent use with the usual dose of OxyContin may result in respiratory depression, profound sedation or coma; reduced dosage (1/3 to 1/2 of the usual dosage) may be necessary).
No products indexed under this heading.

Chlorprothixene Lactate (Concurrent use with the usual dose of OxyContin may result in respiratory depression, profound sedation or coma; reduced dosage (1/3 to 1/2 of the usual dosage) may be necessary).
No products indexed under this heading.

Clorazepate Dipotassium (Concurrent use with the usual dose of OxyContin may result in respiratory depression, profound sedation or coma; reduced dosage (1/3 to 1/2 of the usual dosage) may be necessary). Products include:
Tranxene 2488

Clozapine (Concurrent use with the usual dose of OxyContin may result in respiratory depression, profound sedation or coma; reduced dosage (1/3 to 1/2 of the usual dosage) may be necessary). Products include:
Clozapine Tablets 2141
Clozaril Tablets 2174
FazaClo Orally Disintegrating Tablets 547

Codeine Phosphate (Concurrent use with the usual dose of OxyContin may result in respiratory depression, profound sedation or coma; reduced dosage (1/3 to 1/2 of the usual dosage) may be necessary). Products include:
Tylenol with Codeine 2461

Desflurane (Concurrent use with the usual dose of OxyContin may result in respiratory depression, profound sedation or coma; reduced dosage (1/3 to 1/2 of the usual dosage) may be necessary). Products include:
Suprane Liquid for Inhalation 770

Dezocine (Concurrent use with the usual dose of OxyContin may result in respiratory depression, profound sedation or coma; reduced dosage (1/3 to 1/2 of the usual dosage) may be necessary).
No products indexed under this heading.

Diazepam (Concurrent use with the usual dose of OxyContin may result in respiratory depression, profound sedation or coma; reduced dosage (1/3 to 1/2 of the usual dosage) may be necessary). Products include:
Diastat Rectal Delivery System 3344
Valium Tablets 2822

Droperidol (Concurrent use with the usual dose of OxyContin may result in respiratory depression, profound sedation or coma; reduced dosage (1/3 to 1/2 of the usual dosage) may be necessary).
No products indexed under this heading.

Enflurane (Concurrent use with the usual dose of OxyContin may result in respiratory depression, profound sedation or coma; reduced dosage (1/3 to 1/2 of the usual dosage) may be necessary).
No products indexed under this heading.

Estazolam (Concurrent use with the usual dose of OxyContin may result in respiratory depression, profound sedation or coma; reduced dosage (1/3 to 1/2 of the usual dosage) may be necessary). Products include:
ProSom Tablets 512

Ethanol (Concurrent use with the usual dose of OxyContin may result in respiratory depression, profound sedation or coma; reduced dosage (1/3 to 1/2 of the usual dosage) may be necessary).
No products indexed under this heading.

Ethchlorvynol (Concurrent use with the usual dose of OxyContin may result in respiratory depression, profound sedation or coma; reduced dosage (1/3 to 1/2 of the usual dosage) may be necessary).
No products indexed under this heading.

Ethinamate (Concurrent use with the usual dose of OxyContin may result in respiratory depression, profound sedation or coma; reduced dosage (1/3 to 1/2 of the usual dosage) may be necessary).
No products indexed under this heading.

Ethyl Alcohol (Concurrent use with the usual dose of OxyContin may result in respiratory depression, profound sedation or coma; reduced dosage (1/3 to 1/2 of the usual dosage) may be necessary).
No products indexed under this heading.

Fentanyl (Concurrent use with the usual dose of OxyContin may result in respiratory depression, profound sedation or coma; reduced dosage (1/3 to 1/2 of the usual dosage) may be necessary). Products include:
Duragesic Transdermal System 2448

Fentanyl Citrate (Concurrent use with the usual dose of OxyContin may result in respiratory depression, profound sedation or coma; reduced dosage (1/3 to 1/2 of the usual dosage) may be necessary). Products include:
Actiq 993

Fluphenazine Decanoate (Concurrent use with the usual dose of OxyContin may result in respiratory depression, profound sedation or coma; reduced dosage (1/3 to 1/2 of the usual dosage) may be necessary).
No products indexed under this heading.

Fluphenazine Enanthate (Concurrent use with the usual dose of OxyContin may result in respiratory depression, profound sedation or coma; reduced dosage (1/3 to 1/2 of the usual dosage) may be necessary).
No products indexed under this heading.

Fluphenazine Hydrochloride (Concurrent use with the usual dose of OxyContin may result in respiratory depression, profound sedation or coma; reduced dosage (1/3 to 1/2 of the usual dosage) may be necessary).
No products indexed under this heading.

Flurazepam Hydrochloride (Concurrent use with the usual dose of OxyContin may result in respiratory depression, profound sedation or coma; reduced dosage (1/3 to 1/2 of the usual dosage) may be necessary). Products include:
Dalmane Capsules 3343

Glutethimide (Concurrent use with the usual dose of OxyContin may result in respiratory depression, profound sedation or coma; reduced dosage (1/3 to 1/2 of the usual dosage) may be necessary).
No products indexed under this heading.

Haloperidol (Concurrent use with the usual dose of OxyContin may result in respiratory depression, profound sedation or coma; reduced dosage (1/3 to 1/2 of the usual dosage) may be necessary).
No products indexed under this heading.

Haloperidol Decanoate (Concurrent use with the usual dose of OxyContin may result in respiratory depression, profound sedation or coma; reduced dosage (1/3 to 1/2 of the usual dosage) may be necessary).
No products indexed under this heading.

Hydrocodone Bitartrate (Concurrent use with the usual dose of OxyContin may result in respiratory depression, profound sedation or coma; reduced dosage (1/3 to 1/2 of the usual dosage) may be necessary). Products include:
Hycodan 1104
Hycomine Compound Tablets 1105
Hycotuss Expectorant Syrup 1106
Lortab 3315
Lortab Elixir 3312
Vicodin Tablets 530
Vicodin ES Tablets 531
Vicodin HP Tablets 532
Vicoprofen Tablets 533
Zydone Tablets 1118

Hydrocodone Polistirex (Concurrent use with the usual dose of OxyContin may result in respiratory depression, profound sedation or coma; reduced dosage (1/3 to 1/2 of the usual dosage) may be necessary). Products include:
Tussionex Pennkinetic Extended-Release Suspension 3322

Hydromorphone Hydrochloride (Concurrent use with the usual dose of OxyContin may result in respiratory depression, profound sedation or coma; reduced dosage (1/3 to 1/2 of the usual dosage) may be necessary). Products include:
Dilaudid 439
Dilaudid Oral Liquid 443
Dilaudid Non-Sterile Powder 439
Dilaudid Rectal Suppositories 439
Dilaudid Tablets 439
Dilaudid Tablets - 8 mg 443
Dilaudid-HP 441

Hydroxyzine Hydrochloride (Concurrent use with the usual dose of OxyContin may result in respiratory depression, profound sedation or coma; reduced dosage (1/3 to 1/2 of the usual dosage) may be necessary).
No products indexed under this heading.

Isoflurane (Concurrent use with the usual dose of OxyContin may result in respiratory depression, profound sedation or coma; reduced dosage (1/3 to 1/2 of the usual dosage) may be necessary).
No products indexed under this heading.

Ketamine Hydrochloride (Concurrent use with the usual dose of OxyContin may result in respiratory depression, profound sedation or coma; reduced dosage (1/3 to 1/2 of the usual dosage) may be necessary).
No products indexed under this heading.

Levomethadyl Acetate Hydrochloride (Concurrent use with the usual dose of OxyContin may result in respiratory depression, profound sedation or coma; reduced dosage (1/3 to 1/2 of the usual dosage) may be necessary).
No products indexed under this heading.

Levorphanol Tartrate (Concurrent use with the usual dose of OxyContin may result in respiratory depression, profound sedation or coma; reduced dosage (1/3 to 1/2 of the usual dosage) may be necessary).
No products indexed under this heading.

Lorazepam (Concurrent use with the usual dose of OxyContin may result in respiratory depression, profound sedation or coma; reduced dosage (1/3 to 1/2 of the usual dosage) may be necessary).
No products indexed under this heading.

Loxapine Hydrochloride (Concurrent use with the usual dose of OxyContin may result in respiratory depression, profound sedation or coma; reduced dosage (1/3 to 1/2 of the usual dosage) may be necessary).
No products indexed under this heading.

Loxapine Succinate (Concurrent use with the usual dose of OxyContin may result in respiratory depression, profound sedation or coma; reduced dosage (1/3 to 1/2 of the usual dosage) may be necessary).
No products indexed under this heading.

Meperidine Hydrochloride (Concurrent use with the usual dose of OxyContin may result in respiratory depression, profound sedation or coma; reduced dosage (1/3 to 1/2 of the usual dosage) may be necessary).
No products indexed under this heading.

Mephobarbital (Concurrent use with the usual dose of OxyContin may result in respiratory depression, profound sedation or coma; reduced dosage (1/3 to 1/2 of the usual dosage) may be necessary). Products include:
Mebaral Tablets, USP **2483**

Meprobamate (Concurrent use with the usual dose of OxyContin may result in respiratory depression, profound sedation or coma; reduced dosage (1/3 to 1/2 of the usual dosage) may be necessary).
No products indexed under this heading.

Mesoridazine Besylate (Concurrent use with the usual dose of OxyContin may result in respiratory depression, profound sedation or coma; reduced dosage (1/3 to 1/2 of the usual dosage) may be necessary).
No products indexed under this heading.

Methadone Hydrochloride (Concurrent use with the usual dose of OxyContin may result in respiratory depression, profound sedation or coma; reduced dosage (1/3 to 1/2 of the usual dosage) may be necessary).
No products indexed under this heading.

Methohexital Sodium (Concurrent use with the usual dose of OxyContin may result in respiratory depression, profound sedation or coma; reduced dosage (1/3 to 1/2 of the usual dosage) may be necessary).
No products indexed under this heading.

Methotrimeprazine (Concurrent use with the usual dose of OxyContin may result in respiratory depression, profound sedation or coma; reduced dosage (1/3 to 1/2 of the usual dosage) may be necessary).
No products indexed under this heading.

Methoxyflurane (Concurrent use with the usual dose of OxyContin may result in respiratory depression, profound sedation or coma; reduced dosage (1/3 to 1/2 of the usual dosage) may be necessary).
No products indexed under this heading.

Midazolam Hydrochloride (Concurrent use with the usual dose of OxyContin may result in respiratory depression, profound sedation or coma; reduced dosage (1/3 to 1/2 of the usual dosage) may be necessary).
No products indexed under this heading.

Molindone Hydrochloride (Concurrent use with the usual dose of OxyContin may result in respiratory depression, profound sedation or coma; reduced dosage (1/3 to 1/2 of the usual dosage) may be necessary). Products include:
Moban Tablets **1108**

Morphine Sulfate (Concurrent use with the usual dose of OxyContin may result in respiratory depression, profound sedation or coma; reduced dosage (1/3 to 1/2 of the usual dosage) may be necessary). Products include:
Avinza Capsules **1714**
Kadian Capsules **572**
MS Contin Tablets **2703**

Nalbuphine Hydrochloride (Mixed agonist/antagonist analgesics may reduce the analgesic effect of oxycodone and/or may precipitate withdrawal symptoms). Products include:
Nubain Injection **1111**

Olanzapine (Concurrent use with the usual dose of OxyContin may result in respiratory depression, profound sedation or coma; reduced dosage (1/3 to 1/2 of the usual dosage) may be necessary). Products include:
Symbyax Capsules **1788**
Zyprexa Tablets **1798**
Zyprexa IntraMuscular **1798**
Zyprexa ZYDIS Orally Disintegrating Tablets **1798**

Oxazepam (Concurrent use with the usual dose of OxyContin may result in respiratory depression, profound sedation or coma; reduced dosage (1/3 to 1/2 of the usual dosage) may be necessary).
No products indexed under this heading.

Pentazocine Hydrochloride (Mixed agonist/antagonist analgesics may reduce the analgesic effect of oxycodone and/or may precipitate withdrawal symptoms).
No products indexed under this heading.

Pentazocine Lactate (Mixed agonist/antagonist analgesics may reduce the analgesic effect of oxycodone and/or may precipitate withdrawal symptoms).
No products indexed under this heading.

Pentobarbital Sodium (Concurrent use with the usual dose of OxyContin may result in respiratory depression, profound sedation or coma; reduced dosage (1/3 to 1/2 of the usual dosage) may be necessary). Products include:
Nembutal Sodium Solution, USP **2484**

Perphenazine (Concurrent use with the usual dose of OxyContin may result in respiratory depression, profound sedation or coma; reduced dosage (1/3 to 1/2 of the usual dosage) may be necessary).
No products indexed under this heading.

Phenobarbital (Concurrent use with the usual dose of OxyContin may result in respiratory depression, profound sedation or coma; reduced dosage (1/3 to 1/2 of the usual dosage) may be necessary).
No products indexed under this heading.

Prazepam (Concurrent use with the usual dose of OxyContin may result in respiratory depression, profound sedation or coma; reduced dosage (1/3 to 1/2 of the usual dosage) may be necessary).
No products indexed under this heading.

Prochlorperazine (Concurrent use with the usual dose of OxyContin may result in respiratory depression, profound sedation or coma; reduced dosage (1/3 to 1/2 of the usual dosage) may be necessary).
No products indexed under this heading.

Promethazine Hydrochloride (Concurrent use with the usual dose of OxyContin may result in respiratory depression, profound sedation or coma; reduced dosage (1/3 to 1/2 of the usual dosage) may be necessary). Products include:
Phenergan **3438**

Propofol (Concurrent use with the usual dose of OxyContin may result in respiratory depression, profound sedation or coma; reduced dosage (1/3 to 1/2 of the usual dosage) may be necessary). Products include:
Diprivan Injectable Emulsion **676**

Propoxyphene Hydrochloride (Concurrent use with the usual dose of OxyContin may result in respiratory depression, profound sedation or coma; reduced dosage (1/3 to 1/2 of the usual dosage) may be necessary).
No products indexed under this heading.

Propoxyphene Napsylate (Concurrent use with the usual dose of OxyContin may result in respiratory depression, profound sedation or coma; reduced dosage (1/3 to 1/2 of the usual dosage) may be necessary). Products include:
Darvocet A 500 Tablets **3497**

Quazepam (Concurrent use with the usual dose of OxyContin may result in respiratory depression, profound sedation or coma; reduced dosage (1/3 to 1/2 of the usual dosage) may be necessary).
No products indexed under this heading.

Quetiapine Fumarate (Concurrent use with the usual dose of OxyContin may result in respiratory depression, profound sedation or coma; reduced dosage (1/3 to 1/2 of the usual dosage) may be necessary). Products include:
Seroquel Tablets **691**

Remifentanil Hydrochloride (Concurrent use with the usual dose of OxyContin may result in respiratory depression, profound sedation or coma; reduced dosage (1/3 to 1/2 of the usual dosage) may be necessary).
No products indexed under this heading.

Risperidone (Concurrent use with the usual dose of OxyContin may result in respiratory depression, profound sedation or coma; reduced dosage (1/3 to 1/2 of the usual dosage) may be necessary). Products include:
Risperdal Consta Long-Acting Injection **1664**
Risperdal M-Tab Orally Disintegrating Tablets **1658**
Risperdal **1658**

Secobarbital Sodium (Concurrent use with the usual dose of OxyContin may result in respiratory depression, profound sedation or coma; reduced dosage (1/3 to 1/2 of the usual dosage) may be necessary).
No products indexed under this heading.

Sevoflurane (Concurrent use with the usual dose of OxyContin may result in respiratory depression, profound sedation or coma; reduced dosage (1/3 to 1/2 of the usual dosage) may be necessary). Products include:
Ultane Liquid for Inhalation **526**

Sufentanil Citrate (Concurrent use with the usual dose of OxyContin may result in respiratory depression, profound sedation or coma; reduced dosage (1/3 to 1/2 of the usual dosage) may be necessary).
No products indexed under this heading.

Temazepam (Concurrent use with the usual dose of OxyContin may result in respiratory depression, profound sedation or coma; reduced dosage (1/3 to 1/2 of the usual dosage) may be necessary).
No products indexed under this heading.

Thiamylal Sodium (Concurrent use with the usual dose of OxyContin may result in respiratory depression, profound sedation or coma; reduced dosage (1/3 to 1/2 of the usual dosage) may be necessary).
No products indexed under this heading.

Thioridazine Hydrochloride (Concurrent use with the usual dose of OxyContin may result in respiratory depression, profound sedation or coma; reduced dosage (1/3 to 1/2 of the usual dosage) may be necessary). Products include:
Thioridazine Hydrochloride Tablets **2122**

IMPORTANT NOTE: Always consult each drug listing in the patient's regimen for possible interactions.

Thiothixene (Concurrent use with the usual dose of OxyContin may result in respiratory depression, profound sedation or coma; reduced dosage (1/3 to 1/2 of the usual dosage) may be necessary). Products include:
Thiothixene Capsules **2124**

Triazolam (Concurrent use with the usual dose of OxyContin may result in respiratory depression, profound sedation or coma; reduced dosage (1/3 to 1/2 of the usual dosage) may be necessary).
No products indexed under this heading.

Trifluoperazine Hydrochloride (Concurrent use with the usual dose of OxyContin may result in respiratory depression, profound sedation or coma; reduced dosage (1/3 to 1/2 of the usual dosage) may be necessary).
No products indexed under this heading.

Zaleplon (Concurrent use with the usual dose of OxyContin may result in respiratory depression, profound sedation or coma; reduced dosage (1/3 to 1/2 of the usual dosage) may be necessary). Products include:
Sonata Capsules **1686**

Ziprasidone Hydrochloride (Concurrent use with the usual dose of OxyContin may result in respiratory depression, profound sedation or coma; reduced dosage (1/3 to 1/2 of the usual dosage) may be necessary). Products include:
Geodon Capsules **2514**

Zolpidem Tartrate (Concurrent use with the usual dose of OxyContin may result in respiratory depression, profound sedation or coma; reduced dosage (1/3 to 1/2 of the usual dosage) may be necessary). Products include:
Ambien Tablets **2867**

Food Interactions

Alcohol (Concurrent use with the usual dose of OxyContin may result in respiratory depression, profound sedation or coma).

OXYFAST ORAL CONCENTRATE SOLUTION

(Oxycodone Hydrochloride) **2704**
See OxyIR Capsules

OXYIR CAPSULES

(Oxycodone Hydrochloride) **2704**
May interact with central nervous system depressants, general anesthetics, hypnotics and sedatives, mixed agonist/antagonist opioid analgesics, narcotic analgesics, phenothiazines, tranquilizers, and certain other agents. Compounds in these categories include:

Alfentanil Hydrochloride (Concomitant use may exhibit an additive CNS depression).
No products indexed under this heading.

Alprazolam (Concomitant use may exhibit an additive CNS depression). Products include:
Niravam Orally Disintegrating Tablets **3106**
Xanax XR Tablets **2655**

Aprobarbital (Concomitant use may exhibit an additive CNS depression).
No products indexed under this heading.

Buprenorphine Hydrochloride (Co-administration with mixed agonist/antagonist analgesics may reduce the analgesic effect of oxycodone and/or may precipitate withdrawal symptoms). Products include:
Buprenex Injectable **2718**
Suboxone Tablets **2719**
Subutex Tablets **2719**

Buspirone Hydrochloride (Concomitant use may exhibit an additive CNS depression).
No products indexed under this heading.

Butabarbital (Concomitant use may exhibit an additive CNS depression).
No products indexed under this heading.

Butalbital (Concomitant use may exhibit an additive CNS depression). Products include:
Sedapap Tablets 50 mg/650 mg **2098**

Butorphanol Tartrate (Co-administration with mixed agonist/antagonist analgesics may reduce the analgesic effect of oxycodone and/or may precipitate withdrawal symptoms).
No products indexed under this heading.

Chlordiazepoxide (Concomitant use may exhibit an additive CNS depression).
No products indexed under this heading.

Chlordiazepoxide Hydrochloride (Concomitant use may exhibit an additive CNS depression). Products include:
Librium Capsules **3349**

Chlorpromazine (Concomitant use may exhibit an additive CNS depression).
No products indexed under this heading.

Chlorpromazine Hydrochloride (Concomitant use may exhibit an additive CNS depression).
No products indexed under this heading.

Chlorprothixene (Concomitant use may exhibit an additive CNS depression).
No products indexed under this heading.

Chlorprothixene Hydrochloride (Concomitant use may exhibit an additive CNS depression).
No products indexed under this heading.

Chlorprothixene Lactate (Concomitant use may exhibit an additive CNS depression).
No products indexed under this heading.

Clorazepate Dipotassium (Concomitant use may exhibit an additive CNS depression). Products include:
Tranxene **2488**

Clozapine (Concomitant use may exhibit an additive CNS depression). Products include:
Clozapine Tablets **2141**
Clozaril Tablets **2174**
FazaClo Orally Disintegrating Tablets **547**

Codeine Phosphate (Concomitant use may exhibit an additive CNS depression). Products include:
Tylenol with Codeine **2461**

Desflurane (Concomitant use may exhibit an additive CNS depression). Products include:
Suprane Liquid for Inhalation **770**

Dezocine (Concomitant use may exhibit an additive CNS depression).
No products indexed under this heading.

Diazepam (Concomitant use may exhibit an additive CNS depression). Products include:
Diastat Rectal Delivery System **3344**
Valium Tablets **2822**

Droperidol (Concomitant use may exhibit an additive CNS depression).
No products indexed under this heading.

Enflurane (Concomitant use may exhibit an additive CNS depression).
No products indexed under this heading.

Estazolam (Concomitant use may exhibit an additive CNS depression). Products include:
ProSom Tablets **512**

Ethanol (Concomitant use may exhibit an additive CNS depression).
No products indexed under this heading.

Ethchlorvynol (Concomitant use may exhibit an additive CNS depression).
No products indexed under this heading.

Ethinamate (Concomitant use may exhibit an additive CNS depression).
No products indexed under this heading.

Ethyl Alcohol (Concomitant use may exhibit an additive CNS depression).
No products indexed under this heading.

Fentanyl (Concomitant use may exhibit an additive CNS depression). Products include:
Duragesic Transdermal System **2448**

Fentanyl Citrate (Concomitant use may exhibit an additive CNS depression). Products include:
Actiq **993**

Fluphenazine Decanoate (Concomitant use may exhibit an additive CNS depression).
No products indexed under this heading.

Fluphenazine Enanthate (Concomitant use may exhibit an additive CNS depression).
No products indexed under this heading.

Fluphenazine Hydrochloride (Concomitant use may exhibit an additive CNS depression).
No products indexed under this heading.

Flurazepam Hydrochloride (Concomitant use may exhibit an additive CNS depression). Products include:
Dalmane Capsules **3343**

Glutethimide (Concomitant use may exhibit an additive CNS depression).
No products indexed under this heading.

Haloperidol (Concomitant use may exhibit an additive CNS depression).
No products indexed under this heading.

Haloperidol Decanoate (Concomitant use may exhibit an additive CNS depression).
No products indexed under this heading.

Hydrocodone Bitartrate (Concomitant use may exhibit an additive CNS depression). Products include:
Hycodan **1104**
Hycomine Compound Tablets **1105**
Hycotuss Expectorant Syrup **1106**
Lortab **3315**
Lortab Elixir **3312**
Vicodin Tablets **530**
Vicodin ES Tablets **531**
Vicodin HP Tablets **532**
Vicoprofen Tablets **533**
Zydone Tablets **1118**

Hydrocodone Polistirex (Concomitant use may exhibit an additive CNS depression). Products include:
Tussionex Pennkinetic Extended-Release Suspension **3322**

Hydromorphone Hydrochloride (Concomitant use may exhibit an additive CNS depression). Products include:
Dilaudid **439**
Dilaudid Oral Liquid **443**
Dilaudid Non-Sterile Powder **439**
Dilaudid Rectal Suppositories **439**
Dilaudid Tablets **439**
Dilaudid Tablets - 8 mg **443**
Dilaudid-HP **441**

Hydroxyzine Hydrochloride (Concomitant use may exhibit an additive CNS depression).
No products indexed under this heading.

Isoflurane (Concomitant use may exhibit an additive CNS depression).
No products indexed under this heading.

Ketamine Hydrochloride (Concomitant use may exhibit an additive CNS depression).
No products indexed under this heading.

Levomethadyl Acetate Hydrochloride (Concomitant use may exhibit an additive CNS depression).
No products indexed under this heading.

Levorphanol Tartrate (Concomitant use may exhibit an additive CNS depression).
No products indexed under this heading.

Lorazepam (Concomitant use may exhibit an additive CNS depression).
No products indexed under this heading.

Loxapine Hydrochloride (Concomitant use may exhibit an additive CNS depression).
No products indexed under this heading.

Loxapine Succinate (Concomitant use may exhibit an additive CNS depression).
No products indexed under this heading.

Meperidine Hydrochloride (Concomitant use may exhibit an additive CNS depression).
No products indexed under this heading.

Mephobarbital (Concomitant use may exhibit an additive CNS depression). Products include:
Mebaral Tablets, USP **2483**

Meprobamate (Concomitant use may exhibit an additive CNS depression).
No products indexed under this heading.

Mesoridazine Besylate (Concomitant use may exhibit an additive CNS depression).
No products indexed under this heading.

Methadone Hydrochloride (Concomitant use may exhibit an additive CNS depression).
No products indexed under this heading.

Methohexital Sodium (Concomitant use may exhibit an additive CNS depression).
No products indexed under this heading.

Methotrimeprazine (Concomitant use may exhibit an additive CNS depression).
No products indexed under this heading.

Methoxyflurane (Concomitant use may exhibit an additive CNS depression).
No products indexed under this heading.

Midazolam Hydrochloride (Concomitant use may exhibit an additive CNS depression).
No products indexed under this heading.

Molindone Hydrochloride (Concomitant use may exhibit an additive CNS depression). Products include:
Moban Tablets 1108

Morphine Sulfate (Concomitant use may exhibit an additive CNS depression). Products include:
Avinza Capsules 1714
Kadian Capsules 572
MS Contin Tablets 2703

Nalbuphine Hydrochloride (Co-administration with mixed agonist/antagonist analgesics may reduce the analgesic effect of oxycodone and/or may precipitate withdrawal symptoms). Products include:
Nubain Injection 1111

Olanzapine (Concomitant use may exhibit an additive CNS depression). Products include:
Symbyax Capsules 1788
Zyprexa Tablets 1798
Zyprexa IntraMuscular 1798
Zyprexa ZYDIS Orally Disintegrating Tablets 1798

Oxazepam (Concomitant use may exhibit an additive CNS depression).
No products indexed under this heading.

Pentazocine Hydrochloride (Co-administration with mixed agonist/antagonist analgesics may reduce the analgesic effect of oxycodone and/or may precipitate withdrawal symptoms).
No products indexed under this heading.

Pentazocine Lactate (Co-administration with mixed agonist/antagonist analgesics may reduce the analgesic effect of oxycodone and/or may precipitate withdrawal symptoms).
No products indexed under this heading.

Pentobarbital Sodium (Concomitant use may exhibit an additive CNS depression). Products include:
Nembutal Sodium Solution, USP 2484

Perphenazine (Concomitant use may exhibit an additive CNS depression).
No products indexed under this heading.

Phenobarbital (Concomitant use may exhibit an additive CNS depression).
No products indexed under this heading.

Prazepam (Concomitant use may exhibit an additive CNS depression).
No products indexed under this heading.

Prochlorperazine (Concomitant use may exhibit an additive CNS depression).
No products indexed under this heading.

Promethazine Hydrochloride (Concomitant use may exhibit an additive CNS depression). Products include:
Phenergan 3438

Propofol (Concomitant use may exhibit an additive CNS depression). Products include:
Diprivan Injectable Emulsion 676

Propoxyphene Hydrochloride (Concomitant use may exhibit an additive CNS depression).
No products indexed under this heading.

Propoxyphene Napsylate (Concomitant use may exhibit an additive CNS depression). Products include:
Darvocet A 500 Tablets 3497

Quazepam (Concomitant use may exhibit an additive CNS depression).
No products indexed under this heading.

Quetiapine Fumarate (Concomitant use may exhibit an additive CNS depression). Products include:
Seroquel Tablets 691

Remifentanil Hydrochloride (Concomitant use may exhibit an additive CNS depression).
No products indexed under this heading.

Risperidone (Concomitant use may exhibit an additive CNS depression). Products include:
Risperdal Consta Long-Acting Injection 1664
Risperdal M-Tab Orally Disintegrating Tablets 1658
Risperdal 1658

Secobarbital Sodium (Concomitant use may exhibit an additive CNS depression).
No products indexed under this heading.

Sevoflurane (Concomitant use may exhibit an additive CNS depression). Products include:
Ultane Liquid for Inhalation 526

Sufentanil Citrate (Concomitant use may exhibit an additive CNS depression).
No products indexed under this heading.

Temazepam (Concomitant use may exhibit an additive CNS depression).
No products indexed under this heading.

Thiamylal Sodium (Concomitant use may exhibit an additive CNS depression).
No products indexed under this heading.

Thioridazine Hydrochloride (Concomitant use may exhibit an additive CNS depression). Products include:
Thioridazine Hydrochloride Tablets 2122

Thiothixene (Concomitant use may exhibit an additive CNS depression). Products include:
Thiothixene Capsules 2124

Triazolam (Concomitant use may exhibit an additive CNS depression).
No products indexed under this heading.

Trifluoperazine Hydrochloride (Concomitant use may exhibit an additive CNS depression).
No products indexed under this heading.

Zaleplon (Concomitant use may exhibit an additive CNS depression). Products include:
Sonata Capsules 1686

Ziprasidone Hydrochloride (Concomitant use may exhibit an additive CNS depression). Products include:
Geodon Capsules 2514

Zolpidem Tartrate (Concomitant use may exhibit an additive CNS depression). Products include:
Ambien Tablets 2867

Food Interactions

Alcohol (Concomitant use may exhibit an additive CNS depression).

OXYTROL TRANSDERMAL SYSTEM

(Oxybutynin) 3383
May interact with anticholinergics, bisphosphonates, and certain other agents. Compounds in these categories include:

Alendronate Sodium (Concurrent use with drugs that can cause or exacerbate esophagitis, such as biphosphonates, should be undertaken with caution). Products include:
Fosamax 1949
Fosamax Plus D Tablets 1956

Atropine Sulfate (Co-administration of oxybutynin with other anticholinergic drugs may increase the frequency and/or severity of anticholinergic side effects such as dry mouth, constipation, drowsiness and others).
No products indexed under this heading.

Belladonna Alkaloids (Co-administration of oxybutynin with other anticholinergic drugs may increase the frequency and/or severity of anticholinergic side effects such as dry mouth, constipation, drowsiness and others). Products include:
Hyland's Teething Tablets 736

Benztropine Mesylate (Co-administration of oxybutynin with other anticholinergic drugs may increase the frequency and/or severity of anticholinergic side effects such as dry mouth, constipation, drowsiness and others). Products include:
Cogentin Injection 1903

Biperiden Hydrochloride (Co-administration of oxybutynin with other anticholinergic drugs may increase the frequency and/or severity of anticholinergic side effects such as dry mouth, constipation, drowsiness and others).
No products indexed under this heading.

Clidinium Bromide (Co-administration of oxybutynin with other anticholinergic drugs may increase the frequency and/or severity of anticholinergic side effects such as dry mouth, constipation, drowsiness and others).
No products indexed under this heading.

Dicyclomine Hydrochloride (Co-administration of oxybutynin with other anticholinergic drugs may increase the frequency and/or severity of anticholinergic side effects such as dry mouth, constipation, drowsiness and others). Products include:
Bentyl Capsules 724
Bentyl Injection 724
Bentyl Syrup 724
Bentyl Tablets 724

Etidronate Disodium (Concurrent use with drugs that can cause or exacerbate esophagitis, such as biphosphonates, should be undertaken with caution). Products include:
Didronel Tablets 2693

Glycopyrrolate (Co-administration of oxybutynin with other anticholinergic drugs may increase the frequency and/or severity of anticholinergic side effects such as dry mouth, constipation, drowsiness and others).
No products indexed under this heading.

Hyoscyamine (Co-administration of oxybutynin with other anticholinergic drugs may increase the frequency and/or severity of anticholinergic side effects such as dry mouth, constipation, drowsiness and others).
No products indexed under this heading.

Hyoscyamine Sulfate (Co-administration of oxybutynin with other anticholinergic drugs may increase the frequency and/or severity of anticholinergic side effects such as dry mouth, constipation, drowsiness and others).
No products indexed under this heading.

Ipratropium Bromide (Co-administration of oxybutynin with other anticholinergic drugs may increase the frequency and/or severity of anticholinergic side effects such as dry mouth, constipation, drowsiness and others). Products include:
Atrovent HFA Inhalation Aerosol 872
Atrovent Inhalation Solution 868
Atrovent Nasal Spray 0.03% 869
Atrovent Nasal Spray 0.06% 870
Combivent Inhalation Aerosol 878
DuoNeb Inhalation Solution 1058

Mepenzolate Bromide (Co-administration of oxybutynin with other anticholinergic drugs may increase the frequency and/or severity of anticholinergic side effects such as dry mouth, constipation, drowsiness and others).
No products indexed under this heading.

Procyclidine Hydrochloride (Co-administration of oxybutynin with other anticholinergic drugs may increase the frequency and/or severity of anticholinergic side effects such as dry mouth, constipation, drowsiness and others).
No products indexed under this heading.

Propantheline Bromide (Co-administration of oxybutynin with other anticholinergic drugs may increase the frequency and/or severity of anticholinergic side effects such as dry mouth, constipation, drowsiness and others).
No products indexed under this heading.

Risedronate Sodium (Concurrent use with drugs that can cause or exacerbate esophagitis, such as biphosphonates, should be undertaken with caution). Products include:
Actonel Tablets 2679
Actonel with Calcium Tablets 2684

Scopolamine (Co-administration of oxybutynin with other anticholinergic drugs may increase the frequency and/or severity of anticholinergic

side effects such as dry mouth, constipation, drowsiness and others). Products include:

Transderm Scōp Transdermal Therapeutic System 2166

Scopolamine Hydrobromide (Co-administration of oxybutynin with other anticholinergic drugs may increase the frequency and/or severity of anticholinergic side effects such as dry mouth, constipation, drowsiness and others).

No products indexed under this heading.

Tiludronate Disodium (Concurrent use with drugs that can cause or exacerbate esophagitis, such as biphosphonates, should be undertaken with caution).

No products indexed under this heading.

Tolterodine Tartrate (Co-administration of oxybutynin with other anticholinergic drugs may increase the frequency and/or severity of anticholinergic side effects such as dry mouth, constipation, drowsiness and others). Products include:

Detrol Tablets 2626
Detrol LA Capsules 2629

Tridihexethyl Chloride (Co-administration of oxybutynin with other anticholinergic drugs may increase the frequency and/or severity of anticholinergic side effects such as dry mouth, constipation, drowsiness and others).

No products indexed under this heading.

Trihexyphenidyl Hydrochloride (Co-administration of oxybutynin with other anticholinergic drugs may increase the frequency and/or severity of anticholinergic side effects such as dry mouth, constipation, drowsiness and others).

No products indexed under this heading.

Food Interactions

Alcohol (May enhance drowsiness caused by anticholinergic agents such as oxybutynin).

PACERONE TABLETS

(Amiodarone Hydrochloride) 3337

May interact with azole antifungals, beta blockers, calcium channel blockers, oral anticoagulants, cytochrome p450 1a2 substrates (selected), cytochrome p450 2c9 substrates (selected), cytochrome p450 2d6 substrates (selected), cytochrome p450 3a4 inhibitors (selected), cytochrome p450 3a4 substrates (selected), fluoroquinolone antibiotics, cardiac glycosides, HMG-CoA reductase inhibitors, macrolide antibiotics, phenytoin, protease inhibitors, quinidine, and certain other agents. Compounds in these categories include:

Acarbose (Amiodarone may suppress certain CYP450 enzymes, including CYP2Cp. This inhibition can result in unexpectedly high plasma levels of other drugs which are metabolized by those CYP450 enzymes). Products include:

Precose Tablets 776

Acebutolol Hydrochloride (Possible potentiation of bradycardia, sinus arrest, and AV block when co-administered with beta-blocking agents).

No products indexed under this heading.

Acetaminophen (Amiodarone may suppress certain CYP450 enzymes, including CYP1A2. This inhibition can result in unexpectedly high plasma levels of other drugs which are metabolized by those CYP450 enzymes). Products include:

Benadryl Allergy & Cold Tablets ..... ▣692
Benadryl Allergy & Sinus Headache Caplets & Gelcaps ...... ▣693
Benadryl Maximum Strength Severe Allergy & Sinus Headache Caplets .... ▣694
Contac Severe Cold and Flu Caplets Maximum Strength .... ▣615
Contac Severe Cold and Flu Caplets Non-Drowsy .... ▣615
Darvocet A 500 Tablets 3497
Goody's Body Pain Formula Powder .... ▣621
Goody's Extra Strength Headache Powder .... ▣621
Goody's Extra Strength Pain Relief Tablets .... ▣621
Goody's PM Powder .... ▣622
Hycomine Compound Tablets 1105
Lortab 3315
Lortab Elixir 3312
Percocet Tablets 1114
Robitussin Cough, Cold & Flu Liquid-filled Capsules.................. ▣750
Robitussin Flu Liquid .... ▣752
Sedapap Tablets 50 mg/650 mg 2098
Singlet Caplets .... ▣636
Sudafed Severe Cold .... ▣710
Sudafed Sinus Headache .... ▣711
TheraFlu Cold & Cough Hot Liquid .... ▣680
TheraFlu Cold & Sore Throat Hot Liquid .... ▣680
TheraFlu Flu & Chest Congestion Non-Drowsy Hot Liquid............... ▣681
TheraFlu Flu & Sore Throat Hot Liquid .... ▣681
TheraFlu Severe Cold Non-Drowsy Hot Liquid............... ▣683
TheraFlu Severe Cold & Cough Hot Liquid .... ▣683
TheraFlu Severe Cold Caplets .... ▣679
TheraFlu Severe Cold Hot Liquid .... ▣682
TheraFlu Severe Cold Non-Drowsy Caplets...................... ▣679
Triaminic Cough & Sore Throat Liquid .... ▣687
Triaminic Flu, Cough & Fever Liquid .... ▣685
Triaminic Cough & Sore Throat Softchews .... ▣689
Tylenol 8 Hour Extended Release Geltabs and Caplets 1843
Tylenol Sinus NightTime Caplets .... ▣663
Children's Tylenol Suspension Liquid and Meltaways................... 1850
Children's Tylenol Plus Cold & Allergy Suspension Liquid 1850
Children's Tylenol Plus Cold NightTime Suspension Liquid....... 1851
Children's Tylenol Plus Cold & Cough Suspension Liquid and Chewable Tablets 1851
Children's Tylenol Plus Cold Chewable Tablets 1851
Children's Tylenol Plus Cold Daytime Non-Drowsy Suspension Liquid 1851
Children's Tylenol Plus Flu Suspension Liquid 1853
Concentrated Tylenol Infants' Drops Plus Cold.............................. 1851
Concentrated Tylenol Infants' Drops Plus Cold and Cough 1851
Concentrated Tylenol Infants' Drops.. 1850
Junior Tylenol Meltaways 1850
Tylenol Cold & Flu Severe Daytime Liquid with Cool Bust....... 1846
Tylenol Cold & Flu Severe NightTime Liquid with Cool Burst.. 1846
Tylenol Cold Severe Congestion Non-Drowsy Caplets with Cool Burst.. 1846
Tylenol Cough & Sore Throat Daytime Liquid with Cool Burst...... 1849
Tylenol Cough & Sore Throat NightTime Liquid with Cool Burst.. 1849
Tylenol 1843
Extra Strength Tylenol Rapid Release Gels 1843
Tylenol 1843
Tylenol Allergy Complete Night Time Caplets................................. 1844
Tylenol Allergy Complete Multi-Symptom Caplets and Gelcaps with Cool Burst............... 1844
Tylenol Severe Allergy Caplets 1844
Tylenol Flu NightTime Gelcaps 1846
Tylenol Flu Day Non-Drowsy Gelcaps... 1846
Concentrated Tylenol Infants' Drops Plus Cold Nasal Congestant, Fever Reducer & Pain Reliever .... ▣668
Concentrated Tylenol Infants' Drops Plus Cold & Cough Nasal Decongestant, Fever Reducer & Pain Reliever.............. ▣668
Multi-Symptom Tylenol Cold Night Time Caplets 1845
Multi-Symptom Tylenol Cold Day Non-Drowsy Caplets and Gelcaps... 1845
Extra Strength Tylenol PM Caplets, Geltabs, Gelcaps and Liquid 1847
Tylenol Sinus Day Non-Drowsy 1848
Tylenol Sinus Night Time Caplets 1848
Tylenol Sinus Severe Congestion Caplets with Cool Burst............... 1848
Tylenol Sore Throat Daytime Liquid with Cool Burst.................. 1849
Tylenol Sore Throat NightTime Liquid with Cool Burst.................. 1849
Tylenol with Codeine 2461
Women's Tylenol Menstrual Relief Caplets.. 1849
Ultracet Tablets 2462
Vicks 44M Cough, Cold & Flu Relief.. 2676
Vicks DayQuil LiquiCaps/Liquid Multi-Symptom Cold/Flu Relief..... ▣723
Vicks DayQuil Multi-Symptom Cold/Flu Relief LiquiCaps............. 2675
Vicks DayQuil Multi-Symptom Cold/Flu Relief Liquid.................. 2675
Vicks NyQuil LiquiCaps 2677
Vicks NyQuil LiquiCaps/Liquid Multi-Symptom Cold/Flu Relief..... ▣725
Vicks NyQuil Liquid 2677
Vicodin Tablets 530
Vicodin ES Tablets 531
Vicodin HP Tablets 532
Zydone Tablets 1118

Acetazolamide (Since amiodarone is a substrate for CYP3A4, drugs that inhibit CYP3A4 may decrease the metabolism and increase serum concentration of amiodarone).

No products indexed under this heading.

Alatrofloxacin Mesylate (Fluoroquinolones are known to cause QTc prolongation. There have been reports of QTc prolongation in patients taking amiodarone when fluoroquinolones were administered concomitantly).

No products indexed under this heading.

Alfentanil Hydrochloride (Amiodarone may suppress certain CYP450 enzymes, including CYP3A4. This inhibition can result in unexpectedly high plasma levels of other drugs which are metabolized by those CYP450 enzymes).

No products indexed under this heading.

Alprazolam (Amiodarone may suppress certain CYP450 enzymes, including CYP3A4. This inhibition can result in unexpectedly high plasma levels of other drugs which are metabolized by those CYP450 enzymes). Products include:

Niravam Orally Disintegrating Tablets 3106
Xanax XR Tablets 2655

Amitriptyline Hydrochloride (Amiodarone may suppress certain CYP450 enzymes, including CYP1A2. This inhibition can result in unexpectedly high plasma levels of other drugs which are metabolized by those CYP450 enzymes).

No products indexed under this heading.

Amlodipine Besylate (Possible potentiation of bradycardia, sinus arrest, and AV block when co-administered with calcium antagonists). Products include:

Caduet Tablets 2507
Lotrel Capsules 2238
Norvasc Tablets 2529

Amoxapine (Amiodarone may suppress certain CYP450 enzymes, including CYP1A2. This inhibition can result in unexpectedly high plasma levels of other drugs which are metabolized by those CYP450 enzymes).

No products indexed under this heading.

Amphetamine Aspartate (Amiodarone may suppress certain CYP450 enzymes, including CYP2D6. This inhibition can result in unexpectedly high plasma levels of other drugs which are metabolized by those CYP450 enzymes). Products include:

Adderall Tablets 3168
Adderall XR Capsules 3169

Amphetamine Aspartate Monohydrate (Amiodarone may suppress certain CYP450 enzymes, including CYP2D6. This inhibition can result in unexpectedly high plasma levels of other drugs which are metabolized by those CYP450 enzymes).

No products indexed under this heading.

Amphetamine Sulfate (Amiodarone may suppress certain CYP450 enzymes, including CYP2D6. This inhibition can result in unexpectedly high plasma levels of other drugs which are metabolized by those CYP450 enzymes). Products include:

Adderall Tablets 3168
Adderall XR Capsules 3169

Amprenavir (Protease inhibitors are known to inhibit CYP3A4 to varying degrees. Monitoring for amiodarone toxicity and serial measurement of amiodarone serum concentrations during concomitant protease inhibitor therapy should be considered). Products include:

Agenerase Capsules 1299
Agenerase Oral Solution 1304

Anagrelide Hydrochloride (Amiodarone may suppress certain CYP450 enzymes, including CYP1A2. This inhibition can result in unexpectedly high plasma levels of other drugs which are metabolized by those CYP450 enzymes). Products include:

Agrylin Capsules 3172

Anastrozole (Since amiodarone is a substrate for CYP3A4, drugs that inhibit CYP3A4 may decrease the metabolism and increase serum concentration of amiodarone). Products include:

Arimidex Tablets 665

Anisindione (Co-administration results in potentiation of warfarin-type anticoagulant response and can result in serious bleeding). Products include:

Miradon Tablets 3056

Aprepitant (Since amiodarone is a substrate for CYP3A4, drugs that inhibit CYP3A4 may decrease the metabolism and increase serum concentration of amiodarone). Products include:
- Emend Capsules 1944

Astemizole (Amiodarone may suppress certain CYP450 enzymes, including CYP3A4. This inhibition can result in unexpectedly high plasma levels of other drugs which are metabolized by those CYP450 enzymes).
- No products indexed under this heading.

Atenolol (Possible potentiation of bradycardia, sinus arrest, and AV block when co-administered with beta-blocking agents). Products include:
- Tenormin I.V. Injection 698
- Tenormin Tablets 695

Atomoxetine Hydrochloride (Amiodarone may suppress certain CYP450 enzymes, including CYP2D6. This inhibition can result in unexpectedly high plasma levels of other drugs which are metabolized by those CYP450 enzymes). Products include:
- Strattera Capsules 1784

Atorvastatin Calcium (Simvastatin (CYP3A4 substrate) in combination with amiodarone has been associated with reports of myopathy/rhabdomyolysis). Products include:
- Caduet Tablets 2507
- Lipitor Tablets 2495

Azithromycin Dihydrate (Macrolide antibiotics are known to cause QTc prolongation. There have been reports of QTc prolongation in patients taking amiodarone when Macrolide antibiotics were administered concomitantly). Products include:
- Zithromax 2568
- Zithromax for IV Infusion 2573
- Zithromax for Oral Suspension, 300 mg, 600 mg, 900 mg, 1200 mg 2561
- Zithromax Tablets, 250 mg, 500 mg 2561
- Zithromax Tri-Pak 2561
- Zithromax Z-Pak 2568

Belladonna Ergotamine (Amiodarone may suppress certain CYP450 enzymes, including CYP3A4. This inhibition can result in unexpectedly high plasma levels of other drugs which are metabolized by those CYP450 enzymes).
- No products indexed under this heading.

Bepridil Hydrochloride (Possible potentiation of bradycardia, sinus arrest, and AV block when co-administered with calcium antagonists).
- No products indexed under this heading.

Betaxolol Hydrochloride (Possible potentiation of bradycardia, sinus arrest, and AV block when co-administered with beta-blocking agents). Products include:
- Betoptic S Ophthalmic Suspension 554

Bisoprolol Fumarate (Possible potentiation of bradycardia, sinus arrest, and AV block when co-administered with beta-blocking agents).
- No products indexed under this heading.

Buspirone Hydrochloride (Amiodarone may suppress certain CYP450 enzymes, including CYP3A4. This inhibition can result in unexpectedly high plasma levels of other drugs which are metabolized by those CYP450 enzymes).
- No products indexed under this heading.

Busulfan (Amiodarone may suppress certain CYP450 enzymes, including CYP3A4. This inhibition can result in unexpectedly high plasma levels of other drugs which are metabolized by those CYP450 enzymes). Products include:
- I.V. Busulfex 1125
- Myleran Tablets 1492

Caffeine (Amiodarone may suppress certain CYP450 enzymes, including CYP1A2. This inhibition can result in unexpectedly high plasma levels of other drugs which are metabolized by those CYP450 enzymes). Products include:
- Athena Hair System Shampoo ..... ▣767
- BC Powder ..... ▣612
- Arthritis Strength BC Powder ..... ▣612
- Goody's Extra Strength Headache Powder ..... ▣621
- Goody's Extra Strength Pain Relief Tablets ..... ▣621
- Hycomine Compound Tablets 1105
- Spartan Hair System Shampoo ..... ▣767
- Vivarin ..... ▣639

Caffeine Anhydrous (Amiodarone may suppress certain CYP450 enzymes, including CYP1A2. This inhibition can result in unexpectedly high plasma levels of other drugs which are metabolized by those CYP450 enzymes).
- No products indexed under this heading.

Candesartan Cilexetil (Amiodarone may suppress certain CYP450 enzymes, including CYP2Cp. This inhibition can result in unexpectedly high plasma levels of other drugs which are metabolized by those CYP450 enzymes). Products include:
- Atacand Tablets 634
- Atacand HCT 637

Captopril (Amiodarone may suppress certain CYP450 enzymes, including CYP2D6. This inhibition can result in unexpectedly high plasma levels of other drugs which are metabolized by those CYP450 enzymes). Products include:
- Captopril Tablets 2114

Carbamazepine (Amiodarone may suppress certain CYP450 enzymes, including CYP3A4. This inhibition can result in unexpectedly high plasma levels of other drugs which are metabolized by those CYP450 enzymes). Products include:
- Carbatrol Capsules 3174
- Equetro Extended-Release Capsules 3178
- Tegretol/Tegretol-XR 2278

Carteolol Hydrochloride (Possible potentiation of bradycardia, sinus arrest, and AV block when co-administered with beta-blocking agents). Products include:
- Carteolol Hydrochloride Ophthalmic Solution USP, 1% ..... ⊙246

Carvedilol (Amiodarone may suppress certain CYP450 enzymes, including CYP2Cp. This inhibition can result in unexpectedly high plasma levels of other drugs which are metabolized by those CYP450 enzymes). Products include:
- Coreg Tablets 1376

Celecoxib (Amiodarone may suppress certain CYP450 enzymes, including CYP2Cp. This inhibition can result in unexpectedly high plasma levels of other drugs which are metabolized by those CYP450 enzymes). Products include:
- Celebrex Capsules 3130

Cerivastatin Sodium (Simvastatin (CYP3A4 substrate) in combination with amiodarone has been associated with reports of myopathy/rhabdomyolysis).
- No products indexed under this heading.

Cevimeline Hydrochloride (Amiodarone may suppress certain CYP450 enzymes, including CYP2D6. This inhibition can result in unexpectedly high plasma levels of other drugs which are metabolized by those CYP450 enzymes). Products include:
- Evoxac Capsules 1042

Chlordiazepoxide (Amiodarone may suppress certain CYP450 enzymes, including CYP1A2. This inhibition can result in unexpectedly high plasma levels of other drugs which are metabolized by those CYP450 enzymes).
- No products indexed under this heading.

Chlordiazepoxide Hydrochloride (Amiodarone may suppress certain CYP450 enzymes, including CYP1A2. This inhibition can result in unexpectedly high plasma levels of other drugs which are metabolized by those CYP450 enzymes). Products include:
- Librium Capsules 3349

Chlorpheniramine (Amiodarone may suppress certain CYP450 enzymes, including CYP3A4. This inhibition can result in unexpectedly high plasma levels of other drugs which are metabolized by those CYP450 enzymes).
- No products indexed under this heading.

Chlorpheniramine Maleate (Amiodarone may suppress certain CYP450 enzymes, including CYP3A4. This inhibition can result in unexpectedly high plasma levels of other drugs which are metabolized by those CYP450 enzymes). Products include:
- Advil Allergy Sinus Caplets ..... ▣737
- Advil Multi-Symptom Cold Caplets ..... ▣738
- BC Allergy Sinus Cold Powder ..... ▣612
- Contac Severe Cold and Flu Caplets Maximum Strength ..... ▣615
- Hycomine Compound Tablets 1105
- PediaCare Multi-Symptom Cold Liquid ..... ▣704
- PediaCare NightRest Cough & Cold Liquid ..... ▣704
- Robitussin Flu Liquid ..... ▣752
- Robitussin PM Cough & Cold Liquid ..... ▣752
- Singlet Caplets ..... ▣636
- Sudafed Sinus & Allergy Tablets ..... ▣710
- TheraFlu Cold & Cough Hot Liquid ..... ▣680
- TheraFlu Cold & Sore Throat Hot Liquid ..... ▣680
- TheraFlu Flu & Sore Throat Hot Liquid ..... ▣681
- TheraFlu Severe Cold & Cough Hot Liquid ..... ▣683
- TheraFlu Severe Cold Caplets ..... ▣679
- TheraFlu Severe Cold Hot Liquid ..... ▣682
- Triaminic Cold & Allergy Liquid ..... ▣685
- Triaminic Cold & Cough Liquid ..... ▣685
- Triaminic Flu, Cough & Fever Liquid ..... ▣685
- Triaminic Night Time Cough & Cold Liquid ..... ▣685
- Triaminic Allergy Runny Nose & Congestion Softchews ..... ▣688
- Triaminic Cold & Cough Softchews ..... ▣688
- Children's Tylenol Plus Cold NightTime Suspension Liquid 1851
- Children's Tylenol Plus Cold & Cough Suspension Liquid and Chewable Tablets 1851
- Children's Tylenol Plus Cold Chewable Tablets 1851
- Children's Tylenol Plus Flu Suspension Liquid 1853
- Tylenol Allergy Complete Multi-Symptom Caplets and Gelcaps with Cool Burst 1844
- Multi-Symptom Tylenol Cold Night Time Caplets 1845
- Vicks 44M Cough, Cold & Flu Relief 2676
- Pediatric Vicks 44m Cough & Cold Relief 2673
- Children's Vicks NyQuil Cold/Cough Relief 2671

Chlorpheniramine Polistirex (Amiodarone may suppress certain CYP450 enzymes, including CYP3A4. This inhibition can result in unexpectedly high plasma levels of other drugs which are metabolized by those CYP450 enzymes). Products include:
- Tussionex Pennkinetic Extended-Release Suspension 3322

Chlorpheniramine Tannate (Amiodarone may suppress certain CYP450 enzymes, including CYP3A4. This inhibition can result in unexpectedly high plasma levels of other drugs which are metabolized by those CYP450 enzymes).
- No products indexed under this heading.

Chlorpromazine (Amiodarone may suppress certain CYP450 enzymes, including CYP2D6. This inhibition can result in unexpectedly high plasma levels of other drugs which are metabolized by those CYP450 enzymes).
- No products indexed under this heading.

Chlorpromazine Hydrochloride (Amiodarone may suppress certain CYP450 enzymes, including CYP2D6. This inhibition can result in unexpectedly high plasma levels of other drugs which are metabolized by those CYP450 enzymes).
- No products indexed under this heading.

Chlorpropamide (Amiodarone may suppress certain CYP450 enzymes, including CYP2Cp. This inhibition can result in unexpectedly high plasma levels of other drugs which are metabolized by those CYP450 enzymes).
- No products indexed under this heading.

Cimetidine (Since amiodarone is a substrate for CYP3A4, drugs that inhibit CYP3A4 may decrease the metabolism and increase serum concentration of amiodarone). Products include:
- Tagamet HB 200 Tablets ..... ▣637
- Tagamet Tablets 1547

Cimetidine Hydrochloride (Since amiodarone is a substrate for CYP3A4, drugs that inhibit CYP3A4 may decrease the metabolism and increase serum concentration of amiodarone).
- No products indexed under this heading.

Ciprofloxacin (Fluoroquinolones are known to cause QTc prolonga-

tion. There have been reports of QTc prolongation in patients taking amiodarone when fluoroquinolones were administered concomitantly).
Products include:
Cipro I.V. 2998
Cipro I.V. Pharmacy Bulk Package 3509
Cipro Oral Suspension 2991
Cipro XR Tablets 3004
Ciprodex Otic Suspension 555

Ciprofloxacin Hydrochloride (Fluoroquinolones are known to cause QTc prolongation. There have been reports of QTc prolongation in patients taking amiodarone when fluoroquinolones were administered concomitantly). Products include:
Ciloxan Ophthalmic Ointment 554
Cipro Tablets 2991

Cisapride (Amiodarone may suppress certain CYP450 enzymes, including CYP3A4. This inhibition can result in unexpectedly high plasma levels of other drugs which are metabolized by those CYP450 enzymes).
No products indexed under this heading.

Clarithromycin (Macrolide antibiotics are known to cause QTc prolongation. There have been reports of QTc prolongation in patients taking amiodarone when Macrolide antibiotics were administered concomitantly). Products include:
Biaxin/Biaxin XL 402
PREVPAC 3281

Clomipramine Hydrochloride (Amiodarone may suppress certain CYP450 enzymes, including CYP1A2. This inhibition can result in unexpectedly high plasma levels of other drugs which are metabolized by those CYP450 enzymes).
No products indexed under this heading.

Clopidogrel Bisulfate (Amiodarone may suppress certain CYP450 enzymes, including CYP1A2. This inhibition can result in unexpectedly high plasma levels of other drugs which are metabolized by those CYP450 enzymes). Products include:
Plavix Tablets 940
Plavix Tablets 2942

Clotrimazole (azoles are known to cause QTc prolongation. There have been reports of QTc prolongation in patients taking amiodarone when azoles were administered concomitantly). Products include:
Lotrimin 3053
Lotrisone 3054

Clozapine (Amiodarone may suppress certain CYP450 enzymes, including CYP1A2. This inhibition can result in unexpectedly high plasma levels of other drugs which are metabolized by those CYP450 enzymes). Products include:
Clozapine Tablets 2141
Clozaril Tablets 2174
FazaClo Orally Disintegrating Tablets 547

Codeine Phosphate (Amiodarone may suppress certain CYP450 enzymes, including CYP2D6. This inhibition can result in unexpectedly high plasma levels of other drugs which are metabolized by those CYP450 enzymes). Products include:
Tylenol with Codeine 2461

Codeine Sulfate (Amiodarone may suppress certain CYP450 enzymes, including CYP2D6. This inhibition can result in unexpectedly high plasma levels of other drugs which are metabolized by those CYP450 enzymes).
No products indexed under this heading.

Cyclobenzaprine (Amiodarone may suppress certain CYP450 enzymes, including CYP1A2. This inhibition can result in unexpectedly high plasma levels of other drugs which are metabolized by those CYP450 enzymes).
No products indexed under this heading.

Cyclobenzaprine Hydrochloride (Amiodarone may suppress certain CYP450 enzymes, including CYP1A2. This inhibition can result in unexpectedly high plasma levels of other drugs which are metabolized by those CYP450 enzymes).
Products include:
Flexeril Tablets 1832

Cyclosporine (Co-administration has been reported to produce persistently elevated plasma concentrations of cyclosporine resulting in elevated creatinine, despite reduction in dose of cyclosporine).
Products include:
Gengraf Capsules 458
Neoral Soft Gelatin Capsules 2247
Neoral Oral Solution 2247
Restasis Ophthalmic Emulsion 570
Sandimmune 2259

Dalfopristin (Since amiodarone is a substrate for CYP3A4, drugs that inhibit CYP3A4 may decrease the metabolism and increase serum concentration of amiodarone). Products include:
Synercid I.V. 1690

Danazol (Since amiodarone is a substrate for CYP3A4, drugs that inhibit CYP3A4 may decrease the metabolism and increase serum concentration of amiodarone).
No products indexed under this heading.

Delavirdine Mesylate (Since amiodarone is a substrate for CYP3A4, drugs that inhibit CYP3A4 may decrease the metabolism and increase serum concentration of amiodarone). Products include:
Rescriptor Tablets 2535

Desipramine Hydrochloride (Amiodarone may suppress certain CYP450 enzymes, including CYP1A2. This inhibition can result in unexpectedly high plasma levels of other drugs which are metabolized by those CYP450 enzymes).
No products indexed under this heading.

Deslanoside (Co-administration of amiodarone to patients receiving digitalis therapy regularly results in an increase in the serum digoxin concentration that may reach toxic levels with resultant toxicity).
No products indexed under this heading.

Desogestrel (Amiodarone may suppress certain CYP450 enzymes, including CYP2Cp. This inhibition can result in unexpectedly high plasma levels of other drugs which are metabolized by those CYP450 enzymes). Products include:
Ortho-Cept Tablets 2395

Dexfenfluramine Hydrochloride (Amiodarone may suppress certain CYP450 enzymes, including CYP2D6. This inhibition can result in unexpectedly high plasma levels of other drugs which are metabolized by those CYP450 enzymes).
No products indexed under this heading.

Dextromethorphan (Amiodarone may suppress certain CYP450 enzymes, including CYP2Cp. This inhibition can result in unexpectedly high plasma levels of other drugs which are metabolized by those CYP450 enzymes).
No products indexed under this heading.

Dextromethorphan Hydrobromide (Amiodarone may suppress certain CYP450 enzymes, including CYP2D6. This inhibition can result in unexpectedly high plasma levels of other drugs which are metabolized by those CYP450 enzymes).
Products include:
Alacol DM Syrup 739
Balamine DM 739
Contac Severe Cold and Flu Caplets Maximum Strength ▣ 615
Contac Severe Cold and Flu Caplets Non-Drowsy ▣ 615
Children's Dimetapp DM Cold & Cough Elixir ▣ 745
Children's Dimetapp Long Acting Cough Plus Cold Syrup ▣ 746
Dimetapp Infant Drops Decongestant Plus Cough ▣ 746
Mucinex DM Tablets ▣ 602
PediaCare Decongestant & Cough Infant Drops ▣ 705
PediaCare Freezer Pops Long-Acting Cough-Glacier Grape and Polar Berry Blue ▣ 706
PediaCare Long-Acting Cough Infant Drops ▣ 705
PediaCare Long-Acting Cough Plus Cold Liquid ▣ 704
PediaCare Multi-Symptom Cold Liquid ▣ 704
PediaCare NightRest Cough & Cold Liquid ▣ 704
Robitussin Allergy & Cough Syrup ▣ 750
Robitussin CF Liquid ▣ 755
Robitussin Cough & Cold Liquid-filled Capsules ▣ 750
Robitussin Cough, Cold & Flu Liquid-filled Capsules ▣ 750
Robitussin Cough & Cold Infant Drops ▣ 755
Robitussin DM Infant Drops ▣ 753
Robitussin DM Liquid ▣ 753
Robitussin Flu Liquid ▣ 752
Robitussin Maximum Strength Cough Liquid ▣ 754
Robitussin Maximum Strength Cough & Cold Liquid ▣ 754
Robitussin Pediatric Cough Liquid ▣ 754
Robitussin Pediatric Cough & Cold Liquid ▣ 754
Robitussin PM Cough & Cold Liquid ▣ 752
Robitussin Sugar Free Cough Liquid ▣ 753
Simply Cough Liquid 1840
Sudafed Severe Cold ▣ 710
TheraFlu Cold & Cough Hot Liquid ▣ 680
TheraFlu Flu & Chest Congestion Non-Drowsy Hot Liquid ▣ 681
TheraFlu Severe Cold Non-Drowsy Hot Liquid ▣ 683
TheraFlu Severe Cold & Cough Hot Liquid ▣ 683
TheraFlu Severe Cold Caplets ▣ 679
TheraFlu Severe Cold Hot Liquid ▣ 682
TheraFlu Severe Cold Non-Drowsy Caplets ▣ 679
TheraFlu Thin Strips Long Acting Cough ▣ 684
Triaminic Cold & Cough Liquid ▣ 685
Triaminic Cough Liquid ▣ 687
Triaminic Cough & Nasal Congestion Liquid ▣ 687
Triaminic Cough & Sore Throat Liquid ▣ 687
Triaminic Flu, Cough & Fever Liquid ▣ 685
Triaminic Night Time Cough & Cold Liquid ▣ 685
Triaminic Cold & Cough Softchews ▣ 688
Triaminic Cough & Sore Throat Softchews ▣ 689
Triaminic Thin Strips Long Acting Cough ▣ 689
Children's Tylenol Plus Cold & Cough Suspension Liquid and Chewable Tablets 1851
Children's Tylenol Plus Flu Suspension Liquid 1853
Concentrated Tylenol Infants' Drops Plus Cold and Cough 1851
Tylenol Cold & Flu Severe Daytime Liquid with Cool Bust 1846
Tylenol Cold & Flu Severe NightTime Liquid with Cool Burst 1846
Tylenol Cold Severe Congestion Non-Drowsy Caplets with Cool Burst 1846
Tylenol Cough & Sore Throat Daytime Liquid with Cool Burst 1849
Tylenol Cough & Sore Throat NightTime Liquid with Cool Burst 1849
Tylenol Flu Day Non-Drowsy Gelcaps 1846
Concentrated Tylenol Infants' Drops Plus Cold & Cough Nasal Decongestant, Fever Reducer & Pain Reliever ▣ 668
Multi-Symptom Tylenol Cold Night Time Caplets 1845
Multi-Symptom Tylenol Cold Day Non-Drowsy Caplets and Gelcaps 1845
Vicks 44 Cough Relief 2675
Vicks 44D Cough & Head Congestion Relief 2676
Vicks 44D Cough & Head Congestion Relief Liquid ▣ 721
Vicks 44E Cough & Chest Congestion Relief 2676
Pediatric Vicks 44e Cough & Chest Congestion Relief Liquid 2673
Vicks 44M Cough, Cold & Flu Relief 2676
Pediatric Vicks 44m Cough & Cold Relief 2673
Vicks DayQuil LiquiCaps/Liquid Multi-Symptom Cold/Flu Relief ▣ 723
Vicks DayQuil Multi-Symptom Cold/Flu Relief LiquiCaps 2675
Vicks DayQuil Multi-Symptom Cold/Flu Relief Liquid 2675
Children's Vicks NyQuil Cold/Cough Relief 2671
Vicks NyQuil Cough Liquid 2677
Vicks NyQuil LiquiCaps 2677
Vicks NyQuil LiquiCaps/Liquid Multi-Symptom Cold/Flu Relief ▣ 725
Vicks NyQuil Liquid 2677
Zicam Concentrated Cough Mist for Kids Cool Cherry ▣ 643
Zicam Concentrated Cough Mist for Kids Plus D Cool Cherry ▣ 643
Zicam Concentrated Cough Mist Nite-Cool Cherry ▣ 642
Zicam Concentrated Cough Mist Plus D Cool Cherry ▣ 642
Zicam Concentrated Cough Mist-Honey Lemon & Cool Cherry ▣ 642

Dextromethorphan Polistirex (Amiodarone may suppress certain CYP450 enzymes, including CYP2D6. This inhibition can result in unexpectedly high plasma levels of other drugs which are metabolized by those CYP450 enzymes).
Products include:
Delsym Extended-Release Suspension ▣ 611
Delsym 12 Hour Cough Suppressant for Children ▣ 611

Diazepam (Amiodarone may suppress certain CYP450 enzymes,

including CYP1A2. This inhibition can result in unexpectedly high plasma levels of other drugs which are metabolized by those CYP450 enzymes). Products include:

Diastat Rectal Delivery System **3344**
Valium Tablets **2822**

Diclofenac Potassium (Amiodarone may suppress certain CYP450 enzymes, including CYP2Cp. This inhibition can result in unexpectedly high plasma levels of other drugs which are metabolized by those CYP450 enzymes). Products include:

Cataflam Tablets **2173**

Diclofenac Sodium (Amiodarone may suppress certain CYP450 enzymes, including CYP2Cp. This inhibition can result in unexpectedly high plasma levels of other drugs which are metabolized by those CYP450 enzymes). Products include:

Arthrotec Tablets **3126**
Voltaren Ophthalmic Solution **2300**
Voltaren Tablets **2298**
Voltaren-XR Tablets **2301**

Dicumarol (Co-administration results in potentiation of warfarin-type anticoagulant response and can result in serious bleeding).

No products indexed under this heading.

Digitalis Glycoside Preparations (Co-administration of amiodarone to patients receiving digitalis therapy regularly results in an increase in the serum digoxin concentration that may reach toxic levels with resultant toxicity).

No products indexed under this heading.

Digitoxin (Co-administration of amiodarone to patients receiving digitalis therapy regularly results in an increase in the serum digoxin concentration that may reach toxic levels with resultant toxicity).

No products indexed under this heading.

Digoxin (Co-administration of amiodarone to patients receiving digitalis therapy regularly results in an increase in the serum digoxin concentration that may reach toxic levels with resultant toxicity). Products include:

Digitek Tablets **2146**
Lanoxicaps Capsules **1458**
Lanoxin Injection **1462**
Lanoxin Tablets **1468**
Lanoxin Injection Pediatric **1465**

Dihydroergotamine Mesylate (Amiodarone may suppress certain CYP450 enzymes, including CYP3A4. This inhibition can result in unexpectedly high plasma levels of other drugs which are metabolized by those CYP450 enzymes). Products include:

Migranal Nasal Spray **3350**

Diltiazem Hydrochloride (Possible potentiation of bradycardia, sinus arrest, and AV block when co-administered with calcium antagonists). Products include:

Cardizem LA Extended Release Tablets **1699**
Tiazac Capsules **1204**

Diltiazem Maleate (Since amiodarone is a substrate for CYP3A4, drugs that inhibit CYP3A4 may decrease the metabolism and increase serum concentration of amiodarone).

No products indexed under this heading.

Dirithromycin (Macrolide antibiotics are known to cause QTc prolongation. There have been reports of QTc prolongation in patients taking amiodarone when Macrolide antibiotics were administered concomitantly).

No products indexed under this heading.

Disopyramide (Amiodarone may suppress certain CYP450 enzymes, including CYP3A4. This inhibition can result in unexpectedly high plasma levels of other drugs which are metabolized by those CYP450 enzymes).

No products indexed under this heading.

Disopyramide Phosphate (Amiodarone may suppress certain CYP450 enzymes, including CYP3A4. This inhibition can result in unexpectedly high plasma levels of other drugs which are metabolized by those CYP450 enzymes).

No products indexed under this heading.

Disulfiram (Amiodarone may suppress certain CYP450 enzymes, including CYP3A4. This inhibition can result in unexpectedly high plasma levels of other drugs which are metabolized by those CYP450 enzymes). Products include:

Antabuse Tablets **2343**

Dolasetron Mesylate (Amiodarone may suppress certain CYP450 enzymes, including CYP2D6. This inhibition can result in unexpectedly high plasma levels of other drugs which are metabolized by those CYP450 enzymes). Products include:

Anzemet Injection **2871**
Anzemet Tablets **2874**

Donepezil Hydrochloride (Amiodarone may suppress certain CYP450 enzymes, including CYP2D6. This inhibition can result in unexpectedly high plasma levels of other drugs which are metabolized by those CYP450 enzymes). Products include:

Aricept Tablets **1086**
Aricept ODT Tablets **1086**

Doxepin Hydrochloride (Amiodarone may suppress certain CYP450 enzymes, including CYP1A2. This inhibition can result in unexpectedly high plasma levels of other drugs which are metabolized by those CYP450 enzymes).

No products indexed under this heading.

Doxorubicin Hydrochloride (Amiodarone may suppress certain CYP450 enzymes, including CYP3A4. This inhibition can result in unexpectedly high plasma levels of other drugs which are metabolized by those CYP450 enzymes). Products include:

Adriamycin for Injection, USP **786**
Adriamycin Injection, USP **786**

Dronabinol (Amiodarone may suppress certain CYP450 enzymes, including CYP2Cp. This inhibition can result in unexpectedly high plasma levels of other drugs which are metabolized by those CYP450 enzymes). Products include:

Marinol Capsules **3334**

Efavirenz (Since amiodarone is a substrate for CYP3A4, drugs that inhibit CYP3A4 may decrease the metabolism and increase serum concentration of amiodarone). Products include:

Sustiva Capsules **957**

Encainide Hydrochloride (Amiodarone may suppress certain CYP450 enzymes, including CYP2D6. This inhibition can result in unexpectedly high plasma levels of other drugs which are metabolized by those CYP450 enzymes).

No products indexed under this heading.

Enoxacin (Fluoroquinolones are known to cause QTc prolongation. There have been reports of QTc prolongation in patients taking amiodarone when fluoroquinolones were administered concomitantly).

No products indexed under this heading.

Eprosartan Mesylate (Amiodarone may suppress certain CYP450 enzymes, including CYP2Cp. This inhibition can result in unexpectedly high plasma levels of other drugs which are metabolized by those CYP450 enzymes). Products include:

Teveten Tablets **1707**
Teveten HCT Tablets **1710**

Ergotamine Tartrate (Amiodarone may suppress certain CYP450 enzymes, including CYP3A4. This inhibition can result in unexpectedly high plasma levels of other drugs which are metabolized by those CYP450 enzymes).

No products indexed under this heading.

Erythromycin (Macrolide antibiotics are known to cause QTc prolongation. There have been reports of QTc prolongation in patients taking amiodarone when Macrolide antibiotics were administered concomitantly). Products include:

Erygel Topical Gel **2096**
Ery-Tab Tablets **447**
Erythromycin Base Filmtab Tablets **454**
Erythromycin Delayed-Release Capsules, USP **456**
PCE Dispertab Tablets **510**

Erythromycin Estolate (Macrolide antibiotics are known to cause QTc prolongation. There have been reports of QTc prolongation in patients taking amiodarone when Macrolide antibiotics were administered concomitantly).

No products indexed under this heading.

Erythromycin Ethylsuccinate (Macrolide antibiotics are known to cause QTc prolongation. There have been reports of QTc prolongation in patients taking amiodarone when Macrolide antibiotics were administered concomitantly). Products include:

E.E.S. **449**
EryPed **445**

Erythromycin Gluceptate (Macrolide antibiotics are known to cause QTc prolongation. There have been reports of QTc prolongation in patients taking amiodarone when Macrolide antibiotics were administered concomitantly).

No products indexed under this heading.

Erythromycin Lactobionate (Since amiodarone is a substrate for CYP3A4, drugs that inhibit CYP3A4 may decrease the metabolism and increase serum concentration of amiodarone).

No products indexed under this heading.

Erythromycin Stearate (Macrolide antibiotics are known to cause QTc prolongation. There have been reports of QTc prolongation in patients taking amiodarone when Macrolide antibiotics were administered concomitantly). Products include:

Erythrocin Stearate Filmtab Tablets **452**

Esmolol Hydrochloride (Possible potentiation of bradycardia, sinus arrest, and AV block when co-administered with beta-blocking agents). Products include:

Brevibloc Concentrate **766**
Brevibloc Injection **766**
Brevibloc Double Strength Injection **766**
Brevibloc Premixed Injection **766**
Brevibloc Double Strength Premixed Injection **766**

Esomeprazole Magnesium (Since amiodarone is a substrate for CYP3A4, drugs that inhibit CYP3A4 may decrease the metabolism and increase serum concentration of amiodarone). Products include:

Nexium Delayed-Release Capsules **645**

Estradiol (Amiodarone may suppress certain CYP450 enzymes, including CYP1A2. This inhibition can result in unexpectedly high plasma levels of other drugs which are metabolized by those CYP450 enzymes). Products include:

Activella Tablets **2311**
Climara Transdermal System **795**
Climara Pro Transdermal System **800**
CombiPatch Transdermal System **2180**
Estrogel 0.06% **3200**
Menostar Transdermal System **805**
Prefest Tablets **1069**
Vagifem Tablets **2340**
Vivelle Transdermal System **2288**
Vivelle-Dot Transdermal System **2293**

Estradiol Benzoate (Amiodarone may suppress certain CYP450 enzymes, including CYP1A2. This inhibition can result in unexpectedly high plasma levels of other drugs which are metabolized by those CYP450 enzymes).

No products indexed under this heading.

Estradiol Cypionate (Amiodarone may suppress certain CYP450 enzymes, including CYP1A2. This inhibition can result in unexpectedly high plasma levels of other drugs which are metabolized by those CYP450 enzymes).

No products indexed under this heading.

Estradiol Valerate (Amiodarone may suppress certain CYP450 enzymes, including CYP3A4. This inhibition can result in unexpectedly high plasma levels of other drugs which are metabolized by those CYP450 enzymes).

No products indexed under this heading.

Ethinyl Estradiol (Amiodarone may suppress certain CYP450 enzymes, including CYP3A4. This inhibition can result in unexpectedly high plasma levels of other drugs which are metabolized by those CYP450 enzymes). Products include:

Alesse-28 Tablets 3392
Lo/Ovral-28 Tablets 3423
NuvaRing 2357
Ortho-Cept Tablets 2395
Ortho-Cyclen/Ortho Tri-Cyclen 2414
Ortho Evra Transdermal System 2402
Ortho Tri-Cyclen Lo Tablets 2421
Seasonale Tablets 1073
Triphasil-28 Tablets 3483
Yasmin 28 Tablets 818

Ethosuximide (Amiodarone may suppress certain CYP450 enzymes, including CYP3A4. This inhibition can result in unexpectedly high plasma levels of other drugs which are metabolized by those CYP450 enzymes).
No products indexed under this heading.

Ethynodiol Diacetate (Amiodarone may suppress certain CYP450 enzymes, including CYP3A4. This inhibition can result in unexpectedly high plasma levels of other drugs which are metabolized by those CYP450 enzymes).
No products indexed under this heading.

Etodolac (Amiodarone may suppress certain CYP450 enzymes, including CYP2Cp. This inhibition can result in unexpectedly high plasma levels of other drugs which are metabolized by those CYP450 enzymes).
No products indexed under this heading.

Etoposide (Amiodarone may suppress certain CYP450 enzymes, including CYP3A4. This inhibition can result in unexpectedly high plasma levels of other drugs which are metabolized by those CYP450 enzymes).
No products indexed under this heading.

Etoposide Phosphate (Amiodarone may suppress certain CYP450 enzymes, including CYP3A4. This inhibition can result in unexpectedly high plasma levels of other drugs which are metabolized by those CYP450 enzymes).
No products indexed under this heading.

Felodipine (Possible potentiation of bradycardia, sinus arrest, and AV block when co-administered with calcium antagonists). Products include:
Plendil Extended-Release Tablets 651

Fenoprofen Calcium (Amiodarone may suppress certain CYP450 enzymes, including CYP2Cp. This inhibition can result in unexpectedly high plasma levels of other drugs which are metabolized by those CYP450 enzymes). Products include:
Nalfon Capsules 2504

Fentanyl (Amiodarone may suppress certain CYP450 enzymes, including CYP2D6. This inhibition can result in unexpectedly high plasma levels of other drugs which are metabolized by those CYP450 enzymes). Products include:
Duragesic Transdermal System 2448

Fentanyl Citrate (Amiodarone may suppress certain CYP450 enzymes, including CYP2D6. This inhibition can result in unexpectedly high plasma levels of other drugs which are metabolized by those CYP450 enzymes). Products include:
Actiq 993

Flecainide Acetate (Amiodarone may suppress certain CYP450 enzymes, including CYP2D6. This inhibition can result in unexpectedly high plasma levels of other drugs which are metabolized by those CYP450 enzymes). Products include:
Tambocor Tablets 1824

Fluconazole (azoles are known to cause QTc prolongation. There have been reports of QTc prolongation in patients taking amiodarone when azoles were administered concomitantly).
No products indexed under this heading.

Fluoxetine (Amiodarone may suppress certain CYP450 enzymes, including CYP2D6. This inhibition can result in unexpectedly high plasma levels of other drugs which are metabolized by those CYP450 enzymes).
No products indexed under this heading.

Fluoxetine Hydrochloride (Since amiodarone is a substrate for CYP3A4, drugs that inhibit CYP3A4 may decrease the metabolism and increase serum concentration of amiodarone). Products include:
Prozac Pulvules and Liquid 1771
Symbyax Capsules 1788

Fluphenazine Decanoate (Amiodarone may suppress certain CYP450 enzymes, including CYP2D6. This inhibition can result in unexpectedly high plasma levels of other drugs which are metabolized by those CYP450 enzymes).
No products indexed under this heading.

Fluphenazine Enanthate (Amiodarone may suppress certain CYP450 enzymes, including CYP2D6. This inhibition can result in unexpectedly high plasma levels of other drugs which are metabolized by those CYP450 enzymes).
No products indexed under this heading.

Fluphenazine Hydrochloride (Amiodarone may suppress certain CYP450 enzymes, including CYP2D6. This inhibition can result in unexpectedly high plasma levels of other drugs which are metabolized by those CYP450 enzymes).
No products indexed under this heading.

Flurbiprofen (Amiodarone may suppress certain CYP450 enzymes, including CYP2Cp. This inhibition can result in unexpectedly high plasma levels of other drugs which are metabolized by those CYP450 enzymes).
No products indexed under this heading.

Flurbiprofen Sodium (Amiodarone may suppress certain CYP450 enzymes, including CYP2Cp. This inhibition can result in unexpectedly high plasma levels of other drugs which are metabolized by those CYP450 enzymes). Products include:
Ocufen Ophthalmic Solution .... ⊙230

Flutamide (Amiodarone may suppress certain CYP450 enzymes, including CYP1A2. This inhibition can result in unexpectedly high plasma levels of other drugs which are metabolized by those CYP450 enzymes). Products include:
Eulexin Capsules 3023

Fluticasone Propionate (Amiodarone may suppress certain CYP450 enzymes, including CYP1A2. This inhibition can result in unexpectedly high plasma levels of other drugs which are metabolized by those CYP450 enzymes).
Products include:
Advair Diskus 100/50 1291
Advair Diskus 250/50 1291
Advair Diskus 500/50 1291
Cutivate Cream 1381
Cutivate Lotion 0.05% 1383
Cutivate Ointment 1384
Flonase Nasal Spray 1412
Flovent Diskus 100 mcg 1418
Flovent Diskus 50 mcg 1415

Fluvastatin Sodium (Simvastatin (CYP3A4 substrate) in combination with amiodarone has been associated with reports of myopathy/rhabdomyolysis). Products include:
Lescol Capsules 2227
Lescol 2730
Lescol XL Tablets 2227

Fluvoxamine Maleate (Since amiodarone is a substrate for CYP3A4, drugs that inhibit CYP3A4 may decrease the metabolism and increase serum concentration of amiodarone).
No products indexed under this heading.

Formoterol Fumarate (Amiodarone may suppress certain CYP450 enzymes, including CYP2D6. This inhibition can result in unexpectedly high plasma levels of other drugs which are metabolized by those CYP450 enzymes).
Products include:
Foradil Aerolizer 3024

Fosamprenavir Calcium (Since amiodarone is a substrate for CYP3A4, drugs that inhibit CYP3A4 may decrease the metabolism and increase serum concentration of amiodarone). Products include:
Lexiva Tablets 1473

Fosphenytoin Sodium (Co-administration has resulted in increased steady-state levels of phenytoin).
No products indexed under this heading.

Galantamine Hydrobromide (Amiodarone may suppress certain CYP450 enzymes, including CYP2D6. This inhibition can result in unexpectedly high plasma levels of other drugs which are metabolized by those CYP450 enzymes).
Products include:
Razadyne ER Extended-Release Capsules 2434
Razadyne 2434

Glimepiride (Amiodarone may suppress certain CYP450 enzymes, including CYP2Cp. This inhibition can result in unexpectedly high plasma levels of other drugs which are metabolized by those CYP450 enzymes). Products include:
Amaryl Tablets 2864

Glipizide (Amiodarone may suppress certain CYP450 enzymes, including CYP2Cp. This inhibition can result in unexpectedly high plasma levels of other drugs which are metabolized by those CYP450 enzymes).
No products indexed under this heading.

Grepafloxacin Hydrochloride (Fluoroquinolones are known to cause QTc prolongation. There have been reports of QTc prolongation in patients taking amiodarone when fluoroquinolones were administered concomitantly).
No products indexed under this heading.

Haloperidol (Amiodarone may suppress certain CYP450 enzymes, including CYP1A2. This inhibition can result in unexpectedly high plasma levels of other drugs which are metabolized by those CYP450 enzymes).
No products indexed under this heading.

Haloperidol Decanoate (Amiodarone may suppress certain CYP450 enzymes, including CYP1A2. This inhibition can result in unexpectedly high plasma levels of other drugs which are metabolized by those CYP450 enzymes).
No products indexed under this heading.

Haloperidol Lactate (Amiodarone may suppress certain CYP450 enzymes, including CYP1A2. This inhibition can result in unexpectedly high plasma levels of other drugs which are metabolized by those CYP450 enzymes).
No products indexed under this heading.

Hydrocodone Bitartrate (Amiodarone may suppress certain CYP450 enzymes, including CYP2D6. This inhibition can result in unexpectedly high plasma levels of other drugs which are metabolized by those CYP450 enzymes).
Products include:
Hycodan 1104
Hycomine Compound Tablets 1105
Hycotuss Expectorant Syrup 1106
Lortab 3315
Lortab Elixir 3312
Vicodin Tablets 530
Vicodin ES Tablets 531
Vicodin HP Tablets 532
Vicoprofen Tablets 533
Zydone Tablets 1118

Ibuprofen (Amiodarone may suppress certain CYP450 enzymes, including CYP2Cp. This inhibition can result in unexpectedly high plasma levels of other drugs which are metabolized by those CYP450 enzymes). Products include:
Advil Allergy Sinus Caplets .... ▣737
Advil .... ▣737
Children's Advil Suspension .... ▣742
Children's Advil Chewable Tablets .... ▣741
Advil Cold & Sinus .... ▣739
Advil Flu & Body Ache Caplets .... ▣739
Children's Advil Cold Suspension .... ▣741
Infants' Advil Concentrated Drops .... ▣743
Junior Strength Advil Swallow Tablets .... ▣740
Advil Migraine Liquigels .... ▣740
Advil Multi-Symptom Cold Caplets .... ▣738
Combunox Tablets 1183
Children's Motrin Oral Suspension and Chewable Tablets 1837
Children's Motrin Cold Non-Staining Dye-Free Oral Suspension 1838
Children's Motrin Cold Oral Suspension 1838
Children's Motrin Non-Staining Dye-Free Oral Suspension 1837
Motrin Cold & Sinus Caplets 1836
Motrin IB Tablets and Caplets 1836
Infants' Motrin Concentrated Drops 1837
Infants' Motrin Non-Staining Dye-Free Drops 1837

Junior Strength Motrin Caplets and Chewable Tablets 1837
Vicoprofen Tablets 533

Imipramine Hydrochloride (Amiodarone may suppress certain CYP450 enzymes, including CYP1A2. This inhibition can result in unexpectedly high plasma levels of other drugs which are metabolized by those CYP450 enzymes).
No products indexed under this heading.

Imipramine Pamoate (Amiodarone may suppress certain CYP450 enzymes, including CYP1A2. This inhibition can result in unexpectedly high plasma levels of other drugs which are metabolized by those CYP450 enzymes).
No products indexed under this heading.

Indinavir Sulfate (Protease inhibitors are known to inhibit CYP3A4 to varying degrees. Monitoring for amiodarone toxicity and serial measurement of amiodarone serum concentrations during concomitant protease inhibitor therapy should be considered). Products include:
Crixivan Capsules 1918

Indomethacin (Amiodarone may suppress certain CYP450 enzymes, including CYP2Cp. This inhibition can result in unexpectedly high plasma levels of other drugs which are metabolized by those CYP450 enzymes). Products include:
Indocin 1968

Indomethacin Sodium Trihydrate (Amiodarone may suppress certain CYP450 enzymes, including CYP2Cp. This inhibition can result in unexpectedly high plasma levels of other drugs which are metabolized by those CYP450 enzymes).
Products include:
Indocin I.V. 1973

Indoramin Hydrochloride (Amiodarone may suppress certain CYP450 enzymes, including CYP2D6. This inhibition can result in unexpectedly high plasma levels of other drugs which are metabolized by those CYP450 enzymes).
No products indexed under this heading.

Irbesartan (Amiodarone may suppress certain CYP450 enzymes, including CYP2Cp. This inhibition can result in unexpectedly high plasma levels of other drugs which are metabolized by those CYP450 enzymes). Products include:
Avalide Tablets 922
Avalide Tablets 2889
Avapro Tablets 925
Avapro Tablets 2886

Isoniazid (Since amiodarone is a substrate for CYP3A4, drugs that inhibit CYP3A4 may decrease the metabolism and increase serum concentration of amiodarone).
No products indexed under this heading.

Isradipine (Possible potentiation of bradycardia, sinus arrest, and AV block when co-administered with calcium antagonists). Products include:
DynaCirc CR Tablets 2726

Itraconazole (azoles are known to cause QTc prolongation. There have been reports of QTc prolongation in patients taking amiodarone when azoles were administered concomitantly).
No products indexed under this heading.

Ketoconazole (azoles are known to cause QTc prolongation. There have been reports of QTc prolongation in patients taking amiodarone when azoles were administered concomitantly). Products include:
Nizoral A-D Shampoo, 1% 1839
Nizoral 2% Shampoo 1838

Ketoprofen (Amiodarone may suppress certain CYP450 enzymes, including CYP2Cp. This inhibition can result in unexpectedly high plasma levels of other drugs which are metabolized by those CYP450 enzymes).
No products indexed under this heading.

Ketorolac Tromethamine (Amiodarone may suppress certain CYP450 enzymes, including CYP2Cp. This inhibition can result in unexpectedly high plasma levels of other drugs which are metabolized by those CYP450 enzymes).
Products include:
Acular Ophthalmic Solution 561
Acular LS Ophthalmic Solution 562

Labetalol Hydrochloride (Possible potentiation of bradycardia, sinus arrest, and AV block when co-administered with beta-blocking agents).
No products indexed under this heading.

Lansoprazole (Amiodarone may suppress certain CYP450 enzymes, including CYP2Cp. This inhibition can result in unexpectedly high plasma levels of other drugs which are metabolized by those CYP450 enzymes). Products include:
Prevacid Delayed-Release Capsules 3268
Prevacid for Delayed-Release Oral Suspension 3268
Prevacid I.V. for Injection 3274
Prevacid NapraPAC 3277
Prevacid SoluTab Delayed-Release Orally Disintegrating Tablets 3268
PREVPAC 3281

Levobunolol Hydrochloride (Possible potentiation of bradycardia, sinus arrest, and AV block when co-administered with beta-blocking agents). Products include:
Betagan Ophthalmic Solution, USP .... ⊙217

Levobupivacaine Hydrochloride (Amiodarone may suppress certain CYP450 enzymes, including CYP1A2. This inhibition can result in unexpectedly high plasma levels of other drugs which are metabolized by those CYP450 enzymes).
No products indexed under this heading.

Levonorgestrel (Amiodarone may suppress certain CYP450 enzymes, including CYP3A4. This inhibition can result in unexpectedly high plasma levels of other drugs which are metabolized by those CYP450 enzymes). Products include:
Alesse-28 Tablets 3392
Climara Pro Transdermal System 800
Mirena Intrauterine System 810
Plan B Tablets 1068
Seasonale Tablets 1073
Triphasil-28 Tablets 3483

Lidocaine (Amiodarone may suppress certain CYP450 enzymes, including CYP2D6. This inhibition can result in unexpectedly high plasma levels of other drugs which are metabolized by those CYP450 enzymes). Products include:
Lidoderm Patch 1107

Lidocaine Hydrochloride (Amiodarone may suppress certain CYP450 enzymes, including CYP2D6. This inhibition can result in unexpectedly high plasma levels of other drugs which are metabolized by those CYP450 enzymes).
No products indexed under this heading.

Lomefloxacin Hydrochloride (Fluoroquinolones are known to cause QTc prolongation. There have been reports of QTc prolongation in patients taking amiodarone when fluoroquinolones were administered concomitantly).
No products indexed under this heading.

Lopinavir (Protease inhibitors are known to inhibit CYP3A4 to varying degrees. Monitoring for amiodarone toxicity and serial measurement of amiodarone serum concentrations during concomitant protease inhibitor therapy should be considered). Products include:
Kaletra 474

Loratadine (Since amiodarone is a substrate for CYP3A4, drugs that inhibit CYP3A4 may decrease the metabolism and increase serum concentration of amiodarone). Products include:
Alavert Allergy & Sinus D-12 Hour Tablets 743
Alavert 743
Children's Claritin 24 Hour Non-Drowsy Allergy Syrup 732
Claritin Non-Drowsy 24 Hour Tablets 731
Non-Drowsy Claritin Hives Relief Tablets 733
Claritin Reditabs 24 Hour Non-Drowsy Tablets 732
Claritin-D Non-Drowsy 12 Hour Tablets 731
Claritin-D Non-Drowsy 24 Hour Tablets 731
Children's Dimetapp ND Non-Drowsy Allergy Syrup 746
Triaminic Allerchews 684

Losartan Potassium (Amiodarone may suppress certain CYP450 enzymes, including CYP2Cp. This inhibition can result in unexpectedly high plasma levels of other drugs which are metabolized by those CYP450 enzymes). Products include:
Cozaar Tablets 1913
Hyzaar 1964

Lovastatin (Simvastatin (CYP3A4 substrate) in combination with amiodarone has been associated with reports of myopathy/rhabdomyolysis). Products include:
Advicor Tablets 1694
Altoprev Extended-Release Tablets 1151
Mevacor Tablets 1996

Maprotiline Hydrochloride (Amiodarone may suppress certain CYP450 enzymes, including CYP1A2. This inhibition can result in unexpectedly high plasma levels of other drugs which are metabolized by those CYP450 enzymes).
No products indexed under this heading.

Meclofenamate Sodium (Amiodarone may suppress certain CYP450 enzymes, including CYP2Cp. This inhibition can result in unexpectedly high plasma levels of other drugs which are metabolized by those CYP450 enzymes).
No products indexed under this heading.

Mefenamic Acid (Amiodarone may suppress certain CYP450 enzymes, including CYP2Cp. This inhibition can result in unexpectedly high plasma levels of other drugs which are metabolized by those CYP450 enzymes).
No products indexed under this heading.

Meloxicam (Amiodarone may suppress certain CYP450 enzymes, including CYP2Cp. This inhibition can result in unexpectedly high plasma levels of other drugs which are metabolized by those CYP450 enzymes). Products include:
Mobic Oral Suspension 893
Mobic Tablets 893

Meperidine Hydrochloride (Amiodarone may suppress certain CYP450 enzymes, including CYP2D6. This inhibition can result in unexpectedly high plasma levels of other drugs which are metabolized by those CYP450 enzymes).
No products indexed under this heading.

Mestranol (Amiodarone may suppress certain CYP450 enzymes, including CYP3A4. This inhibition can result in unexpectedly high plasma levels of other drugs which are metabolized by those CYP450 enzymes).
No products indexed under this heading.

Metformin Hydrochloride (Amiodarone may suppress certain CYP450 enzymes, including CYP2Cp. This inhibition can result in unexpectedly high plasma levels of other drugs which are metabolized by those CYP450 enzymes).
Products include:
ActoPlus Met Tablets 3219
Avandamet Tablets 1343
Fortamet Extended-Release Tablets 1156

Methadone Hydrochloride (Amiodarone may suppress certain CYP450 enzymes, including CYP1A2. This inhibition can result in unexpectedly high plasma levels of other drugs which are metabolized by those CYP450 enzymes).
No products indexed under this heading.

Methamphetamine Hydrochloride (Amiodarone may suppress certain CYP450 enzymes, including CYP2D6. This inhibition can result in unexpectedly high plasma levels of other drugs which are metabolized by those CYP450 enzymes).
Products include:
Desoxyn Tablets, USP 2482

Metipranolol Hydrochloride (Possible potentiation of bradycardia, sinus arrest, and AV block when co-administered with beta-blocking agents).
No products indexed under this heading.

Metoprolol Succinate (Possible potentiation of bradycardia, sinus arrest, and AV block when co-administered with beta-blocking agents). Products include:

Toprol-XL Tablets 660

Metoprolol Tartrate (Possible potentiation of bradycardia, sinus arrest, and AV block when co-administered with beta-blocking agents).
No products indexed under this heading.

Metronidazole (Since amiodarone is a substrate for CYP3A4, drugs that inhibit CYP3A4 may decrease the metabolism and increase serum concentration of amiodarone). Products include:
Metrogel 1% 1212
MetroGel-Vaginal Gel 1822
Noritate Cream, 1% 1051

Metronidazole Benzoate (Since amiodarone is a substrate for CYP3A4, drugs that inhibit CYP3A4 may decrease the metabolism and increase serum concentration of amiodarone).
No products indexed under this heading.

Metronidazole Hydrochloride (Since amiodarone is a substrate for CYP3A4, drugs that inhibit CYP3A4 may decrease the metabolism and increase serum concentration of amiodarone).
No products indexed under this heading.

Mexiletine Hydrochloride (Amiodarone may suppress certain CYP450 enzymes, including CYP1A2. This inhibition can result in unexpectedly high plasma levels of other drugs which are metabolized by those CYP450 enzymes).
No products indexed under this heading.

Mibefradil Dihydrochloride (Possible potentiation of bradycardia, sinus arrest, and AV block when co-administered with calcium antagonists).
No products indexed under this heading.

Miconazole (azoles are known to cause QTc prolongation. There have been reports of QTc prolongation in patients taking amiodarone when azoles were administered concomitantly).
No products indexed under this heading.

Miconazole Nitrate (Since amiodarone is a substrate for CYP3A4, drugs that inhibit CYP3A4 may decrease the metabolism and increase serum concentration of amiodarone). Products include:
Desenex .... ▣ 674
Desenex Jock Itch Spray Powder .... ▣ 674

Midazolam Hydrochloride (Amiodarone may suppress certain CYP450 enzymes, including CYP3A4. This inhibition can result in unexpectedly high plasma levels of other drugs which are metabolized by those CYP450 enzymes).
No products indexed under this heading.

Miglitol (Amiodarone may suppress certain CYP450 enzymes, including CYP2Cp. This inhibition can result in unexpectedly high plasma levels of other drugs which are metabolized by those CYP450 enzymes).
No products indexed under this heading.

Mirtazapine (Amiodarone may suppress certain CYP450 enzymes, including CYP1A2. This inhibition can result in unexpectedly high plasma levels of other drugs which are metabolized by those CYP450 enzymes).
No products indexed under this heading.

Montelukast Sodium (Amiodarone may suppress certain CYP450 enzymes, including CYP2Cp. This inhibition can result in unexpectedly high plasma levels of other drugs which are metabolized by those CYP450 enzymes). Products include:
Singulair 2047

Morphine Sulfate (Amiodarone may suppress certain CYP450 enzymes, including CYP2D6. This inhibition can result in unexpectedly high plasma levels of other drugs which are metabolized by those CYP450 enzymes). Products include:
Avinza Capsules 1714
Kadian Capsules 572
MS Contin Tablets 2703

Moxifloxacin Hydrochloride (Fluoroquinolones are known to cause QTc prolongation. There have been reports of QTc prolongation in patients taking amiodarone when fluoroquinolones were administered concomitantly). Products include:
Avelox 2984
Vigamox Ophthalmic Solution .... ⊙ 560

Nabumetone (Amiodarone may suppress certain CYP450 enzymes, including CYP2Cp. This inhibition can result in unexpectedly high plasma levels of other drugs which are metabolized by those CYP450 enzymes). Products include:
Relafen Tablets 1523

Nadolol (Possible potentiation of bradycardia, sinus arrest, and AV block when co-administered with beta-blocking agents). Products include:
Nadolol Tablets 2121

Nafcillin Sodium (Amiodarone may suppress certain CYP450 enzymes, including CYP1A2. This inhibition can result in unexpectedly high plasma levels of other drugs which are metabolized by those CYP450 enzymes).
No products indexed under this heading.

Naproxen (Amiodarone may suppress certain CYP450 enzymes, including CYP1A2. This inhibition can result in unexpectedly high plasma levels of other drugs which are metabolized by those CYP450 enzymes). Products include:
EC-Naprosyn Delayed-Release Tablets 2769
Naprosyn Suspension 2769
Naprosyn Tablets 2769
Prevacid NapraPAC 3277

Naproxen Sodium (Amiodarone may suppress certain CYP450 enzymes, including CYP1A2. This inhibition can result in unexpectedly high plasma levels of other drugs which are metabolized by those CYP450 enzymes). Products include:
Aleve Tablets, Caplets and Gelcaps .... ▣ 605
Anaprox Tablets 2769
Anaprox DS Tablets 2769

Nateglinide (Amiodarone may suppress certain CYP450 enzymes, including CYP2Cp. This inhibition can result in unexpectedly high plasma levels of other drugs which are metabolized by those CYP450 enzymes). Products include:
Starlix Tablets 2276

Nefazodone Hydrochloride (Since amiodarone is a substrate for CYP3A4, drugs that inhibit CYP3A4 may decrease the metabolism and increase serum concentration of amiodarone).
No products indexed under this heading.

Nelfinavir Mesylate (Protease inhibitors are known to inhibit CYP3A4 to varying degrees. Monitoring for amiodarone toxicity and serial measurement of amiodarone serum concentrations during concomitant protease inhibitor therapy should be considered). Products include:
Viracept 2556

Nevirapine (Since amiodarone is a substrate for CYP3A4, drugs that inhibit CYP3A4 may decrease the metabolism and increase serum concentration of amiodarone). Products include:
Viramune Oral Suspension 903
Viramune Tablets 903

Niacinamide (Since amiodarone is a substrate for CYP3A4, drugs that inhibit CYP3A4 may decrease the metabolism and increase serum concentration of amiodarone).
No products indexed under this heading.

Nicardipine Hydrochloride (Possible potentiation of bradycardia, sinus arrest, and AV block when co-administered with calcium antagonists). Products include:
Cardene I.V. 1129

Nicotinamide (Since amiodarone is a substrate for CYP3A4, drugs that inhibit CYP3A4 may decrease the metabolism and increase serum concentration of amiodarone). Products include:
Nicomide Tablets 3190

Nicotine Polacrilex (Amiodarone may suppress certain CYP450 enzymes, including CYP1A2. This inhibition can result in unexpectedly high plasma levels of other drugs which are metabolized by those CYP450 enzymes). Products include:
Commit Lozenges 1625
Nicorette Gum 1632

Nicotine Salicylate (Amiodarone may suppress certain CYP450 enzymes, including CYP1A2. This inhibition can result in unexpectedly high plasma levels of other drugs which are metabolized by those CYP450 enzymes).
No products indexed under this heading.

Nicotine Sulfate (Amiodarone may suppress certain CYP450 enzymes, including CYP1A2. This inhibition can result in unexpectedly high plasma levels of other drugs which are metabolized by those CYP450 enzymes).
No products indexed under this heading.

Nifedipine (Possible potentiation of bradycardia, sinus arrest, and AV block when co-administered with calcium antagonists). Products include:
Adalat CC Tablets 2978

Nimodipine (Possible potentiation of bradycardia, sinus arrest, and AV block when co-administered with calcium antagonists). Products include:
Nimotop Capsules 774

Nisoldipine (Possible potentiation of bradycardia, sinus arrest, and AV block when co-administered with calcium antagonists). Products include:
Sular Tablets 1163

Nitrendipine (Amiodarone may suppress certain CYP450 enzymes, including CYP3A4. This inhibition can result in unexpectedly high plasma levels of other drugs which are metabolized by those CYP450 enzymes).
No products indexed under this heading.

Norethindrone (Amiodarone may suppress certain CYP450 enzymes, including CYP3A4. This inhibition can result in unexpectedly high plasma levels of other drugs which are metabolized by those CYP450 enzymes). Products include:
Ortho Micronor Tablets 2411

Norethindrone Acetate (Amiodarone may suppress certain CYP450 enzymes, including CYP1A2. This inhibition can result in unexpectedly high plasma levels of other drugs which are metabolized by those CYP450 enzymes). Products include:
Activella Tablets 2311
Aygestin Tablets 1062
CombiPatch Transdermal System 2180

Norfloxacin (Fluoroquinolones are known to cause QTc prolongation. There have been reports of QTc prolongation in patients taking amiodarone when fluoroquinolones were administered concomitantly). Products include:
Noroxin Tablets 2009

Norgestrel (Amiodarone may suppress certain CYP450 enzymes, including CYP3A4. This inhibition can result in unexpectedly high plasma levels of other drugs which are metabolized by those CYP450 enzymes). Products include:
Lo/Ovral-28 Tablets 3423

Nortriptyline Hydrochloride (Amiodarone may suppress certain CYP450 enzymes, including CYP1A2. This inhibition can result in unexpectedly high plasma levels of other drugs which are metabolized by those CYP450 enzymes).
No products indexed under this heading.

Ofloxacin (Fluoroquinolones are known to cause QTc prolongation. There have been reports of QTc prolongation in patients taking amiodarone when fluoroquinolones were administered concomitantly). Products include:
Floxin Otic Singles 1045
Floxin Otic Solution 1043

Olanzapine (Amiodarone may suppress certain CYP450 enzymes, including CYP1A2. This inhibition can result in unexpectedly high plasma levels of other drugs which are metabolized by those CYP450 enzymes). Products include:
Symbyax Capsules 1788
Zyprexa Tablets 1798
Zyprexa IntraMuscular 1798
Zyprexa ZYDIS Orally Disintegrating Tablets 1798

Omeprazole (Since amiodarone is a substrate for CYP3A4, drugs that inhibit CYP3A4 may decrease the

metabolism and increase serum concentration of amiodarone). Products include:

Zegerid Powder for Oral Solution 2972

Ondansetron (Amiodarone may suppress certain CYP450 enzymes, including CYP1A2. This inhibition can result in unexpectedly high plasma levels of other drugs which are metabolized by those CYP450 enzymes). Products include:

Zofran ODT Orally Disintegrating Tablets 1613

Ondansetron Hydrochloride (Amiodarone may suppress certain CYP450 enzymes, including CYP1A2. This inhibition can result in unexpectedly high plasma levels of other drugs which are metabolized by those CYP450 enzymes). Products include:

Zofran Injection 1607
Zofran 1613

Oxaprozin (Amiodarone may suppress certain CYP450 enzymes, including CYP2Cp. This inhibition can result in unexpectedly high plasma levels of other drugs which are metabolized by those CYP450 enzymes).

No products indexed under this heading.

Oxiconazole Nitrate (azoles are known to cause QTc prolongation. There have been reports of QTc prolongation in patients taking amiodarone when azoles were administered concomitantly). Products include:

Oxistat 1498

Oxycodone Hydrochloride (Amiodarone may suppress certain CYP450 enzymes, including CYP2D6. This inhibition can result in unexpectedly high plasma levels of other drugs which are metabolized by those CYP450 enzymes). Products include:

Combunox Tablets 1183
OxyContin Tablets 2699
OxyFast Oral Concentrate Solution.. 2704
OxyIR Capsules 2704
Percocet Tablets 1114
Percodan Tablets 1115

Paclitaxel (Amiodarone may suppress certain CYP450 enzymes, including CYP2D6. This inhibition can result in unexpectedly high plasma levels of other drugs which are metabolized by those CYP450 enzymes).

No products indexed under this heading.

Paroxetine Hydrochloride (Since amiodarone is a substrate for CYP3A4, drugs that inhibit CYP3A4 may decrease the metabolism and increase serum concentration of amiodarone). Products include:

Paxil CR Controlled-Release Tablets 1509
Paxil 1501

Penbutolol Sulfate (Possible potentiation of bradycardia, sinus arrest, and AV block when co-administered with beta-blocking agents).

No products indexed under this heading.

Phenobarbital Sodium (Amiodarone may suppress certain CYP450 enzymes, including CYP1A2. This inhibition can result in unexpectedly high plasma levels of other drugs which are metabolized by those CYP450 enzymes).

No products indexed under this heading.

Phenylbutazone (Amiodarone may suppress certain CYP450 enzymes, including CYP2Cp. This inhibition can result in unexpectedly high plasma levels of other drugs which are metabolized by those CYP450 enzymes).

No products indexed under this heading.

Phenytoin (Co-administration has resulted in increased steady-state levels of phenytoin).

No products indexed under this heading.

Phenytoin Sodium (Co-administration has resulted in increased steady-state levels of phenytoin). Products include:

Phenytek Capsules 2153

Pimozide (Amiodarone may suppress certain CYP450 enzymes, including CYP3A4. This inhibition can result in unexpectedly high plasma levels of other drugs which are metabolized by those CYP450 enzymes). Products include:

Orap Tablets 1220

Pindolol (Possible potentiation of bradycardia, sinus arrest, and AV block when co-administered with beta-blocking agents).

No products indexed under this heading.

Pioglitazone Hydrochloride (Amiodarone may suppress certain CYP450 enzymes, including CYP2Cp. This inhibition can result in unexpectedly high plasma levels of other drugs which are metabolized by those CYP450 enzymes). Products include:

ActoPlus Met Tablets 3219
Actos Tablets 3224

Piroxicam (Amiodarone may suppress certain CYP450 enzymes, including CYP2Cp. This inhibition can result in unexpectedly high plasma levels of other drugs which are metabolized by those CYP450 enzymes).

No products indexed under this heading.

Polyestradiol Phosphate (Amiodarone may suppress certain CYP450 enzymes, including CYP3A4. This inhibition can result in unexpectedly high plasma levels of other drugs which are metabolized by those CYP450 enzymes).

No products indexed under this heading.

Pravastatin Sodium (Simvastatin (CYP3A4 substrate) in combination with amiodarone has been associated with reports of myopathy/ rhabdomyolysis). Products include:

Pravachol Tablets 943

Procainamide Hydrochloride (Co-administration has resulted in increased plasma concentration by 55% and NAPA concentration by 33%; dose of procainamide should be reduced by 13%).

No products indexed under this heading.

Propafenone Hydrochloride (Amiodarone may suppress certain CYP450 enzymes, including CYP1A2. This inhibition can result in unexpectedly high plasma levels of other drugs which are metabolized by those CYP450 enzymes). Products include:

Rythmol SR Capsules 2736

Propoxyphene Hydrochloride (Since amiodarone is a substrate for CYP3A4, drugs that inhibit CYP3A4 may decrease the metabolism and increase serum concentration of amiodarone).

No products indexed under this heading.

Propoxyphene Napsylate (Since amiodarone is a substrate for CYP3A4, drugs that inhibit CYP3A4 may decrease the metabolism and increase serum concentration of amiodarone). Products include:

Darvocet A 500 Tablets 3497

Propranolol Hydrochloride (Possible potentiation of bradycardia, sinus arrest, and AV block when co-administered with beta-blocking agents). Products include:

Inderal LA Long-Acting Capsules 3421
InnoPran XL Capsules 2728

Protriptyline Hydrochloride (Amiodarone may suppress certain CYP450 enzymes, including CYP1A2. This inhibition can result in unexpectedly high plasma levels of other drugs which are metabolized by those CYP450 enzymes). Products include:

Vivactil Tablets 2350

Quetiapine Fumarate (Amiodarone may suppress certain CYP450 enzymes, including CYP2D6. This inhibition can result in unexpectedly high plasma levels of other drugs which are metabolized by those CYP450 enzymes). Products include:

Seroquel Tablets 691

Quinidine (Co-administration has resulted in increased serum concentration by 33%; dose of quinidine should be reduced by 1/3 to 1/2).

No products indexed under this heading.

Quinidine Gluconate (Co-administration has resulted in increased serum concentration by 33%; dose of quinidine should be reduced by 1/3 to 1/2).

No products indexed under this heading.

Quinidine Hydrochloride (Co-administration has resulted in increased serum concentration by 33%; dose of quinidine should be reduced by 1/3 to 1/2).

No products indexed under this heading.

Quinidine Polygalacturonate (Co-administration has resulted in increased serum concentration by 33%; dose of quinidine should be reduced by 1/3 to 1/2).

No products indexed under this heading.

Quinidine Sulfate (Co-administration has resulted in increased serum concentration by 33%; dose of quinidine should be reduced by 1/3 to 1/2).

No products indexed under this heading.

Quinine (Since amiodarone is a substrate for CYP3A4, drugs that inhibit CYP3A4 may decrease the metabolism and increase serum concentration of amiodarone).

No products indexed under this heading.

Quinine Sulfate (Since amiodarone is a substrate for CYP3A4, drugs that inhibit CYP3A4 may decrease the metabolism and increase serum concentration of amiodarone).

No products indexed under this heading.

Quinupristin (Since amiodarone is a substrate for CYP3A4, drugs that inhibit CYP3A4 may decrease the metabolism and increase serum concentration of amiodarone). Products include:

Synercid I.V. 1690

Ranitidine Bismuth Citrate (Since amiodarone is a substrate for CYP3A4, drugs that inhibit CYP3A4 may decrease the metabolism and increase serum concentration of amiodarone).

No products indexed under this heading.

Ranitidine Hydrochloride (Since amiodarone is a substrate for CYP3A4, drugs that inhibit CYP3A4 may decrease the metabolism and increase serum concentration of amiodarone). Products include:

Zantac 1597
Zantac Injection 1593
Zantac 75 Tablets 715
Zantac 150 Maximum Strength Tablets... 715
Zantac Injection Pharmacy Bulk Package... 1595

Repaglinide (Amiodarone may suppress certain CYP450 enzymes, including CYP2Cp. This inhibition can result in unexpectedly high plasma levels of other drugs which are metabolized by those CYP450 enzymes). Products include:

Prandin Tablets (0.5, 1, and 2 mg)... 2337

Rifabutin (Amiodarone may suppress certain CYP450 enzymes, including CYP3A4. This inhibition can result in unexpectedly high plasma levels of other drugs which are metabolized by those CYP450 enzymes).

No products indexed under this heading.

Riluzole (Amiodarone may suppress certain CYP450 enzymes, including CYP1A2. This inhibition can result in unexpectedly high plasma levels of other drugs which are metabolized by those CYP450 enzymes). Products include:

Rilutek Tablets 2945

Risperidone (Amiodarone may suppress certain CYP450 enzymes, including CYP2D6. This inhibition can result in unexpectedly high plasma levels of other drugs which are metabolized by those CYP450 enzymes). Products include:

Risperdal Consta Long-Acting Injection 1664
Risperdal M-Tab Orally Disintegrating Tablets.................. 1658
Risperdal 1658

Ritonavir (Protease inhibitors are known to inhibit CYP3A4 to varying degrees. Monitoring for amiodarone toxicity and serial measurement of amiodarone serum concentrations during concomitant protease inhibitor therapy should be considered). Products include:

Kaletra 474
Norvir 499

Rofecoxib (Amiodarone may suppress certain CYP450 enzymes, including CYP2Cp. This inhibition can result in unexpectedly high plasma levels of other drugs which are metabolized by those CYP450 enzymes).
No products indexed under this heading.

Ropinirole Hydrochloride (Amiodarone may suppress certain CYP450 enzymes, including CYP1A2. This inhibition can result in unexpectedly high plasma levels of other drugs which are metabolized by those CYP450 enzymes). Products include:
Requip Tablets 1528

Ropivacaine Hydrochloride (Amiodarone may suppress certain CYP450 enzymes, including CYP1A2. This inhibition can result in unexpectedly high plasma levels of other drugs which are metabolized by those CYP450 enzymes). Products include:
Naropin Injection 640

Rosiglitazone Maleate (Amiodarone may suppress certain CYP450 enzymes, including CYP2Cp. This inhibition can result in unexpectedly high plasma levels of other drugs which are metabolized by those CYP450 enzymes). Products include:
Avandamet Tablets 1343
Avandia Tablets 1348

Saquinavir (Protease inhibitors are known to inhibit CYP3A4 to varying degrees. Monitoring for amiodarone toxicity and serial measurement of amiodarone serum concentrations during concomitant protease inhibitor therapy should be considered).
No products indexed under this heading.

Saquinavir Mesylate (Protease inhibitors are known to inhibit CYP3A4 to varying degrees. Monitoring for amiodarone toxicity and serial measurement of amiodarone serum concentrations during concomitant protease inhibitor therapy should be considered). Products include:
Invirase 2776

Sertraline Hydrochloride (Since amiodarone is a substrate for CYP3A4, drugs that inhibit CYP3A4 may decrease the metabolism and increase serum concentration of amiodarone). Products include:
Zoloft 2581

Sildenafil Citrate (Amiodarone may suppress certain CYP450 enzymes, including CYP2Cp. This inhibition can result in unexpectedly high plasma levels of other drugs which are metabolized by those CYP450 enzymes). Products include:
Revatio Tablets 2541
Viagra Tablets 2552

Simvastatin (Simvastatin (CYP3A4 substrate) in combination with amiodarone has been associated with reports of myopathy/rhabdomyolysis). Products include:
Vytorin 10/10 Tablets 2084
Vytorin 10/10 Tablets 3092
Vytorin 10/20 Tablets 2084
Vytorin 10/20 Tablets 3092
Vytorin 10/40 Tablets 3092
Vytorin 10/40 Tablets 2084
Vytorin 10/80 Tablets 2084
Vytorin 10/80 Tablets 3092
Zocor Tablets 2078

Sirolimus (Amiodarone may suppress certain CYP450 enzymes, including CYP3A4. This inhibition can result in unexpectedly high plasma levels of other drugs which are metabolized by those CYP450 enzymes). Products include:
Rapamune Oral Solution and Tablets 3472

Sotalol Hydrochloride (Possible potentiation of bradycardia, sinus arrest, and AV block when co-administered with beta-blocking agents).
No products indexed under this heading.

Sulfamethoxazole (Amiodarone may suppress certain CYP450 enzymes, including CYP2Cp. This inhibition can result in unexpectedly high plasma levels of other drugs which are metabolized by those CYP450 enzymes).
No products indexed under this heading.

Sulindac (Amiodarone may suppress certain CYP450 enzymes, including CYP2Cp. This inhibition can result in unexpectedly high plasma levels of other drugs which are metabolized by those CYP450 enzymes). Products include:
Clinoril Tablets 1899

Suprofen (Amiodarone may suppress certain CYP450 enzymes, including CYP2Cp. This inhibition can result in unexpectedly high plasma levels of other drugs which are metabolized by those CYP450 enzymes).
No products indexed under this heading.

Tacrine Hydrochloride (Amiodarone may suppress certain CYP450 enzymes, including CYP1A2. This inhibition can result in unexpectedly high plasma levels of other drugs which are metabolized by those CYP450 enzymes).
No products indexed under this heading.

Tacrolimus (Amiodarone may suppress certain CYP450 enzymes, including CYP3A4. This inhibition can result in unexpectedly high plasma levels of other drugs which are metabolized by those CYP450 enzymes). Products include:
Prograf Capsules and Injection 624
Protopic Ointment 629

Tamoxifen Citrate (Amiodarone may suppress certain CYP450 enzymes, including CYP1A2. This inhibition can result in unexpectedly high plasma levels of other drugs which are metabolized by those CYP450 enzymes).
No products indexed under this heading.

Telithromycin (Since amiodarone is a substrate for CYP3A4, drugs that inhibit CYP3A4 may decrease the metabolism and increase serum concentration of amiodarone). Products include:
Ketek Tablets 2920

Telmisartan (Amiodarone may suppress certain CYP450 enzymes, including CYP2Cp. This inhibition can result in unexpectedly high plasma levels of other drugs which are metabolized by those CYP450 enzymes). Products include:
Micardis Tablets 884
Micardis HCT Tablets 886

Teniposide (Amiodarone may suppress certain CYP450 enzymes, including CYP2D6. This inhibition can result in unexpectedly high plasma levels of other drugs which are metabolized by those CYP450 enzymes).
No products indexed under this heading.

Terconazole (azoles are known to cause QTc prolongation. There have been reports of QTc prolongation in patients taking amiodarone when azoles were administered concomitantly).
No products indexed under this heading.

Testosterone (Amiodarone may suppress certain CYP450 enzymes, including CYP2D6. This inhibition can result in unexpectedly high plasma levels of other drugs which are metabolized by those CYP450 enzymes). Products include:
AndroGel 3330
Striant Mucoadhesive 1022
Testim 1% Gel 722

Testosterone Cypionate (Amiodarone may suppress certain CYP450 enzymes, including CYP2D6. This inhibition can result in unexpectedly high plasma levels of other drugs which are metabolized by those CYP450 enzymes).
No products indexed under this heading.

Testosterone Enanthate (Amiodarone may suppress certain CYP450 enzymes, including CYP2D6. This inhibition can result in unexpectedly high plasma levels of other drugs which are metabolized by those CYP450 enzymes). Products include:
Delatestryl Injection 2976

Testosterone Propionate (Amiodarone may suppress certain CYP450 enzymes, including CYP2D6. This inhibition can result in unexpectedly high plasma levels of other drugs which are metabolized by those CYP450 enzymes).
No products indexed under this heading.

Theophylline (Amiodarone may suppress certain CYP450 enzymes, including CYP1A2. This inhibition can result in unexpectedly high plasma levels of other drugs which are metabolized by those CYP450 enzymes).
No products indexed under this heading.

Theophylline Anhydrous (Amiodarone may suppress certain CYP450 enzymes, including CYP1A2. This inhibition can result in unexpectedly high plasma levels of other drugs which are metabolized by those CYP450 enzymes). Products include:
Uniphyl Tablets 2708

Thioridazine (Amiodarone may suppress certain CYP450 enzymes, including CYP2D6. This inhibition can result in unexpectedly high plasma levels of other drugs which are metabolized by those CYP450 enzymes).
No products indexed under this heading.

Thioridazine Hydrochloride (Amiodarone may suppress certain CYP450 enzymes, including CYP2D6. This inhibition can result in unexpectedly high plasma levels of other drugs which are metabolized by those CYP450 enzymes). Products include:
Thioridazine Hydrochloride Tablets 2122

Tiagabine Hydrochloride (Amiodarone may suppress certain CYP450 enzymes, including CYP3A4. This inhibition can result in unexpectedly high plasma levels of other drugs which are metabolized by those CYP450 enzymes). Products include:
Gabitril Tablets 998

Timolol Hemihydrate (Possible potentiation of bradycardia, sinus arrest, and AV block when co-administered with beta-blocking agents). Products include:
Betimol Ophthalmic Solution 3371
Betimol Ophthalmic Solution .... ⊙283

Timolol Maleate (Possible potentiation of bradycardia, sinus arrest, and AV block when co-administered with beta-blocking agents). Products include:
Blocadren Tablets 1891
Cosopt Sterile Ophthalmic Solution 1910
Timolide Tablets 2056
Timoptic in Ocudose 2061
Timoptic Sterile Ophthalmic Solution 2058
Timoptic-XE Sterile Ophthalmic Gel Forming Solution 2062

Tolazamide (Amiodarone may suppress certain CYP450 enzymes, including CYP2Cp. This inhibition can result in unexpectedly high plasma levels of other drugs which are metabolized by those CYP450 enzymes).
No products indexed under this heading.

Tolbutamide (Amiodarone may suppress certain CYP450 enzymes, including CYP2Cp. This inhibition can result in unexpectedly high plasma levels of other drugs which are metabolized by those CYP450 enzymes).
No products indexed under this heading.

Tolbutamide Sodium (Amiodarone may suppress certain CYP450 enzymes, including CYP2Cp. This inhibition can result in unexpectedly high plasma levels of other drugs which are metabolized by those CYP450 enzymes).
No products indexed under this heading.

Tolmetin Sodium (Amiodarone may suppress certain CYP450 enzymes, including CYP2Cp. This inhibition can result in unexpectedly high plasma levels of other drugs which are metabolized by those CYP450 enzymes).
No products indexed under this heading.

Tolterodine Tartrate (Amiodarone may suppress certain CYP450 enzymes, including CYP2D6. This inhibition can result in unexpectedly high plasma levels of other drugs which are metabolized by those CYP450 enzymes). Products include:
Detrol Tablets 2626
Detrol LA Capsules 2629

Torsemide (Amiodarone may suppress certain CYP450 enzymes, including CYP2Cp. This inhibition can result in unexpectedly high plasma levels of other drugs which are metabolized by those CYP450 enzymes).
No products indexed under this heading.

Tramadol Hydrochloride (Amiodarone may suppress certain CYP450 enzymes, including CYP2D6. This inhibition can result in unexpectedly high plasma levels of other drugs which are metabolized by those CYP450 enzymes). Products include:
Ultracet Tablets 2462

Trazodone Hydrochloride (Amiodarone may suppress certain CYP450 enzymes, including CYP2D6. This inhibition can result in unexpectedly high plasma levels of other drugs which are metabolized by those CYP450 enzymes).
No products indexed under this heading.

Triazolam (Amiodarone may suppress certain CYP450 enzymes, including CYP2D6. This inhibition can result in unexpectedly high plasma levels of other drugs which are metabolized by those CYP450 enzymes).
No products indexed under this heading.

Trimethaphan Camsylate (Amiodarone may suppress certain CYP450 enzymes, including CYP1A2. This inhibition can result in unexpectedly high plasma levels of other drugs which are metabolized by those CYP450 enzymes).
No products indexed under this heading.

Trimipramine Maleate (Amiodarone may suppress certain CYP450 enzymes, including CYP1A2. This inhibition can result in unexpectedly high plasma levels of other drugs which are metabolized by those CYP450 enzymes). Products include:
Surmontil Capsules 2347

Troglitazone (Since amiodarone is a substrate for CYP3A4, drugs that inhibit CYP3A4 may decrease the metabolism and increase serum concentration of amiodarone).
No products indexed under this heading.

Troleandomycin (Macrolide antibiotics are known to cause QTc prolongation. There have been reports of QTc prolongation in patients taking amiodarone when Macrolide antibiotics were administered concomitantly).
No products indexed under this heading.

Trovafloxacin Mesylate (Fluoroquinolones are known to cause QTc prolongation. There have been reports of QTc prolongation in patients taking amiodarone when fluoroquinolones were administered concomitantly).
No products indexed under this heading.

Valdecoxib (Amiodarone may suppress certain CYP450 enzymes, including CYP2Cp. This inhibition can result in unexpectedly high plasma levels of other drugs which are metabolized by those CYP450 enzymes).
No products indexed under this heading.

Valproate Sodium (Since amiodarone is a substrate for CYP3A4, drugs that inhibit CYP3A4 may decrease the metabolism and increase serum concentration of amiodarone). Products include:
Depacon Injection 412

Valsartan (Amiodarone may suppress certain CYP450 enzymes, including CYP2Cp. This inhibition can result in unexpectedly high plasma levels of other drugs which are metabolized by those CYP450 enzymes). Products include:
Diovan HCT Tablets 2195
Diovan Tablets 2191

Venlafaxine Hydrochloride (Amiodarone may suppress certain CYP450 enzymes, including CYP2D6. This inhibition can result in unexpectedly high plasma levels of other drugs which are metabolized by those CYP450 enzymes). Products include:
Effexor Tablets 3405
Effexor XR Capsules 3411

Verapamil Hydrochloride (Possible potentiation of bradycardia, sinus arrest, and AV block when co-administered with calcium antagonists). Products include:
Covera-HS Tablets 3135
Tarka Tablets 519
Verelan PM Capsules 3120

Vinblastine Sulfate (Amiodarone may suppress certain CYP450 enzymes, including CYP2D6. This inhibition can result in unexpectedly high plasma levels of other drugs which are metabolized by those CYP450 enzymes).
No products indexed under this heading.

Vincristine Sulfate (Amiodarone may suppress certain CYP450 enzymes, including CYP3A4. This inhibition can result in unexpectedly high plasma levels of other drugs which are metabolized by those CYP450 enzymes).
No products indexed under this heading.

Voriconazole (Since amiodarone is a substrate for CYP3A4, drugs that inhibit CYP3A4 may decrease the metabolism and increase serum concentration of amiodarone). Products include:
VFEND I.V. 2543
VFEND Oral Suspension 2543
VFEND Tablets 2543

Warfarin Sodium (Co-administration results in potentiation of warfarin-type anticoagulant response resulting in increased prothrombin time by 100%; dose of warfarin should be reduced by 1/3 to 1/2). Products include:
Coumadin for Injection 932
Coumadin Tablets 932

Zafirlukast (Since amiodarone is a substrate for CYP3A4, drugs that inhibit CYP3A4 may decrease the metabolism and increase serum concentration of amiodarone). Products include:
Accolate Tablets 663

Zileuton (Since amiodarone is a substrate for CYP3A4, drugs that inhibit CYP3A4 may decrease the metabolism and increase serum concentration of amiodarone).
No products indexed under this heading.

Zolmitriptan (Amiodarone may suppress certain CYP450 enzymes, including CYP1A2. This inhibition can result in unexpectedly high plasma levels of other drugs which are metabolized by those CYP450 enzymes). Products include:
Zomig Nasal Spray 718
Zomig Tablets 714
Zomig-ZMT Tablets 714

Zonisamide (Amiodarone may suppress certain CYP450 enzymes, including CYP2D6. This inhibition can result in unexpectedly high plasma levels of other drugs which are metabolized by those CYP450 enzymes). Products include:
Zonegran Capsules 1089

Food Interactions

Grapefruit (Grapefruit juice given to healthy volunteers increased amiodarone AUC by 50% and Cmax by 84%. Grapefruit juice inhibits CYP3A4-mediated metabolism of oral amiodarone in the intestinal mucosa, resulting in increased plasma levels of amiodarone; therefore, grapefruit juice should not be taken during treatment with oral amiodarone. This information should be considered when changing from intravenous amiodarone to oral amiodarone).

Grapefruit Juice (Grapefruit juice given to healthy volunteers increased amiodarone AUC by 50% and Cmax by 84%. Grapefruit juice inhibits CYP3A4-mediated metabolism of oral amiodarone in the intestinal mucosa, resulting in increased plasma levels of amiodarone; therefore, grapefruit juice should not be taken during treatment with oral amiodarone. This information should be considered when changing from intravenous amiodarone to oral amiodarone).

PANAFIL OINTMENT

(Chlorophyllin Copper Complex Sodium, Papain, Urea)....................... 1637
May interact with:

Heavy metal salts, unspecified (Papain may be inactivated by the salts of heavy metals).
No products indexed under this heading.

Hydrogen Peroxide (May inactivate papain).
No products indexed under this heading.

PANAFIL SPRAY

(Chlorophyllin Copper Complex Sodium, Papain, Urea)....................... 1637
May interact with:

Heavy metal salts, unspecified (Papain may be inactivated by the salts of heavy metals).
No products indexed under this heading.

Hydrogen Peroxide (May inactivate papain).
No products indexed under this heading.

PANCREASE MT CAPSULES

(Pancrelipase) 1839
None cited in PDR database.

PANDEL CREAM, 0.1%

(Hydrocortisone Probutate) 1017
None cited in PDR database.

PANHEMATIN FOR INJECTION

(Hemin) 2487
May interact with barbiturates, oral anticoagulants, and estrogens. Compounds in these categories include:

Anisindione (Hemin exhibits transient, mild anticoagulant effects, therefore, concurrent anticoagulant therapy should be avoided). Products include:
Miradon Tablets 3056

Aprobarbital (Hemin inhibits the enzyme delta-aminolevulinic acid synthetase; concurrent use with drugs that increase the activity of delta-aminolevulinic acid synthetase, such as barbiturates, should be avoided).
No products indexed under this heading.

Butabarbital (Hemin inhibits the enzyme delta-aminolevulinic acid synthetase; concurrent use with drugs that increase the activity of delta-aminolevulinic acid synthetase, such as barbiturates, should be avoided).
No products indexed under this heading.

Butalbital (Hemin inhibits the enzyme delta-aminolevulinic acid synthetase; concurrent use with drugs that increase the activity of delta-aminolevulinic acid synthetase, such as barbiturates, should be avoided). Products include:
Sedapap Tablets 50 mg/650 mg 2098

Chlorotrianisene (Hemin inhibits the enzyme delta-aminolevulinic acid synthetase; concurrent use with drugs that increase the activity of delta-aminolevulinic acid synthetase, such as estrogens, should be avoided).
No products indexed under this heading.

Dicumarol (Hemin exhibits transient, mild anticoagulant effects, therefore, concurrent anticoagulant therapy should be avoided).
No products indexed under this heading.

Dienestrol (Hemin inhibits the enzyme delta-aminolevulinic acid synthetase; concurrent use with drugs that increase the activity of delta-aminolevulinic acid synthetase, such as estrogens, should be avoided).
No products indexed under this heading.

Diethylstilbestrol (Hemin inhibits the enzyme delta-aminolevulinic acid synthetase; concurrent use with drugs that increase the activity of delta-aminolevulinic acid synthetase, such as estrogens, should be avoided).
No products indexed under this heading.

Estradiol (Hemin inhibits the enzyme delta-aminolevulinic acid synthetase; concurrent use with drugs that increase the activity of delta-aminolevulinic acid synthetase, such as estrogens, should be avoided). Products include:
Activella Tablets 2311
Climara Transdermal System 795
Climara Pro Transdermal System 800
CombiPatch Transdermal System 2180

Estrogel 0.06% 3200
Menostar Transdermal System 805
Prefest Tablets 1069
Vagifem Tablets 2340
Vivelle Transdermal System 2288
Vivelle-Dot Transdermal System 2293

Estrogens, Conjugated (Hemin inhibits the enzyme delta-aminolevulinic acid synthetase; concurrent use with drugs that increase the activity of delta-aminolevulinic acid synthetase, such as estrogens, should be avoided). Products include:
Premarin Intravenous 3440
Premarin Tablets 3443
Premarin Vaginal Cream 3449
Premphase Tablets 3452
Prempro Tablets 3452

Estrogens, Esterified (Hemin inhibits the enzyme delta-aminolevulinic acid synthetase; concurrent use with drugs that increase the activity of delta-aminolevulinic acid synthetase, such as estrogens, should be avoided). Products include:
Estratest Tablets 3196
Estratest H.S. Tablets 3196

Estropipate (Hemin inhibits the enzyme delta-aminolevulinic acid synthetase; concurrent use with drugs that increase the activity of delta-aminolevulinic acid synthetase, such as estrogens, should be avoided).
No products indexed under this heading.

Ethinyl Estradiol (Hemin inhibits the enzyme delta-aminolevulinic acid synthetase; concurrent use with drugs that increase the activity of delta-aminolevulinic acid synthetase, such as estrogens, should be avoided). Products include:
Alesse-28 Tablets 3392
Lo/Ovral-28 Tablets 3423
NuvaRing 2357
Ortho-Cept Tablets 2395
Ortho-Cyclen/Ortho Tri-Cyclen 2414
Ortho Evra Transdermal System 2402
Ortho Tri-Cyclen Lo Tablets 2421
Seasonale Tablets 1073
Triphasil-28 Tablets 3483
Yasmin 28 Tablets 818

Mephobarbital (Hemin inhibits the enzyme delta-aminolevulinic acid synthetase; concurrent use with drugs that increase the activity of delta-aminolevulinic acid synthetase, such as barbiturates, should be avoided). Products include:
Mebaral Tablets, USP 2483

Pentobarbital Sodium (Hemin inhibits the enzyme delta-aminolevulinic acid synthetase; concurrent use with drugs that increase the activity of delta-aminolevulinic acid synthetase, such as barbiturates, should be avoided). Products include:
Nembutal Sodium Solution, USP 2484

Phenobarbital (Hemin inhibits the enzyme delta-aminolevulinic acid synthetase; concurrent use with drugs that increase the activity of delta-aminolevulinic acid synthetase, such as barbiturates, should be avoided).
No products indexed under this heading.

Polyestradiol Phosphate (Hemin inhibits the enzyme delta-aminolevulinic acid synthetase; concurrent use with drugs that increase the activity of delta-aminolevulinic acid synthetase, such as estrogens, should be avoided).
No products indexed under this heading.

Quinestrol (Hemin inhibits the enzyme delta-aminolevulinic acid synthetase; concurrent use with drugs that increase the activity of delta-aminolevulinic acid synthetase, such as estrogens, should be avoided).
No products indexed under this heading.

Secobarbital Sodium (Hemin inhibits the enzyme delta-aminolevulinic acid synthetase; concurrent use with drugs that increase the activity of delta-aminolevulinic acid synthetase, such as barbiturates, should be avoided).
No products indexed under this heading.

Thiamylal Sodium (Hemin inhibits the enzyme delta-aminolevulinic acid synthetase; concurrent use with drugs that increase the activity of delta-aminolevulinic acid synthetase, such as barbiturates, should be avoided).
No products indexed under this heading.

Warfarin Sodium (Hemin exhibits transient, mild anticoagulant effects, therefore, concurrent anticoagulant therapy should be avoided). Products include:
Coumadin for Injection 932
Coumadin Tablets 932

PARCOPA ORALLY DISINTEGRATING TABLETS

(Carbidopa, Levodopa) 3111

May interact with antihypertensives, dopamine D2 antagonists, iron salts, nonselective MAO inhibitors, phenytoin, tricyclic antidepressants, and certain other agents. Compounds in these categories include:

Acebutolol Hydrochloride (Symptomatic postural hypotension has occurred with concomitant use; therefore, when therapy with carbidopa/levodopa is started, dosage adjustment of the antihypertensive drug may be required).
No products indexed under this heading.

Amitriptyline Hydrochloride (There have been rare reports of adverse reactions, including hypertension and dyskinesia, resulting from the concomitant use of tricyclic antidepressants and carbidopa/levodopa).
No products indexed under this heading.

Amlodipine Besylate (Symptomatic postural hypotension has occurred with concomitant use; therefore, when therapy with carbidopa/levodopa is started, dosage adjustment of the antihypertensive drug may be required). Products include:
Caduet Tablets 2507
Lotrel Capsules 2238
Norvasc Tablets 2529

Amoxapine (There have been rare reports of adverse reactions, including hypertension and dyskinesia, resulting from the concomitant use of tricyclic antidepressants and carbidopa/levodopa).
No products indexed under this heading.

Atenolol (Symptomatic postural hypotension has occurred with concomitant use; therefore, when therapy with carbidopa/levodopa is started, dosage adjustment of the antihypertensive drug may be required). Products include:
Tenormin I.V. Injection 698
Tenormin Tablets 695

Benazepril Hydrochloride (Symptomatic postural hypotension has occurred with concomitant use; therefore, when therapy with carbidopa/levodopa is started, dosage adjustment of the antihypertensive drug may be required). Products include:
Lotensin Tablets 2232
Lotensin HCT Tablets 2235
Lotrel Capsules 2238

Bendroflumethiazide (Symptomatic postural hypotension has occurred with concomitant use; therefore, when therapy with carbidopa/levodopa is started, dosage adjustment of the antihypertensive drug may be required).
No products indexed under this heading.

Betaxolol Hydrochloride (Symptomatic postural hypotension has occurred with concomitant use; therefore, when therapy with carbidopa/levodopa is started, dosage adjustment of the antihypertensive drug may be required). Products include:
Betoptic S Ophthalmic Suspension 554

Bisoprolol Fumarate (Symptomatic postural hypotension has occurred with concomitant use; therefore, when therapy with carbidopa/levodopa is started, dosage adjustment of the antihypertensive drug may be required).
No products indexed under this heading.

Candesartan Cilexetil (Symptomatic postural hypotension has occurred with concomitant use; therefore, when therapy with carbidopa/levodopa is started, dosage adjustment of the antihypertensive drug may be required). Products include:
Atacand Tablets 634
Atacand HCT 637

Captopril (Symptomatic postural hypotension has occurred with concomitant use; therefore, when therapy with carbidopa/levodopa is started, dosage adjustment of the antihypertensive drug may be required). Products include:
Captopril Tablets 2114

Carteolol Hydrochloride (Symptomatic postural hypotension has occurred with concomitant use; therefore, when therapy with carbidopa/levodopa is started, dosage adjustment of the antihypertensive drug may be required). Products include:
Carteolol Hydrochloride Ophthalmic Solution USP, 1% .... ⊙ 246

Chlorothiazide (Symptomatic postural hypotension has occurred with concomitant use; therefore, when therapy with carbidopa/levodopa is started, dosage adjustment of the antihypertensive drug may be required). Products include:
Aldoclor Tablets 1881
Diuril Oral 1936

Chlorothiazide Sodium (Symptomatic postural hypotension has occurred with concomitant use; therefore, when therapy with carbidopa/levodopa is started, dosage adjustment of the antihypertensive drug may be required). Products include:
Diuril Sodium Intravenous 1934

Chlorpromazine (Dopamine D2 receptor antagonists may reduce the therapeutic effects of levodopa).
No products indexed under this heading.

Chlorpromazine Hydrochloride (Dopamine D2 receptor antagonists may reduce the therapeutic effects of levodopa).
No products indexed under this heading.

Chlorprothixene (Dopamine D2 receptor antagonists may reduce the therapeutic effects of levodopa).
No products indexed under this heading.

Chlorprothixene Hydrochloride (Dopamine D2 receptor antagonists may reduce the therapeutic effects of levodopa).
No products indexed under this heading.

Chlorthalidone (Symptomatic postural hypotension has occurred with concomitant use; therefore, when therapy with carbidopa/levodopa is started, dosage adjustment of the antihypertensive drug may be required). Products include:
Clorpres Tablets 2139

Clomipramine Hydrochloride (There have been rare reports of adverse reactions, including hypertension and dyskinesia, resulting from the concomitant use of tricyclic antidepressants and carbidopa/levodopa).
No products indexed under this heading.

Clonidine (Symptomatic postural hypotension has occurred with concomitant use; therefore, when therapy with carbidopa/levodopa is started, dosage adjustment of the antihypertensive drug may be required). Products include:
Catapres-TTS 875

Clonidine Hydrochloride (Symptomatic postural hypotension has occurred with concomitant use; therefore, when therapy with carbidopa/levodopa is started, dosage adjustment of the antihypertensive drug may be required). Products include:
Catapres Tablets 874
Clorpres Tablets 2139

Deserpidine (Symptomatic postural hypotension has occurred with concomitant use; therefore, when therapy with carbidopa/levodopa is started, dosage adjustment of the antihypertensive drug may be required).
No products indexed under this heading.

Desipramine Hydrochloride (There have been rare reports of adverse reactions, including hypertension and dyskinesia, resulting from the concomitant use of tricyclic antidepressants and carbidopa/levodopa).
No products indexed under this heading.

Diazoxide (Symptomatic postural hypotension has occurred with concomitant use; therefore, when therapy with carbidopa/levodopa is started, dosage adjustment of the antihypertensive drug may be required). Products include:

Hyperstat I.V. Injection 3031

Diltiazem Hydrochloride (Symptomatic postural hypotension has occurred with concomitant use; therefore, when therapy with carbidopa/levodopa is started, dosage adjustment of the antihypertensive drug may be required). Products include:

Cardizem LA Extended Release Tablets 1699
Tiazac Capsules 1204

Doxazosin Mesylate (Symptomatic postural hypotension has occurred with concomitant use; therefore, when therapy with carbidopa/levodopa is started, dosage adjustment of the antihypertensive drug may be required).

No products indexed under this heading.

Doxepin Hydrochloride (There have been rare reports of adverse reactions, including hypertension and dyskinesia, resulting from the concomitant use of tricyclic antidepressants and carbidopa/levodopa).

No products indexed under this heading.

Enalapril Maleate (Symptomatic postural hypotension has occurred with concomitant use; therefore, when therapy with carbidopa/levodopa is started, dosage adjustment of the antihypertensive drug may be required). Products include:

Vaseretic Tablets 2073
Vasotec I.V. Injection 2076

Enalaprilat (Symptomatic postural hypotension has occurred with concomitant use; therefore, when therapy with carbidopa/levodopa is started, dosage adjustment of the antihypertensive drug may be required).

No products indexed under this heading.

Eprosartan Mesylate (Symptomatic postural hypotension has occurred with concomitant use; therefore, when therapy with carbidopa/levodopa is started, dosage adjustment of the antihypertensive drug may be required). Products include:

Teveten Tablets 1707
Teveten HCT Tablets 1710

Esmolol Hydrochloride (Symptomatic postural hypotension has occurred with concomitant use; therefore, when therapy with carbidopa/levodopa is started, dosage adjustment of the antihypertensive drug may be required). Products include:

Brevibloc Concentrate 766
Brevibloc Injection 766
Brevibloc Double Strength Injection...................................... 766
Brevibloc Premixed Injection 766
Brevibloc Double Strength Premixed Injection 766

Felodipine (Symptomatic postural hypotension has occurred with concomitant use; therefore, when therapy with carbidopa/levodopa is started, dosage adjustment of the antihypertensive drug may be required). Products include:

Plendil Extended-Release Tablets 651

Ferrous Fumarate (Iron salts may reduce the bioavailability of levodopa and carbidopa. The clinical relevance is unclear). Products include:

Chromagen Forte Soft Gelatin Capsules 3296
Ferretts Tablets 773
Repliva 21/7 Tablets 3301

Ferrous Gluconate (Iron salts may reduce the bioavailability of levodopa and carbidopa. The clinical relevance is unclear).

No products indexed under this heading.

Ferrous Sulfate (Iron salts may reduce the bioavailability of levodopa and carbidopa. The clinical relevance is unclear). Products include:

Feosol Tablets 1629
Slow Fe Iron Tablets 772
Slow Fe with Folic Acid Tablets 773

Fluphenazine Decanoate (Dopamine D2 receptor antagonists may reduce the therapeutic effects of levodopa).

No products indexed under this heading.

Fluphenazine Enanthate (Dopamine D2 receptor antagonists may reduce the therapeutic effects of levodopa).

No products indexed under this heading.

Fluphenazine Hydrochloride (Dopamine D2 receptor antagonists may reduce the therapeutic effects of levodopa).

No products indexed under this heading.

Fosinopril Sodium (Symptomatic postural hypotension has occurred with concomitant use; therefore, when therapy with carbidopa/levodopa is started, dosage adjustment of the antihypertensive drug may be required).

No products indexed under this heading.

Fosphenytoin Sodium (The beneficial effects of levodopa in Parkinson's disease have been reported to be reversed by phenytoin).

No products indexed under this heading.

Furosemide (Symptomatic postural hypotension has occurred with concomitant use; therefore, when therapy with carbidopa/levodopa is started, dosage adjustment of the antihypertensive drug may be required). Products include:

Furosemide Tablets 2117

Guanabenz Acetate (Symptomatic postural hypotension has occurred with concomitant use; therefore, when therapy with carbidopa/levodopa is started, dosage adjustment of the antihypertensive drug may be required).

No products indexed under this heading.

Guanethidine Monosulfate (Symptomatic postural hypotension has occurred with concomitant use; therefore, when therapy with carbidopa/levodopa is started, dosage adjustment of the antihypertensive drug may be required).

No products indexed under this heading.

Haloperidol (Dopamine D2 receptor antagonists may reduce the therapeutic effects of levodopa).

No products indexed under this heading.

Haloperidol Decanoate (Dopamine D2 receptor antagonists may reduce the therapeutic effects of levodopa).

No products indexed under this heading.

Hydralazine Hydrochloride (Symptomatic postural hypotension has occurred with concomitant use; therefore, when therapy with carbidopa/levodopa is started, dosage adjustment of the antihypertensive drug may be required). Products include:

BiDil Tablets 2161

Hydrochlorothiazide (Symptomatic postural hypotension has occurred with concomitant use; therefore, when therapy with carbidopa/levodopa is started, dosage adjustment of the antihypertensive drug may be required). Products include:

Aldoril Tablets 1884
Atacand HCT 637
Avalide Tablets 2889
Avalide Tablets 922
Benicar HCT Tablets 2852
Diovan HCT Tablets 2195
Dyazide Capsules 1389
Hyzaar 1964
Lotensin HCT Tablets 2235
Maxzide 2150
Micardis HCT Tablets 886
Moduretic Tablets 2003
Prinzide Tablets 2033
Teveten HCT Tablets 1710
Timolide Tablets 2056
Uniretic Tablets 3114
Vaseretic Tablets 2073
Zestoretic Tablets 701

Hydroflumethiazide (Symptomatic postural hypotension has occurred with concomitant use; therefore, when therapy with carbidopa/levodopa is started, dosage adjustment of the antihypertensive drug may be required).

No products indexed under this heading.

Imipramine Hydrochloride (There have been rare reports of adverse reactions, including hypertension and dyskinesia, resulting from the concomitant use of tricyclic antidepressants and carbidopa/levodopa).

No products indexed under this heading.

Imipramine Pamoate (There have been rare reports of adverse reactions, including hypertension and dyskinesia, resulting from the concomitant use of tricyclic antidepressants and carbidopa/levodopa).

No products indexed under this heading.

Indapamide (Symptomatic postural hypotension has occurred with concomitant use; therefore, when therapy with carbidopa/levodopa is started, dosage adjustment of the antihypertensive drug may be required). Products include:

Indapamide Tablets 2119

Irbesartan (Symptomatic postural hypotension has occurred with concomitant use; therefore, when therapy with carbidopa/levodopa is started, dosage adjustment of the antihypertensive drug may be required). Products include:

Avalide Tablets 922
Avalide Tablets 2889
Avapro Tablets 925
Avapro Tablets 2886

Iron (Iron salts may reduce the bioavailability of levodopa and carbidopa. The clinical relevance is unclear). Products include:

Chromagen Forte Soft Gelatin Capsules 3296
Ferretts IPS Liquid 773
OptiNate 1162
Repliva 21/7 Tablets 3301

Iron, Peptonized (Iron salts may reduce the bioavailability of levodopa and carbidopa. The clinical relevance is unclear).

No products indexed under this heading.

Iron Cacodylate (Iron salts may reduce the bioavailability of levodopa and carbidopa. The clinical relevance is unclear).

No products indexed under this heading.

Iron Carbonyl (Iron salts may reduce the bioavailability of levodopa and carbidopa. The clinical relevance is unclear). Products include:

Feosol Caplets 1629

Iron Dextran (Iron salts may reduce the bioavailability of levodopa and carbidopa. The clinical relevance is unclear). Products include:

Infed Injection 3381

Iron Polysaccharide Complex (Iron salts may reduce the bioavailability of levodopa and carbidopa. The clinical relevance is unclear).

No products indexed under this heading.

Iron Sucrose (Iron salts may reduce the bioavailability of levodopa and carbidopa. The clinical relevance is unclear).

No products indexed under this heading.

Iron Supplements (Iron salts may reduce the bioavailability of levodopa and carbidopa. The clinical relevance is unclear).

No products indexed under this heading.

Isocarboxazid (Nonselective MAO inhibitors must be discontinued at least two weeks prior to initiating therapy with carbidopa/levodopa; concurrent use is contraindicated).

No products indexed under this heading.

Isoniazid (Isoniazid may reduce the therapeutic effects of levodopa).

No products indexed under this heading.

Isradipine (Symptomatic postural hypotension has occurred with concomitant use; therefore, when therapy with carbidopa/levodopa is started, dosage adjustment of the antihypertensive drug may be required). Products include:

DynaCirc CR Tablets 2726

Labetalol Hydrochloride (Symptomatic postural hypotension has occurred with concomitant use; therefore, when therapy with carbidopa/levodopa is started, dosage adjustment of the antihypertensive drug may be required).

No products indexed under this heading.

Lisinopril (Symptomatic postural hypotension has occurred with concomitant use; therefore, when therapy with carbidopa/levodopa is started, dosage adjustment of the antihypertensive drug may be required). Products include:

Prinivil Tablets 2029
Prinzide Tablets 2033
Zestoretic Tablets 701
Zestril Tablets 704

Losartan Potassium (Symptomatic postural hypotension has occurred with concomitant use; therefore, when therapy with carbidopa/levodopa is started, dosage adjustment of the antihypertensive drug may be required). Products include:

Cozaar Tablets 1913
Hyzaar 1964

Loxapine Hydrochloride (Dopamine D2 receptor antagonists may reduce the therapeutic effects of levodopa).
No products indexed under this heading.

Loxapine Succinate (Dopamine D2 receptor antagonists may reduce the therapeutic effects of levodopa).
No products indexed under this heading.

Maprotiline Hydrochloride (There have been rare reports of adverse reactions, including hypertension and dyskinesia, resulting from the concomitant use of tricyclic antidepressants and carbidopa/levodopa).
No products indexed under this heading.

Mecamylamine Hydrochloride (Symptomatic postural hypotension has occurred with concomitant use; therefore, when therapy with carbidopa/levodopa is started, dosage adjustment of the antihypertensive drug may be required). Products include:
Inversine Tablets 3286

Mesoridazine Besylate (Dopamine D2 receptor antagonists may reduce the therapeutic effects of levodopa).
No products indexed under this heading.

Methotrimeprazine (Dopamine D2 receptor antagonists may reduce the therapeutic effects of levodopa).
No products indexed under this heading.

Methyclothiazide (Symptomatic postural hypotension has occurred with concomitant use; therefore, when therapy with carbidopa/levodopa is started, dosage adjustment of the antihypertensive drug may be required).
No products indexed under this heading.

Methyldopa (Symptomatic postural hypotension has occurred with concomitant use; therefore, when therapy with carbidopa/levodopa is started, dosage adjustment of the antihypertensive drug may be required). Products include:
Aldoclor Tablets 1881
Aldoril Tablets 1884

Methyldopate Hydrochloride (Symptomatic postural hypotension has occurred with concomitant use; therefore, when therapy with carbidopa/levodopa is started, dosage adjustment of the antihypertensive drug may be required).
No products indexed under this heading.

Metoclopramide Hydrochloride (Metoclopramine may increase the bioavailability of levodopa by increasing gastric emptying and may also adversely affect disease control by its dopamine receptor antagonistic properties).
No products indexed under this heading.

Metolazone (Symptomatic postural hypotension has occurred with concomitant use; therefore, when therapy with carbidopa/levodopa is started, dosage adjustment of the antihypertensive drug may be required).
No products indexed under this heading.

Metoprolol Succinate (Symptomatic postural hypotension has occurred with concomitant use; therefore, when therapy with carbidopa/levodopa is started, dosage adjustment of the antihypertensive drug may be required). Products include:
Toprol-XL Tablets 660

Metoprolol Tartrate (Symptomatic postural hypotension has occurred with concomitant use; therefore, when therapy with carbidopa/levodopa is started, dosage adjustment of the antihypertensive drug may be required).
No products indexed under this heading.

Metyrosine (Symptomatic postural hypotension has occurred with concomitant use; therefore, when therapy with carbidopa/levodopa is started, dosage adjustment of the antihypertensive drug may be required). Products include:
Demser Capsules 1933

Mibefradil Dihydrochloride (Symptomatic postural hypotension has occurred with concomitant use; therefore, when therapy with carbidopa/levodopa is started, dosage adjustment of the antihypertensive drug may be required).
No products indexed under this heading.

Minoxidil (Symptomatic postural hypotension has occurred with concomitant use; therefore, when therapy with carbidopa/levodopa is started, dosage adjustment of the antihypertensive drug may be required). Products include:
Men's Rogaine Extra Strength Topical Solution, Ocean Rush Scent and Original Unscented..... ■ 706
Women's Rogaine Topical Solution, Spring Bloom Scent and Original Unscented.............. ■ 707

Moexipril Hydrochloride (Symptomatic postural hypotension has occurred with concomitant use; therefore, when therapy with carbidopa/levodopa is started, dosage adjustment of the antihypertensive drug may be required). Products include:
Uniretic Tablets 3114
Univasc Tablets 3118

Molindone Hydrochloride (Dopamine D2 receptor antagonists may reduce the therapeutic effects of levodopa). Products include:
Moban Tablets 1108

Nadolol (Symptomatic postural hypotension has occurred with concomitant use; therefore, when therapy with carbidopa/levodopa is started, dosage adjustment of the antihypertensive drug may be required). Products include:
Nadolol Tablets 2121

Nicardipine Hydrochloride (Symptomatic postural hypotension has occurred with concomitant use; therefore, when therapy with carbidopa/levodopa is started, dosage adjustment of the antihypertensive drug may be required). Products include:
Cardene I.V. 1129

Nifedipine (Symptomatic postural hypotension has occurred with concomitant use; therefore, when therapy with carbidopa/levodopa is started, dosage adjustment of the antihypertensive drug may be required). Products include:
Adalat CC Tablets 2978

Nisoldipine (Symptomatic postural hypotension has occurred with concomitant use; therefore, when therapy with carbidopa/levodopa is started, dosage adjustment of the antihypertensive drug may be required). Products include:
Sular Tablets 1163

Nitroglycerin (Symptomatic postural hypotension has occurred with concomitant use; therefore, when therapy with carbidopa/levodopa is started, dosage adjustment of the antihypertensive drug may be required). Products include:
Nitro-Dur Transdermal Infusion System.. 3060
Nitrolingual Pumpspray 1161

Nortriptyline Hydrochloride (There have been rare reports of adverse reactions, including hypertension and dyskinesia, resulting from the concomitant use of tricyclic antidepressants and carbidopa/levodopa).
No products indexed under this heading.

Papaverine (The beneficial effects of levodopa in Parkinson's disease have been reported to be reversed by papaverine).
No products indexed under this heading.

Papaverine Hydrochloride (The beneficial effects of levodopa in Parkinson's disease have been reported to be reversed by papaverine).
No products indexed under this heading.

Pargyline Hydrochloride (Nonselective MAO inhibitors must be discontinued at least two weeks prior to initiating therapy with carbidopa/levodopa; concurrent use is contraindicated).
No products indexed under this heading.

Penbutolol Sulfate (Symptomatic postural hypotension has occurred with concomitant use; therefore, when therapy with carbidopa/levodopa is started, dosage adjustment of the antihypertensive drug may be required).
No products indexed under this heading.

Perindopril Erbumine (Symptomatic postural hypotension has occurred with concomitant use; therefore, when therapy with carbidopa/levodopa is started, dosage adjustment of the antihypertensive drug may be required). Products include:
Aceon Tablets (2 mg, 4 mg, 8 mg).. 3191

Perphenazine (Dopamine D2 receptor antagonists may reduce the therapeutic effects of levodopa).
No products indexed under this heading.

Phenelzine Sulfate (Nonselective MAO inhibitors must be discontinued at least two weeks prior to initiating therapy with carbidopa/levodopa; concurrent use is contraindicated).
No products indexed under this heading.

Phenoxybenzamine Hydrochloride (Symptomatic postural hypotension has occurred with concomitant use; therefore, when therapy with carbidopa/levodopa is started, dosage adjustment of the antihypertensive drug may be required). Products include:
Dibenzyline Capsules 3390

Phentolamine Mesylate (Symptomatic postural hypotension has occurred with concomitant use; therefore, when therapy with carbidopa/levodopa is started, dosage adjustment of the antihypertensive drug may be required).
No products indexed under this heading.

Phenytoin (The beneficial effects of levodopa in Parkinson's disease have been reported to be reversed by phenytoin).
No products indexed under this heading.

Phenytoin Sodium (The beneficial effects of levodopa in Parkinson's disease have been reported to be reversed by phenytoin). Products include:
Phenytek Capsules 2153

Pindolol (Symptomatic postural hypotension has occurred with concomitant use; therefore, when therapy with carbidopa/levodopa is started, dosage adjustment of the antihypertensive drug may be required).
No products indexed under this heading.

Polysaccharide Iron Complex (Iron salts may reduce the bioavailability of levodopa and carbidopa. The clinical relevance is unclear). Products include:
Niferex-150 Forte Capsules 3299
Nu-Iron 150 Capsules 2098

Polythiazide (Symptomatic postural hypotension has occurred with concomitant use; therefore, when therapy with carbidopa/levodopa is started, dosage adjustment of the antihypertensive drug may be required).
No products indexed under this heading.

Prazosin Hydrochloride (Symptomatic postural hypotension has occurred with concomitant use; therefore, when therapy with carbidopa/levodopa is started, dosage adjustment of the antihypertensive drug may be required).
No products indexed under this heading.

Procarbazine Hydrochloride (Nonselective MAO inhibitors must be discontinued at least two weeks prior to initiating therapy with carbidopa/levodopa; concurrent use is contraindicated). Products include:
Matulane Capsules 3188

Prochlorperazine (Dopamine D2 receptor antagonists may reduce the therapeutic effects of levodopa).
No products indexed under this heading.

Promethazine Hydrochloride (Dopamine D2 receptor antagonists may reduce the therapeutic effects of levodopa). Products include:
Phenergan 3438

Propranolol Hydrochloride (Symptomatic postural hypotension has occurred with concomitant use; therefore, when therapy with carbidopa/levodopa is started, dosage adjustment of the antihypertensive drug may be required). Products include:
Inderal LA Long-Acting Capsules 3421
InnoPran XL Capsules 2728

Protriptyline Hydrochloride (There have been rare reports of adverse reactions, including hyper-

tension and dyskinesia, resulting from the concomitant use of tricyclic antidepressants and carbidopa/levodopa). Products include:

Vivactil Tablets 2350

Quetiapine Fumarate (Dopamine D2 receptor antagonists may reduce the therapeutic effects of levodopa). Products include:

Seroquel Tablets 691

Quinapril Hydrochloride (Symptomatic postural hypotension has occurred with concomitant use; therefore, when therapy with carbidopa/levodopa is started, dosage adjustment of the antihypertensive drug may be required).

No products indexed under this heading.

Ramipril (Symptomatic postural hypotension has occurred with concomitant use; therefore, when therapy with carbidopa/levodopa is started, dosage adjustment of the antihypertensive drug may be required). Products include:

Altace Capsules 1673

Rauwolfia Serpentina (Symptomatic postural hypotension has occurred with concomitant use; therefore, when therapy with carbidopa/levodopa is started, dosage adjustment of the antihypertensive drug may be required).

No products indexed under this heading.

Rescinnamine (Symptomatic postural hypotension has occurred with concomitant use; therefore, when therapy with carbidopa/levodopa is started, dosage adjustment of the antihypertensive drug may be required).

No products indexed under this heading.

Reserpine (Symptomatic postural hypotension has occurred with concomitant use; therefore, when therapy with carbidopa/levodopa is started, dosage adjustment of the antihypertensive drug may be required).

No products indexed under this heading.

Risperidone (Dopamine D2 receptor antagonists may reduce the therapeutic effects of levodopa). Products include:

Risperdal Consta Long-Acting Injection 1664
Risperdal M-Tab Orally Disintegrating Tablets.................. 1658
Risperdal 1658

Selegiline Hydrochloride (Concomitant therapy with selegiline may be associated with severe orthostatic hypotension not attributable to carbidopa/levodopa alone). Products include:

Eldepryl Capsules 3209

Sodium Nitroprusside (Symptomatic postural hypotension has occurred with concomitant use; therefore, when therapy with carbidopa/levodopa is started, dosage adjustment of the antihypertensive drug may be required).

No products indexed under this heading.

Sotalol Hydrochloride (Symptomatic postural hypotension has occurred with concomitant use; therefore, when therapy with carbidopa/levodopa is started, dosage adjustment of the antihypertensive drug may be required).

No products indexed under this heading.

Spirapril Hydrochloride (Symptomatic postural hypotension has occurred with concomitant use; therefore, when therapy with carbidopa/levodopa is started, dosage adjustment of the antihypertensive drug may be required).

No products indexed under this heading.

Telmisartan (Symptomatic postural hypotension has occurred with concomitant use; therefore, when therapy with carbidopa/levodopa is started, dosage adjustment of the antihypertensive drug may be required). Products include:

Micardis Tablets 884
Micardis HCT Tablets 886

Terazosin Hydrochloride (Symptomatic postural hypotension has occurred with concomitant use; therefore, when therapy with carbidopa/levodopa is started, dosage adjustment of the antihypertensive drug may be required). Products include:

Hytrin Capsules 469

Thioridazine Hydrochloride (Dopamine D2 receptor antagonists may reduce the therapeutic effects of levodopa). Products include:

Thioridazine Hydrochloride Tablets 2122

Thiothixene (Dopamine D2 receptor antagonists may reduce the therapeutic effects of levodopa). Products include:

Thiothixene Capsules 2124

Timolol Maleate (Symptomatic postural hypotension has occurred with concomitant use; therefore, when therapy with carbidopa/levodopa is started, dosage adjustment of the antihypertensive drug may be required). Products include:

Blocadren Tablets 1891
Cosopt Sterile Ophthalmic Solution.. 1910
Timolide Tablets 2056
Timoptic in Ocudose 2061
Timoptic Sterile Ophthalmic Solution.. 2058
Timoptic-XE Sterile Ophthalmic Gel Forming Solution 2062

Torsemide (Symptomatic postural hypotension has occurred with concomitant use; therefore, when therapy with carbidopa/levodopa is started, dosage adjustment of the antihypertensive drug may be required).

No products indexed under this heading.

Trandolapril (Symptomatic postural hypotension has occurred with concomitant use; therefore, when therapy with carbidopa/levodopa is started, dosage adjustment of the antihypertensive drug may be required). Products include:

Mavik Tablets 482
Tarka Tablets 519

Tranylcypromine Sulfate (Nonselective MAO inhibitors must be discontinued at least two weeks prior to initiating therapy with carbidopa/levodopa; concurrent use is contraindicated). Products include:

Parnate Tablets 1499

Trifluoperazine Hydrochloride (Dopamine D2 receptor antagonists may reduce the therapeutic effects of levodopa).

No products indexed under this heading.

Trimethaphan Camsylate (Symptomatic postural hypotension has occurred with concomitant use; therefore, when therapy with carbidopa/levodopa is started, dosage adjustment of the antihypertensive drug may be required).

No products indexed under this heading.

Trimipramine Maleate (There have been rare reports of adverse reactions, including hypertension and dyskinesia, resulting from the concomitant use of tricyclic antidepressants and carbidopa/levodopa). Products include:

Surmontil Capsules 2347

Valsartan (Symptomatic postural hypotension has occurred with concomitant use; therefore, when therapy with carbidopa/levodopa is started, dosage adjustment of the antihypertensive drug may be required). Products include:

Diovan HCT Tablets 2195
Diovan Tablets 2191

Verapamil Hydrochloride (Symptomatic postural hypotension has occurred with concomitant use; therefore, when therapy with carbidopa/levodopa is started, dosage adjustment of the antihypertensive drug may be required). Products include:

Covera-HS Tablets 3135
Tarka Tablets 519
Verelan PM Capsules 3120

PARNATE TABLETS

(Tranylcypromine Sulfate) 1499

May interact with alpha adrenergic stimulants, amphetamines, anesthetics, anorexiants, antihistamines, antihypertensives, anticholinergic-type antiparkinsonism drugs, dibenzazepines, diuretics, oral hypoglycemic agents, hypnotics and sedatives, insulin, monoamine oxidase inhibitors, narcotic analgesics, phenothiazines, selective serotonin reuptake inhibitors, sympathomimetics, tricyclic antidepressants, and certain other agents. Compounds in these categories include:

Acarbose (Some MAO inhibitors have contributed to hypoglycemic episodes in diabetic patients receiving oral hypoglycemic agents). Products include:

Precose Tablets 776

Acebutolol Hydrochloride (Concurrent use with hypotensive agents is contraindicated; a marked potentiating effect on these classes of drugs has been reported).

No products indexed under this heading.

Acrivastine (Concurrent use is contraindicated).

No products indexed under this heading.

Albuterol (Concurrent and/or sequential use is contraindicated; combination therapy may precipitate hypertension, headache and related symptoms). Products include:

Proventil Inhalation Aerosol 3067

Albuterol Sulfate (Concurrent and/or sequential use is contraindicated; combination therapy may precipitate hypertension, headache and related symptoms). Products include:

AccuNeb Inhalation Solution 1055
Combivent Inhalation Aerosol 878
DuoNeb Inhalation Solution 1058
Proventil Inhalation Solution 0.083%.. 3069
Proventil HFA Inhalation Aerosol 3071
Ventolin HFA Inhalation Aerosol 1576
VoSpire Extended-Release Tablets ... 2352

Alfentanil Hydrochloride (Concurrent use is contraindicated; a marked potentiating effect on these classes of drugs has been reported).

No products indexed under this heading.

Amiloride Hydrochloride (Concurrent use with hypotensive agents is contraindicated; a marked potentiating effect on these classes of drugs has been reported). Products include:

Midamor Tablets 2000
Moduretic Tablets 2003

Amitriptyline Hydrochloride (Concurrent use with dibenzazepine-related entities may result in hypertensive crises or severe convulsive seizures; concurrent and/or sequential use is contraindicated).

No products indexed under this heading.

Amlodipine Besylate (Concurrent use with hypotensive agents is contraindicated; a marked potentiating effect on these classes of drugs has been reported). Products include:

Caduet Tablets 2507
Lotrel Capsules 2238
Norvasc Tablets 2529

Amoxapine (Concurrent use with dibenzazepine-related entities may result in hypertensive crises or severe convulsive seizures; concurrent and/or sequential use is contraindicated).

No products indexed under this heading.

Amphetamine Resins (Concurrent and/or sequential use is contraindicated).

No products indexed under this heading.

Amphetamine Sulfate (Concurrent and/or sequential use is contraindicated). Products include:

Adderall Tablets 3168
Adderall XR Capsules 3169

Astemizole (Concurrent use is contraindicated).

No products indexed under this heading.

Atenolol (Concurrent use with hypotensive agents is contraindicated; a marked potentiating effect on these classes of drugs has been reported). Products include:

Tenormin I.V. Injection 698
Tenormin Tablets 695

Azatadine Maleate (Concurrent use is contraindicated).

No products indexed under this heading.

Benazepril Hydrochloride (Concurrent use with hypotensive agents is contraindicated; a marked potentiating effect on these classes of drugs has been reported). Products include:

Lotensin Tablets 2232
Lotensin HCT Tablets 2235
Lotrel Capsules 2238

Bendroflumethiazide (Concurrent use with hypotensive agents is contraindicated; a marked potentiating effect on these classes of drugs has been reported).

No products indexed under this heading.

Benzphetamine Hydrochloride (Concurrent and/or sequential use is contraindicated).
No products indexed under this heading.

Benztropine Mesylate (Anti-Parkinsonism drugs should be used with caution in patients receiving Parnate since severe reactions have been reported). Products include:
Cogentin Injection 1903

Betaxolol Hydrochloride (Concurrent use with hypotensive agents is contraindicated; a marked potentiating effect on these classes of drugs has been reported). Products include:
Betoptic S Ophthalmic Suspension........................ 554

Biperiden Hydrochloride (Anti-Parkinsonism drugs should be used with caution in patients receiving Parnate since severe reactions have been reported).
No products indexed under this heading.

Bisoprolol Fumarate (Concurrent use with hypotensive agents is contraindicated; a marked potentiating effect on these classes of drugs has been reported).
No products indexed under this heading.

Bromodiphenhydramine Hydrochloride (Concurrent use is contraindicated).
No products indexed under this heading.

Brompheniramine Maleate (Concurrent use is contraindicated). Products include:
Alacol DM Syrup 739
Children's Dimetapp Cold & Allergy Elixir........................ ▣745
Children's Dimetapp DM Cold & Cough Elixir .... ▣745
Robitussin Allergy & Cough Syrup .. ▣750

Bumetanide (Concurrent use with hypotensive agents is contraindicated; a marked potentiating effect on these classes of drugs has been reported).
No products indexed under this heading.

Buprenorphine Hydrochloride (Concurrent use is contraindicated; a marked potentiating effect on these classes of drugs has been reported). Products include:
Buprenex Injectable........................ 2718
Suboxone Tablets........................ 2719
Subutex Tablets 2719

Bupropion Hydrochloride (Concurrent use is contraindicated; at least 14 days should elapse between discontinuation of an MAO inhibitor and initiation of treatment with bupropion). Products include:
Wellbutrin Tablets 1579
Wellbutrin SR Sustained-Release Tablets........................ 1583
Wellbutrin XL Extended-Release Tablets........................ 1588
Zyban Sustained-Release Tablets 1620

Buspirone Hydrochloride (Concurrent use of buspirone and an MAO inhibitor has resulted in several cases of hypertension; concurrent use is contraindicated; at least 10 days should elapse between the discontinuation of Parnate and the initiation of buspirone).
No products indexed under this heading.

Caffeine (Excessive use of caffeine in any form is contraindicated). Products include:
Athena Hair System Shampoo .... ▣767
BC Powder .... ▣612
Arthritis Strength BC Powder .... ▣612
Goody's Extra Strength Headache Powder........................ ▣621
Goody's Extra Strength Pain Relief Tablets........................ ▣621
Hycomine Compound Tablets 1105
Spartan Hair System Shampoo ...... ▣767
Vivarin .... ▣639

Candesartan Cilexetil (Concurrent use with hypotensive agents is contraindicated; a marked potentiating effect on these classes of drugs has been reported). Products include:
Atacand Tablets 634
Atacand HCT 637

Captopril (Concurrent use with hypotensive agents is contraindicated; a marked potentiating effect on these classes of drugs has been reported). Products include:
Captopril Tablets 2114

Carbamazepine (Concurrent use with dibenzazepine-related entities may result in hypertensive crises or severe convulsive seizures; concurrent and/or sequential use is contraindicated). Products include:
Carbatrol Capsules 3174
Equetro Extended-Release Capsules........................ 3178
Tegretol/Tegretol-XR 2278

Carteolol Hydrochloride (Concurrent use with hypotensive agents is contraindicated; a marked potentiating effect on these classes of drugs has been reported). Products include:
Carteolol Hydrochloride Ophthalmic Solution USP, 1%...... ⊙246

Cetirizine Hydrochloride (Concurrent use is contraindicated). Products include:
Zyrtec Chewable Tablets 2589
Zyrtec 2589
Zyrtec-D 12 Hour Extended Release Tablets........................ 2591

Chlorothiazide (Concurrent use with hypotensive agents is contraindicated; a marked potentiating effect on these classes of drugs has been reported). Products include:
Aldoclor Tablets 1881
Diuril Oral 1936

Chlorothiazide Sodium (Concurrent use with hypotensive agents is contraindicated; a marked potentiating effect on these classes of drugs has been reported). Products include:
Diuril Sodium Intravenous 1934

Chlorpheniramine Maleate (Concurrent use is contraindicated). Products include:
Advil Allergy Sinus Caplets .... ▣737
Advil Multi-Symptom Cold Caplets........................ ▣738
BC Allergy Sinus Cold Powder .... ▣612
Contac Severe Cold and Flu Caplets Maximum Strength........ ▣615
Hycomine Compound Tablets 1105
PediaCare Multi-Symptom Cold Liquid .... ▣704
PediaCare NightRest Cough & Cold Liquid........................ ▣704
Robitussin Flu Liquid .... ▣752
Robitussin PM Cough & Cold Liquid .... ▣752
Singlet Caplets .... ▣636
Sudafed Sinus & Allergy Tablets ..... ▣710
TheraFlu Cold & Cough Hot Liquid .... ▣680
TheraFlu Cold & Sore Throat Hot Liquid .... ▣680
TheraFlu Flu & Sore Throat Hot Liquid .... ▣681
TheraFlu Severe Cold & Cough Hot Liquid........................ ▣683
TheraFlu Severe Cold Caplets .... ▣679
TheraFlu Severe Cold Hot Liquid .... ▣682
Triaminic Cold & Allergy Liquid .... ▣685
Triaminic Cold & Cough Liquid .... ▣685
Triaminic Flu, Cough & Fever Liquid .... ▣685
Triaminic Night Time Cough & Cold Liquid........................ ▣685
Triaminic Allergy Runny Nose & Congestion Softchews.............. ▣688
Triaminic Cold & Cough Softchews .... ▣688
Children's Tylenol Plus Cold NightTime Suspension Liquid........ 1851
Children's Tylenol Plus Cold & Cough Suspension Liquid and Chewable Tablets........................ 1851
Children's Tylenol Plus Cold Chewable Tablets........................ 1851
Children's Tylenol Plus Flu Suspension Liquid 1853
Tylenol Allergy Complete Multi-Symptom Caplets and Gelcaps with Cool Burst.............. 1844
Multi-Symptom Tylenol Cold Night Time Caplets........................ 1845
Vicks 44M Cough, Cold & Flu Relief........................ 2676
Pediatric Vicks 44m Cough & Cold Relief........................ 2673
Children's Vicks NyQuil Cold/Cough Relief 2671

Chlorpheniramine Polistirex (Concurrent use is contraindicated). Products include:
Tussionex Pennkinetic Extended-Release Suspension 3322

Chlorpheniramine Tannate (Concurrent use is contraindicated).
No products indexed under this heading.

Chlorpromazine (Possibility of additive hypotensive effects).
No products indexed under this heading.

Chlorpromazine Hydrochloride (Possibility of additive hypotensive effects).
No products indexed under this heading.

Chlorpropamide (Some MAO inhibitors have contributed to hypoglycemic episodes in diabetic patients receiving oral hypoglycemic agents).
No products indexed under this heading.

Chlorthalidone (Concurrent use with hypotensive agents is contraindicated; a marked potentiating effect on these classes of drugs has been reported). Products include:
Clorpres Tablets 2139

Citalopram Hydrobromide (Concurrent and/or sequential use is contraindicated; potential for serious, sometimes fatal, reactions including hyperthermia, rigidity, myoclonus, and other toxicities). Products include:
Celexa 1177

Clemastine Fumarate (Concurrent use is contraindicated).
No products indexed under this heading.

Clomipramine Hydrochloride (Concurrent use with dibenzazepine-related entities may result in hypertensive crises or severe convulsive seizures; concurrent and/or sequential use is contraindicated).
No products indexed under this heading.

Clonidine (Concurrent use with hypotensive agents is contraindicated; a marked potentiating effect on these classes of drugs has been reported). Products include:
Catapres-TTS 875

Clonidine Hydrochloride (Concurrent use with hypotensive agents is contraindicated; a marked potentiating effect on these classes of drugs has been reported). Products include:
Catapres Tablets 874
Clorpres Tablets 2139

Clozapine (Concurrent use with dibenzazepine-related entities may result in hypertensive crises or severe convulsive seizures; concurrent and/or sequential use is contraindicated). Products include:
Clozapine Tablets 2141
Clozaril Tablets 2174
FazaClo Orally Disintegrating Tablets........................ 547

Cocaine Hydrochloride (Concurrent use is contraindicated).
No products indexed under this heading.

Codeine Phosphate (Concurrent use is contraindicated; a marked potentiating effect on these classes of drugs has been reported). Products include:
Tylenol with Codeine 2461

Cyclobenzaprine Hydrochloride (Concurrent use with dibenzazepine-related entities may result in hypertensive crises or severe convulsive seizures; concurrent and/or sequential use is contraindicated). Products include:
Flexeril Tablets 1832

Cyproheptadine Hydrochloride (Concurrent use is contraindicated).
No products indexed under this heading.

Deserpidine (Concurrent use with hypotensive agents is contraindicated; a marked potentiating effect on these classes of drugs has been reported).
No products indexed under this heading.

Desipramine Hydrochloride (Concurrent use with dibenzazepine-related entities may result in hypertensive crises or severe convulsive seizures; concurrent and/or sequential use is contraindicated).
No products indexed under this heading.

Dexchlorpheniramine Maleate (Concurrent use is contraindicated).
No products indexed under this heading.

Dexfenfluramine Hydrochloride (Co-administration with dexfenfluramine, a serotonin releaser and reuptake inhibitor, is contraindicated).
No products indexed under this heading.

Dextroamphetamine Sulfate (Concurrent and/or sequential use is contraindicated). Products include:
Adderall Tablets 3168
Adderall XR Capsules 3169
Dexedrine 1386
DextroStat Tablets 3177

Dextromethorphan Hydrobromide (The combination of dextromethorphan and MAO inhibitors has been reported to cause brief episodes of psychosis or bizzare behavior; concurrent use is contraindicated). Products include:
Alacol DM Syrup 739
Balamine DM 739
Contac Severe Cold and Flu Caplets Maximum Strength........ ▣615
Contac Severe Cold and Flu Caplets Non-Drowsy........................ ▣615
Children's Dimetapp DM Cold & Cough Elixir .... ▣745
Children's Dimetapp Long Acting Cough Plus Cold Syrup................ ▣746

(▣ Described in PDR For Nonprescription Drugs)

(⊙ Described in PDR For Ophthalmic Medicines™)

Dimetapp Infant Drops Decongestant Plus Cough 746
Mucinex DM Tablets 602
PediaCare Decongestant & Cough Infant Drops 705
PediaCare Freezer Pops Long-Acting Cough-Glacier Grape and Polar Berry Blue 706
PediaCare Long-Acting Cough Infant Drops 705
PediaCare Long-Acting Cough Plus Cold Liquid 704
PediaCare Multi-Symptom Cold Liquid 704
PediaCare NightRest Cough & Cold Liquid 704
Robitussin Allergy & Cough Syrup 750
Robitussin CF Liquid 755
Robitussin Cough & Cold Liquid-filled Capsules 750
Robitussin Cough, Cold & Flu Liquid-filled Capsules 750
Robitussin Cough & Cold Infant Drops 755
Robitussin DM Infant Drops 753
Robitussin DM Liquid 753
Robitussin Flu Liquid 752
Robitussin Maximum Strength Cough Liquid 754
Robitussin Maximum Strength Cough & Cold Liquid 754
Robitussin Pediatric Cough Liquid 754
Robitussin Pediatric Cough & Cold Liquid 754
Robitussin PM Cough & Cold Liquid 752
Robitussin Sugar Free Cough Liquid 753
Simply Cough Liquid 1840
Sudafed Severe Cold 710
TheraFlu Cold & Cough Hot Liquid 680
TheraFlu Flu & Chest Congestion Non-Drowsy Hot Liquid 681
TheraFlu Severe Cold Non-Drowsy Hot Liquid 683
TheraFlu Severe Cold & Cough Hot Liquid 683
TheraFlu Severe Cold Caplets 679
TheraFlu Severe Cold Hot Liquid 682
TheraFlu Severe Cold Non-Drowsy Caplets 679
TheraFlu Thin Strips Long Acting Cough 684
Triaminic Cold & Cough Liquid 685
Triaminic Cough Liquid 687
Triaminic Cough & Nasal Congestion Liquid 687
Triaminic Cough & Sore Throat Liquid 687
Triaminic Flu, Cough & Fever Liquid 685
Triaminic Night Time Cough & Cold Liquid 685
Triaminic Cold & Cough Softchews 688
Triaminic Cough & Sore Throat Softchews 689
Triaminic Thin Strips Long Acting Cough 689
Children's Tylenol Plus Cold & Cough Suspension Liquid and Chewable Tablets 1851
Children's Tylenol Plus Flu Suspension Liquid 1853
Concentrated Tylenol Infants' Drops Plus Cold and Cough 1851
Tylenol Cold & Flu Severe Daytime Liquid with Cool Bust 1846
Tylenol Cold & Flu Severe NightTime Liquid with Cool Burst 1846
Tylenol Cold Severe Congestion Non-Drowsy Caplets with Cool Burst 1846
Tylenol Cough & Sore Throat Daytime Liquid with Cool Burst 1849
Tylenol Cough & Sore Throat NightTime Liquid with Cool Burst 1849
Tylenol Flu Day Non-Drowsy Gelcaps 1846
Concentrated Tylenol Infants' Drops Plus Cold & Cough Nasal Decongestant, Fever Reducer & Pain Reliever 668
Multi-Symptom Tylenol Cold Night Time Caplets 1845
Multi-Symptom Tylenol Cold Day Non-Drowsy Caplets and Gelcaps 1845
Vicks 44 Cough Relief 2675
Vicks 44D Cough & Head Congestion Relief 2676
Vicks 44D Cough & Head Congestion Relief Liquid 721
Vicks 44E Cough & Chest Congestion Relief 2676
Pediatric Vicks 44e Cough & Chest Congestion Relief Liquid 2673
Vicks 44M Cough, Cold & Flu Relief 2676
Pediatric Vicks 44m Cough & Cold Relief 2673
Vicks DayQuil LiquiCaps/Liquid Multi-Symptom Cold/Flu Relief 723
Vicks DayQuil Multi-Symptom Cold/Flu Relief LiquiCaps 2675
Vicks DayQuil Multi-Symptom Cold/Flu Relief Liquid 2675
Children's Vicks NyQuil Cold/Cough Relief 2671
Vicks NyQuil Cough Liquid 2677
Vicks NyQuil LiquiCaps 2677
Vicks NyQuil LiquiCaps/Liquid Multi-Symptom Cold/Flu Relief 725
Vicks NyQuil Liquid 2677
Zicam Concentrated Cough Mist for Kids Cool Cherry 643
Zicam Concentrated Cough Mist for Kids Plus D Cool Cherry 643
Zicam Concentrated Cough Mist Nite-Cool Cherry 642
Zicam Concentrated Cough Mist Plus D Cool Cherry 642
Zicam Concentrated Cough Mist-Honey Lemon & Cool Cherry 642

Dextromethorphan Polistirex (The combination of dextromethorphan and MAO inhibitors has been reported to cause brief episodes of psychosis or bizzare behavior; concurrent use is contraindicated). Products include:
Delsym Extended-Release Suspension 611
Delsym 12 Hour Cough Suppressant for Children 611

Dezocine (Concurrent use is contraindicated; a marked potentiating effect on these classes of drugs has been reported).
No products indexed under this heading.

Diazoxide (Concurrent use with hypotensive agents is contraindicated; a marked potentiating effect on these classes of drugs has been reported). Products include:
Hyperstat I.V. Injection 3031

Diethylpropion Hydrochloride (Concurrent and/or sequential use is contraindicated).
No products indexed under this heading.

Diltiazem Hydrochloride (Concurrent use with hypotensive agents is contraindicated; a marked potentiating effect on these classes of drugs has been reported). Products include:
Cardizem LA Extended Release Tablets 1699
Tiazac Capsules 1204

Diphenhydramine Citrate (Concurrent use is contraindicated). Products include:
Children's Benadryl Allergy & Cold Fastmelt Tablets 695
Children's Benadryl D Allergy & Sinus Fastmelt Tablets 694
Children's Benadryl Allergy Fastmelt Tablets 696
Goody's PM Powder 622

Diphenhydramine Hydrochloride (Anti-Parkinsonism drugs should be used with caution in patients receiving Parnate since severe reactions have been reported). Products include:
Benadryl Allergy & Cold Tablets 692
Benadryl Allergy 691
Benadryl Allergy & Sinus Headache Caplets & Gelcaps 693
Children's Benadryl Allergy Liquid 695
Children's Benadryl Dye-Free Allergy Liquid 695
Benadryl Dye-Free Allergy Liqui-Gels Softgels 692
Benadryl Itch Relief Stick Extra Strength 696
Benadryl Itch Stopping Cream Extra Strength 697
Benadryl Itch Stopping Gel Extra Strength 697
Benadryl Itch Stopping Spray Extra Strength 697
Benadryl Maximum Strength Severe Allergy & Sinus Headache Caplets 694
Children's Benadryl D Liquid Medication 693
Benadryl D Tablets 694
Nytol QuickCaps Caplets 635
Maximum Strength Nytol QuickGels Softgels 635
Simply Sleep Caplets 1841
Sominex Original Formula Tablets 637
TheraFlu Thin Strips Multi Symptom 684
Triaminic Thin Strips Cough & Runny Nose 690
Children's Tylenol Plus Cold & Allergy Suspension Liquid 1850
Tylenol Allergy Complete Night Time Caplets 1844
Tylenol Severe Allergy Caplets 1844
Tylenol Flu NightTime Gelcaps 1846
Extra Strength Tylenol PM Caplets, Geltabs, Gelcaps and Liquid 1847
Unisom Maximum Strength SleepGels 712

Diphenylpyraline Hydrochloride (Concurrent use is contraindicated).
No products indexed under this heading.

Disulfiram (Concurrent use requires caution; co-administration in animal models has resulted in severe toxicity, including convulsions and death). Products include:
Antabuse Tablets 2343

Dobutamine Hydrochloride (Concurrent and/or sequential use is contraindicated; combination therapy may precipitate hypertension, headache and related symptoms).
No products indexed under this heading.

Dopamine Hydrochloride (Concurrent and/or sequential use is contraindicated; combination therapy may precipitate hypertension, headache and related symptoms).
No products indexed under this heading.

Doxazosin Mesylate (Concurrent use with hypotensive agents is contraindicated; a marked potentiating effect on these classes of drugs has been reported).
No products indexed under this heading.

Doxepin Hydrochloride (Concurrent use with dibenzazepine-related entities may result in hypertensive crises or severe convulsive seizures; concurrent and/or sequential use is contraindicated).
No products indexed under this heading.

Enalapril Maleate (Concurrent use with hypotensive agents is contraindicated; a marked potentiating effect on these classes of drugs has been reported). Products include:
Vaseretic Tablets 2073
Vasotec I.V. Injection 2076

Enalaprilat (Concurrent use with hypotensive agents is contraindicated; a marked potentiating effect on these classes of drugs has been reported).
No products indexed under this heading.

Enflurane (Patients taking tranylcypromine should not undergo elective surgery requiring general anesthesia; the possible combined hypotensive effects of tranylcypromine should be kept in mind; Parnate should be discontinued at least 10 days prior to elective surgery).
No products indexed under this heading.

Ephedrine Hydrochloride (Concurrent and/or sequential use is contraindicated; combination therapy may precipitate hypertension, headache and related symptoms). Products include:
Primatene Tablets 749

Ephedrine Sulfate (Concurrent and/or sequential use is contraindicated; combination therapy may precipitate hypertension, headache and related symptoms).
No products indexed under this heading.

Ephedrine Tannate (Concurrent and/or sequential use is contraindicated; combination therapy may precipitate hypertension, headache and related symptoms).
No products indexed under this heading.

Epinephrine (Concurrent and/or sequential use is contraindicated; combination therapy may precipitate hypertension, headache and related symptoms). Products include:
EpiPen 1061
Primatene Mist 749

Epinephrine Bitartrate (Concurrent and/or sequential use is contraindicated; combination therapy may precipitate hypertension, headache and related symptoms).
No products indexed under this heading.

Epinephrine Hydrochloride (Concurrent and/or sequential use is contraindicated; combination therapy may precipitate hypertension, headache and related symptoms).
No products indexed under this heading.

Eprosartan Mesylate (Concurrent use with hypotensive agents is contraindicated; a marked potentiating effect on these classes of drugs has been reported). Products include:
Teveten Tablets 1707
Teveten HCT Tablets 1710

Escitalopram Oxalate (Concurrent and/or sequential use is contraindicated; potential for serious, sometimes fatal, reactions including hyperthermia, rigidity, myoclonus, and other toxicities). Products include:
Lexapro Oral Solution 1193
Lexapro Tablets 1193

Esmolol Hydrochloride (Concurrent use with hypotensive agents is contraindicated; a marked potentiating effect on these classes of drugs has been reported). Products include:
Brevibloc Concentrate 766
Brevibloc Injection 766
Brevibloc Double Strength Injection 766
Brevibloc Premixed Injection 766

Brevibloc Double Strength Premixed Injection 766

Estazolam (Concurrent use is contraindicated). Products include:
ProSom Tablets 512

Ethacrynic Acid (Concurrent use with hypotensive agents is contraindicated; a marked potentiating effect on these classes of drugs has been reported). Products include:
Edecrin Tablets 1941

Ethchlorvynol (Concurrent use is contraindicated).
No products indexed under this heading.

Ethinamate (Concurrent use is contraindicated).
No products indexed under this heading.

Felodipine (Concurrent use with hypotensive agents is contraindicated; a marked potentiating effect on these classes of drugs has been reported). Products include:
Plendil Extended-Release Tablets 651

Fenfluramine Hydrochloride (Concurrent and/or sequential use is contraindicated).
No products indexed under this heading.

Fentanyl (Concurrent use is contraindicated; a marked potentiating effect on these classes of drugs has been reported). Products include:
Duragesic Transdermal System 2448

Fentanyl Citrate (Concurrent use is contraindicated; a marked potentiating effect on these classes of drugs has been reported). Products include:
Actiq 993

Fexofenadine Hydrochloride (Concurrent use is contraindicated). Products include:
Allegra 2857
Allegra-D 12 Hour Extended-Release Tablets 2860
Allegra-D 24 Hour Extended-Release Tablets 2862

Fluoxetine Hydrochloride (Concurrent use has resulted in serious, sometimes fatal, reactions, including hyperthermia, rigidity, myoclonus, autonomic instability with possible rapid fluctuations of vital signs and mental status; concurrent use is contraindicated; at least 5 weeks should be allowed after stopping fluoxetine before starting an MAO inhibitor). Products include:
Prozac Pulvules and Liquid 1771
Symbyax Capsules 1788

Fluphenazine Decanoate (Possibility of additive hypotensive effects).
No products indexed under this heading.

Fluphenazine Enanthate (Possibility of additive hypotensive effects).
No products indexed under this heading.

Fluphenazine Hydrochloride (Possibility of additive hypotensive effects).
No products indexed under this heading.

Flurazepam Hydrochloride (Concurrent use is contraindicated). Products include:
Dalmane Capsules 3343

Fluvoxamine Maleate (Concurrent and/or sequential use is contraindicated; potential for serious, sometimes fatal, reactions including hyperthermia, rigidity, myoclonus, and other toxicities).
No products indexed under this heading.

Fosinopril Sodium (Concurrent use with hypotensive agents is contraindicated; a marked potentiating effect on these classes of drugs has been reported).
No products indexed under this heading.

Furazolidone (Concurrent use with another MAO inhibitor may result in hypertensive crises or severe convulsive seizures; concurrent and/or sequential use is contraindicated).
No products indexed under this heading.

Furosemide (Concurrent use with hypotensive agents is contraindicated; a marked potentiating effect on these classes of drugs has been reported). Products include:
Furosemide Tablets 2117

Glimepiride (Some MAO inhibitors have contributed to hypoglycemic episodes in diabetic patients receiving oral hypoglycemic agents). Products include:
Amaryl Tablets 2864

Glipizide (Some MAO inhibitors have contributed to hypoglycemic episodes in diabetic patients receiving oral hypoglycemic agents).
No products indexed under this heading.

Glutethimide (Concurrent use is contraindicated).
No products indexed under this heading.

Glyburide (Some MAO inhibitors have contributed to hypoglycemic episodes in diabetic patients receiving oral hypoglycemic agents).
No products indexed under this heading.

Guanabenz Acetate (Concurrent use with hypotensive agents is contraindicated; a marked potentiating effect on these classes of drugs has been reported).
No products indexed under this heading.

Guanethidine Monosulfate (Concurrent and/or sequential use is contraindicated; combination therapy may precipitate hypertension, headache and related symptoms).
No products indexed under this heading.

Halothane (Patients taking tranylcypromine should not undergo elective surgery requiring general anesthesia; the possible combined hypotensive effects of tranylcypromine should be kept in mind; Parnate should be discontinued at least 10 days prior to elective surgery).
No products indexed under this heading.

Hydralazine Hydrochloride (Concurrent use with hypotensive agents is contraindicated; a marked potentiating effect on these classes of drugs has been reported). Products include:
BiDil Tablets 2161

Hydrochlorothiazide (Concurrent use with hypotensive agents is contraindicated; a marked potentiating effect on these classes of drugs has been reported). Products include:
Aldoril Tablets 1884
Atacand HCT 637
Avalide Tablets 2889
Avalide Tablets 922
Benicar HCT Tablets 2852
Diovan HCT Tablets 2195
Dyazide Capsules 1389
Hyzaar 1964
Lotensin HCT Tablets 2235
Maxzide 2150
Micardis HCT Tablets 886
Moduretic Tablets 2003
Prinzide Tablets 2033
Teveten HCT Tablets 1710
Timolide Tablets 2056
Uniretic Tablets 3114
Vaseretic Tablets 2073
Zestoretic Tablets 701

Hydrocodone Bitartrate (Concurrent use is contraindicated; a marked potentiating effect on these classes of drugs has been reported). Products include:
Hycodan 1104
Hycomine Compound Tablets 1105
Hycotuss Expectorant Syrup 1106
Lortab 3315
Lortab Elixir 3312
Vicodin Tablets 530
Vicodin ES Tablets 531
Vicodin HP Tablets 532
Vicoprofen Tablets 533
Zydone Tablets 1118

Hydrocodone Polistirex (Concurrent use is contraindicated; a marked potentiating effect on these classes of drugs has been reported). Products include:
Tussionex Pennkinetic Extended-Release Suspension 3322

Hydroflumethiazide (Concurrent use with hypotensive agents is contraindicated; a marked potentiating effect on these classes of drugs has been reported).
No products indexed under this heading.

Hydromorphone Hydrochloride (Concurrent use is contraindicated; a marked potentiating effect on these classes of drugs has been reported). Products include:
Dilaudid 439
Dilaudid Oral Liquid 443
Dilaudid Non-Sterile Powder 439
Dilaudid Rectal Suppositories 439
Dilaudid Tablets 439
Dilaudid Tablets - 8 mg 443
Dilaudid-HP 441

Imipramine Hydrochloride (Concurrent use with dibenzazepine-related entities may result in hypertensive crises or severe convulsive seizures; concurrent and/or sequential use is contraindicated).
No products indexed under this heading.

Imipramine Pamoate (Concurrent use with dibenzazepine-related entities may result in hypertensive crises or severe convulsive seizures; concurrent and/or sequential use is contraindicated).
No products indexed under this heading.

Indapamide (Concurrent use with hypotensive agents is contraindicated; a marked potentiating effect on these classes of drugs has been reported). Products include:
Indapamide Tablets 2119

Insulin, Human, Zinc Suspension (Some MAO inhibitors have contributed to hypoglycemic episodes in diabetic patients receiving insulin). Products include:
Humulin L, 100 Units 1763
Humulin U, 100 Units 1770

Insulin, Human NPH (Some MAO inhibitors have contributed to hypoglycemic episodes in diabetic patients receiving insulin). Products include:
Humulin N, 100 Units 1764
Humulin N Pen 1765
Novolin N Human Insulin 10 ml Vials 2322
Novolin N InnoLet 2322
Novolin N PenFill 3 ml Cartridges 2325
Novolin R InnoLet 2322

Insulin, Human Regular (Some MAO inhibitors have contributed to hypoglycemic episodes in diabetic patients receiving insulin). Products include:
Humulin R (U-500) 1768
Humulin R, 100 Units 1767
Novolin R Human Insulin 10 ml Vials 2322
Novolin R PenFill 2325

Insulin, Human Regular and Human NPH Mixture (Some MAO inhibitors have contributed to hypoglycemic episodes in diabetic patients receiving insulin). Products include:
Humulin 50/50, 100 Units 1760
Humulin 70/30 Pen 1761
Novolin 70/30 Human Insulin 10 ml Vials 2321
Novolin 70/30 InnoLet 2322
Novolin 70/30 PenFill 3 ml Cartridges 2325

Insulin, NPH (Some MAO inhibitors have contributed to hypoglycemic episodes in diabetic patients receiving insulin).
No products indexed under this heading.

Insulin, Regular (Some MAO inhibitors have contributed to hypoglycemic episodes in diabetic patients receiving insulin).
No products indexed under this heading.

Insulin, Zinc Crystals (Some MAO inhibitors have contributed to hypoglycemic episodes in diabetic patients receiving insulin).
No products indexed under this heading.

Insulin, Zinc Suspension (Some MAO inhibitors have contributed to hypoglycemic episodes in diabetic patients receiving insulin).
No products indexed under this heading.

Insulin Aspart, Human Regular (Some MAO inhibitors have contributed to hypoglycemic episodes in diabetic patients receiving insulin). Products include:
NovoLog Injection 2326

Insulin glargine (Some MAO inhibitors have contributed to hypoglycemic episodes in diabetic patients receiving insulin). Products include:
Lantus Injection 2925

Insulin Lispro, Human (Some MAO inhibitors have contributed to hypoglycemic episodes in diabetic patients receiving insulin). Products include:
Humalog-Pen 1751
Humalog Mix 75/25-Pen 1754

Insulin Lispro Protamine, Human (Some MAO inhibitors have contributed to hypoglycemic episodes in diabetic patients receiving insulin). Products include:
Humalog Mix 75/25-Pen 1754

Irbesartan (Concurrent use with hypotensive agents is contraindicated; a marked potentiating effect on these classes of drugs has been reported). Products include:

Avalide Tablets 922
Avalide Tablets 2889
Avapro Tablets 925
Avapro Tablets 2886

Isocarboxazid (Concurrent use with another MAO inhibitor may result in hypertensive crises or severe convulsive seizures; concurrent and/or sequential use is contraindicated).
No products indexed under this heading.

Isoflurane (Patients taking tranylcypromine should not undergo elective surgery requiring general anesthesia; the possible combined hypotensive effects of tranylcypromine should be kept in mind; Parnate should be discontinued at least 10 days prior to elective surgery).
No products indexed under this heading.

Isoproterenol Hydrochloride (Concurrent and/or sequential use is contraindicated; combination therapy may precipitate hypertension, headache and related symptoms).
No products indexed under this heading.

Isoproterenol Sulfate (Concurrent and/or sequential use is contraindicated; combination therapy may precipitate hypertension, headache and related symptoms).
No products indexed under this heading.

Isradipine (Concurrent use with hypotensive agents is contraindicated; a marked potentiating effect on these classes of drugs has been reported). Products include:
DynaCirc CR Tablets 2726

Ketamine Hydrochloride (Patients taking tranylcypromine should not undergo elective surgery requiring general anesthesia; the possible combined hypotensive effects of tranylcypromine should be kept in mind; Parnate should be discontinued at least 10 days prior to elective surgery).
No products indexed under this heading.

Labetalol Hydrochloride (Concurrent use with hypotensive agents is contraindicated; a marked potentiating effect on these classes of drugs has been reported).
No products indexed under this heading.

Levalbuterol Hydrochloride (Concurrent and/or sequential use is contraindicated; combination therapy may precipitate hypertension, headache and related symptoms).
Products include:
Xopenex Inhalation Solution 3143
Xopenex Inhalation Solution Concentrate 3147

Levodopa (Concurrent and/or sequential use is contraindicated; combination therapy may precipitate hypertension, headache and related symptoms). Products include:
Parcopa Orally Disintegrating Tablets 3111
Stalevo Tablets 2270

Levorphanol Tartrate (Concurrent use is contraindicated; a marked potentiating effect on these classes of drugs has been reported).
No products indexed under this heading.

Lisinopril (Concurrent use with hypotensive agents is contraindicated; a marked potentiating effect on these classes of drugs has been reported). Products include:
Prinivil Tablets 2029
Prinzide Tablets 2033
Zestoretic Tablets 701
Zestril Tablets 704

Loratadine (Concurrent use is contraindicated). Products include:
Alavert Allergy & Sinus D-12 Hour Tablets 743
Alavert 743
Children's Claritin 24 Hour Non-Drowsy Allergy Syrup 732
Claritin Non-Drowsy 24 Hour Tablets 731
Non-Drowsy Claritin Hives Relief Tablets 733
Claritin Reditabs 24 Hour Non-Drowsy Tablets 732
Claritin-D Non-Drowsy 12 Hour Tablets 731
Claritin-D Non-Drowsy 24 Hour Tablets 731
Children's Dimetapp ND Non-Drowsy Allergy Syrup 746
Triaminic Allerchews 684

Lorazepam (Concurrent use is contraindicated).
No products indexed under this heading.

Losartan Potassium (Concurrent use with hypotensive agents is contraindicated; a marked potentiating effect on these classes of drugs has been reported). Products include:
Cozaar Tablets 1913
Hyzaar 1964

Maprotiline Hydrochloride (Concurrent use with dibenzazepine-related entities may result in hypertensive crises or severe convulsive seizures; concurrent and/or sequential use is contraindicated).
No products indexed under this heading.

Mazindol (Concurrent and/or sequential use is contraindicated).
No products indexed under this heading.

Mecamylamine Hydrochloride (Concurrent use with hypotensive agents is contraindicated; a marked potentiating effect on these classes of drugs has been reported).
Products include:
Inversine Tablets 3286

Meperidine Hydrochloride (Concomitant use or within 2 or 3 weeks following MAOI therapy is contraindicated; serious reactions including coma, severe hypertension or hypotension, convulsion, severe respiratory depression, malignant hyperplexia, excitation, peripheral vascular collapse, and death have been reported with combined use).
No products indexed under this heading.

Mesoridazine Besylate (Possibility of additive hypotensive effects).
No products indexed under this heading.

Metaproterenol Sulfate (Concurrent and/or sequential use is contraindicated; combination therapy may precipitate hypertension, headache and related symptoms). Products include:
Alupent Inhalation Aerosol 858

Metaraminol Bitartrate (Concurrent and/or sequential use is contraindicated; combination therapy may precipitate hypertension, headache and related symptoms). Products include:
Aramine Injection 1889

Metformin Hydrochloride (Some MAO inhibitors have contributed to hypoglycemic episodes in diabetic patients receiving oral hypoglycemic agents). Products include:
ActoPlus Met Tablets 3219
Avandamet Tablets 1343
Fortamet Extended-Release Tablets 1156

Methadone Hydrochloride (Concurrent use is contraindicated; a marked potentiating effect on these classes of drugs has been reported).
No products indexed under this heading.

Methamphetamine Hydrochloride (Concurrent and/or sequential use is contraindicated). Products include:
Desoxyn Tablets, USP 2482

Methdilazine Hydrochloride (Concurrent use is contraindicated).
No products indexed under this heading.

Methohexital Sodium (Patients taking tranylcypromine should not undergo elective surgery requiring general anesthesia; the possible combined hypotensive effects of tranylcypromine should be kept in mind; Parnate should be discontinued at least 10 days prior to elective surgery).
No products indexed under this heading.

Methotrimeprazine (Possibility of additive hypotensive effects).
No products indexed under this heading.

Methoxamine Hydrochloride (Concurrent and/or sequential use is contraindicated; combination therapy may precipitate hypertension, headache and related symptoms).
No products indexed under this heading.

Methyclothiazide (Concurrent use with hypotensive agents is contraindicated; a marked potentiating effect on these classes of drugs has been reported).
No products indexed under this heading.

Methyldopa (Concurrent and/or sequential use is contraindicated; combination therapy may precipitate hypertension, headache and related symptoms). Products include:
Aldoclor Tablets 1881
Aldoril Tablets 1884

Methyldopate Hydrochloride (Concurrent and/or sequential use is contraindicated; combination therapy may precipitate hypertension, headache and related symptoms).
No products indexed under this heading.

Metolazone (Concurrent use with hypotensive agents is contraindicated; a marked potentiating effect on these classes of drugs has been reported).
No products indexed under this heading.

Metoprolol Succinate (Concurrent use with hypotensive agents is contraindicated; a marked potentiating effect on these classes of drugs has been reported). Products include:
Toprol-XL Tablets 660

Metoprolol Tartrate (Concurrent use with hypotensive agents is contraindicated; a marked potentiating effect on these classes of drugs has been reported).
No products indexed under this heading.

Metrizamide (Concurrent use with drugs which lower seizure threshold, including MAO inhibitors, should not be used with metrizamide).
No products indexed under this heading.

Metyrosine (Concurrent use with hypotensive agents is contraindicated; a marked potentiating effect on these classes of drugs has been reported). Products include:
Demser Capsules 1933

Mibefradil Dihydrochloride (Concurrent use with hypotensive agents is contraindicated; a marked potentiating effect on these classes of drugs has been reported).
No products indexed under this heading.

Midazolam Hydrochloride (Patients taking tranylcypromine should not undergo elective surgery requiring general anesthesia; the possible combined hypotensive effects of tranylcypromine should be kept in mind; Parnate should be discontinued at least 10 days prior to elective surgery).
No products indexed under this heading.

Miglitol (Some MAO inhibitors have contributed to hypoglycemic episodes in diabetic patients receiving oral hypoglycemic agents).
No products indexed under this heading.

Minoxidil (Concurrent use with hypotensive agents is contraindicated; a marked potentiating effect on these classes of drugs has been reported). Products include:
Men's Rogaine Extra Strength Topical Solution, Ocean Rush Scent and Original Unscented 706
Women's Rogaine Topical Solution, Spring Bloom Scent and Original Unscented 707

Moclobemide (Concurrent use with another MAO inhibitor may result in hypertensive crises or severe convulsive seizures; concurrent and/or sequential use is contraindicated).
No products indexed under this heading.

Moexipril Hydrochloride (Concurrent use with hypotensive agents is contraindicated; a marked potentiating effect on these classes of drugs has been reported). Products include:
Uniretic Tablets 3114
Univasc Tablets 3118

Morphine Sulfate (Concurrent use is contraindicated; a marked potentiating effect on these classes of drugs has been reported). Products include:
Avinza Capsules 1714
Kadian Capsules 572
MS Contin Tablets 2703

Nadolol (Concurrent use with hypotensive agents is contraindicated; a marked potentiating effect on these classes of drugs has been reported). Products include:
Nadolol Tablets 2121

Naphazoline Hydrochloride (Concurrent and/or sequential use is contraindicated; combination therapy may precipitate hypertension, headache and related symptoms).
Products include:
Albalon Ophthalmic Solution .... ⊙ 216
Visine-A Eye Drops 713

Nicardipine Hydrochloride (Concurrent use with hypotensive agents is contraindicated; a marked potenti-

IMPORTANT NOTE: Always consult each drug listing in the patient's regimen for possible interactions.

ating effect on these classes of drugs has been reported). Products include:

Cardene I.V. 1129

Nifedipine (Concurrent use with hypotensive agents is contraindicated; a marked potentiating effect on these classes of drugs has been reported). Products include:

Adalat CC Tablets 2978

Nisoldipine (Concurrent use with hypotensive agents is contraindicated; a marked potentiating effect on these classes of drugs has been reported). Products include:

Sular Tablets 1163

Nitroglycerin (Concurrent use with hypotensive agents is contraindicated; a marked potentiating effect on these classes of drugs has been reported). Products include:

Nitro-Dur Transdermal Infusion System 3060
Nitrolingual Pumpspray 1161

Norepinephrine Bitartrate (Concurrent and/or sequential use is contraindicated; combination therapy may precipitate hypertension, headache and related symptoms).

No products indexed under this heading.

Nortriptyline Hydrochloride (Concurrent use with dibenzazepine-related entities may result in hypertensive crises or severe convulsive seizures; concurrent and/or sequential use is contraindicated).

No products indexed under this heading.

Oxycodone Hydrochloride (Concurrent use is contraindicated; a marked potentiating effect on these classes of drugs has been reported). Products include:

Combunox Tablets 1183
OxyContin Tablets 2699
OxyFast Oral Concentrate Solution 2704
OxyIR Capsules 2704
Percocet Tablets 1114
Percodan Tablets 1115

Oxymetazoline Hydrochloride (Concurrent and/or sequential use is contraindicated; combination therapy may precipitate hypertension, headache and related symptoms). Products include:

Vicks Sinex 12-Hour Nasal Spray and Ultra Fine Mist for Sinus Relief 2678
Visine L.R. Long Lasting Eye Drops .... ⊙279
Zicam Extreme Congestion Relief Nasal Pump .... ▣
Zicam Sinus Relief Nasal Pump .... ▣

Pargyline Hydrochloride (Concurrent use with another MAO inhibitor may result in hypertensive crises or severe convulsive seizures; concurrent and/or sequential use is contraindicated).

No products indexed under this heading.

Paroxetine Hydrochloride (Concurrent and/or sequential use is contraindicated; potential for serious, sometimes fatal, reactions including hyperthermia, rigidity, myoclonus, and other toxicities; at least 2 weeks should be allowed after stopping paroxetine before starting an MAO inhibitor). Products include:

Paxil CR Controlled-Release Tablets 1509
Paxil 1501

Penbutolol Sulfate (Concurrent use with hypotensive agents is contraindicated; a marked potentiating effect on these classes of drugs has been reported).

No products indexed under this heading.

Perindopril Erbumine (Concurrent use with hypotensive agents is contraindicated; a marked potentiating effect on these classes of drugs has been reported). Products include:

Aceon Tablets (2 mg, 4 mg, 8 mg) 3191

Perphenazine (Possibility of additive hypotensive effects).

No products indexed under this heading.

Phendimetrazine Tartrate (Concurrent and/or sequential use is contraindicated).

No products indexed under this heading.

Phenelzine Sulfate (Concurrent use with another MAO inhibitor may result in hypertensive crises or severe convulsive seizures; concurrent and/or sequential use is contraindicated).

No products indexed under this heading.

Phenmetrazine Hydrochloride (Concurrent and/or sequential use is contraindicated).

No products indexed under this heading.

Phenoxybenzamine Hydrochloride (Concurrent use with hypotensive agents is contraindicated; a marked potentiating effect on these classes of drugs has been reported). Products include:

Dibenzyline Capsules 3390

Phentolamine Mesylate (Concurrent use with hypotensive agents is contraindicated; a marked potentiating effect on these classes of drugs has been reported).

No products indexed under this heading.

Phenylephrine Bitartrate (Concurrent and/or sequential use is contraindicated; combination therapy may precipitate hypertension, headache and related symptoms).

No products indexed under this heading.

Phenylephrine Hydrochloride (Concurrent and/or sequential use is contraindicated; combination therapy may precipitate hypertension, headache and related symptoms). Products include:

Alacol DM Syrup 739
Hycomine Compound Tablets 1105
Preparation H Maximum Strength Cream .... ▣747
Preparation H Cooling Gel .... ▣747
Preparation H .... ▣747
Sudafed PE Tablets .... ▣711
Vicks Sinex Nasal Spray and Ultra Fine Mist for Sinus Relief 2677
Zicam Concentrated Cough Mist for Kids Plus D Cool Cherry .... ▣643
Zicam Concentrated Cough Mist Plus D Cool Cherry .... ▣642

Phenylephrine Tannate (Concurrent and/or sequential use is contraindicated; combination therapy may precipitate hypertension, headache and related symptoms).

No products indexed under this heading.

Phenylpropanolamine Hydrochloride (Concurrent and/or sequential use is contraindicated; combination therapy may precipitate hypertension, headache and related symptoms).

No products indexed under this heading.

Pindolol (Concurrent use with hypotensive agents is contraindicated; a marked potentiating effect on these classes of drugs has been reported).

No products indexed under this heading.

Pioglitazone Hydrochloride (Some MAO inhibitors have contributed to hypoglycemic episodes in diabetic patients receiving oral hypoglycemic agents). Products include:

ActoPlus Met Tablets 3219
Actos Tablets 3224

Pirbuterol Acetate (Concurrent and/or sequential use is contraindicated; combination therapy may precipitate hypertension, headache and related symptoms). Products include:

Maxair Autohaler 1820

Polythiazide (Concurrent use with hypotensive agents is contraindicated; a marked potentiating effect on these classes of drugs has been reported).

No products indexed under this heading.

Prazosin Hydrochloride (Concurrent use with hypotensive agents is contraindicated; a marked potentiating effect on these classes of drugs has been reported).

No products indexed under this heading.

Procarbazine Hydrochloride (Concurrent use with another MAO inhibitor may result in hypertensive crises or severe convulsive seizures; concurrent and/or sequential use is contraindicated). Products include:

Matulane Capsules 3188

Prochlorperazine (Possibility of additive hypotensive effects).

No products indexed under this heading.

Procyclidine Hydrochloride (Anti-Parkinsonism drugs should be used with caution in patients receiving Parnate since severe reactions have been reported).

No products indexed under this heading.

Promethazine Hydrochloride (Concurrent use is contraindicated). Products include:

Phenergan 3438

Propofol (Patients taking tranylcypromine should not undergo elective surgery requiring general anesthesia; the possible combined hypotensive effects of tranylcypromine should be kept in mind; Parnate should be discontinued at least 10 days prior to elective surgery). Products include:

Diprivan Injectable Emulsion 676

Propoxyphene Hydrochloride (Concurrent use is contraindicated; a marked potentiating effect on these classes of drugs has been reported).

No products indexed under this heading.

Propoxyphene Napsylate (Concurrent use is contraindicated; a marked potentiating effect on these classes of drugs has been reported). Products include:

Darvocet A 500 Tablets 3497

Propranolol Hydrochloride (Concurrent use with hypotensive agents is contraindicated; a marked potentiating effect on these classes of drugs has been reported). Products include:

Inderal LA Long-Acting Capsules 3421
InnoPran XL Capsules 2728

Protriptyline Hydrochloride (Concurrent use with dibenzazepine-related entities may result in hypertensive crises or severe convulsive seizures; concurrent and/or sequential use is contraindicated). Products include:

Vivactil Tablets 2350

Pseudoephedrine Hydrochloride (Concurrent and/or sequential use is contraindicated; combination therapy may precipitate hypertension, headache and related symptoms). Products include:

Advil Allergy Sinus Caplets .... ▣737
Advil Cold & Sinus .... ▣739
Advil Flu & Body Ache Caplets .... ▣739
Children's Advil Cold Suspension .... ▣741
Advil Multi-Symptom Cold Caplets .... ▣738
Allegra-D 12 Hour Extended-Release Tablets 2860
Allegra-D 24 Hour Extended-Release Tablets 2862
Balamine DM 739
BC Cold Powder .... ▣612
Benadryl Allergy & Cold Tablets .... ▣692
Benadryl Allergy & Sinus Headache Caplets & Gelcaps .... ▣693
Children's Benadryl Allergy & Cold Fastmelt Tablets .... ▣695
Benadryl Maximum Strength Severe Allergy & Sinus Headache Caplets .... ▣694
Children's Benadryl D Allergy & Sinus Fastmelt Tablets .... ▣694
Children's Benadryl D Liquid Medication .... ▣693
Benadryl D Tablets .... ▣694
Contac Non-Drowsy 12 Hour Cold Caplets .... ▣614
Contac Non-Drowsy Timed Release 12 Hour Cold Caplets .... ▣615
Contac Severe Cold and Flu Caplets Maximum Strength .... ▣615
Contac Severe Cold and Flu Caplets Non-Drowsy .... ▣615
Children's Dimetapp Cold & Allergy Elixir .... ▣745
Children's Dimetapp DM Cold & Cough Elixir .... ▣745
Children's Dimetapp Long Acting Cough Plus Cold Syrup .... ▣746
Dimetapp Infant Drops Decongestant Plus Cough .... ▣746
Children's Motrin Cold Non-Staining Dye-Free Oral Suspension 1838
Children's Motrin Cold Oral Suspension 1838
Motrin Cold & Sinus Caplets 1836
PediaCare Decongestant & Cough Infant Drops .... ▣705
PediaCare Decongestant Infants' Drops .... ▣705
PediaCare Long-Acting Cough Plus Cold Liquid .... ▣704
PediaCare Multi-Symptom Cold Liquid .... ▣704
PediaCare NightRest Cough & Cold Liquid .... ▣704
Robitussin Allergy & Cough Syrup .... ▣750
Robitussin CF Liquid .... ▣755
Robitussin Cough & Cold Liquid-filled Capsules .... ▣750
Robitussin Cough, Cold & Flu Liquid-filled Capsules .... ▣750
Robitussin Cough & Cold Infant Drops .... ▣755
Robitussin Flu Liquid .... ▣752
Robitussin Maximum Strength Cough & Cold Liquid .... ▣754
Robitussin PE Syrup .... ▣753
Robitussin Pediatric Cough & Cold Liquid .... ▣754
Robitussin PM Cough & Cold Liquid .... ▣752

Robitussin Severe Congestion Liquid-filled Capsules 751
Simply Stuffy Liquid 1841
Singlet Caplets 636
Sudafed 12 Hour Caplets 708
Sudafed 24 Hour Tablets 709
Sudafed Nasal Decongestant Tablets 709
Sudafed Severe Cold 710
Sudafed Non-Drying Sinus Liquid Caps 709
Sudafed Sinus & Allergy Tablets 710
Sudafed Sinus Headache 711
TheraFlu Cold & Cough Hot Liquid 680
TheraFlu Cold & Sore Throat Hot Liquid 680
TheraFlu Flu & Chest Congestion Non-Drowsy Hot Liquid 681
TheraFlu Flu & Sore Throat Hot Liquid 681
TheraFlu Severe Cold Non-Drowsy Hot Liquid 683
TheraFlu Severe Cold & Cough Hot Liquid 683
TheraFlu Severe Cold Caplets 679
TheraFlu Severe Cold Hot Liquid 682
TheraFlu Severe Cold Non-Drowsy Caplets 679
Triaminic Chest & Nasal Congestion Liquid 685
Triaminic Cold & Allergy Liquid 685
Triaminic Cold & Cough Liquid 685
Triaminic Cough Liquid 687
Triaminic Cough & Nasal Congestion Liquid 687
Triaminic Cough & Sore Throat Liquid 687
Triaminic Flu, Cough & Fever Liquid 685
Triaminic Night Time Cough & Cold Liquid 685
Triaminic Allergy Runny Nose & Congestion Softchews 688
Triaminic Cold & Cough Softchews 688
Triaminic Cough & Sore Throat Softchews 689
Tylenol Sinus NightTime Caplets 663
Children's Tylenol Plus Cold & Allergy Suspension Liquid 1850
Children's Tylenol Plus Cold NightTime Suspension Liquid 1851
Children's Tylenol Plus Cold & Cough Suspension Liquid and Chewable Tablets 1851
Children's Tylenol Plus Cold Chewable Tablets 1851
Children's Tylenol Plus Cold Daytime Non-Drowsy Suspension Liquid 1851
Children's Tylenol Plus Flu Suspension Liquid 1853
Concentrated Tylenol Infants' Drops Plus Cold 1851
Concentrated Tylenol Infants' Drops Plus Cold and Cough 1851
Tylenol Cold & Flu Severe Daytime Liquid with Cool Bust 1846
Tylenol Cold & Flu Severe NightTime Liquid with Cool Burst 1846
Tylenol Cold Severe Congestion Non-Drowsy Caplets with Cool Burst 1846
Tylenol Allergy Complete Night Time Caplets 1844
Tylenol Allergy Complete Multi-Symptom Caplets and Gelcaps with Cool Burst 1844
Tylenol Flu NightTime Gelcaps 1846
Tylenol Flu Day Non-Drowsy Gelcaps 1846
Concentrated Tylenol Infants' Drops Plus Cold Nasal Congestant, Fever Reducer & Pain Reliever 668
Concentrated Tylenol Infants' Drops Plus Cold & Cough Nasal Decongestant, Fever Reducer & Pain Reliever 668
Multi-Symptom Tylenol Cold Night Time Caplets 1845
Multi-Symptom Tylenol Cold Day Non-Drowsy Caplets and Gelcaps 1845
Tylenol Sinus Day Non-Drowsy 1848
Tylenol Sinus Night Time Caplets 1848
Tylenol Sinus Severe Congestion Caplets with Cool Burst 1848
Vicks 44D Cough & Head Congestion Relief 2676
Vicks 44D Cough & Head Congestion Relief Liquid 721
Vicks 44M Cough, Cold & Flu Relief 2676
Pediatric Vicks 44m Cough & Cold Relief 2673
Vicks DayQuil LiquiCaps/Liquid Multi-Symptom Cold/Flu Relief 723
Vicks DayQuil Multi-Symptom Cold/Flu Relief LiquiCaps 2675
Vicks DayQuil Multi-Symptom Cold/Flu Relief Liquid 2675
Children's Vicks NyQuil Cold/Cough Relief 2671
Vicks NyQuil LiquiCaps 2677
Vicks NyQuil LiquiCaps/Liquid Multi-Symptom Cold/Flu Relief 725
Vicks NyQuil Liquid 2677
Zyrtec-D 12 Hour Extended Release Tablets 2591

Pseudoephedrine Sulfate (Concurrent and/or sequential use is contraindicated; combination therapy may precipitate hypertension, headache and related symptoms). Products include:
Alavert Allergy & Sinus D-12 Hour Tablets 743
Clarinex-D 24-Hour Extended-Release Tablets 3012
Claritin-D Non-Drowsy 12 Hour Tablets 731
Claritin-D Non-Drowsy 24 Hour Tablets 731

Pyrilamine Maleate (Concurrent use is contraindicated).
No products indexed under this heading.

Pyrilamine Tannate (Concurrent use is contraindicated).
No products indexed under this heading.

Quazepam (Concurrent use is contraindicated).
No products indexed under this heading.

Quinapril Hydrochloride (Concurrent use with hypotensive agents is contraindicated; a marked potentiating effect on these classes of drugs has been reported).
No products indexed under this heading.

Ramipril (Concurrent use with hypotensive agents is contraindicated; a marked potentiating effect on these classes of drugs has been reported). Products include:
Altace Capsules 1673

Rauwolfia Serpentina (Concurrent use with hypotensive agents is contraindicated; a marked potentiating effect on these classes of drugs has been reported).
No products indexed under this heading.

Remifentanil Hydrochloride (Concurrent use is contraindicated; a marked potentiating effect on these classes of drugs has been reported).
No products indexed under this heading.

Repaglinide (Some MAO inhibitors have contributed to hypoglycemic episodes in diabetic patients receiving oral hypoglycemic agents). Products include:
Prandin Tablets (0.5, 1, and 2 mg) 2337

Rescinnamine (Concurrent use with hypotensive agents is contraindicated; a marked potentiating effect on these classes of drugs has been reported).
No products indexed under this heading.

Reserpine (Concurrent and/or sequential use is contraindicated; combination therapy may precipitate hypertension, headache and related symptoms).
No products indexed under this heading.

Rosiglitazone Maleate (Some MAO inhibitors have contributed to hypoglycemic episodes in diabetic patients receiving oral hypoglycemic agents). Products include:
Avandamet Tablets 1343
Avandia Tablets 1348

Salmeterol Xinafoate (Concurrent and/or sequential use is contraindicated; combination therapy may precipitate hypertension, headache and related symptoms). Products include:
Advair Diskus 100/50 1291
Advair Diskus 250/50 1291
Advair Diskus 500/50 1291
Serevent Diskus 1540

Secobarbital Sodium (Concurrent use is contraindicated).
No products indexed under this heading.

Selegiline Hydrochloride (Concurrent use with another MAO inhibitor may result in hypertensive crises or severe convulsive seizures; concurrent and/or sequential use is contraindicated). Products include:
Eldepryl Capsules 3209

Sertraline Hydrochloride (Concurrent and/or sequential use is contraindicated; potential for serious, sometimes fatal, reactions, including hyperthermia, rigidity, myoclonus, and other toxicities; at least 2 weeks should be allowed after stopping sertraline before starting an MAOinhibitor). Products include:
Zoloft 2581

Sibutramine Hydrochloride Monohydrate (Concurrent and/or sequential use is contraindicated). Products include:
Meridia Capsules 485

Sodium Nitroprusside (Concurrent use with hypotensive agents is contraindicated; a marked potentiating effect on these classes of drugs has been reported).
No products indexed under this heading.

Sotalol Hydrochloride (Concurrent use with hypotensive agents is contraindicated; a marked potentiating effect on these classes of drugs has been reported).
No products indexed under this heading.

Spirapril Hydrochloride (Concurrent use with hypotensive agents is contraindicated; a marked potentiating effect on these classes of drugs has been reported).
No products indexed under this heading.

Spironolactone (Concurrent use with hypotensive agents is contraindicated; a marked potentiating effect on these classes of drugs has been reported).
No products indexed under this heading.

Sufentanil Citrate (Concurrent use is contraindicated; a marked potentiating effect on these classes of drugs has been reported).
No products indexed under this heading.

Telmisartan (Concurrent use with hypotensive agents is contraindicated; a marked potentiating effect on these classes of drugs has been reported). Products include:
Micardis Tablets 884
Micardis HCT Tablets 886

Temazepam (Concurrent use is contraindicated).
No products indexed under this heading.

Terazosin Hydrochloride (Concurrent use with hypotensive agents is contraindicated; a marked potentiating effect on these classes of drugs has been reported). Products include:
Hytrin Capsules 469

Terbutaline Sulfate (Concurrent and/or sequential use is contraindicated; combination therapy may precipitate hypertension, headache and related symptoms).
No products indexed under this heading.

Terfenadine (Concurrent use is contraindicated).
No products indexed under this heading.

Tetrahydrozoline Hydrochloride (Concurrent and/or sequential use is contraindicated; combination therapy may precipitate hypertension, headache and related symptoms). Products include:
Visine A.C. Seasonal Itching and Redness Relief Drops .... ⊙278
Advanced Relief Visine Eye Drops .... ⊙278

Thiamylal Sodium (Patients taking tranylcypromine should not undergo elective surgery requiring general anesthesia; the possible combined hypotensive effects of tranylcypromine should be kept in mind; Parnate should be discontinued at least 10 days prior to elective surgery).
No products indexed under this heading.

Thioridazine Hydrochloride (Possibility of additive hypotensive effects). Products include:
Thioridazine Hydrochloride Tablets 2122

Timolol Maleate (Concurrent use with hypotensive agents is contraindicated; a marked potentiating effect on these classes of drugs has been reported). Products include:
Blocadren Tablets 1891
Cosopt Sterile Ophthalmic Solution 1910
Timolide Tablets 2056
Timoptic in Ocudose 2061
Timoptic Sterile Ophthalmic Solution 2058
Timoptic-XE Sterile Ophthalmic Gel Forming Solution 2062

Tolazamide (Some MAO inhibitors have contributed to hypoglycemic episodes in diabetic patients receiving oral hypoglycemic agents).
No products indexed under this heading.

Tolbutamide (Some MAO inhibitors have contributed to hypoglycemic episodes in diabetic patients receiving oral hypoglycemic agents).
No products indexed under this heading.

Torsemide (Concurrent use with hypotensive agents is contraindicated; a marked potentiating effect on these classes of drugs has been reported).
No products indexed under this heading.

Trandolapril (Concurrent use with hypotensive agents is contraindi-

cated; a marked potentiating effect on these classes of drugs has been reported). Products include:
- Mavik Tablets ... 482
- Tarka Tablets ... 519

Triamterene (Concurrent use with hypotensive agents is contraindicated; a marked potentiating effect on these classes of drugs has been reported). Products include:
- Dyazide Capsules ... 1389
- Dyrenium Capsules ... 3390
- Maxzide ... 2150

Triazolam (Concurrent use is contraindicated).
No products indexed under this heading.

Tridihexethyl Chloride (Anti-Parkinsonism drugs should be used with caution in patients receiving Parnate since severe reactions have been reported).
No products indexed under this heading.

Trifluoperazine Hydrochloride (Possibility of additive hypotensive effects).
No products indexed under this heading.

Trihexyphenidyl Hydrochloride (Anti-Parkinsonism drugs should be used with caution in patients receiving Parnate since severe reactions have been reported).
No products indexed under this heading.

Trimeprazine Tartrate (Concurrent use is contraindicated).
No products indexed under this heading.

Trimethaphan Camsylate (Concurrent use with hypotensive agents is contraindicated; a marked potentiating effect on these classes of drugs has been reported).
No products indexed under this heading.

Trimipramine Maleate (Concurrent use with dibenzazepine-related entities may result in hypertensive crises or severe convulsive seizures; concurrent and/or sequential use is contraindicated). Products include:
- Surmontil Capsules ... 2347

Tripelennamine Hydrochloride (Concurrent use is contraindicated).
No products indexed under this heading.

Triprolidine Hydrochloride (Concurrent use is contraindicated).
No products indexed under this heading.

Troglitazone (Some MAO inhibitors have contributed to hypoglycemic episodes in diabetic patients receiving oral hypoglycemic agents).
No products indexed under this heading.

L-Tryptophan (Concurrent and/or sequential use is contraindicated; combination therapy may precipitate hypertension, disorientation, memory impairment, other neurologic and behavioral changes, headache and related symptoms).
No products indexed under this heading.

Tyramine (Concurrent use is contraindicated).
No products indexed under this heading.

Valsartan (Concurrent use with hypotensive agents is contraindicated; a marked potentiating effect on these classes of drugs has been reported). Products include:
- Diovan HCT Tablets ... 2195
- Diovan Tablets ... 2191

Verapamil Hydrochloride (Concurrent use with hypotensive agents is contraindicated; a marked potentiating effect on these classes of drugs has been reported). Products include:
- Covera-HS Tablets ... 3135
- Tarka Tablets ... 519
- Verelan PM Capsules ... 3120

Zaleplon (Concurrent use is contraindicated). Products include:
- Sonata Capsules ... 1686

Zolpidem Tartrate (Concurrent use is contraindicated). Products include:
- Ambien Tablets ... 2867

Food Interactions

Alcohol (Concurrent use is contraindicated; a marked potentiating effect on alcohol has been reported).

Anchovies (Potential for hypertensive crisis; concurrent use is contraindicated).

Avocados (Potential for hypertensive crisis; concurrent use is contraindicated).

Bananas (Potential for hypertensive crisis; concurrent use is contraindicated).

Beans, broad (Potential for hypertensive crisis; concurrent use is contraindicated).

Beans, Fava (Potential for hypertensive crisis; concurrent use is contraindicated).

Beer, alcohol-free (Potential for hypertensive crisis; concurrent use is contraindicated).

Beer, unspecified (Potential for hypertensive crisis; concurrent use is contraindicated).

Beverages, caffeine-containing (Potential for hypertensive crisis; concurrent use is contraindicated).

Caviar (Potential for hypertensive crisis; concurrent use is contraindicated).

Cheese, aged (Potential for hypertensive crisis; concurrent use is contraindicated).

Cheese, strong, unpasteurized (Potential for hypertensive crisis; concurrent use is contraindicated).

Cheese, unspecified (Potential for hypertensive crisis; concurrent use is contraindicated).

Chocolate (Potential for hypertensive crisis; concurrent use is contraindicated).

Cream, sour (Potential for hypertensive crisis; concurrent use is contraindicated).

Figs, canned (Potential for hypertensive crisis; concurrent use is contraindicated).

Food with high concentration of tyramine (Potential for hypertensive crisis; concurrent use is contraindicated).

Fruits, dried (Potential for hypertensive crisis; concurrent use is contraindicated).

Fruits, overripe (Potential for hypertensive crisis; concurrent use is contraindicated).

Herring, pickled (Potential for hypertensive crisis; concurrent use is contraindicated).

Liqueurs (Potential for hypertensive crisis; concurrent use is contraindicated).

Liver (Potential for hypertensive crisis; concurrent use is contraindicated).

Meat extracts (Potential for hypertensive crisis; concurrent use is contraindicated).

Meat prepared with tenderizers (Potential for hypertensive crisis; concurrent use is contraindicated).

Prunes (Potential for hypertensive crisis; concurrent use is contraindicated).

Raisins (Potential for hypertensive crisis; concurrent use is contraindicated).

Raspberries (Potential for hypertensive crisis; concurrent use is contraindicated).

Sauerkraut (Potential for hypertensive crisis; concurrent use is contraindicated).

Sherry (Potential for hypertensive crisis; concurrent use is contraindicated).

Soy Sauce (Potential for hypertensive crisis; concurrent use is contraindicated).

Wine, Chianti (Potential for hypertensive crisis; concurrent use is contraindicated).

Yeast Extract (Potential for hypertensive crisis; concurrent use is contraindicated).

Yogurt (Potential for hypertensive crisis; concurrent use is contraindicated).

PASER GRANULES

(Aminosalicylic Acid) ... 1657
May interact with:

Digoxin (Potential for reduced digoxin levels). Products include:
- Digitek Tablets ... 2146
- Lanoxicaps Capsules ... 1458
- Lanoxin Injection ... 1462
- Lanoxin Tablets ... 1468
- Lanoxin Injection Pediatric ... 1465

Isoniazid (Concurrent use with a rapidly available form of aminosalicylic acid has been reported to produce a 20% reduction in the acetylation of INH; the lower serum levels produced by delayed release preparation will result in a reduced effect on the acetylation of INH).
No products indexed under this heading.

Rifampin (May block the absorption of rifampin; PASER granules do not contain excipient that blocks the absorption).
No products indexed under this heading.

Vitamin B_{12} (Reduced absorption of vitamin B_{12} with clinically significant erythrocyte abnormalities developing after depletion). Products include:
- Bevitamel Tablets ... 3392
- Chromagen Forte Soft Gelatin Capsules ... 3296
- Niferex-150 Forte Capsules ... 3299
- Repliva 21/7 Tablets ... 3301

PATANOL OPHTHALMIC SOLUTION

(Olopatadine Hydrochloride) ... 557
None cited in PDR database.

PAXIL CR CONTROLLED-RELEASE TABLETS

(Paroxetine Hydrochloride) ... 1509
See Paxil Tablets

PAXIL ORAL SUSPENSION

(Paroxetine Hydrochloride) ... 1501
See Paxil Tablets

PAXIL TABLETS

(Paroxetine Hydrochloride) ... 1501
May interact with anticoagulants, cytochrome p450 2d6 inhibitors (selected), cytochrome p450 2d6 substrates (selected), lithium preparations, monoamine oxidase inhibitors, non-steroidal anti-inflammatory agents, phenothiazines, phenytoin, highly protein bound drugs (selected), selective serotonin reuptake inhibitors, tricyclic antidepressants, triptans, xanthines, and certain other agents. Compounds in these categories include:

Almotriptan Malate (There have been rare post-marketing reports describing patients with weakness, hyperreflexia, and incoordination following the use of a selective serotonin reuptake inhibitor (SSRI) and sumatriptan. If concomitant treatment with a triptan and an SSRI (eg, paroxetine) is clinically warranted, appropriate observation of the patient is advised). Products include:
- Axert Tablets ... 2430

Aminophylline (There have been reports of elevated theophylline levels associated with co-administration; monitor theophylline levels when these drugs are concurrently administered).
No products indexed under this heading.

Amiodarone Hydrochloride (Paroxetine is metabolized by the cytochrome P450 isoenzyme CYP2D6. Therefore, co-administration of paroxetine with other drugs that inhibit this enzyme should be approached with caution). Products include:
- Pacerone Tablets ... 3337

Amitriptyline Hydrochloride (Caution is indicated in the co-administration of tricyclic antidepressants with paroxetine because paroxetine may inhibit TCA metabolism. Plasma TCA concentrations may need to be monitored and the dose of TCA may need to be reduced if a TCA is co-administered with paroxetine).
No products indexed under this heading.

Amoxapine (Caution is indicated in the co-administration of tricyclic antidepressants with paroxetine because paroxetine may inhibit TCA metabolism. Plasma TCA concentrations may need to be monitored and the dose of TCA may need to be reduced if a TCA is co-administered with paroxetine).
No products indexed under this heading.

Amphetamine Aspartate (Paroxetine may significantly inhibit the activity of the cytochrome P450 2D6 isoenzyme. Concomitant use of paroxetine with other drugs metabolized by cytochrome CYP2D6 has not been formally studied but may require lower doses than usually prescribed for either paroxetine or the other drug. Therefore, co-administration of paroxetine with other drugs that are metabolized by this isozyme should be approached with caution). Products include:
- Adderall Tablets ... 3168
- Adderall XR Capsules ... 3169

Amphetamine Aspartate Monohydrate (Paroxetine may significantly inhibit the activity of the cytochrome P450 2D6 isoenzyme. Concomitant use of paroxetine with other drugs metabolized by cytochrome CYP2D6 has not been for-

mally studied but may require lower doses than usually prescribed for either paroxetine or the other drug. Therefore, co-administration of paroxetine with other drugs that are metabolized by this isozyme should be approached with caution).

No products indexed under this heading.

Amphetamine Sulfate (Paroxetine may significantly inhibit the activity of the cytochrome P450 2D6 isoenzyme. Concomitant use of paroxetine with other drugs metabolized by cytochrome CYP2D6 has not been formally studied but may require lower doses than usually prescribed for either paroxetine or the other drug. Therefore, co-administration of paroxetine with other drugs that are metabolized by this isozyme should be approached with caution). Products include:

Adderall Tablets 3168
Adderall XR Capsules 3169

Anisindione (The combined use of psychotropic drugs that interfere with serotonin reuptake and drugs that affect coagulation has been associated with an increased risk of bleeding; concomitant administration should be undertaken with caution). Products include:

Miradon Tablets 3056

Ardeparin Sodium (The combined use of psychotropic drugs that interfere with serotonin reuptake and drugs that affect coagulation has been associated with an increased risk of bleeding; concomitant administration should be undertaken with caution).

No products indexed under this heading.

Aspirin (The combined use of psychotropic drugs that interfere with serotonin reuptake and drugs that affect coagulation has been associated with an increased risk of bleeding). Products include:

Aggrenox Capsules 855
Bayer, Aspirin Regimen 606
Bayer Aspirin Tablets 3515
BC Powder 612
BC Allergy Sinus Cold Powder 612
Arthritis Strength BC Powder 612
BC Sinus Cold Powder 612
Ecotrin Enteric Coated Aspirin Low, Regular and Maximum Strength Tablets 1627
Goody's Body Pain Formula Powder 621
Goody's Extra Strength Headache Powder 621
Goody's Extra Strength Pain Relief Tablets 621
Percodan Tablets 1115
St. Joseph 81 mg Aspirin Chewable and Enteric Coated Tablets 1841

Aspirin, Enteric Coated (The combined use of psychotropic drugs that interfere with serotonin reuptake and drugs that affect coagulation has been associated with an increased risk of bleeding).

No products indexed under this heading.

Aspirin Buffered (The combined use of psychotropic drugs that interfere with serotonin reuptake and drugs that affect coagulation has been associated with an increased risk of bleeding).

No products indexed under this heading.

Atomoxetine Hydrochloride (Paroxetine may significantly inhibit the activity of the cytochrome P450 2D6 isoenzyme. Concomitant use of paroxetine with other drugs metabolized by cytochrome CYP2D6 has not been formally studied but may require lower doses than usually prescribed for either paroxetine or the other drug. Therefore, co-administration of paroxetine with other drugs that are metabolized by this isozyme should be approached with caution). Products include:

Strattera Capsules 1784

Atovaquone (Co-administration with another drug that is highly protein bound may increase free concentrations of the other drug or paroxetine potentially resulting in adverse events). Products include:

Malarone Tablets 1484
Malarone Pediatric Tablets 1484
Mepron Suspension 1487

Bisoprolol Fumarate (Paroxetine may significantly inhibit the activity of the cytochrome P450 2D6 isoenzyme. Concomitant use of paroxetine with other drugs metabolized by cytochrome CYP2D6 has not been formally studied but may require lower doses than usually prescribed for either paroxetine or the other drug. Therefore, co-administration of paroxetine with other drugs that are metabolized by this isozyme should be approached with caution).

No products indexed under this heading.

Bupropion Hydrochloride (Paroxetine is metabolized by the cytochrome P450 isoenzyme CYP2D6. Therefore, co-administration of paroxetine with other drugs that inhibit this enzyme should be approached with caution). Products include:

Wellbutrin Tablets 1579
Wellbutrin SR Sustained-Release Tablets 1583
Wellbutrin XL Extended-Release Tablets 1588
Zyban Sustained-Release Tablets 1620

Captopril (Paroxetine may significantly inhibit the activity of the cytochrome P450 2D6 isoenzyme. Concomitant use of paroxetine with other drugs metabolized by cytochrome CYP2D6 has not been formally studied but may require lower doses than usually prescribed for either paroxetine or the other drug. Therefore, co-administration of paroxetine with other drugs that are metabolized by this isozyme should be approached with caution). Products include:

Captopril Tablets 2114

Carvedilol (Paroxetine may significantly inhibit the activity of the cytochrome P450 2D6 isoenzyme. Concomitant use of paroxetine with other drugs metabolized by cytochrome CYP2D6 has not been formally studied but may require lower doses than usually prescribed for either paroxetine or the other drug. Therefore, co-administration of paroxetine with other drugs that are metabolized by this isozyme should be approached with caution). Products include:

Coreg Tablets 1376

Cefonicid Sodium (Co-administration with another drug that is highly protein bound may increase free concentrations of the other drug or paroxetine potentially resulting in adverse events).

No products indexed under this heading.

Celecoxib (Paroxetine is metabolized by the cytochrome P450 isoenzyme CYP2D6. Therefore, co-administration of paroxetine with other drugs that inhibit this enzyme should be approached with caution). Products include:

Celebrex Capsules 3130

Cevimeline Hydrochloride (Paroxetine may significantly inhibit the activity of the cytochrome P450 2D6 isoenzyme. Concomitant use of paroxetine with other drugs metabolized by cytochrome CYP2D6 has not been formally studied but may require lower doses than usually prescribed for either paroxetine or the other drug. Therefore, co-administration of paroxetine with other drugs that are metabolized by this isozyme should be approached with caution). Products include:

Evoxac Capsules 1042

Chlordiazepoxide (Co-administration with another drug that is highly protein bound may increase free concentrations of the other drug or paroxetine potentially resulting in adverse events).

No products indexed under this heading.

Chlordiazepoxide Hydrochloride (Co-administration with another drug that is highly protein bound may increase free concentrations of the other drug or paroxetine potentially resulting in adverse events). Products include:

Librium Capsules 3349

Chloroquine Hydrochloride (Paroxetine is metabolized by the cytochrome P450 isoenzyme CYP2D6. Therefore, co-administration of paroxetine with other drugs that inhibit this enzyme should be approached with caution).

No products indexed under this heading.

Chloroquine Phosphate (Paroxetine is metabolized by the cytochrome P450 isoenzyme CYP2D6. Therefore, co-administration of paroxetine with other drugs that inhibit this enzyme should be approached with caution).

No products indexed under this heading.

Chlorpheniramine (Paroxetine is metabolized by the cytochrome P450 isoenzyme CYP2D6. Therefore, co-administration of paroxetine with other drugs that inhibit this enzyme should be approached with caution).

No products indexed under this heading.

Chlorpheniramine Maleate (Paroxetine is metabolized by the cytochrome P450 isoenzyme CYP2D6. Therefore, co-administration of paroxetine with other drugs that inhibit this enzyme should be approached with caution). Products include:

Advil Allergy Sinus Caplets 737
Advil Multi-Symptom Cold Caplets 738
BC Allergy Sinus Cold Powder 612
Contac Severe Cold and Flu Caplets Maximum Strength 615
Hycomine Compound Tablets 1105
PediaCare Multi-Symptom Cold Liquid 704
PediaCare NightRest Cough & Cold Liquid 704
Robitussin Flu Liquid 752
Robitussin PM Cough & Cold Liquid 752
Singlet Caplets 636
Sudafed Sinus & Allergy Tablets 710
TheraFlu Cold & Cough Hot Liquid 680
TheraFlu Cold & Sore Throat Hot Liquid 680
TheraFlu Flu & Sore Throat Hot Liquid 681
TheraFlu Severe Cold & Cough Hot Liquid 683
TheraFlu Severe Cold Caplets 679
TheraFlu Severe Cold Hot Liquid 682
Triaminic Cold & Allergy Liquid 685
Triaminic Cold & Cough Liquid 685
Triaminic Flu, Cough & Fever Liquid 685
Triaminic Night Time Cough & Cold Liquid 685
Triaminic Allergy Runny Nose & Congestion Softchews 688
Triaminic Cold & Cough Softchews 688
Children's Tylenol Plus Cold NightTime Suspension Liquid 1851
Children's Tylenol Plus Cold & Cough Suspension Liquid and Chewable Tablets 1851
Children's Tylenol Plus Cold Chewable Tablets 1851
Children's Tylenol Plus Flu Suspension Liquid 1853
Tylenol Allergy Complete Multi-Symptom Caplets and Gelcaps with Cool Burst 1844
Multi-Symptom Tylenol Cold Night Time Caplets 1845
Vicks 44M Cough, Cold & Flu Relief 2676
Pediatric Vicks 44m Cough & Cold Relief 2673
Children's Vicks NyQuil Cold/Cough Relief 2671

Chlorpheniramine Polistirex (Paroxetine is metabolized by the cytochrome P450 isoenzyme CYP2D6. Therefore, co-administration of paroxetine with other drugs that inhibit this enzyme should be approached with caution). Products include:

Tussionex Pennkinetic Extended-Release Suspension 3322

Chlorpheniramine Tannate (Paroxetine is metabolized by the cytochrome P450 isoenzyme CYP2D6. Therefore, co-administration of paroxetine with other drugs that inhibit this enzyme should be approached with caution).

No products indexed under this heading.

Chlorpromazine (Paroxetine may significantly inhibit the activity of cytochrome P450 2D6 isoenzyme. Concomitant use of paroxetine with other drugs metabolized by cytochrome CYP2D6 has not been formally studied but may require lower doses than usually prescribed for either paroxetine or the other drug. Therefore, co-administration of paroxetine with other drugs that are metabolized by this isozyme should be approached with caution).

No products indexed under this heading.

Chlorpromazine Hydrochloride (Paroxetine may significantly inhibit the activity of cytochrome P450 2D6 isoenzyme. Concomitant use of paroxetine with other drugs metabolized by cytochrome CYP2D6 has not been formally studied but may require lower doses than usually prescribed for either paroxetine or the other drug. Therefore, co-administration of paroxetine with other drugs that are metabolized by this isozyme should be approached with caution).

No products indexed under this heading.

Chlorpropamide (Paroxetine may significantly inhibit the activity of the

cytochrome P450 2D6 isoenzyme. Concomitant use of paroxetine with other drugs metabolized by cytochrome CYP2D6 has not been formally studied but may require lower doses than usually prescribed for either paroxetine or the other drug. Therefore, co-administration of paroxetine with other drugs that are metabolized by this isozyme should be approached with caution).

No products indexed under this heading.

Cimetidine (Co-administration with oral cimetidine has resulted in an increase in steady-state plasma concentrations of paroxetine). Products include:

- Tagamet HB 200 Tablets ▣ 637
- Tagamet Tablets 1547

Cimetidine Hydrochloride (Co-administration with oral cimetidine has resulted in an increase in steady-state plasma concentrations of paroxetine).

No products indexed under this heading.

Citalopram Hydrobromide (Paroxetine is metabolized by the cytochrome P450 isoenzyme CYP2D6. Therefore, co-administration of paroxetine with other drugs that inhibit this enzyme should be approached with caution). Products include:

- Celexa 1177

Clomipramine Hydrochloride (Caution is indicated in the co-administration of tricyclic antidepressants with paroxetine because paroxetine may inhibit TCA metabolism. Plasma TCA concentrations may need to be monitored and the dose of TCA may need to be reduced if a TCA is co-administered with paroxetine).

No products indexed under this heading.

Clozapine (Paroxetine may significantly inhibit the activity of the cytochrome P450 2D6 isoenzyme. Concomitant use of paroxetine with other drugs metabolized by cytochrome CYP2D6 has not been formally studied but may require lower doses than usually prescribed for either paroxetine or the other drug. Therefore, co-administration of paroxetine with other drugs that are metabolized by this isozyme should be approached with caution). Products include:

- Clozapine Tablets 2141
- Clozaril Tablets 2174
- FazaClo Orally Disintegrating Tablets 547

Cocaine Hydrochloride (Paroxetine is metabolized by the cytochrome P450 isoenzyme CYP2D6. Therefore, co-administration of paroxetine with other drugs that inhibit this enzyme should be approached with caution).

No products indexed under this heading.

Codeine Phosphate (Paroxetine may significantly inhibit the activity of the cytochrome P450 2D6 isoenzyme. Concomitant use of paroxetine with other drugs metabolized by cytochrome CYP2D6 has not been formally studied but may require lower doses than usually prescribed for either paroxetine or the other drug. Therefore, co-administration of paroxetine with other drugs that are metabolized by this isozyme should be approached with caution). Products include:

- Tylenol with Codeine 2461

Codeine Sulfate (Paroxetine may significantly inhibit the activity of the cytochrome P450 2D6 isoenzyme. Concomitant use of paroxetine with other drugs metabolized by cytochrome CYP2D6 has not been formally studied but may require lower doses than usually prescribed for either paroxetine or the other drug. Therefore, co-administration of paroxetine with other drugs that are metabolized by this isozyme should be approached with caution).

No products indexed under this heading.

Cyclobenzaprine Hydrochloride (Paroxetine may significantly inhibit the activity of the cytochrome P450 2D6 isoenzyme. Concomitant use of paroxetine with other drugs metabolized by cytochrome CYP2D6 has not been formally studied but may require lower doses than usually prescribed for either paroxetine or the other drug. Therefore, co-administration of paroxetine with other drugs that are metabolized by this isozyme should be approached with caution). Products include:

- Flexeril Tablets 1832

Cyclosporine (Co-administration with another drug that is highly protein bound may increase free concentrations of the other drug or paroxetine potentially resulting in adverse events). Products include:

- Gengraf Capsules 458
- Neoral Soft Gelatin Capsules 2247
- Neoral Oral Solution 2247
- Restasis Ophthalmic Emulsion 570
- Sandimmune 2259

Dalteparin Sodium (The combined use of psychotropic drugs that interfere with serotonin reuptake and drugs that affect coagulation has been associated with an increased risk of bleeding; concomitant administration should be undertaken with caution). Products include:

- Fragmin Injection 2638

Danaparoid Sodium (The combined use of psychotropic drugs that interfere with serotonin reuptake and drugs that affect coagulation has been associated with an increased risk of bleeding; concomitant administration should be undertaken with caution).

No products indexed under this heading.

Desipramine Hydrochloride (Co-administration with desipramine has resulted in an increase in Cmax, AUC and T1/2 by an average of approximately two-, five- and three-fold, respectively).

No products indexed under this heading.

Dexfenfluramine Hydrochloride (Paroxetine may significantly inhibit the activity of the cytochrome P450 2D6 isoenzyme. Concomitant use of paroxetine with other drugs metabolized by cytochrome CYP2D6 has not been formally studied but may require lower doses than usually prescribed for either paroxetine or the other drug. Therefore, co-administration of paroxetine with other drugs that are metabolized by this isozyme should be approached with caution).

No products indexed under this heading.

Dextromethorphan Hydrobromide (Paroxetine may significantly inhibit the activity of the cytochrome P450 2D6 isoenzyme. Concomitant use of paroxetine with other drugs metabolized by cytochrome CYP2D6 has not been formally studied but may require lower doses than usually prescribed for either paroxetine or the other drug. Therefore, co-administration of paroxetine with other drugs that are metabolized by this isozyme should be approached with caution). Products include:

- Alacol DM Syrup 739
- Balamine DM 739
- Contac Severe Cold and Flu Caplets Maximum Strength ▣ 615
- Contac Severe Cold and Flu Caplets Non-Drowsy ▣ 615
- Children's Dimetapp DM Cold & Cough Elixir ▣ 745
- Children's Dimetapp Long Acting Cough Plus Cold Syrup ▣ 746
- Dimetapp Infant Drops Decongestant Plus Cough ▣ 746
- Mucinex DM Tablets ▣ 602
- PediaCare Decongestant & Cough Infant Drops ▣ 705
- PediaCare Freezer Pops Long-Acting Cough-Glacier Grape and Polar Berry Blue ▣ 706
- PediaCare Long-Acting Cough Infant Drops ▣ 705
- PediaCare Long-Acting Cough Plus Cold Liquid ▣ 704
- PediaCare Multi-Symptom Cold Liquid ▣ 704
- PediaCare NightRest Cough & Cold Liquid ▣ 704
- Robitussin Allergy & Cough Syrup ▣ 750
- Robitussin CF Liquid ▣ 755
- Robitussin Cough & Cold Liquid-filled Capsules ▣ 750
- Robitussin Cough, Cold & Flu Liquid-filled Capsules ▣ 750
- Robitussin Cough & Cold Infant Drops ▣ 755
- Robitussin DM Infant Drops ▣ 753
- Robitussin DM Liquid ▣ 753
- Robitussin Flu Liquid ▣ 752
- Robitussin Maximum Strength Cough Liquid ▣ 754
- Robitussin Maximum Strength Cough & Cold Liquid ▣ 754
- Robitussin Pediatric Cough Liquid ▣ 754
- Robitussin Pediatric Cough & Cold Liquid ▣ 754
- Robitussin PM Cough & Cold Liquid ▣ 752
- Robitussin Sugar Free Cough Liquid ▣ 753
- Simply Cough Liquid 1840
- Sudafed Severe Cold ▣ 710
- TheraFlu Cold & Cough Hot Liquid ▣ 680
- TheraFlu Flu & Chest Congestion Non-Drowsy Hot Liquid ▣ 681
- TheraFlu Severe Cold Non-Drowsy Hot Liquid ▣ 683
- TheraFlu Severe Cold & Cough Hot Liquid ▣ 683
- TheraFlu Severe Cold Caplets ▣ 679
- TheraFlu Severe Cold Hot Liquid ▣ 682
- TheraFlu Severe Cold Non-Drowsy Caplets ▣ 679
- TheraFlu Thin Strips Long Acting Cough ▣ 684
- Triaminic Cold & Cough Liquid ▣ 685
- Triaminic Cough Liquid ▣ 687
- Triaminic Cough & Nasal Congestion Liquid ▣ 687
- Triaminic Cough & Sore Throat Liquid ▣ 687
- Triaminic Flu, Cough & Fever Liquid ▣ 685
- Triaminic Night Time Cough & Cold Liquid ▣ 685
- Triaminic Cold & Cough Softchews ▣ 688
- Triaminic Cough & Sore Throat Softchews ▣ 689
- Triaminic Thin Strips Long Acting Cough ▣ 689
- Children's Tylenol Plus Cold & Cough Suspension Liquid and Chewable Tablets 1851
- Children's Tylenol Plus Flu Suspension Liquid 1853
- Concentrated Tylenol Infants' Drops Plus Cold and Cough 1851
- Tylenol Cold & Flu Severe Daytime Liquid with Cool Burst 1846
- Tylenol Cold & Flu Severe NightTime Liquid with Cool Burst 1846
- Tylenol Cold Severe Congestion Non-Drowsy Caplets with Cool Burst 1846
- Tylenol Cough & Sore Throat Daytime Liquid with Cool Burst 1849
- Tylenol Cough & Sore Throat NightTime Liquid with Cool Burst 1849
- Tylenol Flu Day Non-Drowsy Gelcaps 1846
- Concentrated Tylenol Infants' Drops Plus Cold & Cough Nasal Decongestant, Fever Reducer & Pain Reliever ▣ 668
- Multi-Symptom Tylenol Cold Night Time Caplets 1845
- Multi-Symptom Tylenol Cold Day Non-Drowsy Caplets and Gelcaps 1845
- Vicks 44 Cough Relief 2675
- Vicks 44D Cough & Head Congestion Relief 2676
- Vicks 44D Cough & Head Congestion Relief Liquid ▣ 721
- Vicks 44E Cough & Chest Congestion Relief 2676
- Pediatric Vicks 44e Cough & Chest Congestion Relief Liquid 2673
- Vicks 44M Cough, Cold & Flu Relief 2676
- Pediatric Vicks 44m Cough & Cold Relief 2673
- Vicks DayQuil LiquiCaps/Liquid Multi-Symptom Cold/Flu Relief ▣ 723
- Vicks DayQuil Multi-Symptom Cold/Flu Relief LiquiCaps 2675
- Vicks DayQuil Multi-Symptom Cold/Flu Relief Liquid 2675
- Children's Vicks NyQuil Cold/Cough Relief 2671
- Vicks NyQuil Cough Liquid 2677
- Vicks NyQuil LiquiCaps 2677
- Vicks NyQuil LiquiCaps/Liquid Multi-Symptom Cold/Flu Relief ▣ 725
- Vicks NyQuil Liquid 2677
- Zicam Concentrated Cough Mist for Kids Cool Cherry ▣ 643
- Zicam Concentrated Cough Mist for Kids Plus D Cool Cherry ▣ 643
- Zicam Concentrated Cough Mist Nite-Cool Cherry ▣ 642
- Zicam Concentrated Cough Mist Plus D Cool Cherry ▣ 642
- Zicam Concentrated Cough Mist-Honey Lemon & Cool Cherry ▣ 642

Dextromethorphan Polistirex (Paroxetine may significantly inhibit the activity of the cytochrome P450 2D6 isoenzyme. Concomitant use of paroxetine with other drugs metabolized by cytochrome CYP2D6 has not been formally studied but may require lower doses than usually prescribed for either paroxetine or the other drug. Therefore, co-administration of paroxetine with other drugs that are metabolized by this isozyme should be approached with caution). Products include:

- Delsym Extended-Release Suspension ▣ 611
- Delsym 12 Hour Cough Suppressant for Children ▣ 611

Diazepam (Co-administration with another drug that is highly protein bound may increase free concentrations of the other drug or paroxetine potentially resulting in adverse events). Products include:

- Diastat Rectal Delivery System 3344
- Valium Tablets 2822

Diclofenac Potassium (The combined use of psychotropic drugs that interfere with serotonin reuptake and

drugs that affect coagulation has been associated with an increased risk of bleeding). Products include:

Cataflam Tablets ... 2173

Diclofenac Sodium (The combined use of psychotropic drugs that interfere with serotonin reuptake and drugs that affect coagulation has been associated with an increased risk of bleeding). Products include:

Arthrotec Tablets ... 3126
Voltaren Ophthalmic Solution ... 2300
Voltaren Tablets ... 2298
Voltaren-XR Tablets ... 2301

Dicumarol (The combined use of psychotropic drugs that interfere with serotonin reuptake and drugs that affect coagulation has been associated with an increased risk of bleeding; concomitant administration should be undertaken with caution).

No products indexed under this heading.

Digoxin (The steady-state pharmacokinetics of paroxetine was not altered when administered with digoxin at steady state. Mean digoxin AUC at steady state decreased by 15% in the presence of paroxetine. Since there is little clinical experience, the concurrent administration of paroxetine and digoxin should be undertaken with caution). Products include:

Digitek Tablets ... 2146
Lanoxicaps Capsules ... 1458
Lanoxin Injection ... 1462
Lanoxin Tablets ... 1468
Lanoxin Injection Pediatric ... 1465

Diphenhydramine (Paroxetine is metabolized by the cytochrome P450 isoenzyme CYP2D6. Therefore, co-administration of paroxetine with other drugs that inhibit this enzyme should be approached with caution). Products include:

Tylenol Sore Throat NightTime Liquid with Cool Burst ... 1849

Diphenhydramine Hydrochloride (Paroxetine is metabolized by the cytochrome P450 isoenzyme CYP2D6. Therefore, co-administration of paroxetine with other drugs that inhibit this enzyme should be approached with caution). Products include:

Benadryl Allergy & Cold Tablets ... 692
Benadryl Allergy ... 691
Benadryl Allergy & Sinus Headache Caplets & Gelcaps ... 693
Children's Benadryl Allergy Liquid ... 695
Children's Benadryl Dye-Free Allergy Liquid ... 695
Benadryl Dye-Free Allergy Liqui-Gels Softgels ... 692
Benadryl Itch Relief Stick Extra Strength ... 696
Benadryl Itch Stopping Cream Extra Strength ... 697
Benadryl Itch Stopping Gel Extra Strength ... 697
Benadryl Itch Stopping Spray Extra Strength ... 697
Benadryl Maximum Strength Severe Allergy & Sinus Headache Caplets ... 694
Children's Benadryl D Liquid Medication ... 693
Benadryl D Tablets ... 694
Nytol QuickCaps Caplets ... 635
Maximum Strength Nytol QuickGels Softgels ... 635
Simply Sleep Caplets ... 1841
Sominex Original Formula Tablets ... 637
TheraFlu Thin Strips Multi Symptom ... 684
Triaminic Thin Strips Cough & Runny Nose ... 690
Children's Tylenol Plus Cold & Allergy Suspension Liquid ... 1850
Tylenol Allergy Complete Night Time Caplets ... 1844
Tylenol Severe Allergy Caplets ... 1844
Tylenol Flu NightTime Gelcaps ... 1846
Extra Strength Tylenol PM Caplets, Geltabs, Gelcaps and Liquid ... 1847
Unisom Maximum Strength SleepGels ... 712

Dipyridamole (Co-administration with another drug that is highly protein bound may increase free concentrations of the other drug or paroxetine potentially resulting in adverse events). Products include:

Aggrenox Capsules ... 855
Persantine Tablets ... 898

Dolasetron Mesylate (Paroxetine may significantly inhibit the activity of the cytochrome P450 2D6 isoenzyme. Concomitant use of paroxetine with other drugs metabolized by cytochrome CYP2D6 has not been formally studied but may require lower doses than usually prescribed for either paroxetine or the other drug. Therefore, co-administration of paroxetine with other drugs that are metabolized by this isozyme should be approached with caution). Products include:

Anzemet Injection ... 2871
Anzemet Tablets ... 2874

Donepezil Hydrochloride (Paroxetine may significantly inhibit the activity of the cytochrome P450 2D6 isoenzyme. Concomitant use of paroxetine with other drugs metabolized by cytochrome CYP2D6 has not been formally studied but may require lower doses than usually prescribed for either paroxetine or the other drug. Therefore, co-administration of paroxetine with other drugs that are metabolized by this isozyme should be approached with caution). Products include:

Aricept Tablets ... 1086
Aricept ODT Tablets ... 1086

Doxepin Hydrochloride (Caution is indicated in the co-administration of tricyclic antidepressants with paroxetine because paroxetine may inhibit TCA metabolism. Plasma TCA concentrations may need to be monitored and the dose of TCA may need to be reduced if a TCA is co-administered with paroxetine).

No products indexed under this heading.

Dyphylline (There have been reports of elevated theophylline levels associated with co-administration; monitor theophylline levels when these drugs are concurrently administered).

No products indexed under this heading.

Eletriptan Hydrobromide (There have been rare post-marketing reports describing patients with weakness, hyperreflexia, and incoordination following the use of a selective serotonin reuptake inhibitor (SSRI) and sumatriptan. If concomitant treatment with a triptan and an SSRI (eg, paroxetine) is clinically warranted, appropriate observation of the patient is advised). Products include:

Relpax Tablets ... 2531

Encainide Hydrochloride (Paroxetine may significantly inhibit the activity of the cytochrome P450 2D6 isoenzyme. Concomitant use of paroxetine with other drugs metabolized by cytochrome CYP2D6 has not been formally studied but may require lower doses than usually prescribed for either paroxetine or the other drug. Therefore, co-administration of paroxetine with other drugs that are metabolized by this isozyme should be approached with caution).

No products indexed under this heading.

Enoxaparin Sodium (The combined use of psychotropic drugs that interfere with serotonin reuptake and drugs that affect coagulation has been associated with an increased risk of bleeding; concomitant administration should be undertaken with caution). Products include:

Lovenox Injection ... 2931

Escitalopram Oxalate (Paroxetine is metabolized by the cytochrome P450 isoenzyme CYP2D6. Therefore, co-administration of paroxetine with other drugs that inhibit this enzyme should be approached with caution). Products include:

Lexapro Oral Solution ... 1193
Lexapro Tablets ... 1193

Etodolac (The combined use of psychotropic drugs that interfere with serotonin reuptake and drugs that affect coagulation has been associated with an increased risk of bleeding).

No products indexed under this heading.

Fenoprofen Calcium (The combined use of psychotropic drugs that interfere with serotonin reuptake and drugs that affect coagulation has been associated with an increased risk of bleeding). Products include:

Nalfon Capsules ... 2504

Fentanyl (Paroxetine may significantly inhibit the activity of the cytochrome P450 2D6 isoenzyme. Concomitant use of paroxetine with other drugs metabolized by cytochrome CYP2D6 has not been formally studied but may require lower doses than usually prescribed for either paroxetine or the other drug. Therefore, co-administration of paroxetine with other drugs that are metabolized by this isozyme should be approached with caution). Products include:

Duragesic Transdermal System ... 2448

Fentanyl Citrate (Paroxetine may significantly inhibit the activity of the cytochrome P450 2D6 isoenzyme. Concomitant use of paroxetine with other drugs metabolized by cytochrome CYP2D6 has not been formally studied but may require lower doses than usually prescribed for either paroxetine or the other drug. Therefore, co-administration of paroxetine with other drugs that are metabolized by this isozyme should be approached with caution). Products include:

Actiq ... 993

Flecainide Acetate (Paroxetine may significantly inhibit the activity of the cytochrome P450 2D6 isoenzyme. Concomitant use of paroxetine with other drugs metabolized by cytochrome CYP2D6 has not been formally studied but may require lower doses than usually prescribed for either paroxetine or the other drug. Therefore, co-administration of paroxetine with other drugs that are metabolized by this isozyme should be approached with caution). Products include:

Tambocor Tablets ... 1824

Fluoxetine (Paroxetine is metabolized by the cytochrome P450 isoenzyme CYP2D6. Therefore, co-administration of paroxetine with other drugs that inhibit this enzyme should be approached with caution).

No products indexed under this heading.

Fluoxetine Hydrochloride (Paroxetine is metabolized by the cytochrome P450 isoenzyme CYP2D6. Therefore, co-administration of paroxetine with other drugs that inhibit this enzyme should be approached with caution). Products include:

Prozac Pulvules and Liquid ... 1771
Symbyax Capsules ... 1788

Fluphenazine Decanoate (Paroxetine is metabolized by the cytochrome P450 isoenzyme CYP2D6. Therefore, co-administration of paroxetine with other drugs that inhibit this enzyme should be approached with caution).

No products indexed under this heading.

Fluphenazine Enanthate (Paroxetine is metabolized by the cytochrome P450 isoenzyme CYP2D6. Therefore, co-administration of paroxetine with other drugs that inhibit this enzyme should be approached with caution).

No products indexed under this heading.

Fluphenazine Hydrochloride (Paroxetine is metabolized by the cytochrome P450 isoenzyme CYP2D6. Therefore, co-administration of paroxetine with other drugs that inhibit this enzyme should be approached with caution).

No products indexed under this heading.

Flurazepam Hydrochloride (Co-administration with another drug that is highly protein bound may increase free concentrations of the other drug or paroxetine potentially resulting in adverse events). Products include:

Dalmane Capsules ... 3343

Flurbiprofen (The combined use of psychotropic drugs that interfere with serotonin reuptake and drugs that affect coagulation has been associated with an increased risk of bleeding).

No products indexed under this heading.

Fluvoxamine Maleate (Paroxetine is metabolized by the cytochrome P450 isoenzyme CYP2D6. Therefore, co-administration of paroxetine with other drugs that inhibit this enzyme should be approached with caution).

No products indexed under this heading.

Fondaparinux Sodium (The combined use of psychotropic drugs that interfere with serotonin reuptake and drugs that affect coagulation has been associated with an increased risk of bleeding; concomitant administration should be undertaken with caution). Products include:

Arixtra Injection ... 1325

Formoterol Fumarate (Paroxetine may significantly inhibit the activity of the cytochrome P450 2D6 isoenzyme. Concomitant use of paroxetine with other drugs metabolized by cytochrome CYP2D6 has not been formally studied but may require lower doses than usually prescribed for either paroxetine or the other drug. Therefore, co-administration of par-

oxetine with other drugs that are metabolized by this isozyme should be approached with caution). Products include:

Foradil Aerolizer ... 3024

Fosphenytoin Sodium (Co-administration has resulted in reduction of paroxetine AUC and T1/2; potential for elevated phenytoin levels or slight reduction in phenytoin AUC).

No products indexed under this heading.

Frovatriptan Succinate (There have been rare post-marketing reports describing patients with weakness, hyperreflexia, and incoordination following the use of a selective serotonin reuptake inhibitor (SSRI) and sumatriptan. If concomitant treatment with a triptan and an SSRI (eg, paroxetine) is clinically warranted, appropriate observation of the patient is advised). Products include:

Frova Tablets ... 1101

Galantamine Hydrobromide (Paroxetine may significantly inhibit the activity of the cytochrome P450 2D6 isoenzyme. Concomitant use of paroxetine with other drugs metabolized by cytochrome CYP2D6 has not been formally studied but may require lower doses than usually prescribed for either paroxetine or the other drug. Therefore, co-administration of paroxetine with other drugs that are metabolized by this isozyme should be approached with caution). Products include:

Razadyne ER Extended-Release Capsules ... 2434
Razadyne ... 2434

Glipizide (Co-administration with another drug that is highly protein bound may increase free concentrations of the other drug or paroxetine potentially resulting in adverse events).

No products indexed under this heading.

Halofantrine Hydrochloride (Paroxetine is metabolized by the cytochrome P450 isoenzyme CYP2D6. Therefore, co-administration of paroxetine with other drugs that inhibit this enzyme should be approached with caution).

No products indexed under this heading.

Haloperidol (Paroxetine is metabolized by the cytochrome P450 isoenzyme CYP2D6. Therefore, co-administration of paroxetine with other drugs that inhibit this enzyme should be approached with caution).

No products indexed under this heading.

Haloperidol Decanoate (Paroxetine is metabolized by the cytochrome P450 isoenzyme CYP2D6. Therefore, co-administration of paroxetine with other drugs that inhibit this enzyme should be approached with caution).

No products indexed under this heading.

Heparin Calcium (The combined use of psychotropic drugs that interfere with serotonin reuptake and drugs that affect coagulation has been associated with an increased risk of bleeding; concomitant administration should be undertaken with caution).

No products indexed under this heading.

Heparin Sodium (The combined use of psychotropic drugs that interfere with serotonin reuptake and drugs that affect coagulation has been associated with an increased risk of bleeding; concomitant administration should be undertaken with caution).

No products indexed under this heading.

Hydrocodone Bitartrate (Paroxetine may significantly inhibit the activity of the cytochrome P450 2D6 isoenzyme. Concomitant use of paroxetine with other drugs metabolized by cytochrome CYP2D6 has not been formally studied but may require lower doses than usually prescribed for either paroxetine or the other drug. Therefore, co-administration of paroxetine with other drugs that are metabolized by this isozyme should be approached with caution). Products include:

Hycodan ... 1104
Hycomine Compound Tablets ... 1105
Hycotuss Expectorant Syrup ... 1106
Lortab ... 3315
Lortab Elixir ... 3312
Vicodin Tablets ... 530
Vicodin ES Tablets ... 531
Vicodin HP Tablets ... 532
Vicoprofen Tablets ... 533
Zydone Tablets ... 1118

Hydroxychloroquine Sulfate (Paroxetine is metabolized by the cytochrome P450 isoenzyme CYP2D6. Therefore, co-administration of paroxetine with other drugs that inhibit this enzyme should be approached with caution).

No products indexed under this heading.

Hypericum (Based on the mechanism of action of paroxetine and the potential for serotonin syndrome, caution is advised when paroxetine hydrochloride is co-administered with other drugs or agents that may affect the serotonergic neurotransmitter systems, such as St. John's Wort).

No products indexed under this heading.

Ibuprofen (The combined use of psychotropic drugs that interfere with serotonin reuptake and drugs that affect coagulation has been associated with an increased risk of bleeding). Products include:

Advil Allergy Sinus Caplets ... ▣ 737
Advil ... ▣ 737
Children's Advil Suspension ... ▣ 742
Children's Advil Chewable Tablets ... ▣ 741
Advil Cold & Sinus ... ▣ 739
Advil Flu & Body Ache Caplets ... ▣ 739
Children's Advil Cold Suspension ... ▣ 741
Infants' Advil Concentrated Drops ... ▣ 743
Junior Strength Advil Swallow Tablets ... ▣ 740
Advil Migraine Liquigels ... ▣ 740
Advil Multi-Symptom Cold Caplets ... ▣ 738
Combunox Tablets ... 1183
Children's Motrin Oral Suspension and Chewable Tablets ... 1837
Children's Motrin Cold Non-Staining Dye-Free Oral Suspension ... 1838
Children's Motrin Cold Oral Suspension ... 1838
Children's Motrin Non-Staining Dye-Free Oral Suspension ... 1837
Motrin Cold & Sinus Caplets ... 1836
Motrin IB Tablets and Caplets ... 1836
Infants' Motrin Concentrated Drops ... 1837
Infants' Motrin Non-Staining Dye-Free Drops ... 1837
Junior Strength Motrin Caplets and Chewable Tablets ... 1837
Vicoprofen Tablets ... 533

Imatinib Mesylate (Paroxetine is metabolized by the cytochrome P450 isoenzyme CYP2D6. Therefore, co-administration of paroxetine with other drugs that inhibit this enzyme should be approached with caution). Products include:

Gleevec Tablets ... 2221

Imipramine Hydrochloride (Caution is indicated in the co-administration of tricyclic antidepressants with paroxetine because paroxetine may inhibit TCA metabolism. Plasma TCA concentrations may need to be monitored and the dose of TCA may need to be reduced if a TCA is co-administered with paroxetine).

No products indexed under this heading.

Imipramine Pamoate (Caution is indicated in the co-administration of tricyclic antidepressants with paroxetine because paroxetine may inhibit TCA metabolism. Plasma TCA concentrations may need to be monitored and the dose of TCA may need to be reduced if a TCA is co-administered with paroxetine).

No products indexed under this heading.

Indomethacin (The combined use of psychotropic drugs that interfere with serotonin reuptake and drugs that affect coagulation has been associated with an increased risk of bleeding). Products include:

Indocin ... 1968

Indomethacin Sodium Trihydrate (The combined use of psychotropic drugs that interfere with serotonin reuptake and drugs that affect coagulation has been associated with an increased risk of bleeding). Products include:

Indocin I.V. ... 1973

Indoramin Hydrochloride (Paroxetine may significantly inhibit the activity of the cytochrome P450 2D6 isoenzyme. Concomitant use of paroxetine with other drugs metabolized by cytochrome CYP2D6 has not been formally studied but may require lower doses than usually prescribed for either paroxetine or the other drug. Therefore, co-administration of paroxetine with other drugs that are metabolized by this isozyme should be approached with caution).

No products indexed under this heading.

Isocarboxazid (Potential for serious and/or fatal reactions, including hyperthermia, rigidity, myoclonus and other serious reactions; concurrent and/or sequential use is contraindicated).

No products indexed under this heading.

Ketoprofen (The combined use of psychotropic drugs that interfere with serotonin reuptake and drugs that affect coagulation has been associated with an increased risk of bleeding).

No products indexed under this heading.

Ketorolac Tromethamine (The combined use of psychotropic drugs that interfere with serotonin reuptake and drugs that affect coagulation has been associated with an increased risk of bleeding). Products include:

Acular Ophthalmic Solution ... 561
Acular LS Ophthalmic Solution ... 562

Labetalol Hydrochloride (Paroxetine may significantly inhibit the activity of the cytochrome P450 2D6 isoenzyme. Concomitant use of paroxetine with other drugs metabolized by cytochrome CYP2D6 has not been formally studied but may require lower doses than usually prescribed for either paroxetine or the other drug. Therefore, co-administration of paroxetine with other drugs that are metabolized by this isozyme should be approached with caution).

No products indexed under this heading.

Lidocaine (Paroxetine may significantly inhibit the activity of the cytochrome P450 2D6 isoenzyme. Concomitant use of paroxetine with other drugs metabolized by cytochrome CYP2D6 has not been formally studied but may require lower doses than usually prescribed for either paroxetine or the other drug. Therefore, co-administration of paroxetine with other drugs that are metabolized by this isozyme should be approached with caution). Products include:

Lidoderm Patch ... 1107

Lidocaine Hydrochloride (Paroxetine may significantly inhibit the activity of the cytochrome P450 2D6 isoenzyme. Concomitant use of paroxetine with other drugs metabolized by cytochrome CYP2D6 has not been formally studied but may require lower doses than usually prescribed for either paroxetine or the other drug. Therefore, co-administration of paroxetine with other drugs that are metabolized by this isozyme should be approached with caution).

No products indexed under this heading.

Linezolid (Based on the mechanism of action of paroxetine and the potential for serotonin syndrome, caution is advised when paroxetine hydrochloride is co-administered with other drugs or agents that may affect the serotonergic neurotransmitter systems, such as linezolid). Products include:

Zyvox ... 2661

Lithium (A multiple-dose study has shown that there is no pharmacokinetic interaction between paroxetine and lithium carbonate. However, due to the potential for serotonin syndrome, caution is advised when paroxetine is co-administered with lithium).

No products indexed under this heading.

Lithium Carbonate (A multiple-dose study has shown that there is no pharmacokinetic interaction between paroxetine and lithium carbonate. However, due to the potential for serotonin syndrome, caution is advised when paroxetine is co-administered with lithium). Products include:

Eskalith ... 1406
Lithobid Tablets ... 1670

Lithium Citrate (A multiple-dose study has shown that there is no pharmacokinetic interaction between paroxetine and lithium carbonate. However, due to the potential for serotonin syndrome, caution is advised when paroxetine is co-administered with lithium).

No products indexed under this heading.

Low Molecular Weight Heparins (The combined use of psychotropic drugs that interfere with serotonin reuptake and drugs that affect coagulation has been associated with an increased risk of bleeding; concomitant administration should be undertaken with caution).
No products indexed under this heading.

Maprotiline Hydrochloride (Caution is indicated in the co-administration of tricyclic antidepressants with paroxetine because paroxetine may inhibit TCA metabolism. Plasma TCA concentrations may need to be monitored and the dose of TCA may need to be reduced if a TCA is co-administered with paroxetine).
No products indexed under this heading.

Meclofenamate Sodium (The combined use of psychotropic drugs that interfere with serotonin reuptake and drugs that affect coagulation has been associated with an increased risk of bleeding).
No products indexed under this heading.

Mefenamic Acid (The combined use of psychotropic drugs that interfere with serotonin reuptake and drugs that affect coagulation has been associated with an increased risk of bleeding).
No products indexed under this heading.

Meloxicam (The combined use of psychotropic drugs that interfere with serotonin reuptake and drugs that affect coagulation has been associated with an increased risk of bleeding). Products include:
Mobic Oral Suspension **893**
Mobic Tablets **893**

Meperidine Hydrochloride (Paroxetine may significantly inhibit the activity of the cytochrome P450 2D6 isoenzyme. Concomitant use of paroxetine with other drugs metabolized by cytochrome CYP2D6 has not been formally studied but may require lower doses than usually prescribed for either paroxetine or the other drug. Therefore, co-administration of paroxetine with other drugs that are metabolized by this isozyme should be approached with caution).
No products indexed under this heading.

Mesoridazine Besylate (Paroxetine may significantly inhibit the activity of cytochrome P450 2D6 isoenzyme. Concomitant use of paroxetine with other drugs metabolized by cytochrome CYP2D6 has not been formally studied but may require lower doses than usually prescribed for either paroxetine or the other drug. Therefore, co-administration of paroxetine with other drugs that are metabolized by this isozyme should be approached with caution).
No products indexed under this heading.

Methadone Hydrochloride (Paroxetine is metabolized by the cytochrome P450 isoenzyme CYP2D6. Therefore, co-administration of paroxetine with other drugs that inhibit this enzyme should be approached with caution).
No products indexed under this heading.

Methamphetamine Hydrochloride (Paroxetine may significantly inhibit the activity of the cytochrome P450 2D6 isoenzyme. Concomitant use of paroxetine with other drugs metabolized by cytochrome CYP2D6 has not been formally studied but may require lower doses than usually prescribed for either paroxetine or the other drug. Therefore, co-administration of paroxetine with other drugs that are metabolized by this isozyme should be approached with caution). Products include:
Desoxyn Tablets, USP **2482**

Methotrimeprazine (Paroxetine may significantly inhibit the activity of cytochrome P450 2D6 isoenzyme. Concomitant use of paroxetine with other drugs metabolized by cytochrome CYP2D6 has not been formally studied but may require lower doses than usually prescribed for either paroxetine or the other drug. Therefore, co-administration of paroxetine with other drugs that are metabolized by this isozyme should be approached with caution).
No products indexed under this heading.

Metoprolol Succinate (There has been a case report of severe hypotension when immediate-release paroxetine was added to chronic metoprolol treatment). Products include:
Toprol-XL Tablets **660**

Metoprolol Tartrate (There has been a case report of severe hypotension when immediate-release paroxetine was added to chronic metoprolol treatment).
No products indexed under this heading.

Mexiletine Hydrochloride (Paroxetine may significantly inhibit the activity of the cytochrome P450 2D6 isoenzyme. Concomitant use of paroxetine with other drugs metabolized by cytochrome CYP2D6 has not been formally studied but may require lower doses than usually prescribed for either paroxetine or the other drug. Therefore, co-administration of paroxetine with other drugs that are metabolized by this isozyme should be approached with caution).
No products indexed under this heading.

Mibefradil Dihydrochloride (Paroxetine is metabolized by the cytochrome P450 isoenzyme CYP2D6. Therefore, co-administration of paroxetine with other drugs that inhibit this enzyme should be approached with caution).
No products indexed under this heading.

Midazolam Hydrochloride (Co-administration with another drug that is highly protein bound may increase free concentrations of the other drug or paroxetine potentially resulting in adverse events).
No products indexed under this heading.

Mirtazapine (Paroxetine may significantly inhibit the activity of the cytochrome P450 2D6 isoenzyme. Concomitant use of paroxetine with other drugs metabolized by cytochrome CYP2D6 has not been formally studied but may require lower doses than usually prescribed for either paroxetine or the other drug. Therefore, co-administration of paroxetine with other drugs that are metabolized by this isozyme should be approached with caution).
No products indexed under this heading.

Moclobemide (Potential for serious and/or fatal reactions, including hyperthermia, rigidity, myoclonus and other serious reactions; concurrent and/or sequential use is contraindicated).
No products indexed under this heading.

Morphine Sulfate (Paroxetine may significantly inhibit the activity of the cytochrome P450 2D6 isoenzyme. Concomitant use of paroxetine with other drugs metabolized by cytochrome CYP2D6 has not been formally studied but may require lower doses than usually prescribed for either paroxetine or the other drug. Therefore, co-administration of paroxetine with other drugs that are metabolized by this isozyme should be approached with caution). Products include:
Avinza Capsules **1714**
Kadian Capsules **572**
MS Contin Tablets **2703**

Nabumetone (The combined use of psychotropic drugs that interfere with serotonin reuptake and drugs that affect coagulation has been associated with an increased risk of bleeding). Products include:
Relafen Tablets **1523**

Naproxen (The combined use of psychotropic drugs that interfere with serotonin reuptake and drugs that affect coagulation has been associated with an increased risk of bleeding). Products include:
EC-Naprosyn Delayed-Release Tablets **2769**
Naprosyn Suspension **2769**
Naprosyn Tablets **2769**
Prevacid NapraPAC **3277**

Naproxen Sodium (The combined use of psychotropic drugs that interfere with serotonin reuptake and drugs that affect coagulation has been associated with an increased risk of bleeding). Products include:
Aleve Tablets, Caplets and Gelcaps **605**
Anaprox Tablets **2769**
Anaprox DS Tablets **2769**

Naratriptan Hydrochloride (There have been rare post-marketing reports describing patients with weakness, hyperreflexia, and incoordination following the use of a selective serotonin reuptake inhibitor (SSRI) and sumatriptan. If concomitant treatment with a triptan and an SSRI (eg, paroxetine) is clinically warranted, appropriate observation of the patient is advised). Products include:
Amerge Tablets **1312**

Nelfinavir Mesylate (Paroxetine may significantly inhibit the activity of the cytochrome P450 2D6 isoenzyme. Concomitant use of paroxetine with other drugs metabolized by cytochrome CYP2D6 has not been formally studied but may require lower doses than usually prescribed for either paroxetine or the other drug. Therefore, co-administration of paroxetine with other drugs that are metabolized by this isozyme should be approached with caution). Products include:
Viracept **2556**

Nortriptyline Hydrochloride (Caution is indicated in the co-administration of tricyclic antidepressants with paroxetine because paroxetine may inhibit TCA metabolism. Plasma TCA concentrations may need to be monitored and the dose of TCA may need to be reduced if a TCA is co-administered with paroxetine).
No products indexed under this heading.

Olanzapine (Paroxetine may significantly inhibit the activity of the cytochrome P450 2D6 isoenzyme. Concomitant use of paroxetine with other drugs metabolized by cytochrome CYP2D6 has not been formally studied but may require lower doses than usually prescribed for either paroxetine or the other drug. Therefore, co-administration of paroxetine with other drugs that are metabolized by this isozyme should be approached with caution). Products include:
Symbyax Capsules **1788**
Zyprexa Tablets **1798**
Zyprexa IntraMuscular **1798**
Zyprexa ZYDIS Orally Disintegrating Tablets **1798**

Omeprazole (Paroxetine may significantly inhibit the activity of the cytochrome P450 2D6 isoenzyme. Concomitant use of paroxetine with other drugs metabolized by cytochrome CYP2D6 has not been formally studied but may require lower doses than usually prescribed for either paroxetine or the other drug. Therefore, co-administration of paroxetine with other drugs that are metabolized by this isozyme should be approached with caution). Products include:
Zegerid Powder for Oral Solution **2972**

Ondansetron (Paroxetine may significantly inhibit the activity of the cytochrome P450 2D6 isoenzyme. Concomitant use of paroxetine with other drugs metabolized by cytochrome CYP2D6 has not been formally studied but may require lower doses than usually prescribed for either paroxetine or the other drug. Therefore, co-administration of paroxetine with other drugs that are metabolized by this isozyme should be approached with caution). Products include:
Zofran ODT Orally Disintegrating Tablets **1613**

Ondansetron Hydrochloride (Paroxetine may significantly inhibit the activity of the cytochrome P450 2D6 isoenzyme. Concomitant use of paroxetine with other drugs metabolized by cytochrome CYP2D6 has not been formally studied but may require lower doses than usually prescribed for either paroxetine or the other drug. Therefore, co-administration of paroxetine with other drugs that are metabolized by this isozyme should be approached with caution). Products include:
Zofran Injection **1607**
Zofran **1613**

Oxaprozin (The combined use of psychotropic drugs that interfere with serotonin reuptake and drugs that affect coagulation has been associated with an increased risk of bleeding).
No products indexed under this heading.

Oxazepam (Co-administration with another drug that is highly protein bound may increase free concentrations of the other drug or paroxetine potentially resulting in adverse events).
No products indexed under this heading.

Oxycodone Hydrochloride (Paroxetine may significantly inhibit the activity of the cytochrome P450 2D6 isoenzyme. Concomitant use of paroxetine with other drugs metabolized by cytochrome CYP2D6 has not been formally studied but may require lower doses than usually prescribed for either paroxetine or the other drug. Therefore, co-administration of paroxetine with other drugs that are metabolized by this isozyme should be approached with caution). Products include:
Combunox Tablets 1183
OxyContin Tablets 2699
OxyFast Oral Concentrate Solution 2704
OxyIR Capsules 2704
Percocet Tablets 1114
Percodan Tablets 1115

Paclitaxel (Paroxetine may significantly inhibit the activity of the cytochrome P450 2D6 isoenzyme. Concomitant use of paroxetine with other drugs metabolized by cytochrome CYP2D6 has not been formally studied but may require lower doses than usually prescribed for either paroxetine or the other drug. Therefore, co-administration of paroxetine with other drugs that are metabolized by this isozyme should be approached with caution).
No products indexed under this heading.

Pargyline Hydrochloride (Potential for serious and/or fatal reactions, including hyperthermia, rigidity, myoclonus and other serious reactions; concurrent and/or sequential use is contraindicated).
No products indexed under this heading.

Perphenazine (Paroxetine is metabolized by the cytochrome P450 isoenzyme CYP2D6. Therefore, co-administration of paroxetine with other drugs that inhibit this enzyme should be approached with caution).
No products indexed under this heading.

Phenelzine Sulfate (Potential for serious and/or fatal reactions, including hyperthermia, rigidity, myoclonus and other serious reactions; concurrent and/or sequential use is contraindicated).
No products indexed under this heading.

Phenobarbital (Co-administration has resulted in reduction of paroxetine AUC and T1/2).
No products indexed under this heading.

Phenylbutazone (The combined use of psychotropic drugs that interfere with serotonin reuptake and drugs that affect coagulation has been associated with an increased risk of bleeding).
No products indexed under this heading.

Phenytoin (Co-administration has resulted in reduction of paroxetine AUC and T1/2; potential for elevated phenytoin levels or slight reduction in phenytoin AUC).
No products indexed under this heading.

Phenytoin Sodium (Co-administration has resulted in reduction of paroxetine AUC and T1/2; potential for elevated phenytoin levels or slight reduction in phenytoin AUC). Products include:
Phenytek Capsules 2153

Pimozide (Due to the narrow therapeutic index of pimozide and its known ability to prolong the QT interval, concomitant use of pimozide and paroxetine hydrochloride is contraindicated). Products include:
Orap Tablets 1220

Pindolol (Paroxetine may significantly inhibit the activity of the cytochrome P450 2D6 isoenzyme. Concomitant use of paroxetine with other drugs metabolized by cytochrome CYP2D6 has not been formally studied but may require lower doses than usually prescribed for either paroxetine or the other drug. Therefore, co-administration of paroxetine with other drugs that are metabolized by this isozyme should be approached with caution).
No products indexed under this heading.

Piroxicam (The combined use of psychotropic drugs that interfere with serotonin reuptake and drugs that affect coagulation has been associated with an increased risk of bleeding).
No products indexed under this heading.

Procarbazine Hydrochloride (Potential for serious and/or fatal reactions, including hyperthermia, rigidity, myoclonus and other serious reactions; concurrent and/or sequential use is contraindicated). Products include:
Matulane Capsules 3188

Prochlorperazine (Paroxetine may significantly inhibit the activity of cytochrome P450 2D6 isoenzyme. Concomitant use of paroxetine with other drugs metabolized by cytochrome CYP2D6 has not been formally studied but may require lower doses than usually prescribed for either paroxetine or the other drug. Therefore, co-administration of paroxetine with other drugs that are metabolized by this isozyme should be approached with caution).
No products indexed under this heading.

Procyclidine Hydrochloride (Increased steady-state AUC, Cmax and Cmin values of procyclidine with concurrent use).
No products indexed under this heading.

Promethazine Hydrochloride (Paroxetine may significantly inhibit the activity of cytochrome P450 2D6 isoenzyme. Concomitant use of paroxetine with other drugs metabolized by cytochrome CYP2D6 has not been formally studied but may require lower doses than usually prescribed for either paroxetine or the other drug. Therefore, co-administration of paroxetine with other drugs that are metabolized by this isozyme should be approached with caution). Products include:
Phenergan 3438

Propafenone Hydrochloride (Paroxetine is metabolized by the cytochrome P450 isoenzyme CYP2D6. Therefore, co-administration of paroxetine with other drugs that inhibit this enzyme should be approached with caution). Products include:
Rythmol SR Capsules 2736

Propoxyphene Hydrochloride (Paroxetine is metabolized by the cytochrome P450 isoenzyme CYP2D6. Therefore, co-administration of paroxetine with other drugs that inhibit this enzyme should be approached with caution).
No products indexed under this heading.

Propoxyphene Napsylate (Paroxetine is metabolized by the cytochrome P450 isoenzyme CYP2D6. Therefore, co-administration of paroxetine with other drugs that inhibit this enzyme should be approached with caution). Products include:
Darvocet A 500 Tablets 3497

Propranolol Hydrochloride (Paroxetine may significantly inhibit the activity of the cytochrome P450 2D6 isoenzyme. Concomitant use of paroxetine with other drugs metabolized by cytochrome CYP2D6 has not been formally studied but may require lower doses than usually prescribed for either paroxetine or the other drug. Therefore, co-administration of paroxetine with other drugs that are metabolized by this isozyme should be approached with caution). Products include:
Inderal LA Long-Acting Capsules 3421
InnoPran XL Capsules 2728

Protriptyline Hydrochloride (Caution is indicated in the co-administration of tricyclic antidepressants with paroxetine because paroxetine may inhibit TCA metabolism. Plasma TCA concentrations may need to be monitored and the dose of TCA may need to be reduced if a TCA is co-administered with paroxetine). Products include:
Vivactil Tablets 2350

Quetiapine Fumarate (Paroxetine may significantly inhibit the activity of the cytochrome P450 2D6 isoenzyme. Concomitant use of paroxetine with other drugs metabolized by cytochrome CYP2D6 has not been formally studied but may require lower doses than usually prescribed for either paroxetine or the other drug. Therefore, co-administration of paroxetine with other drugs that are metabolized by this isozyme should be approached with caution). Products include:
Seroquel Tablets 691

Quinacrine Hydrochloride (Paroxetine is metabolized by the cytochrome P450 isoenzyme CYP2D6. Therefore, co-administration of paroxetine with other drugs that inhibit this enzyme should be approached with caution).
No products indexed under this heading.

Quinidine Gluconate (Paroxetine is metabolized by the cytochrome P450 isoenzyme CYP2D6. Therefore, co-administration of paroxetine with other drugs that inhibit this enzyme should be approached with caution).
No products indexed under this heading.

Quinidine Hydrochloride (Paroxetine is metabolized by the cytochrome P450 isoenzyme CYP2D6. Therefore, co-administration of paroxetine with other drugs that inhibit this enzyme should be approached with caution).
No products indexed under this heading.

Quinidine Polygalacturonate (Paroxetine is metabolized by the cytochrome P450 isoenzyme CYP2D6. Therefore, co-administration of paroxetine with other drugs that inhibit this enzyme should be approached with caution).
No products indexed under this heading.

Quinidine Sulfate (Paroxetine is metabolized by the cytochrome P450 isoenzyme CYP2D6. Therefore, co-administration of paroxetine with other drugs that inhibit this enzyme should be approached with caution).
No products indexed under this heading.

Ranitidine Bismuth Citrate (Paroxetine is metabolized by the cytochrome P450 isoenzyme CYP2D6. Therefore, co-administration of paroxetine with other drugs that inhibit this enzyme should be approached with caution).
No products indexed under this heading.

Ranitidine Hydrochloride (Paroxetine is metabolized by the cytochrome P450 isoenzyme CYP2D6. Therefore, co-administration of paroxetine with other drugs that inhibit this enzyme should be approached with caution). Products include:
Zantac 1597
Zantac Injection 1593
Zantac 75 Tablets .... ■715
Zantac 150 Maximum Strength Tablets .... ■715
Zantac Injection Pharmacy Bulk Package 1595

Risperidone (Paroxetine may significantly inhibit the activity of the cytochrome P450 2D6 isoenzyme. Concomitant use of paroxetine with other drugs metabolized by cytochrome CYP2D6 has not been formally studied but may require lower doses than usually prescribed for either paroxetine or the other drug. Therefore, co-administration of paroxetine with other drugs that are metabolized by this isozyme should be approached with caution). Products include:
Risperdal Consta Long-Acting Injection 1664
Risperdal M-Tab Orally Disintegrating Tablets 1658
Risperdal 1658

Ritonavir (Paroxetine is metabolized by the cytochrome P450 isoenzyme CYP2D6. Therefore, co-administration of paroxetine with other drugs that inhibit this enzyme should be approached with caution). Products include:
Kaletra 474
Norvir 499

Rizatriptan Benzoate (There have been rare post-marketing reports describing patients with weakness, hyperreflexia, and incoordination following the use of a selective serotonin reuptake inhibitor (SSRI) and sumatriptan. If concomitant treatment with a triptan and an SSRI (eg, paroxetine) is clinically warranted,

appropriate observation of the patient is advised). Products include:
Maxalt Tablets 1983
Maxalt-MLT Orally Disintegrating Tablets 1983

Rofecoxib (The combined use of psychotropic drugs that interfere with serotonin reuptake and drugs that affect coagulation has been associated with an increased risk of bleeding).
No products indexed under this heading.

Selegiline Hydrochloride (Potential for serious and/or fatal reactions, including hyperthermia, rigidity, myoclonus and other serious reactions; concurrent and/or sequential use is contraindicated). Products include:
Eldepryl Capsules 3209

Sertraline Hydrochloride (Paroxetine is metabolized by the cytochrome P450 isoenzyme CYP2D6. Therefore, co-administration of paroxetine with other drugs that inhibit this enzyme should be approached with caution). Products include:
Zoloft 2581

Sulindac (The combined use of psychotropic drugs that interfere with serotonin reuptake and drugs that affect coagulation has been associated with an increased risk of bleeding). Products include:
Clinoril Tablets 1899

Sumatriptan (Co-administration of a selective serotonin reuptake inhibitor (SSRI) and sumatriptan has resulted in weakness, hyperreflexia, and incoordination). Products include:
Imitrex Nasal Spray 1435

Sumatriptan Succinate (Co-administration of a selective serotonin reuptake inhibitor (SSRI) and sumatriptan has resulted in weakness, hyperreflexia, and incoordination). Products include:
Imitrex Injection 1431
Imitrex Tablets 1440

Tamoxifen Citrate (Paroxetine may significantly inhibit the activity of the cytochrome P450 2D6 isoenzyme. Concomitant use of paroxetine with other drugs metabolized by cytochrome CYP2D6 has not been formally studied but may require lower doses than usually prescribed for either paroxetine or the other drug. Therefore, co-administration of paroxetine with other drugs that are metabolized by this isozyme should be approached with caution).
No products indexed under this heading.

Temazepam (Co-administration with another drug that is highly protein bound may increase free concentrations of the other drug or paroxetine potentially resulting in adverse events).
No products indexed under this heading.

Teniposide (Paroxetine may significantly inhibit the activity of the cytochrome P450 2D6 isoenzyme. Concomitant use of paroxetine with other drugs metabolized by cytochrome CYP2D6 has not been formally studied but may require lower doses than usually prescribed for either paroxetine or the other drug. Therefore, co-administration of paroxetine with other drugs that are metabolized by this isozyme should be approached with caution).
No products indexed under this heading.

Terbinafine Hydrochloride (Paroxetine is metabolized by the cytochrome P450 isoenzyme CYP2D6. Therefore, co-administration of paroxetine with other drugs that inhibit this enzyme should be approached with caution). Products include:
Lamisil AT Creams (Athlete's Foot & Jock Itch) 676
Lamisil Tablets 2226

Testosterone (Paroxetine may significantly inhibit the activity of the cytochrome P450 2D6 isoenzyme. Concomitant use of paroxetine with other drugs metabolized by cytochrome CYP2D6 has not been formally studied but may require lower doses than usually prescribed for either paroxetine or the other drug. Therefore, co-administration of paroxetine with other drugs that are metabolized by this isozyme should be approached with caution). Products include:
AndroGel 3330
Striant Mucoadhesive 1022
Testim 1% Gel 722

Testosterone Cypionate (Paroxetine may significantly inhibit the activity of the cytochrome P450 2D6 isoenzyme. Concomitant use of paroxetine with other drugs metabolized by cytochrome CYP2D6 has not been formally studied but may require lower doses than usually prescribed for either paroxetine or the other drug. Therefore, co-administration of paroxetine with other drugs that are metabolized by this isozyme should be approached with caution).
No products indexed under this heading.

Testosterone Enanthate (Paroxetine may significantly inhibit the activity of the cytochrome P450 2D6 isoenzyme. Concomitant use of paroxetine with other drugs metabolized by cytochrome CYP2D6 has not been formally studied but may require lower doses than usually prescribed for either paroxetine or the other drug. Therefore, co-administration of paroxetine with other drugs that are metabolized by this isozyme should be approached with caution). Products include:
Delatestryl Injection 2976

Testosterone Propionate (Paroxetine may significantly inhibit the activity of the cytochrome P450 2D6 isoenzyme. Concomitant use of paroxetine with other drugs metabolized by cytochrome CYP2D6 has not been formally studied but may require lower doses than usually prescribed for either paroxetine or the other drug. Therefore, co-administration of paroxetine with other drugs that are metabolized by this isozyme should be approached with caution).
No products indexed under this heading.

Theophylline (There have been reports of elevated theophylline levels associated with co-administration; monitor theophylline levels when these drugs are concurrently administered).
No products indexed under this heading.

Theophylline Anhydrous (There have been reports of elevated theophylline levels associated with co-administration; monitor theophylline levels when these drugs are concurrently administered). Products include:
Uniphyl Tablets 2708

Theophylline Calcium Salicylate (There have been reports of elevated theophylline levels associated with co-administration; monitor theophylline levels when these drugs are concurrently administered).
No products indexed under this heading.

Theophylline Dihydroxypropyl (Glyceryl) (There have been reports of elevated theophylline levels associated with co-administration; monitor theophylline levels when these drugs are concurrently administered).
No products indexed under this heading.

Theophylline Ethylenediamine (There have been reports of elevated theophylline levels associated with co-administration; monitor theophylline levels when these drugs are concurrently administered).
No products indexed under this heading.

Theophylline Sodium Glycinate (There have been reports of elevated theophylline levels associated with co-administration; monitor theophylline levels when these drugs are concurrently administered).
No products indexed under this heading.

Thioridazine (Co-administration of drugs which inhibit CYP450IID6, such as paroxetine, will elevate plasma levels of thioridazine; because thioridazine administration produces a dose-related prolongation of the QTc interval which is associated with serious ventriculararrhythmias, such as torsade de pointes-type arrhythmias, and sudden death; concurrent use is contraindicated).
No products indexed under this heading.

Thioridazine Hydrochloride (Co-administration of drugs which inhibit CYP450IID6, such as paroxetine, will elevate plasma levels of thioridazine; because thioridazine administration produces a dose-related prolongation of the QTc interval which is associated with serious ventriculararrhythmias, such as torsade de pointes-type arrhythmias, and sudden death; concurrent use is contraindicated). Products include:
Thioridazine Hydrochloride Tablets 2122

Timolol Maleate (Paroxetine may significantly inhibit the activity of the cytochrome P450 2D6 isoenzyme. Concomitant use of paroxetine with other drugs metabolized by cytochrome CYP2D6 has not been formally studied but may require lower doses than usually prescribed for either paroxetine or the other drug. Therefore, co-administration of paroxetine with other drugs that are metabolized by this isozyme should be approached with caution). Products include:
Blocadren Tablets 1891
Cosopt Sterile Ophthalmic Solution 1910
Timolide Tablets 2056
Timoptic in Ocudose 2061
Timoptic Sterile Ophthalmic Solution 2058
Timoptic-XE Sterile Ophthalmic Gel Forming Solution 2062

Tinzaparin Sodium (The combined use of psychotropic drugs that interfere with serotonin reuptake and drugs that affect coagulation has been associated with an increased risk of bleeding; concomitant administration should be undertaken with caution).
No products indexed under this heading.

Tolbutamide (Co-administration with another drug that is highly protein bound may increase free concentrations of the other drug or paroxetine potentially resulting in adverse events).
No products indexed under this heading.

Tolmetin Sodium (The combined use of psychotropic drugs that interfere with serotonin reuptake and drugs that affect coagulation has been associated with an increased risk of bleeding).
No products indexed under this heading.

Tolterodine Tartrate (Paroxetine may significantly inhibit the activity of the cytochrome P450 2D6 isoenzyme. Concomitant use of paroxetine with other drugs metabolized by cytochrome CYP2D6 has not been formally studied but may require lower doses than usually prescribed for either paroxetine or the other drug. Therefore, co-administration of paroxetine with other drugs that are metabolized by this isozyme should be approached with caution). Products include:
Detrol Tablets 2626
Detrol LA Capsules 2629

Tramadol Hydrochloride (Based on the mechanism of action of paroxetine and the potential for serotonin syndrome, caution is advised when paroxetine hydrochloride is co-administered with other drugs or agents that may affect the serotonergic neurotransmitter systems, such as tramadol). Products include:
Ultracet Tablets 2462

Tranylcypromine Sulfate (Potential for serious and/or fatal reactions, including hyperthermia, rigidity, myoclonus and other serious reactions; concurrent and/or sequential use is contraindicated). Products include:
Parnate Tablets 1499

Trazodone Hydrochloride (Paroxetine may significantly inhibit the activity of the cytochrome P450 2D6 isoenzyme. Concomitant use of paroxetine with other drugs metabolized by cytochrome CYP2D6 has not been formally studied but may require lower doses than usually prescribed for either paroxetine or the other drug. Therefore, co-administration of paroxetine with other drugs that are metabolized by this isozyme should be approached with caution).
No products indexed under this heading.

Triazolam (Paroxetine may significantly inhibit the activity of the cytochrome P450 2D6 isoenzyme. Concomitant use of paroxetine with other drugs metabolized by cytochrome CYP2D6 has not been formally studied but may require lower doses than usually prescribed for either paroxetine or the other drug. Therefore, co-administration of paroxetine with other drugs that are metabolized by this isozyme should

be approached with caution).
No products indexed under this heading.

Trifluoperazine Hydrochloride (Paroxetine may significantly inhibit the activity of cytochrome P450 2D6 isoenzyme. Concomitant use of paroxetine with other drugs metabolized by cytochrome CYP2D6 has not been formally studied but may require lower doses than usually prescribed for either paroxetine or the other drug. Therefore, co-administration of paroxetine with other drugs that are metabolized by this isozyme should be approached with caution).
No products indexed under this heading.

Trimipramine Maleate (Caution is indicated in the co-administration of tricyclic antidepressants with paroxetine because paroxetine may inhibit TCA metabolism. Plasma TCA concentrations may need to be monitored and the dose of TCA may need to be reduced if a TCA is co-administered with paroxetine). Products include:
Surmontil Capsules 2347

L-Tryptophan (Potential for headache, nausea, sweating and dizziness; concomitant use is not recommended).
No products indexed under this heading.

Valdecoxib (The combined use of psychotropic drugs that interfere with serotonin reuptake and drugs that affect coagulation has been associated with an increased risk of bleeding).
No products indexed under this heading.

Venlafaxine Hydrochloride (Paroxetine may significantly inhibit the activity of the cytochrome P450 2D6 isoenzyme. Concomitant use of paroxetine with other drugs metabolized by cytochrome CYP2D6 has not been formally studied but may require lower doses than usually prescribed for either paroxetine or the other drug. Therefore, co-administration of paroxetine with other drugs that are metabolized by this isozyme should be approached with caution). Products include:
Effexor Tablets 3405
Effexor XR Capsules 3411

Vinblastine Sulfate (Paroxetine may significantly inhibit the activity of the cytochrome P450 2D6 isoenzyme. Concomitant use of paroxetine with other drugs metabolized by cytochrome CYP2D6 has not been formally studied but may require lower doses than usually prescribed for either paroxetine or the other drug. Therefore, co-administration of paroxetine with other drugs that are metabolized by this isozyme should be approached with caution).
No products indexed under this heading.

Warfarin Sodium (Preliminary data suggest that there may be a pharmacodynamic interaction (that causes an increased bleeding diathesis in the face of unaltered prothrombin time) between paroxetine and warfarin. Since there is little clinical experience, the concomitant administration of paroxetine and warfarin should be undertaken with caution). Products include:
Coumadin for Injection 932
Coumadin Tablets 932

Zolmitriptan (There have been rare post-marketing reports describing patients with weakness, hyperreflexia, and incoordination following the use of a selective serotonin reuptake inhibitor (SSRI) and sumatriptan. If concomitant treatment with a triptan and an SSRI (eg, paroxetine) is clinically warranted, appropriate observation of the patient is advised). Products include:
Zomig Nasal Spray 718
Zomig Tablets 714
Zomig-ZMT Tablets 714

Zonisamide (Paroxetine may significantly inhibit the activity of the cytochrome P450 2D6 isoenzyme. Concomitant use of paroxetine with other drugs metabolized by cytochrome CYP2D6 has not been formally studied but may require lower doses than usually prescribed for either paroxetine or the other drug. Therefore, co-administration of paroxetine with other drugs that are metabolized by this isozyme should be approached with caution). Products include:
Zonegran Capsules 1089

Food Interactions

Alcohol (Concurrent use should be avoided).

Food, unspecified (Co-administration with food resulted in slight increase (6%) in AUC, but Cmax was 29% greater; time to reach peak plasma concentration decreased from 6.4 hours post-dosing to 4.9 hours).

PCE DISPERTAB TABLETS

(Erythromycin) 510
May interact with oral anticoagulants, HMG-CoA reductase inhibitors, phenytoin, triazolobenzodiazepines, valproate, xanthines, and certain other agents. Compounds in these categories include:

Alfentanil Hydrochloride (Concurrent use of erythromycin in patients receiving drugs metabolized by the cytochrome P450 system may be associated with elevation in serum levels of alfentanil).
No products indexed under this heading.

Alprazolam (Erythromycin has been reported to decrease the clearance of triazolam and midazolam; may increase the pharmacologic effect of these benzodiazepines). Products include:
Niravam Orally Disintegrating Tablets 3106
Xanax XR Tablets 2655

Aminophylline (Co-administration in patients who are receiving high doses of theophylline may be associated with an increase in serum theophylline levels and potential theophylline toxicity).
No products indexed under this heading.

Anisindione (Co-administration has resulted in increased anticoagulant effects). Products include:
Miradon Tablets 3056

Astemizole (Concurrent use of erythromycin in patients receiving astemizole has been reported to significantly alter the metabolism of astemizole; rare cases of cardiovascular adverse events, including prolonged QT interval, cardiac arrest, torsade de pointes, and other ventricular arrhythmias have been reported; co-administration is contraindicated).
No products indexed under this heading.

Atorvastatin Calcium (Erythromycin has been reported to increase concentrations of HMG-CoA reductase inhibitors (e.g. lovastatin and simvastatin); rare reports of rhabdomyolysis have been reported in patients taking these drugs concomitantly). Products include:
Caduet Tablets 2507
Lipitor Tablets 2495

Bromocriptine Mesylate (Concurrent use of erythromycin in patients receiving drugs metabolized by the cytochrome P450 system may be associated with elevation in serum levels of bromocriptine).
No products indexed under this heading.

Carbamazepine (Concurrent use of erythromycin in patients receiving drugs metabolized by the cytochrome P450 system may be associated with elevation in serum levels of carbamazepine). Products include:
Carbatrol Capsules 3174
Equetro Extended-Release Capsules 3178
Tegretol/Tegretol-XR 2278

Cerivastatin Sodium (Erythromycin has been reported to increase concentrations of HMG-CoA reductase inhibitors (e.g. lovastatin and simvastatin); rare reports of rhabdomyolysis have been reported in patients taking these drugs concomitantly).
No products indexed under this heading.

Cisapride (Concurrent use of erythromycin in patients receiving cisapride has been reported to inhibit the metabolism of cisapride; cases of cardiovascular adverse events, including prolonged QT interval, torsade de pointes, ventricular tachycardia, and ventricular fibrillation have been reported; co-administration is contraindicated).
No products indexed under this heading.

Cyclosporine (Concurrent use of erythromycin in patients receiving drugs metabolized by the cytochrome P450 system may be associated with elevation in serum levels of cyclosporine). Products include:
Gengraf Capsules 458
Neoral Soft Gelatin Capsules 2247
Neoral Oral Solution 2247
Restasis Ophthalmic Emulsion 570
Sandimmune 2259

Dicumarol (Co-administration has resulted in increased anticoagulant effects).
No products indexed under this heading.

Digoxin (Co-administration has been reported to result in elevated digoxin serum levels). Products include:
Digitek Tablets 2146
Lanoxicaps Capsules 1458
Lanoxin Injection 1462
Lanoxin Tablets 1468
Lanoxin Injection Pediatric 1465

Dihydroergotamine Mesylate (Co-administration has been associated in some patients with acute ergot toxicity characterized by severe peripheral vasospasm and dysesthesia). Products include:
Migranal Nasal Spray 3350

Disopyramide Phosphate (Concurrent use of erythromycin in patients receiving drugs metabolized by the cytochrome P450 system may be associated with elevation in serum levels of disopyramide).
No products indexed under this heading.

Divalproex Sodium (There have been reports of interactions of erythromycin with drugs not thought to be metabolized by CYP3A, including valproate). Products include:
Depakote Sprinkle Capsules 422
Depakote Tablets 427
Depakote ER Tablets 433

Dyphylline (Co-administration in patients who are receiving high doses of theophylline may be associated with an increase in serum theophylline levels and potential theophylline toxicity).
No products indexed under this heading.

Ergotamine Tartrate (Co-administration has been associated in some patients with acute ergot toxicity characterized by severe peripheral vasospasm and dysethesia).
No products indexed under this heading.

Fluvastatin Sodium (Erythromycin has been reported to increase concentrations of HMG-CoA reductase inhibitors (e.g. lovastatin and simvastatin); rare reports of rhabdomyolysis have been reported in patients taking these drugs concomitantly). Products include:
Lescol Capsules 2227
Lescol 2730
Lescol XL Tablets 2227

Fosphenytoin Sodium (There have been reports of interactions of erythromycin with drugs not thought to be metabolized by CYP3A, including phenytoin).
No products indexed under this heading.

Hexobarbital (There have been reports of interactions of erythromycin with drugs not thought to be metabolized by CYP3A, including hexobarbital).
No products indexed under this heading.

Lovastatin (Erythromycin has been reported to increase concentrations of HMG-CoA reductase inhibitors (e.g. lovastatin and simvastatin); rare reports of rhabdomyolysis have been reported in patients taking these drugs concomitantly). Products include:
Advicor Tablets 1694
Altoprev Extended-Release Tablets 1151
Mevacor Tablets 1996

Midazolam Hydrochloride (Erythromycin has been reported to decrease the clearance of triazolam and midazolam; may increase the pharmacologic effect of these benzodiazepines).
No products indexed under this heading.

Phenytoin (There have been reports of interactions of erythromycin with drugs not thought to be metabolized by CYP3A, including phenytoin).
No products indexed under this heading.

Phenytoin Sodium (There have been reports of interactions of erythromycin with drugs not thought to be metabolized by CYP3A, including phenytoin). Products include:
Phenytek Capsules 2153

Pimozide (Concurrent use of erythromycin in patients receiving drugs metabolized by the cytochrome P450 system may be associated with elevation in serum levels of pimozide; co-administration is contraindicated). Products include:
Orap Tablets 1220

Pravastatin Sodium (Erythromycin has been reported to increase concentrations of HMG-CoA reductase inhibitors (e.g. lovastatin and simvastatin); rare reports of rhabdomyolysis have been reported in patients taking these drugs concomitantly). Products include:
Pravachol Tablets 943

Sildenafil Citrate (Erythromycin has been reported to increase the systemic exposure (AUC) of sildenafil). Products include:
Revatio Tablets 2541
Viagra Tablets 2552

Simvastatin (Erythromycin has been reported to increase concentrations of HMG-CoA reductase inhibitors (e.g. lovastatin and simvastatin); rare reports of rhabdomyolysis have been reported in patients taking these drugs concomitantly). Products include:
Vytorin 10/10 Tablets 2084
Vytorin 10/10 Tablets 3092
Vytorin 10/20 Tablets 2084
Vytorin 10/20 Tablets 3092
Vytorin 10/40 Tablets 3092
Vytorin 10/40 Tablets 2084
Vytorin 10/80 Tablets 2084
Vytorin 10/80 Tablets 3092
Zocor Tablets 2078

Tacrolimus (Concurrent use of erythromycin in patients receiving drugs metabolized by the cytochrome P450 system may be associated with elevation in serum levels of tacrolimus). Products include:
Prograf Capsules and Injection 624
Protopic Ointment 629

Terfenadine (Concurrent use of erythromycin in patients receiving terfenadine has been reported to significantly alter the metabolism of terfenadine; rare cases of cardiovascular adverse events, including prolonged QT interval, cardiac arrest, torsade de pointes, other ventricular arrhythmias, and death have been reported; co-administration is contraindicated).
No products indexed under this heading.

Theophylline (Co-administration in patients who are receiving high doses of theophylline may be associated with an increase in serum theophylline levels and potential theophylline toxicity).
No products indexed under this heading.

Theophylline Anhydrous (Co-administration in patients who are receiving high doses of theophylline may be associated with an increase in serum theophylline levels and potential theophylline toxicity). Products include:
Uniphyl Tablets 2708

Theophylline Calcium Salicylate (Co-administration in patients who are receiving high doses of theophylline may be associated with an increase in serum theophylline levels and potential theophylline toxicity).
No products indexed under this heading.

Theophylline Dihydroxypropyl (Glyceryl) (Co-administration in patients who are receiving high doses of theophylline may be associated with an increase in serum theophylline levels and potential theophylline toxicity).
No products indexed under this heading.

Theophylline Ethylenediamine (Co-administration in patients who are receiving high doses of theophylline may be associated with an increase in serum theophylline levels and potential theophylline toxicity).
No products indexed under this heading.

Theophylline Sodium Glycinate (Co-administration in patients who are receiving high doses of theophylline may be associated with an increase in serum theophylline levels and potential theophylline toxicity).
No products indexed under this heading.

Triazolam (Erythromycin has been reported to decrease the clearance of triazolam and midazolam; may increase the pharmacologic effect of these benzodiazepines).
No products indexed under this heading.

Valproate Sodium (There have been reports of interactions of erythromycin with drugs not thought to be metabolized by CYP3A, including valproate). Products include:
Depacon Injection 412

Valproic Acid (There have been reports of interactions of erythromycin with drugs not thought to be metabolized by CYP3A, including valproate). Products include:
Depakene 417

Warfarin Sodium (Co-administration has resulted in increased anticoagulant effects). Products include:
Coumadin for Injection 932
Coumadin Tablets 932

Food Interactions

Meal, unspecified (Presence of food results in lower blood levels; optimal blood levels are obtained when PCE is given in the fasting state (at least ½ hour and preferably 2 hours before meals)).

PEDIACARE DECONGESTANT & COUGH INFANT DROPS

(Dextromethorphan Hydrobromide, Pseudoephedrine Hydrochloride) 705
May interact with monoamine oxidase inhibitors. Compounds in these categories include:

Isocarboxazid (Concurrent and/or sequential use with MAO inhibitors is not recommended).
No products indexed under this heading.

Moclobemide (Concurrent and/or sequential use with MAO inhibitors is not recommended).
No products indexed under this heading.

Pargyline Hydrochloride (Concurrent and/or sequential use with MAO inhibitors is not recommended).
No products indexed under this heading.

Phenelzine Sulfate (Concurrent and/or sequential use with MAO inhibitors is not recommended).
No products indexed under this heading.

Procarbazine Hydrochloride (Concurrent and/or sequential use with MAO inhibitors is not recommended). Products include:
Matulane Capsules 3188

Selegiline Hydrochloride (Concurrent and/or sequential use with MAO inhibitors is not recommended). Products include:
Eldepryl Capsules 3209

Tranylcypromine Sulfate (Concurrent and/or sequential use with MAO inhibitors is not recommended). Products include:
Parnate Tablets 1499

PEDIACARE FREEZER POPS LONG-ACTING COUGH-GLACIER GRAPE AND POLAR BERRY BLUE

(Dextromethorphan Hydrobromide) 706
None cited in PDR database.

PEDIACARE DECONGESTANT INFANTS' DROPS

(Pseudoephedrine Hydrochloride) 705
See PediaCare Long-Acting Cough Plus Cold Liquid

PEDIACARE LONG-ACTING COUGH INFANT DROPS

(Dextromethorphan Hydrobromide) 705
None cited in PDR database.

PEDIACARE LONG-ACTING COUGH PLUS COLD LIQUID

(Dextromethorphan Hydrobromide, Pseudoephedrine Hydrochloride) 704
May interact with monoamine oxidase inhibitors. Compounds in these categories include:

Isocarboxazid (Concurrent and/or sequential use with MAO inhibitors is not recommended).
No products indexed under this heading.

Moclobemide (Concurrent and/or sequential use with MAO inhibitors is not recommended).
No products indexed under this heading.

Pargyline Hydrochloride (Concurrent and/or sequential use with MAO inhibitors is not recommended).
No products indexed under this heading.

Phenelzine Sulfate (Concurrent and/or sequential use with MAO inhibitors is not recommended).
No products indexed under this heading.

Procarbazine Hydrochloride (Concurrent and/or sequential use with MAO inhibitors is not recommended). Products include:
Matulane Capsules 3188

Selegiline Hydrochloride (Concurrent and/or sequential use with MAO inhibitors is not recommended). Products include:
Eldepryl Capsules 3209

Tranylcypromine Sulfate (Concurrent and/or sequential use with MAO inhibitors is not recommended). Products include:
Parnate Tablets 1499

PEDIACARE MULTI-SYMPTOM COLD LIQUID

(Chlorpheniramine Maleate, Dextromethorphan Hydrobromide, Pseudoephedrine Hydrochloride) 704
See PediaCare NightRest Cough & Cold Liquid

PEDIACARE NIGHTREST COUGH & COLD LIQUID

(Chlorpheniramine Maleate, Dextromethorphan Hydrobromide, Pseudoephedrine Hydrochloride) 704
May interact with hypnotics and sedatives, monoamine oxidase inhibitors, and tranquilizers. Compounds in these categories include:

Alprazolam (Increases the drowsiness effect). Products include:
Niravam Orally Disintegrating Tablets 3106
Xanax XR Tablets 2655

Buspirone Hydrochloride (Increases the drowsiness effect).
No products indexed under this heading.

Chlordiazepoxide (Increases the drowsiness effect).
No products indexed under this heading.

Chlordiazepoxide Hydrochloride (Increases the drowsiness effect). Products include:
Librium Capsules 3349

Chlorpromazine (Increases the drowsiness effect).
No products indexed under this heading.

Chlorpromazine Hydrochloride (Increases the drowsiness effect).
No products indexed under this heading.

Chlorprothixene (Increases the drowsiness effect).
No products indexed under this heading.

Chlorprothixene Hydrochloride (Increases the drowsiness effect).
No products indexed under this heading.

Clorazepate Dipotassium (Increases the drowsiness effect). Products include:
Tranxene 2488

Diazepam (Increases the drowsiness effect). Products include:
Diastat Rectal Delivery System 3344
Valium Tablets 2822

Droperidol (Increases the drowsiness effect).
No products indexed under this heading.

Estazolam (Increases the drowsiness effect). Products include:
ProSom Tablets 512

Ethchlorvynol (Increases the drowsiness effect).
No products indexed under this heading.

Ethinamate (Increases the drowsiness effect).
No products indexed under this heading.

Fluphenazine Decanoate (Increases the drowsiness effect).
No products indexed under this heading.

Fluphenazine Enanthate (Increases the drowsiness effect).
No products indexed under this heading.

Fluphenazine Hydrochloride (Increases the drowsiness effect).
No products indexed under this heading.

Flurazepam Hydrochloride (Increases the drowsiness effect). Products include:
Dalmane Capsules 3343

Glutethimide (Increases the drowsiness effect).
No products indexed under this heading.

Haloperidol (Increases the drowsiness effect).
No products indexed under this heading.

Haloperidol Decanoate (Increases the drowsiness effect).
No products indexed under this heading.

Hydroxyzine Hydrochloride (Increases the drowsiness effect).
No products indexed under this heading.

Isocarboxazid (Concurrent and/or sequential use with MAO inhibitors is not recommended).
No products indexed under this heading.

Lorazepam (Increases the drowsiness effect).
No products indexed under this heading.

Loxapine Hydrochloride (Increases the drowsiness effect).
No products indexed under this heading.

Loxapine Succinate (Increases the drowsiness effect).
No products indexed under this heading.

Meprobamate (Increases the drowsiness effect).
No products indexed under this heading.

Mesoridazine Besylate (Increases the drowsiness effect).
No products indexed under this heading.

Midazolam Hydrochloride (Increases the drowsiness effect).
No products indexed under this heading.

Moclobemide (Concurrent and/or sequential use with MAO inhibitors is not recommended).
No products indexed under this heading.

Molindone Hydrochloride (Increases the drowsiness effect). Products include:
Moban Tablets 1108

Oxazepam (Increases the drowsiness effect).
No products indexed under this heading.

Pargyline Hydrochloride (Concurrent and/or sequential use with MAO inhibitors is not recommended).
No products indexed under this heading.

Perphenazine (Increases the drowsiness effect).
No products indexed under this heading.

Phenelzine Sulfate (Concurrent and/or sequential use with MAO inhibitors is not recommended).
No products indexed under this heading.

Prazepam (Increases the drowsiness effect).
No products indexed under this heading.

Procarbazine Hydrochloride (Concurrent and/or sequential use with MAO inhibitors is not recommended). Products include:
Matulane Capsules 3188

Prochlorperazine (Increases the drowsiness effect).
No products indexed under this heading.

Promethazine Hydrochloride (Increases the drowsiness effect). Products include:
Phenergan 3438

Propofol (Increases the drowsiness effect). Products include:
Diprivan Injectable Emulsion 676

Quazepam (Increases the drowsiness effect).
No products indexed under this heading.

Secobarbital Sodium (Increases the drowsiness effect).
No products indexed under this heading.

Selegiline Hydrochloride (Concurrent and/or sequential use with MAO inhibitors is not recommended). Products include:
Eldepryl Capsules 3209

Temazepam (Increases the drowsiness effect).
No products indexed under this heading.

Thioridazine Hydrochloride (Increases the drowsiness effect). Products include:
Thioridazine Hydrochloride Tablets 2122

Thiothixene (Increases the drowsiness effect). Products include:
Thiothixene Capsules 2124

Tranylcypromine Sulfate (Concurrent and/or sequential use with MAO inhibitors is not recommended). Products include:
Parnate Tablets 1499

Triazolam (Increases the drowsiness effect).
No products indexed under this heading.

Trifluoperazine Hydrochloride (Increases the drowsiness effect).
No products indexed under this heading.

Zaleplon (Increases the drowsiness effect). Products include:
Sonata Capsules 1686

Zolpidem Tartrate (Increases the drowsiness effect). Products include:
Ambien Tablets 2867

PEDIALYTE ORAL ELECTROLYTE MAINTENANCE SOLUTION
(Electrolyte Solution) 2842
None cited in PDR database.

PEDIAPRED ORAL SOLUTION
(Prednisolone Sodium Phosphate) 3319
May interact with barbiturates, oral hypoglycemic agents, insulin, and certain other agents. Compounds in these categories include:

Acarbose (Increased requirement of hypoglycemic agents in diabetes). Products include:
Precose Tablets 776

Aprobarbital (Induces hepatic microsomal drug metabolizing enzyme activity which may result in enhanced metabolism of prednisolone; dosage of prednisolone may need to be increased).
No products indexed under this heading.

Aspirin (Aspirin should be used cautiously in conjunction with corticosteroids in hypoprothrobinemia). Products include:
Aggrenox Capsules 855
Bayer, Aspirin Regimen .... ▣606
Bayer Aspirin Tablets 3515
BC Powder .... ▣612
BC Allergy Sinus Cold Powder .... ▣612
Arthritis Strength BC Powder .... ▣612
BC Sinus Cold Powder .... ▣612
Ecotrin Enteric Coated Aspirin Low, Regular and Maximum Strength Tablets 1627
Goody's Body Pain Formula Powder .... ▣621
Goody's Extra Strength Headache Powder .... ▣621
Goody's Extra Strength Pain Relief Tablets .... ▣621
Percodan Tablets 1115
St. Joseph 81 mg Aspirin Chewable and Enteric Coated Tablets 1841

Butabarbital (Induces hepatic microsomal drug metabolizing enzyme activity which may result in enhanced metabolism of prednisolone; dosage of prednisolone may need to be increased).
No products indexed under this heading.

Butalbital (Induces hepatic microsomal drug metabolizing enzyme activity which may result in enhanced metabolism of prednisolone; dosage of prednisolone may need to be increased). Products include:
Sedapap Tablets 50 mg/650 mg 2098

Chlorpropamide (Increased requirement of hypoglycemic agents in diabetes).
No products indexed under this heading.

Glimepiride (Increased requirement of hypoglycemic agents in diabetes). Products include:
Amaryl Tablets 2864

Glipizide (Increased requirement of hypoglycemic agents in diabetes).
No products indexed under this heading.

Glyburide (Increased requirement of hypoglycemic agents in diabetes).
No products indexed under this heading.

Insulin, Human, Zinc Suspension (Increased requirement of insulin in diabetes). Products include:
Humulin L, 100 Units 1763
Humulin U, 100 Units 1770

Insulin, Human NPH (Increased requirement of insulin in diabetes). Products include:
Humulin N, 100 Units 1764
Humulin N Pen 1765
Novolin N Human Insulin 10 ml Vials 2322
Novolin N InnoLet 2322
Novolin N PenFill 3 ml Cartridges 2325
Novolin R InnoLet 2322

Insulin, Human Regular (Increased requirement of insulin in diabetes). Products include:
Humulin R (U-500) 1768
Humulin R, 100 Units 1767
Novolin R Human Insulin 10 ml Vials 2322
Novolin R PenFill 2325

Insulin, Human Regular and Human NPH Mixture (Increased requirement of insulin in diabetes). Products include:
Humulin 50/50, 100 Units 1760
Humulin 70/30 Pen 1761
Novolin 70/30 Human Insulin 10 ml Vials 2321
Novolin 70/30 InnoLet 2322
Novolin 70/30 PenFill 3 ml Cartridges 2325

Insulin, NPH (Increased requirement of insulin in diabetes).
No products indexed under this heading.

Insulin, Regular (Increased requirement of insulin in diabetes).
No products indexed under this heading.

Insulin, Zinc Crystals (Increased requirement of insulin in diabetes).
No products indexed under this heading.

Insulin, Zinc Suspension (Increased requirement of insulin in diabetes).
No products indexed under this heading.

Insulin Aspart, Human Regular (Increased requirement of insulin in diabetes). Products include:
NovoLog Injection 2326

Insulin glargine (Increased requirement of insulin in diabetes). Products include:
Lantus Injection 2925

Insulin Lispro, Human (Increased requirement of insulin in diabetes). Products include:
Humalog-Pen 1751
Humalog Mix 75/25-Pen 1754

Insulin Lispro Protamine, Human (Increased requirement of insulin in diabetes). Products include:
Humalog Mix 75/25-Pen 1754

Mephobarbital (Induces hepatic microsomal drug metabolizing enzyme activity which may result in enhanced metabolism of prednisolone; dosage of prednisolone may need to be increased). Products include:
Mebaral Tablets, USP 2483

Metformin Hydrochloride (Increased requirement of hypoglycemic agents in diabetes). Products include:
ActoPlus Met Tablets 3219
Avandamet Tablets 1343
Fortamet Extended-Release Tablets 1156

Miglitol (Increased requirement of hypoglycemic agents in diabetes).
No products indexed under this heading.

Pentobarbital Sodium (Induces hepatic microsomal drug metabolizing enzyme activity which may result in enhanced metabolism of prednisolone; dosage of prednisolone may need to be increased). Products include:
Nembutal Sodium Solution, USP 2484

Phenobarbital (Induces hepatic microsomal drug metabolizing enzyme activity which may result in enhanced metabolism of prednisolone; dosage of prednisolone may need to be increased).
No products indexed under this heading.

Pioglitazone Hydrochloride (Increased requirement of hypoglycemic agents in diabetes). Products include:
ActoPlus Met Tablets 3219

Actos Tablets 3224

Repaglinide (Increased requirement of hypoglycemic agents in diabetes). Products include:

Prandin Tablets (0.5, 1, and 2 mg).. 2337

Rosiglitazone Maleate (Increased requirement of hypoglycemic agents in diabetes). Products include:

Avandamet Tablets 1343
Avandia Tablets 1348

Secobarbital Sodium (Induces hepatic microsomal drug metabolizing enzyme activity which may result in enhanced metabolism of prednisolone; dosage of prednisolone may need to be increased).

No products indexed under this heading.

Thiamylal Sodium (Induces hepatic microsomal drug metabolizing enzyme activity which may result in enhanced metabolism of prednisolone; dosage of prednisolone may need to be increased).

No products indexed under this heading.

Tolazamide (Increased requirement of hypoglycemic agents in diabetes).

No products indexed under this heading.

Tolbutamide (Increased requirement of hypoglycemic agents in diabetes).

No products indexed under this heading.

Troglitazone (Increased requirement of hypoglycemic agents in diabetes).

No products indexed under this heading.

PEDIARIX VACCINE

(Diphtheria & Tetanus Toxoids and Pertussis Vaccine Adsorbed, Hepatitis B Vaccine, Recombinant, Poliovirus Vaccine Inactivated, Trivalent Types 1,2,3)........................ 1518

May interact with alkylating agents, antimetabolites, corticosteroids, cytotoxic drugs, immunosuppressive agents, and certain other agents. Compounds in these categories include:

Azathioprine (May reduce immune response to vaccines. When administered to patients who are receiving immunosuppressive therapy, who have an immunodeficiency disorder, or who have received a recent injection of immune globulin, an adequate immunologic response may not be obtained). Products include:

Azasan Tablets 2844

Basiliximab (May reduce immune response to vaccines. When administered to patients who are receiving immunosuppressive therapy, who have an immunodeficiency disorder, or who have received a recent injection of immune globulin, an adequate immunologic response may not be obtained). Products include:

Simulect for Injection 2268

Betamethasone Acetate (May reduce immune response to vaccines. When administered to patients who are receiving immunosuppressive therapy, who have an immunodeficiency disorder, or who have received a recent injection of immune globulin, an adequate immunologic response may not be obtained).

No products indexed under this heading.

Betamethasone Sodium Phosphate (May reduce immune response to vaccines. When administered to patients who are receiving immunosuppressive therapy, who have an immunodeficiency disorder, or who have received a recent injection of immune globulin, an adequate immunologic response may not be obtained).

No products indexed under this heading.

Bleomycin Sulfate (May reduce immune response to vaccines. When administered to patients who are receiving immunosuppressive therapy, who have an immunodeficiency disorder, or who have received a recent injection of immune globulin, an adequate immunologic response may not be obtained).

No products indexed under this heading.

Busulfan (May reduce immune response to vaccines. When administered to patients who are receiving immunosuppressive therapy, who have an immunodeficiency disorder, or who have received a recent injection of immune globulin, an adequate immunologic response may not be obtained). Products include:

I.V. Busulfex 1125
Myleran Tablets 1492

Capecitabine (May reduce immune response to vaccines. When administered to patients who are receiving immunosuppressive therapy, who have an immunodeficiency disorder, or who have received a recent injection of immune globulin, an adequate immunologic response may not be obtained). Products include:

Xeloda Tablets 2825

Carmustine (BCNU) (May reduce immune response to vaccines. When administered to patients who are receiving immunosuppressive therapy, who have an immunodeficiency disorder, or who have received a recent injection of immune globulin, an adequate immunologic response may not be obtained).

No products indexed under this heading.

Chlorambucil (May reduce immune response to vaccines. When administered to patients who are receiving immunosuppressive therapy, who have an immunodeficiency disorder, or who have received a recent injection of immune globulin, an adequate immunologic response may not be obtained). Products include:

Leukeran Tablets 1472

Cladribine (May reduce immune response to vaccines. When administered to patients who are receiving immunosuppressive therapy, who have an immunodeficiency disorder, or who have received a recent injection of immune globulin, an adequate immunologic response may not be obtained). Products include:

Leustatin Injection 2368

Cortisone Acetate (May reduce immune response to vaccines. When administered to patients who are receiving immunosuppressive therapy, who have an immunodeficiency disorder, or who have received a recent injection of immune globulin, an adequate immunologic response may not be obtained).

No products indexed under this heading.

Cyclophosphamide (May reduce immune response to vaccines. When administered to patients who are receiving immunosuppressive therapy, who have an immunodeficiency disorder, or who have received a recent injection of immune globulin, an adequate immunologic response may not be obtained).

No products indexed under this heading.

Cyclosporine (May reduce immune response to vaccines. When administered to patients who are receiving immunosuppressive therapy, who have an immunodeficiency disorder, or who have received a recent injection of immune globulin, an adequate immunologic response may not be obtained). Products include:

Gengraf Capsules 458
Neoral Soft Gelatin Capsules 2247
Neoral Oral Solution 2247
Restasis Ophthalmic Emulsion 570
Sandimmune 2259

Cytarabine (May reduce immune response to vaccines. When administered to patients who are receiving immunosuppressive therapy, who have an immunodeficiency disorder, or who have received a recent injection of immune globulin, an adequate immunologic response may not be obtained).

No products indexed under this heading.

Dacarbazine (May reduce immune response to vaccines. When administered to patients who are receiving immunosuppressive therapy, who have an immunodeficiency disorder, or who have received a recent injection of immune globulin, an adequate immunologic response may not be obtained).

No products indexed under this heading.

Daunorubicin Hydrochloride (May reduce immune response to vaccines. When administered to patients who are receiving immunosuppressive therapy, who have an immunodeficiency disorder, or who have received a recent injection of immune globulin, an adequate immunologic response may not be obtained). Products include:

Cerubidine for Injection 788

Dexamethasone (May reduce immune response to vaccines. When administered to patients who are receiving immunosuppressive therapy, who have an immunodeficiency disorder, or who have received a recent injection of immune globulin, an adequate immunologic response may not be obtained). Products include:

Ciprodex Otic Suspension 555
Decadron Tablets 1929
TobraDex Ophthalmic Ointment 558
TobraDex Ophthalmic Suspension ... 558

Dexamethasone Acetate (May reduce immune response to vaccines. When administered to patients who are receiving immunosuppressive therapy, who have an immunodeficiency disorder, or who have received a recent injection of immune globulin, an adequate immunologic response may not be obtained).

No products indexed under this heading.

Dexamethasone Sodium Phosphate (May reduce immune response to vaccines. When administered to patients who are receiving immunosuppressive therapy, who have an immunodeficiency disorder, or who have received a recent injection of immune globulin, an adequate immunologic response may not be obtained). Products include:

Decadron Phosphate Injection 1931

Doxorubicin Hydrochloride (May reduce immune response to vaccines. When administered to patients who are receiving immunosuppressive therapy, who have an immunodeficiency disorder, or who have received a recent injection of immune globulin, an adequate immunologic response may not be obtained). Products include:

Adriamycin for Injection, USP 786
Adriamycin Injection, USP 786

Epirubicin Hydrochloride (May reduce immune response to vaccines. When administered to patients who are receiving immunosuppressive therapy, who have an immunodeficiency disorder, or who have received a recent injection of immune globulin, an adequate immunologic response may not be obtained). Products include:

Ellence Injection 2632

Floxuridine (May reduce immune response to vaccines. When administered to patients who are receiving immunosuppressive therapy, who have an immunodeficiency disorder, or who have received a recent injection of immune globulin, an adequate immunologic response may not be obtained).

No products indexed under this heading.

Fludarabine Phosphate (May reduce immune response to vaccines. When administered to patients who are receiving immunosuppressive therapy, who have an immunodeficiency disorder, or who have received a recent injection of immune globulin, an adequate immunologic response may not be obtained).

No products indexed under this heading.

Fludrocortisone Acetate (May reduce immune response to vaccines. When administered to patients who are receiving immunosuppressive therapy, who have an immunodeficiency disorder, or who have received a recent injection of immune globulin, an adequate immunologic response may not be obtained).

No products indexed under this heading.

Fluorouracil (May reduce immune response to vaccines. When administered to patients who are receiving immunosuppressive therapy, who have an immunodeficiency disorder, or who have received a recent injection of immune globulin, an adequate immunologic response may not be obtained). Products include:

Carac Cream, 0.5% 1048
Efudex 3348

Gemcitabine Hydrochloride (May reduce immune response to vaccines. When administered to patients who are receiving immunosuppressive therapy, who have an immunodeficiency disorder, or who have received a recent injection of immune globulin, an adequate immunologic response may not be obtained). Products include:

Gemzar for Injection 1743

IMPORTANT NOTE: Always consult each drug listing in the patient's regimen for possible interactions.

Hydrocortisone (May reduce immune response to vaccines. When administered to patients who are receiving immunosuppressive therapy, who have an immunodeficiency disorder, or who have received a recent injection of immune globulin, an adequate immunologic response may not be obtained). Products include:

Cortizone•5 Ointment .... ▣ 699
Cortizone•10 Creme .... ▣ 699
Cortizone•10 Ointment .... ▣ 699
Cortizone•10 Plus Creme .... ▣ 700
Cortizone•10 Maximum Strength Quick Shot Spray .... ▣ 700
Hydrocortone Tablets 1963
Preparation H Hydrocortisone Cream .... ▣ 748

Hydrocortisone Acetate (May reduce immune response to vaccines. When administered to patients who are receiving immunosuppressive therapy, who have an immunodeficiency disorder, or who have received a recent injection of immune globulin, an adequate immunologic response may not be obtained). Products include:

Analpram-HC 1136
Pramosone 1139
ProctoFoam-HC 3113
Tucks Anti-Itch Ointment .... ▣ 712
U-cort 1% Cream 3289

Hydrocortisone Sodium Phosphate (May reduce immune response to vaccines. When administered to patients who are receiving immunosuppressive therapy, who have an immunodeficiency disorder, or who have received a recent injection of immune globulin, an adequate immunologic response may not be obtained).

No products indexed under this heading.

Hydrocortisone Sodium Succinate (May reduce immune response to vaccines. When administered to patients who are receiving immunosuppressive therapy, who have an immunodeficiency disorder, or who have received a recent injection of immune globulin, an adequate immunologic response may not be obtained).

No products indexed under this heading.

Hydroxyurea (May reduce immune response to vaccines. When administered to patients who are receiving immunosuppressive therapy, who have an immunodeficiency disorder, or who have received a recent injection of immune globulin, an adequate immunologic response may not be obtained).

No products indexed under this heading.

Immune Globulin Intravenous (Human) (May reduce immune response to vaccines. When administered to patients who are receiving immunosuppressive therapy, who have an immunodeficiency disorder, or who have received a recent injection of immune globulin, an adequate immunologic response may not be obtained). Products include:

Carimune NF 3501
Gammagard Liquid 751
Gammagard S/D 754
Gamunex Immune Globulin I.V., 10% 3232
Iveegam EN 759

Lomustine (CCNU) (May reduce immune response to vaccines. When administered to patients who are receiving immunosuppressive therapy, who have an immunodeficiency disorder, or who have received a recent injection of immune globulin, an adequate immunologic response may not be obtained).

No products indexed under this heading.

Mechlorethamine Hydrochloride (May reduce immune response to vaccines. When administered to patients who are receiving immunosuppressive therapy, who have an immunodeficiency disorder, or who have received a recent injection of immune globulin, an adequate immunologic response may not be obtained). Products include:

Mustargen for Injection 2007

Melphalan (May reduce immune response to vaccines. When administered to patients who are receiving immunosuppressive therapy, who have an immunodeficiency disorder, or who have received a recent injection of immune globulin, an adequate immunologic response may not be obtained). Products include:

Alkeran Tablets 977

Mercaptopurine (May reduce immune response to vaccines. When administered to patients who are receiving immunosuppressive therapy, who have an immunodeficiency disorder, or who have received a recent injection of immune globulin, an adequate immunologic response may not be obtained). Products include:

Purinethol Tablets 1222

Methotrexate (May reduce immune response to vaccines. When administered to patients who are receiving immunosuppressive therapy, who have an immunodeficiency disorder, or who have received a recent injection of immune globulin, an adequate immunologic response may not be obtained).

No products indexed under this heading.

Methotrexate Sodium (May reduce immune response to vaccines. When administered to patients who are receiving immunosuppressive therapy, who have an immunodeficiency disorder, or who have received a recent injection of immune globulin, an adequate immunologic response may not be obtained).

No products indexed under this heading.

Methylprednisolone Acetate (May reduce immune response to vaccines. When administered to patients who are receiving immunosuppressive therapy, who have an immunodeficiency disorder, or who have received a recent injection of immune globulin, an adequate immunologic response may not be obtained). Products include:

Depo-Medrol Injectable Suspension 2615
Depo-Medrol Single-Dose Vial 2617

Methylprednisolone Sodium Succinate (May reduce immune response to vaccines. When administered to patients who are receiving immunosuppressive therapy, who have an immunodeficiency disorder, or who have received a recent injection of immune globulin, an adequate immunologic response may not be obtained).

No products indexed under this heading.

Mitotane (May reduce immune response to vaccines. When administered to patients who are receiving immunosuppressive therapy, who have an immunodeficiency disorder, or who have received a recent injection of immune globulin, an adequate immunologic response may not be obtained).

No products indexed under this heading.

Mitoxantrone Hydrochloride (May reduce immune response to vaccines. When administered to patients who are receiving immunosuppressive therapy, who have an immunodeficiency disorder, or who have received a recent injection of immune globulin, an adequate immunologic response may not be obtained). Products include:

Novantrone for Injection Concentrate 3158

Muromonab-CD3 (May reduce immune response to vaccines. When administered to patients who are receiving immunosuppressive therapy, who have an immunodeficiency disorder, or who have received a recent injection of immune globulin, an adequate immunologic response may not be obtained). Products include:

Orthoclone OKT3 Sterile Solution 2370

Mycophenolate Mofetil (May reduce immune response to vaccines. When administered to patients who are receiving immunosuppressive therapy, who have an immunodeficiency disorder, or who have received a recent injection of immune globulin, an adequate immunologic response may not be obtained). Products include:

CellCept Capsules 2751
CellCept Oral Suspension 2751
CellCept Tablets 2751

Pentostatin (May reduce immune response to vaccines. When administered to patients who are receiving immunosuppressive therapy, who have an immunodeficiency disorder, or who have received a recent injection of immune globulin, an adequate immunologic response may not be obtained). Products include:

Nipent for Injection 3216

Prednisolone Acetate (May reduce immune response to vaccines. When administered to patients who are receiving immunosuppressive therapy, who have an immunodeficiency disorder, or who have received a recent injection of immune globulin, an adequate immunologic response may not be obtained). Products include:

Blephamide Ophthalmic Ointment 563
Blephamide Ophthalmic Suspension 564
Poly-Pred Liquifilm Ophthalmic Suspension .... ⊙ 231
Pred Forte Ophthalmic Suspension .... ⊙ 233
Pred Mild Sterile Ophthalmic Suspension .... ⊙ 236
Pred-G Ophthalmic Suspension .... ⊙ 234
Pred-G Sterile Ophthalmic Ointment .... ⊙ 235

Prednisolone Sodium Phosphate (May reduce immune response to vaccines. When administered to patients who are receiving immunosuppressive therapy, who have an immunodeficiency disorder, or who have received a recent injection of immune globulin, an adequate immunologic response may not be obtained). Products include:

Pediapred Oral Solution 3319

Prednisolone Tebutate (May reduce immune response to vaccines. When administered to patients who are receiving immunosuppressive therapy, who have an immunodeficiency disorder, or who have received a recent injection of immune globulin, an adequate immunologic response may not be obtained).

No products indexed under this heading.

Prednisone (May reduce immune response to vaccines. When administered to patients who are receiving immunosuppressive therapy, who have an immunodeficiency disorder, or who have received a recent injection of immune globulin, an adequate immunologic response may not be obtained).

No products indexed under this heading.

Procarbazine Hydrochloride (May reduce immune response to vaccines. When administered to patients who are receiving immunosuppressive therapy, who have an immunodeficiency disorder, or who have received a recent injection of immune globulin, an adequate immunologic response may not be obtained). Products include:

Matulane Capsules 3188

Sirolimus (May reduce immune response to vaccines. When administered to patients who are receiving immunosuppressive therapy, who have an immunodeficiency disorder, or who have received a recent injection of immune globulin, an adequate immunologic response may not be obtained). Products include:

Rapamune Oral Solution and Tablets 3472

Tacrolimus (May reduce immune response to vaccines. When administered to patients who are receiving immunosuppressive therapy, who have an immunodeficiency disorder, or who have received a recent injection of immune globulin, an adequate immunologic response may not be obtained). Products include:

Prograf Capsules and Injection 624
Protopic Ointment 629

Tamoxifen Citrate (May reduce immune response to vaccines. When administered to patients who are receiving immunosuppressive therapy, who have an immunodeficiency disorder, or who have received a recent injection of immune globulin, an adequate immunologic response may not be obtained).

No products indexed under this heading.

Thioguanine (May reduce immune response to vaccines. When administered to patients who are receiving immunosuppressive therapy, who have an immunodeficiency disorder, or who have received a recent injec-

tion of immune globulin, an adequate immunologic response may not be obtained). Products include:

Tabloid Tablets 1545

Thiotepa (May reduce immune response to vaccines. When administered to patients who are receiving immunosuppressive therapy, who have an immunodeficiency disorder, or who have received a recent injection of immune globulin, an adequate immunologic response may not be obtained).

No products indexed under this heading.

Triamcinolone (May reduce immune response to vaccines. When administered to patients who are receiving immunosuppressive therapy, who have an immunodeficiency disorder, or who have received a recent injection of immune globulin, an adequate immunologic response may not be obtained).

No products indexed under this heading.

Triamcinolone Acetonide (May reduce immune response to vaccines. When administered to patients who are receiving immunosuppressive therapy, who have an immunodeficiency disorder, or who have received a recent injection of immune globulin, an adequate immunologic response may not be obtained). Products include:

Azmacort Inhalation Aerosol 1701
Nasacort HFA Inhalation Aerosol 2939
Nasacort AQ Nasal Spray 2937

Triamcinolone Diacetate (May reduce immune response to vaccines. When administered to patients who are receiving immunosuppressive therapy, who have an immunodeficiency disorder, or who have received a recent injection of immune globulin, an adequate immunologic response may not be obtained).

No products indexed under this heading.

Triamcinolone Hexacetonide (May reduce immune response to vaccines. When administered to patients who are receiving immunosuppressive therapy, who have an immunodeficiency disorder, or who have received a recent injection of immune globulin, an adequate immunologic response may not be obtained).

No products indexed under this heading.

Vincristine Sulfate (May reduce immune response to vaccines. When administered to patients who are receiving immunosuppressive therapy, who have an immunodeficiency disorder, or who have received a recent injection of immune globulin, an adequate immunologic response may not be obtained).

No products indexed under this heading.

PEDIASURE ENTERAL FORMULA

(Entereal Nutrition) 2843
None cited in PDR database.

PEDIASURE FORMULA

(Entereal Nutrition) 2843
None cited in PDR database.

LIQUID PEDVAXHIB

(Haemophilus B Conjugate Vaccine).. 2012
None cited in PDR database.

PEGANONE TABLETS, USP

(Ethotoin) 2487

May interact with oral anticoagulants, drugs that decrease hematopoietic system, and certain other agents. Compounds in these categories include:

Aldesleukin (Avoid, if possible, using ethotoin in combination with other drugs known to adversely affect the hematopoietic system). Products include:

Proleukin for Injection 1007

Alemtuzumab (Avoid, if possible, using ethotoin in combination with other drugs known to adversely affect the hematopoietic system). Products include:

Campath Ampules 826

Altretamine (Avoid, if possible, using ethotoin in combination with other drugs known to adversely affect the hematopoietic system). Products include:

Hexalen Capsules 2101

Amphotericin B (Avoid, if possible, using ethotoin in combination with other drugs known to adversely affect the hematopoietic system).

No products indexed under this heading.

Anisindione (Use caution when administering ethotoin to patients receiving coumarin anticoagulants. Ethotoin may stimulate coumarin metabolism and cause decreased levels of coumarin anticoagulants. Conversely, coumarin anticoagulants may inhibit metabolism of ethotoin causing increased serum levels and prolonged serum half-life). Products include:

Miradon Tablets 3056

Arsenic Trioxide (Avoid, if possible, using ethotoin in combination with other drugs known to adversely affect the hematopoietic system). Products include:

Trisenox Injection 983

Atovaquone (Avoid, if possible, using ethotoin in combination with other drugs known to adversely affect the hematopoietic system). Products include:

Malarone Tablets 1484
Malarone Pediatric Tablets 1484
Mepron Suspension 1487

Aztreonam (Avoid, if possible, using ethotoin in combination with other drugs known to adversely affect the hematopoietic system).

No products indexed under this heading.

Basiliximab (Avoid, if possible, using ethotoin in combination with other drugs known to adversely affect the hematopoietic system). Products include:

Simulect for Injection 2268

BCG, Live (Intravesical) (Avoid, if possible, using ethotoin in combination with other drugs known to adversely affect the hematopoietic system).

No products indexed under this heading.

Bexarotene (Avoid, if possible, using ethotoin in combination with other drugs known to adversely affect the hematopoietic system). Products include:

Targretin Capsules 1719

Bicalutamide (Avoid, if possible, using ethotoin in combination with other drugs known to adversely affect the hematopoietic system). Products include:

Casodex Tablets 670

Bosentan (Avoid, if possible, using ethotoin in combination with other drugs known to adversely affect the hematopoietic system). Products include:

Tracleer Tablets 539

Capecitabine (Avoid, if possible, using ethotoin in combination with other drugs known to adversely affect the hematopoietic system). Products include:

Xeloda Tablets 2825

Carboplatin (Avoid, if possible, using ethotoin in combination with other drugs known to adversely affect the hematopoietic system).

No products indexed under this heading.

Carmustine (BCNU) (Avoid, if possible, using ethotoin in combination with other drugs known to adversely affect the hematopoietic system).

No products indexed under this heading.

Cidofovir (Avoid, if possible, using ethotoin in combination with other drugs known to adversely affect the hematopoietic system).

No products indexed under this heading.

Citalopram Hydrobromide (Avoid, if possible, using ethotoin in combination with other drugs known to adversely affect the hematopoietic system). Products include:

Celexa 1177

Cladribine (Avoid, if possible, using ethotoin in combination with other drugs known to adversely affect the hematopoietic system). Products include:

Leustatin Injection 2368

Clozapine (Avoid, if possible, using ethotoin in combination with other drugs known to adversely affect the hematopoietic system). Products include:

Clozapine Tablets 2141
Clozaril Tablets 2174
FazaClo Orally Disintegrating Tablets 547

Cytarabine Liposome (Avoid, if possible, using ethotoin in combination with other drugs known to adversely affect the hematopoietic system). Products include:

DepoCyt Injection 1121

Daunorubicin Citrate (Avoid, if possible, using ethotoin in combination with other drugs known to adversely affect the hematopoietic system).

No products indexed under this heading.

Delavirdine Mesylate (Avoid, if possible, using ethotoin in combination with other drugs known to adversely affect the hematopoietic system). Products include:

Rescriptor Tablets 2535

Denileukin Diftitox (Avoid, if possible, using ethotoin in combination with other drugs known to adversely affect the hematopoietic system). Products include:

Ontak Vials 1717

Dicumarol (Use caution when administering ethotoin to patients receiving coumarin anticoagulants. Ethotoin may stimulate coumarin metabolism and cause decreased levels of coumarin anticoagulants. Conversely, coumarin anticoagulants may inhibit metabolism of ethotoin causing increased serum levels and prolonged serum half-life).

No products indexed under this heading.

Docetaxel (Avoid, if possible, using ethotoin in combination with other drugs known to adversely affect the hematopoietic system). Products include:

Taxotere Injection Concentrate 2947

Doxorubicin Hydrochloride (Avoid, if possible, using ethotoin in combination with other drugs known to adversely affect the hematopoietic system). Products include:

Adriamycin for Injection, USP 786
Adriamycin Injection, USP 786

Enoxaparin Sodium (Avoid, if possible, using ethotoin in combination with other drugs known to adversely affect the hematopoietic system). Products include:

Lovenox Injection 2931

Epirubicin Hydrochloride (Avoid, if possible, using ethotoin in combination with other drugs known to adversely affect the hematopoietic system). Products include:

Ellence Injection 2632

Filgrastim (Avoid, if possible, using ethotoin in combination with other drugs known to adversely affect the hematopoietic system). Products include:

Neupogen for Injection 598

Floxuridine (Avoid, if possible, using ethotoin in combination with other drugs known to adversely affect the hematopoietic system).

No products indexed under this heading.

Fludarabine Phosphate (Avoid, if possible, using ethotoin in combination with other drugs known to adversely affect the hematopoietic system).

No products indexed under this heading.

Flutamide (Avoid, if possible, using ethotoin in combination with other drugs known to adversely affect the hematopoietic system). Products include:

Eulexin Capsules 3023

Fondaparinux Sodium (Avoid, if possible, using ethotoin in combination with other drugs known to adversely affect the hematopoietic system). Products include:

Arixtra Injection 1325

Foscarnet Sodium (Avoid, if possible, using ethotoin in combination with other drugs known to adversely affect the hematopoietic system).

No products indexed under this heading.

Fulvestrant (Avoid, if possible, using ethotoin in combination with other drugs known to adversely affect the hematopoietic system). Products include:

Faslodex Injection 682

Galantamine Hydrobromide (Avoid, if possible, using ethotoin in combination with other drugs known to adversely affect the hematopoietic system). Products include:

Razadyne ER Extended-Release Capsules ... **2434**
Razadyne ... **2434**

Ganciclovir (Avoid, if possible, using ethotoin in combination with other drugs known to adversely affect the hematopoietic system). Products include:
Cytovene Capsules ... **2763**

Gemcitabine Hydrochloride (Avoid, if possible, using ethotoin in combination with other drugs known to adversely affect the hematopoietic system). Products include:
Gemzar for Injection ... **1743**

Gemtuzumab Ozogamicin (Avoid, if possible, using ethotoin in combination with other drugs known to adversely affect the hematopoietic system). Products include:
Mylotarg for Injection ... **3429**

Granisetron Hydrochloride (Avoid, if possible, using ethotoin in combination with other drugs known to adversely affect the hematopoietic system). Products include:
Kytril Injection ... **2785**
Kytril ... **2788**

Ibritumomab Tiuxetan (Avoid, if possible, using ethotoin in combination with other drugs known to adversely affect the hematopoietic system). Products include:
Zevalin Injection ... **848**

Imatinib Mesylate (Avoid, if possible, using ethotoin in combination with other drugs known to adversely affect the hematopoietic system). Products include:
Gleevec Tablets ... **2221**

Interferon alfa-2a, Recombinant (Avoid, if possible, using ethotoin in combination with other drugs known to adversely affect the hematopoietic system). Products include:
Roferon-A Injection ... **2805**

Interferon alfa-2b, Recombinant (Avoid, if possible, using ethotoin in combination with other drugs known to adversely affect the hematopoietic system). Products include:
Intron A for Injection ... **3038**
Rebetron Combination Therapy ... **3078**

Interferon Beta-1a (Avoid, if possible, using ethotoin in combination with other drugs known to adversely affect the hematopoietic system). Products include:
Avonex ... **839**
Rebif Prefilled Syringe for Injection ... **3163**

Interferon Beta-1b (Avoid, if possible, using ethotoin in combination with other drugs known to adversely affect the hematopoietic system). Products include:
Betaseron for SC Injection ... **791**

Irinotecan Hydrochloride (Avoid, if possible, using ethotoin in combination with other drugs known to adversely affect the hematopoietic system). Products include:
Camptosar Injection ... **2602**

Lamivudine (Avoid, if possible, using ethotoin in combination with other drugs known to adversely affect the hematopoietic system). Products include:
Combivir Tablets ... **1373**
Epivir ... **1394**
Epivir-HBV ... **1398**
Epzicom Tablets ... **1402**
Trizivir Tablets ... **1565**

Lepirudin (Avoid, if possible, using ethotoin in combination with other drugs known to adversely affect the hematopoietic system). Products include:
Refludan for Injection ... **815**

Leuprolide Acetate (Avoid, if possible, using ethotoin in combination with other drugs known to adversely affect the hematopoietic system). Products include:
Eligard 7.5 mg ... **2896**
Eligard 22.5 mg ... **2899**
Eligard 30 mg ... **2901**
Eligard 45 mg ... **2904**
Lupron Depot 3.75 mg ... **3257**
Lupron Depot 7.5 mg ... **3261**
Lupron Depot–3 Month 11.25 mg ... **3262**
Lupron Depot-PED 7.5 mg, 11.25 mg and 15 mg ... **3266**
Lupron Injection Pediatric ... **3256**
Viadur Implant ... **782**

Levamisole Hydrochloride (Avoid, if possible, using ethotoin in combination with other drugs known to adversely affect the hematopoietic system).
No products indexed under this heading.

Levobupivacaine Hydrochloride (Avoid, if possible, using ethotoin in combination with other drugs known to adversely affect the hematopoietic system).
No products indexed under this heading.

Levocarnitine (Avoid, if possible, using ethotoin in combination with other drugs known to adversely affect the hematopoietic system). Products include:
Carnitor Injection ... **3185**
Carnitor Tablets and Oral Solution ... **3187**

Mefenamic Acid (Avoid, if possible, using ethotoin in combination with other drugs known to adversely affect the hematopoietic system).
No products indexed under this heading.

Mitoxantrone Hydrochloride (Avoid, if possible, using ethotoin in combination with other drugs known to adversely affect the hematopoietic system). Products include:
Novantrone for Injection Concentrate ... **3158**

Mycophenolate Mofetil (Avoid, if possible, using ethotoin in combination with other drugs known to adversely affect the hematopoietic system). Products include:
CellCept Capsules ... **2751**
CellCept Oral Suspension ... **2751**
CellCept Tablets ... **2751**

Mycophenolate Mofetil Hydrochloride (Avoid, if possible, using ethotoin in combination with other drugs known to adversely affect the hematopoietic system). Products include:
CellCept Intravenous ... **2751**

Nevirapine (Avoid, if possible, using ethotoin in combination with other drugs known to adversely affect the hematopoietic system). Products include:
Viramune Oral Suspension ... **903**
Viramune Tablets ... **903**

Nilutamide (Avoid, if possible, using ethotoin in combination with other drugs known to adversely affect the hematopoietic system).
No products indexed under this heading.

Nizatidine (Avoid, if possible, using ethotoin in combination with other drugs known to adversely affect the hematopoietic system). Products include:
Axid Oral Solution ... **913**

Octreotide Acetate (Avoid, if possible, using ethotoin in combination with other drugs known to adversely affect the hematopoietic system). Products include:
Sandostatin Injection ... **2263**
Sandostatin LAR Depot ... **2264**

Oprelvekin (Avoid, if possible, using ethotoin in combination with other drugs known to adversely affect the hematopoietic system). Products include:
Neumega for Injection ... **3433**

Oxaliplatin (Avoid, if possible, using ethotoin in combination with other drugs known to adversely affect the hematopoietic system). Products include:
Eloxatin for Injection ... **2908**

Pamidronate Disodium (Avoid, if possible, using ethotoin in combination with other drugs known to adversely affect the hematopoietic system). Products include:
Aredia for Injection ... **2168**

Pegfilgrastim (Avoid, if possible, using ethotoin in combination with other drugs known to adversely affect the hematopoietic system). Products include:
Neulasta Injection ... **596**

Peginterferon alfa-2a (Avoid, if possible, using ethotoin in combination with other drugs known to adversely affect the hematopoietic system). Products include:
Pegasys ... **2793**

Peginterferon Alfa-2b (Avoid, if possible, using ethotoin in combination with other drugs known to adversely affect the hematopoietic system). Products include:
PEG-Intron Powder for Injection ... **3062**

Pentostatin (Avoid, if possible, using ethotoin in combination with other drugs known to adversely affect the hematopoietic system). Products include:
Nipent for Injection ... **3216**

Phenacemide (Use considerable caution when co-administering with phenacemide as paranoid symptoms have been reported).
No products indexed under this heading.

Piroxicam (Avoid, if possible, using ethotoin in combination with other drugs known to adversely affect the hematopoietic system).
No products indexed under this heading.

Porfimer Sodium (Avoid, if possible, using ethotoin in combination with other drugs known to adversely affect the hematopoietic system). Products include:
Photofrin for Injection ... **729**

Prednisolone Acetate (Avoid, if possible, using ethotoin in combination with other drugs known to adversely affect the hematopoietic system). Products include:
Blephamide Ophthalmic Ointment ... **563**
Blephamide Ophthalmic Suspension ... **564**
Poly-Pred Liquifilm Ophthalmic Suspension ... ⊙ **231**
Pred Forte Ophthalmic Suspension ... ⊙ **233**
Pred Mild Sterile Ophthalmic Suspension ... ⊙ **236**
Pred-G Ophthalmic Suspension ... ⊙ **234**
Pred-G Sterile Ophthalmic Ointment ... ⊙ **235**

Progesterone (Avoid, if possible, using ethotoin in combination with other drugs known to adversely affect the hematopoietic system). Products include:
Prochieve 4% Gel ... **1018**
Prochieve 8% Gel ... **1018**
Prometrium Capsules (100 mg, 200 mg) ... **3205**

Ribavirin (Avoid, if possible, using ethotoin in combination with other drugs known to adversely affect the hematopoietic system). Products include:
Copegus Tablets ... **2759**
Rebetol ... **3073**
Rebetron Combination Therapy ... **3078**
Ribavirin, USP Capsules ... **3083**
Virazole for Inhalation Solution ... **3365**

Rifabutin (Avoid, if possible, using ethotoin in combination with other drugs known to adversely affect the hematopoietic system).
No products indexed under this heading.

Rifapentine (Avoid, if possible, using ethotoin in combination with other drugs known to adversely affect the hematopoietic system).
No products indexed under this heading.

Rituximab (Avoid, if possible, using ethotoin in combination with other drugs known to adversely affect the hematopoietic system). Products include:
Rituxan for Infusion ... **845**
Rituxan I.V. ... **1251**

Ropivacaine Hydrochloride (Avoid, if possible, using ethotoin in combination with other drugs known to adversely affect the hematopoietic system). Products include:
Naropin Injection ... **640**

Rosiglitazone Maleate (Avoid, if possible, using ethotoin in combination with other drugs known to adversely affect the hematopoietic system). Products include:
Avandamet Tablets ... **1343**
Avandia Tablets ... **1348**

Sirolimus (Avoid, if possible, using ethotoin in combination with other drugs known to adversely affect the hematopoietic system). Products include:
Rapamune Oral Solution and Tablets ... **3472**

Somatropin (Avoid, if possible, using ethotoin in combination with other drugs known to adversely affect the hematopoietic system). Products include:
Genotropin Lyophilized Powder ... **2642**
Humatrope Vials and Cartridges ... **1756**
Norditropin Cartridges ... **2318**
Nutropin for Injection ... **1238**
Nutropin AQ Injection ... **1241**
Nutropin AQ Pen ... **1241**
Nutropin AQ Pen Cartridge ... **1241**

Stavudine (Avoid, if possible, using ethotoin in combination with other drugs known to adversely affect the hematopoietic system). Products include:
Zerit ... **971**

Tacrolimus (Avoid, if possible, using ethotoin in combination with other drugs known to adversely affect the hematopoietic system). Products include:
Prograf Capsules and Injection ... **624**
Protopic Ointment ... **629**

Thalidomide (Avoid, if possible, using ethotoin in combination with other drugs known to adversely affect the hematopoietic system). Products include:
Thalomid Capsules ... **979**

Topotecan Hydrochloride (Avoid, if possible, using ethotoin in combination with other drugs known to adversely affect the hematopoietic system). Products include:
Hycamtin for Injection 1427

Trastuzumab (Avoid, if possible, using ethotoin in combination with other drugs known to adversely affect the hematopoietic system). Products include:
Herceptin I.V. 1234

Valganciclovir Hydrochloride (Avoid, if possible, using ethotoin in combination with other drugs known to adversely affect the hematopoietic system). Products include:
Valcyte Tablets 2816

Vinorelbine Tartrate (Avoid, if possible, using ethotoin in combination with other drugs known to adversely affect the hematopoietic system). Products include:
Navelbine Injection 1494

Warfarin Sodium (Use caution when administering ethotoin to patients receiving coumarin anticoagulants. Ethotoin may stimulate coumarin metabolism and cause decreased levels of coumarin anticoagulants. Conversely, coumarin anticoagulants may inhibit metabolism of ethotoin causing increased serum levels and prolonged serum half-life). Products include:
Coumadin for Injection 932
Coumadin Tablets 932

Zalacitabine (Avoid, if possible, using ethotoin in combination with other drugs known to adversely affect the hematopoietic system).
No products indexed under this heading.

Zidovudine (Avoid, if possible, using ethotoin in combination with other drugs known to adversely affect the hematopoietic system). Products include:
Combivir Tablets 1373
Retrovir 1533
Retrovir IV Infusion 1537
Trizivir Tablets 1565

Zoledronic acid (Avoid, if possible, using ethotoin in combination with other drugs known to adversely affect the hematopoietic system). Products include:
Zometa for Intravenous Infusion 2306

PEGASYS

(Peginterferon alfa-2a) 2793
May interact with theophyllines and certain other agents. Compounds in these categories include:

Methadone Hydrochloride (In a study of HCV patients concomitantly receiving methadone, treatment with peginterferon alfa-2a once weekly for four weeks was associated with methadone levels that were 10%-15% higher than at baseline. Therefore, patients should be monitored for signs and symptoms of methadone toxicity during co-administration).
No products indexed under this heading.

Theophylline (Inhibition of CYP450 1A2 and a 25% increase in theophylline AUC; monitor theophylline levels and consider appropriate dose adjustments).
No products indexed under this heading.

Theophylline Anhydrous (Inhibition of CYP450 1A2 and a 25% increase in theophylline AUC; monitor theophylline levels and consider appropriate dose adjustments). Products include:
Uniphyl Tablets 2708

Theophylline Calcium Salicylate (Inhibition of CYP450 1A2 and a 25% increase in theophylline AUC; monitor theophylline levels and consider appropriate dose adjustments).
No products indexed under this heading.

Theophylline Dihydroxypropyl (Glyceryl) (Inhibition of CYP450 1A2 and a 25% increase in theophylline AUC; monitor theophylline levels and consider appropriate dose adjustments).
No products indexed under this heading.

Theophylline Ethylenediamine (Inhibition of CYP450 1A2 and a 25% increase in theophylline AUC; monitor theophylline levels and consider appropriate dose adjustments).
No products indexed under this heading.

Theophylline Sodium Glycinate (Inhibition of CYP450 1A2 and a 25% increase in theophylline AUC; monitor theophylline levels and consider appropriate dose adjustments).
No products indexed under this heading.

Zidovudine (Co-administration of zidovudine and Pegasys/Copegus develops sever neutropenia and severe anemia more frequently than similar patients not receiving zidovudine (neutropenia 15% vs. 9%) (anemia 5% vs. 1%)). Products include:
Combivir Tablets 1373
Retrovir 1533
Retrovir IV Infusion 1537
Trizivir Tablets 1565

PEG-INTRON POWDER FOR INJECTION

(Peginterferon Alfa-2b) 3062
May interact with:

Methadone Hydrochloride (In a pharmacokinetic study of 18 chronic hepatitis C patients concomitantly receiving methadone, treatment with PEG-Intron once weekly for four weeks was associated with a mean increase of 16% in methadone AUC. In two out of 18 patients, methadone AUC doubled. The clinical significance of this finding is unknown, however, patients should be monitored for the signs and symptoms of increased narcotic effect).
No products indexed under this heading.

PENLAC NAIL LACQUER, TOPICAL SOLUTION, 8%

(Ciclopirox) 1051
None cited in PDR database.

PENTASA CAPSULES

(Mesalamine) 3182
None cited in PDR database.

PEPCID AC TABLETS, CHEWABLE TABLETS, AND GELCAPS

(Famotidine) 640
None cited in PDR database.

PEPCID AC CHEWABLE TABLETS

(Famotidine) 1672
None cited in PDR database.

PEPCID AC GELCAPS

(Famotidine) 1672
None cited in PDR database.

MAXIMUM STRENGTH PEPCID AC TABLETS

(Famotidine) 640
None cited in PDR database.

PEPCID AC TABLETS

(Famotidine) 1672
None cited in PDR database.

MAXIMUM STRENGTH PEPCID AC TABLETS

(Famotidine) 1672
None cited in PDR database.

PEPCID COMPLETE CHEWABLE TABLETS

(Calcium Carbonate, Famotidine, Magnesium Hydroxide)...................... 641
May interact with:

Prescription Drugs, unspecified (Antacids contained in Pepcid Complete may interact with certain prescription drugs).
No products indexed under this heading.

PEPCID INJECTION

(Famotidine) 2017
None cited in PDR database.

PEPCID INJECTION PREMIXED

(Famotidine) 2017
None cited in PDR database.

PEPCID FOR ORAL SUSPENSION

(Famotidine) 2014
May interact with antacids and certain other agents. Compounds in these categories include:

Aluminum Carbonate (Bioavailability may be slightly decreased by antacids).
No products indexed under this heading.

Aluminum Hydroxide (Bioavailability may be slightly decreased by antacids). Products include:
Gaviscon Regular Strength Liquid .. 620
Gaviscon Regular Strength Tablets... 619
Gaviscon Extra Strength Liquid 620
Gaviscon Extra Strength Tablets 619
Maalox Max Maximum Strength Antacid/Anti-Gas Liquid................. 2165
Maalox Regular Strength Antacid/Antigas Liquid.................. 2164

Magaldrate (Bioavailability may be slightly decreased by antacids).
No products indexed under this heading.

Magnesium Hydroxide (Bioavailability may be slightly decreased by antacids). Products include:
Maalox Max Maximum Strength Antacid/Anti-Gas Liquid................. 2165
Maalox Regular Strength Antacid/Antigas Liquid.................. 2164
Pepcid Complete Chewable Tablets 1672
Rolaids Tablets 707
Extra Strength Rolaids Tablets 707
Rolaids Multi-Symptom Antacid & Antigas Tablets 708

Magnesium Oxide (Bioavailability may be slightly decreased by antacids). Products include:
Beelith Tablets 78
PremCal Light, Regular, and Extra Strength Tablets................ 76
Sodium Bicarbonate (Bioavailability may be slightly decreased by antacids). Products include:
Ceo-Two Evacuant Suppository 607
Colyte with Flavor Packs for Oral Solution....................................... 3102
HalfLytely and Bisacodyl Tablets Bowel Prep Kit with Flavors Packs.. 915
TriLyte with Flavor Packs for Oral Solution....................................... 3114

Food Interactions

Food, unspecified (Bioavailability may be slightly increased by antacids).

PEPCID TABLETS

(Famotidine) 2014
See Pepcid for Oral Suspension

PEPTO-BISMOL MAXIMUM STRENGTH LIQUID

(Bismuth Subsalicylate) 718
May interact with oral anticoagulants, antigout agents, and oral hypoglycemic agents. Compounds in these categories include:

Acarbose (Use cautiously). Products include:
Precose Tablets 776

Allopurinol (Use cautiously).
No products indexed under this heading.

Anisindione (Use cautiously). Products include:
Miradon Tablets 3056

Chlorpropamide (Use cautiously).
No products indexed under this heading.

Dicumarol (Use cautiously).
No products indexed under this heading.

Glimepiride (Use cautiously). Products include:
Amaryl Tablets 2864

Glipizide (Use cautiously).
No products indexed under this heading.

Glyburide (Use cautiously).
No products indexed under this heading.

Metformin Hydrochloride (Use cautiously). Products include:
ActoPlus Met Tablets 3219
Avandamet Tablets 1343
Fortamet Extended-Release Tablets 1156

Miglitol (Use cautiously).
No products indexed under this heading.

Pioglitazone Hydrochloride (Use cautiously). Products include:
ActoPlus Met Tablets 3219
Actos Tablets 3224

Probenecid (Use cautiously).
No products indexed under this heading.

Repaglinide (Use cautiously). Products include:
Prandin Tablets (0.5, 1, and 2 mg).. 2337

Rosiglitazone Maleate (Use cautiously). Products include:
Avandamet Tablets 1343
Avandia Tablets 1348

Sulfinpyrazone (Use cautiously).
No products indexed under this heading.

Tolazamide (Use cautiously).
No products indexed under this heading.

IMPORTANT NOTE: Always consult each drug listing in the patient's regimen for possible interactions.

Tolbutamide (Use cautiously).
No products indexed under this heading.

Troglitazone (Use cautiously).
No products indexed under this heading.

Warfarin Sodium (Use cautiously).
Products include:
Coumadin for Injection 932
Coumadin Tablets 932

PEPTO-BISMOL ORIGINAL LIQUID, MAXIMUM STRENGTH LIQUID, ORIGINAL AND CHERRY TABLETS AND EASY-TO-SWALLOW CAPLETS

(Bismuth Subsalicylate) 2673
May interact with oral anticoagulants, antigout agents, and oral hypoglycemic agents. Compounds in these categories include:

Acarbose (Concurrent use should be undertaken with physician's supervision). Products include:
Precose Tablets 776

Allopurinol (Concurrent use should be undertaken with physician's supervision).
No products indexed under this heading.

Anisindione (Concurrent use should be undertaken with physician's supervision). Products include:
Miradon Tablets 3056

Chlorpropamide (Concurrent use should be undertaken with physician's supervision).
No products indexed under this heading.

Dicumarol (Concurrent use should be undertaken with physician's supervision).
No products indexed under this heading.

Glimepiride (Concurrent use should be undertaken with physician's supervision). Products include:
Amaryl Tablets 2864

Glipizide (Concurrent use should be undertaken with physician's supervision).
No products indexed under this heading.

Glyburide (Concurrent use should be undertaken with physician's supervision).
No products indexed under this heading.

Metformin Hydrochloride (Concurrent use should be undertaken with physician's supervision).
Products include:
ActoPlus Met Tablets 3219
Avandamet Tablets 1343
Fortamet Extended-Release Tablets 1156

Miglitol (Concurrent use should be undertaken with physician's supervision).
No products indexed under this heading.

Pioglitazone Hydrochloride (Concurrent use should be undertaken with physician's supervision).
Products include:
ActoPlus Met Tablets 3219
Actos Tablets 3224

Probenecid (Concurrent use should be undertaken with physician's supervision).
No products indexed under this heading.

Repaglinide (Concurrent use should be undertaken with physician's supervision). Products include:
Prandin Tablets (0.5, 1, and 2 mg) 2337

Rosiglitazone Maleate (Concurrent use should be undertaken with physician's supervision). Products include:
Avandamet Tablets 1343
Avandia Tablets 1348

Sulfinpyrazone (Concurrent use should be undertaken with physician's supervision).
No products indexed under this heading.

Tolazamide (Concurrent use should be undertaken with physician's supervision).
No products indexed under this heading.

Tolbutamide (Concurrent use should be undertaken with physician's supervision).
No products indexed under this heading.

Troglitazone (Concurrent use should be undertaken with physician's supervision).
No products indexed under this heading.

Warfarin Sodium (Concurrent use should be undertaken with physician's supervision). Products include:
Coumadin for Injection 932
Coumadin Tablets 932

PERCOCET TABLETS

(Acetaminophen, Oxycodone Hydrochloride) 1114
May interact with anticholinergics, central nervous system depressants, general anesthetics, hypnotics and sedatives, monoamine oxidase inhibitors, narcotic analgesics, phenothiazines, tranquilizers, tricyclic antidepressants, and certain other agents. Compounds in these categories include:

Alfentanil Hydrochloride (Additive CNS depression; dose of one or both agents should be reduced).
No products indexed under this heading.

Alprazolam (Additive CNS depression; dose of one or both agents should be reduced). Products include:
Niravam Orally Disintegrating Tablets 3106
Xanax XR Tablets 2655

Amitriptyline Hydrochloride (Increased effect of antidepressant or oxycodone).
No products indexed under this heading.

Amoxapine (Increased effect of antidepressant or oxycodone).
No products indexed under this heading.

Aprobarbital (Additive CNS depression; dose of one or both agents should be reduced).
No products indexed under this heading.

Atropine Sulfate (May produce paralytic ileus).
No products indexed under this heading.

Belladonna Alkaloids (May produce paralytic ileus). Products include:
Hyland's Teething Tablets .... ▣736

Benztropine Mesylate (May produce paralytic ileus). Products include:
Cogentin Injection 1903

Biperiden Hydrochloride (May produce paralytic ileus).
No products indexed under this heading.

Buprenorphine Hydrochloride (Additive CNS depression; dose of one or both agents should be reduced). Products include:
Buprenex Injectable 2718
Suboxone Tablets 2719
Subutex Tablets 2719

Buspirone Hydrochloride (Additive CNS depression; dose of one or both agents should be reduced).
No products indexed under this heading.

Butabarbital (Additive CNS depression; dose of one or both agents should be reduced).
No products indexed under this heading.

Butalbital (Additive CNS depression; dose of one or both agents should be reduced). Products include:
Sedapap Tablets 50 mg/650 mg 2098

Chlordiazepoxide (Additive CNS depression; dose of one or both agents should be reduced).
No products indexed under this heading.

Chlordiazepoxide Hydrochloride (Additive CNS depression; dose of one or both agents should be reduced). Products include:
Librium Capsules 3349

Chlorpromazine (Additive CNS depression; dose of one or both agents should be reduced).
No products indexed under this heading.

Chlorpromazine Hydrochloride (Additive CNS depression; dose of one or both agents should be reduced).
No products indexed under this heading.

Chlorprothixene (Additive CNS depression; dose of one or both agents should be reduced).
No products indexed under this heading.

Chlorprothixene Hydrochloride (Additive CNS depression; dose of one or both agents should be reduced).
No products indexed under this heading.

Chlorprothixene Lactate (Additive CNS depression; dose of one or both agents should be reduced).
No products indexed under this heading.

Clidinium Bromide (May produce paralytic ileus).
No products indexed under this heading.

Clomipramine Hydrochloride (Increased effect of antidepressant or oxycodone).
No products indexed under this heading.

Clorazepate Dipotassium (Additive CNS depression; dose of one or both agents should be reduced).
Products include:
Tranxene 2488

Clozapine (Additive CNS depression; dose of one or both agents should be reduced). Products include:
Clozapine Tablets 2141
Clozaril Tablets 2174
FazaClo Orally Disintegrating Tablets 547

Codeine Phosphate (Additive CNS depression; dose of one or both agents should be reduced). Products include:
Tylenol with Codeine 2461

Desflurane (Additive CNS depression; dose of one or both agents should be reduced). Products include:
Suprane Liquid for Inhalation 770

Desipramine Hydrochloride (Increased effect of antidepressant or oxycodone).
No products indexed under this heading.

Dezocine (Additive CNS depression; dose of one or both agents should be reduced).
No products indexed under this heading.

Diazepam (Additive CNS depression; dose of one or both agents should be reduced). Products include:
Diastat Rectal Delivery System 3344
Valium Tablets 2822

Dicyclomine Hydrochloride (May produce paralytic ileus). Products include:
Bentyl Capsules 724
Bentyl Injection 724
Bentyl Syrup 724
Bentyl Tablets 724

Doxepin Hydrochloride (Increased effect of antidepressant or oxycodone).
No products indexed under this heading.

Droperidol (Additive CNS depression; dose of one or both agents should be reduced).
No products indexed under this heading.

Enflurane (Additive CNS depression; dose of one or both agents should be reduced).
No products indexed under this heading.

Estazolam (Additive CNS depression; dose of one or both agents should be reduced). Products include:
ProSom Tablets 512

Ethanol (Additive CNS depression; dose of one or both agents should be reduced).
No products indexed under this heading.

Ethchlorvynol (Additive CNS depression; dose of one or both agents should be reduced).
No products indexed under this heading.

Ethinamate (Additive CNS depression; dose of one or both agents should be reduced).
No products indexed under this heading.

Ethopropazine Hydrochloride (May produce paralytic ileus).
No products indexed under this heading.

Ethyl Alcohol (Additive CNS depression; dose of one or both agents should be reduced).
No products indexed under this heading.

Fentanyl (Additive CNS depression; dose of one or both agents should be reduced). Products include:
Duragesic Transdermal System 2448

Fentanyl Citrate (Additive CNS depression; dose of one or both agents should be reduced). Products include:
Actiq ... 993

Fluphenazine Decanoate (Additive CNS depression; dose of one or both agents should be reduced).
No products indexed under this heading.

Fluphenazine Enanthate (Additive CNS depression; dose of one or both agents should be reduced).
No products indexed under this heading.

Fluphenazine Hydrochloride (Additive CNS depression; dose of one or both agents should be reduced).
No products indexed under this heading.

Flurazepam Hydrochloride (Additive CNS depression; dose of one or both agents should be reduced). Products include:
Dalmane Capsules ... 3343

Glutethimide (Additive CNS depression; dose of one or both agents should be reduced).
No products indexed under this heading.

Glycopyrrolate (May produce paralytic ileus).
No products indexed under this heading.

Haloperidol (Additive CNS depression; dose of one or both agents should be reduced).
No products indexed under this heading.

Haloperidol Decanoate (Additive CNS depression; dose of one or both agents should be reduced).
No products indexed under this heading.

Hydrocodone Bitartrate (Additive CNS depression; dose of one or both agents should be reduced). Products include:
Hycodan ... 1104
Hycomine Compound Tablets ... 1105
Hycotuss Expectorant Syrup ... 1106
Lortab ... 3315
Lortab Elixir ... 3312
Vicodin Tablets ... 530
Vicodin ES Tablets ... 531
Vicodin HP Tablets ... 532
Vicoprofen Tablets ... 533
Zydone Tablets ... 1118

Hydrocodone Polistirex (Additive CNS depression; dose of one or both agents should be reduced). Products include:
Tussionex Pennkinetic Extended-Release Suspension ... 3322

Hydromorphone Hydrochloride (Additive CNS depression; dose of one or both agents should be reduced). Products include:
Dilaudid ... 439
Dilaudid Oral Liquid ... 443
Dilaudid Non-Sterile Powder ... 439
Dilaudid Rectal Suppositories ... 439
Dilaudid Tablets ... 439
Dilaudid Tablets - 8 mg ... 443
Dilaudid-HP ... 441

Hydroxyzine Hydrochloride (Additive CNS depression; dose of one or both agents should be reduced).
No products indexed under this heading.

Hyoscyamine (May produce paralytic ileus).
No products indexed under this heading.

Hyoscyamine Sulfate (May produce paralytic ileus).
No products indexed under this heading.

Imipramine Hydrochloride (Increased effect of antidepressant or oxycodone).
No products indexed under this heading.

Imipramine Pamoate (Increased effect of antidepressant or oxycodone).
No products indexed under this heading.

Ipratropium Bromide (May produce paralytic ileus). Products include:
Atrovent HFA Inhalation Aerosol ... 872
Atrovent Inhalation Solution ... 868
Atrovent Nasal Spray 0.03% ... 869
Atrovent Nasal Spray 0.06% ... 870
Combivent Inhalation Aerosol ... 878
DuoNeb Inhalation Solution ... 1058

Isocarboxazid (Increased effect of either oxycodone or MAO inhibitor).
No products indexed under this heading.

Isoflurane (Additive CNS depression; dose of one or both agents should be reduced).
No products indexed under this heading.

Ketamine Hydrochloride (Additive CNS depression; dose of one or both agents should be reduced).
No products indexed under this heading.

Levomethadyl Acetate Hydrochloride (Additive CNS depression; dose of one or both agents should be reduced).
No products indexed under this heading.

Levorphanol Tartrate (Additive CNS depression; dose of one or both agents should be reduced).
No products indexed under this heading.

Lorazepam (Additive CNS depression; dose of one or both agents should be reduced).
No products indexed under this heading.

Loxapine Hydrochloride (Additive CNS depression; dose of one or both agents should be reduced).
No products indexed under this heading.

Loxapine Succinate (Additive CNS depression; dose of one or both agents should be reduced).
No products indexed under this heading.

Maprotiline Hydrochloride (Increased effect of antidepressant or oxycodone).
No products indexed under this heading.

Mepenzolate Bromide (May produce paralytic ileus).
No products indexed under this heading.

Meperidine Hydrochloride (Additive CNS depression; dose of one or both agents should be reduced).
No products indexed under this heading.

Mephobarbital (Additive CNS depression; dose of one or both agents should be reduced). Products include:
Mebaral Tablets, USP ... 2483

Meprobamate (Additive CNS depression; dose of one or both agents should be reduced).
No products indexed under this heading.

Mesoridazine Besylate (Additive CNS depression; dose of one or both agents should be reduced).
No products indexed under this heading.

Methadone Hydrochloride (Additive CNS depression; dose of one or both agents should be reduced).
No products indexed under this heading.

Methohexital Sodium (Additive CNS depression; dose of one or both agents should be reduced).
No products indexed under this heading.

Methotrimeprazine (Additive CNS depression; dose of one or both agents should be reduced).
No products indexed under this heading.

Methoxyflurane (Additive CNS depression; dose of one or both agents should be reduced).
No products indexed under this heading.

Midazolam Hydrochloride (Additive CNS depression; dose of one or both agents should be reduced).
No products indexed under this heading.

Moclobemide (Increased effect of either oxycodone or MAO inhibitor).
No products indexed under this heading.

Molindone Hydrochloride (Additive CNS depression; dose of one or both agents should be reduced). Products include:
Moban Tablets ... 1108

Morphine Sulfate (Additive CNS depression; dose of one or both agents should be reduced). Products include:
Avinza Capsules ... 1714
Kadian Capsules ... 572
MS Contin Tablets ... 2703

Nortriptyline Hydrochloride (Increased effect of antidepressant or oxycodone).
No products indexed under this heading.

Olanzapine (Additive CNS depression; dose of one or both agents should be reduced). Products include:
Symbyax Capsules ... 1788
Zyprexa Tablets ... 1798
Zyprexa IntraMuscular ... 1798
Zyprexa ZYDIS Orally Disintegrating Tablets ... 1798

Oxazepam (Additive CNS depression; dose of one or both agents should be reduced; increased effect of antidepressant).
No products indexed under this heading.

Oxybutynin Chloride (May produce paralytic ileus). Products include:
Ditropan XL Extended Release Tablets ... 2391

Oxyphenonium Bromide (May produce paralytic ileus).
No products indexed under this heading.

Pargyline Hydrochloride (Increased effect of either oxycodone or MAO inhibitor).
No products indexed under this heading.

Pentobarbital Sodium (Additive CNS depression; dose of one or both agents should be reduced). Products include:
Nembutal Sodium Solution, USP ... 2484

Perphenazine (Additive CNS depression; dose of one or both agents should be reduced).
No products indexed under this heading.

Phenelzine Sulfate (Increased effect of either oxycodone or MAO inhibitor).
No products indexed under this heading.

Phenobarbital (Additive CNS depression; dose of one or both agents should be reduced).
No products indexed under this heading.

Prazepam (Additive CNS depression; dose of one or both agents should be reduced).
No products indexed under this heading.

Procarbazine Hydrochloride (Increased effect of either oxycodone or MAO inhibitor). Products include:
Matulane Capsules ... 3188

Prochlorperazine (Additive CNS depression; dose of one or both agents should be reduced).
No products indexed under this heading.

Procyclidine Hydrochloride (May produce paralytic ileus).
No products indexed under this heading.

Promethazine Hydrochloride (Additive CNS depression; dose of one or both agents should be reduced). Products include:
Phenergan ... 3438

Propantheline Bromide (May produce paralytic ileus).
No products indexed under this heading.

Propofol (Additive CNS depression; dose of one or both agents should be reduced). Products include:
Diprivan Injectable Emulsion ... 676

Propoxyphene Hydrochloride (Additive CNS depression; dose of one or both agents should be reduced).
No products indexed under this heading.

Propoxyphene Napsylate (Additive CNS depression; dose of one or both agents should be reduced). Products include:
Darvocet A 500 Tablets ... 3497

Protriptyline Hydrochloride (Increased effect of antidepressant or oxycodone). Products include:
Vivactil Tablets ... 2350

Quazepam (Additive CNS depression; dose of one or both agents should be reduced).
No products indexed under this heading.

Quetiapine Fumarate (Additive CNS depression; dose of one or both agents should be reduced). Products include:
Seroquel Tablets ... 691

Remifentanil Hydrochloride (Additive CNS depression; dose of one or both agents should be reduced).
No products indexed under this heading.

Risperidone (Additive CNS depression; dose of one or both agents should be reduced). Products include:
Risperdal Consta Long-Acting Injection 1664
Risperdal M-Tab Orally Disintegrating Tablets 1658
Risperdal 1658

Scopolamine (May produce paralytic ileus). Products include:
Transderm Scōp Transdermal Therapeutic System 2166

Scopolamine Hydrobromide (May produce paralytic ileus).
No products indexed under this heading.

Secobarbital Sodium (Additive CNS depression; dose of one or both agents should be reduced).
No products indexed under this heading.

Selegiline Hydrochloride (Increased effect of either oxycodone or MAO inhibitor). Products include:
Eldepryl Capsules 3209

Sevoflurane (Additive CNS depression; dose of one or both agents should be reduced). Products include:
Ultane Liquid for Inhalation 526

Sodium Oxybate (Additive CNS depression; dose of one or both agents should be reduced).
No products indexed under this heading.

Sufentanil Citrate (Additive CNS depression; dose of one or both agents should be reduced).
No products indexed under this heading.

Temazepam (Additive CNS depression; dose of one or both agents should be reduced).
No products indexed under this heading.

Thiamylal Sodium (Additive CNS depression; dose of one or both agents should be reduced).
No products indexed under this heading.

Thioridazine Hydrochloride (Additive CNS depression; dose of one or both agents should be reduced). Products include:
Thioridazine Hydrochloride Tablets 2122

Thiothixene (Additive CNS depression; dose of one or both agents should be reduced). Products include:
Thiothixene Capsules 2124

Tolterodine Tartrate (May produce paralytic ileus). Products include:
Detrol Tablets 2626
Detrol LA Capsules 2629

Tranylcypromine Sulfate (Increased effect of either oxycodone or MAO inhibitor). Products include:
Parnate Tablets 1499

Triazolam (Additive CNS depression; dose of one or both agents should be reduced).
No products indexed under this heading.

Tridihexethyl Chloride (May produce paralytic ileus).
No products indexed under this heading.

Trifluoperazine Hydrochloride (Additive CNS depression; dose of one or both agents should be reduced).
No products indexed under this heading.

Trihexyphenidyl Hydrochloride (May produce paralytic ileus).
No products indexed under this heading.

Trimipramine Maleate (Increased effect of antidepressant or oxycodone). Products include:
Surmontil Capsules 2347

Zaleplon (Additive CNS depression; dose of one or both agents should be reduced). Products include:
Sonata Capsules 1686

Ziprasidone Hydrochloride (Additive CNS depression; dose of one or both agents should be reduced). Products include:
Geodon Capsules 2514

Zolpidem Tartrate (Additive CNS depression; dose of one or both agents should be reduced). Products include:
Ambien Tablets 2867

Food Interactions

Alcohol (Additive CNS depression).

PERCODAN TABLETS

(Aspirin, Oxycodone Hydrochloride, Oxycodone Terephthalate) 1115

May interact with central nervous system depressants, anticoagulants, general anesthetics, hypnotics and sedatives, narcotic analgesics, phenothiazines, tranquilizers, and certain other agents. Compounds in these categories include:

Alfentanil Hydrochloride (Additive CNS depression).
No products indexed under this heading.

Alprazolam (Additive CNS depression). Products include:
Niravam Orally Disintegrating Tablets 3106
Xanax XR Tablets 2655

Anisindione (Enhanced effect of anticoagulant). Products include:
Miradon Tablets 3056

Aprobarbital (Additive CNS depression).
No products indexed under this heading.

Ardeparin Sodium (Enhanced effect of anticoagulant).
No products indexed under this heading.

Buprenorphine Hydrochloride (Additive CNS depression). Products include:
Buprenex Injectable 2718
Suboxone Tablets 2719
Subutex Tablets 2719

Buspirone Hydrochloride (Additive CNS depression).
No products indexed under this heading.

Butabarbital (Additive CNS depression).
No products indexed under this heading.

Butalbital (Additive CNS depression). Products include:
Sedapap Tablets 50 mg/650 mg 2098

Chlordiazepoxide (Additive CNS depression).
No products indexed under this heading.

Chlordiazepoxide Hydrochloride (Additive CNS depression). Products include:
Librium Capsules 3349

Chlorpromazine (Additive CNS depression).
No products indexed under this heading.

Chlorpromazine Hydrochloride (Additive CNS depression).
No products indexed under this heading.

Chlorprothixene (Additive CNS depression).
No products indexed under this heading.

Chlorprothixene Hydrochloride (Additive CNS depression).
No products indexed under this heading.

Chlorprothixene Lactate (Additive CNS depression).
No products indexed under this heading.

Clorazepate Dipotassium (Additive CNS depression). Products include:
Tranxene 2488

Clozapine (Additive CNS depression). Products include:
Clozapine Tablets 2141
Clozaril Tablets 2174
FazaClo Orally Disintegrating Tablets 547

Codeine Phosphate (Additive CNS depression). Products include:
Tylenol with Codeine 2461

Dalteparin Sodium (Enhanced effect of anticoagulant). Products include:
Fragmin Injection 2638

Danaparoid Sodium (Enhanced effect of anticoagulant).
No products indexed under this heading.

Desflurane (Additive CNS depression). Products include:
Suprane Liquid for Inhalation 770

Dezocine (Additive CNS depression).
No products indexed under this heading.

Diazepam (Additive CNS depression). Products include:
Diastat Rectal Delivery System 3344
Valium Tablets 2822

Dicumarol (Enhanced effect of anticoagulant).
No products indexed under this heading.

Droperidol (Additive CNS depression).
No products indexed under this heading.

Enflurane (Additive CNS depression).
No products indexed under this heading.

Enoxaparin Sodium (Enhanced effect of anticoagulant). Products include:
Lovenox Injection 2931

Estazolam (Additive CNS depression). Products include:
ProSom Tablets 512

Ethanol (Additive CNS depression).
No products indexed under this heading.

Ethchlorvynol (Additive CNS depression).
No products indexed under this heading.

Ethinamate (Additive CNS depression).
No products indexed under this heading.

Ethyl Alcohol (Additive CNS depression).
No products indexed under this heading.

Fentanyl (Additive CNS depression). Products include:
Duragesic Transdermal System 2448

Fentanyl Citrate (Additive CNS depression). Products include:
Actiq 993

Fluphenazine Decanoate (Additive CNS depression).
No products indexed under this heading.

Fluphenazine Enanthate (Additive CNS depression).
No products indexed under this heading.

Fluphenazine Hydrochloride (Additive CNS depression).
No products indexed under this heading.

Flurazepam Hydrochloride (Additive CNS depression). Products include:
Dalmane Capsules 3343

Fondaparinux Sodium (Enhanced effect of anticoagulant). Products include:
Arixtra Injection 1325

Glutethimide (Additive CNS depression).
No products indexed under this heading.

Haloperidol (Additive CNS depression).
No products indexed under this heading.

Haloperidol Decanoate (Additive CNS depression).
No products indexed under this heading.

Heparin Calcium (Enhanced effect of anticoagulant).
No products indexed under this heading.

Heparin Sodium (Enhanced effect of anticoagulant).
No products indexed under this heading.

Hydrocodone Bitartrate (Additive CNS depression). Products include:
Hycodan 1104
Hycomine Compound Tablets 1105
Hycotuss Expectorant Syrup 1106
Lortab 3315
Lortab Elixir 3312
Vicodin Tablets 530
Vicodin ES Tablets 531
Vicodin HP Tablets 532
Vicoprofen Tablets 533
Zydone Tablets 1118

Hydrocodone Polistirex (Additive CNS depression). Products include:
Tussionex Pennkinetic Extended-Release Suspension 3322

Hydromorphone Hydrochloride (Additive CNS depression). Products include:
Dilaudid 439
Dilaudid Oral Liquid 443
Dilaudid Non-Sterile Powder 439
Dilaudid Rectal Suppositories 439
Dilaudid Tablets 439
Dilaudid Tablets - 8 mg 443
Dilaudid-HP 441

Hydroxyzine Hydrochloride (Additive CNS depression).
No products indexed under this heading.

Isoflurane (Additive CNS depression).
No products indexed under this heading.

Ketamine Hydrochloride (Additive CNS depression).
No products indexed under this heading.

Levomethadyl Acetate Hydrochloride (Additive CNS depression).
No products indexed under this heading.

Levorphanol Tartrate (Additive CNS depression).
No products indexed under this heading.

Lorazepam (Additive CNS depression).
No products indexed under this heading.

Low Molecular Weight Heparins (Enhanced effect of anticoagulant).
No products indexed under this heading.

Loxapine Hydrochloride (Additive CNS depression).
No products indexed under this heading.

Loxapine Succinate (Additive CNS depression).
No products indexed under this heading.

Meperidine Hydrochloride (Additive CNS depression).
No products indexed under this heading.

Mephobarbital (Additive CNS depression). Products include:
Mebaral Tablets, USP 2483

Meprobamate (Additive CNS depression).
No products indexed under this heading.

Mesoridazine Besylate (Additive CNS depression).
No products indexed under this heading.

Methadone Hydrochloride (Additive CNS depression).
No products indexed under this heading.

Methohexital Sodium (Additive CNS depression).
No products indexed under this heading.

Methotrimeprazine (Additive CNS depression).
No products indexed under this heading.

Methoxyflurane (Additive CNS depression).
No products indexed under this heading.

Midazolam Hydrochloride (Additive CNS depression).
No products indexed under this heading.

Molindone Hydrochloride (Additive CNS depression). Products include:
Moban Tablets 1108

Morphine Sulfate (Additive CNS depression). Products include:
Avinza Capsules 1714
Kadian Capsules 572
MS Contin Tablets 2703

Olanzapine (Additive CNS depression). Products include:
Symbyax Capsules 1788
Zyprexa Tablets 1798
Zyprexa IntraMuscular 1798
Zyprexa ZYDIS Orally Disintegrating Tablets 1798

Oxazepam (Additive CNS depression).
No products indexed under this heading.

Pentobarbital Sodium (Additive CNS depression). Products include:
Nembutal Sodium Solution, USP 2484

Perphenazine (Additive CNS depression).
No products indexed under this heading.

Phenobarbital (Additive CNS depression).
No products indexed under this heading.

Prazepam (Additive CNS depression).
No products indexed under this heading.

Probenecid (Aspirin may inhibit the uricosuric effects).
No products indexed under this heading.

Prochlorperazine (Additive CNS depression).
No products indexed under this heading.

Promethazine Hydrochloride (Additive CNS depression). Products include:
Phenergan 3438

Propofol (Additive CNS depression). Products include:
Diprivan Injectable Emulsion 676

Propoxyphene Hydrochloride (Additive CNS depression).
No products indexed under this heading.

Propoxyphene Napsylate (Additive CNS depression). Products include:
Darvocet A 500 Tablets 3497

Quazepam (Additive CNS depression).
No products indexed under this heading.

Quetiapine Fumarate (Additive CNS depression). Products include:
Seroquel Tablets 691

Remifentanil Hydrochloride (Additive CNS depression).
No products indexed under this heading.

Risperidone (Additive CNS depression). Products include:
Risperdal Consta Long-Acting Injection 1664
Risperdal M-Tab Orally Disintegrating Tablets 1658
Risperdal 1658

Secobarbital Sodium (Additive CNS depression).
No products indexed under this heading.

Sevoflurane (Additive CNS depression). Products include:
Ultane Liquid for Inhalation 526

Sodium Oxybate (Additive CNS depression).
No products indexed under this heading.

Sufentanil Citrate (Additive CNS depression).
No products indexed under this heading.

Sulfinpyrazone (Aspirin may inhibit the uricosuric effects).
No products indexed under this heading.

Temazepam (Additive CNS depression).
No products indexed under this heading.

Thiamylal Sodium (Additive CNS depression).
No products indexed under this heading.

Thioridazine Hydrochloride (Additive CNS depression). Products include:
Thioridazine Hydrochloride Tablets 2122

Thiothixene (Additive CNS depression). Products include:
Thiothixene Capsules 2124

Tinzaparin Sodium (Enhanced effect of anticoagulant).
No products indexed under this heading.

Triazolam (Additive CNS depression).
No products indexed under this heading.

Trifluoperazine Hydrochloride (Additive CNS depression).
No products indexed under this heading.

Warfarin Sodium (Enhanced effect of anticoagulant). Products include:
Coumadin for Injection 932
Coumadin Tablets 932

Zaleplon (Additive CNS depression). Products include:
Sonata Capsules 1686

Ziprasidone Hydrochloride (Additive CNS depression). Products include:
Geodon Capsules 2514

Zolpidem Tartrate (Additive CNS depression). Products include:
Ambien Tablets 2867

Food Interactions

Alcohol (Additive CNS depression).

PERDIEM OVERNIGHT RELIEF PILLS

(Calcium, Sennosides) 2166
None cited in PDR database.

PERI-COLACE TABLETS

(Docusate Sodium, Sennosides) 2716
May interact with:

Mineral Oil (Do not use laxative products if you are presently taking mineral oil, unless told to do so by a doctor). Products include:
Fleet Mineral Oil Enema 1170
Lubriderm Advanced Therapy Moisturizing Lotion .... ▣702
Mineral Oil 2716
Preparation H Ointment .... ▣747
Refresh P.M. Lubricant Eye Ointment .... ⊙239
Tucks Hemorrhoidal Ointment .... ▣711

PERIDIN-C TABLETS

(Bioflavonoids, Hesperidin Complex, Hesperidin Methyl Chalcone, Vitamin C) .... ▣761
None cited in PDR database.

PERMAX TABLETS

(Pergolide Mesylate) 3357
May interact with dopamine antagonists, central nervous system depressants, and certain other agents. Compounds in these categories include:

Alfentanil Hydrochloride (Pergolide may cause somnolence; concurrent use with CNS depressants may result in additive sedative effects).
No products indexed under this heading.

Alprazolam (Pergolide may cause somnolence; concurrent use with CNS depressants may result in additive sedative effects). Products include:
Niravam Orally Disintegrating Tablets 3106
Xanax XR Tablets 2655

Aprobarbital (Pergolide may cause somnolence; concurrent use with CNS depressants may result in additive sedative effects).
No products indexed under this heading.

Buprenorphine Hydrochloride (Pergolide may cause somnolence; concurrent use with CNS depressants may result in additive sedative effects). Products include:
Buprenex Injectable 2718
Suboxone Tablets 2719
Subutex Tablets 2719

Buspirone Hydrochloride (Pergolide may cause somnolence; concurrent use with CNS depressants may result in additive sedative effects).
No products indexed under this heading.

Butabarbital (Pergolide may cause somnolence; concurrent use with CNS depressants may result in additive sedative effects).
No products indexed under this heading.

Butalbital (Pergolide may cause somnolence; concurrent use with CNS depressants may result in additive sedative effects). Products include:
Sedapap Tablets 50 mg/650 mg 2098

Chlordiazepoxide (Pergolide may cause somnolence; concurrent use with CNS depressants may result in additive sedative effects).
No products indexed under this heading.

Chlordiazepoxide Hydrochloride (Pergolide may cause somnolence; concurrent use with CNS depressants may result in additive sedative effects). Products include:
Librium Capsules 3349

Chlorpromazine (May diminish the effectiveness of Permax; caution should be exercised if co-administered).
No products indexed under this heading.

Chlorpromazine Hydrochloride (Concurrent use with dopamine antagonists may diminish the effectiveness of pergolide).
No products indexed under this heading.

Chlorprothixene (Pergolide may cause somnolence; concurrent use with CNS depressants may result in additive sedative effects).
No products indexed under this heading.

Chlorprothixene Hydrochloride (Pergolide may cause somnolence; concurrent use with CNS depressants may result in additive sedative effects).
No products indexed under this heading.

Chlorprothixene Lactate (Pergolide may cause somnolence; concurrent use with CNS depressants may result in additive sedative effects).
No products indexed under this heading.

Clorazepate Dipotassium (Pergolide may cause somnolence; concurrent use with CNS depressants may result in additive sedative effects). Products include:
Tranxene 2488

Clozapine (Concurrent use with dopamine antagonists may diminish the effectiveness of pergolide). Products include:
Clozapine Tablets 2141
Clozaril Tablets 2174
FazaClo Orally Disintegrating Tablets 547

Codeine Phosphate (Pergolide may cause somnolence; concurrent

IMPORTANT NOTE: Always consult each drug listing in the patient's regimen for possible interactions.

use with CNS depressants may result in additive sedative effects). Products include:
Tylenol with Codeine 2461

Desflurane (Pergolide may cause somnolence; concurrent use with CNS depressants may result in additive sedative effects). Products include:
Suprane Liquid for Inhalation 770

Dezocine (Pergolide may cause somnolence; concurrent use with CNS depressants may result in additive sedative effects).
No products indexed under this heading.

Diazepam (Pergolide may cause somnolence; concurrent use with CNS depressants may result in additive sedative effects). Products include:
Diastat Rectal Delivery System 3344
Valium Tablets 2822

Droperidol (Pergolide may cause somnolence; concurrent use with CNS depressants may result in additive sedative effects).
No products indexed under this heading.

Enflurane (Pergolide may cause somnolence; concurrent use with CNS depressants may result in additive sedative effects).
No products indexed under this heading.

Estazolam (Pergolide may cause somnolence; concurrent use with CNS depressants may result in additive sedative effects). Products include:
ProSom Tablets 512

Ethanol (Pergolide may cause somnolence; concurrent use with CNS depressants may result in additive sedative effects).
No products indexed under this heading.

Ethchlorvynol (Pergolide may cause somnolence; concurrent use with CNS depressants may result in additive sedative effects).
No products indexed under this heading.

Ethinamate (Pergolide may cause somnolence; concurrent use with CNS depressants may result in additive sedative effects).
No products indexed under this heading.

Ethyl Alcohol (Pergolide may cause somnolence; concurrent use with CNS depressants may result in additive sedative effects).
No products indexed under this heading.

Fentanyl (Pergolide may cause somnolence; concurrent use with CNS depressants may result in additive sedative effects). Products include:
Duragesic Transdermal System 2448

Fentanyl Citrate (Pergolide may cause somnolence; concurrent use with CNS depressants may result in additive sedative effects). Products include:
Actiq 993

Fluphenazine Decanoate (Concurrent use with dopamine antagonists may diminish the effectiveness of pergolide).
No products indexed under this heading.

Fluphenazine Enanthate (Concurrent use with dopamine antagonists may diminish the effectiveness of pergolide).
No products indexed under this heading.

Fluphenazine Hydrochloride (Concurrent use with dopamine antagonists may diminish the effectiveness of pergolide).
No products indexed under this heading.

Flurazepam Hydrochloride (Pergolide may cause somnolence; concurrent use with CNS depressants may result in additive sedative effects). Products include:
Dalmane Capsules 3343

Glutethimide (Pergolide may cause somnolence; concurrent use with CNS depressants may result in additive sedative effects).
No products indexed under this heading.

Haloperidol (Concurrent use with dopamine antagonists may diminish the effectiveness of pergolide).
No products indexed under this heading.

Haloperidol Decanoate (Concurrent use with dopamine antagonists may diminish the effectiveness of pergolide).
No products indexed under this heading.

Hydrocodone Bitartrate (Pergolide may cause somnolence; concurrent use with CNS depressants may result in additive sedative effects). Products include:
Hycodan 1104
Hycomine Compound Tablets 1105
Hycotuss Expectorant Syrup 1106
Lortab 3315
Lortab Elixir 3312
Vicodin Tablets 530
Vicodin ES Tablets 531
Vicodin HP Tablets 532
Vicoprofen Tablets 533
Zydone Tablets 1118

Hydrocodone Polistirex (Pergolide may cause somnolence; concurrent use with CNS depressants may result in additive sedative effects). Products include:
Tussionex Pennkinetic Extended-Release Suspension 3322

Hydromorphone Hydrochloride (Pergolide may cause somnolence; concurrent use with CNS depressants may result in additive sedative effects). Products include:
Dilaudid 439
Dilaudid Oral Liquid 443
Dilaudid Non-Sterile Powder 439
Dilaudid Rectal Suppositories 439
Dilaudid Tablets 439
Dilaudid Tablets - 8 mg 443
Dilaudid-HP 441

Hydroxyzine Hydrochloride (Pergolide may cause somnolence; concurrent use with CNS depressants may result in additive sedative effects).
No products indexed under this heading.

Isoflurane (Pergolide may cause somnolence; concurrent use with CNS depressants may result in additive sedative effects).
No products indexed under this heading.

Ketamine Hydrochloride (Pergolide may cause somnolence; concurrent use with CNS depressants may result in additive sedative effects).
No products indexed under this heading.

Levodopa (Concomitant use may cause and/or exacerbate preexisting states of confusion and hallucination). Products include:
Parcopa Orally Disintegrating Tablets 3111
Stalevo Tablets 2270

Levomethadyl Acetate Hydrochloride (Pergolide may cause somnolence; concurrent use with CNS depressants may result in additive sedative effects).
No products indexed under this heading.

Levorphanol Tartrate (Pergolide may cause somnolence; concurrent use with CNS depressants may result in additive sedative effects).
No products indexed under this heading.

Lorazepam (Pergolide may cause somnolence; concurrent use with CNS depressants may result in additive sedative effects).
No products indexed under this heading.

Loxapine Hydrochloride (Pergolide may cause somnolence; concurrent use with CNS depressants may result in additive sedative effects).
No products indexed under this heading.

Loxapine Succinate (Pergolide may cause somnolence; concurrent use with CNS depressants may result in additive sedative effects).
No products indexed under this heading.

Meperidine Hydrochloride (Pergolide may cause somnolence; concurrent use with CNS depressants may result in additive sedative effects).
No products indexed under this heading.

Mephobarbital (Pergolide may cause somnolence; concurrent use with CNS depressants may result in additive sedative effects). Products include:
Mebaral Tablets, USP 2483

Meprobamate (Pergolide may cause somnolence; concurrent use with CNS depressants may result in additive sedative effects).
No products indexed under this heading.

Mesoridazine Besylate (Concurrent use with dopamine antagonists may diminish the effectiveness of pergolide).
No products indexed under this heading.

Methadone Hydrochloride (Pergolide may cause somnolence; concurrent use with CNS depressants may result in additive sedative effects).
No products indexed under this heading.

Methohexital Sodium (Pergolide may cause somnolence; concurrent use with CNS depressants may result in additive sedative effects).
No products indexed under this heading.

Methotrimeprazine (Concurrent use with dopamine antagonists may diminish the effectiveness of pergolide).
No products indexed under this heading.

Methoxyflurane (Pergolide may cause somnolence; concurrent use with CNS depressants may result in additive sedative effects).
No products indexed under this heading.

Metoclopramide Hydrochloride (Concurrent use with dopamine antagonists may diminish the effectiveness of pergolide).
No products indexed under this heading.

Midazolam Hydrochloride (Pergolide may cause somnolence; concurrent use with CNS depressants may result in additive sedative effects).
No products indexed under this heading.

Molindone Hydrochloride (Pergolide may cause somnolence; concurrent use with CNS depressants may result in additive sedative effects). Products include:
Moban Tablets 1108

Morphine Sulfate (Pergolide may cause somnolence; concurrent use with CNS depressants may result in additive sedative effects). Products include:
Avinza Capsules 1714
Kadian Capsules 572
MS Contin Tablets 2703

Olanzapine (Concurrent use with dopamine antagonists may diminish the effectiveness of pergolide). Products include:
Symbyax Capsules 1788
Zyprexa Tablets 1798
Zyprexa IntraMuscular 1798
Zyprexa ZYDIS Orally Disintegrating Tablets 1798

Oxazepam (Pergolide may cause somnolence; concurrent use with CNS depressants may result in additive sedative effects).
No products indexed under this heading.

Oxycodone Hydrochloride (Pergolide may cause somnolence; concurrent use with CNS depressants may result in additive sedative effects). Products include:
Combunox Tablets 1183
OxyContin Tablets 2699
OxyFast Oral Concentrate Solution 2704
OxyIR Capsules 2704
Percocet Tablets 1114
Percodan Tablets 1115

Pentobarbital Sodium (Pergolide may cause somnolence; concurrent use with CNS depressants may result in additive sedative effects). Products include:
Nembutal Sodium Solution, USP 2484

Perphenazine (Concurrent use with dopamine antagonists may diminish the effectiveness of pergolide).
No products indexed under this heading.

Phenobarbital (Pergolide may cause somnolence; concurrent use with CNS depressants may result in additive sedative effects).
No products indexed under this heading.

Pimozide (Concurrent use with dopamine antagonists may diminish the effectiveness of pergolide). Products include:

Orap Tablets 1220

Prazepam (Pergolide may cause somnolence; concurrent use with CNS depressants may result in additive sedative effects).
No products indexed under this heading.

Prochlorperazine (Concurrent use with dopamine antagonists may diminish the effectiveness of pergolide).
No products indexed under this heading.

Promethazine Hydrochloride (Concurrent use with dopamine antagonists may diminish the effectiveness of pergolide). Products include:
Phenergan 3438

Propofol (Pergolide may cause somnolence; concurrent use with CNS depressants may result in additive sedative effects). Products include:
Diprivan Injectable Emulsion 676

Propoxyphene Hydrochloride (Pergolide may cause somnolence; concurrent use with CNS depressants may result in additive sedative effects).
No products indexed under this heading.

Propoxyphene Napsylate (Pergolide may cause somnolence; concurrent use with CNS depressants may result in additive sedative effects). Products include:
Darvocet A 500 Tablets 3497

Quazepam (Pergolide may cause somnolence; concurrent use with CNS depressants may result in additive sedative effects).
No products indexed under this heading.

Quetiapine Fumarate (Concurrent use with dopamine antagonists may diminish the effectiveness of pergolide). Products include:
Seroquel Tablets 691

Remifentanil Hydrochloride (Pergolide may cause somnolence; concurrent use with CNS depressants may result in additive sedative effects).
No products indexed under this heading.

Risperidone (Pergolide may cause somnolence; concurrent use with CNS depressants may result in additive sedative effects). Products include:
Risperdal Consta Long-Acting Injection 1664
Risperdal M-Tab Orally Disintegrating Tablets 1658
Risperdal 1658

Secobarbital Sodium (Pergolide may cause somnolence; concurrent use with CNS depressants may result in additive sedative effects).
No products indexed under this heading.

Sevoflurane (Pergolide may cause somnolence; concurrent use with CNS depressants may result in additive sedative effects). Products include:
Ultane Liquid for Inhalation 526

Sodium Oxybate (Pergolide may cause somnolence; concurrent use with CNS depressants may result in additive sedative effects).
No products indexed under this heading.

Sufentanil Citrate (Pergolide may cause somnolence; concurrent use with CNS depressants may result in additive sedative effects).
No products indexed under this heading.

Temazepam (Pergolide may cause somnolence; concurrent use with CNS depressants may result in additive sedative effects).
No products indexed under this heading.

Thiamylal Sodium (Pergolide may cause somnolence; concurrent use with CNS depressants may result in additive sedative effects).
No products indexed under this heading.

Thioridazine Hydrochloride (Concurrent use with dopamine antagonists may diminish the effectiveness of pergolide). Products include:
Thioridazine Hydrochloride Tablets 2122

Thiothixene (May diminish the effectiveness of Permax). Products include:
Thiothixene Capsules 2124

Triazolam (Pergolide may cause somnolence; concurrent use with CNS depressants may result in additive sedative effects).
No products indexed under this heading.

Trifluoperazine Hydrochloride (Concurrent use with dopamine antagonists may diminish the effectiveness of pergolide).
No products indexed under this heading.

Zaleplon (Pergolide may cause somnolence; concurrent use with CNS depressants may result in additive sedative effects). Products include:
Sonata Capsules 1686

Ziprasidone Hydrochloride (Pergolide may cause somnolence; concurrent use with CNS depressants may result in additive sedative effects). Products include:
Geodon Capsules 2514

Zolpidem Tartrate (Pergolide may cause somnolence; concurrent use with CNS depressants may result in additive sedative effects). Products include:
Ambien Tablets 2867

Food Interactions

Alcohol (Pergolide may cause somnolence; concurrent use with alcohol may result in additive sedative effects).

PERMETHRIN LOTION
(Permethrin) .... ▣603
None cited in PDR database.

PERSANTINE TABLETS
(Dipyridamole) 898
May interact with anticholinesterase drugs and certain other agents. Compounds in these categories include:

Adenosine (Dipyridamole has been reported to increase the plasma levels and cardiovascular effects of adenosine. Adjustment of adenosine dosage may be necessary). Products include:
Adenocard Injection 612
Adenoscan 613

Donepezil Hydrochloride (Dipyridamole may counteract the anticholinesterase effect of cholinesterase inhibitors, thereby potentially aggravating myasthenia gravis). Products include:
Aricept Tablets 1086
Aricept ODT Tablets 1086

Galantamine Hydrobromide (Dipyridamole may counteract the anticholinesterase effect of cholinesterase inhibitors, thereby potentially aggravating myasthenia gravis). Products include:
Razadyne ER Extended-Release Capsules 2434
Razadyne 2434

Neostigmine Bromide (Dipyridamole may counteract the anticholinesterase effect of cholinesterase inhibitors, thereby potentially aggravating myasthenia gravis).
No products indexed under this heading.

Neostigmine Methylsulfate (Dipyridamole may counteract the anticholinesterase effect of cholinesterase inhibitors, thereby potentially aggravating myasthenia gravis).
No products indexed under this heading.

Pyridostigmine Bromide (Dipyridamole may counteract the anticholinesterase effect of cholinesterase inhibitors, thereby potentially aggravating myasthenia gravis).
No products indexed under this heading.

Rivastigmine Tartrate (Dipyridamole may counteract the anticholinesterase effect of cholinesterase inhibitors, thereby potentially aggravating myasthenia gravis). Products include:
Exelon Capsules 2204

Tacrine Hydrochloride (Dipyridamole may counteract the anticholinesterase effect of cholinesterase inhibitors, thereby potentially aggravating myasthenia gravis).
No products indexed under this heading.

PHAZYME-125 MG QUICK DISSOLVE CHEWABLE TABLETS
(Simethicone) .... ▣635
None cited in PDR database.

PHAZYME-180 MG ULTRA STRENGTH SOFTGELS
(Simethicone) .... ▣635
None cited in PDR database.

PHENERGAN SUPPOSITORIES
(Promethazine Hydrochloride) 3438
May interact with anticholinergics, barbiturates, central nervous system depressants, monoamine oxidase inhibitors, narcotic analgesics, tricyclic antidepressants, and certain other agents. Compounds in these categories include:

Alfentanil Hydrochloride (Promethazine may increase, prolong, or intensify the sedative action of other CNS depressants; when co-administered with narcotics, the dose of narcotics should be reduced by at least one-quarter to one-half; excessive amount of promethazine relative to narcotic may lead to restlessness and motor hyperactivity in the patient with pain).
No products indexed under this heading.

Alprazolam (Promethazine may increase, prolong, or intensify the sedative action of other CNS depressants; concurrent use should be avoided with other CNS depressants or administered in reduced dosage to patient receiving promethazine). Products include:
Niravam Orally Disintegrating Tablets 3106
Xanax XR Tablets 2655

Amitriptyline Hydrochloride (Promethazine may increase, prolong, or intensify the sedative action of other CNS depressants; concurrent use should be avoided with tricyclic antidepressants or administered in reduced dosage to patient receiving promethazine).
No products indexed under this heading.

Amoxapine (Promethazine may increase, prolong, or intensify the sedative action of other CNS depressants; concurrent use should be avoided with tricyclic antidepressants or administered in reduced dosage to patient receiving promethazine).
No products indexed under this heading.

Aprobarbital (Promethazine may increase, prolong, or intensify the sedative action of other CNS depressants; when co-administered with barbiturates, the dose of barbiturates should be reduced by one-quarter to one-half).
No products indexed under this heading.

Atropine Sulfate (Co-administration with agents with anticholinergic properties should be undertaken with caution).
No products indexed under this heading.

Belladonna Alkaloids (Co-administration with agents with anticholinergic properties should be undertaken with caution). Products include:
Hyland's Teething Tablets .... ▣736

Benztropine Mesylate (Co-administration with agents with anticholinergic properties should be undertaken with caution). Products include:
Cogentin Injection 1903

Biperiden Hydrochloride (Co-administration with agents with anticholinergic properties should be undertaken with caution).
No products indexed under this heading.

Buprenorphine Hydrochloride (Promethazine may increase, prolong, or intensify the sedative action of other CNS depressants; when co-administered with narcotics, the dose of narcotics should be reduced by at least one-quarter to one-half; excessive amount of promethazine relative to narcotic may lead to restlessness and motor hyperactivity in the patient with pain). Products include:
Buprenex Injectable 2718
Suboxone Tablets 2719
Subutex Tablets 2719

Buspirone Hydrochloride (Promethazine may increase, prolong, or intensify the sedative action of other CNS depressants; concurrent use should be avoided with other CNS depressants or administered in reduced dosage to patient receiving promethazine).
No products indexed under this heading.

Butabarbital (Promethazine may increase, prolong, or intensify the sedative action of other CNS depressants; when co-administered with barbiturates, the dose of barbiturates should be reduced by one-quarter to one-half).

No products indexed under this heading.

Butalbital (Promethazine may increase, prolong, or intensify the sedative action of other CNS depressants; when co-administered with barbiturates, the dose of barbiturates should be reduced by one-quarter to one-half). Products include:

Sedapap Tablets 50 mg/650 mg 2098

Chlordiazepoxide (Promethazine may increase, prolong, or intensify the sedative action of other CNS depressants; concurrent use should be avoided with other CNS depressants or administered in reduced dosage to patient receiving promethazine).

No products indexed under this heading.

Chlordiazepoxide Hydrochloride (Promethazine may increase, prolong, or intensify the sedative action of other CNS depressants; concurrent use should be avoided with other CNS depressants or administered in reduced dosage to patient receiving promethazine). Products include:

Librium Capsules 3349

Chlorpromazine (Promethazine may increase, prolong, or intensify the sedative action of other CNS depressants; concurrent use should be avoided with other CNS depressants or administered in reduced dosage to patient receiving promethazine).

No products indexed under this heading.

Chlorpromazine Hydrochloride (Promethazine may increase, prolong, or intensify the sedative action of other CNS depressants; concurrent use should be avoided with other CNS depressants or administered in reduced dosage to patient receiving promethazine).

No products indexed under this heading.

Chlorprothixene (Promethazine may increase, prolong, or intensify the sedative action of other CNS depressants; concurrent use should be avoided with other CNS depressants or administered in reduced dosage to patient receiving promethazine).

No products indexed under this heading.

Chlorprothixene Hydrochloride (Promethazine may increase, prolong, or intensify the sedative action of other CNS depressants; concurrent use should be avoided with other CNS depressants or administered in reduced dosage to patient receiving promethazine).

No products indexed under this heading.

Chlorprothixene Lactate (Promethazine may increase, prolong, or intensify the sedative action of other CNS depressants; concurrent use should be avoided with other CNS depressants or administered in reduced dosage to patient receiving promethazine).

No products indexed under this heading.

Clidinium Bromide (Co-administration with agents with anticholinergic properties should be undertaken with caution).

No products indexed under this heading.

Clomipramine Hydrochloride (Promethazine may increase, prolong, or intensify the sedative action of other CNS depressants; concurrent use should be avoided with tricyclic antidepressants or administered in reduced dosage to patient receiving promethazine).

No products indexed under this heading.

Clorazepate Dipotassium (Promethazine may increase, prolong, or intensify the sedative action of other CNS depressants; concurrent use should be avoided with other CNS depressants or administered in reduced dosage to patient receiving promethazine). Products include:

Tranxene 2488

Clozapine (Promethazine may increase, prolong, or intensify the sedative action of other CNS depressants; concurrent use should be avoided with other CNS depressants or administered in reduced dosage to patient receiving promethazine). Products include:

Clozapine Tablets 2141
Clozaril Tablets 2174
FazaClo Orally Disintegrating Tablets 547

Codeine Phosphate (Promethazine may increase, prolong, or intensify the sedative action of other CNS depressants; when co-administered with narcotics, the dose of narcotics should be reduced by at least one-quarter to one-half; excessive amount of promethazine relative to narcotic may lead to restlessness and motor hyperactivity in the patient with pain). Products include:

Tylenol with Codeine 2461

Desflurane (Promethazine may increase, prolong, or intensify the sedative action of other CNS depressants; concurrent use should be avoided with other CNS depressants or administered in reduced dosage to patient receiving promethazine). Products include:

Suprane Liquid for Inhalation 770

Desipramine Hydrochloride (Promethazine may increase, prolong, or intensify the sedative action of other CNS depressants; concurrent use should be avoided with tricyclic antidepressants or administered in reduced dosage to patient receiving promethazine).

No products indexed under this heading.

Dezocine (Promethazine may increase, prolong, or intensify the sedative action of other CNS depressants; when co-administered with narcotics, the dose of narcotics should be reduced by at least one-quarter to one-half; excessive amount of promethazine relative to narcotic may lead to restlessness and motor hyperactivity in the patient with pain).

No products indexed under this heading.

Diazepam (Promethazine may increase, prolong, or intensify the sedative action of other CNS depressants; concurrent use should be avoided with other CNS depressants or administered in reduced dosage to patient receiving promethazine). Products include:

Diastat Rectal Delivery System 3344
Valium Tablets 2822

Dicyclomine Hydrochloride (Co-administration with agents with anticholinergic properties should be undertaken with caution). Products include:

Bentyl Capsules 724
Bentyl Injection 724
Bentyl Syrup 724
Bentyl Tablets 724

Doxepin Hydrochloride (Promethazine may increase, prolong, or intensify the sedative action of other CNS depressants; concurrent use should be avoided with tricyclic antidepressants or administered in reduced dosage to patient receiving promethazine).

No products indexed under this heading.

Droperidol (Promethazine may increase, prolong, or intensify the sedative action of other CNS depressants; concurrent use should be avoided with other CNS depressants or administered in reduced dosage to patient receiving promethazine).

No products indexed under this heading.

Enflurane (Promethazine may increase, prolong, or intensify the sedative action of other CNS depressants; concurrent use should be avoided with other CNS depressants or administered in reduced dosage to patient receiving promethazine).

No products indexed under this heading.

Estazolam (Promethazine may increase, prolong, or intensify the sedative action of other CNS depressants; concurrent use should be avoided with other CNS depressants or administered in reduced dosage to patient receiving promethazine). Products include:

ProSom Tablets 512

Ethanol (Promethazine may increase, prolong, or intensify the sedative action of other CNS depressants; concurrent use should be avoided with other CNS depressants or administered in reduced dosage to patient receiving promethazine).

No products indexed under this heading.

Ethchlorvynol (Promethazine may increase, prolong, or intensify the sedative action of other CNS depressants; concurrent use should be avoided with other CNS depressants or administered in reduced dosage to patient receiving promethazine).

No products indexed under this heading.

Ethinamate (Promethazine may increase, prolong, or intensify the sedative action of other CNS depressants; concurrent use should be avoided with other CNS depressants or administered in reduced dosage to patient receiving promethazine).

No products indexed under this heading.

Ethyl Alcohol (Promethazine may increase, prolong, or intensify the sedative action of other CNS depressants; concurrent use should be avoided with other CNS depressants or administered in reduced dosage to patient receiving promethazine).

No products indexed under this heading.

Fentanyl (Promethazine may increase, prolong, or intensify the sedative action of other CNS depressants; when co-administered with narcotics, the dose of narcotics should be reduced by at least one-quarter to one-half; excessive amount of promethazine relative to narcotic may lead to restlessness and motor hyperactivity in the patient with pain). Products include:

Duragesic Transdermal System 2448

Fentanyl Citrate (Promethazine may increase, prolong, or intensify the sedative action of other CNS depressants; when co-administered with narcotics, the dose of narcotics should be reduced by at least one-quarter to one-half; excessive amount of promethazine relative to narcotic may lead to restlessness and motor hyperactivity in the patient with pain). Products include:

Actiq 993

Fluphenazine Decanoate (Promethazine may increase, prolong, or intensify the sedative action of other CNS depressants; concurrent use should be avoided with other CNS depressants or administered in reduced dosage to patient receiving promethazine).

No products indexed under this heading.

Fluphenazine Enanthate (Promethazine may increase, prolong, or intensify the sedative action of other CNS depressants; concurrent use should be avoided with other CNS depressants or administered in reduced dosage to patient receiving promethazine).

No products indexed under this heading.

Fluphenazine Hydrochloride (Promethazine may increase, prolong, or intensify the sedative action of other CNS depressants; concurrent use should be avoided with other CNS depressants or administered in reduced dosage to patient receiving promethazine).

No products indexed under this heading.

Flurazepam Hydrochloride (Promethazine may increase, prolong, or intensify the sedative action of other CNS depressants; concurrent use should be avoided with other CNS depressants or administered in reduced dosage to patient receiving promethazine). Products include:

Dalmane Capsules 3343

Glutethimide (Promethazine may increase, prolong, or intensify the sedative action of other CNS depressants; concurrent use should be avoided with other CNS depressants or administered in reduced dosage to patient receiving promethazine).

No products indexed under this heading.

Glycopyrrolate (Co-administration with agents with anticholinergic properties should be undertaken with caution).

No products indexed under this heading.

Haloperidol (Promethazine may increase, prolong, or intensify the sedative action of other CNS depressants; concurrent use should be avoided with other CNS depressants or administered in reduced dosage to patient receiving promethazine).

No products indexed under this heading.

Haloperidol Decanoate (Promethazine may increase, prolong, or intensify the sedative action of other CNS depressants; concurrent use should be avoided with other CNS depressants or administered in reduced dosage to patient receiving promethazine).
No products indexed under this heading.

Hydrocodone Bitartrate (Promethazine may increase, prolong, or intensify the sedative action of other CNS depressants; when co-administered with narcotics, the dose of narcotics should be reduced by at least one-quarter to one-half; excessive amount of promethazine relative to narcotic may lead to restlessness and motor hyperactivity in the patient with pain). Products include:

Hycodan **1104**
Hycomine Compound Tablets **1105**
Hycotuss Expectorant Syrup **1106**
Lortab **3315**
Lortab Elixir **3312**
Vicodin Tablets **530**
Vicodin ES Tablets **531**
Vicodin HP Tablets **532**
Vicoprofen Tablets **533**
Zydone Tablets **1118**

Hydrocodone Polistirex (Promethazine may increase, prolong, or intensify the sedative action of other CNS depressants; when co-administered with narcotics, the dose of narcotics should be reduced by at least one-quarter to one-half; excessive amount of promethazine relative to narcotic may lead to restlessness and motor hyperactivity in the patient with pain). Products include:

Tussionex Pennkinetic Extended-Release Suspension **3322**

Hydromorphone Hydrochloride (Promethazine may increase, prolong, or intensify the sedative action of other CNS depressants; when co-administered with narcotics, the dose of narcotics should be reduced by at least one-quarter to one-half; excessive amount of promethazine relative to narcotic may lead to restlessness and motor hyperactivity in the patient with pain). Products include:

Dilaudid **439**
Dilaudid Oral Liquid **443**
Dilaudid Non-Sterile Powder **439**
Dilaudid Rectal Suppositories **439**
Dilaudid Tablets **439**
Dilaudid Tablets - 8 mg **443**
Dilaudid-HP **441**

Hydroxyzine Hydrochloride (Promethazine may increase, prolong, or intensify the sedative action of other CNS depressants; concurrent use should be avoided with other CNS depressants or administered in reduced dosage to patient receiving promethazine).
No products indexed under this heading.

Hyoscyamine (Co-administration with agents with anticholinergic properties should be undertaken with caution).
No products indexed under this heading.

Hyoscyamine Sulfate (Co-administration with agents with anticholinergic properties should be undertaken with caution).
No products indexed under this heading.

Imipramine Hydrochloride (Promethazine may increase, prolong, or intensify the sedative action of other CNS depressants; concurrent use should be avoided with tricyclic antidepressants or administered in reduced dosage to patient receiving promethazine).
No products indexed under this heading.

Imipramine Pamoate (Promethazine may increase, prolong, or intensify the sedative action of other CNS depressants; concurrent use should be avoided with tricyclic antidepressants or administered in reduced dosage to patient receiving promethazine).
No products indexed under this heading.

Ipratropium Bromide (Co-administration with agents with anticholinergic properties should be undertaken with caution). Products include:

Atrovent HFA Inhalation Aerosol **872**
Atrovent Inhalation Solution **868**
Atrovent Nasal Spray 0.03% **869**
Atrovent Nasal Spray 0.06% **870**
Combivent Inhalation Aerosol **878**
DuoNeb Inhalation Solution **1058**

Isocarboxazid (Co-administration of phenothiazines with MAO inhibitors may increase the incidence of extrapyramidal effects).
No products indexed under this heading.

Isoflurane (Promethazine may increase, prolong, or intensify the sedative action of other CNS depressants; concurrent use should be avoided with other CNS depressants or administered in reduced dosage to patient receiving promethazine).
No products indexed under this heading.

Ketamine Hydrochloride (Promethazine may increase, prolong, or intensify the sedative action of other CNS depressants; concurrent use should be avoided with other CNS depressants or administered in reduced dosage to patient receiving promethazine).
No products indexed under this heading.

Levomethadyl Acetate Hydrochloride (Promethazine may increase, prolong, or intensify the sedative action of other CNS depressants; concurrent use should be avoided with other CNS depressants or administered in reduced dosage to patient receiving promethazine).
No products indexed under this heading.

Levorphanol Tartrate (Promethazine may increase, prolong, or intensify the sedative action of other CNS depressants; when co-administered with narcotics, the dose of narcotics should be reduced by at least one-quarter to one-half; excessive amount of promethazine relative to narcotic may lead to restlessness and motor hyperactivity in the patient with pain).
No products indexed under this heading.

Lorazepam (Promethazine may increase, prolong, or intensify the sedative action of other CNS depressants; concurrent use should be avoided with other CNS depressants or administered in reduced dosage to patient receiving promethazine).
No products indexed under this heading.

Loxapine Hydrochloride (Promethazine may increase, prolong, or intensify the sedative action of other CNS depressants; concurrent use should be avoided with other CNS depressants or administered in reduced dosage to patient receiving promethazine).
No products indexed under this heading.

Loxapine Succinate (Promethazine may increase, prolong, or intensify the sedative action of other CNS depressants; concurrent use should be avoided with other CNS depressants or administered in reduced dosage to patient receiving promethazine).
No products indexed under this heading.

Maprotiline Hydrochloride (Promethazine may increase, prolong, or intensify the sedative action of other CNS depressants; concurrent use should be avoided with tricyclic antidepressants or administered in reduced dosage to patient receiving promethazine).
No products indexed under this heading.

Mepenzolate Bromide (Co-administration with agents with anticholinergic properties should be undertaken with caution).
No products indexed under this heading.

Meperidine Hydrochloride (Promethazine may increase, prolong, or intensify the sedative action of other CNS depressants; when co-administered with narcotics, the dose of narcotics should be reduced by at least one-quarter to one-half; excessive amount of promethazine relative to narcotic may lead to restlessness and motor hyperactivity in the patient with pain).
No products indexed under this heading.

Mephobarbital (Promethazine may increase, prolong, or intensify the sedative action of other CNS depressants; when co-administered with barbiturates, the dose of barbiturates should be reduced by one-quarter to one-half). Products include:

Mebaral Tablets, USP **2483**

Meprobamate (Promethazine may increase, prolong, or intensify the sedative action of other CNS depressants; concurrent use should be avoided with other CNS depressants or administered in reduced dosage to patient receiving promethazine).
No products indexed under this heading.

Mesoridazine Besylate (Promethazine may increase, prolong, or intensify the sedative action of other CNS depressants; concurrent use should be avoided with other CNS depressants or administered in reduced dosage to patient receiving promethazine).
No products indexed under this heading.

Methadone Hydrochloride (Promethazine may increase, prolong, or intensify the sedative action of other CNS depressants; when co-administered with narcotics, the dose of narcotics should be reduced by at least one-quarter to one-half; excessive amount of promethazine relative to narcotic may lead to restlessness and motor hyperactivity in the patient with pain).
No products indexed under this heading.

Methohexital Sodium (Promethazine may increase, prolong, or intensify the sedative action of other CNS depressants; concurrent use should be avoided with other CNS depressants or administered in reduced dosage to patient receiving promethazine).
No products indexed under this heading.

Methotrimeprazine (Promethazine may increase, prolong, or intensify the sedative action of other CNS depressants; concurrent use should be avoided with other CNS depressants or administered in reduced dosage to patient receiving promethazine).
No products indexed under this heading.

Methoxyflurane (Promethazine may increase, prolong, or intensify the sedative action of other CNS depressants; concurrent use should be avoided with other CNS depressants or administered in reduced dosage to patient receiving promethazine).
No products indexed under this heading.

Midazolam Hydrochloride (Promethazine may increase, prolong, or intensify the sedative action of other CNS depressants; concurrent use should be avoided with other CNS depressants or administered in reduced dosage to patient receiving promethazine).
No products indexed under this heading.

Moclobemide (Co-administration of phenothiazines with MAO inhibitors may increase the incidence of extrapyramidal effects).
No products indexed under this heading.

Molindone Hydrochloride (Promethazine may increase, prolong, or intensify the sedative action of other CNS depressants; concurrent use should be avoided with other CNS depressants or administered in reduced dosage to patient receiving promethazine). Products include:

Moban Tablets **1108**

Morphine Sulfate (Promethazine may increase, prolong, or intensify the sedative action of other CNS depressants; when co-administered with narcotics, the dose of narcotics should be reduced by at least one-quarter to one-half; excessive amount of promethazine relative to narcotic may lead to restlessness and motor hyperactivity in the patient with pain). Products include:

Avinza Capsules **1714**
Kadian Capsules **572**
MS Contin Tablets **2703**

Nortriptyline Hydrochloride (Promethazine may increase, prolong, or intensify the sedative action of other CNS depressants; concurrent use should be avoided with tricyclic antidepressants or administered in reduced dosage to patient receiving promethazine).
No products indexed under this heading.

Olanzapine (Promethazine may increase, prolong, or intensify the sedative action of other CNS depressants; concurrent use should be avoided with other CNS depressants or administered in reduced dosage to patient receiving promethazine). Products include:
Symbyax Capsules 1788
Zyprexa Tablets 1798
Zyprexa IntraMuscular 1798
Zyprexa ZYDIS Orally Disintegrating Tablets 1798

Oxazepam (Promethazine may increase, prolong, or intensify the sedative action of other CNS depressants; concurrent use should be avoided with other CNS depressants or administered in reduced dosage to patient receiving promethazine).
No products indexed under this heading.

Oxybutynin Chloride (Co-administration with agents with anticholinergic properties should be undertaken with caution). Products include:
Ditropan XL Extended Release Tablets 2391

Oxycodone Hydrochloride (Promethazine may increase, prolong, or intensify the sedative action of other CNS depressants; when co-administered with narcotics, the dose of narcotics should be reduced by at least one-quarter to one-half; excessive amount of promethazine relative to narcotic may lead to restlessness and motor hyperactivity in the patient with pain). Products include:
Combunox Tablets 1183
OxyContin Tablets 2699
OxyFast Oral Concentrate Solution 2704
OxyIR Capsules 2704
Percocet Tablets 1114
Percodan Tablets 1115

Pargyline Hydrochloride (Co-administration of phenothiazines with MAO inhibitors may increase the incidence of extrapyramidal effects).
No products indexed under this heading.

Pentobarbital Sodium (Promethazine may increase, prolong, or intensify the sedative action of other CNS depressants; when co-administered with barbiturates, the dose of barbiturates should be reduced by one-quarter to one-half). Products include:
Nembutal Sodium Solution, USP 2484

Perphenazine (Promethazine may increase, prolong, or intensify the sedative action of other CNS depressants; concurrent use should be avoided with other CNS depressants or administered in reduced dosage to patient receiving promethazine).
No products indexed under this heading.

Phenelzine Sulfate (Co-administration of phenothiazines with MAO inhibitors may increase the incidence of extrapyramidal effects).
No products indexed under this heading.

Phenobarbital (Promethazine may increase, prolong, or intensify the sedative action of other CNS depressants; when co-administered with barbiturates, the dose of barbiturates should be reduced by one-quarter to one-half).
No products indexed under this heading.

Prazepam (Promethazine may increase, prolong, or intensify the sedative action of other CNS depressants; concurrent use should be avoided with other CNS depressants or administered in reduced dosage to patient receiving promethazine).
No products indexed under this heading.

Procarbazine Hydrochloride (Co-administration of phenothiazines with MAO inhibitors may increase the incidence of extrapyramidal effects). Products include:
Matulane Capsules 3188

Prochlorperazine (Promethazine may increase, prolong, or intensify the sedative action of other CNS depressants; concurrent use should be avoided with other CNS depressants or administered in reduced dosage to patient receiving promethazine).
No products indexed under this heading.

Procyclidine Hydrochloride (Co-administration with agents with anticholinergic properties should be undertaken with caution).
No products indexed under this heading.

Propantheline Bromide (Co-administration with agents with anticholinergic properties should be undertaken with caution).
No products indexed under this heading.

Propofol (Promethazine may increase, prolong, or intensify the sedative action of other CNS depressants; concurrent use should be avoided with other CNS depressants or administered in reduced dosage to patient receiving promethazine). Products include:
Diprivan Injectable Emulsion 676

Propoxyphene Hydrochloride (Promethazine may increase, prolong, or intensify the sedative action of other CNS depressants; when co-administered with narcotics, the dose of narcotics should be reduced by at least one-quarter to one-half; excessive amount of promethazine relative to narcotic may lead to restlessness and motor hyperactivity in the patient with pain).
No products indexed under this heading.

Propoxyphene Napsylate (Promethazine may increase, prolong, or intensify the sedative action of other CNS depressants; when co-administered with narcotics, the dose of narcotics should be reduced by at least one-quarter to one-half; excessive amount of promethazine relative to narcotic may lead to restlessness and motor hyperactivity in the patient with pain). Products include:
Darvocet A 500 Tablets 3497

Protriptyline Hydrochloride (Promethazine may increase, prolong, or intensify the sedative action of other CNS depressants; concurrent use should be avoided with tricyclic antidepressants or administered in reduced dosage to patient receiving promethazine). Products include:
Vivactil Tablets 2350

Quazepam (Promethazine may increase, prolong, or intensify the sedative action of other CNS depressants; concurrent use should be avoided with other CNS depressants or administered in reduced dosage to patient receiving promethazine).
No products indexed under this heading.

Quetiapine Fumarate (Promethazine may increase, prolong, or intensify the sedative action of other CNS depressants; concurrent use should be avoided with other CNS depressants or administered in reduced dosage to patient receiving promethazine). Products include:
Seroquel Tablets 691

Remifentanil Hydrochloride (Promethazine may increase, prolong, or intensify the sedative action of other CNS depressants; when co-administered with narcotics, the dose of narcotics should be reduced by at least one-quarter to one-half; excessive amount of promethazine relative to narcotic may lead to restlessness and motor hyperactivity in the patient with pain).
No products indexed under this heading.

Risperidone (Promethazine may increase, prolong, or intensify the sedative action of other CNS depressants; concurrent use should be avoided with other CNS depressants or administered in reduced dosage to patient receiving promethazine). Products include:
Risperdal Consta Long-Acting Injection 1664
Risperdal M-Tab Orally Disintegrating Tablets 1658
Risperdal 1658

Scopolamine (Co-administration with agents with anticholinergic properties should be undertaken with caution). Products include:
Transderm Scōp Transdermal Therapeutic System 2166

Scopolamine Hydrobromide (Co-administration with agents with anticholinergic properties should be undertaken with caution).
No products indexed under this heading.

Secobarbital Sodium (Promethazine may increase, prolong, or intensify the sedative action of other CNS depressants; when co-administered with barbiturates, the dose of barbiturates should be reduced by one-quarter to one-half).
No products indexed under this heading.

Selegiline Hydrochloride (Co-administration of phenothiazines with MAO inhibitors may increase the incidence of extrapyramidal effects). Products include:
Eldepryl Capsules 3209

Sevoflurane (Promethazine may increase, prolong, or intensify the sedative action of other CNS depressants; concurrent use should be avoided with other CNS depressants or administered in reduced dosage to patient receiving promethazine). Products include:
Ultane Liquid for Inhalation 526

Sufentanil Citrate (Promethazine may increase, prolong, or intensify the sedative action of other CNS depressants; when co-administered with narcotics, the dose of narcotics should be reduced by at least one-quarter to one-half; excessive amount of promethazine relative to narcotic may lead to restlessness and motor hyperactivity in the patient with pain).
No products indexed under this heading.

Temazepam (Promethazine may increase, prolong, or intensify the sedative action of other CNS depressants; concurrent use should be avoided with other CNS depressants or administered in reduced dosage to patient receiving promethazine).
No products indexed under this heading.

Thiamylal Sodium (Promethazine may increase, prolong, or intensify the sedative action of other CNS depressants; when co-administered with barbiturates, the dose of barbiturates should be reduced by one-quarter to one-half).
No products indexed under this heading.

Thioridazine Hydrochloride (Promethazine may increase, prolong, or intensify the sedative action of other CNS depressants; concurrent use should be avoided with other CNS depressants or administered in reduced dosage to patient receiving promethazine). Products include:
Thioridazine Hydrochloride Tablets 2122

Thiothixene (Promethazine may increase, prolong, or intensify the sedative action of other CNS depressants; concurrent use should be avoided with other CNS depressants or administered in reduced dosage to patient receiving promethazine). Products include:
Thiothixene Capsules 2124

Tolterodine Tartrate (Co-administration with agents with anticholinergic properties should be undertaken with caution). Products include:
Detrol Tablets 2626
Detrol LA Capsules 2629

Tranylcypromine Sulfate (Co-administration of phenothiazines with MAO inhibitors may increase the incidence of extrapyramidal effects). Products include:
Parnate Tablets 1499

Triazolam (Promethazine may increase, prolong, or intensify the sedative action of other CNS depressants; concurrent use should be avoided with other CNS depressants or administered in reduced dosage to patient receiving promethazine).
No products indexed under this heading.

Tridihexethyl Chloride (Co-administration with agents with anticholinergic properties should be undertaken with caution).
No products indexed under this heading.

Trifluoperazine Hydrochloride (Promethazine may increase, prolong, or intensify the sedative action of other CNS depressants; concurrent use should be avoided with other CNS depressants or administered in reduced dosage to patient receiving promethazine).
No products indexed under this heading.

Trihexyphenidyl Hydrochloride (Co-administration with agents with anticholinergic properties should be undertaken with caution).
No products indexed under this heading.

Trimipramine Maleate (Promethazine may increase, prolong, or intensify the sedative action of other CNS depressants; concurrent use should be avoided with tricyclic antidepressants or administered in reduced dosage to patient receiving promethazine). Products include:
Surmontil Capsules 2347

Zaleplon (Promethazine may increase, prolong, or intensify the sedative action of other CNS depressants; concurrent use should be avoided with other CNS depressants or administered in reduced dosage to patient receiving promethazine). Products include:
Sonata Capsules 1686

Ziprasidone Hydrochloride (Promethazine may increase, prolong, or intensify the sedative action of other CNS depressants; concurrent use should be avoided with other CNS depressants or administered in reduced dosage to patient receiving promethazine). Products include:
Geodon Capsules 2514

Zolpidem Tartrate (Promethazine may increase, prolong, or intensify the sedative action of other CNS depressants; concurrent use should be avoided with other CNS depressants or administered in reduced dosage to patient receiving promethazine). Products include:
Ambien Tablets 2867

Food Interactions

Alcohol (Promethazine may increase, prolong, or intensify the sedative action of other CNS depressants, such as alcohol).

PHENERGAN TABLETS
(Promethazine Hydrochloride) 3438
See Phenergan Suppositories

PHENYTEK CAPSULES
(Phenytoin Sodium) 2153
May interact with chloramphenicol, corticosteroids, oral anticoagulants, doxycycline, estrogens, histamine H_2-receptor antagonists, oral contraceptives, phenothiazines, quinidine, salicylates, succinimides, tricyclic antidepressants, valproate, xanthines, and certain other agents. Compounds in these categories include:

Aminophylline (Phenytoin impairs efficacy of theophylline).
No products indexed under this heading.

Amiodarone Hydrochloride (May increase phenytoin serum levels). Products include:
Pacerone Tablets 3337

Amitriptyline Hydrochloride (Tricyclic antidepressants may precipitate seizures in susceptible patients and phenytoin dosage may need to be adjusted).
No products indexed under this heading.

Amoxapine (Tricyclic antidepressants may precipitate seizures in susceptible patients and phenytoin dosage may need to be adjusted).
No products indexed under this heading.

Anisindione (Phenytoin impairs efficacy of oral anticoagulants). Products include:
Miradon Tablets 3056

Aspirin (May increase phenytoin serum levels). Products include:
Aggrenox Capsules 855
Bayer, Aspirin Regimen 606
Bayer Aspirin Tablets 3515
BC Powder 612
BC Allergy Sinus Cold Powder 612
Arthritis Strength BC Powder 612
BC Sinus Cold Powder 612
Ecotrin Enteric Coated Aspirin Low, Regular and Maximum Strength Tablets 1627
Goody's Body Pain Formula Powder 621
Goody's Extra Strength Headache Powder 621
Goody's Extra Strength Pain Relief Tablets 621
Percodan Tablets 1115
St. Joseph 81 mg Aspirin Chewable and Enteric Coated Tablets 1841

Aspirin, Enteric Coated (May increase phenytoin serum levels).
No products indexed under this heading.

Aspirin Buffered (May increase phenytoin serum levels).
No products indexed under this heading.

Betamethasone Acetate (Phenytoin impairs efficacy of corticosteroids).
No products indexed under this heading.

Betamethasone Sodium Phosphate (Phenytoin impairs efficacy of corticosteroids).
No products indexed under this heading.

Calcium Carbonate (Ingestion times of phenytoin and antacid preparations containing calcium should be staggered in patients with low phenytoin levels to prevent absorption problems). Products include:
Actonel with Calcium Tablets 2684
Caltrate 600 PLUS Chewables 779
Caltrate 600 PLUS Tablets 779
Caltrate 600 + D Tablets 779
Encora Capsules 3298
Encora AM Tablets 3298
Encora PM Tablets 3298
Gas-X with Maalox 675
Maalox Regular Strength Antacid Tablets 2166
Quick Dissolve Maalox Max Maximum Strength Antacid/Antigas Tablets 2165
Maalox Max Quick Dissolve Maximum Strength Chewable Tablets 678
Os-Cal Chewable Tablets 765
Pepcid Complete Chewable Tablets 1672
PremCal Light, Regular, and Extra Strength Tablets 762
Rolaids Tablets 707
Extra Strength Rolaids Softchews 708
Extra Strength Rolaids Tablets 707
Rolaids Multi-Symptom Antacid & Antigas Tablets 708
Tums 639

Carbamazepine (May increase phenytoin serum levels). Products include:
Carbatrol Capsules 3174
Equetro Extended-Release Capsules 3178
Tegretol/Tegretol-XR 2278

Chloramphenicol (May increase phenytoin serum levels).
No products indexed under this heading.

Chloramphenicol Palmitate (May increase phenytoin serum levels).
No products indexed under this heading.

Chloramphenicol Sodium Succinate (May increase phenytoin serum levels).
No products indexed under this heading.

Chlordiazepoxide (May increase phenytoin serum levels).
No products indexed under this heading.

Chlordiazepoxide Hydrochloride (May increase phenytoin serum levels). Products include:
Librium Capsules 3349

Chlorotrianisene (May increase phenytoin serum levels; phenytoin impairs efficacy of estrogens).
No products indexed under this heading.

Chlorpromazine (Phenothiazines may increase phenytoin serum levels).
No products indexed under this heading.

Chlorpromazine Hydrochloride (Phenothiazines may increase phenytoin serum levels).
No products indexed under this heading.

Choline Magnesium Trisalicylate (May increase phenytoin serum levels).
No products indexed under this heading.

Cimetidine (May increase phenytoin serum levels). Products include:
Tagamet HB 200 Tablets 637
Tagamet Tablets 1547

Cimetidine Hydrochloride (May increase phenytoin serum levels).
No products indexed under this heading.

Clomipramine Hydrochloride (Tricyclic antidepressants may precipitate seizures in susceptible patients and phenytoin dosage may need to be adjusted).
No products indexed under this heading.

Cortisone Acetate (Phenytoin impairs efficacy of corticosteroids).
No products indexed under this heading.

Desipramine Hydrochloride (Tricyclic antidepressants may precipitate seizures in susceptible patients and phenytoin dosage may need to be adjusted).
No products indexed under this heading.

Desogestrel (Phenytoin impairs efficacy of oral contraceptives). Products include:
Ortho-Cept Tablets 2395

Dexamethasone (Phenytoin impairs efficacy of corticosteroids). Products include:
Ciprodex Otic Suspension 555
Decadron Tablets 1929
TobraDex Ophthalmic Ointment 558
TobraDex Ophthalmic Suspension 558

Dexamethasone Acetate (Phenytoin impairs efficacy of corticosteroids).
No products indexed under this heading.

Dexamethasone Sodium Phosphate (Phenytoin impairs efficacy of corticosteroids). Products include:
Decadron Phosphate Injection 1931

Diazepam (May increase phenytoin serum levels). Products include:
Diastat Rectal Delivery System 3344
Valium Tablets 2822

Dicumarol (May increase phenytoin serum levels; phenytoin impairs efficacy of oral anticoagulants).
No products indexed under this heading.

Dienestrol (May increase phenytoin serum levels; phenytoin impairs efficacy of estrogens).
No products indexed under this heading.

Diethylstilbestrol (May increase phenytoin serum levels; phenytoin impairs efficacy of estrogens).
No products indexed under this heading.

Diflunisal (May increase phenytoin serum levels). Products include:
Dolobid Tablets 1937

Digitoxin (Phenytoin impairs efficacy of digitoxin).
No products indexed under this heading.

Disulfiram (May increase phenytoin serum levels). Products include:
Antabuse Tablets 2343

Divalproex Sodium (May decrease or increase phenytoin serum levels; the effect of phenytoin on valproate serum levels is unpredictable). Products include:
Depakote Sprinkle Capsules 422
Depakote Tablets 427
Depakote ER Tablets 433

Doxepin Hydrochloride (Tricyclic antidepressants may precipitate seizures in susceptible patients and phenytoin dosage may need to be adjusted).
No products indexed under this heading.

Doxycycline Calcium (Phenytoin impairs efficacy of doxycycline).
No products indexed under this heading.

Doxycycline Hyclate (Phenytoin impairs efficacy of doxycycline).
No products indexed under this heading.

Doxycycline Monohydrate (Phenytoin impairs efficacy of doxycycline).
No products indexed under this heading.

Dyphylline (Phenytoin impairs efficacy of theophylline).
No products indexed under this heading.

Estradiol (May increase phenytoin serum levels; phenytoin impairs efficacy of estrogens). Products include:
Activella Tablets 2311
Climara Transdermal System 795
Climara Pro Transdermal System 800
CombiPatch Transdermal System 2180
Estrogel 0.06% 3200
Menostar Transdermal System 805
Prefest Tablets 1069
Vagifem Tablets 2340
Vivelle Transdermal System 2288
Vivelle-Dot Transdermal System 2293

Estrogens, Conjugated (May increase phenytoin serum levels; phenytoin impairs efficacy of estrogens). Products include:
Premarin Intravenous 3440
Premarin Tablets 3443
Premarin Vaginal Cream 3449
Premphase Tablets 3452
Prempro Tablets 3452

Estrogens, Esterified (May increase phenytoin serum levels; phenytoin impairs efficacy of estrogens). Products include:
Estratest Tablets 3196
Estratest H.S. Tablets 3196

Estropipate (May increase phenytoin serum levels; phenytoin impairs efficacy of estrogens).
No products indexed under this heading.

Ethinyl Estradiol (May increase phenytoin serum levels; phenytoin impairs efficacy of estrogens).
Products include:
Alesse-28 Tablets 3392
Lo/Ovral-28 Tablets 3423
NuvaRing 2357
Ortho-Cept Tablets 2395
Ortho-Cyclen/Ortho Tri-Cyclen 2414
Ortho Evra Transdermal System 2402
Ortho Tri-Cyclen Lo Tablets 2421
Seasonale Tablets 1073
Triphasil-28 Tablets 3483
Yasmin 28 Tablets 818

Ethosuximide (May increase phenytoin serum levels).
No products indexed under this heading.

Ethynodiol Diacetate (Phenytoin impairs efficacy of oral contraceptives).
No products indexed under this heading.

Famotidine (May increase phenytoin serum levels). Products include:
Pepcid AC Chewable Tablets 1672
Pepcid AC Gelcaps 1672
Pepcid AC Tablets 1672
Maximum Strength Pepcid AC Tablets 1672
Pepcid Complete Chewable Tablets 1672
Pepcid Injection 2017
Pepcid 2014

Fludrocortisone Acetate (Phenytoin impairs efficacy of corticosteroids).
No products indexed under this heading.

Fluphenazine Decanoate (Phenothiazines may increase phenytoin serum levels).
No products indexed under this heading.

Fluphenazine Enanthate (Phenothiazines may increase phenytoin serum levels).
No products indexed under this heading.

Fluphenazine Hydrochloride (Phenothiazines may increase phenytoin serum levels).
No products indexed under this heading.

Furosemide (Phenytoin impairs efficacy of furosemide). Products include:
Furosemide Tablets 2117

Halothane (May increase phenytoin serum levels).
No products indexed under this heading.

Hydrocortisone (Phenytoin impairs efficacy of corticosteroids).
Products include:
Cortizone•5 Ointment .... ▣699
Cortizone•10 Creme .... ▣699
Cortizone•10 Ointment .... ▣699
Cortizone•10 Plus Creme .... ▣700
Cortizone•10 Maximum Strength Quick Shot Spray .... ▣700
Hydrocortone Tablets 1963
Preparation H Hydrocortisone Cream .... ▣748

Hydrocortisone Acetate (Phenytoin impairs efficacy of corticosteroids). Products include:
Analpram-HC 1136
Pramosone 1139
ProctoFoam-HC 3113
Tucks Anti-Itch Ointment .... ▣712
U-cort 1% Cream 3289

Hydrocortisone Sodium Phosphate (Phenytoin impairs efficacy of corticosteroids).
No products indexed under this heading.

Hydrocortisone Sodium Succinate (Phenytoin impairs efficacy of corticosteroids).
No products indexed under this heading.

Imipramine Hydrochloride (Tricyclic antidepressants may precipitate seizures in susceptible patients and phenytoin dosage may need to be adjusted).
No products indexed under this heading.

Imipramine Pamoate (Tricyclic antidepressants may precipitate seizures in susceptible patients and phenytoin dosage may need to be adjusted).
No products indexed under this heading.

Isoniazid (May increase phenytoin serum levels).
No products indexed under this heading.

Levonorgestrel (Phenytoin impairs efficacy of oral contraceptives).
Products include:
Alesse-28 Tablets 3392
Climara Pro Transdermal System 800
Mirena Intrauterine System 810
Plan B Tablets 1068
Seasonale Tablets 1073
Triphasil-28 Tablets 3483

Magnesium Salicylate (May increase phenytoin serum levels).
No products indexed under this heading.

Maprotiline Hydrochloride (Tricyclic antidepressants may precipitate seizures in susceptible patients and phenytoin dosage may need to be adjusted).
No products indexed under this heading.

Mesoridazine Besylate (Phenothiazines may increase phenytoin serum levels).
No products indexed under this heading.

Mestranol (Phenytoin impairs efficacy of oral contraceptives).
No products indexed under this heading.

Methotrimeprazine (Phenothiazines may increase phenytoin serum levels).
No products indexed under this heading.

Methsuximide (May increase phenytoin serum levels).
No products indexed under this heading.

Methylphenidate Hydrochloride (May increase phenytoin serum levels). Products include:
Concerta Extended-Release Tablets 1828
Metadate CD Capsules 3316
Ritalin 2254
Ritalin LA Capsules 2255

Methylprednisolone Acetate (Phenytoin impairs efficacy of corticosteroids). Products include:
Depo-Medrol Injectable Suspension 2615
Depo-Medrol Single-Dose Vial 2617

Methylprednisolone Sodium Succinate (Phenytoin impairs efficacy of corticosteroids).
No products indexed under this heading.

Molindone Hydrochloride (Contains calcium ions which may decrease phenytoin serum levels).
Products include:
Moban Tablets 1108

Nizatidine (May increase phenytoin serum levels). Products include:
Axid Oral Solution 913

Norethindrone (Phenytoin impairs efficacy of oral contraceptives).
Products include:
Ortho Micronor Tablets 2411

Norethynodrel (Phenytoin impairs efficacy of oral contraceptives).
No products indexed under this heading.

Norgestimate (Phenytoin impairs efficacy of oral contraceptives).
Products include:
Ortho-Cyclen/Ortho Tri-Cyclen 2414
Ortho Tri-Cyclen Lo Tablets 2421
Prefest Tablets 1069

Norgestrel (Phenytoin impairs efficacy of oral contraceptives).
Products include:
Lo/Ovral-28 Tablets 3423

Nortriptyline Hydrochloride (Tricyclic antidepressants may precipitate seizures in susceptible patients and phenytoin dosage may need to be adjusted).
No products indexed under this heading.

Perphenazine (Phenothiazines may increase phenytoin serum levels).
No products indexed under this heading.

Phenobarbital (May decrease or increase phenytoin serum levels; the effect of phenytoin on phenobarbital serum levels is unpredictable).
No products indexed under this heading.

Phensuximide (May increase phenytoin serum levels).
No products indexed under this heading.

Phenylbutazone (May increase phenytoin serum levels).
No products indexed under this heading.

Polyestradiol Phosphate (May increase phenytoin serum levels; phenytoin impairs efficacy of estrogens).
No products indexed under this heading.

Prednisolone Acetate (Phenytoin impairs efficacy of corticosteroids).
Products include:
Blephamide Ophthalmic Ointment 563
Blephamide Ophthalmic Suspension 564
Poly-Pred Liquifilm Ophthalmic Suspension .... ⊙231
Pred Forte Ophthalmic Suspension .... ⊙233
Pred Mild Sterile Ophthalmic Suspension .... ⊙236
Pred-G Ophthalmic Suspension .... ⊙234
Pred-G Sterile Ophthalmic Ointment .... ⊙235

Prednisolone Sodium Phosphate (Phenytoin impairs efficacy of corticosteroids). Products include:
Pediapred Oral Solution 3319

Prednisolone Tebutate (Phenytoin impairs efficacy of corticosteroids).
No products indexed under this heading.

Prednisone (Phenytoin impairs efficacy of corticosteroids).
No products indexed under this heading.

Prochlorperazine (Phenothiazines may increase phenytoin serum levels).
No products indexed under this heading.

Promethazine Hydrochloride (Phenothiazines may increase phenytoin serum levels). Products include:
Phenergan 3438

Protriptyline Hydrochloride (Tricyclic antidepressants may precipitate seizures in susceptible patients and phenytoin dosage may need to be adjusted). Products include:
Vivactil Tablets 2350

Quinestrol (May increase phenytoin serum levels; phenytoin impairs efficacy of estrogens).
No products indexed under this heading.

Quinidine (Phenytoin impairs efficacy of quinidine).
No products indexed under this heading.

Quinidine Gluconate (Phenytoin impairs efficacy of quinidine).
No products indexed under this heading.

Quinidine Hydrochloride (Phenytoin impairs efficacy of quinidine).
No products indexed under this heading.

Quinidine Polygalacturonate (Phenytoin impairs efficacy of quinidine).
No products indexed under this heading.

Quinidine Sulfate (Phenytoin impairs efficacy of quinidine).
No products indexed under this heading.

Ranitidine Bismuth Citrate (May increase phenytoin serum levels).
No products indexed under this heading.

Ranitidine Hydrochloride (May increase phenytoin serum levels).
Products include:
Zantac 1597
Zantac Injection 1593
Zantac 75 Tablets .... ▣715
Zantac 150 Maximum Strength Tablets .... ▣715
Zantac Injection Pharmacy Bulk Package 1595

Reserpine (May increase phenytoin serum levels).
No products indexed under this heading.

Rifampin (Phenytoin impairs efficacy of rifampin).
No products indexed under this heading.

Salsalate (May increase phenytoin serum levels).
No products indexed under this heading.

Sucralfate (May increase phenytoin serum levels). Products include:
Carafate Suspension 727
Carafate Tablets 728

Sulfamethizole (May increase phenytoin serum levels).
No products indexed under this heading.

Sulfamethoxazole (May increase phenytoin serum levels).
No products indexed under this heading.

Sulfisoxazole Acetyl (May increase phenytoin serum levels).
No products indexed under this heading.

Theophylline (Phenytoin impairs efficacy of theophylline).
No products indexed under this heading.

Theophylline Anhydrous (Phenytoin impairs efficacy of theophylline). Products include:
Uniphyl Tablets 2708

Theophylline Calcium Salicylate (Phenytoin impairs efficacy of theophylline).
No products indexed under this heading.

Theophylline Dihydroxypropyl (Glyceryl) (Phenytoin impairs efficacy of theophylline).
No products indexed under this heading.

Theophylline Ethylenediamine (Phenytoin impairs efficacy of theophylline).
No products indexed under this heading.

Theophylline Sodium Glycinate (Phenytoin impairs efficacy of theophylline).
No products indexed under this heading.

Thioridazine Hydrochloride (Phenothiazines may increase phenytoin serum levels). Products include:
Thioridazine Hydrochloride Tablets 2122

Tolbutamide (May increase phenytoin serum levels).
No products indexed under this heading.

Trazodone Hydrochloride (May increase phenytoin serum levels).
No products indexed under this heading.

Triamcinolone (Phenytoin impairs efficacy of corticosteroids).
No products indexed under this heading.

Triamcinolone Acetonide (Phenytoin impairs efficacy of corticosteroids). Products include:
Azmacort Inhalation Aerosol 1701
Nasacort HFA Inhalation Aerosol 2939
Nasacort AQ Nasal Spray 2937

Triamcinolone Diacetate (Phenytoin impairs efficacy of corticosteroids).
No products indexed under this heading.

Triamcinolone Hexacetonide (Phenytoin impairs efficacy of corticosteroids).
No products indexed under this heading.

Trifluoperazine Hydrochloride (Phenothiazines may increase phenytoin serum levels).
No products indexed under this heading.

Trimipramine Maleate (Tricyclic antidepressants may precipitate seizures in susceptible patients and phenytoin dosage may need to be adjusted). Products include:
Surmontil Capsules 2347

Valproate Sodium (May decrease or increase phenytoin serum levels; the effect of phenytoin on valproate serum levels is unpredictable). Products include:
Depacon Injection 412

Valproic Acid (May decrease or increase phenytoin serum levels; the effect of phenytoin on valproate serum levels is unpredictable). Products include:
Depakene 417

Vitamin D (Phenytoin impairs efficacy of vitamin D). Products include:
Active Calcium Tablets 3342
Caltrate 600 PLUS Chewables 779
Caltrate 600 PLUS Tablets 779
Caltrate 600 + D Tablets 779
Os-Cal 250 + D Tablets 765
Os-Cal 500 + D Tablets 766

Warfarin Sodium (Phenytoin impairs efficacy of oral anticoagulants). Products include:
Coumadin for Injection 932
Coumadin Tablets 932

Food Interactions

Alcohol (Acute alcohol intake may increase phenytoin serum levels; chronic alcohol abuse may decrease phenytoin serum levels).

PHOSLO GELCAPS

(Calcium Acetate) 2158
May interact with calcium preparations, cardiac glycosides, tetracyclines, and certain other agents. Compounds in these categories include:

Antacids, unspecified (Concurrent use should be avoided).
No products indexed under this heading.

Calcium Carbonate (Potential for increased risk of hypercalcemia; concurrent use with other calcium supplements is not recommended). Products include:
Actonel with Calcium Tablets 2684
Caltrate 600 PLUS Chewables 779
Caltrate 600 PLUS Tablets 779
Caltrate 600 + D Tablets 779
Encora Capsules 3298
Encora AM Tablets 3298
Encora PM Tablets 3298
Gas-X with Maalox 675
Maalox Regular Strength Antacid Tablets 2166
Quick Dissolve Maalox Max Maximum Strength Antacid/Antigas Tablets 2165
Maalox Max Quick Dissolve Maximum Strength Chewable Tablets 678
Os-Cal Chewable Tablets 765
Pepcid Complete Chewable Tablets 1672
PremCal Light, Regular, and Extra Strength Tablets 762
Rolaids Tablets 707
Extra Strength Rolaids Softchews 708
Extra Strength Rolaids Tablets 707
Rolaids Multi-Symptom Antacid & Antigas Tablets 708
Tums 639

Calcium Chloride (Potential for increased risk of hypercalcemia; concurrent use with other calcium supplements is not recommended).
No products indexed under this heading.

Calcium Citrate (Potential for increased risk of hypercalcemia; concurrent use with other calcium supplements is not recommended). Products include:
Active Calcium Tablets 3342
Citracal Tablets 2108

Calcium Glubionate (Potential for increased risk of hypercalcemia; concurrent use with other calcium supplements is not recommended).
No products indexed under this heading.

Demeclocycline Hydrochloride (Bioavailability of oral tetracyclines may be decreased).
No products indexed under this heading.

Deslanoside (Hypercalcemia may precipitate cardiac arrhythmia).
No products indexed under this heading.

Digitalis Glycoside Preparations (Hypercalcemia may precipitate cardiac arrhythmia).
No products indexed under this heading.

Digitoxin (Hypercalcemia may precipitate cardiac arrhythmia).
No products indexed under this heading.

Digoxin (Hypercalcemia may precipitate cardiac arrhythmia). Products include:
Digitek Tablets 2146
Lanoxicaps Capsules 1458
Lanoxin Injection 1462
Lanoxin Tablets 1468
Lanoxin Injection Pediatric 1465

Doxycycline Calcium (Bioavailability of oral tetracyclines may be decreased).
No products indexed under this heading.

Doxycycline Hyclate (Bioavailability of oral tetracyclines may be decreased).
No products indexed under this heading.

Doxycycline Monohydrate (Bioavailability of oral tetracyclines may be decreased).
No products indexed under this heading.

Methacycline Hydrochloride (Bioavailability of oral tetracyclines may be decreased).
No products indexed under this heading.

Minocycline Hydrochloride (Bioavailability of oral tetracyclines may be decreased). Products include:
Dynacin Tablets 1859

Oxytetracycline Hydrochloride (Bioavailability of oral tetracyclines may be decreased).
No products indexed under this heading.

Tetracycline Hydrochloride (Bioavailability of oral tetracyclines may be decreased).
No products indexed under this heading.

PHOTOFRIN FOR INJECTION

(Porfimer Sodium) 729
May interact with calcium channel blockers, glucocorticoids, drugs known to be photosensitizers, inhibitors of endogenous prostaglandin synthesis, and certain other agents. Compounds in these categories include:

Acetazolamide (Co-administration with other photosensitizing agents could increase the photosensitivity reactions).
No products indexed under this heading.

Acitretin (Co-administration with other photosensitizing agents could increase the photosensitivity reactions). Products include:
Soriatane Capsules 1028

Alatrofloxacin Mesylate (Co-administration with other photosensitizing agents could increase the photosensitivity reactions).
No products indexed under this heading.

Allopurinol (Could interfere with porfimer photodynamic therapy).
No products indexed under this heading.

Amlodipine Besylate (Could interfere with porfimer photodynamic therapy). Products include:
Caduet Tablets 2507
Lotrel Capsules 2238
Norvasc Tablets 2529

Anthralin (Co-administration with other photosensitizing agents could increase the photosensitivity reactions). Products include:
Psoriatec Cream 3191

Aspirin (Some prostaglandin synthesis inhibitors could interfere with porfimer photodynamic therapy). Products include:
Aggrenox Capsules 855
Bayer, Aspirin Regimen 606
Bayer Aspirin Tablets 3515
BC Powder 612
BC Allergy Sinus Cold Powder 612
Arthritis Strength BC Powder 612
BC Sinus Cold Powder 612
Ecotrin Enteric Coated Aspirin Low, Regular and Maximum Strength Tablets 1627
Goody's Body Pain Formula Powder 621
Goody's Extra Strength Headache Powder 621
Goody's Extra Strength Pain Relief Tablets 621
Percodan Tablets 1115
St. Joseph 81 mg Aspirin Chewable and Enteric Coated Tablets 1841

Bendroflumethiazide (Co-administration with other photosensitizing agents could increase the photosensitivity reactions).
No products indexed under this heading.

Bepridil Hydrochloride (Could interfere with porfimer photodynamic therapy).
No products indexed under this heading.

Beta-Carotene (Compounds that quench active oxygen species or scavenge radicals, such as b-carotene, would be expected to decrease photodynamic therapy; no human data available to support or rebut this possibility).
No products indexed under this heading.

Betamethasone Acetate (Glucocorticoid hormone given before or concomitantly with photodynamic therapy may decrease the efficacy of the treatment).
No products indexed under this heading.

Betamethasone Sodium Phosphate (Glucocorticoid hormone given before or concomitantly with photodynamic therapy may decrease the efficacy of the treatment).
No products indexed under this heading.

Celecoxib (Some prostaglandin synthesis inhibitors could interfere with porfimer photodynamic therapy). Products include:
Celebrex Capsules 3130

Chlorothiazide (Co-administration with other photosensitizing agents could increase the photosensitivity reactions). Products include:
Aldoclor Tablets 1881
Diuril Oral 1936

Chlorothiazide Sodium (Co-administration with other photosensitizing agents could increase the photosensitivity reactions). Products include:
Diuril Sodium Intravenous 1934

Chlorpromazine (Co-administration with other photosensitizing agents could increase the photosensitivity reactions).
No products indexed under this heading.

Chlorpromazine Hydrochloride (Co-administration with other photosensitizing agents could increase the photosensitivity reactions).
No products indexed under this heading.

Chlorpropamide (Co-administration with other photosensitizing agents could increase the photosensitivity reactions).
No products indexed under this heading.

Ciprofloxacin (Co-administration with other photosensitizing agents could increase the photosensitivity reactions). Products include:
- Cipro I.V. ... 2998
- Cipro I.V. Pharmacy Bulk Package ... 3509
- Cipro Oral Suspension ... 2991
- Cipro XR Tablets ... 3004
- Ciprodex Otic Suspension ... 555

Ciprofloxacin Hydrochloride (Co-administration with other photosensitizing agents could increase the photosensitivity reactions). Products include:
- Ciloxan Ophthalmic Ointment ... 554
- Cipro Tablets ... 2991

Coal Tar (Co-administration with other photosensitizing agents could increase the photosensitivity reactions). Products include:
- Tegrin Dandruff Shampoo - Extra Conditioning ... ■637
- Tegrin Dandruff Shampoo - Fresh Herbal ... ■638
- Tegrin Skin Cream ... ■638

Cortisone Acetate (Glucocorticoid hormone given before or concomitantly with photodynamic therapy may decrease the efficacy of the treatment).
No products indexed under this heading.

Demeclocycline Hydrochloride (Co-administration with other photosensitizing agents could increase the photosensitivity reactions).
No products indexed under this heading.

Dexamethasone (Glucocorticoid hormone given before or concomitantly with photodynamic therapy may decrease the efficacy of the treatment). Products include:
- Ciprodex Otic Suspension ... 555
- Decadron Tablets ... 1929
- TobraDex Ophthalmic Ointment ... 558
- TobraDex Ophthalmic Suspension ... 558

Dexamethasone Acetate (Glucocorticoid hormone given before or concomitantly with photodynamic therapy may decrease the efficacy of the treatment).
No products indexed under this heading.

Dexamethasone Sodium Phosphate (Glucocorticoid hormone given before or concomitantly with photodynamic therapy may decrease the efficacy of the treatment). Products include:
- Decadron Phosphate Injection ... 1931

Diclofenac Potassium (Some prostaglandin synthesis inhibitors could interfere with porfimer photodynamic therapy). Products include:
- Cataflam Tablets ... 2173

Diclofenac Sodium (Some prostaglandin synthesis inhibitors could interfere with porfimer photodynamic therapy). Products include:
- Arthrotec Tablets ... 3126
- Voltaren Ophthalmic Solution ... 2300
- Voltaren Tablets ... 2298
- Voltaren-XR Tablets ... 2301

Diltiazem Hydrochloride (Could interfere with porfimer photodynamic therapy). Products include:
- Cardizem LA Extended Release Tablets ... 1699
- Tiazac Capsules ... 1204

Dimethyl Sulfoxide (Compounds that quench active oxygen species or scavenge radicals, such as DMSO, would be expected to decrease photodynamic therapy; no human data available to support or rebut this possibility).
No products indexed under this heading.

Doxycycline Calcium (Co-administration with other photosensitizing agents could increase the photosensitivity reactions).
No products indexed under this heading.

Doxycycline Hyclate (Co-administration with other photosensitizing agents could increase the photosensitivity reactions).
No products indexed under this heading.

Doxycycline Monohydrate (Co-administration with other photosensitizing agents could increase the photosensitivity reactions).
No products indexed under this heading.

Enoxacin (Co-administration with other photosensitizing agents could increase the photosensitivity reactions).
No products indexed under this heading.

Felodipine (Could interfere with porfimer photodynamic therapy). Products include:
- Plendil Extended-Release Tablets ... 651

Fenoprofen Calcium (Some prostaglandin synthesis inhibitors could interfere with porfimer photodynamic therapy). Products include:
- Nalfon Capsules ... 2504

Fludrocortisone Acetate (Glucocorticoid hormone given before or concomitantly with photodynamic therapy may decrease the efficacy of the treatment).
No products indexed under this heading.

Fluphenazine Decanoate (Co-administration with other photosensitizing agents could increase the photosensitivity reactions).
No products indexed under this heading.

Fluphenazine Enanthate (Co-administration with other photosensitizing agents could increase the photosensitivity reactions).
No products indexed under this heading.

Fluphenazine Hydrochloride (Co-administration with other photosensitizing agents could increase the photosensitivity reactions).
No products indexed under this heading.

Flurbiprofen (Some prostaglandin synthesis inhibitors could interfere with porfimer photodynamic therapy).
No products indexed under this heading.

Furosemide (Co-administration with other photosensitizing agents could increase the photosensitivity reactions). Products include:
- Furosemide Tablets ... 2117

Glipizide (Co-administration with other photosensitizing agents could increase the photosensitivity reactions).
No products indexed under this heading.

Glyburide (Co-administration with other photosensitizing agents could increase the photosensitivity reactions).
No products indexed under this heading.

Grepafloxacin Hydrochloride (Co-administration with other photosensitizing agents could increase the photosensitivity reactions).
No products indexed under this heading.

Griseofulvin (Co-administration with other photosensitizing agents could increase the photosensitivity reactions). Products include:
- Grifulvin V Tablets Microsize and Oral Suspension Microsize ... 2384
- Gris-PEG Tablets ... 2504

Hydrochlorothiazide (Co-administration with other photosensitizing agents could increase the photosensitivity reactions). Products include:
- Aldoril Tablets ... 1884
- Atacand HCT ... 637
- Avalide Tablets ... 2889
- Avalide Tablets ... 922
- Benicar HCT Tablets ... 2852
- Diovan HCT Tablets ... 2195
- Dyazide Capsules ... 1389
- Hyzaar ... 1964
- Lotensin HCT Tablets ... 2235
- Maxzide ... 2150
- Micardis HCT Tablets ... 886
- Moduretic Tablets ... 2003
- Prinzide Tablets ... 2033
- Teveten HCT Tablets ... 1710
- Timolide Tablets ... 2056
- Uniretic Tablets ... 3114
- Vaseretic Tablets ... 2073
- Zestoretic Tablets ... 701

Hydrocortisone (Glucocorticoid hormone given before or concomitantly with photodynamic therapy may decrease the efficacy of the treatment). Products include:
- Cortizone•5 Ointment ... ■699
- Cortizone•10 Creme ... ■699
- Cortizone•10 Ointment ... ■699
- Cortizone•10 Plus Creme ... ■700
- Cortizone•10 Maximum Strength Quick Shot Spray ... ■700
- Hydrocortone Tablets ... 1963
- Preparation H Hydrocortisone Cream ... ■748

Hydrocortisone Acetate (Glucocorticoid hormone given before or concomitantly with photodynamic therapy may decrease the efficacy of the treatment). Products include:
- Analpram-HC ... 1136
- Pramosone ... 1139
- ProctoFoam-HC ... 3113
- Tucks Anti-Itch Ointment ... ■712
- U-cort 1% Cream ... 3289

Hydrocortisone Sodium Phosphate (Glucocorticoid hormone given before or concomitantly with photodynamic therapy may decrease the efficacy of the treatment).
No products indexed under this heading.

Hydrocortisone Sodium Succinate (Glucocorticoid hormone given before or concomitantly with photodynamic therapy may decrease the efficacy of the treatment).
No products indexed under this heading.

Hydroflumethiazide (Co-administration with other photosensitizing agents could increase the photosensitivity reactions).
No products indexed under this heading.

Ibuprofen (Some prostaglandin synthesis inhibitors could interfere with porfimer photodynamic therapy). Products include:
- Advil Allergy Sinus Caplets ... ■737
- Advil ... ■737
- Children's Advil Suspension ... ■742
- Children's Advil Chewable Tablets ... ■741
- Advil Cold & Sinus ... ■739
- Advil Flu & Body Ache Caplets ... ■739
- Children's Advil Cold Suspension ... ■741
- Infants' Advil Concentrated Drops ... ■743
- Junior Strength Advil Swallow Tablets ... ■740
- Advil Migraine Liquigels ... ■740
- Advil Multi-Symptom Cold Caplets ... ■738
- Combunox Tablets ... 1183
- Children's Motrin Oral Suspension and Chewable Tablets ... 1837
- Children's Motrin Cold Non-Staining Dye-Free Oral Suspension ... 1838
- Children's Motrin Cold Oral Suspension ... 1838
- Children's Motrin Non-Staining Dye-Free Oral Suspension ... 1837
- Motrin Cold & Sinus Caplets ... 1836
- Motrin IB Tablets and Caplets ... 1836
- Infants' Motrin Concentrated Drops ... 1837
- Infants' Motrin Non-Staining Dye-Free Drops ... 1837
- Junior Strength Motrin Caplets and Chewable Tablets ... 1837
- Vicoprofen Tablets ... 533

Indomethacin (Some prostaglandin synthesis inhibitors could interfere with porfimer photodynamic therapy). Products include:
- Indocin ... 1968

Indomethacin Sodium Trihydrate (Some prostaglandin synthesis inhibitors could interfere with porfimer photodynamic therapy). Products include:
- Indocin I.V. ... 1973

Isradipine (Could interfere with porfimer photodynamic therapy). Products include:
- DynaCirc CR Tablets ... 2726

Ketoprofen (Some prostaglandin synthesis inhibitors could interfere with porfimer photodynamic therapy).
No products indexed under this heading.

Lomefloxacin Hydrochloride (Co-administration with other photosensitizing agents could increase the photosensitivity reactions).
No products indexed under this heading.

Mannitol (Compounds that quench active oxygen species or scavenge radicals, such as mannitol, would be expected to decrease photodynamic therapy; no human data available to support or rebut this possibility). Products include:
- Trident White Sugarless Gum ... ■611

Meclofenamate Sodium (Some prostaglandin synthesis inhibitors could interfere with porfimer photodynamic therapy).
No products indexed under this heading.

Mefenamic Acid (Some prostaglandin synthesis inhibitors could interfere with porfimer photodynamic therapy).
No products indexed under this heading.

Mesoridazine Besylate (Co-administration with other photosensitizing agents could increase the photosensitivity reactions).
No products indexed under this heading.

Metabromsalan (Co-administration with other photosensitizing agents could increase the photosensitivity reactions).
No products indexed under this heading.

Methacycline Hydrochloride (Co-administration with other photosensitizing agents could increase the photosensitivity reactions).
No products indexed under this heading.

Methotrimeprazine (Co-administration with other photosensitizing agents could increase the photosensitivity reactions).
No products indexed under this heading.

Methyclothiazide (Co-administration with other photosensitizing agents could increase the photosensitivity reactions).
No products indexed under this heading.

Methylprednisolone Acetate (Glucocorticoid hormone given before or concomitantly with photodynamic therapy may decrease the efficacy of the treatment). Products include:
Depo-Medrol Injectable Suspension 2615
Depo-Medrol Single-Dose Vial 2617

Methylprednisolone Sodium Succinate (Glucocorticoid hormone given before or concomitantly with photodynamic therapy may decrease the efficacy of the treatment).
No products indexed under this heading.

Mibefradil Dihydrochloride (Could interfere with porfimer photodynamic therapy).
No products indexed under this heading.

Minocycline Hydrochloride (Co-administration with other photosensitizing agents could increase the photosensitivity reactions). Products include:
Dynacin Tablets 1859

Nalidixic Acid (Co-administration with other photosensitizing agents could increase the photosensitivity reactions).
No products indexed under this heading.

Naproxen (Some prostaglandin synthesis inhibitors could interfere with porfimer photodynamic therapy). Products include:
EC-Naprosyn Delayed-Release Tablets 2769
Naprosyn Suspension 2769
Naprosyn Tablets 2769
Prevacid NapraPAC 3277

Naproxen Sodium (Some prostaglandin synthesis inhibitors could interfere with porfimer photodynamic therapy). Products include:
Aleve Tablets, Caplets and Gelcaps 605
Anaprox Tablets 2769
Anaprox DS Tablets 2769

Nicardipine Hydrochloride (Could interfere with porfimer photodynamic therapy). Products include:
Cardene I.V. 1129

Nifedipine (Could interfere with porfimer photodynamic therapy). Products include:
Adalat CC Tablets 2978

Nimodipine (Could interfere with porfimer photodynamic therapy). Products include:
Nimotop Capsules 774

Nisoldipine (Could interfere with porfimer photodynamic therapy). Products include:
Sular Tablets 1163

Norfloxacin (Co-administration with other photosensitizing agents could increase the photosensitivity reactions). Products include:
Noroxin Tablets 2009

Ofloxacin (Co-administration with other photosensitizing agents could increase the photosensitivity reactions). Products include:
Floxin Otic Singles 1045
Floxin Otic Solution 1043

Oxytetracycline Hydrochloride (Co-administration with other photosensitizing agents could increase the photosensitivity reactions).
No products indexed under this heading.

Perphenazine (Co-administration with other photosensitizing agents could increase the photosensitivity reactions).
No products indexed under this heading.

Phenylbutazone (Some prostaglandin synthesis inhibitors could interfere with porfimer photodynamic therapy).
No products indexed under this heading.

Piroxicam (Some prostaglandin synthesis inhibitors could interfere with porfimer photodynamic therapy).
No products indexed under this heading.

Polythiazide (Co-administration with other photosensitizing agents could increase the photosensitivity reactions).
No products indexed under this heading.

Prednisolone Acetate (Glucocorticoid hormone given before or concomitantly with photodynamic therapy may decrease the efficacy of the treatment). Products include:
Blephamide Ophthalmic Ointment 563
Blephamide Ophthalmic Suspension 564
Poly-Pred Liquifilm Ophthalmic Suspension .... ⊙231
Pred Forte Ophthalmic Suspension .... ⊙233
Pred Mild Sterile Ophthalmic Suspension .... ⊙236
Pred-G Ophthalmic Suspension .... ⊙234
Pred-G Sterile Ophthalmic Ointment .... ⊙235

Prednisolone Sodium Phosphate (Glucocorticoid hormone given before or concomitantly with photodynamic therapy may decrease the efficacy of the treatment). Products include:
Pediapred Oral Solution 3319

Prednisolone Tebutate (Glucocorticoid hormone given before or concomitantly with photodynamic therapy may decrease the efficacy of the treatment).
No products indexed under this heading.

Prednisone (Glucocorticoid hormone given before or concomitantly with photodynamic therapy may decrease the efficacy of the treatment).
No products indexed under this heading.

Prochlorperazine (Co-administration with other photosensitizing agents could increase the photosensitivity reactions).
No products indexed under this heading.

Promethazine Hydrochloride (Co-administration with other photosensitizing agents could increase the photosensitivity reactions). Products include:
Phenergan 3438

Sulfamethizole (Co-administration with other photosensitizing agents could increase the photosensitivity reactions).
No products indexed under this heading.

Sulfamethoxazole (Co-administration with other photosensitizing agents could increase the photosensitivity reactions).
No products indexed under this heading.

Sulfasalazine (Co-administration with other photosensitizing agents could increase the photosensitivity reactions).
No products indexed under this heading.

Sulfinpyrazone (Co-administration with other photosensitizing agents could increase the photosensitivity reactions).
No products indexed under this heading.

Sulfisoxazole (Co-administration with other photosensitizing agents could increase the photosensitivity reactions).
No products indexed under this heading.

Sulfisoxazole Acetyl (Co-administration with other photosensitizing agents could increase the photosensitivity reactions).
No products indexed under this heading.

Sulfisoxazole Diolamine (Co-administration with other photosensitizing agents could increase the photosensitivity reactions).
No products indexed under this heading.

Sulindac (Some prostaglandin synthesis inhibitors could interfere with porfimer photodynamic therapy). Products include:
Clinoril Tablets 1899

Tetrachlorosalicylanilide (Co-administration with other photosensitizing agents could increase the photosensitivity reactions).
No products indexed under this heading.

Tetracycline Hydrochloride (Co-administration with other photosensitizing agents could increase the photosensitivity reactions).
No products indexed under this heading.

Thioridazine Hydrochloride (Co-administration with other photosensitizing agents could increase the photosensitivity reactions). Products include:
Thioridazine Hydrochloride Tablets 2122

Tolazamide (Co-administration with other photosensitizing agents could increase the photosensitivity reactions).
No products indexed under this heading.

Tolbutamide (Co-administration with other photosensitizing agents could increase the photosensitivity reactions).
No products indexed under this heading.

Tolmetin Sodium (Some prostaglandin synthesis inhibitors could interfere with porfimer photodynamic therapy).
No products indexed under this heading.

Triamcinolone (Glucocorticoid hormone given before or concomitantly with photodynamic therapy may decrease the efficacy of the treatment).
No products indexed under this heading.

Triamcinolone Acetonide (Glucocorticoid hormone given before or concomitantly with photodynamic therapy may decrease the efficacy of the treatment). Products include:
Azmacort Inhalation Aerosol 1701
Nasacort HFA Inhalation Aerosol 2939
Nasacort AQ Nasal Spray 2937

Triamcinolone Diacetate (Glucocorticoid hormone given before or concomitantly with photodynamic therapy may decrease the efficacy of the treatment).
No products indexed under this heading.

Triamcinolone Hexacetonide (Glucocorticoid hormone given before or concomitantly with photodynamic therapy may decrease the efficacy of the treatment).
No products indexed under this heading.

Trifluoperazine Hydrochloride (Co-administration with other photosensitizing agents could increase the photosensitivity reactions).
No products indexed under this heading.

Trovafloxacin Mesylate (Co-administration with other photosensitizing agents could increase the photosensitivity reactions).
No products indexed under this heading.

Verapamil Hydrochloride (Could interfere with porfimer photodynamic therapy). Products include:
Covera-HS Tablets 3135
Tarka Tablets 519
Verelan PM Capsules 3120

Food Interactions

Alcohol (Compounds that quench active oxygen species or scavenge radicals, such as ethanol, would be expected to decrease photodynamic therapy; no human data available to support or rebut this possibility).

PLAN B TABLETS
(Levonorgestrel) 1068
May interact with barbiturates and hepatic microsomal enzyme inducers. Compounds in these categories include:

Aprobarbital (Hepatic enzyme-inducing drugs (e.g., barbiturates) may reduce the effectiveness of low-dose progestin-only pills).
No products indexed under this heading.

Butabarbital (Hepatic enzyme-inducing drugs (e.g., barbiturates) may reduce the effectiveness of low-dose progestin-only pills).
No products indexed under this heading.

Butalbital (Hepatic enzyme-inducing drugs (e.g., barbiturates) may reduce the effectiveness of low-dose progestin-only pills). Products include:
Sedapap Tablets 50 mg/650 mg 2098

Carbamazepine (Hepatic enzyme-inducing drugs may reduce the effectiveness of low-dose progestin-only pills). Products include:
Carbatrol Capsules 3174
Equetro Extended-Release Capsules 3178
Tegretol/Tegretol-XR 2278

Chlorpropamide (Hepatic enzyme-inducing drugs may reduce the effectiveness of low-dose progestin-only pills).
No products indexed under this heading.

Ethanol (Hepatic enzyme-inducing drugs may reduce the effectiveness of low-dose progestin-only pills).
No products indexed under this heading.

Fosphenytoin Sodium (Hepatic enzyme-inducing drugs may reduce the effectiveness of low-dose progestin-only pills).
No products indexed under this heading.

Glipizide (Hepatic enzyme-inducing drugs may reduce the effectiveness of low-dose progestin-only pills).
No products indexed under this heading.

Glyburide (Hepatic enzyme-inducing drugs may reduce the effectiveness of low-dose progestin-only pills).
No products indexed under this heading.

Mephobarbital (Hepatic enzyme-inducing drugs (e.g., barbiturates) may reduce the effectiveness of low-dose progestin-only pills). Products include:
Mebaral Tablets, USP 2483

Pentobarbital Sodium (Hepatic enzyme-inducing drugs (e.g., barbiturates) may reduce the effectiveness of low-dose progestin-only pills).
Products include:
Nembutal Sodium Solution, USP 2484

Phenobarbital (Hepatic enzyme-inducing drugs may reduce the effectiveness of low-dose progestin-only pills).
No products indexed under this heading.

Phenylbutazone (Hepatic enzyme-inducing drugs may reduce the effectiveness of low-dose progestin-only pills).
No products indexed under this heading.

Phenytoin (Hepatic enzyme-inducing drugs may reduce the effectiveness of low-dose progestin-only pills).
No products indexed under this heading.

Phenytoin Sodium (Hepatic enzyme-inducing drugs may reduce the effectiveness of low-dose progestin-only pills). Products include:
Phenytek Capsules 2153

Rifampin (Hepatic enzyme-inducing drugs may reduce the effectiveness of low-dose progestin-only pills).
No products indexed under this heading.

Rifapentine (Hepatic enzyme-inducing drugs may reduce the effectiveness of low-dose progestin-only pills).
No products indexed under this heading.

Secobarbital Sodium (Hepatic enzyme-inducing drugs (e.g., barbiturates) may reduce the effectiveness of low-dose progestin-only pills).
No products indexed under this heading.

Thiamylal Sodium (Hepatic enzyme-inducing drugs (e.g., barbiturates) may reduce the effectiveness of low-dose progestin-only pills).
No products indexed under this heading.

Tolazamide (Hepatic enzyme-inducing drugs may reduce the effectiveness of low-dose progestin-only pills).
No products indexed under this heading.

Tolbutamide (Hepatic enzyme-inducing drugs may reduce the effectiveness of low-dose progestin-only pills).
No products indexed under this heading.

PLASBUMIN-5
(Albumin (human)) 3249
None cited in PDR database.

PLASBUMIN-20
(Albumin (human)) 3249
None cited in PDR database.

PLASBUMIN-25
(Albumin (human)) 3251
None cited in PDR database.

PLASMANATE
(Plasma Protein Fraction (Human)) 3252
None cited in PDR database.

PLAVIX TABLETS
(Clopidogrel Bisulfate) 940
May interact with aspirin-acetylsalicylic acid, non-steroidal anti-inflammatory agents, phenytoin, and certain other agents. Compounds in these categories include:

Aspirin (Clopidogrel potentiates the effect of aspirin on collagen-induced platelet aggregation; co-administration did not significantly increase the prolongation of bleeding time induced by clopidogrel but has increased major bleeding). Products include:
Aggrenox Capsules 855
Bayer, Aspirin Regimen .... ▣606
Bayer Aspirin Tablets 3515
BC Powder .... ▣612
BC Allergy Sinus Cold Powder .... ▣612
Arthritis Strength BC Powder .... ▣612
BC Sinus Cold Powder .... ▣612
Ecotrin Enteric Coated Aspirin Low, Regular and Maximum Strength Tablets 1627
Goody's Body Pain Formula Powder .... ▣621
Goody's Extra Strength Headache Powder .... ▣621
Goody's Extra Strength Pain Relief Tablets .... ▣621
Percodan Tablets 1115
St. Joseph 81 mg Aspirin Chewable and Enteric Coated Tablets 1841

Aspirin, Enteric Coated (Clopidogrel potentiates the effect of aspirin on collagen-induced platelet aggregation; co-administration did not significantly increase the prolongation of bleeding time induced by clopidogrel but has increased major bleeding).
No products indexed under this heading.

Aspirin Buffered (Clopidogrel potentiates the effect of aspirin on collagen-induced platelet aggregation; co-administration did not significantly increase the prolongation of bleeding time induced by clopidogrel but has increased major bleeding).
No products indexed under this heading.

Celecoxib (Co-administration can be associated with increased occult gastrointestinal blood loss; at high concentrations in vitro, clopidogrel inhibits P450IIC9; accordingly, it may interfere with the metabolism of many non-steroidal anti-inflammatory agents). Products include:
Celebrex Capsules 3130

Diclofenac Potassium (Co-administration can be associated with increased occult gastrointestinal blood loss; at high concentrations in vitro, clopidogrel inhibits P450IIC9; accordingly, it may interfere with the metabolism of many non-steroidal anti-inflammatory agents). Products include:
Cataflam Tablets 2173

Diclofenac Sodium (Co-administration can be associated with increased occult gastrointestinal blood loss; at high concentrations in vitro, clopidogrel inhibits P450IIC9; accordingly, it may interfere with the metabolism of many non-steroidal anti-inflammatory agents). Products include:
Arthrotec Tablets 3126
Voltaren Ophthalmic Solution 2300
Voltaren Tablets 2298
Voltaren-XR Tablets 2301

Etodolac (Co-administration can be associated with increased occult gastrointestinal blood loss; at high concentrations in vitro, clopidogrel inhibits P450IIC9; accordingly, it may interfere with the metabolism of many non-steroidal anti-inflammatory agents).
No products indexed under this heading.

Fenoprofen Calcium (Co-administration can be associated with increased occult gastrointestinal blood loss; at high concentrations in vitro, clopidogrel inhibits P450IIC9; accordingly, it may interfere with the metabolism of many non-steroidal anti-inflammatory agents). Products include:
Nalfon Capsules 2504

Flurbiprofen (Co-administration can be associated with increased occult gastrointestinal blood loss; at high concentrations in vitro, clopidogrel inhibits P450IIC9; accordingly, it may interfere with the metabolism of many non-steroidal anti-inflammatory agents).
No products indexed under this heading.

Fluvastatin Sodium (At high concentrations in vitro, clopidogrel inhibits P450IIC9; accordingly, it may interfere with the metabolism of fluvastatin). Products include:
Lescol Capsules 2227
Lescol 2730
Lescol XL Tablets 2227

Fosphenytoin Sodium (At high concentrations in vitro, clopidogrel inhibits P450IIC9; accordingly, it may interfere with the metabolism of phenytoin).
No products indexed under this heading.

Heparin Sodium (Co-administration should be undertaken with caution; concomitant heparin has no effect on inhibition of platelet aggregation induced by clopidogrel).
No products indexed under this heading.

Ibuprofen (Co-administration can be associated with increased occult gastrointestinal blood loss; at high concentrations in vitro, clopidogrel inhibits P450IIC9; accordingly, it may interfere with the metabolism of many non-steroidal anti-inflammatory agents). Products include:
Advil Allergy Sinus Caplets .... ▣737
Advil .... ▣737
Children's Advil Suspension .... ▣742
Children's Advil Chewable Tablets .. ▣741
Advil Cold & Sinus .... ▣739
Advil Flu & Body Ache Caplets .... ▣739
Children's Advil Cold Suspension .... ▣741
Infants' Advil Concentrated Drops .. ▣743
Junior Strength Advil Swallow Tablets .... ▣740
Advil Migraine Liquigels .... ▣740
Advil Multi-Symptom Cold Caplets .... ▣738
Combunox Tablets 1183
Children's Motrin Oral Suspension and Chewable Tablets 1837
Children's Motrin Cold Non-Staining Dye-Free Oral Suspension 1838
Children's Motrin Cold Oral Suspension 1838
Children's Motrin Non-Staining Dye-Free Oral Suspension 1837
Motrin Cold & Sinus Caplets 1836
Motrin IB Tablets and Caplets 1836
Infants' Motrin Concentrated Drops 1837
Infants' Motrin Non-Staining Dye-Free Drops 1837
Junior Strength Motrin Caplets and Chewable Tablets 1837
Vicoprofen Tablets 533

Indomethacin (Co-administration can be associated with increased occult gastrointestinal blood loss; at high concentrations in vitro, clopidogrel inhibits P450IIC9; accordingly, it may interfere with the metabolism of many non-steroidal anti-inflammatory agents). Products include:
Indocin 1968

Indomethacin Sodium Trihydrate (Co-administration can be associated with increased occult gastrointestinal blood loss; at high concentrations in vitro, clopidogrel inhibits P450IIC9; accordingly, it

may interfere with the metabolism of many non-steroidal anti-inflammatory agents). Products include:

Indocin I.V. 1973

Ketoprofen (Co-administration can be associated with increased occult gastrointestinal blood loss; at high concentrations in vitro, clopidogrel inhibits P450IIC9; accordingly, it may interfere with the metabolism of many non-steroidal anti-inflammatory agents).

No products indexed under this heading.

Ketorolac Tromethamine (Co-administration can be associated with increased occult gastrointestinal blood loss; at high concentrations in vitro, clopidogrel inhibits P450IIC9; accordingly, it may interfere with the metabolism of many non-steroidal anti-inflammatory agents). Products include:

Acular Ophthalmic Solution 561
Acular LS Ophthalmic Solution 562

Meclofenamate Sodium (Co-administration can be associated with increased occult gastrointestinal blood loss; at high concentrations in vitro, clopidogrel inhibits P450IIC9; accordingly, it may interfere with the metabolism of many non-steroidal anti-inflammatory agents).

No products indexed under this heading.

Mefenamic Acid (Co-administration can be associated with increased occult gastrointestinal blood loss; at high concentrations in vitro, clopidogrel inhibits P450IIC9; accordingly, it may interfere with the metabolism of many non-steroidal anti-inflammatory agents).

No products indexed under this heading.

Meloxicam (Co-administration can be associated with increased occult gastrointestinal blood loss; at high concentrations in vitro, clopidogrel inhibits P450IIC9; accordingly, it may interfere with the metabolism of many non-steroidal anti-inflammatory agents). Products include:

Mobic Oral Suspension 893
Mobic Tablets 893

Nabumetone (Co-administration can be associated with increased occult gastrointestinal blood loss; at high concentrations in vitro, clopidogrel inhibits P450IIC9; accordingly, it may interfere with the metabolism of many non-steroidal anti-inflammatory agents). Products include:

Relafen Tablets 1523

Naproxen (Co-administration can be associated with increased occult gastrointestinal blood loss; at high concentrations in vitro, clopidogrel inhibits P450IIC9; accordingly, it may interfere with the metabolism of many non-steroidal anti-inflammatory agents). Products include:

EC-Naprosyn Delayed-Release Tablets 2769
Naprosyn Suspension 2769
Naprosyn Tablets 2769
Prevacid NapraPAC 3277

Naproxen Sodium (Co-administration can be associated with increased occult gastrointestinal blood loss; at high concentrations in vitro, clopidogrel inhibits P450IIC9; accordingly, it may interfere with the metabolism of many non-steroidal anti-inflammatory agents). Products include:

Aleve Tablets, Caplets and Gelcaps 605
Anaprox Tablets 2769
Anaprox DS Tablets 2769

Oxaprozin (Co-administration can be associated with increased occult gastrointestinal blood loss; at high concentrations in vitro, clopidogrel inhibits P450IIC9; accordingly, it may interfere with the metabolism of many non-steroidal anti-inflammatory agents).

No products indexed under this heading.

Phenylbutazone (Co-administration can be associated with increased occult gastrointestinal blood loss; at high concentrations in vitro, clopidogrel inhibits P450IIC9; accordingly, it may interfere with the metabolism of many non-steroidal anti-inflammatory agents).

No products indexed under this heading.

Phenytoin (At high concentrations in vitro, clopidogrel inhibits P450IIC9; accordingly, it may interfere with the metabolism of phenytoin).

No products indexed under this heading.

Phenytoin Sodium (At high concentrations in vitro, clopidogrel inhibits P450IIC9; accordingly, it may interfere with the metabolism of phenytoin). Products include:

Phenytek Capsules 2153

Piroxicam (Co-administration can be associated with increased occult gastrointestinal blood loss; at high concentrations in vitro, clopidogrel inhibits P450IIC9; accordingly, it may interfere with the metabolism of many non-steroidal anti-inflammatory agents).

No products indexed under this heading.

Rofecoxib (Co-administration can be associated with increased occult gastrointestinal blood loss; at high concentrations in vitro, clopidogrel inhibits P450IIC9; accordingly, it may interfere with the metabolism of many non-steroidal anti-inflammatory agents).

No products indexed under this heading.

Sulindac (Co-administration can be associated with increased occult gastrointestinal blood loss; at high concentrations in vitro, clopidogrel inhibits P450IIC9; accordingly, it may interfere with the metabolism of many non-steroidal anti-inflammatory agents). Products include:

Clinoril Tablets 1899

Tamoxifen Citrate (At high concentrations in vitro, clopidogrel inhibits P450IIC9; accordingly, it may interfere with the metabolism of tamoxifen).

No products indexed under this heading.

Tolbutamide (At high concentrations in vitro, clopidogrel inhibits P450IIC9; accordingly, it may interfere with the metabolism of tolbutamide).

No products indexed under this heading.

Tolmetin Sodium (Co-administration can be associated with increased occult gastrointestinal blood loss; at high concentrations in vitro, clopidogrel inhibits P450IIC9; accordingly, it may interfere with the metabolism of many non-steroidal anti-inflammatory agents).

No products indexed under this heading.

Torsemide (At high concentrations in vitro, clopidogrel inhibits P450IIC9; accordingly, it may interfere with the metabolism of torsemide).

No products indexed under this heading.

Valdecoxib (Co-administration can be associated with increased occult gastrointestinal blood loss; at high concentrations in vitro, clopidogrel inhibits P450IIC9; accordingly, it may interfere with the metabolism of many non-steroidal anti-inflammatory agents).

No products indexed under this heading.

Warfarin Sodium (Co-administration should be undertaken with caution due to the increased risk of bleeding; at high concentrations in vitro, clopidogrel inhibits P450IIC9; accordingly, it may interfere with the metabolism of warfarin). Products include:

Coumadin for Injection 932
Coumadin Tablets 932

PLAVIX TABLETS

(Clopidogrel Bisulfate) 2942

May interact with non-steroidal anti-inflammatory agents, phenytoin, and certain other agents. Compounds in these categories include:

Aspirin (Clopidogrel potentiates the effect of aspirin on collagen-induced platelet aggregation). Products include:

Aggrenox Capsules 855
Bayer, Aspirin Regimen 606
Bayer Aspirin Tablets 3515
BC Powder 612
BC Allergy Sinus Cold Powder 612
Arthritis Strength BC Powder 612
BC Sinus Cold Powder 612
Ecotrin Enteric Coated Aspirin Low, Regular and Maximum Strength Tablets 1627
Goody's Body Pain Formula Powder 621
Goody's Extra Strength Headache Powder 621
Goody's Extra Strength Pain Relief Tablets 621
Percodan Tablets 1115
St. Joseph 81 mg Aspirin Chewable and Enteric Coated Tablets 1841

Celecoxib (Co-administration can be associated with increased occult gastrointestinal blood loss; at high concentrations in vitro, clopidogrel inhibits P450IIC9; accordingly, it may interfere with the metabolism of many non-steroidal anti-inflammatory agents. Use caution when co-adminstering with clopidrogel). Products include:

Celebrex Capsules 3130

Diclofenac Potassium (Co-administration can be associated with increased occult gastrointestinal blood loss; at high concentrations in vitro, clopidogrel inhibits P450IIC9; accordingly, it may interfere with the metabolism of many non-steroidal anti-inflammatory agents. Use caution when co-adminstering with clopidrogel). Products include:

Cataflam Tablets 2173

Diclofenac Sodium (Co-administration can be associated with increased occult gastrointestinal blood loss; at high concentrations in vitro, clopidogrel inhibits P450IIC9; accordingly, it may interfere with the metabolism of many non-steroidal anti-inflammatory agents. Use caution when co-adminstering with clopidrogel). Products include:

Arthrotec Tablets 3126
Voltaren Ophthalmic Solution 2300
Voltaren Tablets 2298
Voltaren-XR Tablets 2301

Etodolac (Co-administration can be associated with increased occult gastrointestinal blood loss; at high concentrations in vitro, clopidogrel inhibits P450IIC9; accordingly, it may interfere with the metabolism of many non-steroidal anti-inflammatory agents. Use caution when co-adminstering with clopidrogel).

No products indexed under this heading.

Fenoprofen Calcium (Co-administration can be associated with increased occult gastrointestinal blood loss; at high concentrations in vitro, clopidogrel inhibits P450IIC9; accordingly, it may interfere with the metabolism of many non-steroidal anti-inflammatory agents. Use caution when co-adminstering with clopidrogel). Products include:

Nalfon Capsules 2504

Flurbiprofen (Co-administration can be associated with increased occult gastrointestinal blood loss; at high concentrations in vitro, clopidogrel inhibits P450IIC9; accordingly, it may interfere with the metabolism of many non-steroidal anti-inflammatory agents. Use caution when co-adminstering with clopidrogel).

No products indexed under this heading.

Fluvastatin Sodium (At high concentrations in vitro, clopidogrel inhibits P450IIC9; accordingly, it may interfere with the metabolism of fluvastatin. Use caution when co-administering with clopidrogel). Products include:

Lescol Capsules 2227
Lescol 2730
Lescol XL Tablets 2227

Fosphenytoin Sodium (At high concentrations in vitro, clopidogrel inhibits P450IIC9; accordingly, it may interfere with the metabolism of phenytoin. Use caution when co-administering with clopidrogel).

No products indexed under this heading.

Ibuprofen (Co-administration can be associated with increased occult gastrointestinal blood loss; at high concentrations in vitro, clopidogrel inhibits P450IIC9; accordingly, it may interfere with the metabolism of many non-steroidal anti-inflammatory agents. Use caution when co-adminstering with clopidrogel). Products include:

Advil Allergy Sinus Caplets 737
Advil 737
Children's Advil Suspension 742
Children's Advil Chewable Tablets .. 741
Advil Cold & Sinus 739
Advil Flu & Body Ache Caplets 739
Children's Advil Cold Suspension ... 741

Infants' Advil Concentrated Drops .. ▣743
Junior Strength Advil Swallow Tablets .... ▣740
Advil Migraine Liquigels .... ▣740
Advil Multi-Symptom Cold Caplets .... ▣738
Combunox Tablets 1183
Children's Motrin Oral Suspension and Chewable Tablets 1837
Children's Motrin Cold Non-Staining Dye-Free Oral Suspension 1838
Children's Motrin Cold Oral Suspension 1838
Children's Motrin Non-Staining Dye-Free Oral Suspension 1837
Motrin Cold & Sinus Caplets 1836
Motrin IB Tablets and Caplets 1836
Infants' Motrin Concentrated Drops 1837
Infants' Motrin Non-Staining Dye-Free Drops 1837
Junior Strength Motrin Caplets and Chewable Tablets 1837
Vicoprofen Tablets 533

Indomethacin (Co-administration can be associated with increased occult gastrointestinal blood loss; at high concentrations in vitro, clopidogrel inhibits P450IIC9; accordingly, it may interfere with the metabolism of many non-steroidal anti-inflammatory agents. Use caution when co-adminstering with clopidrogel). Products include:
Indocin 1968

Indomethacin Sodium Trihydrate (Co-administration can be associated with increased occult gastrointestinal blood loss; at high concentrations in vitro, clopidogrel inhibits P450IIC9; accordingly, it may interfere with the metabolism of many non-steroidal anti-inflammatory agents. Use caution when co-adminstering with clopidrogel). Products include:
Indocin I.V. 1973

Ketoprofen (Co-administration can be associated with increased occult gastrointestinal blood loss; at high concentrations in vitro, clopidogrel inhibits P450IIC9; accordingly, it may interfere with the metabolism of many non-steroidal anti-inflammatory agents. Use caution when co-adminstering with clopidrogel).
No products indexed under this heading.

Ketorolac Tromethamine (Co-administration can be associated with increased occult gastrointestinal blood loss; at high concentrations in vitro, clopidogrel inhibits P450IIC9; accordingly, it may interfere with the metabolism of many non-steroidal anti-inflammatory agents. Use caution when co-adminstering with clopidrogel). Products include:
Acular Ophthalmic Solution 561
Acular LS Ophthalmic Solution 562

Meclofenamate Sodium (Co-administration can be associated with increased occult gastrointestinal blood loss; at high concentrations in vitro, clopidogrel inhibits P450IIC9; accordingly, it may interfere with the metabolism of many non-steroidal anti-inflammatory agents. Use caution when co-adminstering with clopidrogel).
No products indexed under this heading.

Mefenamic Acid (Co-administration can be associated with increased occult gastrointestinal blood loss; at high concentrations in vitro, clopidogrel inhibits P450IIC9; accordingly, it may interfere with the metabolism of many non-steroidal anti-inflammatory agents. Use caution when co-adminstering with clopidrogel).
No products indexed under this heading.

Meloxicam (Co-administration can be associated with increased occult gastrointestinal blood loss; at high concentrations in vitro, clopidogrel inhibits P450IIC9; accordingly, it may interfere with the metabolism of many non-steroidal anti-inflammatory agents. Use caution when co-adminstering with clopidrogel). Products include:
Mobic Oral Suspension 893
Mobic Tablets 893

Nabumetone (Co-administration can be associated with increased occult gastrointestinal blood loss; at high concentrations in vitro, clopidogrel inhibits P450IIC9; accordingly, it may interfere with the metabolism of many non-steroidal anti-inflammatory agents. Use caution when co-adminstering with clopidrogel). Products include:
Relafen Tablets 1523

Naproxen (Co-administration can be associated with increased occult gastrointestinal blood loss; at high concentrations in vitro, clopidogrel inhibits P450IIC9; accordingly, it may interfere with the metabolism of many non-steroidal anti-inflammatory agents. Use caution when co-adminstering with clopidrogel). Products include:
EC-Naprosyn Delayed-Release Tablets 2769
Naprosyn Suspension 2769
Naprosyn Tablets 2769
Prevacid NapraPAC 3277

Naproxen Sodium (Co-administration can be associated with increased occult gastrointestinal blood loss; at high concentrations in vitro, clopidogrel inhibits P450IIC9; accordingly, it may interfere with the metabolism of many non-steroidal anti-inflammatory agents. Use caution when co-adminstering with clopidrogel). Products include:
Aleve Tablets, Caplets and Gelcaps .... ▣605
Anaprox Tablets 2769
Anaprox DS Tablets 2769

Oxaprozin (Co-administration can be associated with increased occult gastrointestinal blood loss; at high concentrations in vitro, clopidogrel inhibits P450IIC9; accordingly, it may interfere with the metabolism of many non-steroidal anti-inflammatory agents. Use caution when co-adminstering with clopidrogel).
No products indexed under this heading.

Phenylbutazone (Co-administration can be associated with increased occult gastrointestinal blood loss; at high concentrations in vitro, clopidogrel inhibits P450IIC9; accordingly, it may interfere with the metabolism of many non-steroidal anti-inflammatory agents. Use caution when co-adminstering with clopidrogel).
No products indexed under this heading.

Phenytoin (At high concentrations in vitro, clopidogrel inhibits P450IIC9; accordingly, it may interfere with the metabolism of phenytoin. Use caution when co-administering with clopidrogel).
No products indexed under this heading.

Phenytoin Sodium (At high concentrations in vitro, clopidogrel inhibits P450IIC9; accordingly, it may interfere with the metabolism of phenytoin. Use caution when co-administering with clopidrogel). Products include:
Phenytek Capsules 2153

Piroxicam (Co-administration can be associated with increased occult gastrointestinal blood loss; at high concentrations in vitro, clopidogrel inhibits P450IIC9; accordingly, it may interfere with the metabolism of many non-steroidal anti-inflammatory agents. Use caution when co-adminstering with clopidrogel).
No products indexed under this heading.

Rofecoxib (Co-administration can be associated with increased occult gastrointestinal blood loss; at high concentrations in vitro, clopidogrel inhibits P450IIC9; accordingly, it may interfere with the metabolism of many non-steroidal anti-inflammatory agents. Use caution when co-adminstering with clopidrogel).
No products indexed under this heading.

Sulindac (Co-administration can be associated with increased occult gastrointestinal blood loss; at high concentrations in vitro, clopidogrel inhibits P450IIC9; accordingly, it may interfere with the metabolism of many non-steroidal anti-inflammatory agents. Use caution when co-adminstering with clopidrogel). Products include:
Clinoril Tablets 1899

Tamoxifen Citrate (At high concentrations in vitro, clopidogrel inhibits P450IIC9; accordingly, it may interfere with the metabolism of tamoxifen. Use caution when co-adminstering with clopidrogel).
No products indexed under this heading.

Tolbutamide (At high concentrations in vitro, clopidogrel inhibits P450IIC9; accordingly, it may interfere with the metabolism of tolbutamide. Use caution when co-adminstering with clopidrogel).
No products indexed under this heading.

Tolmetin Sodium (Co-administration can be associated with increased occult gastrointestinal blood loss; at high concentrations in vitro, clopidogrel inhibits P450IIC9; accordingly, it may interfere with the metabolism of many non-steroidal anti-inflammatory agents. Use caution when co-adminstering with clopidrogel).
No products indexed under this heading.

Torsemide (At high concentrations in vitro, clopidogrel inhibits P450IIC9; accordingly, it may interfere with the metabolism of torsemide. Use caution when co-adminstering with clopidrogel).
No products indexed under this heading.

Valdecoxib (Co-administration can be associated with increased occult gastrointestinal blood loss; at high concentrations in vitro, clopidogrel inhibits P450IIC9; accordingly, it may interfere with the metabolism of many non-steroidal anti-inflammatory agents. Use caution when co-adminstering with clopidrogel).
No products indexed under this heading.

Warfarin Sodium (Because of the increased risk of bleeding, the concomitant administration of warfarin with clopidrogel should be undertaken with caution). Products include:
Coumadin for Injection 932
Coumadin Tablets 932

PLENDIL EXTENDED-RELEASE TABLETS

(Felodipine) 651

May interact with beta blockers, anticonvulsants, erythromycin, and certain other agents. Compounds in these categories include:

Acebutolol Hydrochloride (Caution should be exercised when using Plendil in patients with heart failure or compromised ventricular function, particularly in combination with beta-blocker).
No products indexed under this heading.

Atenolol (Caution should be exercised when using Plendil in patients with heart failure or compromised ventricular function, particularly in combination with beta-blocker). Products include:
Tenormin I.V. Injection 698
Tenormin Tablets 695

Betaxolol Hydrochloride (Caution should be exercised when using Plendil in patients with heart failure or compromised ventricular function, particularly in combination with beta-blocker). Products include:
Betoptic S Ophthalmic Suspension 554

Bisoprolol Fumarate (Caution should be exercised when using Plendil in patients with heart failure or compromised ventricular function, particularly in combination with beta-blocker).
No products indexed under this heading.

Carbamazepine (Potential for low maximum plasma concentrations of felodipine in epileptic patients on long-term anticonvulsant therapy). Products include:
Carbatrol Capsules 3174
Equetro Extended-Release Capsules 3178
Tegretol/Tegretol-XR 2278

Carteolol Hydrochloride (Caution should be exercised when using Plendil in patients with heart failure or compromised ventricular function, particularly in combination with beta-blocker). Products include:
Carteolol Hydrochloride Ophthalmic Solution USP, 1% .... ⊙246

Cimetidine (Increases AUC and Cmax by approximately 50%; low doses of Plendil should be used). Products include:
Tagamet HB 200 Tablets .... ▣637
Tagamet Tablets 1547

Cimetidine Hydrochloride (Increases AUC and Cmax by approximately 50%; low doses of Plendil should be used).
No products indexed under this heading.

Digoxin (Co-administration does not significantly alter the pharmacokinetics of digoxin in patients with heart failure). Products include:
Digitek Tablets **2146**
Lanoxicaps Capsules **1458**
Lanoxin Injection **1462**
Lanoxin Tablets **1468**
Lanoxin Injection Pediatric **1465**

Divalproex Sodium (Potential for low maximum plasma concentrations of felodipine in epileptic patients on long-term anticonvulsant therapy). Products include:
Depakote Sprinkle Capsules **422**
Depakote Tablets **427**
Depakote ER Tablets **433**

Erythromycin (Felodipine is metabolized by CYP3A4; co-administration of felodipine with erythromycin resulted in approximately 2.5-fold increase in the AUC and Cmax, and about 2-fold prolongation in the half-life of felodipine). Products include:
Erygel Topical Gel **2096**
Ery-Tab Tablets **447**
Erythromycin Base Filmtab Tablets **454**
Erythromycin Delayed-Release Capsules, USP **456**
PCE Dispertab Tablets **510**

Erythromycin Estolate (Felodipine is metabolized by CYP3A4; co-administration of felodipine with erythromycin resulted in approximately 2.5-fold increase in the AUC and Cmax, and about 2-fold prolongation in the half-life of felodipine).
No products indexed under this heading.

Erythromycin Ethylsuccinate (Felodipine is metabolized by CYP3A4; co-administration of felodipine with erythromycin resulted in approximately 2.5-fold increase in the AUC and Cmax, and about 2-fold prolongation in the half-life of felodipine). Products include:
E.E.S. **449**
EryPed **445**

Erythromycin Gluceptate (Felodipine is metabolized by CYP3A4; co-administration of felodipine with erythromycin resulted in approximately 2.5-fold increase in the AUC and Cmax, and about 2-fold prolongation in the half-life of felodipine).
No products indexed under this heading.

Erythromycin Lactobionate (Felodipine is metabolized by CYP3A4; co-administration of felodipine with erythromycin resulted in approximately 2.5-fold increase in the AUC and Cmax, and about 2-fold prolongation in the half-life of felodipine).
No products indexed under this heading.

Erythromycin Stearate (Felodipine is metabolized by CYP3A4; co-administration of felodipine with erythromycin resulted in approximately 2.5-fold increase in the AUC and Cmax, and about 2-fold prolongation in the half-life of felodipine). Products include:
Erythrocin Stearate Filmtab Tablets **452**

Esmolol Hydrochloride (Caution should be exercised when using Plendil in patients with heart failure or compromised ventricular function, particularly in combination with beta-blocker). Products include:
Brevibloc Concentrate **766**
Brevibloc Injection **766**
Brevibloc Double Strength Injection **766**
Brevibloc Premixed Injection **766**
Brevibloc Double Strength Premixed Injection **766**

Ethosuximide (Potential for low maximum plasma concentrations of felodipine in epileptic patients on long-term anticonvulsant therapy).
No products indexed under this heading.

Ethotoin (Potential for low maximum plasma concentrations of felodipine in epileptic patients on long-term anticonvulsant therapy). Products include:
Peganone Tablets, USP **2487**

Felbamate (Potential for low maximum plasma concentrations of felodipine in epileptic patients on long-term anticonvulsant therapy).
No products indexed under this heading.

Fosphenytoin (Potential for low maximum plasma concentrations of felodipine in epileptic patients on long-term anticonvulsant therapy).
No products indexed under this heading.

Fosphenytoin Sodium (Potential for low maximum plasma concentrations of felodipine in epileptic patients on long-term anticonvulsant therapy).
No products indexed under this heading.

Gabapentin (Potential for low maximum plasma concentrations of felodipine in epileptic patients on long-term anticonvulsant therapy). Products include:
Neurontin Capsules **2498**
Neurontin Oral Solution **2498**
Neurontin Tablets **2498**

Itraconazole (Felodipine is metabolized by CYP3A4; co-administration of another extended release formulation of felodipine with itraconazole resulted in approximately 8-fold increase in the AUC, more than 6-fold increase in the Cmax, and 2-fold prolongation in the half-life of felodipine).
No products indexed under this heading.

Ketoconazole (Felodipine is metabolized by CYP3A4; co-administration of CYP3A4 inhibitors, such as ketoconazole, with felodipine may lead to several-fold increases in the plasma levels of felodipine, either due to an increase in bioavailability or due to a decrease in metabolism). Products include:
Nizoral A-D Shampoo, 1% **1839**
Nizoral 2% Shampoo **1838**

Labetalol Hydrochloride (Caution should be exercised when using Plendil in patients with heart failure or compromised ventricular function, particularly in combination with beta-blocker).
No products indexed under this heading.

Lamotrigine (Potential for low maximum plasma concentrations of felodipine in epileptic patients on long-term anticonvulsant therapy). Products include:
Lamictal **1449**

Levetiracetam (Potential for low maximum plasma concentrations of felodipine in epileptic patients on long-term anticonvulsant therapy). Products include:
Keppra Oral Solution **3307**
Keppra Tablets **3307**

Levobunolol Hydrochloride (Caution should be exercised when using Plendil in patients with heart failure or compromised ventricular function, particularly in combination with beta-blocker). Products include:
Betagan Ophthalmic Solution, USP .... ⊙**217**

Mephenytoin (Potential for low maximum plasma concentrations of felodipine in epileptic patients on long-term anticonvulsant therapy).
No products indexed under this heading.

Methsuximide (Potential for low maximum plasma concentrations of felodipine in epileptic patients on long-term anticonvulsant therapy).
No products indexed under this heading.

Metipranolol Hydrochloride (Caution should be exercised when using Plendil in patients with heart failure or compromised ventricular function, particularly in combination with beta-blocker).
No products indexed under this heading.

Metoprolol Succinate (Caution should be exercised when using Plendil in patients with heart failure or compromised ventricular function, particularly in combination with beta-blocker). Products include:
Toprol-XL Tablets **660**

Metoprolol Tartrate (Caution should be exercised when using Plendil in patients with heart failure or compromised ventricular function, particularly in combination with beta-blocker).
No products indexed under this heading.

Nadolol (Caution should be exercised when using Plendil in patients with heart failure or compromised ventricular function, particularly in combination with beta-blocker). Products include:
Nadolol Tablets **2121**

Oxcarbazepine (Potential for low maximum plasma concentrations of felodipine in epileptic patients on long-term anticonvulsant therapy). Products include:
Trileptal Oral Suspension **2281**
Trileptal Tablets **2281**

Paramethadione (Potential for low maximum plasma concentrations of felodipine in epileptic patients on long-term anticonvulsant therapy).
No products indexed under this heading.

Penbutolol Sulfate (Caution should be exercised when using Plendil in patients with heart failure or compromised ventricular function, particularly in combination with beta-blocker).
No products indexed under this heading.

Phenacemide (Potential for low maximum plasma concentrations of felodipine in epileptic patients on long-term anticonvulsant therapy).
No products indexed under this heading.

Phenobarbital (Potential for low maximum plasma concentrations of felodipine in epileptic patients on long-term anticonvulsant therapy).
No products indexed under this heading.

Phensuximide (Potential for low maximum plasma concentrations of felodipine in epileptic patients on long-term anticonvulsant therapy).
No products indexed under this heading.

Phenytoin (Potential for low maximum plasma concentrations of felodipine in epileptic patients on long-term anticonvulsant therapy).
No products indexed under this heading.

Phenytoin Sodium (Potential for low maximum plasma concentrations of felodipine in epileptic patients on long-term anticonvulsant therapy). Products include:
Phenytek Capsules **2153**

Pindolol (Caution should be exercised when using Plendil in patients with heart failure or compromised ventricular function, particularly in combination with beta-blocker).
No products indexed under this heading.

Primidone (Potential for low maximum plasma concentrations of felodipine in epileptic patients on long-term anticonvulsant therapy).
No products indexed under this heading.

Propranolol Hydrochloride (Caution should be exercised when using Plendil in patients with heart failure or compromised ventricular function, particularly in combination with beta-blocker). Products include:
Inderal LA Long-Acting Capsules **3421**
InnoPran XL Capsules **2728**

Sotalol Hydrochloride (Caution should be exercised when using Plendil in patients with heart failure or compromised ventricular function, particularly in combination with beta-blocker).
No products indexed under this heading.

Tacrolimus (Felodipine may increase the blood concentration of tacrolimus). Products include:
Prograf Capsules and Injection **624**
Protopic Ointment **629**

Tiagabine Hydrochloride (Potential for low maximum plasma concentrations of felodipine in epileptic patients on long-term anticonvulsant therapy). Products include:
Gabitril Tablets **998**

Timolol Hemihydrate (Caution should be exercised when using Plendil in patients with heart failure or compromised ventricular function, particularly in combination with beta-blocker). Products include:
Betimol Ophthalmic Solution **3371**
Betimol Ophthalmic Solution .... ⊙**283**

Timolol Maleate (Caution should be exercised when using Plendil in patients with heart failure or compromised ventricular function, particularly in combination with beta-blocker). Products include:
Blocadren Tablets **1891**
Cosopt Sterile Ophthalmic Solution **1910**
Timolide Tablets **2056**
Timoptic in Ocudose **2061**
Timoptic Sterile Ophthalmic Solution **2058**
Timoptic-XE Sterile Ophthalmic Gel Forming Solution **2062**

Topiramate (Potential for low maximum plasma concentrations of felodipine in epileptic patients on long-term anticonvulsant therapy). Products include:
Topamax Sprinkle Capsules **2438**

Topamax Tablets 2438

Trimethadione (Potential for low maximum plasma concentrations of felodipine in epileptic patients on long-term anticonvulsant therapy).

No products indexed under this heading.

Valproate Sodium (Potential for low maximum plasma concentrations of felodipine in epileptic patients on long-term anticonvulsant therapy). Products include:

Depacon Injection 412

Valproic Acid (Potential for low maximum plasma concentrations of felodipine in epileptic patients on long-term anticonvulsant therapy). Products include:

Depakene 417

Zonisamide (Potential for low maximum plasma concentrations of felodipine in epileptic patients on long-term anticonvulsant therapy). Products include:

Zonegran Capsules 1089

Food Interactions

Food, unspecified (When Plendil is administered either with a high fat or carbohydrate diet, Cmax is increased by approximately 60%, AUC is unchanged; Plendil should regularly be taken either without food or with a light meal).

Grapefruit Juice (The bioavailability of felodipine is increased more than two-fold when taken with doubly concentrated grapefruit juice).

PLETAL TABLETS

(Cilostazol) 2478

May interact with cytochrome p450 2c9 inhibitors (selected), cytochrome p450 3a4 inhibitors (selected), erythromycin, platelet inhibitors, and certain other agents. Compounds in these categories include:

Acetazolamide (A reduced dose of cilostazol should be considered when taken concomitantly with CYP3A4 inhibitors).

No products indexed under this heading.

Amiodarone Hydrochloride (A reduced dose of cilostazol should be considered when taken concomitantly with CYP3A4 inhibitors). Products include:

Pacerone Tablets 3337

Amprenavir (A reduced dose of cilostazol should be considered when taken concomitantly with CYP3A4 inhibitors). Products include:

Agenerase Capsules 1299
Agenerase Oral Solution 1304

Anastrozole (A reduced dose of cilostazol should be considered when taken concomitantly with CYP3A4 inhibitors). Products include:

Arimidex Tablets 665

Aprepitant (A reduced dose of cilostazol should be considered when taken concomitantly with CYP3A4 inhibitors). Products include:

Emend Capsules 1944

Aspirin (Short-term (less than or equal to 4 days) co-administration has shown a 22% to 37% increase in inhibition of ADP-induced ex vivo platelet aggregation compared to aspirin alone; no clinically significant impact on bleeding time, PT, or aPTT was noted; there was no apparent greater incidence of hemorrhagic adverse effects in patients on cilostazol and aspirin compared to patients taking placebo and aspirin). Products include:

Aggrenox Capsules 855
Bayer, Aspirin Regimen .... ■ 606
Bayer Aspirin Tablets 3515
BC Powder .... ■ 612
BC Allergy Sinus Cold Powder .... ■ 612
Arthritis Strength BC Powder .... ■ 612
BC Sinus Cold Powder .... ■ 612
Ecotrin Enteric Coated Aspirin Low, Regular and Maximum Strength Tablets 1627
Goody's Body Pain Formula Powder .... ■ 621
Goody's Extra Strength Headache Powder .... ■ 621
Goody's Extra Strength Pain Relief Tablets .... ■ 621
Percodan Tablets 1115
St. Joseph 81 mg Aspirin Chewable and Enteric Coated Tablets 1841

Aspirin, Enteric Coated (Caution is advised in patients receiving both cilostazol and any other antiplatelet agent).

No products indexed under this heading.

Aspirin Buffered (Caution is advised in patients receiving both cilostazol and any other antiplatelet agent).

No products indexed under this heading.

Azlocillin Sodium (Caution is advised in patients receiving both cilostazol and any other antiplatelet agent).

No products indexed under this heading.

Bendroflumethiazide (A reduced dose of cilostazol should be considered when taken concomitantly with CYP2C19 inhibitors).

No products indexed under this heading.

Carbenicillin Indanyl Sodium (Caution is advised in patients receiving both cilostazol and any other antiplatelet agent).

No products indexed under this heading.

Chloramphenicol (A reduced dose of cilostazol should be considered when taken concomitantly with CYP2C19 inhibitors).

No products indexed under this heading.

Chlorothiazide (A reduced dose of cilostazol should be considered when taken concomitantly with CYP2C19 inhibitors). Products include:

Aldoclor Tablets 1881
Diuril Oral 1936

Chlorothiazide Sodium (A reduced dose of cilostazol should be considered when taken concomitantly with CYP2C19 inhibitors). Products include:

Diuril Sodium Intravenous 1934

Chlorpropamide (A reduced dose of cilostazol should be considered when taken concomitantly with CYP2C19 inhibitors).

No products indexed under this heading.

Choline Magnesium Trisalicylate (Caution is advised in patients receiving both cilostazol and any other antiplatelet agent).

No products indexed under this heading.

Cimetidine (A reduced dose of cilostazol should be considered when taken concomitantly with CYP3A4 inhibitors). Products include:

Tagamet HB 200 Tablets .... ■ 637
Tagamet Tablets 1547

Cimetidine Hydrochloride (A reduced dose of cilostazol should be considered when taken concomitantly with CYP3A4 inhibitors).

No products indexed under this heading.

Ciprofloxacin (A reduced dose of cilostazol should be considered when taken concomitantly with CYP3A4 inhibitors). Products include:

Cipro I.V. 2998
Cipro I.V. Pharmacy Bulk Package 3509
Cipro Oral Suspension 2991
Cipro XR Tablets 3004
Ciprodex Otic Suspension 555

Clarithromycin (Co-administration of cilostazol with moderate inhibitors of CYP3A4, such as clarithromycin, a macrolide antibiotic, may result in significant increases in the systemic exposure of cilostazol and/or its major metabolites; caution should be exercised if concurrently used). Products include:

Biaxin/Biaxin XL 402
PREVPAC 3281

Clopidogrel Bisulfate (Althought it cannot be determined whether there was an additive effect on bleeding times during concomitant administration, caution should be advised for checking bleeding times). Products include:

Plavix Tablets 940
Plavix Tablets 2942

Clopidogrel Hydrogen Sulfate (Althought it cannot be determined whether there was an additive effect on bleeding times during concomitant administration, caution should be advised for checking bleeding times).

No products indexed under this heading.

Clotrimazole (A reduced dose of cilostazol should be considered when taken concomitantly with CYP3A4 inhibitors). Products include:

Lotrimin 3053
Lotrisone 3054

Cyclosporine (A reduced dose of cilostazol should be considered when taken concomitantly with CYP3A4 inhibitors). Products include:

Gengraf Capsules 458
Neoral Soft Gelatin Capsules 2247
Neoral Oral Solution 2247
Restasis Ophthalmic Emulsion 570
Sandimmune 2259

Dalfopristin (A reduced dose of cilostazol should be considered when taken concomitantly with CYP3A4 inhibitors). Products include:

Synercid I.V. 1690

Danazol (A reduced dose of cilostazol should be considered when taken concomitantly with CYP3A4 inhibitors).

No products indexed under this heading.

Delavirdine Mesylate (A reduced dose of cilostazol should be considered when taken concomitantly with CYP3A4 inhibitors). Products include:

Rescriptor Tablets 2535

Diclofenac Potassium (A reduced dose of cilostazol should be considered when taken concomitantly with CYP2C19 inhibitors). Products include:

Cataflam Tablets 2173

Diclofenac Sodium (A reduced dose of cilostazol should be considered when taken concomitantly with CYP2C19 inhibitors). Products include:

Arthrotec Tablets 3126
Voltaren Ophthalmic Solution 2300
Voltaren Tablets 2298
Voltaren-XR Tablets 2301

Diflunisal (Caution is advised in patients receiving both cilostazol and any other antiplatelet agent). Products include:

Dolobid Tablets 1937

Diltiazem Hydrochloride (Co-administration of cilostazol with moderate inhibitors of CYP3A4, such as diltiazem, has been shown to increase cilostazol plasma concentrations by approximately 30%). Products include:

Cardizem LA Extended Release Tablets 1699
Tiazac Capsules 1204

Diltiazem Maleate (Co-administration of cilostazol with moderate inhibitors of CYP3A4, such as diltiazem, has been shown to increase cilostazol plasma concentrations by approximately 30%).

No products indexed under this heading.

Dipyridamole (Caution is advised in patients receiving both cilostazol and any other antiplatelet agent). Products include:

Aggrenox Capsules 855
Persantine Tablets 898

Disulfiram (A reduced dose of cilostazol should be considered when taken concomitantly with CYP2C19 inhibitors). Products include:

Antabuse Tablets 2343

Efavirenz (A reduced dose of cilostazol should be considered when taken concomitantly with CYP2C19 inhibitors). Products include:

Sustiva Capsules 957

Erythromycin (Co-administration of cilostazol with moderately strong inhibitors of CYP3A4, such as erythromycin, significantly increases the systemic exposure of cilostazol and/or its major metabolites; caution should be exercised if concurrently used). Products include:

Erygel Topical Gel 2096
Ery-Tab Tablets 447
Erythromycin Base Filmtab Tablets 454
Erythromycin Delayed-Release Capsules, USP 456
PCE Dispertab Tablets 510

Erythromycin Estolate (Co-administration of cilostazol with moderately strong inhibitors of CYP3A4, such as erythromycin, significantly increases the systemic exposure of cilostazol and/or its major metabolites; caution should be exercised if concurrently used).

No products indexed under this heading.

Erythromycin Ethylsuccinate (Co-administration of cilostazol with moderately strong inhibitors of CYP3A4, such as erythromycin, significantly increases the systemic exposure of cilostazol and/or its major metabolites; caution should be exercised if concurrently used). Products include:

E.E.S. 449
EryPed 445

Erythromycin Gluceptate (Co-administration of cilostazol with moderately strong inhibitors of CYP3A4, such as erythromycin, significantly increases the systemic exposure of cilostazol and/or its major metabolites; caution should be exercised if concurrently used).
No products indexed under this heading.

Erythromycin Lactobionate (Co-administration of cilostazol with moderately strong inhibitors of CYP3A4, such as erythromycin, significantly increases the systemic exposure of cilostazol and/or its major metabolites; caution should be exercised if concurrently used).
No products indexed under this heading.

Erythromycin Stearate (Co-administration of cilostazol with moderately strong inhibitors of CYP3A4, such as erythromycin, significantly increases the systemic exposure of cilostazol and/or its major metabolites; caution should be exercised if concurrently used). Products include:
Erythrocin Stearate Filmtab Tablets **452**

Esomeprazole Magnesium (A reduced dose of cilostazol should be considered when taken concomitantly with CYP3A4 inhibitors). Products include:
Nexium Delayed-Release Capsules **645**

Fenofibrate (A reduced dose of cilostazol should be considered when taken concomitantly with CYP2C19 inhibitors). Products include:
Antara Capsules **2723**
Lofibra Capsules **1217**
Tricor Tablets **523**
Triglide Tablets **1165**

Fenoprofen Calcium (Caution is advised in patients receiving both cilostazol and any other antiplatelet agent). Products include:
Nalfon Capsules **2504**

Fluconazole (Co-administration of cilostazol with strong inhibitors of CYP3A4, such as fluconazole, would be expected to cause an increase in cilostazol Cmax and AUC).
No products indexed under this heading.

Fluorouracil (A reduced dose of cilostazol should be considered when taken concomitantly with CYP2C19 inhibitors). Products include:
Carac Cream, 0.5% **1048**
Efudex **3348**

Fluoxetine Hydrochloride (Co-administration of cilostazol with strong inhibitors of CYP3A4, such as fluoxetine, would be expected to cause an increase in cilostazol Cmax and AUC). Products include:
Prozac Pulvules and Liquid **1771**
Symbyax Capsules **1788**

Flurbiprofen (A reduced dose of cilostazol should be considered when taken concomitantly with CYP2C19 inhibitors).
No products indexed under this heading.

Flurbiprofen Sodium (A reduced dose of cilostazol should be considered when taken concomitantly with CYP2C19 inhibitors). Products include:
Ocufen Ophthalmic Solution .... ⊙**230**

Fluvastatin Sodium (A reduced dose of cilostazol should be considered when taken concomitantly with CYP2C19 inhibitors). Products include:
Lescol Capsules **2227**
Lescol **2730**
Lescol XL Tablets **2227**

Fluvoxamine Maleate (Co-administration of cilostazol with strong inhibitors of CYP3A4, such as fluvoxamine, would be expected to cause an increase in cilostazol Cmax and AUC).
No products indexed under this heading.

Fosamprenavir Calcium (A reduced dose of cilostazol should be considered when taken concomitantly with CYP3A4 inhibitors). Products include:
Lexiva Tablets **1473**

Gemfibrozil (A reduced dose of cilostazol should be considered when taken concomitantly with CYP2C19 inhibitors).
No products indexed under this heading.

Glipizide (A reduced dose of cilostazol should be considered when taken concomitantly with CYP2C19 inhibitors).
No products indexed under this heading.

Glyburide (A reduced dose of cilostazol should be considered when taken concomitantly with CYP2C19 inhibitors).
No products indexed under this heading.

Hydrochlorothiazide (A reduced dose of cilostazol should be considered when taken concomitantly with CYP2C19 inhibitors). Products include:
Aldoril Tablets **1884**
Atacand HCT **637**
Avalide Tablets **2889**
Avalide Tablets **922**
Benicar HCT Tablets **2852**
Diovan HCT Tablets **2195**
Dyazide Capsules **1389**
Hyzaar **1964**
Lotensin HCT Tablets **2235**
Maxzide **2150**
Micardis HCT Tablets **886**
Moduretic Tablets **2003**
Prinzide Tablets **2033**
Teveten HCT Tablets **1710**
Timolide Tablets **2056**
Uniretic Tablets **3114**
Vaseretic Tablets **2073**
Zestoretic Tablets **701**

Hydroflumethiazide (A reduced dose of cilostazol should be considered when taken concomitantly with CYP2C19 inhibitors).
No products indexed under this heading.

Ibuprofen (Caution is advised in patients receiving both cilostazol and any other antiplatelet agent). Products include:
Advil Allergy Sinus Caplets .... ▣**737**
Advil .... ▣**737**
Children's Advil Suspension .... ▣**742**
Children's Advil Chewable Tablets .. ▣**741**
Advil Cold & Sinus .... ▣**739**
Advil Flu & Body Ache Caplets .... ▣**739**
Children's Advil Cold Suspension ... ▣**741**
Infants' Advil Concentrated Drops .. ▣**743**
Junior Strength Advil Swallow Tablets .... ▣**740**
Advil Migraine Liquigels .... ▣**740**
Advil Multi-Symptom Cold Caplets .... ▣**738**
Combunox Tablets **1183**
Children's Motrin Oral Suspension and Chewable Tablets **1837**
Children's Motrin Cold Non-Staining Dye-Free Oral Suspension **1838**
Children's Motrin Cold Oral Suspension **1838**
Children's Motrin Non-Staining Dye-Free Oral Suspension **1837**
Motrin Cold & Sinus Caplets **1836**
Motrin IB Tablets and Caplets **1836**
Infants' Motrin Concentrated Drops **1837**
Infants' Motrin Non-Staining Dye-Free Drops **1837**
Junior Strength Motrin Caplets and Chewable Tablets **1837**
Vicoprofen Tablets **533**

Imatinib Mesylate (A reduced dose of cilostazol should be considered when taken concomitantly with CYP2C19 inhibitors). Products include:
Gleevec Tablets **2221**

Indinavir Sulfate (A reduced dose of cilostazol should be considered when taken concomitantly with CYP3A4 inhibitors). Products include:
Crixivan Capsules **1918**

Indomethacin (Caution is advised in patients receiving both cilostazol and any other antiplatelet agent). Products include:
Indocin **1968**

Indomethacin Sodium Trihydrate (Caution is advised in patients receiving both cilostazol and any other antiplatelet agent). Products include:
Indocin I.V. **1973**

Isoniazid (A reduced dose of cilostazol should be considered when taken concomitantly with CYP2C19 inhibitors).
No products indexed under this heading.

Itraconazole (Co-administration of cilostazol with strong inhibitors of CYP3A4, such as itraconazole, would be expected to cause an increase in cilostazol Cmax and AUC).
No products indexed under this heading.

Ketoconazole (Co-administration of cilostazol with strong inhibitors of CYP3A4, such as ketoconazole increased cilostazol Cmax and AUC). Products include:
Nizoral A-D Shampoo, 1% **1839**
Nizoral 2% Shampoo **1838**

Ketoprofen (A reduced dose of cilostazol should be considered when taken concomitantly with CYP2C19 inhibitors).
No products indexed under this heading.

Leflunomide (A reduced dose of cilostazol should be considered when taken concomitantly with CYP2C19 inhibitors). Products include:
Arava Tablets **2881**

Lopinavir (A reduced dose of cilostazol should be considered when taken concomitantly with CYP3A4 inhibitors). Products include:
Kaletra **474**

Loratadine (A reduced dose of cilostazol should be considered when taken concomitantly with CYP3A4 inhibitors). Products include:
Alavert Allergy & Sinus D-12 Hour Tablets .... ▣**743**
Alavert .... ▣**743**
Children's Claritin 24 Hour Non-Drowsy Allergy Syrup .... ▣**732**
Claritin Non-Drowsy 24 Hour Tablets .... ▣**731**
Non-Drowsy Claritin Hives Relief Tablets .... ▣**733**
Claritin Reditabs 24 Hour Non-Drowsy Tablets .... ▣**732**
Claritin-D Non-Drowsy 12 Hour Tablets .... ▣**731**
Claritin-D Non-Drowsy 24 Hour Tablets .... ▣**731**
Children's Dimetapp ND Non-Drowsy Allergy Syrup .... ▣**746**
Triaminic Allerchews .... ▣**684**

Lovastatin (A reduced dose of cilostazol should be considered when taken concomitantly with CYP2C19 inhibitors). Products include:
Advicor Tablets **1694**
Altoprev Extended-Release Tablets **1151**
Mevacor Tablets **1996**

Magnesium Salicylate (Caution is advised in patients receiving both cilostazol and any other antiplatelet agent).
No products indexed under this heading.

Meclofenamate Sodium (Caution is advised in patients receiving both cilostazol and any other antiplatelet agent).
No products indexed under this heading.

Mefenamic Acid (Caution is advised in patients receiving both cilostazol and any other antiplatelet agent).
No products indexed under this heading.

Methyclothiazide (A reduced dose of cilostazol should be considered when taken concomitantly with CYP2C19 inhibitors).
No products indexed under this heading.

Metronidazole (A reduced dose of cilostazol should be considered when taken concomitantly with CYP2C19 inhibitors). Products include:
Metrogel 1% **1212**
MetroGel-Vaginal Gel **1822**
Noritate Cream, 1% **1051**

Metronidazole Benzoate (A reduced dose of cilostazol should be considered when taken concomitantly with CYP3A4 inhibitors).
No products indexed under this heading.

Metronidazole Hydrochloride (A reduced dose of cilostazol should be considered when taken concomitantly with CYP2C19 inhibitors).
No products indexed under this heading.

Mezlocillin Sodium (Caution is advised in patients receiving both cilostazol and any other antiplatelet agent).
No products indexed under this heading.

Miconazole (Co-administration of cilostazol with strong inhibitors of CYP3A4, such as miconazole, would be expected to cause an increase in Cmax and AUC).
No products indexed under this heading.

Miconazole Nitrate (A reduced dose of cilostazol should be considered when taken concomitantly with CYP3A4 inhibitors). Products include:
Desenex .... ▣**674**
Desenex Jock Itch Spray Powder ... ▣**674**

Modafinil (A reduced dose of cilostazol should be considered when taken concomitantly with CYP2C19 inhibitors). Products include:

IMPORTANT NOTE: Always consult each drug listing in the patient's regimen for possible interactions.

Provigil Tablets 1002

Nafcillin Sodium (Caution is advised in patients receiving both cilostazol and any other antiplatelet agent).
No products indexed under this heading.

Naproxen (Caution is advised in patients receiving both cilostazol and any other antiplatelet agent). Products include:
EC-Naprosyn Delayed-Release Tablets 2769
Naprosyn Suspension 2769
Naprosyn Tablets 2769
Prevacid NapraPAC 3277

Naproxen Sodium (Caution is advised in patients receiving both cilostazol and any other antiplatelet agent). Products include:
Aleve Tablets, Caplets and Gelcaps .... ▣605
Anaprox Tablets 2769
Anaprox DS Tablets 2769

Nefazodone Hydrochloride (Co-administration of cilostazol with strong inhibitors of CYP3A4, such as nefazodone, would be expected to cause an increase cilostazol Cmax and AUC).
No products indexed under this heading.

Nelfinavir Mesylate (A reduced dose of cilostazol should be considered when taken concomitantly with CYP3A4 inhibitors). Products include:
Viracept 2556

Nevirapine (A reduced dose of cilostazol should be considered when taken concomitantly with CYP3A4 inhibitors). Products include:
Viramune Oral Suspension 903
Viramune Tablets 903

Niacinamide (A reduced dose of cilostazol should be considered when taken concomitantly with CYP3A4 inhibitors).
No products indexed under this heading.

Nicotinamide (A reduced dose of cilostazol should be considered when taken concomitantly with CYP3A4 inhibitors). Products include:
Nicomide Tablets 3190

Nifedipine (A reduced dose of cilostazol should be considered when taken concomitantly with CYP3A4 inhibitors). Products include:
Adalat CC Tablets 2978

Norfloxacin (A reduced dose of cilostazol should be considered when taken concomitantly with CYP3A4 inhibitors). Products include:
Noroxin Tablets 2009

Omeprazole (Co-administration with potent inhibitors of CYP2C19, such as omeprazole, has increased the systemic exposure to 3,4 dehydro-cilostazol by 69%). Products include:
Zegerid Powder for Oral Solution 2972

Oxiconazole Nitrate (A reduced dose of cilostazol should be considered when taken concomitantly with CYP2C19 inhibitors). Products include:
Oxistat 1498

Paroxetine Hydrochloride (A reduced dose of cilostazol should be considered when taken concomitantly with CYP2C19 inhibitors). Products include:
Paxil CR Controlled-Release Tablets 1509
Paxil 1501

Penicillin G Benzathine (Caution is advised in patients receiving both cilostazol and any other antiplatelet agent).
No products indexed under this heading.

Penicillin G Procaine (Caution is advised in patients receiving both cilostazol and any other antiplatelet agent).
No products indexed under this heading.

Phenylbutazone (A reduced dose of cilostazol should be considered when taken concomitantly with CYP2C19 inhibitors).
No products indexed under this heading.

Piroxicam (Caution is advised in patients receiving both cilostazol and any other antiplatelet agent).
No products indexed under this heading.

Polythiazide (A reduced dose of cilostazol should be considered when taken concomitantly with CYP2C19 inhibitors).
No products indexed under this heading.

Propoxyphene Hydrochloride (A reduced dose of cilostazol should be considered when taken concomitantly with CYP3A4 inhibitors).
No products indexed under this heading.

Propoxyphene Napsylate (A reduced dose of cilostazol should be considered when taken concomitantly with CYP3A4 inhibitors). Products include:
Darvocet A 500 Tablets 3497

Quinidine (A reduced dose of cilostazol should be considered when taken concomitantly with CYP3A4 inhibitors).
No products indexed under this heading.

Quinidine Hydrochloride (A reduced dose of cilostazol should be considered when taken concomitantly with CYP3A4 inhibitors).
No products indexed under this heading.

Quinidine Polygalacturonate (A reduced dose of cilostazol should be considered when taken concomitantly with CYP3A4 inhibitors).
No products indexed under this heading.

Quinidine Sulfate (A reduced dose of cilostazol should be considered when taken concomitantly with CYP3A4 inhibitors).
No products indexed under this heading.

Quinine (A reduced dose of cilostazol should be considered when taken concomitantly with CYP3A4 inhibitors).
No products indexed under this heading.

Quinine Sulfate (A reduced dose of cilostazol should be considered when taken concomitantly with CYP3A4 inhibitors).
No products indexed under this heading.

Quinupristin (A reduced dose of cilostazol should be considered when taken concomitantly with CYP3A4 inhibitors). Products include:
Synercid I.V. 1690

Ranitidine Bismuth Citrate (A reduced dose of cilostazol should be considered when taken concomitantly with CYP3A4 inhibitors).
No products indexed under this heading.

Ranitidine Hydrochloride (A reduced dose of cilostazol should be considered when taken concomitantly with CYP3A4 inhibitors). Products include:
Zantac 1597
Zantac Injection 1593
Zantac 75 Tablets .... ▣715
Zantac 150 Maximum Strength Tablets .... ▣715
Zantac Injection Pharmacy Bulk Package 1595

Ritonavir (A reduced dose of cilostazol should be considered when taken concomitantly with CYP2C19 inhibitors). Products include:
Kaletra 474
Norvir 499

Salsalate (Caution is advised in patients receiving both cilostazol and any other antiplatelet agent).
No products indexed under this heading.

Saquinavir (A reduced dose of cilostazol should be considered when taken concomitantly with CYP3A4 inhibitors).
No products indexed under this heading.

Saquinavir Mesylate (A reduced dose of cilostazol should be considered when taken concomitantly with CYP3A4 inhibitors). Products include:
Invirase 2776

Sertraline Hydrochloride (Co-administration of cilostazol with strong inhibitors of CYP3A4, such as sertraline, would be expected to cause an increase in cilostazol Cmax and AUC). Products include:
Zoloft 2581

Sulfacytine (A reduced dose of cilostazol should be considered when taken concomitantly with CYP2C19 inhibitors).
No products indexed under this heading.

Sulfamethizole (A reduced dose of cilostazol should be considered when taken concomitantly with CYP2C19 inhibitors).
No products indexed under this heading.

Sulfamethoxazole (A reduced dose of cilostazol should be considered when taken concomitantly with CYP2C19 inhibitors).
No products indexed under this heading.

Sulfasalazine (A reduced dose of cilostazol should be considered when taken concomitantly with CYP2C19 inhibitors).
No products indexed under this heading.

Sulfinpyrazone (A reduced dose of cilostazol should be considered when taken concomitantly with CYP2C19 inhibitors).
No products indexed under this heading.

Sulfisoxazole (A reduced dose of cilostazol should be considered when taken concomitantly with CYP2C19 inhibitors).
No products indexed under this heading.

Sulfisoxazole Acetyl (A reduced dose of cilostazol should be considered when taken concomitantly with CYP2C19 inhibitors).
No products indexed under this heading.

Sulfisoxazole Diolamine (A reduced dose of cilostazol should be considered when taken concomitantly with CYP2C19 inhibitors).
No products indexed under this heading.

Sulindac (Caution is advised in patients receiving both cilostazol and any other antiplatelet agent). Products include:
Clinoril Tablets 1899

Telithromycin (A reduced dose of cilostazol should be considered when taken concomitantly with CYP3A4 inhibitors). Products include:
Ketek Tablets 2920

Terconazole (A reduced dose of cilostazol should be considered when taken concomitantly with CYP2C19 inhibitors).
No products indexed under this heading.

Ticarcillin Disodium (Caution is advised in patients receiving both cilostazol and any other antiplatelet agent). Products include:
Timentin ADD-Vantage 1556
Timentin Injection Galaxy Container 1559
Timentin IV Infusion 1553
Timentin Pharmacy Bulk Package 1562

Ticlopidine Hydrochloride (A reduced dose of cilostazol should be considered when taken concomitantly with CYP2C19 inhibitors). Products include:
Ticlid Tablets 2813

Tolazamide (A reduced dose of cilostazol should be considered when taken concomitantly with CYP2C19 inhibitors).
No products indexed under this heading.

Tolbutamide (A reduced dose of cilostazol should be considered when taken concomitantly with CYP2C19 inhibitors).
No products indexed under this heading.

Tolbutamide Sodium (A reduced dose of cilostazol should be considered when taken concomitantly with CYP2C19 inhibitors).
No products indexed under this heading.

Tolmetin Sodium (Caution is advised in patients receiving both cilostazol and any other antiplatelet agent).
No products indexed under this heading.

Troglitazone (A reduced dose of cilostazol should be considered when taken concomitantly with CYP2C19 inhibitors).
No products indexed under this heading.

Troleandomycin (A reduced dose of cilostazol should be considered when taken concomitantly with CYP3A4 inhibitors).
No products indexed under this heading.

Valproate Sodium (A reduced dose of cilostazol should be considered when taken concomitantly with CYP3A4 inhibitors). Products include:
Depacon Injection 412

Verapamil Hydrochloride (A reduced dose of cilostazol should be considered when taken concomitantly with CYP3A4 inhibitors). Products include:

Covera-HS Tablets 3135
Tarka Tablets 519
Verelan PM Capsules 3120

Voriconazole (A reduced dose of cilostazol should be considered when taken concomitantly with CYP3A4 inhibitors). Products include:

VFEND I.V. 2543
VFEND Oral Suspension 2543
VFEND Tablets 2543

Zafirlukast (A reduced dose of cilostazol should be considered when taken concomitantly with CYP2C19 inhibitors). Products include:

Accolate Tablets 663

Zileuton (A reduced dose of cilostazol should be considered when taken concomitantly with CYP3A4 inhibitors).

No products indexed under this heading.

Food Interactions

Food, unspecified (Co-administration with a high-fat meal increases absorption, with an approximately 90% increase in Cmax and a 25% increase in AUC; patients should be advised to take Pletal at least one hour before or two hours after breakfast and dinner).

Grapefruit (A reduced dose of cilostazol should be considered when taken concomitantly with CYP3A4 inhibitors).

Grapefruit Juice (Co-administration of cilostazol with inhibitors of CYP3A4, such as grapefruit juice, increase cilostazol plasma concentration by 50%; concurrent consumption of grapefruit juice should be avoided).

PLEXION CLEANSER

(Sodium Sulfacetamide, Sulfur) 1863
None cited in PDR database.

PLEXION CLEANSING CLOTHS

(Sodium Sulfacetamide, Sulfur) 1863
None cited in PDR database.

PLEXION SCT

(Sodium Sulfacetamide, Sulfur) 1863
None cited in PDR database.

PLEXION TOPICAL SUSPENSION

(Sodium Sulfacetamide, Sulfur) 1863
None cited in PDR database.

PLUS WITH AMBROTOSE COMPLEX CAPLETS

(Amino Acid Preparations) .... ■769
None cited in PDR database.

PNEUMOVAX 23

(Pneumococcal Vaccine, Polyvalent) 2020
May interact with:

Azathioprine (Co-administration of vaccine in patients receiving immunosuppressive therapy may not result in expected serum antibody response; potential impairment of future immune responses to pneumoccocal antigens may occur). Products include:

Azasan Tablets 2844

Cyclosporine (Co-administration of vaccine in patients receiving immunosuppressive therapy may not result in expected serum antibody response; potential impairment of future immune responses to pneumoccocal antigens may occur). Products include:

Gengraf Capsules 458
Neoral Soft Gelatin Capsules 2247
Neoral Oral Solution 2247
Restasis Ophthalmic Emulsion 570
Sandimmune 2259

Muromonab-CD3 (Co-administration of vaccine in patients receiving immunosuppressive therapy may not result in expected serum antibody response; potential impairment of future immune responses to pneumoccocal antigens may occur). Products include:

Orthoclone OKT3 Sterile Solution 2370

Mycophenolate Mofetil (Co-administration of vaccine in patients receiving immunosuppressive therapy may not result in expected serum antibody response; potential impairment of future immune responses to pneumoccocal antigens may occur). Products include:

CellCept Capsules 2751
CellCept Oral Suspension 2751
CellCept Tablets 2751

Tacrolimus (Co-administration of vaccine in patients receiving immunosuppressive therapy may not result in expected serum antibody response; potential impairment of future immune responses to pneumoccocal antigens may occur). Products include:

Prograf Capsules and Injection 624
Protopic Ointment 629

POLY-PRED LIQUIFILM OPHTHALMIC SUSPENSION

(Neomycin Sulfate, Polymyxin B Sulfate, Prednisolone Acetate) .... ⊙231
None cited in PDR database.

POLYSPORIN OINTMENT

(Bacitracin, Polymyxin B Sulfate) .... ■706
None cited in PDR database.

POLYTRIM OPHTHALMIC SOLUTION

(Polymyxin B Sulfate, Trimethoprim Sulfate) 570
None cited in PDR database.

POTABA CAPSULES

(Aminobenzoate Potassium) 1634
May interact with sulfonamides. Compounds in these categories include:

Bendroflumethiazide (Co-administration with sulfonamides is contraindicated).

No products indexed under this heading.

Chlorothiazide (Co-administration with sulfonamides is contraindicated). Products include:

Aldoclor Tablets 1881
Diuril Oral 1936

Chlorothiazide Sodium (Co-administration with sulfonamides is contraindicated). Products include:

Diuril Sodium Intravenous 1934

Chlorpropamide (Co-administration with sulfonamides is contraindicated).

No products indexed under this heading.

Glipizide (Co-administration with sulfonamides is contraindicated).

No products indexed under this heading.

Glyburide (Co-administration with sulfonamides is contraindicated).

No products indexed under this heading.

Hydrochlorothiazide (Co-administration with sulfonamides is contraindicated). Products include:

Aldoril Tablets 1884
Atacand HCT 637
Avalide Tablets 2889
Avalide Tablets 922
Benicar HCT Tablets 2852
Diovan HCT Tablets 2195
Dyazide Capsules 1389
Hyzaar 1964
Lotensin HCT Tablets 2235
Maxzide 2150
Micardis HCT Tablets 886
Moduretic Tablets 2003
Prinzide Tablets 2033
Teveten HCT Tablets 1710
Timolide Tablets 2056
Uniretic Tablets 3114
Vaseretic Tablets 2073
Zestoretic Tablets 701

Hydroflumethiazide (Co-administration with sulfonamides is contraindicated).

No products indexed under this heading.

Methyclothiazide (Co-administration with sulfonamides is contraindicated).

No products indexed under this heading.

Polythiazide (Co-administration with sulfonamides is contraindicated).

No products indexed under this heading.

Sulfacytine (Co-administration with sulfonamides is contraindicated).

No products indexed under this heading.

Sulfamethizole (Co-administration with sulfonamides is contraindicated).

No products indexed under this heading.

Sulfamethoxazole (Co-administration with sulfonamides is contraindicated).

No products indexed under this heading.

Sulfasalazine (Co-administration with sulfonamides is contraindicated).

No products indexed under this heading.

Sulfinpyrazone (Co-administration with sulfonamides is contraindicated).

No products indexed under this heading.

Sulfisoxazole (Co-administration with sulfonamides is contraindicated).

No products indexed under this heading.

Sulfisoxazole Acetyl (Co-administration with sulfonamides is contraindicated).

No products indexed under this heading.

Sulfisoxazole Diolamine (Co-administration with sulfonamides is contraindicated).

No products indexed under this heading.

Tolazamide (Co-administration with sulfonamides is contraindicated).

No products indexed under this heading.

Tolbutamide (Co-administration with sulfonamides is contraindicated).

No products indexed under this heading.

POTABA ENVULES

(Aminobenzoate Potassium) 1634
See Potaba Capsules

POTABA TABLETS

(Aminobenzoate Potassium) 1634
See Potaba Capsules

PRAMOSONE CREAM 1% AND 2.5%

(Hydrocortisone Acetate, Pramoxine Hydrochloride) 1139
None cited in PDR database.

PRAMOSONE LOTION 1% AND 2.5%

(Hydrocortisone Acetate, Pramoxine Hydrochloride) 1139
See Pramosone Cream 1% and 2.5%

PRAMOSONE OINTMENT 1% AND 2.5%

(Hydrocortisone Acetate, Pramoxine Hydrochloride) 1139
See Pramosone Cream 1% and 2.5%

PRANDIN TABLETS (0.5, 1, AND 2 MG)

(Repaglinide) 2337
May interact with barbiturates, beta blockers, calcium channel blockers, corticosteroids, oral anticoagulants, diuretics, erythromycin, estrogens, monoamine oxidase inhibitors, nonsteroidal anti-inflammatory agents, phenothiazines, phenytoin, salicylates, sulfonamides, sympathomimetics, thiazides, thyroid preparations, and certain other agents. Compounds in these categories include:

Acebutolol Hydrochloride (The hypoglycemic action of oral antidiabetic agents may be potentiated by beta adrenergic blocking agents; hypoglycemia may be difficult to recognize with co-administration).

No products indexed under this heading.

Albuterol (Sympathomimetics tend to produce hyperglycemia and may lead to loss of glycemic control). Products include:

Proventil Inhalation Aerosol 3067

Albuterol Sulfate (Sympathomimetics tend to produce hyperglycemia and may lead to loss of glycemic control). Products include:

AccuNeb Inhalation Solution 1055
Combivent Inhalation Aerosol 878
DuoNeb Inhalation Solution 1058
Proventil Inhalation Solution 0.083% 3069
Proventil HFA Inhalation Aerosol 3071
Ventolin HFA Inhalation Aerosol 1576
VoSpire Extended-Release Tablets 2352

Amiloride Hydrochloride (Diuretics tend to produce hyperglycemia and may lead to loss of glycemic control). Products include:

Midamor Tablets 2000
Moduretic Tablets 2003

Amlodipine Besylate (Calcium channel blocking agents tend to produce hyperglycemia and may lead to loss of glycemic control). Products include:

Caduet Tablets 2507
Lotrel Capsules 2238
Norvasc Tablets 2529

Anisindione (The hypoglycemic action of oral antidiabetic agents may be potentiated by coumarins). Products include:

Miradon Tablets 3056

IMPORTANT NOTE: Always consult each drug listing in the patient's regimen for possible interactions.

Aprobarbital (Drugs that induce the CYP450 enzyme system 3A4, such as barbiturates, may increase repaglinide metabolism).
No products indexed under this heading.

Aspirin (The hypoglycemic action of oral antidiabetic agents may be potentiated by salicylates). Products include:
Aggrenox Capsules 855
Bayer, Aspirin Regimen .... ▣606
Bayer Aspirin Tablets 3515
BC Powder .... ▣612
BC Allergy Sinus Cold Powder .... ▣612
Arthritis Strength BC Powder .... ▣612
BC Sinus Cold Powder .... ▣612
Ecotrin Enteric Coated Aspirin Low, Regular and Maximum Strength Tablets 1627
Goody's Body Pain Formula Powder .... ▣621
Goody's Extra Strength Headache Powder .... ▣621
Goody's Extra Strength Pain Relief Tablets .... ▣621
Percodan Tablets 1115
St. Joseph 81 mg Aspirin Chewable and Enteric Coated Tablets 1841

Aspirin, Enteric Coated (The hypoglycemic action of oral antidiabetic agents may be potentiated by salicylates).
No products indexed under this heading.

Aspirin Buffered (The hypoglycemic action of oral antidiabetic agents may be potentiated by salicylates).
No products indexed under this heading.

Atenolol (The hypoglycemic action of oral antidiabetic agents may be potentiated by beta adrenergic blocking agents; hypoglycemia may be difficult to recognize with co-administration). Products include:
Tenormin I.V. Injection 698
Tenormin Tablets 695

Bendroflumethiazide (Diuretics tend to produce hyperglycemia and may lead to loss of glycemic control).
No products indexed under this heading.

Bepridil Hydrochloride (Calcium channel blocking agents tend to produce hyperglycemia and may lead to loss of glycemic control).
No products indexed under this heading.

Betamethasone Acetate (Corticosteroids tend to produce hyperglycemia and may lead to loss of glycemic control).
No products indexed under this heading.

Betamethasone Sodium Phosphate (Corticosteroids tend to produce hyperglycemia and may lead to loss of glycemic control).
No products indexed under this heading.

Betaxolol Hydrochloride (The hypoglycemic action of oral antidiabetic agents may be potentiated by beta adrenergic blocking agents; hypoglycemia may be difficult to recognize with co-administration). Products include:
Betoptic S Ophthalmic Suspension 554

Bisoprolol Fumarate (The hypoglycemic action of oral antidiabetic agents may be potentiated by beta adrenergic blocking agents; hypoglycemia may be difficult to recognize with co-administration).
No products indexed under this heading.

Bumetanide (Diuretics tend to produce hyperglycemia and may lead to loss of glycemic control).
No products indexed under this heading.

Butabarbital (Drugs that induce the CYP450 enzyme system 3A4, such as barbiturates, may increase repaglinide metabolism).
No products indexed under this heading.

Butalbital (Drugs that induce the CYP450 enzyme system 3A4, such as barbiturates, may increase repaglinide metabolism). Products include:
Sedapap Tablets 50 mg/650 mg 2098

Carbamazepine (Drugs that induce the CYP450 enzyme system 3A4, such as carbamazepine, may increase repaglinide metabolism). Products include:
Carbatrol Capsules 3174
Equetro Extended-Release Capsules 3178
Tegretol/Tegretol-XR 2278

Carteolol Hydrochloride (The hypoglycemic action of oral antidiabetic agents may be potentiated by beta adrenergic blocking agents; hypoglycemia may be difficult to recognize with co-administration). Products include:
Carteolol Hydrochloride Ophthalmic Solution USP, 1% .... ⊙246

Celecoxib (The hypoglycemic action of oral antidiabetic agents may be potentiated by non-steroidal anti-inflammatory agents). Products include:
Celebrex Capsules 3130

Chloramphenicol Sodium Succinate (The hypoglycemic action of oral antidiabetic agents may be potentiated by chloramphenicol).
No products indexed under this heading.

Chlorothiazide (Diuretics tend to produce hyperglycemia and may lead to loss of glycemic control). Products include:
Aldoclor Tablets 1881
Diuril Oral 1936

Chlorothiazide Sodium (Diuretics tend to produce hyperglycemia and may lead to loss of glycemic control). Products include:
Diuril Sodium Intravenous 1934

Chlorotrianisene (Estrogens and oral contraceptives tend to produce hyperglycemia and may lead to loss of glycemic control).
No products indexed under this heading.

Chlorpromazine (Phenothiazines tend to produce hyperglycemia and may lead to loss of glycemic control).
No products indexed under this heading.

Chlorpromazine Hydrochloride (Phenothiazines tend to produce hyperglycemia and may lead to loss of glycemic control).
No products indexed under this heading.

Chlorpropamide (The hypoglycemic action of oral antidiabetic agents may be potentiated by sulfonamides).
No products indexed under this heading.

Chlorthalidone (Diuretics tend to produce hyperglycemia and may lead to loss of glycemic control). Products include:
Clorpres Tablets 2139

Choline Magnesium Trisalicylate (The hypoglycemic action of oral antidiabetic agents may be potentiated by salicylates).
No products indexed under this heading.

Clarithromycin (Co-administration of clarithromycin (a cytochrome P450 enzyme inhibitor) and Prandin resulted in a clinically significant increase in repaglinide plasma levels. This increase in repaglinide plasma levels may necessitate a Prandin dose adjustment). Products include:
Biaxin/Biaxin XL 402
PREVPAC 3281

Cortisone Acetate (Corticosteroids tend to produce hyperglycemia and may lead to loss of glycemic control).
No products indexed under this heading.

Dexamethasone (Corticosteroids tend to produce hyperglycemia and may lead to loss of glycemic control). Products include:
Ciprodex Otic Suspension 555
Decadron Tablets 1929
TobraDex Ophthalmic Ointment 558
TobraDex Ophthalmic Suspension 558

Dexamethasone Acetate (Corticosteroids tend to produce hyperglycemia and may lead to loss of glycemic control).
No products indexed under this heading.

Dexamethasone Sodium Phosphate (Corticosteroids tend to produce hyperglycemia and may lead to loss of glycemic control). Products include:
Decadron Phosphate Injection 1931

Diclofenac Potassium (The hypoglycemic action of oral antidiabetic agents may be potentiated by non-steroidal anti-inflammatory agents). Products include:
Cataflam Tablets 2173

Diclofenac Sodium (The hypoglycemic action of oral antidiabetic agents may be potentiated by non-steroidal anti-inflammatory agents). Products include:
Arthrotec Tablets 3126
Voltaren Ophthalmic Solution 2300
Voltaren Tablets 2298
Voltaren-XR Tablets 2301

Dicumarol (The hypoglycemic action of oral antidiabetic agents may be potentiated by coumarins).
No products indexed under this heading.

Dienestrol (Estrogens and oral contraceptives tend to produce hyperglycemia and may lead to loss of glycemic control).
No products indexed under this heading.

Diethylstilbestrol (Estrogens and oral contraceptives tend to produce hyperglycemia and may lead to loss of glycemic control).
No products indexed under this heading.

Diflunisal (The hypoglycemic action of oral antidiabetic agents may be potentiated by salicylates). Products include:
Dolobid Tablets 1937

Diltiazem Hydrochloride (Calcium channel blocking agents tend to produce hyperglycemia and may lead to loss of glycemic control). Products include:
Cardizem LA Extended Release Tablets 1699
Tiazac Capsules 1204

Dobutamine Hydrochloride (Sympathomimetics tend to produce hyperglycemia and may lead to loss of glycemic control).
No products indexed under this heading.

Dopamine Hydrochloride (Sympathomimetics tend to produce hyperglycemia and may lead to loss of glycemic control).
No products indexed under this heading.

Ephedrine Hydrochloride (Sympathomimetics tend to produce hyperglycemia and may lead to loss of glycemic control). Products include:
Primatene Tablets .... ▣749

Ephedrine Sulfate (Sympathomimetics tend to produce hyperglycemia and may lead to loss of glycemic control).
No products indexed under this heading.

Ephedrine Tannate (Sympathomimetics tend to produce hyperglycemia and may lead to loss of glycemic control).
No products indexed under this heading.

Epinephrine (Sympathomimetics tend to produce hyperglycemia and may lead to loss of glycemic control). Products include:
EpiPen 1061
Primatene Mist .... ▣749

Epinephrine Bitartrate (Sympathomimetics tend to produce hyperglycemia and may lead to loss of glycemic control).
No products indexed under this heading.

Epinephrine Hydrochloride (Sympathomimetics tend to produce hyperglycemia and may lead to loss of glycemic control).
No products indexed under this heading.

Erythromycin (In vitro data indicate that repaglinide metabolism may be inhibited by erythromycin). Products include:
Erygel Topical Gel 2096
Ery-Tab Tablets 447
Erythromycin Base Filmtab Tablets 454
Erythromycin Delayed-Release Capsules, USP 456
PCE Dispertab Tablets 510

Erythromycin Estolate (In vitro data indicate that repaglinide metabolism may be inhibited by erythromycin).
No products indexed under this heading.

Erythromycin Ethylsuccinate (In vitro data indicate that repaglinide metabolism may be inhibited by erythromycin). Products include:
E.E.S. 449
EryPed 445

Erythromycin Gluceptate (In vitro data indicate that repaglinide metabolism may be inhibited by erythromycin).
No products indexed under this heading.

Erythromycin Lactobionate (In vitro data indicate that repaglinide metabolism may be inhibited by erythromycin).
No products indexed under this heading.

Erythromycin Stearate (In vitro data indicate that repaglinide metabolism may be inhibited by erythromycin). Products include:
Erythrocin Stearate Filmtab Tablets 452

Esmolol Hydrochloride (The hypoglycemic action of oral antidiabetic agents may be potentiated by beta adrenergic blocking agents; hypoglycemia may be difficult to recognize with co-administration). Products include:
Brevibloc Concentrate 766
Brevibloc Injection 766
Brevibloc Double Strength Injection 766
Brevibloc Premixed Injection 766
Brevibloc Double Strength Premixed Injection 766

Estradiol (Estrogens and oral contraceptives tend to produce hyperglycemia and may lead to loss of glycemic control). Products include:
Activella Tablets 2311
Climara Transdermal System 795
Climara Pro Transdermal System 800
CombiPatch Transdermal System 2180
Estrogel 0.06% 3200
Menostar Transdermal System 805
Prefest Tablets 1069
Vagifem Tablets 2340
Vivelle Transdermal System 2288
Vivelle-Dot Transdermal System 2293

Estrogens, Conjugated (Estrogens and oral contraceptives tend to produce hyperglycemia and may lead to loss of glycemic control). Products include:
Premarin Intravenous 3440
Premarin Tablets 3443
Premarin Vaginal Cream 3449
Premphase Tablets 3452
Prempro Tablets 3452

Estrogens, Esterified (Estrogens and oral contraceptives tend to produce hyperglycemia and may lead to loss of glycemic control). Products include:
Estratest Tablets 3196
Estratest H.S. Tablets 3196

Estropipate (Estrogens and oral contraceptives tend to produce hyperglycemia and may lead to loss of glycemic control).
No products indexed under this heading.

Ethacrynic Acid (Diuretics tend to produce hyperglycemia and may lead to loss of glycemic control). Products include:
Edecrin Tablets 1941

Ethinyl Estradiol (Co-administration has resulted in a 20% increase in repaglinide, levonorgestrel and ethinyl estradiol Cmax). Products include:
Alesse-28 Tablets 3392
Lo/Ovral-28 Tablets 3423
NuvaRing 2357
Ortho-Cept Tablets 2395
Ortho-Cyclen/Ortho Tri-Cyclen 2414
Ortho Evra Transdermal System 2402
Ortho Tri-Cyclen Lo Tablets 2421
Seasonale Tablets 1073
Triphasil-28 Tablets 3483
Yasmin 28 Tablets 818

Etodolac (The hypoglycemic action of oral antidiabetic agents may be potentiated by non-steroidal anti-inflammatory agents).
No products indexed under this heading.

Felodipine (Calcium channel blocking agents tend to produce hyperglycemia and may lead to loss of glycemic control). Products include:
Plendil Extended-Release Tablets 651

Fenoprofen Calcium (The hypoglycemic action of oral antidiabetic agents may be potentiated by non-steroidal anti-inflammatory agents). Products include:
Nalfon Capsules 2504

Fludrocortisone Acetate (Corticosteroids tend to produce hyperglycemia and may lead to loss of glycemic control).
No products indexed under this heading.

Fluphenazine Decanoate (Phenothiazines tend to produce hyperglycemia and may lead to loss of glycemic control).
No products indexed under this heading.

Fluphenazine Enanthate (Phenothiazines tend to produce hyperglycemia and may lead to loss of glycemic control).
No products indexed under this heading.

Fluphenazine Hydrochloride (Phenothiazines tend to produce hyperglycemia and may lead to loss of glycemic control).
No products indexed under this heading.

Flurbiprofen (The hypoglycemic action of oral antidiabetic agents may be potentiated by non-steroidal anti-inflammatory agents).
No products indexed under this heading.

Fosphenytoin Sodium (Phenytoin tends to produce hyperglycemia and may lead to loss of glycemic control).
No products indexed under this heading.

Furosemide (Diuretics tend to produce hyperglycemia and may lead to loss of glycemic control). Products include:
Furosemide Tablets 2117

Gemfibrozil (Co-administration of gemfibrozil with repaglinide resulted in a significant increase in repaglinide blood levels. Patients taking repaglinide should not start taking gemfibrozil; patients taking gemfibrozil should not start taking repaglinide. Caution should be used in patients already on repaglinide and gemfibrozil).
No products indexed under this heading.

Glipizide (The hypoglycemic action of oral antidiabetic agents may be potentiated by sulfonamides).
No products indexed under this heading.

Glyburide (The hypoglycemic action of oral antidiabetic agents may be potentiated by sulfonamides).
No products indexed under this heading.

Hydrochlorothiazide (Diuretics tend to produce hyperglycemia and may lead to loss of glycemic control). Products include:
Aldoril Tablets 1884
Atacand HCT 637
Avalide Tablets 2889
Avalide Tablets 922
Benicar HCT Tablets 2852
Diovan HCT Tablets 2195
Dyazide Capsules 1389
Hyzaar 1964
Lotensin HCT Tablets 2235
Maxzide 2150
Micardis HCT Tablets 886
Moduretic Tablets 2003
Prinzide Tablets 2033
Teveten HCT Tablets 1710
Timolide Tablets 2056
Uniretic Tablets 3114
Vaseretic Tablets 2073
Zestoretic Tablets 701

Hydrocortisone (Corticosteroids tend to produce hyperglycemia and may lead to loss of glycemic control). Products include:
Cortizone•5 Ointment 699
Cortizone•10 Creme 699
Cortizone•10 Ointment 699
Cortizone•10 Plus Creme 700
Cortizone•10 Maximum Strength Quick Shot Spray 700
Hydrocortone Tablets 1963
Preparation H Hydrocortisone Cream 748

Hydrocortisone Acetate (Corticosteroids tend to produce hyperglycemia and may lead to loss of glycemic control). Products include:
Analpram-HC 1136
Pramosone 1139
ProctoFoam-HC 3113
Tucks Anti-Itch Ointment 712
U-cort 1% Cream 3289

Hydrocortisone Sodium Phosphate (Corticosteroids tend to produce hyperglycemia and may lead to loss of glycemic control).
No products indexed under this heading.

Hydrocortisone Sodium Succinate (Corticosteroids tend to produce hyperglycemia and may lead to loss of glycemic control).
No products indexed under this heading.

Hydroflumethiazide (Diuretics tend to produce hyperglycemia and may lead to loss of glycemic control).
No products indexed under this heading.

Ibuprofen (The hypoglycemic action of oral antidiabetic agents may be potentiated by non-steroidal anti-inflammatory agents). Products include:
Advil Allergy Sinus Caplets 737
Advil 737
Children's Advil Suspension 742
Children's Advil Chewable Tablets 741
Advil Cold & Sinus 739
Advil Flu & Body Ache Caplets 739
Children's Advil Cold Suspension 741
Infants' Advil Concentrated Drops 743
Junior Strength Advil Swallow Tablets 740
Advil Migraine Liquigels 740
Advil Multi-Symptom Cold Caplets 738
Combunox Tablets 1183
Children's Motrin Oral Suspension and Chewable Tablets 1837
Children's Motrin Cold Non-Staining Dye-Free Oral Suspension 1838
Children's Motrin Cold Oral Suspension 1838
Children's Motrin Non-Staining Dye-Free Oral Suspension 1837
Motrin Cold & Sinus Caplets 1836
Motrin IB Tablets and Caplets 1836
Infants' Motrin Concentrated Drops 1837
Infants' Motrin Non-Staining Dye-Free Drops 1837
Junior Strength Motrin Caplets and Chewable Tablets 1837
Vicoprofen Tablets 533

Indapamide (Diuretics tend to produce hyperglycemia and may lead to loss of glycemic control). Products include:
Indapamide Tablets 2119

Indomethacin (The hypoglycemic action of oral antidiabetic agents may be potentiated by non-steroidal anti-inflammatory agents). Products include:
Indocin 1968

Indomethacin Sodium Trihydrate (The hypoglycemic action of oral antidiabetic agents may be potentiated by non-steroidal anti-inflammatory agents). Products include:
Indocin I.V. 1973

Isocarboxazid (The hypoglycemic action of oral antidiabetic agents may be potentiated by MAO inhibitors).
No products indexed under this heading.

Isoniazid (INH tends to produce hyperglycemia and may lead to loss of glycemic control).
No products indexed under this heading.

Isoproterenol Hydrochloride (Sympathomimetics tend to produce hyperglycemia and may lead to loss of glycemic control).
No products indexed under this heading.

Isoproterenol Sulfate (Sympathomimetics tend to produce hyperglycemia and may lead to loss of glycemic control).
No products indexed under this heading.

Isradipine (Calcium channel blocking agents tend to produce hyperglycemia and may lead to loss of glycemic control). Products include:
DynaCirc CR Tablets 2726

Itraconazole (Gemfibrozil and itraconazole had a synergistic metabolic inhibitory effect on regaglinide. Therefore, patients taking repaglinide and gemfibrozil should not take itraconazole).
No products indexed under this heading.

Ketoconazole (Co-administration has resulted in a 15% and 16% increase in repaglinide AUC and Cmax, respectively). Products include:
Nizoral A-D Shampoo, 1% 1839
Nizoral 2% Shampoo 1838

Ketoprofen (The hypoglycemic action of oral antidiabetic agents may be potentiated by non-steroidal anti-inflammatory agents).
No products indexed under this heading.

Ketorolac Tromethamine (The hypoglycemic action of oral antidiabetic agents may be potentiated by non-steroidal anti-inflammatory agents). Products include:
Acular Ophthalmic Solution 561
Acular LS Ophthalmic Solution 562

Labetalol Hydrochloride (The hypoglycemic action of oral antidiabetic agents may be potentiated by beta adrenergic blocking agents; hypoglycemia may be difficult to recognize with co-administration).
No products indexed under this heading.

Levalbuterol Hydrochloride (Sympathomimetics tend to produce

hyperglycemia and may lead to loss of glycemic control). Products include:

Xopenex Inhalation Solution 3143
Xopenex Inhalation Solution Concentrate 3147

Levobunolol Hydrochloride (The hypoglycemic action of oral antidiabetic agents may be potentiated by beta adrenergic blocking agents; hypoglycemia may be difficult to recognize with co-administration). Products include:

Betagan Ophthalmic Solution, USP............ ⊙217

Levonorgestrel (Co-administration has resulted in a 20% increase in repaglinide, levonorgestrel and ethinyl estradiol Cmax). Products include:

Alesse-28 Tablets 3392
Climara Pro Transdermal System 800
Mirena Intrauterine System 810
Plan B Tablets 1068
Seasonale Tablets 1073
Triphasil-28 Tablets 3483

Levothyroxine Sodium (Thyroid products tend to produce hyperglycemia and may lead to loss of glycemic control). Products include:

Levothroid Tablets 1189
Levoxyl Tablets 1680
Synthroid Tablets 515
Unithroid Tablets 3521

Liothyronine Sodium (Thyroid products tend to produce hyperglycemia and may lead to loss of glycemic control). Products include:

Cytomel Tablets 1678

Liotrix (Thyroid products tend to produce hyperglycemia and may lead to loss of glycemic control). Products include:

Thyrolar 1203

Magnesium Salicylate (The hypoglycemic action of oral antidiabetic agents may be potentiated by salicylates).

No products indexed under this heading.

Meclofenamate Sodium (The hypoglycemic action of oral antidiabetic agents may be potentiated by non-steroidal anti-inflammatory agents).

No products indexed under this heading.

Mefenamic Acid (The hypoglycemic action of oral antidiabetic agents may be potentiated by non-steroidal anti-inflammatory agents).

No products indexed under this heading.

Meloxicam (The hypoglycemic action of oral antidiabetic agents may be potentiated by non-steroidal anti-inflammatory agents). Products include:

Mobic Oral Suspension 893
Mobic Tablets 893

Mephobarbital (Drugs that induce the CYP450 enzyme system 3A4, such as barbiturates, may increase repaglinide metabolism). Products include:

Mebaral Tablets, USP 2483

Mesoridazine Besylate (Phenothiazines tend to produce hyperglycemia and may lead to loss of glycemic control).

No products indexed under this heading.

Metaproterenol Sulfate (Sympathomimetics tend to produce hyperglycemia and may lead to loss of glycemic control). Products include:

Alupent Inhalation Aerosol 858

Metaraminol Bitartrate (Sympathomimetics tend to produce hyperglycemia and may lead to loss of glycemic control). Products include:

Aramine Injection 1889

Methotrimeprazine (Phenothiazines tend to produce hyperglycemia and may lead to loss of glycemic control).

No products indexed under this heading.

Methoxamine Hydrochloride (Sympathomimetics tend to produce hyperglycemia and may lead to loss of glycemic control).

No products indexed under this heading.

Methyclothiazide (Diuretics tend to produce hyperglycemia and may lead to loss of glycemic control).

No products indexed under this heading.

Methylprednisolone Acetate (Corticosteroids tend to produce hyperglycemia and may lead to loss of glycemic control). Products include:

Depo-Medrol Injectable Suspension 2615
Depo-Medrol Single-Dose Vial 2617

Methylprednisolone Sodium Succinate (Corticosteroids tend to produce hyperglycemia and may lead to loss of glycemic control).

No products indexed under this heading.

Metipranolol Hydrochloride (The hypoglycemic action of oral antidiabetic agents may be potentiated by beta adrenergic blocking agents; hypoglycemia may be difficult to recognize with co-administration).

No products indexed under this heading.

Metolazone (Diuretics tend to produce hyperglycemia and may lead to loss of glycemic control).

No products indexed under this heading.

Metoprolol Succinate (The hypoglycemic action of oral antidiabetic agents may be potentiated by beta adrenergic blocking agents; hypoglycemia may be difficult to recognize with co-administration). Products include:

Toprol-XL Tablets 660

Metoprolol Tartrate (The hypoglycemic action of oral antidiabetic agents may be potentiated by beta adrenergic blocking agents; hypoglycemia may be difficult to recognize with co-administration).

No products indexed under this heading.

Mibefradil Dihydrochloride (Calcium channel blocking agents tend to produce hyperglycemia and may lead to loss of glycemic control).

No products indexed under this heading.

Miconazole (In vitro data indicate that repaglinide metabolism may be inhibited by antifungal agent miconazole).

No products indexed under this heading.

Moclobemide (The hypoglycemic action of oral antidiabetic agents may be potentiated by MAO inhibitors).

No products indexed under this heading.

Nabumetone (The hypoglycemic action of oral antidiabetic agents may be potentiated by non-steroidal anti-inflammatory agents). Products include:

Relafen Tablets 1523

Nadolol (The hypoglycemic action of oral antidiabetic agents may be potentiated by beta adrenergic blocking agents; hypoglycemia may be difficult to recognize with co-administration). Products include:

Nadolol Tablets 2121

Naproxen (The hypoglycemic action of oral antidiabetic agents may be potentiated by non-steroidal anti-inflammatory agents). Products include:

EC-Naprosyn Delayed-Release Tablets 2769
Naprosyn Suspension 2769
Naprosyn Tablets 2769
Prevacid NapraPAC 3277

Naproxen Sodium (The hypoglycemic action of oral antidiabetic agents may be potentiated by non-steroidal anti-inflammatory agents). Products include:

Aleve Tablets, Caplets and Gelcaps............ ▣605
Anaprox Tablets 2769
Anaprox DS Tablets 2769

Niacin (Nicotinic acid tends to produce hyperglycemia and may lead to a loss of glycemic control). Products include:

Advicor Tablets 1694
Niaspan Extended-Release Tablets 1703

Nicardipine Hydrochloride (Calcium channel blocking agents tend to produce hyperglycemia and may lead to loss of glycemic control). Products include:

Cardene I.V. 1129

Nifedipine (Calcium channel blocking agents tend to produce hyperglycemia and may lead to loss of glycemic control). Products include:

Adalat CC Tablets 2978

Nimodipine (Calcium channel blocking agents tend to produce hyperglycemia and may lead to loss of glycemic control). Products include:

Nimotop Capsules 774

Nisoldipine (Calcium channel blocking agents tend to produce hyperglycemia and may lead to loss of glycemic control). Products include:

Sular Tablets 1163

Norepinephrine Bitartrate (Sympathomimetics tend to produce hyperglycemia and may lead to loss of glycemic control).

No products indexed under this heading.

Oxaprozin (The hypoglycemic action of oral antidiabetic agents may be potentiated by non-steroidal anti-inflammatory agents).

No products indexed under this heading.

Pargyline Hydrochloride (The hypoglycemic action of oral antidiabetic agents may be potentiated by MAO inhibitors).

No products indexed under this heading.

Penbutolol Sulfate (The hypoglycemic action of oral antidiabetic agents may be potentiated by beta adrenergic blocking agents; hypoglycemia may be difficult to recognize with co-administration).

No products indexed under this heading.

Pentobarbital Sodium (Drugs that induce the CYP450 enzyme system 3A4, such as barbiturates, may increase repaglinide metabolism). Products include:

Nembutal Sodium Solution, USP 2484

Perphenazine (Phenothiazines tend to produce hyperglycemia and may lead to loss of glycemic control).

No products indexed under this heading.

Phenelzine Sulfate (The hypoglycemic action of oral antidiabetic agents may be potentiated by MAO inhibitors).

No products indexed under this heading.

Phenobarbital (Drugs that induce the CYP450 enzyme system 3A4, such as barbiturates, may increase repaglinide metabolism).

No products indexed under this heading.

Phenylbutazone (The hypoglycemic action of oral antidiabetic agents may be potentiated by non-steroidal anti-inflammatory agents).

No products indexed under this heading.

Phenylephrine Bitartrate (Sympathomimetics tend to produce hyperglycemia and may lead to loss of glycemic control).

No products indexed under this heading.

Phenylephrine Hydrochloride (Sympathomimetics tend to produce hyperglycemia and may lead to loss of glycemic control). Products include:

Alacol DM Syrup 739
Hycomine Compound Tablets 1105
Preparation H Maximum Strength Cream .... ▣747
Preparation H Cooling Gel .... ▣747
Preparation H .... ▣747
Sudafed PE Tablets .... ▣711
Vicks Sinex Nasal Spray and Ultra Fine Mist for Sinus Relief............ 2677
Zicam Concentrated Cough Mist for Kids Plus D Cool Cherry............ ▣643
Zicam Concentrated Cough Mist Plus D Cool Cherry............ ▣642

Phenylephrine Tannate (Sympathomimetics tend to produce hyperglycemia and may lead to loss of glycemic control).

No products indexed under this heading.

Phenylpropanolamine Hydrochloride (Sympathomimetics tend to produce hyperglycemia and may lead to loss of glycemic control).

No products indexed under this heading.

Phenytoin (Phenytoin tends to produce hyperglycemia and may lead to loss of glycemic control).

No products indexed under this heading.

Phenytoin Sodium (Phenytoin tends to produce hyperglycemia and may lead to loss of glycemic control). Products include:

Phenytek Capsules 2153

Pindolol (The hypoglycemic action of oral antidiabetic agents may be potentiated by beta adrenergic blocking agents; hypoglycemia may be difficult to recognize with co-administration).

No products indexed under this heading.

Pirbuterol Acetate (Sympathomimetics tend to produce hyperglycemia and may lead to loss of glycemic control). Products include:

Maxair Autohaler 1820

Piroxicam (The hypoglycemic action of oral antidiabetic agents may be potentiated by non-steroidal anti-inflammatory agents).
No products indexed under this heading.

Polyestradiol Phosphate (Estrogens and oral contraceptives tend to produce hyperglycemia and may lead to loss of glycemic control).
No products indexed under this heading.

Polythiazide (Diuretics tend to produce hyperglycemia and may lead to loss of glycemic control).
No products indexed under this heading.

Prednisolone Acetate (Corticosteroids tend to produce hyperglycemia and may lead to loss of glycemic control). Products include:
Blephamide Ophthalmic Ointment 563
Blephamide Ophthalmic Suspension 564
Poly-Pred Liquifilm Ophthalmic Suspension .... ⊙231
Pred Forte Ophthalmic Suspension .... ⊙233
Pred Mild Sterile Ophthalmic Suspension .... ⊙236
Pred-G Ophthalmic Suspension .... ⊙234
Pred-G Sterile Ophthalmic Ointment .... ⊙235

Prednisolone Sodium Phosphate (Corticosteroids tend to produce hyperglycemia and may lead to loss of glycemic control). Products include:
Pediapred Oral Solution 3319

Prednisolone Tebutate (Corticosteroids tend to produce hyperglycemia and may lead to loss of glycemic control).
No products indexed under this heading.

Prednisone (Corticosteroids tend to produce hyperglycemia and may lead to loss of glycemic control).
No products indexed under this heading.

Probenecid (The hypoglycemic action of oral antidiabetic agents may be potentiated by probenecid).
No products indexed under this heading.

Procarbazine Hydrochloride (The hypoglycemic action of oral antidiabetic agents may be potentiated by MAO inhibitors). Products include:
Matulane Capsules 3188

Prochlorperazine (Phenothiazines tend to produce hyperglycemia and may lead to loss of glycemic control).
No products indexed under this heading.

Promethazine Hydrochloride (Phenothiazines tend to produce hyperglycemia and may lead to loss of glycemic control). Products include:
Phenergan 3438

Propranolol Hydrochloride (The hypoglycemic action of oral antidiabetic agents may be potentiated by beta adrenergic blocking agents; hypoglycemia may be difficult to recognize with co-administration). Products include:
Inderal LA Long-Acting Capsules 3421
InnoPran XL Capsules 2728

Pseudoephedrine Hydrochloride (Sympathomimetics tend to produce hyperglycemia and may lead to loss of glycemic control). Products include:
Advil Allergy Sinus Caplets 737
Advil Cold & Sinus 739
Advil Flu & Body Ache Caplets 739
Children's Advil Cold Suspension 741
Advil Multi-Symptom Cold Caplets 738
Allegra-D 12 Hour Extended-Release Tablets 2860
Allegra-D 24 Hour Extended-Release Tablets 2862
Balamine DM 739
BC Cold Powder 612
Benadryl Allergy & Cold Tablets 692
Benadryl Allergy & Sinus Headache Caplets & Gelcaps 693
Children's Benadryl Allergy & Cold Fastmelt Tablets 695
Benadryl Maximum Strength Severe Allergy & Sinus Headache Caplets 694
Children's Benadryl D Allergy & Sinus Fastmelt Tablets 694
Children's Benadryl D Liquid Medication 693
Benadryl D Tablets 694
Contac Non-Drowsy 12 Hour Cold Caplets 614
Contac Non-Drowsy Timed Release 12 Hour Cold Caplets 615
Contac Severe Cold and Flu Caplets Maximum Strength 615
Contac Severe Cold and Flu Caplets Non-Drowsy 615
Children's Dimetapp Cold & Allergy Elixir 745
Children's Dimetapp DM Cold & Cough Elixir 745
Children's Dimetapp Long Acting Cough Plus Cold Syrup 746
Dimetapp Infant Drops Decongestant Plus Cough 746
Children's Motrin Cold Non-Staining Dye-Free Oral Suspension 1838
Children's Motrin Cold Oral Suspension 1838
Motrin Cold & Sinus Caplets 1836
PediaCare Decongestant & Cough Infant Drops 705
PediaCare Decongestant Infants' Drops 705
PediaCare Long-Acting Cough Plus Cold Liquid 704
PediaCare Multi-Symptom Cold Liquid 704
PediaCare NightRest Cough & Cold Liquid 704
Robitussin Allergy & Cough Syrup 750
Robitussin CF Liquid 755
Robitussin Cough & Cold Liquid-filled Capsules 750
Robitussin Cough, Cold & Flu Liquid-filled Capsules 750
Robitussin Cough & Cold Infant Drops 755
Robitussin Flu Liquid 752
Robitussin Maximum Strength Cough & Cold Liquid 754
Robitussin PE Syrup 753
Robitussin Pediatric Cough & Cold Liquid 754
Robitussin PM Cough & Cold Liquid 752
Robitussin Severe Congestion Liquid-filled Capsules 751
Simply Stuffy Liquid 1841
Singlet Caplets 636
Sudafed 12 Hour Caplets 708
Sudafed 24 Hour Tablets 709
Sudafed Nasal Decongestant Tablets 709
Sudafed Severe Cold 710
Sudafed Non-Drying Sinus Liquid Caps 709
Sudafed Sinus & Allergy Tablets 710
Sudafed Sinus Headache 711
TheraFlu Cold & Cough Hot Liquid 680
TheraFlu Cold & Sore Throat Hot Liquid 680
TheraFlu Flu & Chest Congestion Non-Drowsy Hot Liquid 681
TheraFlu Flu & Sore Throat Hot Liquid 681
TheraFlu Severe Cold Non-Drowsy Hot Liquid 683
TheraFlu Severe Cold & Cough Hot Liquid 683
TheraFlu Severe Cold Caplets 679
TheraFlu Severe Cold Hot Liquid 682
TheraFlu Severe Cold Non-Drowsy Caplets 679
Triaminic Chest & Nasal Congestion Liquid 685
Triaminic Cold & Allergy Liquid 685
Triaminic Cold & Cough Liquid 685
Triaminic Cough Liquid 687
Triaminic Cough & Nasal Congestion Liquid 687
Triaminic Cough & Sore Throat Liquid 687
Triaminic Flu, Cough & Fever Liquid 685
Triaminic Night Time Cough & Cold Liquid 685
Triaminic Allergy Runny Nose & Congestion Softchews 688
Triaminic Cold & Cough Softchews 688
Triaminic Cough & Sore Throat Softchews 689
Tylenol Sinus NightTime Caplets 663
Children's Tylenol Plus Cold & Allergy Suspension Liquid 1850
Children's Tylenol Plus Cold NightTime Suspension Liquid 1851
Children's Tylenol Plus Cold & Cough Suspension Liquid and Chewable Tablets 1851
Children's Tylenol Plus Cold Chewable Tablets 1851
Children's Tylenol Plus Cold Daytime Non-Drowsy Suspension Liquid 1851
Children's Tylenol Plus Flu Suspension Liquid 1853
Concentrated Tylenol Infants' Drops Plus Cold 1851
Concentrated Tylenol Infants' Drops Plus Cold and Cough 1851
Tylenol Cold & Flu Severe Daytime Liquid with Cool Burst 1846
Tylenol Cold & Flu Severe NightTime Liquid with Cool Burst 1846
Tylenol Cold Severe Congestion Non-Drowsy Caplets with Cool Burst 1846
Tylenol Allergy Complete Night Time Caplets 1844
Tylenol Allergy Complete Multi-Symptom Caplets and Gelcaps with Cool Burst 1844
Tylenol Flu NightTime Gelcaps 1846
Tylenol Flu Day Non-Drowsy Gelcaps 1846
Concentrated Tylenol Infants' Drops Plus Cold Nasal Congestant, Fever Reducer & Pain Reliever 668
Concentrated Tylenol Infants' Drops Plus Cold & Cough Nasal Decongestant, Fever Reducer & Pain Reliever 668
Multi-Symptom Tylenol Cold Night Time Caplets 1845
Multi-Symptom Tylenol Cold Day Non-Drowsy Caplets and Gelcaps 1845
Tylenol Sinus Day Non-Drowsy 1848
Tylenol Sinus Night Time Caplets 1848
Tylenol Sinus Severe Congestion Caplets with Cool Burst 1848
Vicks 44D Cough & Head Congestion Relief 2676
Vicks 44D Cough & Head Congestion Relief Liquid 721
Vicks 44M Cough, Cold & Flu Relief 2676
Pediatric Vicks 44m Cough & Cold Relief 2673
Vicks DayQuil LiquiCaps/Liquid Multi-Symptom Cold/Flu Relief 723
Vicks DayQuil Multi-Symptom Cold/Flu Relief LiquiCaps 2675
Vicks DayQuil Multi-Symptom Cold/Flu Relief Liquid 2675
Children's Vicks NyQuil Cold/Cough Relief 2671
Vicks NyQuil LiquiCaps 2677
Vicks NyQuil LiquiCaps/Liquid Multi-Symptom Cold/Flu Relief 725
Vicks NyQuil Liquid 2677
Zyrtec-D 12 Hour Extended Release Tablets 2591

Pseudoephedrine Sulfate (Sympathomimetics tend to produce hyperglycemia and may lead to loss of glycemic control). Products include:
Alavert Allergy & Sinus D-12 Hour Tablets 743
Clarinex-D 24-Hour Extended-Release Tablets 3012
Claritin-D Non-Drowsy 12 Hour Tablets 731
Claritin-D Non-Drowsy 24 Hour Tablets 731

Quinestrol (Estrogens and oral contraceptives tend to produce hyperglycemia and may lead to loss of glycemic control).
No products indexed under this heading.

Rifampin (Co-administration has resulted in a 32% and 26% decrease in repaglinide AUC and Cmax respectively).
No products indexed under this heading.

Rofecoxib (The hypoglycemic action of oral antidiabetic agents may be potentiated by non-steroidal anti-inflammatory agents).
No products indexed under this heading.

Salmeterol Xinafoate (Sympathomimetics tend to produce hyperglycemia and may lead to loss of glycemic control). Products include:
Advair Diskus 100/50 1291
Advair Diskus 250/50 1291
Advair Diskus 500/50 1291
Serevent Diskus 1540

Salsalate (The hypoglycemic action of oral antidiabetic agents may be potentiated by salicylates).
No products indexed under this heading.

Secobarbital Sodium (Drugs that induce the CYP450 enzyme system 3A4, such as barbiturates, may increase repaglinide metabolism).
No products indexed under this heading.

Selegiline Hydrochloride (The hypoglycemic action of oral antidiabetic agents may be potentiated by MAO inhibitors). Products include:
Eldepryl Capsules 3209

Simvastatin (Co-administration has resulted in a 26% increase in repaglinide Cmax). Products include:
Vytorin 10/10 Tablets 2084
Vytorin 10/10 Tablets 3092
Vytorin 10/20 Tablets 2084
Vytorin 10/20 Tablets 3092
Vytorin 10/40 Tablets 3092
Vytorin 10/40 Tablets 2084
Vytorin 10/80 Tablets 2084
Vytorin 10/80 Tablets 3092
Zocor Tablets 2078

Sotalol Hydrochloride (The hypoglycemic action of oral antidiabetic agents may be potentiated by beta adrenergic blocking agents; hypoglycemia may be difficult to recognize with co-administration).
No products indexed under this heading.

Spironolactone (Diuretics tend to produce hyperglycemia and may lead to loss of glycemic control).
No products indexed under this heading.

Sulfacytine (The hypoglycemic action of oral antidiabetic agents may be potentiated by sulfonamides).
No products indexed under this heading.

Sulfamethizole (The hypoglycemic action of oral antidiabetic agents may be potentiated by sulfonamides).
No products indexed under this heading.

Sulfamethoxazole (The hypoglycemic action of oral antidiabetic agents may be potentiated by sulfonamides).
No products indexed under this heading.

Sulfasalazine (The hypoglycemic action of oral antidiabetic agents may be potentiated by sulfonamides).
No products indexed under this heading.

Sulfinpyrazone (The hypoglycemic action of oral antidiabetic agents may be potentiated by sulfonamides).
No products indexed under this heading.

Sulfisoxazole (The hypoglycemic action of oral antidiabetic agents may be potentiated by sulfonamides).
No products indexed under this heading.

Sulfisoxazole Acetyl (The hypoglycemic action of oral antidiabetic agents may be potentiated by sulfonamides).
No products indexed under this heading.

Sulfisoxazole Diolamine (The hypoglycemic action of oral antidiabetic agents may be potentiated by sulfonamides).
No products indexed under this heading.

Sulindac (The hypoglycemic action of oral antidiabetic agents may be potentiated by non-steroidal anti-inflammatory agents). Products include:
Clinoril Tablets **1899**

Terbutaline Sulfate (Sympathomimetics tend to produce hyperglycemia and may lead to loss of glycemic control).
No products indexed under this heading.

Thiamylal Sodium (Drugs that induce the CYP450 enzyme system 3A4, such as barbiturates, may increase repaglinide metabolism).
No products indexed under this heading.

Thioridazine Hydrochloride (Phenothiazines tend to produce hyperglycemia and may lead to loss of glycemic control). Products include:
Thioridazine Hydrochloride Tablets **2122**

Thyroglobulin (Thyroid products tend to produce hyperglycemia and may lead to loss of glycemic control).
No products indexed under this heading.

Thyroid (Thyroid products tend to produce hyperglycemia and may lead to loss of glycemic control).
No products indexed under this heading.

Thyroxine (Thyroid products tend to produce hyperglycemia and may lead to loss of glycemic control).
No products indexed under this heading.

Thyroxine Sodium (Thyroid products tend to produce hyperglycemia and may lead to loss of glycemic control).
No products indexed under this heading.

Timolol Hemihydrate (The hypoglycemic action of oral antidiabetic agents may be potentiated by beta adrenergic blocking agents; hypoglycemia may be difficult to recognize with co-administration). Products include:
Betimol Ophthalmic Solution **3371**
Betimol Ophthalmic Solution ..... ⊙**283**

Timolol Maleate (The hypoglycemic action of oral antidiabetic agents may be potentiated by beta adrenergic blocking agents; hypoglycemia may be difficult to recognize with co-administration). Products include:
Blocadren Tablets **1891**
Cosopt Sterile Ophthalmic Solution **1910**
Timolide Tablets **2056**
Timoptic in Ocudose **2061**
Timoptic Sterile Ophthalmic Solution **2058**
Timoptic-XE Sterile Ophthalmic Gel Forming Solution **2062**

Tolazamide (The hypoglycemic action of oral antidiabetic agents may be potentiated by sulfonamides).
No products indexed under this heading.

Tolbutamide (The hypoglycemic action of oral antidiabetic agents may be potentiated by sulfonamides).
No products indexed under this heading.

Tolmetin Sodium (The hypoglycemic action of oral antidiabetic agents may be potentiated by non-steroidal anti-inflammatory agents).
No products indexed under this heading.

Torsemide (Diuretics tend to produce hyperglycemia and may lead to loss of glycemic control).
No products indexed under this heading.

Tranylcypromine Sulfate (The hypoglycemic action of oral antidiabetic agents may be potentiated by MAO inhibitors). Products include:
Parnate Tablets **1499**

Triamcinolone (Corticosteroids tend to produce hyperglycemia and may lead to loss of glycemic control).
No products indexed under this heading.

Triamcinolone Acetonide (Corticosteroids tend to produce hyperglycemia and may lead to loss of glycemic control). Products include:
Azmacort Inhalation Aerosol **1701**
Nasacort HFA Inhalation Aerosol **2939**
Nasacort AQ Nasal Spray **2937**

Triamcinolone Diacetate (Corticosteroids tend to produce hyperglycemia and may lead to loss of glycemic control).
No products indexed under this heading.

Triamcinolone Hexacetonide (Corticosteroids tend to produce hyperglycemia and may lead to loss of glycemic control).
No products indexed under this heading.

Triamterene (Diuretics tend to produce hyperglycemia and may lead to loss of glycemic control). Products include:
Dyazide Capsules **1389**
Dyrenium Capsules **3390**
Maxzide **2150**

Trifluoperazine Hydrochloride (Phenothiazines tend to produce hyperglycemia and may lead to loss of glycemic control).
No products indexed under this heading.

Troglitazone (Drugs that induce the CYP450 enzyme system 3A4, such as troglitazone, may increase repaglinide metabolism).
No products indexed under this heading.

Valdecoxib (The hypoglycemic action of oral antidiabetic agents may be potentiated by non-steroidal anti-inflammatory agents).
No products indexed under this heading.

Verapamil Hydrochloride (Calcium channel blocking agents tend to produce hyperglycemia and may lead to loss of glycemic control). Products include:
Covera-HS Tablets **3135**
Tarka Tablets **519**
Verelan PM Capsules **3120**

Warfarin Sodium (The hypoglycemic action of oral antidiabetic agents may be potentiated by coumarins). Products include:
Coumadin for Injection **932**
Coumadin Tablets **932**

Food Interactions

Food, unspecified (When repaglinide was given with food the mean Cmax and AUC were decreased 20% and 12.4%, respectively; Tmax was unchanged).

PRAVACHOL TABLETS

(Pravastatin Sodium) **943**
May interact with fibrates and certain other agents. Compounds in these categories include:

Cholestyramine (Co-administration has resulted in an approximately 40% to 50% decrease in the mean AUC of pravastatin; Pravachol should be given either 1 hour or more before or at least 4 hours following the resin).
No products indexed under this heading.

Clofibrate (The use of fibrates alone may occasionally be associated with myopathy; the combined use should be avoided).
No products indexed under this heading.

Colestipol Hydrochloride (Co-administration has resulted in an approximately 40% to 50% decrease in the mean AUC of pravastatin; Pravachol should be given either 1 hour or more before or at least 4 hours following the resin).
No products indexed under this heading.

Cyclosporine (The risk of myopathy during treatment with another HMG-CoA reductase inhibitor has increased with concurrent therapy; in one single-dose study, pravastatin levels were found to be increased with concurrent therapy in cardiac transplant patients). Products include:
Gengraf Capsules **458**
Neoral Soft Gelatin Capsules **2247**
Neoral Oral Solution **2247**
Restasis Ophthalmic Emulsion **570**
Sandimmune **2259**

Digoxin (Co-administration indicates that the bioavailability parameters of digoxin are not affected, however, the AUC of pravastatin tends to increase, but the overall bioavailability of pravastatin plus its metabolites are not affected). Products include:
Digitek Tablets **2146**
Lanoxicaps Capsules **1458**
Lanoxin Injection **1462**
Lanoxin Tablets **1468**
Lanoxin Injection Pediatric **1465**

Fenofibrate (The use of fibrates alone may occasionally be associated with myopathy; the combined use should be avoided). Products include:
Antara Capsules **2723**
Lofibra Capsules **1217**
Tricor Tablets **523**
Triglide Tablets **1165**

Gemfibrozil (Co-administration has resulted in a significant decrease in urinary excretion and protein binding of pravastatin; significant increase in AUC, Cmax, and Tmax for the pravastatin metabolite SQ31906; combined therapy has resulted in marked CPK elevation insome patients; combination therapy is not recommended).
No products indexed under this heading.

Itraconazole (Co-administration with itraconazole has resulted in an increase in mean AUC and Cmax for pravastatin by factors of 1.7 and 2.5 respectively compared to placebo; the mean t1/2 was not affected suggesting that the relatively small increases in Cmax and AUCwere solely due to increased bioavailability rather than a decrease in clearance).
No products indexed under this heading.

PRECARE CHEWABLES TABLETS

(Vitamins, Prenatal) **3300**
None cited in PDR database.

PRECARE PRENATAL CAPLETS

(Vitamins, Prenatal) **3300**
None cited in PDR database.

PRECOSE TABLETS

(Acarbose) **776**
May interact with calcium channel blockers, corticosteroids, estrogens, oral contraceptives, phenothiazines, phenytoin, sympathomimetics, thiazides, thyroid preparations, and certain other agents. Compounds in these categories include:

Albuterol (Sympathomimetics tend to produce hyperglycemia leading to loss of control; patients on concurrent therapy should be closely observed for loss of control). Products include:
Proventil Inhalation Aerosol **3067**

Albuterol Sulfate (Sympathomimetics tend to produce hyperglycemia leading to loss of control; patients on concurrent therapy should be closely observed for loss of control). Products include:
AccuNeb Inhalation Solution **1055**
Combivent Inhalation Aerosol **878**
DuoNeb Inhalation Solution **1058**
Proventil Inhalation Solution 0.083% **3069**
Proventil HFA Inhalation Aerosol **3071**
Ventolin HFA Inhalation Aerosol **1576**
VoSpire Extended-Release Tablets **2352**

Amlodipine Besylate (Calcium channel blockers tend to produce hyperglycemia leading to loss of

control; patients on concurrent therapy should be closely observed for loss of control). Products include:
Caduet Tablets 2507
Lotrel Capsules 2238
Norvasc Tablets 2529

Amylase (Amylase, a carbohydrate splitting enzyme, may reduce the effect of acarbose and should not be taken concurrently).
No products indexed under this heading.

Bendroflumethiazide (Thiazide diuretics tend to produce hyperglycemia leading to loss of control; patients on concurrent therapy should be closely observed for loss of control).
No products indexed under this heading.

Bepridil Hydrochloride (Calcium channel blockers tend to produce hyperglycemia leading to loss of control; patients on concurrent therapy should be closely observed for loss of control).
No products indexed under this heading.

Betamethasone Acetate (Corticosteroids tend to produce hyperglycemia leading to loss of control; patients on concurrent therapy should be closely observed for loss of control).
No products indexed under this heading.

Betamethasone Sodium Phosphate (Corticosteroids tend to produce hyperglycemia leading to loss of control; patients on concurrent therapy should be closely observed for loss of control).
No products indexed under this heading.

Charcoal, Activated (Charcoal, an intestinal adsorbent, may reduce the effect of acarbose and should not be taken concurrently).
No products indexed under this heading.

Chlorothiazide (Thiazide diuretics tend to produce hyperglycemia leading to loss of control; patients on concurrent therapy should be closely observed for loss of control).
Products include:
Aldoclor Tablets 1881
Diuril Oral 1936

Chlorothiazide Sodium (Thiazide diuretics tend to produce hyperglycemia leading to loss of control; patients on concurrent therapy should be closely observed for loss of control). Products include:
Diuril Sodium Intravenous 1934

Chlorotrianisene (Estrogens tend to produce hyperglycemia leading to loss of control; patients on concurrent therapy should be closely observed for loss of control).
No products indexed under this heading.

Chlorpromazine (Phenothiazines tend to produce hyperglycemia leading to loss of control; patients on concurrent therapy should be closely observed for loss of control).
No products indexed under this heading.

Chlorpromazine Hydrochloride (Phenothiazines tend to produce hyperglycemia leading to loss of control; patients on concurrent therapy should be closely observed for loss of control).
No products indexed under this heading.

Cortisone Acetate (Corticosteroids tend to produce hyperglycemia leading to loss of control; patients on concurrent therapy should be closely observed for loss of control).
No products indexed under this heading.

Desogestrel (Oral contraceptives tend to produce hyperglycemia leading to loss of control; patients on concurrent therapy should be closely observed for loss of control).
Products include:
Ortho-Cept Tablets 2395

Dexamethasone (Corticosteroids tend to produce hyperglycemia leading to loss of control; patients on concurrent therapy should be closely observed for loss of control).
Products include:
Ciprodex Otic Suspension 555
Decadron Tablets 1929
TobraDex Ophthalmic Ointment 558
TobraDex Ophthalmic Suspension 558

Dexamethasone Acetate (Corticosteroids tend to produce hyperglycemia leading to loss of control; patients on concurrent therapy should be closely observed for loss of control).
No products indexed under this heading.

Dexamethasone Sodium Phosphate (Corticosteroids tend to produce hyperglycemia leading to loss of control; patients on concurrent therapy should be closely observed for loss of control). Products include:
Decadron Phosphate Injection 1931

Dienestrol (Estrogens tend to produce hyperglycemia leading to loss of control; patients on concurrent therapy should be closely observed for loss of control).
No products indexed under this heading.

Diethylstilbestrol (Estrogens tend to produce hyperglycemia leading to loss of control; patients on concurrent therapy should be closely observed for loss of control).
No products indexed under this heading.

Digoxin (Precose has been shown to change the bioavailability of digoxin when they are co-administered, which may require digoxin dose adjustment). Products include:
Digitek Tablets 2146
Lanoxicaps Capsules 1458
Lanoxin Injection 1462
Lanoxin Tablets 1468
Lanoxin Injection Pediatric 1465

Diltiazem Hydrochloride (Calcium channel blockers tend to produce hyperglycemia leading to loss of control; patients on concurrent therapy should be closely observed for loss of control). Products include:
Cardizem LA Extended Release Tablets 1699
Tiazac Capsules 1204

Dobutamine Hydrochloride (Sympathomimetics tend to produce hyperglycemia leading to loss of control; patients on concurrent therapy should be closely observed for loss of control).
No products indexed under this heading.

Dopamine Hydrochloride (Sympathomimetics tend to produce hyperglycemia leading to loss of control; patients on concurrent therapy should be closely observed for loss of control).
No products indexed under this heading.

Ephedrine Hydrochloride (Sympathomimetics tend to produce hyperglycemia leading to loss of control; patients on concurrent therapy should be closely observed for loss of control). Products include:
Primatene Tablets 749

Ephedrine Sulfate (Sympathomimetics tend to produce hyperglycemia leading to loss of control; patients on concurrent therapy should be closely observed for loss of control).
No products indexed under this heading.

Ephedrine Tannate (Sympathomimetics tend to produce hyperglycemia leading to loss of control; patients on concurrent therapy should be closely observed for loss of control).
No products indexed under this heading.

Epinephrine (Sympathomimetics tend to produce hyperglycemia leading to loss of control; patients on concurrent therapy should be closely observed for loss of control).
Products include:
EpiPen 1061
Primatene Mist 749

Epinephrine Bitartrate (Sympathomimetics tend to produce hyperglycemia leading to loss of control; patients on concurrent therapy should be closely observed for loss of control).
No products indexed under this heading.

Epinephrine Hydrochloride (Sympathomimetics tend to produce hyperglycemia leading to loss of control; patients on concurrent therapy should be closely observed for loss of control).
No products indexed under this heading.

Estradiol (Estrogens tend to produce hyperglycemia leading to loss of control; patients on concurrent therapy should be closely observed for loss of control). Products include:
Activella Tablets 2311
Climara Transdermal System 795
Climara Pro Transdermal System 800
CombiPatch Transdermal System 2180
Estrogel 0.06% 3200
Menostar Transdermal System 805
Prefest Tablets 1069
Vagifem Tablets 2340
Vivelle Transdermal System 2288
Vivelle-Dot Transdermal System 2293

Estrogens, Conjugated (Estrogens tend to produce hyperglycemia leading to loss of control; patients on concurrent therapy should be closely observed for loss of control).
Products include:
Premarin Intravenous 3440
Premarin Tablets 3443
Premarin Vaginal Cream 3449
Premphase Tablets 3452
Prempro Tablets 3452

Estrogens, Esterified (Estrogens tend to produce hyperglycemia leading to loss of control; patients on concurrent therapy should be closely observed for loss of control).
Products include:
Estratest Tablets 3196
Estratest H.S. Tablets 3196

Estropipate (Estrogens tend to produce hyperglycemia leading to loss of control; patients on concurrent therapy should be closely observed for loss of control).
No products indexed under this heading.

Ethinyl Estradiol (Estrogens tend to produce hyperglycemia leading to loss of control; patients on concurrent therapy should be closely observed for loss of control).
Products include:
Alesse-28 Tablets 3392
Lo/Ovral-28 Tablets 3423
NuvaRing 2357
Ortho-Cept Tablets 2395
Ortho-Cyclen/Ortho Tri-Cyclen 2414
Ortho Evra Transdermal System 2402
Ortho Tri-Cyclen Lo Tablets 2421
Seasonale Tablets 1073
Triphasil-28 Tablets 3483
Yasmin 28 Tablets 818

Ethynodiol Diacetate (Oral contraceptives tend to produce hyperglycemia leading to loss of control; patients on concurrent therapy should be closely observed for loss of control).
No products indexed under this heading.

Felodipine (Calcium channel blockers tend to produce hyperglycemia leading to loss of control; patients on concurrent therapy should be closely observed for loss of control).
Products include:
Plendil Extended-Release Tablets 651

Fludrocortisone Acetate (Corticosteroids tend to produce hyperglycemia leading to loss of control; patients on concurrent therapy should be closely observed for loss of control).
No products indexed under this heading.

Fluphenazine Decanoate (Phenothiazines tend to produce hyperglycemia leading to loss of control; patients on concurrent therapy should be closely observed for loss of control).
No products indexed under this heading.

Fluphenazine Enanthate (Phenothiazines tend to produce hyperglycemia leading to loss of control; patients on concurrent therapy should be closely observed for loss of control).
No products indexed under this heading.

Fluphenazine Hydrochloride (Phenothiazines tend to produce hyperglycemia leading to loss of control; patients on concurrent therapy should be closely observed for loss of control).
No products indexed under this heading.

Fosphenytoin Sodium (Phenytoin tends to produce hyperglycemia leading to loss of control; patients on concurrent therapy should be closely observed for loss of control).
No products indexed under this heading.

Hydrochlorothiazide (Thiazide diuretics tend to produce hyperglycemia leading to loss of control; patients on concurrent therapy should be closely observed for loss of control). Products include:
Aldoril Tablets 1884
Atacand HCT 637
Avalide Tablets 2889
Avalide Tablets 922
Benicar HCT Tablets 2852
Diovan HCT Tablets 2195
Dyazide Capsules 1389
Hyzaar 1964
Lotensin HCT Tablets 2235
Maxzide 2150
Micardis HCT Tablets 886
Moduretic Tablets 2003

Prinzide Tablets 2033
Teveten HCT Tablets 1710
Timolide Tablets 2056
Uniretic Tablets 3114
Vaseretic Tablets 2073
Zestoretic Tablets 701

Hydrocortisone (Corticosteroids tend to produce hyperglycemia leading to loss of control; patients on concurrent therapy should be closely observed for loss of control). Products include:
Cortizone•5 Ointment 699
Cortizone•10 Creme 699
Cortizone•10 Ointment 699
Cortizone•10 Plus Creme 700
Cortizone•10 Maximum Strength Quick Shot Spray 700
Hydrocortone Tablets 1963
Preparation H Hydrocortisone Cream 748

Hydrocortisone Acetate (Corticosteroids tend to produce hyperglycemia leading to loss of control; patients on concurrent therapy should be closely observed for loss of control). Products include:
Analpram-HC 1136
Pramosone 1139
ProctoFoam-HC 3113
Tucks Anti-Itch Ointment 712
U-cort 1% Cream 3289

Hydrocortisone Sodium Phosphate (Corticosteroids tend to produce hyperglycemia leading to loss of control; patients on concurrent therapy should be closely observed for loss of control).
No products indexed under this heading.

Hydrocortisone Sodium Succinate (Corticosteroids tend to produce hyperglycemia leading to loss of control; patients on concurrent therapy should be closely observed for loss of control).
No products indexed under this heading.

Hydroflumethiazide (Thiazide diuretics tend to produce hyperglycemia leading to loss of control; patients on concurrent therapy should be closely observed for loss of control).
No products indexed under this heading.

Isoniazid (Isoniazid tends to produce hyperglycemia leading to loss of control; patients on concurrent therapy should be closely observed for loss of control).
No products indexed under this heading.

Isoproterenol Hydrochloride (Sympathomimetics tend to produce hyperglycemia leading to loss of control; patients on concurrent therapy should be closely observed for loss of control).
No products indexed under this heading.

Isoproterenol Sulfate (Sympathomimetics tend to produce hyperglycemia leading to loss of control; patients on concurrent therapy should be closely observed for loss of control).
No products indexed under this heading.

Isradipine (Calcium channel blockers tend to produce hyperglycemia leading to loss of control; patients on concurrent therapy should be closely observed for loss of control). Products include:
DynaCirc CR Tablets 2726

Levalbuterol Hydrochloride (Sympathomimetics tend to produce hyperglycemia leading to loss of control; patients on concurrent therapy should be closely observed for loss of control). Products include:
Xopenex Inhalation Solution 3143
Xopenex Inhalation Solution Concentrate 3147

Levonorgestrel (Oral contraceptives tend to produce hyperglycemia leading to loss of control; patients on concurrent therapy should be closely observed for loss of control). Products include:
Alesse-28 Tablets 3392
Climara Pro Transdermal System 800
Mirena Intrauterine System 810
Plan B Tablets 1068
Seasonale Tablets 1073
Triphasil-28 Tablets 3483

Levothyroxine Sodium (Thyroid products tend to produce hyperglycemia leading to loss of control; patients on concurrent therapy should be closely observed for loss of control). Products include:
Levothroid Tablets 1189
Levoxyl Tablets 1680
Synthroid Tablets 515
Unithroid Tablets 3521

Liothyronine Sodium (Thyroid products tend to produce hyperglycemia leading to loss of control; patients on concurrent therapy should be closely observed for loss of control). Products include:
Cytomel Tablets 1678

Liotrix (Thyroid products tend to produce hyperglycemia leading to loss of control; patients on concurrent therapy should be closely observed for loss of control). Products include:
Thyrolar 1203

Mesoridazine Besylate (Phenothiazines tend to produce hyperglycemia leading to loss of control; patients on concurrent therapy should be closely observed for loss of control).
No products indexed under this heading.

Mestranol (Oral contraceptives tend to produce hyperglycemia leading to loss of control; patients on concurrent therapy should be closely observed for loss of control).
No products indexed under this heading.

Metaproterenol Sulfate (Sympathomimetics tend to produce hyperglycemia leading to loss of control; patients on concurrent therapy should be closely observed for loss of control). Products include:
Alupent Inhalation Aerosol 858

Metaraminol Bitartrate (Sympathomimetics tend to produce hyperglycemia leading to loss of control; patients on concurrent therapy should be closely observed for loss of control). Products include:
Aramine Injection 1889

Methotrimeprazine (Phenothiazines tend to produce hyperglycemia leading to loss of control; patients on concurrent therapy should be closely observed for loss of control).
No products indexed under this heading.

Methoxamine Hydrochloride (Sympathomimetics tend to produce hyperglycemia leading to loss of control; patients on concurrent therapy should be closely observed for loss of control).
No products indexed under this heading.

Methyclothiazide (Thiazide diuretics tend to produce hyperglycemia leading to loss of control; patients on concurrent therapy should be closely observed for loss of control).
No products indexed under this heading.

Methylprednisolone Acetate (Corticosteroids tend to produce hyperglycemia leading to loss of control; patients on concurrent therapy should be closely observed for loss of control). Products include:
Depo-Medrol Injectable Suspension 2615
Depo-Medrol Single-Dose Vial 2617

Methylprednisolone Sodium Succinate (Corticosteroids tend to produce hyperglycemia leading to loss of control; patients on concurrent therapy should be closely observed for loss of control).
No products indexed under this heading.

Mibefradil Dihydrochloride (Calcium channel blockers tend to produce hyperglycemia leading to loss of control; patients on concurrent therapy should be closely observed for loss of control).
No products indexed under this heading.

Nicardipine Hydrochloride (Calcium channel blockers tend to produce hyperglycemia leading to loss of control; patients on concurrent therapy should be closely observed for loss of control). Products include:
Cardene I.V. 1129

Nicotinic Acid (Nicotinic acid tends to produce hyperglycemia leading to loss of control; patients on concurrent therapy should be closely observed for loss of control).
No products indexed under this heading.

Nifedipine (Calcium channel blockers tend to produce hyperglycemia leading to loss of control; patients on concurrent therapy should be closely observed for loss of control). Products include:
Adalat CC Tablets 2978

Nimodipine (Calcium channel blockers tend to produce hyperglycemia leading to loss of control; patients on concurrent therapy should be closely observed for loss of control). Products include:
Nimotop Capsules 774

Nisoldipine (Calcium channel blockers tend to produce hyperglycemia leading to loss of control; patients on concurrent therapy should be closely observed for loss of control). Products include:
Sular Tablets 1163

Norepinephrine Bitartrate (Sympathomimetics tend to produce hyperglycemia leading to loss of control; patients on concurrent therapy should be closely observed for loss of control).
No products indexed under this heading.

Norethindrone (Oral contraceptives tend to produce hyperglycemia leading to loss of control; patients on concurrent therapy should be closely observed for loss of control). Products include:
Ortho Micronor Tablets 2411

Norethynodrel (Oral contraceptives tend to produce hyperglycemia leading to loss of control; patients on concurrent therapy should be closely observed for loss of control).
No products indexed under this heading.

Norgestimate (Oral contraceptives tend to produce hyperglycemia leading to loss of control; patients on concurrent therapy should be closely observed for loss of control). Products include:
Ortho-Cyclen/Ortho Tri-Cyclen 2414
Ortho Tri-Cyclen Lo Tablets 2421
Prefest Tablets 1069

Norgestrel (Oral contraceptives tend to produce hyperglycemia leading to loss of control; patients on concurrent therapy should be closely observed for loss of control). Products include:
Lo/Ovral-28 Tablets 3423

Pancreatin (Pancreatin, a carbohydrate splitting enzyme, may reduce the effect of acarbose and should not be taken concurrently).
No products indexed under this heading.

Perphenazine (Phenothiazines tend to produce hyperglycemia leading to loss of control; patients on concurrent therapy should be closely observed for loss of control).
No products indexed under this heading.

Phenylephrine Bitartrate (Sympathomimetics tend to produce hyperglycemia leading to loss of control; patients on concurrent therapy should be closely observed for loss of control).
No products indexed under this heading.

Phenylephrine Hydrochloride (Sympathomimetics tend to produce hyperglycemia leading to loss of control; patients on concurrent therapy should be closely observed for loss of control). Products include:
Alacol DM Syrup 739
Hycomine Compound Tablets 1105
Preparation H Maximum Strength Cream 747
Preparation H Cooling Gel 747
Preparation H 747
Sudafed PE Tablets 711
Vicks Sinex Nasal Spray and Ultra Fine Mist for Sinus Relief 2677
Zicam Concentrated Cough Mist for Kids Plus D Cool Cherry 643
Zicam Concentrated Cough Mist Plus D Cool Cherry 642

Phenylephrine Tannate (Sympathomimetics tend to produce hyperglycemia leading to loss of control; patients on concurrent therapy should be closely observed for loss of control).
No products indexed under this heading.

Phenylpropanolamine Hydrochloride (Sympathomimetics tend to produce hyperglycemia leading to loss of control; patients on concurrent therapy should be closely observed for loss of control).
No products indexed under this heading.

Phenytoin (Phenytoin tends to produce hyperglycemia leading to loss of control; patients on concurrent therapy should be closely observed for loss of control).
No products indexed under this heading.

Phenytoin Sodium (Phenytoin tends to produce hyperglycemia

leading to loss of control; patients on concurrent therapy should be closely observed for loss of control). Products include:
Phenytek Capsules 2153

Pirbuterol Acetate (Sympathomimetics tend to produce hyperglycemia leading to loss of control; patients on concurrent therapy should be closely observed for loss of control). Products include:
Maxair Autohaler 1820

Polyestradiol Phosphate (Estrogens tend to produce hyperglycemia leading to loss of control; patients on concurrent therapy should be closely observed for loss of control).
No products indexed under this heading.

Polythiazide (Thiazide diuretics tend to produce hyperglycemia leading to loss of control; patients on concurrent therapy should be closely observed for loss of control).
No products indexed under this heading.

Prednisolone Acetate (Corticosteroids tend to produce hyperglycemia leading to loss of control; patients on concurrent therapy should be closely observed for loss of control). Products include:
Blephamide Ophthalmic Ointment 563
Blephamide Ophthalmic Suspension 564
Poly-Pred Liquifilm Ophthalmic Suspension ⊙ 231
Pred Forte Ophthalmic Suspension ⊙ 233
Pred Mild Sterile Ophthalmic Suspension ⊙ 236
Pred-G Ophthalmic Suspension ⊙ 234
Pred-G Sterile Ophthalmic Ointment ⊙ 235

Prednisolone Sodium Phosphate (Corticosteroids tend to produce hyperglycemia leading to loss of control; patients on concurrent therapy should be closely observed for loss of control). Products include:
Pediapred Oral Solution 3319

Prednisolone Tebutate (Corticosteroids tend to produce hyperglycemia leading to loss of control; patients on concurrent therapy should be closely observed for loss of control).
No products indexed under this heading.

Prednisone (Corticosteroids tend to produce hyperglycemia leading to loss of control; patients on concurrent therapy should be closely observed for loss of control).
No products indexed under this heading.

Prochlorperazine (Phenothiazines tend to produce hyperglycemia leading to loss of control; patients on concurrent therapy should be closely observed for loss of control).
No products indexed under this heading.

Promethazine Hydrochloride (Phenothiazines tend to produce hyperglycemia leading to loss of control; patients on concurrent therapy should be closely observed for loss of control). Products include:
Phenergan 3438

Pseudoephedrine Hydrochloride (Sympathomimetics tend to produce hyperglycemia leading to loss of control; patients on concurrent therapy should be closely observed for loss of control). Products include:
Advil Allergy Sinus Caplets 737
Advil Cold & Sinus 739
Advil Flu & Body Ache Caplets 739
Children's Advil Cold Suspension 741
Advil Multi-Symptom Cold Caplets 738
Allegra-D 12 Hour Extended-Release Tablets 2860
Allegra-D 24 Hour Extended-Release Tablets 2862
Balamine DM 739
BC Cold Powder 612
Benadryl Allergy & Cold Tablets 692
Benadryl Allergy & Sinus Headache Caplets & Gelcaps 693
Children's Benadryl Allergy & Cold Fastmelt Tablets 695
Benadryl Maximum Strength Severe Allergy & Sinus Headache Caplets 694
Children's Benadryl D Allergy & Sinus Fastmelt Tablets 694
Children's Benadryl D Liquid Medication 693
Benadryl D Tablets 694
Contac Non-Drowsy 12 Hour Cold Caplets 614
Contac Non-Drowsy Timed Release 12 Hour Cold Caplets 615
Contac Severe Cold and Flu Caplets Maximum Strength 615
Contac Severe Cold and Flu Caplets Non-Drowsy 615
Children's Dimetapp Cold & Allergy Elixir 745
Children's Dimetapp DM Cold & Cough Elixir 745
Children's Dimetapp Long Acting Cough Plus Cold Syrup 746
Dimetapp Infant Drops Decongestant Plus Cough 746
Children's Motrin Cold Non-Staining Dye-Free Oral Suspension 1838
Children's Motrin Cold Oral Suspension 1838
Motrin Cold & Sinus Caplets 1836
PediaCare Decongestant & Cough Infant Drops 705
PediaCare Decongestant Infants' Drops 705
PediaCare Long-Acting Cough Plus Cold Liquid 704
PediaCare Multi-Symptom Cold Liquid 704
PediaCare NightRest Cough & Cold Liquid 704
Robitussin Allergy & Cough Syrup 750
Robitussin CF Liquid 755
Robitussin Cough & Cold Liquid-filled Capsules 750
Robitussin Cough, Cold & Flu Liquid-filled Capsules 750
Robitussin Cough & Cold Infant Drops 755
Robitussin Flu Liquid 752
Robitussin Maximum Strength Cough & Cold Liquid 754
Robitussin PE Syrup 753
Robitussin Pediatric Cough & Cold Liquid 754
Robitussin PM Cough & Cold Liquid 752
Robitussin Severe Congestion Liquid-filled Capsules 751
Simply Stuffy Liquid 1841
Singlet Caplets 636
Sudafed 12 Hour Caplets 708
Sudafed 24 Hour Tablets 709
Sudafed Nasal Decongestant Tablets 709
Sudafed Severe Cold 710
Sudafed Non-Drying Sinus Liquid Caps 709
Sudafed Sinus & Allergy Tablets 710
Sudafed Sinus Headache 711
TheraFlu Cold & Cough Hot Liquid 680
TheraFlu Cold & Sore Throat Hot Liquid 680
TheraFlu Flu & Chest Congestion Non-Drowsy Hot Liquid 681
TheraFlu Flu & Sore Throat Hot Liquid 681
TheraFlu Severe Cold Non-Drowsy Hot Liquid 683
TheraFlu Severe Cold & Cough Hot Liquid 683
TheraFlu Severe Cold Caplets 679
TheraFlu Severe Cold Hot Liquid 682
TheraFlu Severe Cold Non-Drowsy Caplets 679
Triaminic Chest & Nasal Congestion Liquid 685
Triaminic Cold & Allergy Liquid 685
Triaminic Cold & Cough Liquid 685
Triaminic Cough Liquid 687
Triaminic Cough & Nasal Congestion Liquid 687
Triaminic Cough & Sore Throat Liquid 687
Triaminic Flu, Cough & Fever Liquid 685
Triaminic Night Time Cough & Cold Liquid 685
Triaminic Allergy Runny Nose & Congestion Softchews 688
Triaminic Cold & Cough Softchews 688
Triaminic Cough & Sore Throat Softchews 689
Tylenol Sinus NightTime Caplets 663
Children's Tylenol Plus Cold & Allergy Suspension Liquid 1850
Children's Tylenol Plus Cold NightTime Suspension Liquid 1851
Children's Tylenol Plus Cold & Cough Suspension Liquid and Chewable Tablets 1851
Children's Tylenol Plus Cold Chewable Tablets 1851
Children's Tylenol Plus Cold Daytime Non-Drowsy Suspension Liquid 1851
Children's Tylenol Plus Flu Suspension Liquid 1853
Concentrated Tylenol Infants' Drops Plus Cold 1851
Concentrated Tylenol Infants' Drops Plus Cold and Cough 1851
Tylenol Cold & Flu Severe Daytime Liquid with Cool Bust 1846
Tylenol Cold & Flu Severe NightTime Liquid with Cool Burst 1846
Tylenol Cold Severe Congestion Non-Drowsy Caplets with Cool Burst 1846
Tylenol Allergy Complete Night Time Caplets 1844
Tylenol Allergy Complete Multi-Symptom Caplets and Gelcaps with Cool Burst 1844
Tylenol Flu NightTime Gelcaps 1846
Tylenol Flu Day Non-Drowsy Gelcaps 1846
Concentrated Tylenol Infants' Drops Plus Cold Nasal Congestant, Fever Reducer & Pain Reliever 668
Concentrated Tylenol Infants' Drops Plus Cold & Cough Nasal Decongestant, Fever Reducer & Pain Reliever 668
Multi-Symptom Tylenol Cold Night Time Caplets 1845
Multi-Symptom Tylenol Cold Day Non-Drowsy Caplets and Gelcaps 1845
Tylenol Sinus Day Non-Drowsy 1848
Tylenol Sinus Night Time Caplets 1848
Tylenol Sinus Severe Congestion Caplets with Cool Burst 1848
Vicks 44D Cough & Head Congestion Relief 2676
Vicks 44D Cough & Head Congestion Relief Liquid 721
Vicks 44M Cough, Cold & Flu Relief 2676
Pediatric Vicks 44m Cough & Cold Relief 2673
Vicks DayQuil LiquiCaps/Liquid Multi-Symptom Cold/Flu Relief 723
Vicks DayQuil Multi-Symptom Cold/Flu Relief LiquiCaps 2675
Vicks DayQuil Multi-Symptom Cold/Flu Relief Liquid 2675
Children's Vicks NyQuil Cold/Cough Relief 2671
Vicks NyQuil LiquiCaps 2677
Vicks NyQuil LiquiCaps/Liquid Multi-Symptom Cold/Flu Relief 725
Vicks NyQuil Liquid 2677
Zyrtec-D 12 Hour Extended Release Tablets 2591

Pseudoephedrine Sulfate (Sympathomimetics tend to produce hyperglycemia leading to loss of control; patients on concurrent therapy should be closely observed for loss of control). Products include:
Alavert Allergy & Sinus D-12 Hour Tablets 743
Clarinex-D 24-Hour Extended-Release Tablets 3012
Claritin-D Non-Drowsy 12 Hour Tablets 731
Claritin-D Non-Drowsy 24 Hour Tablets 731

Quinestrol (Estrogens tend to produce hyperglycemia leading to loss of control; patients on concurrent therapy should be closely observed for loss of control).
No products indexed under this heading.

Salmeterol Xinafoate (Sympathomimetics tend to produce hyperglycemia leading to loss of control; patients on concurrent therapy should be closely observed for loss of control). Products include:
Advair Diskus 100/50 1291
Advair Diskus 250/50 1291
Advair Diskus 500/50 1291
Serevent Diskus 1540

Terbutaline Sulfate (Sympathomimetics tend to produce hyperglycemia leading to loss of control; patients on concurrent therapy should be closely observed for loss of control).
No products indexed under this heading.

Thioridazine Hydrochloride (Phenothiazines tend to produce hyperglycemia leading to loss of control; patients on concurrent therapy should be closely observed for loss of control). Products include:
Thioridazine Hydrochloride Tablets 2122

Thyroglobulin (Thyroid products tend to produce hyperglycemia leading to loss of control; patients on concurrent therapy should be closely observed for loss of control).
No products indexed under this heading.

Thyroid (Thyroid products tend to produce hyperglycemia leading to loss of control; patients on concurrent therapy should be closely observed for loss of control).
No products indexed under this heading.

Thyroxine (Thyroid products tend to produce hyperglycemia leading to loss of control; patients on concurrent therapy should be closely observed for loss of control).
No products indexed under this heading.

Thyroxine Sodium (Thyroid products tend to produce hyperglycemia leading to loss of control; patients on concurrent therapy should be closely observed for loss of control).
No products indexed under this heading.

Triamcinolone (Corticosteroids tend to produce hyperglycemia leading to loss of control; patients on concurrent therapy should be closely observed for loss of control).
No products indexed under this heading.

Triamcinolone Acetonide (Corticosteroids tend to produce hyperglycemia leading to loss of control; patients on concurrent therapy should be closely observed for loss of control). Products include:

Azmacort Inhalation Aerosol 1701
Nasacort HFA Inhalation Aerosol 2939
Nasacort AQ Nasal Spray 2937

Triamcinolone Diacetate (Corticosteroids tend to produce hyperglycemia leading to loss of control; patients on concurrent therapy should be closely observed for loss of control).
No products indexed under this heading.

Triamcinolone Hexacetonide (Corticosteroids tend to produce hyperglycemia leading to loss of control; patients on concurrent therapy should be closely observed for loss of control).
No products indexed under this heading.

Trifluoperazine Hydrochloride (Phenothiazines tend to produce hyperglycemia leading to loss of control; patients on concurrent therapy should be closely observed for loss of control).
No products indexed under this heading.

Verapamil Hydrochloride (Calcium channel blockers tend to produce hyperglycemia leading to loss of control; patients on concurrent therapy should be closely observed for loss of control). Products include:
Covera-HS Tablets 3135
Tarka Tablets 519
Verelan PM Capsules 3120

PRED FORTE OPHTHALMIC SUSPENSION

(Prednisolone Acetate) .... ⊙233
None cited in PDR database.

PRED MILD STERILE OPHTHALMIC SUSPENSION

(Prednisolone Acetate) .... ⊙236
None cited in PDR database.

PRED-G OPHTHALMIC SUSPENSION

(Gentamicin Sulfate, Prednisolone Acetate).. ⊙234
None cited in PDR database.

PRED-G STERILE OPHTHALMIC OINTMENT

(Gentamicin Sulfate, Prednisolone Acetate).. ⊙235
None cited in PDR database.

PREFEST TABLETS

(Estradiol, Norgestimate) 1069
May interact with cytochrome p450 3a4 inducers (selected) and cytochrome p450 3a4 inhibitors (selected). Compounds in these categories include:

Acetazolamide (Inhibitors of CYP3A4 may increase plasma concentrations of estrogens and may result in side effects).
No products indexed under this heading.

Allium sativum (Inducers of CYP3A4 may reduce plasma concentrations of estrogens, possibly resulting in a decrease in therapeutic effects and/or changes in the uterine bleeding profile).
No products indexed under this heading.

Amiodarone Hydrochloride (Inhibitors of CYP3A4 may increase plasma concentrations of estrogens and may result in side effects). Products include:
Pacerone Tablets 3337

Amprenavir (Inhibitors of CYP3A4 may increase plasma concentrations of estrogens and may result in side effects). Products include:
Agenerase Capsules 1299
Agenerase Oral Solution 1304

Anastrozole (Inhibitors of CYP3A4 may increase plasma concentrations of estrogens and may result in side effects). Products include:
Arimidex Tablets 665

Aprepitant (Inhibitors of CYP3A4 may increase plasma concentrations of estrogens and may result in side effects). Products include:
Emend Capsules 1944

Betamethasone Acetate (Inducers of CYP3A4 may reduce plasma concentrations of estrogens, possibly resulting in a decrease in therapeutic effects and/or changes in the uterine bleeding profile).
No products indexed under this heading.

Betamethasone Sodium Phosphate (Inducers of CYP3A4 may reduce plasma concentrations of estrogens, possibly resulting in a decrease in therapeutic effects and/or changes in the uterine bleeding profile).
No products indexed under this heading.

Carbamazepine (Inducers of CYP3A4 may reduce plasma concentrations of estrogens, possibly resulting in a decrease in therapeutic effects and/or changes in the uterine bleeding profile). Products include:
Carbatrol Capsules 3174
Equetro Extended-Release Capsules................................... 3178
Tegretol/Tegretol-XR 2278

Cimetidine (Inhibitors of CYP3A4 may increase plasma concentrations of estrogens and may result in side effects). Products include:
Tagamet HB 200 Tablets .... ▣637
Tagamet Tablets 1547

Cimetidine Hydrochloride (Inhibitors of CYP3A4 may increase plasma concentrations of estrogens and may result in side effects).
No products indexed under this heading.

Ciprofloxacin (Inhibitors of CYP3A4 may increase plasma concentrations of estrogens and may result in side effects). Products include:
Cipro I.V. 2998
Cipro I.V. Pharmacy Bulk Package ... 3509
Cipro Oral Suspension 2991
Cipro XR Tablets 3004
Ciprodex Otic Suspension 555

Ciprofloxacin Hydrochloride (Inducers of CYP3A4 may reduce plasma concentrations of estrogens, possibly resulting in a decrease in therapeutic effects and/or changes in the uterine bleeding profile). Products include:
Ciloxan Ophthalmic Ointment 554
Cipro Tablets 2991

Cisplatin (Inducers of CYP3A4 may reduce plasma concentrations of estrogens, possibly resulting in a decrease in therapeutic effects and/or changes in the uterine bleeding profile).
No products indexed under this heading.

Clarithromycin (Inhibitors of CYP3A4 may increase plasma concentrations of estrogens and may result in side effects). Products include:
Biaxin/Biaxin XL 402
PREVPAC 3281

Clotrimazole (Inhibitors of CYP3A4 may increase plasma concentrations of estrogens and may result in side effects). Products include:
Lotrimin 3053
Lotrisone 3054

Cortisone Acetate (Inducers of CYP3A4 may reduce plasma concentrations of estrogens, possibly resulting in a decrease in therapeutic effects and/or changes in the uterine bleeding profile).
No products indexed under this heading.

Cyclosporine (Inhibitors of CYP3A4 may increase plasma concentrations of estrogens and may result in side effects). Products include:
Gengraf Capsules 458
Neoral Soft Gelatin Capsules 2247
Neoral Oral Solution 2247
Restasis Ophthalmic Emulsion 570
Sandimmune 2259

Dalfopristin (Inhibitors of CYP3A4 may increase plasma concentrations of estrogens and may result in side effects). Products include:
Synercid I.V. 1690

Danazol (Inhibitors of CYP3A4 may increase plasma concentrations of estrogens and may result in side effects).
No products indexed under this heading.

Delavirdine Mesylate (Inhibitors of CYP3A4 may increase plasma concentrations of estrogens and may result in side effects). Products include:
Rescriptor Tablets 2535

Dexamethasone (Inducers of CYP3A4 may reduce plasma concentrations of estrogens, possibly resulting in a decrease in therapeutic effects and/or changes in the uterine bleeding profile). Products include:
Ciprodex Otic Suspension 555
Decadron Tablets 1929
TobraDex Ophthalmic Ointment 558
TobraDex Ophthalmic Suspension ... 558

Dexamethasone Acetate (Inducers of CYP3A4 may reduce plasma concentrations of estrogens, possibly resulting in a decrease in therapeutic effects and/or changes in the uterine bleeding profile).
No products indexed under this heading.

Dexamethasone Sodium Phosphate (Inducers of CYP3A4 may reduce plasma concentrations of estrogens, possibly resulting in a decrease in therapeutic effects and/or changes in the uterine bleeding profile). Products include:
Decadron Phosphate Injection 1931

Diltiazem Hydrochloride (Inhibitors of CYP3A4 may increase plasma concentrations of estrogens and may result in side effects). Products include:
Cardizem LA Extended Release Tablets 1699
Tiazac Capsules 1204

Diltiazem Maleate (Inhibitors of CYP3A4 may increase plasma concentrations of estrogens and may result in side effects).
No products indexed under this heading.

Doxorubicin Hydrochloride (Inducers of CYP3A4 may reduce plasma concentrations of estrogens, possibly resulting in a decrease in therapeutic effects and/or changes in the uterine bleeding profile). Products include:
Adriamycin for Injection, USP 786
Adriamycin Injection, USP 786

Efavirenz (Inhibitors of CYP3A4 may increase plasma concentrations of estrogens and may result in side effects). Products include:
Sustiva Capsules 957

Erythromycin (Inhibitors of CYP3A4 may increase plasma concentrations of estrogens and may result in side effects). Products include:
Erygel Topical Gel 2096
Ery-Tab Tablets 447
Erythromycin Base Filmtab Tablets 454
Erythromycin Delayed-Release Capsules, USP.............................. 456
PCE Dispertab Tablets 510

Erythromycin Estolate (Inhibitors of CYP3A4 may increase plasma concentrations of estrogens and may result in side effects).
No products indexed under this heading.

Erythromycin Ethylsuccinate (Inhibitors of CYP3A4 may increase plasma concentrations of estrogens and may result in side effects). Products include:
E.E.S. 449
EryPed 445

Erythromycin Gluceptate (Inhibitors of CYP3A4 may increase plasma concentrations of estrogens and may result in side effects).
No products indexed under this heading.

Erythromycin Lactobionate (Inhibitors of CYP3A4 may increase plasma concentrations of estrogens and may result in side effects).
No products indexed under this heading.

Erythromycin Stearate (Inhibitors of CYP3A4 may increase plasma concentrations of estrogens and may result in side effects). Products include:
Erythrocin Stearate Filmtab Tablets 452

Esomeprazole Magnesium (Inhibitors of CYP3A4 may increase plasma concentrations of estrogens and may result in side effects). Products include:
Nexium Delayed-Release Capsules 645

Ethosuximide (Inducers of CYP3A4 may reduce plasma concentrations of estrogens, possibly resulting in a decrease in therapeutic effects and/or changes in the uterine bleeding profile).
No products indexed under this heading.

Felbamate (Inducers of CYP3A4 may reduce plasma concentrations of estrogens, possibly resulting in a decrease in therapeutic effects and/or changes in the uterine bleeding profile).
No products indexed under this heading.

Fluconazole (Inhibitors of CYP3A4 may increase plasma concentrations of estrogens and may result in side effects).
No products indexed under this heading.

Fludrocortisone Acetate (Inducers of CYP3A4 may reduce plasma concentrations of estrogens, possibly resulting in a decrease in therapeutic effects and/or changes in the uterine bleeding profile).
No products indexed under this heading.

Fluoxetine Hydrochloride (Inhibitors of CYP3A4 may increase plasma concentrations of estrogens and may result in side effects). Products include:
Prozac Pulvules and Liquid 1771
Symbyax Capsules 1788

Fluvoxamine Maleate (Inhibitors of CYP3A4 may increase plasma concentrations of estrogens and may result in side effects).
No products indexed under this heading.

Fosamprenavir Calcium (Inhibitors of CYP3A4 may increase plasma concentrations of estrogens and may result in side effects). Products include:
Lexiva Tablets 1473

Fosphenytoin Sodium (Inducers of CYP3A4 may reduce plasma concentrations of estrogens, possibly resulting in a decrease in therapeutic effects and/or changes in the uterine bleeding profile).
No products indexed under this heading.

Garlic Extract (Inducers of CYP3A4 may reduce plasma concentrations of estrogens, possibly resulting in a decrease in therapeutic effects and/or changes in the uterine bleeding profile).
No products indexed under this heading.

Garlic Oil (Inducers of CYP3A4 may reduce plasma concentrations of estrogens, possibly resulting in a decrease in therapeutic effects and/or changes in the uterine bleeding profile).
No products indexed under this heading.

Hydrocortisone (Inducers of CYP3A4 may reduce plasma concentrations of estrogens, possibly resulting in a decrease in therapeutic effects and/or changes in the uterine bleeding profile). Products include:
Cortizone•5 Ointment .... ■699
Cortizone•10 Creme .... ■699
Cortizone•10 Ointment .... ■699
Cortizone•10 Plus Creme .... ■700
Cortizone•10 Maximum Strength Quick Shot Spray .... ■700
Hydrocortone Tablets 1963
Preparation H Hydrocortisone Cream .... ■748

Hydrocortisone Acetate (Inducers of CYP3A4 may reduce plasma concentrations of estrogens, possibly resulting in a decrease in therapeutic effects and/or changes in the uterine bleeding profile). Products include:
Analpram-HC 1136
Pramosone 1139
ProctoFoam-HC 3113
Tucks Anti-Itch Ointment .... ■712
U-cort 1% Cream 3289

Hydrocortisone Butyrate (Inducers of CYP3A4 may reduce plasma concentrations of estrogens, possibly resulting in a decrease in therapeutic effects and/or changes in the uterine bleeding profile). Products include:
Locoid 1138
Locoid Lipocream Cream 1138

Hydrocortisone Cypionate (Inducers of CYP3A4 may reduce plasma concentrations of estrogens, possibly resulting in a decrease in therapeutic effects and/or changes in the uterine bleeding profile).
No products indexed under this heading.

Hydrocortisone Hemisuccinate (Inducers of CYP3A4 may reduce plasma concentrations of estrogens, possibly resulting in a decrease in therapeutic effects and/or changes in the uterine bleeding profile).
No products indexed under this heading.

Hydrocortisone Probutate (Inducers of CYP3A4 may reduce plasma concentrations of estrogens, possibly resulting in a decrease in therapeutic effects and/or changes in the uterine bleeding profile). Products include:
Pandel Cream, 0.1% 1017

Hydrocortisone Sodium Phosphate (Inducers of CYP3A4 may reduce plasma concentrations of estrogens, possibly resulting in a decrease in therapeutic effects and/or changes in the uterine bleeding profile).
No products indexed under this heading.

Hydrocortisone Sodium Succinate (Inducers of CYP3A4 may reduce plasma concentrations of estrogens, possibly resulting in a decrease in therapeutic effects and/or changes in the uterine bleeding profile).
No products indexed under this heading.

Hydrocortisone Valerate (Inducers of CYP3A4 may reduce plasma concentrations of estrogens, possibly resulting in a decrease in therapeutic effects and/or changes in the uterine bleeding profile).
No products indexed under this heading.

Hypericum (Inducers of CYP3A4 may reduce plasma concentrations of estrogens, possibly resulting in a decrease in therapeutic effects and/or changes in the uterine bleeding profile).
No products indexed under this heading.

Hypericum Perforatum (Inducers of CYP3A4 may reduce plasma concentrations of estrogens, possibly resulting in a decrease in therapeutic effects and/or changes in the uterine bleeding profile).
No products indexed under this heading.

Indinavir Sulfate (Inhibitors of CYP3A4 may increase plasma concentrations of estrogens and may result in side effects). Products include:
Crixivan Capsules 1918

Isoniazid (Inhibitors of CYP3A4 may increase plasma concentrations of estrogens and may result in side effects).
No products indexed under this heading.

Itraconazole (Inhibitors of CYP3A4 may increase plasma concentrations of estrogens and may result in side effects).
No products indexed under this heading.

Ketoconazole (Inhibitors of CYP3A4 may increase plasma concentrations of estrogens and may result in side effects). Products include:
Nizoral A-D Shampoo, 1% 1839
Nizoral 2% Shampoo 1838

Lopinavir (Inhibitors of CYP3A4 may increase plasma concentrations of estrogens and may result in side effects). Products include:
Kaletra 474

Loratadine (Inhibitors of CYP3A4 may increase plasma concentrations of estrogens and may result in side effects). Products include:
Alavert Allergy & Sinus D-12 Hour Tablets.. ■743
Alavert .... ■743
Children's Claritin 24 Hour Non-Drowsy Allergy Syrup .... ■732
Claritin Non-Drowsy 24 Hour Tablets.. ■731
Non-Drowsy Claritin Hives Relief Tablets.. ■733
Claritin Reditabs 24 Hour Non-Drowsy Tablets .... ■732
Claritin-D Non-Drowsy 12 Hour Tablets.. ■731
Claritin-D Non-Drowsy 24 Hour Tablets.. ■731
Children's Dimetapp ND Non-Drowsy Allergy Syrup .... ■746
Triaminic Allerchews .... ■684

Mephenytoin (Inducers of CYP3A4 may reduce plasma concentrations of estrogens, possibly resulting in a decrease in therapeutic effects and/or changes in the uterine bleeding profile).
No products indexed under this heading.

Methsuximide (Inducers of CYP3A4 may reduce plasma concentrations of estrogens, possibly resulting in a decrease in therapeutic effects and/or changes in the uterine bleeding profile).
No products indexed under this heading.

Methylprednisolone (Inducers of CYP3A4 may reduce plasma concentrations of estrogens, possibly resulting in a decrease in therapeutic effects and/or changes in the uterine bleeding profile).
No products indexed under this heading.

Methylprednisolone Acetate (Inducers of CYP3A4 may reduce plasma concentrations of estrogens, possibly resulting in a decrease in therapeutic effects and/or changes in the uterine bleeding profile). Products include:
Depo-Medrol Injectable Suspension 2615
Depo-Medrol Single-Dose Vial 2617

Methylprednisolone Sodium Succinate (Inducers of CYP3A4 may reduce plasma concentrations of estrogens, possibly resulting in a decrease in therapeutic effects and/or changes in the uterine bleeding profile).
No products indexed under this heading.

Metronidazole (Inhibitors of CYP3A4 may increase plasma concentrations of estrogens and may result in side effects). Products include:
Metrogel 1% 1212
MetroGel-Vaginal Gel 1822
Noritate Cream, 1% 1051

Metronidazole Benzoate (Inhibitors of CYP3A4 may increase plasma concentrations of estrogens and may result in side effects).
No products indexed under this heading.

Metronidazole Hydrochloride (Inhibitors of CYP3A4 may increase plasma concentrations of estrogens and may result in side effects).
No products indexed under this heading.

Miconazole (Inhibitors of CYP3A4 may increase plasma concentrations of estrogens and may result in side effects).
No products indexed under this heading.

Miconazole Nitrate (Inhibitors of CYP3A4 may increase plasma concentrations of estrogens and may result in side effects). Products include:
Desenex .... ■674
Desenex Jock Itch Spray Powder ... ■674

Modafinil (Inducers of CYP3A4 may reduce plasma concentrations of estrogens, possibly resulting in a decrease in therapeutic effects and/or changes in the uterine bleeding profile). Products include:
Provigil Tablets 1002

Nefazodone Hydrochloride (Inhibitors of CYP3A4 may increase plasma concentrations of estrogens and may result in side effects).
No products indexed under this heading.

Nelfinavir Mesylate (Inhibitors of CYP3A4 may increase plasma concentrations of estrogens and may result in side effects). Products include:
Viracept 2556

Nevirapine (Inhibitors of CYP3A4 may increase plasma concentrations of estrogens and may result in side effects). Products include:
Viramune Oral Suspension 903
Viramune Tablets 903

Niacinamide (Inhibitors of CYP3A4 may increase plasma concentrations of estrogens and may result in side effects).
No products indexed under this heading.

Nicotinamide (Inhibitors of CYP3A4 may increase plasma concentrations of estrogens and may result in side effects). Products include:
Nicomide Tablets 3190

Nifedipine (Inhibitors of CYP3A4 may increase plasma concentrations of estrogens and may result in side effects). Products include:
Adalat CC Tablets 2978

Norfloxacin (Inhibitors of CYP3A4 may increase plasma concentrations of estrogens and may result in side effects). Products include:
Noroxin Tablets 2009

Omeprazole (Inhibitors of CYP3A4 may increase plasma concentrations of estrogens and may result in side effects). Products include:
Zegerid Powder for Oral Solution 2972

Oxcarbazepine (Inducers of CYP3A4 may reduce plasma concentrations of estrogens, possibly resulting in a decrease in therapeutic effects and/or changes in the uterine bleeding profile). Products include:
Trileptal Oral Suspension 2281
Trileptal Tablets 2281

Paroxetine Hydrochloride (Inhibitors of CYP3A4 may increase plasma concentrations of estrogens and may result in side effects). Products include:
Paxil CR Controlled-Release Tablets 1509

Paxil 1501

Phenobarbital (Inducers of CYP3A4 may reduce plasma concentrations of estrogens, possibly resulting in a decrease in therapeutic effects and/or changes in the uterine bleeding profile).
No products indexed under this heading.

Phenobarbital Sodium (Inducers of CYP3A4 may reduce plasma concentrations of estrogens, possibly resulting in a decrease in therapeutic effects and/or changes in the uterine bleeding profile).
No products indexed under this heading.

Phenytoin (Inducers of CYP3A4 may reduce plasma concentrations of estrogens, possibly resulting in a decrease in therapeutic effects and/or changes in the uterine bleeding profile).
No products indexed under this heading.

Phenytoin Sodium (Inducers of CYP3A4 may reduce plasma concentrations of estrogens, possibly resulting in a decrease in therapeutic effects and/or changes in the uterine bleeding profile). Products include:
Phenytek Capsules 2153

Prednisolone Acetate (Inducers of CYP3A4 may reduce plasma concentrations of estrogens, possibly resulting in a decrease in therapeutic effects and/or changes in the uterine bleeding profile). Products include:
Blephamide Ophthalmic Ointment 563
Blephamide Ophthalmic Suspension 564
Poly-Pred Liquifilm Ophthalmic Suspension .... ⊙231
Pred Forte Ophthalmic Suspension .... ⊙233
Pred Mild Sterile Ophthalmic Suspension .... ⊙236
Pred-G Ophthalmic Suspension .... ⊙234
Pred-G Sterile Ophthalmic Ointment .... ⊙235

Prednisolone Sodium Phosphate (Inducers of CYP3A4 may reduce plasma concentrations of estrogens, possibly resulting in a decrease in therapeutic effects and/or changes in the uterine bleeding profile). Products include:
Pediapred Oral Solution 3319

Prednisolone Tebutate (Inducers of CYP3A4 may reduce plasma concentrations of estrogens, possibly resulting in a decrease in therapeutic effects and/or changes in the uterine bleeding profile).
No products indexed under this heading.

Prednisone (Inducers of CYP3A4 may reduce plasma concentrations of estrogens, possibly resulting in a decrease in therapeutic effects and/or changes in the uterine bleeding profile).
No products indexed under this heading.

Primidone (Inducers of CYP3A4 may reduce plasma concentrations of estrogens, possibly resulting in a decrease in therapeutic effects and/or changes in the uterine bleeding profile).
No products indexed under this heading.

Propoxyphene Hydrochloride (Inhibitors of CYP3A4 may increase plasma concentrations of estrogens and may result in side effects).
No products indexed under this heading.

Propoxyphene Napsylate (Inhibitors of CYP3A4 may increase plasma concentrations of estrogens and may result in side effects). Products include:
Darvocet A 500 Tablets 3497

Quinidine (Inhibitors of CYP3A4 may increase plasma concentrations of estrogens and may result in side effects).
No products indexed under this heading.

Quinidine Hydrochloride (Inhibitors of CYP3A4 may increase plasma concentrations of estrogens and may result in side effects).
No products indexed under this heading.

Quinidine Polygalacturonate (Inhibitors of CYP3A4 may increase plasma concentrations of estrogens and may result in side effects).
No products indexed under this heading.

Quinidine Sulfate (Inhibitors of CYP3A4 may increase plasma concentrations of estrogens and may result in side effects).
No products indexed under this heading.

Quinine (Inhibitors of CYP3A4 may increase plasma concentrations of estrogens and may result in side effects).
No products indexed under this heading.

Quinine Sulfate (Inhibitors of CYP3A4 may increase plasma concentrations of estrogens and may result in side effects).
No products indexed under this heading.

Quinupristin (Inhibitors of CYP3A4 may increase plasma concentrations of estrogens and may result in side effects). Products include:
Synercid I.V. 1690

Ranitidine Bismuth Citrate (Inhibitors of CYP3A4 may increase plasma concentrations of estrogens and may result in side effects).
No products indexed under this heading.

Ranitidine Hydrochloride (Inhibitors of CYP3A4 may increase plasma concentrations of estrogens and may result in side effects). Products include:
Zantac 1597
Zantac Injection 1593
Zantac 75 Tablets .... ■715
Zantac 150 Maximum Strength Tablets .... ■715
Zantac Injection Pharmacy Bulk Package 1595

Rifabutin (Inducers of CYP3A4 may reduce plasma concentrations of estrogens, possibly resulting in a decrease in therapeutic effects and/or changes in the uterine bleeding profile).
No products indexed under this heading.

Rifampicin (Inducers of CYP3A4 may reduce plasma concentrations of estrogens, possibly resulting in a decrease in therapeutic effects and/or changes in the uterine bleeding profile).
No products indexed under this heading.

Rifampin (Inducers of CYP3A4 may reduce plasma concentrations of estrogens, possibly resulting in a decrease in therapeutic effects and/or changes in the uterine bleeding profile).
No products indexed under this heading.

Rifapentine (Inducers of CYP3A4 may reduce plasma concentrations of estrogens, possibly resulting in a decrease in therapeutic effects and/or changes in the uterine bleeding profile).
No products indexed under this heading.

Ritonavir (Inhibitors of CYP3A4 may increase plasma concentrations of estrogens and may result in side effects). Products include:
Kaletra 474
Norvir 499

Saquinavir (Inhibitors of CYP3A4 may increase plasma concentrations of estrogens and may result in side effects).
No products indexed under this heading.

Saquinavir Mesylate (Inhibitors of CYP3A4 may increase plasma concentrations of estrogens and may result in side effects). Products include:
Invirase 2776

Sertraline Hydrochloride (Inhibitors of CYP3A4 may increase plasma concentrations of estrogens and may result in side effects). Products include:
Zoloft 2581

Sulfinpyrazone (Inducers of CYP3A4 may reduce plasma concentrations of estrogens, possibly resulting in a decrease in therapeutic effects and/or changes in the uterine bleeding profile).
No products indexed under this heading.

Telithromycin (Inhibitors of CYP3A4 may increase plasma concentrations of estrogens and may result in side effects). Products include:
Ketek Tablets 2920

Theophylline (Inducers of CYP3A4 may reduce plasma concentrations of estrogens, possibly resulting in a decrease in therapeutic effects and/or changes in the uterine bleeding profile).
No products indexed under this heading.

Triamcinolone (Inducers of CYP3A4 may reduce plasma concentrations of estrogens, possibly resulting in a decrease in therapeutic effects and/or changes in the uterine bleeding profile).
No products indexed under this heading.

Triamcinolone Acetonide (Inducers of CYP3A4 may reduce plasma concentrations of estrogens, possibly resulting in a decrease in therapeutic effects and/or changes in the uterine bleeding profile). Products include:
Azmacort Inhalation Aerosol 1701
Nasacort HFA Inhalation Aerosol 2939
Nasacort AQ Nasal Spray 2937

Triamcinolone Diacetate (Inducers of CYP3A4 may reduce plasma concentrations of estrogens, possibly resulting in a decrease in therapeutic effects and/or changes in the uterine bleeding profile).
No products indexed under this heading.

Triamcinolone Hexacetonide (Inducers of CYP3A4 may reduce plasma concentrations of estrogens, possibly resulting in a decrease in therapeutic effects and/or changes in the uterine bleeding profile).
No products indexed under this heading.

Troglitazone (Inhibitors of CYP3A4 may increase plasma concentrations of estrogens and may result in side effects).
No products indexed under this heading.

Troleandomycin (Inhibitors of CYP3A4 may increase plasma concentrations of estrogens and may result in side effects).
No products indexed under this heading.

Valproate Sodium (Inhibitors of CYP3A4 may increase plasma concentrations of estrogens and may result in side effects). Products include:
Depacon Injection 412

Verapamil Hydrochloride (Inhibitors of CYP3A4 may increase plasma concentrations of estrogens and may result in side effects). Products include:
Covera-HS Tablets 3135
Tarka Tablets 519
Verelan PM Capsules 3120

Voriconazole (Inhibitors of CYP3A4 may increase plasma concentrations of estrogens and may result in side effects). Products include:
VFEND I.V. 2543
VFEND Oral Suspension 2543
VFEND Tablets 2543

Zafirlukast (Inhibitors of CYP3A4 may increase plasma concentrations of estrogens and may result in side effects). Products include:
Accolate Tablets 663

Zileuton (Inhibitors of CYP3A4 may increase plasma concentrations of estrogens and may result in side effects).
No products indexed under this heading.

Food Interactions

Grapefruit (Inhibitors of CYP3A4 may increase plasma concentrations of estrogens and may result in side effects).

Grapefruit Juice (Inhibitors of CYP3A4 may increase plasma concentrations of estrogens and may result in side effects).

PRELIEF TABLETS AND POWDER

(Calcium Glycerophosphate) .... ■758
May interact with bacteriostatic antibiotics, beta-lactams antibiotics, fluoroquinolone antibiotics, and macrolide antibiotics. Compounds in these categories include:

Alatrofloxacin Mesylate (Calcium may interfere with the availability of some antibiotics).
No products indexed under this heading.

Azithromycin Dihydrate (Calcium may interfere with the availability of some antibiotics). Products include:

Zithromax 2568
Zithromax for IV Infusion 2573
Zithromax for Oral Suspension, 300 mg, 600 mg, 900 mg, 1200 mg.. 2561
Zithromax Tablets, 250 mg, 500 mg.. 2561
Zithromax Tri-Pak 2561
Zithromax Z-Pak 2568

Aztreonam (Calcium may interfere with the availability of some antibiotics).
No products indexed under this heading.

Cefaclor (Calcium may interfere with the availability of some antibiotics).
No products indexed under this heading.

Cefadroxil (Calcium may interfere with the availability of some antibiotics).
No products indexed under this heading.

Cefamandole Nafate (Calcium may interfere with the availability of some antibiotics).
No products indexed under this heading.

Cefazolin Sodium (Calcium may interfere with the availability of some antibiotics). Products include:
Ancef for Injection 1318

Cefixime (Calcium may interfere with the availability of some antibiotics). Products include:
Suprax 1811

Cefmetazole Sodium (Calcium may interfere with the availability of some antibiotics).
No products indexed under this heading.

Cefonicid Sodium (Calcium may interfere with the availability of some antibiotics).
No products indexed under this heading.

Cefoperazone Sodium (Calcium may interfere with the availability of some antibiotics).
No products indexed under this heading.

Ceforanide (Calcium may interfere with the availability of some antibiotics).
No products indexed under this heading.

Cefotaxime Sodium (Calcium may interfere with the availability of some antibiotics).
No products indexed under this heading.

Cefotetan (Calcium may interfere with the availability of some antibiotics).
No products indexed under this heading.

Cefoxitin Sodium (Calcium may interfere with the availability of some antibiotics). Products include:
Mefoxin for Injection 1987
Mefoxin Premixed Intravenous Solution.. 1990

Cefpodoxime Proxetil (Calcium may interfere with the availability of some antibiotics). Products include:
Vantin Tablets and Oral Suspension 2650

Cefprozil (Calcium may interfere with the availability of some antibiotics).
No products indexed under this heading.

Ceftazidime (Calcium may interfere with the availability of some antibiotics). Products include:
Fortaz for Injection 1422

Ceftizoxime Sodium (Calcium may interfere with the availability of some antibiotics).
No products indexed under this heading.

Ceftriaxone Sodium (Calcium may interfere with the availability of some antibiotics). Products include:
Rocephin Injectable Vials, ADD-Vantage, Galaxy, Bulk........... 2801

Cefuroxime Axetil (Calcium may interfere with the availability of some antibiotics). Products include:
Ceftin 1369

Cefuroxime Sodium (Calcium may interfere with the availability of some antibiotics).
No products indexed under this heading.

Cephalexin (Calcium may interfere with the availability of some antibiotics).
No products indexed under this heading.

Cephalothin Sodium (Calcium may interfere with the availability of some antibiotics).
No products indexed under this heading.

Cephapirin Sodium (Calcium may interfere with the availability of some antibiotics).
No products indexed under this heading.

Cephradine (Calcium may interfere with the availability of some antibiotics).
No products indexed under this heading.

Chloramphenicol (Calcium may interfere with the availability of some antibiotics).
No products indexed under this heading.

Chloramphenicol Palmitate (Calcium may interfere with the availability of some antibiotics).
No products indexed under this heading.

Chloramphenicol Sodium Succinate (Calcium may interfere with the availability of some antibiotics).
No products indexed under this heading.

Cilastatin Sodium (Calcium may interfere with the availability of some antibiotics). Products include:
Primaxin I.M. 2022
Primaxin I.V. 2024

Ciprofloxacin (Calcium may interfere with the availability of some antibiotics). Products include:
Cipro I.V. 2998
Cipro I.V. Pharmacy Bulk Package ... 3509
Cipro Oral Suspension 2991
Cipro XR Tablets 3004
Ciprodex Otic Suspension 555

Ciprofloxacin Hydrochloride (Calcium may interfere with the availability of some antibiotics). Products include:
Ciloxan Ophthalmic Ointment 554
Cipro Tablets 2991

Clarithromycin (Calcium may interfere with the availability of some antibiotics). Products include:
Biaxin/Biaxin XL 402
PREVPAC 3281

Demeclocycline Hydrochloride (Calcium may interfere with the availability of some antibiotics).
No products indexed under this heading.

Dirithromycin (Calcium may interfere with the availability of some antibiotics).
No products indexed under this heading.

Doxycycline Calcium (Calcium may interfere with the availability of some antibiotics).
No products indexed under this heading.

Doxycycline Hyclate (Calcium may interfere with the availability of some antibiotics).
No products indexed under this heading.

Doxycycline Monohydrate (Calcium may interfere with the availability of some antibiotics).
No products indexed under this heading.

Enoxacin (Calcium may interfere with the availability of some antibiotics).
No products indexed under this heading.

Erythromycin (Calcium may interfere with the availability of some antibiotics). Products include:
Erygel Topical Gel 2096
Ery-Tab Tablets 447
Erythromycin Base Filmtab Tablets 454
Erythromycin Delayed-Release Capsules, USP.............................. 456
PCE Dispertab Tablets 510

Erythromycin Estolate (Calcium may interfere with the availability of some antibiotics).
No products indexed under this heading.

Erythromycin Ethylsuccinate (Calcium may interfere with the availability of some antibiotics). Products include:
E.E.S. 449
EryPed 445

Erythromycin Gluceptate (Calcium may interfere with the availability of some antibiotics).
No products indexed under this heading.

Erythromycin Stearate (Calcium may interfere with the availability of some antibiotics). Products include:
Erythrocin Stearate Filmtab Tablets 452

Grepafloxacin Hydrochloride (Calcium may interfere with the availability of some antibiotics).
No products indexed under this heading.

Imipenem (Calcium may interfere with the availability of some antibiotics). Products include:
Primaxin I.M. 2022
Primaxin I.V. 2024

Lomefloxacin Hydrochloride (Calcium may interfere with the availability of some antibiotics).
No products indexed under this heading.

Loracarbef (Calcium may interfere with the availability of some antibiotics).
No products indexed under this heading.

Methacycline Hydrochloride (Calcium may interfere with the availability of some antibiotics).
No products indexed under this heading.

Minocycline Hydrochloride (Calcium may interfere with the availability of some antibiotics). Products include:
Dynacin Tablets 1859

Moxifloxacin Hydrochloride (Calcium may interfere with the availability of some antibiotics). Products include:
Avelox 2984
Vigamox Ophthalmic Solution 560

Norfloxacin (Calcium may interfere with the availability of some antibiotics). Products include:
Noroxin Tablets 2009

Ofloxacin (Calcium may interfere with the availability of some antibiotics). Products include:
Floxin Otic Singles 1045
Floxin Otic Solution 1043

Oxytetracycline Hydrochloride (Calcium may interfere with the availability of some antibiotics).
No products indexed under this heading.

Sulfamethizole (Calcium may interfere with the availability of some antibiotics).
No products indexed under this heading.

Sulfamethoxazole (Calcium may interfere with the availability of some antibiotics).
No products indexed under this heading.

Sulfisoxazole (Calcium may interfere with the availability of some antibiotics).
No products indexed under this heading.

Sulfisoxazole Acetyl (Calcium may interfere with the availability of some antibiotics).
No products indexed under this heading.

Tetracycline Hydrochloride (Calcium may interfere with the availability of some antibiotics).
No products indexed under this heading.

Troleandomycin (Calcium may interfere with the availability of some antibiotics).
No products indexed under this heading.

Trovafloxacin Mesylate (Calcium may interfere with the availability of some antibiotics).
No products indexed under this heading.

PREMARIN INTRAVENOUS

(Estrogens, Conjugated) 3440
See Premarin Tablets

PREMARIN TABLETS

(Estrogens, Conjugated) 3443
May interact with cytochrome p450 3a4 inducers (selected), cytochrome p450 3a4 inhibitors (selected), and certain other agents. Compounds in these categories include:

Acetazolamide (Co-administration of inhibitors of CYP3A4 with estrogens may affect estrogen drug metabolism. Inhibitors of CYP3A4 may increase plasma concentrations of estrogens and may result in side effects).
No products indexed under this heading.

Allium sativum (Co-administration of inducers of CYP3A4 with estrogens may affect estrogen drug metabolism. Inducers of CYP3A4 may reduce plasma concentrations of estrogens, possibly resulting in a decrease in therapeutic effects and/or changes in the uterine bleeding profile).

No products indexed under this heading.

Amiodarone Hydrochloride (Co-administration of inhibitors of CYP3A4 with estrogens may affect estrogen drug metabolism. Inhibitors of CYP3A4 may increase plasma concentrations of estrogens and may result in side effects). Products include:

Pacerone Tablets 3337

Amprenavir (Co-administration of inhibitors of CYP3A4 with estrogens may affect estrogen drug metabolism. Inhibitors of CYP3A4 may increase plasma concentrations of estrogens and may result in side effects). Products include:

Agenerase Capsules 1299
Agenerase Oral Solution 1304

Anastrozole (Co-administration of inhibitors of CYP3A4 with estrogens may affect estrogen drug metabolism. Inhibitors of CYP3A4 may increase plasma concentrations of estrogens and may result in side effects). Products include:

Arimidex Tablets 665

Aprepitant (Co-administration of inducers of CYP3A4 with estrogens may affect estrogen drug metabolism. Inducers of CYP3A4 may reduce plasma concentrations of estrogens, possibly resulting in a decrease in therapeutic effects and/or changes in the uterine bleeding profile). Products include:

Emend Capsules 1944

Betamethasone Acetate (Co-administration of inducers of CYP3A4 with estrogens may affect estrogen drug metabolism. Inducers of CYP3A4 may reduce plasma concentrations of estrogens, possibly resulting in a decrease in therapeutic effects and/or changes in the uterine bleeding profile).

No products indexed under this heading.

Betamethasone Sodium Phosphate (Co-administration of inducers of CYP3A4 with estrogens may affect estrogen drug metabolism. Inducers of CYP3A4 may reduce plasma concentrations of estrogens, possibly resulting in a decrease in therapeutic effects and/or changes in the uterine bleeding profile).

No products indexed under this heading.

Carbamazepine (Co-administration of inducers of CYP3A4 with estrogens may affect estrogen drug metabolism. Inducers of CYP3A4 may reduce plasma concentrations of estrogens, possibly resulting in a decrease in therapeutic effects and/or changes in the uterine bleeding profile). Products include:

Carbatrol Capsules 3174
Equetro Extended-Release Capsules 3178
Tegretol/Tegretol-XR 2278

Cimetidine (Co-administration of inhibitors of CYP3A4 with estrogens may affect estrogen drug metabolism. Inhibitors of CYP3A4 may increase plasma concentrations of estrogens and may result in side effects). Products include:

Tagamet HB 200 Tablets .... ■637
Tagamet Tablets 1547

Cimetidine Hydrochloride (Co-administration of inhibitors of CYP3A4 with estrogens may affect estrogen drug metabolism. Inhibitors of CYP3A4 may increase plasma concentrations of estrogens and may result in side effects).

No products indexed under this heading.

Ciprofloxacin (Co-administration of inhibitors of CYP3A4 with estrogens may affect estrogen drug metabolism. Inhibitors of CYP3A4 may increase plasma concentrations of estrogens and may result in side effects). Products include:

Cipro I.V. 2998
Cipro I.V. Pharmacy Bulk Package ... 3509
Cipro Oral Suspension 2991
Cipro XR Tablets 3004
Ciprodex Otic Suspension 555

Ciprofloxacin Hydrochloride (Co-administration of inducers of CYP3A4 with estrogens may affect estrogen drug metabolism. Inducers of CYP3A4 may reduce plasma concentrations of estrogens, possibly resulting in a decrease in therapeutic effects and/or changes in the uterine bleeding profile). Products include:

Ciloxan Ophthalmic Ointment 554
Cipro Tablets 2991

Cisplatin (Co-administration of inducers of CYP3A4 with estrogens may affect estrogen drug metabolism. Inducers of CYP3A4 may reduce plasma concentrations of estrogens, possibly resulting in a decrease in therapeutic effects and/or changes in the uterine bleeding profile).

No products indexed under this heading.

Clarithromycin (Co-administration of inhibitors of CYP3A4 with estrogens may affect estrogen drug metabolism. Inhibitors of CYP3A4 may increase plasma concentrations of estrogens and may result in side effects). Products include:

Biaxin/Biaxin XL 402
PREVPAC 3281

Clotrimazole (Co-administration of inhibitors of CYP3A4 with estrogens may affect estrogen drug metabolism. Inhibitors of CYP3A4 may increase plasma concentrations of estrogens and may result in side effects). Products include:

Lotrimin 3053
Lotrisone 3054

Cortisone Acetate (Co-administration of inducers of CYP3A4 with estrogens may affect estrogen drug metabolism. Inducers of CYP3A4 may reduce plasma concentrations of estrogens, possibly resulting in a decrease in therapeutic effects and/or changes in the uterine bleeding profile).

No products indexed under this heading.

Cyclosporine (Co-administration of inhibitors of CYP3A4 with estrogens may affect estrogen drug metabolism. Inhibitors of CYP3A4 may increase plasma concentrations of estrogens and may result in side effects). Products include:

Gengraf Capsules 458
Neoral Soft Gelatin Capsules 2247
Neoral Oral Solution 2247
Restasis Ophthalmic Emulsion 570
Sandimmune 2259

Dalfopristin (Co-administration of inhibitors of CYP3A4 with estrogens may affect estrogen drug metabolism. Inhibitors of CYP3A4 may increase plasma concentrations of estrogens and may result in side effects). Products include:

Synercid I.V. 1690

Danazol (Co-administration of inhibitors of CYP3A4 with estrogens may affect estrogen drug metabolism. Inhibitors of CYP3A4 may increase plasma concentrations of estrogens and may result in side effects).

No products indexed under this heading.

Delavirdine Mesylate (Co-administration of inhibitors of CYP3A4 with estrogens may affect estrogen drug metabolism. Inhibitors of CYP3A4 may increase plasma concentrations of estrogens and may result in side effects). Products include:

Rescriptor Tablets 2535

Dexamethasone (Co-administration of inducers of CYP3A4 with estrogens may affect estrogen drug metabolism. Inducers of CYP3A4 may reduce plasma concentrations of estrogens, possibly resulting in a decrease in therapeutic effects and/or changes in the uterine bleeding profile). Products include:

Ciprodex Otic Suspension 555
Decadron Tablets 1929
TobraDex Ophthalmic Ointment 558
TobraDex Ophthalmic Suspension ... 558

Dexamethasone Acetate (Co-administration of inducers of CYP3A4 with estrogens may affect estrogen drug metabolism. Inducers of CYP3A4 may reduce plasma concentrations of estrogens, possibly resulting in a decrease in therapeutic effects and/or changes in the uterine bleeding profile).

No products indexed under this heading.

Dexamethasone Sodium Phosphate (Co-administration of inducers of CYP3A4 with estrogens may affect estrogen drug metabolism. Inducers of CYP3A4 may reduce plasma concentrations of estrogens, possibly resulting in a decrease in therapeutic effects and/or changes in the uterine bleeding profile). Products include:

Decadron Phosphate Injection 1931

Diltiazem Hydrochloride (Co-administration of inhibitors of CYP3A4 with estrogens may affect estrogen drug metabolism. Inhibitors of CYP3A4 may increase plasma concentrations of estrogens and may result in side effects). Products include:

Cardizem LA Extended Release Tablets 1699
Tiazac Capsules 1204

Diltiazem Maleate (Co-administration of inhibitors of CYP3A4 with estrogens may affect estrogen drug metabolism. Inhibitors of CYP3A4 may increase plasma concentrations of estrogens and may result in side effects).

No products indexed under this heading.

Doxorubicin Hydrochloride (Co-administration of inducers of CYP3A4 with estrogens may affect estrogen drug metabolism. Inducers of CYP3A4 may reduce plasma concentrations of estrogens, possibly resulting in a decrease in therapeutic effects and/or changes in the uterine bleeding profile). Products include:

Adriamycin for Injection, USP 786
Adriamycin Injection, USP 786

Efavirenz (Co-administration of inducers of CYP3A4 with estrogens may affect estrogen drug metabolism. Inducers of CYP3A4 may reduce plasma concentrations of estrogens, possibly resulting in a decrease in therapeutic effects and/or changes in the uterine bleeding profile). Products include:

Sustiva Capsules 957

Erythromycin (Co-administration of inhibitors of CYP3A4 with estrogens may affect estrogen drug metabolism. Inhibitors of CYP3A4 may increase plasma concentrations of estrogens and may result in side effects). Products include:

Erygel Topical Gel 2096
Ery-Tab Tablets 447
Erythromycin Base Filmtab Tablets 454
Erythromycin Delayed-Release Capsules, USP 456
PCE Dispertab Tablets 510

Erythromycin Estolate (Co-administration of inhibitors of CYP3A4 with estrogens may affect estrogen drug metabolism. Inhibitors of CYP3A4 may increase plasma concentrations of estrogens and may result in side effects).

No products indexed under this heading.

Erythromycin Ethylsuccinate (Co-administration of inhibitors of CYP3A4 with estrogens may affect estrogen drug metabolism. Inhibitors of CYP3A4 may increase plasma concentrations of estrogens and may result in side effects). Products include:

E.E.S. 449
EryPed 445

Erythromycin Gluceptate (Co-administration of inhibitors of CYP3A4 with estrogens may affect estrogen drug metabolism. Inhibitors of CYP3A4 may increase plasma concentrations of estrogens and may result in side effects).

No products indexed under this heading.

Erythromycin Lactobionate (Co-administration of inhibitors of CYP3A4 with estrogens may affect estrogen drug metabolism. Inhibitors of CYP3A4 may increase plasma concentrations of estrogens and may result in side effects).

No products indexed under this heading.

Erythromycin Stearate (Co-administration of inhibitors of CYP3A4 with estrogens may affect estrogen drug metabolism. Inhibitors of CYP3A4 may increase plasma concentrations of estrogens and may result in side effects). Products include:

Erythrocin Stearate Filmtab Tablets 452

Esomeprazole Magnesium (Co-administration of inhibitors of CYP3A4 with estrogens may affect estrogen drug metabolism. Inhibitors of CYP3A4 may increase plasma concentrations of estrogens and may result in side effects). Products include:

Nexium Delayed-Release Capsules 645

Ethosuximide (Co-administration of inducers of CYP3A4 with estrogens may affect estrogen drug metabolism. Inducers of CYP3A4 may reduce plasma concentrations of estrogens, possibly resulting in a decrease in therapeutic effects and/or changes in the uterine bleeding profile).
No products indexed under this heading.

Felbamate (Co-administration of inducers of CYP3A4 with estrogens may affect estrogen drug metabolism. Inducers of CYP3A4 may reduce plasma concentrations of estrogens, possibly resulting in a decrease in therapeutic effects and/or changes in the uterine bleeding profile).
No products indexed under this heading.

Fluconazole (Co-administration of inhibitors of CYP3A4 with estrogens may affect estrogen drug metabolism. Inhibitors of CYP3A4 may increase plasma concentrations of estrogens and may result in side effects).
No products indexed under this heading.

Fludrocortisone Acetate (Co-administration of inducers of CYP3A4 with estrogens may affect estrogen drug metabolism. Inducers of CYP3A4 may reduce plasma concentrations of estrogens, possibly resulting in a decrease in therapeutic effects and/or changes in the uterine bleeding profile).
No products indexed under this heading.

Fluoxetine Hydrochloride (Co-administration of inhibitors of CYP3A4 with estrogens may affect estrogen drug metabolism. Inhibitors of CYP3A4 may increase plasma concentrations of estrogens and may result in side effects). Products include:
Prozac Pulvules and Liquid **1771**
Symbyax Capsules **1788**

Fluvoxamine Maleate (Co-administration of inhibitors of CYP3A4 with estrogens may affect estrogen drug metabolism. Inhibitors of CYP3A4 may increase plasma concentrations of estrogens and may result in side effects).
No products indexed under this heading.

Fosamprenavir Calcium (Co-administration of inhibitors of CYP3A4 with estrogens may affect estrogen drug metabolism. Inhibitors of CYP3A4 may increase plasma concentrations of estrogens and may result in side effects). Products include:
Lexiva Tablets **1473**

Fosphenytoin Sodium (Co-administration of inducers of CYP3A4 with estrogens may affect estrogen drug metabolism. Inducers of CYP3A4 may reduce plasma concentrations of estrogens, possibly resulting in a decrease in therapeutic effects and/or changes in the uterine bleeding profile).
No products indexed under this heading.

Garlic Extract (Co-administration of inducers of CYP3A4 with estrogens may affect estrogen drug metabolism. Inducers of CYP3A4 may reduce plasma concentrations of estrogens, possibly resulting in a decrease in therapeutic effects and/or changes in the uterine bleeding profile).
No products indexed under this heading.

Garlic Oil (Co-administration of inducers of CYP3A4 with estrogens may affect estrogen drug metabolism. Inducers of CYP3A4 may reduce plasma concentrations of estrogens, possibly resulting in a decrease in therapeutic effects and/or changes in the uterine bleeding profile).
No products indexed under this heading.

Hydrocortisone (Co-administration of inducers of CYP3A4 with estrogens may affect estrogen drug metabolism. Inducers of CYP3A4 may reduce plasma concentrations of estrogens, possibly resulting in a decrease in therapeutic effects and/or changes in the uterine bleeding profile). Products include:
Cortizone•5 Ointment **699**
Cortizone•10 Creme **699**
Cortizone•10 Ointment **699**
Cortizone•10 Plus Creme **700**
Cortizone•10 Maximum Strength Quick Shot Spray **700**
Hydrocortone Tablets **1963**
Preparation H Hydrocortisone Cream **748**

Hydrocortisone Acetate (Co-administration of inducers of CYP3A4 with estrogens may affect estrogen drug metabolism. Inducers of CYP3A4 may reduce plasma concentrations of estrogens, possibly resulting in a decrease in therapeutic effects and/or changes in the uterine bleeding profile). Products include:
Analpram-HC **1136**
Pramosone **1139**
ProctoFoam-HC **3113**
Tucks Anti-Itch Ointment **712**
U-cort 1% Cream **3289**

Hydrocortisone Butyrate (Co-administration of inducers of CYP3A4 with estrogens may affect estrogen drug metabolism. Inducers of CYP3A4 may reduce plasma concentrations of estrogens, possibly resulting in a decrease in therapeutic effects and/or changes in the uterine bleeding profile). Products include:
Locoid **1138**
Locoid Lipocream Cream **1138**

Hydrocortisone Cypionate (Co-administration of inducers of CYP3A4 with estrogens may affect estrogen drug metabolism. Inducers of CYP3A4 may reduce plasma concentrations of estrogens, possibly resulting in a decrease in therapeutic effects and/or changes in the uterine bleeding profile).
No products indexed under this heading.

Hydrocortisone Hemisuccinate (Co-administration of inducers of CYP3A4 with estrogens may affect estrogen drug metabolism. Inducers of CYP3A4 may reduce plasma concentrations of estrogens, possibly resulting in a decrease in therapeutic effects and/or changes in the uterine bleeding profile).
No products indexed under this heading.

Hydrocortisone Probutate (Co-administration of inducers of CYP3A4 with estrogens may affect estrogen drug metabolism. Inducers of CYP3A4 may reduce plasma concentrations of estrogens, possibly resulting in a decrease in therapeutic effects and/or changes in the uterine bleeding profile). Products include:
Pandel Cream, 0.1% **1017**

Hydrocortisone Sodium Phosphate (Co-administration of inducers of CYP3A4 with estrogens may affect estrogen drug metabolism. Inducers of CYP3A4 may reduce plasma concentrations of estrogens, possibly resulting in a decrease in therapeutic effects and/or changes in the uterine bleeding profile).
No products indexed under this heading.

Hydrocortisone Sodium Succinate (Co-administration of inducers of CYP3A4 with estrogens may affect estrogen drug metabolism. Inducers of CYP3A4 may reduce plasma concentrations of estrogens, possibly resulting in a decrease in therapeutic effects and/or changes in the uterine bleeding profile).
No products indexed under this heading.

Hydrocortisone Valerate (Co-administration of inducers of CYP3A4 with estrogens may affect estrogen drug metabolism. Inducers of CYP3A4 may reduce plasma concentrations of estrogens, possibly resulting in a decrease in therapeutic effects and/or changes in the uterine bleeding profile).
No products indexed under this heading.

Hypericum (Co-administration of inducers of CYP3A4 with estrogens may affect estrogen drug metabolism. Inducers of CYP3A4 may reduce plasma concentrations of estrogens, possibly resulting in a decrease in therapeutic effects and/or changes in the uterine bleeding profile).
No products indexed under this heading.

Hypericum Perforatum (Co-administration of inducers of CYP3A4 with estrogens may affect estrogen drug metabolism. Inducers of CYP3A4 may reduce plasma concentrations of estrogens, possibly resulting in a decrease in therapeutic effects and/or changes in the uterine bleeding profile).
No products indexed under this heading.

Indinavir Sulfate (Co-administration of inhibitors of CYP3A4 with estrogens may affect estrogen drug metabolism. Inhibitors of CYP3A4 may increase plasma concentrations of estrogens and may result in side effects). Products include:
Crixivan Capsules **1918**

Isoniazid (Co-administration of inhibitors of CYP3A4 with estrogens may affect estrogen drug metabolism. Inhibitors of CYP3A4 may increase plasma concentrations of estrogens and may result in side effects).
No products indexed under this heading.

Itraconazole (Co-administration of inhibitors of CYP3A4 with estrogens may affect estrogen drug metabolism. Inhibitors of CYP3A4 may increase plasma concentrations of estrogens and may result in side effects).
No products indexed under this heading.

Ketoconazole (Co-administration of inhibitors of CYP3A4 with estrogens may affect estrogen drug metabolism. Inhibitors of CYP3A4 may increase plasma concentrations of estrogens and may result in side effects). Products include:
Nizoral A-D Shampoo, 1% **1839**
Nizoral 2% Shampoo **1838**

Lopinavir (Co-administration of inhibitors of CYP3A4 with estrogens may affect estrogen drug metabolism. Inhibitors of CYP3A4 may increase plasma concentrations of estrogens and may result in side effects). Products include:
Kaletra **474**

Loratadine (Co-administration of inhibitors of CYP3A4 with estrogens may affect estrogen drug metabolism. Inhibitors of CYP3A4 may increase plasma concentrations of estrogens and may result in side effects). Products include:
Alavert Allergy & Sinus D-12 Hour Tablets **743**
Alavert **743**
Children's Claritin 24 Hour Non-Drowsy Allergy Syrup **732**
Claritin Non-Drowsy 24 Hour Tablets **731**
Non-Drowsy Claritin Hives Relief Tablets **733**
Claritin Reditabs 24 Hour Non-Drowsy Tablets **732**
Claritin-D Non-Drowsy 12 Hour Tablets **731**
Claritin-D Non-Drowsy 24 Hour Tablets **731**
Children's Dimetapp ND Non-Drowsy Allergy Syrup **746**
Triaminic Allerchews **684**

Mephenytoin (Co-administration of inducers of CYP3A4 with estrogens may affect estrogen drug metabolism. Inducers of CYP3A4 may reduce plasma concentrations of estrogens, possibly resulting in a decrease in therapeutic effects and/or changes in the uterine bleeding profile).
No products indexed under this heading.

Methsuximide (Co-administration of inducers of CYP3A4 with estrogens may affect estrogen drug metabolism. Inducers of CYP3A4 may reduce plasma concentrations of estrogens, possibly resulting in a decrease in therapeutic effects and/or changes in the uterine bleeding profile).
No products indexed under this heading.

Methylprednisolone (Co-administration of inducers of CYP3A4 with estrogens may affect estrogen drug metabolism. Inducers of CYP3A4 may reduce plasma concentrations of estrogens, possibly resulting in a decrease in therapeutic effects and/or changes in the uterine bleeding profile).
No products indexed under this heading.

Methylprednisolone Acetate (Co-administration of inducers of CYP3A4 with estrogens may affect estrogen drug metabolism. Inducers of CYP3A4 may reduce plasma con-

centrations of estrogens, possibly resulting in a decrease in therapeutic effects and/or changes in the uterine bleeding profile). Products include:

- Depo-Medrol Injectable Suspension 2615
- Depo-Medrol Single-Dose Vial 2617

Methylprednisolone Sodium Succinate (Co-administration of inducers of CYP3A4 with estrogens may affect estrogen drug metabolism. Inducers of CYP3A4 may reduce plasma concentrations of estrogens, possibly resulting in a decrease in therapeutic effects and/or changes in the uterine bleeding profile).

No products indexed under this heading.

Metronidazole (Co-administration of inhibitors of CYP3A4 with estrogens may affect estrogen drug metabolism. Inhibitors of CYP3A4 may increase plasma concentrations of estrogens and may result in side effects). Products include:

- Metrogel 1% 1212
- MetroGel-Vaginal Gel 1822
- Noritate Cream, 1% 1051

Metronidazole Benzoate (Co-administration of inhibitors of CYP3A4 with estrogens may affect estrogen drug metabolism. Inhibitors of CYP3A4 may increase plasma concentrations of estrogens and may result in side effects).

No products indexed under this heading.

Metronidazole Hydrochloride (Co-administration of inhibitors of CYP3A4 with estrogens may affect estrogen drug metabolism. Inhibitors of CYP3A4 may increase plasma concentrations of estrogens and may result in side effects).

No products indexed under this heading.

Miconazole (Co-administration of inhibitors of CYP3A4 with estrogens may affect estrogen drug metabolism. Inhibitors of CYP3A4 may increase plasma concentrations of estrogens and may result in side effects).

No products indexed under this heading.

Miconazole Nitrate (Co-administration of inhibitors of CYP3A4 with estrogens may affect estrogen drug metabolism. Inhibitors of CYP3A4 may increase plasma concentrations of estrogens and may result in side effects). Products include:

- Desenex .... ▣674
- Desenex Jock Itch Spray Powder ... ▣674

Modafinil (Co-administration of inducers of CYP3A4 with estrogens may affect estrogen drug metabolism. Inducers of CYP3A4 may reduce plasma concentrations of estrogens, possibly resulting in a decrease in therapeutic effects and/or changes in the uterine bleeding profile). Products include:

- Provigil Tablets 1002

Nefazodone Hydrochloride (Co-administration of inhibitors of CYP3A4 with estrogens may affect estrogen drug metabolism. Inhibitors of CYP3A4 may increase plasma concentrations of estrogens and may result in side effects).

No products indexed under this heading.

Nelfinavir Mesylate (Co-administration of inhibitors of CYP3A4 with estrogens may affect estrogen drug metabolism. Inhibitors of CYP3A4 may increase plasma concentrations of estrogens and may result in side effects). Products include:

- Viracept 2556

Nevirapine (Co-administration of inducers of CYP3A4 with estrogens may affect estrogen drug metabolism. Inducers of CYP3A4 may reduce plasma concentrations of estrogens, possibly resulting in a decrease in therapeutic effects and/or changes in the uterine bleeding profile). Products include:

- Viramune Oral Suspension 903
- Viramune Tablets 903

Niacinamide (Co-administration of inhibitors of CYP3A4 with estrogens may affect estrogen drug metabolism. Inhibitors of CYP3A4 may increase plasma concentrations of estrogens and may result in side effects).

No products indexed under this heading.

Nicotinamide (Co-administration of inhibitors of CYP3A4 with estrogens may affect estrogen drug metabolism. Inhibitors of CYP3A4 may increase plasma concentrations of estrogens and may result in side effects). Products include:

- Nicomide Tablets 3190

Nifedipine (Co-administration of inhibitors of CYP3A4 with estrogens may affect estrogen drug metabolism. Inhibitors of CYP3A4 may increase plasma concentrations of estrogens and may result in side effects). Products include:

- Adalat CC Tablets 2978

Norfloxacin (Co-administration of inhibitors of CYP3A4 with estrogens may affect estrogen drug metabolism. Inhibitors of CYP3A4 may increase plasma concentrations of estrogens and may result in side effects). Products include:

- Noroxin Tablets 2009

Omeprazole (Co-administration of inhibitors of CYP3A4 with estrogens may affect estrogen drug metabolism. Inhibitors of CYP3A4 may increase plasma concentrations of estrogens and may result in side effects). Products include:

- Zegerid Powder for Oral Solution 2972

Oxcarbazepine (Co-administration of inducers of CYP3A4 with estrogens may affect estrogen drug metabolism. Inducers of CYP3A4 may reduce plasma concentrations of estrogens, possibly resulting in a decrease in therapeutic effects and/or changes in the uterine bleeding profile). Products include:

- Trileptal Oral Suspension 2281
- Trileptal Tablets 2281

Paroxetine Hydrochloride (Co-administration of inhibitors of CYP3A4 with estrogens may affect estrogen drug metabolism. Inhibitors of CYP3A4 may increase plasma concentrations of estrogens and may result in side effects). Products include:

- Paxil CR Controlled-Release Tablets 1509
- Paxil 1501

Phenobarbital (Co-administration of inducers of CYP3A4 with estrogens may affect estrogen drug metabolism. Inducers of CYP3A4 may reduce plasma concentrations of estrogens, possibly resulting in a decrease in therapeutic effects and/or changes in the uterine bleeding profile).

No products indexed under this heading.

Phenobarbital Sodium (Co-administration of inducers of CYP3A4 with estrogens may affect estrogen drug metabolism. Inducers of CYP3A4 may reduce plasma concentrations of estrogens, possibly resulting in a decrease in therapeutic effects and/or changes in the uterine bleeding profile).

No products indexed under this heading.

Phenytoin (Co-administration of inducers of CYP3A4 with estrogens may affect estrogen drug metabolism. Inducers of CYP3A4 may reduce plasma concentrations of estrogens, possibly resulting in a decrease in therapeutic effects and/or changes in the uterine bleeding profile).

No products indexed under this heading.

Phenytoin Sodium (Co-administration of inducers of CYP3A4 with estrogens may affect estrogen drug metabolism. Inducers of CYP3A4 may reduce plasma concentrations of estrogens, possibly resulting in a decrease in therapeutic effects and/or changes in the uterine bleeding profile). Products include:

- Phenytek Capsules 2153

Prednisolone Acetate (Co-administration of inducers of CYP3A4 with estrogens may affect estrogen drug metabolism. Inducers of CYP3A4 may reduce plasma concentrations of estrogens, possibly resulting in a decrease in therapeutic effects and/or changes in the uterine bleeding profile). Products include:

- Blephamide Ophthalmic Ointment 563
- Blephamide Ophthalmic Suspension 564
- Poly-Pred Liquifilm Ophthalmic Suspension .... ⊙231
- Pred Forte Ophthalmic Suspension .... ⊙233
- Pred Mild Sterile Ophthalmic Suspension .... ⊙236
- Pred-G Ophthalmic Suspension ...... ⊙234
- Pred-G Sterile Ophthalmic Ointment .... ⊙235

Prednisolone Sodium Phosphate (Co-administration of inducers of CYP3A4 with estrogens may affect estrogen drug metabolism. Inducers of CYP3A4 may reduce plasma concentrations of estrogens, possibly resulting in a decrease in therapeutic effects and/or changes in the uterine bleeding profile). Products include:

- Pediapred Oral Solution 3319

Prednisolone Tebutate (Co-administration of inducers of CYP3A4 with estrogens may affect estrogen drug metabolism. Inducers of CYP3A4 may reduce plasma concentrations of estrogens, possibly resulting in a decrease in therapeutic effects and/or changes in the uterine bleeding profile).

No products indexed under this heading.

Prednisone (Co-administration of inducers of CYP3A4 with estrogens may affect estrogen drug metabolism. Inducers of CYP3A4 may reduce plasma concentrations of estrogens, possibly resulting in a decrease in therapeutic effects and/or changes in the uterine bleeding profile).

No products indexed under this heading.

Primidone (Co-administration of inducers of CYP3A4 with estrogens may affect estrogen drug metabolism. Inducers of CYP3A4 may reduce plasma concentrations of estrogens, possibly resulting in a decrease in therapeutic effects and/or changes in the uterine bleeding profile).

No products indexed under this heading.

Propoxyphene Hydrochloride (Co-administration of inhibitors of CYP3A4 with estrogens may affect estrogen drug metabolism. Inhibitors of CYP3A4 may increase plasma concentrations of estrogens and may result in side effects).

No products indexed under this heading.

Propoxyphene Napsylate (Co-administration of inhibitors of CYP3A4 with estrogens may affect estrogen drug metabolism. Inhibitors of CYP3A4 may increase plasma concentrations of estrogens and may result in side effects). Products include:

- Darvocet A 500 Tablets 3497

Quinidine (Co-administration of inhibitors of CYP3A4 with estrogens may affect estrogen drug metabolism. Inhibitors of CYP3A4 may increase plasma concentrations of estrogens and may result in side effects).

No products indexed under this heading.

Quinidine Hydrochloride (Co-administration of inhibitors of CYP3A4 with estrogens may affect estrogen drug metabolism. Inhibitors of CYP3A4 may increase plasma concentrations of estrogens and may result in side effects).

No products indexed under this heading.

Quinidine Polygalacturonate (Co-administration of inhibitors of CYP3A4 with estrogens may affect estrogen drug metabolism. Inhibitors of CYP3A4 may increase plasma concentrations of estrogens and may result in side effects).

No products indexed under this heading.

Quinidine Sulfate (Co-administration of inhibitors of CYP3A4 with estrogens may affect estrogen drug metabolism. Inhibitors of CYP3A4 may increase plasma concentrations of estrogens and may result in side effects).

No products indexed under this heading.

Quinine (Co-administration of inhibitors of CYP3A4 with estrogens may affect estrogen drug metabolism. Inhibitors of CYP3A4 may increase plasma concentrations of estrogens and may result in side effects).

No products indexed under this heading.

Quinine Sulfate (Co-administration of inhibitors of CYP3A4 with estrogens may affect estrogen drug metabolism. Inhibitors of CYP3A4 may increase plasma concentrations of estrogens and may result in side effects).
No products indexed under this heading.

Quinupristin (Co-administration of inhibitors of CYP3A4 with estrogens may affect estrogen drug metabolism. Inhibitors of CYP3A4 may increase plasma concentrations of estrogens and may result in side effects). Products include:
Synercid I.V. 1690

Ranitidine Bismuth Citrate (Co-administration of inhibitors of CYP3A4 with estrogens may affect estrogen drug metabolism. Inhibitors of CYP3A4 may increase plasma concentrations of estrogens and may result in side effects).
No products indexed under this heading.

Ranitidine Hydrochloride (Co-administration of inhibitors of CYP3A4 with estrogens may affect estrogen drug metabolism. Inhibitors of CYP3A4 may increase plasma concentrations of estrogens and may result in side effects). Products include:
Zantac 1597
Zantac Injection 1593
Zantac 75 Tablets 715
Zantac 150 Maximum Strength Tablets 715
Zantac Injection Pharmacy Bulk Package 1595

Rifabutin (Co-administration of inducers of CYP3A4 with estrogens may affect estrogen drug metabolism. Inducers of CYP3A4 may reduce plasma concentrations of estrogens, possibly resulting in a decrease in therapeutic effects and/or changes in the uterine bleeding profile).
No products indexed under this heading.

Rifampicin (Co-administration of inducers of CYP3A4 with estrogens may affect estrogen drug metabolism. Inducers of CYP3A4 may reduce plasma concentrations of estrogens, possibly resulting in a decrease in therapeutic effects and/or changes in the uterine bleeding profile).
No products indexed under this heading.

Rifampin (Co-administration of inducers of CYP3A4 with estrogens may affect estrogen drug metabolism. Inducers of CYP3A4 may reduce plasma concentrations of estrogens, possibly resulting in a decrease in therapeutic effects and/or changes in the uterine bleeding profile).
No products indexed under this heading.

Rifapentine (Co-administration of inducers of CYP3A4 with estrogens may affect estrogen drug metabolism. Inducers of CYP3A4 may reduce plasma concentrations of estrogens, possibly resulting in a decrease in therapeutic effects and/or changes in the uterine bleeding profile).
No products indexed under this heading.

Ritonavir (Co-administration of inhibitors of CYP3A4 with estrogens may affect estrogen drug metabolism. Inhibitors of CYP3A4 may increase plasma concentrations of estrogens and may result in side effects). Products include:
Kaletra 474
Norvir 499

Saquinavir (Co-administration of inhibitors of CYP3A4 with estrogens may affect estrogen drug metabolism. Inhibitors of CYP3A4 may increase plasma concentrations of estrogens and may result in side effects).
No products indexed under this heading.

Saquinavir Mesylate (Co-administration of inhibitors of CYP3A4 with estrogens may affect estrogen drug metabolism. Inhibitors of CYP3A4 may increase plasma concentrations of estrogens and may result in side effects). Products include:
Invirase 2776

Sertraline Hydrochloride (Co-administration of inhibitors of CYP3A4 with estrogens may affect estrogen drug metabolism. Inhibitors of CYP3A4 may increase plasma concentrations of estrogens and may result in side effects). Products include:
Zoloft 2581

Sulfinpyrazone (Co-administration of inducers of CYP3A4 with estrogens may affect estrogen drug metabolism. Inducers of CYP3A4 may reduce plasma concentrations of estrogens, possibly resulting in a decrease in therapeutic effects and/or changes in the uterine bleeding profile).
No products indexed under this heading.

Telithromycin (Co-administration of inhibitors of CYP3A4 with estrogens may affect estrogen drug metabolism. Inhibitors of CYP3A4 may increase plasma concentrations of estrogens and may result in side effects). Products include:
Ketek Tablets 2920

Theophylline (Co-administration of inducers of CYP3A4 with estrogens may affect estrogen drug metabolism. Inducers of CYP3A4 may reduce plasma concentrations of estrogens, possibly resulting in a decrease in therapeutic effects and/or changes in the uterine bleeding profile).
No products indexed under this heading.

Triamcinolone (Co-administration of inducers of CYP3A4 with estrogens may affect estrogen drug metabolism. Inducers of CYP3A4 may reduce plasma concentrations of estrogens, possibly resulting in a decrease in therapeutic effects and/or changes in the uterine bleeding profile).
No products indexed under this heading.

Triamcinolone Acetonide (Co-administration of inducers of CYP3A4 with estrogens may affect estrogen drug metabolism. Inducers of CYP3A4 may reduce plasma concentrations of estrogens, possibly resulting in a decrease in therapeutic effects and/or changes in the uterine bleeding profile). Products include:
Azmacort Inhalation Aerosol 1701
Nasacort HFA Inhalation Aerosol 2939
Nasacort AQ Nasal Spray 2937

Triamcinolone Diacetate (Co-administration of inducers of CYP3A4 with estrogens may affect estrogen drug metabolism. Inducers of CYP3A4 may reduce plasma concentrations of estrogens, possibly resulting in a decrease in therapeutic effects and/or changes in the uterine bleeding profile).
No products indexed under this heading.

Triamcinolone Hexacetonide (Co-administration of inducers of CYP3A4 with estrogens may affect estrogen drug metabolism. Inducers of CYP3A4 may reduce plasma concentrations of estrogens, possibly resulting in a decrease in therapeutic effects and/or changes in the uterine bleeding profile).
No products indexed under this heading.

Troglitazone (Co-administration of inducers of CYP3A4 with estrogens may affect estrogen drug metabolism. Inducers of CYP3A4 may reduce plasma concentrations of estrogens, possibly resulting in a decrease in therapeutic effects and/or changes in the uterine bleeding profile).
No products indexed under this heading.

Troleandomycin (Co-administration of inhibitors of CYP3A4 with estrogens may affect estrogen drug metabolism. Inhibitors of CYP3A4 may increase plasma concentrations of estrogens and may result in side effects).
No products indexed under this heading.

Valproate Sodium (Co-administration of inhibitors of CYP3A4 with estrogens may affect estrogen drug metabolism. Inhibitors of CYP3A4 may increase plasma concentrations of estrogens and may result in side effects). Products include:
Depacon Injection 412

Verapamil Hydrochloride (Co-administration of inhibitors of CYP3A4 with estrogens may affect estrogen drug metabolism. Inhibitors of CYP3A4 may increase plasma concentrations of estrogens and may result in side effects). Products include:
Covera-HS Tablets 3135
Tarka Tablets 519
Verelan PM Capsules 3120

Voriconazole (Co-administration of inhibitors of CYP3A4 with estrogens may affect estrogen drug metabolism. Inhibitors of CYP3A4 may increase plasma concentrations of estrogens and may result in side effects). Products include:
VFEND I.V. 2543
VFEND Oral Suspension 2543
VFEND Tablets 2543

Zafirlukast (Co-administration of inhibitors of CYP3A4 with estrogens may affect estrogen drug metabolism. Inhibitors of CYP3A4 may increase plasma concentrations of estrogens and may result in side effects). Products include:
Accolate Tablets 663

Zileuton (Co-administration of inhibitors of CYP3A4 with estrogens may affect estrogen drug metabolism. Inhibitors of CYP3A4 may increase plasma concentrations of estrogens and may result in side effects).
No products indexed under this heading.

Food Interactions

Grapefruit (Co-administration of inhibitors of CYP3A4 with estrogens may affect estrogen drug metabolism. Inhibitors of CYP3A4 may increase plasma concentrations of estrogens and may result in side effects).

Grapefruit Juice (Co-administration of grapefruit juice with estrogens may increase plasma concentrations of estrogens and may result in side effects).

PREMARIN VAGINAL CREAM

(Estrogens, Conjugated) 3449
See Premarin Tablets

PREMCAL LIGHT, REGULAR, AND EXTRA STRENGTH TABLETS

(Calcium Carbonate, Magnesium Oxide, Vitamin D_3)............................ 762
None cited in PDR database.

PREMESISRX TABLETS

(Vitamin B_6, Vitamins, Prenatal) 3300
None cited in PDR database.

PREMPHASE TABLETS

(Estrogens, Conjugated, Medroxyprogesterone Acetate)........... 3452
May interact with cytochrome p450 3a4 inducers (selected), cytochrome p450 3a4 inhibitors (selected), and certain other agents. Compounds in these categories include:

Acetazolamide (Co-administration of estrogens with inhibitors of CYP3A4 may increase plasma concentrations of estrogens and may result in side effects).
No products indexed under this heading.

Allium sativum (Co-administration of estrogens with inducers of CYP3A4 may reduce plasma concentrations of estrogens, possibly resulting in a decrease in therapeutic effects and/or changes in the uterine bleeding profile).
No products indexed under this heading.

Aminoglutethimide (Aminoglutethimide administered concomitantly with medroxyprogesterone acetate (MPA) may significantly depress the bioavailability of MPA).
No products indexed under this heading.

Amiodarone Hydrochloride (Co-administration of estrogens with inhibitors of CYP3A4 may increase plasma concentrations of estrogens and may result in side effects). Products include:
Pacerone Tablets 3337

Amprenavir (Co-administration of estrogens with inhibitors of CYP3A4 may increase plasma concentrations of estrogens and may result in side effects). Products include:
Agenerase Capsules 1299
Agenerase Oral Solution 1304

Anastrozole (Co-administration of estrogens with inhibitors of CYP3A4

may increase plasma concentrations of estrogens and may result in side effects). Products include:

Arimidex Tablets 665

Aprepitant (Co-administration of estrogens with inducers of CYP3A4 may reduce plasma concentrations of estrogens, possibly resulting in a decrease in therapeutic effects and/or changes in the uterine bleeding profile). Products include:

Emend Capsules 1944

Betamethasone Acetate (Co-administration of estrogens with inducers of CYP3A4 may reduce plasma concentrations of estrogens, possibly resulting in a decrease in therapeutic effects and/or changes in the uterine bleeding profile).

No products indexed under this heading.

Betamethasone Sodium Phosphate (Co-administration of estrogens with inducers of CYP3A4 may reduce plasma concentrations of estrogens, possibly resulting in a decrease in therapeutic effects and/or changes in the uterine bleeding profile).

No products indexed under this heading.

Carbamazepine (Co-administration of estrogens with inducers of CYP3A4 may reduce plasma concentrations of estrogens, possibly resulting in a decrease in therapeutic effects and/or changes in the uterine bleeding profile). Products include:

Carbatrol Capsules 3174
Equetro Extended-Release Capsules 3178
Tegretol/Tegretol-XR 2278

Cimetidine (Co-administration of estrogens with inhibitors of CYP3A4 may increase plasma concentrations of estrogens and may result in side effects). Products include:

Tagamet HB 200 Tablets .... ▣637
Tagamet Tablets 1547

Cimetidine Hydrochloride (Co-administration of estrogens with inhibitors of CYP3A4 may increase plasma concentrations of estrogens and may result in side effects).

No products indexed under this heading.

Ciprofloxacin (Co-administration of estrogens with inhibitors of CYP3A4 may increase plasma concentrations of estrogens and may result in side effects). Products include:

Cipro I.V. 2998
Cipro I.V. Pharmacy Bulk Package ... 3509
Cipro Oral Suspension 2991
Cipro XR Tablets 3004
Ciprodex Otic Suspension 555

Ciprofloxacin Hydrochloride (Co-administration of estrogens with inducers of CYP3A4 may reduce plasma concentrations of estrogens, possibly resulting in a decrease in therapeutic effects and/or changes in the uterine bleeding profile). Products include:

Ciloxan Ophthalmic Ointment 554
Cipro Tablets 2991

Cisplatin (Co-administration of estrogens with inducers of CYP3A4 may reduce plasma concentrations of estrogens, possibly resulting in a decrease in therapeutic effects and/or changes in the uterine bleeding profile).

No products indexed under this heading.

Clarithromycin (Co-administration of estrogens with inhibitors of CYP3A4 may increase plasma concentrations of estrogens and may result in side effects). Products include:

Biaxin/Biaxin XL 402
PREVPAC 3281

Clotrimazole (Co-administration of estrogens with inhibitors of CYP3A4 may increase plasma concentrations of estrogens and may result in side effects). Products include:

Lotrimin 3053
Lotrisone 3054

Cortisone Acetate (Co-administration of estrogens with inducers of CYP3A4 may reduce plasma concentrations of estrogens, possibly resulting in a decrease in therapeutic effects and/or changes in the uterine bleeding profile).

No products indexed under this heading.

Cyclosporine (Co-administration of estrogens with inhibitors of CYP3A4 may increase plasma concentrations of estrogens and may result in side effects). Products include:

Gengraf Capsules 458
Neoral Soft Gelatin Capsules 2247
Neoral Oral Solution 2247
Restasis Ophthalmic Emulsion 570
Sandimmune 2259

Dalfopristin (Co-administration of estrogens with inhibitors of CYP3A4 may increase plasma concentrations of estrogens and may result in side effects). Products include:

Synercid I.V. 1690

Danazol (Co-administration of estrogens with inhibitors of CYP3A4 may increase plasma concentrations of estrogens and may result in side effects).

No products indexed under this heading.

Delavirdine Mesylate (Co-administration of estrogens with inhibitors of CYP3A4 may increase plasma concentrations of estrogens and may result in side effects). Products include:

Rescriptor Tablets 2535

Dexamethasone (Co-administration of estrogens with inducers of CYP3A4 may reduce plasma concentrations of estrogens, possibly resulting in a decrease in therapeutic effects and/or changes in the uterine bleeding profile). Products include:

Ciprodex Otic Suspension 555
Decadron Tablets 1929
TobraDex Ophthalmic Ointment 558
TobraDex Ophthalmic Suspension ... 558

Dexamethasone Acetate (Co-administration of estrogens with inducers of CYP3A4 may reduce plasma concentrations of estrogens, possibly resulting in a decrease in therapeutic effects and/or changes in the uterine bleeding profile).

No products indexed under this heading.

Dexamethasone Sodium Phosphate (Co-administration of estrogens with inducers of CYP3A4 may reduce plasma concentrations of estrogens, possibly resulting in a decrease in therapeutic effects and/or changes in the uterine bleeding profile). Products include:

Decadron Phosphate Injection 1931

Diltiazem Hydrochloride (Co-administration of estrogens with inhibitors of CYP3A4 may increase plasma concentrations of estrogens and may result in side effects). Products include:

Cardizem LA Extended Release Tablets 1699
Tiazac Capsules 1204

Diltiazem Maleate (Co-administration of estrogens with inhibitors of CYP3A4 may increase plasma concentrations of estrogens and may result in side effects).

No products indexed under this heading.

Doxorubicin Hydrochloride (Co-administration of estrogens with inducers of CYP3A4 may reduce plasma concentrations of estrogens, possibly resulting in a decrease in therapeutic effects and/or changes in the uterine bleeding profile). Products include:

Adriamycin for Injection, USP 786
Adriamycin Injection, USP 786

Efavirenz (Co-administration of estrogens with inducers of CYP3A4 may reduce plasma concentrations of estrogens, possibly resulting in a decrease in therapeutic effects and/or changes in the uterine bleeding profile). Products include:

Sustiva Capsules 957

Erythromycin (Co-administration of estrogens with inhibitors of CYP3A4 may increase plasma concentrations of estrogens and may result in side effects). Products include:

Erygel Topical Gel 2096
Ery-Tab Tablets 447
Erythromycin Base Filmtab Tablets 454
Erythromycin Delayed-Release Capsules, USP 456
PCE Dispertab Tablets 510

Erythromycin Estolate (Co-administration of estrogens with inhibitors of CYP3A4 may increase plasma concentrations of estrogens and may result in side effects).

No products indexed under this heading.

Erythromycin Ethylsuccinate (Co-administration of estrogens with inhibitors of CYP3A4 may increase plasma concentrations of estrogens and may result in side effects). Products include:

E.E.S. 449
EryPed 445

Erythromycin Gluceptate (Co-administration of estrogens with inhibitors of CYP3A4 may increase plasma concentrations of estrogens and may result in side effects).

No products indexed under this heading.

Erythromycin Lactobionate (Co-administration of estrogens with inhibitors of CYP3A4 may increase plasma concentrations of estrogens and may result in side effects).

No products indexed under this heading.

Erythromycin Stearate (Co-administration of estrogens with inhibitors of CYP3A4 may increase plasma concentrations of estrogens and may result in side effects). Products include:

Erythrocin Stearate Filmtab Tablets 452

Esomeprazole Magnesium (Co-administration of estrogens with inhibitors of CYP3A4 may increase plasma concentrations of estrogens and may result in side effects). Products include:

Nexium Delayed-Release Capsules 645

Ethosuximide (Co-administration of estrogens with inducers of CYP3A4 may reduce plasma concentrations of estrogens, possibly resulting in a decrease in therapeutic effects and/or changes in the uterine bleeding profile).

No products indexed under this heading.

Felbamate (Co-administration of estrogens with inducers of CYP3A4 may reduce plasma concentrations of estrogens, possibly resulting in a decrease in therapeutic effects and/or changes in the uterine bleeding profile).

No products indexed under this heading.

Fluconazole (Co-administration of estrogens with inhibitors of CYP3A4 may increase plasma concentrations of estrogens and may result in side effects).

No products indexed under this heading.

Fludrocortisone Acetate (Co-administration of estrogens with inducers of CYP3A4 may reduce plasma concentrations of estrogens, possibly resulting in a decrease in therapeutic effects and/or changes in the uterine bleeding profile).

No products indexed under this heading.

Fluoxetine Hydrochloride (Co-administration of estrogens with inhibitors of CYP3A4 may increase plasma concentrations of estrogens and may result in side effects). Products include:

Prozac Pulvules and Liquid 1771
Symbyax Capsules 1788

Fluvoxamine Maleate (Co-administration of estrogens with inhibitors of CYP3A4 may increase plasma concentrations of estrogens and may result in side effects).

No products indexed under this heading.

Fosamprenavir Calcium (Co-administration of estrogens with inhibitors of CYP3A4 may increase plasma concentrations of estrogens and may result in side effects). Products include:

Lexiva Tablets 1473

Fosphenytoin Sodium (Co-administration of estrogens with inducers of CYP3A4 may reduce plasma concentrations of estrogens, possibly resulting in a decrease in therapeutic effects and/or changes in the uterine bleeding profile).

No products indexed under this heading.

Garlic Extract (Co-administration of estrogens with inducers of CYP3A4 may reduce plasma concentrations of estrogens, possibly resulting in a decrease in therapeutic effects and/or changes in the uterine bleeding profile).

No products indexed under this heading.

Garlic Oil (Co-administration of estrogens with inducers of CYP3A4 may reduce plasma concentrations of estrogens, possibly resulting in a decrease in therapeutic effects and/or changes in the uterine bleeding profile).

No products indexed under this heading.

Hydrocortisone (Co-administration of estrogens with inducers of CYP3A4 may reduce plasma concentrations of estrogens, possibly

resulting in a decrease in therapeutic effects and/or changes in the uterine bleeding profile). Products include:

- Cortizone•5 Ointment 699
- Cortizone•10 Creme 699
- Cortizone•10 Ointment 699
- Cortizone•10 Plus Creme 700
- Cortizone•10 Maximum Strength Quick Shot Spray 700
- Hydrocortone Tablets 1963
- Preparation H Hydrocortisone Cream 748

Hydrocortisone Acetate (Co-administration of estrogens with inducers of CYP3A4 may reduce plasma concentrations of estrogens, possibly resulting in a decrease in therapeutic effects and/or changes in the uterine bleeding profile). Products include:

- Analpram-HC 1136
- Pramosone 1139
- ProctoFoam-HC 3113
- Tucks Anti-Itch Ointment 712
- U-cort 1% Cream 3289

Hydrocortisone Butyrate (Co-administration of estrogens with inducers of CYP3A4 may reduce plasma concentrations of estrogens, possibly resulting in a decrease in therapeutic effects and/or changes in the uterine bleeding profile). Products include:

- Locoid 1138
- Locoid Lipocream Cream 1138

Hydrocortisone Cypionate (Co-administration of estrogens with inducers of CYP3A4 may reduce plasma concentrations of estrogens, possibly resulting in a decrease in therapeutic effects and/or changes in the uterine bleeding profile).

No products indexed under this heading.

Hydrocortisone Hemisuccinate (Co-administration of estrogens with inducers of CYP3A4 may reduce plasma concentrations of estrogens, possibly resulting in a decrease in therapeutic effects and/or changes in the uterine bleeding profile).

No products indexed under this heading.

Hydrocortisone Probutate (Co-administration of estrogens with inducers of CYP3A4 may reduce plasma concentrations of estrogens, possibly resulting in a decrease in therapeutic effects and/or changes in the uterine bleeding profile). Products include:

- Pandel Cream, 0.1% 1017

Hydrocortisone Sodium Phosphate (Co-administration of estrogens with inducers of CYP3A4 may reduce plasma concentrations of estrogens, possibly resulting in a decrease in therapeutic effects and/or changes in the uterine bleeding profile).

No products indexed under this heading.

Hydrocortisone Sodium Succinate (Co-administration of estrogens with inducers of CYP3A4 may reduce plasma concentrations of estrogens, possibly resulting in a decrease in therapeutic effects and/or changes in the uterine bleeding profile).

No products indexed under this heading.

Hydrocortisone Valerate (Co-administration of estrogens with inducers of CYP3A4 may reduce plasma concentrations of estrogens, possibly resulting in a decrease in therapeutic effects and/or changes in the uterine bleeding profile).

No products indexed under this heading.

Hypericum (Co-administration of estrogens with inducers of CYP3A4 may reduce plasma concentrations of estrogens, possibly resulting in a decrease in therapeutic effects and/or changes in the uterine bleeding profile).

No products indexed under this heading.

Hypericum Perforatum (Co-administration of estrogens with inducers of CYP3A4 may reduce plasma concentrations of estrogens, possibly resulting in a decrease in therapeutic effects and/or changes in the uterine bleeding profile).

No products indexed under this heading.

Indinavir Sulfate (Co-administration of estrogens with inhibitors of CYP3A4 may increase plasma concentrations of estrogens and may result in side effects). Products include:

- Crixivan Capsules 1918

Isoniazid (Co-administration of estrogens with inhibitors of CYP3A4 may increase plasma concentrations of estrogens and may result in side effects).

No products indexed under this heading.

Itraconazole (Co-administration of estrogens with inhibitors of CYP3A4 may increase plasma concentrations of estrogens and may result in side effects).

No products indexed under this heading.

Ketoconazole (Co-administration of estrogens with inhibitors of CYP3A4 may increase plasma concentrations of estrogens and may result in side effects). Products include:

- Nizoral A-D Shampoo, 1% 1839
- Nizoral 2% Shampoo 1838

Lopinavir (Co-administration of estrogens with inhibitors of CYP3A4 may increase plasma concentrations of estrogens and may result in side effects). Products include:

- Kaletra 474

Loratadine (Co-administration of estrogens with inhibitors of CYP3A4 may increase plasma concentrations of estrogens and may result in side effects). Products include:

- Alavert Allergy & Sinus D-12 Hour Tablets 743
- Alavert 743
- Children's Claritin 24 Hour Non-Drowsy Allergy Syrup 732
- Claritin Non-Drowsy 24 Hour Tablets 731
- Non-Drowsy Claritin Hives Relief Tablets 733
- Claritin Reditabs 24 Hour Non-Drowsy Tablets 732
- Claritin-D Non-Drowsy 12 Hour Tablets 731
- Claritin-D Non-Drowsy 24 Hour Tablets 731
- Children's Dimetapp ND Non-Drowsy Allergy Syrup 746
- Triaminic Allerchews 684

Mephenytoin (Co-administration of estrogens with inducers of CYP3A4 may reduce plasma concentrations of estrogens, possibly resulting in a decrease in therapeutic effects and/or changes in the uterine bleeding profile).

No products indexed under this heading.

Methsuximide (Co-administration of estrogens with inducers of CYP3A4 may reduce plasma concentrations of estrogens, possibly resulting in a decrease in therapeutic effects and/or changes in the uterine bleeding profile).

No products indexed under this heading.

Methylprednisolone (Co-administration of estrogens with inducers of CYP3A4 may reduce plasma concentrations of estrogens, possibly resulting in a decrease in therapeutic effects and/or changes in the uterine bleeding profile).

No products indexed under this heading.

Methylprednisolone Acetate (Co-administration of estrogens with inducers of CYP3A4 may reduce plasma concentrations of estrogens, possibly resulting in a decrease in therapeutic effects and/or changes in the uterine bleeding profile). Products include:

- Depo-Medrol Injectable Suspension 2615
- Depo-Medrol Single-Dose Vial 2617

Methylprednisolone Sodium Succinate (Co-administration of estrogens with inducers of CYP3A4 may reduce plasma concentrations of estrogens, possibly resulting in a decrease in therapeutic effects and/or changes in the uterine bleeding profile).

No products indexed under this heading.

Metronidazole (Co-administration of estrogens with inhibitors of CYP3A4 may increase plasma concentrations of estrogens and may result in side effects). Products include:

- Metrogel 1% 1212
- MetroGel-Vaginal Gel 1822
- Noritate Cream, 1% 1051

Metronidazole Benzoate (Co-administration of estrogens with inhibitors of CYP3A4 may increase plasma concentrations of estrogens and may result in side effects).

No products indexed under this heading.

Metronidazole Hydrochloride (Co-administration of estrogens with inhibitors of CYP3A4 may increase plasma concentrations of estrogens and may result in side effects).

No products indexed under this heading.

Miconazole (Co-administration of estrogens with inhibitors of CYP3A4 may increase plasma concentrations of estrogens and may result in side effects).

No products indexed under this heading.

Miconazole Nitrate (Co-administration of estrogens with inhibitors of CYP3A4 may increase plasma concentrations of estrogens and may result in side effects). Products include:

- Desenex 674
- Desenex Jock Itch Spray Powder 674

Modafinil (Co-administration of estrogens with inducers of CYP3A4 may reduce plasma concentrations of estrogens, possibly resulting in a decrease in therapeutic effects and/or changes in the uterine bleeding profile). Products include:

- Provigil Tablets 1002

Nefazodone Hydrochloride (Co-administration of estrogens with inhibitors of CYP3A4 may increase plasma concentrations of estrogens and may result in side effects).

No products indexed under this heading.

Nelfinavir Mesylate (Co-administration of estrogens with inhibitors of CYP3A4 may increase plasma concentrations of estrogens and may result in side effects). Products include:

- Viracept 2556

Nevirapine (Co-administration of estrogens with inducers of CYP3A4 may reduce plasma concentrations of estrogens, possibly resulting in a decrease in therapeutic effects and/or changes in the uterine bleeding profile). Products include:

- Viramune Oral Suspension 903
- Viramune Tablets 903

Niacinamide (Co-administration of estrogens with inhibitors of CYP3A4 may increase plasma concentrations of estrogens and may result in side effects).

No products indexed under this heading.

Nicotinamide (Co-administration of estrogens with inhibitors of CYP3A4 may increase plasma concentrations of estrogens and may result in side effects). Products include:

- Nicomide Tablets 3190

Nifedipine (Co-administration of estrogens with inhibitors of CYP3A4 may increase plasma concentrations of estrogens and may result in side effects). Products include:

- Adalat CC Tablets 2978

Norfloxacin (Co-administration of estrogens with inhibitors of CYP3A4 may increase plasma concentrations of estrogens and may result in side effects). Products include:

- Noroxin Tablets 2009

Omeprazole (Co-administration of estrogens with inhibitors of CYP3A4 may increase plasma concentrations of estrogens and may result in side effects). Products include:

- Zegerid Powder for Oral Solution 2972

Oxcarbazepine (Co-administration of estrogens with inducers of CYP3A4 may reduce plasma concentrations of estrogens, possibly resulting in a decrease in therapeutic effects and/or changes in the uterine bleeding profile). Products include:

- Trileptal Oral Suspension 2281
- Trileptal Tablets 2281

Paroxetine Hydrochloride (Co-administration of estrogens with inhibitors of CYP3A4 may increase plasma concentrations of estrogens and may result in side effects). Products include:

- Paxil CR Controlled-Release Tablets 1509
- Paxil 1501

Phenobarbital (Co-administration of estrogens with inducers of CYP3A4 may reduce plasma concentrations of estrogens, possibly resulting in a decrease in therapeutic effects and/or changes in the uterine bleeding profile).
No products indexed under this heading.

Phenobarbital Sodium (Co-administration of estrogens with inducers of CYP3A4 may reduce plasma concentrations of estrogens, possibly resulting in a decrease in therapeutic effects and/or changes in the uterine bleeding profile).
No products indexed under this heading.

Phenytoin (Co-administration of estrogens with inducers of CYP3A4 may reduce plasma concentrations of estrogens, possibly resulting in a decrease in therapeutic effects and/or changes in the uterine bleeding profile).
No products indexed under this heading.

Phenytoin Sodium (Co-administration of estrogens with inducers of CYP3A4 may reduce plasma concentrations of estrogens, possibly resulting in a decrease in therapeutic effects and/or changes in the uterine bleeding profile).
Products include:
Phenytek Capsules 2153

Prednisolone Acetate (Co-administration of estrogens with inducers of CYP3A4 may reduce plasma concentrations of estrogens, possibly resulting in a decrease in therapeutic effects and/or changes in the uterine bleeding profile).
Products include:
Blephamide Ophthalmic Ointment 563
Blephamide Ophthalmic Suspension 564
Poly-Pred Liquifilm Ophthalmic Suspension .... ⊙231
Pred Forte Ophthalmic Suspension .... ⊙233
Pred Mild Sterile Ophthalmic Suspension .... ⊙236
Pred-G Ophthalmic Suspension ...... ⊙234
Pred-G Sterile Ophthalmic Ointment .... ⊙235

Prednisolone Sodium Phosphate (Co-administration of estrogens with inducers of CYP3A4 may reduce plasma concentrations of estrogens, possibly resulting in a decrease in therapeutic effects and/or changes in the uterine bleeding profile).
Products include:
Pediapred Oral Solution 3319

Prednisolone Tebutate (Co-administration of estrogens with inducers of CYP3A4 may reduce plasma concentrations of estrogens, possibly resulting in a decrease in therapeutic effects and/or changes in the uterine bleeding profile).
No products indexed under this heading.

Prednisone (Co-administration of estrogens with inducers of CYP3A4 may reduce plasma concentrations of estrogens, possibly resulting in a decrease in therapeutic effects and/or changes in the uterine bleeding profile).
No products indexed under this heading.

Primidone (Co-administration of estrogens with inducers of CYP3A4 may reduce plasma concentrations of estrogens, possibly resulting in a decrease in therapeutic effects and/or changes in the uterine bleeding profile).
No products indexed under this heading.

Propoxyphene Hydrochloride (Co-administration of estrogens with inhibitors of CYP3A4 may increase plasma concentrations of estrogens and may result in side effects).
No products indexed under this heading.

Propoxyphene Napsylate (Co-administration of estrogens with inhibitors of CYP3A4 may increase plasma concentrations of estrogens and may result in side effects).
Products include:
Darvocet A 500 Tablets 3497

Quinidine (Co-administration of estrogens with inhibitors of CYP3A4 may increase plasma concentrations of estrogens and may result in side effects).
No products indexed under this heading.

Quinidine Hydrochloride (Co-administration of estrogens with inhibitors of CYP3A4 may increase plasma concentrations of estrogens and may result in side effects).
No products indexed under this heading.

Quinidine Polygalacturonate (Co-administration of estrogens with inhibitors of CYP3A4 may increase plasma concentrations of estrogens and may result in side effects).
No products indexed under this heading.

Quinidine Sulfate (Co-administration of estrogens with inhibitors of CYP3A4 may increase plasma concentrations of estrogens and may result in side effects).
No products indexed under this heading.

Quinine (Co-administration of estrogens with inhibitors of CYP3A4 may increase plasma concentrations of estrogens and may result in side effects).
No products indexed under this heading.

Quinine Sulfate (Co-administration of estrogens with inhibitors of CYP3A4 may increase plasma concentrations of estrogens and may result in side effects).
No products indexed under this heading.

Quinupristin (Co-administration of estrogens with inhibitors of CYP3A4 may increase plasma concentrations of estrogens and may result in side effects). Products include:
Synercid I.V. 1690

Ranitidine Bismuth Citrate (Co-administration of estrogens with inhibitors of CYP3A4 may increase plasma concentrations of estrogens and may result in side effects).
No products indexed under this heading.

Ranitidine Hydrochloride (Co-administration of estrogens with inhibitors of CYP3A4 may increase plasma concentrations of estrogens and may result in side effects).
Products include:
Zantac 1597
Zantac Injection 1593
Zantac 75 Tablets .... ■715
Zantac 150 Maximum Strength Tablets .... ■715
Zantac Injection Pharmacy Bulk Package 1595

Rifabutin (Co-administration of estrogens with inducers of CYP3A4 may reduce plasma concentrations of estrogens, possibly resulting in a decrease in therapeutic effects and/or changes in the uterine bleeding profile).
No products indexed under this heading.

Rifampicin (Co-administration of estrogens with inducers of CYP3A4 may reduce plasma concentrations of estrogens, possibly resulting in a decrease in therapeutic effects and/or changes in the uterine bleeding profile).
No products indexed under this heading.

Rifampin (Co-administration of estrogens with inducers of CYP3A4 may reduce plasma concentrations of estrogens, possibly resulting in a decrease in therapeutic effects and/or changes in the uterine bleeding profile).
No products indexed under this heading.

Rifapentine (Co-administration of estrogens with inducers of CYP3A4 may reduce plasma concentrations of estrogens, possibly resulting in a decrease in therapeutic effects and/or changes in the uterine bleeding profile).
No products indexed under this heading.

Ritonavir (Co-administration of estrogens with inhibitors of CYP3A4 may increase plasma concentrations of estrogens and may result in side effects). Products include:
Kaletra 474
Norvir 499

Saquinavir (Co-administration of estrogens with inhibitors of CYP3A4 may increase plasma concentrations of estrogens and may result in side effects).
No products indexed under this heading.

Saquinavir Mesylate (Co-administration of estrogens with inhibitors of CYP3A4 may increase plasma concentrations of estrogens and may result in side effects).
Products include:
Invirase 2776

Sertraline Hydrochloride (Co-administration of estrogens with inhibitors of CYP3A4 may increase plasma concentrations of estrogens and may result in side effects).
Products include:
Zoloft 2581

Sulfinpyrazone (Co-administration of estrogens with inducers of CYP3A4 may reduce plasma concentrations of estrogens, possibly resulting in a decrease in therapeutic effects and/or changes in the uterine bleeding profile).
No products indexed under this heading.

Telithromycin (Co-administration of estrogens with inhibitors of CYP3A4 may increase plasma concentrations of estrogens and may result in side effects). Products include:
Ketek Tablets 2920

Theophylline (Co-administration of estrogens with inducers of CYP3A4 may reduce plasma concentrations of estrogens, possibly resulting in a decrease in therapeutic effects and/or changes in the uterine bleeding profile).
No products indexed under this heading.

Triamcinolone (Co-administration of estrogens with inducers of CYP3A4 may reduce plasma concentrations of estrogens, possibly resulting in a decrease in therapeutic effects and/or changes in the uterine bleeding profile).
No products indexed under this heading.

Triamcinolone Acetonide (Co-administration of estrogens with inducers of CYP3A4 may reduce plasma concentrations of estrogens, possibly resulting in a decrease in therapeutic effects and/or changes in the uterine bleeding profile).
Products include:
Azmacort Inhalation Aerosol 1701
Nasacort HFA Inhalation Aerosol 2939
Nasacort AQ Nasal Spray 2937

Triamcinolone Diacetate (Co-administration of estrogens with inducers of CYP3A4 may reduce plasma concentrations of estrogens, possibly resulting in a decrease in therapeutic effects and/or changes in the uterine bleeding profile).
No products indexed under this heading.

Triamcinolone Hexacetonide (Co-administration of estrogens with inducers of CYP3A4 may reduce plasma concentrations of estrogens, possibly resulting in a decrease in therapeutic effects and/or changes in the uterine bleeding profile).
No products indexed under this heading.

Troglitazone (Co-administration of estrogens with inducers of CYP3A4 may reduce plasma concentrations of estrogens, possibly resulting in a decrease in therapeutic effects and/or changes in the uterine bleeding profile).
No products indexed under this heading.

Troleandomycin (Co-administration of estrogens with inhibitors of CYP3A4 may increase plasma concentrations of estrogens and may result in side effects).
No products indexed under this heading.

Valproate Sodium (Co-administration of estrogens with inhibitors of CYP3A4 may increase plasma concentrations of estrogens and may result in side effects).
Products include:
Depacon Injection 412

Verapamil Hydrochloride (Co-administration of estrogens with inhibitors of CYP3A4 may increase plasma concentrations of estrogens and may result in side effects).
Products include:
Covera-HS Tablets 3135
Tarka Tablets 519
Verelan PM Capsules 3120

Voriconazole (Co-administration of estrogens with inhibitors of CYP3A4 may increase plasma concentrations of estrogens and may result in side effects). Products include:
VFEND I.V. 2543
VFEND Oral Suspension 2543
VFEND Tablets 2543

Zafirlukast (Co-administration of estrogens with inhibitors of CYP3A4 may increase plasma concentrations of estrogens and may result in side effects). Products include:

Accolate Tablets 663

Zileuton (Co-administration of estrogens with inhibitors of CYP3A4 may increase plasma concentrations of estrogens and may result in side effects).

No products indexed under this heading.

Food Interactions

Food, unspecified (Administration with a high fat breakfast decreased total estrone Cmax and increased total equilin Cmax compared to fasting state, no other effect on rate or extent of absorption; administration with food doubles MPA Cmax and increases MPA AUC).

Grapefruit (Co-administration of estrogens with inhibitors of CYP3A4 may increase plasma concentrations of estrogens and may result in side effects).

Grapefruit Juice (Co-administration of estrogens with inhibitors of CYP3A4, such as grapefruit juice, may increase plasma concentrations of estrogens and may result in side effects).

PREMPRO TABLETS

(Estrogens, Conjugated, Medroxyprogesterone Acetate)........... 3452

May interact with cytochrome p450 3a4 inducers (selected), cytochrome p450 3a4 inhibitors (selected), and certain other agents. Compounds in these categories include:

Acetazolamide (Co-administration of estrogens with inhibitors of CYP3A4 may increase plasma concentrations of estrogens and may result in side effects).

No products indexed under this heading.

Allium sativum (Co-administration of estrogens with inducers of CYP3A4 may reduce plasma concentrations of estrogens, possibly resulting in a decrease in therapeutic effects and/or changes in the uterine bleeding profile).

No products indexed under this heading.

Aminoglutethimide (Aminoglutethimide administered concomitantly with medroxyprogesterone acetate (MPA) may significantly depress the bioavailability of MPA).

No products indexed under this heading.

Amiodarone Hydrochloride (Co-administration of estrogens with inhibitors of CYP3A4 may increase plasma concentrations of estrogens and may result in side effects). Products include:

Pacerone Tablets 3337

Amprenavir (Co-administration of estrogens with inhibitors of CYP3A4 may increase plasma concentrations of estrogens and may result in side effects). Products include:

Agenerase Capsules 1299
Agenerase Oral Solution 1304

Anastrozole (Co-administration of estrogens with inhibitors of CYP3A4 may increase plasma concentrations of estrogens and may result in side effects). Products include:

Arimidex Tablets 665

Aprepitant (Co-administration of estrogens with inducers of CYP3A4 may reduce plasma concentrations of estrogens, possibly resulting in a decrease in therapeutic effects and/or changes in the uterine bleeding profile). Products include:

Emend Capsules 1944

Betamethasone Acetate (Co-administration of estrogens with inducers of CYP3A4 may reduce plasma concentrations of estrogens, possibly resulting in a decrease in therapeutic effects and/or changes in the uterine bleeding profile).

No products indexed under this heading.

Betamethasone Sodium Phosphate (Co-administration of estrogens with inducers of CYP3A4 may reduce plasma concentrations of estrogens, possibly resulting in a decrease in therapeutic effects and/or changes in the uterine bleeding profile).

No products indexed under this heading.

Carbamazepine (Co-administration of estrogens with inducers of CYP3A4 may reduce plasma concentrations of estrogens, possibly resulting in a decrease in therapeutic effects and/or changes in the uterine bleeding profile). Products include:

Carbatrol Capsules 3174
Equetro Extended-Release Capsules 3178
Tegretol/Tegretol-XR 2278

Cimetidine (Co-administration of estrogens with inhibitors of CYP3A4 may increase plasma concentrations of estrogens and may result in side effects). Products include:

Tagamet HB 200 Tablets 637
Tagamet Tablets 1547

Cimetidine Hydrochloride (Co-administration of estrogens with inhibitors of CYP3A4 may increase plasma concentrations of estrogens and may result in side effects).

No products indexed under this heading.

Ciprofloxacin (Co-administration of estrogens with inhibitors of CYP3A4 may increase plasma concentrations of estrogens and may result in side effects). Products include:

Cipro I.V. 2998
Cipro I.V. Pharmacy Bulk Package ... 3509
Cipro Oral Suspension 2991
Cipro XR Tablets 3004
Ciprodex Otic Suspension 555

Ciprofloxacin Hydrochloride (Co-administration of estrogens with inducers of CYP3A4 may reduce plasma concentrations of estrogens, possibly resulting in a decrease in therapeutic effects and/or changes in the uterine bleeding profile). Products include:

Ciloxan Ophthalmic Ointment 554
Cipro Tablets 2991

Cisplatin (Co-administration of estrogens with inducers of CYP3A4 may reduce plasma concentrations of estrogens, possibly resulting in a decrease in therapeutic effects and/or changes in the uterine bleeding profile).

No products indexed under this heading.

Clarithromycin (Co-administration of estrogens with inhibitors of CYP3A4 may increase plasma concentrations of estrogens and may result in side effects). Products include:

Biaxin/Biaxin XL 402
PREVPAC 3281

Clotrimazole (Co-administration of estrogens with inhibitors of CYP3A4 may increase plasma concentrations of estrogens and may result in side effects). Products include:

Lotrimin 3053
Lotrisone 3054

Cortisone Acetate (Co-administration of estrogens with inducers of CYP3A4 may reduce plasma concentrations of estrogens, possibly resulting in a decrease in therapeutic effects and/or changes in the uterine bleeding profile).

No products indexed under this heading.

Cyclosporine (Co-administration of estrogens with inhibitors of CYP3A4 may increase plasma concentrations of estrogens and may result in side effects). Products include:

Gengraf Capsules 458
Neoral Soft Gelatin Capsules 2247
Neoral Oral Solution 2247
Restasis Ophthalmic Emulsion 570
Sandimmune 2259

Dalfopristin (Co-administration of estrogens with inhibitors of CYP3A4 may increase plasma concentrations of estrogens and may result in side effects). Products include:

Synercid I.V. 1690

Danazol (Co-administration of estrogens with inhibitors of CYP3A4 may increase plasma concentrations of estrogens and may result in side effects).

No products indexed under this heading.

Delavirdine Mesylate (Co-administration of estrogens with inhibitors of CYP3A4 may increase plasma concentrations of estrogens and may result in side effects). Products include:

Rescriptor Tablets 2535

Dexamethasone (Co-administration of estrogens with inducers of CYP3A4 may reduce plasma concentrations of estrogens, possibly resulting in a decrease in therapeutic effects and/or changes in the uterine bleeding profile). Products include:

Ciprodex Otic Suspension 555
Decadron Tablets 1929
TobraDex Ophthalmic Ointment 558
TobraDex Ophthalmic Suspension ... 558

Dexamethasone Acetate (Co-administration of estrogens with inducers of CYP3A4 may reduce plasma concentrations of estrogens, possibly resulting in a decrease in therapeutic effects and/or changes in the uterine bleeding profile).

No products indexed under this heading.

Dexamethasone Sodium Phosphate (Co-administration of estrogens with inducers of CYP3A4 may reduce plasma concentrations of estrogens, possibly resulting in a decrease in therapeutic effects and/or changes in the uterine bleeding profile). Products include:

Decadron Phosphate Injection 1931

Diltiazem Hydrochloride (Co-administration of estrogens with inhibitors of CYP3A4 may increase plasma concentrations of estrogens and may result in side effects). Products include:

Cardizem LA Extended Release Tablets 1699
Tiazac Capsules 1204

Diltiazem Maleate (Co-administration of estrogens with inhibitors of CYP3A4 may increase plasma concentrations of estrogens and may result in side effects).

No products indexed under this heading.

Doxorubicin Hydrochloride (Co-administration of estrogens with inducers of CYP3A4 may reduce plasma concentrations of estrogens, possibly resulting in a decrease in therapeutic effects and/or changes in the uterine bleeding profile). Products include:

Adriamycin for Injection, USP 786
Adriamycin Injection, USP 786

Efavirenz (Co-administration of estrogens with inducers of CYP3A4 may reduce plasma concentrations of estrogens, possibly resulting in a decrease in therapeutic effects and/or changes in the uterine bleeding profile). Products include:

Sustiva Capsules 957

Erythromycin (Co-administration of estrogens with inhibitors of CYP3A4 may increase plasma concentrations of estrogens and may result in side effects). Products include:

Erygel Topical Gel 2096
Ery-Tab Tablets 447
Erythromycin Base Filmtab Tablets 454
Erythromycin Delayed-Release Capsules, USP 456
PCE Dispertab Tablets 510

Erythromycin Estolate (Co-administration of estrogens with inhibitors of CYP3A4 may increase plasma concentrations of estrogens and may result in side effects).

No products indexed under this heading.

Erythromycin Ethylsuccinate (Co-administration of estrogens with inhibitors of CYP3A4 may increase plasma concentrations of estrogens and may result in side effects). Products include:

E.E.S. 449
EryPed 445

Erythromycin Gluceptate (Co-administration of estrogens with inhibitors of CYP3A4 may increase plasma concentrations of estrogens and may result in side effects).

No products indexed under this heading.

Erythromycin Lactobionate (Co-administration of estrogens with inhibitors of CYP3A4 may increase plasma concentrations of estrogens and may result in side effects).

No products indexed under this heading.

Erythromycin Stearate (Co-administration of estrogens with inhibitors of CYP3A4 may increase plasma concentrations of estrogens and may result in side effects). Products include:

Erythrocin Stearate Filmtab Tablets 452

Esomeprazole Magnesium (Co-administration of estrogens with inhibitors of CYP3A4 may increase plasma concentrations of estrogens and may result in side effects). Products include:

Nexium Delayed-Release Capsules 645

Ethosuximide (Co-administration of estrogens with inducers of CYP3A4 may reduce plasma concentrations of estrogens, possibly resulting in a decrease in therapeutic effects and/or changes in the uterine bleeding profile).

No products indexed under this heading.

Felbamate (Co-administration of estrogens with inducers of CYP3A4 may reduce plasma concentrations of estrogens, possibly resulting in a decrease in therapeutic effects and/or changes in the uterine bleeding profile).

No products indexed under this heading.

Fluconazole (Co-administration of estrogens with inhibitors of CYP3A4 may increase plasma concentrations of estrogens and may result in side effects).

No products indexed under this heading.

Fludrocortisone Acetate (Co-administration of estrogens with inducers of CYP3A4 may reduce plasma concentrations of estrogens, possibly resulting in a decrease in therapeutic effects and/or changes in the uterine bleeding profile).

No products indexed under this heading.

Fluoxetine Hydrochloride (Co-administration of estrogens with inhibitors of CYP3A4 may increase plasma concentrations of estrogens and may result in side effects). Products include:

Prozac Pulvules and Liquid **1771**
Symbyax Capsules **1788**

Fluvoxamine Maleate (Co-administration of estrogens with inhibitors of CYP3A4 may increase plasma concentrations of estrogens and may result in side effects).

No products indexed under this heading.

Fosamprenavir Calcium (Co-administration of estrogens with inhibitors of CYP3A4 may increase plasma concentrations of estrogens and may result in side effects). Products include:

Lexiva Tablets **1473**

Fosphenytoin Sodium (Co-administration of estrogens with inducers of CYP3A4 may reduce plasma concentrations of estrogens, possibly resulting in a decrease in therapeutic effects and/or changes in the uterine bleeding profile).

No products indexed under this heading.

Garlic Extract (Co-administration of estrogens with inducers of CYP3A4 may reduce plasma concentrations of estrogens, possibly resulting in a decrease in therapeutic effects and/or changes in the uterine bleeding profile).

No products indexed under this heading.

Garlic Oil (Co-administration of estrogens with inducers of CYP3A4 may reduce plasma concentrations of estrogens, possibly resulting in a decrease in therapeutic effects and/or changes in the uterine bleeding profile).

No products indexed under this heading.

Hydrocortisone (Co-administration of estrogens with inducers of CYP3A4 may reduce plasma concentrations of estrogens, possibly resulting in a decrease in therapeutic effects and/or changes in the uterine bleeding profile). Products include:

Cortizone•5 Ointment .... ▣ **699**
Cortizone•10 Creme .... ▣ **699**
Cortizone•10 Ointment .... ▣ **699**
Cortizone•10 Plus Creme .... ▣ **700**
Cortizone•10 Maximum Strength Quick Shot Spray .... ▣ **700**
Hydrocortone Tablets **1963**
Preparation H Hydrocortisone Cream .... ▣ **748**

Hydrocortisone Acetate (Co-administration of estrogens with inducers of CYP3A4 may reduce plasma concentrations of estrogens, possibly resulting in a decrease in therapeutic effects and/or changes in the uterine bleeding profile). Products include:

Analpram-HC **1136**
Pramosone **1139**
ProctoFoam-HC **3113**
Tucks Anti-Itch Ointment .... ▣ **712**
U-cort 1% Cream **3289**

Hydrocortisone Butyrate (Co-administration of estrogens with inducers of CYP3A4 may reduce plasma concentrations of estrogens, possibly resulting in a decrease in therapeutic effects and/or changes in the uterine bleeding profile). Products include:

Locoid **1138**
Locoid Lipocream Cream **1138**

Hydrocortisone Cypionate (Co-administration of estrogens with inducers of CYP3A4 may reduce plasma concentrations of estrogens, possibly resulting in a decrease in therapeutic effects and/or changes in the uterine bleeding profile).

No products indexed under this heading.

Hydrocortisone Hemisuccinate (Co-administration of estrogens with inducers of CYP3A4 may reduce plasma concentrations of estrogens, possibly resulting in a decrease in therapeutic effects and/or changes in the uterine bleeding profile).

No products indexed under this heading.

Hydrocortisone Probutate (Co-administration of estrogens with inducers of CYP3A4 may reduce plasma concentrations of estrogens, possibly resulting in a decrease in therapeutic effects and/or changes in the uterine bleeding profile). Products include:

Pandel Cream, 0.1% **1017**

Hydrocortisone Sodium Phosphate (Co-administration of estrogens with inducers of CYP3A4 may reduce plasma concentrations of estrogens, possibly resulting in a decrease in therapeutic effects and/or changes in the uterine bleeding profile).

No products indexed under this heading.

Hydrocortisone Sodium Succinate (Co-administration of estrogens with inducers of CYP3A4 may reduce plasma concentrations of estrogens, possibly resulting in a decrease in therapeutic effects and/or changes in the uterine bleeding profile).

No products indexed under this heading.

Hydrocortisone Valerate (Co-administration of estrogens with inducers of CYP3A4 may reduce plasma concentrations of estrogens, possibly resulting in a decrease in therapeutic effects and/or changes in the uterine bleeding profile).

No products indexed under this heading.

Hypericum (Co-administration of estrogens with inducers of CYP3A4 may reduce plasma concentrations of estrogens, possibly resulting in a decrease in therapeutic effects and/or changes in the uterine bleeding profile).

No products indexed under this heading.

Hypericum Perforatum (Co-administration of estrogens with inducers of CYP3A4 may reduce plasma concentrations of estrogens, possibly resulting in a decrease in therapeutic effects and/or changes in the uterine bleeding profile).

No products indexed under this heading.

Indinavir Sulfate (Co-administration of estrogens with inhibitors of CYP3A4 may increase plasma concentrations of estrogens and may result in side effects). Products include:

Crixivan Capsules **1918**

Isoniazid (Co-administration of estrogens with inhibitors of CYP3A4 may increase plasma concentrations of estrogens and may result in side effects).

No products indexed under this heading.

Itraconazole (Co-administration of estrogens with inhibitors of CYP3A4 may increase plasma concentrations of estrogens and may result in side effects).

No products indexed under this heading.

Ketoconazole (Co-administration of estrogens with inhibitors of CYP3A4 may increase plasma concentrations of estrogens and may result in side effects). Products include:

Nizoral A-D Shampoo, 1% **1839**
Nizoral 2% Shampoo **1838**

Lopinavir (Co-administration of estrogens with inhibitors of CYP3A4 may increase plasma concentrations of estrogens and may result in side effects). Products include:

Kaletra **474**

Loratadine (Co-administration of estrogens with inhibitors of CYP3A4 may increase plasma concentrations of estrogens and may result in side effects). Products include:

Alavert Allergy & Sinus D-12 Hour Tablets .... ▣ **743**
Alavert .... ▣ **743**
Children's Claritin 24 Hour Non-Drowsy Allergy Syrup .... ▣ **732**
Claritin Non-Drowsy 24 Hour Tablets .... ▣ **731**
Non-Drowsy Claritin Hives Relief Tablets .... ▣ **733**
Claritin Reditabs 24 Hour Non-Drowsy Tablets .... ▣ **732**
Claritin-D Non-Drowsy 12 Hour Tablets .... ▣ **731**
Claritin-D Non-Drowsy 24 Hour Tablets .... ▣ **731**
Children's Dimetapp ND Non-Drowsy Allergy Syrup .... ▣ **746**
Triaminic Allerchews .... ▣ **684**

Mephenytoin (Co-administration of estrogens with inducers of CYP3A4 may reduce plasma concentrations of estrogens, possibly resulting in a decrease in therapeutic effects and/or changes in the uterine bleeding profile).

No products indexed under this heading.

Methsuximide (Co-administration of estrogens with inducers of CYP3A4 may reduce plasma concentrations of estrogens, possibly resulting in a decrease in therapeutic effects and/or changes in the uterine bleeding profile).

No products indexed under this heading.

Methylprednisolone (Co-administration of estrogens with inducers of CYP3A4 may reduce plasma concentrations of estrogens, possibly resulting in a decrease in therapeutic effects and/or changes in the uterine bleeding profile).

No products indexed under this heading.

Methylprednisolone Acetate (Co-administration of estrogens with inducers of CYP3A4 may reduce plasma concentrations of estrogens, possibly resulting in a decrease in therapeutic effects and/or changes in the uterine bleeding profile). Products include:

Depo-Medrol Injectable Suspension **2615**
Depo-Medrol Single-Dose Vial **2617**

Methylprednisolone Sodium Succinate (Co-administration of estrogens with inducers of CYP3A4 may reduce plasma concentrations of estrogens, possibly resulting in a decrease in therapeutic effects and/or changes in the uterine bleeding profile).

No products indexed under this heading.

Metronidazole (Co-administration of estrogens with inhibitors of CYP3A4 may increase plasma concentrations of estrogens and may result in side effects). Products include:

Metrogel 1% **1212**
MetroGel-Vaginal Gel **1822**
Noritate Cream, 1% **1051**

Metronidazole Benzoate (Co-administration of estrogens with inhibitors of CYP3A4 may increase plasma concentrations of estrogens and may result in side effects).

No products indexed under this heading.

Metronidazole Hydrochloride (Co-administration of estrogens with inhibitors of CYP3A4 may increase plasma concentrations of estrogens and may result in side effects).

No products indexed under this heading.

Miconazole (Co-administration of estrogens with inhibitors of CYP3A4 may increase plasma concentrations of estrogens and may result in side effects).

No products indexed under this heading.

Miconazole Nitrate (Co-administration of estrogens with inhibitors of CYP3A4 may increase plasma concentrations of estrogens and may result in side effects). Products include:

Desenex .... ▣ **674**
Desenex Jock Itch Spray Powder .... ▣ **674**

Modafinil (Co-administration of estrogens with inducers of CYP3A4 may reduce plasma concentrations of estrogens, possibly resulting in a decrease in therapeutic effects and/or changes in the uterine bleeding profile). Products include:

Provigil Tablets **1002**

Nefazodone Hydrochloride (Co-administration of estrogens with inhibitors of CYP3A4 may increase plasma concentrations of estrogens and may result in side effects).

No products indexed under this heading.

Nelfinavir Mesylate (Co-administration of estrogens with inhibitors of CYP3A4 may increase plasma concentrations of estrogens and may result in side effects). Products include:

Viracept **2556**

Nevirapine (Co-administration of estrogens with inducers of CYP3A4 may reduce plasma concentrations of estrogens, possibly resulting in a decrease in therapeutic effects and/or changes in the uterine bleeding profile). Products include:

Viramune Oral Suspension **903**
Viramune Tablets **903**

Niacinamide (Co-administration of estrogens with inhibitors of CYP3A4 may increase plasma concentrations of estrogens and may result in side effects).

No products indexed under this heading.

Nicotinamide (Co-administration of estrogens with inhibitors of CYP3A4 may increase plasma concentrations of estrogens and may result in side effects). Products include:

Nicomide Tablets **3190**

Nifedipine (Co-administration of estrogens with inhibitors of CYP3A4 may increase plasma concentrations of estrogens and may result in side effects). Products include:

Adalat CC Tablets **2978**

Norfloxacin (Co-administration of estrogens with inhibitors of CYP3A4 may increase plasma concentrations of estrogens and may result in side effects). Products include:

Noroxin Tablets **2009**

Omeprazole (Co-administration of estrogens with inhibitors of CYP3A4 may increase plasma concentrations of estrogens and may result in side effects). Products include:

Zegerid Powder for Oral Solution **2972**

Oxcarbazepine (Co-administration of estrogens with inducers of CYP3A4 may reduce plasma concentrations of estrogens, possibly resulting in a decrease in therapeutic effects and/or changes in the uterine bleeding profile). Products include:

Trileptal Oral Suspension **2281**
Trileptal Tablets **2281**

Paroxetine Hydrochloride (Co-administration of estrogens with inhibitors of CYP3A4 may increase plasma concentrations of estrogens and may result in side effects). Products include:

Paxil CR Controlled-Release Tablets **1509**
Paxil **1501**

Phenobarbital (Co-administration of estrogens with inducers of CYP3A4 may reduce plasma concentrations of estrogens, possibly resulting in a decrease in therapeutic effects and/or changes in the uterine bleeding profile).

No products indexed under this heading.

Phenobarbital Sodium (Co-administration of estrogens with inducers of CYP3A4 may reduce plasma concentrations of estrogens, possibly resulting in a decrease in therapeutic effects and/or changes in the uterine bleeding profile).

No products indexed under this heading.

Phenytoin (Co-administration of estrogens with inducers of CYP3A4 may reduce plasma concentrations of estrogens, possibly resulting in a decrease in therapeutic effects and/or changes in the uterine bleeding profile).

No products indexed under this heading.

Phenytoin Sodium (Co-administration of estrogens with inducers of CYP3A4 may reduce plasma concentrations of estrogens, possibly resulting in a decrease in therapeutic effects and/or changes in the uterine bleeding profile). Products include:

Phenytek Capsules **2153**

Prednisolone Acetate (Co-administration of estrogens with inducers of CYP3A4 may reduce plasma concentrations of estrogens, possibly resulting in a decrease in therapeutic effects and/or changes in the uterine bleeding profile). Products include:

Blephamide Ophthalmic Ointment **563**
Blephamide Ophthalmic Suspension **564**
Poly-Pred Liquifilm Ophthalmic Suspension .... ⊙**231**
Pred Forte Ophthalmic Suspension .... ⊙**233**
Pred Mild Sterile Ophthalmic Suspension .... ⊙**236**
Pred-G Ophthalmic Suspension .... ⊙**234**
Pred-G Sterile Ophthalmic Ointment .... ⊙**235**

Prednisolone Sodium Phosphate (Co-administration of estrogens with inducers of CYP3A4 may reduce plasma concentrations of estrogens, possibly resulting in a decrease in therapeutic effects and/or changes in the uterine bleeding profile). Products include:

Pediapred Oral Solution **3319**

Prednisolone Tebutate (Co-administration of estrogens with inducers of CYP3A4 may reduce plasma concentrations of estrogens, possibly resulting in a decrease in therapeutic effects and/or changes in the uterine bleeding profile).

No products indexed under this heading.

Prednisone (Co-administration of estrogens with inducers of CYP3A4 may reduce plasma concentrations of estrogens, possibly resulting in a decrease in therapeutic effects and/or changes in the uterine bleeding profile).

No products indexed under this heading.

Primidone (Co-administration of estrogens with inducers of CYP3A4 may reduce plasma concentrations of estrogens, possibly resulting in a decrease in therapeutic effects and/or changes in the uterine bleeding profile).

No products indexed under this heading.

Propoxyphene Hydrochloride (Co-administration of estrogens with inhibitors of CYP3A4 may increase plasma concentrations of estrogens and may result in side effects).

No products indexed under this heading.

Propoxyphene Napsylate (Co-administration of estrogens with inhibitors of CYP3A4 may increase plasma concentrations of estrogens and may result in side effects). Products include:

Darvocet A 500 Tablets **3497**

Quinidine (Co-administration of estrogens with inhibitors of CYP3A4 may increase plasma concentrations of estrogens and may result in side effects).

No products indexed under this heading.

Quinidine Hydrochloride (Co-administration of estrogens with inhibitors of CYP3A4 may increase plasma concentrations of estrogens and may result in side effects).

No products indexed under this heading.

Quinidine Polygalacturonate (Co-administration of estrogens with inhibitors of CYP3A4 may increase plasma concentrations of estrogens and may result in side effects).

No products indexed under this heading.

Quinidine Sulfate (Co-administration of estrogens with inhibitors of CYP3A4 may increase plasma concentrations of estrogens and may result in side effects).

No products indexed under this heading.

Quinine (Co-administration of estrogens with inhibitors of CYP3A4 may increase plasma concentrations of estrogens and may result in side effects).

No products indexed under this heading.

Quinine Sulfate (Co-administration of estrogens with inhibitors of CYP3A4 may increase plasma concentrations of estrogens and may result in side effects).

No products indexed under this heading.

Quinupristin (Co-administration of estrogens with inhibitors of CYP3A4 may increase plasma concentrations of estrogens and may result in side effects). Products include:

Synercid I.V. **1690**

Ranitidine Bismuth Citrate (Co-administration of estrogens with inhibitors of CYP3A4 may increase plasma concentrations of estrogens and may result in side effects).

No products indexed under this heading.

Ranitidine Hydrochloride (Co-administration of estrogens with inhibitors of CYP3A4 may increase plasma concentrations of estrogens and may result in side effects). Products include:

Zantac **1597**
Zantac Injection **1593**
Zantac 75 Tablets **715**
Zantac 150 Maximum Strength Tablets **715**
Zantac Injection Pharmacy Bulk Package **1595**

Rifabutin (Co-administration of estrogens with inducers of CYP3A4 may reduce plasma concentrations of estrogens, possibly resulting in a decrease in therapeutic effects and/or changes in the uterine bleeding profile).

No products indexed under this heading.

Rifampicin (Co-administration of estrogens with inducers of CYP3A4 may reduce plasma concentrations of estrogens, possibly resulting in a decrease in therapeutic effects and/or changes in the uterine bleeding profile).

No products indexed under this heading.

Rifampin (Co-administration of estrogens with inducers of CYP3A4 may reduce plasma concentrations of estrogens, possibly resulting in a decrease in therapeutic effects and/or changes in the uterine bleeding profile).

No products indexed under this heading.

Rifapentine (Co-administration of estrogens with inducers of CYP3A4 may reduce plasma concentrations of estrogens, possibly resulting in a decrease in therapeutic effects and/or changes in the uterine bleeding profile).

No products indexed under this heading.

Ritonavir (Co-administration of estrogens with inhibitors of CYP3A4 may increase plasma concentrations of estrogens and may result in side effects). Products include:

Kaletra **474**
Norvir **499**

Saquinavir (Co-administration of estrogens with inhibitors of CYP3A4 may increase plasma concentrations of estrogens and may result in side effects).

No products indexed under this heading.

Saquinavir Mesylate (Co-administration of estrogens with inhibitors of CYP3A4 may increase plasma concentrations of estrogens and may result in side effects). Products include:

Invirase **2776**

Sertraline Hydrochloride (Co-administration of estrogens with inhibitors of CYP3A4 may increase plasma concentrations of estrogens and may result in side effects). Products include:

Zoloft **2581**

Sulfinpyrazone (Co-administration of estrogens with inducers of CYP3A4 may reduce plasma concentrations of estrogens, possibly resulting in a decrease in therapeutic effects and/or changes in the uterine bleeding profile).

No products indexed under this heading.

Telithromycin (Co-administration of estrogens with inhibitors of CYP3A4 may increase plasma concentrations of estrogens and may result in side effects). Products include:

Ketek Tablets **2920**

Theophylline (Co-administration of estrogens with inducers of CYP3A4 may reduce plasma concentrations of estrogens, possibly resulting in a decrease in therapeutic effects and/or changes in the uterine bleeding profile).
No products indexed under this heading.

Triamcinolone (Co-administration of estrogens with inducers of CYP3A4 may reduce plasma concentrations of estrogens, possibly resulting in a decrease in therapeutic effects and/or changes in the uterine bleeding profile).
No products indexed under this heading.

Triamcinolone Acetonide (Co-administration of estrogens with inducers of CYP3A4 may reduce plasma concentrations of estrogens, possibly resulting in a decrease in therapeutic effects and/or changes in the uterine bleeding profile).
Products include:
Azmacort Inhalation Aerosol 1701
Nasacort HFA Inhalation Aerosol 2939
Nasacort AQ Nasal Spray 2937

Triamcinolone Diacetate (Co-administration of estrogens with inducers of CYP3A4 may reduce plasma concentrations of estrogens, possibly resulting in a decrease in therapeutic effects and/or changes in the uterine bleeding profile).
No products indexed under this heading.

Triamcinolone Hexacetonide (Co-administration of estrogens with inducers of CYP3A4 may reduce plasma concentrations of estrogens, possibly resulting in a decrease in therapeutic effects and/or changes in the uterine bleeding profile).
No products indexed under this heading.

Troglitazone (Co-administration of estrogens with inducers of CYP3A4 may reduce plasma concentrations of estrogens, possibly resulting in a decrease in therapeutic effects and/or changes in the uterine bleeding profile).
No products indexed under this heading.

Troleandomycin (Co-administration of estrogens with inhibitors of CYP3A4 may increase plasma concentrations of estrogens and may result in side effects).
No products indexed under this heading.

Valproate Sodium (Co-administration of estrogens with inhibitors of CYP3A4 may increase plasma concentrations of estrogens and may result in side effects).
Products include:
Depacon Injection 412

Verapamil Hydrochloride (Co-administration of estrogens with inhibitors of CYP3A4 may increase plasma concentrations of estrogens and may result in side effects).
Products include:
Covera-HS Tablets 3135
Tarka Tablets 519
Verelan PM Capsules 3120

Voriconazole (Co-administration of estrogens with inhibitors of CYP3A4 may increase plasma concentrations of estrogens and may result in side effects). Products include:
VFEND I.V. 2543
VFEND Oral Suspension 2543
VFEND Tablets 2543

Zafirlukast (Co-administration of estrogens with inhibitors of CYP3A4 may increase plasma concentrations of estrogens and may result in side effects). Products include:
Accolate Tablets 663

Zileuton (Co-administration of estrogens with inhibitors of CYP3A4 may increase plasma concentrations of estrogens and may result in side effects).
No products indexed under this heading.

Food Interactions

Food, unspecified (Administration with food decreased Cmax of total estrone compared to fasting state, no other effect on rate or extent of absorption; administration with food doubles MPA Cmax and increases MPA AUC).

Grapefruit (Co-administration of estrogens with inhibitors of CYP3A4 may increase plasma concentrations of estrogens and may result in side effects).

Grapefruit Juice (Co-administration of estrogens with inhibitors of CYP3A4, such as grapefruit juice, may increase plasma concentrations of estrogens and may result in side effects).

PRENATE ELITE TABLETS

(Vitamins, Prenatal) 1163
None cited in PDR database.

PREPARATION H MAXIMUM STRENGTH CREAM

(Glycerin, Petrolatum, Phenylephrine Hydrochloride, Pramoxine Hydrochloride) .... ■747
None cited in PDR database.

PREPARATION H COOLING GEL

(Phenylephrine Hydrochloride) .... ■747
None cited in PDR database.

PREPARATION H HYDROCORTISONE CREAM

(Hydrocortisone) .... ■748
None cited in PDR database.

PREPARATION H OINTMENT

(Mineral Oil, Petrolatum, Phenylephrine Hydrochloride, Shark Liver Oil) .... ■747
None cited in PDR database.

PREPARATION H SUPPOSITORIES

(Cocoa Butter, Phenylephrine Hydrochloride, Shark Liver Oil) .... ■747
None cited in PDR database.

PREPARATION H MEDICATED WIPES

(Witch Hazel) .... ■748
None cited in PDR database.

PREVACID DELAYED-RELEASE CAPSULES

(Lansoprazole) 3268
May interact with iron containing oral preparations, absorption of drugs where gastric ph is an important determinant in their bioavailability, xanthines, and certain other agents. Compounds in these categories include:

Aminophylline (Co-administration has resulted in a minor increase (10%) in the clearance of theophylline; this interaction is unlikely to be of clinical concern, nonetheless, monitor blood levels).
No products indexed under this heading.

Astemizole (There have been post-marketing reports of drug interactions when clarithromycin and/or erythromycin are co-administered with cisapride, pimozide, astemizole or terfenadine resulting in cardiac arrhythmias most likely due to inhibition of metabolism of these drugs by erythromycin and clarithromycin. Fatalities have been reported).
No products indexed under this heading.

Bacampicillin Hydrochloride (Lansoprazole causes a profound and long-lasting inhibition of gastric acid secretion; therefore, it is theoretically possible that it may interfere with the oral absorption of drugs where gastric pH is an important determinant of bioavailability).
No products indexed under this heading.

Cisapride (There have been post-marketing reports of drug interactions when clarithromycin and/or erythromycin are co-administered with cisapride, pimozide, astemizole or terfenadine resulting in cardiac arrhythmias most likely due to inhibition of metabolism of these drugs by erythromycin and clarithromycin. Fatalities have been reported).
No products indexed under this heading.

Digoxin (Lansoprazole causes a profound and long-lasting inhibition of gastric acid secretion; therefore, it is theoretically possible that it may interfere with the oral absorption of drugs where gastric pH is an important determinant of bioavailability, such as digoxin). Products include:
Digitek Tablets 2146
Lanoxicaps Capsules 1458
Lanoxin Injection 1462
Lanoxin Tablets 1468
Lanoxin Injection Pediatric 1465

Dyphylline (Co-administration has resulted in a minor increase (10%) in the clearance of theophylline; this interaction is unlikely to be of clinical concern, nonetheless, monitor blood levels).
No products indexed under this heading.

Ferrous Fumarate (Lansoprazole causes a profound and long-lasting inhibition of gastric acid secretion; therefore, it is theoretically possible that it may interfere with the absorption of drugs, such as iron salts, where gastric pH is an important determinant of bioavailability).
Products include:
Chromagen Forte Soft Gelatin Capsules 3296
Ferretts Tablets .... ■773
Repliva 21/7 Tablets 3301

Ferrous Gluconate (Lansoprazole causes a profound and long-lasting inhibition of gastric acid secretion; therefore, it is theoretically possible that it may interfere with the absorption of drugs, such as iron salts, where gastric pH is an important determinant of bioavailability).
No products indexed under this heading.

Ferrous Sulfate (Lansoprazole causes a profound and long-lasting inhibition of gastric acid secretion; therefore, it is theoretically possible that it may interfere with the absorption of drugs, such as iron salts, where gastric pH is an important determinant of bioavailability).
Products include:
Feosol Tablets 1629
Slow Fe Iron Tablets .... ■772
Slow Fe with Folic Acid Tablets ...... ■773

Iron (Lansoprazole causes a profound and long-lasting inhibition of gastric acid secretion; therefore, it is theoretically possible that it may interfere with the absorption of drugs, such as iron salts, where gastric pH is an important determinant of bioavailability). Products include:
Chromagen Forte Soft Gelatin Capsules 3296
Ferretts IPS Liquid .... ■773
OptiNate 1162
Repliva 21/7 Tablets 3301

Ketoconazole (Lansoprazole causes a profound and long-lasting inhibition of gastric acid secretion; therefore, it is theoretically possible that it may interfere with the oral absorption of drugs where gastric pH is an important determinant of bioavailability). Products include:
Nizoral A-D Shampoo, 1% 1839
Nizoral 2% Shampoo 1838

Pimozide (There have been post-marketing reports of drug interactions when clarithromycin and/or erythromycin are co-administered with cisapride, pimozide, astemizole or terfenadine resulting in cardiac arrhythmias most likely due to inhibition of metabolism of these drugs by erythromycin and clarithromycin. Fatalities have been reported).
Products include:
Orap Tablets 1220

Polysaccharide Iron Complex (Lansoprazole causes a profound and long-lasting inhibition of gastric acid secretion; therefore, it is theoretically possible that it may interfere with the absorption of drugs, such as iron salts, where gastric pH is an important determinant of bioavailability). Products include:
Niferex-150 Forte Capsules 3299
Nu-Iron 150 Capsules 2098

Sucralfate (Co-administration delays absorption and reduces bioavailability of lansoprazole by about 30%; therefore, lansoprazole should be taken at least 30 minutes prior to sucralfate). Products include:
Carafate Suspension 727
Carafate Tablets 728

Terfenadine (There have been post-marketing reports of drug interactions when clarithromycin and/or erythromycin are co-administered with cisapride, pimozide, astemizole or terfenadine resulting in cardiac arrhythmias most likely due to inhibition of metabolism of these drugs by erythromycin and clarithromycin. Fatalities have been reported).
No products indexed under this heading.

Theophylline (Co-administration has resulted in a minor increase (10%) in the clearance of theophylline; this interaction is unlikely to be of clinical concern, nonetheless, monitor blood levels).
No products indexed under this heading.

Theophylline Anhydrous (Co-administration has resulted in a minor increase (10%) in the clearance of theophylline; this interaction is unlikely to be of clinical concern, nonetheless, monitor blood levels). Products include:
Uniphyl Tablets ... 2708

Theophylline Calcium Salicylate (Co-administration has resulted in a minor increase (10%) in the clearance of theophylline; this interaction is unlikely to be of clinical concern, nonetheless, monitor blood levels).
No products indexed under this heading.

Theophylline Dihydroxypropyl (Glyceryl) (Co-administration has resulted in a minor increase (10%) in the clearance of theophylline; this interaction is unlikely to be of clinical concern, nonetheless, monitor blood levels).
No products indexed under this heading.

Theophylline Ethylenediamine (Co-administration has resulted in a minor increase (10%) in the clearance of theophylline; this interaction is unlikely to be of clinical concern, nonetheless, monitor blood levels).
No products indexed under this heading.

Theophylline Sodium Glycinate (Co-administration has resulted in a minor increase (10%) in the clearance of theophylline; this interaction is unlikely to be of clinical concern, nonetheless, monitor blood levels).
No products indexed under this heading.

Food Interactions

Food, unspecified (Cmax and AUC are diminished by about 50% if the drug is given 30 minutes after food as opposed to the fasting condition; Prevacid should be taken before eating).

PREVACID FOR DELAYED-RELEASE ORAL SUSPENSION

(Lansoprazole) ... 3268
See Prevacid Delayed-Release Capsules

PREVACID I.V. FOR INJECTION

(Lansoprazole) ... 3274
May interact with iron salts, absorption of drugs where gastric ph is an important determinant in their bioavailability, xanthines, and certain other agents. Compounds in these categories include:

Aminophylline (Co-administration has resulted in a minor increase (10%) in the clearance of theophylline; this interaction is unlikely to be of clinical concern; nonetheless, monitor blood levels).
No products indexed under this heading.

Bacampicillin Hydrochloride (Lansoprazole causes a profound and long-lasting inhibition of gastric acid secretion; therefore, it is theoretically possible that it may interfere with the absorption of drugs where gastric pH is an important determinant of bioavailability).
No products indexed under this heading.

Digoxin (Lansoprazole causes a profound and long-lasting inhibition of gastric acid secretion; therefore, it is theoretically possible that it may interfere with the absorption of drugs where gastric pH is an important determinant of bioavailability, such as digoxin). Products include:
Digitek Tablets ... 2146
Lanoxicaps Capsules ... 1458
Lanoxin Injection ... 1462
Lanoxin Tablets ... 1468
Lanoxin Injection Pediatric ... 1465

Dyphylline (Co-administration has resulted in a minor increase (10%) in the clearance of theophylline; this interaction is unlikely to be of clinical concern; nonetheless, monitor blood levels).
No products indexed under this heading.

Ferrous Fumarate (Lansoprazole causes a profound and long-lasting inhibition of gastric acid secretion; therefore, it is theoretically possible that it may interfere with the absorption of drugs, such as iron salts, where gastric pH is an important determinant of bioavailability). Products include:
Chromagen Forte Soft Gelatin Capsules ... 3296
Ferretts Tablets ... 773
Repliva 21/7 Tablets ... 3301

Ferrous Gluconate (Lansoprazole causes a profound and long-lasting inhibition of gastric acid secretion; therefore, it is theoretically possible that it may interfere with the absorption of drugs, such as iron salts, where gastric pH is an important determinant of bioavailability).
No products indexed under this heading.

Ferrous Sulfate (Lansoprazole causes a profound and long-lasting inhibition of gastric acid secretion; therefore, it is theoretically possible that it may interfere with the absorption of drugs, such as iron salts, where gastric pH is an important determinant of bioavailability). Products include:
Feosol Tablets ... 1629
Slow Fe Iron Tablets ... 772
Slow Fe with Folic Acid Tablets ... 773

Iron (Lansoprazole causes a profound and long-lasting inhibition of gastric acid secretion; therefore, it is theoretically possible that it may interfere with the absorption of drugs, such as iron salts, where gastric pH is an important determinant of bioavailability). Products include:
Chromagen Forte Soft Gelatin Capsules ... 3296
Ferretts IPS Liquid ... 773
OptiNate ... 1162
Repliva 21/7 Tablets ... 3301

Iron, Peptonized (Lansoprazole causes a profound and long-lasting inhibition of gastric acid secretion; therefore, it is theoretically possible that it may interfere with the absorption of drugs, such as iron salts, where gastric pH is an important determinant of bioavailability).
No products indexed under this heading.

Iron Cacodylate (Lansoprazole causes a profound and long-lasting inhibition of gastric acid secretion; therefore, it is theoretically possible that it may interfere with the absorption of drugs, such as iron salts, where gastric pH is an important determinant of bioavailability).
No products indexed under this heading.

Iron Carbonyl (Lansoprazole causes a profound and long-lasting inhibition of gastric acid secretion; therefore, it is theoretically possible that it may interfere with the absorption of drugs, such as iron salts, where gastric pH is an important determinant of bioavailability). Products include:
Feosol Caplets ... 1629

Iron Dextran (Lansoprazole causes a profound and long-lasting inhibition of gastric acid secretion; therefore, it is theoretically possible that it may interfere with the absorption of drugs, such as iron salts, where gastric pH is an important determinant of bioavailability). Products include:
Infed Injection ... 3381

Iron Polysaccharide Complex (Lansoprazole causes a profound and long-lasting inhibition of gastric acid secretion; therefore, it is theoretically possible that it may interfere with the absorption of drugs, such as iron salts, where gastric pH is an important determinant of bioavailability).
No products indexed under this heading.

Iron Sucrose (Lansoprazole causes a profound and long-lasting inhibition of gastric acid secretion; therefore, it is theoretically possible that it may interfere with the absorption of drugs, such as iron salts, where gastric pH is an important determinant of bioavailability).
No products indexed under this heading.

Iron Supplements (Lansoprazole causes a profound and long-lasting inhibition of gastric acid secretion; therefore, it is theoretically possible that it may interfere with the absorption of drugs, such as iron salts, where gastric pH is an important determinant of bioavailability).
No products indexed under this heading.

Ketoconazole (Lansoprazole causes a profound and long-lasting inhibition of gastric acid secretion; therefore, it is theoretically possible that it may interfere with the absorption of drugs where gastric pH is an important determinant of bioavailability). Products include:
Nizoral A-D Shampoo, 1% ... 1839
Nizoral 2% Shampoo ... 1838

Polysaccharide Iron Complex (Lansoprazole causes a profound and long-lasting inhibition of gastric acid secretion; therefore, it is theoretically possible that it may interfere with the absorption of drugs, such as iron salts, where gastric pH is an important determinant of bioavailability). Products include:
Niferex-150 Forte Capsules ... 3299
Nu-Iron 150 Capsules ... 2098

Theophylline (Co-administration has resulted in a minor increase (10%) in the clearance of theophylline; this interaction is unlikely to be of clinical concern; nonetheless, monitor blood levels).
No products indexed under this heading.

Theophylline Anhydrous (Co-administration has resulted in a minor increase (10%) in the clearance of theophylline; this interaction is unlikely to be of clinical concern; nonetheless, monitor blood levels). Products include:
Uniphyl Tablets ... 2708

Theophylline Calcium Salicylate (Co-administration has resulted in a minor increase (10%) in the clearance of theophylline; this interaction is unlikely to be of clinical concern; nonetheless, monitor blood levels).
No products indexed under this heading.

Theophylline Dihydroxypropyl (Glyceryl) (Co-administration has resulted in a minor increase (10%) in the clearance of theophylline; this interaction is unlikely to be of clinical concern; nonetheless, monitor blood levels).
No products indexed under this heading.

Theophylline Ethylenediamine (Co-administration has resulted in a minor increase (10%) in the clearance of theophylline; this interaction is unlikely to be of clinical concern; nonetheless, monitor blood levels).
No products indexed under this heading.

Theophylline Sodium Glycinate (Co-administration has resulted in a minor increase (10%) in the clearance of theophylline; this interaction is unlikely to be of clinical concern; nonetheless, monitor blood levels).
No products indexed under this heading.

Warfarin Sodium (There have been reports of increased International Normalized Ratio (INR) and prothrombin time in patients receiving proton pump inhibitors, including lansoprazole, and warfarin concomitantly). Products include:
Coumadin for Injection ... 932
Coumadin Tablets ... 932

PREVACID NAPRAPAC 375

(Lansoprazole, Naproxen) ... 3277
May interact with ACE inhibitors, beta blockers, oral anticoagulants, hydantoin anticonvulsants, lithium preparations, absorption of drugs where gastric ph is an important determinant in their bioavailability, highly protein bound drugs (selected), sulfonamides, sulfonylureas, and certain other agents. Compounds in these categories include:

Acebutolol Hydrochloride (Naproxen can reduce the antihypertensive effect of beta-blockers).
No products indexed under this heading.

Amiodarone Hydrochloride (In vitro studies have shown that naproxen anion, because of its affinity for protein, may displace from their binding sites other drugs that are also albumin-bound). Products include:
Pacerone Tablets ... 3337

Amitriptyline Hydrochloride (In vitro studies have shown that naproxen anion, because of its affinity for protein, may displace from their binding sites other drugs that are also albumin-bound).
No products indexed under this heading.

Anisindione (Short-term studies have failed to show any significant effects of concurrent use on prothrombin time; caution is advised since interactions have been seen with other NSAIDs). Products include:
Miradon Tablets ... 3056

Aspirin (Concomitant administration of naproxen and aspirin is not recommended because naproxen is displaced from its binding sites resulting in lower plasma concentrations and peak plasma levels). Products include:
Aggrenox Capsules ... 855
Bayer, Aspirin Regimen ... ▣606
Bayer Aspirin Tablets ... 3515
BC Powder ... ▣612
BC Allergy Sinus Cold Powder ... ▣612
Arthritis Strength BC Powder ... ▣612
BC Sinus Cold Powder ... ▣612
Ecotrin Enteric Coated Aspirin Low, Regular and Maximum Strength Tablets ... 1627
Goody's Body Pain Formula Powder ... ▣621
Goody's Extra Strength Headache Powder ... ▣621
Goody's Extra Strength Pain Relief Tablets ... ▣621
Percodan Tablets ... 1115
St. Joseph 81 mg Aspirin Chewable and Enteric Coated Tablets ... 1841

Atenolol (Naproxen can reduce the antihypertensive effect of beta-blockers). Products include:
Tenormin I.V. Injection ... 698
Tenormin Tablets ... 695

Atovaquone (In vitro studies have shown that naproxen anion, because of its affinity for protein, may displace from their binding sites other drugs that are also albumin-bound). Products include:
Malarone Tablets ... 1484
Malarone Pediatric Tablets ... 1484
Mepron Suspension ... 1487

Bacampicillin Hydrochloride (Lansoprazole causes a profound and long-lasting inhibition of gastric acid secretion; therefore, it is theoretically possible that lansoprazole may interfere with the absorption of drugs where gastric pH is an important determinant of bioavailability).
No products indexed under this heading.

Benazepril Hydrochloride (Co-administration of NSAIDs and ACE inhibitors may potentiate renal disease states). Products include:
Lotensin Tablets ... 2232
Lotensin HCT Tablets ... 2235
Lotrel Capsules ... 2238

Bendroflumethiazide (Observe signs for sulfonamide toxicity).
No products indexed under this heading.

Betaxolol Hydrochloride (Naproxen can reduce the antihypertensive effect of beta-blockers). Products include:
Betoptic S Ophthalmic Suspension ... 554

Bisoprolol Fumarate (Naproxen can reduce the antihypertensive effect of beta-blockers).
No products indexed under this heading.

Captopril (Co-administration of NSAIDs and ACE inhibitors may potentiate renal disease states). Products include:
Captopril Tablets ... 2114

Carteolol Hydrochloride (Naproxen can reduce the antihypertensive effect of beta-blockers). Products include:
Carteolol Hydrochloride Ophthalmic Solution USP, 1% ... ⊙246

Cefonicid Sodium (In vitro studies have shown that naproxen anion, because of its affinity for protein, may displace from their binding sites other drugs that are also albumin-bound).
No products indexed under this heading.

Celecoxib (In vitro studies have shown that naproxen anion, because of its affinity for protein, may displace from their binding sites other drugs that are also albumin-bound). Products include:
Celebrex Capsules ... 3130

Chlordiazepoxide (In vitro studies have shown that naproxen anion, because of its affinity for protein, may displace from their binding sites other drugs that are also albumin-bound).
No products indexed under this heading.

Chlordiazepoxide Hydrochloride (In vitro studies have shown that naproxen anion, because of its affinity for protein, may displace from their binding sites other drugs that are also albumin-bound). Products include:
Librium Capsules ... 3349

Chlorothiazide (Observe signs for sulfonamide toxicity). Products include:
Aldoclor Tablets ... 1881
Diuril Oral ... 1936

Chlorothiazide Sodium (Observe signs for sulfonamide toxicity). Products include:
Diuril Sodium Intravenous ... 1934

Chlorpromazine (In vitro studies have shown that naproxen anion, because of its affinity for protein, may displace from their binding sites other drugs that are also albumin-bound).
No products indexed under this heading.

Chlorpromazine Hydrochloride (In vitro studies have shown that naproxen anion, because of its affinity for protein, may displace from their binding sites other drugs that are also albumin-bound).
No products indexed under this heading.

Chlorpropamide (Observe signs for sulfonamide toxicity).
No products indexed under this heading.

Clomipramine Hydrochloride (In vitro studies have shown that naproxen anion, because of its affinity for protein, may displace from their binding sites other drugs that are also albumin-bound).
No products indexed under this heading.

Clozapine (In vitro studies have shown that naproxen anion, because of its affinity for protein, may displace from their binding sites other drugs that are also albumin-bound). Products include:
Clozapine Tablets ... 2141
Clozaril Tablets ... 2174
FazaClo Orally Disintegrating Tablets ... 547

Cyclosporine (In vitro studies have shown that naproxen anion, because of its affinity for protein, may displace from their binding sites other drugs that are also albumin-bound). Products include:
Gengraf Capsules ... 458
Neoral Soft Gelatin Capsules ... 2247
Neoral Oral Solution ... 2247
Restasis Ophthalmic Emulsion ... 570
Sandimmune ... 2259

Diazepam (In vitro studies have shown that naproxen anion, because of its affinity for protein, may displace from their binding sites other drugs that are also albumin-bound). Products include:
Diastat Rectal Delivery System ... 3344
Valium Tablets ... 2822

Diclofenac Potassium (In vitro studies have shown that naproxen anion, because of its affinity for protein, may displace from their binding sites other drugs that are also albumin-bound). Products include:
Cataflam Tablets ... 2173

Diclofenac Sodium (In vitro studies have shown that naproxen anion, because of its affinity for protein, may displace from their binding sites other drugs that are also albumin-bound). Products include:
Arthrotec Tablets ... 3126
Voltaren Ophthalmic Solution ... 2300
Voltaren Tablets ... 2298
Voltaren-XR Tablets ... 2301

Dicumarol (Short-term studies have failed to show any significant effects of concurrent use on prothrombin time; caution is advised since interactions have been seen with other NSAIDs).
No products indexed under this heading.

Dipyridamole (In vitro studies have shown that naproxen anion, because of its affinity for protein, may displace from their binding sites other drugs that are also albumin-bound). Products include:
Aggrenox Capsules ... 855
Persantine Tablets ... 898

Enalapril Maleate (Co-administration of NSAIDs and ACE inhibitors may potentiate renal disease states). Products include:
Vaseretic Tablets ... 2073
Vasotec I.V. Injection ... 2076

Enalaprilat (Co-administration of NSAIDs and ACE inhibitors may potentiate renal disease states).
No products indexed under this heading.

Esmolol Hydrochloride (Naproxen can reduce the antihypertensive effect of beta-blockers). Products include:
Brevibloc Concentrate ... 766
Brevibloc Injection ... 766
Brevibloc Double Strength Injection ... 766
Brevibloc Premixed Injection ... 766
Brevibloc Double Strength Premixed Injection ... 766

Ethotoin (Observe signs for hydantoin toxicity). Products include:
Peganone Tablets, USP ... 2487

Fenoprofen Calcium (In vitro studies have shown that naproxen anion, because of its affinity for protein, may displace from their binding sites other drugs that are also albumin-bound). Products include:
Nalfon Capsules ... 2504

Ferrous Fumarate (Lansoprazole causes a profound and long-lasting inhibition of gastric acid secretion; therefore, it is theoretically possible that lansoprazole may interfere with the absorption of drugs where gastric pH is an important determinant of bioavailability). Products include:
Chromagen Forte Soft Gelatin Capsules ... 3296
Ferretts Tablets ... ▣773
Repliva 21/7 Tablets ... 3301

Ferrous Gluconate (Lansoprazole causes a profound and long-lasting inhibition of gastric acid secretion; therefore, it is theoretically possible that lansoprazole may interfere with the absorption of drugs where gastric pH is an important determinant of bioavailability).
No products indexed under this heading.

Ferrous Sulfate (Lansoprazole causes a profound and long-lasting inhibition of gastric acid secretion; therefore, it is theoretically possible that lansoprazole may interfere with the absorption of drugs where gastric pH is an important determinant of bioavailability). Products include:
Feosol Tablets ... 1629
Slow Fe Iron Tablets ... ▣772
Slow Fe with Folic Acid Tablets ... ▣773

Flurazepam Hydrochloride (In vitro studies have shown that naproxen anion, because of its affinity for protein, may displace from their binding sites other drugs that are also albumin-bound). Products include:
Dalmane Capsules ... 3343

Flurbiprofen (In vitro studies have shown that naproxen anion, because of its affinity for protein, may displace from their binding sites other drugs that are also albumin-bound).
No products indexed under this heading.

Fosinopril Sodium (Co-administration of NSAIDs and ACE inhibitors may potentiate renal disease states).
No products indexed under this heading.

Fosphenytoin Sodium (Observe signs for hydantoin toxicity).
No products indexed under this heading.

Furosemide (The natriuretic effect of furosemide has been reported to be inhibited by some NSAIDs). Products include:
Furosemide Tablets ... 2117

Glimepiride (Observe signs for sulfonylurea toxicity). Products include:
Amaryl Tablets ... 2864

Glipizide (Observe signs for sulfonamide toxicity).
No products indexed under this heading.

Glyburide (Observe signs for sulfonamide toxicity).
No products indexed under this heading.

Hydrochlorothiazide (Observe signs for sulfonamide toxicity). Products include:
Aldoril Tablets ... 1884
Atacand HCT ... 637
Avalide Tablets ... 2889
Avalide Tablets ... 922
Benicar HCT Tablets ... 2852
Diovan HCT Tablets ... 2195
Dyazide Capsules ... 1389
Hyzaar ... 1964
Lotensin HCT Tablets ... 2235
Maxzide ... 2150

Micardis HCT Tablets 886
Moduretic Tablets 2003
Prinzide Tablets 2033
Teveten HCT Tablets 1710
Timolide Tablets 2056
Uniretic Tablets 3114
Vaseretic Tablets 2073
Zestoretic Tablets 701

Hydroflumethiazide (Observe signs for sulfonamide toxicity).
No products indexed under this heading.

Ibuprofen (In vitro studies have shown that naproxen anion, because of its affinity for protein, may displace from their binding sites other drugs that are also albumin-bound). Products include:
Advil Allergy Sinus Caplets 737
Advil 737
Children's Advil Suspension 742
Children's Advil Chewable Tablets 741
Advil Cold & Sinus 739
Advil Flu & Body Ache Caplets 739
Children's Advil Cold Suspension 741
Infants' Advil Concentrated Drops 743
Junior Strength Advil Swallow Tablets 740
Advil Migraine Liquigels 740
Advil Multi-Symptom Cold Caplets 738
Combunox Tablets 1183
Children's Motrin Oral Suspension and Chewable Tablets 1837
Children's Motrin Cold Non-Staining Dye-Free Oral Suspension 1838
Children's Motrin Cold Oral Suspension 1838
Children's Motrin Non-Staining Dye-Free Oral Suspension 1837
Motrin Cold & Sinus Caplets 1836
Motrin IB Tablets and Caplets 1836
Infants' Motrin Concentrated Drops 1837
Infants' Motrin Non-Staining Dye-Free Drops 1837
Junior Strength Motrin Caplets and Chewable Tablets 1837
Vicoprofen Tablets 533

Imipramine Hydrochloride (In vitro studies have shown that naproxen anion, because of its affinity for protein, may displace from their binding sites other drugs that are also albumin-bound).
No products indexed under this heading.

Imipramine Pamoate (In vitro studies have shown that naproxen anion, because of its affinity for protein, may displace from their binding sites other drugs that are also albumin-bound).
No products indexed under this heading.

Indomethacin (In vitro studies have shown that naproxen anion, because of its affinity for protein, may displace from their binding sites other drugs that are also albumin-bound). Products include:
Indocin 1968

Indomethacin Sodium Trihydrate (In vitro studies have shown that naproxen anion, because of its affinity for protein, may displace from their binding sites other drugs that are also albumin-bound). Products include:
Indocin I.V. 1973

Ketoconazole (Lansoprazole causes a profound and long-lasting inhibition of gastric acid secretion; therefore, it is theoretically possible that lansoprazole may interfere with the absorption of drugs where gastric pH is an important determinant of bioavailability). Products include:
Nizoral A-D Shampoo, 1% 1839
Nizoral 2% Shampoo 1838

Ketoprofen (In vitro studies have shown that naproxen anion, because of its affinity for protein, may displace from their binding sites other drugs that are also albumin-bound).
No products indexed under this heading.

Ketorolac Tromethamine (In vitro studies have shown that naproxen anion, because of its affinity for protein, may displace from their binding sites other drugs that are also albumin-bound). Products include:
Acular Ophthalmic Solution 561
Acular LS Ophthalmic Solution 562

Labetalol Hydrochloride (Naproxen can reduce the antihypertensive effect of beta-blockers).
No products indexed under this heading.

Levobunolol Hydrochloride (Naproxen can reduce the antihypertensive effect of beta-blockers). Products include:
Betagan Ophthalmic Solution, USP .... ⊙217

Lisinopril (Co-administration of NSAIDs and ACE inhibitors may potentiate renal disease states). Products include:
Prinivil Tablets 2029
Prinzide Tablets 2033
Zestoretic Tablets 701
Zestril Tablets 704

Lithium (Inhibition of renal lithium clearance leading to increases in plasma lithium concentrations has been reported with naproxen).
No products indexed under this heading.

Lithium Carbonate (Inhibition of renal lithium clearance leading to increases in plasma lithium concentrations has been reported with naproxen). Products include:
Eskalith 1406
Lithobid Tablets 1670

Lithium Citrate (Inhibition of renal lithium clearance leading to increases in plasma lithium concentrations has been reported with naproxen).
No products indexed under this heading.

Meclofenamate Sodium (In vitro studies have shown that naproxen anion, because of its affinity for protein, may displace from their binding sites other drugs that are also albumin-bound).
No products indexed under this heading.

Mefenamic Acid (In vitro studies have shown that naproxen anion, because of its affinity for protein, may displace from their binding sites other drugs that are also albumin-bound).
No products indexed under this heading.

Mephenytoin (Observe signs for hydantoin toxicity).
No products indexed under this heading.

Methotrexate Sodium (Naproxen has been reported to reduce the tubular secretion of methotrexate in an animal model, possibly increasing the toxicity of methotrexate; caution is recommended).
No products indexed under this heading.

Methyclothiazide (Observe signs for sulfonamide toxicity).
No products indexed under this heading.

Metipranolol Hydrochloride (Naproxen can reduce the antihypertensive effect of beta-blockers).
No products indexed under this heading.

Metoprolol Succinate (Naproxen can reduce the antihypertensive effect of beta-blockers). Products include:
Toprol-XL Tablets 660

Metoprolol Tartrate (Naproxen can reduce the antihypertensive effect of beta-blockers).
No products indexed under this heading.

Midazolam Hydrochloride (In vitro studies have shown that naproxen anion, because of its affinity for protein, may displace from their binding sites other drugs that are also albumin-bound).
No products indexed under this heading.

Moexipril Hydrochloride (Co-administration of NSAIDs and ACE inhibitors may potentiate renal disease states). Products include:
Uniretic Tablets 3114
Univasc Tablets 3118

Nadolol (Naproxen can reduce the antihypertensive effect of beta-blockers). Products include:
Nadolol Tablets 2121

Naproxen Sodium (In vitro studies have shown that naproxen anion, because of its affinity for protein, may displace from their binding sites other drugs that are also albumin-bound). Products include:
Aleve Tablets, Caplets and Gelcaps 605
Anaprox Tablets 2769
Anaprox DS Tablets 2769

Nortriptyline Hydrochloride (In vitro studies have shown that naproxen anion, because of its affinity for protein, may displace from their binding sites other drugs that are also albumin-bound).
No products indexed under this heading.

Oxaprozin (In vitro studies have shown that naproxen anion, because of its affinity for protein, may displace from their binding sites other drugs that are also albumin-bound).
No products indexed under this heading.

Oxazepam (In vitro studies have shown that naproxen anion, because of its affinity for protein, may displace from their binding sites other drugs that are also albumin-bound).
No products indexed under this heading.

Penbutolol Sulfate (Naproxen can reduce the antihypertensive effect of beta-blockers).
No products indexed under this heading.

Perindopril Erbumine (Co-administration of NSAIDs and ACE inhibitors may potentiate renal disease states). Products include:
Aceon Tablets (2 mg, 4 mg, 8 mg) 3191

Phenylbutazone (In vitro studies have shown that naproxen anion, because of its affinity for protein, may displace from their binding sites other drugs that are also albumin-bound).
No products indexed under this heading.

Phenytoin (Observe signs for hydantoin toxicity).
No products indexed under this heading.

Phenytoin Sodium (Observe signs for hydantoin toxicity). Products include:
Phenytek Capsules 2153

Pindolol (Naproxen can reduce the antihypertensive effect of beta-blockers).
No products indexed under this heading.

Piroxicam (In vitro studies have shown that naproxen anion, because of its affinity for protein, may displace from their binding sites other drugs that are also albumin-bound).
No products indexed under this heading.

Polythiazide (Observe signs for sulfonamide toxicity).
No products indexed under this heading.

Probenecid (Probenecid given concurrently increases naproxen anion plasma levels and extends its plasma half-life significantly).
No products indexed under this heading.

Propranolol Hydrochloride (Naproxen can reduce the antihypertensive effect of beta-blockers). Products include:
Inderal LA Long-Acting Capsules 3421
InnoPran XL Capsules 2728

Quinapril Hydrochloride (Co-administration of NSAIDs and ACE inhibitors may potentiate renal disease states).
No products indexed under this heading.

Ramipril (Co-administration of NSAIDs and ACE inhibitors may potentiate renal disease states). Products include:
Altace Capsules 1673

Sotalol Hydrochloride (Naproxen can reduce the antihypertensive effect of beta-blockers).
No products indexed under this heading.

Spirapril Hydrochloride (Co-administration of NSAIDs and ACE inhibitors may potentiate renal disease states).
No products indexed under this heading.

Sucralfate (In a single-crossover study examining lansoprazole 30 mg given concomitantly with sucralfate 1 gram, absorption was delayed and bioavailability was reduced by 17%; therefore, lansoprazole should be taken at least 30 minutes prior to sucralfate). Products include:
Carafate Suspension 727
Carafate Tablets 728

Sulfacytine (Observe signs for sulfonamide toxicity).
No products indexed under this heading.

Sulfamethizole (Observe signs for sulfonamide toxicity).
No products indexed under this heading.

Sulfamethoxazole (Observe signs for sulfonamide toxicity).
No products indexed under this heading.

Sulfasalazine (Observe signs for sulfonamide toxicity).
No products indexed under this heading.

IMPORTANT NOTE: Always consult each drug listing in the patient's regimen for possible interactions.

Sulfinpyrazone (Observe signs for sulfonamide toxicity).
No products indexed under this heading.

Sulfisoxazole (Observe signs for sulfonamide toxicity).
No products indexed under this heading.

Sulfisoxazole Acetyl (Observe signs for sulfonamide toxicity).
No products indexed under this heading.

Sulfisoxazole Diolamine (Observe signs for sulfonamide toxicity).
No products indexed under this heading.

Sulindac (In vitro studies have shown that naproxen anion, because of its affinity for protein, may displace from their binding sites other drugs that are also albumin-bound). Products include:
Clinoril Tablets 1899

Temazepam (In vitro studies have shown that naproxen anion, because of its affinity for protein, may displace from their binding sites other drugs that are also albumin-bound).
No products indexed under this heading.

Theophylline (Co-administration resulted in a minor increase (10%) in the clearance of theophylline; this interaction is unlikely to be of clinical concern; nonetheless, patients may require additional titration of their theophylline dosage when lansoprazole is started or stopped).
No products indexed under this heading.

Theophylline Anhydrous (Co-administration resulted in a minor increase (10%) in the clearance of theophylline; this interaction is unlikely to be of clinical concern; nonetheless, patients may require additional titration of their theophylline dosage when lansoprazole is started or stopped). Products include:
Uniphyl Tablets 2708

Theophylline Calcium Salicylate (Co-administration resulted in a minor increase (10%) in the clearance of theophylline; this interaction is unlikely to be of clinical concern; nonetheless, patients may require additional titration of their theophylline dosage when lansoprazole is started or stopped).
No products indexed under this heading.

Theophylline Dihydroxypropyl (Glyceryl) (Co-administration resulted in a minor increase (10%) in the clearance of theophylline; this interaction is unlikely to be of clinical concern; nonetheless, patients may require additional titration of their theophylline dosage when lansoprazole is started or stopped).
No products indexed under this heading.

Theophylline Ethylenediamine (Co-administration resulted in a minor increase (10%) in the clearance of theophylline; this interaction is unlikely to be of clinical concern, nonetheless patients may require additional titration of their theophylline dosage when lansoprazole is started or stopped).
No products indexed under this heading.

Theophylline Sodium Glycinate (Co-administration resulted in a minor increase (10%) in the clearance of theophylline; this interaction is unlikely to be of clinical concern; nonetheless, patients may require additional titration of their theophylline dosage when lansoprazole is started or stopped).
No products indexed under this heading.

Timolol Hemihydrate (Naproxen can reduce the antihypertensive effect of beta-blockers). Products include:
Betimol Ophthalmic Solution 3371
Betimol Ophthalmic Solution .... ⊙283

Timolol Maleate (Naproxen can reduce the antihypertensive effect of beta-blockers). Products include:
Blocadren Tablets 1891
Cosopt Sterile Ophthalmic Solution 1910
Timolide Tablets 2056
Timoptic in Ocudose 2061
Timoptic Sterile Ophthalmic Solution 2058
Timoptic-XE Sterile Ophthalmic Gel Forming Solution 2062

Tolazamide (Observe signs for sulfonamide toxicity).
No products indexed under this heading.

Tolbutamide (Observe signs for sulfonamide toxicity).
No products indexed under this heading.

Tolmetin Sodium (In vitro studies have shown that naproxen anion, because of its affinity for protein, may displace from their binding sites other drugs that are also albumin-bound).
No products indexed under this heading.

Trandolapril (Co-administration of NSAIDs and ACE inhibitors may potentiate renal disease states). Products include:
Mavik Tablets 482
Tarka Tablets 519

Trimipramine Maleate (In vitro studies have shown that naproxen anion, because of its affinity for protein, may displace from their binding sites other drugs that are also albumin-bound). Products include:
Surmontil Capsules 2347

Warfarin Sodium (There have been reports of increased INR and prothrombin time in patients receiving proton pump inhibitors, including lansoprazole, and warfarin concomitantly; monitor for these increases). Products include:
Coumadin for Injection 932
Coumadin Tablets 932

PREVACID NAPRAPAC 500

(Lansoprazole, Naproxen) 3277
See Prevacid NapraPAC 375

PREVACID SOLUTAB DELAYED-RELEASE ORALLY DISINTEGRATING TABLETS

(Lansoprazole) 3268
See Prevacid Delayed-Release Capsules

PREVNAR FOR INJECTION

(Pneumococcal vaccine, diphtheria conjugate) 3460
May interact with alkylating agents, antimetabolites, anticoagulants, corticosteroids, cytotoxic drugs, and immunosuppressive agents. Compounds in these categories include:

Anisindione (Prevnar should be given with caution to children on anticoagulant therapy). Products include:
Miradon Tablets 3056

Ardeparin Sodium (Prevnar should be given with caution to children on anticoagulant therapy).
No products indexed under this heading.

Azathioprine (Children receiving immunosuppressive therapy may not respond optimally to active immunization). Products include:
Azasan Tablets 2844

Basiliximab (Children receiving immunosuppressive therapy may not respond optimally to active immunization). Products include:
Simulect for Injection 2268

Betamethasone Acetate (Children receiving large doses of corticosteroids for immunosuppressive therapy may not respond optimally to active immunization).
No products indexed under this heading.

Betamethasone Sodium Phosphate (Children receiving large doses of corticosteroids for immunosuppressive therapy may not respond optimally to active immunization).
No products indexed under this heading.

Bleomycin Sulfate (Children receiving cytotoxic agents may not respond optimally to active immunization).
No products indexed under this heading.

Busulfan (Children receiving alkylating agents may not respond optimally to active immunization). Products include:
I.V. Busulfex 1125
Myleran Tablets 1492

Capecitabine (Children receiving antimetabolite agents may not respond optimally to active immunization). Products include:
Xeloda Tablets 2825

Carmustine (BCNU) (Children receiving alkylating agents may not respond optimally to active immunization).
No products indexed under this heading.

Chlorambucil (Children receiving alkylating agents may not respond optimally to active immunization). Products include:
Leukeran Tablets 1472

Cladribine (Children receiving antimetabolite agents may not respond optimally to active immunization). Products include:
Leustatin Injection 2368

Cortisone Acetate (Children receiving large doses of corticosteroids for immunosuppressive therapy may not respond optimally to active immunization).
No products indexed under this heading.

Cyclophosphamide (Children receiving cytotoxic agents may not respond optimally to active immunization).
No products indexed under this heading.

Cyclosporine (Children receiving immunosuppressive therapy may not respond optimally to active immunization). Products include:
Gengraf Capsules 458
Neoral Soft Gelatin Capsules 2247
Neoral Oral Solution 2247
Restasis Ophthalmic Emulsion 570
Sandimmune 2259

Cytarabine (Children receiving antimetabolite agents may not respond optimally to active immunization).
No products indexed under this heading.

Dacarbazine (Children receiving alkylating agents may not respond optimally to active immunization).
No products indexed under this heading.

Dalteparin Sodium (Prevnar should be given with caution to children on anticoagulant therapy). Products include:
Fragmin Injection 2638

Danaparoid Sodium (Prevnar should be given with caution to children on anticoagulant therapy).
No products indexed under this heading.

Daunorubicin Hydrochloride (Children receiving cytotoxic agents may not respond optimally to active immunization). Products include:
Cerubidine for Injection 788

Dexamethasone (Children receiving large doses of corticosteroids for immunosuppressive therapy may not respond optimally to active immunization). Products include:
Ciprodex Otic Suspension 555
Decadron Tablets 1929
TobraDex Ophthalmic Ointment 558
TobraDex Ophthalmic Suspension ... 558

Dexamethasone Acetate (Children receiving large doses of corticosteroids for immunosuppressive therapy may not respond optimally to active immunization).
No products indexed under this heading.

Dexamethasone Sodium Phosphate (Children receiving large doses of corticosteroids for immunosuppressive therapy may not respond optimally to active immunization). Products include:
Decadron Phosphate Injection 1931

Dicumarol (Prevnar should be given with caution to children on anticoagulant therapy).
No products indexed under this heading.

Doxorubicin Hydrochloride (Children receiving cytotoxic agents may not respond optimally to active immunization). Products include:
Adriamycin for Injection, USP 786
Adriamycin Injection, USP 786

Enoxaparin Sodium (Prevnar should be given with caution to children on anticoagulant therapy). Products include:
Lovenox Injection 2931

Epirubicin Hydrochloride (Children receiving cytotoxic agents may not respond optimally to active immunization). Products include:
Ellence Injection 2632

Floxuridine (Children receiving antimetabolite agents may not respond optimally to active immunization).
No products indexed under this heading.

Fludarabine Phosphate (Children receiving antimetabolite agents may not respond optimally to active immunization).
No products indexed under this heading.

Fludrocortisone Acetate (Children receiving large doses of corticosteroids for immunosuppressive therapy may not respond optimally to active immunization).
No products indexed under this heading.

Fluorouracil (Children receiving cytotoxic agents may not respond optimally to active immunization). Products include:
Carac Cream, 0.5% 1048
Efudex 3348

Fondaparinux Sodium (Prevnar should be given with caution to children on anticoagulant therapy). Products include:
Arixtra Injection 1325

Gemcitabine Hydrochloride (Children receiving antimetabolite agents may not respond optimally to active immunization). Products include:
Gemzar for Injection 1743

Heparin Calcium (Prevnar should be given with caution to children on anticoagulant therapy).
No products indexed under this heading.

Heparin Sodium (Prevnar should be given with caution to children on anticoagulant therapy).
No products indexed under this heading.

Hydrocortisone (Children receiving large doses of corticosteroids for immunosuppressive therapy may not respond optimally to active immunization). Products include:
Cortizone•5 Ointment .... ▣699
Cortizone•10 Creme .... ▣699
Cortizone•10 Ointment .... ▣699
Cortizone•10 Plus Creme .... ▣700
Cortizone•10 Maximum Strength Quick Shot Spray .... ▣700
Hydrocortone Tablets 1963
Preparation H Hydrocortisone Cream .... ▣748

Hydrocortisone Acetate (Children receiving large doses of corticosteroids for immunosuppressive therapy may not respond optimally to active immunization). Products include:
Analpram-HC 1136
Pramosone 1139
ProctoFoam-HC 3113
Tucks Anti-Itch Ointment .... ▣712
U-cort 1% Cream 3289

Hydrocortisone Sodium Phosphate (Children receiving large doses of corticosteroids for immunosuppressive therapy may not respond optimally to active immunization).
No products indexed under this heading.

Hydrocortisone Sodium Succinate (Children receiving large doses of corticosteroids for immunosuppressive therapy may not respond optimally to active immunization).
No products indexed under this heading.

Hydroxyurea (Children receiving cytotoxic agents may not respond optimally to active immunization).
No products indexed under this heading.

Lomustine (CCNU) (Children receiving alkylating agents may not respond optimally to active immunization).
No products indexed under this heading.

Low Molecular Weight Heparins (Prevnar should be given with caution to children on anticoagulant therapy).
No products indexed under this heading.

Mechlorethamine Hydrochloride (Children receiving alkylating agents may not respond optimally to active immunization). Products include:
Mustargen for Injection 2007

Melphalan (Children receiving alkylating agents may not respond optimally to active immunization). Products include:
Alkeran Tablets 977

Mercaptopurine (Children receiving antimetabolite agents may not respond optimally to active immunization). Products include:
Purinethol Tablets 1222

Methotrexate (Children receiving antimetabolite agents may not respond optimally to active immunization).
No products indexed under this heading.

Methotrexate Sodium (Children receiving cytotoxic agents may not respond optimally to active immunization).
No products indexed under this heading.

Methylprednisolone Acetate (Children receiving large doses of corticosteroids for immunosuppressive therapy may not respond optimally to active immunization). Products include:
Depo-Medrol Injectable Suspension 2615
Depo-Medrol Single-Dose Vial 2617

Methylprednisolone Sodium Succinate (Children receiving large doses of corticosteroids for immunosuppressive therapy may not respond optimally to active immunization).
No products indexed under this heading.

Mitotane (Children receiving cytotoxic agents may not respond optimally to active immunization).
No products indexed under this heading.

Mitoxantrone Hydrochloride (Children receiving cytotoxic agents may not respond optimally to active immunization). Products include:
Novantrone for Injection Concentrate 3158

Muromonab-CD3 (Children receiving immunosuppressive therapy may not respond optimally to active immunization). Products include:
Orthoclone OKT3 Sterile Solution 2370

Mycophenolate Mofetil (Children receiving immunosuppressive therapy may not respond optimally to active immunization). Products include:
CellCept Capsules 2751
CellCept Oral Suspension 2751
CellCept Tablets 2751

Pentostatin (Children receiving antimetabolite agents may not respond optimally to active immunization). Products include:
Nipent for Injection 3216

Prednisolone Acetate (Children receiving large doses of corticosteroids for immunosuppressive therapy may not respond optimally to active immunization). Products include:
Blephamide Ophthalmic Ointment 563
Blephamide Ophthalmic Suspension 564
Poly-Pred Liquifilm Ophthalmic Suspension .... ⊙231
Pred Forte Ophthalmic Suspension .... ⊙233
Pred Mild Sterile Ophthalmic Suspension .... ⊙236
Pred-G Ophthalmic Suspension .... ⊙234
Pred-G Sterile Ophthalmic Ointment .... ⊙235

Prednisolone Sodium Phosphate (Children receiving large doses of corticosteroids for immunosuppressive therapy may not respond optimally to active immunization). Products include:
Pediapred Oral Solution 3319

Prednisolone Tebutate (Children receiving large doses of corticosteroids for immunosuppressive therapy may not respond optimally to active immunization).
No products indexed under this heading.

Prednisone (Children receiving large doses of corticosteroids for immunosuppressive therapy may not respond optimally to active immunization).
No products indexed under this heading.

Procarbazine Hydrochloride (Children receiving cytotoxic agents may not respond optimally to active immunization). Products include:
Matulane Capsules 3188

Sirolimus (Children receiving immunosuppressive therapy may not respond optimally to active immunization). Products include:
Rapamune Oral Solution and Tablets 3472

Tacrolimus (Children receiving immunosuppressive therapy may not respond optimally to active immunization). Products include:
Prograf Capsules and Injection 624
Protopic Ointment 629

Tamoxifen Citrate (Children receiving cytotoxic agents may not respond optimally to active immunization).
No products indexed under this heading.

Thioguanine (Children receiving antimetabolite agents may not respond optimally to active immunization). Products include:
Tabloid Tablets 1545

Thiotepa (Children receiving alkylating agents may not respond optimally to active immunization).
No products indexed under this heading.

Tinzaparin Sodium (Prevnar should be given with caution to children on anticoagulant therapy).
No products indexed under this heading.

Triamcinolone (Children receiving large doses of corticosteroids for immunosuppressive therapy may not respond optimally to active immunization).
No products indexed under this heading.

Triamcinolone Acetonide (Children receiving large doses of corticosteroids for immunosuppressive therapy may not respond optimally to active immunization). Products include:
Azmacort Inhalation Aerosol 1701
Nasacort HFA Inhalation Aerosol 2939
Nasacort AQ Nasal Spray 2937

Triamcinolone Diacetate (Children receiving large doses of corticosteroids for immunosuppressive therapy may not respond optimally to active immunization).
No products indexed under this heading.

Triamcinolone Hexacetonide (Children receiving large doses of corticosteroids for immunosuppressive therapy may not respond optimally to active immunization).
No products indexed under this heading.

Vincristine Sulfate (Children receiving cytotoxic agents may not respond optimally to active immunization).
No products indexed under this heading.

Warfarin Sodium (Prevnar should be given with caution to children on anticoagulant therapy). Products include:
Coumadin for Injection 932
Coumadin Tablets 932

PREVPAC

(Amoxicillin, Clarithromycin, Lansoprazole) 3281
May interact with antiarrhythmics, oral anticoagulants, HMG-CoA reductase inhibitors, oral hypoglycemic agents, insulin, iron containing oral preparations, absorption of drugs where gastric ph is an important determinant in their bioavailability, phenytoin, triazolobenzodiazepines, valproate, xanthines, and certain other agents. Compounds in these categories include:

Acarbose (Co-administration has resulted in rare reports of hypoglycemia, some of which occurred in patients taking oral hypoglycemia agents). Products include:
Precose Tablets 776

Acebutolol Hydrochloride (There have been post-marketing reports of torsade de pointes occurring with concurrent use of clarithromycin and quinidine or dispyramide. Electrocardiograms should be monitored for QTc prolongation during co-administration of clarithromycin with these drugs).
No products indexed under this heading.

Adenosine (There have been post-marketing reports of torsade de pointes occurring with concurrent use of clarithromycin and quinidine or dispyramide. Electrocardiograms should be monitored for QTc prolongation during co-administration of clarithromycin with these drugs). Products include:
Adenocard Injection 612
Adenoscan 613

Alfentanil Hydrochloride (There have been reports of CYP3A-based interactions of clarithromycin with alfentanil).
No products indexed under this heading.

Alprazolam (Erythromycin, another macrolide antibiotic, has been reported to decrease the clearance of triazolam and midazolam, and

thus, may increase the pharmacologic effect of these benzodiazepines). Products include:

Niravam Orally Disintegrating Tablets 3106
Xanax XR Tablets 2655

Aminophylline (Co-administration of theophylline with clarithromycin in patients who are receiving high doses of theophylline may be associated with an increase in serum theophylline levels and potential theophylline toxicity).

No products indexed under this heading.

Amiodarone Hydrochloride (There have been post-marketing reports of torsade de pointes occurring with concurrent use of clarithromycin and quinidine or dispyramide. Electrocardiograms should be monitored for QTc prolongation during co-administration of clarithromycin with these drugs). Products include:

Pacerone Tablets 3337

Anisindione (Co-administration of clarithromycin with oral anticoagulants may result in the potentiation of oral coagulant effects). Products include:

Miradon Tablets 3056

Astemizole (Concomitant administration of Prevpac with astemizole is contraindicated. There have been post-marketing reports of drug interactions when clarithromycin is co-administered with astemizole resulting in cardiac arrhythmias (QT prolongation, ventricular tachycardia, ventricular fibrillation, and torsade de pointes) most likely due to inhibition of metabolism of these drugs by clarithromycin. Fatalities have been reported).

No products indexed under this heading.

Atorvastatin Calcium (Clarithromycin has been reported to increase concentrations of HMG-CoA reductase inhibitors. Rare reports of rhabdomyolysis have been reported in patients taking these drugs concomitantly). Products include:

Caduet Tablets 2507
Lipitor Tablets 2495

Bacampicillin Hydrochloride (Lansoprazole causes a profound and long lasting inhibition of gastric secretion; therefore, it is theoretically possible that it may interfere with oral absorption of drugs where gastric pH is an important determinant of bioavailability).

No products indexed under this heading.

Bretylium Tosylate (There have been post-marketing reports of torsade de pointes occurring with concurrent use of clarithromycin and quinidine or dispyramide. Electrocardiograms should be monitored for QTc prolongation during co-administration of clarithromycin with these drugs).

No products indexed under this heading.

Bromocriptine Mesylate (There have been reports of CYP3A-based interactions of clarithromycin with bromocriptine).

No products indexed under this heading.

Carbamazepine (There have been reports of CYP3A-based interactions of clarithromycin with carbamazepine). Products include:

Carbatrol Capsules 3174
Equetro Extended-Release Capsules 3178
Tegretol/Tegretol-XR 2278

Cerivastatin Sodium (Clarithromycin has been reported to increase concentrations of HMG-CoA reductase inhibitors. Rare reports of rhabdomyolysis have been reported in patients taking these drugs concomitantly).

No products indexed under this heading.

Chlorpropamide (Co-administration has resulted in rare reports of hypoglycemia, some of which occurred in patients taking oral hypoglycemia agents).

No products indexed under this heading.

Cilostazol (There have been reports of CYP3A-based interactions of clarithromycin with cilostazol). Products include:

Pletal Tablets 2478

Cisapride (Concomitant administration of Prevpac with cisapride is contraindicated. There have been post-marketing reports of drug interactions when clarithromycin is co-administered with cisapride resulting in cardiac arrhythmias (QT prolongation, ventricular tachycardia, ventricular fibrillation, and torsade de pointes) most likely due to inhibition of metabolism of these drugs by clarithromycin. Fatalities have been reported).

No products indexed under this heading.

Cyclosporine (There have been reports of CYP3A-based interactions of clarithromycin with cyclosporine). Products include:

Gengraf Capsules 458
Neoral Soft Gelatin Capsules 2247
Neoral Oral Solution 2247
Restasis Ophthalmic Emulsion 570
Sandimmune 2259

Dicumarol (Co-administration of clarithromycin with oral anticoagulants may result in the potentiation of oral coagulant effects).

No products indexed under this heading.

Digoxin (Co-administration of clarithromycin and digoxin has resulted in elevated digoxin serum concentrations resulting in clinical signs of digoxin toxicity including potentially fatal arrhythmias; lansoprazole causes profound and long-lasting inhibition of gastric acid secretion; therefore, it is theoretically possible that it may interfere with the absorption of drugs, such as digoxin, where gastric pH is an important determinant of bioavailability). Products include:

Digitek Tablets 2146
Lanoxicaps Capsules 1458
Lanoxin Injection 1462
Lanoxin Tablets 1468
Lanoxin Injection Pediatric 1465

Dihydroergotamine Mesylate (Co-administration of clarithromycin or erythromycin with dihydroergotamine has been associated in some patients with acute ergot toxicity characterized by severe peripheral vasospasm and dysesthesia). Products include:

Migranal Nasal Spray 3350

Disopyramide Phosphate (There have been reports of CYP3A-based interactions of clarithromycin with disopyramide).

No products indexed under this heading.

Divalproex Sodium (Concurrent use of erythromycin or clarithromycin in patients receiving drugs metabolized by the cytochrome P450 system may be associated with elevation in serum levels of valproate). Products include:

Depakote Sprinkle Capsules 422
Depakote Tablets 427
Depakote ER Tablets 433

Dofetilide (There have been post-marketing reports of torsade de pointes occurring with concurrent use of clarithromycin and quinidine or dispyramide. Electrocardiograms should be monitored for QTc prolongation during co-administration of clarithromycin with these drugs).

No products indexed under this heading.

Dyphylline (Co-administration of theophylline with clarithromycin in patients who are receiving high doses of theophylline may be associated with an increase in serum theophylline levels and potential theophylline toxicity).

No products indexed under this heading.

Ergotamine Tartrate (Co-administration of clarithromycin or erythromycin with ergotamine has been associated in some patients with acute ergot toxicity characterized by severe peripheral vasospasm and dysesthesia).

No products indexed under this heading.

Ferrous Fumarate (Lansoprazole causes a profound and long-lasting inhibition of gastric acid secretion; therefore, it is theoretically possible that it may interfere with the absorption of drugs, such as iron salts, where gastric pH is an important determinant of bioavailability). Products include:

Chromagen Forte Soft Gelatin Capsules 3296
Ferretts Tablets .... ▣ 773
Repliva 21/7 Tablets 3301

Ferrous Gluconate (Lansoprazole causes a profound and long-lasting inhibition of gastric acid secretion; therefore, it is theoretically possible that it may interfere with the absorption of drugs, such as iron salts, where gastric pH is an important determinant of bioavailability).

No products indexed under this heading.

Ferrous Sulfate (Lansoprazole causes a profound and long-lasting inhibition of gastric acid secretion; therefore, it is theoretically possible that it may interfere with the absorption of drugs, such as iron salts, where gastric pH is an important determinant of bioavailability). Products include:

Feosol Tablets 1629
Slow Fe Iron Tablets .... ▣ 772
Slow Fe with Folic Acid Tablets .... ▣ 773

Flecainide Acetate (There have been post-marketing reports of torsade de pointes occurring with concurrent use of clarithromycin and quinidine or dispyramide. Electrocardiograms should be monitored for QTc prolongation during co-administration of clarithromycin with these drugs). Products include:

Tambocor Tablets 1824

Fluvastatin Sodium (Clarithromycin has been reported to increase concentrations of HMG-CoA reductase inhibitors. Rare reports of rhabdomyolysis have been reported in patients taking these drugs concomitantly). Products include:

Lescol Capsules 2227
Lescol 2730
Lescol XL Tablets 2227

Fosphenytoin Sodium (Concurrent use of erythromycin or clarithromycin in patients receiving drugs metabolized by the cytochrome P450 system may be associated with elevation in serum levels of phenytoin).

No products indexed under this heading.

Glimepiride (Co-administration has resulted in rare reports of hypoglycemia, some of which occurred in patients taking oral hypoglycemia agents). Products include:

Amaryl Tablets 2864

Glipizide (Co-administration has resulted in rare reports of hypoglycemia, some of which occurred in patients taking oral hypoglycemia agents).

No products indexed under this heading.

Glyburide (Co-administration has resulted in rare reports of hypoglycemia, some of which occurred in patients taking oral hypoglycemia agents).

No products indexed under this heading.

Hexobarbital (Concurrent use of clarithromycin and hexobarbital may be associated with an elevation in the serum levels of hexobarbital).

No products indexed under this heading.

Insulin, Human, Zinc Suspension (Co-administration has resulted in rare reports of hypoglycemia, some of which occurred in patients taking insulin). Products include:

Humulin L, 100 Units 1763
Humulin U, 100 Units 1770

Insulin, Human NPH (Co-administration has resulted in rare reports of hypoglycemia, some of which occurred in patients taking insulin). Products include:

Humulin N, 100 Units 1764
Humulin N Pen 1765
Novolin N Human Insulin 10 ml Vials 2322
Novolin N InnoLet 2322
Novolin N PenFill 3 ml Cartridges 2325
Novolin R InnoLet 2322

Insulin, Human Regular (Co-administration has resulted in rare reports of hypoglycemia, some of which occurred in patients taking insulin). Products include:

Humulin R (U-500) 1768
Humulin R, 100 Units 1767
Novolin R Human Insulin 10 ml Vials 2322
Novolin R PenFill 2325

Insulin, Human Regular and Human NPH Mixture (Co-administration has resulted in rare reports of hypoglycemia, some of which occurred in patients taking insulin). Products include:

Humulin 50/50, 100 Units 1760
Humulin 70/30 Pen 1761
Novolin 70/30 Human Insulin 10 ml Vials 2321
Novolin 70/30 InnoLet 2322
Novolin 70/30 PenFill 3 ml Cartridges 2325

Insulin, NPH (Co-administration has resulted in rare reports of hypoglycemia, some of which occurred in patients taking insulin).
No products indexed under this heading.

Insulin, Regular (Co-administration has resulted in rare reports of hypoglycemia, some of which occurred in patients taking insulin).
No products indexed under this heading.

Insulin, Zinc Crystals (Co-administration has resulted in rare reports of hypoglycemia, some of which occurred in patients taking insulin).
No products indexed under this heading.

Insulin, Zinc Suspension (Co-administration has resulted in rare reports of hypoglycemia, some of which occurred in patients taking insulin).
No products indexed under this heading.

Insulin Aspart, Human Regular (Co-administration has resulted in rare reports of hypoglycemia, some of which occurred in patients taking insulin). Products include:
NovoLog Injection 2326

Insulin glargine (Co-administration has resulted in rare reports of hypoglycemia, some of which occurred in patients taking insulin). Products include:
Lantus Injection 2925

Insulin Lispro, Human (Co-administration has resulted in rare reports of hypoglycemia, some of which occurred in patients taking insulin). Products include:
Humalog-Pen 1751
Humalog Mix 75/25-Pen 1754

Insulin Lispro Protamine, Human (Co-administration has resulted in rare reports of hypoglycemia, some of which occurred in patients taking insulin). Products include:
Humalog Mix 75/25-Pen 1754

Iron (Lansoprazole causes a profound and long-lasting inhibition of gastric acid secretion; therefore, it is theoretically possible that it may interfere with the absorption of drugs, such as iron salts, where gastric pH is an important determinant of bioavailability). Products include:
Chromagen Forte Soft Gelatin Capsules 3296
Ferretts IPS Liquid 773
OptiNate 1162
Repliva 21/7 Tablets 3301

Ketoconazole (Lansoprazole causes a profound and long lasting inhibition of gastric secretion; therefore, it is theoretically possible that it may interfere with oral absorption of drugs where gastric pH is an important determinant of bioavailability). Products include:
Nizoral A-D Shampoo, 1% 1839
Nizoral 2% Shampoo 1838

Lidocaine Hydrochloride (There have been post-marketing reports of torsade de pointes occurring with concurrent use of clarithromycin and quinidine or dispyramide. Electrocardiograms should be monitored for QTc prolongation during co-administration of clarithromycin with these drugs).
No products indexed under this heading.

Lovastatin (Clarithromycin has been reported to increase concentrations of HMG-CoA reductase inhibitors. Rare reports of rhabdomyolysis have been reported in patients taking these drugs concomitantly). Products include:
Advicor Tablets 1694
Altoprev Extended-Release Tablets 1151
Mevacor Tablets 1996

Metformin Hydrochloride (Co-administration has resulted in rare reports of hypoglycemia, some of which occurred in patients taking oral hypoglycemia agents). Products include:
ActoPlus Met Tablets 3219
Avandamet Tablets 1343
Fortamet Extended-Release Tablets 1156

Methylprednisolone (There have been reports of CYP3A-based interactions of clarithromycin with methyprednisolone).
No products indexed under this heading.

Mexiletine Hydrochloride (There have been post-marketing reports of torsade de pointes occurring with concurrent use of clarithromycin and quinidine or dispyramide. Electrocardiograms should be monitored for QTc prolongation during co-administration of clarithromycin with these drugs).
No products indexed under this heading.

Midazolam Hydrochloride (Erythromycin, another macrolide antibiotic, has been reported to decrease the clearance of triazolam and midazolam, and thus, may increase the pharmacologic effect of these benzodiazepines).
No products indexed under this heading.

Miglitol (Co-administration has resulted in rare reports of hypoglycemia, some of which occurred in patients taking oral hypoglycemia agents).
No products indexed under this heading.

Moricizine Hydrochloride (There have been post-marketing reports of torsade de pointes occurring with concurrent use of clarithromycin and quinidine or dispyramide. Electrocardiograms should be monitored for QTc prolongation during co-administration of clarithromycin with these drugs).
No products indexed under this heading.

Phenytoin (Concurrent use of erythromycin or clarithromycin in patients receiving drugs metabolized by the cytochrome P450 system may be associated with elevation in serum levels of phenytoin).
No products indexed under this heading.

Phenytoin Sodium (Concurrent use of erythromycin or clarithromycin in patients receiving drugs metabolized by the cytochrome P450 system may be associated with elevation in serum levels of phenytoin). Products include:
Phenytek Capsules 2153

Pimozide (Concomitant administration of Prevpac with pimozide is contraindicated. There have been post-marketing reports of drug interactions when clarithromycin is co-administered with pimozide resulting in cardiac arrhythmias (QT prolongation, ventricular tachycardia, ventricular fibrillation, and torsade de pointes) most likely due to inhibition of metabolism of these drugs by clarithromycin. Fatalities have been reported). Products include:
Orap Tablets 1220

Pioglitazone Hydrochloride (Co-administration has resulted in rare reports of hypoglycemia, some of which occurred in patients taking oral hypoglycemia agents). Products include:
ActoPlus Met Tablets 3219
Actos Tablets 3224

Polysaccharide Iron Complex (Lansoprazole causes a profound and long-lasting inhibition of gastric acid secretion; therefore, it is theoretically possible that it may interfere with the absorption of drugs, such as iron salts, where gastric pH is an important determinant of bioavailability). Products include:
Niferex-150 Forte Capsules 3299
Nu-Iron 150 Capsules 2098

Pravastatin Sodium (Clarithromycin has been reported to increase concentrations of HMG-CoA reductase inhibitors. Rare reports of rhabdomyolysis have been reported in patients taking these drugs concomitantly). Products include:
Pravachol Tablets 943

Probenecid (Probenecid decreases the renal tubular secretion of amoxicillin. Concurrent use may result in increased and prolonged blood levels of amoxicillin).
No products indexed under this heading.

Procainamide Hydrochloride (There have been post-marketing reports of torsade de pointes occurring with concurrent use of clarithromycin and quinidine or dispyramide. Electrocardiograms should be monitored for QTc prolongation during co-administration of clarithromycin with these drugs).
No products indexed under this heading.

Propafenone Hydrochloride (There have been post-marketing reports of torsade de pointes occurring with concurrent use of clarithromycin and quinidine or dispyramide. Electrocardiograms should be monitored for QTc prolongation during co-administration of clarithromycin with these drugs). Products include:
Rythmol SR Capsules 2736

Propranolol Hydrochloride (There have been post-marketing reports of torsade de pointes occurring with concurrent use of clarithromycin and quinidine or dispyramide. Electrocardiograms should be monitored for QTc prolongation during co-administration of clarithromycin with these drugs). Products include:
Inderal LA Long-Acting Capsules 3421
InnoPran XL Capsules 2728

Quinidine (There have been reports of CYP3A-based interactions of clarithromycin with quinidine).
No products indexed under this heading.

Quinidine Gluconate (There have been post-marketing reports of torsade de pointes occurring with concurrent use of clarithromycin and quinidine or dispyramide. Electrocardiograms should be monitored for QTc prolongation during co-administration of clarithromycin with these drugs).
No products indexed under this heading.

Quinidine Polygalacturonate (There have been post-marketing reports of torsade de pointes occurring with concurrent use of clarithromycin and quinidine or dispyramide. Electrocardiograms should be monitored for QTc prolongation during co-administration of clarithromycin with these drugs).
No products indexed under this heading.

Quinidine Sulfate (There have been post-marketing reports of torsade de pointes occurring with concurrent use of clarithromycin and quinidine or dispyramide. Electrocardiograms should be monitored for QTc prolongation during co-administration of clarithromycin with these drugs).
No products indexed under this heading.

Repaglinide (Co-administration has resulted in rare reports of hypoglycemia, some of which occurred in patients taking oral hypoglycemia agents). Products include:
Prandin Tablets (0.5, 1, and 2 mg) 2337

Rifabutin (There have been reports of CYP3A-based interactions of clarithromycin with rifabutin).
No products indexed under this heading.

Rosiglitazone Maleate (Co-administration has resulted in rare reports of hypoglycemia, some of which occurred in patients taking oral hypoglycemia agents). Products include:
Avandamet Tablets 1343
Avandia Tablets 1348

Sildenafil Citrate (Erythromycin, another macrolide antibiotic, has been reported to increase the systemic exposure (AUC) of sildenafil. A similar interaction may occur with clarithromycin; reduction of sildenafil dosage should be considered). Products include:
Revatio Tablets 2541
Viagra Tablets 2552

Simvastatin (Clarithromycin has been reported to increase concentrations of HMG-CoA reductase inhibitors. Rare reports of rhabdomyolysis have been reported in patients taking these drugs concomitantly). Products include:
Vytorin 10/10 Tablets 2084
Vytorin 10/10 Tablets 3092
Vytorin 10/20 Tablets 2084
Vytorin 10/20 Tablets 3092
Vytorin 10/40 Tablets 3092
Vytorin 10/40 Tablets 2084
Vytorin 10/80 Tablets 2084
Vytorin 10/80 Tablets 3092
Zocor Tablets 2078

Sotalol Hydrochloride (There have been post-marketing reports of torsade de pointes occurring with concurrent use of clarithromycin and quinidine or dispyramide. Electrocardiograms should be monitored for QTc prolongation during co-administration of clarithromycin with these drugs).
No products indexed under this heading.

Sucralfate (Co-administration delays absorption and reduces bioavailability by about 30%; therefore, lansoprazole should be taken at least 30 minutes prior to sucralfate). Products include:
Carafate Suspension 727
Carafate Tablets 728

Tacrolimus (There have been reports of CYP3A-based interactions of clarithromycin with tacrolimus). Products include:
- Prograf Capsules and Injection 624
- Protopic Ointment 629

Terfenadine (Concomitant administration of Prevpac with terfenadine is contraindicated. There have been post-marketing reports of drug interactions when clarithromycin is co-administered with terfenadine resulting in cardiac arrhythmias (QT prolongation, ventricular tachycardia, ventricular fibrillation, and torsade de pointes) most likely due to inhibition of metabolism of these drugs by clarithromycin. Fatalities have been reported).
No products indexed under this heading.

Theophylline (Co-administration of theophylline with clarithromycin in patients who are receiving high doses of theophylline may be associated with an increase in serum theophylline levels and potential theophylline toxicity).
No products indexed under this heading.

Theophylline Anhydrous (Co-administration of theophylline with clarithromycin in patients who are receiving high doses of theophylline may be associated with an increase in serum theophylline levels and potential theophylline toxicity). Products include:
- Uniphyl Tablets 2708

Theophylline Calcium Salicylate (Co-administration of theophylline with clarithromycin in patients who are receiving high doses of theophylline may be associated with an increase in serum theophylline levels and potential theophylline toxicity).
No products indexed under this heading.

Theophylline Dihydroxypropyl (Glyceryl) (Co-administration of theophylline with clarithromycin in patients who are receiving high doses of theophylline may be associated with an increase in serum theophylline levels and potential theophylline toxicity).
No products indexed under this heading.

Theophylline Ethylenediamine (Co-administration of theophylline with clarithromycin in patients who are receiving high doses of theophylline may be associated with an increase in serum theophylline levels and potential theophylline toxicity).
No products indexed under this heading.

Theophylline Sodium Glycinate (Co-administration of theophylline with clarithromycin in patients who are receiving high doses of theophylline may be associated with an increase in serum theophylline levels and potential theophylline toxicity).
No products indexed under this heading.

Tocainide Hydrochloride (There have been post-marketing reports of torsade de pointes occurring with concurrent use of clarithromycin and quinidine or dispyramide. Electrocardiograms should be monitored for QTc prolongation during co-administration of clarithromycin with these drugs).
No products indexed under this heading.

Tolazamide (Co-administration has resulted in rare reports of hypoglycemia, some of which occurred in patients taking oral hypoglycemia agents).
No products indexed under this heading.

Tolbutamide (Co-administration has resulted in rare reports of hypoglycemia, some of which occurred in patients taking oral hypoglycemia agents).
No products indexed under this heading.

Triazolam (Concomitant use of clarithromycin and triazolam has resulted in CNS effects (somnolence and confusion) and drug interactions).
No products indexed under this heading.

Troglitazone (Co-administration has resulted in rare reports of hypoglycemia, some of which occurred in patients taking oral hypoglycemia agents).
No products indexed under this heading.

Valproate Sodium (Concurrent use of erythromycin or clarithromycin in patients receiving drugs metabolized by the cytochrome P450 system may be associated with elevation in serum levels of valproate). Products include:
- Depacon Injection 412

Valproic Acid (Concurrent use of erythromycin or clarithromycin in patients receiving drugs metabolized by the cytochrome P450 system may be associated with elevation in serum levels of valproate). Products include:
- Depakene 417

Verapamil Hydrochloride (There have been post-marketing reports of torsade de pointes occurring with concurrent use of clarithromycin and quinidine or dispyramide. Electrocardiograms should be monitored for QTc prolongation during co-administration of clarithromycin with these drugs). Products include:
- Covera-HS Tablets 3135
- Tarka Tablets 519
- Verelan PM Capsules 3120

Warfarin Sodium (Co-administration of clarithromycin with oral anticoagulants may result in the potentiation of oral coagulant effects. Co-administration of warfarin and proton pump inhibitors, including Prevacid, has resulted in increased International Normalized Ratio (INR) and prothrombin time). Products include:
- Coumadin for Injection 932
- Coumadin Tablets 932

Food Interactions

Food, unspecified (Both Cmax and AUC are diminished by about 50% if the lansoprazole is given 30 minutes after food as opposed to the fasting condition).

PRILOSEC OTC TABLETS

(Omeprazole magnesium) 2674

May interact with benzodiazepines, iron containing oral preparations, phenytoin, and certain other agents. Compounds in these categories include:

Alprazolam (Potential for metabolism interaction via cytochrome P450 system). Products include:
- Niravam Orally Disintegrating Tablets 3106
- Xanax XR Tablets 2655

Astemizole (Co-administration of omeprazole-clarithromycin combination with astemizole is not recommended because clarithromycin, like erythromycin, is also metabolized by cytochrome P450 and there have been reports of QT prolongation and torsade de pointes with concurrent use of erythromycin and astemizole).
No products indexed under this heading.

Bacampicillin Hydrochloride (Omeprazole may interfere with gastric absorption of drugs, such as ampicillin esters, where gastric pH is an important determinant of their bioavailability).
No products indexed under this heading.

Chlordiazepoxide (Potential for metabolism interaction via cytochrome P450 system).
No products indexed under this heading.

Chlordiazepoxide Hydrochloride (Potential for metabolism interaction via cytochrome P450 system). Products include:
- Librium Capsules 3349

Cisapride (Co-administration of omeprazole-clarithromycin combination with cisapride has resulted in cardiac arrhythmias, including QT prolongation, ventricular tachycardia and fibrillation and torsade de points, and fatalities; concomitant use of clarithromycin and cisapride is contraindicated).
No products indexed under this heading.

Clarithromycin (Co-administration may result in increases in plasma levels of omeprazole, clarithromycin, and 14-hydroxy-clarithromycin). Products include:
- Biaxin/Biaxin XL 402
- PREVPAC 3281

Clonazepam (Potential for metabolism interaction via cytochrome P450 system). Products include:
- Klonopin 2782

Clorazepate Dipotassium (Potential for metabolism interaction via cytochrome P450 system). Products include:
- Tranxene 2488

Cyclosporine (Potential for metabolism interaction via cytochrome P450 system). Products include:
- Gengraf Capsules 458
- Neoral Soft Gelatin Capsules 2247
- Neoral Oral Solution 2247
- Restasis Ophthalmic Emulsion 570
- Sandimmune 2259

Diazepam (Potential for metabolism interaction via cytochrome P450 system; prolonged elimination of diazepam). Products include:
- Diastat Rectal Delivery System 3344
- Valium Tablets 2822

Disulfiram (Potential for metabolism interaction via cytochrome P450 system). Products include:
- Antabuse Tablets 2343

Estazolam (Potential for metabolism interaction via cytochrome P450 system). Products include:
- ProSom Tablets 512

Ferrous Fumarate (Omeprazole may interfere with gastric absorption of drugs, such as iron salts, where gastric pH is an important determinant of their bioavailability). Products include:
- Chromagen Forte Soft Gelatin Capsules 3296
- Ferretts Tablets 773
- Repliva 21/7 Tablets 3301

Ferrous Gluconate (Omeprazole may interfere with gastric absorption of drugs, such as iron salts, where gastric pH is an important determinant of their bioavailability).
No products indexed under this heading.

Ferrous Sulfate (Omeprazole may interfere with gastric absorption of drugs, such as iron salts, where gastric pH is an important determinant of their bioavailability). Products include:
- Feosol Tablets 1629
- Slow Fe Iron Tablets 772
- Slow Fe with Folic Acid Tablets 773

Flurazepam Hydrochloride (Potential for metabolism interaction via cytochrome P450 system). Products include:
- Dalmane Capsules 3343

Fosphenytoin Sodium (Prolonged elimination of phenytoin).
No products indexed under this heading.

Halazepam (Potential for metabolism interaction via cytochrome P450 system).
No products indexed under this heading.

Iron (Omeprazole may interfere with gastric absorption of drugs, such as iron salts, where gastric pH is an important determinant of their bioavailability). Products include:
- Chromagen Forte Soft Gelatin Capsules 3296
- Ferretts IPS Liquid 773
- OptiNate 1162
- Repliva 21/7 Tablets 3301

Ketoconazole (Omeprazole may interfere with gastric absorption of drugs, such as ketoconazole, where gastric pH is an important determinant of their bioavailability). Products include:
- Nizoral A-D Shampoo, 1% 1839
- Nizoral 2% Shampoo 1838

Lorazepam (Potential for metabolism interaction via cytochrome P450 system).
No products indexed under this heading.

Midazolam Hydrochloride (Potential for metabolism interaction via cytochrome P450 system).
No products indexed under this heading.

Oxazepam (Potential for metabolism interaction via cytochrome P450 system).
No products indexed under this heading.

Phenytoin (Prolonged elimination of phenytoin).
No products indexed under this heading.

Phenytoin Sodium (Prolonged elimination of phenytoin). Products include:
- Phenytek Capsules 2153

Pimozide (Co-administration of omeprazole-clarithromycin combination with pimozide has resulted in cardiac arrhythmias, including QT prolongation, ventricular tachycardia and fibrillation and torsade de points, and fatalities; concomitant use of clarithromycin and pimozide is contraindicated). Products include:
- Orap Tablets 1220

Polysaccharide Iron Complex (Omeprazole may interfere with gastric absorption of drugs, such as iron salts, where gastric pH is an important determinant of their bioavailability). Products include:
- Niferex-150 Forte Capsules 3299
- Nu-Iron 150 Capsules 2098

Prazepam (Potential for metabolism interaction via cytochrome P450 system).
No products indexed under this heading.

Quazepam (Potential for metabolism interaction via cytochrome P450 system).
No products indexed under this heading.

Temazepam (Potential for metabolism interaction via cytochrome P450 system).
No products indexed under this heading.

Terfenadine (Co-administration of omeprazole-clarithromycin combination with terfenadine has resulted in cardiac arrhythmias, including QT prolongation, ventricular tachycardia and fibrillation and torsade de points, and fatalities; concomitant use of clarithromycin and terfenadine is contraindicated).
No products indexed under this heading.

Triazolam (Potential for metabolism interaction via cytochrome P450 system).
No products indexed under this heading.

Warfarin Sodium (Prolonged elimination of warfarin). Products include:
- Coumadin for Injection 932
- Coumadin Tablets 932

Food Interactions

Food, unspecified (Absorption begins only after the granules leave the stomach; Prilosec should be taken before eating).

PRIMACARE AM CAPSULES

(Vitamins, Prenatal) 3300
None cited in PDR database.

PRIMACARE ONE CAPSULES

(Vitamins, Prenatal) 3301
None cited in PDR database.

PRIMACARE PM TABLETS

(Vitamins, Prenatal) 3300
None cited in PDR database.

PRIMATENE MIST

(Epinephrine) 749
See Primatene Tablets

PRIMATENE TABLETS

(Ephedrine Hydrochloride, Guaifenesin) 749
May interact with monoamine oxidase inhibitors. Compounds in these categories include:

Isocarboxazid (Concurrent and/or sequential use with MAO inhibitors is not recommended).
No products indexed under this heading.

Moclobemide (Concurrent and/or sequential use with MAO inhibitors is not recommended).
No products indexed under this heading.

Pargyline Hydrochloride (Concurrent and/or sequential use with MAO inhibitors is not recommended).
No products indexed under this heading.

Phenelzine Sulfate (Concurrent and/or sequential use with MAO inhibitors is not recommended).
No products indexed under this heading.

Procarbazine Hydrochloride (Concurrent and/or sequential use with MAO inhibitors is not recommended). Products include:
- Matulane Capsules 3188

Selegiline Hydrochloride (Concurrent and/or sequential use with MAO inhibitors is not recommended). Products include:
- Eldepryl Capsules 3209

Tranylcypromine Sulfate (Concurrent and/or sequential use with MAO inhibitors is not recommended). Products include:
- Parnate Tablets 1499

PRIMAXIN I.M.

(Cilastatin Sodium, Imipenem) 2022
See Primaxin I.V.

PRIMAXIN I.V.

(Cilastatin Sodium, Imipenem) 2024
May interact with:

Ganciclovir Sodium (Concomitant administration may result in generalized seizures). Products include:
- Cytovene-IV 2763

Probenecid (Concomitant administration results in only minimal increase in plasma levels of imipenem; concomitant administration not recommended).
No products indexed under this heading.

PRINIVIL TABLETS

(Lisinopril) 2029
May interact with diuretics, lithium preparations, non-steroidal anti-inflammatory agents, potassium preparations, potassium sparing diuretics, thiazides, and certain other agents. Compounds in these categories include:

Amiloride Hydrochloride (Potential for significant hyperkalemia; possibility of excessive reduction in blood pressure). Products include:
- Midamor Tablets 2000
- Moduretic Tablets 2003

Bendroflumethiazide (Thiazide-induced potassium loss attenuated; possibility of excessive reduction in blood pressure).
No products indexed under this heading.

Bumetanide (Possibility of excessive reduction in blood pressure).
No products indexed under this heading.

Celecoxib (Co-administration in some patients with compromised renal function who are being treated with NSAIDs may result in a further deterioration of renal function). Products include:
- Celebrex Capsules 3130

Chlorothiazide (Thiazide-induced potassium loss attenuated; possibility of excessive reduction in blood pressure). Products include:
- Aldoclor Tablets 1881
- Diuril Oral 1936

Chlorothiazide Sodium (Thiazide-induced potassium loss attenuated; possibility of excessive reduction in blood pressure). Products include:
- Diuril Sodium Intravenous 1934

Chlorthalidone (Possibility of excessive reduction in blood pressure). Products include:
- Clorpres Tablets 2139

Diclofenac Potassium (Co-administration in some patients with compromised renal function who are being treated with NSAIDs may result in a further deterioration of renal function). Products include:
- Cataflam Tablets 2173

Diclofenac Sodium (Co-administration in some patients with compromised renal function who are being treated with NSAIDs may result in a further deterioration of renal function). Products include:
- Arthrotec Tablets 3126
- Voltaren Ophthalmic Solution 2300
- Voltaren Tablets 2298
- Voltaren-XR Tablets 2301

Ethacrynic Acid (Possibility of excessive reduction in blood pressure). Products include:
- Edecrin Tablets 1941

Etodolac (Co-administration in some patients with compromised renal function who are being treated with NSAIDs may result in a further deterioration of renal function).
No products indexed under this heading.

Fenoprofen Calcium (Co-administration in some patients with compromised renal function who are being treated with NSAIDs may result in a further deterioration of renal function). Products include:
- Nalfon Capsules 2504

Flurbiprofen (Co-administration in some patients with compromised renal function who are being treated with NSAIDs may result in a further deterioration of renal function).
No products indexed under this heading.

Furosemide (Possibility of excessive reduction in blood pressure). Products include:
- Furosemide Tablets 2117

Hydrochlorothiazide (Thiazide-induced potassium loss attenuated; possibility of excessive reduction in blood pressure). Products include:
- Aldoril Tablets 1884
- Atacand HCT 637
- Avalide Tablets 2889
- Avalide Tablets 922
- Benicar HCT Tablets 2852
- Diovan HCT Tablets 2195
- Dyazide Capsules 1389
- Hyzaar 1964
- Lotensin HCT Tablets 2235
- Maxzide 2150
- Micardis HCT Tablets 886
- Moduretic Tablets 2003
- Prinzide Tablets 2033
- Teveten HCT Tablets 1710
- Timolide Tablets 2056
- Uniretic Tablets 3114
- Vaseretic Tablets 2073
- Zestoretic Tablets 701

Hydroflumethiazide (Thiazide-induced potassium loss attenuated; possibility of excessive reduction in blood pressure).
No products indexed under this heading.

Ibuprofen (Co-administration in some patients with compromised renal function who are being treated with NSAIDs may result in a further deterioration of renal function). Products include:
- Advil Allergy Sinus Caplets 737
- Advil 737
- Children's Advil Suspension 742
- Children's Advil Chewable Tablets .. 741
- Advil Cold & Sinus 739
- Advil Flu & Body Ache Caplets 739
- Children's Advil Cold Suspension ... 741
- Infants' Advil Concentrated Drops .. 743
- Junior Strength Advil Swallow Tablets 740
- Advil Migraine Liquigels 740
- Advil Multi-Symptom Cold Caplets 738
- Combunox Tablets 1183
- Children's Motrin Oral Suspension and Chewable Tablets 1837
- Children's Motrin Cold Non-Staining Dye-Free Oral Suspension 1838
- Children's Motrin Cold Oral Suspension 1838
- Children's Motrin Non-Staining Dye-Free Oral Suspension 1837
- Motrin Cold & Sinus Caplets 1836
- Motrin IB Tablets and Caplets 1836
- Infants' Motrin Concentrated Drops 1837
- Infants' Motrin Non-Staining Dye-Free Drops 1837
- Junior Strength Motrin Caplets and Chewable Tablets 1837
- Vicoprofen Tablets 533

Indapamide (Possibility of excessive reduction in blood pressure). Products include:
- Indapamide Tablets 2119

Indomethacin (Co-administration in some patients with compromised renal function who are being treated with NSAIDs may result in a further deterioration of renal function. In a study, the use of indomethacin was associated with a reduced antihypertensive effect, although the difference between lisinopril alone to lisinopril given concomitantly with indomethacin was not significant). Products include:
- Indocin 1968

Indomethacin Sodium Trihydrate (Co-administration in some patients with compromised renal function who are being treated with NSAIDs may result in a further deterioration of renal function). Products include:
- Indocin I.V. 1973

Ketoprofen (Co-administration in some patients with compromised renal function who are being treated with NSAIDs may result in a further deterioration of renal function).
No products indexed under this heading.

Ketorolac Tromethamine (Co-administration in some patients with compromised renal function who are being treated with NSAIDs may result in a further deterioration of renal function). Products include:
- Acular Ophthalmic Solution 561
- Acular LS Ophthalmic Solution 562

Lithium (Potential for reversible lithium toxicity; frequent monitoring of lithium levels is recommended).
No products indexed under this heading.

Lithium Carbonate (Potential for reversible lithium toxicity; frequent monitoring of lithium levels is recommended). Products include:
- Eskalith 1406
- Lithobid Tablets 1670

Lithium Citrate (Potential for reversible lithium toxicity; frequent monitoring of lithium levels is recommended).
No products indexed under this heading.

Meclofenamate Sodium (Co-administration in some patients with compromised renal function who are being treated with NSAIDs may result in a further deterioration of renal function).
No products indexed under this heading.

Mefenamic Acid (Co-administration in some patients with compromised renal function who are being treated with NSAIDs may result in a further deterioration of renal function).
No products indexed under this heading.

Meloxicam (Co-administration in some patients with compromised renal function who are being treated with NSAIDs may result in a further deterioration of renal function). Products include:
Mobic Oral Suspension 893
Mobic Tablets 893

Methyclothiazide (Thiazide-induced potassium loss attenuated; possibility of excessive reduction in blood pressure).
No products indexed under this heading.

Metolazone (Possibility of excessive reduction in blood pressure).
No products indexed under this heading.

Nabumetone (Co-administration in some patients with compromised renal function who are being treated with NSAIDs may result in a further deterioration of renal function). Products include:
Relafen Tablets 1523

Naproxen (Co-administration in some patients with compromised renal function who are being treated with NSAIDs may result in a further deterioration of renal function). Products include:
EC-Naprosyn Delayed-Release Tablets 2769
Naprosyn Suspension 2769
Naprosyn Tablets 2769
Prevacid NapraPAC 3277

Naproxen Sodium (Co-administration in some patients with compromised renal function who are being treated with NSAIDs may result in a further deterioration of renal function). Products include:
Aleve Tablets, Caplets and Gelcaps .... ▣605
Anaprox Tablets 2769
Anaprox DS Tablets 2769

Oxaprozin (Co-administration in some patients with compromised renal function who are being treated with NSAIDs may result in a further deterioration of renal function).
No products indexed under this heading.

Phenylbutazone (Co-administration in some patients with compromised renal function who are being treated with NSAIDs may result in a further deterioration of renal function).
No products indexed under this heading.

Piroxicam (Co-administration in some patients with compromised renal function who are being treated with NSAIDs may result in a further deterioration of renal function).
No products indexed under this heading.

Polythiazide (Thiazide-induced potassium loss attenuated; possibility of excessive reduction in blood pressure).
No products indexed under this heading.

Potassium Acid Phosphate (Potential for significant hyperkalemia). Products include:
K-Phos Original (Sodium Free) Tablets 785

Potassium Bicarbonate (Potential for significant hyperkalemia).
No products indexed under this heading.

Potassium Chloride (Potential for significant hyperkalemia). Products include:
Colyte with Flavor Packs for Oral Solution 3102
HalfLytely and Bisacodyl Tablets Bowel Prep Kit with Flavors Packs 915
K-Dur Extended-Relase Tablets 3047
K-Lor Powder Packets 472
K-Tab Filmtab Tablets 473
TriLyte with Flavor Packs for Oral Solution 3114

Potassium Citrate (Potential for significant hyperkalemia). Products include:
Urocit-K Tablets 2109

Potassium Gluconate (Potential for significant hyperkalemia).
No products indexed under this heading.

Potassium Phosphate (Potential for significant hyperkalemia). Products include:
K-Phos Neutral Tablets 785

Rofecoxib (Co-administration in some patients with compromised renal function who are being treated with NSAIDs may result in a further deterioration of renal function).
No products indexed under this heading.

Spironolactone (Potential for significant hyperkalemia; possibility of excessive reduction in blood pressure).
No products indexed under this heading.

Sulindac (Co-administration in some patients with compromised renal function who are being treated with NSAIDs may result in a further deterioration of renal function). Products include:
Clinoril Tablets 1899

Tolmetin Sodium (Co-administration in some patients with compromised renal function who are being treated with NSAIDs may result in a further deterioration of renal function).
No products indexed under this heading.

Torsemide (Possibility of excessive reduction in blood pressure).
No products indexed under this heading.

Triamterene (Potential for significant hyperkalemia; possibility of excessive reduction in blood pressure). Products include:
Dyazide Capsules 1389
Dyrenium Capsules 3390
Maxzide 2150

Valdecoxib (Co-administration in some patients with compromised renal function who are being treated with NSAIDs may result in a further deterioration of renal function).
No products indexed under this heading.

PRINZIDE TABLETS

(Hydrochlorothiazide, Lisinopril) 2033

May interact with antihypertensives, barbiturates, corticosteroids, diuretics, cardiac glycosides, oral hypoglycemic agents, insulin, lithium preparations, narcotic analgesics, nondepolarizing neuromuscular blocking agents, non-steroidal anti-inflammatory agents, potassium preparations, potassium sparing diuretics, and certain other agents. Compounds in these categories include:

Acarbose (Hyperglycemia may occur with thiazide diuretics; dosage adjustment of oral hypoglycemic agents may be required). Products include:
Precose Tablets 776

Acebutolol Hydrochloride (Co-administration of thiazide and other antihypertensive agents can lead to additive effect or potentiation).
No products indexed under this heading.

ACTH (Co-administration of thiazide diuretics with ACTH intensifies electrolyte depletion, particularly potassium).
No products indexed under this heading.

Alfentanil Hydrochloride (Co-administration of thiazide and narcotics may potentiate orthostatic hypotension).
No products indexed under this heading.

Amiloride Hydrochloride (Lisinopril attenuates diuretic-induced potassium loss; concomitant use can lead to hyperkalemia; frequent monitoring of serum potassium is recommended if used concurrently; co-administration can result in excessive hypotension). Products include:
Midamor Tablets 2000
Moduretic Tablets 2003

Amlodipine Besylate (Co-administration of thiazide and other antihypertensive agents can lead to additive effect or potentiation). Products include:
Caduet Tablets 2507
Lotrel Capsules 2238
Norvasc Tablets 2529

Aprobarbital (Co-administration of thiazide and barbiturates may potentiate orthostatic hypotension).
No products indexed under this heading.

Atenolol (Co-administration of thiazide and other antihypertensive agents can lead to additive effect or potentiation). Products include:
Tenormin I.V. Injection 698
Tenormin Tablets 695

Atracurium Besylate (Co-administration with nondepolarizing skeletal muscle relaxants may result in possible increased responsiveness to the muscle relaxant).
No products indexed under this heading.

Benazepril Hydrochloride (Co-administration of thiazide and other antihypertensive agents can lead to additive effect or potentiation). Products include:
Lotensin Tablets 2232
Lotensin HCT Tablets 2235
Lotrel Capsules 2238

Bendroflumethiazide (Co-administration of lisinopril in patients on diuretics, especially those in whom diuretic therapy was recently instituted, may occasionally experience excessive hypotension; antihypertensive effects of lisinopril are augmented by antihypertensive agents that cause renin release).
No products indexed under this heading.

Betamethasone Acetate (Co-administration of thiazide diuretics with corticosteroids intensifies electrolyte depletion, particularly potassium).
No products indexed under this heading.

Betamethasone Sodium Phosphate (Co-administration of thiazide diuretics with corticosteroids intensifies electrolyte depletion, particularly potassium).
No products indexed under this heading.

Betaxolol Hydrochloride (Co-administration of thiazide and other antihypertensive agents can lead to additive effect or potentiation). Products include:
Betoptic S Ophthalmic Suspension 554

Bisoprolol Fumarate (Co-administration of thiazide and other antihypertensive agents can lead to additive effect or potentiation).
No products indexed under this heading.

Bumetanide (Co-administration of lisinopril in patients on diuretics, especially those in whom diuretic therapy was recently instituted, may occasionally experience excessive hypotension; antihypertensive effects of lisinopril are augmented by antihypertensive agents that cause renin release).
No products indexed under this heading.

Buprenorphine Hydrochloride (Co-administration of thiazide and narcotics may potentiate orthostatic hypotension). Products include:
Buprenex Injectable 2718
Suboxone Tablets 2719
Subutex Tablets 2719

Butabarbital (Co-administration of thiazide and barbiturates may potentiate orthostatic hypotension).
No products indexed under this heading.

Butalbital (Co-administration of thiazide and barbiturates may potentiate orthostatic hypotension). Products include:
Sedapap Tablets 50 mg/650 mg 2098

Candesartan Cilexetil (Co-administration of thiazide and other antihypertensive agents can lead to additive effect or potentiation). Products include:
Atacand Tablets 634
Atacand HCT 637

Captopril (Co-administration of thiazide and other antihypertensive agents can lead to additive effect or potentiation). Products include:
Captopril Tablets 2114

Carteolol Hydrochloride (Co-administration of thiazide and other antihypertensive agents can lead to additive effect or potentiation). Products include:

Carteolol Hydrochloride Ophthalmic Solution USP, 1%....... ⊙246

Celecoxib (Co-administration in some patients with compromised renal function who are being treated with NSAIDs may result in a further deterioration of renal function: NSAID may reduce the diuretic, natriuretic and antihypertensive effects of thiazide). Products include:
Celebrex Capsules 3130

Chlorothiazide (Co-administration of lisinopril in patients on diuretics, especially those in whom diuretic therapy was recently instituted, may occasionally experience excessive hypotension; antihypertensive effects of lisinopril are augmented by antihypertensive agents that cause renin release). Products include:
Aldoclor Tablets 1881
Diuril Oral 1936

Chlorothiazide Sodium (Co-administration of lisinopril in patients on diuretics, especially those in whom diuretic therapy was recently instituted, may occasionally experience excessive hypotension; antihypertensive effects of lisinopril are augmented by antihypertensive agents that cause renin release). Products include:
Diuril Sodium Intravenous 1934

Chlorpropamide (Hyperglycemia may occur with thiazide diuretics; dosage adjustment of oral hypoglycemic agents may be required).
No products indexed under this heading.

Chlorthalidone (Co-administration of lisinopril in patients on diuretics, especially those in whom diuretic therapy was recently instituted, may occasionally experience excessive hypotension; antihypertensive effects of lisinopril are augmented by antihypertensive agents that cause renin release). Products include:
Clorpres Tablets 2139

Cholestyramine (Absorption of hydrochlorothiazide is impaired in the presence of anionic exchange resins; these resins bind the hydrochlorothiazide and reduce its absorption from GI tract).
No products indexed under this heading.

Cisatracurium Besylate (Co-administration with nondepolarizing skeletal muscle relaxants may result in possible increased responsiveness to the muscle relaxant). Products include:
Nimbex Injection 494

Clonidine (Co-administration of thiazide and other antihypertensive agents can lead to additive effect or potentiation). Products include:
Catapres-TTS 875

Clonidine Hydrochloride (Co-administration of thiazide and other antihypertensive agents can lead to additive effect or potentiation). Products include:
Catapres Tablets 874
Clorpres Tablets 2139

Codeine Phosphate (Co-administration of thiazide and narcotics may potentiate orthostatic hypotension). Products include:
Tylenol with Codeine 2461

Colestipol Hydrochloride (Absorption of hydrochlorothiazide is impaired in the presence of anionic exchange resins; these resins bind the hydrochlorothiazide and reduce its absorption from GI tract).
No products indexed under this heading.

Cortisone Acetate (Co-administration of thiazide diuretics with corticosteroids intensifies electrolyte depletion, particularly potassium).
No products indexed under this heading.

Deserpidine (Co-administration of thiazide and other antihypertensive agents can lead to additive effect or potentiation).
No products indexed under this heading.

Deslanoside (Hypokalemia induced by thiazide diuretics may cause cardiac arrhythmia and may also sensitize or exaggerate the response to the heart to the toxic effects of digitalis, such as ventricular irritability).
No products indexed under this heading.

Dexamethasone (Co-administration of thiazide diuretics with corticosteroids intensifies electrolyte depletion, particularly potassium). Products include:
Ciprodex Otic Suspension 555
Decadron Tablets 1929
TobraDex Ophthalmic Ointment 558
TobraDex Ophthalmic Suspension ... 558

Dexamethasone Acetate (Co-administration of thiazide diuretics with corticosteroids intensifies electrolyte depletion, particularly potassium).
No products indexed under this heading.

Dexamethasone Sodium Phosphate (Co-administration of thiazide diuretics with corticosteroids intensifies electrolyte depletion, particularly potassium). Products include:
Decadron Phosphate Injection 1931

Dezocine (Co-administration of thiazide and narcotics may potentiate orthostatic hypotension).
No products indexed under this heading.

Diazoxide (Co-administration of thiazide and other antihypertensive agents can lead to additive effect or potentiation). Products include:
Hyperstat I.V. Injection 3031

Diclofenac Potassium (Co-administration in some patients with compromised renal function who are being treated with NSAIDs may result in a further deterioration of renal function: NSAID may reduce the diuretic, natriuretic and antihypertensive effects of thiazide). Products include:
Cataflam Tablets 2173

Diclofenac Sodium (Co-administration in some patients with compromised renal function who are being treated with NSAIDs may result in a further deterioration of renal function: NSAID may reduce the diuretic, natriuretic and antihypertensive effects of thiazide). Products include:
Arthrotec Tablets 3126
Voltaren Ophthalmic Solution 2300
Voltaren Tablets 2298
Voltaren-XR Tablets 2301

Digitalis Glycoside Preparations (Hypokalemia induced by thiazide diuretics may cause cardiac arrhythmia and may also sensitize or exaggerate the response to the heart to the toxic effects of digitalis, such as ventricular irritability).
No products indexed under this heading.

Digitoxin (Hypokalemia induced by thiazide diuretics may cause cardiac arrhythmia and may also sensitize or exaggerate the response to the heart to the toxic effects of digitalis, such as ventricular irritability).
No products indexed under this heading.

Digoxin (Hypokalemia induced by thiazide diuretics may cause cardiac arrhythmia and may also sensitize or exaggerate the response to the heart to the toxic effects of digitalis, such as ventricular irritability). Products include:
Digitek Tablets 2146
Lanoxicaps Capsules 1458
Lanoxin Injection 1462
Lanoxin Tablets 1468
Lanoxin Injection Pediatric 1465

Diltiazem Hydrochloride (Co-administration of thiazide and other antihypertensive agents can lead to additive effect or potentiation). Products include:
Cardizem LA Extended Release Tablets 1699
Tiazac Capsules 1204

Doxazosin Mesylate (Co-administration of thiazide and other antihypertensive agents can lead to additive effect or potentiation).
No products indexed under this heading.

Enalapril Maleate (Co-administration of thiazide and other antihypertensive agents can lead to additive effect or potentiation). Products include:
Vaseretic Tablets 2073
Vasotec I.V. Injection 2076

Enalaprilat (Co-administration of thiazide and other antihypertensive agents can lead to additive effect or potentiation).
No products indexed under this heading.

Eprosartan Mesylate (Co-administration of thiazide and other antihypertensive agents can lead to additive effect or potentiation). Products include:
Teveten Tablets 1707
Teveten HCT Tablets 1710

Esmolol Hydrochloride (Co-administration of thiazide and other antihypertensive agents can lead to additive effect or potentiation). Products include:
Brevibloc Concentrate 766
Brevibloc Injection 766
Brevibloc Double Strength Injection.. 766
Brevibloc Premixed Injection 766
Brevibloc Double Strength Premixed Injection........................ 766

Ethacrynic Acid (Co-administration of lisinopril in patients on diuretics, especially those in whom diuretic therapy was recently instituted, may occasionally experience excessive hypotension; antihypertensive effects of lisinopril are augmented by antihypertensive agents that cause renin release). Products include:
Edecrin Tablets 1941

Etodolac (Co-administration in some patients with compromised renal function who are being treated with NSAIDs may result in a further deterioration of renal function: NSAID may reduce the diuretic, natriuretic and antihypertensive effects of thiazide).
No products indexed under this heading.

Felodipine (Co-administration of thiazide and other antihypertensive agents can lead to additive effect or potentiation). Products include:
Plendil Extended-Release Tablets 651

Fenoprofen Calcium (Co-administration in some patients with compromised renal function who are being treated with NSAIDs may result in a further deterioration of renal function: NSAID may reduce the diuretic, natriuretic and antihypertensive effects of thiazide). Products include:
Nalfon Capsules 2504

Fentanyl (Co-administration of thiazide and narcotics may potentiate orthostatic hypotension). Products include:
Duragesic Transdermal System 2448

Fentanyl Citrate (Co-administration of thiazide and narcotics may potentiate orthostatic hypotension). Products include:
Actiq 993

Fludrocortisone Acetate (Co-administration of thiazide diuretics with corticosteroids intensifies electrolyte depletion, particularly potassium).
No products indexed under this heading.

Flurbiprofen (Co-administration in some patients with compromised renal function who are being treated with NSAIDs may result in a further deterioration of renal function: NSAID may reduce the diuretic, natriuretic and antihypertensive effects of thiazide).
No products indexed under this heading.

Fosinopril Sodium (Co-administration of thiazide and other antihypertensive agents can lead to additive effect or potentiation).
No products indexed under this heading.

Furosemide (Co-administration of lisinopril in patients on diuretics, especially those in whom diuretic therapy was recently instituted, may occasionally experience excessive hypotension; antihypertensive effects of lisinopril are augmented by antihypertensive agents that cause renin release). Products include:
Furosemide Tablets 2117

Glimepiride (Hyperglycemia may occur with thiazide diuretics; dosage adjustment of oral hypoglycemic agents may be required). Products include:
Amaryl Tablets 2864

Glipizide (Hyperglycemia may occur with thiazide diuretics; dosage adjustment of oral hypoglycemic agents may be required).
No products indexed under this heading.

Glyburide (Hyperglycemia may occur with thiazide diuretics; dosage adjustment of oral hypoglycemic agents may be required).
No products indexed under this heading.

IMPORTANT NOTE: Always consult each drug listing in the patient's regimen for possible interactions.

Guanabenz Acetate (Co-administration of thiazide and other antihypertensive agents can lead to additive effect or potentiation).
No products indexed under this heading.

Guanethidine Monosulfate (Co-administration of thiazide and other antihypertensive agents can lead to additive effect or potentiation).
No products indexed under this heading.

Hydralazine Hydrochloride (Co-administration of thiazide and other antihypertensive agents can lead to additive effect or potentiation). Products include:
BiDil Tablets 2161

Hydrocodone Bitartrate (Co-administration of thiazide and narcotics may potentiate orthostatic hypotension). Products include:
Hycodan 1104
Hycomine Compound Tablets 1105
Hycotuss Expectorant Syrup 1106
Lortab 3315
Lortab Elixir 3312
Vicodin Tablets 530
Vicodin ES Tablets 531
Vicodin HP Tablets 532
Vicoprofen Tablets 533
Zydone Tablets 1118

Hydrocodone Polistirex (Co-administration of thiazide and narcotics may potentiate orthostatic hypotension). Products include:
Tussionex Pennkinetic Extended-Release Suspension 3322

Hydrocortisone (Co-administration of thiazide diuretics with corticosteroids intensifies electrolyte depletion, particularly potassium). Products include:
Cortizone•5 Ointment .... ▣699
Cortizone•10 Creme .... ▣699
Cortizone•10 Ointment .... ▣699
Cortizone•10 Plus Creme .... ▣700
Cortizone•10 Maximum Strength Quick Shot Spray .... ▣700
Hydrocortone Tablets 1963
Preparation H Hydrocortisone Cream .... ▣748

Hydrocortisone Acetate (Co-administration of thiazide diuretics with corticosteroids intensifies electrolyte depletion, particularly potassium). Products include:
Analpram-HC 1136
Pramosone 1139
ProctoFoam-HC 3113
Tucks Anti-Itch Ointment .... ▣712
U-cort 1% Cream 3289

Hydrocortisone Sodium Phosphate (Co-administration of thiazide diuretics with corticosteroids intensifies electrolyte depletion, particularly potassium).
No products indexed under this heading.

Hydrocortisone Sodium Succinate (Co-administration of thiazide diuretics with corticosteroids intensifies electrolyte depletion, particularly potassium).
No products indexed under this heading.

Hydroflumethiazide (Co-administration of lisinopril in patients on diuretics, especially those in whom diuretic therapy was recently instituted, may occasionally experience excessive hypotension; antihypertensive effects of lisinopril are augmented by antihypertensive agents that cause renin release).
No products indexed under this heading.

Hydromorphone Hydrochloride (Co-administration of thiazide and narcotics may potentiate orthostatic hypotension). Products include:
Dilaudid 439
Dilaudid Oral Liquid 443
Dilaudid Non-Sterile Powder 439
Dilaudid Rectal Suppositories 439
Dilaudid Tablets 439
Dilaudid Tablets - 8 mg 443
Dilaudid-HP 441

Ibuprofen (Co-administration in some patients with compromised renal function who are being treated with NSAIDs may result in a further deterioration of renal function: NSAID may reduce the diuretic, natriuretic and antihypertensive effects of thiazide). Products include:
Advil Allergy Sinus Caplets .... ▣737
Advil .... ▣737
Children's Advil Suspension .... ▣742
Children's Advil Chewable Tablets .. ▣741
Advil Cold & Sinus .... ▣739
Advil Flu & Body Ache Caplets .... ▣739
Children's Advil Cold Suspension ... ▣741
Infants' Advil Concentrated Drops .. ▣743
Junior Strength Advil Swallow Tablets .... ▣740
Advil Migraine Liquigels .... ▣740
Advil Multi-Symptom Cold Caplets .... ▣738
Combunox Tablets 1183
Children's Motrin Oral Suspension and Chewable Tablets 1837
Children's Motrin Cold Non-Staining Dye-Free Oral Suspension 1838
Children's Motrin Cold Oral Suspension 1838
Children's Motrin Non-Staining Dye-Free Oral Suspension 1837
Motrin Cold & Sinus Caplets 1836
Motrin IB Tablets and Caplets 1836
Infants' Motrin Concentrated Drops 1837
Infants' Motrin Non-Staining Dye-Free Drops 1837
Junior Strength Motrin Caplets and Chewable Tablets 1837
Vicoprofen Tablets 533

Indapamide (Co-administration of lisinopril in patients on diuretics, especially those in whom diuretic therapy was recently instituted, may occasionally experience excessive hypotension; antihypertensive effects of lisinopril are augmented by antihypertensive agents that cause renin release). Products include:
Indapamide Tablets 2119

Indomethacin (Co-administration in some patients with compromised renal function who are being treated with NSAIDs may result in a further deterioration of renal function: NSAID may reduce the diuretic, natriuretic and antihypertensive effects of thiazide). Products include:
Indocin 1968

Indomethacin Sodium Trihydrate (Co-administration in some patients with compromised renal function who are being treated with NSAIDs may result in a further deterioration of renal function: NSAID may reduce the diuretic, natriuretic and antihypertensive effects of thiazide). Products include:
Indocin I.V. 1973

Insulin, Human, Zinc Suspension (Hyperglycemia may occur with thiazide diuretics; dosage adjustment of insulin may be required). Products include:
Humulin L, 100 Units 1763
Humulin U, 100 Units 1770

Insulin, Human NPH (Hyperglycemia may occur with thiazide diuretics; dosage adjustment of insulin may be required). Products include:
Humulin N, 100 Units 1764
Humulin N Pen 1765
Novolin N Human Insulin 10 ml Vials 2322
Novolin N InnoLet 2322
Novolin N PenFill 3 ml Cartridges 2325
Novolin R InnoLet 2322

Insulin, Human Regular (Hyperglycemia may occur with thiazide diuretics; dosage adjustment of insulin may be required). Products include:
Humulin R (U-500) 1768
Humulin R, 100 Units 1767
Novolin R Human Insulin 10 ml Vials 2322
Novolin R PenFill 2325

Insulin, Human Regular and Human NPH Mixture (Hyperglycemia may occur with thiazide diuretics; dosage adjustment of insulin may be required). Products include:
Humulin 50/50, 100 Units 1760
Humulin 70/30 Pen 1761
Novolin 70/30 Human Insulin 10 ml Vials 2321
Novolin 70/30 InnoLet 2322
Novolin 70/30 PenFill 3 ml Cartridges 2325

Insulin, NPH (Hyperglycemia may occur with thiazide diuretics; dosage adjustment of insulin may be required).
No products indexed under this heading.

Insulin, Regular (Hyperglycemia may occur with thiazide diuretics; dosage adjustment of insulin may be required).
No products indexed under this heading.

Insulin, Zinc Crystals (Hyperglycemia may occur with thiazide diuretics; dosage adjustment of insulin may be required).
No products indexed under this heading.

Insulin, Zinc Suspension (Hyperglycemia may occur with thiazide diuretics; dosage adjustment of insulin may be required).
No products indexed under this heading.

Insulin Aspart, Human Regular (Hyperglycemia may occur with thiazide diuretics; dosage adjustment of insulin may be required). Products include:
NovoLog Injection 2326

Insulin glargine (Hyperglycemia may occur with thiazide diuretics; dosage adjustment of insulin may be required). Products include:
Lantus Injection 2925

Insulin Lispro, Human (Hyperglycemia may occur with thiazide diuretics; dosage adjustment of insulin may be required). Products include:
Humalog-Pen 1751
Humalog Mix 75/25-Pen 1754

Insulin Lispro Protamine, Human (Hyperglycemia may occur with thiazide diuretics; dosage adjustment of insulin may be required). Products include:
Humalog Mix 75/25-Pen 1754

Irbesartan (Co-administration of thiazide and other antihypertensive agents can lead to additive effect or potentiation). Products include:
Avalide Tablets 922
Avalide Tablets 2889
Avapro Tablets 925
Avapro Tablets 2886

Isradipine (Co-administration of thiazide and other antihypertensive agents can lead to additive effect or potentiation). Products include:
DynaCirc CR Tablets 2726

Ketoprofen (Co-administration in some patients with compromised renal function who are being treated with NSAIDs may result in a further deterioration of renal function: NSAID may reduce the diuretic, natriuretic and antihypertensive effects of thiazide).
No products indexed under this heading.

Ketorolac Tromethamine (Co-administration in some patients with compromised renal function who are being treated with NSAIDs may result in a further deterioration of renal function: NSAID may reduce the diuretic, natriuretic and antihypertensive effects of thiazide). Products include:
Acular Ophthalmic Solution 561
Acular LS Ophthalmic Solution 562

Labetalol Hydrochloride (Co-administration of thiazide and other antihypertensive agents can lead to additive effect or potentiation).
No products indexed under this heading.

Levorphanol Tartrate (Co-administration of thiazide and narcotics may potentiate orthostatic hypotension).
No products indexed under this heading.

Lithium (Co-administration of lithium with drugs that cause elimination of sodium, including ACE inhibitors, can lead to lithium toxicity; diuretics can reduce renal clearance of lithium and add a high risk of lithium toxicity).
No products indexed under this heading.

Lithium Carbonate (Co-administration of lithium with drugs that cause elimination of sodium, including ACE inhibitors, can lead to lithium toxicity; diuretics can reduce renal clearance of lithium and add a high risk of lithium toxicity). Products include:
Eskalith 1406
Lithobid Tablets 1670

Lithium Citrate (Co-administration of lithium with drugs that cause elimination of sodium, including ACE inhibitors, can lead to lithium toxicity; diuretics can reduce renal clearance of lithium and add a high risk of lithium toxicity).
No products indexed under this heading.

Losartan Potassium (Co-administration of thiazide and other antihypertensive agents can lead to additive effect or potentiation). Products include:
Cozaar Tablets 1913
Hyzaar 1964

Mecamylamine Hydrochloride (Co-administration of thiazide and other antihypertensive agents can lead to additive effect or potentiation). Products include:
Inversine Tablets 3286

Meclofenamate Sodium (Co-administration in some patients with compromised renal function who are being treated with NSAIDs may result in a further deterioration of renal function: NSAID may reduce the diuretic, natriuretic and antihypertensive effects of thiazide).
No products indexed under this heading.

Mefenamic Acid (Co-administration in some patients with compromised renal function who are being treated with NSAIDs may result in a further deterioration of renal function: NSAID may reduce the diuretic, natriuretic and antihypertensive effects of thiazide).
No products indexed under this heading.

Meloxicam (Co-administration in some patients with compromised renal function who are being treated with NSAIDs may result in a further deterioration of renal function: NSAID may reduce the diuretic, natriuretic and antihypertensive effects of thiazide). Products include:
Mobic Oral Suspension 893
Mobic Tablets 893

Meperidine Hydrochloride (Co-administration of thiazide and narcotics may potentiate orthostatic hypotension).
No products indexed under this heading.

Mephobarbital (Co-administration of thiazide and barbiturates may potentiate orthostatic hypotension). Products include:
Mebaral Tablets, USP 2483

Metformin Hydrochloride (Hyperglycemia may occur with thiazide diuretics; dosage adjustment of oral hypoglycemic agents may be required). Products include:
ActoPlus Met Tablets 3219
Avandamet Tablets 1343
Fortamet Extended-Release Tablets 1156

Methadone Hydrochloride (Co-administration of thiazide and narcotics may potentiate orthostatic hypotension).
No products indexed under this heading.

Methyclothiazide (Co-administration of lisinopril in patients on diuretics, especially those in whom diuretic therapy was recently instituted, may occasionally experience excessive hypotension; antihypertensive effects of lisinopril are augmented by antihypertensive agents that cause renin release).
No products indexed under this heading.

Methyldopa (Co-administration of thiazide and other antihypertensive agents can lead to additive effect or potentiation). Products include:
Aldoclor Tablets 1881
Aldoril Tablets 1884

Methyldopate Hydrochloride (Co-administration of thiazide and other antihypertensive agents can lead to additive effect or potentiation).
No products indexed under this heading.

Methylprednisolone Acetate (Co-administration of thiazide diuretics with corticosteroids intensifies electrolyte depletion, particularly potassium). Products include:
Depo-Medrol Injectable Suspension 2615
Depo-Medrol Single-Dose Vial 2617

Methylprednisolone Sodium Succinate (Co-administration of thiazide diuretics with corticosteroids intensifies electrolyte depletion, particularly potassium).
No products indexed under this heading.

Metocurine Iodide (Co-administration with nondepolarizing skeletal muscle relaxants may result in possible increased responsiveness to the muscle relaxant).
No products indexed under this heading.

Metolazone (Co-administration of lisinopril in patients on diuretics, especially those in whom diuretic therapy was recently instituted, may occasionally experience excessive hypotension; antihypertensive effects of lisinopril are augmented by antihypertensive agents that cause renin release).
No products indexed under this heading.

Metoprolol Succinate (Co-administration of thiazide and other antihypertensive agents can lead to additive effect or potentiation). Products include:
Toprol-XL Tablets 660

Metoprolol Tartrate (Co-administration of thiazide and other antihypertensive agents can lead to additive effect or potentiation).
No products indexed under this heading.

Metyrosine (Co-administration of thiazide and other antihypertensive agents can lead to additive effect or potentiation). Products include:
Demser Capsules 1933

Mibefradil Dihydrochloride (Co-administration of thiazide and other antihypertensive agents can lead to additive effect or potentiation).
No products indexed under this heading.

Miglitol (Hyperglycemia may occur with thiazide diuretics; dosage adjustment of oral hypoglycemic agents may be required).
No products indexed under this heading.

Minoxidil (Co-administration of thiazide and other antihypertensive agents can lead to additive effect or potentiation). Products include:
Men's Rogaine Extra Strength Topical Solution, Ocean Rush Scent and Original Unscented 706
Women's Rogaine Topical Solution, Spring Bloom Scent and Original Unscented 707

Mivacurium Chloride (Co-administration with nondepolarizing skeletal muscle relaxants may result in possible increased responsiveness to the muscle relaxant). Products include:
Mivacron Injection 489

Moexipril Hydrochloride (Co-administration of thiazide and other antihypertensive agents can lead to additive effect or potentiation). Products include:
Uniretic Tablets 3114
Univasc Tablets 3118

Morphine Sulfate (Co-administration of thiazide and narcotics may potentiate orthostatic hypotension). Products include:
Avinza Capsules 1714
Kadian Capsules 572
MS Contin Tablets 2703

Nabumetone (Co-administration in some patients with compromised renal function who are being treated with NSAIDs may result in a further deterioration of renal function: NSAID may reduce the diuretic, natriuretic and antihypertensive effects of thiazide). Products include:
Relafen Tablets 1523

Nadolol (Co-administration of thiazide and other antihypertensive agents can lead to additive effect or potentiation). Products include:
Nadolol Tablets 2121

Naproxen (Co-administration in some patients with compromised renal function who are being treated with NSAIDs may result in a further deterioration of renal function: NSAID may reduce the diuretic, natriuretic and antihypertensive effects of thiazide). Products include:
EC-Naprosyn Delayed-Release Tablets 2769
Naprosyn Suspension 2769
Naprosyn Tablets 2769
Prevacid NapraPAC 3277

Naproxen Sodium (Co-administration in some patients with compromised renal function who are being treated with NSAIDs may result in a further deterioration of renal function: NSAID may reduce the diuretic, natriuretic and antihypertensive effects of thiazide). Products include:
Aleve Tablets, Caplets and Gelcaps 605
Anaprox Tablets 2769
Anaprox DS Tablets 2769

Nicardipine Hydrochloride (Co-administration of thiazide and other antihypertensive agents can lead to additive effect or potentiation). Products include:
Cardene I.V. 1129

Nifedipine (Co-administration of thiazide and other antihypertensive agents can lead to additive effect or potentiation). Products include:
Adalat CC Tablets 2978

Nisoldipine (Co-administration of thiazide and other antihypertensive agents can lead to additive effect or potentiation). Products include:
Sular Tablets 1163

Nitroglycerin (Co-administration of thiazide and other antihypertensive agents can lead to additive effect or potentiation). Products include:
Nitro-Dur Transdermal Infusion System 3060
Nitrolingual Pumpspray 1161

Norepinephrine Bitartrate (Possible decreased response to pressor amines but not sufficient to preclude pressor amine use).
No products indexed under this heading.

Oxaprozin (Co-administration in some patients with compromised renal function who are being treated with NSAIDs may result in a further deterioration of renal function: NSAID may reduce the diuretic, natriuretic and antihypertensive effects of thiazide).
No products indexed under this heading.

Oxycodone Hydrochloride (Co-administration of thiazide and narcotics may potentiate orthostatic hypotension). Products include:
Combunox Tablets 1183
OxyContin Tablets 2699
OxyFast Oral Concentrate Solution 2704
OxyIR Capsules 2704
Percocet Tablets 1114
Percodan Tablets 1115

Pancuronium Bromide (Co-administration with nondepolarizing skeletal muscle relaxants may result in possible increased responsiveness to the muscle relaxant).
No products indexed under this heading.

Penbutolol Sulfate (Co-administration of thiazide and other antihypertensive agents can lead to additive effect or potentiation).
No products indexed under this heading.

Pentobarbital Sodium (Co-administration of thiazide and barbiturates may potentiate orthostatic hypotension). Products include:
Nembutal Sodium Solution, USP 2484

Perindopril Erbumine (Co-administration of thiazide and other antihypertensive agents can lead to additive effect or potentiation). Products include:
Aceon Tablets (2 mg, 4 mg, 8 mg) 3191

Phenobarbital (Co-administration of thiazide and barbiturates may potentiate orthostatic hypotension).
No products indexed under this heading.

Phenoxybenzamine Hydrochloride (Co-administration of thiazide and other antihypertensive agents can lead to additive effect or potentiation). Products include:
Dibenzyline Capsules 3390

Phentolamine Mesylate (Co-administration of thiazide and other antihypertensive agents can lead to additive effect or potentiation).
No products indexed under this heading.

Phenylbutazone (Co-administration in some patients with compromised renal function who are being treated with NSAIDs may result in a further deterioration of renal function: NSAID may reduce the diuretic, natriuretic and antihypertensive effects of thiazide).
No products indexed under this heading.

Pindolol (Co-administration of thiazide and other antihypertensive agents can lead to additive effect or potentiation).
No products indexed under this heading.

Pioglitazone Hydrochloride (Hyperglycemia may occur with thiazide diuretics; dosage adjustment of oral hypoglycemic agents may be required). Products include:
ActoPlus Met Tablets 3219
Actos Tablets 3224

Piroxicam (Co-administration in some patients with compromised renal function who are being treated with NSAIDs may result in a further deterioration of renal function: NSAID may reduce the diuretic, natriuretic and antihypertensive effects of thiazide).
No products indexed under this heading.

IMPORTANT NOTE: Always consult each drug listing in the patient's regimen for possible interactions.

Polythiazide (Co-administration of lisinopril in patients on diuretics, especially those in whom diuretic therapy was recently instituted, may occasionally experience excessive hypotension; antihypertensive effects of lisinopril are augmented by antihypertensive agents that cause renin release).
No products indexed under this heading.

Potassium Acid Phosphate (Concomitant use of potassium-containing salt substitute or potassium supplements can lead to hyperkalemia; frequent monitoring of serum potassium is recommended if used concurrently). Products include:
K-Phos Original (Sodium Free) Tablets 785

Potassium Bicarbonate (Concomitant use of potassium-containing salt substitute or potassium supplements can lead to hyperkalemia; frequent monitoring of serum potassium is recommended if used concurrently).
No products indexed under this heading.

Potassium Chloride (Concomitant use of potassium-containing salt substitute or potassium supplements can lead to hyperkalemia; frequent monitoring of serum potassium is recommended if used concurrently). Products include:
Colyte with Flavor Packs for Oral Solution 3102
HalfLytely and Bisacodyl Tablets Bowel Prep Kit with Flavors Packs 915
K-Dur Extended-Relase Tablets 3047
K-Lor Powder Packets 472
K-Tab Filmtab Tablets 473
TriLyte with Flavor Packs for Oral Solution 3114

Potassium Citrate (Concomitant use of potassium-containing salt substitute or potassium supplements can lead to hyperkalemia; frequent monitoring of serum potassium is recommended if used concurrently). Products include:
Urocit-K Tablets 2109

Potassium Gluconate (Concomitant use of potassium-containing salt substitute or potassium supplements can lead to hyperkalemia; frequent monitoring of serum potassium is recommended if used concurrently).
No products indexed under this heading.

Potassium Phosphate (Concomitant use of potassium-containing salt substitute or potassium supplements can lead to hyperkalemia; frequent monitoring of serum potassium is recommended if used concurrently). Products include:
K-Phos Neutral Tablets 785

Prazosin Hydrochloride (Co-administration of thiazide and other antihypertensive agents can lead to additive effect or potentiation).
No products indexed under this heading.

Prednisolone Acetate (Co-administration of thiazide diuretics with corticosteroids intensifies electrolyte depletion, particularly potassium). Products include:
Blephamide Ophthalmic Ointment 563
Blephamide Ophthalmic Suspension 564
Poly-Pred Liquifilm Ophthalmic Suspension .... ⊙231
Pred Forte Ophthalmic Suspension .... ⊙233
Pred Mild Sterile Ophthalmic Suspension .... ⊙236
Pred-G Ophthalmic Suspension .... ⊙234
Pred-G Sterile Ophthalmic Ointment .... ⊙235

Prednisolone Sodium Phosphate (Co-administration of thiazide diuretics with corticosteroids intensifies electrolyte depletion, particularly potassium). Products include:
Pediapred Oral Solution 3319

Prednisolone Tebutate (Co-administration of thiazide diuretics with corticosteroids intensifies electrolyte depletion, particularly potassium).
No products indexed under this heading.

Prednisone (Co-administration of thiazide diuretics with corticosteroids intensifies electrolyte depletion, particularly potassium).
No products indexed under this heading.

Propoxyphene Hydrochloride (Co-administration of thiazide and narcotics may potentiate orthostatic hypotension).
No products indexed under this heading.

Propoxyphene Napsylate (Co-administration of thiazide and narcotics may potentiate orthostatic hypotension). Products include:
Darvocet A 500 Tablets 3497

Propranolol Hydrochloride (Co-administration of thiazide and other antihypertensive agents can lead to additive effect or potentiation). Products include:
Inderal LA Long-Acting Capsules 3421
InnoPran XL Capsules 2728

Quinapril Hydrochloride (Co-administration of thiazide and other antihypertensive agents can lead to additive effect or potentiation).
No products indexed under this heading.

Ramipril (Co-administration of thiazide and other antihypertensive agents can lead to additive effect or potentiation). Products include:
Altace Capsules 1673

Rapacuronium Bromide (Co-administration with nondepolarizing skeletal muscle relaxants may result in possible increased responsiveness to the muscle relaxant).
No products indexed under this heading.

Rauwolfia Serpentina (Co-administration of thiazide and other antihypertensive agents can lead to additive effect or potentiation).
No products indexed under this heading.

Remifentanil Hydrochloride (Co-administration of thiazide and narcotics may potentiate orthostatic hypotension).
No products indexed under this heading.

Repaglinide (Hyperglycemia may occur with thiazide diuretics; dosage adjustment of oral hypoglycemic agents may be required). Products include:
Prandin Tablets (0.5, 1, and 2 mg) 2337

Rescinnamine (Co-administration of thiazide and other antihypertensive agents can lead to additive effect or potentiation).
No products indexed under this heading.

Reserpine (Co-administration of thiazide and other antihypertensive agents can lead to additive effect or potentiation).
No products indexed under this heading.

Rocuronium Bromide (Co-administration with nondepolarizing skeletal muscle relaxants may result in possible increased responsiveness to the muscle relaxant). Products include:
Zemuron Injection 2363

Rofecoxib (Co-administration in some patients with compromised renal function who are being treated with NSAIDs may result in a further deterioration of renal function: NSAID may reduce the diuretic, natriuretic and antihypertensive effects of thiazide).
No products indexed under this heading.

Rosiglitazone Maleate (Hyperglycemia may occur with thiazide diuretics; dosage adjustment of oral hypoglycemic agents may be required). Products include:
Avandamet Tablets 1343
Avandia Tablets 1348

Secobarbital Sodium (Co-administration of thiazide and barbiturates may potentiate orthostatic hypotension).
No products indexed under this heading.

Sodium Nitroprusside (Co-administration of thiazide and other antihypertensive agents can lead to additive effect or potentiation).
No products indexed under this heading.

Sotalol Hydrochloride (Co-administration of thiazide and other antihypertensive agents can lead to additive effect or potentiation).
No products indexed under this heading.

Spirapril Hydrochloride (Co-administration of thiazide and other antihypertensive agents can lead to additive effect or potentiation).
No products indexed under this heading.

Spironolactone (Lisinopril attenuates diuretic-induced potassium loss; concomitant use can lead to hyperkalemia; frequent monitoring of serum potassium is recommended if used concurrently; co-administration can result in excessive hypotension).
No products indexed under this heading.

Sufentanil Citrate (Co-administration of thiazide and narcotics may potentiate orthostatic hypotension).
No products indexed under this heading.

Sulindac (Co-administration in some patients with compromised renal function who are being treated with NSAIDs may result in a further deterioration of renal function: NSAID may reduce the diuretic, natriuretic and antihypertensive effects of thiazide). Products include:
Clinoril Tablets 1899

Telmisartan (Co-administration of thiazide and other antihypertensive agents can lead to additive effect or potentiation). Products include:
Micardis Tablets 884
Micardis HCT Tablets 886

Terazosin Hydrochloride (Co-administration of thiazide and other antihypertensive agents can lead to additive effect or potentiation). Products include:
Hytrin Capsules 469

Thiamylal Sodium (Co-administration of thiazide and barbiturates may potentiate orthostatic hypotension).
No products indexed under this heading.

Timolol Maleate (Co-administration of thiazide and other antihypertensive agents can lead to additive effect or potentiation). Products include:
Blocadren Tablets 1891
Cosopt Sterile Ophthalmic Solution 1910
Timolide Tablets 2056
Timoptic in Ocudose 2061
Timoptic Sterile Ophthalmic Solution 2058
Timoptic-XE Sterile Ophthalmic Gel Forming Solution 2062

Tolazamide (Hyperglycemia may occur with thiazide diuretics; dosage adjustment of oral hypoglycemic agents may be required).
No products indexed under this heading.

Tolbutamide (Hyperglycemia may occur with thiazide diuretics; dosage adjustment of oral hypoglycemic agents may be required).
No products indexed under this heading.

Tolmetin Sodium (Co-administration in some patients with compromised renal function who are being treated with NSAIDs may result in a further deterioration of renal function: NSAID may reduce the diuretic, natriuretic and antihypertensive effects of thiazide).
No products indexed under this heading.

Torsemide (Co-administration of lisinopril in patients on diuretics, especially those in whom diuretic therapy was recently instituted, may occasionally experience excessive hypotension; antihypertensive effects of lisinopril are augmented by antihypertensive agents that cause renin release).
No products indexed under this heading.

Trandolapril (Co-administration of thiazide and other antihypertensive agents can lead to additive effect or potentiation). Products include:
Mavik Tablets 482
Tarka Tablets 519

Triamcinolone (Co-administration of thiazide diuretics with corticosteroids intensifies electrolyte depletion, particularly potassium).
No products indexed under this heading.

Triamcinolone Acetonide (Co-administration of thiazide diuretics with corticosteroids intensifies electrolyte depletion, particularly potassium). Products include:
Azmacort Inhalation Aerosol 1701
Nasacort HFA Inhalation Aerosol 2939
Nasacort AQ Nasal Spray 2937

Triamcinolone Diacetate (Co-administration of thiazide diuretics with corticosteroids intensifies electrolyte depletion, particularly potassium).
No products indexed under this heading.

Triamcinolone Hexacetonide (Co-administration of thiazide diuretics with corticosteroids intensifies electrolyte depletion, particularly potassium).
No products indexed under this heading.

Triamterene (Lisinopril attenuates diuretic-induced potassium loss; concomitant use can lead to hyperkalemia; frequent monitoring of serum potassium is recommended if used concurrently; co-administration can result in excessive hypotension). Products include:
- Dyazide Capsules 1389
- Dyrenium Capsules 3390
- Maxzide 2150

Trimethaphan Camsylate (Co-administration of thiazide and other antihypertensive agents can lead to additive effect or potentiation).
No products indexed under this heading.

Troglitazone (Hyperglycemia may occur with thiazide diuretics; dosage adjustment of oral hypoglycemic agents may be required).
No products indexed under this heading.

Valdecoxib (Co-administration in some patients with compromised renal function who are being treated with NSAIDs may result in a further deterioration of renal function: NSAID may reduce the diuretic, natriuretic and antihypertensive effects of thiazide).
No products indexed under this heading.

Valsartan (Co-administration of thiazide and other antihypertensive agents can lead to additive effect or potentiation). Products include:
- Diovan HCT Tablets 2195
- Diovan Tablets 2191

Vecuronium Bromide (Co-administration with nondepolarizing skeletal muscle relaxants may result in possible increased responsiveness to the muscle relaxant).
No products indexed under this heading.

Verapamil Hydrochloride (Co-administration of thiazide and other antihypertensive agents can lead to additive effect or potentiation). Products include:
- Covera-HS Tablets 3135
- Tarka Tablets 519
- Verelan PM Capsules 3120

Food Interactions

Alcohol (Co-administration of thiazide and alcohol may potentiate orthostatic hypotension).

PROAMATINE TABLETS

(Midodrine Hydrochloride) 3183

May interact with alpha adrenergic blockers, cardiac glycosides, quinidine, and certain other agents. Compounds in these categories include:

Cimetidine (The high renal clearance of desglymidodrine is due to active tubular secretion by the base-secreting system also responsible for the secretion of cimetidine; possibility of drug interaction exists with co-administration). Products include:
- Tagamet HB 200 Tablets 637
- Tagamet Tablets 1547

Deslanoside (Co-administration with cardiac glycosides may enhance or precipitate bradycardia, AV block or arrhythmia).
No products indexed under this heading.

Digitalis Glycoside Preparations (Co-administration with cardiac glycosides may enhance or precipitate bradycardia, AV block or arrhythmia).
No products indexed under this heading.

Digitoxin (Co-administration with cardiac glycosides may enhance or precipitate bradycardia, AV block or arrhythmia).
No products indexed under this heading.

Digoxin (Co-administration with cardiac glycosides may enhance or precipitate bradycardia, AV block or arrhythmia). Products include:
- Digitek Tablets 2146
- Lanoxicaps Capsules 1458
- Lanoxin Injection 1462
- Lanoxin Tablets 1468
- Lanoxin Injection Pediatric 1465

Dihydroergotamine Mesylate (Co-administration with alpha-adrenergic receptor stimulants may enhance or potentiate pressor effects of midodrine). Products include:
- Migranal Nasal Spray 3350

Doxazosin Mesylate (Alpha adrenergic blocking agents can antagonize the effects of midodrine).
No products indexed under this heading.

Ephedrine Hydrochloride (Co-administration with alpha-adrenergic receptor stimulants may enhance or potentiate pressor effects of midodrine). Products include:
- Primatene Tablets 749

Ephedrine Sulfate (Co-administration with alpha-adrenergic receptor stimulants may enhance or potentiate pressor effects of midodrine).
No products indexed under this heading.

Ephedrine Tannate (Co-administration with alpha-adrenergic receptor stimulants may enhance or potentiate pressor effects of midodrine).
No products indexed under this heading.

Flecainide Acetate (The high renal clearance of desglymidodrine is due to active tubular secretion by the base-secreting system also responsible for the secretion of flecainide; possibility of drug interaction exists with co-administration). Products include:
- Tambocor Tablets 1824

Fludrocortisone Acetate (Co-administration with salt-retaining steroid therapy increases the potential for supine hypertension; this can be minimized by reducing the dose of fludrocortisone or decreasing salt intake).
No products indexed under this heading.

Metformin (The high renal clearance of desglymidodrine is due to active tubular secretion by the base-secreting system also responsible for the secretion of metformin; possibility of drug interaction exists with co-administration).
No products indexed under this heading.

Phenylephrine Hydrochloride (Co-administration with alpha-adrenergic receptor stimulants may enhance or potentiate pressor effects of midodrine). Products include:
- Alacol DM Syrup 739
- Hycomine Compound Tablets 1105
- Preparation H Maximum Strength Cream 747
- Preparation H Cooling Gel 747
- Preparation H 747
- Sudafed PE Tablets 711
- Vicks Sinex Nasal Spray and Ultra Fine Mist for Sinus Relief 2677
- Zicam Concentrated Cough Mist for Kids Plus D Cool Cherry 643
- Zicam Concentrated Cough Mist Plus D Cool Cherry 642

Phenylephrine Tannate (Co-administration with alpha-adrenergic receptor stimulants may enhance or potentiate pressor effects of midodrine).
No products indexed under this heading.

Prazosin Hydrochloride (Alpha adrenergic blocking agents can antagonize the effects of midodrine).
No products indexed under this heading.

Procainamide Hydrochloride (The high renal clearance of desglymidodrine is due to active tubular secretion by the base-secreting system also responsible for the secretion of procainamide; possibility of drug interaction exists with co-administration).
No products indexed under this heading.

Pseudoephedrine Hydrochloride (Co-administration with alpha-adrenergic receptor stimulants may enhance or potentiate pressor effects of midodrine). Products include:
- Advil Allergy Sinus Caplets 737
- Advil Cold & Sinus 739
- Advil Flu & Body Ache Caplets 739
- Children's Advil Cold Suspension 741
- Advil Multi-Symptom Cold Caplets 738
- Allegra-D 12 Hour Extended-Release Tablets 2860
- Allegra-D 24 Hour Extended-Release Tablets 2862
- Balamine DM 739
- BC Cold Powder 612
- Benadryl Allergy & Cold Tablets 692
- Benadryl Allergy & Sinus Headache Caplets & Gelcaps 693
- Children's Benadryl Allergy & Cold Fastmelt Tablets 695
- Benadryl Maximum Strength Severe Allergy & Sinus Headache Caplets 694
- Children's Benadryl D Allergy & Sinus Fastmelt Tablets 694
- Children's Benadryl D Liquid Medication 693
- Benadryl D Tablets 694
- Contac Non-Drowsy 12 Hour Cold Caplets 614
- Contac Non-Drowsy Timed Release 12 Hour Cold Caplets 615
- Contac Severe Cold and Flu Caplets Maximum Strength 615
- Contac Severe Cold and Flu Caplets Non-Drowsy 615
- Children's Dimetapp Cold & Allergy Elixir 745
- Children's Dimetapp DM Cold & Cough Elixir 745
- Children's Dimetapp Long Acting Cough Plus Cold Syrup 746
- Dimetapp Infant Drops Decongestant Plus Cough 746
- Children's Motrin Cold Non-Staining Dye-Free Oral Suspension 1838
- Children's Motrin Cold Oral Suspension 1838
- Motrin Cold & Sinus Caplets 1836
- PediaCare Decongestant & Cough Infant Drops 705
- PediaCare Decongestant Infants' Drops 705
- PediaCare Long-Acting Cough Plus Cold Liquid 704
- PediaCare Multi-Symptom Cold Liquid 704
- PediaCare NightRest Cough & Cold Liquid 704
- Robitussin Allergy & Cough Syrup 750
- Robitussin CF Liquid 755
- Robitussin Cough & Cold Liquid-filled Capsules 750
- Robitussin Cough, Cold & Flu Liquid-filled Capsules 750
- Robitussin Cough & Cold Infant Drops 755
- Robitussin Flu Liquid 752
- Robitussin Maximum Strength Cough & Cold Liquid 754
- Robitussin PE Syrup 753
- Robitussin Pediatric Cough & Cold Liquid 754
- Robitussin PM Cough & Cold Liquid 752
- Robitussin Severe Congestion Liquid-filled Capsules 751
- Simply Stuffy Liquid 1841
- Singlet Caplets 636
- Sudafed 12 Hour Caplets 708
- Sudafed 24 Hour Tablets 709
- Sudafed Nasal Decongestant Tablets 709
- Sudafed Severe Cold 710
- Sudafed Non-Drying Sinus Liquid Caps 709
- Sudafed Sinus & Allergy Tablets 710
- Sudafed Sinus Headache 711
- TheraFlu Cold & Cough Hot Liquid 680
- TheraFlu Cold & Sore Throat Hot Liquid 680
- TheraFlu Flu & Chest Congestion Non-Drowsy Hot Liquid 681
- TheraFlu Flu & Sore Throat Hot Liquid 681
- TheraFlu Severe Cold Non-Drowsy Hot Liquid 683
- TheraFlu Severe Cold & Cough Hot Liquid 683
- TheraFlu Severe Cold Caplets 679
- TheraFlu Severe Cold Hot Liquid 682
- TheraFlu Severe Cold Non-Drowsy Caplets 679
- Triaminic Chest & Nasal Congestion Liquid 685
- Triaminic Cold & Allergy Liquid 685
- Triaminic Cold & Cough Liquid 685
- Triaminic Cough Liquid 687
- Triaminic Cough & Nasal Congestion Liquid 687
- Triaminic Cough & Sore Throat Liquid 687
- Triaminic Flu, Cough & Fever Liquid 685
- Triaminic Night Time Cough & Cold Liquid 685
- Triaminic Allergy Runny Nose & Congestion Softchews 688
- Triaminic Cold & Cough Softchews 688
- Triaminic Cough & Sore Throat Softchews 689
- Tylenol Sinus NightTime Caplets 663
- Children's Tylenol Plus Cold & Allergy Suspension Liquid 1850
- Children's Tylenol Plus Cold NightTime Suspension Liquid 1851
- Children's Tylenol Plus Cold & Cough Suspension Liquid and Chewable Tablets 1851
- Children's Tylenol Plus Cold Chewable Tablets 1851
- Children's Tylenol Plus Cold Daytime Non-Drowsy Suspension Liquid 1851
- Children's Tylenol Plus Flu Suspension Liquid 1853
- Concentrated Tylenol Infants' Drops Plus Cold 1851
- Concentrated Tylenol Infants' Drops Plus Cold and Cough 1851
- Tylenol Cold & Flu Severe Daytime Liquid with Cool Bust 1846
- Tylenol Cold & Flu Severe NightTime Liquid with Cool Burst 1846
- Tylenol Cold Severe Congestion Non-Drowsy Caplets with Cool Burst 1846

Tylenol Allergy Complete Night Time Caplets 1844
Tylenol Allergy Complete Multi-Symptom Caplets and Gelcaps with Cool Burst 1844
Tylenol Flu NightTime Gelcaps 1846
Tylenol Flu Day Non-Drowsy Gelcaps 1846
Concentrated Tylenol Infants' Drops Plus Cold Nasal Congestant, Fever Reducer & Pain Reliever .... ▣668
Concentrated Tylenol Infants' Drops Plus Cold & Cough Nasal Decongestant, Fever Reducer & Pain Reliever .... ▣668
Multi-Symptom Tylenol Cold Night Time Caplets 1845
Multi-Symptom Tylenol Cold Day Non-Drowsy Caplets and Gelcaps 1845
Tylenol Sinus Day Non-Drowsy 1848
Tylenol Sinus Night Time Caplets 1848
Tylenol Sinus Severe Congestion Caplets with Cool Burst 1848
Vicks 44D Cough & Head Congestion Relief 2676
Vicks 44D Cough & Head Congestion Relief Liquid .... ▣721
Vicks 44M Cough, Cold & Flu Relief 2676
Pediatric Vicks 44m Cough & Cold Relief 2673
Vicks DayQuil LiquiCaps/Liquid Multi-Symptom Cold/Flu Relief .... ▣723
Vicks DayQuil Multi-Symptom Cold/Flu Relief LiquiCaps 2675
Vicks DayQuil Multi-Symptom Cold/Flu Relief Liquid 2675
Children's Vicks NyQuil Cold/Cough Relief 2671
Vicks NyQuil LiquiCaps 2677
Vicks NyQuil LiquiCaps/Liquid Multi-Symptom Cold/Flu Relief .... ▣725
Vicks NyQuil Liquid 2677
Zyrtec-D 12 Hour Extended Release Tablets 2591

Pseudoephedrine Sulfate (Co-administration with alpha-adrenergic receptor stimulants may enhance or potentiate pressor effects of midodrine). Products include:
Alavert Allergy & Sinus D-12 Hour Tablets .... ▣743
Clarinex-D 24-Hour Extended-Release Tablets 3012
Claritin-D Non-Drowsy 12 Hour Tablets .... ▣731
Claritin-D Non-Drowsy 24 Hour Tablets .... ▣731

Quinidine (The high renal clearance of desglymidodrine is due to active tubular secretion by the base-secreting system also responsible for the secretion of quinidine; possibility of drug interaction exists with co-administration).
No products indexed under this heading.

Quinidine Gluconate (The high renal clearance of desglymidodrine is due to active tubular secretion by the base-secreting system also responsible for the secretion of quinidine; possibility of drug interaction exists with co-administration).
No products indexed under this heading.

Quinidine Hydrochloride (The high renal clearance of desglymidodrine is due to active tubular secretion by the base-secreting system also responsible for the secretion of quinidine; possibility of drug interaction exists with co-administration).
No products indexed under this heading.

Quinidine Polygalacturonate (The high renal clearance of desglymidodrine is due to active tubular secretion by the base-secreting system also responsible for the secretion of quinidine; possibility of drug interaction exists with co-administration).
No products indexed under this heading.

Quinidine Sulfate (The high renal clearance of desglymidodrine is due to active tubular secretion by the base-secreting system also responsible for the secretion of quinidine; possibility of drug interaction exists with co-administration).
No products indexed under this heading.

Ranitidine Hydrochloride (The high renal clearance of desglymidodrine is due to active tubular secretion by the base-secreting system also responsible for the secretion of ranitidine; possibility of drug interaction exists with co-administration). Products include:
Zantac 1597
Zantac Injection 1593
Zantac 75 Tablets .... ▣715
Zantac 150 Maximum Strength Tablets .... ▣715
Zantac Injection Pharmacy Bulk Package 1595

Tamsulosin Hydrochloride (Alpha adrenergic blocking agents can antagonize the effects of midodrine). Products include:
Flomax Capsules 881

Terazosin Hydrochloride (Alpha adrenergic blocking agents can antagonize the effects of midodrine). Products include:
Hytrin Capsules 469

Triamterene (The high renal clearance of desglymidodrine is due to active tubular secretion by the base-secreting system also responsible for the secretion of triamterene; possibility of drug interaction exists with co-administration). Products include:
Dyazide Capsules 1389
Dyrenium Capsules 3390
Maxzide 2150

PROCHIEVE 4% GEL
(Progesterone) 1018
None cited in PDR database.

PROCHIEVE 8% GEL
(Progesterone) 1018
None cited in PDR database.

PROCOSA II TABLETS
(Glucosamine Sulfate) 3343
None cited in PDR database.

PROCRIT FOR INJECTION
(Epoetin Alfa) 2374
None cited in PDR database.

PROCTOFOAM-HC
(Hydrocortisone Acetate, Pramoxine Hydrochloride) 3113
None cited in PDR database.

PROFLAVANOL 90 TABLETS
(Dietary Supplement) 3343
None cited in PDR database.

PROGRAF CAPSULES AND INJECTION
(Tacrolimus) 624
May interact with aminoglycosides, cytochrome p450 3a inducers (selected), cytochrome p450 3a inhibitors (selected), erythromycin, methylprednisolone, phenytoin, protease inhibitors, potassium sparing diuretics, vaccines, live, and certain other agents. Compounds in these categories include:

Allium sativum (Since tacrolimus is metabolized mainly by the CYP3A enzyme systems, drugs known to induce these enzymes may result in an increased metabolism of tacrolimus or decreased bioavailability as indicated by decreased whole blood or plasma concentrations. Monitoring of blood concentrations and appropriate dosage adjustments are essential when such drugs are used concomitantly).
No products indexed under this heading.

Aluminum Hydroxide (Co-administration has resulted in a 21% increase in the mean tacrolimus AUC and a 10% decrease in the Cmax). Products include:
Gaviscon Regular Strength Liquid .... ▣620
Gaviscon Regular Strength Tablets .... ▣619
Gaviscon Extra Strength Liquid .... ▣620
Gaviscon Extra Strength Tablets .... ▣619
Maalox Max Maximum Strength Antacid/Anti-Gas Liquid 2165
Maalox Regular Strength Antacid/Antigas Liquid 2164

Amikacin Sulfate (Potential for additive or synergistic impairment of renal function).
No products indexed under this heading.

Amiloride Hydrochloride (Mild to severe hyperkalemia has been reported with tacrolimus; concurrent use with potassium-sparing diuretics should be avoided). Products include:
Midamor Tablets 2000
Moduretic Tablets 2003

Amiodarone Hydrochloride (Since tacrolimus is metabolized mainly by the CYP3A enzyme systems, substances known to inhibit these enzymes may decrease the metabolism or increase bioavailability of tacrolimus as indicated by increased whole blood or plasma concentrations. Monitoringof blood concentrations and appropriate dosage adjustments are essential when such drugs are used concomitantly). Products include:
Pacerone Tablets 3337

Amphotericin B (Potential for additive or synergistic impairment of renal function).
No products indexed under this heading.

Amprenavir (Co-administration with drugs known to inhibit CYP3A enzyme systems, such as protease inhibitors, may increase tacrolimus blood concentrations). Products include:
Agenerase Capsules 1299
Agenerase Oral Solution 1304

Aprepitant (Since tacrolimus is metabolized mainly by the CYP3A enzyme systems, substances known to inhibit these enzymes may decrease the metabolism or increase bioavailability of tacrolimus as indicated by increased whole blood or plasma concentrations. Monitoringof blood concentrations and appropriate dosage adjustments are essential when such drugs are used concomitantly). Products include:
Emend Capsules 1944

BCG Vaccine (Immunosupressants may affect vaccination. Therefore, during treatment with tacrolimus, vaccination may be less effective. The use of live vaccines should be avoided).
No products indexed under this heading.

Bromocriptine Mesylate (Co-administration with drugs known to inhibit CYP3A enzyme systems, such as bromocriptine, may increase tacrolimus blood concentrations).
No products indexed under this heading.

Carbamazepine (Co-administration with drugs known to induce CYP3A enzyme systems, such as carbamazepine, may result in increased metabolism of tacrolimus and decreased blood or plasma concentrations). Products include:
Carbatrol Capsules 3174
Equetro Extended-Release Capsules 3178
Tegretol/Tegretol-XR 2278

Caspofungin acetate (Co-administration has resulted in a significant decrease in oral tacrolimus blood concentrations). Products include:
Cancidas for Injection 1894

Chloramphenicol (Co-administration with drugs known to inhibit CYP3A enzyme systems, such as chloramphenicol, may increase tacrolimus blood concentrations).
No products indexed under this heading.

Chloramphenicol Palmitate (Co-administration with drugs known to inhibit CYP3A enzyme systems, such as chloramphenicol, may increase tacrolimus blood concentrations).
No products indexed under this heading.

Chloramphenicol Sodium Succinate (Co-administration with drugs known to inhibit CYP3A enzyme systems, such as chloramphenicol, may increase tacrolimus blood concentrations).
No products indexed under this heading.

Cimetidine (Co-administration with drugs known to inhibit CYP3A enzyme systems, such as cimetidine, may increase tacrolimus blood concentrations). Products include:
Tagamet HB 200 Tablets .... ▣637
Tagamet Tablets 1547

Cimetidine Hydrochloride (Co-administration with drugs known to inhibit CYP3A enzyme systems, such as cimetidine, may increase tacrolimus blood concentrations).
No products indexed under this heading.

Ciprofloxacin (Since tacrolimus is metabolized mainly by the CYP3A enzyme systems, substances known to inhibit these enzymes may decrease the metabolism or increase bioavailability of tacrolimus as indicated by increased whole blood or plasma concentrations. Monitoringof blood concentrations and appropriate dosage adjustments are essential when such drugs are used concomitantly). Products include:

Cipro I.V. 2998
Cipro I.V. Pharmacy Bulk Package ... 3509
Cipro Oral Suspension 2991
Cipro XR Tablets 3004
Ciprodex Otic Suspension 555

Ciprofloxacin Hydrochloride (Since tacrolimus is metabolized mainly by the CYP3A enzyme systems, substances known to inhibit these enzymes may decrease the metabolism or increase bioavailability of tacrolimus as indicated by increased whole blood or plasma concentrations. Monitoringof blood concentrations and appropriate dosage adjustments are essential when such drugs are used concomitantly). Products include:
Ciloxan Ophthalmic Ointment 554
Cipro Tablets 2991

Cisapride (Co-administration with drugs known to inhibit CYP3A enzyme systems, such as cisapride, may increase tacrolimus blood concentrations).
No products indexed under this heading.

Cisplatin (Potential for additive or synergistic impairment of renal function).
No products indexed under this heading.

Clarithromycin (Co-administration with drugs known to inhibit CYP3A enzyme systems, such as clarithromycin, may increase tacrolimus blood concentrations). Products include:
Biaxin/Biaxin XL 402
PREVPAC 3281

Clotrimazole (Co-administration with drugs known to inhibit CYP3A enzyme systems, such as clotrimazole, may increase tacrolimus blood concentrations). Products include:
Lotrimin 3053
Lotrisone 3054

Cyclosporine (Increases tacrolimus blood levels resulting in additive/synergistic nephrotoxicity; Prograf should not be used simultaneously with cyclosporine; Prograf or cyclosporine should be discontinued at least 24 hours or more prior to initiating the other). Products include:
Gengraf Capsules 458
Neoral Soft Gelatin Capsules 2247
Neoral Oral Solution 2247
Restasis Ophthalmic Emulsion 570
Sandimmune 2259

Danazol (Co-administration with drugs known to inhibit CYP3A enzyme systems, such as danazol, may increase tacrolimus blood concentrations).
No products indexed under this heading.

Delavirdine Mesylate (Since tacrolimus is metabolized mainly by the CYP3A enzyme systems, substances known to inhibit these enzymes may decrease the metabolism or increase bioavailability of tacrolimus as indicated by increased whole blood or plasma concentrations. Monitoringof blood concentrations and appropriate dosage adjustments are essential when such drugs are used concomitantly). Products include:
Rescriptor Tablets 2535

Dexamethasone (Since tacrolimus is metabolized mainly by the CYP3A enzyme systems, drugs known to induce these enzymes may result in an increased metabolism of tacrolimus or decreased bioavailability as indicated by decreased whole blood or plasma concentrations. Monitoring of blood concentrations and appropriate dosage adjustments are essential when such drugs are used concomitantly). Products include:
Ciprodex Otic Suspension 555
Decadron Tablets 1929
TobraDex Ophthalmic Ointment 558
TobraDex Ophthalmic Suspension ... 558

Diltiazem Hydrochloride (Co-administration with drugs known to inhibit CYP3A enzyme systems, such as diltiazem, may increase tacrolimus blood concentrations). Products include:
Cardizem LA Extended Release Tablets 1699
Tiazac Capsules 1204

Diltiazem Maleate (Since tacrolimus is metabolized mainly by the CYP3A enzyme systems, substances known to inhibit these enzymes may decrease the metabolism or increase bioavailability of tacrolimus as indicated by increased whole blood or plasma concentrations. Monitoringof blood concentrations and appropriate dosage adjustments are essential when such drugs are used concomitantly).
No products indexed under this heading.

Efavirenz (Since tacrolimus is metabolized mainly by the CYP3A enzyme systems, substances known to inhibit these enzymes may decrease the metabolism or increase bioavailability of tacrolimus as indicated by increased whole blood or plasma concentrations. Monitoringof blood concentrations and appropriate dosage adjustments are essential when such drugs are used concomitantly). Products include:
Sustiva Capsules 957

Erythromycin (Co-administration with drugs known to inhibit CYP3A enzyme systems, such as erythromycin, may increase tacrolimus blood concentrations). Products include:
Erygel Topical Gel 2096
Ery-Tab Tablets 447
Erythromycin Base Filmtab Tablets 454
Erythromycin Delayed-Release Capsules, USP 456
PCE Dispertab Tablets 510

Erythromycin Estolate (Co-administration with drugs known to inhibit CYP3A enzyme systems, such as erythromycin, may increase tacrolimus blood concentrations).
No products indexed under this heading.

Erythromycin Ethylsuccinate (Co-administration with drugs known to inhibit CYP3A enzyme systems, such as erythromycin, may increase tacrolimus blood concentrations). Products include:
E.E.S. 449
EryPed 445

Erythromycin Gluceptate (Co-administration with drugs known to inhibit CYP3A enzyme systems, such as erythromycin, may increase tacrolimus blood concentrations).
No products indexed under this heading.

Erythromycin Lactobionate (Co-administration with drugs known to inhibit CYP3A enzyme systems, such as erythromycin, may increase tacrolimus blood concentrations).
No products indexed under this heading.

Erythromycin Stearate (Co-administration with drugs known to inhibit CYP3A enzyme systems, such as erythromycin, may increase tacrolimus blood concentrations). Products include:
Erythrocin Stearate Filmtab Tablets 452

Ethinyl Estradiol (May increase tacrolimus blood concentrations). Products include:
Alesse-28 Tablets 3392
Lo/Ovral-28 Tablets 3423
NuvaRing 2357
Ortho-Cept Tablets 2395
Ortho-Cyclen/Ortho Tri-Cyclen 2414
Ortho Evra Transdermal System 2402
Ortho Tri-Cyclen Lo Tablets 2421
Seasonale Tablets 1073
Triphasil-28 Tablets 3483
Yasmin 28 Tablets 818

Ethosuximide (Since tacrolimus is metabolized mainly by the CYP3A enzyme systems, drugs known to induce these enzymes may result in an increased metabolism of tacrolimus or decreased bioavailability as indicated by decreased whole blood or plasma concentrations. Monitoring of blood concentrations and appropriate dosage adjustments are essential when such drugs are used concomitantly).
No products indexed under this heading.

Fluconazole (Co-administration with drugs known to inhibit CYP3A enzyme systems, such as fluconazole, may increase tacrolimus blood concentrations).
No products indexed under this heading.

Fluoxetine (Since tacrolimus is metabolized mainly by the CYP3A enzyme systems, substances known to inhibit these enzymes may decrease the metabolism or increase bioavailability of tacrolimus as indicated by increased whole blood or plasma concentrations. Monitoringof blood concentrations and appropriate dosage adjustments are essential when such drugs are used concomitantly).
No products indexed under this heading.

Fluoxetine Hydrochloride (Since tacrolimus is metabolized mainly by the CYP3A enzyme systems, substances known to inhibit these enzymes may decrease the metabolism or increase bioavailability of tacrolimus as indicated by increased whole blood or plasma concentrations. Monitoringof blood concentrations and appropriate dosage adjustments are essential when such drugs are used concomitantly). Products include:
Prozac Pulvules and Liquid 1771
Symbyax Capsules 1788

Fluvoxamine Maleate (Since tacrolimus is metabolized mainly by the CYP3A enzyme systems, substances known to inhibit these enzymes may decrease the metabolism or increase bioavailability of tacrolimus as indicated by increased whole blood or plasma concentrations. Monitoringof blood concentrations and appropriate dosage adjustments are essential when such drugs are used concomitantly).
No products indexed under this heading.

Fosphenytoin Sodium (Co-administration may result in increased metabolism of tacrolimus and decreased plasma levels; tacrolimus may increase the plasma phenytoin levels).
No products indexed under this heading.

Ganciclovir (May increase nephrotoxicity). Products include:
Cytovene Capsules 2763

Ganciclovir Sodium (May increase nephrotoxicity). Products include:
Cytovene-IV 2763

Gentamicin Sulfate (Potential for additive or synergistic impairment of renal function). Products include:
Garamycin Injectable 3028
Genoptic Sterile Ophthalmic Solution .... ⊙227
Pred-G Ophthalmic Suspension .... ⊙234
Pred-G Sterile Ophthalmic Ointment .... ⊙235

Hypericum (Co-administration with St. John's Wort may result in decreased tacrolimus blood concentrations).
No products indexed under this heading.

Indinavir Sulfate (Co-administration with drugs known to inhibit CYP3A enzyme systems, such as protease inhibitors, may increase tacrolimus blood concentrations). Products include:
Crixivan Capsules 1918

Isoniazid (Since tacrolimus is metabolized mainly by the CYP3A enzyme systems, substances known to inhibit these enzymes may decrease the metabolism or increase bioavailability of tacrolimus as indicated by increased whole blood or plasma concentrations. Monitoringof blood concentrations and appropriate dosage adjustments are essential when such drugs are used concomitantly).
No products indexed under this heading.

Itraconazole (Co-administration with drugs known to inhibit CYP3A enzyme systems, such as itraconazole, may increase tacrolimus blood concentrations).
No products indexed under this heading.

Kanamycin Sulfate (Potential for additive or synergistic impairment of renal function).
No products indexed under this heading.

Ketoconazole (Co-administration has resulted in a significant increase in tacrolimus bioavailability and significant decrease in clearance; overall IV clearance of tacrolimus was not significantly changed by ketoconazole, although it was highly variable between patients). Products include:
Nizoral A-D Shampoo, 1% 1839
Nizoral 2% Shampoo 1838

Lopinavir (Co-administration with drugs known to inhibit CYP3A enzyme systems, such as protease inhibitors, may increase tacrolimus blood concentrations). Products include:

Kaletra ... 474

Magnesium Hydroxide (Co-administration has resulted in a 21% increase in the mean tacrolimus AUC and a 10% decrease in the Cmax). Products include:

Maalox Max Maximum Strength Antacid/Anti-Gas Liquid ... 2165
Maalox Regular Strength Antacid/Antigas Liquid ... 2164
Pepcid Complete Chewable Tablets ... 1672
Rolaids Tablets ... ▣ 707
Extra Strength Rolaids Tablets ... ▣ 707
Rolaids Multi-Symptom Antacid & Antigas Tablets ... ▣ 708

Measles, Mumps & Rubella Virus Vaccine, Live (During treatment with tacrolimus, vaccination may be less effective). Products include:

M-M-R II ... 1980

Measles & Rubella Virus Vaccine Live (During treatment with tacrolimus, vaccination may be less effective).

No products indexed under this heading.

Measles Virus Vaccine Live (During treatment with tacrolimus, vaccination may be less effective). Products include:

Attenuvax ... 1889

Methylprednisolone (May increase tacrolimus blood concentrations).

No products indexed under this heading.

Methylprednisolone Acetate (May increase tacrolimus blood concentrations). Products include:

Depo-Medrol Injectable Suspension ... 2615
Depo-Medrol Single-Dose Vial ... 2617

Methylprednisolone Sodium Succinate (May increase tacrolimus blood concentrations).

No products indexed under this heading.

Metoclopramide Hydrochloride (Co-administration with drugs known to inhibit CYP3A enzyme systems, such as metoclopramide, may increase tacrolimus blood concentrations).

No products indexed under this heading.

Metronidazole (Since tacrolimus is metabolized mainly by the CYP3A enzyme systems, substances known to inhibit these enzymes may decrease the metabolism or increase bioavailability of tacrolimus as indicated by increased whole blood or plasma concentrations. Monitoringof blood concentrations and appropriate dosage adjustments are essential when such drugs are used concomitantly). Products include:

Metrogel 1% ... 1212
MetroGel-Vaginal Gel ... 1822
Noritate Cream, 1% ... 1051

Metronidazole Benzoate (Since tacrolimus is metabolized mainly by the CYP3A enzyme systems, substances known to inhibit these enzymes may decrease the metabolism or increase bioavailability of tacrolimus as indicated by increased whole blood or plasma concentrations. Monitoringof blood concentrations and appropriate dosage adjustments are essential when such drugs are used concomitantly).

No products indexed under this heading.

Metronidazole Hydrochloride (Since tacrolimus is metabolized mainly by the CYP3A enzyme systems, substances known to inhibit these enzymes may decrease the metabolism or increase bioavailability of tacrolimus as indicated by increased whole blood or plasma concentrations. Monitoringof blood concentrations and appropriate dosage adjustments are essential when such drugs are used concomitantly).

No products indexed under this heading.

Miconazole (Since tacrolimus is metabolized mainly by the CYP3A enzyme systems, substances known to inhibit these enzymes may decrease the metabolism or increase bioavailability of tacrolimus as indicated by increased whole blood or plasma concentrations. Monitoringof blood concentrations and appropriate dosage adjustments are essential when such drugs are used concomitantly).

No products indexed under this heading.

Modafinil (Since tacrolimus is metabolized mainly by the CYP3A enzyme systems, drugs known to induce these enzymes may result in an increased metabolism of tacrolimus or decreased bioavailability as indicated by decreased whole blood or plasma concentrations. Monitoring of blood concentrations and appropriate dosage adjustments are essential when such drugs are used concomitantly). Products include:

Provigil Tablets ... 1002

Mumps Virus Vaccine, Live (Immunosupressants may affect vaccination. Therefore, during treatment with tacrolimus, vaccination may be less effective. The use of live vaccines should be avoided). Products include:

Mumpsvax ... 2005

Nefazodone Hydrochloride (May increase tacrolimus blood concentrations).

No products indexed under this heading.

Nelfinavir Mesylate (Co-administration has resulted in a significant increase in oral tacrolimus blood concentrations). Products include:

Viracept ... 2556

Nevirapine (Since tacrolimus is metabolized mainly by the CYP3A enzyme systems, drugs known to induce these enzymes may result in an increased metabolism of tacrolimus or decreased bioavailability as indicated by decreased whole blood or plasma concentrations. Monitoring of blood concentrations and appropriate dosage adjustments are essential when such drugs are used concomitantly). Products include:

Viramune Oral Suspension ... 903
Viramune Tablets ... 903

Nicardipine Hydrochloride (Co-administration with drugs known to inhibit CYP3A enzyme systems, such as nicardipine, may increase tacrolimus blood concentrations). Products include:

Cardene I.V. ... 1129

Nifedipine (Co-administration with drugs known to inhibit CYP3A enzyme systems, such as nifedipine, may increase tacrolimus blood concentrations). Products include:

Adalat CC Tablets ... 2978

Norfloxacin (Since tacrolimus is metabolized mainly by the CYP3A enzyme systems, substances known to inhibit these enzymes may decrease the metabolism or increase bioavailability of tacrolimus as indicated by increased whole blood or plasma concentrations. Monitoringof blood concentrations and appropriate dosage adjustments are essential when such drugs are used concomitantly). Products include:

Noroxin Tablets ... 2009

Omeprazole (May increase tacrolimus blood concentrations). Products include:

Zegerid Powder for Oral Solution ... 2972

Paroxetine Hydrochloride (Since tacrolimus is metabolized mainly by the CYP3A enzyme systems, substances known to inhibit these enzymes may decrease the metabolism or increase bioavailability of tacrolimus as indicated by increased whole blood or plasma concentrations. Monitoringof blood concentrations and appropriate dosage adjustments are essential when such drugs are used concomitantly). Products include:

Paxil CR Controlled-Release Tablets ... 1509
Paxil ... 1501

Phenobarbital (Co-administration with drugs known to induce CYP3A enzyme systems, such as phenobarbital, may result in increased metabolism of tacrolimus and decreased blood or plasma concentrations).

No products indexed under this heading.

Phenytoin (Co-administration may result in increased metabolism of tacrolimus and decreased plasma levels; tacrolimus may increase the plasma phenytoin levels).

No products indexed under this heading.

Phenytoin Sodium (Co-administration may result in increased metabolism of tacrolimus and decreased plasma levels; tacrolimus may increase the plasma phenytoin levels). Products include:

Phenytek Capsules ... 2153

Poliovirus Vaccine, Live, Oral, Trivalent, Types 1,2,3 (Sabin) (During treatment with tacrolimus, vaccination may be less effective).

No products indexed under this heading.

Poliovirus Vaccine Inactivated, Trivalent Types 1,2,3 (During treatment with tacrolimus, vaccination may be less effective). Products include:

Pediarix Vaccine ... 1518

Quinine (Since tacrolimus is metabolized mainly by the CYP3A enzyme systems, substances known to inhibit these enzymes may decrease the metabolism or increase bioavailability of tacrolimus as indicated by increased whole blood or plasma concentrations. Monitoringof blood concentrations and appropriate dosage adjustments are essential when such drugs are used concomitantly).

No products indexed under this heading.

Quinine Sulfate (Since tacrolimus is metabolized mainly by the CYP3A enzyme systems, substances known to inhibit these enzymes may decrease the metabolism or increase bioavailability of tacrolimus as indicated by increased whole blood or plasma concentrations. Monitoringof blood concentrations and appropriate dosage adjustments are essential when such drugs are used concomitantly).

No products indexed under this heading.

Rifabutin (Co-administration with drugs known to induce CYP3A enzyme systems, such as rifabutin, may result in increased metabolism of tacrolimus and decreased blood or plasma concentrations).

No products indexed under this heading.

Rifampicin (Since tacrolimus is metabolized mainly by the CYP3A enzyme systems, drugs known to induce these enzymes may result in an increased metabolism of tacrolimus or decreased bioavailability as indicated by decreased whole blood or plasma concentrations. Monitoring of blood concentrations and appropriate dosage adjustments are essential when such drugs are used concomitantly).

No products indexed under this heading.

Rifampin (Co-administration has resulted in a significant decrease in oral tacrolimus bioavailability and significant increase in clearance).

No products indexed under this heading.

Rifapentine (Since tacrolimus is metabolized mainly by the CYP3A enzyme systems, drugs known to induce these enzymes may result in an increased metabolism of tacrolimus or decreased bioavailability as indicated by decreased whole blood or plasma concentrations. Monitoring of blood concentrations and appropriate dosage adjustments are essential when such drugs are used concomitantly).

No products indexed under this heading.

Ritonavir (Co-administration with drugs known to inhibit CYP3A enzyme systems, such as protease inhibitors, may increase tacrolimus blood concentrations). Products include:

Kaletra ... 474
Norvir ... 499

Rotavirus Vaccine, Live, Oral, Tetravalent (Immunosupressants may affect vaccination. Therefore, during treatment with tacrolimus, vaccination may be less effective. The use of live vaccines should be avoided).

No products indexed under this heading.

Rubella & Mumps Virus Vaccine Live (Immunosupressants may affect vaccination. Therefore, during treatment with tacrolimus, vaccination may be less effective. The use of live vaccines should be avoided).

No products indexed under this heading.

Rubella Virus Vaccine Live (Immunosupressants may affect vaccination. Therefore, during treatment with tacrolimus, vaccination may be

less effective. The use of live vaccines should be avoided). Products include:

Meruvax II 1994

Saquinavir (Co-administration with drugs known to inhibit CYP3A enzyme systems, such as protease inhibitors, may increase tacrolimus blood concentrations).

No products indexed under this heading.

Saquinavir Mesylate (Co-administration with drugs known to inhibit CYP3A enzyme systems, such as protease inhibitors, may increase tacrolimus blood concentrations). Products include:

Invirase 2776

Sertraline Hydrochloride (Since tacrolimus is metabolized mainly by the CYP3A enzyme systems, substances known to inhibit these enzymes may decrease the metabolism or increase bioavailability of tacrolimus as indicated by increased whole blood or plasma concentrations. Monitoringof blood concentrations and appropriate dosage adjustments are essential when such drugs are used concomitantly). Products include:

Zoloft 2581

Sirolimus (Co-administration has resulted in a 30% decrease in oral tacrolimus AUC(0-12) and Cmin). Products include:

Rapamune Oral Solution and Tablets 3472

Smallpox Vaccine (Immunosupressants may affect vaccination. Therefore, during treatment with tacrolimus, vaccination may be less effective. The use of live vaccines should be avoided).

No products indexed under this heading.

Spironolactone (Mild to severe hyperkalemia has been reported with tacrolimus; concurrent use with potassium-sparing diuretics should be avoided).

No products indexed under this heading.

Streptomycin Sulfate (Potential for additive or synergistic impairment of renal function).

No products indexed under this heading.

Tobramycin (Potential for additive or synergistic impairment of renal function). Products include:

TOBI Solution for Inhalation 1015
TobraDex Ophthalmic Ointment 558
TobraDex Ophthalmic Suspension ... 558
Zylet Ophthalmic Suspension 3508

Tobramycin Sulfate (Potential for additive or synergistic impairment of renal function).

No products indexed under this heading.

Triamterene (Mild to severe hyperkalemia has been reported with tacrolimus; concurrent use with potassium-sparing diuretics should be avoided). Products include:

Dyazide Capsules 1389
Dyrenium Capsules 3390
Maxzide 2150

Troleandomycin (Co-administration with drugs known to inhibit CYP3A enzyme systems, such as troleandomycin, may increase tacrolimus blood concentrations).

No products indexed under this heading.

Typhoid Vaccine (Immunosupressants may affect vaccination. Therefore, during treatment with tacrolimus, vaccination may be less effective. The use of live vaccines should be avoided).

No products indexed under this heading.

Typhoid Vaccine Live Oral TY21a (During treatment with tacrolimus, vaccination may be less effective). Products include:

Vivotif 834

Vaccines (Live) (During treatment with tacrolimus, vaccination may be less effective).

No products indexed under this heading.

Varicella Virus Vaccine Live (Immunosupressants may affect vaccination. Therefore, during treatment with tacrolimus, vaccination may be less effective. The use of live vaccines should be avoided). Products include:

Varivax 2070

Venlafaxine Hydrochloride (Since tacrolimus is metabolized mainly by the CYP3A enzyme systems, substances known to inhibit these enzymes may decrease the metabolism or increase bioavailability of tacrolimus as indicated by increased whole blood or plasma concentrations. Monitoringof blood concentrations and appropriate dosage adjustments are essential when such drugs are used concomitantly). Products include:

Effexor Tablets 3405
Effexor XR Capsules 3411

Verapamil Hydrochloride (Co-administration with drugs known to inhibit CYP3A enzyme systems, such as verapamil, may increase tacrolimus blood concentrations). Products include:

Covera-HS Tablets 3135
Tarka Tablets 519
Verelan PM Capsules 3120

Voriconazole (Co-administration with drugs known to inhibit CYP3A enzyme systems, such as voriconazole, may increase tacrolimus blood concentrations). Products include:

VFEND I.V. 2543
VFEND Oral Suspension 2543
VFEND Tablets 2543

Yellow Fever Vaccine (During treatment with tacrolimus, vaccination may be less effective).

No products indexed under this heading.

Zafirlukast (Since tacrolimus is metabolized mainly by the CYP3A enzyme systems, substances known to inhibit these enzymes may decrease the metabolism or increase bioavailability of tacrolimus as indicated by increased whole blood or plasma concentrations. Monitoringof blood concentrations and appropriate dosage adjustments are essential when such drugs are used concomitantly). Products include:

Accolate Tablets 663

Zileuton (Since tacrolimus is metabolized mainly by the CYP3A enzyme systems, substances known to inhibit these enzymes may decrease the metabolism or increase bioavailability of tacrolimus as indicated by increased whole blood or plasma concentrations. Monitoringof blood concentrations and appropriate dosage adjustments are essential when such drugs are used concomitantly).

No products indexed under this heading.

Food Interactions

Food, unspecified (The presence and composition of food has decreased both the rate and extent of tacrolimus absorption; this effect was most pronounced with a high-fat meal; the rate and extent of tacrolimus absorption were greatest under fasted conditions).

Grapefruit (Since tacrolimus is metabolized mainly by the CYP3A enzyme systems, substances known to inhibit these enzymes may decrease the metabolism or increase bioavailability of tacrolimus as indicated by increased whole blood or plasma concentrations. Monitoringof blood concentrations and appropriate dosage adjustments are essential when such drugs are used concomitantly).

Grapefruit Juice (Co-administered grapefruit juice has been reported to increase tacrolimus blood trough concentrations in liver transplant patients; grapefruit juice should be avoided).

PROLASTIN

(Alpha$_1$-Proteinase Inhibitor (Human)) 3252

None cited in PDR database.

PROLEUKIN FOR INJECTION

(Aldesleukin) 1007

May interact with aminoglycosides, antihypertensives, beta blockers, cytotoxic drugs, glucocorticoids, hypnotics and sedatives, narcotic analgesics, radiographic iodinated contrast media, tranquilizers, and certain other agents. Compounds in these categories include:

Acebutolol Hydrochloride (May potentiate the hypotension seen with aldesleukin).

No products indexed under this heading.

Alfentanil Hydrochloride (Potential for unspecified effect on central nervous function).

No products indexed under this heading.

Alprazolam (Potential for unspecified effect on central nervous function). Products include:

Niravam Orally Disintegrating Tablets 3106
Xanax XR Tablets 2655

Amikacin Sulfate (Potential for increased nephrotoxicity).

No products indexed under this heading.

Amlodipine Besylate (May potentiate the hypotension seen with aldesleukin). Products include:

Caduet Tablets 2507
Lotrel Capsules 2238
Norvasc Tablets 2529

Asparaginase (Potential for increased hepatic toxicity). Products include:

Elspar for Injection 1943

Atenolol (May potentiate the hypotension seen with aldesleukin). Products include:

Tenormin I.V. Injection 698
Tenormin Tablets 695

Benazepril Hydrochloride (May potentiate the hypotension seen with aldesleukin). Products include:

Lotensin Tablets 2232
Lotensin HCT Tablets 2235
Lotrel Capsules 2238

Bendroflumethiazide (May potentiate the hypotension seen with aldesleukin).

No products indexed under this heading.

Betamethasone Acetate (May reduce the antitumor effectiveness of aldesleukin).

No products indexed under this heading.

Betamethasone Sodium Phosphate (May reduce the antitumor effectiveness of aldesleukin).

No products indexed under this heading.

Betaxolol Hydrochloride (May potentiate the hypotension seen with aldesleukin). Products include:

Betoptic S Ophthalmic Suspension 554

Bisoprolol Fumarate (May potentiate the hypotension seen with aldesleukin).

No products indexed under this heading.

Bleomycin Sulfate (Potential for increased myelotoxicity).

No products indexed under this heading.

Buprenorphine Hydrochloride (Potential for unspecified effect on central nervous function). Products include:

Buprenex Injectable 2718
Suboxone Tablets 2719
Subutex Tablets 2719

Buspirone Hydrochloride (Potential for unspecified effect on central nervous function).

No products indexed under this heading.

Candesartan Cilexetil (May potentiate the hypotension seen with aldesleukin). Products include:

Atacand Tablets 634
Atacand HCT 637

Captopril (May potentiate the hypotension seen with aldesleukin). Products include:

Captopril Tablets 2114

Carteolol Hydrochloride (May potentiate the hypotension seen with aldesleukin). Products include:

Carteolol Hydrochloride Ophthalmic Solution USP, 1% .... ⊙ 246

Chlordiazepoxide (Potential for unspecified effect on central nervous function).

No products indexed under this heading.

Chlordiazepoxide Hydrochloride (Potential for unspecified effect on central nervous function). Products include:

Librium Capsules 3349

Chlorothiazide (May potentiate the hypotension seen with aldesleukin). Products include:

Aldoclor Tablets 1881
Diuril Oral 1936

Chlorothiazide Sodium (May potentiate the hypotension seen with aldesleukin). Products include:

Diuril Sodium Intravenous 1934

Chlorpromazine (Potential for unspecified effect on central nervous function).
No products indexed under this heading.

Chlorpromazine Hydrochloride (Potential for unspecified effect on central nervous function).
No products indexed under this heading.

Chlorprothixene (Potential for unspecified effect on central nervous function).
No products indexed under this heading.

Chlorprothixene Hydrochloride (Potential for unspecified effect on central nervous function).
No products indexed under this heading.

Chlorthalidone (May potentiate the hypotension seen with aldesleukin). Products include:
Clorpres Tablets 2139

Clonidine (May potentiate the hypotension seen with aldesleukin). Products include:
Catapres-TTS 875

Clonidine Hydrochloride (May potentiate the hypotension seen with aldesleukin). Products include:
Catapres Tablets 874
Clorpres Tablets 2139

Clorazepate Dipotassium (Potential for unspecified effect on central nervous function). Products include:
Tranxene 2488

Codeine Phosphate (Potential for unspecified effect on central nervous function). Products include:
Tylenol with Codeine 2461

Cortisone Acetate (May reduce the antitumor effectiveness of aldesleukin).
No products indexed under this heading.

Cyclophosphamide (Potential for increased myelotoxicity).
No products indexed under this heading.

Daunorubicin Hydrochloride (Potential for increased myelotoxicity). Products include:
Cerubidine for Injection 788

Deserpidine (May potentiate the hypotension seen with aldesleukin).
No products indexed under this heading.

Dexamethasone (May reduce the antitumor effectiveness of aldesleukin). Products include:
Ciprodex Otic Suspension 555
Decadron Tablets 1929
TobraDex Ophthalmic Ointment 558
TobraDex Ophthalmic Suspension 558

Dexamethasone Acetate (May reduce the antitumor effectiveness of aldesleukin).
No products indexed under this heading.

Dexamethasone Sodium Phosphate (May reduce the antitumor effectiveness of aldesleukin). Products include:
Decadron Phosphate Injection 1931

Dezocine (Potential for unspecified effect on central nervous function).
No products indexed under this heading.

Diatrizoate Meglumine (Potential for delayed adverse reactions to iodinated contrast media including fever, chills, nausea, vomiting, pruritus, rash, diarrhea, hypotension, edema, and oliguria).
No products indexed under this heading.

Diatrizoate Sodium (Potential for delayed adverse reactions to iodinated contrast media including fever, chills, nausea, vomiting, pruritus, rash, diarrhea, hypotension, edema, and oliguria).
No products indexed under this heading.

Diazepam (Potential for unspecified effect on central nervous function). Products include:
Diastat Rectal Delivery System 3344
Valium Tablets 2822

Diazoxide (May potentiate the hypotension seen with aldesleukin). Products include:
Hyperstat I.V. Injection 3031

Diltiazem Hydrochloride (May potentiate the hypotension seen with aldesleukin). Products include:
Cardizem LA Extended Release Tablets 1699
Tiazac Capsules 1204

Doxazosin Mesylate (May potentiate the hypotension seen with aldesleukin).
No products indexed under this heading.

Doxorubicin Hydrochloride (Potential for increased cardiotoxicity and myelotoxicity). Products include:
Adriamycin for Injection, USP 786
Adriamycin Injection, USP 786

Droperidol (Potential for unspecified effect on central nervous function).
No products indexed under this heading.

Enalapril Maleate (May potentiate the hypotension seen with aldesleukin). Products include:
Vaseretic Tablets 2073
Vasotec I.V. Injection 2076

Enalaprilat (May potentiate the hypotension seen with aldesleukin).
No products indexed under this heading.

Epirubicin Hydrochloride (Potential for increased myelotoxicity). Products include:
Ellence Injection 2632

Eprosartan Mesylate (May potentiate the hypotension seen with aldesleukin). Products include:
Teveten Tablets 1707
Teveten HCT Tablets 1710

Esmolol Hydrochloride (May potentiate the hypotension seen with aldesleukin). Products include:
Brevibloc Concentrate 766
Brevibloc Injection 766
Brevibloc Double Strength Injection 766
Brevibloc Premixed Injection 766
Brevibloc Double Strength Premixed Injection 766

Estazolam (Potential for unspecified effect on central nervous function). Products include:
ProSom Tablets 512

Ethchlorvynol (Potential for unspecified effect on central nervous function).
No products indexed under this heading.

Ethinamate (Potential for unspecified effect on central nervous function).
No products indexed under this heading.

Ethiodized Oil (Potential for delayed adverse reactions to iodinated contrast media including fever, chills, nausea, vomiting, pruritus, rash, diarrhea, hypotension, edema, and oliguria).
No products indexed under this heading.

Felodipine (May potentiate the hypotension seen with aldesleukin). Products include:
Plendil Extended-Release Tablets 651

Fentanyl (Potential for unspecified effect on central nervous function). Products include:
Duragesic Transdermal System 2448

Fentanyl Citrate (Potential for unspecified effect on central nervous function). Products include:
Actiq 993

Fludrocortisone Acetate (May reduce the antitumor effectiveness of aldesleukin).
No products indexed under this heading.

Fluorouracil (Potential for increased myelotoxicity). Products include:
Carac Cream, 0.5% 1048
Efudex 3348

Fluphenazine Decanoate (Potential for unspecified effect on central nervous function).
No products indexed under this heading.

Fluphenazine Enanthate (Potential for unspecified effect on central nervous function).
No products indexed under this heading.

Fluphenazine Hydrochloride (Potential for unspecified effect on central nervous function).
No products indexed under this heading.

Flurazepam Hydrochloride (Potential for unspecified effect on central nervous function). Products include:
Dalmane Capsules 3343

Fosinopril Sodium (May potentiate the hypotension seen with aldesleukin).
No products indexed under this heading.

Furosemide (May potentiate the hypotension seen with aldesleukin). Products include:
Furosemide Tablets 2117

Gadopentetate Dimeglumine (Potential for delayed adverse reactions to iodinated contrast media including fever, chills, nausea, vomiting, pruritus, rash, diarrhea, hypotension, edema, and oliguria).
No products indexed under this heading.

Gentamicin Sulfate (Potential for increased nephrotoxicity). Products include:
Garamycin Injectable 3028
Genoptic Sterile Ophthalmic Solution .... ⊙ 227
Pred-G Ophthalmic Suspension .... ⊙ 234
Pred-G Sterile Ophthalmic Ointment .... ⊙ 235

Glutethimide (Potential for unspecified effect on central nervous function).
No products indexed under this heading.

Guanabenz Acetate (May potentiate the hypotension seen with aldesleukin).
No products indexed under this heading.

Guanethidine Monosulfate (May potentiate the hypotension seen with aldesleukin).
No products indexed under this heading.

Haloperidol (Potential for unspecified effect on central nervous function).
No products indexed under this heading.

Haloperidol Decanoate (Potential for unspecified effect on central nervous function).
No products indexed under this heading.

Hepatotoxic Drugs, unspecified (Potential for increased hepatic toxicity).
No products indexed under this heading.

Hydralazine Hydrochloride (May potentiate the hypotension seen with aldesleukin). Products include:
BiDil Tablets 2161

Hydrochlorothiazide (May potentiate the hypotension seen with aldesleukin). Products include:
Aldoril Tablets 1884
Atacand HCT 637
Avalide Tablets 2889
Avalide Tablets 922
Benicar HCT Tablets 2852
Diovan HCT Tablets 2195
Dyazide Capsules 1389
Hyzaar 1964
Lotensin HCT Tablets 2235
Maxzide 2150
Micardis HCT Tablets 886
Moduretic Tablets 2003
Prinzide Tablets 2033
Teveten HCT Tablets 1710
Timolide Tablets 2056
Uniretic Tablets 3114
Vaseretic Tablets 2073
Zestoretic Tablets 701

Hydrocodone Bitartrate (Potential for unspecified effect on central nervous function). Products include:
Hycodan 1104
Hycomine Compound Tablets 1105
Hycotuss Expectorant Syrup 1106
Lortab 3315
Lortab Elixir 3312
Vicodin Tablets 530
Vicodin ES Tablets 531
Vicodin HP Tablets 532
Vicoprofen Tablets 533
Zydone Tablets 1118

Hydrocodone Polistirex (Potential for unspecified effect on central nervous function). Products include:
Tussionex Pennkinetic Extended-Release Suspension 3322

Hydrocortisone (May reduce the antitumor effectiveness of aldesleukin). Products include:
Cortizone•5 Ointment .... ▣ 699
Cortizone•10 Creme .... ▣ 699
Cortizone•10 Ointment .... ▣ 699
Cortizone•10 Plus Creme .... ▣ 700
Cortizone•10 Maximum Strength Quick Shot Spray .... ▣ 700
Hydrocortone Tablets 1963
Preparation H Hydrocortisone Cream .... ▣ 748

Hydrocortisone Acetate (May reduce the antitumor effectiveness of aldesleukin). Products include:
Analpram-HC 1136
Pramosone 1139
ProctoFoam-HC 3113
Tucks Anti-Itch Ointment .... ▣ 712
U-cort 1% Cream 3289

Hydrocortisone Sodium Phosphate (May reduce the antitumor effectiveness of aldesleukin).
No products indexed under this heading.

Hydrocortisone Sodium Succinate (May reduce the antitumor effectiveness of aldesleukin).
No products indexed under this heading.

Hydroflumethiazide (May potentiate the hypotension seen with aldesleukin).
No products indexed under this heading.

Hydromorphone Hydrochloride (Potential for unspecified effect on central nervous function). Products include:
Dilaudid ... **439**
Dilaudid Oral Liquid ... **443**
Dilaudid Non-Sterile Powder ... **439**
Dilaudid Rectal Suppositories ... **439**
Dilaudid Tablets ... **439**
Dilaudid Tablets - 8 mg ... **443**
Dilaudid-HP ... **441**

Hydroxyurea (Potential for increased myelotoxicity).
No products indexed under this heading.

Hydroxyzine Hydrochloride (Potential for unspecified effect on central nervous function).
No products indexed under this heading.

Indapamide (May potentiate the hypotension seen with aldesleukin). Products include:
Indapamide Tablets ... **2119**

Indomethacin (Potential for increased nephrotoxicity). Products include:
Indocin ... **1968**

Interferon alfa-2a, Recombinant (Co-administration of Proleukin and interferon-alfa has resulted in increased incidence of myocardial injury, including myocardial infarction, myocarditis, ventricular hypokinesia, and severe rhabdomyolysis; exacerbation or the initial presentation of a number of autoimmune and inflammatory disorders has been observed with concurrent use). Products include:
Roferon-A Injection ... **2805**

Interferon alfa-2b, Recombinant (Co-administration of Proleukin and interferon-alfa has resulted in increased incidence of myocardial injury, including myocardial infarction, myocarditis, ventricular hypokinesia, and severe rhabdomyolysis; exacerbation or the initial presentation of a number of autoimmune and inflammatory disorders has been observed with concurrent use). Products include:
Intron A for Injection ... **3038**
Rebetron Combination Therapy ... **3078**

Iodamide Meglumine (Potential for delayed adverse reactions to iodinated contrast media including fever, chills, nausea, vomiting, pruritus, rash, diarrhea, hypotension, edema, and oliguria).
No products indexed under this heading.

Iohexol (Potential for delayed adverse reactions to iodinated contrast media including fever, chills, nausea, vomiting, pruritus, rash, diarrhea, hypotension, edema, and oliguria).
No products indexed under this heading.

Iopamidol (Potential for delayed adverse reactions to iodinated contrast media including fever, chills, nausea, vomiting, pruritus, rash, diarrhea, hypotension, edema, and oliguria).
No products indexed under this heading.

Iopanoic Acid (Potential for delayed adverse reactions to iodinated contrast media including fever, chills, nausea, vomiting, pruritus, rash, diarrhea, hypotension, edema, and oliguria).
No products indexed under this heading.

Iothalamate Meglumine (Potential for delayed adverse reactions to iodinated contrast media including fever, chills, nausea, vomiting, pruritus, rash, diarrhea, hypotension, edema, and oliguria).
No products indexed under this heading.

Ioxaglate Meglumine (Potential for delayed adverse reactions to iodinated contrast media including fever, chills, nausea, vomiting, pruritus, rash, diarrhea, hypotension, edema, and oliguria).
No products indexed under this heading.

Ioxaglate Sodium (Potential for delayed adverse reactions to iodinated contrast media including fever, chills, nausea, vomiting, pruritus, rash, diarrhea, hypotension, edema, and oliguria).
No products indexed under this heading.

Irbesartan (May potentiate the hypotension seen with aldesleukin). Products include:
Avalide Tablets ... **922**
Avalide Tablets ... **2889**
Avapro Tablets ... **925**
Avapro Tablets ... **2886**

Isradipine (May potentiate the hypotension seen with aldesleukin). Products include:
DynaCirc CR Tablets ... **2726**

Kanamycin Sulfate (Potential for increased nephrotoxicity).
No products indexed under this heading.

Labetalol Hydrochloride (May potentiate the hypotension seen with aldesleukin).
No products indexed under this heading.

Levobunolol Hydrochloride (May potentiate the hypotension seen with aldesleukin). Products include:
Betagan Ophthalmic Solution, USP ... ⊙**217**

Levorphanol Tartrate (Potential for unspecified effect on central nervous function).
No products indexed under this heading.

Lisinopril (May potentiate the hypotension seen with aldesleukin). Products include:
Prinivil Tablets ... **2029**
Prinzide Tablets ... **2033**
Zestoretic Tablets ... **701**
Zestril Tablets ... **704**

Lorazepam (Potential for unspecified effect on central nervous function).
No products indexed under this heading.

Losartan Potassium (May potentiate the hypotension seen with aldesleukin). Products include:
Cozaar Tablets ... **1913**
Hyzaar ... **1964**

Loxapine Hydrochloride (Potential for unspecified effect on central nervous function).
No products indexed under this heading.

Loxapine Succinate (Potential for unspecified effect on central nervous function).
No products indexed under this heading.

Mecamylamine Hydrochloride (May potentiate the hypotension seen with aldesleukin). Products include:
Inversine Tablets ... **3286**

Meperidine Hydrochloride (Potential for unspecified effect on central nervous function).
No products indexed under this heading.

Meprobamate (Potential for unspecified effect on central nervous function).
No products indexed under this heading.

Mesoridazine Besylate (Potential for unspecified effect on central nervous function).
No products indexed under this heading.

Methadone Hydrochloride (Potential for unspecified effect on central nervous function).
No products indexed under this heading.

Methotrexate Sodium (Potential for increased hepatic toxicity and myelotoxicity).
No products indexed under this heading.

Methyclothiazide (May potentiate the hypotension seen with aldesleukin).
No products indexed under this heading.

Methyldopa (May potentiate the hypotension seen with aldesleukin). Products include:
Aldoclor Tablets ... **1881**
Aldoril Tablets ... **1884**

Methyldopate Hydrochloride (May potentiate the hypotension seen with aldesleukin).
No products indexed under this heading.

Methylprednisolone Acetate (May reduce the antitumor effectiveness of aldesleukin). Products include:
Depo-Medrol Injectable Suspension ... **2615**
Depo-Medrol Single-Dose Vial ... **2617**

Methylprednisolone Sodium Succinate (May reduce the antitumor effectiveness of aldesleukin).
No products indexed under this heading.

Metipranolol Hydrochloride (May potentiate the hypotension seen with aldesleukin).
No products indexed under this heading.

Metolazone (May potentiate the hypotension seen with aldesleukin).
No products indexed under this heading.

Metoprolol Succinate (May potentiate the hypotension seen with aldesleukin). Products include:
Toprol-XL Tablets ... **660**

Metoprolol Tartrate (May potentiate the hypotension seen with aldesleukin).
No products indexed under this heading.

Metyrosine (May potentiate the hypotension seen with aldesleukin). Products include:
Demser Capsules ... **1933**

Mibefradil Dihydrochloride (May potentiate the hypotension seen with aldesleukin).
No products indexed under this heading.

Midazolam Hydrochloride (Potential for unspecified effect on central nervous function).
No products indexed under this heading.

Minoxidil (May potentiate the hypotension seen with aldesleukin). Products include:
Men's Rogaine Extra Strength Topical Solution, Ocean Rush Scent and Original Unscented ... **706**
Women's Rogaine Topical Solution, Spring Bloom Scent and Original Unscented ... **707**

Mitotane (Potential for increased myelotoxicity).
No products indexed under this heading.

Mitoxantrone Hydrochloride (Potential for increased myelotoxicity). Products include:
Novantrone for Injection Concentrate ... **3158**

Moexipril Hydrochloride (May potentiate the hypotension seen with aldesleukin). Products include:
Uniretic Tablets ... **3114**
Univasc Tablets ... **3118**

Molindone Hydrochloride (Potential for unspecified effect on central nervous function). Products include:
Moban Tablets ... **1108**

Morphine Sulfate (Potential for unspecified effect on central nervous function). Products include:
Avinza Capsules ... **1714**
Kadian Capsules ... **572**
MS Contin Tablets ... **2703**

Nadolol (May potentiate the hypotension seen with aldesleukin). Products include:
Nadolol Tablets ... **2121**

Nephrotoxic Drugs (Potential for increased nephrotoxicity).
No products indexed under this heading.

Nicardipine Hydrochloride (May potentiate the hypotension seen with aldesleukin). Products include:
Cardene I.V. ... **1129**

Nifedipine (May potentiate the hypotension seen with aldesleukin). Products include:
Adalat CC Tablets ... **2978**

Nisoldipine (May potentiate the hypotension seen with aldesleukin). Products include:
Sular Tablets ... **1163**

Nitroglycerin (May potentiate the hypotension seen with aldesleukin). Products include:
Nitro-Dur Transdermal Infusion System ... **3060**
Nitrolingual Pumpspray ... **1161**

Oxazepam (Potential for unspecified effect on central nervous function).
No products indexed under this heading.

Oxycodone Hydrochloride (Potential for unspecified effect on central nervous function). Products include:

Combunox Tablets 1183
OxyContin Tablets 2699
OxyFast Oral Concentrate Solution 2704
OxyIR Capsules 2704
Percocet Tablets 1114
Percodan Tablets 1115

Penbutolol Sulfate (May potentiate the hypotension seen with aldesleukin).
No products indexed under this heading.

Perindopril Erbumine (May potentiate the hypotension seen with aldesleukin). Products include:
Aceon Tablets (2 mg, 4 mg, 8 mg) 3191

Perphenazine (Potential for unspecified effect on central nervous function).
No products indexed under this heading.

Phenoxybenzamine Hydrochloride (May potentiate the hypotension seen with aldesleukin). Products include:
Dibenzyline Capsules 3390

Phentolamine Mesylate (May potentiate the hypotension seen with aldesleukin).
No products indexed under this heading.

Pindolol (May potentiate the hypotension seen with aldesleukin).
No products indexed under this heading.

Polythiazide (May potentiate the hypotension seen with aldesleukin).
No products indexed under this heading.

Prazepam (Potential for unspecified effect on central nervous function).
No products indexed under this heading.

Prazosin Hydrochloride (May potentiate the hypotension seen with aldesleukin).
No products indexed under this heading.

Prednisolone Acetate (May reduce the antitumor effectiveness of aldesleukin). Products include:
Blephamide Ophthalmic Ointment 563
Blephamide Ophthalmic Suspension 564
Poly-Pred Liquifilm Ophthalmic Suspension .... ⊙231
Pred Forte Ophthalmic Suspension .... ⊙233
Pred Mild Sterile Ophthalmic Suspension .... ⊙236
Pred-G Ophthalmic Suspension .... ⊙234
Pred-G Sterile Ophthalmic Ointment .... ⊙235

Prednisolone Sodium Phosphate (May reduce the antitumor effectiveness of aldesleukin). Products include:
Pediapred Oral Solution 3319

Prednisolone Tebutate (May reduce the antitumor effectiveness of aldesleukin).
No products indexed under this heading.

Prednisone (May reduce the antitumor effectiveness of aldesleukin).
No products indexed under this heading.

Procarbazine Hydrochloride (Potential for increased myelotoxicity). Products include:
Matulane Capsules 3188

Prochlorperazine (Potential for unspecified effect on central nervous function).
No products indexed under this heading.

Promethazine Hydrochloride (Potential for unspecified effect on central nervous function). Products include:
Phenergan 3438

Propofol (Potential for unspecified effect on central nervous function). Products include:
Diprivan Injectable Emulsion 676

Propoxyphene Hydrochloride (Potential for unspecified effect on central nervous function).
No products indexed under this heading.

Propoxyphene Napsylate (Potential for unspecified effect on central nervous function). Products include:
Darvocet A 500 Tablets 3497

Propranolol Hydrochloride (May potentiate the hypotension seen with aldesleukin). Products include:
Inderal LA Long-Acting Capsules 3421
InnoPran XL Capsules 2728

Quazepam (Potential for unspecified effect on central nervous function).
No products indexed under this heading.

Quinapril Hydrochloride (May potentiate the hypotension seen with aldesleukin).
No products indexed under this heading.

Ramipril (May potentiate the hypotension seen with aldesleukin). Products include:
Altace Capsules 1673

Rauwolfia Serpentina (May potentiate the hypotension seen with aldesleukin).
No products indexed under this heading.

Remifentanil Hydrochloride (Potential for unspecified effect on central nervous function).
No products indexed under this heading.

Rescinnamine (May potentiate the hypotension seen with aldesleukin).
No products indexed under this heading.

Reserpine (May potentiate the hypotension seen with aldesleukin).
No products indexed under this heading.

Secobarbital Sodium (Potential for unspecified effect on central nervous function).
No products indexed under this heading.

Sodium Nitroprusside (May potentiate the hypotension seen with aldesleukin).
No products indexed under this heading.

Sotalol Hydrochloride (May potentiate the hypotension seen with aldesleukin).
No products indexed under this heading.

Spirapril Hydrochloride (May potentiate the hypotension seen with aldesleukin).
No products indexed under this heading.

Streptomycin Sulfate (Potential for increased nephrotoxicity).
No products indexed under this heading.

Sufentanil Citrate (Potential for unspecified effect on central nervous function).
No products indexed under this heading.

Tamoxifen Citrate (Potential for increased myelotoxicity).
No products indexed under this heading.

Telmisartan (May potentiate the hypotension seen with aldesleukin). Products include:
Micardis Tablets 884
Micardis HCT Tablets 886

Temazepam (Potential for unspecified effect on central nervous function).
No products indexed under this heading.

Terazosin Hydrochloride (May potentiate the hypotension seen with aldesleukin). Products include:
Hytrin Capsules 469

Thioridazine Hydrochloride (Potential for unspecified effect on central nervous function). Products include:
Thioridazine Hydrochloride Tablets 2122

Thiothixene (Potential for unspecified effect on central nervous function). Products include:
Thiothixene Capsules 2124

Timolol Hemihydrate (May potentiate the hypotension seen with aldesleukin). Products include:
Betimol Ophthalmic Solution 3371
Betimol Ophthalmic Solution .... ⊙283

Timolol Maleate (May potentiate the hypotension seen with aldesleukin). Products include:
Blocadren Tablets 1891
Cosopt Sterile Ophthalmic Solution 1910
Timolide Tablets 2056
Timoptic in Ocudose 2061
Timoptic Sterile Ophthalmic Solution 2058
Timoptic-XE Sterile Ophthalmic Gel Forming Solution 2062

Tobramycin (Potential for increased nephrotoxicity). Products include:
TOBI Solution for Inhalation 1015
TobraDex Ophthalmic Ointment 558
TobraDex Ophthalmic Suspension 558
Zylet Ophthalmic Suspension 3508

Tobramycin Sulfate (Potential for increased nephrotoxicity).
No products indexed under this heading.

Torsemide (May potentiate the hypotension seen with aldesleukin).
No products indexed under this heading.

Trandolapril (May potentiate the hypotension seen with aldesleukin). Products include:
Mavik Tablets 482
Tarka Tablets 519

Triamcinolone (May reduce the antitumor effectiveness of aldesleukin).
No products indexed under this heading.

Triamcinolone Acetonide (May reduce the antitumor effectiveness of aldesleukin). Products include:
Azmacort Inhalation Aerosol 1701
Nasacort HFA Inhalation Aerosol 2939
Nasacort AQ Nasal Spray 2937

Triamcinolone Diacetate (May reduce the antitumor effectiveness of aldesleukin).
No products indexed under this heading.

Triamcinolone Hexacetonide (May reduce the antitumor effectiveness of aldesleukin).
No products indexed under this heading.

Triazolam (Potential for unspecified effect on central nervous function).
No products indexed under this heading.

Trifluoperazine Hydrochloride (Potential for unspecified effect on central nervous function).
No products indexed under this heading.

Trimethaphan Camsylate (May potentiate the hypotension seen with aldesleukin).
No products indexed under this heading.

Tyropanoate Sodium (Potential for delayed adverse reactions to iodinated contrast media including fever, chills, nausea, vomiting, pruritus, rash, diarrhea, hypotension, edema, and oliguria).
No products indexed under this heading.

Valsartan (May potentiate the hypotension seen with aldesleukin). Products include:
Diovan HCT Tablets 2195
Diovan Tablets 2191

Verapamil Hydrochloride (May potentiate the hypotension seen with aldesleukin). Products include:
Covera-HS Tablets 3135
Tarka Tablets 519
Verelan PM Capsules 3120

Vincristine Sulfate (Potential for increased myelotoxicity).
No products indexed under this heading.

Zaleplon (Potential for unspecified effect on central nervous function). Products include:
Sonata Capsules 1686

Zolpidem Tartrate (Potential for unspecified effect on central nervous function). Products include:
Ambien Tablets 2867

PROMETRIUM CAPSULES (100 MG, 200 MG)

(Progesterone) 3205
May interact with:

Estrogens, Conjugated (Coadministration has resulted in an increase in total estrone and equilin concentrations and decrease in circulating 17β estradiol concentrations). Products include:
Premarin Intravenous 3440
Premarin Tablets 3443
Premarin Vaginal Cream 3449
Premphase Tablets 3452
Prempro Tablets 3452

Ketoconazole (The metabolism of progesterone by human liver microsomes is inhibited by ketoconazole, a known inhibitor of CYP4503A4; the clinical relevance of the in vitro findings is unknown). Products include:
Nizoral A-D Shampoo, 1% 1839
Nizoral 2% Shampoo 1838

Food Interactions

Food, unspecified (Concomitant food ingestion increases the bioavailability of Prometrium Capsules relative to the fasting state).

PRONUTRA PROTEIN SUPPLEMENT

(Vitamins with Minerals, Whey Protein Isolate) 1643
None cited in PDR database.

PROPECIA TABLETS
(Finasteride) 2036
None cited in PDR database.

PROPINE OPHTHALMIC SOLUTION
(Dipivefrin Hydrochloride) .... ⊙237
None cited in PDR database.

PROSCAR TABLETS
(Finasteride) 2040
None cited in PDR database.

PROSOM TABLETS
(Estazolam) 512
May interact with antihistamines, barbiturates, central nervous system depressants, anticonvulsants, erythromycin, monoamine oxidase inhibitors, narcotic analgesics, phenothiazines, phenytoin, psychotropics, and certain other agents. Compounds in these categories include:

Acrivastine (Co-administration may result in increased CNS depression).
No products indexed under this heading.

Alfentanil Hydrochloride (Co-administration may result in increased CNS depression).
No products indexed under this heading.

Alprazolam (Co-administration may result in increased CNS depression). Products include:
Niravam Orally Disintegrating Tablets 3106
Xanax XR Tablets 2655

Amitriptyline Hydrochloride (Co-administration may result in increased CNS depression).
No products indexed under this heading.

Amoxapine (Co-administration may result in increased CNS depression).
No products indexed under this heading.

Aprobarbital (Potent CYP3A inducers, such as barbiturates, would be expected to decrease plasma estazolam concentrations and may potentiate the action of estazolam).
No products indexed under this heading.

Astemizole (Co-administration may result in increased CNS depression).
No products indexed under this heading.

Azatadine Maleate (Co-administration may result in increased CNS depression).
No products indexed under this heading.

Bromodiphenhydramine Hydrochloride (Co-administration may result in increased CNS depression).
No products indexed under this heading.

Brompheniramine Maleate (Co-administration may result in increased CNS depression). Products include:
Alacol DM Syrup 739
Children's Dimetapp Cold & Allergy Elixir 745
Children's Dimetapp DM Cold & Cough Elixir 745
Robitussin Allergy & Cough Syrup .. 750

Buprenorphine Hydrochloride (Co-administration may result in increased CNS depression). Products include:
Buprenex Injectable 2718
Suboxone Tablets 2719
Subutex Tablets 2719

Buspirone Hydrochloride (Co-administration may result in increased CNS depression).
No products indexed under this heading.

Butabarbital (Potent CYP3A inducers, such as barbiturates, would be expected to decrease plasma estazolam concentrations and may potentiate the action of estazolam).
No products indexed under this heading.

Butalbital (Potent CYP3A inducers, such as barbiturates, would be expected to decrease plasma estazolam concentrations and may potentiate the action of estazolam). Products include:
Sedapap Tablets 50 mg/650 mg 2098

Carbamazepine (Potent CYP3A inducers, such as carbamazepine, would be expected to decrease plasma estazolam concentrations and may potentiate the action of estazolam). Products include:
Carbatrol Capsules 3174
Equetro Extended-Release Capsules 3178
Tegretol/Tegretol-XR 2278

Cetirizine Hydrochloride (Co-administration may result in increased CNS depression). Products include:
Zyrtec Chewable Tablets 2589
Zyrtec 2589
Zyrtec-D 12 Hour Extended Release Tablets 2591

Chlordiazepoxide (Co-administration may result in increased CNS depression).
No products indexed under this heading.

Chlordiazepoxide Hydrochloride (Co-administration may result in increased CNS depression). Products include:
Librium Capsules 3349

Chlorpheniramine Maleate (Co-administration may result in increased CNS depression). Products include:
Advil Allergy Sinus Caplets 737
Advil Multi-Symptom Cold Caplets 738
BC Allergy Sinus Cold Powder 612
Contac Severe Cold and Flu Caplets Maximum Strength 615
Hycomine Compound Tablets 1105
PediaCare Multi-Symptom Cold Liquid 704
PediaCare NightRest Cough & Cold Liquid 704
Robitussin Flu Liquid 752
Robitussin PM Cough & Cold Liquid 752
Singlet Caplets 636
Sudafed Sinus & Allergy Tablets 710
TheraFlu Cold & Cough Hot Liquid 680
TheraFlu Cold & Sore Throat Hot Liquid 680
TheraFlu Flu & Sore Throat Hot Liquid 681
TheraFlu Severe Cold & Cough Hot Liquid 683
TheraFlu Severe Cold Caplets 679
TheraFlu Severe Cold Hot Liquid 682
Triaminic Cold & Allergy Liquid 685
Triaminic Cold & Cough Liquid 685
Triaminic Flu, Cough & Fever Liquid 685
Triaminic Night Time Cough & Cold Liquid 685
Triaminic Allergy Runny Nose & Congestion Softchews 688
Triaminic Cold & Cough Softchews 688
Children's Tylenol Plus Cold NightTime Suspension Liquid 1851
Children's Tylenol Plus Cold & Cough Suspension Liquid and Chewable Tablets 1851
Children's Tylenol Plus Cold Chewable Tablets 1851
Children's Tylenol Plus Flu Suspension Liquid 1853
Tylenol Allergy Complete Multi-Symptom Caplets and Gelcaps with Cool Burst 1844
Multi-Symptom Tylenol Cold Night Time Caplets 1845
Vicks 44M Cough, Cold & Flu Relief 2676
Pediatric Vicks 44m Cough & Cold Relief 2673
Children's Vicks NyQuil Cold/Cough Relief 2671

Chlorpheniramine Polistirex (Co-administration may result in increased CNS depression). Products include:
Tussionex Pennkinetic Extended-Release Suspension 3322

Chlorpheniramine Tannate (Co-administration may result in increased CNS depression).
No products indexed under this heading.

Chlorpromazine (Co-administration may result in increased CNS depression).
No products indexed under this heading.

Chlorpromazine Hydrochloride (Co-administration may result in increased CNS depression).
No products indexed under this heading.

Chlorprothixene (Co-administration may result in increased CNS depression).
No products indexed under this heading.

Chlorprothixene Hydrochloride (Co-administration may result in increased CNS depression).
No products indexed under this heading.

Chlorprothixene Lactate (Co-administration may result in increased CNS depression).
No products indexed under this heading.

Cimetidine (CYP3A inhibitors, such as cimetidine, would be expected to increase plasma estazolam concentrations). Products include:
Tagamet HB 200 Tablets 637
Tagamet Tablets 1547

Cimetidine Hydrochloride (CYP3A inhibitors, such as cimetidine, would be expected to increase plasma estazolam concentrations).
No products indexed under this heading.

Clemastine Fumarate (Co-administration may result in increased CNS depression).
No products indexed under this heading.

Clonazepam (Co-administration may result in increased CNS depression). Products include:
Klonopin 2782

Clorazepate Dipotassium (Co-administration may result in increased CNS depression). Products include:
Tranxene 2488

Clozapine (Co-administration may result in increased CNS depression). Products include:
Clozapine Tablets 2141
Clozaril Tablets 2174
FazaClo Orally Disintegrating Tablets 547

Codeine Phosphate (Co-administration may result in increased CNS depression). Products include:
Tylenol with Codeine 2461

Cyproheptadine Hydrochloride (Co-administration may result in increased CNS depression).
No products indexed under this heading.

Desflurane (Co-administration may result in increased CNS depression). Products include:
Suprane Liquid for Inhalation 770

Desipramine Hydrochloride (Co-administration may result in increased CNS depression).
No products indexed under this heading.

Dexchlorpheniramine Maleate (Co-administration may result in increased CNS depression).
No products indexed under this heading.

Dezocine (Co-administration may result in increased CNS depression).
No products indexed under this heading.

Diazepam (Co-administration may result in increased CNS depression). Products include:
Diastat Rectal Delivery System 3344
Valium Tablets 2822

Diltiazem Hydrochloride (CYP3A inhibitors, such as diltiazem, would be expected to increase plasma estazolam concentrations). Products include:
Cardizem LA Extended Release Tablets 1699
Tiazac Capsules 1204

Diltiazem Maleate (CYP3A inhibitors, such as diltiazem, would be expected to increase plasma estazolam concentrations).
No products indexed under this heading.

Diphenhydramine Citrate (Co-administration may result in increased CNS depression). Products include:
Children's Benadryl Allergy & Cold Fastmelt Tablets 695
Children's Benadryl D Allergy & Sinus Fastmelt Tablets 694
Children's Benadryl Allergy Fastmelt Tablets 696
Goody's PM Powder 622

Diphenhydramine Hydrochloride (Co-administration may result in increased CNS depression). Products include:
Benadryl Allergy & Cold Tablets 692
Benadryl Allergy 691
Benadryl Allergy & Sinus Headache Caplets & Gelcaps 693
Children's Benadryl Allergy Liquid ... 695
Children's Benadryl Dye-Free Allergy Liquid 695
Benadryl Dye-Free Allergy Liqui-Gels Softgels 692
Benadryl Itch Relief Stick Extra Strength 696
Benadryl Itch Stopping Cream Extra Strength 697
Benadryl Itch Stopping Gel Extra Strength 697
Benadryl Itch Stopping Spray Extra Strength 697
Benadryl Maximum Strength Severe Allergy & Sinus Headache Caplets 694
Children's Benadryl D Liquid Medication 693
Benadryl D Tablets 694
Nytol QuickCaps Caplets 635
Maximum Strength Nytol QuickGels Softgels 635
Simply Sleep Caplets 1841
Sominex Original Formula Tablets .. 637

IMPORTANT NOTE: Always consult each drug listing in the patient's regimen for possible interactions.

TheraFlu Thin Strips Multi Symptom .... ▣684
Triaminic Thin Strips Cough & Runny Nose .... ▣690
Children's Tylenol Plus Cold & Allergy Suspension Liquid 1850
Tylenol Allergy Complete Night Time Caplets 1844
Tylenol Severe Allergy Caplets 1844
Tylenol Flu NightTime Gelcaps 1846
Extra Strength Tylenol PM Caplets, Geltabs, Gelcaps and Liquid 1847
Unisom Maximum Strength SleepGels .... ▣712

Diphenylpyraline Hydrochloride (Co-administration may result in increased CNS depression).
No products indexed under this heading.

Divalproex Sodium (Co-administration may result in increased CNS depression). Products include:
Depakote Sprinkle Capsules 422
Depakote Tablets 427
Depakote ER Tablets 433

Doxepin Hydrochloride (Co-administration may result in increased CNS depression).
No products indexed under this heading.

Droperidol (Co-administration may result in increased CNS depression).
No products indexed under this heading.

Enflurane (Co-administration may result in increased CNS depression).
No products indexed under this heading.

Erythromycin Estolate (Potent CYP3A inhibitors, such as erythromycin, would be expected to increase plasma estazolam concentrations).
No products indexed under this heading.

Erythromycin Ethylsuccinate (Potent CYP3A inhibitors, such as erythromycin, would be expected to increase plasma estazolam concentrations). Products include:
E.E.S. 449
EryPed 445

Erythromycin Gluceptate (Potent CYP3A inhibitors, such as erythromycin, would be expected to increase plasma estazolam concentrations).
No products indexed under this heading.

Erythromycin Lactobionate (Potent CYP3A inhibitors, such as erythromycin, would be expected to increase plasma estazolam concentrations).
No products indexed under this heading.

Erythromycin Stearate (Potent CYP3A inhibitors, such as erythromycin, would be expected to increase plasma estazolam concentrations). Products include:
Erythrocin Stearate Filmtab Tablets 452

Ethanol (Co-administration may result in increased CNS depression).
No products indexed under this heading.

Ethchlorvynol (Co-administration may result in increased CNS depression).
No products indexed under this heading.

Ethinamate (Co-administration may result in increased CNS depression).
No products indexed under this heading.

Ethosuximide (Co-administration may result in increased CNS depression).
No products indexed under this heading.

Ethotoin (Co-administration may result in increased CNS depression). Products include:
Peganone Tablets, USP 2487

Ethyl Alcohol (Co-administration may result in increased CNS depression).
No products indexed under this heading.

Felbamate (Co-administration may result in increased CNS depression).
No products indexed under this heading.

Fentanyl (Co-administration may result in increased CNS depression). Products include:
Duragesic Transdermal System 2448

Fentanyl Citrate (Co-administration may result in increased CNS depression). Products include:
Actiq 993

Fexofenadine Hydrochloride (Co-administration may result in increased CNS depression). Products include:
Allegra 2857
Allegra-D 12 Hour Extended-Release Tablets 2860
Allegra-D 24 Hour Extended-Release Tablets 2862

Fluphenazine Decanoate (Co-administration may result in increased CNS depression).
No products indexed under this heading.

Fluphenazine Enanthate (Co-administration may result in increased CNS depression).
No products indexed under this heading.

Fluphenazine Hydrochloride (Co-administration may result in increased CNS depression).
No products indexed under this heading.

Flurazepam Hydrochloride (Co-administration may result in increased CNS depression). Products include:
Dalmane Capsules 3343

Fluvoxamine (Potent CYP3A inhibitors, such as fluvoxamine, would be expected to increase plasma estazolam concentrations).
No products indexed under this heading.

Fluvoxamine Maleate (Potent CYP3A inhibitors, such as fluvoxamine, would be expected to increase plasma estazolam concentrations).
No products indexed under this heading.

Fosphenytoin (Co-administration may result in increased CNS depression).
No products indexed under this heading.

Fosphenytoin Sodium (Potent CYP3A inducers, such as phenytoin, would be expected to decrease plasma estazolam concentrations and may potentiate the action of estazolam).
No products indexed under this heading.

Gabapentin (Co-administration may result in increased CNS depression). Products include:
Neurontin Capsules 2498
Neurontin Oral Solution 2498
Neurontin Tablets 2498

Glutethimide (Co-administration may result in increased CNS depression).
No products indexed under this heading.

Haloperidol (Co-administration may result in increased CNS depression).
No products indexed under this heading.

Haloperidol Decanoate (Co-administration may result in increased CNS depression).
No products indexed under this heading.

Hydrocodone Bitartrate (Co-administration may result in increased CNS depression). Products include:
Hycodan 1104
Hycomine Compound Tablets 1105
Hycotuss Expectorant Syrup 1106
Lortab 3315
Lortab Elixir 3312
Vicodin Tablets 530
Vicodin ES Tablets 531
Vicodin HP Tablets 532
Vicoprofen Tablets 533
Zydone Tablets 1118

Hydrocodone Polistirex (Co-administration may result in increased CNS depression). Products include:
Tussionex Pennkinetic Extended-Release Suspension 3322

Hydromorphone Hydrochloride (Co-administration may result in increased CNS depression). Products include:
Dilaudid 439
Dilaudid Oral Liquid 443
Dilaudid Non-Sterile Powder 439
Dilaudid Rectal Suppositories 439
Dilaudid Tablets 439
Dilaudid Tablets - 8 mg 443
Dilaudid-HP 441

Hydroxyzine Hydrochloride (Co-administration may result in increased CNS depression).
No products indexed under this heading.

Imipramine Hydrochloride (Co-administration may result in increased CNS depression).
No products indexed under this heading.

Imipramine Pamoate (Co-administration may result in increased CNS depression).
No products indexed under this heading.

Isocarboxazid (Co-administration may result in increased CNS depression).
No products indexed under this heading.

Isoflurane (Co-administration may result in increased CNS depression).
No products indexed under this heading.

Isoniazid (CYP3A inhibitors, such as diltiazem isoniazid, would be expected to increase plasma estazolam concentrations).
No products indexed under this heading.

Itraconazole (Potent CYP3A inhibitors, such as itraconazole, would be expected to increase plasma estazolam concentrations; estazolam should be avoided in patients receiving itraconazole).
No products indexed under this heading.

Ketamine Hydrochloride (Co-administration may result in increased CNS depression).
No products indexed under this heading.

Ketoconazole (Potent CYP3A inhibitors, such as ketoconazole, would be expected to increase plasma estazolam concentrations; estazolam should be avoided in patients receiving ketoconazole). Products include:
Nizoral A-D Shampoo, 1% 1839
Nizoral 2% Shampoo 1838

Lamotrigine (Co-administration may result in increased CNS depression). Products include:
Lamictal 1449

Levetiracetam (Co-administration may result in increased CNS depression). Products include:
Keppra Oral Solution 3307
Keppra Tablets 3307

Levomethadyl Acetate Hydrochloride (Co-administration may result in increased CNS depression).
No products indexed under this heading.

Levorphanol Tartrate (Co-administration may result in increased CNS depression).
No products indexed under this heading.

Lithium Carbonate (Co-administration may result in increased CNS depression). Products include:
Eskalith 1406
Lithobid Tablets 1670

Lithium Citrate (Co-administration may result in increased CNS depression).
No products indexed under this heading.

Loratadine (Co-administration may result in increased CNS depression). Products include:
Alavert Allergy & Sinus D-12 Hour Tablets .... ▣743
Alavert .... ▣743
Children's Claritin 24 Hour Non-Drowsy Allergy Syrup .... ▣732
Claritin Non-Drowsy 24 Hour Tablets .... ▣731
Non-Drowsy Claritin Hives Relief Tablets .... ▣733
Claritin Reditabs 24 Hour Non-Drowsy Tablets .... ▣732
Claritin-D Non-Drowsy 12 Hour Tablets .... ▣731
Claritin-D Non-Drowsy 24 Hour Tablets .... ▣731
Children's Dimetapp ND Non-Drowsy Allergy Syrup .... ▣746
Triaminic Allerchews .... ▣684

Lorazepam (Co-administration may result in increased CNS depression).
No products indexed under this heading.

Loxapine Hydrochloride (Co-administration may result in increased CNS depression).
No products indexed under this heading.

Loxapine Succinate (Co-administration may result in increased CNS depression).
No products indexed under this heading.

Maprotiline Hydrochloride (Co-administration may result in increased CNS depression).
No products indexed under this heading.

Meperidine Hydrochloride (Co-administration may result in increased CNS depression).
No products indexed under this heading.

Mephenytoin (Co-administration may result in increased CNS depression).
No products indexed under this heading.

Mephobarbital (Potent CYP3A inducers, such as barbiturates, would be expected to decrease plasma estazolam concentrations and may potentiate the action of estazolam). Products include:
Mebaral Tablets, USP 2483
Meprobamate (Co-administration may result in increased CNS depression).
No products indexed under this heading.
Mesoridazine Besylate (Co-administration may result in increased CNS depression).
No products indexed under this heading.
Methadone Hydrochloride (Co-administration may result in increased CNS depression).
No products indexed under this heading.
Methdilazine Hydrochloride (Co-administration may result in increased CNS depression).
No products indexed under this heading.
Methohexital Sodium (Co-administration may result in increased CNS depression).
No products indexed under this heading.
Methotrimeprazine (Co-administration may result in increased CNS depression).
No products indexed under this heading.
Methoxyflurane (Co-administration may result in increased CNS depression).
No products indexed under this heading.
Methsuximide (Co-administration may result in increased CNS depression).
No products indexed under this heading.
Midazolam Hydrochloride (Co-administration may result in increased CNS depression).
No products indexed under this heading.
Moclobemide (Co-administration with MAO inhibitors may result in increased CNS depression).
No products indexed under this heading.
Molindone Hydrochloride (Co-administration may result in increased CNS depression). Products include:
Moban Tablets 1108
Morphine Sulfate (Co-administration may result in increased CNS depression). Products include:
Avinza Capsules 1714
Kadian Capsules 572
MS Contin Tablets 2703
Nefazodone Hydrochloride (Potent CYP3A inhibitors, such as nefazodone, would be expected to increase plasma estazolam concentrations).
No products indexed under this heading.
Nortriptyline Hydrochloride (Co-administration may result in increased CNS depression).
No products indexed under this heading.
Olanzapine (Co-administration may result in increased CNS depression). Products include:
Symbyax Capsules 1788
Zyprexa Tablets 1798
Zyprexa IntraMuscular 1798
Zyprexa ZYDIS Orally Disintegrating Tablets 1798
Oxazepam (Co-administration may result in increased CNS depression).
No products indexed under this heading.
Oxcarbazepine (Co-administration may result in increased CNS depression). Products include:
Trileptal Oral Suspension 2281
Trileptal Tablets 2281
Oxycodone Hydrochloride (Co-administration may result in increased CNS depression). Products include:
Combunox Tablets 1183
OxyContin Tablets 2699
OxyFast Oral Concentrate Solution 2704
OxyIR Capsules 2704
Percocet Tablets 1114
Percodan Tablets 1115
Paramethadione (Co-administration may result in increased CNS depression).
No products indexed under this heading.
Pargyline Hydrochloride (Co-administration with MAO inhibitors may result in increased CNS depression).
No products indexed under this heading.
Pentobarbital Sodium (Potent CYP3A inducers, such as barbiturates, would be expected to decrease plasma estazolam concentrations and may potentiate the action of estazolam). Products include:
Nembutal Sodium Solution, USP 2484
Perphenazine (Co-administration may result in increased CNS depression).
No products indexed under this heading.
Phenacemide (Co-administration may result in increased CNS depression).
No products indexed under this heading.
Phenelzine Sulfate (Co-administration may result in increased CNS depression).
No products indexed under this heading.
Phenobarbital (Potent CYP3A inducers, such as barbiturates, would be expected to decrease plasma estazolam concentrations and may potentiate the action of estazolam).
No products indexed under this heading.
Phensuximide (Co-administration may result in increased CNS depression).
No products indexed under this heading.
Phenytoin (Potent CYP3A inducers, such as phenytoin, would be expected to decrease plasma estazolam concentrations and may potentiate the action of estazolam).
No products indexed under this heading.
Phenytoin Sodium (Potent CYP3A inducers, such as phenytoin, would be expected to decrease plasma estazolam concentrations and may potentiate the action of estazolam). Products include:
Phenytek Capsules 2153
Prazepam (Co-administration may result in increased CNS depression).
No products indexed under this heading.
Primidone (Co-administration may result in increased CNS depression).
No products indexed under this heading.
Procarbazine Hydrochloride (Co-administration with MAO inhibitors may result in increased CNS depression). Products include:
Matulane Capsules 3188
Prochlorperazine (Co-administration may result in increased CNS depression).
No products indexed under this heading.
Promethazine Hydrochloride (Co-administration may result in increased CNS depression). Products include:
Phenergan 3438
Propofol (Co-administration may result in increased CNS depression). Products include:
Diprivan Injectable Emulsion 676
Propoxyphene Hydrochloride (Co-administration may result in increased CNS depression).
No products indexed under this heading.
Propoxyphene Napsylate (Co-administration may result in increased CNS depression). Products include:
Darvocet A 500 Tablets 3497
Protriptyline Hydrochloride (Co-administration may result in increased CNS depression). Products include:
Vivactil Tablets 2350
Pyrilamine Maleate (Co-administration may result in increased CNS depression).
No products indexed under this heading.
Pyrilamine Tannate (Co-administration may result in increased CNS depression).
No products indexed under this heading.
Quazepam (Co-administration may result in increased CNS depression).
No products indexed under this heading.
Quetiapine Fumarate (Co-administration may result in increased CNS depression). Products include:
Seroquel Tablets 691
Remifentanil Hydrochloride (Co-administration may result in increased CNS depression).
No products indexed under this heading.
Rifampin (Potent CYP3A inducers, such as rifampin, would be expected to decrease plasma estazolam concentrations).
No products indexed under this heading.
Risperidone (Co-administration may result in increased CNS depression). Products include:
Risperdal Consta Long-Acting Injection 1664
Risperdal M-Tab Orally Disintegrating Tablets.................. 1658
Risperdal 1658
Secobarbital Sodium (Potent CYP3A inducers, such as barbiturates, would be expected to decrease plasma estazolam concentrations and may potentiate the action of estazolam).
No products indexed under this heading.
Selegiline Hydrochloride (Co-administration with MAO inhibitors may result in increased CNS depression). Products include:
Eldepryl Capsules 3209
Sevoflurane (Co-administration may result in increased CNS depression). Products include:
Ultane Liquid for Inhalation 526
Sodium Oxybate (Co-administration may result in increased CNS depression).
No products indexed under this heading.
Sufentanil Citrate (Co-administration may result in increased CNS depression).
No products indexed under this heading.
Temazepam (Co-administration may result in increased CNS depression).
No products indexed under this heading.
Terfenadine (Co-administration may result in increased CNS depression).
No products indexed under this heading.
Thiamylal Sodium (Potent CYP3A inducers, such as barbiturates, would be expected to decrease plasma estazolam concentrations and may potentiate the action of estazolam).
No products indexed under this heading.
Thioridazine Hydrochloride (Co-administration may result in increased CNS depression). Products include:
Thioridazine Hydrochloride Tablets 2122
Thiothixene (Co-administration may result in increased CNS depression). Products include:
Thiothixene Capsules 2124
Tiagabine Hydrochloride (Co-administration may result in increased CNS depression). Products include:
Gabitril Tablets 998
Topiramate (Co-administration may result in increased CNS depression). Products include:
Topamax Sprinkle Capsules 2438
Topamax Tablets 2438
Tranylcypromine Sulfate (Co-administration may result in increased CNS depression). Products include:
Parnate Tablets 1499
Triazolam (Co-administration may result in increased CNS depression).
No products indexed under this heading.
Trifluoperazine Hydrochloride (Co-administration may result in increased CNS depression).
No products indexed under this heading.
Trimeprazine Tartrate (Co-administration may result in increased CNS depression).
No products indexed under this heading.

IMPORTANT NOTE: Always consult each drug listing in the patient's regimen for possible interactions.

Trimethadione (Co-administration may result in increased CNS depression).
No products indexed under this heading.

Trimipramine Maleate (Co-administration may result in increased CNS depression). Products include:
Surmontil Capsules 2347

Tripelennamine Hydrochloride (Co-administration may result in increased CNS depression).
No products indexed under this heading.

Triprolidine Hydrochloride (Co-administration may result in increased CNS depression).
No products indexed under this heading.

Valproate Sodium (Co-administration may result in increased CNS depression). Products include:
Depacon Injection 412

Valproic Acid (Co-administration may result in increased CNS depression). Products include:
Depakene 417

Zaleplon (Co-administration may result in increased CNS depression). Products include:
Sonata Capsules 1686

Ziprasidone Hydrochloride (Co-administration may result in increased CNS depression). Products include:
Geodon Capsules 2514

Zolpidem Tartrate (Co-administration may result in increased CNS depression). Products include:
Ambien Tablets 2867

Zonisamide (Co-administration may result in increased CNS depression). Products include:
Zonegran Capsules 1089

Food Interactions

Alcohol (Co-administration may result in increased CNS depression).

PROTONIX I.V.

(Pantoprazole Sodium) 3468
See Protonix Tablets

PROTONIX TABLETS

(Pantoprazole Sodium) 3465
May interact with iron containing oral preparations and certain other agents. Compounds in these categories include:

Bacampicillin Hydrochloride (Pantoprazole produces sustained inhibition of gastric acid secretion; pantoprazole may interfere with the absorption of certain drugs, such as ampicillin esters, where gastric pH is an important determinant of the bioavailability).
No products indexed under this heading.

Ferrous Fumarate (Pantoprazole produces sustained inhibition of gastric acid secretion; pantoprazole may interfere with the absorption of certain drugs, such as iron salts, where gastric pH is an important determinant of the bioavailability). Products include:
Chromagen Forte Soft Gelatin Capsules 3296
Ferretts Tablets .... ▣773
Repliva 21/7 Tablets 3301

Ferrous Gluconate (Pantoprazole produces sustained inhibition of gastric acid secretion; pantoprazole may interfere with the absorption of certain drugs, such as iron salts, where gastric pH is an important determinant of the bioavailability).
No products indexed under this heading.

Ferrous Sulfate (Pantoprazole produces sustained inhibition of gastric acid secretion; pantoprazole may interfere with the absorption of certain drugs, such as iron salts, where gastric pH is an important determinant of the bioavailability). Products include:
Feosol Tablets 1629
Slow Fe Iron Tablets .... ▣772
Slow Fe with Folic Acid Tablets .... ▣773

Iron (Pantoprazole produces sustained inhibition of gastric acid secretion; pantoprazole may interfere with the absorption of certain drugs, such as iron salts, where gastric pH is an important determinant of the bioavailability). Products include:
Chromagen Forte Soft Gelatin Capsules 3296
Ferretts IPS Liquid .... ▣773
OptiNate 1162
Repliva 21/7 Tablets 3301

Ketoconazole (Pantoprazole produces sustained inhibition of gastric acid secretion; pantoprazole may interfere with the absorption of certain drugs, such as ketoconazole, where gastric pH is an important determinant of the bioavailability). Products include:
Nizoral A-D Shampoo, 1% 1839
Nizoral 2% Shampoo 1838

Polysaccharide Iron Complex (Pantoprazole produces sustained inhibition of gastric acid secretion; pantoprazole may interfere with the absorption of certain drugs, such as iron salts, where gastric pH is an important determinant of the bioavailability). Products include:
Niferex-150 Forte Capsules 3299
Nu-Iron 150 Capsules 2098

Warfarin Sodium (There have been reports of increased INR and prothrombin time in patients receiving proton pump inhibitors, including pantoprazole and warfarin concomitantly. Patients treated with proton pump inhibitors and warfarin concomitantly should be monitored forincreases in INR and prothrombin time). Products include:
Coumadin for Injection 932
Coumadin Tablets 932

PROTOPIC OINTMENT

(Tacrolimus) 629
May interact with calcium channel blockers, erythromycin, and certain other agents. Compounds in these categories include:

Amlodipine Besylate (Co-administration of known CYP3A4 inhibitors, such as calcium channel blockers, in patients with widespread and/or erythrodermic disease should be done with caution; based on its minimal extent of absorption, interactions of Protopic Ointment with systemically administered drugs are unlikely to occur but cannot be ruled out). Products include:
Caduet Tablets 2507
Lotrel Capsules 2238
Norvasc Tablets 2529

Bepridil Hydrochloride (Co-administration of known CYP3A4 inhibitors, such as calcium channel blockers, in patients with widespread and/or erythrodermic disease should be done with caution; based on its minimal extent of absorption, interactions of Protopic Ointment with systemically administered drugs are unlikely to occur but cannot be ruled out).
No products indexed under this heading.

Cimetidine (Co-administration of known CYP3A4 inhibitors, such as cimetidine, in patients with widespread and/or erythrodermic disease should be done with caution; based on its minimal extent of absorption, interactions of Protopic Ointment with systemically administered drugs are unlikely to occur but cannot be ruled out). Products include:
Tagamet HB 200 Tablets .... ▣637
Tagamet Tablets 1547

Cimetidine Hydrochloride (Co-administration of known CYP3A4 inhibitors, such as cimetidine, in patients with widespread and/or erythrodermic disease should be done with caution; based on its minimal extent of absorption, interactions of Protopic Ointment with systemically administered drugs are unlikely to occur but cannot be ruled out).
No products indexed under this heading.

Diltiazem Hydrochloride (Co-administration of known CYP3A4 inhibitors, such as calcium channel blockers, in patients with widespread and/or erythrodermic disease should be done with caution; based on its minimal extent of absorption, interactions of Protopic Ointment with systemically administered drugs are unlikely to occur but cannot be ruled out). Products include:
Cardizem LA Extended Release Tablets 1699
Tiazac Capsules 1204

Erythromycin (Co-administration of known CYP3A4 inhibitors, such as erythromycin, in patients with widespread and/or erythrodermic disease should be done with caution; based on its minimal extent of absorption, interactions of Protopic Ointment with systemically administered drugs are unlikely to occur but cannot be ruled out). Products include:
Erygel Topical Gel 2096
Ery-Tab Tablets 447
Erythromycin Base Filmtab Tablets 454
Erythromycin Delayed-Release Capsules, USP 456
PCE Dispertab Tablets 510

Erythromycin Estolate (Co-administration of known CYP3A4 inhibitors, such as erythromycin, in patients with widespread and/or erythrodermic disease should be done with caution; based on its minimal extent of absorption, interactions of Protopic Ointment with systemically administered drugs are unlikely to occur but cannot be ruled out).
No products indexed under this heading.

Erythromycin Ethylsuccinate (Co-administration of known CYP3A4 inhibitors, such as erythromycin, in patients with widespread and/or erythrodermic disease should be done with caution; based on its minimal extent of absorption, interactions of Protopic Ointment with systemically administered drugs are unlikely to occur but cannot be ruled out). Products include:
E.E.S. 449
EryPed 445

Erythromycin Gluceptate (Co-administration of known CYP3A4 inhibitors, such as erythromycin, in patients with widespread and/or erythrodermic disease should be done with caution; based on its minimal extent of absorption, interactions of Protopic Ointment with systemically administered drugs are unlikely to occur but cannot be ruled out).
No products indexed under this heading.

Erythromycin Lactobionate (Co-administration of known CYP3A4 inhibitors, such as erythromycin, in patients with widespread and/or erythrodermic disease should be done with caution; based on its minimal extent of absorption, interactions of Protopic Ointment with systemically administered drugs are unlikely to occur but cannot be ruled out).
No products indexed under this heading.

Erythromycin Stearate (Co-administration of known CYP3A4 inhibitors, such as erythromycin, in patients with widespread and/or erythrodermic disease should be done with caution; based on its minimal extent of absorption, interactions of Protopic Ointment with systemically administered drugs are unlikely to occur but cannot be ruled out). Products include:
Erythrocin Stearate Filmtab Tablets 452

Felodipine (Co-administration of known CYP3A4 inhibitors, such as calcium channel blockers, in patients with widespread and/or erythrodermic disease should be done with caution; based on its minimal extent of absorption, interactions of Protopic Ointment with systemically administered drugs are unlikely to occur but cannot be ruled out). Products include:
Plendil Extended-Release Tablets 651

Fluconazole (Co-administration of known CYP3A4 inhibitors, such as fluconazole, in patients with widespread and/or erythrodermic disease should be done with caution; based on its minimal extent of absorption, interactions of Protopic Ointment with systemically administered drugs are unlikely to occur but cannot be ruled out).
No products indexed under this heading.

Isradipine (Co-administration of known CYP3A4 inhibitors, such as calcium channel blockers, in patients with widespread and/or erythrodermic disease should be done with caution; based on its minimal extent of absorption, interactions of Protopic Ointment with systemically administered drugs are unlikely to occur but cannot be ruled out). Products include:
DynaCirc CR Tablets 2726

Itraconazole (Co-administration of known CYP3A4 inhibitors, such as itraconazole, in patients with widespread and/or erythrodermic disease should be done with caution; based on its minimal extent of absorption, interactions of Protopic Ointment with systemically administered drugs are unlikely to occur but cannot be ruled out).

No products indexed under this heading.

Ketoconazole (Co-administration of known CYP3A4 inhibitors, such as ketoconazole, in patients with widespread and/or erythrodermic disease should be done with caution; based on its minimal extent of absorption, interactions of Protopic Ointment with systemically administered drugs are unlikely to occur but cannot be ruled out). Products include:

Nizoral A-D Shampoo, 1% ... **1839**
Nizoral 2% Shampoo ... **1838**

Mibefradil Dihydrochloride (Co-administration of known CYP3A4 inhibitors, such as calcium channel blockers, in patients with widespread and/or erythrodermic disease should be done with caution; based on its minimal extent of absorption, interactions of Protopic Ointment with systemically administered drugs are unlikely to occur but cannot be ruled out).

No products indexed under this heading.

Nicardipine Hydrochloride (Co-administration of known CYP3A4 inhibitors, such as calcium channel blockers, in patients with widespread and/or erythrodermic disease should be done with caution; based on its minimal extent of absorption, interactions of Protopic Ointment with systemically administered drugs are unlikely to occur but cannot be ruled out). Products include:

Cardene I.V. ... **1129**

Nifedipine (Co-administration of known CYP3A4 inhibitors, such as calcium channel blockers, in patients with widespread and/or erythrodermic disease should be done with caution; based on its minimal extent of absorption, interactions of Protopic Ointment with systemically administered drugs are unlikely to occur but cannot be ruled out). Products include:

Adalat CC Tablets ... **2978**

Nimodipine (Co-administration of known CYP3A4 inhibitors, such as calcium channel blockers, in patients with widespread and/or erythrodermic disease should be done with caution; based on its minimal extent of absorption, interactions of Protopic Ointment with systemically administered drugs are unlikely to occur but cannot be ruled out). Products include:

Nimotop Capsules ... **774**

Nisoldipine (Co-administration of known CYP3A4 inhibitors, such as calcium channel blockers, in patients with widespread and/or erythrodermic disease should be done with caution; based on its minimal extent of absorption, interactions of Protopic Ointment with systemically administered drugs are unlikely to occur but cannot be ruled out). Products include:

Sular Tablets ... **1163**

Verapamil Hydrochloride (Co-administration of known CYP3A4 inhibitors, such as calcium channel blockers, in patients with widespread and/or erythrodermic disease should be done with caution; based on its minimal extent of absorption, interactions of Protopic Ointment with systemically administered drugs are unlikely to occur but cannot be ruled out). Products include:

Covera-HS Tablets ... **3135**
Tarka Tablets ... **519**
Verelan PM Capsules ... **3120**

PROVENTIL INHALATION AEROSOL

(Albuterol) ... **3067**

May interact with beta blockers, drugs that lower serum potassium (selected), loop diuretics, monoamine oxidase inhibitors, nonpotassium-sparing diuretics, thiazides, tricyclic antidepressants, and certain other agents. Compounds in these categories include:

Acebutolol Hydrochloride (Beta-adrenergic receptor blocking agents not only block the pulmonary effect of beta-agonists, such as albuterol, but may produce severe bronchospasm in asthmatic patients. Therefore, patients with asthma should not normally be treated with beta-blockers. However, under certain circumstances, (e.g., as prophylaxis after myocardial infarction) there may be no acceptable alternatives to the use of beta-adrenergic-blocking agents in patients with asthma. In this setting, cardioselective beta-blockers should be considered, although they should be administered with caution).

No products indexed under this heading.

Amitriptyline Hydrochloride (Albuterol should be administered with extreme caution to patients being treated with tricyclic antidepressants, or within 2 weeks of discontinuation of such agents, because of action of albuterol on the cardiovascular system may be potentiated).

No products indexed under this heading.

Amoxapine (Albuterol should be administered with extreme caution to patients being treated with tricyclic antidepressants, or within 2 weeks of discontinuation of such agents, because of action of albuterol on the cardiovascular system may be potentiated).

No products indexed under this heading.

Atenolol (Beta-adrenergic receptor blocking agents not only block the pulmonary effect of beta-agonists, such as albuterol, but may produce severe bronchospasm in asthmatic patients. Therefore, patients with asthma should not normally be treated with beta-blockers. However, under certain circumstances, (e.g., as prophylaxis after myocardial infarction) there may be no acceptable alternatives to the use of beta-adrenergic-blocking agents in patients with asthma. In this setting, cardioselective beta-blockers should be considered, although they should be administered with caution). Products include:

Tenormin I.V. Injection ... **698**
Tenormin Tablets ... **695**

Bendroflumethiazide (Potential for additive hypokalemic effect with concurrent use).

No products indexed under this heading.

Betamethasone Acetate (Potential for additive hypokalemic effect with concurrent use).

No products indexed under this heading.

Betamethasone Sodium Phosphate (Potential for additive hypokalemic effect with concurrent use).

No products indexed under this heading.

Betaxolol Hydrochloride (Beta-adrenergic receptor blocking agents not only block the pulmonary effect of beta-agonists, such as albuterol, but may produce severe bronchospasm in asthmatic patients. Therefore, patients with asthma should not normally be treated with beta-blockers. However, under certain circumstances, (e.g., as prophylaxis after myocardial infarction) there may be no acceptable alternatives to the use of beta-adrenergic-blocking agents in patients with asthma. In this setting, cardioselective beta-blockers should be considered, although they should be administered with caution). Products include:

Betoptic S Ophthalmic Suspension ... **554**

Bisoprolol Fumarate (Beta-adrenergic receptor blocking agents not only block the pulmonary effect of beta-agonists, such as albuterol, but may produce severe bronchospasm in asthmatic patients. Therefore, patients with asthma should not normally be treated with beta-blockers. However, under certain circumstances, (e.g., as prophylaxis after myocardial infarction) there may be no acceptable alternatives to the use of beta-adrenergic-blocking agents in patients with asthma. In this setting, cardioselective beta-blockers should be considered, although they should be administered with caution).

No products indexed under this heading.

Bumetanide (The ECG changes and/or hypokalemia which may result from the administration of non-potassium sparing diuretics (such as loop or thiazide diuretics) can be acutely worsened by beta agonists, especially when the recommended dose of the beta agonist is exceeded. Although the clinical significance of these effects is not known, caution is advised in the co-administration of beta agonists with non-potassium sparing diuretics).

No products indexed under this heading.

Carteolol Hydrochloride (Beta-adrenergic receptor blocking agents not only block the pulmonary effect of beta-agonists, such as albuterol, but may produce severe bronchospasm in asthmatic patients. Therefore, patients with asthma should not normally be treated with beta-blockers. However, under certain circumstances, (e.g., as prophylaxis after myocardial infarction) there may be no acceptable alternatives to the use of beta-adrenergic-blocking agents in patients with asthma. In this setting, cardioselective beta-blockers should be considered, although they should be administered with caution). Products include:

Carteolol Hydrochloride Ophthalmic Solution USP, 1% ... ⊙ **246**

Chlorothiazide (Potential for additive hypokalemic effect with concurrent use). Products include:

Aldoclor Tablets ... **1881**
Diuril Oral ... **1936**

Chlorothiazide Sodium (Potential for additive hypokalemic effect with concurrent use). Products include:

Diuril Sodium Intravenous ... **1934**

Clomipramine Hydrochloride (Albuterol should be administered with extreme caution to patients being treated with tricyclic antidepressants, or within 2 weeks of discontinuation of such agents, because of action of albuterol on the cardiovascular system may be potentiated).

No products indexed under this heading.

Cortisone Acetate (Potential for additive hypokalemic effect with concurrent use).

No products indexed under this heading.

Desipramine Hydrochloride (Albuterol should be administered with extreme caution to patients being treated with tricyclic antidepressants, or within 2 weeks of discontinuation of such agents, because of action of albuterol on the cardiovascular system may be potentiated).

No products indexed under this heading.

Dexamethasone (Potential for additive hypokalemic effect with concurrent use). Products include:

Ciprodex Otic Suspension ... **555**
Decadron Tablets ... **1929**
TobraDex Ophthalmic Ointment ... **558**
TobraDex Ophthalmic Suspension ... **558**

Dexamethasone Acetate (Potential for additive hypokalemic effect with concurrent use).

No products indexed under this heading.

Dexamethasone Sodium Phosphate (Potential for additive hypokalemic effect with concurrent use). Products include:

Decadron Phosphate Injection ... **1931**

Digoxin (Mean decreases of 16% and 22% in serum digoxin levels were demonstrated after single-dose intravenous and oral administration of albuterol, respectively, to normal volunteers who had received digoxin for 10 days. The clinical significance of these findings for patients with obstructive airway disease who are receiving albuterol and digoxin on a chronic basis is unclear; nevertheless, it would be prudent to carefully evaluate the serum digoxin levels in patients who are currently receiving digoxin and albuterol). Products include:

Digitek Tablets ... **2146**
Lanoxicaps Capsules ... **1458**
Lanoxin Injection ... **1462**
Lanoxin Tablets ... **1468**
Lanoxin Injection Pediatric ... **1465**

Doxepin Hydrochloride (Albuterol should be administered with extreme caution to patients being treated with tricyclic antidepressants, or within 2 weeks of discontinuation of such agents, because of action of albuterol on the cardiovascular system may be potentiated).
No products indexed under this heading.

Esmolol Hydrochloride (Beta-adrenergic receptor blocking agents not only block the pulmonary effect of beta-agonists, such as albuterol, but may produce severe bronchospasm in asthmatic patients. Therefore, patients with asthma should not normally be treated with beta-blockers. However, under certain circumstances, (e.g., as prophylaxis after myocardial infarction) there may be no acceptable alternatives to the use of beta-adrenergic-blocking agents in patients with asthma. In this setting, cardioselective beta-blockers should be considered, although they should be administered with caution). Products include:
Brevibloc Concentrate 766
Brevibloc Injection 766
Brevibloc Double Strength Injection 766
Brevibloc Premixed Injection 766
Brevibloc Double Strength Premixed Injection 766

Ethacrynic Acid (The ECG changes and/or hypokalemia which may result from the administration of non-potassium sparing diuretics (such as loop or thiazide diuretics) can be acutely worsened by beta agonists, especially when the recommended dose of the beta agonist is exceeded. Although the clinical significance of these effects is not known, caution is advised in the co-administration of beta agonists with non-potassium sparing diuretics). Products include:
Edecrin Tablets 1941

Furosemide (The ECG changes and/or hypokalemia which may result from the administration of non-potassium sparing diuretics (such as loop or thiazide diuretics) can be acutely worsened by beta agonists, especially when the recommended dose of the beta agonist is exceeded. Although the clinical significance of these effects is not known, caution is advised in the co-administration of beta agonists with non-potassium sparing diuretics). Products include:
Furosemide Tablets 2117

Hydrochlorothiazide (Potential for additive hypokalemic effect with concurrent use). Products include:
Aldoril Tablets 1884
Atacand HCT 637
Avalide Tablets 2889
Avalide Tablets 922
Benicar HCT Tablets 2852
Diovan HCT Tablets 2195
Dyazide Capsules 1389
Hyzaar 1964
Lotensin HCT Tablets 2235
Maxzide 2150
Micardis HCT Tablets 886
Moduretic Tablets 2003
Prinzide Tablets 2033
Teveten HCT Tablets 1710
Timolide Tablets 2056
Uniretic Tablets 3114
Vaseretic Tablets 2073
Zestoretic Tablets 701

Hydrocortisone (Potential for additive hypokalemic effect with concurrent use). Products include:
Cortizone•5 Ointment .... ▣699
Cortizone•10 Creme .... ▣699
Cortizone•10 Ointment .... ▣699
Cortizone•10 Plus Creme .... ▣700
Cortizone•10 Maximum Strength Quick Shot Spray .... ▣700
Hydrocortone Tablets 1963
Preparation H Hydrocortisone Cream .... ▣748

Hydrocortisone Acetate (Potential for additive hypokalemic effect with concurrent use). Products include:
Analpram-HC 1136
Pramosone 1139
ProctoFoam-HC 3113
Tucks Anti-Itch Ointment .... ▣712
U-cort 1% Cream 3289

Hydrocortisone Sodium Phosphate (Potential for additive hypokalemic effect with concurrent use).
No products indexed under this heading.

Hydrocortisone Sodium Succinate (Potential for additive hypokalemic effect with concurrent use).
No products indexed under this heading.

Hydroflumethiazide (Potential for additive hypokalemic effect with concurrent use).
No products indexed under this heading.

Imipramine Hydrochloride (Albuterol should be administered with extreme caution to patients being treated with tricyclic antidepressants, or within 2 weeks of discontinuation of such agents, because of action of albuterol on the cardiovascular system may be potentiated).
No products indexed under this heading.

Imipramine Pamoate (Albuterol should be administered with extreme caution to patients being treated with tricyclic antidepressants, or within 2 weeks of discontinuation of such agents, because of action of albuterol on the cardiovascular system may be potentiated).
No products indexed under this heading.

Isocarboxazid (Albuterol should be administered with extreme caution to patients being treated with monoamine oxidase inhibitors, or within 2 weeks of discontinuation of such agents, because of action of albuterol on the cardiovascular system may be potentiated).
No products indexed under this heading.

Labetalol Hydrochloride (Beta-adrenergic receptor blocking agents not only block the pulmonary effect of beta-agonists, such as albuterol, but may produce severe bronchospasm in asthmatic patients. Therefore, patients with asthma should not normally be treated with beta-blockers. However, under certain circumstances, (e.g., as prophylaxis after myocardial infarction) there may be no acceptable alternatives to the use of beta-adrenergic-blocking agents in patients with asthma. In this setting, cardioselective beta-blockers should be considered, although they should be administered with caution).
No products indexed under this heading.

Levobunolol Hydrochloride (Beta-adrenergic receptor blocking agents not only block the pulmonary effect of beta-agonists, such as albuterol, but may produce severe bronchospasm in asthmatic patients. Therefore, patients with asthma should not normally be treated with beta-blockers. However, under certain circumstances, (e.g., as prophylaxis after myocardial infarction) there may be no acceptable alternatives to the use of beta-adrenergic-blocking agents in patients with asthma. In this setting, cardioselective beta-blockers should be considered, although they should be administered with caution). Products include:
Betagan Ophthalmic Solution, USP .... ⊙217

Maprotiline Hydrochloride (Albuterol should be administered with extreme caution to patients being treated with tricyclic antidepressants, or within 2 weeks of discontinuation of such agents, because of action of albuterol on the cardiovascular system may be potentiated).
No products indexed under this heading.

Methyclothiazide (Potential for additive hypokalemic effect with concurrent use).
No products indexed under this heading.

Methylprednisolone Acetate (Potential for additive hypokalemic effect with concurrent use). Products include:
Depo-Medrol Injectable Suspension 2615
Depo-Medrol Single-Dose Vial 2617

Methylprednisolone Sodium Succinate (Potential for additive hypokalemic effect with concurrent use).
No products indexed under this heading.

Metipranolol Hydrochloride (Beta-adrenergic receptor blocking agents not only block the pulmonary effect of beta-agonists, such as albuterol, but may produce severe bronchospasm in asthmatic patients. Therefore, patients with asthma should not normally be treated with beta-blockers. However, under certain circumstances, (e.g., as prophylaxis after myocardial infarction) there may be no acceptable alternatives to the use of beta-adrenergic-blocking agents in patients with asthma. In this setting, cardioselective beta-blockers should be considered, although they should be administered with caution).
No products indexed under this heading.

Metoprolol Succinate (Beta-adrenergic receptor blocking agents not only block the pulmonary effect of beta-agonists, such as albuterol, but may produce severe bronchospasm in asthmatic patients. Therefore, patients with asthma should not normally be treated with beta-blockers. However, under certain circumstances, (e.g., as prophylaxis after myocardial infarction) there may be no acceptable alternatives to the use of beta-adrenergic-blocking agents in patients with asthma. In this setting, cardioselective beta-blockers should be considered, although they should be administered with caution). Products include:
Toprol-XL Tablets 660

Metoprolol Tartrate (Beta-adrenergic receptor blocking agents not only block the pulmonary effect of beta-agonists, such as albuterol, but may produce severe bronchospasm in asthmatic patients. Therefore, patients with asthma should not normally be treated with beta-blockers. However, under certain circumstances, (e.g., as prophylaxis after myocardial infarction) there may be no acceptable alternatives to the use of beta-adrenergic-blocking agents in patients with asthma. In this setting, cardioselective beta-blockers should be considered, although they should be administered with caution).
No products indexed under this heading.

Moclobemide (Albuterol should be administered with extreme caution to patients being treated with monoamine oxidase inhibitors, or within 2 weeks of discontinuation of such agents, because of action of albuterol on the cardiovascular system may be potentiated).
No products indexed under this heading.

Nadolol (Beta-adrenergic receptor blocking agents not only block the pulmonary effect of beta-agonists, such as albuterol, but may produce severe bronchospasm in asthmatic patients. Therefore, patients with asthma should not normally be treated with beta-blockers. However, under certain circumstances, (e.g., as prophylaxis after myocardial infarction) there may be no acceptable alternatives to the use of beta-adrenergic-blocking agents in patients with asthma. In this setting, cardioselective beta-blockers should be considered, although they should be administered with caution). Products include:
Nadolol Tablets 2121

Nortriptyline Hydrochloride (Albuterol should be administered with extreme caution to patients being treated with tricyclic antidepressants, or within 2 weeks of discontinuation of such agents, because of action of albuterol on the cardiovascular system may be potentiated).
No products indexed under this heading.

Pargyline Hydrochloride (Albuterol should be administered with extreme caution to patients being treated with monoamine oxidase inhibitors, or within 2 weeks of discontinuation of such agents, because of action of albuterol on the cardiovascular system may be potentiated).
No products indexed under this heading.

Penbutolol Sulfate (Beta-adrenergic receptor blocking agents not only block the pulmonary effect of beta-agonists, such as albuterol, but may produce severe bronchospasm in asthmatic patients. Therefore, patients with asthma should not normally be treated with beta-blockers. However, under certain circumstances, (e.g., as prophylaxis after myocardial infarction) there may be no acceptable alternatives to the use of beta-adrenergic-blocking agents in patients with asthma. In this setting, cardioselective beta-blockers should be considered, although they should

be administered with caution).
No products indexed under this heading.

Phenelzine Sulfate (Albuterol should be administered with extreme caution to patients being treated with monoamine oxidase inhibitors, or within 2 weeks of discontinuation of such agents, because of action of albuterol on the cardiovascular system may be potentiated).
No products indexed under this heading.

Pindolol (Beta-adrenergic receptor blocking agents not only block the pulmonary effect of beta-agonists, such as albuterol, but may produce severe bronchospasm in asthmatic patients. Therefore, patients with asthma should not normally be treated with beta-blockers. However, under certain circumstances, (e.g., as prophylaxis after myocardial infarction) there may be no acceptable alternatives to the use of beta-adrenergic-blocking agents in patients with asthma. In this setting, cardioselective beta-blockers should be considered, although they should be administered with caution).
No products indexed under this heading.

Polythiazide (Potential for additive hypokalemic effect with concurrent use).
No products indexed under this heading.

Prednisolone Acetate (Potential for additive hypokalemic effect with concurrent use). Products include:
Blephamide Ophthalmic Ointment 563
Blephamide Ophthalmic Suspension 564
Poly-Pred Liquifilm Ophthalmic Suspension .... ⊙ 231
Pred Forte Ophthalmic Suspension .... ⊙ 233
Pred Mild Sterile Ophthalmic Suspension .... ⊙ 236
Pred-G Ophthalmic Suspension .... ⊙ 234
Pred-G Sterile Ophthalmic Ointment .... ⊙ 235

Prednisolone Sodium Phosphate (Potential for additive hypokalemic effect with concurrent use). Products include:
Pediapred Oral Solution 3319

Prednisolone Tebutate (Potential for additive hypokalemic effect with concurrent use).
No products indexed under this heading.

Prednisone (Potential for additive hypokalemic effect with concurrent use).
No products indexed under this heading.

Procarbazine Hydrochloride (Albuterol should be administered with extreme caution to patients being treated with monoamine oxidase inhibitors, or within 2 weeks of discontinuation of such agents, because of action of albuterol on the cardiovascular system may be potentiated). Products include:
Matulane Capsules 3188

Propranolol Hydrochloride (Beta-adrenergic receptor blocking agents not only block the pulmonary effect of beta-agonists, such as albuterol, but may produce severe bronchospasm in asthmatic patients. Therefore, patients with asthma should not normally be treated with beta-blockers. However, under certain circumstances, (e.g., as prophylaxis after myocardial infarction) there may be no acceptable alternatives to the use of beta-adrenergic-blocking agents in patients with asthma. In this setting, cardioselective beta-blockers should be considered, although they should be administered with caution). Products include:
Inderal LA Long-Acting Capsules 3421
InnoPran XL Capsules 2728

Protriptyline Hydrochloride (Albuterol should be administered with extreme caution to patients being treated with tricyclic antidepressants, or within 2 weeks of discontinuation of such agents, because of action of albuterol on the cardiovascular system may be potentiated). Products include:
Vivactil Tablets 2350

Selegiline Hydrochloride (Albuterol should be administered with extreme caution to patients being treated with monoamine oxidase inhibitors, or within 2 weeks of discontinuation of such agents, because of action of albuterol on the cardiovascular system may be potentiated). Products include:
Eldepryl Capsules 3209

Sotalol Hydrochloride (Beta-adrenergic receptor blocking agents not only block the pulmonary effect of beta-agonists, such as albuterol, but may produce severe bronchospasm in asthmatic patients. Therefore, patients with asthma should not normally be treated with beta-blockers. However, under certain circumstances, (e.g., as prophylaxis after myocardial infarction) there may be no acceptable alternatives to the use of beta-adrenergic-blocking agents in patients with asthma. In this setting, cardioselective beta-blockers should be considered, although they should be administered with caution).
No products indexed under this heading.

Timolol Hemihydrate (Beta-adrenergic receptor blocking agents not only block the pulmonary effect of beta-agonists, such as albuterol, but may produce severe bronchospasm in asthmatic patients. Therefore, patients with asthma should not normally be treated with beta-blockers. However, under certain circumstances, (e.g., as prophylaxis after myocardial infarction) there may be no acceptable alternatives to the use of beta-adrenergic-blocking agents in patients with asthma. In this setting, cardioselective beta-blockers should be considered, although they should be administered with caution). Products include:
Betimol Ophthalmic Solution 3371
Betimol Ophthalmic Solution .... ⊙ 283

Timolol Maleate (Beta-adrenergic receptor blocking agents not only block the pulmonary effect of beta-agonists, such as albuterol, but may produce severe bronchospasm in asthmatic patients. Therefore, patients with asthma should not normally be treated with beta-blockers. However, under certain circumstances, (e.g., as prophylaxis after myocardial infarction) there may be no acceptable alternatives to the use of beta-adrenergic-blocking agents in patients with asthma. In this setting, cardioselective beta-blockers should be considered, although they should be administered with caution). Products include:
Blocadren Tablets 1891
Cosopt Sterile Ophthalmic Solution 1910
Timolide Tablets 2056
Timoptic in Ocudose 2061
Timoptic Sterile Ophthalmic Solution 2058
Timoptic-XE Sterile Ophthalmic Gel Forming Solution 2062

Torsemide (The ECG changes and/or hypokalemia which may result from the administration of non-potassium sparing diuretics (such as loop or thiazide diuretics) can be acutely worsened by beta agonists, especially when the recommended dose of the beta agonist is exceeded. Although the clinical significance of these effects is not known, caution is advised in the co-administration of beta agonists with non-potassium sparing diuretics).
No products indexed under this heading.

Tranylcypromine Sulfate (Albuterol should be administered with extreme caution to patients being treated with monoamine oxidase inhibitors, or within 2 weeks of discontinuation of such agents, because of action of albuterol on the cardiovascular system may be potentiated). Products include:
Parnate Tablets 1499

Triamcinolone (Potential for additive hypokalemic effect with concurrent use).
No products indexed under this heading.

Triamcinolone Acetonide (Potential for additive hypokalemic effect with concurrent use). Products include:
Azmacort Inhalation Aerosol 1701
Nasacort HFA Inhalation Aerosol 2939
Nasacort AQ Nasal Spray 2937

Triamcinolone Diacetate (Potential for additive hypokalemic effect with concurrent use).
No products indexed under this heading.

Triamcinolone Hexacetonide (Potential for additive hypokalemic effect with concurrent use).
No products indexed under this heading.

Trimipramine Maleate (Albuterol should be administered with extreme caution to patients being treated with tricyclic antidepressants, or within 2 weeks of discontinuation of such agents, because of action of albuterol on the cardiovascular system may be potentiated). Products include:
Surmontil Capsules 2347

PROVENTIL INHALATION SOLUTION 0.083%

(Albuterol Sulfate) 3069
May interact with:

See (Proventil Inhalation Aerosol).

PROVENTIL HFA INHALATION AEROSOL

(Albuterol Sulfate) 3071
May interact with beta blockers, loop diuretics, monoamine oxidase inhibitors, nonpotassium-sparing diuretics, thiazides, tricyclic antidepressants, and certain other agents. Compounds in these categories include:

Acebutolol Hydrochloride (Co-administration with beta adrenergic blocking agent blocks the pulmonary effect of beta agonists and may produce severe bronchospasm in asthmatic patients; co-administer with caution).
No products indexed under this heading.

Amitriptyline Hydrochloride (Action of albuterol on the cardiovascular system may be potentiated by tricyclic antidepressants; co-administer with caution).
No products indexed under this heading.

Amoxapine (Action of albuterol on the cardiovascular system may be potentiated by tricyclic antidepressants; co-administer with caution).
No products indexed under this heading.

Atenolol (Co-administration with beta adrenergic blocking agent blocks the pulmonary effect of beta agonists and may produce severe bronchospasm in asthmatic patients; co-administer with caution). Products include:
Tenormin I.V. Injection 698
Tenormin Tablets 695

Bendroflumethiazide (The ECG changes and hypokalemia which may result from administration of nonpotassium-sparing diuretics can be acutely worsened by beta agonists. Caution is advised in the co-administration of beta agonists with nonpotassium-sparing diuretics).
No products indexed under this heading.

Betaxolol Hydrochloride (Co-administration with beta adrenergic blocking agent blocks the pulmonary effect of beta agonists and may produce severe bronchospasm in asthmatic patients; co-administer with caution). Products include:
Betoptic S Ophthalmic Suspension 554

Bisoprolol Fumarate (Co-administration with beta adrenergic blocking agent blocks the pulmonary effect of beta agonists and may produce severe bronchospasm in asthmatic patients; co-administer with caution).
No products indexed under this heading.

Bumetanide (The ECG changes and hypokalemia which may result from administration of nonpotassium-sparing diuretics can be acutely worsened by beta agonists. Caution is advised in the co-administration of beta agonists with nonpotassium-sparing diuretics).
No products indexed under this heading.

Carteolol Hydrochloride (Co-administration with beta adrenergic blocking agent blocks the pulmonary effect of beta agonists and may produce severe bronchospasm in asthmatic patients; co-administer with caution). Products include:
Carteolol Hydrochloride Ophthalmic Solution USP, 1% .... ⊙ 246

Chlorothiazide (The ECG changes and hypokalemia which may result from administration of nonpotassium-sparing diuretics can be acutely worsened by beta agonists. Caution is advised in the co-administration of beta agonists with nonpotassium-sparing diuretics). Products include:
Aldoclor Tablets 1881
Diuril Oral 1936

Chlorothiazide Sodium (The ECG changes and hypokalemia which may result from administration of nonpotassium-sparing diuretics can be acutely worsened by beta agonists. Caution is advised in the co-administration of beta agonists with nonpotassium-sparing diuretics). Products include:

Diuril Sodium Intravenous 1934

Clomipramine Hydrochloride (Action of albuterol on the cardiovascular system may be potentiated by tricyclic antidepressants; co-administer with caution).

No products indexed under this heading.

Desipramine Hydrochloride (Action of albuterol on the cardiovascular system may be potentiated by tricyclic antidepressants; co-administer with caution).

No products indexed under this heading.

Digoxin (Mean decreases in serum digoxin levels have been demonstrated with intravenous and oral albuterol). Products include:

Digitek Tablets 2146
Lanoxicaps Capsules 1458
Lanoxin Injection 1462
Lanoxin Tablets 1468
Lanoxin Injection Pediatric 1465

Doxepin Hydrochloride (Action of albuterol on the cardiovascular system may be potentiated by tricyclic antidepressants; co-administer with caution).

No products indexed under this heading.

Esmolol Hydrochloride (Co-administration with beta adrenergic blocking agent blocks the pulmonary effect of beta agonists and may produce severe bronchospasm in asthmatic patients; co-administer with caution). Products include:

Brevibloc Concentrate 766
Brevibloc Injection 766
Brevibloc Double Strength Injection 766
Brevibloc Premixed Injection 766
Brevibloc Double Strength Premixed Injection 766

Ethacrynic Acid (The ECG changes and hypokalemia which may result from administration of nonpotassium-sparing diuretics can be acutely worsened by beta agonists. Caution is advised in the co-administration of beta agonists with nonpotassium-sparing diuretics). Products include:

Edecrin Tablets 1941

Furosemide (The ECG changes and hypokalemia which may result from administration of nonpotassium-sparing diuretics can be acutely worsened by beta agonists. Caution is advised in the co-administration of beta agonists with nonpotassium-sparing diuretics). Products include:

Furosemide Tablets 2117

Hydrochlorothiazide (The ECG changes and hypokalemia which may result from administration of nonpotassium-sparing diuretics can be acutely worsened by beta agonists. Caution is advised in the co-administration of beta agonists with nonpotassium-sparing diuretics). Products include:

Aldoril Tablets 1884
Atacand HCT 637
Avalide Tablets 2889
Avalide Tablets 922
Benicar HCT Tablets 2852
Diovan HCT Tablets 2195
Dyazide Capsules 1389
Hyzaar 1964
Lotensin HCT Tablets 2235
Maxzide 2150
Micardis HCT Tablets 886
Moduretic Tablets 2003
Prinzide Tablets 2033
Teveten HCT Tablets 1710
Timolide Tablets 2056
Uniretic Tablets 3114
Vaseretic Tablets 2073
Zestoretic Tablets 701

Hydroflumethiazide (The ECG changes and hypokalemia which may result from administration of nonpotassium-sparing diuretics can be acutely worsened by beta agonists. Caution is advised in the co-administration of beta agonists with nonpotassium-sparing diuretics).

No products indexed under this heading.

Imipramine Hydrochloride (Action of albuterol on the cardiovascular system may be potentiated by tricyclic antidepressants; co-administer with caution).

No products indexed under this heading.

Imipramine Pamoate (Action of albuterol on the cardiovascular system may be potentiated by tricyclic antidepressants; co-administer with caution).

No products indexed under this heading.

Isocarboxazid (Action of albuterol on the cardiovascular system may be potentiated by MAO inhibitors; co-administer with caution).

No products indexed under this heading.

Labetalol Hydrochloride (Co-administration with beta adrenergic blocking agent blocks the pulmonary effect of beta agonists and may produce severe bronchospasm in asthmatic patients; co-administer with caution).

No products indexed under this heading.

Levobunolol Hydrochloride (Co-administration with beta adrenergic blocking agent blocks the pulmonary effect of beta agonists and may produce severe bronchospasm in asthmatic patients; co-administer with caution). Products include:

Betagan Ophthalmic Solution, USP .... ⊙ 217

Maprotiline Hydrochloride (Action of albuterol on the cardiovascular system may be potentiated by tricyclic antidepressants; co-administer with caution).

No products indexed under this heading.

Methyclothiazide (The ECG changes and hypokalemia which may result from administration of nonpotassium-sparing diuretics can be acutely worsened by beta agonists. Caution is advised in the co-administration of beta agonists with nonpotassium-sparing diuretics).

No products indexed under this heading.

Metipranolol Hydrochloride (Co-administration with beta adrenergic blocking agent blocks the pulmonary effect of beta agonists and may produce severe bronchospasm in asthmatic patients; co-administer with caution).

No products indexed under this heading.

Metoprolol Succinate (Co-administration with beta adrenergic blocking agent blocks the pulmonary effect of beta agonists and may produce severe bronchospasm in asthmatic patients; co-administer with caution). Products include:

Toprol-XL Tablets 660

Metoprolol Tartrate (Co-administration with beta adrenergic blocking agent blocks the pulmonary effect of beta agonists and may produce severe bronchospasm in asthmatic patients; co-administer with caution).

No products indexed under this heading.

Moclobemide (Action of albuterol on the cardiovascular system may be potentiated by MAO inhibitors; co-administer with caution).

No products indexed under this heading.

Nadolol (Co-administration with beta adrenergic blocking agent blocks the pulmonary effect of beta agonists and may produce severe bronchospasm in asthmatic patients; co-administer with caution). Products include:

Nadolol Tablets 2121

Nortriptyline Hydrochloride (Action of albuterol on the cardiovascular system may be potentiated by tricyclic antidepressants; co-administer with caution).

No products indexed under this heading.

Pargyline Hydrochloride (Action of albuterol on the cardiovascular system may be potentiated by MAO inhibitors; co-administer with caution).

No products indexed under this heading.

Penbutolol Sulfate (Co-administration with beta adrenergic blocking agent blocks the pulmonary effect of beta agonists and may produce severe bronchospasm in asthmatic patients; co-administer with caution).

No products indexed under this heading.

Phenelzine Sulfate (Action of albuterol on the cardiovascular system may be potentiated by MAO inhibitors; co-administer with caution).

No products indexed under this heading.

Pindolol (Co-administration with beta adrenergic blocking agent blocks the pulmonary effect of beta agonists and may produce severe bronchospasm in asthmatic patients; co-administer with caution).

No products indexed under this heading.

Polythiazide (The ECG changes and hypokalemia which may result from administration of nonpotassium-sparing diuretics can be acutely worsened by beta agonists. Caution is advised in the co-administration of beta agonists with nonpotassium-sparing diuretics).

No products indexed under this heading.

Procarbazine Hydrochloride (Action of albuterol on the cardiovascular system may be potentiated by MAO inhibitors; co-administer with caution). Products include:

Matulane Capsules 3188

Propranolol Hydrochloride (Co-administration with beta adrenergic blocking agent blocks the pulmonary effect of beta agonists and may produce severe bronchospasm in asthmatic patients; co-administer with caution). Products include:

Inderal LA Long-Acting Capsules 3421
InnoPran XL Capsules 2728

Protriptyline Hydrochloride (Action of albuterol on the cardiovascular system may be potentiated by tricyclic antidepressants; co-administer with caution). Products include:

Vivactil Tablets 2350

Selegiline Hydrochloride (Action of albuterol on the cardiovascular system may be potentiated by MAO inhibitors; co-administer with caution). Products include:

Eldepryl Capsules 3209

Sotalol Hydrochloride (Co-administration with beta adrenergic blocking agent blocks the pulmonary effect of beta agonists and may produce severe bronchospasm in asthmatic patients; co-administer with caution).

No products indexed under this heading.

Timolol Hemihydrate (Co-administration with beta adrenergic blocking agent blocks the pulmonary effect of beta agonists and may produce severe bronchospasm in asthmatic patients; co-administer with caution). Products include:

Betimol Ophthalmic Solution 3371
Betimol Ophthalmic Solution .... ⊙ 283

Timolol Maleate (Co-administration with beta adrenergic blocking agent blocks the pulmonary effect of beta agonists and may produce severe bronchospasm in asthmatic patients; co-administer with caution). Products include:

Blocadren Tablets 1891
Cosopt Sterile Ophthalmic Solution 1910
Timolide Tablets 2056
Timoptic in Ocudose 2061
Timoptic Sterile Ophthalmic Solution 2058
Timoptic-XE Sterile Ophthalmic Gel Forming Solution 2062

Torsemide (The ECG changes and hypokalemia which may result from administration of nonpotassium-sparing diuretics can be acutely worsened by beta agonists. Caution is advised in the co-administration of beta agonists with nonpotassium-sparing diuretics).

No products indexed under this heading.

Tranylcypromine Sulfate (Action of albuterol on the cardiovascular system may be potentiated by MAO inhibitors; co-administer with caution). Products include:

Parnate Tablets 1499

Trimipramine Maleate (Action of albuterol on the cardiovascular system may be potentiated by tricyclic antidepressants; co-administer with caution). Products include:

Surmontil Capsules 2347

PROVIGIL TABLETS

(Modafinil) 1002

May interact with cytochrome p450 2c9 substrates (selected), cytochrome p450 3a4 inducers (selected), cytochrome p450 3a4 inhibitors (selected), cytochrome p450 3a4 substrates (selected), monoamine oxidase inhibitors, oral contraceptives, phenytoin, selective serotonin reuptake inhibitors, tricyclic antidepressants, xanthines, and certain other agents. Compounds in these categories include:

Acarbose (An apparent concentration-related suppression of

CYP2C9 activity was observed in human hepatocytes after exposure to modafinil in vitro suggesting that there is a potential for a metabolic interaction between modafinil and substrates of CYP2C9). Products include:

Precose Tablets ... 776

Acetazolamide (Co-administration of potent inhibitors of CYP3A4 could alter the plasma levels of modafinil).

No products indexed under this heading.

Alfentanil Hydrochloride (Chronic administration of modafinil can increase the elimination of substrates of CYP3A4. Dose adjustments may be necessary for patients being treated with these and similar medications).

No products indexed under this heading.

Allium sativum (Co-administration of potent inducers of CYP3A4 could alter the plasma levels of modafinil).

No products indexed under this heading.

Alprazolam (Chronic administration of modafinil can increase the elimination of substrates of CYP3A4. Dose adjustments may be necessary for patients being treated with these and similar medications). Products include:

Niravam Orally Disintegrating Tablets ... 3106
Xanax XR Tablets ... 2655

Aminophylline (Chronic administration of modafinil may cause modest induction of CYP3A4, thus reducing the levels, to a lesser degree, of co-administered substrate for that enzyme system, such as theophylline).

No products indexed under this heading.

Amiodarone Hydrochloride (Co-administration of potent inhibitors of CYP3A4 could alter the plasma levels of modafinil). Products include:

Pacerone Tablets ... 3337

Amitriptyline Hydrochloride (CYP2C19 provides an ancillary pathway for the metabolism of certain tricyclic antidepressants that are primarily metabolized by CYP2D6. In tricyclic-treated patients deficient in CYP2D6, the amount of metabolism by CYP2C19 may be substantially increased. Modafinil may cause elevation of the levels of these tricyclics in this subset of patients. A reduction in the dose of tricyclic agents might be needed in these patients).

No products indexed under this heading.

Amlodipine Besylate (Chronic administration of modafinil can increase the elimination of substrates of CYP3A4. Dose adjustments may be necessary for patients being treated with these and similar medications). Products include:

Caduet Tablets ... 2507
Lotrel Capsules ... 2238
Norvasc Tablets ... 2529

Amoxapine (CYP2C19 provides an ancillary pathway for the metabolism of certain tricyclic antidepressants that are primarily metabolized by CYP2D6. In tricyclic-treated patients deficient in CYP2D6, the amount of metabolism by CYP2C19 may be substantially increased. Modafinil may cause elevation of the levels of these tricyclics in this subset of patients. A reduction in the dose of tricyclic agents might be needed in these patients).

No products indexed under this heading.

Amprenavir (Co-administration of potent inhibitors of CYP3A4 could alter the plasma levels of modafinil). Products include:

Agenerase Capsules ... 1299
Agenerase Oral Solution ... 1304

Anastrozole (Co-administration of potent inhibitors of CYP3A4 could alter the plasma levels of modafinil). Products include:

Arimidex Tablets ... 665

Aprepitant (Chronic administration of modafinil can increase the elimination of substrates of CYP3A4. Dose adjustments may be necessary for patients being treated with these and similar medications). Products include:

Emend Capsules ... 1944

Astemizole (Chronic administration of modafinil can increase the elimination of substrates of CYP3A4. Dose adjustments may be necessary for patients being treated with these and similar medications).

No products indexed under this heading.

Atorvastatin Calcium (Chronic administration of modafinil can increase the elimination of substrates of CYP3A4. Dose adjustments may be necessary for patients being treated with these and similar medications). Products include:

Caduet Tablets ... 2507
Lipitor Tablets ... 2495

Belladonna Ergotamine (Chronic administration of modafinil can increase the elimination of substrates of CYP3A4. Dose adjustments may be necessary for patients being treated with these and similar medications).

No products indexed under this heading.

Betamethasone Acetate (Co-administration of potent inducers of CYP3A4 could alter the plasma levels of modafinil).

No products indexed under this heading.

Betamethasone Sodium Phosphate (Co-administration of potent inducers of CYP3A4 could alter the plasma levels of modafinil).

No products indexed under this heading.

Buspirone Hydrochloride (Chronic administration of modafinil can increase the elimination of substrates of CYP3A4. Dose adjustments may be necessary for patients being treated with these and similar medications).

No products indexed under this heading.

Busulfan (Chronic administration of modafinil can increase the elimination of substrates of CYP3A4. Dose adjustments may be necessary for patients being treated with these and similar medications). Products include:

I.V. Busulfex ... 1125
Myleran Tablets ... 1492

Candesartan Cilexetil (An apparent concentration-related suppression of CYP2C9 activity was observed in human hepatocytes after exposure to modafinil in vitro suggesting that there is a potential for a metabolic interaction between modafinil and substrates of CYP2C9). Products include:

Atacand Tablets ... 634
Atacand HCT ... 637

Carbamazepine (Chronic administration of modafinil may cause induction of its metabolism; co-administration of potent inducers of CYP3A4, such as carbamazepine, could alter the levels of modafinil due to the partial involvement of that enzyme in the metabolic elimination of the compound). Products include:

Carbatrol Capsules ... 3174
Equetro Extended-Release Capsules ... 3178
Tegretol/Tegretol-XR ... 2278

Carvedilol (An apparent concentration-related suppression of CYP2C9 activity was observed in human hepatocytes after exposure to modafinil in vitro suggesting that there is a potential for a metabolic interaction between modafinil and substrates of CYP2C9). Products include:

Coreg Tablets ... 1376

Celecoxib (An apparent concentration-related suppression of CYP2C9 activity was observed in human hepatocytes after exposure to modafinil in vitro suggesting that there is a potential for a metabolic interaction between modafinil and substrates of CYP2C9). Products include:

Celebrex Capsules ... 3130

Cerivastatin Sodium (Chronic administration of modafinil can increase the elimination of substrates of CYP3A4. Dose adjustments may be necessary for patients being treated with these and similar medications).

No products indexed under this heading.

Chlorpheniramine (Chronic administration of modafinil can increase the elimination of substrates of CYP3A4. Dose adjustments may be necessary for patients being treated with these and similar medications).

No products indexed under this heading.

Chlorpheniramine Maleate (Chronic administration of modafinil can increase the elimination of substrates of CYP3A4. Dose adjustments may be necessary for patients being treated with these and similar medications). Products include:

Advil Allergy Sinus Caplets ... 737
Advil Multi-Symptom Cold Caplets ... 738
BC Allergy Sinus Cold Powder ... 612
Contac Severe Cold and Flu Caplets Maximum Strength ... 615
Hycomine Compound Tablets ... 1105
PediaCare Multi-Symptom Cold Liquid ... 704
PediaCare NightRest Cough & Cold Liquid ... 704
Robitussin Flu Liquid ... 752
Robitussin PM Cough & Cold Liquid ... 752
Singlet Caplets ... 636
Sudafed Sinus & Allergy Tablets ... 710
TheraFlu Cold & Cough Hot Liquid ... 680
TheraFlu Cold & Sore Throat Hot Liquid ... 680
TheraFlu Flu & Sore Throat Hot Liquid ... 681
TheraFlu Severe Cold & Cough Hot Liquid ... 683
TheraFlu Severe Cold Caplets ... 679
TheraFlu Severe Cold Hot Liquid ... 682
Triaminic Cold & Allergy Liquid ... 685
Triaminic Cold & Cough Liquid ... 685
Triaminic Flu, Cough & Fever Liquid ... 685
Triaminic Night Time Cough & Cold Liquid ... 685
Triaminic Allergy Runny Nose & Congestion Softchews ... 688
Triaminic Cold & Cough Softchews ... 688
Children's Tylenol Plus Cold NightTime Suspension Liquid ... 1851
Children's Tylenol Plus Cold & Cough Suspension Liquid and Chewable Tablets ... 1851
Children's Tylenol Plus Cold Chewable Tablets ... 1851
Children's Tylenol Plus Flu Suspension Liquid ... 1853
Tylenol Allergy Complete Multi-Symptom Caplets and Gelcaps with Cool Burst ... 1844
Multi-Symptom Tylenol Cold Night Time Caplets ... 1845
Vicks 44M Cough, Cold & Flu Relief ... 2676
Pediatric Vicks 44m Cough & Cold Relief ... 2673
Children's Vicks NyQuil Cold/Cough Relief ... 2671

Chlorpheniramine Polistirex (Chronic administration of modafinil can increase the elimination of substrates of CYP3A4. Dose adjustments may be necessary for patients being treated with these and similar medications). Products include:

Tussionex Pennkinetic Extended-Release Suspension ... 3322

Chlorpheniramine Tannate (Chronic administration of modafinil can increase the elimination of substrates of CYP3A4. Dose adjustments may be necessary for patients being treated with these and similar medications).

No products indexed under this heading.

Chlorpropamide (An apparent concentration-related suppression of CYP2C9 activity was observed in human hepatocytes after exposure to modafinil in vitro suggesting that there is a potential for a metabolic interaction between modafinil and substrates of CYP2C9).

No products indexed under this heading.

Cimetidine (Co-administration of potent inhibitors of CYP3A4 could alter the plasma levels of modafinil). Products include:

Tagamet HB 200 Tablets ... 637
Tagamet Tablets ... 1547

Cimetidine Hydrochloride (Co-administration of potent inhibitors of CYP3A4 could alter the plasma levels of modafinil).

No products indexed under this heading.

Ciprofloxacin (Co-administration of potent inhibitors of CYP3A4 could alter the plasma levels of modafinil). Products include:

Cipro I.V. ... 2998
Cipro I.V. Pharmacy Bulk Package ... 3509
Cipro Oral Suspension ... 2991
Cipro XR Tablets ... 3004
Ciprodex Otic Suspension ... 555

Ciprofloxacin Hydrochloride (Co-administration of potent inducers of CYP3A4 could alter the plasma levels of modafinil). Products include:

Ciloxan Ophthalmic Ointment ... 554
Cipro Tablets ... 2991

Cisapride (Chronic administration of modafinil can increase the elimination of substrates of CYP3A4. Dose adjustments may be necessary for patients being treated with these and similar medications).

No products indexed under this heading.

Cisplatin (Co-administration of potent inducers of CYP3A4 could alter the plasma levels of modafinil).

No products indexed under this heading.

Citalopram Hydrobromide (Modafinil is a reversible inhibitor of the CYP2C19; the levels of CYP2D6 substrates, such as selective serotonin reuptake inhibitors, which have ancillary routes of elimination through CYP2D6, may be increased by co-administration of modafinil). Products include:

Celexa 1177

Clarithromycin (Chronic administration of modafinil can increase the elimination of substrates of CYP3A4. Dose adjustments may be necessary for patients being treated with these and similar medications). Products include:

Biaxin/Biaxin XL 402
PREVPAC 3281

Clomipramine Hydrochloride (Co-administration has resulted in one incident of increased levels of clomipramine and its active metabolite desmethylclomipramine).

No products indexed under this heading.

Clotrimazole (Co-administration of potent inhibitors of CYP3A4 could alter the plasma levels of modafinil). Products include:

Lotrimin 3053
Lotrisone 3054

Cortisone Acetate (Co-administration of potent inducers of CYP3A4 could alter the plasma levels of modafinil).

No products indexed under this heading.

Cyclosporine (One case of an interaction between modafinil and cyclosporine has been reported. After one month of administration of 200mg/day of modafinil, cyclosporine blood levels were decreased by 50%). Products include:

Gengraf Capsules 458
Neoral Soft Gelatin Capsules 2247
Neoral Oral Solution 2247
Restasis Ophthalmic Emulsion 570
Sandimmune 2259

Dalfopristin (Co-administration of potent inhibitors of CYP3A4 could alter the plasma levels of modafinil). Products include:

Synercid I.V. 1690

Danazol (Co-administration of potent inhibitors of CYP3A4 could alter the plasma levels of modafinil).

No products indexed under this heading.

Delavirdine Mesylate (Co-administration of potent inhibitors of CYP3A4 could alter the plasma levels of modafinil). Products include:

Rescriptor Tablets 2535

Desipramine Hydrochloride (CYP2C19 provides an ancillary pathway for the metabolism of certain tricyclic antidepressants that are primarily metabolized by CYP2D6. In tricyclic-treated patients deficient in CYP2D6, the amount of metabolism by CYP2C19 may be substantially increased. Modafinil may cause elevation of the levels of these tricyclics in this subset of patients. A reduction in the dose of tricyclic agents might be needed in these patients).

No products indexed under this heading.

Desogestrel (The effectiveness of steroidal contraceptives may be reduced when used with modafinil tablets and for one month after discontinuation of therapy. Alternative or concomitant methods of contraception are recommended for patients treated with modafinil tablets and for one month after discontinuation of modafinil). Products include:

Ortho-Cept Tablets 2395

Dexamethasone (Co-administration of potent inducers of CYP3A4 could alter the plasma levels of modafinil). Products include:

Ciprodex Otic Suspension 555
Decadron Tablets 1929
TobraDex Ophthalmic Ointment 558
TobraDex Ophthalmic Suspension ... 558

Dexamethasone Acetate (Co-administration of potent inducers of CYP3A4 could alter the plasma levels of modafinil).

No products indexed under this heading.

Dexamethasone Sodium Phosphate (Co-administration of potent inducers of CYP3A4 could alter the plasma levels of modafinil). Products include:

Decadron Phosphate Injection 1931

Dextroamphetamine (Absorption of modafinil may be delayed by approximately one hour when co-administered with dextroamphetamine).

No products indexed under this heading.

Dextroamphetamine Saccharate (Absorption of modafinil may be delayed by approximately one hour when co-administered with dextroamphetamine). Products include:

Adderall Tablets 3168
Adderall XR Capsules 3169

Dextroamphetamine Sulfate (Absorption of modafinil may be delayed by approximately one hour when co-administered with dextroamphetamine). Products include:

Adderall Tablets 3168
Adderall XR Capsules 3169
Dexedrine 1386
DextroStat Tablets 3177

Dextromethorphan (An apparent concentration-related suppression of CYP2C9 activity was observed in human hepatocytes after exposure to modafinil in vitro suggesting that there is a potential for a metabolic interaction between modafinil and substrates of CYP2C9).

No products indexed under this heading.

Diazepam (Modafinil is a reversible inhibitor of the CYP2C19; co-administration with drugs that are largely eliminated via this pathway, such as diazepam, may increase the circulating levels of diazepam). Products include:

Diastat Rectal Delivery System 3344
Valium Tablets 2822

Diclofenac Potassium (An apparent concentration-related suppression of CYP2C9 activity was observed in human hepatocytes after exposure to modafinil in vitro suggesting that there is a potential for a metabolic interaction between modafinil and substrates of CYP2C9). Products include:

Cataflam Tablets 2173

Diclofenac Sodium (An apparent concentration-related suppression of CYP2C9 activity was observed in human hepatocytes after exposure to modafinil in vitro suggesting that there is a potential for a metabolic interaction between modafinil and substrates of CYP2C9). Products include:

Arthrotec Tablets 3126
Voltaren Ophthalmic Solution 2300
Voltaren Tablets 2298
Voltaren-XR Tablets 2301

Dihydroergotamine Mesylate (Chronic administration of modafinil can increase the elimination of substrates of CYP3A4. Dose adjustments may be necessary for patients being treated with these and similar medications). Products include:

Migranal Nasal Spray 3350

Diltiazem Hydrochloride (Chronic administration of modafinil can increase the elimination of substrates of CYP3A4. Dose adjustments may be necessary for patients being treated with these and similar medications). Products include:

Cardizem LA Extended Release Tablets 1699
Tiazac Capsules 1204

Diltiazem Maleate (Chronic administration of modafinil can increase the elimination of substrates of CYP3A4. Dose adjustments may be necessary for patients being treated with these and similar medications).

No products indexed under this heading.

Disopyramide (Chronic administration of modafinil can increase the elimination of substrates of CYP3A4. Dose adjustments may be necessary for patients being treated with these and similar medications).

No products indexed under this heading.

Disopyramide Phosphate (Chronic administration of modafinil can increase the elimination of substrates of CYP3A4. Dose adjustments may be necessary for patients being treated with these and similar medications).

No products indexed under this heading.

Disulfiram (Chronic administration of modafinil can increase the elimination of substrates of CYP3A4. Dose adjustments may be necessary for patients being treated with these and similar medications). Products include:

Antabuse Tablets 2343

Doxepin Hydrochloride (CYP2C19 provides an ancillary pathway for the metabolism of certain tricyclic antidepressants that are primarily metabolized by CYP2D6. In tricyclic-treated patients deficient in CYP2D6, the amount of metabolism by CYP2C19 may be substantially increased. Modafinil may cause elevation of the levels of these tricyclics in this subset of patients. A reduction in the dose of tricyclic agents might be needed in these patients).

No products indexed under this heading.

Doxorubicin Hydrochloride (Chronic administration of modafinil can increase the elimination of substrates of CYP3A4. Dose adjustments may be necessary for patients being treated with these and similar medications). Products include:

Adriamycin for Injection, USP 786
Adriamycin Injection, USP 786

Dronabinol (Chronic administration of modafinil can increase the elimination of substrates of CYP3A4. Dose adjustments may be necessary for patients being treated with these and similar medications). Products include:

Marinol Capsules 3334

Dyphylline (Chronic administration of modafinil may cause modest induction of CYP3A4, thus reducing the levels, to a lesser degree, of co-administered substrate for that enzyme system, such as theophylline).

No products indexed under this heading.

Efavirenz (Co-administration of potent inducers of CYP3A4 could alter the plasma levels of modafinil). Products include:

Sustiva Capsules 957

Eprosartan Mesylate (An apparent concentration-related suppression of CYP2C9 activity was observed in human hepatocytes after exposure to modafinil in vitro suggesting that there is a potential for a metabolic interaction between modafinil and substrates of CYP2C9). Products include:

Teveten Tablets 1707
Teveten HCT Tablets 1710

Ergotamine Tartrate (Chronic administration of modafinil can increase the elimination of substrates of CYP3A4. Dose adjustments may be necessary for patients being treated with these and similar medications).

No products indexed under this heading.

Erythromycin (Chronic administration of modafinil can increase the elimination of substrates of CYP3A4. Dose adjustments may be necessary for patients being treated with these and similar medications). Products include:

Erygel Topical Gel 2096
Ery-Tab Tablets 447
Erythromycin Base Filmtab Tablets 454
Erythromycin Delayed-Release Capsules, USP 456
PCE Dispertab Tablets 510

Erythromycin Estolate (Chronic administration of modafinil can increase the elimination of substrates of CYP3A4. Dose adjustments may be necessary for patients being treated with these and similar medications).

No products indexed under this heading.

Erythromycin Ethylsuccinate (Chronic administration of modafinil can increase the elimination of substrates of CYP3A4. Dose adjustments may be necessary for patients being treated with these and similar medications). Products include:

E.E.S. 449
EryPed 445

Erythromycin Gluceptate (Chronic administration of modafinil can increase the elimination of substrates of CYP3A4. Dose adjustments may be necessary for patients being treated with these and similar medications).
No products indexed under this heading.

Erythromycin Lactobionate (Chronic administration of modafinil can increase the elimination of substrates of CYP3A4. Dose adjustments may be necessary for patients being treated with these and similar medications).
No products indexed under this heading.

Erythromycin Stearate (Chronic administration of modafinil can increase the elimination of substrates of CYP3A4. Dose adjustments may be necessary for patients being treated with these and similar medications). Products include:
Erythrocin Stearate Filmtab Tablets **452**

Escitalopram Oxalate (Modafinil is a reversible inhibitor of the CYP2C19; the levels of CYP2D6 substrates, such as selective serotonin reuptake inhibitors, which have ancillary routes of elimination through CYP2D6, may be increased by co-administration of modafinil). Products include:
Lexapro Oral Solution **1193**
Lexapro Tablets **1193**

Esomeprazole Magnesium (Co-administration of potent inhibitors of CYP3A4 could alter the plasma levels of modafinil). Products include:
Nexium Delayed-Release Capsules **645**

Estradiol (Chronic administration of modafinil can increase the elimination of substrates of CYP3A4. Dose adjustments may be necessary for patients being treated with these and similar medications). Products include:
Activella Tablets **2311**
Climara Transdermal System **795**
Climara Pro Transdermal System **800**
CombiPatch Transdermal System **2180**
Estrogel 0.06% **3200**
Menostar Transdermal System **805**
Prefest Tablets **1069**
Vagifem Tablets **2340**
Vivelle Transdermal System **2288**
Vivelle-Dot Transdermal System **2293**

Estradiol Benzoate (Chronic administration of modafinil can increase the elimination of substrates of CYP3A4. Dose adjustments may be necessary for patients being treated with these and similar medications).
No products indexed under this heading.

Estradiol Cypionate (Chronic administration of modafinil can increase the elimination of substrates of CYP3A4. Dose adjustments may be necessary for patients being treated with these and similar medications).
No products indexed under this heading.

Estradiol Valerate (Chronic administration of modafinil can increase the elimination of substrates of CYP3A4. Dose adjustments may be necessary for patients being treated with these and similar medications).
No products indexed under this heading.

Ethinyl Estradiol (Administration of modafinil to female volunteers resulted in a mean 11% decrease in Cmax and an 18% decrease in AUC of ethinyl estradiol. There was no apparent change in the elimination rate of ethinyl estradiol). Products include:
Alesse-28 Tablets **3392**
Lo/Ovral-28 Tablets **3423**
NuvaRing **2357**
Ortho-Cept Tablets **2395**
Ortho-Cyclen/Ortho Tri-Cyclen **2414**
Ortho Evra Transdermal System **2402**
Ortho Tri-Cyclen Lo Tablets **2421**
Seasonale Tablets **1073**
Triphasil-28 Tablets **3483**
Yasmin 28 Tablets **818**

Ethosuximide (Chronic administration of modafinil can increase the elimination of substrates of CYP3A4. Dose adjustments may be necessary for patients being treated with these and similar medications).
No products indexed under this heading.

Ethynodiol Diacetate (The effectiveness of steroidal contraceptives may be reduced when used with modafinil tablets and for one month after discontinuation of therapy. Alternative or concomitant methods of contraception are recommended for patients treated with modafinil tablets and for one month after discontinuation of modafinil).
No products indexed under this heading.

Etodolac (An apparent concentration-related suppression of CYP2C9 activity was observed in human hepatocytes after exposure to modafinil in vitro suggesting that there is a potential for a metabolic interaction between modafinil and substrates of CYP2C9).
No products indexed under this heading.

Etoposide (Chronic administration of modafinil can increase the elimination of substrates of CYP3A4. Dose adjustments may be necessary for patients being treated with these and similar medications).
No products indexed under this heading.

Etoposide Phosphate (Chronic administration of modafinil can increase the elimination of substrates of CYP3A4. Dose adjustments may be necessary for patients being treated with these and similar medications).
No products indexed under this heading.

Felbamate (Co-administration of potent inducers of CYP3A4 could alter the plasma levels of modafinil).
No products indexed under this heading.

Felodipine (Chronic administration of modafinil can increase the elimination of substrates of CYP3A4. Dose adjustments may be necessary for patients being treated with these and similar medications). Products include:
Plendil Extended-Release Tablets **651**

Fenoprofen Calcium (An apparent concentration-related suppression of CYP2C9 activity was observed in human hepatocytes after exposure to modafinil in vitro suggesting that there is a potential for a metabolic interaction between modafinil and substrates of CYP2C9). Products include:
Nalfon Capsules **2504**

Fentanyl (Chronic administration of modafinil can increase the elimination of substrates of CYP3A4. Dose adjustments may be necessary for patients being treated with these and similar medications). Products include:
Duragesic Transdermal System **2448**

Fentanyl Citrate (Chronic administration of modafinil can increase the elimination of substrates of CYP3A4. Dose adjustments may be necessary for patients being treated with these and similar medications). Products include:
Actiq **993**

Fluconazole (Co-administration of potent inhibitors of CYP3A4 could alter the plasma levels of modafinil).
No products indexed under this heading.

Fludrocortisone Acetate (Co-administration of potent inducers of CYP3A4 could alter the plasma levels of modafinil).
No products indexed under this heading.

Fluoxetine Hydrochloride (Modafinil is a reversible inhibitor of the CYP2C19; the levels of CYP2D6 substrates, such as selective serotonin reuptake inhibitors, which have ancillary routes of elimination through CYP2D6, may be increased by co-administration of modafinil). Products include:
Prozac Pulvules and Liquid **1771**
Symbyax Capsules **1788**

Flurbiprofen (An apparent concentration-related suppression of CYP2C9 activity was observed in human hepatocytes after exposure to modafinil in vitro suggesting that there is a potential for a metabolic interaction between modafinil and substrates of CYP2C9).
No products indexed under this heading.

Flurbiprofen Sodium (An apparent concentration-related suppression of CYP2C9 activity was observed in human hepatocytes after exposure to modafinil in vitro suggesting that there is a potential for a metabolic interaction between modafinil and substrates of CYP2C9). Products include:
Ocufen Ophthalmic Solution .... ⊙**230**

Fluvastatin Sodium (An apparent concentration-related suppression of CYP2C9 activity was observed in human hepatocytes after exposure to modafinil in vitro suggesting that there is a potential for a metabolic interaction between modafinil and substrates of CYP2C9). Products include:
Lescol Capsules **2227**
Lescol **2730**
Lescol XL Tablets **2227**

Fluvoxamine Maleate (Modafinil is a reversible inhibitor of the CYP2C19; the levels of CYP2D6 substrates, such as selective serotonin reuptake inhibitors, which have ancillary routes of elimination through CYP2D6, may be increased by co-administration of modafinil).
No products indexed under this heading.

Fosamprenavir Calcium (Co-administration of potent inhibitors of CYP3A4 could alter the plasma levels of modafinil). Products include:
Lexiva Tablets **1473**

Fosphenytoin Sodium (Modafinil is a reversible inhibitor of the CYP2C19; co-administration with drugs that are largely eliminated via this pathway, such as phenytoin, may increase the circulating levels of phenytoin).
No products indexed under this heading.

Garlic Extract (Co-administration of potent inducers of CYP3A4 could alter the plasma levels of modafinil).
No products indexed under this heading.

Garlic Oil (Co-administration of potent inducers of CYP3A4 could alter the plasma levels of modafinil).
No products indexed under this heading.

Glimepiride (An apparent concentration-related suppression of CYP2C9 activity was observed in human hepatocytes after exposure to modafinil in vitro suggesting that there is a potential for a metabolic interaction between modafinil and substrates of CYP2C9). Products include:
Amaryl Tablets **2864**

Glipizide (An apparent concentration-related suppression of CYP2C9 activity was observed in human hepatocytes after exposure to modafinil in vitro suggesting that there is a potential for a metabolic interaction between modafinil and substrates of CYP2C9).
No products indexed under this heading.

Haloperidol (Chronic administration of modafinil can increase the elimination of substrates of CYP3A4. Dose adjustments may be necessary for patients being treated with these and similar medications).
No products indexed under this heading.

Haloperidol Decanoate (Chronic administration of modafinil can increase the elimination of substrates of CYP3A4. Dose adjustments may be necessary for patients being treated with these and similar medications).
No products indexed under this heading.

Haloperidol Lactate (Chronic administration of modafinil can increase the elimination of substrates of CYP3A4. Dose adjustments may be necessary for patients being treated with these and similar medications).
No products indexed under this heading.

Hydrocortisone (Co-administration of potent inducers of CYP3A4 could alter the plasma levels of modafinil). Products include:
Cortizone•5 Ointment .... ▣**699**
Cortizone•10 Creme .... ▣**699**
Cortizone•10 Ointment .... ▣**699**
Cortizone•10 Plus Creme .... ▣**700**
Cortizone•10 Maximum Strength Quick Shot Spray .... ▣**700**
Hydrocortone Tablets **1963**
Preparation H Hydrocortisone Cream .... ▣**748**

Hydrocortisone Acetate (Co-administration of potent inducers of CYP3A4 could alter the plasma levels of modafinil). Products include:
Analpram-HC **1136**
Pramosone **1139**
ProctoFoam-HC **3113**
Tucks Anti-Itch Ointment .... ▣**712**
U-cort 1% Cream **3289**

IMPORTANT NOTE: Always consult each drug listing in the patient's regimen for possible interactions.

Hydrocortisone Butyrate (Co-administration of potent inducers of CYP3A4 could alter the plasma levels of modafinil). Products include:

Locoid 1138
Locoid Lipocream Cream 1138

Hydrocortisone Cypionate (Co-administration of potent inducers of CYP3A4 could alter the plasma levels of modafinil).

No products indexed under this heading.

Hydrocortisone Hemisuccinate (Co-administration of potent inducers of CYP3A4 could alter the plasma levels of modafinil).

No products indexed under this heading.

Hydrocortisone Probutate (Co-administration of potent inducers of CYP3A4 could alter the plasma levels of modafinil). Products include:

Pandel Cream, 0.1% 1017

Hydrocortisone Sodium Phosphate (Co-administration of potent inducers of CYP3A4 could alter the plasma levels of modafinil).

No products indexed under this heading.

Hydrocortisone Sodium Succinate (Co-administration of potent inducers of CYP3A4 could alter the plasma levels of modafinil).

No products indexed under this heading.

Hydrocortisone Valerate (Co-administration of potent inducers of CYP3A4 could alter the plasma levels of modafinil).

No products indexed under this heading.

Hypericum (Co-administration of potent inducers of CYP3A4 could alter the plasma levels of modafinil).

No products indexed under this heading.

Hypericum Perforatum (Co-administration of potent inducers of CYP3A4 could alter the plasma levels of modafinil).

No products indexed under this heading.

Ibuprofen (An apparent concentration-related suppression of CYP2C9 activity was observed in human hepatocytes after exposure to modafinil in vitro suggesting that there is a potential for a metabolic interaction between modafinil and substrates of CYP2C9). Products include:

Advil Allergy Sinus Caplets .... ▣ 737
Advil .... ▣ 737
Children's Advil Suspension .... ▣ 742
Children's Advil Chewable Tablets .. ▣ 741
Advil Cold & Sinus .... ▣ 739
Advil Flu & Body Ache Caplets .... ▣ 739
Children's Advil Cold Suspension ... ▣ 741
Infants' Advil Concentrated Drops .. ▣ 743
Junior Strength Advil Swallow Tablets .... ▣ 740
Advil Migraine Liquigels .... ▣ 740
Advil Multi-Symptom Cold Caplets .... ▣ 738
Combunox Tablets 1183
Children's Motrin Oral Suspension and Chewable Tablets 1837
Children's Motrin Cold Non-Staining Dye-Free Oral Suspension 1838
Children's Motrin Cold Oral Suspension 1838
Children's Motrin Non-Staining Dye-Free Oral Suspension 1837
Motrin Cold & Sinus Caplets 1836
Motrin IB Tablets and Caplets 1836
Infants' Motrin Concentrated Drops 1837
Infants' Motrin Non-Staining Dye-Free Drops 1837
Junior Strength Motrin Caplets and Chewable Tablets 1837
Vicoprofen Tablets 533

Imipramine Hydrochloride (CYP2C19 provides an ancillary pathway for the metabolism of certain tricyclic antidepressants that are primarily metabolized by CYP2D6. In tricyclic-treated patients deficient in CYP2D6, the amount of metabolism by CYP2C19 may be substantially increased. Modafinil may cause elevation of the levels of these tricyclics in this subset of patients. A reduction in the dose of tricyclic agents might be needed in these patients).

No products indexed under this heading.

Imipramine Pamoate (CYP2C19 provides an ancillary pathway for the metabolism of certain tricyclic antidepressants that are primarily metabolized by CYP2D6. In tricyclic-treated patients deficient in CYP2D6, the amount of metabolism by CYP2C19 may be substantially increased. Modafinil may cause elevation of the levels of these tricyclics in this subset of patients. A reduction in the dose of tricyclic agents might be needed in these patients).

No products indexed under this heading.

Indinavir Sulfate (Chronic administration of modafinil can increase the elimination of substrates of CYP3A4. Dose adjustments may be necessary for patients being treated with these and similar medications). Products include:

Crixivan Capsules 1918

Indomethacin (An apparent concentration-related suppression of CYP2C9 activity was observed in human hepatocytes after exposure to modafinil in vitro suggesting that there is a potential for a metabolic interaction between modafinil and substrates of CYP2C9). Products include:

Indocin 1968

Indomethacin Sodium Trihydrate (An apparent concentration-related suppression of CYP2C9 activity was observed in human hepatocytes after exposure to modafinil in vitro suggesting that there is a potential for a metabolic interaction between modafinil and substrates of CYP2C9). Products include:

Indocin I.V. 1973

Irbesartan (An apparent concentration-related suppression of CYP2C9 activity was observed in human hepatocytes after exposure to modafinil in vitro suggesting that there is a potential for a metabolic interaction between modafinil and substrates of CYP2C9). Products include:

Avalide Tablets 922
Avalide Tablets 2889
Avapro Tablets 925
Avapro Tablets 2886

Isocarboxazid (Co-administration requires caution; no interaction studies have been performed).

No products indexed under this heading.

Isoniazid (Co-administration of potent inhibitors of CYP3A4 could alter the plasma levels of modafinil).

No products indexed under this heading.

Isradipine (Chronic administration of modafinil can increase the elimination of substrates of CYP3A4. Dose adjustments may be necessary for patients being treated with these and similar medications). Products include:

DynaCirc CR Tablets 2726

Itraconazole (Chronic administration of modafinil may cause induction of its metabolism; co-administration of potent inhibitors of CYP3A4, such as itraconazole, could alter the levels of modafinil due to the partial involvement of that enzyme in the metabolic elimination of the compound).

No products indexed under this heading.

Ketoconazole (Chronic administration of modafinil may cause induction of its metabolism; co-administration of potent inhibitors of CYP3A4, such as ketoconazole, could alter the levels of modafinil due to the partial involvement of that enzyme in the metabolic elimination of the compound). Products include:

Nizoral A-D Shampoo, 1% 1839
Nizoral 2% Shampoo 1838

Ketoprofen (An apparent concentration-related suppression of CYP2C9 activity was observed in human hepatocytes after exposure to modafinil in vitro suggesting that there is a potential for a metabolic interaction between modafinil and substrates of CYP2C9).

No products indexed under this heading.

Ketorolac Tromethamine (An apparent concentration-related suppression of CYP2C9 activity was observed in human hepatocytes after exposure to modafinil in vitro suggesting that there is a potential for a metabolic interaction between modafinil and substrates of CYP2C9). Products include:

Acular Ophthalmic Solution 561
Acular LS Ophthalmic Solution 562

Lansoprazole (An apparent concentration-related suppression of CYP2C9 activity was observed in human hepatocytes after exposure to modafinil in vitro suggesting that there is a potential for a metabolic interaction between modafinil and substrates of CYP2C9). Products include:

Prevacid Delayed-Release Capsules 3268
Prevacid for Delayed-Release Oral Suspension 3268
Prevacid I.V. for Injection 3274
Prevacid NapraPAC 3277
Prevacid SoluTab Delayed-Release Orally Disintegrating Tablets 3268
PREVPAC 3281

Levonorgestrel (The effectiveness of steroidal contraceptives may be reduced when used with modafinil tablets and for one month after discontinuation of therapy. Alternative or concomitant methods of contraception are recommended for patients treated with modafinil tablets and for one month after discontinuation of modafinil). Products include:

Alesse-28 Tablets 3392
Climara Pro Transdermal System 800
Mirena Intrauterine System 810
Plan B Tablets 1068
Seasonale Tablets 1073
Triphasil-28 Tablets 3483

Lidocaine (Chronic administration of modafinil can increase the elimination of substrates of CYP3A4. Dose adjustments may be necessary for patients being treated with these and similar medications). Products include:

Lidoderm Patch 1107

Lidocaine Hydrochloride (Chronic administration of modafinil can increase the elimination of substrates of CYP3A4. Dose adjustments may be necessary for patients being treated with these and similar medications).

No products indexed under this heading.

Lopinavir (Co-administration of potent inhibitors of CYP3A4 could alter the plasma levels of modafinil). Products include:

Kaletra 474

Loratadine (Co-administration of potent inhibitors of CYP3A4 could alter the plasma levels of modafinil). Products include:

Alavert Allergy & Sinus D-12 Hour Tablets .... ▣ 743
Alavert .... ▣ 743
Children's Claritin 24 Hour Non-Drowsy Allergy Syrup .... ▣ 732
Claritin Non-Drowsy 24 Hour Tablets .... ▣ 731
Non-Drowsy Claritin Hives Relief Tablets .... ▣ 733
Claritin Reditabs 24 Hour Non-Drowsy Tablets .... ▣ 732
Claritin-D Non-Drowsy 12 Hour Tablets .... ▣ 731
Claritin-D Non-Drowsy 24 Hour Tablets .... ▣ 731
Children's Dimetapp ND Non-Drowsy Allergy Syrup .... ▣ 746
Triaminic Allerchews .... ▣ 684

Losartan Potassium (An apparent concentration-related suppression of CYP2C9 activity was observed in human hepatocytes after exposure to modafinil in vitro suggesting that there is a potential for a metabolic interaction between modafinil and substrates of CYP2C9). Products include:

Cozaar Tablets 1913
Hyzaar 1964

Lovastatin (Chronic administration of modafinil can increase the elimination of substrates of CYP3A4. Dose adjustments may be necessary for patients being treated with these and similar medications). Products include:

Advicor Tablets 1694
Altoprev Extended-Release Tablets 1151
Mevacor Tablets 1996

Maprotiline Hydrochloride (CYP2C19 provides an ancillary pathway for the metabolism of certain tricyclic antidepressants that are primarily metabolized by CYP2D6. In tricyclic-treated patients deficient in CYP2D6, the amount of metabolism by CYP2C19 may be substantially increased. Modafinil may cause elevation of the levels of these tricyclics in this subset of patients. A reduction in the dose of tricyclic agents might be needed in these patients).

No products indexed under this heading.

Meclofenamate Sodium (An apparent concentration-related suppression of CYP2C9 activity was observed in human hepatocytes after exposure to modafinil in vitro suggesting that there is a potential for a metabolic interaction between modafinil and substrates of CYP2C9).
No products indexed under this heading.

Mefenamic Acid (An apparent concentration-related suppression of CYP2C9 activity was observed in human hepatocytes after exposure to modafinil in vitro suggesting that there is a potential for a metabolic interaction between modafinil and substrates of CYP2C9).
No products indexed under this heading.

Meloxicam (An apparent concentration-related suppression of CYP2C9 activity was observed in human hepatocytes after exposure to modafinil in vitro suggesting that there is a potential for a metabolic interaction between modafinil and substrates of CYP2C9). Products include:
Mobic Oral Suspension 893
Mobic Tablets 893

Mephenytoin (Co-administration of potent inducers of CYP3A4 could alter the plasma levels of modafinil).
No products indexed under this heading.

Mestranol (The effectiveness of steroidal contraceptives may be reduced when used with modafinil tablets and for one month after discontinuation of therapy. Alternative or concomitant methods of contraception are recommended for patients treated with modafinil tablets and for one month after discontinuation of modafinil).
No products indexed under this heading.

Metformin Hydrochloride (An apparent concentration-related suppression of CYP2C9 activity was observed in human hepatocytes after exposure to modafinil in vitro suggesting that there is a potential for a metabolic interaction between modafinil and substrates of CYP2C9). Products include:
ActoPlus Met Tablets 3219
Avandamet Tablets 1343
Fortamet Extended-Release Tablets 1156

Methadone Hydrochloride (Chronic administration of modafinil can increase the elimination of substrates of CYP3A4. Dose adjustments may be necessary for patients being treated with these and similar medications).
No products indexed under this heading.

Methsuximide (Co-administration of potent inducers of CYP3A4 could alter the plasma levels of modafinil).
No products indexed under this heading.

Methylphenidate Hydrochloride (May delay absorption of modafinil by approximately one hour; no significant alterations in pharmacokinetics of either drug). Products include:
Concerta Extended-Release Tablets... 1828
Metadate CD Capsules 3316
Ritalin 2254
Ritalin LA Capsules 2255

Methylprednisolone (Co-administration of potent inducers of CYP3A4 could alter the plasma levels of modafinil).
No products indexed under this heading.

Methylprednisolone Acetate (Co-administration of potent inducers of CYP3A4 could alter the plasma levels of modafinil). Products include:
Depo-Medrol Injectable Suspension 2615
Depo-Medrol Single-Dose Vial 2617

Methylprednisolone Sodium Succinate (Co-administration of potent inducers of CYP3A4 could alter the plasma levels of modafinil).
No products indexed under this heading.

Metronidazole (Co-administration of potent inhibitors of CYP3A4 could alter the plasma levels of modafinil). Products include:
Metrogel 1% 1212
MetroGel-Vaginal Gel 1822
Noritate Cream, 1% 1051

Metronidazole Benzoate (Co-administration of potent inhibitors of CYP3A4 could alter the plasma levels of modafinil).
No products indexed under this heading.

Metronidazole Hydrochloride (Co-administration of potent inhibitors of CYP3A4 could alter the plasma levels of modafinil).
No products indexed under this heading.

Miconazole (Co-administration of potent inhibitors of CYP3A4 could alter the plasma levels of modafinil).
No products indexed under this heading.

Miconazole Nitrate (Co-administration of potent inhibitors of CYP3A4 could alter the plasma levels of modafinil). Products include:
Desenex 674
Desenex Jock Itch Spray Powder ... 674

Midazolam Hydrochloride (Chronic administration of modafinil can increase the elimination of substrates of CYP3A4. Dose adjustments may be necessary for patients being treated with these and similar medications).
No products indexed under this heading.

Miglitol (An apparent concentration-related suppression of CYP2C9 activity was observed in human hepatocytes after exposure to modafinil in vitro suggesting that there is a potential for a metabolic interaction between modafinil and substrates of CYP2C9).
No products indexed under this heading.

Mirtazapine (An apparent concentration-related suppression of CYP2C9 activity was observed in human hepatocytes after exposure to modafinil in vitro suggesting that there is a potential for a metabolic interaction between modafinil and substrates of CYP2C9).
No products indexed under this heading.

Moclobemide (Co-administration requires caution; no interaction studies have been performed).
No products indexed under this heading.

Montelukast Sodium (An apparent concentration-related suppression of CYP2C9 activity was observed in human hepatocytes after exposure to modafinil in vitro suggesting that there is a potential for a metabolic interaction between modafinil and substrates of CYP2C9). Products include:
Singulair 2047

Nabumetone (An apparent concentration-related suppression of CYP2C9 activity was observed in human hepatocytes after exposure to modafinil in vitro suggesting that there is a potential for a metabolic interaction between modafinil and substrates of CYP2C9). Products include:
Relafen Tablets 1523

Naproxen (An apparent concentration-related suppression of CYP2C9 activity was observed in human hepatocytes after exposure to modafinil in vitro suggesting that there is a potential for a metabolic interaction between modafinil and substrates of CYP2C9). Products include:
EC-Naprosyn Delayed-Release Tablets... 2769
Naprosyn Suspension 2769
Naprosyn Tablets 2769
Prevacid NapraPAC 3277

Naproxen Sodium (An apparent concentration-related suppression of CYP2C9 activity was observed in human hepatocytes after exposure to modafinil in vitro suggesting that there is a potential for a metabolic interaction between modafinil and substrates of CYP2C9). Products include:
Aleve Tablets, Caplets and Gelcaps 605
Anaprox Tablets 2769
Anaprox DS Tablets 2769

Nateglinide (An apparent concentration-related suppression of CYP2C9 activity was observed in human hepatocytes after exposure to modafinil in vitro suggesting that there is a potential for a metabolic interaction between modafinil and substrates of CYP2C9). Products include:
Starlix Tablets 2276

Nefazodone Hydrochloride (Chronic administration of modafinil can increase the elimination of substrates of CYP3A4. Dose adjustments may be necessary for patients being treated with these and similar medications).
No products indexed under this heading.

Nelfinavir Mesylate (Chronic administration of modafinil can increase the elimination of substrates of CYP3A4. Dose adjustments may be necessary for patients being treated with these and similar medications). Products include:
Viracept 2556

Nevirapine (Co-administration of potent inducers of CYP3A4 could alter the plasma levels of modafinil). Products include:
Viramune Oral Suspension 903
Viramune Tablets 903

Niacinamide (Co-administration of potent inhibitors of CYP3A4 could alter the plasma levels of modafinil).
No products indexed under this heading.

Nicardipine Hydrochloride (Chronic administration of modafinil can increase the elimination of substrates of CYP3A4. Dose adjustments may be necessary for patients being treated with these and similar medications). Products include:
Cardene I.V. 1129

Nicotinamide (Co-administration of potent inhibitors of CYP3A4 could alter the plasma levels of modafinil). Products include:
Nicomide Tablets 3190

Nifedipine (Chronic administration of modafinil can increase the elimination of substrates of CYP3A4. Dose adjustments may be necessary for patients being treated with these and similar medications). Products include:
Adalat CC Tablets 2978

Nimodipine (Chronic administration of modafinil can increase the elimination of substrates of CYP3A4. Dose adjustments may be necessary for patients being treated with these and similar medications). Products include:
Nimotop Capsules 774

Nisoldipine (Chronic administration of modafinil can increase the elimination of substrates of CYP3A4. Dose adjustments may be necessary for patients being treated with these and similar medications). Products include:
Sular Tablets 1163

Nitrendipine (Chronic administration of modafinil can increase the elimination of substrates of CYP3A4. Dose adjustments may be necessary for patients being treated with these and similar medications).
No products indexed under this heading.

Norethindrone (The effectiveness of steroidal contraceptives may be reduced when used with modafinil tablets and for one month after discontinuation of therapy. Alternative or concomitant methods of contraception are recommended for patients treated with modafinil tablets and for one month after discontinuation of modafinil). Products include:
Ortho Micronor Tablets 2411

Norethindrone Acetate (Chronic administration of modafinil can increase the elimination of substrates of CYP3A4. Dose adjustments may be necessary for patients being treated with these and similar medications). Products include:
Activella Tablets 2311
Aygestin Tablets 1062
CombiPatch Transdermal System 2180

Norethynodrel (The effectiveness of steroidal contraceptives may be reduced when used with modafinil tablets and for one month after discontinuation of therapy. Alternative or concomitant methods of contraception are recommended for patients treated with modafinil tablets and for one month after discontinuation of modafinil).
No products indexed under this heading.

Norfloxacin (Co-administration of potent inhibitors of CYP3A4 could alter the plasma levels of modafinil). Products include:
Noroxin Tablets 2009

Norgestimate (The effectiveness of steroidal contraceptives may be reduced when used with modafinil tablets and for one month after discontinuation of therapy. Alternative or concomitant methods of contra-

ception are recommended for patients treated with modafinil tablets and for one month after discontinuation of modafinil). Products include:

Ortho-Cyclen/Ortho Tri-Cyclen **2414**
Ortho Tri-Cyclen Lo Tablets **2421**
Prefest Tablets **1069**

Norgestrel (The effectiveness of steroidal contraceptives may be reduced when used with modafinil tablets and for one month after discontinuation of therapy. Alternative or concomitant methods of contraception are recommended for patients treated with modafinil tablets and for one month after discontinuation of modafinil). Products include:

Lo/Ovral-28 Tablets **3423**

Nortriptyline Hydrochloride (CYP2C19 provides an ancillary pathway for the metabolism of certain tricyclic antidepressants that are primarily metabolized by CYP2D6. In tricyclic-treated patients deficient in CYP2D6, the amount of metabolism by CYP2C19 may be substantially increased. Modafinil may cause elevation of the levels of these tricyclics in this subset of patients. A reduction in the dose of tricyclic agents might be needed in these patients).

No products indexed under this heading.

Omeprazole (An apparent concentration-related suppression of CYP2C9 activity was observed in human hepatocytes after exposure to modafinil in vitro suggesting that there is a potential for a metabolic interaction between modafinil and substrates of CYP2C9). Products include:

Zegerid Powder for Oral Solution **2972**

Ondansetron (Chronic administration of modafinil can increase the elimination of substrates of CYP3A4. Dose adjustments may be necessary for patients being treated with these and similar medications). Products include:

Zofran ODT Orally Disintegrating Tablets **1613**

Ondansetron Hydrochloride (Chronic administration of modafinil can increase the elimination of substrates of CYP3A4. Dose adjustments may be necessary for patients being treated with these and similar medications). Products include:

Zofran Injection **1607**
Zofran **1613**

Oxaprozin (An apparent concentration-related suppression of CYP2C9 activity was observed in human hepatocytes after exposure to modafinil in vitro suggesting that there is a potential for a metabolic interaction between modafinil and substrates of CYP2C9).

No products indexed under this heading.

Oxcarbazepine (Co-administration of potent inducers of CYP3A4 could alter the plasma levels of modafinil). Products include:

Trileptal Oral Suspension **2281**
Trileptal Tablets **2281**

Paclitaxel (Chronic administration of modafinil can increase the elimination of substrates of CYP3A4. Dose adjustments may be necessary for patients being treated with these and similar medications).

No products indexed under this heading.

Pargyline Hydrochloride (Co-administration requires caution; no interaction studies have been performed).

No products indexed under this heading.

Paroxetine Hydrochloride (Modafinil is a reversible inhibitor of the CYP2C19; the levels of CYP2D6 substrates, such as selective serotonin reuptake inhibitors, which have ancillary routes of elimination through CYP2D6, may be increased by co-administration of modafinil). Products include:

Paxil CR Controlled-Release Tablets **1509**
Paxil **1501**

Phenelzine Sulfate (Co-administration requires caution; no interaction studies have been performed).

No products indexed under this heading.

Phenobarbital (Chronic administration of modafinil may cause induction of its metabolism; co-administration of potent inducers of CYP3A4, such as phenobarbital, could alter the levels of modafinil due to the partial involvement of that enzyme in the metabolic elimination of the compound).

No products indexed under this heading.

Phenobarbital Sodium (Co-administration of potent inducers of CYP3A4 could alter the plasma levels of modafinil).

No products indexed under this heading.

Phenylbutazone (An apparent concentration-related suppression of CYP2C9 activity was observed in human hepatocytes after exposure to modafinil in vitro suggesting that there is a potential for a metabolic interaction between modafinil and substrates of CYP2C9).

No products indexed under this heading.

Phenytoin (Modafinil is a reversible inhibitor of the CYP2C19; co-administration with drugs that are largely eliminated via this pathway, such as phenytoin, may increase the circulating levels of phenytoin).

No products indexed under this heading.

Phenytoin Sodium (Modafinil is a reversible inhibitor of the CYP2C19; co-administration with drugs that are largely eliminated via this pathway, such as phenytoin, may increase the circulating levels of phenytoin). Products include:

Phenytek Capsules **2153**

Pimozide (Chronic administration of modafinil can increase the elimination of substrates of CYP3A4. Dose adjustments may be necessary for patients being treated with these and similar medications). Products include:

Orap Tablets **1220**

Pioglitazone Hydrochloride (An apparent concentration-related suppression of CYP2C9 activity was observed in human hepatocytes after exposure to modafinil in vitro suggesting that there is a potential for a metabolic interaction between modafinil and substrates of CYP2C9). Products include:

ActoPlus Met Tablets **3219**
Actos Tablets **3224**

Piroxicam (An apparent concentration-related suppression of CYP2C9 activity was observed in human hepatocytes after exposure to modafinil in vitro suggesting that there is a potential for a metabolic interaction between modafinil and substrates of CYP2C9).

No products indexed under this heading.

Polyestradiol Phosphate (Chronic administration of modafinil can increase the elimination of substrates of CYP3A4. Dose adjustments may be necessary for patients being treated with these and similar medications).

No products indexed under this heading.

Prednisolone Acetate (Co-administration of potent inducers of CYP3A4 could alter the plasma levels of modafinil). Products include:

Blephamide Ophthalmic Ointment **563**
Blephamide Ophthalmic Suspension **564**
Poly-Pred Liquifilm Ophthalmic Suspension .... ⊙**231**
Pred Forte Ophthalmic Suspension .... ⊙**233**
Pred Mild Sterile Ophthalmic Suspension .... ⊙**236**
Pred-G Ophthalmic Suspension ...... ⊙**234**
Pred-G Sterile Ophthalmic Ointment .... ⊙**235**

Prednisolone Sodium Phosphate (Co-administration of potent inducers of CYP3A4 could alter the plasma levels of modafinil). Products include:

Pediapred Oral Solution **3319**

Prednisolone Tebutate (Co-administration of potent inducers of CYP3A4 could alter the plasma levels of modafinil).

No products indexed under this heading.

Prednisone (Co-administration of potent inducers of CYP3A4 could alter the plasma levels of modafinil).

No products indexed under this heading.

Primidone (Co-administration of potent inducers of CYP3A4 could alter the plasma levels of modafinil).

No products indexed under this heading.

Procarbazine Hydrochloride (Co-administration requires caution; no interaction studies have been performed). Products include:

Matulane Capsules **3188**

Propoxyphene Hydrochloride (Co-administration of potent inhibitors of CYP3A4 could alter the plasma levels of modafinil).

No products indexed under this heading.

Propoxyphene Napsylate (Co-administration of potent inhibitors of CYP3A4 could alter the plasma levels of modafinil). Products include:

Darvocet A 500 Tablets **3497**

Propranolol Hydrochloride (Modafinil is a reversible inhibitor of the CYP2C19; co-administration with drugs that are largely eliminated via this pathway, such as propranolol, may increase the circulating levels of propranolol). Products include:

Inderal LA Long-Acting Capsules **3421**
InnoPran XL Capsules **2728**

Protriptyline Hydrochloride (CYP2C19 provides an ancillary pathway for the metabolism of certain tricyclic antidepressants that are primarily metabolized by CYP2D6. In tricyclic-treated patients deficient in CYP2D6, the amount of metabolism by CYP2C19 may be substantially increased. Modafinil may cause elevation of the levels of these tricyclics in this subset of patients. A reduction in the dose of tricyclic agents might be needed in these patients). Products include:

Vivactil Tablets **2350**

Quinidine (Co-administration of potent inhibitors of CYP3A4 could alter the plasma levels of modafinil).

No products indexed under this heading.

Quinidine Gluconate (Chronic administration of modafinil can increase the elimination of substrates of CYP3A4. Dose adjustments may be necessary for patients being treated with these and similar medications).

No products indexed under this heading.

Quinidine Hydrochloride (Co-administration of potent inhibitors of CYP3A4 could alter the plasma levels of modafinil).

No products indexed under this heading.

Quinidine Polygalacturonate (Chronic administration of modafinil can increase the elimination of substrates of CYP3A4. Dose adjustments may be necessary for patients being treated with these and similar medications).

No products indexed under this heading.

Quinidine Sulfate (Chronic administration of modafinil can increase the elimination of substrates of CYP3A4. Dose adjustments may be necessary for patients being treated with these and similar medications).

No products indexed under this heading.

Quinine (Co-administration of potent inhibitors of CYP3A4 could alter the plasma levels of modafinil).

No products indexed under this heading.

Quinine Sulfate (Co-administration of potent inhibitors of CYP3A4 could alter the plasma levels of modafinil).

No products indexed under this heading.

Quinupristin (Co-administration of potent inhibitors of CYP3A4 could alter the plasma levels of modafinil). Products include:

Synercid I.V. **1690**

Ranitidine Bismuth Citrate (Co-administration of potent inhibitors of CYP3A4 could alter the plasma levels of modafinil).

No products indexed under this heading.

Ranitidine Hydrochloride (Co-administration of potent inhibitors of CYP3A4 could alter the plasma levels of modafinil). Products include:

Zantac **1597**
Zantac Injection **1593**
Zantac 75 Tablets .... ▣**715**
Zantac 150 Maximum Strength Tablets .... ▣**715**
Zantac Injection Pharmacy Bulk Package **1595**

Repaglinide (An apparent concentration-related suppression of CYP2C9 activity was observed in human hepatocytes after exposure to modafinil in vitro suggesting that there is a potential for a metabolic interaction between modafinil and substrates of CYP2C9). Products include:

Prandin Tablets (0.5, 1, and 2 mg) 2337

Rifabutin (Chronic administration of modafinil can increase the elimination of substrates of CYP3A4. Dose adjustments may be necessary for patients being treated with these and similar medications).
No products indexed under this heading.

Rifampicin (Co-administration of potent inducers of CYP3A4 could alter the plasma levels of modafinil).
No products indexed under this heading.

Rifampin (Chronic administration of modafinil may cause induction of its metabolism; co-administration of potent inducers of CYP3A4, such as rifampin, could alter the levels of modafinil due to the partial involvement of that enzyme in the metabolic elimination of the compound).
No products indexed under this heading.

Rifapentine (Co-administration of potent inducers of CYP3A4 could alter the plasma levels of modafinil).
No products indexed under this heading.

Ritonavir (Chronic administration of modafinil can increase the elimination of substrates of CYP3A4. Dose adjustments may be necessary for patients being treated with these and similar medications). Products include:
Kaletra 474
Norvir 499

Rofecoxib (An apparent concentration-related suppression of CYP2C9 activity was observed in human hepatocytes after exposure to modafinil in vitro suggesting that there is a potential for a metabolic interaction between modafinil and substrates of CYP2C9).
No products indexed under this heading.

Rosiglitazone Maleate (An apparent concentration-related suppression of CYP2C9 activity was observed in human hepatocytes after exposure to modafinil in vitro suggesting that there is a potential for a metabolic interaction between modafinil and substrates of CYP2C9). Products include:
Avandamet Tablets 1343
Avandia Tablets 1348

Saquinavir (Chronic administration of modafinil can increase the elimination of substrates of CYP3A4. Dose adjustments may be necessary for patients being treated with these and similar medications).
No products indexed under this heading.

Saquinavir Mesylate (Chronic administration of modafinil can increase the elimination of substrates of CYP3A4. Dose adjustments may be necessary for patients being treated with these and similar medications). Products include:
Invirase 2776

Selegiline Hydrochloride (Co-administration requires caution; no interaction studies have been performed). Products include:
Eldepryl Capsules 3209

Sertraline Hydrochloride (Modafinil is a reversible inhibitor of the CYP2C19; the levels of CYP2D6 substrates, such as selective serotonin reuptake inhibitors, which have ancillary routes of elimination through CYP2D6, may be increased by co-administration of modafinil). Products include:
Zoloft 2581

Sildenafil Citrate (Chronic administration of modafinil can increase the elimination of substrates of CYP3A4. Dose adjustments may be necessary for patients being treated with these and similar medications). Products include:
Revatio Tablets 2541
Viagra Tablets 2552

Simvastatin (Chronic administration of modafinil can increase the elimination of substrates of CYP3A4. Dose adjustments may be necessary for patients being treated with these and similar medications). Products include:
Vytorin 10/10 Tablets 2084
Vytorin 10/10 Tablets 3092
Vytorin 10/20 Tablets 2084
Vytorin 10/20 Tablets 3092
Vytorin 10/40 Tablets 3092
Vytorin 10/40 Tablets 2084
Vytorin 10/80 Tablets 2084
Vytorin 10/80 Tablets 3092
Zocor Tablets 2078

Sirolimus (Chronic administration of modafinil can increase the elimination of substrates of CYP3A4. Dose adjustments may be necessary for patients being treated with these and similar medications). Products include:
Rapamune Oral Solution and Tablets 3472

Sulfamethoxazole (An apparent concentration-related suppression of CYP2C9 activity was observed in human hepatocytes after exposure to modafinil in vitro suggesting that there is a potential for a metabolic interaction between modafinil and substrates of CYP2C9).
No products indexed under this heading.

Sulfinpyrazone (Co-administration of potent inducers of CYP3A4 could alter the plasma levels of modafinil).
No products indexed under this heading.

Sulindac (An apparent concentration-related suppression of CYP2C9 activity was observed in human hepatocytes after exposure to modafinil in vitro suggesting that there is a potential for a metabolic interaction between modafinil and substrates of CYP2C9). Products include:
Clinoril Tablets 1899

Suprofen (An apparent concentration-related suppression of CYP2C9 activity was observed in human hepatocytes after exposure to modafinil in vitro suggesting that there is a potential for a metabolic interaction between modafinil and substrates of CYP2C9).
No products indexed under this heading.

Tacrolimus (Chronic administration of modafinil can increase the elimination of substrates of CYP3A4. Dose adjustments may be necessary for patients being treated with these and similar medications). Products include:
Prograf Capsules and Injection 624
Protopic Ointment 629

Tamoxifen Citrate (Chronic administration of modafinil can increase the elimination of substrates of CYP3A4. Dose adjustments may be necessary for patients being treated with these and similar medications).
No products indexed under this heading.

Telithromycin (Co-administration of potent inhibitors of CYP3A4 could alter the plasma levels of modafinil). Products include:
Ketek Tablets 2920

Telmisartan (An apparent concentration-related suppression of CYP2C9 activity was observed in human hepatocytes after exposure to modafinil in vitro suggesting that there is a potential for a metabolic interaction between modafinil and substrates of CYP2C9). Products include:
Micardis Tablets 884
Micardis HCT Tablets 886

Theophylline (Chronic administration of modafinil may cause modest induction of CYP3A4, thus reducing the levels, to a lesser degree, of co-administered substrate for that enzyme system, such as theophylline).
No products indexed under this heading.

Theophylline Anhydrous (Chronic administration of modafinil may cause modest induction of CYP3A4, thus reducing the levels, to a lesser degree, of co-administered substrate for that enzyme system, such as theophylline). Products include:
Uniphyl Tablets 2708

Theophylline Calcium Salicylate (Chronic administration of modafinil may cause modest induction of CYP3A4, thus reducing the levels, to a lesser degree, of co-administered substrate for that enzyme system, such as theophylline).
No products indexed under this heading.

Theophylline Dihydroxypropyl (Glyceryl) (Chronic administration of modafinil may cause modest induction of CYP3A4, thus reducing the levels, to a lesser degree, of co-administered substrate for that enzyme system, such as theophylline).
No products indexed under this heading.

Theophylline Ethylenediamine (Chronic administration of modafinil may cause modest induction of CYP3A4, thus reducing the levels, to a lesser degree, of co-administered substrate for that enzyme system, such as theophylline).
No products indexed under this heading.

Theophylline Sodium Glycinate (Chronic administration of modafinil may cause modest induction of CYP3A4, thus reducing the levels, to a lesser degree, of co-administered substrate for that enzyme system, such as theophylline).
No products indexed under this heading.

Tiagabine Hydrochloride (Chronic administration of modafinil can increase the elimination of substrates of CYP3A4. Dose adjustments may be necessary for patients being treated with these and similar medications). Products include:
Gabitril Tablets 998

Tolazamide (An apparent concentration-related suppression of CYP2C9 activity was observed in human hepatocytes after exposure to modafinil in vitro suggesting that there is a potential for a metabolic interaction between modafinil and substrates of CYP2C9).
No products indexed under this heading.

Tolbutamide (An apparent concentration-related suppression of CYP2C9 activity was observed in human hepatocytes after exposure to modafinil in vitro suggesting that there is a potential for a metabolic interaction between modafinil and substrates of CYP2C9).
No products indexed under this heading.

Tolbutamide Sodium (An apparent concentration-related suppression of CYP2C9 activity was observed in human hepatocytes after exposure to modafinil in vitro suggesting that there is a potential for a metabolic interaction between modafinil and substrates of CYP2C9).
No products indexed under this heading.

Tolmetin Sodium (An apparent concentration-related suppression of CYP2C9 activity was observed in human hepatocytes after exposure to modafinil in vitro suggesting that there is a potential for a metabolic interaction between modafinil and substrates of CYP2C9).
No products indexed under this heading.

Tolterodine Tartrate (Chronic administration of modafinil can increase the elimination of substrates of CYP3A4. Dose adjustments may be necessary for patients being treated with these and similar medications). Products include:
Detrol Tablets 2626
Detrol LA Capsules 2629

Torsemide (An apparent concentration-related suppression of CYP2C9 activity was observed in human hepatocytes after exposure to modafinil in vitro suggesting that there is a potential for a metabolic interaction between modafinil and substrates of CYP2C9).
No products indexed under this heading.

Tranylcypromine Sulfate (Co-administration requires caution; no interaction studies have been performed). Products include:
Parnate Tablets 1499

Trazodone Hydrochloride (Chronic administration of modafinil can increase the elimination of substrates of CYP3A4. Dose adjustments may be necessary for patients being treated with these and similar medications).
No products indexed under this heading.

Triamcinolone (Co-administration of potent inducers of CYP3A4 could alter the plasma levels of modafinil).
No products indexed under this heading.

Triamcinolone Acetonide (Co-administration of potent inducers of CYP3A4 could alter the plasma levels of modafinil). Products include:
Azmacort Inhalation Aerosol 1701
Nasacort HFA Inhalation Aerosol 2939
Nasacort AQ Nasal Spray 2937

Triamcinolone Diacetate (Co-administration of potent inducers of CYP3A4 could alter the plasma levels of modafinil).
No products indexed under this heading.

Triamcinolone Hexacetonide (Co-administration of potent inducers of CYP3A4 could alter the plasma levels of modafinil).
No products indexed under this heading.

Triazolam (When modafinil was administered concurrently with triazolam, mean Cmax and AUC of triazolam were decreased by 42% and 59%, respectively, and its elimination half-life was decreased by approximately an hour after the modafinil treatment).
No products indexed under this heading.

Trimipramine Maleate (CYP2C19 provides an ancillary pathway for the metabolism of certain tricyclic antidepressants that are primarily metabolized by CYP2D6. In tricyclic-treated patients deficient in CYP2D6, the amount of metabolism by CYP2C19 may be substantially increased. Modafinil may cause elevation of the levels of these tricyclics in this subset of patients. A reduction in the dose of tricyclic agents might be needed in these patients). Products include:
Surmontil Capsules ... **2347**

Troglitazone (An apparent concentration-related suppression of CYP2C9 activity was observed in human hepatocytes after exposure to modafinil in vitro suggesting that there is a potential for a metabolic interaction between modafinil and substrates of CYP2C9).
No products indexed under this heading.

Troleandomycin (Co-administration of potent inhibitors of CYP3A4 could alter the plasma levels of modafinil).
No products indexed under this heading.

Valdecoxib (An apparent concentration-related suppression of CYP2C9 activity was observed in human hepatocytes after exposure to modafinil in vitro suggesting that there is a potential for a metabolic interaction between modafinil and substrates of CYP2C9).
No products indexed under this heading.

Valproate Sodium (Co-administration of potent inhibitors of CYP3A4 could alter the plasma levels of modafinil). Products include:
Depacon Injection ... **412**

Valsartan (An apparent concentration-related suppression of CYP2C9 activity was observed in human hepatocytes after exposure to modafinil in vitro suggesting that there is a potential for a metabolic interaction between modafinil and substrates of CYP2C9). Products include:
Diovan HCT Tablets ... **2195**
Diovan Tablets ... **2191**

Verapamil Hydrochloride (Chronic administration of modafinil can increase the elimination of substrates of CYP3A4. Dose adjustments may be necessary for patients being treated with these and similar medications). Products include:
Covera-HS Tablets ... **3135**
Tarka Tablets ... **519**
Verelan PM Capsules ... **3120**

Vinblastine Sulfate (Chronic administration of modafinil can increase the elimination of substrates of CYP3A4. Dose adjustments may be necessary for patients being treated with these and similar medications).
No products indexed under this heading.

Vincristine Sulfate (Chronic administration of modafinil can increase the elimination of substrates of CYP3A4. Dose adjustments may be necessary for patients being treated with these and similar medications).
No products indexed under this heading.

Voriconazole (An apparent concentration-related suppression of CYP2C9 activity was observed in human hepatocytes after exposure to modafinil in vitro suggesting that there is a potential for a metabolic interaction between modafinil and substrates of CYP2C9). Products include:
VFEND I.V. ... **2543**
VFEND Oral Suspension ... **2543**
VFEND Tablets ... **2543**

Warfarin Sodium (There were no significant changes in the pharmacokinetic profile of warfarin in healthy subjects given a single dose of warfarin following chronic administration of modafinil relative to the profiles in subjects given placebo. However, more frequent monitoring of prothrombin times/INR is advisable whenever modafinil is co-administered with warfarin). Products include:
Coumadin for Injection ... **932**
Coumadin Tablets ... **932**

Zafirlukast (An apparent concentration-related suppression of CYP2C9 activity was observed in human hepatocytes after exposure to modafinil in vitro suggesting that there is a potential for a metabolic interaction between modafinil and substrates of CYP2C9). Products include:
Accolate Tablets ... **663**

Zileuton (An apparent concentration-related suppression of CYP2C9 activity was observed in human hepatocytes after exposure to modafinil in vitro suggesting that there is a potential for a metabolic interaction between modafinil and substrates of CYP2C9).
No products indexed under this heading.

Food Interactions

Alcohol (The use of modafinil in combination with alcohol has not been studied. It is advisable to avoid alcohol while taking modafinil).

Food, unspecified (Delays the absorption (tmax) by approximately one hour; no effect on overall bioavailability).

Grapefruit (Co-administration of potent inhibitors of CYP3A4 could alter the plasma levels of modafinil).

Grapefruit Juice (Co-administration of potent inhibitors of CYP3A4 could alter the plasma levels of modafinil).

PROZAC PULVULES AND LIQUID

(Fluoxetine Hydrochloride) ... **1771**
May interact with anticoagulants, cytochrome p450 2d6 substrates (selected), oral hypoglycemic agents, insulin, lithium preparations, monoamine oxidase inhibitors, non-steroidal anti-inflammatory agents, phenytoin, tricyclic antidepressants, and certain other agents. Compounds in these categories include:

Acarbose (Fluoxetine may alter glycemic control in diabetics; hypoglycemia has occurred during therapy with fluoxetine and hyperglycemia has developed following discontinuation of the drug; hypoglycemia dosage may need to be adjusted). Products include:
Precose Tablets ... **776**

Alprazolam (Co-administration has resulted in increased alprazolam plasma concentrations and further psychomotor performance decrement due to increased alprazolam levels). Products include:
Niravam Orally Disintegrating Tablets ... **3106**
Xanax XR Tablets ... **2655**

Amitriptyline Hydrochloride (Fluoxetine inhibits the activity of P450 IID6 isoenzyme making normal metabolizers resemble "poor metabolizers"; therapy with drugs that are predominantly metabolized by the P450 IID6 isoenzyme, such as tricyclic antidepressants, and have a relatively narrow therapeutic index should be initiated at low end of the dose range if a patient is receiving fluoxetine concurrently or has taken it in the previous 5 weeks).
No products indexed under this heading.

Amoxapine (Fluoxetine inhibits the activity of P450 IID6 isoenzyme making normal metabolizers resemble "poor metabolizers"; therapy with drugs that are predominantly metabolized by the P450 IID6 isoenzyme, such as tricyclic antidepressants, and have a relatively narrow therapeutic index should be initiated at low end of the dose range if a patient is receiving fluoxetine concurrently or has taken it in the previous 5 weeks).
No products indexed under this heading.

Amphetamine Aspartate (If fluoxetine is added to the treatment regimen of a patient already receiving a drug metabolized by CYP2D6, the need for decreased dose of the original medication should be considered. Fluoxetine is metabolized by this isoenzyme; thus, both the pharmacokinetic properties and relative proportion of metabolites are altered in poor metabolizers of CYP2D6). Products include:
Adderall Tablets ... **3168**
Adderall XR Capsules ... **3169**

Amphetamine Aspartate Monohydrate (If fluoxetine is added to the treatment regimen of a patient already receiving a drug metabolized by CYP2D6, the need for decreased dose of the original medication should be considered. Fluoxetine is metabolized by this isoenzyme; thus, both the pharmacokinetic properties and relative proportion of metabolites are altered in poor metabolizers of CYP2D6).
No products indexed under this heading.

Amphetamine Sulfate (If fluoxetine is added to the treatment regimen of a patient already receiving a drug metabolized by CYP2D6, the need for decreased dose of the original medication should be considered. Fluoxetine is metabolized by this isoenzyme; thus, both the pharmacokinetic properties and relative proportion of metabolites are altered in poor metabolizers of CYP2D6). Products include:
Adderall Tablets ... **3168**
Adderall XR Capsules ... **3169**

Anisindione (Concurrent use of fluoxetine with drugs that affect coagulation may potentiate the risk of bleeding). Products include:
Miradon Tablets ... **3056**

Ardeparin Sodium (Concurrent use of fluoxetine with drugs that affect coagulation may potentiate the risk of bleeding).
No products indexed under this heading.

Aspirin (Concurrent use of fluoxetine with aspirin potentiated the risk of upper gastrointestinal bleeding and there is a reason to believe that bleeding at other sites may be similarly potentiated. Combined use of psychotropic drugs that interfere with serotonin reuptake and aspirin has been associated with an increased risk of bleeding). Products include:
Aggrenox Capsules ... **855**
Bayer, Aspirin Regimen ... ⊡**606**
Bayer Aspirin Tablets ... **3515**
BC Powder ... ⊡**612**
BC Allergy Sinus Cold Powder ... ⊡**612**
Arthritis Strength BC Powder ... ⊡**612**
BC Sinus Cold Powder ... ⊡**612**
Ecotrin Enteric Coated Aspirin Low, Regular and Maximum Strength Tablets ... **1627**
Goody's Body Pain Formula Powder ... ⊡**621**
Goody's Extra Strength Headache Powder ... ⊡**621**
Goody's Extra Strength Pain Relief Tablets ... ⊡**621**
Percodan Tablets ... **1115**
St. Joseph 81 mg Aspirin Chewable and Enteric Coated Tablets ... **1841**

Aspirin, Enteric Coated (Concurrent use of fluoxetine with aspirin potentiated the risk of upper gastrointestinal bleeding and there is a reason to believe that bleeding at other sites may be similarly potentiated. Combined use of psychotropic drugs that interfere with serotonin reuptake and aspirin has been associated with an increased risk of bleeding).
No products indexed under this heading.

Aspirin Buffered (Concurrent use of fluoxetine with aspirin potentiated the risk of upper gastrointestinal bleeding and there is a reason to believe that bleeding at other sites may be similarly potentiated. Combined use of psychotropic drugs that interfere with serotonin reuptake and aspirin has been associated with an increased risk of bleeding).
No products indexed under this heading.

Atomoxetine Hydrochloride (If fluoxetine is added to the treatment regimen of a patient already receiving a drug metabolized by CYP2D6, the need for decreased dose of the original medication should be considered. Fluoxetine is metabolized by this isoenzyme; thus, both the pharmacokinetic properties and relative

proportion of metabolites are altered in poor metabolizers of CYP2D6). Products include:

Strattera Capsules 1784

Bisoprolol Fumarate (If fluoxetine is added to the treatment regimen of a patient already receiving a drug metabolized by CYP2D6, the need for decreased dose of the original medication should be considered. Fluoxetine is metabolized by this isoenzyme; thus, both the pharmacokinetic properties and relative proportion of metabolites are altered in poor metabolizers of CYP2D6).

No products indexed under this heading.

Captopril (If fluoxetine is added to the treatment regimen of a patient already receiving a drug metabolized by CYP2D6, the need for decreased dose of the original medication should be considered. Fluoxetine is metabolized by this isoenzyme; thus, both the pharmacokinetic properties and relative proportion of metabolites are altered in poor metabolizers of CYP2D6). Products include:

Captopril Tablets 2114

Carbamazepine (Patients stable on doses of carbamazepine have developed elevated plasma carbamazepine concentrations and clinical anticonvulsant toxicity following initiation of concomitant fluoxetine therapy). Products include:

Carbatrol Capsules 3174
Equetro Extended-Release Capsules 3178
Tegretol/Tegretol-XR 2278

Carvedilol (If fluoxetine is added to the treatment regimen of a patient already receiving a drug metabolized by CYP2D6, the need for decreased dose of the original medication should be considered. Fluoxetine is metabolized by this isoenzyme; thus, both the pharmacokinetic properties and relative proportion of metabolites are altered in poor metabolizers of CYP2D6). Products include:

Coreg Tablets 1376

Celecoxib (Concurrent use of fluoxetine with an NSAID potentiated the risk of upper gastrointestinal bleeding and there is a reason to believe that bleeding at other sites may be similarly potentiated. Combined use of psychotropic drugs that interfere with serotonin reuptake and NSAIDs have been associated with an increased risk of bleeding). Products include:

Celebrex Capsules 3130

Cevimeline Hydrochloride (If fluoxetine is added to the treatment regimen of a patient already receiving a drug metabolized by CYP2D6, the need for decreased dose of the original medication should be considered. Fluoxetine is metabolized by this isoenzyme; thus, both the pharmacokinetic properties and relative proportion of metabolites are altered in poor metabolizers of CYP2D6). Products include:

Evoxac Capsules 1042

Chlorpromazine (If fluoxetine is added to the treatment regimen of a patient already receiving a drug metabolized by CYP2D6, the need for decreased dose of the original medication should be considered. Fluoxetine is metabolized by this isoenzyme; thus, both the pharmacokinetic properties and relative proportion of metabolites are altered in poor metabolizers of CYP2D6).

No products indexed under this heading.

Chlorpromazine Hydrochloride (If fluoxetine is added to the treatment regimen of a patient already receiving a drug metabolized by CYP2D6, the need for decreased dose of the original medication should be considered. Fluoxetine is metabolized by this isoenzyme; thus, both the pharmacokinetic properties and relative proportion of metabolites are altered in poor metabolizers of CYP2D6).

No products indexed under this heading.

Chlorpropamide (Fluoxetine may alter glycemic control in diabetics; hypoglycemia has occurred during therapy with fluoxetine and hyperglycemia has developed following discontinuation of the drug; hypoglycemia dosage may need to be adjusted).

No products indexed under this heading.

Clomipramine Hydrochloride (Fluoxetine inhibits the activity of P450 IID6 isoenzyme making normal metabolizers resemble "poor metabolizers"; therapy with drugs that are predominantly metabolized by the P450 IID6 isoenzyme, such as tricyclic antidepressants, and have a relatively narrow therapeutic index should be initiated at low end of the dose range if a patient is receiving fluoxetine concurrently or has taken it in the previous 5 weeks).

No products indexed under this heading.

Clozapine (Co-administration of SSRIs, fluoxetine, and antipsychotics, such as clozapine, has resulted in elevation of blood levels of clozapine). Products include:

Clozapine Tablets 2141
Clozaril Tablets 2174
FazaClo Orally Disintegrating Tablets 547

Codeine Phosphate (If fluoxetine is added to the treatment regimen of a patient already receiving a drug metabolized by CYP2D6, the need for decreased dose of the original medication should be considered. Fluoxetine is metabolized by this isoenzyme; thus, both the pharmacokinetic properties and relative proportion of metabolites are altered in poor metabolizers of CYP2D6). Products include:

Tylenol with Codeine 2461

Codeine Sulfate (If fluoxetine is added to the treatment regimen of a patient already receiving a drug metabolized by CYP2D6, the need for decreased dose of the original medication should be considered. Fluoxetine is metabolized by this isoenzyme; thus, both the pharmacokinetic properties and relative proportion of metabolites are altered in poor metabolizers of CYP2D6).

No products indexed under this heading.

Cyclobenzaprine Hydrochloride (If fluoxetine is added to the treatment regimen of a patient already receiving a drug metabolized by CYP2D6, the need for decreased dose of the original medication should be considered. Fluoxetine is metabolized by this isoenzyme; thus, both the pharmacokinetic properties and relative proportion of metabolites are altered in poor metabolizers of CYP2D6). Products include:

Flexeril Tablets 1832

Dalteparin Sodium (Concurrent use of fluoxetine with drugs that affect coagulation may potentiate the risk of bleeding). Products include:

Fragmin Injection 2638

Danaparoid Sodium (Concurrent use of fluoxetine with drugs that affect coagulation may potentiate the risk of bleeding).

No products indexed under this heading.

Desipramine Hydrochloride (Fluoxetine inhibits the activity of P450 IID6 isoenzyme making normal metabolizers resemble "poor metabolizers"; therapy with drugs that are predominantly metabolized by the P450 IID6 isoenzyme, such as tricyclic antidepressants, and have a relatively narrow therapeutic index should be initiated at low end of the dose range if a patient is receiving fluoxetine concurrently or has taken it in the previous 5 weeks).

No products indexed under this heading.

Dexfenfluramine Hydrochloride (If fluoxetine is added to the treatment regimen of a patient already receiving a drug metabolized by CYP2D6, the need for decreased dose of the original medication should be considered. Fluoxetine is metabolized by this isoenzyme; thus, both the pharmacokinetic properties and relative proportion of metabolites are altered in poor metabolizers of CYP2D6).

No products indexed under this heading.

Dextromethorphan Hydrobromide (If fluoxetine is added to the treatment regimen of a patient already receiving a drug metabolized by CYP2D6, the need for decreased dose of the original medication should be considered. Fluoxetine is metabolized by this isoenzyme; thus, both the pharmacokinetic properties and relative proportion of metabolites are altered in poor metabolizers of CYP2D6). Products include:

Alacol DM Syrup 739
Balamine DM 739
Contac Severe Cold and Flu Caplets Maximum Strength 615
Contac Severe Cold and Flu Caplets Non-Drowsy 615
Children's Dimetapp DM Cold & Cough Elixir 745
Children's Dimetapp Long Acting Cough Plus Cold Syrup 746
Dimetapp Infant Drops Decongestant Plus Cough 746
Mucinex DM Tablets 602
PediaCare Decongestant & Cough Infant Drops 705
PediaCare Freezer Pops Long-Acting Cough-Glacier Grape and Polar Berry Blue 706
PediaCare Long-Acting Cough Infant Drops 705
PediaCare Long-Acting Cough Plus Cold Liquid 704
PediaCare Multi-Symptom Cold Liquid 704
PediaCare NightRest Cough & Cold Liquid 704
Robitussin Allergy & Cough Syrup 750
Robitussin CF Liquid 755
Robitussin Cough & Cold Liquid-filled Capsules 750
Robitussin Cough, Cold & Flu Liquid-filled Capsules 750
Robitussin Cough & Cold Infant Drops 755
Robitussin DM Infant Drops 753
Robitussin DM Liquid 753
Robitussin Flu Liquid 752
Robitussin Maximum Strength Cough Liquid 754
Robitussin Maximum Strength Cough & Cold Liquid 754
Robitussin Pediatric Cough Liquid 754
Robitussin Pediatric Cough & Cold Liquid 754
Robitussin PM Cough & Cold Liquid 752
Robitussin Sugar Free Cough Liquid 753
Simply Cough Liquid 1840
Sudafed Severe Cold 710
TheraFlu Cold & Cough Hot Liquid 680
TheraFlu Flu & Chest Congestion Non-Drowsy Hot Liquid 681
TheraFlu Severe Cold Non-Drowsy Hot Liquid 683
TheraFlu Severe Cold & Cough Hot Liquid 683
TheraFlu Severe Cold Caplets 679
TheraFlu Severe Cold Hot Liquid 682
TheraFlu Severe Cold Non-Drowsy Caplets 679
TheraFlu Thin Strips Long Acting Cough 684
Triaminic Cold & Cough Liquid 685
Triaminic Cough Liquid 687
Triaminic Cough & Nasal Congestion Liquid 687
Triaminic Cough & Sore Throat Liquid 687
Triaminic Flu, Cough & Fever Liquid 685
Triaminic Night Time Cough & Cold Liquid 685
Triaminic Cold & Cough Softchews 688
Triaminic Cough & Sore Throat Softchews 689
Triaminic Thin Strips Long Acting Cough 689
Children's Tylenol Plus Cold & Cough Suspension Liquid and Chewable Tablets 1851
Children's Tylenol Plus Flu Suspension Liquid 1853
Concentrated Tylenol Infants' Drops Plus Cold and Cough 1851
Tylenol Cold & Flu Severe Daytime Liquid with Cool Bust 1846
Tylenol Cold & Flu Severe NightTime Liquid with Cool Burst 1846
Tylenol Cold Severe Congestion Non-Drowsy Caplets with Cool Burst 1846
Tylenol Cough & Sore Throat Daytime Liquid with Cool Burst 1849
Tylenol Cough & Sore Throat NightTime Liquid with Cool Burst 1849
Tylenol Flu Day Non-Drowsy Gelcaps 1846
Concentrated Tylenol Infants' Drops Plus Cold & Cough Nasal Decongestant, Fever Reducer & Pain Reliever 668
Multi-Symptom Tylenol Cold Night Time Caplets 1845
Multi-Symptom Tylenol Cold Day Non-Drowsy Caplets and Gelcaps 1845
Vicks 44 Cough Relief 2675
Vicks 44D Cough & Head Congestion Relief 2676
Vicks 44D Cough & Head Congestion Relief Liquid 721
Vicks 44E Cough & Chest Congestion Relief 2676

Pediatric Vicks 44e Cough & Chest Congestion Relief Liquid...... 2673
Vicks 44M Cough, Cold & Flu Relief...... 2676
Pediatric Vicks 44m Cough & Cold Relief...... 2673
Vicks DayQuil LiquiCaps/Liquid Multi-Symptom Cold/Flu Relief...... ▣ 723
Vicks DayQuil Multi-Symptom Cold/Flu Relief LiquiCaps...... 2675
Vicks DayQuil Multi-Symptom Cold/Flu Relief Liquid...... 2675
Children's Vicks NyQuil Cold/Cough Relief...... 2671
Vicks NyQuil Cough Liquid...... 2677
Vicks NyQuil LiquiCaps...... 2677
Vicks NyQuil LiquiCaps/Liquid Multi-Symptom Cold/Flu Relief...... ▣ 725
Vicks NyQuil Liquid...... 2677
Zicam Concentrated Cough Mist for Kids Cool Cherry...... ▣ 643
Zicam Concentrated Cough Mist for Kids Plus D Cool Cherry...... ▣ 643
Zicam Concentrated Cough Mist Nite-Cool Cherry...... ▣ 642
Zicam Concentrated Cough Mist Plus D Cool Cherry...... ▣ 642
Zicam Concentrated Cough Mist-Honey Lemon & Cool Cherry...... ▣ 642

Dextromethorphan Polistirex (If fluoxetine is added to the treatment regimen of a patient already receiving a drug metabolized by CYP2D6, the need for decreased dose of the original medication should be considered. Fluoxetine is metabolized by this isoenzyme; thus, both the pharmacokinetic properties and relative proportion of metabolites are altered in poor metabolizers of CYP2D6). Products include:
Delsym Extended-Release Suspension...... ▣ 611
Delsym 12 Hour Cough Suppressant for Children...... ▣ 611

Diazepam (Co-administration results in prolonged half-life of diazepam). Products include:
Diastat Rectal Delivery System...... 3344
Valium Tablets...... 2822

Diclofenac Potassium (Concurrent use of fluoxetine with an NSAID potentiated the risk of upper gastrointestinal bleeding and there is a reason to believe that bleeding at other sites may be similarly potentiated. Combined use of psychotropic drugs that interfere with serotonin reuptake and NSAIDs have been associated with an increased risk of bleeding). Products include:
Cataflam Tablets...... 2173

Diclofenac Sodium (Concurrent use of fluoxetine with an NSAID potentiated the risk of upper gastrointestinal bleeding and there is a reason to believe that bleeding at other sites may be similarly potentiated. Combined use of psychotropic drugs that interfere with serotonin reuptake and NSAIDs have been associated with an increased risk of bleeding). Products include:
Arthrotec Tablets...... 3126
Voltaren Ophthalmic Solution...... 2300
Voltaren Tablets...... 2298
Voltaren-XR Tablets...... 2301

Dicumarol (Concurrent use of fluoxetine with drugs that affect coagulation may potentiate the risk of bleeding).
No products indexed under this heading.

Digitoxin (Fluoxetine is tightly bound to protein; co-administration may cause shift in plasma concentrations resulting in potential adverse effects).
No products indexed under this heading.

Dolasetron Mesylate (If fluoxetine is added to the treatment regimen of a patient already receiving a drug metabolized by CYP2D6, the need for decreased dose of the original medication should be considered. Fluoxetine is metabolized by this isoenzyme; thus, both the pharmacokinetic properties and relative proportion of metabolites are altered in poor metabolizers of CYP2D6). Products include:
Anzemet Injection...... 2871
Anzemet Tablets...... 2874

Donepezil Hydrochloride (If fluoxetine is added to the treatment regimen of a patient already receiving a drug metabolized by CYP2D6, the need for decreased dose of the original medication should be considered. Fluoxetine is metabolized by this isoenzyme; thus, both the pharmacokinetic properties and relative proportion of metabolites are altered in poor metabolizers of CYP2D6). Products include:
Aricept Tablets...... 1086
Aricept ODT Tablets...... 1086

Doxepin Hydrochloride (Fluoxetine inhibits the activity of P450 IID6 isoenzyme making normal metabolizers resemble "poor metabolizers"; therapy with drugs that are predominantly metabolized by the P450 IID6 isoenzyme, such as tricyclic antidepressants, and have a relatively narrow therapeutic index should be initiated at low end of the dose range if a patient is receiving fluoxetine concurrently or has taken it in the previous 5 weeks).
No products indexed under this heading.

Encainide Hydrochloride (If fluoxetine is added to the treatment regimen of a patient already receiving a drug metabolized by CYP2D6, the need for decreased dose of the original medication should be considered. Fluoxetine is metabolized by this isoenzyme; thus, both the pharmacokinetic properties and relative proportion of metabolites are altered in poor metabolizers of CYP2D6).
No products indexed under this heading.

Enoxaparin Sodium (Concurrent use of fluoxetine with drugs that affect coagulation may potentiate the risk of bleeding). Products include:
Lovenox Injection...... 2931

Etodolac (Concurrent use of fluoxetine with an NSAID potentiated the risk of upper gastrointestinal bleeding and there is a reason to believe that bleeding at other sites may be similarly potentiated. Combined use of psychotropic drugs that interfere with serotonin reuptake and NSAIDs have been associated with an increased risk of bleeding).
No products indexed under this heading.

Fenoprofen Calcium (Concurrent use of fluoxetine with an NSAID potentiated the risk of upper gastrointestinal bleeding and there is a reason to believe that bleeding at other sites may be similarly potentiated. Combined use of psychotropic drugs that interfere with serotonin reuptake and NSAIDs have been associated with an increased risk of bleeding). Products include:
Nalfon Capsules...... 2504

Fentanyl (If fluoxetine is added to the treatment regimen of a patient already receiving a drug metabolized by CYP2D6, the need for decreased dose of the original medication should be considered. Fluoxetine is metabolized by this isoenzyme; thus, both the pharmacokinetic properties and relative proportion of metabolites are altered in poor metabolizers of CYP2D6). Products include:
Duragesic Transdermal System...... 2448

Fentanyl Citrate (If fluoxetine is added to the treatment regimen of a patient already receiving a drug metabolized by CYP2D6, the need for decreased dose of the original medication should be considered. Fluoxetine is metabolized by this isoenzyme; thus, both the pharmacokinetic properties and relative proportion of metabolites are altered in poor metabolizers of CYP2D6). Products include:
Actiq...... 993

Flecainide Acetate (Fluoxetine inhibits the activity of P450 IID6 isoenzyme making normal metabolizers resemble "poor metabolizers"; therapy with drugs that are predominantly metabolized by the P450 IID6 isoenzyme, such as flecainide, and have a relatively narrow therapeutic index should be initiated at low end of the dose range if a patient is receiving fluoxetine concurrently or has taken it in the previous 5 weeks). Products include:
Tambocor Tablets...... 1824

Fluoxetine (If fluoxetine is added to the treatment regimen of a patient already receiving a drug metabolized by CYP2D6, the need for decreased dose of the original medication should be considered. Fluoxetine is metabolized by this isoenzyme; thus, both the pharmacokinetic properties and relative proportion of metabolites are altered in poor metabolizers of CYP2D6).
No products indexed under this heading.

Fluphenazine Decanoate (If fluoxetine is added to the treatment regimen of a patient already receiving a drug metabolized by CYP2D6, the need for decreased dose of the original medication should be considered. Fluoxetine is metabolized by this isoenzyme; thus, both the pharmacokinetic properties and relative proportion of metabolites are altered in poor metabolizers of CYP2D6).
No products indexed under this heading.

Fluphenazine Enanthate (If fluoxetine is added to the treatment regimen of a patient already receiving a drug metabolized by CYP2D6, the need for decreased dose of the original medication should be considered. Fluoxetine is metabolized by this isoenzyme; thus, both the pharmacokinetic properties and relative proportion of metabolites are altered in poor metabolizers of CYP2D6).
No products indexed under this heading.

Fluphenazine Hydrochloride (If fluoxetine is added to the treatment regimen of a patient already receiving a drug metabolized by CYP2D6, the need for decreased dose of the original medication should be considered. Fluoxetine is metabolized by this isoenzyme; thus, both the pharmacokinetic properties and relative proportion of metabolites are altered in poor metabolizers of CYP2D6).
No products indexed under this heading.

Flurbiprofen (Concurrent use of fluoxetine with an NSAID potentiated the risk of upper gastrointestinal bleeding and there is a reason to believe that bleeding at other sites may be similarly potentiated. Combined use of psychotropic drugs that interfere with serotonin reuptake and NSAIDs have been associated with an increased risk of bleeding).
No products indexed under this heading.

Fluvoxamine Maleate (If fluoxetine is added to the treatment regimen of a patient already receiving a drug metabolized by CYP2D6, the need for decreased dose of the original medication should be considered. Fluoxetine is metabolized by this isoenzyme; thus, both the pharmacokinetic properties and relative proportion of metabolites are altered in poor metabolizers of CYP2D6).
No products indexed under this heading.

Fondaparinux Sodium (Concurrent use of fluoxetine with drugs that affect coagulation may potentiate the risk of bleeding). Products include:
Arixtra Injection...... 1325

Formoterol Fumarate (If fluoxetine is added to the treatment regimen of a patient already receiving a drug metabolized by CYP2D6, the need for decreased dose of the original medication should be considered. Fluoxetine is metabolized by this isoenzyme; thus, both the pharmacokinetic properties and relative proportion of metabolites are altered in poor metabolizers of CYP2D6). Products include:
Foradil Aerolizer...... 3024

Fosphenytoin Sodium (Patients stable on doses of phenytoin have developed elevated plasma phenytoin concentrations and clinical anticonvulsant toxicity following initiation of concomitant fluoxetine therapy).
No products indexed under this heading.

Galantamine Hydrobromide (If fluoxetine is added to the treatment regimen of a patient already receiving a drug metabolized by CYP2D6, the need for decreased dose of the original medication should be considered. Fluoxetine is metabolized by this isoenzyme; thus, both the pharmacokinetic properties and relative proportion of metabolites are altered in poor metabolizers of CYP2D6). Products include:
Razadyne ER Extended-Release Capsules...... 2434
Razadyne...... 2434

Glimepiride (Fluoxetine may alter glycemic control in diabetics; hypoglycemia has occurred during therapy with fluoxetine and hyperglycemia has developed following discontinuation of the drug; hypoglycemia dosage may need to be adjusted). Products include:
Amaryl Tablets...... 2864

Glipizide (Fluoxetine may alter glycemic control in diabetics; hypoglycemia has occurred during therapy with fluoxetine and hyperglycemia has developed following discontinuation of the drug; hypoglycemia dosage may need to be adjusted).
No products indexed under this heading.

Glyburide (Fluoxetine may alter glycemic control in diabetics; hypoglycemia has occurred during therapy with fluoxetine and hyperglycemia has developed following discontinuation of the drug; hypoglycemia dosage may need to be adjusted).
No products indexed under this heading.

Haloperidol (Co-administration of SSRIs, fluoxetine, and antipsychotics, such as haloperidol, has resulted in elevation of blood levels of haloperidol).
No products indexed under this heading.

Haloperidol Decanoate (Co-administration of SSRIs, fluoxetine, and antipsychotics, such as haloperidol, has resulted in elevation of blood levels of haloperidol).
No products indexed under this heading.

Heparin Calcium (Concurrent use of fluoxetine with drugs that affect coagulation may potentiate the risk of bleeding).
No products indexed under this heading.

Heparin Sodium (Concurrent use of fluoxetine with drugs that affect coagulation may potentiate the risk of bleeding).
No products indexed under this heading.

Hydrocodone Bitartrate (If fluoxetine is added to the treatment regimen of a patient already receiving a drug metabolized by CYP2D6, the need for decreased dose of the original medication should be considered. Fluoxetine is metabolized by this isoenzyme; thus, both the pharmacokinetic properties and relative proportion of metabolites are altered in poor metabolizers of CYP2D6). Products include:
- Hycodan **1104**
- Hycomine Compound Tablets **1105**
- Hycotuss Expectorant Syrup **1106**
- Lortab **3315**
- Lortab Elixir **3312**
- Vicodin Tablets **530**
- Vicodin ES Tablets **531**
- Vicodin HP Tablets **532**
- Vicoprofen Tablets **533**
- Zydone Tablets **1118**

Ibuprofen (Concurrent use of fluoxetine with an NSAID potentiated the risk of upper gastrointestinal bleeding and there is a reason to believe that bleeding at other sites may be similarly potentiated. Combined use of psychotropic drugs that interfere with serotonin reuptake and NSAIDs have been associated with an increased risk of bleeding). Products include:
- Advil Allergy Sinus Caplets .... ■ **737**
- Advil .... ■ **737**
- Children's Advil Suspension .... ■ **742**
- Children's Advil Chewable Tablets .... ■ **741**
- Advil Cold & Sinus .... ■ **739**
- Advil Flu & Body Ache Caplets .... ■ **739**
- Children's Advil Cold Suspension .... ■ **741**
- Infants' Advil Concentrated Drops .... ■ **743**
- Junior Strength Advil Swallow Tablets .... ■ **740**
- Advil Migraine Liquigels .... ■ **740**
- Advil Multi-Symptom Cold Caplets .... ■ **738**
- Combunox Tablets **1183**
- Children's Motrin Oral Suspension and Chewable Tablets **1837**
- Children's Motrin Cold Non-Staining Dye-Free Oral Suspension **1838**
- Children's Motrin Cold Oral Suspension **1838**
- Children's Motrin Non-Staining Dye-Free Oral Suspension **1837**
- Motrin Cold & Sinus Caplets **1836**
- Motrin IB Tablets and Caplets **1836**
- Infants' Motrin Concentrated Drops **1837**
- Infants' Motrin Non-Staining Dye-Free Drops **1837**
- Junior Strength Motrin Caplets and Chewable Tablets **1837**
- Vicoprofen Tablets **533**

Imipramine Hydrochloride (Fluoxetine inhibits the activity of P450 IID6 isoenzyme making normal metabolizers resemble "poor metabolizers"; therapy with drugs that are predominantly metabolized by the P450 IID6 isoenzyme, such as tricyclic antidepressants, and have a relatively narrow therapeutic index should be initiated at low end of the dose range if a patient is receiving fluoxetine concurrently or has taken it in the previous 5 weeks).
No products indexed under this heading.

Imipramine Pamoate (Fluoxetine inhibits the activity of P450 IID6 isoenzyme making normal metabolizers resemble "poor metabolizers"; therapy with drugs that are predominantly metabolized by the P450 IID6 isoenzyme, such as tricyclic antidepressants, and have a relatively narrow therapeutic index should be initiated at low end of the dose range if a patient is receiving fluoxetine concurrently or has taken it in the previous 5 weeks).
No products indexed under this heading.

Indomethacin (Concurrent use of fluoxetine with an NSAID potentiated the risk of upper gastrointestinal bleeding and there is a reason to believe that bleeding at other sites may be similarly potentiated. Combined use of psychotropic drugs that interfere with serotonin reuptake and NSAIDs have been associated with an increased risk of bleeding). Products include:
- Indocin **1968**

Indomethacin Sodium Trihydrate (Concurrent use of fluoxetine with an NSAID potentiated the risk of upper gastrointestinal bleeding and there is a reason to believe that bleeding at other sites may be similarly potentiated. Combined use of psychotropic drugs that interfere with serotonin reuptake and NSAIDs have been associated with an increased risk of bleeding). Products include:
- Indocin I.V. **1973**

Indoramin Hydrochloride (If fluoxetine is added to the treatment regimen of a patient already receiving a drug metabolized by CYP2D6, the need for decreased dose of the original medication should be considered. Fluoxetine is metabolized by this isoenzyme; thus, both the pharmacokinetic properties and relative proportion of metabolites are altered in poor metabolizers of CYP2D6).
No products indexed under this heading.

Insulin, Human, Zinc Suspension (Fluoxetine may alter glycemic control in diabetics; hypoglycemia has occurred during therapy with fluoxetine and hyperglycemia has developed following discontinuation of the drug; insulin dosage may need to be adjusted). Products include:
- Humulin L, 100 Units **1763**
- Humulin U, 100 Units **1770**

Insulin, Human NPH (Fluoxetine may alter glycemic control in diabetics; hypoglycemia has occurred during therapy with fluoxetine and hyperglycemia has developed following discontinuation of the drug; insulin dosage may need to be adjusted). Products include:
- Humulin N, 100 Units **1764**
- Humulin N Pen **1765**
- Novolin N Human Insulin 10 ml Vials **2322**
- Novolin N InnoLet **2322**
- Novolin N PenFill 3 ml Cartridges **2325**
- Novolin R InnoLet **2322**

Insulin, Human Regular (Fluoxetine may alter glycemic control in diabetics; hypoglycemia has occurred during therapy with fluoxetine and hyperglycemia has developed following discontinuation of the drug; insulin dosage may need to be adjusted). Products include:
- Humulin R (U-500) **1768**
- Humulin R, 100 Units **1767**
- Novolin R Human Insulin 10 ml Vials **2322**
- Novolin R PenFill **2325**

Insulin, Human Regular and Human NPH Mixture (Fluoxetine may alter glycemic control in diabetics; hypoglycemia has occurred during therapy with fluoxetine and hyperglycemia has developed following discontinuation of the drug; insulin dosage may need to be adjusted). Products include:
- Humulin 50/50, 100 Units **1760**
- Humulin 70/30 Pen **1761**
- Novolin 70/30 Human Insulin 10 ml Vials **2321**
- Novolin 70/30 InnoLet **2322**
- Novolin 70/30 PenFill 3 ml Cartridges **2325**

Insulin, NPH (Fluoxetine may alter glycemic control in diabetics; hypoglycemia has occurred during therapy with fluoxetine and hyperglycemia has developed following discontinuation of the drug; insulin dosage may need to be adjusted).
No products indexed under this heading.

Insulin, Regular (Fluoxetine may alter glycemic control in diabetics; hypoglycemia has occurred during therapy with fluoxetine and hyperglycemia has developed following discontinuation of the drug; insulin dosage may need to be adjusted).
No products indexed under this heading.

Insulin, Zinc Crystals (Fluoxetine may alter glycemic control in diabetics; hypoglycemia has occurred during therapy with fluoxetine and hyperglycemia has developed following discontinuation of the drug; insulin dosage may need to be adjusted).
No products indexed under this heading.

Insulin, Zinc Suspension (Fluoxetine may alter glycemic control in diabetics; hypoglycemia has occurred during therapy with fluoxetine and hyperglycemia has developed following discontinuation of the drug; insulin dosage may need to be adjusted).
No products indexed under this heading.

Insulin Aspart, Human Regular (Fluoxetine may alter glycemic control in diabetics; hypoglycemia has occurred during therapy with fluoxetine and hyperglycemia has developed following discontinuation of the drug; insulin dosage may need to be adjusted). Products include:
- NovoLog Injection **2326**

Insulin glargine (Fluoxetine may alter glycemic control in diabetics; hypoglycemia has occurred during therapy with fluoxetine and hyperglycemia has developed following discontinuation of the drug; insulin dosage may need to be adjusted). Products include:
- Lantus Injection **2925**

Insulin Lispro, Human (Fluoxetine may alter glycemic control in diabetics; hypoglycemia has occurred during therapy with fluoxetine and hyperglycemia has developed following discontinuation of the drug; insulin dosage may need to be adjusted). Products include:
- Humalog-Pen **1751**
- Humalog Mix 75/25-Pen **1754**

Insulin Lispro Protamine, Human (Fluoxetine may alter glycemic control in diabetics; hypoglycemia has occurred during therapy with fluoxetine and hyperglycemia has developed following discontinuation of the drug; insulin dosage may need to be adjusted). Products include:
- Humalog Mix 75/25-Pen **1754**

Isocarboxazid (Co-administration with MAO inhibitors has resulted in serious, sometimes fatal, reactions, including hyperthermia, rigidity, extreme agitation, delirium, coma, and features resembling neuroleptic malignant syndrome; concurrent and/or sequential use is contraindicated).
No products indexed under this heading.

Ketoprofen (Concurrent use of fluoxetine with an NSAID potentiated the risk of upper gastrointestinal bleeding and there is a reason to believe that bleeding at other sites may be similarly potentiated. Combined use of psychotropic drugs that interfere with serotonin reuptake and NSAIDs have been associated with an increased risk of bleeding).
No products indexed under this heading.

Ketorolac Tromethamine (Concurrent use of fluoxetine with an NSAID potentiated the risk of upper gastrointestinal bleeding and there is a reason to believe that bleeding at other sites may be similarly potentiated. Combined use of psychotropic drugs that interfere with serotonin reuptake and NSAIDs have been associated with an increased risk of bleeding). Products include:
- Acular Ophthalmic Solution **561**
- Acular LS Ophthalmic Solution **562**

Labetalol Hydrochloride (If fluoxetine is added to the treatment regimen of a patient already receiving a drug metabolized by CYP2D6, the need for decreased dose of the original medication should be considered. Fluoxetine is metabolized by this isoenzyme; thus, both the pharmacokinetic properties and relative proportion of metabolites are altered in poor metabolizers of CYP2D6).
No products indexed under this heading.

Lidocaine (If fluoxetine is added to the treatment regimen of a patient already receiving a drug metabolized by CYP2D6, the need for decreased dose of the original medication should be considered. Fluoxetine is metabolized by this isoenzyme; thus,

both the pharmacokinetic properties and relative proportion of metabolites are altered in poor metabolizers of CYP2D6). Products include:

Lidoderm Patch 1107

Lidocaine Hydrochloride (If fluoxetine is added to the treatment regimen of a patient already receiving a drug metabolized by CYP2D6, the need for decreased dose of the original medication should be considered. Fluoxetine is metabolized by this isoenzyme; thus, both the pharmacokinetic properties and relative proportion of metabolites are altered in poor metabolizers of CYP2D6).

No products indexed under this heading.

Lithium (Co-administration has resulted in reports of both increased and decreased lithium levels; cases of lithium toxicity have been reported).

No products indexed under this heading.

Lithium Carbonate (Co-administration has resulted in reports of both increased and decreased lithium levels; cases of lithium toxicity have been reported). Products include:

Eskalith 1406
Lithobid Tablets 1670

Lithium Citrate (Co-administration has resulted in reports of both increased and decreased lithium levels; cases of lithium toxicity have been reported).

No products indexed under this heading.

Low Molecular Weight Heparins (Concurrent use of fluoxetine with drugs that affect coagulation may potentiate the risk of bleeding).

No products indexed under this heading.

Maprotiline Hydrochloride (Fluoxetine inhibits the activity of P450 IID6 isoenzyme making normal metabolizers resemble "poor metabolizers"; therapy with drugs that are predominantly metabolized by the P450 IID6 isoenzyme, such as tricyclic antidepressants, and have a relatively narrow therapeutic index should be initiated at low end of the dose range if a patient is receiving fluoxetine concurrently or has taken it in the previous 5 weeks).

No products indexed under this heading.

Meclofenamate Sodium (Concurrent use of fluoxetine with an NSAID potentiated the risk of upper gastrointestinal bleeding and there is a reason to believe that bleeding at other sites may be similarly potentiated. Combined use of psychotropic drugs that interfere with serotonin reuptake and NSAIDs have been associated with an increased risk of bleeding).

No products indexed under this heading.

Mefenamic Acid (Concurrent use of fluoxetine with an NSAID potentiated the risk of upper gastrointestinal bleeding and there is a reason to believe that bleeding at other sites may be similarly potentiated. Combined use of psychotropic drugs that interfere with serotonin reuptake and NSAIDs have been associated with an increased risk of bleeding).

No products indexed under this heading.

Meloxicam (Concurrent use of fluoxetine with an NSAID potentiated the risk of upper gastrointestinal bleeding and there is a reason to believe that bleeding at other sites may be similarly potentiated. Combined use of psychotropic drugs that interfere with serotonin reuptake and NSAIDs have been associated with an increased risk of bleeding). Products include:

Mobic Oral Suspension 893
Mobic Tablets 893

Meperidine Hydrochloride (If fluoxetine is added to the treatment regimen of a patient already receiving a drug metabolized by CYP2D6, the need for decreased dose of the original medication should be considered. Fluoxetine is metabolized by this isoenzyme; thus, both the pharmacokinetic properties and relative proportion of metabolites are altered in poor metabolizers of CYP2D6).

No products indexed under this heading.

Metformin Hydrochloride (Fluoxetine may alter glycemic control in diabetics; hypoglycemia has occurred during therapy with fluoxetine and hyperglycemia has developed following discontinuation of the drug; hypoglycemia dosage may need to be adjusted). Products include:

ActoPlus Met Tablets 3219
Avandamet Tablets 1343
Fortamet Extended-Release Tablets 1156

Methadone Hydrochloride (If fluoxetine is added to the treatment regimen of a patient already receiving a drug metabolized by CYP2D6, the need for decreased dose of the original medication should be considered. Fluoxetine is metabolized by this isoenzyme; thus, both the pharmacokinetic properties and relative proportion of metabolites are altered in poor metabolizers of CYP2D6).

No products indexed under this heading.

Methamphetamine Hydrochloride (If fluoxetine is added to the treatment regimen of a patient already receiving a drug metabolized by CYP2D6, the need for decreased dose of the original medication should be considered. Fluoxetine is metabolized by this isoenzyme; thus, both the pharmacokinetic properties and relative proportion of metabolites are altered in poor metabolizers of CYP2D6). Products include:

Desoxyn Tablets, USP 2482

Metoprolol Succinate (If fluoxetine is added to the treatment regimen of a patient already receiving a drug metabolized by CYP2D6, the need for decreased dose of the original medication should be considered. Fluoxetine is metabolized by this isoenzyme; thus, both the pharmacokinetic properties and relative proportion of metabolites are altered in poor metabolizers of CYP2D6). Products include:

Toprol-XL Tablets 660

Metoprolol Tartrate (If fluoxetine is added to the treatment regimen of a patient already receiving a drug metabolized by CYP2D6, the need for decreased dose of the original medication should be considered. Fluoxetine is metabolized by this isoenzyme; thus, both the pharmacokinetic properties and relative proportion of metabolites are altered in poor metabolizers of CYP2D6).

No products indexed under this heading.

Mexiletine Hydrochloride (If fluoxetine is added to the treatment regimen of a patient already receiving a drug metabolized by CYP2D6, the need for decreased dose of the original medication should be considered. Fluoxetine is metabolized by this isoenzyme; thus, both the pharmacokinetic properties and relative proportion of metabolites are altered in poor metabolizers of CYP2D6).

No products indexed under this heading.

Miglitol (Fluoxetine may alter glycemic control in diabetics; hypoglycemia has occurred during therapy with fluoxetine and hyperglycemia has developed following discontinuation of the drug; hypoglycemia dosage may need to be adjusted).

No products indexed under this heading.

Mirtazapine (If fluoxetine is added to the treatment regimen of a patient already receiving a drug metabolized by CYP2D6, the need for decreased dose of the original medication should be considered. Fluoxetine is metabolized by this isoenzyme; thus, both the pharmacokinetic properties and relative proportion of metabolites are altered in poor metabolizers of CYP2D6).

No products indexed under this heading.

Moclobemide (Co-administration with MAO inhibitors has resulted in serious, sometimes fatal, reactions, including hyperthermia, rigidity, extreme agitation, delirium, coma, and features resembling neuroleptic malignant syndrome; concurrent and/or sequential use is contraindicated).

No products indexed under this heading.

Morphine Sulfate (If fluoxetine is added to the treatment regimen of a patient already receiving a drug metabolized by CYP2D6, the need for decreased dose of the original medication should be considered. Fluoxetine is metabolized by this isoenzyme; thus, both the pharmacokinetic properties and relative proportion of metabolites are altered in poor metabolizers of CYP2D6). Products include:

Avinza Capsules 1714
Kadian Capsules 572
MS Contin Tablets 2703

Nabumetone (Concurrent use of fluoxetine with an NSAID potentiated the risk of upper gastrointestinal bleeding and there is a reason to believe that bleeding at other sites may be similarly potentiated. Combined use of psychotropic drugs that interfere with serotonin reuptake and NSAIDs have been associated with an increased risk of bleeding). Products include:

Relafen Tablets 1523

Naproxen (Concurrent use of fluoxetine with an NSAID potentiated the risk of upper gastrointestinal bleeding and there is a reason to believe that bleeding at other sites may be similarly potentiated. Combined use of psychotropic drugs that interfere with serotonin reuptake and NSAIDs have been associated with an increased risk of bleeding). Products include:

EC-Naprosyn Delayed-Release Tablets 2769
Naprosyn Suspension 2769
Naprosyn Tablets 2769
Prevacid NapraPAC 3277

Naproxen Sodium (Concurrent use of fluoxetine with an NSAID potentiated the risk of upper gastrointestinal bleeding and there is a reason to believe that bleeding at other sites may be similarly potentiated. Combined use of psychotropic drugs that interfere with serotonin reuptake and NSAIDs have been associated with an increased risk of bleeding). Products include:

Aleve Tablets, Caplets and Gelcaps .... ▣605
Anaprox Tablets 2769
Anaprox DS Tablets 2769

Nelfinavir Mesylate (If fluoxetine is added to the treatment regimen of a patient already receiving a drug metabolized by CYP2D6, the need for decreased dose of the original medication should be considered. Fluoxetine is metabolized by this isoenzyme; thus, both the pharmacokinetic properties and relative proportion of metabolites are altered in poor metabolizers of CYP2D6). Products include:

Viracept 2556

Nortriptyline Hydrochloride (Fluoxetine inhibits the activity of P450 IID6 isoenzyme making normal metabolizers resemble "poor metabolizers"; therapy with drugs that are predominantly metabolized by the P450 IID6 isoenzyme, such as tricyclic antidepressants, and have a relatively narrow therapeutic index should be initiated at low end of the dose range if a patient is receiving fluoxetine concurrently or has taken it in the previous 5 weeks).

No products indexed under this heading.

Olanzapine (If fluoxetine is added to the treatment regimen of a patient already receiving a drug metabolized by CYP2D6, the need for decreased dose of the original medication should be considered. Fluoxetine is metabolized by this isoenzyme; thus, both the pharmacokinetic properties and relative proportion of metabolites are altered in poor metabolizers of CYP2D6). Products include:

Symbyax Capsules 1788
Zyprexa Tablets 1798
Zyprexa IntraMuscular 1798
Zyprexa ZYDIS Orally Disintegrating Tablets 1798

Omeprazole (If fluoxetine is added to the treatment regimen of a patient already receiving a drug metabolized by CYP2D6, the need for decreased dose of the original medication should be considered. Fluoxetine is metabolized by this isoenzyme; thus, both the pharmacokinetic properties and relative proportion of metabolites are altered in poor metabolizers of CYP2D6). Products include:

Zegerid Powder for Oral Solution 2972

Ondansetron (If fluoxetine is added to the treatment regimen of a patient already receiving a drug metabolized by CYP2D6, the need for decreased dose of the original medication should be considered. Fluoxetine is metabolized by this isoenzyme; thus, both the pharmacokinetic properties and relative proportion of metabolites are altered in poor metabolizers of CYP2D6). Products include:

Zofran ODT Orally Disintegrating Tablets 1613

Ondansetron Hydrochloride (If fluoxetine is added to the treatment regimen of a patient already receiving a drug metabolized by CYP2D6, the need for decreased dose of the original medication should be considered. Fluoxetine is metabolized by this isoenzyme; thus, both the pharmacokinetic properties and relative proportion of metabolites are altered in poor metabolizers of CYP2D6). Products include:
Zofran Injection 1607
Zofran 1613

Oxaprozin (Concurrent use of fluoxetine with an NSAID potentiated the risk of upper gastrointestinal bleeding and there is a reason to believe that bleeding at other sites may be similarly potentiated. Combined use of psychotropic drugs that interfere with serotonin reuptake and NSAIDs have been associated with an increased risk of bleeding).
No products indexed under this heading.

Oxycodone Hydrochloride (If fluoxetine is added to the treatment regimen of a patient already receiving a drug metabolized by CYP2D6, the need for decreased dose of the original medication should be considered. Fluoxetine is metabolized by this isoenzyme; thus, both the pharmacokinetic properties and relative proportion of metabolites are altered in poor metabolizers of CYP2D6). Products include:
Combunox Tablets 1183
OxyContin Tablets 2699
OxyFast Oral Concentrate Solution 2704
OxyIR Capsules 2704
Percocet Tablets 1114
Percodan Tablets 1115

Paclitaxel (If fluoxetine is added to the treatment regimen of a patient already receiving a drug metabolized by CYP2D6, the need for decreased dose of the original medication should be considered. Fluoxetine is metabolized by this isoenzyme; thus, both the pharmacokinetic properties and relative proportion of metabolites are altered in poor metabolizers of CYP2D6).
No products indexed under this heading.

Pargyline Hydrochloride (Co-administration with MAO inhibitors has resulted in serious, sometimes fatal, reactions, including hyperthermia, rigidity, extreme agitation, delirium, coma, and features resembling neuroleptic malignant syndrome; concurrent and/or sequential use is contraindicated).
No products indexed under this heading.

Paroxetine Hydrochloride (If fluoxetine is added to the treatment regimen of a patient already receiving a drug metabolized by CYP2D6, the need for decreased dose of the original medication should be considered. Fluoxetine is metabolized by this isoenzyme; thus, both the pharmacokinetic properties and relative proportion of metabolites are altered in poor metabolizers of CYP2D6). Products include:
Paxil CR Controlled-Release Tablets 1509
Paxil 1501

Phenelzine Sulfate (Co-administration with MAO inhibitors has resulted in serious, sometimes fatal, reactions, including hyperthermia, rigidity, extreme agitation, delirium, coma, and features resembling neuroleptic malignant syndrome; concurrent and/or sequential use is contraindicated).
No products indexed under this heading.

Phenylbutazone (Concurrent use of fluoxetine with an NSAID potentiated the risk of upper gastrointestinal bleeding and there is a reason to believe that bleeding at other sites may be similarly potentiated. Combined use of psychotropic drugs that interfere with serotonin reuptake and NSAIDs have been associated with an increased risk of bleeding).
No products indexed under this heading.

Phenytoin (Patients stable on doses of phenytoin have developed elevated plasma phenytoin concentrations and clinical anticonvulsant toxicity following initiation of concomitant fluoxetine therapy).
No products indexed under this heading.

Phenytoin Sodium (Patients stable on doses of phenytoin have developed elevated plasma phenytoin concentrations and clinical anticonvulsant toxicity following initiation of concomitant fluoxetine therapy). Products include:
Phenytek Capsules 2153

Pimozide (Co-administration has resulted in a single case report of possible additive effects of pimozide leading to bradycardia). Products include:
Orap Tablets 1220

Pindolol (If fluoxetine is added to the treatment regimen of a patient already receiving a drug metabolized by CYP2D6, the need for decreased dose of the original medication should be considered. Fluoxetine is metabolized by this isoenzyme; thus, both the pharmacokinetic properties and relative proportion of metabolites are altered in poor metabolizers of CYP2D6).
No products indexed under this heading.

Pioglitazone Hydrochloride (Fluoxetine may alter glycemic control in diabetics; hypoglycemia has occurred during therapy with fluoxetine and hyperglycemia has developed following discontinuation of the drug; hypoglycemia dosage may need to be adjusted). Products include:
ActoPlus Met Tablets 3219
Actos Tablets 3224

Piroxicam (Concurrent use of fluoxetine with an NSAID potentiated the risk of upper gastrointestinal bleeding and there is a reason to believe that bleeding at other sites may be similarly potentiated. Combined use of psychotropic drugs that interfere with serotonin reuptake and NSAIDs have been associated with an increased risk of bleeding).
No products indexed under this heading.

Procarbazine Hydrochloride (Co-administration with MAO inhibitors has resulted in serious, sometimes fatal, reactions, including hyperthermia, rigidity, extreme agitation, delirium, coma, and features resembling neuroleptic malignant syndrome; concurrent and/or sequential use is contraindicated). Products include:
Matulane Capsules 3188

Propafenone Hydrochloride (If fluoxetine is added to the treatment regimen of a patient already receiving a drug metabolized by CYP2D6, the need for decreased dose of the original medication should be considered. Fluoxetine is metabolized by this isoenzyme; thus, both the pharmacokinetic properties and relative proportion of metabolites are altered in poor metabolizers of CYP2D6). Products include:
Rythmol SR Capsules 2736

Propoxyphene Hydrochloride (If fluoxetine is added to the treatment regimen of a patient already receiving a drug metabolized by CYP2D6, the need for decreased dose of the original medication should be considered. Fluoxetine is metabolized by this isoenzyme; thus, both the pharmacokinetic properties and relative proportion of metabolites are altered in poor metabolizers of CYP2D6).
No products indexed under this heading.

Propoxyphene Napsylate (If fluoxetine is added to the treatment regimen of a patient already receiving a drug metabolized by CYP2D6, the need for decreased dose of the original medication should be considered. Fluoxetine is metabolized by this isoenzyme; thus, both the pharmacokinetic properties and relative proportion of metabolites are altered in poor metabolizers of CYP2D6). Products include:
Darvocet A 500 Tablets 3497

Propranolol Hydrochloride (If fluoxetine is added to the treatment regimen of a patient already receiving a drug metabolized by CYP2D6, the need for decreased dose of the original medication should be considered. Fluoxetine is metabolized by this isoenzyme; thus, both the pharmacokinetic properties and relative proportion of metabolites are altered in poor metabolizers of CYP2D6). Products include:
Inderal LA Long-Acting Capsules 3421
InnoPran XL Capsules 2728

Protriptyline Hydrochloride (Fluoxetine inhibits the activity of P450 IID6 isoenzyme making normal metabolizers resemble "poor metabolizers"; therapy with drugs that are predominantly metabolized by the P450 IID6 isoenzyme, such as tricyclic antidepressants, and have a relatively narrow therapeutic index should be initiated at low end of the dose range if a patient is receiving fluoxetine concurrently or has taken it in the previous 5 weeks). Products include:
Vivactil Tablets 2350

Quetiapine Fumarate (If fluoxetine is added to the treatment regimen of a patient already receiving a drug metabolized by CYP2D6, the need for decreased dose of the original medication should be considered. Fluoxetine is metabolized by this isoenzyme; thus, both the pharmacokinetic properties and relative proportion of metabolites are altered in poor metabolizers of CYP2D6). Products include:
Seroquel Tablets 691

Quinidine Gluconate (If fluoxetine is added to the treatment regimen of a patient already receiving a drug metabolized by CYP2D6, the need for decreased dose of the original medication should be considered. Fluoxetine is metabolized by this isoenzyme; thus, both the pharmacokinetic properties and relative proportion of metabolites are altered in poor metabolizers of CYP2D6).
No products indexed under this heading.

Quinidine Hydrochloride (If fluoxetine is added to the treatment regimen of a patient already receiving a drug metabolized by CYP2D6, the need for decreased dose of the original medication should be considered. Fluoxetine is metabolized by this isoenzyme; thus, both the pharmacokinetic properties and relative proportion of metabolites are altered in poor metabolizers of CYP2D6).
No products indexed under this heading.

Quinidine Polygalacturonate (If fluoxetine is added to the treatment regimen of a patient already receiving a drug metabolized by CYP2D6, the need for decreased dose of the original medication should be considered. Fluoxetine is metabolized by this isoenzyme; thus, both the pharmacokinetic properties and relative proportion of metabolites are altered in poor metabolizers of CYP2D6).
No products indexed under this heading.

Quinidine Sulfate (If fluoxetine is added to the treatment regimen of a patient already receiving a drug metabolized by CYP2D6, the need for decreased dose of the original medication should be considered. Fluoxetine is metabolized by this isoenzyme; thus, both the pharmacokinetic properties and relative proportion of metabolites are altered in poor metabolizers of CYP2D6).
No products indexed under this heading.

Repaglinide (Fluoxetine may alter glycemic control in diabetics; hypoglycemia has occurred during therapy with fluoxetine and hyperglycemia has developed following discontinuation of the drug; hypoglycemia dosage may need to be adjusted). Products include:
Prandin Tablets (0.5, 1, and 2 mg) 2337

Risperidone (If fluoxetine is added to the treatment regimen of a patient already receiving a drug metabolized by CYP2D6, the need for decreased dose of the original medication should be considered. Fluoxetine is metabolized by this isoenzyme; thus, both the pharmacokinetic properties and relative proportion of metabolites are altered in poor metabolizers of CYP2D6). Products include:
Risperdal Consta Long-Acting Injection 1664
Risperdal M-Tab Orally Disintegrating Tablets 1658
Risperdal 1658

Ritonavir (If fluoxetine is added to the treatment regimen of a patient already receiving a drug metabolized by CYP2D6, the need for decreased dose of the original medication should be considered. Fluoxetine is metabolized by this isoenzyme; thus, both the pharmacokinetic properties

and relative proportion of metabolites are altered in poor metabolizers of CYP2D6). Products include:
Kaletra 474
Norvir 499

Rofecoxib (Concurrent use of fluoxetine with an NSAID potentiated the risk of upper gastrointestinal bleeding and there is a reason to believe that bleeding at other sites may be similarly potentiated. Combined use of psychotropic drugs that interfere with serotonin reuptake and NSAIDs have been associated with an increased risk of bleeding).
No products indexed under this heading.

Rosiglitazone Maleate (Fluoxetine may alter glycemic control in diabetics; hypoglycemia has occurred during therapy with fluoxetine and hyperglycemia has developed following discontinuation of the drug; hypoglycemia dosage may need to be adjusted). Products include:
Avandamet Tablets 1343
Avandia Tablets 1348

Selegiline Hydrochloride (Co-administration with MAO inhibitors has resulted in serious, sometimes fatal, reactions, including hyperthermia, rigidity, extreme agitation, delirium, coma, and features resembling neuroleptic malignant syndrome; concurrent and/or sequential use is contraindicated). Products include:
Eldepryl Capsules 3209

Sulindac (Concurrent use of fluoxetine with an NSAID potentiated the risk of upper gastrointestinal bleeding and there is a reason to believe that bleeding at other sites may be similarly potentiated. Combined use of psychotropic drugs that interfere with serotonin reuptake and NSAIDs have been associated with an increased risk of bleeding). Products include:
Clinoril Tablets 1899

Sumatriptan (Co-administration of SSRIs and sumatriptan has resulted in weakness, hyperreflexia, and incoordination). Products include:
Imitrex Nasal Spray 1435

Sumatriptan Succinate (Co-administration of SSRIs and sumatriptan has resulted in weakness, hyperreflexia, and incoordination). Products include:
Imitrex Injection 1431
Imitrex Tablets 1440

Tamoxifen Citrate (If fluoxetine is added to the treatment regimen of a patient already receiving a drug metabolized by CYP2D6, the need for decreased dose of the original medication should be considered. Fluoxetine is metabolized by this isoenzyme; thus, both the pharmacokinetic properties and relative proportion of metabolites are altered in poor metabolizers of CYP2D6).
No products indexed under this heading.

Teniposide (If fluoxetine is added to the treatment regimen of a patient already receiving a drug metabolized by CYP2D6, the need for decreased dose of the original medication should be considered. Fluoxetine is metabolized by this isoenzyme; thus, both the pharmacokinetic properties and relative proportion of metabolites are altered in poor metabolizers of CYP2D6).
No products indexed under this heading.

Testosterone (If fluoxetine is added to the treatment regimen of a patient already receiving a drug metabolized by CYP2D6, the need for decreased dose of the original medication should be considered. Fluoxetine is metabolized by this isoenzyme; thus, both the pharmacokinetic properties and relative proportion of metabolites are altered in poor metabolizers of CYP2D6). Products include:
AndroGel 3330
Striant Mucoadhesive 1022
Testim 1% Gel 722

Testosterone Cypionate (If fluoxetine is added to the treatment regimen of a patient already receiving a drug metabolized by CYP2D6, the need for decreased dose of the original medication should be considered. Fluoxetine is metabolized by this isoenzyme; thus, both the pharmacokinetic properties and relative proportion of metabolites are altered in poor metabolizers of CYP2D6).
No products indexed under this heading.

Testosterone Enanthate (If fluoxetine is added to the treatment regimen of a patient already receiving a drug metabolized by CYP2D6, the need for decreased dose of the original medication should be considered. Fluoxetine is metabolized by this isoenzyme; thus, both the pharmacokinetic properties and relative proportion of metabolites are altered in poor metabolizers of CYP2D6). Products include:
Delatestryl Injection 2976

Testosterone Propionate (If fluoxetine is added to the treatment regimen of a patient already receiving a drug metabolized by CYP2D6, the need for decreased dose of the original medication should be considered. Fluoxetine is metabolized by this isoenzyme; thus, both the pharmacokinetic properties and relative proportion of metabolites are altered in poor metabolizers of CYP2D6).
No products indexed under this heading.

Thioridazine (If fluoxetine is added to the treatment regimen of a patient already receiving a drug metabolized by CYP2D6, the need for decreased dose of the original medication should be considered. Fluoxetine is metabolized by this isoenzyme; thus, both the pharmacokinetic properties and relative proportion of metabolites are altered in poor metabolizers of CYP2D6).
No products indexed under this heading.

Thioridazine Hydrochloride (Co-administration of fluoxetine with thioridazine has produced a 2.4-fold higher Cmax and a 4.5-fold higher AUC for thioridazine; because thioridazine administration produces a dose-related prolongation of the QTc interval, which is associated with serious ventricular arrhythmias such as torsade de pointes-type arrhythmias and sudden death; concurrent and/or sequential use within a minimum of 5 weeks of Prozac is contraindicated). Products include:
Thioridazine Hydrochloride Tablets 2122

Timolol Maleate (If fluoxetine is added to the treatment regimen of a patient already receiving a drug metabolized by CYP2D6, the need for decreased dose of the original medication should be considered. Fluoxetine is metabolized by this isoenzyme; thus, both the pharmacokinetic properties and relative proportion of metabolites are altered in poor metabolizers of CYP2D6). Products include:
Blocadren Tablets 1891
Cosopt Sterile Ophthalmic Solution 1910
Timolide Tablets 2056
Timoptic in Ocudose 2061
Timoptic Sterile Ophthalmic Solution 2058
Timoptic-XE Sterile Ophthalmic Gel Forming Solution 2062

Tinzaparin Sodium (Concurrent use of fluoxetine with drugs that affect coagulation may potentiate the risk of bleeding).
No products indexed under this heading.

Tolazamide (Fluoxetine may alter glycemic control in diabetics; hypoglycemia has occurred during therapy with fluoxetine and hyperglycemia has developed following discontinuation of the drug; hypoglycemia dosage may need to be adjusted).
No products indexed under this heading.

Tolbutamide (Fluoxetine may alter glycemic control in diabetics; hypoglycemia has occurred during therapy with fluoxetine and hyperglycemia has developed following discontinuation of the drug; hypoglycemia dosage may need to be adjusted).
No products indexed under this heading.

Tolmetin Sodium (Concurrent use of fluoxetine with an NSAID potentiated the risk of upper gastrointestinal bleeding and there is a reason to believe that bleeding at other sites may be similarly potentiated. Combined use of psychotropic drugs that interfere with serotonin reuptake and NSAIDs have been associated with an increased risk of bleeding).
No products indexed under this heading.

Tolterodine Tartrate (If fluoxetine is added to the treatment regimen of a patient already receiving a drug metabolized by CYP2D6, the need for decreased dose of the original medication should be considered. Fluoxetine is metabolized by this isoenzyme; thus, both the pharmacokinetic properties and relative proportion of metabolites are altered in poor metabolizers of CYP2D6). Products include:
Detrol Tablets 2626
Detrol LA Capsules 2629

Tramadol Hydrochloride (If fluoxetine is added to the treatment regimen of a patient already receiving a drug metabolized by CYP2D6, the need for decreased dose of the original medication should be considered. Fluoxetine is metabolized by this isoenzyme; thus, both the pharmacokinetic properties and relative proportion of metabolites are altered in poor metabolizers of CYP2D6). Products include:
Ultracet Tablets 2462

Tranylcypromine Sulfate (Co-administration with MAO inhibitors has resulted in serious, sometimes fatal, reactions, including hyperthermia, rigidity, extreme agitation, delirium, coma, and features resembling neuroleptic malignant syndrome; concurrent and/or sequential use is contraindicated). Products include:
Parnate Tablets 1499

Trazodone Hydrochloride (If fluoxetine is added to the treatment regimen of a patient already receiving a drug metabolized by CYP2D6, the need for decreased dose of the original medication should be considered. Fluoxetine is metabolized by this isoenzyme; thus, both the pharmacokinetic properties and relative proportion of metabolites are altered in poor metabolizers of CYP2D6).
No products indexed under this heading.

Triazolam (If fluoxetine is added to the treatment regimen of a patient already receiving a drug metabolized by CYP2D6, the need for decreased dose of the original medication should be considered. Fluoxetine is metabolized by this isoenzyme; thus, both the pharmacokinetic properties and relative proportion of metabolites are altered in poor metabolizers of CYP2D6).
No products indexed under this heading.

Trimipramine Maleate (Fluoxetine inhibits the activity of P450 IID6 isoenzyme making normal metabolizers resemble "poor metabolizers"; therapy with drugs that are predominantly metabolized by the P450 IID6 isoenzyme, such as tricyclic antidepressants, and have a relatively narrow therapeutic index should be initiated at low end of the dose range if a patient is receiving fluoxetine concurrently or has taken it in the previous 5 weeks). Products include:
Surmontil Capsules 2347

Troglitazone (Fluoxetine may alter glycemic control in diabetics; hypoglycemia has occurred during therapy with fluoxetine and hyperglycemia has developed following discontinuation of the drug; hypoglycemia dosage may need to be adjusted).
No products indexed under this heading.

L-Tryptophan (Co-administration has resulted in adverse reactions, including agitation, restlessness, and gastrointestinal distress).
No products indexed under this heading.

Valdecoxib (Concurrent use of fluoxetine with an NSAID potentiated the risk of upper gastrointestinal bleeding and there is a reason to believe that bleeding at other sites may be similarly potentiated. Combined use of psychotropic drugs that interfere with serotonin reuptake and NSAIDs have been associated with an increased risk of bleeding).
No products indexed under this heading.

Venlafaxine Hydrochloride (If fluoxetine is added to the treatment regimen of a patient already receiving a drug metabolized by CYP2D6, the need for decreased dose of the original medication should be considered. Fluoxetine is metabolized by this isoenzyme; thus, both the pharmacokinetic properties and relative proportion of metabolites are altered in poor metabolizers of CYP2D6). Products include:
Effexor Tablets 3405
Effexor XR Capsules 3411

Vinblastine Sulfate (Fluoxetine inhibits the activity of P450 IID6 isoenzyme making normal metabolizers resemble "poor metabolizers"; therapy with drugs that are predominantly metabolized by the P450 IID6 isoen-

zyme such as vinblastine, and have a relatively narrow therapeutic index, should be initiated at low end of the dose range if a patient is receiving fluoxetine concurrently or has taken it in the previous 5 weeks).

No products indexed under this heading.

Warfarin Sodium (Altered anticoagulant effects, including increased bleeding, have been reported with concomitant use. Patients on warfarin therapy should receive coagulation monitoring when fluoxetine is initiated or stopped). Products include:

Coumadin for Injection 932
Coumadin Tablets 932

Zonisamide (If fluoxetine is added to the treatment regimen of a patient already receiving a drug metabolized by CYP2D6, the need for decreased dose of the original medication should be considered. Fluoxetine is metabolized by this isoenzyme; thus, both the pharmacokinetic properties and relative proportion of metabolites are altered in poor metabolizers of CYP2D6). Products include:

Zonegran Capsules 1089

Food Interactions

Alcohol (Concurrent use with CNS active agents, such as alcohol, requires caution).

Food, unspecified (May delay absorption of fluoxetine inconsequentially; Prozac may be administered with or without food).

PSORIATEC CREAM

(Anthralin) 3191
None cited in PDR database.

PULMICORT RESPULES

(Budesonide) 654
May interact with cytochrome p450 3a4 inhibitors (selected) and certain other agents. Compounds in these categories include:

Acetazolamide (Concomitant administration of budesonide with known inhibitors of CYP3A4 may inhibit the metabolism of, and increase the systemic exposure to, budesonide; care should be exercised).

No products indexed under this heading.

Amiodarone Hydrochloride (Concomitant administration of budesonide with known inhibitors of CYP3A4 may inhibit the metabolism of, and increase the systemic exposure to, budesonide; care should be exercised). Products include:

Pacerone Tablets 3337

Amprenavir (Concomitant administration of budesonide with known inhibitors of CYP3A4 may inhibit the metabolism of, and increase the systemic exposure to, budesonide; care should be exercised). Products include:

Agenerase Capsules 1299
Agenerase Oral Solution 1304

Anastrozole (Concomitant administration of budesonide with known inhibitors of CYP3A4 may inhibit the metabolism of, and increase the systemic exposure to, budesonide; care should be exercised). Products include:

Arimidex Tablets 665

Aprepitant (Concomitant administration of budesonide with known inhibitors of CYP3A4 may inhibit the metabolism of, and increase the systemic exposure to, budesonide; care should be exercised). Products include:

Emend Capsules 1944

Cimetidine (Co-administration of budesonide with cimetidine caused a slight decrease in budesonide clearance and a corresponding increase in its oral bioavailability). Products include:

Tagamet HB 200 Tablets 637
Tagamet Tablets 1547

Cimetidine Hydrochloride (Concomitant administration of budesonide with known inhibitors of CYP3A4 may inhibit the metabolism of, and increase the systemic exposure to, budesonide; care should be exercised).

No products indexed under this heading.

Ciprofloxacin (Concomitant administration of budesonide with known inhibitors of CYP3A4 may inhibit the metabolism of, and increase the systemic exposure to, budesonide; care should be exercised). Products include:

Cipro I.V. 2998
Cipro I.V. Pharmacy Bulk Package ... 3509
Cipro Oral Suspension 2991
Cipro XR Tablets 3004
Ciprodex Otic Suspension 555

Clarithromycin (Concomitant administration of budesonide with known inhibitors of CYP3A4 may inhibit the metabolism of, and increase the systemic exposure to, budesonide; care should be exercised). Products include:

Biaxin/Biaxin XL 402
PREVPAC 3281

Clotrimazole (Concomitant administration of budesonide with known inhibitors of CYP3A4 may inhibit the metabolism of, and increase the systemic exposure to, budesonide; care should be exercised). Products include:

Lotrimin 3053
Lotrisone 3054

Cyclosporine (Concomitant administration of budesonide with known inhibitors of CYP3A4 may inhibit the metabolism of, and increase the systemic exposure to, budesonide; care should be exercised). Products include:

Gengraf Capsules 458
Neoral Soft Gelatin Capsules 2247
Neoral Oral Solution 2247
Restasis Ophthalmic Emulsion 570
Sandimmune 2259

Dalfopristin (Concomitant administration of budesonide with known inhibitors of CYP3A4 may inhibit the metabolism of, and increase the systemic exposure to, budesonide; care should be exercised). Products include:

Synercid I.V. 1690

Danazol (Concomitant administration of budesonide with known inhibitors of CYP3A4 may inhibit the metabolism of, and increase the systemic exposure to, budesonide; care should be exercised).

No products indexed under this heading.

Delavirdine Mesylate (Concomitant administration of budesonide with known inhibitors of CYP3A4 may inhibit the metabolism of, and increase the systemic exposure to, budesonide; care should be exercised). Products include:

Rescriptor Tablets 2535

Diltiazem Hydrochloride (Concomitant administration of budesonide with known inhibitors of CYP3A4 may inhibit the metabolism of, and increase the systemic exposure to, budesonide; care should be exercised). Products include:

Cardizem LA Extended Release Tablets 1699
Tiazac Capsules 1204

Diltiazem Maleate (Concomitant administration of budesonide with known inhibitors of CYP3A4 may inhibit the metabolism of, and increase the systemic exposure to, budesonide; care should be exercised).

No products indexed under this heading.

Efavirenz (Concomitant administration of budesonide with known inhibitors of CYP3A4 may inhibit the metabolism of, and increase the systemic exposure to, budesonide; care should be exercised). Products include:

Sustiva Capsules 957

Erythromycin (Concomitant administration of budesonide with known inhibitors of CYP3A4 may inhibit the metabolism of, and increase the systemic exposure to, budesonide; care should be exercised). Products include:

Erygel Topical Gel 2096
Ery-Tab Tablets 447
Erythromycin Base Filmtab Tablets 454
Erythromycin Delayed-Release Capsules, USP 456
PCE Dispertab Tablets 510

Erythromycin Estolate (Concomitant administration of budesonide with known inhibitors of CYP3A4 may inhibit the metabolism of, and increase the systemic exposure to, budesonide; care should be exercised).

No products indexed under this heading.

Erythromycin Ethylsuccinate (Concomitant administration of budesonide with known inhibitors of CYP3A4 may inhibit the metabolism of, and increase the systemic exposure to, budesonide; care should be exercised). Products include:

E.E.S. 449
EryPed 445

Erythromycin Gluceptate (Concomitant administration of budesonide with known inhibitors of CYP3A4 may inhibit the metabolism of, and increase the systemic exposure to, budesonide; care should be exercised).

No products indexed under this heading.

Erythromycin Lactobionate (Concomitant administration of budesonide with known inhibitors of CYP3A4 may inhibit the metabolism of, and increase the systemic exposure to, budesonide; care should be exercised).

No products indexed under this heading.

Erythromycin Stearate (Concomitant administration of budesonide with known inhibitors of CYP3A4 may inhibit the metabolism of, and increase the systemic exposure to, budesonide; care should be exercised). Products include:

Erythrocin Stearate Filmtab Tablets 452

Esomeprazole Magnesium (Concomitant administration of budesonide with known inhibitors of CYP3A4 may inhibit the metabolism of, and increase the systemic exposure to, budesonide; care should be exercised). Products include:

Nexium Delayed-Release Capsules 645

Fluconazole (Concomitant administration of budesonide with known inhibitors of CYP3A4 may inhibit the metabolism of, and increase the systemic exposure to, budesonide; care should be exercised).

No products indexed under this heading.

Fluoxetine Hydrochloride (Concomitant administration of budesonide with known inhibitors of CYP3A4 may inhibit the metabolism of, and increase the systemic exposure to, budesonide; care should be exercised). Products include:

Prozac Pulvules and Liquid 1771
Symbyax Capsules 1788

Fluvoxamine Maleate (Concomitant administration of budesonide with known inhibitors of CYP3A4 may inhibit the metabolism of, and increase the systemic exposure to, budesonide; care should be exercised).

No products indexed under this heading.

Fosamprenavir Calcium (Concomitant administration of budesonide with known inhibitors of CYP3A4 may inhibit the metabolism of, and increase the systemic exposure to, budesonide; care should be exercised). Products include:

Lexiva Tablets 1473

Indinavir Sulfate (Concomitant administration of budesonide with known inhibitors of CYP3A4 may inhibit the metabolism of, and increase the systemic exposure to, budesonide; care should be exercised). Products include:

Crixivan Capsules 1918

Isoniazid (Concomitant administration of budesonide with known inhibitors of CYP3A4 may inhibit the metabolism of, and increase the systemic exposure to, budesonide; care should be exercised).

No products indexed under this heading.

Itraconazole (Concomitant administration of budesonide with known inhibitors of CYP3A4 may inhibit the metabolism of, and increase the systemic exposure to, budesonide; care should be exercised).

No products indexed under this heading.

Ketoconazole (Concomitant administration of budesonide with known inhibitors of CYP3A4 may inhibit the metabolism of, and increase the systemic exposure to, budesonide; care should be exercised). Products include:

Nizoral A-D Shampoo, 1% 1839
Nizoral 2% Shampoo 1838

Lopinavir (Concomitant administration of budesonide with known inhibitors of CYP3A4 may inhibit the metabolism of, and increase the systemic exposure to, budesonide; care should be exercised). Products include:

Kaletra 474

Loratadine (Concomitant administration of budesonide with known inhibitors of CYP3A4 may inhibit the

metabolism of, and increase the systemic exposure to, budesonide; care should be exercised). Products include:

Alavert Allergy & Sinus D-12 Hour Tablets ..... ▣743
Alavert ..... ▣743
Children's Claritin 24 Hour Non-Drowsy Allergy Syrup ..... ▣732
Claritin Non-Drowsy 24 Hour Tablets ..... ▣731
Non-Drowsy Claritin Hives Relief Tablets ..... ▣733
Claritin Reditabs 24 Hour Non-Drowsy Tablets ..... ▣732
Claritin-D Non-Drowsy 12 Hour Tablets ..... ▣731
Claritin-D Non-Drowsy 24 Hour Tablets ..... ▣731
Children's Dimetapp ND Non-Drowsy Allergy Syrup ..... ▣746
Triaminic Allerchews ..... ▣684

Metronidazole (Concomitant administration of budesonide with known inhibitors of CYP3A4 may inhibit the metabolism of, and increase the systemic exposure to, budesonide; care should be exercised). Products include:

Metrogel 1% 1212
MetroGel-Vaginal Gel 1822
Noritate Cream, 1% 1051

Metronidazole Benzoate (Concomitant administration of budesonide with known inhibitors of CYP3A4 may inhibit the metabolism of, and increase the systemic exposure to, budesonide; care should be exercised).

No products indexed under this heading.

Metronidazole Hydrochloride (Concomitant administration of budesonide with known inhibitors of CYP3A4 may inhibit the metabolism of, and increase the systemic exposure to, budesonide; care should be exercised).

No products indexed under this heading.

Miconazole (Concomitant administration of budesonide with known inhibitors of CYP3A4 may inhibit the metabolism of, and increase the systemic exposure to, budesonide; care should be exercised).

No products indexed under this heading.

Miconazole Nitrate (Concomitant administration of budesonide with known inhibitors of CYP3A4 may inhibit the metabolism of, and increase the systemic exposure to, budesonide; care should be exercised). Products include:

Desenex ..... ▣674
Desenex Jock Itch Spray Powder ..... ▣674

Nefazodone Hydrochloride (Concomitant administration of budesonide with known inhibitors of CYP3A4 may inhibit the metabolism of, and increase the systemic exposure to, budesonide; care should be exercised).

No products indexed under this heading.

Nelfinavir Mesylate (Concomitant administration of budesonide with known inhibitors of CYP3A4 may inhibit the metabolism of, and increase the systemic exposure to, budesonide; care should be exercised). Products include:

Viracept 2556

Nevirapine (Concomitant administration of budesonide with known inhibitors of CYP3A4 may inhibit the metabolism of, and increase the systemic exposure to, budesonide; care should be exercised). Products include:

Viramune Oral Suspension 903
Viramune Tablets 903

Niacinamide (Concomitant administration of budesonide with known inhibitors of CYP3A4 may inhibit the metabolism of, and increase the systemic exposure to, budesonide; care should be exercised).

No products indexed under this heading.

Nicotinamide (Concomitant administration of budesonide with known inhibitors of CYP3A4 may inhibit the metabolism of, and increase the systemic exposure to, budesonide; care should be exercised). Products include:

Nicomide Tablets 3190

Nifedipine (Concomitant administration of budesonide with known inhibitors of CYP3A4 may inhibit the metabolism of, and increase the systemic exposure to, budesonide; care should be exercised). Products include:

Adalat CC Tablets 2978

Norfloxacin (Concomitant administration of budesonide with known inhibitors of CYP3A4 may inhibit the metabolism of, and increase the systemic exposure to, budesonide; care should be exercised). Products include:

Noroxin Tablets 2009

Omeprazole (Concomitant administration of budesonide with known inhibitors of CYP3A4 may inhibit the metabolism of, and increase the systemic exposure to, budesonide; care should be exercised). Products include:

Zegerid Powder for Oral Solution 2972

Paroxetine Hydrochloride (Concomitant administration of budesonide with known inhibitors of CYP3A4 may inhibit the metabolism of, and increase the systemic exposure to, budesonide; care should be exercised). Products include:

Paxil CR Controlled-Release Tablets 1509
Paxil 1501

Propoxyphene Hydrochloride (Concomitant administration of budesonide with known inhibitors of CYP3A4 may inhibit the metabolism of, and increase the systemic exposure to, budesonide; care should be exercised).

No products indexed under this heading.

Propoxyphene Napsylate (Concomitant administration of budesonide with known inhibitors of CYP3A4 may inhibit the metabolism of, and increase the systemic exposure to, budesonide; care should be exercised). Products include:

Darvocet A 500 Tablets 3497

Quinidine (Concomitant administration of budesonide with known inhibitors of CYP3A4 may inhibit the metabolism of, and increase the systemic exposure to, budesonide; care should be exercised).

No products indexed under this heading.

Quinidine Hydrochloride (Concomitant administration of budesonide with known inhibitors of CYP3A4 may inhibit the metabolism of, and increase the systemic exposure to, budesonide; care should be exercised).

No products indexed under this heading.

Quinidine Polygalacturonate (Concomitant administration of budesonide with known inhibitors of CYP3A4 may inhibit the metabolism of, and increase the systemic exposure to, budesonide; care should be exercised).

No products indexed under this heading.

Quinidine Sulfate (Concomitant administration of budesonide with known inhibitors of CYP3A4 may inhibit the metabolism of, and increase the systemic exposure to, budesonide; care should be exercised).

No products indexed under this heading.

Quinine (Concomitant administration of budesonide with known inhibitors of CYP3A4 may inhibit the metabolism of, and increase the systemic exposure to, budesonide; care should be exercised).

No products indexed under this heading.

Quinine Sulfate (Concomitant administration of budesonide with known inhibitors of CYP3A4 may inhibit the metabolism of, and increase the systemic exposure to, budesonide; care should be exercised).

No products indexed under this heading.

Quinupristin (Concomitant administration of budesonide with known inhibitors of CYP3A4 may inhibit the metabolism of, and increase the systemic exposure to, budesonide; care should be exercised). Products include:

Synercid I.V. 1690

Ranitidine Bismuth Citrate (Concomitant administration of budesonide with known inhibitors of CYP3A4 may inhibit the metabolism of, and increase the systemic exposure to, budesonide; care should be exercised).

No products indexed under this heading.

Ranitidine Hydrochloride (Concomitant administration of budesonide with known inhibitors of CYP3A4 may inhibit the metabolism of, and increase the systemic exposure to, budesonide; care should be exercised). Products include:

Zantac 1597
Zantac Injection 1593
Zantac 75 Tablets ..... ▣715
Zantac 150 Maximum Strength Tablets ..... ▣715
Zantac Injection Pharmacy Bulk Package 1595

Ritonavir (Concomitant administration of budesonide with known inhibitors of CYP3A4 may inhibit the metabolism of, and increase the systemic exposure to, budesonide; care should be exercised). Products include:

Kaletra 474
Norvir 499

Saquinavir (Concomitant administration of budesonide with known inhibitors of CYP3A4 may inhibit the metabolism of, and increase the systemic exposure to, budesonide; care should be exercised).

No products indexed under this heading.

Saquinavir Mesylate (Concomitant administration of budesonide with known inhibitors of CYP3A4 may inhibit the metabolism of, and increase the systemic exposure to, budesonide; care should be exercised). Products include:

Invirase 2776

Sertraline Hydrochloride (Concomitant administration of budesonide with known inhibitors of CYP3A4 may inhibit the metabolism of, and increase the systemic exposure to, budesonide; care should be exercised). Products include:

Zoloft 2581

Telithromycin (Concomitant administration of budesonide with known inhibitors of CYP3A4 may inhibit the metabolism of, and increase the systemic exposure to, budesonide; care should be exercised). Products include:

Ketek Tablets 2920

Troglitazone (Concomitant administration of budesonide with known inhibitors of CYP3A4 may inhibit the metabolism of, and increase the systemic exposure to, budesonide; care should be exercised).

No products indexed under this heading.

Troleandomycin (Concomitant administration of budesonide with known inhibitors of CYP3A4 may inhibit the metabolism of, and increase the systemic exposure to, budesonide; care should be exercised).

No products indexed under this heading.

Valproate Sodium (Concomitant administration of budesonide with known inhibitors of CYP3A4 may inhibit the metabolism of, and increase the systemic exposure to, budesonide; care should be exercised). Products include:

Depacon Injection 412

Verapamil Hydrochloride (Concomitant administration of budesonide with known inhibitors of CYP3A4 may inhibit the metabolism of, and increase the systemic exposure to, budesonide; care should be exercised). Products include:

Covera-HS Tablets 3135
Tarka Tablets 519
Verelan PM Capsules 3120

Voriconazole (Concomitant administration of budesonide with known inhibitors of CYP3A4 may inhibit the metabolism of, and increase the systemic exposure to, budesonide; care should be exercised). Products include:

VFEND I.V. 2543
VFEND Oral Suspension 2543
VFEND Tablets 2543

Zafirlukast (Concomitant administration of budesonide with known inhibitors of CYP3A4 may inhibit the metabolism of, and increase the systemic exposure to, budesonide; care should be exercised). Products include:

Accolate Tablets 663

Zileuton (Concomitant administration of budesonide with known inhibitors of CYP3A4 may inhibit the metabolism of, and increase the systemic exposure to, budesonide; care should be exercised).
No products indexed under this heading.

Food Interactions

Grapefruit (Concomitant administration of budesonide with known inhibitors of CYP3A4 may inhibit the metabolism of, and increase the systemic exposure to, budesonide; care should be exercised).

Grapefruit Juice (Concomitant administration of budesonide with known inhibitors of CYP3A4 may inhibit the metabolism of, and increase the systemic exposure to, budesonide; care should be exercised).

PULMOZYME INHALATION SOLUTION

(Dornase Alfa) 1245
None cited in PDR database.

PURE GARDENS CREAM

(Herbals with Vitamins) 760
None cited in PDR database.

PURETRIM WHOLE FOOD WELLNESS SHAKE

(Antioxidants, Fatty Acids, Rice Protein)... 760
None cited in PDR database.

PURINETHOL TABLETS

(Mercaptopurine) 1222
May interact with drugs that inhibit thiopurine methyltransferase (TPMT) and certain other agents. Compounds in these categories include:

Allopurinol (Co-administration may result in life-threatening bone marrow suppression; if used concurrently it is imperative that the dose of mercaptopurine be reduced to one-quarter to one-third of the usual dose; failure to observe this dosage reduction results in a delayed catabolism of mercaptopurine and the strong likelihood of inducing severe toxicity).
No products indexed under this heading.

Doxorubicin Hydrochloride (Potential for increased hepatotoxicity). Products include:
Adriamycin for Injection, USP 786
Adriamycin Injection, USP 786

Hepatotoxic Drugs, unspecified (Co-administration results in increased risk of hepatotoxicity).
No products indexed under this heading.

Mesalamine (Individuals with inherited deficiency of the enzyme TPMT are unusually sensitive to the myelosuppressive effects of mercaptopurine and are prone to developing rapid bone marrow suppression; co-administration with drugs that inhibit TPMT could exacerbate this toxicity). Products include:
Asacol Delayed-Release Tablets 2688
Canasa Rectal Suppositories 726
Pentasa Capsules 3182

Mesalazine (Individuals with inherited deficiency of the enzyme TPMT are unusually sensitive to the myelosuppressive effects of mercaptopurine and are prone to developing rapid bone marrow suppression; co-administration with drugs that inhibit TPMT could exacerbate this toxicity).
No products indexed under this heading.

Olsalazine Sodium (Individuals with inherited deficiency of the enzyme TPMT are unusually sensitive to the myelosuppressive effects of mercaptopurine and are prone to developing rapid bone marrow suppression; co-administration with drugs that inhibit TPMT could exacerbate this toxicity).
No products indexed under this heading.

Sulfamethoxazole (Enhanced bone marrow suppression has been noted in some of the patients also receiving trimethoprim-sulfamethoxazole).
No products indexed under this heading.

Sulphasalazine (Individuals with inherited deficiency of the enzyme TPMT are unusually sensitive to the myelosuppressive effects of mercaptopurine and are prone to developing rapid bone marrow suppression; co-administration with drugs that inhibit TPMT could exacerbate this toxicity).
No products indexed under this heading.

Thioguanine (Complete cross-resistance). Products include:
Tabloid Tablets 1545

Trimethoprim (Enhanced bone marrow suppression has been noted in some of the patients also receiving trimethoprim-sulfamethoxazole).
No products indexed under this heading.

Warfarin Sodium (Co-administration results in inhibition of the anticoagulant effect). Products include:
Coumadin for Injection 932
Coumadin Tablets 932

QUIXIN OPHTHALMIC SOLUTION

(Levofloxacin) 3373
May interact with xanthines and certain other agents. Compounds in these categories include:

Aminophylline (Systemic administration of some quinolones has been shown to elevate plasma concentrations of theophylline).
No products indexed under this heading.

Caffeine (Systemic administration of some quinolones has been shown to interfere with the metabolism of caffeine). Products include:
Athena Hair System Shampoo 767
BC Powder 612
Arthritis Strength BC Powder 612
Goody's Extra Strength Headache Powder....................... 621
Goody's Extra Strength Pain Relief Tablets.............................. 621
Hycomine Compound Tablets 1105
Spartan Hair System Shampoo 767
Vivarin 639

Caffeine Citrate (Systemic administration of some quinolones has been shown to interfere with the metabolism of caffeine). Products include:
Cafcit 1854

Cyclosporine (Systemic administration of some quinolones has been associated with transient elevations of serum creatinine in patients receiving systemic cyclosporine concomitantly). Products include:
Gengraf Capsules 458
Neoral Soft Gelatin Capsules 2247
Neoral Oral Solution 2247
Restasis Ophthalmic Emulsion 570
Sandimmune 2259

Dyphylline (Systemic administration of some quinolones has been shown to elevate plasma concentrations of theophylline).
No products indexed under this heading.

Theophylline (Systemic administration of some quinolones has been shown to elevate plasma concentrations of theophylline).
No products indexed under this heading.

Theophylline Anhydrous (Systemic administration of some quinolones has been shown to elevate plasma concentrations of theophylline). Products include:
Uniphyl Tablets 2708

Theophylline Calcium Salicylate (Systemic administration of some quinolones has been shown to elevate plasma concentrations of theophylline).
No products indexed under this heading.

Theophylline Dihydroxypropyl (Glyceryl) (Systemic administration of some quinolones has been shown to elevate plasma concentrations of theophylline).
No products indexed under this heading.

Theophylline Ethylenediamine (Systemic administration of some quinolones has been shown to elevate plasma concentrations of theophylline).
No products indexed under this heading.

Theophylline Sodium Glycinate (Systemic administration of some quinolones has been shown to elevate plasma concentrations of theophylline).
No products indexed under this heading.

Warfarin Sodium (Systemic administration of some quinolones has been shown to enhance the effects of the oral anticoagulant warfarin). Products include:
Coumadin for Injection 932
Coumadin Tablets 932

QVAR INHALATION AEROSOL

(Beclomethasone Dipropionate) 1654
None cited in PDR database.

RABIES VACCINE RABAVERT

(Rabies Vaccine) 1011
May interact with antimalarials, corticosteroids, immunosuppressive agents, and certain other agents. Compounds in these categories include:

Azathioprine (Immunosuppressive agents can interfere with the development of active immunity after vaccination and may diminish the protective efficacy of the vaccine). Products include:
Azasan Tablets 2844

Basiliximab (Immunosuppressive agents can interfere with the development of active immunity after vaccination and may diminish the protective efficacy of the vaccine). Products include:
Simulect for Injection 2268

Betamethasone Acetate (Corticosteroids can interfere with the development of active immunity after vaccination and may diminish the protective efficacy of the vaccine).
No products indexed under this heading.

Betamethasone Sodium Phosphate (Corticosteroids can interfere with the development of active immunity after vaccination and may diminish the protective efficacy of the vaccine).
No products indexed under this heading.

Chloroquine Hydrochloride (Antimalarials can interfere with the development of active immunity after vaccination and may diminish the protective efficacy of the vaccine).
No products indexed under this heading.

Chloroquine Phosphate (Antimalarials can interfere with the development of active immunity after vaccination and may diminish the protective efficacy of the vaccine).
No products indexed under this heading.

Cortisone Acetate (Corticosteroids can interfere with the development of active immunity after vaccination and may diminish the protective efficacy of the vaccine).
No products indexed under this heading.

Cyclosporine (Immunosuppressive agents can interfere with the development of active immunity after vaccination and may diminish the protective efficacy of the vaccine). Products include:
Gengraf Capsules 458
Neoral Soft Gelatin Capsules 2247
Neoral Oral Solution 2247
Restasis Ophthalmic Emulsion 570
Sandimmune 2259

Dexamethasone (Corticosteroids can interfere with the development of active immunity after vaccination and may diminish the protective efficacy of the vaccine). Products include:
Ciprodex Otic Suspension 555
Decadron Tablets 1929
TobraDex Ophthalmic Ointment 558
TobraDex Ophthalmic Suspension ... 558

Dexamethasone Acetate (Corticosteroids can interfere with the development of active immunity after vaccination and may diminish the protective efficacy of the vaccine).
No products indexed under this heading.

Dexamethasone Sodium Phosphate (Corticosteroids can interfere with the development of active immunity after vaccination and may diminish the protective efficacy of the vaccine). Products include:
Decadron Phosphate Injection 1931

Fludrocortisone Acetate (Corticosteroids can interfere with the development of active immunity after vaccination and may diminish the protective efficacy of the vaccine).
No products indexed under this heading.

Hydrocortisone (Corticosteroids can interfere with the development

of active immunity after vaccination and may diminish the protective efficacy of the vaccine). Products include:
Cortizone•5 Ointment 699
Cortizone•10 Creme 699
Cortizone•10 Ointment 699
Cortizone•10 Plus Creme 700
Cortizone•10 Maximum Strength Quick Shot Spray 700
Hydrocortone Tablets 1963
Preparation H Hydrocortisone Cream 748

Hydrocortisone Acetate (Corticosteroids can interfere with the development of active immunity after vaccination and may diminish the protective efficacy of the vaccine). Products include:
Analpram-HC 1136
Pramosone 1139
ProctoFoam-HC 3113
Tucks Anti-Itch Ointment 712
U-cort 1% Cream 3289

Hydrocortisone Sodium Phosphate (Corticosteroids can interfere with the development of active immunity after vaccination and may diminish the protective efficacy of the vaccine).
No products indexed under this heading.

Hydrocortisone Sodium Succinate (Corticosteroids can interfere with the development of active immunity after vaccination and may diminish the protective efficacy of the vaccine).
No products indexed under this heading.

Mefloquine Hydrochloride (Antimalarials can interfere with the development of active immunity after vaccination and may diminish the protective efficacy of the vaccine). Products include:
Lariam Tablets 2790

Methylprednisolone Acetate (Corticosteroids can interfere with the development of active immunity after vaccination and may diminish the protective efficacy of the vaccine). Products include:
Depo-Medrol Injectable Suspension 2615
Depo-Medrol Single-Dose Vial 2617

Methylprednisolone Sodium Succinate (Corticosteroids can interfere with the development of active immunity after vaccination and may diminish the protective efficacy of the vaccine).
No products indexed under this heading.

Muromonab-CD3 (Immunosuppressive agents can interfere with the development of active immunity after vaccination and may diminish the protective efficacy of the vaccine). Products include:
Orthoclone OKT3 Sterile Solution 2370

Mycophenolate Mofetil (Immunosuppressive agents can interfere with the development of active immunity after vaccination and may diminish the protective efficacy of the vaccine). Products include:
CellCept Capsules 2751
CellCept Oral Suspension 2751
CellCept Tablets 2751

Prednisolone Acetate (Corticosteroids can interfere with the development of active immunity after vaccination and may diminish the protective efficacy of the vaccine). Products include:
Blephamide Ophthalmic Ointment 563
Blephamide Ophthalmic Suspension 564
Poly-Pred Liquifilm Ophthalmic Suspension .... ⊙231
Pred Forte Ophthalmic Suspension .... ⊙233
Pred Mild Sterile Ophthalmic Suspension .... ⊙236
Pred-G Ophthalmic Suspension .... ⊙234
Pred-G Sterile Ophthalmic Ointment .... ⊙235

Prednisolone Sodium Phosphate (Corticosteroids can interfere with the development of active immunity after vaccination and may diminish the protective efficacy of the vaccine). Products include:
Pediapred Oral Solution 3319

Prednisolone Tebutate (Corticosteroids can interfere with the development of active immunity after vaccination and may diminish the protective efficacy of the vaccine).
No products indexed under this heading.

Prednisone (Corticosteroids can interfere with the development of active immunity after vaccination and may diminish the protective efficacy of the vaccine).
No products indexed under this heading.

Pyrimethamine (Antimalarials can interfere with the development of active immunity after vaccination and may diminish the protective efficacy of the vaccine). Products include:
Daraprim Tablets 1385

Rabies Immune Globulin (Human) (Must not be administered at more than the recommended dose since the response to active immunization may be impaired). Products include:
HyperRAB 3239

Radiation (Radiation therapy can interfere with the development of active immunity after vaccination and may diminish the protective efficacy of the vaccine).
No products indexed under this heading.

Sirolimus (Immunosuppressive agents can interfere with the development of active immunity after vaccination and may diminish the protective efficacy of the vaccine). Products include:
Rapamune Oral Solution and Tablets 3472

Tacrolimus (Immunosuppressive agents can interfere with the development of active immunity after vaccination and may diminish the protective efficacy of the vaccine). Products include:
Prograf Capsules and Injection 624
Protopic Ointment 629

Triamcinolone (Corticosteroids can interfere with the development of active immunity after vaccination and may diminish the protective efficacy of the vaccine).
No products indexed under this heading.

Triamcinolone Acetonide (Corticosteroids can interfere with the development of active immunity after vaccination and may diminish the protective efficacy of the vaccine). Products include:
Azmacort Inhalation Aerosol 1701
Nasacort HFA Inhalation Aerosol 2939
Nasacort AQ Nasal Spray 2937

Triamcinolone Diacetate (Corticosteroids can interfere with the development of active immunity after vaccination and may diminish the protective efficacy of the vaccine).
No products indexed under this heading.

Triamcinolone Hexacetonide (Corticosteroids can interfere with the development of active immunity after vaccination and may diminish the protective efficacy of the vaccine).
No products indexed under this heading.

RAPAMUNE ORAL SOLUTION AND TABLETS

(Sirolimus) 3472

May interact with cytochrome p450 3a4 inducers (selected), cytochrome p450 3a4 inhibitors (selected), cytochrome p450 3a4 substrates (selected), erythromycin, fibrates, HMG-CoA reductase inhibitors, phenytoin, protease inhibitors, and certain other agents. Compounds in these categories include:

Acetazolamide (Sirolimus is extensively metabolized by the CYP3A4 isoenzyme in the gut wall and liver. Co-administration with inhibitors of CYP3A4 may decrease the metabolism of sirolimus and increase sirolimus levels. Co-administration with strong inducers of CYP3A4 is not recommended).
No products indexed under this heading.

Alfentanil Hydrochloride (Care should be exercised when drugs or other substances metabolized by CYP3A4 are administered concomitantly with sirolimus).
No products indexed under this heading.

Allium sativum (Sirolimus is extensively metabolized by the CYP3A4 isoenzyme in the gut wall and liver. Co-administration with inducers of CYP3A4 may increase the metabolism of sirolimus and decrease sirolimus levels. Co-administration with strong inducers of CYP3A4 is not recommended).
No products indexed under this heading.

Alprazolam (Care should be exercised when drugs or other substances metabolized by CYP3A4 are administered concomitantly with sirolimus). Products include:
Niravam Orally Disintegrating Tablets 3106
Xanax XR Tablets 2655

Amiodarone Hydrochloride (Sirolimus is extensively metabolized by the CYP3A4 isoenzyme in the gut wall and liver. Co-administration with inhibitors of CYP3A4 may decrease the metabolism of sirolimus and increase sirolimus levels. Co-administration with strong inducers of CYP3A4 is not recommended). Products include:
Pacerone Tablets 3337

Amitriptyline Hydrochloride (Care should be exercised when drugs or other substances metabolized by CYP3A4 are administered concomitantly with sirolimus).
No products indexed under this heading.

Amlodipine Besylate (Care should be exercised when drugs or other substances metabolized by CYP3A4 are administered concomitantly with sirolimus). Products include:
Caduet Tablets 2507
Lotrel Capsules 2238
Norvasc Tablets 2529

Amprenavir (Sirolimus is extensively metabolized by the CYP3A4 isoenzyme in the gut wall and liver. Co-administration with inhibitors of CYP3A4 may decrease the metabolism of sirolimus and increase sirolimus levels. Co-administration with strong inducers of CYP3A4 is not recommended). Products include:
Agenerase Capsules 1299
Agenerase Oral Solution 1304

Anastrozole (Sirolimus is extensively metabolized by the CYP3A4 isoenzyme in the gut wall and liver. Co-administration with inhibitors of CYP3A4 may decrease the metabolism of sirolimus and increase sirolimus levels. Co-administration with strong inducers of CYP3A4 is not recommended). Products include:
Arimidex Tablets 665

Aprepitant (Sirolimus is extensively metabolized by the CYP3A4 isoenzyme in the gut wall and liver. Co-administration with inhibitors of CYP3A4 may decrease the metabolism of sirolimus and increase sirolimus levels. Co-administration with strong inducers of CYP3A4 is not recommended). Products include:
Emend Capsules 1944

Astemizole (Care should be exercised when drugs or other substances metabolized by CYP3A4 are administered concomitantly with sirolimus).
No products indexed under this heading.

Atorvastatin Calcium (Co-administration of sirolimus with cyclosporine in conjunction with HMG-CoA reductase inhibitors should be monitored for the possible development of rhabdomyolysis; in clinical trials, the concurrent use of sirolimus and HMG-CoA reductase inhibitors was well tolerated). Products include:
Caduet Tablets 2507
Lipitor Tablets 2495

Belladonna Ergotamine (Care should be exercised when drugs or other substances metabolized by CYP3A4 are administered concomitantly with sirolimus).
No products indexed under this heading.

Betamethasone Acetate (Sirolimus is extensively metabolized by the CYP3A4 isoenzyme in the gut wall and liver. Co-administration with inducers of CYP3A4 may increase the metabolism of sirolimus and decrease sirolimus levels. Co-administration with strong inducers of CYP3A4 is not recommended).
No products indexed under this heading.

Betamethasone Sodium Phosphate (Sirolimus is extensively metabolized by the CYP3A4 isoenzyme in the gut wall and liver. Co-administration with inducers of CYP3A4 may increase the metabolism of sirolimus and decrease sirolimus levels. Co-administration with strong inducers of CYP3A4 is not recommended).
No products indexed under this heading.

Bromocriptine Mesylate (Sirolimus is extensively metabolized by the CYP3A4 isoenzyme; co-administration with inhibitors of CYP3A4, such as bromocriptine, may decrease the metabolism of sirolimus and increase the plasma levels of sirolimus).
No products indexed under this heading.

Buspirone Hydrochloride (Care should be exercised when drugs or other substances metabolized by CYP3A4 are administered concomitantly with sirolimus).
No products indexed under this heading.

Busulfan (Care should be exercised when drugs or other substances metabolized by CYP3A4 are administered concomitantly with sirolimus). Products include:
I.V. Busulfex 1125
Myleran Tablets 1492

Carbamazepine (Sirolimus is extensively metabolized by the CYP3A4 isoenzyme; co-administration with inducers of CYP3A4, such as carbamazepine, may increase the metabolism of sirolimus and decrease the plasma levels of sirolimus). Products include:
Carbatrol Capsules 3174
Equetro Extended-Release Capsules 3178
Tegretol/Tegretol-XR 2278

Cerivastatin Sodium (Co-administration of sirolimus with cyclosporine in conjunction with HMG-CoA reductase inhibitors should be monitored for the possible development of rhabdomyolysis; in clinical trials, the concurrent use of sirolimus and HMG-CoA reductase inhibitors was well tolerated).
No products indexed under this heading.

Chlorpheniramine (Care should be exercised when drugs or other substances metabolized by CYP3A4 are administered concomitantly with sirolimus).
No products indexed under this heading.

Chlorpheniramine Maleate (Care should be exercised when drugs or other substances metabolized by CYP3A4 are administered concomitantly with sirolimus). Products include:
Advil Allergy Sinus Caplets 737
Advil Multi-Symptom Cold Caplets 738
BC Allergy Sinus Cold Powder 612
Contac Severe Cold and Flu Caplets Maximum Strength 615
Hycomine Compound Tablets 1105
PediaCare Multi-Symptom Cold Liquid 704
PediaCare NightRest Cough & Cold Liquid 704
Robitussin Flu Liquid 752
Robitussin PM Cough & Cold Liquid 752
Singlet Caplets 636
Sudafed Sinus & Allergy Tablets 710
TheraFlu Cold & Cough Hot Liquid 680
TheraFlu Cold & Sore Throat Hot Liquid 680
TheraFlu Flu & Sore Throat Hot Liquid 681
TheraFlu Severe Cold & Cough Hot Liquid 683
TheraFlu Severe Cold Caplets 679
TheraFlu Severe Cold Hot Liquid 682
Triaminic Cold & Allergy Liquid 685
Triaminic Cold & Cough Liquid 685
Triaminic Flu, Cough & Fever Liquid 685
Triaminic Night Time Cough & Cold Liquid 685
Triaminic Allergy Runny Nose & Congestion Softchews 688
Triaminic Cold & Cough Softchews 688
Children's Tylenol Plus Cold NightTime Suspension Liquid 1851
Children's Tylenol Plus Cold & Cough Suspension Liquid and Chewable Tablets 1851
Children's Tylenol Plus Cold Chewable Tablets 1851
Children's Tylenol Plus Flu Suspension Liquid 1853
Tylenol Allergy Complete Multi-Symptom Caplets and Gelcaps with Cool Burst 1844
Multi-Symptom Tylenol Cold Night Time Caplets 1845
Vicks 44M Cough, Cold & Flu Relief 2676
Pediatric Vicks 44m Cough & Cold Relief 2673
Children's Vicks NyQuil Cold/Cough Relief 2671

Chlorpheniramine Polistirex (Care should be exercised when drugs or other substances metabolized by CYP3A4 are administered concomitantly with sirolimus). Products include:
Tussionex Pennkinetic Extended-Release Suspension 3322

Chlorpheniramine Tannate (Care should be exercised when drugs or other substances metabolized by CYP3A4 are administered concomitantly with sirolimus).
No products indexed under this heading.

Cimetidine (Sirolimus is extensively metabolized by the CYP3A4 isoenzyme; co-administration with inhibitors of CYP3A4, such as cimetidine, may decrease the metabolism of sirolimus and increase the plasma levels of sirolimus). Products include:
Tagamet HB 200 Tablets 637
Tagamet Tablets 1547

Cimetidine Hydrochloride (Sirolimus is extensively metabolized by the CYP3A4 isoenzyme; co-administration with inhibitors of CYP3A4, such as cimetidine, may decrease the metabolism of sirolimus and increase the plasma levels of sirolimus).
No products indexed under this heading.

Ciprofloxacin (Sirolimus is extensively metabolized by the CYP3A4 isoenzyme in the gut wall and liver. Co-administration with inhibitors of CYP3A4 may decrease the metabolism of sirolimus and increase sirolimus levels. Co-administration with strong inducers of CYP3A4 is not recommended). Products include:
Cipro I.V. 2998
Cipro I.V. Pharmacy Bulk Package 3509
Cipro Oral Suspension 2991
Cipro XR Tablets 3004
Ciprodex Otic Suspension 555

Ciprofloxacin Hydrochloride (Sirolimus is extensively metabolized by the CYP3A4 isoenzyme in the gut wall and liver. Co-administration with inducers of CYP3A4 may increase the metabolism of sirolimus and decrease sirolimus levels. Co-administration with strong inducers of CYP3A4 is not recommended). Products include:
Ciloxan Ophthalmic Ointment 554
Cipro Tablets 2991

Cisapride (Sirolimus is extensively metabolized by the CYP3A4 isoenzyme; co-administration with inhibitors of CYP3A4, such as cisapride, may decrease the metabolism of sirolimus and increase the plasma levels of sirolimus).
No products indexed under this heading.

Cisplatin (Sirolimus is extensively metabolized by the CYP3A4 isoenzyme in the gut wall and liver. Co-administration with inducers of CYP3A4 may increase the metabolism of sirolimus and decrease sirolimus levels. Co-administration with strong inducers of CYP3A4 is not recommended).
No products indexed under this heading.

Clarithromycin (Sirolimus is extensively metabolized by the CYP3A4 isoenzyme; co-administration with inhibitors of CYP3A4, such as clarithromycin, may decrease the metabolism of sirolimus and increase the plasma levels of sirolimus). Products include:
Biaxin/Biaxin XL 402
PREVPAC 3281

Clofibrate (Co-administration of sirolimus with cyclosporine in conjunction with fibrates should be monitored for the possible development of rhabdomyolysis; in clinical trials, the concurrent use of sirolimus and fibrates was well tolerated).
No products indexed under this heading.

Clotrimazole (Co-administration of sirolimus and clotrimazole may increase sirolimus blood concentrations). Products include:
Lotrimin 3053
Lotrisone 3054

Cortisone Acetate (Sirolimus is extensively metabolized by the CYP3A4 isoenzyme in the gut wall and liver. Co-administration with inducers of CYP3A4 may increase the metabolism of sirolimus and decrease sirolimus levels. Co-administration with strong inducers of CYP3A4 is not recommended).
No products indexed under this heading.

Cyclosporine (Co-administration of sirolimus simultaneously with cyclosporine capsules modified results in increased AUC and Cmax relative to sirolimus alone; because of the effect of cyclosporine capsules, modified, it is recommended that sirolimus should be taken 4 hours after cyclosporine oral solution modified and/or cyclosporine modified capsules; combination use is associated with hepatic artery thrombosis (HAT); the safety and efficacy of Rapamune has not been established in liver transplant patients and, therefore, such use is not recommended). Products include:
Gengraf Capsules 458
Neoral Soft Gelatin Capsules 2247
Neoral Oral Solution 2247
Restasis Ophthalmic Emulsion 570
Sandimmune 2259

Dalfopristin (Sirolimus is extensively metabolized by the CYP3A4 isoenzyme in the gut wall and liver. Co-administration with inhibitors of CYP3A4 may decrease the metabolism of sirolimus and increase sirolimus levels. Co-administration with strong inducers of CYP3A4 is not recommended). Products include:
Synercid I.V. 1690

Danazol (Sirolimus is extensively metabolized by the CYP3A4 isoenzyme; co-administration with inhibitors of CYP3A4, such as danazol, may decrease the metabolism of sirolimus and increase the plasma levels of sirolimus).
No products indexed under this heading.

Delavirdine Mesylate (Sirolimus is extensively metabolized by the CYP3A4 isoenzyme in the gut wall and liver. Co-administration with inhibitors of CYP3A4 may decrease the metabolism of sirolimus and increase sirolimus levels. Co-administration with strong inducers of CYP3A4 is not recommended). Products include:
Rescriptor Tablets 2535

Desogestrel (Care should be exercised when drugs or other substances metabolized by CYP3A4 are administered concomitantly with sirolimus). Products include:
Ortho-Cept Tablets 2395

Dexamethasone (Sirolimus is extensively metabolized by the CYP3A4 isoenzyme in the gut wall and liver. Co-administration with inducers of CYP3A4 may increase the metabolism of sirolimus and decrease sirolimus levels. Co-administration with strong inducers of CYP3A4 is not recommended). Products include:
Ciprodex Otic Suspension 555
Decadron Tablets 1929
TobraDex Ophthalmic Ointment 558
TobraDex Ophthalmic Suspension 558

Dexamethasone Acetate (Sirolimus is extensively metabolized by the CYP3A4 isoenzyme in the gut wall and liver. Co-administration with inducers of CYP3A4 may increase the metabolism of sirolimus and decrease sirolimus levels. Co-administration with strong inducers of CYP3A4 is not recommended).
No products indexed under this heading.

Dexamethasone Sodium Phosphate (Sirolimus is extensively metabolized by the CYP3A4 isoenzyme in the gut wall and liver. Co-administration with inducers of CYP3A4 may increase the metabolism of sirolimus and decrease sirolimus levels. Co-administration with strong inducers of CYP3A4 is not recommended). Products include:
Decadron Phosphate Injection 1931

Diazepam (Care should be exercised when drugs or other substances metabolized by CYP3A4 are administered concomitantly with sirolimus). Products include:
Diastat Rectal Delivery System 3344
Valium Tablets 2822

Dihydroergotamine Mesylate (Care should be exercised when drugs or other substances metabolized by CYP3A4 are administered concomitantly with sirolimus). Products include:
Migranal Nasal Spray 3350

Diltiazem Hydrochloride (Co-administration in healthy individuals significantly affects the bioavailability of sirolimus; monitor sirolimus levels; a dose adjustment may be necessary). Products include:

Cardizem LA Extended Release Tablets 1699
Tiazac Capsules 1204

Diltiazem Maleate (Sirolimus is extensively metabolized by the CYP3A4 isoenzyme in the gut wall and liver. Co-administration with inhibitors of CYP3A4 may decrease the metabolism of sirolimus and increase sirolimus levels. Co-administration with strong inducers of CYP3A4 is not recommended).
No products indexed under this heading.

Disopyramide (Care should be exercised when drugs or other substances metabolized by CYP3A4 are administered concomitantly with sirolimus).
No products indexed under this heading.

Disopyramide Phosphate (Care should be exercised when drugs or other substances metabolized by CYP3A4 are administered concomitantly with sirolimus).
No products indexed under this heading.

Disulfiram (Care should be exercised when drugs or other substances metabolized by CYP3A4 are administered concomitantly with sirolimus). Products include:
Antabuse Tablets 2343

Doxorubicin Hydrochloride (Sirolimus is extensively metabolized by the CYP3A4 isoenzyme in the gut wall and liver. Co-administration with inducers of CYP3A4 may increase the metabolism of sirolimus and decrease sirolimus levels. Co-administration with strong inducers of CYP3A4 is not recommended). Products include:
Adriamycin for Injection, USP 786
Adriamycin Injection, USP 786

Dronabinol (Care should be exercised when drugs or other substances metabolized by CYP3A4 are administered concomitantly with sirolimus). Products include:
Marinol Capsules 3334

Efavirenz (Sirolimus is extensively metabolized by the CYP3A4 isoenzyme in the gut wall and liver. Co-administration with inhibitors of CYP3A4 may decrease the metabolism of sirolimus and increase sirolimus levels. Co-administration with strong inducers of CYP3A4 is not recommended). Products include:
Sustiva Capsules 957

Ergotamine Tartrate (Care should be exercised when drugs or other substances metabolized by CYP3A4 are administered concomitantly with sirolimus).
No products indexed under this heading.

Erythromycin (Sirolimus is extensively metabolized by the CYP3A4 isoenzyme; co-administration with inhibitors of CYP3A4, such as erythromycin, may decrease the metabolism of sirolimus and increase the plasma levels of sirolimus. Co-administration of sirolimus oral solution or tablets and erythromycin is not recommended). Products include:
Erygel Topical Gel 2096
Ery-Tab Tablets 447
Erythromycin Base Filmtab Tablets 454
Erythromycin Delayed-Release Capsules, USP 456
PCE Dispertab Tablets 510

Erythromycin Estolate (Sirolimus is extensively metabolized by the CYP3A4 isoenzyme; co-administration with inhibitors of CYP3A4, such as erythromycin, may decrease the metabolism of sirolimus and increase the plasma levels of sirolimus. Co-administration of sirolimus oral solution or tablets and erythromycin is not recommended).
No products indexed under this heading.

Erythromycin Ethylsuccinate (Sirolimus is extensively metabolized by the CYP3A4 isoenzyme; co-administration with inhibitors of CYP3A4, such as erythromycin, may decrease the metabolism of sirolimus and increase the plasma levels of sirolimus. Co-administration of sirolimus oral solution or tablets and erythromycin is not recommended). Products include:
E.E.S. 449
EryPed 445

Erythromycin Gluceptate (Sirolimus is extensively metabolized by the CYP3A4 isoenzyme; co-administration with inhibitors of CYP3A4, such as erythromycin, may decrease the metabolism of sirolimus and increase the plasma levels of sirolimus. Co-administration of sirolimus oral solution or tablets and erythromycin is not recommended).
No products indexed under this heading.

Erythromycin Lactobionate (Sirolimus is extensively metabolized by the CYP3A4 isoenzyme; co-administration with inhibitors of CYP3A4, such as erythromycin, may decrease the metabolism of sirolimus and increase the plasma levels of sirolimus. Co-administration of sirolimus oral solution or tablets and erythromycin is not recommended).
No products indexed under this heading.

Erythromycin Stearate (Sirolimus is extensively metabolized by the CYP3A4 isoenzyme; co-administration with inhibitors of CYP3A4, such as erythromycin, may decrease the metabolism of sirolimus and increase the plasma levels of sirolimus. Co-administration of sirolimus oral solution or tablets and erythromycin is not recommended). Products include:
Erythrocin Stearate Filmtab Tablets 452

Esomeprazole Magnesium (Sirolimus is extensively metabolized by the CYP3A4 isoenzyme in the gut wall and liver. Co-administration with inhibitors of CYP3A4 may decrease the metabolism of sirolimus and increase sirolimus levels. Co-administration with strong inducers of CYP3A4 is not recommended). Products include:
Nexium Delayed-Release Capsules 645

Estradiol (Care should be exercised when drugs or other substances metabolized by CYP3A4 are administered concomitantly with sirolimus). Products include:
Activella Tablets 2311
Climara Transdermal System 795
Climara Pro Transdermal System 800
CombiPatch Transdermal System 2180
Estrogel 0.06% 3200
Menostar Transdermal System 805
Prefest Tablets 1069
Vagifem Tablets 2340
Vivelle Transdermal System 2288
Vivelle-Dot Transdermal System 2293

Estradiol Benzoate (Care should be exercised when drugs or other substances metabolized by CYP3A4 are administered concomitantly with sirolimus).
No products indexed under this heading.

Estradiol Cypionate (Care should be exercised when drugs or other substances metabolized by CYP3A4 are administered concomitantly with sirolimus).
No products indexed under this heading.

Estradiol Valerate (Care should be exercised when drugs or other substances metabolized by CYP3A4 are administered concomitantly with sirolimus).
No products indexed under this heading.

Ethinyl Estradiol (Care should be exercised when drugs or other substances metabolized by CYP3A4 are administered concomitantly with sirolimus). Products include:
Alesse-28 Tablets 3392
Lo/Ovral-28 Tablets 3423
NuvaRing 2357
Ortho-Cept Tablets 2395
Ortho-Cyclen/Ortho Tri-Cyclen 2414
Ortho Evra Transdermal System 2402
Ortho Tri-Cyclen Lo Tablets 2421
Seasonale Tablets 1073
Triphasil-28 Tablets 3483
Yasmin 28 Tablets 818

Ethosuximide (Sirolimus is extensively metabolized by the CYP3A4 isoenzyme in the gut wall and liver. Co-administration with inducers of CYP3A4 may increase the metabolism of sirolimus and decrease sirolimus levels. Co-administration with strong inducers of CYP3A4 is not recommended).
No products indexed under this heading.

Ethynodiol Diacetate (Care should be exercised when drugs or other substances metabolized by CYP3A4 are administered concomitantly with sirolimus).
No products indexed under this heading.

Etoposide (Care should be exercised when drugs or other substances metabolized by CYP3A4 are administered concomitantly with sirolimus).
No products indexed under this heading.

Etoposide Phosphate (Care should be exercised when drugs or other substances metabolized by CYP3A4 are administered concomitantly with sirolimus).
No products indexed under this heading.

Felbamate (Sirolimus is extensively metabolized by the CYP3A4 isoenzyme in the gut wall and liver. Co-administration with inducers of CYP3A4 may increase the metabolism of sirolimus and decrease sirolimus levels. Co-administration with strong inducers of CYP3A4 is not recommended).
No products indexed under this heading.

Felodipine (Care should be exercised when drugs or other substances metabolized by CYP3A4 are administered concomitantly with sirolimus). Products include:
Plendil Extended-Release Tablets 651

Fenofibrate (Co-administration of sirolimus with cyclosporine in conjunction with fibrates should be monitored for the possible development of rhabdomyolysis; in clinical trials, the concurrent use of sirolimus and fibrates was well tolerated). Products include:
Antara Capsules 2723
Lofibra Capsules 1217
Tricor Tablets 523
Triglide Tablets 1165

Fentanyl (Care should be exercised when drugs or other substances metabolized by CYP3A4 are administered concomitantly with sirolimus). Products include:
Duragesic Transdermal System 2448

Fentanyl Citrate (Care should be exercised when drugs or other substances metabolized by CYP3A4 are administered concomitantly with sirolimus). Products include:
Actiq 993

Fluconazole (Sirolimus is extensively metabolized by the CYP3A4 isoenzyme; co-administration with inhibitors of CYP3A4, such as fluconazole, may decrease the metabolism of sirolimus and increase the plasma levels of sirolimus).
No products indexed under this heading.

Fludrocortisone Acetate (Sirolimus is extensively metabolized by the CYP3A4 isoenzyme in the gut wall and liver. Co-administration with inducers of CYP3A4 may increase the metabolism of sirolimus and decrease sirolimus levels. Co-administration with strong inducers of CYP3A4 is not recommended).
No products indexed under this heading.

Fluoxetine Hydrochloride (Sirolimus is extensively metabolized by the CYP3A4 isoenzyme in the gut wall and liver. Co-administration with inhibitors of CYP3A4 may decrease the metabolism of sirolimus and increase sirolimus levels. Co-administration with strong inducers of CYP3A4 is not recommended). Products include:
Prozac Pulvules and Liquid 1771
Symbyax Capsules 1788

Fluvastatin Sodium (Co-administration of sirolimus with cyclosporine in conjunction with HMG-CoA reductase inhibitors should be monitored for the possible development of rhabdomyolysis; in clinical trials, the concurrent use of sirolimus and HMG-CoA reductase inhibitors was well tolerated). Products include:
Lescol Capsules 2227
Lescol 2730
Lescol XL Tablets 2227

Fluvoxamine Maleate (Sirolimus is extensively metabolized by the CYP3A4 isoenzyme in the gut wall and liver. Co-administration with inhibitors of CYP3A4 may decrease the metabolism of sirolimus and increase sirolimus levels. Co-administration with strong inducers of CYP3A4 is not recommended).
No products indexed under this heading.

Fosamprenavir Calcium (Sirolimus is extensively metabolized by the CYP3A4 isoenzyme in the gut wall and liver. Co-administration with inhibitors of CYP3A4 may decrease the metabolism of sirolimus and increase sirolimus levels. Co-

administration with strong inducers of CYP3A4 is not recommended). Products include:

Lexiva Tablets 1473

Fosphenytoin Sodium (Sirolimus is extensively metabolized by the CYP3A4 isoenzyme; co-administration with inducers of CYP3A4, such as phenytoin, may increase the metabolism of sirolimus and decrease the plasma levels of sirolimus).

No products indexed under this heading.

Garlic Extract (Sirolimus is extensively metabolized by the CYP3A4 isoenzyme in the gut wall and liver. Co-administration with inducers of CYP3A4 may increase the metabolism of sirolimus and decrease sirolimus levels. Co-administration with strong inducers of CYP3A4 is not recommended).

No products indexed under this heading.

Garlic Oil (Sirolimus is extensively metabolized by the CYP3A4 isoenzyme in the gut wall and liver. Co-administration with inducers of CYP3A4 may increase the metabolism of sirolimus and decrease sirolimus levels. Co-administration with strong inducers of CYP3A4 is not recommended).

No products indexed under this heading.

Gemfibrozil (Co-administration of sirolimus with cyclosporine in conjunction with fibrates should be monitored for the possible development of rhabdomyolysis; in clinical trials, the concurrent use of sirolimus and fibrates was well tolerated).

No products indexed under this heading.

Haloperidol (Care should be exercised when drugs or other substances metabolized by CYP3A4 are administered concomitantly with sirolimus).

No products indexed under this heading.

Haloperidol Decanoate (Care should be exercised when drugs or other substances metabolized by CYP3A4 are administered concomitantly with sirolimus).

No products indexed under this heading.

Haloperidol Lactate (Care should be exercised when drugs or other substances metabolized by CYP3A4 are administered concomitantly with sirolimus).

No products indexed under this heading.

Hydrocortisone (Sirolimus is extensively metabolized by the CYP3A4 isoenzyme in the gut wall and liver. Co-administration with inducers of CYP3A4 may increase the metabolism of sirolimus and decrease sirolimus levels. Co-administration with strong inducers of CYP3A4 is not recommended). Products include:

Cortizone•5 Ointment 699
Cortizone•10 Creme 699
Cortizone•10 Ointment 699
Cortizone•10 Plus Creme 700
Cortizone•10 Maximum Strength Quick Shot Spray 700
Hydrocortone Tablets 1963
Preparation H Hydrocortisone Cream 748

Hydrocortisone Acetate (Sirolimus is extensively metabolized by the CYP3A4 isoenzyme in the gut wall and liver. Co-administration with inducers of CYP3A4 may increase the metabolism of sirolimus and decrease sirolimus levels. Co-administration with strong inducers of CYP3A4 is not recommended). Products include:

Analpram-HC 1136
Pramosone 1139
ProctoFoam-HC 3113
Tucks Anti-Itch Ointment 712
U-cort 1% Cream 3289

Hydrocortisone Butyrate (Sirolimus is extensively metabolized by the CYP3A4 isoenzyme in the gut wall and liver. Co-administration with inducers of CYP3A4 may increase the metabolism of sirolimus and decrease sirolimus levels. Co-administration with strong inducers of CYP3A4 is not recommended). Products include:

Locoid 1138
Locoid Lipocream Cream 1138

Hydrocortisone Cypionate (Sirolimus is extensively metabolized by the CYP3A4 isoenzyme in the gut wall and liver. Co-administration with inducers of CYP3A4 may increase the metabolism of sirolimus and decrease sirolimus levels. Co-administration with strong inducers of CYP3A4 is not recommended).

No products indexed under this heading.

Hydrocortisone Hemisuccinate (Sirolimus is extensively metabolized by the CYP3A4 isoenzyme in the gut wall and liver. Co-administration with inducers of CYP3A4 may increase the metabolism of sirolimus and decrease sirolimus levels. Co-administration with strong inducers of CYP3A4 is not recommended).

No products indexed under this heading.

Hydrocortisone Probutate (Sirolimus is extensively metabolized by the CYP3A4 isoenzyme in the gut wall and liver. Co-administration with inducers of CYP3A4 may increase the metabolism of sirolimus and decrease sirolimus levels. Co-administration with strong inducers of CYP3A4 is not recommended). Products include:

Pandel Cream, 0.1% 1017

Hydrocortisone Sodium Phosphate (Sirolimus is extensively metabolized by the CYP3A4 isoenzyme in the gut wall and liver. Co-administration with inducers of CYP3A4 may increase the metabolism of sirolimus and decrease sirolimus levels. Co-administration with strong inducers of CYP3A4 is not recommended).

No products indexed under this heading.

Hydrocortisone Sodium Succinate (Sirolimus is extensively metabolized by the CYP3A4 isoenzyme in the gut wall and liver. Co-administration with inducers of CYP3A4 may increase the metabolism of sirolimus and decrease sirolimus levels. Co-administration with strong inducers of CYP3A4 is not recommended).

No products indexed under this heading.

Hydrocortisone Valerate (Sirolimus is extensively metabolized by the CYP3A4 isoenzyme in the gut wall and liver. Co-administration with inducers of CYP3A4 may increase the metabolism of sirolimus and decrease sirolimus levels. Co-administration with strong inducers of CYP3A4 is not recommended).

No products indexed under this heading.

Hypericum (Potential for reduced sirolimus levels).

No products indexed under this heading.

Hypericum Perforatum (Sirolimus is extensively metabolized by the CYP3A4 isoenzyme in the gut wall and liver. Co-administration with inducers of CYP3A4 may increase the metabolism of sirolimus and decrease sirolimus levels. Co-administration with strong inducers of CYP3A4 is not recommended).

No products indexed under this heading.

Indinavir Sulfate (Sirolimus is extensively metabolized by the CYP3A4 isoenzyme in the gut wall and liver. Co-administration with inhibitors of CYP3A4 may decrease the metabolism of sirolimus and increase sirolimus levels. Co-administration with strong inducers of CYP3A4 is not recommended). Products include:

Crixivan Capsules 1918

Isoniazid (Sirolimus is extensively metabolized by the CYP3A4 isoenzyme in the gut wall and liver. Co-administration with inhibitors of CYP3A4 may decrease the metabolism of sirolimus and increase sirolimus levels. Co-administration with strong inducers of CYP3A4 is not recommended).

No products indexed under this heading.

Isradipine (Care should be exercised when drugs or other substances metabolized by CYP3A4 are administered concomitantly with sirolimus). Products include:

DynaCirc CR Tablets 2726

Itraconazole (Sirolimus is extensively metabolized by the CYP3A4 isoenzyme; co-administration with inhibitors of CYP3A4, such as itraconazole, may decrease the metabolism of sirolimus and increase the plasma levels of sirolimus).

No products indexed under this heading.

Ketoconazole (Multiple-dose ketoconazole administration significantly affected the rate and extent of absorption and sirolimus exposure; sirolimus should not be co-administered with ketoconazole). Products include:

Nizoral A-D Shampoo, 1% 1839
Nizoral 2% Shampoo 1838

Levonorgestrel (Care should be exercised when drugs or other substances metabolized by CYP3A4 are administered concomitantly with sirolimus). Products include:

Alesse-28 Tablets 3392
Climara Pro Transdermal System 800
Mirena Intrauterine System 810
Plan B Tablets 1068
Seasonale Tablets 1073
Triphasil-28 Tablets 3483

Lidocaine (Care should be exercised when drugs or other substances metabolized by CYP3A4 are administered concomitantly with sirolimus). Products include:

Lidoderm Patch 1107

Lidocaine Hydrochloride (Care should be exercised when drugs or other substances metabolized by CYP3A4 are administered concomitantly with sirolimus).

No products indexed under this heading.

Lopinavir (Sirolimus is extensively metabolized by the CYP3A4 isoenzyme in the gut wall and liver. Co-administration with inhibitors of CYP3A4 may decrease the metabolism of sirolimus and increase sirolimus levels. Co-administration with strong inducers of CYP3A4 is not recommended). Products include:

Kaletra 474

Loratadine (Sirolimus is extensively metabolized by the CYP3A4 isoenzyme in the gut wall and liver. Co-administration with inhibitors of CYP3A4 may decrease the metabolism of sirolimus and increase sirolimus levels. Co-administration with strong inducers of CYP3A4 is not recommended). Products include:

Alavert Allergy & Sinus D-12 Hour Tablets.. 743
Alavert 743
Children's Claritin 24 Hour Non-Drowsy Allergy Syrup 732
Claritin Non-Drowsy 24 Hour Tablets.. 731
Non-Drowsy Claritin Hives Relief Tablets.. 733
Claritin Reditabs 24 Hour Non-Drowsy Tablets 732
Claritin-D Non-Drowsy 12 Hour Tablets.. 731
Claritin-D Non-Drowsy 24 Hour Tablets.. 731
Children's Dimetapp ND Non-Drowsy Allergy Syrup 746
Triaminic Allerchews 684

Lovastatin (Co-administration of sirolimus with cyclosporine in conjunction with HMG-CoA reductase inhibitors should be monitored for the possible development of rhabdomyolysis; in clinical trials, the concurrent use of sirolimus and HMG-CoA reductase inhibitors was well tolerated). Products include:

Advicor Tablets 1694
Altoprev Extended-Release Tablets.. 1151
Mevacor Tablets 1996

Mephenytoin (Sirolimus is extensively metabolized by the CYP3A4 isoenzyme in the gut wall and liver. Co-administration with inducers of CYP3A4 may increase the metabolism of sirolimus and decrease sirolimus levels. Co-administration with strong inducers of CYP3A4 is not recommended).

No products indexed under this heading.

Mestranol (Care should be exercised when drugs or other substances metabolized by CYP3A4 are administered concomitantly with sirolimus).

No products indexed under this heading.

Methadone Hydrochloride (Care should be exercised when drugs or other substances metabolized by CYP3A4 are administered concomitantly with sirolimus).

No products indexed under this heading.

Methsuximide (Sirolimus is extensively metabolized by the CYP3A4 isoenzyme in the gut wall and liver. Co-administration with inducers of CYP3A4 may increase the metabolism of sirolimus and decrease sirolimus levels. Co-administration with strong inducers of CYP3A4 is not recommended).
No products indexed under this heading.

Methylprednisolone (Sirolimus is extensively metabolized by the CYP3A4 isoenzyme in the gut wall and liver. Co-administration with inducers of CYP3A4 may increase the metabolism of sirolimus and decrease sirolimus levels. Co-administration with strong inducers of CYP3A4 is not recommended).
No products indexed under this heading.

Methylprednisolone Acetate (Sirolimus is extensively metabolized by the CYP3A4 isoenzyme in the gut wall and liver. Co-administration with inducers of CYP3A4 may increase the metabolism of sirolimus and decrease sirolimus levels. Co-administration with strong inducers of CYP3A4 is not recommended). Products include:
Depo-Medrol Injectable Suspension 2615
Depo-Medrol Single-Dose Vial 2617

Methylprednisolone Sodium Succinate (Sirolimus is extensively metabolized by the CYP3A4 isoenzyme in the gut wall and liver. Co-administration with inducers of CYP3A4 may increase the metabolism of sirolimus and decrease sirolimus levels. Co-administration with strong inducers of CYP3A4 is not recommended).
No products indexed under this heading.

Metoclopramide Hydrochloride (Sirolimus is extensively metabolized by the CYP3A4 isoenzyme; co-administration with inhibitors of CYP3A4, such as metoclopramide, may decrease the metabolism of sirolimus and increase the plasma levels of sirolimus).
No products indexed under this heading.

Metronidazole (Sirolimus is extensively metabolized by the CYP3A4 isoenzyme in the gut wall and liver. Co-administration with inhibitors of CYP3A4 may decrease the metabolism of sirolimus and increase sirolimus levels. Co-administration with strong inducers of CYP3A4 is not recommended). Products include:
Metrogel 1% 1212
MetroGel-Vaginal Gel 1822
Noritate Cream, 1% 1051

Metronidazole Benzoate (Sirolimus is extensively metabolized by the CYP3A4 isoenzyme in the gut wall and liver. Co-administration with inhibitors of CYP3A4 may decrease the metabolism of sirolimus and increase sirolimus levels. Co-administration with strong inducers of CYP3A4 is not recommended).
No products indexed under this heading.

Metronidazole Hydrochloride (Sirolimus is extensively metabolized by the CYP3A4 isoenzyme in the gut wall and liver. Co-administration with inhibitors of CYP3A4 may decrease the metabolism of sirolimus and increase sirolimus levels. Co-administration with strong inducers of CYP3A4 is not recommended).
No products indexed under this heading.

Miconazole (Sirolimus is extensively metabolized by the CYP3A4 isoenzyme in the gut wall and liver. Co-administration with inhibitors of CYP3A4 may decrease the metabolism of sirolimus and increase sirolimus levels. Co-administration with strong inducers of CYP3A4 is not recommended).
No products indexed under this heading.

Miconazole Nitrate (Sirolimus is extensively metabolized by the CYP3A4 isoenzyme in the gut wall and liver. Co-administration with inhibitors of CYP3A4 may decrease the metabolism of sirolimus and increase sirolimus levels. Co-administration with strong inducers of CYP3A4 is not recommended). Products include:
Desenex ..... ▣674
Desenex Jock Itch Spray Powder ..... ▣674

Midazolam Hydrochloride (Care should be exercised when drugs or other substances metabolized by CYP3A4 are administered concomitantly with sirolimus).
No products indexed under this heading.

Modafinil (Sirolimus is extensively metabolized by the CYP3A4 isoenzyme in the gut wall and liver. Co-administration with inducers of CYP3A4 may increase the metabolism of sirolimus and decrease sirolimus levels. Co-administration with strong inducers of CYP3A4 is not recommended). Products include:
Provigil Tablets 1002

Nefazodone Hydrochloride (Sirolimus is extensively metabolized by the CYP3A4 isoenzyme in the gut wall and liver. Co-administration with inhibitors of CYP3A4 may decrease the metabolism of sirolimus and increase sirolimus levels. Co-administration with strong inducers of CYP3A4 is not recommended).
No products indexed under this heading.

Nelfinavir Mesylate (Sirolimus is extensively metabolized by the CYP3A4 isoenzyme in the gut wall and liver. Co-administration with inhibitors of CYP3A4 may decrease the metabolism of sirolimus and increase sirolimus levels. Co-administration with strong inducers of CYP3A4 is not recommended). Products include:
Viracept 2556

Nevirapine (Sirolimus is extensively metabolized by the CYP3A4 isoenzyme in the gut wall and liver. Co-administration with inhibitors of CYP3A4 may decrease the metabolism of sirolimus and increase sirolimus levels. Co-administration with strong inducers of CYP3A4 is not recommended). Products include:
Viramune Oral Suspension 903
Viramune Tablets 903

Niacinamide (Sirolimus is extensively metabolized by the CYP3A4 isoenzyme in the gut wall and liver. Co-administration with inhibitors of CYP3A4 may decrease the metabolism of sirolimus and increase sirolimus levels. Co-administration with strong inducers of CYP3A4 is not recommended).
No products indexed under this heading.

Nicardipine Hydrochloride (Sirolimus is extensively metabolized by the CYP3A4 isoenzyme; co-administration with inhibitors of CYP3A4, such as nicardipine, may decrease the metabolism of sirolimus and increase the plasma levels of sirolimus). Products include:
Cardene I.V. 1129

Nicotinamide (Sirolimus is extensively metabolized by the CYP3A4 isoenzyme in the gut wall and liver. Co-administration with inhibitors of CYP3A4 may decrease the metabolism of sirolimus and increase sirolimus levels. Co-administration with strong inducers of CYP3A4 is not recommended). Products include:
Nicomide Tablets 3190

Nifedipine (Sirolimus is extensively metabolized by the CYP3A4 isoenzyme in the gut wall and liver. Co-administration with inhibitors of CYP3A4 may decrease the metabolism of sirolimus and increase sirolimus levels. Co-administration with strong inducers of CYP3A4 is not recommended). Products include:
Adalat CC Tablets 2978

Nimodipine (Care should be exercised when drugs or other substances metabolized by CYP3A4 are administered concomitantly with sirolimus). Products include:
Nimotop Capsules 774

Nisoldipine (Care should be exercised when drugs or other substances metabolized by CYP3A4 are administered concomitantly with sirolimus). Products include:
Sular Tablets 1163

Nitrendipine (Care should be exercised when drugs or other substances metabolized by CYP3A4 are administered concomitantly with sirolimus).
No products indexed under this heading.

Norethindrone (Care should be exercised when drugs or other substances metabolized by CYP3A4 are administered concomitantly with sirolimus). Products include:
Ortho Micronor Tablets 2411

Norethindrone Acetate (Care should be exercised when drugs or other substances metabolized by CYP3A4 are administered concomitantly with sirolimus). Products include:
Activella Tablets 2311
Aygestin Tablets 1062
CombiPatch Transdermal System 2180

Norfloxacin (Sirolimus is extensively metabolized by the CYP3A4 isoenzyme in the gut wall and liver. Co-administration with inhibitors of CYP3A4 may decrease the metabolism of sirolimus and increase sirolimus levels. Co-administration with strong inducers of CYP3A4 is not recommended). Products include:
Noroxin Tablets 2009

Norgestrel (Care should be exercised when drugs or other substances metabolized by CYP3A4 are administered concomitantly with sirolimus). Products include:
Lo/Ovral-28 Tablets 3423

Omeprazole (Sirolimus is extensively metabolized by the CYP3A4 isoenzyme in the gut wall and liver. Co-administration with inhibitors of CYP3A4 may decrease the metabolism of sirolimus and increase sirolimus levels. Co-administration with strong inducers of CYP3A4 is not recommended). Products include:
Zegerid Powder for Oral Solution 2972

Ondansetron (Care should be exercised when drugs or other substances metabolized by CYP3A4 are administered concomitantly with sirolimus). Products include:
Zofran ODT Orally Disintegrating Tablets 1613

Ondansetron Hydrochloride (Care should be exercised when drugs or other substances metabolized by CYP3A4 are administered concomitantly with sirolimus). Products include:
Zofran Injection 1607
Zofran 1613

Oxcarbazepine (Sirolimus is extensively metabolized by the CYP3A4 isoenzyme in the gut wall and liver. Co-administration with inducers of CYP3A4 may increase the metabolism of sirolimus and decrease sirolimus levels. Co-administration with strong inducers of CYP3A4 is not recommended). Products include:
Trileptal Oral Suspension 2281
Trileptal Tablets 2281

Paclitaxel (Care should be exercised when drugs or other substances metabolized by CYP3A4 are administered concomitantly with sirolimus).
No products indexed under this heading.

Paroxetine Hydrochloride (Sirolimus is extensively metabolized by the CYP3A4 isoenzyme in the gut wall and liver. Co-administration with inhibitors of CYP3A4 may decrease the metabolism of sirolimus and increase sirolimus levels. Co-administration with strong inducers of CYP3A4 is not recommended). Products include:
Paxil CR Controlled-Release Tablets 1509
Paxil 1501

Phenobarbital (Sirolimus is extensively metabolized by the CYP3A4 isoenzyme; co-administration with inducers of CYP3A4, such as phenobarbital, may increase the metabolism of sirolimus and decrease the plasma levels of sirolimus).
No products indexed under this heading.

Phenobarbital Sodium (Sirolimus is extensively metabolized by the CYP3A4 isoenzyme in the gut wall and liver. Co-administration with inducers of CYP3A4 may increase the metabolism of sirolimus and decrease sirolimus levels. Co-administration with strong inducers of CYP3A4 is not recommended).
No products indexed under this heading.

Phenytoin (Sirolimus is extensively metabolized by the CYP3A4 isoenzyme; co-administration with inducers of CYP3A4, such as phenytoin, may increase the metabolism of sirolimus and decrease the plasma levels of sirolimus).
No products indexed under this heading.

Phenytoin Sodium (Sirolimus is extensively metabolized by the CYP3A4 isoenzyme; co-administration with inducers of CYP3A4, such as phenytoin, may increase the metabolism of sirolimus and decrease the plasma levels of sirolimus). Products include:
Phenytek Capsules **2153**

Pimozide (Care should be exercised when drugs or other substances metabolized by CYP3A4 are administered concomitantly with sirolimus). Products include:
Orap Tablets **1220**

Polyestradiol Phosphate (Care should be exercised when drugs or other substances metabolized by CYP3A4 are administered concomitantly with sirolimus).
No products indexed under this heading.

Pravastatin Sodium (Co-administration of sirolimus with cyclosporine in conjunction with HMG-CoA reductase inhibitors should be monitored for the possible development of rhabdomyolysis; in clinical trials, the concurrent use of sirolimus and HMG-CoA reductase inhibitors was well tolerated). Products include:
Pravachol Tablets **943**

Prednisolone Acetate (Sirolimus is extensively metabolized by the CYP3A4 isoenzyme in the gut wall and liver. Co-administration with inducers of CYP3A4 may increase the metabolism of sirolimus and decrease sirolimus levels. Co-administration with strong inducers of CYP3A4 is not recommended). Products include:
Blephamide Ophthalmic Ointment **563**
Blephamide Ophthalmic Suspension.................................. **564**
Poly-Pred Liquifilm Ophthalmic Suspension .... ⊙ **231**
Pred Forte Ophthalmic Suspension .... ⊙ **233**
Pred Mild Sterile Ophthalmic Suspension .... ⊙ **236**
Pred-G Ophthalmic Suspension ...... ⊙ **234**
Pred-G Sterile Ophthalmic Ointment.................................... ⊙ **235**

Prednisolone Sodium Phosphate (Sirolimus is extensively metabolized by the CYP3A4 isoenzyme in the gut wall and liver. Co-administration with inducers of CYP3A4 may increase the metabolism of sirolimus and decrease sirolimus levels. Co-administration with strong inducers of CYP3A4 is not recommended). Products include:
Pediapred Oral Solution **3319**

Prednisolone Tebutate (Sirolimus is extensively metabolized by the CYP3A4 isoenzyme in the gut wall and liver. Co-administration with inducers of CYP3A4 may increase the metabolism of sirolimus and decrease sirolimus levels. Co-administration with strong inducers of CYP3A4 is not recommended).
No products indexed under this heading.

Prednisone (Sirolimus is extensively metabolized by the CYP3A4 isoenzyme in the gut wall and liver. Co-administration with inducers of CYP3A4 may increase the metabolism of sirolimus and decrease sirolimus levels. Co-administration with strong inducers of CYP3A4 is not recommended).
No products indexed under this heading.

Primidone (Sirolimus is extensively metabolized by the CYP3A4 isoenzyme in the gut wall and liver. Co-administration with inducers of CYP3A4 may increase the metabolism of sirolimus and decrease sirolimus levels. Co-administration with strong inducers of CYP3A4 is not recommended).
No products indexed under this heading.

Propoxyphene Hydrochloride (Sirolimus is extensively metabolized by the CYP3A4 isoenzyme in the gut wall and liver. Co-administration with inhibitors of CYP3A4 may decrease the metabolism of sirolimus and increase sirolimus levels. Co-administration with strong inducers of CYP3A4 is not recommended).
No products indexed under this heading.

Propoxyphene Napsylate (Sirolimus is extensively metabolized by the CYP3A4 isoenzyme in the gut wall and liver. Co-administration with inhibitors of CYP3A4 may decrease the metabolism of sirolimus and increase sirolimus levels. Co-administration with strong inducers of CYP3A4 is not recommended). Products include:
Darvocet A 500 Tablets **3497**

Quinidine (Sirolimus is extensively metabolized by the CYP3A4 isoenzyme in the gut wall and liver. Co-administration with inhibitors of CYP3A4 may decrease the metabolism of sirolimus and increase sirolimus levels. Co-administration with strong inducers of CYP3A4 is not recommended).
No products indexed under this heading.

Quinidine Gluconate (Care should be exercised when drugs or other substances metabolized by CYP3A4 are administered concomitantly with sirolimus).
No products indexed under this heading.

Quinidine Hydrochloride (Sirolimus is extensively metabolized by the CYP3A4 isoenzyme in the gut wall and liver. Co-administration with inhibitors of CYP3A4 may decrease the metabolism of sirolimus and increase sirolimus levels. Co-administration with strong inducers of CYP3A4 is not recommended).
No products indexed under this heading.

Quinidine Polygalacturonate (Sirolimus is extensively metabolized by the CYP3A4 isoenzyme in the gut wall and liver. Co-administration with inhibitors of CYP3A4 may decrease the metabolism of sirolimus and increase sirolimus levels. Co-administration with strong inducers of CYP3A4 is not recommended).
No products indexed under this heading.

Quinidine Sulfate (Sirolimus is extensively metabolized by the CYP3A4 isoenzyme in the gut wall and liver. Co-administration with inhibitors of CYP3A4 may decrease the metabolism of sirolimus and increase sirolimus levels. Co-administration with strong inducers of CYP3A4 is not recommended).
No products indexed under this heading.

Quinine (Sirolimus is extensively metabolized by the CYP3A4 isoenzyme in the gut wall and liver. Co-administration with inhibitors of CYP3A4 may decrease the metabolism of sirolimus and increase sirolimus levels. Co-administration with strong inducers of CYP3A4 is not recommended).
No products indexed under this heading.

Quinine Sulfate (Sirolimus is extensively metabolized by the CYP3A4 isoenzyme in the gut wall and liver. Co-administration with inhibitors of CYP3A4 may decrease the metabolism of sirolimus and increase sirolimus levels. Co-administration with strong inducers of CYP3A4 is not recommended).
No products indexed under this heading.

Quinupristin (Sirolimus is extensively metabolized by the CYP3A4 isoenzyme in the gut wall and liver. Co-administration with inhibitors of CYP3A4 may decrease the metabolism of sirolimus and increase sirolimus levels. Co-administration with strong inducers of CYP3A4 is not recommended). Products include:
Synercid I.V. **1690**

Ranitidine Bismuth Citrate (Sirolimus is extensively metabolized by the CYP3A4 isoenzyme in the gut wall and liver. Co-administration with inhibitors of CYP3A4 may decrease the metabolism of sirolimus and increase sirolimus levels. Co-administration with strong inducers of CYP3A4 is not recommended).
No products indexed under this heading.

Ranitidine Hydrochloride (Sirolimus is extensively metabolized by the CYP3A4 isoenzyme in the gut wall and liver. Co-administration with inhibitors of CYP3A4 may decrease the metabolism of sirolimus and increase sirolimus levels. Co-administration with strong inducers of CYP3A4 is not recommended). Products include:
Zantac **1597**
Zantac Injection **1593**
Zantac 75 Tablets .... ▣ **715**
Zantac 150 Maximum Strength Tablets....................................... ▣ **715**
Zantac Injection Pharmacy Bulk Package..................................... **1595**

Rifabutin (Sirolimus is extensively metabolized by the CYP3A4 isoenzyme; co-administration with inducers of CYP3A4, such as rifabutin, may increase the metabolism of sirolimus and decrease the plasma levels of sirolimus).
No products indexed under this heading.

Rifampicin (Sirolimus is extensively metabolized by the CYP3A4 isoenzyme in the gut wall and liver. Co-administration with inducers of CYP3A4 may increase the metabolism of sirolimus and decrease sirolimus levels. Co-administration with strong inducers of CYP3A4 is not recommended).
No products indexed under this heading.

Rifampin (Pretreatment with multiple doses of rifampin greatly increased sirolimus oral dose clearance resulting in mean decrease in AUC and Cmax. Co-administration of sirolimus oral solution or tablets and rifampin is not recommended and alternative therapeutic agents with less enzyme induction potential than rifampin should be considered).
No products indexed under this heading.

Rifapentine (Sirolimus is extensively metabolized by the CYP3A4 isoenzyme; co-administration with inducers of CYP3A4, such as rifapentine, may increase the metabolism of sirolimus and decrease the plasma levels of sirolimus).
No products indexed under this heading.

Ritonavir (Sirolimus is extensively metabolized by the CYP3A4 isoenzyme in the gut wall and liver. Co-administration with inhibitors of CYP3A4 may decrease the metabolism of sirolimus and increase sirolimus levels. Co-administration with strong inducers of CYP3A4 is not recommended). Products include:
Kaletra **474**
Norvir **499**

Saquinavir (Sirolimus is extensively metabolized by the CYP3A4 isoenzyme in the gut wall and liver. Co-administration with inhibitors of CYP3A4 may decrease the metabolism of sirolimus and increase sirolimus levels. Co-administration with strong inducers of CYP3A4 is not recommended).
No products indexed under this heading.

Saquinavir Mesylate (Sirolimus is extensively metabolized by the CYP3A4 isoenzyme in the gut wall and liver. Co-administration with inhibitors of CYP3A4 may decrease the metabolism of sirolimus and increase sirolimus levels. Co-administration with strong inducers of CYP3A4 is not recommended). Products include:
Invirase **2776**

Sertraline Hydrochloride (Sirolimus is extensively metabolized by the CYP3A4 isoenzyme in the gut wall and liver. Co-administration with inhibitors of CYP3A4 may decrease the metabolism of sirolimus and increase sirolimus levels. Co-administration with strong inducers of CYP3A4 is not recommended). Products include:
Zoloft **2581**

Sildenafil Citrate (Care should be exercised when drugs or other substances metabolized by CYP3A4 are administered concomitantly with sirolimus). Products include:
Revatio Tablets **2541**
Viagra Tablets **2552**

Simvastatin (Co-administration of sirolimus with cyclosporine in conjunction with HMG-CoA reductase inhibitors should be monitored for

the possible development of rhabdomyolysis; in clinical trials, the concurrent use of sirolimus and HMG-CoA reductase inhibitors was well tolerated). Products include:
Vytorin 10/10 Tablets 2084
Vytorin 10/10 Tablets 3092
Vytorin 10/20 Tablets 2084
Vytorin 10/20 Tablets 3092
Vytorin 10/40 Tablets 3092
Vytorin 10/40 Tablets 2084
Vytorin 10/80 Tablets 2084
Vytorin 10/80 Tablets 3092
Zocor Tablets 2078

Sulfinpyrazone (Sirolimus is extensively metabolized by the CYP3A4 isoenzyme in the gut wall and liver. Co-administration with inducers of CYP3A4 may increase the metabolism of sirolimus and decrease sirolimus levels. Co-administration with strong inducers of CYP3A4 is not recommended).
No products indexed under this heading.

Tacrolimus (Co-administration was associated with excess mortality and graft loss in de novo liver transplant recipients; combination use is associated with hepatic artery thrombosis (HAT); the safety and efficacy of Rapamune has not been established in liver transplant patients and, therefore, such use is not recommended). Products include:
Prograf Capsules and Injection 624
Protopic Ointment 629

Tamoxifen Citrate (Care should be exercised when drugs or other substances metabolized by CYP3A4 are administered concomitantly with sirolimus).
No products indexed under this heading.

Telithromycin (Sirolimus is extensively metabolized by the CYP3A4 isoenzyme in the gut wall and liver. Co-administration with inhibitors of CYP3A4 may decrease the metabolism of sirolimus and increase sirolimus levels. Co-administration with strong inducers of CYP3A4 is not recommended). Products include:
Ketek Tablets 2920

Theophylline (Sirolimus is extensively metabolized by the CYP3A4 isoenzyme in the gut wall and liver. Co-administration with inducers of CYP3A4 may increase the metabolism of sirolimus and decrease sirolimus levels. Co-administration with strong inducers of CYP3A4 is not recommended).
No products indexed under this heading.

Tiagabine Hydrochloride (Care should be exercised when drugs or other substances metabolized by CYP3A4 are administered concomitantly with sirolimus). Products include:
Gabitril Tablets 998

Tolterodine Tartrate (Care should be exercised when drugs or other substances metabolized by CYP3A4 are administered concomitantly with sirolimus). Products include:
Detrol Tablets 2626
Detrol LA Capsules 2629

Trazodone Hydrochloride (Care should be exercised when drugs or other substances metabolized by CYP3A4 are administered concomitantly with sirolimus).
No products indexed under this heading.

Triamcinolone (Sirolimus is extensively metabolized by the CYP3A4 isoenzyme in the gut wall and liver. Co-administration with inducers of CYP3A4 may increase the metabolism of sirolimus and decrease sirolimus levels. Co-administration with strong inducers of CYP3A4 is not recommended).
No products indexed under this heading.

Triamcinolone Acetonide (Sirolimus is extensively metabolized by the CYP3A4 isoenzyme in the gut wall and liver. Co-administration with inducers of CYP3A4 may increase the metabolism of sirolimus and decrease sirolimus levels. Co-administration with strong inducers of CYP3A4 is not recommended). Products include:
Azmacort Inhalation Aerosol 1701
Nasacort HFA Inhalation Aerosol 2939
Nasacort AQ Nasal Spray 2937

Triamcinolone Diacetate (Sirolimus is extensively metabolized by the CYP3A4 isoenzyme in the gut wall and liver. Co-administration with inducers of CYP3A4 may increase the metabolism of sirolimus and decrease sirolimus levels. Co-administration with strong inducers of CYP3A4 is not recommended).
No products indexed under this heading.

Triamcinolone Hexacetonide (Sirolimus is extensively metabolized by the CYP3A4 isoenzyme in the gut wall and liver. Co-administration with inducers of CYP3A4 may increase the metabolism of sirolimus and decrease sirolimus levels. Co-administration with strong inducers of CYP3A4 is not recommended).
No products indexed under this heading.

Triazolam (Care should be exercised when drugs or other substances metabolized by CYP3A4 are administered concomitantly with sirolimus).
No products indexed under this heading.

Troglitazone (Sirolimus is extensively metabolized by the CYP3A4 isoenzyme in the gut wall and liver. Co-administration with inhibitors of CYP3A4 may decrease the metabolism of sirolimus and increase sirolimus levels. Co-administration with strong inducers of CYP3A4 is not recommended).
No products indexed under this heading.

Troleandomycin (Sirolimus is extensively metabolized by the CYP3A4 isoenzyme; co-administration with inhibitors of CYP3A4, such as troleandomycin, may decrease the metabolism of sirolimus and increase the plasma levels of sirolimus).
No products indexed under this heading.

Valproate Sodium (Sirolimus is extensively metabolized by the CYP3A4 isoenzyme in the gut wall and liver. Co-administration with inhibitors of CYP3A4 may decrease the metabolism of sirolimus and increase sirolimus levels. Co-administration with strong inducers of CYP3A4 is not recommended). Products include:
Depacon Injection 412

Verapamil Hydrochloride (Sirolimus is extensively metabolized by the CYP3A4 isoenzyme; co-administration with inhibitors of CYP3A4, such as verapamil, may decrease the metabolism of sirolimus and increase the plasma levels of sirolimus. Concentrations of sirolimus should be monitored and a dose adjustment may be necessary when co-administered with verapamil). Products include:
Covera-HS Tablets 3135
Tarka Tablets 519
Verelan PM Capsules 3120

Vinblastine Sulfate (Care should be exercised when drugs or other substances metabolized by CYP3A4 are administered concomitantly with sirolimus).
No products indexed under this heading.

Vincristine Sulfate (Care should be exercised when drugs or other substances metabolized by CYP3A4 are administered concomitantly with sirolimus).
No products indexed under this heading.

Voriconazole (Sirolimus is extensively metabolized by the CYP3A4 isoenzyme in the gut wall and liver. Co-administration with inhibitors of CYP3A4 may decrease the metabolism of sirolimus and increase sirolimus levels. Co-administration with strong inducers of CYP3A4 is not recommended). Products include:
VFEND I.V. 2543
VFEND Oral Suspension 2543
VFEND Tablets 2543

Warfarin Sodium (Care should be exercised when drugs or other substances metabolized by CYP3A4 are administered concomitantly with sirolimus). Products include:
Coumadin for Injection 932
Coumadin Tablets 932

Zafirlukast (Sirolimus is extensively metabolized by the CYP3A4 isoenzyme in the gut wall and liver. Co-administration with inhibitors of CYP3A4 may decrease the metabolism of sirolimus and increase sirolimus levels. Co-administration with strong inducers of CYP3A4 is not recommended). Products include:
Accolate Tablets 663

Zileuton (Sirolimus is extensively metabolized by the CYP3A4 isoenzyme in the gut wall and liver. Co-administration with inhibitors of CYP3A4 may decrease the metabolism of sirolimus and increase sirolimus levels. Co-administration with strong inducers of CYP3A4 is not recommended).
No products indexed under this heading.

Food Interactions

Food, unspecified (A high-fat meal altered the bioavailability characteristics of sirolimus compared to fasting; 34% decrease in the peak blood sirolimus concentration, a 3.5-fold increase in the time-to-peak concentration and 35% increase in total exposure; to minimize variability, Rapamune should be taken consistently with or without food).

Grapefruit (Sirolimus is extensively metabolized by the CYP3A4 isoenzyme in the gut wall and liver. Co-administration with inhibitors of CYP3A4 may decrease the metabolism of sirolimus and increase sirolimus levels. Co-administration with strong inducers of CYP3A4 is not recommended).

Grapefruit Juice (Induces CYP3A4-mediated metabolism of sirolimus; Rapamune must not be administered or diluted with grapefruit juice).

RAPTIVA FOR INJECTION

(Efalizumab) 1247
May interact with immunosuppressive agents and vaccines, live. Compounds in these categories include:

Azathioprine (Patients receiving other immunosuppressive agents should not receive concurrent therapy with efalizumab because of the possibility of increased risk of infections and malignancies). Products include:
Azasan Tablets 2844

Basiliximab (Patients receiving other immunosuppressive agents should not receive concurrent therapy with efalizumab because of the possibility of increased risk of infections and malignancies). Products include:
Simulect for Injection 2268

BCG Vaccine (Acellular, live and live-attenuated vaccines should not be administered during efalizumab treatment).
No products indexed under this heading.

Cyclosporine (Patients receiving other immunosuppressive agents should not receive concurrent therapy with efalizumab because of the possibility of increased risk of infections and malignancies). Products include:
Gengraf Capsules 458
Neoral Soft Gelatin Capsules 2247
Neoral Oral Solution 2247
Restasis Ophthalmic Emulsion 570
Sandimmune 2259

Measles, Mumps & Rubella Virus Vaccine, Live (Acellular, live and live-attenuated vaccines should not be administered during efalizumab treatment). Products include:
M-M-R II 1980

Measles & Rubella Virus Vaccine Live (Acellular, live and live-attenuated vaccines should not be administered during efalizumab treatment).
No products indexed under this heading.

Measles Virus Vaccine Live (Acellular, live and live-attenuated vaccines should not be administered during efalizumab treatment). Products include:
Attenuvax 1889

Mumps Virus Vaccine, Live (Acellular, live and live-attenuated vaccines should not be administered during efalizumab treatment). Products include:
Mumpsvax 2005

Muromonab-CD3 (Patients receiving other immunosuppressive agents should not receive concurrent therapy with efalizumab because of the possibility of increased risk of infections and malignancies). Products include:
Orthoclone OKT3 Sterile Solution 2370

Mycophenolate Mofetil (Patients receiving other immunosuppressive agents should not receive concurrent therapy with efalizumab because of the possibility of increased risk of infections and malignancies). Products include:
CellCept Capsules 2751
CellCept Oral Suspension 2751

CellCept Tablets 2751

Poliovirus Vaccine, Live, Oral, Trivalent, Types 1,2,3 (Sabin) (Acellular, live and live-attenuated vaccines should not be administered during efalizumab treatment).
No products indexed under this heading.

Rotavirus Vaccine, Live, Oral, Tetravalent (Acellular, live and live-attenuated vaccines should not be administered during efalizumab treatment).
No products indexed under this heading.

Rubella & Mumps Virus Vaccine Live (Acellular, live and live-attenuated vaccines should not be administered during efalizumab treatment).
No products indexed under this heading.

Rubella Virus Vaccine Live (Acellular, live and live-attenuated vaccines should not be administered during efalizumab treatment). Products include:
Meruvax II 1994

Sirolimus (Patients receiving other immunosuppressive agents should not receive concurrent therapy with efalizumab because of the possibility of increased risk of infections and malignancies). Products include:
Rapamune Oral Solution and Tablets 3472

Smallpox Vaccine (Acellular, live and live-attenuated vaccines should not be administered during efalizumab treatment).
No products indexed under this heading.

Tacrolimus (Patients receiving other immunosuppressive agents should not receive concurrent therapy with efalizumab because of the possibility of increased risk of infections and malignancies). Products include:
Prograf Capsules and Injection 624
Protopic Ointment 629

Typhoid Vaccine (Acellular, live and live-attenuated vaccines should not be administered during efalizumab treatment).
No products indexed under this heading.

Varicella Virus Vaccine Live (Acellular, live and live-attenuated vaccines should not be administered during efalizumab treatment). Products include:
Varivax 2070

Yellow Fever Vaccine (Acellular, live and live-attenuated vaccines should not be administered during efalizumab treatment).
No products indexed under this heading.

RAZADYNE ER EXTENDED-RELEASE CAPSULES

(Galantamine Hydrobromide) 2434
See Razadyne Tablets

RAZADYNE ORAL SOLUTION

(Galantamine Hydrobromide) 2434
See Razadyne Tablets

RAZADYNE TABLETS

(Galantamine Hydrobromide) 2434
May interact with anticholinergics, cholinergic agents, erythromycin, neuromuscular blocking agents, non-steroidal anti-inflammatory agents, and certain other agents. Compounds in these categories include:

Atracurium Besylate (Galantamine is a cholinesterase inhibitor; co-administration with neuromuscular blocking agents may exaggerate neuromuscular blockade).
No products indexed under this heading.

Atropine Sulfate (Galantamine has the potential to interfere with the activity of anticholinergic agents).
No products indexed under this heading.

Belladonna Alkaloids (Galantamine has the potential to interfere with the activity of anticholinergic agents). Products include:
Hyland's Teething Tablets 736

Benztropine Mesylate (Galantamine has the potential to interfere with the activity of anticholinergic agents). Products include:
Cogentin Injection 1903

Bethanechol Chloride (Co-administration with other cholinesterase inhibitors or cholinergic agonists may result in a synergistic effect). Products include:
Urecholine Tablets 2349

Biperiden Hydrochloride (Galantamine has the potential to interfere with the activity of anticholinergic agents).
No products indexed under this heading.

Celecoxib (Cholinomimetics, such as galantamine, may be expected to increase gastric acid secretion; therefore, co-administration in patients with increased risk of developing gastric ulcers or bleeding, such as patients on NSAIDs, should be closely monitored). Products include:
Celebrex Capsules 3130

Cevimeline Hydrochloride (Co-administration with other cholinesterase inhibitors or cholinergic agonists may result in a synergistic effect). Products include:
Evoxac Capsules 1042

Cimetidine (Co-administration with cimetidine has resulted in increased bioavailability galantamine by approximately 16%). Products include:
Tagamet HB 200 Tablets 637
Tagamet Tablets 1547

Cimetidine Hydrochloride (Co-administration with cimetidine has resulted in increased bioavailability galantamine by approximately 16%).
No products indexed under this heading.

Cisatracurium Besylate (Galantamine is a cholinesterase inhibitor; co-administration with neuromuscular blocking agents may exaggerate neuromuscular blockade). Products include:
Nimbex Injection 494

Clidinium Bromide (Galantamine has the potential to interfere with the activity of anticholinergic agents).
No products indexed under this heading.

Diclofenac Potassium (Cholinomimetics, such as galantamine, may be expected to increase gastric acid secretion; therefore, co-administration in patients with increased risk of developing gastric ulcers or bleeding, such as patients on NSAIDs, should be closely monitored). Products include:
Cataflam Tablets 2173

Diclofenac Sodium (Cholinomimetics, such as galantamine, may be expected to increase gastric acid secretion; therefore, co-administration in patients with increased risk of developing gastric ulcers or bleeding, such as patients on NSAIDs, should be closely monitored). Products include:
Arthrotec Tablets 3126
Voltaren Ophthalmic Solution 2300
Voltaren Tablets 2298
Voltaren-XR Tablets 2301

Dicyclomine Hydrochloride (Galantamine has the potential to interfere with the activity of anticholinergic agents). Products include:
Bentyl Capsules 724
Bentyl Injection 724
Bentyl Syrup 724
Bentyl Tablets 724

Digoxin (Co-administration in a healthy subject has resulted in 2nd and 3rd degree heart block and bradycardia). Products include:
Digitek Tablets 2146
Lanoxicaps Capsules 1458
Lanoxin Injection 1462
Lanoxin Tablets 1468
Lanoxin Injection Pediatric 1465

Donepezil Hydrochloride (Co-administration with other cholinesterase inhibitors or cholinergic agonists may result in a synergistic effect). Products include:
Aricept Tablets 1086
Aricept ODT Tablets 1086

Doxacurium Chloride (Galantamine is a cholinesterase inhibitor; co-administration with neuromuscular blocking agents may exaggerate neuromuscular blockade).
No products indexed under this heading.

Edrophonium Chloride (Co-administration with other cholinesterase inhibitors or cholinergic agonists may result in a synergistic effect).
No products indexed under this heading.

Erythromycin (Co-administration with a moderate inhibitor of CYP3A4, such as erythromycin, increases the AUC of galantamine by 10%). Products include:
Erygel Topical Gel 2096
Ery-Tab Tablets 447
Erythromycin Base Filmtab Tablets 454
Erythromycin Delayed-Release Capsules, USP 456
PCE Dispertab Tablets 510

Erythromycin Estolate (Co-administration with a moderate inhibitor of CYP3A4, such as erythromycin, increases the AUC of galantamine by 10%).
No products indexed under this heading.

Erythromycin Ethylsuccinate (Co-administration with a moderate inhibitor of CYP3A4, such as erythromycin, increases the AUC of galantamine by 10%). Products include:
E.E.S. 449
EryPed 445

Erythromycin Gluceptate (Co-administration with a moderate inhibitor of CYP3A4, such as erythromycin, increases the AUC of galantamine by 10%).
No products indexed under this heading.

Erythromycin Lactobionate (Co-administration with a moderate inhibitor of CYP3A4, such as erythromycin, increases the AUC of galantamine by 10%).
No products indexed under this heading.

Erythromycin Stearate (Co-administration with a moderate inhibitor of CYP3A4, such as erythromycin, increases the AUC of galantamine by 10%). Products include:
Erythrocin Stearate Filmtab Tablets 452

Etodolac (Cholinomimetics, such as galantamine, may be expected to increase gastric acid secretion; therefore, co-administration in patients with increased risk of developing gastric ulcers or bleeding, such as patients on NSAIDs, should be closely monitored).
No products indexed under this heading.

Fenoprofen Calcium (Cholinomimetics, such as galantamine, may be expected to increase gastric acid secretion; therefore, co-administration in patients with increased risk of developing gastric ulcers or bleeding, such as patients on NSAIDs, should be closely monitored). Products include:
Nalfon Capsules 2504

Flurbiprofen (Cholinomimetics, such as galantamine, may be expected to increase gastric acid secretion; therefore, co-administration in patients with increased risk of developing gastric ulcers or bleeding, such as patients on NSAIDs, should be closely monitored).
No products indexed under this heading.

Glycopyrrolate (Galantamine has the potential to interfere with the activity of anticholinergic agents).
No products indexed under this heading.

Hyoscyamine (Galantamine has the potential to interfere with the activity of anticholinergic agents).
No products indexed under this heading.

Hyoscyamine Sulfate (Galantamine has the potential to interfere with the activity of anticholinergic agents).
No products indexed under this heading.

Ibuprofen (Cholinomimetics, such as galantamine, may be expected to increase gastric acid secretion; therefore, co-administration in patients with increased risk of developing gastric ulcers or bleeding, such as patients on NSAIDs, should be closely monitored). Products include:
Advil Allergy Sinus Caplets 737
Advil 737
Children's Advil Suspension 742
Children's Advil Chewable Tablets 741
Advil Cold & Sinus 739
Advil Flu & Body Ache Caplets 739
Children's Advil Cold Suspension 741
Infants' Advil Concentrated Drops 743

Junior Strength Advil Swallow Tablets 740
Advil Migraine Liquigels 740
Advil Multi-Symptom Cold Caplets 738
Combunox Tablets 1183
Children's Motrin Oral Suspension and Chewable Tablets 1837
Children's Motrin Cold Non-Staining Dye-Free Oral Suspension 1838
Children's Motrin Cold Oral Suspension 1838
Children's Motrin Non-Staining Dye-Free Oral Suspension 1837
Motrin Cold & Sinus Caplets 1836
Motrin IB Tablets and Caplets 1836
Infants' Motrin Concentrated Drops 1837
Infants' Motrin Non-Staining Dye-Free Drops 1837
Junior Strength Motrin Caplets and Chewable Tablets 1837
Vicoprofen Tablets 533

Indomethacin (Cholinomimetics, such as galantamine, may be expected to increase gastric acid secretion; therefore, co-administration in patients with increased risk of developing gastric ulcers or bleeding, such as patients on NSAIDs, should be closely monitored). Products include:
Indocin 1968

Indomethacin Sodium Trihydrate (Cholinomimetics, such as galantamine, may be expected to increase gastric acid secretion; therefore, co-administration in patients with increased risk of developing gastric ulcers or bleeding, such as patients on NSAIDs, should be closely monitored). Products include:
Indocin I.V. 1973

Ipratropium Bromide (Galantamine has the potential to interfere with the activity of anticholinergic agents). Products include:
Atrovent HFA Inhalation Aerosol 872
Atrovent Inhalation Solution 868
Atrovent Nasal Spray 0.03% 869
Atrovent Nasal Spray 0.06% 870
Combivent Inhalation Aerosol 878
DuoNeb Inhalation Solution 1058

Ketoconazole (Co-administration with a potent inhibitor of CYP3A4, such as ketoconazole, increases the AUC of galantamine by 30%). Products include:
Nizoral A-D Shampoo, 1% 1839
Nizoral 2% Shampoo 1838

Ketoprofen (Cholinomimetics, such as galantamine, may be expected to increase gastric acid secretion; therefore, co-administration in patients with increased risk of developing gastric ulcers or bleeding, such as patients on NSAIDs, should be closely monitored).
No products indexed under this heading.

Ketorolac Tromethamine (Cholinomimetics, such as galantamine, may be expected to increase gastric acid secretion; therefore, co-administration in patients with increased risk of developing gastric ulcers or bleeding, such as patients on NSAIDs, should be closely monitored). Products include:
Acular Ophthalmic Solution 561
Acular LS Ophthalmic Solution 562

Meclofenamate Sodium (Cholinomimetics, such as galantamine, may be expected to increase gastric acid secretion; therefore, co-administration in patients with increased risk of developing gastric ulcers or bleeding, such as patients on NSAIDs, should be closely monitored).
No products indexed under this heading.

Mefenamic Acid (Cholinomimetics, such as galantamine, may be expected to increase gastric acid secretion; therefore, co-administration in patients with increased risk of developing gastric ulcers or bleeding, such as patients on NSAIDs, should be closely monitored).
No products indexed under this heading.

Meloxicam (Cholinomimetics, such as galantamine, may be expected to increase gastric acid secretion; therefore, co-administration in patients with increased risk of developing gastric ulcers or bleeding, such as patients on NSAIDs, should be closely monitored). Products include:
Mobic Oral Suspension 893
Mobic Tablets 893

Mepenzolate Bromide (Galantamine has the potential to interfere with the activity of anticholinergic agents).
No products indexed under this heading.

Metocurine Iodide (Galantamine is a cholinesterase inhibitor; co-administration with neuromuscular blocking agents may exaggerate neuromuscular blockade).
No products indexed under this heading.

Mivacurium Chloride (Galantamine is a cholinesterase inhibitor; co-administration with neuromuscular blocking agents may exaggerate neuromuscular blockade). Products include:
Mivacron Injection 489

Nabumetone (Cholinomimetics, such as galantamine, may be expected to increase gastric acid secretion; therefore, co-administration in patients with increased risk of developing gastric ulcers or bleeding, such as patients on NSAIDs, should be closely monitored). Products include:
Relafen Tablets 1523

Naproxen (Cholinomimetics, such as galantamine, may be expected to increase gastric acid secretion; therefore, co-administration in patients with increased risk of developing gastric ulcers or bleeding, such as patients on NSAIDs, should be closely monitored). Products include:
EC-Naprosyn Delayed-Release Tablets 2769
Naprosyn Suspension 2769
Naprosyn Tablets 2769
Prevacid NapraPAC 3277

Naproxen Sodium (Cholinomimetics, such as galantamine, may be expected to increase gastric acid secretion; therefore, co-administration in patients with increased risk of developing gastric ulcers or bleeding, such as patients on NSAIDs, should be closely monitored). Products include:
Aleve Tablets, Caplets and Gelcaps 605
Anaprox Tablets 2769
Anaprox DS Tablets 2769

Neostigmine Bromide (Co-administration with other cholinesterase inhibitors or cholinergic agonists may result in a synergistic effect).
No products indexed under this heading.

Neostigmine Methylsulfate (Co-administration with other cholinesterase inhibitors or cholinergic agonists may result in a synergistic effect).
No products indexed under this heading.

Oxaprozin (Cholinomimetics, such as galantamine, may be expected to increase gastric acid secretion; therefore, co-administration in patients with increased risk of developing gastric ulcers or bleeding, such as patients on NSAIDs, should be closely monitored).
No products indexed under this heading.

Oxybutynin Chloride (Galantamine has the potential to interfere with the activity of anticholinergic agents). Products include:
Ditropan XL Extended Release Tablets 2391

Pancuronium Bromide (Galantamine is a cholinesterase inhibitor; co-administration with neuromuscular blocking agents may exaggerate neuromuscular blockade).
No products indexed under this heading.

Paroxetine Hydrochloride (Co-administration with a strong inhibitor of CYP2D6, such as paroxetine results in increased AUC of galantamine by 40%). Products include:
Paxil CR Controlled-Release Tablets 1509
Paxil 1501

Phenylbutazone (Cholinomimetics, such as galantamine, may be expected to increase gastric acid secretion; therefore, co-administration in patients with increased risk of developing gastric ulcers or bleeding, such as patients on NSAIDs, should be closely monitored).
No products indexed under this heading.

Piroxicam (Cholinomimetics, such as galantamine, may be expected to increase gastric acid secretion; therefore, co-administration in patients with increased risk of developing gastric ulcers or bleeding, such as patients on NSAIDs, should be closely monitored).
No products indexed under this heading.

Procyclidine Hydrochloride (Galantamine has the potential to interfere with the activity of anticholinergic agents).
No products indexed under this heading.

Propantheline Bromide (Galantamine has the potential to interfere with the activity of anticholinergic agents).
No products indexed under this heading.

Pyridostigmine Bromide (Co-administration with other cholinesterase inhibitors or cholinergic agonists may result in a synergistic effect).
No products indexed under this heading.

Rapacuronium Bromide (Galantamine is a cholinesterase inhibitor; co-administration with neuromuscular blocking agents may exaggerate neuromuscular blockade).
No products indexed under this heading.

Rivastigmine Tartrate (Co-administration with other cholinesterase inhibitors or cholinergic agonists may result in a synergistic effect). Products include:
Exelon Capsules 2204

Rocuronium Bromide (Galantamine is a cholinesterase inhibitor; co-administration with neuromuscular blocking agents may exaggerate neuromuscular blockade). Products include:
Zemuron Injection 2363

Rofecoxib (Cholinomimetics, such as galantamine, may be expected to increase gastric acid secretion; therefore, co-administration in patients with increased risk of developing gastric ulcers or bleeding, such as patients on NSAIDs, should be closely monitored).
No products indexed under this heading.

Scopolamine (Galantamine has the potential to interfere with the activity of anticholinergic agents). Products include:
Transderm Scōp Transdermal Therapeutic System 2166

Scopolamine Hydrobromide (Galantamine has the potential to interfere with the activity of anticholinergic agents).
No products indexed under this heading.

Succinylcholine Chloride (Galantamine is a cholinesterase inhibitor; co-administration with neuromuscular blocking agents may exaggerate neuromuscular blockade).
No products indexed under this heading.

Sulindac (Cholinomimetics, such as galantamine, may be expected to increase gastric acid secretion; therefore, co-administration in patients with increased risk of developing gastric ulcers or bleeding, such as patients on NSAIDs, should be closely monitored). Products include:
Clinoril Tablets 1899

Tacrine Hydrochloride (Co-administration with other cholinesterase inhibitors or cholinergic agonists may result in a synergistic effect).
No products indexed under this heading.

Tolmetin Sodium (Cholinomimetics, such as galantamine, may be expected to increase gastric acid secretion; therefore, co-administration in patients with increased risk of developing gastric ulcers or bleeding, such as patients on NSAIDs, should be closely monitored).
No products indexed under this heading.

Tolterodine Tartrate (Galantamine has the potential to interfere with the activity of anticholinergic agents). Products include:
Detrol Tablets 2626
Detrol LA Capsules 2629

Tridihexethyl Chloride (Galantamine has the potential to interfere with the activity of anticholinergic agents).
No products indexed under this heading.

Trihexyphenidyl Hydrochloride (Galantamine has the potential to interfere with the activity of anticholinergic agents).
No products indexed under this heading.

Valdecoxib (Cholinomimetics, such as galantamine, may be expected to increase gastric acid secretion; therefore, co-administration in patients with increased risk of developing gastric ulcers or bleeding, such as patients on NSAIDs, should be closely monitored).
No products indexed under this heading.

Vecuronium Bromide (Galantamine is a cholinesterase inhibitor; co-administration with neuromuscular blocking agents may exaggerate neuromuscular blockade).
No products indexed under this heading.

REBETOL CAPSULES

(Ribavirin) 3073
May interact with antacids. Compounds in these categories include:

Aluminum Carbonate (Co-administration of ribavirin capsules with an antacid containing magnesium, aluminum and simethicone resulted in a 14% decrease in mean ribavirin AUC. The clinical relevance of results from this study is unknown).
No products indexed under this heading.

Aluminum Hydroxide (Co-administration of ribavirin capsules with an antacid containing magnesium, aluminum and simethicone resulted in a 14% decrease in mean ribavirin AUC. The clinical relevance of results from this study is unknown). Products include:
Gaviscon Regular Strength Liquid .. 620
Gaviscon Regular Strength Tablets 619
Gaviscon Extra Strength Liquid 620
Gaviscon Extra Strength Tablets 619
Maalox Max Maximum Strength Antacid/Anti-Gas Liquid 2165
Maalox Regular Strength Antacid/Antigas Liquid 2164

Magaldrate (Co-administration of ribavirin capsules with an antacid containing magnesium, aluminum and simethicone resulted in a 14% decrease in mean ribavirin AUC. The clinical relevance of results from this study is unknown).
No products indexed under this heading.

Magnesium Hydroxide (Co-administration of ribavirin capsules with an antacid containing magnesium, aluminum and simethicone resulted in a 14% decrease in mean ribavirin AUC. The clinical relevance of results from this study is unknown). Products include:
Maalox Max Maximum Strength Antacid/Anti-Gas Liquid 2165
Maalox Regular Strength Antacid/Antigas Liquid 2164
Pepcid Complete Chewable Tablets 1672
Rolaids Tablets 707
Extra Strength Rolaids Tablets 707
Rolaids Multi-Symptom Antacid & Antigas Tablets 708

Magnesium Oxide (Co-administration of ribavirin capsules with an antacid containing magnesium, aluminum and simethicone resulted in a 14% decrease in mean ribavirin AUC. The clinical relevance of results from this study is unknown). Products include:
Beelith Tablets 784
PremCal Light, Regular, and Extra Strength Tablets 762

Sodium Bicarbonate (Co-administration of ribavirin capsules with an antacid containing magnesium, aluminum and simethicone resulted in a 14% decrease in mean ribavirin AUC. The clinical relevance of results from this study is unknown). Products include:
Ceo-Two Evacuant Suppository 607
Colyte with Flavor Packs for Oral Solution 3102
HalfLytely and Bisacodyl Tablets Bowel Prep Kit with Flavors Packs 915
TriLyte with Flavor Packs for Oral Solution 3114

REBETOL ORAL SOLUTION

(Ribavirin) 3073
May interact with:

See (Rebetol Capsules).

REBETRON COMBINATION THERAPY

(Interferon alfa-2b, Recombinant, Ribavirin) 3078
May interact with:

Abacavir Sulfate (Administration of nucleoside analogues has resulted in fatal and nonfatal lactic acidosis; co-administration of ribavirin and nucleoside analogues should be undertaken with caution and only if the potential benefit outweighs the potential risks). Products include:
Epzicom Tablets 1402
Trizivir Tablets 1565
Ziagen 1600

Didanosine (Administration of nucleoside analogues has resulted in fatal and nonfatal lactic acidosis; co-administration of ribavirin and nucleoside analogues should be undertaken with caution and only if the potential benefit outweighs the potential risks. Exposure to didanosine or its active metabolite is increased when didanosine is co-administered with ribavirin, which could cause or worsen clinical toxicities).
No products indexed under this heading.

Lamivudine (Administration of nucleoside analogues has resulted in fatal and nonfatal lactic acidosis; co-administration of ribavirin and nucleoside analogues should be undertaken with caution and only if the potential benefit outweighs the potential risks). Products include:
Combivir Tablets 1373
Epivir 1394
Epivir-HBV 1398
Epzicom Tablets 1402
Trizivir Tablets 1565

Magnesium Hydroxide (Co-administration with an antacid containing magnesium, aluminum, and simethicone resulted in a 14% decrease in ribavirin AUC; the clinical relevance of results from this single-dose study is unknown). Products include:
Maalox Max Maximum Strength Antacid/Anti-Gas Liquid 2165
Maalox Regular Strength Antacid/Antigas Liquid 2164
Pepcid Complete Chewable Tablets 1672
Rolaids Tablets 707
Extra Strength Rolaids Tablets 707
Rolaids Multi-Symptom Antacid & Antigas Tablets 708

Stavudine (Administration of nucleoside analogues has resulted in fatal and nonfatal lactic acidosis; co-administration of ribavirin and nucleoside analogues should be undertaken with caution and only if the potential benefit outweighs the potential risks. Ribavirin may antagonize the in-vitro antiviral activity of stavudine against HIV; co-administer with caution). Products include:
Zerit 971

Zalacitabine (Administration of nucleoside analogues has resulted in fatal and nonfatal lactic acidosis; co-administration of ribavirin and nucleoside analogues should be undertaken with caution and only if the potential benefit outweighs the potential risks).
No products indexed under this heading.

Zidovudine (Administration of nucleoside analogues has resulted in fatal and nonfatal lactic acidosis; co-administration of ribavirin and nucleoside analogues should be undertaken with caution and only if the potential benefit outweighs the potential risks. Ribavirin may antagonize the in-vitro antiviral activity of zidovudine against HIV; co-administer with caution). Products include:
Combivir Tablets 1373
Retrovir 1533
Retrovir IV Infusion 1537
Trizivir Tablets 1565

Food Interactions

Food, unspecified (Both AUC and Cmax increased by 70% when Rebetron was administered with a high-fat meal in a single-dose pharmacokinetic study; there are insufficient data to address the clinical relevance of these results).

REBIF PREFILLED SYRINGE FOR INJECTION

(Interferon Beta-1a) 3163
None cited in PDR database.

RECOMBINATE

(Antihemophilic Factor (Recombinant)) 762
None cited in PDR database.

RECOMBIVAX HB

(Hepatitis B Vaccine, Recombinant) ... 2045
None cited in PDR database.

REESE'S PINWORM TREATMENTS

(Pyrantel Pamoate) 730
None cited in PDR database.

REFACTO VIALS

(Antihemophilic Factor (Recombinant)) 3479
None cited in PDR database.

REFLUDAN FOR INJECTION

(Lepirudin) 815
May interact with oral anticoagulants, non-steroidal anti-inflammatory agents, thrombolytics, and certain other agents. Compounds in these categories include:

Alteplase (Concomitant therapy with thrombolytics may increase the risk of bleeding complications and considerably enhance the effect of Refludan on aPTT prolongation). Products include:
Activase I.V. 1225
Cathflo Activase 1232

Anisindione (Concomitant therapy with oral anticoagulants may increase the risk of bleeding). Products include:
Miradon Tablets 3056

Anistreplase (Concomitant therapy with thrombolytics may increase the risk of bleeding complications and considerably enhance the effect of Refludan on aPTT prolongation).
No products indexed under this heading.

Aspirin (Concomitant therapy with drugs that affect platelet function, such as aspirin, may increase the risk of bleeding). Products include:
Aggrenox Capsules 855
Bayer, Aspirin Regimen 606
Bayer Aspirin Tablets 3515
BC Powder 612
BC Allergy Sinus Cold Powder 612
Arthritis Strength BC Powder 612
BC Sinus Cold Powder 612
Ecotrin Enteric Coated Aspirin Low, Regular and Maximum Strength Tablets 1627
Goody's Body Pain Formula Powder 621
Goody's Extra Strength Headache Powder 621
Goody's Extra Strength Pain Relief Tablets 621
Percodan Tablets 1115
St. Joseph 81 mg Aspirin Chewable and Enteric Coated Tablets 1841

Celecoxib (Concomitant therapy with drugs that affect platelet function, such as non-steroid anti-inflammatory agents, may increase the risk of bleeding). Products include:
Celebrex Capsules 3130

Clopidogrel Bisulfate (Concomitant therapy with drugs that affect platelet function, such as clopidogrel, may increase the risk of bleeding). Products include:
Plavix Tablets 940
Plavix Tablets 2942

Diclofenac Potassium (Concomitant therapy with drugs that affect platelet function, such as non-steroid anti-inflammatory agents, may increase the risk of bleeding). Products include:
Cataflam Tablets 2173

Diclofenac Sodium (Concomitant therapy with drugs that affect platelet function, such as non-steroid anti-inflammatory agents, may increase the risk of bleeding). Products include:
Arthrotec Tablets 3126
Voltaren Ophthalmic Solution 2300
Voltaren Tablets 2298
Voltaren-XR Tablets 2301

Dicumarol (Concomitant therapy with oral anticoagulants may increase the risk of bleeding).
No products indexed under this heading.

Dipyridamole (Concomitant therapy with drugs that affect platelet function, such as dipyridamole, may increase the risk of bleeding). Products include:
Aggrenox Capsules 855
Persantine Tablets 898

Etodolac (Concomitant therapy with drugs that affect platelet function, such as non-steroid anti-inflammatory agents, may increase the risk of bleeding).
No products indexed under this heading.

Fenoprofen Calcium (Concomitant therapy with drugs that affect platelet function, such as non-steroid anti-inflammatory agents, may increase the risk of bleeding). Products include:
Nalfon Capsules 2504

Flurbiprofen (Concomitant therapy with drugs that affect platelet function, such as non-steroid anti-inflammatory agents, may increase the risk of bleeding).
No products indexed under this heading.

Ibuprofen (Concomitant therapy with drugs that affect platelet function, such as non-steroid anti-inflammatory agents, may increase the risk of bleeding). Products include:
Advil Allergy Sinus Caplets .... ■ 737
Advil .... ■ 737
Children's Advil Suspension .... ■ 742
Children's Advil Chewable Tablets .. ■ 741
Advil Cold & Sinus .... ■ 739
Advil Flu & Body Ache Caplets .... ■ 739
Children's Advil Cold Suspension .... ■ 741
Infants' Advil Concentrated Drops .. ■ 743
Junior Strength Advil Swallow Tablets .... ■ 740
Advil Migraine Liquigels .... ■ 740
Advil Multi-Symptom Cold Caplets .... ■ 738
Combunox Tablets 1183
Children's Motrin Oral Suspension and Chewable Tablets 1837
Children's Motrin Cold Non-Staining Dye-Free Oral Suspension 1838
Children's Motrin Cold Oral Suspension 1838
Children's Motrin Non-Staining Dye-Free Oral Suspension 1837
Motrin Cold & Sinus Caplets 1836
Motrin IB Tablets and Caplets 1836
Infants' Motrin Concentrated Drops 1837
Infants' Motrin Non-Staining Dye-Free Drops 1837
Junior Strength Motrin Caplets and Chewable Tablets 1837
Vicoprofen Tablets 533

Indomethacin (Concomitant therapy with drugs that affect platelet function, such as non-steroid anti-inflammatory agents, may increase the risk of bleeding). Products include:
Indocin 1968

Indomethacin Sodium Trihydrate (Concomitant therapy with drugs that affect platelet function, such as non-steroid anti-inflammatory agents, may increase the risk of bleeding). Products include:
Indocin I.V. 1973

Ketoprofen (Concomitant therapy with drugs that affect platelet function, such as non-steroid anti-inflammatory agents, may increase the risk of bleeding).
No products indexed under this heading.

Ketorolac Tromethamine (Concomitant therapy with drugs that affect platelet function, such as non-steroid anti-inflammatory agents, may increase the risk of bleeding). Products include:
Acular Ophthalmic Solution 561
Acular LS Ophthalmic Solution 562

Meclofenamate Sodium (Concomitant therapy with drugs that affect platelet function, such as non-steroid anti-inflammatory agents, may increase the risk of bleeding).
No products indexed under this heading.

Mefenamic Acid (Concomitant therapy with drugs that affect platelet function, such as non-steroid anti-inflammatory agents, may increase the risk of bleeding).
No products indexed under this heading.

Meloxicam (Concomitant therapy with drugs that affect platelet function, such as non-steroid anti-inflammatory agents, may increase the risk of bleeding). Products include:
Mobic Oral Suspension 893
Mobic Tablets 893

Nabumetone (Concomitant therapy with drugs that affect platelet function, such as non-steroid anti-inflammatory agents, may increase the risk of bleeding). Products include:
Relafen Tablets 1523

Naproxen (Concomitant therapy with drugs that affect platelet function, such as non-steroid anti-inflammatory agents, may increase the risk of bleeding). Products include:
EC-Naprosyn Delayed-Release Tablets 2769
Naprosyn Suspension 2769
Naprosyn Tablets 2769
Prevacid NapraPAC 3277

Naproxen Sodium (Concomitant therapy with drugs that affect platelet function, such as non-steroid anti-inflammatory agents, may increase the risk of bleeding). Products include:
Aleve Tablets, Caplets and Gelcaps .... ■ 605
Anaprox Tablets 2769
Anaprox DS Tablets 2769

Oxaprozin (Concomitant therapy with drugs that affect platelet function, such as non-steroid anti-inflammatory agents, may increase the risk of bleeding).
No products indexed under this heading.

Phenylbutazone (Concomitant therapy with drugs that affect platelet function, such as non-steroid anti-inflammatory agents, may increase the risk of bleeding).
No products indexed under this heading.

Piroxicam (Concomitant therapy with drugs that affect platelet function, such as non-steroid anti-inflammatory agents, may increase the risk of bleeding).
No products indexed under this heading.

Reteplase (Concomitant therapy with thrombolytics may increase the risk of bleeding complications and considerably enhance the effect of Refludan on aPTT prolongation). Products include:
Retavase 1131

Rofecoxib (Concomitant therapy with drugs that affect platelet function, such as non-steroid anti-inflammatory agents, may increase the risk of bleeding).
No products indexed under this heading.

Streptokinase (Concomitant therapy with thrombolytics may increase the risk of bleeding complications and considerably enhance the effect of Refludan on aPTT prolongation).
No products indexed under this heading.

Sulindac (Concomitant therapy with drugs that affect platelet function, such as non-steroid anti-inflammatory agents, may increase the risk of bleeding). Products include:
Clinoril Tablets 1899

Tolmetin Sodium (Concomitant therapy with drugs that affect platelet function, such as non-steroid anti-inflammatory agents, may increase the risk of bleeding).
No products indexed under this heading.

Urokinase (Concomitant therapy with thrombolytics may increase the risk of bleeding complications and considerably enhance the effect of Refludan on aPTT prolongation).
No products indexed under this heading.

Valdecoxib (Concomitant therapy with drugs that affect platelet function, such as non-steroid anti-inflammatory agents, may increase the risk of bleeding).
No products indexed under this heading.

Warfarin Sodium (Concomitant therapy with oral anticoagulants may increase the risk of bleeding). Products include:
Coumadin for Injection 932
Coumadin Tablets 932

REFRESH CELLUVISC LUBRICANT EYE DROPS
(Carboxymethylcellulose Sodium) .... ⊙238
None cited in PDR database.

REFRESH ENDURA LUBRICANT EYE DROPS
(Glycerin, Polysorbate 80) .... ⊙238
None cited in PDR database.

REFRESH LIQUIGEL
(Carboxymethylcellulose Sodium) .... ⊙238
None cited in PDR database.

REFRESH P.M. LUBRICANT EYE OINTMENT
(Mineral Oil, Petrolatum, White) .... ⊙239
None cited in PDR database.

REFRESH PLUS LUBRICANT EYE DROPS
(Carboxymethylcellulose Sodium) .... ⊙238
None cited in PDR database.

REFRESH TEARS LUBRICANT EYE DROPS
(Carboxymethylcellulose Sodium) .... ⊙239
None cited in PDR database.

REISHIMAX CAPSULES
(Ganoderma lucinum mushroom extract) 2669
May interact with oral anticoagulants and immunosuppressive agents. Compounds in these categories include:

Anisindione (Concurrent use with anticoagulants requires consultation with a physician). Products include:
Miradon Tablets 3056

Azathioprine (Concurrent use with immunosuppressive agents requires consultation with a physician). Products include:
Azasan Tablets 2844

Basiliximab (Concurrent use with immunosuppressive agents requires consultation with a physician). Products include:
Simulect for Injection 2268

Cyclosporine (Concurrent use with immunosuppressive agents requires consultation with a physician). Products include:
Gengraf Capsules 458
Neoral Soft Gelatin Capsules 2247
Neoral Oral Solution 2247
Restasis Ophthalmic Emulsion 570
Sandimmune 2259

Dicumarol (Concurrent use with anticoagulants requires consultation with a physician).
No products indexed under this heading.

Muromonab-CD3 (Concurrent use with immunosuppressive agents requires consultation with a physician). Products include:
Orthoclone OKT3 Sterile Solution 2370

Mycophenolate Mofetil (Concurrent use with immunosuppressive agents requires consultation with a physician). Products include:
CellCept Capsules 2751
CellCept Oral Suspension 2751
CellCept Tablets 2751

Sirolimus (Concurrent use with immunosuppressive agents requires consultation with a physician). Products include:
Rapamune Oral Solution and Tablets 3472

Tacrolimus (Concurrent use with immunosuppressive agents requires consultation with a physician). Products include:
Prograf Capsules and Injection 624
Protopic Ointment 629

Warfarin Sodium (Concurrent use with anticoagulants requires consultation with a physician). Products include:
Coumadin for Injection 932
Coumadin Tablets 932

RELAFEN TABLETS
(Nabumetone) 1523
May interact with highly protein bound drugs (selected). Compounds in these categories include:

Amiodarone Hydrochloride (In vitro studies have shown that 6 MNA, an active metabolite of nabumetone, may displace other protein bound drugs from their binding site). Products include:
Pacerone Tablets 3337

Amitriptyline Hydrochloride (In vitro studies have shown that 6 MNA, an active metabolite of nabumetone, may displace other protein bound drugs from their binding site).
No products indexed under this heading.

Atovaquone (In vitro studies have shown that 6 MNA, an active metabolite of nabumetone, may displace other protein bound drugs from their binding site). Products include:
Malarone Tablets 1484
Malarone Pediatric Tablets 1484
Mepron Suspension 1487

Cefonicid Sodium (In vitro studies have shown that 6 MNA, an active metabolite of nabumetone, may displace other protein bound drugs from their binding site).
No products indexed under this heading.

Celecoxib (In vitro studies have shown that 6 MNA, an active metab-

olite of nabumetone, may displace other protein bound drugs from their binding site). Products include:
- Celebrex Capsules 3130

Chlordiazepoxide (In vitro studies have shown that 6 MNA, an active metabolite of nabumetone, may displace other protein bound drugs from their binding site).
- No products indexed under this heading.

Chlordiazepoxide Hydrochloride (In vitro studies have shown that 6 MNA, an active metabolite of nabumetone, may displace other protein bound drugs from their binding site). Products include:
- Librium Capsules 3349

Chlorpromazine (In vitro studies have shown that 6 MNA, an active metabolite of nabumetone, may displace other protein bound drugs from their binding site).
- No products indexed under this heading.

Chlorpromazine Hydrochloride (In vitro studies have shown that 6 MNA, an active metabolite of nabumetone, may displace other protein bound drugs from their binding site).
- No products indexed under this heading.

Clomipramine Hydrochloride (In vitro studies have shown that 6 MNA, an active metabolite of nabumetone, may displace other protein bound drugs from their binding site).
- No products indexed under this heading.

Clozapine (In vitro studies have shown that 6 MNA, an active metabolite of nabumetone, may displace other protein bound drugs from their binding site). Products include:
- Clozapine Tablets 2141
- Clozaril Tablets 2174
- FazaClo Orally Disintegrating Tablets 547

Cyclosporine (In vitro studies have shown that 6 MNA, an active metabolite of nabumetone, may displace other protein bound drugs from their binding site). Products include:
- Gengraf Capsules 458
- Neoral Soft Gelatin Capsules 2247
- Neoral Oral Solution 2247
- Restasis Ophthalmic Emulsion 570
- Sandimmune 2259

Diazepam (In vitro studies have shown that 6 MNA, an active metabolite of nabumetone, may displace other protein bound drugs from their binding site). Products include:
- Diastat Rectal Delivery System 3344
- Valium Tablets 2822

Diclofenac Potassium (In vitro studies have shown that 6 MNA, an active metabolite of nabumetone, may displace other protein bound drugs from their binding site). Products include:
- Cataflam Tablets 2173

Diclofenac Sodium (In vitro studies have shown that 6 MNA, an active metabolite of nabumetone, may displace other protein bound drugs from their binding site). Products include:
- Arthrotec Tablets 3126
- Voltaren Ophthalmic Solution 2300
- Voltaren Tablets 2298
- Voltaren-XR Tablets 2301

Dipyridamole (In vitro studies have shown that 6 MNA, an active metabolite of nabumetone, may displace other protein bound drugs from their binding site). Products include:
- Aggrenox Capsules 855
- Persantine Tablets 898

Fenoprofen Calcium (In vitro studies have shown that 6 MNA, an active metabolite of nabumetone, may displace other protein bound drugs from their binding site). Products include:
- Nalfon Capsules 2504

Flurazepam Hydrochloride (In vitro studies have shown that 6 MNA, an active metabolite of nabumetone, may displace other protein bound drugs from their binding site). Products include:
- Dalmane Capsules 3343

Flurbiprofen (In vitro studies have shown that 6 MNA, an active metabolite of nabumetone, may displace other protein bound drugs from their binding site).
- No products indexed under this heading.

Glipizide (In vitro studies have shown that 6 MNA, an active metabolite of nabumetone, may displace other protein bound drugs from their binding site).
- No products indexed under this heading.

Ibuprofen (In vitro studies have shown that 6 MNA, an active metabolite of nabumetone, may displace other protein bound drugs from their binding site). Products include:
- Advil Allergy Sinus Caplets 737
- Advil 737
- Children's Advil Suspension 742
- Children's Advil Chewable Tablets 741
- Advil Cold & Sinus 739
- Advil Flu & Body Ache Caplets 739
- Children's Advil Cold Suspension 741
- Infants' Advil Concentrated Drops 743
- Junior Strength Advil Swallow Tablets 740
- Advil Migraine Liquigels 740
- Advil Multi-Symptom Cold Caplets 738
- Combunox Tablets 1183
- Children's Motrin Oral Suspension and Chewable Tablets 1837
- Children's Motrin Cold Non-Staining Dye-Free Oral Suspension 1838
- Children's Motrin Cold Oral Suspension 1838
- Children's Motrin Non-Staining Dye-Free Oral Suspension 1837
- Motrin Cold & Sinus Caplets 1836
- Motrin IB Tablets and Caplets 1836
- Infants' Motrin Concentrated Drops 1837
- Infants' Motrin Non-Staining Dye-Free Drops 1837
- Junior Strength Motrin Caplets and Chewable Tablets 1837
- Vicoprofen Tablets 533

Imipramine Hydrochloride (In vitro studies have shown that 6 MNA, an active metabolite of nabumetone, may displace other protein bound drugs from their binding site).
- No products indexed under this heading.

Imipramine Pamoate (In vitro studies have shown that 6 MNA, an active metabolite of nabumetone, may displace other protein bound drugs from their binding site).
- No products indexed under this heading.

Indomethacin (In vitro studies have shown that 6 MNA, an active metabolite of nabumetone, may displace other protein bound drugs from their binding site). Products include:
- Indocin 1968

Indomethacin Sodium Trihydrate (In vitro studies have shown that 6 MNA, an active metabolite of nabumetone, may displace other protein bound drugs from their binding site). Products include:
- Indocin I.V. 1973

Ketoprofen (In vitro studies have shown that 6 MNA, an active metabolite of nabumetone, may displace other protein bound drugs from their binding site).
- No products indexed under this heading.

Ketorolac Tromethamine (In vitro studies have shown that 6 MNA, an active metabolite of nabumetone, may displace other protein bound drugs from their binding site). Products include:
- Acular Ophthalmic Solution 561
- Acular LS Ophthalmic Solution 562

Meclofenamate Sodium (In vitro studies have shown that 6 MNA, an active metabolite of nabumetone, may displace other protein bound drugs from their binding site).
- No products indexed under this heading.

Mefenamic Acid (In vitro studies have shown that 6 MNA, an active metabolite of nabumetone, may displace other protein bound drugs from their binding site).
- No products indexed under this heading.

Midazolam Hydrochloride (In vitro studies have shown that 6 MNA, an active metabolite of nabumetone, may displace other protein bound drugs from their binding site).
- No products indexed under this heading.

Naproxen (In vitro studies have shown that 6 MNA, an active metabolite of nabumetone, may displace other protein bound drugs from their binding site). Products include:
- EC-Naprosyn Delayed-Release Tablets 2769
- Naprosyn Suspension 2769
- Naprosyn Tablets 2769
- Prevacid NapraPAC 3277

Naproxen Sodium (In vitro studies have shown that 6 MNA, an active metabolite of nabumetone, may displace other protein bound drugs from their binding site). Products include:
- Aleve Tablets, Caplets and Gelcaps 605
- Anaprox Tablets 2769
- Anaprox DS Tablets 2769

Nortriptyline Hydrochloride (In vitro studies have shown that 6 MNA, an active metabolite of nabumetone, may displace other protein bound drugs from their binding site).
- No products indexed under this heading.

Oxaprozin (In vitro studies have shown that 6 MNA, an active metabolite of nabumetone, may displace other protein bound drugs from their binding site).
- No products indexed under this heading.

Oxazepam (In vitro studies have shown that 6 MNA, an active metabolite of nabumetone, may displace other protein bound drugs from their binding site).
- No products indexed under this heading.

Phenylbutazone (In vitro studies have shown that 6 MNA, an active metabolite of nabumetone, may displace other protein bound drugs from their binding site).
- No products indexed under this heading.

Piroxicam (In vitro studies have shown that 6 MNA, an active metabolite of nabumetone, may displace other protein bound drugs from their binding site).
- No products indexed under this heading.

Propranolol Hydrochloride (In vitro studies have shown that 6 MNA, an active metabolite of nabumetone, may displace other protein bound drugs from their binding site). Products include:
- Inderal LA Long-Acting Capsules 3421
- InnoPran XL Capsules 2728

Sulindac (In vitro studies have shown that 6 MNA, an active metabolite of nabumetone, may displace other protein bound drugs from their binding site). Products include:
- Clinoril Tablets 1899

Temazepam (In vitro studies have shown that 6 MNA, an active metabolite of nabumetone, may displace other protein bound drugs from their binding site).
- No products indexed under this heading.

Tolbutamide (In vitro studies have shown that 6 MNA, an active metabolite of nabumetone, may displace other protein bound drugs from their binding site).
- No products indexed under this heading.

Tolmetin Sodium (In vitro studies have shown that 6 MNA, an active metabolite of nabumetone, may displace other protein bound drugs from their binding site).
- No products indexed under this heading.

Trimipramine Maleate (In vitro studies have shown that 6 MNA, an active metabolite of nabumetone, may displace other protein bound drugs from their binding site). Products include:
- Surmontil Capsules 2347

Warfarin Sodium (Effects not specified; caution should be exercised; in vitro studies have shown that 6 MNA, an active metabolite of nabumetone, may displace other protein bound drugs from their binding site). Products include:
- Coumadin for Injection 932
- Coumadin Tablets 932

Food Interactions

Dairy products (Potential for more rapid absorption; however, the total amount of GMNA in the plasma is unchanged).

Food, unspecified (Potential for more rapid absorption; however, the total amount of GMNA in the plasma is unchanged).

RELENZA ROTADISK

(Zanamivir) 1525

None cited in PDR database.

RELPAX TABLETS

(Eletriptan Hydrobromide) 2531

May interact with 5HT1-receptor agonists, cytochrome p450 3a4 inhibitors (selected), ergot-containing drugs, and selective serotonin reuptake inhibitors. Compounds in these categories include:

Acetazolamide (Eletriptan should not be used within 72 hours of drugs that have demonstrated potent CYP3A4 inhibition).
- No products indexed under this heading.

Amiodarone Hydrochloride (Eletriptan should not be used within 72

hours of drugs that have demonstrated potent CYP3A4 inhibition). Products include:
- Pacerone Tablets 3337

Amprenavir (Eletriptan should not be used within 72 hours of drugs that have demonstrated potent CYP3A4 inhibition). Products include:
- Agenerase Capsules 1299
- Agenerase Oral Solution 1304

Anastrozole (Eletriptan should not be used within 72 hours of drugs that have demonstrated potent CYP3A4 inhibition). Products include:
- Arimidex Tablets 665

Aprepitant (Eletriptan should not be used within 72 hours of drugs that have demonstrated potent CYP3A4 inhibition). Products include:
- Emend Capsules 1944

Cimetidine (Eletriptan should not be used within 72 hours of drugs that have demonstrated potent CYP3A4 inhibition). Products include:
- Tagamet HB 200 Tablets .... ▣637
- Tagamet Tablets 1547

Cimetidine Hydrochloride (Eletriptan should not be used within 72 hours of drugs that have demonstrated potent CYP3A4 inhibition).
- No products indexed under this heading.

Ciprofloxacin (Eletriptan should not be used within 72 hours of drugs that have demonstrated potent CYP3A4 inhibition). Products include:
- Cipro I.V. 2998
- Cipro I.V. Pharmacy Bulk Package ... 3509
- Cipro Oral Suspension 2991
- Cipro XR Tablets 3004
- Ciprodex Otic Suspension 555

Citalopram Hydrobromide (Selective serotonin reuptake inhibitors (SSRI) have been reported, rarely, to cause weakness, hyperreflexia, and incoordination when co-administered with 5-HT agonists. If concomitant treatment with eletriptan and an SSRI is clinically warranted, appropriate observation of the patient is advised). Products include:
- Celexa 1177

Clarithromycin (Eletriptan should not be used within 72 hours of drugs that have demonstrated potent CYP3A4 inhibition). Products include:
- Biaxin/Biaxin XL 402
- PREVPAC 3281

Clotrimazole (Eletriptan should not be used within 72 hours of drugs that have demonstrated potent CYP3A4 inhibition). Products include:
- Lotrimin 3053
- Lotrisone 3054

Cyclosporine (Eletriptan should not be used within 72 hours of drugs that have demonstrated potent CYP3A4 inhibition). Products include:
- Gengraf Capsules 458
- Neoral Soft Gelatin Capsules 2247
- Neoral Oral Solution 2247
- Restasis Ophthalmic Emulsion 570
- Sandimmune 2259

Dalfopristin (Eletriptan should not be used within 72 hours of drugs that have demonstrated potent CYP3A4 inhibition). Products include:
- Synercid I.V. 1690

Danazol (Eletriptan should not be used within 72 hours of drugs that have demonstrated potent CYP3A4 inhibition).
- No products indexed under this heading.

Delavirdine Mesylate (Eletriptan should not be used within 72 hours of drugs that have demonstrated potent CYP3A4 inhibition). Products include:
- Rescriptor Tablets 2535

Dihydroergotamine Mesylate (Ergot-containing drugs have been reported to cause prolonged vasospastic reactions. Because these effects may be additive, use of ergotamine-containing or ergot-type medications and eletriptan within 24 hours of each other is not recommended). Products include:
- Migranal Nasal Spray 3350

Diltiazem Hydrochloride (Eletriptan should not be used within 72 hours of drugs that have demonstrated potent CYP3A4 inhibition). Products include:
- Cardizem LA Extended Release Tablets 1699
- Tiazac Capsules 1204

Diltiazem Maleate (Eletriptan should not be used within 72 hours of drugs that have demonstrated potent CYP3A4 inhibition).
- No products indexed under this heading.

Efavirenz (Eletriptan should not be used within 72 hours of drugs that have demonstrated potent CYP3A4 inhibition). Products include:
- Sustiva Capsules 957

Ergonovine Maleate (Ergot-containing drugs have been reported to cause prolonged vasospastic reactions. Because these effects may be additive, use of ergotamine-containing or ergot-type medications and eletriptan within 24 hours of each other is not recommended).
- No products indexed under this heading.

Ergotamine Tartrate (Ergot-containing drugs have been reported to cause prolonged vasospastic reactions. Because these effects may be additive, use of ergotamine-containing or ergot-type medications and eletriptan within 24 hours of each other is not recommended).
- No products indexed under this heading.

Erythromycin (Eletriptan should not be used within 72 hours of drugs that have demonstrated potent CYP3A4 inhibition). Products include:
- Erygel Topical Gel 2096
- Ery-Tab Tablets 447
- Erythromycin Base Filmtab Tablets 454
- Erythromycin Delayed-Release Capsules, USP 456
- PCE Dispertab Tablets 510

Erythromycin Estolate (Eletriptan should not be used within 72 hours of drugs that have demonstrated potent CYP3A4 inhibition).
- No products indexed under this heading.

Erythromycin Ethylsuccinate (Eletriptan should not be used within 72 hours of drugs that have demonstrated potent CYP3A4 inhibition). Products include:
- E.E.S. 449
- EryPed 445

Erythromycin Gluceptate (Eletriptan should not be used within 72 hours of drugs that have demonstrated potent CYP3A4 inhibition).
- No products indexed under this heading.

Erythromycin Lactobionate (Eletriptan should not be used within 72 hours of drugs that have demonstrated potent CYP3A4 inhibition).
- No products indexed under this heading.

Erythromycin Stearate (Eletriptan should not be used within 72 hours of drugs that have demonstrated potent CYP3A4 inhibition). Products include:
- Erythrocin Stearate Filmtab Tablets 452

Escitalopram Oxalate (Selective serotonin reuptake inhibitors (SSRI) have been reported, rarely, to cause weakness, hyperreflexia, and incoordination when co-administered with 5-HT agonists. If concomitant treatment with eletriptan and an SSRI is clinically warranted, appropriate observation of the patient is advised). Products include:
- Lexapro Oral Solution 1193
- Lexapro Tablets 1193

Esomeprazole Magnesium (Eletriptan should not be used within 72 hours of drugs that have demonstrated potent CYP3A4 inhibition). Products include:
- Nexium Delayed-Release Capsules 645

Fluconazole (Eletriptan should not be used within 72 hours of drugs that have demonstrated potent CYP3A4 inhibition).
- No products indexed under this heading.

Fluoxetine Hydrochloride (Eletriptan should not be used within 72 hours of drugs that have demonstrated potent CYP3A4 inhibition). Products include:
- Prozac Pulvules and Liquid 1771
- Symbyax Capsules 1788

Fluvoxamine Maleate (Eletriptan should not be used within 72 hours of drugs that have demonstrated potent CYP3A4 inhibition).
- No products indexed under this heading.

Fosamprenavir Calcium (Eletriptan should not be used within 72 hours of drugs that have demonstrated potent CYP3A4 inhibition). Products include:
- Lexiva Tablets 1473

Indinavir Sulfate (Eletriptan should not be used within 72 hours of drugs that have demonstrated potent CYP3A4 inhibition). Products include:
- Crixivan Capsules 1918

Isoniazid (Eletriptan should not be used within 72 hours of drugs that have demonstrated potent CYP3A4 inhibition).
- No products indexed under this heading.

Itraconazole (Eletriptan should not be used within 72 hours of drugs that have demonstrated potent CYP3A4 inhibition).
- No products indexed under this heading.

Ketoconazole (Eletriptan should not be used within 72 hours of drugs that have demonstrated potent CYP3A4 inhibition). Products include:
- Nizoral A-D Shampoo, 1% 1839
- Nizoral 2% Shampoo 1838

Lopinavir (Eletriptan should not be used within 72 hours of drugs that have demonstrated potent CYP3A4 inhibition). Products include:
- Kaletra 474

Loratadine (Eletriptan should not be used within 72 hours of drugs that have demonstrated potent CYP3A4 inhibition). Products include:
- Alavert Allergy & Sinus D-12 Hour Tablets .... ▣743
- Alavert .... ▣743
- Children's Claritin 24 Hour Non-Drowsy Allergy Syrup .... ▣732
- Claritin Non-Drowsy 24 Hour Tablets .... ▣731
- Non-Drowsy Claritin Hives Relief Tablets .... ▣733
- Claritin Reditabs 24 Hour Non-Drowsy Tablets .... ▣732
- Claritin-D Non-Drowsy 12 Hour Tablets .... ▣731
- Claritin-D Non-Drowsy 24 Hour Tablets .... ▣731
- Children's Dimetapp ND Non-Drowsy Allergy Syrup .... ▣746
- Triaminic Allerchews .... ▣684

Methylergonovine Maleate (Ergot-containing drugs have been reported to cause prolonged vasospastic reactions. Because these effects may be additive, use of ergotamine-containing or ergot-type medications and eletriptan within 24 hours of each other is not recommended).
- No products indexed under this heading.

Methysergide Maleate (Ergot-containing drugs have been reported to cause prolonged vasospastic reactions. Because these effects may be additive, use of ergotamine-containing or ergot-type medications and eletriptan within 24 hours of each other is not recommended).
- No products indexed under this heading.

Metronidazole (Eletriptan should not be used within 72 hours of drugs that have demonstrated potent CYP3A4 inhibition). Products include:
- Metrogel 1% 1212
- MetroGel-Vaginal Gel 1822
- Noritate Cream, 1% 1051

Metronidazole Benzoate (Eletriptan should not be used within 72 hours of drugs that have demonstrated potent CYP3A4 inhibition).
- No products indexed under this heading.

Metronidazole Hydrochloride (Eletriptan should not be used within 72 hours of drugs that have demonstrated potent CYP3A4 inhibition).
- No products indexed under this heading.

Miconazole (Eletriptan should not be used within 72 hours of drugs that have demonstrated potent CYP3A4 inhibition).
- No products indexed under this heading.

Miconazole Nitrate (Eletriptan should not be used within 72 hours of drugs that have demonstrated potent CYP3A4 inhibition). Products include:
- Desenex .... ▣674
- Desenex Jock Itch Spray Powder ... ▣674

Naratriptan Hydrochloride (Concomitant use of other 5-HT1 agonists within 24 hours of eletriptan treatment is not recommended). Products include:
- Amerge Tablets 1312

Nefazodone Hydrochloride (Eletriptan should not be used within 72 hours of drugs that have demonstrated potent CYP3A4 inhibition).
- No products indexed under this heading.

Nelfinavir Mesylate (Eletriptan should not be used within 72 hours

of drugs that have demonstrated potent CYP3A4 inhibition). Products include:
- Viracept 2556

Nevirapine (Eletriptan should not be used within 72 hours of drugs that have demonstrated potent CYP3A4 inhibition). Products include:
- Viramune Oral Suspension 903
- Viramune Tablets 903

Niacinamide (Eletriptan should not be used within 72 hours of drugs that have demonstrated potent CYP3A4 inhibition).
- No products indexed under this heading.

Nicotinamide (Eletriptan should not be used within 72 hours of drugs that have demonstrated potent CYP3A4 inhibition). Products include:
- Nicomide Tablets 3190

Nifedipine (Eletriptan should not be used within 72 hours of drugs that have demonstrated potent CYP3A4 inhibition). Products include:
- Adalat CC Tablets 2978

Norfloxacin (Eletriptan should not be used within 72 hours of drugs that have demonstrated potent CYP3A4 inhibition). Products include:
- Noroxin Tablets 2009

Omeprazole (Eletriptan should not be used within 72 hours of drugs that have demonstrated potent CYP3A4 inhibition). Products include:
- Zegerid Powder for Oral Solution 2972

Paroxetine Hydrochloride (Eletriptan should not be used within 72 hours of drugs that have demonstrated potent CYP3A4 inhibition). Products include:
- Paxil CR Controlled-Release Tablets 1509
- Paxil 1501

Propoxyphene Hydrochloride (Eletriptan should not be used within 72 hours of drugs that have demonstrated potent CYP3A4 inhibition).
- No products indexed under this heading.

Propoxyphene Napsylate (Eletriptan should not be used within 72 hours of drugs that have demonstrated potent CYP3A4 inhibition). Products include:
- Darvocet A 500 Tablets 3497

Propranolol Hydrochloride (The Cmax and AUC of eletriptan were increased by 10 and 33% respectively in the presence of propranolol. No interactive increases in blood pressure were observed. No dosage adjustment appears to be needed for patients taking propranolol). Products include:
- Inderal LA Long-Acting Capsules 3421
- InnoPran XL Capsules 2728

Quinidine (Eletriptan should not be used within 72 hours of drugs that have demonstrated potent CYP3A4 inhibition).
- No products indexed under this heading.

Quinidine Hydrochloride (Eletriptan should not be used within 72 hours of drugs that have demonstrated potent CYP3A4 inhibition).
- No products indexed under this heading.

Quinidine Polygalacturonate (Eletriptan should not be used within 72 hours of drugs that have demonstrated potent CYP3A4 inhibition).
- No products indexed under this heading.

Quinidine Sulfate (Eletriptan should not be used within 72 hours of drugs that have demonstrated potent CYP3A4 inhibition).
- No products indexed under this heading.

Quinine (Eletriptan should not be used within 72 hours of drugs that have demonstrated potent CYP3A4 inhibition).
- No products indexed under this heading.

Quinine Sulfate (Eletriptan should not be used within 72 hours of drugs that have demonstrated potent CYP3A4 inhibition).
- No products indexed under this heading.

Quinupristin (Eletriptan should not be used within 72 hours of drugs that have demonstrated potent CYP3A4 inhibition). Products include:
- Synercid I.V. 1690

Ranitidine Bismuth Citrate (Eletriptan should not be used within 72 hours of drugs that have demonstrated potent CYP3A4 inhibition).
- No products indexed under this heading.

Ranitidine Hydrochloride (Eletriptan should not be used within 72 hours of drugs that have demonstrated potent CYP3A4 inhibition). Products include:
- Zantac 1597
- Zantac Injection 1593
- Zantac 75 Tablets 715
- Zantac 150 Maximum Strength Tablets 715
- Zantac Injection Pharmacy Bulk Package 1595

Ritonavir (Eletriptan should not be used within 72 hours of drugs that have demonstrated potent CYP3A4 inhibition). Products include:
- Kaletra 474
- Norvir 499

Rizatriptan Benzoate (Concomitant use of other 5-HT1 agonists within 24 hours of eletriptan treatment is not recommended). Products include:
- Maxalt Tablets 1983
- Maxalt-MLT Orally Disintegrating Tablets 1983

Saquinavir (Eletriptan should not be used within 72 hours of drugs that have demonstrated potent CYP3A4 inhibition).
- No products indexed under this heading.

Saquinavir Mesylate (Eletriptan should not be used within 72 hours of drugs that have demonstrated potent CYP3A4 inhibition). Products include:
- Invirase 2776

Sertraline Hydrochloride (Eletriptan should not be used within 72 hours of drugs that have demonstrated potent CYP3A4 inhibition). Products include:
- Zoloft 2581

Sumatriptan (Concomitant use of other 5-HT1 agonists within 24 hours of eletriptan treatment is not recommended). Products include:
- Imitrex Nasal Spray 1435

Sumatriptan Succinate (Concomitant use of other 5-HT1 agonists within 24 hours of eletriptan treatment is not recommended). Products include:
- Imitrex Injection 1431
- Imitrex Tablets 1440

Telithromycin (Eletriptan should not be used within 72 hours of drugs that have demonstrated potent CYP3A4 inhibition). Products include:
- Ketek Tablets 2920

Troglitazone (Eletriptan should not be used within 72 hours of drugs that have demonstrated potent CYP3A4 inhibition).
- No products indexed under this heading.

Troleandomycin (Eletriptan should not be used within 72 hours of drugs that have demonstrated potent CYP3A4 inhibition).
- No products indexed under this heading.

Valproate Sodium (Eletriptan should not be used within 72 hours of drugs that have demonstrated potent CYP3A4 inhibition). Products include:
- Depacon Injection 412

Verapamil Hydrochloride (Eletriptan should not be used within 72 hours of drugs that have demonstrated potent CYP3A4 inhibition). Products include:
- Covera-HS Tablets 3135
- Tarka Tablets 519
- Verelan PM Capsules 3120

Voriconazole (Eletriptan should not be used within 72 hours of drugs that have demonstrated potent CYP3A4 inhibition). Products include:
- VFEND I.V. 2543
- VFEND Oral Suspension 2543
- VFEND Tablets 2543

Zafirlukast (Eletriptan should not be used within 72 hours of drugs that have demonstrated potent CYP3A4 inhibition). Products include:
- Accolate Tablets 663

Zileuton (Eletriptan should not be used within 72 hours of drugs that have demonstrated potent CYP3A4 inhibition).
- No products indexed under this heading.

Zolmitriptan (Concomitant use of other 5-HT1 agonists within 24 hours of eletriptan treatment is not recommended). Products include:
- Zomig Nasal Spray 718
- Zomig Tablets 714
- Zomig-ZMT Tablets 714

Food Interactions

Grapefruit (Eletriptan should not be used within 72 hours of drugs that have demonstrated potent CYP3A4 inhibition).

Grapefruit Juice (Eletriptan should not be used within 72 hours of drugs that have demonstrated potent CYP3A4 inhibition).

REMICADE FOR IV INJECTION

(Infliximab) 987
May interact with:

Anakinra (Serious infections were seen with concurrent use of anakinra and another TNF2-blocking agent, etanercept. Similar toxicities may also result from the combination of anakinra and other TNF2-blocking agents; therefore, concurrent use of anakinra and infliximab is not recommended). Products include:
- Kineret Injection 594

REMIFEMIN MENOPAUSE TABLETS

(Black Cohosh) 766
None cited in PDR database.

RENAGEL TABLETS

(Sevelamer Hydrochloride) 1268
May interact with:

Ciprofloxacin (Co-administration may decrease the bioavailability of ciprofloxacin by approximately 50%). Products include:
- Cipro I.V. 2998
- Cipro I.V. Pharmacy Bulk Package 3509
- Cipro Oral Suspension 2991
- Cipro XR Tablets 3004
- Ciprodex Otic Suspension 555

RENOVA 0.02% CREAM

(Tretinoin) 2384
See Renova 0.05% Cream

RENOVA 0.05% CREAM

(Tretinoin) 2387
May interact with drugs known to be photosensitizers and certain other agents. Compounds in these categories include:

Acetazolamide (Co-administration with drugs known to be photosensitizers may augment phototoxicity; concurrent use with these agents is not recommended).
- No products indexed under this heading.

Acitretin (Co-administration with drugs known to be photosensitizers may augment phototoxicity; concurrent use with these agents is not recommended). Products include:
- Soriatane Capsules 1028

Alatrofloxacin Mesylate (Co-administration with drugs known to be photosensitizers may augment phototoxicity; concurrent use with these agents is not recommended).
- No products indexed under this heading.

Anthralin (Co-administration with drugs known to be photosensitizers may augment phototoxicity; concurrent use with these agents is not recommended). Products include:
- Psoriatec Cream 3191

Bendroflumethiazide (Co-administration with drugs known to be photosensitizers may augment phototoxicity; concurrent use with these agents is not recommended).
- No products indexed under this heading.

Chlorothiazide (Co-administration with drugs known to be photosensitizers may augment phototoxicity; concurrent use with these agents is not recommended). Products include:
- Aldoclor Tablets 1881
- Diuril Oral 1936

Chlorothiazide Sodium (Co-administration with drugs known to be photosensitizers may augment phototoxicity; concurrent use with these agents is not recommended). Products include:
- Diuril Sodium Intravenous 1934

Chlorpromazine (Co-administration with drugs known to be photosensitizers may augment phototoxicity; concurrent use with these agents is not recommended).
- No products indexed under this heading.

Chlorpromazine Hydrochloride (Co-administration with drugs known to be photosensitizers may augment phototoxicity; concurrent use with these agents is not recommended).
- No products indexed under this heading.

Chlorpropamide (Co-administration with drugs known to be photosensitizers may augment phototoxicity; concurrent use with these agents is not recommended).
No products indexed under this heading.

Ciprofloxacin (Co-administration with drugs known to be photosensitizers may augment phototoxicity; concurrent use with these agents is not recommended). Products include:
Cipro I.V. 2998
Cipro I.V. Pharmacy Bulk Package 3509
Cipro Oral Suspension 2991
Cipro XR Tablets 3004
Ciprodex Otic Suspension 555

Ciprofloxacin Hydrochloride (Co-administration with drugs known to be photosensitizers may augment phototoxicity; concurrent use with these agents is not recommended). Products include:
Ciloxan Ophthalmic Ointment 554
Cipro Tablets 2991

Coal Tar (Co-administration with drugs known to be photosensitizers may augment phototoxicity; concurrent use with these agents is not recommended). Products include:
Tegrin Dandruff Shampoo - Extra Conditioning .... ▣637
Tegrin Dandruff Shampoo - Fresh Herbal .... ▣638
Tegrin Skin Cream .... ▣638

Demeclocycline Hydrochloride (Co-administration with drugs known to be photosensitizers may augment phototoxicity; concurrent use with these agents is not recommended).
No products indexed under this heading.

Doxycycline Calcium (Co-administration with drugs known to be photosensitizers may augment phototoxicity; concurrent use with these agents is not recommended).
No products indexed under this heading.

Doxycycline Hyclate (Co-administration with drugs known to be photosensitizers may augment phototoxicity; concurrent use with these agents is not recommended).
No products indexed under this heading.

Doxycycline Monohydrate (Co-administration with drugs known to be photosensitizers may augment phototoxicity; concurrent use with these agents is not recommended).
No products indexed under this heading.

Enoxacin (Co-administration with drugs known to be photosensitizers may augment phototoxicity; concurrent use with these agents is not recommended).
No products indexed under this heading.

Fluphenazine Decanoate (Co-administration with drugs known to be photosensitizers may augment phototoxicity; concurrent use with these agents is not recommended).
No products indexed under this heading.

Fluphenazine Enanthate (Co-administration with drugs known to be photosensitizers may augment phototoxicity; concurrent use with these agents is not recommended).
No products indexed under this heading.

Fluphenazine Hydrochloride (Co-administration with drugs known to be photosensitizers may augment phototoxicity; concurrent use with these agents is not recommended).
No products indexed under this heading.

Furosemide (Co-administration with drugs known to be photosensitizers may augment phototoxicity; concurrent use with these agents is not recommended). Products include:
Furosemide Tablets 2117

Glipizide (Co-administration with drugs known to be photosensitizers may augment phototoxicity; concurrent use with these agents is not recommended).
No products indexed under this heading.

Glyburide (Co-administration with drugs known to be photosensitizers may augment phototoxicity; concurrent use with these agents is not recommended).
No products indexed under this heading.

Grepafloxacin Hydrochloride (Co-administration with drugs known to be photosensitizers may augment phototoxicity; concurrent use with these agents is not recommended).
No products indexed under this heading.

Griseofulvin (Co-administration with drugs known to be photosensitizers may augment phototoxicity; concurrent use with these agents is not recommended). Products include:
Grifulvin V Tablets Microsize and Oral Suspension Microsize 2384
Gris-PEG Tablets 2504

Hydrochlorothiazide (Co-administration with drugs known to be photosensitizers may augment phototoxicity; concurrent use with these agents is not recommended). Products include:
Aldoril Tablets 1884
Atacand HCT 637
Avalide Tablets 2889
Avalide Tablets 922
Benicar HCT Tablets 2852
Diovan HCT Tablets 2195
Dyazide Capsules 1389
Hyzaar 1964
Lotensin HCT Tablets 2235
Maxzide 2150
Micardis HCT Tablets 886
Moduretic Tablets 2003
Prinzide Tablets 2033
Teveten HCT Tablets 1710
Timolide Tablets 2056
Uniretic Tablets 3114
Vaseretic Tablets 2073
Zestoretic Tablets 701

Hydroflumethiazide (Co-administration with drugs known to be photosensitizers may augment phototoxicity; concurrent use with these agents is not recommended).
No products indexed under this heading.

Lomefloxacin Hydrochloride (Co-administration with drugs known to be photosensitizers may augment phototoxicity; concurrent use with these agents is not recommended).
No products indexed under this heading.

Mesoridazine Besylate (Co-administration with drugs known to be photosensitizers may augment phototoxicity; concurrent use with these agents is not recommended).
No products indexed under this heading.

Metabromsalan (Co-administration with drugs known to be photosensitizers may augment phototoxicity; concurrent use with these agents is not recommended).
No products indexed under this heading.

Methacycline Hydrochloride (Co-administration with drugs known to be photosensitizers may augment phototoxicity; concurrent use with these agents is not recommended).
No products indexed under this heading.

Methotrimeprazine (Co-administration with drugs known to be photosensitizers may augment phototoxicity; concurrent use with these agents is not recommended).
No products indexed under this heading.

Methyclothiazide (Co-administration with drugs known to be photosensitizers may augment phototoxicity; concurrent use with these agents is not recommended).
No products indexed under this heading.

Minocycline Hydrochloride (Co-administration with drugs known to be photosensitizers may augment phototoxicity; concurrent use with these agents is not recommended). Products include:
Dynacin Tablets 1859

Nalidixic Acid (Co-administration with drugs known to be photosensitizers may augment phototoxicity; concurrent use with these agents is not recommended).
No products indexed under this heading.

Norfloxacin (Co-administration with drugs known to be photosensitizers may augment phototoxicity; concurrent use with these agents is not recommended). Products include:
Noroxin Tablets 2009

Ofloxacin (Co-administration with drugs known to be photosensitizers may augment phototoxicity; concurrent use with these agents is not recommended). Products include:
Floxin Otic Singles 1045
Floxin Otic Solution 1043

Oxytetracycline Hydrochloride (Co-administration with drugs known to be photosensitizers may augment phototoxicity; concurrent use with these agents is not recommended).
No products indexed under this heading.

Perphenazine (Co-administration with drugs known to be photosensitizers may augment phototoxicity; concurrent use with these agents is not recommended).
No products indexed under this heading.

Polythiazide (Co-administration with drugs known to be photosensitizers may augment phototoxicity; concurrent use with these agents is not recommended).
No products indexed under this heading.

Prochlorperazine (Co-administration with drugs known to be photosensitizers may augment phototoxicity; concurrent use with these agents is not recommended).
No products indexed under this heading.

Promethazine Hydrochloride (Co-administration with drugs known to be photosensitizers may augment phototoxicity; concurrent use with these agents is not recommended). Products include:
Phenergan 3438

Sulfamethizole (Co-administration with drugs known to be photosensitizers may augment phototoxicity; concurrent use with these agents is not recommended).
No products indexed under this heading.

Sulfamethoxazole (Co-administration with drugs known to be photosensitizers may augment phototoxicity; concurrent use with these agents is not recommended).
No products indexed under this heading.

Sulfasalazine (Co-administration with drugs known to be photosensitizers may augment phototoxicity; concurrent use with these agents is not recommended).
No products indexed under this heading.

Sulfinpyrazone (Co-administration with drugs known to be photosensitizers may augment phototoxicity; concurrent use with these agents is not recommended).
No products indexed under this heading.

Sulfisoxazole (Co-administration with drugs known to be photosensitizers may augment phototoxicity; concurrent use with these agents is not recommended).
No products indexed under this heading.

Sulfisoxazole Acetyl (Co-administration with drugs known to be photosensitizers may augment phototoxicity; concurrent use with these agents is not recommended).
No products indexed under this heading.

Sulfisoxazole Diolamine (Co-administration with drugs known to be photosensitizers may augment phototoxicity; concurrent use with these agents is not recommended).
No products indexed under this heading.

Tetrachlorosalicylanilide (Co-administration with drugs known to be photosensitizers may augment phototoxicity; concurrent use with these agents is not recommended).
No products indexed under this heading.

Tetracycline Hydrochloride (Co-administration with drugs known to be photosensitizers may augment phototoxicity; concurrent use with these agents is not recommended).
No products indexed under this heading.

Thioridazine Hydrochloride (Co-administration with drugs known to be photosensitizers may augment phototoxicity; concurrent use with these agents is not recommended). Products include:
Thioridazine Hydrochloride Tablets 2122

Tolazamide (Co-administration with drugs known to be photosensitizers may augment phototoxicity; concurrent use with these agents is not recommended).
No products indexed under this heading.

Tolbutamide (Co-administration with drugs known to be photosensitizers may augment phototoxicity; concurrent use with these agents is not recommended).
No products indexed under this heading.

Trifluoperazine Hydrochloride (Co-administration with drugs known to be photosensitizers may augment phototoxicity; concurrent use with these agents is not recommended).
No products indexed under this heading.

Trovafloxacin Mesylate (Co-administration with drugs known to be photosensitizers may augment phototoxicity; concurrent use with these agents is not recommended).
No products indexed under this heading.

Food Interactions

Alcohol (Topical products with high concentration of alcohol may increase the irritation when used concurrently).

REOPRO VIALS

(Abciximab) 1779
May interact with anticoagulants, oral anticoagulants, non-steroidal anti-inflammatory agents, thrombolytics, and certain other agents. Compounds in these categories include:

Alteplase (Co-administration with thrombolytics may be associated with an increase in bleeding). Products include:
Activase I.V. 1225
Cathflo Activase 1232

Anisindione (Co-administration of oral anticoagulants within seven days is contraindicated unless prothrombin time is less than or equal to 1.2 times control; concurrent use with other anticoagulant agents may be associated with an increase in bleeding). Products include:
Miradon Tablets 3056

Anistreplase (Co-administration with thrombolytics may be associated with an increase in bleeding).
No products indexed under this heading.

Ardeparin Sodium (Co-administration with other anticoagulant agents may be associated with an increase in bleeding).
No products indexed under this heading.

Aspirin (Co-administration with antiplatelet agents, such as aspirin, may be associated with an increase in bleeding). Products include:
Aggrenox Capsules 855
Bayer, Aspirin Regimen 606
Bayer Aspirin Tablets 3515
BC Powder 612
BC Allergy Sinus Cold Powder 612
Arthritis Strength BC Powder 612
BC Sinus Cold Powder 612
Ecotrin Enteric Coated Aspirin Low, Regular and Maximum Strength Tablets 1627
Goody's Body Pain Formula Powder 621
Goody's Extra Strength Headache Powder 621
Goody's Extra Strength Pain Relief Tablets 621
Percodan Tablets 1115
St. Joseph 81 mg Aspirin Chewable and Enteric Coated Tablets 1841

Celecoxib (Co-administration with antiplatelet agents, such as non-steroidal anti-inflammatory agents, may be associated with an increase in bleeding). Products include:
Celebrex Capsules 3130

Clopidogrel Bisulfate (Co-administration with antiplatelet agents, such as clopidogrel, may be associated with an increase in bleeding). Products include:
Plavix Tablets 940
Plavix Tablets 2942

Dalteparin Sodium (Co-administration with other anticoagulant agents may be associated with an increase in bleeding). Products include:
Fragmin Injection 2638

Danaparoid Sodium (Co-administration with other anticoagulant agents may be associated with an increase in bleeding).
No products indexed under this heading.

Dextran (Co-administration with intravenous dextran before percutaneous coronary intervention, or intent to use it during an intervention is contraindicated).
No products indexed under this heading.

Diclofenac Potassium (Co-administration with antiplatelet agents, such as non-steroidal anti-inflammatory agents, may be associated with an increase in bleeding). Products include:
Cataflam Tablets 2173

Diclofenac Sodium (Co-administration with antiplatelet agents, such as non-steroidal anti-inflammatory agents, may be associated with an increase in bleeding). Products include:
Arthrotec Tablets 3126
Voltaren Ophthalmic Solution 2300
Voltaren Tablets 2298
Voltaren-XR Tablets 2301

Dicumarol (Co-administration of oral anticoagulants within seven days is contraindicated unless prothrombin time is less than or equal to 1.2 times control; concurrent use with other anticoagulant agents may be associated with an increase in bleeding).
No products indexed under this heading.

Dipyridamole (Co-administration with antiplatelet agents, such as dipyridamole, may be associated with an increase in bleeding). Products include:
Aggrenox Capsules 855
Persantine Tablets 898

Enoxaparin Sodium (Co-administration with other anticoagulant agents may be associated with an increase in bleeding). Products include:
Lovenox Injection 2931

Etodolac (Co-administration with antiplatelet agents, such as non-steroidal anti-inflammatory agents, may be associated with an increase in bleeding).
No products indexed under this heading.

Fenoprofen Calcium (Co-administration with antiplatelet agents, such as non-steroidal anti-inflammatory agents, may be associated with an increase in bleeding). Products include:
Nalfon Capsules 2504

Flurbiprofen (Co-administration with antiplatelet agents, such as non-steroidal anti-inflammatory agents, may be associated with an increase in bleeding).
No products indexed under this heading.

Fondaparinux Sodium (Co-administration with other anticoagulant agents may be associated with an increase in bleeding). Products include:
Arixtra Injection 1325

Heparin Calcium (Co-administration with other anticoagulant agents may be associated with an increase in bleeding).
No products indexed under this heading.

Heparin Sodium (Co-administration with other anticoagulant agents may be associated with an increase in bleeding).
No products indexed under this heading.

Ibuprofen (Co-administration with antiplatelet agents, such as non-steroidal anti-inflammatory agents, may be associated with an increase in bleeding). Products include:
Advil Allergy Sinus Caplets 737
Advil 737
Children's Advil Suspension 742
Children's Advil Chewable Tablets 741
Advil Cold & Sinus 739
Advil Flu & Body Ache Caplets 739
Children's Advil Cold Suspension 741
Infants' Advil Concentrated Drops 743
Junior Strength Advil Swallow Tablets 740
Advil Migraine Liquigels 740
Advil Multi-Symptom Cold Caplets 738
Combunox Tablets 1183
Children's Motrin Oral Suspension and Chewable Tablets 1837
Children's Motrin Cold Non-Staining Dye-Free Oral Suspension 1838
Children's Motrin Cold Oral Suspension 1838
Children's Motrin Non-Staining Dye-Free Oral Suspension 1837
Motrin Cold & Sinus Caplets 1836
Motrin IB Tablets and Caplets 1836
Infants' Motrin Concentrated Drops 1837
Infants' Motrin Non-Staining Dye-Free Drops 1837
Junior Strength Motrin Caplets and Chewable Tablets 1837
Vicoprofen Tablets 533

Indomethacin (Co-administration with antiplatelet agents, such as non-steroidal anti-inflammatory agents, may be associated with an increase in bleeding). Products include:
Indocin 1968

Indomethacin Sodium Trihydrate (Co-administration with antiplatelet agents, such as non-steroidal anti-inflammatory agents, may be associated with an increase in bleeding). Products include:
Indocin I.V. 1973

Ketoprofen (Co-administration with antiplatelet agents, such as non-steroidal anti-inflammatory agents, may be associated with an increase in bleeding).
No products indexed under this heading.

Ketorolac Tromethamine (Co-administration with antiplatelet agents, such as non-steroidal anti-inflammatory agents, may be associated with an increase in bleeding). Products include:
Acular Ophthalmic Solution 561
Acular LS Ophthalmic Solution 562

Low Molecular Weight Heparins (Co-administration with other anticoagulant agents may be associated with an increase in bleeding).
No products indexed under this heading.

Meclofenamate Sodium (Co-administration with antiplatelet agents, such as non-steroidal anti-inflammatory agents, may be associated with an increase in bleeding).
No products indexed under this heading.

Mefenamic Acid (Co-administration with antiplatelet agents, such as non-steroidal anti-inflammatory agents, may be associated with an increase in bleeding).
No products indexed under this heading.

Meloxicam (Co-administration with antiplatelet agents, such as non-steroidal anti-inflammatory agents, may be associated with an increase in bleeding). Products include:
Mobic Oral Suspension 893
Mobic Tablets 893

Nabumetone (Co-administration with antiplatelet agents, such as non-steroidal anti-inflammatory agents, may be associated with an increase in bleeding). Products include:
Relafen Tablets 1523

Naproxen (Co-administration with antiplatelet agents, such as non-steroidal anti-inflammatory agents, may be associated with an increase in bleeding). Products include:
EC-Naprosyn Delayed-Release Tablets 2769
Naprosyn Suspension 2769
Naprosyn Tablets 2769
Prevacid NapraPAC 3277

Naproxen Sodium (Co-administration with antiplatelet agents, such as non-steroidal anti-inflammatory agents, may be associated with an increase in bleeding). Products include:
Aleve Tablets, Caplets and Gelcaps 605
Anaprox Tablets 2769
Anaprox DS Tablets 2769

Oxaprozin (Co-administration with antiplatelet agents, such as non-steroidal anti-inflammatory agents, may be associated with an increase in bleeding).
No products indexed under this heading.

Phenylbutazone (Co-administration with antiplatelet agents, such as non-steroidal anti-inflammatory agents, may be associated with an increase in bleeding).
No products indexed under this heading.

Piroxicam (Co-administration with antiplatelet agents, such as non-steroidal anti-inflammatory agents, may be associated with an increase in bleeding).
No products indexed under this heading.

Reteplase (Co-administration with thrombolytics may be associated with an increase in bleeding). Products include:
Retavase 1131

Rofecoxib (Co-administration with antiplatelet agents, such as non-steroidal anti-inflammatory agents, may be associated with an increase in bleeding).
No products indexed under this heading.

Streptokinase (Co-administration with thrombolytics may be associated with an increase in bleeding).
No products indexed under this heading.

Sulindac (Co-administration with antiplatelet agents, such as non-steroidal anti-inflammatory agents, may be associated with an increase in bleeding). Products include:
Clinoril Tablets 1899

Ticlopidine Hydrochloride (Co-administration with antiplatelet agents, such as ticlopidine, may be associated with an increase in bleeding). Products include:
Ticlid Tablets 2813

Tinzaparin Sodium (Co-administration with other anticoagulant agents may be associated with an increase in bleeding).
No products indexed under this heading.

Tolmetin Sodium (Co-administration with antiplatelet agents, such as non-steroidal anti-inflammatory agents, may be associated with an increase in bleeding).
No products indexed under this heading.

Urokinase (Co-administration with thrombolytics may be associated with an increase in bleeding).
No products indexed under this heading.

Valdecoxib (Co-administration with antiplatelet agents, such as non-steroidal anti-inflammatory agents, may be associated with an increase in bleeding).
No products indexed under this heading.

Warfarin Sodium (Co-administration of oral anticoagulants within seven days is contraindicated unless prothrombin time is less than or equal to 1.2 times control; concurrent use with other anticoagulant agents may be associated with an increase in bleeding). Products include:
Coumadin for Injection 932
Coumadin Tablets 932

REPLIVA 21/7 TABLETS

(Ferrous Fumarate, Folic Acid, Iron, Vitamin B_{12}, Vitamin C) 3301
None cited in PDR database.

REPRONEX FOR INTRAMUSCULAR AND SUBCUTANEOUS INJECTION

(Menotropins) 1148
None cited in PDR database.

REQUIP TABLETS

(Ropinirole Hydrochloride) 1528
May interact with central nervous system depressants, cytochrome p450 1a2 inhibitors (selected), antidepressant drugs, dopamine D2 antagonists, and certain other agents. Compounds in these categories include:

Alatrofloxacin Mesylate (If therapy with a drug known to be a potent inhibitor of CYP1A2 is stopped or started during treatment with ropinirole hydrochloride, adjustment of the dose of ropinirole hydrocholoride may be required).
No products indexed under this heading.

Alfentanil Hydrochloride (Possible additive sedative effects).
No products indexed under this heading.

Alprazolam (Possible additive sedative effects). Products include:
Niravam Orally Disintegrating Tablets 3106
Xanax XR Tablets 2655

Amiodarone Hydrochloride (If therapy with a drug known to be a potent inhibitor of CYP1A2 is stopped or started during treatment with ropinirole hydrochloride, adjustment of the dose of ropinirole hydrocholoride may be required). Products include:
Pacerone Tablets 3337

Amitriptyline Hydrochloride (Possible additive sedative effects).
No products indexed under this heading.

Amoxapine (Possible additive sedative effects).
No products indexed under this heading.

Anastrozole (If therapy with a drug known to be a potent inhibitor of CYP1A2 is stopped or started during treatment with ropinirole hydrochloride, adjustment of the dose of ropinirole hydrocholoride may be required). Products include:
Arimidex Tablets 665

Aprobarbital (Possible additive sedative effects).
No products indexed under this heading.

Buprenorphine Hydrochloride (Possible additive sedative effects). Products include:
Buprenex Injectable 2718
Suboxone Tablets 2719
Subutex Tablets 2719

Bupropion Hydrochloride (Possible additive sedative effects). Products include:
Wellbutrin Tablets 1579
Wellbutrin SR Sustained-Release Tablets 1583
Wellbutrin XL Extended-Release Tablets 1588
Zyban Sustained-Release Tablets 1620

Buspirone Hydrochloride (Possible additive sedative effects).
No products indexed under this heading.

Butabarbital (Possible additive sedative effects).
No products indexed under this heading.

Butalbital (Possible additive sedative effects). Products include:
Sedapap Tablets 50 mg/650 mg 2098

Chlordiazepoxide (Possible additive sedative effects).
No products indexed under this heading.

Chlordiazepoxide Hydrochloride (Possible additive sedative effects). Products include:
Librium Capsules 3349

Chlorpromazine (Co-administration with dopamine antagonists may diminish the effectiveness of ropinirole).
No products indexed under this heading.

Chlorpromazine Hydrochloride (Co-administration with dopamine antagonists may diminish the effectiveness of ropinirole).
No products indexed under this heading.

Chlorprothixene (Co-administration with dopamine antagonists may diminish the effectiveness of ropinirole).
No products indexed under this heading.

Chlorprothixene Hydrochloride (Co-administration with dopamine antagonists may diminish the effectiveness of ropinirole).
No products indexed under this heading.

Chlorprothixene Lactate (Possible additive sedative effects).
No products indexed under this heading.

Cimetidine (If therapy with a drug known to be a potent inhibitor of CYP1A2 is stopped or started during treatment with ropinirole hydrochloride, adjustment of the dose of ropinirole hydrocholoride may be required). Products include:
Tagamet HB 200 Tablets .... ▣637
Tagamet Tablets 1547

Cimetidine Hydrochloride (If therapy with a drug known to be a potent inhibitor of CYP1A2 is stopped or started during treatment with ropinirole hydrochloride, adjustment of the dose of ropinirole hydrocholoride may be required).
No products indexed under this heading.

Ciprofloxacin (Co-administration increases ropinirole AUC by 84% on average and Cmax by 60%). Products include:
Cipro I.V. 2998
Cipro I.V. Pharmacy Bulk Package 3509
Cipro Oral Suspension 2991
Cipro XR Tablets 3004
Ciprodex Otic Suspension 555

Ciprofloxacin Hydrochloride (Co-administration increases ropinirole AUC by 84% on average and Cmax by 60%). Products include:
Ciloxan Ophthalmic Ointment 554
Cipro Tablets 2991

Citalopram Hydrobromide (Possible additive sedative effects). Products include:
Celexa 1177

Clarithromycin (If therapy with a drug known to be a potent inhibitor of CYP1A2 is stopped or started during treatment with ropinirole hydrochloride, adjustment of the dose of ropinirole hydrocholoride may be required). Products include:
Biaxin/Biaxin XL 402
PREVPAC 3281

Clorazepate Dipotassium (Possible additive sedative effects). Products include:
Tranxene 2488

Clozapine (Possible additive sedative effects). Products include:
Clozapine Tablets 2141
Clozaril Tablets 2174
FazaClo Orally Disintegrating Tablets 547

Codeine Phosphate (Possible additive sedative effects). Products include:
Tylenol with Codeine 2461

Desflurane (Possible additive sedative effects). Products include:
Suprane Liquid for Inhalation 770

Desipramine Hydrochloride (Possible additive sedative effects).
No products indexed under this heading.

Desogestrel (If therapy with a drug known to be a potent inhibitor of CYP1A2 is stopped or started during treatment with ropinirole hydrochloride, adjustment of the dose of ropinirole hydrocholoride may be required). Products include:
Ortho-Cept Tablets 2395

Dezocine (Possible additive sedative effects).
No products indexed under this heading.

Diazepam (Possible additive sedative effects). Products include:
Diastat Rectal Delivery System 3344
Valium Tablets 2822

Doxepin Hydrochloride (Possible additive sedative effects).
No products indexed under this heading.

Droperidol (Possible additive sedative effects).
No products indexed under this heading.

Enflurane (Possible additive sedative effects).
No products indexed under this heading.

Enoxacin (If therapy with a drug known to be a potent inhibitor of CYP1A2 is stopped or started during treatment with ropinirole hydrochloride, adjustment of the dose of ropinirole hydrocholoride may be required).
No products indexed under this heading.

Escitalopram Oxalate (Possible additive sedative effects). Products include:
Lexapro Oral Solution 1193
Lexapro Tablets 1193

Estazolam (Possible additive sedative effects). Products include:
ProSom Tablets 512

Ethanol (Possible additive sedative effects).
No products indexed under this heading.

Ethchlorvynol (Possible additive sedative effects).
No products indexed under this heading.

Ethinamate (Possible additive sedative effects).
No products indexed under this heading.

Ethinyl Estradiol (Reduces the oral clearance of ropinirole by 36%). Products include:
Alesse-28 Tablets 3392
Lo/Ovral-28 Tablets 3423
NuvaRing 2357
Ortho-Cept Tablets 2395
Ortho-Cyclen/Ortho Tri-Cyclen 2414
Ortho Evra Transdermal System 2402
Ortho Tri-Cyclen Lo Tablets 2421
Seasonale Tablets 1073
Triphasil-28 Tablets 3483
Yasmin 28 Tablets 818

Ethyl Alcohol (Possible additive sedative effects).
No products indexed under this heading.

Fentanyl (Possible additive sedative effects). Products include:
Duragesic Transdermal System 2448

Fentanyl Citrate (Possible additive sedative effects). Products include:
Actiq 993

Fluoxetine Hydrochloride (Possible additive sedative effects). Products include:
Prozac Pulvules and Liquid 1771
Symbyax Capsules 1788

Fluphenazine Decanoate (Co-administration with dopamine antagonists may diminish the effectiveness of ropinirole).
No products indexed under this heading.

Fluphenazine Enanthate (Co-administration with dopamine antagonists may diminish the effectiveness of ropinirole).
No products indexed under this heading.

Fluphenazine Hydrochloride (Co-administration with dopamine antagonists may diminish the effectiveness of ropinirole).
No products indexed under this heading.

Flurazepam Hydrochloride (Possible additive sedative effects). Products include:
Dalmane Capsules **3343**

Fluvoxamine (If therapy with a drug known to be a potent inhibitor of CYP1A2 is stopped or started during treatment with ropinirole hydrochloride, adjustment of the dose of ropinirole hydrocholoride may be required).
No products indexed under this heading.

Fluvoxamine Maleate (If therapy with a drug known to be a potent inhibitor of CYP1A2 is stopped or started during treatment with ropinirole hydrochloride, adjustment of the dose of ropinirole hydrocholoride may be required).
No products indexed under this heading.

Gatifloxacin (If therapy with a drug known to be a potent inhibitor of CYP1A2 is stopped or started during treatment with ropinirole hydrochloride, adjustment of the dose of ropinirole hydrocholoride may be required). Products include:
Tequin Injection **964**
Tequin Tablets **964**
Zymar Ophthalmic Solution **571**

Gemifloxacin Mesylate (If therapy with a drug known to be a potent inhibitor of CYP1A2 is stopped or started during treatment with ropinirole hydrochloride, adjustment of the dose of ropinirole hydrocholoride may be required). Products include:
Factive Tablets **2464**

Glutethimide (Possible additive sedative effects).
No products indexed under this heading.

Grepafloxacin Hydrochloride (If therapy with a drug known to be a potent inhibitor of CYP1A2 is stopped or started during treatment with ropinirole hydrochloride, adjustment of the dose of ropinirole hydrocholoride may be required).
No products indexed under this heading.

Haloperidol (Co-administration with dopamine antagonists may diminish the effectiveness of ropinirole).
No products indexed under this heading.

Haloperidol Decanoate (Co-administration with dopamine antagonists may diminish the effectiveness of ropinirole).
No products indexed under this heading.

Hydrocodone Bitartrate (Possible additive sedative effects). Products include:
Hycodan **1104**
Hycomine Compound Tablets **1105**
Hycotuss Expectorant Syrup **1106**
Lortab **3315**
Lortab Elixir **3312**
Vicodin Tablets **530**
Vicodin ES Tablets **531**
Vicodin HP Tablets **532**
Vicoprofen Tablets **533**
Zydone Tablets **1118**

Hydrocodone Polistirex (Possible additive sedative effects). Products include:
Tussionex Pennkinetic Extended-Release Suspension **3322**

Hydromorphone Hydrochloride (Possible additive sedative effects). Products include:
Dilaudid **439**
Dilaudid Oral Liquid **443**
Dilaudid Non-Sterile Powder **439**
Dilaudid Rectal Suppositories **439**
Dilaudid Tablets **439**
Dilaudid Tablets - 8 mg **443**
Dilaudid-HP **441**

Hydroxyzine Hydrochloride (Possible additive sedative effects).
No products indexed under this heading.

Imipramine Hydrochloride (Possible additive sedative effects).
No products indexed under this heading.

Imipramine Pamoate (Possible additive sedative effects).
No products indexed under this heading.

Isocarboxazid (Possible additive sedative effects).
No products indexed under this heading.

Isoflurane (Possible additive sedative effects).
No products indexed under this heading.

Isoniazid (If therapy with a drug known to be a potent inhibitor of CYP1A2 is stopped or started during treatment with ropinirole hydrochloride, adjustment of the dose of ropinirole hydrocholoride may be required).
No products indexed under this heading.

Ketamine Hydrochloride (Possible additive sedative effects).
No products indexed under this heading.

Ketoconazole (If therapy with a drug known to be a potent inhibitor of CYP1A2 is stopped or started during treatment with ropinirole hydrochloride, adjustment of the dose of ropinirole hydrocholoride may be required). Products include:
Nizoral A-D Shampoo, 1% **1839**
Nizoral 2% Shampoo **1838**

Levodopa (Ropinirole may potentiate the dopaminergic effects of L-dopa and may cause and/or exacerbate pre-existing dyskinesia; increased mean steady state of L-dopa by 20%). Products include:
Parcopa Orally Disintegrating Tablets **3111**
Stalevo Tablets **2270**

Levofloxacin (If therapy with a drug known to be a potent inhibitor of CYP1A2 is stopped or started during treatment with ropinirole hydrochloride, adjustment of the dose of ropinirole hydrocholoride may be required). Products include:
Levaquin in 5% Dextrose Injection **2453**
Levaquin **2453**
Quixin Ophthalmic Solution **3373**

Levomethadyl Acetate Hydrochloride (Possible additive sedative effects).
No products indexed under this heading.

Levonorgestrel (If therapy with a drug known to be a potent inhibitor of CYP1A2 is stopped or started during treatment with ropinirole hydrochloride, adjustment of the dose of ropinirole hydrocholoride may be required). Products include:
Alesse-28 Tablets **3392**
Climara Pro Transdermal System **800**
Mirena Intrauterine System **810**
Plan B Tablets **1068**
Seasonale Tablets **1073**
Triphasil-28 Tablets **3483**

Levorphanol Tartrate (Possible additive sedative effects).
No products indexed under this heading.

Lomefloxacin Hydrochloride (If therapy with a drug known to be a potent inhibitor of CYP1A2 is stopped or started during treatment with ropinirole hydrochloride, adjustment of the dose of ropinirole hydrocholoride may be required).
No products indexed under this heading.

Lorazepam (Possible additive sedative effects).
No products indexed under this heading.

Loxapine Hydrochloride (Co-administration with dopamine antagonists may diminish the effectiveness of ropinirole).
No products indexed under this heading.

Loxapine Succinate (Co-administration with dopamine antagonists may diminish the effectiveness of ropinirole).
No products indexed under this heading.

Maprotiline Hydrochloride (Possible additive sedative effects).
No products indexed under this heading.

Meperidine Hydrochloride (Possible additive sedative effects).
No products indexed under this heading.

Mephobarbital (Possible additive sedative effects). Products include:
Mebaral Tablets, USP **2483**

Meprobamate (Possible additive sedative effects).
No products indexed under this heading.

Mesoridazine Besylate (Co-administration with dopamine antagonists may diminish the effectiveness of ropinirole).
No products indexed under this heading.

Mestranol (If therapy with a drug known to be a potent inhibitor of CYP1A2 is stopped or started during treatment with ropinirole hydrochloride, adjustment of the dose of ropinirole hydrocholoride may be required).
No products indexed under this heading.

Methadone Hydrochloride (Possible additive sedative effects).
No products indexed under this heading.

Methohexital Sodium (Possible additive sedative effects).
No products indexed under this heading.

Methotrimeprazine (Co-administration with dopamine antagonists may diminish the effectiveness of ropinirole).
No products indexed under this heading.

Methoxsalen (If therapy with a drug known to be a potent inhibitor of CYP1A2 is stopped or started during treatment with ropinirole hydrochloride, adjustment of the dose of ropinirole hydrocholoride may be required). Products include:
Oxsoralen Lotion 1% **3354**
Oxsoralen-Ultra Capsules **3354**

Methoxyflurane (Possible additive sedative effects).
No products indexed under this heading.

Metoclopramide Hydrochloride (Co-administration with dopamine antagonists may diminish the effectiveness of ropinirole).
No products indexed under this heading.

Mexiletine Hydrochloride (If therapy with a drug known to be a potent inhibitor of CYP1A2 is stopped or started during treatment with ropinirole hydrochloride, adjustment of the dose of ropinirole hydrocholoride may be required).
No products indexed under this heading.

Mibefradil Dihydrochloride (If therapy with a drug known to be a potent inhibitor of CYP1A2 is stopped or started during treatment with ropinirole hydrochloride, adjustment of the dose of ropinirole hydrocholoride may be required).
No products indexed under this heading.

Midazolam Hydrochloride (Possible additive sedative effects).
No products indexed under this heading.

Mirtazapine (Possible additive sedative effects).
No products indexed under this heading.

Molindone Hydrochloride (Co-administration with dopamine antagonists may diminish the effectiveness of ropinirole). Products include:
Moban Tablets **1108**

Morphine Sulfate (Possible additive sedative effects). Products include:
Avinza Capsules **1714**
Kadian Capsules **572**
MS Contin Tablets **2703**

Moxifloxacin Hydrochloride (If therapy with a drug known to be a potent inhibitor of CYP1A2 is stopped or started during treatment with ropinirole hydrochloride, adjustment of the dose of ropinirole hydrocholoride may be required). Products include:
Avelox **2984**
Vigamox Ophthalmic Solution **560**

Nalidixic Acid (If therapy with a drug known to be a potent inhibitor of CYP1A2 is stopped or started during treatment with ropinirole hydrochloride, adjustment of the dose of ropinirole hydrocholoride may be required).
No products indexed under this heading.

Nefazodone Hydrochloride (Possible additive sedative effects).
No products indexed under this heading.

Norethindrone (If therapy with a drug known to be a potent inhibitor of CYP1A2 is stopped or started during treatment with ropinirole hydrochloride, adjustment of the dose of ropinirole hydrocholoride may be required). Products include:
Ortho Micronor Tablets 2411

Norfloxacin (If therapy with a drug known to be a potent inhibitor of CYP1A2 is stopped or started during treatment with ropinirole hydrochloride, adjustment of the dose of ropinirole hydrocholoride may be required). Products include:
Noroxin Tablets 2009

Norgestrel (If therapy with a drug known to be a potent inhibitor of CYP1A2 is stopped or started during treatment with ropinirole hydrochloride, adjustment of the dose of ropinirole hydrocholoride may be required). Products include:
Lo/Ovral-28 Tablets 3423

Nortriptyline Hydrochloride (Possible additive sedative effects).
No products indexed under this heading.

Ofloxacin (If therapy with a drug known to be a potent inhibitor of CYP1A2 is stopped or started during treatment with ropinirole hydrochloride, adjustment of the dose of ropinirole hydrocholoride may be required). Products include:
Floxin Otic Singles 1045
Floxin Otic Solution 1043

Olanzapine (Possible additive sedative effects). Products include:
Symbyax Capsules 1788
Zyprexa Tablets 1798
Zyprexa IntraMuscular 1798
Zyprexa ZYDIS Orally Disintegrating Tablets 1798

Omeprazole (If therapy with a drug known to be a potent inhibitor of CYP1A2 is stopped or started during treatment with ropinirole hydrochloride, adjustment of the dose of ropinirole hydrocholoride may be required). Products include:
Zegerid Powder for Oral Solution 2972

Oxazepam (Possible additive sedative effects).
No products indexed under this heading.

Oxycodone Hydrochloride (Possible additive sedative effects).
Products include:
Combunox Tablets 1183
OxyContin Tablets 2699
OxyFast Oral Concentrate Solution 2704
OxyIR Capsules 2704
Percocet Tablets 1114
Percodan Tablets 1115

Paroxetine Hydrochloride (Possible additive sedative effects).
Products include:
Paxil CR Controlled-Release Tablets 1509
Paxil 1501

Pentobarbital Sodium (Possible additive sedative effects). Products include:
Nembutal Sodium Solution, USP 2484

Perphenazine (Co-administration with dopamine antagonists may diminish the effectiveness of ropinirole).
No products indexed under this heading.

Phenelzine Sulfate (Possible additive sedative effects).
No products indexed under this heading.

Phenobarbital (Possible additive sedative effects).
No products indexed under this heading.

Prazepam (Possible additive sedative effects).
No products indexed under this heading.

Prochlorperazine (Co-administration with dopamine antagonists may diminish the effectiveness of ropinirole).
No products indexed under this heading.

Promethazine Hydrochloride (Co-administration with dopamine antagonists may diminish the effectiveness of ropinirole). Products include:
Phenergan 3438

Propofol (Possible additive sedative effects). Products include:
Diprivan Injectable Emulsion 676

Propoxyphene Hydrochloride (Possible additive sedative effects).
No products indexed under this heading.

Propoxyphene Napsylate (Possible additive sedative effects).
Products include:
Darvocet A 500 Tablets 3497

Protriptyline Hydrochloride (Possible additive sedative effects).
Products include:
Vivactil Tablets 2350

Quazepam (Possible additive sedative effects).
No products indexed under this heading.

Quetiapine Fumarate (Co-administration with dopamine antagonists may diminish the effectiveness of ropinirole). Products include:
Seroquel Tablets 691

Ranitidine Hydrochloride (If therapy with a drug known to be a potent inhibitor of CYP1A2 is stopped or started during treatment with ropinirole hydrochloride, adjustment of the dose of ropinirole hydrocholoride may be required). Products include:
Zantac 1597
Zantac Injection 1593
Zantac 75 Tablets .... ▣715
Zantac 150 Maximum Strength Tablets .... ▣715
Zantac Injection Pharmacy Bulk Package 1595

Remifentanil Hydrochloride (Possible additive sedative effects).
No products indexed under this heading.

Risperidone (Co-administration with dopamine antagonists may diminish the effectiveness of ropinirole).
Products include:
Risperdal Consta Long-Acting Injection 1664
Risperdal M-Tab Orally Disintegrating Tablets 1658
Risperdal 1658

Ritonavir (If therapy with a drug known to be a potent inhibitor of CYP1A2 is stopped or started during treatment with ropinirole hydrochloride, adjustment of the dose of ropinirole hydrocholoride may be required). Products include:
Kaletra 474
Norvir 499

Secobarbital Sodium (Possible additive sedative effects).
No products indexed under this heading.

Sertraline Hydrochloride (Possible additive sedative effects).
Products include:
Zoloft 2581

Sevoflurane (Possible additive sedative effects). Products include:
Ultane Liquid for Inhalation 526

Sodium Oxybate (Possible additive sedative effects).
No products indexed under this heading.

Sparfloxacin (If therapy with a drug known to be a potent inhibitor of CYP1A2 is stopped or started during treatment with ropinirole hydrochloride, adjustment of the dose of ropinirole hydrocholoride may be required).
No products indexed under this heading.

Sufentanil Citrate (Possible additive sedative effects).
No products indexed under this heading.

Tacrine Hydrochloride (If therapy with a drug known to be a potent inhibitor of CYP1A2 is stopped or started during treatment with ropinirole hydrochloride, adjustment of the dose of ropinirole hydrocholoride may be required).
No products indexed under this heading.

Temazepam (Possible additive sedative effects).
No products indexed under this heading.

Thiamylal Sodium (Possible additive sedative effects).
No products indexed under this heading.

Thioridazine Hydrochloride (Co-administration with dopamine antagonists may diminish the effectiveness of ropinirole). Products include:
Thioridazine Hydrochloride Tablets 2122

Thiothixene (Co-administration with dopamine antagonists may diminish the effectiveness of ropinirole).
Products include:
Thiothixene Capsules 2124

Ticlopidine Hydrochloride (If therapy with a drug known to be a potent inhibitor of CYP1A2 is stopped or started during treatment with ropinirole hydrochloride, adjustment of the dose of ropinirole hydrocholoride may be required). Products include:
Ticlid Tablets 2813

Tobacco (Decreases ropinirole Cmax by 30% and decreases AUC by 38%).
No products indexed under this heading.

Tranylcypromine Sulfate (Possible additive sedative effects).
Products include:
Parnate Tablets 1499

Trazodone Hydrochloride (Possible additive sedative effects).
No products indexed under this heading.

Triazolam (Possible additive sedative effects).
No products indexed under this heading.

Trifluoperazine Hydrochloride (Co-administration with dopamine antagonists may diminish the effectiveness of ropinirole).
No products indexed under this heading.

Trimipramine Maleate (Possible additive sedative effects). Products include:
Surmontil Capsules 2347

Troleandomycin (If therapy with a drug known to be a potent inhibitor of CYP1A2 is stopped or started during treatment with ropinirole hydrochloride, adjustment of the dose of ropinirole hydrocholoride may be required).
No products indexed under this heading.

Trovafloxacin Mesylate (If therapy with a drug known to be a potent inhibitor of CYP1A2 is stopped or started during treatment with ropinirole hydrochloride, adjustment of the dose of ropinirole hydrocholoride may be required).
No products indexed under this heading.

Venlafaxine Hydrochloride (Possible additive sedative effects).
Products include:
Effexor Tablets 3405
Effexor XR Capsules 3411

Zaleplon (Possible additive sedative effects). Products include:
Sonata Capsules 1686

Zileuton (If therapy with a drug known to be a potent inhibitor of CYP1A2 is stopped or started during treatment with ropinirole hydrochloride, adjustment of the dose of ropinirole hydrocholoride may be required).
No products indexed under this heading.

Ziprasidone Hydrochloride (Possible additive sedative effects).
Products include:
Geodon Capsules 2514

Zolpidem Tartrate (Possible additive sedative effects). Products include:
Ambien Tablets 2867

Food Interactions

Alcohol (Possible additive sedative effects).

Food, unspecified (Food does not affect the extent of absorption of ropinirole, although Tmax is increased by 2.5 hours and Cmax is decreased by 25% when taken with a high fat meal).

Grapefruit Juice (If therapy with a drug known to be a potent inhibitor of CYP1A2 is stopped or started during treatment with ropinirole hydrochloride, adjustment of the dose of ropinirole hydrocholoride may be required).

RESCRIPTOR TABLETS

(Delavirdine Mesylate) 2535
May interact with amphetamines, antacids, dexamethasone, dihydropyridine calcium channel blockers, ergot-containing drugs, histamine H_2-receptor antagonists, phenytoin, proton pump inhibitor, quinidine, and certain other agents. Compounds in these categories include:

Alprazolam (Co-administration with drugs that are highly dependent on CYP3A for clearance and for which elevated plasma levels are associated with serious and/or life threatening events, such as prolonged or increased sedation or respiratory depression, is contraindicated).
Products include:
Niravam Orally Disintegrating Tablets 3106
Xanax XR Tablets 2655

Aluminum Carbonate (Co-administration with antacids results in decreased delavirdine concentrations because of reduced absorption; patients taking antacids should be advised to take them at least one hour apart).
No products indexed under this heading.

Aluminum Hydroxide (Co-administration with antacids results in decreased delavirdine concentrations because of reduced absorption; patients taking antacids should be advised to take them at least one hour apart). Products include:
Gaviscon Regular Strength Liquid .. 620
Gaviscon Regular Strength Tablets 619
Gaviscon Extra Strength Liquid 620
Gaviscon Extra Strength Tablets 619
Maalox Max Maximum Strength Antacid/Anti-Gas Liquid 2165
Maalox Regular Strength Antacid/Antigas Liquid 2164

Amiodarone Hydrochloride (Co-administration results in increased amiodarone concentrations). Products include:
Pacerone Tablets 3337

Amlodipine Besylate (Co-administration results in increased dihydropyridine calcium channel blocker concentrations). Products include:
Caduet Tablets 2507
Lotrel Capsules 2238
Norvasc Tablets 2529

Amphetamine Resins (Co-administration results in increased amphetamine concentrations).
No products indexed under this heading.

Amphetamine Sulfate (Co-administration results in increased amphetamine concentrations). Products include:
Adderall Tablets 3168
Adderall XR Capsules 3169

Amprenavir (Co-administration results in increased amprenavir concentrations). Products include:
Agenerase Capsules 1299
Agenerase Oral Solution 1304

Astemizole (Co-administration with drugs that are highly dependent on CYP3A for clearance and for which elevated plasma levels are associated with serious and/or life-threatening events, such as cardiac arrhythmias; concurrent use is contraindicated).
No products indexed under this heading.

Atorvastatin Calcium (The risk of myopathy, including rhabdomolysis, may be increased with concurrent use). Products include:
Caduet Tablets 2507
Lipitor Tablets 2495

Bepridil Hydrochloride (Co-administration results in increased bepridil concentrations; increased bepridil exposure may be associated with life-threatening reactions such as cardiac arrhythmias).
No products indexed under this heading.

Carbamazepine (May lead to loss of virologic response and possible resistance to delavirdine or the class of non-nucleoside reverse transcriptase inhibitors). Products include:
Carbatrol Capsules 3174
Equetro Extended-Release Capsules 3178
Tegretol/Tegretol-XR 2278

Cerivastatin Sodium (The risk of myopathy, including rhabdomyolysis, may be increased with concurrent use).
No products indexed under this heading.

Cimetidine (H2 antagonists increase gastric pH and may reduce the absorption of delavirdine; chronic use of these drugs with delavirdine is not recommended). Products include:
Tagamet HB 200 Tablets 637
Tagamet Tablets 1547

Cimetidine Hydrochloride (H2 antagonists increase gastric pH and may reduce the absorption of delavirdine; chronic use of these drugs with delavirdine is not recommended).
No products indexed under this heading.

Cisapride (Co-administration with drugs that are highly dependent on CYP3A for clearance and for which elevated plasma levels are associated with serious and/or life-threatening events, such as cardiac arrhythmias, is contraindicated).
No products indexed under this heading.

Clarithromycin (Co-administrations results in increased clarithromycin concentrations). Products include:
Biaxin/Biaxin XL 402
PREVPAC 3281

Cyclosporine (Co-administration results in increased cyclosporine concentrations). Products include:
Gengraf Capsules 458
Neoral Soft Gelatin Capsules 2247
Neoral Oral Solution 2247
Restasis Ophthalmic Emulsion 570
Sandimmune 2259

Dexamethasone (Co-administration results in decreased delavirdine concentrations). Products include:
Ciprodex Otic Suspension 555
Decadron Tablets 1929
TobraDex Ophthalmic Ointment 558
TobraDex Ophthalmic Suspension ... 558

Dexamethasone Acetate (Co-administration results in decreased delavirdine concentrations).
No products indexed under this heading.

Dexamethasone Sodium Phosphate (Co-administration results in decreased delavirdine concentrations). Products include:
Decadron Phosphate Injection 1931

Dextroamphetamine Sulfate (Co-administration results in increased amphetamine concentrations). Products include:
Adderall Tablets 3168
Adderall XR Capsules 3169
Dexedrine 1386
DextroStat Tablets 3177

Didanosine (Co-administration results in decreased didanosine and delavirdine plasma concentrations; administration of didanosine (buffered tablets) and delavirdine should be separated by at least one hour).
No products indexed under this heading.

Dihydroergotamine Mesylate (Co-administration with drugs that are highly dependent on CYP3A for clearance and for which elevated plasma levels are associated with serious and/or life-threatening events, such as acute ergot toxicity characterized by peripheral vasospasm and ischemiaof the extremities, is contraindicated). Products include:
Migranal Nasal Spray 3350

Diltiazem Hydrochloride (Co-administration results in increased calcium channel blocker concentrations). Products include:
Cardizem LA Extended Release Tablets 1699
Tiazac Capsules 1204

Ergonovine Maleate (Co-administration with drugs that are highly dependent on CYP3A for clearance and for which elevated plasma levels are associated with serious and/or life-threatening events, such as acute ergot toxicity characterized by peripheral vasospasm and ischemiaof the extremities, is contraindicated).
No products indexed under this heading.

Ergotamine Tartrate (Co-administration with drugs that are highly dependent on CYP3A for clearance and for which elevated plasma levels are associated with serious and/or life-threatening events, such as acute ergot toxicity characterized by peripheral vasospasm and ischemiaof the extremities, is contraindicated).
No products indexed under this heading.

Esomeprazole Magnesium (Proton pump inhibitors increase gastric pH and may reduce the absorption of delavirdine; chronic use of these drugs with delavirdine is not recommended). Products include:
Nexium Delayed-Release Capsules 645

Ethinyl Estradiol (Co-administration results in increased ethinyl estradiol concentrations). Products include:
Alesse-28 Tablets 3392
Lo/Ovral-28 Tablets 3423
NuvaRing 2357
Ortho-Cept Tablets 2395
Ortho-Cyclen/Ortho Tri-Cyclen 2414
Ortho Evra Transdermal System 2402
Ortho Tri-Cyclen Lo Tablets 2421
Seasonale Tablets 1073
Triphasil-28 Tablets 3483
Yasmin 28 Tablets 818

Famotidine (H2 antagonists increase gastric pH and may reduce the absorption of delavirdine; chronic use of these drugs with delavirdine is not recommended). Products include:
Pepcid AC Chewable Tablets 1672
Pepcid AC Gelcaps 1672
Pepcid AC Tablets 1672
Maximum Strength Pepcid AC Tablets 1672
Pepcid Complete Chewable Tablets 1672
Pepcid Injection 2017
Pepcid 2014

Felodipine (Co-administration results in increased dihydropyridine calcium channel blocker concentrations). Products include:
Plendil Extended-Release Tablets 651

Flecainide Acetate (Co-administration results in increased flecainide concentrations). Products include:
Tambocor Tablets 1824

Fluoxetine Hydrochloride (Co-administration has resulted in 50% change in the Cmax). Products include:
Prozac Pulvules and Liquid 1771
Symbyax Capsules 1788

Fluvastatin Sodium (Co-administration results in increased fluvastatin concentrations). Products include:
Lescol Capsules 2227
Lescol 2730
Lescol XL Tablets 2227

Fosphenytoin Sodium (May lead to loss of virologic response and possible resistance to delavirdine or the class of non-nucleoside reverse transcriptase inhibitors).
No products indexed under this heading.

Hypericum (Co-administration with St. John's Wort or St. John's Wort-containing products and delavirdine is expected to substantially decrease delavirdine's concentrations and may result in suboptimal levels of delavirdine and lead to loss of virologic response).
No products indexed under this heading.

Indinavir Sulfate (Co-administration results in increased indinavir concentrations; a dose reduction of indinavir to 600 mg t.i.d. should be considered when used concurrently). Products include:
Crixivan Capsules 1918

Isradipine (Co-administration results in increased dihydropyridine calcium channel blocker concentrations). Products include:
DynaCirc CR Tablets 2726

Lansoprazole (Proton pump inhibitors increase gastric pH and may reduce the absorption of delavirdine; chronic use of these drugs with delavirdine is not recommended). Products include:
Prevacid Delayed-Release Capsules 3268
Prevacid for Delayed-Release Oral Suspension 3268
Prevacid I.V. for Injection 3274
Prevacid NapraPAC 3277
Prevacid SoluTab Delayed-Release Orally Disintegrating Tablets 3268
PREVPAC 3281

Lidocaine Hydrochloride (Co-administration results in increased systemic lidocaine concentrations).
No products indexed under this heading.

Lopinavir (Co-administration results in increased lopinavir concentrations). Products include:
Kaletra 474

Lovastatin (Potential for serious reactions such as myopathy including rhabdomyolysis; concurrent use is not recommended). Products include:
Advicor Tablets 1694
Altoprev Extended-Release Tablets 1151
Mevacor Tablets 1996

Magaldrate (Co-administration with antacids results in decreased delavirdine concentrations because of reduced absorption; patients taking antacids should be advised to take them at least one hour apart).
No products indexed under this heading.

Magnesium Hydroxide (Co-administration with antacids results in decreased delavirdine concentrations because of reduced absorption; patients taking antacids should be advised to take them at least one hour apart). Products include:
Maalox Max Maximum Strength Antacid/Anti-Gas Liquid 2165

IMPORTANT NOTE: Always consult each drug listing in the patient's regimen for possible interactions.

Maalox Regular Strength Antacid/Antigas Liquid 2164
Pepcid Complete Chewable Tablets 1672
Rolaids Tablets .... ■707
Extra Strength Rolaids Tablets .... ■707
Rolaids Multi-Symptom Antacid & Antigas Tablets .... ■708

Magnesium Oxide (Co-administration with antacids results in decreased delavirdine concentrations because of reduced absorption; patients taking antacids should be advised to take them at least one hour apart). Products include:
Beelith Tablets 784
PremCal Light, Regular, and Extra Strength Tablets .... ■762

Methadone Hydrochloride (Co-administration results in increased methadone concentrations).
No products indexed under this heading.

Methamphetamine Hydrochloride (Co-administration results in increased amphetamine concentrations). Products include:
Desoxyn Tablets, USP 2482

Methylergonovine Maleate (Co-administration with drugs that are highly dependent on CYP3A for clearance and for which elevated plasma levels are associated with serious and/or life-threatening events, such as acute ergot toxicity characterized by peripheral vasospasm and ischemiaof the extremities, is contraindicated).
No products indexed under this heading.

Methysergide Maleate (Co-administration with drugs that are highly dependent on CYP3A for clearance and for which elevated plasma levels are associated with serious and/or life-threatening events, such as acute ergot toxicity characterized by peripheral vasospasm and ischemiaof the extremities, is contraindicated).
No products indexed under this heading.

Midazolam Hydrochloride (Co-administration with drugs that are highly dependent on CYP3A for clearance and for which elevated plasma levels are associated with serious and/or life-threatening events, such as cardiac arrhythmias, is contraindicated).
No products indexed under this heading.

Nelfinavir Mesylate (Co-administration results in increased nelfinavir concentrations and decreased delavirdine concentrations). Products include:
Viracept 2556

Nicardipine Hydrochloride (Co-administration results in increased dihydropyridine calcium channel blocker concentrations). Products include:
Cardene I.V. 1129

Nifedipine (Co-administration results in increased dihydropyridine calcium channel blocker concentrations). Products include:
Adalat CC Tablets 2978

Nimodipine (Co-administration results in increased dihydropyridine calcium channel blocker concentrations). Products include:
Nimotop Capsules 774

Nisoldipine (Co-adminstration results in increased calcium channel blocker concentrations). Products include:
Sular Tablets 1163

Nizatidine (H2 antagonists increase gastric pH and may reduce the absorption of delavirdine; chronic use of these drugs with delavirdine is not recommended). Products include:
Axid Oral Solution 913

Omeprazole (Proton pump inhibitors increase gastric pH and may reduce the absorption of delavirdine; chronic use of these drugs with delavirdine is not recommended). Products include:
Zegerid Powder for Oral Solution 2972

Pantoprazole Sodium (Proton pump inhibitors increase gastric pH and may reduce the absorption of delavirdine; chronic use of these drugs with delavirdine is not recommended). Products include:
Protonix I.V. 3468
Protonix Tablets 3465

Phenobarbital (May lead to loss of virologic response and possible resistance to delavirdine or the class of non-nucleoside reverse transcriptase inhibitors).
No products indexed under this heading.

Phenytoin (May lead to loss of virologic response and possible resistance to delavirdine or the class of non-nucleoside reverse transcriptase inhibitors).
No products indexed under this heading.

Phenytoin Sodium (May lead to loss of virologic response and possible resistance to delavirdine or the class of non-nucleoside reverse transcriptase inhibitors). Products include:
Phenytek Capsules 2153

Pimozide (Co-administration with drugs that are highly dependent on CYP3A for clearance and for which elevated plasma levels are associated with serious and/or life-threatening events, such as cardiac arrhythmias, is contraindicated). Products include:
Orap Tablets 1220

Propafenone Hydrochloride (Co-administration results in increased propafenone concentrations). Products include:
Rythmol SR Capsules 2736

Quinidine (Co-administration results in increased quinidine concentrations).
No products indexed under this heading.

Quinidine Gluconate (Co-administration results in increased quinidine concentrations).
No products indexed under this heading.

Quinidine Hydrochloride (Co-administration results in increased quinidine concentrations).
No products indexed under this heading.

Quinidine Polygalacturonate (Co-administration results in increased quinidine concentrations).
No products indexed under this heading.

Quinidine Sulfate (Co-administration results in increased quinidine concentrations).
No products indexed under this heading.

Rabeprazole Sodium (Proton pump inhibitors increase gastric pH and may reduce the absorption of delavirdine; chronic use of these drugs with delavirdine is not recommended). Products include:
Aciphex Tablets 1081

Ranitidine Bismuth Citrate (H2 antagonists increase gastric pH and may reduce the absorption of delavirdine; chronic use of these drugs with delavirdine is not recommended).
No products indexed under this heading.

Ranitidine Hydrochloride (H2 antagonists increase gastric pH and may reduce the absorption of delavirdine; chronic use of these drugs with delavirdine is not recommended). Products include:
Zantac 1597
Zantac Injection 1593
Zantac 75 Tablets .... ■715
Zantac 150 Maximum Strength Tablets .... ■715
Zantac Injection Pharmacy Bulk Package 1595

Rapamycin (Co-administration results in increased rapamycin concentrations).
No products indexed under this heading.

Rifabutin (May lead to loss of virologic response and possible resistance to delavirdine or the class of non-nucleoside reverse transcriptase inhibitors or other co-administered antiviral drugs).
No products indexed under this heading.

Rifampin (May lead to loss or virologic response and possible resistance to delavirdine or the class of non-nucleoside reverse transcriptase inhibitors or other co-administered antiviral drugs).
No products indexed under this heading.

Ritonavir (Co-administration results in increased ritonavir concentrations). Products include:
Kaletra 474
Norvir 499

Saquinavir (Co-administration results in increased saquinavir concentrations).
No products indexed under this heading.

Saquinavir Mesylate (Co-administration results in increased saquinavir concentrations). Products include:
Invirase 2776

Sildenafil Citrate (Co-administration is expected to substantially increase sildenafil concentrations and may result in an increase in sildenafil-associated adverse events, including hypotension, visual changes, and priapism). Products include:
Revatio Tablets 2541
Viagra Tablets 2552

Simvastatin (Potential for serious reactions such as myopathy including rhabdomyolysis; concurrent use is not recommended). Products include:
Vytorin 10/10 Tablets 2084
Vytorin 10/10 Tablets 3092
Vytorin 10/20 Tablets 2084
Vytorin 10/20 Tablets 3092
Vytorin 10/40 Tablets 3092
Vytorin 10/40 Tablets 2084
Vytorin 10/80 Tablets 2084
Vytorin 10/80 Tablets 3092
Zocor Tablets 2078

Sodium Bicarbonate (Co-administration with antacids results in decreased delavirdine concentrations because of reduced absorption; patients taking antacids should be advised to take them at least one hour apart). Products include:
Ceo-Two Evacuant Suppository .... ■607
Colyte with Flavor Packs for Oral Solution 3102
HalfLytely and Bisacodyl Tablets Bowel Prep Kit with Flavors Packs 915
TriLyte with Flavor Packs for Oral Solution 3114

Tacrolimus (Co-administration results in increased tacrolimus concentrations). Products include:
Prograf Capsules and Injection 624
Protopic Ointment 629

Terfenadine (Co-administration with drugs that are highly dependent on CYP3A for clearance and for which elevated plasma levels are associated with serious and/or life-threatening events, such as cardiac arrhythmias, is contraindicated).
No products indexed under this heading.

Triazolam (Co-administration with drugs that are highly dependent on CYP3A for clearance and for which elevated plasma levels are associated with serious and/or life-threatening events, such as prolonged or increased sedation or respiratory depression, is contraindicated).
No products indexed under this heading.

Verapamil Hydrochloride (Co-administration results in increased calcium channel blocker concentrations). Products include:
Covera-HS Tablets 3135
Tarka Tablets 519
Verelan PM Capsules 3120

Warfarin Sodium (Co-administration results in increased warfarin concentrations). Products include:
Coumadin for Injection 932
Coumadin Tablets 932

RESPERATE DEVICE

(Device) 1645
None cited in PDR database.

RESTASIS OPHTHALMIC EMULSION

(Cyclosporine) 570
None cited in PDR database.

RETAVASE

(Reteplase) 1131
May interact with vitamin K antagonists and certain other agents. Compounds in these categories include:

Abciximab (Drugs that alter platelet function, such as abciximab, may increase the risk of bleeding if administered prior to or after reteplase therapy). Products include:
ReoPro Vials 1779

Aspirin (Drugs that alter platelet function, such as aspirin, may increase the risk of bleeding if administered prior to or after reteplase therapy). Products include:
Aggrenox Capsules 855
Bayer, Aspirin Regimen .... ■606
Bayer Aspirin Tablets 3515
BC Powder .... ■612
BC Allergy Sinus Cold Powder .... ■612
Arthritis Strength BC Powder .... ■612
BC Sinus Cold Powder .... ■612
Ecotrin Enteric Coated Aspirin Low, Regular and Maximum Strength Tablets 1627

Goody's Body Pain Formula Powder 621
Goody's Extra Strength Headache Powder 621
Goody's Extra Strength Pain Relief Tablets 621
Percodan Tablets 1115
St. Joseph 81 mg Aspirin Chewable and Enteric Coated Tablets 1841

Clopidogrel Bisulfate (Drugs that alter platelet function, such as clopidogrel, may increase the risk of bleeding if administered prior to or after reteplase therapy). Products include:
Plavix Tablets 940
Plavix Tablets 2942

Dicumarol (Co-administration increases the risk of bleeding).
No products indexed under this heading.

Dipyridamole (Drugs that alter platelet function, such as dipyridamole, may increase the risk of bleeding if administered prior to or after reteplase therapy). Products include:
Aggrenox Capsules 855
Persantine Tablets 898

Eptifibatide (Drugs that alter platelet function, such as eptifibatide, may increase the risk of bleeding if administered prior to or after reteplase therapy). Products include:
Integrilin Injection 3034

Ticlopidine Hydrochloride (Drugs that alter platelet function, such as ticlopidine, may increase the risk of bleeding if administered prior to or after reteplase therapy). Products include:
Ticlid Tablets 2813

Tirofiban Hydrochloride (Drugs that alter platelet function, such as tirofiban, may increase the risk of bleeding if administered prior to or after reteplase therapy). Products include:
Aggrastat 1878

Warfarin Sodium (Co-administration increases the risk of bleeding). Products include:
Coumadin for Injection 932
Coumadin Tablets 932

RETIN-A MICRO 0.1%/ 0.04%

(Tretinoin) 2388
May interact with:

Benzoyl Peroxide (Concurrent use requires caution). Products include:
Benzaclin Topical Gel 1046
Brevoxyl 3212
Brevoxyl 3211
Clinac BPO 7 Gel USP 1137
Duac Topical Gel 3214
Triaz 1864
Triaz Pads 1864

Concomitant Topical Acne Therapy (Effect not specified).
No products indexed under this heading.

Resorcinol (Caution should be exercised).
No products indexed under this heading.

Salicylic Acid (Caution should be exercised).
No products indexed under this heading.

Sulfur (Caution should be exercised). Products include:
Avar Cleanser 3189
Avar Gel 3189
Avar Green 3189
Avar-e Emollient Cream 3189
Avar-e Green Cream 3189
Plexion 1863
Rosac Cream with Sunscreens 3216
Zeel Solution 1639
Zicam Allergy Relief Nasal Pump ....

Topical Medications (Effect not specified).
No products indexed under this heading.

RETISERT IMPLANT

(Fluocinolone Acetonide) 256
None cited in PDR database.

RETROVIR CAPSULES

(Zidovudine) 1533
May interact with cytotoxic drugs, Interferon alpha, phenytoin, valproate, and certain other agents. Compounds in these categories include:

Atovaquone (Co-administration results in increased AUC of zidovudine; routine dose modification of zidovudine is not warranted). Products include:
Malarone Tablets 1484
Malarone Pediatric Tablets 1484
Mepron Suspension 1487

Bleomycin Sulfate (Co-administration with cytotoxic agents may increase the hematologic toxicity of zidovudine).
No products indexed under this heading.

Bone Marrow Suppressants, unspecified (May increase the hematologic toxicity of zidovudine).
No products indexed under this heading.

Cyclophosphamide (Co-administration with cytotoxic agents may increase the hematologic toxicity of zidovudine).
No products indexed under this heading.

Daunorubicin Hydrochloride (Co-administration with cytotoxic agents may increase the hematologic toxicity of zidovudine). Products include:
Cerubidine for Injection 788

Divalproex Sodium (Co-administration results in increased AUC of zidovudine by 80%; routine dose modification of zidovudine is not warranted unless patient is experiencing pronounced anemia or other severe zidovudine-associated events). Products include:
Depakote Sprinkle Capsules 422
Depakote Tablets 427
Depakote ER Tablets 433

Doxorubicin Hydrochloride (Concomitant use should be avoided since an antagonistic relationship has been demonstrated). Products include:
Adriamycin for Injection, USP 786
Adriamycin Injection, USP 786

Epirubicin Hydrochloride (Co-administration with cytotoxic agents may increase the hematologic toxicity of zidovudine). Products include:
Ellence Injection 2632

Fluconazole (Co-administration results in increased AUC of zidovudine by 74%; routine dose modification of zidovudine is not warranted unless patient is experiencing pronounced anemia or other severe zidovudine-associated events).
No products indexed under this heading.

Fluorouracil (Co-administration with cytotoxic agents may increase the hematologic toxicity of zidovudine). Products include:
Carac Cream, 0.5% 1048
Efudex 3348

Fosphenytoin Sodium (Co-administration has resulted in low phenytoin levels in some patients and a high level in one case; a 30% decrease in oral zidovudine clearance was observed with phenytoin).
No products indexed under this heading.

Ganciclovir Sodium (May increase the hematologic toxicity of zidovudine). Products include:
Cytovene-IV 2763

Hydroxyurea (Co-administration with cytotoxic agents may increase the hematologic toxicity of zidovudine).
No products indexed under this heading.

Interferon alfa-2a, Recombinant (May increase the hematologic toxicity of zidovudine). Products include:
Roferon-A Injection 2805

Interferon alfa-2b, Recombinant (May increase the hematologic toxicity of zidovudine). Products include:
Intron A for Injection 3038
Rebetron Combination Therapy 3078

Interferon alfa-N3 (Human Leukocyte Derived) (May increase the hematologic toxicity of zidovudine). Products include:
Alferon N Injection 1640

Methadone Hydrochloride (Co-administration results in increased AUC of zidovudine; routine dose modification of zidovudine is not warranted).
No products indexed under this heading.

Methotrexate Sodium (Co-administration with cytotoxic agents may increase the hematologic toxicity of zidovudine).
No products indexed under this heading.

Mitotane (Co-administration with cytotoxic agents may increase the hematologic toxicity of zidovudine).
No products indexed under this heading.

Mitoxantrone Hydrochloride (Co-administration with cytotoxic agents may increase the hematologic toxicity of zidovudine). Products include:
Novantrone for Injection Concentrate 3158

Nelfinavir Mesylate (Co-administration results in decreased AUC of zidovudine; routine dose modification of zidovudine is not warranted). Products include:
Viracept 2556

Peginterferon Alfa-2b (May increase the hematologic toxicity of zidovudine). Products include:
PEG-Intron Powder for Injection 3062

Phenytoin (Co-administration has resulted in low phenytoin levels in some patients and a high level in one case; a 30% decrease in oral zidovudine clearance was observed with phenytoin).
No products indexed under this heading.

Phenytoin Sodium (Co-administration has resulted in low phenytoin levels in some patients and a high level in one case; a 30% decrease in oral zidovudine clearance was observed with phenytoin). Products include:
Phenytek Capsules 2153

Probenecid (Co-administration results in increased AUC of zidovudine by 106%; routine dose modification of zidovudine is not warranted unless patient is experiencing pronounced anemia or other severe zidovudine-associated events).
No products indexed under this heading.

Procarbazine Hydrochloride (Co-administration with cytotoxic agents may increase the hematologic toxicity of zidovudine). Products include:
Matulane Capsules 3188

Ribavirin (Antagonizes the in vitro antiviral activity of zidovudine against HIV; concomitant use should be avoided). Products include:
Copegus Tablets 2759
Rebetol 3073
Rebetron Combination Therapy 3078
Ribavirin, USP Capsules 3083
Virazole for Inhalation Solution 3365

Rifampin (Co-administration results in decreased AUC of zidovudine; routine dose modification of zidovudine is not warranted).
No products indexed under this heading.

Ritonavir (Co-administration results in decreased AUC of zidovudine; routine dose modification of zidovudine is not warranted). Products include:
Kaletra 474
Norvir 499

Stavudine (Concomitant use should be avoided since an antagonistic relationship has been demonstrated in vitro). Products include:
Zerit 971

Tamoxifen Citrate (Co-administration with cytotoxic agents may increase the hematologic toxicity of zidovudine).
No products indexed under this heading.

Valproate Sodium (Co-administration results in increased AUC of zidovudine by 80%; routine dose modification of zidovudine is not warranted unless patient is experiencing pronounced anemia or other severe zidovudine-associated events). Products include:
Depacon Injection 412

Valproic Acid (Co-administration results in increased AUC of zidovudine by 80%; routine dose modification of zidovudine is not warranted unless patient is experiencing pronounced anemia or other severe zidovudine-associated events). Products include:
Depakene 417

Vincristine Sulfate (Co-administration with cytotoxic agents may increase the hematologic toxicity of zidovudine).
No products indexed under this heading.

RETROVIR IV INFUSION

(Zidovudine) 1537
See Retrovir Capsules

RETROVIR SYRUP

(Zidovudine) 1533
See Retrovir Capsules

RETROVIR TABLETS

(Zidovudine) 1533
See Retrovir Capsules

REVATIO TABLETS
(Sildenafil Citrate) 2541
May interact with cytochrome p450 2c9 inducers (selected), cytochrome p450 2c9 inhibitors (selected), cytochrome p450 3a4 inducers (selected), cytochrome p450 3a4 inhibitors (selected), nitrates and nitrites, vitamin K antagonists, and certain other agents. Compounds in these categories include:

Acetazolamide (Sildenafil metabolism is principally mediated by the CYP3A4 (major route) and CYP2C9 (minor route) cytochrome P450 isoforms. Therefore, inhibitors of these isoenzymes may reduce sildenafil clearance).
No products indexed under this heading.

Allium sativum (Sildenafil metabolism is principally mediated by the CYP3A4 (major route) and CYP2C9 (minor route) cytochrome P450 isoforms. Therefore, inducers of these isoenzymes may increase sildenafil clearance).
No products indexed under this heading.

Amiodarone Hydrochloride (Sildenafil metabolism is principally mediated by the CYP3A4 (major route) and CYP2C9 (minor route) cytochrome P450 isoforms. Therefore, inhibitors of these isoenzymes may reduce sildenafil clearance). Products include:
Pacerone Tablets 3337

Amlodipine Besylate (When sildenafil 100 mg oral was co-administered with amlodipine, 5 mg or 10 mg oral, to hypertensive patients, the mean additional reduction on supine blood pressure was 8mmHg systolic and 7mmHg diastolic). Products include:
Caduet Tablets 2507
Lotrel Capsules 2238
Norvasc Tablets 2529

Amprenavir (Sildenafil metabolism is principally mediated by the CYP3A4 (major route) and CYP2C9 (minor route) cytochrome P450 isoforms. Therefore, inhibitors of these isoenzymes may reduce sildenafil clearance). Products include:
Agenerase Capsules 1299
Agenerase Oral Solution 1304

Amyl Nitrite (Consistent with its known effect on the nitric oxide/cGMP pathway, sildenafil was shown to potentiate the hypotensive effects of nitrates, and its administration to patients who are using organic nitrates, either regularly and/or intermittently, in any form is therefore contraindicated).
No products indexed under this heading.

Anastrozole (Sildenafil metabolism is principally mediated by the CYP3A4 (major route) and CYP2C9 (minor route) cytochrome P450 isoforms. Therefore, inhibitors of these isoenzymes may reduce sildenafil clearance). Products include:
Arimidex Tablets 665

Aprepitant (Sildenafil metabolism is principally mediated by the CYP3A4 (major route) and CYP2C9 (minor route) cytochrome P450 isoforms. Therefore, inducers of these isoenzymes may increase sildenafil clearance). Products include:
Emend Capsules 1944

Bendroflumethiazide (Sildenafil metabolism is principally mediated by the CYP3A4 (major route) and CYP2C9 (minor route) cytochrome P450 isoforms. Therefore, inhibitors of these isoenzymes may reduce sildenafil clearance).
No products indexed under this heading.

Betamethasone Acetate (Sildenafil metabolism is principally mediated by the CYP3A4 (major route) and CYP2C9 (minor route) cytochrome P450 isoforms. Therefore, inducers of these isoenzymes may increase sildenafil clearance).
No products indexed under this heading.

Betamethasone Sodium Phosphate (Sildenafil metabolism is principally mediated by the CYP3A4 (major route) and CYP2C9 (minor route) cytochrome P450 isoforms. Therefore, inducers of these isoenzymes may increase sildenafil clearance).
No products indexed under this heading.

Bosentan (Co-administration of sildenafil at steady state (80 mg t.i.d.) with the endothelin receptor antagonist bosentan (a moderate inducer of CYP3A4, CYP2C9 and possibly of cytochrome p450 2C19) at steady state (125 mg b.i.d.) resulted in a 63% decrease of sildenafil AUC and a 55% decrease in sildenafil Cmax). Products include:
Tracleer Tablets 539

Carbamazepine (Sildenafil metabolism is principally mediated by the CYP3A4 (major route) and CYP2C9 (minor route) cytochrome P450 isoforms. Therefore, inducers of these isoenzymes may increase sildenafil clearance). Products include:
Carbatrol Capsules 3174
Equetro Extended-Release Capsules 3178
Tegretol/Tegretol-XR 2278

Chloramphenicol (Sildenafil metabolism is principally mediated by the CYP3A4 (major route) and CYP2C9 (minor route) cytochrome P450 isoforms. Therefore, inhibitors of these isoenzymes may reduce sildenafil clearance).
No products indexed under this heading.

Chlorothiazide (Sildenafil metabolism is principally mediated by the CYP3A4 (major route) and CYP2C9 (minor route) cytochrome P450 isoforms. Therefore, inhibitors of these isoenzymes may reduce sildenafil clearance). Products include:
Aldoclor Tablets 1881
Diuril Oral 1936

Chlorothiazide Sodium (Sildenafil metabolism is principally mediated by the CYP3A4 (major route) and CYP2C9 (minor route) cytochrome P450 isoforms. Therefore, inhibitors of these isoenzymes may reduce sildenafil clearance). Products include:
Diuril Sodium Intravenous 1934

Chlorpropamide (Sildenafil metabolism is principally mediated by the CYP3A4 (major route) and CYP2C9 (minor route) cytochrome P450 isoforms. Therefore, inhibitors of these isoenzymes may reduce sildenafil clearance).
No products indexed under this heading.

Cimetidine (Cimetidine (800mg), a non-specific CYP inhibitor, caused a 56% increase in plasma sildenafil concentrations when co-administered with sildenafil (50 mg) to healthy volunteers). Products include:
Tagamet HB 200 Tablets .... ▣ 637
Tagamet Tablets 1547

Cimetidine Hydrochloride (Sildenafil metabolism is principally mediated by the CYP3A4 (major route) and CYP2C9 (minor route) cytochrome P450 isoforms. Therefore, inhibitors of these isoenzymes may reduce sildenafil clearance).
No products indexed under this heading.

Ciprofloxacin (Sildenafil metabolism is principally mediated by the CYP3A4 (major route) and CYP2C9 (minor route) cytochrome P450 isoforms. Therefore, inhibitors of these isoenzymes may reduce sildenafil clearance). Products include:
Cipro I.V. 2998
Cipro I.V. Pharmacy Bulk Package 3509
Cipro Oral Suspension 2991
Cipro XR Tablets 3004
Ciprodex Otic Suspension 555

Ciprofloxacin Hydrochloride (Sildenafil metabolism is principally mediated by the CYP3A4 (major route) and CYP2C9 (minor route) cytochrome P450 isoforms. Therefore, inducers of these isoenzymes may increase sildenafil clearance). Products include:
Ciloxan Ophthalmic Ointment 554
Cipro Tablets 2991

Cisplatin (Sildenafil metabolism is principally mediated by the CYP3A4 (major route) and CYP2C9 (minor route) cytochrome P450 isoforms. Therefore, inducers of these isoenzymes may increase sildenafil clearance).
No products indexed under this heading.

Clarithromycin (Sildenafil metabolism is principally mediated by the CYP3A4 (major route) and CYP2C9 (minor route) cytochrome P450 isoforms. Therefore, inhibitors of these isoenzymes may reduce sildenafil clearance). Products include:
Biaxin/Biaxin XL 402
PREVPAC 3281

Clopidogrel Hydrogen Sulfate (Sildenafil metabolism is principally mediated by the CYP3A4 (major route) and CYP2C9 (minor route) cytochrome P450 isoforms. Therefore, inhibitors of these isoenzymes may reduce sildenafil clearance).
No products indexed under this heading.

Clotrimazole (Sildenafil metabolism is principally mediated by the CYP3A4 (major route) and CYP2C9 (minor route) cytochrome P450 isoforms. Therefore, inhibitors of these isoenzymes may reduce sildenafil clearance). Products include:
Lotrimin 3053
Lotrisone 3054

Cortisone Acetate (Sildenafil metabolism is principally mediated by the CYP3A4 (major route) and CYP2C9 (minor route) cytochrome P450 isoforms. Therefore, inducers of these isoenzymes may increase sildenafil clearance).
No products indexed under this heading.

Cyclosporine (Sildenafil metabolism is principally mediated by the CYP3A4 (major route) and CYP2C9 (minor route) cytochrome P450 isoforms. Therefore, inhibitors of these isoenzymes may reduce sildenafil clearance). Products include:
Gengraf Capsules 458
Neoral Soft Gelatin Capsules 2247
Neoral Oral Solution 2247
Restasis Ophthalmic Emulsion 570
Sandimmune 2259

Dalfopristin (Sildenafil metabolism is principally mediated by the CYP3A4 (major route) and CYP2C9 (minor route) cytochrome P450 isoforms. Therefore, inhibitors of these isoenzymes may reduce sildenafil clearance). Products include:
Synercid I.V. 1690

Danazol (Sildenafil metabolism is principally mediated by the CYP3A4 (major route) and CYP2C9 (minor route) cytochrome P450 isoforms. Therefore, inhibitors of these isoenzymes may reduce sildenafil clearance).
No products indexed under this heading.

Delavirdine Mesylate (Sildenafil metabolism is principally mediated by the CYP3A4 (major route) and CYP2C9 (minor route) cytochrome P450 isoforms. Therefore, inhibitors of these isoenzymes may reduce sildenafil clearance). Products include:
Rescriptor Tablets 2535

Dexamethasone (Sildenafil metabolism is principally mediated by the CYP3A4 (major route) and CYP2C9 (minor route) cytochrome P450 isoforms. Therefore, inducers of these isoenzymes may increase sildenafil clearance). Products include:
Ciprodex Otic Suspension 555
Decadron Tablets 1929
TobraDex Ophthalmic Ointment 558
TobraDex Ophthalmic Suspension 558

Dexamethasone Acetate (Sildenafil metabolism is principally mediated by the CYP3A4 (major route) and CYP2C9 (minor route) cytochrome P450 isoforms. Therefore, inducers of these isoenzymes may increase sildenafil clearance).
No products indexed under this heading.

Dexamethasone Sodium Phosphate (Sildenafil metabolism is principally mediated by the CYP3A4 (major route) and CYP2C9 (minor route) cytochrome P450 isoforms. Therefore, inducers of these isoenzymes may increase sildenafil clearance). Products include:
Decadron Phosphate Injection 1931

Diclofenac Potassium (Sildenafil metabolism is principally mediated by the CYP3A4 (major route) and CYP2C9 (minor route) cytochrome P450 isoforms. Therefore, inhibitors of these isoenzymes may reduce sildenafil clearance). Products include:
Cataflam Tablets 2173

Diclofenac Sodium (Sildenafil metabolism is principally mediated by the CYP3A4 (major route) and CYP2C9 (minor route) cytochrome P450 isoforms. Therefore, inhibitors of these isoenzymes may reduce sildenafil clearance). Products include:
Arthrotec Tablets 3126
Voltaren Ophthalmic Solution 2300
Voltaren Tablets 2298
Voltaren-XR Tablets 2301

Dicumarol (In pulmonary arterial hypertension (PAH) patients, the concomitant use of vitamin K antagonists and sildenafil resulted in a greater incidence of reports of bleeding (primarily epistaxis) versus placebo).

No products indexed under this heading.

Diltiazem Hydrochloride (Sildenafil metabolism is principally mediated by the CYP3A4 (major route) and CYP2C9 (minor route) cytochrome P450 isoforms. Therefore, inhibitors of these isoenzymes may reduce sildenafil clearance). Products include:

Cardizem LA Extended Release Tablets 1699
Tiazac Capsules 1204

Diltiazem Maleate (Sildenafil metabolism is principally mediated by the CYP3A4 (major route) and CYP2C9 (minor route) cytochrome P450 isoforms. Therefore, inhibitors of these isoenzymes may reduce sildenafil clearance).

No products indexed under this heading.

Disulfiram (Sildenafil metabolism is principally mediated by the CYP3A4 (major route) and CYP2C9 (minor route) cytochrome P450 isoforms. Therefore, inhibitors of these isoenzymes may reduce sildenafil clearance). Products include:

Antabuse Tablets 2343

Doxazosin Mesylate (In drug-drug interaction studies, co-administration of sildenafil (25 mg, 50mg, or 100mg) and the alpha-blocker doxazosin (4 mg or 8mg) in patients with benign prostatic hyperplasia (BPH) stabilized on doxazosin therapy resulted in mean additional reduction of supine systolic and diastolic blood pressure of 7/7 mmHg, 9/5 mmHg and 8/4 mmHg, respectively, were observed. Mean additional reductions of standing blood pressure of 6/6 mmHg, 11/4 mmHg and 4/5 mmHg, respectively, were also observed. There were infrequent reports of patients who experienced symptomatic postural hypotension. These reports included dizziness and light-headedness, but not syncope).

No products indexed under this heading.

Doxorubicin Hydrochloride (Sildenafil metabolism is principally mediated by the CYP3A4 (major route) and CYP2C9 (minor route) cytochrome P450 isoforms. Therefore, inducers of these isoenzymes may increase sildenafil clearance). Products include:

Adriamycin for Injection, USP 786
Adriamycin Injection, USP 786

Efavirenz (Sildenafil metabolism is principally mediated by the CYP3A4 (major route) and CYP2C9 (minor route) cytochrome P450 isoforms. Therefore, inhibitors of these isoenzymes may reduce sildenafil clearance). Products include:

Sustiva Capsules 957

Erythrityl Tetranitrate (Consistent with its known effect on the nitric oxide/cGMP pathway, sildenafil was shown to potentiate the hypotensive effects of nitrates, and its administration to patients who are using organic nitrates, either regularly and/or intermittently, in any form is therefore contraindicated).

No products indexed under this heading.

Erythromycin (When a single 100 mg dose of sildenafil was co-administered with erythromycin, a CYP3A4 inhibitor, at steady state (500 mg twice daily (b.i.d.) for 5 days), there was a 182% increase in sildenafil systemic exposure (AUC)). Products include:

Erygel Topical Gel 2096
Ery-Tab Tablets 447
Erythromycin Base Filmtab Tablets 454
Erythromycin Delayed-Release Capsules, USP 456
PCE Dispertab Tablets 510

Erythromycin Estolate (Sildenafil metabolism is principally mediated by the CYP3A4 (major route) and CYP2C9 (minor route) cytochrome P450 isoforms. Therefore, inhibitors of these isoenzymes may reduce sildenafil clearance).

No products indexed under this heading.

Erythromycin Ethylsuccinate (Sildenafil metabolism is principally mediated by the CYP3A4 (major route) and CYP2C9 (minor route) cytochrome P450 isoforms. Therefore, inhibitors of these isoenzymes may reduce sildenafil clearance). Products include:

E.E.S. 449
EryPed 445

Erythromycin Gluceptate (Sildenafil metabolism is principally mediated by the CYP3A4 (major route) and CYP2C9 (minor route) cytochrome P450 isoforms. Therefore, inhibitors of these isoenzymes may reduce sildenafil clearance).

No products indexed under this heading.

Erythromycin Lactobionate (Sildenafil metabolism is principally mediated by the CYP3A4 (major route) and CYP2C9 (minor route) cytochrome P450 isoforms. Therefore, inhibitors of these isoenzymes may reduce sildenafil clearance).

No products indexed under this heading.

Erythromycin Stearate (Sildenafil metabolism is principally mediated by the CYP3A4 (major route) and CYP2C9 (minor route) cytochrome P450 isoforms. Therefore, inhibitors of these isoenzymes may reduce sildenafil clearance). Products include:

Erythrocin Stearate Filmtab Tablets 452

Esomeprazole Magnesium (Sildenafil metabolism is principally mediated by the CYP3A4 (major route) and CYP2C9 (minor route) cytochrome P450 isoforms. Therefore, inhibitors of these isoenzymes may reduce sildenafil clearance). Products include:

Nexium Delayed-Release Capsules 645

Ethosuximide (Sildenafil metabolism is principally mediated by the CYP3A4 (major route) and CYP2C9 (minor route) cytochrome P450 isoforms. Therefore, inducers of these isoenzymes may increase sildenafil clearance).

No products indexed under this heading.

Felbamate (Sildenafil metabolism is principally mediated by the CYP3A4 (major route) and CYP2C9 (minor route) cytochrome P450 isoforms. Therefore, inducers of these isoenzymes may increase sildenafil clearance).

No products indexed under this heading.

Fenofibrate (Sildenafil metabolism is principally mediated by the CYP3A4 (major route) and CYP2C9 (minor route) cytochrome P450 isoforms. Therefore, inhibitors of these isoenzymes may reduce sildenafil clearance). Products include:

Antara Capsules 2723
Lofibra Capsules 1217
Tricor Tablets 523
Triglide Tablets 1165

Fluconazole (Sildenafil metabolism is principally mediated by the CYP3A4 (major route) and CYP2C9 (minor route) cytochrome P450 isoforms. Therefore, inhibitors of these isoenzymes may reduce sildenafil clearance).

No products indexed under this heading.

Fludrocortisone Acetate (Sildenafil metabolism is principally mediated by the CYP3A4 (major route) and CYP2C9 (minor route) cytochrome P450 isoforms. Therefore, inducers of these isoenzymes may increase sildenafil clearance).

No products indexed under this heading.

Fluorouracil (Sildenafil metabolism is principally mediated by the CYP3A4 (major route) and CYP2C9 (minor route) cytochrome P450 isoforms. Therefore, inhibitors of these isoenzymes may reduce sildenafil clearance). Products include:

Carac Cream, 0.5% 1048
Efudex 3348

Fluoxetine Hydrochloride (Sildenafil metabolism is principally mediated by the CYP3A4 (major route) and CYP2C9 (minor route) cytochrome P450 isoforms. Therefore, inhibitors of these isoenzymes may reduce sildenafil clearance). Products include:

Prozac Pulvules and Liquid 1771
Symbyax Capsules 1788

Flurbiprofen (Sildenafil metabolism is principally mediated by the CYP3A4 (major route) and CYP2C9 (minor route) cytochrome P450 isoforms. Therefore, inhibitors of these isoenzymes may reduce sildenafil clearance).

No products indexed under this heading.

Flurbiprofen Sodium (Sildenafil metabolism is principally mediated by the CYP3A4 (major route) and CYP2C9 (minor route) cytochrome P450 isoforms. Therefore, inhibitors of these isoenzymes may reduce sildenafil clearance). Products include:

Ocufen Ophthalmic Solution .... ⊙230

Fluvastatin Sodium (Sildenafil metabolism is principally mediated by the CYP3A4 (major route) and CYP2C9 (minor route) cytochrome P450 isoforms. Therefore, inhibitors of these isoenzymes may reduce sildenafil clearance). Products include:

Lescol Capsules 2227
Lescol 2730
Lescol XL Tablets 2227

Fluvoxamine Maleate (Sildenafil metabolism is principally mediated by the CYP3A4 (major route) and CYP2C9 (minor route) cytochrome P450 isoforms. Therefore, inhibitors of these isoenzymes may reduce sildenafil clearance).

No products indexed under this heading.

Fosamprenavir Calcium (Sildenafil metabolism is principally mediated by the CYP3A4 (major route) and CYP2C9 (minor route) cytochrome P450 isoforms. Therefore, inhibitors of these isoenzymes may reduce sildenafil clearance). Products include:

Lexiva Tablets 1473

Fosphenytoin Sodium (Sildenafil metabolism is principally mediated by the CYP3A4 (major route) and CYP2C9 (minor route) cytochrome P450 isoforms. Therefore, inducers of these isoenzymes may increase sildenafil clearance).

No products indexed under this heading.

Garlic Extract (Sildenafil metabolism is principally mediated by the CYP3A4 (major route) and CYP2C9 (minor route) cytochrome P450 isoforms. Therefore, inducers of these isoenzymes may increase sildenafil clearance).

No products indexed under this heading.

Garlic Oil (Sildenafil metabolism is principally mediated by the CYP3A4 (major route) and CYP2C9 (minor route) cytochrome P450 isoforms. Therefore, inducers of these isoenzymes may increase sildenafil clearance).

No products indexed under this heading.

Gemfibrozil (Sildenafil metabolism is principally mediated by the CYP3A4 (major route) and CYP2C9 (minor route) cytochrome P450 isoforms. Therefore, inhibitors of these isoenzymes may reduce sildenafil clearance).

No products indexed under this heading.

Glipizide (Sildenafil metabolism is principally mediated by the CYP3A4 (major route) and CYP2C9 (minor route) cytochrome P450 isoforms. Therefore, inhibitors of these isoenzymes may reduce sildenafil clearance).

No products indexed under this heading.

Glyburide (Sildenafil metabolism is principally mediated by the CYP3A4 (major route) and CYP2C9 (minor route) cytochrome P450 isoforms. Therefore, inhibitors of these isoenzymes may reduce sildenafil clearance).

No products indexed under this heading.

Hydrochlorothiazide (Sildenafil metabolism is principally mediated by the CYP3A4 (major route) and CYP2C9 (minor route) cytochrome P450 isoforms. Therefore, inhibitors of these isoenzymes may reduce sildenafil clearance). Products include:

Aldoril Tablets 1884
Atacand HCT 637
Avalide Tablets 2889
Avalide Tablets 922
Benicar HCT Tablets 2852
Diovan HCT Tablets 2195
Dyazide Capsules 1389

IMPORTANT NOTE: Always consult each drug listing in the patient's regimen for possible interactions.

Hyzaar ... 1964
Lotensin HCT Tablets ... 2235
Maxzide ... 2150
Micardis HCT Tablets ... 886
Moduretic Tablets ... 2003
Prinzide Tablets ... 2033
Teveten HCT Tablets ... 1710
Timolide Tablets ... 2056
Uniretic Tablets ... 3114
Vaseretic Tablets ... 2073
Zestoretic Tablets ... 701

Hydrocortisone (Sildenafil metabolism is principally mediated by the CYP3A4 (major route) and CYP2C9 (minor route) cytochrome P450 isoforms. Therefore, inducers of these isoenzymes may increase sildenafil clearance). Products include:
Cortizone•5 Ointment ... ▣699
Cortizone•10 Creme ... ▣699
Cortizone•10 Ointment ... ▣699
Cortizone•10 Plus Creme ... ▣700
Cortizone•10 Maximum Strength Quick Shot Spray ... ▣700
Hydrocortone Tablets ... 1963
Preparation H Hydrocortisone Cream ... ▣748

Hydrocortisone Acetate (Sildenafil metabolism is principally mediated by the CYP3A4 (major route) and CYP2C9 (minor route) cytochrome P450 isoforms. Therefore, inducers of these isoenzymes may increase sildenafil clearance). Products include:
Analpram-HC ... 1136
Pramosone ... 1139
ProctoFoam-HC ... 3113
Tucks Anti-Itch Ointment ... ▣712
U-cort 1% Cream ... 3289

Hydrocortisone Butyrate (Sildenafil metabolism is principally mediated by the CYP3A4 (major route) and CYP2C9 (minor route) cytochrome P450 isoforms. Therefore, inducers of these isoenzymes may increase sildenafil clearance). Products include:
Locoid ... 1138
Locoid Lipocream Cream ... 1138

Hydrocortisone Cypionate (Sildenafil metabolism is principally mediated by the CYP3A4 (major route) and CYP2C9 (minor route) cytochrome P450 isoforms. Therefore, inducers of these isoenzymes may increase sildenafil clearance).
No products indexed under this heading.

Hydrocortisone Hemisuccinate (Sildenafil metabolism is principally mediated by the CYP3A4 (major route) and CYP2C9 (minor route) cytochrome P450 isoforms. Therefore, inducers of these isoenzymes may increase sildenafil clearance).
No products indexed under this heading.

Hydrocortisone Probutate (Sildenafil metabolism is principally mediated by the CYP3A4 (major route) and CYP2C9 (minor route) cytochrome P450 isoforms. Therefore, inducers of these isoenzymes may increase sildenafil clearance). Products include:
Pandel Cream, 0.1% ... 1017

Hydrocortisone Sodium Phosphate (Sildenafil metabolism is principally mediated by the CYP3A4 (major route) and CYP2C9 (minor route) cytochrome P450 isoforms. Therefore, inducers of these isoenzymes may increase sildenafil clearance).
No products indexed under this heading.

Hydrocortisone Sodium Succinate (Sildenafil metabolism is principally mediated by the CYP3A4 (major route) and CYP2C9 (minor route) cytochrome P450 isoforms. Therefore, inducers of these isoenzymes may increase sildenafil clearance).
No products indexed under this heading.

Hydrocortisone Valerate (Sildenafil metabolism is principally mediated by the CYP3A4 (major route) and CYP2C9 (minor route) cytochrome P450 isoforms. Therefore, inducers of these isoenzymes may increase sildenafil clearance).
No products indexed under this heading.

Hydroflumethiazide (Sildenafil metabolism is principally mediated by the CYP3A4 (major route) and CYP2C9 (minor route) cytochrome P450 isoforms. Therefore, inhibitors of these isoenzymes may reduce sildenafil clearance).
No products indexed under this heading.

Hypericum (Sildenafil metabolism is principally mediated by the CYP3A4 (major route) and CYP2C9 (minor route) cytochrome P450 isoforms. Therefore, inducers of these isoenzymes may increase sildenafil clearance).
No products indexed under this heading.

Hypericum Perforatum (Sildenafil metabolism is principally mediated by the CYP3A4 (major route) and CYP2C9 (minor route) cytochrome P450 isoforms. Therefore, inducers of these isoenzymes may increase sildenafil clearance).
No products indexed under this heading.

Imatinib Mesylate (Sildenafil metabolism is principally mediated by the CYP3A4 (major route) and CYP2C9 (minor route) cytochrome P450 isoforms. Therefore, inhibitors of these isoenzymes may reduce sildenafil clearance). Products include:
Gleevec Tablets ... 2221

Indinavir Sulfate (Sildenafil metabolism is principally mediated by the CYP3A4 (major route) and CYP2C9 (minor route) cytochrome P450 isoforms. Therefore, inhibitors of these isoenzymes may reduce sildenafil clearance). Products include:
Crixivan Capsules ... 1918

Isoniazid (Sildenafil metabolism is principally mediated by the CYP3A4 (major route) and CYP2C9 (minor route) cytochrome P450 isoforms. Therefore, inhibitors of these isoenzymes may reduce sildenafil clearance).
No products indexed under this heading.

Isosorbide Dinitrate (Consistent with its known effect on the nitric oxide/cGMP pathway, sildenafil was shown to potentiate the hypotensive effects of nitrates, and its administration to patients who are using organic nitrates, either regularly and/or intermittently, in any form is therefore contraindicated). Products include:
BiDil Tablets ... 2161

Isosorbide Mononitrate (Consistent with its known effect on the nitric oxide/cGMP pathway, sildenafil was shown to potentiate the hypotensive effects of nitrates, and its administration to patients who are using organic nitrates, either regularly and/or intermittently, in any form is therefore contraindicated). Products include:
Imdur Tablets ... 3032

Itraconazole (Sildenafil metabolism is principally mediated by the CYP3A4 (major route) and CYP2C9 (minor route) cytochrome P450 isoforms. Therefore, inhibitors of these isoenzymes may reduce sildenafil clearance).
No products indexed under this heading.

Ketoconazole (Sildenafil metabolism is principally mediated by the CYP3A4 (major route) and CYP2C9 (minor route) cytochrome P450 isoforms. Therefore, inhibitors of these isoenzymes may reduce sildenafil clearance). Products include:
Nizoral A-D Shampoo, 1% ... 1839
Nizoral 2% Shampoo ... 1838

Ketoprofen (Sildenafil metabolism is principally mediated by the CYP3A4 (major route) and CYP2C9 (minor route) cytochrome P450 isoforms. Therefore, inhibitors of these isoenzymes may reduce sildenafil clearance).
No products indexed under this heading.

Leflunomide (Sildenafil metabolism is principally mediated by the CYP3A4 (major route) and CYP2C9 (minor route) cytochrome P450 isoforms. Therefore, inhibitors of these isoenzymes may reduce sildenafil clearance). Products include:
Arava Tablets ... 2881

Lopinavir (Sildenafil metabolism is principally mediated by the CYP3A4 (major route) and CYP2C9 (minor route) cytochrome P450 isoforms. Therefore, inhibitors of these isoenzymes may reduce sildenafil clearance). Products include:
Kaletra ... 474

Loratadine (Sildenafil metabolism is principally mediated by the CYP3A4 (major route) and CYP2C9 (minor route) cytochrome P450 isoforms. Therefore, inhibitors of these isoenzymes may reduce sildenafil clearance). Products include:
Alavert Allergy & Sinus D-12 Hour Tablets ... ▣743
Alavert ... ▣743
Children's Claritin 24 Hour Non-Drowsy Allergy Syrup ... ▣732
Claritin Non-Drowsy 24 Hour Tablets ... ▣731
Non-Drowsy Claritin Hives Relief Tablets ... ▣733
Claritin Reditabs 24 Hour Non-Drowsy Tablets ... ▣732
Claritin-D Non-Drowsy 12 Hour Tablets ... ▣731
Claritin-D Non-Drowsy 24 Hour Tablets ... ▣731
Children's Dimetapp ND Non-Drowsy Allergy Syrup ... ▣746
Triaminic Allerchews ... ▣684

Lovastatin (Sildenafil metabolism is principally mediated by the CYP3A4 (major route) and CYP2C9 (minor route) cytochrome P450 isoforms. Therefore, inhibitors of these isoenzymes may reduce sildenafil clearance). Products include:
Advicor Tablets ... 1694
Altoprev Extended-Release Tablets ... 1151
Mevacor Tablets ... 1996

Mephenytoin (Sildenafil metabolism is principally mediated by the CYP3A4 (major route) and CYP2C9 (minor route) cytochrome P450 isoforms. Therefore, inducers of these isoenzymes may increase sildenafil clearance).
No products indexed under this heading.

Methsuximide (Sildenafil metabolism is principally mediated by the CYP3A4 (major route) and CYP2C9 (minor route) cytochrome P450 isoforms. Therefore, inducers of these isoenzymes may increase sildenafil clearance).
No products indexed under this heading.

Methyclothiazide (Sildenafil metabolism is principally mediated by the CYP3A4 (major route) and CYP2C9 (minor route) cytochrome P450 isoforms. Therefore, inhibitors of these isoenzymes may reduce sildenafil clearance).
No products indexed under this heading.

Methylprednisolone (Sildenafil metabolism is principally mediated by the CYP3A4 (major route) and CYP2C9 (minor route) cytochrome P450 isoforms. Therefore, inducers of these isoenzymes may increase sildenafil clearance).
No products indexed under this heading.

Methylprednisolone Acetate (Sildenafil metabolism is principally mediated by the CYP3A4 (major route) and CYP2C9 (minor route) cytochrome P450 isoforms. Therefore, inducers of these isoenzymes may increase sildenafil clearance). Products include:
Depo-Medrol Injectable Suspension ... 2615
Depo-Medrol Single-Dose Vial ... 2617

Methylprednisolone Sodium Succinate (Sildenafil metabolism is principally mediated by the CYP3A4 (major route) and CYP2C9 (minor route) cytochrome P450 isoforms. Therefore, inducers of these isoenzymes may increase sildenafil clearance).
No products indexed under this heading.

Metronidazole (Sildenafil metabolism is principally mediated by the CYP3A4 (major route) and CYP2C9 (minor route) cytochrome P450 isoforms. Therefore, inhibitors of these isoenzymes may reduce sildenafil clearance). Products include:
Metrogel 1% ... 1212
MetroGel-Vaginal Gel ... 1822
Noritate Cream, 1% ... 1051

Metronidazole Benzoate (Sildenafil metabolism is principally mediated by the CYP3A4 (major route) and CYP2C9 (minor route) cytochrome P450 isoforms. Therefore, inhibitors of these isoenzymes may reduce sildenafil clearance).
No products indexed under this heading.

Metronidazole Hydrochloride (Sildenafil metabolism is principally mediated by the CYP3A4 (major route) and CYP2C9 (minor route) cytochrome P450 isoforms. Therefore, inhibitors of these isoenzymes may reduce sildenafil clearance).
No products indexed under this heading.

Miconazole (Sildenafil metabolism is principally mediated by the CYP3A4 (major route) and CYP2C9 (minor route) cytochrome P450 isoforms. Therefore, inhibitors of these isoenzymes may reduce sildenafil clearance).
No products indexed under this heading.

Miconazole Nitrate (Sildenafil metabolism is principally mediated by the CYP3A4 (major route) and CYP2C9 (minor route) cytochrome P450 isoforms. Therefore, inhibitors of these isoenzymes may reduce sildenafil clearance). Products include:
Desenex 674
Desenex Jock Itch Spray Powder ... 674

Modafinil (Sildenafil metabolism is principally mediated by the CYP3A4 (major route) and CYP2C9 (minor route) cytochrome P450 isoforms. Therefore, inhibitors of these isoenzymes may reduce sildenafil clearance). Products include:
Provigil Tablets 1002

Nefazodone Hydrochloride (Sildenafil metabolism is principally mediated by the CYP3A4 (major route) and CYP2C9 (minor route) cytochrome P450 isoforms. Therefore, inhibitors of these isoenzymes may reduce sildenafil clearance).
No products indexed under this heading.

Nelfinavir Mesylate (Sildenafil metabolism is principally mediated by the CYP3A4 (major route) and CYP2C9 (minor route) cytochrome P450 isoforms. Therefore, inhibitors of these isoenzymes may reduce sildenafil clearance). Products include:
Viracept 2556

Nevirapine (Sildenafil metabolism is principally mediated by the CYP3A4 (major route) and CYP2C9 (minor route) cytochrome P450 isoforms. Therefore, inducers of these isoenzymes may increase sildenafil clearance). Products include:
Viramune Oral Suspension 903
Viramune Tablets 903

Niacinamide (Sildenafil metabolism is principally mediated by the CYP3A4 (major route) and CYP2C9 (minor route) cytochrome P450 isoforms. Therefore, inhibitors of these isoenzymes may reduce sildenafil clearance).
No products indexed under this heading.

Nicotinamide (Sildenafil metabolism is principally mediated by the CYP3A4 (major route) and CYP2C9 (minor route) cytochrome P450 isoforms. Therefore, inhibitors of these isoenzymes may reduce sildenafil clearance). Products include:
Nicomide Tablets 3190

Nifedipine (Sildenafil metabolism is principally mediated by the CYP3A4 (major route) and CYP2C9 (minor route) cytochrome P450 isoforms. Therefore, inhibitors of these isoenzymes may reduce sildenafil clearance). Products include:
Adalat CC Tablets 2978

Nitroglycerin (Consistent with its known effect on the nitric oxide/cGMP pathway, sildenafil was shown to potentiate the hypotensive effects of nitrates, and its administration to patients who are using organic nitrates, either regularly and/or intermittently, in any form is therefore contraindicated). Products include:
Nitro-Dur Transdermal Infusion System.. 3060
Nitrolingual Pumpspray 1161

Norfloxacin (Sildenafil metabolism is principally mediated by the CYP3A4 (major route) and CYP2C9 (minor route) cytochrome P450 isoforms. Therefore, inhibitors of these isoenzymes may reduce sildenafil clearance). Products include:
Noroxin Tablets 2009

Omeprazole (Sildenafil metabolism is principally mediated by the CYP3A4 (major route) and CYP2C9 (minor route) cytochrome P450 isoforms. Therefore, inhibitors of these isoenzymes may reduce sildenafil clearance). Products include:
Zegerid Powder for Oral Solution 2972

Oxcarbazepine (Sildenafil metabolism is principally mediated by the CYP3A4 (major route) and CYP2C9 (minor route) cytochrome P450 isoforms. Therefore, inducers of these isoenzymes may increase sildenafil clearance). Products include:
Trileptal Oral Suspension 2281
Trileptal Tablets 2281

Oxiconazole Nitrate (Sildenafil metabolism is principally mediated by the CYP3A4 (major route) and CYP2C9 (minor route) cytochrome P450 isoforms. Therefore, inhibitors of these isoenzymes may reduce sildenafil clearance). Products include:
Oxistat 1498

Paroxetine Hydrochloride (Sildenafil metabolism is principally mediated by the CYP3A4 (major route) and CYP2C9 (minor route) cytochrome P450 isoforms. Therefore, inhibitors of these isoenzymes may reduce sildenafil clearance). Products include:
Paxil CR Controlled-Release Tablets.. 1509
Paxil 1501

Pentaerythritol Tetranitrate (Consistent with its known effect on the nitric oxide/cGMP pathway, sildenafil was shown to potentiate the hypotensive effects of nitrates, and its administration to patients who are using organic nitrates, either regularly and/or intermittently, in any form is therefore contraindicated).
No products indexed under this heading.

Phenobarbital (Sildenafil metabolism is principally mediated by the CYP3A4 (major route) and CYP2C9 (minor route) cytochrome P450 isoforms. Therefore, inducers of these isoenzymes may increase sildenafil clearance).
No products indexed under this heading.

Phenobarbital Sodium (Sildenafil metabolism is principally mediated by the CYP3A4 (major route) and CYP2C9 (minor route) cytochrome P450 isoforms. Therefore, inducers of these isoenzymes may increase sildenafil clearance).
No products indexed under this heading.

Phenylbutazone (Sildenafil metabolism is principally mediated by the CYP3A4 (major route) and CYP2C9 (minor route) cytochrome P450 isoforms. Therefore, inhibitors of these isoenzymes may reduce sildenafil clearance).
No products indexed under this heading.

Phenytoin (Sildenafil metabolism is principally mediated by the CYP3A4 (major route) and CYP2C9 (minor route) cytochrome P450 isoforms. Therefore, inducers of these isoenzymes may increase sildenafil clearance).
No products indexed under this heading.

Phenytoin Sodium (Sildenafil metabolism is principally mediated by the CYP3A4 (major route) and CYP2C9 (minor route) cytochrome P450 isoforms. Therefore, inducers of these isoenzymes may increase sildenafil clearance). Products include:
Phenytek Capsules 2153

Polythiazide (Sildenafil metabolism is principally mediated by the CYP3A4 (major route) and CYP2C9 (minor route) cytochrome P450 isoforms. Therefore, inhibitors of these isoenzymes may reduce sildenafil clearance).
No products indexed under this heading.

Prednisolone Acetate (Sildenafil metabolism is principally mediated by the CYP3A4 (major route) and CYP2C9 (minor route) cytochrome P450 isoforms. Therefore, inducers of these isoenzymes may increase sildenafil clearance). Products include:
Blephamide Ophthalmic Ointment 563
Blephamide Ophthalmic Suspension.. 564
Poly-Pred Liquifilm Ophthalmic Suspension .... ⊙231
Pred Forte Ophthalmic Suspension .... ⊙233
Pred Mild Sterile Ophthalmic Suspension .... ⊙236
Pred-G Ophthalmic Suspension ...... ⊙234
Pred-G Sterile Ophthalmic Ointment.................................... ⊙235

Prednisolone Sodium Phosphate (Sildenafil metabolism is principally mediated by the CYP3A4 (major route) and CYP2C9 (minor route) cytochrome P450 isoforms. Therefore, inducers of these isoenzymes may increase sildenafil clearance). Products include:
Pediapred Oral Solution 3319

Prednisolone Tebutate (Sildenafil metabolism is principally mediated by the CYP3A4 (major route) and CYP2C9 (minor route) cytochrome P450 isoforms. Therefore, inducers of these isoenzymes may increase sildenafil clearance).
No products indexed under this heading.

Prednisone (Sildenafil metabolism is principally mediated by the CYP3A4 (major route) and CYP2C9 (minor route) cytochrome P450 isoforms. Therefore, inducers of these isoenzymes may increase sildenafil clearance).
No products indexed under this heading.

Primidone (Sildenafil metabolism is principally mediated by the CYP3A4 (major route) and CYP2C9 (minor route) cytochrome P450 isoforms. Therefore, inducers of these isoenzymes may increase sildenafil clearance).
No products indexed under this heading.

Propoxyphene Hydrochloride (Sildenafil metabolism is principally mediated by the CYP3A4 (major route) and CYP2C9 (minor route) cytochrome P450 isoforms. Therefore, inhibitors of these isoenzymes may reduce sildenafil clearance).
No products indexed under this heading.

Propoxyphene Napsylate (Sildenafil metabolism is principally mediated by the CYP3A4 (major route) and CYP2C9 (minor route) cytochrome P450 isoforms. Therefore, inhibitors of these isoenzymes may reduce sildenafil clearance). Products include:
Darvocet A 500 Tablets 3497

Quinidine (Sildenafil metabolism is principally mediated by the CYP3A4 (major route) and CYP2C9 (minor route) cytochrome P450 isoforms. Therefore, inhibitors of these isoenzymes may reduce sildenafil clearance).
No products indexed under this heading.

Quinidine Hydrochloride (Sildenafil metabolism is principally mediated by the CYP3A4 (major route) and CYP2C9 (minor route) cytochrome P450 isoforms. Therefore, inhibitors of these isoenzymes may reduce sildenafil clearance).
No products indexed under this heading.

Quinidine Polygalacturonate (Sildenafil metabolism is principally mediated by the CYP3A4 (major route) and CYP2C9 (minor route) cytochrome P450 isoforms. Therefore, inhibitors of these isoenzymes may reduce sildenafil clearance).
No products indexed under this heading.

Quinidine Sulfate (Sildenafil metabolism is principally mediated by the CYP3A4 (major route) and CYP2C9 (minor route) cytochrome P450 isoforms. Therefore, inhibitors of these isoenzymes may reduce sildenafil clearance).
No products indexed under this heading.

Quinine (Sildenafil metabolism is principally mediated by the CYP3A4 (major route) and CYP2C9 (minor route) cytochrome P450 isoforms. Therefore, inhibitors of these isoenzymes may reduce sildenafil clearance).
No products indexed under this heading.

Quinine Sulfate (Sildenafil metabolism is principally mediated by the CYP3A4 (major route) and CYP2C9 (minor route) cytochrome P450 isoforms. Therefore, inhibitors of these isoenzymes may reduce sildenafil clearance).
No products indexed under this heading.

Quinupristin (Sildenafil metabolism is principally mediated by the CYP3A4 (major route) and CYP2C9 (minor route) cytochrome P450 iso-

forms. Therefore, inhibitors of these isoenzymes may reduce sildenafil clearance). Products include:

Synercid I.V. 1690

Ranitidine Bismuth Citrate (Sildenafil metabolism is principally mediated by the CYP3A4 (major route) and CYP2C9 (minor route) cytochrome P450 isoforms. Therefore, inhibitors of these isoenzymes may reduce sildenafil clearance).

No products indexed under this heading.

Ranitidine Hydrochloride (Sildenafil metabolism is principally mediated by the CYP3A4 (major route) and CYP2C9 (minor route) cytochrome P450 isoforms. Therefore, inhibitors of these isoenzymes may reduce sildenafil clearance). Products include:

Zantac 1597
Zantac Injection 1593
Zantac 75 Tablets .... ■ 715
Zantac 150 Maximum Strength Tablets.. ■ 715
Zantac Injection Pharmacy Bulk Package.. 1595

Rifabutin (Sildenafil metabolism is principally mediated by the CYP3A4 (major route) and CYP2C9 (minor route) cytochrome P450 isoforms. Therefore, inducers of these isoenzymes may increase sildenafil clearance).

No products indexed under this heading.

Rifampicin (Sildenafil metabolism is principally mediated by the CYP3A4 (major route) and CYP2C9 (minor route) cytochrome P450 isoforms. Therefore, inducers of these isoenzymes may increase sildenafil clearance).

No products indexed under this heading.

Rifampin (Sildenafil metabolism is principally mediated by the CYP3A4 (major route) and CYP2C9 (minor route) cytochrome P450 isoforms. Therefore, inducers of these isoenzymes may increase sildenafil clearance).

No products indexed under this heading.

Rifapentine (Sildenafil metabolism is principally mediated by the CYP3A4 (major route) and CYP2C9 (minor route) cytochrome P450 isoforms. Therefore, inducers of these isoenzymes may increase sildenafil clearance).

No products indexed under this heading.

Ritonavir (In a study in healthy volunteers, co-administration of the HIV protease inhibitor ritonavir, a potent CYP3A4 inhibitor, at steady state (500 mg b.i.d.) with sildenafil (100 mg single dose) resulted in a 300% (4-fold) increase in sildenafil Cmax and a 1000% (11-fold) increase in sildenafil plasma AUC. At 24 hours, the plasma levels of sildenafil were still approximately 200 ng/mL, compared to approximately 5 ng/mL when sildenafil was dosed alone. This is consistent with ritonavir's marked effects on a broad range of P450 substrates). Products include:

Kaletra 474
Norvir 499

Saquinavir (In a study performed in healthy volunteers, co-administration of the HIV protease inhibitor saquinavier, a CYP3A4 inhibitor, at steady state (1200 mg t.i.d.) with sildenafil (100 mg single dose) resulted in a 140% increase in sildenafil Cmax and a 210% increase in sildenafil AUC).

No products indexed under this heading.

Saquinavir Mesylate (Sildenafil metabolism is principally mediated by the CYP3A4 (major route) and CYP2C9 (minor route) cytochrome P450 isoforms. Therefore, inhibitors of these isoenzymes may reduce sildenafil clearance). Products include:

Invirase 2776

Secobarbital Sodium (Sildenafil metabolism is principally mediated by the CYP3A4 (major route) and CYP2C9 (minor route) cytochrome P450 isoforms. Therefore, inducers of these isoenzymes may increase sildenafil clearance).

No products indexed under this heading.

Sertraline Hydrochloride (Sildenafil metabolism is principally mediated by the CYP3A4 (major route) and CYP2C9 (minor route) cytochrome P450 isoforms. Therefore, inhibitors of these isoenzymes may reduce sildenafil clearance). Products include:

Zoloft 2581

Sulfacytine (Sildenafil metabolism is principally mediated by the CYP3A4 (major route) and CYP2C9 (minor route) cytochrome P450 isoforms. Therefore, inhibitors of these isoenzymes may reduce sildenafil clearance).

No products indexed under this heading.

Sulfamethizole (Sildenafil metabolism is principally mediated by the CYP3A4 (major route) and CYP2C9 (minor route) cytochrome P450 isoforms. Therefore, inhibitors of these isoenzymes may reduce sildenafil clearance).

No products indexed under this heading.

Sulfamethoxazole (Sildenafil metabolism is principally mediated by the CYP3A4 (major route) and CYP2C9 (minor route) cytochrome P450 isoforms. Therefore, inhibitors of these isoenzymes may reduce sildenafil clearance).

No products indexed under this heading.

Sulfasalazine (Sildenafil metabolism is principally mediated by the CYP3A4 (major route) and CYP2C9 (minor route) cytochrome P450 isoforms. Therefore, inhibitors of these isoenzymes may reduce sildenafil clearance).

No products indexed under this heading.

Sulfinpyrazone (Sildenafil metabolism is principally mediated by the CYP3A4 (major route) and CYP2C9 (minor route) cytochrome P450 isoforms. Therefore, inhibitors of these isoenzymes may reduce sildenafil clearance).

No products indexed under this heading.

Sulfisoxazole (Sildenafil metabolism is principally mediated by the CYP3A4 (major route) and CYP2C9 (minor route) cytochrome P450 isoforms. Therefore, inhibitors of these isoenzymes may reduce sildenafil clearance).

No products indexed under this heading.

Sulfisoxazole Acetyl (Sildenafil metabolism is principally mediated by the CYP3A4 (major route) and CYP2C9 (minor route) cytochrome P450 isoforms. Therefore, inhibitors of these isoenzymes may reduce sildenafil clearance).

No products indexed under this heading.

Sulfisoxazole Diolamine (Sildenafil metabolism is principally mediated by the CYP3A4 (major route) and CYP2C9 (minor route) cytochrome P450 isoforms. Therefore, inhibitors of these isoenzymes may reduce sildenafil clearance).

No products indexed under this heading.

Telithromycin (Sildenafil metabolism is principally mediated by the CYP3A4 (major route) and CYP2C9 (minor route) cytochrome P450 isoforms. Therefore, inhibitors of these isoenzymes may reduce sildenafil clearance). Products include:

Ketek Tablets 2920

Terconazole (Sildenafil metabolism is principally mediated by the CYP3A4 (major route) and CYP2C9 (minor route) cytochrome P450 isoforms. Therefore, inhibitors of these isoenzymes may reduce sildenafil clearance).

No products indexed under this heading.

Theophylline (Sildenafil metabolism is principally mediated by the CYP3A4 (major route) and CYP2C9 (minor route) cytochrome P450 isoforms. Therefore, inducers of these isoenzymes may increase sildenafil clearance).

No products indexed under this heading.

Ticlopidine Hydrochloride (Sildenafil metabolism is principally mediated by the CYP3A4 (major route) and CYP2C9 (minor route) cytochrome P450 isoforms. Therefore, inhibitors of these isoenzymes may reduce sildenafil clearance). Products include:

Ticlid Tablets 2813

Tolazamide (Sildenafil metabolism is principally mediated by the CYP3A4 (major route) and CYP2C9 (minor route) cytochrome P450 isoforms. Therefore, inhibitors of these isoenzymes may reduce sildenafil clearance).

No products indexed under this heading.

Tolbutamide (Sildenafil metabolism is principally mediated by the CYP3A4 (major route) and CYP2C9 (minor route) cytochrome P450 isoforms. Therefore, inhibitors of these isoenzymes may reduce sildenafil clearance).

No products indexed under this heading.

Tolbutamide Sodium (Sildenafil metabolism is principally mediated by the CYP3A4 (major route) and CYP2C9 (minor route) cytochrome P450 isoforms. Therefore, inhibitors of these isoenzymes may reduce sildenafil clearance).

No products indexed under this heading.

Triamcinolone (Sildenafil metabolism is principally mediated by the CYP3A4 (major route) and CYP2C9 (minor route) cytochrome P450 isoforms. Therefore, inducers of these isoenzymes may increase sildenafil clearance).

No products indexed under this heading.

Triamcinolone Acetonide (Sildenafil metabolism is principally mediated by the CYP3A4 (major route) and CYP2C9 (minor route) cytochrome P450 isoforms. Therefore, inducers of these isoenzymes may increase sildenafil clearance). Products include:

Azmacort Inhalation Aerosol 1701
Nasacort HFA Inhalation Aerosol 2939
Nasacort AQ Nasal Spray 2937

Triamcinolone Diacetate (Sildenafil metabolism is principally mediated by the CYP3A4 (major route) and CYP2C9 (minor route) cytochrome P450 isoforms. Therefore, inducers of these isoenzymes may increase sildenafil clearance).

No products indexed under this heading.

Triamcinolone Hexacetonide (Sildenafil metabolism is principally mediated by the CYP3A4 (major route) and CYP2C9 (minor route) cytochrome P450 isoforms. Therefore, inducers of these isoenzymes may increase sildenafil clearance).

No products indexed under this heading.

Troglitazone (Sildenafil metabolism is principally mediated by the CYP3A4 (major route) and CYP2C9 (minor route) cytochrome P450 isoforms. Therefore, inhibitors of these isoenzymes may reduce sildenafil clearance).

No products indexed under this heading.

Troleandomycin (Sildenafil metabolism is principally mediated by the CYP3A4 (major route) and CYP2C9 (minor route) cytochrome P450 isoforms. Therefore, inhibitors of these isoenzymes may reduce sildenafil clearance).

No products indexed under this heading.

Valproate Sodium (Sildenafil metabolism is principally mediated by the CYP3A4 (major route) and CYP2C9 (minor route) cytochrome P450 isoforms. Therefore, inhibitors of these isoenzymes may reduce sildenafil clearance). Products include:

Depacon Injection 412

Verapamil Hydrochloride (Sildenafil metabolism is principally mediated by the CYP3A4 (major route) and CYP2C9 (minor route) cytochrome P450 isoforms. Therefore, inhibitors of these isoenzymes may reduce sildenafil clearance). Products include:

Covera-HS Tablets 3135
Tarka Tablets 519
Verelan PM Capsules 3120

Voriconazole (Sildenafil metabolism is principally mediated by the

CYP3A4 (major route) and CYP2C9 (minor route) cytochrome P450 isoforms. Therefore, inhibitors of these isoenzymes may reduce sildenafil clearance). Products include:

VFEND I.V. 2543
VFEND Oral Suspension 2543
VFEND Tablets 2543

Warfarin Sodium (In pulmonary arterial hypertension (PAH) patients, the concomitant use of vitamin K antagonists and sildenafil resulted in a greater incidence of reports of bleeding (primarily epistaxis) versus placebo). Products include:

Coumadin for Injection 932
Coumadin Tablets 932

Zafirlukast (Sildenafil metabolism is principally mediated by the CYP3A4 (major route) and CYP2C9 (minor route) cytochrome P450 isoforms. Therefore, inhibitors of these isoenzymes may reduce sildenafil clearance). Products include:

Accolate Tablets 663

Zileuton (Sildenafil metabolism is principally mediated by the CYP3A4 (major route) and CYP2C9 (minor route) cytochrome P450 isoforms. Therefore, inhibitors of these isoenzymes may reduce sildenafil clearance).

No products indexed under this heading.

Food Interactions

Grapefruit (Sildenafil metabolism is principally mediated by the CYP3A4 (major route) and CYP2C9 (minor route) cytochrome P450 isoforms. Therefore, inhibitors of these isoenzymes may reduce sildenafil clearance).

Grapefruit Juice (Sildenafil metabolism is principally mediated by the CYP3A4 (major route) and CYP2C9 (minor route) cytochrome P450 isoforms. Therefore, inhibitors of these isoenzymes may reduce sildenafil clearance).

RĒV-EYES OPHTHALMIC EYEDROPS 0.5%

(Dapiprazole Hydrochloride) .... ⊙256
None cited in PDR database.

REYATAZ CAPSULES

(Atazanavir sulfate) 948
May interact with antacids, cytochrome p450 1a2 substrates (selected), cytochrome p450 2c9 substrates (selected), cytochrome p450 3a inducers (selected), cytochrome p450 3a inhibitors (selected), ergot-containing drugs, histamine H_2-receptor antagonists, immunosuppressive agents, oral contraceptives, protease inhibitors, proton pump inhibitor, and certain other agents. Compounds in these categories include:

Acarbose (Atazanavir sulfate competitively inhibits CYP1A2 and CYP2C9. There is a potential drug-drug interaction between atazanavir sulfate and CYP1A2 or CYP2C9 substrates). Products include:

Precose Tablets 776

Acetaminophen (Atazanavir sulfate competitively inhibits CYP1A2 and CYP2C9. There is a potential drug-drug interaction between atazanavir sulfate and CYP1A2 or CYP2C9 substrates). Products include:

Benadryl Allergy & Cold Tablets .... ◘692
Benadryl Allergy & Sinus Headache Caplets & Gelcaps .... ◘693
Benadryl Maximum Strength Severe Allergy & Sinus Headache Caplets .... ◘694
Contac Severe Cold and Flu Caplets Maximum Strength .... ◘615
Contac Severe Cold and Flu Caplets Non-Drowsy .... ◘615
Darvocet A 500 Tablets 3497
Goody's Body Pain Formula Powder .... ◘621
Goody's Extra Strength Headache Powder .... ◘621
Goody's Extra Strength Pain Relief Tablets .... ◘621
Goody's PM Powder .... ◘622
Hycomine Compound Tablets 1105
Lortab 3315
Lortab Elixir 3312
Percocet Tablets 1114
Robitussin Cough, Cold & Flu Liquid-filled Capsules .... ◘750
Robitussin Flu Liquid .... ◘752
Sedapap Tablets 50 mg/650 mg 2098
Singlet Caplets .... ◘636
Sudafed Severe Cold .... ◘710
Sudafed Sinus Headache .... ◘711
TheraFlu Cold & Cough Hot Liquid .... ◘680
TheraFlu Cold & Sore Throat Hot Liquid .... ◘680
TheraFlu Flu & Chest Congestion Non-Drowsy Hot Liquid .... ◘681
TheraFlu Flu & Sore Throat Hot Liquid .... ◘681
TheraFlu Severe Cold Non-Drowsy Hot Liquid .... ◘683
TheraFlu Severe Cold & Cough Hot Liquid .... ◘683
TheraFlu Severe Cold Caplets .... ◘679
TheraFlu Severe Cold Hot Liquid .... ◘682
TheraFlu Severe Cold Non-Drowsy Caplets .... ◘679
Triaminic Cough & Sore Throat Liquid .... ◘687
Triaminic Flu, Cough & Fever Liquid .... ◘685
Triaminic Cough & Sore Throat Softchews .... ◘689
Tylenol 8 Hour Extended Release Geltabs and Caplets 1843
Tylenol Sinus NightTime Caplets .... ◘663
Children's Tylenol Suspension Liquid and Meltaways 1850
Children's Tylenol Plus Cold & Allergy Suspension Liquid 1850
Children's Tylenol Plus Cold NightTime Suspension Liquid 1851
Children's Tylenol Plus Cold & Cough Suspension Liquid and Chewable Tablets 1851
Children's Tylenol Plus Cold Chewable Tablets 1851
Children's Tylenol Plus Cold Daytime Non-Drowsy Suspension Liquid 1851
Children's Tylenol Plus Flu Suspension Liquid 1853
Concentrated Tylenol Infants' Drops Plus Cold 1851
Concentrated Tylenol Infants' Drops Plus Cold and Cough 1851
Concentrated Tylenol Infants' Drops 1850
Junior Tylenol Meltaways 1850
Tylenol Cold & Flu Severe Daytime Liquid with Cool Bust 1846
Tylenol Cold & Flu Severe NightTime Liquid with Cool Burst 1846
Tylenol Cold Severe Congestion Non-Drowsy Caplets with Cool Burst 1846
Tylenol Cough & Sore Throat Daytime Liquid with Cool Burst 1849
Tylenol Cough & Sore Throat NightTime Liquid with Cool Burst 1849
Tylenol 1843
Extra Strength Tylenol Rapid Release Gels 1843
Tylenol 1843
Tylenol Allergy Complete Night Time Caplets 1844
Tylenol Allergy Complete Multi-Symptom Caplets and Gelcaps with Cool Burst 1844
Tylenol Severe Allergy Caplets 1844
Tylenol Flu NightTime Gelcaps 1846
Tylenol Flu Day Non-Drowsy Gelcaps 1846
Concentrated Tylenol Infants' Drops Plus Cold Nasal Congestant, Fever Reducer & Pain Reliever .... ◘668
Concentrated Tylenol Infants' Drops Plus Cold & Cough Nasal Decongestant, Fever Reducer & Pain Reliever .... ◘668
Multi-Symptom Tylenol Cold Night Time Caplets 1845
Multi-Symptom Tylenol Cold Day Non-Drowsy Caplets and Gelcaps 1845
Extra Strength Tylenol PM Caplets, Geltabs, Gelcaps and Liquid 1847
Tylenol Sinus Day Non-Drowsy 1848
Tylenol Sinus Night Time Caplets 1848
Tylenol Sinus Severe Congestion Caplets with Cool Burst 1848
Tylenol Sore Throat Daytime Liquid with Cool Burst 1849
Tylenol Sore Throat NightTime Liquid with Cool Burst 1849
Tylenol with Codeine 2461
Women's Tylenol Menstrual Relief Caplets 1849
Ultracet Tablets 2462
Vicks 44M Cough, Cold & Flu Relief 2676
Vicks DayQuil LiquiCaps/Liquid Multi-Symptom Cold/Flu Relief .... ◘723
Vicks DayQuil Multi-Symptom Cold/Flu Relief LiquiCaps 2675
Vicks DayQuil Multi-Symptom Cold/Flu Relief Liquid 2675
Vicks NyQuil LiquiCaps 2677
Vicks NyQuil LiquiCaps/Liquid Multi-Symptom Cold/Flu Relief .... ◘725
Vicks NyQuil Liquid 2677
Vicodin Tablets 530
Vicodin ES Tablets 531
Vicodin HP Tablets 532
Zydone Tablets 1118

Alatrofloxacin Mesylate (Atazanavir sulfate competitively inhibits CYP1A2 and CYP2C9. There is a potential drug-drug interaction between atazanavir sulfate and CYP1A2 or CYP2C9 substrates).

No products indexed under this heading.

Allium sativum (Drugs that induce CYP3A activity may increase the clearance of atazanavir sulfate, resulting in lowered plasma concentrations).

No products indexed under this heading.

Aluminum Carbonate (Reduced plasma concentrations of atazanavir are expected if antacids, including buffered medications, are administered with atazanavir sulfate. Atazanavir sulfate should be administered 2 hours before or 1 hour after these medications).

No products indexed under this heading.

Aluminum Hydroxide (Reduced plasma concentrations of atazanavir are expected if antacids, including buffered medications, are administered with atazanavir sulfate. Atazanavir sulfate should be administered 2 hours before or 1 hour after these medications). Products include:

Gaviscon Regular Strength Liquid .... ◘620
Gaviscon Regular Strength Tablets .... ◘619
Gaviscon Extra Strength Liquid .... ◘620
Gaviscon Extra Strength Tablets .... ◘619
Maalox Max Maximum Strength Antacid/Anti-Gas Liquid 2165
Maalox Regular Strength Antacid/Antigas Liquid 2164

Amiodarone Hydrochloride (Co-administration with atazanavir sulfate has the potential to produce serious and/or life-threatening adverse events and has not been studied. Caution is warranted and therapeutic concentration monitoring of these drugs is recommended if they are used concomitantly with atazanavir sulfate). Products include:

Pacerone Tablets 3337

Amitriptyline Hydrochloride (Atazanavir sulfate competitively inhibits CYP1A2 and CYP2C9. There is a potential drug-drug interaction between atazanavir sulfate and CYP1A2 or CYP2C9 substrates).

No products indexed under this heading.

Amoxapine (Atazanavir sulfate competitively inhibits CYP1A2 and CYP2C9. There is a potential drug-drug interaction between atazanavir sulfate and CYP1A2 or CYP2C9 substrates).

No products indexed under this heading.

Amprenavir (Co- administration of atazanavir sulfate/ritonavir and other protease inhibitors would be expected to increase exposure to the other protease inhibitors; co-administration is not recommended). Products include:

Agenerase Capsules 1299
Agenerase Oral Solution 1304

Anagrelide Hydrochloride (Atazanavir sulfate competitively inhibits CYP1A2 and CYP2C9. There is a potential drug-drug interaction between atazanavir sulfate and CYP1A2 or CYP2C9 substrates). Products include:

Agrylin Capsules 3172

Aprepitant (Drugs that induce CYP3A activity may increase the clearance of atazanavir sulfate, resulting in lowered plasma concentrations). Products include:

Emend Capsules 1944

Atorvastatin Calcium (The risk of myopathy, including rhabdomyolysis, may be increased when protease inhibitors, including atazanavir sulfate, are used in combination with atorvastatin. Caution should be exercised). Products include:

Caduet Tablets 2507
Lipitor Tablets 2495

Azathioprine (Therapeutic concentration monitoring is recommended for immunosuppressant agents when co-administered with atazanavir sulfate). Products include:

Azasan Tablets 2844

Basiliximab (Therapeutic concentration monitoring is recommended for immunosuppressant agents when co-administered with atazanavir sulfate). Products include:

Simulect for Injection 2268

Bepridil Hydrochloride (Co-administration with atazanavir sulfate has the potential to produce serious and/or life-threatening adverse events and has not been studied. Caution is warranted and therapeutic concentration monitoring of these drugs is recommended if they are used concomitantly with atazanavir sulfate).

No products indexed under this heading.

Caffeine (Atazanavir sulfate competitively inhibits CYP1A2 and CYP2C9. There is a potential drug-drug interaction between atazanavir sulfate and CYP1A2 or CYP2C9 substrates). Products include:

Athena Hair System Shampoo .... ◘767
BC Powder .... ◘612
Arthritis Strength BC Powder .... ◘612

Goody's Extra Strength Headache Powder .... ▣ 621
Goody's Extra Strength Pain Relief Tablets .... ▣ 621
Hycomine Compound Tablets 1105
Spartan Hair System Shampoo .... ▣ 767
Vivarin .... ▣ 639

Caffeine Anhydrous (Atazanavir sulfate competitively inhibits CYP1A2 and CYP2C9. There is a potential drug-drug interaction between atazanavir sulfate and CYP1A2 or CYP2C9 substrates).
No products indexed under this heading.

Candesartan Cilexetil (Atazanavir sulfate competitively inhibits CYP1A2 and CYP2C9. There is a potential drug-drug interaction between atazanavir sulfate and CYP1A2 or CYP2C9 substrates). Products include:
Atacand Tablets 634
Atacand HCT 637

Carbamazepine (Drugs that induce CYP3A activity may increase the clearance of atazanavir sulfate, resulting in lowered plasma concentrations). Products include:
Carbatrol Capsules 3174
Equetro Extended-Release Capsules 3178
Tegretol/Tegretol-XR 2278

Carvedilol (Atazanavir sulfate competitively inhibits CYP1A2 and CYP2C9. There is a potential drug-drug interaction between atazanavir sulfate and CYP1A2 or CYP2C9 substrates). Products include:
Coreg Tablets 1376

Celecoxib (Atazanavir sulfate competitively inhibits CYP1A2 and CYP2C9. There is a potential drug-drug interaction between atazanavir sulfate and CYP1A2 or CYP2C9 substrates). Products include:
Celebrex Capsules 3130

Chlordiazepoxide (Atazanavir sulfate competitively inhibits CYP1A2 and CYP2C9. There is a potential drug-drug interaction between atazanavir sulfate and CYP1A2 or CYP2C9 substrates).
No products indexed under this heading.

Chlordiazepoxide Hydrochloride (Atazanavir sulfate competitively inhibits CYP1A2 and CYP2C9. There is a potential drug-drug interaction between atazanavir sulfate and CYP1A2 or CYP2C9 substrates). Products include:
Librium Capsules 3349

Chlorpropamide (Atazanavir sulfate competitively inhibits CYP1A2 and CYP2C9. There is a potential drug-drug interaction between atazanavir sulfate and CYP1A2 or CYP2C9 substrates).
No products indexed under this heading.

Cimetidine (Reduced plasma concentrations of atazanavir are expected if H2-receptor antagonists are administered with atazanavir sulfate. This may result in loss of therapeutic effect and development of resistance. To lessen the effect of H2-receptor antagonists on atazanavir exposure, it is recommended that an H2-receptor antagonist and atazanavir sulfate be administered as far apart as possible, preferably 12 hours apart). Products include:
Tagamet HB 200 Tablets .... ▣ 637
Tagamet Tablets 1547

Cimetidine Hydrochloride (Reduced plasma concentrations of atazanavir are expected if H2-receptor antagonists are administered with atazanavir sulfate. This may result in loss of therapeutic effect and development of resistance. To lessen the effect of H2-receptor antagonists on atazanavir exposure, it is recommended that an H2-receptor antagonist and atazanavir sulfate be administered as far apart as possible, preferably 12 hours apart).
No products indexed under this heading.

Ciprofloxacin (Atazanavir sulfate competitively inhibits CYP1A2 and CYP2C9. There is a potential drug-drug interaction between atazanavir sulfate and CYP1A2 or CYP2C9 substrates). Products include:
Cipro I.V. 2998
Cipro I.V. Pharmacy Bulk Package ... 3509
Cipro Oral Suspension 2991
Cipro XR Tablets 3004
Ciprodex Otic Suspension 555

Ciprofloxacin Hydrochloride (Atazanavir sulfate competitively inhibits CYP1A2 and CYP2C9. There is a potential drug-drug interaction between atazanavir sulfate and CYP1A2 or CYP2C9 substrates). Products include:
Ciloxan Ophthalmic Ointment 554
Cipro Tablets 2991

Cisapride (Contraindicated due to potential for serious and/or life-threatening reactions such as cardiac arrhythmias).
No products indexed under this heading.

Clarithromycin (Increased concentrations of clarithromycin may cause QTc prolongations; therefore, a dose reduction of clarithromycin by 50% should be considered when it is co-administered with atazanavir sulfate. In addition, concentrations of the active metabolite 14-OH clarithromycin are significantly reduced; consider alternative therapy for indications other than infections due to Mycobacterium Avium Complex). Products include:
Biaxin/Biaxin XL 402
PREVPAC 3281

Clomipramine Hydrochloride (Atazanavir sulfate competitively inhibits CYP1A2 and CYP2C9. There is a potential drug-drug interaction between atazanavir sulfate and CYP1A2 or CYP2C9 substrates).
No products indexed under this heading.

Clopidogrel Bisulfate (Atazanavir sulfate competitively inhibits CYP1A2 and CYP2C9. There is a potential drug-drug interaction between atazanavir sulfate and CYP1A2 or CYP2C9 substrates). Products include:
Plavix Tablets 940
Plavix Tablets 2942

Clozapine (Atazanavir sulfate competitively inhibits CYP1A2 and CYP2C9. There is a potential drug-drug interaction between atazanavir sulfate and CYP1A2 or CYP2C9 substrates). Products include:
Clozapine Tablets 2141
Clozaril Tablets 2174
FazaClo Orally Disintegrating Tablets 547

Cyclobenzaprine (Atazanavir sulfate competitively inhibits CYP1A2 and CYP2C9. There is a potential drug-drug interaction between atazanavir sulfate and CYP1A2 or CYP2C9 substrates).
No products indexed under this heading.

Cyclobenzaprine Hydrochloride (Atazanavir sulfate competitively inhibits CYP1A2 and CYP2C9. There is a potential drug-drug interaction between atazanavir sulfate and CYP1A2 or CYP2C9 substrates). Products include:
Flexeril Tablets 1832

Cyclosporine (Therapeutic concentration monitoring is recommended for immunosuppressant agents when co-administered with atazanavir sulfate). Products include:
Gengraf Capsules 458
Neoral Soft Gelatin Capsules 2247
Neoral Oral Solution 2247
Restasis Ophthalmic Emulsion 570
Sandimmune 2259

Delavirdine Mesylate (Co-administration of atazanavir sulfate and other drugs that inhibit CYP3A may increase atazanavir sulfate plasma concentrations). Products include:
Rescriptor Tablets 2535

Desipramine Hydrochloride (Atazanavir sulfate competitively inhibits CYP1A2 and CYP2C9. There is a potential drug-drug interaction between atazanavir sulfate and CYP1A2 or CYP2C9 substrates).
No products indexed under this heading.

Desogestrel (Because contraceptive steriod concentrations may be altered when atazanavir sulfate or atazanavir sulfate/ritonavir is co-administered with oral contraceptives or with the contraceptive patch, alternate methods of non-hormonal contraception are recommended). Products include:
Ortho-Cept Tablets 2395

Dexamethasone (Drugs that induce CYP3A activity may increase the clearance of atazanavir sulfate, resulting in lowered plasma concentrations). Products include:
Ciprodex Otic Suspension 555
Decadron Tablets 1929
TobraDex Ophthalmic Ointment 558
TobraDex Ophthalmic Suspension ... 558

Dextromethorphan (Atazanavir sulfate competitively inhibits CYP1A2 and CYP2C9. There is a potential drug-drug interaction between atazanavir sulfate and CYP1A2 or CYP2C9 substrates).
No products indexed under this heading.

Diazepam (Atazanavir sulfate competitively inhibits CYP1A2 and CYP2C9. There is a potential drug-drug interaction between atazanavir sulfate and CYP1A2 or CYP2C9 substrates). Products include:
Diastat Rectal Delivery System 3344
Valium Tablets 2822

Diclofenac Potassium (Atazanavir sulfate competitively inhibits CYP1A2 and CYP2C9. There is a potential drug-drug interaction between atazanavir sulfate and CYP1A2 or CYP2C9 substrates). Products include:
Cataflam Tablets 2173

Diclofenac Sodium (Atazanavir sulfate competitively inhibits CYP1A2 and CYP2C9. There is a potential drug-drug interaction between atazanavir sulfate and CYP1A2 or CYP2C9 substrates). Products include:
Arthrotec Tablets 3126
Voltaren Ophthalmic Solution 2300
Voltaren Tablets 2298
Voltaren-XR Tablets 2301

Didanosine (Presumably due to the increase in gastric pH caused by buffers in the didanosine buffered tablets, exposure to atazanavir sulfate was markedly decreased. Atazanavir sulfate should be given 2 hours before or 1 hour after didanosine buffered formulations. Didanosine EC capsules and atazanavir should also be given at different times).
No products indexed under this heading.

Dihydroergotamine Mesylate (Contraindicated due to potential for serious and/or life-threatening events such as acute ergot toxicity characterized by peripheral vasospasm and ischemia of the extremities and other tissues). Products include:
Migranal Nasal Spray 3350

Diltiazem Hydrochloride (Concomitant administration may lead to increased levels of diltiazem and desacetyl-diltiazem; therefore, caution is warranted and dose reduction of diltiazem by 50% should be considered. ECG monitoring is also recommended). Products include:
Cardizem LA Extended Release Tablets 1699
Tiazac Capsules 1204

Diltiazem Maleate (Atazanavir sulfate competitively inhibits CYP1A2 and CYP2C9. There is a potential drug-drug interaction between atazanavir sulfate and CYP1A2 or CYP2C9 substrates).
No products indexed under this heading.

Doxepin Hydrochloride (Atazanavir sulfate competitively inhibits CYP1A2 and CYP2C9. There is a potential drug-drug interaction between atazanavir sulfate and CYP1A2 or CYP2C9 substrates).
No products indexed under this heading.

Dronabinol (Atazanavir sulfate competitively inhibits CYP1A2 and CYP2C9. There is a potential drug-drug interaction between atazanavir sulfate and CYP1A2 or CYP2C9 substrates). Products include:
Marinol Capsules 3334

Efavirenz (If atazanavir sulfate is to be co-administered with efavirenz, which decreases atazanavir exposure, it is recommended that atazanavir sulfate 300mg with ritonavir 100mg be co-administered with efavirenz 600mg, as this combination results in atazanavir exposure that approximates the mean exposure to atazanavir produced by 400mg of atazanavir sulfate alone. Atazanavir sulfate without ritonavir should not be co-administered with efavirenz). Products include:
Sustiva Capsules 957

Enoxacin (Atazanavir sulfate competitively inhibits CYP1A2 and CYP2C9. There is a potential drug-drug interaction between atazanavir sulfate and CYP1A2 or CYP2C9 substrates).
No products indexed under this heading.

Eprosartan Mesylate (Atazanavir sulfate competitively inhibits CYP1A2

and CYP2C9. There is a potential drug-drug interaction between atazanavir sulfate and CYP1A2 or CYP2C9 substrates). Products include:

Teveten Tablets ... 1707
Teveten HCT Tablets ... 1710

Ergonovine Maleate (Contraindicated due to potential for serious and/or life-threatening events such as acute ergot toxicity characterized by peripheral vasospasm and ischemia of the extremities and other tissues).

No products indexed under this heading.

Ergotamine Tartrate (Contraindicated due to potential for serious and/or life-threatening events such as acute ergot toxicity characterized by peripheral vasospasm and ischemia of the extremities and other tissues).

No products indexed under this heading.

Erythromycin (Atazanavir sulfate competitively inhibits CYP1A2 and CYP2C9. There is a potential drug-drug interaction between atazanavir sulfate and CYP1A2 or CYP2C9 substrates). Products include:

Erygel Topical Gel ... 2096
Ery-Tab Tablets ... 447
Erythromycin Base Filmtab Tablets ... 454
Erythromycin Delayed-Release Capsules, USP ... 456
PCE Dispertab Tablets ... 510

Erythromycin Estolate (Atazanavir sulfate competitively inhibits CYP1A2 and CYP2C9. There is a potential drug-drug interaction between atazanavir sulfate and CYP1A2 or CYP2C9 substrates).

No products indexed under this heading.

Erythromycin Ethylsuccinate (Atazanavir sulfate competitively inhibits CYP1A2 and CYP2C9. There is a potential drug-drug interaction between atazanavir sulfate and CYP1A2 or CYP2C9 substrates). Products include:

E.E.S. ... 449
EryPed ... 445

Erythromycin Gluceptate (Atazanavir sulfate competitively inhibits CYP1A2 and CYP2C9. There is a potential drug-drug interaction between atazanavir sulfate and CYP1A2 or CYP2C9 substrates).

No products indexed under this heading.

Erythromycin Lactobionate (Atazanavir sulfate competitively inhibits CYP1A2 and CYP2C9. There is a potential drug-drug interaction between atazanavir sulfate and CYP1A2 or CYP2C9 substrates).

No products indexed under this heading.

Erythromycin Stearate (Atazanavir sulfate competitively inhibits CYP1A2 and CYP2C9. There is a potential drug-drug interaction between atazanavir sulfate and CYP1A2 or CYP2C9 substrates). Products include:

Erythrocin Stearate Filmtab Tablets ... 452

Esomeprazole Magnesium (Concomitant use of atazanavir sulfate and proton-pump inhibitors is not recommended. Co-administration of atazanavir sulfate with proton-pump inhibitors is expected to substantially decrease atazanavir sulfate plasma concentrations and reduce its therapeutic effect). Products include:

Nexium Delayed-Release Capsules ... 645

Estradiol (Atazanavir sulfate competitively inhibits CYP1A2 and CYP2C9. There is a potential drug-drug interaction between atazanavir sulfate and CYP1A2 or CYP2C9 substrates). Products include:

Activella Tablets ... 2311
Climara Transdermal System ... 795
Climara Pro Transdermal System ... 800
CombiPatch Transdermal System ... 2180
Estrogel 0.06% ... 3200
Menostar Transdermal System ... 805
Prefest Tablets ... 1069
Vagifem Tablets ... 2340
Vivelle Transdermal System ... 2288
Vivelle-Dot Transdermal System ... 2293

Estradiol Benzoate (Atazanavir sulfate competitively inhibits CYP1A2 and CYP2C9. There is a potential drug-drug interaction between atazanavir sulfate and CYP1A2 or CYP2C9 substrates).

No products indexed under this heading.

Estradiol Cypionate (Atazanavir sulfate competitively inhibits CYP1A2 and CYP2C9. There is a potential drug-drug interaction between atazanavir sulfate and CYP1A2 or CYP2C9 substrates).

No products indexed under this heading.

Ethinyl Estradiol (Because contraceptive steriod concentrations may be altered when atazanavir sulfate or atazanavir sulfate/ritonavir is co-administered with oral contraceptives or with the contraceptive patch, alternate methods of non-hormonal contraception are recommended). Products include:

Alesse-28 Tablets ... 3392
Lo/Ovral-28 Tablets ... 3423
NuvaRing ... 2357
Ortho-Cept Tablets ... 2395
Ortho-Cyclen/Ortho Tri-Cyclen ... 2414
Ortho Evra Transdermal System ... 2402
Ortho Tri-Cyclen Lo Tablets ... 2421
Seasonale Tablets ... 1073
Triphasil-28 Tablets ... 3483
Yasmin 28 Tablets ... 818

Ethosuximide (Drugs that induce CYP3A activity may increase the clearance of atazanavir sulfate, resulting in lowered plasma concentrations).

No products indexed under this heading.

Ethynodiol Diacetate (Because contraceptive steriod concentrations may be altered when atazanavir sulfate or atazanavir sulfate/ritonavir is co-administered with oral contraceptives or with the contraceptive patch, alternate methods of non-hormonal contraception are recommended).

No products indexed under this heading.

Etodolac (Atazanavir sulfate competitively inhibits CYP1A2 and CYP2C9. There is a potential drug-drug interaction between atazanavir sulfate and CYP1A2 or CYP2C9 substrates).

No products indexed under this heading.

Famotidine (Reduced plasma concentrations of atazanavir are expected if H2-receptor antagonists are administered with atazanavir sulfate. This may result in loss of therapeutic effect and development of resistance. To lessen the effect of H2-receptor antagonists on atazanavir exposure, it is recommended that an H2-receptor antagonist and atazanavir sulfate be administered as far apart as possible, preferably 12 hours apart). Products include:

Pepcid AC Chewable Tablets ... 1672
Pepcid AC Gelcaps ... 1672
Pepcid AC Tablets ... 1672
Maximum Strength Pepcid AC Tablets ... 1672
Pepcid Complete Chewable Tablets ... 1672
Pepcid Injection ... 2017
Pepcid ... 2014

Fenoprofen Calcium (Atazanavir sulfate competitively inhibits CYP1A2 and CYP2C9. There is a potential drug-drug interaction between atazanavir sulfate and CYP1A2 or CYP2C9 substrates). Products include:

Nalfon Capsules ... 2504

Fluconazole (Co-administration of atazanavir sulfate and other drugs that inhibit CYP3A may increase atazanavir sulfate plasma concentrations).

No products indexed under this heading.

Fluoxetine (Co-administration of atazanavir sulfate and other drugs that inhibit CYP3A may increase atazanavir sulfate plasma concentrations).

No products indexed under this heading.

Fluoxetine Hydrochloride (Atazanavir sulfate competitively inhibits CYP1A2 and CYP2C9. There is a potential drug-drug interaction between atazanavir sulfate and CYP1A2 or CYP2C9 substrates). Products include:

Prozac Pulvules and Liquid ... 1771
Symbyax Capsules ... 1788

Flurbiprofen (Atazanavir sulfate competitively inhibits CYP1A2 and CYP2C9. There is a potential drug-drug interaction between atazanavir sulfate and CYP1A2 or CYP2C9 substrates).

No products indexed under this heading.

Flurbiprofen Sodium (Atazanavir sulfate competitively inhibits CYP1A2 and CYP2C9. There is a potential drug-drug interaction between atazanavir sulfate and CYP1A2 or CYP2C9 substrates). Products include:

Ocufen Ophthalmic Solution ... ⊙230

Flutamide (Atazanavir sulfate competitively inhibits CYP1A2 and CYP2C9. There is a potential drug-drug interaction between atazanavir sulfate and CYP1A2 or CYP2C9 substrates). Products include:

Eulexin Capsules ... 3023

Fluticasone Propionate (A study has shown that ritonavir significantly increases plasma fluticasone propionate exposures, resulting in significantly decreased serum cortisol concentrations. Concomitant use of atazanavir with ritonavir and fluticasone propionate is expected to produce the same effects. Systemic corticosteroid effects, including Cushing's syndrome and adrenal suppression have been reported during postmarketing use in patients receiving ritonavir and inhaled or intranasally administered fluticasone propionate. Therefore, co-administration of fluticasone propionate and atazanavir/ritonavir is not recommended unless the potential benefit to the patient outweighs the risk of systemic corticosteroid side effects). Products include:

Advair Diskus 100/50 ... 1291
Advair Diskus 250/50 ... 1291
Advair Diskus 500/50 ... 1291
Cutivate Cream ... 1381
Cutivate Lotion 0.05% ... 1383
Cutivate Ointment ... 1384
Flonase Nasal Spray ... 1412
Flovent Diskus 100 mcg ... 1418
Flovent Diskus 50 mcg ... 1415

Fluticasone Propionate HFA (A study has shown that ritonavir significantly increases plasma fluticasone propionate exposures, resulting in significantly decreased serum cortisol concentrations. Concomitant use of atazanavir with ritonavir and fluticasone propionate is expected to produce the same effects. Systemic corticosteroid effects, including Cushing's syndrome and adrenal suppression have been reported during postmarketing use in patients receiving ritonavir and inhaled or intranasally administered fluticasone propionate. Therefore, co-administration of fluticasone propionate and atazanavir/ritonavir is not recommended unless the potential benefit to the patient outweighs the risk of systemic corticosteroid side effects). Products include:

Flovent HFA ... 1418

Fluvastatin Sodium (Atazanavir sulfate competitively inhibits CYP1A2 and CYP2C9. There is a potential drug-drug interaction between atazanavir sulfate and CYP1A2 or CYP2C9 substrates). Products include:

Lescol Capsules ... 2227
Lescol ... 2730
Lescol XL Tablets ... 2227

Fluvoxamine Maleate (Atazanavir sulfate competitively inhibits CYP1A2 and CYP2C9. There is a potential drug-drug interaction between atazanavir sulfate and CYP1A2 or CYP2C9 substrates).

No products indexed under this heading.

Glimepiride (Atazanavir sulfate competitively inhibits CYP1A2 and CYP2C9. There is a potential drug-drug interaction between atazanavir sulfate and CYP1A2 or CYP2C9 substrates). Products include:

Amaryl Tablets ... 2864

Glipizide (Atazanavir sulfate competitively inhibits CYP1A2 and CYP2C9. There is a potential drug-drug interaction between atazanavir sulfate and CYP1A2 or CYP2C9 substrates).

No products indexed under this heading.

Grepafloxacin Hydrochloride (Atazanavir sulfate competitively inhibits CYP1A2 and CYP2C9. There is a potential drug-drug interaction between atazanavir sulfate and CYP1A2 or CYP2C9 substrates).

No products indexed under this heading.

Haloperidol (Atazanavir sulfate competitively inhibits CYP1A2 and CYP2C9. There is a potential drug-drug interaction between atazanavir sulfate and CYP1A2 or CYP2C9 substrates).

No products indexed under this heading.

Haloperidol Decanoate (Atazanavir sulfate competitively inhibits CYP1A2 and CYP2C9. There is a potential drug-drug interaction between atazanavir sulfate and CYP1A2 or CYP2C9 substrates).
No products indexed under this heading.

Haloperidol Lactate (Atazanavir sulfate competitively inhibits CYP1A2 and CYP2C9. There is a potential drug-drug interaction between atazanavir sulfate and CYP1A2 or CYP2C9 substrates).
No products indexed under this heading.

Hypericum Perforatum (Concomitant use of atazanavir sulfate and St. John's Wort, or products containing St. John's Wort, is not recommended. Co-administration of protease inhibitors with St. John's Wort is expected to substantially decrease concentrations of the protease inhibitor and may result in suboptimal levels of atazanavir sulfate and lead to loss of virologic response and possible resistance to atazanavir sulfate or to the class of protease inhibitors).
No products indexed under this heading.

Ibuprofen (Atazanavir sulfate competitively inhibits CYP1A2 and CYP2C9. There is a potential drug-drug interaction between atazanavir sulfate and CYP1A2 or CYP2C9 substrates). Products include:
Advil Allergy Sinus Caplets .... ▣ 737
Advil .... ▣ 737
Children's Advil Suspension .... ▣ 742
Children's Advil Chewable Tablets .. ▣ 741
Advil Cold & Sinus .... ▣ 739
Advil Flu & Body Ache Caplets .... ▣ 739
Children's Advil Cold Suspension ... ▣ 741
Infants' Advil Concentrated Drops .. ▣ 743
Junior Strength Advil Swallow Tablets .... ▣ 740
Advil Migraine Liquigels .... ▣ 740
Advil Multi-Symptom Cold Caplets .... ▣ 738
Combunox Tablets 1183
Children's Motrin Oral Suspension and Chewable Tablets 1837
Children's Motrin Cold Non-Staining Dye-Free Oral Suspension 1838
Children's Motrin Cold Oral Suspension 1838
Children's Motrin Non-Staining Dye-Free Oral Suspension 1837
Motrin Cold & Sinus Caplets 1836
Motrin IB Tablets and Caplets 1836
Infants' Motrin Concentrated Drops 1837
Infants' Motrin Non-Staining Dye-Free Drops 1837
Junior Strength Motrin Caplets and Chewable Tablets 1837
Vicoprofen Tablets 533

Imipramine Hydrochloride (Atazanavir sulfate competitively inhibits CYP1A2 and CYP2C9. There is a potential drug-drug interaction between atazanavir sulfate and CYP1A2 or CYP2C9 substrates).
No products indexed under this heading.

Imipramine Pamoate (Atazanavir sulfate competitively inhibits CYP1A2 and CYP2C9. There is a potential drug-drug interaction between atazanavir sulfate and CYP1A2 or CYP2C9 substrates).
No products indexed under this heading.

Indinavir Sulfate (Both atazanavir sulfate and indinavir are associated with indirect hyperbilirubinemia. Combinations of these drugs have not been studied and co-administration is not recommended). Products include:
Crixivan Capsules 1918

Indomethacin (Atazanavir sulfate competitively inhibits CYP1A2 and CYP2C9. There is a potential drug-drug interaction between atazanavir sulfate and CYP1A2 or CYP2C9 substrates). Products include:
Indocin 1968

Indomethacin Sodium Trihydrate (Atazanavir sulfate competitively inhibits CYP1A2 and CYP2C9. There is a potential drug-drug interaction between atazanavir sulfate and CYP1A2 or CYP2C9 substrates). Products include:
Indocin I.V. 1973

Irbesartan (Atazanavir sulfate competitively inhibits CYP1A2 and CYP2C9. There is a potential drug-drug interaction between atazanavir sulfate and CYP1A2 or CYP2C9 substrates). Products include:
Avalide Tablets 922
Avalide Tablets 2889
Avapro Tablets 925
Avapro Tablets 2886

Irinotecan Hydrochloride (Atazanavir inhibits UGT and may interfere with the metabolism of irinotecan, resulting in increased irinotecan toxicity). Products include:
Camptosar Injection 2602

Isoniazid (Co-administration of atazanavir sulfate and other drugs that inhibit CYP3A may increase atazanavir sulfate plasma concentrations).
No products indexed under this heading.

Itraconazole (Due to the effect of ritonavir on ketoconazole, high doses of ketoconazole and itraconazole (greater than 200 mg/day) should be used cautiously with atazanavir sulfate/ritonavir).
No products indexed under this heading.

Ketoconazole (Due to the effect of ritonavir on ketoconazole, high doses of ketoconazole and itraconazole (greater than 200 mg/day) should be used cautiously with atazanavir sulfate/ritonavir). Products include:
Nizoral A-D Shampoo, 1% 1839
Nizoral 2% Shampoo 1838

Ketoprofen (Atazanavir sulfate competitively inhibits CYP1A2 and CYP2C9. There is a potential drug-drug interaction between atazanavir sulfate and CYP1A2 or CYP2C9 substrates).
No products indexed under this heading.

Ketorolac Tromethamine (Atazanavir sulfate competitively inhibits CYP1A2 and CYP2C9. There is a potential drug-drug interaction between atazanavir sulfate and CYP1A2 or CYP2C9 substrates). Products include:
Acular Ophthalmic Solution 561
Acular LS Ophthalmic Solution 562

Lansoprazole (Concomitant use of atazanavir sulfate and proton-pump inhibitors is not recommended. Co-administration of atazanavir sulfate with proton-pump inhibitors is expected to substantially decrease atazanavir sulfate plasma concentrations and reduce its therapeutic effect). Products include:
Prevacid Delayed-Release Capsules 3268
Prevacid for Delayed-Release Oral Suspension 3268
Prevacid I.V. for Injection 3274
Prevacid NapraPAC 3277
Prevacid SoluTab Delayed-Release Orally Disintegrating Tablets 3268
PREVPAC 3281

Levobupivacaine Hydrochloride (Atazanavir sulfate competitively inhibits CYP1A2 and CYP2C9. There is a potential drug-drug interaction between atazanavir sulfate and CYP1A2 or CYP2C9 substrates).
No products indexed under this heading.

Levonorgestrel (Because contraceptive steriod concentrations may be altered when atazanavir sulfate or atazanavir sulfate/ritonavir is co-administered with oral contraceptives or with the contraceptive patch, alternate methods of non-hormonal contraception are recommended). Products include:
Alesse-28 Tablets 3392
Climara Pro Transdermal System 800
Mirena Intrauterine System 810
Plan B Tablets 1068
Seasonale Tablets 1073
Triphasil-28 Tablets 3483

Lidocaine (Co-administration with atazanavir sulfate has the potential to produce serious and/or life-threatening adverse events and has not been studied. Caution is warranted and therapeutic concentration monitoring of these drugs is recommended if they are used concomitantly with atazanavir sulfate). Products include:
Lidoderm Patch 1107

Lidocaine Hydrochloride (Co-administration with atazanavir sulfate has the potential to produce serious and/or life-threatening adverse events and has not been studied. Caution is warranted and therapeutic concentration monitoring of these drugs is recommended if they are used concomitantly with atazanavir sulfate).
No products indexed under this heading.

Lomefloxacin Hydrochloride (Atazanavir sulfate competitively inhibits CYP1A2 and CYP2C9. There is a potential drug-drug interaction between atazanavir sulfate and CYP1A2 or CYP2C9 substrates).
No products indexed under this heading.

Lopinavir (Co- administration of atazanavir sulfate/ritonavir and other protease inhibitors would be expected to increase exposure to the other protease inhibitors; co-administration is not recommended). Products include:
Kaletra 474

Losartan Potassium (Atazanavir sulfate competitively inhibits CYP1A2 and CYP2C9. There is a potential drug-drug interaction between atazanavir sulfate and CYP1A2 or CYP2C9 substrates). Products include:
Cozaar Tablets 1913
Hyzaar 1964

Lovastatin (Concomitant use of atazanavir sulfate with lovastatin is not recommended. Caution should be exercised if HIV protease inhibitors, including atazanavir sulfate, are used concurrently with other HMG-CoA reductase inhibitors that are also metabolized by theCYP3A4 pathway. The risk of myopathy, including rhabdomyolysis, may be increased when HIV protease inhibitors, including atazanavir sulfate, are used in combination with these drugs). Products include:
Advicor Tablets 1694
Altoprev Extended-Release Tablets 1151
Mevacor Tablets 1996

Magaldrate (Reduced plasma concentrations of atazanavir are expected if antacids, including buffered medications, are administered with atazanavir sulfate. Atazanavir sulfate should be administered 2 hours before or 1 hour after these medications).
No products indexed under this heading.

Magnesium Hydroxide (Reduced plasma concentrations of atazanavir are expected if antacids, including buffered medications, are administered with atazanavir sulfate. Atazanavir sulfate should be administered 2 hours before or 1 hour after these medications). Products include:
Maalox Max Maximum Strength Antacid/Anti-Gas Liquid 2165
Maalox Regular Strength Antacid/Antigas Liquid 2164
Pepcid Complete Chewable Tablets 1672
Rolaids Tablets .... ▣ 707
Extra Strength Rolaids Tablets .... ▣ 707
Rolaids Multi-Symptom Antacid & Antigas Tablets .... ▣ 708

Magnesium Oxide (Reduced plasma concentrations of atazanavir are expected if antacids, including buffered medications, are administered with atazanavir sulfate. Atazanavir sulfate should be administered 2 hours before or 1 hour after these medications). Products include:
Beelith Tablets 784
PremCal Light, Regular, and Extra Strength Tablets .... ▣ 762

Maprotiline Hydrochloride (Atazanavir sulfate competitively inhibits CYP1A2 and CYP2C9. There is a potential drug-drug interaction between atazanavir sulfate and CYP1A2 or CYP2C9 substrates).
No products indexed under this heading.

Meclofenamate Sodium (Atazanavir sulfate competitively inhibits CYP1A2 and CYP2C9. There is a potential drug-drug interaction between atazanavir sulfate and CYP1A2 or CYP2C9 substrates).
No products indexed under this heading.

Mefenamic Acid (Atazanavir sulfate competitively inhibits CYP1A2 and CYP2C9. There is a potential drug-drug interaction between atazanavir sulfate and CYP1A2 or CYP2C9 substrates).
No products indexed under this heading.

Meloxicam (Atazanavir sulfate competitively inhibits CYP1A2 and CYP2C9. There is a potential drug-drug interaction between atazanavir sulfate and CYP1A2 or CYP2C9 substrates). Products include:
Mobic Oral Suspension 893
Mobic Tablets 893

Mestranol (Because contraceptive steriod concentrations may be altered when atazanavir sulfate or atazanavir sulfate/ritonavir is co-administered with oral contraceptives or with the contraceptive patch, alternate methods of non-hormonal contraception are recommended).
No products indexed under this heading.

Metformin Hydrochloride (Atazanavir sulfate competitively inhibits CYP1A2 and CYP2C9. There is a potential drug-drug interaction between atazanavir sulfate and CYP1A2 or CYP2C9 substrates). Products include:
ActoPlus Met Tablets 3219
Avandamet Tablets 1343
Fortamet Extended-Release Tablets 1156

Methadone Hydrochloride (Atazanavir sulfate competitively inhibits CYP1A2 and CYP2C9. There is a potential drug-drug interaction between atazanavir sulfate and CYP1A2 or CYP2C9 substrates).
No products indexed under this heading.

Methylergonovine Maleate (Contraindicated due to potential for serious and/or life-threatening events such as acute ergot toxicity characterized by peripheral vasospasm and ischemia of the extremities and other tissues).
No products indexed under this heading.

Methysergide Maleate (Contraindicated due to potential for serious and/or life-threatening events such as acute ergot toxicity characterized by peripheral vasospasm and ischemia of the extremities and other tissues).
No products indexed under this heading.

Metronidazole (Co-administration of atazanavir sulfate and other drugs that inhibit CYP3A may increase atazanavir sulfate plasma concentrations). Products include:
Metrogel 1% 1212
MetroGel-Vaginal Gel 1822
Noritate Cream, 1% 1051

Metronidazole Benzoate (Co-administration of atazanavir sulfate and other drugs that inhibit CYP3A may increase atazanavir sulfate plasma concentrations).
No products indexed under this heading.

Metronidazole Hydrochloride (Co-administration of atazanavir sulfate and other drugs that inhibit CYP3A may increase atazanavir sulfate plasma concentrations).
No products indexed under this heading.

Mexiletine Hydrochloride (Atazanavir sulfate competitively inhibits CYP1A2 and CYP2C9. There is a potential drug-drug interaction between atazanavir sulfate and CYP1A2 or CYP2C9 substrates).
No products indexed under this heading.

Miconazole (Co-administration of atazanavir sulfate and other drugs that inhibit CYP3A may increase atazanavir sulfate plasma concentrations).
No products indexed under this heading.

Midazolam Hydrochloride (Contraindicated due to potential for serious and/or life-threatening events, such as prolonged or increased sedation or respiratory depression).
No products indexed under this heading.

Miglitol (Atazanavir sulfate competitively inhibits CYP1A2 and CYP2C9. There is a potential drug-drug interaction between atazanavir sulfate and CYP1A2 or CYP2C9 substrates).
No products indexed under this heading.

Mirtazapine (Atazanavir sulfate competitively inhibits CYP1A2 and CYP2C9. There is a potential drug-drug interaction between atazanavir sulfate and CYP1A2 or CYP2C9 substrates).
No products indexed under this heading.

Modafinil (Drugs that induce CYP3A activity may increase the clearance of atazanavir sulfate, resulting in lowered plasma concentrations). Products include:
Provigil Tablets 1002

Montelukast Sodium (Atazanavir sulfate competitively inhibits CYP1A2 and CYP2C9. There is a potential drug-drug interaction between atazanavir sulfate and CYP1A2 or CYP2C9 substrates). Products include:
Singulair 2047

Moxifloxacin Hydrochloride (Atazanavir sulfate competitively inhibits CYP1A2 and CYP2C9. There is a potential drug-drug interaction between atazanavir sulfate and CYP1A2 or CYP2C9 substrates). Products include:
Avelox 2984
Vigamox Ophthalmic Solution 560

Muromonab-CD3 (Therapeutic concentration monitoring is recommended for immunosuppressant agents when co-administered with atazanavir sulfate). Products include:
Orthoclone OKT3 Sterile Solution 2370

Mycophenolate Mofetil (Therapeutic concentration monitoring is recommended for immunosuppressant agents when co-administered with atazanavir sulfate). Products include:
CellCept Capsules 2751
CellCept Oral Suspension 2751
CellCept Tablets 2751

Nabumetone (Atazanavir sulfate competitively inhibits CYP1A2 and CYP2C9. There is a potential drug-drug interaction between atazanavir sulfate and CYP1A2 or CYP2C9 substrates). Products include:
Relafen Tablets 1523

Nafcillin Sodium (Atazanavir sulfate competitively inhibits CYP1A2 and CYP2C9. There is a potential drug-drug interaction between atazanavir sulfate and CYP1A2 or CYP2C9 substrates).
No products indexed under this heading.

Naproxen (Atazanavir sulfate competitively inhibits CYP1A2 and CYP2C9. There is a potential drug-drug interaction between atazanavir sulfate and CYP1A2 or CYP2C9 substrates). Products include:
EC-Naprosyn Delayed-Release Tablets 2769
Naprosyn Suspension 2769
Naprosyn Tablets 2769
Prevacid NapraPAC 3277

Naproxen Sodium (Atazanavir sulfate competitively inhibits CYP1A2 and CYP2C9. There is a potential drug-drug interaction between atazanavir sulfate and CYP1A2 or CYP2C9 substrates). Products include:
Aleve Tablets, Caplets and Gelcaps 605
Anaprox Tablets 2769
Anaprox DS Tablets 2769

Nateglinide (Atazanavir sulfate competitively inhibits CYP1A2 and CYP2C9. There is a potential drug-drug interaction between atazanavir sulfate and CYP1A2 or CYP2C9 substrates). Products include:
Starlix Tablets 2276

Nefazodone Hydrochloride (Co-administration of atazanavir sulfate and other drugs that inhibit CYP3A may increase atazanavir sulfate plasma concentrations).
No products indexed under this heading.

Nelfinavir Mesylate (Co- administration of atazanavir sulfate/ritonavir and other protease inhibitors would be expected to increase exposure to the other protease inhibitors; co-administration is not recommended). Products include:
Viracept 2556

Nevirapine (Nevirapine, an inducer of CYP3A, is expected to decrease atazanavir sulfate exposure. In the absence of data, co-administration is not recommended). Products include:
Viramune Oral Suspension 903
Viramune Tablets 903

Nicotine Polacrilex (Atazanavir sulfate competitively inhibits CYP1A2 and CYP2C9. There is a potential drug-drug interaction between atazanavir sulfate and CYP1A2 or CYP2C9 substrates). Products include:
Commit Lozenges 1625
Nicorette Gum 1632

Nicotine Salicylate (Atazanavir sulfate competitively inhibits CYP1A2 and CYP2C9. There is a potential drug-drug interaction between atazanavir sulfate and CYP1A2 or CYP2C9 substrates).
No products indexed under this heading.

Nicotine Sulfate (Atazanavir sulfate competitively inhibits CYP1A2 and CYP2C9. There is a potential drug-drug interaction between atazanavir sulfate and CYP1A2 or CYP2C9 substrates).
No products indexed under this heading.

Nifedipine (Co-administration of atazanavir sulfate and other drugs that inhibit CYP3A may increase atazanavir sulfate plasma concentrations). Products include:
Adalat CC Tablets 2978

Nizatidine (Reduced plasma concentrations of atazanavir are expected if H2-receptor antagonists are administered with atazanavir sulfate. This may result in loss of therapeutic effect and development of resistance. To lessen the effect of H2-receptor antagonists on atazanavir exposure, it is recommended that an H2-receptor antagonist and atazanavir sulfate be administered as far apart as possible, preferably 12 hours apart). Products include:
Axid Oral Solution 913

Norethindrone (Because contraceptive steriod concentrations may be altered when atazanavir sulfate or atazanavir sulfate/ritonavir is co-administered with oral contraceptives or with the contraceptive patch, alternate methods of non-hormonal contraception are recommended). Products include:
Ortho Micronor Tablets 2411

Norethindrone Acetate (Atazanavir sulfate competitively inhibits CYP1A2 and CYP2C9. There is a potential drug-drug interaction between atazanavir sulfate and CYP1A2 or CYP2C9 substrates). Products include:
Activella Tablets 2311
Aygestin Tablets 1062
CombiPatch Transdermal System 2180

Norethynodrel (Because contraceptive steriod concentrations may be altered when atazanavir sulfate or atazanavir sulfate/ritonavir is co-administered with oral contraceptives or with the contraceptive patch, alternate methods of non-hormonal contraception are recommended).
No products indexed under this heading.

Norfloxacin (Atazanavir sulfate competitively inhibits CYP1A2 and CYP2C9. There is a potential drug-drug interaction between atazanavir sulfate and CYP1A2 or CYP2C9 substrates). Products include:
Noroxin Tablets 2009

Norgestimate (Because contraceptive steriod concentrations may be altered when atazanavir sulfate or atazanavir sulfate/ritonavir is co-administered with oral contraceptives or with the contraceptive patch, alternate methods of non-hormonal contraception are recommended). Products include:
Ortho-Cyclen/Ortho Tri-Cyclen 2414
Ortho Tri-Cyclen Lo Tablets 2421
Prefest Tablets 1069

Norgestrel (Because contraceptive steriod concentrations may be altered when atazanavir sulfate or atazanavir sulfate/ritonavir is co-administered with oral contraceptives or with the contraceptive patch, alternate methods of non-hormonal contraception are recommended). Products include:
Lo/Ovral-28 Tablets 3423

Nortriptyline Hydrochloride (Atazanavir sulfate competitively inhibits CYP1A2 and CYP2C9. There is a potential drug-drug interaction between atazanavir sulfate and CYP1A2 or CYP2C9 substrates).
No products indexed under this heading.

Ofloxacin (Atazanavir sulfate competitively inhibits CYP1A2 and CYP2C9. There is a potential drug-drug interaction between atazanavir sulfate and CYP1A2 or CYP2C9 substrates). Products include:
Floxin Otic Singles 1045
Floxin Otic Solution 1043

Olanzapine (Atazanavir sulfate competitively inhibits CYP1A2 and CYP2C9. There is a potential drug-drug interaction between atazanavir sulfate and CYP1A2 or CYP2C9 substrates). Products include:
Symbyax Capsules 1788
Zyprexa Tablets 1798
Zyprexa IntraMuscular 1798
Zyprexa ZYDIS Orally Disintegrating Tablets 1798

Omeprazole (Concomitant use of atazanavir sulfate and proton-pump inhibitors is not recommended. Co-administration of atazanavir sulfate with proton-pump inhibitors is expected to substantially decrease atazanavir sulfate plasma concentrations and reduce its therapeutic effect). Products include:
Zegerid Powder for Oral Solution 2972

Ondansetron (Atazanavir sulfate competitively inhibits CYP1A2 and CYP2C9. There is a potential drug-drug interaction between atazanavir sulfate and CYP1A2 or CYP2C9 substrates). Products include:
Zofran ODT Orally Disintegrating Tablets 1613

Ondansetron Hydrochloride (Atazanavir sulfate competitively inhibits CYP1A2 and CYP2C9. There is a potential drug-drug interaction between atazanavir sulfate and CYP1A2 or CYP2C9 substrates). Products include:
Zofran Injection 1607
Zofran 1613

Oxaprozin (Atazanavir sulfate competitively inhibits CYP1A2 and CYP2C9. There is a potential drug-drug interaction between atazanavir sulfate and CYP1A2 or CYP2C9 substrates).
No products indexed under this heading.

Pantoprazole Sodium (Concomitant use of atazanavir sulfate and proton-pump inhibitors is not recommended. Co-administration of atazanavir sulfate with proton-pump inhibitors is expected to substantially decrease atazanavir sulfate plasma concentrations and reduce its therapeutic effect). Products include:
Protonix I.V. 3468
Protonix Tablets 3465

Paroxetine Hydrochloride (Co-administration of atazanavir sulfate and other drugs that inhibit CYP3A may increase atazanavir sulfate plasma concentrations). Products include:
Paxil CR Controlled-Release Tablets 1509
Paxil 1501

Phenobarbital (Drugs that induce CYP3A activity may increase the clearance of atazanavir sulfate, resulting in lowered plasma concentrations).
No products indexed under this heading.

Phenobarbital Sodium (Atazanavir sulfate competitively inhibits CYP1A2 and CYP2C9. There is a potential drug-drug interaction between atazanavir sulfate and CYP1A2 or CYP2C9 substrates).
No products indexed under this heading.

Phenylbutazone (Atazanavir sulfate competitively inhibits CYP1A2 and CYP2C9. There is a potential drug-drug interaction between atazanavir sulfate and CYP1A2 or CYP2C9 substrates).
No products indexed under this heading.

Phenytoin (Drugs that induce CYP3A activity may increase the clearance of atazanavir sulfate, resulting in lowered plasma concentrations).
No products indexed under this heading.

Phenytoin Sodium (Atazanavir sulfate competitively inhibits CYP1A2 and CYP2C9. There is a potential drug-drug interaction between atazanavir sulfate and CYP1A2 or CYP2C9 substrates). Products include:
Phenytek Capsules 2153

Pimozide (Contraindicated due to potential for serious and/or life-threatening reactions, such as cardiac arrhythmias). Products include:
Orap Tablets 1220

Pioglitazone Hydrochloride (Atazanavir sulfate competitively inhibits CYP1A2 and CYP2C9. There is a potential drug-drug interaction between atazanavir sulfate and CYP1A2 or CYP2C9 substrates). Products include:
ActoPlus Met Tablets 3219
Actos Tablets 3224

Piroxicam (Atazanavir sulfate competitively inhibits CYP1A2 and CYP2C9. There is a potential drug-drug interaction between atazanavir sulfate and CYP1A2 or CYP2C9 substrates).
No products indexed under this heading.

Propafenone Hydrochloride (Atazanavir sulfate competitively inhibits CYP1A2 and CYP2C9. There is a potential drug-drug interaction between atazanavir sulfate and CYP1A2 or CYP2C9 substrates). Products include:
Rythmol SR Capsules 2736

Propranolol Hydrochloride (Atazanavir sulfate competitively inhibits CYP1A2 and CYP2C9. There is a potential drug-drug interaction between atazanavir sulfate and CYP1A2 or CYP2C9 substrates). Products include:
Inderal LA Long-Acting Capsules 3421
InnoPran XL Capsules 2728

Protriptyline Hydrochloride (Atazanavir sulfate competitively inhibits CYP1A2 and CYP2C9. There is a potential drug-drug interaction between atazanavir sulfate and CYP1A2 or CYP2C9 substrates). Products include:
Vivactil Tablets 2350

Quinidine (Co-administration with atazanavir sulfate has the potential to produce serious and/or life-threatening adverse events and has not been studied. Caution is warranted and therapeutic concentration monitoring of these drugs is recommended if they are used concomitantly with atazanavir sulfate).
No products indexed under this heading.

Quinidine Gluconate (Co-administration with atazanavir sulfate has the potential to produce serious and/or life-threatening adverse events and has not been studied. Caution is warranted and therapeutic concentration monitoring of these drugs is recommended if they are used concomitantly with atazanavir sulfate).
No products indexed under this heading.

Quinidine Hydrochloride (Co-administration with atazanavir sulfate has the potential to produce serious and/or life-threatening adverse events and has not been studied. Concentration monitoring of these drugs is recommended if they are used concomitantly with atazanavir sulfate).
No products indexed under this heading.

Quinidine Polygalacturonate (Co-administration with atazanavir sulfate has the potential to produce serious and/or life-threatening adverse events and has not been studied. Caution is warranted and therapeutic concentration monitoring of these drugs is recommended if they are used concomitantly with atazanavir sulfate).
No products indexed under this heading.

Quinidine Sulfate (Co-administration with atazanavir sulfate has the potential to produce serious and/or life-threatening adverse events and has not been studied. Caution is warranted and therapeutic concentration monitoring of these drugs is recommended if they are used concomitantly with atazanavir sulfate).
No products indexed under this heading.

Quinine (Co-administration of atazanavir sulfate and other drugs that inhibit CYP3A may increase atazanavir sulfate plasma concentrations).
No products indexed under this heading.

Quinine Sulfate (Co-administration of atazanavir sulfate and other drugs that inhibit CYP3A may increase atazanavir sulfate plasma concentrations).
No products indexed under this heading.

Rabeprazole Sodium (Concomitant use of atazanavir sulfate and proton-pump inhibitors is not recommended. Co-administration of atazanavir sulfate with proton-pump inhibitors is expected to substantially decrease atazanavir sulfate plasma concentrations and reduce its therapeutic effect). Products include:
Aciphex Tablets 1081

Ranitidine Bismuth Citrate (Reduced plasma concentrations of atazanavir are expected if H2-receptor antagonists are administered with atazanavir sulfate. This may result in loss of therapeutic effect and development of resistance. To lessen the effect of H2-receptor antagonists on atazanavir exposure, it is recommended that an H2-receptor antagonist and atazanavir sulfate be administered as far apart as possible, preferably 12 hours apart).
No products indexed under this heading.

Ranitidine Hydrochloride (Reduced plasma concentrations of atazanavir are expected if H2-receptor antagonists are administered with atazanavir sulfate. This may result in loss of therapeutic effect and development of resistance. To lessen the effect of H2-receptor antagonists on atazanavir exposure, it is recommended that an H2-receptor antagonist and atazanavir sulfate be administered as far apart as possible, preferably 12 hours apart). Products include:
Zantac 1597
Zantac Injection 1593
Zantac 75 Tablets .... ▣715
Zantac 150 Maximum Strength Tablets .... ▣715
Zantac Injection Pharmacy Bulk Package 1595

Repaglinide (Atazanavir sulfate competitively inhibits CYP1A2 and CYP2C9. There is a potential drug-drug interaction between atazanavir sulfate and CYP1A2 or CYP2C9 substrates). Products include:
Prandin Tablets (0.5, 1, and 2 mg) 2337

Rifabutin (A rifabutin dose reduction of up to 75% (e.g., 150mg every other day or three times a week) is recommended).
No products indexed under this heading.

Rifampicin (Drugs that induce CYP3A activity may increase the clearance of atazanavir sulfate, resulting in lowered plasma concentrations).
No products indexed under this heading.

Rifampin (Co-administration of atazanavir sulfate and drugs that induce CYP3A, such as rifampin, may decrease atazanavir plasma concentrations and reduce its therapeutic effect. Rifampin decreases plasma concentrations and AUC of most protease inhibitors by about 90%. This may result in loss of theraputic effect and development of resistance).
No products indexed under this heading.

Rifapentine (Drugs that induce CYP3A activity may increase the clearance of atazanavir sulfate, resulting in lowered plasma concentrations).
No products indexed under this heading.

Riluzole (Atazanavir sulfate competitively inhibits CYP1A2 and CYP2C9. There is a potential drug-drug interaction between atazanavir sulfate and CYP1A2 or CYP2C9 substrates). Products include:
Rilutek Tablets 2945

Ritonavir (If atazanavir sulfate is co-administered with ritonavir, it is recommended that atazanavir sulfate 300 mg once daily be given with ritonavir 100 mg once daily with food). Products include:
Kaletra 474
Norvir 499

Rofecoxib (Atazanavir sulfate competitively inhibits CYP1A2 and CYP2C9. There is a potential drug-drug interaction between atazanavir sulfate and CYP1A2 or CYP2C9 substrates).
No products indexed under this heading.

Ropinirole Hydrochloride (Atazanavir sulfate competitively inhibits CYP1A2 and CYP2C9. There is a potential drug-drug interaction between atazanavir sulfate and CYP1A2 or CYP2C9 substrates). Products include:
Requip Tablets 1528

Ropivacaine Hydrochloride (Atazanavir sulfate competitively inhibits CYP1A2 and CYP2C9. There is a potential drug-drug interaction between atazanavir sulfate and CYP1A2 or CYP2C9 substrates). Products include:
Naropin Injection 640

Rosiglitazone Maleate (Atazanavir sulfate competitively inhibits CYP1A2 and CYP2C9. There is a potential drug-drug interaction between atazanavir sulfate and CYP1A2 or CYP2C9 substrates). Products include:
Avandamet Tablets 1343
Avandia Tablets 1348

Saquinavir (Saquinavir 1200 mg co-administered with atazanavir sulfate 400 mg and tenofovir 300 mg (all given once daily) plus nucleoside analogue reverse transcriptase inhibitors did not provide adequate efficacy).
No products indexed under this heading.

Saquinavir Mesylate (Saquinavir 1200 mg co-administered with atazanavir sulfate 400 mg and tenofovir 300 mg (all given once daily) plus nucleoside analogue reverse transcriptase inhibitors did not provide adequate efficacy). Products include:
Invirase 2776

Sertraline Hydrochloride (Co-administration of atazanavir sulfate and other drugs that inhibit CYP3A may increase atazanavir sulfate plasma concentrations). Products include:
Zoloft 2581

Sildenafil Citrate (Co-administration may result in an increase in PDE5 inhibitor-associated adverse events, including hypertension, visual changes, and priapism. Use sildenafil with caution at reduced doses of 25 mg every 48 hours with increased monitoring for adverse events). Products include:
Revatio Tablets 2541
Viagra Tablets 2552

Simvastatin (Concomitant use of atazanavir sulfate with simvastatin is not recommended. Caution should be exercised if HIV protease inhibitors, including atazanavir sulfate, are used concurrently with other HMG-CoA reductase inhibitors that are also metabolized by the CYP3A4 pathway. The risk of myopathy, including rhabdomyolysis, may be increased when HIV protease inhibitors, including atazanavir sulfate, are used in combination with these drugs). Products include:
Vytorin 10/10 Tablets 2084
Vytorin 10/10 Tablets 3092
Vytorin 10/20 Tablets 2084
Vytorin 10/20 Tablets 3092
Vytorin 10/40 Tablets 3092
Vytorin 10/40 Tablets 2084
Vytorin 10/80 Tablets 2084
Vytorin 10/80 Tablets 3092
Zocor Tablets 2078

Sirolimus (Therapeutic concentration monitoring is recommended for immunosuppressant agents when co-administered with atazanavir sulfate). Products include:
Rapamune Oral Solution and Tablets 3472

Sodium Bicarbonate (Reduced plasma concentrations of atazanavir are expected if antacids, including buffered medications, are administered with atazanavir sulfate. Atazanavir sulfate should be administered 2 hours before or 1 hour after these medications). Products include:
Ceo-Two Evacuant Suppository 607
Colyte with Flavor Packs for Oral Solution 3102
HalfLytely and Bisacodyl Tablets Bowel Prep Kit with Flavors Packs 915
TriLyte with Flavor Packs for Oral Solution 3114

Sulfamethoxazole (Atazanavir sulfate competitively inhibits CYP1A2 and CYP2C9. There is a potential drug-drug interaction between atazanavir sulfate and CYP1A2 or CYP2C9 substrates).
No products indexed under this heading.

Sulindac (Atazanavir sulfate competitively inhibits CYP1A2 and CYP2C9. There is a potential drug-drug interaction between atazanavir sulfate and CYP1A2 or CYP2C9 substrates). Products include:
Clinoril Tablets 1899

Suprofen (Atazanavir sulfate competitively inhibits CYP1A2 and CYP2C9. There is a potential drug-drug interaction between atazanavir sulfate and CYP1A2 or CYP2C9 substrates).
No products indexed under this heading.

Tacrine Hydrochloride (Atazanavir sulfate competitively inhibits CYP1A2 and CYP2C9. There is a potential drug-drug interaction between atazanavir sulfate and CYP1A2 or CYP2C9 substrates).
No products indexed under this heading.

Tacrolimus (Therapeutic concentration monitoring is recommended for immunosuppressant agents when co-administered with atazanavir sulfate). Products include:
Prograf Capsules and Injection 624
Protopic Ointment 629

Tadalafil (Co-administration may result in an increase in PDE5 inhibitor-associated adverse events, including hypertension, visual changes, and priapism. Use tadalafil with caution at reduced doses of 10 mg every 72 hours with increased monitoring of adverse events). Products include:
Cialis Tablets 1806

Tamoxifen Citrate (Atazanavir sulfate competitively inhibits CYP1A2 and CYP2C9. There is a potential drug-drug interaction between atazanavir sulfate and CYP1A2 or CYP2C9 substrates).
No products indexed under this heading.

Telmisartan (Atazanavir sulfate competitively inhibits CYP1A2 and CYP2C9. There is a potential drug-drug interaction between atazanavir sulfate and CYP1A2 or CYP2C9 substrates). Products include:
Micardis Tablets 884
Micardis HCT Tablets 886

Tenofovir Disoproxil Fumarate (Tenofovir may decrease the AUC and Cmin of atazanavir sulfate, while atazanavir sulfate increases tenofovir concentrations. It is recommended to administer tenofovir 300 mg with atazanavir sulfate 300 mg and ritonavir 100 mg as a single dose). Products include:
Truvada Tablets 1279
Viread Tablets 1284

Theophylline (Atazanavir sulfate competitively inhibits CYP1A2 and CYP2C9. There is a potential drug-drug interaction between atazanavir sulfate and CYP1A2 or CYP2C9 substrates).
No products indexed under this heading.

Theophylline Anhydrous (Atazanavir sulfate competitively inhibits CYP1A2 and CYP2C9. There is a potential drug-drug interaction between atazanavir sulfate and CYP1A2 or CYP2C9 substrates). Products include:
Uniphyl Tablets 2708

Tolazamide (Atazanavir sulfate competitively inhibits CYP1A2 and CYP2C9. There is a potential drug-drug interaction between atazanavir sulfate and CYP1A2 or CYP2C9 substrates).
No products indexed under this heading.

Tolbutamide (Atazanavir sulfate competitively inhibits CYP1A2 and CYP2C9. There is a potential drug-drug interaction between atazanavir sulfate and CYP1A2 or CYP2C9 substrates).
No products indexed under this heading.

Tolbutamide Sodium (Atazanavir sulfate competitively inhibits CYP1A2 and CYP2C9. There is a potential drug-drug interaction between atazanavir sulfate and CYP1A2 or CYP2C9 substrates).
No products indexed under this heading.

Tolmetin Sodium (Atazanavir sulfate competitively inhibits CYP1A2 and CYP2C9. There is a potential drug-drug interaction between atazanavir sulfate and CYP1A2 or CYP2C9 substrates).
No products indexed under this heading.

Torsemide (Atazanavir sulfate competitively inhibits CYP1A2 and CYP2C9. There is a potential drug-drug interaction between atazanavir sulfate and CYP1A2 or CYP2C9 substrates).
No products indexed under this heading.

Trazodone Hydrochloride (Concomitant use will increase plasma concentration of trazodone).
No products indexed under this heading.

Triazolam (Contraindicated due to potential for serious and/or life-threatening events, such as prolonged or increased sedation or respiratory depression).
No products indexed under this heading.

Trimethaphan Camsylate (Atazanavir sulfate competitively inhibits CYP1A2 and CYP2C9. There is a potential drug-drug interaction between atazanavir sulfate and CYP1A2 or CYP2C9 substrates).
No products indexed under this heading.

Trimipramine Maleate (Atazanavir sulfate competitively inhibits CYP1A2 and CYP2C9. There is a potential drug-drug interaction between atazanavir sulfate and CYP1A2 or CYP2C9 substrates). Products include:
Surmontil Capsules 2347

Troglitazone (Atazanavir sulfate competitively inhibits CYP1A2 and CYP2C9. There is a potential drug-drug interaction between atazanavir sulfate and CYP1A2 or CYP2C9 substrates).
No products indexed under this heading.

Troleandomycin (Co-administration of atazanavir sulfate and other drugs that inhibit CYP3A may increase atazanavir sulfate plasma concentrations).
No products indexed under this heading.

Trovafloxacin Mesylate (Atazanavir sulfate competitively inhibits CYP1A2 and CYP2C9. There is a potential drug-drug interaction between atazanavir sulfate and CYP1A2 or CYP2C9 substrates).
No products indexed under this heading.

Valdecoxib (Atazanavir sulfate competitively inhibits CYP1A2 and CYP2C9. There is a potential drug-drug interaction between atazanavir sulfate and CYP1A2 or CYP2C9 substrates).
No products indexed under this heading.

Valsartan (Atazanavir sulfate competitively inhibits CYP1A2 and CYP2C9. There is a potential drug-drug interaction between atazanavir sulfate and CYP1A2 or CYP2C9 substrates). Products include:
Diovan HCT Tablets 2195
Diovan Tablets 2191

Vardenafil Hydrochloride (Co-administration may result in an increase in PDE5 inhibitor-associated adverse events, including hypertension, visual changes, and priapism. Use vardenafil with caution at reduced doses of no more than 2.5 mg every 72 hours with increased monitoring of adverse events). Products include:
Levitra Tablets 3048

Venlafaxine Hydrochloride (Co-administration of atazanavir sulfate and other drugs that inhibit CYP3A may increase atazanavir sulfate plasma concentrations). Products include:
Effexor Tablets 3405
Effexor XR Capsules 3411

Verapamil Hydrochloride (Atazanavir sulfate competitively inhibits CYP1A2 and CYP2C9. There is a potential drug-drug interaction between atazanavir sulfate and CYP1A2 or CYP2C9 substrates). Products include:
Covera-HS Tablets 3135
Tarka Tablets 519
Verelan PM Capsules 3120

Voriconazole (Voriconazole with ritonavir 400 mg every 12 hours decreased voriconazole steady state AUC by 82%; therefore, voriconazole should not be co-administered with atazanavir sulfate/ritonavir. Co-administration of voriconazole with atazanavir sulfate (without ritonavir) may increase atazanavir sulfate concentrations; however, no data are available). Products include:
VFEND I.V. 2543
VFEND Oral Suspension 2543
VFEND Tablets 2543

Warfarin Sodium (Atazanavir sulfate competitively inhibits CYP1A2 and CYP2C9. There is a potential drug-drug interaction between atazanavir sulfate and CYP1A2 or CYP2C9 substrates). Products include:
Coumadin for Injection 932
Coumadin Tablets 932

Zafirlukast (Atazanavir sulfate competitively inhibits CYP1A2 and CYP2C9. There is a potential drug-drug interaction between atazanavir sulfate and CYP1A2 or CYP2C9 substrates). Products include:
Accolate Tablets 663

Zileuton (Atazanavir sulfate competitively inhibits CYP1A2 and CYP2C9. There is a potential drug-drug interaction between atazanavir sulfate and CYP1A2 or CYP2C9 substrates).
No products indexed under this heading.

Zolmitriptan (Atazanavir sulfate competitively inhibits CYP1A2 and CYP2C9. There is a potential drug-drug interaction between atazanavir sulfate and CYP1A2 or CYP2C9 substrates). Products include:
Zomig Nasal Spray 718
Zomig Tablets 714
Zomig-ZMT Tablets 714

Food Interactions

Grapefruit (Co-administration of atazanavir sulfate and other drugs that inhibit CYP3A may increase atazanavir sulfate plasma concentrations).

R-GENE 10 FOR INTRAVENOUS USE

(Arginine Hydrochloride) 2647
None cited in PDR database.

RHINOCORT AQUA NASAL SPRAY

(Budesonide) 658
May interact with cytochrome p450 3a4 inhibitors (selected) and certain other agents. Compounds in these categories include:

Acetazolamide (Co-administration with inhibitors of CYP4503A4 may inhibit the metabolism of, and increase the systemic exposure to budesonide).
No products indexed under this heading.

Amiodarone Hydrochloride (Co-administration with inhibitors of CYP4503A4 may inhibit the metabolism of, and increase the systemic exposure to budesonide). Products include:
Pacerone Tablets 3337

Amprenavir (Co-administration with inhibitors of CYP4503A4 may inhibit the metabolism of, and increase the systemic exposure to budesonide). Products include:
Agenerase Capsules 1299
Agenerase Oral Solution 1304

Anastrozole (Co-administration with inhibitors of CYP4503A4 may inhibit the metabolism of, and increase the systemic exposure to budesonide). Products include:
Arimidex Tablets 665

Aprepitant (Co-administration with inhibitors of CYP4503A4 may inhibit the metabolism of, and increase the systemic exposure to budesonide). Products include:
Emend Capsules 1944

Cimetidine (Co-administration with inhibitors of CYP4501A2, such as cimetidine, caused a slight decrease in budesonide clearance and corresponding increase in its oral bioavailability). Products include:
Tagamet HB 200 Tablets .... ■637
Tagamet Tablets 1547

Cimetidine Hydrochloride (Co-administration with inhibitors of CYP4501A2, such as cimetidine, caused a slight decrease in budesonide clearance and corresponding increase in its oral bioavailability).
No products indexed under this heading.

Ciprofloxacin (Co-administration with inhibitors of CYP4503A4 may inhibit the metabolism of, and increase the systemic exposure to budesonide). Products include:
Cipro I.V. 2998
Cipro I.V. Pharmacy Bulk Package 3509
Cipro Oral Suspension 2991
Cipro XR Tablets 3004
Ciprodex Otic Suspension 555

Clarithromycin (Co-administration with inhibitors of CYP4503A4 may inhibit the metabolism of, and increase the systemic exposure to budesonide). Products include:
Biaxin/Biaxin XL 402
PREVPAC 3281

Clotrimazole (Co-administration with inhibitors of CYP4503A4 may inhibit the metabolism of, and increase the systemic exposure to budesonide). Products include:
Lotrimin 3053
Lotrisone 3054

Cyclosporine (Co-administration with inhibitors of CYP4503A4 may inhibit the metabolism of, and increase the systemic exposure to budesonide). Products include:
Gengraf Capsules 458
Neoral Soft Gelatin Capsules 2247
Neoral Oral Solution 2247
Restasis Ophthalmic Emulsion 570
Sandimmune 2259

Dalfopristin (Co-administration with inhibitors of CYP4503A4 may inhibit the metabolism of, and increase the systemic exposure to budesonide). Products include:
Synercid I.V. 1690

Danazol (Co-administration with inhibitors of CYP4503A4 may inhibit the metabolism of, and increase the systemic exposure to budesonide).
No products indexed under this heading.

Delavirdine Mesylate (Co-administration with inhibitors of CYP4503A4 may inhibit the metabolism of, and increase the systemic exposure to budesonide). Products include:
Rescriptor Tablets 2535

Diltiazem Hydrochloride (Co-administration with inhibitors of CYP4503A4 may inhibit the metabolism of, and increase the systemic exposure to budesonide). Products include:
Cardizem LA Extended Release Tablets 1699
Tiazac Capsules 1204

Diltiazem Maleate (Co-administration with inhibitors of CYP4503A4 may inhibit the metabolism of, and increase the systemic exposure to budesonide).
No products indexed under this heading.

Efavirenz (Co-administration with inhibitors of CYP4503A4 may inhibit the metabolism of, and increase the systemic exposure to budesonide). Products include:
Sustiva Capsules 957

Erythromycin (Co-administration with inhibitors of CYP4503A4 may inhibit the metabolism of, and increase the systemic exposure to budesonide). Products include:
Erygel Topical Gel 2096
Ery-Tab Tablets 447
Erythromycin Base Filmtab Tablets 454
Erythromycin Delayed-Release Capsules, USP 456
PCE Dispertab Tablets 510

Erythromycin Estolate (Co-administration with inhibitors of CYP4503A4 may inhibit the metabolism of, and increase the systemic exposure to budesonide).
No products indexed under this heading.

Erythromycin Ethylsuccinate (Co-administration with inhibitors of CYP4503A4 may inhibit the metabolism of, and increase the systemic exposure to budesonide). Products include:
E.E.S. 449
EryPed 445

Erythromycin Gluceptate (Co-administration with inhibitors of CYP4503A4 may inhibit the metabolism of, and increase the systemic exposure to budesonide).
No products indexed under this heading.

Erythromycin Lactobionate (Co-administration with inhibitors of CYP4503A4 may inhibit the metabolism of, and increase the systemic exposure to budesonide).
No products indexed under this heading.

Erythromycin Stearate (Co-administration with inhibitors of CYP4503A4 may inhibit the metabolism of, and increase the systemic exposure to budesonide). Products include:
Erythrocin Stearate Filmtab Tablets 452

Esomeprazole Magnesium (Co-administration with inhibitors of CYP4503A4 may inhibit the metabolism of, and increase the systemic exposure to budesonide). Products include:
Nexium Delayed-Release Capsules 645

Fluconazole (Co-administration with inhibitors of CYP4503A4 may inhibit the metabolism of, and increase the systemic exposure to budesonide).
No products indexed under this heading.

Fluoxetine Hydrochloride (Co-administration with inhibitors of CYP4503A4 may inhibit the metabolism of, and increase the systemic exposure to budesonide). Products include:
Prozac Pulvules and Liquid 1771
Symbyax Capsules 1788

Fluvoxamine Maleate (Co-administration with inhibitors of CYP4503A4 may inhibit the metabolism of, and increase the systemic exposure to budesonide).
No products indexed under this heading.

Fosamprenavir Calcium (Co-administration with inhibitors of CYP4503A4 may inhibit the metabolism of, and increase the systemic exposure to budesonide). Products include:
Lexiva Tablets 1473

Indinavir Sulfate (Co-administration with inhibitors of CYP4503A4 may inhibit the metabolism of, and increase the systemic exposure to budesonide). Products include:
Crixivan Capsules 1918

Isoniazid (Co-administration with inhibitors of CYP4503A4 may inhibit the metabolism of, and increase the systemic exposure to budesonide).
No products indexed under this heading.

Itraconazole (Co-administration with inhibitors of CYP4503A4 may inhibit the metabolism of, and increase the systemic exposure to budesonide).
No products indexed under this heading.

Ketoconazole (The main route of metabolism of budesonide is via CYP4503A4; co-administration with a potent inhibitor of CYP4503A4, such as ketoconazole, has resulted in increased plasma concentration of orally administered budesonide). Products include:
Nizoral A-D Shampoo, 1% 1839
Nizoral 2% Shampoo 1838

Lopinavir (Co-administration with inhibitors of CYP4503A4 may inhibit the metabolism of, and increase the systemic exposure to budesonide). Products include:
Kaletra 474

Loratadine (Co-administration with inhibitors of CYP4503A4 may inhibit the metabolism of, and increase the systemic exposure to budesonide). Products include:
Alavert Allergy & Sinus D-12 Hour Tablets .... ■743
Alavert .... ■743
Children's Claritin 24 Hour Non-Drowsy Allergy Syrup .... ■732
Claritin Non-Drowsy 24 Hour Tablets .... ■731
Non-Drowsy Claritin Hives Relief Tablets .... ■733
Claritin Reditabs 24 Hour Non-Drowsy Tablets .... ■732
Claritin-D Non-Drowsy 12 Hour Tablets .... ■731
Claritin-D Non-Drowsy 24 Hour Tablets .... ■731
Children's Dimetapp ND Non-Drowsy Allergy Syrup .... ■746
Triaminic Allerchews .... ■684

Metronidazole (Co-administration with inhibitors of CYP4503A4 may inhibit the metabolism of, and increase the systemic exposure to budesonide). Products include:
Metrogel 1% 1212
MetroGel-Vaginal Gel 1822
Noritate Cream, 1% 1051

Metronidazole Benzoate (Co-administration with inhibitors of CYP4503A4 may inhibit the metabolism of, and increase the systemic exposure to budesonide).
No products indexed under this heading.

Metronidazole Hydrochloride (Co-administration with inhibitors of CYP4503A4 may inhibit the metabolism of, and increase the systemic exposure to budesonide).
No products indexed under this heading.

Miconazole (Co-administration with inhibitors of CYP4503A4 may inhibit the metabolism of, and increase the systemic exposure to budesonide).
No products indexed under this heading.

Miconazole Nitrate (Co-administration with inhibitors of CYP4503A4 may inhibit the metabolism of, and increase the systemic exposure to budesonide). Products include:
Desenex .... ■674
Desenex Jock Itch Spray Powder .... ■674

Nefazodone Hydrochloride (Co-administration with inhibitors of CYP4503A4 may inhibit the metabolism of, and increase the systemic exposure to budesonide).
No products indexed under this heading.

Nelfinavir Mesylate (Co-administration with inhibitors of CYP4503A4 may inhibit the metabolism of, and increase the systemic exposure to budesonide). Products include:
Viracept 2556

Nevirapine (Co-administration with inhibitors of CYP4503A4 may inhibit the metabolism of, and increase the systemic exposure to budesonide). Products include:
Viramune Oral Suspension 903
Viramune Tablets 903

Niacinamide (Co-administration with inhibitors of CYP4503A4 may inhibit the metabolism of, and increase the systemic exposure to budesonide).
No products indexed under this heading.

Nicotinamide (Co-administration with inhibitors of CYP4503A4 may inhibit the metabolism of, and increase the systemic exposure to budesonide). Products include:
Nicomide Tablets 3190

Nifedipine (Co-administration with inhibitors of CYP4503A4 may inhibit the metabolism of, and increase the systemic exposure to budesonide). Products include:
Adalat CC Tablets 2978

Norfloxacin (Co-administration with inhibitors of CYP4503A4 may inhibit the metabolism of, and increase the systemic exposure to budesonide). Products include:
Noroxin Tablets 2009

Omeprazole (Co-administration with inhibitors of CYP4503A4 may inhibit the metabolism of, and increase the systemic exposure to budesonide). Products include:
Zegerid Powder for Oral Solution 2972

Paroxetine Hydrochloride (Co-administration with inhibitors of CYP4503A4 may inhibit the metabolism of, and increase the systemic exposure to budesonide). Products include:
Paxil CR Controlled-Release Tablets 1509
Paxil 1501

Propoxyphene Hydrochloride (Co-administration with inhibitors of CYP4503A4 may inhibit the metabolism of, and increase the systemic exposure to budesonide).
No products indexed under this heading.

Propoxyphene Napsylate (Co-administration with inhibitors of CYP4503A4 may inhibit the metabolism of, and increase the systemic exposure to budesonide). Products include:
Darvocet A 500 Tablets 3497

Quinidine (Co-administration with inhibitors of CYP4503A4 may inhibit the metabolism of, and increase the systemic exposure to budesonide).
No products indexed under this heading.

Quinidine Hydrochloride (Co-administration with inhibitors of CYP4503A4 may inhibit the metabolism of, and increase the systemic exposure to budesonide).
No products indexed under this heading.

Quinidine Polygalacturonate (Co-administration with inhibitors of CYP4503A4 may inhibit the metabolism of, and increase the systemic exposure to budesonide).
No products indexed under this heading.

Quinidine Sulfate (Co-administration with inhibitors of CYP4503A4 may inhibit the metabolism of, and increase the systemic exposure to budesonide).
No products indexed under this heading.

Quinine (Co-administration with inhibitors of CYP4503A4 may inhibit the metabolism of, and increase the systemic exposure to budesonide).
No products indexed under this heading.

Quinine Sulfate (Co-administration with inhibitors of CYP4503A4 may inhibit the metabolism of, and increase the systemic exposure to budesonide).
No products indexed under this heading.

Quinupristin (Co-administration with inhibitors of CYP4503A4 may inhibit the metabolism of, and increase the systemic exposure to budesonide). Products include:
Synercid I.V. 1690

Ranitidine Bismuth Citrate (Co-administration with inhibitors of CYP4503A4 may inhibit the metabolism of, and increase the systemic exposure to budesonide).
No products indexed under this heading.

Ranitidine Hydrochloride (Co-administration with inhibitors of CYP4503A4 may inhibit the metabolism of, and increase the systemic exposure to budesonide). Products include:
Zantac 1597
Zantac Injection 1593
Zantac 75 Tablets 715
Zantac 150 Maximum Strength Tablets 715
Zantac Injection Pharmacy Bulk Package 1595

Ritonavir (Co-administration with inhibitors of CYP4503A4 may inhibit the metabolism of, and increase the systemic exposure to budesonide). Products include:
Kaletra 474
Norvir 499

Saquinavir (Co-administration with inhibitors of CYP4503A4 may inhibit the metabolism of, and increase the systemic exposure to budesonide).
No products indexed under this heading.

Saquinavir Mesylate (Co-administration with inhibitors of CYP4503A4 may inhibit the metabolism of, and increase the systemic exposure to budesonide). Products include:
Invirase 2776

Sertraline Hydrochloride (Co-administration with inhibitors of CYP4503A4 may inhibit the metabolism of, and increase the systemic exposure to budesonide). Products include:
Zoloft 2581

Telithromycin (Co-administration with inhibitors of CYP4503A4 may inhibit the metabolism of, and increase the systemic exposure to budesonide). Products include:
Ketek Tablets 2920

Troglitazone (Co-administration with inhibitors of CYP4503A4 may inhibit the metabolism of, and increase the systemic exposure to budesonide).
No products indexed under this heading.

Troleandomycin (Co-administration with inhibitors of CYP4503A4 may inhibit the metabolism of, and increase the systemic exposure to budesonide).
No products indexed under this heading.

Valproate Sodium (Co-administration with inhibitors of CYP4503A4 may inhibit the metabolism of, and increase the systemic exposure to budesonide). Products include:
Depacon Injection 412

Verapamil Hydrochloride (Co-administration with inhibitors of CYP4503A4 may inhibit the metabolism of, and increase the systemic exposure to budesonide). Products include:
Covera-HS Tablets 3135
Tarka Tablets 519
Verelan PM Capsules 3120

Voriconazole (Co-administration with inhibitors of CYP4503A4 may inhibit the metabolism of, and increase the systemic exposure to budesonide). Products include:
VFEND I.V. 2543
VFEND Oral Suspension 2543
VFEND Tablets 2543

Zafirlukast (Co-administration with inhibitors of CYP4503A4 may inhibit the metabolism of, and increase the systemic exposure to budesonide). Products include:
Accolate Tablets 663

Zileuton (Co-administration with inhibitors of CYP4503A4 may inhibit the metabolism of, and increase the systemic exposure to budesonide).
No products indexed under this heading.

Food Interactions

Grapefruit (Co-administration with inhibitors of CYP4503A4 may inhibit the metabolism of, and increase the systemic exposure to budesonide).

Grapefruit Juice (Co-administration with inhibitors of CYP4503A4 may inhibit the metabolism of, and increase the systemic exposure to budesonide).

RHOGAM ULTRA-FILTERED

(Rh_o (D) Immune Globulin (Human)) 2429
None cited in PDR database.

RHOPHYLAC

(Rh_o (D) Immune Globulin (Human)) 3504
May interact with:

Measles, Mumps & Rubella Virus Vaccine, Live (Active immunization with live virus vaccines should be postponed until 3 months after the last administration of immunoglobin, as the efficacy of the vaccine may be impaired). Products include:
M-M-R II 1980

Measles & Rubella Virus Vaccine Live (Active immunization with live virus vaccines should be postponed until 3 months after the last administration of immunoglobin, as the efficacy of the vaccine may be impaired).
No products indexed under this heading.

Measles Virus Vaccine Live (Active immunization with live virus vaccines should be postponed until 3 months after the last administration of immunoglobin, as the efficacy of the vaccine may be impaired). Products include:
Attenuvax 1889

Mumps Virus Vaccine, Live (Active immunization with live virus vaccines should be postponed until 3 months after the last administration of immunoglobin, as the efficacy of the vaccine may be impaired). Products include:
Mumpsvax 2005

Rubella & Mumps Virus Vaccine Live (Active immunization with live virus vaccines should be postponed until 3 months after the last administration of immunoglobin, as the efficacy of the vaccine may be impaired).
No products indexed under this heading.

Rubella Virus Vaccine Live (Active immunization with live virus vaccines should be postponed until 3 months after the last administration of immunoglobin, as the efficacy of the vaccine may be impaired). Products include:
Meruvax II 1994

Varicella Virus Vaccine Live (Active immunization with live virus vaccines should be postponed until 3 months after the last administration of immunoglobin, as the efficacy of the vaccine may be impaired). Products include:
Varivax 2070

RIBAVIRIN, USP CAPSULES

(Ribavirin) 3083
May interact with:

Didanosine (Exposure to didanosine or its active metabolite (dideoxyadenosine 5' - triphosphate) is increased when didanosine is co-administered with ribavirin, which could cause or worsen clinical toxicities. Co-administration of ribavirin and didanosine is not recommended).
No products indexed under this heading.

Stavudine (Ribavirin has been shown in vitro to inhibit phosphorylation of zidovudine and stavudine which could lead to decreased antiretroviral activity. Therefore, concomitant use of ribavirin with either of these drugs should be used with caution). Products include:
Zerit 971

Zidovudine (Ribavirin has been shown in vitro to inhibit phosphorylation of zidovudine and stavudine which could lead to decreased antiretroviral activity. Therefore, concomitant use of ribavirin with either of these drugs should be used with caution). Products include:
Combivir Tablets 1373
Retrovir 1533
Retrovir IV Infusion 1537
Trizivir Tablets 1565

RILUTEK TABLETS

(Riluzole) 2945

May interact with quinolones, xanthines, and certain other agents. Compounds in these categories include:

Alatrofloxacin Mesylate (Potential inhibitors of CYP1A2, such as quinolones, could decrease the rate of riluzole elimination).
No products indexed under this heading.

Allopurinol (Riluzole induces hepatic injury; ALS patients on concomitant hepatotoxic drugs, such as allopurinol, were excluded in the clinical trials; if such combination is used, practitioner should exercise caution).
No products indexed under this heading.

Aminophylline (Potential inhibitors of CYP1A2, such as theophylline, could decrease the rate of riluzole elimination).
No products indexed under this heading.

Amitriptyline Hydrochloride (Potential inhibitors of CYP1A2, such as amitriptyline, could decrease the rate of riluzole elimination).
No products indexed under this heading.

Caffeine (Potential inhibitors of CYP1A2, such as caffeine, could decrease the rate of riluzole elimination). Products include:
- Athena Hair System Shampoo .... ▣767
- BC Powder .... ▣612
- Arthritis Strength BC Powder .... ▣612
- Goody's Extra Strength Headache Powder .... ▣621
- Goody's Extra Strength Pain Relief Tablets .... ▣621
- Hycomine Compound Tablets 1105
- Spartan Hair System Shampoo .... ▣767
- Vivarin .... ▣639

Ciprofloxacin (Potential inhibitors of CYP1A2, such as quinolones, could decrease the rate of riluzole elimination). Products include:
- Cipro I.V. 2998
- Cipro I.V. Pharmacy Bulk Package 3509
- Cipro Oral Suspension 2991
- Cipro XR Tablets 3004
- Ciprodex Otic Suspension 555

Ciprofloxacin Hydrochloride (Potential inhibitors of CYP1A2, such as quinolones, could decrease the rate of riluzole elimination). Products include:
- Ciloxan Ophthalmic Ointment 554
- Cipro Tablets 2991

Dyphylline (Potential inhibitors of CYP1A2, such as theophylline, could decrease the rate of riluzole elimination).
No products indexed under this heading.

Enoxacin (Potential inhibitors of CYP1A2, such as quinolones, could decrease the rate of riluzole elimination).
No products indexed under this heading.

Grepafloxacin Hydrochloride (Potential inhibitors of CYP1A2, such as quinolones, could decrease the rate of riluzole elimination).
No products indexed under this heading.

Lomefloxacin Hydrochloride (Potential inhibitors of CYP1A2, such as quinolones, could decrease the rate of riluzole elimination).
No products indexed under this heading.

Methyldopa (Riluzole induces hepatic injury; ALS patients on concomitant hepatotoxic drugs, such as methyldopa, were excluded in the clinical trials; if such combination is used, practitioner should exercise caution). Products include:
- Aldoclor Tablets 1881
- Aldoril Tablets 1884

Moxifloxacin Hydrochloride (Potential inhibitors of CYP1A2, such as quinolones, could decrease the rate of riluzole elimination). Products include:
- Avelox 2984
- Vigamox Ophthalmic Solution 560

Norfloxacin (Potential inhibitors of CYP1A2, such as quinolones, could decrease the rate of riluzole elimination). Products include:
- Noroxin Tablets 2009

Ofloxacin (Potential inhibitors of CYP1A2, such as quinolones, could decrease the rate of riluzole elimination). Products include:
- Floxin Otic Singles 1045
- Floxin Otic Solution 1043

Omeprazole (Potential inducers of CYP1A2, such as theophylline, could increase the rate of riluzole elimination). Products include:
- Zegerid Powder for Oral Solution 2972

Phenacetin (Potential inhibitors of CYP1A2, such as phenacetin, could decrease the rate of riluzole elimination).
No products indexed under this heading.

Rifampin (Potential inducers of CYP1A2, such as theophylline, could increase the rate of riluzole elimination).
No products indexed under this heading.

Sulfasalazine (Riluzole induces hepatic injury; ALS patients on concomitant hepatotoxic drugs, such as sulfasalazine, were excluded in the clinical trials; if such combination is used, practitioner should exercise caution).
No products indexed under this heading.

Tacrine Hydrochloride (CYP1A2 is the principal isoenzyme involved in the initial oxidative metabolism of riluzole; potential interaction may occur when co-administered with other agents, such as tacrine, which are also metabolized primarily by CYP1A2).
No products indexed under this heading.

Theophylline (Potential inhibitors of CYP1A2, such as theophylline, could decrease the rate of riluzole elimination).
No products indexed under this heading.

Theophylline Anhydrous (Potential inhibitors of CYP1A2, such as theophylline, could decrease the rate of riluzole elimination). Products include:
- Uniphyl Tablets 2708

Theophylline Calcium Salicylate (Potential inhibitors of CYP1A2, such as theophylline, could decrease the rate of riluzole elimination).
No products indexed under this heading.

Theophylline Dihydroxypropyl (Glyceryl) (Potential inhibitors of CYP1A2, such as theophylline, could decrease the rate of riluzole elimination).
No products indexed under this heading.

Theophylline Ethylenediamine (Potential inhibitors of CYP1A2, such as theophylline, could decrease the rate of riluzole elimination).
No products indexed under this heading.

Theophylline Sodium Glycinate (Potential inhibitors of CYP1A2, such as theophylline, could decrease the rate of riluzole elimination).
No products indexed under this heading.

Trovafloxacin Mesylate (Potential inhibitors of CYP1A2, such as quinolones, could decrease the rate of riluzole elimination).
No products indexed under this heading.

Food Interactions

Alcohol (Alcohol may increase the risk of hepatotoxicity; patients on riluzole should be discouraged from drinking excessive amounts of alcohol).

Diet, high-lipid (Co-administration with high-fat meal decreases absorption, reduces AUC by about 20% and peak blood levels by about 45%).

Food, charcoal-broiled (Potential inducers of CYP1A2, such as charcoal-broiled food, could increase the rate of riluzole elimination).

RISPERDAL CONSTA LONG-ACTING INJECTION

(Risperidone) 1664
See Risperdal Tablets

RISPERDAL M-TAB ORALLY DISINTEGRATING TABLETS

(Risperidone) 1658
See Risperdal Tablets

RISPERDAL ORAL SOLUTION

(Risperidone) 1658
See Risperdal Tablets

RISPERDAL TABLETS

(Risperidone) 1658

May interact with antihypertensives, central nervous system depressants, dopamine agonists, hepatic microsomal enzyme inducers, and certain other agents. Compounds in these categories include:

Acebutolol Hydrochloride (Because of its potential for inducing hypotension, risperidone may enhance the hypotensive effects of other therapeutic agents with this potential).
No products indexed under this heading.

Alfentanil Hydrochloride (Given the primary CNS effects of risperidone, caution should be taken if used with centrally-acting drugs).
No products indexed under this heading.

Alprazolam (Given the primary CNS effects of risperidone, caution should be taken if used with centrally-acting drugs). Products include:
- Niravam Orally Disintegrating Tablets 3106
- Xanax XR Tablets 2655

Amlodipine Besylate (Because of its potential for inducing hypotension, risperidone may enhance the hypotensive effects of other therapeutic agents with this potential). Products include:
- Caduet Tablets 2507
- Lotrel Capsules 2238
- Norvasc Tablets 2529

Aprobarbital (Given the primary CNS effects of risperidone, caution should be taken if used with centrally-acting drugs).
No products indexed under this heading.

Atenolol (Because of its potential for inducing hypotension, risperidone may enhance the hypotensive effects of other therapeutic agents with this potential). Products include:
- Tenormin I.V. Injection 698
- Tenormin Tablets 695

Benazepril Hydrochloride (Because of its potential for inducing hypotension, risperidone may enhance the hypotensive effects of other therapeutic agents with this potential). Products include:
- Lotensin Tablets 2232
- Lotensin HCT Tablets 2235
- Lotrel Capsules 2238

Bendroflumethiazide (Because of its potential for inducing hypotension, risperidone may enhance the hypotensive effects of other therapeutic agents with this potential).
No products indexed under this heading.

Betaxolol Hydrochloride (Because of its potential for inducing hypotension, risperidone may enhance the hypotensive effects of other therapeutic agents with this potential). Products include:
- Betoptic S Ophthalmic Suspension 554

Bisoprolol Fumarate (Because of its potential for inducing hypotension, risperidone may enhance the hypotensive effects of other therapeutic agents with this potential).
No products indexed under this heading.

Bromocriptine Mesylate (Risperidone may antagonize the effect of dopamine agonists).
No products indexed under this heading.

Buprenorphine Hydrochloride (Given the primary CNS effects of risperidone, caution should be taken if used with centrally-acting drugs). Products include:
- Buprenex Injectable 2718
- Suboxone Tablets 2719
- Subutex Tablets 2719

Buspirone Hydrochloride (Given the primary CNS effects of risperidone, caution should be taken if used with centrally-acting drugs).
No products indexed under this heading.

Butabarbital (Given the primary CNS effects of risperidone, caution should be taken if used with centrally-acting drugs).
No products indexed under this heading.

Butalbital (Given the primary CNS effects of risperidone, caution should be taken if used with centrally-acting drugs). Products include:
- Sedapap Tablets 50 mg/650 mg 2098

Candesartan Cilexetil (Because of its potential for inducing hypotension, risperidone may enhance the hypotensive effects of other therapeutic agents with this potential). Products include:
- Atacand Tablets 634
- Atacand HCT 637

Captopril (Because of its potential for inducing hypotension, risperidone may enhance the hypotensive effects of other therapeutic agents with this potential). Products include:
- Captopril Tablets 2114

Carbamazepine (During co-administration, the plasma concentrations of risperidone and its pharmacologically active metabolite, 9-hydroxyrisperidone, were decreased by about 50%. Plasma concentrations of carbamazepine did not appear to be affected. The dose of risperidone may need to be titrated accordingly for patients receiving carbamazepine, particularly during initiation or discontinuation of carbamazepine therapy). Products include:
- Carbatrol Capsules 3174
- Equetro Extended-Release Capsules 3178
- Tegretol/Tegretol-XR 2278

Carteolol Hydrochloride (Because of its potential for inducing hypotension, risperidone may enhance the hypotensive effects of other therapeutic agents with this potential). Products include:
- Carteolol Hydrochloride Ophthalmic Solution USP, 1%........ ⊙ 246

Chlordiazepoxide (Given the primary CNS effects of risperidone, caution should be taken if used with centrally-acting drugs).
No products indexed under this heading.

Chlordiazepoxide Hydrochloride (Given the primary CNS effects of risperidone, caution should be taken if used with centrally-acting drugs). Products include:
- Librium Capsules 3349

Chlorothiazide (Because of its potential for inducing hypotension, risperidone may enhance the hypotensive effects of other therapeutic agents with this potential). Products include:
- Aldoclor Tablets 1881
- Diuril Oral 1936

Chlorothiazide Sodium (Because of its potential for inducing hypotension, risperidone may enhance the hypotensive effects of other therapeutic agents with this potential). Products include:
- Diuril Sodium Intravenous 1934

Chlorpromazine (Given the primary CNS effects of risperidone, caution should be taken if used with centrally-acting drugs).
No products indexed under this heading.

Chlorpromazine Hydrochloride (Given the primary CNS effects of risperidone, caution should be taken if used with centrally-acting drugs).
No products indexed under this heading.

Chlorpropamide (Co-administration of known enzyme inducers (e.g., phenytoin, rifampin and phenobarbital) with risperidone may cause decreases in the combined plasma concentrations of risperidone and 9-hydroxyrisperidone, which could lead to decreased efficacy. The doseof risperidone may need to be adjusted accordingly, particularly during the initiation or discontinuation of therapy with enzyme inducers).
No products indexed under this heading.

Chlorprothixene (Given the primary CNS effects of risperidone, caution should be taken if used with centrally-acting drugs).
No products indexed under this heading.

Chlorprothixene Hydrochloride (Given the primary CNS effects of risperidone, caution should be taken if used with centrally-acting drugs).
No products indexed under this heading.

Chlorprothixene Lactate (Given the primary CNS effects of risperidone, caution should be taken if used with centrally-acting drugs).
No products indexed under this heading.

Chlorthalidone (Because of its potential for inducing hypotension, risperidone may enhance the hypotensive effects of other therapeutic agents with this potential). Products include:
- Clorpres Tablets 2139

Cimetidine (Cimetidine increased the bioavailability of risperidone, but only marginally increased the plasma concentration of the active anti-psychotic fraction). Products include:
- Tagamet HB 200 Tablets 637
- Tagamet Tablets 1547

Cimetidine Hydrochloride (Cimetidine increased the bioavailability of risperidone, but only marginally increased the plasma concentration of the active anti-psychotic fraction).
No products indexed under this heading.

Clonidine (Because of its potential for inducing hypotension, risperidone may enhance the hypotensive effects of other therapeutic agents with this potential). Products include:
- Catapres-TTS 875

Clonidine Hydrochloride (Because of its potential for inducing hypotension, risperidone may enhance the hypotensive effects of other therapeutic agents with this potential). Products include:
- Catapres Tablets 874
- Clorpres Tablets 2139

Clorazepate Dipotassium (Given the primary CNS effects of risperidone, caution should be taken if used with centrally-acting drugs). Products include:
- Tranxene 2488

Clozapine (Chronic administration of clozapine with risperidone may decrease the clearance of risperidone). Products include:
- Clozapine Tablets 2141
- Clozaril Tablets 2174
- FazaClo Orally Disintegrating Tablets 547

CNS-Active Drugs, unspecified (Given the primary CNS effects of risperidone, caution should be taken if used with centrally-acting drugs).
No products indexed under this heading.

Codeine Phosphate (Given the primary CNS effects of risperidone, caution should be taken if used with centrally-acting drugs). Products include:
- Tylenol with Codeine 2461

Deserpidine (Because of its potential for inducing hypotension, risperidone may enhance the hypotensive effects of other therapeutic agents with this potential).
No products indexed under this heading.

Desflurane (Given the primary CNS effects of risperidone, caution should be taken if used with centrally-acting drugs). Products include:
- Suprane Liquid for Inhalation 770

Dezocine (Given the primary CNS effects of risperidone, caution should be taken if used with centrally-acting drugs).
No products indexed under this heading.

Diazepam (Given the primary CNS effects of risperidone, caution should be taken if used with centrally-acting drugs). Products include:
- Diastat Rectal Delivery System 3344
- Valium Tablets 2822

Diazoxide (Because of its potential for inducing hypotension, risperidone may enhance the hypotensive effects of other therapeutic agents with this potential). Products include:
- Hyperstat I.V. Injection 3031

Diltiazem Hydrochloride (Because of its potential for inducing hypotension, risperidone may enhance the hypotensive effects of other therapeutic agents with this potential). Products include:
- Cardizem LA Extended Release Tablets 1699
- Tiazac Capsules 1204

Dopamine Hydrochloride (Risperidone may antagonize the effect of dopamine agonists).
No products indexed under this heading.

Doxazosin Mesylate (Because of its potential for inducing hypotension, risperidone may enhance the hypotensive effects of other therapeutic agents with this potential).
No products indexed under this heading.

Droperidol (Given the primary CNS effects of risperidone, caution should be taken if used with centrally-acting drugs).
No products indexed under this heading.

Enalapril Maleate (Because of its potential for inducing hypotension, risperidone may enhance the hypotensive effects of other therapeutic agents with this potential). Products include:
- Vaseretic Tablets 2073
- Vasotec I.V. Injection 2076

Enalaprilat (Because of its potential for inducing hypotension, risperidone may enhance the hypotensive effects of other therapeutic agents with this potential).
No products indexed under this heading.

Enflurane (Given the primary CNS effects of risperidone, caution should be taken if used with centrally-acting drugs).
No products indexed under this heading.

Eprosartan Mesylate (Because of its potential for inducing hypotension, risperidone may enhance the hypotensive effects of other therapeutic agents with this potential). Products include:
- Teveten Tablets 1707
- Teveten HCT Tablets 1710

Esmolol Hydrochloride (Because of its potential for inducing hypotension, risperidone may enhance the hypotensive effects of other therapeutic agents with this potential). Products include:
- Brevibloc Concentrate 766
- Brevibloc Injection 766
- Brevibloc Double Strength Injection 766
- Brevibloc Premixed Injection 766
- Brevibloc Double Strength Premixed Injection 766

Estazolam (Given the primary CNS effects of risperidone, caution should be taken if used with centrally-acting drugs). Products include:
- ProSom Tablets 512

Ethanol (Co-administration of known enzyme inducers (e.g., phenytoin, rifampin and phenobarbital) with risperidone may cause decreases in the combined plasma concentrations of risperidone and 9-hydroxyrisperidone, which could lead to decreased efficacy. The doseof risperidone may need to be adjusted accordingly, particularly during the initiation or discontinuation of therapy with enzyme inducers).
No products indexed under this heading.

Ethchlorvynol (Given the primary CNS effects of risperidone, caution should be taken if used with centrally-acting drugs).
No products indexed under this heading.

Ethinamate (Given the primary CNS effects of risperidone, caution should be taken if used with centrally-acting drugs).
No products indexed under this heading.

Ethyl Alcohol (Given the primary CNS effects of risperidone, caution should be taken if used with centrally-acting drugs).
No products indexed under this heading.

Felodipine (Because of its potential for inducing hypotension, risperidone may enhance the hypotensive effects of other therapeutic agents with this potential). Products include:
- Plendil Extended-Release Tablets 651

Fentanyl (Given the primary CNS effects of risperidone, caution should be taken if used with centrally-acting drugs). Products include:
- Duragesic Transdermal System 2448

Fentanyl Citrate (Given the primary CNS effects of risperidone, caution should be taken if used with centrally-acting drugs). Products include:
- Actiq 993

Fluoxetine Hydrochloride (Fluoxetine (20mg QD) has been shown to increase the plasma concentration of risperidone 2.5- to 2.8- fold, while the plasma concentration of 9-hydroxyrisperidone was not affected. When concomitant fluoxetine is initiated or discontinued, the dosage of risperidone should be re-evaluated). Products include:
- Prozac Pulvules and Liquid 1771
- Symbyax Capsules 1788

Fluphenazine Decanoate (Given the primary CNS effects of risperidone, caution should be taken if used with centrally-acting drugs).
No products indexed under this heading.

Fluphenazine Enanthate (Given the primary CNS effects of risperidone, caution should be taken if used with centrally-acting drugs).
No products indexed under this heading.

Fluphenazine Hydrochloride (Given the primary CNS effects of risperidone, caution should be taken if used with centrally-acting drugs).
No products indexed under this heading.

Flurazepam Hydrochloride (Given the primary CNS effects of risperidone, caution should be taken if used with centrally-acting drugs). Products include:
Dalmane Capsules 3343

Fosinopril Sodium (Because of its potential for inducing hypotension, risperidone may enhance the hypotensive effects of other therapeutic agents with this potential).
No products indexed under this heading.

Fosphenytoin Sodium (Co-administration of known enzyme inducers (e.g., phenytoin, rifampin and phenobarbital) with risperidone may cause decreases in the combined plasma concentrations of risperidone and 9-hydroxyrisperidone, which could lead to decreased efficacy. The doseof risperidone may need to be adjusted accordingly, particularly during the initiation or discontinuation of therapy with enzyme inducers).
No products indexed under this heading.

Furosemide (In placebo-controlled trials in elderly patients with dementia-related psychosis, a higher incidence of mortality was observed in patients treated with furosemide plus risperdone (7.3%; mean age 89 years, range 75-97) when compared to patients treated with risperdone alone (3.1%; mean age 84 years, range 70-96) or furosemide alone (4.1%; mean age 80 years, range 67-90). The increase in mortality in patients treated with furosemide plus risperidone was observed in 2 of the 4 clinical trials). Products include:
Furosemide Tablets 2117

Glipizide (Co-administration of known enzyme inducers (e.g., phenytoin, rifampin and phenobarbital) with risperidone may cause decreases in the combined plasma concentrations of risperidone and 9-hydroxyrisperidone, which could lead to decreased efficacy. The doseof risperidone may need to be adjusted accordingly, particularly during the initiation or discontinuation of therapy with enzyme inducers).
No products indexed under this heading.

Glutethimide (Given the primary CNS effects of risperidone, caution should be taken if used with centrally-acting drugs).
No products indexed under this heading.

Glyburide (Co-administration of known enzyme inducers (e.g., phenytoin, rifampin and phenobarbital) with risperidone may cause decreases in the combined plasma concentrations of risperidone and 9-hydroxyrisperidone, which could lead to decreased efficacy. The doseof risperidone may need to be adjusted accordingly, particularly during the initiation or discontinuation of therapy with enzyme inducers).
No products indexed under this heading.

Guanabenz Acetate (Because of its potential for inducing hypotension, risperidone may enhance the hypotensive effects of other therapeutic agents with this potential).
No products indexed under this heading.

Guanethidine Monosulfate (Because of its potential for inducing hypotension, risperidone may enhance the hypotensive effects of other therapeutic agents with this potential).
No products indexed under this heading.

Haloperidol (Given the primary CNS effects of risperidone, caution should be taken if used with centrally-acting drugs).
No products indexed under this heading.

Haloperidol Decanoate (Given the primary CNS effects of risperidone, caution should be taken if used with centrally-acting drugs).
No products indexed under this heading.

Hydralazine Hydrochloride (Because of its potential for inducing hypotension, risperidone may enhance the hypotensive effects of other therapeutic agents with this potential). Products include:
BiDil Tablets 2161

Hydrochlorothiazide (Because of its potential for inducing hypotension, risperidone may enhance the hypotensive effects of other therapeutic agents with this potential). Products include:
Aldoril Tablets 1884
Atacand HCT 637
Avalide Tablets 2889
Avalide Tablets 922
Benicar HCT Tablets 2852
Diovan HCT Tablets 2195
Dyazide Capsules 1389
Hyzaar 1964
Lotensin HCT Tablets 2235
Maxzide 2150
Micardis HCT Tablets 886
Moduretic Tablets 2003
Prinzide Tablets 2033
Teveten HCT Tablets 1710
Timolide Tablets 2056
Uniretic Tablets 3114
Vaseretic Tablets 2073
Zestoretic Tablets 701

Hydrocodone Bitartrate (Given the primary CNS effects of risperidone, caution should be taken if used with centrally-acting drugs). Products include:
Hycodan 1104
Hycomine Compound Tablets 1105
Hycotuss Expectorant Syrup 1106
Lortab 3315
Lortab Elixir 3312
Vicodin Tablets 530
Vicodin ES Tablets 531
Vicodin HP Tablets 532
Vicoprofen Tablets 533
Zydone Tablets 1118

Hydrocodone Polistirex (Given the primary CNS effects of risperidone, caution should be taken if used with centrally-acting drugs). Products include:
Tussionex Pennkinetic Extended-Release Suspension 3322

Hydroflumethiazide (Because of its potential for inducing hypotension, risperidone may enhance the hypotensive effects of other therapeutic agents with this potential).
No products indexed under this heading.

Hydromorphone Hydrochloride (Given the primary CNS effects of risperidone, caution should be taken if used with centrally-acting drugs). Products include:
Dilaudid 439
Dilaudid Oral Liquid 443
Dilaudid Non-Sterile Powder 439
Dilaudid Rectal Suppositories 439
Dilaudid Tablets 439
Dilaudid Tablets - 8 mg 443
Dilaudid-HP 441

Hydroxyzine Hydrochloride (Given the primary CNS effects of risperidone, caution should be taken if used with centrally-acting drugs).
No products indexed under this heading.

Indapamide (Because of its potential for inducing hypotension, risperidone may enhance the hypotensive effects of other therapeutic agents with this potential). Products include:
Indapamide Tablets 2119

Irbesartan (Because of its potential for inducing hypotension, risperidone may enhance the hypotensive effects of other therapeutic agents with this potential). Products include:
Avalide Tablets 922
Avalide Tablets 2889
Avapro Tablets 925
Avapro Tablets 2886

Isoflurane (Given the primary CNS effects of risperidone, caution should be taken if used with centrally-acting drugs).
No products indexed under this heading.

Isradipine (Because of its potential for inducing hypotension, risperidone may enhance the hypotensive effects of other therapeutic agents with this potential). Products include:
DynaCirc CR Tablets 2726

Ketamine Hydrochloride (Given the primary CNS effects of risperidone, caution should be taken if used with centrally-acting drugs).
No products indexed under this heading.

Labetalol Hydrochloride (Because of its potential for inducing hypotension, risperidone may enhance the hypotensive effects of other therapeutic agents with this potential).
No products indexed under this heading.

Levodopa (Risperidone may antagonize the effect of levodopa). Products include:
Parcopa Orally Disintegrating Tablets 3111
Stalevo Tablets 2270

Levomethadyl Acetate Hydrochloride (Given the primary CNS effects of risperidone, caution should be taken if used with centrally-acting drugs).
No products indexed under this heading.

Levorphanol Tartrate (Given the primary CNS effects of risperidone, caution should be taken if used with centrally-acting drugs).
No products indexed under this heading.

Lisinopril (Because of its potential for inducing hypotension, risperidone may enhance the hypotensive effects of other therapeutic agents with this potential). Products include:
Prinivil Tablets 2029
Prinzide Tablets 2033
Zestoretic Tablets 701
Zestril Tablets 704

Lorazepam (Given the primary CNS effects of risperidone, caution should be taken if used with centrally-acting drugs).
No products indexed under this heading.

Losartan Potassium (Because of its potential for inducing hypotension, risperidone may enhance the hypotensive effects of other therapeutic agents with this potential). Products include:
Cozaar Tablets 1913
Hyzaar 1964

Loxapine Hydrochloride (Given the primary CNS effects of risperidone, caution should be taken if used with centrally-acting drugs).
No products indexed under this heading.

Loxapine Succinate (Given the primary CNS effects of risperidone, caution should be taken if used with centrally-acting drugs).
No products indexed under this heading.

Mecamylamine Hydrochloride (Because of its potential for inducing hypotension, risperidone may enhance the hypotensive effects of other therapeutic agents with this potential). Products include:
Inversine Tablets 3286

Meperidine Hydrochloride (Given the primary CNS effects of risperidone, caution should be taken if used with centrally-acting drugs).
No products indexed under this heading.

Mephobarbital (Given the primary CNS effects of risperidone, caution should be taken if used with centrally-acting drugs). Products include:
Mebaral Tablets, USP 2483

Meprobamate (Given the primary CNS effects of risperidone, caution should be taken if used with centrally-acting drugs).
No products indexed under this heading.

Mesoridazine Besylate (Given the primary CNS effects of risperidone, caution should be taken if used with centrally-acting drugs).
No products indexed under this heading.

Methadone Hydrochloride (Given the primary CNS effects of risperidone, caution should be taken if used with centrally-acting drugs).
No products indexed under this heading.

Methohexital Sodium (Given the primary CNS effects of risperidone, caution should be taken if used with centrally-acting drugs).
No products indexed under this heading.

Methotrimeprazine (Given the primary CNS effects of risperidone, caution should be taken if used with centrally-acting drugs).
No products indexed under this heading.

Methoxyflurane (Given the primary CNS effects of risperidone, caution should be taken if used with centrally-acting drugs).
No products indexed under this heading.

Methyclothiazide (Because of its potential for inducing hypotension, risperidone may enhance the hypotensive effects of other therapeutic agents with this potential).
No products indexed under this heading.

Methyldopa (Because of its potential for inducing hypotension, risperidone may enhance the hypotensive effects of other therapeutic agents with this potential). Products include:
Aldoclor Tablets **1881**
Aldoril Tablets **1884**

Methyldopate Hydrochloride (Because of its potential for inducing hypotension, risperidone may enhance the hypotensive effects of other therapeutic agents with this potential).
No products indexed under this heading.

Metolazone (Because of its potential for inducing hypotension, risperidone may enhance the hypotensive effects of other therapeutic agents with this potential).
No products indexed under this heading.

Metoprolol Succinate (Because of its potential for inducing hypotension, risperidone may enhance the hypotensive effects of other therapeutic agents with this potential). Products include:
Toprol-XL Tablets **660**

Metoprolol Tartrate (Because of its potential for inducing hypotension, risperidone may enhance the hypotensive effects of other therapeutic agents with this potential).
No products indexed under this heading.

Metyrosine (Because of its potential for inducing hypotension, risperidone may enhance the hypotensive effects of other therapeutic agents with this potential). Products include:
Demser Capsules **1933**

Mibefradil Dihydrochloride (Because of its potential for inducing hypotension, risperidone may enhance the hypotensive effects of other therapeutic agents with this potential).
No products indexed under this heading.

Midazolam Hydrochloride (Given the primary CNS effects of risperidone, caution should be taken if used with centrally-acting drugs).
No products indexed under this heading.

Minoxidil (Because of its potential for inducing hypotension, risperidone may enhance the hypotensive effects of other therapeutic agents with this potential). Products include:
Men's Rogaine Extra Strength Topical Solution, Ocean Rush Scent and Original Unscented **706**
Women's Rogaine Topical Solution, Spring Bloom Scent and Original Unscented **707**

Moexipril Hydrochloride (Because of its potential for inducing hypotension, risperidone may enhance the hypotensive effects of other therapeutic agents with this potential). Products include:
Uniretic Tablets **3114**
Univasc Tablets **3118**

Molindone Hydrochloride (Given the primary CNS effects of risperidone, caution should be taken if used with centrally-acting drugs). Products include:
Moban Tablets **1108**

Morphine Sulfate (Given the primary CNS effects of risperidone, caution should be taken if used with centrally-acting drugs). Products include:
Avinza Capsules **1714**
Kadian Capsules **572**
MS Contin Tablets **2703**

Nadolol (Because of its potential for inducing hypotension, risperidone may enhance the hypotensive effects of other therapeutic agents with this potential). Products include:
Nadolol Tablets **2121**

Nicardipine Hydrochloride (Because of its potential for inducing hypotension, risperidone may enhance the hypotensive effects of other therapeutic agents with this potential). Products include:
Cardene I.V. **1129**

Nifedipine (Because of its potential for inducing hypotension, risperidone may enhance the hypotensive effects of other therapeutic agents with this potential). Products include:
Adalat CC Tablets **2978**

Nisoldipine (Because of its potential for inducing hypotension, risperidone may enhance the hypotensive effects of other therapeutic agents with this potential). Products include:
Sular Tablets **1163**

Nitroglycerin (Because of its potential for inducing hypotension, risperidone may enhance the hypotensive effects of other therapeutic agents with this potential). Products include:
Nitro-Dur Transdermal Infusion System **3060**
Nitrolingual Pumpspray **1161**

Olanzapine (Given the primary CNS effects of risperidone, caution should be taken if used with centrally-acting drugs). Products include:
Symbyax Capsules **1788**
Zyprexa Tablets **1798**
Zyprexa IntraMuscular **1798**
Zyprexa ZYDIS Orally Disintegrating Tablets **1798**

Oxazepam (Given the primary CNS effects of risperidone, caution should be taken if used with centrally-acting drugs).
No products indexed under this heading.

Oxycodone Hydrochloride (Given the primary CNS effects of risperidone, caution should be taken if used with centrally-acting drugs). Products include:
Combunox Tablets **1183**
OxyContin Tablets **2699**
OxyFast Oral Concentrate Solution **2704**
OxyIR Capsules **2704**
Percocet Tablets **1114**
Percodan Tablets **1115**

Paroxetine Hydrochloride (Paroxetine (20mg QD) has been shown to increase the plasma concentration of risperidone 3- to 9-fold and lower the concentration of 9-hydroxyrisperidone an average of 13%. When concomitant paroxetine is initiated or discontinued, the dosage of risperidone should be re-evaluated). Products include:
Paxil CR Controlled-Release Tablets **1509**
Paxil **1501**

Penbutolol Sulfate (Because of its potential for inducing hypotension, risperidone may enhance the hypotensive effects of other therapeutic agents with this potential).
No products indexed under this heading.

Pentobarbital Sodium (Given the primary CNS effects of risperidone, caution should be taken if used with centrally-acting drugs). Products include:
Nembutal Sodium Solution, USP **2484**

Pergolide Mesylate (Risperidone may antagonize the effect of dopamine agonists). Products include:
Permax Tablets **3357**

Perindopril Erbumine (Because of its potential for inducing hypotension, risperidone may enhance the hypotensive effects of other therapeutic agents with this potential). Products include:
Aceon Tablets (2 mg, 4 mg, 8 mg) **3191**

Perphenazine (Given the primary CNS effects of risperidone, caution should be taken if used with centrally-acting drugs).
No products indexed under this heading.

Phenobarbital (Co-administration of known enzyme inducers (e.g., phenytoin, rifampin and phenobarbital) with risperidone may cause decreases in the combined plasma concentrations of risperidone and 9-hydroxyrisperidone, which could lead to decreased efficacy. The doseof risperidone may need to be adjusted accordingly, particularly during the initiation or discontinuation of therapy with enzyme inducers).
No products indexed under this heading.

Phenoxybenzamine Hydrochloride (Because of its potential for inducing hypotension, risperidone may enhance the hypotensive effects of other therapeutic agents with this potential). Products include:
Dibenzyline Capsules **3390**

Phentolamine Mesylate (Because of its potential for inducing hypotension, risperidone may enhance the hypotensive effects of other therapeutic agents with this potential).
No products indexed under this heading.

Phenylbutazone (Co-administration of known enzyme inducers (e.g., phenytoin, rifampin and phenobarbital) with risperidone may cause decreases in the combined plasma concentrations of risperidone and 9-hydroxyrisperidone, which could lead to decreased efficacy. The doseof risperidone may need to be adjusted accordingly, particularly during the initiation or discontinuation of therapy with enzyme inducers).
No products indexed under this heading.

Phenytoin (Co-administration of known enzyme inducers (e.g., phenytoin, rifampin and phenobarbital) with risperidone may cause decreases in the combined plasma concentrations of risperidone and 9-hydroxyrisperidone, which could lead to decreased efficacy. The doseof risperidone may need to be adjusted accordingly, particularly during the initiation or discontinuation of therapy with enzyme inducers).
No products indexed under this heading.

Phenytoin Sodium (Co-administration of known enzyme inducers (e.g., phenytoin, rifampin and phenobarbital) with risperidone may cause decreases in the combined plasma concentrations of risperidone and 9-hydroxyrisperidone, which could lead to decreased efficacy. The doseof risperidone may need to be adjusted accordingly, particularly during the initiation or discontinuation of therapy with enzyme inducers). Products include:
Phenytek Capsules **2153**

Pindolol (Because of its potential for inducing hypotension, risperidone may enhance the hypotensive effects of other therapeutic agents with this potential).
No products indexed under this heading.

Polythiazide (Because of its potential for inducing hypotension, risperidone may enhance the hypotensive effects of other therapeutic agents with this potential).
No products indexed under this heading.

Pramipexole Dihydrochloride (Risperidone may antagonize the effect of dopamine agonists). Products include:
Mirapex Tablets **889**

Prazepam (Given the primary CNS effects of risperidone, caution should be taken if used with centrally-acting drugs).
No products indexed under this heading.

Prazosin Hydrochloride (Because of its potential for inducing hypotension, risperidone may enhance the hypotensive effects of other therapeutic agents with this potential).
No products indexed under this heading.

Prochlorperazine (Given the primary CNS effects of risperidone, caution should be taken if used with centrally-acting drugs).
No products indexed under this heading.

Promethazine Hydrochloride (Given the primary CNS effects of risperidone, caution should be taken if used with centrally-acting drugs). Products include:
Phenergan **3438**

Propofol (Given the primary CNS effects of risperidone, caution should be taken if used with centrally-acting drugs). Products include:
Diprivan Injectable Emulsion **676**

Propoxyphene Hydrochloride (Given the primary CNS effects of risperidone, caution should be taken if used with centrally-acting drugs).
No products indexed under this heading.

Propoxyphene Napsylate (Given the primary CNS effects of risperidone, caution should be taken if used with centrally-acting drugs). Products include:

Darvocet A 500 Tablets 3497

Propranolol Hydrochloride (Because of its potential for inducing hypotension, risperidone may enhance the hypotensive effects of other therapeutic agents with this potential). Products include:

Inderal LA Long-Acting Capsules 3421
InnoPran XL Capsules 2728

Quazepam (Given the primary CNS effects of risperidone, caution should be taken if used with centrally-acting drugs).

No products indexed under this heading.

Quetiapine Fumarate (Given the primary CNS effects of risperidone, caution should be taken if used with centrally-acting drugs). Products include:

Seroquel Tablets 691

Quinapril Hydrochloride (Because of its potential for inducing hypotension, risperidone may enhance the hypotensive effects of other therapeutic agents with this potential).

No products indexed under this heading.

Ramipril (Because of its potential for inducing hypotension, risperidone may enhance the hypotensive effects of other therapeutic agents with this potential). Products include:

Altace Capsules 1673

Ranitidine Bismuth Citrate (Cimetidine increased the bioavailability of risperidone, but only marginally increased the plasma concentration of the active anti-psychotic fraction).

No products indexed under this heading.

Ranitidine Hydrochloride (Cimetidine increased the bioavailability of risperidone, but only marginally increased the plasma concentration of the active anti-psychotic fraction). Products include:

Zantac 1597
Zantac Injection 1593
Zantac 75 Tablets .... ▣ 715
Zantac 150 Maximum Strength Tablets .... ▣ 715
Zantac Injection Pharmacy Bulk Package 1595

Rauwolfia Serpentina (Because of its potential for inducing hypotension, risperidone may enhance the hypotensive effects of other therapeutic agents with this potential).

No products indexed under this heading.

Remifentanil Hydrochloride (Given the primary CNS effects of risperidone, caution should be taken if used with centrally-acting drugs).

No products indexed under this heading.

Rescinnamine (Because of its potential for inducing hypotension, risperidone may enhance the hypotensive effects of other therapeutic agents with this potential).

No products indexed under this heading.

Reserpine (Because of its potential for inducing hypotension, risperidone may enhance the hypotensive effects of other therapeutic agents with this potential).

No products indexed under this heading.

Rifampin (Co-administration of known enzyme inducers (e.g., phenytoin, rifampin and phenobarbital) with risperidone may cause decreases in the combined plasma concentrations of risperidone and 9-hydroxyrisperidone, which could lead to decreased efficacy. The doseof risperidone may need to be adjusted accordingly, particularly during the initiation or discontinuation of therapy with enzyme inducers).

No products indexed under this heading.

Rifapentine (Co-administration of known enzyme inducers (e.g., phenytoin, rifampin and phenobarbital) with risperidone may cause decreases in the combined plasma concentrations of risperidone and 9-hydroxyrisperidone, which could lead to decreased efficacy. The doseof risperidone may need to be adjusted accordingly, particularly during the initiation or discontinuation of therapy with enzyme inducers).

No products indexed under this heading.

Ropinirole Hydrochloride (Risperidone may antagonize the effect of dopamine agonists). Products include:

Requip Tablets 1528

Secobarbital Sodium (Given the primary CNS effects of risperidone, caution should be taken if used with centrally-acting drugs).

No products indexed under this heading.

Sevoflurane (Given the primary CNS effects of risperidone, caution should be taken if used with centrally-acting drugs). Products include:

Ultane Liquid for Inhalation 526

Sodium Nitroprusside (Because of its potential for inducing hypotension, risperidone may enhance the hypotensive effects of other therapeutic agents with this potential).

No products indexed under this heading.

Sodium Oxybate (Given the primary CNS effects of risperidone, caution should be taken if used with centrally-acting drugs).

No products indexed under this heading.

Sotalol Hydrochloride (Because of its potential for inducing hypotension, risperidone may enhance the hypotensive effects of other therapeutic agents with this potential).

No products indexed under this heading.

Spirapril Hydrochloride (Because of its potential for inducing hypotension, risperidone may enhance the hypotensive effects of other therapeutic agents with this potential).

No products indexed under this heading.

Sufentanil Citrate (Given the primary CNS effects of risperidone, caution should be taken if used with centrally-acting drugs).

No products indexed under this heading.

Telmisartan (Because of its potential for inducing hypotension, risperidone may enhance the hypotensive effects of other therapeutic agents with this potential). Products include:

Micardis Tablets 884
Micardis HCT Tablets 886

Temazepam (Given the primary CNS effects of risperidone, caution should be taken if used with centrally-acting drugs).

No products indexed under this heading.

Terazosin Hydrochloride (Because of its potential for inducing hypotension, risperidone may enhance the hypotensive effects of other therapeutic agents with this potential). Products include:

Hytrin Capsules 469

Thiamylal Sodium (Given the primary CNS effects of risperidone, caution should be taken if used with centrally-acting drugs).

No products indexed under this heading.

Thioridazine Hydrochloride (Given the primary CNS effects of risperidone, caution should be taken if used with centrally-acting drugs). Products include:

Thioridazine Hydrochloride Tablets 2122

Thiothixene (Given the primary CNS effects of risperidone, caution should be taken if used with centrally-acting drugs). Products include:

Thiothixene Capsules 2124

Timolol Maleate (Because of its potential for inducing hypotension, risperidone may enhance the hypotensive effects of other therapeutic agents with this potential). Products include:

Blocadren Tablets 1891
Cosopt Sterile Ophthalmic Solution... 1910
Timolide Tablets 2056
Timoptic in Ocudose 2061
Timoptic Sterile Ophthalmic Solution... 2058
Timoptic-XE Sterile Ophthalmic Gel Forming Solution 2062

Tolazamide (Co-administration of known enzyme inducers (e.g., phenytoin, rifampin and phenobarbital) with risperidone may cause decreases in the combined plasma concentrations of risperidone and 9-hydroxyrisperidone, which could lead to decreased efficacy. The doseof risperidone may need to be adjusted accordingly, particularly during the initiation or discontinuation of therapy with enzyme inducers).

No products indexed under this heading.

Tolbutamide (Co-administration of known enzyme inducers (e.g., phenytoin, rifampin and phenobarbital) with risperidone may cause decreases in the combined plasma concentrations of risperidone and 9-hydroxyrisperidone, which could lead to decreased efficacy. The doseof risperidone may need to be adjusted accordingly, particularly during the initiation or discontinuation of therapy with enzyme inducers).

No products indexed under this heading.

Torsemide (Because of its potential for inducing hypotension, risperidone may enhance the hypotensive effects of other therapeutic agents with this potential).

No products indexed under this heading.

Trandolapril (Because of its potential for inducing hypotension, risperidone may enhance the hypotensive effects of other therapeutic agents with this potential). Products include:

Mavik Tablets 482
Tarka Tablets 519

Triazolam (Given the primary CNS effects of risperidone, caution should be taken if used with centrally-acting drugs).

No products indexed under this heading.

Trifluoperazine Hydrochloride (Given the primary CNS effects of risperidone, caution should be taken if used with centrally-acting drugs).

No products indexed under this heading.

Trimethaphan Camsylate (Because of its potential for inducing hypotension, risperidone may enhance the hypotensive effects of other therapeutic agents with this potential).

No products indexed under this heading.

Valproate Sodium (Repeated oral doses of risperidone (4mg QD) did not affect the pre-dose or average plasma concentrations exposure (AUC) of valproate (1000 mg/day in three divided doses) compared to placebo (n=21). However, there was a 20% increase of valproate peak plasma concentration (Cmax) after concomitant administration of risperidone). Products include:

Depacon Injection 412

Valsartan (Because of its potential for inducing hypotension, risperidone may enhance the hypotensive effects of other therapeutic agents with this potential). Products include:

Diovan HCT Tablets 2195
Diovan Tablets 2191

Verapamil Hydrochloride (Because of its potential for inducing hypotension, risperidone may enhance the hypotensive effects of other therapeutic agents with this potential). Products include:

Covera-HS Tablets 3135
Tarka Tablets 519
Verelan PM Capsules 3120

Zaleplon (Given the primary CNS effects of risperidone, caution should be taken if used with centrally-acting drugs). Products include:

Sonata Capsules 1686

Ziprasidone Hydrochloride (Given the primary CNS effects of risperidone, caution should be taken if used with centrally-acting drugs). Products include:

Geodon Capsules 2514

Zolpidem Tartrate (Given the primary CNS effects of risperidone, caution should be taken if used with centrally-acting drugs). Products include:

Ambien Tablets 2867

Food Interactions

Alcohol (Given the primary CNS effects of risperidone, caution should be taken if used with alcohol).

RITALIN HYDROCHLORIDE TABLETS

(Methylphenidate Hydrochloride) 2254

See Ritalin LA Capsules

RITALIN LA CAPSULES
(Methylphenidate Hydrochloride) 2255
May interact with antacids, oral anticoagulants, histamine H_2-receptor antagonists, monoamine oxidase inhibitors, phenytoin, proton pump inhibitor, tricyclic antidepressants, vasopressors, and certain other agents. Compounds in these categories include:

Aluminum Carbonate (Since the modified release characteristics of Ritalin LA are pH dependent, the co-administration of antacids could alter the release of methylphenidate).
No products indexed under this heading.

Aluminum Hydroxide (Since the modified release characteristics of Ritalin LA are pH dependent, the co-administration of antacids could alter the release of methylphenidate). Products include:
Gaviscon Regular Strength Liquid .. 620
Gaviscon Regular Strength Tablets 619
Gaviscon Extra Strength Liquid 620
Gaviscon Extra Strength Tablets 619
Maalox Max Maximum Strength Antacid/Anti-Gas Liquid 2165
Maalox Regular Strength Antacid/Antigas Liquid 2164

Amitriptyline Hydrochloride (Methylphenidate inhibits the metabolism of tricyclic antidepressants).
No products indexed under this heading.

Amoxapine (Methylphenidate inhibits the metabolism of tricyclic antidepressants).
No products indexed under this heading.

Anisindione (Methylphenidate inhibits the metabolism of coumarin anticoagulants). Products include:
Miradon Tablets 3056

Cimetidine (Since the modified release characteristics of Ritalin LA are pH dependent, the co-administration of acid suppressants could alter the release of methylphenidate). Products include:
Tagamet HB 200 Tablets 637
Tagamet Tablets 1547

Cimetidine Hydrochloride (Since the modified release characteristics of Ritalin LA are pH dependent, the co-administration of acid suppressants could alter the release of methylphenidate).
No products indexed under this heading.

Clomipramine Hydrochloride (Methylphenidate inhibits the metabolism of tricyclic antidepressants).
No products indexed under this heading.

Clonidine (Co-administration has resulted in serious adverse events). Products include:
Catapres-TTS 875

Clonidine Hydrochloride (Co-administration has resulted in serious adverse events). Products include:
Catapres Tablets 874
Clorpres Tablets 2139

Desipramine Hydrochloride (Methylphenidate inhibits the metabolism of tricyclic antidepressants).
No products indexed under this heading.

Dicumarol (Methylphenidate inhibits the metabolism of coumarin anticoagulants).
No products indexed under this heading.

Dobutamine (Possible additive effects on blood pressure with pressor agents if used concurrently).
No products indexed under this heading.

Dobutamine Hydrochloride (Possible additive effects on blood pressure with pressor agents if used concurrently).
No products indexed under this heading.

Dopamine Hydrochloride (Possible additive effects on blood pressure with pressor agents if used concurrently).
No products indexed under this heading.

Doxepin Hydrochloride (Methylphenidate inhibits the metabolism of tricyclic antidepressants).
No products indexed under this heading.

Ephedrine Sulfate (Possible additive effects on blood pressure with pressor agents if used concurrently).
No products indexed under this heading.

Epinephrine Bitartrate (Possible additive effects on blood pressure with pressor agents if used concurrently).
No products indexed under this heading.

Epinephrine Hydrochloride (Possible additive effects on blood pressure with pressor agents if used concurrently).
No products indexed under this heading.

Esomeprazole Magnesium (Since the modified release characteristics of Ritalin LA are pH dependent, the co-administration of acid suppressants could alter the release of methylphenidate). Products include:
Nexium Delayed-Release Capsules 645

Famotidine (Since the modified release characteristics of Ritalin LA are pH dependent, the co-administration of acid suppressants could alter the release of methylphenidate). Products include:
Pepcid AC Chewable Tablets 1672
Pepcid AC Gelcaps 1672
Pepcid AC Tablets 1672
Maximum Strength Pepcid AC Tablets 1672
Pepcid Complete Chewable Tablets 1672
Pepcid Injection 2017
Pepcid 2014

Fosphenytoin Sodium (Methylphenidate inhibits the metabolism of phenytoin).
No products indexed under this heading.

Guanethidine Monosulfate (Decreased hypotensive effect of guanethidine).
No products indexed under this heading.

Imipramine Hydrochloride (Methylphenidate inhibits the metabolism of tricyclic antidepressants).
No products indexed under this heading.

Imipramine Pamoate (Methylphenidate inhibits the metabolism of tricyclic antidepressants).
No products indexed under this heading.

Isocarboxazid (Concurrent and/or sequential use with MAO inhibitors may result in hypertensive crises; concurrent use or use within 14 days following discontinuation of an MAO inhibitor is contraindicated).
No products indexed under this heading.

Isoproterenol Hydrochloride (Possible additive effects on blood pressure with pressor agents if used concurrently).
No products indexed under this heading.

Isoproterenol Sulfate (Possible additive effects on blood pressure with pressor agents if used concurrently).
No products indexed under this heading.

Lansoprazole (Since the modified release characteristics of Ritalin LA are pH dependent, the co-administration of acid suppressants could alter the release of methylphenidate). Products include:
Prevacid Delayed-Release Capsules 3268
Prevacid for Delayed-Release Oral Suspension 3268
Prevacid I.V. for Injection 3274
Prevacid NapraPAC 3277
Prevacid SoluTab Delayed-Release Orally Disintegrating Tablets 3268
PREVPAC 3281

Magaldrate (Since the modified release characteristics of Ritalin LA are pH dependent, the co-administration of antacids could alter the release of methylphenidate).
No products indexed under this heading.

Magnesium Hydroxide (Since the modified release characteristics of Ritalin LA are pH dependent, the co-administration of antacids could alter the release of methylphenidate). Products include:
Maalox Max Maximum Strength Antacid/Anti-Gas Liquid 2165
Maalox Regular Strength Antacid/Antigas Liquid 2164
Pepcid Complete Chewable Tablets 1672
Rolaids Tablets 707
Extra Strength Rolaids Tablets 707
Rolaids Multi-Symptom Antacid & Antigas Tablets 708

Magnesium Oxide (Since the modified release characteristics of Ritalin LA are pH dependent, the co-administration of antacids could alter the release of methylphenidate). Products include:
Beelith Tablets 784
PremCal Light, Regular, and Extra Strength Tablets 762

Maprotiline Hydrochloride (Methylphenidate inhibits the metabolism of tricyclic antidepressants).
No products indexed under this heading.

Mephentermine Sulfate (Possible additive effects on blood pressure with pressor agents if used concurrently).
No products indexed under this heading.

Metaraminol Bitartrate (Possible additive effects on blood pressure with pressor agents if used concurrently). Products include:
Aramine Injection 1889

Methoxamine Hydrochloride (Possible additive effects on blood pressure with pressor agents if used concurrently).
No products indexed under this heading.

Moclobemide (Concurrent and/or sequential use with MAO inhibitors may result in hypertensive crises; concurrent use or use within 14 days following discontinuation of an MAO inhibitor is contraindicated).
No products indexed under this heading.

Nizatidine (Since the modified release characteristics of Ritalin LA are pH dependent, the co-administration of acid suppressants could alter the release of methylphenidate). Products include:
Axid Oral Solution 913

Norepinephrine Bitartrate (Possible additive effects on blood pressure with pressor agents if used concurrently).
No products indexed under this heading.

Nortriptyline Hydrochloride (Methylphenidate inhibits the metabolism of tricyclic antidepressants).
No products indexed under this heading.

Omeprazole (Since the modified release characteristics of Ritalin LA are pH dependent, the co-administration of acid suppressants could alter the release of methylphenidate). Products include:
Zegerid Powder for Oral Solution 2972

Pantoprazole Sodium (Since the modified release characteristics of Ritalin LA are pH dependent, the co-administration of acid suppressants could alter the release of methylphenidate). Products include:
Protonix I.V. 3468
Protonix Tablets 3465

Pargyline Hydrochloride (Concurrent and/or sequential use with MAO inhibitors may result in hypertensive crises; concurrent use or use within 14 days following discontinuation of an MAO inhibitor is contraindicated).
No products indexed under this heading.

Phenelzine Sulfate (Concurrent and/or sequential use with MAO inhibitors may result in hypertensive crises; concurrent use or use within 14 days following discontinuation of an MAO inhibitor is contraindicated).
No products indexed under this heading.

Phenobarbital (Methylphenidate inhibits the metabolism of phenobarbital).
No products indexed under this heading.

Phenylephrine Hydrochloride (Possible additive effects on blood pressure with pressor agents if used concurrently). Products include:
Alacol DM Syrup 739
Hycomine Compound Tablets 1105
Preparation H Maximum Strength Cream 747
Preparation H Cooling Gel 747
Preparation H 747
Sudafed PE Tablets 711
Vicks Sinex Nasal Spray and Ultra Fine Mist for Sinus Relief 2677
Zicam Concentrated Cough Mist for Kids Plus D Cool Cherry 643
Zicam Concentrated Cough Mist Plus D Cool Cherry 642

Phenytoin (Methylphenidate inhibits the metabolism of phenytoin).
No products indexed under this heading.

Phenytoin Sodium (Methylphenidate inhibits the metabolism of phenytoin). Products include:
Phenytek Capsules ... 2153

Primidone (Methylphenidate inhibits the metabolism of primidone).
No products indexed under this heading.

Procarbazine Hydrochloride (Concurrent and/or sequential use with MAO inhibitors may result in hypertensive crises; concurrent use or use within 14 days following discontinuation of an MAO inhibitor is contraindicated). Products include:
Matulane Capsules ... 3188

Protriptyline Hydrochloride (Methylphenidate inhibits the metabolism of tricyclic antidepressants). Products include:
Vivactil Tablets ... 2350

Rabeprazole Sodium (Since the modified release characteristics of Ritalin LA are pH dependent, the co-administration of acid suppressants could alter the release of methylphenidate). Products include:
Aciphex Tablets ... 1081

Ranitidine Bismuth Citrate (Since the modified release characteristics of Ritalin LA are pH dependent, the co-administration of acid suppressants could alter the release of methylphenidate).
No products indexed under this heading.

Ranitidine Hydrochloride (Since the modified release characteristics of Ritalin LA are pH dependent, the co-administration of acid suppressants could alter the release of methylphenidate). Products include:
Zantac ... 1597
Zantac Injection ... 1593
Zantac 75 Tablets ... ▣715
Zantac 150 Maximum Strength Tablets ... ▣715
Zantac Injection Pharmacy Bulk Package ... 1595

Selegiline Hydrochloride (Concurrent and/or sequential use with MAO inhibitors may result in hypertensive crises; concurrent use or use within 14 days following discontinuation of an MAO inhibitor is contraindicated). Products include:
Eldepryl Capsules ... 3209

Sodium Bicarbonate (Since the modified release characteristics of Ritalin LA are pH dependent, the co-administration of antacids could alter the release of methylphenidate). Products include:
Ceo-Two Evacuant Suppository ... ▣607
Colyte with Flavor Packs for Oral Solution ... 3102
HalfLytely and Bisacodyl Tablets Bowel Prep Kit with Flavors Packs ... 915
TriLyte with Flavor Packs for Oral Solution ... 3114

Tranylcypromine Sulfate (Concurrent and/or sequential use with MAO inhibitors may result in hypertensive crises; concurrent use or use within 14 days following discontinuation of an MAO inhibitor is contraindicated). Products include:
Parnate Tablets ... 1499

Trimipramine Maleate (Methylphenidate inhibits the metabolism of tricyclic antidepressants). Products include:
Surmontil Capsules ... 2347

Venlafaxine Hydrochloride (Co-administration of venlafaxine in a patient stabilized on methylphenidate has resulted in an NMS-like event within 45 minutes of ingestion of venlafaxine; it is uncertain whether this case represented a drug-drug interaction, a response to either drug alone, or some other cause). Products include:
Effexor Tablets ... 3405
Effexor XR Capsules ... 3411

Warfarin Sodium (Methylphenidate inhibits the metabolism of coumarin anticoagulants). Products include:
Coumadin for Injection ... 932
Coumadin Tablets ... 932

Food Interactions

Food, unspecified (When Ritalin LA was administered with a high fat breakfast to adults, Ritalin LA had a longer lag time until absorption began and variable delays in the time until the peak concentration, the time until the interpeak minimum, and the time until the second peak; administration times relative to meals and meal composition may need to be individually titrated).

RITALIN-SR TABLETS

(Methylphenidate Hydrochloride) ... 2254
See Ritalin LA Capsules

RITUXAN FOR INFUSION

(Rituximab) ... 845
None cited in PDR database.

RITUXAN I.V.

(Rituximab) ... 1251
May interact with:

Cisplatin (Combination of cisplatin and rituxan is not an approved regimen, extreme caution should be exercised).
No products indexed under this heading.

ROBITUSSIN EXPECTORANT

(Guaifenesin) ... ▣749
None cited in PDR database.

ROBITUSSIN ALLERGY & COUGH SYRUP

(Brompheniramine Maleate, Dextromethorphan Hydrobromide, Pseudoephedrine Hydrochloride) ... ▣750
May interact with hypnotics and sedatives, monoamine oxidase inhibitors, tranquilizers, and certain other agents. Compounds in these categories include:

Alprazolam (May increase drowsiness). Products include:
Niravam Orally Disintegrating Tablets ... 3106
Xanax XR Tablets ... 2655

Buspirone Hydrochloride (May increase drowsiness).
No products indexed under this heading.

Chlordiazepoxide (May increase drowsiness).
No products indexed under this heading.

Chlordiazepoxide Hydrochloride (May increase drowsiness). Products include:
Librium Capsules ... 3349

Chlorpromazine (May increase drowsiness).
No products indexed under this heading.

Chlorpromazine Hydrochloride (May increase drowsiness).
No products indexed under this heading.

Chlorprothixene (May increase drowsiness).
No products indexed under this heading.

Chlorprothixene Hydrochloride (May increase drowsiness).
No products indexed under this heading.

Clorazepate Dipotassium (May increase drowsiness). Products include:
Tranxene ... 2488

Diazepam (May increase drowsiness). Products include:
Diastat Rectal Delivery System ... 3344
Valium Tablets ... 2822

Droperidol (May increase drowsiness).
No products indexed under this heading.

Estazolam (May increase drowsiness). Products include:
ProSom Tablets ... 512

Ethchlorvynol (May increase drowsiness).
No products indexed under this heading.

Ethinamate (May increase drowsiness).
No products indexed under this heading.

Fluphenazine Decanoate (May increase drowsiness).
No products indexed under this heading.

Fluphenazine Enanthate (May increase drowsiness).
No products indexed under this heading.

Fluphenazine Hydrochloride (May increase drowsiness).
No products indexed under this heading.

Flurazepam Hydrochloride (May increase drowsiness). Products include:
Dalmane Capsules ... 3343

Glutethimide (May increase drowsiness).
No products indexed under this heading.

Haloperidol (May increase drowsiness).
No products indexed under this heading.

Haloperidol Decanoate (May increase drowsiness).
No products indexed under this heading.

Hydroxyzine Hydrochloride (May increase drowsiness).
No products indexed under this heading.

Isocarboxazid (Concurrent and/or sequential use with MAO inhibitors is not recommended).
No products indexed under this heading.

Lorazepam (May increase drowsiness).
No products indexed under this heading.

Loxapine Hydrochloride (May increase drowsiness).
No products indexed under this heading.

Loxapine Succinate (May increase drowsiness).
No products indexed under this heading.

Meprobamate (May increase drowsiness).
No products indexed under this heading.

Mesoridazine Besylate (May increase drowsiness).
No products indexed under this heading.

Midazolam Hydrochloride (May increase drowsiness).
No products indexed under this heading.

Moclobemide (Concurrent and/or sequential use with MAO inhibitors is not recommended).
No products indexed under this heading.

Molindone Hydrochloride (May increase drowsiness). Products include:
Moban Tablets ... 1108

Oxazepam (May increase drowsiness).
No products indexed under this heading.

Pargyline Hydrochloride (Concurrent and/or sequential use with MAO inhibitors is not recommended).
No products indexed under this heading.

Perphenazine (May increase drowsiness).
No products indexed under this heading.

Phenelzine Sulfate (Concurrent and/or sequential use with MAO inhibitors is not recommended).
No products indexed under this heading.

Prazepam (May increase drowsiness).
No products indexed under this heading.

Procarbazine Hydrochloride (Concurrent and/or sequential use with MAO inhibitors is not recommended). Products include:
Matulane Capsules ... 3188

Prochlorperazine (May increase drowsiness).
No products indexed under this heading.

Promethazine Hydrochloride (May increase drowsiness). Products include:
Phenergan ... 3438

Propofol (May increase drowsiness). Products include:
Diprivan Injectable Emulsion ... 676

Quazepam (May increase drowsiness).
No products indexed under this heading.

Secobarbital Sodium (May increase drowsiness).
No products indexed under this heading.

Selegiline Hydrochloride (Concurrent and/or sequential use with MAO inhibitors is not recommended). Products include:
Eldepryl Capsules ... 3209

Temazepam (May increase drowsiness).
No products indexed under this heading.

Thioridazine Hydrochloride (May increase drowsiness). Products include:
Thioridazine Hydrochloride Tablets ... 2122

Thiothixene (May increase drowsiness). Products include:
Thiothixene Capsules ... 2124

Tranylcypromine Sulfate (Concurrent and/or sequential use with MAO inhibitors is not recommended). Products include:
Parnate Tablets 1499

Triazolam (May increase drowsiness).
No products indexed under this heading.

Trifluoperazine Hydrochloride (May increase drowsiness).
No products indexed under this heading.

Zaleplon (May increase drowsiness). Products include:
Sonata Capsules 1686

Zolpidem Tartrate (May increase drowsiness). Products include:
Ambien Tablets 2867

Food Interactions

Alcohol (May increase drowsiness effect).

ROBITUSSIN CF LIQUID

(Dextromethorphan Hydrobromide, Guaifenesin, Pseudoephedrine Hydrochloride)....... 755
May interact with monoamine oxidase inhibitors. Compounds in these categories include:

Isocarboxazid (Concurrent and/or sequential use with MAO inhibitors is not recommended).
No products indexed under this heading.

Moclobemide (Concurrent and/or sequential use with MAO inhibitors is not recommended).
No products indexed under this heading.

Pargyline Hydrochloride (Concurrent and/or sequential use with MAO inhibitors is not recommended).
No products indexed under this heading.

Phenelzine Sulfate (Concurrent and/or sequential use with MAO inhibitors is not recommended).
No products indexed under this heading.

Procarbazine Hydrochloride (Concurrent and/or sequential use with MAO inhibitors is not recommended). Products include:
Matulane Capsules 3188

Selegiline Hydrochloride (Concurrent and/or sequential use with MAO inhibitors is not recommended). Products include:
Eldepryl Capsules 3209

Tranylcypromine Sulfate (Concurrent and/or sequential use with MAO inhibitors is not recommended). Products include:
Parnate Tablets 1499

ROBITUSSIN COUGH & COLD LIQUID-FILLED CAPSULES

(Dextromethorphan Hydrobromide, Guaifenesin, Pseudoephedrine Hydrochloride)....... 750
See Robitussin PE Syrup

ROBITUSSIN COUGH, COLD & FLU LIQUID-FILLED CAPSULES

(Acetaminophen, Dextromethorphan Hydrobromide, Guaifenesin, Pseudoephedrine Hydrochloride)................................ 750
May interact with monoamine oxidase inhibitors and certain other agents. Compounds in these categories include:

Isocarboxazid (Concurrent and/or sequential use with MAO inhibitors is not recommended).
No products indexed under this heading.

Moclobemide (Concurrent and/or sequential use with MAO inhibitors is not recommended).
No products indexed under this heading.

Pargyline Hydrochloride (Concurrent and/or sequential use with MAO inhibitors is not recommended).
No products indexed under this heading.

Phenelzine Sulfate (Concurrent and/or sequential use with MAO inhibitors is not recommended).
No products indexed under this heading.

Procarbazine Hydrochloride (Concurrent and/or sequential use with MAO inhibitors is not recommended). Products include:
Matulane Capsules 3188

Selegiline Hydrochloride (Concurrent and/or sequential use with MAO inhibitors is not recommended). Products include:
Eldepryl Capsules 3209

Tranylcypromine Sulfate (Concurrent and/or sequential use with MAO inhibitors is not recommended). Products include:
Parnate Tablets 1499

Food Interactions

Alcohol (Chronic heavy alcohol users, 3 or more drinks per day, should consult their physicians for advice on when and how they should take pain relievers/fever reducers including acetaminophen).

ROBITUSSIN COUGH & COLD INFANT DROPS

(Dextromethorphan Hydrobromide, Guaifenesin, Pseudoephedrine Hydrochloride)....... 755
See Robitussin PE Syrup

ROBITUSSIN COUGH DROPS

(Menthol) 751
None cited in PDR database.

ROBITUSSIN DM INFANT DROPS

(Dextromethorphan Hydrobromide, Guaifenesin).............. 753
See Robitussin DM Liquid

ROBITUSSIN DM LIQUID

(Dextromethorphan Hydrobromide, Guaifenesin).............. 753
May interact with monoamine oxidase inhibitors. Compounds in these categories include:

Isocarboxazid (Concurrent and/or sequential use with MAO inhibitors is not recommended).
No products indexed under this heading.

Moclobemide (Concurrent and/or sequential use with MAO inhibitors is not recommended).
No products indexed under this heading.

Pargyline Hydrochloride (Concurrent and/or sequential use with MAO inhibitors is not recommended).
No products indexed under this heading.

Phenelzine Sulfate (Concurrent and/or sequential use with MAO inhibitors is not recommended).
No products indexed under this heading.

Procarbazine Hydrochloride (Concurrent and/or sequential use with MAO inhibitors is not recommended). Products include:
Matulane Capsules 3188

Selegiline Hydrochloride (Concurrent and/or sequential use with MAO inhibitors is not recommended). Products include:
Eldepryl Capsules 3209

Tranylcypromine Sulfate (Concurrent and/or sequential use with MAO inhibitors is not recommended). Products include:
Parnate Tablets 1499

ROBITUSSIN FLU LIQUID

(Acetaminophen, Chlorpheniramine Maleate, Dextromethorphan Hydrobromide, Pseudoephedrine Hydrochloride)....... 752
May interact with hypnotics and sedatives, monoamine oxidase inhibitors, tranquilizers, and certain other agents. Compounds in these categories include:

Alprazolam (May increase drowsiness). Products include:
Niravam Orally Disintegrating Tablets 3106
Xanax XR Tablets 2655

Buspirone Hydrochloride (May increase drowsiness).
No products indexed under this heading.

Chlordiazepoxide (May increase drowsiness).
No products indexed under this heading.

Chlordiazepoxide Hydrochloride (May increase drowsiness). Products include:
Librium Capsules 3349

Chlorpromazine (May increase drowsiness).
No products indexed under this heading.

Chlorpromazine Hydrochloride (May increase drowsiness).
No products indexed under this heading.

Chlorprothixene (May increase drowsiness).
No products indexed under this heading.

Chlorprothixene Hydrochloride (May increase drowsiness).
No products indexed under this heading.

Clorazepate Dipotassium (May increase drowsiness). Products include:
Tranxene 2488

Diazepam (May increase drowsiness). Products include:
Diastat Rectal Delivery System 3344
Valium Tablets 2822

Droperidol (May increase drowsiness).
No products indexed under this heading.

Estazolam (May increase drowsiness). Products include:
ProSom Tablets 512

Ethchlorvynol (May increase drowsiness).
No products indexed under this heading.

Ethinamate (May increase drowsiness).
No products indexed under this heading.

Fluphenazine Decanoate (May increase drowsiness).
No products indexed under this heading.

Fluphenazine Enanthate (May increase drowsiness).
No products indexed under this heading.

Fluphenazine Hydrochloride (May increase drowsiness).
No products indexed under this heading.

Flurazepam Hydrochloride (May increase drowsiness). Products include:
Dalmane Capsules 3343

Glutethimide (May increase drowsiness).
No products indexed under this heading.

Haloperidol (May increase drowsiness).
No products indexed under this heading.

Haloperidol Decanoate (May increase drowsiness).
No products indexed under this heading.

Hydroxyzine Hydrochloride (May increase drowsiness).
No products indexed under this heading.

Isocarboxazid (Concurrent and/or sequential use with MAO inhibitors is not recommended).
No products indexed under this heading.

Lorazepam (May increase drowsiness).
No products indexed under this heading.

Loxapine Hydrochloride (May increase drowsiness).
No products indexed under this heading.

Loxapine Succinate (May increase drowsiness).
No products indexed under this heading.

Meprobamate (May increase drowsiness).
No products indexed under this heading.

Mesoridazine Besylate (May increase drowsiness).
No products indexed under this heading.

Midazolam Hydrochloride (May increase drowsiness).
No products indexed under this heading.

Moclobemide (Concurrent and/or sequential use with MAO inhibitors is not recommended).
No products indexed under this heading.

Molindone Hydrochloride (May increase drowsiness). Products include:
Moban Tablets 1108

Oxazepam (May increase drowsiness).
No products indexed under this heading.

Pargyline Hydrochloride (Concurrent and/or sequential use with MAO inhibitors is not recommended).
No products indexed under this heading.

Perphenazine (May increase drowsiness).
No products indexed under this heading.

Phenelzine Sulfate (Concurrent and/or sequential use with MAO inhibitors is not recommended).
No products indexed under this heading.

Prazepam (May increase drowsiness).
No products indexed under this heading.

Procarbazine Hydrochloride (Concurrent and/or sequential use with MAO inhibitors is not recommended). Products include:
Matulane Capsules 3188

Prochlorperazine (May increase drowsiness).
No products indexed under this heading.

Promethazine Hydrochloride (May increase drowsiness). Products include:
Phenergan 3438

Propofol (May increase drowsiness). Products include:
Diprivan Injectable Emulsion 676

Quazepam (May increase drowsiness).
No products indexed under this heading.

Secobarbital Sodium (May increase drowsiness).
No products indexed under this heading.

Selegiline Hydrochloride (Concurrent and/or sequential use with MAO inhibitors is not recommended). Products include:
Eldepryl Capsules 3209

Temazepam (May increase drowsiness).
No products indexed under this heading.

Thioridazine Hydrochloride (May increase drowsiness). Products include:
Thioridazine Hydrochloride Tablets 2122

Thiothixene (May increase drowsiness). Products include:
Thiothixene Capsules 2124

Tranylcypromine Sulfate (Concurrent and/or sequential use with MAO inhibitors is not recommended). Products include:
Parnate Tablets 1499

Triazolam (May increase drowsiness).
No products indexed under this heading.

Trifluoperazine Hydrochloride (May increase drowsiness).
No products indexed under this heading.

Zaleplon (May increase drowsiness). Products include:
Sonata Capsules 1686

Zolpidem Tartrate (May increase drowsiness). Products include:
Ambien Tablets 2867

Food Interactions

Alcohol (Chronic heavy alcohol users, 3 or more drinks per day, should consult their physicians for advice on when and how they should take pain relievers/fever reducers including acetaminophen; increases drowsiness effect).

ROBITUSSIN HONEY COUGH DROPS

(Menthol) .... ▣752
None cited in PDR database.

ROBITUSSIN MAXIMUM STRENGTH COUGH LIQUID

(Dextromethorphan Hydrobromide) .... ▣754
See Robitussin Pediatric Cough Liquid

ROBITUSSIN MAXIMUM STRENGTH COUGH & COLD LIQUID

(Dextromethorphan Hydrobromide, Pseudoephedrine Hydrochloride) .... ▣754
May interact with monoamine oxidase inhibitors. Compounds in these categories include:

Isocarboxazid (Concurrent and/or sequential use with MAO inhibitors is not recommended).
No products indexed under this heading.

Moclobemide (Concurrent and/or sequential use with MAO inhibitors is not recommended).
No products indexed under this heading.

Pargyline Hydrochloride (Concurrent and/or sequential use with MAO inhibitors is not recommended).
No products indexed under this heading.

Phenelzine Sulfate (Concurrent and/or sequential use with MAO inhibitors is not recommended).
No products indexed under this heading.

Procarbazine Hydrochloride (Concurrent and/or sequential use with MAO inhibitors is not recommended). Products include:
Matulane Capsules 3188

Selegiline Hydrochloride (Concurrent and/or sequential use with MAO inhibitors is not recommended). Products include:
Eldepryl Capsules 3209

Tranylcypromine Sulfate (Concurrent and/or sequential use with MAO inhibitors is not recommended). Products include:
Parnate Tablets 1499

ROBITUSSIN PE SYRUP

(Guaifenesin, Pseudoephedrine Hydrochloride) .... ▣753
May interact with monoamine oxidase inhibitors. Compounds in these categories include:

Isocarboxazid (Concurrent and/or sequential use with MAO inhibitors is not recommended).
No products indexed under this heading.

Moclobemide (Concurrent and/or sequential use with MAO inhibitors is not recommended).
No products indexed under this heading.

Pargyline Hydrochloride (Concurrent and/or sequential use with MAO inhibitors is not recommended).
No products indexed under this heading.

Phenelzine Sulfate (Concurrent and/or sequential use with MAO inhibitors is not recommended).
No products indexed under this heading.

Procarbazine Hydrochloride (Concurrent and/or sequential use with MAO inhibitors is not recommended). Products include:
Matulane Capsules 3188

Selegiline Hydrochloride (Concurrent and/or sequential use with MAO inhibitors is not recommended). Products include:
Eldepryl Capsules 3209

Tranylcypromine Sulfate (Concurrent and/or sequential use with MAO inhibitors is not recommended). Products include:
Parnate Tablets 1499

ROBITUSSIN PEDIATRIC COUGH LIQUID

(Dextromethorphan Hydrobromide) .... ▣754
May interact with monoamine oxidase inhibitors. Compounds in these categories include:

Isocarboxazid (Concurrent and/or sequential use with MAO inhibitors should be avoided).
No products indexed under this heading.

Moclobemide (Concurrent and/or sequential use with MAO inhibitors should be avoided).
No products indexed under this heading.

Pargyline Hydrochloride (Concurrent and/or sequential use with MAO inhibitors should be avoided).
No products indexed under this heading.

Phenelzine Sulfate (Concurrent and/or sequential use with MAO inhibitors should be avoided).
No products indexed under this heading.

Procarbazine Hydrochloride (Concurrent and/or sequential use with MAO inhibitors should be avoided). Products include:
Matulane Capsules 3188

Selegiline Hydrochloride (Concurrent and/or sequential use with MAO inhibitors should be avoided). Products include:
Eldepryl Capsules 3209

Tranylcypromine Sulfate (Concurrent and/or sequential use with MAO inhibitors should be avoided). Products include:
Parnate Tablets 1499

ROBITUSSIN PEDIATRIC COUGH & COLD LIQUID

(Dextromethorphan Hydrobromide, Pseudoephedrine Hydrochloride) .... ▣754
See Robitussin Maximum Strength Cough & Cold Liquid

ROBITUSSIN PM COUGH & COLD LIQUID

(Chlorpheniramine Maleate, Dextromethorphan Hydrobromide, Pseudoephedrine Hydrochloride) .... ▣752
May interact with hypnotics and sedatives, monoamine oxidase inhibitors, tranquilizers, and certain other agents. Compounds in these categories include:

Alprazolam (May increase drowsiness effect). Products include:
Niravam Orally Disintegrating Tablets 3106
Xanax XR Tablets 2655

Buspirone Hydrochloride (May increase drowsiness effect).
No products indexed under this heading.

Chlordiazepoxide (May increase drowsiness effect).
No products indexed under this heading.

Chlordiazepoxide Hydrochloride (May increase drowsiness effect). Products include:
Librium Capsules 3349

Chlorpromazine (May increase drowsiness effect).
No products indexed under this heading.

Chlorpromazine Hydrochloride (May increase drowsiness effect).
No products indexed under this heading.

Chlorprothixene (May increase drowsiness effect).
No products indexed under this heading.

Chlorprothixene Hydrochloride (May increase drowsiness effect).
No products indexed under this heading.

Clorazepate Dipotassium (May increase drowsiness effect). Products include:
Tranxene 2488

Diazepam (May increase drowsiness effect). Products include:
Diastat Rectal Delivery System 3344
Valium Tablets 2822

Droperidol (May increase drowsiness effect).
No products indexed under this heading.

Estazolam (May increase drowsiness effect). Products include:
ProSom Tablets 512

Ethchlorvynol (May increase drowsiness effect).
No products indexed under this heading.

Ethinamate (May increase drowsiness effect).
No products indexed under this heading.

Fluphenazine Decanoate (May increase drowsiness effect).
No products indexed under this heading.

Fluphenazine Enanthate (May increase drowsiness effect).
No products indexed under this heading.

Fluphenazine Hydrochloride (May increase drowsiness effect).
No products indexed under this heading.

Flurazepam Hydrochloride (May increase drowsiness effect). Products include:
Dalmane Capsules 3343

Glutethimide (May increase drowsiness effect).
No products indexed under this heading.

Haloperidol (May increase drowsiness effect).
No products indexed under this heading.

Haloperidol Decanoate (May increase drowsiness effect).
No products indexed under this heading.

Hydroxyzine Hydrochloride (May increase drowsiness effect).
No products indexed under this heading.

Isocarboxazid (Concurrent and/or sequential use with MAO inhibitors is not recommended).
No products indexed under this heading.

Lorazepam (May increase drowsiness effect).
No products indexed under this heading.

Loxapine Hydrochloride (May increase drowsiness effect).
No products indexed under this heading.

Loxapine Succinate (May increase drowsiness effect).
No products indexed under this heading.

Meprobamate (May increase drowsiness effect).
No products indexed under this heading.

Mesoridazine Besylate (May increase drowsiness effect).
No products indexed under this heading.

Midazolam Hydrochloride (May increase drowsiness effect).
No products indexed under this heading.

Moclobemide (Concurrent and/or sequential use with MAO inhibitors is not recommended).
No products indexed under this heading.

Molindone Hydrochloride (May increase drowsiness effect). Products include:
Moban Tablets 1108

Oxazepam (May increase drowsiness effect).
No products indexed under this heading.

Pargyline Hydrochloride (Concurrent and/or sequential use with MAO inhibitors is not recommended).
No products indexed under this heading.

Perphenazine (May increase drowsiness effect).
No products indexed under this heading.

Phenelzine Sulfate (Concurrent and/or sequential use with MAO inhibitors is not recommended).
No products indexed under this heading.

Prazepam (May increase drowsiness effect).
No products indexed under this heading.

Procarbazine Hydrochloride (Concurrent and/or sequential use with MAO inhibitors is not recommended). Products include:
Matulane Capsules 3188

Prochlorperazine (May increase drowsiness effect).
No products indexed under this heading.

Promethazine Hydrochloride (May increase drowsiness effect). Products include:
Phenergan 3438

Propofol (May increase drowsiness effect). Products include:
Diprivan Injectable Emulsion 676

Quazepam (May increase drowsiness effect).
No products indexed under this heading.

Secobarbital Sodium (May increase drowsiness effect).
No products indexed under this heading.

Selegiline Hydrochloride (Concurrent and/or sequential use with MAO inhibitors is not recommended). Products include:
Eldepryl Capsules 3209

Temazepam (May increase drowsiness effect).
No products indexed under this heading.

Thioridazine Hydrochloride (May increase drowsiness effect). Products include:
Thioridazine Hydrochloride Tablets 2122

Thiothixene (May increase drowsiness effect). Products include:
Thiothixene Capsules 2124

Tranylcypromine Sulfate (Concurrent and/or sequential use with MAO inhibitors is not recommended). Products include:
Parnate Tablets 1499

Triazolam (May increase drowsiness effect).
No products indexed under this heading.

Trifluoperazine Hydrochloride (May increase drowsiness effect).
No products indexed under this heading.

Zaleplon (May increase drowsiness effect). Products include:
Sonata Capsules 1686

Zolpidem Tartrate (May increase drowsiness effect). Products include:
Ambien Tablets 2867

Food Interactions

Alcohol (Chronic heavy alcohol users, 3 or more drinks per day, should consult their physician for advice on when and how they should take pain relievers/ fever reducers including acetaminophen; increases drowsiness effect; avoid alcoholic beverages).

ROBITUSSIN SEVERE CONGESTION LIQUID-FILLED CAPSULES

(Guaifenesin, Pseudoephedrine Hydrochloride) 751
See Robitussin PE Syrup

ROBITUSSIN SUGAR FREE COUGH LIQUID

(Dextromethorphan Hydrobromide, Guaifenesin) 753
May interact with monoamine oxidase inhibitors. Compounds in these categories include:

Isocarboxazid (Concurrent and/or sequential use with MAO inhibitors is not recommended).
No products indexed under this heading.

Moclobemide (Concurrent and/or sequential use with MAO inhibitors is not recommended).
No products indexed under this heading.

Pargyline Hydrochloride (Concurrent and/or sequential use with MAO inhibitors is not recommended).
No products indexed under this heading.

Phenelzine Sulfate (Concurrent and/or sequential use with MAO inhibitors is not recommended).
No products indexed under this heading.

Procarbazine Hydrochloride (Concurrent and/or sequential use with MAO inhibitors is not recommended). Products include:
Matulane Capsules 3188

Selegiline Hydrochloride (Concurrent and/or sequential use with MAO inhibitors is not recommended). Products include:
Eldepryl Capsules 3209

Tranylcypromine Sulfate (Concurrent and/or sequential use with MAO inhibitors is not recommended). Products include:
Parnate Tablets 1499

ROBITUSSIN SUGAR FREE THROAT DROPS

(Menthol) 754
None cited in PDR database.

ROCEPHIN INJECTABLE VIALS, ADD-VANTAGE, GALAXY, BULK

(Ceftriaxone Sodium) 2801
None cited in PDR database.

ROFERON-A INJECTION

(Interferon alfa-2a, Recombinant) 2805
May interact with xanthines and certain other agents. Compounds in these categories include:

Aldesleukin (Co-administration with interleukin-2 may potentiate risks of renal failure). Products include:
Proleukin for Injection 1007

Aminophylline (Co-administration of interferon alfa-2a with theophylline has been reported to reduce the theophylline clearance).
No products indexed under this heading.

Bone Marrow Depressants, unspecified (Caution should be exercised when administered concomitantly with myelosuppressive agents).
No products indexed under this heading.

Dyphylline (Co-administration of interferon alfa-2a with theophylline has been reported to reduce the theophylline clearance).
No products indexed under this heading.

Theophylline (Co-administration of interferon alfa-2a with theophylline has been reported to reduce the theophylline clearance).
No products indexed under this heading.

Theophylline Anhydrous (Co-administration of interferon alfa-2a with theophylline has been reported to reduce the theophylline clearance). Products include:
Uniphyl Tablets 2708

Theophylline Calcium Salicylate (Co-administration of interferon alfa-2a with theophylline has been reported to reduce the theophylline clearance).
No products indexed under this heading.

Theophylline Dihydroxypropyl (Glyceryl) (Co-administration of interferon alfa-2a with theophylline has been reported to reduce the theophylline clearance).
No products indexed under this heading.

Theophylline Ethylenediamine (Co-administration of interferon alfa-2a with theophylline has been reported to reduce the theophylline clearance).
No products indexed under this heading.

Theophylline Sodium Glycinate (Co-administration of interferon alfa-2a with theophylline has been reported to reduce the theophylline clearance).
No products indexed under this heading.

Zidovudine (Co-administration may result in synergistic toxicity, especially hematologic toxicities). Products include:
Combivir Tablets 1373
Retrovir 1533
Retrovir IV Infusion 1537
Trizivir Tablets 1565

MEN'S ROGAINE EXTRA STRENGTH TOPICAL SOLUTION, OCEAN RUSH SCENT AND ORIGINAL UNSCENTED

(Minoxidil) 706
None cited in PDR database.

WOMEN'S ROGAINE TOPICAL SOLUTION, SPRING BLOOM SCENT AND ORIGINAL UNSCENTED

(Minoxidil) 707
None cited in PDR database.

ROLAIDS TABLETS

(Calcium Carbonate, Magnesium Hydroxide) 707
May interact with:

Drugs, Oral, unspecified (Antacids may interact with certain unspecified prescription drugs).

EXTRA STRENGTH ROLAIDS SOFTCHEWS

(Calcium Carbonate) 708
None cited in PDR database.

EXTRA STRENGTH ROLAIDS TABLETS

(Calcium Carbonate, Magnesium Hydroxide) 707
See Rolaids Tablets

ROLAIDS MULTI-SYMPTOM ANTACID & ANTIGAS TABLETS

(Calcium Carbonate, Magnesium Hydroxide, Simethicone) 708
May interact with:

Prescription Drugs, unspecified (Antacids may interact with certain prescription drugs).

ROSAC CREAM WITH SUNSCREENS

(Sodium Sulfacetamide, Sulfur) 3216
None cited in PDR database.

ROZEREM TABLETS

(Ramelteon) 3228
May interact with cytochrome p450 1a2 inducers (selected), cytochrome p450 1a2 inhibitors (selected), cytochrome p450 2c8 inducers (selected), cytochrome p450 2c9 inducers (selected), cytochrome p450 2c9 inhibitors (selected), cytochrome p450 2d6 inducers (selected), cytochrome p450 3a4 inducers (selected), cytochrome p450 3a4 inhibitors (selected), cytochrome p450 3a inducers (selected), and certain other agents. Compounds in these categories include:

Acetazolamide (Ramelteon should be administered with caution in subjects taking strong CYP2C9 inhibitors such as fluconazole).
No products indexed under this heading.

Alatrofloxacin Mesylate (Ramelteon should be administered with caution in subjects taking strong CYP2C9 inhibitors such as fluconazole).
No products indexed under this heading.

Allium sativum (Efficacy may be reduced when ramelteon is used in combination with strong CYP enzyme inducers such as rifampin).
No products indexed under this heading.

Amiodarone Hydrochloride (Ramelteon should be administered with caution in subjects taking strong CYP2C9 inhibitors such as fluconazole). Products include:
Pacerone Tablets 3337

Amprenavir (Ramelteon should be administered with caution in subjects taking strong CYP2C9 inhibitors such as fluconazole). Products include:
Agenerase Capsules 1299
Agenerase Oral Solution 1304

Anastrozole (Ramelteon should be administered with caution in subjects taking strong CYP2C9 inhibitors such as fluconazole). Products include:
Arimidex Tablets 665

Aprepitant (Ramelteon should be administered with caution in subjects taking strong CYP2C9 inhibitors such as fluconazole). Products include:
Emend Capsules 1944

Bendroflumethiazide (Ramelteon should be administered with caution in subjects taking strong CYP2C9 inhibitors such as fluconazole).
No products indexed under this heading.

Betamethasone Acetate (Efficacy may be reduced when ramelteon is used in combination with strong CYP enzyme inducers such as rifampin).
No products indexed under this heading.

Betamethasone Sodium Phosphate (Efficacy may be reduced when ramelteon is used in combination with strong CYP enzyme inducers such as rifampin).
No products indexed under this heading.

Carbamazepine (Efficacy may be reduced when ramelteon is used in combination with strong CYP enzyme inducers such as rifampin). Products include:
Carbatrol Capsules 3174
Equetro Extended-Release Capsules 3178
Tegretol/Tegretol-XR 2278

Chloramphenicol (Ramelteon should be administered with caution in subjects taking strong CYP2C9 inhibitors such as fluconazole).
No products indexed under this heading.

Chlorothiazide (Ramelteon should be administered with caution in subjects taking strong CYP2C9 inhibitors such as fluconazole). Products include:
Aldoclor Tablets 1881
Diuril Oral 1936

Chlorothiazide Sodium (Ramelteon should be administered with caution in subjects taking strong CYP2C9 inhibitors such as fluconazole). Products include:
Diuril Sodium Intravenous 1934

Chlorpropamide (Ramelteon should be administered with caution in subjects taking strong CYP2C9 inhibitors such as fluconazole).
No products indexed under this heading.

Cimetidine (Ramelteon should be administered with caution in subjects taking strong CYP2C9 inhibitors such as fluconazole). Products include:
Tagamet HB 200 Tablets ▣637
Tagamet Tablets 1547

Cimetidine Hydrochloride (Ramelteon should be administered with caution in subjects taking strong CYP2C9 inhibitors such as fluconazole).
No products indexed under this heading.

Ciprofloxacin (Ramelteon should be administered with caution in subjects taking strong CYP2C9 inhibitors such as fluconazole). Products include:
Cipro I.V. 2998
Cipro I.V. Pharmacy Bulk Package 3509
Cipro Oral Suspension 2991
Cipro XR Tablets 3004
Ciprodex Otic Suspension 555

Ciprofloxacin Hydrochloride (Ramelteon should be administered with caution in subjects taking strong CYP2C9 inhibitors such as fluconazole). Products include:
Ciloxan Ophthalmic Ointment 554
Cipro Tablets 2991

Cisplatin (Efficacy may be reduced when ramelteon is used in combination with strong CYP enzyme inducers such as rifampin).
No products indexed under this heading.

Citalopram Hydrobromide (Efficacy may be reduced when ramelteon is used in combination with strong CYP enzyme inducers such as rifampin). Products include:
Celexa 1177

Clarithromycin (Ramelteon should be administered with caution in subjects taking strong CYP2C9 inhibitors such as fluconazole). Products include:
Biaxin/Biaxin XL 402
PREVPAC 3281

Clopidogrel Hydrogen Sulfate (Ramelteon should be administered with caution in subjects taking strong CYP2C9 inhibitors such as fluconazole).
No products indexed under this heading.

Clotrimazole (Ramelteon should be administered with caution in subjects taking strong CYP2C9 inhibitors such as fluconazole). Products include:
Lotrimin 3053
Lotrisone 3054

Cortisone Acetate (Efficacy may be reduced when ramelteon is used in combination with strong CYP enzyme inducers such as rifampin).
No products indexed under this heading.

Cyclosporine (Ramelteon should be administered with caution in subjects taking strong CYP2C9 inhibitors such as fluconazole). Products include:
Gengraf Capsules 458
Neoral Soft Gelatin Capsules 2247
Neoral Oral Solution 2247
Restasis Ophthalmic Emulsion 570
Sandimmune 2259

Dalfopristin (Ramelteon should be administered with caution in subjects taking strong CYP2C9 inhibitors such as fluconazole). Products include:
Synercid I.V. 1690

Danazol (Ramelteon should be administered with caution in subjects taking strong CYP2C9 inhibitors such as fluconazole).
No products indexed under this heading.

Delavirdine Mesylate (Ramelteon should be administered with caution in subjects taking strong CYP2C9 inhibitors such as fluconazole). Products include:
Rescriptor Tablets 2535

Desogestrel (Ramelteon should be administered with caution in subjects taking strong CYP2C9 inhibitors such as fluconazole). Products include:
Ortho-Cept Tablets 2395

Dexamethasone (Efficacy may be reduced when ramelteon is used in combination with strong CYP enzyme inducers such as rifampin). Products include:
Ciprodex Otic Suspension 555
Decadron Tablets 1929
TobraDex Ophthalmic Ointment 558
TobraDex Ophthalmic Suspension 558

Dexamethasone Acetate (Efficacy may be reduced when ramelteon is used in combination with strong CYP enzyme inducers such as rifampin).
No products indexed under this heading.

Dexamethasone Sodium Phosphate (Efficacy may be reduced when ramelteon is used in combination with strong CYP enzyme inducers such as rifampin). Products include:
Decadron Phosphate Injection 1931

Diclofenac Potassium (Ramelteon should be administered with caution in subjects taking strong CYP2C9 inhibitors such as fluconazole). Products include:
Cataflam Tablets 2173

Diclofenac Sodium (Ramelteon should be administered with caution in subjects taking strong CYP2C9 inhibitors such as fluconazole). Products include:
Arthrotec Tablets 3126
Voltaren Ophthalmic Solution 2300
Voltaren Tablets 2298
Voltaren-XR Tablets 2301

Diltiazem Hydrochloride (Ramelteon should be administered with caution in subjects taking strong CYP2C9 inhibitors such as fluconazole). Products include:
Cardizem LA Extended Release Tablets 1699
Tiazac Capsules 1204

Diltiazem Maleate (Ramelteon should be administered with caution in subjects taking strong CYP2C9 inhibitors such as fluconazole).
No products indexed under this heading.

Disulfiram (Ramelteon should be administered with caution in subjects taking strong CYP2C9 inhibitors such as fluconazole). Products include:
Antabuse Tablets 2343

Doxorubicin Hydrochloride (Efficacy may be reduced when ramelteon is used in combination with strong CYP enzyme inducers such as rifampin). Products include:
Adriamycin for Injection, USP 786
Adriamycin Injection, USP 786

Efavirenz (Ramelteon should be administered with caution in subjects taking strong CYP2C9 inhibitors such as fluconazole). Products include:
Sustiva Capsules 957

Enoxacin (Ramelteon should be administered with caution in subjects taking strong CYP2C9 inhibitors such as fluconazole).
No products indexed under this heading.

Erythromycin (Ramelteon should be administered with caution in subjects taking strong CYP2C9 inhibitors such as fluconazole). Products include:
Erygel Topical Gel 2096
Ery-Tab Tablets 447
Erythromycin Base Filmtab Tablets 454
Erythromycin Delayed-Release Capsules, USP 456
PCE Dispertab Tablets 510

Erythromycin Estolate (Ramelteon should be administered with caution in subjects taking strong CYP2C9 inhibitors such as fluconazole).
No products indexed under this heading.

Erythromycin Ethylsuccinate (Ramelteon should be administered with caution in subjects taking strong CYP2C9 inhibitors such as fluconazole). Products include:
E.E.S. 449
EryPed 445

Erythromycin Gluceptate (Ramelteon should be administered with caution in subjects taking strong CYP2C9 inhibitors such as fluconazole).
No products indexed under this heading.

Erythromycin Lactobionate (Ramelteon should be administered with caution in subjects taking strong CYP2C9 inhibitors such as fluconazole).
No products indexed under this heading.

Erythromycin Stearate (Ramelteon should be administered with caution in subjects taking strong CYP2C9 inhibitors such as fluconazole). Products include:
Erythrocin Stearate Filmtab Tablets 452

Esomeprazole Magnesium (Ramelteon should be administered with caution in subjects taking strong CYP2C9 inhibitors such as fluconazole). Products include:
Nexium Delayed-Release Capsules 645

Ethanol (Efficacy may be reduced when ramelteon is used in combination with strong CYP enzyme inducers such as rifampin).
No products indexed under this heading.

Ethinyl Estradiol (Ramelteon should be administered with caution in subjects taking strong CYP2C9 inhibitors such as fluconazole). Products include:
Alesse-28 Tablets 3392
Lo/Ovral-28 Tablets 3423
NuvaRing 2357
Ortho-Cept Tablets 2395
Ortho-Cyclen/Ortho Tri-Cyclen 2414
Ortho Evra Transdermal System 2402
Ortho Tri-Cyclen Lo Tablets 2421
Seasonale Tablets 1073
Triphasil-28 Tablets 3483

Yasmin 28 Tablets **818**

Ethosuximide (Efficacy may be reduced when ramelteon is used in combination with strong CYP enzyme inducers such as rifampin).
No products indexed under this heading.

Felbamate (Efficacy may be reduced when ramelteon is used in combination with strong CYP enzyme inducers such as rifampin).
No products indexed under this heading.

Fenofibrate (Ramelteon should be administered with caution in subjects taking strong CYP2C9 inhibitors such as fluconazole). Products include:
Antara Capsules **2723**
Lofibra Capsules **1217**
Tricor Tablets **523**
Triglide Tablets **1165**

Fluconazole (The total and peak systemic exposure (AUC 0-inf and Cmax) of ramelteon after a single 16 mg dose of ramelteon was increased by approximately 150% when administered with fluconazole. Similar increases were also seen in M-II exposure. Ramelteon should be administered with caution in subjects taking strong CYP2C9 inhibitors such as fluconazole).
No products indexed under this heading.

Fludrocortisone Acetate (Efficacy may be reduced when ramelteon is used in combination with strong CYP enzyme inducers such as rifampin).
No products indexed under this heading.

Fluorouracil (Ramelteon should be administered with caution in subjects taking strong CYP2C9 inhibitors such as fluconazole). Products include:
Carac Cream, 0.5% **1048**
Efudex **3348**

Fluoxetine Hydrochloride (Ramelteon should be administered with caution in subjects taking strong CYP2C9 inhibitors such as fluconazole). Products include:
Prozac Pulvules and Liquid **1771**
Symbyax Capsules **1788**

Flurbiprofen (Ramelteon should be administered with caution in subjects taking strong CYP2C9 inhibitors such as fluconazole).
No products indexed under this heading.

Flurbiprofen Sodium (Ramelteon should be administered with caution in subjects taking strong CYP2C9 inhibitors such as fluconazole). Products include:
Ocufen Ophthalmic Solution .... ⊙**230**

Fluvastatin Sodium (Ramelteon should be administered with caution in subjects taking strong CYP2C9 inhibitors such as fluconazole). Products include:
Lescol Capsules **2227**
Lescol **2730**
Lescol XL Tablets **2227**

Fluvoxamine (When fluvoxamine 100 mg twice daily was administered for 3 days prior to single-dose co-administration of ramelteon 16 mg and fluvoxamine, the AUC 0-inf for ramelteon increased approximately 190-fold, and the Cmax increased approximately 70-fold, compared to ramelteon administered alone. Ramelteon should not be used in combination with fluvoxamine. Other less potent CYP1A2 inhibitors have not been adequately studied. Ramelteon should be administered with caution to patients taking less strong CYP1A2 inhibitors).
No products indexed under this heading.

Fluvoxamine Maleate (Ramelteon should be administered with caution in subjects taking strong CYP2C9 inhibitors such as fluconazole).
No products indexed under this heading.

Fosamprenavir Calcium (Ramelteon should be administered with caution in subjects taking strong CYP2C9 inhibitors such as fluconazole). Products include:
Lexiva Tablets **1473**

Fosphenytoin Sodium (Efficacy may be reduced when ramelteon is used in combination with strong CYP enzyme inducers such as rifampin).
No products indexed under this heading.

Garlic Extract (Efficacy may be reduced when ramelteon is used in combination with strong CYP enzyme inducers such as rifampin).
No products indexed under this heading.

Garlic Oil (Efficacy may be reduced when ramelteon is used in combination with strong CYP enzyme inducers such as rifampin).
No products indexed under this heading.

Gatifloxacin (Ramelteon should be administered with caution in subjects taking strong CYP2C9 inhibitors such as fluconazole). Products include:
Tequin Injection **964**
Tequin Tablets **964**
Zymar Ophthalmic Solution **571**

Gemfibrozil (Ramelteon should be administered with caution in subjects taking strong CYP2C9 inhibitors such as fluconazole).
No products indexed under this heading.

Gemifloxacin Mesylate (Ramelteon should be administered with caution in subjects taking strong CYP2C9 inhibitors such as fluconazole). Products include:
Factive Tablets **2464**

Glipizide (Ramelteon should be administered with caution in subjects taking strong CYP2C9 inhibitors such as fluconazole).
No products indexed under this heading.

Glyburide (Ramelteon should be administered with caution in subjects taking strong CYP2C9 inhibitors such as fluconazole).
No products indexed under this heading.

Grepafloxacin Hydrochloride (Ramelteon should be administered with caution in subjects taking strong CYP2C9 inhibitors such as fluconazole).
No products indexed under this heading.

Hydrochlorothiazide (Ramelteon should be administered with caution in subjects taking strong CYP2C9 inhibitors such as fluconazole). Products include:
Aldoril Tablets **1884**
Atacand HCT **637**
Avalide Tablets **2889**
Avalide Tablets **922**
Benicar HCT Tablets **2852**
Diovan HCT Tablets **2195**
Dyazide Capsules **1389**
Hyzaar **1964**
Lotensin HCT Tablets **2235**
Maxzide **2150**
Micardis HCT Tablets **886**
Moduretic Tablets **2003**
Prinzide Tablets **2033**
Teveten HCT Tablets **1710**
Timolide Tablets **2056**
Uniretic Tablets **3114**
Vaseretic Tablets **2073**
Zestoretic Tablets **701**

Hydrocortisone (Efficacy may be reduced when ramelteon is used in combination with strong CYP enzyme inducers such as rifampin). Products include:
Cortizone•5 Ointment .... ▣**699**
Cortizone•10 Creme .... ▣**699**
Cortizone•10 Ointment .... ▣**699**
Cortizone•10 Plus Creme .... ▣**700**
Cortizone•10 Maximum Strength Quick Shot Spray .... ▣**700**
Hydrocortone Tablets **1963**
Preparation H Hydrocortisone Cream .... ▣**748**

Hydrocortisone Acetate (Efficacy may be reduced when ramelteon is used in combination with strong CYP enzyme inducers such as rifampin). Products include:
Analpram-HC **1136**
Pramosone **1139**
ProctoFoam-HC **3113**
Tucks Anti-Itch Ointment .... ▣**712**
U-cort 1% Cream **3289**

Hydrocortisone Butyrate (Efficacy may be reduced when ramelteon is used in combination with strong CYP enzyme inducers such as rifampin). Products include:
Locoid **1138**
Locoid Lipocream Cream **1138**

Hydrocortisone Cypionate (Efficacy may be reduced when ramelteon is used in combination with strong CYP enzyme inducers such as rifampin).
No products indexed under this heading.

Hydrocortisone Hemisuccinate (Efficacy may be reduced when ramelteon is used in combination with strong CYP enzyme inducers such as rifampin).
No products indexed under this heading.

Hydrocortisone Probutate (Efficacy may be reduced when ramelteon is used in combination with strong CYP enzyme inducers such as rifampin). Products include:
Pandel Cream, 0.1% **1017**

Hydrocortisone Sodium Phosphate (Efficacy may be reduced when ramelteon is used in combination with strong CYP enzyme inducers such as rifampin).
No products indexed under this heading.

Hydrocortisone Sodium Succinate (Efficacy may be reduced when ramelteon is used in combination with strong CYP enzyme inducers such as rifampin).
No products indexed under this heading.

Hydrocortisone Valerate (Efficacy may be reduced when ramelteon is used in combination with strong CYP enzyme inducers such as rifampin).
No products indexed under this heading.

Hydroflumethiazide (Ramelteon should be administered with caution in subjects taking strong CYP2C9 inhibitors such as fluconazole).
No products indexed under this heading.

Hypericum (Efficacy may be reduced when ramelteon is used in combination with strong CYP enzyme inducers such as rifampin).
No products indexed under this heading.

Hypericum Perforatum (Efficacy may be reduced when ramelteon is used in combination with strong CYP enzyme inducers such as rifampin).
No products indexed under this heading.

Imatinib Mesylate (Ramelteon should be administered with caution in subjects taking strong CYP2C9 inhibitors such as fluconazole). Products include:
Gleevec Tablets **2221**

Indinavir Sulfate (Ramelteon should be administered with caution in subjects taking strong CYP2C9 inhibitors such as fluconazole). Products include:
Crixivan Capsules **1918**

Insulin (Efficacy may be reduced when ramelteon is used in combination with strong CYP enzyme inducers such as rifampin).
No products indexed under this heading.

Isoniazid (Ramelteon should be administered with caution in subjects taking strong CYP2C9 inhibitors such as fluconazole).
No products indexed under this heading.

Itraconazole (Ramelteon should be administered with caution in subjects taking strong CYP2C9 inhibitors such as fluconazole).
No products indexed under this heading.

Ketoconazole (The AUC 0-inf and Cmax of ramelteon increased by approximately 84% and 36%, respectively, when a single 16 mg dose of ramelteon was administered on the fourth day of ketoconazole 200 mg twice daily administration, compared to administration of ramelteonalone. Similar increases were seen in M-II pharmacokinetic variables. Ramelteon should be administered with caution in subjects taking strong CYP3A4 inhibitors such as ketoconazole). Products include:
Nizoral A-D Shampoo, 1% **1839**
Nizoral 2% Shampoo **1838**

Ketoprofen (Ramelteon should be administered with caution in subjects taking strong CYP2C9 inhibitors such as fluconazole).
No products indexed under this heading.

Lansoprazole (Efficacy may be reduced when ramelteon is used in combination with strong CYP enzyme inducers such as rifampin). Products include:
Prevacid Delayed-Release Capsules **3268**
Prevacid for Delayed-Release Oral Suspension **3268**
Prevacid I.V. for Injection **3274**
Prevacid NapraPAC **3277**
Prevacid SoluTab Delayed-Release Orally Disintegrating Tablets **3268**
PREVPAC **3281**

Leflunomide (Ramelteon should be administered with caution in subjects taking strong CYP2C9 inhibitors such as fluconazole). Products include:
Arava Tablets **2881**

Levofloxacin (Ramelteon should be administered with caution in subjects taking strong CYP2C9 inhibitors such as fluconazole). Products include:
- Levaquin in 5% Dextrose Injection 2453
- Levaquin 2453
- Quixin Ophthalmic Solution 3373

Levonorgestrel (Ramelteon should be administered with caution in subjects taking strong CYP2C9 inhibitors such as fluconazole). Products include:
- Alesse-28 Tablets 3392
- Climara Pro Transdermal System 800
- Mirena Intrauterine System 810
- Plan B Tablets 1068
- Seasonale Tablets 1073
- Triphasil-28 Tablets 3483

Lomefloxacin Hydrochloride (Ramelteon should be administered with caution in subjects taking strong CYP2C9 inhibitors such as fluconazole).
No products indexed under this heading.

Lopinavir (Ramelteon should be administered with caution in subjects taking strong CYP2C9 inhibitors such as fluconazole). Products include:
- Kaletra 474

Loratadine (Ramelteon should be administered with caution in subjects taking strong CYP2C9 inhibitors such as fluconazole). Products include:
- Alavert Allergy & Sinus D-12 Hour Tablets .... ▣743
- Alavert .... ▣743
- Children's Claritin 24 Hour Non-Drowsy Allergy Syrup .... ▣732
- Claritin Non-Drowsy 24 Hour Tablets .... ▣731
- Non-Drowsy Claritin Hives Relief Tablets .... ▣733
- Claritin Reditabs 24 Hour Non-Drowsy Tablets .... ▣732
- Claritin-D Non-Drowsy 12 Hour Tablets .... ▣731
- Claritin-D Non-Drowsy 24 Hour Tablets .... ▣731
- Children's Dimetapp ND Non-Drowsy Allergy Syrup .... ▣746
- Triaminic Allerchews .... ▣684

Lovastatin (Ramelteon should be administered with caution in subjects taking strong CYP2C9 inhibitors such as fluconazole). Products include:
- Advicor Tablets 1694
- Altoprev Extended-Release Tablets 1151
- Mevacor Tablets 1996

Mephenytoin (Efficacy may be reduced when ramelteon is used in combination with strong CYP enzyme inducers such as rifampin).
No products indexed under this heading.

Mestranol (Ramelteon should be administered with caution in subjects taking strong CYP2C9 inhibitors such as fluconazole).
No products indexed under this heading.

Methoxsalen (Ramelteon should be administered with caution in subjects taking strong CYP2C9 inhibitors such as fluconazole). Products include:
- Oxsoralen Lotion 1% 3354
- Oxsoralen-Ultra Capsules 3354

Methsuximide (Efficacy may be reduced when ramelteon is used in combination with strong CYP enzyme inducers such as rifampin).
No products indexed under this heading.

Methyclothiazide (Ramelteon should be administered with caution in subjects taking strong CYP2C9 inhibitors such as fluconazole).
No products indexed under this heading.

Methylprednisolone (Efficacy may be reduced when ramelteon is used in combination with strong CYP enzyme inducers such as rifampin).
No products indexed under this heading.

Methylprednisolone Acetate (Efficacy may be reduced when ramelteon is used in combination with strong CYP enzyme inducers such as rifampin). Products include:
- Depo-Medrol Injectable Suspension 2615
- Depo-Medrol Single-Dose Vial 2617

Methylprednisolone Sodium Succinate (Efficacy may be reduced when ramelteon is used in combination with strong CYP enzyme inducers such as rifampin).
No products indexed under this heading.

Metronidazole (Ramelteon should be administered with caution in subjects taking strong CYP2C9 inhibitors such as fluconazole). Products include:
- Metrogel 1% 1212
- MetroGel-Vaginal Gel 1822
- Noritate Cream, 1% 1051

Metronidazole Benzoate (Ramelteon should be administered with caution in subjects taking strong CYP2C9 inhibitors such as fluconazole).
No products indexed under this heading.

Metronidazole Hydrochloride (Ramelteon should be administered with caution in subjects taking strong CYP2C9 inhibitors such as fluconazole).
No products indexed under this heading.

Mexiletine Hydrochloride (Ramelteon should be administered with caution in subjects taking strong CYP2C9 inhibitors such as fluconazole).
No products indexed under this heading.

Mibefradil Dihydrochloride (Ramelteon should be administered with caution in subjects taking strong CYP2C9 inhibitors such as fluconazole).
No products indexed under this heading.

Miconazole (Ramelteon should be administered with caution in subjects taking strong CYP2C9 inhibitors such as fluconazole).
No products indexed under this heading.

Miconazole Nitrate (Ramelteon should be administered with caution in subjects taking strong CYP2C9 inhibitors such as fluconazole). Products include:
- Desenex .... ▣674
- Desenex Jock Itch Spray Powder .... ▣674

Modafinil (Ramelteon should be administered with caution in subjects taking strong CYP2C9 inhibitors such as fluconazole). Products include:
- Provigil Tablets 1002

Moxifloxacin Hydrochloride (Ramelteon should be administered with caution in subjects taking strong CYP2C9 inhibitors such as fluconazole). Products include:
- Avelox 2984
- Vigamox Ophthalmic Solution 560

Nafcillin Sodium (Efficacy may be reduced when ramelteon is used in combination with strong CYP enzyme inducers such as rifampin).
No products indexed under this heading.

Nalidixic Acid (Ramelteon should be administered with caution in subjects taking strong CYP2C9 inhibitors such as fluconazole).
No products indexed under this heading.

Nefazodone Hydrochloride (Ramelteon should be administered with caution in subjects taking strong CYP2C9 inhibitors such as fluconazole).
No products indexed under this heading.

Nelfinavir Mesylate (Ramelteon should be administered with caution in subjects taking strong CYP2C9 inhibitors such as fluconazole). Products include:
- Viracept 2556

Nevirapine (Ramelteon should be administered with caution in subjects taking strong CYP2C9 inhibitors such as fluconazole). Products include:
- Viramune Oral Suspension 903
- Viramune Tablets 903

Niacinamide (Ramelteon should be administered with caution in subjects taking strong CYP2C9 inhibitors such as fluconazole).
No products indexed under this heading.

Nicotinamide (Ramelteon should be administered with caution in subjects taking strong CYP2C9 inhibitors such as fluconazole). Products include:
- Nicomide Tablets 3190

Nicotine (Efficacy may be reduced when ramelteon is used in combination with strong CYP enzyme inducers such as rifampin). Products include:
- Nicoderm CQ Patch 1629
- NicoDerm CQ Clear Patch .... ▣627
- Nicotrol Inhaler 2594
- Nicotrol NS 2596

Nicotine Polacrilex (Efficacy may be reduced when ramelteon is used in combination with strong CYP enzyme inducers such as rifampin). Products include:
- Commit Lozenges 1625
- Nicorette Gum 1632

Nicotine Salicylate (Efficacy may be reduced when ramelteon is used in combination with strong CYP enzyme inducers such as rifampin).
No products indexed under this heading.

Nicotine Sulfate (Efficacy may be reduced when ramelteon is used in combination with strong CYP enzyme inducers such as rifampin).
No products indexed under this heading.

Nifedipine (Ramelteon should be administered with caution in subjects taking strong CYP2C9 inhibitors such as fluconazole). Products include:
- Adalat CC Tablets 2978

Norethindrone (Ramelteon should be administered with caution in subjects taking strong CYP2C9 inhibitors such as fluconazole). Products include:
- Ortho Micronor Tablets 2411

Norfloxacin (Ramelteon should be administered with caution in subjects taking strong CYP2C9 inhibitors such as fluconazole). Products include:
- Noroxin Tablets 2009

Norgestrel (Ramelteon should be administered with caution in subjects taking strong CYP2C9 inhibitors such as fluconazole). Products include:
- Lo/Ovral-28 Tablets 3423

Ofloxacin (Ramelteon should be administered with caution in subjects taking strong CYP2C9 inhibitors such as fluconazole). Products include:
- Floxin Otic Singles 1045
- Floxin Otic Solution 1043

Omeprazole (Ramelteon should be administered with caution in subjects taking strong CYP2C9 inhibitors such as fluconazole). Products include:
- Zegerid Powder for Oral Solution 2972

Oxcarbazepine (Efficacy may be reduced when ramelteon is used in combination with strong CYP enzyme inducers such as rifampin). Products include:
- Trileptal Oral Suspension 2281
- Trileptal Tablets 2281

Oxiconazole Nitrate (Ramelteon should be administered with caution in subjects taking strong CYP2C9 inhibitors such as fluconazole). Products include:
- Oxistat 1498

Paroxetine Hydrochloride (Ramelteon should be administered with caution in subjects taking strong CYP2C9 inhibitors such as fluconazole). Products include:
- Paxil CR Controlled-Release Tablets 1509
- Paxil 1501

Phenobarbital (Efficacy may be reduced when ramelteon is used in combination with strong CYP enzyme inducers such as rifampin).
No products indexed under this heading.

Phenobarbital Sodium (Efficacy may be reduced when ramelteon is used in combination with strong CYP enzyme inducers such as rifampin).
No products indexed under this heading.

Phenylbutazone (Ramelteon should be administered with caution in subjects taking strong CYP2C9 inhibitors such as fluconazole).
No products indexed under this heading.

Phenytoin (Efficacy may be reduced when ramelteon is used in combination with strong CYP enzyme inducers such as rifampin).
No products indexed under this heading.

Phenytoin Sodium (Efficacy may be reduced when ramelteon is used in combination with strong CYP enzyme inducers such as rifampin). Products include:
- Phenytek Capsules 2153

Polythiazide (Ramelteon should be administered with caution in subjects taking strong CYP2C9 inhibitors such as fluconazole).
No products indexed under this heading.

Prednisolone Acetate (Efficacy may be reduced when ramelteon is used in combination with strong CYP enzyme inducers such as rifampin). Products include:

Blephamide Ophthalmic Ointment 563
Blephamide Ophthalmic Suspension 564
Poly-Pred Liquifilm Ophthalmic Suspension .... ⊙231
Pred Forte Ophthalmic Suspension .... ⊙233
Pred Mild Sterile Ophthalmic Suspension .... ⊙236
Pred-G Ophthalmic Suspension .... ⊙234
Pred-G Sterile Ophthalmic Ointment .... ⊙235

Prednisolone Sodium Phosphate (Efficacy may be reduced when ramelteon is used in combination with strong CYP enzyme inducers such as rifampin). Products include:
Pediapred Oral Solution 3319

Prednisolone Tebutate (Efficacy may be reduced when ramelteon is used in combination with strong CYP enzyme inducers such as rifampin).
No products indexed under this heading.

Prednisone (Efficacy may be reduced when ramelteon is used in combination with strong CYP enzyme inducers such as rifampin).
No products indexed under this heading.

Primidone (Efficacy may be reduced when ramelteon is used in combination with strong CYP enzyme inducers such as rifampin).
No products indexed under this heading.

Propoxyphene Hydrochloride (Ramelteon should be administered with caution in subjects taking strong CYP2C9 inhibitors such as fluconazole).
No products indexed under this heading.

Propoxyphene Napsylate (Ramelteon should be administered with caution in subjects taking strong CYP2C9 inhibitors such as fluconazole). Products include:
Darvocet A 500 Tablets 3497

Quinidine (Ramelteon should be administered with caution in subjects taking strong CYP2C9 inhibitors such as fluconazole).
No products indexed under this heading.

Quinidine Hydrochloride (Ramelteon should be administered with caution in subjects taking strong CYP2C9 inhibitors such as fluconazole).
No products indexed under this heading.

Quinidine Polygalacturonate (Ramelteon should be administered with caution in subjects taking strong CYP2C9 inhibitors such as fluconazole).
No products indexed under this heading.

Quinidine Sulfate (Ramelteon should be administered with caution in subjects taking strong CYP2C9 inhibitors such as fluconazole).
No products indexed under this heading.

Quinine (Ramelteon should be administered with caution in subjects taking strong CYP2C9 inhibitors such as fluconazole).
No products indexed under this heading.

Quinine Sulfate (Ramelteon should be administered with caution in subjects taking strong CYP2C9 inhibitors such as fluconazole).
No products indexed under this heading.

Quinupristin (Ramelteon should be administered with caution in subjects taking strong CYP2C9 inhibitors such as fluconazole). Products include:
Synercid I.V. 1690

Ranitidine Bismuth Citrate (Ramelteon should be administered with caution in subjects taking strong CYP2C9 inhibitors such as fluconazole).
No products indexed under this heading.

Ranitidine Hydrochloride (Ramelteon should be administered with caution in subjects taking strong CYP2C9 inhibitors such as fluconazole). Products include:
Zantac 1597
Zantac Injection 1593
Zantac 75 Tablets 715
Zantac 150 Maximum Strength Tablets 715
Zantac Injection Pharmacy Bulk Package 1595

Rifabutin (Efficacy may be reduced when ramelteon is used in combination with strong CYP enzyme inducers such as rifampin).
No products indexed under this heading.

Rifampicin (Efficacy may be reduced when ramelteon is used in combination with strong CYP enzyme inducers such as rifampin).
No products indexed under this heading.

Rifampin (Administration of rifampin 600 mg once daily for 11 days resulted in a mean decrease of approximately 80% (40% to 90%) in total exposure to ramelteon and metabolite M-II, (both AUC 0-inf and Cmax) after a single 32 mg dose of ramelteon. Efficacy may be reduced when ramelteon is used in combination with strong CYP enzyme inducers such as rifampin).
No products indexed under this heading.

Rifapentine (Efficacy may be reduced when ramelteon is used in combination with strong CYP enzyme inducers such as rifampin).
No products indexed under this heading.

Ritonavir (Ramelteon should be administered with caution in subjects taking strong CYP2C9 inhibitors such as fluconazole). Products include:
Kaletra 474
Norvir 499

Saquinavir (Ramelteon should be administered with caution in subjects taking strong CYP2C9 inhibitors such as fluconazole).
No products indexed under this heading.

Saquinavir Mesylate (Ramelteon should be administered with caution in subjects taking strong CYP2C9 inhibitors such as fluconazole). Products include:
Invirase 2776

Secobarbital Sodium (Efficacy may be reduced when ramelteon is used in combination with strong CYP enzyme inducers such as rifampin).
No products indexed under this heading.

Sertraline Hydrochloride (Ramelteon should be administered with caution in subjects taking strong CYP2C9 inhibitors such as fluconazole). Products include:
Zoloft 2581

Sparfloxacin (Ramelteon should be administered with caution in subjects taking strong CYP2C9 inhibitors such as fluconazole).
No products indexed under this heading.

Sulfacytine (Ramelteon should be administered with caution in subjects taking strong CYP2C9 inhibitors such as fluconazole).
No products indexed under this heading.

Sulfamethizole (Ramelteon should be administered with caution in subjects taking strong CYP2C9 inhibitors such as fluconazole).
No products indexed under this heading.

Sulfamethoxazole (Ramelteon should be administered with caution in subjects taking strong CYP2C9 inhibitors such as fluconazole).
No products indexed under this heading.

Sulfasalazine (Ramelteon should be administered with caution in subjects taking strong CYP2C9 inhibitors such as fluconazole).
No products indexed under this heading.

Sulfinpyrazone (Ramelteon should be administered with caution in subjects taking strong CYP2C9 inhibitors such as fluconazole).
No products indexed under this heading.

Sulfisoxazole (Ramelteon should be administered with caution in subjects taking strong CYP2C9 inhibitors such as fluconazole).
No products indexed under this heading.

Sulfisoxazole Acetyl (Ramelteon should be administered with caution in subjects taking strong CYP2C9 inhibitors such as fluconazole).
No products indexed under this heading.

Sulfisoxazole Diolamine (Ramelteon should be administered with caution in subjects taking strong CYP2C9 inhibitors such as fluconazole).
No products indexed under this heading.

Tacrine Hydrochloride (Ramelteon should be administered with caution in subjects taking strong CYP2C9 inhibitors such as fluconazole).
No products indexed under this heading.

Telithromycin (Ramelteon should be administered with caution in subjects taking strong CYP2C9 inhibitors such as fluconazole). Products include:
Ketek Tablets 2920

Terconazole (Ramelteon should be administered with caution in subjects taking strong CYP2C9 inhibitors such as fluconazole).
No products indexed under this heading.

Theophylline (Efficacy may be reduced when ramelteon is used in combination with strong CYP enzyme inducers such as rifampin).
No products indexed under this heading.

Ticlopidine Hydrochloride (Ramelteon should be administered with caution in subjects taking strong CYP2C9 inhibitors such as fluconazole). Products include:
Ticlid Tablets 2813

Tobacco (Efficacy may be reduced when ramelteon is used in combination with strong CYP enzyme inducers such as rifampin).
No products indexed under this heading.

Tolazamide (Ramelteon should be administered with caution in subjects taking strong CYP2C9 inhibitors such as fluconazole).
No products indexed under this heading.

Tolbutamide (Ramelteon should be administered with caution in subjects taking strong CYP2C9 inhibitors such as fluconazole).
No products indexed under this heading.

Tolbutamide Sodium (Ramelteon should be administered with caution in subjects taking strong CYP2C9 inhibitors such as fluconazole).
No products indexed under this heading.

Triamcinolone (Efficacy may be reduced when ramelteon is used in combination with strong CYP enzyme inducers such as rifampin).
No products indexed under this heading.

Triamcinolone Acetonide (Efficacy may be reduced when ramelteon is used in combination with strong CYP enzyme inducers such as rifampin). Products include:
Azmacort Inhalation Aerosol 1701
Nasacort HFA Inhalation Aerosol 2939
Nasacort AQ Nasal Spray 2937

Triamcinolone Diacetate (Efficacy may be reduced when ramelteon is used in combination with strong CYP enzyme inducers such as rifampin).
No products indexed under this heading.

Triamcinolone Hexacetonide (Efficacy may be reduced when ramelteon is used in combination with strong CYP enzyme inducers such as rifampin).
No products indexed under this heading.

Troglitazone (Ramelteon should be administered with caution in subjects taking strong CYP2C9 inhibitors such as fluconazole).
No products indexed under this heading.

Troleandomycin (Ramelteon should be administered with caution in subjects taking strong CYP2C9 inhibitors such as fluconazole).
No products indexed under this heading.

Trovafloxacin Mesylate (Ramelteon should be administered with caution in subjects taking strong CYP2C9 inhibitors such as fluconazole).
No products indexed under this heading.

Valproate Sodium (Ramelteon should be administered with caution in subjects taking strong CYP2C9 inhibitors such as fluconazole). Products include:
Depacon Injection 412

Verapamil Hydrochloride (Ramelteon should be administered with caution in subjects taking strong CYP2C9 inhibitors such as fluconazole). Products include:
Covera-HS Tablets 3135
Tarka Tablets 519
Verelan PM Capsules 3120

IMPORTANT NOTE: Always consult each drug listing in the patient's regimen for possible interactions.

Voriconazole (Ramelteon should be administered with caution in subjects taking strong CYP2C9 inhibitors such as fluconazole). Products include:

VFEND I.V. 2543
VFEND Oral Suspension 2543
VFEND Tablets 2543

Zafirlukast (Ramelteon should be administered with caution in subjects taking strong CYP2C9 inhibitors such as fluconazole). Products include:

Accolate Tablets 663

Zileuton (Ramelteon should be administered with caution in subjects taking strong CYP2C9 inhibitors such as fluconazole).

No products indexed under this heading.

Food Interactions

Alcohol (With single-dose, daytime co-administration of ramelteon 32 mg and alcohol (0.6 g/kg), there were no clinically meaningful or statistically significant effects on peak or total exposure to ramelteon. However, an additive effect was seen on some measures of psychomotor performance (ie. the Digit Symbol Substitution Test, the Psychomotor Vigilance Task Test, and a Visual Analog Scale of sedation) at some post-dose time points. No additive effect was seen on the Delayed Word Recognition Test. Because alcohol by itself impairs performance, and the intended effect of ramelteon is to promote sleep, patients should be cautioned not to consume alcohol when using ramelteon).

Broccoli (Efficacy may be reduced when ramelteon is used in combination with strong CYP enzyme inducers such as rifampin).

Brussel Sprouts (Efficacy may be reduced when ramelteon is used in combination with strong CYP enzyme inducers such as rifampin).

Charbroiled Food (Efficacy may be reduced when ramelteon is used in combination with strong CYP enzyme inducers such as rifampin).

Grapefruit (Ramelteon should be administered with caution in subjects taking strong CYP2C9 inhibitors such as fluconazole).

Grapefruit Juice (Ramelteon should be administered with caution in subjects taking strong CYP2C9 inhibitors such as fluconazole).

RYTHMOL SR CAPSULES

(Propafenone Hydrochloride) 2736

May interact with class 1A antiarrhythmics, class III antiarrhythmics, cytochrome p450 1a2 inhibitors (selected), cytochrome p450 2d6 inhibitors (selected), cytochrome p450 3a4 inhibitors (selected), cardiac glycosides, local anesthetics, macrolide antibiotics, drugs that prolong the QT interval, quinidine, xanthines, and certain other agents. Compounds in these categories include:

Acetazolamide (Drugs that inhibit CYP3A4 might lead to increased plasma levels of propafenone; patients should be closely monitored and the propafenone dose adjusted accordingly).

No products indexed under this heading.

Alatrofloxacin Mesylate (Drugs that inhibit CYP1A2 might lead to increased plasma levels of propafenone; patients should be closely monitored and the propafenone dose adjusted accordingly).

No products indexed under this heading.

Aminophylline (Combined therapy may result in an increase in theophylline concentration with the development of theophylline toxicity).

No products indexed under this heading.

Amiodarone Hydrochloride (The use of propafenone in conjunction with other drugs that prolong the QT interval has not been extensively studied and is not recommended). Products include:

Pacerone Tablets 3337

Amitriptyline Hydrochloride (The use of propafenone in conjunction with other drugs that prolong the QT interval has not been extensively studied and is not recommended).

No products indexed under this heading.

Amoxapine (The use of propafenone in conjunction with other drugs that prolong the QT interval has not been extensively studied and is not recommended).

No products indexed under this heading.

Amprenavir (Drugs that inhibit CYP3A4 might lead to increased plasma levels of propafenone; patients should be closely monitored and the propafenone dose adjusted accordingly). Products include:

Agenerase Capsules 1299
Agenerase Oral Solution 1304

Anastrozole (Drugs that inhibit CYP1A2 might lead to increased plasma levels of propafenone; patients should be closely monitored and the propafenone dose adjusted accordingly). Products include:

Arimidex Tablets 665

Aprepitant (Drugs that inhibit CYP3A4 might lead to increased plasma levels of propafenone; patients should be closely monitored and the propafenone dose adjusted accordingly). Products include:

Emend Capsules 1944

Astemizole (The use of propafenone in conjunction with other drugs that prolong the QT interval has not been extensively studied and is not recommended).

No products indexed under this heading.

Azithromycin Dihydrate (The use of propafenone in conjunction with other drugs that prolong the QT interval has not been extensively studied and is not recommended). Products include:

Zithromax 2568
Zithromax for IV Infusion 2573
Zithromax for Oral Suspension, 300 mg, 600 mg, 900 mg, 1200 mg 2561
Zithromax Tablets, 250 mg, 500 mg 2561
Zithromax Tri-Pak 2561
Zithromax Z-Pak 2568

Bepridil Hydrochloride (The use of propafenone in conjunction with other drugs that prolong the QT interval has not been extensively studied and is not recommended).

No products indexed under this heading.

Bretylium Tosylate (The use of propafenone in conjunction with other drugs that prolong the QT interval has not been extensively studied and is not recommended).

No products indexed under this heading.

Bupivacaine Hydrochloride (Concomitant use of local anesthetics may increase the risk of CNS side effects).

No products indexed under this heading.

Bupropion Hydrochloride (Drugs that inhibit CYP2D6 might lead to increased plasma levels of propafenone; patients should be closely monitored and the propafenone dose adjusted accordingly). Products include:

Wellbutrin Tablets 1579
Wellbutrin SR Sustained-Release Tablets 1583
Wellbutrin XL Extended-Release Tablets 1588
Zyban Sustained-Release Tablets 1620

Celecoxib (Drugs that inhibit CYP2D6 might lead to increased plasma levels of propafenone; patients should be closely monitored and the propafenone dose adjusted accordingly). Products include:

Celebrex Capsules 3130

Chloroprocaine Hydrochloride (Concomitant use of local anesthetics may increase the risk of CNS side effects).

No products indexed under this heading.

Chloroquine Hydrochloride (Drugs that inhibit CYP2D6 might lead to increased plasma levels of propafenone; patients should be closely monitored and the propafenone dose adjusted accordingly).

No products indexed under this heading.

Chloroquine Phosphate (Drugs that inhibit CYP2D6 might lead to increased plasma levels of propafenone; patients should be closely monitored and the propafenone dose adjusted accordingly).

No products indexed under this heading.

Chlorpheniramine (Drugs that inhibit CYP2D6 might lead to increased plasma levels of propafenone; patients should be closely monitored and the propafenone dose adjusted accordingly).

No products indexed under this heading.

Chlorpheniramine Maleate (Drugs that inhibit CYP2D6 might lead to increased plasma levels of propafenone; patients should be closely monitored and the propafenone dose adjusted accordingly). Products include:

Advil Allergy Sinus Caplets .... ▣ 737
Advil Multi-Symptom Cold Caplets .... ▣ 738
BC Allergy Sinus Cold Powder .... ▣ 612
Contac Severe Cold and Flu Caplets Maximum Strength .... ▣ 615
Hycomine Compound Tablets 1105
PediaCare Multi-Symptom Cold Liquid .... ▣ 704
PediaCare NightRest Cough & Cold Liquid .... ▣ 704
Robitussin Flu Liquid .... ▣ 752
Robitussin PM Cough & Cold Liquid .... ▣ 752
Singlet Caplets .... ▣ 636
Sudafed Sinus & Allergy Tablets .... ▣ 710
TheraFlu Cold & Cough Hot Liquid .... ▣ 680
TheraFlu Cold & Sore Throat Hot Liquid .... ▣ 680
TheraFlu Flu & Sore Throat Hot Liquid .... ▣ 681
TheraFlu Severe Cold & Cough Hot Liquid .... ▣ 683
TheraFlu Severe Cold Caplets .... ▣ 679
TheraFlu Severe Cold Hot Liquid .... ▣ 682
Triaminic Cold & Allergy Liquid .... ▣ 685
Triaminic Cold & Cough Liquid .... ▣ 685
Triaminic Flu, Cough & Fever Liquid .... ▣ 685
Triaminic Night Time Cough & Cold Liquid .... ▣ 685
Triaminic Allergy Runny Nose & Congestion Softchews .... ▣ 688
Triaminic Cold & Cough Softchews .... ▣ 688
Children's Tylenol Plus Cold NightTime Suspension Liquid 1851
Children's Tylenol Plus Cold & Cough Suspension Liquid and Chewable Tablets 1851
Children's Tylenol Plus Cold Chewable Tablets 1851
Children's Tylenol Plus Flu Suspension Liquid 1853
Tylenol Allergy Complete Multi-Symptom Caplets and Gelcaps with Cool Burst 1844
Multi-Symptom Tylenol Cold Night Time Caplets 1845
Vicks 44M Cough, Cold & Flu Relief 2676
Pediatric Vicks 44m Cough & Cold Relief 2673
Children's Vicks NyQuil Cold/Cough Relief 2671

Chlorpheniramine Polistirex (Drugs that inhibit CYP2D6 might lead to increased plasma levels of propafenone; patients should be closely monitored and the propafenone dose adjusted accordingly). Products include:

Tussionex Pennkinetic Extended-Release Suspension 3322

Chlorpheniramine Tannate (Drugs that inhibit CYP2D6 might lead to increased plasma levels of propafenone; patients should be closely monitored and the propafenone dose adjusted accordingly).

No products indexed under this heading.

Chlorpromazine (The use of propafenone in conjunction with other drugs that prolong the QT interval has not been extensively studied and is not recommended).

No products indexed under this heading.

Chlorpromazine Hydrochloride (The use of propafenone in conjunction with other drugs that prolong the QT interval has not been extensively studied and is not recommended).

No products indexed under this heading.

Cimetidine (Increases steady-state plasma concentrations with no detectable changes in electrocardiographic parameters). Products include:

Tagamet HB 200 Tablets .... ▣ 637
Tagamet Tablets 1547

Cimetidine Hydrochloride (Increases steady-state plasma concentrations with no detectable changes in electrocardiographic parameters).

No products indexed under this heading.

Ciprofloxacin (Drugs that inhibit CYP1A2 might lead to increased plasma levels of propafenone; patients should be closely monitored and the propafenone dose adjusted accordingly). Products include:

Cipro I.V. 2998
Cipro I.V. Pharmacy Bulk Package 3509
Cipro Oral Suspension 2991
Cipro XR Tablets 3004
Ciprodex Otic Suspension 555

Ciprofloxacin Hydrochloride (Drugs that inhibit CYP1A2 might lead to increased plasma levels of propafenone; patients should be closely monitored and the propafenone dose adjusted accordingly). Products include:
Ciloxan Ophthalmic Ointment 554
Cipro Tablets 2991

Cisapride (The use of propafenone in conjunction with other drugs that prolong the QT interval has not been extensively studied and is not recommended).
No products indexed under this heading.

Citalopram Hydrobromide (Drugs that inhibit CYP2D6 might lead to increased plasma levels of propafenone; patients should be closely monitored and the propafenone dose adjusted accordingly). Products include:
Celexa 1177

Clarithromycin (The use of propafenone in conjunction with other drugs that prolong the QT interval has not been extensively studied and is not recommended). Products include:
Biaxin/Biaxin XL 402
PREVPAC 3281

Clomipramine Hydrochloride (The use of propafenone in conjunction with other drugs that prolong the QT interval has not been extensively studied and is not recommended).
No products indexed under this heading.

Clotrimazole (Drugs that inhibit CYP3A4 might lead to increased plasma levels of propafenone; patients should be closely monitored and the propafenone dose adjusted accordingly). Products include:
Lotrimin 3053
Lotrisone 3054

Cocaine Hydrochloride (Drugs that inhibit CYP2D6 might lead to increased plasma levels of propafenone; patients should be closely monitored and the propafenone dose adjusted accordingly).
No products indexed under this heading.

Cyclosporine (Propafenone therapy may increase levels of cyclosporine). Products include:
Gengraf Capsules 458
Neoral Soft Gelatin Capsules 2247
Neoral Oral Solution 2247
Restasis Ophthalmic Emulsion 570
Sandimmune 2259

Dalfopristin (Drugs that inhibit CYP3A4 might lead to increased plasma levels of propafenone; patients should be closely monitored and the propafenone dose adjusted accordingly). Products include:
Synercid I.V. 1690

Danazol (Drugs that inhibit CYP3A4 might lead to increased plasma levels of propafenone; patients should be closely monitored and the propafenone dose adjusted accordingly).
No products indexed under this heading.

Delavirdine Mesylate (Drugs that inhibit CYP3A4 might lead to increased plasma levels of propafenone; patients should be closely monitored and the propafenone dose adjusted accordingly). Products include:
Rescriptor Tablets 2535

Desipramine Hydrochloride (Coadministration may result in elevated serum desipramine levels).
No products indexed under this heading.

Deslanoside (Potential for elevated digoxin levels; dosage reduction of digitalis may be necessary).
No products indexed under this heading.

Desogestrel (Drugs that inhibit CYP1A2 might lead to increased plasma levels of propafenone; patients should be closely monitored and the propafenone dose adjusted accordingly). Products include:
Ortho-Cept Tablets 2395

Digitalis Glycoside Preparations (Potential for elevated digoxin levels; dosage reduction of digitalis may be necessary).
No products indexed under this heading.

Digitoxin (Potential for elevated digoxin levels; dosage reduction of digitalis may be necessary).
No products indexed under this heading.

Digoxin (Potential for elevated digoxin levels; dosage reduction of digitalis may be necessary). Products include:
Digitek Tablets 2146
Lanoxicaps Capsules 1458
Lanoxin Injection 1462
Lanoxin Tablets 1468
Lanoxin Injection Pediatric 1465

Diltiazem Hydrochloride (Drugs that inhibit CYP3A4 might lead to increased plasma levels of propafenone; patients should be closely monitored and the propafenone dose adjusted accordingly). Products include:
Cardizem LA Extended Release Tablets 1699
Tiazac Capsules 1204

Diltiazem Maleate (Drugs that inhibit CYP3A4 might lead to increased plasma levels of propafenone; patients should be closely monitored and the propafenone dose adjusted accordingly).
No products indexed under this heading.

Diphenhydramine (Drugs that inhibit CYP2D6 might lead to increased plasma levels of propafenone; patients should be closely monitored and the propafenone dose adjusted accordingly). Products include:
Tylenol Sore Throat NightTime Liquid with Cool Burst 1849

Diphenhydramine Hydrochloride (Drugs that inhibit CYP2D6 might lead to increased plasma levels of propafenone; patients should be closely monitored and the propafenone dose adjusted accordingly). Products include:
Benadryl Allergy & Cold Tablets 692
Benadryl Allergy 691
Benadryl Allergy & Sinus Headache Caplets & Gelcaps 693
Children's Benadryl Allergy Liquid 695
Children's Benadryl Dye-Free Allergy Liquid 695
Benadryl Dye-Free Allergy Liqui-Gels Softgels 692
Benadryl Itch Relief Stick Extra Strength 696
Benadryl Itch Stopping Cream Extra Strength 697
Benadryl Itch Stopping Gel Extra Strength 697
Benadryl Itch Stopping Spray Extra Strength 697
Benadryl Maximum Strength Severe Allergy & Sinus Headache Caplets 694
Children's Benadryl D Liquid Medication 693
Benadryl D Tablets 694
Nytol QuickCaps Caplets 635
Maximum Strength Nytol QuickGels Softgels 635
Simply Sleep Caplets 1841
Sominex Original Formula Tablets 637
TheraFlu Thin Strips Multi Symptom 684
Triaminic Thin Strips Cough & Runny Nose 690
Children's Tylenol Plus Cold & Allergy Suspension Liquid 1850
Tylenol Allergy Complete Night Time Caplets 1844
Tylenol Severe Allergy Caplets 1844
Tylenol Flu NightTime Gelcaps 1846
Extra Strength Tylenol PM Caplets, Geltabs, Gelcaps and Liquid 1847
Unisom Maximum Strength SleepGels 712

Dirithromycin (The use of propafenone in conjunction with other drugs that prolong the QT interval has not been extensively studied and is not recommended).
No products indexed under this heading.

Disopyramide (Class Ia antiarrythmic agents should be withheld for at least five half-lives prior to dosing with extended release propafenone. The use of propafenone with Class Ia antiarrythmic agents is not recommended).
No products indexed under this heading.

Disopyramide Phosphate (The use of propafenone in conjunction with other drugs that prolong the QT interval has not been extensively studied and is not recommended).
No products indexed under this heading.

Dofetilide (The use of propafenone in conjunction with other drugs that prolong the QT interval has not been extensively studied and is not recommended).
No products indexed under this heading.

Doxepin Hydrochloride (The use of propafenone in conjunction with other drugs that prolong the QT interval has not been extensively studied and is not recommended).
No products indexed under this heading.

Dyphylline (Combined therapy may result in an increase in theophylline concentration with the development of theophylline toxicity).
No products indexed under this heading.

Efavirenz (Drugs that inhibit CYP3A4 might lead to increased plasma levels of propafenone; patients should be closely monitored and the propafenone dose adjusted accordingly). Products include:
Sustiva Capsules 957

Enoxacin (Drugs that inhibit CYP1A2 might lead to increased plasma levels of propafenone; patients should be closely monitored and the propafenone dose adjusted accordingly).
No products indexed under this heading.

Erythromycin (The use of propafenone in conjunction with other drugs that prolong the QT interval has not been extensively studied and is not recommended). Products include:
Erygel Topical Gel 2096
Ery-Tab Tablets 447
Erythromycin Base Filmtab Tablets 454
Erythromycin Delayed-Release Capsules, USP 456
PCE Dispertab Tablets 510

Erythromycin Estolate (The use of propafenone in conjunction with other drugs that prolong the QT interval has not been extensively studied and is not recommended).
No products indexed under this heading.

Erythromycin Ethylsuccinate (The use of propafenone in conjunction with other drugs that prolong the QT interval has not been extensively studied and is not recommended). Products include:
E.E.S. 449
EryPed 445

Erythromycin Gluceptate (The use of propafenone in conjunction with other drugs that prolong the QT interval has not been extensively studied and is not recommended).
No products indexed under this heading.

Erythromycin Lactobionate (Drugs that inhibit CYP3A4 might lead to increased plasma levels of propafenone; patients should be closely monitored and the propafenone dose adjusted accordingly).
No products indexed under this heading.

Erythromycin Stearate (The use of propafenone in conjunction with other drugs that prolong the QT interval has not been extensively studied and is not recommended). Products include:
Erythrocin Stearate Filmtab Tablets 452

Escitalopram Oxalate (Drugs that inhibit CYP2D6 might lead to increased plasma levels of propafenone; patients should be closely monitored and the propafenone dose adjusted accordingly). Products include:
Lexapro Oral Solution 1193
Lexapro Tablets 1193

Esomeprazole Magnesium (Drugs that inhibit CYP3A4 might lead to increased plasma levels of propafenone; patients should be closely monitored and the propafenone dose adjusted accordingly). Products include:
Nexium Delayed-Release Capsules 645

Ethinyl Estradiol (Drugs that inhibit CYP1A2 might lead to increased plasma levels of propafenone; patients should be closely monitored and the propafenone dose adjusted accordingly). Products include:
Alesse-28 Tablets 3392
Lo/Ovral-28 Tablets 3423
NuvaRing 2357
Ortho-Cept Tablets 2395
Ortho-Cyclen/Ortho Tri-Cyclen 2414
Ortho Evra Transdermal System 2402
Ortho Tri-Cyclen Lo Tablets 2421
Seasonale Tablets 1073
Triphasil-28 Tablets 3483
Yasmin 28 Tablets 818

Etidocaine Hydrochloride (Concomitant use of local anesthetics may increase the risk of CNS side effects).
No products indexed under this heading.

Flecainide Acetate (The use of propafenone in conjunction with other drugs that prolong the QT interval has not been extensively studied and is not recommended). Products include:
Tambocor Tablets 1824

Fluconazole (Drugs that inhibit CYP3A4 might lead to increased plasma levels of propafenone; patients should be closely monitored and the propafenone dose adjusted accordingly).
No products indexed under this heading.

Fluoxetine (Drugs that inhibit CYP2D6 might lead to increased plasma levels of propafenone; patients should be closely monitored and the propafenone dose adjusted accordingly).
No products indexed under this heading.

Fluoxetine Hydrochloride (Drugs that inhibit CYP2D6 might lead to increased plasma levels of propafenone; patients should be closely monitored and the propafenone dose adjusted accordingly). Products include:
Prozac Pulvules and Liquid 1771
Symbyax Capsules 1788

Fluphenazine Decanoate (The use of propafenone in conjunction with other drugs that prolong the QT interval has not been extensively studied and is not recommended).
No products indexed under this heading.

Fluphenazine Enanthate (The use of propafenone in conjunction with other drugs that prolong the QT interval has not been extensively studied and is not recommended).
No products indexed under this heading.

Fluphenazine Hydrochloride (The use of propafenone in conjunction with other drugs that prolong the QT interval has not been extensively studied and is not recommended).
No products indexed under this heading.

Fluvoxamine (Drugs that inhibit CYP1A2 might lead to increased plasma levels of propafenone; patients should be closely monitored and the propafenone dose adjusted accordingly).
No products indexed under this heading.

Fluvoxamine Maleate (Drugs that inhibit CYP2D6 might lead to increased plasma levels of propafenone; patients should be closely monitored and the propafenone dose adjusted accordingly).
No products indexed under this heading.

Fosamprenavir Calcium (Drugs that inhibit CYP3A4 might lead to increased plasma levels of propafenone; patients should be closely monitored and the propafenone dose adjusted accordingly). Products include:
Lexiva Tablets 1473

Gatifloxacin (Drugs that inhibit CYP1A2 might lead to increased plasma levels of propafenone; patients should be closely monitored and the propafenone dose adjusted accordingly). Products include:
Tequin Injection 964
Tequin Tablets 964
Zymar Ophthalmic Solution 571

Gemifloxacin Mesylate (Drugs that inhibit CYP1A2 might lead to increased plasma levels of propafenone; patients should be closely monitored and the propafenone dose adjusted accordingly). Products include:
Factive Tablets 2464

Grepafloxacin Hydrochloride (Drugs that inhibit CYP1A2 might lead to increased plasma levels of propafenone; patients should be closely monitored and the propafenone dose adjusted accordingly).
No products indexed under this heading.

Halofantrine Hydrochloride (Drugs that inhibit CYP2D6 might lead to increased plasma levels of propafenone; patients should be closely monitored and the propafenone dose adjusted accordingly).
No products indexed under this heading.

Haloperidol (Drugs that inhibit CYP2D6 might lead to increased plasma levels of propafenone; patients should be closely monitored and the propafenone dose adjusted accordingly).
No products indexed under this heading.

Haloperidol Decanoate (Drugs that inhibit CYP2D6 might lead to increased plasma levels of propafenone; patients should be closely monitored and the propafenone dose adjusted accordingly).
No products indexed under this heading.

Hydroxychloroquine Sulfate (Drugs that inhibit CYP2D6 might lead to increased plasma levels of propafenone; patients should be closely monitored and the propafenone dose adjusted accordingly).
No products indexed under this heading.

Imatinib Mesylate (Drugs that inhibit CYP2D6 might lead to increased plasma levels of propafenone; patients should be closely monitored and the propafenone dose adjusted accordingly). Products include:
Gleevec Tablets 2221

Imipramine Hydrochloride (The use of propafenone in conjunction with other drugs that prolong the QT interval has not been extensively studied and is not recommended).
No products indexed under this heading.

Imipramine Pamoate (The use of propafenone in conjunction with other drugs that prolong the QT interval has not been extensively studied and is not recommended).
No products indexed under this heading.

Indinavir Sulfate (Drugs that inhibit CYP3A4 might lead to increased plasma levels of propafenone; patients should be closely monitored and the propafenone dose adjusted accordingly). Products include:
Crixivan Capsules 1918

Isoniazid (Drugs that inhibit CYP1A2 might lead to increased plasma levels of propafenone; patients should be closely monitored and the propafenone dose adjusted accordingly).
No products indexed under this heading.

Itraconazole (Drugs that inhibit CYP3A4 might lead to increased plasma levels of propafenone; patients should be closely monitored and the propafenone dose adjusted accordingly).
No products indexed under this heading.

Ketoconazole (Drugs that inhibit CYP1A2 might lead to increased plasma levels of propafenone; patients should be closely monitored and the propafenone dose adjusted accordingly). Products include:
Nizoral A-D Shampoo, 1% 1839
Nizoral 2% Shampoo 1838

Levobupivacaine Hydrochloride (Concomitant use of local anesthetics may increase the risk of CNS side effects).
No products indexed under this heading.

Levofloxacin (Drugs that inhibit CYP1A2 might lead to increased plasma levels of propafenone; patients should be closely monitored and the propafenone dose adjusted accordingly). Products include:
Levaquin in 5% Dextrose Injection 2453
Levaquin 2453
Quixin Ophthalmic Solution 3373

Levonorgestrel (Drugs that inhibit CYP1A2 might lead to increased plasma levels of propafenone; patients should be closely monitored and the propafenone dose adjusted accordingly). Products include:
Alesse-28 Tablets 3392
Climara Pro Transdermal System 800
Mirena Intrauterine System 810
Plan B Tablets 1068
Seasonale Tablets 1073
Triphasil-28 Tablets 3483

Lidocaine Hydrochloride (The use of propafenone in conjunction with other drugs that prolong the QT interval has not been extensively studied and is not recommended).
No products indexed under this heading.

Lomefloxacin Hydrochloride (Drugs that inhibit CYP1A2 might lead to increased plasma levels of propafenone; patients should be closely monitored and the propafenone dose adjusted accordingly).
No products indexed under this heading.

Lopinavir (Drugs that inhibit CYP3A4 might lead to increased plasma levels of propafenone; patients should be closely monitored and the propafenone dose adjusted accordingly). Products include:
Kaletra 474

Loratadine (Drugs that inhibit CYP3A4 might lead to increased plasma levels of propafenone; patients should be closely monitored and the propafenone dose adjusted accordingly). Products include:
Alavert Allergy & Sinus D-12 Hour Tablets .... ▣743
Alavert .... ▣743
Children's Claritin 24 Hour Non-Drowsy Allergy Syrup .... ▣732
Claritin Non-Drowsy 24 Hour Tablets .... ▣731
Non-Drowsy Claritin Hives Relief Tablets .... ▣733
Claritin Reditabs 24 Hour Non-Drowsy Tablets .... ▣732
Claritin-D Non-Drowsy 12 Hour Tablets .... ▣731
Claritin-D Non-Drowsy 24 Hour Tablets .... ▣731
Children's Dimetapp ND Non-Drowsy Allergy Syrup .... ▣746
Triaminic Allerchews .... ▣684

Maprotiline Hydrochloride (The use of propafenone in conjunction with other drugs that prolong the QT interval has not been extensively studied and is not recommended).
No products indexed under this heading.

Mepivacaine Hydrochloride (Concomitant use of local anesthetics may increase the risk of CNS side effects).
No products indexed under this heading.

Mesoridazine Besylate (The use of propafenone in conjunction with other drugs that prolong the QT interval has not been extensively studied and is not recommended).
No products indexed under this heading.

Mestranol (Drugs that inhibit CYP1A2 might lead to increased plasma levels of propafenone; patients should be closely monitored and the propafenone dose adjusted accordingly).
No products indexed under this heading.

Methadone Hydrochloride (Drugs that inhibit CYP2D6 might lead to increased plasma levels of propafenone; patients should be closely monitored and the propafenone dose adjusted accordingly).
No products indexed under this heading.

Methoxsalen (Drugs that inhibit CYP1A2 might lead to increased plasma levels of propafenone; patients should be closely monitored and the propafenone dose adjusted accordingly). Products include:
Oxsoralen Lotion 1% 3354
Oxsoralen-Ultra Capsules 3354

Metoprolol Succinate (Coadministration can result in substantial increases in metoprolol concentration and elimination half-life; increased plasma levels of metoprolol could overcome its cardioselectivity). Products include:
Toprol-XL Tablets 660

Metoprolol Tartrate (Coadministration can result in substantial increases in metoprolol concentration and elimination half-life; increased plasma levels of metoprolol could overcome its cardioselectivity).
No products indexed under this heading.

Metronidazole (Drugs that inhibit CYP3A4 might lead to increased plasma levels of propafenone; patients should be closely monitored and the propafenone dose adjusted accordingly). Products include:
Metrogel 1% 1212
MetroGel-Vaginal Gel 1822
Noritate Cream, 1% 1051

Metronidazole Benzoate (Drugs that inhibit CYP3A4 might lead to increased plasma levels of propafenone; patients should be closely monitored and the propafenone dose adjusted accordingly).
No products indexed under this heading.

Metronidazole Hydrochloride (Drugs that inhibit CYP3A4 might lead to increased plasma levels of propafenone; patients should be closely monitored and the propafenone dose adjusted accordingly).
No products indexed under this heading.

Mexiletine Hydrochloride (The use of propafenone in conjunction with other drugs that prolong the QT interval has not been extensively studied and is not recommended).
No products indexed under this heading.

Mibefradil Dihydrochloride (Drugs that inhibit CYP2D6 might lead to increased plasma levels of propafenone; patients should be closely monitored and the propafenone dose adjusted accordingly).
No products indexed under this heading.

Miconazole (Drugs that inhibit CYP3A4 might lead to increased plasma levels of propafenone; patients should be closely monitored and the propafenone dose adjusted accordingly).
No products indexed under this heading.

Miconazole Nitrate (Drugs that inhibit CYP3A4 might lead to increased plasma levels of propafenone; patients should be closely monitored and the propafenone dose adjusted accordingly). Products include:
Desenex 674
Desenex Jock Itch Spray Powder ... 674

Moclobemide (Drugs that inhibit CYP2D6 might lead to increased plasma levels of propafenone; patients should be closely monitored and the propafenone dose adjusted accordingly).
No products indexed under this heading.

Moricizine Hydrochloride (Class Ia antiarrythmic agents should be withheld for at least five half-lives prior to dosing with extended release propafenone. The use of propafenone with Class Ia antiarrythmic agents is not recommended).
No products indexed under this heading.

Moxifloxacin Hydrochloride (Drugs that inhibit CYP1A2 might lead to increased plasma levels of propafenone; patients should be closely monitored and the propafenone dose adjusted accordingly). Products include:
Avelox 2984
Vigamox Ophthalmic Solution 560

Nalidixic Acid (Drugs that inhibit CYP1A2 might lead to increased plasma levels of propafenone; patients should be closely monitored and the propafenone dose adjusted accordingly).
No products indexed under this heading.

Nefazodone Hydrochloride (Drugs that inhibit CYP3A4 might lead to increased plasma levels of propafenone; patients should be closely monitored and the propafenone dose adjusted accordingly).
No products indexed under this heading.

Nelfinavir Mesylate (Drugs that inhibit CYP3A4 might lead to increased plasma levels of propafenone; patients should be closely monitored and the propafenone dose adjusted accordingly). Products include:
Viracept 2556

Nevirapine (Drugs that inhibit CYP3A4 might lead to increased plasma levels of propafenone; patients should be closely monitored and the propafenone dose adjusted accordingly). Products include:
Viramune Oral Suspension 903
Viramune Tablets 903

Niacinamide (Drugs that inhibit CYP3A4 might lead to increased plasma levels of propafenone; patients should be closely monitored and the propafenone dose adjusted accordingly).
No products indexed under this heading.

Nicotinamide (Drugs that inhibit CYP3A4 might lead to increased plasma levels of propafenone; patients should be closely monitored and the propafenone dose adjusted accordingly). Products include:
Nicomide Tablets 3190

Nifedipine (Drugs that inhibit CYP3A4 might lead to increased plasma levels of propafenone; patients should be closely monitored and the propafenone dose adjusted accordingly). Products include:
Adalat CC Tablets 2978

Norethindrone (Drugs that inhibit CYP1A2 might lead to increased plasma levels of propafenone; patients should be closely monitored and the propafenone dose adjusted accordingly). Products include:
Ortho Micronor Tablets 2411

Norfloxacin (Drugs that inhibit CYP1A2 might lead to increased plasma levels of propafenone; patients should be closely monitored and the propafenone dose adjusted accordingly). Products include:
Noroxin Tablets 2009

Norgestrel (Drugs that inhibit CYP1A2 might lead to increased plasma levels of propafenone; patients should be closely monitored and the propafenone dose adjusted accordingly). Products include:
Lo/Ovral-28 Tablets 3423

Nortriptyline Hydrochloride (The use of propafenone in conjunction with other drugs that prolong the QT interval has not been extensively studied and is not recommended).
No products indexed under this heading.

Ofloxacin (Drugs that inhibit CYP1A2 might lead to increased plasma levels of propafenone; patients should be closely monitored and the propafenone dose adjusted accordingly). Products include:
Floxin Otic Singles 1045
Floxin Otic Solution 1043

Omeprazole (Drugs that inhibit CYP1A2 might lead to increased plasma levels of propafenone; patients should be closely monitored and the propafenone dose adjusted accordingly). Products include:
Zegerid Powder for Oral Solution 2972

Paroxetine Hydrochloride (Drugs that inhibit CYP2D6 might lead to increased plasma levels of propafenone; patients should be closely monitored and the propafenone dose adjusted accordingly). Products include:
Paxil CR Controlled-Release Tablets 1509
Paxil 1501

Perphenazine (The use of propafenone in conjunction with other drugs that prolong the QT interval has not been extensively studied and is not recommended).
No products indexed under this heading.

Procainamide (Class Ia antiarrythmic agents should be withheld for at least five half-lives prior to dosing with extended release propafenone. The use of propafenone with Class Ia antiarrythmic agents is not recommended).
No products indexed under this heading.

Procainamide Hydrochloride (The use of propafenone in conjunction with other drugs that prolong the QT interval has not been extensively studied and is not recommended).
No products indexed under this heading.

Procaine Hydrochloride (Concomitant use of local anesthetics may increase the risk of CNS side effects).
No products indexed under this heading.

Prochlorperazine (The use of propafenone in conjunction with other drugs that prolong the QT interval has not been extensively studied and is not recommended).
No products indexed under this heading.

Promethazine Hydrochloride (The use of propafenone in conjunction with other drugs that prolong the QT interval has not been extensively studied and is not recommended). Products include:
Phenergan 3438

Propoxyphene Hydrochloride (Drugs that inhibit CYP2D6 might lead to increased plasma levels of propafenone; patients should be closely monitored and the propafenone dose adjusted accordingly).
No products indexed under this heading.

Propoxyphene Napsylate (Drugs that inhibit CYP2D6 might lead to increased plasma levels of propafenone; patients should be closely monitored and the propafenone dose adjusted accordingly). Products include:
Darvocet A 500 Tablets 3497

Propranolol Hydrochloride (Coadministration has resulted in substantial increases in propranolol concentration and elimination half-life). Products include:
Inderal LA Long-Acting Capsules 3421
InnoPran XL Capsules 2728

Protriptyline Hydrochloride (The use of propafenone in conjunction with other drugs that prolong the QT interval has not been extensively studied and is not recommended). Products include:
Vivactil Tablets 2350

Quinacrine Hydrochloride (Drugs that inhibit CYP2D6 might lead to increased plasma levels of propafenone; patients should be closely monitored and the propafenone dose adjusted accordingly).
No products indexed under this heading.

Quinidine (Class Ia antiarrythmic agents should be withheld for at least five half-lives prior to dosing with extended release propafenone. The use of propafenone with Class Ia antiarrythmic agents is not recommended).
No products indexed under this heading.

Quinidine Gluconate (The use of propafenone in conjunction with other drugs that prolong the QT interval has not been extensively studied and is not recommended).
No products indexed under this heading.

Quinidine Hydrochloride (Small doses of quinidine completely inhibit the hydroxylation metabolic pathway, making all patients, in effect, slow metabolizers; there is too little information to recommend concomitant use).
No products indexed under this heading.

Quinidine Polygalacturonate (The use of propafenone in conjunction with other drugs that prolong the QT interval has not been extensively studied and is not recommended).
No products indexed under this heading.

Quinidine Sulfate (The use of propafenone in conjunction with other drugs that prolong the QT interval has not been extensively studied and is not recommended).
No products indexed under this heading.

Quinine (Drugs that inhibit CYP3A4 might lead to increased plasma levels of propafenone; patients should be closely monitored and the propafenone dose adjusted accordingly).
No products indexed under this heading.

Quinine Sulfate (Drugs that inhibit CYP3A4 might lead to increased plasma levels of propafenone; patients should be closely monitored and the propafenone dose adjusted accordingly).
No products indexed under this heading.

Quinupristin (Drugs that inhibit CYP3A4 might lead to increased plasma levels of propafenone; patients should be closely monitored and the propafenone dose adjusted accordingly). Products include:
Synercid I.V. 1690

Ranitidine Bismuth Citrate (Drugs that inhibit CYP2D6 might lead to increased plasma levels of propafenone; patients should be closely monitored and the propafenone dose adjusted accordingly).
No products indexed under this heading.

Ranitidine Hydrochloride (Drugs that inhibit CYP2D6 might lead to increased plasma levels of pro-

pafenone; patients should be closely monitored and the propafenone dose adjusted accordingly). Products include:

Zantac 1597
Zantac Injection 1593
Zantac 75 Tablets .... ■ 715
Zantac 150 Maximum Strength Tablets.............................. ■ 715
Zantac Injection Pharmacy Bulk Package 1595

Rifampin (May accelerate the metabolism and decrease the plasma levels and antiarythmic efficacy of propafenone).
No products indexed under this heading.

Ritonavir (Drugs that inhibit CYP2D6 might lead to increased plasma levels of propafenone; patients should be closely monitored and the propafenone dose adjusted accordingly). Products include:

Kaletra 474
Norvir 499

Saquinavir (Drugs that inhibit CYP3A4 might lead to increased plasma levels of propafenone; patients should be closely monitored and the propafenone dose adjusted accordingly).
No products indexed under this heading.

Saquinavir Mesylate (Drugs that inhibit CYP3A4 might lead to increased plasma levels of propafenone; patients should be closely monitored and the propafenone dose adjusted accordingly). Products include:

Invirase 2776

Sertraline Hydrochloride (Drugs that inhibit CYP2D6 might lead to increased plasma levels of propafenone; patients should be closely monitored and the propafenone dose adjusted accordingly). Products include:

Zoloft 2581

Sotalol Hydrochloride (Class III antiarrythmic agents should be withheld for at least five half-lives prior to dosing with extended release propafenone. The use of propafenone with Class III antiarrythmic agents is not recommended).
No products indexed under this heading.

Sparfloxacin (Drugs that inhibit CYP1A2 might lead to increased plasma levels of propafenone; patients should be closely monitored and the propafenone dose adjusted accordingly).
No products indexed under this heading.

Tacrine Hydrochloride (Drugs that inhibit CYP1A2 might lead to increased plasma levels of propafenone; patients should be closely monitored and the propafenone dose adjusted accordingly).
No products indexed under this heading.

Telithromycin (Drugs that inhibit CYP3A4 might lead to increased plasma levels of propafenone; patients should be closely monitored and the propafenone dose adjusted accordingly). Products include:

Ketek Tablets 2920

Terbinafine Hydrochloride (Drugs that inhibit CYP2D6 might lead to increased plasma levels of propafenone; patients should be closely monitored and the propafenone dose adjusted accordingly). Products include:

Lamisil[AT] Creams (Athlete's Foot & Jock Itch)........................ ■ 676
Lamisil Tablets 2226

Tetracaine Hydrochloride (Concomitant use of local anesthetics may increase the risk of CNS side effects). Products include:

Cetacaine Topical Anesthetic 1007

Theophylline (Combined therapy may result in an increase in theophylline concentration with the development of theophylline toxicity).
No products indexed under this heading.

Theophylline Anhydrous (Combined therapy may result in an increase in theophylline concentration with the development of theophylline toxicity). Products include:

Uniphyl Tablets 2708

Theophylline Calcium Salicylate (Combined therapy may result in an increase in theophylline concentration with the development of theophylline toxicity).
No products indexed under this heading.

Theophylline Dihydroxypropyl (Glyceryl) (Combined therapy may result in an increase in theophylline concentration with the development of theophylline toxicity).
No products indexed under this heading.

Theophylline Ethylenediamine (Combined therapy may result in an increase in theophylline concentration with the development of theophylline toxicity).
No products indexed under this heading.

Theophylline Sodium Glycinate (Combined therapy may result in an increase in theophylline concentration with the development of theophylline toxicity).
No products indexed under this heading.

Thioridazine Hydrochloride (The use of propafenone in conjunction with other drugs that prolong the QT interval has not been extensively studied and is not recommended). Products include:

Thioridazine Hydrochloride Tablets 2122

Ticlopidine Hydrochloride (Drugs that inhibit CYP1A2 might lead to increased plasma levels of propafenone; patients should be closely monitored and the propafenone dose adjusted accordingly). Products include:

Ticlid Tablets 2813

Tocainide Hydrochloride (The use of propafenone in conjunction with other drugs that prolong the QT interval has not been extensively studied and is not recommended).
No products indexed under this heading.

Trifluoperazine Hydrochloride (The use of propafenone in conjunction with other drugs that prolong the QT interval has not been extensively studied and is not recommended).
No products indexed under this heading.

Trimipramine Maleate (The use of propafenone in conjunction with other drugs that prolong the QT interval has not been extensively studied and is not recommended). Products include:

Surmontil Capsules 2347

Troglitazone (Drugs that inhibit CYP3A4 might lead to increased plasma levels of propafenone; patients should be closely monitored and the propafenone dose adjusted accordingly).
No products indexed under this heading.

Troleandomycin (The use of propafenone in conjunction with other drugs that prolong the QT interval has not been extensively studied and is not recommended).
No products indexed under this heading.

Trovafloxacin Mesylate (Drugs that inhibit CYP1A2 might lead to increased plasma levels of propafenone; patients should be closely monitored and the propafenone dose adjusted accordingly).
No products indexed under this heading.

Valproate Sodium (Drugs that inhibit CYP3A4 might lead to increased plasma levels of propafenone; patients should be closely monitored and the propafenone dose adjusted accordingly). Products include:

Depacon Injection 412

Verapamil Hydrochloride (Drugs that inhibit CYP3A4 might lead to increased plasma levels of propafenone; patients should be closely monitored and the propafenone dose adjusted accordingly). Products include:

Covera-HS Tablets 3135
Tarka Tablets 519
Verelan PM Capsules 3120

Voriconazole (Drugs that inhibit CYP3A4 might lead to increased plasma levels of propafenone; patients should be closely monitored and the propafenone dose adjusted accordingly). Products include:

VFEND I.V. 2543
VFEND Oral Suspension 2543
VFEND Tablets 2543

Warfarin Sodium (Increase in mean steady-state plasma levels of warfarin resulting in increased prothrombin time). Products include:

Coumadin for Injection 932
Coumadin Tablets 932

Zafirlukast (Drugs that inhibit CYP3A4 might lead to increased plasma levels of propafenone; patients should be closely monitored and the propafenone dose adjusted accordingly). Products include:

Accolate Tablets 663

Zileuton (Drugs that inhibit CYP1A2 might lead to increased plasma levels of propafenone; patients should be closely monitored and the propafenone dose adjusted accordingly).
No products indexed under this heading.

Ziprasidone Hydrochloride (The use of propafenone in conjunction with other drugs that prolong the QT interval has not been extensively studied and is not recommended). Products include:

Geodon Capsules 2514

Food Interactions

Food, unspecified (Increased peak blood level and bioavailability in a single dose study).

Grapefruit (Drugs that inhibit CYP3A4 might lead to increased plasma levels of propafenone; patients should be closely monitored and the propafenone dose adjusted accordingly).

Grapefruit Juice (Drugs that inhibit CYP1A2 might lead to increased plasma levels of propafenone; patients should be closely monitored and the propafenone dose adjusted accordingly).

SANCTURA TABLETS

(Trospium Chloride) 1133
May interact with anticholinergics and certain other agents. Compounds in these categories include:

Atropine Sulfate (The concomitant use of trospium with other anticholinergic agents that produce dry mouth, constipation, and other anticholinergic pharmacological effects, may increase the frequency and/or severity of such effects).
No products indexed under this heading.

Belladonna Alkaloids (The concomitant use of trospium with other anticholinergic agents that produce dry mouth, constipation, and other anticholinergic pharmacological effects, may increase the frequency and/or severity of such effects). Products include:

Hyland's Teething Tablets .... ■ 736

Benztropine Mesylate (The concomitant use of trospium with other anticholinergic agents that produce dry mouth, constipation, and other anticholinergic pharmacological effects, may increase the frequency and/or severity of such effects). Products include:

Cogentin Injection 1903

Biperiden Hydrochloride (The concomitant use of trospium with other anticholinergic agents that produce dry mouth, constipation, and other anticholinergic pharmacological effects, may increase the frequency and/or severity of such effects).
No products indexed under this heading.

Clidinium Bromide (The concomitant use of trospium with other anticholinergic agents that produce dry mouth, constipation, and other anticholinergic pharmacological effects, may increase the frequency and/or severity of such effects).
No products indexed under this heading.

Dicyclomine Hydrochloride (The concomitant use of trospium with other anticholinergic agents that produce dry mouth, constipation, and other anticholinergic pharmacological effects, may increase the frequency and/or severity of such effects). Products include:

Bentyl Capsules 724
Bentyl Injection 724
Bentyl Syrup 724
Bentyl Tablets 724

Digoxin (Co-administration with drugs that are eliminated by active renal tubular secretion, like digoxin, may increase the serum concentration of trospium and/or the co-administered drug, due to competition for this elimination pathway). Products include:

Digitek Tablets 2146
Lanoxicaps Capsules 1458
Lanoxin Injection 1462
Lanoxin Tablets 1468
Lanoxin Injection Pediatric 1465

Glycopyrrolate (The concomitant use of trospium with other anticholinergic agents that produce dry mouth, constipation, and other anticholinergic pharmacological effects, may increase the frequency and/or severity of such effects).
No products indexed under this heading.

Hyoscyamine (The concomitant use of trospium with other anticholinergic agents that produce dry mouth, constipation, and other anticholinergic pharmacological effects, may increase the frequency and/or severity of such effects).
No products indexed under this heading.

Hyoscyamine Sulfate (The concomitant use of trospium with other anticholinergic agents that produce dry mouth, constipation, and other anticholinergic pharmacological effects, may increase the frequency and/or severity of such effects).
No products indexed under this heading.

Ipratropium Bromide (The concomitant use of trospium with other anticholinergic agents that produce dry mouth, constipation, and other anticholinergic pharmacological effects, may increase the frequency and/or severity of such effects). Products include:
Atrovent HFA Inhalation Aerosol **872**
Atrovent Inhalation Solution **868**
Atrovent Nasal Spray 0.03% **869**
Atrovent Nasal Spray 0.06% **870**
Combivent Inhalation Aerosol **878**
DuoNeb Inhalation Solution **1058**

Mepenzolate Bromide (The concomitant use of trospium with other anticholinergic agents that produce dry mouth, constipation, and other anticholinergic pharmacological effects, may increase the frequency and/or severity of such effects).
No products indexed under this heading.

Metformin (Co-administration with drugs that are eliminated by active renal tubular secretion, like metformin, may increase the serum concentration of trospium and/or the co-administered drug, due to competition for this elimination pathway).
No products indexed under this heading.

Metformin Hydrochloride (Co-administration with drugs that are eliminated by active renal tubular secretion, like metformin, may increase the serum concentration of trospium and/or the co-administered drug, due to competition for this elimination pathway). Products include:
ActoPlus Met Tablets **3219**
Avandamet Tablets **1343**
Fortamet Extended-Release Tablets **1156**

Morphine Sulfate (Co-administration with drugs that are eliminated by active renal tubular secretion, like morphine, may increase the serum concentration of trospium and/or the co-administered drug, due to competition for this elimination pathway). Products include:
Avinza Capsules **1714**
Kadian Capsules **572**
MS Contin Tablets **2703**

Oxybutynin Chloride (The concomitant use of trospium with other anticholinergic agents that produce dry mouth, constipation, and other anticholinergic pharmacological effects, may increase the frequency and/or severity of such effects). Products include:
Ditropan XL Extended Release Tablets **2391**

Pancuronium Bromide (Co-administration with drugs that are eliminated by active renal tubular secretion, like pancuronium, may increase the serum concentration of trospium and/or the co-administered drug, due to competition for this elimination pathway).
No products indexed under this heading.

Procainamide (Co-administration with drugs that are eliminated by active renal tubular secretion, like procainamide, may increase the serum concentration of trospium and/or the co-administered drug, due to competition for this elimination pathway).
No products indexed under this heading.

Procainamide Hydrochloride (Co-administration with drugs that are eliminated by active renal tubular secretion, like procainamide, may increase the serum concentration of trospium and/or the co-administered drug, due to competition for this elimination pathway).
No products indexed under this heading.

Procyclidine Hydrochloride (The concomitant use of trospium with other anticholinergic agents that produce dry mouth, constipation, and other anticholinergic pharmacological effects, may increase the frequency and/or severity of such effects).
No products indexed under this heading.

Propantheline Bromide (The concomitant use of trospium with other anticholinergic agents that produce dry mouth, constipation, and other anticholinergic pharmacological effects, may increase the frequency and/or severity of such effects).
No products indexed under this heading.

Scopolamine (The concomitant use of trospium with other anticholinergic agents that produce dry mouth, constipation, and other anticholinergic pharmacological effects, may increase the frequency and/or severity of such effects). Products include:
Transderm Scōp Transdermal Therapeutic System **2166**

Scopolamine Hydrobromide (The concomitant use of trospium with other anticholinergic agents that produce dry mouth, constipation, and other anticholinergic pharmacological effects, may increase the frequency and/or severity of such effects).
No products indexed under this heading.

Tenofovir Disoproxil Fumarate (Co-administration with drugs that are eliminated by active renal tubular secretion, like tenofovir, may increase the serum concentration of trospium and/or the co-administered drug, due to competition for this elimination pathway). Products include:
Truvada Tablets **1279**
Viread Tablets **1284**

Tolterodine Tartrate (The concomitant use of trospium with other anticholinergic agents that produce dry mouth, constipation, and other anticholinergic pharmacological effects, may increase the frequency and/or severity of such effects). Products include:
Detrol Tablets **2626**
Detrol LA Capsules **2629**

Tridihexethyl Chloride (The concomitant use of trospium with other anticholinergic agents that produce dry mouth, constipation, and other anticholinergic pharmacological effects, may increase the frequency and/or severity of such effects).
No products indexed under this heading.

Trihexyphenidyl Hydrochloride (The concomitant use of trospium with other anticholinergic agents that produce dry mouth, constipation, and other anticholinergic pharmacological effects, may increase the frequency and/or severity of such effects).
No products indexed under this heading.

Vancomycin Hydrochloride (Co-administration with drugs that are eliminated by active renal tubular secretion, like vancomycin, may increase the serum concentration of trospium and/or the co-administered drug, due to competition for this elimination pathway). Products include:
Vancocin HCl Capsules, USP **3370**

SANDIMMUNE I.V. AMPULS FOR INFUSION

(Cyclosporine) **2259**
May interact with erythromycin, HMG-CoA reductase inhibitors, immunosuppressive agents, methylprednisolone, non-steroidal anti-inflammatory agents, phenytoin, prednisolone, protease inhibitors, potassium sparing diuretics, vaccines, live and certain other agents. Compounds in these categories include:

Allopurinol (Increases cyclosporine concentrations).
No products indexed under this heading.

Amiloride Hydrochloride (Cyclosporine may cause hyperkalemia; concurrent use should be avoided). Products include:
Midamor Tablets **2000**
Moduretic Tablets **2003**

Amiodarone Hydrochloride (Increases cyclosporine concentrations). Products include:
Pacerone Tablets **3337**

Amphotericin B (May potentiate renal dysfunction).
No products indexed under this heading.

Amprenavir (The HIV protease inhibitors are known to inhibit CYP450 3A and, thus, could potentially increase the concentrations of cyclosporine). Products include:
Agenerase Capsules **1299**
Agenerase Oral Solution **1304**

Antibiotics, unspecified (Potential synergies of nephrotoxicity may occur).
No products indexed under this heading.

Atorvastatin Calcium (Cyclosporine may reduce the clearance of HMG-CoA reductase inhibitors (statins). Literature and postmarketing cases of myotoxicity, including muscle pain and weakness, myositis, and rhabdomyolysis have been reported with concomitant administration of cyclosporine and atorvastatin. When concurrently administered with cyclosporine, the dosage of atorvastatin should be reduced. Statin therapy needs to be temporarily withheld or discontinued in patients with signs/symptoms of myopathy or those with risk factors predisposing to severe renal injury). Products include:
Caduet Tablets **2507**
Lipitor Tablets **2495**

Azapropazon (May potentiate renal dysfunction).
No products indexed under this heading.

Azathioprine (Increases susceptibility to infection). Products include:
Azasan Tablets **2844**

Basiliximab (Increases susceptibility to infection). Products include:
Simulect for Injection **2268**

BCG Vaccine (During treatment with cyclosporine, vaccination may be less effective; the use of live vaccines should be avoided).
No products indexed under this heading.

Bromocriptine Mesylate (Increases cyclosporine levels; dosage adjustments are essential).
No products indexed under this heading.

Carbamazepine (Decreases cyclosporine plasma concentrations; dosage adjustments are essential). Products include:
Carbatrol Capsules **3174**
Equetro Extended-Release Capsules **3178**
Tegretol/Tegretol-XR **2278**

Celecoxib (Co-administration with NSAID's, particularly in the setting of dehydration, may potentiate renal dysfunction). Products include:
Celebrex Capsules **3130**

Cerivastatin Sodium (Cyclosporine may reduce the clearance of HMG-CoA reductase inhibitors (statins)).
No products indexed under this heading.

Cimetidine (May potentiate renal dysfunction). Products include:
Tagamet HB 200 Tablets **637**
Tagamet Tablets **1547**

Cimetidine Hydrochloride (May potentiate renal dysfunction).
No products indexed under this heading.

Colchicine (Co-administration results in increased cyclosporine concentrations and potentiation of renal dysfunction. Cyclosporine may reduce the clearance of colchicine. There are reports on the potential of cyclosporine to enhance the toxic effects of colchicine, such as myopathy and neuropathy, especially in patients with renal dysfunction. If colchicine is used concurrently with cyclosporine, close clinical observation is required).
No products indexed under this heading.

Dalfopristin (Co-administration with substrates that inhibit CYP450 3A, such as dalfopristin, could decrease metabolism and increase cyclosporine concentrations). Products include:
Synercid I.V. **1690**

Danazol (Increases cyclosporine plasma concentrations; dosage adjustments are essential).
No products indexed under this heading.

Diclofenac Potassium (Co-administration with NSAID's, particularly in the setting of dehydration, may potentiate renal dysfunction).
Products include:
Cataflam Tablets 2173

Diclofenac Sodium (Co-administration with NSAID's, particularly in the setting of dehydration, may potentiate renal dysfunction).
Products include:
Arthrotec Tablets 3126
Voltaren Ophthalmic Solution 2300
Voltaren Tablets 2298
Voltaren-XR Tablets 2301

Digoxin (Reduced clearance of digoxin and potential for severe digitalis toxicity. If digoxin is used concurrently with cyclosporine, close clinical observation is required).
Products include:
Digitek Tablets 2146
Lanoxicaps Capsules 1458
Lanoxin Injection 1462
Lanoxin Tablets 1468
Lanoxin Injection Pediatric 1465

Diltiazem Hydrochloride (Increases cyclosporine plasma concentrations; dosage adjustments are essential). Products include:
Cardizem LA Extended Release Tablets 1699
Tiazac Capsules 1204

Erythromycin (Co-administration with substrates that inhibit CYP450 3A, such as erythromycin, could decrease metabolism and increase cyclosporine concentrations).
Products include:
Erygel Topical Gel 2096
Ery-Tab Tablets 447
Erythromycin Base Filmtab Tablets 454
Erythromycin Delayed-Release Capsules, USP 456
PCE Dispertab Tablets 510

Erythromycin Estolate (Co-administration with substrates that inhibit CYP450 3A, such as erythromycin, could decrease metabolism and increase cyclosporine concentrations).
No products indexed under this heading.

Erythromycin Ethylsuccinate (Co-administration with substrates that inhibit CYP450 3A, such as erythromycin, could decrease metabolism and increase cyclosporine concentrations). Products include:
E.E.S. 449
EryPed 445

Erythromycin Gluceptate (Co-administration with substrates that inhibit CYP450 3A, such as erythromycin, could decrease metabolism and increase cyclosporine concentrations).
No products indexed under this heading.

Erythromycin Lactobionate (Co-administration with substrates that inhibit CYP450 3A, such as erythromycin, could decrease metabolism and increase cyclosporine concentrations).
No products indexed under this heading.

Erythromycin Stearate (Co-administration with substrates that inhibit CYP450 3A, such as erythromycin, could decrease metabolism and increase cyclosporine concentrations). Products include:
Erythrocin Stearate Filmtab Tablets 452

Etodolac (Co-administration with NSAID's, particularly in the setting of dehydration, may potentiate renal dysfunction).
No products indexed under this heading.

Fenoprofen Calcium (Co-administration with NSAID's, particularly in the setting of dehydration, may potentiate renal dysfunction).
Products include:
Nalfon Capsules 2504

Fluconazole (Increases cyclosporine levels; dosage adjustments are essential).
No products indexed under this heading.

Flurbiprofen (Co-administration with NSAID's, particularly in the setting of dehydration, may potentiate renal dysfunction).
No products indexed under this heading.

Fluvastatin Sodium (Cyclosporine may reduce the clearance of HMG-CoA reductase inhibitors (statins). Literature and postmarketing cases of myotoxicity, including muscle pain and weakness, myositis, and rhabdomyolysis have been reported with concomitant administration of cyclosporine and fluvastatin. When concurrently administered with cyclosporine, the dosage of fluvastatin should be reduced. Statin therapy needs to be temporarily withheld or discontinued in patients with signs/symptoms of myopathy or those with risk factors predisposing to severe renal injury). Products include:
Lescol Capsules 2227
Lescol 2730
Lescol XL Tablets 2227

Fosphenytoin Sodium (Co-administration with agents that are known to induce CYP450 system, such as phenytoin, will increase hepatic metabolism and decrease cyclosporine levels).
No products indexed under this heading.

Gentamicin Sulfate (May potentiate renal dysfunction). Products include:
Garamycin Injectable 3028
Genoptic Sterile Ophthalmic Solution .... ⊙227
Pred-G Ophthalmic Suspension .... ⊙234
Pred-G Sterile Ophthalmic Ointment .... ⊙235

Hypericum (Co-administration has been reported to produce a marked reduction in blood cyclosporine concentrations, resulting in subtherapeutic levels, rejection of transplanted organs, and graft loss).
No products indexed under this heading.

Ibuprofen (Co-administration with NSAID's, particularly in the setting of dehydration, may potentiate renal dysfunction). Products include:
Advil Allergy Sinus Caplets .... ▣737
Advil .... ▣737
Children's Advil Suspension .... ▣742
Children's Advil Chewable Tablets .... ▣741
Advil Cold & Sinus .... ▣739
Advil Flu & Body Ache Caplets .... ▣739
Children's Advil Cold Suspension .... ▣741
Infants' Advil Concentrated Drops .... ▣743
Junior Strength Advil Swallow Tablets .... ▣740
Advil Migraine Liquigels .... ▣740
Advil Multi-Symptom Cold Caplets .... ▣738
Combunox Tablets 1183
Children's Motrin Oral Suspension and Chewable Tablets 1837
Children's Motrin Cold Non-Staining Dye-Free Oral Suspension 1838
Children's Motrin Cold Oral Suspension 1838
Children's Motrin Non-Staining Dye-Free Oral Suspension 1837
Motrin Cold & Sinus Caplets 1836
Motrin IB Tablets and Caplets 1836
Infants' Motrin Concentrated Drops 1837
Infants' Motrin Non-Staining Dye-Free Drops 1837
Junior Strength Motrin Caplets and Chewable Tablets 1837
Vicoprofen Tablets 533

Immune Globulin Intravenous (Human) (Increases susceptibility to infection). Products include:
Carimune NF 3501
Gammagard Liquid 751
Gammagard S/D 754
Gamunex Immune Globulin I.V., 10% 3232
Iveegam EN 759

Indinavir Sulfate (The HIV protease inhibitors are known to inhibit CYP450 3A and, thus, could potentially increase the concentrations of cyclosporine). Products include:
Crixivan Capsules 1918

Indomethacin (Co-administration with NSAID's, particularly in the setting of dehydration, may potentiate renal dysfunction). Products include:
Indocin 1968

Indomethacin Sodium Trihydrate (Co-administration with NSAID's, particularly in the setting of dehydration, may potentiate renal dysfunction). Products include:
Indocin I.V. 1973

Itraconazole (Increases cyclosporine levels; dosage adjustments are essential).
No products indexed under this heading.

Ketoconazole (May potentiate renal dysfunction; co-administration with substrates that inhibit CYP450 3A, such as ketoconazole, could decrease metabolism and increase cyclosporine concentrations).
Products include:
Nizoral A-D Shampoo, 1% 1839
Nizoral 2% Shampoo 1838

Ketoprofen (Co-administration with NSAID's, particularly in the setting of dehydration, may potentiate renal dysfunction).
No products indexed under this heading.

Ketorolac Tromethamine (Co-administration with NSAID's, particularly in the setting of dehydration, may potentiate renal dysfunction).
Products include:
Acular Ophthalmic Solution 561
Acular LS Ophthalmic Solution 562

Lopinavir (The HIV protease inhibitors are known to inhibit CYP450 3A and, thus, could potentially increase the concentrations of cyclosporine).
Products include:
Kaletra 474

Lovastatin (Cyclosporine may reduce the clearance of HMG-CoA reductase inhibitors (statins). Literature and postmarketing cases of myotoxicity, including muscle pain and weakness, myositis, and rhabdomyolysis have been reported with concomitant administration of *cyclosporine and lovastatin. When* concurrently administered with cyclosporine, the dosage of lovastatin should be reduced. Statin therapy needs to be temporarily withheld or discontinued in patients with signs/symptoms of myopathy or those with risk factors predisposing to severe renal injury). Products include:
Advicor Tablets 1694
Altoprev Extended-Release Tablets 1151
Mevacor Tablets 1996

Measles, Mumps & Rubella Virus Vaccine, Live (During treatment with cyclosporine, vaccination may be less effective; the use of live vaccines should be avoided).
Products include:
M-M-R II 1980

Measles & Rubella Virus Vaccine Live (During treatment with cyclosporine, vaccination may be less effective; the use of live vaccines should be avoided).
No products indexed under this heading.

Measles Virus Vaccine Live (During treatment with cyclosporine, vaccination may be less effective; the use of live vaccines should be avoided). Products include:
Attenuvax 1889

Meclofenamate Sodium (Co-administration with NSAID's, particularly in the setting of dehydration, may potentiate renal dysfunction).
No products indexed under this heading.

Mefenamic Acid (Co-administration with NSAID's, particularly in the setting of dehydration, may potentiate renal dysfunction).
No products indexed under this heading.

Meloxicam (Co-administration with NSAID's, particularly in the setting of dehydration, may potentiate renal dysfunction). Products include:
Mobic Oral Suspension 893
Mobic Tablets 893

Melphalan (May potentiate renal dysfunction). Products include:
Alkeran Tablets 977

Methotrexate Sodium (Co-administration in rheumatoid arthritis patients has resulted in increased AUC of methotrexate by approximately 30% and concentration of its metabolite decreased by approximately 80%; the clinical significance is not known).
No products indexed under this heading.

Methylprednisolone (Co-administration with agents that are known to inhibit CYP450 system, such as methylprednisolone, will decrease hepatic metabolism and increase cyclosporine levels; convulsions have been reported with concomitant high doses of methylprednisolone).
No products indexed under this heading.

Methylprednisolone Acetate (Co-administration with agents that are known to inhibit CYP450 system, such as methylprednisolone, will decrease hepatic metabolism and increase cyclosporine levels; convulsions have been reported with concomitant high doses of methylprednisolone). Products include:
Depo-Medrol Injectable Suspension 2615

Depo-Medrol Single-Dose Vial 2617

Methylprednisolone Sodium Succinate (Co-administration with agents that are known to inhibit CYP450 system, such as methylprednisolone, will decrease hepatic metabolism and increase cyclosporine levels; convulsions have been reported with concomitant high doses of methylprednisolone).
No products indexed under this heading.

Metoclopramide Hydrochloride (Increases cyclosporine levels; dosage adjustments are essential).
No products indexed under this heading.

Mumps Virus Vaccine, Live (During treatment with cyclosporine, vaccination may be less effective; the use of live vaccines should be avoided). Products include:
Mumpsvax 2005

Muromonab-CD3 (Increased susceptibility to infection and increased risk for development of lymphomas and malignancies). Products include:
Orthoclone OKT3 Sterile Solution 2370

Mycophenolate Mofetil (Increases susceptibility to infection). Products include:
CellCept Capsules 2751
CellCept Oral Suspension 2751
CellCept Tablets 2751

Nabumetone (Co-administration with NSAID's, particularly in the setting of dehydration, may potentiate renal dysfunction). Products include:
Relafen Tablets 1523

Nafcillin Sodium (Decreases cyclosporine concentrations).
No products indexed under this heading.

Naproxen (Co-administration with NSAID's, particularly in the setting of dehydration, may potentiate renal dysfunction). Products include:
EC-Naprosyn Delayed-Release Tablets 2769
Naprosyn Suspension 2769
Naprosyn Tablets 2769
Prevacid NapraPAC 3277

Naproxen Sodium (Co-administration with NSAID's, particularly in the setting of dehydration, may potentiate renal dysfunction). Products include:
Aleve Tablets, Caplets and Gelcaps .... ◙ 605
Anaprox Tablets 2769
Anaprox DS Tablets 2769

Nelfinavir Mesylate (The HIV protease inhibitors are known to inhibit CYP450 3A and, thus, could potentially increase the concentrations of cyclosporine). Products include:
Viracept 2556

Nephrotoxic Drugs (Potential synergics of nephrotoxicity).
No products indexed under this heading.

Nicardipine Hydrochloride (Increases cyclosporine plasma concentrations; dosage adjustments are essential). Products include:
Cardene I.V. 1129

Nifedipine (Potential for frequent gingival hyperplasia). Products include:
Adalat CC Tablets 2978

Octreotide Acetate (Decreases cyclosporine concentrations). Products include:
Sandostatin Injection 2263
Sandostatin LAR Depot 2264

Orlistat (Co-administration can result in decreased absorption of cyclosporine; concomitant use should be avoided). Products include:
Xenical Capsules 2834

Oxaprozin (Co-administration with NSAID's, particularly in the setting of dehydration, may potentiate renal dysfunction).
No products indexed under this heading.

Phenobarbital (Decreases cyclosporine plasma levels; dosage adjustments are essential).
No products indexed under this heading.

Phenylbutazone (Co-administration with NSAID's, particularly in the setting of dehydration, may potentiate renal dysfunction).
No products indexed under this heading.

Phenytoin (Co-administration with agents that are known to induce CYP450 system, such as phenytoin, will increase hepatic metabolism and decrease cyclosporine levels).
No products indexed under this heading.

Phenytoin Sodium (Co-administration with agents that are known to induce CYP450 system, such as phenytoin, will increase hepatic metabolism and decrease cyclosporine levels). Products include:
Phenytek Capsules 2153

Piroxicam (Co-administration with NSAID's, particularly in the setting of dehydration, may potentiate renal dysfunction).
No products indexed under this heading.

Poliovirus Vaccine, Live, Oral, Trivalent, Types 1,2,3 (Sabin) (During treatment with cyclosporine, vaccination may be less effective; the use of live vaccines should be avoided).
No products indexed under this heading.

Pravastatin Sodium (Cyclosporine may reduce the clearance of HMG-CoA reductase inhibitors (statins). Literature and postmarketing cases of myotoxicity, including muscle pain and weakness, myositis, and rhabdomyolysis have been reported with concomitant administration of cyclosporine and pravastatin. When concurrently administered with cyclosporine, the dosage of pravastatin should be reduced. Statin therapy needs to be temporarily withheld or discontinued in patients with signs/symptoms of myopathy or those with risk factors predisposing to severe renal injury). Products include:
Pravachol Tablets 943

Prednisolone (Co-administration results in reduced clearance of prednisolone).
No products indexed under this heading.

Prednisolone Acetate (Co-administration results in reduced clearance of prednisolone). Products include:
Blephamide Ophthalmic Ointment 563
Blephamide Ophthalmic Suspension 564
Poly-Pred Liquifilm Ophthalmic Suspension .... ⊙ 231
Pred Forte Ophthalmic Suspension .... ⊙ 233
Pred Mild Sterile Ophthalmic Suspension .... ⊙ 236
Pred-G Ophthalmic Suspension ...... ⊙ 234
Pred-G Sterile Ophthalmic Ointment .... ⊙ 235

Prednisolone Sodium Phosphate (Co-administration results in reduced clearance of prednisolone). Products include:
Pediapred Oral Solution 3319

Prednisolone Tebutate (Co-administration results in reduced clearance of prednisolone).
No products indexed under this heading.

Quinupristin (Co-administration with substrates that inhibit CYP450 3A, such as quinupristine, could decrease metabolism and increase cyclosporine concentrations). Products include:
Synercid I.V. 1690

Ranitidine Hydrochloride (May potentiate renal dysfunction). Products include:
Zantac 1597
Zantac Injection 1593
Zantac 75 Tablets .... ◙ 715
Zantac 150 Maximum Strength Tablets .... ◙ 715
Zantac Injection Pharmacy Bulk Package 1595

Rifabutin (Rifabutin is known to increase the metabolism of other drugs metabolized by CYP450 system; the interaction between cyclosporine and rifabutin has not been studied; care should be exercised).
No products indexed under this heading.

Rifampin (Decreases cyclosporine plasma levels; dosage adjustments are essential).
No products indexed under this heading.

Ritonavir (The HIV protease inhibitors are known to inhibit CYP450 3A and, thus, could potentially increase the concentrations of cyclosporine). Products include:
Kaletra 474
Norvir 499

Rofecoxib (Co-administration with NSAID's, particularly in the setting of dehydration, may potentiate renal dysfunction).
No products indexed under this heading.

Rotavirus Vaccine, Live, Oral, Tetravalent (During treatment with cyclosporine, vaccination may be less effective; the use of live vaccines should be avoided).
No products indexed under this heading.

Rubella & Mumps Virus Vaccine Live (During treatment with cyclosporine, vaccination may be less effective; the use of live vaccines should be avoided).
No products indexed under this heading.

Rubella Virus Vaccine Live (During treatment with cyclosporine, vaccination may be less effective; the use of live vaccines should be avoided). Products include:
Meruvax II 1994

Saquinavir (The HIV protease inhibitors are known to inhibit CYP450 3A and, thus, could potentially increase the concentrations of cyclosporine).
No products indexed under this heading.

Saquinavir Mesylate (The HIV protease inhibitors are known to inhibit CYP450 3A and, thus, could potentially increase the concentrations of cyclosporine). Products include:
Invirase 2776

Simvastatin (Cyclosporine may reduce the clearance of HMG-CoA reductase inhibitors (statins). Literature and postmarketing cases of myotoxicity, including muscle pain and weakness, myositis, and rhabdomyolysis have been reported with concomitant administration of cyclosporine and simvastatin. When concurrently administered with cyclosporine, the dosage of simvastatin should be reduced. Statin therapy needs to be temporarily withheld or discontinued in patients with signs/symptoms of myopathy or those with risk factors predisposing to severe renal injury). Products include:
Vytorin 10/10 Tablets 2084
Vytorin 10/10 Tablets 3092
Vytorin 10/20 Tablets 2084
Vytorin 10/20 Tablets 3092
Vytorin 10/40 Tablets 3092
Vytorin 10/40 Tablets 2084
Vytorin 10/80 Tablets 2084
Vytorin 10/80 Tablets 3092
Zocor Tablets 2078

Sirolimus (Increases susceptibility to infection). Products include:
Rapamune Oral Solution and Tablets 3472

Smallpox Vaccine (During treatment with cyclosporine, vaccination may be less effective; the use of live vaccines should be avoided).
No products indexed under this heading.

Spironolactone (Cyclosporine may cause hyperkalemia; concurrent use should be avoided).
No products indexed under this heading.

Sulfamethoxazole (May potentiate renal dysfunction).
No products indexed under this heading.

Sulindac (Co-administration with NSAID's, particularly in the setting of dehydration, may potentiate renal dysfunction). Products include:
Clinoril Tablets 1899

Tacrolimus (May potentiate renal dysfunction). Products include:
Prograf Capsules and Injection 624
Protopic Ointment 629

Ticlopidine Hydrochloride (Decreases cyclosporine concentrations). Products include:
Ticlid Tablets 2813

Tobramycin (May potentiate renal dysfunction). Products include:
TOBI Solution for Inhalation 1015
TobraDex Ophthalmic Ointment 558
TobraDex Ophthalmic Suspension ... 558
Zylet Ophthalmic Suspension 3508

Tobramycin Sulfate (May potentiate renal dysfunction).
No products indexed under this heading.

Tolmetin Sodium (Co-administration with NSAID's, particularly in the setting of dehydration, may potentiate renal dysfunction).
No products indexed under this heading.

Triamterene (Cyclosporine may cause hyperkalemia; concurrent use should be avoided). Products include:
Dyazide Capsules 1389
Dyrenium Capsules 3390
Maxzide 2150

Trimethoprim (May potentiate renal dysfunction).
No products indexed under this heading.

Typhoid Vaccine (During treatment with cyclosporine, vaccination may be less effective; the use of live vaccines should be avoided).
No products indexed under this heading.

Valdecoxib (Co-administration with NSAID's, particularly in the setting of dehydration, may potentiate renal dysfunction).
No products indexed under this heading.

Vancomycin Hydrochloride (May potentiate renal dysfunction). Products include:
Vancocin HCl Capsules, USP 3370

Varicella Virus Vaccine Live (During treatment with cyclosporine, vaccination may be less effective; the use of live vaccines should be avoided). Products include:
Varivax 2070

Verapamil Hydrochloride (Increases cyclosporine levels; dosage adjustments are essential). Products include:
Covera-HS Tablets 3135
Tarka Tablets 519
Verelan PM Capsules 3120

Yellow Fever Vaccine (During treatment with cyclosporine, vaccination may be less effective; the use of live vaccines should be avoided).
No products indexed under this heading.

Food Interactions

Grapefruit (Co-administration results in increased blood concentrations of cyclosporine; concurrent use should be avoided).

Grapefruit Juice (Co-administration results in increased blood concentrations of cyclosporine; concurrent use should be avoided).

SANDIMMUNE ORAL SOLUTION

(Cyclosporine) 2259
See Sandimmune I.V. Ampuls for Infusion

SANDIMMUNE SOFT GELATIN CAPSULES

(Cyclosporine) 2259
See Sandimmune I.V. Ampuls for Infusion

SANDOSTATIN INJECTION

(Octreotide Acetate) 2263
See Sandostatin LAR Depot

SANDOSTATIN LAR DEPOT

(Octreotide Acetate) 2264
May interact with beta blockers, calcium channel blockers, cytochrome p450 3a4 substrates (selected), oral hypoglycemic agents, insulin, and certain other agents. Compounds in these categories include:

Acarbose (Octreotide causes hypo- and hyperglycemia in some patients; dosage adjustments of oral hypoglycemic agents may be required). Products include:
Precose Tablets 776

Acebutolol Hydrochloride (Adjustment of the dosage of beta blockers may be required).
No products indexed under this heading.

Alfentanil Hydrochloride (Data indicates that somatostatin analogs might decrease the metabolic clearance of compounds known to be metabolized by cytochrome P450 enzymes, which may be due to the suppression of growth hormones. Since it cannot be excluded that octreotide may have this effect, other drugs mainly metabolized by CYP3A4, and which have a low therapeutic index should therefore be used with caution).
No products indexed under this heading.

Alprazolam (Data indicates that somatostatin analogs might decrease the metabolic clearance of compounds known to be metabolized by cytochrome P450 enzymes, which may be due to the suppression of growth hormones. Since it cannot be excluded that octreotide may have this effect, other drugs mainly metabolized by CYP3A4, and which have a low therapeutic index should therefore be used with caution). Products include:
Niravam Orally Disintegrating Tablets 3106
Xanax XR Tablets 2655

Amitriptyline Hydrochloride (Data indicates that somatostatin analogs might decrease the metabolic clearance of compounds known to be metabolized by cytochrome P450 enzymes, which may be due to the suppression of growth hormones. Since it cannot be excluded that octreotide may have this effect, other drugs mainly metabolized by CYP3A4, and which have a low therapeutic index should therefore be used with caution).
No products indexed under this heading.

Amlodipine Besylate (Adjustment of the dosage of calcium channel blocker may be required). Products include:
Caduet Tablets 2507
Lotrel Capsules 2238
Norvasc Tablets 2529

Aprepitant (Data indicates that somatostatin analogs might decrease the metabolic clearance of compounds known to be metabolized by cytochrome P450 enzymes, which may be due to the suppression of growth hormones. Since it cannot be excluded that octreotide may have this effect, other drugs mainly metabolized by CYP3A4, and which have a low therapeutic index should therefore be used with caution). Products include:
Emend Capsules 1944

Astemizole (Data indicates that somatostatin analogs might decrease the metabolic clearance of compounds known to be metabolized by cytochrome P450 enzymes, which may be due to the suppression of growth hormones. Since it cannot be excluded that octreotide may have this effect, other drugs mainly metabolized by CYP3A4, and which have a low therapeutic index should therefore be used with caution).
No products indexed under this heading.

Atenolol (Adjustment of the dosage of beta blockers may be required). Products include:
Tenormin I.V. Injection 698
Tenormin Tablets 695

Atorvastatin Calcium (Data indicates that somatostatin analogs might decrease the metabolic clearance of compounds known to be metabolized by cytochrome P450 enzymes, which may be due to the suppression of growth hormones. Since it cannot be excluded that octreotide may have this effect, other drugs mainly metabolized by CYP3A4, and which have a low therapeutic index should therefore be used with caution). Products include:
Caduet Tablets 2507
Lipitor Tablets 2495

Belladonna Ergotamine (Data indicates that somatostatin analogs might decrease the metabolic clearance of compounds known to be metabolized by cytochrome P450 enzymes, which may be due to the suppression of growth hormones. Since it cannot be excluded that octreotide may have this effect, other drugs mainly metabolized by CYP3A4, and which have a low therapeutic index should therefore be used with caution).
No products indexed under this heading.

Bepridil Hydrochloride (Adjustment of the dosage of calcium channel blocker may be required).
No products indexed under this heading.

Betaxolol Hydrochloride (Adjustment of the dosage of beta blockers may be required). Products include:
Betoptic S Ophthalmic Suspension 554

Bisoprolol Fumarate (Adjustment of the dosage of beta blockers may be required).
No products indexed under this heading.

Bromocriptine Mesylate (Co-administration increases the availability of bromocriptine).
No products indexed under this heading.

Buspirone Hydrochloride (Data indicates that somatostatin analogs might decrease the metabolic clearance of compounds known to be metabolized by cytochrome P450 enzymes, which may be due to the suppression of growth hormones. Since it cannot be excluded that octreotide may have this effect, other drugs mainly metabolized by CYP3A4, and which have a low therapeutic index should therefore be used with caution).
No products indexed under this heading.

Busulfan (Data indicates that somatostatin analogs might decrease the metabolic clearance of compounds known to be metabolized by cytochrome P450 enzymes, which may be due to the suppression of growth hormones. Since it cannot be excluded that octreotide may have this effect, other drugs mainly metabolized by CYP3A4, and which have a low therapeutic index should therefore be used with caution). Products include:
I.V. Busulfex 1125
Myleran Tablets 1492

Carbamazepine (Data indicates that somatostatin analogs might decrease the metabolic clearance of compounds known to be metabolized by cytochrome P450 enzymes, which may be due to the suppression of growth hormones. Since it cannot be excluded that octreotide may have this effect, other drugs mainly metabolized by CYP3A4, and which have a low therapeutic index should therefore be used with caution). Products include:
Carbatrol Capsules 3174
Equetro Extended-Release Capsules 3178
Tegretol/Tegretol-XR 2278

Carteolol Hydrochloride (Adjustment of the dosage of beta blockers may be required). Products include:
Carteolol Hydrochloride Ophthalmic Solution USP, 1%....... ⊙246

Cerivastatin Sodium (Data indicates that somatostatin analogs might decrease the metabolic clearance of compounds known to be metabolized by cytochrome P450 enzymes, which may be due to the suppression of growth hormones. Since it cannot be excluded that octreotide may have this effect, other drugs mainly metabolized by CYP3A4, and which have a low therapeutic index should therefore be used with caution).
No products indexed under this heading.

Chlorpheniramine (Data indicates that somatostatin analogs might decrease the metabolic clearance of compounds known to be metabolized by cytochrome P450 enzymes, which may be due to the suppression of growth hormones. Since it cannot be excluded that octreotide may have this effect, other drugs mainly metabolized by CYP3A4, and which have a low therapeutic index should therefore be used with caution).
No products indexed under this heading.

Chlorpheniramine Maleate (Data indicates that somatostatin analogs might decrease the metabolic clearance of compounds known to be metabolized by cytochrome P450 enzymes, which may be due to the suppression of growth hormones. Since it cannot be excluded that octreotide may have this effect, other drugs mainly metabolized by CYP3A4, and which have a low therapeutic index should therefore be used with caution). Products include:
Advil Allergy Sinus Caplets .... ▣737
Advil Multi-Symptom Cold Caplets .... ▣738
BC Allergy Sinus Cold Powder .... ▣612
Contac Severe Cold and Flu Caplets Maximum Strength......... ▣615
Hycomine Compound Tablets 1105
PediaCare Multi-Symptom Cold Liquid .... ▣704
PediaCare NightRest Cough & Cold Liquid...................................... ▣704
Robitussin Flu Liquid .... ▣752
Robitussin PM Cough & Cold Liquid .... ▣752
Singlet Caplets .... ▣636
Sudafed Sinus & Allergy Tablets ..... ▣710
TheraFlu Cold & Cough Hot Liquid .... ▣680
TheraFlu Cold & Sore Throat Hot Liquid .... ▣680
TheraFlu Flu & Sore Throat Hot Liquid .... ▣681
TheraFlu Severe Cold & Cough Hot Liquid .... ▣683
TheraFlu Severe Cold Caplets .... ▣679
TheraFlu Severe Cold Hot Liquid .... ▣682
Triaminic Cold & Allergy Liquid .... ▣685
Triaminic Cold & Cough Liquid .... ▣685
Triaminic Flu, Cough & Fever Liquid .... ▣685
Triaminic Night Time Cough & Cold Liquid....................................... ▣685
Triaminic Allergy Runny Nose & Congestion Softchews.................. ▣688
Triaminic Cold & Cough Softchews .... ▣688

Children's Tylenol Plus Cold NightTime Suspension Liquid........ 1851
Children's Tylenol Plus Cold & Cough Suspension Liquid and Chewable Tablets........................ 1851
Children's Tylenol Plus Cold Chewable Tablets........................ 1851
Children's Tylenol Plus Flu Suspension Liquid........................ 1853
Tylenol Allergy Complete Multi-Symptom Caplets and Gelcaps with Cool Burst................ 1844
Multi-Symptom Tylenol Cold Night Time Caplets........................ 1845
Vicks 44M Cough, Cold & Flu Relief.. 2676
Pediatric Vicks 44m Cough & Cold Relief.................................. 2673
Children's Vicks NyQuil Cold/Cough Relief........................ 2671

Chlorpheniramine Polistirex (Data indicates that somatostatin analogs might decrease the metabolic clearance of compounds known to be metabolized by cytochrome P450 enzymes, which may be due to the suppression of growth hormones. Since it cannot be excluded that octreotide may have this effect, other drugs mainly metabolized by CYP3A4, and which have a low therapeutic index should therefore be used with caution). Products include:
Tussionex Pennkinetic Extended-Release Suspension...... 3322

Chlorpheniramine Tannate (Data indicates that somatostatin analogs might decrease the metabolic clearance of compounds known to be metabolized by cytochrome P450 enzymes, which may be due to the suppression of growth hormones. Since it cannot be excluded that octreotide may have this effect, other drugs mainly metabolized by CYP3A4, and which have a low therapeutic index should therefore be used with caution).
No products indexed under this heading.

Chlorpropamide (Octreotide causes hypo- and hyperglycemia in some patients; dosage adjustments of oral hypoglycemic agents may be required).
No products indexed under this heading.

Cisapride (Data indicates that somatostatin analogs might decrease the metabolic clearance of compounds known to be metabolized by cytochrome P450 enzymes, which may be due to the suppression of growth hormones. Since it cannot be excluded that octreotide may have this effect, other drugs mainly metabolized by CYP3A4, and which have a low therapeutic index should therefore be used with caution).
No products indexed under this heading.

Clarithromycin (Data indicates that somatostatin analogs might decrease the metabolic clearance of compounds known to be metabolized by cytochrome P450 enzymes, which may be due to the suppression of growth hormones. Since it cannot be excluded that octreotide may have this effect, other drugs mainly metabolized by CYP3A4, and which have a low therapeutic index should therefore be used with caution). Products include:
Biaxin/Biaxin XL 402
PREVPAC 3281

Cyclosporine (Co-administration may decrease blood levels of cyclosporine and may result in transplant rejection). Products include:
Gengraf Capsules 458
Neoral Soft Gelatin Capsules 2247
Neoral Oral Solution 2247
Restasis Ophthalmic Emulsion 570
Sandimmune 2259

Desogestrel (Data indicates that somatostatin analogs might decrease the metabolic clearance of compounds known to be metabolized by cytochrome P450 enzymes, which may be due to the suppression of growth hormones. Since it cannot be excluded that octreotide may have this effect, other drugs mainly metabolized by CYP3A4, and which have a low therapeutic index should therefore be used with caution). Products include:
Ortho-Cept Tablets 2395

Diazepam (Data indicates that somatostatin analogs might decrease the metabolic clearance of compounds known to be metabolized by cytochrome P450 enzymes, which may be due to the suppression of growth hormones. Since it cannot be excluded that octreotide may have this effect, other drugs mainly metabolized by CYP3A4, and which have a low therapeutic index should therefore be used with caution). Products include:
Diastat Rectal Delivery System 3344
Valium Tablets 2822

Diazoxide (Adjustment of the dosage of diazoxide may be required). Products include:
Hyperstat I.V. Injection 3031

Dihydroergotamine Mesylate (Data indicates that somatostatin analogs might decrease the metabolic clearance of compounds known to be metabolized by cytochrome P450 enzymes, which may be due to the suppression of growth hormones. Since it cannot be excluded that octreotide may have this effect, other drugs mainly metabolized by CYP3A4, and which have a low therapeutic index should therefore be used with caution). Products include:
Migranal Nasal Spray 3350

Diltiazem Hydrochloride (Adjustment of the dosage of calcium channel blocker may be required). Products include:
Cardizem LA Extended Release Tablets 1699
Tiazac Capsules 1204

Diltiazem Maleate (Data indicates that somatostatin analogs might decrease the metabolic clearance of compounds known to be metabolized by cytochrome P450 enzymes, which may be due to the suppression of growth hormones. Since it cannot be excluded that octreotide may have this effect, other drugs mainly metabolized by CYP3A4, and which have a low therapeutic index should therefore be used with caution).
No products indexed under this heading.

Disopyramide (Data indicates that somatostatin analogs might decrease the metabolic clearance of compounds known to be metabolized by cytochrome P450 enzymes, which may be due to the suppression of growth hormones. Since it cannot be excluded that octreotide may have this effect, other drugs mainly metabolized by CYP3A4, and which have a low therapeutic index should therefore be used with caution).
No products indexed under this heading.

Disopyramide Phosphate (Data indicates that somatostatin analogs might decrease the metabolic clearance of compounds known to be metabolized by cytochrome P450 enzymes, which may be due to the suppression of growth hormones. Since it cannot be excluded that octreotide may have this effect, other drugs mainly metabolized by CYP3A4, and which have a low therapeutic index should therefore be used with caution).
No products indexed under this heading.

Disulfiram (Data indicates that somatostatin analogs might decrease the metabolic clearance of compounds known to be metabolized by cytochrome P450 enzymes, which may be due to the suppression of growth hormones. Since it cannot be excluded that octreotide may have this effect, other drugs mainly metabolized by CYP3A4, and which have a low therapeutic index should therefore be used with caution). Products include:
Antabuse Tablets 2343

Doxorubicin Hydrochloride (Data indicates that somatostatin analogs might decrease the metabolic clearance of compounds known to be metabolized by cytochrome P450 enzymes, which may be due to the suppression of growth hormones. Since it cannot be excluded that octreotide may have this effect, other drugs mainly metabolized by CYP3A4, and which have a low therapeutic index should therefore be used with caution). Products include:
Adriamycin for Injection, USP 786
Adriamycin Injection, USP 786

Dronabinol (Data indicates that somatostatin analogs might decrease the metabolic clearance of compounds known to be metabolized by cytochrome P450 enzymes, which may be due to the suppression of growth hormones. Since it cannot be excluded that octreotide may have this effect, other drugs mainly metabolized by CYP3A4, and which have a low therapeutic index should therefore be used with caution). Products include:
Marinol Capsules 3334

Ergotamine Tartrate (Data indicates that somatostatin analogs might decrease the metabolic clearance of compounds known to be metabolized by cytochrome P450 enzymes, which may be due to the suppression of growth hormones. Since it cannot be excluded that octreotide may have this effect, other drugs mainly metabolized by CYP3A4, and which have a low therapeutic index should therefore be used with caution).
No products indexed under this heading.

Erythromycin (Data indicates that somatostatin analogs might decrease the metabolic clearance of compounds known to be metabolized by cytochrome P450 enzymes, which may be due to the suppression of growth hormones. Since it cannot be excluded that octreotide may have this effect, other drugs mainly metabolized by CYP3A4, and which have a low therapeutic index should therefore be used with caution). Products include:
Erygel Topical Gel 2096
Ery-Tab Tablets 447
Erythromycin Base Filmtab Tablets 454
Erythromycin Delayed-Release Capsules, USP 456
PCE Dispertab Tablets 510

Erythromycin Estolate (Data indicates that somatostatin analogs might decrease the metabolic clearance of compounds known to be metabolized by cytochrome P450 enzymes, which may be due to the suppression of growth hormones. Since it cannot be excluded that octreotide may have this effect, other drugs mainly metabolized by CYP3A4, and which have a low therapeutic index should therefore be used with caution).
No products indexed under this heading.

Erythromycin Ethylsuccinate (Data indicates that somatostatin analogs might decrease the metabolic clearance of compounds known to be metabolized by cytochrome P450 enzymes, which may be due to the suppression of growth hormones. Since it cannot be excluded that octreotide may have this effect, other drugs mainly metabolized by CYP3A4, and which have a low therapeutic index should therefore be used with caution). Products include:
E.E.S. 449
EryPed 445

Erythromycin Gluceptate (Data indicates that somatostatin analogs might decrease the metabolic clearance of compounds known to be metabolized by cytochrome P450 enzymes, which may be due to the suppression of growth hormones. Since it cannot be excluded that octreotide may have this effect, other drugs mainly metabolized by CYP3A4, and which have a low therapeutic index should therefore be used with caution).
No products indexed under this heading.

Erythromycin Lactobionate (Data indicates that somatostatin analogs might decrease the metabolic clearance of compounds known to be metabolized by cytochrome P450 enzymes, which may be due to the suppression of growth hormones. Since it cannot be excluded that octreotide may have this effect, other drugs mainly metabolized by CYP3A4, and which have a low therapeutic index should therefore be used with caution).
No products indexed under this heading.

Erythromycin Stearate (Data indicates that somatostatin analogs might decrease the metabolic clearance of compounds known to be metabolized by cytochrome P450 enzymes, which may be due to the suppression of growth hormones. Since it cannot be excluded that octreotide may have this effect, other drugs mainly metabolized by CYP3A4, and which have a low therapeutic index should therefore be used with caution). Products include:
Erythrocin Stearate Filmtab Tablets 452

Esmolol Hydrochloride (Adjustment of the dosage of beta blockers may be required). Products include:
Brevibloc Concentrate ... 766
Brevibloc Injection ... 766
Brevibloc Double Strength Injection ... 766
Brevibloc Premixed Injection ... 766
Brevibloc Double Strength Premixed Injection ... 766

Estradiol (Data indicates that somatostatin analogs might decrease the metabolic clearance of compounds known to be metabolized by cytochrome P450 enzymes, which may be due to the suppression of growth hormones. Since it cannot be excluded that octreotide may have this effect, other drugs mainly metabolized by CYP3A4, and which have a low therapeutic index should therefore be used with caution). Products include:
Activella Tablets ... 2311
Climara Transdermal System ... 795
Climara Pro Transdermal System ... 800
CombiPatch Transdermal System ... 2180
Estrogel 0.06% ... 3200
Menostar Transdermal System ... 805
Prefest Tablets ... 1069
Vagifem Tablets ... 2340
Vivelle Transdermal System ... 2288
Vivelle-Dot Transdermal System ... 2293

Estradiol Benzoate (Data indicates that somatostatin analogs might decrease the metabolic clearance of compounds known to be metabolized by cytochrome P450 enzymes, which may be due to the suppression of growth hormones. Since it cannot be excluded that octreotide may have this effect, other drugs mainly metabolized by CYP3A4, and which have a low therapeutic index should therefore be used with caution).
No products indexed under this heading.

Estradiol Cypionate (Data indicates that somatostatin analogs might decrease the metabolic clearance of compounds known to be metabolized by cytochrome P450 enzymes, which may be due to the suppression of growth hormones. Since it cannot be excluded that octreotide may have this effect, other drugs mainly metabolized by CYP3A4, and which have a low therapeutic index should therefore be used with caution).
No products indexed under this heading.

Estradiol Valerate (Data indicates that somatostatin analogs might decrease the metabolic clearance of compounds known to be metabolized by cytochrome P450 enzymes, which may be due to the suppression of growth hormones. Since it cannot be excluded that octreotide may have this effect, other drugs mainly metabolized by CYP3A4, and which have a low therapeutic index should therefore be used with caution).
No products indexed under this heading.

Ethinyl Estradiol (Data indicates that somatostatin analogs might decrease the metabolic clearance of compounds known to be metabolized by cytochrome P450 enzymes, which may be due to the suppression of growth hormones. Since it cannot be excluded that octreotide may have this effect, other drugs mainly metabolized by CYP3A4, and which have a low therapeutic index should therefore be used with caution). Products include:
Alesse-28 Tablets ... 3392
Lo/Ovral-28 Tablets ... 3423
NuvaRing ... 2357
Ortho-Cept Tablets ... 2395
Ortho-Cyclen/Ortho Tri-Cyclen ... 2414
Ortho Evra Transdermal System ... 2402
Ortho Tri-Cyclen Lo Tablets ... 2421
Seasonale Tablets ... 1073
Triphasil-28 Tablets ... 3483
Yasmin 28 Tablets ... 818

Ethosuximide (Data indicates that somatostatin analogs might decrease the metabolic clearance of compounds known to be metabolized by cytochrome P450 enzymes, which may be due to the suppression of growth hormones. Since it cannot be excluded that octreotide may have this effect, other drugs mainly metabolized by CYP3A4, and which have a low therapeutic index should therefore be used with caution).
No products indexed under this heading.

Ethynodiol Diacetate (Data indicates that somatostatin analogs might decrease the metabolic clearance of compounds known to be metabolized by cytochrome P450 enzymes, which may be due to the suppression of growth hormones. Since it cannot be excluded that octreotide may have this effect, other drugs mainly metabolized by CYP3A4, and which have a low therapeutic index should therefore be used with caution).
No products indexed under this heading.

Etoposide (Data indicates that somatostatin analogs might decrease the metabolic clearance of compounds known to be metabolized by cytochrome P450 enzymes, which may be due to the suppression of growth hormones. Since it cannot be excluded that octreotide may have this effect, other drugs mainly metabolized by CYP3A4, and which have a low therapeutic index should therefore be used with caution).
No products indexed under this heading.

Etoposide Phosphate (Data indicates that somatostatin analogs might decrease the metabolic clearance of compounds known to be metabolized by cytochrome P450 enzymes, which may be due to the suppression of growth hormones. Since it cannot be excluded that octreotide may have this effect, other drugs mainly metabolized by CYP3A4, and which have a low therapeutic index should therefore be used with caution).
No products indexed under this heading.

Felodipine (Adjustment of the dosage of calcium channel blocker may be required). Products include:
Plendil Extended-Release Tablets ... 651

Fentanyl (Data indicates that somatostatin analogs might decrease the metabolic clearance of compounds known to be metabolized by cytochrome P450 enzymes, which may be due to the suppression of growth hormones. Since it cannot be excluded that octreotide may have this effect, other drugs mainly metabolized by CYP3A4, and which have a low therapeutic index should therefore be used with caution). Products include:
Duragesic Transdermal System ... 2448

Fentanyl Citrate (Data indicates that somatostatin analogs might decrease the metabolic clearance of compounds known to be metabolized by cytochrome P450 enzymes, which may be due to the suppression of growth hormones. Since it cannot be excluded that octreotide may have this effect, other drugs mainly metabolized by CYP3A4, and which have a low therapeutic index should therefore be used with caution). Products include:
Actiq ... 993

Glimepiride (Octreotide causes hypo- and hyperglycemia in some patients; dosage adjustments of oral hypoglycemic agents may be required). Products include:
Amaryl Tablets ... 2864

Glipizide (Octreotide causes hypo- and hyperglycemia in some patients; dosage adjustments of oral hypoglycemic agents may be required).
No products indexed under this heading.

Glyburide (Octreotide causes hypo- and hyperglycemia in some patients; dosage adjustments of oral hypoglycemic agents may be required).
No products indexed under this heading.

Haloperidol (Data indicates that somatostatin analogs might decrease the metabolic clearance of compounds known to be metabolized by cytochrome P450 enzymes, which may be due to the suppression of growth hormones. Since it cannot be excluded that octreotide may have this effect, other drugs mainly metabolized by CYP3A4, and which have a low therapeutic index should therefore be used with caution).
No products indexed under this heading.

Haloperidol Decanoate (Data indicates that somatostatin analogs might decrease the metabolic clearance of compounds known to be metabolized by cytochrome P450 enzymes, which may be due to the suppression of growth hormones. Since it cannot be excluded that octreotide may have this effect, other drugs mainly metabolized by CYP3A4, and which have a low therapeutic index should therefore be used with caution).
No products indexed under this heading.

Haloperidol Lactate (Data indicates that somatostatin analogs might decrease the metabolic clearance of compounds known to be metabolized by cytochrome P450 enzymes, which may be due to the suppression of growth hormones. Since it cannot be excluded that octreotide may have this effect, other drugs mainly metabolized by CYP3A4, and which have a low therapeutic index should therefore be used with caution).
No products indexed under this heading.

Indinavir Sulfate (Data indicates that somatostatin analogs might decrease the metabolic clearance of compounds known to be metabolized by cytochrome P450 enzymes, which may be due to the suppression of growth hormones. Since it cannot be excluded that octreotide may have this effect, other drugs mainly metabolized by CYP3A4, and which have a low therapeutic index should therefore be used with caution). Products include:
Crixivan Capsules ... 1918

Insulin, Human, Zinc Suspension (Octreotide causes hypo- and hyperglycemia in some patients; insulin dosage adjustments may be required). Products include:
Humulin L, 100 Units ... 1763
Humulin U, 100 Units ... 1770

Insulin, Human NPH (Octreotide causes hypo- and hyperglycemia in some patients; insulin dosage adjustments may be required). Products include:
Humulin N, 100 Units ... 1764
Humulin N Pen ... 1765
Novolin N Human Insulin 10 ml Vials ... 2322
Novolin N InnoLet ... 2322
Novolin N PenFill 3 ml Cartridges ... 2325
Novolin R InnoLet ... 2322

Insulin, Human Regular (Octreotide causes hypo- and hyperglycemia in some patients; insulin dosage adjustments may be required). Products include:
Humulin R (U-500) ... 1768
Humulin R, 100 Units ... 1767
Novolin R Human Insulin 10 ml Vials ... 2322
Novolin R PenFill ... 2325

Insulin, Human Regular and Human NPH Mixture (Octreotide causes hypo- and hyperglycemia in some patients; insulin dosage adjustments may be required). Products include:
Humulin 50/50, 100 Units ... 1760
Humulin 70/30 Pen ... 1761
Novolin 70/30 Human Insulin 10 ml Vials ... 2321
Novolin 70/30 InnoLet ... 2322
Novolin 70/30 PenFill 3 ml Cartridges ... 2325

Insulin, NPH (Octreotide causes hypo- and hyperglycemia in some patients; insulin dosage adjustments may be required).
No products indexed under this heading.

Insulin, Regular (Octreotide causes hypo- and hyperglycemia in some patients; insulin dosage adjustments may be required).
No products indexed under this heading.

Insulin, Zinc Crystals (Octreotide causes hypo- and hyperglycemia in some patients; insulin dosage adjustments may be required).
No products indexed under this heading.

Insulin, Zinc Suspension (Octreotide causes hypo- and hyperglycemia in some patients; insulin dosage adjustments may be required).
No products indexed under this heading.

Insulin Aspart, Human Regular (Octreotide causes hypo- and hyperglycemia in some patients; insulin dosage adjustments may be required). Products include:
NovoLog Injection ... 2326

Insulin glargine (Octreotide causes hypo- and hyperglycemia in some patients; insulin dosage adjustments may be required). Products include:
Lantus Injection ... 2925

Insulin Lispro, Human (Octreotide causes hypo- and hyperglycemia in

some patients; insulin dosage adjustments may be required). Products include:
Humalog-Pen 1751
Humalog Mix 75/25-Pen 1754

Insulin Lispro Protamine, Human (Octreotide causes hypo- and hyperglycemia in some patients; insulin dosage adjustments may be required). Products include:
Humalog Mix 75/25-Pen 1754

Isradipine (Adjustment of the dosage of calcium channel blocker may be required). Products include:
DynaCirc CR Tablets 2726

Itraconazole (Data indicates that somatostatin analogs might decrease the metabolic clearance of compounds known to be metabolized by cytochrome P450 enzymes, which may be due to the suppression of growth hormones. Since it cannot be excluded that octreotide may have this effect, other drugs mainly metabolized by CYP3A4, and which have a low therapeutic index should therefore be used with caution).
No products indexed under this heading.

Ketoconazole (Data indicates that somatostatin analogs might decrease the metabolic clearance of compounds known to be metabolized by cytochrome P450 enzymes, which may be due to the suppression of growth hormones. Since it cannot be excluded that octreotide may have this effect, other drugs mainly metabolized by CYP3A4, and which have a low therapeutic index should therefore be used with caution). Products include:
Nizoral A-D Shampoo, 1% 1839
Nizoral 2% Shampoo 1838

Labetalol Hydrochloride (Adjustment of the dosage of beta blockers may be required).
No products indexed under this heading.

Levobunolol Hydrochloride (Adjustment of the dosage of beta blockers may be required). Products include:
Betagan Ophthalmic Solution, USP.. ⊙ 217

Levonorgestrel (Data indicates that somatostatin analogs might decrease the metabolic clearance of compounds known to be metabolized by cytochrome P450 enzymes, which may be due to the suppression of growth hormones. Since it cannot be excluded that octreotide may have this effect, other drugs mainly metabolized by CYP3A4, and which have a low therapeutic index should therefore be used with caution). Products include:
Alesse-28 Tablets 3392
Climara Pro Transdermal System 800
Mirena Intrauterine System 810
Plan B Tablets 1068
Seasonale Tablets 1073
Triphasil-28 Tablets 3483

Lidocaine (Data indicates that somatostatin analogs might decrease the metabolic clearance of compounds known to be metabolized by cytochrome P450 enzymes, which may be due to the suppression of growth hormones. Since it cannot be excluded that octreotide may have this effect, other drugs mainly metabolized by CYP3A4, and which have a low therapeutic index should therefore be used with caution). Products include:
Lidoderm Patch 1107

Lidocaine Hydrochloride (Data indicates that somatostatin analogs might decrease the metabolic clearance of compounds known to be metabolized by cytochrome P450 enzymes, which may be due to the suppression of growth hormones. Since it cannot be excluded that octreotide may have this effect, other drugs mainly metabolized by CYP3A4, and which have a low therapeutic index should therefore be used with caution).
No products indexed under this heading.

Lovastatin (Data indicates that somatostatin analogs might decrease the metabolic clearance of compounds known to be metabolized by cytochrome P450 enzymes, which may be due to the suppression of growth hormones. Since it cannot be excluded that octreotide may have this effect, other drugs mainly metabolized by CYP3A4, and which have a low therapeutic index should therefore be used with caution). Products include:
Advicor Tablets 1694
Altoprev Extended-Release Tablets 1151
Mevacor Tablets 1996

Mestranol (Data indicates that somatostatin analogs might decrease the metabolic clearance of compounds known to be metabolized by cytochrome P450 enzymes, which may be due to the suppression of growth hormones. Since it cannot be excluded that octreotide may have this effect, other drugs mainly metabolized by CYP3A4, and which have a low therapeutic index should therefore be used with caution).
No products indexed under this heading.

Metformin Hydrochloride (Octreotide causes hypo- and hyperglycemia in some patients; dosage adjustments of oral hypoglycemic agents may be required). Products include:
ActoPlus Met Tablets 3219
Avandamet Tablets 1343
Fortamet Extended-Release Tablets 1156

Methadone Hydrochloride (Data indicates that somatostatin analogs might decrease the metabolic clearance of compounds known to be metabolized by cytochrome P450 enzymes, which may be due to the suppression of growth hormones. Since it cannot be excluded that octreotide may have this effect, other drugs mainly metabolized by CYP3A4, and which have a low therapeutic index should therefore be used with caution).
No products indexed under this heading.

Metipranolol Hydrochloride (Adjustment of the dosage of beta blockers may be required).
No products indexed under this heading.

Metoprolol Succinate (Adjustment of the dosage of beta blockers may be required). Products include:
Toprol-XL Tablets 660

Metoprolol Tartrate (Adjustment of the dosage of beta blockers may be required).
No products indexed under this heading.

Mibefradil Dihydrochloride (Adjustment of the dosage of calcium channel blocker may be required).
No products indexed under this heading.

Midazolam Hydrochloride (Data indicates that somatostatin analogs might decrease the metabolic clearance of compounds known to be metabolized by cytochrome P450 enzymes, which may be due to the suppression of growth hormones. Since it cannot be excluded that octreotide may have this effect, other drugs mainly metabolized by CYP3A4, and which have a low therapeutic index should therefore be used with caution).
No products indexed under this heading.

Miglitol (Octreotide causes hypo- and hyperglycemia in some patients; dosage adjustments of oral hypoglycemic agents may be required).
No products indexed under this heading.

Nadolol (Adjustment of the dosage of beta blockers may be required). Products include:
Nadolol Tablets 2121

Nefazodone Hydrochloride (Data indicates that somatostatin analogs might decrease the metabolic clearance of compounds known to be metabolized by cytochrome P450 enzymes, which may be due to the suppression of growth hormones. Since it cannot be excluded that octreotide may have this effect, other drugs mainly metabolized by CYP3A4, and which have a low therapeutic index should therefore be used with caution).
No products indexed under this heading.

Nelfinavir Mesylate (Data indicates that somatostatin analogs might decrease the metabolic clearance of compounds known to be metabolized by cytochrome P450 enzymes, which may be due to the suppression of growth hormones. Since it cannot be excluded that octreotide may have this effect, other drugs mainly metabolized by CYP3A4, and which have a low therapeutic index should therefore be used with caution). Products include:
Viracept 2556

Nicardipine Hydrochloride (Adjustment of the dosage of calcium channel blocker may be required). Products include:
Cardene I.V. 1129

Nifedipine (Adjustment of the dosage of calcium channel blocker may be required). Products include:
Adalat CC Tablets 2978

Nimodipine (Adjustment of the dosage of calcium channel blocker may be required). Products include:
Nimotop Capsules 774

Nisoldipine (Adjustment of the dosage of calcium channel blocker may be required). Products include:
Sular Tablets 1163

Nitrendipine (Data indicates that somatostatin analogs might decrease the metabolic clearance of compounds known to be metabolized by cytochrome P450 enzymes, which may be due to the suppression of growth hormones. Since it cannot be excluded that octreotide may have this effect, other drugs mainly metabolized by CYP3A4, and which have a low therapeutic index should therefore be used with caution).
No products indexed under this heading.

Norethindrone (Data indicates that somatostatin analogs might decrease the metabolic clearance of compounds known to be metabolized by cytochrome P450 enzymes, which may be due to the suppression of growth hormones. Since it cannot be excluded that octreotide may have this effect, other drugs mainly metabolized by CYP3A4, and which have a low therapeutic index should therefore be used with caution). Products include:
Ortho Micronor Tablets 2411

Norethindrone Acetate (Data indicates that somatostatin analogs might decrease the metabolic clearance of compounds known to be metabolized by cytochrome P450 enzymes, which may be due to the suppression of growth hormones. Since it cannot be excluded that octreotide may have this effect, other drugs mainly metabolized by CYP3A4, and which have a low therapeutic index should therefore be used with caution). Products include:
Activella Tablets 2311
Aygestin Tablets 1062
CombiPatch Transdermal System 2180

Norgestrel (Data indicates that somatostatin analogs might decrease the metabolic clearance of compounds known to be metabolized by cytochrome P450 enzymes, which may be due to the suppression of growth hormones. Since it cannot be excluded that octreotide may have this effect, other drugs mainly metabolized by CYP3A4, and which have a low therapeutic index should therefore be used with caution). Products include:
Lo/Ovral-28 Tablets 3423

Ondansetron (Data indicates that somatostatin analogs might decrease the metabolic clearance of compounds known to be metabolized by cytochrome P450 enzymes, which may be due to the suppression of growth hormones. Since it cannot be excluded that octreotide may have this effect, other drugs mainly metabolized by CYP3A4, and which have a low therapeutic index should therefore be used with caution). Products include:
Zofran ODT Orally Disintegrating Tablets 1613

Ondansetron Hydrochloride (Data indicates that somatostatin analogs might decrease the metabolic clearance of compounds known to be metabolized by cytochrome P450 enzymes, which may be due to the suppression of growth hormones. Since it cannot be excluded that octreotide may have this effect, other drugs mainly metabolized by CYP3A4, and which have a low therapeutic index should therefore be used with caution). Products include:
Zofran Injection 1607
Zofran 1613

Paclitaxel (Data indicates that somatostatin analogs might decrease the metabolic clearance of compounds known to be metabolized by cytochrome P450 enzymes, which may be due to the suppression of growth hormones. Since it cannot be excluded that octreotide

may have this effect, other drugs mainly metabolized by CYP3A4, and which have a low therapeutic index should therefore be used with caution).
No products indexed under this heading.

Penbutolol Sulfate (Adjustment of the dosage of beta blockers may be required).
No products indexed under this heading.

Pimozide (Data indicates that somatostatin analogs might decrease the metabolic clearance of compounds known to be metabolized by cytochrome P450 enzymes, which may be due to the suppression of growth hormones. Since it cannot be excluded that octreotide may have this effect, other drugs mainly metabolized by CYP3A4, and which have a low therapeutic index should therefore be used with caution). Products include:
Orap Tablets 1220

Pindolol (Adjustment of the dosage of beta blockers may be required).
No products indexed under this heading.

Pioglitazone Hydrochloride (Octreotide causes hypo- and hyperglycemia in some patients; dosage adjustments of oral hypoglycemic agents may be required). Products include:
ActoPlus Met Tablets 3219
Actos Tablets 3224

Polyestradiol Phosphate (Data indicates that somatostatin analogs might decrease the metabolic clearance of compounds known to be metabolized by cytochrome P450 enzymes, which may be due to the suppression of growth hormones. Since it cannot be excluded that octreotide may have this effect, other drugs mainly metabolized by CYP3A4, and which have a low therapeutic index should therefore be used with caution).
No products indexed under this heading.

Propranolol Hydrochloride (Adjustment of the dosage of beta blockers may be required). Products include:
Inderal LA Long-Acting Capsules 3421
InnoPran XL Capsules 2728

Quinidine (Use caution with drugs mainly metabolized by CYP3A4 and which have a low therapeutic index. Data indicate that somatostatin analogs might decrease the metabolic clearence of compounds metabolized by CYP450 enzymes).
No products indexed under this heading.

Quinidine Gluconate (Use caution with drugs mainly metabolized by CYP3A4 and which have a low therapeutic index. Data indicate that somatostatin analogs might decrease the metabolic clearence of compounds metabolized by CYP450 enzymes).
No products indexed under this heading.

Quinidine Hydrochloride (Use caution with drugs mainly metabolized by CYP3A4 and which have a low therapeutic index. Data indicate that somatostatin analogs might decrease the metabolic clearence of compounds metabolized by CYP450 enzymes).
No products indexed under this heading.

Quinidine Polygalacturonate (Use caution with drugs mainly metabolized by CYP3A4 and which have a low therapeutic index. Data indicate that somatostatin analogs might decrease the metabolic clearence of compounds metabolized by CYP450 enzymes).
No products indexed under this heading.

Quinidine Sulfate (Use caution with drugs mainly metabolized by CYP3A4 and which have a low therapeutic index. Data indicate that somatostatin analogs might decrease the metabolic clearence of compounds metabolized by CYP450 enzymes).
No products indexed under this heading.

Repaglinide (Octreotide causes hypo- and hyperglycemia in some patients; dosage adjustments of oral hypoglycemic agents may be required). Products include:
Prandin Tablets (0.5, 1, and 2 mg) 2337

Rifabutin (Data indicates that somatostatin analogs might decrease the metabolic clearance of compounds known to be metabolized by cytochrome P450 enzymes, which may be due to the suppression of growth hormones. Since it cannot be excluded that octreotide may have this effect, other drugs mainly metabolized by CYP3A4, and which have a low therapeutic index should therefore be used with caution).
No products indexed under this heading.

Ritonavir (Data indicates that somatostatin analogs might decrease the metabolic clearance of compounds known to be metabolized by cytochrome P450 enzymes, which may be due to the suppression of growth hormones. Since it cannot be excluded that octreotide may have this effect, other drugs mainly metabolized by CYP3A4, and which have a low therapeutic index should therefore be used with caution). Products include:
Kaletra 474
Norvir 499

Rosiglitazone Maleate (Octreotide causes hypo- and hyperglycemia in some patients; dosage adjustments of oral hypoglycemic agents may be required). Products include:
Avandamet Tablets 1343
Avandia Tablets 1348

Saquinavir (Data indicates that somatostatin analogs might decrease the metabolic clearance of compounds known to be metabolized by cytochrome P450 enzymes, which may be due to the suppression of growth hormones. Since it cannot be excluded that octreotide may have this effect, other drugs mainly metabolized by CYP3A4, and which have a low therapeutic index should therefore be used with caution).
No products indexed under this heading.

Saquinavir Mesylate (Data indicates that somatostatin analogs might decrease the metabolic clearance of compounds known to be metabolized by cytochrome P450 enzymes, which may be due to the suppression of growth hormones. Since it cannot be excluded that octreotide may have this effect, other drugs mainly metabolized by CYP3A4, and which have a low therapeutic index should therefore be used with caution). Products include:
Invirase 2776

Sertraline Hydrochloride (Data indicates that somatostatin analogs might decrease the metabolic clearance of compounds known to be metabolized by cytochrome P450 enzymes, which may be due to the suppression of growth hormones. Since it cannot be excluded that octreotide may have this effect, other drugs mainly metabolized by CYP3A4, and which have a low therapeutic index should therefore be used with caution). Products include:
Zoloft 2581

Sildenafil Citrate (Data indicates that somatostatin analogs might decrease the metabolic clearance of compounds known to be metabolized by cytochrome P450 enzymes, which may be due to the suppression of growth hormones. Since it cannot be excluded that octreotide may have this effect, other drugs mainly metabolized by CYP3A4, and which have a low therapeutic index should therefore be used with caution). Products include:
Revatio Tablets 2541
Viagra Tablets 2552

Simvastatin (Data indicates that somatostatin analogs might decrease the metabolic clearance of compounds known to be metabolized by cytochrome P450 enzymes, which may be due to the suppression of growth hormones. Since it cannot be excluded that octreotide may have this effect, other drugs mainly metabolized by CYP3A4, and which have a low therapeutic index should therefore be used with caution). Products include:
Vytorin 10/10 Tablets 2084
Vytorin 10/10 Tablets 3092
Vytorin 10/20 Tablets 2084
Vytorin 10/20 Tablets 3092
Vytorin 10/40 Tablets 3092
Vytorin 10/40 Tablets 2084
Vytorin 10/80 Tablets 2084
Vytorin 10/80 Tablets 3092
Zocor Tablets 2078

Sirolimus (Data indicates that somatostatin analogs might decrease the metabolic clearance of compounds known to be metabolized by cytochrome P450 enzymes, which may be due to the suppression of growth hormones. Since it cannot be excluded that octreotide may have this effect, other drugs mainly metabolized by CYP3A4, and which have a low therapeutic index should therefore be used with caution). Products include:
Rapamune Oral Solution and Tablets 3472

Sotalol Hydrochloride (Adjustment of the dosage of beta blockers may be required).
No products indexed under this heading.

Tacrolimus (Data indicates that somatostatin analogs might decrease the metabolic clearance of compounds known to be metabolized by cytochrome P450 enzymes, which may be due to the suppression of growth hormones. Since it cannot be excluded that octreotide may have this effect, other drugs mainly metabolized by CYP3A4, and which have a low therapeutic index should therefore be used with caution). Products include:
Prograf Capsules and Injection 624
Protopic Ointment 629

Tamoxifen Citrate (Data indicates that somatostatin analogs might decrease the metabolic clearance of compounds known to be metabolized by cytochrome P450 enzymes, which may be due to the suppression of growth hormones. Since it cannot be excluded that octreotide may have this effect, other drugs mainly metabolized by CYP3A4, and which have a low therapeutic index should therefore be used with caution).
No products indexed under this heading.

Terfenadine (Use caution with drugs mainly metabolized by CYP3A4 and which have a low therapeutic index. Data indicate that somatostatin analogs might decrease the metabolic clearance of compounds metabolized by CYP450 enzymes).
No products indexed under this heading.

Tiagabine Hydrochloride (Data indicates that somatostatin analogs might decrease the metabolic clearance of compounds known to be metabolized by cytochrome P450 enzymes, which may be due to the suppression of growth hormones. Since it cannot be excluded that octreotide may have this effect, other drugs mainly metabolized by CYP3A4, and which have a low therapeutic index should therefore be used with caution). Products include:
Gabitril Tablets 998

Timolol Hemihydrate (Adjustment of the dosage of beta blockers may be required). Products include:
Betimol Ophthalmic Solution 3371
Betimol Ophthalmic Solution ..... ⊙ 283

Timolol Maleate (Adjustment of the dosage of beta blockers may be required). Products include:
Blocadren Tablets 1891
Cosopt Sterile Ophthalmic Solution 1910
Timolide Tablets 2056
Timoptic in Ocudose 2061
Timoptic Sterile Ophthalmic Solution 2058
Timoptic-XE Sterile Ophthalmic Gel Forming Solution 2062

Tolazamide (Octreotide causes hypo- and hyperglycemia in some patients; dosage adjustments of oral hypoglycemic agents may be required).
No products indexed under this heading.

Tolbutamide (Octreotide causes hypo- and hyperglycemia in some patients; dosage adjustments of oral hypoglycemic agents may be required).
No products indexed under this heading.

Tolterodine Tartrate (Data indicates that somatostatin analogs might decrease the metabolic clearance of compounds known to be metabolized by cytochrome P450 enzymes, which may be due to the suppression of growth hormones. Since it cannot be excluded that octreotide may have this effect, other drugs mainly metabolized by CYP3A4, and which have a low therapeutic index should therefore be used with caution). Products include:
Detrol Tablets 2626
Detrol LA Capsules 2629

Trazodone Hydrochloride (Data indicates that somatostatin analogs might decrease the metabolic clearance of compounds known to be metabolized by cytochrome P450 enzymes, which may be due to the suppression of growth hormones. Since it cannot be excluded that octreotide may have this effect, other drugs mainly metabolized by CYP3A4, and which have a low therapeutic index should therefore be used with caution).
No products indexed under this heading.

Triazolam (Data indicates that somatostatin analogs might decrease the metabolic clearance of compounds known to be metabolized by cytochrome P450 enzymes, which may be due to the suppression of growth hormones. Since it cannot be excluded that octreotide may have this effect, other drugs mainly metabolized by CYP3A4, and which have a low therapeutic index should therefore be used with caution).
No products indexed under this heading.

Troglitazone (Octreotide causes hypo- and hyperglycemia in some patients; dosage adjustments of oral hypoglycemic agents may be required).
No products indexed under this heading.

Verapamil Hydrochloride (Adjustment of the dosage of calcium channel blocker may be required). Products include:
- Covera-HS Tablets ... **3135**
- Tarka Tablets ... **519**
- Verelan PM Capsules ... **3120**

Vinblastine Sulfate (Data indicates that somatostatin analogs might decrease the metabolic clearance of compounds known to be metabolized by cytochrome P450 enzymes, which may be due to the suppression of growth hormones. Since it cannot be excluded that octreotide may have this effect, other drugs mainly metabolized by CYP3A4, and which have a low therapeutic index should therefore be used with caution).
No products indexed under this heading.

Vincristine Sulfate (Data indicates that somatostatin analogs might decrease the metabolic clearance of compounds known to be metabolized by cytochrome P450 enzymes, which may be due to the suppression of growth hormones. Since it cannot be excluded that octreotide may have this effect, other drugs mainly metabolized by CYP3A4, and which have a low therapeutic index should therefore be used with caution).
No products indexed under this heading.

Warfarin Sodium (Data indicates that somatostatin analogs might decrease the metabolic clearance of compounds known to be metabolized by cytochrome P450 enzymes, which may be due to the suppression of growth hormones. Since it cannot be excluded that octreotide may have this effect, other drugs mainly metabolized by CYP3A4, and which have a low therapeutic index should therefore be used with caution). Products include:
- Coumadin for Injection ... **932**
- Coumadin Tablets ... **932**

SEASONALE TABLETS

(Ethinyl Estradiol, Levonorgestrel) **1073**
May interact with barbiturates, cytochrome p450 3a4 inhibitors (selected), phenytoin, protease inhibitors, tetracyclines, xanthines, and certain other agents. Compounds in these categories include:

Acetaminophen (Acetaminophen may increase plasma ethinyl estradiol levels, possibly by inhibition of conjugation. Decreased plasma concentrations of acetaminophen have been noted when co-administered with combination oral contraceptives). Products include:
- Benadryl Allergy & Cold Tablets ... **692**
- Benadryl Allergy & Sinus Headache Caplets & Gelcaps ... **693**
- Benadryl Maximum Strength Severe Allergy & Sinus Headache Caplets ... **694**
- Contac Severe Cold and Flu Caplets Maximum Strength ... **615**
- Contac Severe Cold and Flu Caplets Non-Drowsy ... **615**
- Darvocet A 500 Tablets ... **3497**
- Goody's Body Pain Formula Powder ... **621**
- Goody's Extra Strength Headache Powder ... **621**
- Goody's Extra Strength Pain Relief Tablets ... **621**
- Goody's PM Powder ... **622**
- Hycomine Compound Tablets ... **1105**
- Lortab ... **3315**
- Lortab Elixir ... **3312**
- Percocet Tablets ... **1114**
- Robitussin Cough, Cold & Flu Liquid-filled Capsules ... **750**
- Robitussin Flu Liquid ... **752**
- Sedapap Tablets 50 mg/650 mg ... **2098**
- Singlet Caplets ... **636**
- Sudafed Severe Cold ... **710**
- Sudafed Sinus Headache ... **711**
- TheraFlu Cold & Cough Hot Liquid ... **680**
- TheraFlu Cold & Sore Throat Hot Liquid ... **680**
- TheraFlu Flu & Chest Congestion Non-Drowsy Hot Liquid ... **681**
- TheraFlu Flu & Sore Throat Hot Liquid ... **681**
- TheraFlu Severe Cold Non-Drowsy Hot Liquid ... **683**
- TheraFlu Severe Cold & Cough Hot Liquid ... **683**
- TheraFlu Severe Cold Caplets ... **679**
- TheraFlu Severe Cold Hot Liquid ... **682**
- TheraFlu Severe Cold Non-Drowsy Caplets ... **679**
- Triaminic Cough & Sore Throat Liquid ... **687**
- Triaminic Flu, Cough & Fever Liquid ... **685**
- Triaminic Cough & Sore Throat Softchews ... **689**
- Tylenol 8 Hour Extended Release Geltabs and Caplets ... **1843**
- Tylenol Sinus NightTime Caplets ... **663**
- Children's Tylenol Suspension Liquid and Meltaways ... **1850**
- Children's Tylenol Plus Cold & Allergy Suspension Liquid ... **1850**
- Children's Tylenol Plus Cold NightTime Suspension Liquid ... **1851**
- Children's Tylenol Plus Cold & Cough Suspension Liquid and Chewable Tablets ... **1851**
- Children's Tylenol Plus Cold Chewable Tablets ... **1851**
- Children's Tylenol Plus Cold Daytime Non-Drowsy Suspension Liquid ... **1851**
- Children's Tylenol Plus Flu Suspension Liquid ... **1853**
- Concentrated Tylenol Infants' Drops Plus Cold ... **1851**
- Concentrated Tylenol Infants' Drops Plus Cold and Cough ... **1851**
- Concentrated Tylenol Infants' Drops ... **1850**
- Junior Tylenol Meltaways ... **1850**
- Tylenol Cold & Flu Severe Daytime Liquid with Cool Bust ... **1846**
- Tylenol Cold & Flu Severe NightTime Liquid with Cool Burst ... **1846**
- Tylenol Cold Severe Congestion Non-Drowsy Caplets with Cool Burst ... **1846**
- Tylenol Cough & Sore Throat Daytime Liquid with Cool Burst ... **1849**
- Tylenol Cough & Sore Throat NightTime Liquid with Cool Burst ... **1849**
- Tylenol ... **1843**
- Extra Strength Tylenol Rapid Release Gels ... **1843**
- Tylenol ... **1843**
- Tylenol Allergy Complete Night Time Caplets ... **1844**
- Tylenol Allergy Complete Multi-Symptom Caplets and Gelcaps with Cool Burst ... **1844**
- Tylenol Severe Allergy Caplets ... **1844**
- Tylenol Flu NightTime Gelcaps ... **1846**
- Tylenol Flu Day Non-Drowsy Gelcaps ... **1846**
- Concentrated Tylenol Infants' Drops Plus Cold Nasal Congestant, Fever Reducer & Pain Reliever ... **668**
- Concentrated Tylenol Infants' Drops Plus Cold & Cough Nasal Decongestant, Fever Reducer & Pain Reliever ... **668**
- Multi-Symptom Tylenol Cold Night Time Caplets ... **1845**
- Multi-Symptom Tylenol Cold Day Non-Drowsy Caplets and Gelcaps ... **1845**
- Extra Strength Tylenol PM Caplets, Geltabs, Gelcaps and Liquid ... **1847**
- Tylenol Sinus Day Non-Drowsy ... **1848**
- Tylenol Sinus Night Time Caplets ... **1848**
- Tylenol Sinus Severe Congestion Caplets with Cool Burst ... **1848**
- Tylenol Sore Throat Daytime Liquid with Cool Burst ... **1849**
- Tylenol Sore Throat NightTime Liquid with Cool Burst ... **1849**
- Tylenol with Codeine ... **2461**
- Women's Tylenol Menstrual Relief Caplets ... **1849**
- Ultracet Tablets ... **2462**
- Vicks 44M Cough, Cold & Flu Relief ... **2676**
- Vicks DayQuil LiquiCaps/Liquid Multi-Symptom Cold/Flu Relief ... **723**
- Vicks DayQuil Multi-Symptom Cold/Flu Relief LiquiCaps ... **2675**
- Vicks DayQuil Multi-Symptom Cold/Flu Relief Liquid ... **2675**
- Vicks NyQuil LiquiCaps ... **2677**
- Vicks NyQuil LiquiCaps/Liquid Multi-Symptom Cold/Flu Relief ... **725**
- Vicks NyQuil Liquid ... **2677**
- Vicodin Tablets ... **530**
- Vicodin ES Tablets ... **531**
- Vicodin HP Tablets ... **532**
- Zydone Tablets ... **1118**

Acetazolamide (CYP 3A4 inhibitors may increase plasma ethinyl estradiol levels).
No products indexed under this heading.

Aminophylline (Combination hormonal contraceptives containing some synthetic estrogens (e.g., ethinyl estradiol) may inhibit the metabolism of other compounds. Increased plasma concentrations of theophylline have been reported with concomitant administration of combination oral contraceptives).
No products indexed under this heading.

Amiodarone Hydrochloride (CYP 3A4 inhibitors may increase plasma ethinyl estradiol levels). Products include:
- Pacerone Tablets ... **3337**

Ampicillin (Several cases of contraceptive failure and breakthrough bleeding have been reported in the literature with concomitant administration of antibiotics, such as ampicillin; however, clinical pharmacology studies investigating drug interactions between combined oral contraceptives and these antibiotics have reported inconsistent results).
No products indexed under this heading.

Ampicillin Sodium (Several cases of contraceptive failure and breakthrough bleeding have been reported in the literature with concomitant administration of antibiotics, such as ampicillin; however, clinical pharmacology studies investigating drug interactions between combined oral contraceptives and these antibiotics have reported inconsistent results).
No products indexed under this heading.

Ampicillin Trihydrate (Several cases of contraceptive failure and breakthrough bleeding have been reported in the literature with concomitant administration of antibiotics, such as ampicillin; however, clinical pharmacology studies investigating drug interactions between combined oral contraceptives and these antibiotics have reported inconsistent results).
No products indexed under this heading.

Amprenavir (Several protease inhibitors have been studied with co-administration of oral combination hormonal contraceptives with significant changes (increase and decrease) in the plasma levels of the estrogen and progestin being noted in some cases). Products include:
- Agenerase Capsules ... **1299**
- Agenerase Oral Solution ... **1304**

Anastrozole (CYP 3A4 inhibitors may increase plasma ethinyl estradiol levels). Products include:
- Arimidex Tablets ... **665**

Aprepitant (CYP 3A4 inhibitors may increase plasma ethinyl estradiol levels). Products include:
- Emend Capsules ... **1944**

Aprobarbital (Contraceptive effectiveness may be reduced when hormonal contraceptives are co-administered with drugs that increase the metabolism of contraceptive steroids, such as barbiturates).
No products indexed under this heading.

Ascorbic Acid (Ascorbic acid may increase plasma ethinyl estradiol levels, possibly by inhibition of conjugation).
No products indexed under this heading.

Atorvastatin Calcium (Co-administration of atorvastatin and certain combination oral contraceptives containing ethinyl estradiol increase AUC values for ethinyl estradiol by approximately 20%). Products include:
- Caduet Tablets ... **2507**
- Lipitor Tablets ... **2495**

Butabarbital (Contraceptive effectiveness may be reduced when hormonal contraceptives are co-administered with drugs that increase the metabolism of contraceptive steroids, such as barbiturates).
No products indexed under this heading.

Butalbital (Contraceptive effectiveness may be reduced when hormonal contraceptives are co-administered with drugs that increase the metabolism of contraceptive steroids, such as barbiturates). Products include:
Sedapap Tablets 50 mg/650 mg 2098

Carbamazepine (Contraceptive effectiveness may be reduced when hormonal contraceptives are co-administered with drugs that increase the metabolism of contraceptive steroids, such as carbamazepine). Products include:
Carbatrol Capsules 3174
Equetro Extended-Release Capsules 3178
Tegretol/Tegretol-XR 2278

Cimetidine (CYP 3A4 inhibitors may increase plasma ethinyl estradiol levels). Products include:
Tagamet HB 200 Tablets .... ■637
Tagamet Tablets 1547

Cimetidine Hydrochloride (CYP 3A4 inhibitors may increase plasma ethinyl estradiol levels).
No products indexed under this heading.

Ciprofloxacin (CYP 3A4 inhibitors may increase plasma ethinyl estradiol levels). Products include:
Cipro I.V. 2998
Cipro I.V. Pharmacy Bulk Package ... 3509
Cipro Oral Suspension 2991
Cipro XR Tablets 3004
Ciprodex Otic Suspension 555

Clarithromycin (CYP 3A4 inhibitors may increase plasma ethinyl estradiol levels). Products include:
Biaxin/Biaxin XL 402
PREVPAC 3281

Clofibrate (Increased clearance of clofibric acid due to induction of conjugation has been noted when co-administered with combination oral contraceptives).
No products indexed under this heading.

Clotrimazole (CYP 3A4 inhibitors may increase plasma ethinyl estradiol levels). Products include:
Lotrimin 3053
Lotrisone 3054

Cyclosporine (Combination hormonal contraceptives containing some synthetic estrogens (e.g., ethinyl estradiol) may inhibit the metabolism of other compounds. Increased plasma concentrations of cyclosporine have been reported with concomitant administration of combination oral contraceptives). Products include:
Gengraf Capsules 458
Neoral Soft Gelatin Capsules 2247
Neoral Oral Solution 2247
Restasis Ophthalmic Emulsion 570
Sandimmune 2259

Dalfopristin (CYP 3A4 inhibitors may increase plasma ethinyl estradiol levels). Products include:
Synercid I.V. 1690

Danazol (CYP 3A4 inhibitors may increase plasma ethinyl estradiol levels).
No products indexed under this heading.

Delavirdine Mesylate (CYP 3A4 inhibitors may increase plasma ethinyl estradiol levels). Products include:
Rescriptor Tablets 2535

Demeclocycline Hydrochloride (Several cases of contraceptive failure and breakthrough bleeding have been reported in the literature with concomitant administration of antibiotics, such as tetracyclines; however, clinical pharmacology studies investigating drug interactions between combined oral contraceptives and these antibiotics have reported inconsistent results).
No products indexed under this heading.

Diltiazem Hydrochloride (CYP 3A4 inhibitors may increase plasma ethinyl estradiol levels). Products include:
Cardizem LA Extended Release Tablets 1699
Tiazac Capsules 1204

Diltiazem Maleate (CYP 3A4 inhibitors may increase plasma ethinyl estradiol levels).
No products indexed under this heading.

Doxycycline Calcium (Several cases of contraceptive failure and breakthrough bleeding have been reported in the literature with concomitant administration of antibiotics, such as tetracyclines; however, clinical pharmacology studies investigating drug interactions between combined oral contraceptives and these antibiotics have reported inconsistent results).
No products indexed under this heading.

Doxycycline Hyclate (Several cases of contraceptive failure and breakthrough bleeding have been reported in the literature with concomitant administration of antibiotics, such as tetracyclines; however, clinical pharmacology studies investigating drug interactions between combined oral contraceptives and these antibiotics have reported inconsistent results).
No products indexed under this heading.

Doxycycline Monohydrate (Several cases of contraceptive failure and breakthrough bleeding have been reported in the literature with concomitant administration of antibiotics, such as tetracyclines; however, clinical pharmacology studies investigating drug interactions between combined oral contraceptives and these antibiotics have reported inconsistent results).
No products indexed under this heading.

Dyphylline (Combination hormonal contraceptives containing some synthetic estrogens (e.g., ethinyl estradiol) may inhibit the metabolism of other compounds. Increased plasma concentrations of theophylline have been reported with concomitant administration of combination oral contraceptives).
No products indexed under this heading.

Efavirenz (CYP 3A4 inhibitors may increase plasma ethinyl estradiol levels). Products include:
Sustiva Capsules 957

Erythromycin (CYP 3A4 inhibitors may increase plasma ethinyl estradiol levels). Products include:
Erygel Topical Gel 2096
Ery-Tab Tablets 447
Erythromycin Base Filmtab Tablets 454
Erythromycin Delayed-Release Capsules, USP 456
PCE Dispertab Tablets 510

Erythromycin Estolate (CYP 3A4 inhibitors may increase plasma ethinyl estradiol levels).
No products indexed under this heading.

Erythromycin Ethylsuccinate (CYP 3A4 inhibitors may increase plasma ethinyl estradiol levels). Products include:
E.E.S. 449
EryPed 445

Erythromycin Gluceptate (CYP 3A4 inhibitors may increase plasma ethinyl estradiol levels).
No products indexed under this heading.

Erythromycin Lactobionate (CYP 3A4 inhibitors may increase plasma ethinyl estradiol levels).
No products indexed under this heading.

Erythromycin Stearate (CYP 3A4 inhibitors may increase plasma ethinyl estradiol levels). Products include:
Erythrocin Stearate Filmtab Tablets 452

Esomeprazole Magnesium (CYP 3A4 inhibitors may increase plasma ethinyl estradiol levels). Products include:
Nexium Delayed-Release Capsules 645

Felbamate (Contraceptive effectiveness may be reduced when hormonal contraceptives are co-administered with drugs that increase the metabolism of contraceptive steroids, such as felbamate).
No products indexed under this heading.

Fluconazole (CYP 3A4 inhibitors may increase plasma ethinyl estradiol levels).
No products indexed under this heading.

Fluoxetine Hydrochloride (CYP 3A4 inhibitors may increase plasma ethinyl estradiol levels). Products include:
Prozac Pulvules and Liquid 1771
Symbyax Capsules 1788

Fluvoxamine Maleate (CYP 3A4 inhibitors may increase plasma ethinyl estradiol levels).
No products indexed under this heading.

Fosamprenavir Calcium (CYP 3A4 inhibitors may increase plasma ethinyl estradiol levels). Products include:
Lexiva Tablets 1473

Fosphenytoin Sodium (Contraceptive effectiveness may be reduced when hormonal contraceptives are co-administered with drugs that increase the metabolism of contraceptive steroids, such as phenytoin).
No products indexed under this heading.

Griseofulvin (Contraceptive effectiveness may be reduced when hormonal contraceptives are co-administered with drugs that increase the metabolism of contraceptive steroids, such as griseofulvin). Products include:
Grifulvin V Tablets Microsize and Oral Suspension Microsize 2384
Gris-PEG Tablets 2504

Hypericum (Herbal products containing St. John's Wort (hypericum perforatum) may induce hepatic enzymes (cytochrome P450) and p-glycoprotein transporter and may reduce the effectiveness of contraceptive steroids. This may also result in breakthrough bleeding).
No products indexed under this heading.

Hypericum Perforatum (Herbal products containing St. John's Wort (hypericum perforatum) may induce hepatic enzymes (cytochrome P450) and p-glycoprotein transporter and may reduce the effectiveness of contraceptive steroids. This may also result in breakthrough bleeding).
No products indexed under this heading.

Indinavir Sulfate (Several protease inhibitors have been studied with co-administration of oral combination hormonal contraceptives with significant changes (increase and decrease) in the plasma levels of the estrogen and progestin being noted in some cases). Products include:
Crixivan Capsules 1918

Isoniazid (CYP 3A4 inhibitors may increase plasma ethinyl estradiol levels).
No products indexed under this heading.

Itraconazole (CYP 3A4 inhibitors may increase plasma ethinyl estradiol levels).
No products indexed under this heading.

Ketoconazole (CYP 3A4 inhibitors may increase plasma ethinyl estradiol levels). Products include:
Nizoral A-D Shampoo, 1% 1839
Nizoral 2% Shampoo 1838

Lopinavir (Several protease inhibitors have been studied with co-administration of oral combination hormonal contraceptives with significant changes (increase and decrease) in the plasma levels of the estrogen and progestin being noted in some cases). Products include:
Kaletra 474

Loratadine (CYP 3A4 inhibitors may increase plasma ethinyl estradiol levels). Products include:
Alavert Allergy & Sinus D-12 Hour Tablets .... ■743
Alavert .... ■743
Children's Claritin 24 Hour Non-Drowsy Allergy Syrup .... ■732
Claritin Non-Drowsy 24 Hour Tablets .... ■731
Non-Drowsy Claritin Hives Relief Tablets .... ■733
Claritin Reditabs 24 Hour Non-Drowsy Tablets .... ■732
Claritin-D Non-Drowsy 12 Hour Tablets .... ■731
Claritin-D Non-Drowsy 24 Hour Tablets .... ■731
Children's Dimetapp ND Non-Drowsy Allergy Syrup .... ■746
Triaminic Allerchews .... ■684

Mephobarbital (Contraceptive effectiveness may be reduced when hormonal contraceptives are co-administered with drugs that increase the metabolism of contraceptive steroids, such as barbiturates). Products include:
Mebaral Tablets, USP 2483

Methacycline Hydrochloride (Several cases of contraceptive failure and breakthrough bleeding have been reported in the literature with concomitant administration of antibiotics, such as tetracyclines; however, clinical pharmacology studies investigating drug interactions between combined oral contraceptives and these antibiotics have reported inconsistent results).
No products indexed under this heading.

Metronidazole (CYP 3A4 inhibitors may increase plasma ethinyl estradiol levels). Products include:
Metrogel 1% 1212
MetroGel-Vaginal Gel 1822
Noritate Cream, 1% 1051

Metronidazole Benzoate (CYP 3A4 inhibitors may increase plasma ethinyl estradiol levels).
No products indexed under this heading.

Metronidazole Hydrochloride (CYP 3A4 inhibitors may increase plasma ethinyl estradiol levels).
No products indexed under this heading.

Miconazole (CYP 3A4 inhibitors may increase plasma ethinyl estradiol levels).
No products indexed under this heading.

Miconazole Nitrate (CYP 3A4 inhibitors may increase plasma ethinyl estradiol levels). Products include:
Desenex .... ▣674
Desenex Jock Itch Spray Powder .... ▣674

Minocycline Hydrochloride (Several cases of contraceptive failure and breakthrough bleeding have been reported in the literature with concomitant administration of antibiotics, such as tetracyclines; however, clinical pharmacology studies investigating drug interactions between combined oral contraceptives and these antibiotics have reported inconsistent results). Products include:
Dynacin Tablets 1859

Morphine Sulfate (Increased clearance of morphine due to induction of conjugation has been noted when co-administered with combination oral contraceptives). Products include:
Avinza Capsules 1714
Kadian Capsules 572
MS Contin Tablets 2703

Nefazodone Hydrochloride (CYP 3A4 inhibitors may increase plasma ethinyl estradiol levels).
No products indexed under this heading.

Nelfinavir Mesylate (Several protease inhibitors have been studied with co-administration of oral combination hormonal contraceptives with significant changes (increase and decrease) in the plasma levels of the estrogen and progestin being noted in some cases). Products include:
Viracept 2556

Nevirapine (CYP 3A4 inhibitors may increase plasma ethinyl estradiol levels). Products include:
Viramune Oral Suspension 903
Viramune Tablets 903

Niacinamide (CYP 3A4 inhibitors may increase plasma ethinyl estradiol levels).
No products indexed under this heading.

Nicotinamide (CYP 3A4 inhibitors may increase plasma ethinyl estradiol levels). Products include:
Nicomide Tablets 3190

Nifedipine (CYP 3A4 inhibitors may increase plasma ethinyl estradiol levels). Products include:
Adalat CC Tablets 2978

Norfloxacin (CYP 3A4 inhibitors may increase plasma ethinyl estradiol levels). Products include:
Noroxin Tablets 2009

Omeprazole (CYP 3A4 inhibitors may increase plasma ethinyl estradiol levels). Products include:
Zegerid Powder for Oral Solution 2972

Oxcarbazepine (Contraceptive effectiveness may be reduced when hormonal contraceptives are co-administered with drugs that increase the metabolism of contraceptive steroids, such as oxcarbazepine). Products include:
Trileptal Oral Suspension 2281
Trileptal Tablets 2281

Oxytetracycline Hydrochloride (Several cases of contraceptive failure and breakthrough bleeding have been reported in the literature with concomitant administration of antibiotics, such as tetracyclines; however, clinical pharmacology studies investigating drug interactions between combined oral contraceptives and these antibiotics have reported inconsistent results).
No products indexed under this heading.

Paroxetine Hydrochloride (CYP 3A4 inhibitors may increase plasma ethinyl estradiol levels). Products include:
Paxil CR Controlled-Release Tablets 1509
Paxil 1501

Pentobarbital Sodium (Contraceptive effectiveness may be reduced when hormonal contraceptives are co-administered with drugs that increase the metabolism of contraceptive steroids, such as barbiturates). Products include:
Nembutal Sodium Solution, USP 2484

Phenobarbital (Contraceptive effectiveness may be reduced when hormonal contraceptives are co-administered with drugs that increase the metabolism of contraceptive steroids, such as barbiturates).
No products indexed under this heading.

Phenylbutazone (Contraceptive effectiveness may be reduced when hormonal contraceptives are co-administered with drugs that increase the metabolism of contraceptive steroids, such as phenylbutazone).
No products indexed under this heading.

Phenytoin (Contraceptive effectiveness may be reduced when hormonal contraceptives are co-administered with drugs that increase the metabolism of contraceptive steroids, such as phenytoin).
No products indexed under this heading.

Phenytoin Sodium (Contraceptive effectiveness may be reduced when hormonal contraceptives are co-administered with drugs that increase the metabolism of contraceptive steroids, such as phenytoin). Products include:
Phenytek Capsules 2153

Prednisolone Acetate (Combination hormonal contraceptives containing some synthetic estrogens (e.g., ethinyl estradiol) may inhibit the metabolism of other compounds. Increased plasma concentrations of prednisolone have been reported with concomitant administration of combination oral contraceptives). Products include:
Blephamide Ophthalmic Ointment 563
Blephamide Ophthalmic Suspension 564
Poly-Pred Liquifilm Ophthalmic Suspension .... ⊙231
Pred Forte Ophthalmic Suspension .... ⊙233
Pred Mild Sterile Ophthalmic Suspension .... ⊙236
Pred-G Ophthalmic Suspension .... ⊙234
Pred-G Sterile Ophthalmic Ointment .... ⊙235

Prednisolone Sodium Phosphate (Combination hormonal contraceptives containing some synthetic estrogens (e.g., ethinyl estradiol) may inhibit the metabolism of other compounds. Increased plasma concentrations of prednisolone have been reported with concomitant administration of combination oral contraceptives). Products include:
Pediapred Oral Solution 3319

Prednisolone Tebutate (Combination hormonal contraceptives containing some synthetic estrogens (e.g., ethinyl estradiol) may inhibit the metabolism of other compounds. Increased plasma concentrations of prednisolone have been reported with concomitant administration of combination oral contraceptives).
No products indexed under this heading.

Propoxyphene Hydrochloride (CYP 3A4 inhibitors may increase plasma ethinyl estradiol levels).
No products indexed under this heading.

Propoxyphene Napsylate (CYP 3A4 inhibitors may increase plasma ethinyl estradiol levels). Products include:
Darvocet A 500 Tablets 3497

Quinidine (CYP 3A4 inhibitors may increase plasma ethinyl estradiol levels).
No products indexed under this heading.

Quinidine Hydrochloride (CYP 3A4 inhibitors may increase plasma ethinyl estradiol levels).
No products indexed under this heading.

Quinidine Polygalacturonate (CYP 3A4 inhibitors may increase plasma ethinyl estradiol levels).
No products indexed under this heading.

Quinidine Sulfate (CYP 3A4 inhibitors may increase plasma ethinyl estradiol levels).
No products indexed under this heading.

Quinine (CYP 3A4 inhibitors may increase plasma ethinyl estradiol levels).
No products indexed under this heading.

Quinine Sulfate (CYP 3A4 inhibitors may increase plasma ethinyl estradiol levels).
No products indexed under this heading.

Quinupristin (CYP 3A4 inhibitors may increase plasma ethinyl estradiol levels). Products include:
Synercid I.V. 1690

Ranitidine Bismuth Citrate (CYP 3A4 inhibitors may increase plasma ethinyl estradiol levels).
No products indexed under this heading.

Ranitidine Hydrochloride (CYP 3A4 inhibitors may increase plasma ethinyl estradiol levels). Products include:
Zantac 1597
Zantac Injection 1593
Zantac 75 Tablets .... ▣715
Zantac 150 Maximum Strength Tablets .... ▣715
Zantac Injection Pharmacy Bulk Package 1595

Rifampin (Contraceptive effectiveness may be reduced when hormonal contraceptives are co-administered with drugs that increase the metabolism of contraceptive steroids, such as rifampin).
No products indexed under this heading.

Ritonavir (Several protease inhibitors have been studied with co-administration of oral combination hormonal contraceptives with significant changes (increase and decrease) in the plasma levels of the estrogen and progestin being noted in some cases). Products include:
Kaletra 474
Norvir 499

Salicylic Acid (Increased clearance of salicylic acid due to induction of conjugation has been noted when co-administered with combination oral contraceptives).
No products indexed under this heading.

Saquinavir (Several protease inhibitors have been studied with co-administration of oral combination hormonal contraceptives with significant changes (increase and decrease) in the plasma levels of the estrogen and progestin being noted in some cases).
No products indexed under this heading.

Saquinavir Mesylate (Several protease inhibitors have been studied with co-administration of oral combination hormonal contraceptives with significant changes (increase and decrease) in the plasma levels of the estrogen and progestin being noted in some cases). Products include:
Invirase 2776

Secobarbital Sodium (Contraceptive effectiveness may be reduced when hormonal contraceptives are co-administered with drugs that increase the metabolism of contraceptive steroids, such as barbiturates).
No products indexed under this heading.

Sertraline Hydrochloride (CYP 3A4 inhibitors may increase plasma ethinyl estradiol levels). Products include:
Zoloft 2581

Telithromycin (CYP 3A4 inhibitors may increase plasma ethinyl estradiol levels). Products include:
Ketek Tablets 2920

Temazepam (Increased clearance of temazepam due to induction of conjugation has been noted when co-administered with combination oral contraceptives).
No products indexed under this heading.

Tetracycline Hydrochloride (Several cases of contraceptive failure and breakthrough bleeding have been reported in the literature with concomitant administration of antibiotics, such as tetracyclines; however, clinical pharmacology studies investigating drug interactions between combined oral contraceptives and these antibiotics have reported inconsistent results).
No products indexed under this heading.

Theophylline (Combination hormonal contraceptives containing some synthetic estrogens (e.g., ethinyl estradiol) may inhibit the metabolism of other compounds. Increased plasma concentrations of theophylline have been reported with concomitant administration of combination oral contraceptives).
No products indexed under this heading.

Theophylline Anhydrous (Combination hormonal contraceptives containing some synthetic estrogens (e.g., ethinyl estradiol) may inhibit the metabolism of other compounds. Increased plasma concentrations of theophylline have been reported with concomitant administration of combination oral contraceptives). Products include:
Uniphyl Tablets 2708

Theophylline Calcium Salicylate (Combination hormonal contraceptives containing some synthetic estrogens (e.g., ethinyl estradiol) may inhibit the metabolism of other compounds. Increased plasma concentrations of theophylline have been reported with concomitant administration of combination oral contraceptives).
No products indexed under this heading.

Theophylline Dihydroxypropyl (Glyceryl) (Combination hormonal contraceptives containing some synthetic estrogens (e.g., ethinyl estradiol) may inhibit the metabolism of other compounds. Increased plasma concentrations of theophylline have been reported with concomitant administration of combination oral contraceptives).
No products indexed under this heading.

Theophylline Ethylenediamine (Combination hormonal contraceptives containing some synthetic estrogens (e.g., ethinyl estradiol) may inhibit the metabolism of other compounds. Increased plasma concentrations of theophylline have been reported with concomitant administration of combination oral contraceptives).
No products indexed under this heading.

Theophylline Sodium Glycinate (Combination hormonal contraceptives containing some synthetic estrogens (e.g., ethinyl estradiol) may inhibit the metabolism of other compounds. Increased plasma concentrations of theophylline have been reported with concomitant administration of combination oral contraceptives).
No products indexed under this heading.

Thiamylal Sodium (Contraceptive effectiveness may be reduced when hormonal contraceptives are coadministered with drugs that increase the metabolism of contraceptive steroids, such as barbiturates).
No products indexed under this heading.

Topiramate (Contraceptive effectiveness may be reduced when hormonal contraceptives are coadministered with drugs that increase the metabolism of contraceptive steroids, such as topiramate). Products include:
Topamax Sprinkle Capsules 2438
Topamax Tablets 2438

Troglitazone (CYP 3A4 inhibitors may increase plasma ethinyl estradiol levels).
No products indexed under this heading.

Troleandomycin (CYP 3A4 inhibitors may increase plasma ethinyl estradiol levels).
No products indexed under this heading.

Valproate Sodium (CYP 3A4 inhibitors may increase plasma ethinyl estradiol levels). Products include:
Depacon Injection 412

Verapamil Hydrochloride (CYP 3A4 inhibitors may increase plasma ethinyl estradiol levels). Products include:
Covera-HS Tablets 3135
Tarka Tablets 519
Verelan PM Capsules 3120

Vitamin C (Ascorbic acid may increase plasma ethinyl estradiol levels, possibly by inhibition of conjugation). Products include:
Chromagen Forte Soft Gelatin Capsules 3296
Halls Defense Sugarfree Vitamin C Drops .... ▣611
Niferex-150 Forte Capsules 3299
Peridin-C Tablets .... ▣761
Repliva 21/7 Tablets 3301

Voriconazole (CYP 3A4 inhibitors may increase plasma ethinyl estradiol levels). Products include:
VFEND I.V. 2543
VFEND Oral Suspension 2543
VFEND Tablets 2543

Zafirlukast (CYP 3A4 inhibitors may increase plasma ethinyl estradiol levels). Products include:
Accolate Tablets 663

Zileuton (CYP 3A4 inhibitors may increase plasma ethinyl estradiol levels).
No products indexed under this heading.

Food Interactions

Grapefruit (CYP 3A4 inhibitors may increase plasma ethinyl estradiol levels).

Grapefruit Juice (CYP 3A4 inhibitors may increase plasma ethinyl estradiol levels).

SEDAPAP TABLETS 50 MG/ 650 MG

(Acetaminophen, Butalbital) 2098
May interact with central nervous system depressants, general anesthetics, monoamine oxidase inhibitors, narcotic analgesics, psychotropics, tranquilizers, tricyclic antidepressants, and certain other agents. Compounds in these categories include:

Alfentanil Hydrochloride (Additive CNS depression).
No products indexed under this heading.

Alprazolam (Additive CNS depression). Products include:
Niravam Orally Disintegrating Tablets 3106
Xanax XR Tablets 2655

Amitriptyline Hydrochloride (Additive CNS depression).
No products indexed under this heading.

Amoxapine (Additive CNS depression).
No products indexed under this heading.

Aprobarbital (Additive CNS depression).
No products indexed under this heading.

Buprenorphine Hydrochloride (Additive CNS depression). Products include:
Buprenex Injectable 2718
Suboxone Tablets 2719
Subutex Tablets 2719

Buspirone Hydrochloride (Additive CNS depression).
No products indexed under this heading.

Butabarbital (Additive CNS depression).
No products indexed under this heading.

Chlordiazepoxide (Additive CNS depression).
No products indexed under this heading.

Chlordiazepoxide Hydrochloride (Additive CNS depression). Products include:
Librium Capsules 3349

Chlorpromazine (Additive CNS depression).
No products indexed under this heading.

Chlorpromazine Hydrochloride (Additive CNS depression).
No products indexed under this heading.

Chlorprothixene (Additive CNS depression).
No products indexed under this heading.

Chlorprothixene Hydrochloride (Additive CNS depression).
No products indexed under this heading.

Chlorprothixene Lactate (Additive CNS depression).
No products indexed under this heading.

Clomipramine Hydrochloride (Additive CNS depression).
No products indexed under this heading.

Clorazepate Dipotassium (Additive CNS depression). Products include:
Tranxene 2488

Clozapine (Additive CNS depression). Products include:
Clozapine Tablets 2141
Clozaril Tablets 2174
FazaClo Orally Disintegrating Tablets 547

Codeine Phosphate (Additive CNS depression). Products include:
Tylenol with Codeine 2461

Desflurane (Additive CNS depression). Products include:
Suprane Liquid for Inhalation 770

Desipramine Hydrochloride (Additive CNS depression).
No products indexed under this heading.

Dezocine (Additive CNS depression).
No products indexed under this heading.

Diazepam (Additive CNS depression). Products include:
Diastat Rectal Delivery System 3344
Valium Tablets 2822

Doxepin Hydrochloride (Additive CNS depression).
No products indexed under this heading.

Droperidol (Additive CNS depression).
No products indexed under this heading.

Enflurane (Additive CNS depression).
No products indexed under this heading.

Estazolam (Additive CNS depression). Products include:
ProSom Tablets 512

Ethanol (Additive CNS depression).
No products indexed under this heading.

Ethchlorvynol (Additive CNS depression).
No products indexed under this heading.

Ethinamate (Additive CNS depression).
No products indexed under this heading.

Ethyl Alcohol (Additive CNS depression).
No products indexed under this heading.

Fentanyl (Additive CNS depression). Products include:
Duragesic Transdermal System 2448

Fentanyl Citrate (Additive CNS depression). Products include:
Actiq 993

Fluphenazine Decanoate (Additive CNS depression).
No products indexed under this heading.

Fluphenazine Enanthate (Additive CNS depression).
No products indexed under this heading.

Fluphenazine Hydrochloride (Additive CNS depression).
No products indexed under this heading.

Flurazepam Hydrochloride (Additive CNS depression). Products include:
Dalmane Capsules 3343

Glutethimide (Additive CNS depression).
No products indexed under this heading.

Haloperidol (Additive CNS depression).
No products indexed under this heading.

Haloperidol Decanoate (Additive CNS depression).
No products indexed under this heading.

Hydrocodone Bitartrate (Additive CNS depression). Products include:
Hycodan 1104
Hycomine Compound Tablets 1105
Hycotuss Expectorant Syrup 1106
Lortab 3315
Lortab Elixir 3312
Vicodin Tablets 530
Vicodin ES Tablets 531
Vicodin HP Tablets 532
Vicoprofen Tablets 533
Zydone Tablets 1118

Hydrocodone Polistirex (Additive CNS depression). Products include:
Tussionex Pennkinetic Extended-Release Suspension 3322

Hydromorphone Hydrochloride (Additive CNS depression). Products include:
Dilaudid ... 439
Dilaudid Oral Liquid ... 443
Dilaudid Non-Sterile Powder ... 439
Dilaudid Rectal Suppositories ... 439
Dilaudid Tablets ... 439
Dilaudid Tablets - 8 mg ... 443
Dilaudid-HP ... 441

Hydroxyzine Hydrochloride (Additive CNS depression).
No products indexed under this heading.

Imipramine Hydrochloride (Additive CNS depression).
No products indexed under this heading.

Imipramine Pamoate (Additive CNS depression).
No products indexed under this heading.

Isocarboxazid (The effects of butalbital may be enhanced by MAO inhibitors).
No products indexed under this heading.

Isoflurane (Additive CNS depression).
No products indexed under this heading.

Ketamine Hydrochloride (Additive CNS depression).
No products indexed under this heading.

Levomethadyl Acetate Hydrochloride (Additive CNS depression).
No products indexed under this heading.

Levorphanol Tartrate (Additive CNS depression).
No products indexed under this heading.

Lithium Carbonate (Additive CNS depression). Products include:
Eskalith ... 1406
Lithobid Tablets ... 1670

Lithium Citrate (Additive CNS depression).
No products indexed under this heading.

Lorazepam (Additive CNS depression).
No products indexed under this heading.

Loxapine Hydrochloride (Additive CNS depression).
No products indexed under this heading.

Loxapine Succinate (Additive CNS depression).
No products indexed under this heading.

Maprotiline Hydrochloride (Additive CNS depression).
No products indexed under this heading.

Meperidine Hydrochloride (Additive CNS depression).
No products indexed under this heading.

Mephobarbital (Additive CNS depression). Products include:
Mebaral Tablets, USP ... 2483

Meprobamate (Additive CNS depression).
No products indexed under this heading.

Mesoridazine Besylate (Additive CNS depression).
No products indexed under this heading.

Methadone Hydrochloride (Additive CNS depression).
No products indexed under this heading.

Methohexital Sodium (Additive CNS depression).
No products indexed under this heading.

Methotrimeprazine (Additive CNS depression).
No products indexed under this heading.

Methoxyflurane (Additive CNS depression).
No products indexed under this heading.

Midazolam Hydrochloride (Additive CNS depression).
No products indexed under this heading.

Moclobemide (The effects of butalbital may be enhanced by MAO inhibitors).
No products indexed under this heading.

Molindone Hydrochloride (Additive CNS depression). Products include:
Moban Tablets ... 1108

Morphine Sulfate (Additive CNS depression). Products include:
Avinza Capsules ... 1714
Kadian Capsules ... 572
MS Contin Tablets ... 2703

Nortriptyline Hydrochloride (Additive CNS depression).
No products indexed under this heading.

Olanzapine (Additive CNS depression). Products include:
Symbyax Capsules ... 1788
Zyprexa Tablets ... 1798
Zyprexa IntraMuscular ... 1798
Zyprexa ZYDIS Orally Disintegrating Tablets ... 1798

Oxazepam (Additive CNS depression).
No products indexed under this heading.

Oxycodone Hydrochloride (Additive CNS depression). Products include:
Combunox Tablets ... 1183
OxyContin Tablets ... 2699
OxyFast Oral Concentrate Solution ... 2704
OxyIR Capsules ... 2704
Percocet Tablets ... 1114
Percodan Tablets ... 1115

Pargyline Hydrochloride (The effects of butalbital may be enhanced by MAO inhibitors).
No products indexed under this heading.

Pentobarbital Sodium (Additive CNS depression). Products include:
Nembutal Sodium Solution, USP 2484

Perphenazine (Additive CNS depression).
No products indexed under this heading.

Phenelzine Sulfate (The effects of butalbital may be enhanced by MAO inhibitors).
No products indexed under this heading.

Phenobarbital (Additive CNS depression).
No products indexed under this heading.

Prazepam (Additive CNS depression).
No products indexed under this heading.

Procarbazine Hydrochloride (The effects of butalbital may be enhanced by MAO inhibitors). Products include:
Matulane Capsules ... 3188

Prochlorperazine (Additive CNS depression).
No products indexed under this heading.

Promethazine Hydrochloride (Additive CNS depression). Products include:
Phenergan ... 3438

Propofol (Additive CNS depression). Products include:
Diprivan Injectable Emulsion ... 676

Propoxyphene Hydrochloride (Additive CNS depression).
No products indexed under this heading.

Propoxyphene Napsylate (Additive CNS depression). Products include:
Darvocet A 500 Tablets ... 3497

Protriptyline Hydrochloride (Additive CNS depression; decreased blood levels of the antidepressant). Products include:
Vivactil Tablets ... 2350

Quazepam (Additive CNS depression).
No products indexed under this heading.

Quetiapine Fumarate (Additive CNS depression). Products include:
Seroquel Tablets ... 691

Remifentanil Hydrochloride (Additive CNS depression).
No products indexed under this heading.

Risperidone (Additive CNS depression). Products include:
Risperdal Consta Long-Acting Injection ... 1664
Risperdal M-Tab Orally Disintegrating Tablets ... 1658
Risperdal ... 1658

Secobarbital Sodium (Additive CNS depression).
No products indexed under this heading.

Selegiline Hydrochloride (The effects of butalbital may be enhanced by MAO inhibitors). Products include:
Eldepryl Capsules ... 3209

Sevoflurane (Additive CNS depression). Products include:
Ultane Liquid for Inhalation ... 526

Sufentanil Citrate (Additive CNS depression).
No products indexed under this heading.

Temazepam (Additive CNS depression).
No products indexed under this heading.

Thiamylal Sodium (Additive CNS depression).
No products indexed under this heading.

Thioridazine Hydrochloride (Additive CNS depression). Products include:
Thioridazine Hydrochloride Tablets ... 2122

Thiothixene (Additive CNS depression). Products include:
Thiothixene Capsules ... 2124

Tranylcypromine Sulfate (The effects of butalbital may be enhanced by MAO inhibitors). Products include:
Parnate Tablets ... 1499

Triazolam (Additive CNS depression).
No products indexed under this heading.

Trifluoperazine Hydrochloride (Additive CNS depression).
No products indexed under this heading.

Trimipramine Maleate (Additive CNS depression). Products include:
Surmontil Capsules ... 2347

Zaleplon (Additive CNS depression). Products include:
Sonata Capsules ... 1686

Ziprasidone Hydrochloride (Additive CNS depression). Products include:
Geodon Capsules ... 2514

Zolpidem Tartrate (Additive CNS depression). Products include:
Ambien Tablets ... 2867

Food Interactions

Alcohol (Additive CNS depression).

SENOKOT TABLETS

(Senna) ... 2717
None cited in PDR database.

SENOKOT WHEAT BRAN

(Bran, wheat) ... 2717
May interact with:

Oral Medications, unspecified (Bulk-forming products may affect how medications work. Take Senokot Brand Wheat Bran two or more hours before or after taking oral medications).

SENOKOT-S TABLETS

(Docusate Sodium, Senna) ... 2717
None cited in PDR database.

SEN-SEI-RO LIQUID GOLD

(Dietary Supplement) ... 1713
None cited in PDR database.

SEN-SEI-RO POWDER GOLD

(Dietary Supplement) ... 1713
None cited in PDR database.

SENSIPAR TABLETS

(Cinacalcet Hydrochloride) ... 603
May interact with cytochrome p450 2d6 substrates (selected), cytochrome p450 3a inhibitors (selected), and certain other agents. Compounds in these categories include:

Amiodarone Hydrochloride (Since cinacalcet hydrochloride is metabolized in part by CYP3A4, dose adjustment of cinacalcet hydrochloride may be required and PTH and serum calcium concentrations closely monitored if a patient initiates or discontinues therapy with a strong CYP3A4 inhibitor). Products include:
Pacerone Tablets ... 3337

Amitriptyline Hydrochloride (Administration of 25mg or 100mg cinacalcet with 50mg amitriptyline increased amitriptyline exposure and nortriptyline (active metabolite) exposure by approximately 20% in CYP2D6 extensive metabolizers. Cinacalcet hydrochloride is a strong in vitro inhibitor of CYP2D6. Therefore, dose adjustments of concomitant medications that are predominantly metabolized by CYP2D6 and have a narrow therapeutic index may be required).
No products indexed under this heading.

Amphetamine Aspartate (Cinacalcet hydrochloride is a strong in vitro inhibitor of CYP2D6. Therefore, dose adjustments of concomitant medications that are predominantly metabolized by CYP2D6 and have a narrow therapeutic index may be required). Products include:
Adderall Tablets 3168
Adderall XR Capsules 3169

Amphetamine Aspartate Monohydrate (Cinacalcet hydrochloride is a strong in vitro inhibitor of CYP2D6. Therefore, dose adjustments of concomitant medications that are predominantly metabolized by CYP2D6 and have a narrow therapeutic index may be required).
No products indexed under this heading.

Amphetamine Sulfate (Cinacalcet hydrochloride is a strong in vitro inhibitor of CYP2D6. Therefore, dose adjustments of concomitant medications that are predominantly metabolized by CYP2D6 and have a narrow therapeutic index may be required). Products include:
Adderall Tablets 3168
Adderall XR Capsules 3169

Amprenavir (Since cinacalcet hydrochloride is metabolized in part by CYP3A4, dose adjustment of cinacalcet hydrochloride may be required and PTH and serum calcium concentrations closely monitored if a patient initiates or discontinues therapy with a strong CYP3A4 inhibitor). Products include:
Agenerase Capsules 1299
Agenerase Oral Solution 1304

Aprepitant (Since cinacalcet hydrochloride is metabolized in part by CYP3A4, dose adjustment of cinacalcet hydrochloride may be required and PTH and serum calcium concentrations closely monitored if a patient initiates or discontinues therapy with a strong CYP3A4 inhibitor). Products include:
Emend Capsules 1944

Atomoxetine Hydrochloride (Cinacalcet hydrochloride is a strong in vitro inhibitor of CYP2D6. Therefore, dose adjustments of concomitant medications that are predominantly metabolized by CYP2D6 and have a narrow therapeutic index may be required). Products include:
Strattera Capsules 1784

Bisoprolol Fumarate (Cinacalcet hydrochloride is a strong in vitro inhibitor of CYP2D6. Therefore, dose adjustments of concomitant medications that are predominantly metabolized by CYP2D6 and have a narrow therapeutic index may be required).
No products indexed under this heading.

Captopril (Cinacalcet hydrochloride is a strong in vitro inhibitor of CYP2D6. Therefore, dose adjustments of concomitant medications that are predominantly metabolized by CYP2D6 and have a narrow therapeutic index may be required). Products include:
Captopril Tablets 2114

Carvedilol (Cinacalcet hydrochloride is a strong in vitro inhibitor of CYP2D6. Therefore, dose adjustments of concomitant medications that are predominantly metabolized by CYP2D6 and have a narrow therapeutic index may be required). Products include:
Coreg Tablets 1376

Cevimeline Hydrochloride (Cinacalcet hydrochloride is a strong in vitro inhibitor of CYP2D6. Therefore, dose adjustments of concomitant medications that are predominantly metabolized by CYP2D6 and have a narrow therapeutic index may be required). Products include:
Evoxac Capsules 1042

Chlorpromazine (Cinacalcet hydrochloride is a strong in vitro inhibitor of CYP2D6. Therefore, dose adjustments of concomitant medications that are predominantly metabolized by CYP2D6 and have a narrow therapeutic index may be required).
No products indexed under this heading.

Chlorpromazine Hydrochloride (Cinacalcet hydrochloride is a strong in vitro inhibitor of CYP2D6. Therefore, dose adjustments of concomitant medications that are predominantly metabolized by CYP2D6 and have a narrow therapeutic index may be required).
No products indexed under this heading.

Chlorpropamide (Cinacalcet hydrochloride is a strong in vitro inhibitor of CYP2D6. Therefore, dose adjustments of concomitant medications that are predominantly metabolized by CYP2D6 and have a narrow therapeutic index may be required).
No products indexed under this heading.

Cimetidine (Since cinacalcet hydrochloride is metabolized in part by CYP3A4, dose adjustment of cinacalcet hydrochloride may be required and PTH and serum calcium concentrations closely monitored if a patient initiates or discontinues therapy with a strong CYP3A4 inhibitor). Products include:
Tagamet HB 200 Tablets .... ■637
Tagamet Tablets 1547

Cimetidine Hydrochloride (Since cinacalcet hydrochloride is metabolized in part by CYP3A4, dose adjustment of cinacalcet hydrochloride may be required and PTH and serum calcium concentrations closely monitored if a patient initiates or discontinues therapy with a strong CYP3A4 inhibitor).
No products indexed under this heading.

Ciprofloxacin (Since cinacalcet hydrochloride is metabolized in part by CYP3A4, dose adjustment of cinacalcet hydrochloride may be required and PTH and serum calcium concentrations closely monitored if a patient initiates or discontinues therapy with a strong CYP3A4 inhibitor). Products include:
Cipro I.V. 2998
Cipro I.V. Pharmacy Bulk Package ... 3509
Cipro Oral Suspension 2991
Cipro XR Tablets 3004
Ciprodex Otic Suspension 555

Ciprofloxacin Hydrochloride (Since cinacalcet hydrochloride is metabolized in part by CYP3A4, dose adjustment of cinacalcet hydrochloride may be required and PTH and serum calcium concentrations closely monitored if a patient initiates or discontinues therapy with a strong CYP3A4 inhibitor). Products include:
Ciloxan Ophthalmic Ointment 554
Cipro Tablets 2991

Clarithromycin (Since cinacalcet hydrochloride is metabolized in part by CYP3A4, dose adjustment of cinacalcet hydrochloride may be required and PTH and serum calcium concentrations closely monitored if a patient initiates or discontinues therapy with a strong CYP3A4 inhibitor). Products include:
Biaxin/Biaxin XL 402
PREVPAC 3281

Clomipramine Hydrochloride (Cinacalcet hydrochloride is a strong in vitro inhibitor of CYP2D6. Therefore, dose adjustments of concomitant medications that are predominantly metabolized by CYP2D6 and have a narrow therapeutic index may be required).
No products indexed under this heading.

Clozapine (Cinacalcet hydrochloride is a strong in vitro inhibitor of CYP2D6. Therefore, dose adjustments of concomitant medications that are predominantly metabolized by CYP2D6 and have a narrow therapeutic index may be required). Products include:
Clozapine Tablets 2141
Clozaril Tablets 2174
FazaClo Orally Disintegrating Tablets 547

Codeine Phosphate (Cinacalcet hydrochloride is a strong in vitro inhibitor of CYP2D6. Therefore, dose adjustments of concomitant medications that are predominantly metabolized by CYP2D6 and have a narrow therapeutic index may be required). Products include:
Tylenol with Codeine 2461

Codeine Sulfate (Cinacalcet hydrochloride is a strong in vitro inhibitor of CYP2D6. Therefore, dose adjustments of concomitant medications that are predominantly metabolized by CYP2D6 and have a narrow therapeutic index may be required).
No products indexed under this heading.

Cyclobenzaprine Hydrochloride (Cinacalcet hydrochloride is a strong in vitro inhibitor of CYP2D6. Therefore, dose adjustments of concomitant medications that are predominantly metabolized by CYP2D6 and have a narrow therapeutic index may be required). Products include:
Flexeril Tablets 1832

Cyclosporine (Since cinacalcet hydrochloride is metabolized in part by CYP3A4, dose adjustment of cinacalcet hydrochloride may be required and PTH and serum calcium concentrations closely monitored if a patient initiates or discontinues therapy with a strong CYP3A4 inhibitor). Products include:
Gengraf Capsules 458
Neoral Soft Gelatin Capsules 2247
Neoral Oral Solution 2247
Restasis Ophthalmic Emulsion 570
Sandimmune 2259

Delavirdine Mesylate (Since cinacalcet hydrochloride is metabolized in part by CYP3A4, dose adjustment of cinacalcet hydrochloride may be required and PTH and serum calcium concentrations closely monitored if a patient initiates or discontinues therapy with a strong CYP3A4 inhibitor). Products include:
Rescriptor Tablets 2535

Desipramine Hydrochloride (Cinacalcet hydrochloride is a strong in vitro inhibitor of CYP2D6. Therefore, dose adjustments of concomitant medications that are predominantly metabolized by CYP2D6 and have a narrow therapeutic index may be required).
No products indexed under this heading.

Dexfenfluramine Hydrochloride (Cinacalcet hydrochloride is a strong in vitro inhibitor of CYP2D6. Therefore, dose adjustments of concomitant medications that are predominantly metabolized by CYP2D6 and have a narrow therapeutic index may be required).
No products indexed under this heading.

Dextromethorphan Hydrobromide (Cinacalcet hydrochloride is a strong in vitro inhibitor of CYP2D6. Therefore, dose adjustments of concomitant medications that are predominantly metabolized by CYP2D6 and have a narrow therapeutic index may be required). Products include:
Alacol DM Syrup 739
Balamine DM 739
Contac Severe Cold and Flu Caplets Maximum Strength .... ■615
Contac Severe Cold and Flu Caplets Non-Drowsy .... ■615
Children's Dimetapp DM Cold & Cough Elixir .... ■745
Children's Dimetapp Long Acting Cough Plus Cold Syrup .... ■746
Dimetapp Infant Drops Decongestant Plus Cough .... ■746
Mucinex DM Tablets .... ■602
PediaCare Decongestant & Cough Infant Drops .... ■705
PediaCare Freezer Pops Long-Acting Cough-Glacier Grape and Polar Berry Blue .... ■706
PediaCare Long-Acting Cough Infant Drops .... ■705
PediaCare Long-Acting Cough Plus Cold Liquid .... ■704
PediaCare Multi-Symptom Cold Liquid .... ■704
PediaCare NightRest Cough & Cold Liquid .... ■704
Robitussin Allergy & Cough Syrup .. ■750
Robitussin CF Liquid .... ■755
Robitussin Cough & Cold Liquid-filled Capsules .... ■750
Robitussin Cough, Cold & Flu Liquid-filled Capsules .... ■750
Robitussin Cough & Cold Infant Drops .... ■755
Robitussin DM Infant Drops .... ■753
Robitussin DM Liquid .... ■753
Robitussin Flu Liquid .... ■752
Robitussin Maximum Strength Cough Liquid .... ■754
Robitussin Maximum Strength Cough & Cold Liquid .... ■754
Robitussin Pediatric Cough Liquid .... ■754
Robitussin Pediatric Cough & Cold Liquid .... ■754
Robitussin PM Cough & Cold Liquid .... ■752
Robitussin Sugar Free Cough Liquid .... ■753
Simply Cough Liquid 1840
Sudafed Severe Cold .... ■710
TheraFlu Cold & Cough Hot Liquid .... ■680
TheraFlu Flu & Chest Congestion Non-Drowsy Hot Liquid .... ■681
TheraFlu Severe Cold Non-Drowsy Hot Liquid .... ■683
TheraFlu Severe Cold & Cough Hot Liquid .... ■683
TheraFlu Severe Cold Caplets .... ■679
TheraFlu Severe Cold Hot Liquid .... ■682
TheraFlu Severe Cold Non-Drowsy Caplets .... ■679
TheraFlu Thin Strips Long Acting Cough .... ■684
Triaminic Cold & Cough Liquid .... ■685

Triaminic Cough Liquid 687
Triaminic Cough & Nasal Congestion Liquid 687
Triaminic Cough & Sore Throat Liquid 687
Triaminic Flu, Cough & Fever Liquid 685
Triaminic Night Time Cough & Cold Liquid.................................. 685
Triaminic Cold & Cough Softchews 688
Triaminic Cough & Sore Throat Softchews 689
Triaminic Thin Strips Long Acting Cough.. 689
Children's Tylenol Plus Cold & Cough Suspension Liquid and Chewable Tablets 1851
Children's Tylenol Plus Flu Suspension Liquid 1853
Concentrated Tylenol Infants' Drops Plus Cold and Cough.......... 1851
Tylenol Cold & Flu Severe Daytime Liquid with Cool Bust....... 1846
Tylenol Cold & Flu Severe NightTime Liquid with Cool Burst... 1846
Tylenol Cold Severe Congestion Non-Drowsy Caplets with Cool Burst... 1846
Tylenol Cough & Sore Throat Daytime Liquid with Cool Burst...... 1849
Tylenol Cough & Sore Throat NightTime Liquid with Cool Burst... 1849
Tylenol Flu Day Non-Drowsy Gelcaps.................................... 1846
Concentrated Tylenol Infants' Drops Plus Cold & Cough Nasal Decongestant, Fever Reducer & Pain Reliever............. 668
Multi-Symptom Tylenol Cold Night Time Caplets............................... 1845
Multi-Symptom Tylenol Cold Day Non-Drowsy Caplets and Gelcaps.. 1845
Vicks 44 Cough Relief 2675
Vicks 44D Cough & Head Congestion Relief........................ 2676
Vicks 44D Cough & Head Congestion Relief Liquid............. 721
Vicks 44E Cough & Chest Congestion Relief 2676
Pediatric Vicks 44e Cough & Chest Congestion Relief Liquid...... 2673
Vicks 44M Cough, Cold & Flu Relief... 2676
Pediatric Vicks 44m Cough & Cold Relief................................. 2673
Vicks DayQuil LiquiCaps/Liquid Multi-Symptom Cold/Flu Relief..... 723
Vicks DayQuil Multi-Symptom Cold/Flu Relief LiquiCaps............. 2675
Vicks DayQuil Multi-Symptom Cold/Flu Relief Liquid.................. 2675
Children's Vicks NyQuil Cold/Cough Relief........................ 2671
Vicks NyQuil Cough Liquid 2677
Vicks NyQuil LiquiCaps 2677
Vicks NyQuil LiquiCaps/Liquid Multi-Symptom Cold/Flu Relief..... 725
Vicks NyQuil Liquid 2677
Zicam Concentrated Cough Mist for Kids Cool Cherry.................... 643
Zicam Concentrated Cough Mist for Kids Plus D Cool Cherry......... 643
Zicam Concentrated Cough Mist Nite-Cool Cherry 642
Zicam Concentrated Cough Mist Plus D Cool Cherry..................... 642
Zicam Concentrated Cough Mist-Honey Lemon & Cool Cherry 642

Dextromethorphan Polistirex (Cinacalcet hydrochloride is a strong in vitro inhibitor of CYP2D6. Therefore, dose adjustments of concomitant medications that are predominantly metabolized by CYP2D6 and have a narrow therapeutic index may be required). Products include:
Delsym Extended-Release Suspension.................................. 611
Delsym 12 Hour Cough Suppressant for Children............. 611

Diltiazem Hydrochloride (Since cinacalcet hydrochloride is metabolized in part by CYP3A4, dose adjustment of cinacalcet hydrochloride may be required and PTH and serum calcium concentrations closely monitored if a patient initiates or discontinues therapy with a strong CYP3A4 inhibitor). Products include:
Cardizem LA Extended Release Tablets 1699
Tiazac Capsules 1204

Diltiazem Maleate (Since cinacalcet hydrochloride is metabolized in part by CYP3A4, dose adjustment of cinacalcet hydrochloride may be required and PTH and serum calcium concentrations closely monitored if a patient initiates or discontinues therapy with a strong CYP3A4 inhibitor).
No products indexed under this heading.

Dolasetron Mesylate (Cinacalcet hydrochloride is a strong in vitro inhibitor of CYP2D6. Therefore, dose adjustments of concomitant medications that are predominantly metabolized by CYP2D6 and have a narrow therapeutic index may be required). Products include:
Anzemet Injection 2871
Anzemet Tablets 2874

Donepezil Hydrochloride (Cinacalcet hydrochloride is a strong in vitro inhibitor of CYP2D6. Therefore, dose adjustments of concomitant medications that are predominantly metabolized by CYP2D6 and have a narrow therapeutic index may be required). Products include:
Aricept Tablets 1086
Aricept ODT Tablets 1086

Doxepin Hydrochloride (Cinacalcet hydrochloride is a strong in vitro inhibitor of CYP2D6. Therefore, dose adjustments of concomitant medications that are predominantly metabolized by CYP2D6 and have a narrow therapeutic index may be required).
No products indexed under this heading.

Efavirenz (Since cinacalcet hydrochloride is metabolized in part by CYP3A4, dose adjustment of cinacalcet hydrochloride may be required and PTH and serum calcium concentrations closely monitored if a patient initiates or discontinues therapy with a strong CYP3A4 inhibitor). Products include:
Sustiva Capsules 957

Encainide Hydrochloride (Cinacalcet hydrochloride is a strong in vitro inhibitor of CYP2D6. Therefore, dose adjustments of concomitant medications that are predominantly metabolized by CYP2D6 and have a narrow therapeutic index may be required).
No products indexed under this heading.

Erythromycin (Since cinacalcet hydrochloride is metabolized in part by CYP3A4, dose adjustment of cinacalcet hydrochloride may be required and PTH and serum calcium concentrations closely monitored if a patient initiates or discontinues therapy with a strong CYP3A4 inhibitor). Products include:
Erygel Topical Gel 2096
Ery-Tab Tablets 447
Erythromycin Base Filmtab Tablets 454
Erythromycin Delayed-Release Capsules, USP.............................. 456
PCE Dispertab Tablets 510

Fentanyl (Cinacalcet hydrochloride is a strong in vitro inhibitor of CYP2D6. Therefore, dose adjustments of concomitant medications that are predominantly metabolized by CYP2D6 and have a narrow therapeutic index may be required). Products include:
Duragesic Transdermal System 2448

Fentanyl Citrate (Cinacalcet hydrochloride is a strong in vitro inhibitor of CYP2D6. Therefore, dose adjustments of concomitant medications that are predominantly metabolized by CYP2D6 and have a narrow therapeutic index may be required). Products include:
Actiq 993

Flecainide Acetate (Cinacalcet hydrochloride is a strong in vitro inhibitor of CYP2D6. Therefore, dose adjustments of concomitant medications that are predominantly metabolized by CYP2D6 and have a narrow therapeutic index may be required). Products include:
Tambocor Tablets 1824

Fluconazole (Since cinacalcet hydrochloride is metabolized in part by CYP3A4, dose adjustment of cinacalcet hydrochloride may be required and PTH and serum calcium concentrations closely monitored if a patient initiates or discontinues therapy with a strong CYP3A4 inhibitor).
No products indexed under this heading.

Fluoxetine (Cinacalcet hydrochloride is a strong in vitro inhibitor of CYP2D6. Therefore, dose adjustments of concomitant medications that are predominantly metabolized by CYP2D6 and have a narrow therapeutic index may be required).
No products indexed under this heading.

Fluoxetine Hydrochloride (Cinacalcet hydrochloride is a strong in vitro inhibitor of CYP2D6. Therefore, dose adjustments of concomitant medications that are predominantly metabolized by CYP2D6 and have a narrow therapeutic index may be required). Products include:
Prozac Pulvules and Liquid 1771
Symbyax Capsules 1788

Fluphenazine Decanoate (Cinacalcet hydrochloride is a strong in vitro inhibitor of CYP2D6. Therefore, dose adjustments of concomitant medications that are predominantly metabolized by CYP2D6 and have a narrow therapeutic index may be required).
No products indexed under this heading.

Fluphenazine Enanthate (Cinacalcet hydrochloride is a strong in vitro inhibitor of CYP2D6. Therefore, dose adjustments of concomitant medications that are predominantly metabolized by CYP2D6 and have a narrow therapeutic index may be required).
No products indexed under this heading.

Fluphenazine Hydrochloride (Cinacalcet hydrochloride is a strong in vitro inhibitor of CYP2D6. Therefore, dose adjustments of concomitant medications that are predominantly metabolized by CYP2D6 and have a narrow therapeutic index may be required).
No products indexed under this heading.

Fluvoxamine Maleate (Cinacalcet hydrochloride is a strong in vitro inhibitor of CYP2D6. Therefore, dose adjustments of concomitant medications that are predominantly metabolized by CYP2D6 and have a narrow therapeutic index may be required).
No products indexed under this heading.

Formoterol Fumarate (Cinacalcet hydrochloride is a strong in vitro inhibitor of CYP2D6. Therefore, dose adjustments of concomitant medications that are predominantly metabolized by CYP2D6 and have a narrow therapeutic index may be required). Products include:
Foradil Aerolizer 3024

Galantamine Hydrobromide (Cinacalcet hydrochloride is a strong in vitro inhibitor of CYP2D6. Therefore, dose adjustments of concomitant medications that are predominantly metabolized by CYP2D6 and have a narrow therapeutic index may be required). Products include:
Razadyne ER Extended-Release Capsules.................................... 2434
Razadyne 2434

Haloperidol (Cinacalcet hydrochloride is a strong in vitro inhibitor of CYP2D6. Therefore, dose adjustments of concomitant medications that are predominantly metabolized by CYP2D6 and have a narrow therapeutic index may be required).
No products indexed under this heading.

Haloperidol Decanoate (Cinacalcet hydrochloride is a strong in vitro inhibitor of CYP2D6. Therefore, dose adjustments of concomitant medications that are predominantly metabolized by CYP2D6 and have a narrow therapeutic index may be required).
No products indexed under this heading.

Hydrocodone Bitartrate (Cinacalcet hydrochloride is a strong in vitro inhibitor of CYP2D6. Therefore, dose adjustments of concomitant medications that are predominantly metabolized by CYP2D6 and have a narrow therapeutic index may be required). Products include:
Hycodan 1104
Hycomine Compound Tablets 1105
Hycotuss Expectorant Syrup 1106
Lortab 3315
Lortab Elixir 3312
Vicodin Tablets 530
Vicodin ES Tablets 531
Vicodin HP Tablets 532
Vicoprofen Tablets 533
Zydone Tablets 1118

Imipramine Hydrochloride (Cinacalcet hydrochloride is a strong in vitro inhibitor of CYP2D6. Therefore, dose adjustments of concomitant medications that are predominantly metabolized by CYP2D6 and have a narrow therapeutic index may be required).
No products indexed under this heading.

Imipramine Pamoate (Cinacalcet hydrochloride is a strong in vitro inhibitor of CYP2D6. Therefore, dose adjustments of concomitant medications that are predominantly metabolized by CYP2D6 and have a narrow therapeutic index may be required).
No products indexed under this heading.

Indinavir Sulfate (Since cinacalcet hydrochloride is metabolized in part by CYP3A4, dose adjustment of cinacalcet hydrochloride may be

required and PTH and serum calcium concentrations closely monitored if a patient initiates or discontinues therapy with a strong CYP3A4 inhibitor). Products include:

Crixivan Capsules 1918

Indoramin Hydrochloride (Cinacalcet hydrochloride is a strong in vitro inhibitor of CYP2D6. Therefore, dose adjustments of concomitant medications that are predominantly metabolized by CYP2D6 and have a narrow therapeutic index may be required).

No products indexed under this heading.

Isoniazid (Since cinacalcet hydrochloride is metabolized in part by CYP3A4, dose adjustment of cinacalcet hydrochloride may be required and PTH and serum calcium concentrations closely monitored if a patient initiates or discontinues therapy with a strong CYP3A4 inhibitor).

No products indexed under this heading.

Itraconazole (Since cinacalcet hydrochloride is metabolized in part by CYP3A4, dose adjustment of cinacalcet hydrochloride may be required and PTH and serum calcium concentrations closely monitored if a patient initiates or discontinues therapy with a strong CYP3A4 inhibitor).

No products indexed under this heading.

Ketoconazole (Co-administration of ketoconazole, a strong inhibitor of CYP3A4, increased cinacalcet exposure following a single 90 mg dose of cinacalcet hydrochloride by 2.3 fold. Since cinacalcet hydrochloride is metabolized in part by CYP3A4, dose adjustment of cinacalcet hydrochloride may be required and PTH and serum calcium concentrations closely monitored if a patient initiates or discontinues therapy with a strong CYP3A4 inhibitor). Products include:

Nizoral A-D Shampoo, 1% 1839
Nizoral 2% Shampoo 1838

Labetalol Hydrochloride (Cinacalcet hydrochloride is a strong in vitro inhibitor of CYP2D6. Therefore, dose adjustments of concomitant medications that are predominantly metabolized by CYP2D6 and have a narrow therapeutic index may be required).

No products indexed under this heading.

Lidocaine (Cinacalcet hydrochloride is a strong in vitro inhibitor of CYP2D6. Therefore, dose adjustments of concomitant medications that are predominantly metabolized by CYP2D6 and have a narrow therapeutic index may be required). Products include:

Lidoderm Patch 1107

Lidocaine Hydrochloride (Cinacalcet hydrochloride is a strong in vitro inhibitor of CYP2D6. Therefore, dose adjustments of concomitant medications that are predominantly metabolized by CYP2D6 and have a narrow therapeutic index may be required).

No products indexed under this heading.

Lopinavir (Since cinacalcet hydrochloride is metabolized in part by CYP3A4, dose adjustment of cinacalcet hydrochloride may be required and PTH and serum calcium concentrations closely monitored if a patient initiates or discontinues therapy with a strong CYP3A4 inhibitor). Products include:

Kaletra 474

Maprotiline Hydrochloride (Cinacalcet hydrochloride is a strong in vitro inhibitor of CYP2D6. Therefore, dose adjustments of concomitant medications that are predominantly metabolized by CYP2D6 and have a narrow therapeutic index may be required).

No products indexed under this heading.

Meperidine Hydrochloride (Cinacalcet hydrochloride is a strong in vitro inhibitor of CYP2D6. Therefore, dose adjustments of concomitant medications that are predominantly metabolized by CYP2D6 and have a narrow therapeutic index may be required).

No products indexed under this heading.

Methadone Hydrochloride (Cinacalcet hydrochloride is a strong in vitro inhibitor of CYP2D6. Therefore, dose adjustments of concomitant medications that are predominantly metabolized by CYP2D6 and have a narrow therapeutic index may be required).

No products indexed under this heading.

Methamphetamine Hydrochloride (Cinacalcet hydrochloride is a strong in vitro inhibitor of CYP2D6. Therefore, dose adjustments of concomitant medications that are predominantly metabolized by CYP2D6 and have a narrow therapeutic index may be required). Products include:

Desoxyn Tablets, USP 2482

Metoprolol Succinate (Cinacalcet hydrochloride is a strong in vitro inhibitor of CYP2D6. Therefore, dose adjustments of concomitant medications that are predominantly metabolized by CYP2D6 and have a narrow therapeutic index may be required). Products include:

Toprol-XL Tablets 660

Metoprolol Tartrate (Cinacalcet hydrochloride is a strong in vitro inhibitor of CYP2D6. Therefore, dose adjustments of concomitant medications that are predominantly metabolized by CYP2D6 and have a narrow therapeutic index may be required).

No products indexed under this heading.

Metronidazole (Since cinacalcet hydrochloride is metabolized in part by CYP3A4, dose adjustment of cinacalcet hydrochloride may be required and PTH and serum calcium concentrations closely monitored if a patient initiates or discontinues therapy with a strong CYP3A4 inhibitor). Products include:

Metrogel 1% 1212
MetroGel-Vaginal Gel 1822
Noritate Cream, 1% 1051

Metronidazole Benzoate (Since cinacalcet hydrochloride is metabolized in part by CYP3A4, dose adjustment of cinacalcet hydrochloride may be required and PTH and serum calcium concentrations closely monitored if a patient initiates or discontinues therapy with a strong CYP3A4 inhibitor).

No products indexed under this heading.

Metronidazole Hydrochloride (Since cinacalcet hydrochloride is metabolized in part by CYP3A4, dose adjustment of cinacalcet hydrochloride may be required and PTH and serum calcium concentrations closely monitored if a patient initiates or discontinues therapy with a strong CYP3A4 inhibitor).

No products indexed under this heading.

Mexiletine Hydrochloride (Cinacalcet hydrochloride is a strong in vitro inhibitor of CYP2D6. Therefore, dose adjustments of concomitant medications that are predominantly metabolized by CYP2D6 and have a narrow therapeutic index may be required).

No products indexed under this heading.

Miconazole (Since cinacalcet hydrochloride is metabolized in part by CYP3A4, dose adjustment of cinacalcet hydrochloride may be required and PTH and serum calcium concentrations closely monitored if a patient initiates or discontinues therapy with a strong CYP3A4 inhibitor).

No products indexed under this heading.

Mirtazapine (Cinacalcet hydrochloride is a strong in vitro inhibitor of CYP2D6. Therefore, dose adjustments of concomitant medications that are predominantly metabolized by CYP2D6 and have a narrow therapeutic index may be required).

No products indexed under this heading.

Morphine Sulfate (Cinacalcet hydrochloride is a strong in vitro inhibitor of CYP2D6. Therefore, dose adjustments of concomitant medications that are predominantly metabolized by CYP2D6 and have a narrow therapeutic index may be required). Products include:

Avinza Capsules 1714
Kadian Capsules 572
MS Contin Tablets 2703

Nefazodone Hydrochloride (Since cinacalcet hydrochloride is metabolized in part by CYP3A4, dose adjustment of cinacalcet hydrochloride may be required and PTH and serum calcium concentrations closely monitored if a patient initiates or discontinues therapy with a strong CYP3A4 inhibitor).

No products indexed under this heading.

Nelfinavir Mesylate (Cinacalcet hydrochloride is a strong in vitro inhibitor of CYP2D6. Therefore, dose adjustments of concomitant medications that are predominantly metabolized by CYP2D6 and have a narrow therapeutic index may be required). Products include:

Viracept 2556

Nifedipine (Since cinacalcet hydrochloride is metabolized in part by CYP3A4, dose adjustment of cinacalcet hydrochloride may be required and PTH and serum calcium concentrations closely monitored if a patient initiates or discontinues therapy with a strong CYP3A4 inhibitor). Products include:

Adalat CC Tablets 2978

Norfloxacin (Since cinacalcet hydrochloride is metabolized in part by CYP3A4, dose adjustment of cinacalcet hydrochloride may be required and PTH and serum calcium concentrations closely monitored if a patient initiates or discontinues therapy with a strong CYP3A4 inhibitor). Products include:

Noroxin Tablets 2009

Nortriptyline Hydrochloride (Cinacalcet hydrochloride is a strong in vitro inhibitor of CYP2D6. Therefore, dose adjustments of concomitant medications that are predominantly metabolized by CYP2D6 and have a narrow therapeutic index may be required).

No products indexed under this heading.

Olanzapine (Cinacalcet hydrochloride is a strong in vitro inhibitor of CYP2D6. Therefore, dose adjustments of concomitant medications that are predominantly metabolized by CYP2D6 and have a narrow therapeutic index may be required). Products include:

Symbyax Capsules 1788
Zyprexa Tablets 1798
Zyprexa IntraMuscular 1798
Zyprexa ZYDIS Orally Disintegrating Tablets 1798

Omeprazole (Cinacalcet hydrochloride is a strong in vitro inhibitor of CYP2D6. Therefore, dose adjustments of concomitant medications that are predominantly metabolized by CYP2D6 and have a narrow therapeutic index may be required). Products include:

Zegerid Powder for Oral Solution 2972

Ondansetron (Cinacalcet hydrochloride is a strong in vitro inhibitor of CYP2D6. Therefore, dose adjustments of concomitant medications that are predominantly metabolized by CYP2D6 and have a narrow therapeutic index may be required). Products include:

Zofran ODT Orally Disintegrating Tablets 1613

Ondansetron Hydrochloride (Cinacalcet hydrochloride is a strong in vitro inhibitor of CYP2D6. Therefore, dose adjustments of concomitant medications that are predominantly metabolized by CYP2D6 and have a narrow therapeutic index may be required). Products include:

Zofran Injection 1607
Zofran 1613

Oxycodone Hydrochloride (Cinacalcet hydrochloride is a strong in vitro inhibitor of CYP2D6. Therefore, dose adjustments of concomitant medications that are predominantly metabolized by CYP2D6 and have a narrow therapeutic index may be required). Products include:

Combunox Tablets 1183
OxyContin Tablets 2699
OxyFast Oral Concentrate Solution 2704
OxyIR Capsules 2704
Percocet Tablets 1114
Percodan Tablets 1115

Paclitaxel (Cinacalcet hydrochloride is a strong in vitro inhibitor of CYP2D6. Therefore, dose adjustments of concomitant medications that are predominantly metabolized by CYP2D6 and have a narrow therapeutic index may be required).

No products indexed under this heading.

Paroxetine Hydrochloride (Cinacalcet hydrochloride is a strong in vitro inhibitor of CYP2D6. Therefore, dose adjustments of concomitant medications that are predominantly metabolized by CYP2D6 and have a narrow therapeutic index may be required). Products include:

Paxil CR Controlled-Release Tablets 1509
Paxil 1501

Pindolol (Cinacalcet hydrochloride is a strong in vitro inhibitor of CYP2D6. Therefore, dose adjustments of concomitant medications that are predominantly metabolized by CYP2D6 and have a narrow therapeutic index may be required).
No products indexed under this heading.

Propafenone Hydrochloride (Cinacalcet hydrochloride is a strong in vitro inhibitor of CYP2D6. Therefore, dose adjustments of concomitant medications that are predominantly metabolized by CYP2D6 and have a narrow therapeutic index may be required). Products include:
Rythmol SR Capsules 2736

Propoxyphene Hydrochloride (Cinacalcet hydrochloride is a strong in vitro inhibitor of CYP2D6. Therefore, dose adjustments of concomitant medications that are predominantly metabolized by CYP2D6 and have a narrow therapeutic index may be required).
No products indexed under this heading.

Propoxyphene Napsylate (Cinacalcet hydrochloride is a strong in vitro inhibitor of CYP2D6. Therefore, dose adjustments of concomitant medications that are predominantly metabolized by CYP2D6 and have a narrow therapeutic index may be required). Products include:
Darvocet A 500 Tablets 3497

Propranolol Hydrochloride (Cinacalcet hydrochloride is a strong in vitro inhibitor of CYP2D6. Therefore, dose adjustments of concomitant medications that are predominantly metabolized by CYP2D6 and have a narrow therapeutic index may be required). Products include:
Inderal LA Long-Acting Capsules 3421
InnoPran XL Capsules 2728

Quetiapine Fumarate (Cinacalcet hydrochloride is a strong in vitro inhibitor of CYP2D6. Therefore, dose adjustments of concomitant medications that are predominantly metabolized by CYP2D6 and have a narrow therapeutic index may be required). Products include:
Seroquel Tablets 691

Quinidine Gluconate (Cinacalcet hydrochloride is a strong in vitro inhibitor of CYP2D6. Therefore, dose adjustments of concomitant medications that are predominantly metabolized by CYP2D6 and have a narrow therapeutic index may be required).
No products indexed under this heading.

Quinidine Hydrochloride (Cinacalcet hydrochloride is a strong in vitro inhibitor of CYP2D6. Therefore, dose adjustments of concomitant medications that are predominantly metabolized by CYP2D6 and have a narrow therapeutic index may be required).
No products indexed under this heading.

Quinidine Polygalacturonate (Cinacalcet hydrochloride is a strong in vitro inhibitor of CYP2D6. Therefore, dose adjustments of concomitant medications that are predominantly metabolized by CYP2D6 and have a narrow therapeutic index may be required).
No products indexed under this heading.

Quinidine Sulfate (Cinacalcet hydrochloride is a strong in vitro inhibitor of CYP2D6. Therefore, dose adjustments of concomitant medications that are predominantly metabolized by CYP2D6 and have a narrow therapeutic index may be required).
No products indexed under this heading.

Quinine (Since cinacalcet hydrochloride is metabolized in part by CYP3A4, dose adjustment of cinacalcet hydrochloride may be required and PTH and serum calcium concentrations closely monitored if a patient initiates or discontinues therapy with a strong CYP3A4 inhibitor).
No products indexed under this heading.

Quinine Sulfate (Since cinacalcet hydrochloride is metabolized in part by CYP3A4, dose adjustment of cinacalcet hydrochloride may be required and PTH and serum calcium concentrations closely monitored if a patient initiates or discontinues therapy with a strong CYP3A4 inhibitor).
No products indexed under this heading.

Risperidone (Cinacalcet hydrochloride is a strong in vitro inhibitor of CYP2D6. Therefore, dose adjustments of concomitant medications that are predominantly metabolized by CYP2D6 and have a narrow therapeutic index may be required). Products include:
Risperdal Consta Long-Acting Injection 1664
Risperdal M-Tab Orally Disintegrating Tablets 1658
Risperdal 1658

Ritonavir (Cinacalcet hydrochloride is a strong in vitro inhibitor of CYP2D6. Therefore, dose adjustments of concomitant medications that are predominantly metabolized by CYP2D6 and have a narrow therapeutic index may be required). Products include:
Kaletra 474
Norvir 499

Saquinavir (Since cinacalcet hydrochloride is metabolized in part by CYP3A4, dose adjustment of cinacalcet hydrochloride may be required and PTH and serum calcium concentrations closely monitored if a patient initiates or discontinues therapy with a strong CYP3A4 inhibitor).
No products indexed under this heading.

Saquinavir Mesylate (Since cinacalcet hydrochloride is metabolized in part by CYP3A4, dose adjustment of cinacalcet hydrochloride may be required and PTH and serum calcium concentrations closely monitored if a patient initiates or discontinues therapy with a strong CYP3A4 inhibitor). Products include:
Invirase 2776

Sertraline Hydrochloride (Since cinacalcet hydrochloride is metabolized in part by CYP3A4, dose adjustment of cinacalcet hydrochloride may be required and PTH and serum calcium concentrations closely monitored if a patient initiates or discontinues therapy with a strong CYP3A4 inhibitor). Products include:
Zoloft 2581

Tamoxifen Citrate (Cinacalcet hydrochloride is a strong in vitro inhibitor of CYP2D6. Therefore, dose adjustments of concomitant medications that are predominantly metabolized by CYP2D6 and have a narrow therapeutic index may be required).
No products indexed under this heading.

Teniposide (Cinacalcet hydrochloride is a strong in vitro inhibitor of CYP2D6. Therefore, dose adjustments of concomitant medications that are predominantly metabolized by CYP2D6 and have a narrow therapeutic index may be required).
No products indexed under this heading.

Testosterone (Cinacalcet hydrochloride is a strong in vitro inhibitor of CYP2D6. Therefore, dose adjustments of concomitant medications that are predominantly metabolized by CYP2D6 and have a narrow therapeutic index may be required). Products include:
AndroGel 3330
Striant Mucoadhesive 1022
Testim 1% Gel 722

Testosterone Cypionate (Cinacalcet hydrochloride is a strong in vitro inhibitor of CYP2D6. Therefore, dose adjustments of concomitant medications that are predominantly metabolized by CYP2D6 and have a narrow therapeutic index may be required).
No products indexed under this heading.

Testosterone Enanthate (Cinacalcet hydrochloride is a strong in vitro inhibitor of CYP2D6. Therefore, dose adjustments of concomitant medications that are predominantly metabolized by CYP2D6 and have a narrow therapeutic index may be required). Products include:
Delatestryl Injection 2976

Testosterone Propionate (Cinacalcet hydrochloride is a strong in vitro inhibitor of CYP2D6. Therefore, dose adjustments of concomitant medications that are predominantly metabolized by CYP2D6 and have a narrow therapeutic index may be required).
No products indexed under this heading.

Thioridazine (Cinacalcet hydrochloride is a strong in vitro inhibitor of CYP2D6. Therefore, dose adjustments of concomitant medications that are predominantly metabolized by CYP2D6 and have a narrow therapeutic index may be required).
No products indexed under this heading.

Thioridazine Hydrochloride (Cinacalcet hydrochloride is a strong in vitro inhibitor of CYP2D6. Therefore, dose adjustments of concomitant medications that are predominantly metabolized by CYP2D6 and have a narrow therapeutic index may be required). Products include:
Thioridazine Hydrochloride Tablets 2122

Timolol Maleate (Cinacalcet hydrochloride is a strong in vitro inhibitor of CYP2D6. Therefore, dose adjustments of concomitant medications that are predominantly metabolized by CYP2D6 and have a narrow therapeutic index may be required). Products include:
Blocadren Tablets 1891
Cosopt Sterile Ophthalmic Solution 1910
Timolide Tablets 2056
Timoptic in Ocudose 2061
Timoptic Sterile Ophthalmic Solution 2058
Timoptic-XE Sterile Ophthalmic Gel Forming Solution 2062

Tolterodine Tartrate (Cinacalcet hydrochloride is a strong in vitro inhibitor of CYP2D6. Therefore, dose adjustments of concomitant medications that are predominantly metabolized by CYP2D6 and have a narrow therapeutic index may be required). Products include:
Detrol Tablets 2626
Detrol LA Capsules 2629

Tramadol Hydrochloride (Cinacalcet hydrochloride is a strong in vitro inhibitor of CYP2D6. Therefore, dose adjustments of concomitant medications that are predominantly metabolized by CYP2D6 and have a narrow therapeutic index may be required). Products include:
Ultracet Tablets 2462

Trazodone Hydrochloride (Cinacalcet hydrochloride is a strong in vitro inhibitor of CYP2D6. Therefore, dose adjustments of concomitant medications that are predominantly metabolized by CYP2D6 and have a narrow therapeutic index may be required).
No products indexed under this heading.

Triazolam (Cinacalcet hydrochloride is a strong in vitro inhibitor of CYP2D6. Therefore, dose adjustments of concomitant medications that are predominantly metabolized by CYP2D6 and have a narrow therapeutic index may be required).
No products indexed under this heading.

Trimipramine Maleate (Cinacalcet hydrochloride is a strong in vitro inhibitor of CYP2D6. Therefore, dose adjustments of concomitant medications that are predominantly metabolized by CYP2D6 and have a narrow therapeutic index may be required). Products include:
Surmontil Capsules 2347

Troleandomycin (Since cinacalcet hydrochloride is metabolized in part by CYP3A4, dose adjustment of cinacalcet hydrochloride may be required and PTH and serum calcium concentrations closely monitored if a patient initiates or discontinues therapy with a strong CYP3A4 inhibitor).
No products indexed under this heading.

Venlafaxine Hydrochloride (Cinacalcet hydrochloride is a strong in vitro inhibitor of CYP2D6. Therefore, dose adjustments of concomitant medications that are predominantly metabolized by CYP2D6 and have a narrow therapeutic index may be required). Products include:
Effexor Tablets 3405
Effexor XR Capsules 3411

Verapamil Hydrochloride (Since cinacalcet hydrochloride is metabolized in part by CYP3A4, dose adjustment of cinacalcet hydrochloride may be required and PTH and serum calcium concentrations closely monitored if a patient initiates or discontinues therapy with a strong CYP3A4 inhibitor). Products include:
Covera-HS Tablets 3135
Tarka Tablets 519
Verelan PM Capsules 3120

IMPORTANT NOTE: Always consult each drug listing in the patient's regimen for possible interactions.

Vinblastine Sulfate (Cinacalcet hydrochloride is a strong in vitro inhibitor of CYP2D6. Therefore, dose adjustments of concomitant medications that are predominantly metabolized by CYP2D6 and have a narrow therapeutic index may be required).
No products indexed under this heading.

Voriconazole (Since cinacalcet hydrochloride is metabolized in part by CYP3A4, dose adjustment of cinacalcet hydrochloride may be required and PTH and serum calcium concentrations closely monitored if a patient initiates or discontinues therapy with a strong CYP3A4 inhibitor). Products include:
VFEND I.V. 2543
VFEND Oral Suspension 2543
VFEND Tablets 2543

Zafirlukast (Since cinacalcet hydrochloride is metabolized in part by CYP3A4, dose adjustment of cinacalcet hydrochloride may be required and PTH and serum calcium concentrations closely monitored if a patient initiates or discontinues therapy with a strong CYP3A4 inhibitor). Products include:
Accolate Tablets 663

Zileuton (Since cinacalcet hydrochloride is metabolized in part by CYP3A4, dose adjustment of cinacalcet hydrochloride may be required and PTH and serum calcium concentrations closely monitored if a patient initiates or discontinues therapy with a strong CYP3A4 inhibitor).
No products indexed under this heading.

Zonisamide (Cinacalcet hydrochloride is a strong in vitro inhibitor of CYP2D6. Therefore, dose adjustments of concomitant medications that are predominantly metabolized by CYP2D6 and have a narrow therapeutic index may be required). Products include:
Zonegran Capsules 1089

Food Interactions

Grapefruit (Since cinacalcet hydrochloride is metabolized in part by CYP3A4, dose adjustment of cinacalcet hydrochloride may be required and PTH and serum calcium concentrations closely monitored if a patient initiates or discontinues therapy with a strong CYP3A4 inhibitor).

SENSODYNE ORIGINAL FLAVOR
(Potassium Nitrate, Sodium Fluoride).... ▣636
None cited in PDR database.

SENSODYNE COOL GEL
(Potassium Nitrate, Sodium Fluoride).... ▣636
None cited in PDR database.

SENSODYNE EXTRA WHITENING
(Potassium Nitrate, Sodium Monofluorophosphate).... ▣636
None cited in PDR database.

SENSODYNE FRESH MINT
(Potassium Nitrate, Sodium Fluoride).... ▣636
None cited in PDR database.

SENSODYNE TARTAR CONTROL
(Potassium Nitrate, Sodium Fluoride).... ▣636
None cited in PDR database.

SENSODYNE TARTAR CONTROL PLUS WHITENING
(Potassium Nitrate, Sodium Fluoride).... ▣636
None cited in PDR database.

SENSODYNE WITH BAKING SODA
(Potassium Nitrate, Sodium Fluoride).... ▣636
None cited in PDR database.

SEREVENT DISKUS
(Salmeterol Xinafoate) 1540
May interact with beta blockers, monoamine oxidase inhibitors, non-potassium-sparing diuretics, and tricyclic antidepressants. Compounds in these categories include:

Acebutolol Hydrochloride (Beta-adrenergic blockers may produce severe bronchospasm in asthmatic patients, however, beta blockers do not block the pulmonary effect of beta-agonists).
No products indexed under this heading.

Amitriptyline Hydrochloride (The action of salmeterol on the vascular system may be potentiated by tricyclic antidepressant).
No products indexed under this heading.

Amoxapine (The action of salmeterol on the vascular system may be potentiated by tricyclic antidepressant).
No products indexed under this heading.

Atenolol (Beta-adrenergic blockers may produce severe bronchospasm in asthmatic patients, however, beta blockers do not block the pulmonary effect of beta-agonists). Products include:
Tenormin I.V. Injection 698
Tenormin Tablets 695

Bendroflumethiazide (The ECG changes and/or hypokalemia that may result from the administration of nonpotassium-sparing diuretics can be acutely worsened by beta-agonists, especially when the recommended dose of beta-agonist is exceeded).
No products indexed under this heading.

Betaxolol Hydrochloride (Beta-adrenergic blockers may produce severe bronchospasm in asthmatic patients, however, beta blockers do not block the pulmonary effect of beta-agonists). Products include:
Betoptic S Ophthalmic Suspension 554

Bisoprolol Fumarate (Beta-adrenergic blockers may produce severe bronchospasm in asthmatic patients, however, beta blockers do not block the pulmonary effect of beta-agonists).
No products indexed under this heading.

Bumetanide (The ECG changes and/or hypokalemia that may result from the administration of nonpotassium-sparing diuretics can be acutely worsened by beta-agonists, especially when the recommended dose of beta-agonist is exceeded).
No products indexed under this heading.

Carteolol Hydrochloride (Beta-adrenergic blockers may produce severe bronchospasm in asthmatic patients, however, beta blockers do not block the pulmonary effect of beta-agonists). Products include:
Carteolol Hydrochloride Ophthalmic Solution USP, 1%.... ⊙246

Chlorothiazide (The ECG changes and/or hypokalemia that may result from the administration of nonpotassium-sparing diuretics can be acutely worsened by beta-agonists, especially when the recommended dose of beta-agonist is exceeded). Products include:
Aldoclor Tablets 1881
Diuril Oral 1936

Chlorothiazide Sodium (The ECG changes and/or hypokalemia that may result from the administration of nonpotassium-sparing diuretics can be acutely worsened by beta-agonists, especially when the recommended dose of beta-agonist is exceeded). Products include:
Diuril Sodium Intravenous 1934

Clomipramine Hydrochloride (The action of salmeterol on the vascular system may be potentiated by tricyclic antidepressant).
No products indexed under this heading.

Desipramine Hydrochloride (The action of salmeterol on the vascular system may be potentiated by tricyclic antidepressant).
No products indexed under this heading.

Doxepin Hydrochloride (The action of salmeterol on the vascular system may be potentiated by tricyclic antidepressant).
No products indexed under this heading.

Esmolol Hydrochloride (Beta-adrenergic blockers may produce severe bronchospasm in asthmatic patients, however, beta blockers do not block the pulmonary effect of beta-agonists). Products include:
Brevibloc Concentrate 766
Brevibloc Injection 766
Brevibloc Double Strength Injection 766
Brevibloc Premixed Injection 766
Brevibloc Double Strength Premixed Injection 766

Ethacrynic Acid (The ECG changes and/or hypokalemia that may result from the administration of nonpotassium-sparing diuretics can be acutely worsened by beta-agonists, especially when the recommended dose of beta-agonist is exceeded). Products include:
Edecrin Tablets 1941

Furosemide (The ECG changes and/or hypokalemia that may result from the administration of nonpotassium-sparing diuretics can be acutely worsened by beta-agonists, especially when the recommended dose of beta-agonist is exceeded). Products include:
Furosemide Tablets 2117

Hydrochlorothiazide (The ECG changes and/or hypokalemia that may result from the administration of nonpotassium-sparing diuretics can be acutely worsened by beta-agonists, especially when the recommended dose of beta-agonist is exceeded). Products include:
Aldoril Tablets 1884
Atacand HCT 637
Avalide Tablets 2889
Avalide Tablets 922
Benicar HCT Tablets 2852
Diovan HCT Tablets 2195
Dyazide Capsules 1389
Hyzaar 1964
Lotensin HCT Tablets 2235
Maxzide 2150
Micardis HCT Tablets 886
Moduretic Tablets 2003
Prinzide Tablets 2033
Teveten HCT Tablets 1710
Timolide Tablets 2056
Uniretic Tablets 3114
Vaseretic Tablets 2073
Zestoretic Tablets 701

Hydroflumethiazide (The ECG changes and/or hypokalemia that may result from the administration of nonpotassium-sparing diuretics can be acutely worsened by beta-agonists, especially when the recommended dose of beta-agonist is exceeded).
No products indexed under this heading.

Imipramine Hydrochloride (The action of salmeterol on the vascular system may be potentiated by tricyclic antidepressant).
No products indexed under this heading.

Imipramine Pamoate (The action of salmeterol on the vascular system may be potentiated by tricyclic antidepressant).
No products indexed under this heading.

Isocarboxazid (The action of salmeterol on the vascular system may be potentiated by MAO inhibitor).
No products indexed under this heading.

Labetalol Hydrochloride (Beta-adrenergic blockers may produce severe bronchospasm in asthmatic patients, however, beta blockers do not block the pulmonary effect of beta-agonists).
No products indexed under this heading.

Levobunolol Hydrochloride (Beta-adrenergic blockers may produce severe bronchospasm in asthmatic patients, however, beta blockers do not block the pulmonary effect of beta-agonists). Products include:
Betagan Ophthalmic Solution, USP.... ⊙217

Maprotiline Hydrochloride (The action of salmeterol on the vascular system may be potentiated by tricyclic antidepressant).
No products indexed under this heading.

Methyclothiazide (The ECG changes and/or hypokalemia that may result from the administration of nonpotassium-sparing diuretics can be acutely worsened by beta-agonists, especially when the recommended dose of beta-agonist is exceeded).
No products indexed under this heading.

Metipranolol Hydrochloride (Beta-adrenergic blockers may produce severe bronchospasm in asthmatic patients, however, beta blockers do not block the pulmonary effect of beta-agonists).
No products indexed under this heading.

Metoprolol Succinate (Beta-adrenergic blockers may produce severe bronchospasm in asthmatic patients, however, beta blockers do not block the pulmonary effect of beta-agonists). Products include:
Toprol-XL Tablets 660

Metoprolol Tartrate (Beta-adrenergic blockers may produce severe bronchospasm in asthmatic patients, however, beta blockers do not block the pulmonary effect of beta-agonists).
No products indexed under this heading.

Moclobemide (The action of salmeterol on the vascular system may be potentiated by MAO inhibitor).
No products indexed under this heading.

Nadolol (Beta-adrenergic blockers may produce severe bronchospasm in asthmatic patients, however, beta blockers do not block the pulmonary effect of beta-agonists). Products include:
Nadolol Tablets ... 2121

Nortriptyline Hydrochloride (The action of salmeterol on the vascular system may be potentiated by tricyclic antidepressant).
No products indexed under this heading.

Pargyline Hydrochloride (The action of salmeterol on the vascular system may be potentiated by MAO inhibitor).
No products indexed under this heading.

Penbutolol Sulfate (Beta-adrenergic blockers may produce severe bronchospasm in asthmatic patients, however, beta blockers do not block the pulmonary effect of beta-agonists).
No products indexed under this heading.

Phenelzine Sulfate (The action of salmeterol on the vascular system may be potentiated by MAO inhibitor).
No products indexed under this heading.

Pindolol (Beta-adrenergic blockers may produce severe bronchospasm in asthmatic patients, however, beta blockers do not block the pulmonary effect of beta-agonists).
No products indexed under this heading.

Polythiazide (The ECG changes and/or hypokalemia that may result from the administration of nonpotassium-sparing diuretics can be acutely worsened by beta-agonists, especially when the recommended dose of beta-agonist is exceeded).
No products indexed under this heading.

Procarbazine Hydrochloride (The action of salmeterol on the vascular system may be potentiated by MAO inhibitor). Products include:
Matulane Capsules ... 3188

Propranolol Hydrochloride (Beta-adrenergic blockers may produce severe bronchospasm in asthmatic patients, however, beta blockers do not block the pulmonary effect of beta-agonists). Products include:
Inderal LA Long-Acting Capsules ... 3421
InnoPran XL Capsules ... 2728

Protriptyline Hydrochloride (The action of salmeterol on the vascular system may be potentiated by tricyclic antidepressant). Products include:
Vivactil Tablets ... 2350

Selegiline Hydrochloride (The action of salmeterol on the vascular system may be potentiated by MAO inhibitor). Products include:
Eldepryl Capsules ... 3209

Sotalol Hydrochloride (Beta-adrenergic blockers may produce severe bronchospasm in asthmatic patients, however, beta blockers do not block the pulmonary effect of beta-agonists).
No products indexed under this heading.

Timolol Hemihydrate (Beta-adrenergic blockers may produce severe bronchospasm in asthmatic patients, however, beta blockers do not block the pulmonary effect of beta-agonists). Products include:
Betimol Ophthalmic Solution ... 3371
Betimol Ophthalmic Solution ... ⊙283

Timolol Maleate (Beta-adrenergic blockers may produce severe bronchospasm in asthmatic patients, however, beta blockers do not block the pulmonary effect of beta-agonists). Products include:
Blocadren Tablets ... 1891
Cosopt Sterile Ophthalmic Solution ... 1910
Timolide Tablets ... 2056
Timoptic in Ocudose ... 2061
Timoptic Sterile Ophthalmic Solution ... 2058
Timoptic-XE Sterile Ophthalmic Gel Forming Solution ... 2062

Torsemide (The ECG changes and/or hypokalemia that may result from the administration of nonpotassium-sparing diuretics can be acutely worsened by beta-agonists, especially when the recommended dose of beta-agonist is exceeded).
No products indexed under this heading.

Tranylcypromine Sulfate (The action of salmeterol on the vascular system may be potentiated by MAO inhibitor). Products include:
Parnate Tablets ... 1499

Trimipramine Maleate (The action of salmeterol on the vascular system may be potentiated by tricyclic antidepressant). Products include:
Surmontil Capsules ... 2347

SEROMYCIN CAPSULES

(Cycloserine) ... 1783
May interact with antituberculosis drugs and certain other agents. Compounds in these categories include:

Aminosalicylic Acid (Co-administration has been associated with a few instances of vitamin B_{12} and/or folic acid deficiency, megaloblastic anemia, and sideroblastic anemia). Products include:
Paser Granules ... 1657

p-Aminosalicylic Acid (Co-administration has been associated with a few instances of vitamin B_{12} and/or folic acid deficiency, megaloblastic anemia, and sideroblastic anemia).
No products indexed under this heading.

Ethambutol Hydrochloride (Co-administration has been associated with a few instances of vitamin B_{12} and/or folic acid deficiency, megaloblastic anemia, and sideroblastic anemia).
No products indexed under this heading.

Ethionamide (Co-administration has been reported to potentiate neurotoxic side effects). Products include:
Trecator Tablets ... 3482

Isoniazid (Co-administration may result in increased incidence of CNS effects, such as dizziness or drowsiness).
No products indexed under this heading.

Pyrazinamide (Co-administration has been associated with a few instances of vitamin B_{12} and/or folic acid deficiency, megaloblastic anemia, and sideroblastic anemia).
No products indexed under this heading.

Rifampin (Co-administration has been associated with a few instances of vitamin B_{12} and/or folic acid deficiency, megaloblastic anemia, and sideroblastic anemia).
No products indexed under this heading.

Rifapentine (Co-administration has been associated with a few instances of vitamin B_{12} and/or folic acid deficiency, megaloblastic anemia, and sideroblastic anemia).
No products indexed under this heading.

Food Interactions

Alcohol (Concurrent use increases the possibility and risk of epileptic episodes).

SEROQUEL TABLETS

(Quetiapine Fumarate) ... 691
May interact with antihypertensives, barbiturates, cytochrome p450 3a4 inhibitors (selected), dopamine agonists, glucocorticoids, phenytoin, and certain other agents. Compounds in these categories include:

Acebutolol Hydrochloride (Enhanced effects of certain antihypertensive agents).
No products indexed under this heading.

Acetazolamide (Co-administration with an inhibitor of CYP4503A may reduce oral clearance of quetiapine, resulting in an increase in maximum plasma concentration of quetiapine; dose adjustment of quetiapine will be necessary).
No products indexed under this heading.

Amiodarone Hydrochloride (Co-administration with an inhibitor of CYP4503A may reduce oral clearance of quetiapine, resulting in an increase in maximum plasma concentration of quetiapine; dose adjustment of quetiapine will be necessary). Products include:
Pacerone Tablets ... 3337

Amlodipine Besylate (Enhanced effects of certain antihypertensive agents). Products include:
Caduet Tablets ... 2507
Lotrel Capsules ... 2238
Norvasc Tablets ... 2529

Amprenavir (Co-administration with an inhibitor of CYP4503A may reduce oral clearance of quetiapine, resulting in an increase in maximum plasma concentration of quetiapine; dose adjustment of quetiapine will be necessary). Products include:
Agenerase Capsules ... 1299
Agenerase Oral Solution ... 1304

Anastrozole (Co-administration with an inhibitor of CYP4503A may reduce oral clearance of quetiapine, resulting in an increase in maximum plasma concentration of quetiapine; dose adjustment of quetiapine will be necessary). Products include:
Arimidex Tablets ... 665

Aprepitant (Co-administration with an inhibitor of CYP4503A may reduce oral clearance of quetiapine, resulting in an increase in maximum plasma concentration of quetiapine; dose adjustment of quetiapine will be necessary). Products include:
Emend Capsules ... 1944

Aprobarbital (Co-administration with hepatic enzyme inducers, such as barbiturates, may increase oral clearance).
No products indexed under this heading.

Atenolol (Enhanced effects of certain antihypertensive agents). Products include:
Tenormin I.V. Injection ... 698
Tenormin Tablets ... 695

Benazepril Hydrochloride (Enhanced effects of certain antihypertensive agents). Products include:
Lotensin Tablets ... 2232
Lotensin HCT Tablets ... 2235
Lotrel Capsules ... 2238

Bendroflumethiazide (Enhanced effects of certain antihypertensive agents).
No products indexed under this heading.

Betamethasone Acetate (Co-administration with hepatic enzyme inducers, such as glucocorticosteroids, may increase oral clearance).
No products indexed under this heading.

Betamethasone Sodium Phosphate (Co-administration with hepatic enzyme inducers, such as glucocorticosteroids, may increase oral clearance).
No products indexed under this heading.

Betaxolol Hydrochloride (Enhanced effects of certain antihypertensive agents). Products include:
Betoptic S Ophthalmic Suspension ... 554

Bisoprolol Fumarate (Enhanced effects of certain antihypertensive agents).
No products indexed under this heading.

Bromocriptine Mesylate (Quetiapine may antagonize the effects of dopamine agonists).
No products indexed under this heading.

Butabarbital (Co-administration with hepatic enzyme inducers, such as barbiturates, may increase oral clearance).
No products indexed under this heading.

Butalbital (Co-administration with hepatic enzyme inducers, such as barbiturates, may increase oral clearance). Products include:
Sedapap Tablets 50 mg/650 mg ... 2098

Candesartan Cilexetil (Enhanced effects of certain antihypertensive agents). Products include:
Atacand Tablets ... 634
Atacand HCT ... 637

Captopril (Enhanced effects of certain antihypertensive agents). Products include:
Captopril Tablets ... 2114

Carbamazepine (Co-administration with hepatic enzyme inducers, such as carbamazepine, may increase oral clearance). Products include:
Carbatrol Capsules ... 3174

IMPORTANT NOTE: Always consult each drug listing in the patient's regimen for possible interactions.

Equetro Extended-Release Capsules ... 3178
Tegretol/Tegretol-XR ... 2278

Carteolol Hydrochloride (Enhanced effects of certain antihypertensive agents). Products include:
Carteolol Hydrochloride Ophthalmic Solution USP, 1% ... ⊙ 246

Chlorothiazide (Enhanced effects of certain antihypertensive agents). Products include:
Aldoclor Tablets ... 1881
Diuril Oral ... 1936

Chlorothiazide Sodium (Enhanced effects of certain antihypertensive agents). Products include:
Diuril Sodium Intravenous ... 1934

Chlorthalidone (Enhanced effects of certain antihypertensive agents). Products include:
Clorpres Tablets ... 2139

Cimetidine (Co-administration has resulted in a 20% decrease in the mean oral clearance of quetiapine). Products include:
Tagamet HB 200 Tablets ... ▣ 637
Tagamet Tablets ... 1547

Cimetidine Hydrochloride (Co-administration with an inhibitor of CYP4503A may reduce oral clearance of quetiapine, resulting in an increase in maximum plasma concentration of quetiapine; dose adjustment of quetiapine will be necessary).
No products indexed under this heading.

Ciprofloxacin (Co-administration with an inhibitor of CYP4503A may reduce oral clearance of quetiapine, resulting in an increase in maximum plasma concentration of quetiapine; dose adjustment of quetiapine will be necessary). Products include:
Cipro I.V. ... 2998
Cipro I.V. Pharmacy Bulk Package ... 3509
Cipro Oral Suspension ... 2991
Cipro XR Tablets ... 3004
Ciprodex Otic Suspension ... 555

Clarithromycin (Co-administration with an inhibitor of CYP4503A may reduce oral clearance of quetiapine, resulting in an increase in maximum plasma concentration of quetiapine; dose adjustment of quetiapine will be necessary). Products include:
Biaxin/Biaxin XL ... 402
PREVPAC ... 3281

Clonidine (Enhanced effects of certain antihypertensive agents). Products include:
Catapres-TTS ... 875

Clonidine Hydrochloride (Enhanced effects of certain antihypertensive agents). Products include:
Catapres Tablets ... 874
Clorpres Tablets ... 2139

Clotrimazole (Co-administration with an inhibitor of CYP4503A may reduce oral clearance of quetiapine, resulting in an increase in maximum plasma concentration of quetiapine; dose adjustment of quetiapine will be necessary). Products include:
Lotrimin ... 3053
Lotrisone ... 3054

Cortisone Acetate (Co-administration with hepatic enzyme inducers, such as glucocorticosteroids, may increase oral clearance).
No products indexed under this heading.

Cyclosporine (Co-administration with an inhibitor of CYP4503A may reduce oral clearance of quetiapine, resulting in an increase in maximum plasma concentration of quetiapine; dose adjustment of quetiapine will be necessary). Products include:
Gengraf Capsules ... 458
Neoral Soft Gelatin Capsules ... 2247
Neoral Oral Solution ... 2247
Restasis Ophthalmic Emulsion ... 570
Sandimmune ... 2259

Dalfopristin (Co-administration with an inhibitor of CYP4503A may reduce oral clearance of quetiapine, resulting in an increase in maximum plasma concentration of quetiapine; dose adjustment of quetiapine will be necessary). Products include:
Synercid I.V. ... 1690

Danazol (Co-administration with an inhibitor of CYP4503A may reduce oral clearance of quetiapine, resulting in an increase in maximum plasma concentration of quetiapine; dose adjustment of quetiapine will be necessary).
No products indexed under this heading.

Delavirdine Mesylate (Co-administration with an inhibitor of CYP4503A may reduce oral clearance of quetiapine, resulting in an increase in maximum plasma concentration of quetiapine; dose adjustment of quetiapine will be necessary). Products include:
Rescriptor Tablets ... 2535

Deserpidine (Enhanced effects of certain antihypertensive agents).
No products indexed under this heading.

Dexamethasone (Co-administration with hepatic enzyme inducers, such as glucocorticosteroids, may increase oral clearance). Products include:
Ciprodex Otic Suspension ... 555
Decadron Tablets ... 1929
TobraDex Ophthalmic Ointment ... 558
TobraDex Ophthalmic Suspension ... 558

Dexamethasone Acetate (Co-administration with hepatic enzyme inducers, such as glucocorticosteroids, may increase oral clearance).
No products indexed under this heading.

Dexamethasone Sodium Phosphate (Co-administration with hepatic enzyme inducers, such as glucocorticosteroids, may increase oral clearance). Products include:
Decadron Phosphate Injection ... 1931

Diazoxide (Enhanced effects of certain antihypertensive agents). Products include:
Hyperstat I.V. Injection ... 3031

Diltiazem Hydrochloride (Co-administration with an inhibitor of CYP4503A may reduce oral clearance of quetiapine, resulting in an increase in maximum plasma concentration of quetiapine; dose adjustment of quetiapine will be necessary). Products include:
Cardizem LA Extended Release Tablets ... 1699
Tiazac Capsules ... 1204

Diltiazem Maleate (Co-administration with an inhibitor of CYP4503A may reduce oral clearance of quetiapine, resulting in an increase in maximum plasma concentration of quetiapine; dose adjustment of quetiapine will be necessary).
No products indexed under this heading.

Divalproex Sodium (Co-administration of quetiapine (150 mg bid) and divalproex (500 mg bid) increased the mean maximum plasma concentration of quetiapine at steady state by 17% without affecting the extent of absorption or mean oral clearance. Co-administration also decreased the mean maximum concentration and extent of absorption of total and free valproic acid at steady state by 10% to 12% and increased mean oral clearance of total valproic acid by 11%). Products include:
Depakote Sprinkle Capsules ... 422
Depakote Tablets ... 427
Depakote ER Tablets ... 433

Dopamine Hydrochloride (Quetiapine may antagonize the effects of dopamine agonists).
No products indexed under this heading.

Doxazosin Mesylate (Enhanced effects of certain antihypertensive agents).
No products indexed under this heading.

Efavirenz (Co-administration with an inhibitor of CYP4503A may reduce oral clearance of quetiapine, resulting in an increase in maximum plasma concentration of quetiapine; dose adjustment of quetiapine will be necessary). Products include:
Sustiva Capsules ... 957

Enalapril Maleate (Enhanced effects of certain antihypertensive agents). Products include:
Vaseretic Tablets ... 2073
Vasotec I.V. Injection ... 2076

Enalaprilat (Enhanced effects of certain antihypertensive agents).
No products indexed under this heading.

Eprosartan Mesylate (Enhanced effects of certain antihypertensive agents). Products include:
Teveten Tablets ... 1707
Teveten HCT Tablets ... 1710

Erythromycin (Co-administration with an inhibitor of CYP4503A may reduce oral clearance of quetiapine, resulting in an increase in maximum plasma concentration of quetiapine; dose adjustment of quetiapine will be necessary). Products include:
Erygel Topical Gel ... 2096
Ery-Tab Tablets ... 447
Erythromycin Base Filmtab Tablets ... 454
Erythromycin Delayed-Release Capsules, USP ... 456
PCE Dispertab Tablets ... 510

Erythromycin Estolate (Co-administration with an inhibitor of CYP4503A may reduce oral clearance of quetiapine, resulting in an increase in maximum plasma concentration of quetiapine; dose adjustment of quetiapine will be necessary).
No products indexed under this heading.

Erythromycin Ethylsuccinate (Co-administration with an inhibitor of CYP4503A may reduce oral clearance of quetiapine, resulting in an increase in maximum plasma concentration of quetiapine; dose adjustment of quetiapine will be necessary). Products include:
E.E.S. ... 449
EryPed ... 445

Erythromycin Gluceptate (Co-administration with an inhibitor of CYP4503A may reduce oral clearance of quetiapine, resulting in an increase in maximum plasma concentration of quetiapine; dose adjustment of quetiapine will be necessary).
No products indexed under this heading.

Erythromycin Lactobionate (Co-administration with an inhibitor of CYP4503A may reduce oral clearance of quetiapine, resulting in an increase in maximum plasma concentration of quetiapine; dose adjustment of quetiapine will be necessary).
No products indexed under this heading.

Erythromycin Stearate (Co-administration with an inhibitor of CYP4503A may reduce oral clearance of quetiapine, resulting in an increase in maximum plasma concentration of quetiapine; dose adjustment of quetiapine will be necessary). Products include:
Erythrocin Stearate Filmtab Tablets ... 452

Esmolol Hydrochloride (Enhanced effects of certain antihypertensive agents). Products include:
Brevibloc Concentrate ... 766
Brevibloc Injection ... 766
Brevibloc Double Strength Injection ... 766
Brevibloc Premixed Injection ... 766
Brevibloc Double Strength Premixed Injection ... 766

Esomeprazole Magnesium (Co-administration with an inhibitor of CYP4503A may reduce oral clearance of quetiapine, resulting in an increase in maximum plasma concentration of quetiapine; dose adjustment of quetiapine will be necessary). Products include:
Nexium Delayed-Release Capsules ... 645

Felodipine (Enhanced effects of certain antihypertensive agents). Products include:
Plendil Extended-Release Tablets ... 651

Fludrocortisone Acetate (Co-administration with hepatic enzyme inducers, such as glucocorticosteroids, may increase oral clearance).
No products indexed under this heading.

Fluoxetine Hydrochloride (Co-administration with an inhibitor of CYP4503A may reduce oral clearance of quetiapine, resulting in an increase in maximum plasma concentration of quetiapine; dose adjustment of quetiapine will be necessary). Products include:
Prozac Pulvules and Liquid ... 1771
Symbyax Capsules ... 1788

Fluvoxamine Maleate (Co-administration with an inhibitor of CYP4503A may reduce oral clearance of quetiapine, resulting in an increase in maximum plasma concentration of quetiapine; dose adjustment of quetiapine will be necessary).
No products indexed under this heading.

Fosamprenavir Calcium (Co-administration with an inhibitor of CYP4503A may reduce oral clearance of quetiapine, resulting in an increase in maximum plasma concentration of quetiapine; dose adjustment of quetiapine will be necessary). Products include:

Lexiva Tablets **1473**

Fosinopril Sodium (Enhanced effects of certain antihypertensive agents).
No products indexed under this heading.

Fosphenytoin Sodium (Co-administration has resulted in increased mean oral clearance of quetiapine by 5-fold; increased dose of quetiapine may be required).
No products indexed under this heading.

Furosemide (Enhanced effects of certain antihypertensive agents). Products include:
Furosemide Tablets **2117**

Guanabenz Acetate (Enhanced effects of certain antihypertensive agents).
No products indexed under this heading.

Guanethidine Monosulfate (Enhanced effects of certain antihypertensive agents).
No products indexed under this heading.

Hydralazine Hydrochloride (Enhanced effects of certain antihypertensive agents). Products include:
BiDil Tablets **2161**

Hydrochlorothiazide (Enhanced effects of certain antihypertensive agents). Products include:
Aldoril Tablets **1884**
Atacand HCT **637**
Avalide Tablets **2889**
Avalide Tablets **922**
Benicar HCT Tablets **2852**
Diovan HCT Tablets **2195**
Dyazide Capsules **1389**
Hyzaar **1964**
Lotensin HCT Tablets **2235**
Maxzide **2150**
Micardis HCT Tablets **886**
Moduretic Tablets **2003**
Prinzide Tablets **2033**
Teveten HCT Tablets **1710**
Timolide Tablets **2056**
Uniretic Tablets **3114**
Vaseretic Tablets **2073**
Zestoretic Tablets **701**

Hydrocortisone (Co-administration with hepatic enzyme inducers, such as glucocorticosteroids, may increase oral clearance). Products include:
Cortizone•5 Ointment **699**
Cortizone•10 Creme **699**
Cortizone•10 Ointment **699**
Cortizone•10 Plus Creme **700**
Cortizone•10 Maximum Strength Quick Shot Spray **700**
Hydrocortone Tablets **1963**
Preparation H Hydrocortisone Cream **748**

Hydrocortisone Acetate (Co-administration with hepatic enzyme inducers, such as glucocorticosteroids, may increase oral clearance). Products include:
Analpram-HC **1136**
Pramosone **1139**
ProctoFoam-HC **3113**
Tucks Anti-Itch Ointment **712**
U-cort 1% Cream **3289**

Hydrocortisone Sodium Phosphate (Co-administration with hepatic enzyme inducers, such as glucocorticosteroids, may increase oral clearance).
No products indexed under this heading.

Hydrocortisone Sodium Succinate (Co-administration with hepatic enzyme inducers, such as glucocorticosteroids, may increase oral clearance).
No products indexed under this heading.

Hydroflumethiazide (Enhanced effects of certain antihypertensive agents).
No products indexed under this heading.

Indapamide (Enhanced effects of certain antihypertensive agents). Products include:
Indapamide Tablets **2119**

Indinavir Sulfate (Co-administration with an inhibitor of CYP4503A may reduce oral clearance of quetiapine, resulting in an increase in maximum plasma concentration of quetiapine; dose adjustment of quetiapine will be necessary). Products include:
Crixivan Capsules **1918**

Irbesartan (Enhanced effects of certain antihypertensive agents). Products include:
Avalide Tablets **922**
Avalide Tablets **2889**
Avapro Tablets **925**
Avapro Tablets **2886**

Isoniazid (Co-administration with an inhibitor of CYP4503A may reduce oral clearance of quetiapine, resulting in an increase in maximum plasma concentration of quetiapine; dose adjustment of quetiapine will be necessary).
No products indexed under this heading.

Isradipine (Enhanced effects of certain antihypertensive agents). Products include:
DynaCirc CR Tablets **2726**

Ketoconazole (Co-administration of ketoconazole, a potent inhibitor of CYP4503A, reduced oral clearance of quetiapine by 84%, resulting in a 335% increase in maximum plasma concentration of quetiapine; dose adjustment of quetiapine will be necessary if it is used with ketoconazole). Products include:
Nizoral A-D Shampoo, 1% **1839**
Nizoral 2% Shampoo **1838**

Labetalol Hydrochloride (Enhanced effects of certain antihypertensive agents).
No products indexed under this heading.

Levodopa (Quetiapine may antagonize the effects of levodopa). Products include:
Parcopa Orally Disintegrating Tablets **3111**
Stalevo Tablets **2270**

Lisinopril (Enhanced effects of certain antihypertensive agents). Products include:
Prinivil Tablets **2029**
Prinzide Tablets **2033**
Zestoretic Tablets **701**
Zestril Tablets **704**

Lopinavir (Co-administration with an inhibitor of CYP4503A may reduce oral clearance of quetiapine, resulting in an increase in maximum plasma concentration of quetiapine; dose adjustment of quetiapine will be necessary). Products include:
Kaletra **474**

Loratadine (Co-administration with an inhibitor of CYP4503A may reduce oral clearance of quetiapine, resulting in an increase in maximum plasma concentration of quetiapine; dose adjustment of quetiapine will be necessary). Products include:
Alavert Allergy & Sinus D-12 Hour Tablets **743**
Alavert **743**
Children's Claritin 24 Hour Non-Drowsy Allergy Syrup **732**
Claritin Non-Drowsy 24 Hour Tablets **731**
Non-Drowsy Claritin Hives Relief Tablets **733**
Claritin Reditabs 24 Hour Non-Drowsy Tablets **732**
Claritin-D Non-Drowsy 12 Hour Tablets **731**
Claritin-D Non-Drowsy 24 Hour Tablets **731**
Children's Dimetapp ND Non-Drowsy Allergy Syrup **746**
Triaminic Allerchews **684**

Lorazepam (Co-administration has resulted in reduced (20%) mean oral clearance of lorazepam).
No products indexed under this heading.

Losartan Potassium (Enhanced effects of certain antihypertensive agents). Products include:
Cozaar Tablets **1913**
Hyzaar **1964**

Mecamylamine Hydrochloride (Enhanced effects of certain antihypertensive agents). Products include:
Inversine Tablets **3286**

Mephobarbital (Co-administration with hepatic enzyme inducers, such as barbiturates, may increase oral clearance). Products include:
Mebaral Tablets, USP **2483**

Methyclothiazide (Enhanced effects of certain antihypertensive agents).
No products indexed under this heading.

Methyldopa (Enhanced effects of certain antihypertensive agents). Products include:
Aldoclor Tablets **1881**
Aldoril Tablets **1884**

Methyldopate Hydrochloride (Enhanced effects of certain antihypertensive agents).
No products indexed under this heading.

Methylprednisolone Acetate (Co-administration with hepatic enzyme inducers, such as glucocorticosteroids, may increase oral clearance). Products include:
Depo-Medrol Injectable Suspension **2615**
Depo-Medrol Single-Dose Vial **2617**

Methylprednisolone Sodium Succinate (Co-administration with hepatic enzyme inducers, such as glucocorticosteroids, may increase oral clearance).
No products indexed under this heading.

Metolazone (Enhanced effects of certain antihypertensive agents).
No products indexed under this heading.

Metoprolol Succinate (Enhanced effects of certain antihypertensive agents). Products include:
Toprol-XL Tablets **660**

Metoprolol Tartrate (Enhanced effects of certain antihypertensive agents).
No products indexed under this heading.

Metronidazole (Co-administration with an inhibitor of CYP4503A may reduce oral clearance of quetiapine, resulting in an increase in maximum plasma concentration of quetiapine; dose adjustment of quetiapine will be necessary). Products include:
Metrogel 1% **1212**
MetroGel-Vaginal Gel **1822**
Noritate Cream, 1% **1051**

Metronidazole Benzoate (Co-administration with an inhibitor of CYP4503A may reduce oral clearance of quetiapine, resulting in an increase in maximum plasma concentration of quetiapine; dose adjustment of quetiapine will be necessary).
No products indexed under this heading.

Metronidazole Hydrochloride (Co-administration with an inhibitor of CYP4503A may reduce oral clearance of quetiapine, resulting in an increase in maximum plasma concentration of quetiapine; dose adjustment of quetiapine will be necessary).
No products indexed under this heading.

Metyrosine (Enhanced effects of certain antihypertensive agents). Products include:
Demser Capsules **1933**

Mibefradil Dihydrochloride (Enhanced effects of certain antihypertensive agents).
No products indexed under this heading.

Miconazole (Co-administration with an inhibitor of CYP4503A may reduce oral clearance of quetiapine, resulting in an increase in maximum plasma concentration of quetiapine; dose adjustment of quetiapine will be necessary).
No products indexed under this heading.

Miconazole Nitrate (Co-administration with an inhibitor of CYP4503A may reduce oral clearance of quetiapine, resulting in an increase in maximum plasma concentration of quetiapine; dose adjustment of quetiapine will be necessary). Products include:
Desenex **674**
Desenex Jock Itch Spray Powder **674**

Minoxidil (Enhanced effects of certain antihypertensive agents). Products include:
Men's Rogaine Extra Strength Topical Solution, Ocean Rush Scent and Original Unscented **706**
Women's Rogaine Topical Solution, Spring Bloom Scent and Original Unscented **707**

Moexipril Hydrochloride (Enhanced effects of certain antihypertensive agents). Products include:
Uniretic Tablets **3114**
Univasc Tablets **3118**

Nadolol (Enhanced effects of certain antihypertensive agents). Products include:
Nadolol Tablets **2121**

Nefazodone Hydrochloride (Co-administration with an inhibitor of CYP4503A may reduce oral clearance of quetiapine, resulting in an increase in maximum plasma concentration of quetiapine; dose adjustment of quetiapine will be necessary).
No products indexed under this heading.

Nelfinavir Mesylate (Co-administration with an inhibitor of CYP4503A may reduce oral clearance of quetiapine, resulting in an increase in maximum plasma con-

centration of quetiapine; dose adjustment of quetiapine will be necessary). Products include:
Viracept ... 2556

Nevirapine (Co-administration with an inhibitor of CYP4503A may reduce oral clearance of quetiapine, resulting in an increase in maximum plasma concentration of quetiapine; dose adjustment of quetiapine will be necessary). Products include:
Viramune Oral Suspension ... 903
Viramune Tablets ... 903

Niacinamide (Co-administration with an inhibitor of CYP4503A may reduce oral clearance of quetiapine, resulting in an increase in maximum plasma concentration of quetiapine; dose adjustment of quetiapine will be necessary).
No products indexed under this heading.

Nicardipine Hydrochloride (Enhanced effects of certain antihypertensive agents). Products include:
Cardene I.V. ... 1129

Nicotinamide (Co-administration with an inhibitor of CYP4503A may reduce oral clearance of quetiapine, resulting in an increase in maximum plasma concentration of quetiapine; dose adjustment of quetiapine will be necessary). Products include:
Nicomide Tablets ... 3190

Nifedipine (Co-administration with an inhibitor of CYP4503A may reduce oral clearance of quetiapine, resulting in an increase in maximum plasma concentration of quetiapine; dose adjustment of quetiapine will be necessary). Products include:
Adalat CC Tablets ... 2978

Nisoldipine (Enhanced effects of certain antihypertensive agents). Products include:
Sular Tablets ... 1163

Nitroglycerin (Enhanced effects of certain antihypertensive agents). Products include:
Nitro-Dur Transdermal Infusion System ... 3060
Nitrolingual Pumpspray ... 1161

Norfloxacin (Co-administration with an inhibitor of CYP4503A may reduce oral clearance of quetiapine, resulting in an increase in maximum plasma concentration of quetiapine; dose adjustment of quetiapine will be necessary). Products include:
Noroxin Tablets ... 2009

Omeprazole (Co-administration with an inhibitor of CYP4503A may reduce oral clearance of quetiapine, resulting in an increase in maximum plasma concentration of quetiapine; dose adjustment of quetiapine will be necessary). Products include:
Zegerid Powder for Oral Solution ... 2972

Paroxetine Hydrochloride (Co-administration with an inhibitor of CYP4503A may reduce oral clearance of quetiapine, resulting in an increase in maximum plasma concentration of quetiapine; dose adjustment of quetiapine will be necessary). Products include:
Paxil CR Controlled-Release Tablets ... 1509
Paxil ... 1501

Penbutolol Sulfate (Enhanced effects of certain antihypertensive agents).
No products indexed under this heading.

Pentobarbital Sodium (Co-administration with hepatic enzyme inducers, such as barbiturates, may increase oral clearance). Products include:
Nembutal Sodium Solution, USP ... 2484

Pergolide Mesylate (Quetiapine may antagonize the effects of dopamine agonists). Products include:
Permax Tablets ... 3357

Perindopril Erbumine (Enhanced effects of certain antihypertensive agents). Products include:
Aceon Tablets (2 mg, 4 mg, 8 mg) ... 3191

Phenobarbital (Co-administration with hepatic enzyme inducers, such as barbiturates, may increase oral clearance).
No products indexed under this heading.

Phenoxybenzamine Hydrochloride (Enhanced effects of certain antihypertensive agents). Products include:
Dibenzyline Capsules ... 3390

Phentolamine Mesylate (Enhanced effects of certain antihypertensive agents).
No products indexed under this heading.

Phenytoin (Co-administration has resulted in increased mean oral clearance of quetiapine by 5-fold; increased dose of quetiapine may be required).
No products indexed under this heading.

Phenytoin Sodium (Co-administration has resulted in increased mean oral clearance of quetiapine by 5-fold; increased dose of quetiapine may be required). Products include:
Phenytek Capsules ... 2153

Pindolol (Enhanced effects of certain antihypertensive agents).
No products indexed under this heading.

Polythiazide (Enhanced effects of certain antihypertensive agents).
No products indexed under this heading.

Pramipexole Dihydrochloride (Quetiapine may antagonize the effects of dopamine agonists). Products include:
Mirapex Tablets ... 889

Prazosin Hydrochloride (Enhanced effects of certain antihypertensive agents).
No products indexed under this heading.

Prednisolone Acetate (Co-administration with hepatic enzyme inducers, such as glucocorticosteroids, may increase oral clearance). Products include:
Blephamide Ophthalmic Ointment ... 563
Blephamide Ophthalmic Suspension ... 564
Poly-Pred Liquifilm Ophthalmic Suspension ... ⊙231
Pred Forte Ophthalmic Suspension ... ⊙233
Pred Mild Sterile Ophthalmic Suspension ... ⊙236
Pred-G Ophthalmic Suspension ... ⊙234
Pred-G Sterile Ophthalmic Ointment ... ⊙235

Prednisolone Sodium Phosphate (Co-administration with hepatic enzyme inducers, such as glucocorticosteroids, may increase oral clearance). Products include:
Pediapred Oral Solution ... 3319

Prednisolone Tebutate (Co-administration with hepatic enzyme inducers, such as glucocorticosteroids, may increase oral clearance).
No products indexed under this heading.

Prednisone (Co-administration with hepatic enzyme inducers, such as glucocorticosteroids, may increase oral clearance).
No products indexed under this heading.

Propoxyphene Hydrochloride (Co-administration with an inhibitor of CYP4503A may reduce oral clearance of quetiapine, resulting in an increase in maximum plasma concentration of quetiapine; dose adjustment of quetiapine will be necessary).
No products indexed under this heading.

Propoxyphene Napsylate (Co-administration with an inhibitor of CYP4503A may reduce oral clearance of quetiapine, resulting in an increase in maximum plasma concentration of quetiapine; dose adjustment of quetiapine will be necessary). Products include:
Darvocet A 500 Tablets ... 3497

Propranolol Hydrochloride (Enhanced effects of certain antihypertensive agents). Products include:
Inderal LA Long-Acting Capsules ... 3421
InnoPran XL Capsules ... 2728

Quinapril Hydrochloride (Enhanced effects of certain antihypertensive agents).
No products indexed under this heading.

Quinidine (Co-administration with an inhibitor of CYP4503A may reduce oral clearance of quetiapine, resulting in an increase in maximum plasma concentration of quetiapine; dose adjustment of quetiapine will be necessary).
No products indexed under this heading.

Quinidine Hydrochloride (Co-administration with an inhibitor of CYP4503A may reduce oral clearance of quetiapine, resulting in an increase in maximum plasma concentration of quetiapine; dose adjustment of quetiapine will be necessary).
No products indexed under this heading.

Quinidine Polygalacturonate (Co-administration with an inhibitor of CYP4503A may reduce oral clearance of quetiapine, resulting in an increase in maximum plasma concentration of quetiapine; dose adjustment of quetiapine will be necessary).
No products indexed under this heading.

Quinidine Sulfate (Co-administration with an inhibitor of CYP4503A may reduce oral clearance of quetiapine, resulting in an increase in maximum plasma concentration of quetiapine; dose adjustment of quetiapine will be necessary).
No products indexed under this heading.

Quinine (Co-administration with an inhibitor of CYP4503A may reduce oral clearance of quetiapine, resulting in an increase in maximum plasma concentration of quetiapine; dose adjustment of quetiapine will be necessary).
No products indexed under this heading.

Quinine Sulfate (Co-administration with an inhibitor of CYP4503A may reduce oral clearance of quetiapine, resulting in an increase in maximum plasma concentration of quetiapine; dose adjustment of quetiapine will be necessary).
No products indexed under this heading.

Quinupristin (Co-administration with an inhibitor of CYP4503A may reduce oral clearance of quetiapine, resulting in an increase in maximum plasma concentration of quetiapine; dose adjustment of quetiapine will be necessary). Products include:
Synercid I.V. ... 1690

Ramipril (Enhanced effects of certain antihypertensive agents). Products include:
Altace Capsules ... 1673

Ranitidine Bismuth Citrate (Co-administration with an inhibitor of CYP4503A may reduce oral clearance of quetiapine, resulting in an increase in maximum plasma concentration of quetiapine; dose adjustment of quetiapine will be necessary).
No products indexed under this heading.

Ranitidine Hydrochloride (Co-administration with an inhibitor of CYP4503A may reduce oral clearance of quetiapine, resulting in an increase in maximum plasma concentration of quetiapine; dose adjustment of quetiapine will be necessary). Products include:
Zantac ... 1597
Zantac Injection ... 1593
Zantac 75 Tablets ... ▣715
Zantac 150 Maximum Strength Tablets ... ▣715
Zantac Injection Pharmacy Bulk Package ... 1595

Rauwolfia Serpentina (Enhanced effects of certain antihypertensive agents).
No products indexed under this heading.

Rescinnamine (Enhanced effects of certain antihypertensive agents).
No products indexed under this heading.

Reserpine (Enhanced effects of certain antihypertensive agents).
No products indexed under this heading.

Rifampin (Co-administration with hepatic enzyme inducers, such as rifampin, may increase oral clearance).
No products indexed under this heading.

Ritonavir (Co-administration with an inhibitor of CYP4503A may reduce oral clearance of quetiapine, resulting in an increase in maximum plasma concentration of quetiapine; dose adjustment of quetiapine will be necessary). Products include:
Kaletra ... 474
Norvir ... 499

Ropinirole Hydrochloride (Quetiapine may antagonize the effects of dopamine agonists). Products include:

Requip Tablets 1528

Saquinavir (Co-administration with an inhibitor of CYP4503A may reduce oral clearance of quetiapine, resulting in an increase in maximum plasma concentration of quetiapine; dose adjustment of quetiapine will be necessary).
No products indexed under this heading.

Saquinavir Mesylate (Co-administration with an inhibitor of CYP4503A may reduce oral clearance of quetiapine, resulting in an increase in maximum plasma concentration of quetiapine; dose adjustment of quetiapine will be necessary). Products include:
Invirase 2776

Secobarbital Sodium (Co-administration with hepatic enzyme inducers, such as barbiturates, may increase oral clearance).
No products indexed under this heading.

Sertraline Hydrochloride (Co-administration with an inhibitor of CYP4503A may reduce oral clearance of quetiapine, resulting in an increase in maximum plasma concentration of quetiapine; dose adjustment of quetiapine will be necessary). Products include:
Zoloft 2581

Sodium Nitroprusside (Enhanced effects of certain antihypertensive agents).
No products indexed under this heading.

Sotalol Hydrochloride (Enhanced effects of certain antihypertensive agents).
No products indexed under this heading.

Spirapril Hydrochloride (Enhanced effects of certain antihypertensive agents).
No products indexed under this heading.

Telmisartan (Enhanced effects of certain antihypertensive agents). Products include:
Micardis Tablets 884
Micardis HCT Tablets 886

Terazosin Hydrochloride (Enhanced effects of certain antihypertensive agents). Products include:
Hytrin Capsules 469

Thiamylal Sodium (Co-administration with hepatic enzyme inducers, such as barbiturates, may increase oral clearance).
No products indexed under this heading.

Thioridazine (Increases the oral clearance of quetiapine by 65%).
No products indexed under this heading.

Timolol Maleate (Enhanced effects of certain antihypertensive agents). Products include:
Blocadren Tablets 1891
Cosopt Sterile Ophthalmic Solution 1910
Timolide Tablets 2056
Timoptic in Ocudose 2061
Timoptic Sterile Ophthalmic Solution 2058
Timoptic-XE Sterile Ophthalmic Gel Forming Solution 2062

Torsemide (Enhanced effects of certain antihypertensive agents).
No products indexed under this heading.

Trandolapril (Enhanced effects of certain antihypertensive agents). Products include:
Mavik Tablets 482
Tarka Tablets 519

Triamcinolone (Co-administration with hepatic enzyme inducers, such as glucocorticosteroids, may increase oral clearance).
No products indexed under this heading.

Triamcinolone Acetonide (Co-administration with hepatic enzyme inducers, such as glucocorticosteroids, may increase oral clearance). Products include:
Azmacort Inhalation Aerosol 1701
Nasacort HFA Inhalation Aerosol 2939
Nasacort AQ Nasal Spray 2937

Triamcinolone Diacetate (Co-administration with hepatic enzyme inducers, such as glucocorticosteroids, may increase oral clearance).
No products indexed under this heading.

Triamcinolone Hexacetonide (Co-administration with hepatic enzyme inducers, such as glucocorticosteroids, may increase oral clearance).
No products indexed under this heading.

Trimethaphan Camsylate (Enhanced effects of certain antihypertensive agents).
No products indexed under this heading.

Troglitazone (Co-administration with an inhibitor of CYP4503A may reduce oral clearance of quetiapine, resulting in an increase in maximum plasma concentration of quetiapine; dose adjustment of quetiapine will be necessary).
No products indexed under this heading.

Troleandomycin (Co-administration with an inhibitor of CYP4503A may reduce oral clearance of quetiapine, resulting in an increase in maximum plasma concentration of quetiapine; dose adjustment of quetiapine will be necessary).
No products indexed under this heading.

Valproate Sodium (Co-administration with an inhibitor of CYP4503A may reduce oral clearance of quetiapine, resulting in an increase in maximum plasma concentration of quetiapine; dose adjustment of quetiapine will be necessary). Products include:
Depacon Injection 412

Valsartan (Enhanced effects of certain antihypertensive agents). Products include:
Diovan HCT Tablets 2195
Diovan Tablets 2191

Verapamil Hydrochloride (Co-administration with an inhibitor of CYP4503A may reduce oral clearance of quetiapine, resulting in an increase in maximum plasma concentration of quetiapine; dose adjustment of quetiapine will be necessary). Products include:
Covera-HS Tablets 3135
Tarka Tablets 519
Verelan PM Capsules 3120

Voriconazole (Co-administration with an inhibitor of CYP4503A may reduce oral clearance of quetiapine, resulting in an increase in maximum plasma concentration of quetiapine; dose adjustment of quetiapine will be necessary). Products include:
VFEND I.V. 2543
VFEND Oral Suspension 2543
VFEND Tablets 2543

Zafirlukast (Co-administration with an inhibitor of CYP4503A may reduce oral clearance of quetiapine, resulting in an increase in maximum plasma concentration of quetiapine; dose adjustment of quetiapine will be necessary). Products include:
Accolate Tablets 663

Zileuton (Co-administration with an inhibitor of CYP4503A may reduce oral clearance of quetiapine, resulting in an increase in maximum plasma concentration of quetiapine; dose adjustment of quetiapine will be necessary).
No products indexed under this heading.

Food Interactions

Alcohol (The cognitive and motor effect of alcohol is potentiated; alcohol use should be avoided).

Food, unspecified (The bioavailability of quetiapine is marginally affected by administration with food, with Cmax and AUC values increased by 25% and 15%, respectively).

Grapefruit (Co-administration with an inhibitor of CYP4503A may reduce oral clearance of quetiapine, resulting in an increase in maximum plasma concentration of quetiapine; dose adjustment of quetiapine will be necessary).

Grapefruit Juice (Co-administration with an inhibitor of CYP4503A may reduce oral clearance of quetiapine, resulting in an increase in maximum plasma concentration of quetiapine; dose adjustment of quetiapine will be necessary).

SIMPLY COUGH LIQUID

(Dextromethorphan Hydrobromide) ... 1840
May interact with monoamine oxidase inhibitors. Compounds in these categories include:

Isocarboxazid (Concurrent and/or sequential use with MAO inhibitors is not recommended).
No products indexed under this heading.

Moclobemide (Concurrent and/or sequential use with MAO inhibitors is not recommended).
No products indexed under this heading.

Pargyline Hydrochloride (Concurrent and/or sequential use with MAO inhibitors is not recommended).
No products indexed under this heading.

Phenelzine Sulfate (Concurrent and/or sequential use with MAO inhibitors is not recommended).
No products indexed under this heading.

Procarbazine Hydrochloride (Concurrent and/or sequential use with MAO inhibitors is not recommended). Products include:
Matulane Capsules 3188

Selegiline Hydrochloride (Concurrent and/or sequential use with MAO inhibitors is not recommended). Products include:
Eldepryl Capsules 3209

Tranylcypromine Sulfate (Concurrent and/or sequential use with MAO inhibitors is not recommended). Products include:
Parnate Tablets 1499

SIMPLY SLEEP CAPLETS

(Diphenhydramine Hydrochloride) 1841
May interact with hypnotics and sedatives, tranquilizers, and certain other agents. Compounds in these categories include:

Alprazolam (Diphenhydramine is an antihistamine with sedative properties; concurrent use should be avoided). Products include:
Niravam Orally Disintegrating Tablets 3106
Xanax XR Tablets 2655

Buspirone Hydrochloride (Diphenhydramine is an antihistamine with sedative properties; concurrent use should be avoided).
No products indexed under this heading.

Chlordiazepoxide (Diphenhydramine is an antihistamine with sedative properties; concurrent use should be avoided).
No products indexed under this heading.

Chlordiazepoxide Hydrochloride (Diphenhydramine is an antihistamine with sedative properties; concurrent use should be avoided). Products include:
Librium Capsules 3349

Chlorpromazine (Diphenhydramine is an antihistamine with sedative properties; concurrent use should be avoided).
No products indexed under this heading.

Chlorpromazine Hydrochloride (Diphenhydramine is an antihistamine with sedative properties; concurrent use should be avoided).
No products indexed under this heading.

Chlorprothixene (Diphenhydramine is an antihistamine with sedative properties; concurrent use should be avoided).
No products indexed under this heading.

Chlorprothixene Hydrochloride (Diphenhydramine is an antihistamine with sedative properties; concurrent use should be avoided).
No products indexed under this heading.

Clorazepate Dipotassium (Diphenhydramine is an antihistamine with sedative properties; concurrent use should be avoided). Products include:
Tranxene 2488

Diazepam (Diphenhydramine is an antihistamine with sedative properties; concurrent use should be avoided). Products include:
Diastat Rectal Delivery System 3344
Valium Tablets 2822

Droperidol (Diphenhydramine is an antihistamine with sedative properties; concurrent use should be avoided).
No products indexed under this heading.

Estazolam (Diphenhydramine is an antihistamine with sedative properties; concurrent use should be avoided). Products include:
ProSom Tablets 512

Ethchlorvynol (Diphenhydramine is an antihistamine with sedative properties; concurrent use should be avoided).
No products indexed under this heading.

Ethinamate (Diphenhydramine is an antihistamine with sedative properties; concurrent use should be avoided).
No products indexed under this heading.

Fluphenazine Decanoate (Diphenhydramine is an antihistamine with sedative properties; concurrent use should be avoided).
No products indexed under this heading.

Fluphenazine Enanthate (Diphenhydramine is an antihistamine with sedative properties; concurrent use should be avoided).
No products indexed under this heading.

Fluphenazine Hydrochloride (Diphenhydramine is an antihistamine with sedative properties; concurrent use should be avoided).
No products indexed under this heading.

Flurazepam Hydrochloride (Diphenhydramine is an antihistamine with sedative properties; concurrent use should be avoided). Products include:
Dalmane Capsules 3343

Glutethimide (Diphenhydramine is an antihistamine with sedative properties; concurrent use should be avoided).
No products indexed under this heading.

Haloperidol (Diphenhydramine is an antihistamine with sedative properties; concurrent use should be avoided).
No products indexed under this heading.

Haloperidol Decanoate (Diphenhydramine is an antihistamine with sedative properties; concurrent use should be avoided).
No products indexed under this heading.

Hydroxyzine Hydrochloride (Diphenhydramine is an antihistamine with sedative properties; concurrent use should be avoided).
No products indexed under this heading.

Lorazepam (Diphenhydramine is an antihistamine with sedative properties; concurrent use should be avoided).
No products indexed under this heading.

Loxapine Hydrochloride (Diphenhydramine is an antihistamine with sedative properties; concurrent use should be avoided).
No products indexed under this heading.

Loxapine Succinate (Diphenhydramine is an antihistamine with sedative properties; concurrent use should be avoided).
No products indexed under this heading.

Meprobamate (Diphenhydramine is an antihistamine with sedative properties; concurrent use should be avoided).
No products indexed under this heading.

Mesoridazine Besylate (Diphenhydramine is an antihistamine with sedative properties; concurrent use should be avoided).
No products indexed under this heading.

Midazolam Hydrochloride (Diphenhydramine is an antihistamine with sedative properties; concurrent use should be avoided).
No products indexed under this heading.

Molindone Hydrochloride (Diphenhydramine is an antihistamine with sedative properties; concurrent use should be avoided). Products include:
Moban Tablets 1108

Oxazepam (Diphenhydramine is an antihistamine with sedative properties; concurrent use should be avoided).
No products indexed under this heading.

Perphenazine (Diphenhydramine is an antihistamine with sedative properties; concurrent use should be avoided).
No products indexed under this heading.

Prazepam (Diphenhydramine is an antihistamine with sedative properties; concurrent use should be avoided).
No products indexed under this heading.

Prochlorperazine (Diphenhydramine is an antihistamine with sedative properties; concurrent use should be avoided).
No products indexed under this heading.

Promethazine Hydrochloride (Diphenhydramine is an antihistamine with sedative properties; concurrent use should be avoided). Products include:
Phenergan 3438

Propofol (Diphenhydramine is an antihistamine with sedative properties; concurrent use should be avoided). Products include:
Diprivan Injectable Emulsion 676

Quazepam (Diphenhydramine is an antihistamine with sedative properties; concurrent use should be avoided).
No products indexed under this heading.

Secobarbital Sodium (Diphenhydramine is an antihistamine with sedative properties; concurrent use should be avoided).
No products indexed under this heading.

Temazepam (Diphenhydramine is an antihistamine with sedative properties; concurrent use should be avoided).
No products indexed under this heading.

Thioridazine Hydrochloride (Diphenhydramine is an antihistamine with sedative properties; concurrent use should be avoided). Products include:
Thioridazine Hydrochloride Tablets 2122

Thiothixene (Diphenhydramine is an antihistamine with sedative properties; concurrent use should be avoided). Products include:
Thiothixene Capsules 2124

Triazolam (Diphenhydramine is an antihistamine with sedative properties; concurrent use should be avoided).
No products indexed under this heading.

Trifluoperazine Hydrochloride (Diphenhydramine is an antihistamine with sedative properties; concurrent use should be avoided).
No products indexed under this heading.

Zaleplon (Diphenhydramine is an antihistamine with sedative properties; concurrent use should be avoided). Products include:
Sonata Capsules 1686

Zolpidem Tartrate (Diphenhydramine is an antihistamine with sedative properties; concurrent use should be avoided). Products include:
Ambien Tablets 2867

Food Interactions

Alcohol (Diphenhydramine is an antihistamine with sedative properties; concurrent use with alcoholic beverages should be avoided).

SIMPLY STUFFY LIQUID

(Pseudoephedrine Hydrochloride) 1841
May interact with monoamine oxidase inhibitors. Compounds in these categories include:

Isocarboxazid (Concurrent and/or sequential use with MAO inhibitors is not recommended).
No products indexed under this heading.

Moclobemide (Concurrent and/or sequential use with MAO inhibitors is not recommended).
No products indexed under this heading.

Pargyline Hydrochloride (Concurrent and/or sequential use with MAO inhibitors is not recommended).
No products indexed under this heading.

Phenelzine Sulfate (Concurrent and/or sequential use with MAO inhibitors is not recommended).
No products indexed under this heading.

Procarbazine Hydrochloride (Concurrent and/or sequential use with MAO inhibitors is not recommended). Products include:
Matulane Capsules 3188

Selegiline Hydrochloride (Concurrent and/or sequential use with MAO inhibitors is not recommended). Products include:
Eldepryl Capsules 3209

Tranylcypromine Sulfate (Concurrent and/or sequential use with MAO inhibitors is not recommended). Products include:
Parnate Tablets 1499

SIMULECT FOR INJECTION

(Basiliximab) 2268
None cited in PDR database.

SINECCH CAPSULES

(Arnica montana) .... ■758
May interact with:

Pentazocine Hydrochloride (Avoid concurrent use with Talwin or Talwin NX).
No products indexed under this heading.

SINGLET CAPLETS

(Acetaminophen, Chlorpheniramine Maleate, Pseudoephedrine Hydrochloride) .... ■636
May interact with hypnotics and sedatives, monoamine oxidase inhibitors, tranquilizers, and certain other agents. Compounds in these categories include:

Alprazolam (May increase drowsiness effect). Products include:
Niravam Orally Disintegrating Tablets 3106
Xanax XR Tablets 2655

Buspirone Hydrochloride (May increase drowsiness effect).
No products indexed under this heading.

Chlordiazepoxide (May increase drowsiness effect).
No products indexed under this heading.

Chlordiazepoxide Hydrochloride (May increase drowsiness effect). Products include:
Librium Capsules 3349

Chlorpromazine (May increase drowsiness effect).
No products indexed under this heading.

Chlorpromazine Hydrochloride (May increase drowsiness effect).
No products indexed under this heading.

Chlorprothixene (May increase drowsiness effect).
No products indexed under this heading.

Chlorprothixene Hydrochloride (May increase drowsiness effect).
No products indexed under this heading.

Clorazepate Dipotassium (May increase drowsiness effect). Products include:
Tranxene 2488

Diazepam (May increase drowsiness effect). Products include:
Diastat Rectal Delivery System 3344
Valium Tablets 2822

Droperidol (May increase drowsiness effect).
No products indexed under this heading.

Estazolam (May increase drowsiness effect). Products include:
ProSom Tablets 512

Ethchlorvynol (May increase drowsiness effect).
No products indexed under this heading.

Ethinamate (May increase drowsiness effect).
No products indexed under this heading.

Fluphenazine Decanoate (May increase drowsiness effect).
No products indexed under this heading.

Fluphenazine Enanthate (May increase drowsiness effect).
No products indexed under this heading.

Fluphenazine Hydrochloride (May increase drowsiness effect).
No products indexed under this heading.

Flurazepam Hydrochloride (May increase drowsiness effect). Products include:
Dalmane Capsules 3343

Glutethimide (May increase drowsiness effect).
No products indexed under this heading.

Haloperidol (May increase drowsiness effect).
No products indexed under this heading.

Haloperidol Decanoate (May increase drowsiness effect).
No products indexed under this heading.

Hydroxyzine Hydrochloride (May increase drowsiness effect).
No products indexed under this heading.

Isocarboxazid (Concurrent and/or sequential use with MAO inhibitors is not recommended).
No products indexed under this heading.

Lorazepam (May increase drowsiness effect).
No products indexed under this heading.

Loxapine Hydrochloride (May increase drowsiness effect).
No products indexed under this heading.

Loxapine Succinate (May increase drowsiness effect).
No products indexed under this heading.

Meprobamate (May increase drowsiness effect).
No products indexed under this heading.

Mesoridazine Besylate (May increase drowsiness effect).
No products indexed under this heading.

Midazolam Hydrochloride (May increase drowsiness effect).
No products indexed under this heading.

Moclobemide (Concurrent and/or sequential use with MAO inhibitors is not recommended).
No products indexed under this heading.

Molindone Hydrochloride (May increase drowsiness effect). Products include:
Moban Tablets ... **1108**

Oxazepam (May increase drowsiness effect).
No products indexed under this heading.

Pargyline Hydrochloride (Concurrent and/or sequential use with MAO inhibitors is not recommended).
No products indexed under this heading.

Perphenazine (May increase drowsiness effect).
No products indexed under this heading.

Phenelzine Sulfate (Concurrent and/or sequential use with MAO inhibitors is not recommended).
No products indexed under this heading.

Prazepam (May increase drowsiness effect).
No products indexed under this heading.

Procarbazine Hydrochloride (Concurrent and/or sequential use with MAO inhibitors is not recommended). Products include:
Matulane Capsules ... **3188**

Prochlorperazine (May increase drowsiness effect).
No products indexed under this heading.

Promethazine Hydrochloride (May increase drowsiness effect). Products include:
Phenergan ... **3438**

Propofol (May increase drowsiness effect). Products include:
Diprivan Injectable Emulsion ... **676**

Quazepam (May increase drowsiness effect).
No products indexed under this heading.

Secobarbital Sodium (May increase drowsiness effect).
No products indexed under this heading.

Selegiline Hydrochloride (Concurrent and/or sequential use with MAO inhibitors is not recommended). Products include:
Eldepryl Capsules ... **3209**

Temazepam (May increase drowsiness effect).
No products indexed under this heading.

Thioridazine Hydrochloride (May increase drowsiness effect). Products include:
Thioridazine Hydrochloride Tablets ... **2122**

Thiothixene (May increase drowsiness effect). Products include:
Thiothixene Capsules ... **2124**

Tranylcypromine Sulfate (Concurrent and/or sequential use with MAO inhibitors is not recommended). Products include:
Parnate Tablets ... **1499**

Triazolam (May increase drowsiness effect).
No products indexed under this heading.

Trifluoperazine Hydrochloride (May increase drowsiness effect).
No products indexed under this heading.

Zaleplon (May increase drowsiness effect). Products include:
Sonata Capsules ... **1686**

Zolpidem Tartrate (May increase drowsiness effect). Products include:
Ambien Tablets ... **2867**

Food Interactions

Alcohol (Chronic heavy alcohol users, 3 or more drinks per day, should consult their physicians for advice on when and how they should take pain relievers/fever reducers including acetaminophen; increases drowsiness effect).

SINGULAIR ORAL GRANULES

(Montelukast Sodium) ... **2047**
See Singulair Tablets

SINGULAIR TABLETS

(Montelukast Sodium) ... **2047**
May interact with cytochrome p450 2c8 substrates (selected) and certain other agents. Compounds in these categories include:

Amiodarone Hydrochloride (Montelukast is a potent inhibitor of P450 2C8, but no in vivo drug interaction studies have been conducted between montelukast and cytochrome P450 2C8 substrates. Caution should be exercised when concomitantly administering a cytochrome P450 2C8 substrate). Products include:
Pacerone Tablets ... **3337**

Amitriptyline Hydrochloride (Montelukast is a potent inhibitor of P450 2C8, but no in vivo drug interaction studies have been conducted between montelukast and cytochrome P450 2C8 substrates. Caution should be exercised when concomitantly administering a cytochrome P450 2C8 substrate).
No products indexed under this heading.

Amoxapine (Montelukast is a potent inhibitor of P450 2C8, but no in vivo drug interaction studies have been conducted between montelukast and cytochrome P450 2C8 substrates. Caution should be exercised when concomitantly administering a cytochrome P450 2C8 substrate).
No products indexed under this heading.

Benzphetamine Hydrochloride (Montelukast is a potent inhibitor of P450 2C8, but no in vivo drug interaction studies have been conducted between montelukast and cytochrome P450 2C8 substrates. Caution should be exercised when concomitantly administering a cytochrome P450 2C8 substrate).
No products indexed under this heading.

Carbamazepine (Montelukast is a potent inhibitor of P450 2C8, but no in vivo drug interaction studies have been conducted between montelukast and cytochrome P450 2C8 substrates. Caution should be exercised when concomitantly administering a cytochrome P450 2C8 substrate). Products include:
Carbatrol Capsules ... **3174**
Equetro Extended-Release Capsules ... **3178**
Tegretol/Tegretol-XR ... **2278**

Clomipramine Hydrochloride (Montelukast is a potent inhibitor of P450 2C8, but no in vivo drug interaction studies have been conducted between montelukast and cytochrome P450 2C8 substrates. Caution should be exercised when concomitantly administering a cytochrome P450 2C8 substrate).
No products indexed under this heading.

Desipramine Hydrochloride (Montelukast is a potent inhibitor of P450 2C8, but no in vivo drug interaction studies have been conducted between montelukast and cytochrome P450 2C8 substrates. Caution should be exercised when concomitantly administering a cytochrome P450 2C8 substrate).
No products indexed under this heading.

Diazepam (Montelukast is a potent inhibitor of P450 2C8, but no in vivo drug interaction studies have been conducted between montelukast and cytochrome P450 2C8 substrates. Caution should be exercised when concomitantly administering a cytochrome P450 2C8 substrate). Products include:
Diastat Rectal Delivery System ... **3344**
Valium Tablets ... **2822**

Diclofenac Potassium (Montelukast is a potent inhibitor of P450 2C8, but no in vivo drug interaction studies have been conducted between montelukast and cytochrome P450 2C8 substrates. Caution should be exercised when concomitantly administering a cytochrome P450 2C8 substrate). Products include:
Cataflam Tablets ... **2173**

Diclofenac Sodium (Montelukast is a potent inhibitor of P450 2C8, but no in vivo drug interaction studies have been conducted between montelukast and cytochrome P450 2C8 substrates. Caution should be exercised when concomitantly administering a cytochrome P450 2C8 substrate). Products include:
Arthrotec Tablets ... **3126**
Voltaren Ophthalmic Solution ... **2300**
Voltaren Tablets ... **2298**
Voltaren-XR Tablets ... **2301**

Docetaxel (Montelukast is a potent inhibitor of P450 2C8, but no in vivo drug interaction studies have been conducted between montelukast and cytochrome P450 2C8 substrates. Caution should be exercised when concomitantly administering a cytochrome P450 2C8 substrate). Products include:
Taxotere Injection Concentrate ... **2947**

Doxepin Hydrochloride (Montelukast is a potent inhibitor of P450 2C8, but no in vivo drug interaction studies have been conducted between montelukast and cytochrome P450 2C8 substrates. Caution should be exercised when concomitantly administering a cytochrome P450 2C8 substrate).
No products indexed under this heading.

Fluvastatin Sodium (Montelukast is a potent inhibitor of P450 2C8, but no in vivo drug interaction studies have been conducted between montelukast and cytochrome P450 2C8 substrates. Caution should be exercised when concomitantly administering a cytochrome P450 2C8 substrate). Products include:
Lescol Capsules ... **2227**
Lescol ... **2730**
Lescol XL Tablets ... **2227**

Imipramine Hydrochloride (Montelukast is a potent inhibitor of P450 2C8, but no in vivo drug interaction studies have been conducted between montelukast and cytochrome P450 2C8 substrates. Caution should be exercised when concomitantly administering a cytochrome P450 2C8 substrate).
No products indexed under this heading.

Imipramine Pamoate (Montelukast is a potent inhibitor of P450 2C8, but no in vivo drug interaction studies have been conducted between montelukast and cytochrome P450 2C8 substrates. Caution should be exercised when concomitantly administering a cytochrome P450 2C8 substrate).
No products indexed under this heading.

Isotretinoin (Montelukast is a potent inhibitor of P450 2C8, but no in vivo drug interaction studies have been conducted between montelukast and cytochrome P450 2C8 substrates. Caution should be exercised when concomitantly administering a cytochrome P450 2C8 substrate). Products include:
Accutane Capsules ... **2740**
Amnesteem Capsules ... **2126**

Maprotiline Hydrochloride (Montelukast is a potent inhibitor of P450 2C8, but no in vivo drug interaction studies have been conducted between montelukast and cytochrome P450 2C8 substrates. Caution should be exercised when concomitantly administering a cytochrome P450 2C8 substrate).
No products indexed under this heading.

Mephobarbital (Montelukast is a potent inhibitor of P450 2C8, but no in vivo drug interaction studies have been conducted between montelukast and cytochrome P450 2C8 substrates. Caution should be exercised when concomitantly administering a cytochrome P450 2C8 substrate). Products include:
Mebaral Tablets, USP 2483

Nortriptyline Hydrochloride (Montelukast is a potent inhibitor of P450 2C8, but no in vivo drug interaction studies have been conducted between montelukast and cytochrome P450 2C8 substrates. Caution should be exercised when concomitantly administering a cytochrome P450 2C8 substrate).
No products indexed under this heading.

Omeprazole (Montelukast is a potent inhibitor of P450 2C8, but no in vivo drug interaction studies have been conducted between montelukast and cytochrome P450 2C8 substrates. Caution should be exercised when concomitantly administering a cytochrome P450 2C8 substrate). Products include:
Zegerid Powder for Oral Solution 2972

Paclitaxel (Montelukast is a potent inhibitor of P450 2C8, but no in vivo drug interaction studies have been conducted between montelukast and cytochrome P450 2C8 substrates. Caution should be exercised when concomitantly administering a cytochrome P450 2C8 substrate).
No products indexed under this heading.

Phenobarbital (Induces hepatic metabolism and decreases the AUC of montelukast approximately 40%; no dosage adjustment for Singulair is recommended).
No products indexed under this heading.

Phenytoin (Montelukast is a potent inhibitor of P450 2C8, but no in vivo drug interaction studies have been conducted between montelukast and cytochrome P450 2C8 substrates. Caution should be exercised when concomitantly administering a cytochrome P450 2C8 substrate).
No products indexed under this heading.

Phenytoin Sodium (Montelukast is a potent inhibitor of P450 2C8, but no in vivo drug interaction studies have been conducted between montelukast and cytochrome P450 2C8 substrates. Caution should be exercised when concomitantly administering a cytochrome P450 2C8 substrate). Products include:
Phenytek Capsules 2153

Pioglitazone Hydrochloride (Montelukast is a potent inhibitor of P450 2C8, but no in vivo drug interaction studies have been conducted between montelukast and cytochrome P450 2C8 substrates. Caution should be exercised when concomitantly administering a cytochrome P450 2C8 substrate). Products include:
ActoPlus Met Tablets 3219
Actos Tablets 3224

Protriptyline Hydrochloride (Montelukast is a potent inhibitor of P450 2C8, but no in vivo drug interaction studies have been conducted between montelukast and cytochrome P450 2C8 substrates. Caution should be exercised when concomitantly administering a cytochrome P450 2C8 substrate). Products include:
Vivactil Tablets 2350

Repaglinide (Montelukast is a potent inhibitor of P450 2C8, but no in vivo drug interaction studies have been conducted between montelukast and cytochrome P450 2C8 substrates. Caution should be exercised when concomitantly administering a cytochrome P450 2C8 substrate). Products include:
Prandin Tablets (0.5, 1, and 2 mg) 2337

Rifampin (Co-administration with CYP450 enzyme inducers, such as rifampin, may alter metabolism of montelukast; it is reasonable to employ appropriate clinical monitoring).
No products indexed under this heading.

Rosiglitazone Maleate (Montelukast is a potent inhibitor of P450 2C8, but no in vivo drug interaction studies have been conducted between montelukast and cytochrome P450 2C8 substrates. Caution should be exercised when concomitantly administering a cytochrome P450 2C8 substrate). Products include:
Avandamet Tablets 1343
Avandia Tablets 1348

Rosiglitazone/Metformin (Montelukast is a potent inhibitor of P450 2C8, but no in vivo drug interaction studies have been conducted between montelukast and cytochrome P450 2C8 substrates. Caution should be exercised when concomitantly administering a cytochrome P450 2C8 substrate).
No products indexed under this heading.

Tolbutamide (Montelukast is a potent inhibitor of P450 2C8, but no in vivo drug interaction studies have been conducted between montelukast and cytochrome P450 2C8 substrates. Caution should be exercised when concomitantly administering a cytochrome P450 2C8 substrate).
No products indexed under this heading.

Tolbutamide Sodium (Montelukast is a potent inhibitor of P450 2C8, but no in vivo drug interaction studies have been conducted between montelukast and cytochrome P450 2C8 substrates. Caution should be exercised when concomitantly administering a cytochrome P450 2C8 substrate).
No products indexed under this heading.

Tretinoin (Montelukast is a potent inhibitor of P450 2C8, but no in vivo drug interaction studies have been conducted between montelukast and cytochrome P450 2C8 substrates. Caution should be exercised when concomitantly administering a cytochrome P450 2C8 substrate). Products include:
Avita Cream 2136
Avita Gel 2138
Renova 0.02% Cream 2384
Renova 0.05% Cream 2387
Retin-A Micro 0.1%/0.04% 2388
Solage Topical Solution 740
Tri-Luma Cream 1213
Vesanoid Capsules 2823

Trimipramine Maleate (Montelukast is a potent inhibitor of P450 2C8, but no in vivo drug interaction studies have been conducted between montelukast and cytochrome P450 2C8 substrates. Caution should be exercised when concomitantly administering a cytochrome P450 2C8 substrate). Products include:
Surmontil Capsules 2347

Verapamil Hydrochloride (Montelukast is a potent inhibitor of P450 2C8, but no in vivo drug interaction studies have been conducted between montelukast and cytochrome P450 2C8 substrates. Caution should be exercised when concomitantly administering a cytochrome P450 2C8 substrate). Products include:
Covera-HS Tablets 3135
Tarka Tablets 519
Verelan PM Capsules 3120

Vitamin A (Montelukast is a potent inhibitor of P450 2C8, but no in vivo drug interaction studies have been conducted between montelukast and cytochrome P450 2C8 substrates. Caution should be exercised when concomitantly administering a cytochrome P450 2C8 substrate). Products include:
Visutein Capsules 3328

Vitamin A Acetate (Montelukast is a potent inhibitor of P450 2C8, but no in vivo drug interaction studies have been conducted between montelukast and cytochrome P450 2C8 substrates. Caution should be exercised when concomitantly administering a cytochrome P450 2C8 substrate).
No products indexed under this heading.

Warfarin Sodium (Montelukast is a potent inhibitor of P450 2C8, but no in vivo drug interaction studies have been conducted between montelukast and cytochrome P450 2C8 substrates. Caution should be exercised when concomitantly administering a cytochrome P450 2C8 substrate). Products include:
Coumadin for Injection 932
Coumadin Tablets 932

Zopiclone (Montelukast is a potent inhibitor of P450 2C8, but no in vivo drug interaction studies have been conducted between montelukast and cytochrome P450 2C8 substrates. Caution should be exercised when concomitantly administering a cytochrome P450 2C8 substrate).
No products indexed under this heading.

SINGULAIR CHEWABLE TABLETS

(Montelukast Sodium) 2047
See Singulair Tablets

SKELAXIN TABLETS

(Metaxalone) 1685
May interact with barbiturates, central nervous system depressants, and certain other agents. Compounds in these categories include:

Alfentanil Hydrochloride (Skelaxin may enhance the effects of alcohol, barbiturates and other CNS depressants).
No products indexed under this heading.

Alprazolam (Skelaxin may enhance the effects of alcohol, barbiturates and other CNS depressants). Products include:
Niravam Orally Disintegrating Tablets 3106
Xanax XR Tablets 2655

Aprobarbital (Skelaxin may enhance the effects of alcohol, barbiturates and other CNS depressants).
No products indexed under this heading.

Buprenorphine Hydrochloride (Skelaxin may enhance the effects of alcohol, barbiturates and other CNS depressants). Products include:
Buprenex Injectable 2718
Suboxone Tablets 2719
Subutex Tablets 2719

Buspirone Hydrochloride (Skelaxin may enhance the effects of alcohol, barbiturates and other CNS depressants).
No products indexed under this heading.

Butabarbital (Skelaxin may enhance the effects of alcohol, barbiturates and other CNS depressants).
No products indexed under this heading.

Butalbital (Skelaxin may enhance the effects of alcohol, barbiturates and other CNS depressants). Products include:
Sedapap Tablets 50 mg/650 mg 2098

Chlordiazepoxide (Skelaxin may enhance the effects of alcohol, barbiturates and other CNS depressants).
No products indexed under this heading.

Chlordiazepoxide Hydrochloride (Skelaxin may enhance the effects of alcohol, barbiturates and other CNS depressants). Products include:
Librium Capsules 3349

Chlorpromazine (Skelaxin may enhance the effects of alcohol, barbiturates and other CNS depressants).
No products indexed under this heading.

Chlorpromazine Hydrochloride (Skelaxin may enhance the effects of alcohol, barbiturates and other CNS depressants).
No products indexed under this heading.

Chlorprothixene (Skelaxin may enhance the effects of alcohol, barbiturates and other CNS depressants).
No products indexed under this heading.

Chlorprothixene Hydrochloride (Skelaxin may enhance the effects of alcohol, barbiturates and other CNS depressants).
No products indexed under this heading.

Chlorprothixene Lactate (Skelaxin may enhance the effects of alcohol, barbiturates and other CNS depressants).
No products indexed under this heading.

Clorazepate Dipotassium (Skelaxin may enhance the effects of alcohol, barbiturates and other CNS depressants). Products include:
Tranxene 2488

Clozapine (Skelaxin may enhance the effects of alcohol, barbiturates and other CNS depressants).
Products include:
Clozapine Tablets 2141
Clozaril Tablets 2174
FazaClo Orally Disintegrating Tablets 547

Codeine Phosphate (Skelaxin may enhance the effects of alcohol, barbiturates and other CNS depressants). Products include:
Tylenol with Codeine 2461

Desflurane (Skelaxin may enhance the effects of alcohol, barbiturates and other CNS depressants).
Products include:
Suprane Liquid for Inhalation 770

Dezocine (Skelaxin may enhance the effects of alcohol, barbiturates and other CNS depressants).
No products indexed under this heading.

Diazepam (Skelaxin may enhance the effects of alcohol, barbiturates and other CNS depressants).
Products include:
Diastat Rectal Delivery System 3344
Valium Tablets 2822

Droperidol (Skelaxin may enhance the effects of alcohol, barbiturates and other CNS depressants).
No products indexed under this heading.

Enflurane (Skelaxin may enhance the effects of alcohol, barbiturates and other CNS depressants).
No products indexed under this heading.

Estazolam (Skelaxin may enhance the effects of alcohol, barbiturates and other CNS depressants).
Products include:
ProSom Tablets 512

Ethanol (Skelaxin may enhance the effects of alcohol, barbiturates and other CNS depressants).
No products indexed under this heading.

Ethchlorvynol (Skelaxin may enhance the effects of alcohol, barbiturates and other CNS depressants).
No products indexed under this heading.

Ethinamate (Skelaxin may enhance the effects of alcohol, barbiturates and other CNS depressants).
No products indexed under this heading.

Ethyl Alcohol (Skelaxin may enhance the effects of alcohol, barbiturates and other CNS depressants).
No products indexed under this heading.

Fentanyl (Skelaxin may enhance the effects of alcohol, barbiturates and other CNS depressants). Products include:
Duragesic Transdermal System 2448

Fentanyl Citrate (Skelaxin may enhance the effects of alcohol, barbiturates and other CNS depressants). Products include:
Actiq 993

Fluphenazine Decanoate (Skelaxin may enhance the effects of alcohol, barbiturates and other CNS depressants).
No products indexed under this heading.

Fluphenazine Enanthate (Skelaxin may enhance the effects of alcohol, barbiturates and other CNS depressants).
No products indexed under this heading.

Fluphenazine Hydrochloride (Skelaxin may enhance the effects of alcohol, barbiturates and other CNS depressants).
No products indexed under this heading.

Flurazepam Hydrochloride (Skelaxin may enhance the effects of alcohol, barbiturates and other CNS depressants). Products include:
Dalmane Capsules 3343

Glutethimide (Skelaxin may enhance the effects of alcohol, barbiturates and other CNS depressants).
No products indexed under this heading.

Haloperidol (Skelaxin may enhance the effects of alcohol, barbiturates and other CNS depressants).
No products indexed under this heading.

Haloperidol Decanoate (Skelaxin may enhance the effects of alcohol, barbiturates and other CNS depressants).
No products indexed under this heading.

Hydrocodone Bitartrate (Skelaxin may enhance the effects of alcohol, barbiturates and other CNS depressants). Products include:
Hycodan 1104
Hycomine Compound Tablets 1105
Hycotuss Expectorant Syrup 1106
Lortab 3315
Lortab Elixir 3312
Vicodin Tablets 530
Vicodin ES Tablets 531
Vicodin HP Tablets 532
Vicoprofen Tablets 533
Zydone Tablets 1118

Hydrocodone Polistirex (Skelaxin may enhance the effects of alcohol, barbiturates and other CNS depressants). Products include:
Tussionex Pennkinetic Extended-Release Suspension 3322

Hydromorphone Hydrochloride (Skelaxin may enhance the effects of alcohol, barbiturates and other CNS depressants). Products include:
Dilaudid 439
Dilaudid Oral Liquid 443
Dilaudid Non-Sterile Powder 439
Dilaudid Rectal Suppositories 439
Dilaudid Tablets 439
Dilaudid Tablets - 8 mg 443
Dilaudid-HP 441

Hydroxyzine Hydrochloride (Skelaxin may enhance the effects of alcohol, barbiturates and other CNS depressants).
No products indexed under this heading.

Isoflurane (Skelaxin may enhance the effects of alcohol, barbiturates and other CNS depressants).
No products indexed under this heading.

Ketamine Hydrochloride (Skelaxin may enhance the effects of alcohol, barbiturates and other CNS depressants).
No products indexed under this heading.

Levomethadyl Acetate Hydrochloride (Skelaxin may enhance the effects of alcohol, barbiturates and other CNS depressants).
No products indexed under this heading.

Levorphanol Tartrate (Skelaxin may enhance the effects of alcohol, barbiturates and other CNS depressants).
No products indexed under this heading.

Lorazepam (Skelaxin may enhance the effects of alcohol, barbiturates and other CNS depressants).
No products indexed under this heading.

Loxapine Hydrochloride (Skelaxin may enhance the effects of alcohol, barbiturates and other CNS depressants).
No products indexed under this heading.

Loxapine Succinate (Skelaxin may enhance the effects of alcohol, barbiturates and other CNS depressants).
No products indexed under this heading.

Meperidine Hydrochloride (Skelaxin may enhance the effects of alcohol, barbiturates and other CNS depressants).
No products indexed under this heading.

Mephobarbital (Skelaxin may enhance the effects of alcohol, barbiturates and other CNS depressants). Products include:
Mebaral Tablets, USP 2483

Meprobamate (Skelaxin may enhance the effects of alcohol, barbiturates and other CNS depressants).
No products indexed under this heading.

Mesoridazine Besylate (Skelaxin may enhance the effects of alcohol, barbiturates and other CNS depressants).
No products indexed under this heading.

Methadone Hydrochloride (Skelaxin may enhance the effects of alcohol, barbiturates and other CNS depressants).
No products indexed under this heading.

Methohexital Sodium (Skelaxin may enhance the effects of alcohol, barbiturates and other CNS depressants).
No products indexed under this heading.

Methotrimeprazine (Skelaxin may enhance the effects of alcohol, barbiturates and other CNS depressants).
No products indexed under this heading.

Methoxyflurane (Skelaxin may enhance the effects of alcohol, barbiturates and other CNS depressants).
No products indexed under this heading.

Midazolam Hydrochloride (Skelaxin may enhance the effects of alcohol, barbiturates and other CNS depressants).
No products indexed under this heading.

Molindone Hydrochloride (Skelaxin may enhance the effects of alcohol, barbiturates and other CNS depressants). Products include:
Moban Tablets 1108

Morphine Sulfate (Skelaxin may enhance the effects of alcohol, barbiturates and other CNS depressants). Products include:
Avinza Capsules 1714
Kadian Capsules 572
MS Contin Tablets 2703

Olanzapine (Skelaxin may enhance the effects of alcohol, barbiturates and other CNS depressants).
Products include:
Symbyax Capsules 1788
Zyprexa Tablets 1798
Zyprexa IntraMuscular 1798
Zyprexa ZYDIS Orally Disintegrating Tablets 1798

Oxazepam (Skelaxin may enhance the effects of alcohol, barbiturates and other CNS depressants).
No products indexed under this heading.

Oxycodone Hydrochloride (Skelaxin may enhance the effects of alcohol, barbiturates and other CNS depressants). Products include:
Combunox Tablets 1183
OxyContin Tablets 2699
OxyFast Oral Concentrate Solution 2704
OxyIR Capsules 2704
Percocet Tablets 1114
Percodan Tablets 1115

Pentobarbital Sodium (Skelaxin may enhance the effects of alcohol, barbiturates and other CNS depressants). Products include:
Nembutal Sodium Solution, USP 2484

Perphenazine (Skelaxin may enhance the effects of alcohol, barbiturates and other CNS depressants).
No products indexed under this heading.

Phenobarbital (Skelaxin may enhance the effects of alcohol, barbiturates and other CNS depressants).
No products indexed under this heading.

Prazepam (Skelaxin may enhance the effects of alcohol, barbiturates and other CNS depressants).
No products indexed under this heading.

Prochlorperazine (Skelaxin may enhance the effects of alcohol, barbiturates and other CNS depressants).
No products indexed under this heading.

Promethazine Hydrochloride (Skelaxin may enhance the effects of alcohol, barbiturates and other CNS depressants). Products include:
Phenergan 3438

Propofol (Skelaxin may enhance the effects of alcohol, barbiturates and other CNS depressants). Products include:
Diprivan Injectable Emulsion 676

Propoxyphene Hydrochloride (Skelaxin may enhance the effects of alcohol, barbiturates and other CNS depressants).
No products indexed under this heading.

Propoxyphene Napsylate (Skelaxin may enhance the effects of alcohol, barbiturates and other CNS depressants). Products include:
Darvocet A 500 Tablets 3497

Quazepam (Skelaxin may enhance the effects of alcohol, barbiturates and other CNS depressants).
No products indexed under this heading.

Quetiapine Fumarate (Skelaxin may enhance the effects of alcohol, barbiturates and other CNS depressants). Products include:
Seroquel Tablets 691

Remifentanil Hydrochloride (Skelaxin may enhance the effects of alcohol, barbiturates and other CNS depressants).
No products indexed under this heading.

Risperidone (Skelaxin may enhance the effects of alcohol, barbiturates and other CNS depressants). Products include:
Risperdal Consta Long-Acting Injection 1664
Risperdal M-Tab Orally Disintegrating Tablets.................. 1658
Risperdal 1658

Secobarbital Sodium (Skelaxin may enhance the effects of alcohol, barbiturates and other CNS depressants).
No products indexed under this heading.

Sevoflurane (Skelaxin may enhance the effects of alcohol, barbiturates and other CNS depressants). Products include:
Ultane Liquid for Inhalation 526

Sodium Oxybate (Skelaxin may enhance the effects of alcohol, barbiturates and other CNS depressants).
No products indexed under this heading.

Sufentanil Citrate (Skelaxin may enhance the effects of alcohol, barbiturates and other CNS depressants).
No products indexed under this heading.

Temazepam (Skelaxin may enhance the effects of alcohol, barbiturates and other CNS depressants).
No products indexed under this heading.

Thiamylal Sodium (Skelaxin may enhance the effects of alcohol, barbiturates and other CNS depressants).
No products indexed under this heading.

Thioridazine Hydrochloride (Skelaxin may enhance the effects of alcohol, barbiturates and other CNS depressants). Products include:
Thioridazine Hydrochloride Tablets.. 2122

Thiothixene (Skelaxin may enhance the effects of alcohol, barbiturates and other CNS depressants). Products include:
Thiothixene Capsules 2124

Triazolam (Skelaxin may enhance the effects of alcohol, barbiturates and other CNS depressants).
No products indexed under this heading.

Trifluoperazine Hydrochloride (Skelaxin may enhance the effects of alcohol, barbiturates and other CNS depressants).
No products indexed under this heading.

Zaleplon (Skelaxin may enhance the effects of alcohol, barbiturates and other CNS depressants). Products include:
Sonata Capsules 1686

Ziprasidone Hydrochloride (Skelaxin may enhance the effects of alcohol, barbiturates and other CNS depressants). Products include:
Geodon Capsules 2514

Zolpidem Tartrate (Skelaxin may enhance the effects of alcohol, barbiturates and other CNS depressants). Products include:
Ambien Tablets 2867

Food Interactions

Alcohol (Skelaxin may enhance the effects of alcohol, barbiturates and other CNS depressants).

SLOW FE IRON TABLETS
(Ferrous Sulfate) .... ◘772
May interact with tetracyclines. Compounds in these categories include:

Demeclocycline Hydrochloride (Absorption of oral tetracycline impaired).
No products indexed under this heading.

Doxycycline Calcium (Absorption of oral tetracycline impaired).
No products indexed under this heading.

Doxycycline Hyclate (Absorption of oral tetracycline impaired).
No products indexed under this heading.

Doxycycline Monohydrate (Absorption of oral tetracycline impaired).
No products indexed under this heading.

Methacycline Hydrochloride (Absorption of oral tetracycline impaired).
No products indexed under this heading.

Minocycline Hydrochloride (Absorption of oral tetracycline impaired). Products include:
Dynacin Tablets 1859

Oxytetracycline (Absorption of oral tetracycline impaired).
No products indexed under this heading.

Oxytetracycline Hydrochloride (Absorption of oral tetracycline impaired).
No products indexed under this heading.

Tetracycline Hydrochloride (Absorption of oral tetracycline impaired).
No products indexed under this heading.

SLOW FE WITH FOLIC ACID TABLETS
(Ferrous Sulfate, Folic Acid) .... ◘773
May interact with tetracyclines. Compounds in these categories include:

Demeclocycline Hydrochloride (Oral iron products interfere with oral absorption of tetracycline; do not take within two hours of each other).
No products indexed under this heading.

Doxycycline Calcium (Oral iron products interfere with oral absorption of tetracycline; do not take within two hours of each other).
No products indexed under this heading.

Doxycycline Hyclate (Oral iron products interfere with oral absorption of tetracycline; do not take within two hours of each other).
No products indexed under this heading.

Doxycycline Monohydrate (Oral iron products interfere with oral absorption of tetracycline; do not take within two hours of each other).
No products indexed under this heading.

Methacycline Hydrochloride (Oral iron products interfere with oral absorption of tetracycline; do not take within two hours of each other).
No products indexed under this heading.

Minocycline Hydrochloride (Oral iron products interfere with oral absorption of tetracycline; do not take within two hours of each other). Products include:
Dynacin Tablets 1859

Oxytetracycline Hydrochloride (Oral iron products interfere with oral absorption of tetracycline; do not take within two hours of each other).
No products indexed under this heading.

Tetracycline Hydrochloride (Oral iron products interfere with oral absorption of tetracycline; do not take within two hours of each other).
No products indexed under this heading.

SLOW-MAG TABLETS
(Calcium, Magnesium Chloride) 2717
None cited in PDR database.

SMILE'S PRID SALVE
(Homeopathic Formulations) .... ◘735
None cited in PDR database.

SOLAGE TOPICAL SOLUTION
(Mequinol, Tretinoin) 740
May interact with fluoroquinolone antibiotics, phenothiazines, drugs known to be photosensitizers, sulfonamides, tetracyclines, thiazides, and certain other agents. Compounds in these categories include:

Acetazolamide (Solage should not be administered if the patient is also taking drugs known to be photosensitizers because of the possibility of augmented phototoxicity).
No products indexed under this heading.

Acitretin (Solage should not be administered if the patient is also taking drugs known to be photosensitizers because of the possibility of augmented phototoxicity). Products include:
Soriatane Capsules 1028

Alatrofloxacin Mesylate (Solage should not be administered if the patient is also taking drugs known to be photosensitizers (eg, fluoroquinolones) because of the possibility of augmented phototoxicity).
No products indexed under this heading.

Anthralin (Solage should not be administered if the patient is also taking drugs known to be photosensitizers because of the possibility of augmented phototoxicity). Products include:
Psoriatec Cream 3191

Bendroflumethiazide (Solage should not be administered if the patient is also taking drugs known to be photosensitizers (eg, thiazides) because of the possibility of augmented phototoxicity).
No products indexed under this heading.

Chlorothiazide (Solage should not be administered if the patient is also taking drugs known to be photosensitizers (eg, thiazides) because of the possibility of augmented phototoxicity). Products include:
Aldoclor Tablets 1881
Diuril Oral 1936

Chlorothiazide Sodium (Solage should not be administered if the patient is also taking drugs known to be photosensitizers (eg, thiazides) because of the possibility of augmented phototoxicity). Products include:
Diuril Sodium Intravenous 1934

Chlorpromazine (Solage should not be administered if the patient is also taking drugs known to be photosensitizers (eg, phenothiazines) because of the possibility of augmented phototoxicity).
No products indexed under this heading.

Chlorpromazine Hydrochloride (Solage should not be administered if the patient is also taking drugs known to be photosensitizers (eg, phenothiazines) because of the possibility of augmented phototoxicity).
No products indexed under this heading.

Chlorpropamide (Solage should not be administered if the patient is also taking drugs known to be photosensitizers (eg, sulfonamides) because of the possibility of augmented phototoxicity).
No products indexed under this heading.

Ciprofloxacin (Solage should not be administered if the patient is also taking drugs known to be photosensitizers (eg, fluoroquinolones) because of the possibility of augmented phototoxicity). Products include:
Cipro I.V. 2998
Cipro I.V. Pharmacy Bulk Package ... 3509
Cipro Oral Suspension 2991
Cipro XR Tablets 3004
Ciprodex Otic Suspension 555

Ciprofloxacin Hydrochloride (Solage should not be administered if the patient is also taking drugs known to be photosensitizers (eg, fluoroquinolones) because of the possibility of augmented phototoxicity). Products include:
Ciloxan Ophthalmic Ointment 554
Cipro Tablets 2991

Coal Tar (Solage should not be administered if the patient is also taking drugs known to be photosensitizers because of the possibility of augmented phototoxicity). Products include:
Tegrin Dandruff Shampoo - Extra Conditioning.................................. ◘637
Tegrin Dandruff Shampoo - Fresh Herbal... ◘638
Tegrin Skin Cream .... ◘638

Demeclocycline Hydrochloride (Solage should not be administered if the patient is also taking drugs known to be photosensitizers (eg, tetracyclines) because of the possibility of augmented phototoxicity).
No products indexed under this heading.

Doxycycline Calcium (Solage should not be administered if the patient is also taking drugs known to be photosensitizers (eg, tetracyclines) because of the possibility of augmented phototoxicity).
No products indexed under this heading.

Doxycycline Hyclate (Solage should not be administered if the patient is also taking drugs known to be photosensitizers (eg, tetracyclines) because of the possibility of augmented phototoxicity).
No products indexed under this heading.

Doxycycline Monohydrate (Solage should not be administered if the patient is also taking drugs known to be photosensitizers (eg, tetracyclines) because of the possibility of augmented phototoxicity).
No products indexed under this heading.

Enoxacin (Solage should not be administered if the patient is also taking drugs known to be photosensitizers (eg, fluoroquinolones) because of the possibility of augmented phototoxicity).
No products indexed under this heading.

Fluphenazine Decanoate (Solage should not be administered if the patient is also taking drugs known to be photosensitizers (eg, phenothiazines) because of the possibility of augmented phototoxicity).
No products indexed under this heading.

Fluphenazine Enanthate (Solage should not be administered if the patient is also taking drugs known to be photosensitizers (eg, phenothiazines) because of the possibility of augmented phototoxicity).
No products indexed under this heading.

Fluphenazine Hydrochloride (Solage should not be administered if the patient is also taking drugs known to be photosensitizers (eg, phenothiazines) because of the possibility of augmented phototoxicity).
No products indexed under this heading.

Furosemide (Solage should not be administered if the patient is also taking drugs known to be photosensitizers because of the possibility of augmented phototoxicity). Products include:
Furosemide Tablets **2117**

Glipizide (Solage should not be administered if the patient is also taking drugs known to be photosensitizers (eg, sulfonamides) because of the possibility of augmented phototoxicity).
No products indexed under this heading.

Glyburide (Solage should not be administered if the patient is also taking drugs known to be photosensitizers (eg, sulfonamides) because of the possibility of augmented phototoxicity).
No products indexed under this heading.

Grepafloxacin Hydrochloride (Solage should not be administered if the patient is also taking drugs known to be photosensitizers (eg, fluoroquinolones) because of the possibility of augmented phototoxicity).
No products indexed under this heading.

Griseofulvin (Solage should not be administered if the patient is also taking drugs known to be photosensitizers because of the possibility of augmented phototoxicity). Products include:
Grifulvin V Tablets Microsize and Oral Suspension Microsize **2384**
Gris-PEG Tablets **2504**

Hydrochlorothiazide (Solage should not be administered if the patient is also taking drugs known to be photosensitizers (eg, thiazides) because of the possibility of augmented phototoxicity). Products include:
Aldoril Tablets **1884**
Atacand HCT **637**
Avalide Tablets **2889**
Avalide Tablets **922**
Benicar HCT Tablets **2852**
Diovan HCT Tablets **2195**
Dyazide Capsules **1389**
Hyzaar **1964**
Lotensin HCT Tablets **2235**
Maxzide **2150**
Micardis HCT Tablets **886**
Moduretic Tablets **2003**
Prinzide Tablets **2033**
Teveten HCT Tablets **1710**
Timolide Tablets **2056**
Uniretic Tablets **3114**
Vaseretic Tablets **2073**
Zestoretic Tablets **701**

Hydroflumethiazide (Solage should not be administered if the patient is also taking drugs known to be photosensitizers (eg, thiazides) because of the possibility of augmented phototoxicity).
No products indexed under this heading.

Lomefloxacin Hydrochloride (Solage should not be administered if the patient is also taking drugs known to be photosensitizers (eg, fluoroquinolones) because of the possibility of augmented phototoxicity).
No products indexed under this heading.

Mesoridazine Besylate (Solage should not be administered if the patient is also taking drugs known to be photosensitizers (eg, phenothiazines) because of the possibility of augmented phototoxicity).
No products indexed under this heading.

Metabromsalan (Solage should not be administered if the patient is also taking drugs known to be photosensitizers because of the possibility of augmented phototoxicity).
No products indexed under this heading.

Methacycline Hydrochloride (Solage should not be administered if the patient is also taking drugs known to be photosensitizers (eg, tetracyclines) because of the possibility of augmented phototoxicity).
No products indexed under this heading.

Methotrimeprazine (Solage should not be administered if the patient is also taking drugs known to be photosensitizers (eg, phenothiazines) because of the possibility of augmented phototoxicity).
No products indexed under this heading.

Methyclothiazide (Solage should not be administered if the patient is also taking drugs known to be photosensitizers (eg, thiazides) because of the possibility of augmented phototoxicity).
No products indexed under this heading.

Minocycline Hydrochloride (Solage should not be administered if the patient is also taking drugs known to be photosensitizers (eg, tetracyclines) because of the possibility of augmented phototoxicity). Products include:
Dynacin Tablets **1859**

Moxifloxacin Hydrochloride (Solage should not be administered if the patient is also taking drugs known to be photosensitizers (eg, fluoroquinolones) because of the possibility of augmented phototoxicity). Products include:
Avelox **2984**
Vigamox Ophthalmic Solution **560**

Nalidixic Acid (Solage should not be administered if the patient is also taking drugs known to be photosensitizers because of the possibility of augmented phototoxicity).
No products indexed under this heading.

Norfloxacin (Solage should not be administered if the patient is also taking drugs known to be photosensitizers (eg, fluoroquinolones) because of the possibility of augmented phototoxicity). Products include:
Noroxin Tablets **2009**

Ofloxacin (Solage should not be administered if the patient is also taking drugs known to be photosensitizers (eg, fluoroquinolones) because of the possibility of augmented phototoxicity). Products include:
Floxin Otic Singles **1045**
Floxin Otic Solution **1043**

Oxytetracycline Hydrochloride (Solage should not be administered if the patient is also taking drugs known to be photosensitizers (eg, tetracyclines) because of the possibility of augmented phototoxicity).
No products indexed under this heading.

Perphenazine (Solage should not be administered if the patient is also taking drugs known to be photosensitizers (eg, phenothiazines) because of the possibility of augmented phototoxicity).
No products indexed under this heading.

Polythiazide (Solage should not be administered if the patient is also taking drugs known to be photosensitizers (eg, thiazides) because of the possibility of augmented phototoxicity).
No products indexed under this heading.

Prochlorperazine (Solage should not be administered if the patient is also taking drugs known to be photosensitizers (eg, phenothiazines) because of the possibility of augmented phototoxicity).
No products indexed under this heading.

Promethazine Hydrochloride (Solage should not be administered if the patient is also taking drugs known to be photosensitizers (eg, phenothiazines) because of the possibility of augmented phototoxicity). Products include:
Phenergan **3438**

Sulfacytine (Solage should not be administered if the patient is also taking drugs known to be photosensitizers (eg, sulfonamides) because of the possibility of augmented phototoxicity).
No products indexed under this heading.

Sulfamethizole (Solage should not be administered if the patient is also taking drugs known to be photosensitizers (eg, sulfonamides) because of the possibility of augmented phototoxicity).
No products indexed under this heading.

Sulfamethoxazole (Solage should not be administered if the patient is also taking drugs known to be photosensitizers (eg, sulfonamides) because of the possibility of augmented phototoxicity).
No products indexed under this heading.

Sulfasalazine (Solage should not be administered if the patient is also taking drugs known to be photosensitizers (eg, sulfonamides) because of the possibility of augmented phototoxicity).
No products indexed under this heading.

Sulfinpyrazone (Solage should not be administered if the patient is also taking drugs known to be photosensitizers (eg, sulfonamides) because of the possibility of augmented phototoxicity).
No products indexed under this heading.

Sulfisoxazole (Solage should not be administered if the patient is also taking drugs known to be photosensitizers (eg, sulfonamides) because of the possibility of augmented phototoxicity).
No products indexed under this heading.

Sulfisoxazole Acetyl (Solage should not be administered if the patient is also taking drugs known to be photosensitizers (eg, sulfonamides) because of the possibility of augmented phototoxicity).
No products indexed under this heading.

Sulfisoxazole Diolamine (Solage should not be administered if the patient is also taking drugs known to be photosensitizers (eg, sulfonamides) because of the possibility of augmented phototoxicity).
No products indexed under this heading.

Tetrachlorosalicylanilide (Solage should not be administered if the patient is also taking drugs known to be photosensitizers because of the possibility of augmented phototoxicity).
No products indexed under this heading.

Tetracycline Hydrochloride (Solage should not be administered if the patient is also taking drugs known to be photosensitizers (eg, tetracyclines) because of the possibility of augmented phototoxicity).
No products indexed under this heading.

Thioridazine Hydrochloride (Solage should not be administered if the patient is also taking drugs known to be photosensitizers (eg, phenothiazines) because of the possibility of augmented phototoxicity). Products include:
Thioridazine Hydrochloride Tablets **2122**

Tolazamide (Solage should not be administered if the patient is also taking drugs known to be photosensitizers (eg, sulfonamides) because of the possibility of augmented phototoxicity).
No products indexed under this heading.

Tolbutamide (Solage should not be administered if the patient is also taking drugs known to be photosensitizers (eg, sulfonamides) because of the possibility of augmented phototoxicity).
No products indexed under this heading.

Trifluoperazine Hydrochloride (Solage should not be administered if the patient is also taking drugs known to be photosensitizers (eg, phenothiazines) because of the possibility of augmented phototoxicity).
No products indexed under this heading.

Trovafloxacin Mesylate (Solage should not be administered if the patient is also taking drugs known to be photosensitizers (eg, fluoroquinolones) because of the possibility of augmented phototoxicity).
No products indexed under this heading.

Food Interactions

Alcohol (Concomitant topical products with a strong skin drying effect, such as products with high concentrations of alcohol, should be used with caution in patients being treated with Solage because they may increase irritation when used with Solage).

SOMAVERT INJECTION

(Pegvisomant) **2648**
May interact with oral hypoglycemic agents, insulin, and narcotic analgesics. Compounds in these categories include:

Acarbose (Growth hormone opposes the effects of insulin on carbohydrate metabolism by decreasing insulin sensitivity; therefore, glucose tolerance may increase in some patients treated with pegvisomant. Acromegalic patients with diabetes mellitus being treated with insulin and/or oral hypoglycemic agents may require dose reductions of these therapeutic agents after initiation of therapy with pegvisomant; monitor and reduce dose when necessary). Products include:
Precose Tablets **776**

Alfentanil Hydrochloride (In clinical studies, patients on opioids often needed higher serum pegvisomant concentrations to achieve appropriate IGF-I suppression compared with patients not receiving opioids).
No products indexed under this heading.

Buprenorphine Hydrochloride (In clinical studies, patients on opioids often needed higher serum pegvisomant concentrations to achieve appropriate IGF-I suppression compared with patients not receiving opioids). Products include:
Buprenex Injectable **2718**
Suboxone Tablets **2719**
Subutex Tablets **2719**

Chlorpropamide (Growth hormone opposes the effects of insulin on carbohydrate metabolism by decreasing insulin sensitivity; therefore, glucose tolerance may increase in some patients treated with pegvisomant. Acromegalic patients with diabetes mellitus being treated with insulin and/or oral hypoglycemic agents may require dose reductions of these therapeutic agents after initiation of therapy with pegvisomant; monitor and reduce dose when necessary).
No products indexed under this heading.

Codeine Phosphate (In clinical studies, patients on opioids often needed higher serum pegvisomant concentrations to achieve appropriate IGF-I suppression compared with patients not receiving opioids). Products include:
Tylenol with Codeine **2461**

Dezocine (In clinical studies, patients on opioids often needed higher serum pegvisomant concentrations to achieve appropriate IGF-I suppression compared with patients not receiving opioids).
No products indexed under this heading.

Fentanyl (In clinical studies, patients on opioids often needed higher serum pegvisomant concentrations to achieve appropriate IGF-I suppression compared with patients not receiving opioids). Products include:
Duragesic Transdermal System **2448**

Fentanyl Citrate (In clinical studies, patients on opioids often needed higher serum pegvisomant concentrations to achieve appropriate IGF-I suppression compared with patients not receiving opioids). Products include:
Actiq **993**

Glimepiride (Growth hormone opposes the effects of insulin on carbohydrate metabolism by decreasing insulin sensitivity; therefore, glucose tolerance may increase in some patients treated with pegvisomant. Acromegalic patients with diabetes mellitus being treated with insulin and/or oral hypoglycemic agents may require dose reductions of these therapeutic agents after initiation of therapy with pegvisomant; monitor and reduce dose when necessary). Products include:
Amaryl Tablets **2864**

Glipizide (Growth hormone opposes the effects of insulin on carbohydrate metabolism by decreasing insulin sensitivity; therefore, glucose tolerance may increase in some patients treated with pegvisomant. Acromegalic patients with diabetes mellitus being treated with insulin and/or oral hypoglycemic agents may require dose reductions of these therapeutic agents after initiation of therapy with pegvisomant; monitor and reduce dose when necessary).
No products indexed under this heading.

Glyburide (Growth hormone opposes the effects of insulin on carbohydrate metabolism by decreasing insulin sensitivity; therefore, glucose tolerance may increase in some patients treated with pegvisomant. Acromegalic patients with diabetes mellitus being treated with insulin and/or oral hypoglycemic agents may require dose reductions of these therapeutic agents after initiation of therapy with pegvisomant; monitor and reduce dose when necessary).
No products indexed under this heading.

Hydrocodone Bitartrate (In clinical studies, patients on opioids often needed higher serum pegvisomant concentrations to achieve appropriate IGF-I suppression compared with patients not receiving opioids). Products include:
Hycodan **1104**
Hycomine Compound Tablets **1105**
Hycotuss Expectorant Syrup **1106**
Lortab **3315**
Lortab Elixir **3312**
Vicodin Tablets **530**
Vicodin ES Tablets **531**
Vicodin HP Tablets **532**
Vicoprofen Tablets **533**
Zydone Tablets **1118**

Hydrocodone Polistirex (In clinical studies, patients on opioids often needed higher serum pegvisomant concentrations to achieve appropriate IGF-I suppression compared with patients not receiving opioids). Products include:
Tussionex Pennkinetic Extended-Release Suspension **3322**

Hydromorphone Hydrochloride (In clinical studies, patients on opioids often needed higher serum pegvisomant concentrations to achieve appropriate IGF-I suppression compared with patients not receiving opioids). Products include:
Dilaudid **439**
Dilaudid Oral Liquid **443**
Dilaudid Non-Sterile Powder **439**
Dilaudid Rectal Suppositories **439**
Dilaudid Tablets **439**
Dilaudid Tablets - 8 mg **443**
Dilaudid-HP **441**

Insulin, Human, Zinc Suspension (Growth hormone opposes the effects of insulin on carbohydrate metabolism by decreasing insulin sensitivity; therefore, glucose tolerance may increase in some patients treated with pegvisomant. Acromegalic patients with diabetes mellitus being treated with insulin and/or oral hypoglycemic agents may require dose reductions of these therapeutic agents after initiation of therapy with pegvisomant; monitor and reduce dose when necessary). Products include:
Humulin L, 100 Units **1763**
Humulin U, 100 Units **1770**

Insulin, Human NPH (Growth hormone opposes the effects of insulin on carbohydrate metabolism by decreasing insulin sensitivity; therefore, glucose tolerance may increase in some patients treated with pegvisomant. Acromegalic patients with diabetes mellitus being treated with insulin and/or oral hypoglycemic agents may require dose reductions of these therapeutic agents after initiation of therapy with pegvisomant; monitor and reduce dose when necessary). Products include:
Humulin N, 100 Units **1764**
Humulin N Pen **1765**
Novolin N Human Insulin 10 ml Vials **2322**
Novolin N InnoLet **2322**
Novolin N PenFill 3 ml Cartridges **2325**
Novolin R InnoLet **2322**

Insulin, Human Regular (Growth hormone opposes the effects of insulin on carbohydrate metabolism by decreasing insulin sensitivity; therefore, glucose tolerance may increase in some patients treated with pegvisomant. Acromegalic patients with diabetes mellitus being treated with insulin and/or oral hypoglycemic agents may require dose reductions of these therapeutic agents after initiation of therapy with pegvisomant; monitor and reduce dose when necessary). Products include:
Humulin R (U-500) **1768**
Humulin R, 100 Units **1767**
Novolin R Human Insulin 10 ml Vials **2322**
Novolin R PenFill **2325**

Insulin, Human Regular and Human NPH Mixture (Growth hormone opposes the effects of insulin on carbohydrate metabolism by decreasing insulin sensitivity; therefore, glucose tolerance may increase in some patients treated with pegvisomant. Acromegalic patients with diabetes mellitus being treated with insulin and/or oral hypoglycemic agents may require dose reductions of these therapeutic agents after initiation of therapy with pegvisomant; monitor and reduce dose when necessary). Products include:
Humulin 50/50, 100 Units **1760**
Humulin 70/30 Pen **1761**
Novolin 70/30 Human Insulin 10 ml Vials **2321**
Novolin 70/30 InnoLet **2322**
Novolin 70/30 PenFill 3 ml Cartridges **2325**

Insulin, NPH (Growth hormone opposes the effects of insulin on carbohydrate metabolism by decreasing insulin sensitivity; therefore, glucose tolerance may increase in some patients treated with pegvisomant. Acromegalic patients with diabetes mellitus being treated with insulin and/or oral hypoglycemic agents may require dose reductions of these therapeutic agents after initiation of therapy with pegvisomant; monitor and reduce dose when necessary).
No products indexed under this heading.

Insulin, Regular (Growth hormone opposes the effects of insulin on carbohydrate metabolism by decreasing insulin sensitivity; therefore, glucose tolerance may increase in some patients treated with pegvisomant. Acromegalic patients with diabetes mellitus being treated with insulin and/or oral hypoglycemic agents may require dose reductions of these therapeutic agents after initiation of therapy with

pegvisomant; monitor and reduce dose when necessary).
No products indexed under this heading.

Insulin, Zinc Crystals (Growth hormone opposes the effects of insulin on carbohydrate metabolism by decreasing insulin sensitivity; therefore, glucose tolerance may increase in some patients treated with pegvisomant. Acromegalic patients with diabetes mellitus being treated with insulin and/or oral hypoglycemic agents may require dose reductions of these therapeutic agents after initiation of therapy with pegvisomant; monitor and reduce dose when necessary).
No products indexed under this heading.

Insulin, Zinc Suspension (Growth hormone opposes the effects of insulin on carbohydrate metabolism by decreasing insulin sensitivity; therefore, glucose tolerance may increase in some patients treated with pegvisomant. Acromegalic patients with diabetes mellitus being treated with insulin and/or oral hypoglycemic agents may require dose reductions of these therapeutic agents after initiation of therapy with pegvisomant; monitor and reduce dose when necessary).
No products indexed under this heading.

Insulin Aspart, Human Regular (Growth hormone opposes the effects of insulin on carbohydrate metabolism by decreasing insulin sensitivity; therefore, glucose tolerance may increase in some patients treated with pegvisomant. Acromegalic patients with diabetes mellitus being treated with insulin and/or oral hypoglycemic agents may require dose reductions of these therapeutic agents after initiation of therapy with pegvisomant; monitor and reduce dose when necessary). Products include:
NovoLog Injection 2326

Insulin glargine (Growth hormone opposes the effects of insulin on carbohydrate metabolism by decreasing insulin sensitivity; therefore, glucose tolerance may increase in some patients treated with pegvisomant. Acromegalic patients with diabetes mellitus being treated with insulin and/or oral hypoglycemic agents may require dose reductions of these therapeutic agents after initiation of therapy with pegvisomant; monitor and reduce dose when necessary). Products include:
Lantus Injection 2925

Insulin Lispro, Human (Growth hormone opposes the effects of insulin on carbohydrate metabolism by decreasing insulin sensitivity; therefore, glucose tolerance may increase in some patients treated with pegvisomant. Acromegalic patients with diabetes mellitus being treated with insulin and/or oral hypoglycemic agents may require dose reductions of these therapeutic agents after initiation of therapy with pegvisomant; monitor and reduce dose when necessary). Products include:
Humalog-Pen 1751
Humalog Mix 75/25-Pen 1754

Insulin Lispro Protamine, Human (Growth hormone opposes the effects of insulin on carbohydrate metabolism by decreasing insulin sensitivity; therefore, glucose tolerance may increase in some patients treated with pegvisomant. Acromegalic patients with diabetes mellitus being treated with insulin and/or oral hypoglycemic agents may require dose reductions of these therapeutic agents after initiation of therapy with pegvisomant; monitor and reduce dose when necessary). Products include:
Humalog Mix 75/25-Pen 1754

Levorphanol Tartrate (In clinical studies, patients on opioids often needed higher serum pegvisomant concentrations to achieve appropriate IGF-I suppression compared with patients not receiving opioids).
No products indexed under this heading.

Meperidine Hydrochloride (In clinical studies, patients on opioids often needed higher serum pegvisomant concentrations to achieve appropriate IGF-I suppression compared with patients not receiving opioids).
No products indexed under this heading.

Metformin Hydrochloride (Growth hormone opposes the effects of insulin on carbohydrate metabolism by decreasing insulin sensitivity; therefore, glucose tolerance may increase in some patients treated with pegvisomant. Acromegalic patients with diabetes mellitus being treated with insulin and/or oral hypoglycemic agents may require dose reductions of these therapeutic agents after initiation of therapy with pegvisomant; monitor and reduce dose when necessary). Products include:
ActoPlus Met Tablets 3219
Avandamet Tablets 1343
Fortamet Extended-Release Tablets 1156

Methadone Hydrochloride (In clinical studies, patients on opioids often needed higher serum pegvisomant concentrations to achieve appropriate IGF-I suppression compared with patients not receiving opioids).
No products indexed under this heading.

Miglitol (Growth hormone opposes the effects of insulin on carbohydrate metabolism by decreasing insulin sensitivity; therefore, glucose tolerance may increase in some patients treated with pegvisomant. Acromegalic patients with diabetes mellitus being treated with insulin and/or oral hypoglycemic agents may require dose reductions of these therapeutic agents after initiation of therapy with pegvisomant; monitor and reduce dose when necessary).
No products indexed under this heading.

Morphine Sulfate (In clinical studies, patients on opioids often needed higher serum pegvisomant concentrations to achieve appropriate IGF-I suppression compared with patients not receiving opioids). Products include:
Avinza Capsules 1714
Kadian Capsules 572
MS Contin Tablets 2703

Oxycodone Hydrochloride (In clinical studies, patients on opioids often needed higher serum pegvisomant concentrations to achieve appropriate IGF-I suppression compared with patients not receiving opioids). Products include:
Combunox Tablets 1183
OxyContin Tablets 2699
OxyFast Oral Concentrate Solution 2704
OxyIR Capsules 2704
Percocet Tablets 1114
Percodan Tablets 1115

Pioglitazone Hydrochloride (Growth hormone opposes the effects of insulin on carbohydrate metabolism by decreasing insulin sensitivity; therefore, glucose tolerance may increase in some patients treated with pegvisomant. Acromegalic patients with diabetes mellitus being treated with insulin and/or oral hypoglycemic agents may require dose reductions of these therapeutic agents after initiation of therapy with pegvisomant; monitor and reduce dose when necessary). Products include:
ActoPlus Met Tablets 3219
Actos Tablets 3224

Propoxyphene Hydrochloride (In clinical studies, patients on opioids often needed higher serum pegvisomant concentrations to achieve appropriate IGF-I suppression compared with patients not receiving opioids).
No products indexed under this heading.

Propoxyphene Napsylate (In clinical studies, patients on opioids often needed higher serum pegvisomant concentrations to achieve appropriate IGF-I suppression compared with patients not receiving opioids). Products include:
Darvocet A 500 Tablets 3497

Remifentanil Hydrochloride (In clinical studies, patients on opioids often needed higher serum pegvisomant concentrations to achieve appropriate IGF-I suppression compared with patients not receiving opioids).
No products indexed under this heading.

Repaglinide (Growth hormone opposes the effects of insulin on carbohydrate metabolism by decreasing insulin sensitivity; therefore, glucose tolerance may increase in some patients treated with pegvisomant. Acromegalic patients with diabetes mellitus being treated with insulin and/or oral hypoglycemic agents may require dose reductions of these therapeutic agents after initiation of therapy with pegvisomant; monitor and reduce dose when necessary). Products include:
Prandin Tablets (0.5, 1, and 2 mg) 2337

Rosiglitazone Maleate (Growth hormone opposes the effects of insulin on carbohydrate metabolism by decreasing insulin sensitivity; therefore, glucose tolerance may increase in some patients treated with pegvisomant. Acromegalic patients with diabetes mellitus being treated with insulin and/or oral hypoglycemic agents may require dose reductions of these therapeutic agents after initiation of therapy with pegvisomant; monitor and reduce dose when necessary). Products include:
Avandamet Tablets 1343
Avandia Tablets 1348

Sufentanil Citrate (In clinical studies, patients on opioids often needed higher serum pegvisomant concentrations to achieve appropriate IGF-I suppression compared with patients not receiving opioids).
No products indexed under this heading.

Tolazamide (Growth hormone opposes the effects of insulin on carbohydrate metabolism by decreasing insulin sensitivity; therefore, glucose tolerance may increase in some patients treated with pegvisomant. Acromegalic patients with diabetes mellitus being treated with insulin and/or oral hypoglycemic agents may require dose reductions of these therapeutic agents after initiation of therapy with pegvisomant; monitor and reduce dose when necessary).
No products indexed under this heading.

Tolbutamide (Growth hormone opposes the effects of insulin on carbohydrate metabolism by decreasing insulin sensitivity; therefore, glucose tolerance may increase in some patients treated with pegvisomant. Acromegalic patients with diabetes mellitus being treated with insulin and/or oral hypoglycemic agents may require dose reductions of these therapeutic agents after initiation of therapy with pegvisomant; monitor and reduce dose when necessary).
No products indexed under this heading.

Troglitazone (Growth hormone opposes the effects of insulin on carbohydrate metabolism by decreasing insulin sensitivity; therefore, glucose tolerance may increase in some patients treated with pegvisomant. Acromegalic patients with diabetes mellitus being treated with insulin and/or oral hypoglycemic agents may require dose reductions of these therapeutic agents after initiation of therapy with pegvisomant; monitor and reduce dose when necessary).
No products indexed under this heading.

SOMINEX ORIGINAL FORMULA TABLETS

(Diphenhydramine Hydrochloride) ..... ▣637
May interact with hypnotics and sedatives, tranquilizers, and certain other agents. Compounds in these categories include:

Alprazolam (Concurrent use with tranquilizers is not recommended unless directed by a physician). Products include:
Niravam Orally Disintegrating Tablets 3106
Xanax XR Tablets 2655

Buspirone Hydrochloride (Concurrent use with tranquilizers is not recommended unless directed by a physician).
No products indexed under this heading.

Chlordiazepoxide (Concurrent use with tranquilizers is not recommended unless directed by a physician).
No products indexed under this heading.

Chlordiazepoxide Hydrochloride (Concurrent use with tranquilizers is not recommended unless directed by a physician). Products include:

Librium Capsules 3349

Chlorpromazine (Concurrent use with tranquilizers is not recommended unless directed by a physician).
No products indexed under this heading.

Chlorpromazine Hydrochloride (Concurrent use with tranquilizers is not recommended unless directed by a physician).
No products indexed under this heading.

Chlorprothixene (Concurrent use with tranquilizers is not recommended unless directed by a physician).
No products indexed under this heading.

Chlorprothixene Hydrochloride (Concurrent use with tranquilizers is not recommended unless directed by a physician).
No products indexed under this heading.

Clorazepate Dipotassium (Concurrent use with tranquilizers is not recommended unless directed by a physician). Products include:
Tranxene 2488

Diazepam (Concurrent use with tranquilizers is not recommended unless directed by a physician). Products include:
Diastat Rectal Delivery System 3344
Valium Tablets 2822

Droperidol (Concurrent use with tranquilizers is not recommended unless directed by a physician).
No products indexed under this heading.

Estazolam (Concurrent use with sedatives is not recommended unless directed by a physician). Products include:
ProSom Tablets 512

Ethchlorvynol (Concurrent use with sedatives is not recommended unless directed by a physician).
No products indexed under this heading.

Ethinamate (Concurrent use with sedatives is not recommended unless directed by a physician).
No products indexed under this heading.

Fluphenazine Decanoate (Concurrent use with tranquilizers is not recommended unless directed by a physician).
No products indexed under this heading.

Fluphenazine Enanthate (Concurrent use with tranquilizers is not recommended unless directed by a physician).
No products indexed under this heading.

Fluphenazine Hydrochloride (Concurrent use with tranquilizers is not recommended unless directed by a physician).
No products indexed under this heading.

Flurazepam Hydrochloride (Concurrent use with sedatives is not recommended unless directed by a physician). Products include:
Dalmane Capsules 3343

Glutethimide (Concurrent use with sedatives is not recommended unless directed by a physician).
No products indexed under this heading.

Haloperidol (Concurrent use with tranquilizers is not recommended unless directed by a physician).
No products indexed under this heading.

Haloperidol Decanoate (Concurrent use with tranquilizers is not recommended unless directed by a physician).
No products indexed under this heading.

Hydroxyzine Hydrochloride (Concurrent use with tranquilizers is not recommended unless directed by a physician).
No products indexed under this heading.

Lorazepam (Concurrent use with tranquilizers is not recommended unless directed by a physician).
No products indexed under this heading.

Loxapine Hydrochloride (Concurrent use with tranquilizers is not recommended unless directed by a physician).
No products indexed under this heading.

Loxapine Succinate (Concurrent use with tranquilizers is not recommended unless directed by a physician).
No products indexed under this heading.

Meprobamate (Concurrent use with tranquilizers is not recommended unless directed by a physician).
No products indexed under this heading.

Mesoridazine Besylate (Concurrent use with tranquilizers is not recommended unless directed by a physician).
No products indexed under this heading.

Midazolam Hydrochloride (Concurrent use with sedatives is not recommended unless directed by a physician).
No products indexed under this heading.

Molindone Hydrochloride (Concurrent use with tranquilizers is not recommended unless directed by a physician). Products include:
Moban Tablets 1108

Oxazepam (Concurrent use with tranquilizers is not recommended unless directed by a physician).
No products indexed under this heading.

Perphenazine (Concurrent use with tranquilizers is not recommended unless directed by a physician).
No products indexed under this heading.

Prazepam (Concurrent use with tranquilizers is not recommended unless directed by a physician).
No products indexed under this heading.

Prochlorperazine (Concurrent use with tranquilizers is not recommended unless directed by a physician).
No products indexed under this heading.

Promethazine Hydrochloride (Concurrent use with tranquilizers is not recommended unless directed by a physician). Products include:
Phenergan 3438

Propofol (Concurrent use with sedatives is not recommended unless directed by a physician). Products include:
Diprivan Injectable Emulsion 676

Quazepam (Concurrent use with sedatives is not recommended unless directed by a physician).
No products indexed under this heading.

Secobarbital Sodium (Concurrent use with sedatives is not recommended unless directed by a physician).
No products indexed under this heading.

Temazepam (Concurrent use with sedatives is not recommended unless directed by a physician).
No products indexed under this heading.

Thioridazine Hydrochloride (Concurrent use with tranquilizers is not recommended unless directed by a physician). Products include:
Thioridazine Hydrochloride Tablets 2122

Thiothixene (Concurrent use with tranquilizers is not recommended unless directed by a physician). Products include:
Thiothixene Capsules 2124

Triazolam (Concurrent use with sedatives is not recommended unless directed by a physician).
No products indexed under this heading.

Trifluoperazine Hydrochloride (Concurrent use with tranquilizers is not recommended unless directed by a physician).
No products indexed under this heading.

Zaleplon (Concurrent use with sedatives is not recommended unless directed by a physician). Products include:
Sonata Capsules 1686

Zolpidem Tartrate (Concurrent use with sedatives is not recommended unless directed by a physician). Products include:
Ambien Tablets 2867

Food Interactions

Alcohol (Concurrent use of alcoholic beverages is not recommended).

SON FORMULA TABLETS

(Amino Acid Preparations) 1651
None cited in PDR database.

SONATA CAPSULES

(Zaleplon) 1686
May interact with antihistamines, central nervous system depressants, cytochrome p450 3a4 inducers (selected), cytochrome p450 3a4 inhibitors (selected), anticonvulsants, erythromycin, phenytoin, psychotropics, and certain other agents. Compounds in these categories include:

Acetazolamide (CYP3A4 inhibitors may decrease zaleplon's clearance, possibly increasing its concentration).
No products indexed under this heading.

Acrivastine (Concurrent use may produce additive CNS depressant effects).
No products indexed under this heading.

Alfentanil Hydrochloride (Concurrent use may produce additive CNS depressant effects).
No products indexed under this heading.

Allium sativum (CYP3A4 inhibitors may increase zaleplon's clearance, possibly decreasing its concentration).
No products indexed under this heading.

Alprazolam (Concurrent use may produce additive CNS depressant effects). Products include:
Niravam Orally Disintegrating Tablets 3106
Xanax XR Tablets 2655

Amiodarone Hydrochloride (CYP3A4 inhibitors may decrease zaleplon's clearance, possibly increasing its concentration). Products include:
Pacerone Tablets 3337

Amitriptyline Hydrochloride (Concurrent use may produce additive CNS depressant effects).
No products indexed under this heading.

Amoxapine (Concurrent use may produce additive CNS depressant effects).
No products indexed under this heading.

Amprenavir (CYP3A4 inhibitors may decrease zaleplon's clearance, possibly increasing its concentration). Products include:
Agenerase Capsules 1299
Agenerase Oral Solution 1304

Anastrozole (CYP3A4 inhibitors may decrease zaleplon's clearance, possibly increasing its concentration). Products include:
Arimidex Tablets 665

Aprepitant (CYP3A4 inhibitors may decrease zaleplon's clearance, possibly increasing its concentration). Products include:
Emend Capsules 1944

Aprobarbital (Concurrent use may produce additive CNS depressant effects).
No products indexed under this heading.

Astemizole (Concurrent use may produce additive CNS depressant effects).
No products indexed under this heading.

Azatadine Maleate (Concurrent use may produce additive CNS depressant effects).
No products indexed under this heading.

Betamethasone Acetate (CYP3A4 inhibitors may increase zaleplon's clearance, possibly decreasing its concentration).
No products indexed under this heading.

Betamethasone Sodium Phosphate (CYP3A4 inhibitors may increase zaleplon's clearance, possibly decreasing its concentration).
No products indexed under this heading.

Bromodiphenhydramine Hydrochloride (Concurrent use may produce additive CNS depressant effects).
No products indexed under this heading.

Brompheniramine Maleate (Concurrent use may produce additive CNS depressant effects). Products include:

Alacol DM Syrup 739
Children's Dimetapp Cold & Allergy Elixir 745
Children's Dimetapp DM Cold & Cough Elixir 745
Robitussin Allergy & Cough Syrup .. 750

Buprenorphine Hydrochloride (Concurrent use may produce additive CNS depressant effects). Products include:
Buprenex Injectable 2718
Suboxone Tablets 2719
Subutex Tablets 2719

Buspirone Hydrochloride (Concurrent use may produce additive CNS depressant effects).
No products indexed under this heading.

Butabarbital (Concurrent use may produce additive CNS depressant effects).
No products indexed under this heading.

Butalbital (Concurrent use may produce additive CNS depressant effects). Products include:
Sedapap Tablets 50 mg/650 mg 2098

Carbamazepine (CYP3A4 is ordinarily a minor metabolizing enzyme of zaleplon, the co-administration of a potent inducer, such as carbamazepine, although not posing a safety concern, could lead to ineffectiveness of zaleplon; concurrent use with anticonvulsants may produce additive CNS depressant effects). Products include:
Carbatrol Capsules 3174
Equetro Extended-Release Capsules 3178
Tegretol/Tegretol-XR 2278

Cetirizine Hydrochloride (Concurrent use may produce additive CNS depressant effects). Products include:
Zyrtec Chewable Tablets 2589
Zyrtec 2589
Zyrtec-D 12 Hour Extended Release Tablets 2591

Chlordiazepoxide (Concurrent use may produce additive CNS depressant effects).
No products indexed under this heading.

Chlordiazepoxide Hydrochloride (Concurrent use may produce additive CNS depressant effects). Products include:
Librium Capsules 3349

Chlorpheniramine Maleate (Concurrent use may produce additive CNS depressant effects). Products include:
Advil Allergy Sinus Caplets 737
Advil Multi-Symptom Cold Caplets 738
BC Allergy Sinus Cold Powder 612
Contac Severe Cold and Flu Caplets Maximum Strength 615
Hycomine Compound Tablets 1105
PediaCare Multi-Symptom Cold Liquid 704
PediaCare NightRest Cough & Cold Liquid 704
Robitussin Flu Liquid 752
Robitussin PM Cough & Cold Liquid 752
Singlet Caplets 636
Sudafed Sinus & Allergy Tablets 710
TheraFlu Cold & Cough Hot Liquid 680
TheraFlu Cold & Sore Throat Hot Liquid 680
TheraFlu Flu & Sore Throat Hot Liquid 681
TheraFlu Severe Cold & Cough Hot Liquid 683
TheraFlu Severe Cold Caplets 679
TheraFlu Severe Cold Hot Liquid 682
Triaminic Cold & Allergy Liquid 685
Triaminic Cold & Cough Liquid 685
Triaminic Flu, Cough & Fever Liquid 685
Triaminic Night Time Cough & Cold Liquid 685
Triaminic Allergy Runny Nose & Congestion Softchews 688
Triaminic Cold & Cough Softchews 688
Children's Tylenol Plus Cold NightTime Suspension Liquid 1851
Children's Tylenol Plus Cold & Cough Suspension Liquid and Chewable Tablets 1851
Children's Tylenol Plus Cold Chewable Tablets 1851
Children's Tylenol Plus Flu Suspension Liquid 1853
Tylenol Allergy Complete Multi-Symptom Caplets and Gelcaps with Cool Burst 1844
Multi-Symptom Tylenol Cold Night Time Caplets 1845
Vicks 44M Cough, Cold & Flu Relief 2676
Pediatric Vicks 44m Cough & Cold Relief 2673
Children's Vicks NyQuil Cold/Cough Relief 2671

Chlorpheniramine Polistirex (Concurrent use may produce additive CNS depressant effects). Products include:
Tussionex Pennkinetic Extended-Release Suspension 3322

Chlorpheniramine Tannate (Concurrent use may produce additive CNS depressant effects).
No products indexed under this heading.

Chlorpromazine (Concurrent use may produce additive CNS depressant effects).
No products indexed under this heading.

Chlorpromazine Hydrochloride (Concurrent use may produce additive CNS depressant effects).
No products indexed under this heading.

Chlorprothixene (Concurrent use may produce additive CNS depressant effects).
No products indexed under this heading.

Chlorprothixene Hydrochloride (Concurrent use may produce additive CNS depressant effects).
No products indexed under this heading.

Chlorprothixene Lactate (Concurrent use may produce additive CNS depressant effects).
No products indexed under this heading.

Cimetidine (Co-administration has produced an 85% increase in the mean Cmax and AUC of zaleplon; an initial dose of 5 mg should be given to patients who are concomitantly being treated with cimetidine). Products include:
Tagamet HB 200 Tablets 637
Tagamet Tablets 1547

Cimetidine Hydrochloride (Co-administration has produced an 85% increase in the mean Cmax and AUC of zaleplon; an initial dose of 5 mg should be given to patients who are concomitantly being treated with cimetidine).
No products indexed under this heading.

Ciprofloxacin (CYP3A4 inhibitors may decrease zaleplon's clearance, possibly increasing its concentration). Products include:
Cipro I.V. 2998
Cipro I.V. Pharmacy Bulk Package 3509
Cipro Oral Suspension 2991
Cipro XR Tablets 3004
Ciprodex Otic Suspension 555

Ciprofloxacin Hydrochloride (CYP3A4 inhibitors may increase zaleplon's clearance, possibly decreasing its concentration). Products include:
Ciloxan Ophthalmic Ointment 554
Cipro Tablets 2991

Cisplatin (CYP3A4 inhibitors may increase zaleplon's clearance, possibly decreasing its concentration).
No products indexed under this heading.

Clarithromycin (CYP3A4 inhibitors may decrease zaleplon's clearance, possibly increasing its concentration). Products include:
Biaxin/Biaxin XL 402
PREVPAC 3281

Clemastine Fumarate (Concurrent use may produce additive CNS depressant effects).
No products indexed under this heading.

Clorazepate Dipotassium (Concurrent use may produce additive CNS depressant effects). Products include:
Tranxene 2488

Clotrimazole (CYP3A4 inhibitors may decrease zaleplon's clearance, possibly increasing its concentration). Products include:
Lotrimin 3053
Lotrisone 3054

Clozapine (Concurrent use may produce additive CNS depressant effects). Products include:
Clozapine Tablets 2141
Clozaril Tablets 2174
FazaClo Orally Disintegrating Tablets 547

Codeine Phosphate (Concurrent use may produce additive CNS depressant effects). Products include:
Tylenol with Codeine 2461

Cortisone Acetate (CYP3A4 inhibitors may increase zaleplon's clearance, possibly decreasing its concentration).
No products indexed under this heading.

Cyclosporine (CYP3A4 inhibitors may decrease zaleplon's clearance, possibly increasing its concentration). Products include:
Gengraf Capsules 458
Neoral Soft Gelatin Capsules 2247
Neoral Oral Solution 2247
Restasis Ophthalmic Emulsion 570
Sandimmune 2259

Cyproheptadine Hydrochloride (Concurrent use may produce additive CNS depressant effects).
No products indexed under this heading.

Dalfopristin (CYP3A4 inhibitors may decrease zaleplon's clearance, possibly increasing its concentration). Products include:
Synercid I.V. 1690

Danazol (CYP3A4 inhibitors may decrease zaleplon's clearance, possibly increasing its concentration).
No products indexed under this heading.

Delavirdine Mesylate (CYP3A4 inhibitors may decrease zaleplon's clearance, possibly increasing its concentration). Products include:
Rescriptor Tablets 2535

Desflurane (Concurrent use may produce additive CNS depressant effects). Products include:
Suprane Liquid for Inhalation 770

Desipramine Hydrochloride (Concurrent use may produce additive CNS depressant effects).
No products indexed under this heading.

Dexamethasone (CYP3A4 inhibitors may increase zaleplon's clearance, possibly decreasing its concentration). Products include:
Ciprodex Otic Suspension 555
Decadron Tablets 1929
TobraDex Ophthalmic Ointment 558
TobraDex Ophthalmic Suspension 558

Dexamethasone Acetate (CYP3A4 inhibitors may increase zaleplon's clearance, possibly decreasing its concentration).
No products indexed under this heading.

Dexamethasone Sodium Phosphate (CYP3A4 inhibitors may increase zaleplon's clearance, possibly decreasing its concentration). Products include:
Decadron Phosphate Injection 1931

Dexchlorpheniramine Maleate (Concurrent use may produce additive CNS depressant effects).
No products indexed under this heading.

Dezocine (Concurrent use may produce additive CNS depressant effects).
No products indexed under this heading.

Diazepam (Concurrent use may produce additive CNS depressant effects). Products include:
Diastat Rectal Delivery System 3344
Valium Tablets 2822

Diltiazem Hydrochloride (CYP3A4 inhibitors may decrease zaleplon's clearance, possibly increasing its concentration). Products include:
Cardizem LA Extended Release Tablets 1699
Tiazac Capsules 1204

Diltiazem Maleate (CYP3A4 inhibitors may decrease zaleplon's clearance, possibly increasing its concentration).
No products indexed under this heading.

Diphenhydramine Citrate (Concurrent use may produce additive CNS depressant effects). Products include:
Children's Benadryl Allergy & Cold Fastmelt Tablets 695
Children's Benadryl D Allergy & Sinus Fastmelt Tablets 694
Children's Benadryl Allergy Fastmelt Tablets 696
Goody's PM Powder 622

Diphenhydramine Hydrochloride (Concurrent use may produce additive CNS depressant effects). Products include:
Benadryl Allergy & Cold Tablets 692
Benadryl Allergy 691
Benadryl Allergy & Sinus Headache Caplets & Gelcaps 693
Children's Benadryl Allergy Liquid 695
Children's Benadryl Dye-Free Allergy Liquid 695
Benadryl Dye-Free Allergy Liqui-Gels Softgels 692
Benadryl Itch Relief Stick Extra Strength 696
Benadryl Itch Stopping Cream Extra Strength 697
Benadryl Itch Stopping Gel Extra Strength 697
Benadryl Itch Stopping Spray Extra Strength 697
Benadryl Maximum Strength Severe Allergy & Sinus Headache Caplets 694

Children's Benadryl D Liquid Medication .... ▣693
Benadryl D Tablets .... ▣694
Nytol QuickCaps Caplets .... ▣635
Maximum Strength Nytol QuickGels Softgels .... ▣635
Simply Sleep Caplets 1841
Sominex Original Formula Tablets .. ▣637
TheraFlu Thin Strips Multi Symptom .... ▣684
Triaminic Thin Strips Cough & Runny Nose .... ▣690
Children's Tylenol Plus Cold & Allergy Suspension Liquid 1850
Tylenol Allergy Complete Night Time Caplets 1844
Tylenol Severe Allergy Caplets 1844
Tylenol Flu NightTime Gelcaps 1846
Extra Strength Tylenol PM Caplets, Geltabs, Gelcaps and Liquid 1847
Unisom Maximum Strength SleepGels .... ▣712

Diphenylpyraline Hydrochloride (Concurrent use may produce additive CNS depressant effects).
No products indexed under this heading.

Divalproex Sodium (Concurrent use with anticonvulsants may produce additive CNS depressant effects). Products include:
Depakote Sprinkle Capsules 422
Depakote Tablets 427
Depakote ER Tablets 433

Doxepin Hydrochloride (Concurrent use may produce additive CNS depressant effects).
No products indexed under this heading.

Doxorubicin Hydrochloride (CYP3A4 inhibitors may increase zaleplon's clearance, possibly decreasing its concentration). Products include:
Adriamycin for Injection, USP 786
Adriamycin Injection, USP 786

Droperidol (Concurrent use may produce additive CNS depressant effects).
No products indexed under this heading.

Efavirenz (CYP3A4 inhibitors may decrease zaleplon's clearance, possibly increasing its concentration). Products include:
Sustiva Capsules 957

Enflurane (Concurrent use may produce additive CNS depressant effects).
No products indexed under this heading.

Erythromycin (CYP3A4 is a minor metabolizing enzyme of zaleplon; the co-administration of a strong, selective CYP3A4 inhibitor (erythromycin) produced a 34% increase in zaleplon's plasma concentration. A routine dosage adjustment of zaleplon is not considered necessary). Products include:
Erygel Topical Gel 2096
Ery-Tab Tablets 447
Erythromycin Base Filmtab Tablets 454
Erythromycin Delayed-Release Capsules, USP 456
PCE Dispertab Tablets 510

Erythromycin Estolate (CYP3A4 is a minor metabolizing enzyme of zaleplon; the co-administration of a strong, selective CYP3A4 inhibitor (erythromycin) produced a 34% increase in zaleplon's plasma concentration. A routine dosage adjustment of zaleplon is not considered necessary).
No products indexed under this heading.

Erythromycin Ethylsuccinate (CYP3A4 is a minor metabolizing enzyme of zaleplon; the co-administration of a strong, selective CYP3A4 inhibitor (erythromycin) produced a 34% increase in zaleplon's plasma concentration. A routine dosage adjustment of zaleplon is not considered necessary). Products include:
E.E.S. 449
EryPed 445

Erythromycin Gluceptate (CYP3A4 is a minor metabolizing enzyme of zaleplon; the co-administration of a strong, selective CYP3A4 inhibitor (erythromycin) produced a 34% increase in zaleplon's plasma concentration. A routine dosage adjustment of zaleplon is not considered necessary).
No products indexed under this heading.

Erythromycin Lactobionate (CYP3A4 is a minor metabolizing enzyme of zaleplon; the co-administration of a strong, selective CYP3A4 inhibitor (erythromycin) produced a 34% increase in zaleplon's plasma concentration. A routine dosage adjustment of zaleplon is not considered necessary).
No products indexed under this heading.

Erythromycin Stearate (CYP3A4 is a minor metabolizing enzyme of zaleplon; the co-administration of a strong, selective CYP3A4 inhibitor (erythromycin) produced a 34% increase in zaleplon's plasma concentration. A routine dosage adjustment of zaleplon is not considered necessary). Products include:
Erythrocin Stearate Filmtab Tablets 452

Esomeprazole Magnesium (CYP3A4 inhibitors may decrease zaleplon's clearance, possibly increasing its concentration). Products include:
Nexium Delayed-Release Capsules 645

Estazolam (Concurrent use may produce additive CNS depressant effects). Products include:
ProSom Tablets 512

Ethanol (Concurrent use may produce additive CNS depressant effects).
No products indexed under this heading.

Ethchlorvynol (Concurrent use may produce additive CNS depressant effects).
No products indexed under this heading.

Ethinamate (Concurrent use may produce additive CNS depressant effects).
No products indexed under this heading.

Ethosuximide (Concurrent use with anticonvulsants may produce additive CNS depressant effects).
No products indexed under this heading.

Ethotoin (Concurrent use with anticonvulsants may produce additive CNS depressant effects). Products include:
Peganone Tablets, USP 2487

Ethyl Alcohol (Concurrent use may produce additive CNS depressant effects).
No products indexed under this heading.

Felbamate (Concurrent use with anticonvulsants may produce additive CNS depressant effects).
No products indexed under this heading.

Fentanyl (Concurrent use may produce additive CNS depressant effects). Products include:
Duragesic Transdermal System 2448

Fentanyl Citrate (Concurrent use may produce additive CNS depressant effects). Products include:
Actiq 993

Fexofenadine Hydrochloride (Concurrent use may produce additive CNS depressant effects). Products include:
Allegra 2857
Allegra-D 12 Hour Extended-Release Tablets 2860
Allegra-D 24 Hour Extended-Release Tablets 2862

Fluconazole (CYP3A4 inhibitors may decrease zaleplon's clearance, possibly increasing its concentration).
No products indexed under this heading.

Fludrocortisone Acetate (CYP3A4 inhibitors may increase zaleplon's clearance, possibly decreasing its concentration).
No products indexed under this heading.

Fluoxetine Hydrochloride (CYP3A4 inhibitors may decrease zaleplon's clearance, possibly increasing its concentration). Products include:
Prozac Pulvules and Liquid 1771
Symbyax Capsules 1788

Fluphenazine Decanoate (Concurrent use may produce additive CNS depressant effects).
No products indexed under this heading.

Fluphenazine Enanthate (Concurrent use may produce additive CNS depressant effects).
No products indexed under this heading.

Fluphenazine Hydrochloride (Concurrent use may produce additive CNS depressant effects).
No products indexed under this heading.

Flurazepam Hydrochloride (Concurrent use may produce additive CNS depressant effects). Products include:
Dalmane Capsules 3343

Fluvoxamine Maleate (CYP3A4 inhibitors may decrease zaleplon's clearance, possibly increasing its concentration).
No products indexed under this heading.

Fosamprenavir Calcium (CYP3A4 inhibitors may decrease zaleplon's clearance, possibly increasing its concentration). Products include:
Lexiva Tablets 1473

Fosphenytoin (Concurrent use with anticonvulsants may produce additive CNS depressant effects).
No products indexed under this heading.

Fosphenytoin Sodium (CYP3A4 is ordinarily a minor metabolizing enzyme of zaleplon, the co-administration of a potent inducer, such as phenytoin, although not posing a safety concern, could lead to ineffectiveness of zaleplon; concurrent use with anticonvulsants may produce additive CNS depressant effects).
No products indexed under this heading.

Gabapentin (Concurrent use with anticonvulsants may produce additive CNS depressant effects). Products include:
Neurontin Capsules 2498
Neurontin Oral Solution 2498
Neurontin Tablets 2498

Garlic Extract (CYP3A4 inhibitors may increase zaleplon's clearance, possibly decreasing its concentration).
No products indexed under this heading.

Garlic Oil (CYP3A4 inhibitors may increase zaleplon's clearance, possibly decreasing its concentration).
No products indexed under this heading.

Glutethimide (Concurrent use may produce additive CNS depressant effects).
No products indexed under this heading.

Haloperidol (Concurrent use may produce additive CNS depressant effects).
No products indexed under this heading.

Haloperidol Decanoate (Concurrent use may produce additive CNS depressant effects).
No products indexed under this heading.

Hydrocodone Bitartrate (Concurrent use may produce additive CNS depressant effects). Products include:
Hycodan 1104
Hycomine Compound Tablets 1105
Hycotuss Expectorant Syrup 1106
Lortab 3315
Lortab Elixir 3312
Vicodin Tablets 530
Vicodin ES Tablets 531
Vicodin HP Tablets 532
Vicoprofen Tablets 533
Zydone Tablets 1118

Hydrocodone Polistirex (Concurrent use may produce additive CNS depressant effects). Products include:
Tussionex Pennkinetic Extended-Release Suspension 3322

Hydrocortisone (CYP3A4 inhibitors may increase zaleplon's clearance, possibly decreasing its concentration). Products include:
Cortizone•5 Ointment .... ▣699
Cortizone•10 Creme .... ▣699
Cortizone•10 Ointment .... ▣699
Cortizone•10 Plus Creme .... ▣700
Cortizone•10 Maximum Strength Quick Shot Spray .... ▣700
Hydrocortone Tablets 1963
Preparation H Hydrocortisone Cream .... ▣748

Hydrocortisone Acetate (CYP3A4 inhibitors may increase zaleplon's clearance, possibly decreasing its concentration). Products include:
Analpram-HC 1136
Pramosone 1139
ProctoFoam-HC 3113
Tucks Anti-Itch Ointment .... ▣712
U-cort 1% Cream 3289

Hydrocortisone Butyrate (CYP3A4 inhibitors may increase zaleplon's clearance, possibly decreasing its concentration). Products include:
Locoid ... 1138
Locoid Lipocream Cream ... 1138

Hydrocortisone Cypionate (CYP3A4 inhibitors may increase zaleplon's clearance, possibly decreasing its concentration).
No products indexed under this heading.

Hydrocortisone Hemisuccinate (CYP3A4 inhibitors may increase zaleplon's clearance, possibly decreasing its concentration).
No products indexed under this heading.

Hydrocortisone Probutate (CYP3A4 inhibitors may increase zaleplon's clearance, possibly decreasing its concentration). Products include:
Pandel Cream, 0.1% ... 1017

Hydrocortisone Sodium Phosphate (CYP3A4 inhibitors may increase zaleplon's clearance, possibly decreasing its concentration).
No products indexed under this heading.

Hydrocortisone Sodium Succinate (CYP3A4 inhibitors may increase zaleplon's clearance, possibly decreasing its concentration).
No products indexed under this heading.

Hydrocortisone Valerate (CYP3A4 inhibitors may increase zaleplon's clearance, possibly decreasing its concentration).
No products indexed under this heading.

Hydromorphone Hydrochloride (Concurrent use may produce additive CNS depressant effects). Products include:
Dilaudid ... 439
Dilaudid Oral Liquid ... 443
Dilaudid Non-Sterile Powder ... 439
Dilaudid Rectal Suppositories ... 439
Dilaudid Tablets ... 439
Dilaudid Tablets - 8 mg ... 443
Dilaudid-HP ... 441

Hydroxyzine Hydrochloride (Concurrent use may produce additive CNS depressant effects).
No products indexed under this heading.

Hypericum (CYP3A4 inhibitors may increase zaleplon's clearance, possibly decreasing its concentration).
No products indexed under this heading.

Hypericum Perforatum (CYP3A4 inhibitors may increase zaleplon's clearance, possibly decreasing its concentration).
No products indexed under this heading.

Imipramine Hydrochloride (Concurrent use may produce additive CNS depressant effects).
No products indexed under this heading.

Imipramine Pamoate (Concurrent use may produce additive CNS depressant effects).
No products indexed under this heading.

Indinavir Sulfate (CYP3A4 inhibitors may decrease zaleplon's clearance, possibly increasing its concentration). Products include:
Crixivan Capsules ... 1918

Isocarboxazid (Concurrent use may produce additive CNS depressant effects).
No products indexed under this heading.

Isoflurane (Concurrent use may produce additive CNS depressant effects).
No products indexed under this heading.

Isoniazid (CYP3A4 inhibitors may decrease zaleplon's clearance, possibly increasing its concentration).
No products indexed under this heading.

Itraconazole (CYP3A4 inhibitors may decrease zaleplon's clearance, possibly increasing its concentration).
No products indexed under this heading.

Ketamine Hydrochloride (Concurrent use may produce additive CNS depressant effects).
No products indexed under this heading.

Ketoconazole (CYP3A4 inhibitors may decrease zaleplon's clearance, possibly increasing its concentration). Products include:
Nizoral A-D Shampoo, 1% ... 1839
Nizoral 2% Shampoo ... 1838

Lamotrigine (Concurrent use with anticonvulsants may produce additive CNS depressant effects). Products include:
Lamictal ... 1449

Levetiracetam (Concurrent use with anticonvulsants may produce additive CNS depressant effects). Products include:
Keppra Oral Solution ... 3307
Keppra Tablets ... 3307

Levomethadyl Acetate Hydrochloride (Concurrent use may produce additive CNS depressant effects).
No products indexed under this heading.

Levorphanol Tartrate (Concurrent use may produce additive CNS depressant effects).
No products indexed under this heading.

Lithium Carbonate (Concurrent use may produce additive CNS depressant effects). Products include:
Eskalith ... 1406
Lithobid Tablets ... 1670

Lithium Citrate (Concurrent use may produce additive CNS depressant effects).
No products indexed under this heading.

Lopinavir (CYP3A4 inhibitors may decrease zaleplon's clearance, possibly increasing its concentration). Products include:
Kaletra ... 474

Loratadine (Concurrent use may produce additive CNS depressant effects). Products include:
Alavert Allergy & Sinus D-12 Hour Tablets ... 743
Alavert ... 743
Children's Claritin 24 Hour Non-Drowsy Allergy Syrup ... 732
Claritin Non-Drowsy 24 Hour Tablets ... 731
Non-Drowsy Claritin Hives Relief Tablets ... 733
Claritin Reditabs 24 Hour Non-Drowsy Tablets ... 732
Claritin-D Non-Drowsy 12 Hour Tablets ... 731
Claritin-D Non-Drowsy 24 Hour Tablets ... 731
Children's Dimetapp ND Non-Drowsy Allergy Syrup ... 746
Triaminic Allerchews ... 684

Lorazepam (Concurrent use may produce additive CNS depressant effects).
No products indexed under this heading.

Loxapine Hydrochloride (Concurrent use may produce additive CNS depressant effects).
No products indexed under this heading.

Loxapine Succinate (Concurrent use may produce additive CNS depressant effects).
No products indexed under this heading.

Maprotiline Hydrochloride (Concurrent use may produce additive CNS depressant effects).
No products indexed under this heading.

Meperidine Hydrochloride (Concurrent use may produce additive CNS depressant effects).
No products indexed under this heading.

Mephenytoin (Concurrent use with anticonvulsants may produce additive CNS depressant effects).
No products indexed under this heading.

Mephobarbital (Concurrent use may produce additive CNS depressant effects). Products include:
Mebaral Tablets, USP ... 2483

Meprobamate (Concurrent use may produce additive CNS depressant effects).
No products indexed under this heading.

Mesoridazine Besylate (Concurrent use may produce additive CNS depressant effects).
No products indexed under this heading.

Methadone Hydrochloride (Concurrent use may produce additive CNS depressant effects).
No products indexed under this heading.

Methdilazine Hydrochloride (Concurrent use may produce additive CNS depressant effects).
No products indexed under this heading.

Methohexital Sodium (Concurrent use may produce additive CNS depressant effects).
No products indexed under this heading.

Methotrimeprazine (Concurrent use may produce additive CNS depressant effects).
No products indexed under this heading.

Methoxyflurane (Concurrent use may produce additive CNS depressant effects).
No products indexed under this heading.

Methsuximide (Concurrent use with anticonvulsants may produce additive CNS depressant effects).
No products indexed under this heading.

Methylprednisolone (CYP3A4 inhibitors may increase zaleplon's clearance, possibly decreasing its concentration).
No products indexed under this heading.

Methylprednisolone Acetate (CYP3A4 inhibitors may increase zaleplon's clearance, possibly decreasing its concentration). Products include:
Depo-Medrol Injectable Suspension ... 2615
Depo-Medrol Single-Dose Vial ... 2617

Methylprednisolone Sodium Succinate (CYP3A4 inhibitors may increase zaleplon's clearance, possibly decreasing its concentration).
No products indexed under this heading.

Metronidazole (CYP3A4 inhibitors may decrease zaleplon's clearance, possibly increasing its concentration). Products include:
Metrogel 1% ... 1212
MetroGel-Vaginal Gel ... 1822
Noritate Cream, 1% ... 1051

Metronidazole Benzoate (CYP3A4 inhibitors may decrease zaleplon's clearance, possibly increasing its concentration).
No products indexed under this heading.

Metronidazole Hydrochloride (CYP3A4 inhibitors may decrease zaleplon's clearance, possibly increasing its concentration).
No products indexed under this heading.

Miconazole (CYP3A4 inhibitors may decrease zaleplon's clearance, possibly increasing its concentration).
No products indexed under this heading.

Miconazole Nitrate (CYP3A4 inhibitors may decrease zaleplon's clearance, possibly increasing its concentration). Products include:
Desenex ... 674
Desenex Jock Itch Spray Powder ... 674

Midazolam Hydrochloride (Concurrent use may produce additive CNS depressant effects).
No products indexed under this heading.

Modafinil (CYP3A4 inhibitors may increase zaleplon's clearance, possibly decreasing its concentration). Products include:
Provigil Tablets ... 1002

Molindone Hydrochloride (Concurrent use may produce additive CNS depressant effects). Products include:
Moban Tablets ... 1108

Morphine Sulfate (Concurrent use may produce additive CNS depressant effects). Products include:
Avinza Capsules ... 1714
Kadian Capsules ... 572
MS Contin Tablets ... 2703

Nefazodone Hydrochloride (CYP3A4 inhibitors may decrease zaleplon's clearance, possibly increasing its concentration).
No products indexed under this heading.

Nelfinavir Mesylate (CYP3A4 inhibitors may decrease zaleplon's clearance, possibly increasing its concentration). Products include:
Viracept ... 2556

Nevirapine (CYP3A4 inhibitors may decrease zaleplon's clearance, possibly increasing its concentration). Products include:
Viramune Oral Suspension ... 903
Viramune Tablets ... 903

IMPORTANT NOTE: Always consult each drug listing in the patient's regimen for possible interactions.

Niacinamide (CYP3A4 inhibitors may decrease zaleplon's clearance, possibly increasing its concentration).
No products indexed under this heading.

Nicotinamide (CYP3A4 inhibitors may decrease zaleplon's clearance, possibly increasing its concentration). Products include:
Nicomide Tablets 3190

Nifedipine (CYP3A4 inhibitors may decrease zaleplon's clearance, possibly increasing its concentration). Products include:
Adalat CC Tablets 2978

Norfloxacin (CYP3A4 inhibitors may decrease zaleplon's clearance, possibly increasing its concentration). Products include:
Noroxin Tablets 2009

Nortriptyline Hydrochloride (Concurrent use may produce additive CNS depressant effects).
No products indexed under this heading.

Olanzapine (Concurrent use may produce additive CNS depressant effects). Products include:
Symbyax Capsules 1788
Zyprexa Tablets 1798
Zyprexa IntraMuscular 1798
Zyprexa ZYDIS Orally Disintegrating Tablets 1798

Omeprazole (CYP3A4 inhibitors may decrease zaleplon's clearance, possibly increasing its concentration). Products include:
Zegerid Powder for Oral Solution 2972

Oxazepam (Concurrent use may produce additive CNS depressant effects).
No products indexed under this heading.

Oxcarbazepine (Concurrent use with anticonvulsants may produce additive CNS depressant effects). Products include:
Trileptal Oral Suspension 2281
Trileptal Tablets 2281

Oxycodone Hydrochloride (Concurrent use may produce additive CNS depressant effects). Products include:
Combunox Tablets 1183
OxyContin Tablets 2699
OxyFast Oral Concentrate Solution 2704
OxyIR Capsules 2704
Percocet Tablets 1114
Percodan Tablets 1115

Paramethadione (Concurrent use with anticonvulsants may produce additive CNS depressant effects).
No products indexed under this heading.

Paroxetine Hydrochloride (CYP3A4 inhibitors may decrease zaleplon's clearance, possibly increasing its concentration). Products include:
Paxil CR Controlled-Release Tablets 1509
Paxil 1501

Pentobarbital Sodium (Concurrent use may produce additive CNS depressant effects). Products include:
Nembutal Sodium Solution, USP 2484

Perphenazine (Concurrent use may produce additive CNS depressant effects).
No products indexed under this heading.

Phenacemide (Concurrent use with anticonvulsants may produce additive CNS depressant effects).
No products indexed under this heading.

Phenelzine Sulfate (Concurrent use may produce additive CNS depressant effects).
No products indexed under this heading.

Phenobarbital (CYP3A4 is ordinarily a minor metabolizing enzyme of zaleplon, the co-administration of a potent inducer, such as phenobarbital, although not posing a safety concern, could lead to ineffectiveness of zaleplon; concurrent use with anticonvulsants may produce additive CNS depressant effects).
No products indexed under this heading.

Phenobarbital Sodium (CYP3A4 inhibitors may increase zaleplon's clearance, possibly decreasing its concentration).
No products indexed under this heading.

Phensuximide (Concurrent use with anticonvulsants may produce additive CNS depressant effects).
No products indexed under this heading.

Phenytoin (CYP3A4 is ordinarily a minor metabolizing enzyme of zaleplon, the co-administration of a potent inducer, such as phenytoin, although not posing a safety concern, could lead to ineffectiveness of zaleplon; concurrent use with anticonvulsants may produce additive CNS depressant effects).
No products indexed under this heading.

Phenytoin Sodium (CYP3A4 is ordinarily a minor metabolizing enzyme of zaleplon, the co-administration of a potent inducer, such as phenytoin, although not posing a safety concern, could lead to ineffectiveness of zaleplon; concurrent use with anticonvulsants may produce additive CNS depressant effects). Products include:
Phenytek Capsules 2153

Prazepam (Concurrent use may produce additive CNS depressant effects).
No products indexed under this heading.

Prednisolone Acetate (CYP3A4 inhibitors may increase zaleplon's clearance, possibly decreasing its concentration). Products include:
Blephamide Ophthalmic Ointment 563
Blephamide Ophthalmic Suspension 564
Poly-Pred Liquifilm Ophthalmic Suspension .... ⊙ 231
Pred Forte Ophthalmic Suspension .... ⊙ 233
Pred Mild Sterile Ophthalmic Suspension .... ⊙ 236
Pred-G Ophthalmic Suspension .... ⊙ 234
Pred-G Sterile Ophthalmic Ointment .... ⊙ 235

Prednisolone Sodium Phosphate (CYP3A4 inhibitors may increase zaleplon's clearance, possibly decreasing its concentration). Products include:
Pediapred Oral Solution 3319

Prednisolone Tebutate (CYP3A4 inhibitors may increase zaleplon's clearance, possibly decreasing its concentration).
No products indexed under this heading.

Prednisone (CYP3A4 inhibitors may increase zaleplon's clearance, possibly decreasing its concentration).
No products indexed under this heading.

Primidone (Concurrent use with anticonvulsants may produce additive CNS depressant effects).
No products indexed under this heading.

Prochlorperazine (Concurrent use may produce additive CNS depressant effects).
No products indexed under this heading.

Promethazine Hydrochloride (Co-administration of a single dose of zaleplon and promethazine (10 and 25mg, respectively) resulted in a 15% decrease in maximal plasma concentrations of zalephon, but no change in the area under the plasma curve, however, the pharmacodynamics of co-administration of zalephon and promethazine have not been evaluated. Caution should be exercised when these 2 agents are co-administered). Products include:
Phenergan 3438

Propofol (Concurrent use may produce additive CNS depressant effects). Products include:
Diprivan Injectable Emulsion 676

Propoxyphene Hydrochloride (Concurrent use may produce additive CNS depressant effects).
No products indexed under this heading.

Propoxyphene Napsylate (Concurrent use may produce additive CNS depressant effects). Products include:
Darvocet A 500 Tablets 3497

Protriptyline Hydrochloride (Concurrent use may produce additive CNS depressant effects). Products include:
Vivactil Tablets 2350

Pyrilamine Maleate (Concurrent use may produce additive CNS depressant effects).
No products indexed under this heading.

Pyrilamine Tannate (Concurrent use may produce additive CNS depressant effects).
No products indexed under this heading.

Quazepam (Concurrent use may produce additive CNS depressant effects).
No products indexed under this heading.

Quetiapine Fumarate (Concurrent use may produce additive CNS depressant effects). Products include:
Seroquel Tablets 691

Quinidine (CYP3A4 inhibitors may decrease zaleplon's clearance, possibly increasing its concentration).
No products indexed under this heading.

Quinidine Hydrochloride (CYP3A4 inhibitors may decrease zaleplon's clearance, possibly increasing its concentration).
No products indexed under this heading.

Quinidine Polygalacturonate (CYP3A4 inhibitors may decrease zaleplon's clearance, possibly increasing its concentration).
No products indexed under this heading.

Quinidine Sulfate (CYP3A4 inhibitors may decrease zaleplon's clearance, possibly increasing its concentration).
No products indexed under this heading.

Quinine (CYP3A4 inhibitors may decrease zaleplon's clearance, possibly increasing its concentration).
No products indexed under this heading.

Quinine Sulfate (CYP3A4 inhibitors may decrease zaleplon's clearance, possibly increasing its concentration).
No products indexed under this heading.

Quinupristin (CYP3A4 inhibitors may decrease zaleplon's clearance, possibly increasing its concentration). Products include:
Synercid I.V. 1690

Ranitidine Bismuth Citrate (CYP3A4 inhibitors may decrease zaleplon's clearance, possibly increasing its concentration).
No products indexed under this heading.

Ranitidine Hydrochloride (CYP3A4 inhibitors may decrease zaleplon's clearance, possibly increasing its concentration). Products include:
Zantac 1597
Zantac Injection 1593
Zantac 75 Tablets .... ▣ 715
Zantac 150 Maximum Strength Tablets .... ▣ 715
Zantac Injection Pharmacy Bulk Package 1595

Remifentanil Hydrochloride (Concurrent use may produce additive CNS depressant effects).
No products indexed under this heading.

Rifabutin (CYP3A4 inhibitors may increase zaleplon's clearance, possibly decreasing its concentration).
No products indexed under this heading.

Rifampicin (CYP3A4 inhibitors may increase zaleplon's clearance, possibly decreasing its concentration).
No products indexed under this heading.

Rifampin (The co-administration of a potent CYP3A4 enzyme inducer, although not posing a safety concern, could lead to ineffectiveness of zaleplon).
No products indexed under this heading.

Rifapentine (CYP3A4 inhibitors may increase zaleplon's clearance, possibly decreasing its concentration).
No products indexed under this heading.

Risperidone (Concurrent use may produce additive CNS depressant effects). Products include:
Risperdal Consta Long-Acting Injection 1664
Risperdal M-Tab Orally Disintegrating Tablets 1658
Risperdal 1658

Ritonavir (CYP3A4 inhibitors may decrease zaleplon's clearance, possibly increasing its concentration). Products include:
Kaletra 474
Norvir 499

Saquinavir (CYP3A4 inhibitors may decrease zaleplon's clearance, possibly increasing its concentration).
No products indexed under this heading.

Saquinavir Mesylate (CYP3A4 inhibitors may decrease zaleplon's clearance, possibly increasing its concentration). Products include:
Invirase 2776

Secobarbital Sodium (Concurrent use may produce additive CNS depressant effects).
No products indexed under this heading.

Sertraline Hydrochloride (CYP3A4 inhibitors may decrease zaleplon's clearance, possibly increasing its concentration). Products include:
Zoloft 2581

Sevoflurane (Concurrent use may produce additive CNS depressant effects). Products include:
Ultane Liquid for Inhalation 526

Sodium Oxybate (Concurrent use may produce additive CNS depressant effects).
No products indexed under this heading.

Sufentanil Citrate (Concurrent use may produce additive CNS depressant effects).
No products indexed under this heading.

Sulfinpyrazone (CYP3A4 inhibitors may increase zaleplon's clearance, possibly decreasing its concentration).
No products indexed under this heading.

Telithromycin (CYP3A4 inhibitors may decrease zaleplon's clearance, possibly increasing its concentration). Products include:
Ketek Tablets 2920

Temazepam (Concurrent use may produce additive CNS depressant effects).
No products indexed under this heading.

Terfenadine (Concurrent use may produce additive CNS depressant effects).
No products indexed under this heading.

Theophylline (CYP3A4 inhibitors may increase zaleplon's clearance, possibly decreasing its concentration).
No products indexed under this heading.

Thiamylal Sodium (Concurrent use may produce additive CNS depressant effects).
No products indexed under this heading.

Thioridazine Hydrochloride (Co-administration has produced additive effects of decreased alertness and impaired psychomotor performance for 2 to 4 hours). Products include:
Thioridazine Hydrochloride Tablets 2122

Thiothixene (Concurrent use may produce additive CNS depressant effects). Products include:
Thiothixene Capsules 2124

Tiagabine Hydrochloride (Concurrent use with anticonvulsants may produce additive CNS depressant effects). Products include:
Gabitril Tablets 998

Topiramate (Concurrent use with anticonvulsants may produce additive CNS depressant effects). Products include:
Topamax Sprinkle Capsules 2438
Topamax Tablets 2438

Tranylcypromine Sulfate (Concurrent use may produce additive CNS depressant effects). Products include:
Parnate Tablets 1499

Triamcinolone (CYP3A4 inhibitors may increase zaleplon's clearance, possibly decreasing its concentration).
No products indexed under this heading.

Triamcinolone Acetonide (CYP3A4 inhibitors may increase zaleplon's clearance, possibly decreasing its concentration). Products include:
Azmacort Inhalation Aerosol 1701
Nasacort HFA Inhalation Aerosol 2939
Nasacort AQ Nasal Spray 2937

Triamcinolone Diacetate (CYP3A4 inhibitors may increase zaleplon's clearance, possibly decreasing its concentration).
No products indexed under this heading.

Triamcinolone Hexacetonide (CYP3A4 inhibitors may increase zaleplon's clearance, possibly decreasing its concentration).
No products indexed under this heading.

Triazolam (Concurrent use may produce additive CNS depressant effects).
No products indexed under this heading.

Trifluoperazine Hydrochloride (Concurrent use may produce additive CNS depressant effects).
No products indexed under this heading.

Trimeprazine Tartrate (Concurrent use may produce additive CNS depressant effects).
No products indexed under this heading.

Trimethadione (Concurrent use with anticonvulsants may produce additive CNS depressant effects).
No products indexed under this heading.

Trimipramine Maleate (Concurrent use may produce additive CNS depressant effects). Products include:
Surmontil Capsules 2347

Tripelennamine Hydrochloride (Concurrent use may produce additive CNS depressant effects).
No products indexed under this heading.

Triprolidine Hydrochloride (Concurrent use may produce additive CNS depressant effects).
No products indexed under this heading.

Troglitazone (CYP3A4 inhibitors may decrease zaleplon's clearance, possibly increasing its concentration).
No products indexed under this heading.

Troleandomycin (CYP3A4 inhibitors may decrease zaleplon's clearance, possibly increasing its concentration).
No products indexed under this heading.

Valproate Sodium (Concurrent use with anticonvulsants may produce additive CNS depressant effects). Products include:
Depacon Injection 412

Valproic Acid (Concurrent use with anticonvulsants may produce additive CNS depressant effects). Products include:
Depakene 417

Verapamil Hydrochloride (CYP3A4 inhibitors may decrease zaleplon's clearance, possibly increasing its concentration). Products include:
Covera-HS Tablets 3135
Tarka Tablets 519
Verelan PM Capsules 3120

Voriconazole (CYP3A4 inhibitors may decrease zaleplon's clearance, possibly increasing its concentration). Products include:
VFEND I.V. 2543
VFEND Oral Suspension 2543
VFEND Tablets 2543

Zafirlukast (CYP3A4 inhibitors may decrease zaleplon's clearance, possibly increasing its concentration). Products include:
Accolate Tablets 663

Zileuton (CYP3A4 inhibitors may decrease zaleplon's clearance, possibly increasing its concentration).
No products indexed under this heading.

Ziprasidone Hydrochloride (Concurrent use may produce additive CNS depressant effects). Products include:
Geodon Capsules 2514

Zolpidem Tartrate (Concurrent use may produce additive CNS depressant effects). Products include:
Ambien Tablets 2867

Zonisamide (Concurrent use with anticonvulsants may produce additive CNS depressant effects). Products include:
Zonegran Capsules 1089

Food Interactions

Alcohol (Concurrent use may produce additive CNS depressant effects).

Food, unspecified (A high-fat/heavy meal prolongs the absorption of zaleplon compared to fasting state, delays tmax by approximately 2 hours and reduces Cmax approximately 35%; the effect of Sonata on sleep onset may be reduced if it is taken with or immediately after a high-fat/heavy meal).

Grapefruit (CYP3A4 inhibitors may decrease zaleplon's clearance, possibly increasing its concentration).

Grapefruit Juice (CYP3A4 inhibitors may decrease zaleplon's clearance, possibly increasing its concentration).

SORIATANE CAPSULES

(Acitretin) 1028

May interact with tetracyclines and certain other agents. Compounds in these categories include:

Demeclocycline Hydrochloride (Since both Soriatane and tetracyclines can cause increases in intracranial pressure, their combined use is contraindicated).
No products indexed under this heading.

Doxycycline Calcium (Since both Soriatane and tetracyclines can cause increases in intracranial pressure, their combined use is contraindicated).
No products indexed under this heading.

Doxycycline Hyclate (Since both Soriatane and tetracyclines can cause increases in intracranial pressure, their combined use is contraindicated).
No products indexed under this heading.

Doxycycline Monohydrate (Since both Soriatane and tetracyclines can cause increases in intracranial pressure, their combined use is contraindicated).
No products indexed under this heading.

Glibenclamide (Acitretin treatment potentiated the blood glucose lowering affect of glibenclamide in 3 of the 7 male volunteers).
No products indexed under this heading.

Methacycline Hydrochloride (Since both Soriatane and tetracyclines can cause increases in intracranial pressure, their combined use is contraindicated).
No products indexed under this heading.

Methotrexate (An increased risk of hepatitis has been reported to result from combined use of methotrexate and etretinate).
No products indexed under this heading.

Minocycline Hydrochloride (Since both Soriatane and tetracyclines can cause increases in intracranial pressure, their combined use is contraindicated). Products include:
Dynacin Tablets 1859

Oxytetracycline Hydrochloride (Since both Soriatane and tetracyclines can cause increases in intracranial pressure, their combined use is contraindicated).
No products indexed under this heading.

Phenytoin (If acitretin is given concurrently with phenytoin, the protein binding of phenytoin may be reduced).
No products indexed under this heading.

Tetracycline Hydrochloride (Since both Soriatane and tetracyclines can cause increases in intracranial pressure, their combined use is contraindicated).
No products indexed under this heading.

Vitamin A (Concomitant administration of vitamin A and/or other oral retinoids with acitretin must be avoided because of the risk of hypervitaminosis A). Products include:
Visutein Capsules 3328

Food Interactions

Alcohol (Clinical evidence has shown that etretinate can be formed with concurrent ingestion of acitretin and ethanol).

SPARTAN HAIR SYSTEM SUPPLEMENT

(Herbals with Vitamins) 767

None cited in PDR database.

SPARTAN HAIR SYSTEM SHAMPOO

(Azelaic Acid, Biotin, Caffeine, Lecithin, Panthenol, Phytosterols, Serenoa repens, Tocopherol Acetate, Zinc Sulfate) 767

None cited in PDR database.

SPECTAZOLE CREAM

(Econazole Nitrate) 2390

None cited in PDR database.

SPECTRACEF TABLETS

(Cefditoren Pivoxil) 2706

May interact with histamine H_2-receptor antagonists and certain other agents. Compounds in these categories include:

Aluminum Hydroxide (Co-administration with antacids containing aluminum and magnesium hydroxides reduced oral absorption of cefditoren; clinical significance is not known; Spectracef should not be taken concomitantly with antacids). Products include:
- Gaviscon Regular Strength Liquid ▣620
- Gaviscon Regular Strength Tablets ▣619
- Gaviscon Extra Strength Liquid ▣620
- Gaviscon Extra Strength Tablets ▣619
- Maalox Max Maximum Strength Antacid/Anti-Gas Liquid 2165
- Maalox Regular Strength Antacid/Antigas Liquid 2164

Cimetidine (Co-administration with other H2 receptor antagonists has resulted in reduced oral absorption of cefditoren; Spectracef should not be taken concomitantly with H2 receptor antagonists). Products include:
- Tagamet HB 200 Tablets ▣637
- Tagamet Tablets 1547

Cimetidine Hydrochloride (Co-administration with other H2 receptor antagonists has resulted in reduced oral absorption of cefditoren; Spectracef should not be taken concomitantly with H2 receptor antagonists).

No products indexed under this heading.

Famotidine (Co-administration with famotidine I.V. has resulted in reduced oral absorption of cefditoren; clinical significance is not known; Spectracef should not be taken concomitantly with H2 receptor antagonists). Products include:
- Pepcid AC Chewable Tablets 1672
- Pepcid AC Gelcaps 1672
- Pepcid AC Tablets 1672
- Maximum Strength Pepcid AC Tablets 1672
- Pepcid Complete Chewable Tablets 1672
- Pepcid Injection 2017
- Pepcid 2014

Magnesium Hydroxide (Co-administration with antacids containing aluminum and magnesium hydroxides reduced oral absorption of cefditoren; clinical significance is not known; Spectracef should not be taken concomitantly with H2 receptor antagonists). Products include:
- Maalox Max Maximum Strength Antacid/Anti-Gas Liquid 2165
- Maalox Regular Strength Antacid/Antigas Liquid 2164
- Pepcid Complete Chewable Tablets 1672
- Rolaids Tablets ▣707
- Extra Strength Rolaids Tablets ▣707
- Rolaids Multi-Symptom Antacid & Antigas Tablets ▣708

Nizatidine (Co-administration with other H2 receptor antagonists has resulted in reduced oral absorption of cefditoren; Spectracef should not be taken concomitantly with H2 receptor antagonists). Products include:
- Axid Oral Solution 913

Probenecid (Co-administration has resulted in an increase in the plasma exposure of cefditoren).

No products indexed under this heading.

Ranitidine Bismuth Citrate (Co-administration with other H2 receptor antagonists has resulted in reduced oral absorption of cefditoren; Spectracef should not be taken concomitantly with H2 receptor antagonists).

No products indexed under this heading.

Ranitidine Hydrochloride (Co-administration with other H2 receptor antagonists has resulted in reduced oral absorption of cefditoren; Spectracef should not be taken concomitantly with H2 receptor antagonists). Products include:
- Zantac 1597
- Zantac Injection 1593
- Zantac 75 Tablets ▣715
- Zantac 150 Maximum Strength Tablets ▣715
- Zantac Injection Pharmacy Bulk Package 1595

SPIRIVA HANDIHALER

(Tiotropium bromide) 899

May interact with anticholinergics and certain other agents. Compounds in these categories include:

Atropine Sulfate (Co-administration of tiotropium with other anticholinergic-containing drugs (e.g., ipratropium) has not been studied and is therefore not recommended).

No products indexed under this heading.

Belladonna Alkaloids (Co-administration of tiotropium with other anticholinergic-containing drugs (e.g., ipratropium) has not been studied and is therefore not recommended). Products include:
- Hyland's Teething Tablets ▣736

Benztropine Mesylate (Co-administration of tiotropium with other anticholinergic-containing drugs (e.g., ipratropium) has not been studied and is therefore not recommended). Products include:
- Cogentin Injection 1903

Biperiden Hydrochloride (Co-administration of tiotropium with other anticholinergic-containing drugs (e.g., ipratropium) has not been studied and is therefore not recommended).

No products indexed under this heading.

Cimetidine (Concomitant administration of cimetidine with tiotropium resulted in a 20% increase in the $AUC_{0\text{-}4h}$, a 28% increase in the renal clearance of tiotropium and no significant change in the Cmax and amount excreted in urine over 96 hours. Therefore, no clinically significant interaction occurred between tiotropium and cimetidine). Products include:
- Tagamet HB 200 Tablets ▣637
- Tagamet Tablets 1547

Cimetidine Hydrochloride (Concomitant administration of cimetidine with tiotropium resulted in a 20% increase in the AUC0-4h, a 28% increase in the renal clearance of tiotropium and no significant change in the Cmax and amount excreted in urine over 96 hours. Therefore, no clinically significant interaction occurred between tiotropium and cimetidine).

No products indexed under this heading.

Clidinium Bromide (Co-administration of tiotropium with other anticholinergic-containing drugs (e.g., ipratropium) has not been studied and is therefore not recommended).

No products indexed under this heading.

Dicyclomine Hydrochloride (Co-administration of tiotropium with other anticholinergic-containing drugs (e.g., ipratropium) has not been studied and is therefore not recommended). Products include:
- Bentyl Capsules 724
- Bentyl Injection 724
- Bentyl Syrup 724
- Bentyl Tablets 724

Glycopyrrolate (Co-administration of tiotropium with other anticholinergic-containing drugs (e.g., ipratropium) has not been studied and is therefore not recommended).

No products indexed under this heading.

Hyoscyamine (Co-administration of tiotropium with other anticholinergic-containing drugs (e.g., ipratropium) has not been studied and is therefore not recommended).

No products indexed under this heading.

Hyoscyamine Sulfate (Co-administration of tiotropium with other anticholinergic-containing drugs (e.g., ipratropium) has not been studied and is therefore not recommended).

No products indexed under this heading.

Ipratropium Bromide (Co-administration of tiotropium with other anticholinergic-containing drugs (e.g., ipratropium) has not been studied and is therefore not recommended). Products include:
- Atrovent HFA Inhalation Aerosol 872
- Atrovent Inhalation Solution 868
- Atrovent Nasal Spray 0.03% 869
- Atrovent Nasal Spray 0.06% 870
- Combivent Inhalation Aerosol 878
- DuoNeb Inhalation Solution 1058

Mepenzolate Bromide (Co-administration of tiotropium with other anticholinergic-containing drugs (e.g., ipratropium) has not been studied and is therefore not recommended).

No products indexed under this heading.

Oxybutynin Chloride (Co-administration of tiotropium with other anticholinergic-containing drugs (e.g., ipratropium) has not been studied and is therefore not recommended). Products include:
- Ditropan XL Extended Release Tablets 2391

Procyclidine Hydrochloride (Co-administration of tiotropium with other anticholinergic-containing drugs (e.g., ipratropium) has not been studied and is therefore not recommended).

No products indexed under this heading.

Propantheline Bromide (Co-administration of tiotropium with other anticholinergic-containing drugs (e.g., ipratropium) has not been studied and is therefore not recommended).

No products indexed under this heading.

Scopolamine (Co-administration of tiotropium with other anticholinergic-containing drugs (e.g., ipratropium) has not been studied and is therefore not recommended). Products include:
- Transderm Scōp Transdermal Therapeutic System 2166

Scopolamine Hydrobromide (Co-administration of tiotropium with other anticholinergic-containing drugs (e.g., ipratropium) has not been studied and is therefore not recommended).

No products indexed under this heading.

Tolterodine Tartrate (Co-administration of tiotropium with other anticholinergic-containing drugs (e.g., ipratropium) has not been studied and is therefore not recommended). Products include:
- Detrol Tablets 2626
- Detrol LA Capsules 2629

Tridihexethyl Chloride (Co-administration of tiotropium with other anticholinergic-containing drugs (e.g., ipratropium) has not been studied and is therefore not recommended).

No products indexed under this heading.

Trihexyphenidyl Hydrochloride (Co-administration of tiotropium with other anticholinergic-containing drugs (e.g., ipratropium) has not been studied and is therefore not recommended).

No products indexed under this heading.

ST. JOSEPH 81 MG ASPIRIN

(Aspirin) ▣649

ST. JOSEPH 81 MG ASPIRIN CHEWABLE AND ENTERIC COATED TABLETS

(Aspirin) 1841

May interact with ACE inhibitors, beta blockers, anticoagulants, diuretics, oral hypoglycemic agents, non-steroidal anti-inflammatory agents, phenytoin, valproate, and certain other agents. Compounds in these categories include:

Acarbose (Moderate doses of aspirin may increase the effectiveness of oral hypoglycemic agents leading to hypoglycemia). Products include:
- Precose Tablets 776

Acebutolol Hydrochloride (Decreased hypotensive effects of beta-blockers).

No products indexed under this heading.

Acetazolamide (Co-administration can lead to high serum concentrations of acetazolamide and its toxicity).

No products indexed under this heading.

Acetazolamide Sodium (Co-administration can lead to high serum concentrations of acetazolamide and its toxicity).

No products indexed under this heading.

Amiloride Hydrochloride (Diminished effectiveness of diuretics in patients with underlying renal or cardiovascular disease). Products include:
- Midamor Tablets 2000
- Moduretic Tablets 2003

Anisindione (Patients on anticoagulant therapy are at increased risk of bleeding). Products include:

Miradon Tablets 3056

Ardeparin Sodium (Patients on anticoagulant therapy are at increased risk of bleeding).
No products indexed under this heading.

Atenolol (Decreased hypotensive effects of beta-blockers). Products include:
Tenormin I.V. Injection 698
Tenormin Tablets 695

Benazepril Hydrochloride (Co-administration may result in diminished hyponatremic and hypotensive effects of ACE inhibitors). Products include:
Lotensin Tablets 2232
Lotensin HCT Tablets 2235
Lotrel Capsules 2238

Bendroflumethiazide (Diminished effectiveness of diuretics in patients with underlying renal or cardiovascular disease).
No products indexed under this heading.

Betaxolol Hydrochloride (Decreased hypotensive effects of beta-blockers). Products include:
Betoptic S Ophthalmic Suspension.................................. 554

Bisoprolol Fumarate (Decreased hypotensive effects of beta-blockers).
No products indexed under this heading.

Bumetanide (Diminished effectiveness of diuretics in patients with underlying renal or cardiovascular disease).
No products indexed under this heading.

Captopril (Co-administration may result in diminished hyponatremic and hypotensive effects of ACE inhibitors). Products include:
Captopril Tablets 2114

Carteolol Hydrochloride (Decreased hypotensive effects of beta-blockers). Products include:
Carteolol Hydrochloride Ophthalmic Solution USP, 1%....... ⊙ 246

Celecoxib (Co-administration may increase bleeding or lead to decreased renal function). Products include:
Celebrex Capsules 3130

Chlorothiazide (Diminished effectiveness of diuretics in patients with underlying renal or cardiovascular disease). Products include:
Aldoclor Tablets 1881
Diuril Oral 1936

Chlorothiazide Sodium (Diminished effectiveness of diuretics in patients with underlying renal or cardiovascular disease). Products include:
Diuril Sodium Intravenous 1934

Chlorpropamide (Moderate doses of aspirin may increase the effectiveness of oral hypoglycemic agents leading to hypoglycemia).
No products indexed under this heading.

Chlorthalidone (Diminished effectiveness of diuretics in patients with underlying renal or cardiovascular disease). Products include:
Clorpres Tablets 2139

Dalteparin Sodium (Patients on anticoagulant therapy are at increased risk of bleeding). Products include:
Fragmin Injection 2638

Danaparoid Sodium (Patients on anticoagulant therapy are at increased risk of bleeding).
No products indexed under this heading.

Diclofenac Potassium (Co-administration may increase bleeding or lead to decreased renal function). Products include:
Cataflam Tablets 2173

Diclofenac Sodium (Co-administration may increase bleeding or lead to decreased renal function). Products include:
Arthrotec Tablets 3126
Voltaren Ophthalmic Solution 2300
Voltaren Tablets 2298
Voltaren-XR Tablets 2301

Dicumarol (Patients on anticoagulant therapy are at increased risk of bleeding).
No products indexed under this heading.

Divalproex Sodium (Salicylate can displace protein-bound valproic acid leading to an increase in serum valproic acid levels). Products include:
Depakote Sprinkle Capsules 422
Depakote Tablets 427
Depakote ER Tablets 433

Enalapril Maleate (Co-administration may result in diminished hyponatremic and hypotensive effects of ACE inhibitors). Products include:
Vaseretic Tablets 2073
Vasotec I.V. Injection 2076

Enalaprilat (Co-administration may result in diminished hyponatremic and hypotensive effects of ACE inhibitors).
No products indexed under this heading.

Enoxaparin Sodium (Patients on anticoagulant therapy are at increased risk of bleeding). Products include:
Lovenox Injection 2931

Esmolol Hydrochloride (Decreased hypotensive effects of beta-blockers). Products include:
Brevibloc Concentrate 766
Brevibloc Injection 766
Brevibloc Double Strength Injection.. 766
Brevibloc Premixed Injection 766
Brevibloc Double Strength Premixed Injection......................... 766

Ethacrynic Acid (Diminished effectiveness of diuretics in patients with underlying renal or cardiovascular disease). Products include:
Edecrin Tablets 1941

Etodolac (Co-administration may increase bleeding or lead to decreased renal function).
No products indexed under this heading.

Fenoprofen Calcium (Co-administration may increase bleeding or lead to decreased renal function). Products include:
Nalfon Capsules 2504

Flurbiprofen (Co-administration may increase bleeding or lead to decreased renal function).
No products indexed under this heading.

Fondaparinux Sodium (Patients on anticoagulant therapy are at increased risk of bleeding). Products include:
Arixtra Injection 1325

Fosinopril Sodium (Co-administration may result in diminished hyponatremic and hypotensive effects of ACE inhibitors).
No products indexed under this heading.

Fosphenytoin Sodium (Salicylate can displace protein-bound phenytoin leading to a decrease in the total concentration of phenytoin).
No products indexed under this heading.

Furosemide (Diminished effectiveness of diuretics in patients with underlying renal or cardiovascular disease). Products include:
Furosemide Tablets 2117

Glimepiride (Moderate doses of aspirin may increase the effectiveness of oral hypoglycemic agents leading to hypoglycemia). Products include:
Amaryl Tablets 2864

Glipizide (Moderate doses of aspirin may increase the effectiveness of oral hypoglycemic agents leading to hypoglycemia).
No products indexed under this heading.

Glyburide (Moderate doses of aspirin may increase the effectiveness of oral hypoglycemic agents leading to hypoglycemia).
No products indexed under this heading.

Heparin Calcium (Patients on anticoagulant therapy are at increased risk of bleeding).
No products indexed under this heading.

Heparin Sodium (Aspirin can increase the anticoagulant activity of heparin increasing bleeding risk).
No products indexed under this heading.

Hydrochlorothiazide (Diminished effectiveness of diuretics in patients with underlying renal or cardiovascular disease). Products include:
Aldoril Tablets 1884
Atacand HCT 637
Avalide Tablets 2889
Avalide Tablets 922
Benicar HCT Tablets 2852
Diovan HCT Tablets 2195
Dyazide Capsules 1389
Hyzaar 1964
Lotensin HCT Tablets 2235
Maxzide 2150
Micardis HCT Tablets 886
Moduretic Tablets 2003
Prinzide Tablets 2033
Teveten HCT Tablets 1710
Timolide Tablets 2056
Uniretic Tablets 3114
Vaseretic Tablets 2073
Zestoretic Tablets 701

Hydroflumethiazide (Diminished effectiveness of diuretics in patients with underlying renal or cardiovascular disease).
No products indexed under this heading.

Ibuprofen (Co-administration may increase bleeding or lead to decreased renal function). Products include:
Advil Allergy Sinus Caplets .... ▣ 737
Advil .... ▣ 737
Children's Advil Suspension .... ▣ 742
Children's Advil Chewable Tablets .. ▣ 741
Advil Cold & Sinus .... ▣ 739
Advil Flu & Body Ache Caplets .... ▣ 739
Children's Advil Cold Suspension .... ▣ 741
Infants' Advil Concentrated Drops .. ▣ 743
Junior Strength Advil Swallow Tablets.. ▣ 740
Advil Migraine Liquigels .... ▣ 740
Advil Multi-Symptom Cold Caplets.. ▣ 738
Combunox Tablets 1183
Children's Motrin Oral Suspension and Chewable Tablets.................. 1837
Children's Motrin Cold Non-Staining Dye-Free Oral Suspension 1838
Children's Motrin Cold Oral Suspension 1838
Children's Motrin Non-Staining Dye-Free Oral Suspension............ 1837
Motrin Cold & Sinus Caplets 1836
Motrin IB Tablets and Caplets 1836
Infants' Motrin Concentrated Drops.. 1837
Infants' Motrin Non-Staining Dye-Free Drops............................ 1837
Junior Strength Motrin Caplets and Chewable Tablets.................. 1837
Vicoprofen Tablets 533

Indapamide (Diminished effectiveness of diuretics in patients with underlying renal or cardiovascular disease). Products include:
Indapamide Tablets 2119

Indomethacin (Co-administration may increase bleeding or lead to decreased renal function). Products include:
Indocin 1968

Indomethacin Sodium Trihydrate (Co-administration may increase bleeding or lead to decreased renal function). Products include:
Indocin I.V. 1973

Ketoprofen (Co-administration may increase bleeding or lead to decreased renal function).
No products indexed under this heading.

Ketorolac Tromethamine (Co-administration may increase bleeding or lead to decreased renal function). Products include:
Acular Ophthalmic Solution 561
Acular LS Ophthalmic Solution 562

Labetalol Hydrochloride (Decreased hypotensive effects of beta-blockers).
No products indexed under this heading.

Levobunolol Hydrochloride (Decreased hypotensive effects of beta-blockers). Products include:
Betagan Ophthalmic Solution, USP.. ⊙ 217

Lisinopril (Co-administration may result in diminished hyponatremic and hypotensive effects of ACE inhibitors). Products include:
Prinivil Tablets 2029
Prinzide Tablets 2033
Zestoretic Tablets 701
Zestril Tablets 704

Low Molecular Weight Heparins (Patients on anticoagulant therapy are at increased risk of bleeding).
No products indexed under this heading.

Meclofenamate Sodium (Co-administration may increase bleeding or lead to decreased renal function).
No products indexed under this heading.

Mefenamic Acid (Co-administration may increase bleeding or lead to decreased renal function).
No products indexed under this heading.

Meloxicam (Co-administration may increase bleeding or lead to decreased renal function). Products include:
Mobic Oral Suspension 893

Mobic Tablets 893

Metformin Hydrochloride (Moderate doses of aspirin may increase the effectiveness of oral hypoglycemic agents leading to hypoglycemia). Products include:
ActoPlus Met Tablets 3219
Avandamet Tablets 1343
Fortamet Extended-Release Tablets 1156

Methotrexate Sodium (Salicylate can inhibit renal clearance of methotrexate leading to bone marrow toxicity, especially in the elderly or renal impaired).
No products indexed under this heading.

Methyclothiazide (Diminished effectiveness of diuretics in patients with underlying renal or cardiovascular disease).
No products indexed under this heading.

Metipranolol Hydrochloride (Decreased hypotensive effects of beta-blockers).
No products indexed under this heading.

Metolazone (Diminished effectiveness of diuretics in patients with underlying renal or cardiovascular disease).
No products indexed under this heading.

Metoprolol Succinate (Decreased hypotensive effects of beta-blockers). Products include:
Toprol-XL Tablets 660

Metoprolol Tartrate (Decreased hypotensive effects of beta-blockers).
No products indexed under this heading.

Miglitol (Moderate doses of aspirin may increase the effectiveness of oral hypoglycemic agents leading to hypoglycemia).
No products indexed under this heading.

Moexipril Hydrochloride (Co-administration may result in diminished hyponatremic and hypotensive effects of ACE inhibitors). Products include:
Uniretic Tablets 3114
Univasc Tablets 3118

Nabumetone (Co-administration may increase bleeding or lead to decreased renal function). Products include:
Relafen Tablets 1523

Nadolol (Decreased hypotensive effects of beta-blockers). Products include:
Nadolol Tablets 2121

Naproxen (Co-administration may increase bleeding or lead to decreased renal function). Products include:
EC-Naprosyn Delayed-Release Tablets 2769
Naprosyn Suspension 2769
Naprosyn Tablets 2769
Prevacid NapraPAC 3277

Naproxen Sodium (Co-administration may increase bleeding or lead to decreased renal function). Products include:
Aleve Tablets, Caplets and Gelcaps .... ▣605
Anaprox Tablets 2769
Anaprox DS Tablets 2769

Oxaprozin (Co-administration may increase bleeding or lead to decreased renal function).
No products indexed under this heading.

Penbutolol Sulfate (Decreased hypotensive effects of beta-blockers).
No products indexed under this heading.

Perindopril Erbumine (Co-administration may result in diminished hyponatremic and hypotensive effects of ACE inhibitors). Products include:
Aceon Tablets (2 mg, 4 mg, 8 mg) 3191

Phenylbutazone (Co-administration may increase bleeding or lead to decreased renal function).
No products indexed under this heading.

Phenytoin (Salicylate can displace protein-bound phenytoin leading to a decrease in the total concentration of phenytoin).
No products indexed under this heading.

Phenytoin Sodium (Salicylate can displace protein-bound phenytoin leading to a decrease in the total concentration of phenytoin). Products include:
Phenytek Capsules 2153

Pindolol (Decreased hypotensive effects of beta-blockers).
No products indexed under this heading.

Pioglitazone Hydrochloride (Moderate doses of aspirin may increase the effectiveness of oral hypoglycemic agents leading to hypoglycemia). Products include:
ActoPlus Met Tablets 3219
Actos Tablets 3224

Piroxicam (Co-administration may increase bleeding or lead to decreased renal function).
No products indexed under this heading.

Polythiazide (Diminished effectiveness of diuretics in patients with underlying renal or cardiovascular disease).
No products indexed under this heading.

Probenecid (Salicylate antagonizes the uricosuric action of probenecid).
No products indexed under this heading.

Propranolol Hydrochloride (Decreased hypotensive effects of beta-blockers). Products include:
Inderal LA Long-Acting Capsules 3421
InnoPran XL Capsules 2728

Quinapril Hydrochloride (Co-administration may result in diminished hyponatremic and hypotensive effects of ACE inhibitors).
No products indexed under this heading.

Ramipril (Co-administration may result in diminished hyponatremic and hypotensive effects of ACE inhibitors). Products include:
Altace Capsules 1673

Repaglinide (Moderate doses of aspirin may increase the effectiveness of oral hypoglycemic agents leading to hypoglycemia). Products include:
Prandin Tablets (0.5, 1, and 2 mg) 2337

Rofecoxib (Co-administration may increase bleeding or lead to decreased renal function).
No products indexed under this heading.

Rosiglitazone Maleate (Moderate doses of aspirin may increase the effectiveness of oral hypoglycemic agents leading to hypoglycemia). Products include:
Avandamet Tablets 1343
Avandia Tablets 1348

Sotalol Hydrochloride (Decreased hypotensive effects of beta-blockers).
No products indexed under this heading.

Spirapril Hydrochloride (Co-administration may result in diminished hyponatremic and hypotensive effects of ACE inhibitors).
No products indexed under this heading.

Spironolactone (Diminished effectiveness of diuretics in patients with underlying renal or cardiovascular disease).
No products indexed under this heading.

Sulfinpyrazone (Salicylate antagonizes the uricosuric action of sulfinpyrazone).
No products indexed under this heading.

Sulindac (Co-administration may increase bleeding or lead to decreased renal function). Products include:
Clinoril Tablets 1899

Timolol Hemihydrate (Decreased hypotensive effects of beta-blockers). Products include:
Betimol Ophthalmic Solution 3371
Betimol Ophthalmic Solution .... ⊙283

Timolol Maleate (Decreased hypotensive effects of beta-blockers). Products include:
Blocadren Tablets 1891
Cosopt Sterile Ophthalmic Solution 1910
Timolide Tablets 2056
Timoptic in Ocudose 2061
Timoptic Sterile Ophthalmic Solution 2058
Timoptic-XE Sterile Ophthalmic Gel Forming Solution 2062

Tinzaparin Sodium (Patients on anticoagulant therapy are at increased risk of bleeding).
No products indexed under this heading.

Tolazamide (Moderate doses of aspirin may increase the effectiveness of oral hypoglycemic agents leading to hypoglycemia).
No products indexed under this heading.

Tolbutamide (Moderate doses of aspirin may increase the effectiveness of oral hypoglycemic agents leading to hypoglycemia).
No products indexed under this heading.

Tolmetin Sodium (Co-administration may increase bleeding or lead to decreased renal function).
No products indexed under this heading.

Torsemide (Diminished effectiveness of diuretics in patients with underlying renal or cardiovascular disease).
No products indexed under this heading.

Trandolapril (Co-administration may result in diminished hyponatremic and hypotensive effects of ACE inhibitors). Products include:
Mavik Tablets 482
Tarka Tablets 519

Triamterene (Diminished effectiveness of diuretics in patients with underlying renal or cardiovascular disease). Products include:
Dyazide Capsules 1389
Dyrenium Capsules 3390
Maxzide 2150

Troglitazone (Moderate doses of aspirin may increase the effectiveness of oral hypoglycemic agents leading to hypoglycemia).
No products indexed under this heading.

Valdecoxib (Co-administration may increase bleeding or lead to decreased renal function).
No products indexed under this heading.

Valproate Sodium (Salicylate can displace protein-bound valproic acid leading to an increase in serum valproic acid levels). Products include:
Depacon Injection 412

Valproic Acid (Salicylate can displace protein-bound valproic acid leading to an increase in serum valproic acid levels). Products include:
Depakene 417

Warfarin Sodium (Aspirin can displace Warfarin from protein binding sites leading to prolongation of both the prothrombin time and the bleeding time). Products include:
Coumadin for Injection 932
Coumadin Tablets 932

Food Interactions

Alcohol (Chronic heavy alcohol users, 3 or more drinks per day, in combination with analgesic/antipyretic drug products containing aspirin increases the risk of adverse GI events, including stomach bleeding).

STALEVO TABLETS

(Carbidopa, Entacapone, Levodopa) 2270

May interact with antihypertensives, drugs metabolized by Catechol-*O*-methytransferase, dopamine D2 antagonists, iron containing oral preparations, monoamine oxidase inhibitors, tricyclic antidepressants, and certain other agents. Compounds in these categories include:

Acebutolol Hydrochloride (Symptomatic postural hypotension has occurred when carbidopa-levodopa was added to the treatment of a patient receiving antihypertensive drugs).
No products indexed under this heading.

Amitriptyline Hydrochloride (There have been rare reports of adverse reactions, including hypertension and dyskinesia, resulting from the concomitant use of tricylic antidepressants and carbidopa-levodopa).
No products indexed under this heading.

Amlodipine Besylate (Symptomatic postural hypotension has occurred when carbidopa-levodopa was added to the treatment of a patient receiving antihypertensive drugs). Products include:
Caduet Tablets 2507
Lotrel Capsules 2238
Norvasc Tablets 2529

Amoxapine (There have been rare reports of adverse reactions, including hypertension and dyskinesia, resulting from the concomitant use of tricylic antidepressants and carbidopa-levodopa).
No products indexed under this heading.

Ampicillin (As most entacapone excretion is via the bile, caution should be exercised when drugs known to interfere with biliary excretion, glucuronidation, and intestinal beta-glucuronidase are given concurrently with entacapone).
No products indexed under this heading.

Ampicillin Sodium (As most entacapone excretion is via the bile, caution should be exercised when drugs known to interfere with biliary excretion, glucuronidation, and intestinal beta-glucuronidase are given concurrently with entacapone).
No products indexed under this heading.

Ampicillin Trihydrate (As most entacapone excretion is via the bile, caution should be exercised when drugs known to interfere with biliary excretion, glucuronidation, and intestinal beta-glucuronidase are given concurrently with entacapone).
No products indexed under this heading.

Apomorphine (Drugs known to be metabolized by COMT should be administered with caution in patients receiving entacapone regardless of the route of administration (including inhalation), as their interaction may result in increased heart rates, possibly arrhythmias, and excessive changes in blood pressure).
No products indexed under this heading.

Atenolol (Symptomatic postural hypotension has occurred when carbidopa-levodopa was added to the treatment of a patient receiving antihypertensive drugs). Products include:
Tenormin I.V. Injection 698
Tenormin Tablets 695

Bacampicillin Hydrochloride (As most entacapone excretion is via the bile, caution should be exercised when drugs known to interfere with biliary excretion, glucuronidation, and intestinal beta-glucuronidase are given concurrently with entacapone).
No products indexed under this heading.

Benazepril Hydrochloride (Symptomatic postural hypotension has occurred when carbidopa-levodopa was added to the treatment of a patient receiving antihypertensive drugs). Products include:
Lotensin Tablets 2232
Lotensin HCT Tablets 2235
Lotrel Capsules 2238

Bendroflumethiazide (Symptomatic postural hypotension has occurred when carbidopa-levodopa was added to the treatment of a patient receiving antihypertensive drugs).
No products indexed under this heading.

Betaxolol Hydrochloride (Symptomatic postural hypotension has occurred when carbidopa-levodopa was added to the treatment of a patient receiving antihypertensive drugs). Products include:
Betoptic S Ophthalmic Suspension 554

Bisoprolol Fumarate (Symptomatic postural hypotension has occurred when carbidopa-levodopa was added to the treatment of a patient receiving antihypertensive drugs).
No products indexed under this heading.

Bitolterol Mesylate (Drugs known to be metabolized by COMT should be administered with caution in patients receiving entacapone regardless of the route of administration (including inhalation), as their interaction may result in increased heart rates, possibly arrhythmias, and excessive changes in blood pressure).
No products indexed under this heading.

Candesartan Cilexetil (Symptomatic postural hypotension has occurred when carbidopa-levodopa was added to the treatment of a patient receiving antihypertensive drugs). Products include:
Atacand Tablets 634
Atacand HCT 637

Captopril (Symptomatic postural hypotension has occurred when carbidopa-levodopa was added to the treatment of a patient receiving antihypertensive drugs). Products include:
Captopril Tablets 2114

Carteolol Hydrochloride (Symptomatic postural hypotension has occurred when carbidopa-levodopa was added to the treatment of a patient receiving antihypertensive drugs). Products include:
Carteolol Hydrochloride Ophthalmic Solution USP, 1%....... ⊙246

Chloramphenicol (As most entacapone excretion is via the bile, caution should be exercised when drugs known to interfere with biliary excretion, glucuronidation, and intestinal beta-glucuronidase are given concurrently with entacapone).
No products indexed under this heading.

Chloramphenicol Palmitate (As most entacapone excretion is via the bile, caution should be exercised when drugs known to interfere with biliary excretion, glucuronidation, and intestinal beta-glucuronidase are given concurrently with entacapone).
No products indexed under this heading.

Chloramphenicol Sodium Succinate (As most entacapone excretion is via the bile, caution should be exercised when drugs known to interfere with biliary excretion, glucuronidation, and intestinal beta-glucuronidase are given concurrently with entacapone).
No products indexed under this heading.

Chlorothiazide (Symptomatic postural hypotension has occurred when carbidopa-levodopa was added to the treatment of a patient receiving antihypertensive drugs). Products include:
Aldoclor Tablets 1881
Diuril Oral 1936

Chlorothiazide Sodium (Symptomatic postural hypotension has occurred when carbidopa-levodopa was added to the treatment of a patient receiving antihypertensive drugs). Products include:
Diuril Sodium Intravenous 1934

Chlorpromazine (Dopamine D2 receptor antagonists may reduce the therapeutic effects of levodopa).
No products indexed under this heading.

Chlorpromazine Hydrochloride (Dopamine D2 receptor antagonists may reduce the therapeutic effects of levodopa).
No products indexed under this heading.

Chlorprothixene (Dopamine D2 receptor antagonists may reduce the therapeutic effects of levodopa).
No products indexed under this heading.

Chlorprothixene Hydrochloride (Dopamine D2 receptor antagonists may reduce the therapeutic effects of levodopa).
No products indexed under this heading.

Chlorthalidone (Symptomatic postural hypotension has occurred when carbidopa-levodopa was added to the treatment of a patient receiving antihypertensive drugs). Products include:
Clorpres Tablets 2139

Cholestyramine (As most entacapone excretion is via the bile, caution should be exercised when drugs known to interfere with biliary excretion, glucuronidation, and intestinal beta-glucuronidase are given concurrently with entacapone).
No products indexed under this heading.

Clomipramine Hydrochloride (There have been rare reports of adverse reactions, including hypertension and dyskinesia, resulting from the concomitant use of tricylic antidepressants and carbidopa-levodopa).
No products indexed under this heading.

Clonidine (Symptomatic postural hypotension has occurred when carbidopa-levodopa was added to the treatment of a patient receiving antihypertensive drugs). Products include:
Catapres-TTS 875

Clonidine Hydrochloride (Symptomatic postural hypotension has occurred when carbidopa-levodopa was added to the treatment of a patient receiving antihypertensive drugs). Products include:
Catapres Tablets 874
Clorpres Tablets 2139

Deserpidine (Symptomatic postural hypotension has occurred when carbidopa-levodopa was added to the treatment of a patient receiving antihypertensive drugs).
No products indexed under this heading.

Desipramine Hydrochloride (There have been rare reports of adverse reactions, including hypertension and dyskinesia, resulting from the concomitant use of tricylic antidepressants and carbidopa-levodopa).
No products indexed under this heading.

Diazoxide (Symptomatic postural hypotension has occurred when carbidopa-levodopa was added to the treatment of a patient receiving antihypertensive drugs). Products include:
Hyperstat I.V. Injection 3031

Diltiazem Hydrochloride (Symptomatic postural hypotension has occurred when carbidopa-levodopa was added to the treatment of a patient receiving antihypertensive drugs). Products include:
Cardizem LA Extended Release Tablets 1699
Tiazac Capsules 1204

Dobutamine Hydrochloride (Drugs known to be metabolized by COMT should be administered with caution in patients receiving entacapone regardless of the route of administration (including inhalation), as their interaction may result in increased heart rates, possibly arrhythmias, and excessive changes in blood pressure).
No products indexed under this heading.

Dopamine Hydrochloride (Drugs known to be metabolized by COMT should be administered with caution in patients receiving entacapone regardless of the route of administration (including inhalation), as their interaction may result in increased heart rates, possibly arrhythmias, and excessive changes in blood pressure).
No products indexed under this heading.

Doxazosin Mesylate (Symptomatic postural hypotension has occurred when carbidopa-levodopa was added to the treatment of a patient receiving antihypertensive drugs).
No products indexed under this heading.

Doxepin Hydrochloride (There have been rare reports of adverse reactions, including hypertension and dyskinesia, resulting from the concomitant use of tricylic antidepressants and carbidopa-levodopa).
No products indexed under this heading.

Enalapril Maleate (Symptomatic postural hypotension has occurred when carbidopa-levodopa was added to the treatment of a patient receiving antihypertensive drugs). Products include:
Vaseretic Tablets 2073
Vasotec I.V. Injection 2076

Enalaprilat (Symptomatic postural hypotension has occurred when carbidopa-levodopa was added to the treatment of a patient receiving antihypertensive drugs).
No products indexed under this heading.

Epinephrine (Drugs known to be metabolized by COMT should be administered with caution in patients receiving entacapone regardless of the route of administration (including inhalation), as their interaction may result in increased heart rates, possibly arrhythmias, and excessive changes in blood pressure). Products include:
EpiPen 1061
Primatene Mist .... ▣749

Epinephrine Bitartrate (Drugs known to be metabolized by COMT should be administered with caution in patients receiving entacapone regardless of the route of administration (including inhalation), as their interaction may result in increased heart rates, possibly arrhythmias, and excessive changes in blood pressure).
No products indexed under this heading.

Epinephrine Hydrochloride (Drugs known to be metabolized by COMT should be administered with caution in patients receiving entacapone regardless of the route of administration (including inhalation), as their interaction may result in increased heart rates, possibly arrhythmias, and excessive changes in blood pressure).
No products indexed under this heading.

Eprosartan Mesylate (Symptomatic postural hypotension has occurred when carbidopa-levodopa was added to the treatment of a patient receiving antihypertensive drugs). Products include:
Teveten Tablets 1707
Teveten HCT Tablets 1710

Erythromycin (As most entacapone excretion is via the bile, caution should be exercised when drugs known to interfere with biliary excretion, glucuronidation, and intestinal beta-glucuronidase are given concurrently with entacapone). Products include:
Erygel Topical Gel 2096
Ery-Tab Tablets 447
Erythromycin Base Filmtab Tablets 454
Erythromycin Delayed-Release Capsules, USP 456
PCE Dispertab Tablets 510

Erythromycin Enteric Coated Tablets (As most entacapone excretion is via the bile, caution should be exercised when drugs known to interfere with biliary excretion, glucuronidation, and intestinal beta-glucuronidase are given concurrently with entacapone).
No products indexed under this heading.

Erythromycin Estolate (As most entacapone excretion is via the bile, caution should be exercised when drugs known to interfere with biliary excretion, glucuronidation, and intestinal beta-glucuronidase are given concurrently with entacapone).
No products indexed under this heading.

Erythromycin Ethylsuccinate (As most entacapone excretion is via the bile, caution should be exercised when drugs known to interfere with biliary excretion, glucuronidation, and intestinal beta-glucuronidase are given concurrently with entacapone). Products include:
E.E.S. 449
EryPed 445

Erythromycin Gluceptate (As most entacapone excretion is via the bile, caution should be exercised when drugs known to interfere with biliary excretion, glucuronidation, and intestinal beta-glucuronidase are given concurrently with entacapone).
No products indexed under this heading.

Erythromycin Lactobionate (As most entacapone excretion is via the bile, caution should be exercised when drugs known to interfere with biliary excretion, glucuronidation, and intestinal beta-glucuronidase are given concurrently with entacapone).
No products indexed under this heading.

Erythromycin Stearate (As most entacapone excretion is via the bile, caution should be exercised when drugs known to interfere with biliary excretion, glucuronidation, and intestinal beta-glucuronidase are given concurrently with entacapone). Products include:
Erythrocin Stearate Filmtab Tablets 452

Esmolol Hydrochloride (Symptomatic postural hypotension has occurred when carbidopa-levodopa was added to the treatment of a patient receiving antihypertensive drugs). Products include:
Brevibloc Concentrate 766
Brevibloc Injection 766
Brevibloc Double Strength Injection 766
Brevibloc Premixed Injection 766
Brevibloc Double Strength Premixed Injection 766

Ethylpapaverine Hydrochloride (The beneficial effects of levodopa in Parkinson's disease have been reported to be reversed by papaverine).
No products indexed under this heading.

Felodipine (Symptomatic postural hypotension has occurred when carbidopa-levodopa was added to the treatment of a patient receiving antihypertensive drugs). Products include:
Plendil Extended-Release Tablets 651

Ferrous Fumarate (Iron salts may reduce the bioavailability of levodopa, carbidopa and entacapone). Products include:
Chromagen Forte Soft Gelatin Capsules 3296
Ferretts Tablets .... ▣773
Repliva 21/7 Tablets 3301

Ferrous Gluconate (Iron salts may reduce the bioavailability of levodopa, carbidopa and entacapone).
No products indexed under this heading.

Ferrous Sulfate (Iron salts may reduce the bioavailability of levodopa, carbidopa and entacapone). Products include:
Feosol Tablets 1629
Slow Fe Iron Tablets .... ▣772
Slow Fe with Folic Acid Tablets .... ▣773

Fluphenazine Decanoate (Dopamine D2 receptor antagonists may reduce the therapeutic effects of levodopa).
No products indexed under this heading.

Fluphenazine Enanthate (Dopamine D2 receptor antagonists may reduce the therapeutic effects of levodopa).
No products indexed under this heading.

Fluphenazine Hydrochloride (Dopamine D2 receptor antagonists may reduce the therapeutic effects of levodopa).
No products indexed under this heading.

Fosinopril Sodium (Symptomatic postural hypotension has occurred when carbidopa-levodopa was added to the treatment of a patient receiving antihypertensive drugs).
No products indexed under this heading.

Fosphenytoin (The beneficial effects of levodopa in Parkinson's disease have been reported to be reversed by phenytoin).
No products indexed under this heading.

Fosphenytoin Sodium (The beneficial effects of levodopa in Parkinson's disease have been reported to be reversed by phenytoin).
No products indexed under this heading.

Furosemide (Symptomatic postural hypotension has occurred when carbidopa-levodopa was added to the treatment of a patient receiving antihypertensive drugs). Products include:
Furosemide Tablets 2117

Guanabenz Acetate (Symptomatic postural hypotension has occurred when carbidopa-levodopa was added to the treatment of a patient receiving antihypertensive drugs).
No products indexed under this heading.

Guanethidine Monosulfate (Symptomatic postural hypotension has occurred when carbidopa-levodopa was added to the treatment of a patient receiving antihypertensive drugs).
No products indexed under this heading.

Haloperidol (Dopamine D2 receptor antagonists may reduce the therapeutic effects of levodopa).
No products indexed under this heading.

Haloperidol Decanoate (Dopamine D2 receptor antagonists may reduce the therapeutic effects of levodopa).
No products indexed under this heading.

Hydralazine Hydrochloride (Symptomatic postural hypotension has occurred when carbidopa-levodopa was added to the treatment of a patient receiving antihypertensive drugs). Products include:
BiDil Tablets 2161

Hydrochlorothiazide (Symptomatic postural hypotension has occurred when carbidopa-levodopa was added to the treatment of a patient receiving antihypertensive drugs). Products include:
Aldoril Tablets 1884
Atacand HCT 637
Avalide Tablets 2889
Avalide Tablets 922
Benicar HCT Tablets 2852
Diovan HCT Tablets 2195
Dyazide Capsules 1389
Hyzaar 1964
Lotensin HCT Tablets 2235
Maxzide 2150
Micardis HCT Tablets 886
Moduretic Tablets 2003
Prinzide Tablets 2033
Teveten HCT Tablets 1710
Timolide Tablets 2056
Uniretic Tablets 3114
Vaseretic Tablets 2073
Zestoretic Tablets 701

Hydroflumethiazide (Symptomatic postural hypotension has occurred when carbidopa-levodopa was added to the treatment of a patient receiving antihypertensive drugs).
No products indexed under this heading.

Imipramine Hydrochloride (There have been rare reports of adverse reactions, including hypertension and dyskinesia, resulting from the concomitant use of tricylic antidepressants and carbidopa-levodopa).
No products indexed under this heading.

Imipramine Pamoate (There have been rare reports of adverse reactions, including hypertension and dyskinesia, resulting from the concomitant use of tricylic antidepressants and carbidopa-levodopa).
No products indexed under this heading.

Indapamide (Symptomatic postural hypotension has occurred when carbidopa-levodopa was added to the treatment of a patient receiving antihypertensive drugs). Products include:
Indapamide Tablets 2119

Irbesartan (Symptomatic postural hypotension has occurred when carbidopa-levodopa was added to the treatment of a patient receiving antihypertensive drugs). Products include:
Avalide Tablets 922
Avalide Tablets 2889
Avapro Tablets 925
Avapro Tablets 2886

Iron (Iron salts may reduce the bioavailability of levodopa, carbidopa and entacapone). Products include:
Chromagen Forte Soft Gelatin Capsules 3296
Ferretts IPS Liquid .... ▣773
OptiNate 1162
Repliva 21/7 Tablets 3301

Isocarboxazid (Nonselective monoamine oxidase (MAO) inhibitors are contraindicated for use with Stalevo).
No products indexed under this heading.

Isoetharine (Drugs known to be metabolized by COMT should be administered with caution in patients receiving entacapone regardless of the route of administration (including inhalation), as their interaction may result in increased heart rates, possibly arrhythmias, and excessive changes in blood pressure).
No products indexed under this heading.

Isoniazid (Isoniazid may reduce the therapeutic effects of levodopa).
No products indexed under this heading.

Isoproterenol Hydrochloride (Drugs known to be metabolized by COMT should be administered with caution in patients receiving entacapone regardless of the route of administration (including inhalation), as their interaction may result in increased heart rates, possibly arrhythmias, and excessive changes in blood pressure).
No products indexed under this heading.

Isoproterenol Sulfate (Drugs known to be metabolized by COMT should be administered with caution in patients receiving entacapone regardless of the route of administration (including inhalation), as their interaction may result in increased heart rates, possibly arrhythmias, and excessive changes in blood pressure).
No products indexed under this heading.

Isradipine (Symptomatic postural hypotension has occurred when carbidopa-levodopa was added to the treatment of a patient receiving antihypertensive drugs). Products include:
DynaCirc CR Tablets 2726

Labetalol Hydrochloride (Symptomatic postural hypotension has occurred when carbidopa-levodopa was added to the treatment of a patient receiving antihypertensive drugs).
No products indexed under this heading.

Lisinopril (Symptomatic postural hypotension has occurred when carbidopa-levodopa was added to the treatment of a patient receiving antihypertensive drugs). Products include:
Prinivil Tablets ... 2029
Prinzide Tablets ... 2033
Zestoretic Tablets ... 701
Zestril Tablets ... 704

Losartan Potassium (Symptomatic postural hypotension has occurred when carbidopa-levodopa was added to the treatment of a patient receiving antihypertensive drugs). Products include:
Cozaar Tablets ... 1913
Hyzaar ... 1964

Loxapine Hydrochloride (Dopamine D2 receptor antagonists may reduce the therapeutic effects of levodopa).
No products indexed under this heading.

Loxapine Succinate (Dopamine D2 receptor antagonists may reduce the therapeutic effects of levodopa).
No products indexed under this heading.

Maprotiline Hydrochloride (There have been rare reports of adverse reactions, including hypertension and dyskinesia, resulting from the concomitant use of tricylic antidepressants and carbidopa-levodopa).
No products indexed under this heading.

Mecamylamine Hydrochloride (Symptomatic postural hypotension has occurred when carbidopa-levodopa was added to the treatment of a patient receiving antihypertensive drugs). Products include:
Inversine Tablets ... 3286

Mephenytoin (The beneficial effects of levodopa in Parkinson's disease have been reported to be reversed by phenytoin).
No products indexed under this heading.

Mesoridazine Besylate (Dopamine D2 receptor antagonists may reduce the therapeutic effects of levodopa).
No products indexed under this heading.

Methotrimeprazine (Dopamine D2 receptor antagonists may reduce the therapeutic effects of levodopa).
No products indexed under this heading.

Methyclothiazide (Symptomatic postural hypotension has occurred when carbidopa-levodopa was added to the treatment of a patient receiving antihypertensive drugs).
No products indexed under this heading.

Methyldopa (Drugs known to be metabolized by COMT should be administered with caution in patients receiving entacapone regardless of the route of administration (including inhalation), as their interaction may result in increased heart rates, possibly arrhythmias, and excessive changes in blood pressure). Products include:
Aldoclor Tablets ... 1881
Aldoril Tablets ... 1884

Methyldopate Hydrochloride (Symptomatic postural hypotension has occurred when carbidopa-levodopa was added to the treatment of a patient receiving antihypertensive drugs).
No products indexed under this heading.

Metoclopramide Hydrochloride (Although metoclopramide may increase the bioavailability of levodopa by increasing gastric emptying, metoclopramide may also adversely affect disease control by its dopamine receptor antagonistic properties).
No products indexed under this heading.

Metolazone (Symptomatic postural hypotension has occurred when carbidopa-levodopa was added to the treatment of a patient receiving antihypertensive drugs).
No products indexed under this heading.

Metoprolol Succinate (Symptomatic postural hypotension has occurred when carbidopa-levodopa was added to the treatment of a patient receiving antihypertensive drugs). Products include:
Toprol-XL Tablets ... 660

Metoprolol Tartrate (Symptomatic postural hypotension has occurred when carbidopa-levodopa was added to the treatment of a patient receiving antihypertensive drugs).
No products indexed under this heading.

Metyrosine (Symptomatic postural hypotension has occurred when carbidopa-levodopa was added to the treatment of a patient receiving antihypertensive drugs). Products include:
Demser Capsules ... 1933

Mibefradil Dihydrochloride (Symptomatic postural hypotension has occurred when carbidopa-levodopa was added to the treatment of a patient receiving antihypertensive drugs).
No products indexed under this heading.

Minoxidil (Symptomatic postural hypotension has occurred when carbidopa-levodopa was added to the treatment of a patient receiving antihypertensive drugs). Products include:
Men's Rogaine Extra Strength Topical Solution, Ocean Rush Scent and Original Unscented ... 706
Women's Rogaine Topical Solution, Spring Bloom Scent and Original Unscented ... 707

Moclobemide (Nonselective monoamine oxidase (MAO) inhibitors are contraindicated for use with Stalevo).
No products indexed under this heading.

Moexipril Hydrochloride (Symptomatic postural hypotension has occurred when carbidopa-levodopa was added to the treatment of a patient receiving antihypertensive drugs). Products include:
Uniretic Tablets ... 3114
Univasc Tablets ... 3118

Molindone Hydrochloride (Dopamine D2 receptor antagonists may reduce the therapeutic effects of levodopa). Products include:
Moban Tablets ... 1108

Nadolol (Symptomatic postural hypotension has occurred when carbidopa-levodopa was added to the treatment of a patient receiving antihypertensive drugs). Products include:
Nadolol Tablets ... 2121

Nicardipine Hydrochloride (Symptomatic postural hypotension has occurred when carbidopa-levodopa was added to the treatment of a patient receiving antihypertensive drugs). Products include:
Cardene I.V. ... 1129

Nifedipine (Symptomatic postural hypotension has occurred when carbidopa-levodopa was added to the treatment of a patient receiving antihypertensive drugs). Products include:
Adalat CC Tablets ... 2978

Nisoldipine (Symptomatic postural hypotension has occurred when carbidopa-levodopa was added to the treatment of a patient receiving antihypertensive drugs). Products include:
Sular Tablets ... 1163

Nitroglycerin (Symptomatic postural hypotension has occurred when carbidopa-levodopa was added to the treatment of a patient receiving antihypertensive drugs). Products include:
Nitro-Dur Transdermal Infusion System ... 3060
Nitrolingual Pumpspray ... 1161

Norepinephrine Bitartrate (Drugs known to be metabolized by COMT should be administered with caution in patients receiving entacapone regardless of the route of administration (including inhalation), as their interaction may result in increased heart rates, possibly arrhythmias, and excessive changes in blood pressure).
No products indexed under this heading.

Nortriptyline Hydrochloride (There have been rare reports of adverse reactions, including hypertension and dyskinesia, resulting from the concomitant use of tricylic antidepressants and carbidopa-levodopa).
No products indexed under this heading.

Papaverine (The beneficial effects of levodopa in Parkinson's disease have been reported to be reversed by papaverine).
No products indexed under this heading.

Papaverine Hydrochloride (The beneficial effects of levodopa in Parkinson's disease have been reported to be reversed by papaverine).
No products indexed under this heading.

Pargyline Hydrochloride (Nonselective monoamine oxidase (MAO) inhibitors are contraindicated for use with Stalevo).
No products indexed under this heading.

Penbutolol Sulfate (Symptomatic postural hypotension has occurred when carbidopa-levodopa was added to the treatment of a patient receiving antihypertensive drugs).
No products indexed under this heading.

Perindopril Erbumine (Symptomatic postural hypotension has occurred when carbidopa-levodopa was added to the treatment of a patient receiving antihypertensive drugs). Products include:
Aceon Tablets (2 mg, 4 mg, 8 mg) ... 3191

Perphenazine (Dopamine D2 receptor antagonists may reduce the therapeutic effects of levodopa).
No products indexed under this heading.

Phenelzine Sulfate (Nonselective monoamine oxidase (MAO) inhibitors are contraindicated for use with Stalevo).
No products indexed under this heading.

Phenoxybenzamine Hydrochloride (Symptomatic postural hypotension has occurred when carbidopa-levodopa was added to the treatment of a patient receiving antihypertensive drugs). Products include:
Dibenzyline Capsules ... 3390

Phentolamine Mesylate (Symptomatic postural hypotension has occurred when carbidopa-levodopa was added to the treatment of a patient receiving antihypertensive drugs).
No products indexed under this heading.

Phenytoin (The beneficial effects of levodopa in Parkinson's disease have been reported to be reversed by phenytoin).
No products indexed under this heading.

Phenytoin Sodium (The beneficial effects of levodopa in Parkinson's disease have been reported to be reversed by phenytoin). Products include:
Phenytek Capsules ... 2153

Pindolol (Symptomatic postural hypotension has occurred when carbidopa-levodopa was added to the treatment of a patient receiving antihypertensive drugs).
No products indexed under this heading.

Polysaccharide Iron Complex (Iron salts may reduce the bioavailability of levodopa, carbidopa and entacapone). Products include:
Niferex-150 Forte Capsules ... 3299
Nu-Iron 150 Capsules ... 2098

Polythiazide (Symptomatic postural hypotension has occurred when carbidopa-levodopa was added to the treatment of a patient receiving antihypertensive drugs).
No products indexed under this heading.

Prazosin Hydrochloride (Symptomatic postural hypotension has occurred when carbidopa-levodopa was added to the treatment of a patient receiving antihypertensive drugs).
No products indexed under this heading.

Probenecid (As most entacapone excretion is via the bile, caution should be exercised when drugs known to interfere with biliary excretion, glucuronidation, and intestinal beta-glucuronidase are given concurrently with entacapone).
No products indexed under this heading.

Procarbazine Hydrochloride (Nonselective monoamine oxidase (MAO) inhibitors are contraindicated for use with Stalevo). Products include:

Matulane Capsules 3188

Prochlorperazine (Dopamine D2 receptor antagonists may reduce the therapeutic effects of levodopa).
No products indexed under this heading.

Promethazine Hydrochloride (Dopamine D2 receptor antagonists may reduce the therapeutic effects of levodopa). Products include:
Phenergan 3438

Propranolol Hydrochloride (Symptomatic postural hypotension has occurred when carbidopa-levodopa was added to the treatment of a patient receiving antihypertensive drugs). Products include:
Inderal LA Long-Acting Capsules 3421
InnoPran XL Capsules 2728

Protriptyline Hydrochloride (There have been rare reports of adverse reactions, including hypertension and dyskinesia, resulting from the concomitant use of tricylic antidepressants and carbidopa-levodopa). Products include:
Vivactil Tablets 2350

Quetiapine Fumarate (Dopamine D2 receptor antagonists may reduce the therapeutic effects of levodopa). Products include:
Seroquel Tablets 691

Quinapril Hydrochloride (Symptomatic postural hypotension has occurred when carbidopa-levodopa was added to the treatment of a patient receiving antihypertensive drugs).
No products indexed under this heading.

Ramipril (Symptomatic postural hypotension has occurred when carbidopa-levodopa was added to the treatment of a patient receiving antihypertensive drugs). Products include:
Altace Capsules 1673

Rauwolfia Serpentina (Symptomatic postural hypotension has occurred when carbidopa-levodopa was added to the treatment of a patient receiving antihypertensive drugs).
No products indexed under this heading.

Rescinnamine (Symptomatic postural hypotension has occurred when carbidopa-levodopa was added to the treatment of a patient receiving antihypertensive drugs).
No products indexed under this heading.

Reserpine (Symptomatic postural hypotension has occurred when carbidopa-levodopa was added to the treatment of a patient receiving antihypertensive drugs).
No products indexed under this heading.

Rifampicin (As most entacapone excretion is via the bile, caution should be exercised when drugs known to interfere with biliary excretion, glucuronidation, and intestinal beta-glucuronidase are given concurrently with entacapone).
No products indexed under this heading.

Risperidone (Dopamine D2 receptor antagonists may reduce the therapeutic effects of levodopa). Products include:
Risperdal Consta Long-Acting Injection 1664
Risperdal M-Tab Orally Disintegrating Tablets 1658
Risperdal 1658

Selegiline Hydrochloride (Nonselective monoamine oxidase (MAO) inhibitors are contraindicated for use with Stalevo). Products include:
Eldepryl Capsules 3209

Sodium Nitroprusside (Symptomatic postural hypotension has occurred when carbidopa-levodopa was added to the treatment of a patient receiving antihypertensive drugs).
No products indexed under this heading.

Sotalol Hydrochloride (Symptomatic postural hypotension has occurred when carbidopa-levodopa was added to the treatment of a patient receiving antihypertensive drugs).
No products indexed under this heading.

Spirapril Hydrochloride (Symptomatic postural hypotension has occurred when carbidopa-levodopa was added to the treatment of a patient receiving antihypertensive drugs).
No products indexed under this heading.

Telmisartan (Symptomatic postural hypotension has occurred when carbidopa-levodopa was added to the treatment of a patient receiving antihypertensive drugs). Products include:
Micardis Tablets 884
Micardis HCT Tablets 886

Terazosin Hydrochloride (Symptomatic postural hypotension has occurred when carbidopa-levodopa was added to the treatment of a patient receiving antihypertensive drugs). Products include:
Hytrin Capsules 469

Thioridazine Hydrochloride (Dopamine D2 receptor antagonists may reduce the therapeutic effects of levodopa). Products include:
Thioridazine Hydrochloride Tablets 2122

Thiothixene (Dopamine D2 receptor antagonists may reduce the therapeutic effects of levodopa). Products include:
Thiothixene Capsules 2124

Timolol Maleate (Symptomatic postural hypotension has occurred when carbidopa-levodopa was added to the treatment of a patient receiving antihypertensive drugs). Products include:
Blocadren Tablets 1891
Cosopt Sterile Ophthalmic Solution.. 1910
Timolide Tablets 2056
Timoptic in Ocudose 2061
Timoptic Sterile Ophthalmic Solution.. 2058
Timoptic-XE Sterile Ophthalmic Gel Forming Solution 2062

Torsemide (Symptomatic postural hypotension has occurred when carbidopa-levodopa was added to the treatment of a patient receiving antihypertensive drugs).
No products indexed under this heading.

Trandolapril (Symptomatic postural hypotension has occurred when carbidopa-levodopa was added to the treatment of a patient receiving antihypertensive drugs). Products include:
Mavik Tablets 482
Tarka Tablets 519

Tranylcypromine Sulfate (Nonselective monoamine oxidase (MAO) inhibitors are contraindicated for use with Stalevo). Products include:
Parnate Tablets 1499

Trifluoperazine Hydrochloride (Dopamine D2 receptor antagonists may reduce the therapeutic effects of levodopa).
No products indexed under this heading.

Trimethaphan Camsylate (Symptomatic postural hypotension has occurred when carbidopa-levodopa was added to the treatment of a patient receiving antihypertensive drugs).
No products indexed under this heading.

Trimipramine Maleate (There have been rare reports of adverse reactions, including hypertension and dyskinesia, resulting from the concomitant use of tricylic antidepressants and carbidopa-levodopa). Products include:
Surmontil Capsules 2347

Valsartan (Symptomatic postural hypotension has occurred when carbidopa-levodopa was added to the treatment of a patient receiving antihypertensive drugs). Products include:
Diovan HCT Tablets 2195
Diovan Tablets 2191

Verapamil Hydrochloride (Symptomatic postural hypotension has occurred when carbidopa-levodopa was added to the treatment of a patient receiving antihypertensive drugs). Products include:
Covera-HS Tablets 3135
Tarka Tablets 519
Verelan PM Capsules 3120

STARLIX TABLETS

(Nateglinide) 2276

May interact with beta blockers, corticosteroids, monoamine oxidase inhibitors, non-steroidal anti-inflammatory agents, salicylates, sympathomimetics, thiazides, thyroid preparations, and certain other agents. Compounds in these categories include:

Acebutolol Hydrochloride (The hypoglycemic action of nateglinide may be potentiated by non-selective beta-adrenergic-blocking agents).
No products indexed under this heading.

Albuterol (Co-administration with certain drugs, such as sympathomimetics, may reduce the hypoglycemic action of nateglinide and other oral antidiabetic drugs; when these drugs are administered to or withdrawn from patients receiving nateglinide, the patient should be observed closely for changes in glycemic control). Products include:
Proventil Inhalation Aerosol 3067

Albuterol Sulfate (Co-administration with certain drugs, such as sympathomimetics, may reduce the hypoglycemic action of nateglinide and other oral antidiabetic drugs; when these drugs are administered to or withdrawn from patients receiving nateglinide, the patient should be observed closely for changes in glycemic control). Products include:
AccuNeb Inhalation Solution 1055
Combivent Inhalation Aerosol 878
DuoNeb Inhalation Solution 1058
Proventil Inhalation Solution 0.083%...................................... 3069
Proventil HFA Inhalation Aerosol 3071
Ventolin HFA Inhalation Aerosol 1576
VoSpire Extended-Release Tablets ... 2352

Aspirin (The hypoglycemic action of nateglinide may be potentiated by salicylates). Products include:
Aggrenox Capsules 855
Bayer, Aspirin Regimen .... ▣606
Bayer Aspirin Tablets 3515
BC Powder .... ▣612
BC Allergy Sinus Cold Powder .... ▣612
Arthritis Strength BC Powder .... ▣612
BC Sinus Cold Powder .... ▣612
Ecotrin Enteric Coated Aspirin Low, Regular and Maximum Strength Tablets.......................... 1627
Goody's Body Pain Formula Powder.. ▣621
Goody's Extra Strength Headache Powder....................... ▣621
Goody's Extra Strength Pain Relief Tablets............................. ▣621
Percodan Tablets 1115
St. Joseph 81 mg Aspirin Chewable and Enteric Coated Tablets.. 1841

Aspirin, Enteric Coated (The hypoglycemic action of nateglinide may be potentiated by salicylates).
No products indexed under this heading.

Aspirin Buffered (The hypoglycemic action of nateglinide may be potentiated by salicylates).
No products indexed under this heading.

Atenolol (The hypoglycemic action of nateglinide may be potentiated by non-selective beta-adrenergic-blocking agents). Products include:
Tenormin I.V. Injection 698
Tenormin Tablets 695

Bendroflumethiazide (Co-administration with certain drugs, such as thiazides, may reduce the hypoglycemic action of nateglinide and other oral antidiabetic drugs; when these drugs are administered to or withdrawn from patients receiving nateglinide, the patient should be observed closely for changes in glycemic control).
No products indexed under this heading.

Betamethasone Acetate (Co-administration with certain drugs, such as corticosteroids, may reduce the hypoglycemic action of nateglinide and other oral antidiabetic drugs; when these drugs are administered to or withdrawn from patients receiving nateglinide, the patient should be observed closely for changes in glycemic control).
No products indexed under this heading.

Betamethasone Sodium Phosphate (Co-administration with certain drugs, such as corticosteroids, may reduce the hypoglycemic action of nateglinide and other oral antidiabetic drugs; when these drugs are administered to or withdrawn from patients receiving nateglinide, the patient should be observed closely for changes in glycemic control).
No products indexed under this heading.

Betaxolol Hydrochloride (The hypoglycemic action of nateglinide may be potentiated by non-selective beta-adrenergic-blocking agents). Products include:
Betoptic S Ophthalmic Suspension.................................. 554

Bisoprolol Fumarate (The hypoglycemic action of nateglinide may be potentiated by non-selective beta-adrenergic-blocking agents).
No products indexed under this heading.

Carteolol Hydrochloride (The hypoglycemic action of nateglinide may be potentiated by non-selective beta-adrenergic-blocking agents). Products include:
Carteolol Hydrochloride Ophthalmic Solution USP, 1% ...... ⊙246

Celecoxib (The hypoglycemic action of nateglinide may be potentiated by non-steroidal anti-inflammatory agents). Products include:
Celebrex Capsules 3130

Chlorothiazide (Co-administration with certain drugs, such as thiazides, may reduce the hypoglycemic action of nateglinide and other oral antidiabetic drugs; when these drugs are administered to or withdrawn from patients receiving nateglinide, the patient should be observed closely for changes in glycemic control). Products include:
Aldoclor Tablets 1881
Diuril Oral 1936

Chlorothiazide Sodium (Co-administration with certain drugs, such as thiazides, may reduce the hypoglycemic action of nateglinide and other oral antidiabetic drugs; when these drugs are administered to or withdrawn from patients receiving nateglinide, the patient should be observed closely for changes in glycemic control). Products include:
Diuril Sodium Intravenous 1934

Choline Magnesium Trisalicylate (The hypoglycemic action of nateglinide may be potentiated by salicylates).
No products indexed under this heading.

Cortisone Acetate (Co-administration with certain drugs, such as corticosteroids, may reduce the hypoglycemic action of nateglinide and other oral antidiabetic drugs; when these drugs are administered to or withdrawn from patients receiving nateglinide, the patient should be observed closely for changes in glycemic control).
No products indexed under this heading.

Dexamethasone (Co-administration with certain drugs, such as corticosteroids, may reduce the hypoglycemic action of nateglinide and other oral antidiabetic drugs; when these drugs are administered to or withdrawn from patients receiving nateglinide, the patient should be observed closely for changes in glycemic control). Products include:
Ciprodex Otic Suspension 555
Decadron Tablets 1929
TobraDex Ophthalmic Ointment 558
TobraDex Ophthalmic Suspension ... 558

Dexamethasone Acetate (Co-administration with certain drugs, such as corticosteroids, may reduce the hypoglycemic action of nateglinide and other oral antidiabetic drugs; when these drugs are administered to or withdrawn from patients receiving nateglinide, the patient should be observed closely for changes in glycemic control).
No products indexed under this heading.

Dexamethasone Sodium Phosphate (Co-administration with certain drugs, such as corticosteroids, may reduce the hypoglycemic action of nateglinide and other oral antidiabetic drugs; when these drugs are administered to or withdrawn from patients receiving nateglinide, the patient should be observed closely for changes in glycemic control). Products include:
Decadron Phosphate Injection 1931

Diclofenac Potassium (The hypoglycemic action of nateglinide may be potentiated by non-steroidal anti-inflammatory agents). Products include:
Cataflam Tablets 2173

Diclofenac Sodium (The hypoglycemic action of nateglinide may be potentiated by non-steroidal anti-inflammatory agents). Products include:
Arthrotec Tablets 3126
Voltaren Ophthalmic Solution 2300
Voltaren Tablets 2298
Voltaren-XR Tablets 2301

Diflunisal (The hypoglycemic action of nateglinide may be potentiated by salicylates). Products include:
Dolobid Tablets 1937

Dobutamine Hydrochloride (Co-administration with certain drugs, such as sympathomimetics, may reduce the hypoglycemic action of nateglinide and other oral antidiabetic drugs; when these drugs are administered to or withdrawn from patients receiving nateglinide, the patient should be observed closely for changes in glycemic control).
No products indexed under this heading.

Dopamine Hydrochloride (Co-administration with certain drugs, such as sympathomimetics, may reduce the hypoglycemic action of nateglinide and other oral antidiabetic drugs; when these drugs are administered to or withdrawn from patients receiving nateglinide, the patient should be observed closely for changes in glycemic control).
No products indexed under this heading.

Ephedrine Hydrochloride (Co-administration with certain drugs, such as sympathomimetics, may reduce the hypoglycemic action of nateglinide and other oral antidiabetic drugs; when these drugs are administered to or withdrawn from patients receiving nateglinide, the patient should be observed closely for changes in glycemic control). Products include:
Primatene Tablets 749

Ephedrine Sulfate (Co-administration with certain drugs, such as sympathomimetics, may reduce the hypoglycemic action of nateglinide and other oral antidiabetic drugs; when these drugs are administered to or withdrawn from patients receiving nateglinide, the patient should be observed closely for changes in glycemic control).
No products indexed under this heading.

Ephedrine Tannate (Co-administration with certain drugs, such as sympathomimetics, may reduce the hypoglycemic action of nateglinide and other oral antidiabetic drugs; when these drugs are administered to or withdrawn from patients receiving nateglinide, the patient should be observed closely for changes in glycemic control).
No products indexed under this heading.

Epinephrine (Co-administration with certain drugs, such as sympathomimetics, may reduce the hypoglycemic action of nateglinide and other oral antidiabetic drugs; when these drugs are administered to or withdrawn from patients receiving nateglinide, the patient should be observed closely for changes in glycemic control). Products include:
EpiPen 1061
Primatene Mist 749

Epinephrine Bitartrate (Co-administration with certain drugs, such as sympathomimetics, may reduce the hypoglycemic action of nateglinide and other oral antidiabetic drugs; when these drugs are administered to or withdrawn from patients receiving nateglinide, the patient should be observed closely for changes in glycemic control).
No products indexed under this heading.

Epinephrine Hydrochloride (Co-administration with certain drugs, such as sympathomimetics, may reduce the hypoglycemic action of nateglinide and other oral antidiabetic drugs; when these drugs are administered to or withdrawn from patients receiving nateglinide, the patient should be observed closely for changes in glycemic control).
No products indexed under this heading.

Esmolol Hydrochloride (The hypoglycemic action of nateglinide may be potentiated by non-selective beta-adrenergic-blocking agents). Products include:
Brevibloc Concentrate 766
Brevibloc Injection 766
Brevibloc Double Strength Injection 766
Brevibloc Premixed Injection 766
Brevibloc Double Strength Premixed Injection 766

Etodolac (The hypoglycemic action of nateglinide may be potentiated by non-steroidal anti-inflammatory agents).
No products indexed under this heading.

Fenoprofen Calcium (The hypoglycemic action of nateglinide may be potentiated by non-steroidal anti-inflammatory agents). Products include:
Nalfon Capsules 2504

Fludrocortisone Acetate (Co-administration with certain drugs, such as corticosteroids, may reduce the hypoglycemic action of nateglinide and other oral antidiabetic drugs; when these drugs are administered to or withdrawn from patients receiving nateglinide, the patient should be observed closely for changes in glycemic control).
No products indexed under this heading.

Flurbiprofen (The hypoglycemic action of nateglinide may be potentiated by non-steroidal anti-inflammatory agents).
No products indexed under this heading.

Hydrochlorothiazide (Co-administration with certain drugs, such as thiazides, may reduce the hypoglycemic action of nateglinide and other oral antidiabetic drugs; when these drugs are administered to or withdrawn from patients receiving nateglinide, the patient should be observed closely for changes in glycemic control). Products include:
Aldoril Tablets 1884
Atacand HCT 637
Avalide Tablets 2889
Avalide Tablets 922
Benicar HCT Tablets 2852
Diovan HCT Tablets 2195
Dyazide Capsules 1389
Hyzaar 1964
Lotensin HCT Tablets 2235
Maxzide 2150
Micardis HCT Tablets 886
Moduretic Tablets 2003
Prinzide Tablets 2033
Teveten HCT Tablets 1710
Timolide Tablets 2056
Uniretic Tablets 3114
Vaseretic Tablets 2073
Zestoretic Tablets 701

Hydrocortisone (Co-administration with certain drugs, such as corticosteroids, may reduce the hypoglycemic action of nateglinide and other oral antidiabetic drugs; when these drugs are administered to or withdrawn from patients receiving nateglinide, the patient should be observed closely for changes in glycemic control). Products include:
Cortizone•5 Ointment 699
Cortizone•10 Creme 699
Cortizone•10 Ointment 699
Cortizone•10 Plus Creme 700
Cortizone•10 Maximum Strength Quick Shot Spray 700
Hydrocortone Tablets 1963
Preparation H Hydrocortisone Cream 748

Hydrocortisone Acetate (Co-administration with certain drugs, such as corticosteroids, may reduce the hypoglycemic action of nateglinide and other oral antidiabetic drugs; when these drugs are administered to or withdrawn from patients receiving nateglinide, the patient should be observed closely for changes in glycemic control). Products include:
Analpram-HC 1136
Pramosone 1139
ProctoFoam-HC 3113
Tucks Anti-Itch Ointment 712
U-cort 1% Cream 3289

Hydrocortisone Sodium Phosphate (Co-administration with certain drugs, such as corticosteroids, may reduce the hypoglycemic action of nateglinide and other oral antidiabetic drugs; when these drugs are administered to or withdrawn from patients receiving nateglinide, the patient should be observed closely for changes in glycemic control).
No products indexed under this heading.

Hydrocortisone Sodium Succinate (Co-administration with certain drugs, such as corticosteroids, may reduce the hypoglycemic action of nateglinide and other oral antidiabetic drugs; when these drugs are administered to or withdrawn from patients receiving nateglinide, the patient should be observed closely for changes in glycemic control).
No products indexed under this heading.

Hydroflumethiazide (Co-administration with certain drugs, such as thiazides, may reduce the hypoglycemic action of nateglinide and other oral antidiabetic drugs; when these drugs are administered to or withdrawn from patients receiving nateglinide, the patient should be observed closely for changes in glycemic control).
No products indexed under this heading.

Ibuprofen (The hypoglycemic action of nateglinide may be potentiated by non-steroidal anti-inflammatory agents). Products include:

- Advil Allergy Sinus Caplets .... ■ 737
- Advil .... ■ 737
- Children's Advil Suspension .... ■ 742
- Children's Advil Chewable Tablets .... ■ 741
- Advil Cold & Sinus .... ■ 739
- Advil Flu & Body Ache Caplets .... ■ 739
- Children's Advil Cold Suspension .... ■ 741
- Infants' Advil Concentrated Drops .... ■ 743
- Junior Strength Advil Swallow Tablets .... ■ 740
- Advil Migraine Liquigels .... ■ 740
- Advil Multi-Symptom Cold Caplets .... ■ 738
- Combunox Tablets 1183
- Children's Motrin Oral Suspension and Chewable Tablets 1837
- Children's Motrin Cold Non-Staining Dye-Free Oral Suspension 1838
- Children's Motrin Cold Oral Suspension 1838
- Children's Motrin Non-Staining Dye-Free Oral Suspension 1837
- Motrin Cold & Sinus Caplets 1836
- Motrin IB Tablets and Caplets 1836
- Infants' Motrin Concentrated Drops 1837
- Infants' Motrin Non-Staining Dye-Free Drops 1837
- Junior Strength Motrin Caplets and Chewable Tablets 1837
- Vicoprofen Tablets 533

Indomethacin (The hypoglycemic action of nateglinide may be potentiated by non-steroidal anti-inflammatory agents). Products include:

- Indocin 1968

Indomethacin Sodium Trihydrate (The hypoglycemic action of nateglinide may be potentiated by non-steroidal anti-inflammatory agents). Products include:

- Indocin I.V. 1973

Isocarboxazid (The hypoglycemic action of nateglinide may be potentiated by MAO inhibitors).

No products indexed under this heading.

Isoproterenol Hydrochloride (Co-administration with certain drugs, such as sympathomimetics, may reduce the hypoglycemic action of nateglinide and other oral antidiabetic drugs; when these drugs are administered to or withdrawn from patients receiving nateglinide, the patient should be observed closely for changes in glycemic control).

No products indexed under this heading.

Isoproterenol Sulfate (Co-administration with certain drugs, such as sympathomimetics, may reduce the hypoglycemic action of nateglinide and other oral antidiabetic drugs; when these drugs are administered to or withdrawn from patients receiving nateglinide, the patient should be observed closely for changes in glycemic control).

No products indexed under this heading.

Ketoprofen (The hypoglycemic action of nateglinide may be potentiated by non-steroidal anti-inflammatory agents).

No products indexed under this heading.

Ketorolac Tromethamine (The hypoglycemic action of nateglinide may be potentiated by non-steroidal anti-inflammatory agents). Products include:

- Acular Ophthalmic Solution 561
- Acular LS Ophthalmic Solution 562

Labetalol Hydrochloride (The hypoglycemic action of nateglinide may be potentiated by non-selective beta-adrenergic-blocking agents).

No products indexed under this heading.

Levalbuterol Hydrochloride (Co-administration with certain drugs, such as sympathomimetics, may reduce the hypoglycemic action of nateglinide and other oral antidiabetic drugs; when these drugs are administered to or withdrawn from patients receiving nateglinide, the patient should be observed closely for changes in glycemic control). Products include:

- Xopenex Inhalation Solution 3143
- Xopenex Inhalation Solution Concentrate 3147

Levobunolol Hydrochloride (The hypoglycemic action of nateglinide may be potentiated by non-selective beta-adrenergic-blocking agents). Products include:

- Betagan Ophthalmic Solution, USP .... ⊙ 217

Levothyroxine Sodium (Co-administration with certain drugs, such as thyroid products, may reduce the hypoglycemic action of nateglinide and other oral antidiabetic drugs; when these drugs are administered to or withdrawn from patients receiving nateglinide, the patient should be observed closely for changes in glycemic control). Products include:

- Levothroid Tablets 1189
- Levoxyl Tablets 1680
- Synthroid Tablets 515
- Unithroid Tablets 3521

Liothyronine Sodium (Co-administration with certain drugs, such as thyroid products, may reduce the hypoglycemic action of nateglinide and other oral antidiabetic drugs; when these drugs are administered to or withdrawn from patients receiving nateglinide, the patient should be observed closely for changes in glycemic control). Products include:

- Cytomel Tablets 1678

Liotrix (Co-administration with certain drugs, such as thyroid products, may reduce the hypoglycemic action of nateglinide and other oral antidiabetic drugs; when these drugs are administered to or withdrawn from patients receiving nateglinide, the patient should be observed closely for changes in glycemic control). Products include:

- Thyrolar 1203

Magnesium Salicylate (The hypoglycemic action of nateglinide may be potentiated by salicylates).

No products indexed under this heading.

Meclofenamate Sodium (The hypoglycemic action of nateglinide may be potentiated by non-steroidal anti-inflammatory agents).

No products indexed under this heading.

Mefenamic Acid (The hypoglycemic action of nateglinide may be potentiated by non-steroidal anti-inflammatory agents).

No products indexed under this heading.

Meloxicam (The hypoglycemic action of nateglinide may be potentiated by non-steroidal anti-inflammatory agents). Products include:

- Mobic Oral Suspension 893
- Mobic Tablets 893

Metaproterenol Sulfate (Co-administration with certain drugs, such as sympathomimetics, may reduce the hypoglycemic action of nateglinide and other oral antidiabetic drugs; when these drugs are administered to or withdrawn from patients receiving nateglinide, the patient should be observed closely for changes in glycemic control). Products include:

- Alupent Inhalation Aerosol 858

Metaraminol Bitartrate (Co-administration with certain drugs, such as sympathomimetics, may reduce the hypoglycemic action of nateglinide and other oral antidiabetic drugs; when these drugs are administered to or withdrawn from patients receiving nateglinide, the patient should be observed closely for changes in glycemic control). Products include:

- Aramine Injection 1889

Methoxamine Hydrochloride (Co-administration with certain drugs, such as sympathomimetics, may reduce the hypoglycemic action of nateglinide and other oral antidiabetic drugs; when these drugs are administered to or withdrawn from patients receiving nateglinide, the patient should be observed closely for changes in glycemic control).

No products indexed under this heading.

Methyclothiazide (Co-administration with certain drugs, such as thiazides, may reduce the hypoglycemic action of nateglinide and other oral antidiabetic drugs; when these drugs are administered to or withdrawn from patients receiving nateglinide, the patient should be observed closely for changes in glycemic control).

No products indexed under this heading.

Methylprednisolone Acetate (Co-administration with certain drugs, such as corticosteroids, may reduce the hypoglycemic action of nateglinide and other oral antidiabetic drugs; when these drugs are administered to or withdrawn from patients receiving nateglinide, the patient should be observed closely for changes in glycemic control). Products include:

- Depo-Medrol Injectable Suspension 2615
- Depo-Medrol Single-Dose Vial 2617

Methylprednisolone Sodium Succinate (Co-administration with certain drugs, such as corticosteroids, may reduce the hypoglycemic action of nateglinide and other oral antidiabetic drugs; when these drugs are administered to or withdrawn from patients receiving nateglinide, the patient should be observed closely for changes in glycemic control).

No products indexed under this heading.

Metipranolol Hydrochloride (The hypoglycemic action of nateglinide may be potentiated by non-selective beta-adrenergic-blocking agents).

No products indexed under this heading.

Metoprolol Succinate (The hypoglycemic action of nateglinide may be potentiated by non-selective beta-adrenergic-blocking agents). Products include:

- Toprol-XL Tablets 660

Metoprolol Tartrate (The hypoglycemic action of nateglinide may be potentiated by non-selective beta-adrenergic-blocking agents).

No products indexed under this heading.

Moclobemide (The hypoglycemic action of nateglinide may be potentiated by MAO inhibitors).

No products indexed under this heading.

Nabumetone (The hypoglycemic action of nateglinide may be potentiated by non-steroidal anti-inflammatory agents). Products include:

- Relafen Tablets 1523

Nadolol (The hypoglycemic action of nateglinide may be potentiated by non-selective beta-adrenergic-blocking agents). Products include:

- Nadolol Tablets 2121

Naproxen (The hypoglycemic action of nateglinide may be potentiated by non-steroidal anti-inflammatory agents). Products include:

- EC-Naprosyn Delayed-Release Tablets 2769
- Naprosyn Suspension 2769
- Naprosyn Tablets 2769
- Prevacid NapraPAC 3277

Naproxen Sodium (The hypoglycemic action of nateglinide may be potentiated by non-steroidal anti-inflammatory agents). Products include:

- Aleve Tablets, Caplets and Gelcaps .... ■ 605
- Anaprox Tablets 2769
- Anaprox DS Tablets 2769

Norepinephrine Bitartrate (Co-administration with certain drugs, such as sympathomimetics, may reduce the hypoglycemic action of nateglinide and other oral antidiabetic drugs; when these drugs are administered to or withdrawn from patients receiving nateglinide, the patient should be observed closely for changes in glycemic control).

No products indexed under this heading.

Oxaprozin (The hypoglycemic action of nateglinide may be potentiated by non-steroidal anti-inflammatory agents).

No products indexed under this heading.

Pargyline Hydrochloride (The hypoglycemic action of nateglinide may be potentiated by MAO inhibitors).

No products indexed under this heading.

Penbutolol Sulfate (The hypoglycemic action of nateglinide may be potentiated by non-selective beta-adrenergic-blocking agents).

No products indexed under this heading.

Phenelzine Sulfate (The hypoglycemic action of nateglinide may be potentiated by MAO inhibitors).

No products indexed under this heading.

Phenylbutazone (The hypoglycemic action of nateglinide may be potentiated by non-steroidal anti-inflammatory agents).

No products indexed under this heading.

Phenylephrine Bitartrate (Co-administration with certain drugs, such as sympathomimetics, may reduce the hypoglycemic action of nateglinide and other oral antidiabetic drugs; when these drugs are administered to or withdrawn from patients receiving nateglinide, the patient should be observed closely for changes in glycemic control).
No products indexed under this heading.

Phenylephrine Hydrochloride (Co-administration with certain drugs, such as sympathomimetics, may reduce the hypoglycemic action of nateglinide and other oral antidiabetic drugs; when these drugs are administered to or withdrawn from patients receiving nateglinide, the patient should be observed closely for changes in glycemic control). Products include:
- Alacol DM Syrup 739
- Hycomine Compound Tablets 1105
- Preparation H Maximum Strength Cream .... ■747
- Preparation H Cooling Gel .... ■747
- Preparation H .... ■747
- Sudafed PE Tablets .... ■711
- Vicks Sinex Nasal Spray and Ultra Fine Mist for Sinus Relief 2677
- Zicam Concentrated Cough Mist for Kids Plus D Cool Cherry .... ■643
- Zicam Concentrated Cough Mist Plus D Cool Cherry .... ■642

Phenylephrine Tannate (Co-administration with certain drugs, such as sympathomimetics, may reduce the hypoglycemic action of nateglinide and other oral antidiabetic drugs; when these drugs are administered to or withdrawn from patients receiving nateglinide, the patient should be observed closely for changes in glycemic control).
No products indexed under this heading.

Phenylpropanolamine Hydrochloride (Co-administration with certain drugs, such as sympathomimetics, may reduce the hypoglycemic action of nateglinide and other oral antidiabetic drugs; when these drugs are administered to or withdrawn from patients receiving nateglinide, the patient should be observed closely for changes in glycemic control).
No products indexed under this heading.

Pindolol (The hypoglycemic action of nateglinide may be potentiated by non-selective beta-adrenergic-blocking agents).
No products indexed under this heading.

Pirbuterol Acetate (Co-administration with certain drugs, such as sympathomimetics, may reduce the hypoglycemic action of nateglinide and other oral antidiabetic drugs; when these drugs are administered to or withdrawn from patients receiving nateglinide, the patient should be observed closely for changes in glycemic control). Products include:
- Maxair Autohaler 1820

Piroxicam (The hypoglycemic action of nateglinide may be potentiated by non-steroidal anti-inflammatory agents).
No products indexed under this heading.

Polythiazide (Co-administration with certain drugs, such as thiazides, may reduce the hypoglycemic action of nateglinide and other oral antidiabetic drugs; when these drugs are administered to or withdrawn from patients receiving nateglinide, the patient should be observed closely for changes in glycemic control).
No products indexed under this heading.

Prednisolone Acetate (Co-administration with certain drugs, such as corticosteroids, may reduce the hypoglycemic action of nateglinide and other oral antidiabetic drugs; when these drugs are administered to or withdrawn from patients receiving nateglinide, the patient should be observed closely for changes in glycemic control). Products include:
- Blephamide Ophthalmic Ointment 563
- Blephamide Ophthalmic Suspension 564
- Poly-Pred Liquifilm Ophthalmic Suspension .... ⊙231
- Pred Forte Ophthalmic Suspension .... ⊙233
- Pred Mild Sterile Ophthalmic Suspension .... ⊙236
- Pred-G Ophthalmic Suspension .... ⊙234
- Pred-G Sterile Ophthalmic Ointment .... ⊙235

Prednisolone Sodium Phosphate (Co-administration with certain drugs, such as corticosteroids, may reduce the hypoglycemic action of nateglinide and other oral antidiabetic drugs; when these drugs are administered to or withdrawn from patients receiving nateglinide, the patient should be observed closely for changes in glycemic control). Products include:
- Pediapred Oral Solution 3319

Prednisolone Tebutate (Co-administration with certain drugs, such as corticosteroids, may reduce the hypoglycemic action of nateglinide and other oral antidiabetic drugs; when these drugs are administered to or withdrawn from patients receiving nateglinide, the patient should be observed closely for changes in glycemic control).
No products indexed under this heading.

Prednisone (Co-administration with certain drugs, such as corticosteroids, may reduce the hypoglycemic action of nateglinide and other oral antidiabetic drugs; when these drugs are administered to or withdrawn from patients receiving nateglinide, the patient should be observed closely for changes in glycemic control).
No products indexed under this heading.

Procarbazine Hydrochloride (The hypoglycemic action of nateglinide may be potentiated by MAO inhibitors). Products include:
- Matulane Capsules 3188

Propranolol Hydrochloride (The hypoglycemic action of nateglinide may be potentiated by non-selective beta-adrenergic-blocking agents). Products include:
- Inderal LA Long-Acting Capsules 3421
- InnoPran XL Capsules 2728

Pseudoephedrine Hydrochloride (Co-administration with certain drugs, such as sympathomimetics, may reduce the hypoglycemic action of nateglinide and other oral antidiabetic drugs; when these drugs are administered to or withdrawn from patients receiving nateglinide, the patient should be observed closely for changes in glycemic control). Products include:
- Advil Allergy Sinus Caplets .... ■737
- Advil Cold & Sinus .... ■739
- Advil Flu & Body Ache Caplets .... ■739
- Children's Advil Cold Suspension .... ■741
- Advil Multi-Symptom Cold Caplets .... ■738
- Allegra-D 12 Hour Extended-Release Tablets 2860
- Allegra-D 24 Hour Extended-Release Tablets 2862
- Balamine DM 739
- BC Cold Powder .... ■612
- Benadryl Allergy & Cold Tablets .... ■692
- Benadryl Allergy & Sinus Headache Caplets & Gelcaps .... ■693
- Children's Benadryl Allergy & Cold Fastmelt Tablets .... ■695
- Benadryl Maximum Strength Severe Allergy & Sinus Headache Caplets .... ■694
- Children's Benadryl D Allergy & Sinus Fastmelt Tablets .... ■694
- Children's Benadryl D Liquid Medication .... ■693
- Benadryl D Tablets .... ■694
- Contac Non-Drowsy 12 Hour Cold Caplets .... ■614
- Contac Non-Drowsy Timed Release 12 Hour Cold Caplets .... ■615
- Contac Severe Cold and Flu Caplets Maximum Strength .... ■615
- Contac Severe Cold and Flu Caplets Non-Drowsy .... ■615
- Children's Dimetapp Cold & Allergy Elixir .... ■745
- Children's Dimetapp DM Cold & Cough Elixir .... ■745
- Children's Dimetapp Long Acting Cough Plus Cold Syrup .... ■746
- Dimetapp Infant Drops Decongestant Plus Cough .... ■746
- Children's Motrin Cold Non-Staining Dye-Free Oral Suspension 1838
- Children's Motrin Cold Oral Suspension 1838
- Motrin Cold & Sinus Caplets 1836
- PediaCare Decongestant & Cough Infant Drops .... ■705
- PediaCare Decongestant Infants' Drops .... ■705
- PediaCare Long-Acting Cough Plus Cold Liquid .... ■704
- PediaCare Multi-Symptom Cold Liquid .... ■704
- PediaCare NightRest Cough & Cold Liquid .... ■704
- Robitussin Allergy & Cough Syrup .... ■750
- Robitussin CF Liquid .... ■755
- Robitussin Cough & Cold Liquid-filled Capsules .... ■750
- Robitussin Cough, Cold & Flu Liquid-filled Capsules .... ■750
- Robitussin Cough & Cold Infant Drops .... ■755
- Robitussin Flu Liquid .... ■752
- Robitussin Maximum Strength Cough & Cold Liquid .... ■754
- Robitussin PE Syrup .... ■753
- Robitussin Pediatric Cough & Cold Liquid .... ■754
- Robitussin PM Cough & Cold Liquid .... ■752
- Robitussin Severe Congestion Liquid-filled Capsules .... ■751
- Simply Stuffy Liquid 1841
- Singlet Caplets .... ■636
- Sudafed 12 Hour Caplets .... ■708
- Sudafed 24 Hour Tablets .... ■709
- Sudafed Nasal Decongestant Tablets .... ■709
- Sudafed Severe Cold .... ■710
- Sudafed Non-Drying Sinus Liquid Caps .... ■709
- Sudafed Sinus & Allergy Tablets .... ■710
- Sudafed Sinus Headache .... ■711
- TheraFlu Cold & Cough Hot Liquid .... ■680
- TheraFlu Cold & Sore Throat Hot Liquid .... ■680
- TheraFlu Flu & Chest Congestion Non-Drowsy Hot Liquid .... ■681
- TheraFlu Flu & Sore Throat Hot Liquid .... ■681
- TheraFlu Severe Cold Non-Drowsy Hot Liquid .... ■683
- TheraFlu Severe Cold & Cough Hot Liquid .... ■683
- TheraFlu Severe Cold Caplets .... ■679
- TheraFlu Severe Cold Hot Liquid .... ■682
- TheraFlu Severe Cold Non-Drowsy Caplets .... ■679
- Triaminic Chest & Nasal Congestion Liquid .... ■685
- Triaminic Cold & Allergy Liquid .... ■685
- Triaminic Cold & Cough Liquid .... ■685
- Triaminic Cough Liquid .... ■687
- Triaminic Cough & Nasal Congestion Liquid .... ■687
- Triaminic Cough & Sore Throat Liquid .... ■687
- Triaminic Flu, Cough & Fever Liquid .... ■685
- Triaminic Night Time Cough & Cold Liquid .... ■685
- Triaminic Allergy Runny Nose & Congestion Softchews .... ■688
- Triaminic Cold & Cough Softchews .... ■688
- Triaminic Cough & Sore Throat Softchews .... ■689
- Tylenol Sinus NightTime Caplets .... ■663
- Children's Tylenol Plus Cold & Allergy Suspension Liquid 1850
- Children's Tylenol Plus Cold NightTime Suspension Liquid 1851
- Children's Tylenol Plus Cold & Cough Suspension Liquid and Chewable Tablets 1851
- Children's Tylenol Plus Cold Chewable Tablets 1851
- Children's Tylenol Plus Cold Daytime Non-Drowsy Suspension Liquid 1851
- Children's Tylenol Plus Flu Suspension Liquid 1853
- Concentrated Tylenol Infants' Drops Plus Cold 1851
- Concentrated Tylenol Infants' Drops Plus Cold and Cough 1851
- Tylenol Cold & Flu Severe Daytime Liquid with Cool Burst 1846
- Tylenol Cold & Flu Severe NightTime Liquid with Cool Burst 1846
- Tylenol Cold Severe Congestion Non-Drowsy Caplets with Cool Burst 1846
- Tylenol Allergy Complete Night Time Caplets 1844
- Tylenol Allergy Complete Multi-Symptom Caplets and Gelcaps with Cool Burst 1844
- Tylenol Flu NightTime Gelcaps 1846
- Tylenol Flu Day Non-Drowsy Gelcaps 1846
- Concentrated Tylenol Infants' Drops Plus Cold Nasal Congestant, Fever Reducer & Pain Reliever .... ■668
- Concentrated Tylenol Infants' Drops Plus Cold & Cough Nasal Decongestant, Fever Reducer & Pain Reliever .... ■668
- Multi-Symptom Tylenol Cold Night Time Caplets 1845
- Multi-Symptom Tylenol Cold Day Non-Drowsy Caplets and Gelcaps 1845
- Tylenol Sinus Day Non-Drowsy 1848
- Tylenol Sinus Night Time Caplets 1848
- Tylenol Sinus Severe Congestion Caplets with Cool Burst 1848
- Vicks 44D Cough & Head Congestion Relief 2676
- Vicks 44D Cough & Head Congestion Relief Liquid .... ■721
- Vicks 44M Cough, Cold & Flu Relief 2676
- Pediatric Vicks 44m Cough & Cold Relief 2673
- Vicks DayQuil LiquiCaps/Liquid Multi-Symptom Cold/Flu Relief .... ■723
- Vicks DayQuil Multi-Symptom Cold/Flu Relief LiquiCaps 2675
- Vicks DayQuil Multi-Symptom Cold/Flu Relief Liquid 2675
- Children's Vicks NyQuil Cold/Cough Relief 2671
- Vicks NyQuil LiquiCaps 2677

Vicks NyQuil LiquiCaps/Liquid Multi-Symptom Cold/Flu Relief..... ▣725
Vicks NyQuil Liquid 2677
Zyrtec-D 12 Hour Extended Release Tablets 2591

Pseudoephedrine Sulfate (Co-administration with certain drugs, such as sympathomimetics, may reduce the hypoglycemic action of nateglinide and other oral antidiabetic drugs; when these drugs are administered to or withdrawn from patients receiving nateglinide, the patient should be observed closely for changes in glycemic control). Products include:
Alavert Allergy & Sinus D-12 Hour Tablets .... ▣743
Clarinex-D 24-Hour Extended-Release Tablets 3012
Claritin-D Non-Drowsy 12 Hour Tablets .... ▣731
Claritin-D Non-Drowsy 24 Hour Tablets .... ▣731

Rofecoxib (The hypoglycemic action of nateglinide may be potentiated by non-steroidal anti-inflammatory agents).
No products indexed under this heading.

Salmeterol Xinafoate (Co-administration with certain drugs, such as sympathomimetics, may reduce the hypoglycemic action of nateglinide and other oral antidiabetic drugs; when these drugs are administered to or withdrawn from patients receiving nateglinide, the patient should be observed closely for changes in glycemic control). Products include:
Advair Diskus 100/50 1291
Advair Diskus 250/50 1291
Advair Diskus 500/50 1291
Serevent Diskus 1540

Salsalate (The hypoglycemic action of nateglinide may be potentiated by salicylates).
No products indexed under this heading.

Selegiline Hydrochloride (The hypoglycemic action of nateglinide may be potentiated by MAO inhibitors). Products include:
Eldepryl Capsules 3209

Sotalol Hydrochloride (The hypoglycemic action of nateglinide may be potentiated by non-selective beta-adrenergic-blocking agents).
No products indexed under this heading.

Sulindac (The hypoglycemic action of nateglinide may be potentiated by non-steroidal anti-inflammatory agents). Products include:
Clinoril Tablets 1899

Terbutaline Sulfate (Co-administration with certain drugs, such as sympathomimetics, may reduce the hypoglycemic action of nateglinide and other oral antidiabetic drugs; when these drugs are administered to or withdrawn from patients receiving nateglinide, the patient should be observed closely for changes in glycemic control).
No products indexed under this heading.

Thyroglobulin (Co-administration with certain drugs, such as thyroid products, may reduce the hypoglycemic action of nateglinide and other oral antidiabetic drugs; when these drugs are administered to or withdrawn from patients receiving nateglinide, the patient should be observed closely for changes in glycemic control).
No products indexed under this heading.

Thyroid (Co-administration with certain drugs, such as thyroid products, may reduce the hypoglycemic action of nateglinide and other oral antidiabetic drugs; when these drugs are administered to or withdrawn from patients receiving nateglinide, the patient should be observed closely for changes in glycemic control).
No products indexed under this heading.

Thyroxine (Co-administration with certain drugs, such as thyroid products, may reduce the hypoglycemic action of nateglinide and other oral antidiabetic drugs; when these drugs are administered to or withdrawn from patients receiving nateglinide, the patient should be observed closely for changes in glycemic control).
No products indexed under this heading.

Thyroxine Sodium (Co-administration with certain drugs, such as thyroid products, may reduce the hypoglycemic action of nateglinide and other oral antidiabetic drugs; when these drugs are administered to or withdrawn from patients receiving nateglinide, the patient should be observed closely for changes in glycemic control).
No products indexed under this heading.

Timolol Hemihydrate (The hypoglycemic action of nateglinide may be potentiated by non-selective beta-adrenergic-blocking agents). Products include:
Betimol Ophthalmic Solution 3371
Betimol Ophthalmic Solution .... ⊙283

Timolol Maleate (The hypoglycemic action of nateglinide may be potentiated by non-selective beta-adrenergic-blocking agents). Products include:
Blocadren Tablets 1891
Cosopt Sterile Ophthalmic Solution 1910
Timolide Tablets 2056
Timoptic in Ocudose 2061
Timoptic Sterile Ophthalmic Solution 2058
Timoptic-XE Sterile Ophthalmic Gel Forming Solution 2062

Tolmetin Sodium (The hypoglycemic action of nateglinide may be potentiated by non-steroidal anti-inflammatory agents).
No products indexed under this heading.

Tranylcypromine Sulfate (The hypoglycemic action of nateglinide may be potentiated by MAO inhibitors). Products include:
Parnate Tablets 1499

Triamcinolone (Co-administration with certain drugs, such as corticosteroids, may reduce the hypoglycemic action of nateglinide and other oral antidiabetic drugs; when these drugs are administered to or withdrawn from patients receiving nateglinide, the patient should be observed closely for changes in glycemic control).
No products indexed under this heading.

Triamcinolone Acetonide (Co-administration with certain drugs, such as corticosteroids, may reduce the hypoglycemic action of nateglinide and other oral antidiabetic drugs; when these drugs are administered to or withdrawn from patients receiving nateglinide, the patient should be observed closely for changes in glycemic control). Products include:
Azmacort Inhalation Aerosol 1701
Nasacort HFA Inhalation Aerosol 2939
Nasacort AQ Nasal Spray 2937

Triamcinolone Diacetate (Co-administration with certain drugs, such as corticosteroids, may reduce the hypoglycemic action of nateglinide and other oral antidiabetic drugs; when these drugs are administered to or withdrawn from patients receiving nateglinide, the patient should be observed closely for changes in glycemic control).
No products indexed under this heading.

Triamcinolone Hexacetonide (Co-administration with certain drugs, such as corticosteroids, may reduce the hypoglycemic action of nateglinide and other oral antidiabetic drugs; when these drugs are administered to or withdrawn from patients receiving nateglinide, the patient should be observed closely for changes in glycemic control).
No products indexed under this heading.

Valdecoxib (The hypoglycemic action of nateglinide may be potentiated by non-steroidal anti-inflammatory agents).
No products indexed under this heading.

Food Interactions

Food, unspecified (Administration of nateglinide with liquid meal significantly reduces peak plasma levels).

STRATTERA CAPSULES

(Atomoxetine Hydrochloride) 1784
May interact with beta-adrenergic stimulating agents, cytochrome p450 2d6 inhibitors (selected), monoamine oxidase inhibitors, and certain other agents. Compounds in these categories include:

Albuterol (Atomoxene HCl should be administered with caution to patients being treated with systematically-administered (oral or intravenous) albuterol (or other beta-2 agonists) because the action of albuterol on the cardiovascular system can be potentiated resulting in increases in heart rate and blood pressure). Products include:
Proventil Inhalation Aerosol 3067

Albuterol Sulfate (Atomoxene HCl should be administered with caution to patients being treated with systematically-administered (oral or intravenous) albuterol (or other beta-2 agonists) because the action of albuterol on the cardiovascular system can be potentiated resulting in increases in heart rate and blood pressure). Products include:
AccuNeb Inhalation Solution 1055
Combivent Inhalation Aerosol 878
DuoNeb Inhalation Solution 1058
Proventil Inhalation Solution 0.083% 3069
Proventil HFA Inhalation Aerosol 3071
Ventolin HFA Inhalation Aerosol 1576
VoSpire Extended-Release Tablets 2352

Amiodarone Hydrochloride (CYP2D6 inhibitors increase atomexetine plasma levels; dosage adjustment of atomexetine when co-administered with CYP2D6 inhibitors may be necessary). Products include:
Pacerone Tablets 3337

Amitriptyline Hydrochloride (CYP2D6 inhibitors increase atomexetine plasma levels; dosage adjustment of atomexetine when co-administered with CYP2D6 inhibitors may be necessary).
No products indexed under this heading.

Amoxapine (CYP2D6 inhibitors increase atomexetine plasma levels; dosage adjustment of atomexetine when co-administered with CYP2D6 inhibitors may be necessary).
No products indexed under this heading.

Bitolterol Mesylate (Atomoxene HCl should be administered with caution to patients being treated with systematically-administered (oral or intravenous) albuterol (or other beta-2 agonists) because the action of albuterol on the cardiovascular system can be potentiated resulting in increases in heart rate and blood pressure).
No products indexed under this heading.

Bupropion Hydrochloride (CYP2D6 inhibitors increase atomexetine plasma levels; dosage adjustment of atomexetine when co-administered with CYP2D6 inhibitors may be necessary). Products include:
Wellbutrin Tablets 1579
Wellbutrin SR Sustained-Release Tablets 1583
Wellbutrin XL Extended-Release Tablets 1588
Zyban Sustained-Release Tablets 1620

Celecoxib (CYP2D6 inhibitors increase atomexetine plasma levels; dosage adjustment of atomexetine when co-administered with CYP2D6 inhibitors may be necessary). Products include:
Celebrex Capsules 3130

Chloroquine Hydrochloride (CYP2D6 inhibitors increase atomexetine plasma levels; dosage adjustment of atomexetine when co-administered with CYP2D6 inhibitors may be necessary).
No products indexed under this heading.

Chloroquine Phosphate (CYP2D6 inhibitors increase atomexetine plasma levels; dosage adjustment of atomexetine when co-administered with CYP2D6 inhibitors may be necessary).
No products indexed under this heading.

Chlorpheniramine (CYP2D6 inhibitors increase atomexetine plasma levels; dosage adjustment of atomexetine when co-administered with CYP2D6 inhibitors may be necessary).
No products indexed under this heading.

Chlorpheniramine Maleate (CYP2D6 inhibitors increase atomexetine plasma levels; dosage adjustment of atomexetine when co-administered with CYP2D6 inhibitors may be necessary). Products include:
Advil Allergy Sinus Caplets .... ▣737
Advil Multi-Symptom Cold Caplets .... ▣738
BC Allergy Sinus Cold Powder .... ▣612
Contac Severe Cold and Flu Caplets Maximum Strength .... ▣615
Hycomine Compound Tablets 1105
PediaCare Multi-Symptom Cold Liquid .... ▣704

PediaCare NightRest Cough & Cold Liquid ▣ 704
Robitussin Flu Liquid ▣ 752
Robitussin PM Cough & Cold Liquid ▣ 752
Singlet Caplets ▣ 636
Sudafed Sinus & Allergy Tablets ▣ 710
TheraFlu Cold & Cough Hot Liquid ▣ 680
TheraFlu Cold & Sore Throat Hot Liquid ▣ 680
TheraFlu Flu & Sore Throat Hot Liquid ▣ 681
TheraFlu Severe Cold & Cough Hot Liquid ▣ 683
TheraFlu Severe Cold Caplets ▣ 679
TheraFlu Severe Cold Hot Liquid ▣ 682
Triaminic Cold & Allergy Liquid ▣ 685
Triaminic Cold & Cough Liquid ▣ 685
Triaminic Flu, Cough & Fever Liquid ▣ 685
Triaminic Night Time Cough & Cold Liquid ▣ 685
Triaminic Allergy Runny Nose & Congestion Softchews ▣ 688
Triaminic Cold & Cough Softchews ▣ 688
Children's Tylenol Plus Cold NightTime Suspension Liquid 1851
Children's Tylenol Plus Cold & Cough Suspension Liquid and Chewable Tablets 1851
Children's Tylenol Plus Cold Chewable Tablets 1851
Children's Tylenol Plus Flu Suspension Liquid 1853
Tylenol Allergy Complete Multi-Symptom Caplets and Gelcaps with Cool Burst 1844
Multi-Symptom Tylenol Cold Night Time Caplets 1845
Vicks 44M Cough, Cold & Flu Relief 2676
Pediatric Vicks 44m Cough & Cold Relief 2673
Children's Vicks NyQuil Cold/Cough Relief 2671

Chlorpheniramine Polistirex (CYP2D6 inhibitors increase atomexetine plasma levels; dosage adjustment of atomexetine when co-administered with CYP2D6 inhibitors may be necessary). Products include:

Tussionex Pennkinetic Extended-Release Suspension 3322

Chlorpheniramine Tannate (CYP2D6 inhibitors increase atomexetine plasma levels; dosage adjustment of atomexetine when co-administered with CYP2D6 inhibitors may be necessary).

No products indexed under this heading.

Cimetidine (CYP2D6 inhibitors increase atomexetine plasma levels; dosage adjustment of atomexetine when co-administered with CYP2D6 inhibitors may be necessary). Products include:

Tagamet HB 200 Tablets ▣ 637
Tagamet Tablets 1547

Cimetidine Hydrochloride (CYP2D6 inhibitors increase atomexetine plasma levels; dosage adjustment of atomexetine when co-administered with CYP2D6 inhibitors may be necessary).

No products indexed under this heading.

Citalopram Hydrobromide (CYP2D6 inhibitors increase atomexetine plasma levels; dosage adjustment of atomexetine when co-administered with CYP2D6 inhibitors may be necessary). Products include:

Celexa 1177

Clomipramine Hydrochloride (CYP2D6 inhibitors increase atomexetine plasma levels; dosage adjustment of atomexetine when co-administered with CYP2D6 inhibitors may be necessary).

No products indexed under this heading.

Cocaine Hydrochloride (CYP2D6 inhibitors increase atomexetine plasma levels; dosage adjustment of atomexetine when co-administered with CYP2D6 inhibitors may be necessary).

No products indexed under this heading.

Desipramine Hydrochloride (CYP2D6 inhibitors increase atomexetine plasma levels; dosage adjustment of atomexetine when co-administered with CYP2D6 inhibitors may be necessary).

No products indexed under this heading.

Diphenhydramine (CYP2D6 inhibitors increase atomexetine plasma levels; dosage adjustment of atomexetine when co-administered with CYP2D6 inhibitors may be necessary). Products include:

Tylenol Sore Throat NightTime Liquid with Cool Burst 1849

Diphenhydramine Hydrochloride (CYP2D6 inhibitors increase atomexetine plasma levels; dosage adjustment of atomexetine when co-administered with CYP2D6 inhibitors may be necessary). Products include:

Benadryl Allergy & Cold Tablets ▣ 692
Benadryl Allergy ▣ 691
Benadryl Allergy & Sinus Headache Caplets & Gelcaps ▣ 693
Children's Benadryl Allergy Liquid ▣ 695
Children's Benadryl Dye-Free Allergy Liquid ▣ 695
Benadryl Dye-Free Allergy Liqui-Gels Softgels ▣ 692
Benadryl Itch Relief Stick Extra Strength ▣ 696
Benadryl Itch Stopping Cream Extra Strength ▣ 697
Benadryl Itch Stopping Gel Extra Strength ▣ 697
Benadryl Itch Stopping Spray Extra Strength ▣ 697
Benadryl Maximum Strength Severe Allergy & Sinus Headache Caplets ▣ 694
Children's Benadryl D Liquid Medication ▣ 693
Benadryl D Tablets ▣ 694
Nytol QuickCaps Caplets ▣ 635
Maximum Strength Nytol QuickGels Softgels ▣ 635
Simply Sleep Caplets 1841
Sominex Original Formula Tablets ▣ 637
TheraFlu Thin Strips Multi Symptom ▣ 684
Triaminic Thin Strips Cough & Runny Nose ▣ 690
Children's Tylenol Plus Cold & Allergy Suspension Liquid 1850
Tylenol Allergy Complete Night Time Caplets 1844
Tylenol Severe Allergy Caplets 1844
Tylenol Flu NightTime Gelcaps 1846
Extra Strength Tylenol PM Caplets, Geltabs, Gelcaps and Liquid 1847
Unisom Maximum Strength SleepGels ▣ 712

Dobutamine (Atomoxene HCl should be administered with caution to patients being treated with systematically-administered (oral or intravenous) albuterol (or other beta-2 agonists) because the action of albuterol on the cardiovascular system can be potentiated resulting in increases in heart rate and blood pressure).

No products indexed under this heading.

Dobutamine Hydrochloride (Atomoxene HCl should be administered with caution to patients being treated with systematically-administered (oral or intravenous) albuterol (or other beta-2 agonists) because the action of albuterol on the cardiovascular system can be potentiated resulting in increases in heart rate and blood pressure).

No products indexed under this heading.

Doxepin Hydrochloride (CYP2D6 inhibitors increase atomexetine plasma levels; dosage adjustment of atomexetine when co-administered with CYP2D6 inhibitors may be necessary).

No products indexed under this heading.

Ephedrine Hydrochloride (Atomoxene HCl should be administered with caution to patients being treated with systematically-administered (oral or intravenous) albuterol (or other beta-2 agonists) because the action of albuterol on the cardiovascular system can be potentiated resulting in increases in heart rate and blood pressure). Products include:

Primatene Tablets ▣ 749

Ephedrine Sulfate (Atomoxene HCl should be administered with caution to patients being treated with systematically-administered (oral or intravenous) albuterol (or other beta-2 agonists) because the action of albuterol on the cardiovascular system can be potentiated resulting in increases in heart rate and blood pressure).

No products indexed under this heading.

Ephedrine Tannate (Atomoxene HCl should be administered with caution to patients being treated with systematically-administered (oral or intravenous) albuterol (or other beta-2 agonists) because the action of albuterol on the cardiovascular system can be potentiated resulting in increases in heart rate and blood pressure).

No products indexed under this heading.

Epinephrine (Atomoxene HCl should be administered with caution to patients being treated with systematically-administered (oral or intravenous) albuterol (or other beta-2 agonists) because the action of albuterol on the cardiovascular system can be potentiated resulting in increases in heart rate and blood pressure). Products include:

EpiPen 1061
Primatene Mist ▣ 749

Epinephrine Hydrochloride (Atomoxene HCl should be administered with caution to patients being treated with systematically-administered (oral or intravenous) albuterol (or other beta-2 agonists) because the action of albuterol on the cardiovascular system can be potentiated resulting in increases in heart rate and blood pressure).

No products indexed under this heading.

Escitalopram Oxalate (CYP2D6 inhibitors increase atomexetine plasma levels; dosage adjustment of atomexetine when co-administered with CYP2D6 inhibitors may be necessary). Products include:

Lexapro Oral Solution 1193
Lexapro Tablets 1193

Fluoxetine (CYP2D6 inhibitors increase atomexetine plasma levels; dosage adjustment of atomexetine when co-administered with CYP2D6 inhibitors may be necessary).

No products indexed under this heading.

Fluoxetine Hydrochloride (CYP2D6 inhibitors increase atomexetine plasma levels; dosage adjustment of atomoxetine when co-administered with CYP2D6 inhibitors may be necessary). Products include:

Prozac Pulvules and Liquid 1771
Symbyax Capsules 1788

Fluphenazine Decanoate (CYP2D6 inhibitors increase atomexetine plasma levels; dosage adjustment of atomexetine when co-administered with CYP2D6 inhibitors may be necessary).

No products indexed under this heading.

Fluphenazine Enanthate (CYP2D6 inhibitors increase atomexetine plasma levels; dosage adjustment of atomexetine when co-administered with CYP2D6 inhibitors may be necessary).

No products indexed under this heading.

Fluphenazine Hydrochloride (CYP2D6 inhibitors increase atomexetine plasma levels; dosage adjustment of atomexetine when co-administered with CYP2D6 inhibitors may be necessary).

No products indexed under this heading.

Fluvoxamine Maleate (CYP2D6 inhibitors increase atomexetine plasma levels; dosage adjustment of atomexetine when co-administered with CYP2D6 inhibitors may be necessary).

No products indexed under this heading.

Halofantrine Hydrochloride (CYP2D6 inhibitors increase atomexetine plasma levels; dosage adjustment of atomexetine when co-administered with CYP2D6 inhibitors may be necessary).

No products indexed under this heading.

Haloperidol (CYP2D6 inhibitors increase atomexetine plasma levels; dosage adjustment of atomexetine when co-administered with CYP2D6 inhibitors may be necessary).

No products indexed under this heading.

Haloperidol Decanoate (CYP2D6 inhibitors increase atomexetine plasma levels; dosage adjustment of atomexetine when co-administered with CYP2D6 inhibitors may be necessary).
No products indexed under this heading.

Hydroxychloroquine Sulfate (CYP2D6 inhibitors increase atomexetine plasma levels; dosage adjustment of atomexetine when co-administered with CYP2D6 inhibitors may be necessary).
No products indexed under this heading.

Imatinib Mesylate (CYP2D6 inhibitors increase atomexetine plasma levels; dosage adjustment of atomexetine when co-administered with CYP2D6 inhibitors may be necessary). Products include:
Gleevec Tablets **2221**

Imipramine Hydrochloride (CYP2D6 inhibitors increase atomexetine plasma levels; dosage adjustment of atomexetine when co-administered with CYP2D6 inhibitors may be necessary).
No products indexed under this heading.

Imipramine Pamoate (CYP2D6 inhibitors increase atomexetine plasma levels; dosage adjustment of atomexetine when co-administered with CYP2D6 inhibitors may be necessary).
No products indexed under this heading.

Isocarboxazid (Concurrent use with MAOIs is contraindicated. Atomexetine should not be taken with MAOIs or within two weeks after discontinuing MAOI. Treatment with an MAOI should not be initiated within two weeks after discontinuing atomexetine).
No products indexed under this heading.

Isoetharine (Atomoxene HCl should be administered with caution to patients being treated with systematically-administered (oral or intravenous) albuterol (or other beta-2 agonists) because the action of albuterol on the cardiovascular system can be potentiated resulting in increases in heart rate and blood pressure).
No products indexed under this heading.

Isoproterenol Hydrochloride (Atomoxene HCl should be administered with caution to patients being treated with systematically-administered (oral or intravenous) albuterol (or other beta-2 agonists) because the action of albuterol on the cardiovascular system can be potentiated resulting in increases in heart rate and blood pressure).
No products indexed under this heading.

Isoproterenol Sulfate (Atomoxene HCl should be administered with caution to patients being treated with systematically-administered (oral or intravenous) albuterol (or other beta-2 agonists) because the action of albuterol on the cardiovascular system can be potentiated resulting in increases in heart rate and blood pressure).
No products indexed under this heading.

Levalbuterol Hydrochloride (Atomoxene HCl should be administered with caution to patients being treated with systematically-administered (oral or intravenous) albuterol (or other beta-2 agonists) because the action of albuterol on the cardiovascular system can be potentiated resulting in increases in heart rate and blood pressure). Products include:
Xopenex Inhalation Solution **3143**
Xopenex Inhalation Solution Concentrate **3147**

Maprotiline Hydrochloride (CYP2D6 inhibitors increase atomexetine plasma levels; dosage adjustment of atomexetine when co-administered with CYP2D6 inhibitors may be necessary).
No products indexed under this heading.

Metaproterenol Sulfate (Atomoxene HCl should be administered with caution to patients being treated with systematically-administered (oral or intravenous) albuterol (or other beta-2 agonists) because the action of albuterol on the cardiovascular system can be potentiated resulting in increases in heart rate and blood pressure). Products include:
Alupent Inhalation Aerosol **858**

Methadone Hydrochloride (CYP2D6 inhibitors increase atomexetine plasma levels; dosage adjustment of atomexetine when co-administered with CYP2D6 inhibitors may be necessary).
No products indexed under this heading.

Mibefradil Dihydrochloride (CYP2D6 inhibitors increase atomexetine plasma levels; dosage adjustment of atomexetine when co-administered with CYP2D6 inhibitors may be necessary).
No products indexed under this heading.

Midazolam Hydrochloride (Co-administration of atomexetine with midazolam, resulted in a 15% increase in AUC of midazolam).
No products indexed under this heading.

Moclobemide (Concurrent use with MAOIs is contraindicated. Atomexetine should not be taken with MAOIs or within two weeks after discontinuing MAOI. Treatment with an MAOI should not be initiated within two weeks after discontinuing atomexetine).
No products indexed under this heading.

Nortriptyline Hydrochloride (CYP2D6 inhibitors increase atomexetine plasma levels; dosage adjustment of atomexetine when co-administered with CYP2D6 inhibitors may be necessary).
No products indexed under this heading.

Pargyline Hydrochloride (Concurrent use with MAOIs is contraindicated. Atomexetine should not be taken with MAOIs or within two weeks after discontinuing MAOI. Treatment with an MAOI should not be initiated within two weeks after discontinuing atomexetine).
No products indexed under this heading.

Paroxetine Hydrochloride (CYP2D6 inhibitors increase atomexetine plasma levels; dosage adjustment of atomexetine when co-administered with CYP2D6 inhibitors may be necessary). Products include:
Paxil CR Controlled-Release Tablets **1509**
Paxil **1501**

Perphenazine (CYP2D6 inhibitors increase atomexetine plasma levels; dosage adjustment of atomexetine when co-administered with CYP2D6 inhibitors may be necessary).
No products indexed under this heading.

Phenelzine Sulfate (Concurrent use with MAOIs is contraindicated. Atomexetine should not be taken with MAOIs or within two weeks after discontinuing MAOI. Treatment with an MAOI should not be initiated within two weeks after discontinuing atomexetine).
No products indexed under this heading.

Pirbuterol Acetate (Atomoxene HCl should be administered with caution to patients being treated with systematically-administered (oral or intravenous) albuterol (or other beta-2 agonists) because the action of albuterol on the cardiovascular system can be potentiated resulting in increases in heart rate and blood pressure). Products include:
Maxair Autohaler **1820**

Procarbazine Hydrochloride (Concurrent use with MAOIs is contraindicated. Atomexetine should not be taken with MAOIs or within two weeks after discontinuing MAOI. Treatment with an MAOI should not be initiated within two weeks after discontinuing atomexetine). Products include:
Matulane Capsules **3188**

Propafenone Hydrochloride (CYP2D6 inhibitors increase atomexetine plasma levels; dosage adjustment of atomexetine when co-administered with CYP2D6 inhibitors may be necessary). Products include:
Rythmol SR Capsules **2736**

Propoxyphene Hydrochloride (CYP2D6 inhibitors increase atomexetine plasma levels; dosage adjustment of atomexetine when co-administered with CYP2D6 inhibitors may be necessary).
No products indexed under this heading.

Propoxyphene Napsylate (CYP2D6 inhibitors increase atomexetine plasma levels; dosage adjustment of atomexetine when co-administered with CYP2D6 inhibitors may be necessary). Products include:
Darvocet A 500 Tablets **3497**

Protriptyline Hydrochloride (CYP2D6 inhibitors increase atomexetine plasma levels; dosage adjustment of atomexetine when co-administered with CYP2D6 inhibitors may be necessary). Products include:
Vivactil Tablets **2350**

Quinacrine Hydrochloride (CYP2D6 inhibitors increase atomexetine plasma levels; dosage adjustment of atomexetine when co-administered with CYP2D6 inhibitors may be necessary).
No products indexed under this heading.

Quinidine (CYP2D6 inhibitors increase atomexetine plasma levels; dosage adjustment of atomexetine when co-administered with CYP2D6 inhibitors may be necessary).
No products indexed under this heading.

Quinidine Gluconate (CYP2D6 inhibitors increase atomexetine plasma levels; dosage adjustment of atomexetine when co-administered with CYP2D6 inhibitors may be necessary).
No products indexed under this heading.

Quinidine Hydrochloride (CYP2D6 inhibitors increase atomexetine plasma levels; dosage adjustment of atomexetine when co-administered with CYP2D6 inhibitors may be necessary).
No products indexed under this heading.

Quinidine Polygalacturonate (CYP2D6 inhibitors increase atomexetine plasma levels; dosage adjustment of atomexetine when co-administered with CYP2D6 inhibitors may be necessary).
No products indexed under this heading.

Quinidine Sulfate (CYP2D6 inhibitors increase atomexetine plasma levels; dosage adjustment of atomexetine when co-administered with CYP2D6 inhibitors may be necessary).
No products indexed under this heading.

Ranitidine Bismuth Citrate (CYP2D6 inhibitors increase atomexetine plasma levels; dosage adjustment of atomexetine when co-administered with CYP2D6 inhibitors may be necessary).
No products indexed under this heading.

Ranitidine Hydrochloride (CYP2D6 inhibitors increase atomexetine plasma levels; dosage adjustment of atomexetine when co-administered with CYP2D6 inhibitors may be necessary). Products include:
Zantac **1597**
Zantac Injection **1593**
Zantac 75 Tablets .... ▣**715**
Zantac 150 Maximum Strength Tablets.. ▣**715**
Zantac Injection Pharmacy Bulk Package **1595**

Ritonavir (CYP2D6 inhibitors increase atomexetine plasma levels; dosage adjustment of atomexetine when co-administered with CYP2D6 inhibitors may be necessary). Products include:
Kaletra **474**
Norvir **499**

Salmeterol Xinafoate (Atomoxene HCl should be administered with caution to patients being treated with systematically-administered (oral or intravenous) albuterol (or other beta-2 agonists) because the action of albuterol on the cardiovascular system can be potentiated resulting in increases in heart rate and blood pressure). Products include:
Advair Diskus 100/50 .... **1291**
Advair Diskus 250/50 .... **1291**
Advair Diskus 500/50 .... **1291**
Serevent Diskus **1540**

Selegiline Hydrochloride (Concurrent use with MAOIs is contraindicated. Atomexetine should not be taken with MAOIs or within two

weeks after discontinuing MAOI. Treatment with an MAOI should not be initiated within two weeks after discontinuing atomexetine). Products include:

Eldepryl Capsules 3209

Sertraline Hydrochloride (CYP2D6 inhibitors increase atomexetine plasma levels; dosage adjustment of atomexetine when co-administered with CYP2D6 inhibitors may be necessary). Products include:

Zoloft 2581

Terbinafine Hydrochloride (CYP2D6 inhibitors increase atomexetine plasma levels; dosage adjustment of atomexetine when co-administered with CYP2D6 inhibitors may be necessary). Products include:

Lamisil AT Creams (Athlete's Foot & Jock Itch) .... ▣676
Lamisil Tablets 2226

Terbutaline Sulfate (Atomoxene HCl should be administered with caution to patients being treated with systematically-administered (oral or intravenous) albuterol (or other beta-2 agonists) because the action of albuterol on the cardiovascular system can be potentiated resulting in increases in heart rate and blood pressure).

No products indexed under this heading.

Thioridazine Hydrochloride (CYP2D6 inhibitors increase atomexetine plasma levels; dosage adjustment of atomexetine when co-administered with CYP2D6 inhibitors may be necessary). Products include:

Thioridazine Hydrochloride Tablets 2122

Tranylcypromine Sulfate (Concurrent use with MAOIs is contraindicated. Atomexetine should not be taken with MAOIs or within two weeks after discontinuing MAOI. Treatment with an MAOI should not be initiated within two weeks after discontinuing atomexetine). Products include:

Parnate Tablets 1499

Trimipramine Maleate (CYP2D6 inhibitors increase atomexetine plasma levels; dosage adjustment of atomexetine when co-administered with CYP2D6 inhibitors may be necessary). Products include:

Surmontil Capsules 2347

STRIANT MUCOADHESIVE

(Testosterone) 1022

May interact with corticosteroids, insulin, and certain other agents. Compounds in these categories include:

ACTH (Concurrent administration of testosterone with ACTH or corticosteroids may enhance edema formation and should be administered cautiously, particularly in patients with cardiac or hepatic disease).

No products indexed under this heading.

Betamethasone Acetate (Concurrent administration of testosterone with ACTH or corticosteroids may enhance edema formation and should be administered cautiously, particularly in patients with cardiac or hepatic disease).

No products indexed under this heading.

Betamethasone Sodium Phosphate (Concurrent administration of testosterone with ACTH or corticosteroids may enhance edema formation and should be administered cautiously, particularly in patients with cardiac or hepatic disease).

No products indexed under this heading.

Cortisone Acetate (Concurrent administration of testosterone with ACTH or corticosteroids may enhance edema formation and should be administered cautiously, particularly in patients with cardiac or hepatic disease).

No products indexed under this heading.

Dexamethasone (Concurrent administration of testosterone with ACTH or corticosteroids may enhance edema formation and should be administered cautiously, particularly in patients with cardiac or hepatic disease). Products include:

Ciprodex Otic Suspension 555
Decadron Tablets 1929
TobraDex Ophthalmic Ointment 558
TobraDex Ophthalmic Suspension 558

Dexamethasone Acetate (Concurrent administration of testosterone with ACTH or corticosteroids may enhance edema formation and should be administered cautiously, particularly in patients with cardiac or hepatic disease).

No products indexed under this heading.

Dexamethasone Sodium Phosphate (Concurrent administration of testosterone with ACTH or corticosteroids may enhance edema formation and should be administered cautiously, particularly in patients with cardiac or hepatic disease). Products include:

Decadron Phosphate Injection 1931

Fludrocortisone Acetate (Concurrent administration of testosterone with ACTH or corticosteroids may enhance edema formation and should be administered cautiously, particularly in patients with cardiac or hepatic disease).

No products indexed under this heading.

Hydrocortisone (Concurrent administration of testosterone with ACTH or corticosteroids may enhance edema formation and should be administered cautiously, particularly in patients with cardiac or hepatic disease). Products include:

Cortizone•5 Ointment .... ▣699
Cortizone•10 Creme .... ▣699
Cortizone•10 Ointment .... ▣699
Cortizone•10 Plus Creme .... ▣700
Cortizone•10 Maximum Strength Quick Shot Spray .... ▣700
Hydrocortone Tablets 1963
Preparation H Hydrocortisone Cream .... ▣748

Hydrocortisone Acetate (Concurrent administration of testosterone with ACTH or corticosteroids may enhance edema formation and should be administered cautiously, particularly in patients with cardiac or hepatic disease). Products include:

Analpram-HC 1136
Pramosone 1139
ProctoFoam-HC 3113
Tucks Anti-Itch Ointment .... ▣712
U-cort 1% Cream 3289

Hydrocortisone Sodium Phosphate (Concurrent administration of testosterone with ACTH or corticosteroids may enhance edema formation and should be administered cautiously, particularly in patients with cardiac or hepatic disease).

No products indexed under this heading.

Hydrocortisone Sodium Succinate (Concurrent administration of testosterone with ACTH or corticosteroids may enhance edema formation and should be administered cautiously, particularly in patients with cardiac or hepatic disease).

No products indexed under this heading.

Insulin, Human, Zinc Suspension (In diabetic patients, the metabolic effects of androgens may decrease blood glucose and, therefore, insulin requirements). Products include:

Humulin L, 100 Units 1763
Humulin U, 100 Units 1770

Insulin, Human NPH (In diabetic patients, the metabolic effects of androgens may decrease blood glucose and, therefore, insulin requirements). Products include:

Humulin N, 100 Units 1764
Humulin N Pen 1765
Novolin N Human Insulin 10 ml Vials 2322
Novolin N InnoLet 2322
Novolin N PenFill 3 ml Cartridges 2325
Novolin R InnoLet 2322

Insulin, Human Regular (In diabetic patients, the metabolic effects of androgens may decrease blood glucose and, therefore, insulin requirements). Products include:

Humulin R (U-500) 1768
Humulin R, 100 Units 1767
Novolin R Human Insulin 10 ml Vials 2322
Novolin R PenFill 2325

Insulin, Human Regular and Human NPH Mixture (In diabetic patients, the metabolic effects of androgens may decrease blood glucose and, therefore, insulin requirements). Products include:

Humulin 50/50, 100 Units 1760
Humulin 70/30 Pen 1761
Novolin 70/30 Human Insulin 10 ml Vials 2321
Novolin 70/30 InnoLet 2322
Novolin 70/30 PenFill 3 ml Cartridges 2325

Insulin, NPH (In diabetic patients, the metabolic effects of androgens may decrease blood glucose and, therefore, insulin requirements).

No products indexed under this heading.

Insulin, Regular (In diabetic patients, the metabolic effects of androgens may decrease blood glucose and, therefore, insulin requirements).

No products indexed under this heading.

Insulin, Zinc Crystals (In diabetic patients, the metabolic effects of androgens may decrease blood glucose and, therefore, insulin requirements).

No products indexed under this heading.

Insulin, Zinc Suspension (In diabetic patients, the metabolic effects of androgens may decrease blood glucose and, therefore, insulin requirements).

No products indexed under this heading.

Insulin Aspart, Human Regular (In diabetic patients, the metabolic effects of androgens may decrease blood glucose and, therefore, insulin requirements). Products include:

NovoLog Injection 2326

Insulin glargine (In diabetic patients, the metabolic effects of androgens may decrease blood glucose and, therefore, insulin requirements). Products include:

Lantus Injection 2925

Insulin Lispro, Human (In diabetic patients, the metabolic effects of androgens may decrease blood glucose and, therefore, insulin requirements). Products include:

Humalog-Pen 1751
Humalog Mix 75/25-Pen 1754

Insulin Lispro Protamine, Human (In diabetic patients, the metabolic effects of androgens may decrease blood glucose and, therefore, insulin requirements). Products include:

Humalog Mix 75/25-Pen 1754

Methylprednisolone Acetate (Concurrent administration of testosterone with ACTH or corticosteroids may enhance edema formation and should be administered cautiously, particularly in patients with cardiac or hepatic disease). Products include:

Depo-Medrol Injectable Suspension 2615
Depo-Medrol Single-Dose Vial 2617

Methylprednisolone Sodium Succinate (Concurrent administration of testosterone with ACTH or corticosteroids may enhance edema formation and should be administered cautiously, particularly in patients with cardiac or hepatic disease).

No products indexed under this heading.

Oxyphenbutazone (Concurrent administration of oxyphenbutazone and androgens may result in elevated serum levels of oxyphenbutazone).

No products indexed under this heading.

Prednisolone Acetate (Concurrent administration of testosterone with ACTH or corticosteroids may enhance edema formation and should be administered cautiously, particularly in patients with cardiac or hepatic disease). Products include:

Blephamide Ophthalmic Ointment 563
Blephamide Ophthalmic Suspension 564
Poly-Pred Liquifilm Ophthalmic Suspension .... ⊙231
Pred Forte Ophthalmic Suspension .... ⊙233
Pred Mild Sterile Ophthalmic Suspension .... ⊙236
Pred-G Ophthalmic Suspension .... ⊙234
Pred-G Sterile Ophthalmic Ointment .... ⊙235

Prednisolone Sodium Phosphate (Concurrent administration of testosterone with ACTH or corticosteroids may enhance edema formation and should be administered cautiously, particularly in patients with cardiac or hepatic disease). Products include:

Pediapred Oral Solution 3319

Prednisolone Tebutate (Concurrent administration of testosterone with ACTH or corticosteroids may enhance edema formation and should be administered cautiously, particularly in patients with cardiac or hepatic disease).
No products indexed under this heading.

Prednisone (Concurrent administration of testosterone with ACTH or corticosteroids may enhance edema formation and should be administered cautiously, particularly in patients with cardiac or hepatic disease).
No products indexed under this heading.

Triamcinolone (Concurrent administration of testosterone with ACTH or corticosteroids may enhance edema formation and should be administered cautiously, particularly in patients with cardiac or hepatic disease).
No products indexed under this heading.

Triamcinolone Acetonide (Concurrent administration of testosterone with ACTH or corticosteroids may enhance edema formation and should be administered cautiously, particularly in patients with cardiac or hepatic disease). Products include:
Azmacort Inhalation Aerosol **1701**
Nasacort HFA Inhalation Aerosol **2939**
Nasacort AQ Nasal Spray **2937**

Triamcinolone Diacetate (Concurrent administration of testosterone with ACTH or corticosteroids may enhance edema formation and should be administered cautiously, particularly in patients with cardiac or hepatic disease).
No products indexed under this heading.

Triamcinolone Hexacetonide (Concurrent administration of testosterone with ACTH or corticosteroids may enhance edema formation and should be administered cautiously, particularly in patients with cardiac or hepatic disease).
No products indexed under this heading.

STROMECTOL TABLETS
(Ivermectin) **2053**
None cited in PDR database.

SUBOXONE TABLETS
(Buprenorphine Hydrochloride, Naloxone Hydrochloride).................... **2719**
May interact with cytochrome p450 3a4 inhibitors (selected). Compounds in these categories include:

Acetazolamide (Buprenorphine is metabolized to norbuprenorphine by cytochrome CYP3A4. Because CYP3A4 inhibitors may increase plasma concentrations of buprenorphine, patients already on CYP3A4 inhibitors should have their dose of Subutex or Suboxone adjusted).
No products indexed under this heading.

Amiodarone Hydrochloride (Buprenorphine is metabolized to norbuprenorphine by cytochrome CYP3A4. Because CYP3A4 inhibitors may increase plasma concentrations of buprenorphine, patients already on CYP3A4 inhibitors should have their dose of Subutex or Suboxone adjusted). Products include:
Pacerone Tablets **3337**

Amprenavir (Buprenorphine is metabolized to norbuprenorphine by cytochrome CYP3A4. Because CYP3A4 inhibitors may increase plasma concentrations of buprenorphine, patients already on CYP3A4 inhibitors should have their dose of Subutex or Suboxone adjusted). Products include:
Agenerase Capsules **1299**
Agenerase Oral Solution **1304**

Anastrozole (Buprenorphine is metabolized to norbuprenorphine by cytochrome CYP3A4. Because CYP3A4 inhibitors may increase plasma concentrations of buprenorphine, patients already on CYP3A4 inhibitors should have their dose of Subutex or Suboxone adjusted). Products include:
Arimidex Tablets **665**

Aprepitant (Buprenorphine is metabolized to norbuprenorphine by cytochrome CYP3A4. Because CYP3A4 inhibitors may increase plasma concentrations of buprenorphine, patients already on CYP3A4 inhibitors should have their dose of Subutex or Suboxone adjusted). Products include:
Emend Capsules **1944**

Cimetidine (Buprenorphine is metabolized to norbuprenorphine by cytochrome CYP3A4. Because CYP3A4 inhibitors may increase plasma concentrations of buprenorphine, patients already on CYP3A4 inhibitors should have their dose of Subutex or Suboxone adjusted). Products include:
Tagamet HB 200 Tablets .... ▣ **637**
Tagamet Tablets **1547**

Cimetidine Hydrochloride (Buprenorphine is metabolized to norbuprenorphine by cytochrome CYP3A4. Because CYP3A4 inhibitors may increase plasma concentrations of buprenorphine, patients already on CYP3A4 inhibitors should have their dose of Subutex or Suboxone adjusted).
No products indexed under this heading.

Ciprofloxacin (Buprenorphine is metabolized to norbuprenorphine by cytochrome CYP3A4. Because CYP3A4 inhibitors may increase plasma concentrations of buprenorphine, patients already on CYP3A4 inhibitors should have their dose of Subutex or Suboxone adjusted). Products include:
Cipro I.V. **2998**
Cipro I.V. Pharmacy Bulk Package ... **3509**
Cipro Oral Suspension **2991**
Cipro XR Tablets **3004**
Ciprodex Otic Suspension **555**

Clarithromycin (Buprenorphine is metabolized to norbuprenorphine by cytochrome CYP3A4. Because CYP3A4 inhibitors may increase plasma concentrations of buprenorphine, patients already on CYP3A4 inhibitors should have their dose of Subutex or Suboxone adjusted). Products include:
Biaxin/Biaxin XL **402**
PREVPAC **3281**

Clotrimazole (Buprenorphine is metabolized to norbuprenorphine by cytochrome CYP3A4. Because CYP3A4 inhibitors may increase plasma concentrations of buprenorphine, patients already on CYP3A4 inhibitors should have their dose of Subutex or Suboxone adjusted). Products include:
Lotrimin **3053**
Lotrisone **3054**

Cyclosporine (Buprenorphine is metabolized to norbuprenorphine by cytochrome CYP3A4. Because CYP3A4 inhibitors may increase plasma concentrations of buprenorphine, patients already on CYP3A4 inhibitors should have their dose of Subutex or Suboxone adjusted). Products include:
Gengraf Capsules **458**
Neoral Soft Gelatin Capsules **2247**
Neoral Oral Solution **2247**
Restasis Ophthalmic Emulsion **570**
Sandimmune **2259**

Dalfopristin (Buprenorphine is metabolized to norbuprenorphine by cytochrome CYP3A4. Because CYP3A4 inhibitors may increase plasma concentrations of buprenorphine, patients already on CYP3A4 inhibitors should have their dose of Subutex or Suboxone adjusted). Products include:
Synercid I.V. **1690**

Danazol (Buprenorphine is metabolized to norbuprenorphine by cytochrome CYP3A4. Because CYP3A4 inhibitors may increase plasma concentrations of buprenorphine, patients already on CYP3A4 inhibitors should have their dose of Subutex or Suboxone adjusted).
No products indexed under this heading.

Delavirdine Mesylate (Buprenorphine is metabolized to norbuprenorphine by cytochrome CYP3A4. Because CYP3A4 inhibitors may increase plasma concentrations of buprenorphine, patients already on CYP3A4 inhibitors should have their dose of Subutex or Suboxone adjusted). Products include:
Rescriptor Tablets **2535**

Diltiazem Hydrochloride (Buprenorphine is metabolized to norbuprenorphine by cytochrome CYP3A4. Because CYP3A4 inhibitors may increase plasma concentrations of buprenorphine, patients already on CYP3A4 inhibitors should have their dose of Subutex or Suboxone adjusted). Products include:
Cardizem LA Extended Release Tablets **1699**
Tiazac Capsules **1204**

Diltiazem Maleate (Buprenorphine is metabolized to norbuprenorphine by cytochrome CYP3A4. Because CYP3A4 inhibitors may increase plasma concentrations of buprenorphine, patients already on CYP3A4 inhibitors should have their dose of Subutex or Suboxone adjusted).
No products indexed under this heading.

Efavirenz (Buprenorphine is metabolized to norbuprenorphine by cytochrome CYP3A4. Because CYP3A4 inhibitors may increase plasma concentrations of buprenorphine, patients already on CYP3A4 inhibitors should have their dose of Subutex or Suboxone adjusted). Products include:
Sustiva Capsules **957**

Erythromycin (Buprenorphine is metabolized to norbuprenorphine by cytochrome CYP3A4. Because CYP3A4 inhibitors may increase plasma concentrations of buprenorphine, patients already on CYP3A4 inhibitors should have their dose of Subutex or Suboxone adjusted). Products include:
Erygel Topical Gel **2096**
Ery-Tab Tablets **447**
Erythromycin Base Filmtab Tablets **454**
Erythromycin Delayed-Release Capsules, USP **456**
PCE Dispertab Tablets **510**

Erythromycin Estolate (Buprenorphine is metabolized to norbuprenorphine by cytochrome CYP3A4. Because CYP3A4 inhibitors may increase plasma concentrations of buprenorphine, patients already on CYP3A4 inhibitors should have their dose of Subutex or Suboxone adjusted).
No products indexed under this heading.

Erythromycin Ethylsuccinate (Buprenorphine is metabolized to norbuprenorphine by cytochrome CYP3A4. Because CYP3A4 inhibitors may increase plasma concentrations of buprenorphine, patients already on CYP3A4 inhibitors should have their dose of Subutex or Suboxone adjusted). Products include:
E.E.S. **449**
EryPed **445**

Erythromycin Gluceptate (Buprenorphine is metabolized to norbuprenorphine by cytochrome CYP3A4. Because CYP3A4 inhibitors may increase plasma concentrations of buprenorphine, patients already on CYP3A4 inhibitors should have their dose of Subutex or Suboxone adjusted).
No products indexed under this heading.

Erythromycin Lactobionate (Buprenorphine is metabolized to norbuprenorphine by cytochrome CYP3A4. Because CYP3A4 inhibitors may increase plasma concentrations of buprenorphine, patients already on CYP3A4 inhibitors should have their dose of Subutex or Suboxone adjusted).
No products indexed under this heading.

Erythromycin Stearate (Buprenorphine is metabolized to norbuprenorphine by cytochrome CYP3A4. Because CYP3A4 inhibitors may increase plasma concentrations of buprenorphine, patients already on CYP3A4 inhibitors should have their dose of Subutex or Suboxone adjusted). Products include:
Erythrocin Stearate Filmtab Tablets **452**

Esomeprazole Magnesium (Buprenorphine is metabolized to norbuprenorphine by cytochrome CYP3A4. Because CYP3A4 inhibitors may increase plasma concentrations of buprenorphine, patients already on CYP3A4 inhibitors should have their dose of Subutex or Suboxone adjusted). Products include:
Nexium Delayed-Release Capsules **645**

Fluconazole (Buprenorphine is metabolized to norbuprenorphine by cytochrome CYP3A4. Because CYP3A4 inhibitors may increase plasma concentrations of buprenorphine, patients already on CYP3A4 inhibitors should have their dose of Subutex or Suboxone adjusted).
No products indexed under this heading.

Fluoxetine Hydrochloride (Buprenorphine is metabolized to norbuprenorphine by cytochrome CYP3A4. Because CYP3A4 inhibitors may increase plasma concentrations of buprenorphine, patients already

on CYP3A4 inhibitors should have their dose of Subutex or Subuxone adjusted). Products include:
Prozac Pulvules and Liquid 1771
Symbyax Capsules 1788

Fluvoxamine Maleate (Buprenorphine is metabolized to norbuprenorphine by cytochrome CYP3A4. Because CYP3A4 inhibitors may increase plasma concentrations of buprenorphine, patients already on CYP3A4 inhibitors should have their dose of Subutex or Subuxone adjusted).
No products indexed under this heading.

Fosamprenavir Calcium (Buprenorphine is metabolized to norbuprenorphine by cytochrome CYP3A4. Because CYP3A4 inhibitors may increase plasma concentrations of buprenorphine, patients already on CYP3A4 inhibitors should have their dose of Subutex or Subuxone adjusted). Products include:
Lexiva Tablets 1473

Indinavir Sulfate (Buprenorphine is metabolized to norbuprenorphine by cytochrome CYP3A4. Because CYP3A4 inhibitors may increase plasma concentrations of buprenorphine, patients already on CYP3A4 inhibitors should have their dose of Subutex or Subuxone adjusted). Products include:
Crixivan Capsules 1918

Isoniazid (Buprenorphine is metabolized to norbuprenorphine by cytochrome CYP3A4. Because CYP3A4 inhibitors may increase plasma concentrations of buprenorphine, patients already on CYP3A4 inhibitors should have their dose of Subutex or Subuxone adjusted).
No products indexed under this heading.

Itraconazole (Buprenorphine is metabolized to norbuprenorphine by cytochrome CYP3A4. Because CYP3A4 inhibitors may increase plasma concentrations of buprenorphine, patients already on CYP3A4 inhibitors should have their dose of Subutex or Subuxone adjusted).
No products indexed under this heading.

Ketoconazole (Buprenorphine is metabolized to norbuprenorphine by cytochrome CYP3A4. Because CYP3A4 inhibitors may increase plasma concentrations of buprenorphine, patients already on CYP3A4 inhibitors should have their dose of Subutex or Subuxone adjusted). Products include:
Nizoral A-D Shampoo, 1% 1839
Nizoral 2% Shampoo 1838

Lopinavir (Buprenorphine is metabolized to norbuprenorphine by cytochrome CYP3A4. Because CYP3A4 inhibitors may increase plasma concentrations of buprenorphine, patients already on CYP3A4 inhibitors should have their dose of Subutex or Subuxone adjusted). Products include:
Kaletra 474

Loratadine (Buprenorphine is metabolized to norbuprenorphine by cytochrome CYP3A4. Because CYP3A4 inhibitors may increase plasma concentrations of buprenorphine, patients already on CYP3A4 inhibitors should have their dose of Subutex or Subuxone adjusted). Products include:
Alavert Allergy & Sinus D-12 Hour Tablets 743
Alavert 743
Children's Claritin 24 Hour Non-Drowsy Allergy Syrup 732
Claritin Non-Drowsy 24 Hour Tablets 731
Non-Drowsy Claritin Hives Relief Tablets 733
Claritin Reditabs 24 Hour Non-Drowsy Tablets 732
Claritin-D Non-Drowsy 12 Hour Tablets 731
Claritin-D Non-Drowsy 24 Hour Tablets 731
Children's Dimetapp ND Non-Drowsy Allergy Syrup 746
Triaminic Allerchews 684

Metronidazole (Buprenorphine is metabolized to norbuprenorphine by cytochrome CYP3A4. Because CYP3A4 inhibitors may increase plasma concentrations of buprenorphine, patients already on CYP3A4 inhibitors should have their dose of Subutex or Subuxone adjusted). Products include:
Metrogel 1% 1212
MetroGel-Vaginal Gel 1822
Noritate Cream, 1% 1051

Metronidazole Benzoate (Buprenorphine is metabolized to norbuprenorphine by cytochrome CYP3A4. Because CYP3A4 inhibitors may increase plasma concentrations of buprenorphine, patients already on CYP3A4 inhibitors should have their dose of Subutex or Subuxone adjusted).
No products indexed under this heading.

Metronidazole Hydrochloride (Buprenorphine is metabolized to norbuprenorphine by cytochrome CYP3A4. Because CYP3A4 inhibitors may increase plasma concentrations of buprenorphine, patients already on CYP3A4 inhibitors should have their dose of Subutex or Subuxone adjusted).
No products indexed under this heading.

Miconazole (Buprenorphine is metabolized to norbuprenorphine by cytochrome CYP3A4. Because CYP3A4 inhibitors may increase plasma concentrations of buprenorphine, patients already on CYP3A4 inhibitors should have their dose of Subutex or Subuxone adjusted).
No products indexed under this heading.

Miconazole Nitrate (Buprenorphine is metabolized to norbuprenorphine by cytochrome CYP3A4. Because CYP3A4 inhibitors may increase plasma concentrations of buprenorphine, patients already on CYP3A4 inhibitors should have their dose of Subutex or Subuxone adjusted). Products include:
Desenex 674
Desenex Jock Itch Spray Powder 674

Nefazodone Hydrochloride (Buprenorphine is metabolized to norbuprenorphine by cytochrome CYP3A4. Because CYP3A4 inhibitors may increase plasma concentrations of buprenorphine, patients already on CYP3A4 inhibitors should have their dose of Subutex or Subuxone adjusted).
No products indexed under this heading.

Nelfinavir Mesylate (Buprenorphine is metabolized to norbuprenorphine by cytochrome CYP3A4. Because CYP3A4 inhibitors may increase plasma concentrations of buprenorphine, patients already on CYP3A4 inhibitors should have their dose of Subutex or Subuxone adjusted). Products include:
Viracept 2556

Nevirapine (Buprenorphine is metabolized to norbuprenorphine by cytochrome CYP3A4. Because CYP3A4 inhibitors may increase plasma concentrations of buprenorphine, patients already on CYP3A4 inhibitors should have their dose of Subutex or Subuxone adjusted). Products include:
Viramune Oral Suspension 903
Viramune Tablets 903

Niacinamide (Buprenorphine is metabolized to norbuprenorphine by cytochrome CYP3A4. Because CYP3A4 inhibitors may increase plasma concentrations of buprenorphine, patients already on CYP3A4 inhibitors should have their dose of Subutex or Subuxone adjusted).
No products indexed under this heading.

Nicotinamide (Buprenorphine is metabolized to norbuprenorphine by cytochrome CYP3A4. Because CYP3A4 inhibitors may increase plasma concentrations of buprenorphine, patients already on CYP3A4 inhibitors should have their dose of Subutex or Subuxone adjusted). Products include:
Nicomide Tablets 3190

Nifedipine (Buprenorphine is metabolized to norbuprenorphine by cytochrome CYP3A4. Because CYP3A4 inhibitors may increase plasma concentrations of buprenorphine, patients already on CYP3A4 inhibitors should have their dose of Subutex or Subuxone adjusted). Products include:
Adalat CC Tablets 2978

Norfloxacin (Buprenorphine is metabolized to norbuprenorphine by cytochrome CYP3A4. Because CYP3A4 inhibitors may increase plasma concentrations of buprenorphine, patients already on CYP3A4 inhibitors should have their dose of Subutex or Subuxone adjusted). Products include:
Noroxin Tablets 2009

Omeprazole (Buprenorphine is metabolized to norbuprenorphine by cytochrome CYP3A4. Because CYP3A4 inhibitors may increase plasma concentrations of buprenorphine, patients already on CYP3A4 inhibitors should have their dose of Subutex or Subuxone adjusted). Products include:
Zegerid Powder for Oral Solution 2972

Paroxetine Hydrochloride (Buprenorphine is metabolized to norbuprenorphine by cytochrome CYP3A4. Because CYP3A4 inhibitors may increase plasma concentrations of buprenorphine, patients already on CYP3A4 inhibitors should have their dose of Subutex or Subuxone adjusted). Products include:
Paxil CR Controlled-Release Tablets 1509
Paxil 1501

Propoxyphene Hydrochloride (Buprenorphine is metabolized to norbuprenorphine by cytochrome CYP3A4. Because CYP3A4 inhibitors may increase plasma concentrations of buprenorphine, patients already on CYP3A4 inhibitors should have their dose of Subutex or Subuxone adjusted).
No products indexed under this heading.

Propoxyphene Napsylate (Buprenorphine is metabolized to norbuprenorphine by cytochrome CYP3A4. Because CYP3A4 inhibitors may increase plasma concentrations of buprenorphine, patients already on CYP3A4 inhibitors should have their dose of Subutex or Subuxone adjusted). Products include:
Darvocet A 500 Tablets 3497

Quinidine (Buprenorphine is metabolized to norbuprenorphine by cytochrome CYP3A4. Because CYP3A4 inhibitors may increase plasma concentrations of buprenorphine, patients already on CYP3A4 inhibitors should have their dose of Subutex or Subuxone adjusted).
No products indexed under this heading.

Quinidine Hydrochloride (Buprenorphine is metabolized to norbuprenorphine by cytochrome CYP3A4. Because CYP3A4 inhibitors may increase plasma concentrations of buprenorphine, patients already on CYP3A4 inhibitors should have their dose of Subutex or Subuxone adjusted).
No products indexed under this heading.

Quinidine Polygalacturonate (Buprenorphine is metabolized to norbuprenorphine by cytochrome CYP3A4. Because CYP3A4 inhibitors may increase plasma concentrations of buprenorphine, patients already on CYP3A4 inhibitors should have their dose of Subutex or Subuxone adjusted).
No products indexed under this heading.

Quinidine Sulfate (Buprenorphine is metabolized to norbuprenorphine by cytochrome CYP3A4. Because CYP3A4 inhibitors may increase plasma concentrations of buprenorphine, patients already on CYP3A4 inhibitors should have their dose of Subutex or Subuxone adjusted).
No products indexed under this heading.

Quinine (Buprenorphine is metabolized to norbuprenorphine by cytochrome CYP3A4. Because CYP3A4 inhibitors may increase plasma concentrations of buprenorphine, patients already on CYP3A4 inhibitors should have their dose of Subutex or Subuxone adjusted).
No products indexed under this heading.

Quinine Sulfate (Buprenorphine is metabolized to norbuprenorphine by cytochrome CYP3A4. Because CYP3A4 inhibitors may increase plasma concentrations of buprenorphine, patients already on CYP3A4 inhibitors should have their dose of Subutex or Subuxone adjusted).
No products indexed under this heading.

Quinupristin (Buprenorphine is metabolized to norbuprenorphine by cytochrome CYP3A4. Because CYP3A4 inhibitors may increase plasma concentrations of buprenorphine, patients already on CYP3A4 inhibitors should have their dose of Subutex or Subuxone adjusted). Products include:
Synercid I.V. 1690

Ranitidine Bismuth Citrate (Buprenorphine is metabolized to norbuprenorphine by cytochrome CYP3A4. Because CYP3A4 inhibitors may increase plasma concentrations of buprenorphine, patients already on CYP3A4 inhibitors should have their dose of Subutex or Subuxone adjusted).
No products indexed under this heading.

Ranitidine Hydrochloride (Buprenorphine is metabolized to norbuprenorphine by cytochrome CYP3A4. Because CYP3A4 inhibitors may increase plasma concentrations of buprenorphine, patients already on CYP3A4 inhibitors should have their dose of Subutex or Subuxone adjusted). Products include:
Zantac 1597
Zantac Injection 1593
Zantac 75 Tablets .... ▣715
Zantac 150 Maximum Strength Tablets .... ▣715
Zantac Injection Pharmacy Bulk Package 1595

Ritonavir (Buprenorphine is metabolized to norbuprenorphine by cytochrome CYP3A4. Because CYP3A4 inhibitors may increase plasma concentrations of buprenorphine, patients already on CYP3A4 inhibitors should have their dose of Subutex or Subuxone adjusted). Products include:
Kaletra 474
Norvir 499

Saquinavir (Buprenorphine is metabolized to norbuprenorphine by cytochrome CYP3A4. Because CYP3A4 inhibitors may increase plasma concentrations of buprenorphine, patients already on CYP3A4 inhibitors should have their dose of Subutex or Subuxone adjusted).
No products indexed under this heading.

Saquinavir Mesylate (Buprenorphine is metabolized to norbuprenorphine by cytochrome CYP3A4. Because CYP3A4 inhibitors may increase plasma concentrations of buprenorphine, patients already on CYP3A4 inhibitors should have their dose of Subutex or Subuxone adjusted). Products include:
Invirase 2776

Sertraline Hydrochloride (Buprenorphine is metabolized to norbuprenorphine by cytochrome CYP3A4. Because CYP3A4 inhibitors may increase plasma concentrations of buprenorphine, patients already on CYP3A4 inhibitors should have their dose of Subutex or Subuxone adjusted). Products include:
Zoloft 2581

Telithromycin (Buprenorphine is metabolized to norbuprenorphine by cytochrome CYP3A4. Because CYP3A4 inhibitors may increase plasma concentrations of buprenorphine, patients already on CYP3A4 inhibitors should have their dose of Subutex or Subuxone adjusted). Products include:
Ketek Tablets 2920

Troglitazone (Buprenorphine is metabolized to norbuprenorphine by cytochrome CYP3A4. Because CYP3A4 inhibitors may increase plasma concentrations of buprenorphine, patients already on CYP3A4 inhibitors should have their dose of Subutex or Subuxone adjusted).
No products indexed under this heading.

Troleandomycin (Buprenorphine is metabolized to norbuprenorphine by cytochrome CYP3A4. Because CYP3A4 inhibitors may increase plasma concentrations of buprenorphine, patients already on CYP3A4 inhibitors should have their dose of Subutex or Subuxone adjusted).
No products indexed under this heading.

Valproate Sodium (Buprenorphine is metabolized to norbuprenorphine by cytochrome CYP3A4. Because CYP3A4 inhibitors may increase plasma concentrations of buprenorphine, patients already on CYP3A4 inhibitors should have their dose of Subutex or Subuxone adjusted). Products include:
Depacon Injection 412

Verapamil Hydrochloride (Buprenorphine is metabolized to norbuprenorphine by cytochrome CYP3A4. Because CYP3A4 inhibitors may increase plasma concentrations of buprenorphine, patients already on CYP3A4 inhibitors should have their dose of Subutex or Subuxone adjusted). Products include:
Covera-HS Tablets 3135
Tarka Tablets 519
Verelan PM Capsules 3120

Voriconazole (Buprenorphine is metabolized to norbuprenorphine by cytochrome CYP3A4. Because CYP3A4 inhibitors may increase plasma concentrations of buprenorphine, patients already on CYP3A4 inhibitors should have their dose of Subutex or Subuxone adjusted). Products include:
VFEND I.V. 2543
VFEND Oral Suspension 2543
VFEND Tablets 2543

Zafirlukast (Buprenorphine is metabolized to norbuprenorphine by cytochrome CYP3A4. Because CYP3A4 inhibitors may increase plasma concentrations of buprenorphine, patients already on CYP3A4 inhibitors should have their dose of Subutex or Subuxone adjusted). Products include:
Accolate Tablets 663

Zileuton (Buprenorphine is metabolized to norbuprenorphine by cytochrome CYP3A4. Because CYP3A4 inhibitors may increase plasma concentrations of buprenorphine, patients already on CYP3A4 inhibitors should have their dose of Subutex or Subuxone adjusted).
No products indexed under this heading.

Food Interactions

Grapefruit (Buprenorphine is metabolized to norbuprenorphine by cytochrome CYP3A4. Because CYP3A4 inhibitors may increase plasma concentrations of buprenorphine, patients already on CYP3A4 inhibitors should have their dose of Subutex or Subuxone adjusted).

Grapefruit Juice (Buprenorphine is metabolized to norbuprenorphine by cytochrome CYP3A4. Because CYP3A4 inhibitors may increase plasma concentrations of buprenorphine, patients already on CYP3A4 inhibitors should have their dose of Subutex or Subuxone adjusted).

SUBUTEX TABLETS

(Buprenorphine Hydrochloride) 2719
May interact with cytochrome p450 3a4 inhibitors (selected). Compounds in these categories include:

Acetazolamide (Buprenorphine is metabolized to norbuprenorphine by cytochrome CYP3A4. Because CYP3A4 inhibitors may increase plasma concentrations of buprenorphine, patients already on CYP3A4 inhibitors should have their dose of Subutex or Subuxone adjusted).
No products indexed under this heading.

Amiodarone Hydrochloride (Buprenorphine is metabolized to norbuprenorphine by cytochrome CYP3A4. Because CYP3A4 inhibitors may increase plasma concentrations of buprenorphine, patients already on CYP3A4 inhibitors should have their dose of Subutex or Subuxone adjusted). Products include:
Pacerone Tablets 3337

Amprenavir (Buprenorphine is metabolized to norbuprenorphine by cytochrome CYP3A4. Because CYP3A4 inhibitors may increase plasma concentrations of buprenorphine, patients already on CYP3A4 inhibitors should have their dose of Subutex or Subuxone adjusted). Products include:
Agenerase Capsules 1299
Agenerase Oral Solution 1304

Anastrozole (Buprenorphine is metabolized to norbuprenorphine by cytochrome CYP3A4. Because CYP3A4 inhibitors may increase plasma concentrations of buprenorphine, patients already on CYP3A4 inhibitors should have their dose of Subutex or Subuxone adjusted). Products include:
Arimidex Tablets 665

Aprepitant (Buprenorphine is metabolized to norbuprenorphine by cytochrome CYP3A4. Because CYP3A4 inhibitors may increase plasma concentrations of buprenorphine, patients already on CYP3A4 inhibitors should have their dose of Subutex or Subuxone adjusted). Products include:
Emend Capsules 1944

Cimetidine (Buprenorphine is metabolized to norbuprenorphine by cytochrome CYP3A4. Because CYP3A4 inhibitors may increase plasma concentrations of buprenorphine, patients already on CYP3A4 inhibitors should have their dose of Subutex or Subuxone adjusted). Products include:
Tagamet HB 200 Tablets .... ▣637
Tagamet Tablets 1547

Cimetidine Hydrochloride (Buprenorphine is metabolized to norbuprenorphine by cytochrome CYP3A4. Because CYP3A4 inhibitors may increase plasma concentrations of buprenorphine, patients already on CYP3A4 inhibitors should have their dose of Subutex or Subuxone adjusted).
No products indexed under this heading.

Ciprofloxacin (Buprenorphine is metabolized to norbuprenorphine by cytochrome CYP3A4. Because CYP3A4 inhibitors may increase plasma concentrations of buprenorphine, patients already on CYP3A4 inhibitors should have their dose of Subutex or Subuxone adjusted). Products include:
Cipro I.V. 2998
Cipro I.V. Pharmacy Bulk Package 3509
Cipro Oral Suspension 2991
Cipro XR Tablets 3004
Ciprodex Otic Suspension 555

Clarithromycin (Buprenorphine is metabolized to norbuprenorphine by cytochrome CYP3A4. Because CYP3A4 inhibitors may increase plasma concentrations of buprenorphine, patients already on CYP3A4 inhibitors should have their dose of Subutex or Subuxone adjusted). Products include:
Biaxin/Biaxin XL 402
PREVPAC 3281

Clotrimazole (Buprenorphine is metabolized to norbuprenorphine by cytochrome CYP3A4. Because CYP3A4 inhibitors may increase plasma concentrations of buprenorphine, patients already on CYP3A4 inhibitors should have their dose of Subutex or Subuxone adjusted). Products include:
Lotrimin 3053
Lotrisone 3054

Cyclosporine (Buprenorphine is metabolized to norbuprenorphine by cytochrome CYP3A4. Because CYP3A4 inhibitors may increase plasma concentrations of buprenorphine, patients already on CYP3A4 inhibitors should have their dose of Subutex or Subuxone adjusted). Products include:
Gengraf Capsules 458
Neoral Soft Gelatin Capsules 2247
Neoral Oral Solution 2247
Restasis Ophthalmic Emulsion 570
Sandimmune 2259

Dalfopristin (Buprenorphine is metabolized to norbuprenorphine by cytochrome CYP3A4. Because CYP3A4 inhibitors may increase plasma concentrations of buprenorphine, patients already on CYP3A4 inhibitors should have their dose of Subutex or Subuxone adjusted). Products include:
Synercid I.V. 1690

Danazol (Buprenorphine is metabolized to norbuprenorphine by cytochrome CYP3A4. Because CYP3A4 inhibitors may increase plasma concentrations of buprenorphine, patients already on CYP3A4 inhibitors should have their dose of Subutex or Subuxone adjusted).
No products indexed under this heading.

Delavirdine Mesylate (Buprenorphine is metabolized to norbuprenorphine by cytochrome CYP3A4. Because CYP3A4 inhibitors may increase plasma concentrations of buprenorphine, patients already on CYP3A4 inhibitors should have their dose of Subutex or Subuxone adjusted). Products include:
Rescriptor Tablets 2535

Diltiazem Hydrochloride (Buprenorphine is metabolized to norbuprenorphine by cytochrome CYP3A4. Because CYP3A4 inhibitors may increase plasma concentrations of buprenorphine, patients already on CYP3A4 inhibitors should have their dose of Subutex or Subuxone adjusted). Products include:
Cardizem LA Extended Release Tablets 1699
Tiazac Capsules 1204

Diltiazem Maleate (Buprenorphine is metabolized to norbuprenorphine by cytochrome CYP3A4. Because CYP3A4 inhibitors may increase plasma concentrations of buprenorphine, patients already on CYP3A4 inhibitors should have their dose of Subutex or Subuxone adjusted).

No products indexed under this heading.

Efavirenz (Buprenorphine is metabolized to norbuprenorphine by cytochrome CYP3A4. Because CYP3A4 inhibitors may increase plasma concentrations of buprenorphine, patients already on CYP3A4 inhibitors should have their dose of Subutex or Subuxone adjusted). Products include:

Sustiva Capsules 957

Erythromycin (Buprenorphine is metabolized to norbuprenorphine by cytochrome CYP3A4. Because CYP3A4 inhibitors may increase plasma concentrations of buprenorphine, patients already on CYP3A4 inhibitors should have their dose of Subutex or Subuxone adjusted). Products include:

Erygel Topical Gel 2096
Ery-Tab Tablets 447
Erythromycin Base Filmtab Tablets 454
Erythromycin Delayed-Release Capsules, USP 456
PCE Dispertab Tablets 510

Erythromycin Estolate (Buprenorphine is metabolized to norbuprenorphine by cytochrome CYP3A4. Because CYP3A4 inhibitors may increase plasma concentrations of buprenorphine, patients already on CYP3A4 inhibitors should have their dose of Subutex or Subuxone adjusted).

No products indexed under this heading.

Erythromycin Ethylsuccinate (Buprenorphine is metabolized to norbuprenorphine by cytochrome CYP3A4. Because CYP3A4 inhibitors may increase plasma concentrations of buprenorphine, patients already on CYP3A4 inhibitors should have their dose of Subutex or Subuxone adjusted). Products include:

E.E.S. 449
EryPed 445

Erythromycin Gluceptate (Buprenorphine is metabolized to norbuprenorphine by cytochrome CYP3A4. Because CYP3A4 inhibitors may increase plasma concentrations of buprenorphine, patients already on CYP3A4 inhibitors should have their dose of Subutex or Subuxone adjusted).

No products indexed under this heading.

Erythromycin Lactobionate (Buprenorphine is metabolized to norbuprenorphine by cytochrome CYP3A4. Because CYP3A4 inhibitors may increase plasma concentrations of buprenorphine, patients already on CYP3A4 inhibitors should have their dose of Subutex or Subuxone adjusted).

No products indexed under this heading.

Erythromycin Stearate (Buprenorphine is metabolized to norbuprenorphine by cytochrome CYP3A4. Because CYP3A4 inhibitors may increase plasma concentrations of buprenorphine, patients already on CYP3A4 inhibitors should have their dose of Subutex or Subuxone adjusted). Products include:

Erythrocin Stearate Filmtab Tablets 452

Esomeprazole Magnesium (Buprenorphine is metabolized to norbuprenorphine by cytochrome CYP3A4. Because CYP3A4 inhibitors may increase plasma concentrations of buprenorphine, patients already on CYP3A4 inhibitors should have their dose of Subutex or Subuxone adjusted). Products include:

Nexium Delayed-Release Capsules 645

Fluconazole (Buprenorphine is metabolized to norbuprenorphine by cytochrome CYP3A4. Because CYP3A4 inhibitors may increase plasma concentrations of buprenorphine, patients already on CYP3A4 inhibitors should have their dose of Subutex or Subuxone adjusted).

No products indexed under this heading.

Fluoxetine Hydrochloride (Buprenorphine is metabolized to norbuprenorphine by cytochrome CYP3A4. Because CYP3A4 inhibitors may increase plasma concentrations of buprenorphine, patients already on CYP3A4 inhibitors should have their dose of Subutex or Subuxone adjusted). Products include:

Prozac Pulvules and Liquid 1771
Symbyax Capsules 1788

Fluvoxamine Maleate (Buprenorphine is metabolized to norbuprenorphine by cytochrome CYP3A4. Because CYP3A4 inhibitors may increase plasma concentrations of buprenorphine, patients already on CYP3A4 inhibitors should have their dose of Subutex or Subuxone adjusted).

No products indexed under this heading.

Fosamprenavir Calcium (Buprenorphine is metabolized to norbuprenorphine by cytochrome CYP3A4. Because CYP3A4 inhibitors may increase plasma concentrations of buprenorphine, patients already on CYP3A4 inhibitors should have their dose of Subutex or Subuxone adjusted). Products include:

Lexiva Tablets 1473

Indinavir Sulfate (Buprenorphine is metabolized to norbuprenorphine by cytochrome CYP3A4. Because CYP3A4 inhibitors may increase plasma concentrations of buprenorphine, patients already on CYP3A4 inhibitors should have their dose of Subutex or Subuxone adjusted). Products include:

Crixivan Capsules 1918

Isoniazid (Buprenorphine is metabolized to norbuprenorphine by cytochrome CYP3A4. Because CYP3A4 inhibitors may increase plasma concentrations of buprenorphine, patients already on CYP3A4 inhibitors should have their dose of Subutex or Subuxone adjusted).

No products indexed under this heading.

Itraconazole (Buprenorphine is metabolized to norbuprenorphine by cytochrome CYP3A4. Because CYP3A4 inhibitors may increase plasma concentrations of buprenorphine, patients already on CYP3A4 inhibitors should have their dose of Subutex or Subuxone adjusted).

No products indexed under this heading.

Ketoconazole (Buprenorphine is metabolized to norbuprenorphine by cytochrome CYP3A4. Because CYP3A4 inhibitors may increase plasma concentrations of buprenorphine, patients already on CYP3A4 inhibitors should have their dose of Subutex or Subuxone adjusted). Products include:

Nizoral A-D Shampoo, 1% 1839
Nizoral 2% Shampoo 1838

Lopinavir (Buprenorphine is metabolized to norbuprenorphine by cytochrome CYP3A4. Because CYP3A4 inhibitors may increase plasma concentrations of buprenorphine, patients already on CYP3A4 inhibitors should have their dose of Subutex or Subuxone adjusted). Products include:

Kaletra 474

Loratadine (Buprenorphine is metabolized to norbuprenorphine by cytochrome CYP3A4. Because CYP3A4 inhibitors may increase plasma concentrations of buprenorphine, patients already on CYP3A4 inhibitors should have their dose of Subutex or Subuxone adjusted). Products include:

Alavert Allergy & Sinus D-12 Hour Tablets 743
Alavert 743
Children's Claritin 24 Hour Non-Drowsy Allergy Syrup 732
Claritin Non-Drowsy 24 Hour Tablets 731
Non-Drowsy Claritin Hives Relief Tablets 733
Claritin Reditabs 24 Hour Non-Drowsy Tablets 732
Claritin-D Non-Drowsy 12 Hour Tablets 731
Claritin-D Non-Drowsy 24 Hour Tablets 731
Children's Dimetapp ND Non-Drowsy Allergy Syrup 746
Triaminic Allerchews 684

Metronidazole (Buprenorphine is metabolized to norbuprenorphine by cytochrome CYP3A4. Because CYP3A4 inhibitors may increase plasma concentrations of buprenorphine, patients already on CYP3A4 inhibitors should have their dose of Subutex or Subuxone adjusted). Products include:

Metrogel 1% 1212
MetroGel-Vaginal Gel 1822
Noritate Cream, 1% 1051

Metronidazole Benzoate (Buprenorphine is metabolized to norbuprenorphine by cytochrome CYP3A4. Because CYP3A4 inhibitors may increase plasma concentrations of buprenorphine, patients already on CYP3A4 inhibitors should have their dose of Subutex or Subuxone adjusted).

No products indexed under this heading.

Metronidazole Hydrochloride (Buprenorphine is metabolized to norbuprenorphine by cytochrome CYP3A4. Because CYP3A4 inhibitors may increase plasma concentrations of buprenorphine, patients already on CYP3A4 inhibitors should have their dose of Subutex or Subuxone adjusted).

No products indexed under this heading.

Miconazole (Buprenorphine is metabolized to norbuprenorphine by cytochrome CYP3A4. Because CYP3A4 inhibitors may increase plasma concentrations of buprenorphine, patients already on CYP3A4 inhibitors should have their dose of Subutex or Subuxone adjusted).

No products indexed under this heading.

Miconazole Nitrate (Buprenorphine is metabolized to norbuprenorphine by cytochrome CYP3A4. Because CYP3A4 inhibitors may increase plasma concentrations of buprenorphine, patients already on CYP3A4 inhibitors should have their dose of Subutex or Subuxone adjusted). Products include:

Desenex 674
Desenex Jock Itch Spray Powder 674

Nefazodone Hydrochloride (Buprenorphine is metabolized to norbuprenorphine by cytochrome CYP3A4. Because CYP3A4 inhibitors may increase plasma concentrations of buprenorphine, patients already on CYP3A4 inhibitors should have their dose of Subutex or Subuxone adjusted).

No products indexed under this heading.

Nelfinavir Mesylate (Buprenorphine is metabolized to norbuprenorphine by cytochrome CYP3A4. Because CYP3A4 inhibitors may increase plasma concentrations of buprenorphine, patients already on CYP3A4 inhibitors should have their dose of Subutex or Subuxone adjusted). Products include:

Viracept 2556

Nevirapine (Buprenorphine is metabolized to norbuprenorphine by cytochrome CYP3A4. Because CYP3A4 inhibitors may increase plasma concentrations of buprenorphine, patients already on CYP3A4 inhibitors should have their dose of Subutex or Subuxone adjusted). Products include:

Viramune Oral Suspension 903
Viramune Tablets 903

Niacinamide (Buprenorphine is metabolized to norbuprenorphine by cytochrome CYP3A4. Because CYP3A4 inhibitors may increase plasma concentrations of buprenorphine, patients already on CYP3A4 inhibitors should have their dose of Subutex or Subuxone adjusted).

No products indexed under this heading.

Nicotinamide (Buprenorphine is metabolized to norbuprenorphine by cytochrome CYP3A4. Because CYP3A4 inhibitors may increase plasma concentrations of buprenorphine, patients already on CYP3A4 inhibitors should have their dose of Subutex or Subuxone adjusted). Products include:

Nicomide Tablets 3190

Nifedipine (Buprenorphine is metabolized to norbuprenorphine by cytochrome CYP3A4. Because CYP3A4 inhibitors may increase plasma concentrations of buprenorphine, patients already on CYP3A4 inhibitors should have their dose of Subutex or Subuxone adjusted). Products include:

Adalat CC Tablets 2978

Norfloxacin (Buprenorphine is metabolized to norbuprenorphine by cytochrome CYP3A4. Because CYP3A4 inhibitors may increase

plasma concentrations of buprenorphine, patients already on CYP3A4 inhibitors should have their dose of Subutex or Subuxone adjusted). Products include:

Noroxin Tablets 2009

Omeprazole (Buprenorphine is metabolized to norbuprenorphine by cytochrome CYP3A4. Because CYP3A4 inhibitors may increase plasma concentrations of buprenorphine, patients already on CYP3A4 inhibitors should have their dose of Subutex or Subuxone adjusted). Products include:

Zegerid Powder for Oral Solution 2972

Paroxetine Hydrochloride (Buprenorphine is metabolized to norbuprenorphine by cytochrome CYP3A4. Because CYP3A4 inhibitors may increase plasma concentrations of buprenorphine, patients already on CYP3A4 inhibitors should have their dose of Subutex or Subuxone adjusted). Products include:

Paxil CR Controlled-Release Tablets.............................. 1509
Paxil 1501

Propoxyphene Hydrochloride (Buprenorphine is metabolized to norbuprenorphine by cytochrome CYP3A4. Because CYP3A4 inhibitors may increase plasma concentrations of buprenorphine, patients already on CYP3A4 inhibitors should have their dose of Subutex or Subuxone adjusted).

No products indexed under this heading.

Propoxyphene Napsylate (Buprenorphine is metabolized to norbuprenorphine by cytochrome CYP3A4. Because CYP3A4 inhibitors may increase plasma concentrations of buprenorphine, patients already on CYP3A4 inhibitors should have their dose of Subutex or Subuxone adjusted). Products include:

Darvocet A 500 Tablets 3497

Quinidine (Buprenorphine is metabolized to norbuprenorphine by cytochrome CYP3A4. Because CYP3A4 inhibitors may increase plasma concentrations of buprenorphine, patients already on CYP3A4 inhibitors should have their dose of Subutex or Subuxone adjusted).

No products indexed under this heading.

Quinidine Hydrochloride (Buprenorphine is metabolized to norbuprenorphine by cytochrome CYP3A4. Because CYP3A4 inhibitors may increase plasma concentrations of buprenorphine, patients already on CYP3A4 inhibitors should have their dose of Subutex or Subuxone adjusted).

No products indexed under this heading.

Quinidine Polygalacturonate (Buprenorphine is metabolized to norbuprenorphine by cytochrome CYP3A4. Because CYP3A4 inhibitors may increase plasma concentrations of buprenorphine, patients already on CYP3A4 inhibitors should have their dose of Subutex or Subuxone adjusted).

No products indexed under this heading.

Quinidine Sulfate (Buprenorphine is metabolized to norbuprenorphine by cytochrome CYP3A4. Because CYP3A4 inhibitors may increase plasma concentrations of buprenorphine, patients already on CYP3A4 inhibitors should have their dose of Subutex or Subuxone adjusted).

No products indexed under this heading.

Quinine (Buprenorphine is metabolized to norbuprenorphine by cytochrome CYP3A4. Because CYP3A4 inhibitors may increase plasma concentrations of buprenorphine, patients already on CYP3A4 inhibitors should have their dose of Subutex or Subuxone adjusted).

No products indexed under this heading.

Quinine Sulfate (Buprenorphine is metabolized to norbuprenorphine by cytochrome CYP3A4. Because CYP3A4 inhibitors may increase plasma concentrations of buprenorphine, patients already on CYP3A4 inhibitors should have their dose of Subutex or Subuxone adjusted).

No products indexed under this heading.

Quinupristin (Buprenorphine is metabolized to norbuprenorphine by cytochrome CYP3A4. Because CYP3A4 inhibitors may increase plasma concentrations of buprenorphine, patients already on CYP3A4 inhibitors should have their dose of Subutex or Subuxone adjusted). Products include:

Synercid I.V. 1690

Ranitidine Bismuth Citrate (Buprenorphine is metabolized to norbuprenorphine by cytochrome CYP3A4. Because CYP3A4 inhibitors may increase plasma concentrations of buprenorphine, patients already on CYP3A4 inhibitors should have their dose of Subutex or Subuxone adjusted).

No products indexed under this heading.

Ranitidine Hydrochloride (Buprenorphine is metabolized to norbuprenorphine by cytochrome CYP3A4. Because CYP3A4 inhibitors may increase plasma concentrations of buprenorphine, patients already on CYP3A4 inhibitors should have their dose of Subutex or Subuxone adjusted). Products include:

Zantac 1597
Zantac Injection 1593
Zantac 75 Tablets .... ▣715
Zantac 150 Maximum Strength Tablets.. ▣715
Zantac Injection Pharmacy Bulk Package.. 1595

Ritonavir (Buprenorphine is metabolized to norbuprenorphine by cytochrome CYP3A4. Because CYP3A4 inhibitors may increase plasma concentrations of buprenorphine, patients already on CYP3A4 inhibitors should have their dose of Subutex or Subuxone adjusted). Products include:

Kaletra 474
Norvir 499

Saquinavir (Buprenorphine is metabolized to norbuprenorphine by cytochrome CYP3A4. Because CYP3A4 inhibitors may increase plasma concentrations of buprenorphine, patients already on CYP3A4 inhibitors should have their dose of Subutex or Subuxone adjusted).

No products indexed under this heading.

Saquinavir Mesylate (Buprenorphine is metabolized to norbuprenorphine by cytochrome CYP3A4. Because CYP3A4 inhibitors may increase plasma concentrations of buprenorphine, patients already on CYP3A4 inhibitors should have their dose of Subutex or Subuxone adjusted). Products include:

Invirase 2776

Sertraline Hydrochloride (Buprenorphine is metabolized to norbuprenorphine by cytochrome CYP3A4. Because CYP3A4 inhibitors may increase plasma concentrations of buprenorphine, patients already on CYP3A4 inhibitors should have their dose of Subutex or Subuxone adjusted). Products include:

Zoloft 2581

Telithromycin (Buprenorphine is metabolized to norbuprenorphine by cytochrome CYP3A4. Because CYP3A4 inhibitors may increase plasma concentrations of buprenorphine, patients already on CYP3A4 inhibitors should have their dose of Subutex or Subuxone adjusted). Products include:

Ketek Tablets 2920

Troglitazone (Buprenorphine is metabolized to norbuprenorphine by cytochrome CYP3A4. Because CYP3A4 inhibitors may increase plasma concentrations of buprenorphine, patients already on CYP3A4 inhibitors should have their dose of Subutex or Subuxone adjusted).

No products indexed under this heading.

Troleandomycin (Buprenorphine is metabolized to norbuprenorphine by cytochrome CYP3A4. Because CYP3A4 inhibitors may increase plasma concentrations of buprenorphine, patients already on CYP3A4 inhibitors should have their dose of Subutex or Subuxone adjusted).

No products indexed under this heading.

Valproate Sodium (Buprenorphine is metabolized to norbuprenorphine by cytochrome CYP3A4. Because CYP3A4 inhibitors may increase plasma concentrations of buprenorphine, patients already on CYP3A4 inhibitors should have their dose of Subutex or Subuxone adjusted). Products include:

Depacon Injection 412

Verapamil Hydrochloride (Buprenorphine is metabolized to norbuprenorphine by cytochrome CYP3A4. Because CYP3A4 inhibitors may increase plasma concentrations of buprenorphine, patients already on CYP3A4 inhibitors should have their dose of Subutex or Subuxone adjusted). Products include:

Covera-HS Tablets 3135
Tarka Tablets 519
Verelan PM Capsules 3120

Voriconazole (Buprenorphine is metabolized to norbuprenorphine by cytochrome CYP3A4. Because CYP3A4 inhibitors may increase plasma concentrations of buprenorphine, patients already on CYP3A4 inhibitors should have their dose of Subutex or Subuxone adjusted). Products include:

VFEND I.V. 2543
VFEND Oral Suspension 2543
VFEND Tablets 2543

Zafirlukast (Buprenorphine is metabolized to norbuprenorphine by cytochrome CYP3A4. Because CYP3A4 inhibitors may increase plasma concentrations of buprenorphine, patients already on CYP3A4 inhibitors should have their dose of Subutex or Subuxone adjusted). Products include:

Accolate Tablets 663

Zileuton (Buprenorphine is metabolized to norbuprenorphine by cytochrome CYP3A4. Because CYP3A4 inhibitors may increase plasma concentrations of buprenorphine, patients already on CYP3A4 inhibitors should have their dose of Subutex or Subuxone adjusted).

No products indexed under this heading.

Food Interactions

Grapefruit (Buprenorphine is metabolized to norbuprenorphine by cytochrome CYP3A4. Because CYP3A4 inhibitors may increase plasma concentrations of buprenorphine, patients already on CYP3A4 inhibitors should have their dose of Subutex or Subuxone adjusted).

Grapefruit Juice (Buprenorphine is metabolized to norbuprenorphine by cytochrome CYP3A4. Because CYP3A4 inhibitors may increase plasma concentrations of buprenorphine, patients already on CYP3A4 inhibitors should have their dose of Subutex or Subuxone adjusted).

SUDAFED 12 HOUR CAPLETS

(Pseudoephedrine Hydrochloride) ..... ▣708

May interact with monoamine oxidase inhibitors. Compounds in these categories include:

Isocarboxazid (Concurrent and/or sequential use with MAO inhibitors is not recommended).

No products indexed under this heading.

Moclobemide (Concurrent and/or sequential use with MAO inhibitors is not recommended).

No products indexed under this heading.

Pargyline Hydrochloride (Concurrent and/or sequential use with MAO inhibitors is not recommended).

No products indexed under this heading.

Phenelzine Sulfate (Concurrent and/or sequential use with MAO inhibitors is not recommended).

No products indexed under this heading.

Procarbazine Hydrochloride (Concurrent and/or sequential use with MAO inhibitors is not recommended). Products include:

Matulane Capsules 3188

Selegiline Hydrochloride (Concurrent and/or sequential use with MAO inhibitors is not recommended). Products include:

Eldepryl Capsules 3209

Tranylcypromine Sulfate (Concurrent and/or sequential use with MAO inhibitors is not recommended). Products include:

Parnate Tablets 1499

SUDAFED 24 HOUR TABLETS

(Pseudoephedrine Hydrochloride) ..... ▣709

See Sudafed 12 Hour Caplets

SUDAFED NASAL DECONGESTANT TABLETS
(Pseudoephedrine Hydrochloride) 709
See Sudafed 12 Hour Caplets

SUDAFED NON-DROWSY SEVERE COLD CAPLETS
(Acetaminophen, Dextromethorphan Hydrobromide, Pseudoephedrine Hydrochloride)....... 710
May interact with monoamine oxidase inhibitors and certain other agents. Compounds in these categories include:

Isocarboxazid (Concurrent and/or sequential use with MAO inhibitors is not recommended).
No products indexed under this heading.

Moclobemide (Concurrent and/or sequential use with MAO inhibitors is not recommended).
No products indexed under this heading.

Pargyline Hydrochloride (Concurrent and/or sequential use with MAO inhibitors is not recommended).
No products indexed under this heading.

Phenelzine Sulfate (Concurrent and/or sequential use with MAO inhibitors is not recommended).
No products indexed under this heading.

Procarbazine Hydrochloride (Concurrent and/or sequential use with MAO inhibitors is not recommended). Products include:
Matulane Capsules 3188

Selegiline Hydrochloride (Concurrent and/or sequential use with MAO inhibitors is not recommended).
Products include:
Eldepryl Capsules 3209

Tranylcypromine Sulfate (Concurrent and/or sequential use with MAO inhibitors is not recommended).
Products include:
Parnate Tablets 1499

Food Interactions

Alcohol (Chronic heavy alcohol users, 3 or more drinks per day, should consult their physicians for advice on when and how they should take pain relievers/fever reducers including acetaminophen).

SUDAFED NON-DROWSY SEVERE COLD TABLETS
(Acetaminophen, Dextromethorphan Hydrobromide, Pseudoephedrine Hydrochloride)....... 710
See Sudafed Non-Drowsy Severe Cold Caplets

SUDAFED NON-DRYING SINUS LIQUID CAPS
(Guaifenesin, Pseudoephedrine Hydrochloride).................................. 709
See Sudafed 12 Hour Caplets

SUDAFED PE TABLETS
(Phenylephrine Hydrochloride) 711
May interact with monoamine oxidase inhibitors. Compounds in these categories include:

Isocarboxazid (Avoid use with, or for two weeks after stopping, MAOI drugs).
No products indexed under this heading.

Moclobemide (Avoid use with, or for two weeks after stopping, MAOI drugs).
No products indexed under this heading.

Pargyline Hydrochloride (Avoid use with, or for two weeks after stopping, MAOI drugs).
No products indexed under this heading.

Phenelzine Sulfate (Avoid use with, or for two weeks after stopping, MAOI drugs).
No products indexed under this heading.

Procarbazine Hydrochloride (Avoid use with, or for two weeks after stopping, MAOI drugs). Products include:
Matulane Capsules 3188

Selegiline Hydrochloride (Avoid use with, or for two weeks after stopping, MAOI drugs). Products include:
Eldepryl Capsules 3209

Tranylcypromine Sulfate (Avoid use with, or for two weeks after stopping, MAOI drugs). Products include:
Parnate Tablets 1499

SUDAFED SINUS & ALLERGY TABLETS
(Chlorpheniramine Maleate, Pseudoephedrine Hydrochloride)....... 710
May interact with hypnotics and sedatives, monoamine oxidase inhibitors, tranquilizers, and certain other agents. Compounds in these categories include:

Alprazolam (May increase drowsiness effect). Products include:
Niravam Orally Disintegrating Tablets 3106
Xanax XR Tablets 2655

Buspirone Hydrochloride (May increase drowsiness effect).
No products indexed under this heading.

Chlordiazepoxide (May increase drowsiness effect).
No products indexed under this heading.

Chlordiazepoxide Hydrochloride (May increase drowsiness effect). Products include:
Librium Capsules 3349

Chlorpromazine (May increase drowsiness effect).
No products indexed under this heading.

Chlorpromazine Hydrochloride (May increase drowsiness effect).
No products indexed under this heading.

Chlorprothixene (May increase drowsiness effect).
No products indexed under this heading.

Chlorprothixene Hydrochloride (May increase drowsiness effect).
No products indexed under this heading.

Clorazepate Dipotassium (May increase drowsiness effect). Products include:
Tranxene 2488

Diazepam (May increase drowsiness effect). Products include:
Diastat Rectal Delivery System 3344
Valium Tablets 2822

Droperidol (May increase drowsiness effect).
No products indexed under this heading.

Estazolam (May increase drowsiness effect). Products include:
ProSom Tablets 512

Ethchlorvynol (May increase drowsiness effect).
No products indexed under this heading.

Ethinamate (May increase drowsiness effect).
No products indexed under this heading.

Fluphenazine Decanoate (May increase drowsiness effect).
No products indexed under this heading.

Fluphenazine Enanthate (May increase drowsiness effect).
No products indexed under this heading.

Fluphenazine Hydrochloride (May increase drowsiness effect).
No products indexed under this heading.

Flurazepam Hydrochloride (May increase drowsiness effect). Products include:
Dalmane Capsules 3343

Glutethimide (May increase drowsiness effect).
No products indexed under this heading.

Haloperidol (May increase drowsiness effect).
No products indexed under this heading.

Haloperidol Decanoate (May increase drowsiness effect).
No products indexed under this heading.

Hydroxyzine Hydrochloride (May increase drowsiness effect).
No products indexed under this heading.

Isocarboxazid (Concurrent and/or sequential use with MAO inhibitors is not recommended).
No products indexed under this heading.

Lorazepam (May increase drowsiness effect).
No products indexed under this heading.

Loxapine Hydrochloride (May increase drowsiness effect).
No products indexed under this heading.

Loxapine Succinate (May increase drowsiness effect).
No products indexed under this heading.

Meprobamate (May increase drowsiness effect).
No products indexed under this heading.

Mesoridazine Besylate (May increase drowsiness effect).
No products indexed under this heading.

Midazolam Hydrochloride (May increase drowsiness effect).
No products indexed under this heading.

Moclobemide (Concurrent and/or sequential use with MAO inhibitors is not recommended).
No products indexed under this heading.

Molindone Hydrochloride (May increase drowsiness effect). Products include:
Moban Tablets 1108

Oxazepam (May increase drowsiness effect).
No products indexed under this heading.

Pargyline Hydrochloride (Concurrent and/or sequential use with MAO inhibitors is not recommended).
No products indexed under this heading.

Perphenazine (May increase drowsiness effect).
No products indexed under this heading.

Phenelzine Sulfate (Concurrent and/or sequential use with MAO inhibitors is not recommended).
No products indexed under this heading.

Prazepam (May increase drowsiness effect).
No products indexed under this heading.

Procarbazine Hydrochloride (Concurrent and/or sequential use with MAO inhibitors is not recommended). Products include:
Matulane Capsules 3188

Prochlorperazine (May increase drowsiness effect).
No products indexed under this heading.

Promethazine Hydrochloride (May increase drowsiness effect). Products include:
Phenergan 3438

Propofol (May increase drowsiness effect). Products include:
Diprivan Injectable Emulsion 676

Quazepam (May increase drowsiness effect).
No products indexed under this heading.

Secobarbital Sodium (May increase drowsiness effect).
No products indexed under this heading.

Selegiline Hydrochloride (Concurrent and/or sequential use with MAO inhibitors is not recommended). Products include:
Eldepryl Capsules 3209

Temazepam (May increase drowsiness effect).
No products indexed under this heading.

Thioridazine Hydrochloride (May increase drowsiness effect). Products include:
Thioridazine Hydrochloride Tablets 2122

Thiothixene (May increase drowsiness effect). Products include:
Thiothixene Capsules 2124

Tranylcypromine Sulfate (Concurrent and/or sequential use with MAO inhibitors is not recommended). Products include:
Parnate Tablets 1499

Triazolam (May increase drowsiness effect).
No products indexed under this heading.

Trifluoperazine Hydrochloride (May increase drowsiness effect).
No products indexed under this heading.

Zaleplon (May increase drowsiness effect). Products include:
Sonata Capsules 1686

Zolpidem Tartrate (May increase drowsiness effect). Products include:
Ambien Tablets 2867

Food Interactions

Alcohol (May increase drowsiness effect).

IMPORTANT NOTE: Always consult each drug listing in the patient's regimen for possible interactions.

SUDAFED SINUS HEADACHE CAPLETS

(Acetaminophen, Pseudoephedrine Hydrochloride) .... ▣711

See Sudafed Non-Drowsy Severe Cold Caplets

SUDAFED SINUS HEADACHE TABLETS

(Acetaminophen, Pseudoephedrine Hydrochloride) .... ▣711

See Sudafed Non-Drowsy Severe Cold Caplets

SULAR TABLETS

(Nisoldipine) 1163

May interact with dexamethasone, phenytoin, quinidine, and certain other agents. Compounds in these categories include:

Atenolol (Greater blood pressure effect of Sular with concomitant use). Products include:

- Tenormin I.V. Injection 698
- Tenormin Tablets 695

Carbamazepine (Co-administration of nisoldipine with known CYP3A4 inducer, such as carbamazepine, should be avoided because of possible reduced nisoldipine plasma concentrations). Products include:

- Carbatrol Capsules 3174
- Equetro Extended-Release Capsules 3178
- Tegretol/Tegretol-XR 2278

Cimetidine (Concomitant use increases nisoldipine AUC and Cmax by 30% to 45%). Products include:

- Tagamet HB 200 Tablets .... ▣637
- Tagamet Tablets 1547

Cimetidine Hydrochloride (Concomitant use increases nisoldipine AUC and Cmax by 30% to 45%).

No products indexed under this heading.

Dexamethasone (Co-administration of nisoldipine with known CYP3A4 inducer, such as dexamethasone, should be avoided because of possible reduced nisoldipine plasma concentrations). Products include:

- Ciprodex Otic Suspension 555
- Decadron Tablets 1929
- TobraDex Ophthalmic Ointment 558
- TobraDex Ophthalmic Suspension 558

Dexamethasone Acetate (Co-administration of nisoldipine with known CYP3A4 inducer, such as dexamethasone, should be avoided because of possible reduced nisoldipine plasma concentrations).

No products indexed under this heading.

Dexamethasone Sodium Phosphate (Co-administration of nisoldipine with known CYP3A4 inducer, such as dexamethasone, should be avoided because of possible reduced nisoldipine plasma concentrations). Products include:

- Decadron Phosphate Injection 1931

Fosphenytoin Sodium (Co-administration in epileptic patients has resulted in reduced nisoldipine plasma concentrations to undetectable levels).

No products indexed under this heading.

Phenobarbital (Co-administration of nisoldipine with known CYP3A4 inducer, such as phenobarbital, should be avoided because of possible reduced nisoldipine plasma concentrations).

No products indexed under this heading.

Phenytoin (Co-administration in epileptic patients has resulted in reduced nisoldipine plasma concentrations to undetectable levels).

No products indexed under this heading.

Phenytoin Sodium (Co-administration in epileptic patients has resulted in reduced nisoldipine plasma concentrations to undetectable levels). Products include:

- Phenytek Capsules 2153

Propranolol Hydrochloride (Propranolol attenuates the heart rate increase following the administration of immediate-release nisoldipine). Products include:

- Inderal LA Long-Acting Capsules 3421
- InnoPran XL Capsules 2728

Quinidine (May decrease the bioavailability (AUC) of nisoldipine by 26%, but not the peak concentration; clinical significance is not known).

No products indexed under this heading.

Quinidine Gluconate (May decrease the bioavailability (AUC) of nisoldipine by 26%, but not the peak concentration; clinical significance is not known).

No products indexed under this heading.

Quinidine Hydrochloride (May decrease the bioavailability (AUC) of nisoldipine by 26%, but not the peak concentration; clinical significance is not known).

No products indexed under this heading.

Quinidine Polygalacturonate (May decrease the bioavailability (AUC) of nisoldipine by 26%, but not the peak concentration; clinical significance is not known).

No products indexed under this heading.

Quinidine Sulfate (May decrease the bioavailability (AUC) of nisoldipine by 26%, but not the peak concentration; clinical significance is not known).

No products indexed under this heading.

Ranitidine Hydrochloride (Concomitant use decreases AUC by 15% to 20%). Products include:

- Zantac 1597
- Zantac Injection 1593
- Zantac 75 Tablets .... ▣715
- Zantac 150 Maximum Strength Tablets .... ▣715
- Zantac Injection Pharmacy Bulk Package 1595

Rifampin (Co-administration of nisoldipine with known CYP3A4 inducer, such as rifampin, should be avoided because of possible reduced nisoldipine plasma concentrations).

No products indexed under this heading.

Food Interactions

Diet, high-lipid (Food with a high fat content has a pronounced effect on the release of nisoldipine resulting in a significant increase in peak concentration (Cmax) by up to 300%; concomitant intake of high-fat meal should be avoided).

SULFAMYLON CREAM

(Mafenide Acetate) 2154

None cited in PDR database.

SULFAMYLON FOR 5% TOPICAL SOLUTION

(Mafenide Acetate) 2155

None cited in PDR database.

SUPRANE LIQUID FOR INHALATION

(Desflurane) 770

May interact with:

Atracurium Besylate (Anesthetic concentrations of desflurane reduce the ED_{95} of atracurium by approximately 50%).

No products indexed under this heading.

Fentanyl (Decreases the minimum alveolar concentration (MAC) of desflurane by 50%). Products include:

- Duragesic Transdermal System 2448

Fentanyl Citrate (Decreases the minimum alveolar concentration (MAC) of desflurane by 50%). Products include:

- Actiq 993

Midazolam Hydrochloride (Decreases the minimum alveolar concentration (MAC) of desflurane by 16%).

No products indexed under this heading.

Pancuronium Bromide (Anesthetic concentrations of desflurane reduce the ED_{95} of pancuronium by approximately 50%).

No products indexed under this heading.

Succinylcholine Chloride (Anesthetic concentrations of desflurane reduce the ED_{95} of succinylcholine by approximately 30%).

No products indexed under this heading.

SUPRAX

(Cefixime) 1811

May interact with oral anticoagulants and certain other agents. Compounds in these categories include:

Anisindione (Co-administration has resulted in increased prothrombin time, with or without clinical bleeding). Products include:

- Miradon Tablets 3056

Carbamazepine (Co-administration has resulted in elevated carbamazepine levels). Products include:

- Carbatrol Capsules 3174
- Equetro Extended-Release Capsules 3178
- Tegretol/Tegretol-XR 2278

Dicumarol (Co-administration has resulted in increased prothrombin time, with or without clinical bleeding).

No products indexed under this heading.

Warfarin Sodium (Co-administration has resulted in increased prothrombin time, with or without clinical bleeding). Products include:

- Coumadin for Injection 932
- Coumadin Tablets 932

Food Interactions

Food, unspecified (Increases time to maximal absorption approximately 0.8 hour).

SURMONTIL CAPSULES

(Trimipramine Maleate) 2347

May interact with anticholinergics, monoamine oxidase inhibitors, quinidine, selective serotonin reuptake inhibitors, sympathomimetics, thyroid preparations, and certain other agents. Compounds in these categories include:

Albuterol (Tricyclic antidepressants can potentiate the effects of catecholamines). Products include:

- Proventil Inhalation Aerosol 3067

Albuterol Sulfate (Tricyclic antidepressants can potentiate the effects of catecholamines). Products include:

- AccuNeb Inhalation Solution 1055
- Combivent Inhalation Aerosol 878
- DuoNeb Inhalation Solution 1058
- Proventil Inhalation Solution 0.083% 3069
- Proventil HFA Inhalation Aerosol 3071
- Ventolin HFA Inhalation Aerosol 1576
- VoSpire Extended-Release Tablets 2352

Amiodarone Hydrochloride (Co-administration of tricyclic antidepressant with drugs that can inhibit P450 2D6 may require lower doses than usually prescribed for either the tricyclic antidepressant or the other drug). Products include:

- Pacerone Tablets 3337

Atropine Sulfate (Tricyclic antidepressants can potentiate the atropine-like effects of anticholinergic drugs).

No products indexed under this heading.

Belladonna Alkaloids (Tricyclic antidepressants can potentiate the atropine-like effects of anticholinergic drugs). Products include:

- Hyland's Teething Tablets .... ▣736

Benztropine Mesylate (Tricyclic antidepressants can potentiate the atropine-like effects of anticholinergic drugs). Products include:

- Cogentin Injection 1903

Biperiden Hydrochloride (Tricyclic antidepressants can potentiate the atropine-like effects of anticholinergic drugs).

No products indexed under this heading.

Cimetidine (Inhibits the elimination of tricyclic antidepressants). Products include:

- Tagamet HB 200 Tablets .... ▣637
- Tagamet Tablets 1547

Cimetidine Hydrochloride (Inhibits the elimination of tricyclic antidepressants).

No products indexed under this heading.

Citalopram Hydrobromide (SSRI inhibit P450 2D6; the extent of inhibition varies from one SSRI to another; the extent to which SSRI TCA interactions may pose clinical problems will depend on the degree of inhibition and pharmacokinetics of the SSRI involved; caution is indicated if co-administered). Products include:

- Celexa 1177

Clidinium Bromide (Tricyclic antidepressants can potentiate the atropine-like effects of anticholinergic drugs).

No products indexed under this heading.

Dicyclomine Hydrochloride (Tricyclic antidepressants can potentiate the atropine-like effects of anticholinergic drugs). Products include:

- Bentyl Capsules 724
- Bentyl Injection 724

Bentyl Syrup 724
Bentyl Tablets 724

Dobutamine Hydrochloride (Tricyclic antidepressants can potentiate the effects of catecholamines).
No products indexed under this heading.

Dopamine Hydrochloride (Tricyclic antidepressants can potentiate the effects of catecholamines).
No products indexed under this heading.

Ephedrine Hydrochloride (Tricyclic antidepressants can potentiate the effects of catecholamines). Products include:
Primatene Tablets 749

Ephedrine Sulfate (Tricyclic antidepressants can potentiate the effects of catecholamines).
No products indexed under this heading.

Ephedrine Tannate (Tricyclic antidepressants can potentiate the effects of catecholamines).
No products indexed under this heading.

Epinephrine (Tricyclic antidepressants can potentiate the effects of catecholamines). Products include:
EpiPen 1061
Primatene Mist 749

Epinephrine Bitartrate (Tricyclic antidepressants can potentiate the effects of catecholamines).
No products indexed under this heading.

Epinephrine Hydrochloride (Tricyclic antidepressants can potentiate the effects of catecholamines).
No products indexed under this heading.

Escitalopram Oxalate (SSRI inhibit P450 2D6; the extent of inhibition varies from one SSRI to another; the extent to which SSRI TCA interactions may pose clinical problems will depend on the degree of inhibition and pharmacokinetics of the SSRI involved; caution is indicated if co-administered). Products include:
Lexapro Oral Solution 1193
Lexapro Tablets 1193

Flecainide Acetate (An individual who is stable on a given dose of TCA may become abruptly toxic when given one of the inhibiting drugs or a substrate for P450 2D6). Products include:
Tambocor Tablets 1824

Fluoxetine Hydrochloride (SSRI inhibit P450 2D6; the extent of inhibition varies from one SSRI to another; the extent to which SSRI TCA interactions may pose clinical problems will depend on the degree of inhibition and pharmacokinetics of the SSRI involved; caution is indicated if co-administered). Products include:
Prozac Pulvules and Liquid 1771
Symbyax Capsules 1788

Fluvoxamine Maleate (SSRI inhibit P450 2D6; the extent of inhibition varies from one SSRI to another; the extent to which SSRI TCA interactions may pose clinical problems will depend on the degree of inhibition and pharmacokinetics of the SSRI involved; caution is indicated if co-administered).
No products indexed under this heading.

Glycopyrrolate (Tricyclic antidepressants can potentiate the atropine-like effects of anticholinergic drugs).
No products indexed under this heading.

Guanadrel Sulfate (Trimipramine may block the pharmacologic effects of guanethidine or similar drugs).
No products indexed under this heading.

Guanethidine Monosulfate (Trimipramine may block the pharmacologic effects of guanethidine or similar drugs).
No products indexed under this heading.

Hyoscyamine (Tricyclic antidepressants can potentiate the atropine-like effects of anticholinergic drugs).
No products indexed under this heading.

Hyoscyamine Sulfate (Tricyclic antidepressants can potentiate the atropine-like effects of anticholinergic drugs).
No products indexed under this heading.

Ipratropium Bromide (Tricyclic antidepressants can potentiate the atropine-like effects of anticholinergic drugs). Products include:
Atrovent HFA Inhalation Aerosol 872
Atrovent Inhalation Solution 868
Atrovent Nasal Spray 0.03% 869
Atrovent Nasal Spray 0.06% 870
Combivent Inhalation Aerosol 878
DuoNeb Inhalation Solution 1058

Isocarboxazid (Concurrent and/or sequential use with MAO inhibitors is contraindicated; concurrent use of tricyclic antidepressants and MAO inhibitors has resulted in hyperpyretic reactions, convulsive crises, and death in some patients).
No products indexed under this heading.

Isoproterenol Hydrochloride (Tricyclic antidepressants can potentiate the effects of catecholamines).
No products indexed under this heading.

Isoproterenol Sulfate (Tricyclic antidepressants can potentiate the effects of catecholamines).
No products indexed under this heading.

Levalbuterol Hydrochloride (Tricyclic antidepressants can potentiate the effects of catecholamines). Products include:
Xopenex Inhalation Solution 3143
Xopenex Inhalation Solution Concentrate 3147

Levothyroxine Sodium (Possibility of cardiovascular toxicity). Products include:
Levothroid Tablets 1189
Levoxyl Tablets 1680
Synthroid Tablets 515
Unithroid Tablets 3521

Liothyronine Sodium (Possibility of cardiovascular toxicity). Products include:
Cytomel Tablets 1678

Liotrix (Possibility of cardiovascular toxicity). Products include:
Thyrolar 1203

Mepenzolate Bromide (Tricyclic antidepressants can potentiate the atropine-like effects of anticholinergic drugs).
No products indexed under this heading.

Metaproterenol Sulfate (Tricyclic antidepressants can potentiate the effects of catecholamines). Products include:
Alupent Inhalation Aerosol 858

Metaraminol Bitartrate (Tricyclic antidepressants can potentiate the effects of catecholamines). Products include:
Aramine Injection 1889

Methadone Hydrochloride (Co-administration of tricyclic antidepressant with drugs that can inhibit P450 2D6 may require lower doses than usually prescribed for either the tricyclic antidepressant or the other drug).
No products indexed under this heading.

Methoxamine Hydrochloride (Tricyclic antidepressants can potentiate the effects of catecholamines).
No products indexed under this heading.

Moclobemide (Concurrent and/or sequential use with MAO inhibitors is contraindicated; concurrent use of tricyclic antidepressants and MAO inhibitors has resulted in hyperpyretic reactions, convulsive crises, and death in some patients).
No products indexed under this heading.

Norepinephrine Bitartrate (Tricyclic antidepressants can potentiate the effects of catecholamines).
No products indexed under this heading.

Oxybutynin Chloride (Tricyclic antidepressants can potentiate the atropine-like effects of anticholinergic drugs). Products include:
Ditropan XL Extended Release Tablets 2391

Pargyline Hydrochloride (Concurrent and/or sequential use with MAO inhibitors is contraindicated; concurrent use of tricyclic antidepressants and MAO inhibitors has resulted in hyperpyretic reactions, convulsive crises, and death in some patients).
No products indexed under this heading.

Paroxetine Hydrochloride (SSRI inhibit P450 2D6; the extent of inhibition varies from one SSRI to another; the extent to which SSRI TCA interactions may pose clinical problems will depend on the degree of inhibition and pharmacokinetics of the SSRI involved; caution is indicated if co-administered). Products include:
Paxil CR Controlled-Release Tablets 1509
Paxil 1501

Phenelzine Sulfate (Concurrent and/or sequential use with MAO inhibitors is contraindicated; concurrent use of tricyclic antidepressants and MAO inhibitors has resulted in hyperpyretic reactions, convulsive crises, and death in some patients).
No products indexed under this heading.

Phenylephrine Bitartrate (Tricyclic antidepressants can potentiate the effects of catecholamines).
No products indexed under this heading.

Phenylephrine Hydrochloride (Tricyclic antidepressants can potentiate the effects of catecholamines). Products include:
Alacol DM Syrup 739
Hycomine Compound Tablets 1105
Preparation H Maximum Strength Cream 747
Preparation H Cooling Gel 747
Preparation H 747
Sudafed PE Tablets 711
Vicks Sinex Nasal Spray and Ultra Fine Mist for Sinus Relief 2677
Zicam Concentrated Cough Mist for Kids Plus D Cool Cherry 643
Zicam Concentrated Cough Mist Plus D Cool Cherry 642

Phenylephrine Tannate (Tricyclic antidepressants can potentiate the effects of catecholamines).
No products indexed under this heading.

Phenylpropanolamine Hydrochloride (Tricyclic antidepressants can potentiate the effects of catecholamines).
No products indexed under this heading.

Pirbuterol Acetate (Tricyclic antidepressants can potentiate the effects of catecholamines). Products include:
Maxair Autohaler 1820

Procarbazine Hydrochloride (Concurrent and/or sequential use with MAO inhibitors is contraindicated; concurrent use of tricyclic antidepressants and MAO inhibitors has resulted in hyperpyretic reactions, convulsive crises, and death in some patients). Products include:
Matulane Capsules 3188

Procyclidine Hydrochloride (Tricyclic antidepressants can potentiate the atropine-like effects of anticholinergic drugs).
No products indexed under this heading.

Propafenone Hydrochloride (An individual who is stable on a given dose of TCA may become abruptly toxic when given one of the inhibiting drugs or a substrate for P450 2D6). Products include:
Rythmol SR Capsules 2736

Propantheline Bromide (Tricyclic antidepressants can potentiate the atropine-like effects of anticholinergic drugs).
No products indexed under this heading.

Pseudoephedrine Hydrochloride (Tricyclic antidepressants can potentiate the effects of catecholamines). Products include:
Advil Allergy Sinus Caplets 737
Advil Cold & Sinus 739
Advil Flu & Body Ache Caplets 739
Children's Advil Cold Suspension ... 741
Advil Multi-Symptom Cold Caplets 738
Allegra-D 12 Hour Extended-Release Tablets 2860
Allegra-D 24 Hour Extended-Release Tablets 2862
Balamine DM 739
BC Cold Powder 612
Benadryl Allergy & Cold Tablets 692
Benadryl Allergy & Sinus Headache Caplets & Gelcaps 693
Children's Benadryl Allergy & Cold Fastmelt Tablets 695
Benadryl Maximum Strength Severe Allergy & Sinus Headache Caplets 694
Children's Benadryl D Allergy & Sinus Fastmelt Tablets 694
Children's Benadryl D Liquid Medication 693
Benadryl D Tablets 694
Contac Non-Drowsy 12 Hour Cold Caplets 614
Contac Non-Drowsy Timed Release 12 Hour Cold Caplets 615
Contac Severe Cold and Flu Caplets Maximum Strength 615
Contac Severe Cold and Flu Caplets Non-Drowsy 615

Children's Dimetapp Cold & Allergy Elixir .... ■ 745
Children's Dimetapp DM Cold & Cough Elixir .... ■ 745
Children's Dimetapp Long Acting Cough Plus Cold Syrup .... ■ 746
Dimetapp Infant Drops Decongestant Plus Cough .... ■ 746
Children's Motrin Cold Non-Staining Dye-Free Oral Suspension 1838
Children's Motrin Cold Oral Suspension 1838
Motrin Cold & Sinus Caplets 1836
PediaCare Decongestant & Cough Infant Drops .... ■ 705
PediaCare Decongestant Infants' Drops .... ■ 705
PediaCare Long-Acting Cough Plus Cold Liquid .... ■ 704
PediaCare Multi-Symptom Cold Liquid .... ■ 704
PediaCare NightRest Cough & Cold Liquid .... ■ 704
Robitussin Allergy & Cough Syrup .. ■ 750
Robitussin CF Liquid .... ■ 755
Robitussin Cough & Cold Liquid-filled Capsules .... ■ 750
Robitussin Cough, Cold & Flu Liquid-filled Capsules .... ■ 750
Robitussin Cough & Cold Infant Drops .... ■ 755
Robitussin Flu Liquid .... ■ 752
Robitussin Maximum Strength Cough & Cold Liquid .... ■ 754
Robitussin PE Syrup .... ■ 753
Robitussin Pediatric Cough & Cold Liquid .... ■ 754
Robitussin PM Cough & Cold Liquid .... ■ 752
Robitussin Severe Congestion Liquid-filled Capsules .... ■ 751
Simply Stuffy Liquid 1841
Singlet Caplets .... ■ 636
Sudafed 12 Hour Caplets .... ■ 708
Sudafed 24 Hour Tablets .... ■ 709
Sudafed Nasal Decongestant Tablets .... ■ 709
Sudafed Severe Cold .... ■ 710
Sudafed Non-Drying Sinus Liquid Caps .... ■ 709
Sudafed Sinus & Allergy Tablets ..... ■ 710
Sudafed Sinus Headache .... ■ 711
TheraFlu Cold & Cough Hot Liquid .... ■ 680
TheraFlu Cold & Sore Throat Hot Liquid .... ■ 680
TheraFlu Flu & Chest Congestion Non-Drowsy Hot Liquid .... ■ 681
TheraFlu Flu & Sore Throat Hot Liquid .... ■ 681
TheraFlu Severe Cold Non-Drowsy Hot Liquid .... ■ 683
TheraFlu Severe Cold & Cough Hot Liquid .... ■ 683
TheraFlu Severe Cold Caplets .... ■ 679
TheraFlu Severe Cold Hot Liquid .... ■ 682
TheraFlu Severe Cold Non-Drowsy Caplets .... ■ 679
Triaminic Chest & Nasal Congestion Liquid .... ■ 685
Triaminic Cold & Allergy Liquid .... ■ 685
Triaminic Cold & Cough Liquid .... ■ 685
Triaminic Cough Liquid .... ■ 687
Triaminic Cough & Nasal Congestion Liquid .... ■ 687
Triaminic Cough & Sore Throat Liquid .... ■ 687
Triaminic Flu, Cough & Fever Liquid .... ■ 685
Triaminic Night Time Cough & Cold Liquid .... ■ 685
Triaminic Allergy Runny Nose & Congestion Softchews .... ■ 688
Triaminic Cold & Cough Softchews .... ■ 688
Triaminic Cough & Sore Throat Softchews .... ■ 689
Tylenol Sinus NightTime Caplets .... ■ 663
Children's Tylenol Plus Cold & Allergy Suspension Liquid 1850
Children's Tylenol Plus Cold NightTime Suspension Liquid 1851
Children's Tylenol Plus Cold & Cough Suspension Liquid and Chewable Tablets 1851
Children's Tylenol Plus Cold Chewable Tablets 1851
Children's Tylenol Plus Cold Daytime Non-Drowsy Suspension Liquid 1851
Children's Tylenol Plus Flu Suspension Liquid 1853
Concentrated Tylenol Infants' Drops Plus Cold 1851
Concentrated Tylenol Infants' Drops Plus Cold and Cough 1851
Tylenol Cold & Flu Severe Daytime Liquid with Cool Burst 1846
Tylenol Cold & Flu Severe NightTime Liquid with Cool Burst 1846
Tylenol Cold Severe Congestion Non-Drowsy Caplets with Cool Burst 1846
Tylenol Allergy Complete Night Time Caplets 1844
Tylenol Allergy Complete Multi-Symptom Caplets and Gelcaps with Cool Burst 1844
Tylenol Flu NightTime Gelcaps 1846
Tylenol Flu Day Non-Drowsy Gelcaps 1846
Concentrated Tylenol Infants' Drops Plus Cold Nasal Congestant, Fever Reducer & Pain Reliever .... ■ 668
Concentrated Tylenol Infants' Drops Plus Cold & Cough Nasal Decongestant, Fever Reducer & Pain Reliever .... ■ 668
Multi-Symptom Tylenol Cold Night Time Caplets 1845
Multi-Symptom Tylenol Cold Day Non-Drowsy Caplets and Gelcaps 1845
Tylenol Sinus Day Non-Drowsy 1848
Tylenol Sinus Night Time Caplets 1848
Tylenol Sinus Severe Congestion Caplets with Cool Burst 1848
Vicks 44D Cough & Head Congestion Relief 2676
Vicks 44D Cough & Head Congestion Relief Liquid .... ■ 721
Vicks 44M Cough, Cold & Flu Relief 2676
Pediatric Vicks 44m Cough & Cold Relief 2673
Vicks DayQuil LiquiCaps/Liquid Multi-Symptom Cold/Flu Relief ..... ■ 723
Vicks DayQuil Multi-Symptom Cold/Flu Relief LiquiCaps 2675
Vicks DayQuil Multi-Symptom Cold/Flu Relief Liquid 2675
Children's Vicks NyQuil Cold/Cough Relief 2671
Vicks NyQuil LiquiCaps 2677
Vicks NyQuil LiquiCaps/Liquid Multi-Symptom Cold/Flu Relief ..... ■ 725
Vicks NyQuil Liquid 2677
Zyrtec-D 12 Hour Extended Release Tablets 2591

Pseudoephedrine Sulfate (Tricyclic antidepressants can potentiate the effects of catecholamines). Products include:
Alavert Allergy & Sinus D-12 Hour Tablets .... ■ 743
Clarinex-D 24-Hour Extended-Release Tablets 3012
Claritin-D Non-Drowsy 12 Hour Tablets .... ■ 731
Claritin-D Non-Drowsy 24 Hour Tablets .... ■ 731

Quinidine (Co-administration of tricyclic antidepressant with drugs that can inhibit P450 2D6 may require lower doses than usually prescribed for either the tricyclic antidepressant or the other drug).
No products indexed under this heading.

Quinidine Gluconate (Co-administration of tricyclic antidepressant with drugs that can inhibit P450 2D6 may require lower doses than usually prescribed for either the tricyclic antidepressant or the other drug).
No products indexed under this heading.

Quinidine Hydrochloride (Co-administration of tricyclic antidepressant with drugs that can inhibit P450 2D6 may require lower doses than usually prescribed for either the tricyclic antidepressant or the other drug).
No products indexed under this heading.

Quinidine Polygalacturonate (Co-administration of tricyclic antidepressant with drugs that can inhibit P450 2D6 may require lower doses than usually prescribed for either the tricyclic antidepressant or the other drug).
No products indexed under this heading.

Quinidine Sulfate (Co-administration of tricyclic antidepressant with drugs that can inhibit P450 2D6 may require lower doses than usually prescribed for either the tricyclic antidepressant or the other drug).
No products indexed under this heading.

Ritonavir (Co-administration of tricyclic antidepressant with drugs that can inhibit P450 2D6 may require lower doses than usually prescribed for either the tricyclic antidepressant or the other drug). Products include:
Kaletra 474
Norvir 499

Salmeterol Xinafoate (Tricyclic antidepressants can potentiate the effects of catecholamines). Products include:
Advair Diskus 100/50 1291
Advair Diskus 250/50 1291
Advair Diskus 500/50 1291
Serevent Diskus 1540

Scopolamine (Tricyclic antidepressants can potentiate the atropine-like effects of anticholinergic drugs). Products include:
Transderm Scōp Transdermal Therapeutic System 2166

Scopolamine Hydrobromide (Tricyclic antidepressants can potentiate the atropine-like effects of anticholinergic drugs).
No products indexed under this heading.

Selegiline Hydrochloride (Concurrent and/or sequential use with MAO inhibitors is contraindicated; concurrent use of tricyclic antidepressants and MAO inhibitors has resulted in hyperpyretic reactions, convulsive crises, and death in some patients). Products include:
Eldepryl Capsules 3209

Sertraline Hydrochloride (SSRI inhibit P450 2D6; the extent of inhibition varies from one SSRI to another; the extent to which SSRI TCA interactions may pose clinical problems will depend on the degree of inhibition and pharmacokinetics of the SSRI involved; caution is indicated if co-administered). Products include:
Zoloft 2581

Terbutaline Sulfate (Tricyclic antidepressants can potentiate the effects of catecholamines).
No products indexed under this heading.

Thioridazine Hydrochloride (An individual who is stable on a given dose of TCA may become abruptly toxic when given one of the inhibiting drugs or a substrate for P450 2D6). Products include:
Thioridazine Hydrochloride Tablets 2122

Thyroglobulin (Possibility of cardiovascular toxicity).
No products indexed under this heading.

Thyroid (Possibility of cardiovascular toxicity).
No products indexed under this heading.

Thyroxine (Possibility of cardiovascular toxicity).
No products indexed under this heading.

Thyroxine Sodium (Possibility of cardiovascular toxicity).
No products indexed under this heading.

Tolterodine Tartrate (Tricyclic antidepressants can potentiate the atropine-like effects of anticholinergic drugs). Products include:
Detrol Tablets 2626
Detrol LA Capsules 2629

Tranylcypromine Sulfate (Concurrent and/or sequential use with MAO inhibitors is contraindicated; concurrent use of tricyclic antidepressants and MAO inhibitors has resulted in hyperpyretic reactions, convulsive crises, and death in some patients). Products include:
Parnate Tablets 1499

Tridihexethyl Chloride (Tricyclic antidepressants can potentiate the atropine-like effects of anticholinergic drugs).
No products indexed under this heading.

Trihexyphenidyl Hydrochloride (Tricyclic antidepressants can potentiate the atropine-like effects of anticholinergic drugs).
No products indexed under this heading.

Food Interactions

Alcohol (Concurrent use is associated with exaggerated effects).

SUSTIVA CAPSULES

(Efavirenz) 957

May interact with central nervous system depressants, ergot-containing drugs, phenytoin, and certain other agents. Compounds in these categories include:

Alfentanil Hydrochloride (Potential for additive central nervous system effects when Sustiva is used concomitantly with other CNS depressants).
No products indexed under this heading.

Alprazolam (Potential for additive central nervous system effects when Sustiva is used concomitantly with other CNS depressants). Products include:
Niravam Orally Disintegrating Tablets 3106
Xanax XR Tablets 2655

Amprenavir (Efavirenz has the potential to decrease serum concentrations of amprenavir). Products include:
Agenerase Capsules 1299
Agenerase Oral Solution 1304

Aprobarbital (Potential for additive central nervous system effects when Sustiva is used concomitantly with other CNS depressants).
No products indexed under this heading.

Astemizole (Efavirenz has been shown *in vivo* to induce CYP3A4, other compounds that are substrates of CYP3A4, such as astemizole, may have decreased plasma

concentrations when co-administered; *in vitro* efavirenz inhibits 3A4, co-administration with the drugs primarily metabolized by this isoenzyme, such as astemizole, may result in altered plasma concentrations of astemizole; concurrent use should be avoided).
No products indexed under this heading.

Atazanavir (Co-administration has resulted in decreases in atazanavir Cmax (59%) and AUC (74%)).
No products indexed under this heading.

Azithromycin Dihydrate (Co-administration has resulted in increases in azithromycin Cmax (22%) with no change in AUC; no dosage adjustment is necessary). Products include:
Zithromax **2568**
Zithromax for IV Infusion **2573**
Zithromax for Oral Suspension, 300 mg, 600 mg, 900 mg, 1200 mg **2561**
Zithromax Tablets, 250 mg, 500 mg **2561**
Zithromax Tri-Pak **2561**
Zithromax Z-Pak **2568**

Buprenorphine Hydrochloride (Potential for additive central nervous system effects when Sustiva is used concomitantly with other CNS depressants). Products include:
Buprenex Injectable **2718**
Suboxone Tablets **2719**
Subutex Tablets **2719**

Buspirone Hydrochloride (Potential for additive central nervous system effects when Sustiva is used concomitantly with other CNS depressants).
No products indexed under this heading.

Butabarbital (Potential for additive central nervous system effects when Sustiva is used concomitantly with other CNS depressants).
No products indexed under this heading.

Butalbital (Potential for additive central nervous system effects when Sustiva is used concomitantly with other CNS depressants). Products include:
Sedapap Tablets 50 mg/650 mg **2098**

Carbamazepine (Potential for reduction in anticonvulsant and/or efavirenz plasma levels). Products include:
Carbatrol Capsules **3174**
Equetro Extended-Release Capsules **3178**
Tegretol/Tegretol-XR **2278**

Chlordiazepoxide (Potential for additive central nervous system effects when Sustiva is used concomitantly with other CNS depressants).
No products indexed under this heading.

Chlordiazepoxide Hydrochloride (Potential for additive central nervous system effects when Sustiva is used concomitantly with other CNS depressants). Products include:
Librium Capsules **3349**

Chlorpromazine (Potential for additive central nervous system effects when Sustiva is used concomitantly with other CNS depressants).
No products indexed under this heading.

Chlorpromazine Hydrochloride (Potential for additive central nervous system effects when Sustiva is used concomitantly with other CNS depressants).
No products indexed under this heading.

Chlorprothixene (Potential for additive central nervous system effects when Sustiva is used concomitantly with other CNS depressants).
No products indexed under this heading.

Chlorprothixene Hydrochloride (Potential for additive central nervous system effects when Sustiva is used concomitantly with other CNS depressants).
No products indexed under this heading.

Chlorprothixene Lactate (Potential for additive central nervous system effects when Sustiva is used concomitantly with other CNS depressants).
No products indexed under this heading.

Cisapride (Efavirenz has been shown *in vivo* to induce CYP3A4, other compounds that are substrates of CYP3A4, such as cisapride, may have decreased plasma concentrations when co-administered; *in vitro* efavirenz inhibits 3A4, co-administration with the drugs primarily metabolized by this isoenzyme, such as cisapride, may result in altered plasma concentrations of cisapride; concurrent use should be avoided).
No products indexed under this heading.

Clarithromycin (Decreased plasma concentration of clarithromycin and increased 14-OH metabolite concentration; clinical significance is not known). Products include:
Biaxin/Biaxin XL **402**
PREVPAC **3281**

Clorazepate Dipotassium (Potential for additive central nervous system effects when Sustiva is used concomitantly with other CNS depressants). Products include:
Tranxene **2488**

Clozapine (Potential for additive central nervous system effects when Sustiva is used concomitantly with other CNS depressants). Products include:
Clozapine Tablets **2141**
Clozaril Tablets **2174**
FazaClo Orally Disintegrating Tablets **547**

Codeine Phosphate (Potential for additive central nervous system effects when Sustiva is used concomitantly with other CNS depressants). Products include:
Tylenol with Codeine **2461**

Desflurane (Potential for additive central nervous system effects when Sustiva is used concomitantly with other CNS depressants). Products include:
Suprane Liquid for Inhalation **770**

Dezocine (Potential for additive central nervous system effects when Sustiva is used concomitantly with other CNS depressants).
No products indexed under this heading.

Diazepam (Potential for additive central nervous system effects when Sustiva is used concomitantly with other CNS depressants). Products include:
Diastat Rectal Delivery System **3344**
Valium Tablets **2822**

Dihydroergotamine Mesylate (Efavirenz has been shown *in vivo* to induce CYP3A4, other compounds that are substrates of CYP3A4, such as ergot derivatives, may have decreased plasma concentrations when co-administered; *in vitro* efavirenz inhibits 3A4, co-administration with the drugs primarily metabolized by this isoenzyme, such as ergot derivatives, may result in altered plasma concentrations of ergot derivatives; concurrent use should be avoided). Products include:
Migranal Nasal Spray **3350**

Droperidol (Potential for additive central nervous system effects when Sustiva is used concomitantly with other CNS depressants).
No products indexed under this heading.

Enflurane (Potential for additive central nervous system effects when Sustiva is used concomitantly with other CNS depressants).
No products indexed under this heading.

Ergonovine Maleate (Efavirenz has been shown *in vivo* to induce CYP3A4, other compounds that are substrates of CYP3A4, such as ergot derivatives, may have decreased plasma concentrations when co-administered; *in vitro* efavirenz inhibits 3A4, co-administration with the drugs primarily metabolized by this isoenzyme, such as ergot derivatives, may result in altered plasma concentrations of ergot derivatives; concurrent use should be avoided).
No products indexed under this heading.

Ergotamine Tartrate (Efavirenz has been shown *in vivo* to induce CYP3A4, other compounds that are substrates of CYP3A4, such as ergot derivatives, may have decreased plasma concentrations when co-administered; *in vitro* efavirenz inhibits 3A4, co-administration with the drugs primarily metabolized by this isoenzyme, such as ergot derivatives, may result in altered plasma concentrations of ergot derivatives; concurrent use should be avoided).
No products indexed under this heading.

Estazolam (Potential for additive central nervous system effects when Sustiva is used concomitantly with other CNS depressants). Products include:
ProSom Tablets **512**

Ethanol (Potential for additive central nervous system effects when Sustiva is used concomitantly with other CNS depressants).
No products indexed under this heading.

Ethchlorvynol (Potential for additive central nervous system effects when Sustiva is used concomitantly with other CNS depressants).
No products indexed under this heading.

Ethinamate (Potential for additive central nervous system effects when Sustiva is used concomitantly with other CNS depressants).
No products indexed under this heading.

Ethinyl Estradiol (Co-administration has resulted in increased AUC for ethinyl estradiol; there was no effect on efavirenz AUC or Cmax; clinical significance is unknown). Products include:
Alesse-28 Tablets **3392**
Lo/Ovral-28 Tablets **3423**
NuvaRing **2357**
Ortho-Cept Tablets **2395**
Ortho-Cyclen/Ortho Tri-Cyclen **2414**
Ortho Evra Transdermal System **2402**
Ortho Tri-Cyclen Lo Tablets **2421**
Seasonale Tablets **1073**
Triphasil-28 Tablets **3483**
Yasmin 28 Tablets **818**

Ethyl Alcohol (Potential for additive central nervous system effects when Sustiva is used concomitantly with other CNS depressants).
No products indexed under this heading.

Fentanyl (Potential for additive central nervous system effects when Sustiva is used concomitantly with other CNS depressants). Products include:
Duragesic Transdermal System **2448**

Fentanyl Citrate (Potential for additive central nervous system effects when Sustiva is used concomitantly with other CNS depressants). Products include:
Actiq **993**

Fluconazole (Co-administration has resulted in increase in 16% AUC for efavirenz; there was no change in fluconazole Cmax or AUC).
No products indexed under this heading.

Fluphenazine Decanoate (Potential for additive central nervous system effects when Sustiva is used concomitantly with other CNS depressants).
No products indexed under this heading.

Fluphenazine Enanthate (Potential for additive central nervous system effects when Sustiva is used concomitantly with other CNS depressants).
No products indexed under this heading.

Fluphenazine Hydrochloride (Potential for additive central nervous system effects when Sustiva is used concomitantly with other CNS depressants).
No products indexed under this heading.

Flurazepam Hydrochloride (Potential for additive central nervous system effects when Sustiva is used concomitantly with other CNS depressants). Products include:
Dalmane Capsules **3343**

Fosphenytoin Sodium (Potential for reduction in anticonvulsant and/or efavirenz plasma levels).
No products indexed under this heading.

Glutethimide (Potential for additive central nervous system effects when Sustiva is used concomitantly with other CNS depressants).
No products indexed under this heading.

Haloperidol (Potential for additive central nervous system effects when Sustiva is used concomitantly with other CNS depressants).
No products indexed under this heading.

Haloperidol Decanoate (Potential for additive central nervous system effects when Sustiva is used concomitantly with other CNS depressants).
No products indexed under this heading.

Hydrocodone Bitartrate (Potential for additive central nervous system effects when Sustiva is used concomitantly with other CNS depressants). Products include:
Hycodan 1104
Hycomine Compound Tablets 1105
Hycotuss Expectorant Syrup 1106
Lortab 3315
Lortab Elixir 3312
Vicodin Tablets 530
Vicodin ES Tablets 531
Vicodin HP Tablets 532
Vicoprofen Tablets 533
Zydone Tablets 1118

Hydrocodone Polistirex (Potential for additive central nervous system effects when Sustiva is used concomitantly with other CNS depressants). Products include:
Tussionex Pennkinetic Extended-Release Suspension 3322

Hydromorphone Hydrochloride (Potential for additive central nervous system effects when Sustiva is used concomitantly with other CNS depressants). Products include:
Dilaudid 439
Dilaudid Oral Liquid 443
Dilaudid Non-Sterile Powder 439
Dilaudid Rectal Suppositories 439
Dilaudid Tablets 439
Dilaudid Tablets - 8 mg 443
Dilaudid-HP 441

Hydroxyzine Hydrochloride (Potential for additive central nervous system effects when Sustiva is used concomitantly with other CNS depressants).
No products indexed under this heading.

Hypericum (St. John's Wort is expected to substantially decrease plasma levels of efavirenz; concurrent use is not recommended).
No products indexed under this heading.

Indinavir Sulfate (Decreased plasma concentration of indinavir; indinavir dose should be increased). Products include:
Crixivan Capsules 1918

Isoflurane (Potential for additive central nervous system effects when Sustiva is used concomitantly with other CNS depressants).
No products indexed under this heading.

Itraconazole (Potential for decreased itraconazole concentrations).
No products indexed under this heading.

Ketamine Hydrochloride (Potential for additive central nervous system effects when Sustiva is used concomitantly with other CNS depressants).
No products indexed under this heading.

Ketoconazole (Potential for decreased ketoconazole concentrations). Products include:
Nizoral A-D Shampoo, 1% 1839
Nizoral 2% Shampoo 1838

Levomethadyl Acetate Hydrochloride (Potential for additive central nervous system effects when Sustiva is used concomitantly with other CNS depressants).
No products indexed under this heading.

Levorphanol Tartrate (Potential for additive central nervous system effects when Sustiva is used concomitantly with other CNS depressants).
No products indexed under this heading.

Lorazepam (Potential for additive central nervous system effects when Sustiva is used concomitantly with other CNS depressants).
No products indexed under this heading.

Loxapine Hydrochloride (Potential for additive central nervous system effects when Sustiva is used concomitantly with other CNS depressants).
No products indexed under this heading.

Loxapine Succinate (Potential for additive central nervous system effects when Sustiva is used concomitantly with other CNS depressants).
No products indexed under this heading.

Meperidine Hydrochloride (Potential for additive central nervous system effects when Sustiva is used concomitantly with other CNS depressants).
No products indexed under this heading.

Mephobarbital (Potential for additive central nervous system effects when Sustiva is used concomitantly with other CNS depressants). Products include:
Mebaral Tablets, USP 2483

Meprobamate (Potential for additive central nervous system effects when Sustiva is used concomitantly with other CNS depressants).
No products indexed under this heading.

Mesoridazine Besylate (Potential for additive central nervous system effects when Sustiva is used concomitantly with other CNS depressants).
No products indexed under this heading.

Methadone Hydrochloride (Decreased plasma concentration of methadone; methadone dose may need to be increased).
No products indexed under this heading.

Methohexital Sodium (Potential for additive central nervous system effects when Sustiva is used concomitantly with other CNS depressants).
No products indexed under this heading.

Methotrimeprazine (Potential for additive central nervous system effects when Sustiva is used concomitantly with other CNS depressants).
No products indexed under this heading.

Methoxyflurane (Potential for additive central nervous system effects when Sustiva is used concomitantly with other CNS depressants).
No products indexed under this heading.

Methylergonovine Maleate (Efavirenz has been shown *in vivo* to induce CYP3A4, other compounds that are substrates of CYP3A4, such as ergot derivatives, may have decreased plasma concentrations when co-administered; *in vitro* efavirenz inhibits 3A4, co-administration with the drugs primarily metabolized by this isoenzyme, such as ergot derivatives, may result in altered plasma concentrations of ergot derivatives; concurrent use should be avoided).
No products indexed under this heading.

Methysergide Maleate (Efavirenz has been shown *in vivo* to induce CYP3A4, other compounds that are substrates of CYP3A4, such as ergot derivatives, may have decreased plasma concentrations when co-administered; in vitro efavirenz inhibits 3A4, co-administration with the drugs primarily metabolized by this isoenzyme, such as ergot derivatives, may result in altered plasma concentrations of ergot derivatives; concurrent use should be avoided).
No products indexed under this heading.

Midazolam Hydrochloride (Efavirenz has been shown *in vivo* to induce CYP3A4, other compounds that are substrates of CYP3A4, such as midazolam, may have decreased plasma concentrations when co-administered; *in vitro* efavirenz inhibits 3A4, co-administration with the drugs primarily metabolized by this isoenzyme, such as midazolam, may result in altered plasma concentrations of midazolam; concurrent use should be avoided).
No products indexed under this heading.

Molindone Hydrochloride (Potential for additive central nervous system effects when Sustiva is used concomitantly with other CNS depressants). Products include:
Moban Tablets 1108

Morphine Sulfate (Potential for additive central nervous system effects when Sustiva is used concomitantly with other CNS depressants). Products include:
Avinza Capsules 1714
Kadian Capsules 572
MS Contin Tablets 2703

Nelfinavir Mesylate (Co-administration in uninfected individuals has resulted in increases in AUC (20%) and Cmax (21%) for nelfinavir; no dose adjustment is necessary). Products include:
Viracept 2556

Olanzapine (Potential for additive central nervous system effects when Sustiva is used concomitantly with other CNS depressants). Products include:
Symbyax Capsules 1788
Zyprexa Tablets 1798
Zyprexa IntraMuscular 1798
Zyprexa ZYDIS Orally Disintegrating Tablets 1798

Oxazepam (Potential for additive central nervous system effects when Sustiva is used concomitantly with other CNS depressants).
No products indexed under this heading.

Oxycodone Hydrochloride (Potential for additive central nervous system effects when Sustiva is used concomitantly with other CNS depressants). Products include:
Combunox Tablets 1183
OxyContin Tablets 2699
OxyFast Oral Concentrate Solution 2704
OxyIR Capsules 2704
Percocet Tablets 1114
Percodan Tablets 1115

Pentobarbital Sodium (Potential for additive central nervous system effects when Sustiva is used concomitantly with other CNS depressants). Products include:
Nembutal Sodium Solution, USP 2484

Perphenazine (Potential for additive central nervous system effects when Sustiva is used concomitantly with other CNS depressants).
No products indexed under this heading.

Phenobarbital (Potential for reduction in anticonvulsant and/or efavirenz plasma levels).
No products indexed under this heading.

Phenytoin (Potential for reduction in anticonvulsant and/or efavirenz plasma levels).
No products indexed under this heading.

Phenytoin Sodium (Potential for reduction in anticonvulsant and/or efavirenz plasma levels). Products include:
Phenytek Capsules 2153

Prazepam (Potential for additive central nervous system effects when Sustiva is used concomitantly with other CNS depressants).
No products indexed under this heading.

Prochlorperazine (Potential for additive central nervous system effects when Sustiva is used concomitantly with other CNS depressants).
No products indexed under this heading.

Promethazine Hydrochloride (Potential for additive central nervous system effects when Sustiva is used concomitantly with other CNS depressants). Products include:
Phenergan 3438

Propofol (Potential for additive central nervous system effects when Sustiva is used concomitantly with other CNS depressants). Products include:
Diprivan Injectable Emulsion 676

Propoxyphene Hydrochloride (Potential for additive central nervous system effects when Sustiva is used concomitantly with other CNS depressants).
No products indexed under this heading.

Propoxyphene Napsylate (Potential for additive central nervous system effects when Sustiva is used concomitantly with other CNS depressants). Products include:
Darvocet A 500 Tablets 3497

Quazepam (Potential for additive central nervous system effects when Sustiva is used concomitantly with other CNS depressants).
No products indexed under this heading.

Quetiapine Fumarate (Potential for additive central nervous system effects when Sustiva is used concomitantly with other CNS depressants). Products include:

Seroquel Tablets 691

Remifentanil Hydrochloride (Potential for additive central nervous system effects when Sustiva is used concomitantly with other CNS depressants).
No products indexed under this heading.

Rifabutin (Decreased plasma concentration of rifabutin; rifabutin dose should be increased by 50%).
No products indexed under this heading.

Rifampin (Co-administration has resulted in decreased efavirenz plasma concentrations; clinical significance is unknown).
No products indexed under this heading.

Risperidone (Potential for additive central nervous system effects when Sustiva is used concomitantly with other CNS depressants). Products include:
Risperdal Consta Long-Acting Injection 1664
Risperdal M-Tab Orally Disintegrating Tablets 1658
Risperdal 1658

Ritonavir (Co-administration has resulted in increases in AUC for each drug by 20%; the combination was associated with a higher frequency of adverse clinical experiences including dizziness, nausea, paresthesia, and laboratory abnormalities (elevated liver enzymes)). Products include:
Kaletra 474
Norvir 499

Saquinavir (Co-administration with saquinavir soft gelatin capsule has resulted in decreases in AUC (62%) and Cmax (50%) for saquinavir; saquinavir should not be used as sole protease inhibitor in combination with Sustiva).
No products indexed under this heading.

Saquinavir Mesylate (Co-administration with saquinavir soft gelatin capsule has resulted in decreases in AUC (62%) and Cmax (50%) for saquinavir; saquinavir should not be used as sole protease inhibitor in combination with Sustiva). Products include:
Invirase 2776

Secobarbital Sodium (Potential for additive central nervous system effects when Sustiva is used concomitantly with other CNS depressants).
No products indexed under this heading.

Sevoflurane (Potential for additive central nervous system effects when Sustiva is used concomitantly with other CNS depressants). Products include:
Ultane Liquid for Inhalation 526

Sodium Oxybate (Potential for additive central nervous system effects when Sustiva is used concomitantly with other CNS depressants).
No products indexed under this heading.

Sufentanil Citrate (Potential for additive central nervous system effects when Sustiva is used concomitantly with other CNS depressants).
No products indexed under this heading.

Temazepam (Potential for additive central nervous system effects when Sustiva is used concomitantly with other CNS depressants).
No products indexed under this heading.

Thiamylal Sodium (Potential for additive central nervous system effects when Sustiva is used concomitantly with other CNS depressants).
No products indexed under this heading.

Thioridazine Hydrochloride (Potential for additive central nervous system effects when Sustiva is used concomitantly with other CNS depressants). Products include:
Thioridazine Hydrochloride Tablets 2122

Thiothixene (Potential for additive central nervous system effects when Sustiva is used concomitantly with other CNS depressants). Products include:
Thiothixene Capsules 2124

Triazolam (Efavirenz has been shown *in vivo* to induce CYP3A4, other compounds that are substrates of CYP3A4, such as triazolam, may have decreased plasma concentrations when co-administered; *in vitro* efavirenz inhibits 3A4, co-administration with the drugs primarily metabolized by this isoenzyme, such as triazolam, may result in altered plasma concentrations of triazolam; concurrent use should be avoided).
No products indexed under this heading.

Trifluoperazine Hydrochloride (Potential for additive central nervous system effects when Sustiva is used concomitantly with other CNS depressants).
No products indexed under this heading.

Voriconazole (Co-administration has resulted in increases in voriconazole Cmax (38%) and AUC (44%); efavirenz will significantly decrease voriconazole concentration therefore co-administration is contraindicated). Products include:
VFEND I.V. 2543
VFEND Oral Suspension 2543
VFEND Tablets 2543

Warfarin Sodium (Co-administration may result in increased or decreased plasma concentrations and effects of warfarin). Products include:
Coumadin for Injection 932
Coumadin Tablets 932

Zaleplon (Potential for additive central nervous system effects when Sustiva is used concomitantly with other CNS depressants). Products include:
Sonata Capsules 1686

Ziprasidone Hydrochloride (Potential for additive central nervous system effects when Sustiva is used concomitantly with other CNS depressants). Products include:
Geodon Capsules 2514

Zolpidem Tartrate (Potential for additive central nervous system effects when Sustiva is used concomitantly with other CNS depressants). Products include:
Ambien Tablets 2867

Food Interactions

Alcohol (Potential for additive central nervous system effects when Sustiva is used concomitantly with alcohol).

Food, unspecified (High fat meal may increase the absorption of Sustiva and should be avoided; it can be taken with or without meals of normal composition).

SYMBYAX CAPSULES

(Fluoxetine Hydrochloride, Olanzapine) 1788

May interact with antihypertensives, cytochrome p450 1a2 inducers (selected), cytochrome p450 2d6 substrates (selected), dopamine agonists, monoamine oxidase inhibitors, non-steroidal anti-inflammatory agents, phenytoin, highly protein bound drugs (selected), tricyclic antidepressants, and certain other agents. Compounds in these categories include:

5-hydroxytryptophan (Five patients receiving fluoxetine in combination with tryptophan experienced adverse reactions, including agitation, restlessness, and gastrointestinal distress).
No products indexed under this heading.

Acebutolol Hydrochloride (Because of the potential for olanzapine to induce hypotension, Symbyax may enhance the effects of certain antihypertensive agents).
No products indexed under this heading.

Alprazolam (Co-administration of alprazolam and fluoxetine resulted in increased alprazolam plasma concentrations and in further psychomotor performance decrement due to increased alprazolam levels). Products include:
Niravam Orally Disintegrating Tablets 3106
Xanax XR Tablets 2655

Amiodarone Hydrochloride (Because fluoxetine is tightly bound to plasma protein, the administration of fluoxetine to a patient taking another drug that is tightly bound to protein may cause a shift in plasma concentrations potentially resulting in an adverse effect. Conversely, adverse effects may result from displacement of protein-bound fluoxetine by other tightly bound drugs). Products include:
Pacerone Tablets 3337

Amitriptyline Hydrochloride (In two fluoxetine studies, previously stable plasma levels of imipramine and desipramine have increased >2- to 10-fold when fluoxetine has been administered in combination. This influence may persist for three weeks or longer after fluoxetine is discontinued. Thus, the dose of TCA may need to be reduced and plasma TCA concentrations may need to be monitored temporarily when Symbyax is co-administered or has been recently discontinued).
No products indexed under this heading.

Amlodipine Besylate (Because of the potential for olanzapine to induce hypotension, Symbyax may enhance the effects of certain antihypertensive agents). Products include:
Caduet Tablets 2507
Lotrel Capsules 2238
Norvasc Tablets 2529

Amoxapine (In two fluoxetine studies, previously stable plasma levels of imipramine and desipramine have increased >2- to 10-fold when fluoxetine has been administered in combination. This influence may persist for three weeks or longer after fluoxetine is discontinued. Thus, the dose of TCA may need to be reduced and plasma TCA concentrations may need to be monitored temporarily when Symbyax is co-administered or has been recently discontinued).
No products indexed under this heading.

Amphetamine Aspartate (Fluoxetine, like other agents that are metabolized by CYP2D6, inhibits the activity of this isoenzyme. Therapy with medications that are predominately metabolized by the CYP2D6 system and have a relatively narrow therapeutic index should be initiated at the low end of the dose range if the patient is receiving fluoxetine concurrently or has taken it in the previous five weeks. If fluoxetine is added to the treatment regimen of a patient already receiving a drug metabolized by CYP2D6, the need for a decreased dose of the original medication should be considered). Products include:
Adderall Tablets 3168
Adderall XR Capsules 3169

Amphetamine Aspartate Monohydrate (Fluoxetine, like other agents that are metabolized by CYP2D6, inhibits the activity of this isoenzyme. Therapy with medications that are predominately metabolized by the CYP2D6 system and have a relatively narrow therapeutic index should be initiated at the low end of the dose range if the patient is receiving fluoxetine concurrently or has taken it in the previous five weeks. If fluoxetine is added to the treatment regimen of a patient already receiving a drug metabolized by CYP2D6, the need for a decreased dose of the original medication should be considered).
No products indexed under this heading.

Amphetamine Sulfate (Fluoxetine, like other agents that are metabolized by CYP2D6, inhibits the activity of this isoenzyme. Therapy with medications that are predominately metabolized by the CYP2D6 system and have a relatively narrow therapeutic index should be initiated at the low end of the dose range if the patient is receiving fluoxetine concurrently or has taken it in the previous five weeks. If fluoxetine is added to the treatment regimen of a patient already receiving a drug metabolized by CYP2D6, the need for a decreased dose of the original medication should be considered). Products include:
Adderall Tablets 3168
Adderall XR Capsules 3169

Aspirin (Serotonin release by platelets plays an important role in hemostasis. Studies have demonstrated an association between the use of psychotropic drugs that interfere with serotonin reuptake and the occurrence of upper gastrointestinal bleeding. These studies have also shown that concurrent use of aspirin potentiated the risk of bleeding. Therefore, patients should be cautioned about the use of aspirin concurrently with Symbyax). Products include:
Aggrenox Capsules 855
Bayer, Aspirin Regimen 606
Bayer Aspirin Tablets 3515
BC Powder 612
BC Allergy Sinus Cold Powder 612
Arthritis Strength BC Powder 612

BC Sinus Cold Powder 612
Ecotrin Enteric Coated Aspirin Low, Regular and Maximum Strength Tablets 1627
Goody's Body Pain Formula Powder 621
Goody's Extra Strength Headache Powder 621
Goody's Extra Strength Pain Relief Tablets 621
Percodan Tablets 1115
St. Joseph 81 mg Aspirin Chewable and Enteric Coated Tablets 1841

Aspirin, Enteric Coated (Serotonin release by platelets plays an important role in hemostasis. Studies have demonstrated an association between the use of psychotropic drugs that interfere with serotonin reuptake and the occurrence of upper gastrointestinal bleeding. These studies have also shown that concurrent use of aspirin potentiated the risk of bleeding. Therefore, patients should be cautioned about the use of aspirin concurrently with Symbyax).
No products indexed under this heading.

Aspirin Buffered (Serotonin release by platelets plays an important role in hemostasis. Studies have demonstrated an association between the use of psychotropic drugs that interfere with serotonin reuptake and the occurrence of upper gastrointestinal bleeding. These studies have also shown that concurrent use of aspirin potentiated the risk of bleeding. Therefore, patients should be cautioned about the use of aspirin concurrently with Symbyax).
No products indexed under this heading.

Atenolol (Because of the potential for olanzapine to induce hypotension, Symbyax may enhance the effects of certain antihypertensive agents). Products include:
Tenormin I.V. Injection 698
Tenormin Tablets 695

Atomoxetine Hydrochloride (Fluoxetine, like other agents that are metabolized by CYP2D6, inhibits the activity of this isoenzyme. Therapy with medications that are predominately metabolized by the CYP2D6 system and have a relatively narrow therapeutic index should be initiated at the low end of the dose range if the patient is receiving fluoxetine concurrently or has taken it in the previous five weeks. If fluoxetine is added to the treatment regimen of a patient already receiving a drug metabolized by CYP2D6, the need for a decreased dose of the original medication should be considered). Products include:
Strattera Capsules 1784

Atovaquone (Because fluoxetine is tightly bound to plasma protein, the administration of fluoxetine to a patient taking another drug that is tightly bound to protein may cause a shift in plasma concentrations potentially resulting in an adverse effect. Conversely, adverse effects may result from displacement of protein-bound fluoxetine by other tightly bound drugs). Products include:
Malarone Tablets 1484
Malarone Pediatric Tablets 1484
Mepron Suspension 1487

Benazepril Hydrochloride (Because of the potential for olanzapine to induce hypotension, Symbyax may enhance the effects of certain antihypertensive agents). Products include:
Lotensin Tablets 2232
Lotensin HCT Tablets 2235
Lotrel Capsules 2238

Bendroflumethiazide (Because of the potential for olanzapine to induce hypotension, Symbyax may enhance the effects of certain antihypertensive agents).
No products indexed under this heading.

Betaxolol Hydrochloride (Because of the potential for olanzapine to induce hypotension, Symbyax may enhance the effects of certain antihypertensive agents). Products include:
Betoptic S Ophthalmic Suspension 554

Bisoprolol Fumarate (Because of the potential for olanzapine to induce hypotension, Symbyax may enhance the effects of certain antihypertensive agents).
No products indexed under this heading.

Bromocriptine Mesylate (The olanzapine component of Symbyax may antagonize the effects of levodopa and dopamine agonists).
No products indexed under this heading.

Candesartan Cilexetil (Because of the potential for olanzapine to induce hypotension, Symbyax may enhance the effects of certain antihypertensive agents). Products include:
Atacand Tablets 634
Atacand HCT 637

Captopril (Because of the potential for olanzapine to induce hypotension, Symbyax may enhance the effects of certain antihypertensive agents). Products include:
Captopril Tablets 2114

Carbamazepine (Carbamazepine therapy (200mg bid) causes an approximate 50% increase in the clearance of olanzapine; higher daily doses of carbamazepine may cause an even greater increase in olanzapine clearance. Patients on stable dose of carbamazepine have developed elevated plasma anticonvulsant concentrations and clinical anticonvulsant toxicity following initiation of concomitant fluoxetine treatment). Products include:
Carbatrol Capsules 3174
Equetro Extended-Release Capsules 3178
Tegretol/Tegretol-XR 2278

Carteolol Hydrochloride (Because of the potential for olanzapine to induce hypotension, Symbyax may enhance the effects of certain antihypertensive agents). Products include:
Carteolol Hydrochloride Ophthalmic Solution USP, 1% .... ⊙ 246

Carvedilol (Fluoxetine, like other agents that are metabolized by CYP2D6, inhibits the activity of this isoenzyme. Therapy with medications that are predominately metabolized by the CYP2D6 system and have a relatively narrow therapeutic index should be initiated at the low end of the dose range if the patient is receiving fluoxetine concurrently or has taken it in the previous five weeks. If fluoxetine is added to the treatment regimen of a patient already receiving a drug metabolized by CYP2D6, the need for a decreased dose of the original medication should be considered). Products include:
Coreg Tablets 1376

Cefonicid Sodium (Because fluoxetine is tightly bound to plasma protein, the administration of fluoxetine to a patient taking another drug that is tightly bound to protein may cause a shift in plasma concentrations potentially resulting in an adverse effect. Conversely, adverse effects may result from displacement of protein-bound fluoxetine by other tightly bound drugs).
No products indexed under this heading.

Celecoxib (Serotonin release by platelets plays an important role in hemostasis. Studies have demonstrated an association between the use of psychotropic drugs that interfere with serotonin reuptake and the occurrence of upper gastrointestinal bleeding. These studies have also shown that concurrent use of an NSAID potentiated the risk of bleeding. Therefore, patients should be cautioned about the use of NSAIDs concurrently with Symbyax). Products include:
Celebrex Capsules 3130

Cevimeline Hydrochloride (Fluoxetine, like other agents that are metabolized by CYP2D6, inhibits the activity of this isoenzyme. Therapy with medications that are predominately metabolized by the CYP2D6 system and have a relatively narrow therapeutic index should be initiated at the low end of the dose range if the patient is receiving fluoxetine concurrently or has taken it in the previous five weeks. If fluoxetine is added to the treatment regimen of a patient already receiving a drug metabolized by CYP2D6, the need for a decreased dose of the original medication should be considered). Products include:
Evoxac Capsules 1042

Chlordiazepoxide (Because fluoxetine is tightly bound to plasma protein, the administration of fluoxetine to a patient taking another drug that is tightly bound to protein may cause a shift in plasma concentrations potentially resulting in an adverse effect. Conversely, adverse effects may result from displacement of protein-bound fluoxetine by other tightly bound drugs).
No products indexed under this heading.

Chlordiazepoxide Hydrochloride (Because fluoxetine is tightly bound to plasma protein, the administration of fluoxetine to a patient taking another drug that is tightly bound to protein may cause a shift in plasma concentrations potentially resulting in an adverse effect. Conversely, adverse effects may result from displacement of protein-bound fluoxetine by other tightly bound drugs). Products include:
Librium Capsules 3349

Chlorothiazide (Because of the potential for olanzapine to induce hypotension, Symbyax may enhance the effects of certain antihypertensive agents). Products include:
Aldoclor Tablets 1881
Diuril Oral 1936

Chlorothiazide Sodium (Because of the potential for olanzapine to induce hypotension, Symbyax may enhance the effects of certain antihypertensive agents). Products include:
Diuril Sodium Intravenous 1934

Chlorpromazine (Fluoxetine, like other agents that are metabolized by CYP2D6, inhibits the activity of this isoenzyme. Therapy with medications that are predominately metabolized by the CYP2D6 system and have a relatively narrow therapeutic index should be initiated at the low end of the dose range if the patient is receiving fluoxetine concurrently or has taken it in the previous five weeks. If fluoxetine is added to the treatment regimen of a patient already receiving a drug metabolized by CYP2D6, the need for a decreased dose of the original medication should be considered).
No products indexed under this heading.

Chlorpromazine Hydrochloride (Fluoxetine, like other agents that are metabolized by CYP2D6, inhibits the activity of this isoenzyme. Therapy with medications that are predominately metabolized by the CYP2D6 system and have a relatively narrow therapeutic index should be initiated at the low end of the dose range if the patient is receiving fluoxetine concurrently or has taken it in the previous five weeks. If fluoxetine is added to the treatment regimen of a patient already receiving a drug metabolized by CYP2D6, the need for a decreased dose of the original medication should be considered).
No products indexed under this heading.

Chlorpropamide (Fluoxetine, like other agents that are metabolized by CYP2D6, inhibits the activity of this isoenzyme. Therapy with medications that are predominately metabolized by the CYP2D6 system and have a relatively narrow therapeutic index should be initiated at the low end of the dose range if the patient is receiving fluoxetine concurrently or has taken it in the previous five weeks. If fluoxetine is added to the treatment regimen of a patient already receiving a drug metabolized by CYP2D6, the need for a decreased dose of the original medication should be considered).
No products indexed under this heading.

Chlorthalidone (Because of the potential for olanzapine to induce hypotension, Symbyax may enhance the effects of certain antihypertensive agents). Products include:
Clorpres Tablets 2139

Citalopram Hydrobromide (Agents that induce CYP1A2 or glucuronyl transferase enzymes may cause an increase in olanzapine concentration). Products include:
Celexa 1177

Clomipramine Hydrochloride (In two fluoxetine studies, previously stable plasma levels of imipramine and desipramine have increased >2- to 10-fold when fluoxetine has been administered in combination. This influence may persist for three weeks or longer after fluoxetine is discontinued. Thus, the dose of TCA may need to be reduced and plasma TCA concentrations may need to be monitored temporarily when Symbyax is co-administered or has been

recently discontinued).
No products indexed under this heading.

Clonidine (Because of the potential for olanzapine to induce hypotension, Symbyax may enhance the effects of certain antihypertensive agents). Products include:
Catapres-TTS 875

Clonidine Hydrochloride (Because of the potential for olanzapine to induce hypotension, Symbyax may enhance the effects of certain antihypertensive agents). Products include:
Catapres Tablets 874
Clorpres Tablets 2139

Clozapine (Elevation of blood levels of clozapine has been observed in patients receiving concomitant fluoxetine). Products include:
Clozapine Tablets 2141
Clozaril Tablets 2174
FazaClo Orally Disintegrating Tablets 547

Codeine Phosphate (Fluoxetine, like other agents that are metabolized by CYP2D6, inhibits the activity of this isoenzyme. Therapy with medications that are predominately metabolized by the CYP2D6 system and have a relatively narrow therapeutic index should be initiated at the low end of the dose range if the patient is receiving fluoxetine concurrently or has taken it in the previous five weeks. If fluoxetine is added to the treatment regimen of a patient already receiving a drug metabolized by CYP2D6, the need for a decreased dose of the original medication should be considered). Products include:
Tylenol with Codeine 2461

Codeine Sulfate (Fluoxetine, like other agents that are metabolized by CYP2D6, inhibits the activity of this isoenzyme. Therapy with medications that are predominately metabolized by the CYP2D6 system and have a relatively narrow therapeutic index should be initiated at the low end of the dose range if the patient is receiving fluoxetine concurrently or has taken it in the previous five weeks. If fluoxetine is added to the treatment regimen of a patient already receiving a drug metabolized by CYP2D6, the need for a decreased dose of the original medication should be considered).
No products indexed under this heading.

Cyclobenzaprine Hydrochloride (Fluoxetine, like other agents that are metabolized by CYP2D6, inhibits the activity of this isoenzyme. Therapy with medications that are predominately metabolized by the CYP2D6 system and have a relatively narrow therapeutic index should be initiated at the low end of the dose range if the patient is receiving fluoxetine concurrently or has taken it in the previous five weeks. If fluoxetine is added to the treatment regimen of a patient already receiving a drug metabolized by CYP2D6, the need for a decreased dose of the original medication should be considered). Products include:
Flexeril Tablets 1832

Cyclosporine (Because fluoxetine is tightly bound to plasma protein, the administration of fluoxetine to a patient taking another drug that is tightly bound to protein may cause a shift in plasma concentrations potentially resulting in an adverse effect. Conversely, adverse effects may result from displacement of protein-bound fluoxetine by other tightly bound drugs). Products include:
Gengraf Capsules 458
Neoral Soft Gelatin Capsules 2247
Neoral Oral Solution 2247
Restasis Ophthalmic Emulsion 570
Sandimmune 2259

Deserpidine (Because of the potential for olanzapine to induce hypotension, Symbyax may enhance the effects of certain antihypertensive agents).
No products indexed under this heading.

Desipramine Hydrochloride (In two fluoxetine studies, previously stable plasma levels of imipramine and desipramine have increased >2- to 10-fold when fluoxetine has been administered in combination. This influence may persist for three weeks or longer after fluoxetine is discontinued. Thus, the dose of TCA may need to be reduced and plasma TCA concentrations may need to be monitored temporarily when Symbyax is co-administered or has been recently discontinued).
No products indexed under this heading.

Dexfenfluramine Hydrochloride (Fluoxetine, like other agents that are metabolized by CYP2D6, inhibits the activity of this isoenzyme. Therapy with medications that are predominately metabolized by the CYP2D6 system and have a relatively narrow therapeutic index should be initiated at the low end of the dose range if the patient is receiving fluoxetine concurrently or has taken it in the previous five weeks. If fluoxetine is added to the treatment regimen of a patient already receiving a drug metabolized by CYP2D6, the need for a decreased dose of the original medication should be considered).
No products indexed under this heading.

Dextromethorphan Hydrobromide (Fluoxetine, like other agents that are metabolized by CYP2D6, inhibits the activity of this isoenzyme. Therapy with medications that are predominately metabolized by the CYP2D6 system and have a relatively narrow therapeutic index should be initiated at the low end of the dose range if the patient is receiving fluoxetine concurrently or has taken it in the previous five weeks. If fluoxetine is added to the treatment regimen of a patient already receiving a drug metabolized by CYP2D6, the need for a decreased dose of the original medication should be considered). Products include:
Alacol DM Syrup 739
Balamine DM 739
Contac Severe Cold and Flu Caplets Maximum Strength .... ■ 615
Contac Severe Cold and Flu Caplets Non-Drowsy .... ■ 615
Children's Dimetapp DM Cold & Cough Elixir .... ■ 745
Children's Dimetapp Long Acting Cough Plus Cold Syrup .... ■ 746
Dimetapp Infant Drops Decongestant Plus Cough .... ■ 746
Mucinex DM Tablets .... ■ 602
PediaCare Decongestant & Cough Infant Drops .... ■ 705
PediaCare Freezer Pops Long-Acting Cough-Glacier Grape and Polar Berry Blue .... ■ 706
PediaCare Long-Acting Cough Infant Drops .... ■ 705
PediaCare Long-Acting Cough Plus Cold Liquid .... ■ 704
PediaCare Multi-Symptom Cold Liquid .... ■ 704
PediaCare NightRest Cough & Cold Liquid .... ■ 704
Robitussin Allergy & Cough Syrup .. ■ 750
Robitussin CF Liquid .... ■ 755
Robitussin Cough & Cold Liquid-filled Capsules .... ■ 750
Robitussin Cough, Cold & Flu Liquid-filled Capsules .... ■ 750
Robitussin Cough & Cold Infant Drops .... ■ 755
Robitussin DM Infant Drops .... ■ 753
Robitussin DM Liquid .... ■ 753
Robitussin Flu Liquid .... ■ 752
Robitussin Maximum Strength Cough Liquid .... ■ 754
Robitussin Maximum Strength Cough & Cold Liquid .... ■ 754
Robitussin Pediatric Cough Liquid .... ■ 754
Robitussin Pediatric Cough & Cold Liquid .... ■ 754
Robitussin PM Cough & Cold Liquid .... ■ 752
Robitussin Sugar Free Cough Liquid .... ■ 753
Simply Cough Liquid 1840
Sudafed Severe Cold .... ■ 710
TheraFlu Cold & Cough Hot Liquid .... ■ 680
TheraFlu Flu & Chest Congestion Non-Drowsy Hot Liquid .... ■ 681
TheraFlu Severe Cold Non-Drowsy Hot Liquid .... ■ 683
TheraFlu Severe Cold & Cough Hot Liquid .... ■ 683
TheraFlu Severe Cold Caplets .... ■ 679
TheraFlu Severe Cold Hot Liquid .... ■ 682
TheraFlu Severe Cold Non-Drowsy Caplets .... ■ 679
TheraFlu Thin Strips Long Acting Cough .... ■ 684
Triaminic Cold & Cough Liquid .... ■ 685
Triaminic Cough Liquid .... ■ 687
Triaminic Cough & Nasal Congestion Liquid .... ■ 687
Triaminic Cough & Sore Throat Liquid .... ■ 687
Triaminic Flu, Cough & Fever Liquid .... ■ 685
Triaminic Night Time Cough & Cold Liquid .... ■ 685
Triaminic Cold & Cough Softchews .... ■ 688
Triaminic Cough & Sore Throat Softchews .... ■ 689
Triaminic Thin Strips Long Acting Cough .... ■ 689
Children's Tylenol Plus Cold & Cough Suspension Liquid and Chewable Tablets 1851
Children's Tylenol Plus Flu Suspension Liquid 1853
Concentrated Tylenol Infants' Drops Plus Cold and Cough 1851
Tylenol Cold & Flu Severe Daytime Liquid with Cool Bust 1846
Tylenol Cold & Flu Severe NightTime Liquid with Cool Burst 1846
Tylenol Cold Severe Congestion Non-Drowsy Caplets with Cool Burst 1846
Tylenol Cough & Sore Throat Daytime Liquid with Cool Burst 1849
Tylenol Cough & Sore Throat NightTime Liquid with Cool Burst 1849
Tylenol Flu Day Non-Drowsy Gelcaps 1846
Concentrated Tylenol Infants' Drops Plus Cold & Cough Nasal Decongestant, Fever Reducer & Pain Reliever .... ■ 668
Multi-Symptom Tylenol Cold Night Time Caplets 1845
Multi-Symptom Tylenol Cold Day Non-Drowsy Caplets and Gelcaps 1845
Vicks 44 Cough Relief 2675
Vicks 44D Cough & Head Congestion Relief 2676
Vicks 44D Cough & Head Congestion Relief Liquid .... ■ 721
Vicks 44E Cough & Chest Congestion Relief 2676
Pediatric Vicks 44e Cough & Chest Congestion Relief Liquid 2673
Vicks 44M Cough, Cold & Flu Relief 2676
Pediatric Vicks 44m Cough & Cold Relief 2673
Vicks DayQuil LiquiCaps/Liquid Multi-Symptom Cold/Flu Relief .... ■ 723
Vicks DayQuil Multi-Symptom Cold/Flu Relief LiquiCaps 2675
Vicks DayQuil Multi-Symptom Cold/Flu Relief Liquid 2675
Children's Vicks NyQuil Cold/Cough Relief 2671
Vicks NyQuil Cough Liquid 2677
Vicks NyQuil LiquiCaps 2677
Vicks NyQuil LiquiCaps/Liquid Multi-Symptom Cold/Flu Relief .... ■ 725
Vicks NyQuil Liquid 2677
Zicam Concentrated Cough Mist for Kids Cool Cherry .... ■ 643
Zicam Concentrated Cough Mist for Kids Plus D Cool Cherry .... ■ 643
Zicam Concentrated Cough Mist Nite-Cool Cherry .... ■ 642
Zicam Concentrated Cough Mist Plus D Cool Cherry .... ■ 642
Zicam Concentrated Cough Mist-Honey Lemon & Cool Cherry .... ■ 642

Dextromethorphan Polistirex (Fluoxetine, like other agents that are metabolized by CYP2D6, inhibits the activity of this isoenzyme. Therapy with medications that are predominately metabolized by the CYP2D6 system and have a relatively narrow therapeutic index should be initiated at the low end of the dose range if the patient is receiving fluoxetine concurrently or has taken it in the previous five weeks. If fluoxetine is added to the treatment regimen of a patient already receiving a drug metabolized by CYP2D6, the need for a decreased dose of the original medication should be considered). Products include:
Delsym Extended-Release Suspension .... ■ 611
Delsym 12 Hour Cough Suppressant for Children .... ■ 611

Diazepam (The co-administration of diazepam with olanzapine may potentiate the orthostatic hypotension observed with olanzapine). Products include:
Diastat Rectal Delivery System 3344
Valium Tablets 2822

Diazoxide (Because of the potential for olanzapine to induce hypotension, Symbyax may enhance the effects of certain antihypertensive agents). Products include:
Hyperstat I.V. Injection 3031

Diclofenac Potassium (Serotonin release by platelets plays an important role in hemostasis. Studies have demonstrated an association between the use of psychotropic drugs that interfere with serotonin reuptake and the occurrence of upper gastrointestinal bleeding. These studies have also shown that concurrent use of an NSAID potentiated the risk of bleeding. Therefore, patients should be cautioned about the use of NSAIDs concurrently with Symbyax). Products include:
Cataflam Tablets 2173

Diclofenac Sodium (Serotonin release by platelets plays an important role in hemostasis. Studies have demonstrated an association between the use of psychotropic drugs that interfere with serotonin reuptake and the occurrence of

upper gastrointestinal bleeding. These studies have also shown that concurrent use of an NSAID potentiated the risk of bleeding. Therefore, patients should be cautioned about the use of NSAIDs concurrently with Symbyax). Products include:

Arthrotec Tablets 3126
Voltaren Ophthalmic Solution 2300
Voltaren Tablets 2298
Voltaren-XR Tablets 2301

Diltiazem Hydrochloride (Because of the potential for olanzapine to induce hypotension, Symbyax may enhance the effects of certain antihypertensive agents). Products include:

Cardizem LA Extended Release Tablets 1699
Tiazac Capsules 1204

Diltiazem Maleate (Agents that induce CYP1A2 or glucuronyl transferase enzymes may cause an increase in olanzapine concentration).

No products indexed under this heading.

Dipyridamole (Because fluoxetine is tightly bound to plasma protein, the administration of fluoxetine to a patient taking another drug that is tightly bound to protein may cause a shift in plasma concentrations potentially resulting in an adverse effect. Conversely, adverse effects may result from displacement of protein-bound fluoxetine by other tightly bound drugs). Products include:

Aggrenox Capsules 855
Persantine Tablets 898

Dolasetron Mesylate (Fluoxetine, like other agents that are metabolized by CYP2D6, inhibits the activity of this isoenzyme. Therapy with medications that are predominately metabolized by the CYP2D6 system and have a relatively narrow therapeutic index should be initiated at the low end of the dose range if the patient is receiving fluoxetine concurrently or has taken it in the previous five weeks. If fluoxetine is added to the treatment regimen of a patient already receiving a drug metabolized by CYP2D6, the need for a decreased dose of the original medication should be considered). Products include:

Anzemet Injection 2871
Anzemet Tablets 2874

Donepezil Hydrochloride (Fluoxetine, like other agents that are metabolized by CYP2D6, inhibits the activity of this isoenzyme. Therapy with medications that are predominately metabolized by the CYP2D6 system and have a relatively narrow therapeutic index should be initiated at the low end of the dose range if the patient is receiving fluoxetine concurrently or has taken it in the previous five weeks. If fluoxetine is added to the treatment regimen of a patient already receiving a drug metabolized by CYP2D6, the need for a decreased dose of the original medication should be considered). Products include:

Aricept Tablets 1086
Aricept ODT Tablets 1086

Dopamine Hydrochloride (The olanzapine component of Symbyax may antagonize the effects of levodopa and dopamine agonists).

No products indexed under this heading.

Doxazosin Mesylate (Because of the potential for olanzapine to induce hypotension, Symbyax may enhance the effects of certain antihypertensive agents).

No products indexed under this heading.

Doxepin Hydrochloride (In two fluoxetine studies, previously stable plasma levels of imipramine and desipramine have increased >2- to 10-fold when fluoxetine has been administered in combination. This influence may persist for three weeks or longer after fluoxetine is discontinued. Thus, the dose of TCA may need to be reduced and plasma TCA concentrations may need to be monitored temporarily when Symbyax is co-administered or has been recently discontinued).

No products indexed under this heading.

Enalapril Maleate (Because of the potential for olanzapine to induce hypotension, Symbyax may enhance the effects of certain antihypertensive agents). Products include:

Vaseretic Tablets 2073
Vasotec I.V. Injection 2076

Enalaprilat (Because of the potential for olanzapine to induce hypotension, Symbyax may enhance the effects of certain antihypertensive agents).

No products indexed under this heading.

Encainide Hydrochloride (Fluoxetine, like other agents that are metabolized by CYP2D6, inhibits the activity of this isoenzyme. Therapy with medications that are predominately metabolized by the CYP2D6 system and have a relatively narrow therapeutic index should be initiated at the low end of the dose range if the patient is receiving fluoxetine concurrently or has taken it in the previous five weeks. If fluoxetine is added to the treatment regimen of a patient already receiving a drug metabolized by CYP2D6, the need for a decreased dose of the original medication should be considered).

No products indexed under this heading.

Eprosartan Mesylate (Because of the potential for olanzapine to induce hypotension, Symbyax may enhance the effects of certain antihypertensive agents). Products include:

Teveten Tablets 1707
Teveten HCT Tablets 1710

Erythromycin (Agents that induce CYP1A2 or glucuronyl transferase enzymes may cause an increase in olanzapine concentration). Products include:

Erygel Topical Gel 2096
Ery-Tab Tablets 447
Erythromycin Base Filmtab Tablets 454
Erythromycin Delayed-Release Capsules, USP 456
PCE Dispertab Tablets 510

Erythromycin Estolate (Agents that induce CYP1A2 or glucuronyl transferase enzymes may cause an increase in olanzapine concentration).

No products indexed under this heading.

Erythromycin Ethylsuccinate (Agents that induce CYP1A2 or glucuronyl transferase enzymes may cause an increase in olanzapine concentration). Products include:

E.E.S. 449
EryPed 445

Erythromycin Gluceptate (Agents that induce CYP1A2 or glucuronyl transferase enzymes may cause an increase in olanzapine concentration).

No products indexed under this heading.

Erythromycin Lactobionate (Agents that induce CYP1A2 or glucuronyl transferase enzymes may cause an increase in olanzapine concentration).

No products indexed under this heading.

Erythromycin Stearate (Agents that induce CYP1A2 or glucuronyl transferase enzymes may cause an increase in olanzapine concentration). Products include:

Erythrocin Stearate Filmtab Tablets 452

Esmolol Hydrochloride (Because of the potential for olanzapine to induce hypotension, Symbyax may enhance the effects of certain antihypertensive agents). Products include:

Brevibloc Concentrate 766
Brevibloc Injection 766
Brevibloc Double Strength Injection 766
Brevibloc Premixed Injection 766
Brevibloc Double Strength Premixed Injection 766

Etodolac (Serotonin release by platelets plays an important role in hemostasis. Studies have demonstrated an association between the use of psychotropic drugs that interfere with serotonin reuptake and the occurrence of upper gastrointestinal bleeding. These studies have also shown that concurrent use of an NSAID potentiated the risk of bleeding. Therefore, patients should be cautioned about the use of NSAIDs concurrently with Symbyax).

No products indexed under this heading.

Felodipine (Because of the potential for olanzapine to induce hypotension, Symbyax may enhance the effects of certain antihypertensive agents). Products include:

Plendil Extended-Release Tablets 651

Fenoprofen Calcium (Serotonin release by platelets plays an important role in hemostasis. Studies have demonstrated an association between the use of psychotropic drugs that interfere with serotonin reuptake and the occurrence of upper gastrointestinal bleeding. These studies have also shown that concurrent use of an NSAID potentiated the risk of bleeding. Therefore, patients should be cautioned about the use of NSAIDs concurrently with Symbyax). Products include:

Nalfon Capsules 2504

Fentanyl (Fluoxetine, like other agents that are metabolized by CYP2D6, inhibits the activity of this isoenzyme. Therapy with medications that are predominately metabolized by the CYP2D6 system and have a relatively narrow therapeutic index should be initiated at the low end of the dose range if the patient is receiving fluoxetine concurrently or has taken it in the previous five weeks. If fluoxetine is added to the treatment regimen of a patient already receiving a drug metabolized by CYP2D6, the need for a decreased dose of the original medication should be considered). Products include:

Duragesic Transdermal System 2448

Fentanyl Citrate (Fluoxetine, like other agents that are metabolized by CYP2D6, inhibits the activity of this isoenzyme. Therapy with medications that are predominately metabolized by the CYP2D6 system and have a relatively narrow therapeutic index should be initiated at the low end of the dose range if the patient is receiving fluoxetine concurrently or has taken it in the previous five weeks. If fluoxetine is added to the treatment regimen of a patient already receiving a drug metabolized by CYP2D6, the need for a decreased dose of the original medication should be considered). Products include:

Actiq 993

Flecainide Acetate (Fluoxetine, like other agents that are metabolized by CYP2D6, inhibits the activity of this isoenzyme. Therapy with medications that are predominately metabolized by the CYP2D6 system and have a relatively narrow therapeutic index should be initiated at the low end of the dose range if the patient is receiving fluoxetine concurrently or has taken it in the previous five weeks. If fluoxetine is added to the treatment regimen of a patient already receiving a drug metabolized by CYP2D6, the need for a decreased dose of the original medication should be considered). Products include:

Tambocor Tablets 1824

Fluoxetine (Fluoxetine, like other agents that are metabolized by CYP2D6, inhibits the activity of this isoenzyme. Therapy with medications that are predominately metabolized by the CYP2D6 system and have a relatively narrow therapeutic index should be initiated at the low end of the dose range if the patient is receiving fluoxetine concurrently or has taken it in the previous five weeks. If fluoxetine is added to the treatment regimen of a patient already receiving a drug metabolized by CYP2D6, the need for a decreased dose of the original medication should be considered).

No products indexed under this heading.

Fluphenazine Decanoate (Fluoxetine, like other agents that are metabolized by CYP2D6, inhibits the activity of this isoenzyme. Therapy with medications that are predominately metabolized by the CYP2D6 system and have a relatively narrow therapeutic index should be initiated at the low end of the dose range if the patient is receiving fluoxetine concurrently or has taken it in the previous five weeks. If fluoxetine is added to the treatment regimen of a patient already receiving a drug metabolized by CYP2D6, the need for a decreased dose of the original medication should be considered).

No products indexed under this heading.

Fluphenazine Enanthate (Fluoxetine, like other agents that are metabolized by CYP2D6, inhibits the activity of this isoenzyme. Therapy with medications that are predominately metabolized by the CYP2D6 system and have a relatively narrow therapeutic index should be initiated at

the low end of the dose range if the patient is receiving fluoxetine concurrently or has taken it in the previous five weeks. If fluoxetine is added to the treatment regimen of a patient already receiving a drug metabolized by CYP2D6, the need for a decreased dose of the original medication should be considered).

No products indexed under this heading.

Fluphenazine Hydrochloride (Fluoxetine, like other agents that are metabolized by CYP2D6, inhibits the activity of this isoenzyme. Therapy with medications that are predominately metabolized by the CYP2D6 system and have a relatively narrow therapeutic index should be initiated at the low end of the dose range if the patient is receiving fluoxetine concurrently or has taken it in the previous five weeks. If fluoxetine is added to the treatment regimen of a patient already receiving a drug metabolized by CYP2D6, the need for a decreased dose of the original medication should be considered).

No products indexed under this heading.

Flurazepam Hydrochloride (Because fluoxetine is tightly bound to plasma protein, the administration of fluoxetine to a patient taking another drug that is tightly bound to protein may cause a shift in plasma concentrations potentially resulting in an adverse effect. Conversely, adverse effects may result from displacement of protein-bound fluoxetine by other tightly bound drugs). Products include:

Dalmane Capsules 3343

Flurbiprofen (Serotonin release by platelets plays an important role in hemostasis. Studies have demonstrated an association between the use of psychotropic drugs that interfere with serotonin reuptake and the occurrence of upper gastrointestinal bleeding. These studies have also shown that concurrent use of an NSAID potentiated the risk of bleeding. Therefore, patients should be cautioned about the use of NSAIDs concurrently with Symbyax).

No products indexed under this heading.

Fluvoxamine (Fluvoxamine, a CYP1A2 inhibitor, decreases the clearance of olanzapine. This results in a mean increase in olanzapine Cmax and AUC following fluvoxamine administration. Lower doses of the olanzapine component of Symbyax should be considered in patients receiving concomitant treatment with fluvoxamine).

No products indexed under this heading.

Fluvoxamine Maleate (Fluvoxamine, a CYP1A2 inhibitor, decreases the clearance of olanzapine. This results in a mean increase in olanzapine Cmax and AUC following fluvoxamine administration. Lower doses of the olanzapine component of Symbyax should be considered in patients receiving concomitant treatment with fluvoxamine).

No products indexed under this heading.

Formoterol Fumarate (Fluoxetine, like other agents that are metabolized by CYP2D6, inhibits the activity of this isoenzyme. Therapy with medications that are predominately metabolized by the CYP2D6 system and have a relatively narrow therapeutic index should be initiated at the low end of the dose range if the patient is receiving fluoxetine concurrently or has taken it in the previous five weeks. If fluoxetine is added to the treatment regimen of a patient already receiving a drug metabolized by CYP2D6, the need for a decreased dose of the original medication should be considered). Products include:

Foradil Aerolizer 3024

Fosinopril Sodium (Because of the potential for olanzapine to induce hypotension, Symbyax may enhance the effects of certain antihypertensive agents).

No products indexed under this heading.

Fosphenytoin Sodium (Patients on stable doses of phenytoin have developed elevated plasma levels of phenytoin with clinical pheytoin toxicity following initiation of concomitant fluoxetine).

No products indexed under this heading.

Furosemide (Because of the potential for olanzapine to induce hypotension, Symbyax may enhance the effects of certain antihypertensive agents). Products include:

Furosemide Tablets 2117

Galantamine Hydrobromide (Fluoxetine, like other agents that are metabolized by CYP2D6, inhibits the activity of this isoenzyme. Therapy with medications that are predominately metabolized by the CYP2D6 system and have a relatively narrow therapeutic index should be initiated at the low end of the dose range if the patient is receiving fluoxetine concurrently or has taken it in the previous five weeks. If fluoxetine is added to the treatment regimen of a patient already receiving a drug metabolized by CYP2D6, the need for a decreased dose of the original medication should be considered). Products include:

Razadyne ER Extended-Release Capsules 2434
Razadyne 2434

Glipizide (Because fluoxetine is tightly bound to plasma protein, the administration of fluoxetine to a patient taking another drug that is tightly bound to protein may cause a shift in plasma concentrations potentially resulting in an adverse effect. Conversely, adverse effects may result from displacement of protein-bound fluoxetine by other tightly bound drugs).

No products indexed under this heading.

Guanabenz Acetate (Because of the potential for olanzapine to induce hypotension, Symbyax may enhance the effects of certain antihypertensive agents).

No products indexed under this heading.

Guanethidine Monosulfate (Because of the potential for olanzapine to induce hypotension, Symbyax may enhance the effects of certain antihypertensive agents).

No products indexed under this heading.

Haloperidol (Elevation of blood levels of haloperidol has been observed in patients receiving concomitant fluoxetine).

No products indexed under this heading.

Haloperidol Decanoate (Elevation of blood levels of haloperidol has been observed in patients receiving concomitant fluoxetine).

No products indexed under this heading.

Haloperidol Lactate (Elevation of blood levels of haloperidol have been observed in patients receiving concomitant fluoxetine).

No products indexed under this heading.

Hydralazine Hydrochloride (Because of the potential for olanzapine to induce hypotension, Symbyax may enhance the effects of certain antihypertensive agents). Products include:

BiDil Tablets 2161

Hydrochlorothiazide (Because of the potential for olanzapine to induce hypotension, Symbyax may enhance the effects of certain antihypertensive agents). Products include:

Aldoril Tablets 1884
Atacand HCT 637
Avalide Tablets 2889
Avalide Tablets 922
Benicar HCT Tablets 2852
Diovan HCT Tablets 2195
Dyazide Capsules 1389
Hyzaar 1964
Lotensin HCT Tablets 2235
Maxzide 2150
Micardis HCT Tablets 886
Moduretic Tablets 2003
Prinzide Tablets 2033
Teveten HCT Tablets 1710
Timolide Tablets 2056
Uniretic Tablets 3114
Vaseretic Tablets 2073
Zestoretic Tablets 701

Hydrocodone Bitartrate (Fluoxetine, like other agents that are metabolized by CYP2D6, inhibits the activity of this isoenzyme. Therapy with medications that are predominately metabolized by the CYP2D6 system and have a relatively narrow therapeutic index should be initiated at the low end of the dose range if the patient is receiving fluoxetine concurrently or has taken it in the previous five weeks. If fluoxetine is added to the treatment regimen of a patient already receiving a drug metabolized by CYP2D6, the need for a decreased dose of the original medication should be considered). Products include:

Hycodan 1104
Hycomine Compound Tablets 1105
Hycotuss Expectorant Syrup 1106
Lortab 3315
Lortab Elixir 3312
Vicodin Tablets 530
Vicodin ES Tablets 531
Vicodin HP Tablets 532
Vicoprofen Tablets 533
Zydone Tablets 1118

Hydroflumethiazide (Because of the potential for olanzapine to induce hypotension, Symbyax may enhance the effects of certain antihypertensive agents).

No products indexed under this heading.

Hypericum (Agents that induce CYP1A2 or glucuronyl transferase enzymes may cause an increase in olanzapine concentration).

No products indexed under this heading.

Ibuprofen (Serotonin release by platelets plays an important role in hemostasis. Studies have demonstrated an association between the use of psychotropic drugs that interfere with serotonin reuptake and the occurrence of upper gastrointestinal bleeding. These studies have also shown that concurrent use of an NSAID potentiated the risk of bleeding. Therefore, patients should be cautioned about the use of NSAIDs concurrently with Symbyax). Products include:

Advil Allergy Sinus Caplets 737
Advil 737
Children's Advil Suspension 742
Children's Advil Chewable Tablets 741
Advil Cold & Sinus 739
Advil Flu & Body Ache Caplets 739
Children's Advil Cold Suspension 741
Infants' Advil Concentrated Drops 743
Junior Strength Advil Swallow Tablets 740
Advil Migraine Liquigels 740
Advil Multi-Symptom Cold Caplets 738
Combunox Tablets 1183
Children's Motrin Oral Suspension and Chewable Tablets 1837
Children's Motrin Cold Non-Staining Dye-Free Oral Suspension 1838
Children's Motrin Cold Oral Suspension 1838
Children's Motrin Non-Staining Dye-Free Oral Suspension 1837
Motrin Cold & Sinus Caplets 1836
Motrin IB Tablets and Caplets 1836
Infants' Motrin Concentrated Drops 1837
Infants' Motrin Non-Staining Dye-Free Drops 1837
Junior Strength Motrin Caplets and Chewable Tablets 1837
Vicoprofen Tablets 533

Imipramine Hydrochloride (In two fluoxetine studies, previously stable plasma levels of imipramine and desipramine have increased >2- to 10-fold when fluoxetine has been administered in combination. This influence may persist for three weeks or longer after fluoxetine is discontinued. Thus, the dose of TCA may need to be reduced and plasma TCA concentrations may need to be monitored temporarily when Symbyax is co-administered or has been recently discontinued).

No products indexed under this heading.

Imipramine Pamoate (In two fluoxetine studies, previously stable plasma levels of imipramine and desipramine have increased >2- to 10-fold when fluoxetine has been administered in combination. This influence may persist for three weeks or longer after fluoxetine is discontinued. Thus, the dose of TCA may need to be reduced and plasma TCA concentrations may need to be monitored temporarily when Symbyax is co-administered or has been recently discontinued).

No products indexed under this heading.

Indapamide (Because of the potential for olanzapine to induce hypotension, Symbyax may enhance the effects of certain antihypertensive agents). Products include:

Indapamide Tablets 2119

Indomethacin (Serotonin release by platelets plays an important role in hemostasis. Studies have demonstrated an association between the use of psychotropic drugs that interfere with serotonin reuptake and the occurrence of upper gastrointestinal bleeding. These studies have also shown that concurrent use of an NSAID potentiated the risk of bleeding. Therefore, patients should be

cautioned about the use of NSAIDs concurrently with Symbyax). Products include:

Indocin 1968

Indomethacin Sodium Trihydrate (Serotonin release by platelets plays an important role in hemostasis. Studies have demonstrated an association between the use of psychotropic drugs that interfere with serotonin reuptake and the occurrence of upper gastrointestinal bleeding. These studies have also shown that concurrent use of an NSAID potentiated the risk of bleeding. Therefore, patients should be cautioned about the use of NSAIDs concurrently with Symbyax). Products include:

Indocin I.V. 1973

Indoramin Hydrochloride (Fluoxetine, like other agents that are metabolized by CYP2D6, inhibits the activity of this isoenzyme. Therapy with medications that are predominately metabolized by the CYP2D6 system and have a relatively narrow therapeutic index should be initiated at the low end of the dose range if the patient is receiving fluoxetine concurrently or has taken it in the previous five weeks. If fluoxetine is added to the treatment regimen of a patient already receiving a drug metabolized by CYP2D6, the need for a decreased dose of the original medication should be considered).

No products indexed under this heading.

Insulin (Agents that induce CYP1A2 or glucuronyl transferase enzymes may cause an increase in olanzapine concentration).

No products indexed under this heading.

Irbesartan (Because of the potential for olanzapine to induce hypotension, Symbyax may enhance the effects of certain antihypertensive agents). Products include:

Avalide Tablets 922
Avalide Tablets 2889
Avapro Tablets 925
Avapro Tablets 2886

Isocarboxazid (There have been reports of serious, sometimes fatal, reactions in patients receiving, or who have recently discontinued, fluoxetine and are then started on an MAO inhibitor. Therefore, Symbyax should not be used in combination with, or within a minimum of 14 days of discontinuing, an MAO inhibitor).

No products indexed under this heading.

Isradipine (Because of the potential for olanzapine to induce hypotension, Symbyax may enhance the effects of certain antihypertensive agents). Products include:

DynaCirc CR Tablets 2726

Ketoprofen (Serotonin release by platelets plays an important role in hemostasis. Studies have demonstrated an association between the use of psychotropic drugs that interfere with serotonin reuptake and the occurrence of upper gastrointestinal bleeding. These studies have also shown that concurrent use of an NSAID potentiated the risk of bleeding. Therefore, patients should be cautioned about the use of NSAIDs concurrently with Symbyax).

No products indexed under this heading.

Ketorolac Tromethamine (Serotonin release by platelets plays an important role in hemostasis. Studies have demonstrated an association between the use of psychotropic drugs that interfere with serotonin reuptake and the occurrence of upper gastrointestinal bleeding. These studies have also shown that concurrent use of an NSAID potentiated the risk of bleeding. Therefore, patients should be cautioned about the use of NSAIDs concurrently with Symbyax). Products include:

Acular Ophthalmic Solution 561
Acular LS Ophthalmic Solution 562

Labetalol Hydrochloride (Because of the potential for olanzapine to induce hypotension, Symbyax may enhance the effects of certain antihypertensive agents).

No products indexed under this heading.

Lansoprazole (Agents that induce CYP1A2 or glucuronyl transferase enzymes may cause an increase in olanzapine concentration). Products include:

Prevacid Delayed-Release Capsules 3268
Prevacid for Delayed-Release Oral Suspension 3268
Prevacid I.V. for Injection 3274
Prevacid NapraPAC 3277
Prevacid SoluTab Delayed-Release Orally Disintegrating Tablets 3268
PREVPAC 3281

Levodopa (The olanzapine component of Symbyax may antagonize the effects of levodopa and dopamine agonists). Products include:

Parcopa Orally Disintegrating Tablets 3111
Stalevo Tablets 2270

Lidocaine (Fluoxetine, like other agents that are metabolized by CYP2D6, inhibits the activity of this isoenzyme. Therapy with medications that are predominately metabolized by the CYP2D6 system and have a relatively narrow therapeutic index should be initiated at the low end of the dose range if the patient is receiving fluoxetine concurrently or has taken it in the previous five weeks. If fluoxetine is added to the treatment regimen of a patient already receiving a drug metabolized by CYP2D6, the need for a decreased dose of the original medication should be considered). Products include:

Lidoderm Patch 1107

Lidocaine Hydrochloride (Fluoxetine, like other agents that are metabolized by CYP2D6, inhibits the activity of this isoenzyme. Therapy with medications that are predominately metabolized by the CYP2D6 system and have a relatively narrow therapeutic index should be initiated at the low end of the dose range if the patient is receiving fluoxetine concurrently or has taken it in the previous five weeks. If fluoxetine is added to the treatment regimen of a patient already receiving a drug metabolized by CYP2D6, the need for a decreased dose of the original medication should be considered).

No products indexed under this heading.

Lisinopril (Because of the potential for olanzapine to induce hypotension, Symbyax may enhance the effects of certain antihypertensive agents). Products include:

Prinivil Tablets 2029
Prinzide Tablets 2033
Zestoretic Tablets 701
Zestril Tablets 704

Lithium (There have been reports of both increased and decreased lithium levels when lithium was used concomitantly with fluoxetine. Cases of lithium toxicity and increased serotonergic effects have been reported. Lithium levels should be monitored in patients taking Symbyax concomitantly with lithium).

No products indexed under this heading.

Lithium Carbonate (There have been reports of both increased and decreased lithium levels when lithium was used concomitantly with fluoxetine. Cases of lithium toxicity and increased serotonergic effects have been reported. Lithium levels should be monitored in patients taking Symbyax concomitantly with lithium). Products include:

Eskalith 1406
Lithobid Tablets 1670

Lithium Citrate (There have been reports of both increased and decreased lithium levels when lithium was used concomitantly with fluoxetine. Cases of lithium toxicity and increased serotonergic effects have been reported. Lithium levels should be monitored in patients taking Symbyax concomitantly with lithium).

No products indexed under this heading.

Losartan Potassium (Because of the potential for olanzapine to induce hypotension, Symbyax may enhance the effects of certain antihypertensive agents). Products include:

Cozaar Tablets 1913
Hyzaar 1964

Maprotiline Hydrochloride (In two fluoxetine studies, previously stable plasma levels of imipramine and desipramine have increased >2- to 10-fold when fluoxetine has been administered in combination. This influence may persist for three weeks or longer after fluoxetine is discontinued. Thus, the dose of TCA may need to be reduced and plasma TCA concentrations may need to be monitored temporarily when Symbyax is co-administered or has been recently discontinued).

No products indexed under this heading.

Mecamylamine Hydrochloride (Because of the potential for olanzapine to induce hypotension, Symbyax may enhance the effects of certain antihypertensive agents). Products include:

Inversine Tablets 3286

Meclofenamate Sodium (Serotonin release by platelets plays an important role in hemostasis. Studies have demonstrated an association between the use of psychotropic drugs that interfere with serotonin reuptake and the occurrence of upper gastrointestinal bleeding. These studies have also shown that concurrent use of an NSAID potentiated the risk of bleeding. Therefore, patients should be cautioned about the use of NSAIDs concurrently with Symbyax).

No products indexed under this heading.

Mefenamic Acid (Serotonin release by platelets plays an important role in hemostasis. Studies have demonstrated an association between the use of psychotropic drugs that interfere with serotonin reuptake and the occurrence of upper gastrointestinal bleeding. These studies have also shown that concurrent use of an NSAID potentiated the risk of bleeding. Therefore, patients should be cautioned about the use of NSAIDs concurrently with Symbyax).

No products indexed under this heading.

Meloxicam (Serotonin release by platelets plays an important role in hemostasis. Studies have demonstrated an association between the use of psychotropic drugs that interfere with serotonin reuptake and the occurrence of upper gastrointestinal bleeding. These studies have also shown that concurrent use of an NSAID potentiated the risk of bleeding. Therefore, patients should be cautioned about the use of NSAIDs concurrently with Symbyax). Products include:

Mobic Oral Suspension 893
Mobic Tablets 893

Meperidine Hydrochloride (Fluoxetine, like other agents that are metabolized by CYP2D6, inhibits the activity of this isoenzyme. Therapy with medications that are predominately metabolized by the CYP2D6 system and have a relatively narrow therapeutic index should be initiated at the low end of the dose range if the patient is receiving fluoxetine concurrently or has taken it in the previous five weeks. If fluoxetine is added to the treatment regimen of a patient already receiving a drug metabolized by CYP2D6, the need for a decreased dose of the original medication should be considered).

No products indexed under this heading.

Methadone Hydrochloride (Fluoxetine, like other agents that are metabolized by CYP2D6, inhibits the activity of this isoenzyme. Therapy with medications that are predominately metabolized by the CYP2D6 system and have a relatively narrow therapeutic index should be initiated at the low end of the dose range if the patient is receiving fluoxetine concurrently or has taken it in the previous five weeks. If fluoxetine is added to the treatment regimen of a patient already receiving a drug metabolized by CYP2D6, the need for a decreased dose of the original medication should be considered).

No products indexed under this heading.

Methamphetamine Hydrochloride (Fluoxetine, like other agents that are metabolized by CYP2D6, inhibits the activity of this isoenzyme. Therapy with medications that are predominately metabolized by the CYP2D6 system and have a relatively narrow therapeutic index should be initiated at the low end of the dose range if the patient is receiving fluoxetine concurrently or has taken it in the previous five weeks. If fluoxetine is added to the treatment regimen of a patient already receiving a drug metabolized by CYP2D6, the need for a decreased dose of the original medication should be considered). Products include:

Desoxyn Tablets, USP 2482

Methyclothiazide (Because of the potential for olanzapine to induce hypotension, Symbyax may enhance the effects of certain antihypertensive agents).
No products indexed under this heading.

Methyldopa (Because of the potential for olanzapine to induce hypotension, Symbyax may enhance the effects of certain antihypertensive agents). Products include:
Aldoclor Tablets 1881
Aldoril Tablets 1884

Methyldopate Hydrochloride (Because of the potential for olanzapine to induce hypotension, Symbyax may enhance the effects of certain antihypertensive agents).
No products indexed under this heading.

Metolazone (Because of the potential for olanzapine to induce hypotension, Symbyax may enhance the effects of certain antihypertensive agents).
No products indexed under this heading.

Metoprolol Succinate (Because of the potential for olanzapine to induce hypotension, Symbyax may enhance the effects of certain antihypertensive agents). Products include:
Toprol-XL Tablets 660

Metoprolol Tartrate (Because of the potential for olanzapine to induce hypotension, Symbyax may enhance the effects of certain antihypertensive agents).
No products indexed under this heading.

Metyrosine (Because of the potential for olanzapine to induce hypotension, Symbyax may enhance the effects of certain antihypertensive agents). Products include:
Demser Capsules 1933

Mexiletine Hydrochloride (Fluoxetine, like other agents that are metabolized by CYP2D6, inhibits the activity of this isoenzyme. Therapy with medications that are predominately metabolized by the CYP2D6 system and have a relatively narrow therapeutic index should be initiated at the low end of the dose range if the patient is receiving fluoxetine concurrently or has taken it in the previous five weeks. If fluoxetine is added to the treatment regimen of a patient already receiving a drug metabolized by CYP2D6, the need for a decreased dose of the original medication should be considered).
No products indexed under this heading.

Mibefradil Dihydrochloride (Because of the potential for olanzapine to induce hypotension, Symbyax may enhance the effects of certain antihypertensive agents).
No products indexed under this heading.

Midazolam Hydrochloride (Because fluoxetine is tightly bound to plasma protein, the administration of fluoxetine to a patient taking another drug that is tightly bound to protein may cause a shift in plasma concentrations potentially resulting in an adverse effect. Conversely, adverse effects may result from displacement of protein-bound fluoxetine by other tightly bound drugs).
No products indexed under this heading.

Minoxidil (Because of the potential for olanzapine to induce hypotension, Symbyax may enhance the effects of certain antihypertensive agents). Products include:
Men's Rogaine Extra Strength Topical Solution, Ocean Rush Scent and Original Unscented 706
Women's Rogaine Topical Solution, Spring Bloom Scent and Original Unscented 707

Mirtazapine (Fluoxetine, like other agents that are metabolized by CYP2D6, inhibits the activity of this isoenzyme. Therapy with medications that are predominately metabolized by the CYP2D6 system and have a relatively narrow therapeutic index should be initiated at the low end of the dose range if the patient is receiving fluoxetine concurrently or has taken it in the previous five weeks. If fluoxetine is added to the treatment regimen of a patient already receiving a drug metabolized by CYP2D6, the need for a decreased dose of the original medication should be considered).
No products indexed under this heading.

Moclobemide (There have been reports of serious, sometimes fatal, reactions in patients receiving, or who have recently discontinued, fluoxetine and are then started on an MAO inhibitor. Therefore, Symbyax should not be used in combination with, or within a minimum of 14 days of discontinuing, an MAO inhibitor).
No products indexed under this heading.

Moexipril Hydrochloride (Because of the potential for olanzapine to induce hypotension, Symbyax may enhance the effects of certain antihypertensive agents). Products include:
Uniretic Tablets 3114
Univasc Tablets 3118

Morphine Sulfate (Fluoxetine, like other agents that are metabolized by CYP2D6, inhibits the activity of this isoenzyme. Therapy with medications that are predominately metabolized by the CYP2D6 system and have a relatively narrow therapeutic index should be initiated at the low end of the dose range if the patient is receiving fluoxetine concurrently or has taken it in the previous five weeks. If fluoxetine is added to the treatment regimen of a patient already receiving a drug metabolized by CYP2D6, the need for a decreased dose of the original medication should be considered). Products include:
Avinza Capsules 1714
Kadian Capsules 572
MS Contin Tablets 2703

Nabumetone (Serotonin release by platelets plays an important role in hemostasis. Studies have demonstrated an association between the use of psychotropic drugs that interfere with serotonin reuptake and the occurrence of upper gastrointestinal bleeding. These studies have also shown that concurrent use of an NSAID potentiated the risk of bleeding. Therefore, patients should be cautioned about the use of NSAIDs concurrently with Symbyax). Products include:
Relafen Tablets 1523

Nadolol (Because of the potential for olanzapine to induce hypotension, Symbyax may enhance the effects of certain antihypertensive agents). Products include:
Nadolol Tablets 2121

Nafcillin Sodium (Agents that induce CYP1A2 or glucuronyl transferase enzymes may cause an increase in olanzapine concentration).
No products indexed under this heading.

Naproxen (Serotonin release by platelets plays an important role in hemostasis. Studies have demonstrated an association between the use of psychotropic drugs that interfere with serotonin reuptake and the occurrence of upper gastrointestinal bleeding. These studies have also shown that concurrent use of an NSAID potentiated the risk of bleeding. Therefore, patients should be cautioned about the use of NSAIDs concurrently with Symbyax). Products include:
EC-Naprosyn Delayed-Release Tablets 2769
Naprosyn Suspension 2769
Naprosyn Tablets 2769
Prevacid NapraPAC 3277

Naproxen Sodium (Serotonin release by platelets plays an important role in hemostasis. Studies have demonstrated an association between the use of psychotropic drugs that interfere with serotonin reuptake and the occurrence of upper gastrointestinal bleeding. These studies have also shown that concurrent use of an NSAID potentiated the risk of bleeding. Therefore, patients should be cautioned about the use of NSAIDs concurrently with Symbyax). Products include:
Aleve Tablets, Caplets and Gelcaps 605
Anaprox Tablets 2769
Anaprox DS Tablets 2769

Nelfinavir Mesylate (Fluoxetine, like other agents that are metabolized by CYP2D6, inhibits the activity of this isoenzyme. Therapy with medications that are predominately metabolized by the CYP2D6 system and have a relatively narrow therapeutic index should be initiated at the low end of the dose range if the patient is receiving fluoxetine concurrently or has taken it in the previous five weeks. If fluoxetine is added to the treatment regimen of a patient already receiving a drug metabolized by CYP2D6, the need for a decreased dose of the original medication should be considered). Products include:
Viracept 2556

Nicardipine Hydrochloride (Because of the potential for olanzapine to induce hypotension, Symbyax may enhance the effects of certain antihypertensive agents). Products include:
Cardene I.V. 1129

Nicotine (Agents that induce CYP1A2 or glucuronyl transferase enzymes may cause an increase in olanzapine concentration). Products include:
Nicoderm CQ Patch 1629
NicoDerm CQ Clear Patch 627
Nicotrol Inhaler 2594
Nicotrol NS 2596

Nicotine Polacrilex (Agents that induce CYP1A2 or glucuronyl transferase enzymes may cause an increase in olanzapine concentration). Products include:
Commit Lozenges 1625
Nicorette Gum 1632

Nicotine Salicylate (Agents that induce CYP1A2 or glucuronyl transferase enzymes may cause an increase in olanzapine concentration).
No products indexed under this heading.

Nicotine Sulfate (Agents that induce CYP1A2 or glucuronyl transferase enzymes may cause an increase in olanzapine concentration).
No products indexed under this heading.

Nifedipine (Because of the potential for olanzapine to induce hypotension, Symbyax may enhance the effects of certain antihypertensive agents). Products include:
Adalat CC Tablets 2978

Nisoldipine (Because of the potential for olanzapine to induce hypotension, Symbyax may enhance the effects of certain antihypertensive agents). Products include:
Sular Tablets 1163

Nitroglycerin (Because of the potential for olanzapine to induce hypotension, Symbyax may enhance the effects of certain antihypertensive agents). Products include:
Nitro-Dur Transdermal Infusion System 3060
Nitrolingual Pumpspray 1161

Nortriptyline Hydrochloride (In two fluoxetine studies, previously stable plasma levels of imipramine and desipramine have increased >2- to 10-fold when fluoxetine has been administered in combination. This influence may persist for three weeks or longer after fluoxetine is discontinued. Thus, the dose of TCA may need to be reduced and plasma TCA concentrations may need to be monitored temporarily when Symbyax is co-administered or has been recently discontinued).
No products indexed under this heading.

Omeprazole (Fluoxetine, like other agents that are metabolized by CYP2D6, inhibits the activity of this isoenzyme. Therapy with medications that are predominately metabolized by the CYP2D6 system and have a relatively narrow therapeutic index should be initiated at the low end of the dose range if the patient is receiving fluoxetine concurrently or has taken it in the previous five weeks. If fluoxetine is added to the treatment regimen of a patient already receiving a drug metabolized by CYP2D6, the need for a decreased dose of the original medication should be considered). Products include:
Zegerid Powder for Oral Solution 2972

Ondansetron (Fluoxetine, like other agents that are metabolized by CYP2D6, inhibits the activity of this isoenzyme. Therapy with medications that are predominately metabolized by the CYP2D6 system and have a relatively narrow therapeutic index should be initiated at the low end of the dose range if the patient is receiving fluoxetine concurrently or has taken it in the previous five weeks. If fluoxetine is added to the treatment regimen of a patient already receiving a drug metabolized by CYP2D6, the need for a

decreased dose of the original medication should be considered). Products include:
Zofran ODT Orally Disintegrating Tablets 1613

Ondansetron Hydrochloride (Fluoxetine, like other agents that are metabolized by CYP2D6, inhibits the activity of this isoenzyme. Therapy with medications that are predominately metabolized by the CYP2D6 system and have a relatively narrow therapeutic index should be initiated at the low end of the dose range if the patient is receiving fluoxetine concurrently or has taken it in the previous five weeks. If fluoxetine is added to the treatment regimen of a patient already receiving a drug metabolized by CYP2D6, the need for a decreased dose of the original medication should be considered). Products include:
Zofran Injection 1607
Zofran 1613

Oxaprozin (Serotonin release by platelets plays an important role in hemostasis. Studies have demonstrated an association between the use of psychotropic drugs that interfere with serotonin reuptake and the occurrence of upper gastrointestinal bleeding. These studies have also shown that concurrent use of an NSAID potentiated the risk of bleeding. Therefore, patients should be cautioned about the use of NSAIDs concurrently with Symbyax).
No products indexed under this heading.

Oxazepam (Because fluoxetine is tightly bound to plasma protein, the administration of fluoxetine to a patient taking another drug that is tightly bound to protein may cause a shift in plasma concentrations potentially resulting in an adverse effect. Conversely, adverse effects may result from displacement of protein-bound fluoxetine by other tightly bound drugs).
No products indexed under this heading.

Oxycodone Hydrochloride (Fluoxetine, like other agents that are metabolized by CYP2D6, inhibits the activity of this isoenzyme. Therapy with medications that are predominately metabolized by the CYP2D6 system and have a relatively narrow therapeutic index should be initiated at the low end of the dose range if the patient is receiving fluoxetine concurrently or has taken it in the previous five weeks. If fluoxetine is added to the treatment regimen of a patient already receiving a drug metabolized by CYP2D6, the need for a decreased dose of the original medication should be considered). Products include:
Combunox Tablets 1183
OxyContin Tablets 2699
OxyFast Oral Concentrate Solution 2704
OxyIR Capsules 2704
Percocet Tablets 1114
Percodan Tablets 1115

Paclitaxel (Fluoxetine, like other agents that are metabolized by CYP2D6, inhibits the activity of this isoenzyme. Therapy with medications that are predominately metabolized by the CYP2D6 system and have a relatively narrow therapeutic index should be initiated at the low end of the dose range if the patient is receiving fluoxetine concurrently or has taken it in the previous five weeks. If fluoxetine is added to the treatment regimen of a patient already receiving a drug metabolized by CYP2D6, the need for a decreased dose of the original medication should be considered).
No products indexed under this heading.

Pargyline Hydrochloride (There have been reports of serious, sometimes fatal, reactions in patients receiving, or who have recently discontinued, fluoxetine and are then started on an MAO inhibitor. Therefore, Symbyax should not be used in combination with, or within a minimum of 14 days of discontinuing, an MAO inhibitor).
No products indexed under this heading.

Paroxetine Hydrochloride (Fluoxetine, like other agents that are metabolized by CYP2D6, inhibits the activity of this isoenzyme. Therapy with medications that are predominately metabolized by the CYP2D6 system and have a relatively narrow therapeutic index should be initiated at the low end of the dose range if the patient is receiving fluoxetine concurrently or has taken it in the previous five weeks. If fluoxetine is added to the treatment regimen of a patient already receiving a drug metabolized by CYP2D6, the need for a decreased dose of the original medication should be considered). Products include:
Paxil CR Controlled-Release Tablets 1509
Paxil 1501

Penbutolol Sulfate (Because of the potential for olanzapine to induce hypotension, Symbyax may enhance the effects of certain antihypertensive agents).
No products indexed under this heading.

Pergolide Mesylate (The olanzapine component of Symbyax may antagonize the effects of levodopa and dopamine agonists). Products include:
Permax Tablets 3357

Perindopril Erbumine (Because of the potential for olanzapine to induce hypotension, Symbyax may enhance the effects of certain antihypertensive agents). Products include:
Aceon Tablets (2 mg, 4 mg, 8 mg) 3191

Phenelzine Sulfate (There have been reports of serious, sometimes fatal, reactions in patients receiving, or who have recently discontinued, fluoxetine and are then started on an MAO inhibitor. Therefore, Symbyax should not be used in combination with, or within a minimum of 14 days of discontinuing, an MAO inhibitor).
No products indexed under this heading.

Phenobarbital (Agents that induce CYP1A2 or glucuronyl transferase enzymes may cause an increase in olanzapine concentration).
No products indexed under this heading.

Phenoxybenzamine Hydrochloride (Because of the potential for olanzapine to induce hypotension, Symbyax may enhance the effects of certain antihypertensive agents). Products include:
Dibenzyline Capsules 3390

Phentolamine Mesylate (Because of the potential for olanzapine to induce hypotension, Symbyax may enhance the effects of certain antihypertensive agents).
No products indexed under this heading.

Phenylbutazone (Serotonin release by platelets plays an important role in hemostasis. Studies have demonstrated an association between the use of psychotropic drugs that interfere with serotonin reuptake and the occurrence of upper gastrointestinal bleeding. These studies have also shown that concurrent use of an NSAID potentiated the risk of bleeding. Therefore, patients should be cautioned about the use of NSAIDs concurrently with Symbyax).
No products indexed under this heading.

Phenytoin (Patients on stable doses of phenytoin have developed elevated plasma levels of phenytoin with clinical pheytoin toxicity following initiation of concomitant fluoxetine).
No products indexed under this heading.

Phenytoin Sodium (Patients on stable doses of phenytoin have developed elevated plasma levels of phenytoin with clinical pheytoin toxicity following initiation of concomitant fluoxetine). Products include:
Phenytek Capsules 2153

Pimozide (A single case report has suggested possible additive effects of pimozide and fluoxetine leading to bradycardia). Products include:
Orap Tablets 1220

Pindolol (Because of the potential for olanzapine to induce hypotension, Symbyax may enhance the effects of certain antihypertensive agents).
No products indexed under this heading.

Piroxicam (Serotonin release by platelets plays an important role in hemostasis. Studies have demonstrated an association between the use of psychotropic drugs that interfere with serotonin reuptake and the occurrence of upper gastrointestinal bleeding. These studies have also shown that concurrent use of an NSAID potentiated the risk of bleeding. Therefore, patients should be cautioned about the use of NSAIDs concurrently with Symbyax).
No products indexed under this heading.

Polythiazide (Because of the potential for olanzapine to induce hypotension, Symbyax may enhance the effects of certain antihypertensive agents).
No products indexed under this heading.

Pramipexole Dihydrochloride (The olanzapine component of Symbyax may antagonize the effects of levodopa and dopamine agonists). Products include:
Mirapex Tablets 889

Prazosin Hydrochloride (Because of the potential for olanzapine to induce hypotension, Symbyax may enhance the effects of certain antihypertensive agents).
No products indexed under this heading.

Primidone (Agents that induce CYP1A2 or glucuronyl transferase enzymes may cause an increase in olanzapine concentration).
No products indexed under this heading.

Procarbazine Hydrochloride (There have been reports of serious, sometimes fatal, reactions in patients receiving, or who have recently discontinued, fluoxetine and are then started on an MAO inhibitor. Therefore, Symbyax should not be used in combination with, or within a minimum of 14 days of discontinuing, an MAO inhibitor). Products include:
Matulane Capsules 3188

Propafenone Hydrochloride (Fluoxetine, like other agents that are metabolized by CYP2D6, inhibits the activity of this isoenzyme. Therapy with medications that are predominately metabolized by the CYP2D6 system and have a relatively narrow therapeutic index should be initiated at the low end of the dose range if the patient is receiving fluoxetine concurrently or has taken it in the previous five weeks. If fluoxetine is added to the treatment regimen of a patient already receiving a drug metabolized by CYP2D6, the need for a decreased dose of the original medication should be considered). Products include:
Rythmol SR Capsules 2736

Propoxyphene Hydrochloride (Fluoxetine, like other agents that are metabolized by CYP2D6, inhibits the activity of this isoenzyme. Therapy with medications that are predominately metabolized by the CYP2D6 system and have a relatively narrow therapeutic index should be initiated at the low end of the dose range if the patient is receiving fluoxetine concurrently or has taken it in the previous five weeks. If fluoxetine is added to the treatment regimen of a patient already receiving a drug metabolized by CYP2D6, the need for a decreased dose of the original medication should be considered).
No products indexed under this heading.

Propoxyphene Napsylate (Fluoxetine, like other agents that are metabolized by CYP2D6, inhibits the activity of this isoenzyme. Therapy with medications that are predominately metabolized by the CYP2D6 system and have a relatively narrow therapeutic index should be initiated at the low end of the dose range if the patient is receiving fluoxetine concurrently or has taken it in the previous five weeks. If fluoxetine is added to the treatment regimen of a patient already receiving a drug metabolized by CYP2D6, the need for a decreased dose of the original medication should be considered). Products include:
Darvocet A 500 Tablets 3497

Propranolol Hydrochloride (Because of the potential for olanzapine to induce hypotension, Symbyax may enhance the effects of certain antihypertensive agents). Products include:
Inderal LA Long-Acting Capsules 3421
InnoPran XL Capsules 2728

Protriptyline Hydrochloride (In two fluoxetine studies, previously stable plasma levels of imipramine and desipramine have increased >2- to 10-fold when fluoxetine has been

administered in combination. This influence may persist for three weeks or longer after fluoxetine is discontinued. Thus, the dose of TCA may need to be reduced and plasma TCA concentrations may need to be monitored temporarily when Symbyax is co-administered or has been recently discontinued). Products include:

Vivactil Tablets 2350

Quetiapine Fumarate (Fluoxetine, like other agents that are metabolized by CYP2D6, inhibits the activity of this isoenzyme. Therapy with medications that are predominately metabolized by the CYP2D6 system and have a relatively narrow therapeutic index should be initiated at the low end of the dose range if the patient is receiving fluoxetine concurrently or has taken it in the previous five weeks. If fluoxetine is added to the treatment regimen of a patient already receiving a drug metabolized by CYP2D6, the need for a decreased dose of the original medication should be considered). Products include:

Seroquel Tablets 691

Quinapril Hydrochloride (Because of the potential for olanzapine to induce hypotension, Symbyax may enhance the effects of certain antihypertensive agents).

No products indexed under this heading.

Quinidine Gluconate (Fluoxetine, like other agents that are metabolized by CYP2D6, inhibits the activity of this isoenzyme. Therapy with medications that are predominately metabolized by the CYP2D6 system and have a relatively narrow therapeutic index should be initiated at the low end of the dose range if the patient is receiving fluoxetine concurrently or has taken it in the previous five weeks. If fluoxetine is added to the treatment regimen of a patient already receiving a drug metabolized by CYP2D6, the need for a decreased dose of the original medication should be considered).

No products indexed under this heading.

Quinidine Hydrochloride (Fluoxetine, like other agents that are metabolized by CYP2D6, inhibits the activity of this isoenzyme. Therapy with medications that are predominately metabolized by the CYP2D6 system and have a relatively narrow therapeutic index should be initiated at the low end of the dose range if the patient is receiving fluoxetine concurrently or has taken it in the previous five weeks. If fluoxetine is added to the treatment regimen of a patient already receiving a drug metabolized by CYP2D6, the need for a decreased dose of the original medication should be considered).

No products indexed under this heading.

Quinidine Polygalacturonate (Fluoxetine, like other agents that are metabolized by CYP2D6, inhibits the activity of this isoenzyme. Therapy with medications that are predominately metabolized by the CYP2D6 system and have a relatively narrow therapeutic index should be initiated at the low end of the dose range if the patient is receiving fluoxetine concurrently or has taken it in the previous five weeks. If fluoxetine is added to the treatment regimen of a patient already receiving a drug metabolized by CYP2D6, the need for a decreased dose of the original medication should be considered).

No products indexed under this heading.

Quinidine Sulfate (Fluoxetine, like other agents that are metabolized by CYP2D6, inhibits the activity of this isoenzyme. Therapy with medications that are predominately metabolized by the CYP2D6 system and have a relatively narrow therapeutic index should be initiated at the low end of the dose range if the patient is receiving fluoxetine concurrently or has taken it in the previous five weeks. If fluoxetine is added to the treatment regimen of a patient already receiving a drug metabolized by CYP2D6, the need for a decreased dose of the original medication should be considered).

No products indexed under this heading.

Ramipril (Because of the potential for olanzapine to induce hypotension, Symbyax may enhance the effects of certain antihypertensive agents). Products include:

Altace Capsules 1673

Rauwolfia Serpentina (Because of the potential for olanzapine to induce hypotension, Symbyax may enhance the effects of certain antihypertensive agents).

No products indexed under this heading.

Rescinnamine (Because of the potential for olanzapine to induce hypotension, Symbyax may enhance the effects of certain antihypertensive agents).

No products indexed under this heading.

Reserpine (Because of the potential for olanzapine to induce hypotension, Symbyax may enhance the effects of certain antihypertensive agents).

No products indexed under this heading.

Rifampicin (Agents that induce CYP1A2 or glucuronyl transferase enzymes may cause an increase in olanzapine concentration).

No products indexed under this heading.

Rifampin (Agents that induce CYP1A2 or glucuronyl transferase enzymes may cause an increase in olanzapine concentration).

No products indexed under this heading.

Risperidone (Fluoxetine, like other agents that are metabolized by CYP2D6, inhibits the activity of this isoenzyme. Therapy with medications that are predominately metabolized by the CYP2D6 system and have a relatively narrow therapeutic index should be initiated at the low end of the dose range if the patient is receiving fluoxetine concurrently or has taken it in the previous five weeks. If fluoxetine is added to the treatment regimen of a patient already receiving a drug metabolized by CYP2D6, the need for a decreased dose of the original medication should be considered). Products include:

Risperdal Consta Long-Acting Injection 1664

Risperdal M-Tab Orally Disintegrating Tablets.................. 1658

Risperdal 1658

Ritonavir (Fluoxetine, like other agents that are metabolized by CYP2D6, inhibits the activity of this isoenzyme. Therapy with medications that are predominately metabolized by the CYP2D6 system and have a relatively narrow therapeutic index should be initiated at the low end of the dose range if the patient is receiving fluoxetine concurrently or has taken it in the previous five weeks. If fluoxetine is added to the treatment regimen of a patient already receiving a drug metabolized by CYP2D6, the need for a decreased dose of the original medication should be considered). Products include:

Kaletra 474

Norvir 499

Rofecoxib (Serotonin release by platelets plays an important role in hemostasis. Studies have demonstrated an association between the use of psychotropic drugs that interfere with serotonin reuptake and the occurrence of upper gastrointestinal bleeding. These studies have also shown that concurrent use of an NSAID potentiated the risk of bleeding. Therefore, patients should be cautioned about the use of NSAIDs concurrently with Symbyax).

No products indexed under this heading.

Ropinirole Hydrochloride (The olanzapine component of Symbyax may antagonize the effects of levodopa and dopamine agonists). Products include:

Requip Tablets 1528

Selegiline Hydrochloride (There have been reports of serious, sometimes fatal, reactions in patients receiving, or who have recently discontinued, fluoxetine and are then started on an MAO inhibitor. Therefore, Symbyax should not be used in combination with, or within a minimum of 14 days of discontinuing, an MAO inhibitor). Products include:

Eldepryl Capsules 3209

Sodium Nitroprusside (Because of the potential for olanzapine to induce hypotension, Symbyax may enhance the effects of certain antihypertensive agents).

No products indexed under this heading.

Sotalol Hydrochloride (Because of the potential for olanzapine to induce hypotension, Symbyax may enhance the effects of certain antihypertensive agents).

No products indexed under this heading.

Spirapril Hydrochloride (Because of the potential for olanzapine to induce hypotension, Symbyax may enhance the effects of certain antihypertensive agents).

No products indexed under this heading.

Sulindac (Serotonin release by platelets plays an important role in hemostasis. Studies have demonstrated an association between the use of psychotropic drugs that interfere with serotonin reuptake and the occurrence of upper gastrointestinal bleeding. These studies have also shown that concurrent use of an NSAID potentiated the risk of bleeding. Therefore, patients should be cautioned about the use of NSAIDs concurrently with Symbyax). Products include:

Clinoril Tablets 1899

Sumatriptan (There have been rare postmarketing reports describing patients with weakness, hyperreflexia, and incoordination following the use of an SSRI and sumatriptan. If concomitant treatment with sumatriptan and an SSRI is clinically warranted, appropriate observation of the patient is advised). Products include:

Imitrex Nasal Spray 1435

Sumatriptan Succinate (There have been rare postmarketing reports describing patients with weakness, hyperreflexia, and incoordination following the use of an SSRI and sumatriptan. If concomitant treatment with sumatriptan and an SSRI is clinically warranted, appropriate observation of the patient is advised). Products include:

Imitrex Injection 1431

Imitrex Tablets 1440

Tamoxifen Citrate (Fluoxetine, like other agents that are metabolized by CYP2D6, inhibits the activity of this isoenzyme. Therapy with medications that are predominately metabolized by the CYP2D6 system and have a relatively narrow therapeutic index should be initiated at the low end of the dose range if the patient is receiving fluoxetine concurrently or has taken it in the previous five weeks. If fluoxetine is added to the treatment regimen of a patient already receiving a drug metabolized by CYP2D6, the need for a decreased dose of the original medication should be considered).

No products indexed under this heading.

Telmisartan (Because of the potential for olanzapine to induce hypotension, Symbyax may enhance the effects of certain antihypertensive agents). Products include:

Micardis Tablets 884

Micardis HCT Tablets 886

Temazepam (Because fluoxetine is tightly bound to plasma protein, the administration of fluoxetine to a patient taking another drug that is tightly bound to protein may cause a shift in plasma concentrations potentially resulting in an adverse effect. Conversely, adverse effects may result from displacement of protein-bound fluoxetine by other tightly bound drugs).

No products indexed under this heading.

Teniposide (Fluoxetine, like other agents that are metabolized by CYP2D6, inhibits the activity of this isoenzyme. Therapy with medications that are predominately metabolized by the CYP2D6 system and have a relatively narrow therapeutic index should be initiated at the low end of the dose range if the patient is receiving fluoxetine concurrently or has taken it in the previous five weeks. If fluoxetine is added to the treatment regimen of a patient already receiving a drug metabolized by CYP2D6, the need for a decreased dose of the original medication should be considered).

No products indexed under this heading.

Terazosin Hydrochloride (Because of the potential for olanzapine to induce hypotension, Symbyax may enhance the effects of certain antihypertensive agents). Products include:

Hytrin Capsules ... 469

Testosterone (Fluoxetine, like other agents that are metabolized by CYP2D6, inhibits the activity of this isoenzyme. Therapy with medications that are predominately metabolized by the CYP2D6 system and have a relatively narrow therapeutic index should be initiated at the low end of the dose range if the patient is receiving fluoxetine concurrently or has taken it in the previous five weeks. If fluoxetine is added to the treatment regimen of a patient already receiving a drug metabolized by CYP2D6, the need for a decreased dose of the original medication should be considered). Products include:

AndroGel ... 3330
Striant Mucoadhesive ... 1022
Testim 1% Gel ... 722

Testosterone Cypionate (Fluoxetine, like other agents that are metabolized by CYP2D6, inhibits the activity of this isoenzyme. Therapy with medications that are predominately metabolized by the CYP2D6 system and have a relatively narrow therapeutic index should be initiated at the low end of the dose range if the patient is receiving fluoxetine concurrently or has taken it in the previous five weeks. If fluoxetine is added to the treatment regimen of a patient already receiving a drug metabolized by CYP2D6, the need for a decreased dose of the original medication should be considered).

No products indexed under this heading.

Testosterone Enanthate (Fluoxetine, like other agents that are metabolized by CYP2D6, inhibits the activity of this isoenzyme. Therapy with medications that are predominately metabolized by the CYP2D6 system and have a relatively narrow therapeutic index should be initiated at the low end of the dose range if the patient is receiving fluoxetine concurrently or has taken it in the previous five weeks. If fluoxetine is added to the treatment regimen of a patient already receiving a drug metabolized by CYP2D6, the need for a decreased dose of the original medication should be considered). Products include:

Delatestryl Injection ... 2976

Testosterone Propionate (Fluoxetine, like other agents that are metabolized by CYP2D6, inhibits the activity of this isoenzyme. Therapy with medications that are predominately metabolized by the CYP2D6 system and have a relatively narrow therapeutic index should be initiated at the low end of the dose range if the patient is receiving fluoxetine concurrently or has taken it in the previous five weeks. If fluoxetine is added to the treatment regimen of a patient already receiving a drug metabolized by CYP2D6, the need for a decreased dose of the original medication should be considered).

No products indexed under this heading.

Thioridazine (Thioridazine should not be administered with Symbyax or administered within a minimum of 5 weeks after discontinuation of Symbyax).

No products indexed under this heading.

Thioridazine Hydrochloride (Thioridazine should not be administered with Symbyax or administered within a minimum of 5 weeks after discontinuation of Symbyax). Products include:

Thioridazine Hydrochloride Tablets ... 2122

Timolol Maleate (Because of the potential for olanzapine to induce hypotension, Symbyax may enhance the effects of certain antihypertensive agents). Products include:

Blocadren Tablets ... 1891
Cosopt Sterile Ophthalmic Solution ... 1910
Timolide Tablets ... 2056
Timoptic in Ocudose ... 2061
Timoptic Sterile Ophthalmic Solution ... 2058
Timoptic-XE Sterile Ophthalmic Gel Forming Solution ... 2062

Tobacco (Agents that induce CYP1A2 or glucuronyl transferase enzymes may cause an increase in olanzapine concentration).

No products indexed under this heading.

Tolbutamide (Because fluoxetine is tightly bound to plasma protein, the administration of fluoxetine to a patient taking another drug that is tightly bound to protein may cause a shift in plasma concentrations potentially resulting in an adverse effect. Conversely, adverse effects may result from displacement of protein-bound fluoxetine by other tightly bound drugs).

No products indexed under this heading.

Tolmetin Sodium (Serotonin release by platelets plays an important role in hemostasis. Studies have demonstrated an association between the use of psychotropic drugs that interfere with serotonin reuptake and the occurrence of upper gastrointestinal bleeding. These studies have also shown that concurrent use of an NSAID potentiated the risk of bleeding. Therefore, patients should be cautioned about the use of NSAIDs concurrently with Symbyax).

No products indexed under this heading.

Tolterodine Tartrate (Fluoxetine, like other agents that are metabolized by CYP2D6, inhibits the activity of this isoenzyme. Therapy with medications that are predominately metabolized by the CYP2D6 system and have a relatively narrow therapeutic index should be initiated at the low end of the dose range if the patient is receiving fluoxetine concurrently or has taken it in the previous five weeks. If fluoxetine is added to the treatment regimen of a patient already receiving a drug metabolized by CYP2D6, the need for a decreased dose of the original medication should be considered). Products include:

Detrol Tablets ... 2626
Detrol LA Capsules ... 2629

Torsemide (Because of the potential for olanzapine to induce hypotension, Symbyax may enhance the effects of certain antihypertensive agents).

No products indexed under this heading.

Tramadol Hydrochloride (Fluoxetine, like other agents that are metabolized by CYP2D6, inhibits the activity of this isoenzyme. Therapy with medications that are predominately metabolized by the CYP2D6 system and have a relatively narrow therapeutic index should be initiated at the low end of the dose range if the patient is receiving fluoxetine concurrently or has taken it in the previous five weeks. If fluoxetine is added to the treatment regimen of a patient already receiving a drug metabolized by CYP2D6, the need for a decreased dose of the original medication should be considered). Products include:

Ultracet Tablets ... 2462

Trandolapril (Because of the potential for olanzapine to induce hypotension, Symbyax may enhance the effects of certain antihypertensive agents). Products include:

Mavik Tablets ... 482
Tarka Tablets ... 519

Tranylcypromine Sulfate (There have been reports of serious, sometimes fatal, reactions in patients receiving, or who have recently discontinued, fluoxetine and are then started on an MAO inhibitor. Therefore, Symbyax should not be used in combination with, or within a minimum of 14 days of discontinuing, an MAO inhibitor). Products include:

Parnate Tablets ... 1499

Trazodone Hydrochloride (Fluoxetine, like other agents that are metabolized by CYP2D6, inhibits the activity of this isoenzyme. Therapy with medications that are predominately metabolized by the CYP2D6 system and have a relatively narrow therapeutic index should be initiated at the low end of the dose range if the patient is receiving fluoxetine concurrently or has taken it in the previous five weeks. If fluoxetine is added to the treatment regimen of a patient already receiving a drug metabolized by CYP2D6, the need for a decreased dose of the original medication should be considered).

No products indexed under this heading.

Triazolam (Fluoxetine, like other agents that are metabolized by CYP2D6, inhibits the activity of this isoenzyme. Therapy with medications that are predominately metabolized by the CYP2D6 system and have a relatively narrow therapeutic index should be initiated at the low end of the dose range if the patient is receiving fluoxetine concurrently or has taken it in the previous five weeks. If fluoxetine is added to the treatment regimen of a patient already receiving a drug metabolized by CYP2D6, the need for a decreased dose of the original medication should be considered).

No products indexed under this heading.

Trimethaphan Camsylate (Because of the potential for olanzapine to induce hypotension, Symbyax may enhance the effects of certain antihypertensive agents).

No products indexed under this heading.

Trimipramine Maleate (In two fluoxetine studies, previously stable plasma levels of imipramine and desipramine have increased >2- to 10-fold when fluoxetine has been administered in combination. This influence may persist for three weeks or longer after fluoxetine is discontinued. Thus, the dose of TCA may need to be reduced and plasma TCA concentrations may need to be monitored temporarily when Symbyax is co-administered or has been recently discontinued). Products include:

Surmontil Capsules ... 2347

L-Tryptophan (Five patients receiving fluoxetine in combination with tryptophan experienced adverse reactions, including agitation, restlessness, and gastrointestinal distress).

No products indexed under this heading.

Valdecoxib (Serotonin release by platelets plays an important role in hemostasis. Studies have demonstrated an association between the use of psychotropic drugs that interfere with serotonin reuptake and the occurrence of upper gastrointestinal bleeding. These studies have also shown that concurrent use of an NSAID potentiated the risk of bleeding. Therefore, patients should be cautioned about the use of NSAIDs concurrently with Symbyax).

No products indexed under this heading.

Valsartan (Because of the potential for olanzapine to induce hypotension, Symbyax may enhance the effects of certain antihypertensive agents). Products include:

Diovan HCT Tablets ... 2195
Diovan Tablets ... 2191

Venlafaxine Hydrochloride (Fluoxetine, like other agents that are metabolized by CYP2D6, inhibits the activity of this isoenzyme. Therapy with medications that are predominately metabolized by the CYP2D6 system and have a relatively narrow therapeutic index should be initiated at the low end of the dose range if the patient is receiving fluoxetine concurrently or has taken it in the previous five weeks. If fluoxetine is added to the treatment regimen of a patient already receiving a drug metabolized by CYP2D6, the need for a decreased dose of the original medication should be considered). Products include:

Effexor Tablets ... 3405
Effexor XR Capsules ... 3411

Verapamil Hydrochloride (Because of the potential for olanzapine to induce hypotension, Symbyax may enhance the effects of certain antihypertensive agents). Products include:

Covera-HS Tablets ... 3135
Tarka Tablets ... 519
Verelan PM Capsules ... 3120

Vinblastine Sulfate (Fluoxetine, like other agents that are metabolized by CYP2D6, inhibits the activity of this isoenzyme. Therapy with medications that are predominately metabolized by the CYP2D6 system and have a relatively narrow therapeutic index should be initiated at the low end of the dose range if the patient is receiving fluoxetine concurrently or has taken it in the previous five weeks. If fluoxetine is added to the treatment regimen of a patient already receiving a drug metabolized by CYP2D6, the need for a decreased dose of the original medication should be considered).

No products indexed under this heading.

Warfarin Sodium (Altered anticoagulant effects, including increased bleeding, have been reported when fluoxetine is co-administered with warfarin. Patients receiving warfarin therapy should receive careful coag-

ulation monitoring when Symbyax is initiated or stopped). Products include:

Coumadin for Injection 932
Coumadin Tablets 932

Zonisamide (Fluoxetine, like other agents that are metabolized by CYP2D6, inhibits the activity of this isoenzyme. Therapy with medications that are predominately metabolized by the CYP2D6 system and have a relatively narrow therapeutic index should be initiated at the low end of the dose range if the patient is receiving fluoxetine concurrently or has taken it in the previous five weeks. If fluoxetine is added to the treatment regimen of a patient already receiving a drug metabolized by CYP2D6, the need for a decreased dose of the original medication should be considered). Products include:

Zonegran Capsules 1089

Food Interactions

Alcohol (Alcohol may potentiate the orthostatic effect of olanzapine, increasing the risk of orthostatic hypotension. Therefore, patients should be advised to avoid alcohol while taking Symbyax).

Broccoli (Agents that induce CYP1A2 or glucuronyl transferase enzymes may cause an increase in olanzapine concentration).

Brussel Sprouts (Agents that induce CYP1A2 or glucuronyl transferase enzymes may cause an increase in olanzapine concentration).

Charbroiled Food (Agents that induce CYP1A2 or glucuronyl transferase enzymes may cause an increase in olanzapine concentration).

SYMLIN INJECTION

(Pramlintide Acetate) 608

May interact with ACE inhibitors, anticholinergics, fibrates, drugs affecting gastrointestinal motility, oral hypoglycemic agents, insulin, monoamine oxidase inhibitors, salicylates, sulfonylureas, and certain other agents. Compounds in these categories include:

Acarbose (Due to its effects on gastric emptying, pramlintide acetate therapy should not be considered for patients taking agents that slow the intestinal absorption of nutrients (eg, alpha-glucosidase inhibitors)). Products include:

Precose Tablets 776

Albuterol (Due to its effects on gastric emptying, pramlintide acetate therapy should not be considered for patients taking drugs that alter gastrointestinal motility and agents that slow the intestinal absorption of nutrients). Products include:

Proventil Inhalation Aerosol 3067

Albuterol Sulfate (Due to its effects on gastric emptying, pramlintide acetate therapy should not be considered for patients taking drugs that alter gastrointestinal motility and agents that slow the intestinal absorption of nutrients). Products include:

AccuNeb Inhalation Solution 1055
Combivent Inhalation Aerosol 878
DuoNeb Inhalation Solution 1058
Proventil Inhalation Solution 0.083%....................................... 3069
Proventil HFA Inhalation Aerosol 3071
Ventolin HFA Inhalation Aerosol 1576
VoSpire Extended-Release Tablets ... 2352

Alfentanil Hydrochloride (Due to its effects on gastric emptying, pramlintide acetate therapy should not be considered for patients taking drugs that alter gastrointestinal motility and agents that slow the intestinal absorption of nutrients).

No products indexed under this heading.

Amitriptyline Hydrochloride (Due to its effects on gastric emptying, pramlintide acetate therapy should not be considered for patients taking drugs that alter gastrointestinal motility and agents that slow the intestinal absorption of nutrients).

No products indexed under this heading.

Amlodipine Besylate (Due to its effects on gastric emptying, pramlintide acetate therapy should not be considered for patients taking drugs that alter gastrointestinal motility and agents that slow the intestinal absorption of nutrients). Products include:

Caduet Tablets 2507
Lotrel Capsules 2238
Norvasc Tablets 2529

Amoxapine (Due to its effects on gastric emptying, pramlintide acetate therapy should not be considered for patients taking drugs that alter gastrointestinal motility and agents that slow the intestinal absorption of nutrients).

No products indexed under this heading.

Anti-infectives, oral, unspecified (Pramlintide acetate has the potential to delay the absorption of concomitantly administered oral medications. When the rapid onset of a concomitant orally administered agent is a critical determinant of effectiveness, the agent should be administered at least 1 hr prior to or 2 hrs after pramlintide acetate injection).

No products indexed under this heading.

Aspirin (May increase the blood glucose-lowering effect and susceptibility to hypoglycemia, which may necessitate further insulin dose adjustments and particularly close monitoring of blood glucose). Products include:

Aggrenox Capsules 855
Bayer, Aspirin Regimen 606
Bayer Aspirin Tablets 3515
BC Powder 612
BC Allergy Sinus Cold Powder 612
Arthritis Strength BC Powder 612
BC Sinus Cold Powder 612
Ecotrin Enteric Coated Aspirin Low, Regular and Maximum Strength Tablets 1627
Goody's Body Pain Formula Powder 621
Goody's Extra Strength Headache Powder 621
Goody's Extra Strength Pain Relief Tablets 621
Percodan Tablets 1115
St. Joseph 81 mg Aspirin Chewable and Enteric Coated Tablets 1841

Aspirin, Enteric Coated (May increase the blood glucose-lowering effect and susceptibility to hypoglycemia, which may necessitate further insulin dose adjustments and particularly close monitoring of blood glucose).

No products indexed under this heading.

Aspirin Buffered (May increase the blood glucose-lowering effect and susceptibility to hypoglycemia, which may necessitate further insulin dose adjustments and particularly close monitoring of blood glucose).

No products indexed under this heading.

Astemizole (Due to its effects on gastric emptying, pramlintide acetate therapy should not be considered for patients taking drugs that alter gastrointestinal motility and agents that slow the intestinal absorption of nutrients).

No products indexed under this heading.

Atropine Sulfate (Due to its effects on gastric emptying, pramlintide acetate therapy should not be considered for patients taking drugs that alter gastrointestinal motility and agents that slow the intestinal absorption of nutrients).

No products indexed under this heading.

Azatadine Maleate (Due to its effects on gastric emptying, pramlintide acetate therapy should not be considered for patients taking drugs that alter gastrointestinal motility and agents that slow the intestinal absorption of nutrients).

No products indexed under this heading.

Belladonna Alkaloids (Due to its effects on gastric emptying, pramlintide acetate therapy should not be considered for patients taking drugs that alter gastrointestinal motility and agents that slow the intestinal absorption of nutrients). Products include:

Hyland's Teething Tablets 736

Benazepril Hydrochloride (May increase the blood glucose-lowering effect and susceptibility to hypoglycemia, which may necessitate further insulin dose adjustments and particularly close monitoring of blood glucose). Products include:

Lotensin Tablets 2232
Lotensin HCT Tablets 2235
Lotrel Capsules 2238

Benztropine Mesylate (Due to its effects on gastric emptying, pramlintide acetate therapy should not be considered for patients taking drugs that alter gastrointestinal motility and agents that slow the intestinal absorption of nutrients). Products include:

Cogentin Injection 1903

Bepridil Hydrochloride (Due to its effects on gastric emptying, pramlintide acetate therapy should not be considered for patients taking drugs that alter gastrointestinal motility and agents that slow the intestinal absorption of nutrients).

No products indexed under this heading.

Bethanechol Chloride (Due to its effects on gastric emptying, pramlintide acetate therapy should not be considered for patients taking drugs that alter gastrointestinal motility and agents that slow the intestinal absorption of nutrients). Products include:

Urecholine Tablets 2349

Biperiden Hydrochloride (Due to its effects on gastric emptying, pramlintide acetate therapy should not be considered for patients taking drugs that alter gastrointestinal motility and agents that slow the intestinal absorption of nutrients).

No products indexed under this heading.

Bitolterol Mesylate (Due to its effects on gastric emptying, pramlintide acetate therapy should not be considered for patients taking drugs that alter gastrointestinal motility and agents that slow the intestinal absorption of nutrients).

No products indexed under this heading.

Bromocriptine Mesylate (Due to its effects on gastric emptying, pramlintide acetate therapy should not be considered for patients taking drugs that alter gastrointestinal motility and agents that slow the intestinal absorption of nutrients).

No products indexed under this heading.

Bromodiphenhydramine Hydrochloride (Due to its effects on gastric emptying, pramlintide acetate therapy should not be considered for patients taking drugs that alter gastrointestinal motility and agents that slow the intestinal absorption of nutrients).

No products indexed under this heading.

Brompheniramine Maleate (Due to its effects on gastric emptying, pramlintide acetate therapy should not be considered for patients taking drugs that alter gastrointestinal motility and agents that slow the intestinal absorption of nutrients). Products include:

Alacol DM Syrup 739
Children's Dimetapp Cold & Allergy Elixir 745
Children's Dimetapp DM Cold & Cough Elixir 745
Robitussin Allergy & Cough Syrup .. 750

Buprenorphine Hydrochloride (Due to its effects on gastric emptying, pramlintide acetate therapy should not be considered for patients taking drugs that alter gastrointestinal motility and agents that slow the intestinal absorption of nutrients). Products include:

Buprenex Injectable 2718
Suboxone Tablets 2719
Subutex Tablets 2719

Captopril (May increase the blood glucose-lowering effect and susceptibility to hypoglycemia, which may necessitate further insulin dose adjustments and particularly close monitoring of blood glucose). Products include:

Captopril Tablets 2114

Cevimeline Hydrochloride (Due to its effects on gastric emptying, pramlintide acetate therapy should not be considered for patients taking drugs that alter gastrointestinal motility and agents that slow the intestinal absorption of nutrients). Products include:

Evoxac Capsules 1042

Chlorpheniramine Maleate (Due to its effects on gastric emptying, pramlintide acetate therapy should not be considered for patients taking drugs that alter gastrointestinal motility and agents that slow the intestinal absorption of nutrients). Products include:

Advil Allergy Sinus Caplets .... ■ 737
Advil Multi-Symptom Cold Caplets .... ■ 738
BC Allergy Sinus Cold Powder .... ■ 612
Contac Severe Cold and Flu Caplets Maximum Strength .... ■ 615
Hycomine Compound Tablets 1105
PediaCare Multi-Symptom Cold Liquid .... ■ 704
PediaCare NightRest Cough & Cold Liquid .... ■ 704
Robitussin Flu Liquid .... ■ 752
Robitussin PM Cough & Cold Liquid .... ■ 752
Singlet Caplets .... ■ 636
Sudafed Sinus & Allergy Tablets .... ■ 710
TheraFlu Cold & Cough Hot Liquid .... ■ 680
TheraFlu Cold & Sore Throat Hot Liquid .... ■ 680
TheraFlu Flu & Sore Throat Hot Liquid .... ■ 681
TheraFlu Severe Cold & Cough Hot Liquid .... ■ 683
TheraFlu Severe Cold Caplets .... ■ 679
TheraFlu Severe Cold Hot Liquid .... ■ 682
Triaminic Cold & Allergy Liquid .... ■ 685
Triaminic Cold & Cough Liquid .... ■ 685
Triaminic Flu, Cough & Fever Liquid .... ■ 685
Triaminic Night Time Cough & Cold Liquid .... ■ 685
Triaminic Allergy Runny Nose & Congestion Softchews .... ■ 688
Triaminic Cold & Cough Softchews .... ■ 688
Children's Tylenol Plus Cold NightTime Suspension Liquid 1851
Children's Tylenol Plus Cold & Cough Suspension Liquid and Chewable Tablets 1851
Children's Tylenol Plus Cold Chewable Tablets 1851
Children's Tylenol Plus Flu Suspension Liquid 1853
Tylenol Allergy Complete Multi-Symptom Caplets and Gelcaps with Cool Burst 1844
Multi-Symptom Tylenol Cold Night Time Caplets 1845
Vicks 44M Cough, Cold & Flu Relief 2676
Pediatric Vicks 44m Cough & Cold Relief 2673
Children's Vicks NyQuil Cold/Cough Relief 2671

Chlorpheniramine Polistirex (Due to its effects on gastric emptying, pramlintide acetate therapy should not be considered for patients taking drugs that alter gastrointestinal motility and agents that slow the intestinal absorption of nutrients). Products include:
Tussionex Pennkinetic Extended-Release Suspension 3322

Chlorpheniramine Tannate (Due to its effects on gastric emptying, pramlintide acetate therapy should not be considered for patients taking drugs that alter gastrointestinal motility and agents that slow the intestinal absorption of nutrients).
No products indexed under this heading.

Chlorpropamide (May increase the blood glucose-lowering effect and susceptibility to hypoglycemia, which may necessitate further insulin dose adjustments and particularly close monitoring of blood glucose).
No products indexed under this heading.

Choline Magnesium Trisalicylate (May increase the blood glucose-lowering effect and susceptibility to hypoglycemia, which may necessitate further insulin dose adjustments and particularly close monitoring of blood glucose).
No products indexed under this heading.

Cisapride (Due to its effects on gastric emptying, pramlintide acetate therapy should not be considered for patients taking drugs that alter gastrointestinal motility and agents that slow the intestinal absorption of nutrients).
No products indexed under this heading.

Clemastine Fumarate (Due to its effects on gastric emptying, pramlintide acetate therapy should not be considered for patients taking drugs that alter gastrointestinal motility and agents that slow the intestinal absorption of nutrients).
No products indexed under this heading.

Clidinium Bromide (Due to its effects on gastric emptying, pramlintide acetate therapy should not be considered for patients taking drugs that alter gastrointestinal motility and agents that slow the intestinal absorption of nutrients).
No products indexed under this heading.

Clofibrate (May increase the blood glucose-lowering effect and susceptibility to hypoglycemia, which may necessitate further insulin dose adjustments and particularly close monitoring of blood glucose).
No products indexed under this heading.

Clomipramine Hydrochloride (Due to its effects on gastric emptying, pramlintide acetate therapy should not be considered for patients taking drugs that alter gastrointestinal motility and agents that slow the intestinal absorption of nutrients).
No products indexed under this heading.

Codeine Phosphate (Due to its effects on gastric emptying, pramlintide acetate therapy should not be considered for patients taking drugs that alter gastrointestinal motility and agents that slow the intestinal absorption of nutrients). Products include:
Tylenol with Codeine 2461

Cyproheptadine Hydrochloride (Due to its effects on gastric emptying, pramlintide acetate therapy should not be considered for patients taking drugs that alter gastrointestinal motility and agents that slow the intestinal absorption of nutrients).
No products indexed under this heading.

Desipramine Hydrochloride (Due to its effects on gastric emptying, pramlintide acetate therapy should not be considered for patients taking drugs that alter gastrointestinal motility and agents that slow the intestinal absorption of nutrients).
No products indexed under this heading.

Dexchlorpheniramine Maleate (Due to its effects on gastric emptying, pramlintide acetate therapy should not be considered for patients taking drugs that alter gastrointestinal motility and agents that slow the intestinal absorption of nutrients).
No products indexed under this heading.

Dezocine (Due to its effects on gastric emptying, pramlintide acetate therapy should not be considered for patients taking drugs that alter gastrointestinal motility and agents that slow the intestinal absorption of nutrients).
No products indexed under this heading.

Dicyclomine Hydrochloride (Due to its effects on gastric emptying, pramlintide acetate therapy should not be considered for patients taking drugs that alter gastrointestinal motility and agents that slow the intestinal absorption of nutrients).
Products include:
Bentyl Capsules 724
Bentyl Injection 724
Bentyl Syrup 724
Bentyl Tablets 724

Diflunisal (May increase the blood glucose-lowering effect and susceptibility to hypoglycemia, which may necessitate further insulin dose adjustments and particularly close monitoring of blood glucose).
Products include:
Dolobid Tablets 1937

Diltiazem Hydrochloride (Due to its effects on gastric emptying, pramlintide acetate therapy should not be considered for patients taking drugs that alter gastrointestinal motility and agents that slow the intestinal absorption of nutrients).
Products include:
Cardizem LA Extended Release Tablets 1699
Tiazac Capsules 1204

Diphenhydramine Citrate (Due to its effects on gastric emptying, pramlintide acetate therapy should not be considered for patients taking drugs that alter gastrointestinal motility and agents that slow the intestinal absorption of nutrients).
Products include:
Children's Benadryl Allergy & Cold Fastmelt Tablets .... ■ 695
Children's Benadryl D Allergy & Sinus Fastmelt Tablets .... ■ 694
Children's Benadryl Allergy Fastmelt Tablets .... ■ 696
Goody's PM Powder .... ■ 622

Diphenhydramine Hydrochloride (Due to its effects on gastric emptying, pramlintide acetate therapy should not be considered for patients taking drugs that alter gastrointestinal motility and agents that slow the intestinal absorption of nutrients). Products include:
Benadryl Allergy & Cold Tablets .... ■ 692
Benadryl Allergy .... ■ 691
Benadryl Allergy & Sinus Headache Caplets & Gelcaps .... ■ 693
Children's Benadryl Allergy Liquid .... ■ 695
Children's Benadryl Dye-Free Allergy Liquid .... ■ 695
Benadryl Dye-Free Allergy Liqui-Gels Softgels .... ■ 692
Benadryl Itch Relief Stick Extra Strength .... ■ 696
Benadryl Itch Stopping Cream Extra Strength .... ■ 697
Benadryl Itch Stopping Gel Extra Strength .... ■ 697
Benadryl Itch Stopping Spray Extra Strength .... ■ 697
Benadryl Maximum Strength Severe Allergy & Sinus Headache Caplets .... ■ 694
Children's Benadryl D Liquid Medication .... ■ 693
Benadryl D Tablets .... ■ 694
Nytol QuickCaps Caplets .... ■ 635
Maximum Strength Nytol QuickGels Softgels .... ■ 635
Simply Sleep Caplets 1841
Sominex Original Formula Tablets .... ■ 637
TheraFlu Thin Strips Multi Symptom .... ■ 684
Triaminic Thin Strips Cough & Runny Nose .... ■ 690
Children's Tylenol Plus Cold & Allergy Suspension Liquid 1850
Tylenol Allergy Complete Night Time Caplets 1844
Tylenol Severe Allergy Caplets 1844
Tylenol Flu NightTime Gelcaps 1846
Extra Strength Tylenol PM Caplets, Geltabs, Gelcaps and Liquid 1847
Unisom Maximum Strength SleepGels .... ■ 712

Diphenylpyraline Hydrochloride (Due to its effects on gastric emptying, pramlintide acetate therapy should not be considered for patients taking drugs that alter gastrointestinal motility and agents that slow the intestinal absorption of nutrients).
No products indexed under this heading.

Disopyramide (May increase the blood glucose-lowering effect and susceptibility to hypoglycemia, which may necessitate further insulin dose adjustments and particularly close monitoring of blood glucose).
No products indexed under this heading.

Disopyramide Phosphate (May increase the blood glucose-lowering effect and susceptibility to hypoglycemia, which may necessitate further insulin dose adjustments and particularly close monitoring of blood glucose).
No products indexed under this heading.

Dobutamine (Due to its effects on gastric emptying, pramlintide acetate therapy should not be considered for patients taking drugs that alter gastrointestinal motility and agents that slow the intestinal absorption of nutrients).
No products indexed under this heading.

Dobutamine Hydrochloride (Due to its effects on gastric emptying, pramlintide acetate therapy should not be considered for patients taking drugs that alter gastrointestinal motility and agents that slow the intestinal absorption of nutrients).
No products indexed under this heading.

Domperidone (Due to its effects on gastric emptying, pramlintide acetate therapy should not be considered for patients taking drugs that alter gastrointestinal motility and agents that slow the intestinal absorption of nutrients).
No products indexed under this heading.

Donepezil Hydrochloride (Due to its effects on gastric emptying, pramlintide acetate therapy should not be considered for patients taking drugs that alter gastrointestinal motility and agents that slow the intestinal absorption of nutrients).
Products include:
Aricept Tablets 1086
Aricept ODT Tablets 1086

Dopamine Hydrochloride (Due to its effects on gastric emptying, pramlintide acetate therapy should not be considered for patients taking drugs that alter gastrointestinal motility and agents that slow the intestinal absorption of nutrients).
No products indexed under this heading.

Doxepin Hydrochloride (Due to its effects on gastric emptying, pramlintide acetate therapy should not be considered for patients taking drugs that alter gastrointestinal motility and agents that slow the intestinal absorption of nutrients).
No products indexed under this heading.

Edrophonium Chloride (Due to its effects on gastric emptying, pramlintide acetate therapy should not be considered for patients taking drugs that alter gastrointestinal motility and agents that slow the intestinal absorption of nutrients).
No products indexed under this heading.

Enalapril Maleate (May increase the blood glucose-lowering effect and susceptibility to hypoglycemia, which may necessitate further insulin dose adjustments and particularly close monitoring of blood glucose). Products include:
Vaseretic Tablets 2073
Vasotec I.V. Injection 2076

Enalaprilat (May increase the blood glucose-lowering effect and susceptibility to hypoglycemia, which may necessitate further insulin dose adjustments and particularly close monitoring of blood glucose).
No products indexed under this heading.

Ephedrine Hydrochloride (Due to its effects on gastric emptying, pramlintide acetate therapy should not be considered for patients taking drugs that alter gastrointestinal motility and agents that slow the intestinal absorption of nutrients). Products include:
Primatene Tablets 749

Ephedrine Sulfate (Due to its effects on gastric emptying, pramlintide acetate therapy should not be considered for patients taking drugs that alter gastrointestinal motility and agents that slow the intestinal absorption of nutrients).
No products indexed under this heading.

Ephedrine Tannate (Due to its effects on gastric emptying, pramlintide acetate therapy should not be considered for patients taking drugs that alter gastrointestinal motility and agents that slow the intestinal absorption of nutrients).
No products indexed under this heading.

Epinephrine (Due to its effects on gastric emptying, pramlintide acetate therapy should not be considered for patients taking drugs that alter gastrointestinal motility and agents that slow the intestinal absorption of nutrients). Products include:
EpiPen 1061
Primatene Mist 749

Epinephrine Hydrochloride (Due to its effects on gastric emptying, pramlintide acetate therapy should not be considered for patients taking drugs that alter gastrointestinal motility and agents that slow the intestinal absorption of nutrients).
No products indexed under this heading.

Erythromycin (Due to its effects on gastric emptying, pramlintide acetate therapy should not be considered for patients taking drugs that alter gastrointestinal motility and agents that slow the intestinal absorption of nutrients). Products include:
Erygel Topical Gel 2096
Ery-Tab Tablets 447
Erythromycin Base Filmtab Tablets 454
Erythromycin Delayed-Release Capsules, USP 456
PCE Dispertab Tablets 510

Erythromycin Estolate (Due to its effects on gastric emptying, pramlintide acetate therapy should not be considered for patients taking drugs that alter gastrointestinal motility and agents that slow the intestinal absorption of nutrients).
No products indexed under this heading.

Erythromycin Ethylsuccinate (Due to its effects on gastric emptying, pramlintide acetate therapy should not be considered for patients taking drugs that alter gastrointestinal motility and agents that slow the intestinal absorption of nutrients). Products include:
E.E.S. 449
EryPed 445

Erythromycin Gluceptate (Due to its effects on gastric emptying, pramlintide acetate therapy should not be considered for patients taking drugs that alter gastrointestinal motility and agents that slow the intestinal absorption of nutrients).
No products indexed under this heading.

Erythromycin Stearate (Due to its effects on gastric emptying, pramlintide acetate therapy should not be considered for patients taking drugs that alter gastrointestinal motility and agents that slow the intestinal absorption of nutrients). Products include:
Erythrocin Stearate Filmtab Tablets 452

Felodipine (Due to its effects on gastric emptying, pramlintide acetate therapy should not be considered for patients taking drugs that alter gastrointestinal motility and agents that slow the intestinal absorption of nutrients). Products include:
Plendil Extended-Release Tablets 651

Fenofibrate (May increase the blood glucose-lowering effect and susceptibility to hypoglycemia, which may necessitate further insulin dose adjustments and particularly close monitoring of blood glucose). Products include:
Antara Capsules 2723
Lofibra Capsules 1217
Tricor Tablets 523
Triglide Tablets 1165

Fentanyl (Due to its effects on gastric emptying, pramlintide acetate therapy should not be considered for patients taking drugs that alter gastrointestinal motility and agents that slow the intestinal absorption of nutrients). Products include:
Duragesic Transdermal System 2448

Fentanyl Citrate (Due to its effects on gastric emptying, pramlintide acetate therapy should not be considered for patients taking drugs that alter gastrointestinal motility and agents that slow the intestinal absorption of nutrients). Products include:
Actiq 993

Fluoxetine (May increase the blood glucose-lowering effect and susceptibility to hypoglycemia, which may necessitate further insulin dose adjustments and particularly close monitoring of blood glucose).
No products indexed under this heading.

Fluoxetine Hydrochloride (May increase the blood glucose-lowering effect and susceptibility to hypoglycemia, which may necessitate further insulin dose adjustments and particularly close monitoring of blood glucose). Products include:
Prozac Pulvules and Liquid 1771
Symbyax Capsules 1788

Fosinopril Sodium (May increase the blood glucose-lowering effect and susceptibility to hypoglycemia, which may necessitate further insulin dose adjustments and particularly close monitoring of blood glucose).
No products indexed under this heading.

Galantamine Hydrobromide (Due to its effects on gastric emptying, pramlintide acetate therapy should not be considered for patients taking drugs that alter gastrointestinal motility and agents that slow the intestinal absorption of nutrients). Products include:
Razadyne ER Extended-Release Capsules 2434
Razadyne 2434

Gemfibrozil (May increase the blood glucose-lowering effect and susceptibility to hypoglycemia, which may necessitate further insulin dose adjustments and particularly close monitoring of blood glucose).
No products indexed under this heading.

Glimepiride (May increase the blood glucose-lowering effect and susceptibility to hypoglycemia, which may necessitate further insulin dose adjustments and particularly close monitoring of blood glucose). Products include:
Amaryl Tablets 2864

Glipizide (May increase the blood glucose-lowering effect and susceptibility to hypoglycemia, which may necessitate further insulin dose adjustments and particularly close monitoring of blood glucose).
No products indexed under this heading.

Glyburide (May increase the blood glucose-lowering effect and susceptibility to hypoglycemia, which may necessitate further insulin dose adjustments and particularly close monitoring of blood glucose).
No products indexed under this heading.

Glycopyrrolate (Due to its effects on gastric emptying, pramlintide acetate therapy should not be considered for patients taking drugs that alter gastrointestinal motility and agents that slow the intestinal absorption of nutrients).
No products indexed under this heading.

Hydrocodone Bitartrate (Due to its effects on gastric emptying, pramlintide acetate therapy should not be considered for patients taking drugs that alter gastrointestinal motility and agents that slow the intestinal absorption of nutrients). Products include:
Hycodan 1104
Hycomine Compound Tablets 1105
Hycotuss Expectorant Syrup 1106
Lortab 3315
Lortab Elixir 3312
Vicodin Tablets 530
Vicodin ES Tablets 531
Vicodin HP Tablets 532
Vicoprofen Tablets 533
Zydone Tablets 1118

Hydrocodone Polistirex (Due to its effects on gastric emptying, pramlintide acetate therapy should not be considered for patients taking drugs that alter gastrointestinal motility and agents that slow the intestinal absorption of nutrients). Products include:
Tussionex Pennkinetic Extended-Release Suspension 3322

Hydromorphone Hydrochloride (Due to its effects on gastric emptying, pramlintide acetate therapy should not be considered for patients taking drugs that alter gastrointestinal motility and agents that slow the intestinal absorption of nutrients). Products include:
Dilaudid 439
Dilaudid Oral Liquid 443
Dilaudid Non-Sterile Powder 439
Dilaudid Rectal Suppositories 439
Dilaudid Tablets 439
Dilaudid Tablets - 8 mg 443
Dilaudid-HP 441

Hyoscyamine (Due to its effects on gastric emptying, pramlintide acetate therapy should not be considered for patients taking drugs that alter gastrointestinal motility and agents that slow the intestinal absorption of nutrients).
No products indexed under this heading.

Hyoscyamine Sulfate (Due to its effects on gastric emptying, pramlintide acetate therapy should not be considered for patients taking drugs that alter gastrointestinal motility and agents that slow the intestinal absorption of nutrients).
No products indexed under this heading.

Imipramine Hydrochloride (Due to its effects on gastric emptying, pramlintide acetate therapy should not be considered for patients taking drugs that alter gastrointestinal motility and agents that slow the intestinal absorption of nutrients).
No products indexed under this heading.

Imipramine Pamoate (Due to its effects on gastric emptying, pramlintide acetate therapy should not be considered for patients taking drugs that alter gastrointestinal motility and agents that slow the intestinal absorption of nutrients).
No products indexed under this heading.

Insulin, Human, Zinc Suspension (The addition of any antihyperglycemic agent, such as pramlintide acetate, to an existing regimen of one or more anti-hyperglycemic agents (eg, insulin) may necessitate further insulin dose adjustments and particularly close monitoring of blood glucose). Products include:
Humulin L, 100 Units 1763
Humulin U, 100 Units 1770

Insulin, Human NPH (The addition of any antihyperglycemic agent, such as pramlintide acetate, to an existing regimen of one or more antihyperglycemic agents (eg, insulin) may necessitate further insulin dose

adjustments and particularly close monitoring of blood glucose). Products include:

- Humulin N, 100 Units **1764**
- Humulin N Pen **1765**
- Novolin N Human Insulin 10 ml Vials **2322**
- Novolin N InnoLet **2322**
- Novolin N PenFill 3 ml Cartridges **2325**
- Novolin R InnoLet **2322**

Insulin, Human Regular (The addition of any antihyperglycemic agent, such as pramlintide acetate, to an existing regimen of one or more anti-hyperglycemic agents (eg, insulin) may necessitate further insulin dose adjustments and particularly close monitoring of blood glucose). Products include:

- Humulin R (U-500) **1768**
- Humulin R, 100 Units **1767**
- Novolin R Human Insulin 10 ml Vials **2322**
- Novolin R PenFill **2325**

Insulin, Human Regular and Human NPH Mixture (The addition of any antihyperglycemic agent, such as pramlintide acetate, to an existing regimen of one or more anti-hyperglycemic agents (eg, insulin) may necessitate further insulin dose adjustments and particularly close monitoring of blood glucose). Products include:

- Humulin 50/50, 100 Units **1760**
- Humulin 70/30 Pen **1761**
- Novolin 70/30 Human Insulin 10 ml Vials **2321**
- Novolin 70/30 InnoLet **2322**
- Novolin 70/30 PenFill 3 ml Cartridges **2325**

Insulin, NPH (The addition of any antihyperglycemic agent, such as pramlintide acetate, to an existing regimen of one or more anti-hyperglycemic agents (eg, insulin) may necessitate further insulin dose adjustments and particularly close monitoring of blood glucose).

No products indexed under this heading.

Insulin, Regular (The addition of any antihyperglycemic agent, such as pramlintide acetate, to an existing regimen of one or more anti-hyperglycemic agents (eg, insulin) may necessitate further insulin dose adjustments and particularly close monitoring of blood glucose).

No products indexed under this heading.

Insulin, Zinc Crystals (The addition of any antihyperglycemic agent, such as pramlintide acetate, to an existing regimen of one or more anti-hyperglycemic agents (eg, insulin) may necessitate further insulin dose adjustments and particularly close monitoring of blood glucose).

No products indexed under this heading.

Insulin, Zinc Suspension (The addition of any antihyperglycemic agent, such as pramlintide acetate, to an existing regimen of one or more anti-hyperglycemic agents (eg, insulin) may necessitate further insulin dose adjustments and particularly close monitoring of blood glucose).

No products indexed under this heading.

Insulin Aspart, Human Regular (The addition of any antihyperglycemic agent, such as pramlintide acetate, to an existing regimen of one or more anti-hyperglycemic agents (eg, insulin) may necessitate further insulin dose adjustments and particularly close monitoring of blood glucose). Products include:

- NovoLog Injection **2326**

Insulin glargine (The addition of any antihyperglycemic agent, such as pramlintide acetate, to an existing regimen of one or more anti-hyperglycemic agents (eg, insulin) may necessitate further insulin dose adjustments and particularly close monitoring of blood glucose). Products include:

- Lantus Injection **2925**

Insulin Lispro, Human (The addition of any antihyperglycemic agent, such as pramlintide acetate, to an existing regimen of one or more anti-hyperglycemic agents (eg, insulin) may necessitate further insulin dose adjustments and particularly close monitoring of blood glucose). Products include:

- Humalog-Pen **1751**
- Humalog Mix 75/25-Pen **1754**

Insulin Lispro Protamine, Human (The addition of any antihyperglycemic agent, such as pramlintide acetate, to an existing regimen of one or more anti-hyperglycemic agents (eg, insulin) may necessitate further insulin dose adjustments and particularly close monitoring of blood glucose). Products include:

- Humalog Mix 75/25-Pen **1754**

Ipratropium Bromide (Due to its effects on gastric emptying, pramlintide acetate therapy should not be considered for patients taking drugs that alter gastrointestinal motility and agents that slow the intestinal absorption of nutrients). Products include:

- Atrovent HFA Inhalation Aerosol **872**
- Atrovent Inhalation Solution **868**
- Atrovent Nasal Spray 0.03% **869**
- Atrovent Nasal Spray 0.06% **870**
- Combivent Inhalation Aerosol **878**
- DuoNeb Inhalation Solution **1058**

Isocarboxazid (May increase the blood glucose-lowering effect and susceptibility to hypoglycemia, which may necessitate further insulin dose adjustments and particularly close monitoring of blood glucose).

No products indexed under this heading.

Isoetharine (Due to its effects on gastric emptying, pramlintide acetate therapy should not be considered for patients taking drugs that alter gastrointestinal motility and agents that slow the intestinal absorption of nutrients).

No products indexed under this heading.

Isoproterenol Hydrochloride (Due to its effects on gastric emptying, pramlintide acetate therapy should not be considered for patients taking drugs that alter gastrointestinal motility and agents that slow the intestinal absorption of nutrients).

No products indexed under this heading.

Isoproterenol Sulfate (Due to its effects on gastric emptying, pramlintide acetate therapy should not be considered for patients taking drugs that alter gastrointestinal motility and agents that slow the intestinal absorption of nutrients).

No products indexed under this heading.

Isradipine (Due to its effects on gastric emptying, pramlintide acetate therapy should not be considered for patients taking drugs that alter gastrointestinal motility and agents that slow the intestinal absorption of nutrients). Products include:

- DynaCirc CR Tablets **2726**

Levalbuterol Hydrochloride (Due to its effects on gastric emptying, pramlintide acetate therapy should not be considered for patients taking drugs that alter gastrointestinal motility and agents that slow the intestinal absorption of nutrients). Products include:

- Xopenex Inhalation Solution **3143**
- Xopenex Inhalation Solution Concentrate **3147**

Levorphanol Tartrate (Due to its effects on gastric emptying, pramlintide acetate therapy should not be considered for patients taking drugs that alter gastrointestinal motility and agents that slow the intestinal absorption of nutrients).

No products indexed under this heading.

Lisinopril (May increase the blood glucose-lowering effect and susceptibility to hypoglycemia, which may necessitate further insulin dose adjustments and particularly close monitoring of blood glucose). Products include:

- Prinivil Tablets **2029**
- Prinzide Tablets **2033**
- Zestoretic Tablets **701**
- Zestril Tablets **704**

Magnesium Salicylate (May increase the blood glucose-lowering effect and susceptibility to hypoglycemia, which may necessitate further insulin dose adjustments and particularly close monitoring of blood glucose).

No products indexed under this heading.

Maprotiline Hydrochloride (Due to its effects on gastric emptying, pramlintide acetate therapy should not be considered for patients taking drugs that alter gastrointestinal motility and agents that slow the intestinal absorption of nutrients).

No products indexed under this heading.

Mepenzolate Bromide (Due to its effects on gastric emptying, pramlintide acetate therapy should not be considered for patients taking drugs that alter gastrointestinal motility and agents that slow the intestinal absorption of nutrients).

No products indexed under this heading.

Meperidine Hydrochloride (Due to its effects on gastric emptying, pramlintide acetate therapy should not be considered for patients taking drugs that alter gastrointestinal motility and agents that slow the intestinal absorption of nutrients).

No products indexed under this heading.

Metaproterenol Sulfate (Due to its effects on gastric emptying, pramlintide acetate therapy should not be considered for patients taking drugs that alter gastrointestinal motility and agents that slow the intestinal absorption of nutrients). Products include:

- Alupent Inhalation Aerosol **858**

Metformin Hydrochloride (May increase the blood glucose-lowering effect and susceptibility to hypoglycemia, which may necessitate further insulin dose adjustments and particularly close monitoring of blood glucose). Products include:

- ActoPlus Met Tablets **3219**
- Avandamet Tablets **1343**
- Fortamet Extended-Release Tablets **1156**

Methadone Hydrochloride (Due to its effects on gastric emptying, pramlintide acetate therapy should not be considered for patients taking drugs that alter gastrointestinal motility and agents that slow the intestinal absorption of nutrients).

No products indexed under this heading.

Methdilazine Hydrochloride (Due to its effects on gastric emptying, pramlintide acetate therapy should not be considered for patients taking drugs that alter gastrointestinal motility and agents that slow the intestinal absorption of nutrients).

No products indexed under this heading.

Metoclopramide Hydrochloride (Due to its effects on gastric emptying, pramlintide acetate therapy should not be considered for patients taking drugs that alter gastrointestinal motility and agents that slow the intestinal absorption of nutrients).

No products indexed under this heading.

Mibefradil Dihydrochloride (Due to its effects on gastric emptying, pramlintide acetate therapy should not be considered for patients taking drugs that alter gastrointestinal motility and agents that slow the intestinal absorption of nutrients).

No products indexed under this heading.

Miglitol (Due to its effects on gastric emptying, pramlintide acetate therapy should not be considered for patients taking drugs that slow the intestinal absorption of nutrients (eg, alpha-glucosidase inhibitors)).

No products indexed under this heading.

Moclobemide (May increase the blood glucose-lowering effect and susceptibility to hypoglycemia, which may necessitate further insulin dose adjustments and particularly close monitoring of blood glucose).

No products indexed under this heading.

Moexipril Hydrochloride (May increase the blood glucose-lowering effect and susceptibility to hypoglycemia, which may necessitate further insulin dose adjustments and particularly close monitoring of blood glucose). Products include:

- Uniretic Tablets **3114**
- Univasc Tablets **3118**

Morphine Sulfate (Due to its effects on gastric emptying, pramlintide acetate therapy should not be considered for patients taking drugs that alter gastrointestinal motility and agents that slow the intestinal absorption of nutrients). Products include:

- Avinza Capsules **1714**
- Kadian Capsules **572**
- MS Contin Tablets **2703**

Neostigmine Bromide (Due to its effects on gastric emptying, pramlintide acetate therapy should not be considered for patients taking drugs that alter gastrointestinal motility and agents that slow the intestinal absorption of nutrients).
No products indexed under this heading.

Neostigmine Methylsulfate (Due to its effects on gastric emptying, pramlintide acetate therapy should not be considered for patients taking drugs that alter gastrointestinal motility and agents that slow the intestinal absorption of nutrients).
No products indexed under this heading.

Nicardipine Hydrochloride (Due to its effects on gastric emptying, pramlintide acetate therapy should not be considered for patients taking drugs that alter gastrointestinal motility and agents that slow the intestinal absorption of nutrients). Products include:
Cardene I.V. 1129

Nifedipine (Due to its effects on gastric emptying, pramlintide acetate therapy should not be considered for patients taking drugs that alter gastrointestinal motility and agents that slow the intestinal absorption of nutrients). Products include:
Adalat CC Tablets 2978

Nimodipine (Due to its effects on gastric emptying, pramlintide acetate therapy should not be considered for patients taking drugs that alter gastrointestinal motility and agents that slow the intestinal absorption of nutrients). Products include:
Nimotop Capsules 774

Nisoldipine (Due to its effects on gastric emptying, pramlintide acetate therapy should not be considered for patients taking drugs that alter gastrointestinal motility and agents that slow the intestinal absorption of nutrients). Products include:
Sular Tablets 1163

Nortriptyline Hydrochloride (Due to its effects on gastric emptying, pramlintide acetate therapy should not be considered for patients taking drugs that alter gastrointestinal motility and agents that slow the intestinal absorption of nutrients).
No products indexed under this heading.

Octreotide Acetate (Due to its effects on gastric emptying, pramlintide acetate therapy should not be considered for patients taking drugs that alter gastrointestinal motility and agents that slow the intestinal absorption of nutrients). Products include:
Sandostatin Injection 2263
Sandostatin LAR Depot 2264

Oxybutynin Chloride (Due to its effects on gastric emptying, pramlintide acetate therapy should not be considered for patients taking drugs that alter gastrointestinal motility and agents that slow the intestinal absorption of nutrients). Products include:
Ditropan XL Extended Release Tablets 2391

Oxycodone Hydrochloride (Due to its effects on gastric emptying, pramlintide acetate therapy should not be considered for patients taking drugs that alter gastrointestinal motility and agents that slow the intestinal absorption of nutrients). Products include:
Combunox Tablets 1183
OxyContin Tablets 2699
OxyFast Oral Concentrate Solution 2704
OxyIR Capsules 2704
Percocet Tablets 1114
Percodan Tablets 1115

Oxyphenonium Bromide (Due to its effects on gastric emptying, pramlintide acetate therapy should not be considered for patients taking drugs that alter gastrointestinal motility and agents that slow the intestinal absorption of nutrients).
No products indexed under this heading.

Pargyline Hydrochloride (May increase the blood glucose-lowering effect and susceptibility to hypoglycemia, which may necessitate further insulin dose adjustments and particularly close monitoring of blood glucose).
No products indexed under this heading.

Pentoxifylline (May increase the blood glucose-lowering effect and susceptibility to hypoglycemia, which may necessitate further insulin dose adjustments and particularly close monitoring of blood glucose).
No products indexed under this heading.

Pergolide Mesylate (Due to its effects on gastric emptying, pramlintide acetate therapy should not be considered for patients taking drugs that alter gastrointestinal motility and agents that slow the intestinal absorption of nutrients). Products include:
Permax Tablets 3357

Perindopril Erbumine (May increase the blood glucose-lowering effect and susceptibility to hypoglycemia, which may necessitate further insulin dose adjustments and particularly close monitoring of blood glucose). Products include:
Aceon Tablets (2 mg, 4 mg, 8 mg).. 3191

Phenelzine Sulfate (May increase the blood glucose-lowering effect and susceptibility to hypoglycemia, which may necessitate further insulin dose adjustments and particularly close monitoring of blood glucose).
No products indexed under this heading.

Pioglitazone Hydrochloride (May increase the blood glucose-lowering effect and susceptibility to hypoglycemia, which may necessitate further insulin dose adjustments and particularly close monitoring of blood glucose). Products include:
ActoPlus Met Tablets 3219
Actos Tablets 3224

Pirbuterol Acetate (Due to its effects on gastric emptying, pramlintide acetate therapy should not be considered for patients taking drugs that alter gastrointestinal motility and agents that slow the intestinal absorption of nutrients). Products include:
Maxair Autohaler 1820

Pramipexole Dihydrochloride (Due to its effects on gastric emptying, pramlintide acetate therapy should not be considered for patients taking drugs that alter gastrointestinal motility and agents that slow the intestinal absorption of nutrients). Products include:
Mirapex Tablets 889

Procainamide Hydrochloride (Due to its effects on gastric emptying, pramlintide acetate therapy should not be considered for patients taking drugs that alter gastrointestinal motility and agents that slow the intestinal absorption of nutrients).
No products indexed under this heading.

Procarbazine Hydrochloride (May increase the blood glucose-lowering effect and susceptibility to hypoglycemia, which may necessitate further insulin dose adjustments and particularly close monitoring of blood glucose). Products include:
Matulane Capsules 3188

Procyclidine Hydrochloride (Due to its effects on gastric emptying, pramlintide acetate therapy should not be considered for patients taking drugs that alter gastrointestinal motility and agents that slow the intestinal absorption of nutrients).
No products indexed under this heading.

Promethazine Hydrochloride (Due to its effects on gastric emptying, pramlintide acetate therapy should not be considered for patients taking drugs that alter gastrointestinal motility and agents that slow the intestinal absorption of nutrients). Products include:
Phenergan 3438

Propantheline Bromide (Due to its effects on gastric emptying, pramlintide acetate therapy should not be considered for patients taking drugs that alter gastrointestinal motility and agents that slow the intestinal absorption of nutrients).
No products indexed under this heading.

Propoxyphene Hydrochloride (May increase the blood glucose-lowering effect and susceptibility to hypoglycemia, which may necessitate further insulin dose adjustments and particularly close monitoring of blood glucose).
No products indexed under this heading.

Propoxyphene Napsylate (May increase the blood glucose-lowering effect and susceptibility to hypoglycemia, which may necessitate further insulin dose adjustments and particularly close monitoring of blood glucose). Products include:
Darvocet A 500 Tablets 3497

Protriptyline Hydrochloride (Due to its effects on gastric emptying, pramlintide acetate therapy should not be considered for patients taking drugs that alter gastrointestinal motility and agents that slow the intestinal absorption of nutrients). Products include:
Vivactil Tablets 2350

Pyridostigmine Bromide (Due to its effects on gastric emptying, pramlintide acetate therapy should not be considered for patients taking drugs that alter gastrointestinal motility and agents that slow the intestinal absorption of nutrients).
No products indexed under this heading.

Pyrilamine Maleate (Due to its effects on gastric emptying, pramlintide acetate therapy should not be considered for patients taking drugs that alter gastrointestinal motility and agents that slow the intestinal absorption of nutrients).
No products indexed under this heading.

Pyrilamine Tannate (Due to its effects on gastric emptying, pramlintide acetate therapy should not be considered for patients taking drugs that alter gastrointestinal motility and agents that slow the intestinal absorption of nutrients).
No products indexed under this heading.

Quinapril Hydrochloride (May increase the blood glucose-lowering effect and susceptibility to hypoglycemia, which may necessitate further insulin dose adjustments and particularly close monitoring of blood glucose).
No products indexed under this heading.

Quinidine Gluconate (Due to its effects on gastric emptying, pramlintide acetate therapy should not be considered for patients taking drugs that alter gastrointestinal motility and agents that slow the intestinal absorption of nutrients).
No products indexed under this heading.

Quinidine Polygalacturonate (Due to its effects on gastric emptying, pramlintide acetate therapy should not be considered for patients taking drugs that alter gastrointestinal motility and agents that slow the intestinal absorption of nutrients).
No products indexed under this heading.

Quinidine Sulfate (Due to its effects on gastric emptying, pramlintide acetate therapy should not be considered for patients taking drugs that alter gastrointestinal motility and agents that slow the intestinal absorption of nutrients).
No products indexed under this heading.

Ramipril (May increase the blood glucose-lowering effect and susceptibility to hypoglycemia, which may necessitate further insulin dose adjustments and particularly close monitoring of blood glucose). Products include:
Altace Capsules 1673

Remifentanil Hydrochloride (Due to its effects on gastric emptying, pramlintide acetate therapy should not be considered for patients taking drugs that alter gastrointestinal motility and agents that slow the intestinal absorption of nutrients).
No products indexed under this heading.

Repaglinide (May increase the blood glucose-lowering effect and susceptibility to hypoglycemia, which may necessitate further insulin dose adjustments and particularly close monitoring of blood glucose). Products include:
Prandin Tablets (0.5, 1, and 2 mg).. 2337

Rivastigmine Tartrate (Due to its effects on gastric emptying, pramlintide acetate therapy should not be considered for patients taking drugs that alter gastrointestinal motility

IMPORTANT NOTE: Always consult each drug listing in the patient's regimen for possible interactions.

and agents that slow the intestinal absorption of nutrients). Products include:

Exelon Capsules 2204

Ropinirole Hydrochloride (Due to its effects on gastric emptying, pramlintide acetate therapy should not be considered for patients taking drugs that alter gastrointestinal motility and agents that slow the intestinal absorption of nutrients). Products include:

Requip Tablets 1528

Rosiglitazone Maleate (May increase the blood glucose-lowering effect and susceptibility to hypoglycemia, which may necessitate further insulin dose adjustments and particularly close monitoring of blood glucose). Products include:

Avandamet Tablets 1343
Avandia Tablets 1348

Salmeterol Xinafoate (Due to its effects on gastric emptying, pramlintide acetate therapy should not be considered for patients taking drugs that alter gastrointestinal motility and agents that slow the intestinal absorption of nutrients). Products include:

Advair Diskus 100/50 1291
Advair Diskus 250/50 1291
Advair Diskus 500/50 1291
Serevent Diskus 1540

Salsalate (May increase the blood glucose-lowering effect and susceptibility to hypoglycemia, which may necessitate further insulin dose adjustments and particularly close monitoring of blood glucose).

No products indexed under this heading.

Scopolamine (Due to its effects on gastric emptying, pramlintide acetate therapy should not be considered for patients taking drugs that alter gastrointestinal motility and agents that slow the intestinal absorption of nutrients). Products include:

Transderm Scōp Transdermal Therapeutic System 2166

Scopolamine Hydrobromide (Due to its effects on gastric emptying, pramlintide acetate therapy should not be considered for patients taking drugs that alter gastrointestinal motility and agents that slow the intestinal absorption of nutrients).

No products indexed under this heading.

Selegiline Hydrochloride (May increase the blood glucose-lowering effect and susceptibility to hypoglycemia, which may necessitate further insulin dose adjustments and particularly close monitoring of blood glucose). Products include:

Eldepryl Capsules 3209

Spirapril Hydrochloride (May increase the blood glucose-lowering effect and susceptibility to hypoglycemia, which may necessitate further insulin dose adjustments and particularly close monitoring of blood glucose).

No products indexed under this heading.

Sucralfate (Due to its effects on gastric emptying, pramlintide acetate therapy should not be considered for patients taking drugs that alter gastrointestinal motility and agents that slow the intestinal absorption of nutrients). Products include:

Carafate Suspension 727
Carafate Tablets 728

Sufentanil Citrate (Due to its effects on gastric emptying, pramlintide acetate therapy should not be considered for patients taking drugs that alter gastrointestinal motility and agents that slow the intestinal absorption of nutrients).

No products indexed under this heading.

Sulfamethoxazole (May increase the blood glucose-lowering effect and susceptibility to hypoglycemia, which may necessitate further insulin dose adjustments and particularly close monitoring of blood glucose).

No products indexed under this heading.

Sulfisoxazole (May increase the blood glucose-lowering effect and susceptibility to hypoglycemia, which may necessitate further insulin dose adjustments and particularly close monitoring of blood glucose).

No products indexed under this heading.

Sulfisoxazole Acetyl (May increase the blood glucose-lowering effect and susceptibility to hypoglycemia, which may necessitate further insulin dose adjustments and particularly close monitoring of blood glucose).

No products indexed under this heading.

Sulfisoxazole Diolamine (May increase the blood glucose-lowering effect and susceptibility to hypoglycemia, which may necessitate further insulin dose adjustments and particularly close monitoring of blood glucose).

No products indexed under this heading.

Tacrine Hydrochloride (Due to its effects on gastric emptying, pramlintide acetate therapy should not be considered for patients taking drugs that alter gastrointestinal motility and agents that slow the intestinal absorption of nutrients).

No products indexed under this heading.

Terbutaline Sulfate (Due to its effects on gastric emptying, pramlintide acetate therapy should not be considered for patients taking drugs that alter gastrointestinal motility and agents that slow the intestinal absorption of nutrients).

No products indexed under this heading.

Tolazamide (May increase the blood glucose-lowering effect and susceptibility to hypoglycemia, which may necessitate further insulin dose adjustments and particularly close monitoring of blood glucose).

No products indexed under this heading.

Tolbutamide (May increase the blood glucose-lowering effect and susceptibility to hypoglycemia, which may necessitate further insulin dose adjustments and particularly close monitoring of blood glucose).

No products indexed under this heading.

Tolterodine Tartrate (Due to its effects on gastric emptying, pramlintide acetate therapy should not be considered for patients taking drugs that alter gastrointestinal motility and agents that slow the intestinal absorption of nutrients). Products include:

Detrol Tablets 2626
Detrol LA Capsules 2629

Trandolapril (May increase the blood glucose-lowering effect and susceptibility to hypoglycemia, which may necessitate further insulin dose adjustments and particularly close monitoring of blood glucose). Products include:

Mavik Tablets 482
Tarka Tablets 519

Tranylcypromine Sulfate (May increase the blood glucose-lowering effect and susceptibility to hypoglycemia, which may necessitate further insulin dose adjustments and particularly close monitoring of blood glucose). Products include:

Parnate Tablets 1499

Tridihexethyl Chloride (Due to its effects on gastric emptying, pramlintide acetate therapy should not be considered for patients taking drugs that alter gastrointestinal motility and agents that slow the intestinal absorption of nutrients).

No products indexed under this heading.

Trihexyphenidyl Hydrochloride (Due to its effects on gastric emptying, pramlintide acetate therapy should not be considered for patients taking drugs that alter gastrointestinal motility and agents that slow the intestinal absorption of nutrients).

No products indexed under this heading.

Trimeprazine Tartrate (Due to its effects on gastric emptying, pramlintide acetate therapy should not be considered for patients taking drugs that alter gastrointestinal motility and agents that slow the intestinal absorption of nutrients).

No products indexed under this heading.

Trimipramine Maleate (Due to its effects on gastric emptying, pramlintide acetate therapy should not be considered for patients taking drugs that alter gastrointestinal motility and agents that slow the intestinal absorption of nutrients). Products include:

Surmontil Capsules 2347

Tripelennamine Hydrochloride (Due to its effects on gastric emptying, pramlintide acetate therapy should not be considered for patients taking drugs that alter gastrointestinal motility and agents that slow the intestinal absorption of nutrients).

No products indexed under this heading.

Triprolidine Hydrochloride (Due to its effects on gastric emptying, pramlintide acetate therapy should not be considered for patients taking drugs that alter gastrointestinal motility and agents that slow the intestinal absorption of nutrients).

No products indexed under this heading.

Troglitazone (May increase the blood glucose-lowering effect and susceptibility to hypoglycemia, which may necessitate further insulin dose adjustments and particularly close monitoring of blood glucose).

No products indexed under this heading.

Verapamil Hydrochloride (Due to its effects on gastric emptying, pramlintide acetate therapy should not be considered for patients taking drugs that alter gastrointestinal motility and agents that slow the intestinal absorption of nutrients). Products include:

Covera-HS Tablets 3135
Tarka Tablets 519
Verelan PM Capsules 3120

SYMMETREL SYRUP

(Amantadine Hydrochloride) 1115

See Symmetrel Tablets

SYMMETREL TABLETS

(Amantadine Hydrochloride) 1115

May interact with anticholinergics, central nervous system stimulants, quinidine, and certain other agents. Compounds in these categories include:

Amphetamine Resins (Co-administration with central nervous system stimulants requires careful observation).

No products indexed under this heading.

Atropine Sulfate (Agents with anticholinergic properties may potentiate the anticholinergic-like side effects of amantadine).

No products indexed under this heading.

Belladonna Alkaloids (Agents with anticholinergic properties may potentiate the anticholinergic-like side effects of amantadine). Products include:

Hyland's Teething Tablets .... ■736

Benztropine Mesylate (Agents with anticholinergic properties may potentiate the anticholinergic-like side effects of amantadine). Products include:

Cogentin Injection 1903

Biperiden Hydrochloride (Agents with anticholinergic properties may potentiate the anticholinergic-like side effects of amantadine).

No products indexed under this heading.

Clidinium Bromide (Agents with anticholinergic properties may potentiate the anticholinergic-like side effects of amantadine).

No products indexed under this heading.

Dextroamphetamine Sulfate (Co-administration with central nervous system stimulants requires careful observation). Products include:

Adderall Tablets 3168
Adderall XR Capsules 3169
Dexedrine 1386
DextroStat Tablets 3177

Dicyclomine Hydrochloride (Agents with anticholinergic properties may potentiate the anticholinergic-like side effects of amantadine). Products include:

Bentyl Capsules 724
Bentyl Injection 724
Bentyl Syrup 724
Bentyl Tablets 724

Glycopyrrolate (Agents with anticholinergic properties may potentiate the anticholinergic-like side effects of amantadine).

No products indexed under this heading.

Hydrochlorothiazide (Co-administration with triamterene-hydrochlorothiazide capsules has resulted in a higher plasma amantadine concentration in a patient with Parkinsonism; it is not known which components of triamterene-

hydrochlorothiazide capsules contributed to this interaction). Products include:

Aldoril Tablets **1884**
Atacand HCT **637**
Avalide Tablets **2889**
Avalide Tablets **922**
Benicar HCT Tablets **2852**
Diovan HCT Tablets **2195**
Dyazide Capsules **1389**
Hyzaar **1964**
Lotensin HCT Tablets **2235**
Maxzide **2150**
Micardis HCT Tablets **886**
Moduretic Tablets **2003**
Prinzide Tablets **2033**
Teveten HCT Tablets **1710**
Timolide Tablets **2056**
Uniretic Tablets **3114**
Vaseretic Tablets **2073**
Zestoretic Tablets **701**

Hyoscyamine (Agents with anticholinergic properties may potentiate the anticholinergic-like side effects of amantadine).
No products indexed under this heading.

Hyoscyamine Sulfate (Agents with anticholinergic properties may potentiate the anticholinergic-like side effects of amantadine).
No products indexed under this heading.

Ipratropium Bromide (Agents with anticholinergic properties may potentiate the anticholinergic-like side effects of amantadine). Products include:

Atrovent HFA Inhalation Aerosol **872**
Atrovent Inhalation Solution **868**
Atrovent Nasal Spray 0.03% **869**
Atrovent Nasal Spray 0.06% **870**
Combivent Inhalation Aerosol **878**
DuoNeb Inhalation Solution **1058**

Mepenzolate Bromide (Agents with anticholinergic properties may potentiate the anticholinergic-like side effects of amantadine).
No products indexed under this heading.

Methamphetamine Hydrochloride (Co-administration with central nervous system stimulants requires careful observation). Products include:

Desoxyn Tablets, USP **2482**

Methylphenidate Hydrochloride (Co-administration with central nervous system stimulants requires careful observation). Products include:

Concerta Extended-Release Tablets **1828**
Metadate CD Capsules **3316**
Ritalin **2254**
Ritalin LA Capsules **2255**

Oxybutynin Chloride (Agents with anticholinergic properties may potentiate the anticholinergic-like side effects of amantadine). Products include:

Ditropan XL Extended Release Tablets **2391**

Pemoline (Co-administration with central nervous system stimulants requires careful observation).
No products indexed under this heading.

Procyclidine Hydrochloride (Agents with anticholinergic properties may potentiate the anticholinergic-like side effects of amantadine).
No products indexed under this heading.

Propantheline Bromide (Agents with anticholinergic properties may potentiate the anticholinergic-like side effects of amantadine).
No products indexed under this heading.

Quinidine (Co-administration of quinidine with amantadine has been shown to reduce the renal clearance of amantadine by about 30%).
No products indexed under this heading.

Quinidine Gluconate (Co-administration of quinidine with amantadine has been shown to reduce the renal clearance of amantadine by about 30%).
No products indexed under this heading.

Quinidine Hydrochloride (Co-administration of quinidine with amantadine has been shown to reduce the renal clearance of amantadine by about 30%).
No products indexed under this heading.

Quinidine Polygalacturonate (Co-administration of quinidine with amantadine has been shown to reduce the renal clearance of amantadine by about 30%).
No products indexed under this heading.

Quinidine Sulfate (Co-administration of quinidine with amantadine has been shown to reduce the renal clearance of amantadine by about 30%).
No products indexed under this heading.

Quinine (Co-administration of quinine with amantadine has been shown to reduce the renal clearance of amantadine).
No products indexed under this heading.

Scopolamine (Agents with anticholinergic properties may potentiate the anticholinergic-like side effects of amantadine). Products include:

Transderm Scōp Transdermal Therapeutic System **2166**

Scopolamine Hydrobromide (Agents with anticholinergic properties may potentiate the anticholinergic-like side effects of amantadine).
No products indexed under this heading.

Thioridazine Hydrochloride (Co-administration has been reported to worsen the tremor in elderly patients with Parkinson's disease). Products include:

Thioridazine Hydrochloride Tablets **2122**

Tolterodine Tartrate (Agents with anticholinergic properties may potentiate the anticholinergic-like side effects of amantadine). Products include:

Detrol Tablets **2626**
Detrol LA Capsules **2629**

Triamterene (Co-administration with triamterene-hydrochlorothiazide capsules has resulted in a higher plasma amantadine concentration in a patient with Parkinsonism; it is not known which components of triamterene-hydrochlorothiazide capsules contributed to this interaction). Products include:

Dyazide Capsules **1389**
Dyrenium Capsules **3390**
Maxzide **2150**

Tridihexethyl Chloride (Agents with anticholinergic properties may potentiate the anticholinergic-like side effects of amantadine).
No products indexed under this heading.

Trihexyphenidyl Hydrochloride (Agents with anticholinergic properties may potentiate the anticholinergic-like side effects of amantadine).
No products indexed under this heading.

Food Interactions

Alcohol (May increase the potential for CNS effects such as dizziness, confusion, light-headedness and orthostatic hypotension; avoid excessive alcohol usage).

SYNAGIS INTRAMUSCULAR POWDER
(Palivizumab) **1868**
None cited in PDR database.

SYNAGIS INTRAMUSCULAR SOLUTION
(Palivizumab) **1868**
None cited in PDR database.

SYNERCID I.V.
(Dalfopristin, Quinupristin) **1690**
May interact with:

Cyclosporine (In vitro drug interaction studies have demonstrated that Synercid significantly inhibits cytochrome P450 3A4 metabolism of cyclosporine A). Products include:

Gengraf Capsules **458**
Neoral Soft Gelatin Capsules **2247**
Neoral Oral Solution **2247**
Restasis Ophthalmic Emulsion **570**
Sandimmune **2259**

Midazolam Hydrochloride (In vitro drug interaction studies have demonstrated that Synercid significantly inhibits cytochrome P450 3A4 metabolism of midazolam).
No products indexed under this heading.

Nifedipine (In vitro drug interaction studies have demonstrated that Synercid significantly inhibits cytochrome P450 3A4 metabolism of nifedipine). Products include:

Adalat CC Tablets **2978**

Terfenadine (In vitro drug interaction studies have demonstrated that Synercid significantly inhibits cytochrome P450 3A4 metabolism of terfenadine).
No products indexed under this heading.

SYNERGYDEFENSE CAPSULES
(Herbals, Multiple) **760**
None cited in PDR database.

SYNTHROID TABLETS
(Levothyroxine Sodium) **515**
May interact with androgens, antithyroid agents, beta blockers, oral anticoagulants, cytokines, dopamine agonists, estrogens, glucocorticoids, cardiac glycosides, hepatic microsomal enzyme inducers, oral hypoglycemic agents, insulin, lithium preparations, phenytoin, radiographic iodinated contrast media, salicylates, sulfonamides, sulfonylureas, sympathomimetics, thiazides, tricyclic antidepressants, xanthines, and certain other agents. Compounds in these categories include:

Acarbose (Requirements of oral antidiabetic agents may be reduced in hypothyroid patients with diabetes and may be subsequently increased with initiation of thyroid hormone therapy). Products include:

Precose Tablets **776**

Acebutolol Hydrochloride (Alters thyroid hormone or TSH levels; actions of some beta blockers may be impaired when hypothyroid patients become euthyroid).
No products indexed under this heading.

Albuterol (Possible increased risk of coronary insufficiency in patients with coronary artery disease). Products include:

Proventil Inhalation Aerosol **3067**

Albuterol Sulfate (Possible increased risk of coronary insufficiency in patients with coronary artery disease). Products include:

AccuNeb Inhalation Solution **1055**
Combivent Inhalation Aerosol **878**
DuoNeb Inhalation Solution **1058**
Proventil Inhalation Solution 0.083% **3069**
Proventil HFA Inhalation Aerosol **3071**
Ventolin HFA Inhalation Aerosol **1576**
VoSpire Extended-Release Tablets ... **2352**

Aldesleukin (Cytokines have been reported to induce both hyperthyroidism or hypothyroidism; dosage adjustment may be necessary). Products include:

Proleukin for Injection **1007**

Aluminum Hydroxide (Binds and decreases absorption of levothyroxine sodium from the gastrointestinal tract). Products include:

Gaviscon Regular Strength Liquid .. **620**
Gaviscon Regular Strength Tablets **619**
Gaviscon Extra Strength Liquid **620**
Gaviscon Extra Strength Tablets **619**
Maalox Max Maximum Strength Antacid/Anti-Gas Liquid **2165**
Maalox Regular Strength Antacid/Antigas Liquid **2164**

Aminoglutethimide (Alters thyroid hormone or TSH levels).
No products indexed under this heading.

Aminophylline (Theophylline clearance may be decreased in hypothyroid patients and return toward normal when euthyroid state is achieved).
No products indexed under this heading.

p-Aminosalicylic Acid (Alters thyroid hormone or TSH levels).
No products indexed under this heading.

Amiodarone Hydrochloride (Amiodarone therapy alone can cause hypothyroidism or hyperthyroidism). Products include:

Pacerone Tablets **3337**

Amitriptyline Hydrochloride (Concurrent use may increase the therapeutic and toxic effects of both drugs; onset of action of tricyclics may be accelerated).
No products indexed under this heading.

Amoxapine (Concurrent use may increase the therapeutic and toxic effects of both drugs; onset of action of tricyclics may be accelerated).
No products indexed under this heading.

Anisindione (The hypoprothrombinemic effect of anticoagulants may be potentiated). Products include:

Miradon Tablets **3056**

Asparaginase (May inhibit levothyroxine sodium binding to serum proteins or alter the concentrations of serum proteins). Products include:
- Elspar for Injection ... 1943

Aspirin (May inhibit levothyroxine sodium binding to serum proteins or alter the concentrations of serum proteins). Products include:
- Aggrenox Capsules ... 855
- Bayer, Aspirin Regimen ... ■ 606
- Bayer Aspirin Tablets ... 3515
- BC Powder ... ■ 612
- BC Allergy Sinus Cold Powder ... ■ 612
- Arthritis Strength BC Powder ... ■ 612
- BC Sinus Cold Powder ... ■ 612
- Ecotrin Enteric Coated Aspirin Low, Regular and Maximum Strength Tablets ... 1627
- Goody's Body Pain Formula Powder ... ■ 621
- Goody's Extra Strength Headache Powder ... ■ 621
- Goody's Extra Strength Pain Relief Tablets ... ■ 621
- Percodan Tablets ... 1115
- St. Joseph 81 mg Aspirin Chewable and Enteric Coated Tablets ... 1841

Aspirin, Enteric Coated (May inhibit levothyroxine sodium binding to serum proteins or alter the concentrations of serum proteins).
No products indexed under this heading.

Aspirin Buffered (May inhibit levothyroxine sodium binding to serum proteins or alter the concentrations of serum proteins).
No products indexed under this heading.

Atenolol (Alters thyroid hormone or TSH levels; actions of some beta blockers may be impaired when hypothyroid patients become euthyroid). Products include:
- Tenormin I.V. Injection ... 698
- Tenormin Tablets ... 695

Bendroflumethiazide (Alters thyroid hormone or TSH levels).
No products indexed under this heading.

Betamethasone Acetate (May inhibit levothyroxine sodium binding to serum proteins or alter the concentrations of serum proteins).
No products indexed under this heading.

Betamethasone Sodium Phosphate (May inhibit levothyroxine sodium binding to serum proteins or alter the concentrations of serum proteins).
No products indexed under this heading.

Betaxolol Hydrochloride (Alters thyroid hormone or TSH levels; actions of some beta blockers may be impaired when hypothyroid patients become euthyroid). Products include:
- Betoptic S Ophthalmic Suspension ... 554

Bisoprolol Fumarate (Alters thyroid hormone or TSH levels; actions of some beta blockers may be impaired when hypothyroid patients become euthyroid).
No products indexed under this heading.

Bromocriptine Mesylate (Alters thyroid hormone or TSH levels).
No products indexed under this heading.

Carbamazepine (Alters thyroid hormone or TSH levels). Products include:
- Carbatrol Capsules ... 3174
- Equetro Extended-Release Capsules ... 3178
- Tegretol/Tegretol-XR ... 2278

Carteolol Hydrochloride (Alters thyroid hormone or TSH levels; actions of some beta blockers may be impaired when hypothyroid patients become euthyroid). Products include:
- Carteolol Hydrochloride Ophthalmic Solution USP, 1% ... ⊙ 246

Chloral Hydrate (Alters thyroid hormone or TSH levels).
No products indexed under this heading.

Chlorothiazide (Alters thyroid hormone or TSH levels). Products include:
- Aldoclor Tablets ... 1881
- Diuril Oral ... 1936

Chlorothiazide Sodium (Alters thyroid hormone or TSH levels). Products include:
- Diuril Sodium Intravenous ... 1934

Chlorotrianisene (Estrogens or estrogen-containing compounds may inhibit levothyroxine sodium binding to serum proteins or alter the concentrations of serum proteins).
No products indexed under this heading.

Chlorpropamide (Alters thyroid hormone or TSH levels; requirements of oral antidiabetic agents may be reduced in hypothyroid patients with diabetes and may be subsequently increased with initiation of thyroid hormone therapy).
No products indexed under this heading.

Cholestyramine (Binds and decreases absorption of levothyroxine sodium from the gastrointestinal tract).
No products indexed under this heading.

Choline Magnesium Trisalicylate (May inhibit levothyroxine sodium binding to serum proteins or alter the concentrations of serum proteins).
No products indexed under this heading.

Clofibrate (May inhibit levothyroxine sodium binding to serum proteins or alter the concentrations of serum proteins).
No products indexed under this heading.

Clomipramine Hydrochloride (Concurrent use may increase the therapeutic and toxic effects of both drugs; onset of action of tricyclics may be accelerated).
No products indexed under this heading.

Colestipol Hydrochloride (Binds and decreases absorption of levothyroxine sodium from the gastrointestinal tract).
No products indexed under this heading.

Cortisone Acetate (May inhibit levothyroxine sodium binding to serum proteins or alter the concentrations of serum proteins).
No products indexed under this heading.

Desipramine Hydrochloride (Concurrent use may increase the therapeutic and toxic effects of both drugs; onset of action of tricyclics may be accelerated).
No products indexed under this heading.

Deslanoside (Therapeutic effects of digitalis glycosides may be reduced; serum digitalis levels may be decreased in hyperthyroidism or when a hypothyroid patient becomes euthyroid).
No products indexed under this heading.

Dexamethasone (May inhibit levothyroxine sodium binding to serum proteins or alter the concentrations of serum proteins). Products include:
- Ciprodex Otic Suspension ... 555
- Decadron Tablets ... 1929
- TobraDex Ophthalmic Ointment ... 558
- TobraDex Ophthalmic Suspension ... 558

Dexamethasone Acetate (May inhibit levothyroxine sodium binding to serum proteins or alter the concentrations of serum proteins).
No products indexed under this heading.

Dexamethasone Sodium Phosphate (May inhibit levothyroxine sodium binding to serum proteins or alter the concentrations of serum proteins). Products include:
- Decadron Phosphate Injection ... 1931

Diatrizoate Meglumine (Alters thyroid hormone or TSH levels).
No products indexed under this heading.

Diatrizoate Sodium (Alters thyroid hormone or TSH levels).
No products indexed under this heading.

Diazepam (Alters thyroid hormone or TSH levels). Products include:
- Diastat Rectal Delivery System ... 3344
- Valium Tablets ... 2822

Dicumarol (The hypoprothrombinemic effect of anticoagulants may be potentiated).
No products indexed under this heading.

Dienestrol (Estrogens or estrogen-containing compounds may inhibit levothyroxine sodium binding to serum proteins or alter the concentrations of serum proteins).
No products indexed under this heading.

Diethylstilbestrol (Estrogens or estrogen-containing compounds may inhibit levothyroxine sodium binding to serum proteins or alter the concentrations of serum proteins).
No products indexed under this heading.

Diflunisal (May inhibit levothyroxine sodium binding to serum proteins or alter the concentrations of serum proteins). Products include:
- Dolobid Tablets ... 1937

Digitalis Glycoside Preparations (Therapeutic effects of digitalis glycosides may be reduced; serum digitalis levels may be decreased in hyperthyroidism or when a hypothyroid patient becomes euthyroid).
No products indexed under this heading.

Digitoxin (Therapeutic effects of digitalis glycosides may be reduced; serum digitalis levels may be decreased in hyperthyroidism or when a hypothyroid patient becomes euthyroid).
No products indexed under this heading.

Digoxin (Therapeutic effects of digitalis glycosides may be reduced; serum digitalis levels may be decreased in hyperthyroidism or when a hypothyroid patient becomes euthyroid). Products include:
- Digitek Tablets ... 2146
- Lanoxicaps Capsules ... 1458
- Lanoxin Injection ... 1462
- Lanoxin Tablets ... 1468
- Lanoxin Injection Pediatric ... 1465

Dobutamine Hydrochloride (Possible increased risk of coronary insufficiency in patients with coronary artery disease).
No products indexed under this heading.

Dopamine Hydrochloride (Alters thyroid hormone or TSH levels).
No products indexed under this heading.

Doxepin Hydrochloride (Concurrent use may increase the therapeutic and toxic effects of both drugs; onset of action of tricyclics may be accelerated).
No products indexed under this heading.

Dyphylline (Theophylline clearance may be decreased in hypothyroid patients and return toward normal when euthyroid state is achieved).
No products indexed under this heading.

Ephedrine Hydrochloride (Possible increased risk of coronary insufficiency in patients with coronary artery disease). Products include:
- Primatene Tablets ... ■ 749

Ephedrine Sulfate (Possible increased risk of coronary insufficiency in patients with coronary artery disease).
No products indexed under this heading.

Ephedrine Tannate (Possible increased risk of coronary insufficiency in patients with coronary artery disease).
No products indexed under this heading.

Epinephrine (Possible increased risk of coronary insufficiency in patients with coronary artery disease). Products include:
- EpiPen ... 1061
- Primatene Mist ... ■ 749

Epinephrine Bitartrate (Possible increased risk of coronary insufficiency in patients with coronary artery disease).
No products indexed under this heading.

Epinephrine Hydrochloride (Possible increased risk of coronary insufficiency in patients with coronary artery disease).
No products indexed under this heading.

Esmolol Hydrochloride (Alters thyroid hormone or TSH levels; actions of some beta blockers may be impaired when hypothyroid patients become euthyroid). Products include:
- Brevibloc Concentrate ... 766
- Brevibloc Injection ... 766
- Brevibloc Double Strength Injection ... 766
- Brevibloc Premixed Injection ... 766
- Brevibloc Double Strength Premixed Injection ... 766

Estradiol (Estrogens or estrogen-containing compounds may inhibit levothyroxine sodium binding to serum proteins or alter the concentrations of serum proteins). Products include:
- Activella Tablets ... 2311
- Climara Transdermal System ... 795
- Climara Pro Transdermal System ... 800
- CombiPatch Transdermal System ... 2180
- Estrogel 0.06% ... 3200

(■ Described in PDR For Nonprescription Drugs) (⊙ Described in PDR For Ophthalmic Medicines™)

Menostar Transdermal System 805
Prefest Tablets 1069
Vagifem Tablets 2340
Vivelle Transdermal System 2288
Vivelle-Dot Transdermal System 2293

Estrogens, Conjugated (Estrogens or estrogen-containing compounds may inhibit levothyroxine sodium binding to serum proteins or alter the concentrations of serum proteins). Products include:
Premarin Intravenous 3440
Premarin Tablets 3443
Premarin Vaginal Cream 3449
Premphase Tablets 3452
Prempro Tablets 3452

Estrogens, Esterified (Estrogens or estrogen-containing compounds may inhibit levothyroxine sodium binding to serum proteins or alter the concentrations of serum proteins). Products include:
Estratest Tablets 3196
Estratest H.S. Tablets 3196

Estropipate (Estrogens or estrogen-containing compounds may inhibit levothyroxine sodium binding to serum proteins or alter the concentrations of serum proteins).
No products indexed under this heading.

Ethanol (Alters thyroid hormone or TSH levels).
No products indexed under this heading.

Ethinyl Estradiol (Estrogens or estrogen-containing compounds may inhibit levothyroxine sodium binding to serum proteins or alter the concentrations of serum proteins). Products include:
Alesse-28 Tablets 3392
Lo/Ovral-28 Tablets 3423
NuvaRing 2357
Ortho-Cept Tablets 2395
Ortho-Cyclen/Ortho Tri-Cyclen 2414
Ortho Evra Transdermal System 2402
Ortho Tri-Cyclen Lo Tablets 2421
Seasonale Tablets 1073
Triphasil-28 Tablets 3483
Yasmin 28 Tablets 818

Ethiodized Oil (Alters thyroid hormone or TSH levels).
No products indexed under this heading.

Ethionamide (Alters thyroid hormone or TSH levels). Products include:
Trecator Tablets 3482

Ferrous Sulfate (Binds and decreases absorption of levothyroxine sodium from the gastrointestinal tract). Products include:
Feosol Tablets 1629
Slow Fe Iron Tablets .... ■772
Slow Fe with Folic Acid Tablets .... ■773

Fludrocortisone Acetate (May inhibit levothyroxine sodium binding to serum proteins or alter the concentrations of serum proteins).
No products indexed under this heading.

Fluorouracil (May inhibit levothyroxine sodium binding to serum proteins or alter the concentrations of serum proteins). Products include:
Carac Cream, 0.5% 1048
Efudex 3348

Fluoxymesterone (May inhibit levothyroxine sodium binding to serum proteins or alter the concentrations of serum proteins; alters TSH or thyroid hormone levels).
No products indexed under this heading.

Fosphenytoin Sodium (Alters thyroid hormone or TSH levels).
No products indexed under this heading.

Furosemide (May inhibit levothyroxine sodium binding to serum proteins or alter the concentrations of serum proteins). Products include:
Furosemide Tablets 2117

Gadopentetate Dimeglumine (Alters thyroid hormone or TSH levels).
No products indexed under this heading.

Glimepiride (Alters thyroid hormone or TSH levels; requirements of oral antidiabetic agents may be reduced in hypothyroid patients with diabetes and may be subsequently increased with initiation of thyroid hormone therapy). Products include:
Amaryl Tablets 2864

Glipizide (Alters thyroid hormone or TSH levels; requirements of oral antidiabetic agents may be reduced in hypothyroid patients with diabetes and may be subsequently increased with initiation of thyroid hormone therapy).
No products indexed under this heading.

Glyburide (Alters thyroid hormone or TSH levels; requirements of oral antidiabetic agents may be reduced in hypothyroid patients with diabetes and may be subsequently increased with initiation of thyroid hormone therapy).
No products indexed under this heading.

Heparin Sodium (Alters thyroid hormone or TSH levels).
No products indexed under this heading.

Hydrochlorothiazide (Alters thyroid hormone or TSH levels). Products include:
Aldoril Tablets 1884
Atacand HCT 637
Avalide Tablets 2889
Avalide Tablets 922
Benicar HCT Tablets 2852
Diovan HCT Tablets 2195
Dyazide Capsules 1389
Hyzaar 1964
Lotensin HCT Tablets 2235
Maxzide 2150
Micardis HCT Tablets 886
Moduretic Tablets 2003
Prinzide Tablets 2033
Teveten HCT Tablets 1710
Timolide Tablets 2056
Uniretic Tablets 3114
Vaseretic Tablets 2073
Zestoretic Tablets 701

Hydrocortisone (May inhibit levothyroxine sodium binding to serum proteins or alter the concentrations of serum proteins). Products include:
Cortizone•5 Ointment .... ■699
Cortizone•10 Creme .... ■699
Cortizone•10 Ointment .... ■699
Cortizone•10 Plus Creme .... ■700
Cortizone•10 Maximum Strength Quick Shot Spray .... ■700
Hydrocortone Tablets 1963
Preparation H Hydrocortisone Cream .... ■748

Hydrocortisone Acetate (May inhibit levothyroxine sodium binding to serum proteins or alter the concentrations of serum proteins). Products include:
Analpram-HC 1136
Pramosone 1139
ProctoFoam-HC 3113
Tucks Anti-Itch Ointment .... ■712
U-cort 1% Cream 3289

Hydrocortisone Sodium Phosphate (May inhibit levothyroxine sodium binding to serum proteins or alter the concentrations of serum proteins).
No products indexed under this heading.

Hydrocortisone Sodium Succinate (May inhibit levothyroxine sodium binding to serum proteins or alter the concentrations of serum proteins).
No products indexed under this heading.

Hydroflumethiazide (Alters thyroid hormone or TSH levels).
No products indexed under this heading.

Imipramine Hydrochloride (Concurrent use may increase the therapeutic and toxic effects of both drugs; onset of action of tricyclics may be accelerated).
No products indexed under this heading.

Imipramine Pamoate (Concurrent use may increase the therapeutic and toxic effects of both drugs; onset of action of tricyclics may be accelerated).
No products indexed under this heading.

Insulin, Human, Zinc Suspension (Requirements of insulin may be reduced in hypothyroid patients with diabetes and may be subsequently increased with initiation of thyroid hormone therapy). Products include:
Humulin L, 100 Units 1763
Humulin U, 100 Units 1770

Insulin, Human NPH (Requirements of insulin may be reduced in hypothyroid patients with diabetes and may be subsequently increased with initiation of thyroid hormone therapy). Products include:
Humulin N, 100 Units 1764
Humulin N Pen 1765
Novolin N Human Insulin 10 ml Vials 2322
Novolin N InnoLet 2322
Novolin N PenFill 3 ml Cartridges 2325
Novolin R InnoLet 2322

Insulin, Human Regular (Requirements of insulin may be reduced in hypothyroid patients with diabetes and may be subsequently increased with initiation of thyroid hormone therapy). Products include:
Humulin R (U-500) 1768
Humulin R, 100 Units 1767
Novolin R Human Insulin 10 ml Vials 2322
Novolin R PenFill 2325

Insulin, Human Regular and Human NPH Mixture (Requirements of insulin may be reduced in hypothyroid patients with diabetes and may be subsequently increased with initiation of thyroid hormone therapy). Products include:
Humulin 50/50, 100 Units 1760
Humulin 70/30 Pen 1761
Novolin 70/30 Human Insulin 10 ml Vials 2321
Novolin 70/30 InnoLet 2322
Novolin 70/30 PenFill 3 ml Cartridges 2325

Insulin, NPH (Requirements of insulin may be reduced in hypothyroid patients with diabetes and may be subsequently increased with initiation of thyroid hormone therapy).
No products indexed under this heading.

Insulin, Regular (Requirements of insulin may be reduced in hypothyroid patients with diabetes and may be subsequently increased with initiation of thyroid hormone therapy).
No products indexed under this heading.

Insulin, Zinc Crystals (Requirements of insulin may be reduced in hypothyroid patients with diabetes and may be subsequently increased with initiation of thyroid hormone therapy).
No products indexed under this heading.

Insulin, Zinc Suspension (Requirements of insulin may be reduced in hypothyroid patients with diabetes and may be subsequently increased with initiation of thyroid hormone therapy).
No products indexed under this heading.

Insulin Aspart, Human Regular (Requirements of insulin may be reduced in hypothyroid patients with diabetes and may be subsequently increased with initiation of thyroid hormone therapy). Products include:
NovoLog Injection 2326

Insulin glargine (Requirements of insulin may be reduced in hypothyroid patients with diabetes and may be subsequently increased with initiation of thyroid hormone therapy). Products include:
Lantus Injection 2925

Insulin Lispro, Human (Requirements of insulin may be reduced in hypothyroid patients with diabetes and may be subsequently increased with initiation of thyroid hormone therapy). Products include:
Humalog-Pen 1751
Humalog Mix 75/25-Pen 1754

Insulin Lispro Protamine, Human (Requirements of insulin may be reduced in hypothyroid patients with diabetes and may be subsequently increased with initiation of thyroid hormone therapy). Products include:
Humalog Mix 75/25-Pen 1754

Interferon alfa-2a, Recombinant (Cytokines have been reported to induce both hyperthyroidism or hypothyroidism; dosage adjustment may be necessary). Products include:
Roferon-A Injection 2805

Interferon alfa-2b, Recombinant (Cytokines have been reported to induce both hyperthyroidism or hypothyroidism; dosage adjustment may be necessary). Products include:
Intron A for Injection 3038
Rebetron Combination Therapy 3078

Interferon alfa-N3 (Human Leukocyte Derived) (Cytokines have been reported to induce both hyperthyroidism or hypothyroidism; dosage adjustment may be necessary). Products include:
Alferon N Injection 1640

Interferon Beta-1b (Cytokines have been reported to induce both hyperthyroidism or hypothyroidism; dosage adjustment may be necessary). Products include:
Betaseron for SC Injection 791

Interferon Gamma-1B (Cytokines have been reported to induce both hyperthyroidism or hypothyroidism; dosage adjustment may be necessary). Products include:
Actimmune 1646

Iodamide Meglumine (Alters thyroid hormone or TSH levels).
No products indexed under this heading.

Iodinated Glycerol (Alters thyroid hormone or TSH levels).
No products indexed under this heading.

Iodine, radiolabeled (Uptake of radiolabeled ions may be decreased).
No products indexed under this heading.

Iohexol (Alters thyroid hormone or TSH levels).
No products indexed under this heading.

Iopamidol (Alters thyroid hormone or TSH levels).
No products indexed under this heading.

Iopanoic Acid (Alters thyroid hormone or TSH levels).
No products indexed under this heading.

Iothalamate Meglumine (Alters thyroid hormone or TSH levels).
No products indexed under this heading.

Ioxaglate Meglumine (Alters thyroid hormone or TSH levels).
No products indexed under this heading.

Ioxaglate Sodium (Alters thyroid hormone or TSH levels).
No products indexed under this heading.

Isoproterenol Hydrochloride (Possible increased risk of coronary insufficiency in patients with coronary artery disease).
No products indexed under this heading.

Isoproterenol Sulfate (Possible increased risk of coronary insufficiency in patients with coronary artery disease).
No products indexed under this heading.

Ketamine Hydrochloride (Coadministration produces marked hypertension and tachycardia).
No products indexed under this heading.

Labetalol Hydrochloride (Alters thyroid hormone or TSH levels; actions of some beta blockers may be impaired when hypothyroid patients become euthyroid).
No products indexed under this heading.

Levalbuterol Hydrochloride (Possible increased risk of coronary insufficiency in patients with coronary artery disease). Products include:
Xopenex Inhalation Solution 3143
Xopenex Inhalation Solution Concentrate 3147

Levobunolol Hydrochloride (Alters thyroid hormone or TSH levels; actions of some beta blockers may be impaired when hypothyroid patients become euthyroid).
Products include:
Betagan Ophthalmic Solution, USP .... ⊙ 217

Levodopa (Alters thyroid hormone or TSH levels). Products include:
Parcopa Orally Disintegrating Tablets 3111
Stalevo Tablets 2270

Lithium (Blocks the TSH-mediated release of T4 and T3; thyroid function should therefore be carefully monitored during lithium initiation, stablization, and maintenence; if hypothyroidism occurs during lithium treatment, a higher than usual Synthroid dose may be required).
No products indexed under this heading.

Lithium Carbonate (Blocks the TSH-mediated release of T4 and T3; thyroid function should therefore be carefully monitored during lithium initiation, stablization, and maintenence; if hypothyroidism occurs during lithium treatment, a higher than usual Synthroid dose may be required). Products include:
Eskalith 1406
Lithobid Tablets 1670

Lithium Citrate (Blocks the TSH-mediated release of T4 and T3; thyroid function should therefore be carefully monitored during lithium initiation, stablization, and maintenence; if hypothyroidism occurs during lithium treatment, a higher than usual Synthroid dose may be required).
No products indexed under this heading.

Lovastatin (Alters thyroid hormone or TSH levels). Products include:
Advicor Tablets 1694
Altoprev Extended-Release Tablets 1151
Mevacor Tablets 1996

Magnesium Salicylate (May inhibit levothyroxine sodium binding to serum proteins or alter the concentrations of serum proteins).
No products indexed under this heading.

Maprotiline Hydrochloride (Risk of cardiac arrhythmias may increase).
No products indexed under this heading.

Meclofenamate Sodium (Meclofenamic acid may inhibit levothyroxine sodium binding to serum proteins or alter the concentrations of serum proteins).
No products indexed under this heading.

Mefenamic Acid (May inhibit levothyroxine sodium binding to serum proteins or alter the concentrations of serum proteins).
No products indexed under this heading.

Mercaptopurine (Alters thyroid hormone or TSH levels). Products include:
Purinethol Tablets 1222

Metaproterenol Sulfate (Possible increased risk of coronary insufficiency in patients with coronary artery disease). Products include:
Alupent Inhalation Aerosol 858

Metaraminol Bitartrate (Possible increased risk of coronary insufficiency in patients with coronary artery disease). Products include:
Aramine Injection 1889

Metformin Hydrochloride (Requirements of oral antidiabetic agents may be reduced in hypothyroid patients with diabetes and may be subsequently increased with initiation of thyroid hormone therapy).
Products include:
ActoPlus Met Tablets 3219
Avandamet Tablets 1343
Fortamet Extended-Release Tablets 1156

Methadone Hydrochloride (May inhibit levothyroxine sodium binding to serum proteins or alter the concentrations of serum proteins).
No products indexed under this heading.

Methimazole (Alters thyroid hormone or TSH levels).
No products indexed under this heading.

Methoxamine Hydrochloride (Possible increased risk of coronary insufficiency in patients with coronary artery disease).
No products indexed under this heading.

Methyclothiazide (Alters thyroid hormone or TSH levels).
No products indexed under this heading.

Methylprednisolone Acetate (May inhibit levothyroxine sodium binding to serum proteins or alter the concentrations of serum proteins). Products include:
Depo-Medrol Injectable Suspension 2615
Depo-Medrol Single-Dose Vial 2617

Methylprednisolone Sodium Succinate (May inhibit levothyroxine sodium binding to serum proteins or alter the concentrations of serum proteins).
No products indexed under this heading.

Methyltestosterone (May inhibit levothyroxine sodium binding to serum proteins or alter the concentrations of serum proteins; alters TSH or thyroid hormone levels). Products include:
Estratest Tablets 3196
Estratest H.S. Tablets 3196

Metipranolol Hydrochloride (Alters thyroid hormone or TSH levels; actions of some beta blockers may be impaired when hypothyroid patients become euthyroid).
No products indexed under this heading.

Metoclopramide Hydrochloride (Alters thyroid hormone or TSH levels).
No products indexed under this heading.

Metoprolol Succinate (Alters thyroid hormone or TSH levels; actions of some beta blockers may be impaired when hypothyroid patients become euthyroid). Products include:
Toprol-XL Tablets 660

Metoprolol Tartrate (Alters thyroid hormone or TSH levels; actions of some beta blockers may be impaired when hypothyroid patients become euthyroid).
No products indexed under this heading.

Miglitol (Requirements of oral antidiabetic agents may be reduced in hypothyroid patients with diabetes and may be subsequently increased with initiation of thyroid hormone therapy).
No products indexed under this heading.

Mitotane (Alters thyroid hormone or TSH levels).
No products indexed under this heading.

Nadolol (Alters thyroid hormone or TSH levels; actions of some beta blockers may be impaired when hypothyroid patients become euthyroid). Products include:
Nadolol Tablets 2121

Norepinephrine Bitartrate (Possible increased risk of coronary insufficiency in patients with coronary artery disease).
No products indexed under this heading.

Nortriptyline Hydrochloride (Concurrent use may increase the therapeutic and toxic effects of both drugs; onset of action of tricyclics may be accelerated).
No products indexed under this heading.

Octreotide Acetate (Alters thyroid hormone or TSH levels). Products include:
Sandostatin Injection 2263
Sandostatin LAR Depot 2264

Oxandrolone (May inhibit levothyroxine sodium binding to serum proteins or alter the concentrations of serum proteins; alters TSH or thyroid hormone levels). Products include:
Oxandrin Tablets 2977

Oxymetholone (May inhibit levothyroxine sodium binding to serum proteins or alter the concentrations of serum proteins; alters TSH or thyroid hormone levels). Products include:
Anadrol-50 Tablets 3329

Penbutolol Sulfate (Alters thyroid hormone or TSH levels; actions of some beta blockers may be impaired when hypothyroid patients become euthyroid).
No products indexed under this heading.

Pergolide Mesylate (Alters thyroid hormone or TSH levels). Products include:
Permax Tablets 3357

Perphenazine (May inhibit levothyroxine sodium binding to serum proteins or alter the concentrations of serum proteins).
No products indexed under this heading.

Phenobarbital (Alters thyroid hormone or TSH levels).
No products indexed under this heading.

Phenylbutazone (May inhibit levothyroxine sodium binding to serum proteins or alter the concentrations of serum proteins; alters thyroid hormone or TSH levels).
No products indexed under this heading.

Phenylephrine Bitartrate (Possible increased risk of coronary insufficiency in patients with coronary artery disease).
No products indexed under this heading.

Phenylephrine Hydrochloride (Possible increased risk of coronary insufficiency in patients with coronary artery disease). Products include:
Alacol DM Syrup 739
Hycomine Compound Tablets 1105
Preparation H Maximum Strength Cream .... ▣ 747
Preparation H Cooling Gel .... ▣ 747
Preparation H .... ▣ 747
Sudafed PE Tablets .... ▣ 711
Vicks Sinex Nasal Spray and Ultra Fine Mist for Sinus Relief 2677
Zicam Concentrated Cough Mist for Kids Plus D Cool Cherry .... ▣ 643
Zicam Concentrated Cough Mist Plus D Cool Cherry .... ▣ 642

Phenylephrine Tannate (Possible increased risk of coronary insufficiency in patients with coronary artery disease).
No products indexed under this heading.

Phenylpropanolamine Hydrochloride (Possible increased risk of coronary insufficiency in patients with coronary artery disease).
No products indexed under this heading.

Phenytoin (May inhibit levothyroxine sodium binding to serum proteins or alter the concentrations of serum proteins; alters thyroid hormone or TSH levels).
No products indexed under this heading.

Phenytoin Sodium (May inhibit levothyroxine sodium binding to serum proteins or alter the concentrations of serum proteins; alters thyroid hormone or TSH levels). Products include:
Phenytek Capsules 2153

Pindolol (Alters thyroid hormone or TSH levels; actions of some beta blockers may be impaired when hypothyroid patients become euthyroid).
No products indexed under this heading.

Pioglitazone Hydrochloride (Requirements of oral antidiabetic agents may be reduced in hypothyroid patients with diabetes and may be subsequently increased with initiation of thyroid hormone therapy). Products include:
ActoPlus Met Tablets 3219
Actos Tablets 3224

Pirbuterol Acetate (Possible increased risk of coronary insufficiency in patients with coronary artery disease). Products include:
Maxair Autohaler 1820

Polyestradiol Phosphate (Estrogens or estrogen-containing compounds may inhibit levothyroxine sodium binding to serum proteins or alter the concentrations of serum proteins).
No products indexed under this heading.

Polythiazide (Alters thyroid hormone or TSH levels).
No products indexed under this heading.

Pramipexole Dihydrochloride (Alters thyroid hormone or TSH levels). Products include:
Mirapex Tablets 889

Prednisolone Acetate (May inhibit levothyroxine sodium binding to serum proteins or alter the concentrations of serum proteins). Products include:
Blephamide Ophthalmic Ointment 563
Blephamide Ophthalmic Suspension 564
Poly-Pred Liquifilm Ophthalmic Suspension .... ⊙ 231
Pred Forte Ophthalmic Suspension .... ⊙ 233
Pred Mild Sterile Ophthalmic Suspension .... ⊙ 236
Pred-G Ophthalmic Suspension .... ⊙ 234
Pred-G Sterile Ophthalmic Ointment .... ⊙ 235

Prednisolone Sodium Phosphate (May inhibit levothyroxine sodium binding to serum proteins or alter the concentrations of serum proteins). Products include:
Pediapred Oral Solution 3319

Prednisolone Tebutate (May inhibit levothyroxine sodium binding to serum proteins or alter the concentrations of serum proteins).
No products indexed under this heading.

Prednisone (May inhibit levothyroxine sodium binding to serum proteins or alter the concentrations of serum proteins).
No products indexed under this heading.

Propranolol Hydrochloride (Alters thyroid hormone or TSH levels; actions of some beta blockers may be impaired when hypothyroid patients become euthyroid). Products include:
Inderal LA Long-Acting Capsules 3421
InnoPran XL Capsules 2728

Protriptyline Hydrochloride (Concurrent use may increase the therapeutic and toxic effects of both drugs; onset of action of tricyclics may be accelerated). Products include:
Vivactil Tablets 2350

Pseudoephedrine Hydrochloride (Possible increased risk of coronary insufficiency in patients with coronary artery disease). Products include:
Advil Allergy Sinus Caplets .... ▣ 737
Advil Cold & Sinus .... ▣ 739
Advil Flu & Body Ache Caplets .... ▣ 739
Children's Advil Cold Suspension .... ▣ 741
Advil Multi-Symptom Cold Caplets .... ▣ 738
Allegra-D 12 Hour Extended-Release Tablets 2860
Allegra-D 24 Hour Extended-Release Tablets 2862
Balamine DM 739
BC Cold Powder .... ▣ 612
Benadryl Allergy & Cold Tablets .... ▣ 692
Benadryl Allergy & Sinus Headache Caplets & Gelcaps .... ▣ 693
Children's Benadryl Allergy & Cold Fastmelt Tablets .... ▣ 695
Benadryl Maximum Strength Severe Allergy & Sinus Headache Caplets .... ▣ 694
Children's Benadryl D Allergy & Sinus Fastmelt Tablets .... ▣ 694
Children's Benadryl D Liquid Medication .... ▣ 693
Benadryl D Tablets .... ▣ 694
Contac Non-Drowsy 12 Hour Cold Caplets .... ▣ 614
Contac Non-Drowsy Timed Release 12 Hour Cold Caplets .... ▣ 615
Contac Severe Cold and Flu Caplets Maximum Strength .... ▣ 615
Contac Severe Cold and Flu Caplets Non-Drowsy .... ▣ 615
Children's Dimetapp Cold & Allergy Elixir .... ▣ 745
Children's Dimetapp DM Cold & Cough Elixir .... ▣ 745
Children's Dimetapp Long Acting Cough Plus Cold Syrup .... ▣ 746
Dimetapp Infant Drops Decongestant Plus Cough .... ▣ 746
Children's Motrin Cold Non-Staining Dye-Free Oral Suspension 1838
Children's Motrin Cold Oral Suspension 1838
Motrin Cold & Sinus Caplets 1836
PediaCare Decongestant & Cough Infant Drops .... ▣ 705
PediaCare Decongestant Infants' Drops .... ▣ 705
PediaCare Long-Acting Cough Plus Cold Liquid .... ▣ 704
PediaCare Multi-Symptom Cold Liquid .... ▣ 704
PediaCare NightRest Cough & Cold Liquid .... ▣ 704
Robitussin Allergy & Cough Syrup .... ▣ 750
Robitussin CF Liquid .... ▣ 755
Robitussin Cough & Cold Liquid-filled Capsules .... ▣ 750
Robitussin Cough, Cold & Flu Liquid-filled Capsules .... ▣ 750
Robitussin Cough & Cold Infant Drops .... ▣ 755
Robitussin Flu Liquid .... ▣ 752
Robitussin Maximum Strength Cough & Cold Liquid .... ▣ 754
Robitussin PE Syrup .... ▣ 753
Robitussin Pediatric Cough & Cold Liquid .... ▣ 754
Robitussin PM Cough & Cold Liquid .... ▣ 752
Robitussin Severe Congestion Liquid-filled Capsules .... ▣ 751
Simply Stuffy Liquid 1841
Singlet Caplets .... ▣ 636
Sudafed 12 Hour Caplets .... ▣ 708
Sudafed 24 Hour Tablets .... ▣ 709
Sudafed Nasal Decongestant Tablets .... ▣ 709
Sudafed Severe Cold .... ▣ 710
Sudafed Non-Drying Sinus Liquid Caps .... ▣ 709
Sudafed Sinus & Allergy Tablets .... ▣ 710
Sudafed Sinus Headache .... ▣ 711
TheraFlu Cold & Cough Hot Liquid .... ▣ 680
TheraFlu Cold & Sore Throat Hot Liquid .... ▣ 680
TheraFlu Flu & Chest Congestion Non-Drowsy Hot Liquid .... ▣ 681
TheraFlu Flu & Sore Throat Hot Liquid .... ▣ 681
TheraFlu Severe Cold Non-Drowsy Hot Liquid .... ▣ 683
TheraFlu Severe Cold & Cough Hot Liquid .... ▣ 683
TheraFlu Severe Cold Caplets .... ▣ 679
TheraFlu Severe Cold Hot Liquid .... ▣ 682
TheraFlu Severe Cold Non-Drowsy Caplets .... ▣ 679
Triaminic Chest & Nasal Congestion Liquid .... ▣ 685
Triaminic Cold & Allergy Liquid .... ▣ 685
Triaminic Cold & Cough Liquid .... ▣ 685
Triaminic Cough Liquid .... ▣ 687
Triaminic Cough & Nasal Congestion Liquid .... ▣ 687
Triaminic Cough & Sore Throat Liquid .... ▣ 687
Triaminic Flu, Cough & Fever Liquid .... ▣ 685
Triaminic Night Time Cough & Cold Liquid .... ▣ 685
Triaminic Allergy Runny Nose & Congestion Softchews .... ▣ 688
Triaminic Cold & Cough Softchews .... ▣ 688
Triaminic Cough & Sore Throat Softchews .... ▣ 689
Tylenol Sinus NightTime Caplets .... ▣ 663
Children's Tylenol Plus Cold & Allergy Suspension Liquid 1850
Children's Tylenol Plus Cold NightTime Suspension Liquid 1851
Children's Tylenol Plus Cold & Cough Suspension Liquid and Chewable Tablets 1851
Children's Tylenol Plus Cold Chewable Tablets 1851
Children's Tylenol Plus Cold Daytime Non-Drowsy Suspension Liquid 1851
Children's Tylenol Plus Flu Suspension Liquid 1853
Concentrated Tylenol Infants' Drops Plus Cold 1851
Concentrated Tylenol Infants' Drops Plus Cold and Cough 1851
Tylenol Cold & Flu Severe Daytime Liquid with Cool Burst 1846
Tylenol Cold & Flu Severe NightTime Liquid with Cool Burst 1846
Tylenol Cold Severe Congestion Non-Drowsy Caplets with Cool Burst 1846
Tylenol Allergy Complete Night Time Caplets 1844
Tylenol Allergy Complete Multi-Symptom Caplets and Gelcaps with Cool Burst 1844
Tylenol Flu NightTime Gelcaps 1846
Tylenol Flu Day Non-Drowsy Gelcaps 1846
Concentrated Tylenol Infants' Drops Plus Cold Nasal Congestant, Fever Reducer & Pain Reliever .... ▣ 668
Concentrated Tylenol Infants' Drops Plus Cold & Cough Nasal Decongestant, Fever Reducer & Pain Reliever .... ▣ 668
Multi-Symptom Tylenol Cold Night Time Caplets 1845
Multi-Symptom Tylenol Cold Day Non-Drowsy Caplets and Gelcaps 1845
Tylenol Sinus Day Non-Drowsy 1848
Tylenol Sinus Night Time Caplets 1848
Tylenol Sinus Severe Congestion Caplets with Cool Burst 1848
Vicks 44D Cough & Head Congestion Relief 2676
Vicks 44D Cough & Head Congestion Relief Liquid .... ▣ 721
Vicks 44M Cough, Cold & Flu Relief 2676
Pediatric Vicks 44m Cough & Cold Relief 2673
Vicks DayQuil LiquiCaps/Liquid Multi-Symptom Cold/Flu Relief .... ▣ 723
Vicks DayQuil Multi-Symptom Cold/Flu Relief LiquiCaps 2675
Vicks DayQuil Multi-Symptom Cold/Flu Relief Liquid 2675
Children's Vicks NyQuil Cold/Cough Relief 2671
Vicks NyQuil LiquiCaps 2677
Vicks NyQuil LiquiCaps/Liquid Multi-Symptom Cold/Flu Relief .... ▣ 725
Vicks NyQuil Liquid 2677
Zyrtec-D 12 Hour Extended Release Tablets 2591

Pseudoephedrine Sulfate (Possible increased risk of coronary insufficiency in patients with coronary artery disease). Products include:
Alavert Allergy & Sinus D-12 Hour Tablets .... ▣ 743
Clarinex-D 24-Hour Extended-Release Tablets 3012
Claritin-D Non-Drowsy 12 Hour Tablets .... ▣ 731
Claritin-D Non-Drowsy 24 Hour Tablets .... ▣ 731

Quinestrol (Estrogens or estrogen-containing compounds may inhibit levothyroxine sodium binding to serum proteins or alter the concentrations of serum proteins).
No products indexed under this heading.

Repaglinide (Requirements of oral antidiabetic agents may be reduced in hypothyroid patients with diabetes and may be subsequently increased with initiation of thyroid hormone therapy). Products include:
Prandin Tablets (0.5, 1, and 2 mg) 2337

Resorcinol (Alters thyroid hormone or TSH levels).
No products indexed under this heading.

Rifampin (Alters thyroid hormone or TSH levels).
No products indexed under this heading.

Rifapentine (Alters thyroid hormone or TSH levels).
No products indexed under this heading.

Ropinirole Hydrochloride (Alters thyroid hormone or TSH levels). Products include:
Requip Tablets 1528

Rosiglitazone Maleate (Requirements of oral antidiabetic agents may be reduced in hypothyroid patients with diabetes and may be subsequently increased with initiation of thyroid hormone therapy). Products include:
Avandamet Tablets 1343
Avandia Tablets 1348

Salmeterol Xinafoate (Possible increased risk of coronary insufficiency in patients with coronary artery disease). Products include:
- Advair Diskus 100/50 1291
- Advair Diskus 250/50 1291
- Advair Diskus 500/50 1291
- Serevent Diskus 1540

Salsalate (May inhibit levothyroxine sodium binding to serum proteins or alter the concentrations of serum proteins).
No products indexed under this heading.

Sodium Iodide I 123 (Uptake of radiolabeled ions may be decreased).
No products indexed under this heading.

Sodium Iodide I 131 (Uptake of radiolabeled ions may be decreased).
No products indexed under this heading.

Sodium Nitroprusside (Alters thyroid hormone or TSH levels).
No products indexed under this heading.

Sodium Pertechnetate (Alters thyroid hormone or TSH levels).
No products indexed under this heading.

Sodium Polystyrene Sulfonate (Binds and decreases absorption of levothyroxine sodium from the gastrointestinal tract).
No products indexed under this heading.

Somatrem (Excessive concurrent use of thyroid hormone may accelerate epiphyseal closure; untreated hypothyroidism may interfere with the growth response to somatrem).
No products indexed under this heading.

Somatropin (Excessive concurrent use of thyroid hormone may accelerate epiphyseal closure; untreated hypothyroidism may interfere with the growth response to somatrem). Products include:
- Genotropin Lyophilized Powder 2642
- Humatrope Vials and Cartridges 1756
- Norditropin Cartridges 2318
- Nutropin for Injection 1238
- Nutropin AQ Injection 1241
- Nutropin AQ Pen 1241
- Nutropin AQ Pen Cartridge 1241

Sotalol Hydrochloride (Alters thyroid hormone or TSH levels; actions of some beta blockers may be impaired when hypothyroid patients become euthyroid).
No products indexed under this heading.

Stanozolol (May inhibit levothyroxine sodium binding to serum proteins or alter the concentrations of serum proteins; alters TSH or thyroid hormone levels).
No products indexed under this heading.

Sucralfate (Binds and decreases absorption of levothyroxine sodium from the gastrointestinal tract). Products include:
- Carafate Suspension 727
- Carafate Tablets 728

Sulfacytine (Alters thyroid hormone or TSH levels).
No products indexed under this heading.

Sulfamethizole (Alters thyroid hormone or TSH levels).
No products indexed under this heading.

Sulfamethoxazole (Alters thyroid hormone or TSH levels).
No products indexed under this heading.

Sulfasalazine (Alters thyroid hormone or TSH levels).
No products indexed under this heading.

Sulfinpyrazone (Alters thyroid hormone or TSH levels).
No products indexed under this heading.

Sulfisoxazole (Alters thyroid hormone or TSH levels).
No products indexed under this heading.

Sulfisoxazole Acetyl (Alters thyroid hormone or TSH levels).
No products indexed under this heading.

Sulfisoxazole Diolamine (Alters thyroid hormone or TSH levels).
No products indexed under this heading.

Tamoxifen Citrate (May inhibit levothyroxine sodium binding to serum proteins or alter the concentrations of serum proteins).
No products indexed under this heading.

Terbutaline Sulfate (Possible increased risk of coronary insufficiency in patients with coronary artery disease).
No products indexed under this heading.

Theophylline (Theophylline clearance may be decreased in hypothyroid patients and return toward normal when euthyroid state is achieved).
No products indexed under this heading.

Theophylline Anhydrous (Theophylline clearance may be decreased in hypothyroid patients and return toward normal when euthyroid state is achieved). Products include:
- Uniphyl Tablets 2708

Theophylline Calcium Salicylate (Theophylline clearance may be decreased in hypothyroid patients and return toward normal when euthyroid state is achieved).
No products indexed under this heading.

Theophylline Dihydroxypropyl (Glyceryl) (Theophylline clearance may be decreased in hypothyroid patients and return toward normal when euthyroid state is achieved).
No products indexed under this heading.

Theophylline Ethylenediamine (Theophylline clearance may be decreased in hypothyroid patients and return toward normal when euthyroid state is achieved).
No products indexed under this heading.

Theophylline Sodium Glycinate (Theophylline clearance may be decreased in hypothyroid patients and return toward normal when euthyroid state is achieved).
No products indexed under this heading.

Timolol Hemihydrate (Alters thyroid hormone or TSH levels; actions of some beta blockers may be impaired when hypothyroid patients become euthyroid). Products include:
- Betimol Ophthalmic Solution 3371
- Betimol Ophthalmic Solution .... ⊙283

Timolol Maleate (Alters thyroid hormone or TSH levels; actions of some beta blockers may be impaired when hypothyroid patients become euthyroid). Products include:
- Blocadren Tablets 1891
- Cosopt Sterile Ophthalmic Solution 1910
- Timolide Tablets 2056
- Timoptic in Ocudose 2061
- Timoptic Sterile Ophthalmic Solution 2058
- Timoptic-XE Sterile Ophthalmic Gel Forming Solution 2062

Tolazamide (Alters thyroid hormone or TSH levels; requirements of oral antidiabetic agents may be reduced in hypothyroid patients with diabetes and may be subsequently increased with initiation of thyroid hormone therapy).
No products indexed under this heading.

Tolbutamide (Alters thyroid hormone or TSH levels; requirements of oral antidiabetic agents may be reduced in hypothyroid patients with diabetes and may be subsequently increased with initiation of thyroid hormone therapy).
No products indexed under this heading.

Triamcinolone (May inhibit levothyroxine sodium binding to serum proteins or alter the concentrations of serum proteins).
No products indexed under this heading.

Triamcinolone Acetonide (May inhibit levothyroxine sodium binding to serum proteins or alter the concentrations of serum proteins). Products include:
- Azmacort Inhalation Aerosol 1701
- Nasacort HFA Inhalation Aerosol 2939
- Nasacort AQ Nasal Spray 2937

Triamcinolone Diacetate (May inhibit levothyroxine sodium binding to serum proteins or alter the concentrations of serum proteins).
No products indexed under this heading.

Triamcinolone Hexacetonide (May inhibit levothyroxine sodium binding to serum proteins or alter the concentrations of serum proteins).
No products indexed under this heading.

Trimipramine Maleate (Concurrent use may increase the therapeutic and toxic effects of both drugs; onset of action of tricyclics may be accelerated). Products include:
- Surmontil Capsules 2347

Troglitazone (Requirements of oral antidiabetic agents may be reduced in hypothyroid patients with diabetes and may be subsequently increased with initiation of thyroid hormone therapy).
No products indexed under this heading.

Tyropanoate Sodium (Alters thyroid hormone or TSH levels).
No products indexed under this heading.

Warfarin Sodium (The hypoprothrombinemic effect of anticoagulants may be potentiated). Products include:
- Coumadin for Injection 932
- Coumadin Tablets 932

Food Interactions

Soybean Formula, Children's (Binds and decreases absorption of levothyroxine sodium from the gastrointestinal tract).

SYPRINE CAPSULES
(Trientine Hydrochloride) 2055
None cited in PDR database.

SYSTANE LUBRICANT EYE DROPS
(Polyethylene Glycol, Propylene Glycol) 558
None cited in PDR database.

TABLOID TABLETS
(Thioguanine) 1545
May interact with cytotoxic drugs, drugs that inhibit thiopurine methyltransferase (TPMT), and certain other agents. Compounds in these categories include:

Bleomycin Sulfate (Combination therapy may produce hepatic disease).
No products indexed under this heading.

Busulfan (Potential for esophageal varices associated with abnormal liver function tests). Products include:
- I.V. Busulfex 1125
- Myleran Tablets 1492

Cyclophosphamide (Combination therapy may produce hepatic disease).
No products indexed under this heading.

Daunorubicin Hydrochloride (Combination therapy may produce hepatic disease). Products include:
- Cerubidine for Injection 788

Doxorubicin Hydrochloride (Combination therapy may produce hepatic disease). Products include:
- Adriamycin for Injection, USP 786
- Adriamycin Injection, USP 786

Epirubicin Hydrochloride (Combination therapy may produce hepatic disease). Products include:
- Ellence Injection 2632

Fluorouracil (Combination therapy may produce hepatic disease). Products include:
- Carac Cream, 0.5% 1048
- Efudex 3348

Hydroxyurea (Combination therapy may produce hepatic disease).
No products indexed under this heading.

Mercaptopurine (Complete cross-resistance). Products include:
- Purinethol Tablets 1222

Mesalamine (Individuals with inherited deficiency of the enzyme TPMT are unusually sensitive to the myelosuppressive effects of mercaptopurine and are prone to developing rapid bone marrow suppression; co-administration with drugs that inhibit TPMT could exacerbate this toxicity). Products include:
- Asacol Delayed-Release Tablets 2688
- Canasa Rectal Suppositories 726
- Pentasa Capsules 3182

Mesalazine (Individuals with inherited deficiency of the enzyme TPMT are unusually sensitive to the myelosuppressive effects of mercaptopurine and are prone to developing rapid bone marrow suppression; co-administration with drugs that inhibit TPMT could exacerbate this toxicity).
No products indexed under this heading.

Methotrexate Sodium (Combination therapy may produce hepatic disease).
No products indexed under this heading.

Mitotane (Combination therapy may produce hepatic disease).
No products indexed under this heading.

Mitoxantrone Hydrochloride (Combination therapy may produce hepatic disease). Products include:
Novantrone for Injection Concentrate 3158

Olsalazine Sodium (Individuals with inherited deficiency of the enzyme TPMT are unusually sensitive to the myelosuppressive effects of mercaptopurine and are prone to developing rapid bone marrow suppression; co-administration with drugs that inhibit TPMT could exacerbate this toxicity).
No products indexed under this heading.

Procarbazine Hydrochloride (Combination therapy may produce hepatic disease). Products include:
Matulane Capsules 3188

Sulphasalazine (Individuals with inherited deficiency of the enzyme TPMT are unusually sensitive to the myelosuppressive effects of mercaptopurine and are prone to developing rapid bone marrow suppression; co-administration with drugs that inhibit TPMT could exacerbate this toxicity).
No products indexed under this heading.

Tamoxifen Citrate (Combination therapy may produce hepatic disease).
No products indexed under this heading.

Vincristine Sulfate (Combination therapy may produce hepatic disease).
No products indexed under this heading.

TAGAMET HB 200 TABLETS

(Cimetidine) 637
May interact with dihydropyridine calcium channel blockers, xanthines, and certain other agents. Compounds in these categories include:

Aminophylline (Increased AUC of theophylline by 14% and peak levels by 15% when used concurrently at the maximum recommended OTC dose level; clinically significant pharmacokinetic interactions have been reported at prescription doses).
No products indexed under this heading.

Amlodipine Besylate (Clinically significant pharmacokinetic interactions have been reported with concurrent use at prescription doses of cimetidine; patients are advised to consult their physician). Products include:
Caduet Tablets 2507
Lotrel Capsules 2238
Norvasc Tablets 2529

Dyphylline (Increased AUC of theophylline by 14% and peak levels by 15% when used concurrently at the maximum recommended OTC dose level; clinically significant pharmacokinetic interactions have been reported at prescription doses).
No products indexed under this heading.

Felodipine (Clinically significant pharmacokinetic interactions have been reported with concurrent use at prescription doses of cimetidine; patients are advised to consult their physician). Products include:
Plendil Extended-Release Tablets 651

Isradipine (Clinically significant pharmacokinetic interactions have been reported with concurrent use at prescription doses of cimetidine; patients are advised to consult their physician). Products include:
DynaCirc CR Tablets 2726

Nicardipine Hydrochloride (Clinically significant pharmacokinetic interactions have been reported with concurrent use at prescription doses of cimetidine; patients are advised to consult their physician). Products include:
Cardene I.V. 1129

Nifedipine (Clinically significant pharmacokinetic interactions have been reported with concurrent use at prescription doses of cimetidine; patients are advised to consult their physician). Products include:
Adalat CC Tablets 2978

Nimodipine (Clinically significant pharmacokinetic interactions have been reported with concurrent use at prescription doses of cimetidine; patients are advised to consult their physician). Products include:
Nimotop Capsules 774

Phenytoin (Clinically significant pharmacokinetic interactions have been reported with concurrent use at prescription doses of cimetidine; patients are advised to consult their physician).
No products indexed under this heading.

Phenytoin Sodium (Clinically significant pharmacokinetic interactions have been reported with concurrent use at prescription doses of cimetidine; patients are advised to consult their physician). Products include:
Phenytek Capsules 2153

Theophylline (Increased AUC of theophylline by 14% and peak levels by 15% when used concurrently at the maximum recommended OTC dose level; clinically significant pharmacokinetic interactions have been reported at prescription doses).
No products indexed under this heading.

Theophylline Anhydrous (Increased AUC of theophylline by 14% and peak levels by 15% when used concurrently at the maximum recommended OTC dose level; clinically significant pharmacokinetic interactions have been reported at prescription doses). Products include:
Uniphyl Tablets 2708

Theophylline Calcium Salicylate (Increased AUC of theophylline by 14% and peak levels by 15% when used concurrently at the maximum recommended OTC dose level; clinically significant pharmacokinetic interactions have been reported at prescription doses).
No products indexed under this heading.

Theophylline Dihydroxypropyl (Glyceryl) (Increased AUC of theophylline by 14% and peak levels by 15% when used concurrently at the maximum recommended OTC dose level; clinically significant pharmacokinetic interactions have been reported at prescription doses).
No products indexed under this heading.

Theophylline Ethylenediamine (Increased AUC of theophylline by 14% and peak levels by 15% when used concurrently at the maximum recommended OTC dose level; clinically significant pharmacokinetic interactions have been reported at prescription doses).
No products indexed under this heading.

Theophylline Sodium Glycinate (Increased AUC of theophylline by 14% and peak levels by 15% when used concurrently at the maximum recommended OTC dose level; clinically significant pharmacokinetic interactions have been reported at prescription doses).
No products indexed under this heading.

Triazolam (Potential for increased AUC of triazolam by 26-28% and increased peak levels by 11-23%).
No products indexed under this heading.

Warfarin Sodium (Clinically significant pharmacokinetic interactions have been reported with concurrent use at prescription doses of cimetidine; patients are advised to consult their physician). Products include:
Coumadin for Injection 932
Coumadin Tablets 932

TAGAMET TABLETS

(Cimetidine) 1547
May interact with antacids, oral anticoagulants, tricyclic antidepressants, xanthines, and certain other agents. Compounds in these categories include:

Aluminum Carbonate (Simultaneous administration is not recommended since antacids may interfere with the absorption of cimetidine).
No products indexed under this heading.

Aluminum Hydroxide (Simultaneous administration is not recommended since antacids may interfere with the absorption of cimetidine). Products include:
Gaviscon Regular Strength Liquid .. 620
Gaviscon Regular Strength Tablets....................................... 619
Gaviscon Extra Strength Liquid 620
Gaviscon Extra Strength Tablets 619
Maalox Max Maximum Strength Antacid/Anti-Gas Liquid................. 2165
Maalox Regular Strength Antacid/Antigas Liquid.................. 2164

Aminophylline (Reduces hepatic metabolism of theophylline resulting in delayed elimination and increased blood levels of theophylline).
No products indexed under this heading.

Amitriptyline Hydrochloride (Reduces hepatic metabolism of certain unspecified tricyclic antidepressants resulting in delayed elimination and increased blood levels of these drugs).
No products indexed under this heading.

Amoxapine (Reduces hepatic metabolism of certain unspecified tricyclic antidepressants resulting in delayed elimination and increased blood levels of these drugs).
No products indexed under this heading.

Anisindione (Reduces hepatic metabolism of warfarin-type anticoagulants resulting in clinically significant effects; close monitoring of prothrombin time of these recommended). Products include:
Miradon Tablets 3056

Chlordiazepoxide (Reduces hepatic metabolism of chlordiazepoxide resulting in delayed elimination and increased blood levels of chlordiazepoxide).
No products indexed under this heading.

Chlordiazepoxide Hydrochloride (Reduces hepatic metabolism of chlordiazepoxide resulting in delayed elimination and increased blood levels of chlordiazepoxide). Products include:
Librium Capsules 3349

Clomipramine Hydrochloride (Reduces hepatic metabolism of certain unspecified tricyclic antidepressants resulting in delayed elimination and increased blood levels of these drugs).
No products indexed under this heading.

Desipramine Hydrochloride (Reduces hepatic metabolism of certain unspecified tricyclic antidepressants resulting in delayed elimination and increased blood levels of these drugs).
No products indexed under this heading.

Diazepam (Reduces hepatic metabolism of diazepam resulting in delayed elimination and increased blood levels of diazepam). Products include:
Diastat Rectal Delivery System 3344
Valium Tablets 2822

Dicumarol (Reduces hepatic metabolism of warfarin-type anticoagulants resulting in clinically significant effects; close monitoring of prothrombin time of these recommended).
No products indexed under this heading.

Doxepin Hydrochloride (Reduces hepatic metabolism of certain unspecified tricyclic antidepressants resulting in delayed elimination and increased blood levels of these drugs).
No products indexed under this heading.

Dyphylline (Reduces hepatic metabolism of theophylline resulting in delayed elimination and increased blood levels of theophylline).
No products indexed under this heading.

Imipramine Hydrochloride (Reduces hepatic metabolism of certain unspecified tricyclic antidepressants resulting in delayed elimination and increased blood levels of these drugs).
No products indexed under this heading.

Imipramine Pamoate (Reduces hepatic metabolism of certain unspecified tricyclic antidepressants resulting in delayed elimination and increased blood levels of these drugs).
No products indexed under this heading.

Ketoconazole (Alteration of pH may affect absorption of ketoconazole; administer oral ketoconazole at least 2 hours before cimetidine). Products include:
Nizoral A-D Shampoo, 1% **1839**
Nizoral 2% Shampoo **1838**

Lidocaine Hydrochloride (Reduces hepatic metabolism of lidocaine resulting in delayed elimination and increased blood levels of lidocaine).
No products indexed under this heading.

Magaldrate (Simultaneous administration is not recommended since antacids may interfere with the absorption of cimetidine).
No products indexed under this heading.

Magnesium Hydroxide (Simultaneous administration is not recommended since antacids may interfere with the absorption of cimetidine). Products include:
Maalox Max Maximum Strength Antacid/Anti-Gas Liquid................ **2165**
Maalox Regular Strength Antacid/Antigas Liquid................. **2164**
Pepcid Complete Chewable Tablets **1672**
Rolaids Tablets .... ▣**707**
Extra Strength Rolaids Tablets .... ▣**707**
Rolaids Multi-Symptom Antacid & Antigas Tablets .... ▣**708**

Magnesium Oxide (Simultaneous administration is not recommended since antacids may interfere with the absorption of cimetidine). Products include:
Beelith Tablets **784**
PremCal Light, Regular, and Extra Strength Tablets................. ▣**762**

Maprotiline Hydrochloride (Reduces hepatic metabolism of certain unspecified tricyclic antidepressants resulting in delayed elimination and increased blood levels of these drugs).
No products indexed under this heading.

Metronidazole (Reduces hepatic metabolism of metronidazole resulting in delayed elimination and increased blood levels of metronidazole). Products include:
Metrogel 1% **1212**
MetroGel-Vaginal Gel **1822**
Noritate Cream, 1% **1051**

Metronidazole Hydrochloride (Reduces hepatic metabolism of metronidazole resulting in delayed elimination and increased blood levels of metronidazole).
No products indexed under this heading.

Nifedipine (Reduces hepatic metabolism of nifedipine resulting in delayed elimination and increased blood levels of nifedipine). Products include:
Adalat CC Tablets **2978**

Nortriptyline Hydrochloride (Reduces hepatic metabolism of certain unspecified tricyclic antidepressants resulting in delayed elimination and increased blood levels of these drugs).
No products indexed under this heading.

Phenytoin (Reduces hepatic metabolism of phenytoin resulting in delayed elimination and increased blood levels of phenytoin).
No products indexed under this heading.

Phenytoin Sodium (Reduces hepatic metabolism of phenytoin resulting in delayed elimination and increased blood levels of phenytoin). Products include:
Phenytek Capsules **2153**

Propranolol Hydrochloride (Reduces hepatic metabolism of propranolol resulting in delayed elimination and increased blood levels of propranolol). Products include:
Inderal LA Long-Acting Capsules **3421**
InnoPran XL Capsules **2728**

Protriptyline Hydrochloride (Reduces hepatic metabolism of certain unspecified tricyclic antidepressants resulting in delayed elimination and increased blood levels of these drugs). Products include:
Vivactil Tablets **2350**

Sodium Bicarbonate (Simultaneous administration is not recommended since antacids may interfere with the absorption of cimetidine). Products include:
Ceo-Two Evacuant Suppository ...... ▣**607**
Colyte with Flavor Packs for Oral Solution...................................... **3102**
HalfLytely and Bisacodyl Tablets Bowel Prep Kit with Flavors Packs.. **915**
TriLyte with Flavor Packs for Oral Solution...................................... **3114**

Theophylline (Reduces hepatic metabolism of theophylline resulting in delayed elimination and increased blood levels of theophylline).
No products indexed under this heading.

Theophylline Anhydrous (Reduces hepatic metabolism of theophylline resulting in delayed elimination and increased blood levels of theophylline). Products include:
Uniphyl Tablets **2708**

Theophylline Calcium Salicylate (Reduces hepatic metabolism of theophylline resulting in delayed elimination and increased blood levels of theophylline).
No products indexed under this heading.

Theophylline Dihydroxypropyl (Glyceryl) (Reduces hepatic metabolism of theophylline resulting in delayed elimination and increased blood levels of theophylline).
No products indexed under this heading.

Theophylline Ethylenediamine (Reduces hepatic metabolism of theophylline resulting in delayed elimination and increased blood levels of theophylline).
No products indexed under this heading.

Theophylline Sodium Glycinate (Reduces hepatic metabolism of theophylline resulting in delayed elimination and increased blood levels of theophylline).
No products indexed under this heading.

Trimipramine Maleate (Reduces hepatic metabolism of certain unspecified tricyclic antidepressants resulting in delayed elimination and increased blood levels of these drugs). Products include:
Surmontil Capsules **2347**

Warfarin Sodium (Reduces hepatic metabolism of warfarin-type anticoagulants resulting in clinically significant effects; close monitoring of prothrombin time of these recommended). Products include:
Coumadin for Injection **932**
Coumadin Tablets **932**

TAHITIAN NONI LIQUID

(Dietary Supplement) .... ▣**777**
None cited in PDR database.

TAMBOCOR TABLETS

(Flecainide Acetate) **1824**
May interact with beta blockers, phenytoin, quinidine, and certain other agents. Compounds in these categories include:

Acebutolol Hydrochloride (Co-administration of flecainide with beta adrenergic blocking agents may result in possible additive negative inotropic effects; combined therapy has not resulted in adverse effects).
No products indexed under this heading.

Amiodarone Hydrochloride (When amiodarone is added to flecainide therapy, plasma flecainide levels may increase two-fold or more in some patients, if flecainide dosage is not reduced). Products include:
Pacerone Tablets **3337**

Atenolol (Co-administration of flecainide with beta adrenergic blocking agents may result in possible additive negative inotropic effects; combined therapy has not resulted in adverse effects). Products include:
Tenormin I.V. Injection **698**
Tenormin Tablets **695**

Betaxolol Hydrochloride (Co-administration of flecainide with beta adrenergic blocking agents may result in possible additive negative inotropic effects; combined therapy has not resulted in adverse effects). Products include:
Betoptic S Ophthalmic Suspension.................................... **554**

Bisoprolol Fumarate (Co-administration of flecainide with beta adrenergic blocking agents may result in possible additive negative inotropic effects; combined therapy has not resulted in adverse effects).
No products indexed under this heading.

Carbamazepine (Limited data in patients receiving known enzyme inducers, such as carbamazepine, indicate only a 30% increase in the rate of flecainide elimination). Products include:
Carbatrol Capsules **3174**
Equetro Extended-Release Capsules.................................... **3178**
Tegretol/Tegretol-XR **2278**

Carteolol Hydrochloride (Co-administration of flecainide with beta adrenergic blocking agents may result in possible additive negative inotropic effects; combined therapy has not resulted in adverse effects). Products include:
Carteolol Hydrochloride Ophthalmic Solution USP, 1%....... ⊙**246**

Cimetidine (Increases plasma levels by about 30% and half-life by about 10%). Products include:
Tagamet HB 200 Tablets .... ▣**637**
Tagamet Tablets **1547**

Cimetidine Hydrochloride (Increases plasma levels by about 30% and half-life by about 10%).
No products indexed under this heading.

Digoxin (Co-administration in individuals stabilized on a maintenance dose of digoxin has resulted in increased plasma digoxin levels by 13% to 19% at six hours postdose). Products include:
Digitek Tablets **2146**
Lanoxicaps Capsules **1458**
Lanoxin Injection **1462**
Lanoxin Tablets **1468**
Lanoxin Injection Pediatric **1465**

Disopyramide Phosphate (Co-administration is not recommended because both drugs have negative inotropic properties).
No products indexed under this heading.

Esmolol Hydrochloride (Co-administration of flecainide with beta adrenergic blocking agents may result in possible additive negative inotropic effects; combined therapy has not resulted in adverse effects). Products include:
Brevibloc Concentrate **766**
Brevibloc Injection **766**
Brevibloc Double Strength Injection.. **766**
Brevibloc Premixed Injection **766**
Brevibloc Double Strength Premixed Injection....................... **766**

Fosphenytoin Sodium (Limited data in patients receiving known enzyme inducers, such as phenytoin, indicate only a 30% increase in the rate of flecainide elimination).
No products indexed under this heading.

Labetalol Hydrochloride (Co-administration of flecainide with beta adrenergic blocking agents may result in possible additive negative inotropic effects; combined therapy has not resulted in adverse effects).
No products indexed under this heading.

Levobunolol Hydrochloride (Co-administration of flecainide with beta adrenergic blocking agents may result in possible additive negative inotropic effects; combined therapy has not resulted in adverse effects). Products include:
Betagan Ophthalmic Solution, USP.. ⊙**217**

Metipranolol Hydrochloride (Co-administration of flecainide with beta adrenergic blocking agents may result in possible additive negative inotropic effects; combined therapy has not resulted in adverse effects).
No products indexed under this heading.

Metoprolol Succinate (Co-administration of flecainide with beta adrenergic blocking agents may result in possible additive negative inotropic effects; combined therapy has not resulted in adverse effects). Products include:
Toprol-XL Tablets **660**

Metoprolol Tartrate (Co-administration of flecainide with beta adrenergic blocking agents may result in possible additive negative inotropic effects; combined therapy has not resulted in adverse effects).
No products indexed under this heading.

Nadolol (Co-administration of flecainide with beta adrenergic blocking agents may result in possible additive negative inotropic effects; combined therapy has not resulted in adverse effects). Products include:
Nadolol Tablets 2121

Penbutolol Sulfate (Co-administration of flecainide with beta adrenergic blocking agents may result in possible additive negative inotropic effects; combined therapy has not resulted in adverse effects).
No products indexed under this heading.

Phenobarbital (Limited data in patients receiving known enzyme inducers, such as phenobarbital, indicate only a 30% increase in the rate of flecainide elimination).
No products indexed under this heading.

Phenytoin (Limited data in patients receiving known enzyme inducers, such as phenytoin, indicate only a 30% increase in the rate of flecainide elimination).
No products indexed under this heading.

Phenytoin Sodium (Limited data in patients receiving known enzyme inducers, such as phenytoin, indicate only a 30% increase in the rate of flecainide elimination). Products include:
Phenytek Capsules 2153

Pindolol (Co-administration of flecainide with beta adrenergic blocking agents may result in possible additive negative inotropic effects; combined therapy has not resulted in adverse effects).
No products indexed under this heading.

Propranolol Hydrochloride (Co-administration has resulted in increased flecainide and propranolol levels by about 20% and 30% respectively; concurrent use in this study has resulted in additive negative inotropic effects). Products include:
Inderal LA Long-Acting Capsules 3421
InnoPran XL Capsules 2728

Quinidine (Drugs that inhibit cytochrome P4502D6, such as quinidine, might increase the plasma-concentrations of flecainide in patients who are on chronic flecainide therapy).
No products indexed under this heading.

Quinidine Gluconate (Drugs that inhibit cytochrome P4502D6, such as quinidine, might increase the plasma-concentrations of flecainide in patients who are on chronic flecainide therapy).
No products indexed under this heading.

Quinidine Hydrochloride (Drugs that inhibit cytochrome P4502D6, such as quinidine, might increase the plasma-concentrations of flecainide in patients who are on chronic flecainide therapy).
No products indexed under this heading.

Quinidine Polygalacturonate (Drugs that inhibit cytochrome P4502D6, such as quinidine, might increase the plasma-concentrations of flecainide in patients who are on chronic flecainide therapy).
No products indexed under this heading.

Quinidine Sulfate (Drugs that inhibit cytochrome P4502D6, such as quinidine, might increase the plasma-concentrations of flecainide in patients who are on chronic flecainide therapy).
No products indexed under this heading.

Sotalol Hydrochloride (Co-administration of flecainide with beta adrenergic blocking agents may result in possible additive negative inotropic effects; combined therapy has not resulted in adverse effects).
No products indexed under this heading.

Timolol Hemihydrate (Co-administration of flecainide with beta adrenergic blocking agents may result in possible additive negative inotropic effects; combined therapy has not resulted in adverse effects). Products include:
Betimol Ophthalmic Solution 3371
Betimol Ophthalmic Solution .... ⊙283

Timolol Maleate (Co-administration of flecainide with beta adrenergic blocking agents may result in possible additive negative inotropic effects; combined therapy has not resulted in adverse effects). Products include:
Blocadren Tablets 1891
Cosopt Sterile Ophthalmic Solution 1910
Timolide Tablets 2056
Timoptic in Ocudose 2061
Timoptic Sterile Ophthalmic Solution 2058
Timoptic-XE Sterile Ophthalmic Gel Forming Solution 2062

Verapamil Hydrochloride (Co-administration is not recommended because both drugs have negative inotropic properties). Products include:
Covera-HS Tablets 3135
Tarka Tablets 519
Verelan PM Capsules 3120

Food Interactions

Dairy products (Milk may inhibit absorption in infants; a reduction in Tambocor dosage should be considered when milk is removed from the diet of infants).

TAMIFLU CAPSULES

(Oseltamivir Phosphate) 2810
May interact with:

Probenecid (Co-administration with probenecid results in an approximate two-fold increase in exposure to oseltamivir due to a decrease in active anionic tubular secretion in the kidneys; no dose adjustments are required due to the safety margin of oseltamivir).
No products indexed under this heading.

TAMIFLU ORAL SUSPENSION

(Oseltamivir Phosphate) 2810
See Tamiflu Capsules

TARCEVA TABLETS

(Erlotinib) 2470
May interact with cytochrome p450 3a4 inducers (selected), cytochrome p450 3a4 inhibitors (selected), and certain other agents. Compounds in these categories include:

Acetazolamide (Caution when administering or taking erlotinib with strong CYP3A4 inhibitors such as atazanavir, clarithromycin, indinavir, itraconazole, nefazodone, nelfinavir, ritonavir, saquinavir, telithromycin, troleandomycin, and voriconazole).
No products indexed under this heading.

Amiodarone Hydrochloride (Caution when administering or taking erlotinib with strong CYP3A4 inhibitors such as atazanavir, clarithromycin, indinavir, itraconazole, nefazodone, nelfinavir, ritonavir, saquinavir, telithromycin, troleandomycin, and voriconazole). Products include:
Pacerone Tablets 3337

Amprenavir (Caution when administering or taking erlotinib with strong CYP3A4 inhibitors such as atazanavir, clarithromycin, indinavir, itraconazole, nefazodone, nelfinavir, ritonavir, saquinavir, telithromycin, troleandomycin, and voriconazole). Products include:
Agenerase Capsules 1299
Agenerase Oral Solution 1304

Anastrozole (Caution when administering or taking erlotinib with strong CYP3A4 inhibitors such as atazanavir, clarithromycin, indinavir, itraconazole, nefazodone, nelfinavir, ritonavir, saquinavir, telithromycin, troleandomycin, and voriconazole). Products include:
Arimidex Tablets 665

Aprepitant (Caution when administering or taking erlotinib with strong CYP3A4 inhibitors such as atazanavir, clarithromycin, indinavir, itraconazole, nefazodone, nelfinavir, ritonavir, saquinavir, telithromycin, troleandomycin, and voriconazole). Products include:
Emend Capsules 1944

Atazanavir (Co-treatment with the potent CYP3A4 inhibitor ketoconazole increases erlotinib AUC by 2/3. Caution should be used when administering or taking erlotinib with ketoconazole and other strong CYP3A4 inhibitors such as atazanavir).
No products indexed under this heading.

Atazanavir sulfate (Co-treatment with the potent CYP3A4 inhibitor ketoconazole increases erlotinib AUC by 2/3. Caution should be used when administering or taking erlotinib with ketoconazole and other strong CYP3A4 inhibitors such as atazanavir). Products include:
Reyataz Capsules 948

Cimetidine (Caution when administering or taking erlotinib with strong CYP3A4 inhibitors such as atazanavir, clarithromycin, indinavir, itraconazole, nefazodone, nelfinavir, ritonavir, saquinavir, telithromycin, troleandomycin, and voriconazole). Products include:
Tagamet HB 200 Tablets 637
Tagamet Tablets 1547

Cimetidine Hydrochloride (Caution when administering or taking erlotinib with strong CYP3A4 inhibitors such as atazanavir, clarithromycin, indinavir, itraconazole, nefazodone, nelfinavir, ritonavir, saquinavir, telithromycin, troleandomycin, and voriconazole).
No products indexed under this heading.

Ciprofloxacin (Caution when administering or taking erlotinib with strong CYP3A4 inhibitors such as atazanavir, clarithromycin, indinavir, itraconazole, nefazodone, nelfinavir, ritonavir, saquinavir, telithromycin, troleandomycin, and voriconazole). Products include:
Cipro I.V. 2998
Cipro I.V. Pharmacy Bulk Package 3509
Cipro Oral Suspension 2991
Cipro XR Tablets 3004
Ciprodex Otic Suspension 555

Cisplatin (Pre-treatment with the CYP3A4 inducer rifampicin decreased erlotinib AUC by about 2/3. Alternate treatments lacking CYP3A4 inducing activity should be considered. If and alternative treatment is unavailable, an erlotinib dose greater than 150 mg shouldbe considered. If the erlotinib dose is adjusted upward, the dose will need to be reduced upon discontinuation of rifampicin or otehr CYP3A4 inducers).
No products indexed under this heading.

Clarithromycin (Co-treatment with the potent CYP3A4 inhibitor ketoconazole increases erlotinib AUC by 2/3. Caution should be used when administering or taking erlotinib with ketoconazole and other strong CYP3A4 inhibitors such as clarithromycin). Products include:
Biaxin/Biaxin XL 402
PREVPAC 3281

Clotrimazole (Caution when administering or taking erlotinib with strong CYP3A4 inhibitors such as atazanavir, clarithromycin, indinavir, itraconazole, nefazodone, nelfinavir, ritonavir, saquinavir, telithromycin, troleandomycin, and voriconazole). Products include:
Lotrimin 3053
Lotrisone 3054

Cyclosporine (Caution when administering or taking erlotinib with strong CYP3A4 inhibitors such as atazanavir, clarithromycin, indinavir, itraconazole, nefazodone, nelfinavir, ritonavir, saquinavir, telithromycin, troleandomycin, and voriconazole). Products include:
Gengraf Capsules 458
Neoral Soft Gelatin Capsules 2247
Neoral Oral Solution 2247
Restasis Ophthalmic Emulsion 570
Sandimmune 2259

Dalfopristin (Caution when administering or taking erlotinib with strong CYP3A4 inhibitors such as atazanavir, clarithromycin, indinavir, itraconazole, nefazodone, nelfinavir, ritonavir, saquinavir, telithromycin, troleandomycin, and voriconazole). Products include:
Synercid I.V. 1690

Danazol (Caution when administering or taking erlotinib with strong CYP3A4 inhibitors such as atazanavir, clarithromycin, indinavir, itraconazole, nefazodone, nelfinavir, ritonavir, saquinavir, telithromycin, troleandomycin, and voriconazole).
No products indexed under this heading.

Delavirdine Mesylate (Caution when administering or taking erlotinib with strong CYP3A4 inhibitors such as atazanavir, clarithromycin, indinavir, itraconazole, nefazodone, nelfinavir, ritonavir, saquinavir, telithromycin, troleandomycin, and voriconazole). Products include:

Rescriptor Tablets **2535**

Diltiazem Hydrochloride (Caution when administering or taking erlotinib with strong CYP3A4 inhibitors such as atazanavir, clarithromycin, indinavir, itraconazole, nefazodone, nelfinavir, ritonavir, saquinavir, telithromycin, troleandomycin, and voriconazole). Products include:

Cardizem LA Extended Release Tablets **1699**
Tiazac Capsules **1204**

Diltiazem Maleate (Caution when administering or taking erlotinib with strong CYP3A4 inhibitors such as atazanavir, clarithromycin, indinavir, itraconazole, nefazodone, nelfinavir, ritonavir, saquinavir, telithromycin, troleandomycin, and voriconazole).

No products indexed under this heading.

Doxorubicin Hydrochloride (Pre-treatment with the CYP3A4 inducer rifampicin decreased erlotinib AUC by about 2/3. Alternate treatments lacking CYP3A4 inducing activity should be considered. If and alternative treatment is unavailable, an erlotinib dose greater than 150 mg shouldbe considered. If the erlotinib dose is adjusted upward, the dose will need to be reduced upon discontinuation of rifampicin or otehr CYP3A4 inducers). Products include:

Adriamycin for Injection, USP **786**
Adriamycin Injection, USP **786**

Efavirenz (Caution when administering or taking erlotinib with strong CYP3A4 inhibitors such as atazanavir, clarithromycin, indinavir, itraconazole, nefazodone, nelfinavir, ritonavir, saquinavir, telithromycin, troleandomycin, and voriconazole). Products include:

Sustiva Capsules **957**

Erythromycin (Caution when administering or taking erlotinib with strong CYP3A4 inhibitors such as atazanavir, clarithromycin, indinavir, itraconazole, nefazodone, nelfinavir, ritonavir, saquinavir, telithromycin, troleandomycin, and voriconazole). Products include:

Erygel Topical Gel **2096**
Ery-Tab Tablets **447**
Erythromycin Base Filmtab Tablets **454**
Erythromycin Delayed-Release Capsules, USP **456**
PCE Dispertab Tablets **510**

Erythromycin Estolate (Caution when administering or taking erlotinib with strong CYP3A4 inhibitors such as atazanavir, clarithromycin, indinavir, itraconazole, nefazodone, nelfinavir, ritonavir, saquinavir, telithromycin, troleandomycin, and voriconazole).

No products indexed under this heading.

Erythromycin Ethylsuccinate (Caution when administering or taking erlotinib with strong CYP3A4 inhibitors such as atazanavir, clarithromycin, indinavir, itraconazole, nefazodone, nelfinavir, ritonavir, saquinavir, telithromycin, troleandomycin, and voriconazole). Products include:

E.E.S. **449**
EryPed **445**

Erythromycin Gluceptate (Caution when administering or taking erlotinib with strong CYP3A4 inhibitors such as atazanavir, clarithromycin, indinavir, itraconazole, nefazodone, nelfinavir, ritonavir, saquinavir, telithromycin, troleandomycin, and voriconazole).

No products indexed under this heading.

Erythromycin Lactobionate (Caution when administering or taking erlotinib with strong CYP3A4 inhibitors such as atazanavir, clarithromycin, indinavir, itraconazole, nefazodone, nelfinavir, ritonavir, saquinavir, telithromycin, troleandomycin, and voriconazole).

No products indexed under this heading.

Erythromycin Stearate (Caution when administering or taking erlotinib with strong CYP3A4 inhibitors such as atazanavir, clarithromycin, indinavir, itraconazole, nefazodone, nelfinavir, ritonavir, saquinavir, telithromycin, troleandomycin, and voriconazole). Products include:

Erythrocin Stearate Filmtab Tablets **452**

Esomeprazole Magnesium (Caution when administering or taking erlotinib with strong CYP3A4 inhibitors such as atazanavir, clarithromycin, indinavir, itraconazole, nefazodone, nelfinavir, ritonavir, saquinavir, telithromycin, troleandomycin, and voriconazole). Products include:

Nexium Delayed-Release Capsules **645**

Felbamate (Pre-treatment with the CYP3A4 inducer rifampicin decreased erlotinib AUC by about 2/3. Alternate treatments lacking CYP3A4 inducing activity should be considered. If and alternative treatment is unavailable, an erlotinib dose greater than 150 mg shouldbe considered. If the erlotinib dose is adjusted upward, the dose will need to be reduced upon discontinuation of rifampicin or otehr CYP3A4 inducers).

No products indexed under this heading.

Fluconazole (Caution when administering or taking erlotinib with strong CYP3A4 inhibitors such as atazanavir, clarithromycin, indinavir, itraconazole, nefazodone, nelfinavir, ritonavir, saquinavir, telithromycin, troleandomycin, and voriconazole).

No products indexed under this heading.

Fluoxetine Hydrochloride (Caution when administering or taking erlotinib with strong CYP3A4 inhibitors such as atazanavir, clarithromycin, indinavir, itraconazole, nefazodone, nelfinavir, ritonavir, saquinavir, telithromycin, troleandomycin, and voriconazole). Products include:

Prozac Pulvules and Liquid **1771**
Symbyax Capsules **1788**

Fluvoxamine Maleate (Caution when administering or taking erlotinib with strong CYP3A4 inhibitors such as atazanavir, clarithromycin, indinavir, itraconazole, nefazodone, nelfinavir, ritonavir, saquinavir, telithromycin, troleandomycin, and voriconazole).

No products indexed under this heading.

Fosamprenavir Calcium (Caution when administering or taking erlotinib with strong CYP3A4 inhibitors such as atazanavir, clarithromycin, indinavir, itraconazole, nefazodone, nelfinavir, ritonavir, saquinavir, telithromycin, troleandomycin, and voriconazole). Products include:

Lexiva Tablets **1473**

Indinavir Sulfate (Co-treatment with the potent CYP3A4 inhibitor ketoconazole increases erlotinib AUC by 2/3. Caution should be used when administering or taking erlotinib with ketoconazole and other strong CYP3A4 inhibitors such as indinavir). Products include:

Crixivan Capsules **1918**

Isoniazid (Caution when administering or taking erlotinib with strong CYP3A4 inhibitors such as atazanavir, clarithromycin, indinavir, itraconazole, nefazodone, nelfinavir, ritonavir, saquinavir, telithromycin, troleandomycin, and voriconazole).

No products indexed under this heading.

Itraconazole (Co-treatment with the potent CYP3A4 inhibitor ketoconazole increases erlotinib AUC by 2/3. Caution should be used when administering or taking erlotinib with ketoconazole and other strong CYP3A4 inhibitors such as itraconazole).

No products indexed under this heading.

Ketoconazole (Co-treatment with the potent CYP3A4 inhibitor ketoconazole increases erlotinib AUC by 2/3. Caution should be used when administering or taking erlotinib with ketoconazole and other strong CYP3A4 inhibitors). Products include:

Nizoral A-D Shampoo, 1% **1839**
Nizoral 2% Shampoo **1838**

Lopinavir (Caution when administering or taking erlotinib with strong CYP3A4 inhibitors such as atazanavir, clarithromycin, indinavir, itraconazole, nefazodone, nelfinavir, ritonavir, saquinavir, telithromycin, troleandomycin, and voriconazole). Products include:

Kaletra **474**

Loratadine (Caution when administering or taking erlotinib with strong CYP3A4 inhibitors such as atazanavir, clarithromycin, indinavir, itraconazole, nefazodone, nelfinavir, ritonavir, saquinavir, telithromycin, troleandomycin, and voriconazole). Products include:

Alavert Allergy & Sinus D-12 Hour Tablets .... ▣**743**
Alavert .... ▣**743**
Children's Claritin 24 Hour Non-Drowsy Allergy Syrup .... ▣**732**
Claritin Non-Drowsy 24 Hour Tablets .... ▣**731**
Non-Drowsy Claritin Hives Relief Tablets .... ▣**733**
Claritin Reditabs 24 Hour Non-Drowsy Tablets .... ▣**732**
Claritin-D Non-Drowsy 12 Hour Tablets .... ▣**731**
Claritin-D Non-Drowsy 24 Hour Tablets .... ▣**731**
Children's Dimetapp ND Non-Drowsy Allergy Syrup .... ▣**746**
Triaminic Allerchews .... ▣**684**

Methsuximide (Pre-treatment with the CYP3A4 inducer rifampicin decreased erlotinib AUC by about 2/3. Alternate treatments lacking CYP3A4 inducing activity should be considered. If and alternative treatment is unavailable, an erlotinib dose greater than 150 mg shouldbe considered. If the erlotinib dose is adjusted upward, the dose will need to be reduced upon discontinuation of rifampicin or otehr CYP3A4 inducers).

No products indexed under this heading.

Metronidazole (Caution when administering or taking erlotinib with strong CYP3A4 inhibitors such as atazanavir, clarithromycin, indinavir, itraconazole, nefazodone, nelfinavir, ritonavir, saquinavir, telithromycin, troleandomycin, and voriconazole). Products include:

Metrogel 1% **1212**
MetroGel-Vaginal Gel **1822**
Noritate Cream, 1% **1051**

Metronidazole Benzoate (Caution when administering or taking erlotinib with strong CYP3A4 inhibitors such as atazanavir, clarithromycin, indinavir, itraconazole, nefazodone, nelfinavir, ritonavir, saquinavir, telithromycin, troleandomycin, and voriconazole).

No products indexed under this heading.

Metronidazole Hydrochloride (Caution when administering or taking erlotinib with strong CYP3A4 inhibitors such as atazanavir, clarithromycin, indinavir, itraconazole, nefazodone, nelfinavir, ritonavir, saquinavir, telithromycin, troleandomycin, and voriconazole).

No products indexed under this heading.

Miconazole (Caution when administering or taking erlotinib with strong CYP3A4 inhibitors such as atazanavir, clarithromycin, indinavir, itraconazole, nefazodone, nelfinavir, ritonavir, saquinavir, telithromycin, troleandomycin, and voriconazole).

No products indexed under this heading.

Miconazole Nitrate (Caution when administering or taking erlotinib with strong CYP3A4 inhibitors such as atazanavir, clarithromycin, indinavir, itraconazole, nefazodone, nelfinavir, ritonavir, saquinavir, telithromycin, troleandomycin, and voriconazole). Products include:

Desenex .... ▣**674**
Desenex Jock Itch Spray Powder .... ▣**674**

Nefazodone Hydrochloride (Co-treatment with the potent CYP3A4 inhibitor ketoconazole increases erlotinib AUC by 2/3. Caution should be used when administering or taking erlotinib with ketoconazole and other strong CYP3A4 inhibitors such as nefazodone).

No products indexed under this heading.

Nelfinavir Mesylate (Co-treatment with the potent CYP3A4 inhibitor ketoconazole increases erlotinib AUC by 2/3. Caution should be used when administering or taking erlotinib with ketoconazole and other strong CYP3A4 inhibitors such as nelfinavir). Products include:

Viracept **2556**

Nevirapine (Caution when administering or taking erlotinib with strong CYP3A4 inhibitors such as atazanavir, clarithromycin, indinavir, itraconazole, nefazodone, nelfinavir, ritonavir, saquinavir, telithromycin, troleandomycin, and voriconazole). Products include:

Viramune Oral Suspension **903**
Viramune Tablets **903**

Niacinamide (Caution when administering or taking erlotinib with strong CYP3A4 inhibitors such as atazanavir, clarithromycin, indinavir, itraconazole, nefazodone, nelfinavir, ritonavir, saquinavir, telithromycin, troleandomycin, and voriconazole).
No products indexed under this heading.

Nicotinamide (Caution when administering or taking erlotinib with strong CYP3A4 inhibitors such as atazanavir, clarithromycin, indinavir, itraconazole, nefazodone, nelfinavir, ritonavir, saquinavir, telithromycin, troleandomycin, and voriconazole). Products include:
Nicomide Tablets 3190

Nifedipine (Caution when administering or taking erlotinib with strong CYP3A4 inhibitors such as atazanavir, clarithromycin, indinavir, itraconazole, nefazodone, nelfinavir, ritonavir, saquinavir, telithromycin, troleandomycin, and voriconazole). Products include:
Adalat CC Tablets 2978

Norfloxacin (Caution when administering or taking erlotinib with strong CYP3A4 inhibitors such as atazanavir, clarithromycin, indinavir, itraconazole, nefazodone, nelfinavir, ritonavir, saquinavir, telithromycin, troleandomycin, and voriconazole). Products include:
Noroxin Tablets 2009

Omeprazole (Caution when administering or taking erlotinib with strong CYP3A4 inhibitors such as atazanavir, clarithromycin, indinavir, itraconazole, nefazodone, nelfinavir, ritonavir, saquinavir, telithromycin, troleandomycin, and voriconazole). Products include:
Zegerid Powder for Oral Solution 2972

Paroxetine Hydrochloride (Caution when administering or taking erlotinib with strong CYP3A4 inhibitors such as atazanavir, clarithromycin, indinavir, itraconazole, nefazodone, nelfinavir, ritonavir, saquinavir, telithromycin, troleandomycin, and voriconazole). Products include:
Paxil CR Controlled-Release Tablets 1509
Paxil 1501

Propoxyphene Hydrochloride (Caution when administering or taking erlotinib with strong CYP3A4 inhibitors such as atazanavir, clarithromycin, indinavir, itraconazole, nefazodone, nelfinavir, ritonavir, saquinavir, telithromycin, troleandomycin, and voriconazole).
No products indexed under this heading.

Propoxyphene Napsylate (Caution when administering or taking erlotinib with strong CYP3A4 inhibitors such as atazanavir, clarithromycin, indinavir, itraconazole, nefazodone, nelfinavir, ritonavir, saquinavir, telithromycin, troleandomycin, and voriconazole). Products include:
Darvocet A 500 Tablets 3497

Quinidine (Caution when administering or taking erlotinib with strong CYP3A4 inhibitors such as atazanavir, clarithromycin, indinavir, itraconazole, nefazodone, nelfinavir, ritonavir, saquinavir, telithromycin, troleandomycin, and voriconazole).
No products indexed under this heading.

Quinidine Hydrochloride (Caution when administering or taking erlotinib with strong CYP3A4 inhibitors such as atazanavir, clarithromycin, indinavir, itraconazole, nefazodone, nelfinavir, ritonavir, saquinavir, telithromycin, troleandomycin, and voriconazole).
No products indexed under this heading.

Quinidine Polygalacturonate (Caution when administering or taking erlotinib with strong CYP3A4 inhibitors such as atazanavir, clarithromycin, indinavir, itraconazole, nefazodone, nelfinavir, ritonavir, saquinavir, telithromycin, troleandomycin, and voriconazole).
No products indexed under this heading.

Quinidine Sulfate (Caution when administering or taking erlotinib with strong CYP3A4 inhibitors such as atazanavir, clarithromycin, indinavir, itraconazole, nefazodone, nelfinavir, ritonavir, saquinavir, telithromycin, troleandomycin, and voriconazole).
No products indexed under this heading.

Quinine (Caution when administering or taking erlotinib with strong CYP3A4 inhibitors such as atazanavir, clarithromycin, indinavir, itraconazole, nefazodone, nelfinavir, ritonavir, saquinavir, telithromycin, troleandomycin, and voriconazole).
No products indexed under this heading.

Quinine Sulfate (Caution when administering or taking erlotinib with strong CYP3A4 inhibitors such as atazanavir, clarithromycin, indinavir, itraconazole, nefazodone, nelfinavir, ritonavir, saquinavir, telithromycin, troleandomycin, and voriconazole).
No products indexed under this heading.

Quinupristin (Caution when administering or taking erlotinib with strong CYP3A4 inhibitors such as atazanavir, clarithromycin, indinavir, itraconazole, nefazodone, nelfinavir, ritonavir, saquinavir, telithromycin, troleandomycin, and voriconazole). Products include:
Synercid I.V. 1690

Ranitidine Bismuth Citrate (Caution when administering or taking erlotinib with strong CYP3A4 inhibitors such as atazanavir, clarithromycin, indinavir, itraconazole, nefazodone, nelfinavir, ritonavir, saquinavir, telithromycin, troleandomycin, and voriconazole).
No products indexed under this heading.

Ranitidine Hydrochloride (Caution when administering or taking erlotinib with strong CYP3A4 inhibitors such as atazanavir, clarithromycin, indinavir, itraconazole, nefazodone, nelfinavir, ritonavir, saquinavir, telithromycin, troleandomycin, and voriconazole). Products include:
Zantac 1597
Zantac Injection 1593
Zantac 75 Tablets 715
Zantac 150 Maximum Strength Tablets 715
Zantac Injection Pharmacy Bulk Package 1595

Rifampicin (Pre-treatment with the CYP3A4 inducer rifampicin decreased erlotinib AUC by about 2/3. Alternate treatments lacking CYP3A4 inducing activity should be considered. If and alternative treatment is unavailable, an erlotinib dose greater than 150 mg shouldbe considered. If the erlotinib dose is adjusted upward, the dose will need to be reduced upon discontinuation of rifampicin or otehr CYP3A4 inducers).
No products indexed under this heading.

Rifapentine (Pre-treatment with the CYP3A4 inducer rifampicin decreased erlotinib AUC by about 2/3. Alternate treatments lacking CYP3A4 inducing activity should be considered. If and alternative treatment is unavailable, an erlotinib dose greater than 150 mg shouldbe considered. If the erlotinib dose is adjusted upward, the dose will need to be reduced upon discontinuation of rifampicin or otehr CYP3A4 inducers).
No products indexed under this heading.

Ritonavir (Co-treatment with the potent CYP3A4 inhibitor ketoconazole increases erlotinib AUC by 2/3. Caution should be used when administering or taking erlotinib with ketoconazole and other strong CYP3A4 inhibitors such as ritonavir). Products include:
Kaletra 474
Norvir 499

Saquinavir (Co-treatment with the potent CYP3A4 inhibitor ketoconazole increases erlotinib AUC by 2/3. Caution should be used when administering or taking erlotinib with ketoconazole and other strong CYP3A4 inhibitors such as saquinavir).
No products indexed under this heading.

Saquinavir Mesylate (Co-treatment with the potent CYP3A4 inhibitor ketoconazole increases erlotinib AUC by 2/3. Caution should be used when administering or taking erlotinib with ketoconazole and other strong CYP3A4 inhibitors such as saquinavir). Products include:
Invirase 2776

Sertraline Hydrochloride (Caution when administering or taking erlotinib with strong CYP3A4 inhibitors such as atazanavir, clarithromycin, indinavir, itraconazole, nefazodone, nelfinavir, ritonavir, saquinavir, telithromycin, troleandomycin, and voriconazole). Products include:
Zoloft 2581

Telithromycin (Co-treatment with the potent CYP3A4 inhibitor ketoconazole increases erlotinib AUC by 2/3. Caution should be used when administering or taking erlotinib with ketoconazole and other strong CYP3A4 inhibitors such as telithromycin). Products include:
Ketek Tablets 2920

Theophylline (Pre-treatment with the CYP3A4 inducer rifampicin decreased erlotinib AUC by about 2/3. Alternate treatments lacking CYP3A4 inducing activity should be considered. If and alternative treatment is unavailable, an erlotinib dose greater than 150 mg shouldbe considered. If the erlotinib dose is adjusted upward, the dose will need to be reduced upon discontinuation of rifampicin or otehr CYP3A4 inducers).
No products indexed under this heading.

Troglitazone (Caution when administering or taking erlotinib with strong CYP3A4 inhibitors such as atazanavir, clarithromycin, indinavir, itraconazole, nefazodone, nelfinavir, ritonavir, saquinavir, telithromycin, troleandomycin, and voriconazole).
No products indexed under this heading.

Troleandomycin (Co-treatment with the potent CYP3A4 inhibitor ketoconazole increases erlotinib AUC by 2/3. Caution should be used when administering or taking erlotinib with ketoconazole and other strong CYP3A4 inhibitors such as troleandomycin).
No products indexed under this heading.

Valproate Sodium (Caution when administering or taking erlotinib with strong CYP3A4 inhibitors such as atazanavir, clarithromycin, indinavir, itraconazole, nefazodone, nelfinavir, ritonavir, saquinavir, telithromycin, troleandomycin, and voriconazole). Products include:
Depacon Injection 412

Verapamil Hydrochloride (Caution when administering or taking erlotinib with strong CYP3A4 inhibitors such as atazanavir, clarithromycin, indinavir, itraconazole, nefazodone, nelfinavir, ritonavir, saquinavir, telithromycin, troleandomycin, and voriconazole). Products include:
Covera-HS Tablets 3135
Tarka Tablets 519
Verelan PM Capsules 3120

Voriconazole (Co-treatment with the potent CYP3A4 inhibitor ketoconazole increases erlotinib AUC by 2/3. Caution should be used when administering or taking erlotinib with ketoconazole and other strong CYP3A4 inhibitors such as voriconazole). Products include:
VFEND I.V. 2543
VFEND Oral Suspension 2543
VFEND Tablets 2543

Zafirlukast (Caution when administering or taking erlotinib with strong CYP3A4 inhibitors such as atazanavir, clarithromycin, indinavir, itraconazole, nefazodone, nelfinavir, ritonavir, saquinavir, telithromycin, troleandomycin, and voriconazole). Products include:
Accolate Tablets 663

Zileuton (Caution when administering or taking erlotinib with strong CYP3A4 inhibitors such as atazanavir, clarithromycin, indinavir, itraconazole, nefazodone, nelfinavir, ritonavir, saquinavir, telithromycin, troleandomycin, and voriconazole).
No products indexed under this heading.

Food Interactions

Grapefruit (Caution when administering or taking erlotinib with strong CYP3A4 inhibitors such as atazanavir, clarithromycin, indinavir, itraconazole, nefazodone, nelfinavir, ritonavir, saquinavir, telithromycin, troleandomycin, and voriconazole).

Grapefruit Juice (Caution when administering or taking erlotinib with strong CYP3A4 inhibitors such as atazanavir, clarithromycin, indinavir, itraconazole, nefazodone, nelfinavir, ritonavir, saquinavir, telithromycin, troleandomycin, and voriconazole).

TARCEVA TABLETS
(Erlotinib) 1254
May interact with cytochrome p450 3a4 inducers (selected), cytochrome p450 3a4 inhibitors (selected), and certain other agents. Compounds in these categories include:

Acetazolamide (Caution when administering or taking erlotinib with strong CYP3A4 inhibitors such as atazanavir, clarithromycin, indinavir, itraconazole, nefazodone, nelfinavir, ritonavir, saquinavir, telithromycin, troleandomycin, and voriconazole).
No products indexed under this heading.

Amiodarone Hydrochloride (Caution when administering or taking erlotinib with strong CYP3A4 inhibitors such as atazanavir, clarithromycin, indinavir, itraconazole, nefazodone, nelfinavir, ritonavir, saquinavir, telithromycin, troleandomycin, and voriconazole). Products include:
Pacerone Tablets 3337

Amprenavir (Caution when administering or taking erlotinib with strong CYP3A4 inhibitors such as atazanavir, clarithromycin, indinavir, itraconazole, nefazodone, nelfinavir, ritonavir, saquinavir, telithromycin, troleandomycin, and voriconazole). Products include:
Agenerase Capsules 1299
Agenerase Oral Solution 1304

Anastrozole (Caution when administering or taking erlotinib with strong CYP3A4 inhibitors such as atazanavir, clarithromycin, indinavir, itraconazole, nefazodone, nelfinavir, ritonavir, saquinavir, telithromycin, troleandomycin, and voriconazole). Products include:
Arimidex Tablets 665

Aprepitant (Caution when administering or taking erlotinib with strong CYP3A4 inhibitors such as atazanavir, clarithromycin, indinavir, itraconazole, nefazodone, nelfinavir, ritonavir, saquinavir, telithromycin, troleandomycin, and voriconazole). Products include:
Emend Capsules 1944

Atazanavir (Co-treatment with the potent CYP3A4 inhibitor ketoconazole increases erlotinib AUC by 2/3. Caution should be used when administering or taking erlotinib with ketoconazole and other strong CYP3A4 inhibitors such as atazanavir).
No products indexed under this heading.

Atazanavir sulfate (Co-treatment with the potent CYP3A4 inhibitor ketoconazole increases erlotinib AUC by 2/3. Caution should be used when administering or taking erlotinib with ketoconazole and other strong CYP3A4 inhibitors such as atazanavir). Products include:
Reyataz Capsules 948

Cimetidine (Caution when administering or taking erlotinib with strong CYP3A4 inhibitors such as atazanavir, clarithromycin, indinavir, itraconazole, nefazodone, nelfinavir, ritonavir, saquinavir, telithromycin, troleandomycin, and voriconazole). Products include:
Tagamet HB 200 Tablets .... ▣ 637
Tagamet Tablets 1547

Cimetidine Hydrochloride (Caution when administering or taking erlotinib with strong CYP3A4 inhibitors such as atazanavir, clarithromycin, indinavir, itraconazole, nefazodone, nelfinavir, ritonavir, saquinavir, telithromycin, troleandomycin, and voriconazole).
No products indexed under this heading.

Ciprofloxacin (Caution when administering or taking erlotinib with strong CYP3A4 inhibitors such as atazanavir, clarithromycin, indinavir, itraconazole, nefazodone, nelfinavir, ritonavir, saquinavir, telithromycin, troleandomycin, and voriconazole). Products include:
Cipro I.V. 2998
Cipro I.V. Pharmacy Bulk Package ... 3509
Cipro Oral Suspension 2991
Cipro XR Tablets 3004
Ciprodex Otic Suspension 555

Cisplatin (Pre-treatment with the CYP3A4 inducer rifampicin decreased erlotinib AUC by about 2/3. Alternate treatments lacking CYP3A4 inducing activity should be considered. If and alternative treatment is unavailable, an erlotinib dose greater than 150 mg shouldbe considered. If the erlotinib dose is adjusted upward, the dose will need to be reduced upon discontinuation of rifampicin or otehr CYP3A4 inducers).
No products indexed under this heading.

Clarithromycin (Co-treatment with the potent CYP3A4 inhibitor ketoconazole increases erlotinib AUC by 2/3. Caution should be used when administering or taking erlotinib with ketoconazole and other strong CYP3A4 inhibitors such as clarithromycin). Products include:
Biaxin/Biaxin XL 402
PREVPAC 3281

Clotrimazole (Caution when administering or taking erlotinib with strong CYP3A4 inhibitors such as atazanavir, clarithromycin, indinavir, itraconazole, nefazodone, nelfinavir, ritonavir, saquinavir, telithromycin, troleandomycin, and voriconazole). Products include:
Lotrimin 3053
Lotrisone 3054

Cyclosporine (Caution when administering or taking erlotinib with strong CYP3A4 inhibitors such as atazanavir, clarithromycin, indinavir, itraconazole, nefazodone, nelfinavir, ritonavir, saquinavir, telithromycin, troleandomycin, and voriconazole). Products include:
Gengraf Capsules 458
Neoral Soft Gelatin Capsules 2247
Neoral Oral Solution 2247
Restasis Ophthalmic Emulsion 570
Sandimmune 2259

Dalfopristin (Caution when administering or taking erlotinib with strong CYP3A4 inhibitors such as atazanavir, clarithromycin, indinavir, itraconazole, nefazodone, nelfinavir, ritonavir, saquinavir, telithromycin, troleandomycin, and voriconazole). Products include:
Synercid I.V. 1690

Danazol (Caution when administering or taking erlotinib with strong CYP3A4 inhibitors such as atazanavir, clarithromycin, indinavir, itraconazole, nefazodone, nelfinavir, ritonavir, saquinavir, telithromycin, troleandomycin, and voriconazole).
No products indexed under this heading.

Delavirdine Mesylate (Caution when administering or taking erlotinib with strong CYP3A4 inhibitors such as atazanavir, clarithromycin, indinavir, itraconazole, nefazodone, nelfinavir, ritonavir, saquinavir, telithromycin, troleandomycin, and voriconazole). Products include:
Rescriptor Tablets 2535

Diltiazem Hydrochloride (Caution when administering or taking erlotinib with strong CYP3A4 inhibitors such as atazanavir, clarithromycin, indinavir, itraconazole, nefazodone, nelfinavir, ritonavir, saquinavir, telithromycin, troleandomycin, and voriconazole). Products include:
Cardizem LA Extended Release Tablets 1699
Tiazac Capsules 1204

Diltiazem Maleate (Caution when administering or taking erlotinib with strong CYP3A4 inhibitors such as atazanavir, clarithromycin, indinavir, itraconazole, nefazodone, nelfinavir, ritonavir, saquinavir, telithromycin, troleandomycin, and voriconazole).
No products indexed under this heading.

Doxorubicin Hydrochloride (Pre-treatment with the CYP3A4 inducer rifampicin decreased erlotinib AUC by about 2/3. Alternate treatments lacking CYP3A4 inducing activity should be considered. If and alternative treatment is unavailable, an erlotinib dose greater than 150 mg shouldbe considered. If the erlotinib dose is adjusted upward, the dose will need to be reduced upon discontinuation of rifampicin or otehr CYP3A4 inducers). Products include:
Adriamycin for Injection, USP 786
Adriamycin Injection, USP 786

Efavirenz (Caution when administering or taking erlotinib with strong CYP3A4 inhibitors such as atazanavir, clarithromycin, indinavir, itraconazole, nefazodone, nelfinavir, ritonavir, saquinavir, telithromycin, troleandomycin, and voriconazole). Products include:
Sustiva Capsules 957

Erythromycin (Caution when administering or taking erlotinib with strong CYP3A4 inhibitors such as atazanavir, clarithromycin, indinavir, itraconazole, nefazodone, nelfinavir, ritonavir, saquinavir, telithromycin, troleandomycin, and voriconazole). Products include:
Erygel Topical Gel 2096
Ery-Tab Tablets 447
Erythromycin Base Filmtab Tablets 454
Erythromycin Delayed-Release Capsules, USP 456
PCE Dispertab Tablets 510

Erythromycin Estolate (Caution when administering or taking erlotinib with strong CYP3A4 inhibitors such as atazanavir, clarithromycin, indinavir, itraconazole, nefazodone, nelfinavir, ritonavir, saquinavir, telithromycin, troleandomycin, and voriconazole).
No products indexed under this heading.

Erythromycin Ethylsuccinate (Caution when administering or taking erlotinib with strong CYP3A4 inhibitors such as atazanavir, clarithromycin, indinavir, itraconazole, nefazodone, nelfinavir, ritonavir, saquinavir, telithromycin, troleandomycin, and voriconazole). Products include:
E.E.S. 449
EryPed 445

Erythromycin Gluceptate (Caution when administering or taking erlotinib with strong CYP3A4 inhibitors such as atazanavir, clarithromycin, indinavir, itraconazole, nefazodone, nelfinavir, ritonavir, saquinavir, telithromycin, troleandomycin, and voriconazole).
No products indexed under this heading.

Erythromycin Lactobionate (Caution when administering or taking erlotinib with strong CYP3A4 inhibitors such as atazanavir, clarithromycin, indinavir, itraconazole, nefazodone, nelfinavir, ritonavir, saquinavir, telithromycin, troleandomycin, and voriconazole).
No products indexed under this heading.

Erythromycin Stearate (Caution when administering or taking erlotinib with strong CYP3A4 inhibitors such as atazanavir, clarithromycin, indinavir, itraconazole, nefazodone, nelfinavir, ritonavir, saquinavir, telithromycin, troleandomycin, and voriconazole). Products include:
Erythrocin Stearate Filmtab Tablets 452

Esomeprazole Magnesium (Caution when administering or taking erlotinib with strong CYP3A4 inhibitors such as atazanavir, clarithromycin, indinavir, itraconazole, nefazodone, nelfinavir, ritonavir, saquinavir, telithromycin, troleandomycin, and voriconazole). Products include:
Nexium Delayed-Release Capsules 645

Felbamate (Pre-treatment with the CYP3A4 inducer rifampicin decreased erlotinib AUC by about 2/3. Alternate treatments lacking CYP3A4 inducing activity should be considered. If and alternative treatment is unavailable, an erlotinib dose greater than 150 mg shouldbe considered. If the erlotinib dose is adjusted upward, the dose will need to be reduced upon discontinuation of rifampicin or otehr CYP3A4 inducers).
No products indexed under this heading.

Fluconazole (Caution when administering or taking erlotinib with strong CYP3A4 inhibitors such as atazanavir, clarithromycin, indinavir, itraconazole, nefazodone, nelfinavir, ritonavir, saquinavir, telithromycin, troleandomycin, and voriconazole).
No products indexed under this heading.

Fluoxetine Hydrochloride (Caution when administering or taking erlotinib with strong CYP3A4 inhibitors such as atazanavir, clarithromycin, indinavir, itraconazole, nefazodone, nelfinavir, ritonavir, saquinavir, telithromycin, troleandomycin, and voriconazole). Products include:
Prozac Pulvules and Liquid 1771
Symbyax Capsules 1788

Fluvoxamine Maleate (Caution when administering or taking erlotinib with strong CYP3A4 inhibitors such as atazanavir, clarithromycin, indinavir, itraconazole, nefazodone, nelfinavir, ritonavir, saquinavir, telithromycin, troleandomycin, and voriconazole).
No products indexed under this heading.

Fosamprenavir Calcium (Caution when administering or taking erlotinib with strong CYP3A4 inhibitors such as atazanavir, clarithromycin, indinavir, itraconazole, nefazodone, nelfinavir, ritonavir, saquinavir, telithromycin, troleandomycin, and voriconazole). Products include:

Lexiva Tablets 1473

Indinavir Sulfate (Co-treatment with the potent CYP3A4 inhibitor ketoconazole increases erlotinib AUC by 2/3. Caution should be used when administering or taking erlotinib with ketoconazole and other strong CYP3A4 inhibitors such as indinavir). Products include:

Crixivan Capsules 1918

Isoniazid (Caution when administering or taking erlotinib with strong CYP3A4 inhibitors such as atazanavir, clarithromycin, indinavir, itraconazole, nefazodone, nelfinavir, ritonavir, saquinavir, telithromycin, troleandomycin, and voriconazole).

No products indexed under this heading.

Itraconazole (Co-treatment with the potent CYP3A4 inhibitor ketoconazole increases erlotinib AUC by 2/3. Caution should be used when administering or taking erlotinib with ketoconazole and other strong CYP3A4 inhibitors such as itraconazole).

No products indexed under this heading.

Ketoconazole (Co-treatment with the potent CYP3A4 inhibitor ketoconazole increases erlotinib AUC by 2/3. Caution should be used when administering or taking erlotinib with ketoconazole and other strong CYP3A4 inhibitors). Products include:

Nizoral A-D Shampoo, 1% 1839
Nizoral 2% Shampoo 1838

Lopinavir (Caution when administering or taking erlotinib with strong CYP3A4 inhibitors such as atazanavir, clarithromycin, indinavir, itraconazole, nefazodone, nelfinavir, ritonavir, saquinavir, telithromycin, troleandomycin, and voriconazole). Products include:

Kaletra 474

Loratadine (Caution when administering or taking erlotinib with strong CYP3A4 inhibitors such as atazanavir, clarithromycin, indinavir, itraconazole, nefazodone, nelfinavir, ritonavir, saquinavir, telithromycin, troleandomycin, and voriconazole). Products include:

Alavert Allergy & Sinus D-12 Hour Tablets 743
Alavert 743
Children's Claritin 24 Hour Non-Drowsy Allergy Syrup 732
Claritin Non-Drowsy 24 Hour Tablets 731
Non-Drowsy Claritin Hives Relief Tablets 733
Claritin Reditabs 24 Hour Non-Drowsy Tablets 732
Claritin-D Non-Drowsy 12 Hour Tablets 731
Claritin-D Non-Drowsy 24 Hour Tablets 731
Children's Dimetapp ND Non-Drowsy Allergy Syrup 746
Triaminic Allerchews 684

Methsuximide (Pre-treatment with the CYP3A4 inducer rifampicin decreased erlotinib AUC by about 2/3. Alternate treatments lacking CYP3A4 inducing activity should be considered. If and alternative treatment is unavailable, an erlotinib dose greater than 150 mg shouldbe considered. If the erlotinib dose is adjusted upward, the dose will need to be reduced upon discontinuation of rifampicin or otehr CYP3A4 inducers).

No products indexed under this heading.

Metronidazole (Caution when administering or taking erlotinib with strong CYP3A4 inhibitors such as atazanavir, clarithromycin, indinavir, itraconazole, nefazodone, nelfinavir, ritonavir, saquinavir, telithromycin, troleandomycin, and voriconazole). Products include:

Metrogel 1% 1212
MetroGel-Vaginal Gel 1822
Noritate Cream, 1% 1051

Metronidazole Benzoate (Caution when administering or taking erlotinib with strong CYP3A4 inhibitors such as atazanavir, clarithromycin, indinavir, itraconazole, nefazodone, nelfinavir, ritonavir, saquinavir, telithromycin, troleandomycin, and voriconazole).

No products indexed under this heading.

Metronidazole Hydrochloride (Caution when administering or taking erlotinib with strong CYP3A4 inhibitors such as atazanavir, clarithromycin, indinavir, itraconazole, nefazodone, nelfinavir, ritonavir, saquinavir, telithromycin, troleandomycin, and voriconazole).

No products indexed under this heading.

Miconazole (Caution when administering or taking erlotinib with strong CYP3A4 inhibitors such as atazanavir, clarithromycin, indinavir, itraconazole, nefazodone, nelfinavir, ritonavir, saquinavir, telithromycin, troleandomycin, and voriconazole).

No products indexed under this heading.

Miconazole Nitrate (Caution when administering or taking erlotinib with strong CYP3A4 inhibitors such as atazanavir, clarithromycin, indinavir, itraconazole, nefazodone, nelfinavir, ritonavir, saquinavir, telithromycin, troleandomycin, and voriconazole). Products include:

Desenex 674
Desenex Jock Itch Spray Powder ... 674

Nefazodone Hydrochloride (Co-treatment with the potent CYP3A4 inhibitor ketoconazole increases erlotinib AUC by 2/3. Caution should be used when administering or taking erlotinib with ketoconazole and other strong CYP3A4 inhibitors such as nefazodone).

No products indexed under this heading.

Nelfinavir Mesylate (Co-treatment with the potent CYP3A4 inhibitor ketoconazole increases erlotinib AUC by 2/3. Caution should be used when administering or taking erlotinib with ketoconazole and other strong CYP3A4 inhibitors such as nelfinavir). Products include:

Viracept 2556

Nevirapine (Caution when administering or taking erlotinib with strong CYP3A4 inhibitors such as atazanavir, clarithromycin, indinavir, itraconazole, nefazodone, nelfinavir, ritonavir, saquinavir, telithromycin, troleandomycin, and voriconazole). Products include:

Viramune Oral Suspension 903
Viramune Tablets 903

Niacinamide (Caution when administering or taking erlotinib with strong CYP3A4 inhibitors such as atazanavir, clarithromycin, indinavir, itraconazole, nefazodone, nelfinavir, ritonavir, saquinavir, telithromycin, troleandomycin, and voriconazole).

No products indexed under this heading.

Nicotinamide (Caution when administering or taking erlotinib with strong CYP3A4 inhibitors such as atazanavir, clarithromycin, indinavir, itraconazole, nefazodone, nelfinavir, ritonavir, saquinavir, telithromycin, troleandomycin, and voriconazole). Products include:

Nicomide Tablets 3190

Nifedipine (Caution when administering or taking erlotinib with strong CYP3A4 inhibitors such as atazanavir, clarithromycin, indinavir, itraconazole, nefazodone, nelfinavir, ritonavir, saquinavir, telithromycin, troleandomycin, and voriconazole). Products include:

Adalat CC Tablets 2978

Norfloxacin (Caution when administering or taking erlotinib with strong CYP3A4 inhibitors such as atazanavir, clarithromycin, indinavir, itraconazole, nefazodone, nelfinavir, ritonavir, saquinavir, telithromycin, troleandomycin, and voriconazole). Products include:

Noroxin Tablets 2009

Omeprazole (Caution when administering or taking erlotinib with strong CYP3A4 inhibitors such as atazanavir, clarithromycin, indinavir, itraconazole, nefazodone, nelfinavir, ritonavir, saquinavir, telithromycin, troleandomycin, and voriconazole). Products include:

Zegerid Powder for Oral Solution 2972

Paroxetine Hydrochloride (Caution when administering or taking erlotinib with strong CYP3A4 inhibitors such as atazanavir, clarithromycin, indinavir, itraconazole, nefazodone, nelfinavir, ritonavir, saquinavir, telithromycin, troleandomycin, and voriconazole). Products include:

Paxil CR Controlled-Release Tablets 1509
Paxil 1501

Propoxyphene Hydrochloride (Caution when administering or taking erlotinib with strong CYP3A4 inhibitors such as atazanavir, clarithromycin, indinavir, itraconazole, nefazodone, nelfinavir, ritonavir, saquinavir, telithromycin, troleandomycin, and voriconazole).

No products indexed under this heading.

Propoxyphene Napsylate (Caution when administering or taking erlotinib with strong CYP3A4 inhibitors such as atazanavir, clarithromycin, indinavir, itraconazole, nefazodone, nelfinavir, ritonavir, saquinavir, telithromycin, troleandomycin, and voriconazole). Products include:

Darvocet A 500 Tablets 3497

Quinidine (Caution when administering or taking erlotinib with strong CYP3A4 inhibitors such as atazanavir, clarithromycin, indinavir, itraconazole, nefazodone, nelfinavir, ritonavir, saquinavir, telithromycin, troleandomycin, and voriconazole).

No products indexed under this heading.

Quinidine Hydrochloride (Caution when administering or taking erlotinib with strong CYP3A4 inhibitors such as atazanavir, clarithromycin, indinavir, itraconazole, nefazodone, nelfinavir, ritonavir, saquinavir, telithromycin, troleandomycin, and voriconazole).

No products indexed under this heading.

Quinidine Polygalacturonate (Caution when administering or taking erlotinib with strong CYP3A4 inhibitors such as atazanavir, clarithromycin, indinavir, itraconazole, nefazodone, nelfinavir, ritonavir, saquinavir, telithromycin, troleandomycin, and voriconazole).

No products indexed under this heading.

Quinidine Sulfate (Caution when administering or taking erlotinib with strong CYP3A4 inhibitors such as atazanavir, clarithromycin, indinavir, itraconazole, nefazodone, nelfinavir, ritonavir, saquinavir, telithromycin, troleandomycin, and voriconazole).

No products indexed under this heading.

Quinine (Caution when administering or taking erlotinib with strong CYP3A4 inhibitors such as atazanavir, clarithromycin, indinavir, itraconazole, nefazodone, nelfinavir, ritonavir, saquinavir, telithromycin, troleandomycin, and voriconazole).

No products indexed under this heading.

Quinine Sulfate (Caution when administering or taking erlotinib with strong CYP3A4 inhibitors such as atazanavir, clarithromycin, indinavir, itraconazole, nefazodone, nelfinavir, ritonavir, saquinavir, telithromycin, troleandomycin, and voriconazole).

No products indexed under this heading.

Quinupristin (Caution when administering or taking erlotinib with strong CYP3A4 inhibitors such as atazanavir, clarithromycin, indinavir, itraconazole, nefazodone, nelfinavir, ritonavir, saquinavir, telithromycin, troleandomycin, and voriconazole). Products include:

Synercid I.V. 1690

Ranitidine Bismuth Citrate (Caution when administering or taking erlotinib with strong CYP3A4 inhibitors such as atazanavir, clarithromycin, indinavir, itraconazole, nefazodone, nelfinavir, ritonavir, saquinavir, telithromycin, troleandomycin, and voriconazole).

No products indexed under this heading.

Ranitidine Hydrochloride (Caution when administering or taking erlotinib with strong CYP3A4 inhibitors such as atazanavir, clarithromycin, indinavir, itraconazole, nefazodone, nelfinavir, ritonavir, saquinavir, telithromycin, troleandomycin, and voriconazole). Products include:

Zantac 1597
Zantac Injection 1593
Zantac 75 Tablets 715
Zantac 150 Maximum Strength Tablets 715
Zantac Injection Pharmacy Bulk Package 1595

Rifampicin (Pre-treatment with the CYP3A4 inducer rifampicin decreased erlotinib AUC by about 2/3. Alternate treatments lacking CYP3A4 inducing activity should be considered. If and alternative treat-

IMPORTANT NOTE: Always consult each drug listing in the patient's regimen for possible interactions.

ment is unavailable, an erlotinib dose greater than 150 mg shouldbe considered. If the erlotinib dose is adjusted upward, the dose will need to be reduced upon discontinuation of rifampicin or otehr CYP3A4 inducers).
No products indexed under this heading.

Rifapentine (Pre-treatment with the CYP3A4 inducer rifampicin decreased erlotinib AUC by about 2/3. Alternate treatments lacking CYP3A4 inducing activity should be considered. If and alternative treatment is unavailable, an erlotinib dose greater than 150 mg shouldbe considered. If the erlotinib dose is adjusted upward, the dose will need to be reduced upon discontinuation of rifampicin or otehr CYP3A4 inducers).
No products indexed under this heading.

Ritonavir (Co-treatment with the potent CYP3A4 inhibitor ketoconazole increases erlotinib AUC by 2/3. Caution should be used when administering or taking erlotinib with ketoconazole and other strong CYP3A4 inhibitors such as ritonavir). Products include:
Kaletra 474
Norvir 499

Saquinavir (Co-treatment with the potent CYP3A4 inhibitor ketoconazole increases erlotinib AUC by 2/3. Caution should be used when administering or taking erlotinib with ketoconazole and other strong CYP3A4 inhibitors such as saquinavir).
No products indexed under this heading.

Saquinavir Mesylate (Co-treatment with the potent CYP3A4 inhibitor ketoconazole increases erlotinib AUC by 2/3. Caution should be used when administering or taking erlotinib with ketoconazole and other strong CYP3A4 inhibitors such as saquinavir). Products include:
Invirase 2776

Sertraline Hydrochloride (Caution when administering or taking erlotinib with strong CYP3A4 inhibitors such as atazanavir, clarithromycin, indinavir, itraconazole, nefazodone, nelfinavir, ritonavir, saquinavir, telithromycin, troleandomycin, and voriconazole). Products include:
Zoloft 2581

Telithromycin (Co-treatment with the potent CYP3A4 inhibitor ketoconazole increases erlotinib AUC by 2/3. Caution should be used when administering or taking erlotinib with ketoconazole and other strong CYP3A4 inhibitors such as telithromycin). Products include:
Ketek Tablets 2920

Theophylline (Pre-treatment with the CYP3A4 inducer rifampicin decreased erlotinib AUC by about 2/3. Alternate treatments lacking CYP3A4 inducing activity should be considered. If and alternative treatment is unavailable, an erlotinib dose greater than 150 mg shouldbe considered. If the erlotinib dose is adjusted upward, the dose will need to be reduced upon discontinuation of rifampicin or otehr CYP3A4 inducers).
No products indexed under this heading.

Troglitazone (Caution when administering or taking erlotinib with strong CYP3A4 inhibitors such as atazanavir, clarithromycin, indinavir, itraconazole, nefazodone, nelfinavir, ritonavir, saquinavir, telithromycin, troleandomycin, and voriconazole).
No products indexed under this heading.

Troleandomycin (Co-treatment with the potent CYP3A4 inhibitor ketoconazole increases erlotinib AUC by 2/3. Caution should be used when administering or taking erlotinib with ketoconazole and other strong CYP3A4 inhibitors such as troleandomycin).
No products indexed under this heading.

Valproate Sodium (Caution when administering or taking erlotinib with strong CYP3A4 inhibitors such as atazanavir, clarithromycin, indinavir, itraconazole, nefazodone, nelfinavir, ritonavir, saquinavir, telithromycin, troleandomycin, and voriconazole). Products include:
Depacon Injection 412

Verapamil Hydrochloride (Caution when administering or taking erlotinib with strong CYP3A4 inhibitors such as atazanavir, clarithromycin, indinavir, itraconazole, nefazodone, nelfinavir, ritonavir, saquinavir, telithromycin, troleandomycin, and voriconazole). Products include:
Covera-HS Tablets 3135
Tarka Tablets 519
Verelan PM Capsules 3120

Voriconazole (Co-treatment with the potent CYP3A4 inhibitor ketoconazole increases erlotinib AUC by 2/3. Caution should be used when administering or taking erlotinib with ketoconazole and other strong CYP3A4 inhibitors such as voriconazole). Products include:
VFEND I.V. 2543
VFEND Oral Suspension 2543
VFEND Tablets 2543

Zafirlukast (Caution when administering or taking erlotinib with strong CYP3A4 inhibitors such as atazanavir, clarithromycin, indinavir, itraconazole, nefazodone, nelfinavir, ritonavir, saquinavir, telithromycin, troleandomycin, and voriconazole). Products include:
Accolate Tablets 663

Zileuton (Caution when administering or taking erlotinib with strong CYP3A4 inhibitors such as atazanavir, clarithromycin, indinavir, itraconazole, nefazodone, nelfinavir, ritonavir, saquinavir, telithromycin, troleandomycin, and voriconazole).
No products indexed under this heading.

Food Interactions

Grapefruit (Caution when administering or taking erlotinib with strong CYP3A4 inhibitors such as atazanavir, clarithromycin, indinavir, itraconazole, nefazodone, nelfinavir, ritonavir, saquinavir, telithromycin, troleandomycin, and voriconazole).

Grapefruit Juice (Caution when administering or taking erlotinib with strong CYP3A4 inhibitors such as atazanavir, clarithromycin, indinavir, itraconazole, nefazodone, nelfinavir, ritonavir, saquinavir, telithromycin, troleandomycin, and voriconazole).

TARGRETIN CAPSULES

(Bexarotene) 1719
May interact with erythromycin, oral hypoglycemic agents, insulin, oral contraceptives, phenytoin, protease inhibitors, and certain other agents. Compounds in these categories include:

Acarbose (Bexarotene could enhance the action of hypoglycemic agents resulting in hypoglycemia). Products include:
Precose Tablets 776

Amiodarone Hydrochloride (Bexarotene is metabolized by CYP4503A4; co-administration with inhibitors of CYP4503A4, such as amiodarone, would be expected to lead to an increase in plasma bexarotene concentrations). Products include:
Pacerone Tablets 3337

Amprenavir (Bexarotene is metabolized by CYP4503A4; co-administration with inhibitors of CYP4503A4, such as protease inhibitors, would be expected to lead to an increase in plasma bexarotene concentrations). Products include:
Agenerase Capsules 1299
Agenerase Oral Solution 1304

Carbamazepine (Bexarotene is metabolized by CYP4503A4; co-administration with inducers of CYP4503A4, such as carbamazepine, may cause a reduction in plasma bexarotene concentrations). Products include:
Carbatrol Capsules 3174
Equetro Extended-Release Capsules 3178
Tegretol/Tegretol-XR 2278

Chlorpropamide (Bexarotene could enhance the action of hypoglycemic agents resulting in hypoglycemia).
No products indexed under this heading.

Desogestrel (Bexarotene may theoretically increase the rate of metabolism and reduce plasma concentrations of other substrates metabolized by CYP4503A4, including hormonal contraceptives; it is strongly recommended that two reliable forms of contraception be used concurrently, one of which should be non-hormonal). Products include:
Ortho-Cept Tablets 2395

Erythromycin (Bexarotene is metabolized by CYP4503A4; co-administration with inhibitors of CYP4503A4, such as erythromycin, would be expected to lead to an increase in plasma bexarotene concentrations). Products include:
Erygel Topical Gel 2096
Ery-Tab Tablets 447
Erythromycin Base Filmtab Tablets 454
Erythromycin Delayed-Release Capsules, USP 456
PCE Dispertab Tablets 510

Erythromycin Estolate (Bexarotene is metabolized by CYP4503A4; co-administration with inhibitors of CYP4503A4, such as erythromycin, would be expected to lead to an increase in plasma bexarotene concentrations).
No products indexed under this heading.

Erythromycin Ethylsuccinate (Bexarotene is metabolized by CYP4503A4; co-administration with inhibitors of CYP4503A4, such as erythromycin, would be expected to lead to an increase in plasma bexarotene concentrations). Products include:
E.E.S. 449
EryPed 445

Erythromycin Gluceptate (Bexarotene is metabolized by CYP4503A4; co-administration with inhibitors of CYP4503A4, such as erythromycin, would be expected to lead to an increase in plasma bexarotene concentrations).
No products indexed under this heading.

Erythromycin Lactobionate (Bexarotene is metabolized by CYP4503A4; co-administration with inhibitors of CYP4503A4, such as erythromycin, would be expected to lead to an increase in plasma bexarotene concentrations).
No products indexed under this heading.

Erythromycin Stearate (Bexarotene is metabolized by CYP4503A4; co-administration with inhibitors of CYP4503A4, such as erythromycin, would be expected to lead to an increase in plasma bexarotene concentrations). Products include:
Erythrocin Stearate Filmtab Tablets 452

Ethinyl Estradiol (Bexarotene may theoretically increase the rate of metabolism and reduce plasma concentrations of other substrates metabolized by CYP4503A4, including hormonal contraceptives; it is strongly recommended that two reliable forms of contraception be used concurrently, one of which should be non-hormonal). Products include:
Alesse-28 Tablets 3392
Lo/Ovral-28 Tablets 3423
NuvaRing 2357
Ortho-Cept Tablets 2395
Ortho-Cyclen/Ortho Tri-Cyclen 2414
Ortho Evra Transdermal System 2402
Ortho Tri-Cyclen Lo Tablets 2421
Seasonale Tablets 1073
Triphasil-28 Tablets 3483
Yasmin 28 Tablets 818

Ethynodiol Diacetate (Bexarotene may theoretically increase the rate of metabolism and reduce plasma concentrations of other substrates metabolized by CYP4503A4, including hormonal contraceptives; it is strongly recommended that two reliable forms of contraception be used concurrently, one of which should be non-hormonal).
No products indexed under this heading.

Fosphenytoin Sodium (Bexarotene is metabolized by CYP4503A4; co-administration with inducers of CYP4503A4, such as phenytoin, may cause a reduction in plasma bexarotene concentrations).
No products indexed under this heading.

Gemfibrozil (Co-administration has resulted in substantial increases in plasma bexarotene concentrations; concomitant administration is not recommended).
No products indexed under this heading.

Glimepiride (Bexarotene could enhance the action of hypoglycemic agents resulting in hypoglycemia). Products include:
Amaryl Tablets 2864

Glipizide (Bexarotene could enhance the action of hypoglycemic agents resulting in hypoglycemia).
No products indexed under this heading.

Glyburide (Bexarotene could enhance the action of hypoglycemic agents resulting in hypoglycemia).
No products indexed under this heading.

Hypericum (Bexarotene is metabolized by CYP4503A4; co-administration with inducers of CYP4503A4, such as St. John's Wort, may cause a reduction in plasma bexarotene concentrations).
No products indexed under this heading.

Indinavir Sulfate (Bexarotene is metabolized by CYP4503A4; co-administration with inhibitors of CYP4503A4, such as protease inhibitors, would be expected to lead to an increase in plasma bexarotene concentrations). Products include:
Crixivan Capsules ... 1918

Insulin, Human, Zinc Suspension (Bexarotene could enhance the action of insulin resulting in hypoglycemia). Products include:
Humulin L, 100 Units ... 1763
Humulin U, 100 Units ... 1770

Insulin, Human NPH (Bexarotene could enhance the action of insulin resulting in hypoglycemia). Products include:
Humulin N, 100 Units ... 1764
Humulin N Pen ... 1765
Novolin N Human Insulin 10 ml Vials ... 2322
Novolin N InnoLet ... 2322
Novolin N PenFill 3 ml Cartridges ... 2325
Novolin R InnoLet ... 2322

Insulin, Human Regular (Bexarotene could enhance the action of insulin resulting in hypoglycemia). Products include:
Humulin R (U-500) ... 1768
Humulin R, 100 Units ... 1767
Novolin R Human Insulin 10 ml Vials ... 2322
Novolin R PenFill ... 2325

Insulin, Human Regular and Human NPH Mixture (Bexarotene could enhance the action of insulin resulting in hypoglycemia). Products include:
Humulin 50/50, 100 Units ... 1760
Humulin 70/30 Pen ... 1761
Novolin 70/30 Human Insulin 10 ml Vials ... 2321
Novolin 70/30 InnoLet ... 2322
Novolin 70/30 PenFill 3 ml Cartridges ... 2325

Insulin, NPH (Bexarotene could enhance the action of insulin resulting in hypoglycemia).
No products indexed under this heading.

Insulin, Regular (Bexarotene could enhance the action of insulin resulting in hypoglycemia).
No products indexed under this heading.

Insulin, Zinc Crystals (Bexarotene could enhance the action of insulin resulting in hypoglycemia).
No products indexed under this heading.

Insulin, Zinc Suspension (Bexarotene could enhance the action of insulin resulting in hypoglycemia).
No products indexed under this heading.

Insulin Aspart, Human Regular (Bexarotene could enhance the action of insulin resulting in hypoglycemia). Products include:
NovoLog Injection ... 2326

Insulin glargine (Bexarotene could enhance the action of insulin resulting in hypoglycemia). Products include:
Lantus Injection ... 2925

Insulin Lispro, Human (Bexarotene could enhance the action of insulin resulting in hypoglycemia). Products include:
Humalog-Pen ... 1751
Humalog Mix 75/25-Pen ... 1754

Insulin Lispro Protamine, Human (Bexarotene could enhance the action of insulin resulting in hypoglycemia). Products include:
Humalog Mix 75/25-Pen ... 1754

Itraconazole (Bexarotene is metabolized by CYP4503A4; co-administration with inhibitors of CYP4503A4, such as itraconazole, would be expected to lead to an increase in plasma bexarotene concentrations).
No products indexed under this heading.

Ketoconazole (Bexarotene is metabolized by CYP4503A4; co-administration with inhibitors of CYP4503A4, such as ketoconazole, would be expected to lead to an increase in plasma concentrations). Products include:
Nizoral A-D Shampoo, 1% ... 1839
Nizoral 2% Shampoo ... 1838

Levonorgestrel (Bexarotene may theoretically increase the rate of metabolism and reduce plasma concentrations of other substrates metabolized by CYP4503A4, including hormonal contraceptives; it is strongly recommended that two reliable forms of contraception be used concurrently, one of which should be non-hormonal). Products include:
Alesse-28 Tablets ... 3392
Climara Pro Transdermal System ... 800
Mirena Intrauterine System ... 810
Plan B Tablets ... 1068
Seasonale Tablets ... 1073
Triphasil-28 Tablets ... 3483

Lopinavir (Bexarotene is metabolized by CYP4503A4; co-administration with inhibitors of CYP4503A4, such as protease inhibitors, would be expected to lead to an increase in plasma bexarotene concentrations). Products include:
Kaletra ... 474

Mestranol (Bexarotene may theoretically increase the rate of metabolism and reduce plasma concentrations of other substrates metabolized by CYP4503A4, including hormonal contraceptives; it is strongly recommended that two reliable forms of contraception be used concurrently, one of which should be non-hormonal).
No products indexed under this heading.

Metformin Hydrochloride (Bexarotene could enhance the action of hypoglycemic agents resulting in hypoglycemia). Products include:
ActoPlus Met Tablets ... 3219
Avandamet Tablets ... 1343
Fortamet Extended-Release Tablets ... 1156

Miglitol (Bexarotene could enhance the action of hypoglycemic agents resulting in hypoglycemia).
No products indexed under this heading.

Nefazodone Hydrochloride (Bexarotene is metabolized by CYP4503A4; co-administration with inhibitors of CYP4503A4, such as nefazodone, would be expected to lead to an increase in plasma bexarotene concentrations).
No products indexed under this heading.

Nelfinavir Mesylate (Bexarotene is metabolized by CYP4503A4; co-administration with inhibitors of CYP4503A4, such as protease inhibitors, would be expected to lead to an increase in plasma bexarotene concentrations). Products include:
Viracept ... 2556

Norethindrone (Bexarotene may theoretically increase the rate of metabolism and reduce plasma concentrations of other substrates metabolized by CYP4503A4, including hormonal contraceptives; it is strongly recommended that two reliable forms of contraception be used concurrently, one of which should be non-hormonal). Products include:
Ortho Micronor Tablets ... 2411

Norethynodrel (Bexarotene may theoretically increase the rate of metabolism and reduce plasma concentrations of other substrates metabolized by CYP4503A4, including hormonal contraceptives; it is strongly recommended that two reliable forms of contraception be used concurrently, one of which should be non-hormonal).
No products indexed under this heading.

Norgestimate (Bexarotene may theoretically increase the rate of metabolism and reduce plasma concentrations of other substrates metabolized by CYP4503A4, including hormonal contraceptives; it is strongly recommended that two reliable forms of contraception be used concurrently, one of which should be non-hormonal). Products include:
Ortho-Cyclen/Ortho Tri-Cyclen ... 2414
Ortho Tri-Cyclen Lo Tablets ... 2421
Prefest Tablets ... 1069

Norgestrel (Bexarotene may theoretically increase the rate of metabolism and reduce plasma concentrations of other substrates metabolized by CYP4503A4, including hormonal contraceptives; it is strongly recommended that two reliable forms of contraception be used concurrently, one of which should be non-hormonal). Products include:
Lo/Ovral-28 Tablets ... 3423

Phenobarbital (Bexarotene is metabolized by CYP4503A4; co-administration with inducers of CYP4503A4, such as phenobarbital, may cause a reduction in plasma bexarotene concentrations).
No products indexed under this heading.

Phenytoin (Bexarotene is metabolized by CYP4503A4; co-administration with inducers of CYP4503A4, such as phenytoin, may cause a reduction in plasma bexarotene concentrations).
No products indexed under this heading.

Phenytoin Sodium (Bexarotene is metabolized by CYP4503A4; co-administration with inducers of CYP4503A4, such as phenytoin, may cause a reduction in plasma bexarotene concentrations). Products include:
Phenytek Capsules ... 2153

Pioglitazone Hydrochloride (Bexarotene could enhance the action of hypoglycemic agents resulting in hypoglycemia). Products include:
ActoPlus Met Tablets ... 3219
Actos Tablets ... 3224

Repaglinide (Bexarotene could enhance the action of hypoglycemic agents resulting in hypoglycemia). Products include:
Prandin Tablets (0.5, 1, and 2 mg) ... 2337

Rifampin (Bexarotene is metabolized by CYP4503A4; co-administration with inducers of CYP4503A4, such as rifampin, may cause a reduction in plasma bexarotene concentrations).
No products indexed under this heading.

Ritonavir (Bexarotene is metabolized by CYP4503A4; co-administration with inhibitors of CYP4503A4, such as protease inhibitors, would be expected to lead to an increase in plasma bexarotene concentrations). Products include:
Kaletra ... 474
Norvir ... 499

Rosiglitazone Maleate (Bexarotene could enhance the action of hypoglycemic agents resulting in hypoglycemia). Products include:
Avandamet Tablets ... 1343
Avandia Tablets ... 1348

Saquinavir (Bexarotene is metabolized by CYP4503A4; co-administration with inhibitors of CYP4503A4, such as protease inhibitors, would be expected to lead to an increase in plasma bexarotene concentrations).
No products indexed under this heading.

Saquinavir Mesylate (Bexarotene is metabolized by CYP4503A4; co-administration with inhibitors of CYP4503A4, such as protease inhibitors, would be expected to lead to an increase in plasma bexarotene concentrations). Products include:
Invirase ... 2776

Tamoxifen Citrate (Co-administration has resulted in a modest decrease in plasma concentrations of tamoxifen).
No products indexed under this heading.

Tolazamide (Bexarotene could enhance the action of hypoglycemic agents resulting in hypoglycemia).
No products indexed under this heading.

Tolbutamide (Bexarotene could enhance the action of hypoglycemic agents resulting in hypoglycemia).
No products indexed under this heading.

Troglitazone (Bexarotene could enhance the action of hypoglycemic agents resulting in hypoglycemia).
No products indexed under this heading.

Vitamin A (Potential for additive toxic effects because of the relationship of bexarotene to vitamin A; patients should be advised to limit their vitamin A intake). Products include:
Visutein Capsules ... 3328

Food Interactions

Food, unspecified (Co-administration with a fat-containing meal has resulted in higher plasma bexarotene AUC and Cmax values; because safety and effica-

cy data are based upon administration with food, it is recommended that Targretin capsules be administered with or immediately following a meal).

Grapefruit Juice (Bexarotene is metabolized by CYP403A4; co-administration with inhibitors of CYP4503A4, such as grapefruit juice, would be expected to lead to an increase in plasma bexarotene concentrations).

TARKA TABLETS
(Trandolapril, Verapamil Hydrochloride)................................. 519
May interact with beta blockers, diuretics, cardiac glycosides, inhalant anesthetics, lithium preparations, neuromuscular blocking agents, potassium preparations, potassium sparing diuretics, quinidine, xanthines, and certain other agents. Compounds in these categories include:

Acebutolol Hydrochloride (Co-administration of beta blockers and verapamil may result in additive effects on heart rate, atrioventricular conduction, and/or cardiac contractility).
No products indexed under this heading.

Amiloride Hydrochloride (Increased risk of hyperkalemia; patients on diuretics, especially those on recently instituted diuretic therapy, may occasionally experience an excessive reduction of blood pressure after initiation of therapy with Tarka). Products include:
Midamor Tablets 2000
Moduretic Tablets 2003

Aminophylline (Verapamil may inhibit the clearance and increase the plasma levels of theophylline).
No products indexed under this heading.

Atenolol (Co-administration of beta blockers and verapamil may result in additive effects on heart rate, atrioventricular conduction, and/or cardiac contractility). Products include:
Tenormin I.V. Injection 698
Tenormin Tablets 695

Atracurium Besylate (Verapamil may potentiate the activity of neuromuscular blocking agents).
No products indexed under this heading.

Bendroflumethiazide (Patients on diuretics, especially those on recently instituted diuretic therapy, may occasionally experience an excessive reduction of blood pressure after initiation of therapy with Tarka).
No products indexed under this heading.

Betaxolol Hydrochloride (Co-administration of beta blockers and verapamil may result in additive effects on heart rate, atrioventricular conduction, and/or cardiac contractility). Products include:
Betoptic S Ophthalmic Suspension.................................. 554

Bisoprolol Fumarate (Co-administration of beta blockers and verapamil may result in additive effects on heart rate, atrioventricular conduction, and/or cardiac contractility).
No products indexed under this heading.

Bumetanide (Patients on diuretics, especially those on recently instituted diuretic therapy, may occasionally experience an excessive reduction of blood pressure after initiation of therapy with Tarka).
No products indexed under this heading.

Carbamazepine (Combined therapy of verapamil and carbamazepine may increase carbamazepine concentrations resulting in side effects such as diplopia, ataxia, and headache). Products include:
Carbatrol Capsules 3174
Equetro Extended-Release Capsules............................... 3178
Tegretol/Tegretol-XR 2278

Carteolol Hydrochloride (Co-administration of beta blockers and verapamil may result in additive effects on heart rate, atrioventricular conduction, and/or cardiac contractility). Products include:
Carteolol Hydrochloride Ophthalmic Solution USP, 1%....... ⊙246

Chlorothiazide (Patients on diuretics, especially those on recently instituted diuretic therapy, may occasionally experience an excessive reduction of blood pressure after initiation of therapy with Tarka). Products include:
Aldoclor Tablets 1881
Diuril Oral 1936

Chlorothiazide Sodium (Patients on diuretics, especially those on recently instituted diuretic therapy, may occasionally experience an excessive reduction of blood pressure after initiation of therapy with Tarka). Products include:
Diuril Sodium Intravenous 1934

Chlorthalidone (Patients on diuretics, especially those on recently instituted diuretic therapy, may occasionally experience an excessive reduction of blood pressure after initiation of therapy with Tarka). Products include:
Clorpres Tablets 2139

Cimetidine (Variable results on clearance have been obtained in acute studies during concomitant therapy; clearance of verapamil may be reduced or unchanged). Products include:
Tagamet HB 200 Tablets .... ▣637
Tagamet Tablets 1547

Cimetidine Hydrochloride (Variable results on clearance have been obtained in acute studies during concomitant therapy; clearance of verapamil may be reduced or unchanged).
No products indexed under this heading.

Cisatracurium Besylate (Verapamil may potentiate the activity of neuromuscular blocking agents). Products include:
Nimbex Injection 494

Cyclosporine (Increased serum levels of cyclosporine). Products include:
Gengraf Capsules 458
Neoral Soft Gelatin Capsules 2247
Neoral Oral Solution 2247
Restasis Ophthalmic Emulsion 570
Sandimmune 2259

Desflurane (Potential for excessive cardiovascular depression). Products include:
Suprane Liquid for Inhalation 770

Deslanoside (Chronic verapamil therapy can increase serum digoxin levels by 50% to 75% during the first week, and this can result in digoxin toxicity; patient should be carefully monitored to avoid over- or under-digitalization).
No products indexed under this heading.

Digitalis Glycoside Preparations (Chronic verapamil therapy can increase serum digoxin levels by 50% to 75% during the first week, and this can result in digoxin toxicity; patient should be carefully monitored to avoid over- or under-digitalization).
No products indexed under this heading.

Digitoxin (Chronic verapamil therapy can increase serum digoxin levels by 50% to 75% during the first week, and this can result in digoxin toxicity; patient should be carefully monitored to avoid over- or under-digitalization).
No products indexed under this heading.

Digoxin (Chronic verapamil therapy can increase serum digoxin levels by 50% to 75% during the first week, and this can result in digoxin toxicity; patient should be carefully monitored to avoid over- or under-digitalization). Products include:
Digitek Tablets 2146
Lanoxicaps Capsules 1458
Lanoxin Injection 1462
Lanoxin Tablets 1468
Lanoxin Injection Pediatric 1465

Doxacurium Chloride (Verapamil may potentiate the activity of neuromuscular blocking agents).
No products indexed under this heading.

Dyphylline (Verapamil may inhibit the clearance and increase the plasma levels of theophylline).
No products indexed under this heading.

Enflurane (Potential for excessive cardiovascular depression).
No products indexed under this heading.

Esmolol Hydrochloride (Co-administration of beta blockers and verapamil may result in additive effects on heart rate, atrioventricular conduction, and/or cardiac contractility). Products include:
Brevibloc Concentrate 766
Brevibloc Injection 766
Brevibloc Double Strength Injection.................................. 766
Brevibloc Premixed Injection 766
Brevibloc Double Strength Premixed Injection 766

Ethacrynic Acid (Patients on diuretics, especially those on recently instituted diuretic therapy, may occasionally experience an excessive reduction of blood pressure after initiation of therapy with Tarka). Products include:
Edecrin Tablets 1941

Flecainide Acetate (Concomitant use may result in additive effects on myocardial contractility, AV conduction and repolarization; concurrent use of flecainide and verapamil may result in additive inotropic effect and prolongation of atrioventricular conduction). Products include:
Tambocor Tablets 1824

Furosemide (Patients on diuretics, especially those on recently instituted diuretic therapy, may occasionally experience an excessive reduction of blood pressure after initiation of therapy with Tarka). Products include:
Furosemide Tablets 2117

Halothane (Potential for excessive cardiovascular depression).
No products indexed under this heading.

Hydrochlorothiazide (Patients on diuretics, especially those on recently instituted diuretic therapy, may occasionally experience an excessive reduction of blood pressure after initiation of therapy with Tarka). Products include:
Aldoril Tablets 1884
Atacand HCT 637
Avalide Tablets 2889
Avalide Tablets 922
Benicar HCT Tablets 2852
Diovan HCT Tablets 2195
Dyazide Capsules 1389
Hyzaar 1964
Lotensin HCT Tablets 2235
Maxzide 2150
Micardis HCT Tablets 886
Moduretic Tablets 2003
Prinzide Tablets 2033
Teveten HCT Tablets 1710
Timolide Tablets 2056
Uniretic Tablets 3114
Vaseretic Tablets 2073
Zestoretic Tablets 701

Hydroflumethiazide (Patients on diuretics, especially those on recently instituted diuretic therapy, may occasionally experience an excessive reduction of blood pressure after initiation of therapy with Tarka).
No products indexed under this heading.

Indapamide (Patients on diuretics, especially those on recently instituted diuretic therapy, may occasionally experience an excessive reduction of blood pressure after initiation of therapy with Tarka). Products include:
Indapamide Tablets 2119

Isoflurane (Potential for excessive cardiovascular depression).
No products indexed under this heading.

Labetalol Hydrochloride (Co-administration of beta blockers and verapamil may result in additive effects on heart rate, atrioventricular conduction, and/or cardiac contractility).
No products indexed under this heading.

Levobunolol Hydrochloride (Co-administration of beta blockers and verapamil may result in additive effects on heart rate, atrioventricular conduction, and/or cardiac contractility). Products include:
Betagan Ophthalmic Solution, USP.. ⊙217

Lithium (Co-administration results in increased sensitivity to the effects of lithium (neurotoxicity) with either no change or increase in serum lithium levels; increased lithium levels have been reported in patients receiving lithium and ACE inhibitor).
No products indexed under this heading.

Lithium Carbonate (Co-administration results in increased sensitivity to the effects of lithium (neurotoxicity) with either no change or increase in serum lithium levels; increased lithium levels have been reported in patients receiving lithium and ACE inhibitor). Products include:
Eskalith 1406
Lithobid Tablets 1670

Lithium Citrate (Co-administration results in increased sensitivity to the effects of lithium (neurotoxicity) with either no change or increase in serum lithium levels; increased lithium levels have been reported in patients receiving lithium and ACE inhibitor).
No products indexed under this heading.

Methoxyflurane (Potential for excessive cardiovascular depression).
No products indexed under this heading.

Methyclothiazide (Patients on diuretics, especially those on recently instituted diuretic therapy, may occasionally experience an excessive reduction of blood pressure after initiation of therapy with Tarka).
No products indexed under this heading.

Metipranolol Hydrochloride (Co-administration of beta blockers and verapamil may result in additive effects on heart rate, atrioventricular conduction, and/or cardiac contractility).
No products indexed under this heading.

Metocurine Iodide (Verapamil may potentiate the activity of neuromuscular blocking agents).
No products indexed under this heading.

Metolazone (Patients on diuretics, especially those on recently instituted diuretic therapy, may occasionally experience an excessive reduction of blood pressure after initiation of therapy with Tarka).
No products indexed under this heading.

Metoprolol Succinate (Co-administration of beta blockers and verapamil may result in additive effects on heart rate, atrioventricular conduction, and/or cardiac contractility). Products include:
Toprol-XL Tablets 660

Metoprolol Tartrate (Co-administration of beta blockers and verapamil may result in additive effects on heart rate, atrioventricular conduction, and/or cardiac contractility).
No products indexed under this heading.

Mivacurium Chloride (Verapamil may potentiate the activity of neuromuscular blocking agents). Products include:
Mivacron Injection 489

Nadolol (Co-administration of beta blockers and verapamil may result in additive effects on heart rate, atrioventricular conduction, and/or cardiac contractility). Products include:
Nadolol Tablets 2121

Pancuronium Bromide (Verapamil may potentiate the activity of neuromuscular blocking agents).
No products indexed under this heading.

Penbutolol Sulfate (Co-administration of beta blockers and verapamil may result in additive effects on heart rate, atrioventricular conduction, and/or cardiac contractility).
No products indexed under this heading.

Phenobarbital (May increase verapamil clearance).
No products indexed under this heading.

Pindolol (Co-administration of beta blockers and verapamil may result in additive effects on heart rate, atrioventricular conduction, and/or cardiac contractility).
No products indexed under this heading.

Polythiazide (Patients on diuretics, especially those on recently instituted diuretic therapy, may occasionally experience an excessive reduction of blood pressure after initiation of therapy with Tarka).
No products indexed under this heading.

Potassium Acid Phosphate (Increased risk of hyperkalemia). Products include:
K-Phos Original (Sodium Free) Tablets 785

Potassium Bicarbonate (Increased risk of hyperkalemia).
No products indexed under this heading.

Potassium Chloride (Increased risk of hyperkalemia). Products include:
Colyte with Flavor Packs for Oral Solution 3102
HalfLytely and Bisacodyl Tablets Bowel Prep Kit with Flavors Packs 915
K-Dur Extended-Relase Tablets 3047
K-Lor Powder Packets 472
K-Tab Filmtab Tablets 473
TriLyte with Flavor Packs for Oral Solution 3114

Potassium Citrate (Increased risk of hyperkalemia). Products include:
Urocit-K Tablets 2109

Potassium Gluconate (Increased risk of hyperkalemia).
No products indexed under this heading.

Potassium Phosphate (Increased risk of hyperkalemia). Products include:
K-Phos Neutral Tablets 785

Propranolol Hydrochloride (Co-administration of beta blockers and verapamil may result in additive effects on heart rate, atrioventricular conduction, and/or cardiac contractility). Products include:
Inderal LA Long-Acting Capsules 3421
InnoPran XL Capsules 2728

Quinidine (Concomitant use of verapamil and quinidine has resulted in significant hypotension and/or increased quinidine levels during verapamil therapy).
No products indexed under this heading.

Quinidine Gluconate (Concomitant use of verapamil and quinidine has resulted in significant hypotension and/or increased quinidine levels during verapamil therapy).
No products indexed under this heading.

Quinidine Hydrochloride (Concomitant use of verapamil and quinidine has resulted in significant hypotension and/or increased quinidine levels during verapamil therapy).
No products indexed under this heading.

Quinidine Polygalacturonate (Concomitant use of verapamil and quinidine has resulted in significant hypotension and/or increased quinidine levels during verapamil therapy).
No products indexed under this heading.

Quinidine Sulfate (Concomitant use of verapamil and quinidine has resulted in significant hypotension and/or increased quinidine levels during verapamil therapy).
No products indexed under this heading.

Rapacuronium Bromide (Verapamil may potentiate the activity of neuromuscular blocking agents).
No products indexed under this heading.

Rifampin (May markedly reduce oral verapamil bioavailability).
No products indexed under this heading.

Rocuronium Bromide (Verapamil may potentiate the activity of neuromuscular blocking agents). Products include:
Zemuron Injection 2363

Sotalol Hydrochloride (Co-administration of beta blockers and verapamil may result in additive effects on heart rate, atrioventricular conduction, and/or cardiac contractility).
No products indexed under this heading.

Spironolactone (Increased risk of hyperkalemia; patients on diuretics, especially those on recently instituted diuretic therapy, may occasionally experience an excessive reduction of blood pressure after initiation of therapy with Tarka).
No products indexed under this heading.

Succinylcholine Chloride (Verapamil may potentiate the activity of neuromuscular blocking agents).
No products indexed under this heading.

Theophylline (Verapamil may inhibit the clearance and increase the plasma levels of theophylline).
No products indexed under this heading.

Theophylline Anhydrous (Verapamil may inhibit the clearance and increase the plasma levels of theophylline). Products include:
Uniphyl Tablets 2708

Theophylline Calcium Salicylate (Verapamil may inhibit the clearance and increase the plasma levels of theophylline).
No products indexed under this heading.

Theophylline Dihydroxypropyl (Glyceryl) (Verapamil may inhibit the clearance and increase the plasma levels of theophylline).
No products indexed under this heading.

Theophylline Ethylenediamine (Verapamil may inhibit the clearance and increase the plasma levels of theophylline).
No products indexed under this heading.

Theophylline Sodium Glycinate (Verapamil may inhibit the clearance and increase the plasma levels of theophylline).
No products indexed under this heading.

Timolol Hemihydrate (Concomitant use of timolol eye drops and verapamil has resulted in asymptomatic bradycardia with wandering atrial pacemaker). Products include:
Betimol Ophthalmic Solution 3371
Betimol Ophthalmic Solution ..... ⊙283

Timolol Maleate (Concomitant use of timolol eye drops and verapamil has resulted in asymptomatic bradycardia with wandering atrial pacemaker). Products include:
Blocadren Tablets 1891
Cosopt Sterile Ophthalmic Solution 1910
Timolide Tablets 2056
Timoptic in Ocudose 2061
Timoptic Sterile Ophthalmic Solution 2058
Timoptic-XE Sterile Ophthalmic Gel Forming Solution 2062

Torsemide (Patients on diuretics, especially those on recently instituted diuretic therapy, may occasionally experience an excessive reduction of blood pressure after initiation of therapy with Tarka).
No products indexed under this heading.

Triamterene (Increased risk of hyperkalemia; patients on diuretics, especially those on recently instituted diuretic therapy, may occasionally experience an excessive reduction of blood pressure after initiation of therapy with Tarka). Products include:
Dyazide Capsules 1389
Dyrenium Capsules 3390
Maxzide 2150

Vecuronium Bromide (Verapamil may potentiate the activity of neuromuscular blocking agents).
No products indexed under this heading.

Food Interactions

Food, unspecified (Co-administration with food decreases verapamil bioavailability and the time to peak plasma concentration is delayed; bioavailability of trandolapril is not altered; Tarka should be administered with food).

TASMAR TABLETS

(Tolcapone) 3360

May interact with central nervous system depressants, nonselective MAO inhibitors, and certain other agents. Compounds in these categories include:

Alfentanil Hydrochloride (Possible additive sedative effects when used in combination with CNS depressants).
No products indexed under this heading.

Alprazolam (Possible additive sedative effects when used in combination with CNS depressants). Products include:
Niravam Orally Disintegrating Tablets 3106
Xanax XR Tablets 2655

Apomorphine (Tolcapone may influence the pharmacokinetics of drugs metabolized by COMT; dosage adjustments should be considered when co-administered).
No products indexed under this heading.

Aprobarbital (Possible additive sedative effects when used in combination with CNS depressants).
No products indexed under this heading.

Buprenorphine Hydrochloride (Possible additive sedative effects when used in combination with CNS depressants). Products include:
Buprenex Injectable 2718
Suboxone Tablets 2719
Subutex Tablets 2719

Buspirone Hydrochloride (Possible additive sedative effects when used in combination with CNS depressants).
No products indexed under this heading.

Butabarbital (Possible additive sedative effects when used in combination with CNS depressants).
No products indexed under this heading.

Butalbital (Possible additive sedative effects when used in combination with CNS depressants).
Products include:
Sedapap Tablets 50 mg/650 mg 2098

Chlordiazepoxide (Possible additive sedative effects when used in combination with CNS depressants).
No products indexed under this heading.

Chlordiazepoxide Hydrochloride (Possible additive sedative effects when used in combination with CNS depressants). Products include:
Librium Capsules 3349

Chlorpromazine (Possible additive sedative effects when used in combination with CNS depressants).
No products indexed under this heading.

Chlorpromazine Hydrochloride (Possible additive sedative effects when used in combination with CNS depressants).
No products indexed under this heading.

Chlorprothixene (Possible additive sedative effects when used in combination with CNS depressants).
No products indexed under this heading.

Chlorprothixene Hydrochloride (Possible additive sedative effects when used in combination with CNS depressants).
No products indexed under this heading.

Chlorprothixene Lactate (Possible additive sedative effects when used in combination with CNS depressants).
No products indexed under this heading.

Clorazepate Dipotassium (Possible additive sedative effects when used in combination with CNS depressants). Products include:
Tranxene 2488

Clozapine (Possible additive sedative effects when used in combination with CNS depressants).
Products include:
Clozapine Tablets 2141
Clozaril Tablets 2174
FazaClo Orally Disintegrating Tablets 547

Codeine Phosphate (Possible additive sedative effects when used in combination with CNS depressants). Products include:
Tylenol with Codeine 2461

Desflurane (Possible additive sedative effects when used in combination with CNS depressants).
Products include:
Suprane Liquid for Inhalation 770

Desipramine Hydrochloride (Co-administration of tolcapone with levodopa/carbidopa and desipramine has resulted in slight increase in frequency of adverse events; caution should be exercised when co-administered).
No products indexed under this heading.

Dezocine (Possible additive sedative effects when used in combination with CNS depressants).
No products indexed under this heading.

Diazepam (Possible additive sedative effects when used in combination with CNS depressants).
Products include:
Diastat Rectal Delivery System 3344
Valium Tablets 2822

Dobutamine Hydrochloride (Tolcapone may influence the pharmacokinetics of drugs metabolized by COMT; dosage adjustments should be considered when co-administered).
No products indexed under this heading.

Droperidol (Possible additive sedative effects when used in combination with CNS depressants).
No products indexed under this heading.

Enflurane (Possible additive sedative effects when used in combination with CNS depressants).
No products indexed under this heading.

Estazolam (Possible additive sedative effects when used in combination with CNS depressants).
Products include:
ProSom Tablets 512

Ethanol (Possible additive sedative effects when used in combination with CNS depressants).
No products indexed under this heading.

Ethchlorvynol (Possible additive sedative effects when used in combination with CNS depressants).
No products indexed under this heading.

Ethinamate (Possible additive sedative effects when used in combination with CNS depressants).
No products indexed under this heading.

Ethyl Alcohol (Possible additive sedative effects when used in combination with CNS depressants).
No products indexed under this heading.

Fentanyl (Possible additive sedative effects when used in combination with CNS depressants). Products include:
Duragesic Transdermal System 2448

Fentanyl Citrate (Possible additive sedative effects when used in combination with CNS depressants).
Products include:
Actiq 993

Fluphenazine Decanoate (Possible additive sedative effects when used in combination with CNS depressants).
No products indexed under this heading.

Fluphenazine Enanthate (Possible additive sedative effects when used in combination with CNS depressants).
No products indexed under this heading.

Fluphenazine Hydrochloride (Possible additive sedative effects when used in combination with CNS depressants).
No products indexed under this heading.

Flurazepam Hydrochloride (Possible additive sedative effects when used in combination with CNS depressants). Products include:
Dalmane Capsules 3343

Glutethimide (Possible additive sedative effects when used in combination with CNS depressants).
No products indexed under this heading.

Haloperidol (Possible additive sedative effects when used in combination with CNS depressants).
No products indexed under this heading.

Haloperidol Decanoate (Possible additive sedative effects when used in combination with CNS depressants).
No products indexed under this heading.

Hydrocodone Bitartrate (Possible additive sedative effects when used in combination with CNS depressants). Products include:
Hycodan 1104
Hycomine Compound Tablets 1105
Hycotuss Expectorant Syrup 1106
Lortab 3315
Lortab Elixir 3312
Vicodin Tablets 530
Vicodin ES Tablets 531
Vicodin HP Tablets 532
Vicoprofen Tablets 533
Zydone Tablets 1118

Hydrocodone Polistirex (Possible additive sedative effects when used in combination with CNS depressants). Products include:
Tussionex Pennkinetic Extended-Release Suspension 3322

Hydromorphone Hydrochloride (Possible additive sedative effects when used in combination with CNS depressants). Products include:
Dilaudid 439
Dilaudid Oral Liquid 443
Dilaudid Non-Sterile Powder 439
Dilaudid Rectal Suppositories 439
Dilaudid Tablets 439
Dilaudid Tablets - 8 mg 443
Dilaudid-HP 441

Hydroxyzine Hydrochloride (Possible additive sedative effects when used in combination with CNS depressants).
No products indexed under this heading.

Isocarboxazid (The combination, in theory, of tolcapone and non-selective MAO inhibitor may result in inhibition of the majority of the pathways responsible for normal catecholamine metabolism; patients should ordinarily not be treated concomitantly).
No products indexed under this heading.

Isoflurane (Possible additive sedative effects when used in combination with CNS depressants).
No products indexed under this heading.

Isoproterenol Hydrochloride (Tolcapone may influence the pharmacokinetics of drugs metabolized by COMT; dosage adjustments should be considered when co-administered).
No products indexed under this heading.

Ketamine Hydrochloride (Possible additive sedative effects when used in combination with CNS depressants).
No products indexed under this heading.

Levodopa (Tolcapone enhances levodopa bioavailability and, therefore, may increase the occurence of orthostatic hypotension; tolcapone may potentiate the dopaminergic side effects of levodopa and may cause and/or exacerbate preexisting dyskinesia). Products include:
Parcopa Orally Disintegrating Tablets 3111
Stalevo Tablets 2270

Levomethadyl Acetate Hydrochloride (Possible additive sedative effects when used in combination with CNS depressants).
No products indexed under this heading.

Levorphanol Tartrate (Possible additive sedative effects when used in combination with CNS depressants).
No products indexed under this heading.

Lorazepam (Possible additive sedative effects when used in combination with CNS depressants).
No products indexed under this heading.

Loxapine Hydrochloride (Possible additive sedative effects when used in combination with CNS depressants).
No products indexed under this heading.

Loxapine Succinate (Possible additive sedative effects when used in combination with CNS depressants).
No products indexed under this heading.

Meperidine Hydrochloride (Possible additive sedative effects when used in combination with CNS depressants).
No products indexed under this heading.

Mephobarbital (Possible additive sedative effects when used in combination with CNS depressants).
Products include:
Mebaral Tablets, USP 2483

Meprobamate (Possible additive sedative effects when used in combination with CNS depressants).
No products indexed under this heading.

Mesoridazine Besylate (Possible additive sedative effects when used in combination with CNS depressants).
No products indexed under this heading.

Methadone Hydrochloride (Possible additive sedative effects when used in combination with CNS depressants).
No products indexed under this heading.

Methohexital Sodium (Possible additive sedative effects when used in combination with CNS depressants).
No products indexed under this heading.

Methotrimeprazine (Possible additive sedative effects when used in combination with CNS depressants).
No products indexed under this heading.

Methoxyflurane (Possible additive sedative effects when used in combination with CNS depressants).
No products indexed under this heading.

Methyldopa (Tolcapone may influence the pharmacokinetics of drugs metabolized by COMT; dosage adjustments should be considered when co-administered). Products include:

Aldoclor Tablets 1881
Aldoril Tablets 1884

Midazolam Hydrochloride (Possible additive sedative effects when used in combination with CNS depressants).
No products indexed under this heading.

Molindone Hydrochloride (Possible additive sedative effects when used in combination with CNS depressants). Products include:
Moban Tablets 1108

Morphine Sulfate (Possible additive sedative effects when used in combination with CNS depressants). Products include:
Avinza Capsules 1714
Kadian Capsules 572
MS Contin Tablets 2703

Olanzapine (Possible additive sedative effects when used in combination with CNS depressants). Products include:
Symbyax Capsules 1788
Zyprexa Tablets 1798
Zyprexa IntraMuscular 1798
Zyprexa ZYDIS Orally Disintegrating Tablets 1798

Oxazepam (Possible additive sedative effects when used in combination with CNS depressants).
No products indexed under this heading.

Oxycodone Hydrochloride (Possible additive sedative effects when used in combination with CNS depressants). Products include:
Combunox Tablets 1183
OxyContin Tablets 2699
OxyFast Oral Concentrate Solution 2704
OxyIR Capsules 2704
Percocet Tablets 1114
Percodan Tablets 1115

Pargyline Hydrochloride (The combination, in theory, of tolcapone and non-selective MAO inhibitor may result in inhibition of the majority of the pathways responsible for normal catecholamine metabolism; patients should ordinarily not be treated concomitantly).
No products indexed under this heading.

Pentobarbital Sodium (Possible additive sedative effects when used in combination with CNS depressants). Products include:
Nembutal Sodium Solution, USP 2484

Perphenazine (Possible additive sedative effects when used in combination with CNS depressants).
No products indexed under this heading.

Phenelzine Sulfate (The combination, in theory, of tolcapone and non-selective MAO inhibitor may result in inhibition of the majority of the pathways responsible for normal catecholamine metabolism; patients should ordinarily not be treated concomitantly).
No products indexed under this heading.

Phenobarbital (Possible additive sedative effects when used in combination with CNS depressants).
No products indexed under this heading.

Prazepam (Possible additive sedative effects when used in combination with CNS depressants).
No products indexed under this heading.

Procarbazine Hydrochloride (The combination, in theory, of tolcapone and non-selective MAO inhibitor may result in inhibition of the majority of the pathways responsible for normal catecholamine metabolism; patients should ordinarily not be treated concomitantly). Products include:
Matulane Capsules 3188

Prochlorperazine (Possible additive sedative effects when used in combination with CNS depressants).
No products indexed under this heading.

Promethazine Hydrochloride (Possible additive sedative effects when used in combination with CNS depressants). Products include:
Phenergan 3438

Propofol (Possible additive sedative effects when used in combination with CNS depressants). Products include:
Diprivan Injectable Emulsion 676

Propoxyphene Hydrochloride (Possible additive sedative effects when used in combination with CNS depressants).
No products indexed under this heading.

Propoxyphene Napsylate (Possible additive sedative effects when used in combination with CNS depressants). Products include:
Darvocet A 500 Tablets 3497

Quazepam (Possible additive sedative effects when used in combination with CNS depressants).
No products indexed under this heading.

Quetiapine Fumarate (Possible additive sedative effects when used in combination with CNS depressants). Products include:
Seroquel Tablets 691

Remifentanil Hydrochloride (Possible additive sedative effects when used in combination with CNS depressants).
No products indexed under this heading.

Risperidone (Possible additive sedative effects when used in combination with CNS depressants). Products include:
Risperdal Consta Long-Acting Injection 1664
Risperdal M-Tab Orally Disintegrating Tablets 1658
Risperdal 1658

Secobarbital Sodium (Possible additive sedative effects when used in combination with CNS depressants).
No products indexed under this heading.

Sevoflurane (Possible additive sedative effects when used in combination with CNS depressants). Products include:
Ultane Liquid for Inhalation 526

Sufentanil Citrate (Possible additive sedative effects when used in combination with CNS depressants).
No products indexed under this heading.

Temazepam (Possible additive sedative effects when used in combination with CNS depressants).
No products indexed under this heading.

Thiamylal Sodium (Possible additive sedative effects when used in combination with CNS depressants).
No products indexed under this heading.

Thioridazine Hydrochloride (Possible additive sedative effects when used in combination with CNS depressants). Products include:
Thioridazine Hydrochloride Tablets 2122

Thiothixene (Possible additive sedative effects when used in combination with CNS depressants). Products include:
Thiothixene Capsules 2124

Tranylcypromine Sulfate (The combination, in theory, of tolcapone and non-selective MAO inhibitor may result in inhibition of the majority of the pathways responsible for normal catecholamine metabolism; patients should ordinarily not be treated concomitantly). Products include:
Parnate Tablets 1499

Triazolam (Possible additive sedative effects when used in combination with CNS depressants).
No products indexed under this heading.

Trifluoperazine Hydrochloride (Possible additive sedative effects when used in combination with CNS depressants).
No products indexed under this heading.

Zaleplon (Possible additive sedative effects when used in combination with CNS depressants). Products include:
Sonata Capsules 1686

Ziprasidone Hydrochloride (Possible additive sedative effects when used in combination with CNS depressants). Products include:
Geodon Capsules 2514

Zolpidem Tartrate (Possible additive sedative effects when used in combination with CNS depressants). Products include:
Ambien Tablets 2867

Food Interactions

Alcohol (Possible additive sedative effects when used in combination with CNS depressants, such as alcohol).

Food, unspecified (Food given within 1 hour before and 2 hours after dosing of tolcapone decreases the relative bioavailability by 10% to 20%; Tasmar may be taken with or without food).

TAXOTERE INJECTION CONCENTRATE

(Docetaxel) 2947

May interact with cytochrome p450 3a4 inhibitors (selected). Compounds in these categories include:

Acetazolamide (Metabolism of docetaxel may be inhibited by co-administration with CYP3A4 inhibitors, thereby leading to substantial increases in docetaxel blood concentrations).
No products indexed under this heading.

Amiodarone Hydrochloride (Metabolism of docetaxel may be inhibited by co-administration with CYP3A4 inhibitors, thereby leading to substantial increases in docetaxel blood concentrations). Products include:
Pacerone Tablets 3337

Amprenavir (Metabolism of docetaxel may be inhibited by co-administration with CYP3A4 inhibitors, thereby leading to substantial increases in docetaxel blood concentrations). Products include:
Agenerase Capsules 1299
Agenerase Oral Solution 1304

Anastrozole (Metabolism of docetaxel may be inhibited by co-administration with CYP3A4 inhibitors, thereby leading to substantial increases in docetaxel blood concentrations). Products include:
Arimidex Tablets 665

Aprepitant (Metabolism of docetaxel may be inhibited by co-administration with CYP3A4 inhibitors, thereby leading to substantial increases in docetaxel blood concentrations). Products include:
Emend Capsules 1944

Cimetidine (Metabolism of docetaxel may be inhibited by co-administration with CYP3A4 inhibitors, thereby leading to substantial increases in docetaxel blood concentrations). Products include:
Tagamet HB 200 Tablets 637
Tagamet Tablets 1547

Cimetidine Hydrochloride (Metabolism of docetaxel may be inhibited by co-administration with CYP3A4 inhibitors, thereby leading to substantial increases in docetaxel blood concentrations).
No products indexed under this heading.

Ciprofloxacin (Metabolism of docetaxel may be inhibited by co-administration with CYP3A4 inhibitors, thereby leading to substantial increases in docetaxel blood concentrations). Products include:
Cipro I.V. 2998
Cipro I.V. Pharmacy Bulk Package ... 3509
Cipro Oral Suspension 2991
Cipro XR Tablets 3004
Ciprodex Otic Suspension 555

Clarithromycin (Metabolism of docetaxel may be inhibited by co-administration with CYP3A4 inhibitors, thereby leading to substantial increases in docetaxel blood concentrations). Products include:
Biaxin/Biaxin XL 402
PREVPAC 3281

Clotrimazole (Metabolism of docetaxel may be inhibited by co-administration with CYP3A4 inhibitors, thereby leading to substantial increases in docetaxel blood concentrations). Products include:
Lotrimin 3053
Lotrisone 3054

Cyclosporine (Metabolism of docetaxel may be inhibited by co-administration with CYP3A4 inhibitors, thereby leading to substantial increases in docetaxel blood concentrations). Products include:
Gengraf Capsules 458
Neoral Soft Gelatin Capsules 2247
Neoral Oral Solution 2247
Restasis Ophthalmic Emulsion 570
Sandimmune 2259

Dalfopristin (Metabolism of docetaxel may be inhibited by co-administration with CYP3A4 inhibitors, thereby leading to substantial increases in docetaxel blood concentrations). Products include:
Synercid I.V. 1690

Danazol (Metabolism of docetaxel may be inhibited by co-administration with CYP3A4 inhibitors, thereby leading to substantial increases in docetaxel blood concentrations).
No products indexed under this heading.

Delavirdine Mesylate (Metabolism of docetaxel may be inhibited by co-administration with CYP3A4 inhibi-

tors, thereby leading to substantial increases in docetaxel blood concentrations). Products include:
- Rescriptor Tablets 2535

Diltiazem Hydrochloride (Metabolism of docetaxel may be inhibited by co-administration with CYP3A4 inhibitors, thereby leading to substantial increases in docetaxel blood concentrations). Products include:
- Cardizem LA Extended Release Tablets 1699
- Tiazac Capsules 1204

Diltiazem Maleate (Metabolism of docetaxel may be inhibited by co-administration with CYP3A4 inhibitors, thereby leading to substantial increases in docetaxel blood concentrations).
- No products indexed under this heading.

Efavirenz (Metabolism of docetaxel may be inhibited by co-administration with CYP3A4 inhibitors, thereby leading to substantial increases in docetaxel blood concentrations). Products include:
- Sustiva Capsules 957

Erythromycin (Metabolism of docetaxel may be inhibited by co-administration with CYP3A4 inhibitors, thereby leading to substantial increases in docetaxel blood concentrations). Products include:
- Erygel Topical Gel 2096
- Ery-Tab Tablets 447
- Erythromycin Base Filmtab Tablets 454
- Erythromycin Delayed-Release Capsules, USP 456
- PCE Dispertab Tablets 510

Erythromycin Estolate (Metabolism of docetaxel may be inhibited by co-administration with CYP3A4 inhibitors, thereby leading to substantial increases in docetaxel blood concentrations).
- No products indexed under this heading.

Erythromycin Ethylsuccinate (Metabolism of docetaxel may be inhibited by co-administration with CYP3A4 inhibitors, thereby leading to substantial increases in docetaxel blood concentrations). Products include:
- E.E.S. 449
- EryPed 445

Erythromycin Gluceptate (Metabolism of docetaxel may be inhibited by co-administration with CYP3A4 inhibitors, thereby leading to substantial increases in docetaxel blood concentrations).
- No products indexed under this heading.

Erythromycin Lactobionate (Metabolism of docetaxel may be inhibited by co-administration with CYP3A4 inhibitors, thereby leading to substantial increases in docetaxel blood concentrations).
- No products indexed under this heading.

Erythromycin Stearate (Metabolism of docetaxel may be inhibited by co-administration with CYP3A4 inhibitors, thereby leading to substantial increases in docetaxel blood concentrations). Products include:
- Erythrocin Stearate Filmtab Tablets 452

Esomeprazole Magnesium (Metabolism of docetaxel may be inhibited by co-administration with CYP3A4 inhibitors, thereby leading to substantial increases in docetaxel blood concentrations). Products include:
- Nexium Delayed-Release Capsules 645

Fluconazole (Metabolism of docetaxel may be inhibited by co-administration with CYP3A4 inhibitors, thereby leading to substantial increases in docetaxel blood concentrations).
- No products indexed under this heading.

Fluoxetine Hydrochloride (Metabolism of docetaxel may be inhibited by co-administration with CYP3A4 inhibitors, thereby leading to substantial increases in docetaxel blood concentrations). Products include:
- Prozac Pulvules and Liquid 1771
- Symbyax Capsules 1788

Fluvoxamine Maleate (Metabolism of docetaxel may be inhibited by co-administration with CYP3A4 inhibitors, thereby leading to substantial increases in docetaxel blood concentrations).
- No products indexed under this heading.

Fosamprenavir Calcium (Metabolism of docetaxel may be inhibited by co-administration with CYP3A4 inhibitors, thereby leading to substantial increases in docetaxel blood concentrations). Products include:
- Lexiva Tablets 1473

Indinavir Sulfate (Metabolism of docetaxel may be inhibited by co-administration with CYP3A4 inhibitors, thereby leading to substantial increases in docetaxel blood concentrations). Products include:
- Crixivan Capsules 1918

Isoniazid (Metabolism of docetaxel may be inhibited by co-administration with CYP3A4 inhibitors, thereby leading to substantial increases in docetaxel blood concentrations).
- No products indexed under this heading.

Itraconazole (Metabolism of docetaxel may be inhibited by co-administration with CYP3A4 inhibitors, thereby leading to substantial increases in docetaxel blood concentrations).
- No products indexed under this heading.

Ketoconazole (Metabolism of docetaxel may be inhibited by co-administration with CYP3A4 inhibitors, thereby leading to substantial increases in docetaxel blood concentrations). Products include:
- Nizoral A-D Shampoo, 1% 1839
- Nizoral 2% Shampoo 1838

Lopinavir (Metabolism of docetaxel may be inhibited by co-administration with CYP3A4 inhibitors, thereby leading to substantial increases in docetaxel blood concentrations). Products include:
- Kaletra 474

Loratadine (Metabolism of docetaxel may be inhibited by co-administration with CYP3A4 inhibitors, thereby leading to substantial increases in docetaxel blood concentrations). Products include:
- Alavert Allergy & Sinus D-12 Hour Tablets .... ▣743
- Alavert .... ▣743
- Children's Claritin 24 Hour Non-Drowsy Allergy Syrup .... ▣732
- Claritin Non-Drowsy 24 Hour Tablets .... ▣731
- Non-Drowsy Claritin Hives Relief Tablets .... ▣733
- Claritin Reditabs 24 Hour Non-Drowsy Tablets .... ▣732
- Claritin-D Non-Drowsy 12 Hour Tablets .... ▣731
- Claritin-D Non-Drowsy 24 Hour Tablets .... ▣731
- Children's Dimetapp ND Non-Drowsy Allergy Syrup .... ▣746
- Triaminic Allerchews .... ▣684

Metronidazole (Metabolism of docetaxel may be inhibited by co-administration with CYP3A4 inhibitors, thereby leading to substantial increases in docetaxel blood concentrations). Products include:
- Metrogel 1% 1212
- MetroGel-Vaginal Gel 1822
- Noritate Cream, 1% 1051

Metronidazole Benzoate (Metabolism of docetaxel may be inhibited by co-administration with CYP3A4 inhibitors, thereby leading to substantial increases in docetaxel blood concentrations).
- No products indexed under this heading.

Metronidazole Hydrochloride (Metabolism of docetaxel may be inhibited by co-administration with CYP3A4 inhibitors, thereby leading to substantial increases in docetaxel blood concentrations).
- No products indexed under this heading.

Miconazole (Metabolism of docetaxel may be inhibited by co-administration with CYP3A4 inhibitors, thereby leading to substantial increases in docetaxel blood concentrations).
- No products indexed under this heading.

Miconazole Nitrate (Metabolism of docetaxel may be inhibited by co-administration with CYP3A4 inhibitors, thereby leading to substantial increases in docetaxel blood concentrations). Products include:
- Desenex .... ▣674
- Desenex Jock Itch Spray Powder ... ▣674

Nefazodone Hydrochloride (Metabolism of docetaxel may be inhibited by co-administration with CYP3A4 inhibitors, thereby leading to substantial increases in docetaxel blood concentrations).
- No products indexed under this heading.

Nelfinavir Mesylate (Metabolism of docetaxel may be inhibited by co-administration with CYP3A4 inhibitors, thereby leading to substantial increases in docetaxel blood concentrations). Products include:
- Viracept 2556

Nevirapine (Metabolism of docetaxel may be inhibited by co-administration with CYP3A4 inhibitors, thereby leading to substantial increases in docetaxel blood concentrations). Products include:
- Viramune Oral Suspension 903
- Viramune Tablets 903

Niacinamide (Metabolism of docetaxel may be inhibited by co-administration with CYP3A4 inhibitors, thereby leading to substantial increases in docetaxel blood concentrations).
- No products indexed under this heading.

Nicotinamide (Metabolism of docetaxel may be inhibited by co-administration with CYP3A4 inhibitors, thereby leading to substantial increases in docetaxel blood concentrations). Products include:
- Nicomide Tablets 3190

Nifedipine (Metabolism of docetaxel may be inhibited by co-administration with CYP3A4 inhibitors, thereby leading to substantial increases in docetaxel blood concentrations). Products include:
- Adalat CC Tablets 2978

Norfloxacin (Metabolism of docetaxel may be inhibited by co-administration with CYP3A4 inhibitors, thereby leading to substantial increases in docetaxel blood concentrations). Products include:
- Noroxin Tablets 2009

Omeprazole (Metabolism of docetaxel may be inhibited by co-administration with CYP3A4 inhibitors, thereby leading to substantial increases in docetaxel blood concentrations). Products include:
- Zegerid Powder for Oral Solution 2972

Paroxetine Hydrochloride (Metabolism of docetaxel may be inhibited by co-administration with CYP3A4 inhibitors, thereby leading to substantial increases in docetaxel blood concentrations). Products include:
- Paxil CR Controlled-Release Tablets 1509
- Paxil 1501

Propoxyphene Hydrochloride (Metabolism of docetaxel may be inhibited by co-administration with CYP3A4 inhibitors, thereby leading to substantial increases in docetaxel blood concentrations).
- No products indexed under this heading.

Propoxyphene Napsylate (Metabolism of docetaxel may be inhibited by co-administration with CYP3A4 inhibitors, thereby leading to substantial increases in docetaxel blood concentrations). Products include:
- Darvocet A 500 Tablets 3497

Quinidine (Metabolism of docetaxel may be inhibited by co-administration with CYP3A4 inhibitors, thereby leading to substantial increases in docetaxel blood concentrations).
- No products indexed under this heading.

Quinidine Hydrochloride (Metabolism of docetaxel may be inhibited by co-administration with CYP3A4 inhibitors, thereby leading to substantial increases in docetaxel blood concentrations).
- No products indexed under this heading.

Quinidine Polygalacturonate (Metabolism of docetaxel may be inhibited by co-administration with CYP3A4 inhibitors, thereby leading to substantial increases in docetaxel blood concentrations).
- No products indexed under this heading.

Quinidine Sulfate (Metabolism of docetaxel may be inhibited by co-administration with CYP3A4 inhibitors, thereby leading to substantial increases in docetaxel blood concentrations).
- No products indexed under this heading.

Quinine (Metabolism of docetaxel may be inhibited by co-administration with CYP3A4 inhibitors, thereby leading to substantial increases in docetaxel blood concentrations).
No products indexed under this heading.

Quinine Sulfate (Metabolism of docetaxel may be inhibited by co-administration with CYP3A4 inhibitors, thereby leading to substantial increases in docetaxel blood concentrations).
No products indexed under this heading.

Quinupristin (Metabolism of docetaxel may be inhibited by co-administration with CYP3A4 inhibitors, thereby leading to substantial increases in docetaxel blood concentrations). Products include:
Synercid I.V. 1690

Ranitidine Bismuth Citrate (Metabolism of docetaxel may be inhibited by co-administration with CYP3A4 inhibitors, thereby leading to substantial increases in docetaxel blood concentrations).
No products indexed under this heading.

Ranitidine Hydrochloride (Metabolism of docetaxel may be inhibited by co-administration with CYP3A4 inhibitors, thereby leading to substantial increases in docetaxel blood concentrations). Products include:
Zantac 1597
Zantac Injection 1593
Zantac 75 Tablets 715
Zantac 150 Maximum Strength Tablets 715
Zantac Injection Pharmacy Bulk Package 1595

Ritonavir (Metabolism of docetaxel may be inhibited by co-administration with CYP3A4 inhibitors, thereby leading to substantial increases in docetaxel blood concentrations). Products include:
Kaletra 474
Norvir 499

Saquinavir (Metabolism of docetaxel may be inhibited by co-administration with CYP3A4 inhibitors, thereby leading to substantial increases in docetaxel blood concentrations).
No products indexed under this heading.

Saquinavir Mesylate (Metabolism of docetaxel may be inhibited by co-administration with CYP3A4 inhibitors, thereby leading to substantial increases in docetaxel blood concentrations). Products include:
Invirase 2776

Sertraline Hydrochloride (Metabolism of docetaxel may be inhibited by co-administration with CYP3A4 inhibitors, thereby leading to substantial increases in docetaxel blood concentrations). Products include:
Zoloft 2581

Telithromycin (Metabolism of docetaxel may be inhibited by co-administration with CYP3A4 inhibitors, thereby leading to substantial increases in docetaxel blood concentrations). Products include:
Ketek Tablets 2920

Troglitazone (Metabolism of docetaxel may be inhibited by co-administration with CYP3A4 inhibitors, thereby leading to substantial increases in docetaxel blood concentrations).
No products indexed under this heading.

Troleandomycin (Metabolism of docetaxel may be inhibited by co-administration with CYP3A4 inhibitors, thereby leading to substantial increases in docetaxel blood concentrations).
No products indexed under this heading.

Valproate Sodium (Metabolism of docetaxel may be inhibited by co-administration with CYP3A4 inhibitors, thereby leading to substantial increases in docetaxel blood concentrations). Products include:
Depacon Injection 412

Verapamil Hydrochloride (Metabolism of docetaxel may be inhibited by co-administration with CYP3A4 inhibitors, thereby leading to substantial increases in docetaxel blood concentrations). Products include:
Covera-HS Tablets 3135
Tarka Tablets 519
Verelan PM Capsules 3120

Voriconazole (Metabolism of docetaxel may be inhibited by co-administration with CYP3A4 inhibitors, thereby leading to substantial increases in docetaxel blood concentrations). Products include:
VFEND I.V. 2543
VFEND Oral Suspension 2543
VFEND Tablets 2543

Zafirlukast (Metabolism of docetaxel may be inhibited by co-administration with CYP3A4 inhibitors, thereby leading to substantial increases in docetaxel blood concentrations). Products include:
Accolate Tablets 663

Zileuton (Metabolism of docetaxel may be inhibited by co-administration with CYP3A4 inhibitors, thereby leading to substantial increases in docetaxel blood concentrations).
No products indexed under this heading.

Food Interactions

Grapefruit (Metabolism of docetaxel may be inhibited by co-administration with CYP3A4 inhibitors, thereby leading to substantial increases in docetaxel blood concentrations).

Grapefruit Juice (Metabolism of docetaxel may be inhibited by co-administration with CYP3A4 inhibitors, thereby leading to substantial increases in docetaxel blood concentrations).

TĒGREEN 97 CAPSULES

(Camellia sinensis) 2669
May interact with oral anticoagulants. Compounds in these categories include:

Anisindione (Concurrent use with anticoagulants requires consultation with a physician). Products include:
Miradon Tablets 3056

Dicumarol (Concurrent use with anticoagulants requires consultation with a physician).
No products indexed under this heading.

Warfarin Sodium (Concurrent use with anticoagulants requires consultation with a physician). Products include:
Coumadin for Injection 932
Coumadin Tablets 932

TEGRETOL CHEWABLE TABLETS

(Carbamazepine) 2278
See Tegretol-XR Tablets

TEGRETOL SUSPENSION

(Carbamazepine) 2278
See Tegretol-XR Tablets

TEGRETOL TABLETS

(Carbamazepine) 2278
See Tegretol-XR Tablets

TEGRETOL-XR TABLETS

(Carbamazepine) 2278
May interact with calcium channel blockers, corticosteroids, doxycycline, anticonvulsants, erythromycin, lithium preparations, macrolide antibiotics, monoamine oxidase inhibitors, oral contraceptives, phenytoin, protease inhibitors, tricyclic antidepressants, valproate, xanthines, and certain other agents. Compounds in these categories include:

Acetaminophen (Carbamazepine induces hepatic CYP activity; carbamazepine causes, or would be expected to cause, decreased levels of acetaminophen). Products include:
Benadryl Allergy & Cold Tablets 692
Benadryl Allergy & Sinus Headache Caplets & Gelcaps 693
Benadryl Maximum Strength Severe Allergy & Sinus Headache Caplets 694
Contac Severe Cold and Flu Caplets Maximum Strength 615
Contac Severe Cold and Flu Caplets Non-Drowsy 615
Darvocet A 500 Tablets 3497
Goody's Body Pain Formula Powder 621
Goody's Extra Strength Headache Powder 621
Goody's Extra Strength Pain Relief Tablets 621
Goody's PM Powder 622
Hycomine Compound Tablets 1105
Lortab 3315
Lortab Elixir 3312
Percocet Tablets 1114
Robitussin Cough, Cold & Flu Liquid-filled Capsules 750
Robitussin Flu Liquid 752
Sedapap Tablets 50 mg/650 mg 2098
Singlet Caplets 636
Sudafed Severe Cold 710
Sudafed Sinus Headache 711
TheraFlu Cold & Cough Hot Liquid 680
TheraFlu Cold & Sore Throat Hot Liquid 680
TheraFlu Flu & Chest Congestion Non-Drowsy Hot Liquid 681
TheraFlu Flu & Sore Throat Hot Liquid 681
TheraFlu Severe Cold Non-Drowsy Hot Liquid 683
TheraFlu Severe Cold & Cough Hot Liquid 683
TheraFlu Severe Cold Caplets 679
TheraFlu Severe Cold Hot Liquid 682
TheraFlu Severe Cold Non-Drowsy Caplets 679
Triaminic Cough & Sore Throat Liquid 687
Triaminic Flu, Cough & Fever Liquid 685
Triaminic Cough & Sore Throat Softchews 689
Tylenol 8 Hour Extended Release Geltabs and Caplets 1843
Tylenol Sinus NightTime Caplets 663
Children's Tylenol Suspension Liquid and Meltaways 1850
Children's Tylenol Plus Cold & Allergy Suspension Liquid 1850
Children's Tylenol Plus Cold NightTime Suspension Liquid 1851
Children's Tylenol Plus Cold & Cough Suspension Liquid and Chewable Tablets 1851
Children's Tylenol Plus Cold Chewable Tablets 1851
Children's Tylenol Plus Cold Daytime Non-Drowsy Suspension Liquid 1851
Children's Tylenol Plus Flu Suspension Liquid 1853
Concentrated Tylenol Infants' Drops Plus Cold 1851
Concentrated Tylenol Infants' Drops Plus Cold and Cough 1851
Concentrated Tylenol Infants' Drops 1850
Junior Tylenol Meltaways 1850
Tylenol Cold & Flu Severe Daytime Liquid with Cool Bust 1846
Tylenol Cold & Flu Severe NightTime Liquid with Cool Burst 1846
Tylenol Cold Severe Congestion Non-Drowsy Caplets with Cool Burst 1846
Tylenol Cough & Sore Throat Daytime Liquid with Cool Burst 1849
Tylenol Cough & Sore Throat NightTime Liquid with Cool Burst 1849
Tylenol 1843
Extra Strength Tylenol Rapid Release Gels 1843
Tylenol 1843
Tylenol Allergy Complete Night Time Caplets 1844
Tylenol Allergy Complete Multi-Symptom Caplets and Gelcaps with Cool Burst 1844
Tylenol Severe Allergy Caplets 1844
Tylenol Flu NightTime Gelcaps 1846
Tylenol Flu Day Non-Drowsy Gelcaps 1846
Concentrated Tylenol Infants' Drops Plus Cold Nasal Congestant, Fever Reducer & Pain Reliever 668
Concentrated Tylenol Infants' Drops Plus Cold & Cough Nasal Decongestant, Fever Reducer & Pain Reliever 668
Multi-Symptom Tylenol Cold Night Time Caplets 1845
Multi-Symptom Tylenol Cold Day Non-Drowsy Caplets and Gelcaps 1845
Extra Strength Tylenol PM Caplets, Geltabs, Gelcaps and Liquid 1847
Tylenol Sinus Day Non-Drowsy 1848
Tylenol Sinus Night Time Caplets 1848
Tylenol Sinus Severe Congestion Caplets with Cool Burst 1848
Tylenol Sore Throat Daytime Liquid with Cool Burst 1849
Tylenol Sore Throat NightTime Liquid with Cool Burst 1849
Tylenol with Codeine 2461
Women's Tylenol Menstrual Relief Caplets 1849
Ultracet Tablets 2462
Vicks 44M Cough, Cold & Flu Relief 2676
Vicks DayQuil LiquiCaps/Liquid Multi-Symptom Cold/Flu Relief 723
Vicks DayQuil Multi-Symptom Cold/Flu Relief LiquiCaps 2675
Vicks DayQuil Multi-Symptom Cold/Flu Relief Liquid 2675
Vicks NyQuil LiquiCaps 2677
Vicks NyQuil LiquiCaps/Liquid Multi-Symptom Cold/Flu Relief 725
Vicks NyQuil Liquid 2677
Vicodin Tablets 530
Vicodin ES Tablets 531
Vicodin HP Tablets 532
Zydone Tablets 1118

Alprazolam (Carbamazepine induces hepatic CYP activity; carbamazepine causes, or would be expected to cause, decreased levels of alprazolam). Products include:
Niravam Orally Disintegrating Tablets 3106
Xanax XR Tablets 2655

Aminophylline (Co-administration with CYP3A4 inducers, such as theophylline, has been shown, or that would be expected, to decrease carbamazepine plasma levels; carbamazepine induces hepatic CYP activity; carbamazepine causes, or would be expected to cause decreased levels of theophylline).
No products indexed under this heading.

Amitriptyline Hydrochloride (Since carbamazepine induces hepatic CYP activity, carbamazepine may cause decreased levels of tricyclic antidepressants).
No products indexed under this heading.

Amlodipine Besylate (Since carbamazepine induces hepatic CYP activity, carbamazepine may cause decreased levels of the dihydropyridine calcium channel blockers).
Products include:
Caduet Tablets 2507
Lotrel Capsules 2238
Norvasc Tablets 2529

Amoxapine (Since carbamazepine induces hepatic CYP activity, carbamazepine may cause decreased levels of tricyclic antidepressants).
No products indexed under this heading.

Amprenavir (Since carbamazepine induces hepatic CYP activity, carbamazepine may cause decreased levels of protease inhibitors).
Products include:
Agenerase Capsules 1299
Agenerase Oral Solution 1304

Azithromycin Dihydrate (Co-administration with CYP3A4 inhibitors, such as macrolides, inhibits carbamazepine metabolism and has been shown, or would be expected to increase carbamazepine plasma levels). Products include:
Zithromax 2568
Zithromax for IV Infusion 2573
Zithromax for Oral Suspension, 300 mg, 600 mg, 900 mg, 1200 mg 2561
Zithromax Tablets, 250 mg, 500 mg 2561
Zithromax Tri-Pak 2561
Zithromax Z-Pak 2568

Bepridil Hydrochloride (Since carbamazepine induces hepatic CYP activity, carbamazepine may cause decreased levels of the dihydropyridine calcium channel blockers).
No products indexed under this heading.

Betamethasone Acetate (Since carbamazepine induces hepatic CYP activity, carbamazepine may cause decreased levels of corticosteroids).
No products indexed under this heading.

Betamethasone Sodium Phosphate (Since carbamazepine induces hepatic CYP activity, carbamazepine may cause decreased levels of corticosteroids).
No products indexed under this heading.

Chlorpromazine Hydrochloride (Concurrent use of Thorazine solution and Tegretol Suspension has resulted in an orange rubbery precipitate in stool; Tegretol Suspension should not be administered simultaneously with other liquid medications).
No products indexed under this heading.

Cimetidine (Co-administration with CYP3A4 inhibitors, such as cimetidine, inhibits carbamazepine metabolism and has been shown, or would be expected to increase carbamazepine plasma levels). Products include:
Tagamet HB 200 Tablets .... ▣ 637
Tagamet Tablets 1547

Cimetidine Hydrochloride (Co-administration with CYP3A4 inhibitors, such as cimetidine inhibits carbamazepine metabolism and has been shown, or would be expected to increase carbamazepine plasma levels).
No products indexed under this heading.

Cisplatin (Co-administration with CYP3A4 inducers, such as cisplatin, has been shown, or that would be expected, to decrease carbamazepine plasma levels).
No products indexed under this heading.

Clarithromycin (Co-administration with CYP3A4 inhibitors, such as macrolides, inhibits carbamazepine metabolism and has been shown, or would be expected to increase carbamazepine plasma levels).
Products include:
Biaxin/Biaxin XL 402
PREVPAC 3281

Clomipramine Hydrochloride (Carbamazepine increases clomipramine plasma levels).
No products indexed under this heading.

Clonazepam (Carbamazepine induces hepatic CYP activity; carbamazepine causes, or would be expected to cause, decreased levels of clonazepam; combination therapy with other anticonvulsant drugs has resulted in alterations in thyroid function). Products include:
Klonopin 2782

Clozapine (Carbamazepine induces hepatic CYP activity: carbamazepine causes, or would be expected to cause decreased levels of clozapine). Products include:
Clozapine Tablets 2141
Clozaril Tablets 2174
FazaClo Orally Disintegrating Tablets 547

Cortisone Acetate (Since carbamazepine induces hepatic CYP activity, carbamazepine may cause decreased levels of corticosteroids).
No products indexed under this heading.

Cyclosporine (Since carbamazepine induces hepatic CYP activity, carbamazepine may cause decreased levels of cyclosporine).
Products include:
Gengraf Capsules 458
Neoral Soft Gelatin Capsules 2247
Neoral Oral Solution 2247
Restasis Ophthalmic Emulsion 570
Sandimmune 2259

Danazol (Co-administration with CYP3A4 inhibitors, such as danazol, inhibits carbamazepine metabolism and has been shown, or would be expected to increase carbamazepine plasma levels).
No products indexed under this heading.

Desipramine Hydrochloride (Since carbamazepine induces hepatic CYP activity, carbamazepine may cause decreased levels of tricyclic antidepressants).
No products indexed under this heading.

Desogestrel (Carbamazepine induces hepatic CYP activity; carbamazepine causes, or would be expected to cause, decreased levels of oral contraceptives; breakthrough bleeding has been reported among patients receiving concomitant oral and subdermal contraceptives and their reliability may be adversely affected). Products include:
Ortho-Cept Tablets 2395

Dexamethasone (Since carbamazepine induces hepatic CYP activity, carbamazepine may cause decreased levels of corticosteroids).
Products include:
Ciprodex Otic Suspension 555
Decadron Tablets 1929
TobraDex Ophthalmic Ointment 558
TobraDex Ophthalmic Suspension 558

Dexamethasone Acetate (Since carbamazepine induces hepatic CYP activity, carbamazepine may cause decreased levels of corticosteroids).
No products indexed under this heading.

Dexamethasone Sodium Phosphate (Since carbamazepine induces hepatic CYP activity, carbamazepine may cause decreased levels of corticosteroids). Products include:
Decadron Phosphate Injection 1931

Dicumarol (Carbamazepine induces hepatic CYP activity; carbamazepine causes, or would be expected to cause, decreased levels of dicumarol).
No products indexed under this heading.

Diltiazem Hydrochloride (Co-administration with CYP3A4 inhibitors, such as diltiazem, inhibits carbamazepine metabolism and has been shown, or would be expected to increase carbamazepine plasma levels). Products include:
Cardizem LA Extended Release Tablets 1699
Tiazac Capsules 1204

Dirithromycin (Co-administration with CYP3A4 inhibitors, such as macrolides, inhibits carbamazepine metabolism and has been shown, or would be expected to increase carbamazepine plasma levels).
No products indexed under this heading.

Divalproex Sodium (Co-administration with CYP3A4 inhibitors, such as valproate, inhibits carbamazepine metabolism and has been shown, or would be expected to increase carbamazepine (active 10, 11-epoxide) plasma levels; carbamazepine causes, or would be expected to cause, decreased levels of valproate; combination therapy with other anticonvulsant drugs has resulted in alterations in thyroid function). Products include:
Depakote Sprinkle Capsules 422
Depakote Tablets 427
Depakote ER Tablets 433

Doxepin Hydrochloride (Since carbamazepine induces hepatic CYP activity, carbamazepine may cause decreased levels of tricyclic antidepressants).
No products indexed under this heading.

Doxorubicin Hydrochloride (Co-administration with CYP3A4 inducers, such as doxorubicin, has been shown, or that would be expected, to decrease carbamazepine plasma levels). Products include:
Adriamycin for Injection, USP 786
Adriamycin Injection, USP 786

Doxycycline Calcium (Carbamazepine induces hepatic CYP activity; carbamazepine causes, or would be expected to cause, decreased levels of doxycycline).
No products indexed under this heading.

Doxycycline Hyclate (Carbamazepine induces hepatic CYP activity; carbamazepine causes, or would be expected to cause, decreased levels of doxycycline).
No products indexed under this heading.

Doxycycline Monohydrate (Carbamazepine induces hepatic CYP activity; carbamazepine causes, or would be expected to cause, decreased levels of doxycycline).
No products indexed under this heading.

Dyphylline (Co-administration with CYP3A4 inducers, such as theophylline, has been shown, or that would be expected, to decrease carbamazepine plasma levels; carbamazepine induces hepatic CYP activity; carbamazepine causes, or would be expected to cause decreased levels of theophylline).
No products indexed under this heading.

Erythromycin (Co-administration with CYP3A4 inhibitors, such as erythromycin, inhibits carbamazepine metabolism and has been shown, or would be expected to increase carbamazepine plasma levels). Products include:
Erygel Topical Gel 2096
Ery-Tab Tablets 447
Erythromycin Base Filmtab Tablets 454
Erythromycin Delayed-Release Capsules, USP 456
PCE Dispertab Tablets 510

Erythromycin Estolate (Co-administration with CYP3A4 inhibitors, such as erythromycin, inhibits carbamazepine metabolism and has been shown, or would be expected to increase carbamazepine plasma levels).
No products indexed under this heading.

Erythromycin Ethylsuccinate (Co-administration with CYP3A4 inhibitors, such as erythromycin, inhibits carbamazepine metabolism and has been shown, or would be expected to increase carbamazepine plasma levels). Products include:
E.E.S. 449
EryPed 445

Erythromycin Gluceptate (Co-administration with CYP3A4 inhibitors, such as erythromycin, inhibits carbamazepine metabolism and has been shown, or would be expected to increase carbamazepine plasma levels).
No products indexed under this heading.

Erythromycin Lactobionate (Co-administration with CYP3A4 inhibitors, such as erythromycin, inhibits carbamazepine metabolism and has been shown, or would be expected to increase carbamazepine plasma levels).
No products indexed under this heading.

Erythromycin Stearate (Co-administration with CYP3A4 inhibitors, such as erythromycin, inhibits carbamazepine metabolism and has

been shown, or would be expected to increase carbamazepine plasma levels). Products include:

Erythrocin Stearate Filmtab Tablets 452

Ethinyl Estradiol (Carbamazepine induces hepatic CYP activity; carbamazepine causes, or would be expected to cause, decreased levels of oral contraceptives; breakthrough bleeding has been reported among patients receiving concomitant oral and subdermal contraceptives and their reliability may be adversely affected). Products include:

Alesse-28 Tablets 3392
Lo/Ovral-28 Tablets 3423
NuvaRing 2357
Ortho-Cept Tablets 2395
Ortho-Cyclen/Ortho Tri-Cyclen 2414
Ortho Evra Transdermal System 2402
Ortho Tri-Cyclen Lo Tablets 2421
Seasonale Tablets 1073
Triphasil-28 Tablets 3483
Yasmin 28 Tablets 818

Ethosuximide (Carbamazepine induces hepatic CYP activity; carbamazepine causes, or would be expected to cause, decreased levels of ethosuximide; combination therapy with other anticonvulsant drugs has resulted in alterations in thyroid function).

No products indexed under this heading.

Ethotoin (Combination therapy with other anticonvulsant drugs has resulted in alterations in thyroid function. Since carbamazepine induces hepatic CYP activity, carbamazepine may cause decreased levels of zonisamide). Products include:

Peganone Tablets, USP 2487

Ethynodiol Diacetate (Carbamazepine induces hepatic CYP activity; carbamazepine causes, or would be expected to cause, decreased levels of oral contraceptives; breakthrough bleeding has been reported among patients receiving concomitant oral and subdermal contraceptives and their reliability may be adversely affected).

No products indexed under this heading.

Felbamate (Co-administration with CYP3A4 inducers, such as felbamate, has been shown, or that would be expected, to decrease carbamazepine and increased levels of the 10, 11-epoxide plasma levels; combination therapy with other anticonvulsant drugs has resulted in alterations in thyroid function).

No products indexed under this heading.

Felodipine (Since carbamazepine induces hepatic CYP activity, carbamazepine may cause decreased levels of the dihydropyridine calcium channel blockers). Products include:

Plendil Extended-Release Tablets 651

Fludrocortisone Acetate (Since carbamazepine induces hepatic CYP activity, carbamazepine may cause decreased levels of corticosteroids).

No products indexed under this heading.

Fluoxetine Hydrochloride (Co-administration with CYP3A4 inhibitors, such as fluoxetine, inhibits carbamazepine metabolism and has been shown, or would be expected to increase carbamazepine plasma levels). Products include:

Prozac Pulvules and Liquid 1771
Symbyax Capsules 1788

Fosphenytoin (Combination therapy with other anticonvulsant drugs has resulted in alterations in thyroid function. Since carbamazepine induces hepatic CYP activity, carbamazepine may cause decreased levels of zonisamide).

No products indexed under this heading.

Fosphenytoin Sodium (Co-administration with CYP3A4 inducers, such as phenytoin, has been shown, or that would be expected, to decrease carbamazepine plasma levels; carbamazepine increases phenytoin plasma levels; carbamazepine induces hepatic CYP activity; carbamazepine causes, or would be expected to cause, decreased levels of phenytoin; combination therapy with other anticonvulsant drugs has resulted in alterations in thyroid function).

No products indexed under this heading.

Gabapentin (Combination therapy with other anticonvulsant drugs has resulted in alterations in thyroid function. Since carbamazepine induces hepatic CYP activity, carbamazepine may cause decreased levels of zonisamide). Products include:

Neurontin Capsules 2498
Neurontin Oral Solution 2498
Neurontin Tablets 2498

Haloperidol (Carbamazepine induces hepatic CYP activity; carbamazepine causes, or would be expected to cause, decreased levels of haloperidol).

No products indexed under this heading.

Haloperidol Decanoate (Carbamazepine induces hepatic CYP activity; carbamazepine causes, or would be expected to cause, decreased levels of haloperidol).

No products indexed under this heading.

Hydrocortisone (Since carbamazepine induces hepatic CYP activity, carbamazepine may cause decreased levels of corticosteroids). Products include:

Cortizone•5 Ointment 699
Cortizone•10 Creme 699
Cortizone•10 Ointment 699
Cortizone•10 Plus Creme 700
Cortizone•10 Maximum Strength Quick Shot Spray 700
Hydrocortone Tablets 1963
Preparation H Hydrocortisone Cream 748

Hydrocortisone Acetate (Since carbamazepine induces hepatic CYP activity, carbamazepine may cause decreased levels of corticosteroids). Products include:

Analpram-HC 1136
Pramosone 1139
ProctoFoam-HC 3113
Tucks Anti-Itch Ointment 712
U-cort 1% Cream 3289

Hydrocortisone Sodium Phosphate (Since carbamazepine induces hepatic CYP activity, carbamazepine may cause decreased levels of corticosteroids).

No products indexed under this heading.

Hydrocortisone Sodium Succinate (Since carbamazepine induces hepatic CYP activity, carbamazepine may cause decreased levels of corticosteroids).

No products indexed under this heading.

Imipramine Hydrochloride (Since carbamazepine induces hepatic CYP activity, carbamazepine may cause decreased levels of tricyclic antidepressants).

No products indexed under this heading.

Imipramine Pamoate (Since carbamazepine induces hepatic CYP activity, carbamazepine may cause decreased levels of tricyclic antidepressants).

No products indexed under this heading.

Indinavir Sulfate (Since carbamazepine induces hepatic CYP activity, carbamazepine may cause decreased levels of protease inhibitors). Products include:

Crixivan Capsules 1918

Isocarboxazid (Because of the relationship of carbamazepine to other tricyclic compounds, on theoretical grounds, co-administration with MAO inhibitors is contraindicated).

No products indexed under this heading.

Isoniazid (Co-administration with CYP3A4 inhibitors, such as isoniazid, inhibits carbamazepine metabolism and has been shown, or would be expected to increase carbamazepine plasma levels).

No products indexed under this heading.

Isradipine (Since carbamazepine induces hepatic CYP activity, carbamazepine may cause decreased levels of the dihydropyridine calcium channel blockers). Products include:

DynaCirc CR Tablets 2726

Itraconazole (Co-administration with CYP3A4 inhibitors, such as itraconazole, inhibits carbamazepine metabolism and has been shown, or would be expected to increase carbamazepine plasma levels. Since carbamazepine induces hepatic CYP activity, carbamazepine may cause decreased levels of itraconazole).

No products indexed under this heading.

Ketoconazole (Co-administration with CYP3A4 inhibitors, such as ketoconazole, inhibits carbamazepine metabolism and has been shown, or would be expected to increase carbamazepine plasma levels). Products include:

Nizoral A-D Shampoo, 1% 1839
Nizoral 2% Shampoo 1838

Lamotrigine (Carbamazepine induces hepatic CYP activity; carbamazepine causes, or would be expected to cause, decreased levels of lamotrigine; combination therapy with other anticonvulsant drugs has resulted in alterations in thyroid function). Products include:

Lamictal 1449

Levetiracetam (Combination therapy with other anticonvulsant drugs has resulted in alterations in thyroid function. Since carbamazepine induces hepatic CYP activity, carbamazepine may cause decreased levels of zonisamide). Products include:

Keppra Oral Solution 3307
Keppra Tablets 3307

Levonorgestrel (Carbamazepine induces hepatic CYP activity; carbamazepine causes, or would be expected to cause, decreased levels of oral contraceptives; breakthrough bleeding has been reported among patients receiving concomitant oral and subdermal contraceptives and their reliability may be adversely affected). Products include:

Alesse-28 Tablets 3392
Climara Pro Transdermal System 800
Mirena Intrauterine System 810
Plan B Tablets 1068
Seasonale Tablets 1073
Triphasil-28 Tablets 3483

Levothyroxine Sodium (Since carbamazepine induces hepatic CYP activity, carbamazepine may cause decreased levels of levothyroxine). Products include:

Levothroid Tablets 1189
Levoxyl Tablets 1680
Synthroid Tablets 515
Unithroid Tablets 3521

Lithium (Co-administration may increase the risk of nuerotoxic side effects).

No products indexed under this heading.

Lithium Carbonate (Co-administration may increase the risk of nuerotoxic side effects). Products include:

Eskalith 1406
Lithobid Tablets 1670

Lithium Citrate (Co-administration may increase the risk of nuerotoxic side effects).

No products indexed under this heading.

Lopinavir (Since carbamazepine induces hepatic CYP activity, carbamazepine may cause decreased levels of protease inhibitors). Products include:

Kaletra 474

Loratadine (Co-administration with CYP3A4 inhibitors, such as loratadine, inhibits carbamazepine metabolism and has been shown, or would be expected to increase carbamazepine plasma levels). Products include:

Alavert Allergy & Sinus D-12 Hour Tablets 743
Alavert 743
Children's Claritin 24 Hour Non-Drowsy Allergy Syrup 732
Claritin Non-Drowsy 24 Hour Tablets 731
Non-Drowsy Claritin Hives Relief Tablets 733
Claritin Reditabs 24 Hour Non-Drowsy Tablets 732
Claritin-D Non-Drowsy 12 Hour Tablets 731
Claritin-D Non-Drowsy 24 Hour Tablets 731
Children's Dimetapp ND Non-Drowsy Allergy Syrup 746
Triaminic Allerchews 684

Maprotiline Hydrochloride (Since carbamazepine induces hepatic CYP activity, carbamazepine may cause decreased levels of tricyclic antidepressants).

No products indexed under this heading.

Mephenytoin (Combination therapy with other anticonvulsant drugs has resulted in alterations in thyroid function. Since carbamazepine induces hepatic CYP activity, carbamazepine may cause decreased levels of zonisamide).

No products indexed under this heading.

Mestranol (Carbamazepine induces hepatic CYP activity; carbamazepine causes, or would be expected to cause, decreased levels of oral contraceptives; breakthrough bleeding has been reported among patients receiving concomitant oral and subdermal contraceptives and their reliability may be adversely affected).
No products indexed under this heading.

Methadone Hydrochloride (Since carbamazepine induces hepatic CYP activity, carbamazepine may cause decreased levels of methadone).
No products indexed under this heading.

Methsuximide (Carbamazepine induces hepatic CYP activity; carbamazepine causes, or would be expected to cause, decreased levels of methsuximide; combination therapy with other anticonvulsant drugs has resulted in alterations in thyroid function).
No products indexed under this heading.

Methylprednisolone Acetate (Since carbamazepine induces hepatic CYP activity, carbamazepine may cause decreased levels of corticosteroids). Products include:
Depo-Medrol Injectable Suspension 2615
Depo-Medrol Single-Dose Vial 2617

Methylprednisolone Sodium Succinate (Since carbamazepine induces hepatic CYP activity, carbamazepine may cause decreased levels of corticosteroids).
No products indexed under this heading.

Mibefradil Dihydrochloride (Since carbamazepine induces hepatic CYP activity, carbamazepine may cause decreased levels of the dihydropyridine calcium channel blockers).
No products indexed under this heading.

Midazolam Hydrochloride (Since carbamazepine induces hepatic CYP activity, carbamazepine may cause decreased levels of midazolam).
No products indexed under this heading.

Moclobemide (Because of the relationship of carbamazepine to other tricyclic compounds, on theoretical grounds, co-administration with MAO inhibitors is contraindicated).
No products indexed under this heading.

Nelfinavir Mesylate (Since carbamazepine induces hepatic CYP activity, carbamazepine may cause decreased levels of protease inhibitors). Products include:
Viracept 2556

Niacinamide (Co-administration with CYP3A4 inhibitors, such as niacinamide, inhibits carbamazepine metabolism and has been shown, or would be expected to increase carbamazepine plasma levels).
No products indexed under this heading.

Nicardipine Hydrochloride (Since carbamazepine induces hepatic CYP activity, carbamazepine may cause decreased levels of the dihydropyridine calcium channel blockers). Products include:
Cardene I.V. 1129

Nicotinamide (Co-administration with CYP3A4 inhibitors, such as nicotinamide, inhibits carbamazepine metabolism and has been shown, or would be expected to increase carbamazepine plasma levels). Products include:
Nicomide Tablets 3190

Nifedipine (Since carbamazepine induces hepatic CYP activity, carbamazepine may cause decreased levels of the dihydropyridine calcium channel blockers). Products include:
Adalat CC Tablets 2978

Nimodipine (Since carbamazepine induces hepatic CYP activity, carbamazepine may cause decreased levels of the dihydropyridine calcium channel blockers). Products include:
Nimotop Capsules 774

Nisoldipine (Since carbamazepine induces hepatic CYP activity, carbamazepine may cause decreased levels of the dihydropyridine calcium channel blockers). Products include:
Sular Tablets 1163

Norethindrone (Carbamazepine induces hepatic CYP activity; carbamazepine causes, or would be expected to cause, decreased levels of oral contraceptives; breakthrough bleeding has been reported among patients receiving concomitant oral and subdermal contraceptives and their reliability may be adversely affected). Products include:
Ortho Micronor Tablets 2411

Norethynodrel (Carbamazepine induces hepatic CYP activity; carbamazepine causes, or would be expected to cause, decreased levels of oral contraceptives; breakthrough bleeding has been reported among patients receiving concomitant oral and subdermal contraceptives and their reliability may be adversely affected).
No products indexed under this heading.

Norgestimate (Carbamazepine induces hepatic CYP activity; carbamazepine causes, or would be expected to cause, decreased levels of oral contraceptives; breakthrough bleeding has been reported among patients receiving concomitant oral and subdermal contraceptives and their reliability may be adversely affected). Products include:
Ortho-Cyclen/Ortho Tri-Cyclen 2414
Ortho Tri-Cyclen Lo Tablets 2421
Prefest Tablets 1069

Norgestrel (Carbamazepine induces hepatic CYP activity; carbamazepine causes, or would be expected to cause, decreased levels of oral contraceptives; breakthrough bleeding has been reported among patients receiving concomitant oral and subdermal contraceptives and their reliability may be adversely affected). Products include:
Lo/Ovral-28 Tablets 3423

Nortriptyline Hydrochloride (Since carbamazepine induces hepatic CYP activity, carbamazepine may cause decreased levels of tricyclic antidepressants).
No products indexed under this heading.

Olanzapine (Since carbamazepine induces hepatic CYP activity, carbamazepine may cause decreased levels of olanzapine). Products include:
Symbyax Capsules 1788
Zyprexa Tablets 1798
Zyprexa IntraMuscular 1798
Zyprexa ZYDIS Orally Disintegrating Tablets 1798

Oxcarbazepine (Combination therapy with other anticonvulsant drugs has resulted in alterations in thyroid function. Since carbamazepine induces hepatic CYP activity, carbamazepine may cause decreased levels of oxcarbazepine). Products include:
Trileptal Oral Suspension 2281
Trileptal Tablets 2281

Paramethadione (Combination therapy with other anticonvulsant drugs has resulted in alterations in thyroid function. Since carbamazepine induces hepatic CYP activity, carbamazepine may cause decreased levels of zonisamide).
No products indexed under this heading.

Pargyline Hydrochloride (Because of the relationship of carbamazepine to other tricyclic compounds, on theoretical grounds, co-administration with MAO inhibitors is contraindicated).
No products indexed under this heading.

Phenacemide (Combination therapy with other anticonvulsant drugs has resulted in alterations in thyroid function. Since carbamazepine induces hepatic CYP activity, carbamazepine may cause decreased levels of zonisamide).
No products indexed under this heading.

Phenelzine Sulfate (Because of the relationship of carbamazepine to other tricyclic compounds, on theoretical grounds, co-administration with MAO inhibitors is contraindicated).
No products indexed under this heading.

Phenobarbital (Co-administration with CYP3A4 inducers, such as phenobarbital, has been shown, or that would be expected, to decrease carbamazepine plasma levels; carbamezepine increases phenobarbital plasma levels; combination therapy with other anticonvulsant drugs has resulted in alterations of thyroid function).
No products indexed under this heading.

Phensuximide (Carbamazepine induces hepatic CYP activity; carbamazepine causes, or would be expected to cause, decreased levels of phensuximide; combination therapy with other anticonvulsant drugs has resulted in alterations in thyroid function).
No products indexed under this heading.

Phenytoin (Co-administration with CYP3A4 inducers, such as phenytoin, has been shown, or that would be expected, to decrease carbamazepine plasma levels; carbamazepine increases phenytoin plasma levels; carbamazepine induces hepatic CYP activity; carbamazepine causes, or would be expected to cause, decreased levels of phenytoin; combination therapy with other anticonvulsant drugs has resulted in alterations in thyroid function).
No products indexed under this heading.

Phenytoin Sodium (Co-administration with CYP3A4 inducers, such as phenytoin, has been shown, or that would be expected, to decrease carbamazepine plasma levels; carbamazepine increases phenytoin plasma levels; carbamazepine induces hepatic CYP activity; carbamazepine causes, or would be expected to cause, decreased levels of phenytoin; combination therapy with other anticonvulsant drugs has resulted in alterations in thyroid function). Products include:
Phenytek Capsules 2153

Praziquantel (Since carbamazepine induces hepatic CYP activity, carbamazepine may cause decreased levels of praziquantel). Products include:
Biltricide Tablets 2990

Prednisolone Acetate (Since carbamazepine induces hepatic CYP activity, carbamazepine may cause decreased levels of corticosteroids). Products include:
Blephamide Ophthalmic Ointment 563
Blephamide Ophthalmic Suspension 564
Poly-Pred Liquifilm Ophthalmic Suspension .... ⊙231
Pred Forte Ophthalmic Suspension .... ⊙233
Pred Mild Sterile Ophthalmic Suspension .... ⊙236
Pred-G Ophthalmic Suspension .... ⊙234
Pred-G Sterile Ophthalmic Ointment .... ⊙235

Prednisolone Sodium Phosphate (Since carbamazepine induces hepatic CYP activity, carbamazepine may cause decreased levels of corticosteroids). Products include:
Pediapred Oral Solution 3319

Prednisolone Tebutate (Since carbamazepine induces hepatic CYP activity, carbamazepine may cause decreased levels of corticosteroids).
No products indexed under this heading.

Prednisone (Since carbamazepine induces hepatic CYP activity, carbamazepine may cause decreased levels of corticosteroids).
No products indexed under this heading.

Primidone (Co-administration with CYP3A4 inducers, such as primidone, has been shown, or that would be expected, to decrease carbamazepine plasma levels; carbamazepine increases primidone plasma levels; combination therapy with other anticonvulsant drugs has resulted in alterations in thyroid function).
No products indexed under this heading.

Procarbazine Hydrochloride (Because of the relationship of carbamazepine to other tricyclic compounds, on theoretical grounds, co-administration with MAO inhibitors is contraindicated). Products include:
Matulane Capsules 3188

Propoxyphene Hydrochloride (Co-administration with CYP3A4 inhibitors, such as propoxyphene, inhibits carbamazepine metabolism and has been shown, or would be expected to increase carbamazepine plasma levels).
No products indexed under this heading.

Propoxyphene Napsylate (Co-administration with CYP3A4 inhibitors, such as propoxyphene, inhibits carbamazepine metabolism and has been shown, or would be expected to increase carbamazepine plasma levels). Products include:
Darvocet A 500 Tablets 3497

Protriptyline Hydrochloride (Since carbamazepine induces hepatic CYP activity, carbamazepine

may cause decreased levels of tricyclic antidepressants). Products include:
Vivactil Tablets 2350

Rifampin (Co-administration with CYP3A4 inducers, such as rifampin, has been shown, or that would be expected, to decrease carbamazepine plasma levels).
No products indexed under this heading.

Risperidone (Since carbamazepine induces hepatic CYP activity, carbamazepine may cause decreased levels of risperidone). Products include:
Risperdal Consta Long-Acting Injection 1664
Risperdal M-Tab Orally Disintegrating Tablets 1658
Risperdal 1658

Ritonavir (Since carbamazepine induces hepatic CYP activity, carbamazepine may cause decreased levels of protease inhibitors). Products include:
Kaletra 474
Norvir 499

Saquinavir (Since carbamazepine induces hepatic CYP activity, carbamazepine may cause decreased levels of protease inhibitors).
No products indexed under this heading.

Saquinavir Mesylate (Since carbamazepine induces hepatic CYP activity, carbamazepine may cause decreased levels of protease inhibitors). Products include:
Invirase 2776

Selegiline Hydrochloride (Because of the relationship of carbamazepine to other tricyclic compounds, on theoretical grounds, co-administration with MAO inhibitors is contraindicated). Products include:
Eldepryl Capsules 3209

Terfenadine (Co-administration with CYP3A4 inhibitors, such as terfenadine, inhibits carbamazepine metabolism and has been shown, or would be expected to increase carbamazepine plasma levels).
No products indexed under this heading.

Theophylline (Co-administration with CYP3A4 inducers, such as theophylline, has been shown, or that would be expected, to decrease carbamazepine plasma levels; carbamazepine induces hepatic CYP activity; carbamazepine causes, or would be expected to cause decreased levels of theophylline).
No products indexed under this heading.

Theophylline Anhydrous (Co-administration with CYP3A4 inducers, such as theophylline, has been shown, or that would be expected, to decrease carbamazepine plasma levels; carbamazepine induces hepatic CYP activity; carbamazepine causes, or would be expected to cause decreased levels of theophylline). Products include:
Uniphyl Tablets 2708

Theophylline Calcium Salicylate (Co-administration with CYP3A4 inducers, such as theophylline, has been shown, or that would be expected, to decrease carbamazepine plasma levels; carbamazepine induces hepatic CYP activity; carbamazepine causes, or would be expected to cause decreased levels of theophylline).
No products indexed under this heading.

Theophylline Dihydroxypropyl (Glyceryl) (Co-administration with CYP3A4 inducers, such as theophylline, has been shown, or that would be expected, to decrease carbamazepine plasma levels; carbamazepine induces hepatic CYP activity; carbamazepine causes, or would be expected to cause decreased levels of theophylline).
No products indexed under this heading.

Theophylline Ethylenediamine (Co-administration with CYP3A4 inducers, such as theophylline, has been shown, or that would be expected, to decrease carbamazepine plasma levels; carbamazepine induces hepatic CYP activity; carbamazepine causes, or would be expected to cause decreased levels of theophylline).
No products indexed under this heading.

Theophylline Sodium Glycinate (Co-administration with CYP3A4 inducers, such as theophylline, has been shown, or that would be expected, to decrease carbamazepine plasma levels; carbamazepine induces hepatic CYP activity; carbamazepine causes, or would be expected to cause decreased levels of theophylline).
No products indexed under this heading.

Thioridazine Hydrochloride (Concurrent use of Mellaril Solution and Tegretol Suspension has resulted in an orange rubbery precipitate in stool; Tegretol Suspension should not be administered simultaneously with other liquid medications). Products include:
Thioridazine Hydrochloride Tablets 2122

Tiagabine Hydrochloride (Carbamazepine induces hepatic CYP activity; carbamazepine causes, or would be expected to cause, decreased levels of tiagabine; combination therapy with other anticonvulsant drugs has resulted in alterations in thyroid function). Products include:
Gabitril Tablets 998

Topiramate (Carbamazepine induces hepatic CYP activity; carbamazepine causes, or would be expected to cause, decreased levels of topiramate; combination therapy with other anticonvulsant drugs has resulted in alterations in thyroid function). Products include:
Topamax Sprinkle Capsules 2438
Topamax Tablets 2438

Tramadol Hydrochloride (Since carbamazepine induces hepatic CYP activity, carbamazepine may cause decreased levels of tramadol). Products include:
Ultracet Tablets 2462

Tranylcypromine Sulfate (Because of the relationship of carbamazepine to other tricyclic compounds, on theoretical grounds, co-administration with MAO inhibitors is contraindicated). Products include:
Parnate Tablets 1499

Triamcinolone (Since carbamazepine induces hepatic CYP activity, carbamazepine may cause decreased levels of corticosteroids).
No products indexed under this heading.

Triamcinolone Acetonide (Since carbamazepine induces hepatic CYP activity, carbamazepine may cause decreased levels of corticosteroids). Products include:
Azmacort Inhalation Aerosol 1701
Nasacort HFA Inhalation Aerosol 2939
Nasacort AQ Nasal Spray 2937

Triamcinolone Diacetate (Since carbamazepine induces hepatic CYP activity, carbamazepine may cause decreased levels of corticosteroids).
No products indexed under this heading.

Triamcinolone Hexacetonide (Since carbamazepine induces hepatic CYP activity, carbamazepine may cause decreased levels of corticosteroids).
No products indexed under this heading.

Trimethadione (Combination therapy with other anticonvulsant drugs has resulted in alterations in thyroid function. Since carbamazepine induces hepatic CYP activity, carbamazepine may cause decreased levels of zonisamide).
No products indexed under this heading.

Trimipramine Maleate (Since carbamazepine induces hepatic CYP activity, carbamazepine may cause decreased levels of tricyclic antidepressants). Products include:
Surmontil Capsules 2347

Troleandomycin (Co-administration with CYP3A4 inhibitors, such as macrolides, inhibits carbamazepine metabolism and has been shown, or would be expected to increase carbamazepine plasma levels).
No products indexed under this heading.

Valproate Sodium (Co-administration with CYP3A4 inhibitors, such as valproate, inhibits carbamazepine metabolism and has been shown, or would be expected to increase carbamazepine (active 10, 11-epoxide) plasma levels; carbamazepine causes, or would be expected to cause, decreased levels of valproate; combination therapy with other anticonvulsant drugs has resulted in alterations in thyroid function). Products include:
Depacon Injection 412

Valproic Acid (Co-administration with CYP3A4 inhibitors, such as valproate, inhibits carbamazepine metabolism and has been shown, or would be expected to increase carbamazepine (active 10, 11-epoxide) plasma levels; carbamazepine causes, or would be expected to cause, decreased levels of valproate; combination therapy with other anticonvulsant drugs has resulted in alterations in thyroid function). Products include:
Depakene 417

Verapamil Hydrochloride (Co-administration with CYP3A4 inhibitors, such as verapamil, inhibits carbamazepine metabolism and has been shown, or would be expected to increase carbamazepine plasma levels). Products include:
Covera-HS Tablets 3135
Tarka Tablets 519
Verelan PM Capsules 3120

Warfarin Sodium (Carbamazepine induces hepatic CYP activity; carbamazepine causes, or would be expected to cause, decreased levels of warfarin). Products include:
Coumadin for Injection 932
Coumadin Tablets 932

Zonisamide (Combination therapy with other anticonvulsant drugs has resulted in alterations in thyroid function. Since carbamazepine induces hepatic CYP activity, carbamazepine may cause decreased levels of zonisamide). Products include:
Zonegran Capsules 1089

TEGRIN DANDRUFF SHAMPOO - EXTRA CONDITIONING

(Coal Tar) 637
May interact with:

Antipsoriatic Agents (Concurrent use should be directed by physician).
No products indexed under this heading.

Ultraviolet radiation (Concurrent use should be directed by physician).

TEGRIN DANDRUFF SHAMPOO - FRESH HERBAL

(Coal Tar) 638
None cited in PDR database.

TEGRIN SKIN CREAM

(Coal Tar) 638
None cited in PDR database.

TEMODAR CAPSULES

(Temozolomide) 3088
May interact with valproate and certain other agents. Compounds in these categories include:

Divalproex Sodium (Co-administration with valproic acid decreases oral clearance of temozolomide by about 5%; the clinical implication of this effect is not known). Products include:
Depakote Sprinkle Capsules 422
Depakote Tablets 427
Depakote ER Tablets 433

Valproate Sodium (Co-administration with valproic acid decreases oral clearance of temozolomide by about 5%; the clinical implication of this effect is not known). Products include:
Depacon Injection 412

Valproic Acid (Co-administration with valproic acid decreases oral clearance of temozolomide by about 5%; the clinical implication of this effect is not known). Products include:
Depakene 417

Food Interactions

Food, unspecified (Co-administration with a modified high-fat breakfast has resulted in decrease in mean plasma concentration and AUC by 32% and 9%, respectively, and 2-fold increase in Tmax).

TEMOVATE CREAM

(Clobetasol Propionate) 1549
None cited in PDR database.

TEMOVATE GEL

(Clobetasol Propionate) 1550
None cited in PDR database.

TEMOVATE OINTMENT

(Clobetasol Propionate) 1549
None cited in PDR database.

TEMOVATE SCALP APPLICATION

(Clobetasol Propionate) 1551
None cited in PDR database.

TEMOVATE E EMOLLIENT

(Clobetasol Propionate) 1552
None cited in PDR database.

TENORMIN I.V. INJECTION
(Atenolol) 698
May interact with calcium channel blockers and certain other agents. Compounds in these categories include:

Amlodipine Besylate (Calcium channel blockers may also have an additive effect when given with Tenormin). Products include:
Caduet Tablets 2507
Lotrel Capsules 2238
Norvasc Tablets 2529

Bepridil Hydrochloride (Calcium channel blockers may also have an additive effect when given with Tenormin).
No products indexed under this heading.

Clonidine (Beta-blockers may exacerbate the rebound hypertension which can follow the withdrawal of clonidine). Products include:
Catapres-TTS 875

Clonidine Hydrochloride (Beta-blockers may exacerbate the rebound hypertension which can follow the withdrawal of clonidine). Products include:
Catapres Tablets 874
Clorpres Tablets 2139

Diltiazem Hydrochloride (Co-administration of beta-blockers with diltiazem may result in bradycardia and heart block and the left ventricular and end diastolic pressure can rise). Products include:
Cardizem LA Extended Release Tablets 1699
Tiazac Capsules 1204

Epinephrine (While taking beta-blockers, patients with a history of anaphylactic reaction may be unresponsive to the usual dose of epinephrine). Products include:
EpiPen 1061
Primatene Mist .... ▣749

Epinephrine Hydrochloride (While taking beta-blockers, patients with a history of anaphylactic reaction may be unresponsive to the usual dose of epinephrine).
No products indexed under this heading.

Felodipine (Calcium channel blockers may also have an additive effect when given with Tenormin). Products include:
Plendil Extended-Release Tablets 651

Indomethacin (Co-administration of prostaglandin synthase inhibiting drugs, such as indomethacin, may decrease the hypotensive effects of beta-blockers). Products include:
Indocin 1968

Isradipine (Calcium channel blockers may also have an additive effect when given with Tenormin). Products include:
DynaCirc CR Tablets 2726

Mibefradil Dihydrochloride (Calcium channel blockers may also have an additive effect when given with Tenormin).
No products indexed under this heading.

Nicardipine Hydrochloride (Calcium channel blockers may also have an additive effect when given with Tenormin). Products include:
Cardene I.V. 1129

Nifedipine (Calcium channel blockers may also have an additive effect when given with Tenormin). Products include:
Adalat CC Tablets 2978

Nimodipine (Calcium channel blockers may also have an additive effect when given with Tenormin). Products include:
Nimotop Capsules 774

Nisoldipine (Calcium channel blockers may also have an additive effect when given with Tenormin). Products include:
Sular Tablets 1163

Reserpine (Co-administration of catecholamine depletors, such as reserpine, may result in hypotension and/or marked tachycardia which may produce vertigo, syncope or postural hypotension).
No products indexed under this heading.

Verapamil Hydrochloride (Co-administration of beta-blockers with verapamil may result in bradycardia and heart block and the left ventricular and end diastolic pressure can rise; caution should be exercised with Tenormin I.V. Injection when given in close proximity with drugs that may also have a depressant effect on myocardial contractility). Products include:
Covera-HS Tablets 3135
Tarka Tablets 519
Verelan PM Capsules 3120

TENORMIN TABLETS
(Atenolol) 695
See Tenormin I.V. Injection

TEQUIN INJECTION
(Gatifloxacin) 964
See Tequin Tablets

TEQUIN TABLETS
(Gatifloxacin) 964
May interact with corticosteroids, erythromycin, oral hypoglycemic agents, insulin, iron containing oral preparations, magnesium-containing antacids, non-steroidal anti-inflammatory agents, psychotropics, quinidine, tricyclic antidepressants, and certain other agents. Compounds in these categories include:

Acarbose (During the postmarketing period, co-administration has resulted in hypoglycemic episodes, in some cases severe). Products include:
Precose Tablets 776

Alprazolam (Gatifloxacin may have the potential to prolong the QTc interval; co-administration with drugs known to prolong QT interval should be avoided). Products include:
Niravam Orally Disintegrating Tablets 3106
Xanax XR Tablets 2655

Aluminum Hydroxide (Systemic exposure to Tequin Tablets is reduced by co-administration of Tequin Tablets with antacids containing aluminum salts; Tequin Tablets can be administered 4 hours before the administration of antacids). Products include:
Gaviscon Regular Strength Liquid .. ▣620
Gaviscon Regular Strength Tablets .... ▣619
Gaviscon Extra Strength Liquid ...... ▣620
Gaviscon Extra Strength Tablets ..... ▣619
Maalox Max Maximum Strength Antacid/Anti-Gas Liquid 2165
Maalox Regular Strength Antacid/Antigas Liquid 2164

Amiodarone Hydrochloride (Gatifloxacin may have the potential to prolong the QTc interval; co-administration with drugs known to prolong QT interval should be avoided). Products include:
Pacerone Tablets 3337

Amitriptyline Hydrochloride (Gatifloxacin may have the potential to prolong the QTc interval; co-administration with drugs known to prolong QT interval should be avoided).
No products indexed under this heading.

Amoxapine (Gatifloxacin may have the potential to prolong the QTc interval; co-administration with drugs known to prolong QT interval should be avoided).
No products indexed under this heading.

Arsenic Trioxide (Gatifloxacin may have the potential to prolong the QTc interval; co-administration with drugs known to prolong QT interval should be avoided). Products include:
Trisenox Injection 983

Betamethasone Acetate (Post-marketing surveillance reports indicate that this risk may be increased in patients receiving concomitant corticosteroids, especially the elderly).
No products indexed under this heading.

Betamethasone Sodium Phosphate (Post-marketing surveillance reports indicate that this risk may be increased in patients receiving concomitant corticosteroids, especially the elderly).
No products indexed under this heading.

Buspirone Hydrochloride (Gatifloxacin may have the potential to prolong the QTc interval; co-administration with drugs known to prolong QT interval should be avoided).
No products indexed under this heading.

Celecoxib (Co-administration of non-steroidal anti-inflammatory agents with quinolones may increase the risks of CNS stimulation and convulsions; these events have not been observed with gatifloxacin in pre-clinical and clinical trials). Products include:
Celebrex Capsules 3130

Chlordiazepoxide (Gatifloxacin may have the potential to prolong the QTc interval; co-administration with drugs known to prolong QT interval should be avoided).
No products indexed under this heading.

Chlordiazepoxide Hydrochloride (Gatifloxacin may have the potential to prolong the QTc interval; co-administration with drugs known to prolong QT interval should be avoided). Products include:
Librium Capsules 3349

Chlorpromazine (Gatifloxacin may have the potential to prolong the QTc interval; co-administration with drugs known to prolong QT interval should be avoided).
No products indexed under this heading.

Chlorpromazine Hydrochloride (Gatifloxacin may have the potential to prolong the QTc interval; co-administration with drugs known to prolong QT interval should be avoided).
No products indexed under this heading.

Chlorpropamide (During the post-marketing period, co-administration has resulted in hypoglycemic episodes, in some cases severe).
No products indexed under this heading.

Chlorprothixene (Gatifloxacin may have the potential to prolong the QTc interval; co-administration with drugs known to prolong QT interval should be avoided).
No products indexed under this heading.

Chlorprothixene Hydrochloride (Gatifloxacin may have the potential to prolong the QTc interval; co-administration with drugs known to prolong QT interval should be avoided).
No products indexed under this heading.

Cisapride (Gatifloxacin may have the potential to prolong the QTc interval; co-administration with drugs known to prolong QT interval should be avoided).
No products indexed under this heading.

Clomipramine Hydrochloride (Gatifloxacin may have the potential to prolong the QTc interval; co-administration with drugs known to prolong QT interval should be avoided).
No products indexed under this heading.

Clorazepate Dipotassium (Gatifloxacin may have the potential to prolong the QTc interval; co-administration with drugs known to prolong QT interval should be avoided). Products include:
Tranxene 2488

Clozapine (Gatifloxacin may have the potential to prolong the QTc interval; co-administration with drugs known to prolong QT interval should be avoided). Products include:
Clozapine Tablets 2141
Clozaril Tablets 2174
FazaClo Orally Disintegrating Tablets 547

Cortisone Acetate (Post-marketing surveillance reports indicate that this risk may be increased in patients receiving concomitant corticosteroids, especially the elderly).
No products indexed under this heading.

Desipramine Hydrochloride (Gatifloxacin may have the potential to prolong the QTc interval; co-administration with drugs known to prolong QT interval should be avoided).
No products indexed under this heading.

Dexamethasone (Post-marketing surveillance reports indicate that this risk may be increased in patients receiving concomitant corticosteroids, especially the elderly). Products include:
Ciprodex Otic Suspension 555
Decadron Tablets 1929
TobraDex Ophthalmic Ointment 558
TobraDex Ophthalmic Suspension ... 558

Dexamethasone Acetate (Post-marketing surveillance reports indicate that this risk may be increased in patients receiving concomitant corticosteroids, especially the elderly).
No products indexed under this heading.

Dexamethasone Sodium Phosphate (Post-marketing surveillance

reports indicate that this risk may be increased in patients receiving concomitant corticosteroids, especially the elderly). Products include:
- Decadron Phosphate Injection ... 1931

Diazepam (Gatifloxacin may have the potential to prolong the QTc interval; co-administration with drugs known to prolong QT interval should be avoided). Products include:
- Diastat Rectal Delivery System ... 3344
- Valium Tablets ... 2822

Diclofenac Potassium (Co-administration of non-steroidal anti-inflammatory agents with quinolones may increase the risks of CNS stimulation and convulsions; these events have not been observed with gatifloxacin in pre-clinical and clinical trials). Products include:
- Cataflam Tablets ... 2173

Diclofenac Sodium (Co-administration of non-steroidal anti-inflammatory agents with quinolones may increase the risks of CNS stimulation and convulsions; these events have not been observed with gatifloxacin in pre-clinical and clinical trials). Products include:
- Arthrotec Tablets ... 3126
- Voltaren Ophthalmic Solution ... 2300
- Voltaren Tablets ... 2298
- Voltaren-XR Tablets ... 2301

Digoxin (Co-administration has resulted in modest increases in Cmax and AUC of digoxin; although dose adjustments for digoxin are not warranted with initiation of gatifloxacin treatment; patients taking digoxin should be monitored for signs and symptoms of toxicity). Products include:
- Digitek Tablets ... 2146
- Lanoxicaps Capsules ... 1458
- Lanoxin Injection ... 1462
- Lanoxin Tablets ... 1468
- Lanoxin Injection Pediatric ... 1465

Doxepin Hydrochloride (Gatifloxacin may have the potential to prolong the QTc interval; co-administration with drugs known to prolong QT interval should be avoided).
No products indexed under this heading.

Droperidol (Gatifloxacin may have the potential to prolong the QTc interval; co-administration with drugs known to prolong QT interval should be avoided).
No products indexed under this heading.

Erythromycin (Gatifloxacin may have the potential to prolong the QTc interval; co-administration with drugs known to prolong QT interval should be avoided). Products include:
- Erygel Topical Gel ... 2096
- Ery-Tab Tablets ... 447
- Erythromycin Base Filmtab Tablets ... 454
- Erythromycin Delayed-Release Capsules, USP ... 456
- PCE Dispertab Tablets ... 510

Erythromycin Estolate (Gatifloxacin may have the potential to prolong the QTc interval; co-administration with drugs known to prolong QT interval should be avoided).
No products indexed under this heading.

Erythromycin Ethylsuccinate (Gatifloxacin may have the potential to prolong the QTc interval; co-administration with drugs known to prolong QT interval should be avoided). Products include:
- E.E.S. ... 449
- EryPed ... 445

Erythromycin Gluceptate (Gatifloxacin may have the potential to prolong the QTc interval; co-administration with drugs known to prolong QT interval should be avoided).
No products indexed under this heading.

Erythromycin Lactobionate (Gatifloxacin may have the potential to prolong the QTc interval; co-administration with drugs known to prolong QT interval should be avoided).
No products indexed under this heading.

Erythromycin Stearate (Gatifloxacin may have the potential to prolong the QTc interval; co-administration with drugs known to prolong QT interval should be avoided). Products include:
- Erythrocin Stearate Filmtab Tablets ... 452

Etodolac (Co-administration of non-steroidal anti-inflammatory agents with quinolones may increase the risks of CNS stimulation and convulsions; these events have not been observed with gatifloxacin in pre-clinical and clinical trials).
No products indexed under this heading.

Fenoprofen Calcium (Co-administration of non-steroidal anti-inflammatory agents with quinolones may increase the risks of CNS stimulation and convulsions; these events have not been observed with gatifloxacin in pre-clinical and clinical trials). Products include:
- Nalfon Capsules ... 2504

Ferrous Fumarate (Systemic exposure to gatifloxacin is reduced by co-administration of gatifloxacin with iron-containing products; Tequin can be administered 4 hours before the administration of iron-containing products). Products include:
- Chromagen Forte Soft Gelatin Capsules ... 3296
- Ferretts Tablets ... 773
- Repliva 21/7 Tablets ... 3301

Ferrous Gluconate (Systemic exposure to gatifloxacin is reduced by co-administration of gatifloxacin with iron-containing products; Tequin can be administered 4 hours before the administration of iron-containing products).
No products indexed under this heading.

Ferrous Sulfate (Systemic exposure to Tequin Tablets is reduced by co-administration of Tequin Tablets with ferrous sulfate; Tequin Tablets can be administered 4 hours before the administration of iron-containing products). Products include:
- Feosol Tablets ... 1629
- Slow Fe Iron Tablets ... 772
- Slow Fe with Folic Acid Tablets ... 773

Fludrocortisone Acetate (Post-marketing surveillance reports indicate that this risk may be increased in patients receiving concomitant corticosteroids, especially the elderly).
No products indexed under this heading.

Fluphenazine Decanoate (Gatifloxacin may have the potential to prolong the QTc interval; co-administration with drugs known to prolong QT interval should be avoided).
No products indexed under this heading.

Fluphenazine Enanthate (Gatifloxacin may have the potential to prolong the QTc interval; co-administration with drugs known to prolong QT interval should be avoided).
No products indexed under this heading.

Fluphenazine Hydrochloride (Gatifloxacin may have the potential to prolong the QTc interval; co-administration with drugs known to prolong QT interval should be avoided).
No products indexed under this heading.

Flurbiprofen (Co-administration of non-steroidal anti-inflammatory agents with quinolones may increase the risks of CNS stimulation and convulsions; these events have not been observed with gatifloxacin in pre-clinical and clinical trials).
No products indexed under this heading.

Glimepiride (During the postmarketing period, co-administration has resulted in hypoglycemic episodes, in some cases severe). Products include:
- Amaryl Tablets ... 2864

Glipizide (During the postmarketing period, co-administration has resulted in hypoglycemic episodes, in some cases severe).
No products indexed under this heading.

Glyburide (During the postmarketing period, co-administration has resulted in hypoglycemic episodes, in some cases severe).
No products indexed under this heading.

Haloperidol (Gatifloxacin may have the potential to prolong the QTc interval; co-administration with drugs known to prolong QT interval should be avoided).
No products indexed under this heading.

Haloperidol Decanoate (Gatifloxacin may have the potential to prolong the QTc interval; co-administration with drugs known to prolong QT interval should be avoided).
No products indexed under this heading.

Hydrocortisone (Post-marketing surveillance reports indicate that this risk may be increased in patients receiving concomitant corticosteroids, especially the elderly). Products include:
- Cortizone•5 Ointment ... 699
- Cortizone•10 Creme ... 699
- Cortizone•10 Ointment ... 699
- Cortizone•10 Plus Creme ... 700
- Cortizone•10 Maximum Strength Quick Shot Spray ... 700
- Hydrocortone Tablets ... 1963
- Preparation H Hydrocortisone Cream ... 748

Hydrocortisone Acetate (Post-marketing surveillance reports indicate that this risk may be increased in patients receiving concomitant corticosteroids, especially the elderly). Products include:
- Analpram-HC ... 1136
- Pramosone ... 1139
- ProctoFoam-HC ... 3113
- Tucks Anti-Itch Ointment ... 712
- U-cort 1% Cream ... 3289

Hydrocortisone Sodium Phosphate (Post-marketing surveillance reports indicate that this risk may be increased in patients receiving concomitant corticosteroids, especially the elderly).
No products indexed under this heading.

Hydrocortisone Sodium Succinate (Post-marketing surveillance reports indicate that this risk may be increased in patients receiving concomitant corticosteroids, especially the elderly).
No products indexed under this heading.

Hydroxyzine Hydrochloride (Gatifloxacin may have the potential to prolong the QTc interval; co-administration with drugs known to prolong QT interval should be avoided).
No products indexed under this heading.

Ibuprofen (Co-administration of non-steroidal anti-inflammatory agents with quinolones may increase the risks of CNS stimulation and convulsions; these events have not been observed with gatifloxacin in pre-clinical and clinical trials). Products include:
- Advil Allergy Sinus Caplets ... 737
- Advil ... 737
- Children's Advil Suspension ... 742
- Children's Advil Chewable Tablets ... 741
- Advil Cold & Sinus ... 739
- Advil Flu & Body Ache Caplets ... 739
- Children's Advil Cold Suspension ... 741
- Infants' Advil Concentrated Drops ... 743
- Junior Strength Advil Swallow Tablets ... 740
- Advil Migraine Liquigels ... 740
- Advil Multi-Symptom Cold Caplets ... 738
- Combunox Tablets ... 1183
- Children's Motrin Oral Suspension and Chewable Tablets ... 1837
- Children's Motrin Cold Non-Staining Dye-Free Oral Suspension ... 1838
- Children's Motrin Cold Oral Suspension ... 1838
- Children's Motrin Non-Staining Dye-Free Oral Suspension ... 1837
- Motrin Cold & Sinus Caplets ... 1836
- Motrin IB Tablets and Caplets ... 1836
- Infants' Motrin Concentrated Drops ... 1837
- Infants' Motrin Non-Staining Dye-Free Drops ... 1837
- Junior Strength Motrin Caplets and Chewable Tablets ... 1837
- Vicoprofen Tablets ... 533

Imipramine Hydrochloride (Gatifloxacin may have the potential to prolong the QTc interval; co-administration with drugs known to prolong QT interval should be avoided).
No products indexed under this heading.

Imipramine Pamoate (Gatifloxacin may have the potential to prolong the QTc interval; co-administration with drugs known to prolong QT interval should be avoided).
No products indexed under this heading.

Indomethacin (Co-administration of non-steroidal anti-inflammatory agents with quinolones may increase the risks of CNS stimulation and convulsions; these events have not been observed with gatifloxacin in pre-clinical and clinical trials). Products include:
- Indocin ... 1968

Indomethacin Sodium Trihydrate (Co-administration of non-

steroidal anti-inflammatory agents with quinolones may increase the risks of CNS stimulation and convulsions; these events have not been observed with gatifloxacin in pre-clinical and clinical trials). Products include:
Indocin I.V. 1973

Insulin, Human, Zinc Suspension (As with other quinolones, disturbances of blood glucose, including symptomatic hyper- and hypoglycemia have been reported, usually in diabetic patients receiving insulin). Products include:
Humulin L, 100 Units 1763
Humulin U, 100 Units 1770

Insulin, Human NPH (As with other quinolones, disturbances of blood glucose, including symptomatic hyper- and hypoglycemia have been reported, usually in diabetic patients receiving insulin). Products include:
Humulin N, 100 Units 1764
Humulin N Pen 1765
Novolin N Human Insulin 10 ml Vials 2322
Novolin N InnoLet 2322
Novolin N PenFill 3 ml Cartridges 2325
Novolin R InnoLet 2322

Insulin, Human Regular (As with other quinolones, disturbances of blood glucose, including symptomatic hyper- and hypoglycemia have been reported, usually in diabetic patients receiving insulin). Products include:
Humulin R (U-500) 1768
Humulin R, 100 Units 1767
Novolin R Human Insulin 10 ml Vials 2322
Novolin R PenFill 2325

Insulin, Human Regular and Human NPH Mixture (As with other quinolones, disturbances of blood glucose, including symptomatic hyper- and hypoglycemia have been reported, usually in diabetic patients receiving insulin). Products include:
Humulin 50/50, 100 Units 1760
Humulin 70/30 Pen 1761
Novolin 70/30 Human Insulin 10 ml Vials 2321
Novolin 70/30 InnoLet 2322
Novolin 70/30 PenFill 3 ml Cartridges 2325

Insulin, NPH (As with other quinolones, disturbances of blood glucose, including symptomatic hyper- and hypoglycemia have been reported, usually in diabetic patients receiving insulin).
No products indexed under this heading.

Insulin, Regular (As with other quinolones, disturbances of blood glucose, including symptomatic hyper- and hypoglycemia have been reported, usually in diabetic patients receiving insulin).
No products indexed under this heading.

Insulin, Zinc Crystals (As with other quinolones, disturbances of blood glucose, including symptomatic hyper- and hypoglycemia have been reported, usually in diabetic patients receiving insulin).
No products indexed under this heading.

Insulin, Zinc Suspension (As with other quinolones, disturbances of blood glucose, including symptomatic hyper- and hypoglycemia have been reported, usually in diabetic patients receiving insulin).
No products indexed under this heading.

Insulin Aspart, Human Regular (As with other quinolones, disturbances of blood glucose, including symptomatic hyper- and hypoglycemia have been reported, usually in diabetic patients receiving insulin). Products include:
NovoLog Injection 2326

Insulin glargine (As with other quinolones, disturbances of blood glucose, including symptomatic hyper- and hypoglycemia have been reported, usually in diabetic patients receiving insulin). Products include:
Lantus Injection 2925

Insulin Lispro, Human (As with other quinolones, disturbances of blood glucose, including symptomatic hyper- and hypoglycemia have been reported, usually in diabetic patients receiving insulin). Products include:
Humalog-Pen 1751
Humalog Mix 75/25-Pen 1754

Insulin Lispro Protamine, Human (As with other quinolones, disturbances of blood glucose, including symptomatic hyper- and hypoglycemia have been reported, usually in diabetic patients receiving insulin). Products include:
Humalog Mix 75/25-Pen 1754

Iron (Systemic exposure to gatifloxacin is reduced by co-administration of gatifloxacin with iron-containing products; Tequin can be administered 4 hours before the administration of iron-containing products). Products include:
Chromagen Forte Soft Gelatin Capsules 3296
Ferretts IPS Liquid .... ■773
OptiNate 1162
Repliva 21/7 Tablets 3301

Isocarboxazid (Gatifloxacin may have the potential to prolong the QTc interval; co-administration with drugs known to prolong QT interval should be avoided).
No products indexed under this heading.

Ketoprofen (Co-administration of non-steroidal anti-inflammatory agents with quinolones may increase the risks of CNS stimulation and convulsions; these events have not been observed with gatifloxacin in pre-clinical and clinical trials).
No products indexed under this heading.

Ketorolac Tromethamine (Co-administration of non-steroidal anti-inflammatory agents with quinolones may increase the risks of CNS stimulation and convulsions; these events have not been observed with gatifloxacin in pre-clinical and clinical trials). Products include:
Acular Ophthalmic Solution 561
Acular LS Ophthalmic Solution 562

Lithium Carbonate (Gatifloxacin may have the potential to prolong the QTc interval; co-administration with drugs known to prolong QT interval should be avoided). Products include:
Eskalith 1406
Lithobid Tablets 1670

Lithium Citrate (Gatifloxacin may have the potential to prolong the QTc interval; co-administration with drugs known to prolong QT interval should be avoided).
No products indexed under this heading.

Lorazepam (Gatifloxacin may have the potential to prolong the QTc interval; co-administration with drugs known to prolong QT interval should be avoided).
No products indexed under this heading.

Loxapine Hydrochloride (Gatifloxacin may have the potential to prolong the QTc interval; co-administration with drugs known to prolong QT interval should be avoided).
No products indexed under this heading.

Loxapine Succinate (Gatifloxacin may have the potential to prolong the QTc interval; co-administration with drugs known to prolong QT interval should be avoided).
No products indexed under this heading.

Magaldrate (Systemic exposure to Tequin Tablets is reduced by co-administration of Tequin Tablets with antacids containing magnesium salts; Tequin Tablets can be administered 4 hours before the administration of antacids).
No products indexed under this heading.

Magnesium Carbonate (Systemic exposure to gatifloxacin is reduced by concomitant administration of gatifloxacin and antacids containing magnesium). Products include:
Gaviscon Regular Strength Liquid .... ■620
Gaviscon Extra Strength Liquid .... ■620
Gaviscon Extra Strength Tablets .... ■619

Magnesium Hydroxide (Systemic exposure to Tequin Tablets is reduced by co-administration of Tequin Tablets with antacids containing magnesium salts; Tequin Tablets can be administered 4 hours before the administration of antacids). Products include:
Maalox Max Maximum Strength Antacid/Anti-Gas Liquid 2165
Maalox Regular Strength Antacid/Antigas Liquid 2164
Pepcid Complete Chewable Tablets 1672
Rolaids Tablets .... ■707
Extra Strength Rolaids Tablets .... ■707
Rolaids Multi-Symptom Antacid & Antigas Tablets .... ■708

Magnesium Oxide (Systemic exposure to Tequin Tablets is reduced by co-administration of Tequin Tablets with antacids containing magnesium salts; Tequin Tablets can be administered 4 hours before the administration of antacids). Products include:
Beelith Tablets 784
PremCal Light, Regular, and Extra Strength Tablets .... ■762

Magnesium Trisilicate (Systemic exposure to gatifloxacin is reduced by concomitant administration of gatifloxacin and antacids containing magnesium). Products include:
Gaviscon Regular Strength Tablets .... ■619

Maprotiline Hydrochloride (Gatifloxacin may have the potential to prolong the QTc interval; co-administration with drugs known to prolong QT interval should be avoided).
No products indexed under this heading.

Meclofenamate Sodium (Co-administration of non-steroidal anti-inflammatory agents with quinolones may increase the risks of CNS stimulation and convulsions; these events have not been observed with gatifloxacin in pre-clinical and clinical trials).
No products indexed under this heading.

Mefenamic Acid (Co-administration of non-steroidal anti-inflammatory agents with quinolones may increase the risks of CNS stimulation and convulsions; these events have not been observed with gatifloxacin in pre-clinical and clinical trials).
No products indexed under this heading.

Meloxicam (Co-administration of non-steroidal anti-inflammatory agents with quinolones may increase the risks of CNS stimulation and convulsions; these events have not been observed with gatifloxacin in pre-clinical and clinical trials). Products include:
Mobic Oral Suspension 893
Mobic Tablets 893

Meprobamate (Gatifloxacin may have the potential to prolong the QTc interval; co-administration with drugs known to prolong QT interval should be avoided).
No products indexed under this heading.

Mesoridazine Besylate (Gatifloxacin may have the potential to prolong the QTc interval; co-administration with drugs known to prolong QT interval should be avoided).
No products indexed under this heading.

Metformin Hydrochloride (During the postmarketing period, co-administration has resulted in hypoglycemic episodes, in some cases severe). Products include:
ActoPlus Met Tablets 3219
Avandamet Tablets 1343
Fortamet Extended-Release Tablets 1156

Methylprednisolone Acetate (Post-marketing surveillance reports indicate that this risk may be increased in patients receiving concomitant corticosteroids, especially the elderly). Products include:
Depo-Medrol Injectable Suspension 2615
Depo-Medrol Single-Dose Vial 2617

Methylprednisolone Sodium Succinate (Post-marketing surveillance reports indicate that this risk may be increased in patients receiving concomitant corticosteroids, especially the elderly).
No products indexed under this heading.

Midazolam Hydrochloride (Gatifloxacin may have the potential to prolong the QTc interval; co-administration with drugs known to prolong QT interval should be avoided).
No products indexed under this heading.

Miglitol (During the postmarketing period, co-administration has resulted in hypoglycemic episodes, in some cases severe).
No products indexed under this heading.

Molindone Hydrochloride (Gatifloxacin may have the potential to prolong the QTc interval; co-

administration with drugs known to prolong QT interval should be avoided). Products include:

Moban Tablets 1108

Multivitamins (Systemic exposure to gatifloxacin is reduced by concomitant administration of gatifloxacin and ferrous sulfate. Gatifloxacin can be administered 4 hours before the administration of dietary supplements containing zinc, magnesium, or iron (such as multivitamins)).

No products indexed under this heading.

Nabumetone (Co-administration of non-steroidal anti-inflammatory agents with quinolones may increase the risks of CNS stimulation and convulsions; these events have not been observed with gatifloxacin in pre-clinical and clinical trials). Products include:

Relafen Tablets 1523

Naproxen (Co-administration of non-steroidal anti-inflammatory agents with quinolones may increase the risks of CNS stimulation and convulsions; these events have not been observed with gatifloxacin in pre-clinical and clinical trials). Products include:

EC-Naprosyn Delayed-Release Tablets 2769
Naprosyn Suspension 2769
Naprosyn Tablets 2769
Prevacid NapraPAC 3277

Naproxen Sodium (Co-administration of non-steroidal anti-inflammatory agents with quinolones may increase the risks of CNS stimulation and convulsions; these events have not been observed with gatifloxacin in pre-clinical and clinical trials). Products include:

Aleve Tablets, Caplets and Gelcaps .... ▣605
Anaprox Tablets 2769
Anaprox DS Tablets 2769

Nortriptyline Hydrochloride (Gatifloxacin may have the potential to prolong the QTc interval; co-administration with drugs known to prolong QT interval should be avoided).

No products indexed under this heading.

Olanzapine (Gatifloxacin may have the potential to prolong the QTc interval; co-administration with drugs known to prolong QT interval should be avoided). Products include:

Symbyax Capsules 1788
Zyprexa Tablets 1798
Zyprexa IntraMuscular 1798
Zyprexa ZYDIS Orally Disintegrating Tablets 1798

Oxaprozin (Co-administration of non-steroidal anti-inflammatory agents with quinolones may increase the risks of CNS stimulation and convulsions; these events have not been observed with gatifloxacin in pre-clinical and clinical trials).

No products indexed under this heading.

Oxazepam (Gatifloxacin may have the potential to prolong the QTc interval; co-administration with drugs known to prolong QT interval should be avoided).

No products indexed under this heading.

Perphenazine (Gatifloxacin may have the potential to prolong the QTc interval; co-administration with drugs known to prolong QT interval should be avoided).

No products indexed under this heading.

Phenelzine Sulfate (Gatifloxacin may have the potential to prolong the QTc interval; co-administration with drugs known to prolong QT interval should be avoided).

No products indexed under this heading.

Phenylbutazone (Co-administration of non-steroidal anti-inflammatory agents with quinolones may increase the risks of CNS stimulation and convulsions; these events have not been observed with gatifloxacin in pre-clinical and clinical trials).

No products indexed under this heading.

Pimozide (Gatifloxacin may have the potential to prolong the QTc interval; co-administration with drugs known to prolong QT interval should be avoided). Products include:

Orap Tablets 1220

Pioglitazone Hydrochloride (During the postmarketing period, co-administration has resulted in hypoglycemic episodes, in some cases severe). Products include:

ActoPlus Met Tablets 3219
Actos Tablets 3224

Piroxicam (Co-administration of non-steroidal anti-inflammatory agents with quinolones may increase the risks of CNS stimulation and convulsions; these events have not been observed with gatifloxacin in pre-clinical and clinical trials).

No products indexed under this heading.

Polysaccharide Iron Complex (Systemic exposure to gatifloxacin is reduced by co-administration of gatifloxacin with iron-containing products; Tequin can be administered 4 hours before the administration of iron-containing products). Products include:

Niferex-150 Forte Capsules 3299
Nu-Iron 150 Capsules 2098

Prazepam (Gatifloxacin may have the potential to prolong the QTc interval; co-administration with drugs known to prolong QT interval should be avoided).

No products indexed under this heading.

Prednisolone Acetate (Post-marketing surveillance reports indicate that this risk may be increased in patients receiving concomitant corticosteroids, especially the elderly). Products include:

Blephamide Ophthalmic Ointment 563
Blephamide Ophthalmic Suspension 564
Poly-Pred Liquifilm Ophthalmic Suspension .... ⊙231
Pred Forte Ophthalmic Suspension .... ⊙233
Pred Mild Sterile Ophthalmic Suspension .... ⊙236
Pred-G Ophthalmic Suspension ...... ⊙234
Pred-G Sterile Ophthalmic Ointment .... ⊙235

Prednisolone Sodium Phosphate (Post-marketing surveillance reports indicate that this risk may be increased in patients receiving concomitant corticosteroids, especially the elderly). Products include:

Pediapred Oral Solution 3319

Prednisolone Tebutate (Post-marketing surveillance reports indicate that this risk may be increased in patients receiving concomitant corticosteroids, especially the elderly).

No products indexed under this heading.

Prednisone (Post-marketing surveillance reports indicate that this risk may be increased in patients receiving concomitant corticosteroids, especially the elderly).

No products indexed under this heading.

Probenecid (Systemic exposure to gatifloxacin is increased following co-administration of gatifloxacin with probenecid resulting in a 42% increase in AUC and a 44% longer half-life of gatifloxacin).

No products indexed under this heading.

Procainamide Hydrochloride (Gatifloxacin may have the potential to prolong the QTc interval; co-administration with drugs known to prolong QT interval should be avoided).

No products indexed under this heading.

Prochlorperazine (Gatifloxacin may have the potential to prolong the QTc interval; co-administration with drugs known to prolong QT interval should be avoided).

No products indexed under this heading.

Promethazine Hydrochloride (Gatifloxacin may have the potential to prolong the QTc interval; co-administration with drugs known to prolong QT interval should be avoided). Products include:

Phenergan 3438

Protriptyline Hydrochloride (Gatifloxacin may have the potential to prolong the QTc interval; co-administration with drugs known to prolong QT interval should be avoided). Products include:

Vivactil Tablets 2350

Quetiapine Fumarate (Gatifloxacin may have the potential to prolong the QTc interval; co-administration with drugs known to prolong QT interval should be avoided). Products include:

Seroquel Tablets 691

Quinidine (Gatifloxacin may have the potential to prolong the QTc interval; co-administration with drugs known to prolong QT interval should be avoided).

No products indexed under this heading.

Quinidine Gluconate (Gatifloxacin may have the potential to prolong the QTc interval; co-administration with drugs known to prolong QT interval should be avoided).

No products indexed under this heading.

Quinidine Hydrochloride (Gatifloxacin may have the potential to prolong the QTc interval; co-administration with drugs known to prolong QT interval should be avoided).

No products indexed under this heading.

Quinidine Polygalacturonate (Gatifloxacin may have the potential to prolong the QTc interval; co-administration with drugs known to prolong QT interval should be avoided).

No products indexed under this heading.

Quinidine Sulfate (Gatifloxacin may have the potential to prolong the QTc interval; co-administration with drugs known to prolong QT interval should be avoided).

No products indexed under this heading.

Repaglinide (During the postmarketing period, co-administration has resulted in hypoglycemic episodes, in some cases severe). Products include:

Prandin Tablets (0.5, 1, and 2 mg) 2337

Risperidone (Gatifloxacin may have the potential to prolong the QTc interval; co-administration with drugs known to prolong QT interval should be avoided). Products include:

Risperdal Consta Long-Acting Injection 1664
Risperdal M-Tab Orally Disintegrating Tablets 1658
Risperdal 1658

Rofecoxib (Co-administration of non-steroidal anti-inflammatory agents with quinolones may increase the risks of CNS stimulation and convulsions; these events have not been observed with gatifloxacin in pre-clinical and clinical trials).

No products indexed under this heading.

Rosiglitazone Maleate (During the postmarketing period, co-administration has resulted in hypoglycemic episodes, in some cases severe). Products include:

Avandamet Tablets 1343
Avandia Tablets 1348

Sotalol Hydrochloride (Gatifloxacin may have the potential to prolong the QTc interval; co-administration with drugs known to prolong QT interval should be avoided).

No products indexed under this heading.

Sulindac (Co-administration of non-steroidal anti-inflammatory agents with quinolones may increase the risks of CNS stimulation and convulsions; these events have not been observed with gatifloxacin in pre-clinical and clinical trials). Products include:

Clinoril Tablets 1899

Thioridazine Hydrochloride (Gatifloxacin may have the potential to prolong the QTc interval; co-administration with drugs known to prolong QT interval should be avoided). Products include:

Thioridazine Hydrochloride Tablets 2122

Thiothixene (Gatifloxacin may have the potential to prolong the QTc interval; co-administration with drugs known to prolong QT interval should be avoided). Products include:

Thiothixene Capsules 2124

Tolazamide (During the postmarketing period, co-administration has resulted in hypoglycemic episodes, in some cases severe).

No products indexed under this heading.

IMPORTANT NOTE: Always consult each drug listing in the patient's regimen for possible interactions.

Tolbutamide (During the postmarketing period, co-administration has resulted in hypoglycemic episodes, in some cases severe).
No products indexed under this heading.

Tolmetin Sodium (Co-administration of non-steroidal anti-inflammatory agents with quinolones may increase the risks of CNS stimulation and convulsions; these events have not been observed with gatifloxacin in pre-clinical and clinical trials).
No products indexed under this heading.

Tranylcypromine Sulfate (Gatifloxacin may have the potential to prolong the QTc interval; co-administration with drugs known to prolong QT interval should be avoided). Products include:
Parnate Tablets 1499

Triamcinolone (Post-marketing surveillance reports indicate that this risk may be increased in patients receiving concomitant corticosteroids, especially the elderly).
No products indexed under this heading.

Triamcinolone Acetonide (Post-marketing surveillance reports indicate that this risk may be increased in patients receiving concomitant corticosteroids, especially the elderly). Products include:
Azmacort Inhalation Aerosol 1701
Nasacort HFA Inhalation Aerosol 2939
Nasacort AQ Nasal Spray 2937

Triamcinolone Diacetate (Post-marketing surveillance reports indicate that this risk may be increased in patients receiving concomitant corticosteroids, especially the elderly).
No products indexed under this heading.

Triamcinolone Hexacetonide (Post-marketing surveillance reports indicate that this risk may be increased in patients receiving concomitant corticosteroids, especially the elderly).
No products indexed under this heading.

Trifluoperazine Hydrochloride (Gatifloxacin may have the potential to prolong the QTc interval; co-administration with drugs known to prolong QT interval should be avoided).
No products indexed under this heading.

Trimipramine Maleate (Gatifloxacin may have the potential to prolong the QTc interval; co-administration with drugs known to prolong QT interval should be avoided). Products include:
Surmontil Capsules 2347

Troglitazone (During the postmarketing period, co-administration has resulted in hypoglycemic episodes, in some cases severe).
No products indexed under this heading.

Valdecoxib (Co-administration of non-steroidal anti-inflammatory agents with quinolones may increase the risks of CNS stimulation and convulsions; these events have not been observed with gatifloxacin in pre-clinical and clinical trials).
No products indexed under this heading.

Zinc-Containing Multivitamins (Systemic exposure to gatifloxacin is reduced by concomitant administration of gatifloxacin and ferrous sulfate. Gatifloxacin can be administered 4 hours before the administration of dietary supplements containing zinc, magnesium, or iron (such as multivitamins)).
No products indexed under this heading.

Zinc Sulfate (Gatifloxacin can be administered 4 hours before the administration of zinc-containing supplements). Products include:
Athena Hair System Shampoo .... ▣ 767
Spartan Hair System Shampoo .... ▣ 767
Visine A.C. Seasonal Itching and Redness Relief Drops .... ⊙ 278
Zinc-220 Capsules 576

Ziprasidone Hydrochloride (Gatifloxacin may have the potential to prolong the QTc interval; co-administration with drugs known to prolong QT interval should be avoided). Products include:
Geodon Capsules 2514

TESSALON CAPSULES

(Benzonatate) 1202
None cited in PDR database.

TESSALON PERLES

(Benzonatate) 1202
None cited in PDR database.

TESTIM 1% GEL

(Testosterone) 722
May interact with corticosteroids, insulin, and certain other agents. Compounds in these categories include:

ACTH (Co-administration of testosterone with ACTH may enhance edema formation).
No products indexed under this heading.

Betamethasone Acetate (Co-administration of testosterone with corticosteroids may enhance edema formation).
No products indexed under this heading.

Betamethasone Sodium Phosphate (Co-administration of testosterone with corticosteroids may enhance edema formation).
No products indexed under this heading.

Cortisone Acetate (Co-administration of testosterone with corticosteroids may enhance edema formation).
No products indexed under this heading.

Dexamethasone (Co-administration of testosterone with corticosteroids may enhance edema formation). Products include:
Ciprodex Otic Suspension 555
Decadron Tablets 1929
TobraDex Ophthalmic Ointment 558
TobraDex Ophthalmic Suspension 558

Dexamethasone Acetate (Co-administration of testosterone with corticosteroids may enhance edema formation).
No products indexed under this heading.

Dexamethasone Sodium Phosphate (Co-administration of testosterone with corticosteroids may enhance edema formation). Products include:
Decadron Phosphate Injection 1931

Fludrocortisone Acetate (Co-administration of testosterone with corticosteroids may enhance edema formation).
No products indexed under this heading.

Hydrocortisone (Co-administration of testosterone with corticosteroids may enhance edema formation). Products include:
Cortizone•5 Ointment .... ▣ 699
Cortizone•10 Creme .... ▣ 699
Cortizone•10 Ointment .... ▣ 699
Cortizone•10 Plus Creme .... ▣ 700
Cortizone•10 Maximum Strength Quick Shot Spray .... ▣ 700
Hydrocortone Tablets 1963
Preparation H Hydrocortisone Cream .... ▣ 748

Hydrocortisone Acetate (Co-administration of testosterone with corticosteroids may enhance edema formation). Products include:
Analpram-HC 1136
Pramosone 1139
ProctoFoam-HC 3113
Tucks Anti-Itch Ointment .... ▣ 712
U-cort 1% Cream 3289

Hydrocortisone Sodium Phosphate (Co-administration of testosterone with corticosteroids may enhance edema formation).
No products indexed under this heading.

Hydrocortisone Sodium Succinate (Co-administration of testosterone with corticosteroids may enhance edema formation).
No products indexed under this heading.

Insulin, Human, Zinc Suspension (In diabetic patients, the metabolic effects of androgens may decrease blood glucose and, therefore, insulin requirements). Products include:
Humulin L, 100 Units 1763
Humulin U, 100 Units 1770

Insulin, Human NPH (In diabetic patients, the metabolic effects of androgens may decrease blood glucose and, therefore, insulin requirements). Products include:
Humulin N, 100 Units 1764
Humulin N Pen 1765
Novolin N Human Insulin 10 ml Vials 2322
Novolin N InnoLet 2322
Novolin N PenFill 3 ml Cartridges 2325
Novolin R InnoLet 2322

Insulin, Human Regular (In diabetic patients, the metabolic effects of androgens may decrease blood glucose and, therefore, insulin requirements). Products include:
Humulin R (U-500) 1768
Humulin R, 100 Units 1767
Novolin R Human Insulin 10 ml Vials 2322
Novolin R PenFill 2325

Insulin, Human Regular and Human NPH Mixture (In diabetic patients, the metabolic effects of androgens may decrease blood glucose and, therefore, insulin requirements). Products include:
Humulin 50/50, 100 Units 1760
Humulin 70/30 Pen 1761
Novolin 70/30 Human Insulin 10 ml Vials 2321
Novolin 70/30 InnoLet 2322
Novolin 70/30 PenFill 3 ml Cartridges 2325

Insulin, NPH (In diabetic patients, the metabolic effects of androgens may decrease blood glucose and, therefore, insulin requirements).
No products indexed under this heading.

Insulin, Regular (In diabetic patients, the metabolic effects of androgens may decrease blood glucose and, therefore, insulin requirements).
No products indexed under this heading.

Insulin, Zinc Crystals (In diabetic patients, the metabolic effects of androgens may decrease blood glucose and, therefore, insulin requirements).
No products indexed under this heading.

Insulin, Zinc Suspension (In diabetic patients, the metabolic effects of androgens may decrease blood glucose and, therefore, insulin requirements).
No products indexed under this heading.

Insulin Aspart, Human Regular (In diabetic patients, the metabolic effects of androgens may decrease blood glucose and, therefore, insulin requirements). Products include:
NovoLog Injection 2326

Insulin glargine (In diabetic patients, the metabolic effects of androgens may decrease blood glucose and, therefore, insulin requirements). Products include:
Lantus Injection 2925

Insulin Lispro, Human (In diabetic patients, the metabolic effects of androgens may decrease blood glucose and, therefore, insulin requirements). Products include:
Humalog-Pen 1751
Humalog Mix 75/25-Pen 1754

Insulin Lispro Protamine, Human (In diabetic patients, the metabolic effects of androgens may decrease blood glucose and, therefore, insulin requirements). Products include:
Humalog Mix 75/25-Pen 1754

Methylprednisolone Acetate (Co-administration of testosterone with corticosteroids may enhance edema formation). Products include:
Depo-Medrol Injectable Suspension 2615
Depo-Medrol Single-Dose Vial 2617

Methylprednisolone Sodium Succinate (Co-administration of testosterone with corticosteroids may enhance edema formation).
No products indexed under this heading.

Oxyphenbutazone (Co-administration of androgens and oxyphenbutazone may result in elevated serum levels of oxyphenbutazone).
No products indexed under this heading.

Prednisolone Acetate (Co-administration of testosterone with corticosteroids may enhance edema formation). Products include:
Blephamide Ophthalmic Ointment 563
Blephamide Ophthalmic Suspension 564
Poly-Pred Liquifilm Ophthalmic Suspension .... ⊙ 231
Pred Forte Ophthalmic Suspension .... ⊙ 233
Pred Mild Sterile Ophthalmic Suspension .... ⊙ 236
Pred-G Ophthalmic Suspension .... ⊙ 234
Pred-G Sterile Ophthalmic Ointment .... ⊙ 235

Prednisolone Sodium Phosphate (Co-administration of testosterone with corticosteroids may enhance edema formation). Products include:
Pediapred Oral Solution 3319

Prednisolone Tebutate (Co-administration of testosterone with corticosteroids may enhance edema formation).
No products indexed under this heading.

Prednisone (Co-administration of testosterone with corticosteroids may enhance edema formation).
No products indexed under this heading.

Propranolol Hydrochloride (Co-administration of injectable testosterone cypionate has resulted in an increased clearance of propranolol). Products include:
Inderal LA Long-Acting Capsules 3421
InnoPran XL Capsules 2728

Triamcinolone (Co-administration of testosterone with corticosteroids may enhance edema formation).
No products indexed under this heading.

Triamcinolone Acetonide (Co-administration of testosterone with corticosteroids may enhance edema formation). Products include:
Azmacort Inhalation Aerosol 1701
Nasacort HFA Inhalation Aerosol 2939
Nasacort AQ Nasal Spray 2937

Triamcinolone Diacetate (Co-administration of testosterone with corticosteroids may enhance edema formation).
No products indexed under this heading.

Triamcinolone Hexacetonide (Co-administration of testosterone with corticosteroids may enhance edema formation).
No products indexed under this heading.

TEVETEN TABLETS

(Eprosartan Mesylate) 1707

Food Interactions

Food, unspecified (Co-administration with food delays absorption and causes variable changes in Cmax and AUC values which do not appear clinically important).

TEVETEN HCT TABLETS

(Eprosartan Mesylate, Hydrochlorothiazide)........................... 1710

May interact with antihypertensives, barbiturates, corticosteroids, cardiac glycosides, oral hypoglycemic agents, insulin, lithium preparations, narcotic analgesics, nondepolarizing neuromuscular blocking agents, non-steroidal anti-inflammatory agents, potassium preparations, potassium sparing diuretics, and certain other agents. Compounds in these categories include:

Acarbose (Hyperglycemia may occur with thiazide diuretics; oral hypoglycemic dosage may need to be adjusted). Products include:
Precose Tablets 776

Acebutolol Hydrochloride (Co-administration of thiazides with other antihypertensive agents may lead to additive effects or potentiation).
No products indexed under this heading.

ACTH (Intensifies the electrolyte balance, particularly hypokalemia).
No products indexed under this heading.

Alfentanil Hydrochloride (Narcotics may potentiate orthostatic hypotension).
No products indexed under this heading.

Amiloride Hydrochloride (Concomitant use of potassium sparing diuretics with eprosartan may lead to hyperkalemia). Products include:
Midamor Tablets 2000
Moduretic Tablets 2003

Amlodipine Besylate (Co-administration of thiazides with other antihypertensive agents may lead to additive effects or potentiation). Products include:
Caduet Tablets 2507
Lotrel Capsules 2238
Norvasc Tablets 2529

Aprobarbital (Barbiturates may potentiate orthostatic hypotension).
No products indexed under this heading.

Atenolol (Co-administration of thiazides with other antihypertensive agents may lead to additive effects or potentiation). Products include:
Tenormin I.V. Injection 698
Tenormin Tablets 695

Atracurium Besylate (Possible increased responsiveness to muscle relaxants).
No products indexed under this heading.

Benazepril Hydrochloride (Co-administration of thiazides with other antihypertensive agents may lead to additive effects or potentiation). Products include:
Lotensin Tablets 2232
Lotensin HCT Tablets 2235
Lotrel Capsules 2238

Bendroflumethiazide (Co-administration of thiazides with other antihypertensive agents may lead to additive effects or potentiation).
No products indexed under this heading.

Betamethasone Acetate (Corticosteroids intensify the electrolyte imbalance, particularly hypokalemia).
No products indexed under this heading.

Betamethasone Sodium Phosphate (Corticosteroids intensify the electrolyte imbalance, particularly hypokalemia).
No products indexed under this heading.

Betaxolol Hydrochloride (Co-administration of thiazides with other antihypertensive agents may lead to additive effects or potentiation). Products include:
Betoptic S Ophthalmic Suspension................................. 554

Bisoprolol Fumarate (Co-administration of thiazides with other antihypertensive agents may lead to additive effects or potentiation).
No products indexed under this heading.

Buprenorphine Hydrochloride (Narcotics may potentiate orthostatic hypotension). Products include:
Buprenex Injectable 2718
Suboxone Tablets 2719
Subutex Tablets 2719

Butabarbital (Barbiturates may potentiate orthostatic hypotension).
No products indexed under this heading.

Butalbital (Barbiturates may potentiate orthostatic hypotension). Products include:
Sedapap Tablets 50 mg/650 mg 2098

Candesartan Cilexetil (Co-administration of thiazides with other antihypertensive agents may lead to additive effects or potentiation). Products include:
Atacand Tablets 634
Atacand HCT 637

Captopril (Co-administration of thiazides with other antihypertensive agents may lead to additive effects or potentiation). Products include:
Captopril Tablets 2114

Carteolol Hydrochloride (Co-administration of thiazides with other antihypertensive agents may lead to additive effects or potentiation). Products include:
Carteolol Hydrochloride Ophthalmic Solution USP, 1%....... ⊙246

Celecoxib (Nonsteroidal anti-inflammatory agents can reduce the natriuretic, diuretic, and antihypertensive effects). Products include:
Celebrex Capsules 3130

Chlorothiazide (Co-administration of thiazides with other antihypertensive agents may lead to additive effects or potentiation). Products include:
Aldoclor Tablets 1881
Diuril Oral 1936

Chlorothiazide Sodium (Co-administration of thiazides with other antihypertensive agents may lead to additive effects or potentiation). Products include:
Diuril Sodium Intravenous 1934

Chlorpropamide (Hyperglycemia may occur with thiazide diuretics; oral hypoglycemic dosage may need to be adjusted).
No products indexed under this heading.

Chlorthalidone (Co-administration of thiazides with other antihypertensive agents may lead to additive effects or potentiation). Products include:
Clorpres Tablets 2139

Cholestyramine (Binds hydrochlorothiazide and reduces its absorption from gastrointestinal tract by 85%).
No products indexed under this heading.

Cisatracurium Besylate (Possible increased responsiveness to muscle relaxants). Products include:
Nimbex Injection 494

Clonidine (Co-administration of thiazides with other antihypertensive agents may lead to additive effects or potentiation). Products include:
Catapres-TTS 875

Clonidine Hydrochloride (Co-administration of thiazides with other antihypertensive agents may lead to additive effects or potentiation). Products include:
Catapres Tablets 874
Clorpres Tablets 2139

Codeine Phosphate (Narcotics may potentiate orthostatic hypotension). Products include:
Tylenol with Codeine 2461

Colestipol Hydrochloride (Binds hydrochlorothiazide and reduces its absorption from gastrointestinal tract by 43%).
No products indexed under this heading.

Cortisone Acetate (Corticosteroids intensify the electrolyte imbalance, particularly hypokalemia).
No products indexed under this heading.

Deserpidine (Co-administration of thiazides with other antihypertensive agents may lead to additive effects or potentiation).
No products indexed under this heading.

Deslanoside (Thiazide-induced hypokalemia may cause cardiac arrhythmias and may also sensitize or exaggerate response of the heart to the toxic effects of digitalis).
No products indexed under this heading.

Dexamethasone (Corticosteroids intensify the electrolyte imbalance, particularly hypokalemia). Products include:
Ciprodex Otic Suspension 555
Decadron Tablets 1929
TobraDex Ophthalmic Ointment 558
TobraDex Ophthalmic Suspension ... 558

Dexamethasone Acetate (Corticosteroids intensify the electrolyte imbalance, particularly hypokalemia).
No products indexed under this heading.

Dexamethasone Sodium Phosphate (Corticosteroids intensify the electrolyte imbalance, particularly hypokalemia). Products include:
Decadron Phosphate Injection 1931

Dezocine (Narcotics may potentiate orthostatic hypotension).
No products indexed under this heading.

Diazoxide (Co-administration of thiazides with other antihypertensive agents may lead to additive effects or potentiation). Products include:
Hyperstat I.V. Injection 3031

Diclofenac Potassium (Nonsteroidal anti-inflammatory agents can reduce the natriuretic, diuretic, and antihypertensive effects). Products include:
Cataflam Tablets 2173

Diclofenac Sodium (Nonsteroidal anti-inflammatory agents can reduce the natriuretic, diuretic, and antihypertensive effects). Products include:
Arthrotec Tablets 3126
Voltaren Ophthalmic Solution 2300
Voltaren Tablets 2298
Voltaren-XR Tablets 2301

Digitalis Glycoside Preparations (Thiazide-induced hypokalemia may cause cardiac arrhythmias and may also sensitize or exaggerate response of the heart to the toxic effects of digitalis).
No products indexed under this heading.

Digitoxin (Thiazide-induced hypokalemia may cause cardiac arrhythmias and may also sensitize or exaggerate response of the heart to the toxic effects of digitalis).
No products indexed under this heading.

Digoxin (Thiazide-induced hypokalemia may cause cardiac arrhythmias and may also sensitize or exaggerate response of the heart to the toxic effects of digitalis). Products include:
Digitek Tablets 2146
Lanoxicaps Capsules 1458
Lanoxin Injection 1462
Lanoxin Tablets 1468
Lanoxin Injection Pediatric 1465

Diltiazem Hydrochloride (Co-administration of thiazides with other antihypertensive agents may lead to additive effects or potentiation). Products include:

Cardizem LA Extended Release Tablets 1699
Tiazac Capsules 1204

Doxazosin Mesylate (Co-administration of thiazides with other antihypertensive agents may lead to additive effects or potentiation).
No products indexed under this heading.

Enalapril Maleate (Co-administration of thiazides with other antihypertensive agents may lead to additive effects or potentiation). Products include:
Vaseretic Tablets 2073
Vasotec I.V. Injection 2076

Enalaprilat (Co-administration of thiazides with other antihypertensive agents may lead to additive effects or potentiation).
No products indexed under this heading.

Esmolol Hydrochloride (Co-administration of thiazides with other antihypertensive agents may lead to additive effects or potentiation). Products include:
Brevibloc Concentrate 766
Brevibloc Injection 766
Brevibloc Double Strength Injection 766
Brevibloc Premixed Injection 766
Brevibloc Double Strength Premixed Injection 766

Etodolac (Nonsteroidal anti-inflammatory agents can reduce the natriuretic, diuretic, and antihypertensive effects).
No products indexed under this heading.

Felodipine (Co-administration of thiazides with other antihypertensive agents may lead to additive effects or potentiation). Products include:
Plendil Extended-Release Tablets 651

Fenoprofen Calcium (Nonsteroidal anti-inflammatory agents can reduce the natriuretic, diuretic, and antihypertensive effects). Products include:
Nalfon Capsules 2504

Fentanyl (Narcotics may potentiate orthostatic hypotension). Products include:
Duragesic Transdermal System 2448

Fentanyl Citrate (Narcotics may potentiate orthostatic hypotension). Products include:
Actiq 993

Fludrocortisone Acetate (Corticosteroids intensify the electrolyte imbalance, particularly hypokalemia).
No products indexed under this heading.

Flurbiprofen (Nonsteroidal anti-inflammatory agents can reduce the natriuretic, diuretic, and antihypertensive effects).
No products indexed under this heading.

Fosinopril Sodium (Co-administration of thiazides with other antihypertensive agents may lead to additive effects or potentiation).
No products indexed under this heading.

Furosemide (Co-administration of thiazides with other antihypertensive agents may lead to additive effects or potentiation). Products include:
Furosemide Tablets 2117

Glimepiride (Hyperglycemia may occur with thiazide diuretics; oral hypoglycemic dosage may need to be adjusted). Products include:
Amaryl Tablets 2864

Glipizide (Hyperglycemia may occur with thiazide diuretics; oral hypoglycemic dosage may need to be adjusted).
No products indexed under this heading.

Glyburide (Hyperglycemia may occur with thiazide diuretics; oral hypoglycemic dosage may need to be adjusted).
No products indexed under this heading.

Guanabenz Acetate (Co-administration of thiazides with other antihypertensive agents may lead to additive effects or potentiation).
No products indexed under this heading.

Guanethidine Monosulfate (Co-administration of thiazides with other antihypertensive agents may lead to additive effects or potentiation).
No products indexed under this heading.

Hydralazine Hydrochloride (Co-administration of thiazides with other antihypertensive agents may lead to additive effects or potentiation). Products include:
BiDil Tablets 2161

Hydrocodone Bitartrate (Narcotics may potentiate orthostatic hypotension). Products include:
Hycodan 1104
Hycomine Compound Tablets 1105
Hycotuss Expectorant Syrup 1106
Lortab 3315
Lortab Elixir 3312
Vicodin Tablets 530
Vicodin ES Tablets 531
Vicodin HP Tablets 532
Vicoprofen Tablets 533
Zydone Tablets 1118

Hydrocodone Polistirex (Narcotics may potentiate orthostatic hypotension). Products include:
Tussionex Pennkinetic Extended-Release Suspension 3322

Hydrocortisone (Corticosteroids intensify the electrolyte imbalance, particularly hypokalemia). Products include:
Cortizone•5 Ointment .... ▣699
Cortizone•10 Creme .... ▣699
Cortizone•10 Ointment .... ▣699
Cortizone•10 Plus Creme .... ▣700
Cortizone•10 Maximum Strength Quick Shot Spray .... ▣700
Hydrocortone Tablets 1963
Preparation H Hydrocortisone Cream .... ▣748

Hydrocortisone Acetate (Corticosteroids intensify the electrolyte imbalance, particularly hypokalemia). Products include:
Analpram-HC 1136
Pramosone 1139
ProctoFoam-HC 3113
Tucks Anti-Itch Ointment .... ▣712
U-cort 1% Cream 3289

Hydrocortisone Sodium Phosphate (Corticosteroids intensify the electrolyte imbalance, particularly hypokalemia).
No products indexed under this heading.

Hydrocortisone Sodium Succinate (Corticosteroids intensify the electrolyte imbalance, particularly hypokalemia).
No products indexed under this heading.

Hydroflumethiazide (Co-administration of thiazides with other antihypertensive agents may lead to additive effects or potentiation).
No products indexed under this heading.

Hydromorphone Hydrochloride (Narcotics may potentiate orthostatic hypotension). Products include:
Dilaudid 439
Dilaudid Oral Liquid 443
Dilaudid Non-Sterile Powder 439
Dilaudid Rectal Suppositories 439
Dilaudid Tablets 439
Dilaudid Tablets - 8 mg 443
Dilaudid-HP 441

Ibuprofen (Nonsteroidal anti-inflammatory agents can reduce the natriuretic, diuretic, and antihypertensive effects). Products include:
Advil Allergy Sinus Caplets .... ▣737
Advil .... ▣737
Children's Advil Suspension .... ▣742
Children's Advil Chewable Tablets .... ▣741
Advil Cold & Sinus .... ▣739
Advil Flu & Body Ache Caplets .... ▣739
Children's Advil Cold Suspension .... ▣741
Infants' Advil Concentrated Drops .... ▣743
Junior Strength Advil Swallow Tablets .... ▣740
Advil Migraine Liquigels .... ▣740
Advil Multi-Symptom Cold Caplets .... ▣738
Combunox Tablets 1183
Children's Motrin Oral Suspension and Chewable Tablets 1837
Children's Motrin Cold Non-Staining Dye-Free Oral Suspension 1838
Children's Motrin Cold Oral Suspension 1838
Children's Motrin Non-Staining Dye-Free Oral Suspension 1837
Motrin Cold & Sinus Caplets 1836
Motrin IB Tablets and Caplets 1836
Infants' Motrin Concentrated Drops 1837
Infants' Motrin Non-Staining Dye-Free Drops 1837
Junior Strength Motrin Caplets and Chewable Tablets 1837
Vicoprofen Tablets 533

Indapamide (Co-administration of thiazides with other antihypertensive agents may lead to additive effects or potentiation). Products include:
Indapamide Tablets 2119

Indomethacin (Nonsteroidal anti-inflammatory agents can reduce the natriuretic, diuretic, and antihypertensive effects). Products include:
Indocin 1968

Indomethacin Sodium Trihydrate (Nonsteroidal anti-inflammatory agents can reduce the natriuretic, diuretic, and antihypertensive effects). Products include:
Indocin I.V. 1973

Insulin, Human, Zinc Suspension (Hyperglycemia may occur with thiazide diuretics; insulin dosage may need to be adjusted): Products include:
Humulin L, 100 Units 1763
Humulin U, 100 Units 1770

Insulin, Human NPH (Hyperglycemia may occur with thiazide diuretics; insulin dosage may need to be adjusted). Products include:
Humulin N, 100 Units 1764
Humulin N Pen 1765
Novolin N Human Insulin 10 ml Vials 2322
Novolin N InnoLet 2322
Novolin N PenFill 3 ml Cartridges 2325
Novolin R InnoLet 2322

Insulin, Human Regular (Hyperglycemia may occur with thiazide diuretics; insulin dosage may need to be adjusted). Products include:
Humulin R (U-500) 1768
Humulin R, 100 Units 1767
Novolin R Human Insulin 10 ml Vials 2322
Novolin R PenFill 2325

Insulin, Human Regular and Human NPH Mixture (Hyperglycemia may occur with thiazide diuretics; insulin dosage may need to be adjusted). Products include:
Humulin 50/50, 100 Units 1760
Humulin 70/30 Pen 1761
Novolin 70/30 Human Insulin 10 ml Vials 2321
Novolin 70/30 InnoLet 2322
Novolin 70/30 PenFill 3 ml Cartridges 2325

Insulin, NPH (Hyperglycemia may occur with thiazide diuretics; insulin dosage may need to be adjusted).
No products indexed under this heading.

Insulin, Regular (Hyperglycemia may occur with thiazide diuretics; insulin dosage may need to be adjusted).
No products indexed under this heading.

Insulin, Zinc Crystals (Hyperglycemia may occur with thiazide diuretics; insulin dosage may need to be adjusted).
No products indexed under this heading.

Insulin, Zinc Suspension (Hyperglycemia may occur with thiazide diuretics; insulin dosage may need to be adjusted).
No products indexed under this heading.

Insulin Aspart, Human Regular (Hyperglycemia may occur with thiazide diuretics; insulin dosage may need to be adjusted). Products include:
NovoLog Injection 2326

Insulin glargine (Hyperglycemia may occur with thiazide diuretics; insulin dosage may need to be adjusted). Products include:
Lantus Injection 2925

Insulin Lispro, Human (Hyperglycemia may occur with thiazide diuretics; insulin dosage may need to be adjusted). Products include:
Humalog-Pen 1751
Humalog Mix 75/25-Pen 1754

Insulin Lispro Protamine, Human (Hyperglycemia may occur with thiazide diuretics; insulin dosage may need to be adjusted). Products include:
Humalog Mix 75/25-Pen 1754

Irbesartan (Co-administration of thiazides with other antihypertensive agents may lead to additive effects or potentiation). Products include:
Avalide Tablets 922
Avalide Tablets 2889
Avapro Tablets 925
Avapro Tablets 2886

Isradipine (Co-administration of thiazides with other antihypertensive agents may lead to additive effects or potentiation). Products include:
DynaCirc CR Tablets 2726

Ketoprofen (Nonsteroidal anti-inflammatory agents can reduce the natriuretic, diuretic, and antihypertensive effects).
No products indexed under this heading.

Ketorolac Tromethamine (Nonsteroidal anti-inflammatory agents can reduce the natriuretic, diuretic, and antihypertensive effects). Products include:
Acular Ophthalmic Solution 561
Acular LS Ophthalmic Solution 562

Labetalol Hydrochloride (Co-administration of thiazides with other antihypertensive agents may lead to additive effects or potentiation).
No products indexed under this heading.

Levorphanol Tartrate (Narcotics may potentiate orthostatic hypotension).
No products indexed under this heading.

Lisinopril (Co-administration of thiazides with other antihypertensive agents may lead to additive effects or potentiation). Products include:
Prinivil Tablets **2029**
Prinzide Tablets **2033**
Zestoretic Tablets **701**
Zestril Tablets **704**

Lithium (Diuretics reduce the renal clearance of lithium and add a high risk of lithium toxicity).
No products indexed under this heading.

Lithium Carbonate (Diuretics reduce the renal clearance of lithium and add a high risk of lithium toxicity). Products include:
Eskalith **1406**
Lithobid Tablets **1670**

Lithium Citrate (Diuretics reduce the renal clearance of lithium and add a high risk of lithium toxicity).
No products indexed under this heading.

Losartan Potassium (Co-administration of thiazides with other antihypertensive agents may lead to additive effects or potentiation). Products include:
Cozaar Tablets **1913**
Hyzaar **1964**

Mecamylamine Hydrochloride (Co-administration of thiazides with other antihypertensive agents may lead to additive effects or potentiation). Products include:
Inversine Tablets **3286**

Meclofenamate Sodium (Nonsteroidal anti-inflammatory agents can reduce the natriuretic, diuretic, and antihypertensive effects).
No products indexed under this heading.

Mefenamic Acid (Nonsteroidal anti-inflammatory agents can reduce the natriuretic, diuretic, and antihypertensive effects).
No products indexed under this heading.

Meloxicam (Nonsteroidal anti-inflammatory agents can reduce the natriuretic, diuretic, and antihypertensive effects). Products include:
Mobic Oral Suspension **893**
Mobic Tablets **893**

Meperidine Hydrochloride (Narcotics may potentiate orthostatic hypotension).
No products indexed under this heading.

Mephobarbital (Barbiturates may potentiate orthostatic hypotension). Products include:
Mebaral Tablets, USP **2483**

Metformin Hydrochloride (Hyperglycemia may occur with thiazide diuretics; oral hypoglycemic dosage may need to be adjusted). Products include:
ActoPlus Met Tablets **3219**
Avandamet Tablets **1343**
Fortamet Extended-Release Tablets **1156**

Methadone Hydrochloride (Narcotics may potentiate orthostatic hypotension).
No products indexed under this heading.

Methyclothiazide (Co-administration of thiazides with other antihypertensive agents may lead to additive effects or potentiation).
No products indexed under this heading.

Methyldopa (Co-administration of thiazides with other antihypertensive agents may lead to additive effects or potentiation). Products include:
Aldoclor Tablets **1881**
Aldoril Tablets **1884**

Methyldopate Hydrochloride (Co-administration of thiazides with other antihypertensive agents may lead to additive effects or potentiation).
No products indexed under this heading.

Methylprednisolone Acetate (Corticosteroids intensify the electrolyte imbalance, particularly hypokalemia). Products include:
Depo-Medrol Injectable Suspension **2615**
Depo-Medrol Single-Dose Vial **2617**

Methylprednisolone Sodium Succinate (Corticosteroids intensify the electrolyte imbalance, particularly hypokalemia).
No products indexed under this heading.

Metocurine Iodide (Possible increased responsiveness to muscle relaxants).
No products indexed under this heading.

Metolazone (Co-administration of thiazides with other antihypertensive agents may lead to additive effects or potentiation).
No products indexed under this heading.

Metoprolol Succinate (Co-administration of thiazides with other antihypertensive agents may lead to additive effects or potentiation). Products include:
Toprol-XL Tablets **660**

Metoprolol Tartrate (Co-administration of thiazides with other antihypertensive agents may lead to additive effects or potentiation).
No products indexed under this heading.

Metyrosine (Co-administration of thiazides with other antihypertensive agents may lead to additive effects or potentiation). Products include:
Demser Capsules **1933**

Mibefradil Dihydrochloride (Co-administration of thiazides with other antihypertensive agents may lead to additive effects or potentiation).
No products indexed under this heading.

Miglitol (Hyperglycemia may occur with thiazide diuretics; oral hypoglycemic dosage may need to be adjusted).
No products indexed under this heading.

Minoxidil (Co-administration of thiazides with other antihypertensive agents may lead to additive effects or potentiation). Products include:
Men's Rogaine Extra Strength Topical Solution, Ocean Rush Scent and Original Unscented **706**
Women's Rogaine Topical Solution, Spring Bloom Scent and Original Unscented **707**

Mivacurium Chloride (Possible increased responsiveness to muscle relaxants). Products include:
Mivacron Injection **489**

Moexipril Hydrochloride (Co-administration of thiazides with other antihypertensive agents may lead to additive effects or potentiation). Products include:
Uniretic Tablets **3114**
Univasc Tablets **3118**

Morphine Sulfate (Narcotics may potentiate orthostatic hypotension). Products include:
Avinza Capsules **1714**
Kadian Capsules **572**
MS Contin Tablets **2703**

Nabumetone (Nonsteroidal anti-inflammatory agents can reduce the natriuretic, diuretic, and antihypertensive effects). Products include:
Relafen Tablets **1523**

Nadolol (Co-administration of thiazides with other antihypertensive agents may lead to additive effects or potentiation). Products include:
Nadolol Tablets **2121**

Naproxen (Nonsteroidal anti-inflammatory agents can reduce the natriuretic, diuretic, and antihypertensive effects). Products include:
EC-Naprosyn Delayed-Release Tablets **2769**
Naprosyn Suspension **2769**
Naprosyn Tablets **2769**
Prevacid NapraPAC **3277**

Naproxen Sodium (Nonsteroidal anti-inflammatory agents can reduce the natriuretic, diuretic, and antihypertensive effects). Products include:
Aleve Tablets, Caplets and Gelcaps **605**
Anaprox Tablets **2769**
Anaprox DS Tablets **2769**

Nicardipine Hydrochloride (Co-administration of thiazides with other antihypertensive agents may lead to additive effects or potentiation). Products include:
Cardene I.V. **1129**

Nifedipine (Co-administration of thiazides with other antihypertensive agents may lead to additive effects or potentiation). Products include:
Adalat CC Tablets **2978**

Nisoldipine (Co-administration of thiazides with other antihypertensive agents may lead to additive effects or potentiation). Products include:
Sular Tablets **1163**

Nitroglycerin (Co-administration of thiazides with other antihypertensive agents may lead to additive effects or potentiation). Products include:
Nitro-Dur Transdermal Infusion System **3060**
Nitrolingual Pumpspray **1161**

Norepinephrine Bitartrate (Possible decreased response to pressor amines).
No products indexed under this heading.

Oxaprozin (Nonsteroidal anti-inflammatory agents can reduce the natriuretic, diuretic, and antihypertensive effects).
No products indexed under this heading.

Oxycodone Hydrochloride (Narcotics may potentiate orthostatic hypotension). Products include:
Combunox Tablets **1183**
OxyContin Tablets **2699**
OxyFast Oral Concentrate Solution **2704**
OxyIR Capsules **2704**
Percocet Tablets **1114**
Percodan Tablets **1115**

Pancuronium Bromide (Possible increased responsiveness to muscle relaxants).
No products indexed under this heading.

Penbutolol Sulfate (Co-administration of thiazides with other antihypertensive agents may lead to additive effects or potentiation).
No products indexed under this heading.

Pentobarbital Sodium (Barbiturates may potentiate orthostatic hypotension). Products include:
Nembutal Sodium Solution, USP **2484**

Perindopril Erbumine (Co-administration of thiazides with other antihypertensive agents may lead to additive effects or potentiation). Products include:
Aceon Tablets (2 mg, 4 mg, 8 mg) **3191**

Phenobarbital (Barbiturates may potentiate orthostatic hypotension).
No products indexed under this heading.

Phenoxybenzamine Hydrochloride (Co-administration of thiazides with other antihypertensive agents may lead to additive effects or potentiation). Products include:
Dibenzyline Capsules **3390**

Phentolamine Mesylate (Co-administration of thiazides with other antihypertensive agents may lead to additive effects or potentiation).
No products indexed under this heading.

Phenylbutazone (Nonsteroidal anti-inflammatory agents can reduce the natriuretic, diuretic, and antihypertensive effects).
No products indexed under this heading.

Pindolol (Co-administration of thiazides with other antihypertensive agents may lead to additive effects or potentiation).
No products indexed under this heading.

Pioglitazone Hydrochloride (Hyperglycemia may occur with thiazide diuretics; oral hypoglycemic dosage may need to be adjusted). Products include:
ActoPlus Met Tablets **3219**
Actos Tablets **3224**

Piroxicam (Nonsteroidal anti-inflammatory agents can reduce the natriuretic, diuretic, and antihypertensive effects).
No products indexed under this heading.

Polythiazide (Co-administration of thiazides with other antihypertensive agents may lead to additive effects or potentiation).
No products indexed under this heading.

Potassium Acid Phosphate (Concomitant use of potassium supplements with eprosartan may lead to hyperkalemia). Products include:
K-Phos Original (Sodium Free) Tablets **785**

Potassium Bicarbonate (Concomitant use of potassium supplements with eprosartan may lead to hyperkalemia).
No products indexed under this heading.

IMPORTANT NOTE: Always consult each drug listing in the patient's regimen for possible interactions.

Potassium Chloride (Concomitant use of potassium supplements with eprosartan may lead to hyperkalemia). Products include:
Colyte with Flavor Packs for Oral Solution 3102
HalfLytely and Bisacodyl Tablets Bowel Prep Kit with Flavors Packs 915
K-Dur Extended-Relase Tablets 3047
K-Lor Powder Packets 472
K-Tab Filmtab Tablets 473
TriLyte with Flavor Packs for Oral Solution 3114

Potassium Citrate (Concomitant use of potassium supplements with eprosartan may lead to hyperkalemia). Products include:
Urocit-K Tablets 2109

Potassium Gluconate (Concomitant use of potassium supplements with eprosartan may lead to hyperkalemia).
No products indexed under this heading.

Potassium Phosphate (Concomitant use of potassium supplements with eprosartan may lead to hyperkalemia). Products include:
K-Phos Neutral Tablets 785

Prazosin Hydrochloride (Co-administration of thiazides with other antihypertensive agents may lead to additive effects or potentiation).
No products indexed under this heading.

Prednisolone Acetate (Corticosteroids intensify the electrolyte imbalance, particularly hypokalemia). Products include:
Blephamide Ophthalmic Ointment 563
Blephamide Ophthalmic Suspension 564
Poly-Pred Liquifilm Ophthalmic Suspension .... ⊙231
Pred Forte Ophthalmic Suspension .... ⊙233
Pred Mild Sterile Ophthalmic Suspension .... ⊙236
Pred-G Ophthalmic Suspension .... ⊙234
Pred-G Sterile Ophthalmic Ointment .... ⊙235

Prednisolone Sodium Phosphate (Corticosteroids intensify the electrolyte imbalance, particularly hypokalemia). Products include:
Pediapred Oral Solution 3319

Prednisolone Tebutate (Corticosteroids intensify the electrolyte imbalance, particularly hypokalemia).
No products indexed under this heading.

Prednisone (Corticosteroids intensify the electrolyte imbalance, particularly hypokalemia).
No products indexed under this heading.

Propoxyphene Hydrochloride (Narcotics may potentiate orthostatic hypotension).
No products indexed under this heading.

Propoxyphene Napsylate (Narcotics may potentiate orthostatic hypotension). Products include:
Darvocet A 500 Tablets 3497

Propranolol Hydrochloride (Co-administration of thiazides with other antihypertensive agents may lead to additive effects or potentiation). Products include:
Inderal LA Long-Acting Capsules 3421
InnoPran XL Capsules 2728

Quinapril Hydrochloride (Co-administration of thiazides with other antihypertensive agents may lead to additive effects or potentiation).
No products indexed under this heading.

Ramipril (Co-administration of thiazides with other antihypertensive agents may lead to additive effects or potentiation). Products include:
Altace Capsules 1673

Rapacuronium Bromide (Possible increased responsiveness to muscle relaxants).
No products indexed under this heading.

Rauwolfia Serpentina (Co-administration of thiazides with other antihypertensive agents may lead to additive effects or potentiation).
No products indexed under this heading.

Remifentanil Hydrochloride (Narcotics may potentiate orthostatic hypotension).
No products indexed under this heading.

Repaglinide (Hyperglycemia may occur with thiazide diuretics; oral hypoglycemic dosage may need to be adjusted). Products include:
Prandin Tablets (0.5, 1, and 2 mg) 2337

Rescinnamine (Co-administration of thiazides with other antihypertensive agents may lead to additive effects or potentiation).
No products indexed under this heading.

Reserpine (Co-administration of thiazides with other antihypertensive agents may lead to additive effects or potentiation).
No products indexed under this heading.

Rocuronium Bromide (Possible increased responsiveness to muscle relaxants). Products include:
Zemuron Injection 2363

Rofecoxib (Nonsteroidal anti-inflammatory agents can reduce the natriuretic, diuretic, and antihypertensive effects).
No products indexed under this heading.

Rosiglitazone Maleate (Hyperglycemia may occur with thiazide diuretics; oral hypoglycemic dosage may need to be adjusted). Products include:
Avandamet Tablets 1343
Avandia Tablets 1348

Secobarbital Sodium (Barbiturates may potentiate orthostatic hypotension).
No products indexed under this heading.

Sodium Nitroprusside (Co-administration of thiazides with other antihypertensive agents may lead to additive effects or potentiation).
No products indexed under this heading.

Sotalol Hydrochloride (Co-administration of thiazides with other antihypertensive agents may lead to additive effects or potentiation).
No products indexed under this heading.

Spirapril Hydrochloride (Co-administration of thiazides with other antihypertensive agents may lead to additive effects or potentiation).
No products indexed under this heading.

Spironolactone (Concomitant use of potassium sparing diuretics with eprosartan may lead to hyperkalemia).
No products indexed under this heading.

Sufentanil Citrate (Narcotics may potentiate orthostatic hypotension).
No products indexed under this heading.

Sulindac (Nonsteroidal anti-inflammatory agents can reduce the natriuretic, diuretic, and antihypertensive effects). Products include:
Clinoril Tablets 1899

Telmisartan (Co-administration of thiazides with other antihypertensive agents may lead to additive effects or potentiation). Products include:
Micardis Tablets 884
Micardis HCT Tablets 886

Terazosin Hydrochloride (Co-administration of thiazides with other antihypertensive agents may lead to additive effects or potentiation). Products include:
Hytrin Capsules 469

Thiamylal Sodium (Barbiturates may potentiate orthostatic hypotension).
No products indexed under this heading.

Timolol Maleate (Co-administration of thiazides with other antihypertensive agents may lead to additive effects or potentiation). Products include:
Blocadren Tablets 1891
Cosopt Sterile Ophthalmic Solution 1910
Timolide Tablets 2056
Timoptic in Ocudose 2061
Timoptic Sterile Ophthalmic Solution 2058
Timoptic-XE Sterile Ophthalmic Gel Forming Solution 2062

Tolazamide (Hyperglycemia may occur with thiazide diuretics; oral hypoglycemic dosage may need to be adjusted).
No products indexed under this heading.

Tolbutamide (Hyperglycemia may occur with thiazide diuretics; oral hypoglycemic dosage may need to be adjusted).
No products indexed under this heading.

Tolmetin Sodium (Nonsteroidal anti-inflammatory agents can reduce the natriuretic, diuretic, and antihypertensive effects).
No products indexed under this heading.

Torsemide (Co-administration of thiazides with other antihypertensive agents may lead to additive effects or potentiation).
No products indexed under this heading.

Trandolapril (Co-administration of thiazides with other antihypertensive agents may lead to additive effects or potentiation). Products include:
Mavik Tablets 482
Tarka Tablets 519

Triamcinolone (Corticosteroids intensify the electrolyte imbalance, particularly hypokalemia).
No products indexed under this heading.

Triamcinolone Acetonide (Corticosteroids intensify the electrolyte imbalance, particularly hypokalemia). Products include:
Azmacort Inhalation Aerosol 1701
Nasacort HFA Inhalation Aerosol 2939
Nasacort AQ Nasal Spray 2937

Triamcinolone Diacetate (Corticosteroids intensify the electrolyte imbalance, particularly hypokalemia).
No products indexed under this heading.

Triamcinolone Hexacetonide (Corticosteroids intensify the electrolyte imbalance, particularly hypokalemia).
No products indexed under this heading.

Triamterene (Concomitant use of potassium sparing diuretics with eprosartan may lead to hyperkalemia). Products include:
Dyazide Capsules 1389
Dyrenium Capsules 3390
Maxzide 2150

Trimethaphan Camsylate (Co-administration of thiazides with other antihypertensive agents may lead to additive effects or potentiation).
No products indexed under this heading.

Troglitazone (Hyperglycemia may occur with thiazide diuretics; oral hypoglycemic dosage may need to be adjusted).
No products indexed under this heading.

Tubocurarine Chloride (Possible increased responsiveness to muscle relaxant).
No products indexed under this heading.

Valdecoxib (Nonsteroidal anti-inflammatory agents can reduce the natriuretic, diuretic, and antihypertensive effects).
No products indexed under this heading.

Valsartan (Co-administration of thiazides with other antihypertensive agents may lead to additive effects or potentiation). Products include:
Diovan HCT Tablets 2195
Diovan Tablets 2191

Vecuronium Bromide (Possible increased responsiveness to muscle relaxants).
No products indexed under this heading.

Verapamil Hydrochloride (Co-administration of thiazides with other antihypertensive agents may lead to additive effects or potentiation). Products include:
Covera-HS Tablets 3135
Tarka Tablets 519
Verelan PM Capsules 3120

Food Interactions

Alcohol (May potentiate orthostatic hypotension).

TEV-TROPIN FOR INJECTION

(Somatropin (rDNA Origin)) 1224
May interact with glucocorticoids. Compounds in these categories include:

Betamethasone Acetate (Glucocorticoid therapy may inhibit the growth-promoting effect of human growth hormone. Patients with co-existing ACTH deficiency should have their glucocorticoid replacement dose carefully adjusted to avoid an inhibitory effect on growth).
No products indexed under this heading.

Betamethasone Sodium Phosphate (Glucocorticoid therapy may inhibit the growth-promoting effect of human growth hormone. Patients with co-existing ACTH deficiency should have their glucocorticoid replacement dose carefully adjusted to avoid an inhibitory effect on growth).
No products indexed under this heading.

Cortisone Acetate (Glucocorticoid therapy may inhibit the growth-promoting effect of human growth hormone. Patients with co-existing ACTH deficiency should have their glucocorticoid replacement dose carefully adjusted to avoid an inhibitory effect on growth).
No products indexed under this heading.

Dexamethasone (Glucocorticoid therapy may inhibit the growth-promoting effect of human growth hormone. Patients with co-existing ACTH deficiency should have their glucocorticoid replacement dose carefully adjusted to avoid an inhibitory effect on growth). Products include:
- Ciprodex Otic Suspension **555**
- Decadron Tablets **1929**
- TobraDex Ophthalmic Ointment **558**
- TobraDex Ophthalmic Suspension ... **558**

Dexamethasone Acetate (Glucocorticoid therapy may inhibit the growth-promoting effect of human growth hormone. Patients with co-existing ACTH deficiency should have their glucocorticoid replacement dose carefully adjusted to avoid an inhibitory effect on growth).
No products indexed under this heading.

Dexamethasone Sodium Phosphate (Glucocorticoid therapy may inhibit the growth-promoting effect of human growth hormone. Patients with co-existing ACTH deficiency should have their glucocorticoid replacement dose carefully adjusted to avoid an inhibitory effect on growth). Products include:
- Decadron Phosphate Injection **1931**

Fludrocortisone Acetate (Glucocorticoid therapy may inhibit the growth-promoting effect of human growth hormone. Patients with co-existing ACTH deficiency should have their glucocorticoid replacement dose carefully adjusted to avoid an inhibitory effect on growth).
No products indexed under this heading.

Hydrocortisone (Glucocorticoid therapy may inhibit the growth-promoting effect of human growth hormone. Patients with co-existing ACTH deficiency should have their glucocorticoid replacement dose carefully adjusted to avoid an inhibitory effect on growth). Products include:
- Cortizone•5 Ointment **699**
- Cortizone•10 Creme **699**
- Cortizone•10 Ointment **699**
- Cortizone•10 Plus Creme **700**
- Cortizone•10 Maximum Strength Quick Shot Spray **700**
- Hydrocortone Tablets **1963**
- Preparation H Hydrocortisone Cream **748**

Hydrocortisone Acetate (Glucocorticoid therapy may inhibit the growth-promoting effect of human growth hormone. Patients with co-existing ACTH deficiency should have their glucocorticoid replacement dose carefully adjusted to avoid an inhibitory effect on growth). Products include:
- Analpram-HC **1136**
- Pramosone **1139**
- ProctoFoam-HC **3113**
- Tucks Anti-Itch Ointment **712**
- U-cort 1% Cream **3289**

Hydrocortisone Sodium Phosphate (Glucocorticoid therapy may inhibit the growth-promoting effect of human growth hormone. Patients with co-existing ACTH deficiency should have their glucocorticoid replacement dose carefully adjusted to avoid an inhibitory effect on growth).
No products indexed under this heading.

Hydrocortisone Sodium Succinate (Glucocorticoid therapy may inhibit the growth-promoting effect of human growth hormone. Patients with co-existing ACTH deficiency should have their glucocorticoid replacement dose carefully adjusted to avoid an inhibitory effect on growth).
No products indexed under this heading.

Methylprednisolone Acetate (Glucocorticoid therapy may inhibit the growth-promoting effect of human growth hormone. Patients with co-existing ACTH deficiency should have their glucocorticoid replacement dose carefully adjusted to avoid an inhibitory effect on growth). Products include:
- Depo-Medrol Injectable Suspension **2615**
- Depo-Medrol Single-Dose Vial **2617**

Methylprednisolone Sodium Succinate (Glucocorticoid therapy may inhibit the growth-promoting effect of human growth hormone. Patients with co-existing ACTH deficiency should have their glucocorticoid replacement dose carefully adjusted to avoid an inhibitory effect on growth).
No products indexed under this heading.

Prednisolone Acetate (Glucocorticoid therapy may inhibit the growth-promoting effect of human growth hormone. Patients with co-existing ACTH deficiency should have their glucocorticoid replacement dose carefully adjusted to avoid an inhibitory effect on growth). Products include:
- Blephamide Ophthalmic Ointment **563**
- Blephamide Ophthalmic Suspension **564**
- Poly-Pred Liquifilm Ophthalmic Suspension .... ⊙**231**
- Pred Forte Ophthalmic Suspension .... ⊙**233**
- Pred Mild Sterile Ophthalmic Suspension .... ⊙**236**
- Pred-G Ophthalmic Suspension ...... ⊙**234**
- Pred-G Sterile Ophthalmic Ointment .... ⊙**235**

Prednisolone Sodium Phosphate (Glucocorticoid therapy may inhibit the growth-promoting effect of human growth hormone. Patients with co-existing ACTH deficiency should have their glucocorticoid replacement dose carefully adjusted to avoid an inhibitory effect on growth). Products include:
- Pediapred Oral Solution **3319**

Prednisolone Tebutate (Glucocorticoid therapy may inhibit the growth-promoting effect of human growth hormone. Patients with co-existing ACTH deficiency should have their glucocorticoid replacement dose carefully adjusted to avoid an inhibitory effect on growth).
No products indexed under this heading.

Prednisone (Glucocorticoid therapy may inhibit the growth-promoting effect of human growth hormone. Patients with co-existing ACTH deficiency should have their glucocorticoid replacement dose carefully adjusted to avoid an inhibitory effect on growth).
No products indexed under this heading.

Triamcinolone (Glucocorticoid therapy may inhibit the growth-promoting effect of human growth hormone. Patients with co-existing ACTH deficiency should have their glucocorticoid replacement dose carefully adjusted to avoid an inhibitory effect on growth).
No products indexed under this heading.

Triamcinolone Acetonide (Glucocorticoid therapy may inhibit the growth-promoting effect of human growth hormone. Patients with co-existing ACTH deficiency should have their glucocorticoid replacement dose carefully adjusted to avoid an inhibitory effect on growth). Products include:
- Azmacort Inhalation Aerosol **1701**
- Nasacort HFA Inhalation Aerosol **2939**
- Nasacort AQ Nasal Spray **2937**

Triamcinolone Diacetate (Glucocorticoid therapy may inhibit the growth-promoting effect of human growth hormone. Patients with co-existing ACTH deficiency should have their glucocorticoid replacement dose carefully adjusted to avoid an inhibitory effect on growth).
No products indexed under this heading.

Triamcinolone Hexacetonide (Glucocorticoid therapy may inhibit the growth-promoting effect of human growth hormone. Patients with co-existing ACTH deficiency should have their glucocorticoid replacement dose carefully adjusted to avoid an inhibitory effect on growth).
No products indexed under this heading.

THALOMID CAPSULES

(Thalidomide) **979**

May interact with barbiturates, drugs that may exacerbate peripheral neuropathy (selected), phenytoin, protease inhibitors, and certain other agents. Compounds in these categories include:

Amprenavir (Concomitant use of HIV-protease inhibitors with hormonal contraceptives may reduce the effectiveness of contraception; women requiring treatment with HIV-protease inhibitors must use two other highly effective methods of contraception or abstain from heterosexual sexual intercourse during treatment with thalidomide). Products include:
- Agenerase Capsules **1299**
- Agenerase Oral Solution **1304**

Aprobarbital (Thalidomide has been reported to enhance the sedative activity of barbiturates).
No products indexed under this heading.

Butabarbital (Thalidomide has been reported to enhance the sedative activity of barbiturates).
No products indexed under this heading.

Butalbital (Thalidomide has been reported to enhance the sedative activity of barbiturates). Products include:
- Sedapap Tablets 50 mg/650 mg **2098**

Carbamazepine (Concomitant use of carbamazepine with hormonal contraceptives may reduce the effectiveness of contraception; women requiring treatment with carbamazepine must use two other highly effective methods of contraception or abstain from heterosexual sexual intercourse during treatment with thalidomide). Products include:
- Carbatrol Capsules **3174**
- Equetro Extended-Release Capsules **3178**
- Tegretol/Tegretol-XR **2278**

Carboplatin (Peripheral neuropathy is a common, potentially severe, side effect of treatment with thalidomide; therefore, concomitant use of drugs known to be associated with peripheral neuropathy should be undertaken with caution).
No products indexed under this heading.

Chlorpromazine (Thalidomide has been reported to enhance the sedative activity of chlorpromazine).
No products indexed under this heading.

Chlorpromazine Hydrochloride (Thalidomide has been reported to enhance the sedative activity of chlorpromazine).
No products indexed under this heading.

Didanosine (Peripheral neuropathy is a common, potentially severe, side effect of treatment with thalidomide; therefore, concomitant use of drugs known to be associated with peripheral neuropathy should be undertaken with caution).
No products indexed under this heading.

Fosphenytoin Sodium (Concomitant use of phenytoin with hormonal contraceptives may reduce the effectiveness of contraception; women requiring treatment with phenytoin must use two other highly effective methods of contraception or abstain from heterosexual sexual intercourse during treatment with thalidomide).
No products indexed under this heading.

Griseofulvin (Concomitant use of griseofulvin with hormonal contraceptives may reduce the effectiveness of contraception; women requiring treatment with griseofulvin must use two other highly effective methods of contraception or abstain from heterosexual sexual intercourse during treatment with thalidomide). Products include:
- Grifulvin V Tablets Microsize and Oral Suspension Microsize............ **2384**
- Gris-PEG Tablets **2504**

Indinavir Sulfate (Concomitant use of HIV-protease inhibitors with hormonal contraceptives may reduce the effectiveness of contraception;

women requiring treatment with HIV-protease inhibitors must use two other highly effective methods of contraception or abstain from heterosexual sexual intercourse during treatment with thalidomide).
Products include:
Crixivan Capsules 1918

Isoniazid (Peripheral neuropathy is a common, potentially severe, side effect of treatment with thalidomide; therefore, concomitant use of drugs known to be associated with peripheral neuropathy should be undertaken with caution).
No products indexed under this heading.

Lopinavir (Concomitant use of HIV-protease inhibitors with hormonal contraceptives may reduce the effectiveness of contraception; women requiring treatment with HIV-protease inhibitors must use two other highly effective methods of contraception or abstain from heterosexual sexual intercourse during treatment with thalidomide).
Products include:
Kaletra 474

Mephobarbital (Thalidomide has been reported to enhance the sedative activity of barbiturates).
Products include:
Mebaral Tablets, USP 2483

Nelfinavir Mesylate (Concomitant use of HIV-protease inhibitors with hormonal contraceptives may reduce the effectiveness of contraception; women requiring treatment with HIV-protease inhibitors must use two other highly effective methods of contraception or abstain from heterosexual sexual intercourse during treatment with thalidomide).
Products include:
Viracept 2556

Paclitaxel (Peripheral neuropathy is a common, potentially severe, side effect of treatment with thalidomide; therefore, concomitant use of drugs known to be associated with peripheral neuropathy should be undertaken with caution).
No products indexed under this heading.

Pentobarbital Sodium (Thalidomide has been reported to enhance the sedative activity of barbiturates).
Products include:
Nembutal Sodium Solution, USP 2484

Phenobarbital (Thalidomide has been reported to enhance the sedative activity of barbiturates).
No products indexed under this heading.

Phenytoin (Concomitant use of phenytoin with hormonal contraceptives may reduce the effectiveness of contraception; women requiring treatment with phenytoin must use two other highly effective methods of contraception or abstain from heterosexual sexual intercourse during treatment with thalidomide).
No products indexed under this heading.

Phenytoin Sodium (Concomitant use of phenytoin with hormonal contraceptives may reduce the effectiveness of contraception; women requiring treatment with phenytoin must use two other highly effective methods of contraception or abstain from heterosexual sexual intercourse during treatment with thalidomide).
Products include:
Phenytek Capsules 2153

Reserpine (Thalidomide has been reported to enhance the sedative activity of reserpine).
No products indexed under this heading.

Rifabutin (Concomitant use of rifabutin with hormonal contraceptives may reduce the effectiveness of contraception; women requiring treatment with rifabutin must use two other highly effective methods of contraception or abstain from heterosexual sexual intercourse during treatment with thalidomide).
No products indexed under this heading.

Rifampin (Concomitant use of rifampin with hormonal contraceptives may reduce the effectiveness of contraception; women requiring treatment with rifampin must use two other highly effective methods of contraception or abstain from heterosexual sexual intercourse during treatment with thalidomide).
No products indexed under this heading.

Ritonavir (Concomitant use of HIV-protease inhibitors with hormonal contraceptives may reduce the effectiveness of contraception; women requiring treatment with HIV-protease inhibitors must use two other highly effective methods of contraception or abstain from heterosexual sexual intercourse during treatment with thalidomide).
Products include:
Kaletra 474
Norvir 499

Saquinavir (Concomitant use of HIV-protease inhibitors with hormonal contraceptives may reduce the effectiveness of contraception; women requiring treatment with HIV-protease inhibitors must use two other highly effective methods of contraception or abstain from heterosexual sexual intercourse during treatment with thalidomide).
No products indexed under this heading.

Saquinavir Mesylate (Concomitant use of HIV-protease inhibitors with hormonal contraceptives may reduce the effectiveness of contraception; women requiring treatment with HIV-protease inhibitors must use two other highly effective methods of contraception or abstain from heterosexual sexual intercourse during treatment with thalidomide).
Products include:
Invirase 2776

Secobarbital Sodium (Thalidomide has been reported to enhance the sedative activity of barbiturates).
No products indexed under this heading.

Stavudine (Peripheral neuropathy is a common, potentially severe, side effect of treatment with thalidomide; therefore, concomitant use of drugs known to be associated with peripheral neuropathy should be undertaken with caution). Products include:
Zerit 971

Thiamylal Sodium (Thalidomide has been reported to enhance the sedative activity of barbiturates).
No products indexed under this heading.

Zalcitabine (Peripheral neuropathy is a common, potentially severe, side effect of treatment with thalidomide; therefore, concomitant use of drugs known to be associated with peripheral neuropathy should be undertaken with caution).
No products indexed under this heading.

Food Interactions

Alcohol (Thalidomide has been reported to enhance the sedative activity of alcohol).

Food, unspecified (Co-administration of Thalomid with a high fat meal causes minor changes in the observed AUC and Cmax values; however, it causes an increase in Tmax to approximately 6 hours).

THERAFLU COLD & COUGH HOT LIQUID

(Acetaminophen, Chlorpheniramine Maleate, Dextromethorphan Hydrobromide, Pseudoephedrine Hydrochloride)....... ▣680
May interact with hypnotics and sedatives, monoamine oxidase inhibitors, tranquilizers, and certain other agents. Compounds in these categories include:

Alprazolam (Concurrent use with tranquilizers may increase drowsiness; use caution when co-administering). Products include:
Niravam Orally Disintegrating Tablets 3106
Xanax XR Tablets 2655

Buspirone Hydrochloride (Concurrent use with tranquilizers may increase drowsiness; use caution when co-administering).
No products indexed under this heading.

Chlordiazepoxide (Concurrent use with tranquilizers may increase drowsiness; use caution when co-administering).
No products indexed under this heading.

Chlordiazepoxide Hydrochloride (Concurrent use with tranquilizers may increase drowsiness; use caution when co-administering).
Products include:
Librium Capsules 3349

Chlorpromazine (Concurrent use with tranquilizers may increase drowsiness; use caution when co-administering).
No products indexed under this heading.

Chlorpromazine Hydrochloride (Concurrent use with tranquilizers may increase drowsiness; use caution when co-administering).
No products indexed under this heading.

Chlorprothixene (Concurrent use with tranquilizers may increase drowsiness; use caution when co-administering).
No products indexed under this heading.

Chlorprothixene Hydrochloride (Concurrent use with tranquilizers may increase drowsiness; use caution when co-administering).
No products indexed under this heading.

Clorazepate Dipotassium (Concurrent use with tranquilizers may increase drowsiness; use caution when co-administering). Products include:
Tranxene 2488

Diazepam (Concurrent use with tranquilizers may increase drowsiness; use caution when co-administering). Products include:
Diastat Rectal Delivery System 3344
Valium Tablets 2822

Droperidol (Concurrent use with tranquilizers may increase drowsiness; use caution when co-administering).
No products indexed under this heading.

Estazolam (Concurrent use with sedatives may increase drowsiness; use caution when co-administering).
Products include:
ProSom Tablets 512

Ethchlorvynol (Concurrent use with sedatives may increase drowsiness; use caution when co-administering).
No products indexed under this heading.

Ethinamate (Concurrent use with sedatives may increase drowsiness; use caution when co-administering).
No products indexed under this heading.

Fluphenazine Decanoate (Concurrent use with tranquilizers may increase drowsiness; use caution when co-administering).
No products indexed under this heading.

Fluphenazine Enanthate (Concurrent use with tranquilizers may increase drowsiness; use caution when co-administering).
No products indexed under this heading.

Fluphenazine Hydrochloride (Concurrent use with tranquilizers may increase drowsiness; use caution when co-administering).
No products indexed under this heading.

Flurazepam Hydrochloride (Concurrent use with sedatives may increase drowsiness; use caution when co-administering). Products include:
Dalmane Capsules 3343

Glutethimide (Concurrent use with sedatives may increase drowsiness; use caution when co-administering).
No products indexed under this heading.

Haloperidol (Concurrent use with tranquilizers may increase drowsiness; use caution when co-administering).
No products indexed under this heading.

Haloperidol Decanoate (Concurrent use with tranquilizers may increase drowsiness; use caution when co-administering).
No products indexed under this heading.

Hydroxyzine Hydrochloride (Concurrent use with tranquilizers may increase drowsiness; use caution when co-administering).
No products indexed under this heading.

Isocarboxazid (Do not use while taking, or for two weeks after stopping, MAO inhibitors).
No products indexed under this heading.

Lorazepam (Concurrent use with sedatives may increase drowsiness; use caution when co-administering).
No products indexed under this heading.

Loxapine Hydrochloride (Concurrent use with tranquilizers may increase drowsiness; use caution when co-administering).
No products indexed under this heading.

Loxapine Succinate (Concurrent use with tranquilizers may increase drowsiness; use caution when co-administering).
No products indexed under this heading.

Meprobamate (Concurrent use with tranquilizers may increase drowsiness; use caution when co-administering).
No products indexed under this heading.

Mesoridazine Besylate (Concurrent use with tranquilizers may increase drowsiness; use caution when co-administering).
No products indexed under this heading.

Midazolam Hydrochloride (Concurrent use with sedatives may increase drowsiness; use caution when co-administering).
No products indexed under this heading.

Moclobemide (Do not use while taking, or for two weeks after stopping, MAO inhibitors).
No products indexed under this heading.

Molindone Hydrochloride (Concurrent use with tranquilizers may increase drowsiness; use caution when co-administering). Products include:
Moban Tablets 1108

Oxazepam (Concurrent use with tranquilizers may increase drowsiness; use caution when co-administering).
No products indexed under this heading.

Pargyline Hydrochloride (Do not use while taking, or for two weeks after stopping, MAO inhibitors).
No products indexed under this heading.

Perphenazine (Concurrent use with tranquilizers may increase drowsiness; use caution when co-administering).
No products indexed under this heading.

Phenelzine Sulfate (Do not use while taking, or for two weeks after stopping, MAO inhibitors).
No products indexed under this heading.

Prazepam (Concurrent use with tranquilizers may increase drowsiness; use caution when co-administering).
No products indexed under this heading.

Procarbazine Hydrochloride (Do not use while taking, or for two weeks after stopping, MAO inhibitors). Products include:
Matulane Capsules 3188

Prochlorperazine (Concurrent use with tranquilizers may increase drowsiness; use caution when co-administering).
No products indexed under this heading.

Promethazine Hydrochloride (Concurrent use with tranquilizers may increase drowsiness; use caution when co-administering). Products include:
Phenergan 3438

Propofol (Concurrent use with sedatives may increase drowsiness; use caution when co-administering). Products include:
Diprivan Injectable Emulsion 676

Quazepam (Concurrent use with sedatives may increase drowsiness; use caution when co-administering).
No products indexed under this heading.

Secobarbital Sodium (Concurrent use with sedatives may increase drowsiness; use caution when co-administering).
No products indexed under this heading.

Selegiline Hydrochloride (Do not use while taking, or for two weeks after stopping, MAO inhibitors). Products include:
Eldepryl Capsules 3209

Temazepam (Concurrent use with sedatives may increase drowsiness; use caution when co-administering).
No products indexed under this heading.

Thioridazine Hydrochloride (Concurrent use with tranquilizers may increase drowsiness; use caution when co-administering). Products include:
Thioridazine Hydrochloride Tablets 2122

Thiothixene (Concurrent use with tranquilizers may increase drowsiness; use caution when co-administering). Products include:
Thiothixene Capsules 2124

Tranylcypromine Sulfate (Do not use while taking, or for two weeks after stopping, MAO inhibitors). Products include:
Parnate Tablets 1499

Triazolam (Concurrent use with sedatives may increase drowsiness; use caution when co-administering).
No products indexed under this heading.

Trifluoperazine Hydrochloride (Concurrent use with tranquilizers may increase drowsiness; use caution when co-administering).
No products indexed under this heading.

Zaleplon (Concurrent use with sedatives may increase drowsiness; use caution when co-administering). Products include:
Sonata Capsules 1686

Zolpidem Tartrate (Concurrent use with sedatives may increase drowsiness; use caution when co-administering). Products include:
Ambien Tablets 2867

Food Interactions

Alcohol (Concurrent use may increase drowsiness; avoid alcoholic drinks).

THERAFLU COLD & SORE THROAT HOT LIQUID

(Acetaminophen, Chlorpheniramine Maleate, Pseudoephedrine Hydrochloride)....... 680
May interact with hypnotics and sedatives, monoamine oxidase inhibitors, tranquilizers, and certain other agents. Compounds in these categories include:

Alprazolam (Concurrent use with tranquilizers may increase drowsiness; use caution when co-administering). Products include:
Niravam Orally Disintegrating Tablets 3106
Xanax XR Tablets 2655

Buspirone Hydrochloride (Concurrent use with tranquilizers may increase drowsiness; use caution when co-administering).
No products indexed under this heading.

Chlordiazepoxide (Concurrent use with tranquilizers may increase drowsiness; use caution when co-administering).
No products indexed under this heading.

Chlordiazepoxide Hydrochloride (Concurrent use with tranquilizers may increase drowsiness; use caution when co-administering). Products include:
Librium Capsules 3349

Chlorpromazine (Concurrent use with tranquilizers may increase drowsiness; use caution when co-administering).
No products indexed under this heading.

Chlorpromazine Hydrochloride (Concurrent use with tranquilizers may increase drowsiness; use caution when co-administering).
No products indexed under this heading.

Chlorprothixene (Concurrent use with tranquilizers may increase drowsiness; use caution when co-administering).
No products indexed under this heading.

Chlorprothixene Hydrochloride (Concurrent use with tranquilizers may increase drowsiness; use caution when co-administering).
No products indexed under this heading.

Clorazepate Dipotassium (Concurrent use with tranquilizers may increase drowsiness; use caution when co-administering). Products include:
Tranxene 2488

Diazepam (Concurrent use with tranquilizers may increase drowsiness; use caution when co-administering). Products include:
Diastat Rectal Delivery System 3344
Valium Tablets 2822

Droperidol (Concurrent use with tranquilizers may increase drowsiness; use caution when co-administering).
No products indexed under this heading.

Estazolam (Concurrent use with sedatives may increase drowsiness; use caution when co-administering). Products include:
ProSom Tablets 512

Ethchlorvynol (Concurrent use with sedatives may increase drowsiness; use caution when co-administering).
No products indexed under this heading.

Ethinamate (Concurrent use with sedatives may increase drowsiness; use caution when co-administering).
No products indexed under this heading.

Fluphenazine Decanoate (Concurrent use with tranquilizers may increase drowsiness; use caution when co-administering).
No products indexed under this heading.

Fluphenazine Enanthate (Concurrent use with tranquilizers may increase drowsiness; use caution when co-administering).
No products indexed under this heading.

Fluphenazine Hydrochloride (Concurrent use with tranquilizers may increase drowsiness; use caution when co-administering).
No products indexed under this heading.

Flurazepam Hydrochloride (Concurrent use with sedatives may increase drowsiness; use caution when co-administering). Products include:
Dalmane Capsules 3343

Glutethimide (Concurrent use with sedatives may increase drowsiness; use caution when co-administering).
No products indexed under this heading.

Haloperidol (Concurrent use with tranquilizers may increase drowsiness; use caution when co-administering).
No products indexed under this heading.

Haloperidol Decanoate (Concurrent use with tranquilizers may increase drowsiness; use caution when co-administering).
No products indexed under this heading.

Hydroxyzine Hydrochloride (Concurrent use with tranquilizers may increase drowsiness; use caution when co-administering).
No products indexed under this heading.

Isocarboxazid (Do not use while taking, or for two weeks after stopping, MAO inhibitors).
No products indexed under this heading.

Lorazepam (Concurrent use with sedatives may increase drowsiness; use caution when co-administering).
No products indexed under this heading.

Loxapine Hydrochloride (Concurrent use with tranquilizers may increase drowsiness; use caution when co-administering).
No products indexed under this heading.

Loxapine Succinate (Concurrent use with tranquilizers may increase drowsiness; use caution when co-administering).
No products indexed under this heading.

Meprobamate (Concurrent use with tranquilizers may increase drowsiness; use caution when co-administering).
No products indexed under this heading.

Mesoridazine Besylate (Concurrent use with tranquilizers may increase drowsiness; use caution when co-administering).
No products indexed under this heading.

Midazolam Hydrochloride (Concurrent use with sedatives may increase drowsiness; use caution when co-administering).
No products indexed under this heading.

Moclobemide (Do not use while taking, or for two weeks after stopping, MAO inhibitors).
No products indexed under this heading.

Molindone Hydrochloride (Concurrent use with tranquilizers may increase drowsiness; use caution when co-administering). Products include:
Moban Tablets 1108

Oxazepam (Concurrent use with tranquilizers may increase drowsiness; use caution when co-administering).
No products indexed under this heading.

Pargyline Hydrochloride (Do not use while taking, or for two weeks after stopping, MAO inhibitors).
No products indexed under this heading.

Perphenazine (Concurrent use with tranquilizers may increase drowsiness; use caution when co-administering).
No products indexed under this heading.

Phenelzine Sulfate (Do not use while taking, or for two weeks after stopping, MAO inhibitors).
No products indexed under this heading.

Prazepam (Concurrent use with tranquilizers may increase drowsiness; use caution when co-administering).
No products indexed under this heading.

Procarbazine Hydrochloride (Do not use while taking, or for two weeks after stopping, MAO inhibitors). Products include:
Matulane Capsules 3188

Prochlorperazine (Concurrent use with tranquilizers may increase drowsiness; use caution when co-administering).
No products indexed under this heading.

Promethazine Hydrochloride (Concurrent use with tranquilizers may increase drowsiness; use caution when co-administering).
Products include:
Phenergan 3438

Propofol (Concurrent use with sedatives may increase drowsiness; use caution when co-administering).
Products include:
Diprivan Injectable Emulsion 676

Quazepam (Concurrent use with sedatives may increase drowsiness; use caution when co-administering).
No products indexed under this heading.

Secobarbital Sodium (Concurrent use with sedatives may increase drowsiness; use caution when co-administering).
No products indexed under this heading.

Selegiline Hydrochloride (Do not use while taking, or for two weeks after stopping, MAO inhibitors).
Products include:
Eldepryl Capsules 3209

Temazepam (Concurrent use with sedatives may increase drowsiness; use caution when co-administering).
No products indexed under this heading.

Thioridazine Hydrochloride (Concurrent use with tranquilizers may increase drowsiness; use caution when co-administering). Products include:
Thioridazine Hydrochloride Tablets 2122

Thiothixene (Concurrent use with tranquilizers may increase drowsiness; use caution when co-administering). Products include:
Thiothixene Capsules 2124

Tranylcypromine Sulfate (Do not use while taking, or for two weeks after stopping, MAO inhibitors).
Products include:
Parnate Tablets 1499

Triazolam (Concurrent use with sedatives may increase drowsiness; use caution when co-administering).
No products indexed under this heading.

Trifluoperazine Hydrochloride (Concurrent use with tranquilizers may increase drowsiness; use caution when co-administering).
No products indexed under this heading.

Zaleplon (Concurrent use with sedatives may increase drowsiness; use caution when co-administering).
Products include:
Sonata Capsules 1686

Zolpidem Tartrate (Concurrent use with sedatives may increase drowsiness; use caution when co-administering). Products include:
Ambien Tablets 2867

Food Interactions

Alcohol (Concurrent use may increase drowsiness; avoid alcoholic drinks).

THERAFLU FLU & CHEST CONGESTION NON-DROWSY HOT LIQUID

(Acetaminophen, Dextromethorphan Hydrobromide, Guaifenesin, Pseudoephedrine Hydrochloride) .... ▣681
May interact with monoamine oxidase inhibitors and certain other agents. Compounds in these categories include:

Isocarboxazid (Do not use while taking, or for two weeks after stopping, MAO inhibitors).
No products indexed under this heading.

Moclobemide (Do not use while taking, or for two weeks after stopping, MAO inhibitors).
No products indexed under this heading.

Pargyline Hydrochloride (Do not use while taking, or for two weeks after stopping, MAO inhibitors).
No products indexed under this heading.

Phenelzine Sulfate (Do not use while taking, or for two weeks after stopping, MAO inhibitors).
No products indexed under this heading.

Procarbazine Hydrochloride (Do not use while taking, or for two weeks after stopping, MAO inhibitors). Products include:
Matulane Capsules 3188

Selegiline Hydrochloride (Do not use while taking, or for two weeks after stopping, MAO inhibitors).
Products include:
Eldepryl Capsules 3209

Tranylcypromine Sulfate (Do not use while taking, or for two weeks after stopping, MAO inhibitors).
Products include:
Parnate Tablets 1499

Food Interactions

Alcohol (Concurrent use may increase drowsiness; avoid alcoholic drinks).

THERAFLU FLU & SORE THROAT HOT LIQUID

(Acetaminophen, Chlorpheniramine Maleate, Pseudoephedrine Hydrochloride) .... ▣681
May interact with hypnotics and sedatives, monoamine oxidase inhibitors, tranquilizers, and certain other agents. Compounds in these categories include:

Alprazolam (Concurrent use with tranquilizers may increase drowsiness; use caution when co-administering). Products include:
Niravam Orally Disintegrating Tablets 3106
Xanax XR Tablets 2655

Buspirone Hydrochloride (Concurrent use with tranquilizers may increase drowsiness; use caution when co-administering).
No products indexed under this heading.

Chlordiazepoxide (Concurrent use with tranquilizers may increase drowsiness; use caution when co-administering).
No products indexed under this heading.

Chlordiazepoxide Hydrochloride (Concurrent use with tranquilizers may increase drowsiness; use caution when co-administering).
Products include:
Librium Capsules 3349

Chlorpromazine (Concurrent use with tranquilizers may increase drowsiness; use caution when co-administering).
No products indexed under this heading.

Chlorpromazine Hydrochloride (Concurrent use with tranquilizers may increase drowsiness; use caution when co-administering).
No products indexed under this heading.

Chlorprothixene (Concurrent use with tranquilizers may increase drowsiness; use caution when co-administering).
No products indexed under this heading.

Chlorprothixene Hydrochloride (Concurrent use with tranquilizers may increase drowsiness; use caution when co-administering).
No products indexed under this heading.

Clorazepate Dipotassium (Concurrent use with tranquilizers may increase drowsiness; use caution when co-administering). Products include:
Tranxene 2488

Diazepam (Concurrent use with tranquilizers may increase drowsiness; use caution when co-administering). Products include:
Diastat Rectal Delivery System 3344
Valium Tablets 2822

Droperidol (Concurrent use with tranquilizers may increase drowsiness; use caution when co-administering).
No products indexed under this heading.

Estazolam (Concurrent use with sedatives may increase drowsiness; use caution when co-administering).
Products include:
ProSom Tablets 512

Ethchlorvynol (Concurrent use with sedatives may increase drowsiness; use caution when co-administering).
No products indexed under this heading.

Ethinamate (Concurrent use with sedatives may increase drowsiness; use caution when co-administering).
No products indexed under this heading.

Fluphenazine Decanoate (Concurrent use with tranquilizers may increase drowsiness; use caution when co-administering).
No products indexed under this heading.

Fluphenazine Enanthate (Concurrent use with tranquilizers may increase drowsiness; use caution when co-administering).
No products indexed under this heading.

Fluphenazine Hydrochloride (Concurrent use with tranquilizers may increase drowsiness; use caution when co-administering).
No products indexed under this heading.

Flurazepam Hydrochloride (Concurrent use with sedatives may increase drowsiness; use caution when co-administering). Products include:
Dalmane Capsules 3343

Glutethimide (Concurrent use with sedatives may increase drowsiness; use caution when co-administering).
No products indexed under this heading.

Haloperidol (Concurrent use with tranquilizers may increase drowsiness; use caution when co-administering).
No products indexed under this heading.

Haloperidol Decanoate (Concurrent use with tranquilizers may increase drowsiness; use caution when co-administering).
No products indexed under this heading.

Hydroxyzine Hydrochloride (Concurrent use with tranquilizers may increase drowsiness; use caution when co-administering).
No products indexed under this heading.

Isocarboxazid (Do not use while taking, or for two weeks after stopping, MAO inhibitors).
No products indexed under this heading.

Lorazepam (Concurrent use with sedatives may increase drowsiness; use caution when co-administering).
No products indexed under this heading.

Loxapine Hydrochloride (Concurrent use with tranquilizers may increase drowsiness; use caution when co-administering).
No products indexed under this heading.

Loxapine Succinate (Concurrent use with tranquilizers may increase drowsiness; use caution when co-administering).
No products indexed under this heading.

Meprobamate (Concurrent use with tranquilizers may increase drowsiness; use caution when co-administering).
No products indexed under this heading.

Mesoridazine Besylate (Concurrent use with tranquilizers may increase drowsiness; use caution when co-administering).
No products indexed under this heading.

Midazolam Hydrochloride (Concurrent use with sedatives may increase drowsiness; use caution when co-administering).
No products indexed under this heading.

Moclobemide (Do not use while taking, or for two weeks after stopping, MAO inhibitors).
No products indexed under this heading.

Molindone Hydrochloride (Concurrent use with tranquilizers may increase drowsiness; use caution when co-administering). Products include:
Moban Tablets 1108

Oxazepam (Concurrent use with tranquilizers may increase drowsiness; use caution when co-administering).
No products indexed under this heading.

Pargyline Hydrochloride (Do not use while taking, or for two weeks after stopping, MAO inhibitors).
No products indexed under this heading.

Perphenazine (Concurrent use with tranquilizers may increase drowsiness; use caution when co-administering).
No products indexed under this heading.

Phenelzine Sulfate (Do not use while taking, or for two weeks after stopping, MAO inhibitors).
No products indexed under this heading.

Prazepam (Concurrent use with tranquilizers may increase drowsiness; use caution when co-administering).
No products indexed under this heading.

Procarbazine Hydrochloride (Do not use while taking, or for two weeks after stopping, MAO inhibitors). Products include:
Matulane Capsules 3188

Prochlorperazine (Concurrent use with tranquilizers may increase drowsiness; use caution when co-administering).
No products indexed under this heading.

Promethazine Hydrochloride (Concurrent use with tranquilizers may increase drowsiness; use caution when co-administering). Products include:
Phenergan 3438

Propofol (Concurrent use with sedatives may increase drowsiness; use caution when co-administering). Products include:
Diprivan Injectable Emulsion 676

Quazepam (Concurrent use with sedatives may increase drowsiness; use caution when co-administering).
No products indexed under this heading.

Secobarbital Sodium (Concurrent use with sedatives may increase drowsiness; use caution when co-administering).
No products indexed under this heading.

Selegiline Hydrochloride (Do not use while taking, or for two weeks after stopping, MAO inhibitors). Products include:
Eldepryl Capsules 3209

Temazepam (Concurrent use with sedatives may increase drowsiness; use caution when co-administering).
No products indexed under this heading.

Thioridazine Hydrochloride (Concurrent use with tranquilizers may increase drowsiness; use caution when co-administering). Products include:
Thioridazine Hydrochloride Tablets 2122

Thiothixene (Concurrent use with tranquilizers may increase drowsiness; use caution when co-administering). Products include:
Thiothixene Capsules 2124

Tranylcypromine Sulfate (Do not use while taking, or for two weeks after stopping, MAO inhibitors). Products include:
Parnate Tablets 1499

Triazolam (Concurrent use with sedatives may increase drowsiness; use caution when co-administering).
No products indexed under this heading.

Trifluoperazine Hydrochloride (Concurrent use with tranquilizers may increase drowsiness; use caution when co-administering).
No products indexed under this heading.

Zaleplon (Concurrent use with sedatives may increase drowsiness; use caution when co-administering). Products include:
Sonata Capsules 1686

Zolpidem Tartrate (Concurrent use with sedatives may increase drowsiness; use caution when co-administering). Products include:
Ambien Tablets 2867

Food Interactions

Alcohol (Concurrent use may increase drowsiness; avoid alcoholic drinks).

THERAFLU SEVERE COLD NON-DROWSY HOT LIQUID

(Acetaminophen, Dextromethorphan Hydrobromide, Pseudoephedrine Hydrochloride) 683

May interact with monoamine oxidase inhibitors and certain other agents. Compounds in these categories include:

Isocarboxazid (Concurrent and/or sequential use with MAO inhibitors is not recommended).
No products indexed under this heading.

Moclobemide (Concurrent and/or sequential use with MAO inhibitors is not recommended).
No products indexed under this heading.

Pargyline Hydrochloride (Concurrent and/or sequential use with MAO inhibitors is not recommended).
No products indexed under this heading.

Phenelzine Sulfate (Concurrent and/or sequential use with MAO inhibitors is not recommended).
No products indexed under this heading.

Procarbazine Hydrochloride (Concurrent and/or sequential use with MAO inhibitors is not recommended). Products include:
Matulane Capsules 3188

Selegiline Hydrochloride (Concurrent and/or sequential use with MAO inhibitors is not recommended). Products include:
Eldepryl Capsules 3209

Tranylcypromine Sulfate (Concurrent and/or sequential use with MAO inhibitors is not recommended). Products include:
Parnate Tablets 1499

Food Interactions

Alcohol (Chronic heavy alcohol users, 3 or more drinks per day, should consult their physicians for advice on when and how they should take pain relievers/fever reducers, including acetaminophen; may increase the drowsiness effect).

THERAFLU SEVERE COLD & COUGH HOT LIQUID

(Acetaminophen, Chlorpheniramine Maleate, Dextromethorphan Hydrobromide, Pseudoephedrine Hydrochloride) 683

May interact with hypnotics and sedatives, monoamine oxidase inhibitors, tranquilizers, and certain other agents. Compounds in these categories include:

Alprazolam (Concurrent use with tranquilizers may increase drowsiness; use caution when co-administering). Products include:
Niravam Orally Disintegrating Tablets 3106
Xanax XR Tablets 2655

Buspirone Hydrochloride (Concurrent use with tranquilizers may increase drowsiness; use caution when co-administering).
No products indexed under this heading.

Chlordiazepoxide (Concurrent use with tranquilizers may increase drowsiness; use caution when co-administering).
No products indexed under this heading.

Chlordiazepoxide Hydrochloride (Concurrent use with tranquilizers may increase drowsiness; use caution when co-administering). Products include:
Librium Capsules 3349

Chlorpromazine (Concurrent use with tranquilizers may increase drowsiness; use caution when co-administering).
No products indexed under this heading.

Chlorpromazine Hydrochloride (Concurrent use with tranquilizers may increase drowsiness; use caution when co-administering).
No products indexed under this heading.

Chlorprothixene (Concurrent use with tranquilizers may increase drowsiness; use caution when co-administering).
No products indexed under this heading.

Chlorprothixene Hydrochloride (Concurrent use with tranquilizers may increase drowsiness; use caution when co-administering).
No products indexed under this heading.

Clorazepate Dipotassium (Concurrent use with tranquilizers may increase drowsiness; use caution when co-administering). Products include:
Tranxene 2488

Diazepam (Concurrent use with tranquilizers may increase drowsiness; use caution when co-administering). Products include:
Diastat Rectal Delivery System 3344
Valium Tablets 2822

Droperidol (Concurrent use with tranquilizers may increase drowsiness; use caution when co-administering).
No products indexed under this heading.

Estazolam (Concurrent use with sedatives may increase drowsiness; use caution when co-administering). Products include:
ProSom Tablets 512

Ethchlorvynol (Concurrent use with sedatives may increase drowsiness; use caution when co-administering).
No products indexed under this heading.

Ethinamate (Concurrent use with sedatives may increase drowsiness; use caution when co-administering).
No products indexed under this heading.

Fluphenazine Decanoate (Concurrent use with tranquilizers may increase drowsiness; use caution when co-administering).
No products indexed under this heading.

Fluphenazine Enanthate (Concurrent use with tranquilizers may increase drowsiness; use caution when co-administering).
No products indexed under this heading.

Fluphenazine Hydrochloride (Concurrent use with tranquilizers may increase drowsiness; use caution when co-administering).
No products indexed under this heading.

Flurazepam Hydrochloride (Concurrent use with sedatives may increase drowsiness; use caution when co-administering). Products include:
Dalmane Capsules 3343

Glutethimide (Concurrent use with sedatives may increase drowsiness; use caution when co-administering).
No products indexed under this heading.

Haloperidol (Concurrent use with tranquilizers may increase drowsiness; use caution when co-administering).
No products indexed under this heading.

Haloperidol Decanoate (Concurrent use with tranquilizers may increase drowsiness; use caution when co-administering).
No products indexed under this heading.

Hydroxyzine Hydrochloride (Concurrent use with tranquilizers may increase drowsiness; use caution when co-administering).
No products indexed under this heading.

Isocarboxazid (Do not use while taking, or for two weeks after stopping, MAO inhibitors).
No products indexed under this heading.

Lorazepam (Concurrent use with sedatives may increase drowsiness; use caution when co-administering).
No products indexed under this heading.

Loxapine Hydrochloride (Concurrent use with tranquilizers may increase drowsiness; use caution when co-administering).
No products indexed under this heading.

Loxapine Succinate (Concurrent use with tranquilizers may increase drowsiness; use caution when co-administering).
No products indexed under this heading.

Meprobamate (Concurrent use with tranquilizers may increase drowsiness; use caution when co-administering).
No products indexed under this heading.

Mesoridazine Besylate (Concurrent use with tranquilizers may increase drowsiness; use caution when co-administering).
No products indexed under this heading.

Midazolam Hydrochloride (Concurrent use with sedatives may increase drowsiness; use caution when co-administering).
No products indexed under this heading.

Moclobemide (Do not use while taking, or for two weeks after stopping, MAO inhibitors).
No products indexed under this heading.

Molindone Hydrochloride (Concurrent use with tranquilizers may increase drowsiness; use caution when co-administering). Products include:
Moban Tablets 1108

Oxazepam (Concurrent use with tranquilizers may increase drowsiness; use caution when co-administering).
No products indexed under this heading.

Pargyline Hydrochloride (Do not use while taking, or for two weeks after stopping, MAO inhibitors).
No products indexed under this heading.

Perphenazine (Concurrent use with tranquilizers may increase drowsiness; use caution when co-administering).
No products indexed under this heading.

Phenelzine Sulfate (Do not use while taking, or for two weeks after stopping, MAO inhibitors).
No products indexed under this heading.

Prazepam (Concurrent use with tranquilizers may increase drowsiness; use caution when co-administering).
No products indexed under this heading.

Procarbazine Hydrochloride (Do not use while taking, or for two weeks after stopping, MAO inhibitors). Products include:
Matulane Capsules 3188

Prochlorperazine (Concurrent use with tranquilizers may increase drowsiness; use caution when co-administering).
No products indexed under this heading.

Promethazine Hydrochloride (Concurrent use with tranquilizers may increase drowsiness; use caution when co-administering). Products include:
Phenergan 3438

Propofol (Concurrent use with sedatives may increase drowsiness; use caution when co-administering). Products include:
Diprivan Injectable Emulsion 676

Quazepam (Concurrent use with sedatives may increase drowsiness; use caution when co-administering).
No products indexed under this heading.

Secobarbital Sodium (Concurrent use with sedatives may increase drowsiness; use caution when co-administering).
No products indexed under this heading.

Selegiline Hydrochloride (Do not use while taking, or for two weeks after stopping, MAO inhibitors). Products include:
Eldepryl Capsules 3209

Temazepam (Concurrent use with sedatives may increase drowsiness; use caution when co-administering).
No products indexed under this heading.

Thioridazine Hydrochloride (Concurrent use with tranquilizers may increase drowsiness; use caution when co-administering). Products include:
Thioridazine Hydrochloride Tablets 2122

Thiothixene (Concurrent use with tranquilizers may increase drowsiness; use caution when co-administering). Products include:
Thiothixene Capsules 2124

Tranylcypromine Sulfate (Do not use while taking, or for two weeks after stopping, MAO inhibitors). Products include:
Parnate Tablets 1499

Triazolam (Concurrent use with sedatives may increase drowsiness; use caution when co-administering).
No products indexed under this heading.

Trifluoperazine Hydrochloride (Concurrent use with tranquilizers may increase drowsiness; use caution when co-administering).
No products indexed under this heading.

Zaleplon (Concurrent use with sedatives may increase drowsiness; use caution when co-administering). Products include:
Sonata Capsules 1686

Zolpidem Tartrate (Concurrent use with sedatives may increase drowsiness; use caution when co-administering). Products include:
Ambien Tablets 2867

Food Interactions

Alcohol (Concurrent use may increase drowsiness; avoid alcoholic drinks).

THERAFLU SEVERE COLD CAPLETS

(Acetaminophen, Chlorpheniramine Maleate, Dextromethorphan Hydrobromide, Pseudoephedrine Hydrochloride)....... ▣ 679

May interact with hypnotics and sedatives, monoamine oxidase inhibitors, tranquilizers, and certain other agents. Compounds in these categories include:

Alprazolam (Concurrent use with tranquilizers may increase drowsiness; use caution when co-administering). Products include:
Niravam Orally Disintegrating Tablets 3106
Xanax XR Tablets 2655

Buspirone Hydrochloride (Concurrent use with tranquilizers may increase drowsiness; use caution when co-administering).
No products indexed under this heading.

Chlordiazepoxide (Concurrent use with tranquilizers may increase drowsiness; use caution when co-administering).
No products indexed under this heading.

Chlordiazepoxide Hydrochloride (Concurrent use with tranquilizers may increase drowsiness; use caution when co-administering). Products include:
Librium Capsules 3349

Chlorpromazine (Concurrent use with tranquilizers may increase drowsiness; use caution when co-administering).
No products indexed under this heading.

Chlorpromazine Hydrochloride (Concurrent use with tranquilizers may increase drowsiness; use caution when co-administering).
No products indexed under this heading.

Chlorprothixene (Concurrent use with tranquilizers may increase drowsiness; use caution when co-administering).
No products indexed under this heading.

Chlorprothixene Hydrochloride (Concurrent use with tranquilizers may increase drowsiness; use caution when co-administering).
No products indexed under this heading.

Clorazepate Dipotassium (Concurrent use with tranquilizers may increase drowsiness; use caution when co-administering). Products include:
Tranxene 2488

Diazepam (Concurrent use with tranquilizers may increase drowsiness; use caution when co-administering). Products include:
Diastat Rectal Delivery System 3344
Valium Tablets 2822

Droperidol (Concurrent use with tranquilizers may increase drowsiness; use caution when co-administering).
No products indexed under this heading.

Estazolam (Concurrent use with sedatives may increase drowsiness; use caution when co-administering). Products include:
ProSom Tablets 512

Ethchlorvynol (Concurrent use with sedatives may increase drowsiness; use caution when co-administering).
No products indexed under this heading.

Ethinamate (Concurrent use with sedatives may increase drowsiness; use caution when co-administering).
No products indexed under this heading.

Fluphenazine Decanoate (Concurrent use with tranquilizers may increase drowsiness; use caution when co-administering).
No products indexed under this heading.

Fluphenazine Enanthate (Concurrent use with tranquilizers may increase drowsiness; use caution when co-administering).
No products indexed under this heading.

Fluphenazine Hydrochloride (Concurrent use with tranquilizers may increase drowsiness; use caution when co-administering).
No products indexed under this heading.

Flurazepam Hydrochloride (Concurrent use with sedatives may increase drowsiness; use caution when co-administering). Products include:
Dalmane Capsules 3343

Glutethimide (Concurrent use with sedatives may increase drowsiness; use caution when co-administering).
No products indexed under this heading.

Haloperidol (Concurrent use with tranquilizers may increase drowsiness; use caution when co-administering).
No products indexed under this heading.

Haloperidol Decanoate (Concurrent use with tranquilizers may increase drowsiness; use caution when co-administering).
No products indexed under this heading.

Hydroxyzine Hydrochloride (Concurrent use with tranquilizers may increase drowsiness; use caution when co-administering).
No products indexed under this heading.

Isocarboxazid (Do not use while taking, or for two weeks after stopping, MAO inhibitors).
No products indexed under this heading.

Lorazepam (Concurrent use with sedatives may increase drowsiness; use caution when co-administering).
No products indexed under this heading.

Loxapine Hydrochloride (Concurrent use with tranquilizers may increase drowsiness; use caution when co-administering).
No products indexed under this heading.

Loxapine Succinate (Concurrent use with tranquilizers may increase drowsiness; use caution when co-administering).
No products indexed under this heading.

Meprobamate (Concurrent use with tranquilizers may increase drowsiness; use caution when co-administering).
No products indexed under this heading.

Mesoridazine Besylate (Concurrent use with tranquilizers may increase drowsiness; use caution when co-administering).
No products indexed under this heading.

Midazolam Hydrochloride (Concurrent use with sedatives may increase drowsiness; use caution when co-administering).
No products indexed under this heading.

Moclobemide (Do not use while taking, or for two weeks after stopping, MAO inhibitors).
No products indexed under this heading.

Molindone Hydrochloride (Concurrent use with tranquilizers may increase drowsiness; use caution when co-administering). Products include:
Moban Tablets 1108

Oxazepam (Concurrent use with tranquilizers may increase drowsiness; use caution when co-administering).
No products indexed under this heading.

Pargyline Hydrochloride (Do not use while taking, or for two weeks after stopping, MAO inhibitors).
No products indexed under this heading.

Perphenazine (Concurrent use with tranquilizers may increase drowsiness; use caution when co-administering).
No products indexed under this heading.

Phenelzine Sulfate (Do not use while taking, or for two weeks after stopping, MAO inhibitors).
No products indexed under this heading.

Prazepam (Concurrent use with tranquilizers may increase drowsiness; use caution when co-administering).
No products indexed under this heading.

Procarbazine Hydrochloride (Do not use while taking, or for two weeks after stopping, MAO inhibitors). Products include:
Matulane Capsules 3188

Prochlorperazine (Concurrent use with tranquilizers may increase drowsiness; use caution when co-administering).
No products indexed under this heading.

Promethazine Hydrochloride (Concurrent use with tranquilizers may increase drowsiness; use caution when co-administering). Products include:
Phenergan 3438

Propofol (Concurrent use with sedatives may increase drowsiness; use caution when co-administering). Products include:
Diprivan Injectable Emulsion 676

Quazepam (Concurrent use with sedatives may increase drowsiness; use caution when co-administering).
No products indexed under this heading.

Secobarbital Sodium (Concurrent use with sedatives may increase drowsiness; use caution when co-administering).
No products indexed under this heading.

Selegiline Hydrochloride (Do not use while taking, or for two weeks after stopping, MAO inhibitors). Products include:
Eldepryl Capsules 3209

Temazepam (Concurrent use with sedatives may increase drowsiness; use caution when co-administering).
No products indexed under this heading.

Thioridazine Hydrochloride (Concurrent use with tranquilizers may increase drowsiness; use caution when co-administering). Products include:
Thioridazine Hydrochloride Tablets 2122

Thiothixene (Concurrent use with tranquilizers may increase drowsiness; use caution when co-administering). Products include:
Thiothixene Capsules 2124

Tranylcypromine Sulfate (Do not use while taking, or for two weeks after stopping, MAO inhibitors). Products include:
Parnate Tablets 1499

Triazolam (Concurrent use with sedatives may increase drowsiness; use caution when co-administering).
No products indexed under this heading.

Trifluoperazine Hydrochloride (Concurrent use with tranquilizers may increase drowsiness; use caution when co-administering).
No products indexed under this heading.

Zaleplon (Concurrent use with sedatives may increase drowsiness; use caution when co-administering). Products include:
Sonata Capsules 1686

Zolpidem Tartrate (Concurrent use with sedatives may increase drowsiness; use caution when co-administering). Products include:
Ambien Tablets 2867

Food Interactions

Alcohol (Concurrent use may increase drowsiness; avoid alcoholic drinks).

THERAFLU SEVERE COLD HOT LIQUID
(Acetaminophen, Chlorpheniramine Maleate, Dextromethorphan Hydrobromide, Pseudoephedrine Hydrochloride)........ 682
May interact with hypnotics and sedatives, monoamine oxidase inhibitors, tranquilizers, and certain other agents. Compounds in these categories include:

Alprazolam (Concurrent use with tranquilizers may increase drowsiness; use caution when co-administering). Products include:
Niravam Orally Disintegrating Tablets 3106
Xanax XR Tablets 2655

Buspirone Hydrochloride (Concurrent use with tranquilizers may increase drowsiness; use caution when co-administering).
No products indexed under this heading.

Chlordiazepoxide (Concurrent use with tranquilizers may increase drowsiness; use caution when co-administering).
No products indexed under this heading.

Chlordiazepoxide Hydrochloride (Concurrent use with tranquilizers may increase drowsiness; use caution when co-administering). Products include:
Librium Capsules 3349

Chlorpromazine (Concurrent use with tranquilizers may increase drowsiness; use caution when co-administering).
No products indexed under this heading.

Chlorpromazine Hydrochloride (Concurrent use with tranquilizers may increase drowsiness; use caution when co-administering).
No products indexed under this heading.

Chlorprothixene (Concurrent use with tranquilizers may increase drowsiness; use caution when co-administering).
No products indexed under this heading.

Chlorprothixene Hydrochloride (Concurrent use with tranquilizers may increase drowsiness; use caution when co-administering).
No products indexed under this heading.

Clorazepate Dipotassium (Concurrent use with tranquilizers may increase drowsiness; use caution when co-administering). Products include:
Tranxene 2488

Diazepam (Concurrent use with tranquilizers may increase drowsiness; use caution when co-administering). Products include:
Diastat Rectal Delivery System 3344
Valium Tablets 2822

Droperidol (Concurrent use with tranquilizers may increase drowsiness; use caution when co-administering).
No products indexed under this heading.

Estazolam (Concurrent use with sedatives may increase drowsiness; use caution when co-administering). Products include:
ProSom Tablets 512

Ethchlorvynol (Concurrent use with sedatives may increase drowsiness; use caution when co-administering).
No products indexed under this heading.

Ethinamate (Concurrent use with sedatives may increase drowsiness; use caution when co-administering).
No products indexed under this heading.

Fluphenazine Decanoate (Concurrent use with tranquilizers may increase drowsiness; use caution when co-administering).
No products indexed under this heading.

Fluphenazine Enanthate (Concurrent use with tranquilizers may increase drowsiness; use caution when co-administering).
No products indexed under this heading.

Fluphenazine Hydrochloride (Concurrent use with tranquilizers may increase drowsiness; use caution when co-administering).
No products indexed under this heading.

Flurazepam Hydrochloride (Concurrent use with sedatives may increase drowsiness; use caution when co-administering). Products include:
Dalmane Capsules 3343

Glutethimide (Concurrent use with sedatives may increase drowsiness; use caution when co-administering).
No products indexed under this heading.

Haloperidol (Concurrent use with tranquilizers may increase drowsiness; use caution when co-administering).
No products indexed under this heading.

Haloperidol Decanoate (Concurrent use with tranquilizers may increase drowsiness; use caution when co-administering).
No products indexed under this heading.

Hydroxyzine Hydrochloride (Concurrent use with tranquilizers may increase drowsiness; use caution when co-administering).
No products indexed under this heading.

Isocarboxazid (Do not use while taking, or for two weeks after stopping, MAO inhibitors).
No products indexed under this heading.

Lorazepam (Concurrent use with sedatives may increase drowsiness; use caution when co-administering).
No products indexed under this heading.

Loxapine Hydrochloride (Concurrent use with tranquilizers may increase drowsiness; use caution when co-administering).
No products indexed under this heading.

Loxapine Succinate (Concurrent use with tranquilizers may increase drowsiness; use caution when co-administering).
No products indexed under this heading.

Meprobamate (Concurrent use with tranquilizers may increase drowsiness; use caution when co-administering).
No products indexed under this heading.

Mesoridazine Besylate (Concurrent use with tranquilizers may increase drowsiness; use caution when co-administering).
No products indexed under this heading.

Midazolam Hydrochloride (Concurrent use with sedatives may increase drowsiness; use caution when co-administering).
No products indexed under this heading.

Moclobemide (Do not use while taking, or for two weeks after stopping, MAO inhibitors).
No products indexed under this heading.

Molindone Hydrochloride (Concurrent use with tranquilizers may increase drowsiness; use caution when co-administering). Products include:
Moban Tablets 1108

Oxazepam (Concurrent use with tranquilizers may increase drowsiness; use caution when co-administering).
No products indexed under this heading.

Pargyline Hydrochloride (Do not use while taking, or for two weeks after stopping, MAO inhibitors).
No products indexed under this heading.

Perphenazine (Concurrent use with tranquilizers may increase drowsiness; use caution when co-administering).
No products indexed under this heading.

Phenelzine Sulfate (Do not use while taking, or for two weeks after stopping, MAO inhibitors).
No products indexed under this heading.

Prazepam (Concurrent use with tranquilizers may increase drowsiness; use caution when co-administering).
No products indexed under this heading.

Procarbazine Hydrochloride (Do not use while taking, or for two weeks after stopping, MAO inhibitors). Products include:
Matulane Capsules 3188

Prochlorperazine (Concurrent use with tranquilizers may increase drowsiness; use caution when co-administering).
No products indexed under this heading.

Promethazine Hydrochloride (Concurrent use with tranquilizers may increase drowsiness; use caution when co-administering). Products include:
Phenergan 3438

Propofol (Concurrent use with sedatives may increase drowsiness; use caution when co-administering). Products include:
Diprivan Injectable Emulsion 676

Quazepam (Concurrent use with sedatives may increase drowsiness; use caution when co-administering).
No products indexed under this heading.

Secobarbital Sodium (Concurrent use with sedatives may increase drowsiness; use caution when co-administering).
No products indexed under this heading.

Selegiline Hydrochloride (Do not use while taking, or for two weeks after stopping, MAO inhibitors). Products include:
Eldepryl Capsules 3209

Temazepam (Concurrent use with sedatives may increase drowsiness; use caution when co-administering).
No products indexed under this heading.

Thioridazine Hydrochloride (Concurrent use with tranquilizers may increase drowsiness; use caution when co-administering). Products include:
Thioridazine Hydrochloride Tablets 2122

Thiothixene (Concurrent use with tranquilizers may increase drowsiness; use caution when co-administering). Products include:
Thiothixene Capsules 2124

Tranylcypromine Sulfate (Do not use while taking, or for two weeks after stopping, MAO inhibitors). Products include:
Parnate Tablets 1499

Triazolam (Concurrent use with sedatives may increase drowsiness; use caution when co-administering).
No products indexed under this heading.

Trifluoperazine Hydrochloride (Concurrent use with tranquilizers may increase drowsiness; use caution when co-administering).
No products indexed under this heading.

Zaleplon (Concurrent use with sedatives may increase drowsiness; use caution when co-administering). Products include:
Sonata Capsules 1686

Zolpidem Tartrate (Concurrent use with sedatives may increase drowsiness; use caution when co-administering). Products include:
Ambien Tablets 2867

Food Interactions

Alcohol (Concurrent use may increase drowsiness; avoid alcoholic drinks).

THERAFLU SEVERE COLD NON-DROWSY CAPLETS

(Acetaminophen, Dextromethorphan Hydrobromide, Pseudoephedrine Hydrochloride)....... ▣ 679
See TheraFlu Severe Cold Non-Drowsy Hot Liquid

THERAFLU THIN STRIPS LONG ACTING COUGH

(Dextromethorphan Hydrobromide) .... ▣ 684
May interact with monoamine oxidase inhibitors. Compounds in these categories include:

Isocarboxazid (Do not use concurrently with, or for two weeks after stopping, MAO Inhibitors).
No products indexed under this heading.

Moclobemide (Do not use concurrently with, or for two weeks after stopping, MAO Inhibitors).
No products indexed under this heading.

Pargyline Hydrochloride (Do not use concurrently with, or for two weeks after stopping, MAO Inhibitors).
No products indexed under this heading.

Phenelzine Sulfate (Do not use concurrently with, or for two weeks after stopping, MAO Inhibitors).
No products indexed under this heading.

Procarbazine Hydrochloride (Do not use concurrently with, or for two weeks after stopping, MAO Inhibitors). Products include:
Matulane Capsules 3188

Selegiline Hydrochloride (Do not use concurrently with, or for two weeks after stopping, MAO Inhibitors). Products include:
Eldepryl Capsules 3209

Tranylcypromine Sulfate (Do not use concurrently with, or for two weeks after stopping, MAO Inhibitors). Products include:
Parnate Tablets 1499

THERAFLU THIN STRIPS MULTI SYMPTOM

(Diphenhydramine Hydrochloride) ..... ▣ 684
May interact with hypnotics and sedatives, tranquilizers, and certain other agents. Compounds in these categories include:

Alprazolam (Co-administration with tranquilizers may increase drowsiness). Products include:
Niravam Orally Disintegrating Tablets 3106
Xanax XR Tablets 2655

Buspirone Hydrochloride (Co-administration with tranquilizers may increase drowsiness).
No products indexed under this heading.

Chlordiazepoxide (Co-administration with tranquilizers may increase drowsiness).
No products indexed under this heading.

Chlordiazepoxide Hydrochloride (Co-administration with tranquilizers may increase drowsiness). Products include:
Librium Capsules 3349

Chlorpromazine (Co-administration with tranquilizers may increase drowsiness).
No products indexed under this heading.

Chlorpromazine Hydrochloride (Co-administration with tranquilizers may increase drowsiness).
No products indexed under this heading.

Chlorprothixene (Co-administration with tranquilizers may increase drowsiness).
No products indexed under this heading.

Chlorprothixene Hydrochloride (Co-administration with tranquilizers may increase drowsiness).
No products indexed under this heading.

Clorazepate Dipotassium (Co-administration with tranquilizers may increase drowsiness). Products include:
Tranxene 2488

Diazepam (Co-administration with tranquilizers may increase drowsiness). Products include:
Diastat Rectal Delivery System 3344
Valium Tablets 2822

Droperidol (Co-administration with tranquilizers may increase drowsiness).
No products indexed under this heading.

Estazolam (Co-administration with sedatives may increase drowsiness). Products include:
ProSom Tablets 512

Ethchlorvynol (Co-administration with sedatives may increase drowsiness).
No products indexed under this heading.

Ethinamate (Co-administration with sedatives may increase drowsiness).
No products indexed under this heading.

Fluphenazine Decanoate (Co-administration with tranquilizers may increase drowsiness).
No products indexed under this heading.

Fluphenazine Enanthate (Co-administration with tranquilizers may increase drowsiness).
No products indexed under this heading.

Fluphenazine Hydrochloride (Co-administration with tranquilizers may increase drowsiness).
No products indexed under this heading.

Flurazepam Hydrochloride (Co-administration with sedatives may increase drowsiness). Products include:
Dalmane Capsules 3343

Glutethimide (Co-administration with sedatives may increase drowsiness).
No products indexed under this heading.

Haloperidol (Co-administration with tranquilizers may increase drowsiness).
No products indexed under this heading.

Haloperidol Decanoate (Co-administration with tranquilizers may increase drowsiness).
No products indexed under this heading.

Hydroxyzine Hydrochloride (Co-administration with tranquilizers may increase drowsiness).
No products indexed under this heading.

Lorazepam (Co-administration with sedatives may increase drowsiness).
No products indexed under this heading.

Loxapine Hydrochloride (Co-administration with tranquilizers may increase drowsiness).
No products indexed under this heading.

Loxapine Succinate (Co-administration with tranquilizers may increase drowsiness).
No products indexed under this heading.

Meprobamate (Co-administration with tranquilizers may increase drowsiness).
No products indexed under this heading.

Mesoridazine Besylate (Co-administration with tranquilizers may increase drowsiness).
No products indexed under this heading.

Midazolam Hydrochloride (Co-administration with sedatives may increase drowsiness).
No products indexed under this heading.

Molindone Hydrochloride (Co-administration with tranquilizers may increase drowsiness). Products include:
Moban Tablets 1108

Oxazepam (Co-administration with tranquilizers may increase drowsiness).
No products indexed under this heading.

Perphenazine (Co-administration with tranquilizers may increase drowsiness).
No products indexed under this heading.

Prazepam (Co-administration with tranquilizers may increase drowsiness).
No products indexed under this heading.

Prochlorperazine (Co-administration with tranquilizers may increase drowsiness).
No products indexed under this heading.

Promethazine Hydrochloride (Co-administration with tranquilizers may increase drowsiness). Products include:
Phenergan 3438

Propofol (Co-administration with sedatives may increase drowsiness). Products include:
Diprivan Injectable Emulsion 676

Quazepam (Co-administration with sedatives may increase drowsiness).
No products indexed under this heading.

Secobarbital Sodium (Co-administration with sedatives may increase drowsiness).
No products indexed under this heading.

Temazepam (Co-administration with sedatives may increase drowsiness).
No products indexed under this heading.

Thioridazine Hydrochloride (Co-administration with tranquilizers may increase drowsiness). Products include:
Thioridazine Hydrochloride Tablets 2122

Thiothixene (Co-administration with tranquilizers may increase drowsiness). Products include:

Thiothixene Capsules 2124

Triazolam (Co-administration with sedatives may increase drowsiness).
No products indexed under this heading.

Trifluoperazine Hydrochloride (Co-administration with tranquilizers may increase drowsiness).
No products indexed under this heading.

Zaleplon (Co-administration with sedatives may increase drowsiness). Products include:
Sonata Capsules 1686

Zolpidem Tartrate (Co-administration with sedatives may increase drowsiness). Products include:
Ambien Tablets 2867

Food Interactions

Alcohol (Co-administration with alcohol may increase drowsiness).

THERA-GESIC CREME

(Menthol, Methyl Salicylate) 2108
None cited in PDR database.

THERA-GESIC PLUS CREME

(Menthol, Methyl Salicylate) 673
None cited in PDR database.

THERMACARE HEAT WRAPS

(Device) 2674
None cited in PDR database.

THIORIDAZINE HYDROCHLORIDE TABLETS

(Thioridazine Hydrochloride) 2122
May interact with central nervous system depressants, erythromycin, potassium-depleting diuretics, quinidine, and certain other agents. Compounds in these categories include:

Alfentanil Hydrochloride (Thioridazine is capable of potentiating CNS depressants).
No products indexed under this heading.

Alprazolam (Thioridazine is capable of potentiating CNS depressants). Products include:
Niravam Orally Disintegrating Tablets 3106
Xanax XR Tablets 2655

Amiodarone Hydrochloride (Thioridazine has been shown to prolong QTc interval in a dose-related manner; drugs with this potential have been associated with Torsade de pointes-type arrhythmias and sudden death; co-administration with other drugs that are known to prolong QTc interval is contraindicated). Products include:
Pacerone Tablets 3337

Aprobarbital (Thioridazine is capable of potentiating CNS depressants).
No products indexed under this heading.

Arsenic Trioxide (Thioridazine has been shown to prolong QTc interval in a dose-related manner; drugs with this potential have been associated with torsade de pointes-type arrhythmias and sudden death; co-administration with other drugs that are known to prolong QTc interval is contraindicated). Products include:
Trisenox Injection 983

Atropine Sulfate (Thioridazine is capable of potentiating atropine).
No products indexed under this heading.

Bendroflumethiazide (Hypokalemia may result from diuretic therapy and this may increase the risk of QT prolongation and arrhythmias; co-administration may increase the risk of serious, potentially fatal, cardiac arrhythmias).
No products indexed under this heading.

Bepridil Hydrochloride (Thioridazine has been shown to prolong QTc interval in a dose-related manner; drugs with this potential have been associated with torsade de pointes-type arrhythmias and sudden death; co-administration with other drugs that are known to prolong QTc interval is contraindicated).
No products indexed under this heading.

Bumetanide (Hypokalemia may result from diuretic therapy and this may increase the risk of QT prolongation and arrhythmias; co-administration may increase the risk of serious, potentially fatal, cardiac arrhythmias).
No products indexed under this heading.

Buprenorphine Hydrochloride (Thioridazine is capable of potentiating CNS depressants). Products include:
Buprenex Injectable 2718
Suboxone Tablets 2719
Subutex Tablets 2719

Buspirone Hydrochloride (Thioridazine is capable of potentiating CNS depressants).
No products indexed under this heading.

Butabarbital (Thioridazine is capable of potentiating CNS depressants).
No products indexed under this heading.

Butalbital (Thioridazine is capable of potentiating CNS depressants). Products include:
Sedapap Tablets 50 mg/650 mg 2098

Chlordiazepoxide (Thioridazine is capable of potentiating CNS depressants).
No products indexed under this heading.

Chlordiazepoxide Hydrochloride (Thioridazine is capable of potentiating CNS depressants). Products include:
Librium Capsules 3349

Chlorothiazide (Hypokalemia may result from diuretic therapy and this may increase the risk of QT prolongation and arrhythmias; co-administration may increase the risk of serious, potentially fatal, cardiac arrhythmias). Products include:
Aldoclor Tablets 1881
Diuril Oral 1936

Chlorothiazide Sodium (Hypokalemia may result from diuretic therapy and this may increase the risk of QT prolongation and arrhythmias; co-administration may increase the risk of serious, potentially fatal, cardiac arrhythmias). Products include:
Diuril Sodium Intravenous 1934

Chlorpromazine (Thioridazine is capable of potentiating CNS depressants).
No products indexed under this heading.

Chlorpromazine Hydrochloride (Thioridazine is capable of potentiating CNS depressants).
No products indexed under this heading.

Chlorprothixene (Thioridazine is capable of potentiating CNS depressants).
No products indexed under this heading.

Chlorprothixene Hydrochloride (Thioridazine is capable of potentiating CNS depressants).
No products indexed under this heading.

Chlorprothixene Lactate (Thioridazine is capable of potentiating CNS depressants).
No products indexed under this heading.

Clorazepate Dipotassium (Thioridazine is capable of potentiating CNS depressants). Products include:
Tranxene 2488

Clozapine (Thioridazine is capable of potentiating CNS depressants). Products include:
Clozapine Tablets 2141
Clozaril Tablets 2174
FazaClo Orally Disintegrating Tablets 547

Codeine Phosphate (Thioridazine is capable of potentiating CNS depressants). Products include:
Tylenol with Codeine 2461

Desflurane (Thioridazine is capable of potentiating CNS depressants). Products include:
Suprane Liquid for Inhalation 770

Desipramine Hydrochloride (Thioridazine has been shown to prolong QTc interval in a dose-related manner; drugs with this potential have been associated with torsade de pointes-type arrhythmias and sudden death; co-administration with other drugs that are known to prolong QTc interval is contraindicated).
No products indexed under this heading.

Dezocine (Thioridazine is capable of potentiating CNS depressants).
No products indexed under this heading.

Diazepam (Thioridazine is capable of potentiating CNS depressants). Products include:
Diastat Rectal Delivery System 3344
Valium Tablets 2822

Disopyramide Phosphate (Thioridazine has been shown to prolong QTc interval in a dose-related manner; drugs with this potential have been associated with torsade de pointes-type arrhythmias and sudden death; co-administration with other drugs that are known to prolong QTc interval is contraindicated).
No products indexed under this heading.

Dofetilide (Thioridazine has been shown to prolong QTc interval in a dose-related manner; drugs with this potential have been associated with Torsade de pointes-type arrhythmias and sudden death; co-administration with other drugs that are known to prolong QTc interval is contraindicated).
No products indexed under this heading.

Dolasetron Mesylate (Thioridazine has been shown to prolong QTc interval in a dose-related manner; drugs with this potential have been associated with Torsade de pointes-type arrhythmias and sudden death; co-administration with other drugs that are known to prolong QTc interval is contraindicated). Products include:
Anzemet Injection 2871
Anzemet Tablets 2874

Droperidol (Thioridazine has been shown to prolong QTc interval in a dose-related manner; drugs with this potential have been associated with torsade de pointes-type arrhythmias and sudden death; co-administration with other drugs that are known to prolong QTc interval is contraindicated).
No products indexed under this heading.

Enflurane (Thioridazine is capable of potentiating CNS depressants).
No products indexed under this heading.

Epinephrine (Thioridazine causes orthostatic hypotension, especially in female patients; use of epinephrine should be avoided in view of the fact that phenothiazines may induce a reversed epinephrine effect). Products include:
EpiPen 1061
Primatene Mist 749

Epinephrine Hydrochloride (Thioridazine causes orthostatic hypotension, especially in female patients; use of epinephrine should be avoided in view of the fact that phenothiazines may induce a reversed epinephrine effect).
No products indexed under this heading.

Erythromycin (Thioridazine has been shown to prolong QTc interval in a dose-related manner; drugs with this potential have been associated with torsade de pointes-type arrhythmias and sudden death; co-administration with other drugs that are known to prolong QTc interval is contraindicated). Products include:
Erygel Topical Gel 2096
Ery-Tab Tablets 447
Erythromycin Base Filmtab Tablets 454
Erythromycin Delayed-Release Capsules, USP 456
PCE Dispertab Tablets 510

Erythromycin Estolate (Thioridazine has been shown to prolong QTc interval in a dose-related manner; drugs with this potential have been associated with torsade de pointes-type arrhythmias and sudden death; co-administration with other drugs that are known to prolong QTc interval is contraindicated).
No products indexed under this heading.

Erythromycin Ethylsuccinate (Thioridazine has been shown to prolong QTc interval in a dose-related manner; drugs with this potential have been associated with torsade de pointes-type arrhythmias and sudden death; co-administration with other drugs that are known to prolong QTc interval is contraindicated). Products include:
E.E.S. 449
EryPed 445

Erythromycin Gluceptate (Thioridazine has been shown to prolong QTc interval in a dose-related manner; drugs with this potential have been associated with torsade de pointes-type arrhythmias and sudden death; co-administration with other drugs that are known to prolong QTc interval is contraindicated).
No products indexed under this heading.

Erythromycin Lactobionate (Thioridazine has been shown to prolong QTc interval in a dose-related manner; drugs with this potential have been associated with torsade de pointes-type arrhythmias and sudden death; co-administration with other drugs that are known to prolong QTc interval is contraindicated).
No products indexed under this heading.

Erythromycin Stearate (Thioridazine has been shown to prolong QTc interval in a dose-related manner; drugs with this potential have been associated with torsade de pointes-type arrhythmias and sudden death; co-administration with other drugs that are known to prolong QTc interval is contraindicated). Products include:
Erythrocin Stearate Filmtab Tablets 452

Estazolam (Thioridazine is capable of potentiating CNS depressants). Products include:
ProSom Tablets 512

Ethacrynic Acid (Hypokalemia may result from diuretic therapy and this may increase the risk of QT prolongation and arrhythmias; co-administration may increase the risk of serious, potentially fatal, cardiac arrhythmias). Products include:
Edecrin Tablets 1941

Ethanol (Thioridazine is capable of potentiating CNS depressants).
No products indexed under this heading.

Ethchlorvynol (Thioridazine is capable of potentiating CNS depressants).
No products indexed under this heading.

Ethinamate (Thioridazine is capable of potentiating CNS depressants).
No products indexed under this heading.

Ethyl Alcohol (Thioridazine is capable of potentiating CNS depressants).
No products indexed under this heading.

Fentanyl (Thioridazine is capable of potentiating CNS depressants). Products include:
Duragesic Transdermal System 2448

Fentanyl Citrate (Thioridazine is capable of potentiating CNS depressants). Products include:
Actiq 993

Flecainide Acetate (Thioridazine has been shown to prolong QTc interval in a dose-related manner; drugs with this potential have been associated with Torsade de pointes-type arrhythmias and sudden death; co-administration with other drugs that are known to prolong QTc interval is contraindicated). Products include:
Tambocor Tablets 1824

Fluoxetine Hydrochloride (Co-administration with drugs that inhibit CYP450 2D6 isoenzyme will appreciably inhibit metabolism of thioridazine and resulting elevated levels of thioridazine would be expected to augment the prolongation of QTc interval and may increase the risk of serious, potentially fatal, cardiac arrhythmias; concurrent use is contraindicated). Products include:
Prozac Pulvules and Liquid 1771
Symbyax Capsules 1788

Fluphenazine Decanoate (Thioridazine is capable of potentiating CNS depressants).
No products indexed under this heading.

Fluphenazine Enanthate (Thioridazine is capable of potentiating CNS depressants).
No products indexed under this heading.

Fluphenazine Hydrochloride (Thioridazine is capable of potentiating CNS depressants).
No products indexed under this heading.

Flurazepam Hydrochloride (Thioridazine is capable of potentiating CNS depressants). Products include:
Dalmane Capsules 3343

Fluvoxamine Maleate (Co-administration with drugs that inhibit CYP450 2D6 isoenzyme will appreciably inhibit metabolism of thioridazine and resulting elevated levels of thioridazine would be expected to augment the prolongation of QTc interval and may increase the risk of serious, potentially fatal, cardiac arrhythmias; concurrent use is contraindicated).
No products indexed under this heading.

Furosemide (Hypokalemia may result from diuretic therapy and this may increase the risk of QT prolongation and arrhythmias; co-administration may increase the risk of serious, potentially fatal, cardiac arrhythmias). Products include:
Furosemide Tablets 2117

Gatifloxacin (Thioridazine has been shown to prolong QTc interval in a dose-related manner; drugs with this potential have been associated with torsade de pointes-type arrhythmias and sudden death; co-administration with other drugs that are known to prolong QTc interval is contraindicated). Products include:
Tequin Injection 964
Tequin Tablets 964
Zymar Ophthalmic Solution 571

Glutethimide (Thioridazine is capable of potentiating CNS depressants).
No products indexed under this heading.

Halofantrine (Thioridazine has been shown to prolong QTc interval in a dose-related manner; drugs with this potential have been associated with Torsade de pointes-type arrhythmias and sudden death; co-administration with other drugs that are known to prolong QTc interval is contraindicated).
No products indexed under this heading.

Haloperidol (Thioridazine is capable of potentiating CNS depressants).
No products indexed under this heading.

Haloperidol Decanoate (Thioridazine is capable of potentiating CNS depressants).
No products indexed under this heading.

Hydrochlorothiazide (Hypokalemia may result from diuretic therapy and this may increase the risk of QT prolongation and arrhythmias; co-administration may increase the risk of serious, potentially fatal, cardiac arrhythmias). Products include:
Aldoril Tablets 1884
Atacand HCT 637
Avalide Tablets 2889
Avalide Tablets 922
Benicar HCT Tablets 2852
Diovan HCT Tablets 2195
Dyazide Capsules 1389
Hyzaar 1964
Lotensin HCT Tablets 2235
Maxzide 2150
Micardis HCT Tablets 886
Moduretic Tablets 2003
Prinzide Tablets 2033
Teveten HCT Tablets 1710
Timolide Tablets 2056
Uniretic Tablets 3114
Vaseretic Tablets 2073
Zestoretic Tablets 701

Hydrocodone Bitartrate (Thioridazine is capable of potentiating CNS depressants). Products include:
Hycodan 1104
Hycomine Compound Tablets 1105
Hycotuss Expectorant Syrup 1106
Lortab 3315
Lortab Elixir 3312
Vicodin Tablets 530
Vicodin ES Tablets 531
Vicodin HP Tablets 532
Vicoprofen Tablets 533
Zydone Tablets 1118

Hydrocodone Polistirex (Thioridazine is capable of potentiating CNS depressants). Products include:
Tussionex Pennkinetic Extended-Release Suspension 3322

Hydroflumethiazide (Hypokalemia may result from diuretic therapy and this may increase the risk of QT prolongation and arrhythmias; co-administration may increase the risk of serious, potentially fatal, cardiac arrhythmias).
No products indexed under this heading.

Hydromorphone Hydrochloride (Thioridazine is capable of potentiating CNS depressants). Products include:
Dilaudid 439
Dilaudid Oral Liquid 443
Dilaudid Non-Sterile Powder 439
Dilaudid Rectal Suppositories 439
Dilaudid Tablets 439
Dilaudid Tablets - 8 mg 443
Dilaudid-HP 441

Hydroxyzine Hydrochloride (Thioridazine is capable of potentiating CNS depressants).
No products indexed under this heading.

Ibutilide Fumarate (Thioridazine has been shown to prolong QTc interval in a dose-related manner; drugs with this potential have been associated with torsade de pointes-type arrhythmias and sudden death; co-administration with other drugs that are known to prolong QTc interval is contraindicated).
No products indexed under this heading.

Isoflurane (Thioridazine is capable of potentiating CNS depressants).
No products indexed under this heading.

Ketamine Hydrochloride (Thioridazine is capable of potentiating CNS depressants).
No products indexed under this heading.

Levomethadyl Acetate Hydrochloride (Thioridazine has been shown to prolong QTc interval in a dose-related manner; drugs with this potential have been associated with torsade de pointes-type arrhythmias and sudden death; co-administration with other drugs that are known to prolong QTc interval is contraindicated).
No products indexed under this heading.

Levorphanol Tartrate (Thioridazine is capable of potentiating CNS depressants).
No products indexed under this heading.

Lorazepam (Thioridazine is capable of potentiating CNS depressants).
No products indexed under this heading.

Loxapine Hydrochloride (Thioridazine is capable of potentiating CNS depressants).
No products indexed under this heading.

Loxapine Succinate (Thioridazine is capable of potentiating CNS depressants).
No products indexed under this heading.

Mefloquine Hydrochloride (Thioridazine has been shown to prolong QTc interval in a dose-related manner; drugs with this potential have been associated with Torsade de pointes-type arrhythmias and sudden death; co-administration with other drugs that are known to prolong QTc interval is contraindicated). Products include:
Lariam Tablets 2790

Meperidine Hydrochloride (Thioridazine is capable of potentiating CNS depressants).
No products indexed under this heading.

Mephobarbital (Thioridazine is capable of potentiating CNS depressants). Products include:
Mebaral Tablets, USP 2483

Meprobamate (Thioridazine is capable of potentiating CNS depressants).
No products indexed under this heading.

Mesoridazine Besylate (Thioridazine is capable of potentiating CNS depressants).
No products indexed under this heading.

Methadone Hydrochloride (Thioridazine is capable of potentiating CNS depressants).
No products indexed under this heading.

Methohexital Sodium (Thioridazine is capable of potentiating CNS depressants).
No products indexed under this heading.

Methotrimeprazine (Thioridazine is capable of potentiating CNS depressants).
No products indexed under this heading.

Methoxyflurane (Thioridazine is capable of potentiating CNS depressants).
No products indexed under this heading.

Methyclothiazide (Hypokalemia may result from diuretic therapy and this may increase the risk of QT prolongation and arrhythmias; co-administration may increase the risk of serious, potentially fatal, cardiac arrhythmias).
No products indexed under this heading.

Midazolam Hydrochloride (Thioridazine is capable of potentiating CNS depressants).
No products indexed under this heading.

Molindone Hydrochloride (Thioridazine is capable of potentiating CNS depressants). Products include:
Moban Tablets ... 1108

Morphine Sulfate (Thioridazine is capable of potentiating CNS depressants). Products include:
Avinza Capsules ... 1714
Kadian Capsules ... 572
MS Contin Tablets ... 2703

Moxifloxacin Hydrochloride (Thioridazine has been shown to prolong QTc interval in a dose-related manner; drugs with this potential have been associated with torsade de pointes-type arrhythmias and sudden death; co-administration with other drugs that are known to prolong QTc interval is contraindicated). Products include:
Avelox ... 2984
Vigamox Ophthalmic Solution ... 560

Olanzapine (Thioridazine is capable of potentiating CNS depressants). Products include:
Symbyax Capsules ... 1788
Zyprexa Tablets ... 1798
Zyprexa IntraMuscular ... 1798
Zyprexa ZYDIS Orally Disintegrating Tablets ... 1798

Oxazepam (Thioridazine is capable of potentiating CNS depressants).
No products indexed under this heading.

Oxycodone Hydrochloride (Thioridazine is capable of potentiating CNS depressants). Products include:
Combunox Tablets ... 1183
OxyContin Tablets ... 2699
OxyFast Oral Concentrate Solution ... 2704
OxyIR Capsules ... 2704
Percocet Tablets ... 1114
Percodan Tablets ... 1115

Paroxetine Hydrochloride (Co-administration with drugs that inhibit CYP450 2D6 isoenzyme will appreciably inhibit metabolism of thioridazine and resulting elevated levels of thioridazine would be expected to augment the prolongation of QTc interval and may increase the risk of serious, potentially fatal, cardiac arrhythmias; concurrent use is contraindicated). Products include:
Paxil CR Controlled-Release Tablets ... 1509
Paxil ... 1501

Pentamidine Isethionate (Thioridazine has been shown to prolong QTc interval in a dose-related manner; drugs with this potential have been associated with torsade de pointes-type arrhythmias and sudden death; co-administration with other drugs that are known to prolong QTc interval is contraindicated).
No products indexed under this heading.

Pentobarbital Sodium (Thioridazine is capable of potentiating CNS depressants). Products include:
Nembutal Sodium Solution, USP ... 2484

Perphenazine (Thioridazine is capable of potentiating CNS depressants).
No products indexed under this heading.

Phenobarbital (Thioridazine is capable of potentiating CNS depressants).
No products indexed under this heading.

Pimozide (Thioridazine has been shown to prolong QTc interval in a dose-related manner; drugs with this potential have been associated with torsade de pointes-type arrhythmias and sudden death; co-administration with other drugs that are known to prolong QTc interval is contraindicated). Products include:
Orap Tablets ... 1220

Pindolol (Co-administration with drugs that inhibit CYP450 2D6 isoenzyme will appreciably inhibit metabolism of thioridazine and resulting elevated levels of thioridazine would be expected to augment the prolongation of QTc interval and may increase the risk of serious, potentially fatal, cardiac arrhythmias; concurrent use is contraindicated).
No products indexed under this heading.

Polythiazide (Hypokalemia may result from diuretic therapy and this may increase the risk of QT prolongation and arrhythmias; co-administration may increase the risk of serious, potentially fatal, cardiac arrhythmias).
No products indexed under this heading.

Prazepam (Thioridazine is capable of potentiating CNS depressants).
No products indexed under this heading.

Procainamide Hydrochloride (Thioridazine has been shown to prolong QTc interval in a dose-related manner; drugs with this potential have been associated with torsade de pointes-type arrhythmias and sudden death; co-administration with other drugs that are known to prolong QTc interval is contraindicated).
No products indexed under this heading.

Prochlorperazine (Thioridazine is capable of potentiating CNS depressants).
No products indexed under this heading.

Promethazine Hydrochloride (Thioridazine is capable of potentiating CNS depressants). Products include:
Phenergan ... 3438

Propofol (Thioridazine is capable of potentiating CNS depressants). Products include:
Diprivan Injectable Emulsion ... 676

Propoxyphene Hydrochloride (Thioridazine is capable of potentiating CNS depressants).
No products indexed under this heading.

Propoxyphene Napsylate (Thioridazine is capable of potentiating CNS depressants). Products include:
Darvocet A 500 Tablets ... 3497

Propranolol Hydrochloride (Co-administration with drugs that inhibit CYP450 2D6 isoenzyme will appreciably inhibit metabolism of thioridazine and resulting elevated levels of thioridazine would be expected to augment the prolongation of QTc interval and may increase the risk of serious, potentially fatal, cardiac arrhythmias; concurrent use is contraindicated). Products include:
Inderal LA Long-Acting Capsules ... 3421
InnoPran XL Capsules ... 2728

Quazepam (Thioridazine is capable of potentiating CNS depressants).
No products indexed under this heading.

Quetiapine Fumarate (Thioridazine is capable of potentiating CNS depressants). Products include:
Seroquel Tablets ... 691

Quinidine (Thioridazine has been shown to prolong QTc interval in a dose-related manner; drugs with this potential have been associated with torsade de pointes-type arrhythmias and sudden death; co-administration with other drugs that are known to prolong QTc interval is contraindicated).
No products indexed under this heading.

Quinidine Gluconate (Thioridazine has been shown to prolong QTc interval in a dose-related manner; drugs with this potential have been associated with torsade de pointes-type arrhythmias and sudden death; co-administration with other drugs that are known to prolong QTc interval is contraindicated).
No products indexed under this heading.

Quinidine Hydrochloride (Thioridazine has been shown to prolong QTc interval in a dose-related manner; drugs with this potential have been associated with torsade de pointes-type arrhythmias and sudden death; co-administration with other drugs that are known to prolong QTc interval is contraindicated).
No products indexed under this heading.

Quinidine Polygalacturonate (Thioridazine has been shown to prolong QTc interval in a dose-related manner; drugs with this potential have been associated with torsade de pointes-type arrhythmias and sudden death; co-administration with other drugs that are known to prolong QTc interval is contraindicated).
No products indexed under this heading.

Quinidine Sulfate (Thioridazine has been shown to prolong QTc interval in a dose-related manner; drugs with this potential have been associated with torsade de pointes-type arrhythmias and sudden death; co-administration with other drugs that are known to prolong QTc interval is contraindicated).
No products indexed under this heading.

Remifentanil Hydrochloride (Thioridazine is capable of potentiating CNS depressants).
No products indexed under this heading.

Risperidone (Thioridazine is capable of potentiating CNS depressants). Products include:
Risperdal Consta Long-Acting Injection ... 1664
Risperdal M-Tab Orally Disintegrating Tablets ... 1658
Risperdal ... 1658

Secobarbital Sodium (Thioridazine is capable of potentiating CNS depressants).
No products indexed under this heading.

Sevoflurane (Thioridazine is capable of potentiating CNS depressants). Products include:
Ultane Liquid for Inhalation ... 526

Sotalol Hydrochloride (Thioridazine has been shown to prolong QTc interval in a dose-related manner; drugs with this potential have been associated with torsade de pointes-type arrhythmias and sudden death; co-administration with other drugs that are known to prolong QTc interval is contraindicated).
No products indexed under this heading.

Sparfloxacin (Thioridazine has been shown to prolong QTc interval in a dose-related manner; drugs with this potential have been associated with torsade de pointes-type arrhythmias and sudden death; co-administration with other drugs that are known to prolong QTc interval is contraindicated).
No products indexed under this heading.

Sufentanil Citrate (Thioridazine is capable of potentiating CNS depressants).
No products indexed under this heading.

Tacrolimus (Thioridazine has been shown to prolong QTc interval in a dose-related manner; drugs with this potential have been associated with torsade de pointes-type arrhythmias and sudden death; co-administration with other drugs that are known to prolong QTc interval is contraindicated). Products include:
Prograf Capsules and Injection ... 624
Protopic Ointment ... 629

Temazepam (Thioridazine is capable of potentiating CNS depressants).
No products indexed under this heading.

Thiamylal Sodium (Thioridazine is capable of potentiating CNS depressants).
No products indexed under this heading.

Thiothixene (Thioridazine is capable of potentiating CNS depressants). Products include:
Thiothixene Capsules ... 2124

Torsemide (Hypokalemia may result from diuretic therapy and this may increase the risk of QT prolongation and arrhythmias; co-administration may increase the risk of serious, potentially fatal, cardiac arrhythmias).
No products indexed under this heading.

Triazolam (Thioridazine is capable of potentiating CNS depressants).
No products indexed under this heading.

Trifluoperazine Hydrochloride (Thioridazine is capable of potentiating CNS depressants).
No products indexed under this heading.

Zaleplon (Thioridazine is capable of potentiating CNS depressants). Products include:
Sonata Capsules ... 1686

Ziprasidone Hydrochloride (Thioridazine has been shown to prolong QTc interval in a dose-related manner; drugs with this potential have been associated with torsade de pointes-type arrhythmias and sudden death; co-administration with other

drugs that are known to prolong QTc interval is contraindicated). Products include:

Geodon Capsules 2514

Ziprasidone Mesylate (Thioridazine has been shown to prolong QTc interval in a dose-related manner; drugs with this potential have been associated with torsade de pointes-type arrhythmias and sudden death; co-administration with other drugs that are known to prolong QTc interval is contraindicated). Products include:

Geodon for Injection 2514

Zolpidem Tartrate (Thioridazine is capable of potentiating CNS depressants). Products include:

Ambien Tablets 2867

Food Interactions

Alcohol (Thioridazine is capable of potentiating CNS depressants).

THIOTHIXENE CAPSULES

(Thiothixene) 2124

May interact with belladona products, central nervous system depressants, and certain other agents. Compounds in these categories include:

Alfentanil Hydrochloride (Possible additive effects which may include hypotension).

No products indexed under this heading.

Alprazolam (Possible additive effects which may include hypotension). Products include:

Niravam Orally Disintegrating Tablets 3106

Xanax XR Tablets 2655

Aprobarbital (Possible additive effects which may include hypotension).

No products indexed under this heading.

Atropine Sulfate (Thiothixene exhibits weak anticholinergic properties; concurrent use with atropine or related drugs requires caution).

No products indexed under this heading.

Belladonna Alkaloids (Thiothixene exhibits weak anticholinergic properties; concurrent use with atropine or related drugs requires caution). Products include:

Hyland's Teething Tablets .... ▣736

Buprenorphine Hydrochloride (Possible additive effects which may include hypotension). Products include:

Buprenex Injectable 2718

Suboxone Tablets 2719

Subutex Tablets 2719

Buspirone Hydrochloride (Possible additive effects which may include hypotension).

No products indexed under this heading.

Butabarbital (Possible additive effects which may include hypotension).

No products indexed under this heading.

Butalbital (Possible additive effects which may include hypotension). Products include:

Sedapap Tablets 50 mg/650 mg 2098

Chlordiazepoxide (Possible additive effects which may include hypotension).

No products indexed under this heading.

Chlordiazepoxide Hydrochloride (Possible additive effects which may include hypotension). Products include:

Librium Capsules 3349

Chlorpromazine (Possible additive effects which may include hypotension).

No products indexed under this heading.

Chlorpromazine Hydrochloride (Possible additive effects which may include hypotension).

No products indexed under this heading.

Chlorprothixene (Possible additive effects which may include hypotension).

No products indexed under this heading.

Chlorprothixene Hydrochloride (Possible additive effects which may include hypotension).

No products indexed under this heading.

Chlorprothixene Lactate (Possible additive effects which may include hypotension).

No products indexed under this heading.

Clorazepate Dipotassium (Possible additive effects which may include hypotension). Products include:

Tranxene 2488

Clozapine (Possible additive effects which may include hypotension). Products include:

Clozapine Tablets 2141

Clozaril Tablets 2174

FazaClo Orally Disintegrating Tablets 547

Codeine Phosphate (Possible additive effects which may include hypotension). Products include:

Tylenol with Codeine 2461

Desflurane (Possible additive effects which may include hypotension). Products include:

Suprane Liquid for Inhalation 770

Dezocine (Possible additive effects which may include hypotension).

No products indexed under this heading.

Diazepam (Possible additive effects which may include hypotension). Products include:

Diastat Rectal Delivery System 3344

Valium Tablets 2822

Droperidol (Possible additive effects which may include hypotension).

No products indexed under this heading.

Enflurane (Possible additive effects which may include hypotension).

No products indexed under this heading.

Estazolam (Possible additive effects which may include hypotension). Products include:

ProSom Tablets 512

Ethanol (Possible additive effects which may include hypotension).

No products indexed under this heading.

Ethchlorvynol (Possible additive effects which may include hypotension).

No products indexed under this heading.

Ethinamate (Possible additive effects which may include hypotension).

No products indexed under this heading.

Ethyl Alcohol (Possible additive effects which may include hypotension).

No products indexed under this heading.

Fentanyl (Possible additive effects which may include hypotension). Products include:

Duragesic Transdermal System 2448

Fentanyl Citrate (Possible additive effects which may include hypotension). Products include:

Actiq 993

Fluphenazine Decanoate (Possible additive effects which may include hypotension).

No products indexed under this heading.

Fluphenazine Enanthate (Possible additive effects which may include hypotension).

No products indexed under this heading.

Fluphenazine Hydrochloride (Possible additive effects which may include hypotension).

No products indexed under this heading.

Flurazepam Hydrochloride (Possible additive effects which may include hypotension). Products include:

Dalmane Capsules 3343

Glutethimide (Possible additive effects which may include hypotension).

No products indexed under this heading.

Haloperidol (Possible additive effects which may include hypotension).

No products indexed under this heading.

Haloperidol Decanoate (Possible additive effects which may include hypotension).

No products indexed under this heading.

Hydrocodone Bitartrate (Possible additive effects which may include hypotension). Products include:

Hycodan 1104

Hycomine Compound Tablets 1105

Hycotuss Expectorant Syrup 1106

Lortab 3315

Lortab Elixir 3312

Vicodin Tablets 530

Vicodin ES Tablets 531

Vicodin HP Tablets 532

Vicoprofen Tablets 533

Zydone Tablets 1118

Hydrocodone Polistirex (Possible additive effects which may include hypotension). Products include:

Tussionex Pennkinetic Extended-Release Suspension 3322

Hydromorphone Hydrochloride (Possible additive effects which may include hypotension). Products include:

Dilaudid 439

Dilaudid Oral Liquid 443

Dilaudid Non-Sterile Powder 439

Dilaudid Rectal Suppositories 439

Dilaudid Tablets 439

Dilaudid Tablets - 8 mg 443

Dilaudid-HP 441

Hydroxyzine Hydrochloride (Possible additive effects which may include hypotension).

No products indexed under this heading.

Hyoscyamine (Thiothixene exhibits weak anticholinergic properties; concurrent use with atropine or related drugs requires caution).

No products indexed under this heading.

Hyoscyamine Sulfate (Thiothixene exhibits weak anticholinergic properties; concurrent use with atropine or related drugs requires caution).

No products indexed under this heading.

Isoflurane (Possible additive effects which may include hypotension).

No products indexed under this heading.

Ketamine Hydrochloride (Possible additive effects which may include hypotension).

No products indexed under this heading.

Levomethadyl Acetate Hydrochloride (Possible additive effects which may include hypotension).

No products indexed under this heading.

Levorphanol Tartrate (Possible additive effects which may include hypotension).

No products indexed under this heading.

Lorazepam (Possible additive effects which may include hypotension).

No products indexed under this heading.

Loxapine Hydrochloride (Possible additive effects which may include hypotension).

No products indexed under this heading.

Loxapine Succinate (Possible additive effects which may include hypotension).

No products indexed under this heading.

Meperidine Hydrochloride (Possible additive effects which may include hypotension).

No products indexed under this heading.

Mephobarbital (Possible additive effects which may include hypotension). Products include:

Mebaral Tablets, USP 2483

Meprobamate (Possible additive effects which may include hypotension).

No products indexed under this heading.

Mesoridazine Besylate (Possible additive effects which may include hypotension).

No products indexed under this heading.

Methadone Hydrochloride (Possible additive effects which may include hypotension).

No products indexed under this heading.

Methohexital Sodium (Possible additive effects which may include hypotension).

No products indexed under this heading.

Methotrimeprazine (Possible additive effects which may include hypotension).

No products indexed under this heading.

Methoxyflurane (Possible additive effects which may include hypotension).

No products indexed under this heading.

Midazolam Hydrochloride (Possible additive effects which may include hypotension).
No products indexed under this heading.

Molindone Hydrochloride (Possible additive effects which may include hypotension). Products include:
Moban Tablets 1108

Morphine Sulfate (Possible additive effects which may include hypotension). Products include:
Avinza Capsules 1714
Kadian Capsules 572
MS Contin Tablets 2703

Olanzapine (Possible additive effects which may include hypotension). Products include:
Symbyax Capsules 1788
Zyprexa Tablets 1798
Zyprexa IntraMuscular 1798
Zyprexa ZYDIS Orally Disintegrating Tablets 1798

Oxazepam (Possible additive effects which may include hypotension).
No products indexed under this heading.

Oxycodone Hydrochloride (Possible additive effects which may include hypotension). Products include:
Combunox Tablets 1183
OxyContin Tablets 2699
OxyFast Oral Concentrate Solution 2704
OxyIR Capsules 2704
Percocet Tablets 1114
Percodan Tablets 1115

Pentobarbital Sodium (Possible additive effects which may include hypotension). Products include:
Nembutal Sodium Solution, USP 2484

Perphenazine (Possible additive effects which may include hypotension).
No products indexed under this heading.

Phenobarbital (Possible additive effects which may include hypotension).
No products indexed under this heading.

Prazepam (Possible additive effects which may include hypotension).
No products indexed under this heading.

Prochlorperazine (Possible additive effects which may include hypotension).
No products indexed under this heading.

Promethazine Hydrochloride (Possible additive effects which may include hypotension). Products include:
Phenergan 3438

Propofol (Possible additive effects which may include hypotension). Products include:
Diprivan Injectable Emulsion 676

Propoxyphene Hydrochloride (Possible additive effects which may include hypotension).
No products indexed under this heading.

Propoxyphene Napsylate (Possible additive effects which may include hypotension). Products include:
Darvocet A 500 Tablets 3497

Quazepam (Possible additive effects which may include hypotension).
No products indexed under this heading.

Quetiapine Fumarate (Possible additive effects which may include hypotension). Products include:
Seroquel Tablets 691

Remifentanil Hydrochloride (Possible additive effects which may include hypotension).
No products indexed under this heading.

Risperidone (Possible additive effects which may include hypotension). Products include:
Risperdal Consta Long-Acting Injection 1664
Risperdal M-Tab Orally Disintegrating Tablets 1658
Risperdal 1658

Scopolamine (Thiothixene exhibits weak anticholinergic properties; concurrent use with atropine or related drugs requires caution). Products include:
Transderm Scōp Transdermal Therapeutic System 2166

Scopolamine Hydrobromide (Thiothixene exhibits weak anticholinergic properties; concurrent use with atropine or related drugs requires caution).
No products indexed under this heading.

Secobarbital Sodium (Possible additive effects which may include hypotension).
No products indexed under this heading.

Sevoflurane (Possible additive effects which may include hypotension). Products include:
Ultane Liquid for Inhalation 526

Sufentanil Citrate (Possible additive effects which may include hypotension).
No products indexed under this heading.

Temazepam (Possible additive effects which may include hypotension).
No products indexed under this heading.

Thiamylal Sodium (Possible additive effects which may include hypotension).
No products indexed under this heading.

Thioridazine Hydrochloride (Possible additive effects which may include hypotension). Products include:
Thioridazine Hydrochloride Tablets 2122

Triazolam (Possible additive effects which may include hypotension).
No products indexed under this heading.

Trifluoperazine Hydrochloride (Possible additive effects which may include hypotension).
No products indexed under this heading.

Zaleplon (Possible additive effects which may include hypotension). Products include:
Sonata Capsules 1686

Ziprasidone Hydrochloride (Possible additive effects which may include hypotension). Products include:
Geodon Capsules 2514

Zolpidem Tartrate (Possible additive effects which may include hypotension). Products include:
Ambien Tablets 2867

Food Interactions

Alcohol (Possible additive effects which may include hypotension).

THROMBATE III
(Antithrombin III) 3254
May interact with:

Heparin Sodium (The anticoagulant effect of heparin is enhanced by concurrent treatment with antithrombin III; reduced dosage of heparin may be required).
No products indexed under this heading.

THROMBIN-JMI
(Thrombin) 1693
None cited in PDR database.

THYMOGLOBULIN FOR INJECTION
(Anti-thymocyte Globulin) 2848
May interact with immunosuppressive agents and certain other agents. Compounds in these categories include:

Azathioprine (Co-administration with standard immunosuppressive regimen may predispose patients to over-immunosuppression; decrease in maintenance immunosuppression therapy during the period of antibody therapy may be needed). Products include:
Azasan Tablets 2844

Basiliximab (Co-administration with standard immunosuppressive regimen may predispose patients to over-immunosuppression; decrease in maintenance immunosuppression therapy during the period of antibody therapy may be needed). Products include:
Simulect for Injection 2268

Cyclosporine (Co-administration with standard immunosuppressive regimen may predispose patients to over-immunosuppression; decrease in maintenance immunosuppression therapy during the period of antibody therapy may be needed). Products include:
Gengraf Capsules 458
Neoral Soft Gelatin Capsules 2247
Neoral Oral Solution 2247
Restasis Ophthalmic Emulsion 570
Sandimmune 2259

Globulin, immune (rabbit) (Thymoglobulin can stimulate the production of antibodies which cross-react with rabbit immune globulin).
No products indexed under this heading.

Muromonab-CD3 (Co-administration with standard immunosuppressive regimen may predispose patients to over-immunosuppression; decrease in maintenance immunosuppression therapy during the period of antibody therapy may be needed). Products include:
Orthoclone OKT3 Sterile Solution 2370

Mycophenolate Mofetil (Co-administration with standard immunosuppressive regimen may predispose patients to over-immunosuppression; decrease in maintenance immunosuppression therapy during the period of antibody therapy may be needed). Products include:
CellCept Capsules 2751
CellCept Oral Suspension 2751
CellCept Tablets 2751

Sirolimus (Co-administration with standard immunosuppressive regimen may predispose patients to over-immunosuppression; decrease in maintenance immunosuppression therapy during the period of antibody therapy may be needed). Products include:
Rapamune Oral Solution and Tablets 3472

Tacrolimus (Co-administration with standard immunosuppressive regimen may predispose patients to over-immunosuppression; decrease in maintenance immunosuppression therapy during the period of antibody therapy may be needed). Products include:
Prograf Capsules and Injection 624
Protopic Ointment 629

THYROGEN FOR INJECTION
(Thyrotropin alfa) 1270
None cited in PDR database.

THYROLAR
(Liotrix) 1203
May interact with oral anticoagulants, estrogens, oral hypoglycemic agents, insulin, oral contraceptives, and certain other agents. Compounds in these categories include:

Acarbose (Initiating thyroid replacement therapy may cause increases in roal hypoglycemic requirements. The effects seen are poorly understood and depend upon a variety of factors such as dose and type of thyroid preparations and endocrine status of the patient. Patients receiving oral hypoglycemics should be closely watched during initiation of thyroid replacement therapy). Products include:
Precose Tablets 776

Anisindione (Thyroid hormones appear to increase catabolism of vitamin K-dependent clotting factoes. If oral anticoagulants are also being given, compensatory increases in clotting factor synthesis are impaired. Patients stabilized on oral anticoagulants who are found to require thyroid replacement therapy should be watched very closely when thyroid is started. If a patient is truly hypothyroid, it is likely that a reduction in anticoagulant dosage will be required. No special precautions appear to be necessary when oral anticoagulant therapy is begun in a patient already stabilized on maintenance thyroid replacement therapy). Products include:
Miradon Tablets 3056

Chlorotrianisene (Estrogens tend to increase serum thyroxine-binding globulin (TBg). In a patient with a nonfunctioning thyroid gland who is reveiving thyroid replacement therapy, free levothyroxine may be decreased when estrogens are started, thus increasing thyroid requirements. However, if the patient's thyroid gland has sufficient function, the decreased free thyroxine will result in a compensatory increase in thyroxine output by the thyroid. Therefore, patients without a functioning thyroid gland who are on thyroid replacement therapy may need to increase their thyroid dose if estrogens or estrogen-containing oral

contraceptives are given).
No products indexed under this heading.

Chlorpropamide (Initiating thyroid replacement therapy may cause increases in roal hypoglycemic requirements. The effects seen are poorly understood and depend upon a variety of factors such as dose and type of thyroid preparations and endocrine status of the patient. Patients receiving oral hypoglycemics should be closely watched during initiation of thyroid replacement therapy).
No products indexed under this heading.

Cholestyramine (Cholestyramine binds both T4 and T3 in the intesting thus impairing absorption of these thyroid hormones. In vitro studues indicate that the binding is not easily removed. Therefore, 4-5 hours should elapse between the administration of cholestyramine and thyroid hormones).
No products indexed under this heading.

Colestipol (Colestipol binds both T4 and T3 in the intesting thus impairing absorption of these thyroid hormones. In vitro studues indicate that the binding is not easily removed. Therefore, 4-5 hours should elapse between the administration of colestipol and thyroid hormones).
No products indexed under this heading.

Colestipol Hydrochloride (Colestipol binds both T4 and T3 in the intesting thus impairing absorption of these thyroid hormones. In vitro studues indicate that the binding is not easily removed. Therefore, 4-5 hours should elapse between the administration of colestipol and thyroid hormones).
No products indexed under this heading.

Desogestrel (Estrogens tend to increase serum thyroxine-binding globulin (TBg). In a patient with a nonfunctioning thyroid gland who is receiving thyroid replacement therapy, free levothyroxine may be decreased when estrogens are started, thus increasing thyroid requirements. However, if the patient's thyroid gland has sufficient function, the decreased free thyroxine will result in a compensatory increase in thyroxine output by the thyroid. Therefore, patients without a functioning thyroid gland who are on thyroid replacement therapy may need to increase their thyroid dose if estrogens or estrogen-containing oral contraceptives are given). Products include:
Ortho-Cept Tablets **2395**

Dicumarol (Thyroid hormones appear to increase catabolism of vitamin K-dependent clotting factoes. If oral anticoagulants are also being given, compensatory increases in clotting factor synthesis are impaired. Patients stabilized on oral anticoagulants who are found to require thyroid replacement therapy should be watched very closely when thyroid is started. If a patient is truly hypothyroid, it is likely that a reduction in anticoagulant dosage will be required. No special precautions appear to be necessary when oral anticoagulant therapy is begun in a patient already stabilized on maintenance thyroid replacement therapy).
No products indexed under this heading.

Dienestrol (Estrogens tend to increase serum thyroxine-binding globulin (TBg). In a patient with a nonfunctioning thyroid gland who is reveiving thyroid replacement therapy, free levothyroxine may be decreased when estrogens are started, thus increasing thyroid requirements. However, if the patient's thyroid gland has sufficient function, the decreased free thyroxine will result in a compensatory increase in thyroxine output by the thyroid. Therefore, patients without a functioning thyroid gland who are on thyroid replacement therapy may need to increase their thyroid dose if estrogens or estrogen-containing oral contraceptives are given).
No products indexed under this heading.

Diethylstilbestrol (Estrogens tend to increase serum thyroxine-binding globulin (TBg). In a patient with a nonfunctioning thyroid gland who is reveiving thyroid replacement therapy, free levothyroxine may be decreased when estrogens are started, thus increasing thyroid requirements. However, if the patient's thyroid gland has sufficient function, the decreased free thyroxine will result in a compensatory increase in thyroxine output by the thyroid. Therefore, patients without a functioning thyroid gland who are on thyroid replacement therapy may need to increase their thyroid dose if estrogens or estrogen-containing oral contraceptives are given).
No products indexed under this heading.

Estradiol (Estrogens tend to increase serum thyroxine-binding globulin (TBg). In a patient with a nonfunctioning thyroid gland who is reveiving thyroid replacement therapy, free levothyroxine may be decreased when estrogens are started, thus increasing thyroid requirements. However, if the patient's thyroid gland has sufficient function, the decreased free thyroxine will result in a compensatory increase in thyroxine output by the thyroid. Therefore, patients without a functioning thyroid gland who are on thyroid replacement therapy may need to increase their thyroid dose if estrogens or estrogen-containing oral contraceptives are given). Products include:
Activella Tablets **2311**
Climara Transdermal System **795**
Climara Pro Transdermal System **800**
CombiPatch Transdermal System **2180**
Estrogel 0.06% **3200**
Menostar Transdermal System **805**
Prefest Tablets **1069**
Vagifem Tablets **2340**
Vivelle Transdermal System **2288**
Vivelle-Dot Transdermal System **2293**

Estrogens, Conjugated (Estrogens tend to increase serum thyroxine-binding globulin (TBg). In a patient with a nonfunctioning thyroid gland who is reveiving thyroid replacement therapy, free levothyroxine may be decreased when estrogens are started, thus increasing thyroid requirements. However, if the patient's thyroid gland has sufficient function, the decreased free thyroxine will result in a compensatory increase in thyroxine output by the thyroid. Therefore, patients without a functioning thyroid gland who are on thyroid replacement therapy may need to increase their thyroid dose if estrogens or estrogen-containing oral contraceptives are given). Products include:
Premarin Intravenous **3440**
Premarin Tablets **3443**
Premarin Vaginal Cream **3449**
Premphase Tablets **3452**
Prempro Tablets **3452**

Estrogens, Esterified (Estrogens tend to increase serum thyroxine-binding globulin (TBg). In a patient with a nonfunctioning thyroid gland who is reveiving thyroid replacement therapy, free levothyroxine may be decreased when estrogens are started, thus increasing thyroid requirements. However, if the patient's thyroid gland has sufficient function, the decreased free thyroxine will result in a compensatory increase in thyroxine output by the thyroid. Therefore, patients without a functioning thyroid gland who are on thyroid replacement therapy may need to increase their thyroid dose if estrogens or estrogen-containing oral contraceptives are given). Products include:
Estratest Tablets **3196**
Estratest H.S. Tablets **3196**

Estropipate (Estrogens tend to increase serum thyroxine-binding globulin (TBg). In a patient with a nonfunctioning thyroid gland who is reveiving thyroid replacement therapy, free levothyroxine may be decreased when estrogens are started, thus increasing thyroid requirements. However, if the patient's thyroid gland has sufficient function, the decreased free thyroxine will result in a compensatory increase in thyroxine output by the thyroid. Therefore, patients without a functioning thyroid gland who are on thyroid replacement therapy may need to increase their thyroid dose if estrogens or estrogen-containing oral contraceptives are given).
No products indexed under this heading.

Ethinyl Estradiol (Estrogens tend to increase serum thyroxine-binding globulin (TBg). In a patient with a nonfunctioning thyroid gland who is reveiving thyroid replacement therapy, free levothyroxine may be decreased when estrogens are started, thus increasing thyroid requirements. However, if the patient's thyroid gland has sufficient function, the decreased free thyroxine will result in a compensatory increase in thyroxine output by the thyroid. Therefore, patients without a functioning thyroid gland who are on thyroid replacement therapy may need to increase their thyroid dose if estrogens or estrogen-containing oral contraceptives are given). Products include:
Alesse-28 Tablets **3392**
Lo/Ovral-28 Tablets **3423**
NuvaRing **2357**
Ortho-Cept Tablets **2395**
Ortho-Cyclen/Ortho Tri-Cyclen **2414**
Ortho Evra Transdermal System **2402**
Ortho Tri-Cyclen Lo Tablets **2421**
Seasonale Tablets **1073**
Triphasil-28 Tablets **3483**
Yasmin 28 Tablets **818**

Ethynodiol Diacetate (Estrogens tend to increase serum thyroxine-binding globulin (TBg). In a patient with a nonfunctioning thyroid gland who is receiving thyroid replacement therapy, free levothyroxine may be decreased when estrogens are started, thus increasing thyroid requirements. However, if the patient's thyroid gland has sufficient function, the decreased free thyroxine will result in a compensatory increase in thyroxine output by the thyroid. Therefore, patients without a functioning thyroid gland who are on thyroid replacement therapy may need to increase their thyroid dose if estrogens or estrogen-containing oral contraceptives are given).
No products indexed under this heading.

Glimepiride (Initiating thyroid replacement therapy may cause increases in roal hypoglycemic requirements. The effects seen are poorly understood and depend upon a variety of factors such as dose and type of thyroid preparations and endocrine status of the patient. Patients receiving oral hypoglycemics should be closely watched during initiation of thyroid replacement therapy). Products include:
Amaryl Tablets **2864**

Glipizide (Initiating thyroid replacement therapy may cause increases in roal hypoglycemic requirements. The effects seen are poorly understood and depend upon a variety of factors such as dose and type of thyroid preparations and endocrine status of the patient. Patients receiving oral hypoglycemics should be closely watched during initiation of thyroid replacement therapy).
No products indexed under this heading.

Glyburide (Initiating thyroid replacement therapy may cause increases in roal hypoglycemic requirements. The effects seen are poorly understood and depend upon a variety of factors such as dose and type of thyroid preparations and endocrine status of the patient. Patients receiving oral hypoglycemics should be closely watched during initiation of thyroid replacement therapy).
No products indexed under this heading.

Insulin, Human, Zinc Suspension (Initiating thyroid replacement therapy may cause increases in requirements. The effects seen are poorly understood and depend upon a variety of factors such as dose and type of thyroid preparations and endocrine status of the patient. Patients receivinginsulin should be closely watched during initiation of thyroid replacement therapy). Products include:
Humulin L, 100 Units **1763**
Humulin U, 100 Units **1770**

Insulin, Human NPH (Initiating thyroid replacement therapy may cause increases in requirements. The effects seen are poorly understood and depend upon a variety of factors such as dose and type of thyroid preparations and endocrine status of the patient. Patients receivinginsulin should be closely watched during initiation of thyroid replacement therapy). Products include:
Humulin N, 100 Units **1764**
Humulin N Pen **1765**
Novolin N Human Insulin 10 ml Vials **2322**
Novolin N InnoLet **2322**
Novolin N PenFill 3 ml Cartridges **2325**
Novolin R InnoLet **2322**

Insulin, Human Regular (Initiating thyroid replacement therapy may cause increases in requirements. The effects seen are poorly understood and depend upon a variety of factors such as dose and type of thyroid preparations and endocrine status of the patient. Patients receivinginsulin should be closely watched during initiation of thyroid replacement therapy). Products include:

Humulin R (U-500) 1768
Humulin R, 100 Units 1767
Novolin R Human Insulin 10 ml Vials 2322
Novolin R PenFill 2325

Insulin, Human Regular and Human NPH Mixture (Initiating thyroid replacement therapy may cause increases in requirements. The effects seen are poorly understood and depend upon a variety of factors such as dose and type of thyroid preparations and endocrine status of the patient. Patients receivinginsulin should be closely watched during initiation of thyroid replacement therapy). Products include:

Humulin 50/50, 100 Units 1760
Humulin 70/30 Pen 1761
Novolin 70/30 Human Insulin 10 ml Vials 2321
Novolin 70/30 InnoLet 2322
Novolin 70/30 PenFill 3 ml Cartridges 2325

Insulin, NPH (Initiating thyroid replacement therapy may cause increases in requirements. The effects seen are poorly understood and depend upon a variety of factors such as dose and type of thyroid preparations and endocrine status of the patient. Patients receivinginsulin should be closely watched during initiation of thyroid replacement therapy).

No products indexed under this heading.

Insulin, Regular (Initiating thyroid replacement therapy may cause increases in requirements. The effects seen are poorly understood and depend upon a variety of factors such as dose and type of thyroid preparations and endocrine status of the patient. Patients receivinginsulin should be closely watched during initiation of thyroid replacement therapy).

No products indexed under this heading.

Insulin, Zinc Crystals (Initiating thyroid replacement therapy may cause increases in requirements. The effects seen are poorly understood and depend upon a variety of factors such as dose and type of thyroid preparations and endocrine status of the patient. Patients receivinginsulin should be closely watched during initiation of thyroid replacement therapy).

No products indexed under this heading.

Insulin, Zinc Suspension (Initiating thyroid replacement therapy may cause increases in requirements. The effects seen are poorly understood and depend upon a variety of factors such as dose and type of thyroid preparations and endocrine status of the patient. Patients receivinginsulin should be closely watched during initiation of thyroid replacement therapy).

No products indexed under this heading.

Insulin Aspart, Human Regular (Initiating thyroid replacement therapy may cause increases in requirements. The effects seen are poorly understood and depend upon a variety of factors such as dose and type of thyroid preparations and endocrine status of the patient. Patients receivinginsulin should be closely watched during initiation of thyroid replacement therapy). Products include:

NovoLog Injection 2326

Insulin glargine (Initiating thyroid replacement therapy may cause increases in requirements. The effects seen are poorly understood and depend upon a variety of factors such as dose and type of thyroid preparations and endocrine status of the patient. Patients receivinginsulin should be closely watched during initiation of thyroid replacement therapy). Products include:

Lantus Injection 2925

Insulin Lispro, Human (Initiating thyroid replacement therapy may cause increases in requirements. The effects seen are poorly understood and depend upon a variety of factors such as dose and type of thyroid preparations and endocrine status of the patient. Patients receivinginsulin should be closely watched during initiation of thyroid replacement therapy). Products include:

Humalog-Pen 1751
Humalog Mix 75/25-Pen 1754

Insulin Lispro Protamine, Human (Initiating thyroid replacement therapy may cause increases in requirements. The effects seen are poorly understood and depend upon a variety of factors such as dose and type of thyroid preparations and endocrine status of the patient. Patients receivinginsulin should be closely watched during initiation of thyroid replacement therapy). Products include:

Humalog Mix 75/25-Pen 1754

Levonorgestrel (Estrogens tend to increase serum thyroxine-binding globulin (TBg). In a patient with a nonfunctioning thyroid gland who is receiving thyroid replacement therapy, free levothyroxine may be decreased when estrogens are started, thus increasing thyroid requirements. However, if the patient's thyroid gland has sufficient function, the decreased free thyroxine will result in a compensatory increase in thyroxine output by the thyroid. Therefore, patients without a functioning thyroid gland who are on thyroid replacement therapy may need to increase their thyroid dose if estrogens or estrogen-containing oral contraceptives are given). Products include:

Alesse-28 Tablets 3392
Climara Pro Transdermal System 800
Mirena Intrauterine System 810
Plan B Tablets 1068
Seasonale Tablets 1073
Triphasil-28 Tablets 3483

Mestranol (Estrogens tend to increase serum thyroxine-binding globulin (TBg). In a patient with a nonfunctioning thyroid gland who is receiving thyroid replacement therapy, free levothyroxine may be decreased when estrogens are started, thus increasing thyroid requirements. However, if the patient's thyroid gland has sufficient function, the decreased free thyroxine will result in a compensatory increase in thyroxine output by the thyroid. Therefore, patients without a functioning thyroid gland who are on thyroid replacement therapy may need to increase their thyroid dose if estrogens or estrogen-containing oral contraceptives are given).

No products indexed under this heading.

Metformin Hydrochloride (Initiating thyroid replacement therapy may cause increases in roal hypoglycemic requirements. The effects seen are poorly understood and depend upon a variety of factors such as dose and type of thyroid preparations and endocrine status of the patient. Patients receiving oral hypoglycemics should be closely watched during initiation of thyroid replacement therapy). Products include:

ActoPlus Met Tablets 3219
Avandamet Tablets 1343
Fortamet Extended-Release Tablets 1156

Miglitol (Initiating thyroid replacement therapy may cause increases in roal hypoglycemic requirements. The effects seen are poorly understood and depend upon a variety of factors such as dose and type of thyroid preparations and endocrine status of the patient. Patients receiving oral hypoglycemics should be closely watched during initiation of thyroid replacement therapy).

No products indexed under this heading.

Norethindrone (Estrogens tend to increase serum thyroxine-binding globulin (TBg). In a patient with a nonfunctioning thyroid gland who is receiving thyroid replacement therapy, free levothyroxine may be decreased when estrogens are started, thus increasing thyroid requirements. However, if the patient's thyroid gland has sufficient function, the decreased free thyroxine will result in a compensatory increase in thyroxine output by the thyroid. Therefore, patients without a functioning thyroid gland who are on thyroid replacement therapy may need to increase their thyroid dose if estrogens or estrogen-containing oral contraceptives are given). Products include:

Ortho Micronor Tablets 2411

Norethynodrel (Estrogens tend to increase serum thyroxine-binding globulin (TBg). In a patient with a nonfunctioning thyroid gland who is receiving thyroid replacement therapy, free levothyroxine may be decreased when estrogens are started, thus increasing thyroid requirements. However, if the patient's thyroid gland has sufficient function, the decreased free thyroxine will result in a compensatory increase in thyroxine output by the thyroid. Therefore, patients without a functioning thyroid gland who are on thyroid replacement therapy may need to increase their thyroid dose if estrogens or estrogen-containing oral contraceptives are given).

No products indexed under this heading.

Norgestimate (Estrogens tend to increase serum thyroxine-binding globulin (TBg). In a patient with a nonfunctioning thyroid gland who is receiving thyroid replacement therapy, free levothyroxine may be decreased when estrogens are started, thus increasing thyroid requirements. However, if the patient's thyroid gland has sufficient function, the decreased free thyroxine will result in a compensatory increase in thyroxine output by the thyroid. Therefore, patients without a functioning thyroid gland who are on thyroid replacement therapy may need to increase their thyroid dose if estrogens or estrogen-containing oral contraceptives are given). Products include:

Ortho-Cyclen/Ortho Tri-Cyclen 2414
Ortho Tri-Cyclen Lo Tablets 2421
Prefest Tablets 1069

Norgestrel (Estrogens tend to increase serum thyroxine-binding globulin (TBg). In a patient with a nonfunctioning thyroid gland who is receiving thyroid replacement therapy, free levothyroxine may be decreased when estrogens are started, thus increasing thyroid requirements. However, if the patient's thyroid gland has sufficient function, the decreased free thyroxine will result in a compensatory increase in thyroxine output by the thyroid. Therefore, patients without a functioning thyroid gland who are on thyroid replacement therapy may need to increase their thyroid dose if estrogens or estrogen-containing oral contraceptives are given). Products include:

Lo/Ovral-28 Tablets 3423

Pioglitazone Hydrochloride (Initiating thyroid replacement therapy may cause increases in roal hypoglycemic requirements. The effects seen are poorly understood and depend upon a variety of factors such as dose and type of thyroid preparations and endocrine status of the patient. Patients receiving oral hypoglycemics should be closely watched during initiation of thyroid replacement therapy). Products include:

ActoPlus Met Tablets 3219
Actos Tablets 3224

Polyestradiol Phosphate (Estrogens tend to increase serum thyroxine-binding globulin (TBg). In a patient with a nonfunctioning thyroid gland who is reveiving thyroid replacement therapy, free levothyroxine may be decreased when estrogens are started, thus increasing thyroid requirements. However, if the patient's thyroid gland has sufficient function, the decreased free thyroxine will result in a compensatory increase in thyroxine output by the thyroid. Therefore, patients without a functioning thyroid gland who are on thyroid replacement therapy may need to increase their thyroid dose if estrogens or estrogen-containing oral contraceptives are given).

No products indexed under this heading.

Quinestrol (Estrogens tend to increase serum thyroxine-binding globulin (TBg). In a patient with a nonfunctioning thyroid gland who is reveiving thyroid replacement therapy, free levothyroxine may be decreased when estrogens are started, thus increasing thyroid requirements. However, if the patient's thyroid gland has sufficient function, the decreased free thyroxine will result in a compensatory increase in thyroxine output by the thyroid. Therefore, patients without a functioning thyroid gland who are on thyroid replacement therapy may need to

increase their thyroid dose if estrogens or estrogen-containing oral contraceptives are given).

No products indexed under this heading.

Repaglinide (Initiating thyroid replacement therapy may cause increases in roal hypoglycemic requirements. The effects seen are poorly understood and depend upon a variety of factors such as dose and type of thyroid preparations and endocrine status of the patient. Patients receiving oral hypoglycemics should be closely watched during initiation of thyroid replacement therapy). Products include:

- Prandin Tablets (0.5, 1, and 2 mg) ... 2337

Rosiglitazone Maleate (Initiating thyroid replacement therapy may cause increases in roal hypoglycemic requirements. The effects seen are poorly understood and depend upon a variety of factors such as dose and type of thyroid preparations and endocrine status of the patient. Patients receiving oral hypoglycemics should be closely watched during initiation of thyroid replacement therapy). Products include:

- Avandamet Tablets ... 1343
- Avandia Tablets ... 1348

Tolazamide (Initiating thyroid replacement therapy may cause increases in roal hypoglycemic requirements. The effects seen are poorly understood and depend upon a variety of factors such as dose and type of thyroid preparations and endocrine status of the patient. Patients receiving oral hypoglycemics should be closely watched during initiation of thyroid replacement therapy).

No products indexed under this heading.

Tolbutamide (Initiating thyroid replacement therapy may cause increases in roal hypoglycemic requirements. The effects seen are poorly understood and depend upon a variety of factors such as dose and type of thyroid preparations and endocrine status of the patient. Patients receiving oral hypoglycemics should be closely watched during initiation of thyroid replacement therapy).

No products indexed under this heading.

Troglitazone (Initiating thyroid replacement therapy may cause increases in roal hypoglycemic requirements. The effects seen are poorly understood and depend upon a variety of factors such as dose and type of thyroid preparations and endocrine status of the patient. Patients receiving oral hypoglycemics should be closely watched during initiation of thyroid replacement therapy).

No products indexed under this heading.

Warfarin Sodium (Thyroid hormones appear to increase catabolism of vitamin K-dependent clotting factoes. If oral anticoagulants are also being given, compensatory increases in clotting factor synthesis are impaired. Patients stabilized on oral anticoagulants who are found to require thyroid replacement therapy should be watched very closely when thyroid is started. If a patient is truly hypothyroid, it is likely that a reduction in anticoagulant dosage will be required. No special precautions appear to be necessary when oral anticoagulant therapy is begun in a patient already stabilized on maintenance thyroid replacement therapy). Products include:

- Coumadin for Injection ... 932
- Coumadin Tablets ... 932

TIAZAC CAPSULES

(Diltiazem Hydrochloride) ... 1204

May interact with anesthetics, beta blockers, erythromycin, cardiac glycosides, phenytoin, and certain other agents. Compounds in these categories include:

Acebutolol Hydrochloride (Concomitant use of diltiazem with beta blockers may result in additive effects on cardiac conduction).

No products indexed under this heading.

Alfentanil Hydrochloride (Calcium channel blockers potentiate the depression of cardiac contractility, conductivity, and automaticity as well as vascular dilation associated with anesthetics).

No products indexed under this heading.

Amiodarone Hydrochloride (Agents known to affect cardiac contractility, such as amiodarone, may produce additive inhibition of cardiac conduction leading to increased risk of AV block). Products include:

- Pacerone Tablets ... 3337

Atenolol (Concomitant use of diltiazem with beta blockers may result in additive effects on cardiac conduction). Products include:

- Tenormin I.V. Injection ... 698
- Tenormin Tablets ... 695

Betaxolol Hydrochloride (Concomitant use of diltiazem with beta blockers may result in additive effects on cardiac conduction). Products include:

- Betoptic S Ophthalmic Suspension ... 554

Bisoprolol Fumarate (Concomitant use of diltiazem with beta blockers may result in additive effects on cardiac conduction).

No products indexed under this heading.

Carbamazepine (Co-administration has resulted in increased serum levels of carbamazepine resulting in toxicity in some patients). Products include:

- Carbatrol Capsules ... 3174
- Equetro Extended-Release Capsules ... 3178
- Tegretol/Tegretol-XR ... 2278

Carteolol Hydrochloride (Concomitant use of diltiazem with beta blockers may result in additive effects on cardiac conduction). Products include:

- Carteolol Hydrochloride Ophthalmic Solution USP, 1% ... ⊙246

Cimetidine (Co-administration has resulted in inhibition of hepatic cytochrome P450 by cimetidine producing significant increase in peak diltiazem plasma levels and AUC; am adjustment in diltiazem dosage may be warranted). Products include:

- Tagamet HB 200 Tablets ... ▣637
- Tagamet Tablets ... 1547

Cimetidine Hydrochloride (Co-administration has resulted in inhibition of hepatic cytochrome P450 by cimetidine producing significant increase in peak diltiazem plasma levels and AUC; am adjustment in diltiazem dosage may be warranted).

No products indexed under this heading.

Cyclosporine (Diltiazem inhibits cytochrome P450 3A enzyme and co-administration may result in increased cyclosporine concentrations; a reduction in cyclosporine dose may be required, especially in renal and cardiac transplant recipients). Products include:

- Gengraf Capsules ... 458
- Neoral Soft Gelatin Capsules ... 2247
- Neoral Oral Solution ... 2247
- Restasis Ophthalmic Emulsion ... 570
- Sandimmune ... 2259

Deslanoside (Concomitant use of diltiazem with digitalis may result in additive effects on cardiac conduction).

No products indexed under this heading.

Digitalis Glycoside Preparations (Concomitant use of diltiazem with digitalis may result in additive effects on cardiac conduction).

No products indexed under this heading.

Digitoxin (Concomitant use of diltiazem with digitalis may result in additive effects on cardiac conduction).

No products indexed under this heading.

Digoxin (Co-administration has resulted in increased plasma digoxin concentrations in some patients; concomitant use of diltiazem with digitalis may result in additive effects on cardiac conduction). Products include:

- Digitek Tablets ... 2146
- Lanoxicaps Capsules ... 1458
- Lanoxin Injection ... 1462
- Lanoxin Tablets ... 1468
- Lanoxin Injection Pediatric ... 1465

Enflurane (Calcium channel blockers potentiate the depression of cardiac contractility, conductivity, and automaticity as well as vascular dilation associated with anesthetics).

No products indexed under this heading.

Erythromycin (Diltiazem is both a substrate and inhibitor of the CYP4503A4; co-administration with inhibitors of this enzyme system, such as erythromycin, may have significant impact on the side effect profile of diltiazem). Products include:

- Erygel Topical Gel ... 2096
- Ery-Tab Tablets ... 447
- Erythromycin Base Filmtab Tablets ... 454
- Erythromycin Delayed-Release Capsules, USP ... 456
- PCE Dispertab Tablets ... 510

Erythromycin Estolate (Diltiazem is both a substrate and inhibitor of the CYP4503A4; co-administration with inhibitors of this enzyme system, such as erythromycin, may have significant impact on the side effect profile of diltiazem).

No products indexed under this heading.

Erythromycin Ethylsuccinate (Diltiazem is both a substrate and inhibitor of the CYP4503A4; co-administration with inhibitors of this enzyme system, such as erythromycin, may have significant impact on the side effect profile of diltiazem). Products include:

- E.E.S. ... 449
- EryPed ... 445

Erythromycin Gluceptate (Diltiazem is both a substrate and inhibitor of the CYP4503A4; co-administration with inhibitors of this enzyme system, such as erythromycin, may have significant impact on the side effect profile of diltiazem).

No products indexed under this heading.

Erythromycin Lactobionate (Diltiazem is both a substrate and inhibitor of the CYP4503A4; co-administration with inhibitors of this enzyme system, such as erythromycin, may have significant impact on the side effect profile of diltiazem).

No products indexed under this heading.

Erythromycin Stearate (Diltiazem is both a substrate and inhibitor of the CYP4503A4; co-administration with inhibitors of this enzyme system, such as erythromycin, may have significant impact on the side effect profile of diltiazem). Products include:

- Erythrocin Stearate Filmtab Tablets ... 452

Esmolol Hydrochloride (Concomitant use of diltiazem with beta blockers may result in additive effects on cardiac conduction). Products include:

- Brevibloc Concentrate ... 766
- Brevibloc Injection ... 766
- Brevibloc Double Strength Injection ... 766
- Brevibloc Premixed Injection ... 766
- Brevibloc Double Strength Premixed Injection ... 766

Fentanyl Citrate (Calcium channel blockers potentiate the depression of cardiac contractility, conductivity, and automaticity as well as vascular dilation associated with anesthetics). Products include:

- Actiq ... 993

Fluoxetine Hydrochloride (Diltiazem undergoes biotransformation by cytochrome P450 mixed funciton oxidase; co-administration with other agents which follow the same route of biotransformation may result in competitve inhibition of metabolism). Products include:

- Prozac Pulvules and Liquid ... 1771
- Symbyax Capsules ... 1788

Fluvoxamine Maleate (Diltiazem undergoes biotransformation by cytochrome P450 mixed funciton oxidase; co-administration with other agents which follow the same route of biotransformation may result in competitve inhibition of metabolism).

No products indexed under this heading.

Fosphenytoin Sodium (Diltiazem is both a substrate and inhibitor of the CYP4503A4; co-administration with inducers of this enzyme system, such as phenytoin, may have significant impact on the efficacy of diltiazem).

No products indexed under this heading.

Halothane (Calcium channel blockers potentiate the depression of cardiac contractility, conductivity, and automaticity as well as vascular dilation associated with anesthetics).

No products indexed under this heading.

Isoflurane (Calcium channel blockers potentiate the depression of cardiac contractility, conductivity, and automaticity as well as vascular dilation associated with anesthetics).
No products indexed under this heading.

Ketamine Hydrochloride (Calcium channel blockers potentiate the depression of cardiac contractility, conductivity, and automaticity as well as vascular dilation associated with anesthetics).
No products indexed under this heading.

Ketoconazole (Diltiazem is both a substrate and inhibitor of the CYP4503A4; co-administration with inhibitors of this enzyme system, such as ketoconazole, may have significant impact on the side effect profile of diltiazem). Products include:
Nizoral A-D Shampoo, 1% 1839
Nizoral 2% Shampoo 1838

Labetalol Hydrochloride (Concomitant use of diltiazem with beta blockers may result in additive effects on cardiac conduction).
No products indexed under this heading.

Levobunolol Hydrochloride (Concomitant use of diltiazem with beta blockers may result in additive effects on cardiac conduction). Products include:
Betagan Ophthalmic Solution, USP .... ⊙217

Lovastatin (Co-administration has resulted in a 3-4 times increase in mean lovastatin AUC and Cmax). Products include:
Advicor Tablets 1694
Altoprev Extended-Release Tablets 1151
Mevacor Tablets 1996

Methohexital Sodium (Calcium channel blockers potentiate the depression of cardiac contractility, conductivity, and automaticity as well as vascular dilation associated with anesthetics).
No products indexed under this heading.

Metipranolol Hydrochloride (Concomitant use of diltiazem with beta blockers may result in additive effects on cardiac conduction).
No products indexed under this heading.

Metoprolol Succinate (Concomitant use of diltiazem with beta blockers may result in additive effects on cardiac conduction). Products include:
Toprol-XL Tablets 660

Metoprolol Tartrate (Concomitant use of diltiazem with beta blockers may result in additive effects on cardiac conduction).
No products indexed under this heading.

Midazolam Hydrochloride (Co-administration has resulted in increased AUC of midazolam by 3-4 fold and the Cmax by 2-fold; the elimination half-life of midazolam also increased during co-administration).
No products indexed under this heading.

Nadolol (Concomitant use of diltiazem with beta blockers may result in additive effects on cardiac conduction). Products include:
Nadolol Tablets 2121

Penbutolol Sulfate (Concomitant use of diltiazem with beta blockers may result in additive effects on cardiac conduction).
No products indexed under this heading.

Phenobarbital (Diltiazem is both a substrate and inhibitor of the CYP4503A4; co-administration with inducers of this enzyme system, such as phenobarbital, may have significant impact on the efficacy of diltiazem).
No products indexed under this heading.

Phenytoin (Diltiazem is both a substrate and inhibitor of the CYP4503A4; co-administration with inducers of this enzyme system, such as phenytoin, may have significant impact on the efficacy of diltiazem).
No products indexed under this heading.

Phenytoin Sodium (Diltiazem is both a substrate and inhibitor of the CYP4503A4; co-administration with inducers of this enzyme system, such as phenytoin, may have significant impact on the efficacy of diltiazem). Products include:
Phenytek Capsules 2153

Pindolol (Concomitant use of diltiazem with beta blockers may result in additive effects on cardiac conduction).
No products indexed under this heading.

Propofol (Calcium channel blockers potentiate the depression of cardiac contractility, conductivity, and automaticity as well as vascular dilation associated with anesthetics). Products include:
Diprivan Injectable Emulsion 676

Propranolol Hydrochloride (Concomitant use of diltiazem with propranolol resulted in increased propranolol levels and bioavailability of propanolol was increased by approximately 50%; Concurrent therapy of diltiazem with beta blockers may result in additive effects on cardiac conduction). Products include:
Inderal LA Long-Acting Capsules 3421
InnoPran XL Capsules 2728

Ranitidine Hydrochloride (Co-administration produces smaller, nonsignificant increase in diltiazem plasma levels). Products include:
Zantac 1597
Zantac Injection 1593
Zantac 75 Tablets .... ▣715
Zantac 150 Maximum Strength Tablets.. ▣715
Zantac Injection Pharmacy Bulk Package 1595

Remifentanil Hydrochloride (Calcium channel blockers potentiate the depression of cardiac contractility, conductivity, and automaticity as well as vascular dilation associated with anesthetics).
No products indexed under this heading.

Rifampin (Co-administration has resulted in lowered diltiazem plasma concentrations to undetectable levels; co-administration should be avoided).
No products indexed under this heading.

Ritonavir (Diltiazem is both a substrate and inhibitor of the CYP4503A4; co-administration with inhibitors of this enzyme system, such as ritonavir, may have significant impact on the side effect profile of diltiazem). Products include:
Kaletra 474
Norvir 499

Sotalol Hydrochloride (Concomitant use of diltiazem with beta blockers may result in additive effects on cardiac conduction).
No products indexed under this heading.

Sufentanil Citrate (Calcium channel blockers potentiate the depression of cardiac contractility, conductivity, and automaticity as well as vascular dilation associated with anesthetics).
No products indexed under this heading.

Thiamylal Sodium (Calcium channel blockers potentiate the depression of cardiac contractility, conductivity, and automaticity as well as vascular dilation associated with anesthetics).
No products indexed under this heading.

Timolol Hemihydrate (Concomitant use of diltiazem with beta blockers may result in additive effects on cardiac conduction). Products include:
Betimol Ophthalmic Solution 3371
Betimol Ophthalmic Solution .... ⊙283

Timolol Maleate (Concomitant use of diltiazem with beta blockers may result in additive effects on cardiac conduction). Products include:
Blocadren Tablets 1891
Cosopt Sterile Ophthalmic Solution 1910
Timolide Tablets 2056
Timoptic in Ocudose 2061
Timoptic Sterile Ophthalmic Solution 2058
Timoptic-XE Sterile Ophthalmic Gel Forming Solution 2062

Triazolam (Co-administration has resulted in increased AUC of triazolam by 3-4 fold and the Cmax by 2-fold; the elimination half-life of triazolam also increased during co-administration).
No products indexed under this heading.

TICLID TABLETS

(Ticlopidine Hydrochloride) 2813
May interact with antacids, anticoagulants, non-steroidal anti-inflammatory agents, phenytoin, xanthines, and certain other agents. Compounds in these categories include:

Aluminum Carbonate (18% decrease in plasma levels of ticlopidine when administered after antacids).
No products indexed under this heading.

Aluminum Hydroxide (18% decrease in plasma levels of ticlopidine when administered after antacids). Products include:
Gaviscon Regular Strength Liquid .. ▣620
Gaviscon Regular Strength Tablets.. ▣619
Gaviscon Extra Strength Liquid ...... ▣620
Gaviscon Extra Strength Tablets .... ▣619
Maalox Max Maximum Strength Antacid/Anti-Gas Liquid................. 2165
Maalox Regular Strength Antacid/Antigas Liquid.................. 2164

Aminophylline (Co-administration may result in significant increase in the theophylline elimination half-life and a comparable reduction in total plasma clearance of theophylline).
No products indexed under this heading.

Anisindione (The tolerance and safety of co-administration has not been established; anticoagulant should be discontinued prior to Ticlid administration). Products include:
Miradon Tablets 3056

Ardeparin Sodium (The tolerance and safety of co-administration has not been established; anticoagulant should be discontinued prior to Ticlid administration).
No products indexed under this heading.

Aspirin (Ticlopidine potentiates the effect of aspirin on collagen-induced platelet aggregation; concurrent use is not recommended). Products include:
Aggrenox Capsules 855
Bayer, Aspirin Regimen .... ▣606
Bayer Aspirin Tablets 3515
BC Powder .... ▣612
BC Allergy Sinus Cold Powder .... ▣612
Arthritis Strength BC Powder .... ▣612
BC Sinus Cold Powder .... ▣612
Ecotrin Enteric Coated Aspirin Low, Regular and Maximum Strength Tablets.......................... 1627
Goody's Body Pain Formula Powder.. ▣621
Goody's Extra Strength Headache Powder....................... ▣621
Goody's Extra Strength Pain Relief Tablets.............................. ▣621
Percodan Tablets 1115
St. Joseph 81 mg Aspirin Chewable and Enteric Coated Tablets.. 1841

Celecoxib (Ticlopidine potentiates the effect of NSAIDS on platelet aggregation). Products include:
Celebrex Capsules 3130

Cimetidine (Chronic administration of cimetidine reduces the clearance of a single dose of ticlopidine by 50%). Products include:
Tagamet HB 200 Tablets .... ▣637
Tagamet Tablets 1547

Cimetidine Hydrochloride (Chronic administration of cimetidine reduces the clearance of a single dose of ticlopidine by 50%).
No products indexed under this heading.

Dalteparin Sodium (The tolerance and safety of co-administration has not been established; anticoagulant should be discontinued prior to Ticlid administration). Products include:
Fragmin Injection 2638

Danaparoid Sodium (The tolerance and safety of co-administration has not been established; anticoagulant should be discontinued prior to Ticlid administration).
No products indexed under this heading.

Diclofenac Potassium (Ticlopidine potentiates the effect of NSAIDS on platelet aggregation). Products include:
Cataflam Tablets 2173

Diclofenac Sodium (Ticlopidine potentiates the effect of NSAIDS on platelet aggregation). Products include:
Arthrotec Tablets 3126
Voltaren Ophthalmic Solution 2300
Voltaren Tablets 2298
Voltaren-XR Tablets 2301

Dicumarol (The tolerance and safety of co-administration has not been established; anticoagulant should be discontinued prior to Ticlid administration).
No products indexed under this heading.

Digoxin (Co-administration resulted in slight decrease in digoxin plasma levels; little or no change in efficacy of digoxin). Products include:
Digitek Tablets 2146
Lanoxicaps Capsules 1458
Lanoxin Injection 1462
Lanoxin Tablets 1468
Lanoxin Injection Pediatric 1465

Dyphylline (Co-administration may result in significant increase in the theophylline elimination half-life and a comparable reduction in total plasma clearance of theophylline).
No products indexed under this heading.

Enoxaparin Sodium (The tolerance and safety of co-administration has not been established; anticoagulant should be discontinued prior to Ticlid administration). Products include:
Lovenox Injection 2931

Etodolac (Ticlopidine potentiates the effect of NSAIDS on platelet aggregation).
No products indexed under this heading.

Fenoprofen Calcium (Ticlopidine potentiates the effect of NSAIDS on platelet aggregation). Products include:
Nalfon Capsules 2504

Flurbiprofen (Ticlopidine potentiates the effect of NSAIDS on platelet aggregation).
No products indexed under this heading.

Fondaparinux Sodium (The tolerance and safety of co-administration has not been established; anticoagulant should be discontinued prior to Ticlid administration). Products include:
Arixtra Injection 1325

Fosphenytoin Sodium (Co-administration has resulted in several cases of elevated phenytoin plasma levels with associated somnolence and lethargy; caution is advised).
No products indexed under this heading.

Heparin Calcium (The tolerance and safety of co-administration has not been established; anticoagulant should be discontinued prior to Ticlid administration).
No products indexed under this heading.

Heparin Sodium (The tolerance and safety of co-administration has not been established; anticoagulant should be discontinued prior to Ticlid administration).
No products indexed under this heading.

Ibuprofen (Ticlopidine potentiates the effect of NSAIDS on platelet aggregation). Products include:
Advil Allergy Sinus Caplets .... ▣737
Advil .... ▣737
Children's Advil Suspension .... ▣742
Children's Advil Chewable Tablets .. ▣741
Advil Cold & Sinus .... ▣739
Advil Flu & Body Ache Caplets .... ▣739
Children's Advil Cold Suspension .... ▣741
Infants' Advil Concentrated Drops .. ▣743
Junior Strength Advil Swallow Tablets .... ▣740
Advil Migraine Liquigels .... ▣740
Advil Multi-Symptom Cold Caplets .... ▣738
Combunox Tablets 1183
Children's Motrin Oral Suspension and Chewable Tablets 1837
Children's Motrin Cold Non-Staining Dye-Free Oral Suspension 1838
Children's Motrin Cold Oral Suspension 1838
Children's Motrin Non-Staining Dye-Free Oral Suspension 1837
Motrin Cold & Sinus Caplets 1836
Motrin IB Tablets and Caplets 1836
Infants' Motrin Concentrated Drops 1837
Infants' Motrin Non-Staining Dye-Free Drops 1837
Junior Strength Motrin Caplets and Chewable Tablets 1837
Vicoprofen Tablets 533

Indomethacin (Ticlopidine potentiates the effect of NSAIDS on platelet aggregation). Products include:
Indocin 1968

Indomethacin Sodium Trihydrate (Ticlopidine potentiates the effect of NSAIDS on platelet aggregation). Products include:
Indocin I.V. 1973

Ketoprofen (Ticlopidine potentiates the effect of NSAIDS on platelet aggregation).
No products indexed under this heading.

Ketorolac Tromethamine (Ticlopidine potentiates the effect of NSAIDS on platelet aggregation). Products include:
Acular Ophthalmic Solution 561
Acular LS Ophthalmic Solution 562

Low Molecular Weight Heparins (The tolerance and safety of co-administration has not been established; anticoagulant should be discontinued prior to Ticlid administration).
No products indexed under this heading.

Magaldrate (18% decrease in plasma levels of ticlopidine when administered after antacids).
No products indexed under this heading.

Magnesium Hydroxide (18% decrease in plasma levels of ticlopidine when administered after antacids). Products include:
Maalox Max Maximum Strength Antacid/Anti-Gas Liquid 2165
Maalox Regular Strength Antacid/Antigas Liquid 2164
Pepcid Complete Chewable Tablets 1672
Rolaids Tablets .... ▣707
Extra Strength Rolaids Tablets .... ▣707
Rolaids Multi-Symptom Antacid & Antigas Tablets .... ▣708

Magnesium Oxide (18% decrease in plasma levels of ticlopidine when administered after antacids). Products include:
Beelith Tablets 784
PremCal Light, Regular, and Extra Strength Tablets .... ▣762

Meclofenamate Sodium (Ticlopidine potentiates the effect of NSAIDS on platelet aggregation).
No products indexed under this heading.

Mefenamic Acid (Ticlopidine potentiates the effect of NSAIDS on platelet aggregation).
No products indexed under this heading.

Meloxicam (Ticlopidine potentiates the effect of NSAIDS on platelet aggregation). Products include:
Mobic Oral Suspension 893
Mobic Tablets 893

Nabumetone (Ticlopidine potentiates the effect of NSAIDS on platelet aggregation). Products include:
Relafen Tablets 1523

Naproxen (Ticlopidine potentiates the effect of NSAIDS on platelet aggregation). Products include:
EC-Naprosyn Delayed-Release Tablets 2769
Naprosyn Suspension 2769
Naprosyn Tablets 2769
Prevacid NapraPAC 3277

Naproxen Sodium (Ticlopidine potentiates the effect of NSAIDS on platelet aggregation). Products include:
Aleve Tablets, Caplets and Gelcaps .... ▣605
Anaprox Tablets 2769
Anaprox DS Tablets 2769

Oxaprozin (Ticlopidine potentiates the effect of NSAIDS on platelet aggregation).
No products indexed under this heading.

Phenylbutazone (Ticlopidine potentiates the effect of NSAIDS on platelet aggregation).
No products indexed under this heading.

Phenytoin (Co-administration has resulted in several cases of elevated phenytoin plasma levels with associated somnolence and lethargy; caution is advised).
No products indexed under this heading.

Phenytoin Sodium (Co-administration has resulted in several cases of elevated phenytoin plasma levels with associated somnolence and lethargy; caution is advised). Products include:
Phenytek Capsules 2153

Piroxicam (Ticlopidine potentiates the effect of NSAIDS on platelet aggregation).
No products indexed under this heading.

Propranolol Hydrochloride (Exercise caution if co-administered; *in vitro* studies indicate no alteration of plasma protein binding of propranolol). Products include:
Inderal LA Long-Acting Capsules 3421
InnoPran XL Capsules 2728

Rofecoxib (Ticlopidine potentiates the effect of NSAIDS on platelet aggregation).
No products indexed under this heading.

Sodium Bicarbonate (18% decrease in plasma levels of ticlopidine when administered after antacids). Products include:
Ceo-Two Evacuant Suppository .... ▣607
Colyte with Flavor Packs for Oral Solution 3102
HalfLytely and Bisacodyl Tablets Bowel Prep Kit with Flavors Packs 915
TriLyte with Flavor Packs for Oral Solution 3114

Sulindac (Ticlopidine potentiates the effect of NSAIDS on platelet aggregation). Products include:
Clinoril Tablets 1899

Theophylline (Co-administration may result in significant increase in the theophylline elimination half-life and a comparable reduction in total plasma clearance of theophylline).
No products indexed under this heading.

Theophylline Anhydrous (Co-administration may result in significant increase in the theophylline elimination half-life and a comparable reduction in total plasma clearance of theophylline). Products include:
Uniphyl Tablets 2708

Theophylline Calcium Salicylate (Co-administration may result in significant increase in the theophylline elimination half-life and a comparable reduction in total plasma clearance of theophylline).
No products indexed under this heading.

Theophylline Dihydroxypropyl (Glyceryl) (Co-administration may result in significant increase in the theophylline elimination half-life and a comparable reduction in total plasma clearance of theophylline).
No products indexed under this heading.

Theophylline Ethylenediamine (Co-administration may result in significant increase in the theophylline elimination half-life and a comparable reduction in total plasma clearance of theophylline).
No products indexed under this heading.

Theophylline Sodium Glycinate (Co-administration may result in significant increase in the theophylline elimination half-life and a comparable reduction in total plasma clearance of theophylline).
No products indexed under this heading.

Tinzaparin Sodium (The tolerance and safety of co-administration has not been established; anticoagulant should be discontinued prior to Ticlid administration).
No products indexed under this heading.

Tolmetin Sodium (Ticlopidine potentiates the effect of NSAIDS on platelet aggregation).
No products indexed under this heading.

Valdecoxib (Ticlopidine potentiates the effect of NSAIDS on platelet aggregation).
No products indexed under this heading.

Warfarin Sodium (The tolerance and safety of co-administration has not been established; anticoagulant should be discontinued prior to Ticlid administration). Products include:
Coumadin for Injection 932
Coumadin Tablets 932

Food Interactions

Meal, unspecified (Administration after meals results in a 20% increase in the AUC of ticlopidine).

TIMENTIN ADD-VANTAGE

(Clavulanate Potassium, Ticarcillin Disodium) 1556
See Timentin IV Infusion

TIMENTIN INJECTION GALAXY CONTAINER

(Clavulanate Potassium, Ticarcillin Disodium) 1559
See Timentin IV Infusion

TIMENTIN IV INFUSION
(Clavulanate Potassium, Ticarcillin Disodium).. 1553
May interact with aminoglycosides and certain other agents. Compounds in these categories include:

Amikacin Sulfate (The mixing of Timentin with an aminoglycoside in solutions for parental administration can result in substantial inactivation of the aminoglycoside).
No products indexed under this heading.

Gentamicin Sulfate (The mixing of Timentin with an aminoglycoside in solutions for parental administration can result in substantial inactivation of the aminoglycoside). Products include:
Garamycin Injectable 3028
Genoptic Sterile Ophthalmic Solution.. ⊙227
Pred-G Ophthalmic Suspension ...... ⊙234
Pred-G Sterile Ophthalmic Ointment.. ⊙235

Kanamycin Sulfate (The mixing of Timentin with an aminoglycoside in solutions for parental administration can result in substantial inactivation of the aminoglycoside).
No products indexed under this heading.

Probenecid (Interferes with the renal tubular secretion of ticarcillin, thereby increasing serum concentrations and prolonged serum half-life of the antibiotic).
No products indexed under this heading.

Streptomycin Sulfate (The mixing of Timentin with an aminoglycoside in solutions for parental administration can result in substantial inactivation of the aminoglycoside).
No products indexed under this heading.

Tobramycin (The mixing of Timentin with an aminoglycoside in solutions for parental administration can result in substantial inactivation of the aminoglycoside). Products include:
TOBI Solution for Inhalation 1015
TobraDex Ophthalmic Ointment 558
TobraDex Ophthalmic Suspension ... 558
Zylet Ophthalmic Suspension 3508

Tobramycin Sulfate (The mixing of Timentin with an aminoglycoside in solutions for parental administration can result in substantial inactivation of the aminoglycoside).
No products indexed under this heading.

TIMENTIN PHARMACY BULK PACKAGE
(Clavulanate Potassium, Ticarcillin Disodium).. 1562
See Timentin IV Infusion

TIMOLIDE TABLETS
(Hydrochlorothiazide, Timolol Maleate).. 2056
May interact with antihypertensives, catecholamine depleting drugs, calcium channel blockers, cardiac glycosides, oral hypoglycemic agents, insulin, lithium preparations, non-steroidal anti-inflammatory agents, quinidine, and certain other agents. Compounds in these categories include:

Acarbose (Beta-blockers may mask the signs and symptoms of hypoglycemia). Products include:
Precose Tablets 776

Acebutolol Hydrochloride (Timolide may potentiate the action of other antihypertensive agents used concomitantly).
No products indexed under this heading.

Amlodipine Besylate (Hypotension, AV conduction disturbances, and left ventricular failure have been reported in some patients receiving beta-adrenergic blocking agents when an oral calcium antagonist was added to the treatment regimen). Products include:
Caduet Tablets 2507
Lotrel Capsules 2238
Norvasc Tablets 2529

Atenolol (Timolide may potentiate the action of other antihypertensive agents used concomitantly). Products include:
Tenormin I.V. Injection 698
Tenormin Tablets 695

Benazepril Hydrochloride (Timolide may potentiate the action of other antihypertensive agents used concomitantly). Products include:
Lotensin Tablets 2232
Lotensin HCT Tablets 2235
Lotrel Capsules 2238

Bendroflumethiazide (Timolide may potentiate the action of other antihypertensive agents used concomitantly).
No products indexed under this heading.

Bepridil Hydrochloride (Hypotension, AV conduction disturbances, and left ventricular failure have been reported in some patients receiving beta-adrenergic blocking agents when an oral calcium antagonist was added to the treatment regimen).
No products indexed under this heading.

Betaxolol Hydrochloride (Timolide may potentiate the action of other antihypertensive agents used concomitantly). Products include:
Betoptic S Ophthalmic Suspension.. 554

Bisoprolol Fumarate (Timolide may potentiate the action of other antihypertensive agents used concomitantly).
No products indexed under this heading.

Candesartan Cilexetil (Timolide may potentiate the action of other antihypertensive agents used concomitantly). Products include:
Atacand Tablets 634
Atacand HCT 637

Captopril (Timolide may potentiate the action of other antihypertensive agents used concomitantly). Products include:
Captopril Tablets 2114

Carteolol Hydrochloride (Timolide may potentiate the action of other antihypertensive agents used concomitantly). Products include:
Carteolol Hydrochloride Ophthalmic Solution USP, 1%....... ⊙246

Celecoxib (NSAIDs reduce the diuretic, natriuretic, and antihypertensive effects of Timolide). Products include:
Celebrex Capsules 3130

Chlorothiazide (Timolide may potentiate the action of other antihypertensive agents used concomitantly). Products include:
Aldoclor Tablets 1881
Diuril Oral 1936

Chlorothiazide Sodium (Timolide may potentiate the action of other antihypertensive agents used concomitantly). Products include:
Diuril Sodium Intravenous 1934

Chlorpropamide (Beta-blockers may mask the signs and symptoms of hypoglycemia).
No products indexed under this heading.

Chlorthalidone (Timolide may potentiate the action of other antihypertensive agents used concomitantly). Products include:
Clorpres Tablets 2139

Cholestyramine (Cholestyramine resin has potential of binding hydrochlorothiazide and reducing its absorption from the GI tract by up to 85%).
No products indexed under this heading.

Clonidine (Beta adrenergic blocking agents may exacerbate the rebound hypertension which can follow the withdrawal of clonidine). Products include:
Catapres-TTS 875

Clonidine Hydrochloride (Beta adrenergic blocking agents may exacerbate the rebound hypertension which can follow the withdrawal of clonidine). Products include:
Catapres Tablets 874
Clorpres Tablets 2139

Colestipol Hydrochloride (Colestipol resin has potential of binding hydrochlorothiazide and reducing its absorption from the GI tract by up to 43%).
No products indexed under this heading.

Deserpidine (Close observation of the patient is recommended when Timolide is administered to patients receiving catecholamine-depleting drugs such as reserpine, because of possible additive effects and the production of hypotension and/or marked bradycardia, which may produce vertigo, syncope, or postural hypotension).
No products indexed under this heading.

Deslanoside (The concomitant use of beta-adrenergic blocking agents with digitalis and either diltiazem or verapamil may have additive effects in prolonging AV conduction time. Hypokalemia may develop during thiazide therapy and may cause cardiac arrhythmia and may also sensitize or exaggerate the response of the heart to the toxic effects of digitalis (e.g., increased ventricular irritability)).
No products indexed under this heading.

Diazoxide (Timolide may potentiate the action of other antihypertensive agents used concomitantly). Products include:
Hyperstat I.V. Injection 3031

Diclofenac Potassium (NSAIDs reduce the diuretic, natriuretic, and antihypertensive effects of Timolide). Products include:
Cataflam Tablets 2173

Diclofenac Sodium (NSAIDs reduce the diuretic, natriuretic, and antihypertensive effects of Timolide). Products include:
Arthrotec Tablets 3126
Voltaren Ophthalmic Solution 2300
Voltaren Tablets 2298
Voltaren-XR Tablets 2301

Digitalis Glycoside Preparations (The concomitant use of beta-adrenergic blocking agents with digitalis and either diltiazem or verapamil may have additive effects in prolonging AV conduction time. Hypokalemia may develop during thiazide therapy and may cause cardiac arrhythmia and may also sensitize or exaggerate the response of the heart to the toxic effects of digitalis (e.g., increased ventricular irritability)).
No products indexed under this heading.

Digitoxin (The concomitant use of beta-adrenergic blocking agents with digitalis and either diltiazem or verapamil may have additive effects in prolonging AV conduction time. Hypokalemia may develop during thiazide therapy and may cause cardiac arrhythmia and may also sensitize or exaggerate the response of the heart to the toxic effects of digitalis (e.g., increased ventricular irritability)).
No products indexed under this heading.

Digoxin (The concomitant use of beta-adrenergic blocking agents with digitalis and either diltiazem or verapamil may have additive effects in prolonging AV conduction time. Hypokalemia may develop during thiazide therapy and may cause cardiac arrhythmia and may also sensitize or exaggerate the response of the heart to the toxic effects of digitalis (e.g., increased ventricular irritability)). Products include:
Digitek Tablets 2146
Lanoxicaps Capsules 1458
Lanoxin Injection 1462
Lanoxin Tablets 1468
Lanoxin Injection Pediatric 1465

Diltiazem Hydrochloride (Left ventricular failure and AV conduction disturbances). Products include:
Cardizem LA Extended Release Tablets.. 1699
Tiazac Capsules 1204

Doxazosin Mesylate (Timolide may potentiate the action of other antihypertensive agents used concomitantly).
No products indexed under this heading.

Enalapril Maleate (Timolide may potentiate the action of other antihypertensive agents used concomitantly). Products include:
Vaseretic Tablets 2073
Vasotec I.V. Injection 2076

Enalaprilat (Timolide may potentiate the action of other antihypertensive agents used concomitantly).
No products indexed under this heading.

Eprosartan Mesylate (Timolide may potentiate the action of other antihypertensive agents used concomitantly). Products include:
Teveten Tablets 1707
Teveten HCT Tablets 1710

Esmolol Hydrochloride (Timolide may potentiate the action of other antihypertensive agents used concomitantly). Products include:
Brevibloc Concentrate 766
Brevibloc Injection 766
Brevibloc Double Strength Injection.. 766
Brevibloc Premixed Injection 766
Brevibloc Double Strength Premixed Injection 766

Etodolac (NSAIDs reduce the diuretic, natriuretic, and antihypertensive effects of Timolide).
No products indexed under this heading.

Felodipine (Hypotension, AV conduction disturbances, and left ventricular failure have been reported in some patients receiving beta-adrenergic blocking agents when an oral calcium antagonist was added to the treatment regimen). Products include:
Plendil Extended-Release Tablets 651

Fenoprofen Calcium (NSAIDs reduce the diuretic, natriuretic, and antihypertensive effects of Timolide). Products include:
Nalfon Capsules 2504

Flurbiprofen (NSAIDs reduce the diuretic, natriuretic, and antihypertensive effects of Timolide).
No products indexed under this heading.

Fosinopril Sodium (Timolide may potentiate the action of other antihypertensive agents used concomitantly).
No products indexed under this heading.

Furosemide (Timolide may potentiate the action of other antihypertensive agents used concomitantly). Products include:
Furosemide Tablets 2117

Glimepiride (Beta-blockers may mask the signs and symptoms of hypoglycemia). Products include:
Amaryl Tablets 2864

Glipizide (Beta-blockers may mask the signs and symptoms of hypoglycemia).
No products indexed under this heading.

Glyburide (Beta-blockers may mask the signs and symptoms of hypoglycemia).
No products indexed under this heading.

Guanabenz Acetate (Timolide may potentiate the action of other antihypertensive agents used concomitantly).
No products indexed under this heading.

Guanethidine Monosulfate (Close observation of the patient is recommended when Timolide is administered to patients receiving catecholamine-depleting drugs such as reserpine, because of possible additive effects and the production of hypotension and/or marked bradycardia, which may produce vertigo, syncope, or postural hypotension).
No products indexed under this heading.

Hydralazine Hydrochloride (Timolide may potentiate the action of other antihypertensive agents used concomitantly). Products include:
BiDil Tablets 2161

Hydroflumethiazide (Timolide may potentiate the action of other antihypertensive agents used concomitantly).
No products indexed under this heading.

Ibuprofen (NSAIDs reduce the diuretic, natriuretic, and antihypertensive effects of Timolide). Products include:
Advil Allergy Sinus Caplets ..... ◘ 737
Advil ..... ◘ 737
Children's Advil Suspension ..... ◘ 742
Children's Advil Chewable Tablets ..... ◘ 741
Advil Cold & Sinus ..... ◘ 739
Advil Flu & Body Ache Caplets ..... ◘ 739
Children's Advil Cold Suspension ..... ◘ 741
Infants' Advil Concentrated Drops ..... ◘ 743
Junior Strength Advil Swallow Tablets ..... ◘ 740
Advil Migraine Liquigels ..... ◘ 740
Advil Multi-Symptom Cold Caplets ..... ◘ 738
Combunox Tablets 1183
Children's Motrin Oral Suspension and Chewable Tablets 1837
Children's Motrin Cold Non-Staining Dye-Free Oral Suspension 1838
Children's Motrin Cold Oral Suspension 1838
Children's Motrin Non-Staining Dye-Free Oral Suspension 1837
Motrin Cold & Sinus Caplets 1836
Motrin IB Tablets and Caplets 1836
Infants' Motrin Concentrated Drops 1837
Infants' Motrin Non-Staining Dye-Free Drops 1837
Junior Strength Motrin Caplets and Chewable Tablets 1837
Vicoprofen Tablets 533

Indapamide (Timolide may potentiate the action of other antihypertensive agents used concomitantly). Products include:
Indapamide Tablets 2119

Indomethacin (NSAIDs reduce the diuretic, natriuretic, and antihypertensive effects of Timolide). Products include:
Indocin 1968

Indomethacin Sodium Trihydrate (NSAIDs reduce the diuretic, natriuretic, and antihypertensive effects of Timolide). Products include:
Indocin I.V. 1973

Insulin, Human, Zinc Suspension (Beta-blockers may mask the signs and symptoms of acute hypoglycemia. Insulin requirements may be altered). Products include:
Humulin L, 100 Units 1763
Humulin U, 100 Units 1770

Insulin, Human NPH (Beta-blockers may mask the signs and symptoms of acute hypoglycemia. Insulin requirements may be altered). Products include:
Humulin N, 100 Units 1764
Humulin N Pen 1765
Novolin N Human Insulin 10 ml Vials 2322
Novolin N InnoLet 2322
Novolin N PenFill 3 ml Cartridges 2325
Novolin R InnoLet 2322

Insulin, Human Regular (Beta-blockers may mask the signs and symptoms of acute hypoglycemia. Insulin requirements may be altered). Products include:
Humulin R (U-500) 1768
Humulin R, 100 Units 1767
Novolin R Human Insulin 10 ml Vials 2322
Novolin R PenFill 2325

Insulin, Human Regular and Human NPH Mixture (Beta-blockers may mask the signs and symptoms of acute hypoglycemia. Insulin requirements may be altered). Products include:
Humulin 50/50, 100 Units 1760
Humulin 70/30 Pen 1761
Novolin 70/30 Human Insulin 10 ml Vials 2321
Novolin 70/30 InnoLet 2322
Novolin 70/30 PenFill 3 ml Cartridges 2325

Insulin, NPH (Beta-blockers may mask the signs and symptoms of acute hypoglycemia. Insulin requirements may be altered).
No products indexed under this heading.

Insulin, Regular (Beta-blockers may mask the signs and symptoms of acute hypoglycemia. Insulin requirements may be altered).
No products indexed under this heading.

Insulin, Zinc Crystals (Beta-blockers may mask the signs and symptoms of acute hypoglycemia. Insulin requirements may be altered).
No products indexed under this heading.

Insulin, Zinc Suspension (Beta-blockers may mask the signs and symptoms of acute hypoglycemia. Insulin requirements may be altered).
No products indexed under this heading.

Insulin Aspart, Human Regular (Beta-blockers may mask the signs and symptoms of acute hypoglycemia. Insulin requirements may be altered). Products include:
NovoLog Injection 2326

Insulin glargine (Beta-blockers may mask the signs and symptoms of acute hypoglycemia. Insulin requirements may be altered). Products include:
Lantus Injection 2925

Insulin Lispro, Human (Beta-blockers may mask the signs and symptoms of acute hypoglycemia. Insulin requirements may be altered). Products include:
Humalog-Pen 1751
Humalog Mix 75/25-Pen 1754

Insulin Lispro Protamine, Human (Beta-blockers may mask the signs and symptoms of acute hypoglycemia. Insulin requirements may be altered). Products include:
Humalog Mix 75/25-Pen 1754

Irbesartan (Timolide may potentiate the action of other antihypertensive agents used concomitantly). Products include:
Avalide Tablets 922
Avalide Tablets 2889
Avapro Tablets 925
Avapro Tablets 2886

Isradipine (Hypotension, AV conduction disturbances, and left ventricular failure have been reported in some patients receiving beta-adrenergic blocking agents when an oral calcium antagonist was added to the treatment regimen). Products include:
DynaCirc CR Tablets 2726

Ketoprofen (NSAIDs reduce the diuretic, natriuretic, and antihypertensive effects of Timolide).
No products indexed under this heading.

Ketorolac Tromethamine (NSAIDs reduce the diuretic, natriuretic, and antihypertensive effects of Timolide). Products include:
Acular Ophthalmic Solution 561
Acular LS Ophthalmic Solution 562

Labetalol Hydrochloride (Timolide may potentiate the action of other antihypertensive agents used concomitantly).
No products indexed under this heading.

Lisinopril (Timolide may potentiate the action of other antihypertensive agents used concomitantly). Products include:
Prinivil Tablets 2029
Prinzide Tablets 2033
Zestoretic Tablets 701
Zestril Tablets 704

Lithium (Lithium generally should not be given with diuretics because they reduce its renal clearance and add a high risk of lithium toxicity).
No products indexed under this heading.

Lithium Carbonate (Lithium generally should not be given with diuretics because they reduce its renal clearance and add a high risk of lithium toxicity). Products include:
Eskalith 1406
Lithobid Tablets 1670

Lithium Citrate (Lithium generally should not be given with diuretics because they reduce its renal clearance and add a high risk of lithium toxicity).
No products indexed under this heading.

Losartan Potassium (Timolide may potentiate the action of other antihypertensive agents used concomitantly). Products include:
Cozaar Tablets 1913
Hyzaar 1964

Mecamylamine Hydrochloride (Timolide may potentiate the action of other antihypertensive agents used concomitantly). Products include:
Inversine Tablets 3286

Meclofenamate Sodium (NSAIDs reduce the diuretic, natriuretic, and antihypertensive effects of Timolide).
No products indexed under this heading.

Mefenamic Acid (NSAIDs reduce the diuretic, natriuretic, and antihypertensive effects of Timolide).
No products indexed under this heading.

Meloxicam (NSAIDs reduce the diuretic, natriuretic, and antihypertensive effects of Timolide). Products include:
Mobic Oral Suspension 893
Mobic Tablets 893

Metformin Hydrochloride (Beta-blockers may mask the signs and symptoms of hypoglycemia). Products include:
ActoPlus Met Tablets 3219
Avandamet Tablets 1343
Fortamet Extended-Release Tablets 1156

Methyclothiazide (Timolide may potentiate the action of other antihypertensive agents used concomitantly).
No products indexed under this heading.

Methyldopa (Timolide may potentiate the action of other antihypertensive agents used concomitantly). Products include:
Aldoclor Tablets 1881
Aldoril Tablets 1884

Methyldopate Hydrochloride (Timolide may potentiate the action of other antihypertensive agents used concomitantly).
No products indexed under this heading.

Metolazone (Timolide may potentiate the action of other antihypertensive agents used concomitantly).
No products indexed under this heading.

Metoprolol Succinate (Timolide may potentiate the action of other antihypertensive agents used concomitantly). Products include:

Toprol-XL Tablets 660

Metoprolol Tartrate (Timolide may potentiate the action of other antihypertensive agents used concomitantly).
No products indexed under this heading.

Metyrosine (Timolide may potentiate the action of other antihypertensive agents used concomitantly). Products include:
Demser Capsules 1933

Mibefradil Dihydrochloride (Hypotension, AV conduction disturbances, and left ventricular failure have been reported in some patients receiving beta-adrenergic blocking agents when an oral calcium antagonist was added to the treatment regimen).
No products indexed under this heading.

Miglitol (Beta-blockers may mask the signs and symptoms of hypoglycemia).
No products indexed under this heading.

Minoxidil (Timolide may potentiate the action of other antihypertensive agents used concomitantly). Products include:
Men's Rogaine Extra Strength Topical Solution, Ocean Rush Scent and Original Unscented 706
Women's Rogaine Topical Solution, Spring Bloom Scent and Original Unscented 707

Moexipril Hydrochloride (Timolide may potentiate the action of other antihypertensive agents used concomitantly). Products include:
Uniretic Tablets 3114
Univasc Tablets 3118

Nabumetone (NSAIDs reduce the diuretic, natriuretic, and antihypertensive effects of Timolide). Products include:
Relafen Tablets 1523

Nadolol (Timolide may potentiate the action of other antihypertensive agents used concomitantly). Products include:
Nadolol Tablets 2121

Naproxen (NSAIDs reduce the diuretic, natriuretic, and antihypertensive effects of Timolide). Products include:
EC-Naprosyn Delayed-Release Tablets 2769
Naprosyn Suspension 2769
Naprosyn Tablets 2769
Prevacid NapraPAC 3277

Naproxen Sodium (NSAIDs reduce the diuretic, natriuretic, and antihypertensive effects of Timolide). Products include:
Aleve Tablets, Caplets and Gelcaps 605
Anaprox Tablets 2769
Anaprox DS Tablets 2769

Nicardipine Hydrochloride (Hypotension, AV conduction disturbances, and left ventricular failure have been reported in some patients receiving beta-adrenergic blocking agents when an oral calcium antagonist was added to the treatment regimen). Products include:
Cardene I.V. 1129

Nifedipine (Hypotension, AV conduction disturbances, and left ventricular failure have been reported in some patients receiving beta-adrenergic blocking agents when an oral calcium antagonist was added to the treatment regimen). Products include:
Adalat CC Tablets 2978

Nimodipine (Hypotension, AV conduction disturbances, and left ventricular failure have been reported in some patients receiving beta-adrenergic blocking agents when an oral calcium antagonist was added to the treatment regimen). Products include:
Nimotop Capsules 774

Nisoldipine (Hypotension, AV conduction disturbances, and left ventricular failure have been reported in some patients receiving beta-adrenergic blocking agents when an oral calcium antagonist was added to the treatment regimen). Products include:
Sular Tablets 1163

Nitroglycerin (Timolide may potentiate the action of other antihypertensive agents used concomitantly). Products include:
Nitro-Dur Transdermal Infusion System 3060
Nitrolingual Pumpspray 1161

Norepinephrine Bitartrate (Decreased arterial responsiveness to norepinephrine).
No products indexed under this heading.

Oxaprozin (NSAIDs reduce the diuretic, natriuretic, and antihypertensive effects of Timolide).
No products indexed under this heading.

Penbutolol Sulfate (Timolide may potentiate the action of other antihypertensive agents used concomitantly).
No products indexed under this heading.

Perindopril Erbumine (Timolide may potentiate the action of other antihypertensive agents used concomitantly). Products include:
Aceon Tablets (2 mg, 4 mg, 8 mg) 3191

Phenoxybenzamine Hydrochloride (Timolide may potentiate the action of other antihypertensive agents used concomitantly). Products include:
Dibenzyline Capsules 3390

Phentolamine Mesylate (Timolide may potentiate the action of other antihypertensive agents used concomitantly).
No products indexed under this heading.

Phenylbutazone (NSAIDs reduce the diuretic, natriuretic, and antihypertensive effects of Timolide).
No products indexed under this heading.

Pindolol (Timolide may potentiate the action of other antihypertensive agents used concomitantly).
No products indexed under this heading.

Pioglitazone Hydrochloride (Beta-blockers may mask the signs and symptoms of hypoglycemia). Products include:
ActoPlus Met Tablets 3219
Actos Tablets 3224

Piroxicam (NSAIDs reduce the diuretic, natriuretic, and antihypertensive effects of Timolide).
No products indexed under this heading.

Polythiazide (Timolide may potentiate the action of other antihypertensive agents used concomitantly).
No products indexed under this heading.

Prazosin Hydrochloride (Timolide may potentiate the action of other antihypertensive agents used concomitantly).
No products indexed under this heading.

Propranolol Hydrochloride (Timolide may potentiate the action of other antihypertensive agents used concomitantly). Products include:
Inderal LA Long-Acting Capsules 3421
InnoPran XL Capsules 2728

Quinapril Hydrochloride (Timolide may potentiate the action of other antihypertensive agents used concomitantly).
No products indexed under this heading.

Quinidine (Co-administration has resulted in potentiated systemic beta-blockade, e.g., decreased heart rate).
No products indexed under this heading.

Quinidine Gluconate (Co-administration has resulted in potentiated systemic beta-blockade, e.g., decreased heart rate).
No products indexed under this heading.

Quinidine Hydrochloride (Co-administration has resulted in potentiated systemic beta-blockade, e.g., decreased heart rate).
No products indexed under this heading.

Quinidine Polygalacturonate (Co-administration has resulted in potentiated systemic beta-blockade, e.g., decreased heart rate).
No products indexed under this heading.

Quinidine Sulfate (Co-administration has resulted in potentiated systemic beta-blockade, e.g., decreased heart rate).
No products indexed under this heading.

Ramipril (Timolide may potentiate the action of other antihypertensive agents used concomitantly). Products include:
Altace Capsules 1673

Rauwolfia Serpentina (Close observation of the patient is recommended when Timolide is administered to patients receiving catecholamine-depleting drugs such as reserpine, because of possible additive effects and the production of hypotension and/or marked bradycardia, which may produce vertigo, syncope, or postural hypotension).
No products indexed under this heading.

Repaglinide (Beta-blockers may mask the signs and symptoms of hypoglycemia). Products include:
Prandin Tablets (0.5, 1, and 2 mg) 2337

Rescinnamine (Close observation of the patient is recommended when Timolide is administered to patients receiving catecholamine-depleting drugs such as reserpine, because of possible additive effects and the production of hypotension and/or marked bradycardia, which may produce vertigo, syncope, or postural hypotension).
No products indexed under this heading.

Reserpine (Close observation of the patient is recommended when Timolide is administered to patients receiving catecholamine-depleting drugs such as reserpine, because of possible additive effects and the production of hypotension and/or marked bradycardia, which may produce vertigo, syncope, or postural hypotension).
No products indexed under this heading.

Rofecoxib (NSAIDs reduce the diuretic, natriuretic, and antihypertensive effects of Timolide).
No products indexed under this heading.

Rosiglitazone Maleate (Beta-blockers may mask the signs and symptoms of hypoglycemia). Products include:
Avandamet Tablets 1343
Avandia Tablets 1348

Sodium Nitroprusside (Timolide may potentiate the action of other antihypertensive agents used concomitantly).
No products indexed under this heading.

Sotalol Hydrochloride (Timolide may potentiate the action of other antihypertensive agents used concomitantly).
No products indexed under this heading.

Spirapril Hydrochloride (Timolide may potentiate the action of other antihypertensive agents used concomitantly).
No products indexed under this heading.

Sulindac (NSAIDs reduce the diuretic, natriuretic, and antihypertensive effects of Timolide). Products include:
Clinoril Tablets 1899

Telmisartan (Timolide may potentiate the action of other antihypertensive agents used concomitantly). Products include:
Micardis Tablets 884
Micardis HCT Tablets 886

Terazosin Hydrochloride (Potentiation of other antihypertensives). Products include:
Hytrin Capsules 469

Tolazamide (Beta-blockers may mask the signs and symptoms of hypoglycemia).
No products indexed under this heading.

Tolbutamide (Beta-blockers may mask the signs and symptoms of hypoglycemia).
No products indexed under this heading.

Tolmetin Sodium (NSAIDs reduce the diuretic, natriuretic, and antihypertensive effects of Timolide).
No products indexed under this heading.

Torsemide (Timolide may potentiate the action of other antihypertensive agents used concomitantly).
No products indexed under this heading.

Trandolapril (Timolide may potentiate the action of other antihypertensive agents used concomitantly). Products include:
Mavik Tablets 482
Tarka Tablets 519

Trimethaphan Camsylate (Timolide may potentiate the action of other antihypertensive agents used concomitantly).
No products indexed under this heading.

Troglitazone (Beta-blockers may mask the signs and symptoms of hypoglycemia).
No products indexed under this heading.

Tubocurarine Chloride (Increased responsiveness to tubocurarine).
No products indexed under this heading.

Valdecoxib (NSAIDs reduce the diuretic, natriuretic, and antihypertensive effects of Timolide).
No products indexed under this heading.

Valsartan (Timolide may potentiate the action of other antihypertensive agents used concomitantly). Products include:
Diovan HCT Tablets **2195**
Diovan Tablets **2191**

Verapamil Hydrochloride (Left ventricular failure and AV conduction disturbances). Products include:
Covera-HS Tablets **3135**
Tarka Tablets **519**
Verelan PM Capsules **3120**

TIMOPTIC IN OCUDOSE

(Timolol Maleate) **2061**
May interact with beta blockers, catecholamine depleting drugs, calcium channel blockers, cardiac glycosides, oral hypoglycemic agents, insulin, quinidine, and certain other agents. Compounds in these categories include:

Acarbose (Beta blocking agents, usually systemic, may mask the sign and symptoms of acute hypoglycemia). Products include:
Precose Tablets **776**

Acebutolol Hydrochloride (Concurrent use with systemic beta blocker may have additive effects of beta blockade, both systemic and on intraocular pressure).
No products indexed under this heading.

Amlodipine Besylate (Possible atrioventricular conduction disturbances, left ventricular failure, or hypotension when used concurrently). Products include:
Caduet Tablets **2507**
Lotrel Capsules **2238**
Norvasc Tablets **2529**

Atenolol (Concurrent use with systemic beta blocker may have additive effects of beta blockade, both systemic and on intraocular pressure). Products include:
Tenormin I.V. Injection **698**
Tenormin Tablets **695**

Bepridil Hydrochloride (Possible atrioventricular conduction disturbances, left ventricular failure, or hypotension when used concurrently).
No products indexed under this heading.

Betaxolol Hydrochloride (Concurrent use with systemic beta blocker may have additive effects of beta blockade, both systemic and on intraocular pressure; concurrent use of two topical beta blockers is not recommended). Products include:
Betoptic S Ophthalmic Suspension **554**

Bisoprolol Fumarate (Concurrent use with systemic beta blocker may have additive effects of beta blockade, both systemic and on intraocular pressure).
No products indexed under this heading.

Carteolol Hydrochloride (Concurrent use with systemic beta blocker may have additive effects of beta blockade, both systemic and on intraocular pressure; concurrent use of two topical beta blockers is not recommended). Products include:
Carteolol Hydrochloride Ophthalmic Solution USP, 1% .... ⊙**246**

Chlorpropamide (Beta blocking agents, usually systemic, may mask the sign and symptoms of acute hypoglycemia).
No products indexed under this heading.

Clonidine (Oral beta-adrenergic blocking agents may exacerbate the rebound hypertension which can follow the withdrawal of clonidine; there have been no reports of exacerbation of rebound hypertension with ophthalmic timolol). Products include:
Catapres-TTS **875**

Clonidine Hydrochloride (Oral beta-adrenergic blocking agents may exacerbate the rebound hypertension which can follow the withdrawal of clonidine; there have been no reports of exacerbation of rebound hypertension with ophthalmic timolol). Products include:
Catapres Tablets **874**
Clorpres Tablets **2139**

Deserpidine (Possible additive effects and the production of hypotension and/or bradycardia).
No products indexed under this heading.

Deslanoside (Co-administration with digitalis and calcium antagonists may have additive effects in prolonging atrioventricular conduction time).
No products indexed under this heading.

Digitalis Glycoside Preparations (Co-administration with digitalis and calcium antagonists may have additive effects in prolonging atrioventricular conduction time).
No products indexed under this heading.

Digitoxin (Co-administration with digitalis and calcium antagonists may have additive effects in prolonging atrioventricular conduction time).
No products indexed under this heading.

Digoxin (Co-administration with digitalis and calcium antagonists may have additive effects in prolonging atrioventricular conduction time). Products include:
Digitek Tablets **2146**
Lanoxicaps Capsules **1458**
Lanoxin Injection **1462**
Lanoxin Tablets **1468**
Lanoxin Injection Pediatric **1465**

Diltiazem Hydrochloride (Possible atrioventricular conduction disturbances, left ventricular failure, or hypotension when used concurrently). Products include:
Cardizem LA Extended Release Tablets **1699**
Tiazac Capsules **1204**

Epinephrine (Patients with a history of atopy or anaphylactic reactions to a variety of allergens may be unresponsive to the usual dose of injectable epinephrine used to treat allergic reactions). Products include:
EpiPen **1061**
Primatene Mist .... ▣**749**

Epinephrine Bitartrate (Patients with a history of atopy or anaphylactic reactions to a variety of allergens may be unresponsive to the usual dose of injectable epinephrine used to treat allergic reactions).
No products indexed under this heading.

Esmolol Hydrochloride (Concurrent use with systemic beta blocker may have additive effects of beta blockade, both systemic and on intraocular pressure). Products include:
Brevibloc Concentrate **766**
Brevibloc Injection **766**
Brevibloc Double Strength Injection **766**
Brevibloc Premixed Injection **766**
Brevibloc Double Strength Premixed Injection **766**

Felodipine (Possible atrioventricular conduction disturbances, left ventricular failure, or hypotension when used concurrently). Products include:
Plendil Extended-Release Tablets **651**

Glimepiride (Beta blocking agents, usually systemic, may mask the sign and symptoms of acute hypoglycemia). Products include:
Amaryl Tablets **2864**

Glipizide (Beta blocking agents, usually systemic, may mask the sign and symptoms of acute hypoglycemia).
No products indexed under this heading.

Glyburide (Beta blocking agents, usually systemic, may mask the sign and symptoms of acute hypoglycemia).
No products indexed under this heading.

Guanethidine Monosulfate (Possible additive effects and the production of hypotension and/or bradycardia).
No products indexed under this heading.

Insulin, Human, Zinc Suspension (Beta blocking agents, usually systemic, may mask the sign and symptoms of acute hypoglycemia). Products include:
Humulin L, 100 Units **1763**
Humulin U, 100 Units **1770**

Insulin, Human NPH (Beta blocking agents, usually systemic, may mask the sign and symptoms of acute hypoglycemia). Products include:
Humulin N, 100 Units **1764**
Humulin N Pen **1765**
Novolin N Human Insulin 10 ml Vials **2322**
Novolin N InnoLet **2322**
Novolin N PenFill 3 ml Cartridges **2325**
Novolin R InnoLet **2322**

Insulin, Human Regular (Beta blocking agents, usually systemic, may mask the sign and symptoms of acute hypoglycemia). Products include:
Humulin R (U-500) **1768**
Humulin R, 100 Units **1767**
Novolin R Human Insulin 10 ml Vials **2322**
Novolin R PenFill **2325**

Insulin, Human Regular and Human NPH Mixture (Beta blocking agents, usually systemic, may mask the sign and symptoms of acute hypoglycemia). Products include:
Humulin 50/50, 100 Units **1760**
Humulin 70/30 Pen **1761**
Novolin 70/30 Human Insulin 10 ml Vials **2321**
Novolin 70/30 InnoLet **2322**
Novolin 70/30 PenFill 3 ml Cartridges **2325**

Insulin, NPH (Beta blocking agents, usually systemic, may mask the sign and symptoms of acute hypoglycemia).
No products indexed under this heading.

Insulin, Regular (Beta blocking agents, usually systemic, may mask the sign and symptoms of acute hypoglycemia).
No products indexed under this heading.

Insulin, Zinc Crystals (Beta blocking agents, usually systemic, may mask the sign and symptoms of acute hypoglycemia).
No products indexed under this heading.

Insulin, Zinc Suspension (Beta blocking agents, usually systemic, may mask the sign and symptoms of acute hypoglycemia).
No products indexed under this heading.

Insulin Aspart, Human Regular (Beta blocking agents, usually systemic, may mask the sign and symptoms of acute hypoglycemia). Products include:
NovoLog Injection **2326**

Insulin glargine (Beta blocking agents, usually systemic, may mask the sign and symptoms of acute hypoglycemia). Products include:
Lantus Injection **2925**

Insulin Lispro, Human (Beta blocking agents, usually systemic, may mask the sign and symptoms of acute hypoglycemia). Products include:
Humalog-Pen **1751**
Humalog Mix 75/25-Pen **1754**

Insulin Lispro Protamine, Human (Beta blocking agents, usually systemic, may mask the sign and symptoms of acute hypoglycemia). Products include:
Humalog Mix 75/25-Pen **1754**

Isradipine (Possible atrioventricular conduction disturbances, left ventricular failure, or hypotension when used concurrently). Products include:
DynaCirc CR Tablets **2726**

Labetalol Hydrochloride (Concurrent use with systemic beta blocker may have additive effects of beta blockade, both systemic and on intraocular pressure).
No products indexed under this heading.

Levobunolol Hydrochloride (Concurrent use of two topical beta blockers is not recommended). Products include:
Betagan Ophthalmic Solution, USP .... ⊙**217**

Metformin Hydrochloride (Beta blocking agents, usually systemic, may mask the sign and symptoms of acute hypoglycemia). Products include:
ActoPlus Met Tablets **3219**
Avandamet Tablets **1343**
Fortamet Extended-Release Tablets **1156**

Metipranolol Hydrochloride (Concurrent use of two topical beta blockers is not recommended).
No products indexed under this heading.

Metoprolol Succinate (Concurrent use with systemic beta blocker may have additive effects of beta blockade, both systemic and on intraocular pressure). Products include:
Toprol-XL Tablets 660

Metoprolol Tartrate (Concurrent use with systemic beta blocker may have additive effects of beta blockade, both systemic and on intraocular pressure).
No products indexed under this heading.

Mibefradil Dihydrochloride (Possible atrioventricular conduction disturbances, left ventricular failure, or hypotension when used concurrently).
No products indexed under this heading.

Miglitol (Beta blocking agents, usually systemic, may mask the sign and symptoms of acute hypoglycemia).
No products indexed under this heading.

Nadolol (Concurrent use with systemic beta blocker may have additive effects of beta blockade, both systemic and on intraocular pressure). Products include:
Nadolol Tablets 2121

Nicardipine Hydrochloride (Possible atrioventricular conduction disturbances, left ventricular failure, or hypotension when used concurrently). Products include:
Cardene I.V. 1129

Nifedipine (Possible atrioventricular conduction disturbances, left ventricular failure, or hypotension when used concurrently). Products include:
Adalat CC Tablets 2978

Nimodipine (Possible atrioventricular conduction disturbances, left ventricular failure, or hypotension when used concurrently). Products include:
Nimotop Capsules 774

Nisoldipine (Possible atrioventricular conduction disturbances, left ventricular failure, or hypotension when used concurrently). Products include:
Sular Tablets 1163

Penbutolol Sulfate (Concurrent use with systemic beta blocker may have additive effects of beta blockade, both systemic and on intraocular pressure).
No products indexed under this heading.

Pindolol (Concurrent use with systemic beta blocker may have additive effects of beta blockade, both systemic and on intraocular pressure).
No products indexed under this heading.

Pioglitazone Hydrochloride (Beta blocking agents, usually systemic, may mask the sign and symptoms of acute hypoglycemia). Products include:
ActoPlus Met Tablets 3219
Actos Tablets 3224

Propranolol Hydrochloride (Concurrent use with systemic beta blocker may have additive effects of beta blockade, both systemic and on intraocular pressure). Products include:
Inderal LA Long-Acting Capsules 3421
InnoPran XL Capsules 2728

Quinidine (Co-administration has resulted in potentiated systemic beta-blockade, e.g., decreased heart rate).
No products indexed under this heading.

Quinidine Gluconate (Co-administration has resulted in potentiated systemic beta-blockade, e.g., decreased heart rate).
No products indexed under this heading.

Quinidine Hydrochloride (Co-administration has resulted in potentiated systemic beta-blockade, e.g., decreased heart rate).
No products indexed under this heading.

Quinidine Polygalacturonate (Co-administration has resulted in potentiated systemic beta-blockade, e.g., decreased heart rate).
No products indexed under this heading.

Quinidine Sulfate (Co-administration has resulted in potentiated systemic beta-blockade, e.g., decreased heart rate).
No products indexed under this heading.

Rauwolfia Serpentina (Possible additive effects and the production of hypotension and/or bradycardia).
No products indexed under this heading.

Repaglinide (Beta blocking agents, usually systemic, may mask the sign and symptoms of acute hypoglycemia). Products include:
Prandin Tablets (0.5, 1, and 2 mg) 2337

Rescinnamine (Possible additive effects and the production of hypotension and/or bradycardia).
No products indexed under this heading.

Reserpine (Possible additive effects and the production of hypotension and/or bradycardia).
No products indexed under this heading.

Rosiglitazone Maleate (Beta blocking agents, usually systemic, may mask the sign and symptoms of acute hypoglycemia). Products include:
Avandamet Tablets 1343
Avandia Tablets 1348

Sotalol Hydrochloride (Concurrent use with systemic beta blocker may have additive effects of beta blockade, both systemic and on intraocular pressure).
No products indexed under this heading.

Timolol Hemihydrate (Concurrent use of two topical beta blockers is not recommended). Products include:
Betimol Ophthalmic Solution 3371
Betimol Ophthalmic Solution .... ⊙283

Tolazamide (Beta blocking agents, usually systemic, may mask the sign and symptoms of acute hypoglycemia).
No products indexed under this heading.

Tolbutamide (Beta blocking agents, usually systemic, may mask the sign and symptoms of acute hypoglycemia).
No products indexed under this heading.

Troglitazone (Beta blocking agents, usually systemic, may mask the sign and symptoms of acute hypoglycemia).
No products indexed under this heading.

Verapamil Hydrochloride (Possible atrioventricular conduction disturbances, left ventricular failure, or hypotension when used concurrently). Products include:
Covera-HS Tablets 3135
Tarka Tablets 519
Verelan PM Capsules 3120

TIMOPTIC STERILE OPHTHALMIC SOLUTION

(Timolol Maleate) 2058
See Timoptic in Ocudose

TIMOPTIC-XE STERILE OPHTHALMIC GEL FORMING SOLUTION

(Timolol Maleate) 2062
See Timoptic in Ocudose

TINDAMAX

(Tinidazole) 2670
May interact with oral anticoagulants, lithium preparations, and phenytoin. Compounds in these categories include:

Anisindione (May enhance the effect of warfarin and other coumarin anticoagulants resulting in a prolongation of prothrombin time. The dosage of oral anticoagulants may need to be adjusted during co-administration and up to 8 days after tinidazole discontinuation). Products include:
Miradon Tablets 3056

Cholestyramine (It is advisable to separate dosing of cholestyramine and tinidazole to minimize any potential effect on the oral bioavailability of tinidazole).
No products indexed under this heading.

Cimetidine (Co-administration with drugs that inhibit the activity of liver microsomal enzymes, such as cimetidine, may prolong the half-life and decrease the plasma clearance of tinidazole, increasing the plasma level of tinidazole). Products include:
Tagamet HB 200 Tablets .... ▣637
Tagamet Tablets 1547

Cimetidine Hydrochloride (Co-administration with drugs that inhibit the activity of liver microsomal enzymes, such as cimetidine, may prolong the half-life and decrease the plasma clearance of tinidazole, increasing the plasma level of tinidazole).
No products indexed under this heading.

Cyclosporine (Metronidazole has the potential to increase the levels of cyclosporine. During tinidazole co-administration, the patient should be monitored for signs of calcineurin-inhibitor associated toxicities). Products include:
Gengraf Capsules 458
Neoral Soft Gelatin Capsules 2247
Neoral Oral Solution 2247
Restasis Ophthalmic Emulsion 570
Sandimmune 2259

Dicumarol (May enhance the effect of warfarin and other coumarin anticoagulants resulting in a prolongation of prothrombin time. The dosage of oral anticoagulants may need to be adjusted during co-administration and up to 8 days after tinidazole discontinuation).
No products indexed under this heading.

Disulfiram (Psychotic reactions have been reported in alcoholic patients using metronidazole and disulfiram concurrently. Though no similar reactions have been reported with tinidazole, tinidazole should not be given to patients who have taken disulfiram within the last two weeks). Products include:
Antabuse Tablets 2343

Ethanol (Alcoholic beverages and preparations containing ethanol should be avoided during tinidazole therapy and for three days afterward because abdominal cramps, nausea, vomiting, headaches and flushing may occur).
No products indexed under this heading.

Fluorouracil (Metronidazole was shown to decrease the clearance of fluorouracil, resulting in side-effects without an increase in therapeutic benefits. If the concomitant use of tinidazole and fluorouracil cannot be avoided, the patient should be monitored for fluorouracil-associated toxicities). Products include:
Carac Cream, 0.5% 1048
Efudex 3348

Fosphenytoin Sodium (Concomitant administration of oral metronidazole and IV phenytoin was reported to result in prolongation of the half-life and reduction in the clearance of phenytoin. This may occur with tinidazole. Phenytoin and fosphenytoin may accelerate the elimination of tinidazole, decreasing the plasma level of tinidazole).
No products indexed under this heading.

Ketoconazole (Co-administration with drugs that inhibit the activity of liver microsomal enzymes, such as ketoconazole, may prolong the half-life and decrease the plasma clearance of tinidazole, increasing the plasma level of tinidazole). Products include:
Nizoral A-D Shampoo, 1% 1839
Nizoral 2% Shampoo 1838

Lithium (Consideration should be given to measuring serum lithium creatinine levels after several days of simultaneous lithium and tinidazole treatment to detect potential lithium intoxication).
No products indexed under this heading.

Lithium Carbonate (Consideration should be given to measuring serum lithium creatinine levels after several days of simultaneous lithium and tinidazole treatment to detect potential lithium intoxication). Products include:
Eskalith 1406
Lithobid Tablets 1670

Lithium Citrate (Consideration should be given to measuring serum lithium creatinine levels after several days of simultaneous lithium and tinidazole treatment to detect potential lithium intoxication).
No products indexed under this heading.

Oxytetracycline (Oxytetracycline was reported to antagonize the therapeutic effect of metronidazole and may potentially have the same effect on tinidazole).
No products indexed under this heading.

Oxytetracycline Hydrochloride (Oxytetracycline was reported to antagonize the therapeutic effect of metronidazole and may potentially have the same effect on tinidazole).
No products indexed under this heading.

Phenobarbital (Co-administration with drugs that induce liver microsomal enzymes, such as phenobarbital, may accelerate the elimination of tinidazole, decreasing the plasma level of tinidazole).
No products indexed under this heading.

Phenobarbital Sodium (Co-administration with drugs that induce liver microsomal enzymes, such as phenobarbital, may accelerate the elimination of tinidazole, decreasing the plasma level of tinidazole).
No products indexed under this heading.

Phenytoin (Concomitant administration of oral metronidazole and IV phenytoin was reported to result in prolongation of the half-life and reduction in the clearance of phenytoin. This may occur with tinidazole. Phenytoin and fosphenytoin may accelerate the elimination of tinidazole, decreasing the plasma level of tinidazole).
No products indexed under this heading.

Phenytoin Sodium (Concomitant administration of oral metronidazole and IV phenytoin was reported to result in prolongation of the half-life and reduction in the clearance of phenytoin. This may occur with tinidazole. Phenytoin and fosphenytoin may accelerate the elimination of tinidazole, decreasing the plasma level of tinidazole). Products include:
Phenytek Capsules 2153

Propylene Glycol (Preparations containing propylene glycol should be avoided during tinidazole therapy and for three days afterward because abdominal cramps, nausea, vomiting, headaches and flushing may occur). Products include:
Biafine Topical Emulsion 2382
Systane Lubricant Eye Drops 558

Propylene Glycol-containing Solutions (Preparations containing propylene glycol should be avoided during tinidazole therapy and for three days afterward because abdominal cramps, nausea, vomiting, headaches and flushing may occur).
No products indexed under this heading.

Rifampin (Co-administration with drugs that induce liver microsomal enzymes, such as rifampin, may accelerate the elimination of tinidazole, decreasing the plasma level of tinidazole).
No products indexed under this heading.

Tacrolimus (Metronidazole has the potential to increase the levels of tacrolimus. During tinidazole co-administration, the patient should be monitored for signs of calcineurin-inhibitor associated toxins). Products include:
Prograf Capsules and Injection 624
Protopic Ointment 629

Warfarin Sodium (May enhance the effect of warfarin and other coumarin anticoagulants resulting in a prolongation of prothrombin time. The dosage of oral anticoagulants may need to be adjusted during co-administration and up to 8 days after tinidazole discontinuation). Products include:
Coumadin for Injection 932
Coumadin Tablets 932

Food Interactions

Alcohol (Alcoholic beverages should be avoided during tinidazole therapy and for three days afterward because abdominal cramps, nausea, vomiting, headaches and flushing may occur).

TNKASE I.V.

(Tenecteplase) 1256
May interact with vitamin K antagonists and certain other agents. Compounds in these categories include:

Abciximab (Drugs that alter platelet function, such as abciximab, may increase the risk of bleeding if administered prior to or after tenecteplase therapy). Products include:
ReoPro Vials 1779

Aspirin (Drugs that alter platelet function, such as aspirin, may increase the risk of bleeding if administered prior to or after tenecteplase therapy). Products include:
Aggrenox Capsules 855
Bayer, Aspirin Regimen .... ▣606
Bayer Aspirin Tablets 3515
BC Powder .... ▣612
BC Allergy Sinus Cold Powder .... ▣612
Arthritis Strength BC Powder .... ▣612
BC Sinus Cold Powder .... ▣612
Ecotrin Enteric Coated Aspirin Low, Regular and Maximum Strength Tablets 1627
Goody's Body Pain Formula Powder .... ▣621
Goody's Extra Strength Headache Powder .... ▣621
Goody's Extra Strength Pain Relief Tablets .... ▣621
Percodan Tablets 1115
St. Joseph 81 mg Aspirin Chewable and Enteric Coated Tablets 1841

Clopidogrel Bisulfate (Drugs that alter platelet function, such as clopidogrel, may increase the risk of bleeding if administered prior to or after tenecteplase therapy). Products include:
Plavix Tablets 940
Plavix Tablets 2942

Dicumarol (Co-administration increases the risk of bleeding).
No products indexed under this heading.

Dipyridamole (Drugs that alter platelet function, such as dipyridamole, may increase the risk of bleeding if administered prior to or after tenecteplase therapy). Products include:
Aggrenox Capsules 855
Persantine Tablets 898

Epitifibatide (Drugs that alter platelet function, such as epitifibatide, may increase the risk of bleeding if administered prior to or after tenecteplase therapy).
No products indexed under this heading.

Ticlopidine Hydrochloride (Drugs that alter platelet function, such as ticlopidine, may increase the risk of bleeding if administered prior to or after tenecteplase therapy). Products include:
Ticlid Tablets 2813

Tirofiban Hydrochloride (Drugs that alter platelet function, such as tirofiban, may increase the risk of bleeding if administered prior to or after tenecteplase therapy). Products include:
Aggrastat 1878

Warfarin Sodium (Co-administration increases the risk of bleeding). Products include:
Coumadin for Injection 932
Coumadin Tablets 932

TOBI SOLUTION FOR INHALATION

(Tobramycin) 1015
May interact with aminoglycosides and certain other agents. Compounds in these categories include:

Amikacin Sulfate (Co-administration in some patients receiving TOBI and extensive previous or concomitant parenteral aminoglycosides has resulted in hearing loss; potential for increased risk of neurotoxicity and/or ototoxicity).
No products indexed under this heading.

Ethacrynic Acid (Some diuretics, such as ethacrynic acid, can enhance aminoglycoside toxicity by altering antibiotic concentrations in serum and tissue; TOBI should not be administered with ethacrynic acid). Products include:
Edecrin Tablets 1941

Furosemide (Some diuretics, such as furosemide, can enhance aminoglycoside toxicity by altering antibiotic concentrations in serum and tissue; TOBI should not be administered with furosemide). Products include:
Furosemide Tablets 2117

Gentamicin Sulfate (Co-administration in some patients receiving TOBI and extensive previous or concomitant parenteral aminoglycosides has resulted in hearing loss; potential for increased risk of neurotoxicity and/or ototoxicity). Products include:
Garamycin Injectable 3028
Genoptic Sterile Ophthalmic Solution .... ⊙227
Pred-G Ophthalmic Suspension .... ⊙234
Pred-G Sterile Ophthalmic Ointment .... ⊙235

Kanamycin Sulfate (Co-administration in some patients receiving TOBI and extensive previous or concomitant parenteral aminoglycosides has resulted in hearing loss; potential for increased risk of neurotoxicity and/or ototoxicity).
No products indexed under this heading.

Mannitol (Some diuretics, such as mannitol, can enhance aminoglycoside toxicity by altering antibiotic concentrations in serum and tissue; TOBI should not be administered with mannitol). Products include:
Trident White Sugarless Gum .... ▣611

Streptomycin Sulfate (Co-administration in some patients receiving TOBI and extensive previous or concomitant parenteral aminoglycosides has resulted in hearing loss; potential for increased risk of neurotoxicity and/or ototoxicity).
No products indexed under this heading.

Tobramycin Sulfate (Co-administration in some patients receiving TOBI and extensive previous or concomitant parenteral aminoglycosides has resulted in hearing loss; potential for increased risk of neurotoxicity and/or ototoxicity).
No products indexed under this heading.

Urea (Some diuretics, such as systemic urea, can enhance aminoglycoside toxicity by altering antibiotic concentrations in serum and tissue; TOBI should not be administered with urea). Products include:
Accuzyme Debriding Ointment 1636
Accuzyme Spray 1637
Panafil Ointment 1637
Panafil Spray 1637
U-Kera Cream 3290
Ultralytic 2 Cream 20% 1651
Ultralytic 2 Foam 20% 1652

TOBRADEX OPHTHALMIC OINTMENT

(Dexamethasone, Tobramycin) 558
May interact with aminoglycosides. Compounds in these categories include:

Amikacin Sulfate (Monitor the total serum concentration if administered with systemic aminoglycoside).
No products indexed under this heading.

Gentamicin Sulfate (Monitor the total serum concentration if administered with systemic aminoglycoside). Products include:
Garamycin Injectable 3028
Genoptic Sterile Ophthalmic Solution .... ⊙227
Pred-G Ophthalmic Suspension .... ⊙234
Pred-G Sterile Ophthalmic Ointment .... ⊙235

Kanamycin Sulfate (Monitor the total serum concentration if administered with systemic aminoglycoside).
No products indexed under this heading.

Streptomycin Sulfate (Monitor the total serum concentration if administered with systemic aminoglycoside).
No products indexed under this heading.

Tobramycin Sulfate (Monitor the total serum concentration if administered with systemic aminoglycoside).
No products indexed under this heading.

TOBRADEX OPHTHALMIC SUSPENSION

(Dexamethasone, Tobramycin) 558
See TobraDex Ophthalmic Ointment

TOPAMAX SPRINKLE CAPSULES

(Topiramate) 2438
See Topamax Tablets

TOPAMAX TABLETS

(Topiramate) 2438
May interact with carbonic anhydrase inhibitors, central nervous system depressants, lithium preparations, oral contraceptives, phenytoin, valproate, and certain other agents. Compounds in these categories include:

Acetazolamide (Co-administration of topiramate with carbonic anhydrase inhibitors may create a physiological environment that increases the risk of kidney stone formation; concurrent use should be avoided).
No products indexed under this heading.

Alfentanil Hydrochloride (Potential for increased CNS depression).
No products indexed under this heading.

Alprazolam (Potential for increased CNS depression). Products include:
Niravam Orally Disintegrating Tablets 3106
Xanax XR Tablets 2655

Amitriptyline Hydrochloride (There was a 12% increase in AUC and Cmax for amitriptyline (25mg per day) in 18 normal subjects receiving 200mg/day of topiramate. Some subjects may experience a large increase in amitriptyline concentration in the presence of topiramate and any adjustments in amitriptyline dose should be made according to the patient's clinical response and not on the basis of plasma levels).
No products indexed under this heading.

Aprobarbital (Potential for increased CNS depression).
No products indexed under this heading.

Buprenorphine Hydrochloride (Potential for increased CNS depression). Products include:
Buprenex Injectable 2718
Suboxone Tablets 2719
Subutex Tablets 2719

Buspirone Hydrochloride (Potential for increased CNS depression).
No products indexed under this heading.

Butabarbital (Potential for increased CNS depression).
No products indexed under this heading.

Butalbital (Potential for increased CNS depression). Products include:
Sedapap Tablets 50 mg/650 mg 2098

Carbamazepine (Co-administration has resulted in 40% decrease in topiramate concentration and no change in carbamazepine concentration). Products include:
Carbatrol Capsules 3174
Equetro Extended-Release Capsules 3178
Tegretol/Tegretol-XR 2278

Chlordiazepoxide (Potential for increased CNS depression).
No products indexed under this heading.

Chlordiazepoxide Hydrochloride (Potential for increased CNS depression). Products include:
Librium Capsules 3349

Chlorpromazine (Potential for increased CNS depression).
No products indexed under this heading.

Chlorpromazine Hydrochloride (Potential for increased CNS depression).
No products indexed under this heading.

Chlorprothixene (Potential for increased CNS depression).
No products indexed under this heading.

Chlorprothixene Hydrochloride (Potential for increased CNS depression).
No products indexed under this heading.

Chlorprothixene Lactate (Potential for increased CNS depression).
No products indexed under this heading.

Clorazepate Dipotassium (Potential for increased CNS depression). Products include:
Tranxene 2488

Clozapine (Potential for increased CNS depression). Products include:
Clozapine Tablets 2141
Clozaril Tablets 2174
FazaClo Orally Disintegrating Tablets 547

Codeine Phosphate (Potential for increased CNS depression). Products include:
Tylenol with Codeine 2461

Desflurane (Potential for increased CNS depression). Products include:
Suprane Liquid for Inhalation 770

Desogestrel (The possibility of decreased contraceptive efficacy and increased breakthrough bleeding should be considered in patients taking combination oral contraceptive products with topiramate). Products include:
Ortho-Cept Tablets 2395

Dezocine (Potential for increased CNS depression).
No products indexed under this heading.

Diazepam (Potential for increased CNS depression). Products include:
Diastat Rectal Delivery System 3344
Valium Tablets 2822

Dichlorphenamide (Co-administration of topiramate with carbonic anhydrase inhibitors may create a physiological environment that increases the risk of kidney stone formation; concurrent use should be avoided). Products include:
Daranide Tablets 1928

Digoxin (Co-administration has resulted in decreased serum digoxin AUC by 12%; clinical significance of this interaction is unknown). Products include:
Digitek Tablets 2146
Lanoxicaps Capsules 1458
Lanoxin Injection 1462
Lanoxin Tablets 1468
Lanoxin Injection Pediatric 1465

Divalproex Sodium (Co-administration resulted in an 11% decrease in valproic acid concentration and a 14% decrease in topiramate concentration. Concomitant administration of topiramate and valproic acid has been associated with hyperammonemia, with or without encephalopathy, in patients who have tolerated either drug alone). Products include:
Depakote Sprinkle Capsules 422
Depakote Tablets 427
Depakote ER Tablets 433

Dorzolamide Hydrochloride (Co-administration of topiramate with carbonic anhydrase inhibitors may create a physiological environment that increases the risk of kidney stone formation; concurrent use should be avoided). Products include:
Cosopt Sterile Ophthalmic Solution 1910
Trusopt Sterile Ophthalmic Solution 2065

Droperidol (Potential for increased CNS depression).
No products indexed under this heading.

Enflurane (Potential for increased CNS depression).
No products indexed under this heading.

Estazolam (Potential for increased CNS depression). Products include:
ProSom Tablets 512

Ethanol (Potential for increased CNS depression).
No products indexed under this heading.

Ethchlorvynol (Potential for increased CNS depression).
No products indexed under this heading.

Ethinamate (Potential for increased CNS depression).
No products indexed under this heading.

Ethinyl Estradiol (The possibility of decreased contraceptive efficacy and increased breakthrough bleeding should be considered in patients taking combination oral contraceptive products with topiramate). Products include:
Alesse-28 Tablets 3392
Lo/Ovral-28 Tablets 3423
NuvaRing 2357
Ortho-Cept Tablets 2395
Ortho-Cyclen/Ortho Tri-Cyclen 2414
Ortho Evra Transdermal System 2402
Ortho Tri-Cyclen Lo Tablets 2421
Seasonale Tablets 1073
Triphasil-28 Tablets 3483
Yasmin 28 Tablets 818

Ethyl Alcohol (Potential for increased CNS depression).
No products indexed under this heading.

Ethynodiol Diacetate (The possibility of decreased contraceptive efficacy and increased breakthrough bleeding should be considered in patients taking combination oral contraceptive products with topiramate).
No products indexed under this heading.

Fentanyl (Potential for increased CNS depression). Products include:
Duragesic Transdermal System 2448

Fentanyl Citrate (Potential for increased CNS depression). Products include:
Actiq 993

Fluphenazine Decanoate (Potential for increased CNS depression).
No products indexed under this heading.

Fluphenazine Enanthate (Potential for increased CNS depression).
No products indexed under this heading.

Fluphenazine Hydrochloride (Potential for increased CNS depression).
No products indexed under this heading.

Flurazepam Hydrochloride (Potential for increased CNS depression). Products include:
Dalmane Capsules 3343

Fosphenytoin Sodium (Co-administration has resulted in 48% decrease in topiramate concentration and no change or 25% increase in phenytoin concentration).
No products indexed under this heading.

Glutethimide (Potential for increased CNS depression).
No products indexed under this heading.

Haloperidol (Potential for increased CNS depression).
No products indexed under this heading.

Haloperidol Decanoate (Potential for increased CNS depression).
No products indexed under this heading.

Hydrochlorothiazide (A study done in healthy volunteers indicated that topiramate Cmax increased by 27% and AUC increased by 29% when HCTZ was added to topiramate. The addition of HCTZ to topiramate therapy may require an adjustment of the topiramate dose. The steady state pharmacokinetics of HCTZ were not significantly influenced by the concomitant administration of topiramate. Clinical laboratory results indicated decreases in serum potassium after topiramate of HCTZ administration, which were greater when HCTZ and topiramate were administered in combination). Products include:
Aldoril Tablets 1884
Atacand HCT 637
Avalide Tablets 2889
Avalide Tablets 922
Benicar HCT Tablets 2852
Diovan HCT Tablets 2195
Dyazide Capsules 1389
Hyzaar 1964
Lotensin HCT Tablets 2235
Maxzide 2150
Micardis HCT Tablets 886
Moduretic Tablets 2003
Prinzide Tablets 2033
Teveten HCT Tablets 1710
Timolide Tablets 2056
Uniretic Tablets 3114
Vaseretic Tablets 2073
Zestoretic Tablets 701

Hydrochlorothiazide Hydrochloride (A study done in healthy volunteers indicated that topiramate Cmax increased by 27% and AUC increased by 29% when HCTZ was added to topiramate. The addition of HCTZ to topiramate therapy may require an adjustment of the topiramate dose. The steady state pharmacokinetics of HCTZ were not significantly influenced by the concomitant administration of topiramate. Clinical laboratory results indicated decreases in serum potassium after topiramate of HCTZ administration, which were greater when HCTZ and topiramate were administered in combination).
No products indexed under this heading.

Hydrocodone Bitartrate (Potential for increased CNS depression). Products include:
Hycodan 1104
Hycomine Compound Tablets 1105
Hycotuss Expectorant Syrup 1106
Lortab 3315
Lortab Elixir 3312
Vicodin Tablets 530
Vicodin ES Tablets 531
Vicodin HP Tablets 532
Vicoprofen Tablets 533
Zydone Tablets 1118

Hydrocodone Polistirex (Potential for increased CNS depression). Products include:
Tussionex Pennkinetic Extended-Release Suspension 3322

Hydromorphone Hydrochloride (Potential for increased CNS depression). Products include:
Dilaudid 439
Dilaudid Oral Liquid 443
Dilaudid Non-Sterile Powder 439
Dilaudid Rectal Suppositories 439
Dilaudid Tablets 439
Dilaudid Tablets - 8 mg 443
Dilaudid-HP 441

Hydroxyzine Hydrochloride (Potential for increased CNS depression).
No products indexed under this heading.

Isoflurane (Potential for increased CNS depression).
No products indexed under this heading.

Ketamine Hydrochloride (Potential for increased CNS depression).
No products indexed under this heading.

Levomethadyl Acetate Hydrochloride (Potential for increased CNS depression).
No products indexed under this heading.

Levonorgestrel (The possibility of decreased contraceptive efficacy and increased breakthrough bleeding should be considered in patients taking combination oral contraceptive products with topiramate).
Products include:
Alesse-28 Tablets ... 3392
Climara Pro Transdermal System ... 800
Mirena Intrauterine System ... 810
Plan B Tablets ... 1068
Seasonale Tablets ... 1073
Triphasil-28 Tablets ... 3483

Levorphanol Tartrate (Potential for increased CNS depression).
No products indexed under this heading.

Lithium (Multiple dosing of topiramate 100mg every 12 hours has decreased the AUC and Cmax of lithium (300mg every 8 hrs) by 20%).
No products indexed under this heading.

Lithium Carbonate (Multiple dosing of topiramate 100mg every 12 hours has decreased the AUC and Cmax of lithium (300mg every 8 hrs) by 20%). Products include:
Eskalith ... 1406
Lithobid Tablets ... 1670

Lithium Citrate (Multiple dosing of topiramate 100mg every 12 hours has decreased the AUC and Cmax of lithium (300mg every 8 hrs) by 20%).
No products indexed under this heading.

Lorazepam (Potential for increased CNS depression).
No products indexed under this heading.

Loxapine Hydrochloride (Potential for increased CNS depression).
No products indexed under this heading.

Loxapine Succinate (Potential for increased CNS depression).
No products indexed under this heading.

Meperidine Hydrochloride (Potential for increased CNS depression).
No products indexed under this heading.

Mephobarbital (Potential for increased CNS depression).
Products include:
Mebaral Tablets, USP ... 2483

Meprobamate (Potential for increased CNS depression).
No products indexed under this heading.

Mesoridazine Besylate (Potential for increased CNS depression).
No products indexed under this heading.

Mestranol (The possibility of decreased contraceptive efficacy and increased breakthrough bleeding should be considered in patients taking combination oral contraceptive products with topiramate).
No products indexed under this heading.

Metformin (Co-administration has resulted in increased metformin mean AUC and Cmax and decreased CL/F; oral plasma clearance of Topiramate appears to be reduced with co-administration; clinical significance of these findings is unclear).
No products indexed under this heading.

Methadone Hydrochloride (Potential for increased CNS depression).
No products indexed under this heading.

Methazolamide (Co-administration of topiramate with carbonic anhydrase inhibitors may create a physiological environment that increases the risk of kidney stone formation; concurrent use should be avoided).
No products indexed under this heading.

Methohexital Sodium (Potential for increased CNS depression).
No products indexed under this heading.

Methotrimeprazine (Potential for increased CNS depression).
No products indexed under this heading.

Methoxyflurane (Potential for increased CNS depression).
No products indexed under this heading.

Midazolam Hydrochloride (Potential for increased CNS depression).
No products indexed under this heading.

Molindone Hydrochloride (Potential for increased CNS depression).
Products include:
Moban Tablets ... 1108

Morphine Sulfate (Potential for increased CNS depression).
Products include:
Avinza Capsules ... 1714
Kadian Capsules ... 572
MS Contin Tablets ... 2703

Norethindrone (The possibility of decreased contraceptive efficacy and increased breakthrough bleeding should be considered in patients taking combination oral contraceptive products with topiramate).
Products include:
Ortho Micronor Tablets ... 2411

Norethynodrel (The possibility of decreased contraceptive efficacy and increased breakthrough bleeding should be considered in patients taking combination oral contraceptive products with topiramate).
No products indexed under this heading.

Norgestimate (The possibility of decreased contraceptive efficacy and increased breakthrough bleeding should be considered in patients taking combination oral contraceptive products with topiramate).
Products include:
Ortho-Cyclen/Ortho Tri-Cyclen ... 2414
Ortho Tri-Cyclen Lo Tablets ... 2421
Prefest Tablets ... 1069

Norgestrel (The possibility of decreased contraceptive efficacy and increased breakthrough bleeding should be considered in patients taking combination oral contraceptive products with topiramate).
Products include:
Lo/Ovral-28 Tablets ... 3423

Olanzapine (Potential for increased CNS depression). Products include:
Symbyax Capsules ... 1788
Zyprexa Tablets ... 1798
Zyprexa IntraMuscular ... 1798
Zyprexa ZYDIS Orally Disintegrating Tablets ... 1798

Oxazepam (Potential for increased CNS depression).
No products indexed under this heading.

Oxycodone Hydrochloride (Potential for increased CNS depression). Products include:
Combunox Tablets ... 1183
OxyContin Tablets ... 2699
OxyFast Oral Concentrate Solution ... 2704
OxyIR Capsules ... 2704
Percocet Tablets ... 1114
Percodan Tablets ... 1115

Pentobarbital Sodium (Potential for increased CNS depression).
Products include:
Nembutal Sodium Solution, USP ... 2484

Perphenazine (Potential for increased CNS depression).
No products indexed under this heading.

Phenobarbital (Potential for increased CNS depression).
No products indexed under this heading.

Phenytoin (Co-administration has resulted in 48% decrease in topiramate concentration and no change or 25% increase in phenytoin concentration).
No products indexed under this heading.

Phenytoin Sodium (Co-administration has resulted in 48% decrease in topiramate concentration and no change or 25% increase in phenytoin concentration).
Products include:
Phenytek Capsules ... 2153

Pioglitazone Hydrochloride (When topiramate is added to pioglitazone therapy or pioglitazone is added to topiramate therapy, careful attention should be given to the routine monitoring of patients for adequate control of their diabetic disease status). Products include:
ActoPlus Met Tablets ... 3219
Actos Tablets ... 3224

Prazepam (Potential for increased CNS depression).
No products indexed under this heading.

Prochlorperazine (Potential for increased CNS depression).
No products indexed under this heading.

Promethazine Hydrochloride (Potential for increased CNS depression). Products include:
Phenergan ... 3438

Propofol (Potential for increased CNS depression). Products include:
Diprivan Injectable Emulsion ... 676

Propoxyphene Hydrochloride (Potential for increased CNS depression).
No products indexed under this heading.

Propoxyphene Napsylate (Potential for increased CNS depression).
Products include:
Darvocet A 500 Tablets ... 3497

Quazepam (Potential for increased CNS depression).
No products indexed under this heading.

Quetiapine Fumarate (Potential for increased CNS depression).
Products include:
Seroquel Tablets ... 691

Remifentanil Hydrochloride (Potential for increased CNS depression).
No products indexed under this heading.

Risperidone (There was a 25% decrease in exposure to risperidone (2mg single dose) in 12 healthy volunteers receiving 200mg/day of topiramate. Therefore, patients receiving risperidone in combination with topiramate should be closely monitored for clinical response).
Products include:
Risperdal Consta Long-Acting Injection ... 1664
Risperdal M-Tab Orally Disintegrating Tablets ... 1658
Risperdal ... 1658

Secobarbital Sodium (Potential for increased CNS depression).
No products indexed under this heading.

Sevoflurane (Potential for increased CNS depression).
Products include:
Ultane Liquid for Inhalation ... 526

Sodium Oxybate (Potential for increased CNS depression).
No products indexed under this heading.

Sufentanil Citrate (Potential for increased CNS depression).
No products indexed under this heading.

Temazepam (Potential for increased CNS depression).
No products indexed under this heading.

Thiamylal Sodium (Potential for increased CNS depression).
No products indexed under this heading.

Thioridazine Hydrochloride (Potential for increased CNS depression). Products include:
Thioridazine Hydrochloride Tablets ... 2122

Thiothixene (Potential for increased CNS depression). Products include:
Thiothixene Capsules ... 2124

Torsemide (Co-administration of topiramate with carbonic anhydrase inhibitors may create a physiological environment that increases the risk of kidney stone formation; concurrent use should be avoided).
No products indexed under this heading.

Triazolam (Potential for increased CNS depression).
No products indexed under this heading.

Trifluoperazine Hydrochloride (Potential for increased CNS depression).
No products indexed under this heading.

Valproate Sodium (Co-administration resulted in an 11% decrease in valproic acid concentration and a 14% decrease in topiramate concentration. Concomitant administration of topiramate and valproic acid has been associated with hyperammonemia, with or without encephalopathy, in patients who have tolerated either drug alone).
Products include:

Depacon Injection 412

Valproic Acid (Co-administration resulted in an 11% decrease in valproic acid concentration and a 14% decrease in topiramate concentration. Concomitant administration of topiramate and valproic acid has been associated with hyperammonemia, with or without encephalopathy, in patients who have tolerated either drug alone). Products include:

Depakene 417

Zaleplon (Potential for increased CNS depression). Products include:

Sonata Capsules 1686

Ziprasidone Hydrochloride (Potential for increased CNS depression). Products include:

Geodon Capsules 2514

Zolpidem Tartrate (Potential for increased CNS depression). Products include:

Ambien Tablets 2867

Food Interactions

Alcohol (Potential for increased CNS depression).

TOPICORT .05% GEL

(Desoximetasone) 3288

None cited in PDR database.

TOPICORT .25% CREAM

(Desoximetasone) 3288

None cited in PDR database.

TOPICORT .25% OINTMENT

(Desoximetasone) 3288

None cited in PDR database.

TOPICORT LP .05% CREAM

(Desoximetasone) 3288

None cited in PDR database.

TOPROL-XL TABLETS

(Metoprolol Succinate) 660

May interact with catecholamine depleting drugs, cytochrome p450 2d6 inhibitors (selected), monoamine oxidase inhibitors, and certain other agents. Compounds in these categories include:

Amiodarone Hydrochloride (Co-administration of metoprolol with drugs that inhibit CYP2D6, such as quinidine, is likely to increase metoprolol concentration; this increase in plasma concentration would decrease the cardioselectivity of metoprolol). Products include:

Pacerone Tablets 3337

Amitriptyline Hydrochloride (Co-administration of metoprolol with drugs that inhibit CYP2D6, such as quinidine, is likely to increase metoprolol concentration; this increase in plasma concentration would decrease the cardioselectivity of metoprolol).

No products indexed under this heading.

Amoxapine (Co-administration of metoprolol with drugs that inhibit CYP2D6, such as quinidine, is likely to increase metoprolol concentration; this increase in plasma concentration would decrease the cardioselectivity of metoprolol).

No products indexed under this heading.

Bupropion Hydrochloride (Co-administration of metoprolol with drugs that inhibit CYP2D6, such as quinidine, is likely to increase metoprolol concentration; this increase in plasma concentration would decrease the cardioselectivity of metoprolol). Products include:

Wellbutrin Tablets 1579

Wellbutrin SR Sustained-Release Tablets 1583

Wellbutrin XL Extended-Release Tablets 1588

Zyban Sustained-Release Tablets 1620

Celecoxib (Co-administration of metoprolol with drugs that inhibit CYP2D6, such as quinidine, is likely to increase metoprolol concentration; this increase in plasma concentration would decrease the cardioselectivity of metoprolol). Products include:

Celebrex Capsules 3130

Chloroquine Hydrochloride (Co-administration of metoprolol with drugs that inhibit CYP2D6, such as quinidine, is likely to increase metoprolol concentration; this increase in plasma concentration would decrease the cardioselectivity of metoprolol).

No products indexed under this heading.

Chloroquine Phosphate (Co-administration of metoprolol with drugs that inhibit CYP2D6, such as quinidine, is likely to increase metoprolol concentration; this increase in plasma concentration would decrease the cardioselectivity of metoprolol).

No products indexed under this heading.

Chlorpheniramine (Co-administration of metoprolol with drugs that inhibit CYP2D6, such as quinidine, is likely to increase metoprolol concentration; this increase in plasma concentration would decrease the cardioselectivity of metoprolol).

No products indexed under this heading.

Chlorpheniramine Maleate (Co-administration of metoprolol with drugs that inhibit CYP2D6, such as quinidine, is likely to increase metoprolol concentration; this increase in plasma concentration would decrease the cardioselectivity of metoprolol). Products include:

Advil Allergy Sinus Caplets 737

Advil Multi-Symptom Cold Caplets 738

BC Allergy Sinus Cold Powder 612

Contac Severe Cold and Flu Caplets Maximum Strength......... 615

Hycomine Compound Tablets 1105

PediaCare Multi-Symptom Cold Liquid 704

PediaCare NightRest Cough & Cold Liquid....................................... 704

Robitussin Flu Liquid 752

Robitussin PM Cough & Cold Liquid 752

Singlet Caplets 636

Sudafed Sinus & Allergy Tablets 710

TheraFlu Cold & Cough Hot Liquid 680

TheraFlu Cold & Sore Throat Hot Liquid 680

TheraFlu Flu & Sore Throat Hot Liquid 681

TheraFlu Severe Cold & Cough Hot Liquid 683

TheraFlu Severe Cold Caplets 679

TheraFlu Severe Cold Hot Liquid 682

Triaminic Cold & Allergy Liquid 685

Triaminic Cold & Cough Liquid 685

Triaminic Flu, Cough & Fever Liquid 685

Triaminic Night Time Cough & Cold Liquid 685

Triaminic Allergy Runny Nose & Congestion Softchews................ 688

Triaminic Cold & Cough Softchews 688

Children's Tylenol Plus Cold NightTime Suspension Liquid........ 1851

Children's Tylenol Plus Cold & Cough Suspension Liquid and Chewable Tablets 1851

Children's Tylenol Plus Cold Chewable Tablets 1851

Children's Tylenol Plus Flu Suspension Liquid 1853

Tylenol Allergy Complete Multi-Symptom Caplets and Gelcaps with Cool Burst............... 1844

Multi-Symptom Tylenol Cold Night Time Caplets 1845

Vicks 44M Cough, Cold & Flu Relief.. 2676

Pediatric Vicks 44m Cough & Cold Relief.................................. 2673

Children's Vicks NyQuil Cold/Cough Relief....................... 2671

Chlorpheniramine Polistirex (Co-administration of metoprolol with drugs that inhibit CYP2D6, such as quinidine, is likely to increase metoprolol concentration; this increase in plasma concentration would decrease the cardioselectivity of metoprolol). Products include:

Tussionex Pennkinetic Extended-Release Suspension...... 3322

Chlorpheniramine Tannate (Co-administration of metoprolol with drugs that inhibit CYP2D6, such as quinidine, is likely to increase metoprolol concentration; this increase in plasma concentration would decrease the cardioselectivity of metoprolol).

No products indexed under this heading.

Cimetidine (Co-administration of metoprolol with drugs that inhibit CYP2D6, such as quinidine, is likely to increase metoprolol concentration; this increase in plasma concentration would decrease the cardioselectivity of metoprolol). Products include:

Tagamet HB 200 Tablets 637

Tagamet Tablets 1547

Cimetidine Hydrochloride (Co-administration of metoprolol with drugs that inhibit CYP2D6, such as quinidine, is likely to increase metoprolol concentration; this increase in plasma concentration would decrease the cardioselectivity of metoprolol).

No products indexed under this heading.

Citalopram Hydrobromide (Co-administration of metoprolol with drugs that inhibit CYP2D6, such as quinidine, is likely to increase metoprolol concentration; this increase in plasma concentration would decrease the cardioselectivity of metoprolol). Products include:

Celexa 1177

Clomipramine Hydrochloride (Co-administration of metoprolol with drugs that inhibit CYP2D6, such as quinidine, is likely to increase metoprolol concentration; this increase in plasma concentration would decrease the cardioselectivity of metoprolol).

No products indexed under this heading.

Clonidine (Beta-blockers may exacerbate the rebound hypertension which can follow the withdrawal of clonidine. If co-administered, withdraw beta-blockers several days before the gradual withdrawal of clonidine. If replacing clonidine by beta-blocker therapy, delay start of beta-blockers for several days after clonidine administration has stopped). Products include:

Catapres-TTS 875

Cocaine Hydrochloride (Co-administration of metoprolol with drugs that inhibit CYP2D6, such as quinidine, is likely to increase metoprolol concentration; this increase in plasma concentration would decrease the cardioselectivity of metoprolol).

No products indexed under this heading.

Deserpidine (Catecholamine-depleting drugs may have an additive effect when given with beta-blocking agents; monitor closely for signs of hypotension or marked bradycardia).

No products indexed under this heading.

Desipramine Hydrochloride (Co-administration of metoprolol with drugs that inhibit CYP2D6, such as quinidine, is likely to increase metoprolol concentration; this increase in plasma concentration would decrease the cardioselectivity of metoprolol).

No products indexed under this heading.

Diltiazem Hydrochloride (Because of significant inotropic and chronotropic effects in patients treated with beta-blockers and calcium-channel blockers of the diltiazem type, caution should be exercised in patients treated with these agents concomitantly). Products include:

Cardizem LA Extended Release Tablets 1699

Tiazac Capsules 1204

Diphenhydramine (Co-administration of metoprolol with drugs that inhibit CYP2D6, such as quinidine, is likely to increase metoprolol concentration; this increase in plasma concentration would decrease the cardioselectivity of metoprolol). Products include:

Tylenol Sore Throat NightTime Liquid with Cool Burst.................. 1849

Diphenhydramine Hydrochloride (Co-administration of metoprolol with drugs that inhibit CYP2D6, such as quinidine, is likely to increase metoprolol concentration; this increase in plasma concentration would decrease the cardioselectivity of metoprolol). Products include:

Benadryl Allergy & Cold Tablets 692

Benadryl Allergy 691

Benadryl Allergy & Sinus Headache Caplets & Gelcaps...... 693

Children's Benadryl Allergy Liquid ... 695

Children's Benadryl Dye-Free Allergy Liquid 695

Benadryl Dye-Free Allergy Liqui-Gels Softgels...................... 692

Benadryl Itch Relief Stick Extra Strength 696

Benadryl Itch Stopping Cream Extra Strength 697

Benadryl Itch Stopping Gel Extra Strength 697

Benadryl Itch Stopping Spray Extra Strength 697

Benadryl Maximum Strength Severe Allergy & Sinus Headache Caplets....................... 694

Children's Benadryl D Liquid Medication.................................. 693

Benadryl D Tablets 694

Nytol QuickCaps Caplets 635

Maximum Strength Nytol QuickGels Softgels 635

Simply Sleep Caplets 1841

Sominex Original Formula Tablets .. 637

TheraFlu Thin Strips Multi Symptom.................................... 684

Triaminic Thin Strips Cough & Runny Nose 690

Children's Tylenol Plus Cold & Allergy Suspension Liquid............ 1850

IMPORTANT NOTE: Always consult each drug listing in the patient's regimen for possible interactions.

Tylenol Allergy Complete Night Time Caplets 1844
Tylenol Severe Allergy Caplets 1844
Tylenol Flu NightTime Gelcaps 1846
Extra Strength Tylenol PM Caplets, Geltabs, Gelcaps and Liquid 1847
Unisom Maximum Strength SleepGels ..... ▣712

Doxepin Hydrochloride (Co-administration of metoprolol with drugs that inhibit CYP2D6, such as quinidine, is likely to increase metoprolol concentration; this increase in plasma concentration would decrease the cardioselectivity of metoprolol).
No products indexed under this heading.

Epinephrine Hydrochloride (Potential unresponsiveness to the usual dose of epinephrine to treat allergic reactions in certain patients).
No products indexed under this heading.

Escitalopram Oxalate (Co-administration of metoprolol with drugs that inhibit CYP2D6, such as quinidine, is likely to increase metoprolol concentration; this increase in plasma concentration would decrease the cardioselectivity of metoprolol). Products include:
Lexapro Oral Solution 1193
Lexapro Tablets 1193

Fluoxetine (Co-administration of metoprolol with drugs that inhibit CYP2D6, such as quinidine, is likely to increase metoprolol concentration; this increase in plasma concentration would decrease the cardioselectivity of metoprolol).
No products indexed under this heading.

Fluoxetine Hydrochloride (Co-administration with drugs that inhibit CYP2D6, such as fluoxetine, are likely to increase metoprolol concentrations; these increases in plasma concentration would decrease the cardioselectivity of metoprolol). Products include:
Prozac Pulvules and Liquid 1771
Symbyax Capsules 1788

Fluphenazine Decanoate (Co-administration of metoprolol with drugs that inhibit CYP2D6, such as quinidine, is likely to increase metoprolol concentration; this increase in plasma concentration would decrease the cardioselectivity of metoprolol).
No products indexed under this heading.

Fluphenazine Enanthate (Co-administration of metoprolol with drugs that inhibit CYP2D6, such as quinidine, is likely to increase metoprolol concentration; this increase in plasma concentration would decrease the cardioselectivity of metoprolol).
No products indexed under this heading.

Fluphenazine Hydrochloride (Co-administration of metoprolol with drugs that inhibit CYP2D6, such as quinidine, is likely to increase metoprolol concentration; this increase in plasma concentration would decrease the cardioselectivity of metoprolol).
No products indexed under this heading.

Fluvoxamine Maleate (Co-administration of metoprolol with drugs that inhibit CYP2D6, such as quinidine, is likely to increase metoprolol concentration; this increase in plasma concentration would decrease the cardioselectivity of metoprolol).
No products indexed under this heading.

Guanethidine Monosulfate (Catecholamine-depleting drugs may have an additive effect when given with beta-blocking agents; monitor closely for signs of hypotension or marked bradycardia).
No products indexed under this heading.

Halofantrine Hydrochloride (Co-administration of metoprolol with drugs that inhibit CYP2D6, such as quinidine, is likely to increase metoprolol concentration; this increase in plasma concentration would decrease the cardioselectivity of metoprolol).
No products indexed under this heading.

Haloperidol (Co-administration of metoprolol with drugs that inhibit CYP2D6, such as quinidine, is likely to increase metoprolol concentration; this increase in plasma concentration would decrease the cardioselectivity of metoprolol).
No products indexed under this heading.

Haloperidol Decanoate (Co-administration of metoprolol with drugs that inhibit CYP2D6, such as quinidine, is likely to increase metoprolol concentration; this increase in plasma concentration would decrease the cardioselectivity of metoprolol).
No products indexed under this heading.

Hydroxychloroquine Sulfate (Co-administration of metoprolol with drugs that inhibit CYP2D6, such as quinidine, is likely to increase metoprolol concentration; this increase in plasma concentration would decrease the cardioselectivity of metoprolol).
No products indexed under this heading.

Imatinib Mesylate (Co-administration of metoprolol with drugs that inhibit CYP2D6, such as quinidine, is likely to increase metoprolol concentration; this increase in plasma concentration would decrease the cardioselectivity of metoprolol). Products include:
Gleevec Tablets 2221

Imipramine Hydrochloride (Co-administration of metoprolol with drugs that inhibit CYP2D6, such as quinidine, is likely to increase metoprolol concentration; this increase in plasma concentration would decrease the cardioselectivity of metoprolol).
No products indexed under this heading.

Imipramine Pamoate (Co-administration of metoprolol with drugs that inhibit CYP2D6, such as quinidine, is likely to increase metoprolol concentration; this increase in plasma concentration would decrease the cardioselectivity of metoprolol).
No products indexed under this heading.

Isocarboxazid (Catecholamine-depleting drugs may have an additive effect when given with beta-blocking agents; monitor closely for signs of hypotension or marked bradycardia).
No products indexed under this heading.

Maprotiline Hydrochloride (Co-administration of metoprolol with drugs that inhibit CYP2D6, such as quinidine, is likely to increase metoprolol concentration; this increase in plasma concentration would decrease the cardioselectivity of metoprolol).
No products indexed under this heading.

Methadone Hydrochloride (Co-administration of metoprolol with drugs that inhibit CYP2D6, such as quinidine, is likely to increase metoprolol concentration; this increase in plasma concentration would decrease the cardioselectivity of metoprolol).
No products indexed under this heading.

Mibefradil Dihydrochloride (Co-administration of metoprolol with drugs that inhibit CYP2D6, such as quinidine, is likely to increase metoprolol concentration; this increase in plasma concentration would decrease the cardioselectivity of metoprolol).
No products indexed under this heading.

Moclobemide (Catecholamine-depleting drugs may have an additive effect when given with beta-blocking agents; monitor closely for signs of hypotension or marked bradycardia).
No products indexed under this heading.

Nortriptyline Hydrochloride (Co-administration of metoprolol with drugs that inhibit CYP2D6, such as quinidine, is likely to increase metoprolol concentration; this increase in plasma concentration would decrease the cardioselectivity of metoprolol).
No products indexed under this heading.

Pargyline Hydrochloride (Catecholamine-depleting drugs may have an additive effect when given with beta-blocking agents; monitor closely for signs of hypotension or marked bradycardia).
No products indexed under this heading.

Paroxetine Hydrochloride (Co-administration with drugs that inhibit CYP2D6, such as paroxetine, are likely to increase metoprolol concentrations; these increases in plasma concentration would decrease the cardioselectivity of metoprolol). Products include:
Paxil CR Controlled-Release Tablets 1509
Paxil 1501

Perphenazine (Co-administration of metoprolol with drugs that inhibit CYP2D6, such as quinidine, is likely to increase metoprolol concentration; this increase in plasma concentration would decrease the cardioselectivity of metoprolol).
No products indexed under this heading.

Phenelzine Sulfate (Catecholamine-depleting drugs may have an additive effect when given with beta-blocking agents; monitor closely for signs of hypotension or marked bradycardia).
No products indexed under this heading.

Procarbazine Hydrochloride (Catecholamine-depleting drugs may have an additive effect when given with beta-blocking agents; monitor closely for signs of hypotension or marked bradycardia). Products include:
Matulane Capsules 3188

Propafenone Hydrochloride (Co-administration with drugs that inhibit CYP2D6, such as propafenone, are likely to increase metoprolol concentrations; these increases in plasma concentration would decrease the cardioselectivity of metoprolol). Products include:
Rythmol SR Capsules 2736

Propoxyphene Hydrochloride (Co-administration of metoprolol with drugs that inhibit CYP2D6, such as quinidine, is likely to increase metoprolol concentration; this increase in plasma concentration would decrease the cardioselectivity of metoprolol).
No products indexed under this heading.

Propoxyphene Napsylate (Co-administration of metoprolol with drugs that inhibit CYP2D6, such as quinidine, is likely to increase metoprolol concentration; this increase in plasma concentration would decrease the cardioselectivity of metoprolol). Products include:
Darvocet A 500 Tablets 3497

Protriptyline Hydrochloride (Co-administration of metoprolol with drugs that inhibit CYP2D6, such as quinidine, is likely to increase metoprolol concentration; this increase in plasma concentration would decrease the cardioselectivity of metoprolol). Products include:
Vivactil Tablets 2350

Quinacrine Hydrochloride (Co-administration of metoprolol with drugs that inhibit CYP2D6, such as quinidine, is likely to increase metoprolol concentration; this increase in plasma concentration would decrease the cardioselectivity of metoprolol).
No products indexed under this heading.

Quinidine Gluconate (Co-administration of metoprolol with drugs that inhibit CYP2D6, such as quinidine, is likely to increase metoprolol concentration; this increase in plasma concentration would decrease the cardioselectivity of metoprolol).
No products indexed under this heading.

Quinidine Hydrochloride (Co-administration of metoprolol with drugs that inhibit CYP2D6, such as quinidine, is likely to increase metoprolol concentration; this increase in plasma concentration would decrease the cardioselectivity of metoprolol).
No products indexed under this heading.

Quinidine Polygalacturonate (Co-administration of metoprolol with drugs that inhibit CYP2D6, such as quinidine, is likely to increase metoprolol concentration; this increase in plasma concentration would decrease the cardioselectivity of metoprolol).
No products indexed under this heading.

Quinidine Sulfate (Co-administration of metoprolol with drugs that inhibit CYP2D6, such as quinidine, is likely to increase metoprolol concentration; this increase in plasma concentration would decrease the cardioselectivity of metoprolol).
No products indexed under this heading.

Ranitidine Bismuth Citrate (Co-administration of metoprolol with drugs that inhibit CYP2D6, such as quinidine, is likely to increase metoprolol concentration; this increase in plasma concentration would decrease the cardioselectivity of metoprolol).
No products indexed under this heading.

Ranitidine Hydrochloride (Co-administration of metoprolol with drugs that inhibit CYP2D6, such as quinidine, is likely to increase metoprolol concentration; this increase in plasma concentration would decrease the cardioselectivity of metoprolol). Products include:
Zantac ... **1597**
Zantac Injection ... **1593**
Zantac 75 Tablets ... **715**
Zantac 150 Maximum Strength Tablets ... **715**
Zantac Injection Pharmacy Bulk Package ... **1595**

Rauwolfia Serpentina (Catecholamine-depleting drugs may have an additive effect when given with beta-blocking agents; monitor closely for signs of hypotension or marked bradycardia).
No products indexed under this heading.

Rescinnamine (Catecholamine-depleting drugs may have an additive effect when given with beta-blocking agents; monitor closely for signs of hypotension or marked bradycardia).
No products indexed under this heading.

Reserpine (Catecholamine-depleting drugs may have an additive effect when given with beta-blocking agents; monitor closely for signs of hypotension or marked bradycardia).
No products indexed under this heading.

Ritonavir (Co-administration of metoprolol with drugs that inhibit CYP2D6, such as quinidine, is likely to increase metoprolol concentration; this increase in plasma concentration would decrease the cardioselectivity of metoprolol). Products include:
Kaletra ... **474**
Norvir ... **499**

Selegiline Hydrochloride (Catecholamine-depleting drugs may have an additive effect when given with beta-blocking agents; monitor closely for signs of hypotension or marked bradycardia). Products include:
Eldepryl Capsules ... **3209**

Sertraline Hydrochloride (Co-administration of metoprolol with drugs that inhibit CYP2D6, such as quinidine, is likely to increase metoprolol concentration; this increase in plasma concentration would decrease the cardioselectivity of metoprolol). Products include:
Zoloft ... **2581**

Terbinafine Hydrochloride (Co-administration of metoprolol with drugs that inhibit CYP2D6, such as quinidine, is likely to increase metoprolol concentration; this increase in plasma concentration would decrease the cardioselectivity of metoprolol). Products include:
Lamisil AT Creams (Athlete's Foot & Jock Itch) ... **676**
Lamisil Tablets ... **2226**

Thioridazine Hydrochloride (Co-administration of metoprolol with drugs that inhibit CYP2D6, such as quinidine, is likely to increase metoprolol concentration; this increase in plasma concentration would decrease the cardioselectivity of metoprolol). Products include:
Thioridazine Hydrochloride Tablets ... **2122**

Tranylcypromine Sulfate (Catecholamine-depleting drugs may have an additive effect when given with beta-blocking agents; monitor closely for signs of hypotension or marked bradycardia). Products include:
Parnate Tablets ... **1499**

Trimipramine Maleate (Co-administration of metoprolol with drugs that inhibit CYP2D6, such as quinidine, is likely to increase metoprolol concentration; this increase in plasma concentration would decrease the cardioselectivity of metoprolol). Products include:
Surmontil Capsules ... **2347**

Verapamil Hydrochloride (Because of significant inotropic and chronotropic effects in patients treated with beta-blockers and calcium-channel blockers of the verapamil type, caution should be exercised in patients treated with these agents concomitantly). Products include:
Covera-HS Tablets ... **3135**
Tarka Tablets ... **519**
Verelan PM Capsules ... **3120**

TRACLEER TABLETS

(Bosentan) ... **539**
May interact with oral contraceptives and certain other agents. Compounds in these categories include:

Atorvastatin Calcium (Bosentan is expected to reduce plasma concentrations of statins that have significant metabolism by CYP3A4, such as atorvastatin). Products include:
Caduet Tablets ... **2507**
Lipitor Tablets ... **2495**

Cyclosporine (Co-administration has resulted in markedly increased plasma concentrations of bosentan; concurrent use is contraindicated). Products include:
Gengraf Capsules ... **458**
Neoral Soft Gelatin Capsules ... **2247**
Neoral Oral Solution ... **2247**
Restasis Ophthalmic Emulsion ... **570**
Sandimmune ... **2259**

Desogestrel (Co-administration increases the possibility of failure of contraception. Women should practice additional methods of contraception). Products include:
Ortho-Cept Tablets ... **2395**

Ethinyl Estradiol (Co-administration increases the possibility of failure of contraception. Women should practice additional methods of contraception). Products include:
Alesse-28 Tablets ... **3392**
Lo/Ovral-28 Tablets ... **3423**
NuvaRing ... **2357**
Ortho-Cept Tablets ... **2395**
Ortho-Cyclen/Ortho Tri-Cyclen ... **2414**
Ortho Evra Transdermal System ... **2402**
Ortho Tri-Cyclen Lo Tablets ... **2421**
Seasonale Tablets ... **1073**
Triphasil-28 Tablets ... **3483**
Yasmin 28 Tablets ... **818**

Ethynodiol Diacetate (Co-administration increases the possibility of failure of contraception. Women should practice additional methods of contraception).
No products indexed under this heading.

Glyburide (Co-administration increases the risk of liver enzyme elevation; concurrent use is contraindicated).
No products indexed under this heading.

Ketoconazole (Co-administration increases the plasma concentrations of bosentan by approximately two-fold). Products include:
Nizoral A-D Shampoo, 1% ... **1839**
Nizoral 2% Shampoo ... **1838**

Levonorgestrel (Co-administration increases the possibility of failure of contraception. Women should practice additional methods of contraception). Products include:
Alesse-28 Tablets ... **3392**
Climara Pro Transdermal System ... **800**
Mirena Intrauterine System ... **810**
Plan B Tablets ... **1068**
Seasonale Tablets ... **1073**
Triphasil-28 Tablets ... **3483**

Lovastatin (Bosentan is expected to reduce plasma concentrations of statins that have significant metabolism by CYP3A4, such as lovastatin). Products include:
Advicor Tablets ... **1694**
Altoprev Extended-Release Tablets ... **1151**
Mevacor Tablets ... **1996**

Mestranol (Co-administration increases the possibility of failure of contraception. Women should practice additional methods of contraception).
No products indexed under this heading.

Norethindrone (Co-administration increases the possibility of failure of contraception. Women should practice additional methods of contraception). Products include:
Ortho Micronor Tablets ... **2411**

Norethynodrel (Co-administration increases the possibility of failure of contraception. Women should practice additional methods of contraception).
No products indexed under this heading.

Norgestimate (Co-administration increases the possibility of failure of contraception. Women should practice additional methods of contraception). Products include:
Ortho-Cyclen/Ortho Tri-Cyclen ... **2414**
Ortho Tri-Cyclen Lo Tablets ... **2421**
Prefest Tablets ... **1069**

Norgestrel (Co-administration increases the possibility of failure of contraception. Women should practice additional methods of contraception). Products include:
Lo/Ovral-28 Tablets ... **3423**

Simvastatin (Co-administration decreases plasma concentrations of simvastatin and its active metabolite by 50%). Products include:
Vytorin 10/10 Tablets ... **2084**
Vytorin 10/10 Tablets ... **3092**
Vytorin 10/20 Tablets ... **2084**
Vytorin 10/20 Tablets ... **3092**
Vytorin 10/40 Tablets ... **3092**
Vytorin 10/40 Tablets ... **2084**
Vytorin 10/80 Tablets ... **2084**
Vytorin 10/80 Tablets ... **3092**
Zocor Tablets ... **2078**

Tacrolimus (Caution should be exercised if tacrolimus and bosentan are used together). Products include:
Prograf Capsules and Injection ... **624**
Protopic Ointment ... **629**

TRANSDERM SCOP TRANSDERMAL THERAPEUTIC SYSTEM

(Scopolamine) ... **2166**
May interact with anticholinergics, antihistamines, central nervous system depressants, tricyclic antidepressants, and certain other agents. Compounds in these categories include:

Acrivastine (Antihistamines have anticholinergic properties and co-administration may result in additive effects).
No products indexed under this heading.

Alfentanil Hydrochloride (Scopolamine is an anticholinergic agent and causes certain CNS effects, such as drowsiness and dizziness, and hence it should be used with care in patients on concomitant therapy).
No products indexed under this heading.

Alprazolam (Scopolamine is an anticholinergic agent and causes certain CNS effects, such as drowsiness and dizziness, and hence it should be used with care in patients on concomitant therapy). Products include:
Niravam Orally Disintegrating Tablets ... **3106**
Xanax XR Tablets ... **2655**

Amitriptyline Hydrochloride (Tricyclic antidepressants have anticholinergic properties and co-administration may result in additive effects).
No products indexed under this heading.

Amoxapine (Tricyclic antidepressants have anticholinergic properties and co-administration may result in additive effects).
No products indexed under this heading.

Aprobarbital (Scopolamine is an anticholinergic agent and causes certain CNS effects, such as drowsiness and dizziness, and hence it should be used with care in patients on concomitant therapy).
No products indexed under this heading.

Astemizole (Antihistamines have anticholinergic properties and co-administration may result in additive effects).
No products indexed under this heading.

Atropine Sulfate (Co-administration may result in additive anticholinergic effects).
No products indexed under this heading.

Azatadine Maleate (Antihistamines have anticholinergic properties and co-administration may result in additive effects).
No products indexed under this heading.

Belladonna Alkaloids (Co-administration may result in additive anticholinergic effects). Products include:
Hyland's Teething Tablets .... ▣736

Benztropine Mesylate (Co-administration may result in additive anticholinergic effects). Products include:
Cogentin Injection 1903

Biperiden Hydrochloride (Co-administration may result in additive anticholinergic effects).
No products indexed under this heading.

Bromodiphenhydramine Hydrochloride (Antihistamines have anticholinergic properties and co-administration may result in additive effects).
No products indexed under this heading.

Brompheniramine Maleate (Antihistamines have anticholinergic properties and co-administration may result in additive effects). Products include:
Alacol DM Syrup 739
Children's Dimetapp Cold & Allergy Elixir .... ▣745
Children's Dimetapp DM Cold & Cough Elixir .... ▣745
Robitussin Allergy & Cough Syrup .. ▣750

Buprenorphine Hydrochloride (Scopolamine is an anticholinergic agent and causes certain CNS effects, such as drowsiness and dizziness, and hence it should be used with care in patients on concomitant therapy). Products include:
Buprenex Injectable 2718
Suboxone Tablets 2719
Subutex Tablets 2719

Buspirone Hydrochloride (Scopolamine is an anticholinergic agent and causes certain CNS effects, such as drowsiness and dizziness, and hence it should be used with care in patients on concomitant therapy).
No products indexed under this heading.

Butabarbital (Scopolamine is an anticholinergic agent and causes certain CNS effects, such as drowsiness and dizziness, and hence it should be used with care in patients on concomitant therapy).
No products indexed under this heading.

Butalbital (Scopolamine is an anticholinergic agent and causes certain CNS effects, such as drowsiness and dizziness, and hence it should be used with care in patients on concomitant therapy). Products include:
Sedapap Tablets 50 mg/650 mg 2098

Cetirizine Hydrochloride (Antihistamines have anticholinergic properties and co-administration may result in additive effects). Products include:
Zyrtec Chewable Tablets 2589
Zyrtec 2589
Zyrtec-D 12 Hour Extended Release Tablets 2591

Chlordiazepoxide (Scopolamine is an anticholinergic agent and causes certain CNS effects, such as drowsiness and dizziness, and hence it should be used with care in patients on concomitant therapy).
No products indexed under this heading.

Chlordiazepoxide Hydrochloride (Scopolamine is an anticholinergic agent and causes certain CNS effects, such as drowsiness and dizziness, and hence it should be used with care in patients on concomitant therapy). Products include:
Librium Capsules 3349

Chlorpheniramine Maleate (Antihistamines have anticholinergic properties and co-administration may result in additive effects). Products include:
Advil Allergy Sinus Caplets .... ▣737
Advil Multi-Symptom Cold Caplets .... ▣738
BC Allergy Sinus Cold Powder .... ▣612
Contac Severe Cold and Flu Caplets Maximum Strength .... ▣615
Hycomine Compound Tablets 1105
PediaCare Multi-Symptom Cold Liquid .... ▣704
PediaCare NightRest Cough & Cold Liquid .... ▣704
Robitussin Flu Liquid .... ▣752
Robitussin PM Cough & Cold Liquid .... ▣752
Singlet Caplets .... ▣636
Sudafed Sinus & Allergy Tablets ..... ▣710
TheraFlu Cold & Cough Hot Liquid .... ▣680
TheraFlu Cold & Sore Throat Hot Liquid .... ▣680
TheraFlu Flu & Sore Throat Hot Liquid .... ▣681
TheraFlu Severe Cold & Cough Hot Liquid .... ▣683
TheraFlu Severe Cold Caplets .... ▣679
TheraFlu Severe Cold Hot Liquid ..... ▣682
Triaminic Cold & Allergy Liquid .... ▣685
Triaminic Cold & Cough Liquid .... ▣685
Triaminic Flu, Cough & Fever Liquid .... ▣685
Triaminic Night Time Cough & Cold Liquid .... ▣685
Triaminic Allergy Runny Nose & Congestion Softchews .... ▣688
Triaminic Cold & Cough Softchews .... ▣688
Children's Tylenol Plus Cold NightTime Suspension Liquid 1851
Children's Tylenol Plus Cold & Cough Suspension Liquid and Chewable Tablets 1851
Children's Tylenol Plus Cold Chewable Tablets 1851
Children's Tylenol Plus Flu Suspension Liquid 1853
Tylenol Allergy Complete Multi-Symptom Caplets and Gelcaps with Cool Burst 1844
Multi-Symptom Tylenol Cold Night Time Caplets 1845
Vicks 44M Cough, Cold & Flu Relief 2676
Pediatric Vicks 44m Cough & Cold Relief 2673
Children's Vicks NyQuil Cold/Cough Relief 2671

Chlorpheniramine Polistirex (Antihistamines have anticholinergic properties and co-administration may result in additive effects). Products include:
Tussionex Pennkinetic Extended-Release Suspension 3322

Chlorpheniramine Tannate (Antihistamines have anticholinergic properties and co-administration may result in additive effects).
No products indexed under this heading.

Chlorpromazine (Scopolamine is an anticholinergic agent and causes certain CNS effects, such as drowsiness and dizziness, and hence it should be used with care in patients on concomitant therapy).
No products indexed under this heading.

Chlorpromazine Hydrochloride (Scopolamine is an anticholinergic agent and causes certain CNS effects, such as drowsiness and dizziness, and hence it should be used with care in patients on concomitant therapy).
No products indexed under this heading.

Chlorprothixene (Scopolamine is an anticholinergic agent and causes certain CNS effects, such as drowsiness and dizziness, and hence it should be used with care in patients on concomitant therapy).
No products indexed under this heading.

Chlorprothixene Hydrochloride (Scopolamine is an anticholinergic agent and causes certain CNS effects, such as drowsiness and dizziness, and hence it should be used with care in patients on concomitant therapy).
No products indexed under this heading.

Chlorprothixene Lactate (Scopolamine is an anticholinergic agent and causes certain CNS effects, such as drowsiness and dizziness, and hence it should be used with care in patients on concomitant therapy).
No products indexed under this heading.

Clemastine Fumarate (Antihistamines have anticholinergic properties and co-administration may result in additive effects).
No products indexed under this heading.

Clidinium Bromide (Co-administration may result in additive anticholinergic effects).
No products indexed under this heading.

Clomipramine Hydrochloride (Tricyclic antidepressants have anticholinergic properties and co-administration may result in additive effects).
No products indexed under this heading.

Clorazepate Dipotassium (Scopolamine is an anticholinergic agent and causes certain CNS effects, such as drowsiness and dizziness, and hence it should be used with care in patients on concomitant therapy). Products include:
Tranxene 2488

Clozapine (Scopolamine is an anticholinergic agent and causes certain CNS effects, such as drowsiness and dizziness, and hence it should be used with care in patients on concomitant therapy). Products include:
Clozapine Tablets 2141
Clozaril Tablets 2174
FazaClo Orally Disintegrating Tablets 547

Codeine Phosphate (Scopolamine is an anticholinergic agent and causes certain CNS effects, such as drowsiness and dizziness, and hence it should be used with care in patients on concomitant therapy). Products include:
Tylenol with Codeine 2461

Cyproheptadine Hydrochloride (Antihistamines have anticholinergic properties and co-administration may result in additive effects).
No products indexed under this heading.

Desflurane (Scopolamine is an anticholinergic agent and causes certain CNS effects, such as drowsiness and dizziness, and hence it should be used with care in patients on concomitant therapy). Products include:
Suprane Liquid for Inhalation 770

Desipramine Hydrochloride (Tricyclic antidepressants have anticholinergic properties and co-administration may result in additive effects).
No products indexed under this heading.

Dexchlorpheniramine Maleate (Antihistamines have anticholinergic properties and co-administration may result in additive effects).
No products indexed under this heading.

Dezocine (Scopolamine is an anticholinergic agent and causes certain CNS effects, such as drowsiness and dizziness, and hence it should be used with care in patients on concomitant therapy).
No products indexed under this heading.

Diazepam (Scopolamine is an anticholinergic agent and causes certain CNS effects, such as drowsiness and dizziness, and hence it should be used with care in patients on concomitant therapy). Products include:
Diastat Rectal Delivery System 3344
Valium Tablets 2822

Dicyclomine Hydrochloride (Co-administration may result in additive anticholinergic effects). Products include:
Bentyl Capsules 724
Bentyl Injection 724
Bentyl Syrup 724
Bentyl Tablets 724

Diphenhydramine Citrate (Antihistamines have anticholinergic properties and co-administration may result in additive effects). Products include:
Children's Benadryl Allergy & Cold Fastmelt Tablets .... ▣695
Children's Benadryl D Allergy & Sinus Fastmelt Tablets .... ▣694
Children's Benadryl Allergy Fastmelt Tablets .... ▣696
Goody's PM Powder .... ▣622

Diphenhydramine Hydrochloride (Antihistamines have anticholinergic properties and co-administration may result in additive effects). Products include:
Benadryl Allergy & Cold Tablets ..... ▣692
Benadryl Allergy .... ▣691
Benadryl Allergy & Sinus Headache Caplets & Gelcaps .... ▣693
Children's Benadryl Allergy Liquid ... ▣695
Children's Benadryl Dye-Free Allergy Liquid .... ▣695
Benadryl Dye-Free Allergy Liqui-Gels Softgels .... ▣692
Benadryl Itch Relief Stick Extra Strength .... ▣696
Benadryl Itch Stopping Cream Extra Strength .... ▣697
Benadryl Itch Stopping Gel Extra Strength .... ▣697
Benadryl Itch Stopping Spray Extra Strength .... ▣697
Benadryl Maximum Strength Severe Allergy & Sinus Headache Caplets .... ▣694
Children's Benadryl D Liquid Medication .... ▣693
Benadryl D Tablets .... ▣694
Nytol QuickCaps Caplets .... ▣635

Maximum Strength Nytol QuickGels Softgels .... ▣ **635**
Simply Sleep Caplets **1841**
Sominex Original Formula Tablets .. ▣ **637**
TheraFlu Thin Strips Multi Symptom..................... ▣ **684**
Triaminic Thin Strips Cough & Runny Nose .... ▣ **690**
Children's Tylenol Plus Cold & Allergy Suspension Liquid............ **1850**
Tylenol Allergy Complete Night Time Caplets..................... **1844**
Tylenol Severe Allergy Caplets **1844**
Tylenol Flu NightTime Gelcaps **1846**
Extra Strength Tylenol PM Caplets, Geltabs, Gelcaps and Liquid..................... **1847**
Unisom Maximum Strength SleepGels..................... ▣ **712**

Diphenylpyraline Hydrochloride (Antihistamines have anticholinergic properties and co-administration may result in additive effects).
No products indexed under this heading.

Doxepin Hydrochloride (Tricyclic antidepressants have anticholinergic properties and co-administration may result in additive effects).
No products indexed under this heading.

Droperidol (Scopolamine is an anticholinergic agent and causes certain CNS effects, such as drowsiness and dizziness, and hence it should be used with care in patients on concomitant therapy).
No products indexed under this heading.

Enflurane (Scopolamine is an anticholinergic agent and causes certain CNS effects, such as drowsiness and dizziness, and hence it should be used with care in patients on concomitant therapy).
No products indexed under this heading.

Estazolam (Scopolamine is an anticholinergic agent and causes certain CNS effects, such as drowsiness and dizziness, and hence it should be used with care in patients on concomitant therapy). Products include:
ProSom Tablets **512**

Ethanol (Scopolamine is an anticholinergic agent and causes certain CNS effects, such as drowsiness and dizziness, and hence it should be used with care in patients on concomitant therapy).
No products indexed under this heading.

Ethchlorvynol (Scopolamine is an anticholinergic agent and causes certain CNS effects, such as drowsiness and dizziness, and hence it should be used with care in patients on concomitant therapy).
No products indexed under this heading.

Ethinamate (Scopolamine is an anticholinergic agent and causes certain CNS effects, such as drowsiness and dizziness, and hence it should be used with care in patients on concomitant therapy).
No products indexed under this heading.

Ethyl Alcohol (Scopolamine is an anticholinergic agent and causes certain CNS effects, such as drowsiness and dizziness, and hence it should be used with care in patients on concomitant therapy).
No products indexed under this heading.

Fentanyl (Scopolamine is an anticholinergic agent and causes certain CNS effects, such as drowsiness and dizziness, and hence it should be used with care in patients on concomitant therapy). Products include:
Duragesic Transdermal System **2448**

Fentanyl Citrate (Scopolamine is an anticholinergic agent and causes certain CNS effects, such as drowsiness and dizziness, and hence it should be used with care in patients on concomitant therapy). Products include:
Actiq **993**

Fexofenadine Hydrochloride (Antihistamines have anticholinergic properties and co-administration may result in additive effects). Products include:
Allegra **2857**
Allegra-D 12 Hour Extended-Release Tablets............ **2860**
Allegra-D 24 Hour Extended-Release Tablets............ **2862**

Fluphenazine Decanoate (Scopolamine is an anticholinergic agent and causes certain CNS effects, such as drowsiness and dizziness, and hence it should be used with care in patients on concomitant therapy).
No products indexed under this heading.

Fluphenazine Enanthate (Scopolamine is an anticholinergic agent and causes certain CNS effects, such as drowsiness and dizziness, and hence it should be used with care in patients on concomitant therapy).
No products indexed under this heading.

Fluphenazine Hydrochloride (Scopolamine is an anticholinergic agent and causes certain CNS effects, such as drowsiness and dizziness, and hence it should be used with care in patients on concomitant therapy).
No products indexed under this heading.

Flurazepam Hydrochloride (Scopolamine is an anticholinergic agent and causes certain CNS effects, such as drowsiness and dizziness, and hence it should be used with care in patients on concomitant therapy). Products include:
Dalmane Capsules **3343**

Glutethimide (Scopolamine is an anticholinergic agent and causes certain CNS effects, such as drowsiness and dizziness, and hence it should be used with care in patients on concomitant therapy).
No products indexed under this heading.

Glycopyrrolate (Co-administration may result in additive anticholinergic effects).
No products indexed under this heading.

Haloperidol (Scopolamine is an anticholinergic agent and causes certain CNS effects, such as drowsiness and dizziness, and hence it should be used with care in patients on concomitant therapy).
No products indexed under this heading.

Haloperidol Decanoate (Scopolamine is an anticholinergic agent and causes certain CNS effects, such as drowsiness and dizziness, and hence it should be used with care in patients on concomitant therapy).
No products indexed under this heading.

Hydrocodone Bitartrate (Scopolamine is an anticholinergic agent and causes certain CNS effects, such as drowsiness and dizziness, and hence it should be used with care in patients on concomitant therapy). Products include:
Hycodan **1104**
Hycomine Compound Tablets **1105**
Hycotuss Expectorant Syrup **1106**
Lortab **3315**
Lortab Elixir **3312**
Vicodin Tablets **530**
Vicodin ES Tablets **531**
Vicodin HP Tablets **532**
Vicoprofen Tablets **533**
Zydone Tablets **1118**

Hydrocodone Polistirex (Scopolamine is an anticholinergic agent and causes certain CNS effects, such as drowsiness and dizziness, and hence it should be used with care in patients on concomitant therapy). Products include:
Tussionex Pennkinetic Extended-Release Suspension...... **3322**

Hydromorphone Hydrochloride (Scopolamine is an anticholinergic agent and causes certain CNS effects, such as drowsiness and dizziness, and hence it should be used with care in patients on concomitant therapy). Products include:
Dilaudid **439**
Dilaudid Oral Liquid **443**
Dilaudid Non-Sterile Powder **439**
Dilaudid Rectal Suppositories **439**
Dilaudid Tablets **439**
Dilaudid Tablets - 8 mg **443**
Dilaudid-HP **441**

Hydroxyzine Hydrochloride (Scopolamine is an anticholinergic agent and causes certain CNS effects, such as drowsiness and dizziness, and hence it should be used with care in patients on concomitant therapy).
No products indexed under this heading.

Hyoscyamine (Co-administration may result in additive anticholinergic effects).
No products indexed under this heading.

Hyoscyamine Sulfate (Co-administration may result in additive anticholinergic effects).
No products indexed under this heading.

Imipramine Hydrochloride (Tricyclic antidepressants have anticholinergic properties and co-administration may result in additive effects).
No products indexed under this heading.

Imipramine Pamoate (Tricyclic antidepressants have anticholinergic properties and co-administration may result in additive effects).
No products indexed under this heading.

Ipratropium Bromide (Co-administration may result in additive anticholinergic effects). Products include:
Atrovent HFA Inhalation Aerosol **872**
Atrovent Inhalation Solution **868**
Atrovent Nasal Spray 0.03% **869**
Atrovent Nasal Spray 0.06% **870**
Combivent Inhalation Aerosol **878**
DuoNeb Inhalation Solution **1058**

Isoflurane (Scopolamine is an anticholinergic agent and causes certain CNS effects, such as drowsiness and dizziness, and hence it should be used with care in patients on concomitant therapy).
No products indexed under this heading.

Ketamine Hydrochloride (Scopolamine is an anticholinergic agent and causes certain CNS effects, such as drowsiness and dizziness, and hence it should be used with care in patients on concomitant therapy).
No products indexed under this heading.

Levomethadyl Acetate Hydrochloride (Scopolamine is an anticholinergic agent and causes certain CNS effects, such as drowsiness and dizziness, and hence it should be used with care in patients on concomitant therapy).
No products indexed under this heading.

Levorphanol Tartrate (Scopolamine is an anticholinergic agent and causes certain CNS effects, such as drowsiness and dizziness, and hence it should be used with care in patients on concomitant therapy).
No products indexed under this heading.

Loratadine (Antihistamines have anticholinergic properties and co-administration may result in additive effects). Products include:
Alavert Allergy & Sinus D-12 Hour Tablets..................... ▣ **743**
Alavert .... ▣ **743**
Children's Claritin 24 Hour Non-Drowsy Allergy Syrup.......... ▣ **732**
Claritin Non-Drowsy 24 Hour Tablets..................... ▣ **731**
Non-Drowsy Claritin Hives Relief Tablets..................... ▣ **733**
Claritin Reditabs 24 Hour Non-Drowsy Tablets..................... ▣ **732**
Claritin-D Non-Drowsy 12 Hour Tablets..................... ▣ **731**
Claritin-D Non-Drowsy 24 Hour Tablets..................... ▣ **731**
Children's Dimetapp ND Non-Drowsy Allergy Syrup........... ▣ **746**
Triaminic Allerchews .... ▣ **684**

Lorazepam (Scopolamine is an anticholinergic agent and causes certain CNS effects, such as drowsiness and dizziness, and hence it should be used with care in patients on concomitant therapy).
No products indexed under this heading.

Loxapine Hydrochloride (Scopolamine is an anticholinergic agent and causes certain CNS effects, such as drowsiness and dizziness, and hence it should be used with care in patients on concomitant therapy).
No products indexed under this heading.

Loxapine Succinate (Scopolamine is an anticholinergic agent and causes certain CNS effects, such as drowsiness and dizziness, and hence it should be used with care in patients on concomitant therapy).
No products indexed under this heading.

Maprotiline Hydrochloride (Tricyclic antidepressants have anticholinergic properties and co-administration may result in additive effects).
No products indexed under this heading.

Meclizine Hydrochloride (Antihistamines have anticholinergic properties and co-administration may result in additive effects).
No products indexed under this heading.

Mepenzolate Bromide (Co-administration may result in additive anticholinergic effects).
No products indexed under this heading.

Meperidine Hydrochloride (Scopolamine is an anticholinergic agent and causes certain CNS effects, such as drowsiness and dizziness, and hence it should be used with care in patients on concomitant therapy).
No products indexed under this heading.

Mephobarbital (Scopolamine is an anticholinergic agent and causes certain CNS effects, such as drowsiness and dizziness, and hence it should be used with care in patients on concomitant therapy). Products include:
Mebaral Tablets, USP 2483

Meprobamate (Scopolamine is an anticholinergic agent and causes certain CNS effects, such as drowsiness and dizziness, and hence it should be used with care in patients on concomitant therapy).
No products indexed under this heading.

Mesoridazine Besylate (Scopolamine is an anticholinergic agent and causes certain CNS effects, such as drowsiness and dizziness, and hence it should be used with care in patients on concomitant therapy).
No products indexed under this heading.

Methadone Hydrochloride (Scopolamine is an anticholinergic agent and causes certain CNS effects, such as drowsiness and dizziness, and hence it should be used with care in patients on concomitant therapy).
No products indexed under this heading.

Methdilazine Hydrochloride (Antihistamines have anticholinergic properties and co-administration may result in additive effects).
No products indexed under this heading.

Methohexital Sodium (Scopolamine is an anticholinergic agent and causes certain CNS effects, such as drowsiness and dizziness, and hence it should be used with care in patients on concomitant therapy).
No products indexed under this heading.

Methotrimeprazine (Scopolamine is an anticholinergic agent and causes certain CNS effects, such as drowsiness and dizziness, and hence it should be used with care in patients on concomitant therapy).
No products indexed under this heading.

Methoxyflurane (Scopolamine is an anticholinergic agent and causes certain CNS effects, such as drowsiness and dizziness, and hence it should be used with care in patients on concomitant therapy).
No products indexed under this heading.

Midazolam Hydrochloride (Scopolamine is an anticholinergic agent and causes certain CNS effects, such as drowsiness and dizziness, and hence it should be used with care in patients on concomitant therapy).
No products indexed under this heading.

Molindone Hydrochloride (Scopolamine is an anticholinergic agent and causes certain CNS effects, such as drowsiness and dizziness, and hence it should be used with care in patients on concomitant therapy). Products include:
Moban Tablets 1108

Morphine Sulfate (Scopolamine is an anticholinergic agent and causes certain CNS effects, such as drowsiness and dizziness, and hence it should be used with care in patients on concomitant therapy). Products include:
Avinza Capsules 1714
Kadian Capsules 572
MS Contin Tablets 2703

Nortriptyline Hydrochloride (Tricyclic antidepressants have anticholinergic properties and co-administration may result in additive effects).
No products indexed under this heading.

Olanzapine (Scopolamine is an anticholinergic agent and causes certain CNS effects, such as drowsiness and dizziness, and hence it should be used with care in patients on concomitant therapy). Products include:
Symbyax Capsules 1788
Zyprexa Tablets 1798
Zyprexa IntraMuscular 1798
Zyprexa ZYDIS Orally Disintegrating Tablets 1798

Oxazepam (Scopolamine is an anticholinergic agent and causes certain CNS effects, such as drowsiness and dizziness, and hence it should be used with care in patients on concomitant therapy).
No products indexed under this heading.

Oxybutynin Chloride (Co-administration may result in additive anticholinergic effects). Products include:
Ditropan XL Extended Release Tablets 2391

Oxycodone Hydrochloride (Scopolamine is an anticholinergic agent and causes certain CNS effects, such as drowsiness and dizziness, and hence it should be used with care in patients on concomitant therapy). Products include:
Combunox Tablets 1183
OxyContin Tablets 2699
OxyFast Oral Concentrate Solution 2704
OxyIR Capsules 2704
Percocet Tablets 1114
Percodan Tablets 1115

Pentobarbital Sodium (Scopolamine is an anticholinergic agent and causes certain CNS effects, such as drowsiness and dizziness, and hence it should be used with care in patients on concomitant therapy). Products include:
Nembutal Sodium Solution, USP 2484

Perphenazine (Scopolamine is an anticholinergic agent and causes certain CNS effects, such as drowsiness and dizziness, and hence it should be used with care in patients on concomitant therapy).
No products indexed under this heading.

Phenobarbital (Scopolamine is an anticholinergic agent and causes certain CNS effects, such as drowsiness and dizziness, and hence it should be used with care in patients on concomitant therapy).
No products indexed under this heading.

Prazepam (Scopolamine is an anticholinergic agent and causes certain CNS effects, such as drowsiness and dizziness, and hence it should be used with care in patients on concomitant therapy).
No products indexed under this heading.

Prochlorperazine (Scopolamine is an anticholinergic agent and causes certain CNS effects, such as drowsiness and dizziness, and hence it should be used with care in patients on concomitant therapy).
No products indexed under this heading.

Procyclidine Hydrochloride (Co-administration may result in additive anticholinergic effects).
No products indexed under this heading.

Promethazine Hydrochloride (Antihistamines have anticholinergic properties and co-administration may result in additive effects). Products include:
Phenergan 3438

Propantheline Bromide (Co-administration may result in additive anticholinergic effects).
No products indexed under this heading.

Propofol (Scopolamine is an anticholinergic agent and causes certain CNS effects, such as drowsiness and dizziness, and hence it should be used with care in patients on concomitant therapy). Products include:
Diprivan Injectable Emulsion 676

Propoxyphene Hydrochloride (Scopolamine is an anticholinergic agent and causes certain CNS effects, such as drowsiness and dizziness, and hence it should be used with care in patients on concomitant therapy).
No products indexed under this heading.

Propoxyphene Napsylate (Scopolamine is an anticholinergic agent and causes certain CNS effects, such as drowsiness and dizziness, and hence it should be used with care in patients on concomitant therapy). Products include:
Darvocet A 500 Tablets 3497

Protriptyline Hydrochloride (Tricyclic antidepressants have anticholinergic properties and co-administration may result in additive effects). Products include:
Vivactil Tablets 2350

Pyrilamine Maleate (Antihistamines have anticholinergic properties and co-administration may result in additive effects).
No products indexed under this heading.

Pyrilamine Tannate (Antihistamines have anticholinergic properties and co-administration may result in additive effects).
No products indexed under this heading.

Quazepam (Scopolamine is an anticholinergic agent and causes certain CNS effects, such as drowsiness and dizziness, and hence it should be used with care in patients on concomitant therapy).
No products indexed under this heading.

Quetiapine Fumarate (Scopolamine is an anticholinergic agent and causes certain CNS effects, such as drowsiness and dizziness, and hence it should be used with care in patients on concomitant therapy). Products include:
Seroquel Tablets 691

Remifentanil Hydrochloride (Scopolamine is an anticholinergic agent and causes certain CNS effects, such as drowsiness and dizziness, and hence it should be used with care in patients on concomitant therapy).
No products indexed under this heading.

Risperidone (Scopolamine is an anticholinergic agent and causes certain CNS effects, such as drowsiness and dizziness, and hence it should be used with care in patients on concomitant therapy). Products include:
Risperdal Consta Long-Acting Injection 1664
Risperdal M-Tab Orally Disintegrating Tablets 1658
Risperdal 1658

Scopolamine Hydrobromide (Co-administration may result in additive anticholinergic effects).
No products indexed under this heading.

Secobarbital Sodium (Scopolamine is an anticholinergic agent and causes certain CNS effects, such as drowsiness and dizziness, and hence it should be used with care in patients on concomitant therapy).
No products indexed under this heading.

Sevoflurane (Scopolamine is an anticholinergic agent and causes certain CNS effects, such as drowsiness and dizziness, and hence it should be used with care in patients on concomitant therapy). Products include:
Ultane Liquid for Inhalation 526

Sufentanil Citrate (Scopolamine is an anticholinergic agent and causes certain CNS effects, such as drowsiness and dizziness, and hence it should be used with care in patients on concomitant therapy).
No products indexed under this heading.

Temazepam (Scopolamine is an anticholinergic agent and causes certain CNS effects, such as drowsiness and dizziness, and hence it should be used with care in patients on concomitant therapy).
No products indexed under this heading.

Terfenadine (Antihistamines have anticholinergic properties and co-administration may result in additive effects).
No products indexed under this heading.

Thiamylal Sodium (Scopolamine is an anticholinergic agent and causes certain CNS effects, such as drowsiness and dizziness, and hence it should be used with care in patients on concomitant therapy).
No products indexed under this heading.

Thioridazine Hydrochloride (Scopolamine is an anticholinergic agent and causes certain CNS effects, such as drowsiness and dizziness, and hence it should be used with care in patients on concomitant therapy). Products include:
Thioridazine Hydrochloride Tablets 2122

Thiothixene (Scopolamine is an anticholinergic agent and causes

certain CNS effects, such as drowsiness and dizziness, and hence it should be used with care in patients on concomitant therapy). Products include:
Thiothixene Capsules 2124

Tolterodine Tartrate (Co-administration may result in additive anticholinergic effects). Products include:
Detrol Tablets 2626
Detrol LA Capsules 2629

Triazolam (Scopolamine is an anticholinergic agent and causes certain CNS effects, such as drowsiness and dizziness, and hence it should be used with care in patients on concomitant therapy).
No products indexed under this heading.

Tridihexethyl Chloride (Co-administration may result in additive anticholinergic effects).
No products indexed under this heading.

Trifluoperazine Hydrochloride (Scopolamine is an anticholinergic agent and causes certain CNS effects, such as drowsiness and dizziness, and hence it should be used with care in patients on concomitant therapy).
No products indexed under this heading.

Trihexyphenidyl Hydrochloride (Co-administration may result in additive anticholinergic effects).
No products indexed under this heading.

Trimeprazine Tartrate (Antihistamines have anticholinergic properties and co-administration may result in additive effects).
No products indexed under this heading.

Trimipramine Maleate (Tricyclic antidepressants have anticholinergic properties and co-administration may result in additive effects). Products include:
Surmontil Capsules 2347

Tripelennamine Hydrochloride (Antihistamines have anticholinergic properties and co-administration may result in additive effects).
No products indexed under this heading.

Triprolidine Hydrochloride (Antihistamines have anticholinergic properties and co-administration may result in additive effects).
No products indexed under this heading.

Zaleplon (Scopolamine is an anticholinergic agent and causes certain CNS effects, such as drowsiness and dizziness, and hence it should be used with care in patients on concomitant therapy). Products include:
Sonata Capsules 1686

Ziprasidone Hydrochloride (Scopolamine is an anticholinergic agent and causes certain CNS effects, such as drowsiness and dizziness, and hence it should be used with care in patients on concomitant therapy). Products include:
Geodon Capsules 2514

Zolpidem Tartrate (Scopolamine is an anticholinergic agent and causes certain CNS effects, such as drowsiness and dizziness, and hence it should be used with care in patients on concomitant therapy). Products include:
Ambien Tablets 2867

Food Interactions

Alcohol (Scopolamine is an anticholinergic agent and causes certain CNS effects, such as drowsiness and dizziness, and hence it should be used with care in patients on concomitant therapy).

4LIFE TRANSFER FACTOR PLUS ADVANCED FORMULA CAPSULES
(Amino Acid Preparations) 763
None cited in PDR database.

TRANXENE T-TAB TABLETS
(Clorazepate Dipotassium) 2488
May interact with narcotic analgesics, phenothiazines, and certain other agents. Compounds in these categories include:

Alfentanil Hydrochloride (Actions of benzodiazepines may be potentiated).
No products indexed under this heading.

Alprazolam (Actions of benzodiazepines may be potentiated). Products include:
Niravam Orally Disintegrating Tablets 3106
Xanax XR Tablets 2655

Amitriptyline Hydrochloride (Actions of benzodiazepines may be potentiated).
No products indexed under this heading.

Amoxapine (Actions of benzodiazepines may be potentiated).
No products indexed under this heading.

Aprobarbital (Actions of benzodiazepines may be potentiated).
No products indexed under this heading.

Buprenorphine Hydrochloride (Actions of benzodiazepines may be potentiated). Products include:
Buprenex Injectable 2718
Suboxone Tablets 2719
Subutex Tablets 2719

Bupropion Hydrochloride (Actions of benzodiazepines may be potentiated). Products include:
Wellbutrin Tablets 1579
Wellbutrin SR Sustained-Release Tablets 1583
Wellbutrin XL Extended-Release Tablets 1588
Zyban Sustained-Release Tablets 1620

Buspirone Hydrochloride (Actions of benzodiazepines may be potentiated).
No products indexed under this heading.

Butabarbital (Actions of benzodiazepines may be potentiated).
No products indexed under this heading.

Butalbital (Actions of benzodiazepines may be potentiated). Products include:
Sedapap Tablets 50 mg/650 mg 2098

Chlordiazepoxide (Actions of benzodiazepines may be potentiated).
No products indexed under this heading.

Chlordiazepoxide Hydrochloride (Actions of benzodiazepines may be potentiated). Products include:
Librium Capsules 3349

Chlorpromazine (Actions of benzodiazepines may be potentiated).
No products indexed under this heading.

Chlorpromazine Hydrochloride (Actions of benzodiazepines may be potentiated).
No products indexed under this heading.

Chlorprothixene (Actions of benzodiazepines may be potentiated).
No products indexed under this heading.

Chlorprothixene Hydrochloride (Actions of benzodiazepines may be potentiated).
No products indexed under this heading.

Chlorprothixene Lactate (Actions of benzodiazepines may be potentiated).
No products indexed under this heading.

Citalopram Hydrobromide (Actions of benzodiazepines may be potentiated). Products include:
Celexa 1177

Clozapine (Actions of benzodiazepines may be potentiated). Products include:
Clozapine Tablets 2141
Clozaril Tablets 2174
FazaClo Orally Disintegrating Tablets 547

Codeine Phosphate (Actions of benzodiazepines may be potentiated). Products include:
Tylenol with Codeine 2461

Desflurane (Actions of benzodiazepines may be potentiated). Products include:
Suprane Liquid for Inhalation 770

Desipramine Hydrochloride (Actions of benzodiazepines may be potentiated).
No products indexed under this heading.

Dezocine (Actions of benzodiazepines may be potentiated).
No products indexed under this heading.

Diazepam (Actions of benzodiazepines may be potentiated). Products include:
Diastat Rectal Delivery System 3344
Valium Tablets 2822

Doxepin Hydrochloride (Actions of benzodiazepines may be potentiated).
No products indexed under this heading.

Droperidol (Actions of benzodiazepines may be potentiated).
No products indexed under this heading.

Enflurane (Actions of benzodiazepines may be potentiated).
No products indexed under this heading.

Estazolam (Actions of benzodiazepines may be potentiated; increased sedation with concurrent use). Products include:
ProSom Tablets 512

Ethanol (Actions of benzodiazepines may be potentiated).
No products indexed under this heading.

Ethchlorvynol (Actions of benzodiazepines may be potentiated; increased sedation with concurrent use).
No products indexed under this heading.

Ethinamate (Actions of benzodiazepines may be potentiated; increased sedation with concurrent use).
No products indexed under this heading.

Ethyl Alcohol (Actions of benzodiazepines may be potentiated).
No products indexed under this heading.

Fentanyl (Actions of benzodiazepines may be potentiated). Products include:
Duragesic Transdermal System 2448

Fentanyl Citrate (Actions of benzodiazepines may be potentiated). Products include:
Actiq 993

Fluoxetine Hydrochloride (Actions of benzodiazepines may be potentiated). Products include:
Prozac Pulvules and Liquid 1771
Symbyax Capsules 1788

Fluphenazine Decanoate (Actions of benzodiazepines may be potentiated).
No products indexed under this heading.

Fluphenazine Enanthate (Actions of benzodiazepines may be potentiated).
No products indexed under this heading.

Fluphenazine Hydrochloride (Actions of benzodiazepines may be potentiated).
No products indexed under this heading.

Flurazepam Hydrochloride (Actions of benzodiazepines may be potentiated; increased sedation with concurrent use). Products include:
Dalmane Capsules 3343

Glutethimide (Actions of benzodiazepines may be potentiated; increased sedation with concurrent use).
No products indexed under this heading.

Haloperidol (Actions of benzodiazepines may be potentiated).
No products indexed under this heading.

Haloperidol Decanoate (Actions of benzodiazepines may be potentiated).
No products indexed under this heading.

Hydrocodone Bitartrate (Actions of benzodiazepines may be potentiated). Products include:
Hycodan 1104
Hycomine Compound Tablets 1105
Hycotuss Expectorant Syrup 1106
Lortab 3315
Lortab Elixir 3312
Vicodin Tablets 530
Vicodin ES Tablets 531
Vicodin HP Tablets 532
Vicoprofen Tablets 533
Zydone Tablets 1118

Hydrocodone Polistirex (Actions of benzodiazepines may be potentiated). Products include:
Tussionex Pennkinetic Extended-Release Suspension 3322

Hydromorphone Hydrochloride (Actions of benzodiazepines may be potentiated). Products include:
Dilaudid 439
Dilaudid Oral Liquid 443
Dilaudid Non-Sterile Powder 439
Dilaudid Rectal Suppositories 439
Dilaudid Tablets 439
Dilaudid Tablets - 8 mg 443
Dilaudid-HP 441

Hydroxyzine Hydrochloride (Actions of benzodiazepines may be potentiated).
No products indexed under this heading.

Imipramine Hydrochloride (Actions of benzodiazepines may be potentiated).
No products indexed under this heading.

Imipramine Pamoate (Actions of benzodiazepines may be potentiated).
No products indexed under this heading.

Isocarboxazid (Actions of benzodiazepines may be potentiated).
No products indexed under this heading.

Isoflurane (Actions of benzodiazepines may be potentiated).
No products indexed under this heading.

Ketamine Hydrochloride (Actions of benzodiazepines may be potentiated).
No products indexed under this heading.

Levomethadyl Acetate Hydrochloride (Actions of benzodiazepines may be potentiated).
No products indexed under this heading.

Levorphanol Tartrate (Actions of benzodiazepines may be potentiated).
No products indexed under this heading.

Lorazepam (Actions of benzodiazepines may be potentiated; increased sedation with concurrent use).
No products indexed under this heading.

Loxapine Hydrochloride (Actions of benzodiazepines may be potentiated).
No products indexed under this heading.

Loxapine Succinate (Actions of benzodiazepines may be potentiated).
No products indexed under this heading.

Maprotiline Hydrochloride (Actions of benzodiazepines may be potentiated).
No products indexed under this heading.

Meperidine Hydrochloride (Actions of benzodiazepines may be potentiated).
No products indexed under this heading.

Mephobarbital (Actions of benzodiazepines may be potentiated). Products include:
Mebaral Tablets, USP **2483**

Meprobamate (Actions of benzodiazepines may be potentiated).
No products indexed under this heading.

Mesoridazine Besylate (Actions of benzodiazepines may be potentiated).
No products indexed under this heading.

Methadone Hydrochloride (Actions of benzodiazepines may be potentiated).
No products indexed under this heading.

Methohexital Sodium (Actions of benzodiazepines may be potentiated).
No products indexed under this heading.

Methotrimeprazine (Actions of benzodiazepines may be potentiated).
No products indexed under this heading.

Methoxyflurane (Actions of benzodiazepines may be potentiated).
No products indexed under this heading.

Midazolam Hydrochloride (Actions of benzodiazepines may be potentiated; increased sedation with concurrent use).
No products indexed under this heading.

Mirtazapine (Actions of benzodiazepines may be potentiated).
No products indexed under this heading.

Moclobemide (Actions of benzodiazepines may be potentiated).
No products indexed under this heading.

Molindone Hydrochloride (Actions of benzodiazepines may be potentiated). Products include:
Moban Tablets **1108**

Morphine Sulfate (Actions of benzodiazepines may be potentiated). Products include:
Avinza Capsules **1714**
Kadian Capsules **572**
MS Contin Tablets **2703**

Nefazodone Hydrochloride (Actions of benzodiazepines may be potentiated).
No products indexed under this heading.

Nortriptyline Hydrochloride (Actions of benzodiazepines may be potentiated).
No products indexed under this heading.

Olanzapine (Actions of benzodiazepines may be potentiated). Products include:
Symbyax Capsules **1788**
Zyprexa Tablets **1798**
Zyprexa IntraMuscular **1798**
Zyprexa ZYDIS Orally Disintegrating Tablets **1798**

Oxazepam (Actions of benzodiazepines may be potentiated).
No products indexed under this heading.

Oxycodone Hydrochloride (Actions of benzodiazepines may be potentiated). Products include:
Combunox Tablets **1183**
OxyContin Tablets **2699**
OxyFast Oral Concentrate Solution **2704**
OxyIR Capsules **2704**
Percocet Tablets **1114**
Percodan Tablets **1115**

Pargyline Hydrochloride (Actions of benzodiazepines may be potentiated).
No products indexed under this heading.

Paroxetine Hydrochloride (Actions of benzodiazepines may be potentiated). Products include:
Paxil CR Controlled-Release Tablets **1509**
Paxil **1501**

Pentobarbital Sodium (Actions of benzodiazepines may be potentiated). Products include:
Nembutal Sodium Solution, USP **2484**

Perphenazine (Actions of benzodiazepines may be potentiated).
No products indexed under this heading.

Phenelzine Sulfate (Actions of benzodiazepines may be potentiated).
No products indexed under this heading.

Phenobarbital (Actions of benzodiazepines may be potentiated).
No products indexed under this heading.

Prazepam (Actions of benzodiazepines may be potentiated).
No products indexed under this heading.

Procarbazine Hydrochloride (Actions of benzodiazepines may be potentiated). Products include:
Matulane Capsules **3188**

Prochlorperazine (Actions of benzodiazepines may be potentiated).
No products indexed under this heading.

Promethazine Hydrochloride (Actions of benzodiazepines may be potentiated). Products include:
Phenergan **3438**

Propofol (Actions of benzodiazepines may be potentiated; increased sedation with concurrent use). Products include:
Diprivan Injectable Emulsion **676**

Propoxyphene Hydrochloride (Actions of benzodiazepines may be potentiated).
No products indexed under this heading.

Propoxyphene Napsylate (Actions of benzodiazepines may be potentiated). Products include:
Darvocet A 500 Tablets **3497**

Protriptyline Hydrochloride (Actions of benzodiazepines may be potentiated). Products include:
Vivactil Tablets **2350**

Quazepam (Actions of benzodiazepines may be potentiated; increased sedation with concurrent use).
No products indexed under this heading.

Quetiapine Fumarate (Actions of benzodiazepines may be potentiated). Products include:
Seroquel Tablets **691**

Remifentanil Hydrochloride (Actions of benzodiazepines may be potentiated).
No products indexed under this heading.

Risperidone (Actions of benzodiazepines may be potentiated). Products include:
Risperdal Consta Long-Acting Injection **1664**
Risperdal M-Tab Orally Disintegrating Tablets **1658**
Risperdal **1658**

Secobarbital Sodium (Actions of benzodiazepines may be potentiated).
No products indexed under this heading.

Selegiline Hydrochloride (Actions of benzodiazepines may be potentiated). Products include:
Eldepryl Capsules **3209**

Sertraline Hydrochloride (Actions of benzodiazepines may be potentiated). Products include:
Zoloft **2581**

Sevoflurane (Actions of benzodiazepines may be potentiated). Products include:
Ultane Liquid for Inhalation **526**

Sufentanil Citrate (Actions of benzodiazepines may be potentiated).
No products indexed under this heading.

Temazepam (Actions of benzodiazepines may be potentiated; increased sedation with concurrent use).
No products indexed under this heading.

Thiamylal Sodium (Actions of benzodiazepines may be potentiated).
No products indexed under this heading.

Thioridazine Hydrochloride (Actions of benzodiazepines may be potentiated). Products include:
Thioridazine Hydrochloride Tablets **2122**

Thiothixene (Actions of benzodiazepines may be potentiated). Products include:
Thiothixene Capsules **2124**

Tranylcypromine Sulfate (Actions of benzodiazepines may be potentiated). Products include:
Parnate Tablets **1499**

Trazodone Hydrochloride (Actions of benzodiazepines may be potentiated).
No products indexed under this heading.

Triazolam (Actions of benzodiazepines may be potentiated; increased sedation with concurrent use).
No products indexed under this heading.

Trifluoperazine Hydrochloride (Actions of benzodiazepines may be potentiated).
No products indexed under this heading.

Trimipramine Maleate (Actions of benzodiazepines may be potentiated). Products include:
Surmontil Capsules **2347**

Venlafaxine Hydrochloride (Actions of benzodiazepines may be potentiated). Products include:
Effexor Tablets **3405**
Effexor XR Capsules **3411**

Zaleplon (Actions of benzodiazepines may be potentiated). Products include:
Sonata Capsules **1686**

Ziprasidone Hydrochloride (Actions of benzodiazepines may be potentiated). Products include:
Geodon Capsules **2514**

Zolpidem Tartrate (Actions of benzodiazepines may be potentiated; increased sedation with concurrent use). Products include:
Ambien Tablets **2867**

Food Interactions

Alcohol (Actions of benzodiazepines may be potentiated; prolonged sleeping time).

TRANXENE-SD TABLETS
(Clorazepate Dipotassium) **2488**
May interact with:

See (Tranxene T-TAB Tablets).

TRANXENE-SD HALF STRENGTH TABLETS
(Clorazepate Dipotassium) **2488**
May interact with:

See (Tranxene T-TAB Tablets).

TRASYLOL INJECTION

(Aprotinin) 779

May interact with fibrinolytic agents and certain other agents. Compounds in these categories include:

Alteplase (Aprotinin may inhibit the effects of fibrinolytic agents). Products include:

Activase I.V. 1225
Cathflo Activase 1232

Anistreplase (Aprotinin may inhibit the effects of fibrinolytic agents).

No products indexed under this heading.

Captopril (Aprotinin may block the acute hypotensive effects of captopril). Products include:

Captopril Tablets 2114

Heparin Sodium (Aprotinin, in the presence of heparin, has been found to prolong the activated clotting time (ACT) as measured by surface activation methods).

No products indexed under this heading.

Streptokinase (Aprotinin may inhibit the effects of fibrinolytic agents).

No products indexed under this heading.

Urokinase (Aprotinin may inhibit the effects of fibrinolytic agents).

No products indexed under this heading.

TRAUMEEL INJECTION SOLUTION

(Homeopathic Formulations) 1638

None cited in PDR database.

TRAVATAN OPHTHALMIC SOLUTION

(Travoprost) 559

None cited in PDR database.

TRECATOR TABLETS

(Ethionamide) 3482

May interact with antituberculosis drugs and certain other agents. Compounds in these categories include:

Aminosalicylic Acid (Ethionamide may potentiate the adverse effects of other antituberculous drugs administered concomitantly). Products include:

Paser Granules 1657

p-Aminosalicylic Acid (Ethionamide may potentiate the adverse effects of other antituberculous drugs administered concomitantly).

No products indexed under this heading.

Cycloserine (Ethionamide may potentiate the adverse effects of other antituberculous drugs administered concomitantly. In particular, convulsions have been reported when ethionamide is administered with cycloserine and special care should be taken when the treatment regimen includes both of these drugs). Products include:

Seromycin Capsules 1783

Ethambutol Hydrochloride (Ethionamide may potentiate the adverse effects of other antituberculous drugs administered concomitantly).

No products indexed under this heading.

Ethanol (Excessive ethanol ingestion should be avoided because a psychotic reaction has been reported).

No products indexed under this heading.

Isoniazid (Ethionamide has been found to temporarily raise serum concentrations of isoniazid).

No products indexed under this heading.

Pyrazinamide (Ethionamide may potentiate the adverse effects of other antituberculous drugs administered concomitantly).

No products indexed under this heading.

Rifampin (Ethionamide may potentiate the adverse effects of other antituberculous drugs administered concomitantly).

No products indexed under this heading.

Rifapentine (Ethionamide may potentiate the adverse effects of other antituberculous drugs administered concomitantly).

No products indexed under this heading.

Food Interactions

Alcohol (Excessive ethanol ingestion should be avoided because a psychotic reaction has been reported).

TRELSTAR DEPOT

(Triptorelin Pamoate) 3385

May interact with drugs which may cause hyperprolactinemia. Compounds in these categories include:

Alprazolam (Hyperprolactinemic drugs should not be prescribed concomitantly with triptorelin, since hyperprolactinemia reduces the number of pituitary GnRH receptors). Products include:

Niravam Orally Disintegrating Tablets 3106
Xanax XR Tablets 2655

Chlorpromazine (Hyperprolactinemic drugs should not be prescribed concomitantly with triptorelin, since hyperprolactinemia reduces the number of pituitary GnRH receptors).

No products indexed under this heading.

Chlorpromazine Hydrochloride (Hyperprolactinemic drugs should not be prescribed concomitantly with triptorelin, since hyperprolactinemia reduces the number of pituitary GnRH receptors).

No products indexed under this heading.

Chlorprothixene (Hyperprolactinemic drugs should not be prescribed concomitantly with triptorelin, since hyperprolactinemia reduces the number of pituitary GnRH receptors).

No products indexed under this heading.

Chlorprothixene Hydrochloride (Hyperprolactinemic drugs should not be prescribed concomitantly with triptorelin, since hyperprolactinemia reduces the number of pituitary GnRH receptors).

No products indexed under this heading.

Fluoxetine Hydrochloride (Hyperprolactinemic drugs should not be prescribed concomitantly with triptorelin, since hyperprolactinemia reduces the number of pituitary GnRH receptors). Products include:

Prozac Pulvules and Liquid 1771
Symbyax Capsules 1788

Fluphenazine Decanoate (Hyperprolactinemic drugs should not be prescribed concomitantly with triptorelin, since hyperprolactinemia reduces the number of pituitary GnRH receptors).

No products indexed under this heading.

Fluphenazine Enanthate (Hyperprolactinemic drugs should not be prescribed concomitantly with triptorelin, since hyperprolactinemia reduces the number of pituitary GnRH receptors).

No products indexed under this heading.

Fluphenazine Hydrochloride (Hyperprolactinemic drugs should not be prescribed concomitantly with triptorelin, since hyperprolactinemia reduces the number of pituitary GnRH receptors).

No products indexed under this heading.

Haloperidol (Hyperprolactinemic drugs should not be prescribed concomitantly with triptorelin, since hyperprolactinemia reduces the number of pituitary GnRH receptors).

No products indexed under this heading.

Haloperidol Decanoate (Hyperprolactinemic drugs should not be prescribed concomitantly with triptorelin, since hyperprolactinemia reduces the number of pituitary GnRH receptors).

No products indexed under this heading.

Loxapine Hydrochloride (Hyperprolactinemic drugs should not be prescribed concomitantly with triptorelin, since hyperprolactinemia reduces the number of pituitary GnRH receptors).

No products indexed under this heading.

Loxapine Succinate (Hyperprolactinemic drugs should not be prescribed concomitantly with triptorelin, since hyperprolactinemia reduces the number of pituitary GnRH receptors).

No products indexed under this heading.

Mesoridazine Besylate (Hyperprolactinemic drugs should not be prescribed concomitantly with triptorelin, since hyperprolactinemia reduces the number of pituitary GnRH receptors).

No products indexed under this heading.

Methotrimeprazine (Hyperprolactinemic drugs should not be prescribed concomitantly with triptorelin, since hyperprolactinemia reduces the number of pituitary GnRH receptors).

No products indexed under this heading.

Methyldopa (Hyperprolactinemic drugs should not be prescribed concomitantly with triptorelin, since hyperprolactinemia reduces the number of pituitary GnRH receptors). Products include:

Aldoclor Tablets 1881
Aldoril Tablets 1884

Metoclopramide Hydrochloride (Hyperprolactinemic drugs should not be prescribed concomitantly with triptorelin, since hyperprolactinemia reduces the number of pituitary GnRH receptors).

No products indexed under this heading.

Molindone Hydrochloride (Hyperprolactinemic drugs should not be prescribed concomitantly with triptorelin, since hyperprolactinemia reduces the number of pituitary GnRH receptors). Products include:

Moban Tablets 1108

Olanzapine (Hyperprolactinemic drugs should not be prescribed concomitantly with triptorelin, since hyperprolactinemia reduces the number of pituitary GnRH receptors). Products include:

Symbyax Capsules 1788
Zyprexa Tablets 1798
Zyprexa IntraMuscular 1798
Zyprexa ZYDIS Orally Disintegrating Tablets 1798

Perphenazine (Hyperprolactinemic drugs should not be prescribed concomitantly with triptorelin, since hyperprolactinemia reduces the number of pituitary GnRH receptors).

No products indexed under this heading.

Prochlorperazine (Hyperprolactinemic drugs should not be prescribed concomitantly with triptorelin, since hyperprolactinemia reduces the number of pituitary GnRH receptors).

No products indexed under this heading.

Promethazine Hydrochloride (Hyperprolactinemic drugs should not be prescribed concomitantly with triptorelin, since hyperprolactinemia reduces the number of pituitary GnRH receptors). Products include:

Phenergan 3438

Quetiapine Fumarate (Hyperprolactinemic drugs should not be prescribed concomitantly with triptorelin, since hyperprolactinemia reduces the number of pituitary GnRH receptors). Products include:

Seroquel Tablets 691

Risperidone (Hyperprolactinemic drugs should not be prescribed concomitantly with triptorelin, since hyperprolactinemia reduces the number of pituitary GnRH receptors). Products include:

Risperdal Consta Long-Acting Injection 1664
Risperdal M-Tab Orally Disintegrating Tablets 1658
Risperdal 1658

Sertraline Hydrochloride (Hyperprolactinemic drugs should not be prescribed concomitantly with triptorelin, since hyperprolactinemia reduces the number of pituitary GnRH receptors). Products include:

Zoloft 2581

Thioridazine Hydrochloride (Hyperprolactinemic drugs should not be prescribed concomitantly with triptorelin, since hyperprolactinemia reduces the number of pituitary GnRH receptors). Products include:

Thioridazine Hydrochloride Tablets 2122

Thiothixene (Hyperprolactinemic drugs should not be prescribed concomitantly with triptorelin, since hyperprolactinemia reduces the number of pituitary GnRH receptors). Products include:

Thiothixene Capsules 2124

Trifluoperazine Hydrochloride (Hyperprolactinemic drugs should not be prescribed concomitantly with triptorelin, since hyperprolactinemia reduces the number of pituitary GnRH receptors).

No products indexed under this heading.

Verapamil Hydrochloride (Hyperprolactinemic drugs should not be prescribed concomitantly with triptorelin, since hyperprolactinemia reduces the number of pituitary GnRH receptors). Products include:
- Covera-HS Tablets 3135
- Tarka Tablets 519
- Verelan PM Capsules 3120

Ziprasidone Hydrochloride (Hyperprolactinemic drugs should not be prescribed concomitantly with triptorelin, since hyperprolactinemia reduces the number of pituitary GnRH receptors). Products include:
- Geodon Capsules 2514

Ziprasidone Mesylate (Hyperprolactinemic drugs should not be prescribed concomitantly with triptorelin, since hyperprolactinemia reduces the number of pituitary GnRH receptors). Products include:
- Geodon for Injection 2514

TRELSTAR LA SUSPENSION

(Triptorelin Pamoate) 3387

May interact with drugs which may cause hyperprolactinemia. Compounds in these categories include:

Alprazolam (Hyperprolactinemic drugs should not be prescribed concomitantly with triptorelin pamoate since hyperprolactinemia reduces the number of pituitary GnRH receptors). Products include:
- Niravam Orally Disintegrating Tablets 3106
- Xanax XR Tablets 2655

Chlorpromazine (Hyperprolactinemic drugs should not be prescribed concomitantly with triptorelin pamoate since hyperprolactinemia reduces the number of pituitary GnRH receptors).
No products indexed under this heading.

Chlorpromazine Hydrochloride (Hyperprolactinemic drugs should not be prescribed concomitantly with triptorelin pamoate since hyperprolactinemia reduces the number of pituitary GnRH receptors).
No products indexed under this heading.

Chlorprothixene (Hyperprolactinemic drugs should not be prescribed concomitantly with triptorelin pamoate since hyperprolactinemia reduces the number of pituitary GnRH receptors).
No products indexed under this heading.

Chlorprothixene Hydrochloride (Hyperprolactinemic drugs should not be prescribed concomitantly with triptorelin pamoate since hyperprolactinemia reduces the number of pituitary GnRH receptors).
No products indexed under this heading.

Fluoxetine Hydrochloride (Hyperprolactinemic drugs should not be prescribed concomitantly with triptorelin pamoate since hyperprolactinemia reduces the number of pituitary GnRH receptors). Products include:
- Prozac Pulvules and Liquid 1771
- Symbyax Capsules 1788

Fluphenazine Decanoate (Hyperprolactinemic drugs should not be prescribed concomitantly with triptorelin pamoate since hyperprolactinemia reduces the number of pituitary GnRH receptors).
No products indexed under this heading.

Fluphenazine Enanthate (Hyperprolactinemic drugs should not be prescribed concomitantly with triptorelin pamoate since hyperprolactinemia reduces the number of pituitary GnRH receptors).
No products indexed under this heading.

Fluphenazine Hydrochloride (Hyperprolactinemic drugs should not be prescribed concomitantly with triptorelin pamoate since hyperprolactinemia reduces the number of pituitary GnRH receptors).
No products indexed under this heading.

Haloperidol (Hyperprolactinemic drugs should not be prescribed concomitantly with triptorelin pamoate since hyperprolactinemia reduces the number of pituitary GnRH receptors).
No products indexed under this heading.

Haloperidol Decanoate (Hyperprolactinemic drugs should not be prescribed concomitantly with triptorelin pamoate since hyperprolactinemia reduces the number of pituitary GnRH receptors).
No products indexed under this heading.

Loxapine Hydrochloride (Hyperprolactinemic drugs should not be prescribed concomitantly with triptorelin pamoate since hyperprolactinemia reduces the number of pituitary GnRH receptors).
No products indexed under this heading.

Loxapine Succinate (Hyperprolactinemic drugs should not be prescribed concomitantly with triptorelin pamoate since hyperprolactinemia reduces the number of pituitary GnRH receptors).
No products indexed under this heading.

Mesoridazine Besylate (Hyperprolactinemic drugs should not be prescribed concomitantly with triptorelin pamoate since hyperprolactinemia reduces the number of pituitary GnRH receptors).
No products indexed under this heading.

Methotrimeprazine (Hyperprolactinemic drugs should not be prescribed concomitantly with triptorelin pamoate since hyperprolactinemia reduces the number of pituitary GnRH receptors).
No products indexed under this heading.

Methyldopa (Hyperprolactinemic drugs should not be prescribed concomitantly with triptorelin pamoate since hyperprolactinemia reduces the number of pituitary GnRH receptors). Products include:
- Aldoclor Tablets 1881
- Aldoril Tablets 1884

Metoclopramide Hydrochloride (Hyperprolactinemic drugs should not be prescribed concomitantly with triptorelin pamoate since hyperprolactinemia reduces the number of pituitary GnRH receptors).
No products indexed under this heading.

Molindone Hydrochloride (Hyperprolactinemic drugs should not be prescribed concomitantly with triptorelin pamoate since hyperprolactinemia reduces the number of pituitary GnRH receptors). Products include:
- Moban Tablets 1108

Olanzapine (Hyperprolactinemic drugs should not be prescribed concomitantly with triptorelin pamoate since hyperprolactinemia reduces the number of pituitary GnRH receptors). Products include:
- Symbyax Capsules 1788
- Zyprexa Tablets 1798
- Zyprexa IntraMuscular 1798
- Zyprexa ZYDIS Orally Disintegrating Tablets 1798

Perphenazine (Hyperprolactinemic drugs should not be prescribed concomitantly with triptorelin pamoate since hyperprolactinemia reduces the number of pituitary GnRH receptors).
No products indexed under this heading.

Prochlorperazine (Hyperprolactinemic drugs should not be prescribed concomitantly with triptorelin pamoate since hyperprolactinemia reduces the number of pituitary GnRH receptors).
No products indexed under this heading.

Promethazine Hydrochloride (Hyperprolactinemic drugs should not be prescribed concomitantly with triptorelin pamoate since hyperprolactinemia reduces the number of pituitary GnRH receptors). Products include:
- Phenergan 3438

Quetiapine Fumarate (Hyperprolactinemic drugs should not be prescribed concomitantly with triptorelin pamoate since hyperprolactinemia reduces the number of pituitary GnRH receptors). Products include:
- Seroquel Tablets 691

Risperidone (Hyperprolactinemic drugs should not be prescribed concomitantly with triptorelin pamoate since hyperprolactinemia reduces the number of pituitary GnRH receptors). Products include:
- Risperdal Consta Long-Acting Injection 1664
- Risperdal M-Tab Orally Disintegrating Tablets 1658
- Risperdal 1658

Sertraline Hydrochloride (Hyperprolactinemic drugs should not be prescribed concomitantly with triptorelin pamoate since hyperprolactinemia reduces the number of pituitary GnRH receptors). Products include:
- Zoloft 2581

Thioridazine Hydrochloride (Hyperprolactinemic drugs should not be prescribed concomitantly with triptorelin pamoate since hyperprolactinemia reduces the number of pituitary GnRH receptors). Products include:
- Thioridazine Hydrochloride Tablets 2122

Thiothixene (Hyperprolactinemic drugs should not be prescribed concomitantly with triptorelin pamoate since hyperprolactinemia reduces the number of pituitary GnRH receptors). Products include:
- Thiothixene Capsules 2124

Trifluoperazine Hydrochloride (Hyperprolactinemic drugs should not be prescribed concomitantly with triptorelin pamoate since hyperprolactinemia reduces the number of pituitary GnRH receptors).
No products indexed under this heading.

Verapamil Hydrochloride (Hyperprolactinemic drugs should not be prescribed concomitantly with triptorelin pamoate since hyperprolactinemia reduces the number of pituitary GnRH receptors). Products include:
- Covera-HS Tablets 3135
- Tarka Tablets 519
- Verelan PM Capsules 3120

Ziprasidone Hydrochloride (Hyperprolactinemic drugs should not be prescribed concomitantly with triptorelin pamoate since hyperprolactinemia reduces the number of pituitary GnRH receptors). Products include:
- Geodon Capsules 2514

Ziprasidone Mesylate (Hyperprolactinemic drugs should not be prescribed concomitantly with triptorelin pamoate since hyperprolactinemia reduces the number of pituitary GnRH receptors). Products include:
- Geodon for Injection 2514

TRIAMINIC ALLERCHEWS

(Loratadine) .... ▣684

None cited in PDR database.

TRIAMINIC CHEST & NASAL CONGESTION LIQUID

(Guaifenesin, Pseudoephedrine Hydrochloride) .... ▣685

May interact with monoamine oxidase inhibitors. Compounds in these categories include:

Isocarboxazid (Concurrent and/or sequential use with MAO inhibitors is not recommended).
No products indexed under this heading.

Moclobemide (Concurrent and/or sequential use with MAO inhibitors is not recommended).
No products indexed under this heading.

Pargyline Hydrochloride (Concurrent and/or sequential use with MAO inhibitors is not recommended).
No products indexed under this heading.

Phenelzine Sulfate (Concurrent and/or sequential use with MAO inhibitors is not recommended).
No products indexed under this heading.

Procarbazine Hydrochloride (Concurrent and/or sequential use with MAO inhibitors is not recommended). Products include:
- Matulane Capsules 3188

Selegiline Hydrochloride (Concurrent and/or sequential use with MAO inhibitors is not recommended). Products include:
- Eldepryl Capsules 3209

Tranylcypromine Sulfate (Concurrent and/or sequential use with MAO inhibitors is not recommended). Products include:

Parnate Tablets 1499

TRIAMINIC COLD & ALLERGY LIQUID
(Chlorpheniramine Maleate, Pseudoephedrine Hydrochloride)....... 685
May interact with:

See (Triaminic Night Time Cough & Cold Liquid).

TRIAMINIC COLD & COUGH LIQUID
(Chlorpheniramine Maleate, Dextromethorphan Hydrobromide, Pseudoephedrine Hydrochloride)....... 685

TRIAMINIC COUGH LIQUID
(Dextromethorphan Hydrobromide, Pseudoephedrine Hydrochloride)................................. 687
See Triaminic Cough & Sore Throat Liquid

TRIAMINIC COUGH & NASAL CONGESTION LIQUID
(Dextromethorphan Hydrobromide, Pseudoephedrine Hydrochloride)................................. 687
See Triaminic Cough & Sore Throat Liquid

TRIAMINIC COUGH & SORE THROAT LIQUID
(Acetaminophen, Dextromethorphan Hydrobromide, Pseudoephedrine Hydrochloride)....... 687
May interact with monoamine oxidase inhibitors. Compounds in these categories include:

Isocarboxazid (Concurrent and/or sequential use with MAO inhibitors is not recommened).
No products indexed under this heading.

Moclobemide (Concurrent and/or sequential use with MAO inhibitors is not recommened).
No products indexed under this heading.

Pargyline Hydrochloride (Concurrent and/or sequential use with MAO inhibitors is not recommened).
No products indexed under this heading.

Phenelzine Sulfate (Concurrent and/or sequential use with MAO inhibitors is not recommened).
No products indexed under this heading.

Procarbazine Hydrochloride (Concurrent and/or sequential use with MAO inhibitors is not recommened). Products include:
Matulane Capsules 3188

Selegiline Hydrochloride (Concurrent and/or sequential use with MAO inhibitors is not recommened). Products include:
Eldepryl Capsules 3209

Tranylcypromine Sulfate (Concurrent and/or sequential use with MAO inhibitors is not recommened). Products include:
Parnate Tablets 1499

TRIAMINIC FLU, COUGH & FEVER LIQUID
(Acetaminophen, Chlorpheniramine Maleate, Dextromethorphan Hydrobromide, Pseudoephedrine Hydrochloride)....... 685

TRIAMINIC NIGHT TIME COUGH & COLD LIQUID
(Chlorpheniramine Maleate, Dextromethorphan Hydrobromide, Pseudoephedrine Hydrochloride)....... 685
May interact with hypnotics and sedatives, monoamine oxidase inhibitors, and tranquilizers. Compounds in these categories include:

Alprazolam (May increase drowsiness). Products include:
Niravam Orally Disintegrating Tablets 3106
Xanax XR Tablets 2655

Buspirone Hydrochloride (May increase drowsiness).
No products indexed under this heading.

Chlordiazepoxide (May increase drowsiness).
No products indexed under this heading.

Chlordiazepoxide Hydrochloride (May increase drowsiness). Products include:
Librium Capsules 3349

Chlorpromazine (May increase drowsiness).
No products indexed under this heading.

Chlorpromazine Hydrochloride (May increase drowsiness).
No products indexed under this heading.

Chlorprothixene (May increase drowsiness).
No products indexed under this heading.

Chlorprothixene Hydrochloride (May increase drowsiness).
No products indexed under this heading.

Clorazepate Dipotassium (May increase drowsiness). Products include:
Tranxene 2488

Diazepam (May increase drowsiness). Products include:
Diastat Rectal Delivery System 3344
Valium Tablets 2822

Droperidol (May increase drowsiness).
No products indexed under this heading.

Estazolam (May increase drowsiness). Products include:
ProSom Tablets 512

Ethchlorvynol (May increase drowsiness).
No products indexed under this heading.

Ethinamate (May increase drowsiness).
No products indexed under this heading.

Fluphenazine Decanoate (May increase drowsiness).
No products indexed under this heading.

Fluphenazine Enanthate (May increase drowsiness).
No products indexed under this heading.

Fluphenazine Hydrochloride (May increase drowsiness).
No products indexed under this heading.

Flurazepam Hydrochloride (May increase drowsiness). Products include:
Dalmane Capsules 3343

Glutethimide (May increase drowsiness).
No products indexed under this heading.

Haloperidol (May increase drowsiness).
No products indexed under this heading.

Haloperidol Decanoate (May increase drowsiness).
No products indexed under this heading.

Hydroxyzine Hydrochloride (May increase drowsiness).
No products indexed under this heading.

Isocarboxazid (Concurrent and/or sequential use with MAO inhibitors is not recommended).
No products indexed under this heading.

Lorazepam (May increase drowsiness).
No products indexed under this heading.

Loxapine Hydrochloride (May increase drowsiness).
No products indexed under this heading.

Loxapine Succinate (May increase drowsiness).
No products indexed under this heading.

Meprobamate (May increase drowsiness).
No products indexed under this heading.

Mesoridazine Besylate (May increase drowsiness).
No products indexed under this heading.

Midazolam Hydrochloride (May increase drowsiness).
No products indexed under this heading.

Moclobemide (Concurrent and/or sequential use with MAO inhibitors is not recommended).
No products indexed under this heading.

Molindone Hydrochloride (May increase drowsiness). Products include:
Moban Tablets 1108

Oxazepam (May increase drowsiness).
No products indexed under this heading.

Pargyline Hydrochloride (Concurrent and/or sequential use with MAO inhibitors is not recommended).
No products indexed under this heading.

Perphenazine (May increase drowsiness).
No products indexed under this heading.

Phenelzine Sulfate (Concurrent and/or sequential use with MAO inhibitors is not recommended).
No products indexed under this heading.

Prazepam (May increase drowsiness).
No products indexed under this heading.

Procarbazine Hydrochloride (Concurrent and/or sequential use with MAO inhibitors is not recommended). Products include:
Matulane Capsules 3188

Prochlorperazine (May increase drowsiness).
No products indexed under this heading.

Promethazine Hydrochloride (May increase drowsiness). Products include:
Phenergan 3438

Propofol (May increase drowsiness). Products include:
Diprivan Injectable Emulsion 676

Quazepam (May increase drowsiness).
No products indexed under this heading.

Secobarbital Sodium (May increase drowsiness).
No products indexed under this heading.

Selegiline Hydrochloride (Concurrent and/or sequential use with MAO inhibitors is not recommended). Products include:
Eldepryl Capsules 3209

Temazepam (May increase drowsiness).
No products indexed under this heading.

Thioridazine Hydrochloride (May increase drowsiness). Products include:
Thioridazine Hydrochloride Tablets 2122

Thiothixene (May increase drowsiness). Products include:
Thiothixene Capsules 2124

Tranylcypromine Sulfate (Concurrent and/or sequential use with MAO inhibitors is not recommended). Products include:
Parnate Tablets 1499

Triazolam (May increase drowsiness).
No products indexed under this heading.

Trifluoperazine Hydrochloride (May increase drowsiness).
No products indexed under this heading.

Zaleplon (May increase drowsiness). Products include:
Sonata Capsules 1686

Zolpidem Tartrate (May increase drowsiness). Products include:
Ambien Tablets 2867

TRIAMINIC ALLERGY RUNNY NOSE & CONGESTION SOFTCHEWS
(Chlorpheniramine Maleate, Pseudoephedrine Hydrochloride)....... 688
May interact with hypnotics and sedatives, monoamine oxidase inhibitors, and tranquilizers. Compounds in these categories include:

Alprazolam (May increase drowsiness effect). Products include:
Niravam Orally Disintegrating Tablets 3106
Xanax XR Tablets 2655

Buspirone Hydrochloride (May increase drowsiness effect).
No products indexed under this heading.

Chlordiazepoxide (May increase drowsiness effect).
No products indexed under this heading.

Chlordiazepoxide Hydrochloride (May increase drowsiness effect). Products include:
Librium Capsules 3349

Chlorpromazine (May increase drowsiness effect).
No products indexed under this heading.

Chlorpromazine Hydrochloride (May increase drowsiness effect).
No products indexed under this heading.

Chlorprothixene (May increase drowsiness effect).
No products indexed under this heading.

Chlorprothixene Hydrochloride (May increase drowsiness effect).
No products indexed under this heading.

Clorazepate Dipotassium (May increase drowsiness effect). Products include:
Tranxene 2488

Diazepam (May increase drowsiness effect). Products include:
Diastat Rectal Delivery System 3344
Valium Tablets 2822

Droperidol (May increase drowsiness effect).
No products indexed under this heading.

Estazolam (May increase drowsiness effect). Products include:
ProSom Tablets 512

Ethchlorvynol (May increase drowsiness effect).
No products indexed under this heading.

Ethinamate (May increase drowsiness effect).
No products indexed under this heading.

Fluphenazine Decanoate (May increase drowsiness effect).
No products indexed under this heading.

Fluphenazine Enanthate (May increase drowsiness effect).
No products indexed under this heading.

Fluphenazine Hydrochloride (May increase drowsiness effect).
No products indexed under this heading.

Flurazepam Hydrochloride (May increase drowsiness effect). Products include:
Dalmane Capsules 3343

Glutethimide (May increase drowsiness effect).
No products indexed under this heading.

Haloperidol (May increase drowsiness effect).
No products indexed under this heading.

Haloperidol Decanoate (May increase drowsiness effect).
No products indexed under this heading.

Hydroxyzine Hydrochloride (May increase drowsiness effect).
No products indexed under this heading.

Isocarboxazid (Concurrent and/or sequential use with MAO inhibitors is not recommended).
No products indexed under this heading.

Lorazepam (May increase drowsiness effect).
No products indexed under this heading.

Loxapine Hydrochloride (May increase drowsiness effect).
No products indexed under this heading.

Loxapine Succinate (May increase drowsiness effect).
No products indexed under this heading.

Meprobamate (May increase drowsiness effect).
No products indexed under this heading.

Mesoridazine Besylate (May increase drowsiness effect).
No products indexed under this heading.

Midazolam Hydrochloride (May increase drowsiness effect).
No products indexed under this heading.

Moclobemide (Concurrent and/or sequential use with MAO inhibitors is not recommended).
No products indexed under this heading.

Molindone Hydrochloride (May increase drowsiness effect). Products include:
Moban Tablets 1108

Oxazepam (May increase drowsiness effect).
No products indexed under this heading.

Pargyline Hydrochloride (Concurrent and/or sequential use with MAO inhibitors is not recommended).
No products indexed under this heading.

Perphenazine (May increase drowsiness effect).
No products indexed under this heading.

Phenelzine Sulfate (Concurrent and/or sequential use with MAO inhibitors is not recommended).
No products indexed under this heading.

Prazepam (May increase drowsiness effect).
No products indexed under this heading.

Procarbazine Hydrochloride (Concurrent and/or sequential use with MAO inhibitors is not recommended). Products include:
Matulane Capsules 3188

Prochlorperazine (May increase drowsiness effect).
No products indexed under this heading.

Promethazine Hydrochloride (May increase drowsiness effect). Products include:
Phenergan 3438

Propofol (May increase drowsiness effect). Products include:
Diprivan Injectable Emulsion 676

Quazepam (May increase drowsiness effect).
No products indexed under this heading.

Secobarbital Sodium (May increase drowsiness effect).
No products indexed under this heading.

Selegiline Hydrochloride (Concurrent and/or sequential use with MAO inhibitors is not recommended). Products include:
Eldepryl Capsules 3209

Temazepam (May increase drowsiness effect).
No products indexed under this heading.

Thioridazine Hydrochloride (May increase drowsiness effect). Products include:
Thioridazine Hydrochloride Tablets 2122

Thiothixene (May increase drowsiness effect). Products include:
Thiothixene Capsules 2124

Tranylcypromine Sulfate (Concurrent and/or sequential use with MAO inhibitors is not recommended). Products include:
Parnate Tablets 1499

Triazolam (May increase drowsiness effect).
No products indexed under this heading.

Trifluoperazine Hydrochloride (May increase drowsiness effect).
No products indexed under this heading.

Zaleplon (May increase drowsiness effect). Products include:
Sonata Capsules 1686

Zolpidem Tartrate (May increase drowsiness effect). Products include:
Ambien Tablets 2867

TRIAMINIC COLD & COUGH SOFTCHEWS
(Chlorpheniramine Maleate, Dextromethorphan Hydrobromide, Pseudoephedrine Hydrochloride)....... ▣688
May interact with hypnotics and sedatives, monoamine oxidase inhibitors, tranquilizers, and certain other agents. Compounds in these categories include:

Alprazolam (May increase drowsiness effect). Products include:
Niravam Orally Disintegrating Tablets 3106
Xanax XR Tablets 2655

Buspirone Hydrochloride (May increase drowsiness effect).
No products indexed under this heading.

Chlordiazepoxide (May increase drowsiness effect).
No products indexed under this heading.

Chlordiazepoxide Hydrochloride (May increase drowsiness effect). Products include:
Librium Capsules 3349

Chlorpromazine (May increase drowsiness effect).
No products indexed under this heading.

Chlorpromazine Hydrochloride (May increase drowsiness effect).
No products indexed under this heading.

Chlorprothixene (May increase drowsiness effect).
No products indexed under this heading.

Chlorprothixene Hydrochloride (May increase drowsiness effect).
No products indexed under this heading.

Clorazepate Dipotassium (May increase drowsiness effect). Products include:
Tranxene 2488

Diazepam (May increase drowsiness effect). Products include:
Diastat Rectal Delivery System 3344
Valium Tablets 2822

Droperidol (May increase drowsiness effect).
No products indexed under this heading.

Estazolam (May increase drowsiness effect). Products include:
ProSom Tablets 512

Ethchlorvynol (May increase drowsiness effect).
No products indexed under this heading.

Ethinamate (May increase drowsiness effect).
No products indexed under this heading.

Fluphenazine Decanoate (May increase drowsiness effect).
No products indexed under this heading.

Fluphenazine Enanthate (May increase drowsiness effect).
No products indexed under this heading.

Fluphenazine Hydrochloride (May increase drowsiness effect).
No products indexed under this heading.

Flurazepam Hydrochloride (May increase drowsiness effect). Products include:
Dalmane Capsules 3343

Glutethimide (May increase drowsiness effect).
No products indexed under this heading.

Haloperidol (May increase drowsiness effect).
No products indexed under this heading.

Haloperidol Decanoate (May increase drowsiness effect).
No products indexed under this heading.

Hydroxyzine Hydrochloride (May increase drowsiness effect).
No products indexed under this heading.

Isocarboxazid (Concurrent and/or sequential use with MAO inhibitors is not recommended).
No products indexed under this heading.

Lorazepam (May increase drowsiness effect).
No products indexed under this heading.

Loxapine Hydrochloride (May increase drowsiness effect).
No products indexed under this heading.

Loxapine Succinate (May increase drowsiness effect).
No products indexed under this heading.

Meprobamate (May increase drowsiness effect).
No products indexed under this heading.

Mesoridazine Besylate (May increase drowsiness effect).
No products indexed under this heading.

Midazolam Hydrochloride (May increase drowsiness effect).
No products indexed under this heading.

Moclobemide (Concurrent and/or sequential use with MAO inhibitors is not recommended).
No products indexed under this heading.

Molindone Hydrochloride (May increase drowsiness effect). Products include:
Moban Tablets 1108

Oxazepam (May increase drowsiness effect).
No products indexed under this heading.

Pargyline Hydrochloride (Concurrent and/or sequential use with MAO inhibitors is not recommended).
No products indexed under this heading.

Perphenazine (May increase drowsiness effect).
No products indexed under this heading.

Phenelzine Sulfate (Concurrent and/or sequential use with MAO inhibitors is not recommended).
No products indexed under this heading.

Prazepam (May increase drowsiness effect).
No products indexed under this heading.

Procarbazine Hydrochloride (Concurrent and/or sequential use with MAO inhibitors is not recommended). Products include:
Matulane Capsules 3188

Prochlorperazine (May increase drowsiness effect).
No products indexed under this heading.

Promethazine Hydrochloride (May increase drowsiness effect). Products include:
Phenergan 3438

Propofol (May increase drowsiness effect). Products include:
Diprivan Injectable Emulsion 676

Quazepam (May increase drowsiness effect).
No products indexed under this heading.

Secobarbital Sodium (May increase drowsiness effect).
No products indexed under this heading.

Selegiline Hydrochloride (Concurrent and/or sequential use with MAO inhibitors is not recommended). Products include:
Eldepryl Capsules 3209

Temazepam (May increase drowsiness effect).
No products indexed under this heading.

Thioridazine Hydrochloride (May increase drowsiness effect). Products include:
Thioridazine Hydrochloride Tablets 2122

Thiothixene (May increase drowsiness effect). Products include:
Thiothixene Capsules 2124

Tranylcypromine Sulfate (Concurrent and/or sequential use with MAO inhibitors is not recommended). Products include:
Parnate Tablets 1499

Triazolam (May increase drowsiness effect).
No products indexed under this heading.

Trifluoperazine Hydrochloride (May increase drowsiness effect).
No products indexed under this heading.

Zaleplon (May increase drowsiness effect). Products include:
Sonata Capsules 1686

Zolpidem Tartrate (May increase drowsiness effect). Products include:
Ambien Tablets 2867

Food Interactions

Alcohol (May increase drowsiness effect).

TRIAMINIC COUGH & SORE THROAT SOFTCHEWS

(Acetaminophen, Dextromethorphan Hydrobromide, Pseudoephedrine Hydrochloride)....... 689
May interact with monoamine oxidase inhibitors. Compounds in these categories include:

Isocarboxazid (Concurrent and/or sequential use with MAO inhibitors is not recommended).
No products indexed under this heading.

Moclobemide (Concurrent and/or sequential use with MAO inhibitors is not recommended).
No products indexed under this heading.

Pargyline Hydrochloride (Concurrent and/or sequential use with MAO inhibitors is not recommended).
No products indexed under this heading.

Phenelzine Sulfate (Concurrent and/or sequential use with MAO inhibitors is not recommended).
No products indexed under this heading.

Procarbazine Hydrochloride (Concurrent and/or sequential use with MAO inhibitors is not recommended). Products include:
Matulane Capsules 3188

Selegiline Hydrochloride (Concurrent and/or sequential use with MAO inhibitors is not recommended). Products include:
Eldepryl Capsules 3209

Tranylcypromine Sulfate (Concurrent and/or sequential use with MAO inhibitors is not recommended). Products include:
Parnate Tablets 1499

TRIAMINIC SORE THROAT SPRAY

(Phenol) 689
None cited in PDR database.

TRIAMINIC THIN STRIPS COUGH & RUNNY NOSE

(Diphenhydramine Hydrochloride) 690
May interact with hypnotics and sedatives and tranquilizers. Compounds in these categories include:

Alprazolam (Co-administration with sedatives/tranquilizers may increase the drowsiness effect). Products include:
Niravam Orally Disintegrating Tablets 3106
Xanax XR Tablets 2655

Buspirone Hydrochloride (Co-administration with sedatives/tranquilizers may increase the drowsiness effect).
No products indexed under this heading.

Chlordiazepoxide (Co-administration with sedatives/tranquilizers may increase the drowsiness effect).
No products indexed under this heading.

Chlordiazepoxide Hydrochloride (Co-administration with sedatives/tranquilizers may increase the drowsiness effect). Products include:
Librium Capsules 3349

Chlorpromazine (Co-administration with sedatives/tranquilizers may increase the drowsiness effect).
No products indexed under this heading.

Chlorpromazine Hydrochloride (Co-administration with sedatives/tranquilizers may increase the drowsiness effect).
No products indexed under this heading.

Chlorprothixene (Co-administration with sedatives/tranquilizers may increase the drowsiness effect).
No products indexed under this heading.

Chlorprothixene Hydrochloride (Co-administration with sedatives/tranquilizers may increase the drowsiness effect).
No products indexed under this heading.

Clorazepate Dipotassium (Co-administration with sedatives/tranquilizers may increase the drowsiness effect). Products include:
Tranxene 2488

Diazepam (Co-administration with sedatives/tranquilizers may increase the drowsiness effect). Products include:
Diastat Rectal Delivery System 3344
Valium Tablets 2822

Droperidol (Co-administration with sedatives/tranquilizers may increase the drowsiness effect).
No products indexed under this heading.

Estazolam (Co-administration with sedatives/tranquilizers may increase the drowsiness effect). Products include:
ProSom Tablets 512

Ethchlorvynol (Co-administration with sedatives/tranquilizers may increase the drowsiness effect).
No products indexed under this heading.

Ethinamate (Co-administration with sedatives/tranquilizers may increase the drowsiness effect).
No products indexed under this heading.

Fluphenazine Decanoate (Co-administration with sedatives/tranquilizers may increase the drowsiness effect).
No products indexed under this heading.

Fluphenazine Enanthate (Co-administration with sedatives/tranquilizers may increase the drowsiness effect).
No products indexed under this heading.

Fluphenazine Hydrochloride (Co-administration with sedatives/tranquilizers may increase the drowsiness effect).
No products indexed under this heading.

Flurazepam Hydrochloride (Co-administration with sedatives/tranquilizers may increase the drowsiness effect). Products include:
Dalmane Capsules 3343

Glutethimide (Co-administration with sedatives/tranquilizers may increase the drowsiness effect).
No products indexed under this heading.

Haloperidol (Co-administration with sedatives/tranquilizers may increase the drowsiness effect).
No products indexed under this heading.

Haloperidol Decanoate (Co-administration with sedatives/tranquilizers may increase the drowsiness effect).
No products indexed under this heading.

Hydroxyzine Hydrochloride (Co-administration with sedatives/tranquilizers may increase the drowsiness effect).
No products indexed under this heading.

Lorazepam (Co-administration with sedatives/tranquilizers may increase the drowsiness effect).
No products indexed under this heading.

Loxapine Hydrochloride (Co-administration with sedatives/tranquilizers may increase the drowsiness effect).
No products indexed under this heading.

Loxapine Succinate (Co-administration with sedatives/tranquilizers may increase the drowsiness effect).
No products indexed under this heading.

Meprobamate (Co-administration with sedatives/tranquilizers may increase the drowsiness effect).
No products indexed under this heading.

Mesoridazine Besylate (Co-administration with sedatives/tranquilizers may increase the drowsiness effect).
No products indexed under this heading.

Midazolam Hydrochloride (Co-administration with sedatives/tranquilizers may increase the drowsiness effect).
No products indexed under this heading.

Molindone Hydrochloride (Co-administration with sedatives/tranquilizers may increase the drowsiness effect). Products include:
Moban Tablets 1108

Oxazepam (Co-administration with sedatives/tranquilizers may increase the drowsiness effect).
No products indexed under this heading.

Perphenazine (Co-administration with sedatives/tranquilizers may increase the drowsiness effect).
No products indexed under this heading.

Prazepam (Co-administration with sedatives/tranquilizers may increase the drowsiness effect).
No products indexed under this heading.

Prochlorperazine (Co-administration with sedatives/tranquilizers may increase the drowsiness effect).
No products indexed under this heading.

Promethazine Hydrochloride (Co-administration with sedatives/tranquilizers may increase the drowsiness effect). Products include:
Phenergan 3438

Propofol (Co-administration with sedatives/tranquilizers may increase the drowsiness effect). Products include:
Diprivan Injectable Emulsion 676

Quazepam (Co-administration with sedatives/tranquilizers may increase the drowsiness effect).
No products indexed under this heading.

Secobarbital Sodium (Co-administration with sedatives/tranquilizers may increase the drowsiness effect).
No products indexed under this heading.

Temazepam (Co-administration with sedatives/tranquilizers may increase the drowsiness effect).
No products indexed under this heading.

Thioridazine Hydrochloride (Co-administration with sedatives/tranquilizers may increase the drowsiness effect). Products include:
Thioridazine Hydrochloride Tablets 2122

Thiothixene (Co-administration with sedatives/tranquilizers may increase the drowsiness effect). Products include:
Thiothixene Capsules 2124

Triazolam (Co-administration with sedatives/tranquilizers may increase the drowsiness effect).
No products indexed under this heading.

Trifluoperazine Hydrochloride (Co-administration with sedatives/tranquilizers may increase the drowsiness effect).
No products indexed under this heading.

Zaleplon (Co-administration with sedatives/tranquilizers may increase the drowsiness effect). Products include:
Sonata Capsules 1686

Zolpidem Tartrate (Co-administration with sedatives/tranquilizers may increase the drowsiness effect). Products include:
Ambien Tablets 2867

TRIAMINIC THIN STRIPS LONG ACTING COUGH

(Dextromethorphan Hydrobromide) .... ▣689
May interact with monoamine oxidase inhibitors. Compounds in these categories include:

Isocarboxazid (Avoid use with, or for two weeks after stopping, MAOI drugs).
No products indexed under this heading.

Moclobemide (Avoid use with, or for two weeks after stopping, MAOI drugs).
No products indexed under this heading.

Pargyline Hydrochloride (Avoid use with, or for two weeks after stopping, MAOI drugs).
No products indexed under this heading.

Phenelzine Sulfate (Avoid use with, or for two weeks after stopping, MAOI drugs).
No products indexed under this heading.

Procarbazine Hydrochloride (Avoid use with, or for two weeks after stopping, MAOI drugs). Products include:
Matulane Capsules 3188

Selegiline Hydrochloride (Avoid use with, or for two weeks after stopping, MAOI drugs). Products include:
Eldepryl Capsules 3209

Tranylcypromine Sulfate (Avoid use with, or for two weeks after stopping, MAOI drugs). Products include:
Parnate Tablets 1499

TRIAMINIC VAPOR PATCH-CHERRY SCENT

(Camphor, Menthol) .... ▣690
None cited in PDR database.

TRIAMINIC VAPOR PATCH-MENTHOL SCENT

(Camphor, Menthol) .... ▣690
None cited in PDR database.

TRIAZ CLEANSER

(Benzoyl Peroxide) 1864
None cited in PDR database.

TRIAZ GEL

(Benzoyl Peroxide) 1864
None cited in PDR database.

TRIAZ PADS

(Benzoyl Peroxide) 1864
None cited in PDR database.

TRICOR TABLETS

(Fenofibrate) 523
May interact with bile acid sequestering agents, oral anticoagulants, HMG-CoA reductase inhibitors, immunosuppressive agents, nephrotoxic agents, and certain other agents. Compounds in these categories include:

Abacavir Sulfate (The benefits and risks of using fenofibrate tablets with immunosuppressants and other potentially nephrotoxic agents should be carefully considered and the lowest effective dose employed). Products include:
Epzicom Tablets 1402
Trizivir Tablets 1565
Ziagen 1600

Acyclovir (The benefits and risks of using fenofibrate tablets with immunosuppressants and other potentially nephrotoxic agents should be carefully considered and the lowest effective dose employed). Products include:
Zovirax 1616
Zovirax Cream 853
Zovirax Ointment 854

Acyclovir Sodium (The benefits and risks of using fenofibrate tablets with immunosuppressants and other potentially nephrotoxic agents should be carefully considered and the lowest effective dose employed). Products include:
Zovirax for Injection 1618

Alatrofloxacin Mesylate (The benefits and risks of using fenofibrate tablets with immunosuppressants and other potentially nephrotoxic agents should be carefully considered and the lowest effective dose employed).
No products indexed under this heading.

Aldesleukin (The benefits and risks of using fenofibrate tablets with immunosuppressants and other potentially nephrotoxic agents should be carefully considered and the lowest effective dose employed). Products include:
Proleukin for Injection 1007

Amikacin Sulfate (The benefits and risks of using fenofibrate tablets with immunosuppressants and other potentially nephrotoxic agents should be carefully considered and the lowest effective dose employed).
No products indexed under this heading.

Amoxicillin (The benefits and risks of using fenofibrate tablets with immunosuppressants and other potentially nephrotoxic agents should be carefully considered and the lowest effective dose employed). Products include:
Amoxil Capsules 1315
Amoxil Chewable Tablets 1315
Amoxil Pediatric Drops for Oral Suspension 1315
Amoxil Powder for Oral Suspension 1315
Amoxil Tablets 1315
Augmentin 1331
Augmentin Tablets 1334
Augmentin XR Extended-Release Tablets 1340
Augmentin ES-600 Powder for Oral Suspension 1337
PREVPAC 3281

Amoxicillin Trihydrate (The benefits and risks of using fenofibrate tablets with immunosuppressants and other potentially nephrotoxic agents should be carefully considered and the lowest effective dose employed).
No products indexed under this heading.

Amphotericin B (The benefits and risks of using fenofibrate tablets with immunosuppressants and other potentially nephrotoxic agents should be carefully considered and the lowest effective dose employed).
No products indexed under this heading.

Amphotericin B, liposomal (The benefits and risks of using fenofibrate tablets with immunosuppressants and other potentially nephrotoxic agents should be carefully considered and the lowest effective dose employed). Products include:
AmBisome for Injection 615

Amphotericin B Cholesteryl Sulfate (The benefits and risks of using fenofibrate tablets with immunosuppressants and other potentially nephrotoxic agents should be carefully considered and the lowest effective dose employed).
No products indexed under this heading.

Amphotericin B Lipid Complex (The benefits and risks of using fenofibrate tablets with immunosuppressants and other potentially nephrotoxic agents should be carefully considered and the lowest effective dose employed). Products include:
Abelcet Injection 1119

Ampicillin (The benefits and risks of using fenofibrate tablets with immunosuppressants and other potentially nephrotoxic agents should be carefully considered and the lowest effective dose employed).
No products indexed under this heading.

Ampicillin Sodium (The benefits and risks of using fenofibrate tablets with immunosuppressants and other potentially nephrotoxic agents should be carefully considered and the lowest effective dose employed).
No products indexed under this heading.

Ampicillin Trihydrate (The benefits and risks of using fenofibrate tablets with immunosuppressants and other potentially nephrotoxic agents should be carefully considered and the lowest effective dose employed).
No products indexed under this heading.

Amprenavir (The benefits and risks of using fenofibrate tablets with immunosuppressants and other potentially nephrotoxic agents should be carefully considered and the lowest effective dose employed). Products include:
Agenerase Capsules 1299
Agenerase Oral Solution 1304

Anisindione (Caution should be exercised when anticoagulants are given in conjunction with fenofibrate because of the potentiation of coumarin-type anticoagulants in prolonging the PT/INR. The dosage of the anticoagulant should be reduced to maintain the PT/INR at the desired level to prevent bleeding complications. Frequent PT/INR determinations are advisable until it has been definitely determined that the PT/INR has stabilized). Products include:
Miradon Tablets 3056

Aspirin (The benefits and risks of using fenofibrate tablets with immunosuppressants and other potentially nephrotoxic agents should be carefully considered and the lowest effective dose employed). Products include:
Aggrenox Capsules 855
Bayer, Aspirin Regimen .... ▣606
Bayer Aspirin Tablets 3515
BC Powder .... ▣612
BC Allergy Sinus Cold Powder .... ▣612
Arthritis Strength BC Powder .... ▣612
BC Sinus Cold Powder .... ▣612
Ecotrin Enteric Coated Aspirin Low, Regular and Maximum Strength Tablets 1627
Goody's Body Pain Formula Powder .... ▣621
Goody's Extra Strength Headache Powder .... ▣621
Goody's Extra Strength Pain Relief Tablets .... ▣621
Percodan Tablets 1115
St. Joseph 81 mg Aspirin Chewable and Enteric Coated Tablets 1841

Atazanavir (The benefits and risks of using fenofibrate tablets with immunosuppressants and other potentially nephrotoxic agents should be carefully considered and the lowest effective dose employed).
No products indexed under this heading.

Atorvastatin Calcium (Co-administration of fibric acid derivatives and HMG-CoA reductase inhibitors has been associated with rhabdomyolysis, markedly elevated creatine kinase levels and myoglobulinuria, leading in a high proportion of cases to acute renal failure; the combined use should be avoided unless the benefit of further alterations in lipid levels is likely to outweigh the increased risk of this combination). Products include:
Caduet Tablets 2507
Lipitor Tablets 2495

Azathioprine (The benefits and risks of using fenofibrate tablets with immunosuppressants and other potentially nephrotoxic agents should be carefully considered and the lowest effective dose employed). Products include:
Azasan Tablets 2844

Azithromycin Dihydrate (The benefits and risks of using fenofibrate tablets with immunosuppressants and other potentially nephrotoxic agents should be carefully considered and the lowest effective dose employed). Products include:
Zithromax 2568
Zithromax for IV Infusion 2573
Zithromax for Oral Suspension, 300 mg, 600 mg, 900 mg, 1200 mg 2561
Zithromax Tablets, 250 mg, 500 mg 2561
Zithromax Tri-Pak 2561
Zithromax Z-Pak 2568

Azlocillin Sodium (The benefits and risks of using fenofibrate tablets with immunosuppressants and other potentially nephrotoxic agents should be carefully considered and the lowest effective dose employed).
No products indexed under this heading.

Aztreonam (The benefits and risks of using fenofibrate tablets with immunosuppressants and other potentially nephrotoxic agents should be carefully considered and the lowest effective dose employed).
No products indexed under this heading.

Bacampicillin Hydrochloride (The benefits and risks of using fenofibrate tablets with immunosuppressants and other potentially nephrotoxic agents should be carefully considered and the lowest effective dose employed).
No products indexed under this heading.

Balsalazide Disodium (The benefits and risks of using fenofibrate tablets with immunosuppressants and other potentially nephrotoxic agents should be carefully considered and the lowest effective dose employed). Products include:
Colazal Capsules 2845

Basiliximab (The benefits and risks of using fenofibrate tablets with immunosuppressants and other potentially nephrotoxic agents should be carefully considered and the lowest effective dose employed). Products include:
Simulect for Injection 2268

Benazepril Hydrochloride (The benefits and risks of using fenofibrate tablets with immunosuppressants and other potentially nephrotoxic agents should be carefully considered and the lowest effective dose employed). Products include:
Lotensin Tablets 2232
Lotensin HCT Tablets 2235
Lotrel Capsules 2238

Bendroflumethiazide (The benefits and risks of using fenofibrate tablets with immunosuppressants and other potentially nephrotoxic agents should be carefully considered and the lowest effective dose employed).
No products indexed under this heading.

Caffeine (The benefits and risks of using fenofibrate tablets with immunosuppressants and other potentially nephrotoxic agents should be carefully considered and the lowest effective dose employed). Products include:
Athena Hair System Shampoo 767
BC Powder 612
Arthritis Strength BC Powder 612
Goody's Extra Strength Headache Powder 621
Goody's Extra Strength Pain Relief Tablets 621
Hycomine Compound Tablets 1105
Spartan Hair System Shampoo 767
Vivarin 639

Captopril (The benefits and risks of using fenofibrate tablets with immunosuppressants and other potentially nephrotoxic agents should be carefully considered and the lowest effective dose employed). Products include:
Captopril Tablets 2114

Carbenicillin Disodium (The benefits and risks of using fenofibrate tablets with immunosuppressants and other potentially nephrotoxic agents should be carefully considered and the lowest effective dose employed).
No products indexed under this heading.

Carbenicillin Indanyl Sodium (The benefits and risks of using fenofibrate tablets with immunosuppressants and other potentially nephrotoxic agents should be carefully considered and the lowest effective dose employed).
No products indexed under this heading.

Carboplatin (The benefits and risks of using fenofibrate tablets with immunosuppressants and other potentially nephrotoxic agents should be carefully considered and the lowest effective dose employed).
No products indexed under this heading.

Carmustine (BCNU) (The benefits and risks of using fenofibrate tablets with immunosuppressants and other potentially nephrotoxic agents should be carefully considered and the lowest effective dose employed).
No products indexed under this heading.

Cefaclor (The benefits and risks of using fenofibrate tablets with immunosuppressants and other potentially nephrotoxic agents should be carefully considered and the lowest effective dose employed).
No products indexed under this heading.

Cefadroxil (The benefits and risks of using fenofibrate tablets with immunosuppressants and other potentially nephrotoxic agents should be carefully considered and the lowest effective dose employed).
No products indexed under this heading.

Cefamandole Nafate (The benefits and risks of using fenofibrate tablets with immunosuppressants and other potentially nephrotoxic agents should be carefully considered and the lowest effective dose employed).
No products indexed under this heading.

Cefazolin Sodium (The benefits and risks of using fenofibrate tablets with immunosuppressants and other potentially nephrotoxic agents should be carefully considered and the lowest effective dose employed). Products include:
Ancef for Injection 1318

Cefdinir (The benefits and risks of using fenofibrate tablets with immunosuppressants and other potentially nephrotoxic agents should be carefully considered and the lowest effective dose employed). Products include:
Omnicef Capsules 506
Omnicef for Oral Suspension 506

Cefepime Hydrochloride (The benefits and risks of using fenofibrate tablets with immunosuppressants and other potentially nephrotoxic agents should be carefully considered and the lowest effective dose employed). Products include:
Maxipime for Injection 1093

Cefixime (The benefits and risks of using fenofibrate tablets with immunosuppressants and other potentially nephrotoxic agents should be carefully considered and the lowest effective dose employed). Products include:
Suprax 1811

Cefmetazole Sodium (The benefits and risks of using fenofibrate tablets with immunosuppressants and other potentially nephrotoxic agents should be carefully considered and the lowest effective dose employed).
No products indexed under this heading.

Cefonicid Sodium (The benefits and risks of using fenofibrate tablets with immunosuppressants and other potentially nephrotoxic agents should be carefully considered and the lowest effective dose employed).
No products indexed under this heading.

Cefoperazone Sodium (The benefits and risks of using fenofibrate tablets with immunosuppressants and other potentially nephrotoxic agents should be carefully considered and the lowest effective dose employed).
No products indexed under this heading.

Ceforanide (The benefits and risks of using fenofibrate tablets with immunosuppressants and other potentially nephrotoxic agents should be carefully considered and the lowest effective dose employed).
No products indexed under this heading.

Cefotaxime Sodium (The benefits and risks of using fenofibrate tablets with immunosuppressants and other potentially nephrotoxic agents should be carefully considered and the lowest effective dose employed).
No products indexed under this heading.

Cefotetan (The benefits and risks of using fenofibrate tablets with immunosuppressants and other potentially nephrotoxic agents should be carefully considered and the lowest effective dose employed).
No products indexed under this heading.

Cefoxitin Sodium (The benefits and risks of using fenofibrate tablets with immunosuppressants and other potentially nephrotoxic agents should be carefully considered and the lowest effective dose employed). Products include:
Mefoxin for Injection 1987
Mefoxin Premixed Intravenous Solution 1990

Cefpodoxime Proxetil (The benefits and risks of using fenofibrate tablets with immunosuppressants and other potentially nephrotoxic agents should be carefully considered and the lowest effective dose employed). Products include:
Vantin Tablets and Oral Suspension 2650

Cefprozil (The benefits and risks of using fenofibrate tablets with immunosuppressants and other potentially nephrotoxic agents should be carefully considered and the lowest effective dose employed).
No products indexed under this heading.

Ceftazidime (The benefits and risks of using fenofibrate tablets with immunosuppressants and other potentially nephrotoxic agents should be carefully considered and the lowest effective dose employed). Products include:
Fortaz for Injection 1422

Ceftizoxime Sodium (The benefits and risks of using fenofibrate tablets with immunosuppressants and other potentially nephrotoxic agents should be carefully considered and the lowest effective dose employed).
No products indexed under this heading.

Ceftriaxone Sodium (The benefits and risks of using fenofibrate tablets with immunosuppressants and other potentially nephrotoxic agents should be carefully considered and the lowest effective dose employed). Products include:
Rocephin Injectable Vials, ADD-Vantage, Galaxy, Bulk 2801

Cefuroxime Axetil (The benefits and risks of using fenofibrate tablets with immunosuppressants and other potentially nephrotoxic agents should be carefully considered and the lowest effective dose employed). Products include:
Ceftin 1369

Cefuroxime Sodium (The benefits and risks of using fenofibrate tablets with immunosuppressants and other potentially nephrotoxic agents should be carefully considered and the lowest effective dose employed).
No products indexed under this heading.

Celecoxib (The benefits and risks of using fenofibrate tablets with immunosuppressants and other potentially nephrotoxic agents should be carefully considered and the lowest effective dose employed). Products include:
Celebrex Capsules 3130

Cephalexin (The benefits and risks of using fenofibrate tablets with immunosuppressants and other potentially nephrotoxic agents should be carefully considered and the lowest effective dose employed).
No products indexed under this heading.

Cephalothin Sodium (The benefits and risks of using fenofibrate tablets with immunosuppressants and other potentially nephrotoxic agents should be carefully considered and the lowest effective dose employed).
No products indexed under this heading.

Cephapirin Sodium (The benefits and risks of using fenofibrate tablets with immunosuppressants and other potentially nephrotoxic agents should be carefully considered and the lowest effective dose employed).
No products indexed under this heading.

Cephradine (The benefits and risks of using fenofibrate tablets with immunosuppressants and other potentially nephrotoxic agents should be carefully considered and the lowest effective dose employed).
No products indexed under this heading.

Cerivastatin Sodium (Co-administration of fibric acid derivatives and HMG-CoA reductase inhibitors has been associated with rhabdomyolysis, markedly elevated creatine kinase levels and myoglobulinuria, leading in a high proportion of cases to acute renal failure; the combined use should be avoided unless the benefit of further alterations in

lipid levels is likely to outweigh the increased risk of this combination).
No products indexed under this heading.

Chlorothiazide (The benefits and risks of using fenofibrate tablets with immunosuppressants and other potentially nephrotoxic agents should be carefully considered and the lowest effective dose employed). Products include:
Aldoclor Tablets **1881**
Diuril Oral **1936**

Chlorothiazide Sodium (The benefits and risks of using fenofibrate tablets with immunosuppressants and other potentially nephrotoxic agents should be carefully considered and the lowest effective dose employed). Products include:
Diuril Sodium Intravenous **1934**

Chlorpropamide (The benefits and risks of using fenofibrate tablets with immunosuppressants and other potentially nephrotoxic agents should be carefully considered and the lowest effective dose employed).
No products indexed under this heading.

Cholestyramine (Bile acid sequestrants may bind fenofibrate; fenofibrate should be taken at least 1 hours before or 4-6 hours after a bile acid binding resin to avoid impeding its absorption).
No products indexed under this heading.

Cidofovir (The benefits and risks of using fenofibrate tablets with immunosuppressants and other potentially nephrotoxic agents should be carefully considered and the lowest effective dose employed).
No products indexed under this heading.

Cilastatin Sodium (The benefits and risks of using fenofibrate tablets with immunosuppressants and other potentially nephrotoxic agents should be carefully considered and the lowest effective dose employed). Products include:
Primaxin I.M. **2022**
Primaxin I.V. **2024**

Cimetidine (The benefits and risks of using fenofibrate tablets with immunosuppressants and other potentially nephrotoxic agents should be carefully considered and the lowest effective dose employed). Products include:
Tagamet HB 200 Tablets .... ▣**637**
Tagamet Tablets **1547**

Cimetidine Hydrochloride (The benefits and risks of using fenofibrate tablets with immunosuppressants and other potentially nephrotoxic agents should be carefully considered and the lowest effective dose employed).
No products indexed under this heading.

Cisplatin (The benefits and risks of using fenofibrate tablets with immunosuppressants and other potentially nephrotoxic agents should be carefully considered and the lowest effective dose employed).
No products indexed under this heading.

Cladribine (The benefits and risks of using fenofibrate tablets with immunosuppressants and other potentially nephrotoxic agents should be carefully considered and the lowest effective dose employed). Products include:
Leustatin Injection **2368**

Clozapine (The benefits and risks of using fenofibrate tablets with immunosuppressants and other potentially nephrotoxic agents should be carefully considered and the lowest effective dose employed). Products include:
Clozapine Tablets **2141**
Clozaril Tablets **2174**
FazaClo Orally Disintegrating Tablets **547**

Colesevelam Hydrochloride (Bile acid sequestrants may bind fenofibrate; fenofibrate should be taken at least 1 hours before or 4-6 hours after a bile acid binding resin to avoid impeding its absorption). Products include:
WelChol Tablets **2855**

Colestipol Hydrochloride (Bile acid sequestrants may bind fenofibrate; fenofibrate should be taken at least 1 hours before or 4-6 hours after a bile acid binding resin to avoid impeding its absorption).
No products indexed under this heading.

Colistimethate Sodium (The benefits and risks of using fenofibrate tablets with immunosuppressants and other potentially nephrotoxic agents should be carefully considered and the lowest effective dose employed).
No products indexed under this heading.

Colistin Sulfate (The benefits and risks of using fenofibrate tablets with immunosuppressants and other potentially nephrotoxic agents should be carefully considered and the lowest effective dose employed).
No products indexed under this heading.

Cyclophosphamide (The benefits and risks of using fenofibrate tablets with immunosuppressants and other potentially nephrotoxic agents should be carefully considered and the lowest effective dose employed).
No products indexed under this heading.

Cyclosporine (Because Cyclosporine can produce nephrotoxicity with decreases in creatinine clearance and rises in serum creatinine, and because renal excretion is the primary elimination route of fibrate drugs including fenofibrate, there is a risk that an interactionwill lead to deterioration. The benefits and risks of using fenofibrate tablets with immunosuppressants and other potentially nephrotoxic agents should be carefully considered and the lowest effective dose employed). Products include:
Gengraf Capsules **458**
Neoral Soft Gelatin Capsules **2247**
Neoral Oral Solution **2247**
Restasis Ophthalmic Emulsion **570**
Sandimmune **2259**

Cytarabine (The benefits and risks of using fenofibrate tablets with immunosuppressants and other potentially nephrotoxic agents should be carefully considered and the lowest effective dose employed).
No products indexed under this heading.

Cytarabine Liposome (The benefits and risks of using fenofibrate tablets with immunosuppressants and other potentially nephrotoxic agents should be carefully considered and the lowest effective dose employed). Products include:
DepoCyt Injection **1121**

Delavirdine Mesylate (The benefits and risks of using fenofibrate tablets with immunosuppressants and other potentially nephrotoxic agents should be carefully considered and the lowest effective dose employed). Products include:
Rescriptor Tablets **2535**

Diatrizoate Meglumine (The benefits and risks of using fenofibrate tablets with immunosuppressants and other potentially nephrotoxic agents should be carefully considered and the lowest effective dose employed).
No products indexed under this heading.

Diatrizoate Sodium (The benefits and risks of using fenofibrate tablets with immunosuppressants and other potentially nephrotoxic agents should be carefully considered and the lowest effective dose employed).
No products indexed under this heading.

Diclofenac Potassium (The benefits and risks of using fenofibrate tablets with immunosuppressants and other potentially nephrotoxic agents should be carefully considered and the lowest effective dose employed). Products include:
Cataflam Tablets **2173**

Diclofenac Sodium (The benefits and risks of using fenofibrate tablets with immunosuppressants and other potentially nephrotoxic agents should be carefully considered and the lowest effective dose employed). Products include:
Arthrotec Tablets **3126**
Voltaren Ophthalmic Solution **2300**
Voltaren Tablets **2298**
Voltaren-XR Tablets **2301**

Dicloxacillin Sodium (The benefits and risks of using fenofibrate tablets with immunosuppressants and other potentially nephrotoxic agents should be carefully considered and the lowest effective dose employed).
No products indexed under this heading.

Dicumarol (Caution should be exercised when anticoagulants are given in conjunction with fenofibrate because of the potentiation of coumarin-type anticoagulants in prolonging the PT/INR. The dosage of the anticoagulant should be reduced to maintain the PT/INR at the desired level to prevent bleeding complications. Frequent PT/INR determinations are advisable until it has been definitely determined that the PT/INR has stabilized).
No products indexed under this heading.

Didanosine (The benefits and risks of using fenofibrate tablets with immunosuppressants and other potentially nephrotoxic agents should be carefully considered and the lowest effective dose employed).
No products indexed under this heading.

Efavirenz (The benefits and risks of using fenofibrate tablets with immunosuppressants and other potentially nephrotoxic agents should be carefully considered and the lowest effective dose employed). Products include:
Sustiva Capsules **957**

Emtricitabine (The benefits and risks of using fenofibrate tablets with immunosuppressants and other potentially nephrotoxic agents should be carefully considered and the lowest effective dose employed). Products include:
Emtriva Capsules **1272**
Truvada Tablets **1279**

Enalapril Maleate (The benefits and risks of using fenofibrate tablets with immunosuppressants and other potentially nephrotoxic agents should be carefully considered and the lowest effective dose employed). Products include:
Vaseretic Tablets **2073**
Vasotec I.V. Injection **2076**

Enalaprilat (The benefits and risks of using fenofibrate tablets with immunosuppressants and other potentially nephrotoxic agents should be carefully considered and the lowest effective dose employed).
No products indexed under this heading.

Enfuvirtide (The benefits and risks of using fenofibrate tablets with immunosuppressants and other potentially nephrotoxic agents should be carefully considered and the lowest effective dose employed). Products include:
Fuzeon Injection **2772**

Ethiodized Oil (The benefits and risks of using fenofibrate tablets with immunosuppressants and other potentially nephrotoxic agents should be carefully considered and the lowest effective dose employed).
No products indexed under this heading.

Etodolac (The benefits and risks of using fenofibrate tablets with immunosuppressants and other potentially nephrotoxic agents should be carefully considered and the lowest effective dose employed).
No products indexed under this heading.

Fenoprofen Calcium (The benefits and risks of using fenofibrate tablets with immunosuppressants and other potentially nephrotoxic agents should be carefully considered and the lowest effective dose employed). Products include:
Nalfon Capsules **2504**

Filgrastim (The benefits and risks of using fenofibrate tablets with immunosuppressants and other potentially nephrotoxic agents should be carefully considered and the lowest effective dose employed). Products include:
Neupogen for Injection **598**

Fluorouracil (The benefits and risks of using fenofibrate tablets with immunosuppressants and other potentially nephrotoxic agents should be carefully considered and the lowest effective dose employed). Products include:
Carac Cream, 0.5% **1048**
Efudex **3348**

Flurbiprofen (The benefits and risks of using fenofibrate tablets with immunosuppressants and other potentially nephrotoxic agents should be carefully considered and the lowest effective dose employed).
No products indexed under this heading.

Fluvastatin Sodium (Co-administration of fibric acid derivatives and HMG-CoA reductase inhibitors has been associated with rhabdomyolysis, markedly elevated creatine kinase levels and myoglobulinuria, leading in a high proportion of

cases to acute renal failure; the combined use should be avoided unless the benefit of further alterations in lipid levels is likely to outweigh the increased risk of this combination). Products include:

- Lescol Capsules 2227
- Lescol 2730
- Lescol XL Tablets 2227

Foscarnet Sodium (The benefits and risks of using fenofibrate tablets with immunosuppressants and other potentially nephrotoxic agents should be carefully considered and the lowest effective dose employed).
No products indexed under this heading.

Fosinopril Sodium (The benefits and risks of using fenofibrate tablets with immunosuppressants and other potentially nephrotoxic agents should be carefully considered and the lowest effective dose employed).
No products indexed under this heading.

Furosemide (The benefits and risks of using fenofibrate tablets with immunosuppressants and other potentially nephrotoxic agents should be carefully considered and the lowest effective dose employed). Products include:

- Furosemide Tablets 2117

Gadopentetate Dimeglumine (The benefits and risks of using fenofibrate tablets with immunosuppressants and other potentially nephrotoxic agents should be carefully considered and the lowest effective dose employed).
No products indexed under this heading.

Gentamicin (The benefits and risks of using fenofibrate tablets with immunosuppressants and other potentially nephrotoxic agents should be carefully considered and the lowest effective dose employed).
No products indexed under this heading.

Gentamicin Sulfate (The benefits and risks of using fenofibrate tablets with immunosuppressants and other potentially nephrotoxic agents should be carefully considered and the lowest effective dose employed). Products include:

- Garamycin Injectable 3028
- Genoptic Sterile Ophthalmic Solution .... ⊙227
- Pred-G Ophthalmic Suspension .... ⊙234
- Pred-G Sterile Ophthalmic Ointment .... ⊙235

Glipizide (The benefits and risks of using fenofibrate tablets with immunosuppressants and other potentially nephrotoxic agents should be carefully considered and the lowest effective dose employed).
No products indexed under this heading.

Globulin, Immune (Human) (The benefits and risks of using fenofibrate tablets with immunosuppressants and other potentially nephrotoxic agents should be carefully considered and the lowest effective dose employed). Products include:

- GamaSTAN 3231

Glyburide (The benefits and risks of using fenofibrate tablets with immunosuppressants and other potentially nephrotoxic agents should be carefully considered and the lowest effective dose employed).
No products indexed under this heading.

Gold Therapy (The benefits and risks of using fenofibrate tablets with immunosuppressants and other potentially nephrotoxic agents should be carefully considered and the lowest effective dose employed).
No products indexed under this heading.

HMG-CoA Reductase Inhibitors (The benefits and risks of using fenofibrate tablets with immunosuppressants and other potentially nephrotoxic agents should be carefully considered and the lowest effective dose employed).
No products indexed under this heading.

Hydrochlorothiazide (The benefits and risks of using fenofibrate tablets with immunosuppressants and other potentially nephrotoxic agents should be carefully considered and the lowest effective dose employed). Products include:

- Aldoril Tablets 1884
- Atacand HCT 637
- Avalide Tablets 2889
- Avalide Tablets 922
- Benicar HCT Tablets 2852
- Diovan HCT Tablets 2195
- Dyazide Capsules 1389
- Hyzaar 1964
- Lotensin HCT Tablets 2235
- Maxzide 2150
- Micardis HCT Tablets 886
- Moduretic Tablets 2003
- Prinzide Tablets 2033
- Teveten HCT Tablets 1710
- Timolide Tablets 2056
- Uniretic Tablets 3114
- Vaseretic Tablets 2073
- Zestoretic Tablets 701

Hydroflumethiazide (The benefits and risks of using fenofibrate tablets with immunosuppressants and other potentially nephrotoxic agents should be carefully considered and the lowest effective dose employed).
No products indexed under this heading.

Ibuprofen (The benefits and risks of using fenofibrate tablets with immunosuppressants and other potentially nephrotoxic agents should be carefully considered and the lowest effective dose employed). Products include:

- Advil Allergy Sinus Caplets 737
- Advil 737
- Children's Advil Suspension 742
- Children's Advil Chewable Tablets 741
- Advil Cold & Sinus 739
- Advil Flu & Body Ache Caplets 739
- Children's Advil Cold Suspension 741
- Infants' Advil Concentrated Drops 743
- Junior Strength Advil Swallow Tablets 740
- Advil Migraine Liquigels 740
- Advil Multi-Symptom Cold Caplets 738
- Combunox Tablets 1183
- Children's Motrin Oral Suspension and Chewable Tablets 1837
- Children's Motrin Cold Non-Staining Dye-Free Oral Suspension 1838
- Children's Motrin Cold Oral Suspension 1838
- Children's Motrin Non-Staining Dye-Free Oral Suspension 1837
- Motrin Cold & Sinus Caplets 1836
- Motrin IB Tablets and Caplets 1836
- Infants' Motrin Concentrated Drops 1837
- Infants' Motrin Non-Staining Dye-Free Drops 1837
- Junior Strength Motrin Caplets and Chewable Tablets 1837
- Vicoprofen Tablets 533

Idarubicin Hydrochloride (The benefits and risks of using fenofibrate tablets with immunosuppressants and other potentially nephrotoxic agents should be carefully considered and the lowest effective dose employed). Products include:

- Idamycin PFS Injection 2645

Ifosfamide (The benefits and risks of using fenofibrate tablets with immunosuppressants and other potentially nephrotoxic agents should be carefully considered and the lowest effective dose employed).
No products indexed under this heading.

Imipenem (The benefits and risks of using fenofibrate tablets with immunosuppressants and other potentially nephrotoxic agents should be carefully considered and the lowest effective dose employed). Products include:

- Primaxin I.M. 2022
- Primaxin I.V. 2024

Immune Globulin Intravenous (Human) (The benefits and risks of using fenofibrate tablets with immunosuppressants and other potentially nephrotoxic agents should be carefully considered and the lowest effective dose employed). Products include:

- Carimune NF 3501
- Gammagard Liquid 751
- Gammagard S/D 754
- Gamunex Immune Globulin I.V., 10% 3232
- Iveegam EN 759

Indinavir Sulfate (The benefits and risks of using fenofibrate tablets with immunosuppressants and other potentially nephrotoxic agents should be carefully considered and the lowest effective dose employed). Products include:

- Crixivan Capsules 1918

Indomethacin (The benefits and risks of using fenofibrate tablets with immunosuppressants and other potentially nephrotoxic agents should be carefully considered and the lowest effective dose employed). Products include:

- Indocin 1968

Indomethacin Sodium Trihydrate (The benefits and risks of using fenofibrate tablets with immunosuppressants and other potentially nephrotoxic agents should be carefully considered and the lowest effective dose employed). Products include:

- Indocin I.V. 1973

Interferon Beta-1b (The benefits and risks of using fenofibrate tablets with immunosuppressants and other potentially nephrotoxic agents should be carefully considered and the lowest effective dose employed). Products include:

- Betaseron for SC Injection 791

Interleuken-2 (The benefits and risks of using fenofibrate tablets with immunosuppressants and other potentially nephrotoxic agents should be carefully considered and the lowest effective dose employed).
No products indexed under this heading.

Iodamide Meglumine (The benefits and risks of using fenofibrate tablets with immunosuppressants and other potentially nephrotoxic agents should be carefully considered and the lowest effective dose employed).
No products indexed under this heading.

Iohexol (The benefits and risks of using fenofibrate tablets with immunosuppressants and other potentially nephrotoxic agents should be carefully considered and the lowest effective dose employed).
No products indexed under this heading.

Iopamidol (The benefits and risks of using fenofibrate tablets with immunosuppressants and other potentially nephrotoxic agents should be carefully considered and the lowest effective dose employed).
No products indexed under this heading.

Iopanoic Acid (The benefits and risks of using fenofibrate tablets with immunosuppressants and other potentially nephrotoxic agents should be carefully considered and the lowest effective dose employed).
No products indexed under this heading.

Iothalamate Meglumine (The benefits and risks of using fenofibrate tablets with immunosuppressants and other potentially nephrotoxic agents should be carefully considered and the lowest effective dose employed).
No products indexed under this heading.

Ioxaglate Meglumine (The benefits and risks of using fenofibrate tablets with immunosuppressants and other potentially nephrotoxic agents should be carefully considered and the lowest effective dose employed).
No products indexed under this heading.

Ioxaglate Sodium (The benefits and risks of using fenofibrate tablets with immunosuppressants and other potentially nephrotoxic agents should be carefully considered and the lowest effective dose employed).
No products indexed under this heading.

Kanamycin Sulfate (The benefits and risks of using fenofibrate tablets with immunosuppressants and other potentially nephrotoxic agents should be carefully considered and the lowest effective dose employed).
No products indexed under this heading.

Ketoprofen (The benefits and risks of using fenofibrate tablets with immunosuppressants and other potentially nephrotoxic agents should be carefully considered and the lowest effective dose employed).
No products indexed under this heading.

Ketorolac Tromethamine (The benefits and risks of using fenofibrate tablets with immunosuppressants and other potentially nephrotoxic agents should be carefully considered and the lowest effective dose employed). Products include:

- Acular Ophthalmic Solution 561
- Acular LS Ophthalmic Solution 562

Lamium album (The benefits and risks of using fenofibrate tablets with immunosuppressants and other potentially nephrotoxic agents should be carefully considered and the lowest effective dose employed).
No products indexed under this heading.

Lisinopril (The benefits and risks of using fenofibrate tablets with immunosuppressants and other potentially nephrotoxic agents should be care-

fully considered and the lowest effective dose employed). Products include:

- Prinivil Tablets 2029
- Prinzide Tablets 2033
- Zestoretic Tablets 701
- Zestril Tablets 704

Lithium (The benefits and risks of using fenofibrate tablets with immunosuppressants and other potentially nephrotoxic agents should be carefully considered and the lowest effective dose employed).

No products indexed under this heading.

Lithium Carbonate (The benefits and risks of using fenofibrate tablets with immunosuppressants and other potentially nephrotoxic agents should be carefully considered and the lowest effective dose employed). Products include:

- Eskalith 1406
- Lithobid Tablets 1670

Lithium Citrate (The benefits and risks of using fenofibrate tablets with immunosuppressants and other potentially nephrotoxic agents should be carefully considered and the lowest effective dose employed).

No products indexed under this heading.

Lopinavir (The benefits and risks of using fenofibrate tablets with immunosuppressants and other potentially nephrotoxic agents should be carefully considered and the lowest effective dose employed). Products include:

- Kaletra 474

Loracarbef (The benefits and risks of using fenofibrate tablets with immunosuppressants and other potentially nephrotoxic agents should be carefully considered and the lowest effective dose employed).

No products indexed under this heading.

Lovastatin (Co-administration of fibric acid derivatives and HMG-CoA reductase inhibitors has been associated with rhabdomyolysis, markedly elevated creatine kinase levels and myoglobulinuria, leading in a high proportion of cases to acute renal failure; the combined use should be avoided unless the benefit of further alterations in lipid levels is likely to outweigh the increased risk of this combination). Products include:

- Advicor Tablets 1694
- Altoprev Extended-Release Tablets 1151
- Mevacor Tablets 1996

Meclofenamate Sodium (The benefits and risks of using fenofibrate tablets with immunosuppressants and other potentially nephrotoxic agents should be carefully considered and the lowest effective dose employed).

No products indexed under this heading.

Mefenamic Acid (The benefits and risks of using fenofibrate tablets with immunosuppressants and other potentially nephrotoxic agents should be carefully considered and the lowest effective dose employed).

No products indexed under this heading.

Meloxicam (The benefits and risks of using fenofibrate tablets with immunosuppressants and other potentially nephrotoxic agents should be carefully considered and the lowest effective dose employed). Products include:

- Mobic Oral Suspension 893
- Mobic Tablets 893

Melphalan Hydrochloride (The benefits and risks of using fenofibrate tablets with immunosuppressants and other potentially nephrotoxic agents should be carefully considered and the lowest effective dose employed). Products include:

- Alkeran for Injection 976

Mesalamine (The benefits and risks of using fenofibrate tablets with immunosuppressants and other potentially nephrotoxic agents should be carefully considered and the lowest effective dose employed). Products include:

- Asacol Delayed-Release Tablets 2688
- Canasa Rectal Suppositories 726
- Pentasa Capsules 3182

Methimazole (The benefits and risks of using fenofibrate tablets with immunosuppressants and other potentially nephrotoxic agents should be carefully considered and the lowest effective dose employed).

No products indexed under this heading.

Methotrexate (The benefits and risks of using fenofibrate tablets with immunosuppressants and other potentially nephrotoxic agents should be carefully considered and the lowest effective dose employed).

No products indexed under this heading.

Methotrexate Sodium (The benefits and risks of using fenofibrate tablets with immunosuppressants and other potentially nephrotoxic agents should be carefully considered and the lowest effective dose employed).

No products indexed under this heading.

Methyclothiazide (The benefits and risks of using fenofibrate tablets with immunosuppressants and other potentially nephrotoxic agents should be carefully considered and the lowest effective dose employed).

No products indexed under this heading.

Mezlocillin Sodium (The benefits and risks of using fenofibrate tablets with immunosuppressants and other potentially nephrotoxic agents should be carefully considered and the lowest effective dose employed).

No products indexed under this heading.

Minocycline Hydrochloride (The benefits and risks of using fenofibrate tablets with immunosuppressants and other potentially nephrotoxic agents should be carefully considered and the lowest effective dose employed). Products include:

- Dynacin Tablets 1859

Mitomycin (Mitomycin-C) (The benefits and risks of using fenofibrate tablets with immunosuppressants and other potentially nephrotoxic agents should be carefully considered and the lowest effective dose employed).

No products indexed under this heading.

Moexipril Hydrochloride (The benefits and risks of using fenofibrate tablets with immunosuppressants and other potentially nephrotoxic agents should be carefully considered and the lowest effective dose employed). Products include:

- Uniretic Tablets 3114
- Univasc Tablets 3118

Muromonab-CD3 (The benefits and risks of using fenofibrate tablets with immunosuppressants and other potentially nephrotoxic agents should be carefully considered and the lowest effective dose employed). Products include:

- Orthoclone OKT3 Sterile Solution 2370

Mycophenolate Mofetil (The benefits and risks of using fenofibrate tablets with immunosuppressants and other potentially nephrotoxic agents should be carefully considered and the lowest effective dose employed). Products include:

- CellCept Capsules 2751
- CellCept Oral Suspension 2751
- CellCept Tablets 2751

Nabumetone (The benefits and risks of using fenofibrate tablets with immunosuppressants and other potentially nephrotoxic agents should be carefully considered and the lowest effective dose employed). Products include:

- Relafen Tablets 1523

Nafcillin Sodium (The benefits and risks of using fenofibrate tablets with immunosuppressants and other potentially nephrotoxic agents should be carefully considered and the lowest effective dose employed).

No products indexed under this heading.

Naproxen (The benefits and risks of using fenofibrate tablets with immunosuppressants and other potentially nephrotoxic agents should be carefully considered and the lowest effective dose employed). Products include:

- EC-Naprosyn Delayed-Release Tablets 2769
- Naprosyn Suspension 2769
- Naprosyn Tablets 2769
- Prevacid NapraPAC 3277

Naproxen Sodium (The benefits and risks of using fenofibrate tablets with immunosuppressants and other potentially nephrotoxic agents should be carefully considered and the lowest effective dose employed). Products include:

- Aleve Tablets, Caplets and Gelcaps .... ■ 605
- Anaprox Tablets 2769
- Anaprox DS Tablets 2769

Nelfinavir Mesylate (The benefits and risks of using fenofibrate tablets with immunosuppressants and other potentially nephrotoxic agents should be carefully considered and the lowest effective dose employed). Products include:

- Viracept 2556

Neomycin (The benefits and risks of using fenofibrate tablets with immunosuppressants and other potentially nephrotoxic agents should be carefully considered and the lowest effective dose employed). Products include:

- Neosporin Ointment .... ■ 702
- Neosporin + Pain Relief Maximum Strength Cream .... ■ 703
- Neosporin + Pain Relief Maximum Strength Ointment .... ■ 703

Neomycin, oral (The benefits and risks of using fenofibrate tablets with immunosuppressants and other potentially nephrotoxic agents should be carefully considered and the lowest effective dose employed).

No products indexed under this heading.

Neomycin Sulfate (The benefits and risks of using fenofibrate tablets with immunosuppressants and other potentially nephrotoxic agents should be carefully considered and the lowest effective dose employed). Products include:

- Poly-Pred Liquifilm Ophthalmic Suspension .... ⊙ 231

Nevirapine (The benefits and risks of using fenofibrate tablets with immunosuppressants and other potentially nephrotoxic agents should be carefully considered and the lowest effective dose employed). Products include:

- Viramune Oral Suspension 903
- Viramune Tablets 903

Norfloxacin (The benefits and risks of using fenofibrate tablets with immunosuppressants and other potentially nephrotoxic agents should be carefully considered and the lowest effective dose employed). Products include:

- Noroxin Tablets 2009

Olsalazine Sodium (The benefits and risks of using fenofibrate tablets with immunosuppressants and other potentially nephrotoxic agents should be carefully considered and the lowest effective dose employed).

No products indexed under this heading.

Omeprazole (The benefits and risks of using fenofibrate tablets with immunosuppressants and other potentially nephrotoxic agents should be carefully considered and the lowest effective dose employed). Products include:

- Zegerid Powder for Oral Solution 2972

Oxaprozin (The benefits and risks of using fenofibrate tablets with immunosuppressants and other potentially nephrotoxic agents should be carefully considered and the lowest effective dose employed).

No products indexed under this heading.

Pamidronate Disodium (The benefits and risks of using fenofibrate tablets with immunosuppressants and other potentially nephrotoxic agents should be carefully considered and the lowest effective dose employed). Products include:

- Aredia for Injection 2168

Paroxetine Hydrochloride (The benefits and risks of using fenofibrate tablets with immunosuppressants and other potentially nephrotoxic agents should be carefully considered and the lowest effective dose employed). Products include:

- Paxil CR Controlled-Release Tablets 1509
- Paxil 1501

Penicillamine (The benefits and risks of using fenofibrate tablets with immunosuppressants and other potentially nephrotoxic agents should be carefully considered and the lowest effective dose employed). Products include:

- Cuprimine Capsules 1925

Penicillin G Benzathine (The benefits and risks of using fenofibrate tablets with immunosuppressants and other potentially nephrotoxic agents should be carefully considered and the lowest effective dose employed).

No products indexed under this heading.

Penicillin G Potassium (The benefits and risks of using fenofibrate tablets with immunosuppressants and other potentially nephrotoxic agents should be carefully considered and the lowest effective dose employed).
No products indexed under this heading.

Penicillin G Procaine (The benefits and risks of using fenofibrate tablets with immunosuppressants and other potentially nephrotoxic agents should be carefully considered and the lowest effective dose employed).
No products indexed under this heading.

Penicillin G Sodium (The benefits and risks of using fenofibrate tablets with immunosuppressants and other potentially nephrotoxic agents should be carefully considered and the lowest effective dose employed).
No products indexed under this heading.

Penicillin V Potassium (The benefits and risks of using fenofibrate tablets with immunosuppressants and other potentially nephrotoxic agents should be carefully considered and the lowest effective dose employed).
No products indexed under this heading.

Pentamidine Isethionate (The benefits and risks of using fenofibrate tablets with immunosuppressants and other potentially nephrotoxic agents should be carefully considered and the lowest effective dose employed).
No products indexed under this heading.

Perindopril Erbumine (The benefits and risks of using fenofibrate tablets with immunosuppressants and other potentially nephrotoxic agents should be carefully considered and the lowest effective dose employed). Products include:
Aceon Tablets (2 mg, 4 mg, 8 mg) 3191

Phenylbutazone (The benefits and risks of using fenofibrate tablets with immunosuppressants and other potentially nephrotoxic agents should be carefully considered and the lowest effective dose employed).
No products indexed under this heading.

Piroxicam (The benefits and risks of using fenofibrate tablets with immunosuppressants and other potentially nephrotoxic agents should be carefully considered and the lowest effective dose employed).
No products indexed under this heading.

Plicamycin (The benefits and risks of using fenofibrate tablets with immunosuppressants and other potentially nephrotoxic agents should be carefully considered and the lowest effective dose employed).
No products indexed under this heading.

Polymyxin (The benefits and risks of using fenofibrate tablets with immunosuppressants and other potentially nephrotoxic agents should be carefully considered and the lowest effective dose employed).
No products indexed under this heading.

Polymyxin B Sulfate (The benefits and risks of using fenofibrate tablets with immunosuppressants and other potentially nephrotoxic agents should be carefully considered and the lowest effective dose employed). Products include:
Neosporin Ointment 702
Neosporin + Pain Relief Maximum Strength Cream 703
Neosporin + Pain Relief Maximum Strength Ointment 703
Poly-Pred Liquifilm Ophthalmic Suspension .... ⊙ 231
Polysporin Ointment 706
Polytrim Ophthalmic Solution 570

Polythiazide (The benefits and risks of using fenofibrate tablets with immunosuppressants and other potentially nephrotoxic agents should be carefully considered and the lowest effective dose employed).
No products indexed under this heading.

Pravastatin Sodium (Co-administration of fibric acid derivatives and HMG-CoA reductase inhibitors has been associated with rhabdomyolysis, markedly elevated creatine kinase levels and myoglobulinuria, leading in a high proportion of cases to acute renal failure; the combined use should be avoided unless the benefit of further alterations in lipid levels is likely to outweigh the increased risk of this combination). Products include:
Pravachol Tablets 943

Probenecid (The benefits and risks of using fenofibrate tablets with immunosuppressants and other potentially nephrotoxic agents should be carefully considered and the lowest effective dose employed).
No products indexed under this heading.

Quinapril Hydrochloride (The benefits and risks of using fenofibrate tablets with immunosuppressants and other potentially nephrotoxic agents should be carefully considered and the lowest effective dose employed).
No products indexed under this heading.

Rabeprazole Sodium (The benefits and risks of using fenofibrate tablets with immunosuppressants and other potentially nephrotoxic agents should be carefully considered and the lowest effective dose employed). Products include:
Aciphex Tablets 1081

Ramipril (The benefits and risks of using fenofibrate tablets with immunosuppressants and other potentially nephrotoxic agents should be carefully considered and the lowest effective dose employed). Products include:
Altace Capsules 1673

Rifampin (The benefits and risks of using fenofibrate tablets with immunosuppressants and other potentially nephrotoxic agents should be carefully considered and the lowest effective dose employed).
No products indexed under this heading.

Riluzole (The benefits and risks of using fenofibrate tablets with immunosuppressants and other potentially nephrotoxic agents should be carefully considered and the lowest effective dose employed). Products include:
Rilutek Tablets 2945

Ritonavir (The benefits and risks of using fenofibrate tablets with immunosuppressants and other potentially nephrotoxic agents should be carefully considered and the lowest effective dose employed). Products include:
Kaletra 474
Norvir 499

Rofecoxib (The benefits and risks of using fenofibrate tablets with immunosuppressants and other potentially nephrotoxic agents should be carefully considered and the lowest effective dose employed).
No products indexed under this heading.

Saquinavir (The benefits and risks of using fenofibrate tablets with immunosuppressants and other potentially nephrotoxic agents should be carefully considered and the lowest effective dose employed).
No products indexed under this heading.

Sibutramine Hydrochloride Monohydrate (The benefits and risks of using fenofibrate tablets with immunosuppressants and other potentially nephrotoxic agents should be carefully considered and the lowest effective dose employed). Products include:
Meridia Capsules 485

Simvastatin (Co-administration of fibric acid derivatives and HMG-CoA reductase inhibitors has been associated with rhabdomyolysis, markedly elevated creatine kinase levels and myoglobulinuria, leading in a high proportion of cases to acute renal failure; the combined use should be avoided unless the benefit of further alterations in lipid levels is likely to outweigh the increased risk of this combination). Products include:
Vytorin 10/10 Tablets 2084
Vytorin 10/10 Tablets 3092
Vytorin 10/20 Tablets 2084
Vytorin 10/20 Tablets 3092
Vytorin 10/40 Tablets 3092
Vytorin 10/40 Tablets 2084
Vytorin 10/80 Tablets 2084
Vytorin 10/80 Tablets 3092
Zocor Tablets 2078

Sirolimus (The benefits and risks of using fenofibrate tablets with immunosuppressants and other potentially nephrotoxic agents should be carefully considered and the lowest effective dose employed). Products include:
Rapamune Oral Solution and Tablets 3472

Spirapril Hydrochloride (The benefits and risks of using fenofibrate tablets with immunosuppressants and other potentially nephrotoxic agents should be carefully considered and the lowest effective dose employed).
No products indexed under this heading.

Stavudine (The benefits and risks of using fenofibrate tablets with immunosuppressants and other potentially nephrotoxic agents should be carefully considered and the lowest effective dose employed). Products include:
Zerit 971

Streptomycin Sulfate (The benefits and risks of using fenofibrate tablets with immunosuppressants and other potentially nephrotoxic agents should be carefully considered and the lowest effective dose employed).
No products indexed under this heading.

Streptozocin (The benefits and risks of using fenofibrate tablets with immunosuppressants and other potentially nephrotoxic agents should be carefully considered and the lowest effective dose employed).
No products indexed under this heading.

Sulfacytine (The benefits and risks of using fenofibrate tablets with immunosuppressants and other potentially nephrotoxic agents should be carefully considered and the lowest effective dose employed).
No products indexed under this heading.

Sulfamethizole (The benefits and risks of using fenofibrate tablets with immunosuppressants and other potentially nephrotoxic agents should be carefully considered and the lowest effective dose employed).
No products indexed under this heading.

Sulfamethoxazole (The benefits and risks of using fenofibrate tablets with immunosuppressants and other potentially nephrotoxic agents should be carefully considered and the lowest effective dose employed).
No products indexed under this heading.

Sulfasalazine (The benefits and risks of using fenofibrate tablets with immunosuppressants and other potentially nephrotoxic agents should be carefully considered and the lowest effective dose employed).
No products indexed under this heading.

Sulfinpyrazone (The benefits and risks of using fenofibrate tablets with immunosuppressants and other potentially nephrotoxic agents should be carefully considered and the lowest effective dose employed).
No products indexed under this heading.

Sulfisoxazole (The benefits and risks of using fenofibrate tablets with immunosuppressants and other potentially nephrotoxic agents should be carefully considered and the lowest effective dose employed).
No products indexed under this heading.

Sulfisoxazole Acetyl (The benefits and risks of using fenofibrate tablets with immunosuppressants and other potentially nephrotoxic agents should be carefully considered and the lowest effective dose employed).
No products indexed under this heading.

Sulfisoxazole Diolamine (The benefits and risks of using fenofibrate tablets with immunosuppressants and other potentially nephrotoxic agents should be carefully considered and the lowest effective dose employed).
No products indexed under this heading.

Sulindac (The benefits and risks of using fenofibrate tablets with immunosuppressants and other potentially nephrotoxic agents should be carefully considered and the lowest effective dose employed). Products include:
Clinoril Tablets 1899

Tacrolimus (The benefits and risks of using fenofibrate tablets with immunosuppressants and other potentially nephrotoxic agents

should be carefully considered and the lowest effective dose employed). Products include:

Prograf Capsules and Injection 624
Protopic Ointment 629

Tenofovir Disoproxil Fumarate (The benefits and risks of using fenofibrate tablets with immunosuppressants and other potentially nephrotoxic agents should be carefully considered and the lowest effective dose employed). Products include:

Truvada Tablets 1279
Viread Tablets 1284

Thioguanine (The benefits and risks of using fenofibrate tablets with immunosuppressants and other potentially nephrotoxic agents should be carefully considered and the lowest effective dose employed). Products include:

Tabloid Tablets 1545

Ticarcillin Disodium (The benefits and risks of using fenofibrate tablets with immunosuppressants and other potentially nephrotoxic agents should be carefully considered and the lowest effective dose employed). Products include:

Timentin ADD-Vantage 1556
Timentin Injection Galaxy Container 1559
Timentin IV Infusion 1553
Timentin Pharmacy Bulk Package 1562

Tobramycin (The benefits and risks of using fenofibrate tablets with immunosuppressants and other potentially nephrotoxic agents should be carefully considered and the lowest effective dose employed). Products include:

TOBI Solution for Inhalation 1015
TobraDex Ophthalmic Ointment 558
TobraDex Ophthalmic Suspension ... 558
Zylet Ophthalmic Suspension 3508

Tobramycin Sulfate (The benefits and risks of using fenofibrate tablets with immunosuppressants and other potentially nephrotoxic agents should be carefully considered and the lowest effective dose employed).

No products indexed under this heading.

Tolazamide (The benefits and risks of using fenofibrate tablets with immunosuppressants and other potentially nephrotoxic agents should be carefully considered and the lowest effective dose employed).

No products indexed under this heading.

Tolbutamide (The benefits and risks of using fenofibrate tablets with immunosuppressants and other potentially nephrotoxic agents should be carefully considered and the lowest effective dose employed).

No products indexed under this heading.

Tolmetin Sodium (The benefits and risks of using fenofibrate tablets with immunosuppressants and other potentially nephrotoxic agents should be carefully considered and the lowest effective dose employed).

No products indexed under this heading.

Trandolapril (The benefits and risks of using fenofibrate tablets with immunosuppressants and other potentially nephrotoxic agents should be carefully considered and the lowest effective dose employed). Products include:

Mavik Tablets 482
Tarka Tablets 519

Triamterene (The benefits and risks of using fenofibrate tablets with immunosuppressants and other potentially nephrotoxic agents should be carefully considered and the lowest effective dose employed). Products include:

Dyazide Capsules 1389
Dyrenium Capsules 3390
Maxzide 2150

Trimethadione (The benefits and risks of using fenofibrate tablets with immunosuppressants and other potentially nephrotoxic agents should be carefully considered and the lowest effective dose employed).

No products indexed under this heading.

Trovafloxacin Mesylate (The benefits and risks of using fenofibrate tablets with immunosuppressants and other potentially nephrotoxic agents should be carefully considered and the lowest effective dose employed).

No products indexed under this heading.

Tyropanoate Sodium (The benefits and risks of using fenofibrate tablets with immunosuppressants and other potentially nephrotoxic agents should be carefully considered and the lowest effective dose employed).

No products indexed under this heading.

Valacyclovir Hydrochloride (The benefits and risks of using fenofibrate tablets with immunosuppressants and other potentially nephrotoxic agents should be carefully considered and the lowest effective dose employed). Products include:

Valtrex Caplets 1573

Valdecoxib (The benefits and risks of using fenofibrate tablets with immunosuppressants and other potentially nephrotoxic agents should be carefully considered and the lowest effective dose employed).

No products indexed under this heading.

Vancomycin Hydrochloride (The benefits and risks of using fenofibrate tablets with immunosuppressants and other potentially nephrotoxic agents should be carefully considered and the lowest effective dose employed). Products include:

Vancocin HCl Capsules, USP 3370

Voriconazole (The benefits and risks of using fenofibrate tablets with immunosuppressants and other potentially nephrotoxic agents should be carefully considered and the lowest effective dose employed). Products include:

VFEND I.V. 2543
VFEND Oral Suspension 2543
VFEND Tablets 2543

Warfarin Sodium (Caution should be exercised when anticoagulants are given in conjunction with fenofibrate because of the potentiation of coumarin-type anticoagulants in prolonging the PT/INR. The dosage of the anticoagulant should be reduced to maintain the PT/INR at the desired level to prevent bleeding complications. Frequent PT/INR determinations are advisable until it has been definitely determined that the PT/INR has stabilized). Products include:

Coumadin for Injection 932
Coumadin Tablets 932

Zalcitabine (The benefits and risks of using fenofibrate tablets with immunosuppressants and other potentially nephrotoxic agents should be carefully considered and the lowest effective dose employed).

No products indexed under this heading.

Zidovudine (The benefits and risks of using fenofibrate tablets with immunosuppressants and other potentially nephrotoxic agents should be carefully considered and the lowest effective dose employed). Products include:

Combivir Tablets 1373
Retrovir 1533
Retrovir IV Infusion 1537
Trizivir Tablets 1565

Zoledronic acid (The benefits and risks of using fenofibrate tablets with immunosuppressants and other potentially nephrotoxic agents should be carefully considered and the lowest effective dose employed). Products include:

Zometa for Intravenous Infusion 2306

Food Interactions

Food, unspecified (The absorption of fenofibrate is increased when administered with food; Tricor should be given with meals).

TRIDENT WHITE SUGARLESS GUM

(Mannitol, Sorbitol) .... ▣611
None cited in PDR database.

TRIGLIDE TABLETS

(Fenofibrate) 1165

May interact with bile acid sequestering agents, oral anticoagulants, cytochrome p450 2c19 substrates (selected), cytochrome p450 2c9 substrates (selected), HMG-CoA reductase inhibitors, immunosuppressive agents, nephrotoxic agents, and certain other agents. Compounds in these categories include:

Abacavir Sulfate (The benefits and risks of using fenofibrate with immunosuppressants and other potentially nephrotoxic agents should be carefully considered, and the lowest effective dose employed). Products include:

Epzicom Tablets 1402
Trizivir Tablets 1565
Ziagen 1600

Acarbose (Fenofibrates are mild-moderate inhibitors of CYP2C9 at therapeutic concentrations). Products include:

Precose Tablets 776

Acyclovir (The benefits and risks of using fenofibrate with immunosuppressants and other potentially nephrotoxic agents should be carefully considered, and the lowest effective dose employed). Products include:

Zovirax 1616
Zovirax Cream 853
Zovirax Ointment 854

Acyclovir Sodium (The benefits and risks of using fenofibrate with immunosuppressants and other potentially nephrotoxic agents should be carefully considered, and the lowest effective dose employed). Products include:

Zovirax for Injection 1618

Alatrofloxacin Mesylate (The benefits and risks of using fenofibrate with immunosuppressants and other potentially nephrotoxic agents should be carefully considered, and the lowest effective dose employed).

No products indexed under this heading.

Aldesleukin (The benefits and risks of using fenofibrate with immunosuppressants and other potentially nephrotoxic agents should be carefully considered, and the lowest effective dose employed). Products include:

Proleukin for Injection 1007

Amikacin Sulfate (The benefits and risks of using fenofibrate with immunosuppressants and other potentially nephrotoxic agents should be carefully considered, and the lowest effective dose employed).

No products indexed under this heading.

Amitriptyline Hydrochloride (Fenofibrates are mild-moderate inhibitors of CYP2C9 at therapeutic concentrations).

No products indexed under this heading.

Amoxapine (Fenofibrates are weak inhibitors of CYP2C19 at therapeutic concentrations).

No products indexed under this heading.

Amoxicillin (The benefits and risks of using fenofibrate with immunosuppressants and other potentially nephrotoxic agents should be carefully considered, and the lowest effective dose employed). Products include:

Amoxil Capsules 1315
Amoxil Chewable Tablets 1315
Amoxil Pediatric Drops for Oral Suspension 1315
Amoxil Powder for Oral Suspension 1315
Amoxil Tablets 1315
Augmentin 1331
Augmentin Tablets 1334
Augmentin XR Extended-Release Tablets 1340
Augmentin ES-600 Powder for Oral Suspension 1337
PREVPAC 3281

Amoxicillin Trihydrate (The benefits and risks of using fenofibrate with immunosuppressants and other potentially nephrotoxic agents should be carefully considered, and the lowest effective dose employed).

No products indexed under this heading.

Amphotericin B (The benefits and risks of using fenofibrate with immunosuppressants and other potentially nephrotoxic agents should be carefully considered, and the lowest effective dose employed).

No products indexed under this heading.

Amphotericin B, liposomal (The benefits and risks of using fenofibrate with immunosuppressants and other potentially nephrotoxic agents should be carefully considered, and the lowest effective dose employed). Products include:

AmBisome for Injection 615

Amphotericin B Cholesteryl Sulfate (The benefits and risks of using fenofibrate with immunosuppressants and other potentially nephrotoxic agents should be carefully considered, and the lowest effective dose employed).

No products indexed under this heading.

Amphotericin B Lipid Complex (The benefits and risks of using fenofibrate with immunosuppressants and other potentially nephrotoxic agents should be carefully considered, and the lowest effective dose employed). Products include:
Abelcet Injection 1119

Ampicillin (The benefits and risks of using fenofibrate with immunosuppressants and other potentially nephrotoxic agents should be carefully considered, and the lowest effective dose employed).
No products indexed under this heading.

Ampicillin Sodium (The benefits and risks of using fenofibrate with immunosuppressants and other potentially nephrotoxic agents should be carefully considered, and the lowest effective dose employed).
No products indexed under this heading.

Ampicillin Trihydrate (The benefits and risks of using fenofibrate with immunosuppressants and other potentially nephrotoxic agents should be carefully considered, and the lowest effective dose employed).
No products indexed under this heading.

Amprenavir (The benefits and risks of using fenofibrate with immunosuppressants and other potentially nephrotoxic agents should be carefully considered, and the lowest effective dose employed). Products include:
Agenerase Capsules 1299
Agenerase Oral Solution 1304

Anisindione (Caution should be exercised when anticoagulants are given in conjunction with fenofibrate because of the potentiation of coumarin-type anticoagulants in prolonging the prothrombin time/INR. The dosage of the anticoagulant should be reduced to maintain the prothrombin time/INR at the desired level to prevent bleeding complications. Frequent prothrombin time/INR determinations are advisably until it has been definitely determined that the prothrombin time/INR has stabilized). Products include:
Miradon Tablets 3056

Aspirin (The benefits and risks of using fenofibrate with immunosuppressants and other potentially nephrotoxic agents should be carefully considered, and the lowest effective dose employed). Products include:
Aggrenox Capsules 855
Bayer, Aspirin Regimen 606
Bayer Aspirin Tablets 3515
BC Powder 612
BC Allergy Sinus Cold Powder 612
Arthritis Strength BC Powder 612
BC Sinus Cold Powder 612
Ecotrin Enteric Coated Aspirin Low, Regular and Maximum Strength Tablets 1627
Goody's Body Pain Formula Powder 621
Goody's Extra Strength Headache Powder 621
Goody's Extra Strength Pain Relief Tablets 621
Percodan Tablets 1115
St. Joseph 81 mg Aspirin Chewable and Enteric Coated Tablets 1841

Atazanavir (The benefits and risks of using fenofibrate with immunosuppressants and other potentially nephrotoxic agents should be carefully considered, and the lowest effective dose employed).
No products indexed under this heading.

Atorvastatin Calcium (The combined use of fenofibrates and HMG-CoA reductase inhibitors should be avoided unless the benefit of further alterations in lipid levels is likely to outweigh the increased risk of this drug combination. The combined use of fibric acid derivatives and HMG-CoA reductase inhibitors has been associated, in the absence of a marked pharmacokinetic interaction, in numerous case reports, with rhabdomyolysis, markedly elevated creatine kinase (CK) levels and myoglobinuria, leading in a high proportion of cases to acute renal failure). Products include:
Caduet Tablets 2507
Lipitor Tablets 2495

Azathioprine (The benefits and risks of using fenofibrate with immunosuppressants and other potentially nephrotoxic agents should be carefully considered, and the lowest effective dose employed). Products include:
Azasan Tablets 2844

Azithromycin Dihydrate (The benefits and risks of using fenofibrate with immunosuppressants and other potentially nephrotoxic agents should be carefully considered, and the lowest effective dose employed). Products include:
Zithromax 2568
Zithromax for IV Infusion 2573
Zithromax for Oral Suspension, 300 mg, 600 mg, 900 mg, 1200 mg.................................... 2561
Zithromax Tablets, 250 mg, 500 mg... 2561
Zithromax Tri-Pak 2561
Zithromax Z-Pak 2568

Azlocillin Sodium (The benefits and risks of using fenofibrate with immunosuppressants and other potentially nephrotoxic agents should be carefully considered, and the lowest effective dose employed).
No products indexed under this heading.

Aztreonam (The benefits and risks of using fenofibrate with immunosuppressants and other potentially nephrotoxic agents should be carefully considered, and the lowest effective dose employed).
No products indexed under this heading.

Bacampicillin Hydrochloride (The benefits and risks of using fenofibrate with immunosuppressants and other potentially nephrotoxic agents should be carefully considered, and the lowest effective dose employed).
No products indexed under this heading.

Balsalazide Disodium (The benefits and risks of using fenofibrate with immunosuppressants and other potentially nephrotoxic agents should be carefully considered, and the lowest effective dose employed). Products include:
Colazal Capsules 2845

Basiliximab (The benefits and risks of using fenofibrate with immunosuppressants and other potentially nephrotoxic agents should be carefully considered, and the lowest effective dose employed). Products include:
Simulect for Injection 2268

Benazepril Hydrochloride (The benefits and risks of using fenofibrate with immunosuppressants and other potentially nephrotoxic agents should be carefully considered, and the lowest effective dose employed). Products include:
Lotensin Tablets 2232
Lotensin HCT Tablets 2235
Lotrel Capsules 2238

Bendroflumethiazide (The benefits and risks of using fenofibrate with immunosuppressants and other potentially nephrotoxic agents should be carefully considered, and the lowest effective dose employed).
No products indexed under this heading.

Caffeine (The benefits and risks of using fenofibrate with immunosuppressants and other potentially nephrotoxic agents should be carefully considered, and the lowest effective dose employed). Products include:
Athena Hair System Shampoo 767
BC Powder 612
Arthritis Strength BC Powder 612
Goody's Extra Strength Headache Powder...................... 621
Goody's Extra Strength Pain Relief Tablets 621
Hycomine Compound Tablets 1105
Spartan Hair System Shampoo 767
Vivarin 639

Candesartan Cilexetil (Fenofibrates are mild-moderate inhibitors of CYP2C9 at therapeutic concentrations). Products include:
Atacand Tablets 634
Atacand HCT 637

Captopril (The benefits and risks of using fenofibrate with immunosuppressants and other potentially nephrotoxic agents should be carefully considered, and the lowest effective dose employed). Products include:
Captopril Tablets 2114

Carbenicillin Disodium (The benefits and risks of using fenofibrate with immunosuppressants and other potentially nephrotoxic agents should be carefully considered, and the lowest effective dose employed).
No products indexed under this heading.

Carbenicillin Indanyl Sodium (The benefits and risks of using fenofibrate with immunosuppressants and other potentially nephrotoxic agents should be carefully considered, and the lowest effective dose employed).
No products indexed under this heading.

Carboplatin (The benefits and risks of using fenofibrate with immunosuppressants and other potentially nephrotoxic agents should be carefully considered, and the lowest effective dose employed).
No products indexed under this heading.

Carisoprodol (Fenofibrates are weak inhibitors of CYP2C19 at therapeutic concentrations).
No products indexed under this heading.

Carmustine (BCNU) (The benefits and risks of using fenofibrate with immunosuppressants and other potentially nephrotoxic agents should be carefully considered, and the lowest effective dose employed).
No products indexed under this heading.

Carvedilol (Fenofibrates are mild-moderate inhibitors of CYP2C9 at therapeutic concentrations). Products include:
Coreg Tablets 1376

Cefaclor (The benefits and risks of using fenofibrate with immunosuppressants and other potentially nephrotoxic agents should be carefully considered, and the lowest effective dose employed).
No products indexed under this heading.

Cefadroxil (The benefits and risks of using fenofibrate with immunosuppressants and other potentially nephrotoxic agents should be carefully considered, and the lowest effective dose employed).
No products indexed under this heading.

Cefamandole Nafate (The benefits and risks of using fenofibrate with immunosuppressants and other potentially nephrotoxic agents should be carefully considered, and the lowest effective dose employed).
No products indexed under this heading.

Cefazolin Sodium (The benefits and risks of using fenofibrate with immunosuppressants and other potentially nephrotoxic agents should be carefully considered, and the lowest effective dose employed). Products include:
Ancef for Injection 1318

Cefdinir (The benefits and risks of using fenofibrate with immunosuppressants and other potentially nephrotoxic agents should be carefully considered, and the lowest effective dose employed). Products include:
Omnicef Capsules 506
Omnicef for Oral Suspension 506

Cefepime Hydrochloride (The benefits and risks of using fenofibrate with immunosuppressants and other potentially nephrotoxic agents should be carefully considered, and the lowest effective dose employed). Products include:
Maxipime for Injection 1093

Cefixime (The benefits and risks of using fenofibrate with immunosuppressants and other potentially nephrotoxic agents should be carefully considered, and the lowest effective dose employed). Products include:
Suprax 1811

Cefmetazole Sodium (The benefits and risks of using fenofibrate with immunosuppressants and other potentially nephrotoxic agents should be carefully considered, and the lowest effective dose employed).
No products indexed under this heading.

Cefonicid Sodium (The benefits and risks of using fenofibrate with immunosuppressants and other potentially nephrotoxic agents should be carefully considered, and the lowest effective dose employed).
No products indexed under this heading.

IMPORTANT NOTE: Always consult each drug listing in the patient's regimen for possible interactions.

Cefoperazone Sodium (The benefits and risks of using fenofibrate with immunosuppressants and other potentially nephrotoxic agents should be carefully considered, and the lowest effective dose employed).
No products indexed under this heading.

Ceforanide (The benefits and risks of using fenofibrate with immunosuppressants and other potentially nephrotoxic agents should be carefully considered, and the lowest effective dose employed).
No products indexed under this heading.

Cefotaxime Sodium (The benefits and risks of using fenofibrate with immunosuppressants and other potentially nephrotoxic agents should be carefully considered, and the lowest effective dose employed).
No products indexed under this heading.

Cefotetan (The benefits and risks of using fenofibrate with immunosuppressants and other potentially nephrotoxic agents should be carefully considered, and the lowest effective dose employed).
No products indexed under this heading.

Cefoxitin Sodium (The benefits and risks of using fenofibrate with immunosuppressants and other potentially nephrotoxic agents should be carefully considered, and the lowest effective dose employed). Products include:
Mefoxin for Injection 1987
Mefoxin Premixed Intravenous Solution.. 1990

Cefpodoxime Proxetil (The benefits and risks of using fenofibrate with immunosuppressants and other potentially nephrotoxic agents should be carefully considered, and the lowest effective dose employed). Products include:
Vantin Tablets and Oral Suspension 2650

Cefprozil (The benefits and risks of using fenofibrate with immunosuppressants and other potentially nephrotoxic agents should be carefully considered, and the lowest effective dose employed).
No products indexed under this heading.

Ceftazidime (The benefits and risks of using fenofibrate with immunosuppressants and other potentially nephrotoxic agents should be carefully considered, and the lowest effective dose employed). Products include:
Fortaz for Injection 1422

Ceftizoxime Sodium (The benefits and risks of using fenofibrate with immunosuppressants and other potentially nephrotoxic agents should be carefully considered, and the lowest effective dose employed).
No products indexed under this heading.

Ceftriaxone Sodium (The benefits and risks of using fenofibrate with immunosuppressants and other potentially nephrotoxic agents should be carefully considered, and the lowest effective dose employed). Products include:
Rocephin Injectable Vials, ADD-Vantage, Galaxy, Bulk............ 2801

Cefuroxime Axetil (The benefits and risks of using fenofibrate with immunosuppressants and other potentially nephrotoxic agents should be carefully considered, and the lowest effective dose employed). Products include:
Ceftin 1369

Cefuroxime Sodium (The benefits and risks of using fenofibrate with immunosuppressants and other potentially nephrotoxic agents should be carefully considered, and the lowest effective dose employed).
No products indexed under this heading.

Celecoxib (Fenofibrates are mild-moderate inhibitors of CYP2C9 at therapeutic concentrations). Products include:
Celebrex Capsules 3130

Cephalexin (The benefits and risks of using fenofibrate with immunosuppressants and other potentially nephrotoxic agents should be carefully considered, and the lowest effective dose employed).
No products indexed under this heading.

Cephalothin Sodium (The benefits and risks of using fenofibrate with immunosuppressants and other potentially nephrotoxic agents should be carefully considered, and the lowest effective dose employed).
No products indexed under this heading.

Cephapirin Sodium (The benefits and risks of using fenofibrate with immunosuppressants and other potentially nephrotoxic agents should be carefully considered, and the lowest effective dose employed).
No products indexed under this heading.

Cephradine (The benefits and risks of using fenofibrate with immunosuppressants and other potentially nephrotoxic agents should be carefully considered, and the lowest effective dose employed).
No products indexed under this heading.

Cerivastatin Sodium (The combined use of fenofibrates and HMG-CoA reductase inhibitors should be avoided unless the benefit of further alterations in lipid levels is likely to outweigh the increased risk of this drug combination. The combined use of fibric acid derivatives and HMG-CoA reductase inhibitors has been associated, in the absence of a marked pharmacokinetic interaction, in numerous case reports, with rhabdomyolysis, markedly elevated creatine kinase (CK) levels and myoglobinuria, leading in a high proportion of cases to acute renal failure).
No products indexed under this heading.

Chlorothiazide (The benefits and risks of using fenofibrate with immunosuppressants and other potentially nephrotoxic agents should be carefully considered, and the lowest effective dose employed). Products include:
Aldoclor Tablets 1881
Diuril Oral 1936

Chlorothiazide Sodium (The benefits and risks of using fenofibrate with immunosuppressants and other potentially nephrotoxic agents should be carefully considered, and the lowest effective dose employed). Products include:
Diuril Sodium Intravenous 1934

Chlorpropamide (Fenofibrates are mild-moderate inhibitors of CYP2C9 at therapeutic concentrations).
No products indexed under this heading.

Cholestyramine (Bile acid sequestrants have been shown to bind to other drugs given concurrently. Therefore, fenofibrates should be taken at least 1 hour before, or 4-6 hours after a bile acid binding resin to avoid impeding its absorption).
No products indexed under this heading.

Cidofovir (The benefits and risks of using fenofibrate with immunosuppressants and other potentially nephrotoxic agents should be carefully considered, and the lowest effective dose employed).
No products indexed under this heading.

Cilastatin Sodium (The benefits and risks of using fenofibrate with immunosuppressants and other potentially nephrotoxic agents should be carefully considered, and the lowest effective dose employed). Products include:
Primaxin I.M. 2022
Primaxin I.V. 2024

Cilostazol (Fenofibrates are weak inhibitors of CYP2C19 at therapeutic concentrations). Products include:
Pletal Tablets 2478

Cimetidine (The benefits and risks of using fenofibrate with immunosuppressants and other potentially nephrotoxic agents should be carefully considered, and the lowest effective dose employed). Products include:
Tagamet HB 200 Tablets .... ▣637
Tagamet Tablets 1547

Cimetidine Hydrochloride (The benefits and risks of using fenofibrate with immunosuppressants and other potentially nephrotoxic agents should be carefully considered, and the lowest effective dose employed).
No products indexed under this heading.

Cisplatin (The benefits and risks of using fenofibrate with immunosuppressants and other potentially nephrotoxic agents should be carefully considered, and the lowest effective dose employed).
No products indexed under this heading.

Citalopram Hydrobromide (Fenofibrates are weak inhibitors of CYP2C19 at therapeutic concentrations). Products include:
Celexa 1177

Cladribine (The benefits and risks of using fenofibrate with immunosuppressants and other potentially nephrotoxic agents should be carefully considered, and the lowest effective dose employed). Products include:
Leustatin Injection 2368

Clomipramine Hydrochloride (Fenofibrates are mild-moderate inhibitors of CYP2C9 at therapeutic concentrations).
No products indexed under this heading.

Clozapine (The benefits and risks of using fenofibrate with immunosuppressants and other potentially nephrotoxic agents should be carefully considered, and the lowest effective dose employed). Products include:
Clozapine Tablets 2141
Clozaril Tablets 2174
FazaClo Orally Disintegrating Tablets 547

Colesevelam Hydrochloride (Bile acid sequestrants have been shown to bind to other drugs given concurrently. Therefore, fenofibrates should be taken at least 1 hour before, or 4-6 hours after a bile acid binding resin to avoid impeding its absorption). Products include:
WelChol Tablets 2855

Colestipol Hydrochloride (Bile acid sequestrants have been shown to bind to other drugs given concurrently. Therefore, fenofibrates should be taken at least 1 hour before, or 4-6 hours after a bile acid binding resin to avoid impeding its absorption).
No products indexed under this heading.

Colistimethate Sodium (The benefits and risks of using fenofibrate with immunosuppressants and other potentially nephrotoxic agents should be carefully considered, and the lowest effective dose employed).
No products indexed under this heading.

Colistin Sulfate (The benefits and risks of using fenofibrate with immunosuppressants and other potentially nephrotoxic agents should be carefully considered, and the lowest effective dose employed).
No products indexed under this heading.

Cyclophosphamide (Fenofibrates are weak inhibitors of CYP2C19 at therapeutic concentrations).
No products indexed under this heading.

Cyclosporine (Because cyclosporine can produce nephrotoxicity with decreases in creatinine clearance and rises in serum creatinine, and because renal excretion is the primary elimination route of fibrate drugs including fenofibrate, there is a risk that an interactionwill lead to deterioration). Products include:
Gengraf Capsules 458
Neoral Soft Gelatin Capsules 2247
Neoral Oral Solution 2247
Restasis Ophthalmic Emulsion 570
Sandimmune 2259

Cytarabine (The benefits and risks of using fenofibrate with immunosuppressants and other potentially nephrotoxic agents should be carefully considered, and the lowest effective dose employed).
No products indexed under this heading.

Cytarabine Liposome (The benefits and risks of using fenofibrate with immunosuppressants and other potentially nephrotoxic agents should be carefully considered, and the lowest effective dose employed). Products include:
DepoCyt Injection 1121

Delavirdine Mesylate (The benefits and risks of using fenofibrate with immunosuppressants and other potentially nephrotoxic agents should be carefully considered, and the lowest effective dose employed). Products include:
Rescriptor Tablets 2535

Desipramine Hydrochloride (Fenofibrates are weak inhibitors of CYP2C19 at therapeutic concentrations).
No products indexed under this heading.

Desogestrel (Fenofibrates are mild-moderate inhibitors of CYP2C9 at therapeutic concentrations). Products include:

Ortho-Cept Tablets ... 2395

Dextromethorphan (Fenofibrates are mild-moderate inhibitors of CYP2C9 at therapeutic concentrations).

No products indexed under this heading.

Dextromethorphan Hydrobromide (Fenofibrates are weak inhibitors of CYP2C19 at therapeutic concentrations). Products include:

Alacol DM Syrup ... 739
Balamine DM ... 739
Contac Severe Cold and Flu Caplets Maximum Strength ... 615
Contac Severe Cold and Flu Caplets Non-Drowsy ... 615
Children's Dimetapp DM Cold & Cough Elixir ... 745
Children's Dimetapp Long Acting Cough Plus Cold Syrup ... 746
Dimetapp Infant Drops Decongestant Plus Cough ... 746
Mucinex DM Tablets ... 602
PediaCare Decongestant & Cough Infant Drops ... 705
PediaCare Freezer Pops Long-Acting Cough-Glacier Grape and Polar Berry Blue ... 706
PediaCare Long-Acting Cough Infant Drops ... 705
PediaCare Long-Acting Cough Plus Cold Liquid ... 704
PediaCare Multi-Symptom Cold Liquid ... 704
PediaCare NightRest Cough & Cold Liquid ... 704
Robitussin Allergy & Cough Syrup ... 750
Robitussin CF Liquid ... 755
Robitussin Cough & Cold Liquid-filled Capsules ... 750
Robitussin Cough, Cold & Flu Liquid-filled Capsules ... 750
Robitussin Cough & Cold Infant Drops ... 755
Robitussin DM Infant Drops ... 753
Robitussin DM Liquid ... 753
Robitussin Flu Liquid ... 752
Robitussin Maximum Strength Cough Liquid ... 754
Robitussin Maximum Strength Cough & Cold Liquid ... 754
Robitussin Pediatric Cough Liquid ... 754
Robitussin Pediatric Cough & Cold Liquid ... 754
Robitussin PM Cough & Cold Liquid ... 752
Robitussin Sugar Free Cough Liquid ... 753
Simply Cough Liquid ... 1840
Sudafed Severe Cold ... 710
TheraFlu Cold & Cough Hot Liquid ... 680
TheraFlu Flu & Chest Congestion Non-Drowsy Hot Liquid ... 681
TheraFlu Severe Cold Non-Drowsy Hot Liquid ... 683
TheraFlu Severe Cold & Cough Hot Liquid ... 683
TheraFlu Severe Cold Caplets ... 679
TheraFlu Severe Cold Hot Liquid ... 682
TheraFlu Severe Cold Non-Drowsy Caplets ... 679
TheraFlu Thin Strips Long Acting Cough ... 684
Triaminic Cold & Cough Liquid ... 685
Triaminic Cough Liquid ... 687
Triaminic Cough & Nasal Congestion Liquid ... 687
Triaminic Cough & Sore Throat Liquid ... 687
Triaminic Flu, Cough & Fever Liquid ... 685
Triaminic Night Time Cough & Cold Liquid ... 685
Triaminic Cold & Cough Softchews ... 688
Triaminic Cough & Sore Throat Softchews ... 689
Triaminic Thin Strips Long Acting Cough ... 689
Children's Tylenol Plus Cold & Cough Suspension Liquid and Chewable Tablets ... 1851
Children's Tylenol Plus Flu Suspension Liquid ... 1853
Concentrated Tylenol Infants' Drops Plus Cold and Cough ... 1851
Tylenol Cold & Flu Severe Daytime Liquid with Cool Bust ... 1846
Tylenol Cold & Flu Severe NightTime Liquid with Cool Burst ... 1846
Tylenol Cold Severe Congestion Non-Drowsy Caplets with Cool Burst ... 1846
Tylenol Cough & Sore Throat Daytime Liquid with Cool Burst ... 1849
Tylenol Cough & Sore Throat NightTime Liquid with Cool Burst ... 1849
Tylenol Flu Day Non-Drowsy Gelcaps ... 1846
Concentrated Tylenol Infants' Drops Plus Cold & Cough Nasal Decongestant, Fever Reducer & Pain Reliever ... 668
Multi-Symptom Tylenol Cold Night Time Caplets ... 1845
Multi-Symptom Tylenol Cold Day Non-Drowsy Caplets and Gelcaps ... 1845
Vicks 44 Cough Relief ... 2675
Vicks 44D Cough & Head Congestion Relief ... 2676
Vicks 44D Cough & Head Congestion Relief Liquid ... 721
Vicks 44E Cough & Chest Congestion Relief ... 2676
Pediatric Vicks 44e Cough & Chest Congestion Relief Liquid ... 2673
Vicks 44M Cough, Cold & Flu Relief ... 2676
Pediatric Vicks 44m Cough & Cold Relief ... 2673
Vicks DayQuil LiquiCaps/Liquid Multi-Symptom Cold/Flu Relief ... 723
Vicks DayQuil Multi-Symptom Cold/Flu Relief LiquiCaps ... 2675
Vicks DayQuil Multi-Symptom Cold/Flu Relief Liquid ... 2675
Children's Vicks NyQuil Cold/Cough Relief ... 2671
Vicks NyQuil Cough Liquid ... 2677
Vicks NyQuil LiquiCaps ... 2677
Vicks NyQuil LiquiCaps/Liquid Multi-Symptom Cold/Flu Relief ... 725
Vicks NyQuil Liquid ... 2677
Zicam Concentrated Cough Mist for Kids Cool Cherry ... 643
Zicam Concentrated Cough Mist for Kids Plus D Cool Cherry ... 643
Zicam Concentrated Cough Mist Nite-Cool Cherry ... 642
Zicam Concentrated Cough Mist Plus D Cool Cherry ... 642
Zicam Concentrated Cough Mist-Honey Lemon & Cool Cherry ... 642

Diatrizoate Meglumine (The benefits and risks of using fenofibrate with immunosuppressants and other potentially nephrotoxic agents should be carefully considered, and the lowest effective dose employed).

No products indexed under this heading.

Diatrizoate Sodium (The benefits and risks of using fenofibrate with immunosuppressants and other potentially nephrotoxic agents should be carefully considered, and the lowest effective dose employed).

No products indexed under this heading.

Diazepam (Fenofibrates are mild-moderate inhibitors of CYP2C9 at therapeutic concentrations). Products include:

Diastat Rectal Delivery System ... 3344
Valium Tablets ... 2822

Diclofenac Potassium (Fenofibrates are mild-moderate inhibitors of CYP2C9 at therapeutic concentrations). Products include:

Cataflam Tablets ... 2173

Diclofenac Sodium (Fenofibrates are mild-moderate inhibitors of CYP2C9 at therapeutic concentrations). Products include:

Arthrotec Tablets ... 3126
Voltaren Ophthalmic Solution ... 2300
Voltaren Tablets ... 2298
Voltaren-XR Tablets ... 2301

Dicloxacillin Sodium (The benefits and risks of using fenofibrate with immunosuppressants and other potentially nephrotoxic agents should be carefully considered, and the lowest effective dose employed).

No products indexed under this heading.

Dicumarol (Caution should be exercised when anticoagulants are given in conjunction with fenofibrate because of the potentiation of coumarin-type anticoagulants in prolonging the prothrombin time/INR. The dosage of the anticoagulant should be reduced to maintain the prothrombin time/INR at the desired level to prevent bleeding complications. Frequent prothrombin time/INR determinations are advisably until it has been definitely determined that the prothrombin time/INR has stabilized).

No products indexed under this heading.

Didanosine (The benefits and risks of using fenofibrate with immunosuppressants and other potentially nephrotoxic agents should be carefully considered, and the lowest effective dose employed).

No products indexed under this heading.

Divalproex Sodium (Fenofibrates are weak inhibitors of CYP2C19 at therapeutic concentrations). Products include:

Depakote Sprinkle Capsules ... 422
Depakote Tablets ... 427
Depakote ER Tablets ... 433

Doxepin Hydrochloride (Fenofibrates are weak inhibitors of CYP2C19 at therapeutic concentrations).

No products indexed under this heading.

Dronabinol (Fenofibrates are mild-moderate inhibitors of CYP2C9 at therapeutic concentrations). Products include:

Marinol Capsules ... 3334

Efavirenz (The benefits and risks of using fenofibrate with immunosuppressants and other potentially nephrotoxic agents should be carefully considered, and the lowest effective dose employed). Products include:

Sustiva Capsules ... 957

Emtricitabine (The benefits and risks of using fenofibrate with immunosuppressants and other potentially nephrotoxic agents should be carefully considered, and the lowest effective dose employed). Products include:

Emtriva Capsules ... 1272
Truvada Tablets ... 1279

Enalapril Maleate (The benefits and risks of using fenofibrate with immunosuppressants and other potentially nephrotoxic agents should be carefully considered, and the lowest effective dose employed). Products include:

Vaseretic Tablets ... 2073
Vasotec I.V. Injection ... 2076

Enalaprilat (The benefits and risks of using fenofibrate with immunosuppressants and other potentially nephrotoxic agents should be carefully considered, and the lowest effective dose employed).

No products indexed under this heading.

Enfuvirtide (The benefits and risks of using fenofibrate with immunosuppressants and other potentially nephrotoxic agents should be carefully considered, and the lowest effective dose employed). Products include:

Fuzeon Injection ... 2772

Eprosartan Mesylate (Fenofibrates are mild-moderate inhibitors of CYP2C9 at therapeutic concentrations). Products include:

Teveten Tablets ... 1707
Teveten HCT Tablets ... 1710

Esomeprazole Magnesium (Fenofibrates are weak inhibitors of CYP2C19 at therapeutic concentrations). Products include:

Nexium Delayed-Release Capsules ... 645

Ethiodized Oil (The benefits and risks of using fenofibrate with immunosuppressants and other potentially nephrotoxic agents should be carefully considered, and the lowest effective dose employed).

No products indexed under this heading.

Ethosuximide (Fenofibrates are weak inhibitors of CYP2C19 at therapeutic concentrations).

No products indexed under this heading.

Ethotoin (Fenofibrates are weak inhibitors of CYP2C19 at therapeutic concentrations). Products include:

Peganone Tablets, USP ... 2487

Etodolac (Fenofibrates are mild-moderate inhibitors of CYP2C9 at therapeutic concentrations).

No products indexed under this heading.

Felbamate (Fenofibrates are weak inhibitors of CYP2C19 at therapeutic concentrations).

No products indexed under this heading.

Fenoprofen Calcium (Fenofibrates are mild-moderate inhibitors of CYP2C9 at therapeutic concentrations). Products include:

Nalfon Capsules ... 2504

Filgrastim (The benefits and risks of using fenofibrate with immunosuppressants and other potentially nephrotoxic agents should be carefully considered, and the lowest effective dose employed). Products include:

Neupogen for Injection ... 598

Fluorouracil (The benefits and risks of using fenofibrate with immunosuppressants and other potentially nephrotoxic agents should be carefully considered, and the lowest effective dose employed). Products include:

Carac Cream, 0.5% ... 1048
Efudex ... 3348

Fluoxetine Hydrochloride (Fenofibrates are mild-moderate inhibitors of CYP2C9 at therapeutic concentrations). Products include:

Prozac Pulvules and Liquid ... 1771
Symbyax Capsules ... 1788

Flurbiprofen (Fenofibrates are mild-moderate inhibitors of CYP2C9 at therapeutic concentrations).
No products indexed under this heading.

Flurbiprofen Sodium (Fenofibrates are mild-moderate inhibitors of CYP2C9 at therapeutic concentrations). Products include:
Ocufen Ophthalmic Solution .... ⊙230

Fluvastatin Sodium (The combined use of fenofibrates and HMG-CoA reductase inhibitors should be avoided unless the benefit of further alterations in lipid levels is likely to outweigh the increased risk of this drug combination. The combined use of fibric acid derivatives and HMG-CoA reductase inhibitors has been associated, in the absence of a marked pharmacokinetic interaction, in numerous case reports, with rhabdomyolysis, markedly elevated creatine kinase (CK) levels and myoglobinuria, leading in a high proportion of cases to acute renal failure). Products include:
Lescol Capsules 2227
Lescol 2730
Lescol XL Tablets 2227

Formoterol Fumarate (Fenofibrates are weak inhibitors of CYP2C19 at therapeutic concentrations). Products include:
Foradil Aerolizer 3024

Foscarnet Sodium (The benefits and risks of using fenofibrate with immunosuppressants and other potentially nephrotoxic agents should be carefully considered, and the lowest effective dose employed).
No products indexed under this heading.

Fosinopril Sodium (The benefits and risks of using fenofibrate with immunosuppressants and other potentially nephrotoxic agents should be carefully considered, and the lowest effective dose employed).
No products indexed under this heading.

Fosphenytoin (Fenofibrates are weak inhibitors of CYP2C19 at therapeutic concentrations).
No products indexed under this heading.

Fosphenytoin Sodium (Fenofibrates are weak inhibitors of CYP2C19 at therapeutic concentrations).
No products indexed under this heading.

Furosemide (The benefits and risks of using fenofibrate with immunosuppressants and other potentially nephrotoxic agents should be carefully considered, and the lowest effective dose employed). Products include:
Furosemide Tablets 2117

Gabapentin (Fenofibrates are weak inhibitors of CYP2C19 at therapeutic concentrations). Products include:
Neurontin Capsules 2498
Neurontin Oral Solution 2498
Neurontin Tablets 2498

Gadopentetate Dimeglumine (The benefits and risks of using fenofibrate with immunosuppressants and other potentially nephrotoxic agents should be carefully considered, and the lowest effective dose employed).
No products indexed under this heading.

Gentamicin (The benefits and risks of using fenofibrate with immunosuppressants and other potentially nephrotoxic agents should be carefully considered, and the lowest effective dose employed).
No products indexed under this heading.

Gentamicin Sulfate (The benefits and risks of using fenofibrate with immunosuppressants and other potentially nephrotoxic agents should be carefully considered, and the lowest effective dose employed). Products include:
Garamycin Injectable 3028
Genoptic Sterile Ophthalmic Solution .... ⊙227
Pred-G Ophthalmic Suspension .... ⊙234
Pred-G Sterile Ophthalmic Ointment .... ⊙235

Glimepiride (Fenofibrates are mild-moderate inhibitors of CYP2C9 at therapeutic concentrations). Products include:
Amaryl Tablets 2864

Glipizide (Fenofibrates are mild-moderate inhibitors of CYP2C9 at therapeutic concentrations).
No products indexed under this heading.

Globulin, Immune (Human) (The benefits and risks of using fenofibrate with immunosuppressants and other potentially nephrotoxic agents should be carefully considered, and the lowest effective dose employed). Products include:
GamaSTAN 3231

Glyburide (The benefits and risks of using fenofibrate with immunosuppressants and other potentially nephrotoxic agents should be carefully considered, and the lowest effective dose employed).
No products indexed under this heading.

Gold Therapy (The benefits and risks of using fenofibrate with immunosuppressants and other potentially nephrotoxic agents should be carefully considered, and the lowest effective dose employed).
No products indexed under this heading.

HMG-CoA Reductase Inhibitors (The benefits and risks of using fenofibrate with immunosuppressants and other potentially nephrotoxic agents should be carefully considered, and the lowest effective dose employed).
No products indexed under this heading.

Hydrochlorothiazide (The benefits and risks of using fenofibrate with immunosuppressants and other potentially nephrotoxic agents should be carefully considered, and the lowest effective dose employed). Products include:
Aldoril Tablets 1884
Atacand HCT 637
Avalide Tablets 2889
Avalide Tablets 922
Benicar HCT Tablets 2852
Diovan HCT Tablets 2195
Dyazide Capsules 1389
Hyzaar 1964
Lotensin HCT Tablets 2235
Maxzide 2150
Micardis HCT Tablets 886
Moduretic Tablets 2003
Prinzide Tablets 2033
Teveten HCT Tablets 1710
Timolide Tablets 2056
Uniretic Tablets 3114
Vaseretic Tablets 2073
Zestoretic Tablets 701

Hydroflumethiazide (The benefits and risks of using fenofibrate with immunosuppressants and other potentially nephrotoxic agents should be carefully considered, and the lowest effective dose employed).
No products indexed under this heading.

Ibuprofen (Fenofibrates are mild-moderate inhibitors of CYP2C9 at therapeutic concentrations). Products include:
Advil Allergy Sinus Caplets .... ▣737
Advil .... ▣737
Children's Advil Suspension .... ▣742
Children's Advil Chewable Tablets .... ▣741
Advil Cold & Sinus .... ▣739
Advil Flu & Body Ache Caplets .... ▣739
Children's Advil Cold Suspension .... ▣741
Infants' Advil Concentrated Drops .... ▣743
Junior Strength Advil Swallow Tablets .... ▣740
Advil Migraine Liquigels .... ▣740
Advil Multi-Symptom Cold Caplets .... ▣738
Combunox Tablets 1183
Children's Motrin Oral Suspension and Chewable Tablets 1837
Children's Motrin Cold Non-Staining Dye-Free Oral Suspension 1838
Children's Motrin Cold Oral Suspension 1838
Children's Motrin Non-Staining Dye-Free Oral Suspension 1837
Motrin Cold & Sinus Caplets 1836
Motrin IB Tablets and Caplets 1836
Infants' Motrin Concentrated Drops 1837
Infants' Motrin Non-Staining Dye-Free Drops 1837
Junior Strength Motrin Caplets and Chewable Tablets 1837
Vicoprofen Tablets 533

Idarubicin Hydrochloride (The benefits and risks of using fenofibrate with immunosuppressants and other potentially nephrotoxic agents should be carefully considered, and the lowest effective dose employed). Products include:
Idamycin PFS Injection 2645

Ifosfamide (The benefits and risks of using fenofibrate with immunosuppressants and other potentially nephrotoxic agents should be carefully considered, and the lowest effective dose employed).
No products indexed under this heading.

Imipenem (The benefits and risks of using fenofibrate with immunosuppressants and other potentially nephrotoxic agents should be carefully considered, and the lowest effective dose employed). Products include:
Primaxin I.M. 2022
Primaxin I.V. 2024

Imipramine Hydrochloride (Fenofibrates are mild-moderate inhibitors of CYP2C9 at therapeutic concentrations).
No products indexed under this heading.

Imipramine Pamoate (Fenofibrates are weak inhibitors of CYP2C19 at therapeutic concentrations).
No products indexed under this heading.

Immune Globulin Intravenous (Human) (The benefits and risks of using fenofibrate with immunosuppressants and other potentially nephrotoxic agents should be carefully considered, and the lowest effective dose employed). Products include:
Carimune NF 3501
Gammagard Liquid 751
Gammagard S/D 754
Gamunex Immune Globulin I.V., 10% 3232
Iveegam EN 759

Indinavir Sulfate (The benefits and risks of using fenofibrate with immunosuppressants and other potentially nephrotoxic agents should be carefully considered, and the lowest effective dose employed). Products include:
Crixivan Capsules 1918

Indomethacin (Fenofibrates are mild-moderate inhibitors of CYP2C9 at therapeutic concentrations). Products include:
Indocin 1968

Indomethacin Sodium Trihydrate (Fenofibrates are mild-moderate inhibitors of CYP2C9 at therapeutic concentrations). Products include:
Indocin I.V. 1973

Interferon Beta-1b (The benefits and risks of using fenofibrate with immunosuppressants and other potentially nephrotoxic agents should be carefully considered, and the lowest effective dose employed). Products include:
Betaseron for SC Injection 791

Interleuken-2 (The benefits and risks of using fenofibrate with immunosuppressants and other potentially nephrotoxic agents should be carefully considered, and the lowest effective dose employed).
No products indexed under this heading.

Iodamide Meglumine (The benefits and risks of using fenofibrate with immunosuppressants and other potentially nephrotoxic agents should be carefully considered, and the lowest effective dose employed).
No products indexed under this heading.

Iohexol (The benefits and risks of using fenofibrate with immunosuppressants and other potentially nephrotoxic agents should be carefully considered, and the lowest effective dose employed).
No products indexed under this heading.

Iopamidol (The benefits and risks of using fenofibrate with immunosuppressants and other potentially nephrotoxic agents should be carefully considered, and the lowest effective dose employed).
No products indexed under this heading.

Iopanoic Acid (The benefits and risks of using fenofibrate with immunosuppressants and other potentially nephrotoxic agents should be carefully considered, and the lowest effective dose employed).
No products indexed under this heading.

Iothalamate Meglumine (The benefits and risks of using fenofibrate with immunosuppressants and other potentially nephrotoxic agents should be carefully considered, and the lowest effective dose employed).
No products indexed under this heading.

Ioxaglate Meglumine (The benefits and risks of using fenofibrate with immunosuppressants and other potentially nephrotoxic agents should be carefully considered, and the lowest effective dose employed).
No products indexed under this heading.

Ioxaglate Sodium (The benefits and risks of using fenofibrate with immunosuppressants and other potentially nephrotoxic agents should be carefully considered, and the lowest effective dose employed).
No products indexed under this heading.

Irbesartan (Fenofibrates are mild-moderate inhibitors of CYP2C9 at therapeutic concentrations).
Products include:
Avalide Tablets 922
Avalide Tablets 2889
Avapro Tablets 925
Avapro Tablets 2886

Kanamycin Sulfate (The benefits and risks of using fenofibrate with immunosuppressants and other potentially nephrotoxic agents should be carefully considered, and the lowest effective dose employed).
No products indexed under this heading.

Ketoprofen (Fenofibrates are mild-moderate inhibitors of CYP2C9 at therapeutic concentrations).
No products indexed under this heading.

Ketorolac Tromethamine (Fenofibrates are mild-moderate inhibitors of CYP2C9 at therapeutic concentrations). Products include:
Acular Ophthalmic Solution 561
Acular LS Ophthalmic Solution 562

Lamium album (The benefits and risks of using fenofibrate with immunosuppressants and other potentially nephrotoxic agents should be carefully considered, and the lowest effective dose employed).
No products indexed under this heading.

Lamotrigine (Fenofibrates are weak inhibitors of CYP2C19 at therapeutic concentrations). Products include:
Lamictal 1449

Lansoprazole (Fenofibrates are mild-moderate inhibitors of CYP2C9 at therapeutic concentrations).
Products include:
Prevacid Delayed-Release Capsules 3268
Prevacid for Delayed-Release Oral Suspension 3268
Prevacid I.V. for Injection 3274
Prevacid NapraPAC 3277
Prevacid SoluTab Delayed-Release Orally Disintegrating Tablets 3268
PREVPAC 3281

Levetiracetam (Fenofibrates are weak inhibitors of CYP2C19 at therapeutic concentrations). Products include:
Keppra Oral Solution 3307
Keppra Tablets 3307

Lisinopril (The benefits and risks of using fenofibrate with immunosuppressants and other potentially nephrotoxic agents should be carefully considered, and the lowest effective dose employed). Products include:
Prinivil Tablets 2029
Prinzide Tablets 2033
Zestoretic Tablets 701
Zestril Tablets 704

Lithium (The benefits and risks of using fenofibrate with immunosuppressants and other potentially nephrotoxic agents should be carefully considered, and the lowest effective dose employed).
No products indexed under this heading.

Lithium Carbonate (The benefits and risks of using fenofibrate with immunosuppressants and other potentially nephrotoxic agents should be carefully considered, and the lowest effective dose employed).
Products include:
Eskalith 1406
Lithobid Tablets 1670

Lithium Citrate (The benefits and risks of using fenofibrate with immunosuppressants and other potentially nephrotoxic agents should be carefully considered, and the lowest effective dose employed).
No products indexed under this heading.

Lopinavir (The benefits and risks of using fenofibrate with immunosuppressants and other potentially nephrotoxic agents should be carefully considered, and the lowest effective dose employed). Products include:
Kaletra 474

Loracarbef (The benefits and risks of using fenofibrate with immunosuppressants and other potentially nephrotoxic agents should be carefully considered, and the lowest effective dose employed).
No products indexed under this heading.

Losartan Potassium (Fenofibrates are mild-moderate inhibitors of CYP2C9 at therapeutic concentrations). Products include:
Cozaar Tablets 1913
Hyzaar 1964

Lovastatin (The combined use of fenofibrates and HMG-CoA reductase inhibitors should be avoided unless the benefit of further alterations in lipid levels is likely to outweigh the increased risk of this drug combination. The combined use of fibric acid derivatives and HMG-CoA reductase inhibitors has been associated, in the absence of a marked pharmacokinetic interaction, in numerous case reports, with rhabdomyolysis, markedly elevated creatine kinase (CK) levels and myoglobinuria, leading in a high proportion of cases to acute renal failure). Products include:
Advicor Tablets 1694
Altoprev Extended-Release Tablets 1151
Mevacor Tablets 1996

Maprotiline Hydrochloride (Fenofibrates are weak inhibitors of CYP2C19 at therapeutic concentrations).
No products indexed under this heading.

Meclofenamate Sodium (Fenofibrates are mild-moderate inhibitors of CYP2C9 at therapeutic concentrations).
No products indexed under this heading.

Mefenamic Acid (Fenofibrates are mild-moderate inhibitors of CYP2C9 at therapeutic concentrations).
No products indexed under this heading.

Meloxicam (Fenofibrates are mild-moderate inhibitors of CYP2C9 at therapeutic concentrations).
Products include:
Mobic Oral Suspension 893
Mobic Tablets 893

Melphalan Hydrochloride (The benefits and risks of using fenofibrate with immunosuppressants and other potentially nephrotoxic agents should be carefully considered, and the lowest effective dose employed).
Products include:
Alkeran for Injection 976

Mephenytoin (Fenofibrates are weak inhibitors of CYP2C19 at therapeutic concentrations).
No products indexed under this heading.

Mephobarbital (Fenofibrates are weak inhibitors of CYP2C19 at therapeutic concentrations). Products include:
Mebaral Tablets, USP 2483

Meprobamate (Fenofibrates are weak inhibitors of CYP2C19 at therapeutic concentrations).
No products indexed under this heading.

Mesalamine (The benefits and risks of using fenofibrate with immunosuppressants and other potentially nephrotoxic agents should be carefully considered, and the lowest effective dose employed). Products include:
Asacol Delayed-Release Tablets 2688
Canasa Rectal Suppositories 726
Pentasa Capsules 3182

Metformin Hydrochloride (Fenofibrates are mild-moderate inhibitors of CYP2C9 at therapeutic concentrations). Products include:
ActoPlus Met Tablets 3219
Avandamet Tablets 1343
Fortamet Extended-Release Tablets 1156

Methimazole (The benefits and risks of using fenofibrate with immunosuppressants and other potentially nephrotoxic agents should be carefully considered, and the lowest effective dose employed).
No products indexed under this heading.

Methotrexate (The benefits and risks of using fenofibrate with immunosuppressants and other potentially nephrotoxic agents should be carefully considered, and the lowest effective dose employed).
No products indexed under this heading.

Methotrexate Sodium (The benefits and risks of using fenofibrate with immunosuppressants and other potentially nephrotoxic agents should be carefully considered, and the lowest effective dose employed).
No products indexed under this heading.

Methsuximide (Fenofibrates are weak inhibitors of CYP2C19 at therapeutic concentrations).
No products indexed under this heading.

Methyclothiazide (The benefits and risks of using fenofibrate with immunosuppressants and other potentially nephrotoxic agents should be carefully considered, and the lowest effective dose employed).
No products indexed under this heading.

Mezlocillin Sodium (The benefits and risks of using fenofibrate with immunosuppressants and other potentially nephrotoxic agents should be carefully considered, and the lowest effective dose employed).
No products indexed under this heading.

Midazolam Hydrochloride (Fenofibrates are weak inhibitors of CYP2C19 at therapeutic concentrations).
No products indexed under this heading.

Miglitol (Fenofibrates are mild-moderate inhibitors of CYP2C9 at therapeutic concentrations).
No products indexed under this heading.

Minocycline Hydrochloride (The benefits and risks of using fenofibrate with immunosuppressants and other potentially nephrotoxic agents should be carefully considered, and the lowest effective dose employed).
Products include:
Dynacin Tablets 1859

Mirtazapine (Fenofibrates are mild-moderate inhibitors of CYP2C9 at therapeutic concentrations).
No products indexed under this heading.

Mitomycin (Mitomycin-C) (The benefits and risks of using fenofibrate with immunosuppressants and other potentially nephrotoxic agents should be carefully considered, and the lowest effective dose employed).
No products indexed under this heading.

Moexipril Hydrochloride (The benefits and risks of using fenofibrate with immunosuppressants and other potentially nephrotoxic agents should be carefully considered, and the lowest effective dose employed).
Products include:
Uniretic Tablets 3114
Univasc Tablets 3118

Montelukast Sodium (Fenofibrates are mild-moderate inhibitors of CYP2C9 at therapeutic concentrations). Products include:
Singulair 2047

Muromonab-CD3 (The benefits and risks of using fenofibrate with immunosuppressants and other potentially nephrotoxic agents should be carefully considered, and the lowest effective dose employed).
Products include:
Orthoclone OKT3 Sterile Solution 2370

Mycophenolate Mofetil (The benefits and risks of using fenofibrate with immunosuppressants and other potentially nephrotoxic agents should be carefully considered, and the lowest effective dose employed).
Products include:
CellCept Capsules 2751
CellCept Oral Suspension 2751
CellCept Tablets 2751

Nabumetone (Fenofibrates are mild-moderate inhibitors of CYP2C9 at therapeutic concentrations).
Products include:
Relafen Tablets 1523

Nafcillin Sodium (The benefits and risks of using fenofibrate with immunosuppressants and other potentially nephrotoxic agents should be carefully considered, and the lowest effective dose employed).
No products indexed under this heading.

Naproxen (Fenofibrates are mild-moderate inhibitors of CYP2C9 at therapeutic concentrations).
Products include:
EC-Naprosyn Delayed-Release Tablets 2769
Naprosyn Suspension 2769
Naprosyn Tablets 2769
Prevacid NapraPAC 3277

Naproxen Sodium (Fenofibrates are mild-moderate inhibitors of CYP2C9 at therapeutic concentrations). Products include:
Aleve Tablets, Caplets and Gelcaps 605
Anaprox Tablets 2769

IMPORTANT NOTE: Always consult each drug listing in the patient's regimen for possible interactions.

Anaprox DS Tablets 2769

Nateglinide (Fenofibrates are mild-moderate inhibitors of CYP2C9 at therapeutic concentrations). Products include:
Starlix Tablets 2276

Nelfinavir Mesylate (Fenofibrates are weak inhibitors of CYP2C19 at therapeutic concentrations). Products include:
Viracept 2556

Neomycin (The benefits and risks of using fenofibrate with immunosuppressants and other potentially nephrotoxic agents should be carefully considered, and the lowest effective dose employed). Products include:
Neosporin Ointment .... ■□702
Neosporin + Pain Relief Maximum Strength Cream........... ■□703
Neosporin + Pain Relief Maximum Strength Ointment....... ■□703

Neomycin, oral (The benefits and risks of using fenofibrate with immunosuppressants and other potentially nephrotoxic agents should be carefully considered, and the lowest effective dose employed).
No products indexed under this heading.

Neomycin Sulfate (The benefits and risks of using fenofibrate with immunosuppressants and other potentially nephrotoxic agents should be carefully considered, and the lowest effective dose employed). Products include:
Poly-Pred Liquifilm Ophthalmic Suspension .... ⊙231

Nevirapine (The benefits and risks of using fenofibrate with immunosuppressants and other potentially nephrotoxic agents should be carefully considered, and the lowest effective dose employed). Products include:
Viramune Oral Suspension 903
Viramune Tablets 903

Nilutamide (Fenofibrates are weak inhibitors of CYP2C19 at therapeutic concentrations).
No products indexed under this heading.

Norfloxacin (The benefits and risks of using fenofibrate with immunosuppressants and other potentially nephrotoxic agents should be carefully considered, and the lowest effective dose employed). Products include:
Noroxin Tablets 2009

Nortriptyline Hydrochloride (Fenofibrates are weak inhibitors of CYP2C19 at therapeutic concentrations).
No products indexed under this heading.

Olsalazine Sodium (The benefits and risks of using fenofibrate with immunosuppressants and other potentially nephrotoxic agents should be carefully considered, and the lowest effective dose employed).
No products indexed under this heading.

Omeprazole (Fenofibrates are mild-moderate inhibitors of CYP2C9 at therapeutic concentrations). Products include:
Zegerid Powder for Oral Solution 2972

Oxaprozin (Fenofibrates are mild-moderate inhibitors of CYP2C9 at therapeutic concentrations).
No products indexed under this heading.

Oxcarbazepine (Fenofibrates are weak inhibitors of CYP2C19 at therapeutic concentrations). Products include:
Trileptal Oral Suspension 2281
Trileptal Tablets 2281

Pamidronate Disodium (The benefits and risks of using fenofibrate with immunosuppressants and other potentially nephrotoxic agents should be carefully considered, and the lowest effective dose employed). Products include:
Aredia for Injection 2168

Pantoprazole Sodium (Fenofibrates are weak inhibitors of CYP2C19 at therapeutic concentrations). Products include:
Protonix I.V. 3468
Protonix Tablets 3465

Paramethadione (Fenofibrates are weak inhibitors of CYP2C19 at therapeutic concentrations).
No products indexed under this heading.

Paroxetine Hydrochloride (The benefits and risks of using fenofibrate with immunosuppressants and other potentially nephrotoxic agents should be carefully considered, and the lowest effective dose employed). Products include:
Paxil CR Controlled-Release Tablets 1509
Paxil 1501

Penicillamine (The benefits and risks of using fenofibrate with immunosuppressants and other potentially nephrotoxic agents should be carefully considered, and the lowest effective dose employed). Products include:
Cuprimine Capsules 1925

Penicillin G Benzathine (The benefits and risks of using fenofibrate with immunosuppressants and other potentially nephrotoxic agents should be carefully considered, and the lowest effective dose employed).
No products indexed under this heading.

Penicillin G Potassium (The benefits and risks of using fenofibrate with immunosuppressants and other potentially nephrotoxic agents should be carefully considered, and the lowest effective dose employed).
No products indexed under this heading.

Penicillin G Procaine (The benefits and risks of using fenofibrate with immunosuppressants and other potentially nephrotoxic agents should be carefully considered, and the lowest effective dose employed).
No products indexed under this heading.

Penicillin G Sodium (The benefits and risks of using fenofibrate with immunosuppressants and other potentially nephrotoxic agents should be carefully considered, and the lowest effective dose employed).
No products indexed under this heading.

Penicillin V Potassium (The benefits and risks of using fenofibrate with immunosuppressants and other potentially nephrotoxic agents should be carefully considered, and the lowest effective dose employed).
No products indexed under this heading.

Pentamidine Isethionate (Fenofibrates are weak inhibitors of CYP2C19 at therapeutic concentrations).
No products indexed under this heading.

Perindopril Erbumine (The benefits and risks of using fenofibrate with immunosuppressants and other potentially nephrotoxic agents should be carefully considered, and the lowest effective dose employed). Products include:
Aceon Tablets (2 mg, 4 mg, 8 mg).. 3191

Phenacemide (Fenofibrates are weak inhibitors of CYP2C19 at therapeutic concentrations).
No products indexed under this heading.

Phenobarbital (Fenofibrates are weak inhibitors of CYP2C19 at therapeutic concentrations).
No products indexed under this heading.

Phenobarbital Sodium (Fenofibrates are weak inhibitors of CYP2C19 at therapeutic concentrations).
No products indexed under this heading.

Phensuximide (Fenofibrates are weak inhibitors of CYP2C19 at therapeutic concentrations).
No products indexed under this heading.

Phenylbutazone (Fenofibrates are mild-moderate inhibitors of CYP2C9 at therapeutic concentrations).
No products indexed under this heading.

Phenytoin (Fenofibrates are weak inhibitors of CYP2C19 at therapeutic concentrations).
No products indexed under this heading.

Phenytoin Sodium (Fenofibrates are mild-moderate inhibitors of CYP2C9 at therapeutic concentrations). Products include:
Phenytek Capsules 2153

Pioglitazone Hydrochloride (Fenofibrates are mild-moderate inhibitors of CYP2C9 at therapeutic concentrations). Products include:
ActoPlus Met Tablets 3219
Actos Tablets 3224

Piroxicam (Fenofibrates are mild-moderate inhibitors of CYP2C9 at therapeutic concentrations).
No products indexed under this heading.

Plicamycin (The benefits and risks of using fenofibrate with immunosuppressants and other potentially nephrotoxic agents should be carefully considered, and the lowest effective dose employed).
No products indexed under this heading.

Polymyxin (The benefits and risks of using fenofibrate with immunosuppressants and other potentially nephrotoxic agents should be carefully considered, and the lowest effective dose employed).
No products indexed under this heading.

Polymyxin B Sulfate (The benefits and risks of using fenofibrate with immunosuppressants and other potentially nephrotoxic agents should be carefully considered, and the lowest effective dose employed). Products include:
Neosporin Ointment .... ■□702
Neosporin + Pain Relief Maximum Strength Cream........... ■□703
Neosporin + Pain Relief Maximum Strength Ointment....... ■□703
Poly-Pred Liquifilm Ophthalmic Suspension .... ⊙231
Polysporin Ointment .... ■□706
Polytrim Ophthalmic Solution 570

Polythiazide (The benefits and risks of using fenofibrate with immunosuppressants and other potentially nephrotoxic agents should be carefully considered, and the lowest effective dose employed).
No products indexed under this heading.

Pravastatin Sodium (The combined use of fenofibrates and HMG-CoA reductase inhibitors should be avoided unless the benefit of further alterations in lipid levels is likely to outweigh the increased risk of this drug combination. The combined use of fibric acid derivatives and HMG-CoA reductase inhibitors has been associated, in the absence of a marked pharmacokinetic interaction, in numerous case reports, with rhabdomyolysis, markedly elevated creatine kinase (CK) levels and myoglobinuria, leading in a high proportion of cases to acute renal failure). Products include:
Pravachol Tablets 943

Primidone (Fenofibrates are weak inhibitors of CYP2C19 at therapeutic concentrations).
No products indexed under this heading.

Probenecid (The benefits and risks of using fenofibrate with immunosuppressants and other potentially nephrotoxic agents should be carefully considered, and the lowest effective dose employed).
No products indexed under this heading.

Progesterone (Fenofibrates are weak inhibitors of CYP2C19 at therapeutic concentrations). Products include:
Prochieve 4% Gel 1018
Prochieve 8% Gel 1018
Prometrium Capsules (100 mg, 200 mg).. 3205

Proguanil Hydrochloride (Fenofibrates are weak inhibitors of CYP2C19 at therapeutic concentrations). Products include:
Malarone Tablets 1484
Malarone Pediatric Tablets 1484

Propranolol Hydrochloride (Fenofibrates are weak inhibitors of CYP2C19 at therapeutic concentrations). Products include:
Inderal LA Long-Acting Capsules 3421
InnoPran XL Capsules 2728

Protriptyline Hydrochloride (Fenofibrates are weak inhibitors of CYP2C19 at therapeutic concentrations). Products include:
Vivactil Tablets 2350

Quinapril Hydrochloride (The benefits and risks of using fenofibrate with immunosuppressants and other potentially nephrotoxic agents should be carefully considered, and the lowest effective dose employed).
No products indexed under this heading.

Rabeprazole Sodium (Fenofibrates are weak inhibitors of CYP2C19 at therapeutic concentrations). Products include:
Aciphex Tablets 1081

Ramipril (The benefits and risks of using fenofibrate with immunosuppressants and other potentially nephrotoxic agents should be carefully considered, and the lowest effective dose employed). Products include:
Altace Capsules 1673

Repaglinide (Fenofibrates are mild-moderate inhibitors of CYP2C9 at therapeutic concentrations). Products include:
Prandin Tablets (0.5, 1, and 2 mg) ... 2337

Rifampin (The benefits and risks of using fenofibrate with immunosuppressants and other potentially nephrotoxic agents should be carefully considered, and the lowest effective dose employed).
No products indexed under this heading.

Riluzole (The benefits and risks of using fenofibrate with immunosuppressants and other potentially nephrotoxic agents should be carefully considered, and the lowest effective dose employed). Products include:
Rilutek Tablets ... 2945

Ritonavir (The benefits and risks of using fenofibrate with immunosuppressants and other potentially nephrotoxic agents should be carefully considered, and the lowest effective dose employed). Products include:
Kaletra ... 474
Norvir ... 499

Rofecoxib (Fenofibrates are mild-moderate inhibitors of CYP2C9 at therapeutic concentrations).
No products indexed under this heading.

Rosiglitazone Maleate (Fenofibrates are mild-moderate inhibitors of CYP2C9 at therapeutic concentrations). Products include:
Avandamet Tablets ... 1343
Avandia Tablets ... 1348

Saquinavir (The benefits and risks of using fenofibrate with immunosuppressants and other potentially nephrotoxic agents should be carefully considered, and the lowest effective dose employed).
No products indexed under this heading.

Sertraline Hydrochloride (Fenofibrates are weak inhibitors of CYP2C19 at therapeutic concentrations). Products include:
Zoloft ... 2581

Sibutramine Hydrochloride Monohydrate (The benefits and risks of using fenofibrate with immunosuppressants and other potentially nephrotoxic agents should be carefully considered, and the lowest effective dose employed). Products include:
Meridia Capsules ... 485

Sildenafil Citrate (Fenofibrates are mild-moderate inhibitors of CYP2C9 at therapeutic concentrations). Products include:
Revatio Tablets ... 2541
Viagra Tablets ... 2552

Simvastatin (The combined use of fenofibrates and HMG-CoA reductase inhibitors should be avoided unless the benefit of further alterations in lipid levels is likely to outweigh the increased risk of this drug combination. The combined use of fibric acid derivatives and HMG-CoA reductase inhibitors has been associated, in the absence of a marked pharmacokinetic interaction, in numerous case reports, with rhabdomyolysis, markedly elevated creatine kinase (CK) levels and myoglobinuria, leading in a high proportion of cases to acute renal failure). Products include:
Vytorin 10/10 Tablets ... 2084
Vytorin 10/10 Tablets ... 3092
Vytorin 10/20 Tablets ... 2084
Vytorin 10/20 Tablets ... 3092
Vytorin 10/40 Tablets ... 3092
Vytorin 10/40 Tablets ... 2084
Vytorin 10/80 Tablets ... 2084
Vytorin 10/80 Tablets ... 3092
Zocor Tablets ... 2078

Sirolimus (The benefits and risks of using fenofibrate with immunosuppressants and other potentially nephrotoxic agents should be carefully considered, and the lowest effective dose employed). Products include:
Rapamune Oral Solution and Tablets ... 3472

Spirapril Hydrochloride (The benefits and risks of using fenofibrate with immunosuppressants and other potentially nephrotoxic agents should be carefully considered, and the lowest effective dose employed).
No products indexed under this heading.

Stavudine (The benefits and risks of using fenofibrate with immunosuppressants and other potentially nephrotoxic agents should be carefully considered, and the lowest effective dose employed). Products include:
Zerit ... 971

Streptomycin Sulfate (The benefits and risks of using fenofibrate with immunosuppressants and other potentially nephrotoxic agents should be carefully considered, and the lowest effective dose employed).
No products indexed under this heading.

Streptozocin (The benefits and risks of using fenofibrate with immunosuppressants and other potentially nephrotoxic agents should be carefully considered, and the lowest effective dose employed).
No products indexed under this heading.

Sulfacytine (The benefits and risks of using fenofibrate with immunosuppressants and other potentially nephrotoxic agents should be carefully considered, and the lowest effective dose employed).
No products indexed under this heading.

Sulfamethizole (The benefits and risks of using fenofibrate with immunosuppressants and other potentially nephrotoxic agents should be carefully considered, and the lowest effective dose employed).
No products indexed under this heading.

Sulfamethoxazole (Fenofibrates are mild-moderate inhibitors of CYP2C9 at therapeutic concentrations).
No products indexed under this heading.

Sulfasalazine (The benefits and risks of using fenofibrate with immunosuppressants and other potentially nephrotoxic agents should be carefully considered, and the lowest effective dose employed).
No products indexed under this heading.

Sulfinpyrazone (The benefits and risks of using fenofibrate with immunosuppressants and other potentially nephrotoxic agents should be carefully considered, and the lowest effective dose employed).
No products indexed under this heading.

Sulfisoxazole (The benefits and risks of using fenofibrate with immunosuppressants and other potentially nephrotoxic agents should be carefully considered, and the lowest effective dose employed).
No products indexed under this heading.

Sulfisoxazole Acetyl (The benefits and risks of using fenofibrate with immunosuppressants and other potentially nephrotoxic agents should be carefully considered, and the lowest effective dose employed).
No products indexed under this heading.

Sulfisoxazole Diolamine (The benefits and risks of using fenofibrate with immunosuppressants and other potentially nephrotoxic agents should be carefully considered, and the lowest effective dose employed).
No products indexed under this heading.

Sulindac (Fenofibrates are mild-moderate inhibitors of CYP2C9 at therapeutic concentrations). Products include:
Clinoril Tablets ... 1899

Suprofen (Fenofibrates are mild-moderate inhibitors of CYP2C9 at therapeutic concentrations).
No products indexed under this heading.

Tacrolimus (The benefits and risks of using fenofibrate with immunosuppressants and other potentially nephrotoxic agents should be carefully considered, and the lowest effective dose employed). Products include:
Prograf Capsules and Injection ... 624
Protopic Ointment ... 629

Tamoxifen Citrate (Fenofibrates are mild-moderate inhibitors of CYP2C9 at therapeutic concentrations).
No products indexed under this heading.

Telmisartan (Fenofibrates are mild-moderate inhibitors of CYP2C9 at therapeutic concentrations). Products include:
Micardis Tablets ... 884
Micardis HCT Tablets ... 886

Teniposide (Fenofibrates are weak inhibitors of CYP2C19 at therapeutic concentrations).
No products indexed under this heading.

Tenofovir Disoproxil Fumarate (The benefits and risks of using fenofibrate with immunosuppressants and other potentially nephrotoxic agents should be carefully considered, and the lowest effective dose employed). Products include:
Truvada Tablets ... 1279
Viread Tablets ... 1284

Thioguanine (The benefits and risks of using fenofibrate with immunosuppressants and other potentially nephrotoxic agents should be carefully considered, and the lowest effective dose employed). Products include:
Tabloid Tablets ... 1545

Thioridazine (Fenofibrates are weak inhibitors of CYP2C19 at therapeutic concentrations).
No products indexed under this heading.

Thioridazine Hydrochloride (Fenofibrates are weak inhibitors of CYP2C19 at therapeutic concentrations). Products include:
Thioridazine Hydrochloride Tablets ... 2122

Tiagabine Hydrochloride (Fenofibrates are weak inhibitors of CYP2C19 at therapeutic concentrations). Products include:
Gabitril Tablets ... 998

Ticarcillin Disodium (The benefits and risks of using fenofibrate with immunosuppressants and other potentially nephrotoxic agents should be carefully considered, and the lowest effective dose employed). Products include:
Timentin ADD-Vantage ... 1556
Timentin Injection Galaxy Container ... 1559
Timentin IV Infusion ... 1553
Timentin Pharmacy Bulk Package ... 1562

Tobramycin (The benefits and risks of using fenofibrate with immunosuppressants and other potentially nephrotoxic agents should be carefully considered, and the lowest effective dose employed). Products include:
TOBI Solution for Inhalation ... 1015
TobraDex Ophthalmic Ointment ... 558
TobraDex Ophthalmic Suspension ... 558
Zylet Ophthalmic Suspension ... 3508

Tobramycin Sulfate (The benefits and risks of using fenofibrate with immunosuppressants and other potentially nephrotoxic agents should be carefully considered, and the lowest effective dose employed).
No products indexed under this heading.

Tolazamide (Fenofibrates are mild-moderate inhibitors of CYP2C9 at therapeutic concentrations).
No products indexed under this heading.

Tolbutamide (Fenofibrates are mild-moderate inhibitors of CYP2C9 at therapeutic concentrations).
No products indexed under this heading.

Tolbutamide Sodium (Fenofibrates are mild-moderate inhibitors of CYP2C9 at therapeutic concentrations).
No products indexed under this heading.

Tolmetin Sodium (Fenofibrates are mild-moderate inhibitors of CYP2C9 at therapeutic concentrations).
No products indexed under this heading.

Topiramate (Fenofibrates are weak inhibitors of CYP2C19 at therapeutic concentrations). Products include:
Topamax Sprinkle Capsules ... 2438
Topamax Tablets ... 2438

Torsemide (Fenofibrates are mild-moderate inhibitors of CYP2C9 at therapeutic concentrations).
No products indexed under this heading.

Trandolapril (The benefits and risks of using fenofibrate with immunosuppressants and other potentially nephrotoxic agents should be carefully considered, and the lowest effective dose employed). Products include:
Mavik Tablets ... 482
Tarka Tablets ... 519

Triamterene (The benefits and risks of using fenofibrate with immunosuppressants and other potentially nephrotoxic agents should be carefully considered, and the lowest effective dose employed). Products include:
Dyazide Capsules ... 1389
Dyrenium Capsules ... 3390
Maxzide ... 2150

Trimethadione (Fenofibrates are weak inhibitors of CYP2C19 at therapeutic concentrations).
No products indexed under this heading.

Trimipramine Maleate (Fenofibrates are weak inhibitors of CYP2C19 at therapeutic concentrations). Products include:
Surmontil Capsules **2347**

Troglitazone (Fenofibrates are mild-moderate inhibitors of CYP2C9 at therapeutic concentrations).
No products indexed under this heading.

Trovafloxacin Mesylate (The benefits and risks of using fenofibrate with immunosuppressants and other potentially nephrotoxic agents should be carefully considered, and the lowest effective dose employed).
No products indexed under this heading.

Tyropanoate Sodium (The benefits and risks of using fenofibrate with immunosuppressants and other potentially nephrotoxic agents should be carefully considered, and the lowest effective dose employed).
No products indexed under this heading.

Valacyclovir Hydrochloride (The benefits and risks of using fenofibrate with immunosuppressants and other potentially nephrotoxic agents should be carefully considered, and the lowest effective dose employed). Products include:
Valtrex Caplets **1573**

Valdecoxib (Fenofibrates are mild-moderate inhibitors of CYP2C9 at therapeutic concentrations).
No products indexed under this heading.

Valproate Sodium (Fenofibrates are weak inhibitors of CYP2C19 at therapeutic concentrations). Products include:
Depacon Injection **412**

Valproic Acid (Fenofibrates are weak inhibitors of CYP2C19 at therapeutic concentrations). Products include:
Depakene **417**

Valsartan (Fenofibrates are mild-moderate inhibitors of CYP2C9 at therapeutic concentrations). Products include:
Diovan HCT Tablets **2195**
Diovan Tablets **2191**

Vancomycin Hydrochloride (The benefits and risks of using fenofibrate with immunosuppressants and other potentially nephrotoxic agents should be carefully considered, and the lowest effective dose employed). Products include:
Vancocin HCl Capsules, USP **3370**

Verapamil Hydrochloride (Fenofibrates are mild-moderate inhibitors of CYP2C9 at therapeutic concentrations). Products include:
Covera-HS Tablets **3135**
Tarka Tablets **519**
Verelan PM Capsules **3120**

Voriconazole (Fenofibrates are mild-moderate inhibitors of CYP2C9 at therapeutic concentrations). Products include:
VFEND I.V. **2543**
VFEND Oral Suspension **2543**
VFEND Tablets **2543**

Warfarin Sodium (Caution should be exercised when anticoagulants are given in conjunction with fenofibrate because of the potentiation of coumarin-type anticoagulants in prolonging the prothrombin time/INR. The dosage of the anticoagulant should be reduced to maintain the prothrombin time/INR at the desired level to prevent bleeding complications. Frequent prothrombin time/INR determinations are advisably until it has been definitely determined that the prothrombin time/INR has stabilized). Products include:
Coumadin for Injection **932**
Coumadin Tablets **932**

Zafirlukast (Fenofibrates are mild-moderate inhibitors of CYP2C9 at therapeutic concentrations). Products include:
Accolate Tablets **663**

Zalcitabine (The benefits and risks of using fenofibrate with immunosuppressants and other potentially nephrotoxic agents should be carefully considered, and the lowest effective dose employed).
No products indexed under this heading.

Zidovudine (The benefits and risks of using fenofibrate with immunosuppressants and other potentially nephrotoxic agents should be carefully considered, and the lowest effective dose employed). Products include:
Combivir Tablets **1373**
Retrovir **1533**
Retrovir IV Infusion **1537**
Trizivir Tablets **1565**

Zileuton (Fenofibrates are mild-moderate inhibitors of CYP2C9 at therapeutic concentrations).
No products indexed under this heading.

Zoledronic acid (The benefits and risks of using fenofibrate with immunosuppressants and other potentially nephrotoxic agents should be carefully considered, and the lowest effective dose employed). Products include:
Zometa for Intravenous Infusion **2306**

Zonisamide (Fenofibrates are weak inhibitors of CYP2C19 at therapeutic concentrations). Products include:
Zonegran Capsules **1089**

TRILEPTAL ORAL SUSPENSION

(Oxcarbazepine) **2281**
See Trileptal Tablets

TRILEPTAL TABLETS

(Oxcarbazepine) **2281**
May interact with dihydropyridine calcium channel blockers, phenytoin, valproate, and certain other agents. Compounds in these categories include:

Amlodipine Besylate (Oxcarbazepine and MHD induce a subgroup of the CYP4503A family responsible for the metabolism of dihydropyridine calcium channel antagonists, resulting in a lower plasma concentration of these drugs). Products include:
Caduet Tablets **2507**
Lotrel Capsules **2238**
Norvasc Tablets **2529**

Carbamazepine (Co-administration with carbamazepine decreases the plasma levels of MHD (29% to 40%)). Products include:
Carbatrol Capsules **3174**
Equetro Extended-Release
Capsules **3178**
Tegretol/Tegretol-XR **2278**

Divalproex Sodium (Co-administration decreases MHD concentration by 18%). Products include:
Depakote Sprinkle Capsules **422**
Depakote Tablets **427**
Depakote ER Tablets **433**

Ethinyl Estradiol (Co-administration with an oral contraceptive containing ethinyl estradiol and levonorgestrel results in the decreased mean AUC value of EE by 48% to 52%, therefore, concurrent use of Trileptal with hormonal contraceptives may render these contraceptives less effective; studies with other oral or implant contraceptives have not been studied). Products include:
Alesse-28 Tablets **3392**
Lo/Ovral-28 Tablets **3423**
NuvaRing **2357**
Ortho-Cept Tablets **2395**
Ortho-Cyclen/Ortho Tri-Cyclen **2414**
Ortho Evra Transdermal System **2402**
Ortho Tri-Cyclen Lo Tablets **2421**
Seasonale Tablets **1073**
Triphasil-28 Tablets **3483**
Yasmin 28 Tablets **818**

Felodipine (Repeated co-administration of Trileptal lowers felodipine AUC by 28%). Products include:
Plendil Extended-Release Tablets **651**

Fosphenytoin Sodium (Co-administration increases the plasma phenytoin levels by up to 40%; phenytoin decreases the plasma levels of its active metabolite monohydroxy metabolite (MHD); a decrease in the dose of phenytoin may be required).
No products indexed under this heading.

Isradipine (Oxcarbazepine and MHD induce a subgroup of the CYP4503A family responsible for the metabolism of dihydropyridine calcium channel antagonists, resulting in a lower plasma concentration of these drugs). Products include:
DynaCirc CR Tablets **2726**

Levonorgestrel (Co-administration with an oral contraceptive containing ethinyl estradiol and levonorgestrel results in the decreased mean AUC value of EE by 48% to 52%, therefore, concurrent use of Trileptal with hormonal contraceptives may render these contraceptives less effective; studies with other oral or implant contraceptives have not been studied). Products include:
Alesse-28 Tablets **3392**
Climara Pro Transdermal System **800**
Mirena Intrauterine System **810**
Plan B Tablets **1068**
Seasonale Tablets **1073**
Triphasil-28 Tablets **3483**

Nicardipine Hydrochloride (Oxcarbazepine and MHD induce a subgroup of the CYP4503A family responsible for the metabolism of dihydropyridine calcium channel antagonists, resulting in a lower plasma concentration of these drugs). Products include:
Cardene I.V. **1129**

Nifedipine (Oxcarbazepine and MHD induce a subgroup of the CYP4503A family responsible for the metabolism of dihydropyridine calcium channel antagonists, resulting in a lower plasma concentration of these drugs). Products include:
Adalat CC Tablets **2978**

Nimodipine (Oxcarbazepine and MHD induce a subgroup of the CYP4503A family responsible for the metabolism of dihydropyridine calcium channel antagonists, resulting in a lower plasma concentration of these drugs). Products include:
Nimotop Capsules **774**

Phenobarbital (Co-administration with phenobarbital decreases the plasma levels of MHD (29% to 40%); concurrent use increases the phenobarbital level by approximately 15%).
No products indexed under this heading.

Phenytoin (Co-administration increases the plasma phenytoin levels by up to 40%; phenytoin decreases the plasma levels of its active metabolite monohydroxy metabolite (MHD); a decrease in the dose of phenytoin may be required).
No products indexed under this heading.

Phenytoin Sodium (Co-administration increases the plasma phenytoin levels by up to 40%; phenytoin decreases the plasma levels of its active metabolite monohydroxy metabolite (MHD); a decrease in the dose of phenytoin may be required). Products include:
Phenytek Capsules **2153**

Valproate Sodium (Co-administration decreases MHD concentration by 18%). Products include:
Depacon Injection **412**

Valproic Acid (Co-administration decreases MHD concentration by 18%). Products include:
Depakene **417**

Verapamil Hydrochloride (Produces a decrease of 20% of the plasma levels of MHD). Products include:
Covera-HS Tablets **3135**
Tarka Tablets **519**
Verelan PM Capsules **3120**

Food Interactions

Alcohol (Oxcarbazepine causes dizziness and somnolence, concurrent use with alcohol could result in possible additive sedative effect).

TRI-LUMA CREAM

(Fluocinolone Acetonide, Hydroquinone, Tretinoin) **1213**
May interact with drugs known to be photosensitizers and certain other agents. Compounds in these categories include:

Acetazolamide (Patients should be cautioned on concomitant use of medications that are known to be photosensitizing).
No products indexed under this heading.

Acitretin (Patients should be cautioned on concomitant use of medications that are known to be photosensitizing). Products include:
Soriatane Capsules **1028**

Alatrofloxacin Mesylate (Patients should be cautioned on concomitant use of medications that are known to be photosensitizing).
No products indexed under this heading.

Anthralin (Patients should be cautioned on concomitant use of medications that are known to be photosensitizing). Products include:
Psoriatec Cream **3191**

Bendroflumethiazide (Patients should be cautioned on concomitant use of medications that are known to be photosensitizing).
No products indexed under this heading.

Chlorothiazide (Patients should be cautioned on concomitant use of medications that are known to be photosensitizing). Products include:
Aldoclor Tablets 1881
Diuril Oral 1936

Chlorothiazide Sodium (Patients should be cautioned on concomitant use of medications that are known to be photosensitizing). Products include:
Diuril Sodium Intravenous 1934

Chlorpromazine (Patients should be cautioned on concomitant use of medications that are known to be photosensitizing).
No products indexed under this heading.

Chlorpromazine Hydrochloride (Patients should be cautioned on concomitant use of medications that are known to be photosensitizing).
No products indexed under this heading.

Chlorpropamide (Patients should be cautioned on concomitant use of medications that are known to be photosensitizing).
No products indexed under this heading.

Ciprofloxacin (Patients should be cautioned on concomitant use of medications that are known to be photosensitizing). Products include:
Cipro I.V. 2998
Cipro I.V. Pharmacy Bulk Package ... 3509
Cipro Oral Suspension 2991
Cipro XR Tablets 3004
Ciprodex Otic Suspension 555

Ciprofloxacin Hydrochloride (Patients should be cautioned on concomitant use of medications that are known to be photosensitizing). Products include:
Ciloxan Ophthalmic Ointment 554
Cipro Tablets 2991

Coal Tar (Patients should be cautioned on concomitant use of medications that are known to be photosensitizing). Products include:
Tegrin Dandruff Shampoo - Extra Conditioning 637
Tegrin Dandruff Shampoo - Fresh Herbal 638
Tegrin Skin Cream 638

Demeclocycline Hydrochloride (Patients should be cautioned on concomitant use of medications that are known to be photosensitizing).
No products indexed under this heading.

Doxycycline Calcium (Patients should be cautioned on concomitant use of medications that are known to be photosensitizing).
No products indexed under this heading.

Doxycycline Hyclate (Patients should be cautioned on concomitant use of medications that are known to be photosensitizing).
No products indexed under this heading.

Doxycycline Monohydrate (Patients should be cautioned on concomitant use of medications that are known to be photosensitizing).
No products indexed under this heading.

Enoxacin (Patients should be cautioned on concomitant use of medications that are known to be photosensitizing).
No products indexed under this heading.

Fluphenazine Decanoate (Patients should be cautioned on concomitant use of medications that are known to be photosensitizing).
No products indexed under this heading.

Fluphenazine Enanthate (Patients should be cautioned on concomitant use of medications that are known to be photosensitizing).
No products indexed under this heading.

Fluphenazine Hydrochloride (Patients should be cautioned on concomitant use of medications that are known to be photosensitizing).
No products indexed under this heading.

Furosemide (Patients should be cautioned on concomitant use of medications that are known to be photosensitizing). Products include:
Furosemide Tablets 2117

Glipizide (Patients should be cautioned on concomitant use of medications that are known to be photosensitizing).
No products indexed under this heading.

Glyburide (Patients should be cautioned on concomitant use of medications that are known to be photosensitizing).
No products indexed under this heading.

Grepafloxacin Hydrochloride (Patients should be cautioned on concomitant use of medications that are known to be photosensitizing).
No products indexed under this heading.

Griseofulvin (Patients should be cautioned on concomitant use of medications that are known to be photosensitizing). Products include:
Grifulvin V Tablets Microsize and Oral Suspension Microsize 2384
Gris-PEG Tablets 2504

Hydrochlorothiazide (Patients should be cautioned on concomitant use of medications that are known to be photosensitizing). Products include:
Aldoril Tablets 1884
Atacand HCT 637
Avalide Tablets 2889
Avalide Tablets 922
Benicar HCT Tablets 2852
Diovan HCT Tablets 2195
Dyazide Capsules 1389
Hyzaar 1964
Lotensin HCT Tablets 2235
Maxzide 2150
Micardis HCT Tablets 886
Moduretic Tablets 2003
Prinzide Tablets 2033
Teveten HCT Tablets 1710
Timolide Tablets 2056
Uniretic Tablets 3114
Vaseretic Tablets 2073
Zestoretic Tablets 701

Hydroflumethiazide (Patients should be cautioned on concomitant use of medications that are known to be photosensitizing).
No products indexed under this heading.

Lomefloxacin Hydrochloride (Patients should be cautioned on concomitant use of medications that are known to be photosensitizing).
No products indexed under this heading.

Mesoridazine Besylate (Patients should be cautioned on concomitant use of medications that are known to be photosensitizing).
No products indexed under this heading.

Metabromsalan (Patients should be cautioned on concomitant use of medications that are known to be photosensitizing).
No products indexed under this heading.

Methacycline Hydrochloride (Patients should be cautioned on concomitant use of medications that are known to be photosensitizing).
No products indexed under this heading.

Methotrimeprazine (Patients should be cautioned on concomitant use of medications that are known to be photosensitizing).
No products indexed under this heading.

Methyclothiazide (Patients should be cautioned on concomitant use of medications that are known to be photosensitizing).
No products indexed under this heading.

Minocycline Hydrochloride (Patients should be cautioned on concomitant use of medications that are known to be photosensitizing). Products include:
Dynacin Tablets 1859

Nalidixic Acid (Patients should be cautioned on concomitant use of medications that are known to be photosensitizing).
No products indexed under this heading.

Norfloxacin (Patients should be cautioned on concomitant use of medications that are known to be photosensitizing). Products include:
Noroxin Tablets 2009

Ofloxacin (Patients should be cautioned on concomitant use of medications that are known to be photosensitizing). Products include:
Floxin Otic Singles 1045
Floxin Otic Solution 1043

Oxytetracycline Hydrochloride (Patients should be cautioned on concomitant use of medications that are known to be photosensitizing).
No products indexed under this heading.

Perphenazine (Patients should be cautioned on concomitant use of medications that are known to be photosensitizing).
No products indexed under this heading.

Polythiazide (Patients should be cautioned on concomitant use of medications that are known to be photosensitizing).
No products indexed under this heading.

Prochlorperazine (Patients should be cautioned on concomitant use of medications that are known to be photosensitizing).
No products indexed under this heading.

Promethazine Hydrochloride (Patients should be cautioned on concomitant use of medications that are known to be photosensitizing). Products include:
Phenergan 3438

Salicylic Acid (Patients should avoid products containing keratolytic agents).
No products indexed under this heading.

Sulfamethizole (Patients should be cautioned on concomitant use of medications that are known to be photosensitizing).
No products indexed under this heading.

Sulfamethoxazole (Patients should be cautioned on concomitant use of medications that are known to be photosensitizing).
No products indexed under this heading.

Sulfasalazine (Patients should be cautioned on concomitant use of medications that are known to be photosensitizing).
No products indexed under this heading.

Sulfinpyrazone (Patients should be cautioned on concomitant use of medications that are known to be photosensitizing).
No products indexed under this heading.

Sulfisoxazole (Patients should be cautioned on concomitant use of medications that are known to be photosensitizing).
No products indexed under this heading.

Sulfisoxazole Acetyl (Patients should be cautioned on concomitant use of medications that are known to be photosensitizing).
No products indexed under this heading.

Sulfisoxazole Diolamine (Patients should be cautioned on concomitant use of medications that are known to be photosensitizing).
No products indexed under this heading.

Tetrachlorosalicylanilide (Patients should be cautioned on concomitant use of medications that are known to be photosensitizing).
No products indexed under this heading.

Tetracycline Hydrochloride (Patients should be cautioned on concomitant use of medications that are known to be photosensitizing).
No products indexed under this heading.

Thioridazine Hydrochloride (Patients should be cautioned on concomitant use of medications that are known to be photosensitizing). Products include:
Thioridazine Hydrochloride Tablets 2122

Tolazamide (Patients should be cautioned on concomitant use of medications that are known to be photosensitizing).
No products indexed under this heading.

Tolbutamide (Patients should be cautioned on concomitant use of medications that are known to be photosensitizing).
No products indexed under this heading.

Trifluoperazine Hydrochloride (Patients should be cautioned on concomitant use of medications that are known to be photosensitizing).
No products indexed under this heading.

Trovafloxacin Mesylate (Patients should be cautioned on concomitant use of medications that are known to be photosensitizing).
No products indexed under this heading.

Food Interactions

Alcohol (Patients should avoid topical products containing high alcohol concentrations).

TRILYTE WITH FLAVOR PACKS FOR ORAL SOLUTION

(PEG-3350, Potassium Chloride, Sodium Bicarbonate, Sodium Chloride)........ 3114
May interact with:

Oral Medications, unspecified (Oral medication administered within one hour of the start of administration of TriLyte with flavor packs may be flushed from the gastrointestinal tract and not absorbed).

TRIPHASIL-28 TABLETS

(Ethinyl Estradiol, Levonorgestrel) 3483
May interact with barbiturates, corticosteroids, penicillins, phenytoin, protease inhibitors, tetracyclines, xanthines, and certain other agents. Compounds in these categories include:

Acetaminophen (Co-administration increases plasma ethinyl estradiol levels possibly by inhibition of conjugation; decreased plasma levels of acetaminophen). Products include:
- Benadryl Allergy & Cold Tablets ..... ▣692
- Benadryl Allergy & Sinus Headache Caplets & Gelcaps...... ▣693
- Benadryl Maximum Strength Severe Allergy & Sinus Headache Caplets........ ▣694
- Contac Severe Cold and Flu Caplets Maximum Strength........ ▣615
- Contac Severe Cold and Flu Caplets Non-Drowsy........ ▣615
- Darvocet A 500 Tablets 3497
- Goody's Body Pain Formula Powder........ ▣621
- Goody's Extra Strength Headache Powder........ ▣621
- Goody's Extra Strength Pain Relief Tablets .... ▣621
- Goody's PM Powder .... ▣622
- Hycomine Compound Tablets 1105
- Lortab 3315
- Lortab Elixir 3312
- Percocet Tablets 1114
- Robitussin Cough, Cold & Flu Liquid-filled Capsules........ ▣750
- Robitussin Flu Liquid .... ▣752
- Sedapap Tablets 50 mg/650 mg 2098
- Singlet Caplets .... ▣636
- Sudafed Severe Cold .... ▣710
- Sudafed Sinus Headache .... ▣711
- TheraFlu Cold & Cough Hot Liquid .... ▣680
- TheraFlu Cold & Sore Throat Hot Liquid .... ▣680
- TheraFlu Flu & Chest Congestion Non-Drowsy Hot Liquid........ ▣681
- TheraFlu Flu & Sore Throat Hot Liquid .... ▣681
- TheraFlu Severe Cold Non-Drowsy Hot Liquid........ ▣683
- TheraFlu Severe Cold & Cough Hot Liquid........ ▣683
- TheraFlu Severe Cold Caplets .... ▣679
- TheraFlu Severe Cold Hot Liquid .... ▣682
- TheraFlu Severe Cold Non-Drowsy Caplets........ ▣679
- Triaminic Cough & Sore Throat Liquid .... ▣687
- Triaminic Flu, Cough & Fever Liquid .... ▣685
- Triaminic Cough & Sore Throat Softchews .... ▣689
- Tylenol 8 Hour Extended Release Geltabs and Caplets 1843
- Tylenol Sinus NightTime Caplets .... ▣663
- Children's Tylenol Suspension Liquid and Meltaways........ 1850
- Children's Tylenol Plus Cold & Allergy Suspension Liquid 1850
- Children's Tylenol Plus Cold NightTime Suspension Liquid........ 1851
- Children's Tylenol Plus Cold & Cough Suspension Liquid and Chewable Tablets 1851
- Children's Tylenol Plus Cold Chewable Tablets 1851
- Children's Tylenol Plus Cold Daytime Non-Drowsy Suspension Liquid 1851
- Children's Tylenol Plus Flu Suspension Liquid 1853
- Concentrated Tylenol Infants' Drops Plus Cold........ 1851
- Concentrated Tylenol Infants' Drops Plus Cold and Cough 1851
- Concentrated Tylenol Infants' Drops........ 1850
- Junior Tylenol Meltaways 1850
- Tylenol Cold & Flu Severe Daytime Liquid with Cool Bust....... 1846
- Tylenol Cold & Flu Severe NightTime Liquid with Cool Burst........ 1846
- Tylenol Cold Severe Congestion Non-Drowsy Caplets with Cool Burst........ 1846
- Tylenol Cough & Sore Throat Daytime Liquid with Cool Burst...... 1849
- Tylenol Cough & Sore Throat NightTime Liquid with Cool Burst........ 1849
- Tylenol 1843
- Extra Strength Tylenol Rapid Release Gels 1843
- Tylenol 1843
- Tylenol Allergy Complete Night Time Caplets 1844
- Tylenol Allergy Complete Multi-Symptom Caplets and Gelcaps with Cool Burst........ 1844
- Tylenol Severe Allergy Caplets 1844
- Tylenol Flu NightTime Gelcaps 1846
- Tylenol Flu Day Non-Drowsy Gelcaps........ 1846
- Concentrated Tylenol Infants' Drops Plus Cold Nasal Congestant, Fever Reducer & Pain Reliever .... ▣668
- Concentrated Tylenol Infants' Drops Plus Cold & Cough Nasal Decongestant, Fever Reducer & Pain Reliever........ ▣668
- Multi-Symptom Tylenol Cold Night Time Caplets........ 1845
- Multi-Symptom Tylenol Cold Day Non-Drowsy Caplets and Gelcaps........ 1845
- Extra Strength Tylenol PM Caplets, Geltabs, Gelcaps and Liquid........ 1847
- Tylenol Sinus Day Non-Drowsy 1848
- Tylenol Sinus Night Time Caplets 1848
- Tylenol Sinus Severe Congestion Caplets with Cool Burst........ 1848
- Tylenol Sore Throat Daytime Liquid with Cool Burst........ 1849
- Tylenol Sore Throat NightTime Liquid with Cool Burst........ 1849
- Tylenol with Codeine 2461
- Women's Tylenol Menstrual Relief Caplets........ 1849
- Ultracet Tablets 2462
- Vicks 44M Cough, Cold & Flu Relief........ 2676
- Vicks DayQuil LiquiCaps/Liquid Multi-Symptom Cold/Flu Relief..... ▣723
- Vicks DayQuil Multi-Symptom Cold/Flu Relief LiquiCaps........ 2675
- Vicks DayQuil Multi-Symptom Cold/Flu Relief Liquid........ 2675
- Vicks NyQuil LiquiCaps 2677
- Vicks NyQuil LiquiCaps/Liquid Multi-Symptom Cold/Flu Relief..... ▣725
- Vicks NyQuil Liquid 2677
- Vicodin Tablets 530
- Vicodin ES Tablets 531
- Vicodin HP Tablets 532
- Zydone Tablets 1118

Aminophylline (Co-administration increases the plasma concentrations of theophylline).
No products indexed under this heading.

Amoxicillin (Ampicillin, another penicillin may decrease plasma ethinyl estradiol concentrations by a decrease of enterohepatic circulation of estrogens leading to reduced contraceptive effectiveness, increased incidence of breakthrough bleeding and menstrual irregularities). Products include:
- Amoxil Capsules 1315
- Amoxil Chewable Tablets 1315
- Amoxil Pediatric Drops for Oral Suspension 1315
- Amoxil Powder for Oral Suspension 1315
- Amoxil Tablets 1315
- Augmentin 1331
- Augmentin Tablets 1334
- Augmentin XR Extended-Release Tablets 1340
- Augmentin ES-600 Powder for Oral Suspension 1337
- PREVPAC 3281

Amoxicillin Trihydrate (Ampicillin, another penicillin may decrease plasma ethinyl estradiol concentrations by a decrease of enterohepatic circulation of estrogens leading to reduced contraceptive effectiveness, increased incidence of breakthrough bleeding and menstrual irregularities).
No products indexed under this heading.

Ampicillin (May decrease plasma ethinyl estradiol concentrations by a decrease of enterohepatic circulation of estrogens leading to reduced contraceptive effectiveness, increased incidence of breakthrough bleeding and menstrual irregularities).
No products indexed under this heading.

Ampicillin Sodium (May decrease plasma ethinyl estradiol concentrations by a decrease of enterohepatic circulation of estrogens leading to reduced contraceptive effectiveness, increased incidence of breakthrough bleeding and menstrual irregularities).
No products indexed under this heading.

Ampicillin Trihydrate (Ampicillin, another penicillin may decrease plasma ethinyl estradiol concentrations by a decrease of enterohepatic circulation of estrogens leading to reduced contraceptive effectiveness, increased incidence of breakthrough bleeding and menstrual irregularities).
No products indexed under this heading.

Amprenavir (Some protease inhibitors increase the metabolism of ethinyl estradiol resulting in decreased plasma concentrations leading to reduced contraceptive effectiveness, increased incidence of breakthrough bleeding and menstrual irregularities). Products include:
- Agenerase Capsules 1299
- Agenerase Oral Solution 1304

Aprobarbital (Barbiturates increase the metabolism of ethinyl estradiol resulting in decreased plasma concentrations leading to reduced contraceptive effectiveness, increased incidence of breakthrough bleeding and menstrual irregularities).
No products indexed under this heading.

Atorvastatin Calcium (Co-administration may result in increased ethinyl estradiol plasma concentrations). Products include:
- Caduet Tablets 2507
- Lipitor Tablets 2495

Azlocillin Sodium (Ampicillin, another penicillin may decrease plasma ethinyl estradiol concentrations by a decrease of enterohepatic circulation of estrogens leading to reduced contraceptive effectiveness, increased incidence of breakthrough bleeding and menstrual irregularities).
No products indexed under this heading.

Bacampicillin Hydrochloride (Ampicillin, another penicillin may decrease plasma ethinyl estradiol concentrations by a decrease of enterohepatic circulation of estrogens leading to reduced contraceptive effectiveness, increased incidence of breakthrough bleeding and menstrual irregularities).
No products indexed under this heading.

Betamethasone Acetate (Co-administration with corticosteroids increases the plasma concentrations of corticosteroids).
No products indexed under this heading.

Betamethasone Sodium Phosphate (Co-administration with corticosteroids increases the plasma concentrations of corticosteroids).
No products indexed under this heading.

Butabarbital (Barbiturates increase the metabolism of ethinyl estradiol resulting in decreased plasma concentrations leading to reduced contraceptive effectiveness, increased incidence of breakthrough bleeding and menstrual irregularities).
No products indexed under this heading.

Butalbital (Barbiturates increase the metabolism of ethinyl estradiol resulting in decreased plasma concentrations leading to reduced contraceptive effectiveness, increased incidence of breakthrough bleeding and menstrual irregularities). Products include:
- Sedapap Tablets 50 mg/650 mg 2098

Carbenicillin Disodium (Ampicillin, another penicillin may decrease plasma ethinyl estradiol concentrations by a decrease of enterohepatic circulation of estrogens leading to reduced contraceptive effectiveness, increased incidence of breakthrough bleeding and menstrual irregularities).
No products indexed under this heading.

(▣ Described in PDR For Nonprescription Drugs) (⊙ Described in PDR For Ophthalmic Medicines™)

Carbenicillin Indanyl Sodium (Ampicillin, another penicillin may decrease plasma ethinyl estradiol concentrations by a decrease of enterohepatic circulation of estrogens leading to reduced contraceptive effectiveness, increased incidence of breakthrough bleeding and menstrual irregularities).
No products indexed under this heading.

Cortisone Acetate (Co-administration with corticosteroids increases the plasma concentrations of corticosteroids).
No products indexed under this heading.

Cyclosporine (Co-administration increases the plasma concentrations of cyclosporine). Products include:
- Gengraf Capsules 458
- Neoral Soft Gelatin Capsules 2247
- Neoral Oral Solution 2247
- Restasis Ophthalmic Emulsion 570
- Sandimmune 2259

Demeclocycline Hydrochloride (May decrease plasma ethinyl estradiol concentrations by a decrease of enterohepatic circulation of estrogens leading to reduced contraceptive effectiveness, increased incidence of breakthrough bleeding and menstrual irregularities).
No products indexed under this heading.

Dexamethasone (Co-administration with corticosteroids increases the plasma concentrations of corticosteroids). Products include:
- Ciprodex Otic Suspension 555
- Decadron Tablets 1929
- TobraDex Ophthalmic Ointment 558
- TobraDex Ophthalmic Suspension 558

Dexamethasone Acetate (Co-administration with corticosteroids increases the plasma concentrations of corticosteroids).
No products indexed under this heading.

Dexamethasone Sodium Phosphate (Co-administration with corticosteroids increases the plasma concentrations of corticosteroids). Products include:
- Decadron Phosphate Injection 1931

Dicloxacillin Sodium (Ampicillin, another penicillin may decrease plasma ethinyl estradiol concentrations by a decrease of enterohepatic circulation of estrogens leading to reduced contraceptive effectiveness, increased incidence of breakthrough bleeding and menstrual irregularities).
No products indexed under this heading.

Doxycycline Calcium (May decrease plasma ethinyl estradiol concentrations by a decrease of enterohepatic circulation of estrogens leading to reduced contraceptive effectiveness, increased incidence of breakthrough bleeding and menstrual irregularities).
No products indexed under this heading.

Doxycycline Hyclate (May decrease plasma ethinyl estradiol concentrations by a decrease of enterohepatic circulation of estrogens leading to reduced contraceptive effectiveness, increased incidence of breakthrough bleeding and menstrual irregularities).
No products indexed under this heading.

Doxycycline Monohydrate (May decrease plasma ethinyl estradiol concentrations by a decrease of enterohepatic circulation of estrogens leading to reduced contraceptive effectiveness, increased incidence of breakthrough bleeding and menstrual irregularities).
No products indexed under this heading.

Dyphylline (Co-administration increases the plasma concentrations of theophylline).
No products indexed under this heading.

Edrophonium Chloride (Co-administration with drugs that increases gastrointestinal motility and reduces gut transit time may reduce ethinyl estradiol plasma concentrations).
No products indexed under this heading.

Fluconazole (Co-administration with CYP 3A4 inhibitors may increase plasma ethinyl estradiol levels).
No products indexed under this heading.

Fludrocortisone Acetate (Co-administration with corticosteroids increases the plasma concentrations of corticosteroids).
No products indexed under this heading.

Fosphenytoin Sodium (Increases the metabolism of ethinyl estradiol resulting in decreased plasma concentrations leading to reduced contraceptive effectiveness, increased incidence of breakthrough bleeding and menstrual irregularities).
No products indexed under this heading.

Griseofulvin (Increases the metabolism of ethinyl estradiol resulting in decreased plasma concentrations leading to reduced contraceptive effectiveness, increased incidence of breakthrough bleeding and menstrual irregularities). Products include:
- Grifulvin V Tablets Microsize and Oral Suspension Microsize 2384
- Gris-PEG Tablets 2504

Hydrocortisone (Co-administration with corticosteroids increases the plasma concentrations of corticosteroids). Products include:
- Cortizone•5 Ointment 699
- Cortizone•10 Creme 699
- Cortizone•10 Ointment 699
- Cortizone•10 Plus Creme 700
- Cortizone•10 Maximum Strength Quick Shot Spray 700
- Hydrocortone Tablets 1963
- Preparation H Hydrocortisone Cream 748

Hydrocortisone Acetate (Co-administration with corticosteroids increases the plasma concentrations of corticosteroids). Products include:
- Analpram-HC 1136
- Pramosone 1139
- ProctoFoam-HC 3113
- Tucks Anti-Itch Ointment 712
- U-cort 1% Cream 3289

Hydrocortisone Sodium Phosphate (Co-administration with corticosteroids increases the plasma concentrations of corticosteroids).
No products indexed under this heading.

Hydrocortisone Sodium Succinate (Co-administration with corticosteroids increases the plasma concentrations of corticosteroids).
No products indexed under this heading.

Hypericum (Increases the metabolism of ethinyl estradiol resulting in decreased plasma concentrations leading to reduced contraceptive effectiveness, increased incidence of breakthrough bleeding and menstrual irregularities).
No products indexed under this heading.

Indinavir Sulfate (Co-administration with CYP 3A4 inhibitors may increase plasma ethinyl estradiol levels). Products include:
- Crixivan Capsules 1918

Itraconazole (Co-administration with CYP 3A4 inhibitors may increase plasma ethinyl estradiol levels).
No products indexed under this heading.

Ketoconazole (Co-administration with CYP 3A4 inhibitors may increase plasma ethinyl estradiol levels). Products include:
- Nizoral A-D Shampoo, 1% 1839
- Nizoral 2% Shampoo 1838

Lopinavir (Some protease inhibitors increase the metabolism of ethinyl estradiol resulting in decreased plasma concentrations leading to reduced contraceptive effectiveness, increased incidence of breakthrough bleeding and menstrual irregularities). Products include:
- Kaletra 474

Mephobarbital (Barbiturates increase the metabolism of ethinyl estradiol resulting in decreased plasma concentrations leading to reduced contraceptive effectiveness, increased incidence of breakthrough bleeding and menstrual irregularities). Products include:
- Mebaral Tablets, USP 2483

Methacycline Hydrochloride (May decrease plasma ethinyl estradiol concentrations by a decrease of enterohepatic circulation of estrogens leading to reduced contraceptive effectiveness, increased incidence of breakthrough bleeding and menstrual irregularities).
No products indexed under this heading.

Methylprednisolone Acetate (Co-administration with corticosteroids increases the plasma concentrations of corticosteroids). Products include:
- Depo-Medrol Injectable Suspension 2615
- Depo-Medrol Single-Dose Vial 2617

Methylprednisolone Sodium Succinate (Co-administration with corticosteroids increases the plasma concentrations of corticosteroids).
No products indexed under this heading.

Mezlocillin Sodium (Ampicillin, another penicillin may decrease plasma ethinyl estradiol concentrations by a decrease of enterohepatic circulation of estrogens leading to reduced contraceptive effectiveness, increased incidence of breakthrough bleeding and menstrual irregularities).
No products indexed under this heading.

Minocycline Hydrochloride (May decrease plasma ethinyl estradiol concentrations by a decrease of enterohepatic circulation of estrogens leading to reduced contraceptive effectiveness, increased incidence of breakthrough bleeding and menstrual irregularities). Products include:
- Dynacin Tablets 1859

Modafinil (Increases the metabolism of ethinyl estradiol resulting in decreased plasma concentrations leading to reduced contraceptive effectiveness, increased incidence of breakthrough bleeding and menstrual irregularities). Products include:
- Provigil Tablets 1002

Nafcillin Sodium (Ampicillin, another penicillin may decrease plasma ethinyl estradiol concentrations by a decrease of enterohepatic circulation of estrogens leading to reduced contraceptive effectiveness, increased incidence of breakthrough bleeding and menstrual irregularities).
No products indexed under this heading.

Nelfinavir Mesylate (Some protease inhibitors increase the metabolism of ethinyl estradiol resulting in decreased plasma concentrations leading to reduced contraceptive effectiveness, increased incidence of breakthrough bleeding and menstrual irregularities). Products include:
- Viracept 2556

Neostigmine Bromide (Co-administration with drugs that increases gastrointestinal motility and reduces gut transit time may reduce ethinyl estradiol plasma concentrations).
No products indexed under this heading.

Neostigmine Methylsulfate (Co-administration with drugs that increases gastrointestinal motility and reduces gut transit time may reduce ethinyl estradiol plasma concentrations).
No products indexed under this heading.

Oxytetracycline Hydrochloride (May decrease plasma ethinyl estradiol concentrations by a decrease of enterohepatic circulation of estrogens leading to reduced contraceptive effectiveness, increased incidence of breakthrough bleeding and menstrual irregularities).
No products indexed under this heading.

Penicillin G Benzathine (Ampicillin, another penicillin may decrease plasma ethinyl estradiol concentrations by a decrease of enterohepatic circulation of estrogens leading to reduced contraceptive effectiveness, increased incidence of breakthrough bleeding and menstrual irregularities).
No products indexed under this heading.

Penicillin G Potassium (Ampicillin, another penicillin may decrease plasma ethinyl estradiol concentrations by a decrease of enterohepatic circulation of estrogens leading to reduced contraceptive effectiveness, increased incidence of breakthrough bleeding and menstrual irregularities).
No products indexed under this heading.

Penicillin G Procaine (Ampicillin, another penicillin may decrease plasma ethinyl estradiol concentrations by a decrease of enterohepatic circulation of estrogens leading to reduced contraceptive effectiveness, increased incidence of breakthrough bleeding and menstrual irregularities).
No products indexed under this heading.

Penicillin G Sodium (Ampicillin, another penicillin may decrease plasma ethinyl estradiol concentrations by a decrease of enterohepatic circulation of estrogens leading to reduced contraceptive effectiveness, increased incidence of breakthrough bleeding and menstrual irregularities).
No products indexed under this heading.

Penicillin V Potassium (Ampicillin, another penicillin may decrease plasma ethinyl estradiol concentrations by a decrease of enterohepatic circulation of estrogens leading to reduced contraceptive effectiveness, increased incidence of breakthrough bleeding and menstrual irregularities).
No products indexed under this heading.

Pentobarbital Sodium (Barbiturates increase the metabolism of ethinyl estradiol resulting in decreased plasma concentrations leading to reduced contraceptive effectiveness, increased incidence of breakthrough bleeding and menstrual irregularities). Products include:
Nembutal Sodium Solution, USP...... **2484**

Phenobarbital (Barbiturates increase the metabolism of ethinyl estradiol resulting in decreased plasma concentrations leading to reduced contraceptive effectiveness, increased incidence of breakthrough bleeding and menstrual irregularities).
No products indexed under this heading.

Phenylbutazone (Increases the metabolism of ethinyl estradiol resulting in decreased plasma concentrations leading to reduced contraceptive effectiveness, increased incidence of breakthrough bleeding and menstrual irregularities).
No products indexed under this heading.

Phenytoin (Increases the metabolism of ethinyl estradiol resulting in decreased plasma concentrations leading to reduced contraceptive effectiveness, increased incidence of breakthrough bleeding and menstrual irregularities).
No products indexed under this heading.

Phenytoin Sodium (Increases the metabolism of ethinyl estradiol resulting in decreased plasma concentrations leading to reduced contraceptive effectiveness, increased incidence of breakthrough bleeding and menstrual irregularities). Products include:
Phenytek Capsules.......................... **2153**

Prednisolone Acetate (Co-administration with corticosteroids increases the plasma concentrations of corticosteroids). Products include:
Blephamide Ophthalmic Ointment.... **563**
Blephamide Ophthalmic Suspension.................................. **564**
Poly-Pred Liquifilm Ophthalmic Suspension................................ ⊙ **231**
Pred Forte Ophthalmic Suspension................................ ⊙ **233**
Pred Mild Sterile Ophthalmic Suspension................................ ⊙ **236**
Pred-G Ophthalmic Suspension ...... ⊙ **234**
Pred-G Sterile Ophthalmic Ointment.................................. ⊙ **235**

Prednisolone Sodium Phosphate (Co-administration with corticosteroids increases the plasma concentrations of corticosteroids). Products include:
Pediapred Oral Solution.................. **3319**

Prednisolone Tebutate (Co-administration with corticosteroids increases the plasma concentrations of corticosteroids).
No products indexed under this heading.

Prednisone (Co-administration with corticosteroids increases the plasma concentrations of corticosteroids).
No products indexed under this heading.

Pyridostigmine Bromide (Co-administration with drugs that increases gastrointestinal motility and reduces gut transit time may reduce ethinyl estradiol plasma concentrations).
No products indexed under this heading.

Rifabutin (Increases the metabolism of ethinyl estradiol resulting in decreased plasma concentrations leading to reduced contraceptive effectiveness, increased incidence of breakthrough bleeding and menstrual irregularities).
No products indexed under this heading.

Rifampin (Increases the metabolism of ethinyl estradiol resulting in decreased plasma concentrations leading to reduced contraceptive effectiveness, increased incidence of breakthrough bleeding and menstrual irregularities).
No products indexed under this heading.

Ritonavir (Some protease inhibitors increase the metabolism of ethinyl estradiol resulting in decreased plasma concentrations leading to reduced contraceptive effectiveness, increased incidence of breakthrough bleeding and menstrual irregularities). Products include:
Kaletra.. **474**
Norvir.. **499**

Saquinavir (Some protease inhibitors increase the metabolism of ethinyl estradiol resulting in decreased plasma concentrations leading to reduced contraceptive effectiveness, increased incidence of breakthrough bleeding and menstrual irregularities).
No products indexed under this heading.

Saquinavir Mesylate (Some protease inhibitors increase the metabolism of ethinyl estradiol resulting in decreased plasma concentrations leading to reduced contraceptive effectiveness, increased incidence of breakthrough bleeding and menstrual irregularities). Products include:
Invirase.. **2776**

Secobarbital Sodium (Barbiturates increase the metabolism of ethinyl estradiol resulting in decreased plasma concentrations leading to reduced contraceptive effectiveness, increased incidence of breakthrough bleeding and menstrual irregularities).
No products indexed under this heading.

Tetracycline Hydrochloride (May decrease plasma ethinyl estradiol concentrations by a decrease of enterohepatic circulation of estrogens leading to reduced contraceptive effectiveness, increased incidence of breakthrough bleeding and menstrual irregularities).
No products indexed under this heading.

Theophylline (Co-administration increases the plasma concentrations of theophylline).
No products indexed under this heading.

Theophylline Anhydrous (Co-administration increases the plasma concentrations of theophylline). Products include:
Uniphyl Tablets.............................. **2708**

Theophylline Calcium Salicylate (Co-administration increases the plasma concentrations of theophylline).
No products indexed under this heading.

Theophylline Dihydroxypropyl (Glyceryl) (Co-administration increases the plasma concentrations of theophylline).
No products indexed under this heading.

Theophylline Ethylenediamine (Co-administration increases the plasma concentrations of theophylline).
No products indexed under this heading.

Theophylline Sodium Glycinate (Co-administration increases the plasma concentrations of theophylline).
No products indexed under this heading.

Thiamylal Sodium (Barbiturates increase the metabolism of ethinyl estradiol resulting in decreased plasma concentrations leading to reduced contraceptive effectiveness, increased incidence of breakthrough bleeding and menstrual irregularities).
No products indexed under this heading.

Ticarcillin Disodium (Ampicillin, another penicillin may decrease plasma ethinyl estradiol concentrations by a decrease of enterohepatic circulation of estrogens leading to reduced contraceptive effectiveness, increased incidence of breakthrough bleeding and menstrual irregularities). Products include:
Timentin ADD-Vantage.................... **1556**
Timentin Injection Galaxy Container.................................. **1559**
Timentin IV Infusion **1553**
Timentin Pharmacy Bulk Package.... **1562**

Topiramate (Increases the metabolism of ethinyl estradiol resulting in decreased plasma concentrations leading to reduced contraceptive effectiveness, increased incidence of breakthrough bleeding and menstrual irregularities). Products include:
Topamax Sprinkle Capsules............ **2438**
Topamax Tablets............................ **2438**

Triamcinolone (Co-administration with corticosteroids increases the plasma concentrations of corticosteroids).
No products indexed under this heading.

Triamcinolone Acetonide (Co-administration with corticosteroids increases the plasma concentrations of corticosteroids). Products include:
Azmacort Inhalation Aerosol........... **1701**
Nasacort HFA Inhalation Aerosol...... **2939**
Nasacort AQ Nasal Spray.............. **2937**

Triamcinolone Diacetate (Co-administration with corticosteroids increases the plasma concentrations of corticosteroids).
No products indexed under this heading.

Triamcinolone Hexacetonide (Co-administration with corticosteroids increases the plasma concentrations of corticosteroids).
No products indexed under this heading.

Troleandomycin (Co-administration with CYP 3A4 inhibitors may increase plasma ethinyl estradiol levels; increased risk of intrahepatic cholestasis).
No products indexed under this heading.

Vitamin C (Co-administration increases plasma ethinyl estradiol levels possibly by inhibition of conjugation). Products include:
Chromagen Forte Soft Gelatin Capsules...................................... **3296**
Halls Defense Sugarfree Vitamin C Drops.................................... ▣ **611**
Niferex-150 Forte Capsules............ **3299**
Peridin-C Tablets............................ ▣ **761**
Repliva 21/7 Tablets...................... **3301**

TRISENOX INJECTION

(Arsenic Trioxide) **983**
May interact with potassium-depleting diuretics, quinidine, and certain other agents. Compounds in these categories include:

Amiodarone Hydrochloride (Arsenic trioxide can cause QT interval prolongation and complete AV block; QT prolongation can lead to torsade de pointes-type ventricular arrhythmias, which can be fatal; co-administration with other drugs that can prolong the QT interval, such as certain anti-arrhythmics, increases the risk and extent of QT prolongation). Products include:
Pacerone Tablets............................ **3337**

Amphotericin B (Arsenic trioxide can cause QT interval prolongation and complete AV block; QT prolongation can lead to torsade de pointes-type ventricular arrhythmias, which can be fatal; co-administration with other drugs that can prolong the QT interval, such as amphotericin B, increases the risk and extent of QT prolongation).
No products indexed under this heading.

Bendroflumethiazide (Arsenic trioxide can cause QT interval prolongation and complete AV block; QT prolongation can lead to torsade de pointes-type ventricular arrhythmias, which can be fatal; co-administration with other drugs that cause hypokalemia or hypomagnesemia resulting in prolongation of the QT interval, such as potassium-wasting diuretics, increases the risk and extent of QT

prolongation).
No products indexed under this heading.

Bumetanide (Arsenic trioxide can cause QT interval prolongation and complete AV block; QT prolongation can lead to torsade de pointes-type ventricular arrhythmias, which can be fatal; co-administration with other drugs that cause hypokalemia or hypomagnesemia resulting in prolongation of the QT interval, such as potassium-wasting diuretics, increases the risk and extent of QT prolongation).
No products indexed under this heading.

Chlorothiazide (Arsenic trioxide can cause QT interval prolongation and complete AV block; QT prolongation can lead to torsade de pointes-type ventricular arrhythmias, which can be fatal; co-administration with other drugs that cause hypokalemia or hypomagnesemia resulting in prolongation of the QT interval, such as potassium-wasting diuretics, increases the risk and extent of QT prolongation). Products include:
- Aldoclor Tablets 1881
- Diuril Oral 1936

Chlorothiazide Sodium (Arsenic trioxide can cause QT interval prolongation and complete AV block; QT prolongation can lead to torsade de pointes-type ventricular arrhythmias, which can be fatal; co-administration with other drugs that cause hypokalemia or hypomagnesemia resulting in prolongation of the QT interval, such as potassium-wasting diuretics, increases the risk and extent of QT prolongation). Products include:
- Diuril Sodium Intravenous 1934

Ethacrynic Acid (Arsenic trioxide can cause QT interval prolongation and complete AV block; QT prolongation can lead to torsade de pointes-type ventricular arrhythmias, which can be fatal; co-administration with other drugs that cause hypokalemia or hypomagnesemia resulting in prolongation of the QT interval, such as potassium-wasting diuretics, increases the risk and extent of QT prolongation). Products include:
- Edecrin Tablets 1941

Furosemide (Arsenic trioxide can cause QT interval prolongation and complete AV block; QT prolongation can lead to torsade de pointes-type ventricular arrhythmias, which can be fatal; co-administration with other drugs that cause hypokalemia or hypomagnesemia resulting in prolongation of the QT interval, such as potassium-wasting diuretics, increases the risk and extent of QT prolongation). Products include:
- Furosemide Tablets 2117

Hydrochlorothiazide (Arsenic trioxide can cause QT interval prolongation and complete AV block; QT prolongation can lead to torsade de pointes-type ventricular arrhythmias, which can be fatal; co-administration with other drugs that cause hypokalemia or hypomagnesemia resulting in prolongation of the QT interval, such as potassium-wasting diuretics, increases the risk and extent of QT prolongation). Products include:
- Aldoril Tablets 1884
- Atacand HCT 637
- Avalide Tablets 2889
- Avalide Tablets 922
- Benicar HCT Tablets 2852
- Diovan HCT Tablets 2195
- Dyazide Capsules 1389
- Hyzaar 1964
- Lotensin HCT Tablets 2235
- Maxzide 2150
- Micardis HCT Tablets 886
- Moduretic Tablets 2003
- Prinzide Tablets 2033
- Teveten HCT Tablets 1710
- Timolide Tablets 2056
- Uniretic Tablets 3114
- Vaseretic Tablets 2073
- Zestoretic Tablets 701

Hydroflumethiazide (Arsenic trioxide can cause QT interval prolongation and complete AV block; QT prolongation can lead to torsade de pointes-type ventricular arrhythmias, which can be fatal; co-administration with other drugs that cause hypokalemia or hypomagnesemia resulting in prolongation of the QT interval, such as potassium-wasting diuretics, increases the risk and extent of QT prolongation).
No products indexed under this heading.

Methyclothiazide (Arsenic trioxide can cause QT interval prolongation and complete AV block; QT prolongation can lead to torsade de pointes-type ventricular arrhythmias, which can be fatal; co-administration with other drugs that cause hypokalemia or hypomagnesemia resulting in prolongation of the QT interval, such as potassium-wasting diuretics, increases the risk and extent of QT prolongation).
No products indexed under this heading.

Polythiazide (Arsenic trioxide can cause QT interval prolongation and complete AV block; QT prolongation can lead to torsade de pointes-type ventricular arrhythmias, which can be fatal; co-administration with other drugs that cause hypokalemia or hypomagnesemia resulting in prolongation of the QT interval, such as potassium-wasting diuretics, increases the risk and extent of QT prolongation).
No products indexed under this heading.

Procainamide Hydrochloride (Arsenic trioxide can cause QT interval prolongation and complete AV block; QT prolongation can lead to torsade de pointes-type ventricular arrhythmias, which can be fatal; co-administration with other drugs that can prolong the QT interval, such as certain antiarrhythmics, increases the risk and extent of QT prolongation).
No products indexed under this heading.

Quinidine (Arsenic trioxide can cause QT interval prolongation and complete AV block; QT prolongation can lead to torsade de pointes-type ventricular arrhythmias, which can be fatal; co-administration with other drugs that can prolong the QT interval, such as certain anti-arrhythmic quinidine, increases the risk and extent of QT prolongation).
No products indexed under this heading.

Quinidine Gluconate (Arsenic trioxide can cause QT interval prolongation and complete AV block; QT prolongation can lead to torsade de pointes-type ventricular arrhythmias, which can be fatal; co-administration with other drugs that can prolong the QT interval, such as certain anti-arrhythmic quinidine, increases the risk and extent of QT prolongation).
No products indexed under this heading.

Quinidine Hydrochloride (Arsenic trioxide can cause QT interval prolongation and complete AV block; QT prolongation can lead to torsade de pointes-type ventricular arrhythmias, which can be fatal; co-administration with other drugs that can prolong the QT interval, such as certain anti-arrhythmic quinidine, increases the risk and extent of QT prolongation).
No products indexed under this heading.

Quinidine Polygalacturonate (Arsenic trioxide can cause QT interval prolongation and complete AV block; QT prolongation can lead to torsade de pointes-type ventricular arrhythmias, which can be fatal; co-administration with other drugs that can prolong the QT interval, such as certain anti-arrhythmic quinidine, increases the risk and extent of QT prolongation).
No products indexed under this heading.

Quinidine Sulfate (Arsenic trioxide can cause QT interval prolongation and complete AV block; QT prolongation can lead to torsade de pointes-type ventricular arrhythmias, which can be fatal; co-administration with other drugs that can prolong the QT interval, such as certain anti-arrhythmic quinidine, increases the risk and extent of QT prolongation).
No products indexed under this heading.

Sotalol Hydrochloride (Arsenic trioxide can cause QT interval prolongation and complete AV block; QT prolongation can lead to torsade de pointes-type ventricular arrhythmias, which can be fatal; co-administration with other drugs that can prolong the QT interval, such as certain anti-arrhythmics, increases the risk and extent of QT prolongation).
No products indexed under this heading.

Thioridazine Hydrochloride (Arsenic trioxide can cause QT interval prolongation and complete AV block; QT prolongation can lead to torsade de pointes-type ventricular arrhythmias, which can be fatal; co-administration with other drugs that can prolong the QT interval, such as thioridazine, increases the risk and extent of QT prolongation). Products include:
- Thioridazine Hydrochloride Tablets 2122

Torsemide (Arsenic trioxide can cause QT interval prolongation and complete AV block; QT prolongation can lead to torsade de pointes-type ventricular arrhythmias, which can be fatal; co-administration with other drugs that cause hypokalemia or hypomagnesemia resulting in prolongation of the QT interval, such as potassium-wasting diuretics, increases the risk and extent of QT prolongation).
No products indexed under this heading.

TRIZIVIR TABLETS

(Abacavir Sulfate, Lamivudine, Zidovudine) 1565

May interact with cytotoxic drugs, valproate, and certain other agents. Compounds in these categories include:

Atovaquone (Co-administration may alter zidovudine blood concentrations; routine dose modification is not warranted). Products include:
- Malarone Tablets 1484
- Malarone Pediatric Tablets 1484
- Mepron Suspension 1487

Bleomycin Sulfate (Co-administration with cytotoxic agents may increase the hematologic toxicity of zidovudine).
No products indexed under this heading.

Cyclophosphamide (Co-administration with cytotoxic agents may increase the hematologic toxicity of zidovudine).
No products indexed under this heading.

Daunorubicin Hydrochloride (Co-administration with cytotoxic agents may increase the hematologic toxicity of zidovudine). Products include:
- Cerubidine for Injection 788

Divalproex Sodium (Co-administration may alter zidovudine blood concentrations; routine dose modification is not warranted). Products include:
- Depakote Sprinkle Capsules 422
- Depakote Tablets 427
- Depakote ER Tablets 433

Doxorubicin Hydrochloride (Co-administration with cytotoxic agents may increase the hematologic toxicity of zidovudine). Products include:
- Adriamycin for Injection, USP 786
- Adriamycin Injection, USP 786

Emtricitabine (Trizir should not be administered concomitantly with emtricitabine). Products include:
- Emtriva Capsules 1272
- Truvada Tablets 1279

Epirubicin Hydrochloride (Co-administration with cytotoxic agents may increase the hematologic toxicity of zidovudine). Products include:
- Ellence Injection 2632

Fluconazole (Co-administration may alter zidovudine blood concentrations; routine dose modification is not warranted).
No products indexed under this heading.

Fluorouracil (Co-administration with cytotoxic agents may increase the hematologic toxicity of zidovudine). Products include:
- Carac Cream, 0.5% 1048
- Efudex 3348

Ganciclovir (Co-administration may increase the hematologic toxicity of zidovudine). Products include:
- Cytovene Capsules 2763

Ganciclovir Sodium (Co-administration may increase the hematologic toxicity of zidovudine). Products include:
- Cytovene-IV 2763

Hydroxyurea (Co-administration with cytotoxic agents may increase the hematologic toxicity of zidovudine).
No products indexed under this heading.

Interferon alfa-2a, Recombinant (Co-administration may increase the hematologic toxicity of zidovudine). Products include:

Roferon-A Injection 2805

Interferon alfa-2b, Recombinant (Co-administration may increase the hematologic toxicity of zidovudine). Products include:
Intron A for Injection 3038
Rebetron Combination Therapy 3078

Methadone Hydrochloride (Co-administration may alter zidovudine blood concentrations; routine dose modification is not warranted).
No products indexed under this heading.

Methotrexate Sodium (Co-administration with cytotoxic agents may increase the hematologic toxicity of zidovudine).
No products indexed under this heading.

Mitotane (Co-administration with cytotoxic agents may increase the hematologic toxicity of zidovudine).
No products indexed under this heading.

Mitoxantrone Hydrochloride (Co-administration with cytotoxic agents may increase the hematologic toxicity of zidovudine). Products include:
Novantrone for Injection Concentrate 3158

Nelfinavir Mesylate (Co-administration may alter lamivudine and zidovudine blood concentrations; routine dose modification is not warranted). Products include:
Viracept 2556

Probenecid (Co-administration may alter zidovudine blood concentrations; routine dose modification is not warranted).
No products indexed under this heading.

Procarbazine Hydrochloride (Co-administration with cytotoxic agents may increase the hematologic toxicity of zidovudine). Products include:
Matulane Capsules 3188

Ribavirin (Co-administration of zidovudine with ribavirin should be avoided since an antagonistic relationship has been demonstrated in vitro). Products include:
Copegus Tablets 2759
Rebetol 3073
Rebetron Combination Therapy 3078
Ribavirin, USP Capsules 3083
Virazole for Inhalation Solution 3365

Ritonavir (Co-administration may alter zidovudine blood concentrations; routine dose modification is not warranted). Products include:
Kaletra 474
Norvir 499

Stavudine (Co-administration of zidovudine with stavudine should be avoided since an antagonistic relationship has been demonstrated in vitro). Products include:
Zerit 971

Sulfamethoxazole (Co-administration with trimethoprim/sulfamethoxazole may alter lamivudine blood concentrations; routine dose modification is not warranted).
No products indexed under this heading.

Tamoxifen Citrate (Co-administration with cytotoxic agents may increase the hematologic toxicity of zidovudine).
No products indexed under this heading.

Trimethoprim (Co-administration with trimethoprim/sulfamethoxazole may alter lamivudine blood concentrations; routine dose modification is not warranted).
No products indexed under this heading.

Valproate Sodium (Co-administration may alter zidovudine blood concentrations; routine dose modification is not warranted). Products include:
Depacon Injection 412

Valproic Acid (Co-administration may alter zidovudine blood concentrations; routine dose modification is not warranted). Products include:
Depakene 417

Vincristine Sulfate (Co-administration with cytotoxic agents may increase the hematologic toxicity of zidovudine).
No products indexed under this heading.

Zalacitabine (Lamivudine and zalcitabine may inhibit the intracellular phosphorylation of one another; co-administration is not recommended).
No products indexed under this heading.

Food Interactions

Alcohol (Concurrent use decreases the elimination of abacavir causing an increase in overall exposure).

TRUSOPT STERILE OPHTHALMIC SOLUTION
(Dorzolamide Hydrochloride) 2065
May interact with carbonic anhydrase inhibitors and certain other agents. Compounds in these categories include:

Acetazolamide (Potential for an additive effect on the known systemic effects of carbonic anhydrase inhibition in patients receiving a systemic carbonic anhydrase inhibitor and Trusopt).
No products indexed under this heading.

Acetazolamide Sodium (Potential for an additive effect on the known systemic effects of carbonic anhydrase inhibition in patients receiving a systemic carbonic anhydrase inhibitor and Trusopt).
No products indexed under this heading.

Aspirin (Potential for acid-base and electrolyte disturbances with concomitant use; these disturbances have been reported with oral agent and have not been reported during clinical trials with Trusopt). Products include:
Aggrenox Capsules 855
Bayer, Aspirin Regimen .... ▣606
Bayer Aspirin Tablets 3515
BC Powder .... ▣612
BC Allergy Sinus Cold Powder .... ▣612
Arthritis Strength BC Powder .... ▣612
BC Sinus Cold Powder .... ▣612
Ecotrin Enteric Coated Aspirin Low, Regular and Maximum Strength Tablets 1627
Goody's Body Pain Formula Powder .... ▣621
Goody's Extra Strength Headache Powder .... ▣621
Goody's Extra Strength Pain Relief Tablets .... ▣621
Percodan Tablets 1115
St. Joseph 81 mg Aspirin Chewable and Enteric Coated Tablets 1841

Dichlorphenamide (Potential for an additive effect on the known systemic effects of carbonic anhydrase inhibition in patients receiving a systemic carbonic anhydrase inhibitor and Trusopt). Products include:
Daranide Tablets 1928

Methazolamide (Potential for an additive effect on the known systemic effects of carbonic anhydrase inhibition in patients receiving a systemic carbonic anhydrase inhibitor and Trusopt).
No products indexed under this heading.

TRUVADA TABLETS
(Emtricitabine, Tenofovir Disoproxil Fumarate).. 1279
May interact with cationic drugs that are eliminated by renal tubular and certain other agents. Compounds in these categories include:

Acyclovir (Since emtricitabine and tenofovir are primarily eliminated by the kidneys, co-administration of Truvada with drugs that reduce renal function or compete for active tubular secretion, may increase serum concentrations of emtricitabine, tenofovir, and/or other renally eliminated drugs, such as acyclovir). Products include:
Zovirax 1616
Zovirax Cream 853
Zovirax Ointment 854

Acyclovir Sodium (Since emtricitabine and tenofovir are primarily eliminated by the kidneys, co-administration of Truvada with drugs that reduce renal function or compete for active tubular secretion, may increase serum concentrations of emtricitabine, tenofovir, and/or other renally eliminated drugs, such as acyclovir). Products include:
Zovirax for Injection 1618

Adefovir dipivoxil (Since emtricitabine and tenofovir are primarily eliminated by the kidneys, co-administration of Truvada with drugs that reduce renal function or compete for active tubular secretion, may increase serum concentrations of emtricitabine, tenofovir, and/or other renally eliminated drugs, such as adefovir dipivoxil). Products include:
Hepsera Tablets 1275

Amiloride Hydrochloride (Co-administration of Truvada with drugs that are eliminated by active tubular secretion, may increase concentrations of emtricitabine, tenofovir, and/or the co-administered drug). Products include:
Midamor Tablets 2000
Moduretic Tablets 2003

Atazanavir (Atazanavir and lopinavir/ritonavir have been shown to increase tenofovir concentrations. Patients receiving atazanavir and lopinavir/ritonavir and Truvada should be monitored for Truvada-associated adverse events. Truvada should be discontinued in patients who develop Truvada-associated adverse events. Tenofovir decreases the AUC and Cmin of atazanavir. When co-administered with Truvada, it is recommended that atazanavir 300 mg is given with ritonavir 100 mg. Atazanavir without ritonavir should not be co-administered with Truvada).
No products indexed under this heading.

Atazanavir sulfate (Atazanavir and lopinavir/ritonavir have been shown to increase tenofovir concentrations. Patients receiving atazanavir and lopinavir/ritonavir and Truvada should be monitored for Truvada-associated adverse events. Truvada should be discontinued in patients who develop Truvada-associated adverse events. Tenofovir decreases the AUC and Cmin of atazanavir. When co-administered with Truvada, it is recommended that atazanavir 300 mg is given with ritonavir 100 mg. Atazanavir without ritonavir should not be co-administered with Truvada). Products include:
Reyataz Capsules 948

Cidofovir (Since emtricitabine and tenofovir are primarily eliminated by the kidneys, co-administration of Truvada with drugs that reduce renal function or compete for active tubular secretion, may increase serum concentrations of emtricitabine, tenofovir, and/or other renally eliminated drugs, such as cidofovir).
No products indexed under this heading.

Didanosine (When tenofovir disoproxil fumarate was administered with didanosine, the Cmax and AUC of didanosine, administered as either the buffered or enteric-coated formulation, increased significantly. Higher didanosine concentrations could potentiate didanosine-associated adverse events. Co-administration of Truvada and didanosine should be undertaken with caution, and patients receiving this combination should be monitored closely for didanosine-associated adverse events. Didanosine should be discontinued in patients who develop didanosine-associated adverse events).
No products indexed under this heading.

Digoxin (Co-administration of Truvada with drugs that are eliminated by active tubular secretion, may increase concentrations of emtricitabine, tenofovir, and/or the co-administered drug). Products include:
Digitek Tablets 2146
Lanoxicaps Capsules 1458
Lanoxin Injection 1462
Lanoxin Tablets 1468
Lanoxin Injection Pediatric 1465

Ganciclovir (Since emtricitabine and tenofovir are primarily eliminated by the kidneys, co-administration of Truvada with drugs that reduce renal function or compete for active tubular secretion, may increase serum concentrations of emtricitabine, tenofovir, and/or other renally eliminated drugs, such as ganciclovir). Products include:
Cytovene Capsules 2763

Ganciclovir Sodium (Since emtricitabine and tenofovir are primarily eliminated by the kidneys, co-administration of Truvada with drugs that reduce renal function or compete for active tubular secretion, may increase serum concentrations of emtricitabine, tenofovir, and/or other renally eliminated drugs, such as ganciclovir). Products include:
Cytovene-IV 2763

Lamivudine (Due to similarities between emtricitabine and lamivudine, Truvada should not be co-administered with other drugs containing lamivudine). Products include:
Combivir Tablets 1373
Epivir 1394

Epivir-HBV 1398
Epzicom Tablets 1402
Trizivir Tablets 1565

Lopinavir (Atazanavir and lopinavir/ritonavir have been shown to increase tenofovir concentrations. Patients receiving atazanavir and lopinavir/ritonavir and Truvada should be monitored for Truvada-associated adverse events. Truvada should be discontinued in patients who develop Truvada-associated adverse events). Products include:
Kaletra 474

Morphine Sulfate (Co-administration of Truvada with drugs that are eliminated by active tubular secretion, may increase concentrations of emtricitabine, tenofovir, and/or the co-administered drug). Products include:
Avinza Capsules 1714
Kadian Capsules 572
MS Contin Tablets 2703

Procainamide Hydrochloride (Co-administration of Truvada with drugs that are eliminated by active tubular secretion, may increase concentrations of emtricitabine, tenofovir, and/or the co-administered drug).
No products indexed under this heading.

Quinidine Gluconate (Co-administration of Truvada with drugs that are eliminated by active tubular secretion, may increase concentrations of emtricitabine, tenofovir, and/or the co-administered drug).
No products indexed under this heading.

Quinidine Polygalacturonate (Co-administration of Truvada with drugs that are eliminated by active tubular secretion, may increase concentrations of emtricitabine, tenofovir, and/or the co-administered drug).
No products indexed under this heading.

Quinidine Sulfate (Co-administration of Truvada with drugs that are eliminated by active tubular secretion, may increase concentrations of emtricitabine, tenofovir, and/or the co-administered drug).
No products indexed under this heading.

Quinine Sulfate (Co-administration of Truvada with drugs that are eliminated by active tubular secretion, may increase concentrations of emtricitabine, tenofovir, and/or the co-administered drug).
No products indexed under this heading.

Ranitidine Hydrochloride (Co-administration of Truvada with drugs that are eliminated by active tubular secretion, may increase concentrations of emtricitabine, tenofovir, and/or the co-administered drug). Products include:
Zantac 1597
Zantac Injection 1593
Zantac 75 Tablets 715
Zantac 150 Maximum Strength Tablets 715
Zantac Injection Pharmacy Bulk Package 1595

Ritonavir (Atazanavir and lopinavir/ritonavir have been shown to increase tenofovir concentrations. Patients receiving atazanavir and lopinavir/ritonavir and Truvada should be monitored for Truvada-associated adverse events. Truvada should be discontinued in patients who develop Truvada-associated adverse events). Products include:
Kaletra 474
Norvir 499

Triamterene (Co-administration of Truvada with drugs that are eliminated by active tubular secretion, may increase concentrations of emtricitabine, tenofovir, and/or the co-administered drug). Products include:
Dyazide Capsules 1389
Dyrenium Capsules 3390
Maxzide 2150

Trimethoprim (Co-administration of Truvada with drugs that are eliminated by active tubular secretion, may increase concentrations of emtricitabine, tenofovir, and/or the co-administered drug).
No products indexed under this heading.

Trimethoprim Sulfate (Co-administration of Truvada with drugs that are eliminated by active tubular secretion, may increase concentrations of emtricitabine, tenofovir, and/or the co-administered drug). Products include:
Polytrim Ophthalmic Solution 570

Valacyclovir Hydrochloride (Since emtricitabine and tenofovir are primarily eliminated by the kidneys, co-administration of Truvada with drugs that reduce renal function or compete for active tubular secretion, may increase serum concentrations of emtricitabine, tenofovir, and/or other renally eliminated drugs, such as valacyclovir). Products include:
Valtrex Caplets 1573

Valganciclovir Hydrochloride (Since emtricitabine and tenofovir are primarily eliminated by the kidneys, co-administration of Truvada with drugs that reduce renal function or compete for active tubular secretion, may increase serum concentrations of emtricitabine, tenofovir, and/or other renally eliminated drugs, such as valganciclovir). Products include:
Valcyte Tablets 2816

Vancomycin Hydrochloride (Co-administration of Truvada with drugs that are eliminated by active tubular secretion, may increase concentrations of emtricitabine, tenofovir, and/or the co-administered drug). Products include:
Vancocin HCl Capsules, USP 3370

TUCKS ANTI-ITCH OINTMENT
(Hydrocortisone Acetate) 712
None cited in PDR database.

TUCKS HEMORRHOIDAL OINTMENT
(Mineral Oil, Pramoxine Hydrochloride, Zinc Oxide) 711
None cited in PDR database.

TUCKS HEMORRHOIDAL SUPPOSITORIES
(Starch, topical) 712
None cited in PDR database.

TUCKS WITCH HAZEL HEMORRHOIDAL PAD
(Witch Hazel) 712
None cited in PDR database.

TUMS E-X ANTACID/CALCIUM TABLETS
(Calcium Carbonate) 639
See Tums Regular Antacid/Calcium Tablets

TUMS E-X SUGAR FREE ANTACID/CALCIUM TABLETS
(Calcium Carbonate) 639
See Tums Regular Antacid/Calcium Tablets

TUMS REGULAR ANTACID/CALCIUM TABLETS
(Calcium Carbonate) 639
May interact with:

Prescription Drugs, unspecified (Antacids may interact with certain unspecified prescription drugs).

TUMS ULTRA ANTACID/CALCIUM TABLETS
(Calcium Carbonate) 639
See Tums Regular Antacid/Calcium Tablets

TUSSIONEX PENNKINETIC EXTENDED-RELEASE SUSPENSION
(Chlorpheniramine Polistirex, Hydrocodone Polistirex) 3322
May interact with tricyclic antidepressants and certain other agents. Compounds in these categories include:

Acrivastine (Combined therapy may result in additive CNS depression).
No products indexed under this heading.

Alfentanil Hydrochloride (Combined therapy may result in additive CNS depression).
No products indexed under this heading.

Alprazolam (Combined therapy may result in additive CNS depression). Products include:
Niravam Orally Disintegrating Tablets 3106
Xanax XR Tablets 2655

Amitriptyline Hydrochloride (Co-administration of hydrocodone with MAO inhibitors may increase the effect of tricyclic antidepressant or hydrocodone).
No products indexed under this heading.

Amoxapine (Co-administration of hydrocodone with MAO inhibitors may increase the effect of tricyclic antidepressant or hydrocodone).
No products indexed under this heading.

Aprobarbital (Combined therapy may result in additive CNS depression).
No products indexed under this heading.

Astemizole (Combined therapy may result in additive CNS depression).
No products indexed under this heading.

Atropine Sulfate (Concurrent use of other anticholinergic agents with hydrocodone may produce paralytic ileus).
No products indexed under this heading.

Azatadine Maleate (Combined therapy may result in additive CNS depression).
No products indexed under this heading.

Belladonna Alkaloids (Concurrent use of other anticholinergic agents with hydrocodone may produce paralytic ileus). Products include:
Hyland's Teething Tablets 736

Benztropine Mesylate (Concurrent use of other anticholinergic agents with hydrocodone may produce paralytic ileus). Products include:
Cogentin Injection 1903

Biperiden Hydrochloride (Concurrent use of other anticholinergic agents with hydrocodone may produce paralytic ileus).
No products indexed under this heading.

Bromodiphenhydramine Hydrochloride (Combined therapy may result in additive CNS depression).
No products indexed under this heading.

Brompheniramine Maleate (Combined therapy may result in additive CNS depression). Products include:
Alacol DM Syrup 739
Children's Dimetapp Cold & Allergy Elixir 745
Children's Dimetapp DM Cold & Cough Elixir 745
Robitussin Allergy & Cough Syrup 750

Buprenorphine Hydrochloride (Combined therapy may result in additive CNS depression). Products include:
Buprenex Injectable 2718
Suboxone Tablets 2719
Subutex Tablets 2719

Buspirone Hydrochloride (Combined therapy may result in additive CNS depression).
No products indexed under this heading.

Butabarbital (Combined therapy may result in additive CNS depression).
No products indexed under this heading.

Butalbital (Combined therapy may result in additive CNS depression). Products include:
Sedapap Tablets 50 mg/650 mg 2098

Cetirizine Hydrochloride (Combined therapy may result in additive CNS depression). Products include:
Zyrtec Chewable Tablets 2589
Zyrtec 2589
Zyrtec-D 12 Hour Extended Release Tablets 2591

Chlordiazepoxide (Combined therapy may result in additive CNS depression).
No products indexed under this heading.

Chlordiazepoxide Hydrochloride (Combined therapy may result in additive CNS depression). Products include:
Librium Capsules 3349

Chlorpheniramine Maleate (Combined therapy may result in additive CNS depression). Products include:
Advil Allergy Sinus Caplets 737
Advil Multi-Symptom Cold Caplets 738
BC Allergy Sinus Cold Powder 612
Contac Severe Cold and Flu Caplets Maximum Strength 615
Hycomine Compound Tablets 1105
PediaCare Multi-Symptom Cold Liquid 704
PediaCare NightRest Cough & Cold Liquid 704
Robitussin Flu Liquid 752
Robitussin PM Cough & Cold Liquid 752
Singlet Caplets 636
Sudafed Sinus & Allergy Tablets 710

TheraFlu Cold & Cough Hot Liquid .... ▣680
TheraFlu Cold & Sore Throat Hot Liquid .... ▣680
TheraFlu Flu & Sore Throat Hot Liquid .... ▣681
TheraFlu Severe Cold & Cough Hot Liquid .... ▣683
TheraFlu Severe Cold Caplets .... ▣679
TheraFlu Severe Cold Hot Liquid .... ▣682
Triaminic Cold & Allergy Liquid .... ▣685
Triaminic Cold & Cough Liquid .... ▣685
Triaminic Flu, Cough & Fever Liquid .... ▣685
Triaminic Night Time Cough & Cold Liquid .... ▣685
Triaminic Allergy Runny Nose & Congestion Softchews .... ▣688
Triaminic Cold & Cough Softchews .... ▣688
Children's Tylenol Plus Cold NightTime Suspension Liquid 1851
Children's Tylenol Plus Cold & Cough Suspension Liquid and Chewable Tablets 1851
Children's Tylenol Plus Cold Chewable Tablets 1851
Children's Tylenol Plus Flu Suspension Liquid 1853
Tylenol Allergy Complete Multi-Symptom Caplets and Gelcaps with Cool Burst 1844
Multi-Symptom Tylenol Cold Night Time Caplets 1845
Vicks 44M Cough, Cold & Flu Relief 2676
Pediatric Vicks 44m Cough & Cold Relief 2673
Children's Vicks NyQuil Cold/Cough Relief 2671

Chlorpheniramine Tannate (Combined therapy may result in additive CNS depression).
No products indexed under this heading.

Chlorpromazine (Combined therapy may result in additive CNS depression).
No products indexed under this heading.

Chlorpromazine Hydrochloride (Combined therapy may result in additive CNS depression).
No products indexed under this heading.

Chlorprothixene (Combined therapy may result in additive CNS depression).
No products indexed under this heading.

Chlorprothixene Hydrochloride (Combined therapy may result in additive CNS depression).
No products indexed under this heading.

Chlorprothixene Lactate (Combined therapy may result in additive CNS depression).
No products indexed under this heading.

Clemastine Fumarate (Combined therapy may result in additive CNS depression).
No products indexed under this heading.

Clidinium Bromide (Concurrent use of other anticholinergic agents with hydrocodone may produce paralytic ileus).
No products indexed under this heading.

Clomipramine Hydrochloride (Co-administration of hydrocodone with MAO inhibitors may increase the effect of tricyclic antidepressant or hydrocodone).
No products indexed under this heading.

Clorazepate Dipotassium (Combined therapy may result in additive CNS depression). Products include:
Tranxene 2488

Clozapine (Combined therapy may result in additive CNS depression). Products include:
Clozapine Tablets 2141
Clozaril Tablets 2174
FazaClo Orally Disintegrating Tablets 547

Codeine Phosphate (Combined therapy may result in additive CNS depression). Products include:
Tylenol with Codeine 2461

Cyproheptadine Hydrochloride (Combined therapy may result in additive CNS depression).
No products indexed under this heading.

Desflurane (Combined therapy may result in additive CNS depression). Products include:
Suprane Liquid for Inhalation 770

Desipramine Hydrochloride (Co-administration of hydrocodone with MAO inhibitors may increase the effect of tricyclic antidepressant or hydrocodone).
No products indexed under this heading.

Dexchlorpheniramine Maleate (Combined therapy may result in additive CNS depression).
No products indexed under this heading.

Dezocine (Combined therapy may result in additive CNS depression).
No products indexed under this heading.

Diazepam (Combined therapy may result in additive CNS depression). Products include:
Diastat Rectal Delivery System 3344
Valium Tablets 2822

Dicyclomine Hydrochloride (Concurrent use of other anticholinergic agents with hydrocodone may produce paralytic ileus). Products include:
Bentyl Capsules 724
Bentyl Injection 724
Bentyl Syrup 724
Bentyl Tablets 724

Diphenhydramine Citrate (Combined therapy may result in additive CNS depression). Products include:
Children's Benadryl Allergy & Cold Fastmelt Tablets .... ▣695
Children's Benadryl D Allergy & Sinus Fastmelt Tablets .... ▣694
Children's Benadryl Allergy Fastmelt Tablets .... ▣696
Goody's PM Powder .... ▣622

Diphenhydramine Hydrochloride (Combined therapy may result in additive CNS depression). Products include:
Benadryl Allergy & Cold Tablets .... ▣692
Benadryl Allergy .... ▣691
Benadryl Allergy & Sinus Headache Caplets & Gelcaps .... ▣693
Children's Benadryl Allergy Liquid .... ▣695
Children's Benadryl Dye-Free Allergy Liquid .... ▣695
Benadryl Dye-Free Allergy Liqui-Gels Softgels .... ▣692
Benadryl Itch Relief Stick Extra Strength .... ▣696
Benadryl Itch Stopping Cream Extra Strength .... ▣697
Benadryl Itch Stopping Gel Extra Strength .... ▣697
Benadryl Itch Stopping Spray Extra Strength .... ▣697
Benadryl Maximum Strength Severe Allergy & Sinus Headache Caplets .... ▣694
Children's Benadryl D Liquid Medication .... ▣693
Benadryl D Tablets .... ▣694
Nytol QuickCaps Caplets .... ▣635
Maximum Strength Nytol QuickGels Softgels .... ▣635
Simply Sleep Caplets 1841
Sominex Original Formula Tablets .... ▣637
TheraFlu Thin Strips Multi Symptom .... ▣684
Triaminic Thin Strips Cough & Runny Nose .... ▣690
Children's Tylenol Plus Cold & Allergy Suspension Liquid 1850
Tylenol Allergy Complete Night Time Caplets 1844
Tylenol Severe Allergy Caplets 1844
Tylenol Flu NightTime Gelcaps 1846
Extra Strength Tylenol PM Caplets, Geltabs, Gelcaps and Liquid 1847
Unisom Maximum Strength SleepGels .... ▣712

Diphenylpyraline Hydrochloride (Combined therapy may result in additive CNS depression).
No products indexed under this heading.

Doxepin Hydrochloride (Co-administration of hydrocodone with MAO inhibitors may increase the effect of tricyclic antidepressant or hydrocodone).
No products indexed under this heading.

Droperidol (Combined therapy may result in additive CNS depression).
No products indexed under this heading.

Enflurane (Combined therapy may result in additive CNS depression).
No products indexed under this heading.

Estazolam (Combined therapy may result in additive CNS depression). Products include:
ProSom Tablets 512

Ethanol (Combined therapy may result in additive CNS depression).
No products indexed under this heading.

Ethchlorvynol (Combined therapy may result in additive CNS depression).
No products indexed under this heading.

Ethinamate (Combined therapy may result in additive CNS depression).
No products indexed under this heading.

Ethyl Alcohol (Combined therapy may result in additive CNS depression).
No products indexed under this heading.

Fentanyl (Combined therapy may result in additive CNS depression). Products include:
Duragesic Transdermal System 2448

Fentanyl Citrate (Combined therapy may result in additive CNS depression). Products include:
Actiq 993

Fexofenadine Hydrochloride (Combined therapy may result in additive CNS depression). Products include:
Allegra 2857
Allegra-D 12 Hour Extended-Release Tablets 2860
Allegra-D 24 Hour Extended-Release Tablets 2862

Fluphenazine Decanoate (Combined therapy may result in additive CNS depression).
No products indexed under this heading.

Fluphenazine Enanthate (Combined therapy may result in additive CNS depression).
No products indexed under this heading.

Fluphenazine Hydrochloride (Combined therapy may result in additive CNS depression).
No products indexed under this heading.

Flurazepam Hydrochloride (Combined therapy may result in additive CNS depression). Products include:
Dalmane Capsules 3343

Glutethimide (Combined therapy may result in additive CNS depression).
No products indexed under this heading.

Glycopyrrolate (Concurrent use of other anticholinergic agents with hydrocodone may produce paralytic ileus).
No products indexed under this heading.

Haloperidol (Combined therapy may result in additive CNS depression).
No products indexed under this heading.

Haloperidol Decanoate (Combined therapy may result in additive CNS depression).
No products indexed under this heading.

Hydrocodone Bitartrate (Combined therapy may result in additive CNS depression). Products include:
Hycodan 1104
Hycomine Compound Tablets 1105
Hycotuss Expectorant Syrup 1106
Lortab 3315
Lortab Elixir 3312
Vicodin Tablets 530
Vicodin ES Tablets 531
Vicodin HP Tablets 532
Vicoprofen Tablets 533
Zydone Tablets 1118

Hydromorphone Hydrochloride (Combined therapy may result in additive CNS depression). Products include:
Dilaudid 439
Dilaudid Oral Liquid 443
Dilaudid Non-Sterile Powder 439
Dilaudid Rectal Suppositories 439
Dilaudid Tablets 439
Dilaudid Tablets - 8 mg 443
Dilaudid-HP 441

Hydroxyzine Hydrochloride (Combined therapy may result in additive CNS depression).
No products indexed under this heading.

Hyoscyamine (Concurrent use of other anticholinergic agents with hydrocodone may produce paralytic ileus).
No products indexed under this heading.

Hyoscyamine Sulfate (Concurrent use of other anticholinergic agents with hydrocodone may produce paralytic ileus).
No products indexed under this heading.

Imipramine Hydrochloride (Co-administration of hydrocodone with MAO inhibitors may increase the effect of tricyclic antidepressant or hydrocodone).
No products indexed under this heading.

Imipramine Pamoate (Co-administration of hydrocodone with MAO inhibitors may increase the effect of tricyclic antidepressant or hydrocodone).
No products indexed under this heading.

Ipratropium Bromide (Concurrent use of other anticholinergic agents with hydrocodone may produce paralytic ileus). Products include:
Atrovent HFA Inhalation Aerosol 872
Atrovent Inhalation Solution 868
Atrovent Nasal Spray 0.03% 869
Atrovent Nasal Spray 0.06% 870
Combivent Inhalation Aerosol 878
DuoNeb Inhalation Solution 1058

Isocarboxazid (Co-administration of hydrocodone with MAO inhibitors may increase the effect of MAOI or hydrocodone).
No products indexed under this heading.

Isoflurane (Combined therapy may result in additive CNS depression).
No products indexed under this heading.

Ketamine Hydrochloride (Combined therapy may result in additive CNS depression).
No products indexed under this heading.

Levomethadyl Acetate Hydrochloride (Combined therapy may result in additive CNS depression).
No products indexed under this heading.

Levorphanol Tartrate (Combined therapy may result in additive CNS depression).
No products indexed under this heading.

Loratadine (Combined therapy may result in additive CNS depression). Products include:
Alavert Allergy & Sinus D-12 Hour Tablets 743
Alavert 743
Children's Claritin 24 Hour Non-Drowsy Allergy Syrup 732
Claritin Non-Drowsy 24 Hour Tablets 731
Non-Drowsy Claritin Hives Relief Tablets 733
Claritin Reditabs 24 Hour Non-Drowsy Tablets 732
Claritin-D Non-Drowsy 12 Hour Tablets 731
Claritin-D Non-Drowsy 24 Hour Tablets 731
Children's Dimetapp ND Non-Drowsy Allergy Syrup 746
Triaminic Allerchews 684

Lorazepam (Combined therapy may result in additive CNS depression).
No products indexed under this heading.

Loxapine Hydrochloride (Combined therapy may result in additive CNS depression).
No products indexed under this heading.

Loxapine Succinate (Combined therapy may result in additive CNS depression).
No products indexed under this heading.

Maprotiline Hydrochloride (Co-administration of hydrocodone with MAO inhibitors may increase the effect of tricyclic antidepressant or hydrocodone).
No products indexed under this heading.

Mepenzolate Bromide (Concurrent use of other anticholinergic agents with hydrocodone may produce paralytic ileus).
No products indexed under this heading.

Meperidine Hydrochloride (Combined therapy may result in additive CNS depression).
No products indexed under this heading.

Mephobarbital (Combined therapy may result in additive CNS depression). Products include:
Mebaral Tablets, USP 2483

Meprobamate (Combined therapy may result in additive CNS depression).
No products indexed under this heading.

Mesoridazine Besylate (Combined therapy may result in additive CNS depression).
No products indexed under this heading.

Methadone Hydrochloride (Combined therapy may result in additive CNS depression).
No products indexed under this heading.

Methdilazine Hydrochloride (Combined therapy may result in additive CNS depression).
No products indexed under this heading.

Methohexital Sodium (Combined therapy may result in additive CNS depression).
No products indexed under this heading.

Methotrimeprazine (Combined therapy may result in additive CNS depression).
No products indexed under this heading.

Methoxyflurane (Combined therapy may result in additive CNS depression).
No products indexed under this heading.

Midazolam Hydrochloride (Combined therapy may result in additive CNS depression).
No products indexed under this heading.

Moclobemide (Co-administration of hydrocodone with MAO inhibitors may increase the effect of MAOI or hydrocodone).
No products indexed under this heading.

Molindone Hydrochloride (Combined therapy may result in additive CNS depression). Products include:
Moban Tablets 1108

Morphine Sulfate (Combined therapy may result in additive CNS depression). Products include:
Avinza Capsules 1714
Kadian Capsules 572
MS Contin Tablets 2703

Nortriptyline Hydrochloride (Co-administration of hydrocodone with MAO inhibitors may increase the effect of tricyclic antidepressant or hydrocodone).
No products indexed under this heading.

Olanzapine (Combined therapy may result in additive CNS depression). Products include:
Symbyax Capsules 1788
Zyprexa Tablets 1798
Zyprexa IntraMuscular 1798
Zyprexa ZYDIS Orally Disintegrating Tablets 1798

Oxazepam (Combined therapy may result in additive CNS depression).
No products indexed under this heading.

Oxybutynin Chloride (Concurrent use of other anticholinergic agents with hydrocodone may produce paralytic ileus). Products include:
Ditropan XL Extended Release Tablets 2391

Oxycodone Hydrochloride (Combined therapy may result in additive CNS depression). Products include:
Combunox Tablets 1183
OxyContin Tablets 2699
OxyFast Oral Concentrate Solution 2704
OxyIR Capsules 2704
Percocet Tablets 1114
Percodan Tablets 1115

Pargyline Hydrochloride (Co-administration of hydrocodone with MAO inhibitors may increase the effect of MAOI or hydrocodone).
No products indexed under this heading.

Pentobarbital Sodium (Combined therapy may result in additive CNS depression). Products include:
Nembutal Sodium Solution, USP 2484

Perphenazine (Combined therapy may result in additive CNS depression).
No products indexed under this heading.

Phenelzine Sulfate (Co-administration of hydrocodone with MAO inhibitors may increase the effect of MAOI or hydrocodone).
No products indexed under this heading.

Phenobarbital (Combined therapy may result in additive CNS depression).
No products indexed under this heading.

Prazepam (Combined therapy may result in additive CNS depression).
No products indexed under this heading.

Procarbazine Hydrochloride (Co-administration of hydrocodone with MAO inhibitors may increase the effect of MAOI or hydrocodone). Products include:
Matulane Capsules 3188

Prochlorperazine (Combined therapy may result in additive CNS depression).
No products indexed under this heading.

Procyclidine Hydrochloride (Concurrent use of other anticholinergic agents with hydrocodone may produce paralytic ileus).
No products indexed under this heading.

Promethazine Hydrochloride (Combined therapy may result in additive CNS depression). Products include:
Phenergan 3438

Propantheline Bromide (Concurrent use of other anticholinergic agents with hydrocodone may produce paralytic ileus).
No products indexed under this heading.

Propofol (Combined therapy may result in additive CNS depression). Products include:
Diprivan Injectable Emulsion 676

Propoxyphene Hydrochloride (Combined therapy may result in additive CNS depression).
No products indexed under this heading.

Propoxyphene Napsylate (Combined therapy may result in additive CNS depression). Products include:
Darvocet A 500 Tablets 3497

Protriptyline Hydrochloride (Co-administration of hydrocodone with MAO inhibitors may increase the effect of tricyclic antidepressant or hydrocodone). Products include:
Vivactil Tablets 2350

Pyrilamine Maleate (Combined therapy may result in additive CNS depression).
No products indexed under this heading.

Pyrilamine Tannate (Combined therapy may result in additive CNS depression).
No products indexed under this heading.

Quazepam (Combined therapy may result in additive CNS depression).
No products indexed under this heading.

Quetiapine Fumarate (Combined therapy may result in additive CNS depression). Products include:
Seroquel Tablets 691

Remifentanil Hydrochloride (Combined therapy may result in additive CNS depression).
No products indexed under this heading.

Risperidone (Combined therapy may result in additive CNS depression). Products include:
Risperdal Consta Long-Acting Injection 1664
Risperdal M-Tab Orally Disintegrating Tablets 1658
Risperdal 1658

Scopolamine (Concurrent use of other anticholinergic agents with hydrocodone may produce paralytic ileus). Products include:
Transderm Scōp Transdermal Therapeutic System 2166

Scopolamine Hydrobromide (Concurrent use of other anticholinergic agents with hydrocodone may produce paralytic ileus).
No products indexed under this heading.

Secobarbital Sodium (Combined therapy may result in additive CNS depression).
No products indexed under this heading.

Selegiline Hydrochloride (Co-administration of hydrocodone with MAO inhibitors may increase the effect of MAOI or hydrocodone). Products include:
Eldepryl Capsules 3209

Sevoflurane (Combined therapy may result in additive CNS depression). Products include:
Ultane Liquid for Inhalation 526

Sodium Oxybate (Combined therapy may result in additive CNS depression).
No products indexed under this heading.

Sufentanil Citrate (Combined therapy may result in additive CNS depression).
No products indexed under this heading.

IMPORTANT NOTE: Always consult each drug listing in the patient's regimen for possible interactions.

Temazepam (Combined therapy may result in additive CNS depression).
No products indexed under this heading.

Terfenadine (Combined therapy may result in additive CNS depression).
No products indexed under this heading.

Thiamylal Sodium (Combined therapy may result in additive CNS depression).
No products indexed under this heading.

Thioridazine Hydrochloride (Combined therapy may result in additive CNS depression). Products include:
Thioridazine Hydrochloride Tablets 2122

Thiothixene (Combined therapy may result in additive CNS depression). Products include:
Thiothixene Capsules 2124

Tolterodine Tartrate (Concurrent use of other anticholinergic agents with hydrocodone may produce paralytic ileus). Products include:
Detrol Tablets 2626
Detrol LA Capsules 2629

Tranylcypromine Sulfate (Co-administration of hydrocodone with MAO inhibitors may increase the effect of MAOI or hydrocodone). Products include:
Parnate Tablets 1499

Triazolam (Combined therapy may result in additive CNS depression).
No products indexed under this heading.

Tridihexethyl Chloride (Concurrent use of other anticholinergic agents with hydrocodone may produce paralytic ileus).
No products indexed under this heading.

Trifluoperazine Hydrochloride (Combined therapy may result in additive CNS depression).
No products indexed under this heading.

Trihexyphenidyl Hydrochloride (Concurrent use of other anticholinergic agents with hydrocodone may produce paralytic ileus).
No products indexed under this heading.

Trimeprazine Tartrate (Combined therapy may result in additive CNS depression).
No products indexed under this heading.

Trimipramine Maleate (Co-administration of hydrocodone with MAO inhibitors may increase the effect of tricyclic antidepressant or hydrocodone). Products include:
Surmontil Capsules 2347

Tripelennamine Hydrochloride (Combined therapy may result in additive CNS depression).
No products indexed under this heading.

Triprolidine Hydrochloride (Combined therapy may result in additive CNS depression).
No products indexed under this heading.

Zaleplon (Combined therapy may result in additive CNS depression). Products include:
Sonata Capsules 1686

Ziprasidone Hydrochloride (Combined therapy may result in additive CNS depression). Products include:
Geodon Capsules 2514

Zolpidem Tartrate (Combined therapy may result in additive CNS depression). Products include:
Ambien Tablets 2867

Food Interactions

Alcohol (Combined use may result in additive CNS depression).

TWINRIX VACCINE

(Hepatitis A Vaccine, Inactivated, Hepatitis B Vaccine, Recombinant) 1571
None cited in PDR database.

TYGACIL FOR INJECTION

(Tigecycline) 3489
May interact with oral contraceptives and certain other agents. Compounds in these categories include:

Desogestrel (Concurrent use of antibacterial drugs with oral contraceptives may render oral contraceptives less effective). Products include:
Ortho-Cept Tablets 2395

Ethinyl Estradiol (Concurrent use of antibacterial drugs with oral contraceptives may render oral contraceptives less effective). Products include:
Alesse-28 Tablets 3392
Lo/Ovral-28 Tablets 3423
NuvaRing 2357
Ortho-Cept Tablets 2395
Ortho-Cyclen/Ortho Tri-Cyclen 2414
Ortho Evra Transdermal System 2402
Ortho Tri-Cyclen Lo Tablets 2421
Seasonale Tablets 1073
Triphasil-28 Tablets 3483
Yasmin 28 Tablets 818

Ethynodiol Diacetate (Concurrent use of antibacterial drugs with oral contraceptives may render oral contraceptives less effective).
No products indexed under this heading.

Levonorgestrel (Concurrent use of antibacterial drugs with oral contraceptives may render oral contraceptives less effective). Products include:
Alesse-28 Tablets 3392
Climara Pro Transdermal System 800
Mirena Intrauterine System 810
Plan B Tablets 1068
Seasonale Tablets 1073
Triphasil-28 Tablets 3483

Mestranol (Concurrent use of antibacterial drugs with oral contraceptives may render oral contraceptives less effective).
No products indexed under this heading.

Norethindrone (Concurrent use of antibacterial drugs with oral contraceptives may render oral contraceptives less effective). Products include:
Ortho Micronor Tablets 2411

Norethynodrel (Concurrent use of antibacterial drugs with oral contraceptives may render oral contraceptives less effective).
No products indexed under this heading.

Norgestimate (Concurrent use of antibacterial drugs with oral contraceptives may render oral contraceptives less effective). Products include:
Ortho-Cyclen/Ortho Tri-Cyclen 2414
Ortho Tri-Cyclen Lo Tablets 2421
Prefest Tablets 1069

Norgestrel (Concurrent use of antibacterial drugs with oral contraceptives may render oral contraceptives less effective). Products include:
Lo/Ovral-28 Tablets 3423

Warfarin Sodium (Prothrombin time or other suitable anticoagulation test should be monitored if tigecycline is administered with warfarin). Products include:
Coumadin for Injection 932
Coumadin Tablets 932

TYLENOL 8 HOUR EXTENDED RELEASE GELTABS AND CAPLETS

(Acetaminophen) 1843
See Regular Strength Tylenol Tablets

TYLENOL COLD & FLU SEVERE NIGHTTIME LIQUID WITH COOL BURST

(Acetaminophen, Dextromethorphan Hydrobromide, Doxylamine Succinate, Pseudoephedrine Hydrochloride) ...... ▣660

TYLENOL COUGH & SORE THROAT DAYTIME LIQUID WITH COOL BURST

(Acetaminophen, Dextromethorphan Hydrobromide) .... ▣664
May interact with monoamine oxidase inhibitors. Compounds in these categories include:

Isocarboxazid (Avoid use with, or for two weeks after stopping, MAOI drugs).
No products indexed under this heading.

Moclobemide (Avoid use with, or for two weeks after stopping, MAOI drugs).
No products indexed under this heading.

Pargyline Hydrochloride (Avoid use with, or for two weeks after stopping, MAOI drugs).
No products indexed under this heading.

Phenelzine Sulfate (Avoid use with, or for two weeks after stopping, MAOI drugs).
No products indexed under this heading.

Procarbazine Hydrochloride (Avoid use with, or for two weeks after stopping, MAOI drugs). Products include:
Matulane Capsules 3188

Selegiline Hydrochloride (Avoid use with, or for two weeks after stopping, MAOI drugs). Products include:
Eldepryl Capsules 3209

Tranylcypromine Sulfate (Avoid use with, or for two weeks after stopping, MAOI drugs). Products include:
Parnate Tablets 1499

TYLENOL COUGH & SORE THROAT NIGHTTIME LIQUID WITH COOL BURST

(Acetaminophen, Dextromethorphan Hydrobromide, Doxylamine Succinate) .... ▣664
May interact with hypnotics and sedatives, monoamine oxidase inhibitors, tranquilizers, and certain other agents. Compounds in these categories include:

Alprazolam (Co-administration with tranquilizers may increase drowsiness). Products include:
Niravam Orally Disintegrating Tablets 3106
Xanax XR Tablets 2655

Buspirone Hydrochloride (Co-administration with tranquilizers may increase drowsiness).
No products indexed under this heading.

Chlordiazepoxide (Co-administration with tranquilizers may increase drowsiness).
No products indexed under this heading.

Chlordiazepoxide Hydrochloride (Co-administration with tranquilizers may increase drowsiness). Products include:
Librium Capsules 3349

Chlorpromazine (Co-administration with tranquilizers may increase drowsiness).
No products indexed under this heading.

Chlorpromazine Hydrochloride (Co-administration with tranquilizers may increase drowsiness).
No products indexed under this heading.

Chlorprothixene (Co-administration with tranquilizers may increase drowsiness).
No products indexed under this heading.

Chlorprothixene Hydrochloride (Co-administration with tranquilizers may increase drowsiness).
No products indexed under this heading.

Clorazepate Dipotassium (Co-administration with tranquilizers may increase drowsiness). Products include:
Tranxene 2488

Diazepam (Co-administration with tranquilizers may increase drowsiness). Products include:
Diastat Rectal Delivery System 3344
Valium Tablets 2822

Droperidol (Co-administration with tranquilizers may increase drowsiness).
No products indexed under this heading.

Estazolam (Co-administration with sedatives may increase drowsiness). Products include:
ProSom Tablets 512

Ethchlorvynol (Co-administration with sedatives may increase drowsiness).
No products indexed under this heading.

Ethinamate (Co-administration with sedatives may increase drowsiness).
No products indexed under this heading.

Fluphenazine Decanoate (Co-administration with tranquilizers may increase drowsiness).
No products indexed under this heading.

Fluphenazine Enanthate (Co-administration with tranquilizers may increase drowsiness).
No products indexed under this heading.

Fluphenazine Hydrochloride (Co-administration with tranquilizers may increase drowsiness).
No products indexed under this heading.

Flurazepam Hydrochloride (Co-administration with sedatives may increase drowsiness). Products include:
Dalmane Capsules **3343**

Glutethimide (Co-administration with sedatives may increase drowsiness).
No products indexed under this heading.

Haloperidol (Co-administration with tranquilizers may increase drowsiness).
No products indexed under this heading.

Haloperidol Decanoate (Co-administration with tranquilizers may increase drowsiness).
No products indexed under this heading.

Hydroxyzine Hydrochloride (Co-administration with tranquilizers may increase drowsiness).
No products indexed under this heading.

Isocarboxazid (Avoid use with, or for two weeks after stopping, MAOI drugs).
No products indexed under this heading.

Lorazepam (Co-administration with sedatives may increase drowsiness).
No products indexed under this heading.

Loxapine Hydrochloride (Co-administration with tranquilizers may increase drowsiness).
No products indexed under this heading.

Loxapine Succinate (Co-administration with tranquilizers may increase drowsiness).
No products indexed under this heading.

Meprobamate (Co-administration with tranquilizers may increase drowsiness).
No products indexed under this heading.

Mesoridazine Besylate (Co-administration with tranquilizers may increase drowsiness).
No products indexed under this heading.

Midazolam Hydrochloride (Co-administration with sedatives may increase drowsiness).
No products indexed under this heading.

Moclobemide (Avoid use with, or for two weeks after stopping, MAOI drugs).
No products indexed under this heading.

Molindone Hydrochloride (Co-administration with tranquilizers may increase drowsiness). Products include:
Moban Tablets **1108**

Oxazepam (Co-administration with tranquilizers may increase drowsiness).
No products indexed under this heading.

Pargyline Hydrochloride (Avoid use with, or for two weeks after stopping, MAOI drugs).
No products indexed under this heading.

Perphenazine (Co-administration with tranquilizers may increase drowsiness).
No products indexed under this heading.

Phenelzine Sulfate (Avoid use with, or for two weeks after stopping, MAOI drugs).
No products indexed under this heading.

Prazepam (Co-administration with tranquilizers may increase drowsiness).
No products indexed under this heading.

Procarbazine Hydrochloride (Avoid use with, or for two weeks after stopping, MAOI drugs). Products include:
Matulane Capsules **3188**

Prochlorperazine (Co-administration with tranquilizers may increase drowsiness).
No products indexed under this heading.

Promethazine Hydrochloride (Co-administration with tranquilizers may increase drowsiness). Products include:
Phenergan **3438**

Propofol (Co-administration with sedatives may increase drowsiness). Products include:
Diprivan Injectable Emulsion **676**

Quazepam (Co-administration with sedatives may increase drowsiness).
No products indexed under this heading.

Secobarbital Sodium (Co-administration with sedatives may increase drowsiness).
No products indexed under this heading.

Selegiline Hydrochloride (Avoid use with, or for two weeks after stopping, MAOI drugs). Products include:
Eldepryl Capsules **3209**

Temazepam (Co-administration with sedatives may increase drowsiness).
No products indexed under this heading.

Thioridazine Hydrochloride (Co-administration with tranquilizers may increase drowsiness). Products include:
Thioridazine Hydrochloride Tablets **2122**

Thiothixene (Co-administration with tranquilizers may increase drowsiness). Products include:
Thiothixene Capsules **2124**

Tranylcypromine Sulfate (Avoid use with, or for two weeks after stopping, MAOI drugs). Products include:
Parnate Tablets **1499**

Triazolam (Co-administration with sedatives may increase drowsiness).
No products indexed under this heading.

Trifluoperazine Hydrochloride (Co-administration with tranquilizers may increase drowsiness).
No products indexed under this heading.

Zaleplon (Co-administration with sedatives may increase drowsiness). Products include:
Sonata Capsules **1686**

Zolpidem Tartrate (Co-administration with sedatives may increase drowsiness). Products include:
Ambien Tablets **2867**

Food Interactions

Alcohol (Co-administration with alcohol may increase drowsiness; avoid concurrent alcohol use).

CHILDREN'S TYLENOL SUSPENSION LIQUID AND MELTAWAYS

(Acetaminophen) **1850**
None cited in PDR database.

CHILDREN'S TYLENOL PLUS COLD & ALLERGY SUSPENSION LIQUID

(Acetaminophen, Diphenhydramine Hydrochloride, Pseudoephedrine Hydrochloride).................................. **1850**
See Children's Tylenol Plus Flu Suspension Liquid

CHILDREN'S TYLENOL PLUS COLD NIGHTTIME SUSPENSION LIQUID

(Acetaminophen, Chlorpheniramine Maleate, Pseudoephedrine Hydrochloride).................................. **1851**
See Children's Tylenol Plus Flu Suspension Liquid

CHILDREN'S TYLENOL PLUS COLD & COUGH SUSPENSION LIQUID AND CHEWABLE TABLETS

(Acetaminophen, Chlorpheniramine Maleate, Dextromethorphan Hydrobromide, Pseudoephedrine Hydrochloride).................................. **1851**
See Children's Tylenol Plus Flu Suspension Liquid

CHILDREN'S TYLENOL PLUS COLD CHEWABLE TABLETS

(Acetaminophen, Chlorpheniramine Maleate, Pseudoephedrine Hydrochloride).................................. **1851**
See Children's Tylenol Plus Cold NightTime Suspension Liquid

CHILDREN'S TYLENOL PLUS COLD DAYTIME NON-DROWSY SUSPENSION LIQUID

(Acetaminophen, Pseudoephedrine Hydrochloride).................................. **1851**
See Concentrated Tylenol Infants' Drops Plus Cold and Cough

CHILDREN'S TYLENOL PLUS FLU SUSPENSION LIQUID

(Acetaminophen, Chlorpheniramine Maleate, Dextromethorphan Hydrobromide, Pseudoephedrine Hydrochloride).................................. **1853**
May interact with hypnotics and sedatives, monoamine oxidase inhibitors, and tranquilizers. Compounds in these categories include:

Alprazolam (May increase the drowsiness effect). Products include:
Niravam Orally Disintegrating Tablets **3106**
Xanax XR Tablets **2655**

Buspirone Hydrochloride (May increase the drowsiness effect).
No products indexed under this heading.

Chlordiazepoxide (May increase the drowsiness effect).
No products indexed under this heading.

Chlordiazepoxide Hydrochloride (May increase the drowsiness effect). Products include:
Librium Capsules **3349**

Chlorpromazine (May increase the drowsiness effect).
No products indexed under this heading.

Chlorpromazine Hydrochloride (May increase the drowsiness effect).
No products indexed under this heading.

Chlorprothixene (May increase the drowsiness effect).
No products indexed under this heading.

Chlorprothixene Hydrochloride (May increase the drowsiness effect).
No products indexed under this heading.

Clorazepate Dipotassium (May increase the drowsiness effect). Products include:
Tranxene **2488**

Diazepam (May increase the drowsiness effect). Products include:
Diastat Rectal Delivery System **3344**
Valium Tablets **2822**

Droperidol (May increase the drowsiness effect).
No products indexed under this heading.

Estazolam (May increase the drowsiness effect). Products include:
ProSom Tablets **512**

Ethchlorvynol (May increase the drowsiness effect).
No products indexed under this heading.

Ethinamate (May increase the drowsiness effect).
No products indexed under this heading.

Fluphenazine Decanoate (May increase the drowsiness effect).
No products indexed under this heading.

Fluphenazine Enanthate (May increase the drowsiness effect).
No products indexed under this heading.

Fluphenazine Hydrochloride (May increase the drowsiness effect).
No products indexed under this heading.

Flurazepam Hydrochloride (May increase the drowsiness effect). Products include:
Dalmane Capsules **3343**

Glutethimide (May increase the drowsiness effect).
No products indexed under this heading.

Haloperidol (May increase the drowsiness effect).
No products indexed under this heading.

Haloperidol Decanoate (May increase the drowsiness effect).
No products indexed under this heading.

Hydroxyzine Hydrochloride (May increase the drowsiness effect).
No products indexed under this heading.

Isocarboxazid (Concurrent and/or sequential use with MAO inhibitor is not recommended).
No products indexed under this heading.

Lorazepam (May increase the drowsiness effect).
No products indexed under this heading.

Loxapine Hydrochloride (May increase the drowsiness effect).
No products indexed under this heading.

Loxapine Succinate (May increase the drowsiness effect).
No products indexed under this heading.

Meprobamate (May increase the drowsiness effect).
No products indexed under this heading.

Mesoridazine Besylate (May increase the drowsiness effect).
No products indexed under this heading.

Midazolam Hydrochloride (May increase the drowsiness effect).
No products indexed under this heading.

Moclobemide (Concurrent and/or sequential use with MAO inhibitor is not recommended).
No products indexed under this heading.

Molindone Hydrochloride (May increase the drowsiness effect). Products include:
Moban Tablets 1108

Oxazepam (May increase the drowsiness effect).
No products indexed under this heading.

Pargyline Hydrochloride (Concurrent and/or sequential use with MAO inhibitor is not recommended).
No products indexed under this heading.

Perphenazine (May increase the drowsiness effect).
No products indexed under this heading.

Phenelzine Sulfate (Concurrent and/or sequential use with MAO inhibitor is not recommended).
No products indexed under this heading.

Prazepam (May increase the drowsiness effect).
No products indexed under this heading.

Procarbazine Hydrochloride (Concurrent and/or sequential use with MAO inhibitor is not recommended). Products include:
Matulane Capsules 3188

Prochlorperazine (May increase the drowsiness effect).
No products indexed under this heading.

Promethazine Hydrochloride (May increase the drowsiness effect). Products include:
Phenergan 3438

Propofol (May increase the drowsiness effect). Products include:
Diprivan Injectable Emulsion 676

Quazepam (May increase the drowsiness effect).
No products indexed under this heading.

Secobarbital Sodium (May increase the drowsiness effect).
No products indexed under this heading.

Selegiline Hydrochloride (Concurrent and/or sequential use with MAO inhibitor is not recommended). Products include:
Eldepryl Capsules 3209

Temazepam (May increase the drowsiness effect).
No products indexed under this heading.

Thioridazine Hydrochloride (May increase the drowsiness effect). Products include:
Thioridazine Hydrochloride Tablets 2122

Thiothixene (May increase the drowsiness effect). Products include:
Thiothixene Capsules 2124

Tranylcypromine Sulfate (Concurrent and/or sequential use with MAO inhibitor is not recommended). Products include:
Parnate Tablets 1499

Triazolam (May increase the drowsiness effect).
No products indexed under this heading.

Trifluoperazine Hydrochloride (May increase the drowsiness effect).
No products indexed under this heading.

Zaleplon (May increase the drowsiness effect). Products include:
Sonata Capsules 1686

Zolpidem Tartrate (May increase the drowsiness effect). Products include:
Ambien Tablets 2867

CONCENTRATED TYLENOL INFANTS' DROPS PLUS COLD

(Acetaminophen, Pseudoephedrine Hydrochloride)................................. 1851
See Concentrated Tylenol Infants' Drops Plus Cold and Cough

CONCENTRATED TYLENOL INFANTS' DROPS PLUS COLD AND COUGH

(Acetaminophen, Dextromethorphan Hydrobromide, Pseudoephedrine Hydrochloride)........ 1851
May interact with monoamine oxidase inhibitors. Compounds in these categories include:

Isocarboxazid (Concurrent and/or sequential use with MAO inhibitors is contraindicated).
No products indexed under this heading.

Moclobemide (Concurrent and/or sequential use with MAO inhibitors is contraindicated).
No products indexed under this heading.

Pargyline Hydrochloride (Concurrent and/or sequential use with MAO inhibitors is contraindicated).
No products indexed under this heading.

Phenelzine Sulfate (Concurrent and/or sequential use with MAO inhibitors is contraindicated).
No products indexed under this heading.

Procarbazine Hydrochloride (Concurrent and/or sequential use with MAO inhibitors is contraindicated). Products include:
Matulane Capsules 3188

Selegiline Hydrochloride (Concurrent and/or sequential use with MAO inhibitors is contraindicated). Products include:
Eldepryl Capsules 3209

Tranylcypromine Sulfate (Concurrent and/or sequential use with MAO inhibitors is contraindicated). Products include:
Parnate Tablets 1499

CONCENTRATED TYLENOL INFANTS' DROPS

(Acetaminophen) 1850
None cited in PDR database.

JUNIOR TYLENOL MELTAWAYS

(Acetaminophen) 1850
None cited in PDR database.

TYLENOL COLD & FLU SEVERE DAYTIME LIQUID WITH COOL BUST

(Acetaminophen, Dextromethorphan Hydrobromide, Pseudoephedrine Hydrochloride)........ 1846
See Tylenol Flu NightTime Gelcaps

TYLENOL COLD & FLU SEVERE NIGHTTIME LIQUID WITH COOL BURST

(Acetaminophen, Dextromethorphan Hydrobromide, Doxylamine Succinate, Pseudoephedrine Hydrochloride)........ 1846
See Tylenol Flu NightTime Gelcaps

TYLENOL COLD SEVERE CONGESTION NON-DROWSY CAPLETS WITH COOL BURST

(Acetaminophen, Dextromethorphan Hydrobromide, Guaifenesin, Pseudoephedrine Hydrochloride)................................. 1846
May interact with monoamine oxidase inhibitors and certain other agents. Compounds in these categories include:

Isocarboxazid (Concurrent and/or sequential use with MAO inhibitors is not recommended).
No products indexed under this heading.

Moclobemide (Concurrent and/or sequential use with MAO inhibitors is not recommended).
No products indexed under this heading.

Pargyline Hydrochloride (Concurrent and/or sequential use with MAO inhibitors is not recommended).
No products indexed under this heading.

Phenelzine Sulfate (Concurrent and/or sequential use with MAO inhibitors is not recommended).
No products indexed under this heading.

Procarbazine Hydrochloride (Concurrent and/or sequential use with MAO inhibitors is not recommended). Products include:
Matulane Capsules 3188

Selegiline Hydrochloride (Concurrent and/or sequential use with MAO inhibitors is not recommended). Products include:
Eldepryl Capsules 3209

Tranylcypromine Sulfate (Concurrent and/or sequential use with MAO inhibitors is not recommended). Products include:
Parnate Tablets 1499

Food Interactions

Alcohol (Chronic heavy alcohol abusers, 3 or more drinks per day, may be at increased risk of liver toxicity from acetaminophen use).

TYLENOL COUGH & SORE THROAT DAYTIME LIQUID WITH COOL BURST

(Acetaminophen, Dextromethorphan Hydrobromide)...... 1849
May interact with monoamine oxidase inhibitors. Compounds in these categories include:

Isocarboxazid (Avoid use with, or for two weeks after stopping, MAOI drugs).
No products indexed under this heading.

Moclobemide (Avoid use with, or for two weeks after stopping, MAOI drugs).
No products indexed under this heading.

Pargyline Hydrochloride (Avoid use with, or for two weeks after stopping, MAOI drugs).
No products indexed under this heading.

Phenelzine Sulfate (Avoid use with, or for two weeks after stopping, MAOI drugs).
No products indexed under this heading.

Procarbazine Hydrochloride (Avoid use with, or for two weeks after stopping, MAOI drugs). Products include:
Matulane Capsules 3188

Selegiline Hydrochloride (Avoid use with, or for two weeks after stopping, MAOI drugs). Products include:
Eldepryl Capsules 3209

Tranylcypromine Sulfate (Avoid use with, or for two weeks after stopping, MAOI drugs). Products include:
Parnate Tablets 1499

TYLENOL COUGH & SORE THROAT NIGHTTIME LIQUID WITH COOL BURST

(Acetaminophen, Dextromethorphan Hydrobromide, Doxylamine Succinate)....................... 1849
May interact with hypnotics and sedatives, monoamine oxidase inhibitors, tranquilizers, and certain other agents. Compounds in these categories include:

Alprazolam (Co-administration with tranquilizers may increase drowsiness). Products include:
Niravam Orally Disintegrating Tablets 3106
Xanax XR Tablets 2655

Buspirone Hydrochloride (Co-administration with tranquilizers may increase drowsiness).
No products indexed under this heading.

Chlordiazepoxide (Co-administration with tranquilizers may increase drowsiness).
No products indexed under this heading.

Chlordiazepoxide Hydrochloride (Co-administration with tranquilizers may increase drowsiness). Products include:
Librium Capsules 3349

Chlorpromazine (Co-administration with tranquilizers may increase drowsiness).
No products indexed under this heading.

Chlorpromazine Hydrochloride (Co-administration with tranquilizers may increase drowsiness).
No products indexed under this heading.

Chlorprothixene (Co-administration with tranquilizers may increase drowsiness).
No products indexed under this heading.

Chlorprothixene Hydrochloride (Co-administration with tranquilizers may increase drowsiness).
No products indexed under this heading.

Clorazepate Dipotassium (Co-administration with tranquilizers may increase drowsiness). Products include:
Tranxene 2488

Diazepam (Co-administration with tranquilizers may increase drowsiness). Products include:
Diastat Rectal Delivery System 3344
Valium Tablets 2822

Droperidol (Co-administration with tranquilizers may increase drowsiness).
No products indexed under this heading.

Estazolam (Co-administration with sedatives may increase drowsiness). Products include:
ProSom Tablets 512

Ethchlorvynol (Co-administration with sedatives may increase drowsiness).
No products indexed under this heading.

Ethinamate (Co-administration with sedatives may increase drowsiness).
No products indexed under this heading.

Fluphenazine Decanoate (Co-administration with tranquilizers may increase drowsiness).
No products indexed under this heading.

Fluphenazine Enanthate (Co-administration with tranquilizers may increase drowsiness).
No products indexed under this heading.

Fluphenazine Hydrochloride (Co-administration with tranquilizers may increase drowsiness).
No products indexed under this heading.

Flurazepam Hydrochloride (Co-administration with sedatives may increase drowsiness). Products include:
Dalmane Capsules 3343

Glutethimide (Co-administration with sedatives may increase drowsiness).
No products indexed under this heading.

Haloperidol (Co-administration with tranquilizers may increase drowsiness).
No products indexed under this heading.

Haloperidol Decanoate (Co-administration with tranquilizers may increase drowsiness).
No products indexed under this heading.

Hydroxyzine Hydrochloride (Co-administration with tranquilizers may increase drowsiness).
No products indexed under this heading.

Isocarboxazid (Avoid use with, or for two weeks after stopping, MAOI drugs).
No products indexed under this heading.

Lorazepam (Co-administration with sedatives may increase drowsiness).
No products indexed under this heading.

Loxapine Hydrochloride (Co-administration with tranquilizers may increase drowsiness).
No products indexed under this heading.

Loxapine Succinate (Co-administration with tranquilizers may increase drowsiness).
No products indexed under this heading.

Meprobamate (Co-administration with tranquilizers may increase drowsiness).
No products indexed under this heading.

Mesoridazine Besylate (Co-administration with tranquilizers may increase drowsiness).
No products indexed under this heading.

Midazolam Hydrochloride (Co-administration with sedatives may increase drowsiness).
No products indexed under this heading.

Moclobemide (Avoid use with, or for two weeks after stopping, MAOI drugs).
No products indexed under this heading.

Molindone Hydrochloride (Co-administration with tranquilizers may increase drowsiness). Products include:
Moban Tablets 1108

Oxazepam (Co-administration with tranquilizers may increase drowsiness).
No products indexed under this heading.

Pargyline Hydrochloride (Avoid use with, or for two weeks after stopping, MAOI drugs).
No products indexed under this heading.

Perphenazine (Co-administration with tranquilizers may increase drowsiness).
No products indexed under this heading.

Phenelzine Sulfate (Avoid use with, or for two weeks after stopping, MAOI drugs).
No products indexed under this heading.

Prazepam (Co-administration with tranquilizers may increase drowsiness).
No products indexed under this heading.

Procarbazine Hydrochloride (Avoid use with, or for two weeks after stopping, MAOI drugs). Products include:
Matulane Capsules 3188

Prochlorperazine (Co-administration with tranquilizers may increase drowsiness).
No products indexed under this heading.

Promethazine Hydrochloride (Co-administration with tranquilizers may increase drowsiness). Products include:
Phenergan 3438

Propofol (Co-administration with sedatives may increase drowsiness). Products include:
Diprivan Injectable Emulsion 676

Quazepam (Co-administration with sedatives may increase drowsiness).
No products indexed under this heading.

Secobarbital Sodium (Co-administration with sedatives may increase drowsiness).
No products indexed under this heading.

Selegiline Hydrochloride (Avoid use with, or for two weeks after stopping, MAOI drugs). Products include:
Eldepryl Capsules 3209

Temazepam (Co-administration with sedatives may increase drowsiness).
No products indexed under this heading.

Thioridazine Hydrochloride (Co-administration with tranquilizers may increase drowsiness). Products include:
Thioridazine Hydrochloride Tablets 2122

Thiothixene (Co-administration with tranquilizers may increase drowsiness). Products include:
Thiothixene Capsules 2124

Tranylcypromine Sulfate (Avoid use with, or for two weeks after stopping, MAOI drugs). Products include:
Parnate Tablets 1499

Triazolam (Co-administration with sedatives may increase drowsiness).
No products indexed under this heading.

Trifluoperazine Hydrochloride (Co-administration with tranquilizers may increase drowsiness).
No products indexed under this heading.

Zaleplon (Co-administration with sedatives may increase drowsiness). Products include:
Sonata Capsules 1686

Zolpidem Tartrate (Co-administration with sedatives may increase drowsiness). Products include:
Ambien Tablets 2867

Food Interactions

Alcohol (Co-administration with alcohol may increase drowsiness; avoid concurrent alcohol use).

EXTRA STRENGTH TYLENOL ADULT LIQUID PAIN RELIEVER

(Acetaminophen) 1843
See Regular Strength Tylenol Tablets

EXTRA STRENGTH TYLENOL GELTABS, CAPLETS, COOL CAPLETS AND EZ TABS

(Acetaminophen) 1843
See Regular Strength Tylenol Tablets

EXTRA STRENGTH TYLENOL RAPID RELEASE GELS

(Acetaminophen) 1843
See Regular Strength Tylenol Tablets

REGULAR STRENGTH TYLENOL TABLETS

(Acetaminophen) 1843

Food Interactions

Alcohol (Chronic heavy alcohol users, 3 or more drinks per day, should consult their physicians for advice on when and how they should take pain relievers including acetaminophen).

TYLENOL ALLERGY COMPLETE NIGHT TIME CAPLETS

(Acetaminophen, Diphenhydramine Hydrochloride, Pseudoephedrine Hydrochloride) 1844

May interact with hypnotics and sedatives, monoamine oxidase inhibitors, tranquilizers, and certain other agents. Compounds in these categories include:

Alprazolam (Concurrent use may increase drowsiness effect). Products include:
Niravam Orally Disintegrating Tablets 3106
Xanax XR Tablets 2655

Buspirone Hydrochloride (Concurrent use may increase drowsiness effect).
No products indexed under this heading.

Chlordiazepoxide (Concurrent use may increase drowsiness effect).
No products indexed under this heading.

Chlordiazepoxide Hydrochloride (Concurrent use may increase drowsiness effect). Products include:
Librium Capsules 3349

Chlorpromazine (Concurrent use may increase drowsiness effect).
No products indexed under this heading.

Chlorpromazine Hydrochloride (Concurrent use may increase drowsiness effect).
No products indexed under this heading.

Chlorprothixene (Concurrent use may increase drowsiness effect).
No products indexed under this heading.

Chlorprothixene Hydrochloride (Concurrent use may increase drowsiness effect).
No products indexed under this heading.

Clorazepate Dipotassium (Concurrent use may increase drowsiness effect). Products include:
Tranxene 2488

Diazepam (Concurrent use may increase drowsiness effect). Products include:
Diastat Rectal Delivery System 3344
Valium Tablets 2822

Droperidol (Concurrent use may increase drowsiness effect).
No products indexed under this heading.

Estazolam (Concurrent use may increase drowsiness effect). Products include:
ProSom Tablets 512

Ethchlorvynol (Concurrent use may increase drowsiness effect).
No products indexed under this heading.

Ethinamate (Concurrent use may increase drowsiness effect).
No products indexed under this heading.

Fluphenazine Decanoate (Concurrent use may increase drowsiness effect).
No products indexed under this heading.

Fluphenazine Enanthate (Concurrent use may increase drowsiness effect).
No products indexed under this heading.

Fluphenazine Hydrochloride (Concurrent use may increase drowsiness effect).
No products indexed under this heading.

Flurazepam Hydrochloride (Concurrent use may increase drowsiness effect). Products include:
Dalmane Capsules 3343

Glutethimide (Concurrent use may increase drowsiness effect).
No products indexed under this heading.

Haloperidol (Concurrent use may increase drowsiness effect).
No products indexed under this heading.

Haloperidol Decanoate (Concurrent use may increase drowsiness effect).
No products indexed under this heading.

Hydroxyzine Hydrochloride (Concurrent use may increase drowsiness effect).
No products indexed under this heading.

Isocarboxazid (Concurrent and/or sequential use with MAO inhibitors is not recommended).
No products indexed under this heading.

Lorazepam (Concurrent use may increase drowsiness effect).
No products indexed under this heading.

Loxapine Hydrochloride (Concurrent use may increase drowsiness effect).
No products indexed under this heading.

Loxapine Succinate (Concurrent use may increase drowsiness effect).
No products indexed under this heading.

Meprobamate (Concurrent use may increase drowsiness effect).
No products indexed under this heading.

Mesoridazine Besylate (Concurrent use may increase drowsiness effect).
No products indexed under this heading.

Midazolam Hydrochloride (Concurrent use may increase drowsiness effect).
No products indexed under this heading.

Moclobemide (Concurrent and/or sequential use with MAO inhibitors is not recommended).
No products indexed under this heading.

Molindone Hydrochloride (Concurrent use may increase drowsiness effect). Products include:
Moban Tablets 1108

Oxazepam (Concurrent use may increase drowsiness effect).
No products indexed under this heading.

Pargyline Hydrochloride (Concurrent and/or sequential use with MAO inhibitors is not recommended).
No products indexed under this heading.

Perphenazine (Concurrent use may increase drowsiness effect).
No products indexed under this heading.

Phenelzine Sulfate (Concurrent and/or sequential use with MAO inhibitors is not recommended).
No products indexed under this heading.

Prazepam (Concurrent use may increase drowsiness effect).
No products indexed under this heading.

Procarbazine Hydrochloride (Concurrent and/or sequential use with MAO inhibitors is not recommended). Products include:
Matulane Capsules 3188

Prochlorperazine (Concurrent use may increase drowsiness effect).
No products indexed under this heading.

Promethazine Hydrochloride (Concurrent use may increase drowsiness effect). Products include:
Phenergan 3438

Propofol (Concurrent use may increase drowsiness effect).
Products include:
Diprivan Injectable Emulsion 676

Quazepam (Concurrent use may increase drowsiness effect).
No products indexed under this heading.

Secobarbital Sodium (Concurrent use may increase drowsiness effect).
No products indexed under this heading.

Selegiline Hydrochloride (Concurrent and/or sequential use with MAO inhibitors is not recommended).
Products include:
Eldepryl Capsules 3209

Temazepam (Concurrent use may increase drowsiness effect).
No products indexed under this heading.

Thioridazine Hydrochloride (Concurrent use may increase drowsiness effect). Products include:
Thioridazine Hydrochloride Tablets 2122

Thiothixene (Concurrent use may increase drowsiness effect).
Products include:
Thiothixene Capsules 2124

Tranylcypromine Sulfate (Concurrent and/or sequential use with MAO inhibitors is not recommended).
Products include:
Parnate Tablets 1499

Triazolam (Concurrent use may increase drowsiness effect).
No products indexed under this heading.

Trifluoperazine Hydrochloride (Concurrent use may increase drowsiness effect).
No products indexed under this heading.

Zaleplon (Concurrent use may increase drowsiness effect).
Products include:
Sonata Capsules 1686

Zolpidem Tartrate (Concurrent use may increase drowsiness effect).
Products include:
Ambien Tablets 2867

Food Interactions

Alcohol (Concurrent use may increase drowsiness effect; chronic heavy alcohol abusers, 3 or more drinks per day, may be at increased risk of liver toxicity from excessive acetaminophen use).

TYLENOL ALLERGY COMPLETE MULTI-SYMPTOM CAPLETS AND GELCAPS WITH COOL BURST

(Acetaminophen, Chlorpheniramine Maleate, Pseudoephedrine Hydrochloride)................................ 1844
See Tylenol Allergy Complete Night Time Caplets

TYLENOL SEVERE ALLERGY CAPLETS

(Acetaminophen, Diphenhydramine Hydrochloride)................................ 1844
See Tylenol Allergy Complete Night Time Caplets

TYLENOL ARTHRITIS PAIN EXTENDED RELEASE CAPLETS AND GELTABS

(Acetaminophen) 1843
See Regular Strength Tylenol Tablets

TYLENOL FLU NIGHTTIME GELCAPS

(Acetaminophen, Diphenhydramine Hydrochloride, Pseudoephedrine Hydrochloride)................................ 1846

May interact with hypnotics and sedatives, monoamine oxidase inhibitors, tranquilizers, and certain other agents. Compounds in these categories include:

Alprazolam (Concurrent use may increase drowsiness effect).
Products include:
Niravam Orally Disintegrating Tablets 3106
Xanax XR Tablets 2655

Buspirone Hydrochloride (Concurrent use may increase drowsiness effect).
No products indexed under this heading.

Chlordiazepoxide (Concurrent use may increase drowsiness effect).
No products indexed under this heading.

Chlordiazepoxide Hydrochloride (Concurrent use may increase drowsiness effect). Products include:
Librium Capsules 3349

Chlorpromazine (Concurrent use may increase drowsiness effect).
No products indexed under this heading.

Chlorpromazine Hydrochloride (Concurrent use may increase drowsiness effect).
No products indexed under this heading.

Chlorprothixene (Concurrent use may increase drowsiness effect).
No products indexed under this heading.

Chlorprothixene Hydrochloride (Concurrent use may increase drowsiness effect).
No products indexed under this heading.

Clorazepate Dipotassium (Concurrent use may increase drowsiness effect). Products include:
Tranxene 2488

Diazepam (Concurrent use may increase drowsiness effect).
Products include:
Diastat Rectal Delivery System 3344
Valium Tablets 2822

Droperidol (Concurrent use may increase drowsiness effect).
No products indexed under this heading.

Estazolam (Concurrent use may increase drowsiness effect).
Products include:
ProSom Tablets 512

Ethchlorvynol (Concurrent use may increase drowsiness effect).
No products indexed under this heading.

Ethinamate (Concurrent use may increase drowsiness effect).
No products indexed under this heading.

Fluphenazine Decanoate (Concurrent use may increase drowsiness effect).
No products indexed under this heading.

Fluphenazine Enanthate (Concurrent use may increase drowsiness effect).
No products indexed under this heading.

Fluphenazine Hydrochloride (Concurrent use may increase drowsiness effect).
No products indexed under this heading.

Flurazepam Hydrochloride (Concurrent use may increase drowsiness effect). Products include:
Dalmane Capsules 3343

Glutethimide (Concurrent use may increase drowsiness effect).
No products indexed under this heading.

Haloperidol (Concurrent use may increase drowsiness effect).
No products indexed under this heading.

Haloperidol Decanoate (Concurrent use may increase drowsiness effect).
No products indexed under this heading.

Hydroxyzine Hydrochloride (Concurrent use may increase drowsiness effect).
No products indexed under this heading.

Isocarboxazid (Concurrent and/or sequential use with MAO inhibitors is not recommended).
No products indexed under this heading.

Lorazepam (Concurrent use may increase drowsiness effect).
No products indexed under this heading.

Loxapine Hydrochloride (Concurrent use may increase drowsiness effect).
No products indexed under this heading.

Loxapine Succinate (Concurrent use may increase drowsiness effect).
No products indexed under this heading.

Meprobamate (Concurrent use may increase drowsiness effect).
No products indexed under this heading.

Mesoridazine Besylate (Concurrent use may increase drowsiness effect).
No products indexed under this heading.

Midazolam Hydrochloride (Concurrent use may increase drowsiness effect).
No products indexed under this heading.

Moclobemide (Concurrent and/or sequential use with MAO inhibitors is not recommended).
No products indexed under this heading.

Molindone Hydrochloride (Concurrent use may increase drowsiness effect). Products include:
Moban Tablets 1108

Oxazepam (Concurrent use may increase drowsiness effect).
No products indexed under this heading.

Pargyline Hydrochloride (Concurrent and/or sequential use with MAO inhibitors is not recommended).
No products indexed under this heading.

Perphenazine (Concurrent use may increase drowsiness effect).
No products indexed under this heading.

Phenelzine Sulfate (Concurrent and/or sequential use with MAO inhibitors is not recommended).
No products indexed under this heading.

Prazepam (Concurrent use may increase drowsiness effect).
No products indexed under this heading.

Procarbazine Hydrochloride (Concurrent and/or sequential use with MAO inhibitors is not recommended). Products include:
Matulane Capsules 3188

Prochlorperazine (Concurrent use may increase drowsiness effect).
No products indexed under this heading.

Promethazine Hydrochloride (Concurrent use may increase drowsiness effect). Products include:
Phenergan 3438

Propofol (Concurrent use may increase drowsiness effect). Products include:
Diprivan Injectable Emulsion 676

Quazepam (Concurrent use may increase drowsiness effect).
No products indexed under this heading.

Secobarbital Sodium (Concurrent use may increase drowsiness effect).
No products indexed under this heading.

Selegiline Hydrochloride (Concurrent and/or sequential use with MAO inhibitors is not recommended). Products include:
Eldepryl Capsules 3209

Temazepam (Concurrent use may increase drowsiness effect).
No products indexed under this heading.

Thioridazine Hydrochloride (Concurrent use may increase drowsiness effect). Products include:
Thioridazine Hydrochloride Tablets 2122

Thiothixene (Concurrent use may increase drowsiness effect). Products include:
Thiothixene Capsules 2124

Tranylcypromine Sulfate (Concurrent and/or sequential use with MAO inhibitors is not recommended). Products include:
Parnate Tablets 1499

Triazolam (Concurrent use may increase drowsiness effect).
No products indexed under this heading.

Trifluoperazine Hydrochloride (Concurrent use may increase drowsiness effect).
No products indexed under this heading.

Zaleplon (Concurrent use may increase drowsiness effect). Products include:
Sonata Capsules 1686

Zolpidem Tartrate (Concurrent use may increase drowsiness effect). Products include:
Ambien Tablets 2867

Food Interactions

Alcohol (Concurrent use may increase drowsiness effect; chronic heavy alcohol abusers, 3 or more drinks per day, may be at increased risk of liver toxicity from excessive acetaminophen use).

TYLENOL FLU DAY NON-DROWSY GELCAPS

(Acetaminophen, Dextromethorphan Hydrobromide, Pseudoephedrine Hydrochloride)........ 1846
See Tylenol Flu NightTime Gelcaps

CONCENTRATED TYLENOL INFANTS' DROPS PLUS COLD NASAL CONGESTANT, FEVER REDUCER & PAIN RELIEVER

(Acetaminophen, Pseudoephedrine Hydrochloride)....... 668
May interact with monoamine oxidase inhibitors. Compounds in these categories include:

Isocarboxazid (Avoid concurrent use while taking, or for up to 2 weeks after stopping, MAO inhibitors).
No products indexed under this heading.

Moclobemide (Avoid concurrent use while taking, or for up to 2 weeks after stopping, MAO inhibitors).
No products indexed under this heading.

Pargyline Hydrochloride (Avoid concurrent use while taking, or for up to 2 weeks after stopping, MAO inhibitors).
No products indexed under this heading.

Phenelzine Sulfate (Avoid concurrent use while taking, or for up to 2 weeks after stopping, MAO inhibitors).
No products indexed under this heading.

Procarbazine Hydrochloride (Avoid concurrent use while taking, or for up to 2 weeks after stopping, MAO inhibitors). Products include:
Matulane Capsules 3188

Selegiline Hydrochloride (Avoid concurrent use while taking, or for up to 2 weeks after stopping, MAO inhibitors). Products include:
Eldepryl Capsules 3209

Tranylcypromine Sulfate (Avoid concurrent use while taking, or for up to 2 weeks after stopping, MAO inhibitors). Products include:
Parnate Tablets 1499

CONCENTRATED TYLENOL INFANTS' DROPS PLUS COLD & COUGH NASAL DECONGESTANT, FEVER REDUCER & PAIN RELIEVER

(Acetaminophen, Dextromethorphan Hydrobromide, Pseudoephedrine Hydrochloride)....... 668
May interact with monoamine oxidase inhibitors. Compounds in these categories include:

Isocarboxazid (Avoid concurrent use while taking, or for up to 2 weeks after stopping, MAO inhibitors).
No products indexed under this heading.

Moclobemide (Avoid concurrent use while taking, or for up to 2 weeks after stopping, MAO inhibitors).
No products indexed under this heading.

Pargyline Hydrochloride (Avoid concurrent use while taking, or for up to 2 weeks after stopping, MAO inhibitors).
No products indexed under this heading.

Phenelzine Sulfate (Avoid concurrent use while taking, or for up to 2 weeks after stopping, MAO inhibitors).
No products indexed under this heading.

Procarbazine Hydrochloride (Avoid concurrent use while taking, or for up to 2 weeks after stopping, MAO inhibitors). Products include:
Matulane Capsules 3188

Selegiline Hydrochloride (Avoid concurrent use while taking, or for up to 2 weeks after stopping, MAO inhibitors). Products include:
Eldepryl Capsules 3209

Tranylcypromine Sulfate (Avoid concurrent use while taking, or for up to 2 weeks after stopping, MAO inhibitors). Products include:
Parnate Tablets 1499

MULTI-SYMPTOM TYLENOL COLD NIGHT TIME CAPLETS

(Acetaminophen, Chlorpheniramine Maleate, Dextromethorphan Hydrobromide, Pseudoephedrine Hydrochloride).................................. 1845
See Tylenol Allergy Complete Night Time Caplets

MULTI-SYMPTOM TYLENOL COLD DAY NON-DROWSY CAPLETS AND GELCAPS

(Acetaminophen, Dextromethorphan Hydrobromide, Pseudoephedrine Hydrochloride)........ 1845
See Tylenol Allergy Complete Night Time Caplets

EXTRA STRENGTH TYLENOL PM CAPLETS, GELTABS, GELCAPS AND LIQUID

(Acetaminophen, Diphenhydramine Hydrochloride).................................. 1847
May interact with hypnotics and sedatives, tranquilizers, and certain other agents. Compounds in these categories include:

Alprazolam (Tylenol PM causes drowsiness; concurrent use may increase the drowsiness effect). Products include:
Niravam Orally Disintegrating Tablets 3106
Xanax XR Tablets 2655

Buspirone Hydrochloride (Tylenol PM causes drowsiness; concurrent use may increase the drowsiness effect).
No products indexed under this heading.

Chlordiazepoxide (Tylenol PM causes drowsiness; concurrent use may increase the drowsiness effect).
No products indexed under this heading.

Chlordiazepoxide Hydrochloride (Tylenol PM causes drowsiness; concurrent use may increase the drowsiness effect). Products include:
Librium Capsules 3349

Chlorpromazine (Tylenol PM causes drowsiness; concurrent use may increase the drowsiness effect).
No products indexed under this heading.

Chlorpromazine Hydrochloride (Tylenol PM causes drowsiness; concurrent use may increase the drowsiness effect).
No products indexed under this heading.

Chlorprothixene (Tylenol PM causes drowsiness; concurrent use may increase the drowsiness effect).
No products indexed under this heading.

Chlorprothixene Hydrochloride (Tylenol PM causes drowsiness; concurrent use may increase the drowsiness effect).
No products indexed under this heading.

Clorazepate Dipotassium (Tylenol PM causes drowsiness; concurrent use may increase the drowsiness effect). Products include:
Tranxene 2488

Diazepam (Tylenol PM causes drowsiness; concurrent use may increase the drowsiness effect). Products include:
Diastat Rectal Delivery System 3344
Valium Tablets 2822

Droperidol (Tylenol PM causes drowsiness; concurrent use may increase the drowsiness effect).
No products indexed under this heading.

Estazolam (Tylenol PM causes drowsiness; concurrent use may increase the drowsiness effect). Products include:
ProSom Tablets 512

Ethchlorvynol (Tylenol PM causes drowsiness; concurrent use may increase the drowsiness effect).
No products indexed under this heading.

Ethinamate (Tylenol PM causes drowsiness; concurrent use may increase the drowsiness effect).
No products indexed under this heading.

IMPORTANT NOTE: Always consult each drug listing in the patient's regimen for possible interactions.

Fluphenazine Decanoate (Tylenol PM causes drowsiness; concurrent use may increase the drowsiness effect).
No products indexed under this heading.

Fluphenazine Enanthate (Tylenol PM causes drowsiness; concurrent use may increase the drowsiness effect).
No products indexed under this heading.

Fluphenazine Hydrochloride (Tylenol PM causes drowsiness; concurrent use may increase the drowsiness effect).
No products indexed under this heading.

Flurazepam Hydrochloride (Tylenol PM causes drowsiness; concurrent use may increase the drowsiness effect). Products include:
Dalmane Capsules 3343

Glutethimide (Tylenol PM causes drowsiness; concurrent use may increase the drowsiness effect).
No products indexed under this heading.

Haloperidol (Tylenol PM causes drowsiness; concurrent use may increase the drowsiness effect).
No products indexed under this heading.

Haloperidol Decanoate (Tylenol PM causes drowsiness; concurrent use may increase the drowsiness effect).
No products indexed under this heading.

Hydroxyzine Hydrochloride (Tylenol PM causes drowsiness; concurrent use may increase the drowsiness effect).
No products indexed under this heading.

Lorazepam (Tylenol PM causes drowsiness; concurrent use may increase the drowsiness effect).
No products indexed under this heading.

Loxapine Hydrochloride (Tylenol PM causes drowsiness; concurrent use may increase the drowsiness effect).
No products indexed under this heading.

Loxapine Succinate (Tylenol PM causes drowsiness; concurrent use may increase the drowsiness effect).
No products indexed under this heading.

Meprobamate (Tylenol PM causes drowsiness; concurrent use may increase the drowsiness effect).
No products indexed under this heading.

Mesoridazine Besylate (Tylenol PM causes drowsiness; concurrent use may increase the drowsiness effect).
No products indexed under this heading.

Midazolam Hydrochloride (Tylenol PM causes drowsiness; concurrent use may increase the drowsiness effect).
No products indexed under this heading.

Molindone Hydrochloride (Tylenol PM causes drowsiness; concurrent use may increase the drowsiness effect). Products include:
Moban Tablets 1108

Oxazepam (Tylenol PM causes drowsiness; concurrent use may increase the drowsiness effect).
No products indexed under this heading.

Perphenazine (Tylenol PM causes drowsiness; concurrent use may increase the drowsiness effect).
No products indexed under this heading.

Prazepam (Tylenol PM causes drowsiness; concurrent use may increase the drowsiness effect).
No products indexed under this heading.

Prochlorperazine (Tylenol PM causes drowsiness; concurrent use may increase the drowsiness effect).
No products indexed under this heading.

Promethazine Hydrochloride (Tylenol PM causes drowsiness; concurrent use may increase the drowsiness effect). Products include:
Phenergan 3438

Propofol (Tylenol PM causes drowsiness; concurrent use may increase the drowsiness effect). Products include:
Diprivan Injectable Emulsion 676

Quazepam (Tylenol PM causes drowsiness; concurrent use may increase the drowsiness effect).
No products indexed under this heading.

Secobarbital Sodium (Tylenol PM causes drowsiness; concurrent use may increase the drowsiness effect).
No products indexed under this heading.

Temazepam (Tylenol PM causes drowsiness; concurrent use may increase the drowsiness effect).
No products indexed under this heading.

Thioridazine Hydrochloride (Tylenol PM causes drowsiness; concurrent use may increase the drowsiness effect). Products include:
Thioridazine Hydrochloride Tablets 2122

Thiothixene (Tylenol PM causes drowsiness; concurrent use may increase the drowsiness effect). Products include:
Thiothixene Capsules 2124

Triazolam (Tylenol PM causes drowsiness; concurrent use may increase the drowsiness effect).
No products indexed under this heading.

Trifluoperazine Hydrochloride (Tylenol PM causes drowsiness; concurrent use may increase the drowsiness effect).
No products indexed under this heading.

Zaleplon (Tylenol PM causes drowsiness; concurrent use may increase the drowsiness effect). Products include:
Sonata Capsules 1686

Zolpidem Tartrate (Tylenol PM causes drowsiness; concurrent use may increase the drowsiness effect). Products include:
Ambien Tablets 2867

Food Interactions

Alcohol (Avoid concurrent use; chronic heavy alcohol abusers, 3 or more drinks per day, may be at increased risk of liver toxicity from acetaminophen use).

TYLENOL SINUS DAY NON-DROWSY CAPLETS

(Acetaminophen, Pseudoephedrine Hydrochloride) 1848
May interact with monoamine oxidase inhibitors. Compounds in these categories include:

Isocarboxazid (Concurrent and/or sequential use with MAO inhibitors is not recommended).
No products indexed under this heading.

Moclobemide (Concurrent and/or sequential use with MAO inhibitors is not recommended).
No products indexed under this heading.

Pargyline Hydrochloride (Concurrent and/or sequential use with MAO inhibitors is not recommended).
No products indexed under this heading.

Phenelzine Sulfate (Concurrent and/or sequential use with MAO inhibitors is not recommended).
No products indexed under this heading.

Procarbazine Hydrochloride (Concurrent and/or sequential use with MAO inhibitors is not recommended). Products include:
Matulane Capsules 3188

Selegiline Hydrochloride (Concurrent and/or sequential use with MAO inhibitors is not recommended). Products include:
Eldepryl Capsules 3209

Tranylcypromine Sulfate (Concurrent and/or sequential use with MAO inhibitors is not recommended). Products include:
Parnate Tablets 1499

TYLENOL SINUS DAY NON-DROWSY GELCAPS

(Acetaminophen, Pseudoephedrine Hydrochloride) 1848
May interact with monoamine oxidase inhibitors. Compounds in these categories include:

Isocarboxazid (Concurrent and/or sequential use with MAO inhibitors is not recommended).
No products indexed under this heading.

Moclobemide (Concurrent and/or sequential use with MAO inhibitors is not recommended).
No products indexed under this heading.

Pargyline Hydrochloride (Concurrent and/or sequential use with MAO inhibitors is not recommended).
No products indexed under this heading.

Phenelzine Sulfate (Concurrent and/or sequential use with MAO inhibitors is not recommended).
No products indexed under this heading.

Procarbazine Hydrochloride (Concurrent and/or sequential use with MAO inhibitors is not recommended). Products include:
Matulane Capsules 3188

Selegiline Hydrochloride (Concurrent and/or sequential use with MAO inhibitors is not recommended). Products include:
Eldepryl Capsules 3209

Tranylcypromine Sulfate (Concurrent and/or sequential use with MAO inhibitors is not recommended). Products include:
Parnate Tablets 1499

TYLENOL SINUS NIGHT TIME CAPLETS

(Acetaminophen, Doxylamine Succinate, Pseudoephedrine Hydrochloride) 1848
May interact with hypnotics and sedatives, monoamine oxidase inhibitors, tranquilizers, and certain other agents. Compounds in these categories include:

Alprazolam (May increase drowsiness effect). Products include:
Niravam Orally Disintegrating Tablets 3106
Xanax XR Tablets 2655

Buspirone Hydrochloride (May increase drowsiness effect).
No products indexed under this heading.

Chlordiazepoxide (May increase drowsiness effect).
No products indexed under this heading.

Chlordiazepoxide Hydrochloride (May increase drowsiness effect). Products include:
Librium Capsules 3349

Chlorpromazine (May increase drowsiness effect).
No products indexed under this heading.

Chlorpromazine Hydrochloride (May increase drowsiness effect).
No products indexed under this heading.

Chlorprothixene (May increase drowsiness effect).
No products indexed under this heading.

Chlorprothixene Hydrochloride (May increase drowsiness effect).
No products indexed under this heading.

Clorazepate Dipotassium (May increase drowsiness effect). Products include:
Tranxene 2488

Diazepam (May increase drowsiness effect). Products include:
Diastat Rectal Delivery System 3344
Valium Tablets 2822

Droperidol (May increase drowsiness effect).
No products indexed under this heading.

Estazolam (May increase drowsiness effect). Products include:
ProSom Tablets 512

Ethchlorvynol (May increase drowsiness effect).
No products indexed under this heading.

Ethinamate (May increase drowsiness effect).
No products indexed under this heading.

Fluphenazine Decanoate (May increase drowsiness effect).
No products indexed under this heading.

Fluphenazine Enanthate (May increase drowsiness effect).
No products indexed under this heading.

Fluphenazine Hydrochloride (May increase drowsiness effect).
No products indexed under this heading.

Flurazepam Hydrochloride (May increase drowsiness effect). Products include:
Dalmane Capsules 3343

Glutethimide (May increase drowsiness effect).
No products indexed under this heading.

Haloperidol (May increase drowsiness effect).
No products indexed under this heading.

Haloperidol Decanoate (May increase drowsiness effect).
No products indexed under this heading.

Hydroxyzine Hydrochloride (May increase drowsiness effect).
No products indexed under this heading.

Isocarboxazid (Concurrent and/or sequential use with MAO inhibitors is not recommended).
No products indexed under this heading.

Lorazepam (May increase drowsiness effect).
No products indexed under this heading.

Loxapine Hydrochloride (May increase drowsiness effect).
No products indexed under this heading.

Loxapine Succinate (May increase drowsiness effect).
No products indexed under this heading.

Meprobamate (May increase drowsiness effect).
No products indexed under this heading.

Mesoridazine Besylate (May increase drowsiness effect).
No products indexed under this heading.

Midazolam Hydrochloride (May increase drowsiness effect).
No products indexed under this heading.

Moclobemide (Concurrent and/or sequential use with MAO inhibitors is not recommended).
No products indexed under this heading.

Molindone Hydrochloride (May increase drowsiness effect). Products include:
Moban Tablets 1108

Oxazepam (May increase drowsiness effect).
No products indexed under this heading.

Pargyline Hydrochloride (Concurrent and/or sequential use with MAO inhibitors is not recommended).
No products indexed under this heading.

Perphenazine (May increase drowsiness effect).
No products indexed under this heading.

Phenelzine Sulfate (Concurrent and/or sequential use with MAO inhibitors is not recommended).
No products indexed under this heading.

Prazepam (May increase drowsiness effect).
No products indexed under this heading.

Procarbazine Hydrochloride (Concurrent and/or sequential use with MAO inhibitors is not recommended). Products include:
Matulane Capsules 3188

Prochlorperazine (May increase drowsiness effect).
No products indexed under this heading.

Promethazine Hydrochloride (May increase drowsiness effect). Products include:
Phenergan 3438

Propofol (May increase drowsiness effect). Products include:
Diprivan Injectable Emulsion 676

Quazepam (May increase drowsiness effect).
No products indexed under this heading.

Secobarbital Sodium (May increase drowsiness effect).
No products indexed under this heading.

Selegiline Hydrochloride (Concurrent and/or sequential use with MAO inhibitors is not recommended). Products include:
Eldepryl Capsules 3209

Temazepam (May increase drowsiness effect).
No products indexed under this heading.

Thioridazine Hydrochloride (May increase drowsiness effect). Products include:
Thioridazine Hydrochloride Tablets 2122

Thiothixene (May increase drowsiness effect). Products include:
Thiothixene Capsules 2124

Tranylcypromine Sulfate (Concurrent and/or sequential use with MAO inhibitors is not recommended). Products include:
Parnate Tablets 1499

Triazolam (May increase drowsiness effect).
No products indexed under this heading.

Trifluoperazine Hydrochloride (May increase drowsiness effect).
No products indexed under this heading.

Zaleplon (May increase drowsiness effect). Products include:
Sonata Capsules 1686

Zolpidem Tartrate (May increase drowsiness effect). Products include:
Ambien Tablets 2867

Food Interactions

Alcohol (May increase drowsiness effect).

TYLENOL SINUS SEVERE CONGESTION CAPLETS WITH COOL BURST
(Acetaminophen, Doxylamine Succinate, Pseudoephedrine Hydrochloride) 1848
See Tylenol Sinus Night Time Caplets

TYLENOL SORE THROAT DAYTIME LIQUID WITH COOL BURST
(Acetaminophen) 1849
See Tylenol Cough & Sore Throat Daytime Liquid with Cool Burst

TYLENOL SORE THROAT NIGHTTIME LIQUID WITH COOL BURST
(Acetaminophen, Diphenhydramine) 1849
See Tylenol Cough & Sore Throat Night-Time Liquid with Cool Burst

TYLENOL WITH CODEINE ELIXIR
(Acetaminophen, Codeine Phosphate) 2461
May interact with anticholinergics and central nervous system depressants. Compounds in these categories include:

Alfentanil Hydrochloride (Co-administration with other CNS depressants may exhibit an additive CNS depression).
No products indexed under this heading.

Alprazolam (Co-administration with other CNS depressants may exhibit an additive CNS depression). Products include:
Niravam Orally Disintegrating Tablets 3106
Xanax XR Tablets 2655

Aprobarbital (Co-administration with other CNS depressants may exhibit an additive CNS depression).
No products indexed under this heading.

Atropine Sulfate (Co-administration of codeine with anticholinergics may produce paralytic ileus).
No products indexed under this heading.

Belladonna Alkaloids (Co-administration of codeine with anticholinergics may produce paralytic ileus). Products include:
Hyland's Teething Tablets .... ▣ 736

Benztropine Mesylate (Co-administration of codeine with anticholinergics may produce paralytic ileus). Products include:
Cogentin Injection 1903

Biperiden Hydrochloride (Co-administration of codeine with anticholinergics may produce paralytic ileus).
No products indexed under this heading.

Buprenorphine Hydrochloride (Co-administration with other CNS depressants may exhibit an additive CNS depression). Products include:
Buprenex Injectable 2718
Suboxone Tablets 2719
Subutex Tablets 2719

Buspirone Hydrochloride (Co-administration with other CNS depressants may exhibit an additive CNS depression).
No products indexed under this heading.

Butabarbital (Co-administration with other CNS depressants may exhibit an additive CNS depression).
No products indexed under this heading.

Butalbital (Co-administration with other CNS depressants may exhibit an additive CNS depression). Products include:
Sedapap Tablets 50 mg/650 mg 2098

Chlordiazepoxide (Co-administration with other CNS depressants may exhibit an additive CNS depression).
No products indexed under this heading.

Chlordiazepoxide Hydrochloride (Co-administration with other CNS depressants may exhibit an additive CNS depression). Products include:
Librium Capsules 3349

Chlorpromazine (Co-administration with other CNS depressants may exhibit an additive CNS depression).
No products indexed under this heading.

Chlorpromazine Hydrochloride (Co-administration with other CNS depressants may exhibit an additive CNS depression).
No products indexed under this heading.

Chlorprothixene (Co-administration with other CNS depressants may exhibit an additive CNS depression).
No products indexed under this heading.

Chlorprothixene Hydrochloride (Co-administration with other CNS depressants may exhibit an additive CNS depression).
No products indexed under this heading.

Chlorprothixene Lactate (Co-administration with other CNS depressants may exhibit an additive CNS depression).
No products indexed under this heading.

Clidinium Bromide (Co-administration of codeine with anticholinergics may produce paralytic ileus).
No products indexed under this heading.

Clorazepate Dipotassium (Co-administration with other CNS depressants may exhibit an additive CNS depression). Products include:
Tranxene 2488

Clozapine (Co-administration with other CNS depressants may exhibit an additive CNS depression). Products include:
Clozapine Tablets 2141
Clozaril Tablets 2174
FazaClo Orally Disintegrating Tablets 547

Desflurane (Co-administration with other CNS depressants may exhibit an additive CNS depression). Products include:
Suprane Liquid for Inhalation 770

Dezocine (Co-administration with other CNS depressants may exhibit an additive CNS depression).
No products indexed under this heading.

Diazepam (Co-administration with other CNS depressants may exhibit an additive CNS depression). Products include:
Diastat Rectal Delivery System 3344
Valium Tablets 2822

Dicyclomine Hydrochloride (Co-administration of codeine with anticholinergics may produce paralytic ileus). Products include:
Bentyl Capsules 724
Bentyl Injection 724
Bentyl Syrup 724
Bentyl Tablets 724

Droperidol (Co-administration with other CNS depressants may exhibit an additive CNS depression).
No products indexed under this heading.

Enflurane (Co-administration with other CNS depressants may exhibit an additive CNS depression).
No products indexed under this heading.

Estazolam (Co-administration with other CNS depressants may exhibit an additive CNS depression). Products include:
ProSom Tablets 512

Ethanol (Co-administration with other CNS depressants may exhibit an additive CNS depression).
No products indexed under this heading.

Ethchlorvynol (Co-administration with other CNS depressants may exhibit an additive CNS depression).
No products indexed under this heading.

Ethinamate (Co-administration with other CNS depressants may exhibit an additive CNS depression).
No products indexed under this heading.

Ethyl Alcohol (Co-administration with other CNS depressants may exhibit an additive CNS depression).
No products indexed under this heading.

Fentanyl (Co-administration with other CNS depressants may exhibit an additive CNS depression).
Products include:
Duragesic Transdermal System **2448**

Fentanyl Citrate (Co-administration with other CNS depressants may exhibit an additive CNS depression).
Products include:
Actiq **993**

Fluphenazine Decanoate (Co-administration with other CNS depressants may exhibit an additive CNS depression).
No products indexed under this heading.

Fluphenazine Enanthate (Co-administration with other CNS depressants may exhibit an additive CNS depression).
No products indexed under this heading.

Fluphenazine Hydrochloride (Co-administration with other CNS depressants may exhibit an additive CNS depression).
No products indexed under this heading.

Flurazepam Hydrochloride (Co-administration with other CNS depressants may exhibit an additive CNS depression). Products include:
Dalmane Capsules **3343**

Glutethimide (Co-administration with other CNS depressants may exhibit an additive CNS depression).
No products indexed under this heading.

Glycopyrrolate (Co-administration of codeine with anticholinergics may produce paralytic ileus).
No products indexed under this heading.

Haloperidol (Co-administration with other CNS depressants may exhibit an additive CNS depression).
No products indexed under this heading.

Haloperidol Decanoate (Co-administration with other CNS depressants may exhibit an additive CNS depression).
No products indexed under this heading.

Hydrocodone Bitartrate (Co-administration with other CNS depressants may exhibit an additive CNS depression). Products include:
Hycodan **1104**
Hycomine Compound Tablets **1105**
Hycotuss Expectorant Syrup **1106**
Lortab **3315**
Lortab Elixir **3312**
Vicodin Tablets **530**
Vicodin ES Tablets **531**
Vicodin HP Tablets **532**
Vicoprofen Tablets **533**
Zydone Tablets **1118**

Hydrocodone Polistirex (Co-administration with other CNS depressants may exhibit an additive CNS depression). Products include:
Tussionex Pennkinetic Extended-Release Suspension **3322**

Hydromorphone Hydrochloride (Co-administration with other CNS depressants may exhibit an additive CNS depression). Products include:
Dilaudid **439**
Dilaudid Oral Liquid **443**
Dilaudid Non-Sterile Powder **439**
Dilaudid Rectal Suppositories **439**
Dilaudid Tablets **439**
Dilaudid Tablets - 8 mg **443**
Dilaudid-HP **441**

Hydroxyzine Hydrochloride (Co-administration with other CNS depressants may exhibit an additive CNS depression).
No products indexed under this heading.

Hyoscyamine (Co-administration of codeine with anticholinergics may produce paralytic ileus).
No products indexed under this heading.

Hyoscyamine Sulfate (Co-administration of codeine with anticholinergics may produce paralytic ileus).
No products indexed under this heading.

Ipratropium Bromide (Co-administration of codeine with anticholinergics may produce paralytic ileus). Products include:
Atrovent HFA Inhalation Aerosol **872**
Atrovent Inhalation Solution **868**
Atrovent Nasal Spray 0.03% **869**
Atrovent Nasal Spray 0.06% **870**
Combivent Inhalation Aerosol **878**
DuoNeb Inhalation Solution **1058**

Isoflurane (Co-administration with other CNS depressants may exhibit an additive CNS depression).
No products indexed under this heading.

Ketamine Hydrochloride (Co-administration with other CNS depressants may exhibit an additive CNS depression).
No products indexed under this heading.

Levomethadyl Acetate Hydrochloride (Co-administration with other CNS depressants may exhibit an additive CNS depression).
No products indexed under this heading.

Levorphanol Tartrate (Co-administration with other CNS depressants may exhibit an additive CNS depression).
No products indexed under this heading.

Lorazepam (Co-administration with other CNS depressants may exhibit an additive CNS depression).
No products indexed under this heading.

Loxapine Hydrochloride (Co-administration with other CNS depressants may exhibit an additive CNS depression).
No products indexed under this heading.

Loxapine Succinate (Co-administration with other CNS depressants may exhibit an additive CNS depression).
No products indexed under this heading.

Mepenzolate Bromide (Co-administration of codeine with anticholinergics may produce paralytic ileus).
No products indexed under this heading.

Meperidine Hydrochloride (Co-administration with other CNS depressants may exhibit an additive CNS depression).
No products indexed under this heading.

Mephobarbital (Co-administration with other CNS depressants may exhibit an additive CNS depression).
Products include:
Mebaral Tablets, USP **2483**

Meprobamate (Co-administration with other CNS depressants may exhibit an additive CNS depression).
No products indexed under this heading.

Mesoridazine Besylate (Co-administration with other CNS depressants may exhibit an additive CNS depression).
No products indexed under this heading.

Methadone Hydrochloride (Co-administration with other CNS depressants may exhibit an additive CNS depression).
No products indexed under this heading.

Methohexital Sodium (Co-administration with other CNS depressants may exhibit an additive CNS depression).
No products indexed under this heading.

Methotrimeprazine (Co-administration with other CNS depressants may exhibit an additive CNS depression).
No products indexed under this heading.

Methoxyflurane (Co-administration with other CNS depressants may exhibit an additive CNS depression).
No products indexed under this heading.

Midazolam Hydrochloride (Co-administration with other CNS depressants may exhibit an additive CNS depression).
No products indexed under this heading.

Molindone Hydrochloride (Co-administration with other CNS depressants may exhibit an additive CNS depression). Products include:
Moban Tablets **1108**

Morphine Sulfate (Co-administration with other CNS depressants may exhibit an additive CNS depression). Products include:
Avinza Capsules **1714**
Kadian Capsules **572**
MS Contin Tablets **2703**

Olanzapine (Co-administration with other CNS depressants may exhibit an additive CNS depression).
Products include:
Symbyax Capsules **1788**
Zyprexa Tablets **1798**
Zyprexa IntraMuscular **1798**
Zyprexa ZYDIS Orally Disintegrating Tablets **1798**

Oxazepam (Co-administration with other CNS depressants may exhibit an additive CNS depression).
No products indexed under this heading.

Oxybutynin Chloride (Co-administration of codeine with anticholinergics may produce paralytic ileus). Products include:
Ditropan XL Extended Release Tablets **2391**

Oxycodone Hydrochloride (Co-administration with other CNS depressants may exhibit an additive CNS depression). Products include:
Combunox Tablets **1183**
OxyContin Tablets **2699**
OxyFast Oral Concentrate Solution **2704**
OxyIR Capsules **2704**
Percocet Tablets **1114**
Percodan Tablets **1115**

Pentobarbital Sodium (Co-administration with other CNS depressants may exhibit an additive CNS depression). Products include:
Nembutal Sodium Solution, USP **2484**

Perphenazine (Co-administration with other CNS depressants may exhibit an additive CNS depression).
No products indexed under this heading.

Phenobarbital (Co-administration with other CNS depressants may exhibit an additive CNS depression).
No products indexed under this heading.

Prazepam (Co-administration with other CNS depressants may exhibit an additive CNS depression).
No products indexed under this heading.

Prochlorperazine (Co-administration with other CNS depressants may exhibit an additive CNS depression).
No products indexed under this heading.

Procyclidine Hydrochloride (Co-administration of codeine with anticholinergics may produce paralytic ileus).
No products indexed under this heading.

Promethazine Hydrochloride (Co-administration with other CNS depressants may exhibit an additive CNS depression). Products include:
Phenergan **3438**

Propantheline Bromide (Co-administration of codeine with anticholinergics may produce paralytic ileus).
No products indexed under this heading.

Propofol (Co-administration with other CNS depressants may exhibit an additive CNS depression).
Products include:
Diprivan Injectable Emulsion **676**

Propoxyphene Hydrochloride (Co-administration with other CNS depressants may exhibit an additive CNS depression).
No products indexed under this heading.

Propoxyphene Napsylate (Co-administration with other CNS depressants may exhibit an additive CNS depression). Products include:
Darvocet A 500 Tablets **3497**

Quazepam (Co-administration with other CNS depressants may exhibit an additive CNS depression).
No products indexed under this heading.

Quetiapine Fumarate (Co-administration with other CNS depressants may exhibit an additive CNS depression). Products include:
Seroquel Tablets **691**

Remifentanil Hydrochloride (Co-administration with other CNS depressants may exhibit an additive CNS depression).
No products indexed under this heading.

Risperidone (Co-administration with other CNS depressants may exhibit an additive CNS depression). Products include:
Risperdal Consta Long-Acting Injection 1664
Risperdal M-Tab Orally Disintegrating Tablets 1658
Risperdal 1658

Scopolamine (Co-administration of codeine with anticholinergics may produce paralytic ileus). Products include:
Transderm Scōp Transdermal Therapeutic System 2166

Scopolamine Hydrobromide (Co-administration of codeine with anticholinergics may produce paralytic ileus).
No products indexed under this heading.

Secobarbital Sodium (Co-administration with other CNS depressants may exhibit an additive CNS depression).
No products indexed under this heading.

Sevoflurane (Co-administration with other CNS depressants may exhibit an additive CNS depression). Products include:
Ultane Liquid for Inhalation 526

Sufentanil Citrate (Co-administration with other CNS depressants may exhibit an additive CNS depression).
No products indexed under this heading.

Temazepam (Co-administration with other CNS depressants may exhibit an additive CNS depression).
No products indexed under this heading.

Thiamylal Sodium (Co-administration with other CNS depressants may exhibit an additive CNS depression).
No products indexed under this heading.

Thioridazine Hydrochloride (Co-administration with other CNS depressants may exhibit an additive CNS depression). Products include:
Thioridazine Hydrochloride Tablets 2122

Thiothixene (Co-administration with other CNS depressants may exhibit an additive CNS depression). Products include:
Thiothixene Capsules 2124

Tolterodine Tartrate (Co-administration of codeine with anticholinergics may produce paralytic ileus). Products include:
Detrol Tablets 2626
Detrol LA Capsules 2629

Triazolam (Co-administration with other CNS depressants may exhibit an additive CNS depression).
No products indexed under this heading.

Tridihexethyl Chloride (Co-administration of codeine with anticholinergics may produce paralytic ileus).
No products indexed under this heading.

Trifluoperazine Hydrochloride (Co-administration with other CNS depressants may exhibit an additive CNS depression).
No products indexed under this heading.

Trihexyphenidyl Hydrochloride (Co-administration of codeine with anticholinergics may produce paralytic ileus).
No products indexed under this heading.

Zaleplon (Co-administration with other CNS depressants may exhibit an additive CNS depression). Products include:
Sonata Capsules 1686

Ziprasidone Hydrochloride (Co-administration with other CNS depressants may exhibit an additive CNS depression). Products include:
Geodon Capsules 2514

Zolpidem Tartrate (Co-administration with other CNS depressants may exhibit an additive CNS depression). Products include:
Ambien Tablets 2867

Food Interactions

Alcohol (Concurrent use with other CNS depressants may exhibit an additive CNS depression).

TYLENOL WITH CODEINE TABLETS

(Acetaminophen, Codeine Phosphate) 2461
See Tylenol with Codeine Elixir

WOMEN'S TYLENOL MENSTRUAL RELIEF CAPLETS

(Acetaminophen, Pamabrom) 1849

Food Interactions

Alcohol (Chronic heavy alcohol users, 3 or more drinks per day, should consult their physicians for advice on when and how they should take pain relievers, including acetaminophen).

U-CORT 1% CREAM

(Hydrocortisone Acetate) 3289
None cited in PDR database.

U-KERA CREAM

(Urea) 3290
None cited in PDR database.

ULTANE LIQUID FOR INHALATION

(Sevoflurane) 526
May interact with benzodiazepines, narcotic analgesics, nondepolarizing neuromuscular blocking agents, and certain other agents. Compounds in these categories include:

Alfentanil Hydrochloride (Benzodiazepines would be expected to decrease the MAC of sevoflurane in the same manner as with other inhalational anesthetics. Sevoflurane administration is compatible with benzodiazepines and opioids as commonly used in surgical practice).
No products indexed under this heading.

Alprazolam (Benzodiazepines would be expected to decrease the MAC of sevoflurane in the same manner as with other inhalational anesthetics. Sevoflurane administration is compatible with benzodiazepines and opioids as commonly used in surgical practice). Products include:
Niravam Orally Disintegrating Tablets 3106
Xanax XR Tablets 2655

Atracurium Besylate (Sevoflurane increases both the intensity and duration of neuromuscular blockade induced by non-depolarizing muscle relaxants. When used to supplement alfentanil-nitrous oxide anesthesia, sevoflurane and isoflurane equally potentiate neuromuscular block induced with pancuronium, vecuronium or atracurium. Among available non-depolarizing agents, only vecuronium, pancuronium and atracurium interactions have been studied during sevoflurane anesthesia. In the absence of specific guidelines: 1) For endotracheal intubation, do not reduce the dose of non-depolarizing muscle relaxants. 2) During maintenance of anesthesia, the required dose of non-depolarizing muscle relaxants is likely to be reduced compared to that during nitrous oxide/opioid anesthesia).
No products indexed under this heading.

Buprenorphine Hydrochloride (Benzodiazepines would be expected to decrease the MAC of sevoflurane in the same manner as with other inhalational anesthetics. Sevoflurane administration is compatible with benzodiazepines and opioids as commonly used in surgical practice). Products include:
Buprenex Injectable 2718
Suboxone Tablets 2719
Subutex Tablets 2719

Chlordiazepoxide (Benzodiazepines would be expected to decrease the MAC of sevoflurane in the same manner as with other inhalational anesthetics. Sevoflurane administration is compatible with benzodiazepines and opioids as commonly used in surgical practice).
No products indexed under this heading.

Chlordiazepoxide Hydrochloride (Benzodiazepines would be expected to decrease the MAC of sevoflurane in the same manner as with other inhalational anesthetics. Sevoflurane administration is compatible with benzodiazepines and opioids as commonly used in surgical practice). Products include:
Librium Capsules 3349

Cisatracurium Besylate (Sevoflurane increases both the intensity and duration of neuromuscular blockade induced by non-depolarizing muscle relaxants. When used to supplement alfentanil-nitrous oxide anesthesia, sevoflurane and isoflurane equally potentiate neuromuscular block induced with pancuronium, vecuronium or atracurium. Among available non-depolarizing agents, only vecuronium, pancuronium and atracurium interactions have been studied during sevoflurane anesthesia. In the absence of specific guidelines: 1) For endotracheal intubation, do not reduce the dose of non-depolarizing muscle relaxants. 2) During maintenance of anesthesia, the required dose of non-depolarizing muscle relaxants is likely to be reduced compared to that during nitrous oxide/opioid anesthesia). Products include:
Nimbex Injection 494

Clorazepate Dipotassium (Benzodiazepines would be expected to decrease the MAC of sevoflurane in the same manner as with other inhalational anesthetics. Sevoflurane administration is compatible with benzodiazepines and opioids as commonly used in surgical practice). Products include:
Tranxene 2488

Codeine Phosphate (Benzodiazepines would be expected to decrease the MAC of sevoflurane in the same manner as with other inhalational anesthetics. Sevoflurane administration is compatible with benzodiazepines and opioids as commonly used in surgical practice). Products include:
Tylenol with Codeine 2461

Dezocine (Benzodiazepines would be expected to decrease the MAC of sevoflurane in the same manner as with other inhalational anesthetics. Sevoflurane administration is compatible with benzodiazepines and opioids as commonly used in surgical practice).
No products indexed under this heading.

Diazepam (Benzodiazepines would be expected to decrease the MAC of sevoflurane in the same manner as with other inhalational anesthetics. Sevoflurane administration is compatible with benzodiazepines and opioids as commonly used in surgical practice). Products include:
Diastat Rectal Delivery System 3344
Valium Tablets 2822

Estazolam (Benzodiazepines would be expected to decrease the MAC of sevoflurane in the same manner as with other inhalational anesthetics. Sevoflurane administration is compatible with benzodiazepines and opioids as commonly used in surgical practice). Products include:
ProSom Tablets 512

Fentanyl (Benzodiazepines would be expected to decrease the MAC of sevoflurane in the same manner as with other inhalational anesthetics. Sevoflurane administration is compatible with benzodiazepines and opioids as commonly used in surgical practice). Products include:
Duragesic Transdermal System 2448

Fentanyl Citrate (Benzodiazepines would be expected to decrease the MAC of sevoflurane in the same manner as with other inhalational anesthetics. Sevoflurane administration is compatible with benzodiazepines and opioids as commonly used in surgical practice). Products include:
Actiq 993

Flurazepam Hydrochloride (Benzodiazepines would be expected to decrease the MAC of sevoflurane in the same manner as with other inhalational anesthetics. Sevoflurane administration is compatible with benzodiazepines and opioids as commonly used in surgical practice). Products include:
Dalmane Capsules 3343

Halazepam (Benzodiazepines would be expected to decrease the MAC of sevoflurane in the same manner as with other inhalational anesthetics. Sevoflurane administration is compatible with benzodiazepines and opioids as commonly used in surgical practice).
No products indexed under this heading.

Hydrocodone Bitartrate (Benzodiazepines would be expected to decrease the MAC of sevoflurane in the same manner as with other inhalational anesthetics. Sevoflurane administration is compatible with benzodiazepines and opioids as commonly used in surgical practice).
Products include:
Hycodan **1104**
Hycomine Compound Tablets **1105**
Hycotuss Expectorant Syrup **1106**
Lortab **3315**
Lortab Elixir **3312**
Vicodin Tablets **530**
Vicodin ES Tablets **531**
Vicodin HP Tablets **532**
Vicoprofen Tablets **533**
Zydone Tablets **1118**

Hydrocodone Polistirex (Benzodiazepines would be expected to decrease the MAC of sevoflurane in the same manner as with other inhalational anesthetics. Sevoflurane administration is compatible with benzodiazepines and opioids as commonly used in surgical practice).
Products include:
Tussionex Pennkinetic Extended-Release Suspension **3322**

Hydromorphone Hydrochloride (Benzodiazepines would be expected to decrease the MAC of sevoflurane in the same manner as with other inhalational anesthetics. Sevoflurane administration is compatible with benzodiazepines and opioids as commonly used in surgical practice).
Products include:
Dilaudid **439**
Dilaudid Oral Liquid **443**
Dilaudid Non-Sterile Powder **439**
Dilaudid Rectal Suppositories **439**
Dilaudid Tablets **439**
Dilaudid Tablets - 8 mg **443**
Dilaudid-HP **441**

Levorphanol Tartrate (Benzodiazepines would be expected to decrease the MAC of sevoflurane in the same manner as with other inhalational anesthetics. Sevoflurane administration is compatible with benzodiazepines and opioids as commonly used in surgical practice).
No products indexed under this heading.

Lorazepam (Benzodiazepines would be expected to decrease the MAC of sevoflurane in the same manner as with other inhalational anesthetics. Sevoflurane administration is compatible with benzodiazepines and opioids as commonly used in surgical practice).
No products indexed under this heading.

Meperidine Hydrochloride (Benzodiazepines would be expected to decrease the MAC of sevoflurane in the same manner as with other inhalational anesthetics. Sevoflurane administration is compatible with benzodiazepines and opioids as commonly used in surgical practice).
No products indexed under this heading.

Methadone Hydrochloride (Benzodiazepines would be expected to decrease the MAC of sevoflurane in the same manner as with other inhalational anesthetics. Sevoflurane administration is compatible with benzodiazepines and opioids as commonly used in surgical practice).
No products indexed under this heading.

Metocurine Iodide (Sevoflurane increases both the intensity and duration of neuromuscular blockade induced by non-depolarizing muscle relaxants. When used to supplement alfentanil-nitrous oxide anesthesia, sevoflurane and isoflurane equally potentiate neuromuscular block induced with pancuronium, vecuronium or atracurium. Among available non-depolarizing agents, only vecuronium, pancuronium and atracurium interactions have been studied during sevoflurane anesthesia. In the absence of specific guidelines: 1) For endotracheal intubation, do not reduce the dose of non-depolarizing muscle relaxants. 2) During maintenance of anesthesia, the required dose of non-depolarizing muscle relaxants is likely to be reduced compared to that during nitrous oxide/opioid anesthesia).
No products indexed under this heading.

Midazolam Hydrochloride (Benzodiazepines would be expected to decrease the MAC of sevoflurane in the same manner as with other inhalational anesthetics. Sevoflurane administration is compatible with benzodiazepines and opioids as commonly used in surgical practice).
No products indexed under this heading.

Mivacurium Chloride (Sevoflurane increases both the intensity and duration of neuromuscular blockade induced by non-depolarizing muscle relaxants. When used to supplement alfentanil-nitrous oxide anesthesia, sevoflurane and isoflurane equally potentiate neuromuscular block induced with pancuronium, vecuronium or atracurium. Among available non-depolarizing agents, only vecuronium, pancuronium and atracurium interactions have been studied during sevoflurane anesthesia. In the absence of specific guidelines: 1) For endotracheal intubation, do not reduce the dose of non-depolarizing muscle relaxants. 2) During maintenance of anesthesia, the required dose of non-depolarizing muscle relaxants is likely to be reduced compared to that during nitrous oxide/opioid anesthesia). Products include:
Mivacron Injection **489**

Morphine Sulfate (Benzodiazepines would be expected to decrease the MAC of sevoflurane in the same manner as with other inhalational anesthetics. Sevoflurane administration is compatible with benzodiazepines and opioids as commonly used in surgical practice).
Products include:
Avinza Capsules **1714**
Kadian Capsules **572**
MS Contin Tablets **2703**

Nitrous Oxide (As with other halogenated volatile anesthetics, the anesthetic requirement for sevoflurane is decreased when administered in combination with nitrous oxide. Using 50% nitrous oxide, the MAC equivalent dose requirement is reduced approximately 50% in adults and approximately 25% in pediatrics patients).
No products indexed under this heading.

Oxazepam (Benzodiazepines would be expected to decrease the MAC of sevoflurane in the same manner as with other inhalational anesthetics. Sevoflurane administration is compatible with benzodiazepines and opioids as commonly used in surgical practice).
No products indexed under this heading.

Oxycodone Hydrochloride (Benzodiazepines would be expected to decrease the MAC of sevoflurane in the same manner as with other inhalational anesthetics. Sevoflurane administration is compatible with benzodiazepines and opioids as commonly used in surgical practice).
Products include:
Combunox Tablets **1183**
OxyContin Tablets **2699**
OxyFast Oral Concentrate Solution **2704**
OxyIR Capsules **2704**
Percocet Tablets **1114**
Percodan Tablets **1115**

Pancuronium Bromide (Sevoflurane increases both the intensity and duration of neuromuscular blockade induced by non-depolarizing muscle relaxants. When used to supplement alfentanil-nitrous oxide anesthesia, sevoflurane and isoflurane equally potentiate neuromuscular block induced with pancuronium, vecuronium or atracurium. Among available non-depolarizing agents, only vecuronium, pancuronium and atracurium interactions have been studied during sevoflurane anesthesia. In the absence of specific guidelines: 1) For endotracheal intubation, do not reduce the dose of non-depolarizing muscle relaxants. 2) During maintenance of anesthesia, the required dose of non-depolarizing muscle relaxants is likely to be reduced compared to that during nitrous oxide/opioid anesthesia).
No products indexed under this heading.

Prazepam (Benzodiazepines would be expected to decrease the MAC of sevoflurane in the same manner as with other inhalational anesthetics. Sevoflurane administration is compatible with benzodiazepines and opioids as commonly used in surgical practice).
No products indexed under this heading.

Propoxyphene Hydrochloride (Benzodiazepines would be expected to decrease the MAC of sevoflurane in the same manner as with other inhalational anesthetics. Sevoflurane administration is compatible with benzodiazepines and opioids as commonly used in surgical practice).
No products indexed under this heading.

Propoxyphene Napsylate (Benzodiazepines would be expected to decrease the MAC of sevoflurane in the same manner as with other inhalational anesthetics. Sevoflurane administration is compatible with benzodiazepines and opioids as commonly used in surgical practice).
Products include:
Darvocet A 500 Tablets **3497**

Quazepam (Benzodiazepines would be expected to decrease the MAC of sevoflurane in the same manner as with other inhalational anesthetics. Sevoflurane administration is compatible with benzodiazepines and opioids as commonly used in surgical practice).
No products indexed under this heading.

Rapacuronium Bromide (Sevoflurane increases both the intensity and duration of neuromuscular blockade induced by non-depolarizing muscle relaxants. When used to supplement alfentanil-nitrous oxide anesthesia, sevoflurane and isoflurane equally potentiate neuromuscular block induced with pancuronium, vecuronium or atracurium. Among available non-depolarizing agents, only vecuronium, pancuronium and atracurium interactions have been studied during sevoflurane anesthesia. In the absence of specific guidelines: 1) For endotracheal intubation, do not reduce the dose of non-depolarizing muscle relaxants. 2) During maintenance of anesthesia, the required dose of non-depolarizing muscle relaxants is likely to be reduced compared to that during nitrous oxide/opioid anesthesia).
No products indexed under this heading.

Remifentanil Hydrochloride (Benzodiazepines would be expected to decrease the MAC of sevoflurane in the same manner as with other inhalational anesthetics. Sevoflurane administration is compatible with benzodiazepines and opioids as commonly used in surgical practice).
No products indexed under this heading.

Rocuronium Bromide (Sevoflurane increases both the intensity and duration of neuromuscular blockade induced by non-depolarizing muscle relaxants. When used to supplement alfentanil-nitrous oxide anesthesia, sevoflurane and isoflurane equally potentiate neuromuscular block induced with pancuronium, vecuronium or atracurium. Among available non-depolarizing agents, only vecuronium, pancuronium and atracurium interactions have been studied during sevoflurane anesthesia. In the absence of specific guidelines: 1) For endotracheal intubation, do not reduce the dose of non-depolarizing muscle relaxants. 2) During maintenance of anesthesia, the required dose of non-depolarizing muscle relaxants is likely to be reduced compared to that during nitrous oxide/opioid anesthesia). Products include:
Zemuron Injection **2363**

Sufentanil Citrate (Benzodiazepines would be expected to decrease the MAC of sevoflurane in the same manner as with other inhalational anesthetics. Sevoflurane administration is compatible with benzodiazepines and opioids as commonly used in surgical practice).
No products indexed under this heading.

Temazepam (Benzodiazepines would be expected to decrease the MAC of sevoflurane in the same manner as with other inhalational anesthetics. Sevoflurane administration is compatible with benzodiazepines and opioids as commonly used in surgical practice).
No products indexed under this heading.

Triazolam (Benzodiazepines would be expected to decrease the MAC of sevoflurane in the same manner as with other inhalational anesthetics. Sevoflurane administration is compatible with benzodiazepines and opioids as commonly used in surgical practice).
No products indexed under this heading.

Vecuronium Bromide (Sevoflurane increases both the intensity and duration of neuromuscular blockade induced by non-depolarizing muscle relaxants. When used to supplement alfentanil-nitrous oxide anesthesia, sevoflurane and isoflurane equally potentiate neuromuscular block induced with pancuronium, vecuronium or atracurium. Among available non-depolarizing agents, only vecuronium, pancuronium and atracurium interactions have been studied during sevoflurane anesthesia. In the absence of specific guidelines: 1) For endotracheal intubation, do not reduce the dose of non-depolarizing muscle relaxants. 2) During maintenance of anesthesia, the required dose of non-depolarizing muscle relaxants is likely to be reduced compared to that during nitrous oxide/opioid anesthesia).
No products indexed under this heading.

ULTRACET TABLETS

(Acetaminophen, Tramadol Hydrochloride).................................... 2462

May interact with central nervous system depressants, monoamine oxidase inhibitors, narcotic analgesics, antipsychotic agents, phenothiazines, quinidine, drugs which lower seizure threshold, selective serotonin reuptake inhibitors, and tricyclic antidepressants. Compounds in these categories include:

Acetaminophen-containing products (Due to the potential for acetaminophen hepatotoxicity at doses higher than the recommended dose, Ultracet should not be used concomitantly with other acetaminophen-containing products).
No products indexed under this heading.

Alfentanil Hydrochloride (Co-administration increases the risk of CNS and respiratory depression).
No products indexed under this heading.

Alprazolam (Co-administration enhances the risk of seizures). Products include:
Niravam Orally Disintegrating Tablets.. 3106
Xanax XR Tablets.............................. 2655

Amitriptyline Hydrochloride (Co-administration with tricyclic antidepressants may enhance the risk of seizures; inhibitors of CYP2D6, such as amitriptyline could inhibit metabolism of tramadol).
No products indexed under this heading.

Amoxapine (Co-administration with tricyclic antidepressants may enhance the risk of seizures).
No products indexed under this heading.

Aprobarbital (Co-administration increases the risk of CNS and respiratory depression).
No products indexed under this heading.

Aripiprazole (Co-administration enhances the risk of seizures; increased risk of CNS and respiratory depression). Products include:
Abilify Tablets.................................. 2472
Abilify Tablets.................................. 916

Buprenorphine Hydrochloride (Co-administration increases the risk of CNS and respiratory depression). Products include:
Buprenex Injectable........................ 2718
Suboxone Tablets........................... 2719
Subutex Tablets............................. 2719

Buspirone Hydrochloride (Co-administration increases the risk of CNS and respiratory depression).
No products indexed under this heading.

Butabarbital (Co-administration increases the risk of CNS and respiratory depression).
No products indexed under this heading.

Butalbital (Co-administration increases the risk of CNS and respiratory depression). Products include:
Sedapap Tablets 50 mg/650 mg 2098

Carbamazepine (Co-administration may result in a significant reduction in analgesic effect of tramadol due to increased tramadol metabolism; concurrent use is not recommended). Products include:
Carbatrol Capsules......................... 3174
Equetro Extended-Release Capsules.. 3178
Tegretol/Tegretol-XR...................... 2278

Chlordiazepoxide (Co-administration enhances the risk of seizures).
No products indexed under this heading.

Chlordiazepoxide Hydrochloride (Co-administration enhances the risk of seizures). Products include:
Librium Capsules........................... 3349

Chlorpromazine (Co-administration enhances the risk of seizures; increased risk of CNS and respiratory depression).
No products indexed under this heading.

Chlorpromazine Hydrochloride (Co-administration enhances the risk of seizures; increased risk of CNS and respiratory depression).
No products indexed under this heading.

Chlorprothixene (Co-administration enhances the risk of seizures; increased risk of CNS and respiratory depression).
No products indexed under this heading.

Chlorprothixene Hydrochloride (Co-administration enhances the risk of seizures; increased risk of CNS and respiratory depression).
No products indexed under this heading.

Chlorprothixene Lactate (Co-administration increases the risk of CNS and respiratory depression).
No products indexed under this heading.

Citalopram Hydrobromide (Co-administration with SSRI may enhance the risk of seizures). Products include:
Celexa.. 1177

Clomipramine Hydrochloride (Co-administration with tricyclic antidepressants may enhance the risk of seizures).
No products indexed under this heading.

Clorazepate Dipotassium (Co-administration increases the risk of CNS and respiratory depression). Products include:
Tranxene.. 2488

Clozapine (Co-administration enhances the risk of seizures; increased risk of CNS and respiratory depression). Products include:
Clozapine Tablets........................... 2141
Clozaril Tablets.............................. 2174
FazaClo Orally Disintegrating Tablets... 547

Codeine Phosphate (Co-administration increases the risk of CNS and respiratory depression). Products include:
Tylenol with Codeine....................... 2461

Desflurane (Co-administration increases the risk of CNS and respiratory depression). Products include:
Suprane Liquid for Inhalation 770

Desipramine Hydrochloride (Co-administration with tricyclic antidepressants may enhance the risk of seizures).
No products indexed under this heading.

Dezocine (Co-administration increases the risk of CNS and respiratory depression).
No products indexed under this heading.

Diazepam (Co-administration enhances the risk of seizures). Products include:
Diastat Rectal Delivery System........ 3344
Valium Tablets................................ 2822

Digoxin (Post-marketing surveillance of tramadol has revealed rare reports of digoxin toxicity). Products include:
Digitek Tablets................................ 2146
Lanoxicaps Capsules....................... 1458
Lanoxin Injection............................ 1462
Lanoxin Tablets.............................. 1468
Lanoxin Injection Pediatric.............. 1465

Doxepin Hydrochloride (Co-administration with tricyclic antidepressants may enhance the risk of seizures).
No products indexed under this heading.

Droperidol (Co-administration increases the risk of CNS and respiratory depression).
No products indexed under this heading.

Enflurane (Co-administration increases the risk of CNS and respiratory depression).
No products indexed under this heading.

Estazolam (Co-administration increases the risk of CNS and respiratory depression). Products include:
ProSom Tablets.............................. 512

Ethanol (Co-administration increases the risk of CNS and respiratory depression).
No products indexed under this heading.

Ethchlorvynol (Co-administration increases the risk of CNS and respiratory depression).
No products indexed under this heading.

Ethinamate (Co-administration increases the risk of CNS and respiratory depression).
No products indexed under this heading.

Ethyl Alcohol (Co-administration increases the risk of CNS and respiratory depression).
No products indexed under this heading.

Fentanyl (Co-administration increases the risk of CNS and respiratory depression). Products include:
Duragesic Transdermal System....... 2448

Fentanyl Citrate (Co-administration increases the risk of CNS and respiratory depression). Products include:
Actiq... 993

Fluoxetine Hydrochloride (Co-administration with SSRI may enhance the risk of seizures; inhibitors of CYP2D6, such as fluoxetine, could inhibit metabolism of tramadol). Products include:
Prozac Pulvules and Liquid............. 1771
Symbyax Capsules.......................... 1788

Fluphenazine Decanoate (Co-administration enhances the risk of seizures; increased risk of CNS and respiratory depression).
No products indexed under this heading.

Fluphenazine Enanthate (Co-administration enhances the risk of seizures; increased risk of CNS and respiratory depression).
No products indexed under this heading.

Fluphenazine Hydrochloride (Co-administration enhances the risk of seizures; increased risk of CNS and respiratory depression).
No products indexed under this heading.

Flurazepam Hydrochloride (Co-administration increases the risk of CNS and respiratory depression). Products include:
Dalmane Capsules.......................... 3343

Fluvoxamine Maleate (Co-administration with SSRI may enhance the risk of seizures).
No products indexed under this heading.

Glutethimide (Co-administration increases the risk of CNS and respiratory depression).
No products indexed under this heading.

Haloperidol (Co-administration enhances the risk of seizures).
No products indexed under this heading.

Haloperidol Decanoate (Co-administration enhances the risk of seizures).
No products indexed under this heading.

Hydrocodone Bitartrate (Co-administration increases the risk of CNS and respiratory depression). Products include:
Hycodan.. 1104
Hycomine Compound Tablets.......... 1105
Hycotuss Expectorant Syrup........... 1106
Lortab... 3315
Lortab Elixir.................................... 3312
Vicodin Tablets............................... 530
Vicodin ES Tablets.......................... 531
Vicodin HP Tablets.......................... 532
Vicoprofen Tablets.......................... 533

Zydone Tablets 1118

Hydrocodone Polistirex (Co-administration increases the risk of CNS and respiratory depression). Products include:
Tussionex Pennkinetic Extended-Release Suspension 3322

Hydromorphone Hydrochloride (Co-administration increases the risk of CNS and respiratory depression). Products include:
Dilaudid 439
Dilaudid Oral Liquid 443
Dilaudid Non-Sterile Powder 439
Dilaudid Rectal Suppositories 439
Dilaudid Tablets 439
Dilaudid Tablets - 8 mg 443
Dilaudid-HP 441

Hydroxyzine Hydrochloride (Co-administration increases the risk of CNS and respiratory depression).
No products indexed under this heading.

Imipramine Hydrochloride (Co-administration with tricyclic antidepressants may enhance the risk of seizures).
No products indexed under this heading.

Imipramine Pamoate (Co-administration with tricyclic antidepressants may enhance the risk of seizures).
No products indexed under this heading.

Isocarboxazid (Co-administration with MAO inhibitors may enhance the risk of seizures; animal studies have shown increased deaths with combined use; interference with detoxification mechanism has been reported with combined use of MAO inhibitors and centrally acting drugs).
No products indexed under this heading.

Isoflurane (Co-administration increases the risk of CNS and respiratory depression).
No products indexed under this heading.

Ketamine Hydrochloride (Co-administration increases the risk of CNS and respiratory depression).
No products indexed under this heading.

Levomethadyl Acetate Hydrochloride (Co-administration increases the risk of CNS and respiratory depression).
No products indexed under this heading.

Levorphanol Tartrate (Co-administration increases the risk of CNS and respiratory depression).
No products indexed under this heading.

Lithium Carbonate (Co-administration enhances the risk of seizures; increased risk of CNS and respiratory depression). Products include:
Eskalith 1406
Lithobid Tablets 1670

Lithium Citrate (Co-administration enhances the risk of seizures; increased risk of CNS and respiratory depression).
No products indexed under this heading.

Lorazepam (Co-administration enhances the risk of seizures).
No products indexed under this heading.

Loxapine Hydrochloride (Co-administration enhances the risk of seizures; increased risk of CNS and respiratory depression).
No products indexed under this heading.

Loxapine Succinate (Co-administration enhances the risk of seizures; increased risk of CNS and respiratory depression).
No products indexed under this heading.

Maprotiline Hydrochloride (Co-administration with tricyclic antidepressants may enhance the risk of seizures).
No products indexed under this heading.

Meperidine Hydrochloride (Co-administration increases the risk of CNS and respiratory depression).
No products indexed under this heading.

Mephobarbital (Co-administration increases the risk of CNS and respiratory depression). Products include:
Mebaral Tablets, USP 2483

Meprobamate (Co-administration increases the risk of CNS and respiratory depression).
No products indexed under this heading.

Mesoridazine Besylate (Co-administration enhances the risk of seizures; increased risk of CNS and respiratory depression).
No products indexed under this heading.

Methadone Hydrochloride (Co-administration increases the risk of CNS and respiratory depression).
No products indexed under this heading.

Methohexital Sodium (Co-administration increases the risk of CNS and respiratory depression).
No products indexed under this heading.

Methotrimeprazine (Co-administration enhances the risk of seizures; increased risk of CNS and respiratory depression).
No products indexed under this heading.

Methoxyflurane (Co-administration increases the risk of CNS and respiratory depression).
No products indexed under this heading.

Midazolam Hydrochloride (Co-administration increases the risk of CNS and respiratory depression).
No products indexed under this heading.

Moclobemide (Co-administration with MAO inhibitors may enhance the risk of seizures; animal studies have shown increased deaths with combined use; interference with detoxification mechanism has been reported with combined use of MAO inhibitors and centrally acting drugs).
No products indexed under this heading.

Molindone Hydrochloride (Co-administration enhances the risk of seizures; increased risk of CNS and respiratory depression). Products include:
Moban Tablets 1108

Morphine Sulfate (Co-administration increases the risk of CNS and respiratory depression). Products include:
Avinza Capsules 1714
Kadian Capsules 572
MS Contin Tablets 2703

Nortriptyline Hydrochloride (Co-administration with tricyclic antidepressants may enhance the risk of seizures).
No products indexed under this heading.

Olanzapine (Co-administration enhances the risk of seizures; increased risk of CNS and respiratory depression). Products include:
Symbyax Capsules 1788
Zyprexa Tablets 1798
Zyprexa IntraMuscular 1798
Zyprexa ZYDIS Orally Disintegrating Tablets 1798

Oxazepam (Co-administration enhances the risk of seizures).
No products indexed under this heading.

Oxycodone Hydrochloride (Co-administration increases the risk of CNS and respiratory depression). Products include:
Combunox Tablets 1183
OxyContin Tablets 2699
OxyFast Oral Concentrate Solution 2704
OxyIR Capsules 2704
Percocet Tablets 1114
Percodan Tablets 1115

Pargyline Hydrochloride (Co-administration with MAO inhibitors may enhance the risk of seizures; animal studies have shown increased deaths with combined use; interference with detoxification mechanism has been reported with combined use of MAO inhibitors and centrally acting drugs).
No products indexed under this heading.

Paroxetine Hydrochloride (Co-administration with SSRI may enhance the risk of seizures; inhibitors of CYP2D6, such as paroxetine, could inhibit metabolism of tramadol). Products include:
Paxil CR Controlled-Release Tablets 1509
Paxil 1501

Pentobarbital Sodium (Co-administration increases the risk of CNS and respiratory depression). Products include:
Nembutal Sodium Solution, USP 2484

Perphenazine (Co-administration enhances the risk of seizures; increased risk of CNS and respiratory depression).
No products indexed under this heading.

Phenelzine Sulfate (Co-administration with MAO inhibitors may enhance the risk of seizures; animal studies have shown increased deaths with combined use; interference with detoxification mechanism has been reported with combined use of MAO inhibitors and centrally acting drugs).
No products indexed under this heading.

Phenobarbital (Co-administration increases the risk of CNS and respiratory depression).
No products indexed under this heading.

Pimozide (Co-administration enhances the risk of seizures; increased risk of CNS and respiratory depression). Products include:
Orap Tablets 1220

Prazepam (Co-administration enhances the risk of seizures).
No products indexed under this heading.

Procarbazine Hydrochloride (Co-administration with MAO inhibitors may enhance the risk of seizures; animal studies have shown increased deaths with combined use; interference with detoxification mechanism has been reported with combined use of MAO inhibitors and centrally acting drugs). Products include:
Matulane Capsules 3188

Prochlorperazine (Co-administration enhances the risk of seizures; increased risk of CNS and respiratory depression).
No products indexed under this heading.

Promethazine Hydrochloride (Co-administration enhances the risk of seizures; increased risk of CNS and respiratory depression). Products include:
Phenergan 3438

Propofol (Co-administration increases the risk of CNS and respiratory depression). Products include:
Diprivan Injectable Emulsion 676

Propoxyphene Hydrochloride (Co-administration increases the risk of CNS and respiratory depression).
No products indexed under this heading.

Propoxyphene Napsylate (Co-administration increases the risk of CNS and respiratory depression). Products include:
Darvocet A 500 Tablets 3497

Protriptyline Hydrochloride (Co-administration with tricyclic antidepressants may enhance the risk of seizures). Products include:
Vivactil Tablets 2350

Quazepam (Co-administration increases the risk of CNS and respiratory depression).
No products indexed under this heading.

Quetiapine Fumarate (Co-administration enhances the risk of seizures; increased risk of CNS and respiratory depression). Products include:
Seroquel Tablets 691

Quinidine (Co-administration results in increased concentrations of tramadol and reduced concentrations of its metabolite, M1).
No products indexed under this heading.

Quinidine Gluconate (Co-administration results in increased concentrations of tramadol and reduced concentrations of its metabolite, M1).
No products indexed under this heading.

Quinidine Hydrochloride (Co-administration results in increased concentrations of tramadol and reduced concentrations of its metabolite, M1).
No products indexed under this heading.

Quinidine Polygalacturonate (Co-administration results in increased concentrations of tramadol and reduced concentrations of its metabolite, M1).
No products indexed under this heading.

Quinidine Sulfate (Co-administration results in increased concentrations of tramadol and reduced concentrations of its metabolite, M1).
No products indexed under this heading.

Remifentanil Hydrochloride (Co-administration increases the risk of CNS and respiratory depression).
No products indexed under this heading.

Risperidone (Co-administration enhances the risk of seizures; increased risk of CNS and respiratory depression). Products include:
Risperdal Consta Long-Acting Injection 1664
Risperdal M-Tab Orally Disintegrating Tablets 1658
Risperdal 1658

Secobarbital Sodium (Co-administration increases the risk of CNS and respiratory depression).
No products indexed under this heading.

Selegiline Hydrochloride (Co-administration with MAO inhibitors may enhance the risk of seizures; animal studies have shown increased deaths with combined use; interference with detoxification mechanism has been reported with combined use of MAO inhibitors and centrally acting drugs). Products include:
Eldepryl Capsules 3209

Sertraline Hydrochloride (Co-administration with SSRI may enhance the risk of seizures). Products include:
Zoloft 2581

Sevoflurane (Co-administration increases the risk of CNS and respiratory depression). Products include:
Ultane Liquid for Inhalation 526

Sufentanil Citrate (Co-administration increases the risk of CNS and respiratory depression).
No products indexed under this heading.

Temazepam (Co-administration increases the risk of CNS and respiratory depression).
No products indexed under this heading.

Thiamylal Sodium (Co-administration increases the risk of CNS and respiratory depression).
No products indexed under this heading.

Thioridazine Hydrochloride (Co-administration enhances the risk of seizures; increased risk of CNS and respiratory depression). Products include:
Thioridazine Hydrochloride Tablets 2122

Thiothixene (Co-administration enhances the risk of seizures; increased risk of CNS and respiratory depression). Products include:
Thiothixene Capsules 2124

Tranylcypromine Sulfate (Co-administration with MAO inhibitors may enhance the risk of seizures; animal studies have shown increased deaths with combined use; interference with detoxification mechanism has been reported with combined use of MAO inhibitors and centrally acting drugs). Products include:
Parnate Tablets 1499

Trazodone Hydrochloride (Co-administration enhances the risk of seizures).
No products indexed under this heading.

Triazolam (Co-administration increases the risk of CNS and respiratory depression).
No products indexed under this heading.

Trifluoperazine Hydrochloride (Co-administration enhances the risk of seizures; increased risk of CNS and respiratory depression).
No products indexed under this heading.

Trimipramine Maleate (Co-administration with tricyclic antidepressants may enhance the risk of seizures). Products include:
Surmontil Capsules 2347

Warfarin Sodium (Post-marketing surveillance of both tramadol and acetaminophen individual products has revealed rare alterations of warfarin effect, including elevation of prothrombin time). Products include:
Coumadin for Injection 932
Coumadin Tablets 932

Zaleplon (Co-administration increases the risk of CNS and respiratory depression). Products include:
Sonata Capsules 1686

Ziprasidone Hydrochloride (Co-administration enhances the risk of seizures; increased risk of CNS and respiratory depression). Products include:
Geodon Capsules 2514

Zolpidem Tartrate (Co-administration increases the risk of CNS and respiratory depression). Products include:
Ambien Tablets 2867

Food Interactions

Alcohol (Tramadol increases the risk of CNS and respiratory depression with concurrent use; alcohol consumption with Ultracet is not recommended).

ULTRALYTIC 2 CREAM 20%
(Urea) 1651
None cited in PDR database.

ULTRALYTIC 2 FOAM 20%
(Urea) 1652
None cited in PDR database.

ULTRASE CAPSULES
(Pancrelipase) 735

Food Interactions

Food having a pH greater than 5.5 (Can dissolve the protective coating resulting in early release of enzymes, irritation of oral mucosa, and/or loss of enzyme activity).

ULTRASE MT CAPSULES
(Pancrelipase) 736

Food Interactions

Food having a pH greater than 5.5 (Can dissolve the protective enteric shell).

UNIPHYL TABLETS
(Theophylline Anhydrous) 2708
May interact with erythromycin, lithium preparations, and certain other agents. Compounds in these categories include:

Adenosine (Theophylline blocks adenosine receptors; higher doses of adenosine may be required to achieve desired effect). Products include:
Adenocard Injection 612
Adenoscan 613

Allopurinol (Decreases theophylline clearance at allopurinol doses greater than or equal to 600 mg/day).
No products indexed under this heading.

Aminoglutethimide (Increases theophylline clearance by induction of microsomal enzyme).
No products indexed under this heading.

Carbamazepine (Increases theophylline clearance by induction of microsomal enzyme). Products include:
Carbatrol Capsules 3174
Equetro Extended-Release Capsules 3178
Tegretol/Tegretol-XR 2278

Cimetidine (Decreases theophylline clearance by inhibiting cytochrome P450 1A2). Products include:
Tagamet HB 200 Tablets 637
Tagamet Tablets 1547

Cimetidine Hydrochloride (Decreases theophylline clearance by inhibiting cytochrome P450 1A2).
No products indexed under this heading.

Ciprofloxacin (Decreases theophylline clearance by inhibiting cytochrome P450 1A2). Products include:
Cipro I.V. 2998
Cipro I.V. Pharmacy Bulk Package ... 3509
Cipro Oral Suspension 2991
Cipro XR Tablets 3004
Ciprodex Otic Suspension 555

Ciprofloxacin Hydrochloride (Decreases theophylline clearance by inhibiting cytochrome P450 1A2). Products include:
Ciloxan Ophthalmic Ointment 554
Cipro Tablets 2991

Clarithromycin (Decreases theophylline clearance by inhibiting cytochrome P450 3A3). Products include:
Biaxin/Biaxin XL 402
PREVPAC 3281

Diazepam (Benzodiazepines increase CNS concentrations of adenosine, a potent CNS depressant, while theophylline blocks adenosine receptors; larger diazepam doses may be required to produce desired level of sedation; discontinuation of theophylline without reduction of diazepam dose may result in respiratory depression). Products include:
Diastat Rectal Delivery System 3344
Valium Tablets 2822

Disulfiram (Decreases theophylline clearance by inhibiting hydroxylation and demethylation). Products include:
Antabuse Tablets 2343

Enoxacin (Decreases theophylline clearance by inhibiting cytochrome P450 1A2).
No products indexed under this heading.

Ephedrine Hydrochloride (Co-administration results in synergistic CNS effects resulting in increased frequency of nausea, nervousness, and insomnia). Products include:
Primatene Tablets 749

Ephedrine Sulfate (Co-administration results in synergistic CNS effects resulting in increased frequency of nausea, nervousness, and insomnia).
No products indexed under this heading.

Ephedrine Tannate (Co-administration results in synergistic CNS effects resulting in increased frequency of nausea, nervousness, and insomnia).
No products indexed under this heading.

Erythromycin (Erythromycin metabolite decreases theophylline clearance by inhibiting cytochrome P450 3A3; decreased erythromycin steady-state serum concentrations). Products include:
Erygel Topical Gel 2096
Ery-Tab Tablets 447
Erythromycin Base Filmtab Tablets 454
Erythromycin Delayed-Release Capsules, USP 456
PCE Dispertab Tablets 510

Erythromycin Estolate (Erythromycin metabolite decreases theophylline clearance by inhibiting cytochrome P450 3A3; decreased erythromycin steady-state serum concentrations).
No products indexed under this heading.

Erythromycin Ethylsuccinate (Erythromycin metabolite decreases theophylline clearance by inhibiting cytochrome P450 3A3; decreased erythromycin steady-state serum concentrations). Products include:
E.E.S. 449
EryPed 445

Erythromycin Gluceptate (Erythromycin metabolite decreases theophylline clearance by inhibiting cytochrome P450 3A3; decreased erythromycin steady-state serum concentrations).
No products indexed under this heading.

Erythromycin Lactobionate (Erythromycin metabolite decreases theophylline clearance by inhibiting cytochrome P450 3A3; decreased erythromycin steady-state serum concentrations).
No products indexed under this heading.

Erythromycin Stearate (Erythromycin metabolite decreases theophylline clearance by inhibiting cytochrome P450 3A3; decreased erythromycin steady-state serum concentrations). Products include:
Erythrocin Stearate Filmtab Tablets 452

Ethinyl Estradiol (Estrogen containing oral contraceptives decreases theophylline clearance in dose dependent fashion). Products include:
Alesse-28 Tablets 3392
Lo/Ovral-28 Tablets 3423
NuvaRing 2357
Ortho-Cept Tablets 2395
Ortho-Cyclen/Ortho Tri-Cyclen 2414
Ortho Evra Transdermal System 2402
Ortho Tri-Cyclen Lo Tablets 2421
Seasonale Tablets 1073
Triphasil-28 Tablets 3483
Yasmin 28 Tablets 818

Flurazepam Hydrochloride (Benzodiazepines increase CNS concentrations of adenosine, a potent CNS depressant, while theophylline blocks adenosine receptors; larger flurazepam doses may be required to produce desired level of sedation; discontinuation of theophylline without reduction of flurazepam dose may result in respiratory depression). Products include:
Dalmane Capsules 3343

Fluvoxamine Maleate (Decreases theophylline clearance by inhibiting cytochrome P450 1A2).
No products indexed under this heading.

Halothane (Halothane sensitizes the myocardium to catecholamines; theophylline increases release of endogenous catecholamines resulting in increased risk of ventricular arrhythmias).
No products indexed under this heading.

Hypericum (Increases theophylline clearance; higher doses of theophylline may be required to achieve desired effect; stopping St. John's Wort may result in theophylline toxicity).
No products indexed under this heading.

Interferon alfa-2a, Recombinant (Decreases theophylline clearance). Products include:
Roferon-A Injection 2805

Isoproterenol Hydrochloride (Co-administration with intravenous isoproterenol decreases theophylline clearance).
No products indexed under this heading.

Ketamine Hydrochloride (May lower theophylline seizure threshold).
No products indexed under this heading.

Lithium (Theophylline increases renal lithium clearance; increase in lithium dose may be required to achieve a therapeutic serum concentration).
No products indexed under this heading.

Lithium Carbonate (Theophylline increases renal lithium clearance; increase in lithium dose may be required to achieve a therapeutic serum concentration). Products include:
Eskalith 1406
Lithobid Tablets 1670

Lithium Citrate (Theophylline increases renal lithium clearance; increase in lithium dose may be required to achieve a therapeutic serum concentration).
No products indexed under this heading.

Lorazepam (Benzodiazepines increase CNS concentrations of adenosine, a potent CNS depressant, while theophylline blocks adenosine receptors; larger lorazepam doses may be required to produce desired level of sedation; discontinuation of theophylline without reduction of lorazepam dose may result in respiratory depression).
No products indexed under this heading.

Mestranol (Estrogen containing oral contraceptives decreases theophylline clearance in dose dependent fashion).
No products indexed under this heading.

Methotrexate Sodium (Decreases theophylline clearance).
No products indexed under this heading.

Mexiletine Hydrochloride (Decreases theophylline clearance by inhibiting hydroxylation and demethylation).
No products indexed under this heading.

Midazolam Hydrochloride (Benzodiazepines increase CNS concentrations of adenosine, a potent CNS depressant, while theophylline blocks adenosine receptors; larger midazolam doses may be required to produce desired level of sedation; discontinuation of theophylline without reduction of midazolam dose may result in respiratory depression).
No products indexed under this heading.

Moricizine Hydrochloride (Increases theophylline clearance).
No products indexed under this heading.

Pancuronium Bromide (Theophylline may antagonize non-depolarizing neuromuscular blocking effects; possibly due to phosphodiesterase inhibition; larger pancuronium doses may be required to achieve neuromuscular blockade).
No products indexed under this heading.

Pentoxifylline (Decreases theophylline clearance).
No products indexed under this heading.

Phenobarbital (Increases theophylline clearance by induction of microsomal enzyme).
No products indexed under this heading.

Phenytoin (Phenytoin increases theophylline clearance by increasing microsomal enzyme activity; theophylline decreases phenytoin absorption).
No products indexed under this heading.

Phenytoin Sodium (Phenytoin increases theophylline clearance by increasing microsomal enzyme activity; theophylline decreases phenytoin absorption). Products include:
Phenytek Capsules 2153

Propafenone Hydrochloride (Decreases theophylline clearance). Products include:
Rythmol SR Capsules 2736

Propranolol Hydrochloride (Decreases theophylline clearance by inhibiting cytochrome P450 1A2). Products include:
Inderal LA Long-Acting Capsules 3421
InnoPran XL Capsules 2728

Rifampin (Increases theophylline clearance by increasing cytochrome P450 1A2 and 3A3 activity).
No products indexed under this heading.

Sulfinpyrazone (Increases theophylline clearance by increasing demethylation and hydroxylation; decreases renal clearance of theophylline).
No products indexed under this heading.

Tacrine Hydrochloride (Decreases theophylline clearance by inhibiting cytochrome P450 1A2 and also increases renal clearance of theophylline).
No products indexed under this heading.

Thiabendazole (Decreases theophylline clearance). Products include:
Mintezol 2002

Ticlopidine Hydrochloride (Decreases theophylline clearance). Products include:
Ticlid Tablets 2813

Troleandomycin (Decreases theophylline clearance by inhibiting cytochrome P450 3A3).
No products indexed under this heading.

Verapamil Hydrochloride (Decreases theophylline clearance by inhibiting hydroxylation and demethylation). Products include:
Covera-HS Tablets 3135
Tarka Tablets 519
Verelan PM Capsules 3120

Food Interactions

Alcohol (Concurrent use with a single dose of alcohol (3mL/kg of whiskey) decreases theophylline clearance for up to 24 hours).

Diet, high-lipid (Co-administration with a standardized high-fat meal results in increased peak plasma concentration and bioavailability; however, a precipitous increase in the rate and extent of absorption was not evident; the dosing should be ideally administered consistently either with or without food).

UNIQUE E VITAMIN E CONCENTRATE CAPSULES

(Vitamin E) .... ■□602
None cited in PDR database.

UNIRETIC TABLETS

(Hydrochlorothiazide, Moexipril Hydrochloride)................................. 3114
May interact with barbiturates, beta blockers, corticosteroids, oral hypoglycemic agents, insulin, lithium preparations, narcotic analgesics, non-steroidal anti-inflammatory agents, potassium preparations, potassium sparing diuretics, and certain other agents. Compounds in these categories include:

Acarbose (Thiazide diuretic may reduce glucose tolerance; concomitant use may require dosage adjustment of oral hypoglycemic agents). Products include:
Precose Tablets 776

Acebutolol Hydrochloride (ACE inhibitors have less than additive effects with beta-adrenergic blockers, presumably because both work by inhibiting the renin-angiotension system).
No products indexed under this heading.

ACTH (Concomitant use of thiazides with ACTH may intensify electrolyte depletion, particularly hypokalemia).
No products indexed under this heading.

Alfentanil Hydrochloride (Co-administration of narcotics with thiazide diuretics may result in potentiation of orthostatic hypotension).
No products indexed under this heading.

Amiloride Hydrochloride (Potassium-sparing diuretics can increase the risk of hyperkalemia). Products include:
Midamor Tablets 2000
Moduretic Tablets 2003

Aprobarbital (Co-administration of barbiturate with thiazide diuretics may result in potentiation of orthostatic hypotension).
No products indexed under this heading.

Atenolol (ACE inhibitors have less than additive effects with beta-adrenergic blockers, presumably because both work by inhibiting the renin-angiotension system). Products include:
Tenormin I.V. Injection 698
Tenormin Tablets 695

Betamethasone Acetate (Concomitant use of thiazides with corticosteroids may intensify electrolyte depletion, particularly hypokalemia).
No products indexed under this heading.

Betamethasone Sodium Phosphate (Concomitant use of thiazides with corticosteroids may intensify electrolyte depletion, particularly hypokalemia).
No products indexed under this heading.

Betaxolol Hydrochloride (ACE inhibitors have less than additive effects with beta-adrenergic blockers, presumably because both work by inhibiting the renin-angiotension system). Products include:
Betoptic S Ophthalmic Suspension............................... 554

Bisoprolol Fumarate (ACE inhibitors have less than additive effects with beta-adrenergic blockers, presumably because both work by inhibiting the renin-angiotension system).
No products indexed under this heading.

Buprenorphine Hydrochloride (Co-administration of narcotics with thiazide diuretics may result in potentiation of orthostatic hypotension). Products include:
Buprenex Injectable 2718
Suboxone Tablets 2719
Subutex Tablets 2719

Butabarbital (Co-administration of barbiturate with thiazide diuretics may result in potentiation of orthostatic hypotension).
No products indexed under this heading.

Butalbital (Co-administration of barbiturate with thiazide diuretics may result in potentiation of orthostatic hypotension). Products include:
Sedapap Tablets 50 mg/650 mg 2098

Carteolol Hydrochloride (ACE inhibitors have less than additive effects with beta-adrenergic blockers, presumably because both work by inhibiting the renin-angiotension system). Products include:
Carteolol Hydrochloride Ophthalmic Solution USP, 1%....... ⊙246

Celecoxib (NSAIDs can reduce the diuretic, natriuretic, and antihypertensive effects of thiazides). Products include:
Celebrex Capsules 3130

Chlorpropamide (Thiazide diuretic may reduce glucose tolerance; concomitant use may require dosage adjustment of oral hypoglycemic agents).
No products indexed under this heading.

Cholestyramine (Absorption of hydrochlorothiazide is impaired in the presence of anionic exchange resins; binds the hydrochlorothiazide and reduces its absorption from GI tract by up to 85%).
No products indexed under this heading.

Codeine Phosphate (Co-administration of narcotics with thiazide diuretics may result in potentiation of orthostatic hypotension). Products include:
Tylenol with Codeine 2461

Colestipol Hydrochloride (Absorption of hydrochlorothiazide is impaired in the presence of anionic exchange resins; binds the hydrochlorothiazide and reduces its absorption from GI tract by up to 43%).
No products indexed under this heading.

Cortisone Acetate (Concomitant use of thiazides with corticosteroids may intensify electrolyte depletion, particularly hypokalemia).
No products indexed under this heading.

Dexamethasone (Concomitant use of thiazides with corticosteroids may intensify electrolyte depletion, particularly hypokalemia). Products include:
Ciprodex Otic Suspension ... 555
Decadron Tablets ... 1929
TobraDex Ophthalmic Ointment ... 558
TobraDex Ophthalmic Suspension ... 558

Dexamethasone Acetate (Concomitant use of thiazides with corticosteroids may intensify electrolyte depletion, particularly hypokalemia).
No products indexed under this heading.

Dexamethasone Sodium Phosphate (Concomitant use of thiazides with corticosteroids may intensify electrolyte depletion, particularly hypokalemia). Products include:
Decadron Phosphate Injection ... 1931

Dezocine (Co-administration of narcotics with thiazide diuretics may result in potentiation of orthostatic hypotension).
No products indexed under this heading.

Diclofenac Potassium (NSAIDs can reduce the diuretic, natriuretic, and antihypertensive effects of thiazides). Products include:
Cataflam Tablets ... 2173

Diclofenac Sodium (NSAIDs can reduce the diuretic, natriuretic, and antihypertensive effects of thiazides). Products include:
Arthrotec Tablets ... 3126
Voltaren Ophthalmic Solution ... 2300
Voltaren Tablets ... 2298
Voltaren-XR Tablets ... 2301

Esmolol Hydrochloride (ACE inhibitors have less than additive effects with beta-adrenergic blockers, presumably because both work by inhibiting the renin-angiotension system). Products include:
Brevibloc Concentrate ... 766
Brevibloc Injection ... 766
Brevibloc Double Strength Injection ... 766
Brevibloc Premixed Injection ... 766
Brevibloc Double Strength Premixed Injection ... 766

Etodolac (NSAIDs can reduce the diuretic, natriuretic, and antihypertensive effects of thiazides).
No products indexed under this heading.

Fenoprofen Calcium (NSAIDs can reduce the diuretic, natriuretic, and antihypertensive effects of thiazides). Products include:
Nalfon Capsules ... 2504

Fentanyl (Co-administration of narcotics with thiazide diuretics may result in potentiation of orthostatic hypotension). Products include:
Duragesic Transdermal System ... 2448

Fentanyl Citrate (Co-administration of narcotics with thiazide diuretics may result in potentiation of orthostatic hypotension). Products include:
Actiq ... 993

Fludrocortisone Acetate (Concomitant use of thiazides with corticosteroids may intensify electrolyte depletion, particularly hypokalemia).
No products indexed under this heading.

Flurbiprofen (NSAIDs can reduce the diuretic, natriuretic, and antihypertensive effects of thiazides).
No products indexed under this heading.

Glimepiride (Thiazide diuretic may reduce glucose tolerance; concomitant use may require dosage adjustment of oral hypoglycemic agents). Products include:
Amaryl Tablets ... 2864

Glipizide (Thiazide diuretic may reduce glucose tolerance; concomitant use may require dosage adjustment of oral hypoglycemic agents).
No products indexed under this heading.

Glyburide (Thiazide diuretic may reduce glucose tolerance; concomitant use may require dosage adjustment of oral hypoglycemic agents).
No products indexed under this heading.

Guanabenz Acetate (Co-administration increases the absorption of hydrochlorothiazide).
No products indexed under this heading.

Hydrocodone Bitartrate (Co-administration of narcotics with thiazide diuretics may result in potentiation of orthostatic hypotension). Products include:
Hycodan ... 1104
Hycomine Compound Tablets ... 1105
Hycotuss Expectorant Syrup ... 1106
Lortab ... 3315
Lortab Elixir ... 3312
Vicodin Tablets ... 530
Vicodin ES Tablets ... 531
Vicodin HP Tablets ... 532
Vicoprofen Tablets ... 533
Zydone Tablets ... 1118

Hydrocodone Polistirex (Co-administration of narcotics with thiazide diuretics may result in potentiation of orthostatic hypotension). Products include:
Tussionex Pennkinetic Extended-Release Suspension ... 3322

Hydrocortisone (Concomitant use of thiazides with corticosteroids may intensify electrolyte depletion, particularly hypokalemia). Products include:
Cortizone•5 Ointment ... 699
Cortizone•10 Creme ... 699
Cortizone•10 Ointment ... 699
Cortizone•10 Plus Creme ... 700
Cortizone•10 Maximum Strength Quick Shot Spray ... 700
Hydrocortone Tablets ... 1963
Preparation H Hydrocortisone Cream ... 748

Hydrocortisone Acetate (Concomitant use of thiazides with corticosteroids may intensify electrolyte depletion, particularly hypokalemia). Products include:
Analpram-HC ... 1136
Pramosone ... 1139
ProctoFoam-HC ... 3113
Tucks Anti-Itch Ointment ... 712
U-cort 1% Cream ... 3289

Hydrocortisone Sodium Phosphate (Concomitant use of thiazides with corticosteroids may intensify electrolyte depletion, particularly hypokalemia).
No products indexed under this heading.

Hydrocortisone Sodium Succinate (Concomitant use of thiazides with corticosteroids may intensify electrolyte depletion, particularly hypokalemia).
No products indexed under this heading.

Hydromorphone Hydrochloride (Co-administration of narcotics with thiazide diuretics may result in potentiation of orthostatic hypotension). Products include:
Dilaudid ... 439
Dilaudid Oral Liquid ... 443
Dilaudid Non-Sterile Powder ... 439
Dilaudid Rectal Suppositories ... 439
Dilaudid Tablets ... 439
Dilaudid Tablets - 8 mg ... 443
Dilaudid-HP ... 441

Ibuprofen (NSAIDs can reduce the diuretic, natriuretic, and antihypertensive effects of thiazides). Products include:
Advil Allergy Sinus Caplets ... 737
Advil ... 737
Children's Advil Suspension ... 742
Children's Advil Chewable Tablets ... 741
Advil Cold & Sinus ... 739
Advil Flu & Body Ache Caplets ... 739
Children's Advil Cold Suspension ... 741
Infants' Advil Concentrated Drops ... 743
Junior Strength Advil Swallow Tablets ... 740
Advil Migraine Liquigels ... 740
Advil Multi-Symptom Cold Caplets ... 738
Combunox Tablets ... 1183
Children's Motrin Oral Suspension and Chewable Tablets ... 1837
Children's Motrin Cold Non-Staining Dye-Free Oral Suspension ... 1838
Children's Motrin Cold Oral Suspension ... 1838
Children's Motrin Non-Staining Dye-Free Oral Suspension ... 1837
Motrin Cold & Sinus Caplets ... 1836
Motrin IB Tablets and Caplets ... 1836
Infants' Motrin Concentrated Drops ... 1837
Infants' Motrin Non-Staining Dye-Free Drops ... 1837
Junior Strength Motrin Caplets and Chewable Tablets ... 1837
Vicoprofen Tablets ... 533

Indomethacin (NSAIDs can reduce the diuretic, natriuretic, and antihypertensive effects of thiazides). Products include:
Indocin ... 1968

Indomethacin Sodium Trihydrate (NSAIDs can reduce the diuretic, natriuretic, and antihypertensive effects of thiazides). Products include:
Indocin I.V. ... 1973

Insulin, Human, Zinc Suspension (Thiazide diuretic may reduce glucose tolerance; concomitant use may require dosage adjustment of insulin). Products include:
Humulin L, 100 Units ... 1763
Humulin U, 100 Units ... 1770

Insulin, Human NPH (Thiazide diuretic may reduce glucose tolerance; concomitant use may require dosage adjustment of insulin). Products include:
Humulin N, 100 Units ... 1764
Humulin N Pen ... 1765
Novolin N Human Insulin 10 ml Vials ... 2322
Novolin N InnoLet ... 2322
Novolin N PenFill 3 ml Cartridges ... 2325
Novolin R InnoLet ... 2322

Insulin, Human Regular (Thiazide diuretic may reduce glucose tolerance; concomitant use may require dosage adjustment of insulin). Products include:
Humulin R (U-500) ... 1768
Humulin R, 100 Units ... 1767
Novolin R Human Insulin 10 ml Vials ... 2322
Novolin R PenFill ... 2325

Insulin, Human Regular and Human NPH Mixture (Thiazide diuretic may reduce glucose tolerance; concomitant use may require dosage adjustment of insulin). Products include:
Humulin 50/50, 100 Units ... 1760
Humulin 70/30 Pen ... 1761
Novolin 70/30 Human Insulin 10 ml Vials ... 2321
Novolin 70/30 InnoLet ... 2322
Novolin 70/30 PenFill 3 ml Cartridges ... 2325

Insulin, NPH (Thiazide diuretic may reduce glucose tolerance; concomitant use may require dosage adjustment of insulin).
No products indexed under this heading.

Insulin, Regular (Thiazide diuretic may reduce glucose tolerance; concomitant use may require dosage adjustment of insulin).
No products indexed under this heading.

Insulin, Zinc Crystals (Thiazide diuretic may reduce glucose tolerance; concomitant use may require dosage adjustment of insulin).
No products indexed under this heading.

Insulin, Zinc Suspension (Thiazide diuretic may reduce glucose tolerance; concomitant use may require dosage adjustment of insulin).
No products indexed under this heading.

Insulin Aspart, Human Regular (Thiazide diuretic may reduce glucose tolerance; concomitant use may require dosage adjustment of insulin). Products include:
NovoLog Injection ... 2326

Insulin glargine (Thiazide diuretic may reduce glucose tolerance; concomitant use may require dosage adjustment of insulin). Products include:
Lantus Injection ... 2925

Insulin Lispro, Human (Thiazide diuretic may reduce glucose tolerance; concomitant use may require dosage adjustment of insulin). Products include:
Humalog-Pen ... 1751
Humalog Mix 75/25-Pen ... 1754

Insulin Lispro Protamine, Human (Thiazide diuretic may reduce glucose tolerance; concomitant use may require dosage adjustment of insulin). Products include:
Humalog Mix 75/25-Pen ... 1754

Ketoprofen (NSAIDs can reduce the diuretic, natriuretic, and antihypertensive effects of thiazides).
No products indexed under this heading.

Ketorolac Tromethamine (NSAIDs can reduce the diuretic, natriuretic, and antihypertensive effects of thiazides). Products include:
Acular Ophthalmic Solution ... 561
Acular LS Ophthalmic Solution ... 562

IMPORTANT NOTE: Always consult each drug listing in the patient's regimen for possible interactions.

Labetalol Hydrochloride (ACE inhibitors have less than additive effects with beta-adrenergic blockers, presumably because both work by inhibiting the renin-angiotension system).
No products indexed under this heading.

Levobunolol Hydrochloride (ACE inhibitors have less than additive effects with beta-adrenergic blockers, presumably because both work by inhibiting the renin-angiotension system). Products include:
Betagan Ophthalmic Solution, USP ⊙ 217

Levorphanol Tartrate (Co-administration of narcotics with thiazide diuretics may result in potentiation of orthostatic hypotension).
No products indexed under this heading.

Lithium (Co-administration of ACE inhibitors and lithium has resulted in increased serum lithium levels and symptoms of lithium toxicity).
No products indexed under this heading.

Lithium Carbonate (Co-administration of ACE inhibitors and lithium has resulted in increased serum lithium levels and symptoms of lithium toxicity). Products include:
Eskalith 1406
Lithobid Tablets 1670

Lithium Citrate (Co-administration of ACE inhibitors and lithium has resulted in increased serum lithium levels and symptoms of lithium toxicity).
No products indexed under this heading.

Meclofenamate Sodium (NSAIDs can reduce the diuretic, natriuretic, and antihypertensive effects of thiazides).
No products indexed under this heading.

Mefenamic Acid (NSAIDs can reduce the diuretic, natriuretic, and antihypertensive effects of thiazides).
No products indexed under this heading.

Meloxicam (NSAIDs can reduce the diuretic, natriuretic, and antihypertensive effects of thiazides). Products include:
Mobic Oral Suspension 893
Mobic Tablets 893

Meperidine Hydrochloride (Co-administration of narcotics with thiazide diuretics may result in potentiation of orthostatic hypotension).
No products indexed under this heading.

Mephobarbital (Co-administration of barbiturate with thiazide diuretics may result in potentiation of orthostatic hypotension). Products include:
Mebaral Tablets, USP 2483

Metformin Hydrochloride (Thiazide diuretic may reduce glucose tolerance; concomitant use may require dosage adjustment of oral hypoglycemic agents). Products include:
ActoPlus Met Tablets 3219
Avandamet Tablets 1343
Fortamet Extended-Release Tablets 1156

Methadone Hydrochloride (Co-administration of narcotics with thiazide diuretics may result in potentiation of orthostatic hypotension).
No products indexed under this heading.

Methylprednisolone Acetate (Concomitant use of thiazides with corticosteroids may intensify electrolyte depletion, particularly hypokalemia). Products include:
Depo-Medrol Injectable Suspension 2615
Depo-Medrol Single-Dose Vial 2617

Methylprednisolone Sodium Succinate (Concomitant use of thiazides with corticosteroids may intensify electrolyte depletion, particularly hypokalemia).
No products indexed under this heading.

Metipranolol Hydrochloride (ACE inhibitors have less than additive effects with beta-adrenergic blockers, presumably because both work by inhibiting the renin-angiotension system).
No products indexed under this heading.

Metoprolol Succinate (ACE inhibitors have less than additive effects with beta-adrenergic blockers, presumably because both work by inhibiting the renin-angiotension system). Products include:
Toprol-XL Tablets 660

Metoprolol Tartrate (ACE inhibitors have less than additive effects with beta-adrenergic blockers, presumably because both work by inhibiting the renin-angiotension system).
No products indexed under this heading.

Miglitol (Thiazide diuretic may reduce glucose tolerance; concomitant use may require dosage adjustment of oral hypoglycemic agents).
No products indexed under this heading.

Morphine Sulfate (Co-administration of narcotics with thiazide diuretics may result in potentiation of orthostatic hypotension). Products include:
Avinza Capsules 1714
Kadian Capsules 572
MS Contin Tablets 2703

Nabumetone (NSAIDs can reduce the diuretic, natriuretic, and antihypertensive effects of thiazides). Products include:
Relafen Tablets 1523

Nadolol (ACE inhibitors have less than additive effects with beta-adrenergic blockers, presumably because both work by inhibiting the renin-angiotension system). Products include:
Nadolol Tablets 2121

Naproxen (NSAIDs can reduce the diuretic, natriuretic, and antihypertensive effects of thiazides). Products include:
EC-Naprosyn Delayed-Release Tablets 2769
Naprosyn Suspension 2769
Naprosyn Tablets 2769
Prevacid NapraPAC 3277

Naproxen Sodium (NSAIDs can reduce the diuretic, natriuretic, and antihypertensive effects of thiazides). Products include:
Aleve Tablets, Caplets and Gelcaps ▣ 605
Anaprox Tablets 2769
Anaprox DS Tablets 2769

Norepinephrine Bitartrate (Thiazide diuretics may decrease arterial responsiveness to pressor amines).
No products indexed under this heading.

Oxaprozin (NSAIDs can reduce the diuretic, natriuretic, and antihypertensive effects of thiazides).
No products indexed under this heading.

Oxycodone Hydrochloride (Co-administration of narcotics with thiazide diuretics may result in potentiation of orthostatic hypotension). Products include:
Combunox Tablets 1183
OxyContin Tablets 2699
OxyFast Oral Concentrate Solution 2704
OxyIR Capsules 2704
Percocet Tablets 1114
Percodan Tablets 1115

Penbutolol Sulfate (ACE inhibitors have less than additive effects with beta-adrenergic blockers, presumably because both work by inhibiting the renin-angiotension system).
No products indexed under this heading.

Pentobarbital Sodium (Co-administration of barbiturate with thiazide diuretics may result in potentiation of orthostatic hypotension). Products include:
Nembutal Sodium Solution, USP 2484

Phenobarbital (Co-administration of barbiturate with thiazide diuretics may result in potentiation of orthostatic hypotension).
No products indexed under this heading.

Phenylbutazone (NSAIDs can reduce the diuretic, natriuretic, and antihypertensive effects of thiazides).
No products indexed under this heading.

Pindolol (ACE inhibitors have less than additive effects with beta-adrenergic blockers, presumably because both work by inhibiting the renin-angiotension system).
No products indexed under this heading.

Pioglitazone Hydrochloride (Thiazide diuretic may reduce glucose tolerance; concomitant use may require dosage adjustment of oral hypoglycemic agents). Products include:
ActoPlus Met Tablets 3219
Actos Tablets 3224

Piroxicam (NSAIDs can reduce the diuretic, natriuretic, and antihypertensive effects of thiazides).
No products indexed under this heading.

Potassium Acid Phosphate (Potassium supplements can increase the risk of hyperkalemia). Products include:
K-Phos Original (Sodium Free) Tablets 785

Potassium Bicarbonate (Potassium supplements can increase the risk of hyperkalemia).
No products indexed under this heading.

Potassium Chloride (Potassium supplements can increase the risk of hyperkalemia). Products include:
Colyte with Flavor Packs for Oral Solution 3102
HalfLytely and Bisacodyl Tablets Bowel Prep Kit with Flavors Packs 915
K-Dur Extended-Relase Tablets 3047
K-Lor Powder Packets 472
K-Tab Filmtab Tablets 473
TriLyte with Flavor Packs for Oral Solution 3114

Potassium Citrate (Potassium supplements can increase the risk of hyperkalemia). Products include:
Urocit-K Tablets 2109

Potassium Gluconate (Potassium supplements can increase the risk of hyperkalemia).
No products indexed under this heading.

Potassium Phosphate (Potassium supplements can increase the risk of hyperkalemia). Products include:
K-Phos Neutral Tablets 785

Prednisolone Acetate (Concomitant use of thiazides with corticosteroids may intensify electrolyte depletion, particularly hypokalemia). Products include:
Blephamide Ophthalmic Ointment 563
Blephamide Ophthalmic Suspension 564
Poly-Pred Liquifilm Ophthalmic Suspension ⊙ 231
Pred Forte Ophthalmic Suspension ⊙ 233
Pred Mild Sterile Ophthalmic Suspension ⊙ 236
Pred-G Ophthalmic Suspension ⊙ 234
Pred-G Sterile Ophthalmic Ointment ⊙ 235

Prednisolone Sodium Phosphate (Concomitant use of thiazides with corticosteroids may intensify electrolyte depletion, particularly hypokalemia). Products include:
Pediapred Oral Solution 3319

Prednisolone Tebutate (Concomitant use of thiazides with corticosteroids may intensify electrolyte depletion, particularly hypokalemia).
No products indexed under this heading.

Prednisone (Concomitant use of thiazides with corticosteroids may intensify electrolyte depletion, particularly hypokalemia).
No products indexed under this heading.

Propantheline Bromide (Co-administration increases the absorption of hydrochlorothiazide).
No products indexed under this heading.

Propoxyphene Hydrochloride (Co-administration of narcotics with thiazide diuretics may result in potentiation of orthostatic hypotension).
No products indexed under this heading.

Propoxyphene Napsylate (Co-administration of narcotics with thiazide diuretics may result in potentiation of orthostatic hypotension). Products include:
Darvocet A 500 Tablets 3497

Propranolol Hydrochloride (ACE inhibitors have less than additive effects with beta-adrenergic blockers, presumably because both work by inhibiting the renin-angiotension system). Products include:
Inderal LA Long-Acting Capsules 3421
InnoPran XL Capsules 2728

Remifentanil Hydrochloride (Co-administration of narcotics with thiazide diuretics may result in potentiation of orthostatic hypotension).
No products indexed under this heading.

Repaglinide (Thiazide diuretic may reduce glucose tolerance; concomitant use may require dosage adjustment of oral hypoglycemic agents). Products include:

Prandin Tablets (0.5, 1, and 2 mg) 2337

Rofecoxib (NSAIDs can reduce the diuretic, natriuretic, and antihypertensive effects of thiazides).
No products indexed under this heading.

Rosiglitazone Maleate (Thiazide diuretic may reduce glucose tolerance; concomitant use may require dosage adjustment of oral hypoglycemic agents). Products include:
Avandamet Tablets 1343
Avandia Tablets 1348

Secobarbital Sodium (Co-administration of barbiturate with thiazide diuretics may result in potentiation of orthostatic hypotension).
No products indexed under this heading.

Sotalol Hydrochloride (ACE inhibitors have less than additive effects with beta-adrenergic blockers, presumably because both work by inhibiting the renin-angiotension system).
No products indexed under this heading.

Spironolactone (Potassium-sparing diuretics can increase the risk of hyperkalemia).
No products indexed under this heading.

Sufentanil Citrate (Co-administration of narcotics with thiazide diuretics may result in potentiation of orthostatic hypotension).
No products indexed under this heading.

Sulindac (NSAIDs can reduce the diuretic, natriuretic, and antihypertensive effects of thiazides). Products include:
Clinoril Tablets 1899

Thiamylal Sodium (Co-administration of barbiturate with thiazide diuretics may result in potentiation of orthostatic hypotension).
No products indexed under this heading.

Timolol Hemihydrate (ACE inhibitors have less than additive effects with beta-adrenergic blockers, presumably because both work by inhibiting the renin-angiotension system). Products include:
Betimol Ophthalmic Solution 3371
Betimol Ophthalmic Solution .... ⊙283

Timolol Maleate (ACE inhibitors have less than additive effects with beta-adrenergic blockers, presumably because both work by inhibiting the renin-angiotension system). Products include:
Blocadren Tablets 1891
Cosopt Sterile Ophthalmic Solution 1910
Timolide Tablets 2056
Timoptic in Ocudose 2061
Timoptic Sterile Ophthalmic Solution 2058
Timoptic-XE Sterile Ophthalmic Gel Forming Solution 2062

Tolazamide (Thiazide diuretic may reduce glucose tolerance; concomitant use may require dosage adjustment of oral hypoglycemic agents).
No products indexed under this heading.

Tolbutamide (Thiazide diuretic may reduce glucose tolerance; concomitant use may require dosage adjustment of oral hypoglycemic agents).
No products indexed under this heading.

Tolmetin Sodium (NSAIDs can reduce the diuretic, natriuretic, and antihypertensive effects of thiazides).
No products indexed under this heading.

Triamcinolone (Concomitant use of thiazides with corticosteroids may intensify electrolyte depletion, particularly hypokalemia).
No products indexed under this heading.

Triamcinolone Acetonide (Concomitant use of thiazides with corticosteroids may intensify electrolyte depletion, particularly hypokalemia). Products include:
Azmacort Inhalation Aerosol 1701
Nasacort HFA Inhalation Aerosol 2939
Nasacort AQ Nasal Spray 2937

Triamcinolone Diacetate (Concomitant use of thiazides with corticosteroids may intensify electrolyte depletion, particularly hypokalemia).
No products indexed under this heading.

Triamcinolone Hexacetonide (Concomitant use of thiazides with corticosteroids may intensify electrolyte depletion, particularly hypokalemia).
No products indexed under this heading.

Triamterene (Potassium-sparing diuretics can increase the risk of hyperkalemia). Products include:
Dyazide Capsules 1389
Dyrenium Capsules 3390
Maxzide 2150

Troglitazone (Thiazide diuretic may reduce glucose tolerance; concomitant use may require dosage adjustment of oral hypoglycemic agents).
No products indexed under this heading.

Tubocurarine Chloride (Thiazide diuretics may increase the responsiveness to tubocurarine).
No products indexed under this heading.

Valdecoxib (NSAIDs can reduce the diuretic, natriuretic, and antihypertensive effects of thiazides).
No products indexed under this heading.

Food Interactions

Alcohol (Co-administration of alcohol with thiazide diuretics may result in potentiation of orthostatic hypotension).

Food, unspecified (Bioavailability varies with formulation and food intake which reduces Cmax and AUC of moexiprilat by about 70% and 40% respectively after ingestion of low-fat breakfast or by 80% and 50% respectively after the ingestion of a high-fat breakfast; patients should be advised to take Uniretic one hour before a meal).

UNISOM SLEEPTABS

(Doxylamine Succinate) .... ▣713

Food Interactions

Alcohol (Use Unisom cautiously).

UNISOM MAXIMUM STRENGTH SLEEPGELS

(Diphenhydramine Hydrochloride) .... ▣712
May interact with hypnotics and sedatives, tranquilizers, and certain other agents. Compounds in these categories include:

Alprazolam (Concurrent use with tranquilizers should be avoided). Products include:
Niravam Orally Disintegrating Tablets 3106
Xanax XR Tablets 2655

Buspirone Hydrochloride (Concurrent use with tranquilizers should be avoided).
No products indexed under this heading.

Chlordiazepoxide (Concurrent use with tranquilizers should be avoided).
No products indexed under this heading.

Chlordiazepoxide Hydrochloride (Concurrent use with tranquilizers should be avoided). Products include:
Librium Capsules 3349

Chlorpromazine (Concurrent use with tranquilizers should be avoided).
No products indexed under this heading.

Chlorpromazine Hydrochloride (Concurrent use with tranquilizers should be avoided).
No products indexed under this heading.

Chlorprothixene (Concurrent use with tranquilizers should be avoided).
No products indexed under this heading.

Chlorprothixene Hydrochloride (Concurrent use with tranquilizers should be avoided).
No products indexed under this heading.

Clorazepate Dipotassium (Concurrent use with tranquilizers should be avoided). Products include:
Tranxene 2488

Diazepam (Concurrent use with tranquilizers should be avoided). Products include:
Diastat Rectal Delivery System 3344
Valium Tablets 2822

Droperidol (Concurrent use with tranquilizers should be avoided).
No products indexed under this heading.

Estazolam (Concurrent use with sedatives should be avoided). Products include:
ProSom Tablets 512

Ethchlorvynol (Concurrent use with sedatives should be avoided).
No products indexed under this heading.

Ethinamate (Concurrent use with sedatives should be avoided).
No products indexed under this heading.

Fluphenazine Decanoate (Concurrent use with tranquilizers should be avoided).
No products indexed under this heading.

Fluphenazine Enanthate (Concurrent use with tranquilizers should be avoided).
No products indexed under this heading.

Fluphenazine Hydrochloride (Concurrent use with tranquilizers should be avoided).
No products indexed under this heading.

Flurazepam Hydrochloride (Concurrent use with sedatives should be avoided). Products include:
Dalmane Capsules 3343

Glutethimide (Concurrent use with sedatives should be avoided).
No products indexed under this heading.

Haloperidol (Concurrent use with tranquilizers should be avoided).
No products indexed under this heading.

Haloperidol Decanoate (Concurrent use with tranquilizers should be avoided).
No products indexed under this heading.

Hydroxyzine Hydrochloride (Concurrent use with tranquilizers should be avoided).
No products indexed under this heading.

Lorazepam (Concurrent use with sedatives should be avoided).
No products indexed under this heading.

Loxapine Hydrochloride (Concurrent use with tranquilizers should be avoided).
No products indexed under this heading.

Loxapine Succinate (Concurrent use with tranquilizers should be avoided).
No products indexed under this heading.

Meprobamate (Concurrent use with tranquilizers should be avoided).
No products indexed under this heading.

Mesoridazine Besylate (Concurrent use with tranquilizers should be avoided).
No products indexed under this heading.

Midazolam Hydrochloride (Concurrent use with sedatives should be avoided).
No products indexed under this heading.

Molindone Hydrochloride (Concurrent use with tranquilizers should be avoided). Products include:
Moban Tablets 1108

Oxazepam (Concurrent use with tranquilizers should be avoided).
No products indexed under this heading.

Perphenazine (Concurrent use with tranquilizers should be avoided).
No products indexed under this heading.

Prazepam (Concurrent use with tranquilizers should be avoided).
No products indexed under this heading.

Prochlorperazine (Concurrent use with tranquilizers should be avoided).
No products indexed under this heading.

Promethazine Hydrochloride (Concurrent use with tranquilizers should be avoided). Products include:
Phenergan 3438

Propofol (Concurrent use with sedatives should be avoided). Products include:
Diprivan Injectable Emulsion 676

Quazepam (Concurrent use with sedatives should be avoided).
No products indexed under this heading.

Secobarbital Sodium (Concurrent use with sedatives should be avoided).
No products indexed under this heading.

Temazepam (Concurrent use with sedatives should be avoided).
No products indexed under this heading.

Thioridazine Hydrochloride (Concurrent use with tranquilizers should be avoided). Products include:
Thioridazine Hydrochloride Tablets 2122

Thiothixene (Concurrent use with tranquilizers should be avoided). Products include:
Thiothixene Capsules 2124

Triazolam (Concurrent use with sedatives should be avoided).
No products indexed under this heading.

Trifluoperazine Hydrochloride (Concurrent use with tranquilizers should be avoided).
No products indexed under this heading.

Zaleplon (Concurrent use with sedatives should be avoided). Products include:
Sonata Capsules 1686

Zolpidem Tartrate (Concurrent use with sedatives should be avoided). Products include:
Ambien Tablets 2867

Food Interactions

Alcohol (Concurrent use with alcoholic beverages should be avoided).

UNITHROID TABLETS

(Levothyroxine Sodium) 3521

May interact with androgens, antacids containing aluminum, calcium and magnesium, beta blockers, oral anticoagulants, dopamine agonists, estrogens, glucocorticoids, cardiac glycosides, hydantoin anticonvulsants, oral hypoglycemic agents, insulin, lithium preparations, phenytoin, radiographic iodinated contrast media, salicylates, sympathomimetics, thiazides, tricyclic antidepressants, xanthines, and certain other agents. Compounds in these categories include:

Acarbose (Addition of levothyroxine to antidiabetic therapy may result in increased antidiabetic agent requirements). Products include:
Precose Tablets 776

Acebutolol Hydrochloride (Co-administration with beta-blockers may decrease T_4 5'-deiodinase activity; action of beta-blocker may be impaired when the hypothyroid patient is converted to euthyroid).
No products indexed under this heading.

Albuterol (Co-administration of sympathomimetic agents may increase the effects of sympathomimetics or thyroid hormone; thyroid hormones may increase risk of coronary insufficiency when sympathomimetic agents are administered to patients with coronary disease). Products include:
Proventil Inhalation Aerosol 3067

Albuterol Sulfate (Co-administration of sympathomimetic agents may increase the effects of sympathomimetics or thyroid hormone; thyroid hormones may increase risk of coronary insufficiency when sympathomimetic agents are administered to patients with coronary disease). Products include:
AccuNeb Inhalation Solution 1055
Combivent Inhalation Aerosol 878
DuoNeb Inhalation Solution 1058
Proventil Inhalation Solution 0.083% 3069
Proventil HFA Inhalation Aerosol 3071
Ventolin HFA Inhalation Aerosol 1576
VoSpire Extended-Release Tablets 2352

Aldesleukin (Co-administration has been associated with transient painless thyroiditis in 20% of patients). Products include:
Proleukin for Injection 1007

Aluminum Carbonate (Co-administration with antacids may reduce the efficacy of levothyroxine by binding and delaying or preventing absorption, potentially resulting in hypothyroidism; administer levothyroxine at least 4 hours apart from these agents).
No products indexed under this heading.

Aluminum Hydroxide (Co-administration with antacids may reduce the efficacy of levothyroxine by binding and delaying or preventing absorption, potentially resulting in hypothyroidism; administer levothyroxine at least 4 hours apart from these agents). Products include:
Gaviscon Regular Strength Liquid .... ▣620
Gaviscon Regular Strength Tablets .... ▣619
Gaviscon Extra Strength Liquid .... ▣620
Gaviscon Extra Strength Tablets .... ▣619
Maalox Max Maximum Strength Antacid/Anti-Gas Liquid 2165
Maalox Regular Strength Antacid/Antigas Liquid 2164

Aminoglutethimide (May decrease thyroid hormone secretion which may result in hypothyrodism).
No products indexed under this heading.

Aminophylline (Decreased theophylline clearance may occur in hypothyroid patients; clearance returns to normal when euthyroid state is achieved).
No products indexed under this heading.

p-Aminosalicylic Acid (Co-administration has been associated with thyroid hormone and/or TSH level alterations by various mechanisms).
No products indexed under this heading.

Amiodarone Hydrochloride (May decrease thyroid hormone secretion which may result in hypothyrodism; amiodarone is slowly excreted producing more prolonged hypothyroidism; amiodarone may induce hyperthyroidism by causing thyroiditis). Products include:
Pacerone Tablets 3337

Amitriptyline Hydrochloride (Co-administration may increase the therapeutic and toxic effects of both drugs possibly due to increased receptor sensitivity to catecholamines; toxic effects may include increased risk of arrhythmias and CNS stimulation; onset of tricyclics may be accelerated).
No products indexed under this heading.

Amoxapine (Co-administration may increase the therapeutic and toxic effects of both drugs possibly due to increased receptor sensitivity to catecholamines; toxic effects may include increased risk of arrhythmias and CNS stimulation; onset of tricyclics may be accelerated).
No products indexed under this heading.

Anisindione (Thyroid hormones appear to increase the catabolism of vitamin K-dependent clotting factors, thereby increasing the anticoagulant activity of oral anticoagulants). Products include:
Miradon Tablets 3056

Asparaginase (Co-administration may result in decreased serum TBG concentration). Products include:
Elspar for Injection 1943

Aspirin (Co-administration with salicylates at greater than 2 gm inhibit binding of T4 and T3 to TBG and transthyrelin; an initial increase in serum FT4 is followed by return of FT4 to normal levels with sustained therapeutic salicylate concentrations although total T4 levels may decrease by as much as 30%). Products include:
Aggrenox Capsules 855
Bayer, Aspirin Regimen .... ▣606
Bayer Aspirin Tablets 3515
BC Powder .... ▣612
BC Allergy Sinus Cold Powder .... ▣612
Arthritis Strength BC Powder .... ▣612
BC Sinus Cold Powder .... ▣612
Ecotrin Enteric Coated Aspirin Low, Regular and Maximum Strength Tablets 1627
Goody's Body Pain Formula Powder .... ▣621
Goody's Extra Strength Headache Powder .... ▣621
Goody's Extra Strength Pain Relief Tablets .... ▣621
Percodan Tablets 1115
St. Joseph 81 mg Aspirin Chewable and Enteric Coated Tablets 1841

Aspirin, Enteric Coated (Co-administration with salicylates at greater than 2 gm inhibit binding of T4 and T3 to TBG and transthyrelin; an initial increase in serum FT4 is followed by return of FT4 to normal levels with sustained therapeutic salicylate concentrations although total T4 levels may decrease by as much as 30%).
No products indexed under this heading.

Aspirin Buffered (Co-administration with salicylates at greater than 2 gm inhibit binding of T4 and T3 to TBG and transthyrelin; an initial increase in serum FT4 is followed by return of FT4 to normal levels with sustained therapeutic salicylate concentrations although total T4 levels may decrease by as much as 30%).
No products indexed under this heading.

Atenolol (Co-administration with beta-blockers may decrease T_4 5'-deiodinase activity; action of beta-blocker may be impaired when the hypothyroid patient is converted to euthyroid). Products include:
Tenormin I.V. Injection 698
Tenormin Tablets 695

Bendroflumethiazide (Co-administration has been associated with thyroid hormone and/or TSH level alterations by various mechanisms).
No products indexed under this heading.

Betamethasone Acetate (Co-administration with glucocorticoids may result in a transient reduction in TSH secretion; the reduction is not sustained; therefore, hypothyroidism does not occur. Glucocorticoids may decrease serum TBG concentration).
No products indexed under this heading.

Betamethasone Sodium Phosphate (Co-administration with glucocorticoids may result in a transient reduction in TSH secretion; the reduction is not sustained; therefore, hypothyroidism does not occur. Glucocorticoids may decrease serum TBG concentration).
No products indexed under this heading.

Betaxolol Hydrochloride (Co-administration with beta-blockers may decrease T_4 5'-deiodinase activity; action of beta-blocker may be impaired when the hypothyroid patient is converted to euthyroid). Products include:
Betoptic S Ophthalmic Suspension 554

Bisoprolol Fumarate (Co-administration with beta-blockers may decrease T_4 5'-deiodinase activity; action of beta-blocker may be impaired when the hypothyroid patient is converted to euthyroid).
No products indexed under this heading.

Bromocriptine Mesylate (Co-administration with dopamine agonists may result in a transient reduction in TSH secretion; the reduction is not sustained; therefore, hypothyroidism does not occur).
No products indexed under this heading.

Calcium Carbonate (Co-administration with calcium carbonate may form insoluble chelate with levothyroxine which may result in hypothyroidism; administer levothyroxine at least 4 hours apart from these agents). Products include:
Actonel with Calcium Tablets 2684
Caltrate 600 PLUS Chewables .... ▣779
Caltrate 600 PLUS Tablets .... ▣779
Caltrate 600 + D Tablets .... ▣779
Encora Capsules 3298
Encora AM Tablets 3298
Encora PM Tablets 3298
Gas-X with Maalox .... ▣675
Maalox Regular Strength Antacid Tablets 2166
Quick Dissolve Maalox Max Maximum Strength Antacid/Antigas Tablets 2165
Maalox Max Quick Dissolve Maximum Strength Chewable Tablets .... ▣678
Os-Cal Chewable Tablets .... ▣765
Pepcid Complete Chewable Tablets 1672
PremCal Light, Regular, and Extra Strength Tablets .... ▣762
Rolaids Tablets .... ▣707
Extra Strength Rolaids Softchews .... ▣708
Extra Strength Rolaids Tablets .... ▣707
Rolaids Multi-Symptom Antacid & Antigas Tablets .... ▣708
Tums .... ▣639

Carbamazepine (Co-administration may increase hepatic metabolism which may result in hypothyroidism, resulting in increased levothyroxine requirements; carbamazepine reduces serum protein binding of levothyroxine, and total- and free-T4 may be reduced by 20% to 40%, but most patients have normal serum TSH levels and are clinically euthyroid). Products include:
Carbatrol Capsules 3174
Equetro Extended-Release Capsules 3178
Tegretol/Tegretol-XR 2278

Carteolol Hydrochloride (Co-administration with beta-blockers may decrease T_4 5'-deiodinase activity; action of beta-blocker may be

impaired when the hypothyroid patient is converted to euthyroid). Products include:

Carteolol Hydrochloride Ophthalmic Solution USP, 1%....... ⊙ **246**

Chloral Hydrate (Co-administration has been associated with thyroid hormone and/or TSH level alterations by various mechanisms).

No products indexed under this heading.

Chlorothiazide (Co-administration has been associated with thyroid hormone and/or TSH level alterations by various mechanisms). Products include:

Aldoclor Tablets **1881**
Diuril Oral **1936**

Chlorothiazide Sodium (Co-administration has been associated with thyroid hormone and/or TSH level alterations by various mechanisms). Products include:

Diuril Sodium Intravenous **1934**

Chlorotrianisene (Co-administration with oral estrogens may result in increased serum TBG concentrations).

No products indexed under this heading.

Chlorpropamide (Addition of levothyroxine to antidiabetic therapy may result in increased antidiabetic agent requirements).

No products indexed under this heading.

Cholestyramine (Co-administration may result in decreased T4 absorption which may result in hypothyroidism; administer levothyroxine at least 4 hours apart from these agents).

No products indexed under this heading.

Choline Magnesium Trisalicylate (Co-administration with salicylates at greater than 2 gm inhibit binding of T4 and T3 to TBG and transthyrelin; an initial increase in serum FT4 is followed by return of FT4 to normal levels with sustained therapeutic salicylate concentrations although total T4 levels may decrease by as much as 30%).

No products indexed under this heading.

Clofibrate (Co-administration may result in increased serum TBG concentrations).

No products indexed under this heading.

Clomipramine Hydrochloride (Co-administration may increase the therapeutic and toxic effects of both drugs possibly due to increased receptor sensitivity to catecholamines; toxic effects may include increased risk of arrhythmias and CNS stimulation; onset of tricyclics may be accelerated).

No products indexed under this heading.

Colestipol Hydrochloride (Co-administration may result in decreased T4 absorption which may result in hypothyroidism; administer levothyroxine at least 4 hours apart from these agents).

No products indexed under this heading.

Cortisone Acetate (Co-administration with glucocorticoids may result in a transient reduction in TSH secretion; the reduction is not sustained; therefore, hypothyroidism does not occur. Glucocorticoids may decrease serum TBG concentration).

No products indexed under this heading.

Desipramine Hydrochloride (Co-administration may increase the therapeutic and toxic effects of both drugs possibly due to increased receptor sensitivity to catecholamines; toxic effects may include increased risk of arrhythmias and CNS stimulation; onset of tricyclics may be accelerated).

No products indexed under this heading.

Deslanoside (Co-administration may result in reduced serum digitalis glycosides in hyperthyroidism or when the hypothyroid patient is converted to euthyroid state; therapeutic effect of digitalis glycoside may be reduced).

No products indexed under this heading.

Dexamethasone (Co-administration with glucocorticoids may result in a transient reduction in TSH secretion; the reduction is not sustained; therefore, hypothyroidism does not occur. Glucocorticoids may decrease serum TBG concentration). Products include:

Ciprodex Otic Suspension **555**
Decadron Tablets **1929**
TobraDex Ophthalmic Ointment **558**
TobraDex Ophthalmic Suspension ... **558**

Dexamethasone Acetate (Co-administration with glucocorticoids may result in a transient reduction in TSH secretion; the reduction is not sustained; therefore, hypothyroidism does not occur. Glucocorticoids may decrease serum TBG concentration).

No products indexed under this heading.

Dexamethasone Sodium Phosphate (Co-administration with glucocorticoids may result in a transient reduction in TSH secretion; the reduction is not sustained; therefore, hypothyroidism does not occur. Glucocorticoids may decrease serum TBG concentration). Products include:

Decadron Phosphate Injection **1931**

Diatrizoate Meglumine (May decrease thyroid hormone secretion, which may result in hypothyrodism; the fetus, elderly, and euthyroid patients with underlying thyroid disease are among those individuals who are susceptible to iodine-induced hypothyroidism; oral cholecytographic agents slowly excreted, producing more prolonged hypothyroidism; iodide drugs that contain pharmacologic amounts of iodide may cause hypothyroidism in euthyroid patients with Grave's disease previously treated with thyroid autonomy; hyperthyroidism may develop over several weeks and may persist for several months after therapy discontinuation).

No products indexed under this heading.

Diatrizoate Sodium (May decrease thyroid hormone secretion, which may result in hypothyrodism; the fetus, elderly, and euthyroid patients with underlying thyroid disease are among those individuals who are susceptible to iodine-induced hypothyroidism; oral cholecytographic agents slowly excreted, producing more prolonged hypothyroidism; iodide drugs that contain pharmacologic amounts of iodide may cause hypothyroidism in euthyroid patients with Grave's disease previously treated with thyroid autonomy; hyperthyroidism may develop over several weeks and may persist for several months after therapy discontinuation).

No products indexed under this heading.

Diazepam (Co-administration has been associated with thyroid hormone and/or TSH level alterations by various mechanisms). Products include:

Diastat Rectal Delivery System **3344**
Valium Tablets **2822**

Dicumarol (Thyroid hormones appear to increase the catabolism of vitamin K-dependent clotting factors, thereby increasing the anticoagulant activity of oral anticoagulants).

No products indexed under this heading.

Dienestrol (Co-administration with oral estrogens may result in increased serum TBG concentrations).

No products indexed under this heading.

Diethylstilbestrol (Co-administration with oral estrogens may result in increased serum TBG concentrations).

No products indexed under this heading.

Diflunisal (Co-administration with salicylates at greater than 2 gm inhibit binding of T4 and T3 to TBG and transthyrelin; an initial increase in serum FT4 is followed by return of FT4 to normal levels with sustained therapeutic salicylate concentrations although total T4 levels may decrease by as much as 30%). Products include:

Dolobid Tablets **1937**

Digitalis Glycoside Preparations (Co-administration may result in reduced serum digitalis glycosides in hyperthyroidism or when the hypothyroid patient is converted to euthyroid state; therapeutic effect of digitalis glycoside may be reduced).

No products indexed under this heading.

Digitoxin (Co-administration may result in reduced serum digitalis glycosides in hyperthyroidism or when the hypothyroid patient is converted to euthyroid state; therapeutic effect of digitalis glycoside may be reduced).

No products indexed under this heading.

Digoxin (Co-administration may result in reduced serum digitalis glycosides in hyperthyroidism or when the hypothyroid patient is converted to euthyroid state; therapeutic effect of digitalis glycoside may be reduced). Products include:

Digitek Tablets **2146**
Lanoxicaps Capsules **1458**
Lanoxin Injection **1462**
Lanoxin Tablets **1468**
Lanoxin Injection Pediatric **1465**

Dobutamine Hydrochloride (Co-administration of sympathomimetic agents may increase the effects of sympathomimetics or thyroid hormone; thyroid hormones may increase risk of coronary insufficiency when sympathomimetic agents are administered to patients with coronary disease).

No products indexed under this heading.

Dopamine Hydrochloride (Co-administration with dopamine may result in a transient reduction in TSH secretion; the reduction is not sustained; therefore, hypothyroidism does not occur).

No products indexed under this heading.

Doxepin Hydrochloride (Co-administration may increase the therapeutic and toxic effects of both drugs possibly due to increased receptor sensitivity to catecholamines; toxic effects may include increased risk of arrhythmias and CNS stimulation; onset of tricyclics may be accelerated).

No products indexed under this heading.

Dyphylline (Decreased theophylline clearance may occur in hypothyroid patients; clearance returns to normal when euthyroid state is achieved).

No products indexed under this heading.

Ephedrine Hydrochloride (Co-administration of sympathomimetic agents may increase the effects of sympathomimetics or thyroid hormone; thyroid hormones may increase risk of coronary insufficiency when sympathomimetic agents are administered to patients with coronary disease). Products include:

Primatene Tablets **749**

Ephedrine Sulfate (Co-administration of sympathomimetic agents may increase the effects of sympathomimetics or thyroid hormone; thyroid hormones may increase risk of coronary insufficiency when sympathomimetic agents are administered to patients with coronary disease).

No products indexed under this heading.

Ephedrine Tannate (Co-administration of sympathomimetic agents may increase the effects of sympathomimetics or thyroid hormone; thyroid hormones may increase risk of coronary insufficiency when sympathomimetic agents are administered to patients with coronary disease).

No products indexed under this heading.

Epinephrine (Co-administration of sympathomimetic agents may increase the effects of sympathomimetics or thyroid hormone; thyroid hormones may increase risk of coronary insufficiency when sympathomimetic agents are administered to patients with coronary disease). Products include:

EpiPen **1061**
Primatene Mist **749**

Epinephrine Bitartrate (Co-administration of sympathomimetic agents may increase the effects of sympathomimetics or thyroid hormone; thyroid hormones may increase risk of coronary insufficiency when sympathomimetic agents are administered to patients with coronary disease).
No products indexed under this heading.

Epinephrine Hydrochloride (Co-administration of sympathomimetic agents may increase the effects of sympathomimetics or thyroid hormone; thyroid hormones may increase risk of coronary insufficiency when sympathomimetic agents are administered to patients with coronary disease).
No products indexed under this heading.

Esmolol Hydrochloride (Co-administration with beta-blockers may decrease T_4 5'-deiodinase activity; action of beta-blocker may be impaired when the hypothyroid patient is converted to euthyroid). Products include:
Brevibloc Concentrate 766
Brevibloc Injection 766
Brevibloc Double Strength Injection 766
Brevibloc Premixed Injection 766
Brevibloc Double Strength Premixed Injection 766

Estradiol (Co-administration with oral estrogens may result in increased serum TBG concentrations). Products include:
Activella Tablets 2311
Climara Transdermal System 795
Climara Pro Transdermal System 800
CombiPatch Transdermal System 2180
Estrogel 0.06% 3200
Menostar Transdermal System 805
Prefest Tablets 1069
Vagifem Tablets 2340
Vivelle Transdermal System 2288
Vivelle-Dot Transdermal System 2293

Estrogens, Conjugated (Co-administration with oral estrogens may result in increased serum TBG concentrations). Products include:
Premarin Intravenous 3440
Premarin Tablets 3443
Premarin Vaginal Cream 3449
Premphase Tablets 3452
Prempro Tablets 3452

Estrogens, Esterified (Co-administration with oral estrogens may result in increased serum TBG concentrations). Products include:
Estratest Tablets 3196
Estratest H.S. Tablets 3196

Estropipate (Co-administration with oral estrogens may result in increased serum TBG concentrations).
No products indexed under this heading.

Ethinyl Estradiol (Co-administration with estrogen containing oral contraceptives may result in increased serum TBG concentrations). Products include:
Alesse-28 Tablets 3392
Lo/Ovral-28 Tablets 3423
NuvaRing 2357
Ortho-Cept Tablets 2395
Ortho-Cyclen/Ortho Tri-Cyclen 2414
Ortho Evra Transdermal System 2402
Ortho Tri-Cyclen Lo Tablets 2421
Seasonale Tablets 1073
Triphasil-28 Tablets 3483
Yasmin 28 Tablets 818

Ethiodized Oil (May decrease thyroid hormone secretion, which may result in hypothyrodism; the fetus, elderly, and euthyroid patients with underlying thyroid disease are among those individuals who are susceptible to iodine-induced hypothyroidism; oral cholecytographic agents slowly excreted, producing more prolonged hypothyroidism; iodide drugs that contain pharmacologic amounts of iodide may cause hypothyroidism in euthyroid patients with Grave's disease previously treated with thyroid autonomy; hyperthyroidism may develop over several weeks and may persist for several months after therapy discontinuation).
No products indexed under this heading.

Ethionamide (Co-administration has been associated with thyroid hormone and/or TSH level alterations by various mechanisms). Products include:
Trecator Tablets 3482

Ethotoin (Hydantoins may cause protein-binding site displacement; co-administration results in an initial transient increase in FT_4; continued administration results in a decrease in serum T_4 and normal FT_4 and TSH concentrations and, therefore, patients are clinically euthyroid). Products include:
Peganone Tablets, USP 2487

Ferrous Sulfate (Co-administration may result in decreased T4 absorption which may result in hypothyroidism; ferrous sulfate may form a ferric-thyroxine complex; administer levothyroxine at least 4 hours apart from these agents). Products include:
Feosol Tablets 1629
Slow Fe Iron Tablets .... ◘772
Slow Fe with Folic Acid Tablets .... ◘773

Fiber Supplement (Concurrent use of dietary fiber may bind and decrease the absorption of levothyroxine sodium from GI tract).
No products indexed under this heading.

Fludrocortisone Acetate (Co-administration with glucocorticoids may result in a transient reduction in TSH secretion; the reduction is not sustained; therefore, hypothyroidism does not occur. Glucocorticoids may decrease serum TBG concentration).
No products indexed under this heading.

Fluorouracil (Co-administration with 5-FU may result in increased serum TBG concentrations). Products include:
Carac Cream, 0.5% 1048
Efudex 3348

Fluoxymesterone (Co-administration with androgens/anabolic steroids may result in decreased serum TBG concentration).
No products indexed under this heading.

Fosphenytoin Sodium (Hydantoins may cause protein-binding site displacement; co-administration results in an initial transient increase in FT4; co-administration may increase hepatic metabolism, which may result in hypothyroidism, resulting in increased levothyroxine requirements; phenytoin reduces serum protein binding of levothyroxine, and total- and free-T4 may be reduced by 20% to 40%, but most patients have normal serum TSH levels and are clinically euthyroid).
No products indexed under this heading.

Furosemide (May cause protein-binding site displacement at greater than 80 mg IV; co-administration results in an initial transient increase in FT_4; continued administration results in a decrease in serum T_4 and normal FT_4 and TSH concentrations and, therefore, patients are clinically euthyroid). Products include:
Furosemide Tablets 2117

Gadopentetate Dimeglumine (May decrease thyroid hormone secretion, which may result in hypothyrodism; the fetus, elderly, and euthyroid patients with underlying thyroid disease are among those individuals who are susceptible to iodine-induced hypothyroidism; oral cholecytographic agents slowly excreted, producing more prolonged hypothyroidism; iodide drugs that contain pharmacologic amounts of iodide may cause hypothyroidism in euthyroid patients with Grave's disease previously treated with thyroid autonomy; hyperthyroidism may develop over several weeks and may persist for several months after therapy discontinuation).
No products indexed under this heading.

Glimepiride (Addition of levothyroxine to antidiabetic therapy may result in increased antidiabetic agent requirements). Products include:
Amaryl Tablets 2864

Glipizide (Addition of levothyroxine to antidiabetic therapy may result in increased antidiabetic agent requirements).
No products indexed under this heading.

Glyburide (Addition of levothyroxine to antidiabetic therapy may result in increased antidiabetic agent requirements).
No products indexed under this heading.

Heparin Sodium (May cause protein-binding site displacement; co-administration results in an initial transient increase in FT_4; continued administration results in a decrease in serum T_4 and normal FT_4 and TSH concentrations and, therefore, patients are clinically euthyroid).
No products indexed under this heading.

Heroin (Co-administration may result in increased serum TBG concentrations).
No products indexed under this heading.

Hydrochlorothiazide (Co-administration has been associated with thyroid hormone and/or TSH level alterations by various mechanisms). Products include:
Aldoril Tablets 1884
Atacand HCT 637
Avalide Tablets 2889
Avalide Tablets 922
Benicar HCT Tablets 2852
Diovan HCT Tablets 2195
Dyazide Capsules 1389
Hyzaar 1964
Lotensin HCT Tablets 2235
Maxzide 2150
Micardis HCT Tablets 886
Moduretic Tablets 2003
Prinzide Tablets 2033
Teveten HCT Tablets 1710
Timolide Tablets 2056
Uniretic Tablets 3114
Vaseretic Tablets 2073
Zestoretic Tablets 701

Hydrocortisone (Co-administration with glucocorticoids may result in a transient reduction in TSH secretion; the reduction is not sustained; therefore, hypothyroidism does not occur. Glucocorticoids may decrease serum TBG concentration). Products include:
Cortizone•5 Ointment .... ◘699
Cortizone•10 Creme .... ◘699
Cortizone•10 Ointment .... ◘699
Cortizone•10 Plus Creme .... ◘700
Cortizone•10 Maximum Strength Quick Shot Spray .... ◘700
Hydrocortone Tablets 1963
Preparation H Hydrocortisone Cream .... ◘748

Hydrocortisone Acetate (Co-administration with glucocorticoids may result in a transient reduction in TSH secretion; the reduction is not sustained; therefore, hypothyroidism does not occur. Glucocorticoids may decrease serum TBG concentration). Products include:
Analpram-HC 1136
Pramosone 1139
ProctoFoam-HC 3113
Tucks Anti-Itch Ointment .... ◘712
U-cort 1% Cream 3289

Hydrocortisone Sodium Phosphate (Co-administration with glucocorticoids may result in a transient reduction in TSH secretion; the reduction is not sustained; therefore, hypothyroidism does not occur. Glucocorticoids may decrease serum TBG concentration).
No products indexed under this heading.

Hydrocortisone Sodium Succinate (Co-administration with glucocorticoids may result in a transient reduction in TSH secretion; the reduction is not sustained; therefore, hypothyroidism does not occur. Glucocorticoids may decrease serum TBG concentration).
No products indexed under this heading.

Hydroflumethiazide (Co-administration has been associated with thyroid hormone and/or TSH level alterations by various mechanisms).
No products indexed under this heading.

Imipramine Hydrochloride (Co-administration may increase the therapeutic and toxic effects of both drugs possibly due to increased receptor sensitivity to catecholamines; toxic effects may include increased risk of arrhythmias and CNS stimulation; onset of tricyclics may be accelerated).
No products indexed under this heading.

Imipramine Pamoate (Co-administration may increase the therapeutic and toxic effects of both drugs possibly due to increased receptor sensitivity to catecholamines; toxic effects may include increased risk of arrhythmias and CNS stimulation; onset of tricyclics may be accelerated).
No products indexed under this heading.

Infant Formula (Concurrent use of soybean flour may bind and decrease the absorption of levothyroxine sodium from GI tract).
No products indexed under this heading.

Insulin, Human, Zinc Suspension (Addition of levothyroxine to insulin therapy may result in increased insulin requirements). Products include:
Humulin L, 100 Units 1763
Humulin U, 100 Units 1770

Insulin, Human NPH (Addition of levothyroxine to insulin therapy may result in increased insulin requirements). Products include:
Humulin N, 100 Units 1764
Humulin N Pen 1765
Novolin N Human Insulin 10 ml Vials 2322
Novolin N InnoLet 2322
Novolin N PenFill 3 ml Cartridges 2325
Novolin R InnoLet 2322

Insulin, Human Regular (Addition of levothyroxine to insulin therapy may result in increased insulin requirements). Products include:
Humulin R (U-500) 1768
Humulin R, 100 Units 1767
Novolin R Human Insulin 10 ml Vials 2322
Novolin R PenFill 2325

Insulin, Human Regular and Human NPH Mixture (Addition of levothyroxine to insulin therapy may result in increased insulin requirements). Products include:
Humulin 50/50, 100 Units 1760
Humulin 70/30 Pen 1761
Novolin 70/30 Human Insulin 10 ml Vials 2321
Novolin 70/30 InnoLet 2322
Novolin 70/30 PenFill 3 ml Cartridges 2325

Insulin, NPH (Addition of levothyroxine to insulin therapy may result in increased insulin requirements).
No products indexed under this heading.

Insulin, Regular (Addition of levothyroxine to insulin therapy may result in increased insulin requirements).
No products indexed under this heading.

Insulin, Zinc Crystals (Addition of levothyroxine to insulin therapy may result in increased insulin requirements).
No products indexed under this heading.

Insulin, Zinc Suspension (Addition of levothyroxine to insulin therapy may result in increased insulin requirements).
No products indexed under this heading.

Insulin Aspart, Human Regular (Addition of levothyroxine to insulin therapy may result in increased insulin requirements). Products include:
NovoLog Injection 2326

Insulin glargine (Addition of levothyroxine to insulin therapy may result in increased insulin requirements). Products include:
Lantus Injection 2925

Insulin Lispro, Human (Addition of levothyroxine to insulin therapy may result in increased insulin requirements). Products include:
Humalog-Pen 1751
Humalog Mix 75/25-Pen 1754

Insulin Lispro Protamine, Human (Addition of levothyroxine to insulin therapy may result in increased insulin requirements). Products include:
Humalog Mix 75/25-Pen 1754

Interferon alfa-2a, Recombinant (Co-administration with interferon alpha has been associated with the development of antithyroid microsomal antibodies in 20% of patients and some have transient hypothyroidism, hyperthyroidism, or both; patients who have antithyroid antibodies before treatment are at higher risk for thyroid dysfunction). Products include:
Roferon-A Injection 2805

Interferon alfa-2b, Recombinant (Co-administration with interferon alpha has been associated with the development of antithyroid microsomal antibodies in 20% of patients and some have transient hypothyroidism, hyperthyroidism, or both; patients who have antithyroid antibodies before treatment are at higher risk for thyroid dysfunction). Products include:
Intron A for Injection 3038
Rebetron Combination Therapy 3078

Interferon alfa-N3 (Human Leukocyte Derived) (Co-administration with interferon alpha has been associated with the development of antithyroid microsomal antibodies in 20% of patients and some have transient hypothyroidism, hyperthyroidism, or both; patients who have antithyroid antibodies before treatment are at higher risk for thyroid dysfunction). Products include:
Alferon N Injection 1640

Iodamide Meglumine (May decrease thyroid hormone secretion, which may result in hypothyrodism; the fetus, elderly, and euthyroid patients with underlying thyroid disease are among those individuals who are susceptible to iodine-induced hypothyroidism; oral cholecytographic agents slowly excreted, producing more prolonged hypothyroidism; iodide drugs that contain pharmacologic amounts of iodide may cause hypothyroidism in euthyroid patients with Grave's disease previously treated with thyroid autonomy; hyperthyroidism may develop over several weeks and may persist for several months after therapy discontinuation).
No products indexed under this heading.

Iohexol (May decrease thyroid hormone secretion, which may result in hypothyrodism; the fetus, elderly, and euthyroid patients with underlying thyroid disease are among those individuals who are susceptible to iodine-induced hypothyroidism; oral cholecytographic agents slowly excreted, producing more prolonged hypothyroidism; iodide drugs that contain pharmacologic amounts of iodide may cause hypothyroidism in euthyroid patients with Grave's disease previously treated with thyroid autonomy; hyperthyroidism may develop over several weeks and may persist for several months after therapy discontinuation).
No products indexed under this heading.

Iopamidol (May decrease thyroid hormone secretion, which may result in hypothyrodism; the fetus, elderly, and euthyroid patients with underlying thyroid disease are among those individuals who are susceptible to iodine-induced hypothyroidism; oral cholecytographic agents slowly excreted, producing more prolonged hypothyroidism; iodide drugs that contain pharmacologic amounts of iodide may cause hypothyroidism in euthyroid patients with Grave's disease previously treated with thyroid autonomy; hyperthyroidism may develop over several weeks and may persist for several months after therapy discontinuation).
No products indexed under this heading.

Iopanoic Acid (May decrease thyroid hormone secretion, which may result in hypothyrodism; the fetus, elderly, and euthyroid patients with underlying thyroid disease are among those individuals who are susceptible to iodine-induced hypothyroidism; oral cholecytographic agents slowly excreted, producing more prolonged hypothyroidism; iodide drugs that contain pharmacologic amounts of iodide may cause hypothyroidism in euthyroid patients with Grave's disease previously treated with thyroid autonomy; hyperthyroidism may develop over several weeks and may persist for several months after therapy discontinuation).
No products indexed under this heading.

Iothalamate Meglumine (May decrease thyroid hormone secretion, which may result in hypothyrodism; the fetus, elderly, and euthyroid patients with underlying thyroid disease are among those individuals who are susceptible to iodine-induced hypothyroidism; oral cholecytographic agents slowly excreted, producing more prolonged hypothyroidism; iodide drugs that contain pharmacologic amounts of iodide may cause hypothyroidism in euthyroid patients with Grave's disease previously treated with thyroid autonomy; hyperthyroidism may develop over several weeks and may persist for several months after therapy discontinuation).
No products indexed under this heading.

Ioxaglate Meglumine (May decrease thyroid hormone secretion, which may result in hypothyrodism; the fetus, elderly, and euthyroid patients with underlying thyroid disease are among those individuals who are susceptible to iodine-induced hypothyroidism; oral cholecytographic agents slowly excreted, producing more prolonged hypothyroidism; iodide drugs that contain pharmacologic amounts of iodide may cause hypothyroidism in euthyroid patients with Grave's disease previously treated with thyroid autonomy; hyperthyroidism may develop over several weeks and may persist for several months after therapy discontinuation).
No products indexed under this heading.

Ioxaglate Sodium (May decrease thyroid hormone secretion, which may result in hypothyrodism; the fetus, elderly, and euthyroid patients with underlying thyroid disease are among those individuals who are susceptible to iodine-induced hypothyroidism; oral cholecytographic agents slowly excreted, producing more prolonged hypothyroidism; iodide drugs that contain pharmacologic amounts of iodide may cause hypothyroidism in euthyroid patients with Grave's disease previously treated with thyroid autonomy; hyperthyroidism may develop over several weeks and may persist for several months after therapy discontinuation).
No products indexed under this heading.

Isoproterenol Hydrochloride (Co-administration of sympathomimetic agents may increase the effects of sympathomimetics or thyroid hormone; thyroid hormones may increase risk of coronary insufficiency when sympathomimetic agents are administered to patients with coronary disease).
No products indexed under this heading.

Isoproterenol Sulfate (Co-administration of sympathomimetic agents may increase the effects of sympathomimetics or thyroid hormone; thyroid hormones may increase risk of coronary insufficiency when sympathomimetic agents are administered to patients with coronary disease).
No products indexed under this heading.

Ketamine Hydrochloride (Co-administration may produce marked hypertension and tachycardia).
No products indexed under this heading.

Labetalol Hydrochloride (Co-administration with beta-blockers may decrease T_4 5'-deiodinase activity; action of beta-blocker may be impaired when the hypothyroid patient is converted to euthyroid).
No products indexed under this heading.

Levalbuterol Hydrochloride (Co-administration of sympathomimetic agents may increase the effects of sympathomimetics or thyroid hormone; thyroid hormones may increase risk of coronary insufficiency when sympathomimetic agents are administered to patients with coronary disease). Products include:
Xopenex Inhalation Solution 3143
Xopenex Inhalation Solution Concentrate 3147

Levobunolol Hydrochloride (Co-administration with beta-blockers may decrease T_4 5'-deiodinase activity; action of beta-blocker may be impaired when the hypothyroid patient is converted to euthyroid). Products include:
Betagan Ophthalmic Solution, USP .... ⊙217

Lithium (May decrease thyroid hormone secretion, which may result in hypothyrodism; long-term lithium therapy can result in goiter in up to 50% of patients, and either subclinical or overt hypothyroidism, each in up to 20% of patients).
No products indexed under this heading.

Lithium Carbonate (May decrease thyroid hormone secretion, which may result in hypothyrodism; long-term lithium therapy can result in goiter in up to 50% of patients, and either subclinical or overt hypothyroidism, each in up to 20% of patients). Products include:
Eskalith 1406
Lithobid Tablets 1670

Lithium Citrate (May decrease thyroid hormone secretion, which may result in hypothyrodism; long-term lithium therapy can result in goiter in up to 50% of patients, and either subclinical or overt hypothyroidism, each in up to 20% of patients).
No products indexed under this heading.

Lovastatin (Co-administration has been associated with thyroid hor-

mone and/or TSH level alterations by various mechanisms). Products include:

- Advicor Tablets 1694
- Altoprev Extended-Release Tablets 1151
- Mevacor Tablets 1996

Magaldrate (Co-administration with antacids may reduce the efficacy of levothyroxine by binding and delaying or preventing absorption, potentially resulting in hypothyroidism; administer levothyroxine at least 4 hours apart from these agents).
No products indexed under this heading.

Magnesium Hydroxide (Co-administration with antacids may reduce the efficacy of levothyroxine by binding and delaying or preventing absorption, potentially resulting in hypothyroidism; administer levothyroxine at least 4 hours apart from these agents). Products include:

- Maalox Max Maximum Strength Antacid/Anti-Gas Liquid 2165
- Maalox Regular Strength Antacid/Antigas Liquid 2164
- Pepcid Complete Chewable Tablets 1672
- Rolaids Tablets .... ▣ 707
- Extra Strength Rolaids Tablets .... ▣ 707
- Rolaids Multi-Symptom Antacid & Antigas Tablets .... ▣ 708

Magnesium Oxide (Co-administration with antacids may reduce the efficacy of levothyroxine by binding and delaying or preventing absorption, potentially resulting in hypothyroidism; administer levothyroxine at least 4 hours apart from these agents). Products include:

- Beelith Tablets 784
- PremCal Light, Regular, and Extra Strength Tablets .... ▣ 762

Magnesium Salicylate (Co-administration with salicylates at greater than 2 gm inhibit binding of T4 and T3 to TBG and transthyrelin; an initial increase in serum FT4 is followed by return of FT4 to normal levels with sustained therapeutic salicylate concentrations although total T4 levels may decrease by as much as 30%).
No products indexed under this heading.

Maprotiline Hydrochloride (Co-administration may increase the therapeutic and toxic effects of both drugs possibly due to increased receptor sensitivity to catecholamines; toxic effects may include increased risk of arrhythmias and CNS stimulation; onset of tricyclics may be accelerated).
No products indexed under this heading.

Meclofenamate Sodium (Co-administration with fenamate NSAID may result in decreased serum TBG concentration).
No products indexed under this heading.

Mefenamic Acid (Co-administration with fenamate NSAID may result in decreased serum TBG concentration).
No products indexed under this heading.

Mephenytoin (Hydantoins may cause protein-binding site displacement; co-administration results in an initial transient increase in FT_4; continued administration results in a decrease in serum T_4 and normal FT_4 and TSH concentrations and, therefore, patients are clinically euthyroid).
No products indexed under this heading.

Mercaptopurine (Co-administration has been associated with thyroid hormone and/or TSH level alterations by various mechanisms). Products include:

- Purinethol Tablets 1222

Mestranol (Co-administration with estrogen containing oral contraceptives may result in increased serum TBG concentrations).
No products indexed under this heading.

Metaproterenol Sulfate (Co-administration of sympathomimetic agents may increase the effects of sympathomimetics or thyroid hormone; thyroid hormones may increase risk of coronary insufficiency when sympathomimetic agents are administered to patients with coronary disease). Products include:

- Alupent Inhalation Aerosol 858

Metaraminol Bitartrate (Co-administration of sympathomimetic agents may increase the effects of sympathomimetics or thyroid hormone; thyroid hormones may increase risk of coronary insufficiency when sympathomimetic agents are administered to patients with coronary disease). Products include:

- Aramine Injection 1889

Metformin Hydrochloride (Addition of levothyroxine to antidiabetic therapy may result in increased antidiabetic agent requirements). Products include:

- ActoPlus Met Tablets 3219
- Avandamet Tablets 1343
- Fortamet Extended-Release Tablets 1156

Methadone Hydrochloride (Co-administration may result in increased serum TBG concentrations).
No products indexed under this heading.

Methimazole (May decrease thyroid hormone secretion which may result in hypothyrodism).
No products indexed under this heading.

Methoxamine Hydrochloride (Co-administration of sympathomimetic agents may increase the effects of sympathomimetics or thyroid hormone; thyroid hormones may increase risk of coronary insufficiency when sympathomimetic agents are administered to patients with coronary disease).
No products indexed under this heading.

Methyclothiazide (Co-administration has been associated with thyroid hormone and/or TSH level alterations by various mechanisms).
No products indexed under this heading.

Methylprednisolone Acetate (Co-administration with glucocorticoids may result in a transient reduction in TSH secretion; the reduction is not sustained; therefore, hypothyroidism does not occur. Glucocorticoids may decrease serum TBG concentration). Products include:

- Depo-Medrol Injectable Suspension 2615
- Depo-Medrol Single-Dose Vial 2617

Methylprednisolone Sodium Succinate (Co-administration with glucocorticoids may result in a transient reduction in TSH secretion; the reduction is not sustained; therefore, hypothyroidism does not occur. Glucocorticoids may decrease serum TBG concentration).
No products indexed under this heading.

Methyltestosterone (Co-administration with androgens/anabolic steroids may result in decreased serum TBG concentration). Products include:

- Estratest Tablets 3196
- Estratest H.S. Tablets 3196

Metipranolol Hydrochloride (Co-administration with beta-blockers may decrease T_4 5'-deiodinase activity; action of beta-blocker may be impaired when the hypothyroid patient is converted to euthyroid).
No products indexed under this heading.

Metoclopramide Hydrochloride (Co-administration has been associated with thyroid hormone and/or TSH level alterations by various mechanisms).
No products indexed under this heading.

Metoprolol Succinate (Co-administration with beta-blockers may decrease T_4 5'-deiodinase activity; action of beta-blocker may be impaired when the hypothyroid patient is converted to euthyroid). Products include:

- Toprol-XL Tablets 660

Metoprolol Tartrate (Co-administration with beta-blockers may decrease T_4 5'-deiodinase activity; action of beta-blocker may be impaired when the hypothyroid patient is converted to euthyroid).
No products indexed under this heading.

Miglitol (Addition of levothyroxine to antidiabetic therapy may result in increased antidiabetic agent requirements).
No products indexed under this heading.

Mitotane (Co-administration may result in increased serum TBG concentrations).
No products indexed under this heading.

Nadolol (Co-administration with beta-blockers may decrease T_4 5'-deiodinase activity; action of beta-blocker may be impaired when the hypothyroid patient is converted to euthyroid). Products include:

- Nadolol Tablets 2121

Niacin (Co-administration with slow-release nicotinic acid may result in decreased serum TBG concentration). Products include:

- Advicor Tablets 1694
- Niaspan Extended-Release Tablets 1703

Norepinephrine Bitartrate (Co-administration of sympathomimetic agents may increase the effects of sympathomimetics or thyroid hormone; thyroid hormones may increase risk of coronary insufficiency when sympathomimetic agents are administered to patients with coronary disease).
No products indexed under this heading.

Nortriptyline Hydrochloride (Co-administration may increase the therapeutic and toxic effects of both drugs possibly due to increased receptor sensitivity to catecholamines; toxic effects may include increased risk of arrhythmias and CNS stimulation; onset of tricyclics may be accelerated).
No products indexed under this heading.

Octreotide Acetate (Co-administration with octreotide may result in a transient reduction in TSH secretion; the reduction is not sustained, therefore, hypothyroidism does not occur). Products include:

- Sandostatin Injection 2263
- Sandostatin LAR Depot 2264

Oxandrolone (Co-administration with androgens/anabolic steroids may result in decreased serum TBG concentration). Products include:

- Oxandrin Tablets 2977

Oxymetholone (Co-administration with androgens/anabolic steroids may result in decreased serum TBG concentration). Products include:

- Anadrol-50 Tablets 3329

Penbutolol Sulfate (Co-administration with beta-blockers may decrease T_4 5'-deiodinase activity; action of beta-blocker may be impaired when the hypothyroid patient is converted to euthyroid).
No products indexed under this heading.

Pergolide Mesylate (Co-administration with dopamine agonists may result in a transient reduction in TSH secretion; the reduction is not sustained; therefore, hypothyroidism does not occur). Products include:

- Permax Tablets 3357

Perphenazine (Co-administration has been associated with thyroid hormone and/or TSH level alterations by various mechanisms).
No products indexed under this heading.

Phenobarbital (Co-administration may increase hepatic metabolism which may result in hypothyroidism; resulting in increased levothyroxine requirements).
No products indexed under this heading.

Phenylbutazone (Co-administration may cause protein-binding site displacement).
No products indexed under this heading.

Phenylephrine Bitartrate (Co-administration of sympathomimetic agents may increase the effects of sympathomimetics or thyroid hormone; thyroid hormones may increase risk of coronary insufficiency when sympathomimetic agents are administered to patients with coronary disease).
No products indexed under this heading.

Phenylephrine Hydrochloride (Co-administration of sympathomi-

metic agents may increase the effects of sympathomimetics or thyroid hormone; thyroid hormones may increase risk of coronary insufficiency when sympathomimetic agents are administered to patients with coronary disease). Products include:

- Alacol DM Syrup 739
- Hycomine Compound Tablets 1105
- Preparation H Maximum Strength Cream .... ▣747
- Preparation H Cooling Gel .... ▣747
- Preparation H .... ▣747
- Sudafed PE Tablets .... ▣711
- Vicks Sinex Nasal Spray and Ultra Fine Mist for Sinus Relief 2677
- Zicam Concentrated Cough Mist for Kids Plus D Cool Cherry .... ▣643
- Zicam Concentrated Cough Mist Plus D Cool Cherry .... ▣642

Phenylephrine Tannate (Co-administration of sympathomimetic agents may increase the effects of sympathomimetics or thyroid hormone; thyroid hormones may increase risk of coronary insufficiency when sympathomimetic agents are administered to patients with coronary disease).

No products indexed under this heading.

Phenylpropanolamine Hydrochloride (Co-administration of sympathomimetic agents may increase the effects of sympathomimetics or thyroid hormone; thyroid hormones may increase risk of coronary insufficiency when sympathomimetic agents are administered to patients with coronary disease).

No products indexed under this heading.

Phenytoin (Hydantoins may cause protein-binding site displacement; co-administration results in an initial transient increase in FT4; co-administration may increase hepatic metabolism, which may result in hypothyroidism, resulting in increased levothyroxine requirements; phenytoin reduces serum protein binding of levothyroxine, and total- and free-T4 may be reduced by 20% to 40%, but most patients have normal serum TSH levels and are clinically euthyroid).

No products indexed under this heading.

Phenytoin Sodium (Hydantoins may cause protein-binding site displacement; co-administration results in an initial transient increase in FT4; co-administration may increase hepatic metabolism, which may result in hypothyroidism, resulting in increased levothyroxine requirements; phenytoin reduces serum protein binding of levothyroxine, and total- and free-T4 may be reduced by 20% to 40%, but most patients have normal serum TSH levels and are clinically euthyroid). Products include:

- Phenytek Capsules 2153

Pindolol (Co-administration with beta-blockers may decrease T_4 5'-deiodinase activity; action of beta-blocker may be impaired when the hypothyroid patient is converted to euthyroid).

No products indexed under this heading.

Pioglitazone Hydrochloride (Addition of levothyroxine to antidiabetic therapy may result in increased antidiabetic agent requirements). Products include:

- ActoPlus Met Tablets 3219
- Actos Tablets 3224

Pirbuterol Acetate (Co-administration of sympathomimetic agents may increase the effects of sympathomimetics or thyroid hormone; thyroid hormones may increase risk of coronary insufficiency when sympathomimetic agents are administered to patients with coronary disease). Products include:

- Maxair Autohaler 1820

Polyestradiol Phosphate (Co-administration with oral estrogens may result in increased serum TBG concentrations).

No products indexed under this heading.

Polythiazide (Co-administration has been associated with thyroid hormone and/or TSH level alterations by various mechanisms).

No products indexed under this heading.

Potassium Iodide (May decrease thyroid hormone secretion which may result in hypothyrodism; iodide drugs that contain pharmacologic amounts of iodide may cause hypothyroidism in euthyroid patients with Grave's disease previously treated with thyroid autonomy; hyperthyroidism may develop over several weeks and may persist for several months after therapy discontinuation).

No products indexed under this heading.

Pramipexole Dihydrochloride (Co-administration with dopamine agonists may result in a transient reduction in TSH secretion; the reduction is not sustained; therefore, hypothyroidism does not occur). Products include:

- Mirapex Tablets 889

Prednisolone Acetate (Co-administration with glucocorticoids may result in a transient reduction in TSH secretion; the reduction is not sustained; therefore, hypothyroidism does not occur. Glucocorticoids may decrease serum TBG concentration). Products include:

- Blephamide Ophthalmic Ointment 563
- Blephamide Ophthalmic Suspension 564
- Poly-Pred Liquifilm Ophthalmic Suspension .... ⊙231
- Pred Forte Ophthalmic Suspension .... ⊙233
- Pred Mild Sterile Ophthalmic Suspension .... ⊙236
- Pred-G Ophthalmic Suspension .... ⊙234
- Pred-G Sterile Ophthalmic Ointment .... ⊙235

Prednisolone Sodium Phosphate (Co-administration with glucocorticoids may result in a transient reduction in TSH secretion; the reduction is not sustained; therefore, hypothyroidism does not occur. Glucocorticoids may decrease serum TBG concentration). Products include:

- Pediapred Oral Solution 3319

Prednisolone Tebutate (Co-administration with glucocorticoids may result in a transient reduction in TSH secretion; the reduction is not sustained; therefore, hypothyroidism does not occur. Glucocorticoids may decrease serum TBG concentration).

No products indexed under this heading.

Prednisone (Co-administration with glucocorticoids may result in a transient reduction in TSH secretion; the reduction is not sustained; therefore, hypothyroidism does not occur. Glucocorticoids may decrease serum TBG concentration).

No products indexed under this heading.

Propranolol Hydrochloride (Co-administration with beta-blockers may decrease T_4 5'-deiodinase activity; in patients treated with large doses of propranolol, greater than 160 mg/day, T_3 and T_4 levels change slightly, TSH levels remain normal, and patients are clinically euthyroid; action of beta-blocker may be impaired when the hypothyroid patient is converted to euthyroid). Products include:

- Inderal LA Long-Acting Capsules 3421
- InnoPran XL Capsules 2728

Propylthiouracil (May decrease thyroid hormone secretion which may result in hypothyrodism).

No products indexed under this heading.

Protriptyline Hydrochloride (Co-administration may increase the therapeutic and toxic effects of both drugs possibly due to increased receptor sensitivity to catecholamines; toxic effects may include increased risk of arrhythmias and CNS stimulation; onset of tricyclics may be accelerated). Products include:

- Vivactil Tablets 2350

Pseudoephedrine Hydrochloride (Co-administration of sympathomimetic agents may increase the effects of sympathomimetics or thyroid hormone; thyroid hormones may increase risk of coronary insufficiency when sympathomimetic agents are administered to patients with coronary disease). Products include:

- Advil Allergy Sinus Caplets .... ▣737
- Advil Cold & Sinus .... ▣739
- Advil Flu & Body Ache Caplets .... ▣739
- Children's Advil Cold Suspension .... ▣741
- Advil Multi-Symptom Cold Caplets .... ▣738
- Allegra-D 12 Hour Extended-Release Tablets 2860
- Allegra-D 24 Hour Extended-Release Tablets 2862
- Balamine DM 739
- BC Cold Powder .... ▣612
- Benadryl Allergy & Cold Tablets .... ▣692
- Benadryl Allergy & Sinus Headache Caplets & Gelcaps .... ▣693
- Children's Benadryl Allergy & Cold Fastmelt Tablets .... ▣695
- Benadryl Maximum Strength Severe Allergy & Sinus Headache Caplets .... ▣694
- Children's Benadryl D Allergy & Sinus Fastmelt Tablets .... ▣694
- Children's Benadryl D Liquid Medication .... ▣693
- Benadryl D Tablets .... ▣694
- Contac Non-Drowsy 12 Hour Cold Caplets .... ▣614
- Contac Non-Drowsy Timed Release 12 Hour Cold Caplets .... ▣615
- Contac Severe Cold and Flu Caplets Maximum Strength .... ▣615
- Contac Severe Cold and Flu Caplets Non-Drowsy .... ▣615
- Children's Dimetapp Cold & Allergy Elixir .... ▣745
- Children's Dimetapp DM Cold & Cough Elixir .... ▣745
- Children's Dimetapp Long Acting Cough Plus Cold Syrup .... ▣746
- Dimetapp Infant Drops Decongestant Plus Cough .... ▣746
- Children's Motrin Cold Non-Staining Dye-Free Oral Suspension 1838
- Children's Motrin Cold Oral Suspension 1838
- Motrin Cold & Sinus Caplets 1836
- PediaCare Decongestant & Cough Infant Drops .... ▣705
- PediaCare Decongestant Infants' Drops .... ▣705
- PediaCare Long-Acting Cough Plus Cold Liquid .... ▣704
- PediaCare Multi-Symptom Cold Liquid .... ▣704
- PediaCare NightRest Cough & Cold Liquid .... ▣704
- Robitussin Allergy & Cough Syrup .... ▣750
- Robitussin CF Liquid .... ▣755
- Robitussin Cough & Cold Liquid-filled Capsules .... ▣750
- Robitussin Cough, Cold & Flu Liquid-filled Capsules .... ▣750
- Robitussin Cough & Cold Infant Drops .... ▣755
- Robitussin Flu Liquid .... ▣752
- Robitussin Maximum Strength Cough & Cold Liquid .... ▣754
- Robitussin PE Syrup .... ▣753
- Robitussin Pediatric Cough & Cold Liquid .... ▣754
- Robitussin PM Cough & Cold Liquid .... ▣752
- Robitussin Severe Congestion Liquid-filled Capsules .... ▣751
- Simply Stuffy Liquid 1841
- Singlet Caplets .... ▣636
- Sudafed 12 Hour Caplets .... ▣708
- Sudafed 24 Hour Tablets .... ▣709
- Sudafed Nasal Decongestant Tablets .... ▣709
- Sudafed Severe Cold .... ▣710
- Sudafed Non-Drying Sinus Liquid Caps .... ▣709
- Sudafed Sinus & Allergy Tablets .... ▣710
- Sudafed Sinus Headache .... ▣711
- TheraFlu Cold & Cough Hot Liquid .... ▣680
- TheraFlu Cold & Sore Throat Hot Liquid .... ▣680
- TheraFlu Flu & Chest Congestion Non-Drowsy Hot Liquid .... ▣681
- TheraFlu Flu & Sore Throat Hot Liquid .... ▣681
- TheraFlu Severe Cold Non-Drowsy Hot Liquid .... ▣683
- TheraFlu Severe Cold & Cough Hot Liquid .... ▣683
- TheraFlu Severe Cold Caplets .... ▣679
- TheraFlu Severe Cold Hot Liquid .... ▣682
- TheraFlu Severe Cold Non-Drowsy Caplets .... ▣679
- Triaminic Chest & Nasal Congestion Liquid .... ▣685
- Triaminic Cold & Allergy Liquid .... ▣685
- Triaminic Cold & Cough Liquid .... ▣685
- Triaminic Cough Liquid .... ▣687
- Triaminic Cough & Nasal Congestion Liquid .... ▣687
- Triaminic Cough & Sore Throat Liquid .... ▣687
- Triaminic Flu, Cough & Fever Liquid .... ▣685
- Triaminic Night Time Cough & Cold Liquid .... ▣685
- Triaminic Allergy Runny Nose & Congestion Softchews .... ▣688
- Triaminic Cold & Cough Softchews .... ▣688
- Triaminic Cough & Sore Throat Softchews .... ▣689
- Tylenol Sinus NightTime Caplets .... ▣663
- Children's Tylenol Plus Cold & Allergy Suspension Liquid 1850
- Children's Tylenol Plus Cold NightTime Suspension Liquid 1851
- Children's Tylenol Plus Cold & Cough Suspension Liquid and Chewable Tablets 1851
- Children's Tylenol Plus Cold Chewable Tablets 1851
- Children's Tylenol Plus Cold Daytime Non-Drowsy Suspension Liquid 1851
- Children's Tylenol Plus Flu Suspension Liquid 1853
- Concentrated Tylenol Infants' Drops Plus Cold 1851

IMPORTANT NOTE: Always consult each drug listing in the patient's regimen for possible interactions.

Concentrated Tylenol Infants' Drops Plus Cold and Cough 1851
Tylenol Cold & Flu Severe Daytime Liquid with Cool Bust....... 1846
Tylenol Cold & Flu Severe NightTime Liquid with Cool Burst.. 1846
Tylenol Cold Severe Congestion Non-Drowsy Caplets with Cool Burst.. 1846
Tylenol Allergy Complete Night Time Caplets.............................. 1844
Tylenol Allergy Complete Multi-Symptom Caplets and Gelcaps with Cool Burst............... 1844
Tylenol Flu NightTime Gelcaps 1846
Tylenol Flu Day Non-Drowsy Gelcaps.................................... 1846
Concentrated Tylenol Infants' Drops Plus Cold Nasal Congestant, Fever Reducer & Pain Reliever............................. ▣ 668
Concentrated Tylenol Infants' Drops Plus Cold & Cough Nasal Decongestant, Fever Reducer & Pain Reliever.............. ▣ 668
Multi-Symptom Tylenol Cold Night Time Caplets.............................. 1845
Multi-Symptom Tylenol Cold Day Non-Drowsy Caplets and Gelcaps.................................... 1845
Tylenol Sinus Day Non-Drowsy 1848
Tylenol Sinus Night Time Caplets 1848
Tylenol Sinus Severe Congestion Caplets with Cool Burst............... 1848
Vicks 44D Cough & Head Congestion Relief......................... 2676
Vicks 44D Cough & Head Congestion Relief Liquid.............. ▣ 721
Vicks 44M Cough, Cold & Flu Relief.. 2676
Pediatric Vicks 44m Cough & Cold Relief.................................. 2673
Vicks DayQuil LiquiCaps/Liquid Multi-Symptom Cold/Flu Relief..... ▣ 723
Vicks DayQuil Multi-Symptom Cold/Flu Relief LiquiCaps............. 2675
Vicks DayQuil Multi-Symptom Cold/Flu Relief Liquid................... 2675
Children's Vicks NyQuil Cold/Cough Relief........................ 2671
Vicks NyQuil LiquiCaps 2677
Vicks NyQuil LiquiCaps/Liquid Multi-Symptom Cold/Flu Relief..... ▣ 725
Vicks NyQuil Liquid 2677
Zyrtec-D 12 Hour Extended Release Tablets........................... 2591

Pseudoephedrine Sulfate (Co-administration of sympathomimetic agents may increase the effects of sympathomimetics or thyroid hormone; thyroid hormones may increase risk of coronary insufficiency when sympathomimetic agents are administered to patients with coronary disease). Products include:

Alavert Allergy & Sinus D-12 Hour Tablets.. ▣ 743
Clarinex-D 24-Hour Extended-Release Tablets............ 3012
Claritin-D Non-Drowsy 12 Hour Tablets.. ▣ 731
Claritin-D Non-Drowsy 24 Hour Tablets.. ▣ 731

Quinestrol (Co-administration with oral estrogens may result in increased serum TBG concentrations).
No products indexed under this heading.

Repaglinide (Addition of levothyroxine to antidiabetic therapy may result in increased antidiabetic agent requirements). Products include:

Prandin Tablets (0.5, 1, and 2 mg)... 2337

Resorcinol (Co-administration of excessive topical use of resorcinol has been associated with thyroid hormone and/or TSH level alterations by various mechanisms).
No products indexed under this heading.

Rifampin (Co-administration may increase hepatic metabolism which may result in hypothyroidism, resulting in increased levothyroxine requirements).
No products indexed under this heading.

Ropinirole Hydrochloride (Co-administration with dopamine agonists may result in a transient reduction in TSH secretion; the reduction is not sustained; therefore, hypothyroidism does not occur). Products include:

Requip Tablets 1528

Rosiglitazone Maleate (Addition of levothyroxine to antidiabetic therapy may result in increased antidiabetic agent requirements). Products include:

Avandamet Tablets 1343
Avandia Tablets 1348

Salmeterol Xinafoate (Co-administration of sympathomimetic agents may increase the effects of sympathomimetics or thyroid hormone; thyroid hormones may increase risk of coronary insufficiency when sympathomimetic agents are administered to patients with coronary disease). Products include:

Advair Diskus 100/50 1291
Advair Diskus 250/50 1291
Advair Diskus 500/50 1291
Serevent Diskus 1540

Salsalate (Co-administration with salicylates at greater than 2 gm inhibit binding of T4 and T3 to TBG and transthyrelin; an initial increase in serum FT4 is followed by return of FT4 to normal levels with sustained therapeutic salicylate concentrations although total T4 levels may decrease by as much as 30%).
No products indexed under this heading.

Sertraline Hydrochloride (Co-administration of sertraline in patients stabilized on levothyroxine may result in increased levothyroxine requirements). Products include:

Zoloft 2581

Sodium Nitroprusside (Co-administration has been associated with thyroid hormone and/or TSH level alterations by various mechanisms).
No products indexed under this heading.

Sodium Polystyrene Sulfonate (Co-administration may result in decreased T4 absorption which may result in hypothyroidism; administer levothyroxine at least 4 hours apart from these agents).
No products indexed under this heading.

Somatrem (Excessive use of thyroid hormone with growth hormones may accelerate epiphyseal closure; however, untreated hypothyroidism may interfere with growth response to growth hormone).
No products indexed under this heading.

Somatropin (Excessive use of thyroid hormone with growth hormones may accelerate epiphyseal closure; however, untreated hypothyroidism may interfere with growth response to growth hormone). Products include:

Genotropin Lyophilized Powder 2642
Humatrope Vials and Cartridges 1756
Norditropin Cartridges 2318
Nutropin for Injection 1238
Nutropin AQ Injection 1241
Nutropin AQ Pen 1241
Nutropin AQ Pen Cartridge 1241

Sotalol Hydrochloride (Co-administration with beta-blockers may decrease T_4 5'-deiodinase activity; action of beta-blocker may be impaired when the hypothyroid patient is converted to euthyroid).
No products indexed under this heading.

Soybean Preparations (Concurrent use of soybean flour may bind and decrease the absorption of levothyroxine sodium from GI tract).
No products indexed under this heading.

Stanozolol (Co-administration with androgens/anabolic steroids may result in decreased serum TBG concentration).
No products indexed under this heading.

Sucralfate (Co-administration may result in decreased T4 absorption which may result in hypothyroidism; administer levothyroxine at least 4 hours apart from these agents). Products include:

Carafate Suspension 727
Carafate Tablets 728

Sulfamethoxazole (May decrease thyroid hormone secretion which may result in hypothyrodism).
No products indexed under this heading.

Sulfisoxazole Acetyl (May decrease thyroid hormone secretion which may result in hypothyrodism).
No products indexed under this heading.

Tamoxifen Citrate (Co-administration may result in increased serum TBG concentrations).
No products indexed under this heading.

Terbutaline Sulfate (Co-administration of sympathomimetic agents may increase the effects of sympathomimetics or thyroid hormone; thyroid hormones may increase risk of coronary insufficiency when sympathomimetic agents are administered to patients with coronary disease).
No products indexed under this heading.

Theophylline (Decreased theophylline clearance may occur in hypothyroid patients; clearance returns to normal when euthyroid state is achieved).
No products indexed under this heading.

Theophylline Anhydrous (Decreased theophylline clearance may occur in hypothyroid patients; clearance returns to normal when euthyroid state is achieved). Products include:

Uniphyl Tablets 2708

Theophylline Calcium Salicylate (Decreased theophylline clearance may occur in hypothyroid patients; clearance returns to normal when euthyroid state is achieved).
No products indexed under this heading.

Theophylline Dihydroxypropyl (Glyceryl) (Decreased theophylline clearance may occur in hypothyroid patients; clearance returns to normal when euthyroid state is achieved).
No products indexed under this heading.

Theophylline Ethylenediamine (Decreased theophylline clearance may occur in hypothyroid patients; clearance returns to normal when euthyroid state is achieved).
No products indexed under this heading.

Theophylline Sodium Glycinate (Decreased theophylline clearance may occur in hypothyroid patients; clearance returns to normal when euthyroid state is achieved).
No products indexed under this heading.

Timolol Hemihydrate (Co-administration with beta-blockers may decrease T_4 5'-deiodinase activity; action of beta-blocker may be impaired when the hypothyroid patient is converted to euthyroid). Products include:

Betimol Ophthalmic Solution 3371
Betimol Ophthalmic Solution .... ⊙ 283

Timolol Maleate (Co-administration with beta-blockers may decrease T_4 5'-deiodinase activity; action of beta-blocker may be impaired when the hypothyroid patient is converted to euthyroid). Products include:

Blocadren Tablets 1891
Cosopt Sterile Ophthalmic Solution.. 1910
Timolide Tablets 2056
Timoptic in Ocudose 2061
Timoptic Sterile Ophthalmic Solution.. 2058
Timoptic-XE Sterile Ophthalmic Gel Forming Solution 2062

Tolazamide (Addition of levothyroxine to antidiabetic therapy may result in increased antidiabetic agent requirements).
No products indexed under this heading.

Tolbutamide (May decrease thyroid hormone secretion which may result in hypothyrodism).
No products indexed under this heading.

Triamcinolone (Co-administration with glucocorticoids may result in a transient reduction in TSH secretion; the reduction is not sustained; therefore, hypothyroidism does not occur. Glucocorticoids may decrease serum TBG concentration).
No products indexed under this heading.

Triamcinolone Acetonide (Co-administration with glucocorticoids may result in a transient reduction in TSH secretion; the reduction is not sustained; therefore, hypothyroidism does not occur. Glucocorticoids may decrease serum TBG concentration). Products include:

Azmacort Inhalation Aerosol 1701
Nasacort HFA Inhalation Aerosol 2939
Nasacort AQ Nasal Spray 2937

Triamcinolone Diacetate (Co-administration with glucocorticoids may result in a transient reduction in TSH secretion; the reduction is not sustained; therefore, hypothyroidism does not occur. Glucocorticoids may decrease serum TBG concentration).
No products indexed under this heading.

Triamcinolone Hexacetonide (Co-administration with glucocorticoids may result in a transient reduction in TSH secretion; the reduction is not sustained; therefore, hypothyroidism does not occur. Glucocorticoids may decrease serum TBG concentration).
No products indexed under this heading.

Trimipramine Maleate (Co-administration may increase the therapeutic and toxic effects of both drugs possibly due to increased receptor sensitivity to catecholamines; toxic effects may include increased risk of arrhythmias and CNS stimulation; onset of tricyclics may be accelerated). Products include:

Surmontil Capsules 2347

Troglitazone (Addition of levothyroxine to antidiabetic therapy may result in increased antidiabetic agent requirements).

No products indexed under this heading.

Tyropanoate Sodium (May decrease thyroid hormone secretion, which may result in hypothyrodism; the fetus, elderly, and euthyroid patients with underlying thyroid disease are among those individuals who are susceptible to iodine-induced hypothyroidism; oral cholecytographic agents slowly excreted, producing more prolonged hypothyroidism; iodide drugs that contain pharmacologic amounts of iodide may cause hypothyroidism in euthyroid patients with Grave's disease previously treated with thyroid autonomy; hyperthyroidism may develop over several weeks and may persist for several months after therapy discontinuation).

No products indexed under this heading.

Warfarin Sodium (Thyroid hormones appear to increase the catabolism of vitamin K-dependent clotting factors, thereby increasing the anticoagulant activity of oral anticoagulants). Products include:

Coumadin for Injection 932
Coumadin Tablets 932

Food Interactions

Cotton seed meal (Concurrent use of cotton seed meal may bind and decrease the absorption of levothyroxine sodium from GI tract).

Dietary Fiber (Concurrent use of dietary fiber may bind and decrease the absorption of levothyroxine sodium from GI tract).

Soybean Formula, Children's (Concurrent use of soybean flour may bind and decrease the absorption of levothyroxine sodium from GI tract).

Walnuts (Concurrent use of walnuts may bind and decrease the absorption of levothyroxine sodium from GI tract).

UNIVASC TABLETS

(Moexipril Hydrochloride) 3118

May interact with diuretics, lithium preparations, potassium preparations, potassium sparing diuretics, and certain other agents. Compounds in these categories include:

Amiloride Hydrochloride (Co-administration can increase the risk of hyperkalemia; therefore, potassium-sparing diuretics should be given with caution, and serum potassium should be monitored). Products include:

Midamor Tablets 2000
Moduretic Tablets 2003

Bendroflumethiazide (Co-administration may result in excessive reductions in blood pressure. This can be minimized by discontinuing diuretic therapy for several days or cautiously increasing salt intake before initiating with moexipril. If this is not possible, the starting dose of moexipril should be reduced).

No products indexed under this heading.

Bumetanide (Co-administration may result in excessive reductions in blood pressure. This can be minimized by discontinuing diuretic therapy for several days or cautiously increasing salt intake before initiating with moexipril. If this is not possible, the starting dose of moexipril should be reduced).

No products indexed under this heading.

Chlorothiazide (Co-administration may result in excessive reductions in blood pressure. This can be minimized by discontinuing diuretic therapy for several days or cautiously increasing salt intake before initiating with moexipril. If this is not possible, the starting dose of moexipril should be reduced). Products include:

Aldoclor Tablets 1881
Diuril Oral 1936

Chlorothiazide Sodium (Co-administration may result in excessive reductions in blood pressure. This can be minimized by discontinuing diuretic therapy for several days or cautiously increasing salt intake before initiating with moexipril. If this is not possible, the starting dose of moexipril should be reduced). Products include:

Diuril Sodium Intravenous 1934

Chlorthalidone (Co-administration may result in excessive reductions in blood pressure. This can be minimized by discontinuing diuretic therapy for several days or cautiously increasing salt intake before initiating with moexipril. If this is not possible, the starting dose of moexipril should be reduced). Products include:

Clorpres Tablets 2139

Ethacrynic Acid (Co-administration may result in excessive reductions in blood pressure. This can be minimized by discontinuing diuretic therapy for several days or cautiously increasing salt intake before initiating with moexipril. If this is not possible, the starting dose of moexipril should be reduced). Products include:

Edecrin Tablets 1941

Furosemide (Co-administration may result in excessive reductions in blood pressure. This can be minimized by discontinuing diuretic therapy for several days or cautiously increasing salt intake before initiating with moexipril. If this is not possible, the starting dose of moexipril should be reduced). Products include:

Furosemide Tablets 2117

Hydrochlorothiazide (Co-administration may result in excessive reductions in blood pressure. This can be minimized by discontinuing diuretic therapy for several days or cautiously increasing salt intake before initiating with moexipril. If this is not possible, the starting dose of moexipril should be reduced). Products include:

Aldoril Tablets 1884
Atacand HCT 637
Avalide Tablets 2889
Avalide Tablets 922
Benicar HCT Tablets 2852
Diovan HCT Tablets 2195
Dyazide Capsules 1389
Hyzaar 1964
Lotensin HCT Tablets 2235
Maxzide 2150
Micardis HCT Tablets 886
Moduretic Tablets 2003
Prinzide Tablets 2033
Teveten HCT Tablets 1710
Timolide Tablets 2056
Uniretic Tablets 3114
Vaseretic Tablets 2073
Zestoretic Tablets 701

Hydroflumethiazide (Co-administration may result in excessive reductions in blood pressure. This can be minimized by discontinuing diuretic therapy for several days or cautiously increasing salt intake before initiating with moexipril. If this is not possible, the starting dose of moexipril should be reduced).

No products indexed under this heading.

Indapamide (Co-administration may result in excessive reductions in blood pressure. This can be minimized by discontinuing diuretic therapy for several days or cautiously increasing salt intake before initiating with moexipril. If this is not possible, the starting dose of moexipril should be reduced). Products include:

Indapamide Tablets 2119

Lithium (Increased serum lithium levels and symptoms of lithium toxicity have been reported during concomitant use. Lithium should be co-administered with caution, and frequent monitoring of serum lithium levels is recommended).

Lithium Carbonate (Increased serum lithium levels and symptoms of lithium toxicity have been reported during concomitant use. Lithium should be co-administered with caution, and frequent monitoring of serum lithium levels is recommended). Products include:

Eskalith 1406
Lithobid Tablets 1670

Lithium Citrate (Increased serum lithium levels and symptoms of lithium toxicity have been reported during concomitant use. Lithium should be co-administered with caution, and frequent monitoring of serum lithium levels is recommended).

No products indexed under this heading.

Methyclothiazide (Co-administration may result in excessive reductions in blood pressure. This can be minimized by discontinuing diuretic therapy for several days or cautiously increasing salt intake before initiating with moexipril. If this is not possible, the starting dose of moexipril should be reduced).

No products indexed under this heading.

Metolazone (Co-administration may result in excessive reductions in blood pressure. This can be minimized by discontinuing diuretic therapy for several days or cautiously increasing salt intake before initiating with moexipril. If this is not possible, the starting dose of moexipril should be reduced).

No products indexed under this heading.

Polythiazide (Co-administration may result in excessive reductions in blood pressure. This can be minimized by discontinuing diuretic therapy for several days or cautiously increasing salt intake before initiating with moexipril. If this is not possible, the starting dose of moexipril should be reduced).

No products indexed under this heading.

Potassium Acid Phosphate (Co-administration can increase the risk of hyperkalemia; therefore, potassium supplements should be given with caution, and serum potassium should be monitored). Products include:

K-Phos Original (Sodium Free) Tablets 785

Potassium Bicarbonate (Co-administration can increase the risk of hyperkalemia; therefore, potassium supplements should be given with caution, and serum potassium should be monitored).

No products indexed under this heading.

Potassium Chloride (Co-administration can increase the risk of hyperkalemia; therefore, potassium supplements should be given with caution, and serum potassium should be monitored). Products include:

Colyte with Flavor Packs for Oral Solution.. 3102
HalfLytely and Bisacodyl Tablets Bowel Prep Kit with Flavors Packs.. 915
K-Dur Extended-Relase Tablets 3047
K-Lor Powder Packets 472
K-Tab Filmtab Tablets 473
TriLyte with Flavor Packs for Oral Solution.. 3114

Potassium Citrate (Co-administration can increase the risk of hyperkalemia; therefore, potassium supplements should be given with caution, and serum potassium should be monitored). Products include:

Urocit-K Tablets 2109

Potassium Gluconate (Co-administration can increase the risk of hyperkalemia; therefore, potassium supplements should be given with caution, and serum potassium should be monitored).

No products indexed under this heading.

Potassium Phosphate (Co-administration can increase the risk of hyperkalemia; therefore, potassium supplements should be given with caution, and serum potassium should be monitored). Products include:

K-Phos Neutral Tablets 785

Spironolactone (Co-administration can increase the risk of hyperkalemia; therefore, potassium-sparing diuretics should be given with caution, and serum potassium should be monitored).

No products indexed under this heading.

Torsemide (Co-administration may result in excessive reductions in blood pressure. This can be minimized by discontinuing diuretic therapy for several days or cautiously increasing salt intake before initiating with moexipril. If this is not possible, the starting dose of moexipril should be reduced).

No products indexed under this heading.

Triamterene (Co-administration can increase the risk of hyperkalemia; therefore, potassium-sparing diuretics should be given with caution, and serum potassium should be monitored). Products include:

- Dyazide Capsules 1389
- Dyrenium Capsules 3390
- Maxzide 2150

Food Interactions

Food, unspecified (Food reduces Cmax and AUC by about 70% and 40% respectively after ingestion of a low-fat breakfast or by 80% and 50% respectively after the ingestion of high-fat breakfast).

URECHOLINE TABLETS

(Bethanechol Chloride) 2349

May interact with ganglionic blocking agents. Compounds in these categories include:

Mecamylamine Hydrochloride (Co-administration with ganglion blocking compounds may result in a critical fall in blood pressure). Products include:

- Inversine Tablets 3286

Trimethaphan Camsylate (Co-administration with ganglion blocking compounds may result in a critical fall in blood pressure).

No products indexed under this heading.

UROCIT-K TABLETS

(Potassium Citrate) 2109

May interact with anticholinergics and potassium sparing diuretics. Compounds in these categories include:

Amiloride Hydrochloride (Co-administration can produce severe hyperkalemia; concurrent use should be avoided). Products include:

- Midamor Tablets 2000
- Moduretic Tablets 2003

Atropine Sulfate (Co-administration with drugs that slow gastrointestinal transit time, such as anticholinergics, can be expected to increase the gastrointestinal irritation produced by potassium salts; concurrent use is contraindicated).

No products indexed under this heading.

Belladonna Alkaloids (Co-administration with drugs that slow gastrointestinal transit time, such as anticholinergics, can be expected to increase the gastrointestinal irritation produced by potassium salts; concurrent use is contraindicated). Products include:

- Hyland's Teething Tablets ▣736

Benztropine Mesylate (Co-administration with drugs that slow gastrointestinal transit time, such as anticholinergics, can be expected to increase the gastrointestinal irritation produced by potassium salts; concurrent use is contraindicated). Products include:

- Cogentin Injection 1903

Biperiden Hydrochloride (Co-administration with drugs that slow gastrointestinal transit time, such as anticholinergics, can be expected to increase the gastrointestinal irritation produced by potassium salts; concurrent use is contraindicated).

No products indexed under this heading.

Clidinium Bromide (Co-administration with drugs that slow gastrointestinal transit time, such as anticholinergics, can be expected to increase the gastrointestinal irritation produced by potassium salts; concurrent use is contraindicated).

No products indexed under this heading.

Dicyclomine Hydrochloride (Co-administration with drugs that slow gastrointestinal transit time, such as anticholinergics, can be expected to increase the gastrointestinal irritation produced by potassium salts; concurrent use is contraindicated). Products include:

- Bentyl Capsules 724
- Bentyl Injection 724
- Bentyl Syrup 724
- Bentyl Tablets 724

Glycopyrrolate (Co-administration with drugs that slow gastrointestinal transit time, such as anticholinergics, can be expected to increase the gastrointestinal irritation produced by potassium salts; concurrent use is contraindicated).

No products indexed under this heading.

Hyoscyamine (Co-administration with drugs that slow gastrointestinal transit time, such as anticholinergics, can be expected to increase the gastrointestinal irritation produced by potassium salts; concurrent use is contraindicated).

No products indexed under this heading.

Hyoscyamine Sulfate (Co-administration with drugs that slow gastrointestinal transit time, such as anticholinergics, can be expected to increase the gastrointestinal irritation produced by potassium salts; concurrent use is contraindicated).

No products indexed under this heading.

Ipratropium Bromide (Co-administration with drugs that slow gastrointestinal transit time, such as anticholinergics, can be expected to increase the gastrointestinal irritation produced by potassium salts; concurrent use is contraindicated). Products include:

- Atrovent HFA Inhalation Aerosol 872
- Atrovent Inhalation Solution 868
- Atrovent Nasal Spray 0.03% 869
- Atrovent Nasal Spray 0.06% 870
- Combivent Inhalation Aerosol 878
- DuoNeb Inhalation Solution 1058

Mepenzolate Bromide (Co-administration with drugs that slow gastrointestinal transit time, such as anticholinergics, can be expected to increase the gastrointestinal irritation produced by potassium salts; concurrent use is contraindicated).

No products indexed under this heading.

Oxybutynin Chloride (Co-administration with drugs that slow gastrointestinal transit time, such as anticholinergics, can be expected to increase the gastrointestinal irritation produced by potassium salts; concurrent use is contraindicated). Products include:

- Ditropan XL Extended Release Tablets 2391

Procyclidine Hydrochloride (Co-administration with drugs that slow gastrointestinal transit time, such as anticholinergics, can be expected to increase the gastrointestinal irritation produced by potassium salts; concurrent use is contraindicated).

No products indexed under this heading.

Propantheline Bromide (Co-administration with drugs that slow gastrointestinal transit time, such as anticholinergics, can be expected to increase the gastrointestinal irritation produced by potassium salts; concurrent use is contraindicated).

No products indexed under this heading.

Scopolamine (Co-administration with drugs that slow gastrointestinal transit time, such as anticholinergics, can be expected to increase the gastrointestinal irritation produced by potassium salts; concurrent use is contraindicated). Products include:

- Transderm Scōp Transdermal Therapeutic System 2166

Scopolamine Hydrobromide (Co-administration with drugs that slow gastrointestinal transit time, such as anticholinergics, can be expected to increase the gastrointestinal irritation produced by potassium salts; concurrent use is contraindicated).

No products indexed under this heading.

Spironolactone (Co-administration can produce severe hyperkalemia; concurrent use should be avoided).

No products indexed under this heading.

Tolterodine Tartrate (Co-administration with drugs that slow gastrointestinal transit time, such as anticholinergics, can be expected to increase the gastrointestinal irritation produced by potassium salts; concurrent use is contraindicated). Products include:

- Detrol Tablets 2626
- Detrol LA Capsules 2629

Triamterene (Co-administration can produce severe hyperkalemia; concurrent use should be avoided). Products include:

- Dyazide Capsules 1389
- Dyrenium Capsules 3390
- Maxzide 2150

Tridihexethyl Chloride (Co-administration with drugs that slow gastrointestinal transit time, such as anticholinergics, can be expected to increase the gastrointestinal irritation produced by potassium salts; concurrent use is contraindicated).

No products indexed under this heading.

Trihexyphenidyl Hydrochloride (Co-administration with drugs that slow gastrointestinal transit time, such as anticholinergics, can be expected to increase the gastrointestinal irritation produced by potassium salts; concurrent use is contraindicated).

No products indexed under this heading.

UROQID-ACID NO. 2 TABLETS

(Methenamine Mandelate, Sodium Acid Phosphate) 785

May interact with:

Acetazolamide (Reduces the effectiveness of methenamine by causing urine to become alkaline).

No products indexed under this heading.

ACTH (Concurrent use with sodium phosphate may result in hypernatremia).

No products indexed under this heading.

Aluminum Carbonate (Reduces the effectiveness of methenamine by causing urine to become alkaline).

No products indexed under this heading.

Aluminum Hydroxide (Reduces the effectiveness of methenamine by causing urine to become alkaline). Products include:

- Gaviscon Regular Strength Liquid ▣620
- Gaviscon Regular Strength Tablets ▣619
- Gaviscon Extra Strength Liquid ▣620
- Gaviscon Extra Strength Tablets ▣619
- Maalox Max Maximum Strength Antacid/Anti-Gas Liquid 2165
- Maalox Regular Strength Antacid/Antigas Liquid 2164

Aspirin (Concurrent use may lead to increased serum salicylate levels since excretion of salicylates is reduced in acidic urine). Products include:

- Aggrenox Capsules 855
- Bayer, Aspirin Regimen ▣606
- Bayer Aspirin Tablets 3515
- BC Powder ▣612
- BC Allergy Sinus Cold Powder ▣612
- Arthritis Strength BC Powder ▣612
- BC Sinus Cold Powder ▣612
- Ecotrin Enteric Coated Aspirin Low, Regular and Maximum Strength Tablets 1627
- Goody's Body Pain Formula Powder ▣621
- Goody's Extra Strength Headache Powder ▣621
- Goody's Extra Strength Pain Relief Tablets ▣621
- Percodan Tablets 1115
- St. Joseph 81 mg Aspirin Chewable and Enteric Coated Tablets 1841

Bendroflumethiazide (Reduces the effectiveness of methenamine by causing urine to become alkaline).

No products indexed under this heading.

Betamethasone Acetate (Concurrent use with sodium phosphate may result in hypernatremia).

No products indexed under this heading.

Betamethasone Sodium Phosphate (Concurrent use with sodium phosphate may result in hypernatremia).

No products indexed under this heading.

Chlorothiazide (Reduces the effectiveness of methenamine by causing urine to become alkaline). Products include:

- Aldoclor Tablets 1881
- Diuril Oral 1936

Chlorothiazide Sodium (Reduces the effectiveness of methenamine by causing urine to become alkaline). Products include:

- Diuril Sodium Intravenous 1934

Choline Magnesium Trisalicylate (Concurrent use may lead to increased serum salicylate levels since excretion of salicylates is reduced in acidic urine).
No products indexed under this heading.

Cortisone Acetate (Concurrent use with sodium phosphate may result in hypernatremia).
No products indexed under this heading.

Deserpidine (Concurrent use with sodium phosphate may result in hypernatremia).
No products indexed under this heading.

Desoxycorticosterone Acetate (Concurrent use with sodium phosphate may result in hypernatremia).
No products indexed under this heading.

Desoxycorticosterone Pivalate (Concurrent use with sodium phosphate may result in hypernatremia).
No products indexed under this heading.

Dexamethasone (Concurrent use with sodium phosphate may result in hypernatremia). Products include:
Ciprodex Otic Suspension **555**
Decadron Tablets **1929**
TobraDex Ophthalmic Ointment **558**
TobraDex Ophthalmic Suspension ... **558**

Dexamethasone Acetate (Concurrent use with sodium phosphate may result in hypernatremia).
No products indexed under this heading.

Dexamethasone Sodium Phosphate (Concurrent use with sodium phosphate may result in hypernatremia). Products include:
Decadron Phosphate Injection **1931**

Diazoxide (Concurrant use with sodium phosphate may result in hypernatremia). Products include:
Hyperstat I.V. Injection **3031**

Dichlorphenamide (Reduces the effectiveness of methenamine by causing urine to become alkaline). Products include:
Daranide Tablets **1928**

Diflunisal (Concurrent use may lead to increased serum salicylate levels since excretion of salicylates is reduced in acidic urine). Products include:
Dolobid Tablets **1937**

Fludrocortisone Acetate (Concurrent use with sodium phosphate may result in hypernatremia).
No products indexed under this heading.

Guanethidine Monosulfate (Concurrent use with sodium phosphate may result in hypernatremia).
No products indexed under this heading.

Hydralazine Hydrochloride (Concurrent use with sodium phosphate may result in hypernatremia). Products include:
BiDil Tablets **2161**

Hydrochlorothiazide (Reduces the effectiveness of methenamine by causing urine to become alkaline). Products include:
Aldoril Tablets **1884**
Atacand HCT **637**
Avalide Tablets **2889**
Avalide Tablets **922**
Benicar HCT Tablets **2852**
Diovan HCT Tablets **2195**
Dyazide Capsules **1389**
Hyzaar **1964**
Lotensin HCT Tablets **2235**
Maxzide **2150**
Micardis HCT Tablets **886**
Moduretic Tablets **2003**
Prinzide Tablets **2033**
Teveten HCT Tablets **1710**
Timolide Tablets **2056**
Uniretic Tablets **3114**
Vaseretic Tablets **2073**
Zestoretic Tablets **701**

Hydrocortisone (Concurrent use with sodium phosphate may result in hypernatremia). Products include:
Cortizone•5 Ointment **699**
Cortizone•10 Creme **699**
Cortizone•10 Ointment **699**
Cortizone•10 Plus Creme **700**
Cortizone•10 Maximum Strength Quick Shot Spray **700**
Hydrocortone Tablets **1963**
Preparation H Hydrocortisone Cream **748**

Hydrocortisone Acetate (Concurrent use with sodium phosphate may result in hypernatremia). Products include:
Analpram-HC **1136**
Pramosone **1139**
ProctoFoam-HC **3113**
Tucks Anti-Itch Ointment **712**
U-cort 1% Cream **3289**

Hydrocortisone Sodium Phosphate (Concurrent use with sodium phosphate may result in hypernatremia).
No products indexed under this heading.

Hydrocortisone Sodium Succinate (Concurrent use with sodium phosphate may result in hypernatremia).
No products indexed under this heading.

Hydroflumethiazide (Reduces the effectiveness of methenamine by causing urine to become alkaline).
No products indexed under this heading.

Magaldrate (Reduces the effectiveness of methenamine by causing urine to become alkaline).
No products indexed under this heading.

Magnesium Hydroxide (Reduces the effectiveness of methenamine by causing urine to become alkaline). Products include:
Maalox Max Maximum Strength Antacid/Anti-Gas Liquid................. **2165**
Maalox Regular Strength Antacid/Antigas Liquid.................. **2164**
Pepcid Complete Chewable Tablets **1672**
Rolaids Tablets **707**
Extra Strength Rolaids Tablets **707**
Rolaids Multi-Symptom Antacid & Antigas Tablets **708**

Magnesium Oxide (Reduces the effectiveness of methenamine by causing urine to become alkaline). Products include:
Beelith Tablets **784**
PremCal Light, Regular, and Extra Strength Tablets................. **762**

Magnesium Salicylate (Concurrent use may lead to increased serum salicylate levels since excretion of salicylates is reduced in acidic urine).
No products indexed under this heading.

Methazolamide (Reduces the effectiveness of methenamine by causing urine to become alkaline).
No products indexed under this heading.

Methyclothiazide (Reduces the effectiveness of methenamine by causing urine to become alkaline).
No products indexed under this heading.

Methyldopa (Concurrent use with sodium phosphate may result in hypernatremia). Products include:
Aldoclor Tablets **1881**
Aldoril Tablets **1884**

Methylprednisolone Acetate (Concurrent use with sodium phosphate may result in hypernatremia). Products include:
Depo-Medrol Injectable Suspension **2615**
Depo-Medrol Single-Dose Vial **2617**

Methylprednisolone Sodium Succinate (Concurrent use with sodium phosphate may result in hypernatremia).
No products indexed under this heading.

Polythiazide (Reduces the effectiveness of methenamine by causing urine to become alkaline).
No products indexed under this heading.

Potassium Citrate (Reduces the effectiveness of methenamine by causing urine to become alkaline). Products include:
Urocit-K Tablets **2109**

Prednisolone Acetate (Concurrent use with sodium phosphate may result in hypernatremia). Products include:
Blephamide Ophthalmic Ointment **563**
Blephamide Ophthalmic Suspension................................. **564**
Poly-Pred Liquifilm Ophthalmic Suspension .... ⊙ **231**
Pred Forte Ophthalmic Suspension .... ⊙ **233**
Pred Mild Sterile Ophthalmic Suspension .... ⊙ **236**
Pred-G Ophthalmic Suspension ...... ⊙ **234**
Pred-G Sterile Ophthalmic Ointment.................................... ⊙ **235**

Prednisolone Sodium Phosphate (Concurrent use with sodium phosphate may result in hypernatremia). Products include:
Pediapred Oral Solution **3319**

Prednisolone Tebutate (Concurrent use with sodium phosphate may result in hypernatremia).
No products indexed under this heading.

Prednisone (Concurrent use with sodium phosphate may result in hypernatremia).
No products indexed under this heading.

Rauwolfia Serpentina (Concurrent use with sodium phosphate may result in hypernatremia).
No products indexed under this heading.

Rescinnamine (Concurrent use with sodium phosphate may result in hypernatremia).
No products indexed under this heading.

Reserpine (Concurrent use with sodium phosphate may result in hypernatremia).
No products indexed under this heading.

Salsalate (Concurrent use may lead to increased serum salicylate levels since excretion of salicylates is reduced in acidic urine).
No products indexed under this heading.

Sodium Bicarbonate (Reduces the effectiveness of methenamine by causing urine to become alkaline). Products include:
Ceo-Two Evacuant Suppository **607**
Colyte with Flavor Packs for Oral Solution.. **3102**
HalfLytely and Bisacodyl Tablets Bowel Prep Kit with Flavors Packs **915**
TriLyte with Flavor Packs for Oral Solution.. **3114**

Sodium Citrate (Reduces the effectiveness of methenamine by causing urine to become alkaline).
No products indexed under this heading.

Sulfamethizole (Concurrent use with sulfamethizole and formaldehyde forms an insoluble precipitate in acid urine and increases the risk of crystaluria).
No products indexed under this heading.

Triamcinolone (Concurrent use with sodium phosphate may result in hypernatremia).
No products indexed under this heading.

Triamcinolone Acetonide (Concurrent use with sodium phosphate may result in hypernatremia). Products include:
Azmacort Inhalation Aerosol **1701**
Nasacort HFA Inhalation Aerosol **2939**
Nasacort AQ Nasal Spray **2937**

Triamcinolone Diacetate (Concurrent use with sodium phosphate may result in hypernatremia).
No products indexed under this heading.

Triamcinolone Hexacetonide (Concurrent use with sodium phosphate may result in hypernatremia).
No products indexed under this heading.

UROXATRAL TABLETS

(Alfuzosin Hydrochloride) **2957**
May interact with alpha adrenergic blockers and cytochrome p450 3a4 inhibitors (selected). Compounds in these categories include:

Acetazolamide (Uroxatral should not be co-administered with potent CYP3A4 inhibitors such as ketoconazole, itraconazole, and ritonavir, since alfuzosin blood levels are increased).
No products indexed under this heading.

Amiodarone Hydrochloride (Uroxatral should not be co-administered with potent CYP3A4 inhibitors such as ketoconazole, itraconazole, and ritonavir, since alfuzosin blood levels are increased). Products include:
Pacerone Tablets **3337**

Amprenavir (Uroxatral should not be co-administered with potent CYP3A4 inhibitors such as ketoconazole, itraconazole, and ritonavir, since alfuzosin blood levels are increased). Products include:
Agenerase Capsules **1299**
Agenerase Oral Solution **1304**

Anastrozole (Uroxatral should not be co-administered with potent CYP3A4 inhibitors such as ketoconazole, itraconazole, and ritonavir, since alfuzosin blood levels are increased). Products include:
Arimidex Tablets **665**

Aprepitant (Uroxatral should not be co-administered with potent CYP3A4 inhibitors such as ketoconazole, itra-

conazole, and ritonavir, since alfuzosin blood levels are increased). Products include:
- Emend Capsules ... **1944**

Cimetidine (Uroxatral should not be co-administered with potent CYP3A4 inhibitors such as ketoconazole, itraconazole, and ritonavir, since alfuzosin blood levels are increased). Products include:
- Tagamet HB 200 Tablets ... ▣**637**
- Tagamet Tablets ... **1547**

Cimetidine Hydrochloride (Uroxatral should not be co-administered with potent CYP3A4 inhibitors such as ketoconazole, itraconazole, and ritonavir, since alfuzosin blood levels are increased).
No products indexed under this heading.

Ciprofloxacin (Uroxatral should not be co-administered with potent CYP3A4 inhibitors such as ketoconazole, itraconazole, and ritonavir, since alfuzosin blood levels are increased). Products include:
- Cipro I.V. ... **2998**
- Cipro I.V. Pharmacy Bulk Package ... **3509**
- Cipro Oral Suspension ... **2991**
- Cipro XR Tablets ... **3004**
- Ciprodex Otic Suspension ... **555**

Clarithromycin (Uroxatral should not be co-administered with potent CYP3A4 inhibitors such as ketoconazole, itraconazole, and ritonavir, since alfuzosin blood levels are increased). Products include:
- Biaxin/Biaxin XL ... **402**
- PREVPAC ... **3281**

Clotrimazole (Uroxatral should not be co-administered with potent CYP3A4 inhibitors such as ketoconazole, itraconazole, and ritonavir, since alfuzosin blood levels are increased). Products include:
- Lotrimin ... **3053**
- Lotrisone ... **3054**

Cyclosporine (Uroxatral should not be co-administered with potent CYP3A4 inhibitors such as ketoconazole, itraconazole, and ritonavir, since alfuzosin blood levels are increased). Products include:
- Gengraf Capsules ... **458**
- Neoral Soft Gelatin Capsules ... **2247**
- Neoral Oral Solution ... **2247**
- Restasis Ophthalmic Emulsion ... **570**
- Sandimmune ... **2259**

Dalfopristin (Uroxatral should not be co-administered with potent CYP3A4 inhibitors such as ketoconazole, itraconazole, and ritonavir, since alfuzosin blood levels are increased). Products include:
- Synercid I.V. ... **1690**

Danazol (Uroxatral should not be co-administered with potent CYP3A4 inhibitors such as ketoconazole, itraconazole, and ritonavir, since alfuzosin blood levels are increased).
No products indexed under this heading.

Delavirdine Mesylate (Uroxatral should not be co-administered with potent CYP3A4 inhibitors such as ketoconazole, itraconazole, and ritonavir, since alfuzosin blood levels are increased). Products include:
- Rescriptor Tablets ... **2535**

Diltiazem Hydrochloride (Uroxatral should not be co-administered with potent CYP3A4 inhibitors such as ketoconazole, itraconazole, and ritonavir, since alfuzosin blood levels are increased). Products include:
- Cardizem LA Extended Release Tablets ... **1699**
- Tiazac Capsules ... **1204**

Diltiazem Maleate (Uroxatral should not be co-administered with potent CYP3A4 inhibitors such as ketoconazole, itraconazole, and ritonavir, since alfuzosin blood levels are increased).
No products indexed under this heading.

Doxazosin Mesylate (Interactions may be expected; uroxatral should not be used in combination with other alpha-blockers).
No products indexed under this heading.

Efavirenz (Uroxatral should not be co-administered with potent CYP3A4 inhibitors such as ketoconazole, itraconazole, and ritonavir, since alfuzosin blood levels are increased). Products include:
- Sustiva Capsules ... **957**

Erythromycin (Uroxatral should not be co-administered with potent CYP3A4 inhibitors such as ketoconazole, itraconazole, and ritonavir, since alfuzosin blood levels are increased). Products include:
- Erygel Topical Gel ... **2096**
- Ery-Tab Tablets ... **447**
- Erythromycin Base Filmtab Tablets ... **454**
- Erythromycin Delayed-Release Capsules, USP ... **456**
- PCE Dispertab Tablets ... **510**

Erythromycin Estolate (Uroxatral should not be co-administered with potent CYP3A4 inhibitors such as ketoconazole, itraconazole, and ritonavir, since alfuzosin blood levels are increased).
No products indexed under this heading.

Erythromycin Ethylsuccinate (Uroxatral should not be co-administered with potent CYP3A4 inhibitors such as ketoconazole, itraconazole, and ritonavir, since alfuzosin blood levels are increased). Products include:
- E.E.S. ... **449**
- EryPed ... **445**

Erythromycin Gluceptate (Uroxatral should not be co-administered with potent CYP3A4 inhibitors such as ketoconazole, itraconazole, and ritonavir, since alfuzosin blood levels are increased).
No products indexed under this heading.

Erythromycin Lactobionate (Uroxatral should not be co-administered with potent CYP3A4 inhibitors such as ketoconazole, itraconazole, and ritonavir, since alfuzosin blood levels are increased).
No products indexed under this heading.

Erythromycin Stearate (Uroxatral should not be co-administered with potent CYP3A4 inhibitors such as ketoconazole, itraconazole, and ritonavir, since alfuzosin blood levels are increased). Products include:
- Erythrocin Stearate Filmtab Tablets ... **452**

Esomeprazole Magnesium (Uroxatral should not be co-administered with potent CYP3A4 inhibitors such as ketoconazole, itraconazole, and ritonavir, since alfuzosin blood levels are increased). Products include:
- Nexium Delayed-Release Capsules ... **645**

Fluconazole (Uroxatral should not be co-administered with potent CYP3A4 inhibitors such as ketoconazole, itraconazole, and ritonavir, since alfuzosin blood levels are increased).
No products indexed under this heading.

Fluoxetine Hydrochloride (Uroxatral should not be co-administered with potent CYP3A4 inhibitors such as ketoconazole, itraconazole, and ritonavir, since alfuzosin blood levels are increased). Products include:
- Prozac Pulvules and Liquid ... **1771**
- Symbyax Capsules ... **1788**

Fluvoxamine Maleate (Uroxatral should not be co-administered with potent CYP3A4 inhibitors such as ketoconazole, itraconazole, and ritonavir, since alfuzosin blood levels are increased).
No products indexed under this heading.

Fosamprenavir Calcium (Uroxatral should not be co-administered with potent CYP3A4 inhibitors such as ketoconazole, itraconazole, and ritonavir, since alfuzosin blood levels are increased). Products include:
- Lexiva Tablets ... **1473**

Indinavir Sulfate (Uroxatral should not be co-administered with potent CYP3A4 inhibitors such as ketoconazole, itraconazole, and ritonavir, since alfuzosin blood levels are increased). Products include:
- Crixivan Capsules ... **1918**

Isoniazid (Uroxatral should not be co-administered with potent CYP3A4 inhibitors such as ketoconazole, itraconazole, and ritonavir, since alfuzosin blood levels are increased).
No products indexed under this heading.

Itraconazole (Uroxatral should not be co-administered with potent CYP3A4 inhibitors such as ketoconazole, itraconazole, and ritonavir, since alfuzosin blood levels are increased).
No products indexed under this heading.

Ketoconazole (Uroxatral should not be co-administered with potent CYP3A4 inhibitors such as ketoconazole, itraconazole, and ritonavir, since alfuzosin blood levels are increased). Products include:
- Nizoral A-D Shampoo, 1% ... **1839**
- Nizoral 2% Shampoo ... **1838**

Lopinavir (Uroxatral should not be co-administered with potent CYP3A4 inhibitors such as ketoconazole, itraconazole, and ritonavir, since alfuzosin blood levels are increased). Products include:
- Kaletra ... **474**

Loratadine (Uroxatral should not be co-administered with potent CYP3A4 inhibitors such as ketoconazole, itraconazole, and ritonavir, since alfuzosin blood levels are increased). Products include:
- Alavert Allergy & Sinus D-12 Hour Tablets ... ▣**743**
- Alavert ... ▣**743**
- Children's Claritin 24 Hour Non-Drowsy Allergy Syrup ... ▣**732**
- Claritin Non-Drowsy 24 Hour Tablets ... ▣**731**
- Non-Drowsy Claritin Hives Relief Tablets ... ▣**733**
- Claritin Reditabs 24 Hour Non-Drowsy Tablets ... ▣**732**
- Claritin-D Non-Drowsy 12 Hour Tablets ... ▣**731**
- Claritin-D Non-Drowsy 24 Hour Tablets ... ▣**731**
- Children's Dimetapp ND Non-Drowsy Allergy Syrup ... ▣**746**
- Triaminic Allerchews ... ▣**684**

Metronidazole (Uroxatral should not be co-administered with potent CYP3A4 inhibitors such as ketoconazole, itraconazole, and ritonavir, since alfuzosin blood levels are increased). Products include:
- Metrogel 1% ... **1212**
- MetroGel-Vaginal Gel ... **1822**
- Noritate Cream, 1% ... **1051**

Metronidazole Benzoate (Uroxatral should not be co-administered with potent CYP3A4 inhibitors such as ketoconazole, itraconazole, and ritonavir, since alfuzosin blood levels are increased).
No products indexed under this heading.

Metronidazole Hydrochloride (Uroxatral should not be co-administered with potent CYP3A4 inhibitors such as ketoconazole, itraconazole, and ritonavir, since alfuzosin blood levels are increased).
No products indexed under this heading.

Miconazole (Uroxatral should not be co-administered with potent CYP3A4 inhibitors such as ketoconazole, itraconazole, and ritonavir, since alfuzosin blood levels are increased).
No products indexed under this heading.

Miconazole Nitrate (Uroxatral should not be co-administered with potent CYP3A4 inhibitors such as ketoconazole, itraconazole, and ritonavir, since alfuzosin blood levels are increased). Products include:
- Desenex ... ▣**674**
- Desenex Jock Itch Spray Powder ... ▣**674**

Nefazodone Hydrochloride (Uroxatral should not be co-administered with potent CYP3A4 inhibitors such as ketoconazole, itraconazole, and ritonavir, since alfuzosin blood levels are increased).
No products indexed under this heading.

Nelfinavir Mesylate (Uroxatral should not be co-administered with potent CYP3A4 inhibitors such as ketoconazole, itraconazole, and ritonavir, since alfuzosin blood levels are increased). Products include:
- Viracept ... **2556**

Nevirapine (Uroxatral should not be co-administered with potent CYP3A4 inhibitors such as ketoconazole, itraconazole, and ritonavir, since alfuzosin blood levels are increased). Products include:
- Viramune Oral Suspension ... **903**
- Viramune Tablets ... **903**

Niacinamide (Uroxatral should not be co-administered with potent CYP3A4 inhibitors such as ketoconazole, itraconazole, and ritonavir, since alfuzosin blood levels are increased).
No products indexed under this heading.

Nicotinamide (Uroxatral should not be co-administered with potent CYP3A4 inhibitors such as ketoconazole, itraconazole, and ritonavir, since alfuzosin blood levels are increased). Products include:
- Nicomide Tablets ... **3190**

Nifedipine (Uroxatral should not be co-administered with potent CYP3A4 inhibitors such as ketoconazole, itra-

conazole, and ritonavir, since alfuzosin blood levels are increased). Products include:
Adalat CC Tablets 2978

Norfloxacin (Uroxatral should not be co-administered with potent CYP3A4 inhibitors such as ketoconazole, itraconazole, and ritonavir, since alfuzosin blood levels are increased). Products include:
Noroxin Tablets 2009

Omeprazole (Uroxatral should not be co-administered with potent CYP3A4 inhibitors such as ketoconazole, itraconazole, and ritonavir, since alfuzosin blood levels are increased). Products include:
Zegerid Powder for Oral Solution 2972

Paroxetine Hydrochloride (Uroxatral should not be co-administered with potent CYP3A4 inhibitors such as ketoconazole, itraconazole, and ritonavir, since alfuzosin blood levels are increased). Products include:
Paxil CR Controlled-Release Tablets 1509
Paxil 1501

Prazosin Hydrochloride (Interactions may be expected; uroxatral should not be used in combination with other alpha-blockers).
No products indexed under this heading.

Propoxyphene Hydrochloride (Uroxatral should not be co-administered with potent CYP3A4 inhibitors such as ketoconazole, itraconazole, and ritonavir, since alfuzosin blood levels are increased).
No products indexed under this heading.

Propoxyphene Napsylate (Uroxatral should not be co-administered with potent CYP3A4 inhibitors such as ketoconazole, itraconazole, and ritonavir, since alfuzosin blood levels are increased). Products include:
Darvocet A 500 Tablets 3497

Quinidine (Uroxatral should not be co-administered with potent CYP3A4 inhibitors such as ketoconazole, itraconazole, and ritonavir, since alfuzosin blood levels are increased).
No products indexed under this heading.

Quinidine Hydrochloride (Uroxatral should not be co-administered with potent CYP3A4 inhibitors such as ketoconazole, itraconazole, and ritonavir, since alfuzosin blood levels are increased).
No products indexed under this heading.

Quinidine Polygalacturonate (Uroxatral should not be co-administered with potent CYP3A4 inhibitors such as ketoconazole, itraconazole, and ritonavir, since alfuzosin blood levels are increased).
No products indexed under this heading.

Quinidine Sulfate (Uroxatral should not be co-administered with potent CYP3A4 inhibitors such as ketoconazole, itraconazole, and ritonavir, since alfuzosin blood levels are increased).
No products indexed under this heading.

Quinine (Uroxatral should not be co-administered with potent CYP3A4 inhibitors such as ketoconazole, itraconazole, and ritonavir, since alfuzosin blood levels are increased).
No products indexed under this heading.

Quinine Sulfate (Uroxatral should not be co-administered with potent CYP3A4 inhibitors such as ketoconazole, itraconazole, and ritonavir, since alfuzosin blood levels are increased).
No products indexed under this heading.

Quinupristin (Uroxatral should not be co-administered with potent CYP3A4 inhibitors such as ketoconazole, itraconazole, and ritonavir, since alfuzosin blood levels are increased). Products include:
Synercid I.V. 1690

Ranitidine Bismuth Citrate (Uroxatral should not be co-administered with potent CYP3A4 inhibitors such as ketoconazole, itraconazole, and ritonavir, since alfuzosin blood levels are increased).
No products indexed under this heading.

Ranitidine Hydrochloride (Uroxatral should not be co-administered with potent CYP3A4 inhibitors such as ketoconazole, itraconazole, and ritonavir, since alfuzosin blood levels are increased). Products include:
Zantac 1597
Zantac Injection 1593
Zantac 75 Tablets 715
Zantac 150 Maximum Strength Tablets 715
Zantac Injection Pharmacy Bulk Package 1595

Ritonavir (Uroxatral should not be co-administered with potent CYP3A4 inhibitors such as ketoconazole, itraconazole, and ritonavir, since alfuzosin blood levels are increased). Products include:
Kaletra 474
Norvir 499

Saquinavir (Uroxatral should not be co-administered with potent CYP3A4 inhibitors such as ketoconazole, itraconazole, and ritonavir, since alfuzosin blood levels are increased).
No products indexed under this heading.

Saquinavir Mesylate (Uroxatral should not be co-administered with potent CYP3A4 inhibitors such as ketoconazole, itraconazole, and ritonavir, since alfuzosin blood levels are increased). Products include:
Invirase 2776

Sertraline Hydrochloride (Uroxatral should not be co-administered with potent CYP3A4 inhibitors such as ketoconazole, itraconazole, and ritonavir, since alfuzosin blood levels are increased). Products include:
Zoloft 2581

Tamsulosin Hydrochloride (Interactions may be expected; uroxatral should not be used in combination with other alpha-blockers). Products include:
Flomax Capsules 881

Telithromycin (Uroxatral should not be co-administered with potent CYP3A4 inhibitors such as ketoconazole, itraconazole, and ritonavir, since alfuzosin blood levels are increased). Products include:
Ketek Tablets 2920

Terazosin Hydrochloride (Interactions may be expected; uroxatral should not be used in combination with other alpha-blockers). Products include:
Hytrin Capsules 469

Troglitazone (Uroxatral should not be co-administered with potent CYP3A4 inhibitors such as ketoconazole, itraconazole, and ritonavir, since alfuzosin blood levels are increased).
No products indexed under this heading.

Troleandomycin (Uroxatral should not be co-administered with potent CYP3A4 inhibitors such as ketoconazole, itraconazole, and ritonavir, since alfuzosin blood levels are increased).
No products indexed under this heading.

Valproate Sodium (Uroxatral should not be co-administered with potent CYP3A4 inhibitors such as ketoconazole, itraconazole, and ritonavir, since alfuzosin blood levels are increased). Products include:
Depacon Injection 412

Verapamil Hydrochloride (Uroxatral should not be co-administered with potent CYP3A4 inhibitors such as ketoconazole, itraconazole, and ritonavir, since alfuzosin blood levels are increased). Products include:
Covera-HS Tablets 3135
Tarka Tablets 519
Verelan PM Capsules 3120

Voriconazole (Uroxatral should not be co-administered with potent CYP3A4 inhibitors such as ketoconazole, itraconazole, and ritonavir, since alfuzosin blood levels are increased). Products include:
VFEND I.V. 2543
VFEND Oral Suspension 2543
VFEND Tablets 2543

Zafirlukast (Uroxatral should not be co-administered with potent CYP3A4 inhibitors such as ketoconazole, itraconazole, and ritonavir, since alfuzosin blood levels are increased). Products include:
Accolate Tablets 663

Zileuton (Uroxatral should not be co-administered with potent CYP3A4 inhibitors such as ketoconazole, itraconazole, and ritonavir, since alfuzosin blood levels are increased).
No products indexed under this heading.

Food Interactions

Grapefruit (Uroxatral should not be co-administered with potent CYP3A4 inhibitors such as ketoconazole, itraconazole, and ritonavir, since alfuzosin blood levels are increased).

Grapefruit Juice (Uroxatral should not be co-administered with potent CYP3A4 inhibitors such as ketoconazole, itraconazole, and ritonavir, since alfuzosin blood levels are increased).

URSO 250 TABLETS

(Ursodiol) 737
May interact with bile acid sequestering agents, estrogens, lipid-lowering drugs, oral contraceptives, and certain other agents. Compounds in these categories include:

Aluminum Hydroxide (Aluminum-based antacids have been shown to adsorb bile acid in vitro and may be expected to interfere with ursodiol in the same manner as the bile acid sequestering agents). Products include:
Gaviscon Regular Strength Liquid 620
Gaviscon Regular Strength Tablets 619
Gaviscon Extra Strength Liquid 620
Gaviscon Extra Strength Tablets 619
Maalox Max Maximum Strength Antacid/Anti-Gas Liquid 2165
Maalox Regular Strength Antacid/Antigas Liquid 2164

Atorvastatin Calcium (Lipid-lowering drugs increase hepatic cholesterol secretion and encourage cholesterol gallstone formation and hence may counteract the effectiveness of ursodiol). Products include:
Caduet Tablets 2507
Lipitor Tablets 2495

Cerivastatin Sodium (Lipid-lowering drugs increase hepatic cholesterol secretion and encourage cholesterol gallstone formation and hence may counteract the effectiveness of ursodiol).
No products indexed under this heading.

Chlorotrianisene (Estrogens and oral contraceptives increase hepatic cholesterol excretion and encourage cholesterol gallstone formation and hence may counteract the effectiveness of ursodiol).
No products indexed under this heading.

Cholestyramine (Lipid-lowering drugs increase hepatic cholesterol secretion and encourage cholesterol gallstone formation and hence may counteract the effectiveness of ursodiol).
No products indexed under this heading.

Clofibrate (Lipid-lowering drugs increase hepatic cholesterol secretion and encourage cholesterol gallstone formation and hence may counteract the effectiveness of ursodiol).
No products indexed under this heading.

Colesevelam Hydrochloride (Bile sequestering agents may interfere with the action of ursodiol by reducing its absorption). Products include:
WelChol Tablets 2855

Colestipol Hydrochloride (Lipid-lowering drugs increase hepatic cholesterol secretion and encourage cholesterol gallstone formation and hence may counteract the effectiveness of ursodiol).
No products indexed under this heading.

Desogestrel (Estrogens and oral contraceptives increase hepatic cholesterol secretion and encourage cholesterol gallstone formation and hence may counteract the effectiveness of ursodiol). Products include:
Ortho-Cept Tablets 2395

Dienestrol (Estrogens and oral contraceptives increase hepatic cholesterol excretion and encourage cholesterol gallstone formation and hence may counteract the effectiveness of ursodiol).
No products indexed under this heading.

Diethylstilbestrol (Estrogens and oral contraceptives increase hepatic cholesterol excretion and encourage cholesterol gallstone formation and hence may counteract the effectiveness of ursodiol).
No products indexed under this heading.

Estradiol (Estrogens and oral contraceptives increase hepatic cholesterol excretion and encourage cholesterol gallstone formation and hence may counteract the effectiveness of ursodiol). Products include:
Activella Tablets 2311

Climara Transdermal System 795
Climara Pro Transdermal System 800
CombiPatch Transdermal System 2180
Estrogel 0.06% 3200
Menostar Transdermal System 805
Prefest Tablets 1069
Vagifem Tablets 2340
Vivelle Transdermal System 2288
Vivelle-Dot Transdermal System 2293

Estrogens, Conjugated (Estrogens and oral contraceptives increase hepatic cholesterol excretion and encourage cholesterol gallstone formation and hence may counteract the effectiveness of ursodiol). Products include:
Premarin Intravenous 3440
Premarin Tablets 3443
Premarin Vaginal Cream 3449
Premphase Tablets 3452
Prempro Tablets 3452

Estrogens, Esterified (Estrogens and oral contraceptives increase hepatic cholesterol excretion and encourage cholesterol gallstone formation and hence may counteract the effectiveness of ursodiol). Products include:
Estratest Tablets 3196
Estratest H.S. Tablets 3196

Estropipate (Estrogens and oral contraceptives increase hepatic cholesterol excretion and encourage cholesterol gallstone formation and hence may counteract the effectiveness of ursodiol).
No products indexed under this heading.

Ethinyl Estradiol (Estrogens and oral contraceptives increase hepatic cholesterol secretion and encourage cholesterol gallstone formation and hence may counteract the effectiveness of ursodiol). Products include:
Alesse-28 Tablets 3392
Lo/Ovral-28 Tablets 3423
NuvaRing 2357
Ortho-Cept Tablets 2395
Ortho-Cyclen/Ortho Tri-Cyclen 2414
Ortho Evra Transdermal System 2402
Ortho Tri-Cyclen Lo Tablets 2421
Seasonale Tablets 1073
Triphasil-28 Tablets 3483
Yasmin 28 Tablets 818

Ethynodiol Diacetate (Estrogens and oral contraceptives increase hepatic cholesterol secretion and encourage cholesterol gallstone formation and hence may counteract the effectiveness of ursodiol).
No products indexed under this heading.

Fenofibrate (Lipid-lowering drugs increase hepatic cholesterol secretion and encourage cholesterol gallstone formation and hence may counteract the effectiveness of ursodiol). Products include:
Antara Capsules 2723
Lofibra Capsules 1217
Tricor Tablets 523
Triglide Tablets 1165

Fluvastatin Sodium (Lipid-lowering drugs increase hepatic cholesterol secretion and encourage cholesterol gallstone formation and hence may counteract the effectiveness of ursodiol). Products include:
Lescol Capsules 2227
Lescol 2730
Lescol XL Tablets 2227

Gemfibrozil (Lipid-lowering drugs increase hepatic cholesterol secretion and encourage cholesterol gallstone formation and hence may counteract the effectiveness of ursodiol).
No products indexed under this heading.

Levonorgestrel (Estrogens and oral contraceptives increase hepatic cholesterol secretion and encourage cholesterol gallstone formation and hence may counteract the effectiveness of ursodiol). Products include:
Alesse-28 Tablets 3392
Climara Pro Transdermal System 800
Mirena Intrauterine System 810
Plan B Tablets 1068
Seasonale Tablets 1073
Triphasil-28 Tablets 3483

Lovastatin (Lipid-lowering drugs increase hepatic cholesterol secretion and encourage cholesterol gallstone formation and hence may counteract the effectiveness of ursodiol). Products include:
Advicor Tablets 1694
Altoprev Extended-Release Tablets 1151
Mevacor Tablets 1996

Mestranol (Estrogens and oral contraceptives increase hepatic cholesterol secretion and encourage cholesterol gallstone formation and hence may counteract the effectiveness of ursodiol).
No products indexed under this heading.

Norethindrone (Estrogens and oral contraceptives increase hepatic cholesterol secretion and encourage cholesterol gallstone formation and hence may counteract the effectiveness of ursodiol). Products include:
Ortho Micronor Tablets 2411

Norethynodrel (Estrogens and oral contraceptives increase hepatic cholesterol secretion and encourage cholesterol gallstone formation and hence may counteract the effectiveness of ursodiol).
No products indexed under this heading.

Norgestimate (Estrogens and oral contraceptives increase hepatic cholesterol secretion and encourage cholesterol gallstone formation and hence may counteract the effectiveness of ursodiol). Products include:
Ortho-Cyclen/Ortho Tri-Cyclen 2414
Ortho Tri-Cyclen Lo Tablets 2421
Prefest Tablets 1069

Norgestrel (Estrogens and oral contraceptives increase hepatic cholesterol secretion and encourage cholesterol gallstone formation and hence may counteract the effectiveness of ursodiol). Products include:
Lo/Ovral-28 Tablets 3423

Polyestradiol Phosphate (Estrogens and oral contraceptives increase hepatic cholesterol excretion and encourage cholesterol gallstone formation and hence may counteract the effectiveness of ursodiol).
No products indexed under this heading.

Pravastatin Sodium (Lipid-lowering drugs increase hepatic cholesterol secretion and encourage cholesterol gallstone formation and hence may counteract the effectiveness of ursodiol). Products include:
Pravachol Tablets 943

Probucol (Lipid-lowering drugs increase hepatic cholesterol secretion and encourage cholesterol gallstone formation and hence may counteract the effectiveness of ursodiol).
No products indexed under this heading.

Quinestrol (Estrogens and oral contraceptives increase hepatic cholesterol secretion and encourage cholesterol gallstone formation and hence may counteract the effectiveness of ursodiol).
No products indexed under this heading.

Simvastatin (Lipid-lowering drugs increase hepatic cholesterol secretion and encourage cholesterol gallstone formation and hence may counteract the effectiveness of ursodiol). Products include:
Vytorin 10/10 Tablets 2084
Vytorin 10/10 Tablets 3092
Vytorin 10/20 Tablets 2084
Vytorin 10/20 Tablets 3092
Vytorin 10/40 Tablets 3092
Vytorin 10/40 Tablets 2084
Vytorin 10/80 Tablets 2084
Vytorin 10/80 Tablets 3092
Zocor Tablets 2078

URSO FORTE TABLETS

(Ursodiol) 737
See Urso 250 Tablets

VAGIFEM TABLETS

(Estradiol) 2340
None cited in PDR database.

VALCYTE TABLETS

(Valganciclovir Hydrochloride) 2816
May interact with:

Didanosine (Valganciclovir is extensively converted to ganciclovir; co-administration of ganciclovir with didanosine has resulted in decreased AUC of ganciclovir and increased AUC of didanosine; patients should be monitored for didanosine toxicity).
No products indexed under this heading.

Mycophenolate Mofetil (Valganciclovir is extensively converted to ganciclovir; co-administration of ganciclovir with mycophenolate in patients with normal renal function has not resulted in any effect on PK parameters, however, patients with renal impairment should be monitored carefully as levels of metabolites or both drugs may increase). Products include:
CellCept Capsules 2751
CellCept Oral Suspension 2751
CellCept Tablets 2751

Probenecid (Valganciclovir is extensively converted to ganciclovir; co-administration of ganciclovir with probenecid results in increase in AUC of ganciclovir and decrease in ganciclovir renal cleareance; patients on concomitant therapy should be monitored for evidence of ganciclovir toxicity).
No products indexed under this heading.

Trimethoprim (Valganciclovir is extensively converted to ganciclovir; co-administration of ganciclovir with trimethoprim has resulted in decreased renal clearance and increased half-life of ganciclovir and an increase in Cmax of trimethoprim; effects of this interaction are not likely to be clinically significant).
No products indexed under this heading.

Zalcitabine (Valganciclovir is extensively converted to ganciclovir; co-administration of ganciclovir with zalcitabine has resulted in increased AUC of ganciclovir; effects of this interaction are not likely to be clinically significant).
No products indexed under this heading.

Zidovudine (Valganciclovir is extensively converted to ganciclovir; co-administration of ganciclovir with zidovudine has resulted in decreased AUC of ganciclovir and increased AUC of zidovudine; zidovudine and valganciclovir each have the potential to cause neutropenia and anemia; some patients may not tolerate concomitant therapy at full dosage). Products include:
Combivir Tablets 1373
Retrovir 1533
Retrovir IV Infusion 1537
Trizivir Tablets 1565

Food Interactions

Food, unspecified (Co-administration with high fat meals has resulted in increased steady-state ganciclovir AUC and Cmax without any prolongation in time to peak plasma concentrations; Valcyte should be administered with food).

VALIUM TABLETS

(Diazepam) 2822
May interact with barbiturates, central nervous system depressants, antidepressant drugs, anticonvulsants, monoamine oxidase inhibitors, narcotic analgesics, phenothiazines, and certain other agents. Compounds in these categories include:

Alfentanil Hydrochloride (May potentiate the actions of diazepam).
No products indexed under this heading.

Alprazolam (May potentiate the actions of diazepam). Products include:
Niravam Orally Disintegrating Tablets 3106
Xanax XR Tablets 2655

Amitriptyline Hydrochloride (May potentiate the actions of diazepam).
No products indexed under this heading.

Amoxapine (May potentiate the actions of diazepam).
No products indexed under this heading.

Aprobarbital (May potentiate the actions of diazepam).
No products indexed under this heading.

Buprenorphine Hydrochloride (May potentiate the actions of diazepam). Products include:
Buprenex Injectable 2718
Suboxone Tablets 2719
Subutex Tablets 2719

Bupropion Hydrochloride (May potentiate the actions of diazepam). Products include:
Wellbutrin Tablets 1579
Wellbutrin SR Sustained-Release Tablets 1583
Wellbutrin XL Extended-Release Tablets 1588
Zyban Sustained-Release Tablets 1620

Buspirone Hydrochloride (May potentiate the actions of diazepam).
No products indexed under this heading.

Butabarbital (May potentiate the actions of diazepam).
No products indexed under this heading.

Butalbital (May potentiate the actions of diazepam). Products include:
Sedapap Tablets 50 mg/650 mg 2098

Carbamazepine (Co-administration of diazepam as an adjunct in treating convulsive disorders results in possibility of an increase in the frequency and/or severity of grand mal seizures which may require an increase in the dosage of standard anticonvulsant agent). Products include:
Carbatrol Capsules 3174
Equetro Extended-Release Capsules 3178
Tegretol/Tegretol-XR 2278

Chlordiazepoxide (May potentiate the actions of diazepam).
No products indexed under this heading.

Chlordiazepoxide Hydrochloride (May potentiate the actions of diazepam). Products include:
Librium Capsules 3349

Chlorpromazine (May potentiate the actions of diazepam).
No products indexed under this heading.

Chlorpromazine Hydrochloride (May potentiate the actions of diazepam).
No products indexed under this heading.

Chlorprothixene (May potentiate the actions of diazepam).
No products indexed under this heading.

Chlorprothixene Hydrochloride (May potentiate the actions of diazepam).
No products indexed under this heading.

Chlorprothixene Lactate (May potentiate the actions of diazepam).
No products indexed under this heading.

Cimetidine (Co-administration delays diazepam clearance; clinical significance of this interaction is unclear). Products include:
Tagamet HB 200 Tablets 637
Tagamet Tablets 1547

Cimetidine Hydrochloride (Co-administration delays diazepam clearance; clinical significance of this interaction is unclear).
No products indexed under this heading.

Citalopram Hydrobromide (May potentiate the actions of diazepam). Products include:
Celexa 1177

Clonazepam (Co-administration of diazepam as an adjunct in treating convulsive disorders results in possibility of an increase in the frequency and/or severity of grand mal seizures which may require an increase in the dosage of standard anticonvulsant agent; may potentiate the CNS depression caused by diazepam). Products include:
Klonopin 2782

Clorazepate Dipotassium (May potentiate the actions of diazepam). Products include:
Tranxene 2488

Clozapine (May potentiate the actions of diazepam). Products include:
Clozapine Tablets 2141
Clozaril Tablets 2174

FazaClo Orally Disintegrating Tablets 547

Codeine Phosphate (May potentiate the actions of diazepam). Products include:
Tylenol with Codeine 2461

Desflurane (May potentiate the actions of diazepam). Products include:
Suprane Liquid for Inhalation 770

Desipramine Hydrochloride (May potentiate the actions of diazepam).
No products indexed under this heading.

Dezocine (May potentiate the actions of diazepam).
No products indexed under this heading.

Divalproex Sodium (Co-administration of diazepam as an adjunct in treating convulsive disorders results in possibility of an increase in the frequency and/or severity of grand mal seizures which may require an increase in the dosage of standard anticonvulsant agent). Products include:
Depakote Sprinkle Capsules 422
Depakote Tablets 427
Depakote ER Tablets 433

Doxepin Hydrochloride (May potentiate the actions of diazepam).
No products indexed under this heading.

Droperidol (May potentiate the actions of diazepam).
No products indexed under this heading.

Enflurane (May potentiate the actions of diazepam).
No products indexed under this heading.

Estazolam (May potentiate the actions of diazepam). Products include:
ProSom Tablets 512

Ethanol (May potentiate the actions of diazepam).
No products indexed under this heading.

Ethchlorvynol (May potentiate the actions of diazepam).
No products indexed under this heading.

Ethinamate (May potentiate the actions of diazepam).
No products indexed under this heading.

Ethosuximide (Co-administration of diazepam as an adjunct in treating convulsive disorders results in possibility of an increase in the frequency and/or severity of grand mal seizures which may require an increase in the dosage of standard anticonvulsant agent).
No products indexed under this heading.

Ethotoin (Co-administration of diazepam as an adjunct in treating convulsive disorders results in possibility of an increase in the frequency and/or severity of grand mal seizures which may require an increase in the dosage of standard anticonvulsant agent). Products include:
Peganone Tablets, USP 2487

Ethyl Alcohol (May potentiate the actions of diazepam).
No products indexed under this heading.

Felbamate (Co-administration of diazepam as an adjunct in treating convulsive disorders results in possibility of an increase in the frequency and/or severity of grand mal seizures which may require an increase in the dosage of standard anticonvulsant agent).
No products indexed under this heading.

Fentanyl (May potentiate the actions of diazepam). Products include:
Duragesic Transdermal System 2448

Fentanyl Citrate (May potentiate the actions of diazepam). Products include:
Actiq 993

Fluoxetine Hydrochloride (May potentiate the actions of diazepam). Products include:
Prozac Pulvules and Liquid 1771
Symbyax Capsules 1788

Fluphenazine Decanoate (May potentiate the actions of diazepam).
No products indexed under this heading.

Fluphenazine Enanthate (May potentiate the actions of diazepam).
No products indexed under this heading.

Fluphenazine Hydrochloride (May potentiate the actions of diazepam).
No products indexed under this heading.

Flurazepam Hydrochloride (May potentiate the actions of diazepam). Products include:
Dalmane Capsules 3343

Fosphenytoin (Co-administration of diazepam as an adjunct in treating convulsive disorders results in possibility of an increase in the frequency and/or severity of grand mal seizures which may require an increase in the dosage of standard anticonvulsant agent).
No products indexed under this heading.

Fosphenytoin Sodium (Co-administration of diazepam as an adjunct in treating convulsive disorders results in possibility of an increase in the frequency and/or severity of grand mal seizures which may require an increase in the dosage of standard anticonvulsant agent).
No products indexed under this heading.

Gabapentin (Co-administration of diazepam as an adjunct in treating convulsive disorders results in possibility of an increase in the frequency and/or severity of grand mal seizures which may require an increase in the dosage of standard anticonvulsant agent). Products include:
Neurontin Capsules 2498
Neurontin Oral Solution 2498
Neurontin Tablets 2498

Glutethimide (May potentiate the actions of diazepam).
No products indexed under this heading.

Haloperidol (May potentiate the actions of diazepam).
No products indexed under this heading.

Haloperidol Decanoate (May potentiate the actions of diazepam).
No products indexed under this heading.

Hydrocodone Bitartrate (May potentiate the actions of diazepam). Products include:
Hycodan 1104
Hycomine Compound Tablets 1105
Hycotuss Expectorant Syrup 1106
Lortab 3315
Lortab Elixir 3312
Vicodin Tablets 530
Vicodin ES Tablets 531
Vicodin HP Tablets 532
Vicoprofen Tablets 533
Zydone Tablets 1118

Hydrocodone Polistirex (May potentiate the actions of diazepam). Products include:
Tussionex Pennkinetic Extended-Release Suspension 3322

Hydromorphone Hydrochloride (May potentiate the actions of diazepam). Products include:
Dilaudid 439
Dilaudid Oral Liquid 443
Dilaudid Non-Sterile Powder 439
Dilaudid Rectal Suppositories 439
Dilaudid Tablets 439
Dilaudid Tablets - 8 mg 443
Dilaudid-HP 441

Hydroxyzine Hydrochloride (May potentiate the actions of diazepam).
No products indexed under this heading.

Imipramine Hydrochloride (May potentiate the actions of diazepam).
No products indexed under this heading.

Imipramine Pamoate (May potentiate the actions of diazepam).
No products indexed under this heading.

Isocarboxazid (May potentiate the actions of diazepam).
No products indexed under this heading.

Isoflurane (May potentiate the actions of diazepam).
No products indexed under this heading.

Ketamine Hydrochloride (May potentiate the actions of diazepam).
No products indexed under this heading.

Lamotrigine (Co-administration of diazepam as an adjunct in treating convulsive disorders results in possibility of an increase in the frequency and/or severity of grand mal seizures which may require an increase in the dosage of standard anticonvulsant agent). Products include:
Lamictal 1449

Levetiracetam (Co-administration of diazepam as an adjunct in treating convulsive disorders results in possibility of an increase in the frequency and/or severity of grand mal seizures which may require an increase in the dosage of standard anticonvulsant agent). Products include:
Keppra Oral Solution 3307
Keppra Tablets 3307

Levomethadyl Acetate Hydrochloride (May potentiate the actions of diazepam).
No products indexed under this heading.

Levorphanol Tartrate (May potentiate the actions of diazepam).
No products indexed under this heading.

Lorazepam (May potentiate the actions of diazepam).
No products indexed under this heading.

Loxapine Hydrochloride (May potentiate the actions of diazepam).
No products indexed under this heading.

Loxapine Succinate (May potentiate the actions of diazepam).
No products indexed under this heading.

Maprotiline Hydrochloride (May potentiate the actions of diazepam).
No products indexed under this heading.

Meperidine Hydrochloride (May potentiate the actions of diazepam).
No products indexed under this heading.

Mephenytoin (Co-administration of diazepam as an adjunct in treating convulsive disorders results in possibility of an increase in the frequency and/or severity of grand mal seizures which may require an increase in the dosage of standard anticonvulsant agent).
No products indexed under this heading.

Mephobarbital (May potentiate the actions of diazepam). Products include:
Mebaral Tablets, USP **2483**

Meprobamate (May potentiate the actions of diazepam).
No products indexed under this heading.

Mesoridazine Besylate (May potentiate the actions of diazepam).
No products indexed under this heading.

Methadone Hydrochloride (May potentiate the actions of diazepam).
No products indexed under this heading.

Methohexital Sodium (May potentiate the actions of diazepam).
No products indexed under this heading.

Methotrimeprazine (May potentiate the actions of diazepam).
No products indexed under this heading.

Methoxyflurane (May potentiate the actions of diazepam).
No products indexed under this heading.

Methsuximide (Co-administration of diazepam as an adjunct in treating convulsive disorders results in possibility of an increase in the frequency and/or severity of grand mal seizures which may require an increase in the dosage of standard anticonvulsant agent).
No products indexed under this heading.

Midazolam Hydrochloride (May potentiate the actions of diazepam).
No products indexed under this heading.

Mirtazapine (May potentiate the actions of diazepam).
No products indexed under this heading.

Moclobemide (May potentiate the actions of diazepam).
No products indexed under this heading.

Molindone Hydrochloride (May potentiate the actions of diazepam). Products include:
Moban Tablets **1108**

Morphine Sulfate (May potentiate the actions of diazepam). Products include:
Avinza Capsules **1714**
Kadian Capsules **572**
MS Contin Tablets **2703**

Nefazodone Hydrochloride (May potentiate the actions of diazepam).
No products indexed under this heading.

Nortriptyline Hydrochloride (May potentiate the actions of diazepam).
No products indexed under this heading.

Olanzapine (May potentiate the actions of diazepam). Products include:
Symbyax Capsules **1788**
Zyprexa Tablets **1798**
Zyprexa IntraMuscular **1798**
Zyprexa ZYDIS Orally Disintegrating Tablets **1798**

Oxazepam (May potentiate the actions of diazepam).
No products indexed under this heading.

Oxcarbazepine (Co-administration of diazepam as an adjunct in treating convulsive disorders results in possibility of an increase in the frequency and/or severity of grand mal seizures which may require an increase in the dosage of standard anticonvulsant agent). Products include:
Trileptal Oral Suspension **2281**
Trileptal Tablets **2281**

Oxycodone Hydrochloride (May potentiate the actions of diazepam). Products include:
Combunox Tablets **1183**
OxyContin Tablets **2699**
OxyFast Oral Concentrate Solution **2704**
OxyIR Capsules **2704**
Percocet Tablets **1114**
Percodan Tablets **1115**

Paramethadione (Co-administration of diazepam as an adjunct in treating convulsive disorders results in possibility of an increase in the frequency and/or severity of grand mal seizures which may require an increase in the dosage of standard anticonvulsant agent).
No products indexed under this heading.

Pargyline Hydrochloride (May potentiate the actions of diazepam).
No products indexed under this heading.

Paroxetine Hydrochloride (May potentiate the actions of diazepam). Products include:
Paxil CR Controlled-Release Tablets **1509**
Paxil **1501**

Pentobarbital Sodium (May potentiate the actions of diazepam). Products include:
Nembutal Sodium Solution, USP **2484**

Perphenazine (May potentiate the actions of diazepam).
No products indexed under this heading.

Phenacemide (Co-administration of diazepam as an adjunct in treating convulsive disorders results in possibility of an increase in the frequency and/or severity of grand mal seizures which may require an increase in the dosage of standard anticonvulsant agent).
No products indexed under this heading.

Phenelzine Sulfate (May potentiate the actions of diazepam).
No products indexed under this heading.

Phenobarbital (Co-administration of diazepam as an adjunct in treating convulsive disorders results in possibility of an increase in the frequency and/or severity of grand mal seizures which may require an increase in the dosage of standard anticonvulsant agent; may potentiate the CNS depression caused by diazepam).
No products indexed under this heading.

Phensuximide (Co-administration of diazepam as an adjunct in treating convulsive disorders results in possibility of an increase in the frequency and/or severity of grand mal seizures which may require an increase in the dosage of standard anticonvulsant agent).
No products indexed under this heading.

Phenytoin (Co-administration of diazepam as an adjunct in treating convulsive disorders results in possibility of an increase in the frequency and/or severity of grand mal seizures which may require an increase in the dosage of standard anticonvulsant agent).
No products indexed under this heading.

Phenytoin Sodium (Co-administration of diazepam as an adjunct in treating convulsive disorders results in possibility of an increase in the frequency and/or severity of grand mal seizures which may require an increase in the dosage of standard anticonvulsant agent). Products include:
Phenytek Capsules **2153**

Prazepam (May potentiate the actions of diazepam).
No products indexed under this heading.

Primidone (Co-administration of diazepam as an adjunct in treating convulsive disorders results in possibility of an increase in the frequency and/or severity of grand mal seizures which may require an increase in the dosage of standard anticonvulsant agent).
No products indexed under this heading.

Procarbazine Hydrochloride (May potentiate the actions of diazepam). Products include:
Matulane Capsules **3188**

Prochlorperazine (May potentiate the actions of diazepam).
No products indexed under this heading.

Promethazine Hydrochloride (May potentiate the actions of diazepam). Products include:
Phenergan **3438**

Propofol (May potentiate the actions of diazepam). Products include:
Diprivan Injectable Emulsion **676**

Propoxyphene Hydrochloride (May potentiate the actions of diazepam).
No products indexed under this heading.

Propoxyphene Napsylate (May potentiate the actions of diazepam). Products include:
Darvocet A 500 Tablets **3497**

Protriptyline Hydrochloride (May potentiate the actions of diazepam). Products include:
Vivactil Tablets **2350**

Quazepam (May potentiate the actions of diazepam).
No products indexed under this heading.

Quetiapine Fumarate (May potentiate the actions of diazepam). Products include:
Seroquel Tablets **691**

Remifentanil Hydrochloride (May potentiate the actions of diazepam).
No products indexed under this heading.

Risperidone (May potentiate the actions of diazepam). Products include:
Risperdal Consta Long-Acting Injection **1664**
Risperdal M-Tab Orally Disintegrating Tablets **1658**
Risperdal **1658**

Secobarbital Sodium (May potentiate the actions of diazepam).
No products indexed under this heading.

Selegiline Hydrochloride (May potentiate the actions of diazepam). Products include:
Eldepryl Capsules **3209**

Sertraline Hydrochloride (May potentiate the actions of diazepam). Products include:
Zoloft **2581**

Sevoflurane (May potentiate the actions of diazepam). Products include:
Ultane Liquid for Inhalation **526**

Sufentanil Citrate (May potentiate the actions of diazepam).
No products indexed under this heading.

Temazepam (May potentiate the actions of diazepam).
No products indexed under this heading.

Thiamylal Sodium (May potentiate the actions of diazepam).
No products indexed under this heading.

Thioridazine Hydrochloride (May potentiate the actions of diazepam). Products include:
Thioridazine Hydrochloride Tablets **2122**

Thiothixene (May potentiate the actions of diazepam). Products include:
Thiothixene Capsules **2124**

Tiagabine Hydrochloride (Co-administration of diazepam as an adjunct in treating convulsive disorders results in possibility of an increase in the frequency and/or severity of grand mal seizures which may require an increase in the dosage of standard anticonvulsant agent). Products include:
Gabitril Tablets **998**

Topiramate (Co-administration of diazepam as an adjunct in treating convulsive disorders results in possibility of an increase in the frequency and/or severity of grand mal seizures which may require an increase in the dosage of standard anticonvulsant agent). Products include:
Topamax Sprinkle Capsules **2438**
Topamax Tablets **2438**

Tranylcypromine Sulfate (May potentiate the actions of diazepam). Products include:
Parnate Tablets **1499**

Trazodone Hydrochloride (May potentiate the actions of diazepam).
No products indexed under this heading.

Triazolam (May potentiate the actions of diazepam).
No products indexed under this heading.

Trifluoperazine Hydrochloride (May potentiate the actions of diazepam).
No products indexed under this heading.

Trimethadione (Co-administration of diazepam as an adjunct in treating convulsive disorders results in possibility of an increase in the frequency and/or severity of grand mal seizures which may require an increase in the dosage of standard anticonvulsant agent).
No products indexed under this heading.

Trimipramine Maleate (May potentiate the actions of diazepam). Products include:
Surmontil Capsules **2347**

Valproate Sodium (Co-administration of diazepam as an adjunct in treating convulsive disorders results in possibility of an increase in the frequency and/or severity of grand mal seizures which may require an increase in the dosage of standard anticonvulsant agent). Products include:
Depacon Injection **412**

Valproic Acid (Co-administration of diazepam as an adjunct in treating convulsive disorders results in possibility of an increase in the frequency and/or severity of grand mal seizures which may require an increase in the dosage of standard anticonvulsant agent). Products include:
Depakene **417**

Venlafaxine Hydrochloride (May potentiate the actions of diazepam). Products include:
Effexor Tablets **3405**
Effexor XR Capsules **3411**

Zaleplon (May potentiate the actions of diazepam). Products include:
Sonata Capsules **1686**

Ziprasidone Hydrochloride (May potentiate the actions of diazepam). Products include:
Geodon Capsules **2514**

Zolpidem Tartrate (May potentiate the actions of diazepam). Products include:
Ambien Tablets **2867**

Zonisamide (Co-administration of diazepam as an adjunct in treating convulsive disorders results in possibility of an increase in the frequency and/or severity of grand mal seizures which may require an increase in the dosage of standard anticonvulsant agent). Products include:
Zonegran Capsules **1089**

Food Interactions

Alcohol (May potentiate the actions of diazepam).

VALTREX CAPLETS

(Valacyclovir Hydrochloride) **1573**
May interact with:

Cimetidine (Co-administration reduces renal clearance of acyclovir causing an increase in acyclovir AUC and Cmax). Products include:
Tagamet HB 200 Tablets .... ▣**637**
Tagamet Tablets **1547**

Cimetidine Hydrochloride (Co-administration reduces renal clearance of acyclovir causing an increase in acyclovir AUC and Cmax).
No products indexed under this heading.

Probenecid (Co-administration reduces renal clearance of acyclovir causing an increase in acyclovir AUC and Cmax).
No products indexed under this heading.

VANCOCIN HCL CAPSULES, USP

(Vancomycin Hydrochloride) **3370**
May interact with aminoglycosides, anesthetics, and certain other agents. Compounds in these categories include:

Alfentanil Hydrochloride (Co-administration with anesthetic agents has been associated with erythema and histamine-like flushing in children).
No products indexed under this heading.

Amikacin Sulfate (Concurrent and/or sequential use may result in increased potential for neurotoxicity and/or nephrotoxicity).
No products indexed under this heading.

Amphotericin B (Concurrent and/or sequential use may result in increased potential for neurotoxicity and/or nephrotoxicity).
No products indexed under this heading.

Bacitracin Zinc (Concurrent and/or sequential use may result in increased potential for neurotoxicity and/or nephrotoxicity).
No products indexed under this heading.

Cisplatin (Concurrent and/or sequential use may result in increased potential for neurotoxicity and/or nephrotoxicity).
No products indexed under this heading.

Colistin Sulfate (Concurrent and/or sequential use may result in increased potential for neurotoxicity and/or nephrotoxicity).
No products indexed under this heading.

Enflurane (Co-administration with anesthetic agents has been associated with erythema and histamine-like flushing in children).
No products indexed under this heading.

Fentanyl Citrate (Co-administration with anesthetic agents has been associated with erythema and histamine-like flushing in children). Products include:
Actiq **993**

Gentamicin Sulfate (Concurrent and/or sequential use may result in increased potential for neurotoxicity and/or nephrotoxicity). Products include:
Garamycin Injectable **3028**
Genoptic Sterile Ophthalmic Solution .... ⊙**227**
Pred-G Ophthalmic Suspension ...... ⊙**234**
Pred-G Sterile Ophthalmic Ointment .... ⊙**235**

Halothane (Co-administration with anesthetic agents has been associated with erythema and histamine-like flushing in children).
No products indexed under this heading.

Isoflurane (Co-administration with anesthetic agents has been associated with erythema and histamine-like flushing in children).
No products indexed under this heading.

Kanamycin Sulfate (Concurrent and/or sequential use may result in increased potential for neurotoxicity and/or nephrotoxicity).
No products indexed under this heading.

Ketamine Hydrochloride (Co-administration with anesthetic agents has been associated with erythema and histamine-like flushing in children).
No products indexed under this heading.

Methohexital Sodium (Co-administration with anesthetic agents has been associated with erythema and histamine-like flushing in children).
No products indexed under this heading.

Midazolam Hydrochloride (Co-administration with anesthetic agents has been associated with erythema and histamine-like flushing in children).
No products indexed under this heading.

Polymyxin B Sulfate (Concurrent and/or sequential use may result in increased potential for neurotoxicity and/or nephrotoxicity). Products include:
Neosporin Ointment .... ▣**702**
Neosporin + Pain Relief Maximum Strength Cream........... ▣**703**
Neosporin + Pain Relief Maximum Strength Ointment....... ▣**703**
Poly-Pred Liquifilm Ophthalmic Suspension .... ⊙**231**
Polysporin Ointment .... ▣**706**
Polytrim Ophthalmic Solution **570**

Propofol (Co-administration with anesthetic agents has been associated with erythema and histamine-like flushing in children). Products include:
Diprivan Injectable Emulsion **676**

Remifentanil Hydrochloride (Co-administration with anesthetic agents has been associated with erythema and histamine-like flushing in children).
No products indexed under this heading.

Streptomycin Sulfate (Concurrent and/or sequential use may result in increased potential for neurotoxicity and/or nephrotoxicity).
No products indexed under this heading.

Sufentanil Citrate (Co-administration with anesthetic agents has been associated with erythema and histamine-like flushing in children).
No products indexed under this heading.

Thiamylal Sodium (Co-administration with anesthetic agents has been associated with erythema and histamine-like flushing in children).
No products indexed under this heading.

Tobramycin (Concurrent and/or sequential use may result in increased potential for neurotoxicity and/or nephrotoxicity). Products include:
TOBI Solution for Inhalation **1015**
TobraDex Ophthalmic Ointment **558**
TobraDex Ophthalmic Suspension ... **558**
Zylet Ophthalmic Suspension **3508**

Tobramycin Sulfate (Concurrent and/or sequential use may result in increased potential for neurotoxicity and/or nephrotoxicity).
No products indexed under this heading.

Viomycin (Concurrent and/or sequential use may result in increased potential for neurotoxicity and/or nephrotoxicity).
No products indexed under this heading.

VANOS CREAM

(Fluocinonide) **1864**
None cited in PDR database.

VANTAS

(Histrelin Acetate) **3367**
None cited in PDR database.

VANTIN TABLETS AND ORAL SUSPENSION

(Cefpodoxime Proxetil) **2650**
May interact with aminoglycosides, antacids, anticholinergics, histamine H_2-receptor antagonists, and certain other agents. Compounds in these categories include:

Aluminum Carbonate (High doses of antacids reduces peak plasma levels by 24% and the extent of absorption by 27%; the rate of absorption is not altered).
No products indexed under this heading.

Aluminum Hydroxide (High doses of antacids reduces peak plasma levels by 24% and the extent of absorption by 27%; the rate of absorption is not altered). Products include:
Gaviscon Regular Strength Liquid .. ▣**620**
Gaviscon Regular Strength Tablets.. ▣**619**
Gaviscon Extra Strength Liquid ...... ▣**620**
Gaviscon Extra Strength Tablets .... ▣**619**
Maalox Max Maximum Strength Antacid/Anti-Gas Liquid................ **2165**
Maalox Regular Strength Antacid/Antigas Liquid................. **2164**

Amikacin Sulfate (Close monitoring of renal function is required when co-administered with compounds of known nephrotoxicity potential, such as aminoglycosides).
No products indexed under this heading.

Atropine Sulfate (Oral anti-cholinergics delay peak plasma levels but do not affect the extent of absorption).
No products indexed under this heading.

Belladonna Alkaloids (Oral anti-cholinergics delay peak plasma levels but do not affect the extent of absorption). Products include:
Hyland's Teething Tablets .... ▣**736**

Benztropine Mesylate (Oral anti-cholinergics delay peak plasma levels but do not affect the extent of absorption). Products include:
Cogentin Injection **1903**

Biperiden Hydrochloride (Oral anti-cholinergics delay peak plasma levels but do not affect the extent of absorption).
No products indexed under this heading.

IMPORTANT NOTE: Always consult each drug listing in the patient's regimen for possible interactions.

Cimetidine (High doses of H_2 blockers reduces peak plasma levels by 42% and the extent of absorption by 32%; the rate of absorption is not altered). Products include:

Tagamet HB 200 Tablets .... ▣637
Tagamet Tablets 1547

Cimetidine Hydrochloride (High doses of H_2 blockers reduces peak plasma levels by 42% and the extent of absorption by 32%; the rate of absorption is not altered).

No products indexed under this heading.

Clidinium Bromide (Oral anti-cholinergics delay peak plasma levels but do not affect the extent of absorption).

No products indexed under this heading.

Dicyclomine Hydrochloride (Oral anti-cholinergics delay peak plasma levels but do not affect the extent of absorption). Products include:

Bentyl Capsules 724
Bentyl Injection 724
Bentyl Syrup 724
Bentyl Tablets 724

Famotidine (High doses of H_2 blockers reduces peak plasma levels by 42% and the extent of absorption by 32%; the rate of absorption is not altered). Products include:

Pepcid AC Chewable Tablets 1672
Pepcid AC Gelcaps 1672
Pepcid AC Tablets 1672
Maximum Strength Pepcid AC Tablets 1672
Pepcid Complete Chewable Tablets 1672
Pepcid Injection 2017
Pepcid 2014

Gentamicin Sulfate (Close monitoring of renal function is required when co-administered with compounds of known nephrotoxicity potential, such as aminoglycosides). Products include:

Garamycin Injectable 3028
Genoptic Sterile Ophthalmic Solution .... ⊙227
Pred-G Ophthalmic Suspension ...... ⊙234
Pred-G Sterile Ophthalmic Ointment .... ⊙235

Glycopyrrolate (Oral anti-cholinergics delay peak plasma levels but do not affect the extent of absorption).

No products indexed under this heading.

Hyoscyamine (Oral anti-cholinergics delay peak plasma levels but do not affect the extent of absorption).

No products indexed under this heading.

Hyoscyamine Sulfate (Oral anti-cholinergics delay peak plasma levels but do not affect the extent of absorption).

No products indexed under this heading.

Ipratropium Bromide (Oral anti-cholinergics delay peak plasma levels but do not affect the extent of absorption). Products include:

Atrovent HFA Inhalation Aerosol 872
Atrovent Inhalation Solution 868
Atrovent Nasal Spray 0.03% 869
Atrovent Nasal Spray 0.06% 870
Combivent Inhalation Aerosol 878
DuoNeb Inhalation Solution 1058

Kanamycin Sulfate (Close monitoring of renal function is required when co-administered with compounds of known nephrotoxicity potential, such as aminoglycosides).

No products indexed under this heading.

Magaldrate (High doses of antacids reduces peak plasma levels by 24% and the extent of absorption by 27%; the rate of absorption is not altered).

No products indexed under this heading.

Magnesium Hydroxide (High doses of antacids reduces peak plasma levels by 24% and the extent of absorption by 27%; the rate of absorption is not altered). Products include:

Maalox Max Maximum Strength Antacid/Anti-Gas Liquid 2165
Maalox Regular Strength Antacid/Antigas Liquid 2164
Pepcid Complete Chewable Tablets 1672
Rolaids Tablets .... ▣707
Extra Strength Rolaids Tablets .... ▣707
Rolaids Multi-Symptom Antacid & Antigas Tablets .... ▣708

Magnesium Oxide (High doses of antacids reduces peak plasma levels by 24% and the extent of absorption by 27%; the rate of absorption is not altered). Products include:

Beelith Tablets 784
PremCal Light, Regular, and Extra Strength Tablets .... ▣762

Mepenzolate Bromide (Oral anti-cholinergics delay peak plasma levels but do not affect the extent of absorption).

No products indexed under this heading.

Nephrotoxic Drugs (Close monitoring of renal function is required when co-administered with compounds of known nephrotoxicity potential).

No products indexed under this heading.

Nizatidine (High doses of H_2 blockers reduces peak plasma levels by 42% and the extent of absorption by 32%; the rate of absorption is not altered). Products include:

Axid Oral Solution 913

Oxybutynin Chloride (Oral anti-cholinergics delay peak plasma levels but do not affect the extent of absorption). Products include:

Ditropan XL Extended Release Tablets 2391

Probenecid (Renal excretion of cefpodoxime is inhibited by probenecid and resulting in an approximately 31% increase in AUC and 20% increase in peak plasma levels).

No products indexed under this heading.

Procyclidine Hydrochloride (Oral anti-cholinergics delay peak plasma levels but do not affect the extent of absorption).

No products indexed under this heading.

Propantheline Bromide (Oral anti-cholinergics delay peak plasma levels but do not affect the extent of absorption).

No products indexed under this heading.

Ranitidine Bismuth Citrate (High doses of H_2 blockers reduces peak plasma levels by 42% and the extent of absorption by 32%; the rate of absorption is not altered).

No products indexed under this heading.

Ranitidine Hydrochloride (High doses of H_2 blockers reduces peak plasma levels by 42% and the extent of absorption by 32%; the rate of absorption is not altered). Products include:

Zantac 1597
Zantac Injection 1593
Zantac 75 Tablets .... ▣715
Zantac 150 Maximum Strength Tablets .... ▣715
Zantac Injection Pharmacy Bulk Package 1595

Scopolamine (Oral anti-cholinergics delay peak plasma levels but do not affect the extent of absorption). Products include:

Transderm Scōp Transdermal Therapeutic System 2166

Scopolamine Hydrobromide (Oral anti-cholinergics delay peak plasma levels but do not affect the extent of absorption).

No products indexed under this heading.

Sodium Bicarbonate (High doses of antacids reduces peak plasma levels by 24% and the extent of absorption by 27%; the rate of absorption is not altered). Products include:

Ceo-Two Evacuant Suppository ...... ▣607
Colyte with Flavor Packs for Oral Solution 3102
HalfLytely and Bisacodyl Tablets Bowel Prep Kit with Flavors Packs 915
TriLyte with Flavor Packs for Oral Solution 3114

Streptomycin Sulfate (Close monitoring of renal function is required when co-administered with compounds of known nephrotoxicity potential, such as aminoglycosides).

No products indexed under this heading.

Tobramycin (Close monitoring of renal function is required when co-administered with compounds of known nephrotoxicity potential, such as aminoglycosides). Products include:

TOBI Solution for Inhalation 1015
TobraDex Ophthalmic Ointment 558
TobraDex Ophthalmic Suspension ... 558
Zylet Ophthalmic Suspension 3508

Tobramycin Sulfate (Close monitoring of renal function is required when co-administered with compounds of known nephrotoxicity potential, such as aminoglycosides).

No products indexed under this heading.

Tolterodine Tartrate (Oral anti-cholinergics delay peak plasma levels but do not affect the extent of absorption). Products include:

Detrol Tablets 2626
Detrol LA Capsules 2629

Tridihexethyl Chloride (Oral anti-cholinergics delay peak plasma levels but do not affect the extent of absorption).

No products indexed under this heading.

Trihexyphenidyl Hydrochloride (Oral anti-cholinergics delay peak plasma levels but do not affect the extent of absorption).

No products indexed under this heading.

Food Interactions

Food, unspecified (The extent of absorption and the mean peak plasma concentration increased when film-coated tablets were administered with food).

VAQTA

(Hepatitis A Vaccine, Inactivated) 2067

May interact with typhoid vaccine and certain other agents. Compounds in these categories include:

Typhoid Vaccine (Co-administration of Vaqta, typhoid and yellow fever vaccines has resulted in reduced GMTs for hepatitis A compared to Vaqta alone; however, following the receipt of the booster dose of Vaqta the GMTs for hepatits A in these two groups were observed to be comparable).

No products indexed under this heading.

Typhoid Vaccine Live Oral TY21a (Co-administration of Vaqta, typhoid and yellow fever vaccines has resulted in reduced GMTs for hepatitis A compared to Vaqta alone; however, following the receipt of the booster dose of Vaqta the GMTs for hepatits A in these two groups were observed to be comparable). Products include:

Vivotif 834

Typhoid Vi Polysaccharide Vaccine (Co-administration of Vaqta, typhoid and yellow fever vaccines has resulted in reduced GMTs for hepatitis A compared to Vaqta alone; however, following the receipt of the booster dose of Vaqta the GMTs for hepatits A in these two groups were observed to be comparable).

No products indexed under this heading.

Yellow Fever Vaccine (Co-administration of Vaqta, typhoid and yellow fever vaccines has resulted in reduced GMTs for hepatitis A compared to Vaqta alone; however, following the receipt of the booster dose of Vaqta the GMTs for hepatitis A in these two groups were observed to be comparable).

No products indexed under this heading.

VARIVAX

(Varicella Virus Vaccine Live) 2070

May interact with corticosteroids, salicylates, and certain other agents. Compounds in these categories include:

Aspirin (Vaccine recipients should avoid use of salicylates for 6 weeks after vaccination with Varivax because of the potential for Reye's syndrome). Products include:

Aggrenox Capsules 855
Bayer, Aspirin Regimen .... ▣606
Bayer Aspirin Tablets 3515
BC Powder .... ▣612
BC Allergy Sinus Cold Powder .... ▣612
Arthritis Strength BC Powder .... ▣612
BC Sinus Cold Powder .... ▣612
Ecotrin Enteric Coated Aspirin Low, Regular and Maximum Strength Tablets 1627
Goody's Body Pain Formula Powder .... ▣621
Goody's Extra Strength Headache Powder .... ▣621
Goody's Extra Strength Pain Relief Tablets .... ▣621
Percodan Tablets 1115
St. Joseph 81 mg Aspirin Chewable and Enteric Coated Tablets 1841

Aspirin, Enteric Coated (Vaccine recipients should avoid use of salicylates for 6 weeks after vaccination with Varivax because of the potential for Reye's syndrome).
No products indexed under this heading.

Aspirin Buffered (Vaccine recipients should avoid use of salicylates for 6 weeks after vaccination with Varivax because of the potential for Reye's syndrome).
No products indexed under this heading.

Azathioprine (Concurrent use in individuals who are on immunosuppressant drugs can result in greater susceptibility to infections; co-administration is contraindicated). Products include:
Azasan Tablets 2844

Betamethasone Acetate (Co-administration in individuals on immunosuppressant doses of corticosteroids can result in more extensive vaccine-associated rash or disseminated disease).
No products indexed under this heading.

Betamethasone Sodium Phosphate (Co-administration in individuals on immunosuppressant doses of corticosteroids can result in more extensive vaccine-associated rash or disseminated disease).
No products indexed under this heading.

Choline Magnesium Trisalicylate (Vaccine recipients should avoid use of salicylates for 6 weeks after vaccination with Varivax because of the potential for Reye's syndrome).
No products indexed under this heading.

Cortisone Acetate (Co-administration in individuals on immunosuppressant doses of corticosteroids can result in more extensive vaccine-associated rash or disseminated disease).
No products indexed under this heading.

Cyclosporine (Concurrent use in individuals who are on immunosuppressant drugs can result in greater susceptibility to infections; co-administration is contraindicated). Products include:
Gengraf Capsules 458
Neoral Soft Gelatin Capsules 2247
Neoral Oral Solution 2247
Restasis Ophthalmic Emulsion 570
Sandimmune 2259

Dexamethasone (Co-administration in individuals on immunosuppressant doses of corticosteroids can result in more extensive vaccine-associated rash or disseminated disease). Products include:
Ciprodex Otic Suspension 555
Decadron Tablets 1929
TobraDex Ophthalmic Ointment 558
TobraDex Ophthalmic Suspension ... 558

Dexamethasone Acetate (Co-administration in individuals on immunosuppressant doses of corticosteroids can result in more extensive vaccine-associated rash or disseminated disease).
No products indexed under this heading.

Dexamethasone Sodium Phosphate (Co-administration in individuals on immunosuppressant doses of corticosteroids can result in more extensive vaccine-associated rash or disseminated disease). Products include:
Decadron Phosphate Injection 1931

Diflunisal (Vaccine recipients should avoid use of salicylates for 6 weeks after vaccination with Varivax because of the potential for Reye's syndrome). Products include:
Dolobid Tablets 1937

Fludrocortisone Acetate (Co-administration in individuals on immunosuppressant doses of corticosteroids can result in more extensive vaccine-associated rash or disseminated disease).
No products indexed under this heading.

Globulin, Immune (Human) (Vaccination should be deferred for at least 5 months following immune globulin administration; following administration of Varivax, immune globulin should not be given for 2 months). Products include:
GamaSTAN 3231

Hydrocortisone (Co-administration in individuals on immunosuppressant doses of corticosteroids can result in more extensive vaccine-associated rash or disseminated disease). Products include:
Cortizone•5 Ointment .... ▣699
Cortizone•10 Creme .... ▣699
Cortizone•10 Ointment .... ▣699
Cortizone•10 Plus Creme .... ▣700
Cortizone•10 Maximum Strength Quick Shot Spray .... ▣700
Hydrocortone Tablets 1963
Preparation H Hydrocortisone Cream .... ▣748

Hydrocortisone Acetate (Co-administration in individuals on immunosuppressant doses of corticosteroids can result in more extensive vaccine-associated rash or disseminated disease). Products include:
Analpram-HC 1136
Pramosone 1139
ProctoFoam-HC 3113
Tucks Anti-Itch Ointment .... ▣712
U-cort 1% Cream 3289

Hydrocortisone Sodium Phosphate (Co-administration in individuals on immunosuppressant doses of corticosteroids can result in more extensive vaccine-associated rash or disseminated disease).
No products indexed under this heading.

Hydrocortisone Sodium Succinate (Co-administration in individuals on immunosuppressant doses of corticosteroids can result in more extensive vaccine-associated rash or disseminated disease).
No products indexed under this heading.

Magnesium Salicylate (Vaccine recipients should avoid use of salicylates for 6 weeks after vaccination with Varivax because of the potential for Reye's syndrome).
No products indexed under this heading.

Methylprednisolone Acetate (Co-administration in individuals on immunosuppressant doses of corticosteroids can result in more extensive vaccine-associated rash or disseminated disease). Products include:
Depo-Medrol Injectable Suspension 2615
Depo-Medrol Single-Dose Vial 2617

Methylprednisolone Sodium Succinate (Co-administration in individuals on immunosuppressant doses of corticosteroids can result in more extensive vaccine-associated rash or disseminated disease).
No products indexed under this heading.

Muromonab-CD3 (Concurrent use in individuals who are on immunosuppressant drugs can result in greater susceptibility to infections; co-administration is contraindicated). Products include:
Orthoclone OKT3 Sterile Solution 2370

Mycophenolate Mofetil (Concurrent use in individuals who are on immunosuppressant drugs can result in greater susceptibility to infections; co-administration is contraindicated). Products include:
CellCept Capsules 2751
CellCept Oral Suspension 2751
CellCept Tablets 2751

Prednisolone Acetate (Co-administration in individuals on immunosuppressant doses of corticosteroids can result in more extensive vaccine-associated rash or disseminated disease). Products include:
Blephamide Ophthalmic Ointment 563
Blephamide Ophthalmic Suspension 564
Poly-Pred Liquifilm Ophthalmic Suspension .... ⊙231
Pred Forte Ophthalmic Suspension .... ⊙233
Pred Mild Sterile Ophthalmic Suspension .... ⊙236
Pred-G Ophthalmic Suspension ...... ⊙234
Pred-G Sterile Ophthalmic Ointment .... ⊙235

Prednisolone Sodium Phosphate (Co-administration in individuals on immunosuppressant doses of corticosteroids can result in more extensive vaccine-associated rash or disseminated disease). Products include:
Pediapred Oral Solution 3319

Prednisolone Tebutate (Co-administration in individuals on immunosuppressant doses of corticosteroids can result in more extensive vaccine-associated rash or disseminated disease).
No products indexed under this heading.

Prednisone (Co-administration in individuals on immunosuppressant doses of corticosteroids can result in more extensive vaccine-associated rash or disseminated disease).
No products indexed under this heading.

Salsalate (Vaccine recipients should avoid use of salicylates for 6 weeks after vaccination with Varivax because of the potential for Reye's syndrome).
No products indexed under this heading.

Tacrolimus (Concurrent use in individuals who are on immunosuppressant drugs can result in greater susceptibility to infections; co-administration is contraindicated). Products include:
Prograf Capsules and Injection 624
Protopic Ointment 629

Triamcinolone (Co-administration in individuals on immunosuppressant doses of corticosteroids can result in more extensive vaccine-associated rash or disseminated disease).
No products indexed under this heading.

Triamcinolone Acetonide (Co-administration in individuals on immunosuppressant doses of corticosteroids can result in more extensive vaccine-associated rash or disseminated disease). Products include:
Azmacort Inhalation Aerosol 1701
Nasacort HFA Inhalation Aerosol 2939
Nasacort AQ Nasal Spray 2937

Triamcinolone Diacetate (Co-administration in individuals on immunosuppressant doses of corticosteroids can result in more extensive vaccine-associated rash or disseminated disease).
No products indexed under this heading.

Triamcinolone Hexacetonide (Co-administration in individuals on immunosuppressant doses of corticosteroids can result in more extensive vaccine-associated rash or disseminated disease).
No products indexed under this heading.

VASERETIC TABLETS

(Enalapril Maleate, Hydrochlorothiazide) 2073
May interact with antihypertensives, barbiturates, corticosteroids, diuretics, cardiac glycosides, oral hypoglycemic agents, insulin, lithium preparations, narcotic analgesics, nondepolarizing neuromuscular blocking agents, non-steroidal anti-inflammatory agents, potassium preparations, potassium sparing diuretics, and certain other agents. Compounds in these categories include:

Acarbose (Hyperglycemia may occur with thiazide diuretics; dosage adjustment of oral hypoglycemic agents may be required). Products include:
Precose Tablets 776

Acebutolol Hydrochloride (Co-administration of thiazide and other antihypertensive agents can lead to additive effect or potentiation).
No products indexed under this heading.

ACTH (Co-administration of thiazide diuretics with ACTH intensifies electrolyte depletion, particularly potassium).
No products indexed under this heading.

Alfentanil Hydrochloride (Co-administration of thiazide and narcotics may potentiate orthostatic hypotension).
No products indexed under this heading.

Amiloride Hydrochloride (Enalapril attenuates diuretic-induced potassium loss; concomitant use can lead to hyperkalemia; frequent monitoring of serum potassium is recommended if used concurrently; co-administration can result in excessive hypotension). Products include:
Midamor Tablets 2000
Moduretic Tablets 2003

Amlodipine Besylate (Co-administration of thiazide and other

antihypertensive agents can lead to additive effect or potentiation). Products include:
Caduet Tablets ... 2507
Lotrel Capsules ... 2238
Norvasc Tablets ... 2529

Aprobarbital (Co-administration of thiazide and barbiturates may potentiate orthostatic hypotension).
No products indexed under this heading.

Atenolol (Co-administration of thiazide and other antihypertensive agents can lead to additive effect or potentiation). Products include:
Tenormin I.V. Injection ... 698
Tenormin Tablets ... 695

Atracurium Besylate (Co-administration with nondepolarizing skeletal muscle relaxants may result in possible increased responsiveness to the muscle relaxant).
No products indexed under this heading.

Benazepril Hydrochloride (Co-administration of thiazide and other antihypertensive agents can lead to additive effect or potentiation). Products include:
Lotensin Tablets ... 2232
Lotensin HCT Tablets ... 2235
Lotrel Capsules ... 2238

Bendroflumethiazide (Co-administration of enalapril in patients on diuretics, especially those in whom diuretic therapy was recently instituted, may occasionally experience excessive hypotension; antihypertensive effects of enalapril are augmented by antihypertensive agents that cause renin release).
No products indexed under this heading.

Betamethasone Acetate (Co-administration of thiazide diuretics with corticosteroids intensifies electrolyte depletion, particularly potassium).
No products indexed under this heading.

Betamethasone Sodium Phosphate (Co-administration of thiazide diuretics with corticosteroids intensifies electrolyte depletion, particularly potassium).
No products indexed under this heading.

Betaxolol Hydrochloride (Co-administration of thiazide and other antihypertensive agents can lead to additive effect or potentiation). Products include:
Betoptic S Ophthalmic Suspension... 554

Bisoprolol Fumarate (Co-administration of thiazide and other antihypertensive agents can lead to additive effect or potentiation).
No products indexed under this heading.

Bumetanide (Co-administration of enalapril in patients on diuretics, especially those in whom diuretic therapy was recently instituted, may occasionally experience excessive hypotension; antihypertensive effects of enalapril are augmented by antihypertensive agents that cause renin release).
No products indexed under this heading.

Buprenorphine Hydrochloride (Co-administration of thiazide and narcotics may potentiate orthostatic hypotension). Products include:
Buprenex Injectable ... 2718
Suboxone Tablets ... 2719
Subutex Tablets ... 2719

Butabarbital (Co-administration of thiazide and barbiturates may potentiate orthostatic hypotension).
No products indexed under this heading.

Butalbital (Co-administration of thiazide and barbiturates may potentiate orthostatic hypotension). Products include:
Sedapap Tablets 50 mg/650 mg ... 2098

Candesartan Cilexetil (Co-administration of thiazide and other antihypertensive agents can lead to additive effect or potentiation). Products include:
Atacand Tablets ... 634
Atacand HCT ... 637

Captopril (Co-administration of thiazide and other antihypertensive agents can lead to additive effect or potentiation). Products include:
Captopril Tablets ... 2114

Carteolol Hydrochloride (Co-administration of thiazide and other antihypertensive agents can lead to additive effect or potentiation). Products include:
Carteolol Hydrochloride Ophthalmic Solution USP, 1% ... ⊙246

Celecoxib (Co-administration in some patients with compromised renal function who are being treated with NSAIDS may result in a further deterioration of renal function; NSAID may reduce the diuretic, natriuretic and antihypertensive effects of thiazide). Products include:
Celebrex Capsules ... 3130

Chlorothiazide (Co-administration of enalapril in patients on diuretics, especially those in whom diuretic therapy was recently instituted, may occasionally experience excessive hypotension; antihypertensive effects of enalapril are augmented by antihypertensive agents that cause renin release). Products include:
Aldoclor Tablets ... 1881
Diuril Oral ... 1936

Chlorothiazide Sodium (Co-administration of enalapril in patients on diuretics, especially those in whom diuretic therapy was recently instituted, may occasionally experience excessive hypotension; antihypertensive effects of enalapril are augmented by antihypertensive agents that cause renin release). Products include:
Diuril Sodium Intravenous ... 1934

Chlorpropamide (Hyperglycemia may occur with thiazide diuretics; dosage adjustment of oral hypoglycemic agents may be required).
No products indexed under this heading.

Chlorthalidone (Co-administration of enalapril in patients on diuretics, especially those in whom diuretic therapy was recently instituted, may occasionally experience excessive hypotension; antihypertensive effects of enalapril are augmented by antihypertensive agents that cause renin release). Products include:
Clorpres Tablets ... 2139

Cholestyramine (Absorption of hydrochlorothiazide is impaired in the presence of anionic exchange resins; these resins bind the hydrochlorothiazide and reduce its absorption from GI tract).
No products indexed under this heading.

Cisatracurium Besylate (Co-administration with nondepolarizing skeletal muscle relaxants may result in possible increased responsiveness to the muscle relaxant). Products include:
Nimbex Injection ... 494

Clonidine (Co-administration of thiazide and other antihypertensive agents can lead to additive effect or potentiation). Products include:
Catapres-TTS ... 875

Clonidine Hydrochloride (Co-administration of thiazide and other antihypertensive agents can lead to additive effect or potentiation). Products include:
Catapres Tablets ... 874
Clorpres Tablets ... 2139

Codeine Phosphate (Co-administration of thiazide and narcotics may potentiate orthostatic hypotension). Products include:
Tylenol with Codeine ... 2461

Colestipol Hydrochloride (Absorption of hydrochlorothiazide is impaired in the presence of anionic exchange resins; these resins bind the hydrochlorothiazide and reduce its absorption from GI tract).
No products indexed under this heading.

Cortisone Acetate (Co-administration of thiazide diuretics with corticosteroids intensifies electrolyte depletion, particularly potassium).
No products indexed under this heading.

Deserpidine (Co-administration of thiazide and other antihypertensive agents can lead to additive effect or potentiation).
No products indexed under this heading.

Deslanoside (Hypokalemia induced by thiazide diuretics may cause cardiac arrhythmia and may also sensitize or exaggerate the response to the heart to the toxic effects of digitalis, such as ventricular irritability).
No products indexed under this heading.

Dexamethasone (Co-administration of thiazide diuretics with corticosteroids intensifies electrolyte depletion, particularly potassium). Products include:
Ciprodex Otic Suspension ... 555
Decadron Tablets ... 1929
TobraDex Ophthalmic Ointment ... 558
TobraDex Ophthalmic Suspension ... 558

Dexamethasone Acetate (Co-administration of thiazide diuretics with corticosteroids intensifies electrolyte depletion, particularly potassium).
No products indexed under this heading.

Dexamethasone Sodium Phosphate (Co-administration of thiazide diuretics with corticosteroids intensifies electrolyte depletion, particularly potassium). Products include:
Decadron Phosphate Injection ... 1931

Dezocine (Co-administration of thiazide and narcotics may potentiate orthostatic hypotension).
No products indexed under this heading.

Diazoxide (Co-administration of thiazide and other antihypertensive agents can lead to additive effect or potentiation). Products include:
Hyperstat I.V. Injection ... 3031

Diclofenac Potassium (Co-administration in some patients with compromised renal function who are being treated with NSAIDS may result in a further deterioration of renal function; NSAID may reduce the diuretic, natriuretic and antihypertensive effects of thiazide). Products include:
Cataflam Tablets ... 2173

Diclofenac Sodium (Co-administration in some patients with compromised renal function who are being treated with NSAIDS may result in a further deterioration of renal function; NSAID may reduce the diuretic, natriuretic and antihypertensive effects of thiazide). Products include:
Arthrotec Tablets ... 3126
Voltaren Ophthalmic Solution ... 2300
Voltaren Tablets ... 2298
Voltaren-XR Tablets ... 2301

Digitalis Glycoside Preparations (Hypokalemia induced by thiazide diuretics may cause cardiac arrhythmia and may also sensitize or exaggerate the response to the heart to the toxic effects of digitalis, such as ventricular irritability).
No products indexed under this heading.

Digitoxin (Hypokalemia induced by thiazide diuretics may cause cardiac arrhythmia and may also sensitize or exaggerate the response to the heart to the toxic effects of digitalis, such as ventricular irritability).
No products indexed under this heading.

Digoxin (Hypokalemia induced by thiazide diuretics may cause cardiac arrhythmia and may also sensitize or exaggerate the response to the heart to the toxic effects of digitalis, such as ventricular irritability). Products include:
Digitek Tablets ... 2146
Lanoxicaps Capsules ... 1458
Lanoxin Injection ... 1462
Lanoxin Tablets ... 1468
Lanoxin Injection Pediatric ... 1465

Diltiazem Hydrochloride (Co-administration of thiazide and other antihypertensive agents can lead to additive effect or potentiation). Products include:
Cardizem LA Extended Release Tablets ... 1699
Tiazac Capsules ... 1204

Doxazosin Mesylate (Co-administration of thiazide and other antihypertensive agents can lead to additive effect or potentiation).
No products indexed under this heading.

Enalaprilat (Co-administration of thiazide and other antihypertensive agents can lead to additive effect or potentiation).
No products indexed under this heading.

Eprosartan Mesylate (Co-administration of thiazide and other antihypertensive agents can lead to additive effect or potentiation). Products include:
Teveten Tablets ... 1707
Teveten HCT Tablets ... 1710

Esmolol Hydrochloride (Co-administration of thiazide and other antihypertensive agents can lead to additive effect or potentiation). Products include:
Brevibloc Concentrate ... 766
Brevibloc Injection ... 766
Brevibloc Double Strength Injection ... 766

Brevibloc Premixed Injection 766
Brevibloc Double Strength Premixed Injection 766

Ethacrynic Acid (Co-administration of enalapril in patients on diuretics, especially those in whom diuretic therapy was recently instituted, may occasionally experience excessive hypotension; antihypertensive effects of enalapril are augmented by antihypertensive agents that cause renin release). Products include:
Edecrin Tablets 1941

Etodolac (Co-administration in some patients with compromised renal function who are being treated with NSAIDS may result in a further deterioration of renal function; NSAID may reduce the diuretic, natriuretic and antihypertensive effects of thiazide).
No products indexed under this heading.

Felodipine (Co-administration of thiazide and other antihypertensive agents can lead to additive effect or potentiation). Products include:
Plendil Extended-Release Tablets 651

Fenoprofen Calcium (Co-administration in some patients with compromised renal function who are being treated with NSAIDS may result in a further deterioration of renal function; NSAID may reduce the diuretic, natriuretic and antihypertensive effects of thiazide). Products include:
Nalfon Capsules 2504

Fentanyl (Co-administration of thiazide and narcotics may potentiate orthostatic hypotension). Products include:
Duragesic Transdermal System 2448

Fentanyl Citrate (Co-administration of thiazide and narcotics may potentiate orthostatic hypotension). Products include:
Actiq 993

Fludrocortisone Acetate (Co-administration of thiazide diuretics with corticosteroids intensifies electrolyte depletion, particularly potassium).
No products indexed under this heading.

Flurbiprofen (Co-administration in some patients with compromised renal function who are being treated with NSAIDS may result in a further deterioration of renal function; NSAID may reduce the diuretic, natriuretic and antihypertensive effects of thiazide).
No products indexed under this heading.

Fosinopril Sodium (Co-administration of thiazide and other antihypertensive agents can lead to additive effect or potentiation).
No products indexed under this heading.

Furosemide (Co-administration of enalapril in patients on diuretics, especially those in whom diuretic therapy was recently instituted, may occasionally experience excessive hypotension; antihypertensive effects of enalapril are augmented by antihypertensive agents that cause renin release). Products include:
Furosemide Tablets 2117

Glimepiride (Hyperglycemia may occur with thiazide diuretics; dosage adjustment of oral hypoglycemic agents may be required). Products include:
Amaryl Tablets 2864

Glipizide (Hyperglycemia may occur with thiazide diuretics; dosage adjustment of oral hypoglycemic agents may be required).
No products indexed under this heading.

Glyburide (Hyperglycemia may occur with thiazide diuretics; dosage adjustment of oral hypoglycemic agents may be required).
No products indexed under this heading.

Guanabenz Acetate (Co-administration of thiazide and other antihypertensive agents can lead to additive effect or potentiation).
No products indexed under this heading.

Guanethidine Monosulfate (Co-administration of thiazide and other antihypertensive agents can lead to additive effect or potentiation).
No products indexed under this heading.

Hydralazine Hydrochloride (Co-administration of thiazide and other antihypertensive agents can lead to additive effect or potentiation). Products include:
BiDil Tablets 2161

Hydrocodone Bitartrate (Co-administration of thiazide and narcotics may potentiate orthostatic hypotension). Products include:
Hycodan 1104
Hycomine Compound Tablets 1105
Hycotuss Expectorant Syrup 1106
Lortab 3315
Lortab Elixir 3312
Vicodin Tablets 530
Vicodin ES Tablets 531
Vicodin HP Tablets 532
Vicoprofen Tablets 533
Zydone Tablets 1118

Hydrocodone Polistirex (Co-administration of thiazide and narcotics may potentiate orthostatic hypotension). Products include:
Tussionex Pennkinetic Extended-Release Suspension 3322

Hydrocortisone (Co-administration of thiazide diuretics with corticosteroids intensifies electrolyte depletion, particularly potassium). Products include:
Cortizone•5 Ointment 699
Cortizone•10 Creme 699
Cortizone•10 Ointment 699
Cortizone•10 Plus Creme 700
Cortizone•10 Maximum Strength Quick Shot Spray 700
Hydrocortone Tablets 1963
Preparation H Hydrocortisone Cream 748

Hydrocortisone Acetate (Co-administration of thiazide diuretics with corticosteroids intensifies electrolyte depletion, particularly potassium). Products include:
Analpram-HC 1136
Pramosone 1139
ProctoFoam-HC 3113
Tucks Anti-Itch Ointment 712
U-cort 1% Cream 3289

Hydrocortisone Sodium Phosphate (Co-administration of thiazide diuretics with corticosteroids intensifies electrolyte depletion, particularly potassium).
No products indexed under this heading.

Hydrocortisone Sodium Succinate (Co-administration of thiazide diuretics with corticosteroids intensifies electrolyte depletion, particularly potassium).
No products indexed under this heading.

Hydroflumethiazide (Co-administration of enalapril in patients on diuretics, especially those in whom diuretic therapy was recently instituted, may occasionally experience excessive hypotension; antihypertensive effects of enalapril are augmented by antihypertensive agents that cause renin release).
No products indexed under this heading.

Hydromorphone Hydrochloride (Co-administration of thiazide and narcotics may potentiate orthostatic hypotension). Products include:
Dilaudid 439
Dilaudid Oral Liquid 443
Dilaudid Non-Sterile Powder 439
Dilaudid Rectal Suppositories 439
Dilaudid Tablets 439
Dilaudid Tablets - 8 mg 443
Dilaudid-HP 441

Ibuprofen (Co-administration in some patients with compromised renal function who are being treated with NSAIDS may result in a further deterioration of renal function; NSAID may reduce the diuretic, natriuretic and antihypertensive effects of thiazide). Products include:
Advil Allergy Sinus Caplets 737
Advil 737
Children's Advil Suspension 742
Children's Advil Chewable Tablets 741
Advil Cold & Sinus 739
Advil Flu & Body Ache Caplets 739
Children's Advil Cold Suspension 741
Infants' Advil Concentrated Drops 743
Junior Strength Advil Swallow Tablets 740
Advil Migraine Liquigels 740
Advil Multi-Symptom Cold Caplets 738
Combunox Tablets 1183
Children's Motrin Oral Suspension and Chewable Tablets 1837
Children's Motrin Cold Non-Staining Dye-Free Oral Suspension 1838
Children's Motrin Cold Oral Suspension 1838
Children's Motrin Non-Staining Dye-Free Oral Suspension 1837
Motrin Cold & Sinus Caplets 1836
Motrin IB Tablets and Caplets 1836
Infants' Motrin Concentrated Drops 1837
Infants' Motrin Non-Staining Dye-Free Drops 1837
Junior Strength Motrin Caplets and Chewable Tablets 1837
Vicoprofen Tablets 533

Indapamide (Co-administration of enalapril in patients on diuretics, especially those in whom diuretic therapy was recently instituted, may occasionally experience excessive hypotension; antihypertensive effects of enalapril are augmented by antihypertensive agents that cause renin release). Products include:
Indapamide Tablets 2119

Indomethacin (Co-administration in some patients with compromised renal function who are being treated with NSAIDS may result in a further deterioration of renal function; NSAID may reduce the diuretic, natriuretic and antihypertensive effects of thiazide). Products include:
Indocin 1968

Indomethacin Sodium Trihydrate (Co-administration in some patients with compromised renal function who are being treated with NSAIDS may result in a further deterioration of renal function; NSAID may reduce the diuretic, natriuretic and antihypertensive effects of thiazide). Products include:
Indocin I.V. 1973

Insulin, Human, Zinc Suspension (Hyperglycemia may occur with thiazide diuretics; dosage adjustment of insulin may be required). Products include:
Humulin L, 100 Units 1763
Humulin U, 100 Units 1770

Insulin, Human NPH (Hyperglycemia may occur with thiazide diuretics; dosage adjustment of insulin may be required). Products include:
Humulin N, 100 Units 1764
Humulin N Pen 1765
Novolin N Human Insulin 10 ml Vials 2322
Novolin N InnoLet 2322
Novolin N PenFill 3 ml Cartridges 2325
Novolin R InnoLet 2322

Insulin, Human Regular (Hyperglycemia may occur with thiazide diuretics; dosage adjustment of insulin may be required). Products include:
Humulin R (U-500) 1768
Humulin R, 100 Units 1767
Novolin R Human Insulin 10 ml Vials 2322
Novolin R PenFill 2325

Insulin, Human Regular and Human NPH Mixture (Hyperglycemia may occur with thiazide diuretics; dosage adjustment of insulin may be required). Products include:
Humulin 50/50, 100 Units 1760
Humulin 70/30 Pen 1761
Novolin 70/30 Human Insulin 10 ml Vials 2321
Novolin 70/30 InnoLet 2322
Novolin 70/30 PenFill 3 ml Cartridges 2325

Insulin, NPH (Hyperglycemia may occur with thiazide diuretics; dosage adjustment of insulin may be required).
No products indexed under this heading.

Insulin, Regular (Hyperglycemia may occur with thiazide diuretics; dosage adjustment of insulin may be required).
No products indexed under this heading.

Insulin, Zinc Crystals (Hyperglycemia may occur with thiazide diuretics; dosage adjustment of insulin may be required).
No products indexed under this heading.

Insulin, Zinc Suspension (Hyperglycemia may occur with thiazide diuretics; dosage adjustment of insulin may be required).
No products indexed under this heading.

Insulin Aspart, Human Regular (Hyperglycemia may occur with thiazide diuretics; dosage adjustment of insulin may be required). Products include:
NovoLog Injection 2326

Insulin glargine (Hyperglycemia may occur with thiazide diuretics; dosage adjustment of insulin may be required). Products include:
Lantus Injection 2925

Insulin Lispro, Human (Hyperglycemia may occur with thiazide diuretics; dosage adjustment of insulin may be required). Products include:

Humalog-Pen 1751
Humalog Mix 75/25-Pen 1754

Insulin Lispro Protamine, Human (Hyperglycemia may occur with thiazide diuretics; dosage adjustment of insulin may be required). Products include:
Humalog Mix 75/25-Pen 1754

Irbesartan (Co-administration of thiazide and other antihypertensive agents can lead to additive effect or potentiation). Products include:
Avalide Tablets 922
Avalide Tablets 2889
Avapro Tablets 925
Avapro Tablets 2886

Isradipine (Co-administration of thiazide and other antihypertensive agents can lead to additive effect or potentiation). Products include:
DynaCirc CR Tablets 2726

Ketoprofen (Co-administration in some patients with compromised renal function who are being treated with NSAIDS may result in a further deterioration of renal function; NSAID may reduce the diuretic, natriuretic and antihypertensive effects of thiazide).
No products indexed under this heading.

Ketorolac Tromethamine (Co-administration in some patients with compromised renal function who are being treated with NSAIDS may result in a further deterioration of renal function; NSAID may reduce the diuretic, natriuretic and antihypertensive effects of thiazide). Products include:
Acular Ophthalmic Solution 561
Acular LS Ophthalmic Solution 562

Labetalol Hydrochloride (Co-administration of thiazide and other antihypertensive agents can lead to additive effect or potentiation).
No products indexed under this heading.

Levorphanol Tartrate (Co-administration of thiazide and narcotics may potentiate orthostatic hypotension).
No products indexed under this heading.

Lisinopril (Co-administration of thiazide and other antihypertensive agents can lead to additive effect or potentiation). Products include:
Prinivil Tablets 2029
Prinzide Tablets 2033
Zestoretic Tablets 701
Zestril Tablets 704

Lithium (Co-administration of lithium with drugs that cause elimination of sodium, including ACE inhibitors, can lead to lithium toxicity; diuretics can reduce renal clearance of lithium and add a high risk of lithium toxicity).
No products indexed under this heading.

Lithium Carbonate (Co-administration of lithium with drugs that cause elimination of sodium, including ACE inhibitors, can lead to lithium toxicity; diuretics can reduce renal clearance of lithium and add a high risk of lithium toxicity). Products include:
Eskalith 1406
Lithobid Tablets 1670

Lithium Citrate (Co-administration of lithium with drugs that cause elimination of sodium, including ACE inhibitors, can lead to lithium toxicity; diuretics can reduce renal clearance of lithium and add a high risk of lithium toxicity).
No products indexed under this heading.

Losartan Potassium (Co-administration of thiazide and other antihypertensive agents can lead to additive effect or potentiation). Products include:
Cozaar Tablets 1913
Hyzaar 1964

Mecamylamine Hydrochloride (Co-administration of thiazide and other antihypertensive agents can lead to additive effect or potentiation). Products include:
Inversine Tablets 3286

Meclofenamate Sodium (Co-administration in some patients with compromised renal function who are being treated with NSAIDS may result in a further deterioration of renal function; NSAID may reduce the diuretic, natriuretic and antihypertensive effects of thiazide).
No products indexed under this heading.

Mefenamic Acid (Co-administration in some patients with compromised renal function who are being treated with NSAIDS may result in a further deterioration of renal function; NSAID may reduce the diuretic, natriuretic and antihypertensive effects of thiazide).
No products indexed under this heading.

Meloxicam (Co-administration in some patients with compromised renal function who are being treated with NSAIDS may result in a further deterioration of renal function; NSAID may reduce the diuretic, natriuretic and antihypertensive effects of thiazide). Products include:
Mobic Oral Suspension 893
Mobic Tablets 893

Meperidine Hydrochloride (Co-administration of thiazide and narcotics may potentiate orthostatic hypotension).
No products indexed under this heading.

Mephobarbital (Co-administration of thiazide and barbiturates may potentiate orthostatic hypotension). Products include:
Mebaral Tablets, USP 2483

Metformin Hydrochloride (Hyperglycemia may occur with thiazide diuretics; dosage adjustment of oral hypoglycemic agents may be required). Products include:
ActoPlus Met Tablets 3219
Avandamet Tablets 1343
Fortamet Extended-Release Tablets 1156

Methadone Hydrochloride (Co-administration of thiazide and narcotics may potentiate orthostatic hypotension).
No products indexed under this heading.

Methyclothiazide (Co-administration of enalapril in patients on diuretics, especially those in whom diuretic therapy was recently instituted, may occasionally experience excessive hypotension; antihypertensive effects of enalapril are augmented by antihypertensive agents that cause renin release).
No products indexed under this heading.

Methyldopa (Co-administration of thiazide and other antihypertensive agents can lead to additive effect or potentiation). Products include:
Aldoclor Tablets 1881
Aldoril Tablets 1884

Methyldopate Hydrochloride (Co-administration of thiazide and other antihypertensive agents can lead to additive effect or potentiation).
No products indexed under this heading.

Methylprednisolone Acetate (Co-administration of thiazide diuretics with corticosteroids intensifies electrolyte depletion, particularly potassium). Products include:
Depo-Medrol Injectable Suspension 2615
Depo-Medrol Single-Dose Vial 2617

Methylprednisolone Sodium Succinate (Co-administration of thiazide diuretics with corticosteroids intensifies electrolyte depletion, particularly potassium).
No products indexed under this heading.

Metocurine Iodide (Co-administration with nondepolarizing skeletal muscle relaxants may result in possible increased responsiveness to the muscle relaxant).
No products indexed under this heading.

Metolazone (Co-administration of enalapril in patients on diuretics, especially those in whom diuretic therapy was recently instituted, may occasionally experience excessive hypotension; antihypertensive effects of enalapril are augmented by antihypertensive agents that cause renin release).
No products indexed under this heading.

Metoprolol Succinate (Co-administration of thiazide and other antihypertensive agents can lead to additive effect or potentiation). Products include:
Toprol-XL Tablets 660

Metoprolol Tartrate (Co-administration of thiazide and other antihypertensive agents can lead to additive effect or potentiation).
No products indexed under this heading.

Metyrosine (Co-administration of thiazide and other antihypertensive agents can lead to additive effect or potentiation). Products include:
Demser Capsules 1933

Mibefradil Dihydrochloride (Co-administration of thiazide and other antihypertensive agents can lead to additive effect or potentiation).
No products indexed under this heading.

Miglitol (Hyperglycemia may occur with thiazide diuretics; dosage adjustment of oral hypoglycemic agents may be required).
No products indexed under this heading.

Minoxidil (Co-administration of thiazide and other antihypertensive agents can lead to additive effect or potentiation). Products include:
Men's Rogaine Extra Strength Topical Solution, Ocean Rush Scent and Original Unscented .... ■□706
Women's Rogaine Topical Solution, Spring Bloom Scent and Original Unscented .... ■□707

Mivacurium Chloride (Co-administration with nondepolarizing skeletal muscle relaxants may result in possible increased responsiveness to the muscle relaxant). Products include:
Mivacron Injection 489

Moexipril Hydrochloride (Co-administration of thiazide and other antihypertensive agents can lead to additive effect or potentiation). Products include:
Uniretic Tablets 3114
Univasc Tablets 3118

Morphine Sulfate (Co-administration of thiazide and narcotics may potentiate orthostatic hypotension). Products include:
Avinza Capsules 1714
Kadian Capsules 572
MS Contin Tablets 2703

Nabumetone (Co-administration in some patients with compromised renal function who are being treated with NSAIDS may result in a further deterioration of renal function; NSAID may reduce the diuretic, natriuretic and antihypertensive effects of thiazide). Products include:
Relafen Tablets 1523

Nadolol (Co-administration of thiazide and other antihypertensive agents can lead to additive effect or potentiation). Products include:
Nadolol Tablets 2121

Naproxen (Co-administration in some patients with compromised renal function who are being treated with NSAIDS may result in a further deterioration of renal function; NSAID may reduce the diuretic, natriuretic and antihypertensive effects of thiazide). Products include:
EC-Naprosyn Delayed-Release Tablets 2769
Naprosyn Suspension 2769
Naprosyn Tablets 2769
Prevacid NapraPAC 3277

Naproxen Sodium (Co-administration in some patients with compromised renal function who are being treated with NSAIDS may result in a further deterioration of renal function; NSAID may reduce the diuretic, natriuretic and antihypertensive effects of thiazide). Products include:
Aleve Tablets, Caplets and Gelcaps .... ■□605
Anaprox Tablets 2769
Anaprox DS Tablets 2769

Nicardipine Hydrochloride (Co-administration of thiazide and other antihypertensive agents can lead to additive effect or potentiation). Products include:
Cardene I.V. 1129

Nifedipine (Co-administration of thiazide and other antihypertensive agents can lead to additive effect or potentiation). Products include:
Adalat CC Tablets 2978

Nisoldipine (Co-administration of thiazide and other antihypertensive agents can lead to additive effect or potentiation). Products include:
Sular Tablets 1163

Nitroglycerin (Co-administration of thiazide and other antihypertensive agents can lead to additive effect or potentiation). Products include:
- Nitro-Dur Transdermal Infusion System 3060
- Nitrolingual Pumpspray 1161

Norepinephrine Bitartrate (Possible decreased response to pressor amines but not sufficient to preclude pressor amine use).
- No products indexed under this heading.

Oxaprozin (Co-administration in some patients with compromised renal function who are being treated with NSAIDS may result in a further deterioration of renal function; NSAID may reduce the diuretic, natriuretic and antihypertensive effects of thiazide).
- No products indexed under this heading.

Oxycodone Hydrochloride (Co-administration of thiazide and narcotics may potentiate orthostatic hypotension). Products include:
- Combunox Tablets 1183
- OxyContin Tablets 2699
- OxyFast Oral Concentrate Solution 2704
- OxyIR Capsules 2704
- Percocet Tablets 1114
- Percodan Tablets 1115

Pancuronium Bromide (Co-administration with nondepolarizing skeletal muscle relaxants may result in possible increased responsiveness to the muscle relaxant).
- No products indexed under this heading.

Penbutolol Sulfate (Co-administration of thiazide and other antihypertensive agents can lead to additive effect or potentiation).
- No products indexed under this heading.

Pentobarbital Sodium (Co-administration of thiazide and barbiturates may potentiate orthostatic hypotension). Products include:
- Nembutal Sodium Solution, USP 2484

Perindopril Erbumine (Co-administration of thiazide and other antihypertensive agents can lead to additive effect or potentiation). Products include:
- Aceon Tablets (2 mg, 4 mg, 8 mg) 3191

Phenobarbital (Co-administration of thiazide and barbiturates may potentiate orthostatic hypotension).
- No products indexed under this heading.

Phenoxybenzamine Hydrochloride (Co-administration of thiazide and other antihypertensive agents can lead to additive effect or potentiation). Products include:
- Dibenzyline Capsules 3390

Phentolamine Mesylate (Co-administration of thiazide and other antihypertensive agents can lead to additive effect or potentiation).
- No products indexed under this heading.

Phenylbutazone (Co-administration in some patients with compromised renal function who are being treated with NSAIDS may result in a further deterioration of renal function; NSAID may reduce the diuretic, natriuretic and antihypertensive effects of thiazide).
- No products indexed under this heading.

Pindolol (Co-administration of thiazide and other antihypertensive agents can lead to additive effect or potentiation).
- No products indexed under this heading.

Pioglitazone Hydrochloride (Hyperglycemia may occur with thiazide diuretics; dosage adjustment of oral hypoglycemic agents may be required). Products include:
- ActoPlus Met Tablets 3219
- Actos Tablets 3224

Piroxicam (Co-administration in some patients with compromised renal function who are being treated with NSAIDS may result in a further deterioration of renal function; NSAID may reduce the diuretic, natriuretic and antihypertensive effects of thiazide).
- No products indexed under this heading.

Polythiazide (Co-administration of enalapril in patients on diuretics, especially those in whom diuretic therapy was recently instituted, may occasionally experience excessive hypotension; antihypertensive effects of enalapril are augmented by antihypertensive agents that cause renin release).
- No products indexed under this heading.

Potassium Acid Phosphate (Concomitant use of potassium-containing salt substitute or potassium supplements can lead to hyperkalemia; frequent monitoring of serum potassium is recommended if used concurrently). Products include:
- K-Phos Original (Sodium Free) Tablets 785

Potassium Bicarbonate (Concomitant use of potassium-containing salt substitute or potassium supplements can lead to hyperkalemia; frequent monitoring of serum potassium is recommended if used concurrently).
- No products indexed under this heading.

Potassium Chloride (Concomitant use of potassium-containing salt substitute or potassium supplements can lead to hyperkalemia; frequent monitoring of serum potassium is recommended if used concurrently). Products include:
- Colyte with Flavor Packs for Oral Solution 3102
- HalfLytely and Bisacodyl Tablets Bowel Prep Kit with Flavors Packs 915
- K-Dur Extended-Relase Tablets 3047
- K-Lor Powder Packets 472
- K-Tab Filmtab Tablets 473
- TriLyte with Flavor Packs for Oral Solution 3114

Potassium Citrate (Concomitant use of potassium-containing salt substitute or potassium supplements can lead to hyperkalemia; frequent monitoring of serum potassium is recommended if used concurrently). Products include:
- Urocit-K Tablets 2109

Potassium Gluconate (Concomitant use of potassium-containing salt substitute or potassium supplements can lead to hyperkalemia; frequent monitoring of serum potassium is recommended if used concurrently).
- No products indexed under this heading.

Potassium Phosphate (Concomitant use of potassium-containing salt substitute or potassium supplements can lead to hyperkalemia; frequent monitoring of serum potassium is recommended if used concurrently). Products include:
- K-Phos Neutral Tablets 785

Prazosin Hydrochloride (Co-administration of thiazide and other antihypertensive agents can lead to additive effect or potentiation).
- No products indexed under this heading.

Prednisolone Acetate (Co-administration of thiazide diuretics with corticosteroids intensifies electrolyte depletion, particularly potassium). Products include:
- Blephamide Ophthalmic Ointment 563
- Blephamide Ophthalmic Suspension 564
- Poly-Pred Liquifilm Ophthalmic Suspension .... ⊙ 231
- Pred Forte Ophthalmic Suspension .... ⊙ 233
- Pred Mild Sterile Ophthalmic Suspension .... ⊙ 236
- Pred-G Ophthalmic Suspension .... ⊙ 234
- Pred-G Sterile Ophthalmic Ointment .... ⊙ 235

Prednisolone Sodium Phosphate (Co-administration of thiazide diuretics with corticosteroids intensifies electrolyte depletion, particularly potassium). Products include:
- Pediapred Oral Solution 3319

Prednisolone Tebutate (Co-administration of thiazide diuretics with corticosteroids intensifies electrolyte depletion, particularly potassium).
- No products indexed under this heading.

Prednisone (Co-administration of thiazide diuretics with corticosteroids intensifies electrolyte depletion, particularly potassium).
- No products indexed under this heading.

Propoxyphene Hydrochloride (Co-administration of thiazide and narcotics may potentiate orthostatic hypotension).
- No products indexed under this heading.

Propoxyphene Napsylate (Co-administration of thiazide and narcotics may potentiate orthostatic hypotension). Products include:
- Darvocet A 500 Tablets 3497

Propranolol Hydrochloride (Co-administration of thiazide and other antihypertensive agents can lead to additive effect or potentiation). Products include:
- Inderal LA Long-Acting Capsules 3421
- InnoPran XL Capsules 2728

Quinapril Hydrochloride (Co-administration of thiazide and other antihypertensive agents can lead to additive effect or potentiation).
- No products indexed under this heading.

Ramipril (Co-administration of thiazide and other antihypertensive agents can lead to additive effect or potentiation). Products include:
- Altace Capsules 1673

Rapacuronium Bromide (Co-administration with nondepolarizing skeletal muscle relaxants may result in possible increased responsiveness to the muscle relaxant).
- No products indexed under this heading.

Rauwolfia Serpentina (Co-administration of thiazide and other antihypertensive agents can lead to additive effect or potentiation).
- No products indexed under this heading.

Remifentanil Hydrochloride (Co-administration of thiazide and narcotics may potentiate orthostatic hypotension).
- No products indexed under this heading.

Repaglinide (Hyperglycemia may occur with thiazide diuretics; dosage adjustment of oral hypoglycemic agents may be required). Products include:
- Prandin Tablets (0.5, 1, and 2 mg) 2337

Rescinnamine (Co-administration of thiazide and other antihypertensive agents can lead to additive effect or potentiation).
- No products indexed under this heading.

Reserpine (Co-administration of thiazide and other antihypertensive agents can lead to additive effect or potentiation).
- No products indexed under this heading.

Rocuronium Bromide (Co-administration with nondepolarizing skeletal muscle relaxants may result in possible increased responsiveness to the muscle relaxant). Products include:
- Zemuron Injection 2363

Rofecoxib (Co-administration in some patients with compromised renal function who are being treated with NSAIDS may result in a further deterioration of renal function; NSAID may reduce the diuretic, natriuretic and antihypertensive effects of thiazide).
- No products indexed under this heading.

Rosiglitazone Maleate (Hyperglycemia may occur with thiazide diuretics; dosage adjustment of oral hypoglycemic agents may be required). Products include:
- Avandamet Tablets 1343
- Avandia Tablets 1348

Secobarbital Sodium (Co-administration of thiazide and barbiturates may potentiate orthostatic hypotension).
- No products indexed under this heading.

Sodium Nitroprusside (Co-administration of thiazide and other antihypertensive agents can lead to additive effect or potentiation).
- No products indexed under this heading.

Sotalol Hydrochloride (Co-administration of thiazide and other antihypertensive agents can lead to additive effect or potentiation).
- No products indexed under this heading.

Spirapril Hydrochloride (Co-administration of thiazide and other antihypertensive agents can lead to additive effect or potentiation).
- No products indexed under this heading.

Spironolactone (Enalapril attenuates diuretic-induced potassium loss; concomitant use can lead to hyperkalemia; frequent monitoring of serum potassium is recommended if used concurrently; co-administration can result in excessive hypotension).
No products indexed under this heading.

Sufentanil Citrate (Co-administration of thiazide and narcotics may potentiate orthostatic hypotension).
No products indexed under this heading.

Sulindac (Co-administration in some patients with compromised renal function who are being treated with NSAIDS may result in a further deterioration of renal function; NSAID may reduce the diuretic, natriuretic and antihypertensive effects of thiazide). Products include:
Clinoril Tablets ... 1899

Telmisartan (Co-administration of thiazide and other antihypertensive agents can lead to additive effect or potentiation). Products include:
Micardis Tablets ... 884
Micardis HCT Tablets ... 886

Terazosin Hydrochloride (Co-administration of thiazide and other antihypertensive agents can lead to additive effect or potentiation). Products include:
Hytrin Capsules ... 469

Thiamylal Sodium (Co-administration of thiazide and barbiturates may potentiate orthostatic hypotension).
No products indexed under this heading.

Timolol Maleate (Co-administration of thiazide and other antihypertensive agents can lead to additive effect or potentiation). Products include:
Blocadren Tablets ... 1891
Cosopt Sterile Ophthalmic Solution ... 1910
Timolide Tablets ... 2056
Timoptic in Ocudose ... 2061
Timoptic Sterile Ophthalmic Solution ... 2058
Timoptic-XE Sterile Ophthalmic Gel Forming Solution ... 2062

Tolazamide (Hyperglycemia may occur with thiazide diuretics; dosage adjustment of oral hypoglycemic agents may be required).
No products indexed under this heading.

Tolbutamide (Hyperglycemia may occur with thiazide diuretics; dosage adjustment of oral hypoglycemic agents may be required).
No products indexed under this heading.

Tolmetin Sodium (Co-administration in some patients with compromised renal function who are being treated with NSAIDS may result in a further deterioration of renal function; NSAID may reduce the diuretic, natriuretic and antihypertensive effects of thiazide).
No products indexed under this heading.

Torsemide (Co-administration of enalapril in patients on diuretics, especially those in whom diuretic therapy was recently instituted, may occasionally experience excessive hypotension; antihypertensive effects of enalapril are augmented by antihypertensive agents that cause renin release).
No products indexed under this heading.

Trandolapril (Co-administration of thiazide and other antihypertensive agents can lead to additive effect or potentiation). Products include:
Mavik Tablets ... 482
Tarka Tablets ... 519

Triamcinolone (Co-administration of thiazide diuretics with corticosteroids intensifies electrolyte depletion, particularly potassium).
No products indexed under this heading.

Triamcinolone Acetonide (Co-administration of thiazide diuretics with corticosteroids intensifies electrolyte depletion, particularly potassium). Products include:
Azmacort Inhalation Aerosol ... 1701
Nasacort HFA Inhalation Aerosol ... 2939
Nasacort AQ Nasal Spray ... 2937

Triamcinolone Diacetate (Co-administration of thiazide diuretics with corticosteroids intensifies electrolyte depletion, particularly potassium).
No products indexed under this heading.

Triamcinolone Hexacetonide (Co-administration of thiazide diuretics with corticosteroids intensifies electrolyte depletion, particularly potassium).
No products indexed under this heading.

Triamterene (Enalapril attenuates diuretic-induced potassium loss; concomitant use can lead to hyperkalemia; frequent monitoring of serum potassium is recommended if used concurrently; co-administration can result in excessive hypotension). Products include:
Dyazide Capsules ... 1389
Dyrenium Capsules ... 3390
Maxzide ... 2150

Trimethaphan Camsylate (Co-administration of thiazide and other antihypertensive agents can lead to additive effect or potentiation).
No products indexed under this heading.

Troglitazone (Hyperglycemia may occur with thiazide diuretics; dosage adjustment of oral hypoglycemic agents may be required).
No products indexed under this heading.

Valdecoxib (Co-administration in some patients with compromised renal function who are being treated with NSAIDS may result in a further deterioration of renal function; NSAID may reduce the diuretic, natriuretic and antihypertensive effects of thiazide).
No products indexed under this heading.

Valsartan (Co-administration of thiazide and other antihypertensive agents can lead to additive effect or potentiation). Products include:
Diovan HCT Tablets ... 2195
Diovan Tablets ... 2191

Vecuronium Bromide (Co-administration with nondepolarizing skeletal muscle relaxants may result in possible increased responsiveness to the muscle relaxant).
No products indexed under this heading.

Verapamil Hydrochloride (Co-administration of thiazide and other antihypertensive agents can lead to additive effect or potentiation). Products include:
Covera-HS Tablets ... 3135
Tarka Tablets ... 519
Verelan PM Capsules ... 3120

Food Interactions

Alcohol (Co-administration of thiazide and alcohol may potentiate orthostatic hypotension).

VASOTEC I.V. INJECTION

(Enalapril Maleate) ... 2076
May interact with diuretics, lithium preparations, non-steroidal anti-inflammatory agents, potassium preparations, and potassium sparing diuretics. Compounds in these categories include:

Amiloride Hydrochloride (Enalapril attenuates diuretic-induced potassium loss; concomitant use can lead to hyperkalemia; frequent monitoring of serum potassium is recommended if used concurrently; co-administration can result in excessive hypotension). Products include:
Midamor Tablets ... 2000
Moduretic Tablets ... 2003

Bendroflumethiazide (Co-administration of enalapril in patients on diuretics, especially those in whom diuretic therapy was recently instituted, may occasionally experience excessive hypotension; antihypertensive effects of enalapril are augmented by antihypertensive agents that cause renin release).
No products indexed under this heading.

Bumetanide (Co-administration of enalapril in patients on diuretics, especially those in whom diuretic therapy was recently instituted, may occasionally experience excessive hypotension; antihypertensive effects of enalapril are augmented by antihypertensive agents that cause renin release).
No products indexed under this heading.

Celecoxib (Co-administration with NSAIDs may diminish the antihypertensive effect of ACE inhibitors; potential for further deterioration of renal function in patients with compromised renal function when used concurrently). Products include:
Celebrex Capsules ... 3130

Chlorothiazide (Co-administration of enalapril in patients on diuretics, especially those in whom diuretic therapy was recently instituted, may occasionally experience excessive hypotension; antihypertensive effects of enalapril are augmented by antihypertensive agents that cause renin release). Products include:
Aldoclor Tablets ... 1881
Diuril Oral ... 1936

Chlorothiazide Sodium (Co-administration of enalapril in patients on diuretics, especially those in whom diuretic therapy was recently instituted, may occasionally experience excessive hypotension; antihypertensive effects of enalapril are augmented by antihypertensive agents that cause renin release). Products include:
Diuril Sodium Intravenous ... 1934

Chlorthalidone (Co-administration of enalapril in patients on diuretics, especially those in whom diuretic therapy was recently instituted, may occasionally experience excessive hypotension; antihypertensive effects of enalapril are augmented by antihypertensive agents that cause renin release). Products include:
Clorpres Tablets ... 2139

Diclofenac Potassium (Co-administration with NSAIDs may diminish the antihypertensive effect of ACE inhibitors; potential for further deterioration of renal function in patients with compromised renal function when used concurrently). Products include:
Cataflam Tablets ... 2173

Diclofenac Sodium (Co-administration with NSAIDs may diminish the antihypertensive effect of ACE inhibitors; potential for further deterioration of renal function in patients with compromised renal function when used concurrently). Products include:
Arthrotec Tablets ... 3126
Voltaren Ophthalmic Solution ... 2300
Voltaren Tablets ... 2298
Voltaren-XR Tablets ... 2301

Ethacrynic Acid (Co-administration of enalapril in patients on diuretics, especially those in whom diuretic therapy was recently instituted, may occasionally experience excessive hypotension; antihypertensive effects of enalapril are augmented by antihypertensive agents that cause renin release). Products include:
Edecrin Tablets ... 1941

Etodolac (Co-administration with NSAIDs may diminish the antihypertensive effect of ACE inhibitors; potential for further deterioration of renal function in patients with compromised renal function when used concurrently).
No products indexed under this heading.

Fenoprofen Calcium (Co-administration with NSAIDs may diminish the antihypertensive effect of ACE inhibitors; potential for further deterioration of renal function in patients with compromised renal function when used concurrently). Products include:
Nalfon Capsules ... 2504

Flurbiprofen (Co-administration with NSAIDs may diminish the antihypertensive effect of ACE inhibitors; potential for further deterioration of renal function in patients with compromised renal function when used concurrently).
No products indexed under this heading.

Furosemide (Co-administration of enalapril in patients on diuretics, especially those in whom diuretic therapy was recently instituted, may occasionally experience excessive hypotension; antihypertensive effects of enalapril are augmented by antihypertensive agents that cause renin release). Products include:
Furosemide Tablets ... 2117

Hydrochlorothiazide (Co-administration of enalapril in patients

on diuretics, especially those in whom diuretic therapy was recently instituted, may occasionally experience excessive hypotension; antihypertensive effects of enalapril are augmented by antihypertensive agents that cause renin release). Products include:

- Aldoril Tablets 1884
- Atacand HCT 637
- Avalide Tablets 2889
- Avalide Tablets 922
- Benicar HCT Tablets 2852
- Diovan HCT Tablets 2195
- Dyazide Capsules 1389
- Hyzaar 1964
- Lotensin HCT Tablets 2235
- Maxzide 2150
- Micardis HCT Tablets 886
- Moduretic Tablets 2003
- Prinzide Tablets 2033
- Teveten HCT Tablets 1710
- Timolide Tablets 2056
- Uniretic Tablets 3114
- Vaseretic Tablets 2073
- Zestoretic Tablets 701

Hydroflumethiazide (Co-administration of enalapril in patients on diuretics, especially those in whom diuretic therapy was recently instituted, may occasionally experience excessive hypotension; antihypertensive effects of enalapril are augmented by antihypertensive agents that cause renin release).
No products indexed under this heading.

Ibuprofen (Co-administration with NSAIDs may diminish the antihypertensive effect of ACE inhibitors; potential for further deterioration of renal function in patients with compromised renal function when used concurrently). Products include:

- Advil Allergy Sinus Caplets 737
- Advil 737
- Children's Advil Suspension 742
- Children's Advil Chewable Tablets 741
- Advil Cold & Sinus 739
- Advil Flu & Body Ache Caplets 739
- Children's Advil Cold Suspension 741
- Infants' Advil Concentrated Drops 743
- Junior Strength Advil Swallow Tablets 740
- Advil Migraine Liquigels 740
- Advil Multi-Symptom Cold Caplets 738
- Combunox Tablets 1183
- Children's Motrin Oral Suspension and Chewable Tablets 1837
- Children's Motrin Cold Non-Staining Dye-Free Oral Suspension 1838
- Children's Motrin Cold Oral Suspension 1838
- Children's Motrin Non-Staining Dye-Free Oral Suspension 1837
- Motrin Cold & Sinus Caplets 1836
- Motrin IB Tablets and Caplets 1836
- Infants' Motrin Concentrated Drops 1837
- Infants' Motrin Non-Staining Dye-Free Drops 1837
- Junior Strength Motrin Caplets and Chewable Tablets 1837
- Vicoprofen Tablets 533

Indapamide (Co-administration of enalapril in patients on diuretics, especially those in whom diuretic therapy was recently instituted, may occasionally experience excessive hypotension; antihypertensive effects of enalapril are augmented by antihypertensive agents that cause renin release). Products include:

- Indapamide Tablets 2119

Indomethacin (Co-administration with NSAIDs may diminish the antihypertensive effect of ACE inhibitors; potential for further deterioration of renal function in patients with compromised renal function when used concurrently). Products include:

- Indocin 1968

Indomethacin Sodium Trihydrate (Co-administration with NSAIDs may diminish the antihypertensive effect of ACE inhibitors; potential for further deterioration of renal function in patients with compromised renal function when used concurrently). Products include:

- Indocin I.V. 1973

Ketoprofen (Co-administration with NSAIDs may diminish the antihypertensive effect of ACE inhibitors; potential for further deterioration of renal function in patients with compromised renal function when used concurrently).
No products indexed under this heading.

Ketorolac Tromethamine (Co-administration with NSAIDs may diminish the antihypertensive effect of ACE inhibitors; potential for further deterioration of renal function in patients with compromised renal function when used concurrently). Products include:

- Acular Ophthalmic Solution 561
- Acular LS Ophthalmic Solution 562

Lithium (Co-administration of lithium with drugs that cause elimination of sodium, including ACE inhibitors, can lead to lithium toxicity).
No products indexed under this heading.

Lithium Carbonate (Co-administration of lithium with drugs that cause elimination of sodium, including ACE inhibitors, can lead to lithium toxicity). Products include:

- Eskalith 1406
- Lithobid Tablets 1670

Lithium Citrate (Co-administration of lithium with drugs that cause elimination of sodium, including ACE inhibitors, can lead to lithium toxicity).
No products indexed under this heading.

Meclofenamate Sodium (Co-administration with NSAIDs may diminish the antihypertensive effect of ACE inhibitors; potential for further deterioration of renal function in patients with compromised renal function when used concurrently).
No products indexed under this heading.

Mefenamic Acid (Co-administration with NSAIDs may diminish the antihypertensive effect of ACE inhibitors; potential for further deterioration of renal function in patients with compromised renal function when used concurrently).
No products indexed under this heading.

Meloxicam (Co-administration with NSAIDs may diminish the antihypertensive effect of ACE inhibitors; potential for further deterioration of renal function in patients with compromised renal function when used concurrently). Products include:

- Mobic Oral Suspension 893
- Mobic Tablets 893

Methyclothiazide (Co-administration of enalapril in patients on diuretics, especially those in whom diuretic therapy was recently instituted, may occasionally experience excessive hypotension; antihypertensive effects of enalapril are augmented by antihypertensive agents that cause renin release).
No products indexed under this heading.

Metolazone (Co-administration of enalapril in patients on diuretics, especially those in whom diuretic therapy was recently instituted, may occasionally experience excessive hypotension; antihypertensive effects of enalapril are augmented by antihypertensive agents that cause renin release).
No products indexed under this heading.

Nabumetone (Co-administration with NSAIDs may diminish the antihypertensive effect of ACE inhibitors; potential for further deterioration of renal function in patients with compromised renal function when used concurrently). Products include:

- Relafen Tablets 1523

Naproxen (Co-administration with NSAIDs may diminish the antihypertensive effect of ACE inhibitors; potential for further deterioration of renal function in patients with compromised renal function when used concurrently). Products include:

- EC-Naprosyn Delayed-Release Tablets 2769
- Naprosyn Suspension 2769
- Naprosyn Tablets 2769
- Prevacid NapraPAC 3277

Naproxen Sodium (Co-administration with NSAIDs may diminish the antihypertensive effect of ACE inhibitors; potential for further deterioration of renal function in patients with compromised renal function when used concurrently). Products include:

- Aleve Tablets, Caplets and Gelcaps 605
- Anaprox Tablets 2769
- Anaprox DS Tablets 2769

Oxaprozin (Co-administration with NSAIDs may diminish the antihypertensive effect of ACE inhibitors; potential for further deterioration of renal function in patients with compromised renal function when used concurrently).
No products indexed under this heading.

Phenylbutazone (Co-administration with NSAIDs may diminish the antihypertensive effect of ACE inhibitors; potential for further deterioration of renal function in patients with compromised renal function when used concurrently).
No products indexed under this heading.

Piroxicam (Co-administration with NSAIDs may diminish the antihypertensive effect of ACE inhibitors; potential for further deterioration of renal function in patients with compromised renal function when used concurrently).
No products indexed under this heading.

Polythiazide (Co-administration of enalapril in patients on diuretics, especially those in whom diuretic therapy was recently instituted, may occasionally experience excessive hypotension; antihypertensive effects of enalapril are augmented by antihypertensive agents that cause renin release).
No products indexed under this heading.

Potassium Acid Phosphate (Concomitant use of potassium-containing salt substitute or potassium supplements can lead to hyperkalemia; frequent monitoring of serum potassium is recommended if used concurrently). Products include:

- K-Phos Original (Sodium Free) Tablets 785

Potassium Bicarbonate (Concomitant use of potassium-containing salt substitute or potassium supplements can lead to hyperkalemia; frequent monitoring of serum potassium is recommended if used concurrently).
No products indexed under this heading.

Potassium Chloride (Concomitant use of potassium-containing salt substitute or potassium supplements can lead to hyperkalemia; frequent monitoring of serum potassium is recommended if used concurrently). Products include:

- Colyte with Flavor Packs for Oral Solution 3102
- HalfLytely and Bisacodyl Tablets Bowel Prep Kit with Flavors Packs 915
- K-Dur Extended-Relase Tablets 3047
- K-Lor Powder Packets 472
- K-Tab Filmtab Tablets 473
- TriLyte with Flavor Packs for Oral Solution 3114

Potassium Citrate (Concomitant use of potassium-containing salt substitute or potassium supplements can lead to hyperkalemia; frequent monitoring of serum potassium is recommended if used concurrently). Products include:

- Urocit-K Tablets 2109

Potassium Gluconate (Concomitant use of potassium-containing salt substitute or potassium supplements can lead to hyperkalemia; frequent monitoring of serum potassium is recommended if used concurrently).
No products indexed under this heading.

Potassium Phosphate (Concomitant use of potassium-containing salt substitute or potassium supplements can lead to hyperkalemia; frequent monitoring of serum potassium is recommended if used concurrently). Products include:

- K-Phos Neutral Tablets 785

Rofecoxib (Co-administration with NSAIDs may diminish the antihypertensive effect of ACE inhibitors; potential for further deterioration of renal function in patients with compromised renal function when used concurrently).
No products indexed under this heading.

Spironolactone (Enalapril attenuates diuretic-induced potassium loss; concomitant use can lead to hyperkalemia; frequent monitoring of serum potassium is recommended if used concurrently; co-administration can result in excessive hypotension).
No products indexed under this heading.

Sulindac (Co-administration with NSAIDs may diminish the antihypertensive effect of ACE inhibitors; potential for further deterioration of renal function in patients with compromised renal function when used concurrently). Products include:
Clinoril Tablets 1899

Tolmetin Sodium (Co-administration with NSAIDs may diminish the antihypertensive effect of ACE inhibitors; potential for further deterioration of renal function in patients with compromised renal function when used concurrently).
No products indexed under this heading.

Torsemide (Co-administration of enalapril in patients on diuretics, especially those in whom diuretic therapy was recently instituted, may occasionally experience excessive hypotension; antihypertensive effects of enalapril are augmented by antihypertensive agents that cause renin release).
No products indexed under this heading.

Triamterene (Enalapril attenuates diuretic-induced potassium loss; concomitant use can lead to hyperkalemia; frequent monitoring of serum potassium is recommended if used concurrently; co-administration can result in excessive hypotension). Products include:
Dyazide Capsules 1389
Dyrenium Capsules 3390
Maxzide 2150

Valdecoxib (Co-administration with NSAIDs may diminish the antihypertensive effect of ACE inhibitors; potential for further deterioration of renal function in patients with compromised renal function when used concurrently).
No products indexed under this heading.

VELCADE FOR INJECTION

(Bortezomib) 2102
May interact with cytochrome p450 2c19 substrates (selected), cytochrome p450 3a4 inducers (selected), cytochrome p450 3a4 inhibitors (selected), and oral hypoglycemic agents. Compounds in these categories include:

Acarbose (Patients on oral antidiabetic agents receiving bortezomib treatment may require close monitoring of their blood glucose levels and adjustment of the dose of their antidiabetic medication; during clinical trials, hypoglycemia and hyperglycemia were reported in diabetic patients receiving oral hypoglycemics). Products include:
Precose Tablets 776

Acetazolamide (Patients who are concomitantly receiving Velcade and drugs that are inhibitors or inducers of cytochrome P450 3A4 should be closely monitored for either toxicities or reduced efficacy).
No products indexed under this heading.

Allium sativum (Patients who are concomitantly receiving Velcade and drugs that are inhibitors or inducers of cytochrome P450 3A4 should be closely monitored for either toxicities or reduced efficacy).
No products indexed under this heading.

Amiodarone Hydrochloride (Patients who are concomitantly receiving Velcade and drugs that are inhibitors or inducers of cytochrome P450 3A4 should be closely monitored for either toxicities or reduced efficacy). Products include:
Pacerone Tablets 3337

Amitriptyline Hydrochloride (Bortezomib may inhibit 2C19 activity and increase exposure to drugs that are substrates for this enzyme).
No products indexed under this heading.

Amoxapine (Bortezomib may inhibit 2C19 activity and increase exposure to drugs that are substrates for this enzyme).
No products indexed under this heading.

Amprenavir (Patients who are concomitantly receiving Velcade and drugs that are inhibitors or inducers of cytochrome P450 3A4 should be closely monitored for either toxicities or reduced efficacy). Products include:
Agenerase Capsules 1299
Agenerase Oral Solution 1304

Anastrozole (Patients who are concomitantly receiving Velcade and drugs that are inhibitors or inducers of cytochrome P450 3A4 should be closely monitored for either toxicities or reduced efficacy). Products include:
Arimidex Tablets 665

Aprepitant (Patients who are concomitantly receiving Velcade and drugs that are inhibitors or inducers of cytochrome P450 3A4 should be closely monitored for either toxicities or reduced efficacy). Products include:
Emend Capsules 1944

Betamethasone Acetate (Patients who are concomitantly receiving Velcade and drugs that are inhibitors or inducers of cytochrome P450 3A4 should be closely monitored for either toxicities or reduced efficacy).
No products indexed under this heading.

Betamethasone Sodium Phosphate (Patients who are concomitantly receiving Velcade and drugs that are inhibitors or inducers of cytochrome P450 3A4 should be closely monitored for either toxicities or reduced efficacy).
No products indexed under this heading.

Carbamazepine (Patients who are concomitantly receiving Velcade and drugs that are inhibitors or inducers of cytochrome P450 3A4 should be closely monitored for either toxicities or reduced efficacy). Products include:
Carbatrol Capsules 3174
Equetro Extended-Release Capsules 3178
Tegretol/Tegretol-XR 2278

Carisoprodol (Bortezomib may inhibit 2C19 activity and increase exposure to drugs that are substrates for this enzyme).
No products indexed under this heading.

Chlorpropamide (Patients on oral antidiabetic agents receiving bortezomib treatment may require close monitoring of their blood glucose levels and adjustment of the dose of their antidiabetic medication; during clinical trials, hypoglycemia and hyperglycemia were reported in diabetic patients receiving oral hypoglycemics).
No products indexed under this heading.

Cilostazol (Bortezomib may inhibit 2C19 activity and increase exposure to drugs that are substrates for this enzyme). Products include:
Pletal Tablets 2478

Cimetidine (Patients who are concomitantly receiving Velcade and drugs that are inhibitors or inducers of cytochrome P450 3A4 should be closely monitored for either toxicities or reduced efficacy). Products include:
Tagamet HB 200 Tablets .... ▣ 637
Tagamet Tablets 1547

Cimetidine Hydrochloride (Patients who are concomitantly receiving Velcade and drugs that are inhibitors or inducers of cytochrome P450 3A4 should be closely monitored for either toxicities or reduced efficacy).
No products indexed under this heading.

Ciprofloxacin (Patients who are concomitantly receiving Velcade and drugs that are inhibitors or inducers of cytochrome P450 3A4 should be closely monitored for either toxicities or reduced efficacy). Products include:
Cipro I.V. 2998
Cipro I.V. Pharmacy Bulk Package ... 3509
Cipro Oral Suspension 2991
Cipro XR Tablets 3004
Ciprodex Otic Suspension 555

Ciprofloxacin Hydrochloride (Patients who are concomitantly receiving Velcade and drugs that are inhibitors or inducers of cytochrome P450 3A4 should be closely monitored for either toxicities or reduced efficacy). Products include:
Ciloxan Ophthalmic Ointment 554
Cipro Tablets 2991

Cisplatin (Patients who are concomitantly receiving Velcade and drugs that are inhibitors or inducers of cytochrome P450 3A4 should be closely monitored for either toxicities or reduced efficacy).
No products indexed under this heading.

Citalopram Hydrobromide (Bortezomib may inhibit 2C19 activity and increase exposure to drugs that are substrates for this enzyme). Products include:
Celexa 1177

Clarithromycin (Patients who are concomitantly receiving Velcade and drugs that are inhibitors or inducers of cytochrome P450 3A4 should be closely monitored for either toxicities or reduced efficacy). Products include:
Biaxin/Biaxin XL 402
PREVPAC 3281

Clomipramine Hydrochloride (Bortezomib may inhibit 2C19 activity and increase exposure to drugs that are substrates for this enzyme).
No products indexed under this heading.

Clotrimazole (Patients who are concomitantly receiving Velcade and drugs that are inhibitors or inducers of cytochrome P450 3A4 should be closely monitored for either toxicities or reduced efficacy). Products include:
Lotrimin 3053
Lotrisone 3054

Cortisone Acetate (Patients who are concomitantly receiving Velcade and drugs that are inhibitors or inducers of cytochrome P450 3A4 should be closely monitored for either toxicities or reduced efficacy).
No products indexed under this heading.

Cyclophosphamide (Bortezomib may inhibit 2C19 activity and increase exposure to drugs that are substrates for this enzyme).
No products indexed under this heading.

Cyclosporine (Patients who are concomitantly receiving Velcade and drugs that are inhibitors or inducers of cytochrome P450 3A4 should be closely monitored for either toxicities or reduced efficacy). Products include:
Gengraf Capsules 458
Neoral Soft Gelatin Capsules 2247
Neoral Oral Solution 2247
Restasis Ophthalmic Emulsion 570
Sandimmune 2259

Dalfopristin (Patients who are concomitantly receiving Velcade and drugs that are inhibitors or inducers of cytochrome P450 3A4 should be closely monitored for either toxicities or reduced efficacy). Products include:
Synercid I.V. 1690

Danazol (Patients who are concomitantly receiving Velcade and drugs that are inhibitors or inducers of cytochrome P450 3A4 should be closely monitored for either toxicities or reduced efficacy).
No products indexed under this heading.

Delavirdine Mesylate (Patients who are concomitantly receiving Velcade and drugs that are inhibitors or inducers of cytochrome P450 3A4 should be closely monitored for either toxicities or reduced efficacy). Products include:
Rescriptor Tablets 2535

Desipramine Hydrochloride (Bortezomib may inhibit 2C19 activity and increase exposure to drugs that are substrates for this enzyme).
No products indexed under this heading.

Dexamethasone (Patients who are concomitantly receiving Velcade and drugs that are inhibitors or inducers of cytochrome P450 3A4 should be closely monitored for either toxicities or reduced efficacy). Products include:
Ciprodex Otic Suspension 555
Decadron Tablets 1929
TobraDex Ophthalmic Ointment 558
TobraDex Ophthalmic Suspension ... 558

Dexamethasone Acetate (Patients who are concomitantly receiving Velcade and drugs that are inhibitors or inducers of cytochrome P450 3A4 should be closely monitored for either toxicities or reduced efficacy).
No products indexed under this heading.

Dexamethasone Sodium Phosphate (Patients who are concomitantly receiving Velcade and drugs that are inhibitors or inducers of cytochrome P450 3A4 should be closely monitored for either toxicities or reduced efficacy). Products include:
Decadron Phosphate Injection 1931

Dextromethorphan (Bortezomib may inhibit 2C19 activity and increase exposure to drugs that are substrates for this enzyme).
No products indexed under this heading.

Dextromethorphan Hydrobromide (Bortezomib may inhibit 2C19 activity and increase exposure to drugs that are substrates for this enzyme). Products include:
Alacol DM Syrup ... 739
Balamine DM ... 739
Contac Severe Cold and Flu Caplets Maximum Strength ... 615
Contac Severe Cold and Flu Caplets Non-Drowsy ... 615
Children's Dimetapp DM Cold & Cough Elixir ... 745
Children's Dimetapp Long Acting Cough Plus Cold Syrup ... 746
Dimetapp Infant Drops Decongestant Plus Cough ... 746
Mucinex DM Tablets ... 602
PediaCare Decongestant & Cough Infant Drops ... 705
PediaCare Freezer Pops Long-Acting Cough-Glacier Grape and Polar Berry Blue ... 706
PediaCare Long-Acting Cough Infant Drops ... 705
PediaCare Long-Acting Cough Plus Cold Liquid ... 704
PediaCare Multi-Symptom Cold Liquid ... 704
PediaCare NightRest Cough & Cold Liquid ... 704
Robitussin Allergy & Cough Syrup ... 750
Robitussin CF Liquid ... 755
Robitussin Cough & Cold Liquid-filled Capsules ... 750
Robitussin Cough, Cold & Flu Liquid-filled Capsules ... 750
Robitussin Cough & Cold Infant Drops ... 755
Robitussin DM Infant Drops ... 753
Robitussin DM Liquid ... 753
Robitussin Flu Liquid ... 752
Robitussin Maximum Strength Cough Liquid ... 754
Robitussin Maximum Strength Cough & Cold Liquid ... 754
Robitussin Pediatric Cough Liquid ... 754
Robitussin Pediatric Cough & Cold Liquid ... 754
Robitussin PM Cough & Cold Liquid ... 752
Robitussin Sugar Free Cough Liquid ... 753
Simply Cough Liquid ... 1840
Sudafed Severe Cold ... 710
TheraFlu Cold & Cough Hot Liquid ... 680
TheraFlu Flu & Chest Congestion Non-Drowsy Hot Liquid ... 681
TheraFlu Severe Cold Non-Drowsy Hot Liquid ... 683
TheraFlu Severe Cold & Cough Hot Liquid ... 683
TheraFlu Severe Cold Caplets ... 679
TheraFlu Severe Cold Hot Liquid ... 682
TheraFlu Severe Cold Non-Drowsy Caplets ... 679
TheraFlu Thin Strips Long Acting Cough ... 684
Triaminic Cold & Cough Liquid ... 685
Triaminic Cough Liquid ... 687
Triaminic Cough & Nasal Congestion Liquid ... 687
Triaminic Cough & Sore Throat Liquid ... 687
Triaminic Flu, Cough & Fever Liquid ... 685
Triaminic Night Time Cough & Cold Liquid ... 685
Triaminic Cold & Cough Softchews ... 688
Triaminic Cough & Sore Throat Softchews ... 689
Triaminic Thin Strips Long Acting Cough ... 689
Children's Tylenol Plus Cold & Cough Suspension Liquid and Chewable Tablets ... 1851
Children's Tylenol Plus Flu Suspension Liquid ... 1853
Concentrated Tylenol Infants' Drops Plus Cold and Cough ... 1851
Tylenol Cold & Flu Severe Daytime Liquid with Cool Burst ... 1846
Tylenol Cold & Flu Severe NightTime Liquid with Cool Burst ... 1846
Tylenol Cold Severe Congestion Non-Drowsy Caplets with Cool Burst ... 1846
Tylenol Cough & Sore Throat Daytime Liquid with Cool Burst ... 1849
Tylenol Cough & Sore Throat NightTime Liquid with Cool Burst ... 1849
Tylenol Flu Day Non-Drowsy Gelcaps ... 1846
Concentrated Tylenol Infants' Drops Plus Cold & Cough Nasal Decongestant, Fever Reducer & Pain Reliever ... 668
Multi-Symptom Tylenol Cold Night Time Caplets ... 1845
Multi-Symptom Tylenol Cold Day Non-Drowsy Caplets and Gelcaps ... 1845
Vicks 44 Cough Relief ... 2675
Vicks 44D Cough & Head Congestion Relief ... 2676
Vicks 44D Cough & Head Congestion Relief Liquid ... 721
Vicks 44E Cough & Chest Congestion Relief ... 2676
Pediatric Vicks 44e Cough & Chest Congestion Relief Liquid ... 2673
Vicks 44M Cough, Cold & Flu Relief ... 2676
Pediatric Vicks 44m Cough & Cold Relief ... 2673
Vicks DayQuil LiquiCaps/Liquid Multi-Symptom Cold/Flu Relief ... 723
Vicks DayQuil Multi-Symptom Cold/Flu Relief LiquiCaps ... 2675
Vicks DayQuil Multi-Symptom Cold/Flu Relief Liquid ... 2675
Children's Vicks NyQuil Cold/Cough Relief ... 2671
Vicks NyQuil Cough Liquid ... 2677
Vicks NyQuil LiquiCaps ... 2677
Vicks NyQuil LiquiCaps/Liquid Multi-Symptom Cold/Flu Relief ... 725
Vicks NyQuil Liquid ... 2677
Zicam Concentrated Cough Mist for Kids Cool Cherry ... 643
Zicam Concentrated Cough Mist for Kids Plus D Cool Cherry ... 643
Zicam Concentrated Cough Mist Nite-Cool Cherry ... 642
Zicam Concentrated Cough Mist Plus D Cool Cherry ... 642
Zicam Concentrated Cough Mist-Honey Lemon & Cool Cherry ... 642

Diazepam (Bortezomib may inhibit 2C19 activity and increase exposure to drugs that are substrates for this enzyme). Products include:
Diastat Rectal Delivery System ... 3344
Valium Tablets ... 2822

Diltiazem Hydrochloride (Patients who are concomitantly receiving Velcade and drugs that are inhibitors or inducers of cytochrome P450 3A4 should be closely monitored for either toxicities or reduced efficacy). Products include:
Cardizem LA Extended Release Tablets ... 1699
Tiazac Capsules ... 1204

Diltiazem Maleate (Patients who are concomitantly receiving Velcade and drugs that are inhibitors or inducers of cytochrome P450 3A4 should be closely monitored for either toxicities or reduced efficacy).
No products indexed under this heading.

Divalproex Sodium (Bortezomib may inhibit 2C19 activity and increase exposure to drugs that are substrates for this enzyme). Products include:
Depakote Sprinkle Capsules ... 422
Depakote Tablets ... 427
Depakote ER Tablets ... 433

Doxepin Hydrochloride (Bortezomib may inhibit 2C19 activity and increase exposure to drugs that are substrates for this enzyme).
No products indexed under this heading.

Doxorubicin Hydrochloride (Patients who are concomitantly receiving Velcade and drugs that are inhibitors or inducers of cytochrome P450 3A4 should be closely monitored for either toxicities or reduced efficacy). Products include:
Adriamycin for Injection, USP ... 786
Adriamycin Injection, USP ... 786

Efavirenz (Patients who are concomitantly receiving Velcade and drugs that are inhibitors or inducers of cytochrome P450 3A4 should be closely monitored for either toxicities or reduced efficacy). Products include:
Sustiva Capsules ... 957

Erythromycin (Patients who are concomitantly receiving Velcade and drugs that are inhibitors or inducers of cytochrome P450 3A4 should be closely monitored for either toxicities or reduced efficacy). Products include:
Erygel Topical Gel ... 2096
Ery-Tab Tablets ... 447
Erythromycin Base Filmtab Tablets ... 454
Erythromycin Delayed-Release Capsules, USP ... 456
PCE Dispertab Tablets ... 510

Erythromycin Estolate (Patients who are concomitantly receiving Velcade and drugs that are inhibitors or inducers of cytochrome P450 3A4 should be closely monitored for either toxicities or reduced efficacy).
No products indexed under this heading.

Erythromycin Ethylsuccinate (Patients who are concomitantly receiving Velcade and drugs that are inhibitors or inducers of cytochrome P450 3A4 should be closely monitored for either toxicities or reduced efficacy). Products include:
E.E.S. ... 449
EryPed ... 445

Erythromycin Gluceptate (Patients who are concomitantly receiving Velcade and drugs that are inhibitors or inducers of cytochrome P450 3A4 should be closely monitored for either toxicities or reduced efficacy).
No products indexed under this heading.

Erythromycin Lactobionate (Patients who are concomitantly receiving Velcade and drugs that are inhibitors or inducers of cytochrome P450 3A4 should be closely monitored for either toxicities or reduced efficacy).
No products indexed under this heading.

Erythromycin Stearate (Patients who are concomitantly receiving Velcade and drugs that are inhibitors or inducers of cytochrome P450 3A4 should be closely monitored for either toxicities or reduced efficacy). Products include:
Erythrocin Stearate Filmtab Tablets ... 452

Esomeprazole Magnesium (Patients who are concomitantly receiving Velcade and drugs that are inhibitors or inducers of cytochrome P450 3A4 should be closely monitored for either toxicities or reduced efficacy). Products include:
Nexium Delayed-Release Capsules ... 645

Ethosuximide (Patients who are concomitantly receiving Velcade and drugs that are inhibitors or inducers of cytochrome P450 3A4 should be closely monitored for either toxicities or reduced efficacy).
No products indexed under this heading.

Ethotoin (Bortezomib may inhibit 2C19 activity and increase exposure to drugs that are substrates for this enzyme). Products include:
Peganone Tablets, USP ... 2487

Felbamate (Patients who are concomitantly receiving Velcade and drugs that are inhibitors or inducers of cytochrome P450 3A4 should be closely monitored for either toxicities or reduced efficacy).
No products indexed under this heading.

Fluconazole (Patients who are concomitantly receiving Velcade and drugs that are inhibitors or inducers of cytochrome P450 3A4 should be closely monitored for either toxicities or reduced efficacy).
No products indexed under this heading.

Fludrocortisone Acetate (Patients who are concomitantly receiving Velcade and drugs that are inhibitors or inducers of cytochrome P450 3A4 should be closely monitored for either toxicities or reduced efficacy).
No products indexed under this heading.

Fluoxetine Hydrochloride (Patients who are concomitantly receiving Velcade and drugs that are inhibitors or inducers of cytochrome P450 3A4 should be closely monitored for either toxicities or reduced efficacy). Products include:
Prozac Pulvules and Liquid ... 1771
Symbyax Capsules ... 1788

Fluvoxamine Maleate (Patients who are concomitantly receiving Velcade and drugs that are inhibitors or inducers of cytochrome P450 3A4 should be closely monitored for either toxicities or reduced efficacy).
No products indexed under this heading.

Formoterol Fumarate (Bortezomib may inhibit 2C19 activity and increase exposure to drugs that are substrates for this enzyme). Products include:
Foradil Aerolizer ... 3024

Fosamprenavir Calcium (Patients who are concomitantly receiving Velcade and drugs that are inhibitors or inducers of cytochrome P450 3A4 should be closely monitored for either toxicities or reduced efficacy). Products include:
Lexiva Tablets ... 1473

Fosphenytoin (Bortezomib may inhibit 2C19 activity and increase exposure to drugs that are substrates for this enzyme).
No products indexed under this heading.

Fosphenytoin Sodium (Patients who are concomitantly receiving Velcade and drugs that are inhibitors or inducers of cytochrome P450 3A4 should be closely monitored for either toxicities or reduced efficacy).
No products indexed under this heading.

IMPORTANT NOTE: Always consult each drug listing in the patient's regimen for possible interactions.

Gabapentin (Bortezomib may inhibit 2C19 activity and increase exposure to drugs that are substrates for this enzyme). Products include:
- Neuronti Capsules 2498
- Neurontin Oral Solution 2498
- Neurontin Tablets 2498

Garlic Extract (Patients who are concomitantly receiving Velcade and drugs that are inhibitors or inducers of cytochrome P450 3A4 should be closely monitored for either toxicities or reduced efficacy).
No products indexed under this heading.

Garlic Oil (Patients who are concomitantly receiving Velcade and drugs that are inhibitors or inducers of cytochrome P450 3A4 should be closely monitored for either toxicities or reduced efficacy).
No products indexed under this heading.

Glimepiride (Patients on oral antidiabetic agents receiving bortezomib treatment may require close monitoring of their blood glucose levels and adjustment of the dose of their antidiabetic medication; during clinical trials, hypoglycemia and hyperglycemia were reported in diabetic patients receiving oral hypoglycemics). Products include:
- Amaryl Tablets 2864

Glipizide (Patients on oral antidiabetic agents receiving bortezomib treatment may require close monitoring of their blood glucose levels and adjustment of the dose of their antidiabetic medication; during clinical trials, hypoglycemia and hyperglycemia were reported in diabetic patients receiving oral hypoglycemics).
No products indexed under this heading.

Glyburide (Patients on oral antidiabetic agents receiving bortezomib treatment may require close monitoring of their blood glucose levels and adjustment of the dose of their antidiabetic medication; during clinical trials, hypoglycemia and hyperglycemia were reported in diabetic patients receiving oral hypoglycemics).
No products indexed under this heading.

Hydrocortisone (Patients who are concomitantly receiving Velcade and drugs that are inhibitors or inducers of cytochrome P450 3A4 should be closely monitored for either toxicities or reduced efficacy). Products include:
- Cortizone•5 Ointment .... ▣699
- Cortizone•10 Creme .... ▣699
- Cortizone•10 Ointment .... ▣699
- Cortizone•10 Plus Creme .... ▣700
- Cortizone•10 Maximum Strength Quick Shot Spray .... ▣700
- Hydrocortone Tablets 1963
- Preparation H Hydrocortisone Cream .... ▣748

Hydrocortisone Acetate (Patients who are concomitantly receiving Velcade and drugs that are inhibitors or inducers of cytochrome P450 3A4 should be closely monitored for either toxicities or reduced efficacy). Products include:
- Analpram-HC 1136
- Pramosone 1139
- ProctoFoam-HC 3113
- Tucks Anti-Itch Ointment .... ▣712
- U-cort 1% Cream 3289

Hydrocortisone Butyrate (Patients who are concomitantly receiving Velcade and drugs that are inhibitors or inducers of cytochrome P450 3A4 should be closely monitored for either toxicities or reduced efficacy). Products include:
- Locoid 1138
- Locoid Lipocream Cream 1138

Hydrocortisone Cypionate (Patients who are concomitantly receiving Velcade and drugs that are inhibitors or inducers of cytochrome P450 3A4 should be closely monitored for either toxicities or reduced efficacy).
No products indexed under this heading.

Hydrocortisone Hemisuccinate (Patients who are concomitantly receiving Velcade and drugs that are inhibitors or inducers of cytochrome P450 3A4 should be closely monitored for either toxicities or reduced efficacy).
No products indexed under this heading.

Hydrocortisone Probutate (Patients who are concomitantly receiving Velcade and drugs that are inhibitors or inducers of cytochrome P450 3A4 should be closely monitored for either toxicities or reduced efficacy). Products include:
- Pandel Cream, 0.1% 1017

Hydrocortisone Sodium Phosphate (Patients who are concomitantly receiving Velcade and drugs that are inhibitors or inducers of cytochrome P450 3A4 should be closely monitored for either toxicities or reduced efficacy).
No products indexed under this heading.

Hydrocortisone Sodium Succinate (Patients who are concomitantly receiving Velcade and drugs that are inhibitors or inducers of cytochrome P450 3A4 should be closely monitored for either toxicities or reduced efficacy).
No products indexed under this heading.

Hydrocortisone Valerate (Patients who are concomitantly receiving Velcade and drugs that are inhibitors or inducers of cytochrome P450 3A4 should be closely monitored for either toxicities or reduced efficacy).
No products indexed under this heading.

Hypericum (Patients who are concomitantly receiving Velcade and drugs that are inhibitors or inducers of cytochrome P450 3A4 should be closely monitored for either toxicities or reduced efficacy).
No products indexed under this heading.

Hypericum Perforatum (Patients who are concomitantly receiving Velcade and drugs that are inhibitors or inducers of cytochrome P450 3A4 should be closely monitored for either toxicities or reduced efficacy).
No products indexed under this heading.

Imipramine Hydrochloride (Bortezomib may inhibit 2C19 activity and increase exposure to drugs that are substrates for this enzyme).
No products indexed under this heading.

Imipramine Pamoate (Bortezomib may inhibit 2C19 activity and increase exposure to drugs that are substrates for this enzyme).
No products indexed under this heading.

Indinavir Sulfate (Patients who are concomitantly receiving Velcade and drugs that are inhibitors or inducers of cytochrome P450 3A4 should be closely monitored for either toxicities or reduced efficacy). Products include:
- Crixivan Capsules 1918

Indomethacin (Bortezomib may inhibit 2C19 activity and increase exposure to drugs that are substrates for this enzyme). Products include:
- Indocin 1968

Indomethacin Sodium Trihydrate (Bortezomib may inhibit 2C19 activity and increase exposure to drugs that are substrates for this enzyme). Products include:
- Indocin I.V. 1973

Isoniazid (Patients who are concomitantly receiving Velcade and drugs that are inhibitors or inducers of cytochrome P450 3A4 should be closely monitored for either toxicities or reduced efficacy).
No products indexed under this heading.

Itraconazole (Patients who are concomitantly receiving Velcade and drugs that are inhibitors or inducers of cytochrome P450 3A4 should be closely monitored for either toxicities or reduced efficacy).
No products indexed under this heading.

Ketoconazole (Patients who are concomitantly receiving Velcade and drugs that are inhibitors or inducers of cytochrome P450 3A4 should be closely monitored for either toxicities or reduced efficacy). Products include:
- Nizoral A-D Shampoo, 1% 1839
- Nizoral 2% Shampoo 1838

Lamotrigine (Bortezomib may inhibit 2C19 activity and increase exposure to drugs that are substrates for this enzyme). Products include:
- Lamictal 1449

Lansoprazole (Bortezomib may inhibit 2C19 activity and increase exposure to drugs that are substrates for this enzyme). Products include:
- Prevacid Delayed-Release Capsules 3268
- Prevacid for Delayed-Release Oral Suspension 3268
- Prevacid I.V. for Injection 3274
- Prevacid NapraPAC 3277
- Prevacid SoluTab Delayed-Release Orally Disintegrating Tablets 3268
- PREVPAC 3281

Levetiracetam (Bortezomib may inhibit 2C19 activity and increase exposure to drugs that are substrates for this enzyme). Products include:
- Keppra Oral Solution 3307
- Keppra Tablets 3307

Lopinavir (Patients who are concomitantly receiving Velcade and drugs that are inhibitors or inducers of cytochrome P450 3A4 should be closely monitored for either toxicities or reduced efficacy). Products include:
- Kaletra 474

Loratadine (Patients who are concomitantly receiving Velcade and drugs that are inhibitors or inducers of cytochrome P450 3A4 should be closely monitored for either toxicities or reduced efficacy). Products include:
- Alavert Allergy & Sinus D-12 Hour Tablets .... ▣743
- Alavert .... ▣743
- Children's Claritin 24 Hour Non-Drowsy Allergy Syrup .... ▣732
- Claritin Non-Drowsy 24 Hour Tablets .... ▣731
- Non-Drowsy Claritin Hives Relief Tablets .... ▣733
- Claritin Reditabs 24 Hour Non-Drowsy Tablets .... ▣732
- Claritin-D Non-Drowsy 12 Hour Tablets .... ▣731
- Claritin-D Non-Drowsy 24 Hour Tablets .... ▣731
- Children's Dimetapp ND Non-Drowsy Allergy Syrup .... ▣746
- Triaminic Allerchews .... ▣684

Maprotiline Hydrochloride (Bortezomib may inhibit 2C19 activity and increase exposure to drugs that are substrates for this enzyme).
No products indexed under this heading.

Mephenytoin (Patients who are concomitantly receiving Velcade and drugs that are inhibitors or inducers of cytochrome P450 3A4 should be closely monitored for either toxicities or reduced efficacy).
No products indexed under this heading.

Mephobarbital (Bortezomib may inhibit 2C19 activity and increase exposure to drugs that are substrates for this enzyme). Products include:
- Mebaral Tablets, USP 2483

Meprobamate (Bortezomib may inhibit 2C19 activity and increase exposure to drugs that are substrates for this enzyme).
No products indexed under this heading.

Metformin Hydrochloride (Patients on oral antidiabetic agents receiving bortezomib treatment may require close monitoring of their blood glucose levels and adjustment of the dose of their antidiabetic medication; during clinical trials, hypoglycemia and hyperglycemia were reported in diabetic patients receiving oral hypoglycemics). Products include:
- ActoPlus Met Tablets 3219
- Avandamet Tablets 1343
- Fortamet Extended-Release Tablets 1156

Methsuximide (Patients who are concomitantly receiving Velcade and drugs that are inhibitors or inducers of cytochrome P450 3A4 should be closely monitored for either toxicities or reduced efficacy).
No products indexed under this heading.

Methylprednisolone (Patients who are concomitantly receiving Velcade and drugs that are inhibitors or inducers of cytochrome P450 3A4 should be closely monitored for either toxicities or reduced efficacy).
No products indexed under this heading.

Methylprednisolone Acetate (Patients who are concomitantly receiving Velcade and drugs that are inhibitors or inducers of cytochrome P450 3A4 should be closely monitored for either toxicities or reduced efficacy). Products include:
- Depo-Medrol Injectable Suspension 2615
- Depo-Medrol Single-Dose Vial 2617

Methylprednisolone Sodium Succinate (Patients who are concomitantly receiving Velcade and drugs that are inhibitors or inducers of cytochrome P450 3A4 should be closely monitored for either toxicities or reduced efficacy).
No products indexed under this heading.

Metronidazole (Patients who are concomitantly receiving Velcade and drugs that are inhibitors or inducers of cytochrome P450 3A4 should be closely monitored for either toxicities or reduced efficacy). Products include:
Metrogel 1% 1212
MetroGel-Vaginal Gel 1822
Noritate Cream, 1% 1051

Metronidazole Benzoate (Patients who are concomitantly receiving Velcade and drugs that are inhibitors or inducers of cytochrome P450 3A4 should be closely monitored for either toxicities or reduced efficacy).
No products indexed under this heading.

Metronidazole Hydrochloride (Patients who are concomitantly receiving Velcade and drugs that are inhibitors or inducers of cytochrome P450 3A4 should be closely monitored for either toxicities or reduced efficacy).
No products indexed under this heading.

Miconazole (Patients who are concomitantly receiving Velcade and drugs that are inhibitors or inducers of cytochrome P450 3A4 should be closely monitored for either toxicities or reduced efficacy).
No products indexed under this heading.

Miconazole Nitrate (Patients who are concomitantly receiving Velcade and drugs that are inhibitors or inducers of cytochrome P450 3A4 should be closely monitored for either toxicities or reduced efficacy). Products include:
Desenex 674
Desenex Jock Itch Spray Powder 674

Midazolam Hydrochloride (Bortezomib may inhibit 2C19 activity and increase exposure to drugs that are substrates for this enzyme).
No products indexed under this heading.

Miglitol (Patients on oral antidiabetic agents receiving bortezomib treatment may require close monitoring of their blood glucose levels and adjustment of the dose of their antidiabetic medication; during clinical trials, hypoglycemia and hyperglycemia were reported in diabetic patients receiving oral hypoglycemics).
No products indexed under this heading.

Modafinil (Patients who are concomitantly receiving Velcade and drugs that are inhibitors or inducers of cytochrome P450 3A4 should be closely monitored for either toxicities or reduced efficacy). Products include:
Provigil Tablets 1002

Nefazodone Hydrochloride (Patients who are concomitantly receiving Velcade and drugs that are inhibitors or inducers of cytochrome P450 3A4 should be closely monitored for either toxicities or reduced efficacy).
No products indexed under this heading.

Nelfinavir Mesylate (Patients who are concomitantly receiving Velcade and drugs that are inhibitors or inducers of cytochrome P450 3A4 should be closely monitored for either toxicities or reduced efficacy). Products include:
Viracept 2556

Nevirapine (Patients who are concomitantly receiving Velcade and drugs that are inhibitors or inducers of cytochrome P450 3A4 should be closely monitored for either toxicities or reduced efficacy). Products include:
Viramune Oral Suspension 903
Viramune Tablets 903

Niacinamide (Patients who are concomitantly receiving Velcade and drugs that are inhibitors or inducers of cytochrome P450 3A4 should be closely monitored for either toxicities or reduced efficacy).
No products indexed under this heading.

Nicotinamide (Patients who are concomitantly receiving Velcade and drugs that are inhibitors or inducers of cytochrome P450 3A4 should be closely monitored for either toxicities or reduced efficacy). Products include:
Nicomide Tablets 3190

Nifedipine (Patients who are concomitantly receiving Velcade and drugs that are inhibitors or inducers of cytochrome P450 3A4 should be closely monitored for either toxicities or reduced efficacy). Products include:
Adalat CC Tablets 2978

Nilutamide (Bortezomib may inhibit 2C19 activity and increase exposure to drugs that are substrates for this enzyme).
No products indexed under this heading.

Norfloxacin (Patients who are concomitantly receiving Velcade and drugs that are inhibitors or inducers of cytochrome P450 3A4 should be closely monitored for either toxicities or reduced efficacy). Products include:
Noroxin Tablets 2009

Nortriptyline Hydrochloride (Bortezomib may inhibit 2C19 activity and increase exposure to drugs that are substrates for this enzyme).
No products indexed under this heading.

Omeprazole (Patients who are concomitantly receiving Velcade and drugs that are inhibitors or inducers of cytochrome P450 3A4 should be closely monitored for either toxicities or reduced efficacy). Products include:
Zegerid Powder for Oral Solution 2972

Oxcarbazepine (Patients who are concomitantly receiving Velcade and drugs that are inhibitors or inducers of cytochrome P450 3A4 should be closely monitored for either toxicities or reduced efficacy). Products include:
Trileptal Oral Suspension 2281
Trileptal Tablets 2281

Pantoprazole Sodium (Bortezomib may inhibit 2C19 activity and increase exposure to drugs that are substrates for this enzyme). Products include:
Protonix I.V. 3468
Protonix Tablets 3465

Paramethadione (Bortezomib may inhibit 2C19 activity and increase exposure to drugs that are substrates for this enzyme).
No products indexed under this heading.

Paroxetine Hydrochloride (Patients who are concomitantly receiving Velcade and drugs that are inhibitors or inducers of cytochrome P450 3A4 should be closely monitored for either toxicities or reduced efficacy). Products include:
Paxil CR Controlled-Release Tablets 1509
Paxil 1501

Pentamidine Isethionate (Bortezomib may inhibit 2C19 activity and increase exposure to drugs that are substrates for this enzyme).
No products indexed under this heading.

Phenacemide (Bortezomib may inhibit 2C19 activity and increase exposure to drugs that are substrates for this enzyme).
No products indexed under this heading.

Phenobarbital (Patients who are concomitantly receiving Velcade and drugs that are inhibitors or inducers of cytochrome P450 3A4 should be closely monitored for either toxicities or reduced efficacy).
No products indexed under this heading.

Phenobarbital Sodium (Patients who are concomitantly receiving Velcade and drugs that are inhibitors or inducers of cytochrome P450 3A4 should be closely monitored for either toxicities or reduced efficacy).
No products indexed under this heading.

Phensuximide (Bortezomib may inhibit 2C19 activity and increase exposure to drugs that are substrates for this enzyme).
No products indexed under this heading.

Phenytoin (Patients who are concomitantly receiving Velcade and drugs that are inhibitors or inducers of cytochrome P450 3A4 should be closely monitored for either toxicities or reduced efficacy).
No products indexed under this heading.

Phenytoin Sodium (Patients who are concomitantly receiving Velcade and drugs that are inhibitors or inducers of cytochrome P450 3A4 should be closely monitored for either toxicities or reduced efficacy). Products include:
Phenytek Capsules 2153

Pioglitazone Hydrochloride (Patients on oral antidiabetic agents receiving bortezomib treatment may require close monitoring of their blood glucose levels and adjustment of the dose of their antidiabetic medication; during clinical trials, hypoglycemia and hyperglycemia were reported in diabetic patients receiving oral hypoglycemics). Products include:
ActoPlus Met Tablets 3219
Actos Tablets 3224

Prednisolone Acetate (Patients who are concomitantly receiving Velcade and drugs that are inhibitors or inducers of cytochrome P450 3A4 should be closely monitored for either toxicities or reduced efficacy). Products include:
Blephamide Ophthalmic Ointment 563
Blephamide Ophthalmic Suspension 564
Poly-Pred Liquifilm Ophthalmic Suspension .... ⊙231
Pred Forte Ophthalmic Suspension .... ⊙233
Pred Mild Sterile Ophthalmic Suspension .... ⊙236
Pred-G Ophthalmic Suspension .... ⊙234
Pred-G Sterile Ophthalmic Ointment .... ⊙235

Prednisolone Sodium Phosphate (Patients who are concomitantly receiving Velcade and drugs that are inhibitors or inducers of cytochrome P450 3A4 should be closely monitored for either toxicities or reduced efficacy). Products include:
Pediapred Oral Solution 3319

Prednisolone Tebutate (Patients who are concomitantly receiving Velcade and drugs that are inhibitors or inducers of cytochrome P450 3A4 should be closely monitored for either toxicities or reduced efficacy).
No products indexed under this heading.

Prednisone (Patients who are concomitantly receiving Velcade and drugs that are inhibitors or inducers of cytochrome P450 3A4 should be closely monitored for either toxicities or reduced efficacy).
No products indexed under this heading.

Primidone (Patients who are concomitantly receiving Velcade and drugs that are inhibitors or inducers of cytochrome P450 3A4 should be closely monitored for either toxicities or reduced efficacy).
No products indexed under this heading.

Progesterone (Bortezomib may inhibit 2C19 activity and increase exposure to drugs that are substrates for this enzyme). Products include:
Prochieve 4% Gel 1018
Prochieve 8% Gel 1018
Prometrium Capsules (100 mg, 200 mg) 3205

Proguanil Hydrochloride (Bortezomib may inhibit 2C19 activity and increase exposure to drugs that are substrates for this enzyme). Products include:
Malarone Tablets 1484
Malarone Pediatric Tablets 1484

Propoxyphene Hydrochloride (Patients who are concomitantly receiving Velcade and drugs that are inhibitors or inducers of cytochrome P450 3A4 should be closely monitored for either toxicities or reduced efficacy).
No products indexed under this heading.

Propoxyphene Napsylate (Patients who are concomitantly receiving Velcade and drugs that are inhibitors or inducers of cytochrome P450 3A4 should be closely monitored for either toxicities or reduced efficacy). Products include:
Darvocet A 500 Tablets 3497

Propranolol Hydrochloride (Bortezomib may inhibit 2C19 activity and

increase exposure to drugs that are substrates for this enzyme). Products include:
Inderal LA Long-Acting Capsules 3421
InnoPran XL Capsules 2728

Protriptyline Hydrochloride (Bortezomib may inhibit 2C19 activity and increase exposure to drugs that are substrates for this enzyme). Products include:
Vivactil Tablets 2350

Quinidine (Patients who are concomitantly receiving Velcade and drugs that are inhibitors or inducers of cytochrome P450 3A4 should be closely monitored for either toxicities or reduced efficacy).
No products indexed under this heading.

Quinidine Hydrochloride (Patients who are concomitantly receiving Velcade and drugs that are inhibitors or inducers of cytochrome P450 3A4 should be closely monitored for either toxicities or reduced efficacy).
No products indexed under this heading.

Quinidine Polygalacturonate (Patients who are concomitantly receiving Velcade and drugs that are inhibitors or inducers of cytochrome P450 3A4 should be closely monitored for either toxicities or reduced efficacy).
No products indexed under this heading.

Quinidine Sulfate (Patients who are concomitantly receiving Velcade and drugs that are inhibitors or inducers of cytochrome P450 3A4 should be closely monitored for either toxicities or reduced efficacy).
No products indexed under this heading.

Quinine (Patients who are concomitantly receiving Velcade and drugs that are inhibitors or inducers of cytochrome P450 3A4 should be closely monitored for either toxicities or reduced efficacy).
No products indexed under this heading.

Quinine Sulfate (Patients who are concomitantly receiving Velcade and drugs that are inhibitors or inducers of cytochrome P450 3A4 should be closely monitored for either toxicities or reduced efficacy).
No products indexed under this heading.

Quinupristin (Patients who are concomitantly receiving Velcade and drugs that are inhibitors or inducers of cytochrome P450 3A4 should be closely monitored for either toxicities or reduced efficacy). Products include:
Synercid I.V. 1690

Rabeprazole Sodium (Bortezomib may inhibit 2C19 activity and increase exposure to drugs that are substrates for this enzyme). Products include:
Aciphex Tablets 1081

Ranitidine Bismuth Citrate (Patients who are concomitantly receiving Velcade and drugs that are inhibitors or inducers of cytochrome P450 3A4 should be closely monitored for either toxicities or reduced efficacy).
No products indexed under this heading.

Ranitidine Hydrochloride (Patients who are concomitantly receiving Velcade and drugs that are inhibitors or inducers of cytochrome P450 3A4 should be closely monitored for either toxicities or reduced efficacy). Products include:
Zantac 1597
Zantac Injection 1593
Zantac 75 Tablets .... ▣715
Zantac 150 Maximum Strength Tablets .... ▣715
Zantac Injection Pharmacy Bulk Package 1595

Repaglinide (Patients on oral antidiabetic agents receiving bortezomib treatment may require close monitoring of their blood glucose levels and adjustment of the dose of their antidiabetic medication; during clinical trials, hypoglycemia and hyperglycemia were reported in diabetic patients receiving oral hypoglycemics). Products include:
Prandin Tablets (0.5, 1, and 2 mg) 2337

Rifabutin (Patients who are concomitantly receiving Velcade and drugs that are inhibitors or inducers of cytochrome P450 3A4 should be closely monitored for either toxicities or reduced efficacy).
No products indexed under this heading.

Rifampicin (Patients who are concomitantly receiving Velcade and drugs that are inhibitors or inducers of cytochrome P450 3A4 should be closely monitored for either toxicities or reduced efficacy).
No products indexed under this heading.

Rifampin (Patients who are concomitantly receiving Velcade and drugs that are inhibitors or inducers of cytochrome P450 3A4 should be closely monitored for either toxicities or reduced efficacy).
No products indexed under this heading.

Rifapentine (Patients who are concomitantly receiving Velcade and drugs that are inhibitors or inducers of cytochrome P450 3A4 should be closely monitored for either toxicities or reduced efficacy).
No products indexed under this heading.

Ritonavir (Patients who are concomitantly receiving Velcade and drugs that are inhibitors or inducers of cytochrome P450 3A4 should be closely monitored for either toxicities or reduced efficacy). Products include:
Kaletra 474
Norvir 499

Rosiglitazone Maleate (Patients on oral antidiabetic agents receiving bortezomib treatment may require close monitoring of their blood glucose levels and adjustment of the dose of their antidiabetic medication; during clinical trials, hypoglycemia and hyperglycemia were reported in diabetic patients receiving oral hypoglycemics). Products include:
Avandamet Tablets 1343
Avandia Tablets 1348

Saquinavir (Patients who are concomitantly receiving Velcade and drugs that are inhibitors or inducers of cytochrome P450 3A4 should be closely monitored for either toxicities or reduced efficacy).
No products indexed under this heading.

Saquinavir Mesylate (Patients who are concomitantly receiving Velcade and drugs that are inhibitors or inducers of cytochrome P450 3A4 should be closely monitored for either toxicities or reduced efficacy). Products include:
Invirase 2776

Sertraline Hydrochloride (Patients who are concomitantly receiving Velcade and drugs that are inhibitors or inducers of cytochrome P450 3A4 should be closely monitored for either toxicities or reduced efficacy). Products include:
Zoloft 2581

Sulfinpyrazone (Patients who are concomitantly receiving Velcade and drugs that are inhibitors or inducers of cytochrome P450 3A4 should be closely monitored for either toxicities or reduced efficacy).
No products indexed under this heading.

Telithromycin (Patients who are concomitantly receiving Velcade and drugs that are inhibitors or inducers of cytochrome P450 3A4 should be closely monitored for either toxicities or reduced efficacy). Products include:
Ketek Tablets 2920

Teniposide (Bortezomib may inhibit 2C19 activity and increase exposure to drugs that are substrates for this enzyme).
No products indexed under this heading.

Theophylline (Patients who are concomitantly receiving Velcade and drugs that are inhibitors or inducers of cytochrome P450 3A4 should be closely monitored for either toxicities or reduced efficacy).
No products indexed under this heading.

Thioridazine (Bortezomib may inhibit 2C19 activity and increase exposure to drugs that are substrates for this enzyme).
No products indexed under this heading.

Thioridazine Hydrochloride (Bortezomib may inhibit 2C19 activity and increase exposure to drugs that are substrates for this enzyme). Products include:
Thioridazine Hydrochloride Tablets 2122

Tiagabine Hydrochloride (Bortezomib may inhibit 2C19 activity and increase exposure to drugs that are substrates for this enzyme). Products include:
Gabitril Tablets 998

Tolazamide (Patients on oral antidiabetic agents receiving bortezomib treatment may require close monitoring of their blood glucose levels and adjustment of the dose of their antidiabetic medication; during clinical trials, hypoglycemia and hyperglycemia were reported in diabetic patients receiving oral hypoglycemics).
No products indexed under this heading.

Tolbutamide (Bortezomib may inhibit 2C19 activity and increase exposure to drugs that are substrates for this enzyme).
No products indexed under this heading.

Tolbutamide Sodium (Bortezomib may inhibit 2C19 activity and increase exposure to drugs that are substrates for this enzyme).
No products indexed under this heading.

Topiramate (Bortezomib may inhibit 2C19 activity and increase exposure to drugs that are substrates for this enzyme). Products include:
Topamax Sprinkle Capsules 2438
Topamax Tablets 2438

Triamcinolone (Patients who are concomitantly receiving Velcade and drugs that are inhibitors or inducers of cytochrome P450 3A4 should be closely monitored for either toxicities or reduced efficacy).
No products indexed under this heading.

Triamcinolone Acetonide (Patients who are concomitantly receiving Velcade and drugs that are inhibitors or inducers of cytochrome P450 3A4 should be closely monitored for either toxicities or reduced efficacy). Products include:
Azmacort Inhalation Aerosol 1701
Nasacort HFA Inhalation Aerosol 2939
Nasacort AQ Nasal Spray 2937

Triamcinolone Diacetate (Patients who are concomitantly receiving Velcade and drugs that are inhibitors or inducers of cytochrome P450 3A4 should be closely monitored for either toxicities or reduced efficacy).
No products indexed under this heading.

Triamcinolone Hexacetonide (Patients who are concomitantly receiving Velcade and drugs that are inhibitors or inducers of cytochrome P450 3A4 should be closely monitored for either toxicities or reduced efficacy).
No products indexed under this heading.

Trimethadione (Bortezomib may inhibit 2C19 activity and increase exposure to drugs that are substrates for this enzyme).
No products indexed under this heading.

Trimipramine Maleate (Bortezomib may inhibit 2C19 activity and increase exposure to drugs that are substrates for this enzyme). Products include:
Surmontil Capsules 2347

Troglitazone (Patients who are concomitantly receiving Velcade and drugs that are inhibitors or inducers of cytochrome P450 3A4 should be closely monitored for either toxicities or reduced efficacy).
No products indexed under this heading.

Troleandomycin (Patients who are concomitantly receiving Velcade and drugs that are inhibitors or inducers of cytochrome P450 3A4 should be closely monitored for either toxicities or reduced efficacy).
No products indexed under this heading.

Valproate Sodium (Patients who are concomitantly receiving Velcade and drugs that are inhibitors or inducers of cytochrome P450 3A4 should be closely monitored for either toxicities or reduced efficacy). Products include:
Depacon Injection 412

Valproic Acid (Bortezomib may inhibit 2C19 activity and increase exposure to drugs that are substrates for this enzyme). Products include:
Depakene 417

Verapamil Hydrochloride (Patients who are concomitantly receiving Velcade and drugs that are

inhibitors or inducers of cytochrome P450 3A4 should be closely monitored for either toxicities or reduced efficacy). Products include:
- Covera-HS Tablets 3135
- Tarka Tablets 519
- Verelan PM Capsules 3120

Voriconazole (Patients who are concomitantly receiving Velcade and drugs that are inhibitors or inducers of cytochrome P450 3A4 should be closely monitored for either toxicities or reduced efficacy). Products include:
- VFEND I.V. 2543
- VFEND Oral Suspension 2543
- VFEND Tablets 2543

Warfarin Sodium (Bortezomib may inhibit 2C19 activity and increase exposure to drugs that are substrates for this enzyme). Products include:
- Coumadin for Injection 932
- Coumadin Tablets 932

Zafirlukast (Patients who are concomitantly receiving Velcade and drugs that are inhibitors or inducers of cytochrome P450 3A4 should be closely monitored for either toxicities or reduced efficacy). Products include:
- Accolate Tablets 663

Zileuton (Patients who are concomitantly receiving Velcade and drugs that are inhibitors or inducers of cytochrome P450 3A4 should be closely monitored for either toxicities or reduced efficacy).
No products indexed under this heading.

Zonisamide (Bortezomib may inhibit 2C19 activity and increase exposure to drugs that are substrates for this enzyme). Products include:
- Zonegran Capsules 1089

Food Interactions

Grapefruit (Patients who are concomitantly receiving Velcade and drugs that are inhibitors or inducers of cytochrome P450 3A4 should be closely monitored for either toxicities or reduced efficacy).

Grapefruit Juice (Patients who are concomitantly receiving Velcade and drugs that are inhibitors or inducers of cytochrome P450 3A4 should be closely monitored for either toxicities or reduced efficacy).

VEMMA NUTRITION PROGRAM - ESSENTIAL MINERALS
(Minerals, Multiple) 778
None cited in PDR database.

VEMMA NUTRITION PROGRAM - MANGOSTEEN PLUS
(Aloe vera, Herbals with Vitamins, Phytonutrients) 778
None cited in PDR database.

VENTAVIS INHALATION SOLUTION
(Iloprost) 1036
May interact with antihypertensives, anticoagulants, and vasodilators. Compounds in these categories include:

Acebutolol Hydrochloride (Iloprost has the potential to increase the hypotensive effect of vasodilators and antihypertensive agents).
No products indexed under this heading.

Amlodipine Besylate (Iloprost has the potential to increase the hypotensive effect of vasodilators and antihypertensive agents). Products include:
- Caduet Tablets 2507
- Lotrel Capsules 2238
- Norvasc Tablets 2529

Amyl Nitrite (Iloprost has the potential to increase the hypotensive effect of vasodilators and antihypertensive agents).
No products indexed under this heading.

Anisindione (Since iloprost inhibits platelet function, there is a potential for increased risk of bleeding, particularly in patients maintained on anticoagulants). Products include:
- Miradon Tablets 3056

Ardeparin Sodium (Since iloprost inhibits platelet function, there is a potential for increased risk of bleeding, particularly in patients maintained on anticoagulants).
No products indexed under this heading.

Atenolol (Iloprost has the potential to increase the hypotensive effect of vasodilators and antihypertensive agents). Products include:
- Tenormin I.V. Injection 698
- Tenormin Tablets 695

Benazepril Hydrochloride (Iloprost has the potential to increase the hypotensive effect of vasodilators and antihypertensive agents). Products include:
- Lotensin Tablets 2232
- Lotensin HCT Tablets 2235
- Lotrel Capsules 2238

Bendroflumethiazide (Iloprost has the potential to increase the hypotensive effect of vasodilators and antihypertensive agents).
No products indexed under this heading.

Betaxolol Hydrochloride (Iloprost has the potential to increase the hypotensive effect of vasodilators and antihypertensive agents). Products include:
- Betoptic S Ophthalmic Suspension 554

Bisoprolol Fumarate (Iloprost has the potential to increase the hypotensive effect of vasodilators and antihypertensive agents).
No products indexed under this heading.

Candesartan Cilexetil (Iloprost has the potential to increase the hypotensive effect of vasodilators and antihypertensive agents). Products include:
- Atacand Tablets 634
- Atacand HCT 637

Captopril (Iloprost has the potential to increase the hypotensive effect of vasodilators and antihypertensive agents). Products include:
- Captopril Tablets 2114

Carteolol Hydrochloride (Iloprost has the potential to increase the hypotensive effect of vasodilators and antihypertensive agents). Products include:
- Carteolol Hydrochloride Ophthalmic Solution USP, 1% .... ⊙246

Chlorothiazide (Iloprost has the potential to increase the hypotensive effect of vasodilators and antihypertensive agents). Products include:
- Aldoclor Tablets 1881
- Diuril Oral 1936

Chlorothiazide Sodium (Iloprost has the potential to increase the hypotensive effect of vasodilators and antihypertensive agents). Products include:
- Diuril Sodium Intravenous 1934

Chlorthalidone (Iloprost has the potential to increase the hypotensive effect of vasodilators and antihypertensive agents). Products include:
- Clorpres Tablets 2139

Clonidine (Iloprost has the potential to increase the hypotensive effect of vasodilators and antihypertensive agents). Products include:
- Catapres-TTS 875

Clonidine Hydrochloride (Iloprost has the potential to increase the hypotensive effect of vasodilators and antihypertensive agents). Products include:
- Catapres Tablets 874
- Clorpres Tablets 2139

Dalteparin Sodium (Since iloprost inhibits platelet function, there is a potential for increased risk of bleeding, particularly in patients maintained on anticoagulants). Products include:
- Fragmin Injection 2638

Danaparoid Sodium (Since iloprost inhibits platelet function, there is a potential for increased risk of bleeding, particularly in patients maintained on anticoagulants).
No products indexed under this heading.

Deserpidine (Iloprost has the potential to increase the hypotensive effect of vasodilators and antihypertensive agents).
No products indexed under this heading.

Diazoxide (Iloprost has the potential to increase the hypotensive effect of vasodilators and antihypertensive agents). Products include:
- Hyperstat I.V. Injection 3031

Dicumarol (Since iloprost inhibits platelet function, there is a potential for increased risk of bleeding, particularly in patients maintained on anticoagulants).
No products indexed under this heading.

Diltiazem Hydrochloride (Iloprost has the potential to increase the hypotensive effect of vasodilators and antihypertensive agents). Products include:
- Cardizem LA Extended Release Tablets 1699
- Tiazac Capsules 1204

Doxazosin Mesylate (Iloprost has the potential to increase the hypotensive effect of vasodilators and antihypertensive agents).
No products indexed under this heading.

Enalapril Maleate (Iloprost has the potential to increase the hypotensive effect of vasodilators and antihypertensive agents). Products include:
- Vaseretic Tablets 2073
- Vasotec I.V. Injection 2076

Enalaprilat (Iloprost has the potential to increase the hypotensive effect of vasodilators and antihypertensive agents).
No products indexed under this heading.

Enoxaparin Sodium (Since iloprost inhibits platelet function, there is a potential for increased risk of bleeding, particularly in patients maintained on anticoagulants). Products include:
- Lovenox Injection 2931

Epoprostenol Sodium (Iloprost has the potential to increase the hypotensive effect of vasodilators and antihypertensive agents). Products include:
- Flolan for Injection 1408

Eprosartan Mesylate (Iloprost has the potential to increase the hypotensive effect of vasodilators and antihypertensive agents). Products include:
- Teveten Tablets 1707
- Teveten HCT Tablets 1710

Esmolol Hydrochloride (Iloprost has the potential to increase the hypotensive effect of vasodilators and antihypertensive agents). Products include:
- Brevibloc Concentrate 766
- Brevibloc Injection 766
- Brevibloc Double Strength Injection 766
- Brevibloc Premixed Injection 766
- Brevibloc Double Strength Premixed Injection 766

Ethaverine Hydrochloride (Iloprost has the potential to increase the hypotensive effect of vasodilators and antihypertensive agents).
No products indexed under this heading.

Felodipine (Iloprost has the potential to increase the hypotensive effect of vasodilators and antihypertensive agents). Products include:
- Plendil Extended-Release Tablets 651

Fondaparinux Sodium (Since iloprost inhibits platelet function, there is a potential for increased risk of bleeding, particularly in patients maintained on anticoagulants). Products include:
- Arixtra Injection 1325

Fosinopril Sodium (Iloprost has the potential to increase the hypotensive effect of vasodilators and antihypertensive agents).
No products indexed under this heading.

Furosemide (Iloprost has the potential to increase the hypotensive effect of vasodilators and antihypertensive agents). Products include:
- Furosemide Tablets 2117

Guanabenz Acetate (Iloprost has the potential to increase the hypotensive effect of vasodilators and antihypertensive agents).
No products indexed under this heading.

Guanethidine Monosulfate (Iloprost has the potential to increase the hypotensive effect of vasodilators and antihypertensive agents).
No products indexed under this heading.

Heparin Calcium (Since iloprost inhibits platelet function, there is a potential for increased risk of bleeding, particularly in patients maintained on anticoagulants).
No products indexed under this heading.

Heparin Sodium (Since iloprost inhibits platelet function, there is a potential for increased risk of bleeding, particularly in patients maintained on anticoagulants).
No products indexed under this heading.

Hydralazine Hydrochloride (Iloprost has the potential to increase the hypotensive effect of vasodilators and antihypertensive agents). Products include:
- BiDil Tablets 2161

Hydrochlorothiazide (Iloprost has the potential to increase the hypotensive effect of vasodilators and antihypertensive agents). Products include:
Aldoril Tablets 1884
Atacand HCT 637
Avalide Tablets 2889
Avalide Tablets 922
Benicar HCT Tablets 2852
Diovan HCT Tablets 2195
Dyazide Capsules 1389
Hyzaar 1964
Lotensin HCT Tablets 2235
Maxzide 2150
Micardis HCT Tablets 886
Moduretic Tablets 2003
Prinzide Tablets 2033
Teveten HCT Tablets 1710
Timolide Tablets 2056
Uniretic Tablets 3114
Vaseretic Tablets 2073
Zestoretic Tablets 701

Hydroflumethiazide (Iloprost has the potential to increase the hypotensive effect of vasodilators and antihypertensive agents).
No products indexed under this heading.

Indapamide (Iloprost has the potential to increase the hypotensive effect of vasodilators and antihypertensive agents). Products include:
Indapamide Tablets 2119

Irbesartan (Iloprost has the potential to increase the hypotensive effect of vasodilators and antihypertensive agents). Products include:
Avalide Tablets 922
Avalide Tablets 2889
Avapro Tablets 925
Avapro Tablets 2886

Isosorbide Dinitrate (Iloprost has the potential to increase the hypotensive effect of vasodilators and antihypertensive agents). Products include:
BiDil Tablets 2161

Isosorbide Mononitrate (Iloprost has the potential to increase the hypotensive effect of vasodilators and antihypertensive agents). Products include:
Imdur Tablets 3032

Isoxsuprine Hydrochloride (Iloprost has the potential to increase the hypotensive effect of vasodilators and antihypertensive agents).
No products indexed under this heading.

Isradipine (Iloprost has the potential to increase the hypotensive effect of vasodilators and antihypertensive agents). Products include:
DynaCirc CR Tablets 2726

Labetalol Hydrochloride (Iloprost has the potential to increase the hypotensive effect of vasodilators and antihypertensive agents).
No products indexed under this heading.

Lisinopril (Iloprost has the potential to increase the hypotensive effect of vasodilators and antihypertensive agents). Products include:
Prinivil Tablets 2029
Prinzide Tablets 2033
Zestoretic Tablets 701
Zestril Tablets 704

Losartan Potassium (Iloprost has the potential to increase the hypotensive effect of vasodilators and antihypertensive agents). Products include:
Cozaar Tablets 1913
Hyzaar 1964

Low Molecular Weight Heparins (Since iloprost inhibits platelet function, there is a potential for increased risk of bleeding, particularly in patients maintained on anticoagulants).
No products indexed under this heading.

Mecamylamine Hydrochloride (Iloprost has the potential to increase the hypotensive effect of vasodilators and antihypertensive agents). Products include:
Inversine Tablets 3286

Methyclothiazide (Iloprost has the potential to increase the hypotensive effect of vasodilators and antihypertensive agents).
No products indexed under this heading.

Methyldopa (Iloprost has the potential to increase the hypotensive effect of vasodilators and antihypertensive agents). Products include:
Aldoclor Tablets 1881
Aldoril Tablets 1884

Methyldopate Hydrochloride (Iloprost has the potential to increase the hypotensive effect of vasodilators and antihypertensive agents).
No products indexed under this heading.

Metolazone (Iloprost has the potential to increase the hypotensive effect of vasodilators and antihypertensive agents).
No products indexed under this heading.

Metoprolol Succinate (Iloprost has the potential to increase the hypotensive effect of vasodilators and antihypertensive agents). Products include:
Toprol-XL Tablets 660

Metoprolol Tartrate (Iloprost has the potential to increase the hypotensive effect of vasodilators and antihypertensive agents).
No products indexed under this heading.

Metyrosine (Iloprost has the potential to increase the hypotensive effect of vasodilators and antihypertensive agents). Products include:
Demser Capsules 1933

Mibefradil Dihydrochloride (Iloprost has the potential to increase the hypotensive effect of vasodilators and antihypertensive agents).
No products indexed under this heading.

Minoxidil (Iloprost has the potential to increase the hypotensive effect of vasodilators and antihypertensive agents). Products include:
Men's Rogaine Extra Strength Topical Solution, Ocean Rush Scent and Original Unscented .... ▣ 706
Women's Rogaine Topical Solution, Spring Bloom Scent and Original Unscented .... ▣ 707

Moexipril Hydrochloride (Iloprost has the potential to increase the hypotensive effect of vasodilators and antihypertensive agents). Products include:
Uniretic Tablets 3114
Univasc Tablets 3118

Nadolol (Iloprost has the potential to increase the hypotensive effect of vasodilators and antihypertensive agents). Products include:
Nadolol Tablets 2121

Nicardipine Hydrochloride (Iloprost has the potential to increase the hypotensive effect of vasodilators and antihypertensive agents). Products include:
Cardene I.V. 1129

Nifedipine (Iloprost has the potential to increase the hypotensive effect of vasodilators and antihypertensive agents). Products include:
Adalat CC Tablets 2978

Nisoldipine (Iloprost has the potential to increase the hypotensive effect of vasodilators and antihypertensive agents). Products include:
Sular Tablets 1163

Nitroglycerin (Iloprost has the potential to increase the hypotensive effect of vasodilators and antihypertensive agents). Products include:
Nitro-Dur Transdermal Infusion System 3060
Nitrolingual Pumpspray 1161

Nitroglycerin, long-acting formulations (Iloprost has the potential to increase the hypotensive effect of vasodilators and antihypertensive agents).
No products indexed under this heading.

Nitroglycerin Intravenous (Iloprost has the potential to increase the hypotensive effect of vasodilators and antihypertensive agents).
No products indexed under this heading.

Papaverine (Iloprost has the potential to increase the hypotensive effect of vasodilators and antihypertensive agents).
No products indexed under this heading.

Papaverine Hydrochloride (Iloprost has the potential to increase the hypotensive effect of vasodilators and antihypertensive agents).
No products indexed under this heading.

Penbutolol Sulfate (Iloprost has the potential to increase the hypotensive effect of vasodilators and antihypertensive agents).
No products indexed under this heading.

Perindopril Erbumine (Iloprost has the potential to increase the hypotensive effect of vasodilators and antihypertensive agents). Products include:
Aceon Tablets (2 mg, 4 mg, 8 mg) 3191

Phenoxybenzamine Hydrochloride (Iloprost has the potential to increase the hypotensive effect of vasodilators and antihypertensive agents). Products include:
Dibenzyline Capsules 3390

Phentolamine Mesylate (Iloprost has the potential to increase the hypotensive effect of vasodilators and antihypertensive agents).
No products indexed under this heading.

Pindolol (Iloprost has the potential to increase the hypotensive effect of vasodilators and antihypertensive agents).
No products indexed under this heading.

Polythiazide (Iloprost has the potential to increase the hypotensive effect of vasodilators and antihypertensive agents).
No products indexed under this heading.

Prazosin Hydrochloride (Iloprost has the potential to increase the hypotensive effect of vasodilators and antihypertensive agents).
No products indexed under this heading.

Propranolol Hydrochloride (Iloprost has the potential to increase the hypotensive effect of vasodilators and antihypertensive agents). Products include:
Inderal LA Long-Acting Capsules 3421
InnoPran XL Capsules 2728

Quinapril Hydrochloride (Iloprost has the potential to increase the hypotensive effect of vasodilators and antihypertensive agents).
No products indexed under this heading.

Ramipril (Iloprost has the potential to increase the hypotensive effect of vasodilators and antihypertensive agents). Products include:
Altace Capsules 1673

Rauwolfia Serpentina (Iloprost has the potential to increase the hypotensive effect of vasodilators and antihypertensive agents).
No products indexed under this heading.

Rescinnamine (Iloprost has the potential to increase the hypotensive effect of vasodilators and antihypertensive agents).
No products indexed under this heading.

Reserpine (Iloprost has the potential to increase the hypotensive effect of vasodilators and antihypertensive agents).
No products indexed under this heading.

Sodium Nitroprusside (Iloprost has the potential to increase the hypotensive effect of vasodilators and antihypertensive agents).
No products indexed under this heading.

Sotalol Hydrochloride (Iloprost has the potential to increase the hypotensive effect of vasodilators and antihypertensive agents).
No products indexed under this heading.

Spirapril Hydrochloride (Iloprost has the potential to increase the hypotensive effect of vasodilators and antihypertensive agents).
No products indexed under this heading.

Telmisartan (Iloprost has the potential to increase the hypotensive effect of vasodilators and antihypertensive agents). Products include:
Micardis Tablets 884
Micardis HCT Tablets 886

Terazosin Hydrochloride (Iloprost has the potential to increase the hypotensive effect of vasodilators and antihypertensive agents). Products include:
Hytrin Capsules 469

Timolol Maleate (Iloprost has the potential to increase the hypotensive effect of vasodilators and antihypertensive agents). Products include:
Blocadren Tablets 1891
Cosopt Sterile Ophthalmic Solution 1910
Timolide Tablets 2056
Timoptic in Ocudose 2061
Timoptic Sterile Ophthalmic Solution 2058
Timoptic-XE Sterile Ophthalmic Gel Forming Solution 2062

Tinzaparin Sodium (Since iloprost inhibits platelet function, there is a potential for increased risk of bleeding, particularly in patients maintained on anticoagulants).
No products indexed under this heading.

Tolazoline Hydrochloride (Iloprost has the potential to increase the hypotensive effect of vasodilators and antihypertensive agents).
No products indexed under this heading.

Torsemide (Iloprost has the potential to increase the hypotensive effect of vasodilators and antihypertensive agents).
No products indexed under this heading.

Trandolapril (Iloprost has the potential to increase the hypotensive effect of vasodilators and antihypertensive agents). Products include:
Mavik Tablets 482
Tarka Tablets 519

Trimethaphan Camsylate (Iloprost has the potential to increase the hypotensive effect of vasodilators and antihypertensive agents).
No products indexed under this heading.

Valsartan (Iloprost has the potential to increase the hypotensive effect of vasodilators and antihypertensive agents). Products include:
Diovan HCT Tablets 2195
Diovan Tablets 2191

Verapamil Hydrochloride (Iloprost has the potential to increase the hypotensive effect of vasodilators and antihypertensive agents). Products include:
Covera-HS Tablets 3135
Tarka Tablets 519
Verelan PM Capsules 3120

Warfarin Sodium (Since iloprost inhibits platelet function, there is a potential for increased risk of bleeding, particularly in patients maintained on anticoagulants). Products include:
Coumadin for Injection 932
Coumadin Tablets 932

Food Interactions

Alcohol (Iloprost has the potential to increase the hypotensive effect of vasodilators and antihypertensive agents).

VENTOLIN HFA INHALATION AEROSOL

(Albuterol Sulfate) 1576
May interact with monoamine oxidase inhibitors, nonpotassium-sparing diuretics, sympathomimetic bronchodilators, sympathomimetics, tricyclic antidepressants, and certain other agents. Compounds in these categories include:

Albuterol (Co-administration with other short-acting sympathomimetic aerosol bronchodilators should not be used concomitantly with albuterol). Products include:
Proventil Inhalation Aerosol 3067

Amitriptyline Hydrochloride (Co-administration with tricyclic antidepressants may potentiate action of albuterol on the vascular system).
No products indexed under this heading.

Amoxapine (Co-administration with tricyclic antidepressants may potentiate action of albuterol on the vascular system).
No products indexed under this heading.

Bendroflumethiazide (The ECG changes and/or hypokalemia that may result from the adminstration of nonpotassium-sparing diuretics can be acutely worsened by beta-agonists, especially when the recommended dose of beta-agonist is exceeded).
No products indexed under this heading.

Bitolterol Mesylate (Co-administration with other short-acting sympathomimetic aerosol bronchodilators should not be used concomitantly with albuterol).
No products indexed under this heading.

Bumetanide (The ECG changes and/or hypokalemia that may result from the adminstration of nonpotassium-sparing diuretics can be acutely worsened by beta-agonists, especially when the recommended dose of beta-agonist is exceeded).
No products indexed under this heading.

Chlorothiazide (The ECG changes and/or hypokalemia that may result from the adminstration of nonpotassium-sparing diuretics can be acutely worsened by beta-agonists, especially when the recommended dose of beta-agonist is exceeded). Products include:
Aldoclor Tablets 1881
Diuril Oral 1936

Chlorothiazide Sodium (The ECG changes and/or hypokalemia that may result from the adminstration of nonpotassium-sparing diuretics can be acutely worsened by beta-agonists, especially when the recommended dose of beta-agonist is exceeded). Products include:
Diuril Sodium Intravenous 1934

Clomipramine Hydrochloride (Co-administration with tricyclic antidepressants may potentiate action of albuterol on the vascular system).
No products indexed under this heading.

Desipramine Hydrochloride (Co-administration with tricyclic antidepressants may potentiate action of albuterol on the vascular system).
No products indexed under this heading.

Digoxin (Co-administration of intravenous and oral administration of albuterol to volunteers who had received digoxin for 10 days has resulted in mean decrease in digoxin levels; the clinical significance of this finding is unknown). Products include:
Digitek Tablets 2146
Lanoxicaps Capsules 1458
Lanoxin Injection 1462
Lanoxin Tablets 1468
Lanoxin Injection Pediatric 1465

Dobutamine Hydrochloride (Co-administration with other adrenergic agents may result in deleterious cardiovascular events).
No products indexed under this heading.

Dopamine Hydrochloride (Co-administration with other adrenergic agents may result in deleterious cardiovascular events).
No products indexed under this heading.

Doxepin Hydrochloride (Co-administration with tricyclic antidepressants may potentiate action of albuterol on the vascular system).
No products indexed under this heading.

Ephedrine Hydrochloride (Co-administration with other short-acting sympathomimetic aerosol bronchodilators should not be used concomitantly with albuterol). Products include:
Primatene Tablets 749

Ephedrine Sulfate (Co-administration with other short-acting sympathomimetic aerosol bronchodilators should not be used concomitantly with albuterol).
No products indexed under this heading.

Ephedrine Tannate (Co-administration with other short-acting sympathomimetic aerosol bronchodilators should not be used concomitantly with albuterol).
No products indexed under this heading.

Epinephrine (Co-administration with other short-acting sympathomimetic aerosol bronchodilators should not be used concomitantly with albuterol). Products include:
EpiPen 1061
Primatene Mist 749

Epinephrine Bitartrate (Co-administration with other adrenergic agents may result in deleterious cardiovascular events).
No products indexed under this heading.

Epinephrine Hydrochloride (Co-administration with other short-acting sympathomimetic aerosol bronchodilators should not be used concomitantly with albuterol).
No products indexed under this heading.

Ethacrynic Acid (The ECG changes and/or hypokalemia that may result from the adminstration of nonpotassium-sparing diuretics can be acutely worsened by beta-agonists, especially when the recommended dose of beta-agonist is exceeded). Products include:
Edecrin Tablets 1941

Furosemide (The ECG changes and/or hypokalemia that may result from the adminstration of nonpotassium-sparing diuretics can be acutely worsened by beta-agonists, especially when the recommended dose of beta-agonist is exceeded). Products include:
Furosemide Tablets 2117

Hydrochlorothiazide (The ECG changes and/or hypokalemia that may result from the adminstration of nonpotassium-sparing diuretics can be acutely worsened by beta-agonists, especially when the recommended dose of beta-agonist is exceeded). Products include:
Aldoril Tablets 1884
Atacand HCT 637
Avalide Tablets 2889
Avalide Tablets 922
Benicar HCT Tablets 2852
Diovan HCT Tablets 2195
Dyazide Capsules 1389
Hyzaar 1964
Lotensin HCT Tablets 2235
Maxzide 2150
Micardis HCT Tablets 886
Moduretic Tablets 2003
Prinzide Tablets 2033
Teveten HCT Tablets 1710
Timolide Tablets 2056
Uniretic Tablets 3114
Vaseretic Tablets 2073
Zestoretic Tablets 701

Hydroflumethiazide (The ECG changes and/or hypokalemia that may result from the adminstration of nonpotassium-sparing diuretics can be acutely worsened by beta-agonists, especially when the recommended dose of beta-agonist is exceeded).
No products indexed under this heading.

Imipramine Hydrochloride (Co-administration with tricyclic antidepressants may potentiate action of albuterol on the vascular system).
No products indexed under this heading.

Imipramine Pamoate (Co-administration with tricyclic antidepressants may potentiate action of albuterol on the vascular system).
No products indexed under this heading.

Isocarboxazid (Co-administration with MAO inhibitors may potentiate action of albuterol on the vascular system).
No products indexed under this heading.

Isoetharine (Co-administration with other short-acting sympathomimetic aerosol bronchodilators should not be used concomitantly with albuterol).
No products indexed under this heading.

Isoproterenol Hydrochloride (Co-administration with other short-acting sympathomimetic aerosol bronchodilators should not be used concomitantly with albuterol).
No products indexed under this heading.

Isoproterenol Sulfate (Co-administration with other short-acting sympathomimetic aerosol bronchodilators should not be used concomitantly with albuterol).
No products indexed under this heading.

Levalbuterol Hydrochloride (Co-administration with other short-acting sympathomimetic aerosol bronchodilators should not be used concomitantly with albuterol). Products include:
Xopenex Inhalation Solution 3143
Xopenex Inhalation Solution Concentrate 3147

Maprotiline Hydrochloride (Co-administration with tricyclic antidepressants may potentiate action of albuterol on the vascular system).
No products indexed under this heading.

Metaproterenol Sulfate (Co-administration with other short-acting sympathomimetic aerosol bronchodilators should not be used concomitantly with albuterol). Products include:
Alupent Inhalation Aerosol 858

Metaraminol Bitartrate (Co-administration with other adrenergic agents may result in deleterious cardiovascular events). Products include:
Aramine Injection 1889

Methoxamine Hydrochloride (Co-administration with other adrenergic agents may result in deleterious cardiovascular events).
No products indexed under this heading.

Methyclothiazide (The ECG changes and/or hypokalemia that may result from the adminstration of nonpotassium-sparing diuretics can be acutely worsened by beta-agonists, especially when the recommended dose of beta-agonist is exceeded).
No products indexed under this heading.

Moclobemide (Co-administration with MAO inhibitors may potentiate action of albuterol on the vascular system).
No products indexed under this heading.

Norepinephrine Bitartrate (Co-administration with other adrenergic agents may result in deleterious cardiovascular events).
No products indexed under this heading.

Nortriptyline Hydrochloride (Co-administration with tricyclic antidepressants may potentiate action of albuterol on the vascular system).
No products indexed under this heading.

Pargyline Hydrochloride (Co-administration with MAO inhibitors may potentiate action of albuterol on the vascular system).
No products indexed under this heading.

Phenelzine Sulfate (Co-administration with MAO inhibitors may potentiate action of albuterol on the vascular system).
No products indexed under this heading.

Phenylephrine Bitartrate (Co-administration with other adrenergic agents may result in deleterious cardiovascular events).
No products indexed under this heading.

Phenylephrine Hydrochloride (Co-administration with other adrenergic agents may result in deleterious cardiovascular events). Products include:
- Alacol DM Syrup ... 739
- Hycomine Compound Tablets ... 1105
- Preparation H Maximum Strength Cream ... ▣747
- Preparation H Cooling Gel ... ▣747
- Preparation H ... ▣747
- Sudafed PE Tablets ... ▣711
- Vicks Sinex Nasal Spray and Ultra Fine Mist for Sinus Relief ... 2677
- Zicam Concentrated Cough Mist for Kids Plus D Cool Cherry ... ▣643
- Zicam Concentrated Cough Mist Plus D Cool Cherry ... ▣642

Phenylephrine Tannate (Co-administration with other adrenergic agents may result in deleterious cardiovascular events).
No products indexed under this heading.

Phenylpropanolamine Hydrochloride (Co-administration with other adrenergic agents may result in deleterious cardiovascular events).
No products indexed under this heading.

Pirbuterol Acetate (Co-administration with other short-acting sympathomimetic aerosol bronchodilators should not be used concomitantly with albuterol). Products include:
- Maxair Autohaler ... 1820

Polythiazide (The ECG changes and/or hypokalemia that may result from the adminstration of nonpotassium-sparing diuretics can be acutely worsened by beta-agonists, especially when the recommended dose of beta-agonist is exceeded).
No products indexed under this heading.

Procarbazine Hydrochloride (Co-administration with MAO inhibitors may potentiate action of albuterol on the vascular system). Products include:
- Matulane Capsules ... 3188

Protriptyline Hydrochloride (Co-administration with tricyclic antidepressants may potentiate action of albuterol on the vascular system). Products include:
- Vivactil Tablets ... 2350

Pseudoephedrine Hydrochloride (Co-administration with other adrenergic agents may result in deleterious cardiovascular events). Products include:
- Advil Allergy Sinus Caplets ... ▣737
- Advil Cold & Sinus ... ▣739
- Advil Flu & Body Ache Caplets ... ▣739
- Children's Advil Cold Suspension ... ▣741
- Advil Multi-Symptom Cold Caplets ... ▣738
- Allegra-D 12 Hour Extended-Release Tablets ... 2860
- Allegra-D 24 Hour Extended-Release Tablets ... 2862
- Balamine DM ... 739
- BC Cold Powder ... ▣612
- Benadryl Allergy & Cold Tablets ... ▣692
- Benadryl Allergy & Sinus Headache Caplets & Gelcaps ... ▣693
- Children's Benadryl Allergy & Cold Fastmelt Tablets ... ▣695
- Benadryl Maximum Strength Severe Allergy & Sinus Headache Caplets ... ▣694
- Children's Benadryl D Allergy & Sinus Fastmelt Tablets ... ▣694
- Children's Benadryl D Liquid Medication ... ▣693
- Benadryl D Tablets ... ▣694
- Contac Non-Drowsy 12 Hour Cold Caplets ... ▣614
- Contac Non-Drowsy Timed Release 12 Hour Cold Caplets ... ▣615
- Contac Severe Cold and Flu Caplets Maximum Strength ... ▣615
- Contac Severe Cold and Flu Caplets Non-Drowsy ... ▣615
- Children's Dimetapp Cold & Allergy Elixir ... ▣745
- Children's Dimetapp DM Cold & Cough Elixir ... ▣745
- Children's Dimetapp Long Acting Cough Plus Cold Syrup ... ▣746
- Dimetapp Infant Drops Decongestant Plus Cough ... ▣746
- Children's Motrin Cold Non-Staining Dye-Free Oral Suspension ... 1838
- Children's Motrin Cold Oral Suspension ... 1838
- Motrin Cold & Sinus Caplets ... 1836
- PediaCare Decongestant & Cough Infant Drops ... ▣705
- PediaCare Decongestant Infants' Drops ... ▣705
- PediaCare Long-Acting Cough Plus Cold Liquid ... ▣704
- PediaCare Multi-Symptom Cold Liquid ... ▣704
- PediaCare NightRest Cough & Cold Liquid ... ▣704
- Robitussin Allergy & Cough Syrup ... ▣750
- Robitussin CF Liquid ... ▣755
- Robitussin Cough & Cold Liquid-filled Capsules ... ▣750
- Robitussin Cough, Cold & Flu Liquid-filled Capsules ... ▣750
- Robitussin Cough & Cold Infant Drops ... ▣755
- Robitussin Flu Liquid ... ▣752
- Robitussin Maximum Strength Cough & Cold Liquid ... ▣754
- Robitussin PE Syrup ... ▣753
- Robitussin Pediatric Cough & Cold Liquid ... ▣754
- Robitussin PM Cough & Cold Liquid ... ▣752
- Robitussin Severe Congestion Liquid-filled Capsules ... ▣751
- Simply Stuffy Liquid ... 1841
- Singlet Caplets ... ▣636
- Sudafed 12 Hour Caplets ... ▣708
- Sudafed 24 Hour Tablets ... ▣709
- Sudafed Nasal Decongestant Tablets ... ▣709
- Sudafed Severe Cold ... ▣710
- Sudafed Non-Drying Sinus Liquid Caps ... ▣709
- Sudafed Sinus & Allergy Tablets ... ▣710
- Sudafed Sinus Headache ... ▣711
- TheraFlu Cold & Cough Hot Liquid ... ▣680
- TheraFlu Cold & Sore Throat Hot Liquid ... ▣680
- TheraFlu Flu & Chest Congestion Non-Drowsy Hot Liquid ... ▣681
- TheraFlu Flu & Sore Throat Hot Liquid ... ▣681
- TheraFlu Severe Cold Non-Drowsy Hot Liquid ... ▣683
- TheraFlu Severe Cold & Cough Hot Liquid ... ▣683
- TheraFlu Severe Cold Caplets ... ▣679
- TheraFlu Severe Cold Hot Liquid ... ▣682
- TheraFlu Severe Cold Non-Drowsy Caplets ... ▣679
- Triaminic Chest & Nasal Congestion Liquid ... ▣685
- Triaminic Cold & Allergy Liquid ... ▣685
- Triaminic Cold & Cough Liquid ... ▣685
- Triaminic Cough Liquid ... ▣687
- Triaminic Cough & Nasal Congestion Liquid ... ▣687
- Triaminic Cough & Sore Throat Liquid ... ▣687
- Triaminic Flu, Cough & Fever Liquid ... ▣685
- Triaminic Night Time Cough & Cold Liquid ... ▣685
- Triaminic Allergy Runny Nose & Congestion Softchews ... ▣688
- Triaminic Cold & Cough Softchews ... ▣688
- Triaminic Cough & Sore Throat Softchews ... ▣689
- Tylenol Sinus NightTime Caplets ... ▣663
- Children's Tylenol Plus Cold & Allergy Suspension Liquid ... 1850
- Children's Tylenol Plus Cold NightTime Suspension Liquid ... 1851
- Children's Tylenol Plus Cold & Cough Suspension Liquid and Chewable Tablets ... 1851
- Children's Tylenol Plus Cold Chewable Tablets ... 1851
- Children's Tylenol Plus Cold Daytime Non-Drowsy Suspension Liquid ... 1851
- Children's Tylenol Plus Flu Suspension Liquid ... 1853
- Concentrated Tylenol Infants' Drops Plus Cold ... 1851
- Concentrated Tylenol Infants' Drops Plus Cold and Cough ... 1851
- Tylenol Cold & Flu Severe Daytime Liquid with Cool Bust ... 1846
- Tylenol Cold & Flu Severe NightTime Liquid with Cool Burst ... 1846
- Tylenol Cold Severe Congestion Non-Drowsy Caplets with Cool Burst ... 1846
- Tylenol Allergy Complete Night Time Caplets ... 1844
- Tylenol Allergy Complete Multi-Symptom Caplets and Gelcaps with Cool Burst ... 1844
- Tylenol Flu NightTime Gelcaps ... 1846
- Tylenol Flu Day Non-Drowsy Gelcaps ... 1846
- Concentrated Tylenol Infants' Drops Plus Cold Nasal Congestant, Fever Reducer & Pain Reliever ... ▣668
- Concentrated Tylenol Infants' Drops Plus Cold & Cough Nasal Decongestant, Fever Reducer & Pain Reliever ... ▣668
- Multi-Symptom Tylenol Cold Night Time Caplets ... 1845
- Multi-Symptom Tylenol Cold Day Non-Drowsy Caplets and Gelcaps ... 1845
- Tylenol Sinus Day Non-Drowsy ... 1848
- Tylenol Sinus Night Time Caplets ... 1848
- Tylenol Sinus Severe Congestion Caplets with Cool Burst ... 1848
- Vicks 44D Cough & Head Congestion Relief ... 2676
- Vicks 44D Cough & Head Congestion Relief Liquid ... ▣721
- Vicks 44M Cough, Cold & Flu Relief ... 2676
- Pediatric Vicks 44m Cough & Cold Relief ... 2673
- Vicks DayQuil LiquiCaps/Liquid Multi-Symptom Cold/Flu Relief ... ▣723
- Vicks DayQuil Multi-Symptom Cold/Flu Relief LiquiCaps ... 2675
- Vicks DayQuil Multi-Symptom Cold/Flu Relief Liquid ... 2675
- Children's Vicks NyQuil Cold/Cough Relief ... 2671
- Vicks NyQuil LiquiCaps ... 2677
- Vicks NyQuil LiquiCaps/Liquid Multi-Symptom Cold/Flu Relief ... ▣725
- Vicks NyQuil Liquid ... 2677
- Zyrtec-D 12 Hour Extended Release Tablets ... 2591

Pseudoephedrine Sulfate (Co-administration with other adrenergic agents may result in deleterious cardiovascular events). Products include:
- Alavert Allergy & Sinus D-12 Hour Tablets ... ▣743
- Clarinex-D 24-Hour Extended-Release Tablets ... 3012
- Claritin-D Non-Drowsy 12 Hour Tablets ... ▣731
- Claritin-D Non-Drowsy 24 Hour Tablets ... ▣731

Salmeterol Xinafoate (Co-administration with other short-acting sympathomimetic aerosol bronchodilators should not be used concomitantly with albuterol). Products include:
- Advair Diskus 100/50 ... 1291
- Advair Diskus 250/50 ... 1291
- Advair Diskus 500/50 ... 1291
- Serevent Diskus ... 1540

Selegiline Hydrochloride (Co-administration with MAO inhibitors may potentiate action of albuterol on the vascular system). Products include:
- Eldepryl Capsules ... 3209

Terbutaline Sulfate (Co-administration with other short-acting sympathomimetic aerosol bronchodilators should not be used concomitantly with albuterol).
No products indexed under this heading.

Torsemide (The ECG changes and/or hypokalemia that may result from the adminstration of nonpotassium-sparing diuretics can be acutely worsened by beta-agonists, especially when the recommended dose of beta-agonist is exceeded).
No products indexed under this heading.

Tranylcypromine Sulfate (Co-administration with MAO inhibitors may potentiate action of albuterol on the vascular system). Products include:
- Parnate Tablets ... 1499

Trimipramine Maleate (Co-administration with tricyclic antidepressants may potentiate action of albuterol on the vascular system). Products include:
- Surmontil Capsules ... 2347

VERELAN PM CAPSULES

(Verapamil Hydrochloride) 3120

May interact with ACE inhibitors, antihypertensives, beta blockers, cytochrome p450 3a4 inducers (selected), cytochrome p450 3a4 inhibitors (selected), diuretics, cardiac glycosides, inhalant anesthetics, lithium preparations, neuromuscular blocking agents, quinidine, theophyllines, vasodilators, and certain other agents. Compounds in these categories include:

Acebutolol Hydrochloride (Concomitant therapy with beta-adrenergic blockers and verapamil may result in additive negative effects on heart rate, A-V conduction, and/or cardiac contractility; excessive bradycardia and A-V block have been reported with concurrent use in hypertensive patients. This combination should be used only with caution and close monitoring).
No products indexed under this heading.

Acetazolamide (Clinically significant interactions have been reported with inhibitors of cytochrome P450 3A4 causing elevation of plasma levels of verapamil).
No products indexed under this heading.

Allium sativum (Clinically significant interactions have been reported with inducers of cytochrome P450 3A4 causing a lowering of plasma levels of verapamil).
No products indexed under this heading.

Amiloride Hydrochloride (Co-administration with oral antihypertensive agents (eg, diuretics) will usually have an additive effect on lowering blood pressure). Products include:
Midamor Tablets 2000
Moduretic Tablets 2003

Amiodarone Hydrochloride (Clinically significant interactions have been reported with inhibitors of cytochrome P450 3A4 causing elevation of plasma levels of verapamil). Products include:
Pacerone Tablets 3337

Amlodipine Besylate (Co-administration with oral antihypertensive agents will usually have an additive effect on lowering blood pressure). Products include:
Caduet Tablets 2507
Lotrel Capsules 2238
Norvasc Tablets 2529

Amprenavir (Clinically significant interactions have been reported with inhibitors of cytochrome P450 3A4 causing elevation of plasma levels of verapamil). Products include:
Agenerase Capsules 1299
Agenerase Oral Solution 1304

Amyl Nitrite (Co-administration with oral antihypertensive agents (eg, vasodilators) will usually have an additive effect on lowering blood pressure).
No products indexed under this heading.

Anastrozole (Clinically significant interactions have been reported with inhibitors of cytochrome P450 3A4 causing elevation of plasma levels of verapamil). Products include:
Arimidex Tablets 665

Aprepitant (Clinically significant interactions have been reported with inducers of cytochrome P450 3A4 causing a lowering of plasma levels of verapamil). Products include:
Emend Capsules 1944

Aspirin (Co-administration, in a few reported cases, has led to increased bleeding times greater than those observed with aspirin alone). Products include:
Aggrenox Capsules 855
Bayer, Aspirin Regimen 606
Bayer Aspirin Tablets 3515
BC Powder 612
BC Allergy Sinus Cold Powder 612
Arthritis Strength BC Powder 612
BC Sinus Cold Powder 612
Ecotrin Enteric Coated Aspirin Low, Regular and Maximum Strength Tablets 1627
Goody's Body Pain Formula Powder 621
Goody's Extra Strength Headache Powder 621
Goody's Extra Strength Pain Relief Tablets 621
Percodan Tablets 1115
St. Joseph 81 mg Aspirin Chewable and Enteric Coated Tablets 1841

Aspirin, Enteric Coated (Co-administration, in a few reported cases, has led to increased bleeding times greater than those observed with aspirin alone).
No products indexed under this heading.

Aspirin Buffered (Co-administration, in a few reported cases, has led to increased bleeding times greater than those observed with aspirin alone).
No products indexed under this heading.

Atenolol (Concomitant therapy with beta-adrenergic blockers and verapamil may result in additive negative effects on heart rate, A-V conduction, and/or cardiac contractility; excessive bradycardia and A-V block have been reported with concurrent use in hypertensive patients. This combination should be used only with caution and close monitoring). Products include:
Tenormin I.V. Injection 698
Tenormin Tablets 695

Atracurium Besylate (Clinical data and animal studies suggest that verapamil may potentiate the activity of neuromuscular blocking agents (curare-like and depolarizing). It may be necessary to decrease the dose of verapamil and/or the dose of the neuromuscular blocking agent when the drugs are used concomitantly).
No products indexed under this heading.

Benazepril Hydrochloride (Co-administration with oral antihypertensive agents will usually have an additive effect on lowering blood pressure). Products include:
Lotensin Tablets 2232
Lotensin HCT Tablets 2235
Lotrel Capsules 2238

Bendroflumethiazide (Co-administration with oral antihypertensive agents will usually have an additive effect on lowering blood pressure).
No products indexed under this heading.

Betamethasone Acetate (Clinically significant interactions have been reported with inducers of cytochrome P450 3A4 causing a lowering of plasma levels of verapamil).
No products indexed under this heading.

Betamethasone Sodium Phosphate (Clinically significant interactions have been reported with inducers of cytochrome P450 3A4 causing a lowering of plasma levels of verapamil).
No products indexed under this heading.

Betaxolol Hydrochloride (Concomitant therapy with beta-adrenergic blockers and verapamil may result in additive negative effects on heart rate, A-V conduction, and/or cardiac contractility; excessive bradycardia and A-V block have been reported with concurrent use in hypertensive patients. This combination should be used only with caution and close monitoring). Products include:
Betoptic S Ophthalmic Suspension 554

Bisoprolol Fumarate (Concomitant therapy with beta-adrenergic blockers and verapamil may result in additive negative effects on heart rate, A-V conduction, and/or cardiac contractility; excessive bradycardia and A-V block have been reported with concurrent use in hypertensive patients. This combination should be used only with caution and close monitoring).
No products indexed under this heading.

Bumetanide (Co-administration with oral antihypertensive agents (eg, diuretics) will usually have an additive effect on lowering blood pressure).
No products indexed under this heading.

Candesartan Cilexetil (Co-administration with oral antihypertensive agents will usually have an additive effect on lowering blood pressure). Products include:
Atacand Tablets 634
Atacand HCT 637

Captopril (Co-administration with oral antihypertensive agents will usually have an additive effect on lowering blood pressure). Products include:
Captopril Tablets 2114

Carbamazepine (Verapamil therapy may increase carbamazepine concentrations during combined therapy resulting in side effects such as diplopia, headache, ataxia, or dizziness). Products include:
Carbatrol Capsules 3174
Equetro Extended-Release Capsules 3178
Tegretol/Tegretol-XR 2278

Carteolol Hydrochloride (Concomitant therapy with beta-adrenergic blockers and verapamil may result in additive negative effects on heart rate, A-V conduction, and/or cardiac contractility; excessive bradycardia and A-V block have been reported with concurrent use in hypertensive patients. This combination should be used only with caution and close monitoring). Products include:
Carteolol Hydrochloride Ophthalmic Solution USP, 1% .... ⊙ 246

Chlorothiazide (Co-administration with oral antihypertensive agents will usually have an additive effect on lowering blood pressure). Products include:
Aldoclor Tablets 1881
Diuril Oral 1936

Chlorothiazide Sodium (Co-administration with oral antihypertensive agents will usually have an additive effect on lowering blood pressure). Products include:
Diuril Sodium Intravenous 1934

Chlorthalidone (Co-administration with oral antihypertensive agents will usually have an additive effect on lowering blood pressure). Products include:
Clorpres Tablets 2139

Cimetidine (The interaction between cimetidine and chronically administered verapamil has not been studied. Variable results on clearance have been obtained in acute studies of healthy volunteers; clearance of verapamil was either reduced or unchanged). Products include:
Tagamet HB 200 Tablets 637
Tagamet Tablets 1547

Cimetidine Hydrochloride (The interaction between cimetidine and chronically administered verapamil has not been studied. Variable results on clearance have been obtained in acute studies of healthy volunteers; clearance of verapamil was either reduced or unchanged).
No products indexed under this heading.

Ciprofloxacin (Clinically significant interactions have been reported with inhibitors of cytochrome P450 3A4 causing elevation of plasma levels of verapamil). Products include:
Cipro I.V. 2998
Cipro I.V. Pharmacy Bulk Package 3509
Cipro Oral Suspension 2991
Cipro XR Tablets 3004
Ciprodex Otic Suspension 555

Ciprofloxacin Hydrochloride (Clinically significant interactions have been reported with inducers of cytochrome P450 3A4 causing a lowering of plasma levels of verapamil). Products include:
Ciloxan Ophthalmic Ointment 554
Cipro Tablets 2991

Cisatracurium Besylate (Clinical data and animal studies suggest that verapamil may potentiate the activity of neuromuscular blocking agents (curare-like and depolarizing). It may be necessary to decrease the dose of verapamil and/or the dose of the neuromuscular blocking agent when the drugs are used concomitantly). Products include:
Nimbex Injection 494

Cisplatin (Clinically significant interactions have been reported with inducers of cytochrome P450 3A4 causing a lowering of plasma levels of verapamil).
No products indexed under this heading.

Clarithromycin (Clinically significant interactions have been reported with inhibitors of cytochrome P450 3A4 causing elevation of plasma levels of verapamil). Products include:
Biaxin/Biaxin XL 402
PREVPAC 3281

Clonidine (Co-administration with oral antihypertensive agents will usually have an additive effect on lowering blood pressure). Products include:
Catapres-TTS 875

Clonidine Hydrochloride (Co-administration with oral antihypertensive agents will usually have an additive effect on lowering blood pressure). Products include:
Catapres Tablets 874

Clorpres Tablets 2139

Clotrimazole (Clinically significant interactions have been reported with inhibitors of cytochrome P450 3A4 causing elevation of plasma levels of verapamil). Products include:

Lotrimin 3053
Lotrisone 3054

Cortisone Acetate (Clinically significant interactions have been reported with inducers of cytochrome P450 3A4 causing a lowering of plasma levels of verapamil).

No products indexed under this heading.

Cyclosporine (Verapamil therapy may increase serum levels of cyclosporine). Products include:

Gengraf Capsules 458
Neoral Soft Gelatin Capsules 2247
Neoral Oral Solution 2247
Restasis Ophthalmic Emulsion 570
Sandimmune 2259

Dalfopristin (Clinically significant interactions have been reported with inhibitors of cytochrome P450 3A4 causing elevation of plasma levels of verapamil). Products include:

Synercid I.V. 1690

Danazol (Clinically significant interactions have been reported with inhibitors of cytochrome P450 3A4 causing elevation of plasma levels of verapamil).

No products indexed under this heading.

Delavirdine Mesylate (Clinically significant interactions have been reported with inhibitors of cytochrome P450 3A4 causing elevation of plasma levels of verapamil). Products include:

Rescriptor Tablets 2535

Deserpidine (Co-administration with oral antihypertensive agents will usually have an additive effect on lowering blood pressure).

No products indexed under this heading.

Desflurane (When used concomitantly, inhalation anesthetics and calcium antagonists, such as verapamil, should each be titrated carefully to avoid excessive cardiovascular depression). Products include:

Suprane Liquid for Inhalation 770

Deslanoside (Chronic verapamil treatment can increase serum digoxin levels by 50% to 70% during the first week of therapy and this may result in digitalis toxicity.The influence of verapamil on digoxin kinetics is magnified in hepatic cirrhosis patients).

No products indexed under this heading.

Dexamethasone (Clinically significant interactions have been reported with inducers of cytochrome P450 3A4 causing a lowering of plasma levels of verapamil). Products include:

Ciprodex Otic Suspension 555
Decadron Tablets 1929
TobraDex Ophthalmic Ointment 558
TobraDex Ophthalmic Suspension ... 558

Dexamethasone Acetate (Clinically significant interactions have been reported with inducers of cytochrome P450 3A4 causing a lowering of plasma levels of verapamil).

No products indexed under this heading.

Dexamethasone Sodium Phosphate (Clinically significant interactions have been reported with inducers of cytochrome P450 3A4 causing a lowering of plasma levels of verapamil). Products include:

Decadron Phosphate Injection 1931

Diazoxide (Co-administration with oral antihypertensive agents will usually have an additive effect on lowering blood pressure). Products include:

Hyperstat I.V. Injection 3031

Digitalis Glycoside Preparations (Chronic verapamil treatment can increase serum digoxin levels by 50% to 70% during the first week of therapy and this may result in digitalis toxicity.The influence of verapamil on digoxin kinetics is magnified in hepatic cirrhosis patients).

No products indexed under this heading.

Digitoxin (Chronic verapamil treatment can increase serum digoxin levels by 50% to 70% during the first week of therapy and this may result in digitalis toxicity.The influence of verapamil on digoxin kinetics is magnified in hepatic cirrhosis patients).

No products indexed under this heading.

Digoxin (Chronic verapamil treatment can increase serum digoxin levels by 50% to 70% during the first week of therapy and this may result in digitalis toxicity.The influence of verapamil on digoxin kinetics is magnified in hepatic cirrhosis patients). Products include:

Digitek Tablets 2146
Lanoxicaps Capsules 1458
Lanoxin Injection 1462
Lanoxin Tablets 1468
Lanoxin Injection Pediatric 1465

Diltiazem Hydrochloride (Co-administration with oral antihypertensive agents will usually have an additive effect on lowering blood pressure). Products include:

Cardizem LA Extended Release Tablets 1699
Tiazac Capsules 1204

Diltiazem Maleate (Clinically significant interactions have been reported with inhibitors of cytochrome P450 3A4 causing elevation of plasma levels of verapamil).

No products indexed under this heading.

Disopyramide (Disopyramide should not be administered within 48 hours before, or 24 hours after, verapamil administration).

No products indexed under this heading.

Disopyramide Phosphate (Disopyramide should not be administered within 48 hours before or 24 hours after verapamil administration).

No products indexed under this heading.

Doxacurium Chloride (Clinical data and animal studies suggest that verapamil may potentiate the activity of neuromuscular blocking agents (curare-like and depolarizing). It may be necessary to decrease the dose of verapamil and/or the dose of the neuromuscular blocking agent when the drugs are used concomitantly).

No products indexed under this heading.

Doxazosin Mesylate (Concomitant use of agents that attenuate alpha-adrenergic function, such as doxazosin, may result in excessive reduction in blood pressure).

No products indexed under this heading.

Doxorubicin Hydrochloride (Verapamil can increase the efficacy of doxorubicin both in tissue culture systems and in patients. It raises the serum doxorubicin levels). Products include:

Adriamycin for Injection, USP 786
Adriamycin Injection, USP 786

Doxorubicin Hydrochloride Liposome (Verapamil can increase the efficacy of doxorubicin both in tissue culture systems and in patients. It raises the serum doxorubicin levels). Products include:

Doxil Injection 3302

Efavirenz (Clinically significant interactions have been reported with inducers of cytochrome P450 3A4 causing a lowering of plasma levels of verapamil). Products include:

Sustiva Capsules 957

Enalapril Maleate (Co-administration with oral antihypertensive agents will usually have an additive effect on lowering blood pressure). Products include:

Vaseretic Tablets 2073
Vasotec I.V. Injection 2076

Enalaprilat (Co-administration with oral antihypertensive agents will usually have an additive effect on lowering blood pressure).

No products indexed under this heading.

Enflurane (When used concomitantly, inhalation anesthetics and calcium antagonists, such as verapamil, should each be titrated carefully to avoid excessive cardiovascular depression).

No products indexed under this heading.

Epoprostenol Sodium (Co-administration with oral antihypertensive agents (eg, vasodilators) will usually have an additive effect on lowering blood pressure). Products include:

Flolan for Injection 1408

Eprosartan Mesylate (Co-administration with oral antihypertensive agents will usually have an additive effect on lowering blood pressure). Products include:

Teveten Tablets 1707
Teveten HCT Tablets 1710

Erythromycin (Clinically significant interactions have been reported with inhibitors of cytochrome P450 3A4 causing elevation of plasma levels of verapamil). Products include:

Erygel Topical Gel 2096
Ery-Tab Tablets 447
Erythromycin Base Filmtab Tablets 454
Erythromycin Delayed-Release Capsules, USP 456
PCE Dispertab Tablets 510

Erythromycin Estolate (Clinically significant interactions have been reported with inhibitors of cytochrome P450 3A4 causing elevation of plasma levels of verapamil).

No products indexed under this heading.

Erythromycin Ethylsuccinate (Clinically significant interactions have been reported with inhibitors of cytochrome P450 3A4 causing elevation of plasma levels of verapamil). Products include:

E.E.S. 449
EryPed 445

Erythromycin Gluceptate (Clinically significant interactions have been reported with inhibitors of cytochrome P450 3A4 causing elevation of plasma levels of verapamil).

No products indexed under this heading.

Erythromycin Lactobionate (Clinically significant interactions have been reported with inhibitors of cytochrome P450 3A4 causing elevation of plasma levels of verapamil).

No products indexed under this heading.

Erythromycin Stearate (Clinically significant interactions have been reported with inhibitors of cytochrome P450 3A4 causing elevation of plasma levels of verapamil). Products include:

Erythrocin Stearate Filmtab Tablets 452

Esmolol Hydrochloride (Concomitant therapy with beta-adrenergic blockers and verapamil may result in additive negative effects on heart rate, A-V conduction, and/or cardiac contractility; excessive bradycardia and A-V block have been reported with concurrent use in hypertensive patients.This combination should be used only with caution and close monitoring). Products include:

Brevibloc Concentrate 766
Brevibloc Injection 766
Brevibloc Double Strength Injection 766
Brevibloc Premixed Injection 766
Brevibloc Double Strength Premixed Injection 766

Esomeprazole Magnesium (Clinically significant interactions have been reported with inhibitors of cytochrome P450 3A4 causing elevation of plasma levels of verapamil). Products include:

Nexium Delayed-Release Capsules 645

Ethacrynic Acid (Co-administration with oral antihypertensive agents (eg, diuretics) will usually have an additive effect on lowering blood pressure). Products include:

Edecrin Tablets 1941

Ethaverine Hydrochloride (Co-administration with oral antihypertensive agents (eg, vasodilators) will usually have an additive effect on lowering blood pressure).

No products indexed under this heading.

Ethosuximide (Clinically significant interactions have been reported with inducers of cytochrome P450 3A4 causing a lowering of plasma levels of verapamil).

No products indexed under this heading.

Felbamate (Clinically significant interactions have been reported with inducers of cytochrome P450 3A4 causing a lowering of plasma levels of verapamil).

No products indexed under this heading.

Felodipine (Co-administration with oral antihypertensive agents will usually have an additive effect on lowering blood pressure). Products include:

Plendil Extended-Release Tablets 651

Flecainide Acetate (Concomitant administration of flecainide and verapamil may have additive effects on myocardial contractility, A-V conduction, and repolarization). Products include:

Tambocor Tablets 1824

Fluconazole (Clinically significant interactions have been reported with inhibitors of cytochrome P450 3A4 causing elevation of plasma levels of verapamil).
No products indexed under this heading.

Fludrocortisone Acetate (Clinically significant interactions have been reported with inducers of cytochrome P450 3A4 causing a lowering of plasma levels of verapamil).
No products indexed under this heading.

Fluoxetine Hydrochloride (Clinically significant interactions have been reported with inhibitors of cytochrome P450 3A4 causing elevation of plasma levels of verapamil). Products include:
Prozac Pulvules and Liquid 1771
Symbyax Capsules 1788

Fluvoxamine Maleate (Clinically significant interactions have been reported with inhibitors of cytochrome P450 3A4 causing elevation of plasma levels of verapamil).
No products indexed under this heading.

Fosamprenavir Calcium (Clinically significant interactions have been reported with inhibitors of cytochrome P450 3A4 causing elevation of plasma levels of verapamil). Products include:
Lexiva Tablets 1473

Fosinopril Sodium (Co-administration with oral antihypertensive agents will usually have an additive effect on lowering blood pressure).
No products indexed under this heading.

Fosphenytoin Sodium (Clinically significant interactions have been reported with inducers of cytochrome P450 3A4 causing a lowering of plasma levels of verapamil).
No products indexed under this heading.

Furosemide (Co-administration with oral antihypertensive agents will usually have an additive effect on lowering blood pressure). Products include:
Furosemide Tablets 2117

Garlic Extract (Clinically significant interactions have been reported with inducers of cytochrome P450 3A4 causing a lowering of plasma levels of verapamil).
No products indexed under this heading.

Garlic Oil (Clinically significant interactions have been reported with inducers of cytochrome P450 3A4 causing a lowering of plasma levels of verapamil).
No products indexed under this heading.

Guanabenz Acetate (Co-administration with oral antihypertensive agents will usually have an additive effect on lowering blood pressure).
No products indexed under this heading.

Guanethidine Monosulfate (Co-administration with oral antihypertensive agents will usually have an additive effect on lowering blood pressure).
No products indexed under this heading.

Halothane (When used concomitantly, inhalation anesthetics and calcium antagonists, such as verapamil, should each be titrated carefully to avoid excessive cardiovascular depression).
No products indexed under this heading.

Hydralazine Hydrochloride (Co-administration with oral antihypertensive agents will usually have an additive effect on lowering blood pressure). Products include:
BiDil Tablets 2161

Hydrochlorothiazide (Co-administration with oral antihypertensive agents will usually have an additive effect on lowering blood pressure). Products include:
Aldoril Tablets 1884
Atacand HCT 637
Avalide Tablets 2889
Avalide Tablets 922
Benicar HCT Tablets 2852
Diovan HCT Tablets 2195
Dyazide Capsules 1389
Hyzaar 1964
Lotensin HCT Tablets 2235
Maxzide 2150
Micardis HCT Tablets 886
Moduretic Tablets 2003
Prinzide Tablets 2033
Teveten HCT Tablets 1710
Timolide Tablets 2056
Uniretic Tablets 3114
Vaseretic Tablets 2073
Zestoretic Tablets 701

Hydrocortisone (Clinically significant interactions have been reported with inducers of cytochrome P450 3A4 causing a lowering of plasma levels of verapamil). Products include:
Cortizone•5 Ointment 699
Cortizone•10 Creme 699
Cortizone•10 Ointment 699
Cortizone•10 Plus Creme 700
Cortizone•10 Maximum Strength Quick Shot Spray 700
Hydrocortone Tablets 1963
Preparation H Hydrocortisone Cream 748

Hydrocortisone Acetate (Clinically significant interactions have been reported with inducers of cytochrome P450 3A4 causing a lowering of plasma levels of verapamil). Products include:
Analpram-HC 1136
Pramosone 1139
ProctoFoam-HC 3113
Tucks Anti-Itch Ointment 712
U-cort 1% Cream 3289

Hydrocortisone Butyrate (Clinically significant interactions have been reported with inducers of cytochrome P450 3A4 causing a lowering of plasma levels of verapamil). Products include:
Locoid 1138
Locoid Lipocream Cream 1138

Hydrocortisone Cypionate (Clinically significant interactions have been reported with inducers of cytochrome P450 3A4 causing a lowering of plasma levels of verapamil).
No products indexed under this heading.

Hydrocortisone Hemisuccinate (Clinically significant interactions have been reported with inducers of cytochrome P450 3A4 causing a lowering of plasma levels of verapamil).
No products indexed under this heading.

Hydrocortisone Probutate (Clinically significant interactions have been reported with inducers of cytochrome P450 3A4 causing a lowering of plasma levels of verapamil). Products include:
Pandel Cream, 0.1% 1017

Hydrocortisone Sodium Phosphate (Clinically significant interactions have been reported with inducers of cytochrome P450 3A4 causing a lowering of plasma levels of verapamil).
No products indexed under this heading.

Hydrocortisone Sodium Succinate (Clinically significant interactions have been reported with inducers of cytochrome P450 3A4 causing a lowering of plasma levels of verapamil).
No products indexed under this heading.

Hydrocortisone Valerate (Clinically significant interactions have been reported with inducers of cytochrome P450 3A4 causing a lowering of plasma levels of verapamil).
No products indexed under this heading.

Hydroflumethiazide (Co-administration with oral antihypertensive agents will usually have an additive effect on lowering blood pressure).
No products indexed under this heading.

Hypericum (Clinically significant interactions have been reported with inducers of cytochrome P450 3A4 causing a lowering of plasma levels of verapamil).
No products indexed under this heading.

Hypericum Perforatum (Clinically significant interactions have been reported with inducers of cytochrome P450 3A4 causing a lowering of plasma levels of verapamil).
No products indexed under this heading.

Indapamide (Co-administration with oral antihypertensive agents will usually have an additive effect on lowering blood pressure). Products include:
Indapamide Tablets 2119

Indinavir Sulfate (Clinically significant interactions have been reported with inhibitors of cytochrome P450 3A4 causing elevation of plasma levels of verapamil). Products include:
Crixivan Capsules 1918

Irbesartan (Co-administration with oral antihypertensive agents will usually have an additive effect on lowering blood pressure). Products include:
Avalide Tablets 922
Avalide Tablets 2889
Avapro Tablets 925
Avapro Tablets 2886

Isoflurane (When used concomitantly, inhalation anesthetics and calcium antagonists, such as verapamil, should each be titrated carefully to avoid excessive cardiovascular depression).
No products indexed under this heading.

Isoniazid (Clinically significant interactions have been reported with inhibitors of cytochrome P450 3A4 causing elevation of plasma levels of verapamil).
No products indexed under this heading.

Isosorbide Dinitrate (Co-administration with oral antihypertensive agents (eg, vasodilators) will usually have an additive effect on lowering blood pressure). Products include:
BiDil Tablets 2161

Isosorbide Mononitrate (Co-administration with oral antihypertensive agents (eg, vasodilators) will usually have an additive effect on lowering blood pressure). Products include:
Imdur Tablets 3032

Isoxsuprine Hydrochloride (Co-administration with oral antihypertensive agents (eg, vasodilators) will usually have an additive effect on lowering blood pressure).
No products indexed under this heading.

Isradipine (Co-administration with oral antihypertensive agents will usually have an additive effect on lowering blood pressure). Products include:
DynaCirc CR Tablets 2726

Itraconazole (Clinically significant interactions have been reported with inhibitors of cytochrome P450 3A4 causing elevation of plasma levels of verapamil).
No products indexed under this heading.

Ketoconazole (Clinically significant interactions have been reported with inhibitors of cytochrome P450 3A4 causing elevation of plasma levels of verapamil). Products include:
Nizoral A-D Shampoo, 1% 1839
Nizoral 2% Shampoo 1838

Labetalol Hydrochloride (Concomitant therapy with beta-adrenergic blockers and verapamil may result in additive negative effects on heart rate, A-V conduction, and/or cardiac contractility; excessive bradycardia and A-V block have been reported with concurrent use in hypertensive patients.This combination should be used only with caution and close monitoring).
No products indexed under this heading.

Levobunolol Hydrochloride (Concomitant therapy with beta-adrenergic blockers and verapamil may result in additive negative effects on heart rate, A-V conduction, and/or cardiac contractility; excessive bradycardia and A-V block have been reported with concurrent use in hypertensive patients.This combination should be used only with caution and close monitoring). Products include:
Betagan Ophthalmic Solution, USP .... ⊙ 217

Lisinopril (Co-administration with oral antihypertensive agents will usually have an additive effect on lowering blood pressure). Products include:
Prinivil Tablets 2029
Prinzide Tablets 2033
Zestoretic Tablets 701
Zestril Tablets 704

Lithium (Increased sensitivity to the effects of lithium (neurotoxicity) has been reported during concomitant verapamil-lithium therapy with either no change or an increase in serum lithium levels. However, the addition of verapamil has also resulted in the lowering of serum lithium levels in patients receiving chronic stable oral lithium. Patients receiving both drugs

must be monitored carefully).
No products indexed under this heading.

Lithium Carbonate (Increased sensitivity to the effects of lithium (neurotoxicity) has been reported during concomitant verapamil-lithium therapy with either no change or an increase in serum lithium levels. However, the addition of verapamil has also resulted in the lowering of serum lithium levels in patients receiving chronic stable oral lithium. Patients receiving both drugs must be monitored carefully). Products include:
Eskalith 1406
Lithobid Tablets 1670

Lithium Citrate (Increased sensitivity to the effects of lithium (neurotoxicity) has been reported during concomitant verapamil-lithium therapy with either no change or an increase in serum lithium levels. However, the addition of verapamil has also resulted in the lowering of serum lithium levels in patients receiving chronic stable oral lithium. Patients receiving both drugs must be monitored carefully).
No products indexed under this heading.

Lopinavir (Clinically significant interactions have been reported with inhibitors of cytochrome P450 3A4 causing elevation of plasma levels of verapamil). Products include:
Kaletra 474

Loratadine (Clinically significant interactions have been reported with inhibitors of cytochrome P450 3A4 causing elevation of plasma levels of verapamil). Products include:
Alavert Allergy & Sinus D-12 Hour Tablets .... ▣743
Alavert .... ▣743
Children's Claritin 24 Hour Non-Drowsy Allergy Syrup .... ▣732
Claritin Non-Drowsy 24 Hour Tablets .... ▣731
Non-Drowsy Claritin Hives Relief Tablets .... ▣733
Claritin Reditabs 24 Hour Non-Drowsy Tablets .... ▣732
Claritin-D Non-Drowsy 12 Hour Tablets .... ▣731
Claritin-D Non-Drowsy 24 Hour Tablets .... ▣731
Children's Dimetapp ND Non-Drowsy Allergy Syrup .... ▣746
Triaminic Allerchews .... ▣684

Losartan Potassium (Co-administration with oral antihypertensive agents will usually have an additive effect on lowering blood pressure). Products include:
Cozaar Tablets 1913
Hyzaar 1964

Mecamylamine Hydrochloride (Co-administration with oral antihypertensive agents will usually have an additive effect on lowering blood pressure). Products include:
Inversine Tablets 3286

Mephenytoin (Clinically significant interactions have been reported with inducers of cytochrome P450 3A4 causing a lowering of plasma levels of verapamil).
No products indexed under this heading.

Methoxyflurane (When used concomitantly, inhalation anesthetics and calcium antagonists, such as verapamil, should each be titrated carefully to avoid excessive cardiovascular depression).
No products indexed under this heading.

Methsuximide (Clinically significant interactions have been reported with inducers of cytochrome P450 3A4 causing a lowering of plasma levels of verapamil).
No products indexed under this heading.

Methyclothiazide (Co-administration with oral antihypertensive agents will usually have an additive effect on lowering blood pressure).
No products indexed under this heading.

Methyldopa (Co-administration with oral antihypertensive agents will usually have an additive effect on lowering blood pressure). Products include:
Aldoclor Tablets 1881
Aldoril Tablets 1884

Methyldopate Hydrochloride (Co-administration with oral antihypertensive agents will usually have an additive effect on lowering blood pressure).
No products indexed under this heading.

Methylprednisolone (Clinically significant interactions have been reported with inducers of cytochrome P450 3A4 causing a lowering of plasma levels of verapamil).
No products indexed under this heading.

Methylprednisolone Acetate (Clinically significant interactions have been reported with inducers of cytochrome P450 3A4 causing a lowering of plasma levels of verapamil). Products include:
Depo-Medrol Injectable Suspension 2615
Depo-Medrol Single-Dose Vial 2617

Methylprednisolone Sodium Succinate (Clinically significant interactions have been reported with inducers of cytochrome P450 3A4 causing a lowering of plasma levels of verapamil).
No products indexed under this heading.

Metipranolol Hydrochloride (Concomitant therapy with beta-adrenergic blockers and verapamil may result in additive negative effects on heart rate, A-V conduction, and/or cardiac contractility; excessive bradycardia and A-V block have been reported with concurrent use in hypertensive patients.This combination should be used only with caution and close monitoring).
No products indexed under this heading.

Metocurine Iodide (Clinical data and animal studies suggest that verapamil may potentiate the activity of neuromuscular blocking agents (curare-like and depolarizing). It may be necessary to decrease the dose of verapamil and/or the dose of the neuromuscular blocking agent when the drugs are used concomitantly).
No products indexed under this heading.

Metolazone (Co-administration with oral antihypertensive agents will usually have an additive effect on lowering blood pressure).
No products indexed under this heading.

Metoprolol Succinate (Co-administration has resulted in a decrease in metoprolol clearance; concomitant therapy may result in additive negative effects on heart rate, A-V conduction, and/or cardiac contractility; excessive bradycardia and A-V block have been reported with concurrent use in hypertensive patients). Products include:
Toprol-XL Tablets 660

Metoprolol Tartrate (Co-administration has resulted in a decrease in metoprolol clearance; concomitant therapy may result in additive negative effects on heart rate, A-V conduction, and/or cardiac contractility; excessive bradycardia and A-V block have been reported with concurrent use in hypertensive patients).
No products indexed under this heading.

Metronidazole (Clinically significant interactions have been reported with inhibitors of cytochrome P450 3A4 causing elevation of plasma levels of verapamil). Products include:
Metrogel 1% 1212
MetroGel-Vaginal Gel 1822
Noritate Cream, 1% 1051

Metronidazole Benzoate (Clinically significant interactions have been reported with inhibitors of cytochrome P450 3A4 causing elevation of plasma levels of verapamil).
No products indexed under this heading.

Metronidazole Hydrochloride (Clinically significant interactions have been reported with inhibitors of cytochrome P450 3A4 causing elevation of plasma levels of verapamil).
No products indexed under this heading.

Metyrosine (Co-administration with oral antihypertensive agents will usually have an additive effect on lowering blood pressure). Products include:
Demser Capsules 1933

Mibefradil Dihydrochloride (Co-administration with oral antihypertensive agents will usually have an additive effect on lowering blood pressure).
No products indexed under this heading.

Miconazole (Clinically significant interactions have been reported with inhibitors of cytochrome P450 3A4 causing elevation of plasma levels of verapamil).
No products indexed under this heading.

Miconazole Nitrate (Clinically significant interactions have been reported with inhibitors of cytochrome P450 3A4 causing elevation of plasma levels of verapamil). Products include:
Desenex .... ▣674
Desenex Jock Itch Spray Powder ... ▣674

Minoxidil (Co-administration with oral antihypertensive agents will usually have an additive effect on lowering blood pressure). Products include:
Men's Rogaine Extra Strength Topical Solution, Ocean Rush Scent and Original Unscented ..... ▣706
Women's Rogaine Topical Solution, Spring Bloom Scent and Original Unscented .... ▣707

Mivacurium Chloride (Clinical data and animal studies suggest that verapamil may potentiate the activity of neuromuscular blocking agents (curare-like and depolarizing). It may be necessary to decrease the dose of verapamil and/or the dose of the neuromuscular blocking agent when the drugs are used concomitantly). Products include:
Mivacron Injection 489

Modafinil (Clinically significant interactions have been reported with inducers of cytochrome P450 3A4 causing a lowering of plasma levels of verapamil). Products include:
Provigil Tablets 1002

Moexipril Hydrochloride (Co-administration with oral antihypertensive agents will usually have an additive effect on lowering blood pressure). Products include:
Uniretic Tablets 3114
Univasc Tablets 3118

Nadolol (Concomitant therapy with beta-adrenergic blockers and verapamil may result in additive negative effects on heart rate, A-V conduction, and/or cardiac contractility; excessive bradycardia and A-V block have been reported with concurrent use in hypertensive patients.This combination should be used only with caution and close monitoring). Products include:
Nadolol Tablets 2121

Nefazodone Hydrochloride (Clinically significant interactions have been reported with inhibitors of cytochrome P450 3A4 causing elevation of plasma levels of verapamil).
No products indexed under this heading.

Nelfinavir Mesylate (Clinically significant interactions have been reported with inhibitors of cytochrome P450 3A4 causing elevation of plasma levels of verapamil). Products include:
Viracept 2556

Nevirapine (Clinically significant interactions have been reported with inducers of cytochrome P450 3A4 causing a lowering of plasma levels of verapamil). Products include:
Viramune Oral Suspension 903
Viramune Tablets 903

Niacinamide (Clinically significant interactions have been reported with inhibitors of cytochrome P450 3A4 causing elevation of plasma levels of verapamil).
No products indexed under this heading.

Nicardipine Hydrochloride (Co-administration with oral antihypertensive agents will usually have an additive effect on lowering blood pressure). Products include:
Cardene I.V. 1129

Nicotinamide (Clinically significant interactions have been reported with inhibitors of cytochrome P450 3A4 causing elevation of plasma levels of verapamil). Products include:
Nicomide Tablets 3190

Nifedipine (Co-administration with oral antihypertensive agents will usually have an additive effect on lowering blood pressure). Products include:
Adalat CC Tablets 2978

Nisoldipine (Co-administration with oral antihypertensive agents will usually have an additive effect on lowering blood pressure). Products include:
Sular Tablets 1163

Nitroglycerin (Verapamil has been given concomitantly with short- and long-acting nitrates without any undesirable drug interactions. The pharmacologic profile of both drugs and

the clinical experience suggest beneficial interactions). Products include:
Nitro-Dur Transdermal Infusion System ... 3060
Nitrolingual Pumpspray ... 1161

Nitroglycerin, long-acting formulations (Co-administration with oral antihypertensive agents (eg, vasodilators) will usually have an additive effect on lowering blood pressure).
No products indexed under this heading.

Nitroglycerin Intravenous (Co-administration with oral antihypertensive agents (eg, vasodilators) will usually have an additive effect on lowering blood pressure).
No products indexed under this heading.

Norfloxacin (Clinically significant interactions have been reported with inhibitors of cytochrome P450 3A4 causing elevation of plasma levels of verapamil). Products include:
Noroxin Tablets ... 2009

Omeprazole (Clinically significant interactions have been reported with inhibitors of cytochrome P450 3A4 causing elevation of plasma levels of verapamil). Products include:
Zegerid Powder for Oral Solution ... 2972

Oxcarbazepine (Clinically significant interactions have been reported with inducers of cytochrome P450 3A4 causing a lowering of plasma levels of verapamil). Products include:
Trileptal Oral Suspension ... 2281
Trileptal Tablets ... 2281

Paclitaxel (Concomitant administration of R-verapamil can decrease the clearance of paclitaxel).
No products indexed under this heading.

Paclitaxel, protein-bound (Concomitant administration of verapamil can decrease the clearance of paclitaxel).
No products indexed under this heading.

Pancuronium Bromide (Clinical data and animal studies suggest that verapamil may potentiate the activity of neuromuscular blocking agents (curare-like and depolarizing). It may be necessary to decrease the dose of verapamil and/or the dose of the neuromuscular blocking agent when the drugs are used concomitantly).
No products indexed under this heading.

Papaverine (Co-administration with oral antihypertensive agents (eg, vasodilators) will usually have an additive effect on lowering blood pressure).
No products indexed under this heading.

Papaverine Hydrochloride (Co-administration with oral antihypertensive agents (eg, vasodilators) will usually have an additive effect on lowering blood pressure).
No products indexed under this heading.

Paroxetine Hydrochloride (Clinically significant interactions have been reported with inhibitors of cytochrome P450 3A4 causing elevation of plasma levels of verapamil). Products include:
Paxil CR Controlled-Release Tablets ... 1509
Paxil ... 1501

Penbutolol Sulfate (Concomitant therapy with beta-adrenergic blockers and verapamil may result in additive negative effects on heart rate, A-V conduction, and/or cardiac contractility; excessive bradycardia and A-V block have been reported with concurrent use in hypertensive patients.This combination should be used only with caution and close monitoring).
No products indexed under this heading.

Perindopril Erbumine (Co-administration with oral antihypertensive agents will usually have an additive effect on lowering blood pressure). Products include:
Aceon Tablets (2 mg, 4 mg, 8 mg) ... 3191

Phenobarbital (Combined therapy with phenobarbital may increase verapamil clearance).
No products indexed under this heading.

Phenobarbital Sodium (Clinically significant interactions have been reported with inducers of cytochrome P450 3A4 causing a lowering of plasma levels of verapamil).
No products indexed under this heading.

Phenoxybenzamine Hydrochloride (Co-administration with oral antihypertensive agents will usually have an additive effect on lowering blood pressure). Products include:
Dibenzyline Capsules ... 3390

Phentolamine Mesylate (Co-administration with oral antihypertensive agents will usually have an additive effect on lowering blood pressure).
No products indexed under this heading.

Phenytoin (Clinically significant interactions have been reported with inducers of cytochrome P450 3A4 causing a lowering of plasma levels of verapamil).
No products indexed under this heading.

Phenytoin Sodium (Clinically significant interactions have been reported with inducers of cytochrome P450 3A4 causing a lowering of plasma levels of verapamil). Products include:
Phenytek Capsules ... 2153

Pindolol (Concomitant therapy with beta-adrenergic blockers and verapamil may result in additive negative effects on heart rate, A-V conduction, and/or cardiac contractility; excessive bradycardia and A-V block have been reported with concurrent use in hypertensive patients.This combination should be used only with caution and close monitoring).
No products indexed under this heading.

Polythiazide (Co-administration with oral antihypertensive agents will usually have an additive effect on lowering blood pressure).
No products indexed under this heading.

Prazosin Hydrochloride (Concomitant use of agents that attenuate alpha-adrenergic function, such as prazosin, may result in excessive reduction in blood pressure).
No products indexed under this heading.

Prednisolone Acetate (Clinically significant interactions have been reported with inducers of cytochrome P450 3A4 causing a lowering of plasma levels of verapamil). Products include:
Blephamide Ophthalmic Ointment ... 563
Blephamide Ophthalmic Suspension ... 564
Poly-Pred Liquifilm Ophthalmic Suspension ... ⊙231
Pred Forte Ophthalmic Suspension ... ⊙233
Pred Mild Sterile Ophthalmic Suspension ... ⊙236
Pred-G Ophthalmic Suspension ... ⊙234
Pred-G Sterile Ophthalmic Ointment ... ⊙235

Prednisolone Sodium Phosphate (Clinically significant interactions have been reported with inducers of cytochrome P450 3A4 causing a lowering of plasma levels of verapamil). Products include:
Pediapred Oral Solution ... 3319

Prednisolone Tebutate (Clinically significant interactions have been reported with inducers of cytochrome P450 3A4 causing a lowering of plasma levels of verapamil).
No products indexed under this heading.

Prednisone (Clinically significant interactions have been reported with inducers of cytochrome P450 3A4 causing a lowering of plasma levels of verapamil).
No products indexed under this heading.

Primidone (Clinically significant interactions have been reported with inducers of cytochrome P450 3A4 causing a lowering of plasma levels of verapamil).
No products indexed under this heading.

Propoxyphene Hydrochloride (Clinically significant interactions have been reported with inhibitors of cytochrome P450 3A4 causing elevation of plasma levels of verapamil).
No products indexed under this heading.

Propoxyphene Napsylate (Clinically significant interactions have been reported with inhibitors of cytochrome P450 3A4 causing elevation of plasma levels of verapamil). Products include:
Darvocet A 500 Tablets ... 3497

Propranolol Hydrochloride (Concomitant therapy with beta-adrenergic blockers and verapamil may result in additive negative effects on heart rate, A-V conduction, and/or cardiac contractility; excessive bradycardia and A-V block have been reported with concurrent use in hypertensive patients.This combination should be used only with caution and close monitoring). Products include:
Inderal LA Long-Acting Capsules ... 3421
InnoPran XL Capsules ... 2728

Quinapril Hydrochloride (Co-administration with oral antihypertensive agents will usually have an additive effect on lowering blood pressure).
No products indexed under this heading.

Quinidine (In a small number of patients with hypertrophic cardiomyopathy, co-administration has resulted in significant hypotension; combined use in these patients should probably be avoided).
No products indexed under this heading.

Quinidine Gluconate (In a small number of patients with hypertrophic cardiomyopathy, co-administration has resulted in significant hypotension; combined use in these patients should probably be avoided).
No products indexed under this heading.

Quinidine Hydrochloride (In a small number of patients with hypertrophic cardiomyopathy, co-administration has resulted in significant hypotension; combined use in these patients should probably be avoided).
No products indexed under this heading.

Quinidine Polygalacturonate (In a small number of patients with hypertrophic cardiomyopathy, co-administration has resulted in significant hypotension; combined use in these patients should probably be avoided).
No products indexed under this heading.

Quinidine Sulfate (In a small number of patients with hypertrophic cardiomyopathy, co-administration has resulted in significant hypotension; combined use in these patients should probably be avoided).
No products indexed under this heading.

Quinine (Clinically significant interactions have been reported with inhibitors of cytochrome P450 3A4 causing elevation of plasma levels of verapamil).
No products indexed under this heading.

Quinine Sulfate (Clinically significant interactions have been reported with inhibitors of cytochrome P450 3A4 causing elevation of plasma levels of verapamil).
No products indexed under this heading.

Quinupristin (Clinically significant interactions have been reported with inhibitors of cytochrome P450 3A4 causing elevation of plasma levels of verapamil). Products include:
Synercid I.V. ... 1690

Ramipril (Co-administration with oral antihypertensive agents will usually have an additive effect on lowering blood pressure). Products include:
Altace Capsules ... 1673

Ranitidine Bismuth Citrate (Clinically significant interactions have been reported with inhibitors of cytochrome P450 3A4 causing elevation of plasma levels of verapamil).
No products indexed under this heading.

Ranitidine Hydrochloride (Clinically significant interactions have been reported with inhibitors of cytochrome P450 3A4 causing elevation of plasma levels of verapamil). Products include:
Zantac ... 1597
Zantac Injection ... 1593
Zantac 75 Tablets ... 715
Zantac 150 Maximum Strength Tablets ... 715
Zantac Injection Pharmacy Bulk Package ... 1595

IMPORTANT NOTE: Always consult each drug listing in the patient's regimen for possible interactions.

Rapacuronium Bromide (Clinical data and animal studies suggest that verapamil may potentiate the activity of neuromuscular blocking agents (curare-like and depolarizing). It may be necessary to decrease the dose of verapamil and/or the dose of the neuromuscular blocking agent when the drugs are used concomitantly).
No products indexed under this heading.

Rauwolfia Serpentina (Co-administration with oral antihypertensive agents will usually have an additive effect on lowering blood pressure).
No products indexed under this heading.

Rescinnamine (Co-administration with oral antihypertensive agents will usually have an additive effect on lowering blood pressure).
No products indexed under this heading.

Reserpine (Co-administration with oral antihypertensive agents will usually have an additive effect on lowering blood pressure).
No products indexed under this heading.

Rifabutin (Clinically significant interactions have been reported with inducers of cytochrome P450 3A4 causing a lowering of plasma levels of verapamil).
No products indexed under this heading.

Rifampicin (Clinically significant interactions have been reported with inducers of cytochrome P450 3A4 causing a lowering of plasma levels of verapamil).
No products indexed under this heading.

Rifampin (Combined therapy with rifampin may markedly reduce oral verapamil bioavailability).
No products indexed under this heading.

Rifapentine (Clinically significant interactions have been reported with inducers of cytochrome P450 3A4 causing a lowering of plasma levels of verapamil).
No products indexed under this heading.

Ritonavir (Clinically significant interactions have been reported with inhibitors of cytochrome P450 3A4 causing elevation of plasma levels of verapamil). Products include:
Kaletra **474**
Norvir **499**

Rocuronium Bromide (Clinical data and animal studies suggest that verapamil may potentiate the activity of neuromuscular blocking agents (curare-like and depolarizing). It may be necessary to decrease the dose of verapamil and/or the dose of the neuromuscular blocking agent when the drugs are used concomitantly). Products include:
Zemuron Injection **2363**

Saquinavir (Clinically significant interactions have been reported with inhibitors of cytochrome P450 3A4 causing elevation of plasma levels of verapamil).
No products indexed under this heading.

Saquinavir Mesylate (Clinically significant interactions have been reported with inhibitors of cytochrome P450 3A4 causing elevation of plasma levels of verapamil). Products include:
Invirase **2776**

Sertraline Hydrochloride (Clinically significant interactions have been reported with inhibitors of cytochrome P450 3A4 causing elevation of plasma levels of verapamil). Products include:
Zoloft **2581**

Sodium Nitroprusside (Co-administration with oral antihypertensive agents will usually have an additive effect on lowering blood pressure).
No products indexed under this heading.

Sotalol Hydrochloride (Concomitant therapy with beta-adrenergic blockers and verapamil may result in additive negative effects on heart rate, A-V conduction, and/or cardiac contractility; excessive bradycardia and A-V block have been reported with concurrent use in hypertensive patients.This combination should be used only with caution and close monitoring).
No products indexed under this heading.

Spirapril Hydrochloride (Co-administration with oral antihypertensive agents will usually have an additive effect on lowering blood pressure).
No products indexed under this heading.

Spironolactone (Co-administration with oral antihypertensive agents (eg, diuretics) will usually have an additive effect on lowering blood pressure).
No products indexed under this heading.

Succinylcholine Chloride (Clinical data and animal studies suggest that verapamil may potentiate the activity of neuromuscular blocking agents (curare-like and depolarizing). It may be necessary to decrease the dose of verapamil and/or the dose of the neuromuscular blocking agent when the drugs are used concomitantly).
No products indexed under this heading.

Sulfinpyrazone (Clinically significant interactions have been reported with inducers of cytochrome P450 3A4 causing a lowering of plasma levels of verapamil).
No products indexed under this heading.

Telithromycin (Clinically significant interactions have been reported with inhibitors of cytochrome P450 3A4 causing elevation of plasma levels of verapamil). Products include:
Ketek Tablets **2920**

Telmisartan (Co-administration with oral antihypertensive agents will usually have an additive effect on lowering blood pressure). Products include:
Micardis Tablets **884**
Micardis HCT Tablets **886**

Terazosin Hydrochloride (Concomitant use of agents that attenuate alpha-adrenergic function, such as terazosin, may result in excessive reduction in blood pressure). Products include:
Hytrin Capsules **469**

Theophylline (Clinically significant interactions have been reported with inducers of cytochrome P450 3A4 causing a lowering of plasma levels of verapamil).
No products indexed under this heading.

Theophylline Anhydrous (Verapamil may inhibit the clearance and increase the plasma levels of theophylline). Products include:
Uniphyl Tablets **2708**

Theophylline Calcium Salicylate (Verapamil may inhibit the clearance and increase the plasma levels of theophylline).
No products indexed under this heading.

Theophylline Dihydroxypropyl (Glyceryl) (Verapamil may inhibit the clearance and increase the plasma levels of theophylline).
No products indexed under this heading.

Theophylline Ethylenediamine (Verapamil may inhibit the clearance and increase the plasma levels of theophylline).
No products indexed under this heading.

Theophylline Sodium Glycinate (Verapamil may inhibit the clearance and increase the plasma levels of theophylline).
No products indexed under this heading.

Timolol Hemihydrate (Co-administration of oral verapamil and timolol eye drops has resulted in asymptomatic bradycardia with a wandering atrial pacemaker). Products include:
Betimol Ophthalmic Solution **3371**
Betimol Ophthalmic Solution .... ⊙ **283**

Timolol Maleate (Co-administration of oral verapamil and timolol eye drops has resulted in asymptomatic bradycardia with a wandering atrial pacemaker; concomitant therapy may result in additive negative effects on heart rate, A-V conduction, and/or cardiac contractility;excessive bradycardia and A-V block have been reported with concurrent use in hypertensive patients). Products include:
Blocadren Tablets **1891**
Cosopt Sterile Ophthalmic Solution **1910**
Timolide Tablets **2056**
Timoptic in Ocudose **2061**
Timoptic Sterile Ophthalmic Solution **2058**
Timoptic-XE Sterile Ophthalmic Gel Forming Solution **2062**

Tolazoline Hydrochloride (Co-administration with oral antihypertensive agents (eg, vasodilators) will usually have an additive effect on lowering blood pressure).
No products indexed under this heading.

Torsemide (Co-administration with oral antihypertensive agents will usually have an additive effect on lowering blood pressure).
No products indexed under this heading.

Trandolapril (Co-administration with oral antihypertensive agents will usually have an additive effect on lowering blood pressure). Products include:
Mavik Tablets **482**
Tarka Tablets **519**

Triamcinolone (Clinically significant interactions have been reported with inducers of cytochrome P450 3A4 causing a lowering of plasma levels of verapamil).
No products indexed under this heading.

Triamcinolone Acetonide (Clinically significant interactions have been reported with inducers of cytochrome P450 3A4 causing a lowering of plasma levels of verapamil). Products include:
Azmacort Inhalation Aerosol **1701**
Nasacort HFA Inhalation Aerosol **2939**
Nasacort AQ Nasal Spray **2937**

Triamcinolone Diacetate (Clinically significant interactions have been reported with inducers of cytochrome P450 3A4 causing a lowering of plasma levels of verapamil).
No products indexed under this heading.

Triamcinolone Hexacetonide (Clinically significant interactions have been reported with inducers of cytochrome P450 3A4 causing a lowering of plasma levels of verapamil).
No products indexed under this heading.

Triamterene (Co-administration with oral antihypertensive agents (eg, diuretics) will usually have an additive effect on lowering blood pressure). Products include:
Dyazide Capsules **1389**
Dyrenium Capsules **3390**
Maxzide **2150**

Trimethaphan Camsylate (Co-administration with oral antihypertensive agents will usually have an additive effect on lowering blood pressure).
No products indexed under this heading.

Troglitazone (Clinically significant interactions have been reported with inducers of cytochrome P450 3A4 causing a lowering of plasma levels of verapamil).
No products indexed under this heading.

Troleandomycin (Clinically significant interactions have been reported with inhibitors of cytochrome P450 3A4 causing elevation of plasma levels of verapamil).
No products indexed under this heading.

Tubocurarine Chloride (Verapamil may potentiate the activity of neuromuscular blocking drugs).
No products indexed under this heading.

Valproate Sodium (Clinically significant interactions have been reported with inhibitors of cytochrome P450 3A4 causing elevation of plasma levels of verapamil). Products include:
Depacon Injection **412**

Valsartan (Co-administration with oral antihypertensive agents will usually have an additive effect on lowering blood pressure). Products include:
Diovan HCT Tablets **2195**
Diovan Tablets **2191**

Vecuronium Bromide (Clinical data and animal studies suggest that verapamil may potentiate the activity of neuromuscular blocking agents (curare-like and depolarizing). It may be necessary to decrease the dose of verapamil and/or the dose of the neuromuscular blocking agent when the drugs are used concomitantly).
No products indexed under this heading.

Voriconazole (Clinically significant interactions have been reported with inhibitors of cytochrome P450 3A4 causing elevation of plasma levels of verapamil). Products include:

VFEND I.V. **2543**
VFEND Oral Suspension **2543**
VFEND Tablets **2543**

Zafirlukast (Clinically significant interactions have been reported with inhibitors of cytochrome P450 3A4 causing elevation of plasma levels of verapamil). Products include:
Accolate Tablets **663**

Zileuton (Clinically significant interactions have been reported with inhibitors of cytochrome P450 3A4 causing elevation of plasma levels of verapamil).
No products indexed under this heading.

Food Interactions

Alcohol (Verapamil has been found to significantly inhibit ethanol elimination resulting in elevated blood ethanol concentration that may prolong the intoxicating effects of alcohol).

Grapefruit (Grapefruit juice may significantly increase concentrations of verapamil).

Grapefruit Juice (Grapefruit juice may significantly increase concentrations of verapamil).

VERMOX CHEWABLE TABLETS

(Mebendazole) **1853**
May interact with:

Cimetidine (Inhibits mebendazole metabolism and may result in an increase in plasma concentrations of mebendazole). Products include:
Tagamet HB 200 Tablets **637**
Tagamet Tablets **1547**

Cimetidine Hydrochloride (Inhibits mebendazole metabolism and may result in an increase in plasma concentrations of mebendazole).
No products indexed under this heading.

VESANOID CAPSULES

(Tretinoin) **2823**
May interact with cytochrome p450 3a4 inducers (selected), cytochrome p450 3a4 inhibitors (selected), erythromycin, glucocorticoids, tetracyclines, and certain other agents. Compounds in these categories include:

Acetazolamide (Tretinoin is metaboized by the hepatic P450 system; therefore, there is a potential for alteration of pharmacokinetic parameters in patients administered concomitant medications that are also inducers of this system. To date, there is no data to suggestthat co-use with these medications increases or decreases either efficacy or toxicity of tretinoin).
No products indexed under this heading.

Allium sativum (Tretinoin is metaboized by the hepatic P450 system; therefore, there is a potential for alteration of pharmacokinetic parameters in patients administered concomitant medications that are also inducers of this system. To date, there is no data to suggestthat co-use with these medications increases or decreases either efficacy or toxicity of tretinoin).
No products indexed under this heading.

Aminocaproic Acid (Cases of fatal thrombotic complications have been reported rarely in patients concomitantly treated with tretinoin and antifibrinolytic agents. Therefore, caution should be exercised when administering tretinoin concomitantly with these agents).
No products indexed under this heading.

Amiodarone Hydrochloride (Tretinoin is metaboized by the hepatic P450 system; therefore, there is a potential for alteration of pharmacokinetic parameters in patients administered concomitant medications that are also inducers of this system. To date, there is no data to suggest that co-use with these medications increases or decreases either efficacy or toxicity of tretinoin). Products include:
Pacerone Tablets **3337**

Amprenavir (Tretinoin is metaboized by the hepatic P450 system; therefore, there is a potential for alteration of pharmacokinetic parameters in patients administered concomitant medications that are also inducers of this system. To date, there is no data to suggestthat co-use with these medications increases or decreases either efficacy or toxicity of tretinoin). Products include:
Agenerase Capsules **1299**
Agenerase Oral Solution **1304**

Anastrozole (Tretinoin is metaboized by the hepatic P450 system; therefore, there is a potential for alteration of pharmacokinetic parameters in patients administered concomitant medications that are also inducers of this system. To date, there is no data to suggestthat co-use with these medications increases or decreases either efficacy or toxicity of tretinoin). Products include:
Arimidex Tablets **665**

Aprepitant (Tretinoin is metaboized by the hepatic P450 system; therefore, there is a potential for alteration of pharmacokinetic parameters in patients administered concomitant medications that are also inducers of this system. To date, there is no data to suggestthat co-use with these medications increases or decreases either efficacy or toxicity of tretinoin). Products include:
Emend Capsules **1944**

Aprotinin (Cases of fatal thrombotic complications have been reported rarely in patients concomitantly treated with tretinoin and anti-fibrinolytic agents. Therefore, caution should be exercised when administering tretinoin concomitantly with these agents). Products include:
Trasylol Injection **779**

Betamethasone Acetate (Potential for alteration of pharmacokinetic parameters in patients on concomitant drugs that are inducers of hepatic CYP enzymes).
No products indexed under this heading.

Betamethasone Sodium Phosphate (Potential for alteration of pharmacokinetic parameters in patients on concomitant drugs that are inducers of hepatic CYP enzymes).
No products indexed under this heading.

Carbamazepine (Tretinoin is metaboized by the hepatic P450 system; therefore, there is a potential for alteration of pharmacokinetic parameters in patients administered concomitant medications that are also inducers of this system. To date, there is no data to suggestthat co-use with these medications increases or decreases either efficacy or toxicity of tretinoin). Products include:
Carbatrol Capsules **3174**
Equetro Extended-Release Capsules **3178**
Tegretol/Tegretol-XR **2278**

Cimetidine (Potential for alteration of pharmacokinetic parameters in patients on concomitant drugs that inhibit hepatic CYP enzymes). Products include:
Tagamet HB 200 Tablets **637**
Tagamet Tablets **1547**

Cimetidine Hydrochloride (Potential for alteration of pharmacokinetic parameters in patients on concomitant drugs that inhibit hepatic CYP enzymes).
No products indexed under this heading.

Ciprofloxacin (Tretinoin is metaboized by the hepatic P450 system; therefore, there is a potential for alteration of pharmacokinetic parameters in patients administered concomitant medications that are also inducers of this system. To date, there is no data to suggestthat co-use with these medications increases or decreases either efficacy or toxicity of tretinoin). Products include:
Cipro I.V. **2998**
Cipro I.V. Pharmacy Bulk Package ... **3509**
Cipro Oral Suspension **2991**
Cipro XR Tablets **3004**
Ciprodex Otic Suspension **555**

Ciprofloxacin Hydrochloride (Tretinoin is metaboized by the hepatic P450 system; therefore, there is a potential for alteration of pharmacokinetic parameters in patients administered concomitant medications that are also inducers of this system. To date, there is no data to suggest that co-use with these medications increases or decreases either efficacy or toxicity of tretinoin). Products include:
Ciloxan Ophthalmic Ointment **554**
Cipro Tablets **2991**

Cisplatin (Tretinoin is metaboized by the hepatic P450 system; therefore, there is a potential for alteration of pharmacokinetic parameters in patients administered concomitant medications that are also inducers of this system. To date, there is no data to suggestthat co-use with these medications increases or decreases either efficacy or toxicity of tretinoin).
No products indexed under this heading.

Clarithromycin (Tretinoin is metaboized by the hepatic P450 system; therefore, there is a potential for alteration of pharmacokinetic parameters in patients administered concomitant medications that are also inducers of this system. To date, there is no data to suggestthat co-use with these medications increases or decreases either efficacy or toxicity of tretinoin). Products include:
Biaxin/Biaxin XL **402**
PREVPAC **3281**

Clotrimazole (Tretinoin is metaboized by the hepatic P450 system; therefore, there is a potential for alteration of pharmacokinetic parameters in patients administered concomitant medications that are also inducers of this system. To date, there is no data to suggestthat co-use with these medications increases or decreases either efficacy or toxicity of tretinoin). Products include:
Lotrimin **3053**
Lotrisone **3054**

Cortisone Acetate (Potential for alteration of pharmacokinetic parameters in patients on concomitant drugs that are inducers of hepatic CYP enzymes).
No products indexed under this heading.

Cyclosporine (Potential for alteration of pharmacokinetic parameters in patients on concomitant drugs that inhibit hepatic CYP enzymes). Products include:
Gengraf Capsules **458**
Neoral Soft Gelatin Capsules **2247**
Neoral Oral Solution **2247**
Restasis Ophthalmic Emulsion **570**
Sandimmune **2259**

Dalfopristin (Tretinoin is metaboized by the hepatic P450 system; therefore, there is a potential for alteration of pharmacokinetic parameters in patients administered concomitant medications that are also inducers of this system. To date, there is no data to suggestthat co-use with these medications increases or decreases either efficacy or toxicity of tretinoin). Products include:
Synercid I.V. **1690**

Danazol (Tretinoin is metaboized by the hepatic P450 system; therefore, there is a potential for alteration of pharmacokinetic parameters in patients administered concomitant medications that are also inducers of this system. To date, there is no data to suggestthat co-use with these medications increases or decreases either efficacy or toxicity of tretinoin).
No products indexed under this heading.

Delavirdine Mesylate (Tretinoin is metaboized by the hepatic P450 system; therefore, there is a potential for alteration of pharmacokinetic parameters in patients administered concomitant medications that are also inducers of this system. To date, there is no data to suggestthat co-use with these medications increases or decreases either efficacy or toxicity of tretinoin). Products include:
Rescriptor Tablets **2535**

Demeclocycline Hydrochloride (Tretinoin may cause pseudotumor cerebri/intracranial hypertension. Concomitant administration of tretinoin and agents known to cause pseudotumor cerebri/intracranial hypertension as well might increase the risk of this condition).
No products indexed under this heading.

Dexamethasone (Potential for alteration of pharmacokinetic parameters in patients on concomitant drugs that are inducers of hepatic CYP enzymes). Products include:
Ciprodex Otic Suspension **555**
Decadron Tablets **1929**
TobraDex Ophthalmic Ointment **558**
TobraDex Ophthalmic Suspension ... **558**

IMPORTANT NOTE: Always consult each drug listing in the patient's regimen for possible interactions.

Dexamethasone Acetate (Potential for alteration of pharmacokinetic parameters in patients on concomitant drugs that are inducers of hepatic CYP enzymes).
No products indexed under this heading.

Dexamethasone Sodium Phosphate (Potential for alteration of pharmacokinetic parameters in patients on concomitant drugs that are inducers of hepatic CYP enzymes). Products include:
Decadron Phosphate Injection **1931**

Diltiazem Hydrochloride (Potential for alteration of pharmacokinetic parameters in patients on concomitant drugs that inhibit hepatic CYP enzymes). Products include:
Cardizem LA Extended Release Tablets **1699**
Tiazac Capsules **1204**

Diltiazem Maleate (Tretinoin is metaboized by the hepatic P450 system; therefore, there is a potential for alteration of pharmacokinetic parameters in patients administered concomitant medications that are also inducers of this system. To date, there is no data to suggestthat co-use with these medications increases or decreases either efficacy or toxicity of tretinoin).
No products indexed under this heading.

Doxorubicin Hydrochloride (Tretinoin is metaboized by the hepatic P450 system; therefore, there is a potential for alteration of pharmacokinetic parameters in patients administered concomitant medications that are also inducers of this system. To date, there is no data to suggestthat co-use with these medications increases or decreases either efficacy or toxicity of tretinoin). Products include:
Adriamycin for Injection, USP **786**
Adriamycin Injection, USP **786**

Doxycycline Calcium (Tretinoin may cause pseudotumor cerebri/intracranial hypertension. Concomitant administration of tretinoin and agents known to cause pseudotumor cerebri/intracranial hypertension as well might increase the risk of this condition).
No products indexed under this heading.

Doxycycline Hyclate (Tretinoin may cause pseudotumor cerebri/intracranial hypertension. Concomitant administration of tretinoin and agents known to cause pseudotumor cerebri/intracranial hypertension as well might increase the risk of this condition).
No products indexed under this heading.

Doxycycline Monohydrate (Tretinoin may cause pseudotumor cerebri/intracranial hypertension. Concomitant administration of tretinoin and agents known to cause pseudotumor cerebri/intracranial hypertension as well might increase the risk of this condition).
No products indexed under this heading.

Efavirenz (Tretinoin is metaboized by the hepatic P450 system; therefore, there is a potential for alteration of pharmacokinetic parameters in patients administered concomitant medications that are also inducers of this system. To date, there is no data to suggestthat co-use with these medications increases or decreases either efficacy or toxicity of tretinoin). Products include:
Sustiva Capsules **957**

Erythromycin (Potential for alteration of pharmacokinetic parameters in patients on concomitant drugs that inhibit hepatic CYP enzymes). Products include:
Erygel Topical Gel **2096**
Ery-Tab Tablets **447**
Erythromycin Base Filmtab Tablets **454**
Erythromycin Delayed-Release Capsules, USP **456**
PCE Dispertab Tablets **510**

Erythromycin Estolate (Potential for alteration of pharmacokinetic parameters in patients on concomitant drugs that inhibit hepatic CYP enzymes).
No products indexed under this heading.

Erythromycin Ethylsuccinate (Potential for alteration of pharmacokinetic parameters in patients on concomitant drugs that inhibit hepatic CYP enzymes). Products include:
E.E.S. **449**
EryPed **445**

Erythromycin Gluceptate (Potential for alteration of pharmacokinetic parameters in patients on concomitant drugs that inhibit hepatic CYP enzymes).
No products indexed under this heading.

Erythromycin Lactobionate (Potential for alteration of pharmacokinetic parameters in patients on concomitant drugs that inhibit hepatic CYP enzymes).
No products indexed under this heading.

Erythromycin Stearate (Potential for alteration of pharmacokinetic parameters in patients on concomitant drugs that inhibit hepatic CYP enzymes). Products include:
Erythrocin Stearate Filmtab Tablets **452**

Esomeprazole Magnesium (Tretinoin is metaboized by the hepatic P450 system; therefore, there is a potential for alteration of pharmacokinetic parameters in patients administered concomitant medications that are also inducers of this system. To date, there is no data to suggestthat co-use with these medications increases or decreases either efficacy or toxicity of tretinoin). Products include:
Nexium Delayed-Release Capsules **645**

Ethosuximide (Tretinoin is metaboized by the hepatic P450 system; therefore, there is a potential for alteration of pharmacokinetic parameters in patients administered concomitant medications that are also inducers of this system. To date, there is no data to suggestthat co-use with these medications increases or decreases either efficacy or toxicity of tretinoin).
No products indexed under this heading.

Felbamate (Tretinoin is metaboized by the hepatic P450 system; therefore, there is a potential for alteration of pharmacokinetic parameters in patients administered concomitant medications that are also inducers of this system. To date, there is no data to suggestthat co-use with these medications increases or decreases either efficacy or toxicity of tretinoin).
No products indexed under this heading.

Fluconazole (Tretinoin is metaboized by the hepatic P450 system; therefore, there is a potential for alteration of pharmacokinetic parameters in patients administered concomitant medications that are also inducers of this system. To date, there is no data to suggestthat co-use with these medications increases or decreases either efficacy or toxicity of tretinoin).
No products indexed under this heading.

Fludrocortisone Acetate (Potential for alteration of pharmacokinetic parameters in patients on concomitant drugs that are inducers of hepatic CYP enzymes).
No products indexed under this heading.

Fluoxetine Hydrochloride (Tretinoin is metaboized by the hepatic P450 system; therefore, there is a potential for alteration of pharmacokinetic parameters in patients administered concomitant medications that are also inducers of this system. To date, there is no data to suggest-that co-use with these medications increases or decreases either efficacy or toxicity of tretinoin). Products include:
Prozac Pulvules and Liquid **1771**
Symbyax Capsules **1788**

Fluvoxamine Maleate (Tretinoin is metaboized by the hepatic P450 system; therefore, there is a potential for alteration of pharmacokinetic parameters in patients administered concomitant medications that are also inducers of this system. To date, there is no data to suggestthat co-use with these medications increases or decreases either efficacy or toxicity of tretinoin).
No products indexed under this heading.

Fosamprenavir Calcium (Tretinoin is metaboized by the hepatic P450 system; therefore, there is a potential for alteration of pharmacokinetic parameters in patients administered concomitant medications that are also inducers of this system. To date, there is no data to suggestthat co-use with these medications increases or decreases either efficacy or toxicity of tretinoin). Products include:
Lexiva Tablets **1473**

Fosphenytoin Sodium (Tretinoin is metaboized by the hepatic P450 system; therefore, there is a potential for alteration of pharmacokinetic parameters in patients administered concomitant medications that are also inducers of this system. To date, there is no data to suggestthat co-use with these medications increases or decreases either efficacy or toxicity of tretinoin).
No products indexed under this heading.

Garlic Extract (Tretinoin is metaboized by the hepatic P450 system; therefore, there is a potential for alteration of pharmacokinetic parameters in patients administered concomitant medications that are also inducers of this system. To date, there is no data to suggestthat co-use with these medications increases or decreases either efficacy or toxicity of tretinoin).
No products indexed under this heading.

Garlic Oil (Tretinoin is metaboized by the hepatic P450 system; therefore, there is a potential for alteration of pharmacokinetic parameters in patients administered concomitant medications that are also inducers of this system. To date, there is no data to suggestthat co-use with these medications increases or decreases either efficacy or toxicity of tretinoin).
No products indexed under this heading.

Hydrocortisone (Potential for alteration of pharmacokinetic parameters in patients on concomitant drugs that are inducers of hepatic CYP enzymes). Products include:
Cortizone•5 Ointment .... ▣ **699**
Cortizone•10 Creme .... ▣ **699**
Cortizone•10 Ointment .... ▣ **699**
Cortizone•10 Plus Creme .... ▣ **700**
Cortizone•10 Maximum Strength Quick Shot Spray .... ▣ **700**
Hydrocortone Tablets **1963**
Preparation H Hydrocortisone Cream .... ▣ **748**

Hydrocortisone Acetate (Potential for alteration of pharmacokinetic parameters in patients on concomitant drugs that are inducers of hepatic CYP enzymes). Products include:
Analpram-HC **1136**
Pramosone **1139**
ProctoFoam-HC **3113**
Tucks Anti-Itch Ointment .... ▣ **712**
U-cort 1% Cream **3289**

Hydrocortisone Butyrate (Tretinoin is metaboized by the hepatic P450 system; therefore, there is a potential for alteration of pharmacokinetic parameters in patients administered concomitant medications that are also inducers of this system. To date, there is no data to suggest-that co-use with these medications increases or decreases either efficacy or toxicity of tretinoin). Products include:
Locoid **1138**
Locoid Lipocream Cream **1138**

Hydrocortisone Cypionate (Tretinoin is metaboized by the hepatic P450 system; therefore, there is a potential for alteration of pharmacokinetic parameters in patients administered concomitant medications that are also inducers of this system. To date, there is no data to suggest-that co-use with these medications increases or decreases either efficacy or toxicity of tretinoin).
No products indexed under this heading.

Hydrocortisone Hemisuccinate (Tretinoin is metaboized by the hepatic P450 system; therefore, there is a potential for alteration of pharmacokinetic parameters in patients administered concomitant medications that are also inducers of this system. To date, there is no data to suggestthat co-use with these medications increases or decreases either efficacy or toxicity of tretinoin).
No products indexed under this heading.

Hydrocortisone Probutate (Tretinoin is metaboized by the hepatic P450 system; therefore, there is a potential for alteration of pharmacokinetic parameters in patients administered concomitant medications that are also inducers of this system. To date, there is no data to suggestthat co-use with these medications increases or decreases either efficacy or toxicity of tretinoin). Products include:
Pandel Cream, 0.1% 1017

Hydrocortisone Sodium Phosphate (Potential for alteration of pharmacokinetic parameters in patients on concomitant drugs that are inducers of hepatic CYP enzymes).
No products indexed under this heading.

Hydrocortisone Sodium Succinate (Potential for alteration of pharmacokinetic parameters in patients on concomitant drugs that are inducers of hepatic CYP enzymes).
No products indexed under this heading.

Hydrocortisone Valerate (Tretinoin is metaboized by the hepatic P450 system; therefore, there is a potential for alteration of pharmacokinetic parameters in patients administered concomitant medications that are also inducers of this system. To date, there is no data to suggestthat co-use with these medications increases or decreases either efficacy or toxicity of tretinoin).
No products indexed under this heading.

Hypericum (Tretinoin is metaboized by the hepatic P450 system; therefore, there is a potential for alteration of pharmacokinetic parameters in patients administered concomitant medications that are also inducers of this system. To date, there is no data to suggestthat co-use with these medications increases or decreases either efficacy or toxicity of tretinoin).
No products indexed under this heading.

Hypericum Perforatum (Tretinoin is metaboized by the hepatic P450 system; therefore, there is a potential for alteration of pharmacokinetic parameters in patients administered concomitant medications that are also inducers of this system. To date, there is no data to suggestthat co-use with these medications increases or decreases either efficacy or toxicity of tretinoin).
No products indexed under this heading.

Indinavir Sulfate (Tretinoin is metaboized by the hepatic P450 system; therefore, there is a potential for alteration of pharmacokinetic parameters in patients administered concomitant medications that are also inducers of this system. To date, there is no data to suggestthat co-use with these medications increases or decreases either efficacy or toxicity of tretinoin). Products include:
Crixivan Capsules 1918

Isoniazid (Tretinoin is metaboized by the hepatic P450 system; therefore, there is a potential for alteration of pharmacokinetic parameters in patients administered concomitant medications that are also inducers of this system. To date, there is no data to suggestthat co-use with these medications increases or decreases either efficacy or toxicity of tretinoin).
No products indexed under this heading.

Itraconazole (Tretinoin is metaboized by the hepatic P450 system; therefore, there is a potential for alteration of pharmacokinetic parameters in patients administered concomitant medications that are also inducers of this system. To date, there is no data to suggestthat co-use with these medications increases or decreases either efficacy or toxicity of tretinoin).
No products indexed under this heading.

Ketoconazole (Potential for alteration of pharmacokinetic parameters in patients on concomitant drugs that inhibit hepatic CYP enzymes). Products include:
Nizoral A-D Shampoo, 1% 1839
Nizoral 2% Shampoo 1838

Lopinavir (Tretinoin is metaboized by the hepatic P450 system; therefore, there is a potential for alteration of pharmacokinetic parameters in patients administered concomitant medications that are also inducers of this system. To date, there is no data to suggestthat co-use with these medications increases or decreases either efficacy or toxicity of tretinoin). Products include:
Kaletra 474

Loratadine (Tretinoin is metaboized by the hepatic P450 system; therefore, there is a potential for alteration of pharmacokinetic parameters in patients administered concomitant medications that are also inducers of this system. To date, there is no data to suggestthat co-use with these medications increases or decreases either efficacy or toxicity of tretinoin). Products include:
Alavert Allergy & Sinus D-12 Hour Tablets 743
Alavert 743
Children's Claritin 24 Hour Non-Drowsy Allergy Syrup 732
Claritin Non-Drowsy 24 Hour Tablets 731
Non-Drowsy Claritin Hives Relief Tablets 733
Claritin Reditabs 24 Hour Non-Drowsy Tablets 732
Claritin-D Non-Drowsy 12 Hour Tablets 731
Claritin-D Non-Drowsy 24 Hour Tablets 731
Children's Dimetapp ND Non-Drowsy Allergy Syrup 746
Triaminic Allerchews 684

Mephenytoin (Tretinoin is metaboized by the hepatic P450 system; therefore, there is a potential for alteration of pharmacokinetic parameters in patients administered concomitant medications that are also inducers of this system. To date, there is no data to suggestthat co-use with these medications increases or decreases either efficacy or toxicity of tretinoin).
No products indexed under this heading.

Methacycline Hydrochloride (Tretinoin may cause pseudotumor cerebri/intracranial hypertension. Concomitant administration of tretinoin and agents known to cause pseudotumor cerebri/intracranial hypertension as well might increase the risk of this condition).
No products indexed under this heading.

Methsuximide (Tretinoin is metaboized by the hepatic P450 system; therefore, there is a potential for alteration of pharmacokinetic parameters in patients administered concomitant medications that are also inducers of this system. To date, there is no data to suggestthat co-use with these medications increases or decreases either efficacy or toxicity of tretinoin).
No products indexed under this heading.

Methylprednisolone (Tretinoin is metaboized by the hepatic P450 system; therefore, there is a potential for alteration of pharmacokinetic parameters in patients administered concomitant medications that are also inducers of this system. To date, there is no data to suggestthat co-use with these medications increases or decreases either efficacy or toxicity of tretinoin).
No products indexed under this heading.

Methylprednisolone Acetate (Potential for alteration of pharmacokinetic parameters in patients on concomitant drugs that are inducers of hepatic CYP enzymes). Products include:
Depo-Medrol Injectable Suspension 2615
Depo-Medrol Single-Dose Vial 2617

Methylprednisolone Sodium Succinate (Potential for alteration of pharmacokinetic parameters in patients on concomitant drugs that are inducers of hepatic CYP enzymes).
No products indexed under this heading.

Metronidazole (Tretinoin is metaboized by the hepatic P450 system; therefore, there is a potential for alteration of pharmacokinetic parameters in patients administered concomitant medications that are also inducers of this system. To date, there is no data to suggestthat co-use with these medications increases or decreases either efficacy or toxicity of tretinoin). Products include:
Metrogel 1% 1212
MetroGel-Vaginal Gel 1822
Noritate Cream, 1% 1051

Metronidazole Benzoate (Tretinoin is metaboized by the hepatic P450 system; therefore, there is a potential for alteration of pharmacokinetic parameters in patients administered concomitant medications that are also inducers of this system. To date, there is no data to suggestthat co-use with these medications increases or decreases either efficacy or toxicity of tretinoin).
No products indexed under this heading.

Metronidazole Hydrochloride (Tretinoin is metaboized by the hepatic P450 system; therefore, there is a potential for alteration of pharmacokinetic parameters in patients administered concomitant medications that are also inducers of this system. To date, there is no data to suggestthat co-use with these medications increases or decreases either efficacy or toxicity of tretinoin).
No products indexed under this heading.

Miconazole (Tretinoin is metaboized by the hepatic P450 system; therefore, there is a potential for alteration of pharmacokinetic parameters in patients administered concomitant medications that are also inducers of this system. To date, there is no data to suggestthat co-use with these medications increases or decreases either efficacy or toxicity of tretinoin).
No products indexed under this heading.

Miconazole Nitrate (Tretinoin is metaboized by the hepatic P450 system; therefore, there is a potential for alteration of pharmacokinetic parameters in patients administered concomitant medications that are also inducers of this system. To date, there is no data to suggestthat co-use with these medications increases or decreases either efficacy or toxicity of tretinoin). Products include:
Desenex 674
Desenex Jock Itch Spray Powder ... 674

Minocycline Hydrochloride (Tretinoin may cause pseudotumor cerebri/intracranial hypertension. Concomitant administration of tretinoin and agents known to cause pseudotumor cerebri/intracranial hypertension as well might increase the risk of this condition). Products include:
Dynacin Tablets 1859

Modafinil (Tretinoin is metaboized by the hepatic P450 system; therefore, there is a potential for alteration of pharmacokinetic parameters in patients administered concomitant medications that are also inducers of this system. To date, there is no data to suggestthat co-use with these medications increases or decreases either efficacy or toxicity of tretinoin). Products include:
Provigil Tablets 1002

Nefazodone Hydrochloride (Tretinoin is metaboized by the hepatic P450 system; therefore, there is a potential for alteration of pharmacokinetic parameters in patients administered concomitant medications that are also inducers of this system. To date, there is no data to suggestthat co-use with these medications increases or decreases either efficacy or toxicity of tretinoin).
No products indexed under this heading.

Nelfinavir Mesylate (Tretinoin is metaboized by the hepatic P450 system; therefore, there is a potential for alteration of pharmacokinetic parameters in patients administered concomitant medications that are also inducers of this system. To date, there is no data to suggestthat co-use with these medications increases or decreases either efficacy or toxicity of tretinoin). Products include:

Viracept **2556**

Nevirapine (Tretinoin is metaboized by the hepatic P450 system; therefore, there is a potential for alteration of pharmacokinetic parameters in patients administered concomitant medications that are also inducers of this system. To date, there is no data to suggestthat co-use with these medications increases or decreases either efficacy or toxicity of tretinoin). Products include:

Viramune Oral Suspension **903**
Viramune Tablets **903**

Niacinamide (Tretinoin is metaboized by the hepatic P450 system; therefore, there is a potential for alteration of pharmacokinetic parameters in patients administered concomitant medications that are also inducers of this system. To date, there is no data to suggestthat co-use with these medications increases or decreases either efficacy or toxicity of tretinoin).

No products indexed under this heading.

Nicotinamide (Tretinoin is metaboized by the hepatic P450 system; therefore, there is a potential for alteration of pharmacokinetic parameters in patients administered concomitant medications that are also inducers of this system. To date, there is no data to suggestthat co-use with these medications increases or decreases either efficacy or toxicity of tretinoin). Products include:

Nicomide Tablets **3190**

Nifedipine (Tretinoin is metaboized by the hepatic P450 system; therefore, there is a potential for alteration of pharmacokinetic parameters in patients administered concomitant medications that are also inducers of this system. To date, there is no data to suggestthat co-use with these medications increases or decreases either efficacy or toxicity of tretinoin). Products include:

Adalat CC Tablets **2978**

Norfloxacin (Tretinoin is metaboized by the hepatic P450 system; therefore, there is a potential for alteration of pharmacokinetic parameters in patients administered concomitant medications that are also inducers of this system. To date, there is no data to suggestthat co-use with these medications increases or decreases either efficacy or toxicity of tretinoin). Products include:

Noroxin Tablets **2009**

Omeprazole (Tretinoin is metaboized by the hepatic P450 system; therefore, there is a potential for alteration of pharmacokinetic parameters in patients administered concomitant medications that are also inducers of this system. To date, there is no data to suggestthat co-use with these medications increases or decreases either efficacy or toxicity of tretinoin). Products include:

Zegerid Powder for Oral Solution **2972**

Oxcarbazepine (Tretinoin is metaboized by the hepatic P450 system; therefore, there is a potential for alteration of pharmacokinetic parameters in patients administered concomitant medications that are also inducers of this system. To date, there is no data to suggestthat co-use with these medications increases or decreases either efficacy or toxicity of tretinoin). Products include:

Trileptal Oral Suspension **2281**
Trileptal Tablets **2281**

Oxytetracycline Hydrochloride (Tretinoin may cause pseudotumor cerebri/intracranial hypertension. Concomitant administration of tretinoin and agents known to cause pseudotumor cerebri/intracranial hypertension as well might increase the risk of this condition).

No products indexed under this heading.

Paroxetine Hydrochloride (Tretinoin is metaboized by the hepatic P450 system; therefore, there is a potential for alteration of pharmacokinetic parameters in patients administered concomitant medications that are also inducers of this system. To date, there is no data to suggestthat co-use with these medications increases or decreases either efficacy or toxicity of tretinoin). Products include:

Paxil CR Controlled-Release Tablets **1509**
Paxil **1501**

Pentobarbital Sodium (Potential for alteration of pharmacokinetic parameters in patients on concomitant drugs that are inducers of hepatic CYP enzymes). Products include:

Nembutal Sodium Solution, USP **2484**

Phenobarbital (Potential for alteration of pharmacokinetic parameters in patients on concomitant drugs that are inducers of hepatic CYP enzymes).

No products indexed under this heading.

Phenobarbital Sodium (Tretinoin is metaboized by the hepatic P450 system; therefore, there is a potential for alteration of pharmacokinetic parameters in patients administered concomitant medications that are also inducers of this system. To date, there is no data to suggestthat co-use with these medications increases or decreases either efficacy or toxicity of tretinoin).

No products indexed under this heading.

Phenytoin (Tretinoin is metaboized by the hepatic P450 system; therefore, there is a potential for alteration of pharmacokinetic parameters in patients administered concomitant medications that are also inducers of this system. To date, there is no data to suggestthat co-use with these medications increases or decreases either efficacy or toxicity of tretinoin).

No products indexed under this heading.

Phenytoin Sodium (Tretinoin is metaboized by the hepatic P450 system; therefore, there is a potential for alteration of pharmacokinetic parameters in patients administered concomitant medications that are also inducers of this system. To date, there is no data to suggestthat co-use with these medications increases or decreases either efficacy or toxicity of tretinoin). Products include:

Phenytek Capsules **2153**

Prednisolone Acetate (Potential for alteration of pharmacokinetic parameters in patients on concomitant drugs that are inducers of hepatic CYP enzymes). Products include:

Blephamide Ophthalmic Ointment **563**
Blephamide Ophthalmic Suspension................................. **564**
Poly-Pred Liquifilm Ophthalmic Suspension .... ⊙ **231**
Pred Forte Ophthalmic Suspension .... ⊙ **233**
Pred Mild Sterile Ophthalmic Suspension .... ⊙ **236**
Pred-G Ophthalmic Suspension ...... ⊙ **234**
Pred-G Sterile Ophthalmic Ointment .... ⊙ **235**

Prednisolone Sodium Phosphate (Potential for alteration of pharmacokinetic parameters in patients on concomitant drugs that are inducers of hepatic CYP enzymes). Products include:

Pediapred Oral Solution **3319**

Prednisolone Tebutate (Potential for alteration of pharmacokinetic parameters in patients on concomitant drugs that are inducers of hepatic CYP enzymes).

No products indexed under this heading.

Prednisone (Potential for alteration of pharmacokinetic parameters in patients on concomitant drugs that are inducers of hepatic CYP enzymes).

No products indexed under this heading.

Primidone (Tretinoin is metaboized by the hepatic P450 system; therefore, there is a potential for alteration of pharmacokinetic parameters in patients administered concomitant medications that are also inducers of this system. To date, there is no data to suggestthat co-use with these medications increases or decreases either efficacy or toxicity of tretinoin).

No products indexed under this heading.

Propoxyphene Hydrochloride (Tretinoin is metaboized by the hepatic P450 system; therefore, there is a potential for alteration of pharmacokinetic parameters in patients administered concomitant medications that are also inducers of this system. To date, there is no data to suggestthat co-use with these medications increases or decreases either efficacy or toxicity of tretinoin).

No products indexed under this heading.

Propoxyphene Napsylate (Tretinoin is metaboized by the hepatic P450 system; therefore, there is a potential for alteration of pharmacokinetic parameters in patients administered concomitant medications that are also inducers of this system. To date, there is no data to suggestthat co-use with these medications increases or decreases either efficacy or toxicity of tretinoin). Products include:

Darvocet A 500 Tablets **3497**

Quinidine (Tretinoin is metaboized by the hepatic P450 system; therefore, there is a potential for alteration of pharmacokinetic parameters in patients administered concomitant medications that are also inducers of this system. To date, there is no data to suggestthat co-use with these medications increases or decreases either efficacy or toxicity of tretinoin).

No products indexed under this heading.

Quinidine Hydrochloride (Tretinoin is metaboized by the hepatic P450 system; therefore, there is a potential for alteration of pharmacokinetic parameters in patients administered concomitant medications that are also inducers of this system. To date, there is no data to suggestthat co-use with these medications increases or decreases either efficacy or toxicity of tretinoin).

No products indexed under this heading.

Quinidine Polygalacturonate (Tretinoin is metaboized by the hepatic P450 system; therefore, there is a potential for alteration of pharmacokinetic parameters in patients administered concomitant medications that are also inducers of this system. To date, there is no data to suggestthat co-use with these medications increases or decreases either efficacy or toxicity of tretinoin).

No products indexed under this heading.

Quinidine Sulfate (Tretinoin is metaboized by the hepatic P450 system; therefore, there is a potential for alteration of pharmacokinetic parameters in patients administered concomitant medications that are also inducers of this system. To date, there is no data to suggestthat co-use with these medications increases or decreases either efficacy or toxicity of tretinoin).

No products indexed under this heading.

Quinine (Tretinoin is metaboized by the hepatic P450 system; therefore, there is a potential for alteration of pharmacokinetic parameters in patients administered concomitant medications that are also inducers of this system. To date, there is no data to suggestthat co-use with these medications increases or decreases either efficacy or toxicity of tretinoin).

No products indexed under this heading.

Quinine Sulfate (Tretinoin is metaboized by the hepatic P450 system; therefore, there is a potential for alteration of pharmacokinetic parameters in patients administered concomitant medications that are also inducers of this system. To date, there is no data to suggestthat co-use with these medications increases or decreases either efficacy or toxicity of tretinoin).

No products indexed under this heading.

Quinupristin (Tretinoin is metaboized by the hepatic P450 system; therefore, there is a potential for alteration of pharmacokinetic parameters in patients administered concomitant medications that are also inducers of this system. To date, there is no data to suggestthat co-use with these medications

increases or decreases either efficacy or toxicity of tretinoin). Products include:

Synercid I.V. 1690

Ranitidine Bismuth Citrate (Tretinoin is metaboized by the hepatic P450 system; therefore, there is a potential for alteration of pharmacokinetic parameters in patients administered concomitant medications that are also inducers of this system. To date, there is no data to suggest that co-use with these medications increases or decreases either efficacy or toxicity of tretinoin).

No products indexed under this heading.

Ranitidine Hydrochloride (Tretinoin is metaboized by the hepatic P450 system; therefore, there is a potential for alteration of pharmacokinetic parameters in patients administered concomitant medications that are also inducers of this system. To date, there is no data to suggest that co-use with these medications increases or decreases either efficacy or toxicity of tretinoin). Products include:

Zantac 1597
Zantac Injection 1593
Zantac 75 Tablets 715
Zantac 150 Maximum Strength Tablets.. 715
Zantac Injection Pharmacy Bulk Package.. 1595

Rifabutin (Tretinoin is metaboized by the hepatic P450 system; therefore, there is a potential for alteration of pharmacokinetic parameters in patients administered concomitant medications that are also inducers of this system. To date, there is no data to suggestthat co-use with these medications increases or decreases either efficacy or toxicity of tretinoin).

No products indexed under this heading.

Rifampicin (Tretinoin is metaboized by the hepatic P450 system; therefore, there is a potential for alteration of pharmacokinetic parameters in patients administered concomitant medications that are also inducers of this system. To date, there is no data to suggestthat co-use with these medications increases or decreases either efficacy or toxicity of tretinoin).

No products indexed under this heading.

Rifampin (Potential for alteration of pharmacokinetic parameters in patients on concomitant drugs that are inducers of hepatic CYP enzymes).

No products indexed under this heading.

Rifapentine (Tretinoin is metaboized by the hepatic P450 system; therefore, there is a potential for alteration of pharmacokinetic parameters in patients administered concomitant medications that are also inducers of this system. To date, there is no data to suggestthat co-use with these medications increases or decreases either efficacy or toxicity of tretinoin).

No products indexed under this heading.

Ritonavir (Tretinoin is metaboized by the hepatic P450 system; therefore, there is a potential for alteration of pharmacokinetic parameters in patients administered concomitant medications that are also inducers of this system. To date, there is no data to suggestthat co-use with these medications increases or decreases either efficacy or toxicity of tretinoin). Products include:

Kaletra 474
Norvir 499

Saquinavir (Tretinoin is metaboized by the hepatic P450 system; therefore, there is a potential for alteration of pharmacokinetic parameters in patients administered concomitant medications that are also inducers of this system. To date, there is no data to suggestthat co-use with these medications increases or decreases either efficacy or toxicity of tretinoin).

No products indexed under this heading.

Saquinavir Mesylate (Tretinoin is metaboized by the hepatic P450 system; therefore, there is a potential for alteration of pharmacokinetic parameters in patients administered concomitant medications that are also inducers of this system. To date, there is no data to suggestthat co-use with these medications increases or decreases either efficacy or toxicity of tretinoin). Products include:

Invirase 2776

Sertraline Hydrochloride (Tretinoin is metaboized by the hepatic P450 system; therefore, there is a potential for alteration of pharmacokinetic parameters in patients administered concomitant medications that are also inducers of this system. To date, there is no data to suggest that co-use with these medications increases or decreases either efficacy or toxicity of tretinoin). Products include:

Zoloft 2581

Sulfinpyrazone (Tretinoin is metaboized by the hepatic P450 system; therefore, there is a potential for alteration of pharmacokinetic parameters in patients administered concomitant medications that are also inducers of this system. To date, there is no data to suggestthat co-use with these medications increases or decreases either efficacy or toxicity of tretinoin).

No products indexed under this heading.

Telithromycin (Tretinoin is metaboized by the hepatic P450 system; therefore, there is a potential for alteration of pharmacokinetic parameters in patients administered concomitant medications that are also inducers of this system. To date, there is no data to suggestthat co-use with these medications increases or decreases either efficacy or toxicity of tretinoin). Products include:

Ketek Tablets 2920

Tetracycline Hydrochloride (Tretinoin may cause pseudotumor cerebri/intracranial hypertension. Concomitant administration of tretinoin and agents known to cause pseudotumor cerebri/intracranial hypertension as well might increase the risk of this condition).

No products indexed under this heading.

Theophylline (Tretinoin is metaboized by the hepatic P450 system; therefore, there is a potential for alteration of pharmacokinetic parameters in patients administered concomitant medications that are also inducers of this system. To date, there is no data to suggestthat co-use with these medications increases or decreases either efficacy or toxicity of tretinoin).

No products indexed under this heading.

Tranexamic Acid (Cases of fatal thrombotic complications have been reported rarely in patients concomitantly treated with tretinoin and antifibrinolytic agents. Therefore, caution should be exercised when administering tretinoin concomitantly with these agents).

No products indexed under this heading.

Triamcinolone (Potential for alteration of pharmacokinetic parameters in patients on concomitant drugs that are inducers of hepatic CYP enzymes).

No products indexed under this heading.

Triamcinolone Acetonide (Potential for alteration of pharmacokinetic parameters in patients on concomitant drugs that are inducers of hepatic CYP enzymes). Products include:

Azmacort Inhalation Aerosol 1701
Nasacort HFA Inhalation Aerosol 2939
Nasacort AQ Nasal Spray 2937

Triamcinolone Diacetate (Potential for alteration of pharmacokinetic parameters in patients on concomitant drugs that are inducers of hepatic CYP enzymes).

No products indexed under this heading.

Triamcinolone Hexacetonide (Potential for alteration of pharmacokinetic parameters in patients on concomitant drugs that are inducers of hepatic CYP enzymes).

No products indexed under this heading.

Troglitazone (Tretinoin is metaboized by the hepatic P450 system; therefore, there is a potential for alteration of pharmacokinetic parameters in patients administered concomitant medications that are also inducers of this system. To date, there is no data to suggestthat co-use with these medications increases or decreases either efficacy or toxicity of tretinoin).

No products indexed under this heading.

Troleandomycin (Tretinoin is metaboized by the hepatic P450 system; therefore, there is a potential for alteration of pharmacokinetic parameters in patients administered concomitant medications that are also inducers of this system. To date, there is no data to suggestthat co-use with these medications increases or decreases either efficacy or toxicity of tretinoin).

No products indexed under this heading.

Valproate Sodium (Tretinoin is metaboized by the hepatic P450 system; therefore, there is a potential for alteration of pharmacokinetic parameters in patients administered concomitant medications that are also inducers of this system. To date, there is no data to suggestthat co-use with these medications increases or decreases either efficacy or toxicity of tretinoin). Products include:

Depacon Injection 412

Verapamil Hydrochloride (Potential for alteration of pharmacokinetic parameters in patients on concomitant drugs that inhibit hepatic CYP enzymes). Products include:

Covera-HS Tablets 3135
Tarka Tablets 519
Verelan PM Capsules 3120

Vitamin A (Vesanoid must not be administered in combination with vitamin A because of symptoms of hypervitaminosis A could be aggravated). Products include:

Visutein Capsules 3328

Voriconazole (Tretinoin is metaboized by the hepatic P450 system; therefore, there is a potential for alteration of pharmacokinetic parameters in patients administered concomitant medications that are also inducers of this system. To date, there is no data to suggestthat co-use with these medications increases or decreases either efficacy or toxicity of tretinoin). Products include:

VFEND I.V. 2543
VFEND Oral Suspension 2543
VFEND Tablets 2543

Zafirlukast (Tretinoin is metaboized by the hepatic P450 system; therefore, there is a potential for alteration of pharmacokinetic parameters in patients administered concomitant medications that are also inducers of this system. To date, there is no data to suggestthat co-use with these medications increases or decreases either efficacy or toxicity of tretinoin). Products include:

Accolate Tablets 663

Zileuton (Tretinoin is metaboized by the hepatic P450 system; therefore, there is a potential for alteration of pharmacokinetic parameters in patients administered concomitant medications that are also inducers of this system. To date, there is no data to suggestthat co-use with these medications increases or decreases either efficacy or toxicity of tretinoin).

No products indexed under this heading.

Food Interactions

Food, unspecified (The absorption of retinoids as a class has been shown to be enhanced when taken with food).

Grapefruit (Tretinoin is metaboized by the hepatic P450 system; therefore, there is a potential for alteration of pharmacokinetic parameters in patients administered concomitant medications that are also inducers of this system. To date, there is no data to suggestthat co-use with these medications increases or decreases either efficacy or toxicity of tretinoin).

Grapefruit Juice (Tretinoin is metaboized by the hepatic P450 system; therefore, there is a potential for alteration of pharmacokinetic parameters in patients administered concomitant medications that are also inducers of this system. To date, there is no data to suggestthat co-use with these medications increases or decreases either efficacy or toxicity of tretinoin).

VESICARE TABLETS
(Solifenacin Succinate) 631
May interact with cytochrome p450 3a4 inhibitors, potent and drugs that prolong the QT interval. Compounds in these categories include:

Amiodarone Hydrochloride (In a study of the effect of solifenacin on the QT interval in 76 healthy women, the QT prolonging effect appered less with solifenacin 10 mg than with 30 mg (three times the maximum recommended dose), and the effect of solifenacin 30 mg did not appear as large as that of the positive control moxifloxacin at its therapeutic dose. This observation should be considered in clinical decisions to prescribe solifenacin succinate for patients with a known history of QT prolongation or patients who are taking medications known to prolong the QT interval). Products include:
Pacerone Tablets 3337

Amitriptyline Hydrochloride (In a study of the effect of solifenacin on the QT interval in 76 healthy women, the QT prolonging effect appered less with solifenacin 10 mg than with 30 mg (three times the maximum recommended dose), and the effect of solifenacin 30 mg did not appear as large as that of the positive control moxifloxacin at its therapeutic dose. This observation should be considered in clinical decisions to prescribe solifenacin succinate for patients with a known history of QT prolongation or patients who are taking medications known to prolong the QT interval).
No products indexed under this heading.

Amoxapine (In a study of the effect of solifenacin on the QT interval in 76 healthy women, the QT prolonging effect appered less with solifenacin 10 mg than with 30 mg (three times the maximum recommended dose), and the effect of solifenacin 30 mg did not appear as large as that of the positive control moxifloxacin at its therapeutic dose. This observation should be considered in clinical decisions to prescribe solifenacin succinate for patients with a known history of QT prolongation or patients who are taking medications known to prolong the QT interval).
No products indexed under this heading.

Amprenavir (Do not exceed a 5 mg daily dose of solifenacin succinate when administered with therapeutic doses of ketoconazole or other potent CYP3A4 inhibitors). Products include:
Agenerase Capsules 1299
Agenerase Oral Solution 1304

Astemizole (In a study of the effect of solifenacin on the QT interval in 76 healthy women, the QT prolonging effect appered less with solifenacin 10 mg than with 30 mg (three times the maximum recommended dose), and the effect of solifenacin 30 mg did not appear as large as that of the positive control moxifloxacin at its therapeutic dose. This observation should be considered in clinical decisions to prescribe solifenacin succinate for patients with a known history of QT prolongation or patients who are taking medications known to prolong the QT interval).
No products indexed under this heading.

Atazanavir (Do not exceed a 5 mg daily dose of solifenacin succinate when administered with therapeutic doses of ketoconazole or other potent CYP3A4 inhibitors).
No products indexed under this heading.

Atazanavir sulfate (Do not exceed a 5 mg daily dose of solifenacin succinate when administered with therapeutic doses of ketoconazole or other potent CYP3A4 inhibitors). Products include:
Reyataz Capsules 948

Bretylium Tosylate (In a study of the effect of solifenacin on the QT interval in 76 healthy women, the QT prolonging effect appered less with solifenacin 10 mg than with 30 mg (three times the maximum recommended dose), and the effect of solifenacin 30 mg did not appear as large as that of the positive control moxifloxacin at its therapeutic dose. This observation should be considered in clinical decisions to prescribe solifenacin succinate for patients with a known history of QT prolongation or patients who are taking medications known to prolong the QT interval).
No products indexed under this heading.

Chlorpromazine (In a study of the effect of solifenacin on the QT interval in 76 healthy women, the QT prolonging effect appered less with solifenacin 10 mg than with 30 mg (three times the maximum recommended dose), and the effect of solifenacin 30 mg did not appear as large as that of the positive control moxifloxacin at its therapeutic dose. This observation should be considered in clinical decisions to prescribe solifenacin succinate for patients with a known history of QT prolongation or patients who are taking medications known to prolong the QT interval).
No products indexed under this heading.

Chlorpromazine Hydrochloride (In a study of the effect of solifenacin on the QT interval in 76 healthy women, the QT prolonging effect appered less with solifenacin 10 mg than with 30 mg (three times the maximum recommended dose), and the effect of solifenacin 30 mg did not appear as large as that of the positive control moxifloxacin at its therapeutic dose. This observation should be considered in clinical decisions to prescribe solifenacin succinate for patients with a known history of QT prolongation or patients who are taking medications known to prolong the QT interval).
No products indexed under this heading.

Clarithromycin (Do not exceed a 5 mg daily dose of solifenacin succinate when administered with therapeutic doses of ketoconazole or other potent CYP3A4 inhibitors). Products include:
Biaxin/Biaxin XL 402
PREVPAC 3281

Clomipramine Hydrochloride (In a study of the effect of solifenacin on the QT interval in 76 healthy women, the QT prolonging effect appered less with solifenacin 10 mg than with 30 mg (three times the maximum recommended dose), and the effect of solifenacin 30 mg did not appear as large as that of the positive control moxifloxacin at its therapeutic dose. This observation should be considered in clinical decisions to prescribe solifenacin succinate for patients with a known history of QT prolongation or patients who are taking medications known to prolong the QT interval).
No products indexed under this heading.

Desipramine Hydrochloride (In a study of the effect of solifenacin on the QT interval in 76 healthy women, the QT prolonging effect appered less with solifenacin 10 mg than with 30 mg (three times the maximum recommended dose), and the effect of solifenacin 30 mg did not appear as large as that of the positive control moxifloxacin at its therapeutic dose. This observation should be considered in clinical decisions to prescribe solifenacin succinate for patients with a known history of QT prolongation or patients who are taking medications known to prolong the QT interval).
No products indexed under this heading.

Disopyramide Phosphate (In a study of the effect of solifenacin on the QT interval in 76 healthy women, the QT prolonging effect appered less with solifenacin 10 mg than with 30 mg (three times the maximum recommended dose), and the effect of solifenacin 30 mg did not appear as large as that of the positive control moxifloxacin at its therapeutic dose. This observation should be considered in clinical decisions to prescribe solifenacin succinate for patients with a known history of QT prolongation or patients who are taking medications known to prolong the QT interval).
No products indexed under this heading.

Dofetilide (In a study of the effect of solifenacin on the QT interval in 76 healthy women, the QT prolonging effect appered less with solifenacin 10 mg than with 30 mg (three times the maximum recommended dose), and the effect of solifenacin 30 mg did not appear as large as that of the positive control moxifloxacin at its therapeutic dose. This observation should be considered in clinical decisions to prescribe solifenacin succinate for patients with a known history of QT prolongation or patients who are taking medications known to prolong the QT interval).
No products indexed under this heading.

Doxepin Hydrochloride (In a study of the effect of solifenacin on the QT interval in 76 healthy women, the QT prolonging effect appered less with solifenacin 10 mg than with 30 mg (three times the maximum recommended dose), and the effect of solifenacin 30 mg did not appear as large as that of the positive control moxifloxacin at its therapeutic dose. This observation should be considered in clinical decisions to prescribe solifenacin succinate for patients with a known history of QT prolongation or patients who are taking medications known to prolong the QT interval).
No products indexed under this heading.

Flecainide Acetate (In a study of the effect of solifenacin on the QT interval in 76 healthy women, the QT prolonging effect appered less with solifenacin 10 mg than with 30 mg (three times the maximum recommended dose), and the effect of solifenacin 30 mg did not appear as large as that of the positive control moxifloxacin at its therapeutic dose. This observation should be considered in clinical decisions to prescribe solifenacin succinate for patients with a known history of QT prolongation or patients who are taking medications known to prolong the QT interval). Products include:
Tambocor Tablets 1824

Fluphenazine Decanoate (In a study of the effect of solifenacin on the QT interval in 76 healthy women, the QT prolonging effect appered less with solifenacin 10 mg than with 30 mg (three times the maximum recommended dose), and the effect of solifenacin 30 mg did not appear as large as that of the positive control moxifloxacin at its therapeutic dose. This observation should be considered in clinical decisions to prescribe solifenacin succinate for patients with a known history of QT prolongation or patients who are taking medications known to prolong the QT interval).
No products indexed under this heading.

Fluphenazine Enanthate (In a study of the effect of solifenacin on the QT interval in 76 healthy women, the QT prolonging effect appered less with solifenacin 10 mg than with 30 mg (three times the maximum recommended dose), and the effect of solifenacin 30 mg did not appear as large as that of the positive control moxifloxacin at its therapeutic dose. This observation should be considered in clinical decisions to prescribe solifenacin succinate for patients with a known history of QT prolongation or patients who are taking medications known to prolong the QT interval).
No products indexed under this heading.

Fluphenazine Hydrochloride (In a study of the effect of solifenacin on the QT interval in 76 healthy women, the QT prolonging effect appered less with solifenacin 10 mg than with 30 mg (three times the maximum recommended dose), and the effect of solifenacin 30 mg did not appear as large as that of the positive control moxifloxacin at its therapeutic dose. This observation should be considered in clinical decisions to prescribe solifenacin succinate for patients with a known history of QT prolongation or patients who are taking medications known to prolong the QT interval).
No products indexed under this heading.

Fosamprenavir Calcium (Do not exceed a 5 mg daily dose of solifenacin succinate when administered with therapeutic doses of ketoconazole or other potent CYP3A4 inhibitors). Products include:
Lexiva Tablets 1473

Imipramine Hydrochloride (In a study of the effect of solifenacin on the QT interval in 76 healthy women, the QT prolonging effect appered less with solifenacin 10 mg than with 30 mg (three times the maximum recommended dose), and the effect of solifenacin 30 mg did not appear as large as that of the positive con-

trol moxifloxacin at its therapeutic dose. This observation should be considered in clinical decisions to prescribe solifenacin succinate for patients with a known history of QT prolongation or patients who are taking medications known to prolong the QT interval).
No products indexed under this heading.

Imipramine Pamoate (In a study of the effect of solifenacin on the QT interval in 76 healthy women, the QT prolonging effect appered less with solifenacin 10 mg than with 30 mg (three times the maximum recommended dose), and the effect of solifenacin 30 mg did not appear as large as that of the positive control moxifloxacin at its therapeutic dose. This observation should be considered in clinical decisions to prescribe solifenacin succinate for patients with a known history of QT prolongation or patients who are taking medications known to prolong the QT interval).
No products indexed under this heading.

Indinavir Sulfate (Do not exceed a 5 mg daily dose of solifenacin succinate when administered with therapeutic doses of ketoconazole or other potent CYP3A4 inhibitors). Products include:
Crixivan Capsules 1918

Itraconazole (Do not exceed a 5 mg daily dose of solifenacin succinate when administered with therapeutic doses of ketoconazole or other potent CYP3A4 inhibitors).
No products indexed under this heading.

Ketoconazole (Do not exceed a 5 mg daily dose of solifenacin succinate when administered with therapeutic doses of ketoconazole or other potent CYP3A4 inhibitors). Products include:
Nizoral A-D Shampoo, 1% 1839
Nizoral 2% Shampoo 1838

Lidocaine Hydrochloride (In a study of the effect of solifenacin on the QT interval in 76 healthy women, the QT prolonging effect appered less with solifenacin 10 mg than with 30 mg (three times the maximum recommended dose), and the effect of solifenacin 30 mg did not appear as large as that of the positive control moxifloxacin at its therapeutic dose. This observation should be considered in clinical decisions to prescribe solifenacin succinate for patients with a known history of QT prolongation or patients who are taking medications known to prolong the QT interval).
No products indexed under this heading.

Lopinavir (Do not exceed a 5 mg daily dose of solifenacin succinate when administered with therapeutic doses of ketoconazole or other potent CYP3A4 inhibitors). Products include:
Kaletra 474

Maprotiline Hydrochloride (In a study of the effect of solifenacin on the QT interval in 76 healthy women, the QT prolonging effect appered less with solifenacin 10 mg than with 30 mg (three times the maximum recommended dose), and the effect of solifenacin 30 mg did not appear as large as that of the positive control moxifloxacin at its therapeutic dose. This observation should be considered in clinical decisions to prescribe solifenacin succinate for patients with a known history of QT prolongation or patients who are taking medications known to prolong the QT interval).
No products indexed under this heading.

Mesoridazine Besylate (In a study of the effect of solifenacin on the QT interval in 76 healthy women, the QT prolonging effect appered less with solifenacin 10 mg than with 30 mg (three times the maximum recommended dose), and the effect of solifenacin 30 mg did not appear as large as that of the positive control moxifloxacin at its therapeutic dose. This observation should be considered in clinical decisions to prescribe solifenacin succinate for patients with a known history of QT prolongation or patients who are taking medications known to prolong the QT interval).
No products indexed under this heading.

Mexiletine Hydrochloride (In a study of the effect of solifenacin on the QT interval in 76 healthy women, the QT prolonging effect appered less with solifenacin 10 mg than with 30 mg (three times the maximum recommended dose), and the effect of solifenacin 30 mg did not appear as large as that of the positive control moxifloxacin at its therapeutic dose. This observation should be considered in clinical decisions to prescribe solifenacin succinate for patients with a known history of QT prolongation or patients who are taking medications known to prolong the QT interval).
No products indexed under this heading.

Nefazodone Hydrochloride (Do not exceed a 5 mg daily dose of solifenacin succinate when administered with therapeutic doses of ketoconazole or other potent CYP3A4 inhibitors).
No products indexed under this heading.

Nelfinavir Mesylate (Do not exceed a 5 mg daily dose of solifenacin succinate when administered with therapeutic doses of ketoconazole or other potent CYP3A4 inhibitors). Products include:
Viracept 2556

Nortriptyline Hydrochloride (In a study of the effect of solifenacin on the QT interval in 76 healthy women, the QT prolonging effect appered less with solifenacin 10 mg than with 30 mg (three times the maximum recommended dose), and the effect of solifenacin 30 mg did not appear as large as that of the positive control moxifloxacin at its therapeutic dose. This observation should be considered in clinical decisions to prescribe solifenacin succinate for patients with a known history of QT prolongation or patients who are taking medications known to prolong the QT interval).
No products indexed under this heading.

Perphenazine (In a study of the effect of solifenacin on the QT interval in 76 healthy women, the QT prolonging effect appered less with solifenacin 10 mg than with 30 mg (three times the maximum recommended dose), and the effect of solifenacin 30 mg did not appear as large as that of the positive control moxifloxacin at its therapeutic dose. This observation should be considered in clinical decisions to prescribe solifenacin succinate for patients with a known history of QT prolongation or patients who are taking medications known to prolong the QT interval).
No products indexed under this heading.

Procainamide Hydrochloride (In a study of the effect of solifenacin on the QT interval in 76 healthy women, the QT prolonging effect appered less with solifenacin 10 mg than with 30 mg (three times the maximum recommended dose), and the effect of solifenacin 30 mg did not appear as large as that of the positive control moxifloxacin at its therapeutic dose. This observation should be considered in clinical decisions to prescribe solifenacin succinate for patients with a known history of QT prolongation or patients who are taking medications known to prolong the QT interval).
No products indexed under this heading.

Prochlorperazine (In a study of the effect of solifenacin on the QT interval in 76 healthy women, the QT prolonging effect appered less with solifenacin 10 mg than with 30 mg (three times the maximum recommended dose), and the effect of solifenacin 30 mg did not appear as large as that of the positive control moxifloxacin at its therapeutic dose. This observation should be considered in clinical decisions to prescribe solifenacin succinate for patients with a known history of QT prolongation or patients who are taking medications known to prolong the QT interval).
No products indexed under this heading.

Promethazine Hydrochloride (In a study of the effect of solifenacin on the QT interval in 76 healthy women, the QT prolonging effect appered less with solifenacin 10 mg than with 30 mg (three times the maximum recommended dose), and the effect of solifenacin 30 mg did not appear as large as that of the positive control moxifloxacin at its therapeutic dose. This observation should be considered in clinical decisions to prescribe solifenacin succinate for patients with a known history of QT prolongation or patients who are taking medications known to prolong the QT interval). Products include:
Phenergan 3438

Propafenone Hydrochloride (In a study of the effect of solifenacin on the QT interval in 76 healthy women, the QT prolonging effect appered less with solifenacin 10 mg than with 30 mg (three times the maximum recommended dose), and the effect of solifenacin 30 mg did not appear as large as that of the positive control moxifloxacin at its therapeutic dose. This observation should be considered in clinical decisions to prescribe solifenacin succinate for patients with a known history of QT prolongation or patients who are taking medications known to prolong the QT interval). Products include:
Rythmol SR Capsules 2736

Protriptyline Hydrochloride (In a study of the effect of solifenacin on the QT interval in 76 healthy women, the QT prolonging effect appered less with solifenacin 10 mg than with 30 mg (three times the maximum recommended dose), and the effect of solifenacin 30 mg did not appear as large as that of the positive control moxifloxacin at its therapeutic dose. This observation should be considered in clinical decisions to prescribe solifenacin succinate for patients with a known history of QT prolongation or patients who are taking medications known to prolong the QT interval). Products include:
Vivactil Tablets 2350

Quinidine Gluconate (In a study of the effect of solifenacin on the QT interval in 76 healthy women, the QT prolonging effect appered less with solifenacin 10 mg than with 30 mg (three times the maximum recommended dose), and the effect of solifenacin 30 mg did not appear as large as that of the positive control moxifloxacin at its therapeutic dose. This observation should be considered in clinical decisions to prescribe solifenacin succinate for patients with a known history of QT prolongation or patients who are taking medications known to prolong the QT interval).
No products indexed under this heading.

Quinidine Polygalacturonate (In a study of the effect of solifenacin on the QT interval in 76 healthy women, the QT prolonging effect appered less with solifenacin 10 mg than with 30 mg (three times the maximum recommended dose), and the effect of solifenacin 30 mg did not appear as large as that of the positive control moxifloxacin at its therapeutic dose. This observation should be considered in clinical decisions to prescribe solifenacin succinate for patients with a known history of QT prolongation or patients who are taking medications known to prolong the QT interval).
No products indexed under this heading.

Quinidine Sulfate (In a study of the effect of solifenacin on the QT interval in 76 healthy women, the QT prolonging effect appered less with solifenacin 10 mg than with 30 mg (three times the maximum recommended dose), and the effect of solifenacin 30 mg did not appear as large as that of the positive control moxifloxacin at its therapeutic dose. This observation should be considered in clinical decisions to prescribe solifenacin succinate for patients with a known history of QT prolongation or patients who are taking medications known to prolong the QT interval).
No products indexed under this heading.

Ritonavir (Do not exceed a 5 mg daily dose of solifenacin succinate when administered with therapeutic doses of ketoconazole or other potent CYP3A4 inhibitors). Products include:
Kaletra 474
Norvir 499

Saquinavir (Do not exceed a 5 mg daily dose of solifenacin succinate when administered with therapeutic doses of ketoconazole or other potent CYP3A4 inhibitors).
No products indexed under this heading.

Saquinavir Mesylate (Do not exceed a 5 mg daily dose of solifenacin succinate when administered with therapeutic doses of ketoconazole or other potent CYP3A4 inhibitors). Products include:
Invirase 2776
Telithromycin (Do not exceed a 5 mg daily dose of solifenacin succinate when administered with therapeutic doses of ketoconazole or other potent CYP3A4 inhibitors). Products include:
Ketek Tablets 2920
Thioridazine Hydrochloride (In a study of the effect of solifenacin on the QT interval in 76 healthy women, the QT prolonging effect appered less with solifenacin 10 mg than with 30 mg (three times the maximum recommended dose), and the effect of solifenacin 30 mg did not appear as large as that of the positive control moxifloxacin at its therapeutic dose. This observation should be considered in clinical decisions to prescribe solifenacin succinate for patients with a known history of QT prolongation or patients who are taking medications known to prolong the QT interval). Products include:
Thioridazine Hydrochloride Tablets 2122
Tocainide Hydrochloride (In a study of the effect of solifenacin on the QT interval in 76 healthy women, the QT prolonging effect appered less with solifenacin 10 mg than with 30 mg (three times the maximum recommended dose), and the effect of solifenacin 30 mg did not appear as large as that of the positive control moxifloxacin at its therapeutic dose. This observation should be considered in clinical decisions to prescribe solifenacin succinate for patients with a known history of QT prolongation or patients who are taking medications known to prolong the QT interval).
No products indexed under this heading.
Trifluoperazine Hydrochloride (In a study of the effect of solifenacin on the QT interval in 76 healthy women, the QT prolonging effect appered less with solifenacin 10 mg than with 30 mg (three times the maximum recommended dose), and the effect of solifenacin 30 mg did not appear as large as that of the positive control moxifloxacin at its therapeutic dose. This observation should be considered in clinical decisions to prescribe solifenacin succinate for patients with a known history of QT prolongation or patients who are taking medications known to prolong the QT interval).
No products indexed under this heading.
Trimipramine Maleate (In a study of the effect of solifenacin on the QT interval in 76 healthy women, the QT prolonging effect appered less with solifenacin 10 mg than with 30 mg (three times the maximum recommended dose), and the effect of solifenacin 30 mg did not appear as large as that of the positive control moxifloxacin at its therapeutic dose. This observation should be considered in clinical decisions to prescribe solifenacin succinate for patients with a known history of QT prolongation or patients who are taking medications known to prolong the QT interval). Products include:
Surmontil Capsules 2347
Troleandomycin (Do not exceed a 5 mg daily dose of solifenacin succinate when administered with therapeutic doses of ketoconazole or other potent CYP3A4 inhibitors).
No products indexed under this heading.
Voriconazole (Do not exceed a 5 mg daily dose of solifenacin succinate when administered with therapeutic doses of ketoconazole or other potent CYP3A4 inhibitors). Products include:
VFEND I.V. 2543
VFEND Oral Suspension 2543
VFEND Tablets 2543
Ziprasidone Hydrochloride (In a study of the effect of solifenacin on the QT interval in 76 healthy women, the QT prolonging effect appered less with solifenacin 10 mg than with 30 mg (three times the maximum recommended dose), and the effect of solifenacin 30 mg did not appear as large as that of the positive control moxifloxacin at its therapeutic dose. This observation should be considered in clinical decisions to prescribe solifenacin succinate for patients with a known history of QT prolongation or patients who are taking medications known to prolong the QT interval). Products include:
Geodon Capsules 2514

VFEND I.V.

(Voriconazole) 2543
See VFEND Tablets

VFEND ORAL SUSPENSION

(Voriconazole) 2543
See VFEND Tablets

VFEND TABLETS

(Voriconazole) 2543
May interact with barbiturates, benzodiazepine that are metabolized by CYP3A4, calcium channel blockers that are metabolized by CYP3A4, oral anticoagulants, cytochrome p450 2c19 inducers (selected), cytochrome p450 2c19 inhibitors (selected), cytochrome p450 2c9 inducers (selected), cytochrome p450 2c9 inhibitors (selected), cytochrome p450 3a4 inducers (selected), cytochrome p450 3a4 inhibitors (selected), ergot-containing drugs, Non-nucleoside reverse transcriptase inhibitors, phenytoin, prednisolone, proton pump inhibitor, quinidine, statins that are metabolized by CYP3A4, sulfonylureas that are substrate of CYP2C9, vinca alkaloids, and certain other agents. Compounds in these categories include:

Acetazolamide (CYP3A4 inhibitors may increase voriconazole systemic exposure (plasma concentrations)).
No products indexed under this heading.
Allium sativum (CYP3A4 inducers may decrease voriconazole systemic exposure (plasma concentrations)).
No products indexed under this heading.
Alprazolam (Co-administration may increase plasma concentrations of benzodiazepines that are metabolized by CYP3A4). Products include:
Niravam Orally Disintegrating Tablets 3106
Xanax XR Tablets 2655
Amiodarone Hydrochloride (CYP2C9 inhibitors may increase voriconazole systemic exposure (plasma concentrations)). Products include:
Pacerone Tablets 3337
Amlodipine Besylate (Co-administration may increase plasma concentrations of calcium channel blockers that are metabolized by CYP3A4). Products include:
Caduet Tablets 2507
Lotrel Capsules 2238
Norvasc Tablets 2529
Amprenavir (Voriconazole may inhibit the metabolism of amprenavir; amprenavir may inhibit the metabolism of voriconazole). Products include:
Agenerase Capsules 1299
Agenerase Oral Solution 1304
Anastrozole (CYP2C9 inhibitors may increase voriconazole systemic exposure (plasma concentrations)). Products include:
Arimidex Tablets 665
Anisindione (Co-administration may increase prothrombin time). Products include:
Miradon Tablets 3056
Aprepitant (CYP2C9 inducers may decrease voriconazole systemic exposure (plasma concentrations)). Products include:
Emend Capsules 1944
Aprobarbital (Long-acting barbiturates are likely to significantly decrease plasma voriconazole concentrations. Co-administration of voriconazole with long-acting barbiturates is contraindicated).
No products indexed under this heading.
Astemizole (Co-administration with a CYP3A4 substrate, such as astemizole may result in inhibition of the metabolism of astemizole; increased plasma concentrations of astemizole can lead to QT prolongation and rare occurrence of torsade de pointes; co-administration is contraindicated).
No products indexed under this heading.
Atorvastatin Calcium (Co-administration may increase plasma concentrations of statins that are metabolized by CYP3A4). Products include:
Caduet Tablets 2507
Lipitor Tablets 2495
Bendroflumethiazide (CYP2C9 inhibitors may increase voriconazole systemic exposure (plasma concentrations)).
No products indexed under this heading.
Betamethasone Acetate (CYP3A4 inducers may decrease voriconazole systemic exposure (plasma concentrations)).
No products indexed under this heading.
Betamethasone Sodium Phosphate (CYP3A4 inducers may decrease voriconazole systemic exposure (plasma concentrations)).
No products indexed under this heading.
Butabarbital (Long-acting barbiturates are likely to significantly decrease plasma voriconazole concentrations. Co-administration of voriconazole with long-acting barbiturates is contraindicated).
No products indexed under this heading.
Butalbital (Long-acting barbiturates are likely to significantly decrease plasma voriconazole concentrations. Co-administration of voriconazole with long-acting barbiturates is contraindicated). Products include:
Sedapap Tablets 50 mg/650 mg 2098
Carbamazepine (Co-administration with potent inducer of CYP450, such as carbamazepine, is likely to significantly decrease plasma voriconazole concentrations; co-administration is contraindicated). Products include:
Carbatrol Capsules 3174
Equetro Extended-Release Capsules 3178
Tegretol/Tegretol-XR 2278
Chloramphenicol (CYP2C9 inhibitors may increase voriconazole systemic exposure (plasma concentrations)).
No products indexed under this heading.
Chlorothiazide (CYP2C9 inhibitors may increase voriconazole systemic exposure (plasma concentrations)). Products include:
Aldoclor Tablets 1881
Diuril Oral 1936
Chlorothiazide Sodium (CYP2C9 inhibitors may increase voriconazole systemic exposure (plasma concentrations)). Products include:
Diuril Sodium Intravenous 1934
Chlorpropamide (CYP2C9 inhibitors may increase voriconazole systemic exposure (plasma concentrations)).
No products indexed under this heading.
Cimetidine (Increases voriconazole steady state Cmax and AUC by an average of 18% and 23% respectively; no dosage adjustment required). Products include:
Tagamet HB 200 Tablets .... ▣637
Tagamet Tablets 1547
Cimetidine Hydrochloride (Increases voriconazole steady state Cmax and AUC by an average of 18% and 23% respectively; no dosage adjustment required).
No products indexed under this heading.
Ciprofloxacin (CYP3A4 inhibitors may increase voriconazole systemic exposure (plasma concentrations)). Products include:
Cipro I.V. 2998
Cipro I.V. Pharmacy Bulk Package ... 3509
Cipro Oral Suspension 2991
Cipro XR Tablets 3004
Ciprodex Otic Suspension 555
Ciprofloxacin Hydrochloride (CYP3A4 inducers may decrease voriconazole systemic exposure (plasma concentrations)). Products include:
Ciloxan Ophthalmic Ointment 554
Cipro Tablets 2991
Cisapride (Co-administration with a CYP3A4 substrate, such as cisapride may result in inhibition of the metabolism of cisapride; increased plasma concentrations of cisapride can lead to QT prolongation and rare occurrence of torsade de pointes; co-administration is contraindicated).
No products indexed under this heading.
Cisplatin (CYP3A4 inducers may decrease voriconazole systemic exposure (plasma concentrations)).
No products indexed under this heading.
Citalopram Hydrobromide (CYP2C19 inhibitors may increase

voriconazole systemic exposure (plasma concentrations)). Products include:
- Celexa 1177

Clarithromycin (CYP3A4 inhibitors may increase voriconazole systemic exposure (plasma concentrations)). Products include:
- Biaxin/Biaxin XL 402
- PREVPAC 3281

Clopidogrel Hydrogen Sulfate (CYP2C9 inhibitors may increase voriconazole systemic exposure (plasma concentrations)).
- No products indexed under this heading.

Clotrimazole (CYP2C9 inhibitors may increase voriconazole systemic exposure (plasma concentrations)). Products include:
- Lotrimin 3053
- Lotrisone 3054

Cortisone Acetate (CYP3A4 inducers may decrease voriconazole systemic exposure (plasma concentrations)).
- No products indexed under this heading.

Cyclosporine (Co-administration results in increased exposure to cyclosporine; it is recommended that the cyclosporine dose be reduced by one-half when initiating the therapy; close and frequent monitoring of cyclosporine levels is recommended when voriconazole is discontinued). Products include:
- Gengraf Capsules 458
- Neoral Soft Gelatin Capsules 2247
- Neoral Oral Solution 2247
- Restasis Ophthalmic Emulsion 570
- Sandimmune 2259

Dalfopristin (CYP3A4 inhibitors may increase voriconazole systemic exposure (plasma concentrations)). Products include:
- Synercid I.V. 1690

Danazol (CYP3A4 inhibitors may increase voriconazole systemic exposure (plasma concentrations)).
- No products indexed under this heading.

Delavirdine Mesylate (May inhibit the metabolism of voriconazole; voriconazole may inhibit the metabolism of delavirdine). Products include:
- Rescriptor Tablets 2535

Desogestrel (CYP2C19 inhibitors may increase voriconazole systemic exposure (plasma concentrations)). Products include:
- Ortho-Cept Tablets 2395

Dexamethasone (CYP2C9 inducers may decrease voriconazole systemic exposure (plasma concentrations)). Products include:
- Ciprodex Otic Suspension 555
- Decadron Tablets 1929
- TobraDex Ophthalmic Ointment 558
- TobraDex Ophthalmic Suspension ... 558

Dexamethasone Acetate (CYP3A4 inducers may decrease voriconazole systemic exposure (plasma concentrations)).
- No products indexed under this heading.

Dexamethasone Sodium Phosphate (CYP3A4 inducers may decrease voriconazole systemic exposure (plasma concentrations)). Products include:
- Decadron Phosphate Injection 1931

Diazepam (Co-administration may increase plasma concentrations of benzodiazepines that are metabolized by CYP3A4). Products include:
- Diastat Rectal Delivery System 3344
- Valium Tablets 2822

Diclofenac Potassium (CYP2C9 inhibitors may increase voriconazole systemic exposure (plasma concentrations)). Products include:
- Cataflam Tablets 2173

Diclofenac Sodium (CYP2C9 inhibitors may increase voriconazole systemic exposure (plasma concentrations)). Products include:
- Arthrotec Tablets 3126
- Voltaren Ophthalmic Solution 2300
- Voltaren Tablets 2298
- Voltaren-XR Tablets 2301

Dicumarol (Co-administration may increase prothrombin time).
- No products indexed under this heading.

Dihydroergotamine Mesylate (Co-administration may result in increased plasma concentrations of ergot alkaloids and this can lead to ergotism; co-administration is contraindicated). Products include:
- Migranal Nasal Spray 3350

Diltiazem Hydrochloride (Co-administration may increase plasma concentrations of calcium channel blockers that are metabolized by CYP3A4). Products include:
- Cardizem LA Extended Release Tablets 1699
- Tiazac Capsules 1204

Diltiazem Maleate (CYP3A4 inhibitors may increase voriconazole systemic exposure (plasma concentrations)).
- No products indexed under this heading.

Disulfiram (CYP2C9 inhibitors may increase voriconazole systemic exposure (plasma concentrations)). Products include:
- Antabuse Tablets 2343

Doxorubicin Hydrochloride (CYP3A4 inducers may decrease voriconazole systemic exposure (plasma concentrations)). Products include:
- Adriamycin for Injection, USP 786
- Adriamycin Injection, USP 786

Efavirenz (May inhibit the metabolism of voriconazole; the metabolism of voriconazole may be induced by efavirenz. Co-administration is contraindicated). Products include:
- Sustiva Capsules 957

Ergonovine Maleate (Co-administration may result in increased plasma concentrations of ergot alkaloids and this can lead to ergotism; co-administration is contraindicated).
- No products indexed under this heading.

Ergotamine Tartrate (Co-administration may result in increased plasma concentrations of ergot alkaloids and this can lead to ergotism; co-administration is contraindicated).
- No products indexed under this heading.

Erythromycin (CYP3A4 inhibitors may increase voriconazole systemic exposure (plasma concentrations)). Products include:
- Erygel Topical Gel 2096
- Ery-Tab Tablets 447
- Erythromycin Base Filmtab Tablets 454
- Erythromycin Delayed-Release Capsules, USP 456
- PCE Dispertab Tablets 510

Erythromycin Estolate (CYP3A4 inhibitors may increase voriconazole systemic exposure (plasma concentrations)).
- No products indexed under this heading.

Erythromycin Ethylsuccinate (CYP3A4 inhibitors may increase voriconazole systemic exposure (plasma concentrations)). Products include:
- E.E.S. 449
- EryPed 445

Erythromycin Gluceptate (CYP3A4 inhibitors may increase voriconazole systemic exposure (plasma concentrations)).
- No products indexed under this heading.

Erythromycin Lactobionate (CYP3A4 inhibitors may increase voriconazole systemic exposure (plasma concentrations)).
- No products indexed under this heading.

Erythromycin Stearate (CYP3A4 inhibitors may increase voriconazole systemic exposure (plasma concentrations)). Products include:
- Erythrocin Stearate Filmtab Tablets 452

Esomeprazole Magnesium (The metabolism of other proton pump inhibitors may also be inhibited by voriconazole and may result in increased plasma concentrations of other proton pump inhibitors). Products include:
- Nexium Delayed-Release Capsules 645

Ethinyl Estradiol (CYP2C19 inhibitors may increase voriconazole systemic exposure (plasma concentrations)). Products include:
- Alesse-28 Tablets 3392
- Lo/Ovral-28 Tablets 3423
- NuvaRing 2357
- Ortho-Cept Tablets 2395
- Ortho-Cyclen/Ortho Tri-Cyclen 2414
- Ortho Evra Transdermal System 2402
- Ortho Tri-Cyclen Lo Tablets 2421
- Seasonale Tablets 1073
- Triphasil-28 Tablets 3483
- Yasmin 28 Tablets 818

Ethosuximide (CYP3A4 inducers may decrease voriconazole systemic exposure (plasma concentrations)).
- No products indexed under this heading.

Ethynodiol Diacetate (CYP2C19 inhibitors may increase voriconazole systemic exposure (plasma concentrations)).
- No products indexed under this heading.

Felbamate (CYP2C19 inhibitors may increase voriconazole systemic exposure (plasma concentrations)).
- No products indexed under this heading.

Felodipine (Co-administration may increase plasma concentrations of calcium channel blockers that are metabolized by CYP3A4). Products include:
- Plendil Extended-Release Tablets 651

Fenofibrate (CYP2C9 inhibitors may increase voriconazole systemic exposure (plasma concentrations)). Products include:
- Antara Capsules 2723
- Lofibra Capsules 1217
- Tricor Tablets 523
- Triglide Tablets 1165

Fluconazole (CYP2C9 inhibitors may increase voriconazole systemic exposure (plasma concentrations)).
- No products indexed under this heading.

Fludrocortisone Acetate (CYP3A4 inducers may decrease voriconazole systemic exposure (plasma concentrations)).
- No products indexed under this heading.

Fluorouracil (CYP2C9 inhibitors may increase voriconazole systemic exposure (plasma concentrations)). Products include:
- Carac Cream, 0.5% 1048
- Efudex 3348

Fluoxetine (CYP2C19 inhibitors may increase voriconazole systemic exposure (plasma concentrations)).
- No products indexed under this heading.

Fluoxetine Hydrochloride (CYP2C19 inhibitors may increase voriconazole systemic exposure (plasma concentrations)). Products include:
- Prozac Pulvules and Liquid 1771
- Symbyax Capsules 1788

Flurbiprofen (CYP2C9 inhibitors may increase voriconazole systemic exposure (plasma concentrations)).
- No products indexed under this heading.

Flurbiprofen Sodium (CYP2C9 inhibitors may increase voriconazole systemic exposure (plasma concentrations)). Products include:
- Ocufen Ophthalmic Solution .... ⊙230

Fluvastatin Sodium (CYP2C19 inhibitors may increase voriconazole systemic exposure (plasma concentrations)). Products include:
- Lescol Capsules 2227
- Lescol 2730
- Lescol XL Tablets 2227

Fluvoxamine (CYP2C19 inhibitors may increase voriconazole systemic exposure (plasma concentrations)).
- No products indexed under this heading.

Fluvoxamine Maleate (CYP2C19 inhibitors may increase voriconazole systemic exposure (plasma concentrations)).
- No products indexed under this heading.

Fosamprenavir Calcium (CYP3A4 inhibitors may increase voriconazole systemic exposure (plasma concentrations)). Products include:
- Lexiva Tablets 1473

Fosphenytoin Sodium (Co-administration results in decreased steady-state Cmax and AUC of orally administered voriconazole and increased steady-state Cmax and AUC of phenytoin; frequent monitoring of plasma phenytoin levels and related adverse events is recommended).
- No products indexed under this heading.

Garlic Extract (CYP3A4 inducers may decrease voriconazole systemic exposure (plasma concentrations)).
- No products indexed under this heading.

Garlic Oil (CYP3A4 inducers may decrease voriconazole systemic exposure (plasma concentrations)).
- No products indexed under this heading.

Gemfibrozil (CYP2C9 inhibitors may increase voriconazole systemic exposure (plasma concentrations)).
No products indexed under this heading.

Glipizide (Co-administration may increase plasma concentrations of sulfonylureas that are metabolized by CYP2C9 and, therefore, cause hypoglycemia).
No products indexed under this heading.

Glyburide (Co-administration may increase plasma concentrations of sulfonylureas that are metabolized by CYP2C9 and, therefore, cause hypoglycemia).
No products indexed under this heading.

Hydrochlorothiazide (CYP2C9 inhibitors may increase voriconazole systemic exposure (plasma concentrations)). Products include:
Aldoril Tablets 1884
Atacand HCT 637
Avalide Tablets 2889
Avalide Tablets 922
Benicar HCT Tablets 2852
Diovan HCT Tablets 2195
Dyazide Capsules 1389
Hyzaar 1964
Lotensin HCT Tablets 2235
Maxzide 2150
Micardis HCT Tablets 886
Moduretic Tablets 2003
Prinzide Tablets 2033
Teveten HCT Tablets 1710
Timolide Tablets 2056
Uniretic Tablets 3114
Vaseretic Tablets 2073
Zestoretic Tablets 701

Hydrocortisone (CYP3A4 inducers may decrease voriconazole systemic exposure (plasma concentrations)). Products include:
Cortizone•5 Ointment .... ▣ 699
Cortizone•10 Creme .... ▣ 699
Cortizone•10 Ointment .... ▣ 699
Cortizone•10 Plus Creme .... ▣ 700
Cortizone•10 Maximum Strength Quick Shot Spray .... ▣ 700
Hydrocortone Tablets 1963
Preparation H Hydrocortisone Cream .... ▣ 748

Hydrocortisone Acetate (CYP3A4 inducers may decrease voriconazole systemic exposure (plasma concentrations)). Products include:
Analpram-HC 1136
Pramosone 1139
ProctoFoam-HC 3113
Tucks Anti-Itch Ointment .... ▣ 712
U-cort 1% Cream 3289

Hydrocortisone Butyrate (CYP3A4 inducers may decrease voriconazole systemic exposure (plasma concentrations)). Products include:
Locoid 1138
Locoid Lipocream Cream 1138

Hydrocortisone Cypionate (CYP3A4 inducers may decrease voriconazole systemic exposure (plasma concentrations)).
No products indexed under this heading.

Hydrocortisone Hemisuccinate (CYP3A4 inducers may decrease voriconazole systemic exposure (plasma concentrations)).
No products indexed under this heading.

Hydrocortisone Probutate (CYP3A4 inducers may decrease voriconazole systemic exposure (plasma concentrations)). Products include:
Pandel Cream, 0.1% 1017

Hydrocortisone Sodium Phosphate (CYP3A4 inducers may decrease voriconazole systemic exposure (plasma concentrations)).
No products indexed under this heading.

Hydrocortisone Sodium Succinate (CYP3A4 inducers may decrease voriconazole systemic exposure (plasma concentrations)).
No products indexed under this heading.

Hydrocortisone Valerate (CYP3A4 inducers may decrease voriconazole systemic exposure (plasma concentrations)).
No products indexed under this heading.

Hydroflumethiazide (CYP2C9 inhibitors may increase voriconazole systemic exposure (plasma concentrations)).
No products indexed under this heading.

Hypericum (CYP3A4 inducers may decrease voriconazole systemic exposure (plasma concentrations)).
No products indexed under this heading.

Hypericum Perforatum (CYP3A4 inducers may decrease voriconazole systemic exposure (plasma concentrations)).
No products indexed under this heading.

Imatinib Mesylate (CYP2C9 inhibitors may increase voriconazole systemic exposure (plasma concentrations)). Products include:
Gleevec Tablets 2221

Indinavir Sulfate (CYP3A4 inhibitors may increase voriconazole systemic exposure (plasma concentrations)). Products include:
Crixivan Capsules 1918

Indomethacin (CYP2C19 inhibitors may increase voriconazole systemic exposure (plasma concentrations)). Products include:
Indocin 1968

Indomethacin Sodium Trihydrate (CYP2C19 inhibitors may increase voriconazole systemic exposure (plasma concentrations)). Products include:
Indocin I.V. 1973

Isoniazid (CYP2C19 inhibitors may increase voriconazole systemic exposure (plasma concentrations)).
No products indexed under this heading.

Itraconazole (CYP2C9 inhibitors may increase voriconazole systemic exposure (plasma concentrations)).
No products indexed under this heading.

Ketoconazole (CYP2C19 inhibitors may increase voriconazole systemic exposure (plasma concentrations)). Products include:
Nizoral A-D Shampoo, 1% 1839
Nizoral 2% Shampoo 1838

Ketoprofen (CYP2C9 inhibitors may increase voriconazole systemic exposure (plasma concentrations)).
No products indexed under this heading.

Lansoprazole (The metabolism of other proton pump inhibitors may also be inhibited by voriconazole and may result in increased plasma concentrations of other proton pump inhibitors). Products include:
Prevacid Delayed-Release Capsules 3268
Prevacid for Delayed-Release Oral Suspension 3268
Prevacid I.V. for Injection 3274
Prevacid NapraPAC 3277
Prevacid SoluTab Delayed-Release Orally Disintegrating Tablets 3268
PREVPAC 3281

Leflunomide (CYP2C9 inhibitors may increase voriconazole systemic exposure (plasma concentrations)). Products include:
Arava Tablets 2881

Letrozole (CYP2C19 inhibitors may increase voriconazole systemic exposure (plasma concentrations)). Products include:
Femara Tablets 2210

Levonorgestrel (CYP2C19 inhibitors may increase voriconazole systemic exposure (plasma concentrations)). Products include:
Alesse-28 Tablets 3392
Climara Pro Transdermal System 800
Mirena Intrauterine System 810
Plan B Tablets 1068
Seasonale Tablets 1073
Triphasil-28 Tablets 3483

Lopinavir (CYP3A4 inhibitors may increase voriconazole systemic exposure (plasma concentrations)). Products include:
Kaletra 474

Loratadine (CYP3A4 inhibitors may increase voriconazole systemic exposure (plasma concentrations)). Products include:
Alavert Allergy & Sinus D-12 Hour Tablets .... ▣ 743
Alavert .... ▣ 743
Children's Claritin 24 Hour Non-Drowsy Allergy Syrup .... ▣ 732
Claritin Non-Drowsy 24 Hour Tablets .... ▣ 731
Non-Drowsy Claritin Hives Relief Tablets .... ▣ 733
Claritin Reditabs 24 Hour Non-Drowsy Tablets .... ▣ 732
Claritin-D Non-Drowsy 12 Hour Tablets .... ▣ 731
Claritin-D Non-Drowsy 24 Hour Tablets .... ▣ 731
Children's Dimetapp ND Non-Drowsy Allergy Syrup .... ▣ 746
Triaminic Allerchews .... ▣ 684

Lovastatin (Co-administration may increase plasma concentrations of statins that are metabolized by CYP3A4). Products include:
Advicor Tablets 1694
Altoprev Extended-Release Tablets 1151
Mevacor Tablets 1996

Mephenytoin (CYP3A4 inducers may decrease voriconazole systemic exposure (plasma concentrations)).
No products indexed under this heading.

Mephobarbital (Co-administration with potent inducer of CYP450, such as long-acting barbiturates- mephobarbital, is likely to significantly decrease plasma voriconazole concentrations; co-administration is contraindicated). Products include:
Mebaral Tablets, USP 2483

Mestranol (CYP2C19 inhibitors may increase voriconazole systemic exposure (plasma concentrations)).
No products indexed under this heading.

Methadone Hydrochloride (Increased plasma concentrations of methadone have been associated with toxicity, including QT prolongation. Frequent monitoring for adverse events and toxicity related to methadone is recommended during co-administration. Dose reduction of methadone may be needed).
No products indexed under this heading.

Methsuximide (CYP3A4 inducers may decrease voriconazole systemic exposure (plasma concentrations)).
No products indexed under this heading.

Methyclothiazide (CYP2C9 inhibitors may increase voriconazole systemic exposure (plasma concentrations)).
No products indexed under this heading.

Methylergonovine Maleate (Co-administration may result in increased plasma concentrations of ergot alkaloids and this can lead to ergotism; co-administration is contraindicated).
No products indexed under this heading.

Methylprednisolone (CYP3A4 inducers may decrease voriconazole systemic exposure (plasma concentrations)).
No products indexed under this heading.

Methylprednisolone Acetate (CYP3A4 inducers may decrease voriconazole systemic exposure (plasma concentrations)). Products include:
Depo-Medrol Injectable Suspension 2615
Depo-Medrol Single-Dose Vial 2617

Methylprednisolone Sodium Succinate (CYP3A4 inducers may decrease voriconazole systemic exposure (plasma concentrations)).
No products indexed under this heading.

Methysergide Maleate (Co-administration may result in increased plasma concentrations of ergot alkaloids and this can lead to ergotism; co-administration is contraindicated).
No products indexed under this heading.

Metronidazole (CYP2C9 inhibitors may increase voriconazole systemic exposure (plasma concentrations)). Products include:
Metrogel 1% 1212
MetroGel-Vaginal Gel 1822
Noritate Cream, 1% 1051

Metronidazole Benzoate (CYP2C9 inhibitors may increase voriconazole systemic exposure (plasma concentrations)).
No products indexed under this heading.

Metronidazole Hydrochloride (CYP2C9 inhibitors may increase voriconazole systemic exposure (plasma concentrations)).
No products indexed under this heading.

Miconazole (CYP2C9 inhibitors may increase voriconazole systemic exposure (plasma concentrations)).
No products indexed under this heading.

Miconazole Nitrate (CYP3A4 inhibitors may increase voriconazole systemic exposure (plasma concentrations)). Products include:

Desenex .... ▣674
Desenex Jock Itch Spray Powder ... ▣674

Midazolam Hydrochloride (Co-administration may increase plasma concentrations of benzodiazepines that are metabolized by CYP3A4).
No products indexed under this heading.

Modafinil (CYP2C19 inhibitors may increase voriconazole systemic exposure (plasma concentrations)). Products include:
Provigil Tablets 1002

Nefazodone Hydrochloride (CYP3A4 inhibitors may increase voriconazole systemic exposure (plasma concentrations)).
No products indexed under this heading.

Nelfinavir Mesylate (Voriconazole may inhibit the metabolism of nelfinavir). Products include:
Viracept 2556

Nevirapine (The metabolism of voriconazole may be induced by nevirapine). Products include:
Viramune Oral Suspension 903
Viramune Tablets 903

Niacinamide (CYP3A4 inhibitors may increase voriconazole systemic exposure (plasma concentrations)).
No products indexed under this heading.

Nicotinamide (CYP3A4 inhibitors may increase voriconazole systemic exposure (plasma concentrations)). Products include:
Nicomide Tablets 3190

Nifedipine (Co-administration may increase plasma concentrations of calcium channel blockers that are metabolized by CYP3A4). Products include:
Adalat CC Tablets 2978

Nisoldipine (Co-administration may increase plasma concentrations of calcium channel blockers that are metabolized by CYP3A4). Products include:
Sular Tablets 1163

Norethindrone (CYP2C19 inducers may decrease voriconazole systemic exposure (plasma concentrations)). Products include:
Ortho Micronor Tablets 2411

Norethindrone Acetate (CYP2C19 inducers may decrease voriconazole systemic exposure (plasma concentrations)). Products include:
Activella Tablets 2311
Aygestin Tablets 1062
CombiPatch Transdermal System 2180

Norethynodrel (CYP2C19 inhibitors may increase voriconazole systemic exposure (plasma concentrations)).
No products indexed under this heading.

Norfloxacin (CYP3A4 inhibitors may increase voriconazole systemic exposure (plasma concentrations)). Products include:
Noroxin Tablets 2009

Norgestimate (CYP2C19 inhibitors may increase voriconazole systemic exposure (plasma concentrations)). Products include:
Ortho-Cyclen/Ortho Tri-Cyclen 2414
Ortho Tri-Cyclen Lo Tablets 2421
Prefest Tablets 1069

Norgestrel (CYP2C19 inhibitors may increase voriconazole systemic exposure (plasma concentrations)). Products include:
Lo/Ovral-28 Tablets 3423

Omeprazole (Co-administration results in a significant increase in omeprazole plasma exposure; when initiating therapy with VFEND in patients already receiving omeprazole doses of 40 mg or greater, reduce the omeprazole dose by one-half). Products include:
Zegerid Powder for Oral Solution 2972

Oxcarbazepine (CYP2C19 inhibitors may increase voriconazole systemic exposure (plasma concentrations)). Products include:
Trileptal Oral Suspension 2281
Trileptal Tablets 2281

Oxiconazole Nitrate (CYP2C9 inhibitors may increase voriconazole systemic exposure (plasma concentrations)). Products include:
Oxistat 1498

Pantoprazole Sodium (The metabolism of other proton pump inhibitors may also be inhibited by voriconazole and may result in increased plasma concentrations of other proton pump inhibitors). Products include:
Protonix I.V. 3468
Protonix Tablets 3465

Paroxetine Hydrochloride (CYP2C19 inhibitors may increase voriconazole systemic exposure (plasma concentrations)). Products include:
Paxil CR Controlled-Release Tablets 1509
Paxil 1501

Pentobarbital Sodium (Long-acting barbiturates are likely to significantly decrease plasma voriconazole concentrations. Co-administration of voriconazole with long-acting barbiturates is contraindicated). Products include:
Nembutal Sodium Solution, USP 2484

Phenobarbital (Co-administration with potent inducer of CYP450, such as long-acting barbiturates- phenobarbital, are likely to significantly decrease plasma voriconazole concentrations; co-administration is contraindicated).
No products indexed under this heading.

Phenobarbital Sodium (CYP2C19 inducers may decrease voriconazole systemic exposure (plasma concentrations)).
No products indexed under this heading.

Phenylbutazone (CYP2C9 inhibitors may increase voriconazole systemic exposure (plasma concentrations)).
No products indexed under this heading.

Phenytoin (Co-administration results in decreased steady-state Cmax and AUC of orally administered voriconazole and increased steady-state Cmax and AUC of phenytoin; frequent monitoring of plasma phenytoin levels and related adverse events is recommended).
No products indexed under this heading.

Phenytoin Sodium (Co-administration results in decreased steady-state Cmax and AUC of orally administered voriconazole and increased steady-state Cmax and AUC of phenytoin; frequent monitoring of plasma phenytoin levels and related adverse events is recommended). Products include:
Phenytek Capsules 2153

Pimozide (Co-administration with a CYP3A4 substrate, such as pimozide may result in inhibition of the metabolism of pimozide; increased plasma concentrations of pimozide can lead to QT prolongation and rare occurrence of torsade de pointes; co-administration is contraindicated). Products include:
Orap Tablets 1220

Polythiazide (CYP2C9 inhibitors may increase voriconazole systemic exposure (plasma concentrations)).
No products indexed under this heading.

Prednisolone (Increased Cmax and AUC of prednisolone by 11% and 34%, respectively; no dosage adjustments of prednisolone are needed).
No products indexed under this heading.

Prednisolone Acetate (Increased Cmax and AUC of prednisolone by 11% and 34%, respectively; no dosage adjustments of prednisolone are needed). Products include:
Blephamide Ophthalmic Ointment 563
Blephamide Ophthalmic Suspension 564
Poly-Pred Liquifilm Ophthalmic Suspension .... ⊙231
Pred Forte Ophthalmic Suspension .... ⊙233
Pred Mild Sterile Ophthalmic Suspension .... ⊙236
Pred-G Ophthalmic Suspension ...... ⊙234
Pred-G Sterile Ophthalmic Ointment .... ⊙235

Prednisolone Sodium Phosphate (Increased Cmax and AUC of prednisolone by 11% and 34%, respectively; no dosage adjustments of prednisolone are needed). Products include:
Pediapred Oral Solution 3319

Prednisolone Tebutate (Increased Cmax and AUC of prednisolone by 11% and 34%, respectively; no dosage adjustments of prednisolone are needed).
No products indexed under this heading.

Prednisone (CYP2C19 inducers may decrease voriconazole systemic exposure (plasma concentrations)).
No products indexed under this heading.

Primidone (CYP2C9 inducers may decrease voriconazole systemic exposure (plasma concentrations)).
No products indexed under this heading.

Propoxyphene Hydrochloride (CYP3A4 inhibitors may increase voriconazole systemic exposure (plasma concentrations)).
No products indexed under this heading.

Propoxyphene Napsylate (CYP3A4 inhibitors may increase voriconazole systemic exposure (plasma concentrations)). Products include:
Darvocet A 500 Tablets 3497

Quinidine (Co-administration with a CYP3A4 substrate, such as quinidine, may result in inhibition of the metabolism of quinidine; increased plasma concentrations of quinidine can lead to QT prolongation and rare occurrence of torsade de pointes; co-administration is contraindicated).
No products indexed under this heading.

Quinidine Gluconate (Co-administration with a CYP3A4 substrate, such as quinidine, may result in inhibition of the metabolism of quinidine; increased plasma concentrations of quinidine can lead to QT prolongation and rare occurrence of torsade de pointes; co-administration is contraindicated).
No products indexed under this heading.

Quinidine Hydrochloride (Co-administration with a CYP3A4 substrate, such as quinidine, may result in inhibition of the metabolism of quinidine; increased plasma concentrations of quinidine can lead to QT prolongation and rare occurrence of torsade de pointes; co-administration is contraindicated).
No products indexed under this heading.

Quinidine Polygalacturonate (Co-administration with a CYP3A4 substrate, such as quinidine, may result in inhibition of the metabolism of quinidine; increased plasma concentrations of quinidine can lead to QT prolongation and rare occurrence of torsade de pointes; co-administration is contraindicated).
No products indexed under this heading.

Quinidine Sulfate (Co-administration with a CYP3A4 substrate, such as quinidine, may result in inhibition of the metabolism of quinidine; increased plasma concentrations of quinidine can lead to QT prolongation and rare occurrence of torsade de pointes; co-administration is contraindicated).
No products indexed under this heading.

Quinine (CYP3A4 inhibitors may increase voriconazole systemic exposure (plasma concentrations)).
No products indexed under this heading.

Quinine Sulfate (CYP3A4 inhibitors may increase voriconazole systemic exposure (plasma concentrations)).
No products indexed under this heading.

Quinupristin (CYP3A4 inhibitors may increase voriconazole systemic exposure (plasma concentrations)). Products include:
Synercid I.V. 1690

Rabeprazole Sodium (The metabolism of other proton pump inhibitors may also be inhibited by voriconazole and may result in increased plasma concentrations of other proton pump inhibitors). Products include:
Aciphex Tablets 1081

Ranitidine Bismuth Citrate (CYP3A4 inhibitors may increase voriconazole systemic exposure (plasma concentrations)).
No products indexed under this heading.

Ranitidine Hydrochloride (CYP3A4 inhibitors may increase voriconazole systemic exposure (plasma concentrations)). Products include:
Zantac 1597
Zantac Injection 1593
Zantac 75 Tablets .... ▣715
Zantac 150 Maximum Strength Tablets .... ▣715
Zantac Injection Pharmacy Bulk Package 1595

Rifabutin (Co-administration results in a significant increase in rifabutin plasma exposure; co-administration is contraindicated).
No products indexed under this heading.

Rifampicin (CYP3A4 inducers may decrease voriconazole systemic exposure (plasma concentrations)).
No products indexed under this heading.

Rifampin (Co-administration with potent inducer of CYP450, such as rifampin, can significantly reduce the systemic exposure; doubling the dose of voriconazole does not restore adequate exposure to voriconazole; co-administration is contraindicated).
No products indexed under this heading.

Rifapentine (CYP2C9 inducers may decrease voriconazole systemic exposure (plasma concentrations)).
No products indexed under this heading.

Ritonavir (May inhibit the metabolism of voriconazole. Co-administration of voriconazole and ritonavir (400 mg every 12 hours) is contraindicated). Products include:
Kaletra 474
Norvir 499

Saquinavir (Voriconazole may inhibit the metabolism of saquinavir; saquinavir may inhibit the metabolism of voriconazole).
No products indexed under this heading.

Saquinavir Mesylate (Voriconazole may inhibit the metabolism of saquinavir; saquinavir may inhibit the metabolism of voriconazole).
Products include:
Invirase 2776

Secobarbital Sodium (Long-acting barbiturates are likely to significantly decrease plasma voriconazole concentrations. Co-administration of voriconazole with long-acting barbiturates is contraindicated).
No products indexed under this heading.

Sertraline Hydrochloride (CYP2C19 inhibitors may increase voriconazole systemic exposure (plasma concentrations)). Products include:
Zoloft 2581

Simvastatin (Co-administration may increase plasma concentrations of statins that are metabolized by CYP3A4). Products include:
Vytorin 10/10 Tablets 2084
Vytorin 10/10 Tablets 3092
Vytorin 10/20 Tablets 2084
Vytorin 10/20 Tablets 3092
Vytorin 10/40 Tablets 3092
Vytorin 10/40 Tablets 2084
Vytorin 10/80 Tablets 2084
Vytorin 10/80 Tablets 3092
Zocor Tablets 2078

Sirolimus (Co-administration with a CYP3A4 substrate, such as sirolimus, can significantly increase the systemic exposure of sirolimus; co-administration is contraindicated).
Products include:
Rapamune Oral Solution and Tablets 3472

Sulfacytine (CYP2C9 inhibitors may increase voriconazole systemic exposure (plasma concentrations)).
No products indexed under this heading.

Sulfamethizole (CYP2C9 inhibitors may increase voriconazole systemic exposure (plasma concentrations)).
No products indexed under this heading.

Sulfamethoxazole (CYP2C9 inhibitors may increase voriconazole systemic exposure (plasma concentrations)).
No products indexed under this heading.

Sulfaphenazole (CYP2C19 inhibitors may increase voriconazole systemic exposure (plasma concentrations)).
No products indexed under this heading.

Sulfasalazine (CYP2C9 inhibitors may increase voriconazole systemic exposure (plasma concentrations)).
No products indexed under this heading.

Sulfinpyrazone (CYP2C9 inhibitors may increase voriconazole systemic exposure (plasma concentrations)).
No products indexed under this heading.

Sulfisoxazole (CYP2C9 inhibitors may increase voriconazole systemic exposure (plasma concentrations)).
No products indexed under this heading.

Sulfisoxazole Acetyl (CYP2C9 inhibitors may increase voriconazole systemic exposure (plasma concentrations)).
No products indexed under this heading.

Sulfisoxazole Diolamine (CYP2C9 inhibitors may increase voriconazole systemic exposure (plasma concentrations)).
No products indexed under this heading.

Tacrolimus (Co-administration results in increased exposure to tacrolimus; it is recommended that the tacrolimus dose be reduced by one-half when initiating the therapy; close and frequent monitoring of tacrolimus levels is recommended when voriconazole is discontinued).
Products include:
Prograf Capsules and Injection 624
Protopic Ointment 629

Telithromycin (CYP3A4 inhibitors may increase voriconazole systemic exposure (plasma concentrations)).
Products include:
Ketek Tablets 2920

Telmisartan (CYP2C19 inhibitors may increase voriconazole systemic exposure (plasma concentrations)).
Products include:
Micardis Tablets 884
Micardis HCT Tablets 886

Terconazole (CYP2C9 inhibitors may increase voriconazole systemic exposure (plasma concentrations)).
No products indexed under this heading.

Terfenadine (Co-administration with a CYP3A4 substrate, such as terfenadine may result in inhibition of the metabolism of terfenadine; increased plasma concentrations of terfenadine can lead to QT prolongation and rare occurrence of torsade de pointes; co-administration is contraindicated).
No products indexed under this heading.

Theophylline (CYP3A4 inducers may decrease voriconazole systemic exposure (plasma concentrations)).
No products indexed under this heading.

Thiamylal Sodium (Long-acting barbiturates are likely to significantly decrease plasma voriconazole concentrations. Co-administration of voriconazole with long-acting barbiturates is contraindicated).
No products indexed under this heading.

Ticlopidine Hydrochloride (CYP2C19 inhibitors may increase voriconazole systemic exposure (plasma concentrations)). Products include:
Ticlid Tablets 2813

Tolazamide (CYP2C9 inhibitors may increase voriconazole systemic exposure (plasma concentrations)).
No products indexed under this heading.

Tolbutamide (Co-administration may increase plasma concentrations of sulfonylureas that are metabolized by CYP2C9 and, therefore, cause hypoglycemia).
No products indexed under this heading.

Tolbutamide Sodium (CYP2C19 inhibitors may increase voriconazole systemic exposure (plasma concentrations)).
No products indexed under this heading.

Topiramate (CYP2C19 inhibitors may increase voriconazole systemic exposure (plasma concentrations)).
Products include:
Topamax Sprinkle Capsules 2438
Topamax Tablets 2438

Triamcinolone (CYP3A4 inducers may decrease voriconazole systemic exposure (plasma concentrations)).
No products indexed under this heading.

Triamcinolone Acetonide (CYP3A4 inducers may decrease voriconazole systemic exposure (plasma concentrations)). Products include:
Azmacort Inhalation Aerosol 1701
Nasacort HFA Inhalation Aerosol 2939
Nasacort AQ Nasal Spray 2937

Triamcinolone Diacetate (CYP3A4 inducers may decrease voriconazole systemic exposure (plasma concentrations)).
No products indexed under this heading.

Triamcinolone Hexacetonide (CYP3A4 inducers may decrease voriconazole systemic exposure (plasma concentrations)).
No products indexed under this heading.

Triazolam (Co-administration may increase plasma concentrations of benzodiazepines that are metabolized by CYP3A4).
No products indexed under this heading.

Troglitazone (CYP2C9 inhibitors may increase voriconazole systemic exposure (plasma concentrations)).
No products indexed under this heading.

Troleandomycin (CYP3A4 inhibitors may increase voriconazole systemic exposure (plasma concentrations)).
No products indexed under this heading.

Valproate Sodium (CYP3A4 inhibitors may increase voriconazole systemic exposure (plasma concentrations)). Products include:
Depacon Injection 412

Verapamil Hydrochloride (Co-administration may increase plasma concentrations of calcium channel blockers that are metabolized by CYP3A4). Products include:
Covera-HS Tablets 3135
Tarka Tablets 519
Verelan PM Capsules 3120

Vinblastine Sulfate (Co-administration may increase plasma concentrations of vinca alkaloids and lead to neurotoxicity).
No products indexed under this heading.

Vincristine Sulfate (Co-administration may increase plasma concentrations of vinca alkaloids and lead to neurotoxicity).
No products indexed under this heading.

Vinorelbine Tartrate (Co-administration may increase plasma concentrations of vinca alkaloids and lead to neurotoxicity). Products include:
Navelbine Injection 1494

Warfarin Sodium (Co-administration significantly increases maximum prothrombin time by 2-times). Products include:
Coumadin for Injection 932
Coumadin Tablets 932

Zafirlukast (CYP2C9 inhibitors may increase voriconazole systemic exposure (plasma concentrations)).
Products include:
Accolate Tablets 663

Zileuton (CYP3A4 inhibitors may increase voriconazole systemic exposure (plasma concentrations)).
No products indexed under this heading.

Food Interactions

Food, unspecified (When multiple doses of voriconazole are administered with high fat meals, the mean Cmax and AUC are reduced; VFEND tablets should be taken at least one hour before or one hour following a meal).

Grapefruit (CYP3A4 inhibitors may increase voriconazole systemic exposure (plasma concentrations)).

Grapefruit Juice (CYP3A4 inhibitors may increase voriconazole systemic exposure (plasma concentrations)).

VIADUR IMPLANT

(Leuprolide Acetate) 782
None cited in PDR database.

VIAGRA TABLETS

(Sildenafil Citrate) 2552
May interact with alpha adrenergic blockers, nonspecific beta-blockers, erythromycin, loop diuretics, nitrates and nitrites, protease inhibitors, potassium sparing diuretics, and certain other agents. Compounds in these categories include:

Alprostadil (The safety and efficacy of combinations of Viagra with other treatments for erectile dysfunction have not been studied; therefore, the use of such combinations is not recommended). Products include:
Caverject Impulse Injection 2610
Edex Injection 3103

Amiloride Hydrochloride (The AUC of the active metabolite, N-desmethyl sildenafil, was increased 62% by potassium-sparing

diuretics; these effects on the metabolite are not expected to be of clinical consequence). Products include:
- Midamor Tablets ... 2000
- Moduretic Tablets ... 2003

Amlodipine Besylate (Co-administration in hypertensive patients has resulted in mean additional reduction on supine blood pressure by 8 mmHg systolic and 7 mmHg diastolic). Products include:
- Caduet Tablets ... 2507
- Lotrel Capsules ... 2238
- Norvasc Tablets ... 2529

Amprenavir (Although the interaction between other protease inhibitors and sildenafil has not been studied, their concomitant use is expected to increase sildenafil levels). Products include:
- Agenerase Capsules ... 1299
- Agenerase Oral Solution ... 1304

Amyl Nitrite (Viagra has been shown to potentiate the hypotensive effects of nitrates, and its administration to patients who are using organic nitrates, either regularly and/or intermittently, in any form is therefore contraindicated).
No products indexed under this heading.

Bumetanide (The AUC of the active metabolite, N-desmethyl sildenafil, was increased 62% by loop diuretics; these effects on the metabolite are not expected to be of clinical consequence).
No products indexed under this heading.

Cimetidine (Co-administration of sildenafil with non-specific CYP inhibitors, such as cimetidine, has caused a 56% increase in plasma sildenafil concentrations; potential for reduction in sildenafil clearance). Products include:
- Tagamet HB 200 Tablets ... 637
- Tagamet Tablets ... 1547

Cimetidine Hydrochloride (Co-administration of sildenafil with non-specific CYP inhibitors, such as cimetidine, has caused a 56% increase in plasma sildenafil concentrations; potential for reduction in sildenafil clearance).
No products indexed under this heading.

Doxazosin Mesylate (Simultaneous administration of sildenafil citrate doses above 25mg and an alpha-blocker may lead to symptomatic hypotension in some patients. Therefore, Viagra doses above 25mg should not be taken within four hours of taking alpha-blockers).
No products indexed under this heading.

Erythrityl Tetranitrate (Viagra has been shown to potentiate the hypotensive effects of nitrates, and its administration to patients who are using organic nitrates, either regularly and/or intermittently, in any form is therefore contraindicated).
No products indexed under this heading.

Erythromycin (Co-administration of sildenafil with a specific CYP3A4 inhibitor, such as erythromycin, at steady state has resulted in a 182% increase in sildenafil systemic exposure; potential for reduction in sildenafil clearance). Products include:
- Erygel Topical Gel ... 2096
- Ery-Tab Tablets ... 447
- Erythromycin Base Filmtab Tablets ... 454
- Erythromycin Delayed-Release Capsules, USP ... 456
- PCE Dispertab Tablets ... 510

Erythromycin Estolate (Co-administration of sildenafil with a specific CYP3A4 inhibitor, such as erythromycin, at steady state has resulted in a 182% increase in sildenafil systemic exposure; potential for reduction in sildenafil clearance).
No products indexed under this heading.

Erythromycin Ethylsuccinate (Co-administration of sildenafil with a specific CYP3A4 inhibitor, such as erythromycin, at steady state has resulted in a 182% increase in sildenafil systemic exposure; potential for reduction in sildenafil clearance). Products include:
- E.E.S. ... 449
- EryPed ... 445

Erythromycin Gluceptate (Co-administration of sildenafil with a specific CYP3A4 inhibitor, such as erythromycin, at steady state has resulted in a 182% increase in sildenafil systemic exposure; potential for reduction in sildenafil clearance).
No products indexed under this heading.

Erythromycin Lactobionate (Co-administration of sildenafil with a specific CYP3A4 inhibitor, such as erythromycin, at steady state has resulted in a 182% increase in sildenafil systemic exposure; potential for reduction in sildenafil clearance).
No products indexed under this heading.

Erythromycin Stearate (Co-administration of sildenafil with a specific CYP3A4 inhibitor, such as erythromycin, at steady state has resulted in a 182% increase in sildenafil systemic exposure; potential for reduction in sildenafil clearance). Products include:
- Erythrocin Stearate Filmtab Tablets ... 452

Ethacrynic Acid (The AUC of the active metabolite, N-desmethyl sildenafil, was increased 62% by loop diuretics; these effects on the metabolite are not expected to be of clinical consequence). Products include:
- Edecrin Tablets ... 1941

Furosemide (The AUC of the active metabolite, N-desmethyl sildenafil, was increased 62% by loop diuretics; these effects on the metabolite are not expected to be of clinical consequence). Products include:
- Furosemide Tablets ... 2117

Indinavir Sulfate (Although the interaction between other protease inhibitors and sildenafil has not been studied, their concomitant use is expected to increase sildenafil levels). Products include:
- Crixivan Capsules ... 1918

Isosorbide Dinitrate (Viagra has been shown to potentiate the hypotensive effects of nitrates, and its administration to patients who are using organic nitrates, either regularly and/or intermittently, in any form is therefore contraindicated). Products include:
- BiDil Tablets ... 2161

Isosorbide Mononitrate (Viagra has been shown to potentiate the hypotensive effects of nitrates, and its administration to patients who are using organic nitrates, either regularly and/or intermittently, in any form is therefore contraindicated). Products include:
- Imdur Tablets ... 3032

Itraconazole (Co-administration of sildenafil with a stronger CYP3A4 inhibitor, such as itraconazole, would be expected to have a greater effect on the increase in sildenafil systemic exposure and a reduction in sildenafil clearance).
No products indexed under this heading.

Ketoconazole (Co-administration of sildenafil with a stronger CYP3A4 inhibitor, such as ketoconazole, would be expected to have a greater effect on the increase in sildenafil systemic exposure and a reduction in sildenafil clearance). Products include:
- Nizoral A-D Shampoo, 1% ... 1839
- Nizoral 2% Shampoo ... 1838

Labetalol Hydrochloride (Co-administration with nonspecific beta-blockers has resulted in the AUC of the active metabolite, N-desmethyl sildenafil by 102%; these effects on the metabolite are not expected to be of clinical consequences).
No products indexed under this heading.

Lopinavir (Although the interaction between other protease inhibitors and sildenafil has not been studied, their concomitant use is expected to increase sildenafil levels). Products include:
- Kaletra ... 474

Nadolol (Co-administration with nonspecific beta-blockers has resulted in the AUC of the active metabolite, N-desmethyl sildenafil by 102%; these effects on the metabolite are not expected to be of clinical consequences). Products include:
- Nadolol Tablets ... 2121

Nelfinavir Mesylate (Although the interaction between other protease inhibitors and sildenafil has not been studied, their concomitant use is expected to increase sildenafil levels). Products include:
- Viracept ... 2556

Nitroglycerin (Viagra has been shown to potentiate the hypotensive effects of nitrates, and its administration to patients who are using organic nitrates, either regularly and/or intermittently, in any form is therefore contraindicated). Products include:
- Nitro-Dur Transdermal Infusion System ... 3060
- Nitrolingual Pumpspray ... 1161

Pentaerythritol Tetranitrate (Viagra has been shown to potentiate the hypotensive effects of nitrates, and its administration to patients who are using organic nitrates, either regularly and/or intermittently, in any form is therefore contraindicated).
No products indexed under this heading.

Pindolol (Co-administration with nonspecific beta-blockers has resulted in the AUC of the active metabolite, N-desmethyl sildenafil by 102%; these effects on the metabolite are not expected to be of clinical consequences).
No products indexed under this heading.

Prazosin Hydrochloride (Simultaneous administration of sildenafil citrate doses above 25mg and an alpha-blocker may lead to symptomatic hypotension in some patients. Therefore, Viagra doses above 25mg should not be taken within four hours of taking alpha-blockers).
No products indexed under this heading.

Propranolol Hydrochloride (Co-administration with nonspecific beta-blockers has resulted in the AUC of the active metabolite, N-desmethyl sildenafil by 102%; these effects on the metabolite are not expected to be of clinical consequences). Products include:
- Inderal LA Long-Acting Capsules ... 3421
- InnoPran XL Capsules ... 2728

Rifampin (Co-administration of sildenafil with CYP3A4 inducers, such as rifampin, would be expected to result in decreased plasma levels of sildenafil).
No products indexed under this heading.

Ritonavir (Co-administration of ritonavir substantially increases serum concentrations of sildenafil, 11-fold increase in AUC; visual disturbances have occurred more commonly at higher systemic levels of sildenafil; decreased blood pressure, syncope, and prolonged erection have been reported in some healthy subjects exposed to high doses of sildenafil; a decrease in sildenafil dosage is recommended). Products include:
- Kaletra ... 474
- Norvir ... 499

Saquinavir (Co-administration of HIV protease inhibitor saquinavir, CYP3A4 inhibitor, at steady-state has resulted in a 140% increase in sildenafil Cmax and a 210% increase in sildenafil plasma AUC).
No products indexed under this heading.

Saquinavir Mesylate (Although the interaction between other protease inhibitors and sildenafil has not been studied, their concomitant use is expected to increase sildenafil levels). Products include:
- Invirase ... 2776

Spironolactone (The AUC of the active metabolite, N-desmethyl sildenafil, was increased 62% by potassium-sparing diuretics; these effects on the metabolite are not expected to be of clinical consequence).
No products indexed under this heading.

Tamsulosin Hydrochloride (Simultaneous administration of sildenafil citrate doses above 25mg and an alpha-blocker may lead to symptomatic hypotension in some patients. Therefore, Viagra doses above 25mg should not be taken within four hours of taking alpha-blockers). Products include:
- Flomax Capsules ... 881

Terazosin Hydrochloride (Simultaneous administration of sildenafil

citrate doses above 25mg and an alpha-blocker may lead to symptomatic hypotension in some patients. Therefore, Viagra doses above 25mg should not be taken within four hours of taking alpha-blockers). Products include:
Hytrin Capsules 469

Timolol Maleate (Co-administration with nonspecific beta-blockers has resulted in the AUC of the active metabolite, N-desmethyl sildenafil by 102%; these effects on the metabolite are not expected to be of clinical consequences). Products include:
Blocadren Tablets 1891
Cosopt Sterile Ophthalmic Solution 1910
Timolide Tablets 2056
Timoptic in Ocudose 2061
Timoptic Sterile Ophthalmic Solution 2058
Timoptic-XE Sterile Ophthalmic Gel Forming Solution 2062

Torsemide (The AUC of the active metabolite, N-desmethyl sildenafil, was increased 62% by loop diuretics; these effects on the metabolite are not expected to be of clinical consequence).
No products indexed under this heading.

Triamterene (The AUC of the active metabolite, N-desmethyl sildenafil, was increased 62% by potassium-sparing diuretics; these effects on the metabolite are not expected to be of clinical consequence). Products include:
Dyazide Capsules 1389
Dyrenium Capsules 3390
Maxzide 2150

Food Interactions

Food, unspecified (When Viagra is taken with a high fat meal, the rate of absorption is reduced with a mean delay in Tmax of 60 minutes and a mean reduction in Cmax of 29%).

VICKS 44 COUGH RELIEF

(Dextromethorphan Hydrobromide) ... 2675
See Vicks 44E Cough & Chest Congestion Relief

VICKS 44D COUGH & HEAD CONGESTION RELIEF

(Dextromethorphan Hydrobromide, Pseudoephedrine Hydrochloride) 2676
See Vicks 44E Cough & Chest Congestion Relief

VICKS 44D COUGH & HEAD CONGESTION RELIEF LIQUID

(Dextromethorphan Hydrobromide, Pseudoephedrine Hydrochloride) 721
See Vicks 44E Cough & Chest Congestion Relief Liquid

VICKS 44E COUGH & CHEST CONGESTION RELIEF

(Dextromethorphan Hydrobromide, Guaifenesin) 2676
May interact with monoamine oxidase inhibitors. Compounds in these categories include:

Isocarboxazid (Concurrent and/or sequential use with MAO inhibitors is not recommended).
No products indexed under this heading.

Moclobemide (Concurrent and/or sequential use with MAO inhibitors is not recommended).
No products indexed under this heading.

Pargyline Hydrochloride (Concurrent and/or sequential use with MAO inhibitors is not recommended).
No products indexed under this heading.

Phenelzine Sulfate (Concurrent and/or sequential use with MAO inhibitors is not recommended).
No products indexed under this heading.

Procarbazine Hydrochloride (Concurrent and/or sequential use with MAO inhibitors is not recommended). Products include:
Matulane Capsules 3188

Selegiline Hydrochloride (Concurrent and/or sequential use with MAO inhibitors is not recommended). Products include:
Eldepryl Capsules 3209

Tranylcypromine Sulfate (Concurrent and/or sequential use with MAO inhibitors is not recommended). Products include:
Parnate Tablets 1499

PEDIATRIC VICKS 44E COUGH & CHEST CONGESTION RELIEF LIQUID

(Dextromethorphan Hydrobromide, Guaifenesin) 2673
See Vicks 44E Cough & Chest Congestion Relief

VICKS 44M COUGH, COLD & FLU RELIEF

(Acetaminophen, Chlorpheniramine Maleate, Dextromethorphan Hydrobromide, Pseudoephedrine Hydrochloride) 2676
May interact with hypnotics and sedatives, monoamine oxidase inhibitors, tranquilizers, and certain other agents. Compounds in these categories include:

Alprazolam (May increase drowsiness effect). Products include:
Niravam Orally Disintegrating Tablets 3106
Xanax XR Tablets 2655

Buspirone Hydrochloride (May increase drowsiness effect).
No products indexed under this heading.

Chlordiazepoxide (May increase drowsiness effect).
No products indexed under this heading.

Chlordiazepoxide Hydrochloride (May increase drowsiness effect). Products include:
Librium Capsules 3349

Chlorpromazine (May increase drowsiness effect).
No products indexed under this heading.

Chlorpromazine Hydrochloride (May increase drowsiness effect).
No products indexed under this heading.

Chlorprothixene (May increase drowsiness effect).
No products indexed under this heading.

Chlorprothixene Hydrochloride (May increase drowsiness effect).
No products indexed under this heading.

Clorazepate Dipotassium (May increase drowsiness effect). Products include:
Tranxene 2488

Diazepam (May increase drowsiness effect). Products include:
Diastat Rectal Delivery System 3344
Valium Tablets 2822

Droperidol (May increase drowsiness effect).
No products indexed under this heading.

Estazolam (May increase drowsiness effect). Products include:
ProSom Tablets 512

Ethchlorvynol (May increase drowsiness effect).
No products indexed under this heading.

Ethinamate (May increase drowsiness effect).
No products indexed under this heading.

Fluphenazine Decanoate (May increase drowsiness effect).
No products indexed under this heading.

Fluphenazine Enanthate (May increase drowsiness effect).
No products indexed under this heading.

Fluphenazine Hydrochloride (May increase drowsiness effect).
No products indexed under this heading.

Flurazepam Hydrochloride (May increase drowsiness effect). Products include:
Dalmane Capsules 3343

Glutethimide (May increase drowsiness effect).
No products indexed under this heading.

Haloperidol (May increase drowsiness effect).
No products indexed under this heading.

Haloperidol Decanoate (May increase drowsiness effect).
No products indexed under this heading.

Hydroxyzine Hydrochloride (May increase drowsiness effect).
No products indexed under this heading.

Isocarboxazid (Concurrent and/or sequential use with MAO inhibitors is not recommended).
No products indexed under this heading.

Lorazepam (May increase drowsiness effect).
No products indexed under this heading.

Loxapine Hydrochloride (May increase drowsiness effect).
No products indexed under this heading.

Loxapine Succinate (May increase drowsiness effect).
No products indexed under this heading.

Meprobamate (May increase drowsiness effect).
No products indexed under this heading.

Mesoridazine Besylate (May increase drowsiness effect).
No products indexed under this heading.

Midazolam Hydrochloride (May increase drowsiness effect).
No products indexed under this heading.

Moclobemide (Concurrent and/or sequential use with MAO inhibitors is not recommended).
No products indexed under this heading.

Molindone Hydrochloride (May increase drowsiness effect). Products include:
Moban Tablets 1108

Oxazepam (May increase drowsiness effect).
No products indexed under this heading.

Pargyline Hydrochloride (Concurrent and/or sequential use with MAO inhibitors is not recommended).
No products indexed under this heading.

Perphenazine (May increase drowsiness effect).
No products indexed under this heading.

Phenelzine Sulfate (Concurrent and/or sequential use with MAO inhibitors is not recommended).
No products indexed under this heading.

Prazepam (May increase drowsiness effect).
No products indexed under this heading.

Procarbazine Hydrochloride (Concurrent and/or sequential use with MAO inhibitors is not recommended). Products include:
Matulane Capsules 3188

Prochlorperazine (May increase drowsiness effect).
No products indexed under this heading.

Promethazine Hydrochloride (May increase drowsiness effect). Products include:
Phenergan 3438

Propofol (May increase drowsiness effect). Products include:
Diprivan Injectable Emulsion 676

Quazepam (May increase drowsiness effect).
No products indexed under this heading.

Secobarbital Sodium (May increase drowsiness effect).
No products indexed under this heading.

Selegiline Hydrochloride (Concurrent and/or sequential use with MAO inhibitors is not recommended). Products include:
Eldepryl Capsules 3209

Temazepam (May increase drowsiness effect).
No products indexed under this heading.

Thioridazine Hydrochloride (May increase drowsiness effect). Products include:
Thioridazine Hydrochloride Tablets 2122

Thiothixene (May increase drowsiness effect). Products include:
Thiothixene Capsules 2124

Tranylcypromine Sulfate (Concurrent and/or sequential use with MAO inhibitors is not recommended). Products include:
Parnate Tablets 1499

Triazolam (May increase drowsiness effect).
No products indexed under this heading.

Trifluoperazine Hydrochloride (May increase drowsiness effect).
No products indexed under this heading.

Zaleplon (May increase drowsiness effect). Products include:
Sonata Capsules 1686

Zolpidem Tartrate (May increase drowsiness effect). Products include:
Ambien Tablets 2867

Food Interactions

Alcohol (May increase drowsiness effect; patients consuming 3 or more alcoholic drinks per day should consult their physician for advice on when and how they should take this medication).

PEDIATRIC VICKS 44M COUGH & COLD RELIEF

(Chlorpheniramine Maleate, Dextromethorphan Hydrobromide, Pseudoephedrine Hydrochloride)........ 2673
May interact with hypnotics and sedatives, monoamine oxidase inhibitors, tranquilizers, and certain other agents. Compounds in these categories include:

Alprazolam (May increase drowsiness effect). Products include:
Niravam Orally Disintegrating Tablets 3106
Xanax XR Tablets 2655

Buspirone Hydrochloride (May increase drowsiness effect).
No products indexed under this heading.

Chlordiazepoxide (May increase drowsiness effect).
No products indexed under this heading.

Chlordiazepoxide Hydrochloride (May increase drowsiness effect). Products include:
Librium Capsules 3349

Chlorpromazine (May increase drowsiness effect).
No products indexed under this heading.

Chlorpromazine Hydrochloride (May increase drowsiness effect).
No products indexed under this heading.

Chlorprothixene (May increase drowsiness effect).
No products indexed under this heading.

Chlorprothixene Hydrochloride (May increase drowsiness effect).
No products indexed under this heading.

Clorazepate Dipotassium (May increase drowsiness effect). Products include:
Tranxene 2488

Diazepam (May increase drowsiness effect). Products include:
Diastat Rectal Delivery System 3344
Valium Tablets 2822

Droperidol (May increase drowsiness effect).
No products indexed under this heading.

Estazolam (May increase drowsiness effect). Products include:
ProSom Tablets 512

Ethchlorvynol (May increase drowsiness effect).
No products indexed under this heading.

Ethinamate (May increase drowsiness effect).
No products indexed under this heading.

Fluphenazine Decanoate (May increase drowsiness effect).
No products indexed under this heading.

Fluphenazine Enanthate (May increase drowsiness effect).
No products indexed under this heading.

Fluphenazine Hydrochloride (May increase drowsiness effect).
No products indexed under this heading.

Flurazepam Hydrochloride (May increase drowsiness effect). Products include:
Dalmane Capsules 3343

Glutethimide (May increase drowsiness effect).
No products indexed under this heading.

Haloperidol (May increase drowsiness effect).
No products indexed under this heading.

Haloperidol Decanoate (May increase drowsiness effect).
No products indexed under this heading.

Hydroxyzine Hydrochloride (May increase drowsiness effect).
No products indexed under this heading.

Isocarboxazid (Concurrent and/or sequential use with MAO inhibitors is not recommended).
No products indexed under this heading.

Lorazepam (May increase drowsiness effect).
No products indexed under this heading.

Loxapine Hydrochloride (May increase drowsiness effect).
No products indexed under this heading.

Loxapine Succinate (May increase drowsiness effect).
No products indexed under this heading.

Meprobamate (May increase drowsiness effect).
No products indexed under this heading.

Mesoridazine Besylate (May increase drowsiness effect).
No products indexed under this heading.

Midazolam Hydrochloride (May increase drowsiness effect).
No products indexed under this heading.

Moclobemide (Concurrent and/or sequential use with MAO inhibitors is not recommended).
No products indexed under this heading.

Molindone Hydrochloride (May increase drowsiness effect). Products include:
Moban Tablets 1108

Oxazepam (May increase drowsiness effect).
No products indexed under this heading.

Pargyline Hydrochloride (Concurrent and/or sequential use with MAO inhibitors is not recommended).
No products indexed under this heading.

Perphenazine (May increase drowsiness effect).
No products indexed under this heading.

Phenelzine Sulfate (Concurrent and/or sequential use with MAO inhibitors is not recommended).
No products indexed under this heading.

Prazepam (May increase drowsiness effect).
No products indexed under this heading.

Procarbazine Hydrochloride (Concurrent and/or sequential use with MAO inhibitors is not recommended). Products include:
Matulane Capsules 3188

Prochlorperazine (May increase drowsiness effect).
No products indexed under this heading.

Promethazine Hydrochloride (May increase drowsiness effect). Products include:
Phenergan 3438

Propofol (May increase drowsiness effect). Products include:
Diprivan Injectable Emulsion 676

Quazepam (May increase drowsiness effect).
No products indexed under this heading.

Secobarbital Sodium (May increase drowsiness effect).
No products indexed under this heading.

Selegiline Hydrochloride (Concurrent and/or sequential use with MAO inhibitors is not recommended). Products include:
Eldepryl Capsules 3209

Temazepam (May increase drowsiness effect).
No products indexed under this heading.

Thioridazine Hydrochloride (May increase drowsiness effect). Products include:
Thioridazine Hydrochloride Tablets 2122

Thiothixene (May increase drowsiness effect). Products include:
Thiothixene Capsules 2124

Tranylcypromine Sulfate (Concurrent and/or sequential use with MAO inhibitors is not recommended). Products include:
Parnate Tablets 1499

Triazolam (May increase drowsiness effect).
No products indexed under this heading.

Trifluoperazine Hydrochloride (May increase drowsiness effect).
No products indexed under this heading.

Zaleplon (May increase drowsiness effect). Products include:
Sonata Capsules 1686

Zolpidem Tartrate (May increase drowsiness effect). Products include:
Ambien Tablets 2867

Food Interactions

Alcohol (May increase drowsiness effect).

VICKS COUGH DROPS, MENTHOL & CHERRY FLAVORS

(Menthol) 2675
None cited in PDR database.

VICKS DAYQUIL MULTI-SYMPTOM COLD/ FLU RELIEF LIQUICAPS

(Acetaminophen, Dextromethorphan Hydrobromide, Pseudoephedrine Hydrochloride)........ 2675
See Vicks DayQuil Multi-Symptom Cold/Flu Relief Liquid

VICKS DAYQUIL MULTI-SYMPTOM COLD/ FLU RELIEF LIQUID

(Acetaminophen, Dextromethorphan Hydrobromide, Pseudoephedrine Hydrochloride)........ 2675
May interact with monoamine oxidase inhibitors and certain other agents. Compounds in these categories include:

Isocarboxazid (Concurrent and/or sequential use with MAO inhibitors is not recommended).
No products indexed under this heading.

Moclobemide (Concurrent and/or sequential use with MAO inhibitors is not recommended).
No products indexed under this heading.

Pargyline Hydrochloride (Concurrent and/or sequential use with MAO inhibitors is not recommended).
No products indexed under this heading.

Phenelzine Sulfate (Concurrent and/or sequential use with MAO inhibitors is not recommended).
No products indexed under this heading.

Procarbazine Hydrochloride (Concurrent and/or sequential use with MAO inhibitors is not recommended). Products include:
Matulane Capsules 3188

Selegiline Hydrochloride (Concurrent and/or sequential use with MAO inhibitors is not recommended). Products include:
Eldepryl Capsules 3209

Tranylcypromine Sulfate (Concurrent and/or sequential use with MAO inhibitors is not recommended). Products include:
Parnate Tablets 1499

Food Interactions

Alcohol (Patients consuming 3 or more alcoholic drinks per day should consult their physician for advice on when and how they should take this medication).

CHILDREN'S VICKS NYQUIL COLD/COUGH RELIEF

(Chlorpheniramine Maleate, Dextromethorphan Hydrobromide, Pseudoephedrine Hydrochloride)........ 2671
May interact with hypnotics and sedatives, monoamine oxidase inhibitors, tranquilizers, and certain other agents. Compounds in these categories include:

Alprazolam (May increase drowsiness effect). Products include:
Niravam Orally Disintegrating Tablets 3106

Xanax XR Tablets 2655

Buspirone Hydrochloride (May increase drowsiness effect).
No products indexed under this heading.

Chlordiazepoxide (May increase drowsiness effect).
No products indexed under this heading.

Chlordiazepoxide Hydrochloride (May increase drowsiness effect).
Products include:
Librium Capsules 3349

Chlorpromazine (May increase drowsiness effect).
No products indexed under this heading.

Chlorpromazine Hydrochloride (May increase drowsiness effect).
No products indexed under this heading.

Chlorprothixene (May increase drowsiness effect).
No products indexed under this heading.

Chlorprothixene Hydrochloride (May increase drowsiness effect).
No products indexed under this heading.

Clorazepate Dipotassium (May increase drowsiness effect).
Products include:
Tranxene 2488

Diazepam (May increase drowsiness effect). Products include:
Diastat Rectal Delivery System 3344
Valium Tablets 2822

Droperidol (May increase drowsiness effect).
No products indexed under this heading.

Estazolam (May increase drowsiness effect). Products include:
ProSom Tablets 512

Ethchlorvynol (May increase drowsiness effect).
No products indexed under this heading.

Ethinamate (May increase drowsiness effect).
No products indexed under this heading.

Fluphenazine Decanoate (May increase drowsiness effect).
No products indexed under this heading.

Fluphenazine Enanthate (May increase drowsiness effect).
No products indexed under this heading.

Fluphenazine Hydrochloride (May increase drowsiness effect).
No products indexed under this heading.

Flurazepam Hydrochloride (May increase drowsiness effect).
Products include:
Dalmane Capsules 3343

Glutethimide (May increase drowsiness effect).
No products indexed under this heading.

Haloperidol (May increase drowsiness effect).
No products indexed under this heading.

Haloperidol Decanoate (May increase drowsiness effect).
No products indexed under this heading.

Hydroxyzine Hydrochloride (May increase drowsiness effect).
No products indexed under this heading.

Isocarboxazid (Concurrent and/or sequential use with MAO inhibitors is not recommended).
No products indexed under this heading.

Lorazepam (May increase drowsiness effect).
No products indexed under this heading.

Loxapine Hydrochloride (May increase drowsiness effect).
No products indexed under this heading.

Loxapine Succinate (May increase drowsiness effect).
No products indexed under this heading.

Meprobamate (May increase drowsiness effect).
No products indexed under this heading.

Mesoridazine Besylate (May increase drowsiness effect).
No products indexed under this heading.

Midazolam Hydrochloride (May increase drowsiness effect).
No products indexed under this heading.

Moclobemide (Concurrent and/or sequential use with MAO inhibitors is not recommended).
No products indexed under this heading.

Molindone Hydrochloride (May increase drowsiness effect).
Products include:
Moban Tablets 1108

Oxazepam (May increase drowsiness effect).
No products indexed under this heading.

Pargyline Hydrochloride (Concurrent and/or sequential use with MAO inhibitors is not recommended).
No products indexed under this heading.

Perphenazine (May increase drowsiness effect).
No products indexed under this heading.

Phenelzine Sulfate (Concurrent and/or sequential use with MAO inhibitors is not recommended).
No products indexed under this heading.

Prazepam (May increase drowsiness effect).
No products indexed under this heading.

Procarbazine Hydrochloride (Concurrent and/or sequential use with MAO inhibitors is not recommended). Products include:
Matulane Capsules 3188

Prochlorperazine (May increase drowsiness effect).
No products indexed under this heading.

Promethazine Hydrochloride (May increase drowsiness effect).
Products include:
Phenergan 3438

Propofol (May increase drowsiness effect). Products include:
Diprivan Injectable Emulsion 676

Quazepam (May increase drowsiness effect).
No products indexed under this heading.

Secobarbital Sodium (May increase drowsiness effect).
No products indexed under this heading.

Selegiline Hydrochloride (Concurrent and/or sequential use with MAO inhibitors is not recommended).
Products include:
Eldepryl Capsules 3209

Temazepam (May increase drowsiness effect).
No products indexed under this heading.

Thioridazine Hydrochloride (May increase drowsiness effect).
Products include:
Thioridazine Hydrochloride Tablets 2122

Thiothixene (May increase drowsiness effect). Products include:
Thiothixene Capsules 2124

Tranylcypromine Sulfate (Concurrent and/or sequential use with MAO inhibitors is not recommended).
Products include:
Parnate Tablets 1499

Triazolam (May increase drowsiness effect).
No products indexed under this heading.

Trifluoperazine Hydrochloride (May increase drowsiness effect).
No products indexed under this heading.

Zaleplon (May increase drowsiness effect). Products include:
Sonata Capsules 1686

Zolpidem Tartrate (May increase drowsiness effect). Products include:
Ambien Tablets 2867

Food Interactions

Alcohol (May increase drowsiness effect).

VICKS NYQUIL COUGH LIQUID
(Dextromethorphan Hydrobromide, Doxylamine Succinate)........................ 2677
See Vicks NyQuil LiquiCaps

VICKS NYQUIL LIQUICAPS
(Acetaminophen, Dextromethorphan Hydrobromide, Doxylamine Succinate, Pseudoephedrine Hydrochloride)........ 2677
May interact with hypnotics and sedatives, monoamine oxidase inhibitors, tranquilizers, and certain other agents. Compounds in these categories include:

Alprazolam (May increase drowsiness effect). Products include:
Niravam Orally Disintegrating Tablets 3106
Xanax XR Tablets 2655

Buspirone Hydrochloride (May increase drowsiness effect).
No products indexed under this heading.

Chlordiazepoxide (May increase drowsiness effect).
No products indexed under this heading.

Chlordiazepoxide Hydrochloride (May increase drowsiness effect).
Products include:
Librium Capsules 3349

Chlorpromazine (May increase drowsiness effect).
No products indexed under this heading.

Chlorpromazine Hydrochloride (May increase drowsiness effect).
No products indexed under this heading.

Chlorprothixene (May increase drowsiness effect).
No products indexed under this heading.

Chlorprothixene Hydrochloride (May increase drowsiness effect).
No products indexed under this heading.

Clorazepate Dipotassium (May increase drowsiness effect).
Products include:
Tranxene 2488

Diazepam (May increase drowsiness effect). Products include:
Diastat Rectal Delivery System 3344
Valium Tablets 2822

Droperidol (May increase drowsiness effect).
No products indexed under this heading.

Estazolam (May increase drowsiness effect). Products include:
ProSom Tablets 512

Ethchlorvynol (May increase drowsiness effect).
No products indexed under this heading.

Ethinamate (May increase drowsiness effect).
No products indexed under this heading.

Fluphenazine Decanoate (May increase drowsiness effect).
No products indexed under this heading.

Fluphenazine Enanthate (May increase drowsiness effect).
No products indexed under this heading.

Fluphenazine Hydrochloride (May increase drowsiness effect).
No products indexed under this heading.

Flurazepam Hydrochloride (May increase drowsiness effect).
Products include:
Dalmane Capsules 3343

Glutethimide (May increase drowsiness effect).
No products indexed under this heading.

Haloperidol (May increase drowsiness effect).
No products indexed under this heading.

Haloperidol Decanoate (May increase drowsiness effect).
No products indexed under this heading.

Hydroxyzine Hydrochloride (May increase drowsiness effect).
No products indexed under this heading.

Isocarboxazid (Concurrent and/or sequential use with MAO inhibitors is not recommended).
No products indexed under this heading.

Lorazepam (May increase drowsiness effect).
No products indexed under this heading.

Loxapine Hydrochloride (May increase drowsiness effect).
No products indexed under this heading.

Loxapine Succinate (May increase drowsiness effect).
No products indexed under this heading.

Meprobamate (May increase drowsiness effect).
No products indexed under this heading.

Mesoridazine Besylate (May increase drowsiness effect).
No products indexed under this heading.

Midazolam Hydrochloride (May increase drowsiness effect).
No products indexed under this heading.

Moclobemide (Concurrent and/or sequential use with MAO inhibitors is not recommended).
No products indexed under this heading.

Molindone Hydrochloride (May increase drowsiness effect). Products include:
Moban Tablets 1108

Oxazepam (May increase drowsiness effect).
No products indexed under this heading.

Pargyline Hydrochloride (Concurrent and/or sequential use with MAO inhibitors is not recommended).
No products indexed under this heading.

Perphenazine (May increase drowsiness effect).
No products indexed under this heading.

Phenelzine Sulfate (Concurrent and/or sequential use with MAO inhibitors is not recommended).
No products indexed under this heading.

Prazepam (May increase drowsiness effect).
No products indexed under this heading.

Procarbazine Hydrochloride (Concurrent and/or sequential use with MAO inhibitors is not recommended). Products include:
Matulane Capsules 3188

Prochlorperazine (May increase drowsiness effect).
No products indexed under this heading.

Promethazine Hydrochloride (May increase drowsiness effect). Products include:
Phenergan 3438

Propofol (May increase drowsiness effect). Products include:
Diprivan Injectable Emulsion 676

Quazepam (May increase drowsiness effect).
No products indexed under this heading.

Secobarbital Sodium (May increase drowsiness effect).
No products indexed under this heading.

Selegiline Hydrochloride (Concurrent and/or sequential use with MAO inhibitors is not recommended). Products include:
Eldepryl Capsules 3209

Temazepam (May increase drowsiness effect).
No products indexed under this heading.

Thioridazine Hydrochloride (May increase drowsiness effect). Products include:
Thioridazine Hydrochloride Tablets 2122

Thiothixene (May increase drowsiness effect). Products include:
Thiothixene Capsules 2124

Tranylcypromine Sulfate (Concurrent and/or sequential use with MAO inhibitors is not recommended). Products include:
Parnate Tablets 1499

Triazolam (May increase drowsiness effect).
No products indexed under this heading.

Trifluoperazine Hydrochloride (May increase drowsiness effect).
No products indexed under this heading.

Zaleplon (May increase drowsiness effect). Products include:
Sonata Capsules 1686

Zolpidem Tartrate (May increase drowsiness effect). Products include:
Ambien Tablets 2867

Food Interactions

Alcohol (May increase drowsiness effect; patients consuming 3 or more alcoholic drinks per day should consult their physician for advice on when and how they should take this medication).

VICKS NYQUIL LIQUICAPS/LIQUID MULTI-SYMPTOM COLD/FLU RELIEF

(Acetaminophen, Dextromethorphan Hydrobromide, Doxylamine Succinate, Pseudoephedrine Hydrochloride)....... 725

May interact with hypnotics and sedatives, monoamine oxidase inhibitors, tranquilizers, and certain other agents. Compounds in these categories include:

Alprazolam (May increase drowsiness effect). Products include:
Niravam Orally Disintegrating Tablets 3106
Xanax XR Tablets 2655

Buspirone Hydrochloride (May increase drowsiness effect).
No products indexed under this heading.

Chlordiazepoxide (May increase drowsiness effect).
No products indexed under this heading.

Chlordiazepoxide Hydrochloride (May increase drowsiness effect). Products include:
Librium Capsules 3349

Chlorpromazine (May increase drowsiness effect).
No products indexed under this heading.

Chlorpromazine Hydrochloride (May increase drowsiness effect).
No products indexed under this heading.

Chlorprothixene (May increase drowsiness effect).
No products indexed under this heading.

Chlorprothixene Hydrochloride (May increase drowsiness effect).
No products indexed under this heading.

Clorazepate Dipotassium (May increase drowsiness effect). Products include:
Tranxene 2488

Diazepam (May increase drowsiness effect). Products include:
Diastat Rectal Delivery System 3344
Valium Tablets 2822

Droperidol (May increase drowsiness effect).
No products indexed under this heading.

Estazolam (May increase drowsiness effect). Products include:
ProSom Tablets 512

Ethchlorvynol (May increase drowsiness effect).
No products indexed under this heading.

Ethinamate (May increase drowsiness effect).
No products indexed under this heading.

Fluphenazine Decanoate (May increase drowsiness effect).
No products indexed under this heading.

Fluphenazine Enanthate (May increase drowsiness effect).
No products indexed under this heading.

Fluphenazine Hydrochloride (May increase drowsiness effect).
No products indexed under this heading.

Flurazepam Hydrochloride (May increase drowsiness effect). Products include:
Dalmane Capsules 3343

Glutethimide (May increase drowsiness effect).
No products indexed under this heading.

Haloperidol (May increase drowsiness effect).
No products indexed under this heading.

Haloperidol Decanoate (May increase drowsiness effect).
No products indexed under this heading.

Hydroxyzine Hydrochloride (May increase drowsiness effect).
No products indexed under this heading.

Isocarboxazid (Do not use while taking, or for 2 weeks after stopping, MAO inhibitors).
No products indexed under this heading.

Lorazepam (May increase drowsiness effect).
No products indexed under this heading.

Loxapine Hydrochloride (May increase drowsiness effect).
No products indexed under this heading.

Loxapine Succinate (May increase drowsiness effect).
No products indexed under this heading.

Meprobamate (May increase drowsiness effect).
No products indexed under this heading.

Mesoridazine Besylate (May increase drowsiness effect).
No products indexed under this heading.

Midazolam Hydrochloride (May increase drowsiness effect).
No products indexed under this heading.

Moclobemide (Do not use while taking, or for 2 weeks after stopping, MAO inhibitors).
No products indexed under this heading.

Molindone Hydrochloride (May increase drowsiness effect). Products include:
Moban Tablets 1108

Oxazepam (May increase drowsiness effect).
No products indexed under this heading.

Pargyline Hydrochloride (Do not use while taking, or for 2 weeks after stopping, MAO inhibitors).
No products indexed under this heading.

Perphenazine (May increase drowsiness effect).
No products indexed under this heading.

Phenelzine Sulfate (Do not use while taking, or for 2 weeks after stopping, MAO inhibitors).
No products indexed under this heading.

Prazepam (May increase drowsiness effect).
No products indexed under this heading.

Procarbazine Hydrochloride (Do not use while taking, or for 2 weeks after stopping, MAO inhibitors). Products include:
Matulane Capsules 3188

Prochlorperazine (May increase drowsiness effect).
No products indexed under this heading.

Promethazine Hydrochloride (May increase drowsiness effect). Products include:
Phenergan 3438

Propofol (May increase drowsiness effect). Products include:
Diprivan Injectable Emulsion 676

Quazepam (May increase drowsiness effect).
No products indexed under this heading.

Secobarbital Sodium (May increase drowsiness effect).
No products indexed under this heading.

Selegiline Hydrochloride (Do not use while taking, or for 2 weeks after stopping, MAO inhibitors). Products include:
Eldepryl Capsules 3209

Temazepam (May increase drowsiness effect).
No products indexed under this heading.

Thioridazine Hydrochloride (May increase drowsiness effect). Products include:
Thioridazine Hydrochloride Tablets 2122

Thiothixene (May increase drowsiness effect). Products include:
Thiothixene Capsules 2124

Tranylcypromine Sulfate (Do not use while taking, or for 2 weeks after stopping, MAO inhibitors). Products include:
Parnate Tablets 1499

Triazolam (May increase drowsiness effect).
No products indexed under this heading.

Trifluoperazine Hydrochloride (May increase drowsiness effect).
No products indexed under this heading.

Zaleplon (May increase drowsiness effect). Products include:
Sonata Capsules 1686

Zolpidem Tartrate (May increase drowsiness effect). Products include:
Ambien Tablets 2867

Food Interactions

Alcohol (Chronic heavy alcohol users, 3 or more drinks per day, are at increased risk of liver toxicity from excessive acetaminophen use; alcohol increases drowsiness effect and concurrent use of alcoholic beverages should be avoided).

VICKS NYQUIL LIQUID
(Acetaminophen, Dextromethorphan Hydrobromide, Doxylamine Succinate, Pseudoephedrine Hydrochloride) 2677
See Vicks NyQuil LiquiCaps

VICKS SINEX 12-HOUR NASAL SPRAY AND ULTRA FINE MIST FOR SINUS RELIEF
(Oxymetazoline Hydrochloride) 2678
None cited in PDR database.

VICKS SINEX NASAL SPRAY AND ULTRA FINE MIST FOR SINUS RELIEF
(Phenylephrine Hydrochloride) 2677
None cited in PDR database.

VICKS VAPOR INHALER
(Levmetamfetamine) 2678
None cited in PDR database.

VICKS VAPORUB CREAM
(Camphor, Menthol) 2678
None cited in PDR database.

VICKS VAPORUB OINTMENT
(Camphor, Eucalyptus, Oil of, Menthol) 2678
None cited in PDR database.

VICKS VAPOSTEAM
(Camphor) 2679
None cited in PDR database.

VICODIN TABLETS
(Acetaminophen, Hydrocodone Bitartrate) 530
May interact with antihistamines, central nervous system depressants, monoamine oxidase inhibitors, narcotic analgesics, tricyclic antidepressants, and certain other agents. Compounds in these categories include:

Acrivastine (May exhibit an additive CNS depression).
No products indexed under this heading.

Alfentanil Hydrochloride (May exhibit an additive CNS depression).
No products indexed under this heading.

Alprazolam (May exhibit an additive CNS depression). Products include:
Niravam Orally Disintegrating Tablets 3106
Xanax XR Tablets 2655

Amitriptyline Hydrochloride (Co-administration may increase the effect of either antidepressant or hydrocodone).
No products indexed under this heading.

Amoxapine (Co-administration may increase the effect of either antidepressant or hydrocodone).
No products indexed under this heading.

Aprobarbital (May exhibit an additive CNS depression).
No products indexed under this heading.

Astemizole (May exhibit an additive CNS depression).
No products indexed under this heading.

Azatadine Maleate (May exhibit an additive CNS depression).
No products indexed under this heading.

Bromodiphenhydramine Hydrochloride (May exhibit an additive CNS depression).
No products indexed under this heading.

Brompheniramine Maleate (May exhibit an additive CNS depression). Products include:
Alacol DM Syrup 739
Children's Dimetapp Cold & Allergy Elixir .... ▣ 745
Children's Dimetapp DM Cold & Cough Elixir .... ▣ 745
Robitussin Allergy & Cough Syrup .. ▣ 750

Buprenorphine Hydrochloride (May exhibit an additive CNS depression). Products include:
Buprenex Injectable 2718
Suboxone Tablets 2719
Subutex Tablets 2719

Buspirone Hydrochloride (May exhibit an additive CNS depression).
No products indexed under this heading.

Butabarbital (May exhibit an additive CNS depression).
No products indexed under this heading.

Butalbital (May exhibit an additive CNS depression). Products include:
Sedapap Tablets 50 mg/650 mg 2098

Cetirizine Hydrochloride (May exhibit an additive CNS depression). Products include:
Zyrtec Chewable Tablets 2589
Zyrtec 2589
Zyrtec-D 12 Hour Extended Release Tablets 2591

Chlordiazepoxide (May exhibit an additive CNS depression).
No products indexed under this heading.

Chlordiazepoxide Hydrochloride (May exhibit an additive CNS depression). Products include:
Librium Capsules 3349

Chlorpheniramine Maleate (May exhibit an additive CNS depression). Products include:
Advil Allergy Sinus Caplets .... ▣ 737
Advil Multi-Symptom Cold Caplets .... ▣ 738
BC Allergy Sinus Cold Powder .... ▣ 612
Contac Severe Cold and Flu Caplets Maximum Strength .... ▣ 615
Hycomine Compound Tablets 1105
PediaCare Multi-Symptom Cold Liquid .... ▣ 704
PediaCare NightRest Cough & Cold Liquid .... ▣ 704
Robitussin Flu Liquid .... ▣ 752
Robitussin PM Cough & Cold Liquid .... ▣ 752
Singlet Caplets .... ▣ 636
Sudafed Sinus & Allergy Tablets ..... ▣ 710
TheraFlu Cold & Cough Hot Liquid .... ▣ 680
TheraFlu Cold & Sore Throat Hot Liquid .... ▣ 680
TheraFlu Flu & Sore Throat Hot Liquid .... ▣ 681
TheraFlu Severe Cold & Cough Hot Liquid .... ▣ 683
TheraFlu Severe Cold Caplets .... ▣ 679
TheraFlu Severe Cold Hot Liquid .... ▣ 682
Triaminic Cold & Allergy Liquid ...... ▣ 685
Triaminic Cold & Cough Liquid .... ▣ 685
Triaminic Flu, Cough & Fever Liquid .... ▣ 685
Triaminic Night Time Cough & Cold Liquid .... ▣ 685
Triaminic Allergy Runny Nose & Congestion Softchews .... ▣ 688
Triaminic Cold & Cough Softchews .... ▣ 688
Children's Tylenol Plus Cold NightTime Suspension Liquid 1851
Children's Tylenol Plus Cold & Cough Suspension Liquid and Chewable Tablets 1851
Children's Tylenol Plus Cold Chewable Tablets 1851
Children's Tylenol Plus Flu Suspension Liquid 1853
Tylenol Allergy Complete Multi-Symptom Caplets and Gelcaps with Cool Burst 1844
Multi-Symptom Tylenol Cold Night Time Caplets 1845
Vicks 44M Cough, Cold & Flu Relief 2676
Pediatric Vicks 44m Cough & Cold Relief 2673
Children's Vicks NyQuil Cold/Cough Relief 2671

Chlorpheniramine Polistirex (May exhibit an additive CNS depression). Products include:
Tussionex Pennkinetic Extended-Release Suspension 3322

Chlorpheniramine Tannate (May exhibit an additive CNS depression).
No products indexed under this heading.

Chlorpromazine (May exhibit an additive CNS depression).
No products indexed under this heading.

Chlorpromazine Hydrochloride (May exhibit an additive CNS depression).
No products indexed under this heading.

Chlorprothixene (May exhibit an additive CNS depression).
No products indexed under this heading.

Chlorprothixene Hydrochloride (May exhibit an additive CNS depression).
No products indexed under this heading.

Chlorprothixene Lactate (May exhibit an additive CNS depression).
No products indexed under this heading.

Clemastine Fumarate (May exhibit an additive CNS depression).
No products indexed under this heading.

Clomipramine Hydrochloride (Co-administration may increase the effect of either antidepressant or hydrocodone).
No products indexed under this heading.

Clorazepate Dipotassium (May exhibit an additive CNS depression). Products include:
Tranxene 2488

Clozapine (May exhibit an additive CNS depression). Products include:
Clozapine Tablets 2141
Clozaril Tablets 2174
FazaClo Orally Disintegrating Tablets 547

Codeine Phosphate (May exhibit an additive CNS depression). Products include:
Tylenol with Codeine 2461

Cyproheptadine Hydrochloride (May exhibit an additive CNS depression).
No products indexed under this heading.

Desflurane (May exhibit an additive CNS depression). Products include:
Suprane Liquid for Inhalation 770

Desipramine Hydrochloride (Co-administration may increase the effect of either antidepressant or hydrocodone).
No products indexed under this heading.

Dexchlorpheniramine Maleate (May exhibit an additive CNS depression).
No products indexed under this heading.

Dezocine (May exhibit an additive CNS depression).
No products indexed under this heading.

Diazepam (May exhibit an additive CNS depression). Products include:
Diastat Rectal Delivery System 3344
Valium Tablets 2822

Diphenhydramine Citrate (May exhibit an additive CNS depression). Products include:
Children's Benadryl Allergy & Cold Fastmelt Tablets .... ▣ 695
Children's Benadryl D Allergy & Sinus Fastmelt Tablets .... ▣ 694
Children's Benadryl Allergy Fastmelt Tablets .... ▣ 696
Goody's PM Powder .... ▣ 622

Diphenhydramine Hydrochloride (May exhibit an additive CNS depression). Products include:
Benadryl Allergy & Cold Tablets ..... ▣ 692
Benadryl Allergy .... ▣ 691
Benadryl Allergy & Sinus Headache Caplets & Gelcaps ...... ▣ 693
Children's Benadryl Allergy Liquid ... ▣ 695
Children's Benadryl Dye-Free Allergy Liquid .... ▣ 695
Benadryl Dye-Free Allergy Liqui-Gels Softgels .... ▣ 692
Benadryl Itch Relief Stick Extra Strength .... ▣ 696
Benadryl Itch Stopping Cream Extra Strength .... ▣ 697
Benadryl Itch Stopping Gel Extra Strength .... ▣ 697
Benadryl Itch Stopping Spray Extra Strength .... ▣ 697
Benadryl Maximum Strength Severe Allergy & Sinus Headache Caplets .... ▣ 694
Children's Benadryl D Liquid Medication .... ▣ 693
Benadryl D Tablets .... ▣ 694
Nytol QuickCaps Caplets .... ▣ 635
Maximum Strength Nytol QuickGels Softgels .... ▣ 635
Simply Sleep Caplets 1841
Sominex Original Formula Tablets .. ▣ 637
TheraFlu Thin Strips Multi Symptom .... ▣ 684
Triaminic Thin Strips Cough & Runny Nose .... ▣ 690
Children's Tylenol Plus Cold & Allergy Suspension Liquid 1850
Tylenol Allergy Complete Night Time Caplets 1844
Tylenol Severe Allergy Caplets 1844
Tylenol Flu NightTime Gelcaps 1846
Extra Strength Tylenol PM Caplets, Geltabs, Gelcaps and Liquid 1847
Unisom Maximum Strength SleepGels .... ▣ 712

Diphenylpyraline Hydrochloride (May exhibit an additive CNS depression).
No products indexed under this heading.

Doxepin Hydrochloride (Co-administration may increase the effect of either antidepressant or hydrocodone).
No products indexed under this heading.

Droperidol (May exhibit an additive CNS depression).
No products indexed under this heading.

Enflurane (May exhibit an additive CNS depression).
No products indexed under this heading.

Estazolam (May exhibit an additive CNS depression). Products include:
ProSom Tablets 512

Ethanol (May exhibit an additive CNS depression).
No products indexed under this heading.

Ethchlorvynol (May exhibit an additive CNS depression).
No products indexed under this heading.

Ethinamate (May exhibit an additive CNS depression).
No products indexed under this heading.

Ethyl Alcohol (May exhibit an additive CNS depression).
No products indexed under this heading.

Fentanyl (May exhibit an additive CNS depression). Products include:
Duragesic Transdermal System **2448**

Fentanyl Citrate (May exhibit an additive CNS depression). Products include:
Actiq **993**

Fexofenadine Hydrochloride (May exhibit an additive CNS depression). Products include:
Allegra **2857**
Allegra-D 12 Hour Extended-Release Tablets **2860**
Allegra-D 24 Hour Extended-Release Tablets **2862**

Fluphenazine Decanoate (May exhibit an additive CNS depression).
No products indexed under this heading.

Fluphenazine Enanthate (May exhibit an additive CNS depression).
No products indexed under this heading.

Fluphenazine Hydrochloride (May exhibit an additive CNS depression).
No products indexed under this heading.

Flurazepam Hydrochloride (May exhibit an additive CNS depression). Products include:
Dalmane Capsules **3343**

Glutethimide (May exhibit an additive CNS depression).
No products indexed under this heading.

Haloperidol (May exhibit an additive CNS depression).
No products indexed under this heading.

Haloperidol Decanoate (May exhibit an additive CNS depression).
No products indexed under this heading.

Hydrocodone Polistirex (May exhibit an additive CNS depression). Products include:
Tussionex Pennkinetic Extended-Release Suspension **3322**

Hydromorphone Hydrochloride (May exhibit an additive CNS depression). Products include:
Dilaudid **439**
Dilaudid Oral Liquid **443**
Dilaudid Non-Sterile Powder **439**
Dilaudid Rectal Suppositories **439**
Dilaudid Tablets **439**
Dilaudid Tablets - 8 mg **443**
Dilaudid-HP **441**

Hydroxyzine Hydrochloride (May exhibit an additive CNS depression).
No products indexed under this heading.

Imipramine Hydrochloride (Co-administration may increase the effect of either antidepressant or hydrocodone).
No products indexed under this heading.

Imipramine Pamoate (Co-administration may increase the effect of either antidepressant or hydrocodone).
No products indexed under this heading.

Isocarboxazid (Co-administration may increase the effect of either the MAO inhibitor or hydrocodone).
No products indexed under this heading.

Isoflurane (May exhibit an additive CNS depression).
No products indexed under this heading.

Ketamine Hydrochloride (May exhibit an additive CNS depression).
No products indexed under this heading.

Levomethadyl Acetate Hydrochloride (May exhibit an additive CNS depression).
No products indexed under this heading.

Levorphanol Tartrate (May exhibit an additive CNS depression).
No products indexed under this heading.

Loratadine (May exhibit an additive CNS depression). Products include:
Alavert Allergy & Sinus D-12 Hour Tablets **743**
Alavert **743**
Children's Claritin 24 Hour Non-Drowsy Allergy Syrup **732**
Claritin Non-Drowsy 24 Hour Tablets **731**
Non-Drowsy Claritin Hives Relief Tablets **733**
Claritin Reditabs 24 Hour Non-Drowsy Tablets **732**
Claritin-D Non-Drowsy 12 Hour Tablets **731**
Claritin-D Non-Drowsy 24 Hour Tablets **731**
Children's Dimetapp ND Non-Drowsy Allergy Syrup **746**
Triaminic Allerchews **684**

Lorazepam (May exhibit an additive CNS depression).
No products indexed under this heading.

Loxapine Hydrochloride (May exhibit an additive CNS depression).
No products indexed under this heading.

Loxapine Succinate (May exhibit an additive CNS depression).
No products indexed under this heading.

Maprotiline Hydrochloride (Co-administration may increase the effect of either antidepressant or hydrocodone).
No products indexed under this heading.

Meperidine Hydrochloride (May exhibit an additive CNS depression).
No products indexed under this heading.

Mephobarbital (May exhibit an additive CNS depression). Products include:
Mebaral Tablets, USP **2483**

Meprobamate (May exhibit an additive CNS depression).
No products indexed under this heading.

Mesoridazine Besylate (May exhibit an additive CNS depression).
No products indexed under this heading.

Methadone Hydrochloride (May exhibit an additive CNS depression).
No products indexed under this heading.

Methdilazine Hydrochloride (May exhibit an additive CNS depression).
No products indexed under this heading.

Methohexital Sodium (May exhibit an additive CNS depression).
No products indexed under this heading.

Methotrimeprazine (May exhibit an additive CNS depression).
No products indexed under this heading.

Methoxyflurane (May exhibit an additive CNS depression).
No products indexed under this heading.

Midazolam Hydrochloride (May exhibit an additive CNS depression).
No products indexed under this heading.

Moclobemide (Co-administration may increase the effect of either the MAO inhibitor or hydrocodone).
No products indexed under this heading.

Molindone Hydrochloride (May exhibit an additive CNS depression). Products include:
Moban Tablets **1108**

Morphine Sulfate (May exhibit an additive CNS depression). Products include:
Avinza Capsules **1714**
Kadian Capsules **572**
MS Contin Tablets **2703**

Nortriptyline Hydrochloride (Co-administration may increase the effect of either antidepressant or hydrocodone).
No products indexed under this heading.

Olanzapine (May exhibit an additive CNS depression). Products include:
Symbyax Capsules **1788**
Zyprexa Tablets **1798**
Zyprexa IntraMuscular **1798**
Zyprexa ZYDIS Orally Disintegrating Tablets **1798**

Oxazepam (May exhibit an additive CNS depression).
No products indexed under this heading.

Oxycodone Hydrochloride (May exhibit an additive CNS depression). Products include:
Combunox Tablets **1183**
OxyContin Tablets **2699**
OxyFast Oral Concentrate Solution **2704**
OxyIR Capsules **2704**
Percocet Tablets **1114**
Percodan Tablets **1115**

Pargyline Hydrochloride (Co-administration may increase the effect of either the MAO inhibitor or hydrocodone).
No products indexed under this heading.

Pentobarbital Sodium (May exhibit an additive CNS depression). Products include:
Nembutal Sodium Solution, USP **2484**

Perphenazine (May exhibit an additive CNS depression).
No products indexed under this heading.

Phenelzine Sulfate (Co-administration may increase the effect of either the MAO inhibitor or hydrocodone).
No products indexed under this heading.

Phenobarbital (May exhibit an additive CNS depression).
No products indexed under this heading.

Prazepam (May exhibit an additive CNS depression).
No products indexed under this heading.

Procarbazine Hydrochloride (Co-administration may increase the effect of either the MAO inhibitor or hydrocodone). Products include:
Matulane Capsules **3188**

Prochlorperazine (May exhibit an additive CNS depression).
No products indexed under this heading.

Promethazine Hydrochloride (May exhibit an additive CNS depression). Products include:
Phenergan **3438**

Propofol (May exhibit an additive CNS depression). Products include:
Diprivan Injectable Emulsion **676**

Propoxyphene Hydrochloride (May exhibit an additive CNS depression).
No products indexed under this heading.

Propoxyphene Napsylate (May exhibit an additive CNS depression). Products include:
Darvocet A 500 Tablets **3497**

Protriptyline Hydrochloride (Co-administration may increase the effect of either antidepressant or hydrocodone). Products include:
Vivactil Tablets **2350**

Pyrilamine Maleate (May exhibit an additive CNS depression).
No products indexed under this heading.

Pyrilamine Tannate (May exhibit an additive CNS depression).
No products indexed under this heading.

Quazepam (May exhibit an additive CNS depression).
No products indexed under this heading.

Quetiapine Fumarate (May exhibit an additive CNS depression). Products include:
Seroquel Tablets **691**

Remifentanil Hydrochloride (May exhibit an additive CNS depression).
No products indexed under this heading.

Risperidone (May exhibit an additive CNS depression). Products include:
Risperdal Consta Long-Acting Injection **1664**
Risperdal M-Tab Orally Disintegrating Tablets **1658**
Risperdal **1658**

Secobarbital Sodium (May exhibit an additive CNS depression).
No products indexed under this heading.

Selegiline Hydrochloride (Co-administration may increase the effect of either the MAO inhibitor or hydrocodone). Products include:
Eldepryl Capsules **3209**

Sevoflurane (May exhibit an additive CNS depression). Products include:
Ultane Liquid for Inhalation **526**

Sufentanil Citrate (May exhibit an additive CNS depression).
No products indexed under this heading.

Temazepam (May exhibit an additive CNS depression).
No products indexed under this heading.

IMPORTANT NOTE: Always consult each drug listing in the patient's regimen for possible interactions.

Terfenadine (May exhibit an additive CNS depression).
No products indexed under this heading.

Thiamylal Sodium (May exhibit an additive CNS depression).
No products indexed under this heading.

Thioridazine Hydrochloride (May exhibit an additive CNS depression). Products include:
Thioridazine Hydrochloride Tablets 2122

Thiothixene (May exhibit an additive CNS depression). Products include:
Thiothixene Capsules 2124

Tranylcypromine Sulfate (Co-administration may increase the effect of either the MAO inhibitor or hydrocodone). Products include:
Parnate Tablets 1499

Triazolam (May exhibit an additive CNS depression).
No products indexed under this heading.

Trifluoperazine Hydrochloride (May exhibit an additive CNS depression).
No products indexed under this heading.

Trimeprazine Tartrate (May exhibit an additive CNS depression).
No products indexed under this heading.

Trimipramine Maleate (Co-administration may increase the effect of either antidepressant or hydrocodone). Products include:
Surmontil Capsules 2347

Tripelennamine Hydrochloride (May exhibit an additive CNS depression).
No products indexed under this heading.

Triprolidine Hydrochloride (May exhibit an additive CNS depression).
No products indexed under this heading.

Zaleplon (May exhibit an additive CNS depression). Products include:
Sonata Capsules 1686

Ziprasidone Hydrochloride (May exhibit an additive CNS depression). Products include:
Geodon Capsules 2514

Zolpidem Tartrate (May exhibit an additive CNS depression). Products include:
Ambien Tablets 2867

Food Interactions

Alcohol (May exhibit an additive CNS depression).

VICODIN ES TABLETS

(Acetaminophen, Hydrocodone Bitartrate) 531

May interact with anticholinergics, central nervous system depressants, narcotic analgesics, psychotropics, tranquilizers, tricyclic antidepressants, and certain other agents. Compounds in these categories include:

Alfentanil Hydrochloride (Additive CNS depression; the dose of one or both agents should be reduced).
No products indexed under this heading.

Alprazolam (Additive CNS depression; the dose of one or both agents should be reduced). Products include:
Niravam Orally Disintegrating Tablets 3106
Xanax XR Tablets 2655

Amitriptyline Hydrochloride (Concurrent use of tricyclic antidepressants and hydrocodone preparations may increase the effect of either the antidepressant or hydrocodone).
No products indexed under this heading.

Amoxapine (Concurrent use of tricyclic antidepressants and hydrocodone preparations may increase the effect of either the antidepressant or hydrocodone).
No products indexed under this heading.

Aprobarbital (Additive CNS depression; the dose of one or both agents should be reduced).
No products indexed under this heading.

Atropine Sulfate (May produce paralytic ileus).
No products indexed under this heading.

Belladonna Alkaloids (May produce paralytic ileus). Products include:
Hyland's Teething Tablets .... ▣ 736

Benztropine Mesylate (May produce paralytic ileus). Products include:
Cogentin Injection 1903

Biperiden Hydrochloride (May produce paralytic ileus).
No products indexed under this heading.

Buprenorphine Hydrochloride (Additive CNS depression; the dose of one or both agents should be reduced). Products include:
Buprenex Injectable 2718
Suboxone Tablets 2719
Subutex Tablets 2719

Buspirone Hydrochloride (Additive CNS depression; the dose of one or both agents should be reduced).
No products indexed under this heading.

Butabarbital (Additive CNS depression; the dose of one or both agents should be reduced).
No products indexed under this heading.

Butalbital (Additive CNS depression; the dose of one or both agents should be reduced). Products include:
Sedapap Tablets 50 mg/650 mg 2098

Chlordiazepoxide (Additive CNS depression; the dose of one or both agents should be reduced).
No products indexed under this heading.

Chlordiazepoxide Hydrochloride (Additive CNS depression; the dose of one or both agents should be reduced). Products include:
Librium Capsules 3349

Chlorpromazine (Additive CNS depression; the dose of one or both agents should be reduced).
No products indexed under this heading.

Chlorpromazine Hydrochloride (Additive CNS depression; the dose of one or both agents should be reduced).
No products indexed under this heading.

Chlorprothixene (Additive CNS depression; the dose of one or both agents should be reduced).
No products indexed under this heading.

Chlorprothixene Hydrochloride (Additive CNS depression; the dose of one or both agents should be reduced).
No products indexed under this heading.

Chlorprothixene Lactate (Additive CNS depression; the dose of one or both agents should be reduced).
No products indexed under this heading.

Clidinium Bromide (May produce paralytic ileus).
No products indexed under this heading.

Clomipramine Hydrochloride (Concurrent use of tricyclic antidepressants and hydrocodone preparations may increase the effect of either the antidepressant or hydrocodone).
No products indexed under this heading.

Clorazepate Dipotassium (Additive CNS depression; the dose of one or both agents should be reduced). Products include:
Tranxene 2488

Clozapine (Additive CNS depression; the dose of one or both agents should be reduced). Products include:
Clozapine Tablets 2141
Clozaril Tablets 2174
FazaClo Orally Disintegrating Tablets 547

Codeine Phosphate (Additive CNS depression; the dose of one or both agents should be reduced). Products include:
Tylenol with Codeine 2461

Desflurane (Additive CNS depression; the dose of one or both agents should be reduced). Products include:
Suprane Liquid for Inhalation 770

Desipramine Hydrochloride (Concurrent use of tricyclic antidepressants and hydrocodone preparations may increase the effect of either the antidepressant or hydrocodone).
No products indexed under this heading.

Dezocine (Additive CNS depression; the dose of one or both agents should be reduced).
No products indexed under this heading.

Diazepam (Additive CNS depression; the dose of one or both agents should be reduced). Products include:
Diastat Rectal Delivery System 3344
Valium Tablets 2822

Dicyclomine Hydrochloride (May produce paralytic ileus). Products include:
Bentyl Capsules 724
Bentyl Injection 724
Bentyl Syrup 724
Bentyl Tablets 724

Doxepin Hydrochloride (Concurrent use of tricyclic antidepressants and hydrocodone preparations may increase the effect of either the antidepressant or hydrocodone).
No products indexed under this heading.

Droperidol (Additive CNS depression; the dose of one or both agents should be reduced).
No products indexed under this heading.

Enflurane (Additive CNS depression; the dose of one or both agents should be reduced).
No products indexed under this heading.

Estazolam (Additive CNS depression; the dose of one or both agents should be reduced). Products include:
ProSom Tablets 512

Ethanol (Additive CNS depression; the dose of one or both agents should be reduced).
No products indexed under this heading.

Ethchlorvynol (Additive CNS depression; the dose of one or both agents should be reduced).
No products indexed under this heading.

Ethinamate (Additive CNS depression; the dose of one or both agents should be reduced).
No products indexed under this heading.

Ethyl Alcohol (Additive CNS depression; the dose of one or both agents should be reduced).
No products indexed under this heading.

Fentanyl (Additive CNS depression; the dose of one or both agents should be reduced). Products include:
Duragesic Transdermal System 2448

Fentanyl Citrate (Additive CNS depression; the dose of one or both agents should be reduced). Products include:
Actiq 993

Fluphenazine Decanoate (Additive CNS depression; the dose of one or both agents should be reduced).
No products indexed under this heading.

Fluphenazine Enanthate (Additive CNS depression; the dose of one or both agents should be reduced).
No products indexed under this heading.

Fluphenazine Hydrochloride (Additive CNS depression; the dose of one or both agents should be reduced).
No products indexed under this heading.

Flurazepam Hydrochloride (Additive CNS depression; the dose of one or both agents should be reduced). Products include:
Dalmane Capsules 3343

Glutethimide (Additive CNS depression; the dose of one or both agents should be reduced).
No products indexed under this heading.

Glycopyrrolate (May produce paralytic ileus).
No products indexed under this heading.

Haloperidol (Additive CNS depression; the dose of one or both agents should be reduced).
No products indexed under this heading.

Haloperidol Decanoate (Additive CNS depression; the dose of one or both agents should be reduced).
No products indexed under this heading.

Hydrocodone Polistirex (Additive CNS depression; the dose of one or both agents should be reduced). Products include:

Tussionex Pennkinetic Extended-Release Suspension **3322**

Hydromorphone Hydrochloride (Additive CNS depression; the dose of one or both agents should be reduced). Products include:

Dilaudid **439**
Dilaudid Oral Liquid **443**
Dilaudid Non-Sterile Powder **439**
Dilaudid Rectal Suppositories **439**
Dilaudid Tablets **439**
Dilaudid Tablets - 8 mg **443**
Dilaudid-HP **441**

Hydroxyzine Hydrochloride (Additive CNS depression; the dose of one or both agents should be reduced).
No products indexed under this heading.

Hyoscyamine (May produce paralytic ileus).
No products indexed under this heading.

Hyoscyamine Sulfate (May produce paralytic ileus).
No products indexed under this heading.

Imipramine Hydrochloride (Concurrent use of tricyclic antidepressants and hydrocodone preparations may increase the effect of either the antidepressant or hydrocodone).
No products indexed under this heading.

Imipramine Pamoate (Concurrent use of tricyclic antidepressants and hydrocodone preparations may increase the effect of either the antidepressant or hydrocodone).
No products indexed under this heading.

Ipratropium Bromide (May produce paralytic ileus). Products include:

Atrovent HFA Inhalation Aerosol **872**
Atrovent Inhalation Solution **868**
Atrovent Nasal Spray 0.03% **869**
Atrovent Nasal Spray 0.06% **870**
Combivent Inhalation Aerosol **878**
DuoNeb Inhalation Solution **1058**

Isocarboxazid (Concurrent use of MAO inhibitor and hydrocodone preparations may increase the effect of either the MAO inhibitor or hydrocodone).
No products indexed under this heading.

Isoflurane (Additive CNS depression; the dose of one or both agents should be reduced).
No products indexed under this heading.

Ketamine Hydrochloride (Additive CNS depression; the dose of one or both agents should be reduced).
No products indexed under this heading.

Levomethadyl Acetate Hydrochloride (Additive CNS depression; the dose of one or both agents should be reduced).
No products indexed under this heading.

Levorphanol Tartrate (Additive CNS depression; the dose of one or both agents should be reduced).
No products indexed under this heading.

Lithium Carbonate (Additive CNS depression; the dose of one or both agents should be reduced). Products include:

Eskalith **1406**
Lithobid Tablets **1670**

Lithium Citrate (Additive CNS depression; the dose of one or both agents should be reduced).
No products indexed under this heading.

Lorazepam (Additive CNS depression; the dose of one or both agents should be reduced).
No products indexed under this heading.

Loxapine Hydrochloride (Additive CNS depression; the dose of one or both agents should be reduced).
No products indexed under this heading.

Loxapine Succinate (Additive CNS depression; the dose of one or both agents should be reduced).
No products indexed under this heading.

Maprotiline Hydrochloride (Concurrent use of tricyclic antidepressants and hydrocodone preparations may increase the effect of either the antidepressant or hydrocodone).
No products indexed under this heading.

Mepenzolate Bromide (May produce paralytic ileus).
No products indexed under this heading.

Meperidine Hydrochloride (Additive CNS depression; the dose of one or both agents should be reduced).
No products indexed under this heading.

Mephobarbital (Additive CNS depression; the dose of one or both agents should be reduced). Products include:

Mebaral Tablets, USP **2483**

Meprobamate (Additive CNS depression; the dose of one or both agents should be reduced).
No products indexed under this heading.

Mesoridazine Besylate (Additive CNS depression; the dose of one or both agents should be reduced).
No products indexed under this heading.

Methadone Hydrochloride (Additive CNS depression; the dose of one or both agents should be reduced).
No products indexed under this heading.

Methohexital Sodium (Additive CNS depression; the dose of one or both agents should be reduced).
No products indexed under this heading.

Methotrimeprazine (Additive CNS depression; the dose of one or both agents should be reduced).
No products indexed under this heading.

Methoxyflurane (Additive CNS depression; the dose of one or both agents should be reduced).
No products indexed under this heading.

Midazolam Hydrochloride (Additive CNS depression; the dose of one or both agents should be reduced).
No products indexed under this heading.

Molindone Hydrochloride (Additive CNS depression; the dose of one or both agents should be reduced). Products include:

Moban Tablets **1108**

Morphine Sulfate (Additive CNS depression; the dose of one or both agents should be reduced). Products include:

Avinza Capsules **1714**
Kadian Capsules **572**
MS Contin Tablets **2703**

Nortriptyline Hydrochloride (Concurrent use of tricyclic antidepressants and hydrocodone preparations may increase the effect of either the antidepressant or hydrocodone).
No products indexed under this heading.

Olanzapine (Additive CNS depression; the dose of one or both agents should be reduced). Products include:

Symbyax Capsules **1788**
Zyprexa Tablets **1798**
Zyprexa IntraMuscular **1798**
Zyprexa ZYDIS Orally Disintegrating Tablets **1798**

Oxazepam (Additive CNS depression; the dose of one or both agents should be reduced).
No products indexed under this heading.

Oxybutynin Chloride (May produce paralytic ileus). Products include:

Ditropan XL Extended Release Tablets **2391**

Oxycodone Hydrochloride (Additive CNS depression; the dose of one or both agents should be reduced). Products include:

Combunox Tablets **1183**
OxyContin Tablets **2699**
OxyFast Oral Concentrate Solution **2704**
OxyIR Capsules **2704**
Percocet Tablets **1114**
Percodan Tablets **1115**

Pentobarbital Sodium (Additive CNS depression; the dose of one or both agents should be reduced). Products include:

Nembutal Sodium Solution, USP **2484**

Perphenazine (Additive CNS depression; the dose of one or both agents should be reduced).
No products indexed under this heading.

Phenelzine Sulfate (Concurrent use of MAO inhibitor and hydrocodone preparations may increase the effect of either the MAO inhibitor or hydrocodone).
No products indexed under this heading.

Phenobarbital (Additive CNS depression; the dose of one or both agents should be reduced).
No products indexed under this heading.

Prazepam (Additive CNS depression; the dose of one or both agents should be reduced).
No products indexed under this heading.

Prochlorperazine (Additive CNS depression; the dose of one or both agents should be reduced).
No products indexed under this heading.

Procyclidine Hydrochloride (May produce paralytic ileus).
No products indexed under this heading.

Promethazine Hydrochloride (Additive CNS depression; the dose of one or both agents should be reduced). Products include:

Phenergan **3438**

Propantheline Bromide (May produce paralytic ileus).
No products indexed under this heading.

Propofol (Additive CNS depression; the dose of one or both agents should be reduced). Products include:

Diprivan Injectable Emulsion **676**

Propoxyphene Hydrochloride (Additive CNS depression; the dose of one or both agents should be reduced).
No products indexed under this heading.

Propoxyphene Napsylate (Additive CNS depression; the dose of one or both agents should be reduced). Products include:

Darvocet A 500 Tablets **3497**

Protriptyline Hydrochloride (Concurrent use of tricyclic antidepressants and hydrocodone preparations may increase the effect of either the antidepressant or hydrocodone). Products include:

Vivactil Tablets **2350**

Quazepam (Additive CNS depression; the dose of one or both agents should be reduced).
No products indexed under this heading.

Quetiapine Fumarate (Additive CNS depression; the dose of one or both agents should be reduced). Products include:

Seroquel Tablets **691**

Remifentanil Hydrochloride (Additive CNS depression; the dose of one or both agents should be reduced).
No products indexed under this heading.

Risperidone (Additive CNS depression; the dose of one or both agents should be reduced). Products include:

Risperdal Consta Long-Acting Injection **1664**
Risperdal M-Tab Orally Disintegrating Tablets **1658**
Risperdal **1658**

Scopolamine (May produce paralytic ileus). Products include:

Transderm Scōp Transdermal Therapeutic System **2166**

Scopolamine Hydrobromide (May produce paralytic ileus).
No products indexed under this heading.

Secobarbital Sodium (Additive CNS depression; the dose of one or both agents should be reduced).
No products indexed under this heading.

Selegiline Hydrochloride (Concurrent use of MAO inhibitor and hydrocodone preparations may increase the effect of either the MAO inhibitor or hydrocodone). Products include:

Eldepryl Capsules **3209**

Sevoflurane (Additive CNS depression; the dose of one or both agents should be reduced). Products include:

Ultane Liquid for Inhalation **526**

Sufentanil Citrate (Additive CNS depression; the dose of one or both agents should be reduced).
No products indexed under this heading.

Temazepam (Additive CNS depression; the dose of one or both agents should be reduced).
No products indexed under this heading.

Thiamylal Sodium (Additive CNS depression; the dose of one or both agents should be reduced).
No products indexed under this heading.

Thioridazine Hydrochloride (Additive CNS depression; the dose of one or both agents should be reduced). Products include:
Thioridazine Hydrochloride Tablets 2122

Thiothixene (Additive CNS depression; the dose of one or both agents should be reduced). Products include:
Thiothixene Capsules 2124

Tolterodine Tartrate (May produce paralytic ileus). Products include:
Detrol Tablets 2626
Detrol LA Capsules 2629

Tranylcypromine Sulfate (Concurrent use of MAO inhibitor and hydrocodone preparations may increase the effect of either the MAO inhibitor or hydrocodone). Products include:
Parnate Tablets 1499

Triazolam (Additive CNS depression; the dose of one or both agents should be reduced).
No products indexed under this heading.

Tridihexethyl Chloride (May produce paralytic ileus).
No products indexed under this heading.

Trifluoperazine Hydrochloride (Additive CNS depression; the dose of one or both agents should be reduced).
No products indexed under this heading.

Trihexyphenidyl Hydrochloride (May produce paralytic ileus).
No products indexed under this heading.

Trimipramine Maleate (Concurrent use of tricyclic antidepressants and hydrocodone preparations may increase the effect of either the antidepressant or hydrocodone). Products include:
Surmontil Capsules 2347

Zaleplon (Additive CNS depression; the dose of one or both agents should be reduced). Products include:
Sonata Capsules 1686

Ziprasidone Hydrochloride (Additive CNS depression; the dose of one or both agents should be reduced). Products include:
Geodon Capsules 2514

Zolpidem Tartrate (Additive CNS depression; the dose of one or both agents should be reduced). Products include:
Ambien Tablets 2867

Food Interactions

Alcohol (Additive CNS depression).

VICODIN HP TABLETS

(Acetaminophen, Hydrocodone Bitartrate) 532

May interact with antihistamines, central nervous system depressants, monoamine oxidase inhibitors, narcotic analgesics, tranquilizers, tricyclic antidepressants, and certain other agents. Compounds in these categories include:

Acrivastine (Co-administration may result in an additive CNS depression).
No products indexed under this heading.

Alfentanil Hydrochloride (Co-administration may result in an additive CNS depression).
No products indexed under this heading.

Alprazolam (Co-administration may result in an additive CNS depression). Products include:
Niravam Orally Disintegrating Tablets 3106
Xanax XR Tablets 2655

Amitriptyline Hydrochloride (Co-administration with tricyclic antidepressants may increase the effect of either hydrocodone or the tricyclic antidepressant).
No products indexed under this heading.

Amoxapine (Co-administration with tricyclic antidepressants may increase the effect of either hydrocodone or the tricyclic antidepressant).
No products indexed under this heading.

Aprobarbital (Co-administration may result in an additive CNS depression).
No products indexed under this heading.

Astemizole (Co-administration may result in an additive CNS depression).
No products indexed under this heading.

Azatadine Maleate (Co-administration may result in an additive CNS depression).
No products indexed under this heading.

Bromodiphenhydramine Hydrochloride (Co-administration may result in an additive CNS depression).
No products indexed under this heading.

Brompheniramine Maleate (Co-administration may result in an additive CNS depression). Products include:
Alacol DM Syrup 739
Children's Dimetapp Cold & Allergy Elixir .... ▣745
Children's Dimetapp DM Cold & Cough Elixir .... ▣745
Robitussin Allergy & Cough Syrup .. ▣750

Buprenorphine Hydrochloride (Co-administration may result in an additive CNS depression). Products include:
Buprenex Injectable 2718
Suboxone Tablets 2719
Subutex Tablets 2719

Buspirone Hydrochloride (Co-administration may result in an additive CNS depression).
No products indexed under this heading.

Butabarbital (Co-administration may result in an additive CNS depression).
No products indexed under this heading.

Butalbital (Co-administration may result in an additive CNS depression). Products include:
Sedapap Tablets 50 mg/650 mg 2098

Cetirizine Hydrochloride (Co-administration may result in an additive CNS depression). Products include:
Zyrtec Chewable Tablets 2589
Zyrtec 2589
Zyrtec-D 12 Hour Extended Release Tablets 2591

Chlordiazepoxide (Co-administration may result in an additive CNS depression).
No products indexed under this heading.

Chlordiazepoxide Hydrochloride (Co-administration may result in an additive CNS depression). Products include:
Librium Capsules 3349

Chlorpheniramine Maleate (Co-administration may result in an additive CNS depression). Products include:
Advil Allergy Sinus Caplets .... ▣737
Advil Multi-Symptom Cold Caplets .... ▣738
BC Allergy Sinus Cold Powder .... ▣612
Contac Severe Cold and Flu Caplets Maximum Strength .... ▣615
Hycomine Compound Tablets 1105
PediaCare Multi-Symptom Cold Liquid .... ▣704
PediaCare NightRest Cough & Cold Liquid .... ▣704
Robitussin Flu Liquid .... ▣752
Robitussin PM Cough & Cold Liquid .... ▣752
Singlet Caplets .... ▣636
Sudafed Sinus & Allergy Tablets .... ▣710
TheraFlu Cold & Cough Hot Liquid .... ▣680
TheraFlu Cold & Sore Throat Hot Liquid .... ▣680
TheraFlu Flu & Sore Throat Hot Liquid .... ▣681
TheraFlu Severe Cold & Cough Hot Liquid .... ▣683
TheraFlu Severe Cold Caplets .... ▣679
TheraFlu Severe Cold Hot Liquid .... ▣682
Triaminic Cold & Allergy Liquid .... ▣685
Triaminic Cold & Cough Liquid .... ▣685
Triaminic Flu, Cough & Fever Liquid .... ▣685
Triaminic Night Time Cough & Cold Liquid .... ▣685
Triaminic Allergy Runny Nose & Congestion Softchews .... ▣688
Triaminic Cold & Cough Softchews .... ▣688
Children's Tylenol Plus Cold NightTime Suspension Liquid 1851
Children's Tylenol Plus Cold & Cough Suspension Liquid and Chewable Tablets 1851
Children's Tylenol Plus Cold Chewable Tablets 1851
Children's Tylenol Plus Flu Suspension Liquid 1853
Tylenol Allergy Complete Multi-Symptom Caplets and Gelcaps with Cool Burst 1844
Multi-Symptom Tylenol Cold Night Time Caplets 1845
Vicks 44M Cough, Cold & Flu Relief 2676
Pediatric Vicks 44m Cough & Cold Relief 2673
Children's Vicks NyQuil Cold/Cough Relief 2671

Chlorpheniramine Polistirex (Co-administration may result in an additive CNS depression). Products include:
Tussionex Pennkinetic Extended-Release Suspension 3322

Chlorpheniramine Tannate (Co-administration may result in an additive CNS depression).
No products indexed under this heading.

Chlorpromazine (Co-administration may result in an additive CNS depression).
No products indexed under this heading.

Chlorpromazine Hydrochloride (Co-administration may result in an additive CNS depression).
No products indexed under this heading.

Chlorprothixene (Co-administration may result in an additive CNS depression).
No products indexed under this heading.

Chlorprothixene Hydrochloride (Co-administration may result in an additive CNS depression).
No products indexed under this heading.

Chlorprothixene Lactate (Co-administration may result in an additive CNS depression).
No products indexed under this heading.

Clemastine Fumarate (Co-administration may result in an additive CNS depression).
No products indexed under this heading.

Clomipramine Hydrochloride (Co-administration with tricyclic antidepressants may increase the effect of either hydrocodone or the tricyclic antidepressant).
No products indexed under this heading.

Clorazepate Dipotassium (Co-administration may result in an additive CNS depression). Products include:
Tranxene 2488

Clozapine (Co-administration may result in an additive CNS depression). Products include:
Clozapine Tablets 2141
Clozaril Tablets 2174
FazaClo Orally Disintegrating Tablets 547

Codeine Phosphate (Co-administration may result in an additive CNS depression). Products include:
Tylenol with Codeine 2461

Cyproheptadine Hydrochloride (Co-administration may result in an additive CNS depression).
No products indexed under this heading.

Desflurane (Co-administration may result in an additive CNS depression). Products include:
Suprane Liquid for Inhalation 770

Desipramine Hydrochloride (Co-administration with tricyclic antidepressants may increase the effect of either hydrocodone or the tricyclic antidepressant).
No products indexed under this heading.

Dexchlorpheniramine Maleate (Co-administration may result in an additive CNS depression).
No products indexed under this heading.

Dezocine (Co-administration may result in an additive CNS depression).
No products indexed under this heading.

Diazepam (Co-administration may result in an additive CNS depression). Products include:
Diastat Rectal Delivery System 3344
Valium Tablets 2822

Diphenhydramine Citrate (Co-administration may result in an additive CNS depression). Products include:
Children's Benadryl Allergy & Cold Fastmelt Tablets .... ▣695
Children's Benadryl D Allergy & Sinus Fastmelt Tablets .... ▣694
Children's Benadryl Allergy Fastmelt Tablets .... ▣696
Goody's PM Powder .... ▣622

Diphenhydramine Hydrochloride (Co-administration may result in an additive CNS depression). Products include:
- Benadryl Allergy & Cold Tablets 692
- Benadryl Allergy 691
- Benadryl Allergy & Sinus Headache Caplets & Gelcaps 693
- Children's Benadryl Allergy Liquid 695
- Children's Benadryl Dye-Free Allergy Liquid 695
- Benadryl Dye-Free Allergy Liqui-Gels Softgels 692
- Benadryl Itch Relief Stick Extra Strength 696
- Benadryl Itch Stopping Cream Extra Strength 697
- Benadryl Itch Stopping Gel Extra Strength 697
- Benadryl Itch Stopping Spray Extra Strength 697
- Benadryl Maximum Strength Severe Allergy & Sinus Headache Caplets 694
- Children's Benadryl D Liquid Medication 693
- Benadryl D Tablets 694
- Nytol QuickCaps Caplets 635
- Maximum Strength Nytol QuickGels Softgels 635
- Simply Sleep Caplets 1841
- Sominex Original Formula Tablets 637
- TheraFlu Thin Strips Multi Symptom 684
- Triaminic Thin Strips Cough & Runny Nose 690
- Children's Tylenol Plus Cold & Allergy Suspension Liquid 1850
- Tylenol Allergy Complete Night Time Caplets 1844
- Tylenol Severe Allergy Caplets 1844
- Tylenol Flu NightTime Gelcaps 1846
- Extra Strength Tylenol PM Caplets, Geltabs, Gelcaps and Liquid 1847
- Unisom Maximum Strength SleepGels 712

Diphenylpyraline Hydrochloride (Co-administration may result in an additive CNS depression).
No products indexed under this heading.

Doxepin Hydrochloride (Co-administration with tricyclic antidepressants may increase the effect of either hydrocodone or the tricyclic antidepressant).
No products indexed under this heading.

Droperidol (Co-administration may result in an additive CNS depression).
No products indexed under this heading.

Enflurane (Co-administration may result in an additive CNS depression).
No products indexed under this heading.

Estazolam (Co-administration may result in an additive CNS depression). Products include:
- ProSom Tablets 512

Ethanol (Co-administration may result in an additive CNS depression).
No products indexed under this heading.

Ethchlorvynol (Co-administration may result in an additive CNS depression).
No products indexed under this heading.

Ethinamate (Co-administration may result in an additive CNS depression).
No products indexed under this heading.

Ethyl Alcohol (Co-administration may result in an additive CNS depression).
No products indexed under this heading.

Fentanyl (Co-administration may result in an additive CNS depression). Products include:
- Duragesic Transdermal System 2448

Fentanyl Citrate (Co-administration may result in an additive CNS depression). Products include:
- Actiq 993

Fexofenadine Hydrochloride (Co-administration may result in an additive CNS depression). Products include:
- Allegra 2857
- Allegra-D 12 Hour Extended-Release Tablets 2860
- Allegra-D 24 Hour Extended-Release Tablets 2862

Fluphenazine Decanoate (Co-administration may result in an additive CNS depression).
No products indexed under this heading.

Fluphenazine Enanthate (Co-administration may result in an additive CNS depression).
No products indexed under this heading.

Fluphenazine Hydrochloride (Co-administration may result in an additive CNS depression).
No products indexed under this heading.

Flurazepam Hydrochloride (Co-administration may result in an additive CNS depression). Products include:
- Dalmane Capsules 3343

Glutethimide (Co-administration may result in an additive CNS depression).
No products indexed under this heading.

Haloperidol (Co-administration may result in an additive CNS depression).
No products indexed under this heading.

Haloperidol Decanoate (Co-administration may result in an additive CNS depression).
No products indexed under this heading.

Hydrocodone Polistirex (Co-administration may result in an additive CNS depression). Products include:
- Tussionex Pennkinetic Extended-Release Suspension 3322

Hydromorphone Hydrochloride (Co-administration may result in an additive CNS depression). Products include:
- Dilaudid 439
- Dilaudid Oral Liquid 443
- Dilaudid Non-Sterile Powder 439
- Dilaudid Rectal Suppositories 439
- Dilaudid Tablets 439
- Dilaudid Tablets - 8 mg 443
- Dilaudid-HP 441

Hydroxyzine Hydrochloride (Co-administration may result in an additive CNS depression).
No products indexed under this heading.

Imipramine Hydrochloride (Co-administration with tricyclic antidepressants may increase the effect of either hydrocodone or the tricyclic antidepressant).
No products indexed under this heading.

Imipramine Pamoate (Co-administration with tricyclic antidepressants may increase the effect of either hydrocodone or the tricyclic antidepressant).
No products indexed under this heading.

Isocarboxazid (Co-administration with an MAO inhibitor may increase the effect of either hydrocodone or the MAO inhibitor).
No products indexed under this heading.

Isoflurane (Co-administration may result in an additive CNS depression).
No products indexed under this heading.

Ketamine Hydrochloride (Co-administration may result in an additive CNS depression).
No products indexed under this heading.

Levomethadyl Acetate Hydrochloride (Co-administration may result in an additive CNS depression).
No products indexed under this heading.

Levorphanol Tartrate (Co-administration may result in an additive CNS depression).
No products indexed under this heading.

Loratadine (Co-administration may result in an additive CNS depression). Products include:
- Alavert Allergy & Sinus D-12 Hour Tablets 743
- Alavert 743
- Children's Claritin 24 Hour Non-Drowsy Allergy Syrup 732
- Claritin Non-Drowsy 24 Hour Tablets 731
- Non-Drowsy Claritin Hives Relief Tablets 733
- Claritin Reditabs 24 Hour Non-Drowsy Tablets 732
- Claritin-D Non-Drowsy 12 Hour Tablets 731
- Claritin-D Non-Drowsy 24 Hour Tablets 731
- Children's Dimetapp ND Non-Drowsy Allergy Syrup 746
- Triaminic Allerchews 684

Lorazepam (Co-administration may result in an additive CNS depression).
No products indexed under this heading.

Loxapine Hydrochloride (Co-administration may result in an additive CNS depression).
No products indexed under this heading.

Loxapine Succinate (Co-administration may result in an additive CNS depression).
No products indexed under this heading.

Maprotiline Hydrochloride (Co-administration with tricyclic antidepressants may increase the effect of either hydrocodone or the tricyclic antidepressant).
No products indexed under this heading.

Meperidine Hydrochloride (Co-administration may result in an additive CNS depression).
No products indexed under this heading.

Mephobarbital (Co-administration may result in an additive CNS depression). Products include:
- Mebaral Tablets, USP 2483

Meprobamate (Co-administration may result in an additive CNS depression).
No products indexed under this heading.

Mesoridazine Besylate (Co-administration may result in an additive CNS depression).
No products indexed under this heading.

Methadone Hydrochloride (Co-administration may result in an additive CNS depression).
No products indexed under this heading.

Methdilazine Hydrochloride (Co-administration may result in an additive CNS depression).
No products indexed under this heading.

Methohexital Sodium (Co-administration may result in an additive CNS depression).
No products indexed under this heading.

Methotrimeprazine (Co-administration may result in an additive CNS depression).
No products indexed under this heading.

Methoxyflurane (Co-administration may result in an additive CNS depression).
No products indexed under this heading.

Midazolam Hydrochloride (Co-administration may result in an additive CNS depression).
No products indexed under this heading.

Moclobemide (Co-administration with an MAO inhibitor may increase the effect of either hydrocodone or the MAO inhibitor).
No products indexed under this heading.

Molindone Hydrochloride (Co-administration may result in an additive CNS depression). Products include:
- Moban Tablets 1108

Morphine Sulfate (Co-administration may result in an additive CNS depression). Products include:
- Avinza Capsules 1714
- Kadian Capsules 572
- MS Contin Tablets 2703

Nortriptyline Hydrochloride (Co-administration with tricyclic antidepressants may increase the effect of either hydrocodone or the tricyclic antidepressant).
No products indexed under this heading.

Olanzapine (Co-administration may result in an additive CNS depression). Products include:
- Symbyax Capsules 1788
- Zyprexa Tablets 1798
- Zyprexa IntraMuscular 1798
- Zyprexa ZYDIS Orally Disintegrating Tablets 1798

Oxazepam (Co-administration may result in an additive CNS depression).
No products indexed under this heading.

Oxycodone Hydrochloride (Co-administration may result in an additive CNS depression). Products include:
- Combunox Tablets 1183
- OxyContin Tablets 2699
- OxyFast Oral Concentrate Solution 2704

OxyIR Capsules 2704
Percocet Tablets 1114
Percodan Tablets 1115

Pargyline Hydrochloride (Co-administration with an MAO inhibitor may increase the effect of either hydrocodone or the MAO inhibitor).
No products indexed under this heading.

Pentobarbital Sodium (Co-administration may result in an additive CNS depression). Products include:
Nembutal Sodium Solution, USP 2484

Perphenazine (Co-administration may result in an additive CNS depression).
No products indexed under this heading.

Phenelzine Sulfate (Co-administration with an MAO inhibitor may increase the effect of either hydrocodone or the MAO inhibitor).
No products indexed under this heading.

Phenobarbital (Co-administration may result in an additive CNS depression).
No products indexed under this heading.

Prazepam (Co-administration may result in an additive CNS depression).
No products indexed under this heading.

Procarbazine Hydrochloride (Co-administration with an MAO inhibitor may increase the effect of either hydrocodone or the MAO inhibitor). Products include:
Matulane Capsules 3188

Prochlorperazine (Co-administration may result in an additive CNS depression).
No products indexed under this heading.

Promethazine Hydrochloride (Co-administration may result in an additive CNS depression). Products include:
Phenergan 3438

Propofol (Co-administration may result in an additive CNS depression). Products include:
Diprivan Injectable Emulsion 676

Propoxyphene Hydrochloride (Co-administration may result in an additive CNS depression).
No products indexed under this heading.

Propoxyphene Napsylate (Co-administration may result in an additive CNS depression). Products include:
Darvocet A 500 Tablets 3497

Protriptyline Hydrochloride (Co-administration with tricyclic antidepressants may increase the effect of either hydrocodone or the tricyclic antidepressant). Products include:
Vivactil Tablets 2350

Pyrilamine Maleate (Co-administration may result in an additive CNS depression).
No products indexed under this heading.

Pyrilamine Tannate (Co-administration may result in an additive CNS depression).
No products indexed under this heading.

Quazepam (Co-administration may result in an additive CNS depression).
No products indexed under this heading.

Quetiapine Fumarate (Co-administration may result in an additive CNS depression). Products include:
Seroquel Tablets 691

Remifentanil Hydrochloride (Co-administration may result in an additive CNS depression).
No products indexed under this heading.

Risperidone (Co-administration may result in an additive CNS depression). Products include:
Risperdal Consta Long-Acting Injection 1664
Risperdal M-Tab Orally Disintegrating Tablets 1658
Risperdal 1658

Secobarbital Sodium (Co-administration may result in an additive CNS depression).
No products indexed under this heading.

Selegiline Hydrochloride (Co-administration with an MAO inhibitor may increase the effect of either hydrocodone or the MAO inhibitor). Products include:
Eldepryl Capsules 3209

Sevoflurane (Co-administration may result in an additive CNS depression). Products include:
Ultane Liquid for Inhalation 526

Sufentanil Citrate (Co-administration may result in an additive CNS depression).
No products indexed under this heading.

Temazepam (Co-administration may result in an additive CNS depression).
No products indexed under this heading.

Terfenadine (Co-administration may result in an additive CNS depression).
No products indexed under this heading.

Thiamylal Sodium (Co-administration may result in an additive CNS depression).
No products indexed under this heading.

Thioridazine Hydrochloride (Co-administration may result in an additive CNS depression). Products include:
Thioridazine Hydrochloride Tablets 2122

Thiothixene (Co-administration may result in an additive CNS depression). Products include:
Thiothixene Capsules 2124

Tranylcypromine Sulfate (Co-administration with an MAO inhibitor may increase the effect of either hydrocodone or the MAO inhibitor). Products include:
Parnate Tablets 1499

Triazolam (Co-administration may result in an additive CNS depression).
No products indexed under this heading.

Trifluoperazine Hydrochloride (Co-administration may result in an additive CNS depression).
No products indexed under this heading.

Trimeprazine Tartrate (Co-administration may result in an additive CNS depression).
No products indexed under this heading.

Trimipramine Maleate (Co-administration with tricyclic antidepressants may increase the effect of either hydrocodone or the tricyclic antidepressant). Products include:
Surmontil Capsules 2347

Tripelennamine Hydrochloride (Co-administration may result in an additive CNS depression).
No products indexed under this heading.

Triprolidine Hydrochloride (Co-administration may result in an additive CNS depression).
No products indexed under this heading.

Zaleplon (Co-administration may result in an additive CNS depression). Products include:
Sonata Capsules 1686

Ziprasidone Hydrochloride (Co-administration may result in an additive CNS depression). Products include:
Geodon Capsules 2514

Zolpidem Tartrate (Co-administration may result in an additive CNS depression). Products include:
Ambien Tablets 2867

Food Interactions

Alcohol (Concurrent use results in an additive CNS depression).

VICOPROFEN TABLETS

(Hydrocodone Bitartrate, Ibuprofen).. 533

May interact with ACE inhibitors, anticholinergics, central nervous system depressants, lithium preparations, monoamine oxidase inhibitors, thiazides, tricyclic antidepressants, and certain other agents. Compounds in these categories include:

Alfentanil Hydrochloride (May exhibit additive CNS depression).
No products indexed under this heading.

Alprazolam (May exhibit additive CNS depression). Products include:
Niravam Orally Disintegrating Tablets 3106
Xanax XR Tablets 2655

Amitriptyline Hydrochloride (Co-administration of tricyclic antidepressants with hydrocodone preparations may increase the effect of either the antidepressant or hydrocodone).
No products indexed under this heading.

Amoxapine (Co-administration of tricyclic antidepressants with hydrocodone preparations may increase the effect of either the antidepressant or hydrocodone).
No products indexed under this heading.

Aprobarbital (May exhibit additive CNS depression).
No products indexed under this heading.

Aspirin (Co-administration of Vicoprofen and aspirin may increase the risk of adverse effects; concurrent use should be avoided). Products include:
Aggrenox Capsules 855
Bayer, Aspirin Regimen .... ▣ 606
Bayer Aspirin Tablets 3515
BC Powder .... ▣ 612
BC Allergy Sinus Cold Powder .... ▣ 612
Arthritis Strength BC Powder .... ▣ 612
BC Sinus Cold Powder .... ▣ 612
Ecotrin Enteric Coated Aspirin Low, Regular and Maximum Strength Tablets 1627
Goody's Body Pain Formula Powder .... ▣ 621
Goody's Extra Strength Headache Powder .... ▣ 621
Goody's Extra Strength Pain Relief Tablets .... ▣ 621
Percodan Tablets 1115
St. Joseph 81 mg Aspirin Chewable and Enteric Coated Tablets 1841

Aspirin, Enteric Coated (Co-administration of Vicoprofen and aspirin may increase the risk of adverse effects; concurrent use should be avoided).
No products indexed under this heading.

Aspirin Buffered (Co-administration of Vicoprofen and aspirin may increase the risk of adverse effects; concurrent use should be avoided).
No products indexed under this heading.

Atropine Sulfate (Concurrent use of anticholinergics with hydrocodone preparations may produce paralytic ileus).
No products indexed under this heading.

Belladonna Alkaloids (Concurrent use of anticholinergics with hydrocodone preparations may produce paralytic ileus). Products include:
Hyland's Teething Tablets .... ▣ 736

Benazepril Hydrochloride (NSAIDs may diminish the antihypertensive effect of ACE inhibitors). Products include:
Lotensin Tablets 2232
Lotensin HCT Tablets 2235
Lotrel Capsules 2238

Bendroflumethiazide (Ibuprofen has been shown to reduce the natriuretic effect of thiazides in some patients).
No products indexed under this heading.

Benztropine Mesylate (Concurrent use of anticholinergics with hydrocodone preparations may produce paralytic ileus). Products include:
Cogentin Injection 1903

Biperiden Hydrochloride (Concurrent use of anticholinergics with hydrocodone preparations may produce paralytic ileus).
No products indexed under this heading.

Buprenorphine Hydrochloride (May exhibit additive CNS depression). Products include:
Buprenex Injectable 2718
Suboxone Tablets 2719
Subutex Tablets 2719

Buspirone Hydrochloride (May exhibit additive CNS depression).
No products indexed under this heading.

Butabarbital (May exhibit additive CNS depression).
No products indexed under this heading.

Butalbital (May exhibit additive CNS depression). Products include:
Sedapap Tablets 50 mg/650 mg 2098

Captopril (NSAIDs may diminish the antihypertensive effect of ACE inhibitors). Products include:
Captopril Tablets 2114

Chlordiazepoxide (May exhibit additive CNS depression).
No products indexed under this heading.

Chlordiazepoxide Hydrochloride (May exhibit additive CNS depression). Products include:

Librium Capsules 3349

Chlorothiazide (Ibuprofen has been shown to reduce the natriuretic effect of thiazides in some patients). Products include:

Aldoclor Tablets 1881
Diuril Oral 1936

Chlorothiazide Sodium (Ibuprofen has been shown to reduce the natriuretic effect of thiazides in some patients). Products include:

Diuril Sodium Intravenous 1934

Chlorpromazine (May exhibit additive CNS depression).

No products indexed under this heading.

Chlorpromazine Hydrochloride (May exhibit additive CNS depression).

No products indexed under this heading.

Chlorprothixene (May exhibit additive CNS depression).

No products indexed under this heading.

Chlorprothixene Hydrochloride (May exhibit additive CNS depression).

No products indexed under this heading.

Chlorprothixene Lactate (May exhibit additive CNS depression).

No products indexed under this heading.

Clidinium Bromide (Concurrent use of anticholinergics with hydrocodone preparations may produce paralytic ileus).

No products indexed under this heading.

Clomipramine Hydrochloride (Co-administration of tricyclic antidepressants with hydrocodone preparations may increase the effect of either the antidepressant or hydrocodone).

No products indexed under this heading.

Clorazepate Dipotassium (May exhibit additive CNS depression). Products include:

Tranxene 2488

Clozapine (May exhibit additive CNS depression). Products include:

Clozapine Tablets 2141
Clozaril Tablets 2174
FazaClo Orally Disintegrating Tablets 547

Codeine Phosphate (May exhibit additive CNS depression). Products include:

Tylenol with Codeine 2461

Desflurane (May exhibit additive CNS depression). Products include:

Suprane Liquid for Inhalation 770

Desipramine Hydrochloride (Co-administration of tricyclic antidepressants with hydrocodone preparations may increase the effect of either the antidepressant or hydrocodone).

No products indexed under this heading.

Dezocine (May exhibit additive CNS depression).

No products indexed under this heading.

Diazepam (May exhibit additive CNS depression). Products include:

Diastat Rectal Delivery System 3344
Valium Tablets 2822

Dicyclomine Hydrochloride (Concurrent use of anticholinergics with hydrocodone preparations may produce paralytic ileus). Products include:

Bentyl Capsules 724
Bentyl Injection 724
Bentyl Syrup 724
Bentyl Tablets 724

Doxepin Hydrochloride (Co-administration of tricyclic antidepressants with hydrocodone preparations may increase the effect of either the antidepressant or hydrocodone).

No products indexed under this heading.

Droperidol (May exhibit additive CNS depression).

No products indexed under this heading.

Enalapril Maleate (NSAIDs may diminish the antihypertensive effect of ACE inhibitors). Products include:

Vaseretic Tablets 2073
Vasotec I.V. Injection 2076

Enalaprilat (NSAIDs may diminish the antihypertensive effect of ACE inhibitors).

No products indexed under this heading.

Enflurane (May exhibit additive CNS depression).

No products indexed under this heading.

Estazolam (May exhibit additive CNS depression). Products include:

ProSom Tablets 512

Ethanol (May exhibit additive CNS depression).

No products indexed under this heading.

Ethchlorvynol (May exhibit additive CNS depression).

No products indexed under this heading.

Ethinamate (May exhibit additive CNS depression).

No products indexed under this heading.

Ethyl Alcohol (May exhibit additive CNS depression).

No products indexed under this heading.

Fentanyl (May exhibit additive CNS depression). Products include:

Duragesic Transdermal System 2448

Fentanyl Citrate (May exhibit additive CNS depression). Products include:

Actiq 993

Fluphenazine Decanoate (May exhibit additive CNS depression).

No products indexed under this heading.

Fluphenazine Enanthate (May exhibit additive CNS depression).

No products indexed under this heading.

Fluphenazine Hydrochloride (May exhibit additive CNS depression).

No products indexed under this heading.

Flurazepam Hydrochloride (May exhibit additive CNS depression). Products include:

Dalmane Capsules 3343

Fosinopril Sodium (NSAIDs may diminish the antihypertensive effect of ACE inhibitors).

No products indexed under this heading.

Furosemide (Ibuprofen has been shown to reduce the natriuretic effect of furosemide). Products include:

Furosemide Tablets 2117

Glutethimide (May exhibit additive CNS depression).

No products indexed under this heading.

Glycopyrrolate (Concurrent use of anticholinergics with hydrocodone preparations may produce paralytic ileus).

No products indexed under this heading.

Haloperidol (May exhibit additive CNS depression).

No products indexed under this heading.

Haloperidol Decanoate (May exhibit additive CNS depression).

No products indexed under this heading.

Hydrochlorothiazide (Ibuprofen has been shown to reduce the natriuretic effect of thiazides in some patients). Products include:

Aldoril Tablets 1884
Atacand HCT 637
Avalide Tablets 2889
Avalide Tablets 922
Benicar HCT Tablets 2852
Diovan HCT Tablets 2195
Dyazide Capsules 1389
Hyzaar 1964
Lotensin HCT Tablets 2235
Maxzide 2150
Micardis HCT Tablets 886
Moduretic Tablets 2003
Prinzide Tablets 2033
Teveten HCT Tablets 1710
Timolide Tablets 2056
Uniretic Tablets 3114
Vaseretic Tablets 2073
Zestoretic Tablets 701

Hydrocodone Polistirex (May exhibit additive CNS depression). Products include:

Tussionex Pennkinetic Extended-Release Suspension 3322

Hydroflumethiazide (Ibuprofen has been shown to reduce the natriuretic effect of thiazides in some patients).

No products indexed under this heading.

Hydromorphone Hydrochloride (May exhibit additive CNS depression). Products include:

Dilaudid 439
Dilaudid Oral Liquid 443
Dilaudid Non-Sterile Powder 439
Dilaudid Rectal Suppositories 439
Dilaudid Tablets 439
Dilaudid Tablets - 8 mg 443
Dilaudid-HP 441

Hydroxyzine Hydrochloride (May exhibit additive CNS depression).

No products indexed under this heading.

Hyoscyamine (Concurrent use of anticholinergics with hydrocodone preparations may produce paralytic ileus).

No products indexed under this heading.

Hyoscyamine Sulfate (Concurrent use of anticholinergics with hydrocodone preparations may produce paralytic ileus).

No products indexed under this heading.

Imipramine Hydrochloride (Co-administration of tricyclic antidepressants with hydrocodone preparations may increase the effect of either the antidepressant or hydrocodone).

No products indexed under this heading.

Imipramine Pamoate (Co-administration of tricyclic antidepressants with hydrocodone preparations may increase the effect of either the antidepressant or hydrocodone).

No products indexed under this heading.

Ipratropium Bromide (Concurrent use of anticholinergics with hydrocodone preparations may produce paralytic ileus). Products include:

Atrovent HFA Inhalation Aerosol 872
Atrovent Inhalation Solution 868
Atrovent Nasal Spray 0.03% 869
Atrovent Nasal Spray 0.06% 870
Combivent Inhalation Aerosol 878
DuoNeb Inhalation Solution 1058

Isocarboxazid (Co-administration of MAO inhibitors with hydrocodone preparations may increase the effect of either the MAO inhibitors or hydrocodone).

No products indexed under this heading.

Isoflurane (May exhibit additive CNS depression).

No products indexed under this heading.

Ketamine Hydrochloride (May exhibit additive CNS depression).

No products indexed under this heading.

Levomethadyl Acetate Hydrochloride (May exhibit additive CNS depression).

No products indexed under this heading.

Levorphanol Tartrate (May exhibit additive CNS depression).

No products indexed under this heading.

Lisinopril (NSAIDs may diminish the antihypertensive effect of ACE inhibitors). Products include:

Prinivil Tablets 2029
Prinzide Tablets 2033
Zestoretic Tablets 701
Zestril Tablets 704

Lithium (Ibuprofen has been shown to elevate plasma lithium concentration and reduce renal clearance).

No products indexed under this heading.

Lithium Carbonate (Ibuprofen has been shown to elevate plasma lithium concentration and reduce renal clearance). Products include:

Eskalith 1406
Lithobid Tablets 1670

Lithium Citrate (Ibuprofen has been shown to elevate plasma lithium concentration and reduce renal clearance).

No products indexed under this heading.

Lorazepam (May exhibit additive CNS depression).

No products indexed under this heading.

Loxapine Hydrochloride (May exhibit additive CNS depression).

No products indexed under this heading.

Loxapine Succinate (May exhibit additive CNS depression).

No products indexed under this heading.

Maprotiline Hydrochloride (Co-administration of tricyclic antidepressants with hydrocodone preparations may increase the effect of either the antidepressant or hydrocodone).

No products indexed under this heading.

Mepenzolate Bromide (Concurrent use of anticholinergics with hydrocodone preparations may produce paralytic ileus).
No products indexed under this heading.

Meperidine Hydrochloride (May exhibit additive CNS depression).
No products indexed under this heading.

Mephobarbital (May exhibit additive CNS depression). Products include:
Mebaral Tablets, USP 2483

Meprobamate (May exhibit additive CNS depression).
No products indexed under this heading.

Mesoridazine Besylate (May exhibit additive CNS depression).
No products indexed under this heading.

Methadone Hydrochloride (May exhibit additive CNS depression).
No products indexed under this heading.

Methohexital Sodium (May exhibit additive CNS depression).
No products indexed under this heading.

Methotrexate Sodium (Ibuprofen, in animal studies, has been reported to competitively inhibit methotrexate accumulation; this could lead to enhanced toxicity of methotrexate).
No products indexed under this heading.

Methotrimeprazine (May exhibit additive CNS depression).
No products indexed under this heading.

Methoxyflurane (May exhibit additive CNS depression).
No products indexed under this heading.

Methyclothiazide (Ibuprofen has been shown to reduce the natriuretic effect of thiazides in some patients).
No products indexed under this heading.

Midazolam Hydrochloride (May exhibit additive CNS depression).
No products indexed under this heading.

Moclobemide (Co-administration of MAO inhibitors with hydrocodone preparations may increase the effect of either the MAO inhibitors or hydrocodone).
No products indexed under this heading.

Moexipril Hydrochloride (NSAIDs may diminish the antihypertensive effect of ACE inhibitors). Products include:
Uniretic Tablets 3114
Univasc Tablets 3118

Molindone Hydrochloride (May exhibit additive CNS depression). Products include:
Moban Tablets 1108

Morphine Sulfate (May exhibit additive CNS depression). Products include:
Avinza Capsules 1714
Kadian Capsules 572
MS Contin Tablets 2703

Nortriptyline Hydrochloride (Co-administration of tricyclic antidepressants with hydrocodone preparations may increase the effect of either the antidepressant or hydrocodone).
No products indexed under this heading.

Olanzapine (May exhibit additive CNS depression). Products include:
Symbyax Capsules 1788
Zyprexa Tablets 1798
Zyprexa IntraMuscular 1798
Zyprexa ZYDIS Orally Disintegrating Tablets 1798

Oxazepam (May exhibit additive CNS depression).
No products indexed under this heading.

Oxybutynin Chloride (Concurrent use of anticholinergics with hydrocodone preparations may produce paralytic ileus). Products include:
Ditropan XL Extended Release Tablets 2391

Oxycodone Hydrochloride (May exhibit additive CNS depression). Products include:
Combunox Tablets 1183
OxyContin Tablets 2699
OxyFast Oral Concentrate Solution 2704
OxyIR Capsules 2704
Percocet Tablets 1114
Percodan Tablets 1115

Pargyline Hydrochloride (Co-administration of MAO inhibitors with hydrocodone preparations may increase the effect of either the MAO inhibitors or hydrocodone).
No products indexed under this heading.

Pentobarbital Sodium (May exhibit additive CNS depression). Products include:
Nembutal Sodium Solution, USP 2484

Perindopril Erbumine (NSAIDs may diminish the antihypertensive effect of ACE inhibitors). Products include:
Aceon Tablets (2 mg, 4 mg, 8 mg) 3191

Perphenazine (May exhibit additive CNS depression).
No products indexed under this heading.

Phenelzine Sulfate (Co-administration of MAO inhibitors with hydrocodone preparations may increase the effect of either the MAO inhibitors or hydrocodone).
No products indexed under this heading.

Phenobarbital (May exhibit additive CNS depression).
No products indexed under this heading.

Polythiazide (Ibuprofen has been shown to reduce the natriuretic effect of thiazides in some patients).
No products indexed under this heading.

Prazepam (May exhibit additive CNS depression).
No products indexed under this heading.

Procarbazine Hydrochloride (Co-administration of MAO inhibitors with hydrocodone preparations may increase the effect of either the MAO inhibitors or hydrocodone). Products include:
Matulane Capsules 3188

Prochlorperazine (May exhibit additive CNS depression).
No products indexed under this heading.

Procyclidine Hydrochloride (Concurrent use of anticholinergics with hydrocodone preparations may produce paralytic ileus).
No products indexed under this heading.

Promethazine Hydrochloride (May exhibit additive CNS depression). Products include:
Phenergan 3438

Propantheline Bromide (Concurrent use of anticholinergics with hydrocodone preparations may produce paralytic ileus).
No products indexed under this heading.

Propofol (May exhibit additive CNS depression). Products include:
Diprivan Injectable Emulsion 676

Propoxyphene Hydrochloride (May exhibit additive CNS depression).
No products indexed under this heading.

Propoxyphene Napsylate (May exhibit additive CNS depression). Products include:
Darvocet A 500 Tablets 3497

Protriptyline Hydrochloride (Co-administration of tricyclic antidepressants with hydrocodone preparations may increase the effect of either the antidepressant or hydrocodone). Products include:
Vivactil Tablets 2350

Quazepam (May exhibit additive CNS depression).
No products indexed under this heading.

Quetiapine Fumarate (May exhibit additive CNS depression). Products include:
Seroquel Tablets 691

Quinapril Hydrochloride (NSAIDs may diminish the antihypertensive effect of ACE inhibitors).
No products indexed under this heading.

Ramipril (NSAIDs may diminish the antihypertensive effect of ACE inhibitors). Products include:
Altace Capsules 1673

Remifentanil Hydrochloride (May exhibit additive CNS depression).
No products indexed under this heading.

Risperidone (May exhibit additive CNS depression). Products include:
Risperdal Consta Long-Acting Injection 1664
Risperdal M-Tab Orally Disintegrating Tablets 1658
Risperdal 1658

Scopolamine (Concurrent use of anticholinergics with hydrocodone preparations may produce paralytic ileus). Products include:
Transderm Scōp Transdermal Therapeutic System 2166

Scopolamine Hydrobromide (Concurrent use of anticholinergics with hydrocodone preparations may produce paralytic ileus).
No products indexed under this heading.

Secobarbital Sodium (May exhibit additive CNS depression).
No products indexed under this heading.

Selegiline Hydrochloride (Co-administration of MAO inhibitors with hydrocodone preparations may increase the effect of either the MAO inhibitors or hydrocodone). Products include:
Eldepryl Capsules 3209

Sevoflurane (May exhibit additive CNS depression). Products include:
Ultane Liquid for Inhalation 526

Spirapril Hydrochloride (NSAIDs may diminish the antihypertensive effect of ACE inhibitors).
No products indexed under this heading.

Sufentanil Citrate (May exhibit additive CNS depression).
No products indexed under this heading.

Temazepam (May exhibit additive CNS depression).
No products indexed under this heading.

Thiamylal Sodium (May exhibit additive CNS depression).
No products indexed under this heading.

Thioridazine Hydrochloride (May exhibit additive CNS depression). Products include:
Thioridazine Hydrochloride Tablets 2122

Thiothixene (May exhibit additive CNS depression). Products include:
Thiothixene Capsules 2124

Tolterodine Tartrate (Concurrent use of anticholinergics with hydrocodone preparations may produce paralytic ileus). Products include:
Detrol Tablets 2626
Detrol LA Capsules 2629

Trandolapril (NSAIDs may diminish the antihypertensive effect of ACE inhibitors). Products include:
Mavik Tablets 482
Tarka Tablets 519

Tranylcypromine Sulfate (Co-administration of MAO inhibitors with hydrocodone preparations may increase the effect of either the MAO inhibitors or hydrocodone). Products include:
Parnate Tablets 1499

Triazolam (May exhibit additive CNS depression).
No products indexed under this heading.

Tridihexethyl Chloride (Concurrent use of anticholinergics with hydrocodone preparations may produce paralytic ileus).
No products indexed under this heading.

Trifluoperazine Hydrochloride (May exhibit additive CNS depression).
No products indexed under this heading.

Trihexyphenidyl Hydrochloride (Concurrent use of anticholinergics with hydrocodone preparations may produce paralytic ileus).
No products indexed under this heading.

Trimipramine Maleate (Co-administration of tricyclic antidepressants with hydrocodone preparations may increase the effect of either the antidepressant or hydrocodone). Products include:
Surmontil Capsules 2347

Warfarin Sodium (The effects of warfarin and NSAIDs on GI bleeding are synergistic). Products include:
Coumadin for Injection 932
Coumadin Tablets 932

Zaleplon (May exhibit additive CNS depression). Products include:
Sonata Capsules 1686

Ziprasidone Hydrochloride (May exhibit additive CNS depression). Products include:
Geodon Capsules 2514

Zolpidem Tartrate (May exhibit additive CNS depression). Products include:
Ambien Tablets 2867

Food Interactions

Alcohol (May exhibit additive CNS depression).

VIGAMOX OPHTHALMIC SOLUTION

(Moxifloxacin Hydrochloride) 560
None cited in PDR database.

VIOKASE POWDER

(Pancrelipase) 738
None cited in PDR database.

VIOKASE TABLETS

(Pancrelipase) 738
None cited in PDR database.

VIRACEPT ORAL POWDER

(Nelfinavir Mesylate) 2556
See Viracept Tablets

VIRACEPT TABLETS

(Nelfinavir Mesylate) 2556
May interact with cytochrome p450 2c19 inducers (selected), cytochrome p450 2c19 inhibitors (selected), cytochrome p450 3a inducers (selected), cytochrome p450 3a inhibitors (selected), dihydropyridine calcium channel blockers, ergot-containing drugs, oral contraceptives, phenytoin, quinidine, statins that are metabolized by CYP3A4, and certain other agents. Compounds in these categories include:

Allium sativum (Nelfinavir is metabolized by CYP3A and CYP2C19; co-administration of Viracept and drugs that induce CYP3A or CYP2C19 may decrease nelfinavir plasma concentrations and reduce its therapeutic effect).
No products indexed under this heading.

Amiodarone Hydrochloride (Nelfinavir is an inhibitor of CYP3A and co-administration with drugs primarily metabolized by CYP3A, such as amiodarone, could result in competition for CYP3A by nelfinavir; contraindicated due to potential for serious and/or life-threatening reactions, such as cardiac arrhythmias). Products include:
Pacerone Tablets 3337

Amlodipine Besylate (Nelfinavir is an inhibitor of CYP450 3A enzymes which are responsible for the metabolism of dihydropyridine calcium channel blockers; co-administration may result in increased plasma concentrations of these calcium channel blockers). Products include:
Caduet Tablets 2507
Lotrel Capsules 2238
Norvasc Tablets 2529

Amprenavir (Nelfinavir is metabolized by CYP3A and CYP2C19; co-administration of Viracept and drugs that inhibit CYP3A or CYP2C19 may increase nelfinavir plasma concentrations). Products include:
Agenerase Capsules 1299
Agenerase Oral Solution 1304

Aprepitant (Nelfinavir is metabolized by CYP3A and CYP2C19; co-administration of Viracept and drugs that induce CYP3A or CYP2C19 may decrease nelfinavir plasma concentrations and reduce its therapeutic effect). Products include:
Emend Capsules 1944

Atorvastatin Calcium (Nelfinavir is an inhibitor of CYP3A and co-administration with drugs primarily metabolized by CYP3A could increase the risk of myopathy including rhabdomyolysis). Products include:
Caduet Tablets 2507
Lipitor Tablets 2495

Azithromycin Dihydrate (Co-administration results in increases in azithromycin plasma concentrations). Products include:
Zithromax 2568
Zithromax for IV Infusion 2573
Zithromax for Oral Suspension, 300 mg, 600 mg, 900 mg, 1200 mg 2561
Zithromax Tablets, 250 mg, 500 mg 2561
Zithromax Tri-Pak 2561
Zithromax Z-Pak 2568

Carbamazepine (May decrease nelfinavir plasma concentrations; Viracept may not be effective due to decreased nelfinavir plasma concentrations in patients taking carbamazepine). Products include:
Carbatrol Capsules 3174
Equetro Extended-Release Capsules 3178
Tegretol/Tegretol-XR 2278

Cerivastatin Sodium (Nelfinavir is an inhibitor of CYP3A and co-administration with drugs primarily metabolized by CYP3A, such as cerivastatin, could increase the risk of myopathy including rhabdomyolysis).
No products indexed under this heading.

Cimetidine (Nelfinavir is metabolized by CYP3A and CYP2C19; co-administration of Viracept and drugs that inhibit CYP3A or CYP2C19 may increase nelfinavir plasma concentrations). Products include:
Tagamet HB 200 Tablets 637
Tagamet Tablets 1547

Cimetidine Hydrochloride (Nelfinavir is metabolized by CYP3A and CYP2C19; co-administration of Viracept and drugs that inhibit CYP3A or CYP2C19 may increase nelfinavir plasma concentrations).
No products indexed under this heading.

Ciprofloxacin (Nelfinavir is metabolized by CYP3A and CYP2C19; co-administration of Viracept and drugs that inhibit CYP3A or CYP2C19 may increase nelfinavir plasma concentrations). Products include:
Cipro I.V. 2998
Cipro I.V. Pharmacy Bulk Package ... 3509
Cipro Oral Suspension 2991
Cipro XR Tablets 3004
Ciprodex Otic Suspension 555

Ciprofloxacin Hydrochloride (Nelfinavir is metabolized by CYP3A and CYP2C19; co-administration of Viracept and drugs that inhibit CYP3A or CYP2C19 may increase nelfinavir plasma concentrations). Products include:
Ciloxan Ophthalmic Ointment 554
Cipro Tablets 2991

Cisapride (Nelfinavir is an inhibitor of CYP3A and co-administration with drugs primarily metabolized by CYP3A, such as cisapride, could affect hepatic metabolism of cisapride and create the potential for serious and/or life-threatening adverse events; concurrent use is contraindicated).
No products indexed under this heading.

Citalopram Hydrobromide (Nelfinavir is metabolized by CYP3A and CYP2C19; co-administration of Viracept and drugs that inhibit CYP3A or CYP2C19 may increase nelfinavir plasma concentrations). Products include:
Celexa 1177

Clarithromycin (Nelfinavir is metabolized by CYP3A and CYP2C19; co-administration of Viracept and drugs that inhibit CYP3A or CYP2C19 may increase nelfinavir plasma concentrations). Products include:
Biaxin/Biaxin XL 402
PREVPAC 3281

Cyclosporine (Nelfinavir is an inhibitor of CYP450 3A enzymes which are responsible for the metabolism of immunosuppressants, such as cyclosporine; co-administration may result in increased plasma concentrations of immunosuppressants). Products include:
Gengraf Capsules 458
Neoral Soft Gelatin Capsules 2247
Neoral Oral Solution 2247
Restasis Ophthalmic Emulsion 570
Sandimmune 2259

Delavirdine Mesylate (Co-administration results in increases in nelfinavir plasma concentrations and decreases in delavirdine plasma concentrations; appropriate doses for these combinations, with respect to safety and efficacy, have not been established). Products include:
Rescriptor Tablets 2535

Desogestrel (Nelfinavir is metabolized by CYP3A and CYP2C19; co-administration of Viracept and drugs that inhibit CYP3A or CYP2C19 may increase nelfinavir plasma concentrations). Products include:
Ortho-Cept Tablets 2395

Dexamethasone (Nelfinavir is metabolized by CYP3A and CYP2C19; co-administration of Viracept and drugs that induce CYP3A or CYP2C19 may decrease nelfinavir plasma concentrations and reduce its therapeutic effect). Products include:
Ciprodex Otic Suspension 555
Decadron Tablets 1929
TobraDex Ophthalmic Ointment 558
TobraDex Ophthalmic Suspension ... 558

Didanosine (Co-administration with didanosine indicates no change in AUC or Cmax of nelfinavir; however, it is recommended that didanosine be administered on an empty stomach; therefore, nelfinavir should be administered with food one hour after or more than 2 hours before didanosine).
No products indexed under this heading.

Dihydroergotamine Mesylate (Nelfinavir is an inhibitor of CYP3A and co-administration with drugs primarily metabolized by CYP3A, such as ergot derivatives, could result in competition for CYP3A by nelfinavir; inhibition of the metabolism of ergot derivatives could create a potential for serious cardiac arrhythmias or prolong adverse events; contraindicated due to potential for serious and/or life-threatening reactions, such as acute ergot toxicity characterized by peripheral vasospasm and ischemia of the extremities and other tissues). Products include:
Migranal Nasal Spray 3350

Diltiazem Hydrochloride (Nelfinavir is metabolized by CYP3A and CYP2C19; co-administration of Viracept and drugs that inhibit CYP3A or CYP2C19 may increase nelfinavir plasma concentrations). Products include:
Cardizem LA Extended Release Tablets 1699
Tiazac Capsules 1204

Diltiazem Maleate (Nelfinavir is metabolized by CYP3A and CYP2C19; co-administration of Viracept and drugs that inhibit CYP3A or CYP2C19 may increase nelfinavir plasma concentrations).
No products indexed under this heading.

Efavirenz (Nelfinavir is metabolized by CYP3A and CYP2C19; co-administration of Viracept and drugs that inhibit CYP3A or CYP2C19 may increase nelfinavir plasma concentrations). Products include:
Sustiva Capsules 957

Ergonovine Maleate (Nelfinavir is an inhibitor of CYP3A and co-administration with drugs primarily metabolized by CYP3A, such as ergot derivatives, could result in competition for CYP3A by nelfinavir; inhibition of the metabolism of ergot derivatives could create a potential for serious cardiac arrhythmias or prolong adverse events; contraindicated due to potential for serious and/or life-threatening reactions, such as acute ergot toxicity characterized by peripheral vasospasm and ischemia of the extremities and other tissues).
No products indexed under this heading.

Ergotamine Tartrate (Nelfinavir is an inhibitor of CYP3A and co-administration with drugs primarily metabolized by CYP3A, such as ergot derivatives, could result in competition for CYP3A by nelfinavir; inhibition of the metabolism of ergot derivatives could create a potential for serious cardiac arrhythmias or prolong adverse events; contraindicated due to potential for serious and/or life-threatening reactions, such as acute ergot toxicity characterized by peripheral vasospasm and ischemia of the extremities and other tissues).
No products indexed under this heading.

Erythromycin (Nelfinavir is metabolized by CYP3A and CYP2C19; co-administration of Viracept and drugs that inhibit CYP3A or CYP2C19 may increase nelfinavir plasma concentrations). Products include:
Erygel Topical Gel 2096
Ery-Tab Tablets 447
Erythromycin Base Filmtab Tablets 454
Erythromycin Delayed-Release Capsules, USP 456
PCE Dispertab Tablets 510

Ethinyl Estradiol (Co-administration with oral contraceptives containing ethinyl estradiol results in decreased ethinyl estradiol plasma concentrations; alternative or additional contraceptive measures should be used when oral contraceptives and Viracept are co-administered). Products include:
Alesse-28 Tablets 3392
Lo/Ovral-28 Tablets 3423
NuvaRing 2357
Ortho-Cept Tablets 2395
Ortho-Cyclen/Ortho Tri-Cyclen 2414
Ortho Evra Transdermal System 2402
Ortho Tri-Cyclen Lo Tablets 2421
Seasonale Tablets 1073
Triphasil-28 Tablets 3483
Yasmin 28 Tablets 818

Ethosuximide (Nelfinavir is metabolized by CYP3A and CYP2C19; co-administration of Viracept and drugs that induce CYP3A or CYP2C19 may decrease nelfinavir plasma concentrations and reduce its therapeutic effect).
No products indexed under this heading.

Ethynodiol Diacetate (Nelfinavir is metabolized by CYP3A and CYP2C19; co-administration of Viracept and drugs that inhibit CYP3A or CYP2C19 may increase nelfinavir plasma concentrations).
No products indexed under this heading.

Felbamate (Nelfinavir is metabolized by CYP3A and CYP2C19; co-administration of Viracept and drugs that inhibit CYP3A or CYP2C19 may increase nelfinavir plasma concentrations).
No products indexed under this heading.

Felodipine (Nelfinavir is an inhibitor of CYP450 3A enzymes which are responsible for the metabolism of dihydropyridine calcium channel blockers; co-administration may result in increased plasma concentrations of these calcium channel blockers). Products include:
Plendil Extended-Release Tablets 651

Fluconazole (Nelfinavir is metabolized by CYP3A and CYP2C19; co-administration of Viracept and drugs that inhibit CYP3A or CYP2C19 may increase nelfinavir plasma concentrations).
No products indexed under this heading.

Fluoxetine (Nelfinavir is metabolized by CYP3A and CYP2C19; co-administration of Viracept and drugs that inhibit CYP3A or CYP2C19 may increase nelfinavir plasma concentrations).
No products indexed under this heading.

Fluoxetine Hydrochloride (Nelfinavir is metabolized by CYP3A and CYP2C19; co-administration of Viracept and drugs that inhibit CYP3A or CYP2C19 may increase nelfinavir plasma concentrations). Products include:
Prozac Pulvules and Liquid 1771
Symbyax Capsules 1788

Fluvastatin Sodium (Nelfinavir is metabolized by CYP3A and CYP2C19; co-administration of Viracept and drugs that inhibit CYP3A or CYP2C19 may increase nelfinavir plasma concentrations). Products include:
Lescol Capsules 2227
Lescol 2730
Lescol XL Tablets 2227

Fluvoxamine (Nelfinavir is metabolized by CYP3A and CYP2C19; co-administration of Viracept and drugs that inhibit CYP3A or CYP2C19 may increase nelfinavir plasma concentrations).
No products indexed under this heading.

Fluvoxamine Maleate (Nelfinavir is metabolized by CYP3A and CYP2C19; co-administration of Viracept and drugs that inhibit CYP3A or CYP2C19 may increase nelfinavir plasma concentrations).
No products indexed under this heading.

Fosphenytoin Sodium (May decrease nelfinavir plasma concentrations; Viracept may not be effective due to decreased nelfinavir plasma concentrations in patients taking phenytoin).
No products indexed under this heading.

Hypericum (Concomitant use of St. John's Wort or products containing St. John's Wort and nelfinavir is expected to substantially decrease protease inhibitor concentrations and may result in sub-optimal levels of nelfinavir and lead to loss of virologic response andpossible resistance to nelfinavir or other co-administered antiretroviral agents).
No products indexed under this heading.

Indinavir Sulfate (Co-administration results in increases in both nelfinavir and indinavir plasma concentrations; appropriate doses for this combination, with respect to safety and efficacy, have not been established). Products include:
Crixivan Capsules 1918

Indomethacin (Nelfinavir is metabolized by CYP3A and CYP2C19; co-administration of Viracept and drugs that inhibit CYP3A or CYP2C19 may increase nelfinavir plasma concentrations). Products include:
Indocin 1968

Indomethacin Sodium Trihydrate (Nelfinavir is metabolized by CYP3A and CYP2C19; co-administration of Viracept and drugs that inhibit CYP3A or CYP2C19 may increase nelfinavir plasma concentrations). Products include:
Indocin I.V. 1973

Isoniazid (Nelfinavir is metabolized by CYP3A and CYP2C19; co-administration of Viracept and drugs that inhibit CYP3A or CYP2C19 may increase nelfinavir plasma concentrations).
No products indexed under this heading.

Isradipine (Nelfinavir is an inhibitor of CYP450 3A enzymes which are responsible for the metabolism of dihydropyridine calcium channel blockers; co-administration may result in increased plasma concentrations of these calcium channel blockers). Products include:
DynaCirc CR Tablets 2726

Itraconazole (Nelfinavir is metabolized by CYP3A and CYP2C19; co-administration of Viracept and drugs that inhibit CYP3A or CYP2C19 may increase nelfinavir plasma concentrations).
No products indexed under this heading.

Ketoconazole (Nelfinavir is metabolized by CYP3A and CYP2C19; co-administration of Viracept and drugs that inhibit CYP3A or CYP2C19 may increase nelfinavir plasma concentrations). Products include:
Nizoral A-D Shampoo, 1% 1839
Nizoral 2% Shampoo 1838

Lamivudine (Nelfinavir increases lamivudine's AUC and Cmax by 10% and 31%, respectively). Products include:
Combivir Tablets 1373
Epivir 1394
Epivir-HBV 1398
Epzicom Tablets 1402
Trizivir Tablets 1565

Lansoprazole (Nelfinavir is metabolized by CYP3A and CYP2C19; co-administration of Viracept and drugs that inhibit CYP3A or CYP2C19 may increase nelfinavir plasma concentrations). Products include:
Prevacid Delayed-Release Capsules 3268
Prevacid for Delayed-Release Oral Suspension 3268
Prevacid I.V. for Injection 3274
Prevacid NapraPAC 3277
Prevacid SoluTab Delayed-Release Orally Disintegrating Tablets 3268
PREVPAC 3281

Letrozole (Nelfinavir is metabolized by CYP3A and CYP2C19; co-administration of Viracept and drugs that inhibit CYP3A or CYP2C19 may increase nelfinavir plasma concentrations). Products include:
Femara Tablets 2210

Levonorgestrel (Nelfinavir is metabolized by CYP3A and CYP2C19; co-administration of Viracept and drugs that inhibit CYP3A or CYP2C19 may increase nelfinavir plasma concentrations). Products include:
Alesse-28 Tablets 3392
Climara Pro Transdermal System 800
Mirena Intrauterine System 810
Plan B Tablets 1068
Seasonale Tablets 1073
Triphasil-28 Tablets 3483

Lopinavir (Nelfinavir is metabolized by CYP3A and CYP2C19; co-administration of Viracept and drugs that inhibit CYP3A or CYP2C19 may increase nelfinavir plasma concentrations). Products include:
Kaletra 474

Lovastatin (Concurrent use is contraindicated). Products include:
Advicor Tablets 1694
Altoprev Extended-Release Tablets 1151
Mevacor Tablets 1996

Mestranol (Nelfinavir is metabolized by CYP3A and CYP2C19; co-administration of Viracept and drugs that inhibit CYP3A or CYP2C19 may increase nelfinavir plasma concentrations).
No products indexed under this heading.

Methylergonovine Maleate (Nelfinavir is an inhibitor of CYP3A and co-administration with drugs primarily metabolized by CYP3A, such as ergot derivatives, could result in competition for CYP3A by nelfinavir; inhibition of the metabolism of ergot derivatives could create a potential for serious cardiac arrhythmias or prolong adverse events; contraindicated due to potential for serious and/or life-threatening reactions, such as acute ergot toxicity characterized by peripheral vasospasm and ischemia of the extremities and other tissues).
No products indexed under this heading.

Methysergide Maleate (Nelfinavir is an inhibitor of CYP3A and co-administration with drugs primarily metabolized by CYP3A, such as ergot derivatives, could result in competition for CYP3A by nelfinavir; inhibition of the metabolism of ergot derivatives could create a potential for serious cardiac arrhythmias or prolong adverse events; contraindicated due to potential for serious and/or life-threatening reactions, such as acute ergot toxicity characterized by peripheral vasospasm and ischemia of the extremities and other tissues).
No products indexed under this heading.

Metronidazole (Nelfinavir is metabolized by CYP3A and CYP2C19; co-administration of Viracept and drugs that inhibit CYP3A or CYP2C19 may increase nelfinavir plasma concentrations). Products include:
Metrogel 1% 1212
MetroGel-Vaginal Gel 1822
Noritate Cream, 1% 1051

Metronidazole Benzoate (Nelfinavir is metabolized by CYP3A and CYP2C19; co-administration of Viracept and drugs that inhibit CYP3A or CYP2C19 may increase nelfinavir plasma concentrations).
No products indexed under this heading.

Metronidazole Hydrochloride (Nelfinavir is metabolized by CYP3A and CYP2C19; co-administration of Viracept and drugs that inhibit CYP3A or CYP2C19 may increase nelfinavir plasma concentrations).
No products indexed under this heading.

Miconazole (Nelfinavir is metabolized by CYP3A and CYP2C19; co-administration of Viracept and drugs that inhibit CYP3A or CYP2C19 may increase nelfinavir plasma concentrations).
No products indexed under this heading.

Midazolam Hydrochloride (Nelfinavir is an inhibitor of CYP3A and co-administration with drugs primarily metabolized by CYP3A, such as midazolam, could affect hepatic metabolism of midazolam; contraindicated due to potential for serious and/or life-threatening reactions, such as prolonged or increased sedation or respiratory depression).
No products indexed under this heading.

Modafinil (Nelfinavir is metabolized by CYP3A and CYP2C19; co-administration of Viracept and drugs that inhibit CYP3A or CYP2C19 may increase nelfinavir plasma concentrations). Products include:
Provigil Tablets 1002

Nefazodone Hydrochloride (Nelfinavir is metabolized by CYP3A and CYP2C19; co-administration of Viracept and drugs that inhibit CYP3A or CYP2C19 may increase nelfinavir plasma concentrations).
No products indexed under this heading.

Nevirapine (Nelfinavir is metabolized by CYP3A and CYP2C19; co-administration of Viracept and drugs that induce CYP3A or CYP2C19 may decrease nelfinavir plasma concentrations and reduce its therapeutic effect). Products include:
Viramune Oral Suspension 903
Viramune Tablets 903

Nicardipine Hydrochloride (Nelfinavir is an inhibitor of CYP450 3A enzymes which are responsible for the metabolism of dihydropyridine calcium channel blockers; co-administration may result in increased plasma concentrations of these calcium channel blockers). Products include:
Cardene I.V. 1129

Nifedipine (Nelfinavir is an inhibitor of CYP450 3A enzymes which are responsible for the metabolism of dihydropyridine calcium channel blockers; co-administration may

result in increased plasma concentrations of these calcium channel blockers). Products include:
Adalat CC Tablets 2978

Nimodipine (Nelfinavir is an inhibitor of CYP450 3A enzymes which are responsible for the metabolism of dihydropyridine calcium channel blockers; co-administration may result in increased plasma concentrations of these calcium channel blockers). Products include:
Nimotop Capsules 774

Norethindrone (Co-administration with oral contraceptives containing norethindrone results in decreased norethindrone AUC by approximately 18%; alternative or additional contraceptive measures should be used when oral contraceptives and Viracept are co-administered). Products include:
Ortho Micronor Tablets 2411

Norethindrone Acetate (Co-administration with oral contraceptives containing norethindrone results in decreased norethindrone AUC by approximately 18%; alternative or additional contraceptive measures should be used when oral contraceptives and Viracept are co-administered). Products include:
Activella Tablets 2311
Aygestin Tablets 1062
CombiPatch Transdermal System 2180

Norethynodrel (Nelfinavir is metabolized by CYP3A and CYP2C19; co-administration of Viracept and drugs that inhibit CYP3A or CYP2C19 may increase nelfinavir plasma concentrations).
No products indexed under this heading.

Norfloxacin (Nelfinavir is metabolized by CYP3A and CYP2C19; co-administration of Viracept and drugs that inhibit CYP3A or CYP2C19 may increase nelfinavir plasma concentrations). Products include:
Noroxin Tablets 2009

Norgestimate (Nelfinavir is metabolized by CYP3A and CYP2C19; co-administration of Viracept and drugs that inhibit CYP3A or CYP2C19 may increase nelfinavir plasma concentrations). Products include:
Ortho-Cyclen/Ortho Tri-Cyclen 2414
Ortho Tri-Cyclen Lo Tablets 2421
Prefest Tablets 1069

Norgestrel (Nelfinavir is metabolized by CYP3A and CYP2C19; co-administration of Viracept and drugs that inhibit CYP3A or CYP2C19 may increase nelfinavir plasma concentrations). Products include:
Lo/Ovral-28 Tablets 3423

Omeprazole (Nelfinavir is metabolized by CYP3A and CYP2C19; co-administration of Viracept and drugs that inhibit CYP3A or CYP2C19 may increase nelfinavir plasma concentrations). Products include:
Zegerid Powder for Oral Solution 2972

Oxcarbazepine (Nelfinavir is metabolized by CYP3A and CYP2C19; co-administration of Viracept and drugs that inhibit CYP3A or CYP2C19 may increase nelfinavir plasma concentrations). Products include:
Trileptal Oral Suspension 2281
Trileptal Tablets 2281

Paroxetine Hydrochloride (Nelfinavir is metabolized by CYP3A and CYP2C19; co-administration of Viracept and drugs that inhibit CYP3A or CYP2C19 may increase nelfinavir plasma concentrations). Products include:
Paxil CR Controlled-Release Tablets 1509
Paxil 1501

Phenobarbital (May decrease nelfinavir plasma concentrations; Viracept may not be effective due to decreased nelfinavir plasma concentrations in patients taking phenobarbital).
No products indexed under this heading.

Phenobarbital Sodium (Nelfinavir is metabolized by CYP3A and CYP2C19; co-administration of Viracept and drugs that induce CYP3A or CYP2C19 may decrease nelfinavir plasma concentrations and reduce its therapeutic effect).
No products indexed under this heading.

Phenytoin (May decrease nelfinavir plasma concentrations; Viracept may not be effective due to decreased nelfinavir plasma concentrations in patients taking phenytoin).
No products indexed under this heading.

Phenytoin Sodium (May decrease nelfinavir plasma concentrations; Viracept may not be effective due to decreased nelfinavir plasma concentrations in patients taking phenytoin). Products include:
Phenytek Capsules 2153

Pimozide (Concurrent use with nelfinavir is contraindicted due to potential for serious and/or life-threatening reactions, such as cardiac arrhythmias). Products include:
Orap Tablets 1220

Prednisone (Nelfinavir is metabolized by CYP3A and CYP2C19; co-administration of Viracept and drugs that induce CYP3A or CYP2C19 may decrease nelfinavir plasma concentrations and reduce its therapeutic effect).
No products indexed under this heading.

Quinidine (Nelfinavir is an inhibitor of CYP3A and co-administration with drugs primarily metabolized by CYP3A, such as quinidine, could result in competition for CYP3A by nelfinavir; contraindicated due to potential for serious and/or life-threatening reactions, such as cardiac arrhythmias).
No products indexed under this heading.

Quinidine Gluconate (Nelfinavir is an inhibitor of CYP3A and co-administration with drugs primarily metabolized by CYP3A, such as quinidine, could result in competition for CYP3A by nelfinavir; contraindicated due to potential for serious and/or life-threatening reactions, such as cardiac arrhythmias).
No products indexed under this heading.

Quinidine Hydrochloride (Nelfinavir is an inhibitor of CYP3A and co-administration with drugs primarily metabolized by CYP3A, such as quinidine, could result in competition for CYP3A by nelfinavir; contraindicated due to potential for serious and/or life-threatening reactions, such as cardiac arrhythmias).
No products indexed under this heading.

Quinidine Polygalacturonate (Nelfinavir is an inhibitor of CYP3A and co-administration with drugs primarily metabolized by CYP3A, such as quinidine, could result in competition for CYP3A by nelfinavir; contraindicated due to potential for serious and/or life-threatening reactions, such as cardiac arrhythmias).
No products indexed under this heading.

Quinidine Sulfate (Nelfinavir is an inhibitor of CYP3A and co-administration with drugs primarily metabolized by CYP3A, such as quinidine, could result in competition for CYP3A by nelfinavir; contraindicated due to potential for serious and/or life-threatening reactions, such as cardiac arrhythmias).
No products indexed under this heading.

Quinine (Nelfinavir is metabolized by CYP3A and CYP2C19; co-administration of Viracept and drugs that inhibit CYP3A or CYP2C19 may increase nelfinavir plasma concentrations).
No products indexed under this heading.

Quinine Sulfate (Nelfinavir is metabolized by CYP3A and CYP2C19; co-administration of Viracept and drugs that inhibit CYP3A or CYP2C19 may increase nelfinavir plasma concentrations).
No products indexed under this heading.

Rifabutin (It is recommended that the dose of rifabutin be reduced to one-half the usual dose when administered with nelfinavir; co-administration results in no change or a decrease in nelfinavir plasma concentrations (depending upon dosage) and increases in rifabutin plasma concentrations).
No products indexed under this heading.

Rifampicin (Nelfinavir is metabolized by CYP3A and CYP2C19; co-administration of Viracept and drugs that induce CYP3A or CYP2C19 may decrease nelfinavir plasma concentrations and reduce its therapeutic effect).
No products indexed under this heading.

Rifampin (Co-administration with rifampin results in decreased nelfinavir AUC and Cmax; may lead to loss of virologic response and possible resistance to nelfinavir or other co-administered antiretroviral agents).
No products indexed under this heading.

Rifapentine (Nelfinavir is metabolized by CYP3A and CYP2C19; co-administration of Viracept and drugs that induce CYP3A or CYP2C19 may decrease nelfinavir plasma concentrations and reduce its therapeutic effect).
No products indexed under this heading.

Ritonavir (Co-administration results in increased nelfinavir plasma concentrations; appropriate doses for this combination, with respect to safety and efficacy, have not been established). Products include:
Kaletra 474
Norvir 499

Saquinavir (Co-administration results in increase in saquinavir plasma concentrations; appropriate doses for this combination, with respect to safety and efficacy, have not been established).
No products indexed under this heading.

Saquinavir Mesylate (Co-administration results in increase in saquinavir plasma concentrations; appropriate doses for this combination, with respect to safety and efficacy, have not been established). Products include:
Invirase 2776

Sertraline Hydrochloride (Nelfinavir is metabolized by CYP3A and CYP2C19; co-administration of Viracept and drugs that inhibit CYP3A or CYP2C19 may increase nelfinavir plasma concentrations). Products include:
Zoloft 2581

Sildenafil Citrate (Co-administration of a protease inhibitor with sildenafil is expected to substantially increase sildenafil concentrations and may result in an increase in sildenafil-associated adverse events, including hypotension, visual changes, and priapism; sildenafil should not exceed a maximum single dose of 25 mg in a 48 hour period when administered in patients receiving protease inhibitors). Products include:
Revatio Tablets 2541
Viagra Tablets 2552

Simvastatin (Concurrent use is contraindicated). Products include:
Vytorin 10/10 Tablets 2084
Vytorin 10/10 Tablets 3092
Vytorin 10/20 Tablets 2084
Vytorin 10/20 Tablets 3092
Vytorin 10/40 Tablets 3092
Vytorin 10/40 Tablets 2084
Vytorin 10/80 Tablets 2084
Vytorin 10/80 Tablets 3092
Zocor Tablets 2078

Sirolimus (Nelfinavir is an inhibitor of CYP450 3A enzymes which are responsible for the metabolism of immunosuppressants, such as sirolimus; co-administration may result in increased plasma concentrations of immunosuppressants). Products include:
Rapamune Oral Solution and Tablets 3472

Sulfaphenazole (Nelfinavir is metabolized by CYP3A and CYP2C19; co-administration of Viracept and drugs that inhibit CYP3A or CYP2C19 may increase nelfinavir plasma concentrations).
No products indexed under this heading.

Tacrolimus (Nelfinavir is an inhibitor of CYP450 3A enzymes which are responsible for the metabolism of immunosuppressants, such as tacrolimus; co-administration may result in increased plasma concentrations of immunosuppressants). Products include:
Prograf Capsules and Injection 624
Protopic Ointment 629

Telmisartan (Nelfinavir is metabolized by CYP3A and CYP2C19; co-administration of Viracept and drugs that inhibit CYP3A or CYP2C19 may increase nelfinavir plasma concentrations). Products include:
Micardis Tablets 884
Micardis HCT Tablets 886

Ticlopidine Hydrochloride (Nelfinavir is metabolized by CYP3A and

CYP2C19; co-administration of Viracept and drugs that inhibit CYP3A or CYP2C19 may increase nelfinavir plasma concentrations). Products include:

Ticlid Tablets 2813

Tolbutamide (Nelfinavir is metabolized by CYP3A and CYP2C19; co-administration of Viracept and drugs that inhibit CYP3A or CYP2C19 may increase nelfinavir plasma concentrations).

No products indexed under this heading.

Tolbutamide Sodium (Nelfinavir is metabolized by CYP3A and CYP2C19; co-administration of Viracept and drugs that inhibit CYP3A or CYP2C19 may increase nelfinavir plasma concentrations).

No products indexed under this heading.

Topiramate (Nelfinavir is metabolized by CYP3A and CYP2C19; co-administration of Viracept and drugs that inhibit CYP3A or CYP2C19 may increase nelfinavir plasma concentrations). Products include:

Topamax Sprinkle Capsules 2438
Topamax Tablets 2438

Triazolam (Nelfinavir is an inhibitor of CYP3A and co-administration with drugs primarily metabolized by CYP3A, such as triazolam, could affect hepatic metabolism of triazolam; contraindicated due to potential for serious and/or life-threatening reactions, such as prolonged or increased sedation or respiratory depression).

No products indexed under this heading.

Troleandomycin (Nelfinavir is metabolized by CYP3A and CYP2C19; co-administration of Viracept and drugs that inhibit CYP3A or CYP2C19 may increase nelfinavir plasma concentrations).

No products indexed under this heading.

Venlafaxine Hydrochloride (Nelfinavir is metabolized by CYP3A and CYP2C19; co-administration of Viracept and drugs that inhibit CYP3A or CYP2C19 may increase nelfinavir plasma concentrations). Products include:

Effexor Tablets 3405
Effexor XR Capsules 3411

Verapamil Hydrochloride (Nelfinavir is metabolized by CYP3A and CYP2C19; co-administration of Viracept and drugs that inhibit CYP3A or CYP2C19 may increase nelfinavir plasma concentrations). Products include:

Covera-HS Tablets 3135
Tarka Tablets 519
Verelan PM Capsules 3120

Voriconazole (Nelfinavir is metabolized by CYP3A and CYP2C19; co-administration of Viracept and drugs that inhibit CYP3A or CYP2C19 may increase nelfinavir plasma concentrations). Products include:

VFEND I.V. 2543
VFEND Oral Suspension 2543
VFEND Tablets 2543

Zafirlukast (Nelfinavir is metabolized by CYP3A and CYP2C19; co-administration of Viracept and drugs that inhibit CYP3A or CYP2C19 may increase nelfinavir plasma concentrations). Products include:

Accolate Tablets 663

Zidovudine (Nelfinavir decreases zidovudine's AUC and Cmax by 35% and 31%, respectively). Products include:

Combivir Tablets 1373
Retrovir 1533
Retrovir IV Infusion 1537
Trizivir Tablets 1565

Zileuton (Nelfinavir is metabolized by CYP3A and CYP2C19; co-administration of Viracept and drugs that inhibit CYP3A or CYP2C19 may increase nelfinavir plasma concentrations).

No products indexed under this heading.

Food Interactions

Food, unspecified (Maximum plasma concentrations and AUC were 2- to 3-fold higher under fed conditions compared to fasting; Viracept should be taken with a meal or light snack).

Grapefruit (Nelfinavir is metabolized by CYP3A and CYP2C19; co-administration of Viracept and drugs that inhibit CYP3A or CYP2C19 may increase nelfinavir plasma concentrations).

VIRAMUNE ORAL SUSPENSION

(Nevirapine) 903

See Viramune Tablets

VIRAMUNE TABLETS

(Nevirapine) 903

May interact with antiarrhythmics, azole antifungals, calcium channel blockers, antineoplastics, anticoagulants, anticonvulsants, ergot-containing drugs, drugs affecting gastrointestinal motility, immunosuppressive agents, narcotic analgesics, oral contraceptives, and certain other agents. Compounds in these categories include:

Acebutolol Hydrochloride (Plasma concentrations of antiarrhythmics may be decreased by co-administration with nevirapine. Dose adjustment of co-administered drug may be needed due to possible decrease in clinical effect).

No products indexed under this heading.

Adenosine (Plasma concentrations of antiarrhythmics may be decreased by co-administration with nevirapine. Dose adjustment of co-administered drug may be needed due to possible decrease in clinical effect). Products include:

Adenocard Injection 612
Adenoscan 613

Albuterol (Plasma concentrations of GI motility agents may be decreased by co-administration with nevirapine. Dose adjustment of co-administered drug may be needed due to possible decrease in clinical effect). Products include:

Proventil Inhalation Aerosol 3067

Albuterol Sulfate (Plasma concentrations of GI motility agents may be decreased by co-administration with nevirapine. Dose adjustment of co-administered drug may be needed due to possible decrease in clinical effect). Products include:

AccuNeb Inhalation Solution 1055
Combivent Inhalation Aerosol 878
DuoNeb Inhalation Solution 1058
Proventil Inhalation Solution 0.083% 3069
Proventil HFA Inhalation Aerosol 3071
Ventolin HFA Inhalation Aerosol 1576
VoSpire Extended-Release Tablets ... 2352

Alfentanil Hydrochloride (Plasma concentrations of GI motility agents may be decreased by co-administration with nevirapine. Dose adjustment of co-administered drug may be needed due to possible decrease in clinical effect).

No products indexed under this heading.

Altretamine (Plasma concentrations of cancer chemotherapeutic agents may be decreased by co-administration with nevirapine. Dose adjustment of co-administered drug may be needed due to possible decrease in clinical effect). Products include:

Hexalen Capsules 2101

Amiodarone Hydrochloride (Plasma concentrations of antiarrhythmics may be decreased by co-administration with nevirapine. Dose adjustment of co-administered drug may be needed due to possible decrease in clinical effect). Products include:

Pacerone Tablets 3337

Amitriptyline Hydrochloride (Plasma concentrations of GI motility agents may be decreased by co-administration with nevirapine. Dose adjustment of co-administered drug may be needed due to possible decrease in clinical effect).

No products indexed under this heading.

Amlodipine Besylate (Plasma concentrations of calcium channel blockers may be decreased by co-administration with nevirapine. Dose adjustment of co-administered drug may be needed due to possible decrease in clinical effect). Products include:

Caduet Tablets 2507
Lotrel Capsules 2238
Norvasc Tablets 2529

Amoxapine (Plasma concentrations of GI motility agents may be decreased by co-administration with nevirapine. Dose adjustment of co-administered drug may be needed due to possible decrease in clinical effect).

No products indexed under this heading.

Anastrozole (Plasma concentrations of cancer chemotherapeutic agents may be decreased by co-administration with nevirapine. Dose adjustment of co-administered drug may be needed due to possible decrease in clinical effect). Products include:

Arimidex Tablets 665

Anisindione (Plasma concentrations of antithrombotics may be increased by co-administration with nevirapine. Dose adjustment of co-administered drug may be needed due to possible decrease in clinical effect). Products include:

Miradon Tablets 3056

Ardeparin Sodium (Plasma concentrations of antithrombotics may be increased by co-administration with nevirapine. Dose adjustment of co-administered drug may be needed due to possible decrease in clinical effect).

No products indexed under this heading.

Asparaginase (Plasma concentrations of cancer chemotherapeutic agents may be decreased by co-administration with nevirapine. Dose adjustment of co-administered drug may be needed due to possible decrease in clinical effect). Products include:

Elspar for Injection 1943

Astemizole (Plasma concentrations of GI motility agents may be decreased by co-administration with nevirapine. Dose adjustment of co-administered drug may be needed due to possible decrease in clinical effect).

No products indexed under this heading.

Atropine Sulfate (Plasma concentrations of GI motility agents may be decreased by co-administration with nevirapine. Dose adjustment of co-administered drug may be needed due to possible decrease in clinical effect).

No products indexed under this heading.

Azatadine Maleate (Plasma concentrations of GI motility agents may be decreased by co-administration with nevirapine. Dose adjustment of co-administered drug may be needed due to possible decrease in clinical effect).

No products indexed under this heading.

Azathioprine (Plasma concentrations of immunosuppressants may be decreased by co-administration with nevirapine. Dose adjustment of co-administered drug may be needed due to possible decrease in clinical effect). Products include:

Azasan Tablets 2844

Basiliximab (Plasma concentrations of immunosuppressants may be decreased by co-administration with nevirapine. Dose adjustment of co-administered drug may be needed due to possible decrease in clinical effect). Products include:

Simulect for Injection 2268

Belladonna Alkaloids (Plasma concentrations of GI motility agents may be decreased by co-administration with nevirapine. Dose adjustment of co-administered drug may be needed due to possible decrease in clinical effect). Products include:

Hyland's Teething Tablets .... ■ 736

Benztropine Mesylate (Plasma concentrations of GI motility agents may be decreased by co-administration with nevirapine. Dose adjustment of co-administered drug may be needed due to possible decrease in clinical effect). Products include:

Cogentin Injection 1903

Bepridil Hydrochloride (Plasma concentrations of calcium channel blockers may be decreased by co-administration with nevirapine. Dose adjustment of co-administered drug may be needed due to possible decrease in clinical effect).

No products indexed under this heading.

Bethanechol Chloride (Plasma concentrations of GI motility agents may be decreased by co-administration with nevirapine. Dose adjustment of co-administered drug may be needed due to possible decrease in clinical effect). Products include:

Urecholine Tablets 2349

Bicalutamide (Plasma concentrations of cancer chemotherapeutic agents may be decreased by co-administration with nevirapine. Dose

adjustment of co-administered drug may be needed due to possible decrease in clinical effect). Products include:
- Casodex Tablets 670

Biperiden Hydrochloride (Plasma concentrations of GI motility agents may be decreased by co-administration with nevirapine. Dose adjustment of co-administered drug may be needed due to possible decrease in clinical effect).
No products indexed under this heading.

Bitolterol Mesylate (Plasma concentrations of GI motility agents may be decreased by co-administration with nevirapine. Dose adjustment of co-administered drug may be needed due to possible decrease in clinical effect).
No products indexed under this heading.

Bleomycin Sulfate (Plasma concentrations of cancer chemotherapeutic agents may be decreased by co-administration with nevirapine. Dose adjustment of co-administered drug may be needed due to possible decrease in clinical effect).
No products indexed under this heading.

Bretylium Tosylate (Plasma concentrations of antiarrhythmics may be decreased by co-administration with nevirapine. Dose adjustment of co-administered drug may be needed due to possible decrease in clinical effect).
No products indexed under this heading.

Bromocriptine Mesylate (Plasma concentrations of GI motility agents may be decreased by co-administration with nevirapine. Dose adjustment of co-administered drug may be needed due to possible decrease in clinical effect).
No products indexed under this heading.

Bromodiphenhydramine Hydrochloride (Plasma concentrations of GI motility agents may be decreased by co-administration with nevirapine. Dose adjustment of co-administered drug may be needed due to possible decrease in clinical effect).
No products indexed under this heading.

Brompheniramine Maleate (Plasma concentrations of GI motility agents may be decreased by co-administration with nevirapine. Dose adjustment of co-administered drug may be needed due to possible decrease in clinical effect). Products include:
- Alacol DM Syrup 739
- Children's Dimetapp Cold & Allergy Elixir .... ■745
- Children's Dimetapp DM Cold & Cough Elixir .... ■745
- Robitussin Allergy & Cough Syrup .. ■750

Buprenorphine Hydrochloride (Plasma concentrations of GI motility agents may be decreased by co-administration with nevirapine. Dose adjustment of co-administered drug may be needed due to possible decrease in clinical effect). Products include:
- Buprenex Injectable 2718
- Suboxone Tablets 2719
- Subutex Tablets 2719

Busulfan (Plasma concentrations of cancer chemotherapeutic agents may be decreased by co-administration with nevirapine. Dose adjustment of co-administered drug may be needed due to possible decrease in clinical effect). Products include:
- I.V. Busulfex 1125
- Myleran Tablets 1492

Carbamazepine (Plasma concentrations of anticonvulsants may be decreased by co-administration with nevirapine. Dose adjustment of co-administered drug may be needed due to possible decrease in clinical effect). Products include:
- Carbatrol Capsules 3174
- Equetro Extended-Release Capsules 3178
- Tegretol/Tegretol-XR 2278

Carboplatin (Plasma concentrations of cancer chemotherapeutic agents may be decreased by co-administration with nevirapine. Dose adjustment of co-administered drug may be needed due to possible decrease in clinical effect).
No products indexed under this heading.

Carmustine (BCNU) (Plasma concentrations of cancer chemotherapeutic agents may be decreased by co-administration with nevirapine. Dose adjustment of co-administered drug may be needed due to possible decrease in clinical effect).
No products indexed under this heading.

Cevimeline Hydrochloride (Plasma concentrations of GI motility agents may be decreased by co-administration with nevirapine. Dose adjustment of co-administered drug may be needed due to possible decrease in clinical effect). Products include:
- Evoxac Capsules 1042

Chlorambucil (Plasma concentrations of cancer chemotherapeutic agents may be decreased by co-administration with nevirapine. Dose adjustment of co-administered drug may be needed due to possible decrease in clinical effect). Products include:
- Leukeran Tablets 1472

Chlorpheniramine Maleate (Plasma concentrations of GI motility agents may be decreased by co-administration with nevirapine. Dose adjustment of co-administered drug may be needed due to possible decrease in clinical effect). Products include:
- Advil Allergy Sinus Caplets .... ■737
- Advil Multi-Symptom Cold Caplets .... ■738
- BC Allergy Sinus Cold Powder .... ■612
- Contac Severe Cold and Flu Caplets Maximum Strength .... ■615
- Hycomine Compound Tablets 1105
- PediaCare Multi-Symptom Cold Liquid .... ■704
- PediaCare NightRest Cough & Cold Liquid .... ■704
- Robitussin Flu Liquid .... ■752
- Robitussin PM Cough & Cold Liquid .... ■752
- Singlet Caplets .... ■636
- Sudafed Sinus & Allergy Tablets ..... ■710
- TheraFlu Cold & Cough Hot Liquid .... ■680
- TheraFlu Cold & Sore Throat Hot Liquid .... ■680
- TheraFlu Flu & Sore Throat Hot Liquid .... ■681
- TheraFlu Severe Cold & Cough Hot Liquid .... ■683
- TheraFlu Severe Cold Caplets .... ■679
- TheraFlu Severe Cold Hot Liquid .... ■682
- Triaminic Cold & Allergy Liquid .... ■685
- Triaminic Cold & Cough Liquid .... ■685
- Triaminic Flu, Cough & Fever Liquid .... ■685
- Triaminic Night Time Cough & Cold Liquid .... ■685
- Triaminic Allergy Runny Nose & Congestion Softchews .... ■688
- Triaminic Cold & Cough Softchews .... ■688
- Children's Tylenol Plus Cold NightTime Suspension Liquid 1851
- Children's Tylenol Plus Cold & Cough Suspension Liquid and Chewable Tablets 1851
- Children's Tylenol Plus Cold Chewable Tablets 1851
- Children's Tylenol Plus Flu Suspension Liquid 1853
- Tylenol Allergy Complete Multi-Symptom Caplets and Gelcaps with Cool Burst 1844
- Multi-Symptom Tylenol Cold Night Time Caplets 1845
- Vicks 44M Cough, Cold & Flu Relief 2676
- Pediatric Vicks 44m Cough & Cold Relief 2673
- Children's Vicks NyQuil Cold/Cough Relief 2671

Chlorpheniramine Polistirex (Plasma concentrations of GI motility agents may be decreased by co-administration with nevirapine. Dose adjustment of co-administered drug may be needed due to possible decrease in clinical effect). Products include:
- Tussionex Pennkinetic Extended-Release Suspension 3322

Chlorpheniramine Tannate (Plasma concentrations of GI motility agents may be decreased by co-administration with nevirapine. Dose adjustment of co-administered drug may be needed due to possible decrease in clinical effect).
No products indexed under this heading.

Cisapride (Plasma concentrations of GI motility agents may be decreased by co-administration with nevirapine. Dose adjustment of co-administered drug may be needed due to possible decrease in clinical effect).
No products indexed under this heading.

Cisplatin (Plasma concentrations of cancer chemotherapeutic agents may be decreased by co-administration with nevirapine. Dose adjustment of co-administered drug may be needed due to possible decrease in clinical effect).
No products indexed under this heading.

Clarithromycin (Clarithromycin exposure was significantly decreased by nevirapine; however, 14-OH-metabolite concentrations were increased. Because clarithromycin active metabolite has reduced activity against Mycobacterium Avium-Intracellulare Complex, overall activity against this pathogen may be altered. Alternatives to clarithromycin, such as azithromycin, should be considered). Products include:
- Biaxin/Biaxin XL 402
- PREVPAC 3281

Clemastine Fumarate (Plasma concentrations of GI motility agents may be decreased by co-administration with nevirapine. Dose adjustment of co-administered drug may be needed due to possible decrease in clinical effect).
No products indexed under this heading.

Clidinium Bromide (Plasma concentrations of GI motility agents may be decreased by co-administration with nevirapine. Dose adjustment of co-administered drug may be needed due to possible decrease in clinical effect).
No products indexed under this heading.

Clomipramine Hydrochloride (Plasma concentrations of GI motility agents may be decreased by co-administration with nevirapine. Dose adjustment of co-administered drug may be needed due to possible decrease in clinical effect).
No products indexed under this heading.

Clotrimazole (Plasma concentrations of antifungals may be decreased by co-administration with nevirapine. Dose adjustment of co-administered drug may be needed due to possible decrease in clinical effect). Products include:
- Lotrimin 3053
- Lotrisone 3054

Codeine Phosphate (Plasma concentrations of GI motility agents may be decreased by co-administration with nevirapine. Dose adjustment of co-administered drug may be needed due to possible decrease in clinical effect). Products include:
- Tylenol with Codeine 2461

Cyclophosphamide (Plasma concentrations of cancer chemotherapeutic agents may be decreased by co-administration with nevirapine. Dose adjustment of co-administered drug may be needed due to possible decrease in clinical effect).
No products indexed under this heading.

Cyclosporine (Plasma concentrations of immunosuppressants may be decreased by co-administration with nevirapine. Dose adjustment of co-administered drug may be needed due to possible decrease in clinical effect). Products include:
- Gengraf Capsules 458
- Neoral Soft Gelatin Capsules 2247
- Neoral Oral Solution 2247
- Restasis Ophthalmic Emulsion 570
- Sandimmune 2259

Cyproheptadine Hydrochloride (Plasma concentrations of GI motility agents may be decreased by co-administration with nevirapine. Dose adjustment of co-administered drug may be needed due to possible decrease in clinical effect).
No products indexed under this heading.

Dacarbazine (Plasma concentrations of cancer chemotherapeutic agents may be decreased by co-administration with nevirapine. Dose adjustment of co-administered drug may be needed due to possible decrease in clinical effect).
No products indexed under this heading.

Dalteparin Sodium (Plasma concentrations of antithrombotics may be increased by co-administration with nevirapine. Dose adjustment of co-administered drug may be needed due to possible decrease in clinical effect). Products include:
- Fragmin Injection 2638

Danaparoid Sodium (Plasma concentrations of antithrombotics may be increased by co-administration with nevirapine. Dose adjustment of co-administered drug may be needed due to possible decrease in clinical effect).
No products indexed under this heading.

Daunorubicin Citrate (Plasma concentrations of cancer chemotherapeutic agents may be decreased by co-administration with nevirapine. Dose adjustment of co-administered drug may be needed due to possible decrease in clinical effect).
No products indexed under this heading.

Daunorubicin Hydrochloride (Plasma concentrations of cancer chemotherapeutic agents may be decreased by co-administration with nevirapine. Dose adjustment of co-administered drug may be needed due to possible decrease in clinical effect). Products include:
Cerubidine for Injection **788**

Denileukin Diftitox (Plasma concentrations of cancer chemotherapeutic agents may be decreased by co-administration with nevirapine. Dose adjustment of co-administered drug may be needed due to possible decrease in clinical effect). Products include:
Ontak Vials **1717**

Desipramine Hydrochloride (Plasma concentrations of GI motility agents may be decreased by co-administration with nevirapine. Dose adjustment of co-administered drug may be needed due to possible decrease in clinical effect).
No products indexed under this heading.

Desogestrel (Oral contraceptives and other hormonal methods of birth control should not be used as the sole method of contraception in women taking nevirapine, may lower plasma levels of these medications. An alternative or additional method of contraception is recommended). Products include:
Ortho-Cept Tablets **2395**

Dexchlorpheniramine Maleate (Plasma concentrations of GI motility agents may be decreased by co-administration with nevirapine. Dose adjustment of co-administered drug may be needed due to possible decrease in clinical effect).
No products indexed under this heading.

Dezocine (Plasma concentrations of GI motility agents may be decreased by co-administration with nevirapine. Dose adjustment of co-administered drug may be needed due to possible decrease in clinical effect).
No products indexed under this heading.

Dicumarol (Plasma concentrations of antithrombotics may be increased by co-administration with nevirapine. Dose adjustment of co-administered drug may be needed due to possible decrease in clinical effect).
No products indexed under this heading.

Dicyclomine Hydrochloride (Plasma concentrations of GI motility agents may be decreased by co-administration with nevirapine. Dose adjustment of co-administered drug may be needed due to possible decrease in clinical effect). Products include:
Bentyl Capsules **724**
Bentyl Injection **724**
Bentyl Syrup **724**
Bentyl Tablets **724**

Dihydroergotamine Mesylate (Plasma concentrations of ergot alkaloids may be decreased by co-administration with nevirapine. Dose adjustment of co-administered drug may be needed due to possible decrease in clinical effect). Products include:
Migranal Nasal Spray **3350**

Diltiazem Hydrochloride (Plasma concentrations of calcium channel blockers may be decreased by co-administration with nevirapine. Dose adjustment of co-administered drug may be needed due to possible decrease in clinical effect). Products include:
Cardizem LA Extended Release Tablets **1699**
Tiazac Capsules **1204**

Diphenhydramine Citrate (Plasma concentrations of GI motility agents may be decreased by co-administration with nevirapine. Dose adjustment of co-administered drug may be needed due to possible decrease in clinical effect). Products include:
Children's Benadryl Allergy & Cold Fastmelt Tablets................. ■ **695**
Children's Benadryl D Allergy & Sinus Fastmelt Tablets............... ■ **694**
Children's Benadryl Allergy Fastmelt Tablets .... ■ **696**
Goody's PM Powder .... ■ **622**

Diphenhydramine Hydrochloride (Plasma concentrations of GI motility agents may be decreased by co-administration with nevirapine. Dose adjustment of co-administered drug may be needed due to possible decrease in clinical effect). Products include:
Benadryl Allergy & Cold Tablets ..... ■ **692**
Benadryl Allergy .... ■ **691**
Benadryl Allergy & Sinus Headache Caplets & Gelcaps...... ■ **693**
Children's Benadryl Allergy Liquid ... ■ **695**
Children's Benadryl Dye-Free Allergy Liquid .... ■ **695**
Benadryl Dye-Free Allergy Liqui-Gels Softgels.................... ■ **692**
Benadryl Itch Relief Stick Extra Strength .... ■ **696**
Benadryl Itch Stopping Cream Extra Strength .... ■ **697**
Benadryl Itch Stopping Gel Extra Strength .... ■ **697**
Benadryl Itch Stopping Spray Extra Strength .... ■ **697**
Benadryl Maximum Strength Severe Allergy & Sinus Headache Caplets....................... ■ **694**
Children's Benadryl D Liquid Medication................................ ■ **693**
Benadryl D Tablets .... ■ **694**
Nytol QuickCaps Caplets .... ■ **635**
Maximum Strength Nytol QuickGels Softgels .... ■ **635**
Simply Sleep Caplets **1841**
Sominex Original Formula Tablets .. ■ **637**
TheraFlu Thin Strips Multi Symptom.................................. ■ **684**
Triaminic Thin Strips Cough & Runny Nose .... ■ **690**
Children's Tylenol Plus Cold & Allergy Suspension Liquid............ **1850**
Tylenol Allergy Complete Night Time Caplets **1844**
Tylenol Severe Allergy Caplets **1844**
Tylenol Flu NightTime Gelcaps **1846**
Extra Strength Tylenol PM Caplets, Geltabs, Gelcaps and Liquid.. **1847**
Unisom Maximum Strength SleepGels.................................. ■ **712**

Diphenylpyraline Hydrochloride (Plasma concentrations of GI motility agents may be decreased by co-administration with nevirapine. Dose adjustment of co-administered drug may be needed due to possible decrease in clinical effect).
No products indexed under this heading.

Disopyramide Phosphate (Plasma concentrations of antiarrhythmics may be decreased by co-administration with nevirapine. Dose adjustment of co-administered drug may be needed due to possible decrease in clinical effect).
No products indexed under this heading.

Divalproex Sodium (Plasma concentrations of anticonvulsants may be decreased by co-administration with nevirapine. Dose adjustment of co-administered drug may be needed due to possible decrease in clinical effect). Products include:
Depakote Sprinkle Capsules **422**
Depakote Tablets **427**
Depakote ER Tablets **433**

Dobutamine (Plasma concentrations of GI motility agents may be decreased by co-administration with nevirapine. Dose adjustment of co-administered drug may be needed due to possible decrease in clinical effect).
No products indexed under this heading.

Dobutamine Hydrochloride (Plasma concentrations of GI motility agents may be decreased by co-administration with nevirapine. Dose adjustment of co-administered drug may be needed due to possible decrease in clinical effect).
No products indexed under this heading.

Docetaxel (Plasma concentrations of cancer chemotherapeutic agents may be decreased by co-administration with nevirapine. Dose adjustment of co-administered drug may be needed due to possible decrease in clinical effect). Products include:
Taxotere Injection Concentrate **2947**

Dofetilide (Plasma concentrations of antiarrhythmics may be decreased by co-administration with nevirapine. Dose adjustment of co-administered drug may be needed due to possible decrease in clinical effect).
No products indexed under this heading.

Domperidone (Plasma concentrations of GI motility agents may be decreased by co-administration with nevirapine. Dose adjustment of co-administered drug may be needed due to possible decrease in clinical effect).
No products indexed under this heading.

Donepezil Hydrochloride (Plasma concentrations of GI motility agents may be decreased by co-administration with nevirapine. Dose adjustment of co-administered drug may be needed due to possible decrease in clinical effect). Products include:
Aricept Tablets **1086**
Aricept ODT Tablets **1086**

Dopamine Hydrochloride (Plasma concentrations of GI motility agents may be decreased by co-administration with nevirapine. Dose adjustment of co-administered drug may be needed due to possible decrease in clinical effect).
No products indexed under this heading.

Doxepin Hydrochloride (Plasma concentrations of GI motility agents may be decreased by co-administration with nevirapine. Dose adjustment of co-administered drug may be needed due to possible decrease in clinical effect).
No products indexed under this heading.

Doxorubicin Hydrochloride (Plasma concentrations of cancer chemotherapeutic agents may be decreased by co-administration with nevirapine. Dose adjustment of co-administered drug may be needed due to possible decrease in clinical effect). Products include:
Adriamycin for Injection, USP **786**
Adriamycin Injection, USP **786**

Edrophonium Chloride (Plasma concentrations of GI motility agents may be decreased by co-administration with nevirapine. Dose adjustment of co-administered drug may be needed due to possible decrease in clinical effect).
No products indexed under this heading.

Efavirenz (Efavirenz plasma concentration levels are decreased when used concomitantly with nevirapine. Appropriate doses for this combination are not established). Products include:
Sustiva Capsules **957**

Enoxaparin Sodium (Plasma concentrations of antithrombotics may be increased by co-administration with nevirapine. Dose adjustment of co-administered drug may be needed due to possible decrease in clinical effect). Products include:
Lovenox Injection **2931**

Ephedrine Hydrochloride (Plasma concentrations of GI motility agents may be decreased by co-administration with nevirapine. Dose adjustment of co-administered drug may be needed due to possible decrease in clinical effect). Products include:
Primatene Tablets .... ■ **749**

Ephedrine Sulfate (Plasma concentrations of GI motility agents may be decreased by co-administration with nevirapine. Dose adjustment of co-administered drug may be needed due to possible decrease in clinical effect).
No products indexed under this heading.

Ephedrine Tannate (Plasma concentrations of GI motility agents may be decreased by co-administration with nevirapine. Dose adjustment of co-administered drug may be needed due to possible decrease in clinical effect).
No products indexed under this heading.

Epinephrine (Plasma concentrations of GI motility agents may be decreased by co-administration with nevirapine. Dose adjustment of co-administered drug may be needed due to possible decrease in clinical effect). Products include:
EpiPen **1061**

Primatene Mist .... ▭749

Epinephrine Hydrochloride (Plasma concentrations of GI motility agents may be decreased by co-administration with nevirapine. Dose adjustment of co-administered drug may be needed due to possible decrease in clinical effect).
No products indexed under this heading.

Epirubicin Hydrochloride (Plasma concentrations of cancer chemotherapeutic agents may be decreased by co-administration with nevirapine. Dose adjustment of co-administered drug may be needed due to possible decrease in clinical effect). Products include:
Ellence Injection 2632

Ergonovine Maleate (Plasma concentrations of ergot alkaloids may be decreased by co-administration with nevirapine. Dose adjustment of co-administered drug may be needed due to possible decrease in clinical effect).
No products indexed under this heading.

Ergotamine Tartrate (Plasma concentrations of ergot alkaloids may be decreased by co-administration with nevirapine. Dose adjustment of co-administered drug may be needed due to possible decrease in clinical effect).
No products indexed under this heading.

Erythromycin (Plasma concentrations of GI motility agents may be decreased by co-administration with nevirapine. Dose adjustment of co-administered drug may be needed due to possible decrease in clinical effect). Products include:
Erygel Topical Gel 2096
Ery-Tab Tablets 447
Erythromycin Base Filmtab Tablets 454
Erythromycin Delayed-Release Capsules, USP 456
PCE Dispertab Tablets 510

Erythromycin Estolate (Plasma concentrations of GI motility agents may be decreased by co-administration with nevirapine. Dose adjustment of co-administered drug may be needed due to possible decrease in clinical effect).
No products indexed under this heading.

Erythromycin Ethylsuccinate (Plasma concentrations of GI motility agents may be decreased by co-administration with nevirapine. Dose adjustment of co-administered drug may be needed due to possible decrease in clinical effect). Products include:
E.E.S. 449
EryPed 445

Erythromycin Gluceptate (Plasma concentrations of GI motility agents may be decreased by co-administration with nevirapine. Dose adjustment of co-administered drug may be needed due to possible decrease in clinical effect).
No products indexed under this heading.

Erythromycin Stearate (Plasma concentrations of GI motility agents may be decreased by co-administration with nevirapine. Dose adjustment of co-administered drug may be needed due to possible decrease in clinical effect). Products include:
Erythrocin Stearate Filmtab Tablets 452

Estramustine Phosphate Sodium (Plasma concentrations of cancer chemotherapeutic agents may be decreased by co-administration with nevirapine. Dose adjustment of co-administered drug may be needed due to possible decrease in clinical effect). Products include:
Emcyt Capsules 3137

Ethinyl Estradiol (When ethinyl estradiol and Viramune are co-administered, the AUC for ethinyl estradiol is decreased by 20%). Products include:
Alesse-28 Tablets 3392
Lo/Ovral-28 Tablets 3423
NuvaRing 2357
Ortho-Cept Tablets 2395
Ortho-Cyclen/Ortho Tri-Cyclen 2414
Ortho Evra Transdermal System 2402
Ortho Tri-Cyclen Lo Tablets 2421
Seasonale Tablets 1073
Triphasil-28 Tablets 3483
Yasmin 28 Tablets 818

Ethosuximide (Plasma concentrations of anticonvulsants may be decreased by co-administration with nevirapine. Dose adjustment of co-administered drug may be needed due to possible decrease in clinical effect).
No products indexed under this heading.

Ethotoin (Plasma concentrations of anticonvulsants may be decreased by co-administration with nevirapine. Dose adjustment of co-administered drug may be needed due to possible decrease in clinical effect). Products include:
Peganone Tablets, USP 2487

Ethynodiol Diacetate (Oral contraceptives and other hormonal methods of birth control should not be used as the sole method of contraception in women taking nevirapine, may lower plasma levels of these medications. An alternative or additional method of contraception is recommended).
No products indexed under this heading.

Etoposide (Plasma concentrations of cancer chemotherapeutic agents may be decreased by co-administration with nevirapine. Dose adjustment of co-administered drug may be needed due to possible decrease in clinical effect).
No products indexed under this heading.

Exemestane (Plasma concentrations of cancer chemotherapeutic agents may be decreased by co-administration with nevirapine. Dose adjustment of co-administered drug may be needed due to possible decrease in clinical effect). Products include:
Aromasin Tablets 2600

Felbamate (Plasma concentrations of anticonvulsants may be decreased by co-administration with nevirapine. Dose adjustment of co-administered drug may be needed due to possible decrease in clinical effect).
No products indexed under this heading.

Felodipine (Plasma concentrations of calcium channel blockers may be decreased by co-administration with nevirapine. Dose adjustment of co-administered drug may be needed due to possible decrease in clinical effect). Products include:
Plendil Extended-Release Tablets 651

Fentanyl (Plasma concentrations of GI motility agents may be decreased by co-administration with nevirapine. Dose adjustment of co-administered drug may be needed due to possible decrease in clinical effect). Products include:
Duragesic Transdermal System 2448

Fentanyl Citrate (Plasma concentrations of GI motility agents may be decreased by co-administration with nevirapine. Dose adjustment of co-administered drug may be needed due to possible decrease in clinical effect). Products include:
Actiq 993

Flecainide Acetate (Plasma concentrations of antiarrhythmics may be decreased by co-administration with nevirapine. Dose adjustment of co-administered drug may be needed due to possible decrease in clinical effect). Products include:
Tambocor Tablets 1824

Floxuridine (Plasma concentrations of cancer chemotherapeutic agents may be decreased by co-administration with nevirapine. Dose adjustment of co-administered drug may be needed due to possible decrease in clinical effect).
No products indexed under this heading.

Fluconazole (Administration of fluconazole resulted in an approximate 100% increase in nevirapine exposure, based on a comparison to historic data. Because of the risk of increased exposure to nevirapine, caution should be used in concomitant administration, and patients should be monitored closely for nevirapine associated adverse events).
No products indexed under this heading.

Fluorouracil (Plasma concentrations of cancer chemotherapeutic agents may be decreased by co-administration with nevirapine. Dose adjustment of co-administered drug may be needed due to possible decrease in clinical effect). Products include:
Carac Cream, 0.5% 1048
Efudex 3348

Flutamide (Plasma concentrations of cancer chemotherapeutic agents may be decreased by co-administration with nevirapine. Dose adjustment of co-administered drug may be needed due to possible decrease in clinical effect). Products include:
Eulexin Capsules 3023

Fondaparinux Sodium (Plasma concentrations of antithrombotics may be increased by co-administration with nevirapine. Dose adjustment of co-administered drug may be needed due to possible decrease in clinical effect). Products include:
Arixtra Injection 1325

Fosphenytoin (Plasma concentrations of anticonvulsants may be decreased by co-administration with nevirapine. Dose adjustment of co-administered drug may be needed due to possible decrease in clinical effect).
No products indexed under this heading.

Fosphenytoin Sodium (Plasma concentrations of anticonvulsants may be decreased by co-administration with nevirapine. Dose adjustment of co-administered drug may be needed due to possible decrease in clinical effect).
No products indexed under this heading.

Gabapentin (Plasma concentrations of anticonvulsants may be decreased by co-administration with nevirapine. Dose adjustment of co-administered drug may be needed due to possible decrease in clinical effect). Products include:
Neurontin Capsules 2498
Neurontin Oral Solution 2498
Neurontin Tablets 2498

Galantamine Hydrobromide (Plasma concentrations of GI motility agents may be decreased by co-administration with nevirapine. Dose adjustment of co-administered drug may be needed due to possible decrease in clinical effect). Products include:
Razadyne ER Extended-Release Capsules 2434
Razadyne 2434

Gemcitabine Hydrochloride (Plasma concentrations of cancer chemotherapeutic agents may be decreased by co-administration with nevirapine. Dose adjustment of co-administered drug may be needed due to possible decrease in clinical effect). Products include:
Gemzar for Injection 1743

Glycopyrrolate (Plasma concentrations of GI motility agents may be decreased by co-administration with nevirapine. Dose adjustment of co-administered drug may be needed due to possible decrease in clinical effect).
No products indexed under this heading.

Heparin Calcium (Plasma concentrations of antithrombotics may be increased by co-administration with nevirapine. Dose adjustment of co-administered drug may be needed due to possible decrease in clinical effect).
No products indexed under this heading.

Heparin Sodium (Plasma concentrations of antithrombotics may be increased by co-administration with nevirapine. Dose adjustment of co-administered drug may be needed due to possible decrease in clinical effect).
No products indexed under this heading.

Hydrocodone Bitartrate (Plasma concentrations of GI motility agents may be decreased by co-administration with nevirapine. Dose adjustment of co-administered drug may be needed due to possible decrease in clinical effect). Products include:
Hycodan 1104
Hycomine Compound Tablets 1105
Hycotuss Expectorant Syrup 1106
Lortab 3315
Lortab Elixir 3312
Vicodin Tablets 530
Vicodin ES Tablets 531
Vicodin HP Tablets 532
Vicoprofen Tablets 533
Zydone Tablets 1118

Hydrocodone Polistirex (Plasma concentrations of GI motility agents may be decreased by co-administration with nevirapine. Dose

adjustment of co-administered drug may be needed due to possible decrease in clinical effect). Products include:
Tussionex Pennkinetic Extended-Release Suspension 3322

Hydromorphone Hydrochloride (Plasma concentrations of GI motility agents may be decreased by co-administration with nevirapine. Dose adjustment of co-administered drug may be needed due to possible decrease in clinical effect). Products include:
Dilaudid 439
Dilaudid Oral Liquid 443
Dilaudid Non-Sterile Powder 439
Dilaudid Rectal Suppositories 439
Dilaudid Tablets 439
Dilaudid Tablets - 8 mg 443
Dilaudid-HP 441

Hydroxyurea (Plasma concentrations of cancer chemotherapeutic agents may be decreased by co-administration with nevirapine. Dose adjustment of co-administered drug may be needed due to possible decrease in clinical effect).
No products indexed under this heading.

Hyoscyamine (Plasma concentrations of GI motility agents may be decreased by co-administration with nevirapine. Dose adjustment of co-administered drug may be needed due to possible decrease in clinical effect).
No products indexed under this heading.

Hyoscyamine Sulfate (Plasma concentrations of GI motility agents may be decreased by co-administration with nevirapine. Dose adjustment of co-administered drug may be needed due to possible decrease in clinical effect).
No products indexed under this heading.

Idarubicin Hydrochloride (Plasma concentrations of cancer chemotherapeutic agents may be decreased by co-administration with nevirapine. Dose adjustment of co-administered drug may be needed due to possible decrease in clinical effect). Products include:
Idamycin PFS Injection 2645

Ifosfamide (Plasma concentrations of cancer chemotherapeutic agents may be decreased by co-administration with nevirapine. Dose adjustment of co-administered drug may be needed due to possible decrease in clinical effect).
No products indexed under this heading.

Imipramine Hydrochloride (Plasma concentrations of GI motility agents may be decreased by co-administration with nevirapine. Dose adjustment of co-administered drug may be needed due to possible decrease in clinical effect).
No products indexed under this heading.

Imipramine Pamoate (Plasma concentrations of GI motility agents may be decreased by co-administration with nevirapine. Dose adjustment of co-administered drug may be needed due to possible decrease in clinical effect).
No products indexed under this heading.

Indinavir Sulfate (Appropriate doses for this combination are not established, but an increase in the dosage of indinavir may be required). Products include:
Crixivan Capsules 1918

Interferon alfa-2a, Recombinant (Plasma concentrations of cancer chemotherapeutic agents may be decreased by co-administration with nevirapine. Dose adjustment of co-administered drug may be needed due to possible decrease in clinical effect). Products include:
Roferon-A Injection 2805

Interferon alfa-2b, Recombinant (Plasma concentrations of cancer chemotherapeutic agents may be decreased by co-administration with nevirapine. Dose adjustment of co-administered drug may be needed due to possible decrease in clinical effect). Products include:
Intron A for Injection 3038
Rebetron Combination Therapy 3078

Ipratropium Bromide (Plasma concentrations of GI motility agents may be decreased by co-administration with nevirapine. Dose adjustment of co-administered drug may be needed due to possible decrease in clinical effect). Products include:
Atrovent HFA Inhalation Aerosol 872
Atrovent Inhalation Solution 868
Atrovent Nasal Spray 0.03% 869
Atrovent Nasal Spray 0.06% 870
Combivent Inhalation Aerosol 878
DuoNeb Inhalation Solution 1058

Irinotecan Hydrochloride (Plasma concentrations of cancer chemotherapeutic agents may be decreased by co-administration with nevirapine. Dose adjustment of co-administered drug may be needed due to possible decrease in clinical effect). Products include:
Camptosar Injection 2602

Isoetharine (Plasma concentrations of GI motility agents may be decreased by co-administration with nevirapine. Dose adjustment of co-administered drug may be needed due to possible decrease in clinical effect).
No products indexed under this heading.

Isoproterenol Hydrochloride (Plasma concentrations of GI motility agents may be decreased by co-administration with nevirapine. Dose adjustment of co-administered drug may be needed due to possible decrease in clinical effect).
No products indexed under this heading.

Isoproterenol Sulfate (Plasma concentrations of GI motility agents may be decreased by co-administration with nevirapine. Dose adjustment of co-administered drug may be needed due to possible decrease in clinical effect).
No products indexed under this heading.

Isradipine (Plasma concentrations of calcium channel blockers may be decreased by co-administration with nevirapine. Dose adjustment of co-administered drug may be needed due to possible decrease in clinical effect). Products include:
DynaCirc CR Tablets 2726

Itraconazole (Plasma concentrations of antifungals may be decreased by co-administration with nevirapine. Dose adjustment of co-administered drug may be needed due to possible decrease in clinical effect).
No products indexed under this heading.

Ketoconazole (Nevirapine and ketoconazole should not be administered concomitantly because decreases in ketoconazole plasma concentrations may reduce the efficacy of the drug). Products include:
Nizoral A-D Shampoo, 1% 1839
Nizoral 2% Shampoo 1838

Lamotrigine (Plasma concentrations of anticonvulsants may be decreased by co-administration with nevirapine. Dose adjustment of co-administered drug may be needed due to possible decrease in clinical effect). Products include:
Lamictal 1449

Levalbuterol Hydrochloride (Plasma concentrations of GI motility agents may be decreased by co-administration with nevirapine. Dose adjustment of co-administered drug may be needed due to possible decrease in clinical effect). Products include:
Xopenex Inhalation Solution 3143
Xopenex Inhalation Solution Concentrate 3147

Levamisole Hydrochloride (Plasma concentrations of cancer chemotherapeutic agents may be decreased by co-administration with nevirapine. Dose adjustment of co-administered drug may be needed due to possible decrease in clinical effect).
No products indexed under this heading.

Levetiracetam (Plasma concentrations of anticonvulsants may be decreased by co-administration with nevirapine. Dose adjustment of co-administered drug may be needed due to possible decrease in clinical effect). Products include:
Keppra Oral Solution 3307
Keppra Tablets 3307

Levonorgestrel (Oral contraceptives and other hormonal methods of birth control should not be used as the sole method of contraception in women taking nevirapine, may lower plasma levels of these medications. An alternative or additional method of contraception is recommended). Products include:
Alesse-28 Tablets 3392
Climara Pro Transdermal System 800
Mirena Intrauterine System 810
Plan B Tablets 1068
Seasonale Tablets 1073
Triphasil-28 Tablets 3483

Levorphanol Tartrate (Plasma concentrations of GI motility agents may be decreased by co-administration with nevirapine. Dose adjustment of co-administered drug may be needed due to possible decrease in clinical effect).
No products indexed under this heading.

Lidocaine Hydrochloride (Plasma concentrations of antiarrhythmics may be decreased by co-administration with nevirapine. Dose adjustment of co-administered drug may be needed due to possible decrease in clinical effect).
No products indexed under this heading.

Lomustine (CCNU) (Plasma concentrations of cancer chemotherapeutic agents may be decreased by co-administration with nevirapine. Dose adjustment of co-administered drug may be needed due to possible decrease in clinical effect).
No products indexed under this heading.

Lopinavir (A dose increase of lopinavir/ritonavir to 533/133 mg twice daily with food is recommended in combination with nevirapine). Products include:
Kaletra 474

Low Molecular Weight Heparins (Plasma concentrations of antithrombotics may be increased by co-administration with nevirapine. Dose adjustment of co-administered drug may be needed due to possible decrease in clinical effect).
No products indexed under this heading.

Maprotiline Hydrochloride (Plasma concentrations of GI motility agents may be decreased by co-administration with nevirapine. Dose adjustment of co-administered drug may be needed due to possible decrease in clinical effect).
No products indexed under this heading.

Mechlorethamine Hydrochloride (Plasma concentrations of cancer chemotherapeutic agents may be decreased by co-administration with nevirapine. Dose adjustment of co-administered drug may be needed due to possible decrease in clinical effect). Products include:
Mustargen for Injection 2007

Megestrol Acetate (Plasma concentrations of cancer chemotherapeutic agents may be decreased by co-administration with nevirapine. Dose adjustment of co-administered drug may be needed due to possible decrease in clinical effect). Products include:
Megace ES Oral Suspension 2492

Melphalan (Plasma concentrations of cancer chemotherapeutic agents may be decreased by co-administration with nevirapine. Dose adjustment of co-administered drug may be needed due to possible decrease in clinical effect). Products include:
Alkeran Tablets 977

Mepenzolate Bromide (Plasma concentrations of GI motility agents may be decreased by co-administration with nevirapine. Dose adjustment of co-administered drug may be needed due to possible decrease in clinical effect).
No products indexed under this heading.

Meperidine Hydrochloride (Plasma concentrations of GI motility agents may be decreased by co-administration with nevirapine. Dose adjustment of co-administered drug may be needed due to possible decrease in clinical effect).
No products indexed under this heading.

Mephenytoin (Plasma concentrations of anticonvulsants may be decreased by co-administration with nevirapine. Dose adjustment of co-administered drug may be needed due to possible decrease in clinical effect).
No products indexed under this heading.

Mercaptopurine (Plasma concentrations of cancer chemotherapeutic agents may be decreased by co-administration with nevirapine. Dose adjustment of co-administered drug may be needed due to possible decrease in clinical effect). Products include:
Purinethol Tablets 1222

Mestranol (Oral contraceptives and other hormonal methods of birth control should not be used as the sole method of contraception in women taking nevirapine, may lower plasma levels of these medications. An alternative or additional method of contraception is recommended).
No products indexed under this heading.

Metaproterenol Sulfate (Plasma concentrations of GI motility agents may be decreased by co-administration with nevirapine. Dose adjustment of co-administered drug may be needed due to possible decrease in clinical effect). Products include:
Alupent Inhalation Aerosol 858

Methadone Hydrochloride (Methadone levels may be decreased; increased dosages may be required to prevent symptoms of opiate withdrawal. Methadone maintained patients beginning nevirapine therapy should be monitored for evidence of withdrawal and methadone dose should be adjusted accordingly).
No products indexed under this heading.

Methdilazine Hydrochloride (Plasma concentrations of GI motility agents may be decreased by co-administration with nevirapine. Dose adjustment of co-administered drug may be needed due to possible decrease in clinical effect).
No products indexed under this heading.

Methotrexate Sodium (Plasma concentrations of cancer chemotherapeutic agents may be decreased by co-administration with nevirapine. Dose adjustment of co-administered drug may be needed due to possible decrease in clinical effect).
No products indexed under this heading.

Methsuximide (Plasma concentrations of anticonvulsants may be decreased by co-administration with nevirapine. Dose adjustment of co-administered drug may be needed due to possible decrease in clinical effect).
No products indexed under this heading.

Methylergonovine Maleate (Plasma concentrations of ergot alkaloids may be decreased by co-administration with nevirapine. Dose adjustment of co-administered drug may be needed due to possible decrease in clinical effect).
No products indexed under this heading.

Methysergide Maleate (Plasma concentrations of ergot alkaloids may be decreased by co-administration with nevirapine. Dose adjustment of co-administered drug may be needed due to possible decrease in clinical effect).
No products indexed under this heading.

Metoclopramide Hydrochloride (Plasma concentrations of GI motility agents may be decreased by co-administration with nevirapine. Dose adjustment of co-administered drug may be needed due to possible decrease in clinical effect).
No products indexed under this heading.

Mexiletine Hydrochloride (Plasma concentrations of antiarrhythmics may be decreased by co-administration with nevirapine. Dose adjustment of co-administered drug may be needed due to possible decrease in clinical effect).
No products indexed under this heading.

Mibefradil Dihydrochloride (Plasma concentrations of calcium channel blockers may be decreased by co-administration with nevirapine. Dose adjustment of co-administered drug may be needed due to possible decrease in clinical effect).
No products indexed under this heading.

Miconazole (Plasma concentrations of antifungals may be decreased by co-administration with nevirapine. Dose adjustment of co-administered drug may be needed due to possible decrease in clinical effect).
No products indexed under this heading.

Mitomycin (Mitomycin-C) (Plasma concentrations of cancer chemotherapeutic agents may be decreased by co-administration with nevirapine. Dose adjustment of co-administered drug may be needed due to possible decrease in clinical effect).
No products indexed under this heading.

Mitotane (Plasma concentrations of cancer chemotherapeutic agents may be decreased by co-administration with nevirapine. Dose adjustment of co-administered drug may be needed due to possible decrease in clinical effect).
No products indexed under this heading.

Mitoxantrone Hydrochloride (Plasma concentrations of cancer chemotherapeutic agents may be decreased by co-administration with nevirapine. Dose adjustment of co-administered drug may be needed due to possible decrease in clinical effect). Products include:
Novantrone for Injection Concentrate 3158

Moricizine Hydrochloride (Plasma concentrations of antiarrhythmics may be decreased by co-administration with nevirapine. Dose adjustment of co-administered drug may be needed due to possible decrease in clinical effect).
No products indexed under this heading.

Morphine Sulfate (Plasma concentrations of GI motility agents may be decreased by co-administration with nevirapine. Dose adjustment of co-administered drug may be needed due to possible decrease in clinical effect). Products include:
Avinza Capsules 1714
Kadian Capsules 572
MS Contin Tablets 2703

Muromonab-CD3 (Plasma concentrations of immunosuppressants may be decreased by co-administration with nevirapine. Dose adjustment of co-administered drug may be needed due to possible decrease in clinical effect). Products include:
Orthoclone OKT3 Sterile Solution 2370

Mycophenolate Mofetil (Plasma concentrations of immunosuppressants may be decreased by co-administration with nevirapine. Dose adjustment of co-administered drug may be needed due to possible decrease in clinical effect). Products include:
CellCept Capsules 2751
CellCept Oral Suspension 2751
CellCept Tablets 2751

Nelfinavir Mesylate (When nelfinavir and Viramune are co-administered, the plasma concentrations of nelfinavir and the nelfinavir-M8 metabolite are decreased. The appropriate dose for nelfinavir in combination with nevirapine, with respect to safety and efficacy, has not been established). Products include:
Viracept 2556

Neostigmine Bromide (Plasma concentrations of GI motility agents may be decreased by co-administration with nevirapine. Dose adjustment of co-administered drug may be needed due to possible decrease in clinical effect).
No products indexed under this heading.

Neostigmine Methylsulfate (Plasma concentrations of GI motility agents may be decreased by co-administration with nevirapine. Dose adjustment of co-administered drug may be needed due to possible decrease in clinical effect).
No products indexed under this heading.

Nicardipine Hydrochloride (Plasma concentrations of calcium channel blockers may be decreased by co-administration with nevirapine. Dose adjustment of co-administered drug may be needed due to possible decrease in clinical effect). Products include:
Cardene I.V. 1129

Nifedipine (Plasma concentrations of calcium channel blockers may be decreased by co-administration with nevirapine. Dose adjustment of co-administered drug may be needed due to possible decrease in clinical effect). Products include:
Adalat CC Tablets 2978

Nimodipine (Plasma concentrations of calcium channel blockers may be decreased by co-administration with nevirapine. Dose adjustment of co-administered drug may be needed due to possible decrease in clinical effect). Products include:
Nimotop Capsules 774

Nisoldipine (Plasma concentrations of calcium channel blockers may be decreased by co-administration with nevirapine. Dose adjustment of co-administered drug may be needed due to possible decrease in clinical effect). Products include:
Sular Tablets 1163

Norethindrone (When norethindrone and Viramune are co-administered, the AUC and Cmax for norethindrone are decreased by 19% and 16%, respectively). Products include:
Ortho Micronor Tablets 2411

Norethynodrel (Oral contraceptives and other hormonal methods of birth control should not be used as the sole method of contraception in women taking nevirapine, may lower plasma levels of these medications. An alternative or additional method of contraception is recommended).
No products indexed under this heading.

Norgestimate (Oral contraceptives and other hormonal methods of birth control should not be used as the sole method of contraception in women taking nevirapine, may lower plasma levels of these medications. An alternative or additional method of contraception is recommended). Products include:
Ortho-Cyclen/Ortho Tri-Cyclen 2414
Ortho Tri-Cyclen Lo Tablets 2421
Prefest Tablets 1069

Norgestrel (Oral contraceptives and other hormonal methods of birth control should not be used as the sole method of contraception in women taking nevirapine, may lower plasma levels of these medications. An alternative or additional method of contraception is recommended). Products include:
Lo/Ovral-28 Tablets 3423

Nortriptyline Hydrochloride (Plasma concentrations of GI motility agents may be decreased by co-administration with nevirapine. Dose adjustment of co-administered drug may be needed due to possible decrease in clinical effect).
No products indexed under this heading.

Octreotide Acetate (Plasma concentrations of GI motility agents may be decreased by co-administration with nevirapine. Dose adjustment of co-administered drug may be needed due to possible decrease in clinical effect). Products include:
Sandostatin Injection 2263
Sandostatin LAR Depot 2264

Oxaliplatin (Plasma concentrations of cancer chemotherapeutic agents may be decreased by co-administration with nevirapine. Dose adjustment of co-administered drug may be needed due to possible decrease in clinical effect). Products include:
Eloxatin for Injection 2908

Oxcarbazepine (Plasma concentrations of anticonvulsants may be decreased by co-administration with nevirapine. Dose adjustment of co-administered drug may be needed due to possible decrease in clinical effect). Products include:
Trileptal Oral Suspension 2281
Trileptal Tablets 2281

Oxiconazole Nitrate (Plasma concentrations of antifungals may be decreased by co-administration with nevirapine. Dose adjustment of co-administered drug may be needed due to possible decrease in clinical effect). Products include:
Oxistat 1498

Oxybutynin Chloride (Plasma concentrations of GI motility agents may be decreased by co-administration with nevirapine. Dose adjustment of co-administered drug may be needed due to possible decrease in clinical effect). Products include:
Ditropan XL Extended Release Tablets 2391

Oxycodone Hydrochloride (Plasma concentrations of GI motility

agents may be decreased by co-administration with nevirapine. Dose adjustment of co-administered drug may be needed due to possible decrease in clinical effect). Products include:
Combunox Tablets 1183
OxyContin Tablets 2699
OxyFast Oral Concentrate Solution........................ 2704
OxyIR Capsules 2704
Percocet Tablets 1114
Percodan Tablets 1115

Oxyphenonium Bromide (Plasma concentrations of GI motility agents may be decreased by co-administration with nevirapine. Dose adjustment of co-administered drug may be needed due to possible decrease in clinical effect).
No products indexed under this heading.

Paclitaxel (Plasma concentrations of cancer chemotherapeutic agents may be decreased by co-administration with nevirapine. Dose adjustment of co-administered drug may be needed due to possible decrease in clinical effect).
No products indexed under this heading.

Paramethadione (Plasma concentrations of anticonvulsants may be decreased by co-administration with nevirapine. Dose adjustment of co-administered drug may be needed due to possible decrease in clinical effect).
No products indexed under this heading.

Pergolide Mesylate (Plasma concentrations of GI motility agents may be decreased by co-administration with nevirapine. Dose adjustment of co-administered drug may be needed due to possible decrease in clinical effect). Products include:
Permax Tablets 3357

Phenacemide (Plasma concentrations of anticonvulsants may be decreased by co-administration with nevirapine. Dose adjustment of co-administered drug may be needed due to possible decrease in clinical effect).
No products indexed under this heading.

Phenobarbital (Plasma concentrations of anticonvulsants may be decreased by co-administration with nevirapine. Dose adjustment of co-administered drug may be needed due to possible decrease in clinical effect).
No products indexed under this heading.

Phensuximide (Plasma concentrations of anticonvulsants may be decreased by co-administration with nevirapine. Dose adjustment of co-administered drug may be needed due to possible decrease in clinical effect).
No products indexed under this heading.

Phenytoin (Plasma concentrations of anticonvulsants may be decreased by co-administration with nevirapine. Dose adjustment of co-administered drug may be needed due to possible decrease in clinical effect).
No products indexed under this heading.

Phenytoin Sodium (Plasma concentrations of anticonvulsants may be decreased by co-administration with nevirapine. Dose adjustment of co-administered drug may be needed due to possible decrease in clinical effect). Products include:
Phenytek Capsules 2153

Pirbuterol Acetate (Plasma concentrations of GI motility agents may be decreased by co-administration with nevirapine. Dose adjustment of co-administered drug may be needed due to possible decrease in clinical effect). Products include:
Maxair Autohaler 1820

Pramipexole Dihydrochloride (Plasma concentrations of GI motility agents may be decreased by co-administration with nevirapine. Dose adjustment of co-administered drug may be needed due to possible decrease in clinical effect). Products include:
Mirapex Tablets 889

Primidone (Plasma concentrations of anticonvulsants may be decreased by co-administration with nevirapine. Dose adjustment of co-administered drug may be needed due to possible decrease in clinical effect).
No products indexed under this heading.

Procainamide Hydrochloride (Plasma concentrations of antiarrhythmics may be decreased by co-administration with nevirapine. Dose adjustment of co-administered drug may be needed due to possible decrease in clinical effect).
No products indexed under this heading.

Procarbazine Hydrochloride (Plasma concentrations of cancer chemotherapeutic agents may be decreased by co-administration with nevirapine. Dose adjustment of co-administered drug may be needed due to possible decrease in clinical effect). Products include:
Matulane Capsules 3188

Procyclidine Hydrochloride (Plasma concentrations of GI motility agents may be decreased by co-administration with nevirapine. Dose adjustment of co-administered drug may be needed due to possible decrease in clinical effect).
No products indexed under this heading.

Promethazine Hydrochloride (Plasma concentrations of GI motility agents may be decreased by co-administration with nevirapine. Dose adjustment of co-administered drug may be needed due to possible decrease in clinical effect). Products include:
Phenergan 3438

Propafenone Hydrochloride (Plasma concentrations of antiarrhythmics may be decreased by co-administration with nevirapine. Dose adjustment of co-administered drug may be needed due to possible decrease in clinical effect). Products include:
Rythmol SR Capsules 2736

Propantheline Bromide (Plasma concentrations of GI motility agents may be decreased by co-administration with nevirapine. Dose adjustment of co-administered drug may be needed due to possible decrease in clinical effect).
No products indexed under this heading.

Propoxyphene Hydrochloride (Plasma concentrations of GI motility agents may be decreased by co-administration with nevirapine. Dose adjustment of co-administered drug may be needed due to possible decrease in clinical effect).
No products indexed under this heading.

Propoxyphene Napsylate (Plasma concentrations of GI motility agents may be decreased by co-administration with nevirapine. Dose adjustment of co-administered drug may be needed due to possible decrease in clinical effect). Products include:
Darvocet A 500 Tablets 3497

Propranolol Hydrochloride (Plasma concentrations of antiarrhythmics may be decreased by co-administration with nevirapine. Dose adjustment of co-administered drug may be needed due to possible decrease in clinical effect). Products include:
Inderal LA Long-Acting Capsules 3421
InnoPran XL Capsules 2728

Protriptyline Hydrochloride (Plasma concentrations of GI motility agents may be decreased by co-administration with nevirapine. Dose adjustment of co-administered drug may be needed due to possible decrease in clinical effect). Products include:
Vivactil Tablets 2350

Pyridostigmine Bromide (Plasma concentrations of GI motility agents may be decreased by co-administration with nevirapine. Dose adjustment of co-administered drug may be needed due to possible decrease in clinical effect).
No products indexed under this heading.

Pyrilamine Maleate (Plasma concentrations of GI motility agents may be decreased by co-administration with nevirapine. Dose adjustment of co-administered drug may be needed due to possible decrease in clinical effect).
No products indexed under this heading.

Pyrilamine Tannate (Plasma concentrations of GI motility agents may be decreased by co-administration with nevirapine. Dose adjustment of co-administered drug may be needed due to possible decrease in clinical effect).
No products indexed under this heading.

Quinidine Gluconate (Plasma concentrations of antiarrhythmics may be decreased by co-administration with nevirapine. Dose adjustment of co-administered drug may be needed due to possible decrease in clinical effect).
No products indexed under this heading.

Quinidine Polygalacturonate (Plasma concentrations of antiarrhythmics may be decreased by co-administration with nevirapine. Dose adjustment of co-administered drug may be needed due to possible decrease in clinical effect).
No products indexed under this heading.

Quinidine Sulfate (Plasma concentrations of antiarrhythmics may be decreased by co-administration with nevirapine. Dose adjustment of co-administered drug may be needed due to possible decrease in clinical effect).
No products indexed under this heading.

Remifentanil Hydrochloride (Plasma concentrations of GI motility agents may be decreased by co-administration with nevirapine. Dose adjustment of co-administered drug may be needed due to possible decrease in clinical effect).
No products indexed under this heading.

Rifabutin (Rifabutin and its metabolite concentrations were moderately increased. Due to high intersubject variability, however, some patients may experience large increases in rifabutin exposure and may be at higher risk for rifabutin toxicity. Therefore, caution should be used in concomitant administration).
No products indexed under this heading.

Rifampin (Nevirapine and rifampin should not be administered concomitantly because decreases in nevirapine plasma concentrations may reduce the efficacy of the drug. Physicians needing to treat patients co-infected with tuberculosis and using a nevirapine containing regimen may use rifabutin instead).
No products indexed under this heading.

Rivastigmine Tartrate (Plasma concentrations of GI motility agents may be decreased by co-administration with nevirapine. Dose adjustment of co-administered drug may be needed due to possible decrease in clinical effect). Products include:
Exelon Capsules 2204

Ropinirole Hydrochloride (Plasma concentrations of GI motility agents may be decreased by co-administration with nevirapine. Dose adjustment of co-administered drug may be needed due to possible decrease in clinical effect). Products include:
Requip Tablets 1528

Salmeterol Xinafoate (Plasma concentrations of GI motility agents may be decreased by co-administration with nevirapine. Dose adjustment of co-administered drug may be needed due to possible decrease in clinical effect). Products include:
Advair Diskus 100/50 1291
Advair Diskus 250/50 1291
Advair Diskus 500/50 1291
Serevent Diskus 1540

Saquinavir (Saquinavir concentrations may be decreased when used concomitantly with nevirapine. Appropriate doses for this combination are not established, but an increase in the dosage of saquinavir may be required).
No products indexed under this heading.

Scopolamine (Plasma concentrations of GI motility agents may be decreased by co-administration with nevirapine. Dose adjustment of co-administered drug may be needed due to possible decrease in clinical effect). Products include:

Transderm Scōp Transdermal Therapeutic System 2166

Scopolamine Hydrobromide (Plasma concentrations of GI motility agents may be decreased by co-administration with nevirapine. Dose adjustment of co-administered drug may be needed due to possible decrease in clinical effect).
No products indexed under this heading.

Sirolimus (Plasma concentrations of immunosuppressants may be decreased by co-administration with nevirapine. Dose adjustment of co-administered drug may be needed due to possible decrease in clinical effect). Products include:
Rapamune Oral Solution and Tablets 3472

Sotalol Hydrochloride (Plasma concentrations of antiarrhythmics may be decreased by co-administration with nevirapine. Dose adjustment of co-administered drug may be needed due to possible decrease in clinical effect).
No products indexed under this heading.

Streptozocin (Plasma concentrations of cancer chemotherapeutic agents may be decreased by co-administration with nevirapine. Dose adjustment of co-administered drug may be needed due to possible decrease in clinical effect).
No products indexed under this heading.

Sucralfate (Plasma concentrations of GI motility agents may be decreased by co-administration with nevirapine. Dose adjustment of co-administered drug may be needed due to possible decrease in clinical effect). Products include:
Carafate Suspension 727
Carafate Tablets 728

Sufentanil Citrate (Plasma concentrations of GI motility agents may be decreased by co-administration with nevirapine. Dose adjustment of co-administered drug may be needed due to possible decrease in clinical effect).
No products indexed under this heading.

Tacrine Hydrochloride (Plasma concentrations of GI motility agents may be decreased by co-administration with nevirapine. Dose adjustment of co-administered drug may be needed due to possible decrease in clinical effect).
No products indexed under this heading.

Tacrolimus (Plasma concentrations of immunosuppressants may be decreased by co-administration with nevirapine. Dose adjustment of co-administered drug may be needed due to possible decrease in clinical effect). Products include:
Prograf Capsules and Injection 624
Protopic Ointment 629

Tamoxifen Citrate (Plasma concentrations of cancer chemotherapeutic agents may be decreased by co-administration with nevirapine. Dose adjustment of co-administered drug may be needed due to possible decrease in clinical effect).
No products indexed under this heading.

Teniposide (Plasma concentrations of cancer chemotherapeutic agents may be decreased by co-administration with nevirapine. Dose adjustment of co-administered drug may be needed due to possible decrease in clinical effect).
No products indexed under this heading.

Terbutaline Sulfate (Plasma concentrations of GI motility agents may be decreased by co-administration with nevirapine. Dose adjustment of co-administered drug may be needed due to possible decrease in clinical effect).
No products indexed under this heading.

Terconazole (Plasma concentrations of antifungals may be decreased by co-administration with nevirapine. Dose adjustment of co-administered drug may be needed due to possible decrease in clinical effect).
No products indexed under this heading.

Thioguanine (Plasma concentrations of cancer chemotherapeutic agents may be decreased by co-administration with nevirapine. Dose adjustment of co-administered drug may be needed due to possible decrease in clinical effect). Products include:
Tabloid Tablets 1545

Thiotepa (Plasma concentrations of cancer chemotherapeutic agents may be decreased by co-administration with nevirapine. Dose adjustment of co-administered drug may be needed due to possible decrease in clinical effect).
No products indexed under this heading.

Tiagabine Hydrochloride (Plasma concentrations of anticonvulsants may be decreased by co-administration with nevirapine. Dose adjustment of co-administered drug may be needed due to possible decrease in clinical effect). Products include:
Gabitril Tablets 998

Tinzaparin Sodium (Plasma concentrations of antithrombotics may be increased by co-administration with nevirapine. Dose adjustment of co-administered drug may be needed due to possible decrease in clinical effect).
No products indexed under this heading.

Tocainide Hydrochloride (Plasma concentrations of antiarrhythmics may be decreased by co-administration with nevirapine. Dose adjustment of co-administered drug may be needed due to possible decrease in clinical effect).
No products indexed under this heading.

Tolterodine Tartrate (Plasma concentrations of GI motility agents may be decreased by co-administration with nevirapine. Dose adjustment of co-administered drug may be needed due to possible decrease in clinical effect). Products include:
Detrol Tablets 2626
Detrol LA Capsules 2629

Topiramate (Plasma concentrations of anticonvulsants may be decreased by co-administration with nevirapine. Dose adjustment of co-administered drug may be needed due to possible decrease in clinical effect). Products include:
Topamax Sprinkle Capsules 2438
Topamax Tablets 2438

Topotecan Hydrochloride (Plasma concentrations of cancer chemotherapeutic agents may be decreased by co-administration with nevirapine. Dose adjustment of co-administered drug may be needed due to possible decrease in clinical effect). Products include:
Hycamtin for Injection 1427

Toremifene Citrate (Plasma concentrations of cancer chemotherapeutic agents may be decreased by co-administration with nevirapine. Dose adjustment of co-administered drug may be needed due to possible decrease in clinical effect).
No products indexed under this heading.

Tridihexethyl Chloride (Plasma concentrations of GI motility agents may be decreased by co-administration with nevirapine. Dose adjustment of co-administered drug may be needed due to possible decrease in clinical effect).
No products indexed under this heading.

Trihexyphenidyl Hydrochloride (Plasma concentrations of GI motility agents may be decreased by co-administration with nevirapine. Dose adjustment of co-administered drug may be needed due to possible decrease in clinical effect).
No products indexed under this heading.

Trimeprazine Tartrate (Plasma concentrations of GI motility agents may be decreased by co-administration with nevirapine. Dose adjustment of co-administered drug may be needed due to possible decrease in clinical effect).
No products indexed under this heading.

Trimethadione (Plasma concentrations of anticonvulsants may be decreased by co-administration with nevirapine. Dose adjustment of co-administered drug may be needed due to possible decrease in clinical effect).
No products indexed under this heading.

Trimipramine Maleate (Plasma concentrations of GI motility agents may be decreased by co-administration with nevirapine. Dose adjustment of co-administered drug may be needed due to possible decrease in clinical effect). Products include:
Surmontil Capsules 2347

Tripelennamine Hydrochloride (Plasma concentrations of GI motility agents may be decreased by co-administration with nevirapine. Dose adjustment of co-administered drug may be needed due to possible decrease in clinical effect).
No products indexed under this heading.

Triprolidine Hydrochloride (Plasma concentrations of GI motility agents may be decreased by co-administration with nevirapine. Dose adjustment of co-administered drug may be needed due to possible decrease in clinical effect).
No products indexed under this heading.

Valproate Sodium (Plasma concentrations of anticonvulsants may be decreased by co-administration with nevirapine. Dose adjustment of co-administered drug may be needed due to possible decrease in clinical effect). Products include:
Depacon Injection 412

Valproic Acid (Plasma concentrations of anticonvulsants may be decreased by co-administration with nevirapine. Dose adjustment of co-administered drug may be needed due to possible decrease in clinical effect). Products include:
Depakene 417

Valrubicin (Plasma concentrations of cancer chemotherapeutic agents may be decreased by co-administration with nevirapine. Dose adjustment of co-administered drug may be needed due to possible decrease in clinical effect).
No products indexed under this heading.

Verapamil Hydrochloride (Plasma concentrations of antiarrhythmics may be decreased by co-administration with nevirapine. Dose adjustment of co-administered drug may be needed due to possible decrease in clinical effect). Products include:
Covera-HS Tablets 3135
Tarka Tablets 519
Verelan PM Capsules 3120

Vincristine Sulfate (Plasma concentrations of cancer chemotherapeutic agents may be decreased by co-administration with nevirapine. Dose adjustment of co-administered drug may be needed due to possible decrease in clinical effect).
No products indexed under this heading.

Vinorelbine Tartrate (Plasma concentrations of cancer chemotherapeutic agents may be decreased by co-administration with nevirapine. Dose adjustment of co-administered drug may be needed due to possible decrease in clinical effect). Products include:
Navelbine Injection 1494

Warfarin Sodium (Plasma concentrations of antithrombotics may be increased by co-administration with nevirapine. Dose adjustment of co-administered drug may be needed due to possible decrease in clinical effect). Products include:
Coumadin for Injection 932
Coumadin Tablets 932

Zidovudine (When zidovudine and Viramune are co-administered the AUC and Cmax for zidovudine are decreased by 28% and 30%, respectively). Products include:
Combivir Tablets 1373
Retrovir 1533
Retrovir IV Infusion 1537
Trizivir Tablets 1565

Zonisamide (Plasma concentrations of anticonvulsants may be decreased by co-administration with nevirapine. Dose adjustment of co-administered drug may be needed due to possible decrease in clinical effect). Products include:
Zonegran Capsules 1089

VIRAZOLE FOR INHALATION SOLUTION

(Ribavirin) 3365
None cited in PDR database.

VIREAD TABLETS
(Tenofovir Disoproxil Fumarate) 1284
May interact with:

Acyclovir (Co-administration with drugs that reduce renal function or compete for active tubular secretion may increase serum concentrations of tenofovir and/or increase the concentrations of other renally eliminated drugs, such as acyclovir).
Products include:
Zovirax 1616
Zovirax Cream 853
Zovirax Ointment 854

Acyclovir Sodium (Co-administration with drugs that reduce renal function or compete for active tubular secretion may increase serum concentrations of tenofovir and/or increase the concentrations of other renally eliminated drugs, such as acyclovir).
Products include:
Zovirax for Injection 1618

Atazanavir (Tenofovir decreases the AUC and Cmin of atazanavir. When co-administered with tenofovir, it is recommended that atazanavir 300mg is given with ritonavir 100mg. Atazanavir without ritonavir should not be co-administered with tenofovir. Atazanavir may increase the Cmax, AUC and Cmin of tenofovir).
No products indexed under this heading.

Atazanavir sulfate (Tenofovir decreases the AUC and Cmin of atazanavir. When co-administered with tenofovir, it is recommended that atazanavir 300mg is given with ritonavir 100mg. Atazanavir without ritonavir should not be co-administered with tenofovir. Atazanavir may increase the Cmax, AUC and Cmin of tenofovir). Products include:
Reyataz Capsules 948

Cidofovir (Co-administration with drugs that reduce renal function or compete for active tubular secretion may increase serum concentrations of tenofovir and/or increase the concentrations of other renally eliminated drugs, such as cidofovir).
No products indexed under this heading.

Didanosine (Co-administration results in increased AUC and Cmax of didanosine and could potentiate didanosine-associated adverse events. Discontinue didanosine if didanosine-associated adverse events develop).
No products indexed under this heading.

Ganciclovir (Co-administration with drugs that reduce renal function or compete for active tubular secretion may increase serum concentrations of tenofovir and/or increase the concentrations of other renally eliminated drugs, such as ganciclovir).
Products include:
Cytovene Capsules 2763

Indinavir Sulfate (Co-administration of tenofovir with indinavir has resulted in increased Cmax tenofovir and decreased Cmax for indinavir). Products include:
Crixivan Capsules 1918

Lamivudine (Co-administration of tenofovir with lamivudine has resulted in decreased Cmax for lamivudine). Products include:
Combivir Tablets 1373
Epivir 1394
Epivir-HBV 1398
Epzicom Tablets 1402
Trizivir Tablets 1565

Lopinavir (Co-administration of tenofovir with lopinavir has resulted in increased Cmax, AUC, and Cmin for tenofovir and decreased AUC, Cmax, and Cmin for lopinavir).
Products include:
Kaletra 474

Ritonavir (Co-administration of tenofovir with ritonavir has resulted in increased Cmax, AUC, and Cmin for tenofovir and decreased AUC and Cmax, and increased Cmin for ritonavir). Products include:
Kaletra 474
Norvir 499

Valacyclovir Hydrochloride (Co-administration with drugs that reduce renal function or compete for active tubular secretion may increase serum concentrations of tenofovir and/or increase the concentrations of other renally eliminated drugs, such as valacyclovir).
Products include:
Valtrex Caplets 1573

Valganciclovir Hydrochloride (Co-administration with drugs that reduce renal function or compete for active tubular secretion may increase serum concentrations of tenofovir and/or increase the concentrations of other renally eliminated drugs, such as valganciclovir).
Products include:
Valcyte Tablets 2816

Food Interactions

Food, unspecified (Increases the bioavailability and delays the time to tenofovir Cmax; Viread should be taken with a meal).

VISINE A.C. SEASONAL ITCHING AND REDNESS RELIEF DROPS
(Tetrahydrozoline Hydrochloride, Zinc Sulfate) .... ⊙278
None cited in PDR database.

ADVANCED RELIEF VISINE EYE DROPS
(Dextran 70, Polyethylene Glycol, Povidone, Tetrahydrozoline Hydrochloride) .... ⊙278
None cited in PDR database.

VISINE FOR CONTACTS REWETTING DROPS
(Glycerin, Hydroxypropyl Methylcellulose) .... ⊙278
None cited in PDR database.

VISINE L.R. LONG LASTING EYE DROPS
(Oxymetazoline Hydrochloride) .... ⊙279
None cited in PDR database.

VISINE PURE TEARS EYE DROPS SINGLE DROP DISPENSER
(Glycerin, Hypromellose, Polyethylene Glycol) .... ⊙280
None cited in PDR database.

VISINE PURE TEARS PORTABLES
(Glycerin, Hypromellose, Polyethylene Glycol) .... ⊙280
None cited in PDR database.

VISINE TEARS EYE DROPS
(Glycerin, Hypromellose, Polyethylene Glycol) .... ⊙279
None cited in PDR database.

VISINE-A EYE ALLERGY RELIEF EYE DROPS
(Naphazoline Hydrochloride, Pheniramine Maleate) .... ⊙278
None cited in PDR database.

VISINE-A EYE DROPS
(Naphazoline Hydrochloride, Pheniramine Maleate) .... ▣713
None cited in PDR database.

VISUDYNE FOR INJECTION
(Verteporfin) 2286
May interact with calcium channel blockers, anticoagulants, phenothiazines, sulfonamides, sulfonylureas, tetracyclines, thiazides, and certain other agents. Compounds in these categories include:

Amlodipine Besylate (Co-administration with calcium channel blockers could enhance the rate of verteporfin's uptake by the vascular endothelium). Products include:
Caduet Tablets 2507
Lotrel Capsules 2238
Norvasc Tablets 2529

Anisindione (Co-administration with drugs that decrease clotting would be expected to decrease verteporfin activity). Products include:
Miradon Tablets 3056

Ardeparin Sodium (Co-administration with drugs that decrease clotting would be expected to decrease verteporfin activity).
No products indexed under this heading.

Aspirin (Co-administration with drugs that decrease platelet aggregation would be expected to decrease verteporfin activity).
Products include:
Aggrenox Capsules 855
Bayer, Aspirin Regimen .... ▣606
Bayer Aspirin Tablets 3515
BC Powder .... ▣612
BC Allergy Sinus Cold Powder .... ▣612
Arthritis Strength BC Powder .... ▣612
BC Sinus Cold Powder .... ▣612
Ecotrin Enteric Coated Aspirin Low, Regular and Maximum Strength Tablets 1627
Goody's Body Pain Formula Powder .... ▣621
Goody's Extra Strength Headache Powder .... ▣621
Goody's Extra Strength Pain Relief Tablets .... ▣621
Percodan Tablets 1115
St. Joseph 81 mg Aspirin Chewable and Enteric Coated Tablets 1841

Bendroflumethiazide (Co-administration with other photosensitizing agents, such as thiazide diuretics, could increase the potential for skin photosensitivity reactions).
No products indexed under this heading.

Bepridil Hydrochloride (Co-administration with calcium channel blockers could enhance the rate of verteporfin's uptake by the vascular endothelium).
No products indexed under this heading.

Chlorothiazide (Co-administration with other photosensitizing agents, such as thiazide diuretics, could increase the potential for skin photosensitivity reactions). Products include:
Aldoclor Tablets 1881
Diuril Oral 1936

Chlorothiazide Sodium (Co-administration with other photosensitizing agents, such as thiazide diuretics, could increase the potential for skin photosensitivity reactions).
Products include:
Diuril Sodium Intravenous 1934

Chlorpromazine (Co-administration with other photosensitizing agents, such as phenothiazines, could increase the potential for skin photosensitivity reactions).
No products indexed under this heading.

Chlorpromazine Hydrochloride (Co-administration with other photosensitizing agents, such as phenothiazines, could increase the potential for skin photosensitivity reactions).
No products indexed under this heading.

Chlorpropamide (Co-administration with other photosensitizing agents, such as sulfonylurea hypoglycemic agents, could increase the potential for skin photosensitivity reactions).
No products indexed under this heading.

Clopidogrel Bisulfate (Co-administration with drugs that decrease platelet aggregation would be expected to decrease verteporfin activity). Products include:
Plavix Tablets 940
Plavix Tablets 2942

Dalteparin Sodium (Co-administration with drugs that decrease clotting would be expected to decrease verteporfin activity).
Products include:
Fragmin Injection 2638

Danaparoid Sodium (Co-administration with drugs that decrease clotting would be expected to decrease verteporfin activity).
No products indexed under this heading.

Demeclocycline Hydrochloride (Co-administration with other photosensitizing agents, such as tetracyclines, could increase the potential for skin photosensitivity reactions).
No products indexed under this heading.

Dicumarol (Co-administration with drugs that decrease clotting would be expected to decrease verteporfin activity).
No products indexed under this heading.

Diltiazem Hydrochloride (Co-administration with calcium channel blockers could enhance the rate of verteporfin's uptake by the vascular endothelium). Products include:
Cardizem LA Extended Release Tablets 1699
Tiazac Capsules 1204

Dimethyl Sulfoxide (Co-administration with compounds that quench active oxygen species or scavenge radicals, such as dimethyl sulfoxide, would be expected to decrease verteporfin activity).
No products indexed under this heading.

Dipyridamole (Co-administration with drugs that decrease platelet aggregation would be expected to decrease verteporfin activity).
Products include:

Aggrenox Capsules 855
Persantine Tablets 898

Doxycycline Calcium (Co-administration with other photosensitizing agents, such as tetracyclines, could increase the potential for skin photosensitivity reactions).
No products indexed under this heading.

Doxycycline Hyclate (Co-administration with other photosensitizing agents, such as tetracyclines, could increase the potential for skin photosensitivity reactions).
No products indexed under this heading.

Doxycycline Monohydrate (Co-administration with other photosensitizing agents, such as tetracyclines, could increase the potential for skin photosensitivity reactions).
No products indexed under this heading.

Enoxaparin Sodium (Co-administration with drugs that decrease clotting would be expected to decrease verteporfin activity). Products include:
Lovenox Injection 2931

Felodipine (Co-administration with calcium channel blockers could enhance the rate of verteporfin's uptake by the vascular endothelium). Products include:
Plendil Extended-Release Tablets 651

Fluphenazine Decanoate (Co-administration with other photosensitizing agents, such as phenothiazines, could increase the potential for skin photosensitivity reactions).
No products indexed under this heading.

Fluphenazine Enanthate (Co-administration with other photosensitizing agents, such as phenothiazines, could increase the potential for skin photosensitivity reactions).
No products indexed under this heading.

Fluphenazine Hydrochloride (Co-administration with other photosensitizing agents, such as phenothiazines, could increase the potential for skin photosensitivity reactions).
No products indexed under this heading.

Fondaparinux Sodium (Co-administration with drugs that decrease clotting would be expected to decrease verteporfin activity). Products include:
Arixtra Injection 1325

Glimepiride (Co-administration with other photosensitizing agents, such as sulfonylurea hypoglycemic agents, could increase the potential for skin photosensitivity reactions). Products include:
Amaryl Tablets 2864

Glipizide (Co-administration with other photosensitizing agents, such as sulfonylurea hypoglycemic agents, could increase the potential for skin photosensitivity reactions).
No products indexed under this heading.

Glyburide (Co-administration with other photosensitizing agents, such as sulfonylurea hypoglycemic agents, could increase the potential for skin photosensitivity reactions).
No products indexed under this heading.

Griseofulvin (Co-administration with other photosensitizing agents, such as griseofulvin, could increase the potential for skin photosensitivity reactions). Products include:
Grifulvin V Tablets Microsize and Oral Suspension Microsize........... 2384
Gris-PEG Tablets 2504

Heparin Calcium (Co-administration with drugs that decrease clotting would be expected to decrease verteporfin activity).
No products indexed under this heading.

Heparin Sodium (Co-administration with drugs that decrease clotting would be expected to decrease verteporfin activity).
No products indexed under this heading.

Hydrochlorothiazide (Co-administration with other photosensitizing agents, such as thiazide diuretics, could increase the potential for skin photosensitivity reactions). Products include:
Aldoril Tablets 1884
Atacand HCT 637
Avalide Tablets 2889
Avalide Tablets 922
Benicar HCT Tablets 2852
Diovan HCT Tablets 2195
Dyazide Capsules 1389
Hyzaar 1964
Lotensin HCT Tablets 2235
Maxzide 2150
Micardis HCT Tablets 886
Moduretic Tablets 2003
Prinzide Tablets 2033
Teveten HCT Tablets 1710
Timolide Tablets 2056
Uniretic Tablets 3114
Vaseretic Tablets 2073
Zestoretic Tablets 701

Hydroflumethiazide (Co-administration with other photosensitizing agents, such as thiazide diuretics, could increase the potential for skin photosensitivity reactions).
No products indexed under this heading.

Isradipine (Co-administration with calcium channel blockers could enhance the rate of verteporfin's uptake by the vascular endothelium). Products include:
DynaCirc CR Tablets 2726

Low Molecular Weight Heparins (Co-administration with drugs that decrease clotting would be expected to decrease verteporfin activity).
No products indexed under this heading.

Mannitol (Co-administration with compounds that quench active oxygen species or scavenge radicals, such as mannitol, would be expected to decrease verteporfin activity). Products include:
Trident White Sugarless Gum .... ■ 611

Mesoridazine Besylate (Co-administration with other photosensitizing agents, such as phenothiazines, could increase the potential for skin photosensitivity reactions).
No products indexed under this heading.

Methacycline Hydrochloride (Co-administration with other photosensitizing agents, such as tetracyclines, could increase the potential for skin photosensitivity reactions).
No products indexed under this heading.

Methotrimeprazine (Co-administration with other photosensitizing agents, such as phenothiazines, could increase the potential for skin photosensitivity reactions).
No products indexed under this heading.

Methyclothiazide (Co-administration with other photosensitizing agents, such as thiazide diuretics, could increase the potential for skin photosensitivity reactions).
No products indexed under this heading.

Mibefradil Dihydrochloride (Co-administration with calcium channel blockers could enhance the rate of verteporfin's uptake by the vascular endothelium).
No products indexed under this heading.

Minocycline Hydrochloride (Co-administration with other photosensitizing agents, such as tetracyclines, could increase the potential for skin photosensitivity reactions). Products include:
Dynacin Tablets 1859

Nicardipine Hydrochloride (Co-administration with calcium channel blockers could enhance the rate of verteporfin's uptake by the vascular endothelium). Products include:
Cardene I.V. 1129

Nifedipine (Co-administration with calcium channel blockers could enhance the rate of verteporfin's uptake by the vascular endothelium). Products include:
Adalat CC Tablets 2978

Nimodipine (Co-administration with calcium channel blockers could enhance the rate of verteporfin's uptake by the vascular endothelium). Products include:
Nimotop Capsules 774

Nisoldipine (Co-administration with calcium channel blockers could enhance the rate of verteporfin's uptake by the vascular endothelium). Products include:
Sular Tablets 1163

Oxytetracycline Hydrochloride (Co-administration with other photosensitizing agents, such as tetracyclines, could increase the potential for skin photosensitivity reactions).
No products indexed under this heading.

Perphenazine (Co-administration with other photosensitizing agents, such as phenothiazines, could increase the potential for skin photosensitivity reactions).
No products indexed under this heading.

Polymyxin B Sulfate (Co-administration with polymyxin B could enhance the rate of verteporfin's uptake by the vascular endothelium). Products include:
Neosporin Ointment .... ■ 702
Neosporin + Pain Relief Maximum Strength Cream........... ■ 703
Neosporin + Pain Relief Maximum Strength Ointment....... ■ 703
Poly-Pred Liquifilm Ophthalmic Suspension .... ⊙ 231
Polysporin Ointment .... ■ 706
Polytrim Ophthalmic Solution 570

Polythiazide (Co-administration with other photosensitizing agents, such as thiazide diuretics, could increase the potential for skin photosensitivity reactions).
No products indexed under this heading.

Prochlorperazine (Co-administration with other photosensitizing agents, such as phenothiazines, could increase the potential for skin photosensitivity reactions).
No products indexed under this heading.

Promethazine Hydrochloride (Co-administration with other photosensitizing agents, such as phenothiazines, could increase the potential for skin photosensitivity reactions). Products include:
Phenergan 3438

Sulfacytine (Co-administration with other photosensitizing agents, such as sulfonamides, could increase the potential for skin photosensitivity reactions).
No products indexed under this heading.

Sulfamethizole (Co-administration with other photosensitizing agents, such as sulfonamides, could increase the potential for skin photosensitivity reactions).
No products indexed under this heading.

Sulfamethoxazole (Co-administration with other photosensitizing agents, such as sulfonamides, could increase the potential for skin photosensitivity reactions).
No products indexed under this heading.

Sulfasalazine (Co-administration with other photosensitizing agents, such as sulfonamides, could increase the potential for skin photosensitivity reactions).
No products indexed under this heading.

Sulfinpyrazone (Co-administration with other photosensitizing agents, such as sulfonamides, could increase the potential for skin photosensitivity reactions).
No products indexed under this heading.

Sulfisoxazole (Co-administration with other photosensitizing agents, such as sulfonamides, could increase the potential for skin photosensitivity reactions).
No products indexed under this heading.

Sulfisoxazole Acetyl (Co-administration with other photosensitizing agents, such as sulfonamides, could increase the potential for skin photosensitivity reactions).
No products indexed under this heading.

Sulfisoxazole Diolamine (Co-administration with other photosensitizing agents, such as sulfonamides, could increase the potential for skin photosensitivity reactions).
No products indexed under this heading.

Tetracycline Hydrochloride (Co-administration with other photosensitizing agents, such as tetracyclines, could increase the potential for skin photosensitivity reactions).
No products indexed under this heading.

Thioridazine Hydrochloride (Co-administration with other photosensitizing agents, such as phenothiazines, could increase the potential for skin photosensitivity reactions). Products include:
Thioridazine Hydrochloride Tablets 2122

Tinzaparin Sodium (Co-administration with drugs that decrease clotting would be expected to decrease verteporfin activity).
No products indexed under this heading.

Tolazamide (Co-administration with other photosensitizing agents, such as sulfonylurea hypoglycemic agents, could increase the potential for skin photosensitivity reactions).
No products indexed under this heading.

Tolbutamide (Co-administration with other photosensitizing agents, such as sulfonylurea hypoglycemic agents, could increase the potential for skin photosensitivity reactions).
No products indexed under this heading.

Trifluoperazine Hydrochloride (Co-administration with other photosensitizing agents, such as phenothiazines, could increase the potential for skin photosensitivity reactions).
No products indexed under this heading.

Verapamil Hydrochloride (Co-administration with calcium channel blockers could enhance the rate of verteporfin's uptake by the vascular endothelium). Products include:
Covera-HS Tablets 3135
Tarka Tablets 519
Verelan PM Capsules 3120

Warfarin Sodium (Co-administration with drugs that decrease clotting would be expected to decrease verteporfin activity). Products include:
Coumadin for Injection 932
Coumadin Tablets 932

Food Interactions

Alcohol (Co-administration with compounds that quench active oxygen species or scavenge radicals, such as ethanol, would be expected to decrease verteporfin activity).

VISUTEIN CAPSULES

(Acetylcysteine, Carotenoids, Lutein, Vitamin A, Vitamin B_2, Zinc)...... 3328
None cited in PDR database.

VIVA EYE DROPS

(Polysorbate 80) .... ⊙282
None cited in PDR database.

VIVACTIL TABLETS

(Protriptyline Hydrochloride) 2350
May interact with anticholinergics, barbiturates, central nervous system depressants, antidepressant drugs, monoamine oxidase inhibitors, phenothiazines, quinidine, selective serotonin reuptake inhibitors, sympathomimetics, thyroid preparations, and certain other agents. Compounds in these categories include:

Albuterol (Effects of concurrent use not specified; careful adjustment of dosage and close supervision are required). Products include:
Proventil Inhalation Aerosol 3067

Albuterol Sulfate (Effects of concurrent use not specified; careful adjustment of dosage and close supervision are required). Products include:
AccuNeb Inhalation Solution 1055
Combivent Inhalation Aerosol 878
DuoNeb Inhalation Solution 1058
Proventil Inhalation Solution 0.083%.......... 3069
Proventil HFA Inhalation Aerosol 3071
Ventolin HFA Inhalation Aerosol 1576
VoSpire Extended-Release Tablets 2352

Alfentanil Hydrochloride (Co-administration results in enhanced response to CNS depressants).
No products indexed under this heading.

Alprazolam (Co-administration results in enhanced response to CNS depressants). Products include:
Niravam Orally Disintegrating Tablets 3106
Xanax XR Tablets 2655

Amitriptyline Hydrochloride (Co-administration with cytochrome P4502D6 inhibitors, such as antidepressants, may make normal metabolizer resemble poor metabolizer leading to higher than expected plasma concentration of TCA with resultant toxicity; lower than usual doses of either drug may be required).
No products indexed under this heading.

Amoxapine (Co-administration with cytochrome P4502D6 inhibitors, such as antidepressants, may make normal metabolizer resemble poor metabolizer leading to higher than expected plasma concentration of TCA with resultant toxicity; lower than usual doses of either drug may be required).
No products indexed under this heading.

Aprobarbital (Co-administration results in enhanced response to CNS depressants).
No products indexed under this heading.

Atropine Sulfate (Co-administration may result in hyperpyrexia, particularly during hot weather).
No products indexed under this heading.

Belladonna Alkaloids (Co-administration may result in hyperpyrexia, particularly during hot weather). Products include:
Hyland's Teething Tablets .... ▣736

Benztropine Mesylate (Co-administration may result in hyperpyrexia, particularly during hot weather). Products include:
Cogentin Injection 1903

Biperiden Hydrochloride (Co-administration may result in hyperpyrexia, particularly during hot weather).
No products indexed under this heading.

Buprenorphine Hydrochloride (Co-administration results in enhanced response to CNS depressants). Products include:
Buprenex Injectable 2718
Suboxone Tablets 2719
Subutex Tablets 2719

Bupropion Hydrochloride (Co-administration with cytochrome P4502D6 inhibitors, such as antidepressants, may make normal metabolizer resemble poor metabolizer leading to higher than expected plasma concentration of TCA with resultant toxicity; lower than usual doses of either drug may be required). Products include:
Wellbutrin Tablets 1579
Wellbutrin SR Sustained-Release Tablets 1583
Wellbutrin XL Extended-Release Tablets 1588
Zyban Sustained-Release Tablets 1620

Buspirone Hydrochloride (Co-administration results in enhanced response to CNS depressants).
No products indexed under this heading.

Butabarbital (Co-administration results in enhanced response to CNS depressants).
No products indexed under this heading.

Butalbital (Co-administration results in enhanced response to CNS depressants). Products include:
Sedapap Tablets 50 mg/650 mg 2098

Chlordiazepoxide (Co-administration results in enhanced response to CNS depressants).
No products indexed under this heading.

Chlordiazepoxide Hydrochloride (Co-administration results in enhanced response to CNS depressants). Products include:
Librium Capsules 3349

Chlorpromazine (Co-administration with cytochrome P4502D6 inhibitors, such as phenothiazines, may make normal metabolizer resemble poor metabolizer leading to higher than expected plasma concentration of TCA with resultant toxicity; lower than usual doses of either drug may be required; co-administration results in enhanced response to CNS depressants).
No products indexed under this heading.

Chlorpromazine Hydrochloride (Co-administration with cytochrome P4502D6 inhibitors, such as phenothiazines, may make normal metabolizer resemble poor metabolizer leading to higher than expected plasma concentration of TCA with resultant toxicity; lower than usual doses of either drug may be required; co-administration results in enhanced response to CNS depressants).
No products indexed under this heading.

Chlorprothixene (Co-administration results in enhanced response to CNS depressants).
No products indexed under this heading.

Chlorprothixene Hydrochloride (Co-administration results in enhanced response to CNS depressants).
No products indexed under this heading.

Chlorprothixene Lactate (Co-administration results in enhanced response to CNS depressants).
No products indexed under this heading.

Cimetidine (Co-administration has been reported to reduce hepatic metabolism of certain tricyclic antidepressants, thereby delaying elimination and increasing steady-state concentrations of TCA resulting in the frequency and severity of side effects, particularly anticholinergic). Products include:
Tagamet HB 200 Tablets .... ▣637
Tagamet Tablets 1547

Cimetidine Hydrochloride (Co-administration has been reported to reduce hepatic metabolism of certain tricyclic antidepressants, thereby delaying elimination and increasing steady-state concentrations of TCA resulting in the frequency and severity of side effects, particularly anticholinergic).
No products indexed under this heading.

Cisapride (Co-administration can result in possible adverse cardiac interactions including prolongation of the QT interval, cardiac arrhythmias and conduction system disturbances; concurrent use in contraindicated).
No products indexed under this heading.

Citalopram Hydrobromide (Co-administration with cytochrome P4502D6 inhibitors, such as antidepressants, may make normal metabolizer resemble poor metabolizer leading to higher than expected plasma concentration of TCA with resultant toxicity; lower than usual doses of either drug may be required). Products include:
Celexa 1177

Clidinium Bromide (Co-administration may result in hyperpyrexia, particularly during hot weather).
No products indexed under this heading.

Clorazepate Dipotassium (Co-administration results in enhanced response to CNS depressants). Products include:
Tranxene 2488

Clozapine (Co-administration results in enhanced response to CNS depressants). Products include:
Clozapine Tablets 2141
Clozaril Tablets 2174
FazaClo Orally Disintegrating Tablets 547

Codeine Phosphate (Co-administration results in enhanced response to CNS depressants). Products include:
Tylenol with Codeine 2461

Desflurane (Co-administration results in enhanced response to CNS depressants). Products include:
Suprane Liquid for Inhalation 770

Desipramine Hydrochloride (Co-administration with cytochrome P4502D6 inhibitors, such as antidepressants, may make normal metabolizer resemble poor metabolizer leading to higher than expected plasma concentration of TCA with resultant toxicity; lower than usual doses of either drug may be required).
No products indexed under this heading.

Dezocine (Co-administration results in enhanced response to CNS depressants).
No products indexed under this heading.

Diazepam (Co-administration results in enhanced response to CNS depressants). Products include:
Diastat Rectal Delivery System 3344
Valium Tablets 2822

Dicyclomine Hydrochloride (Co-administration may result in hyperpyrexia, particularly during hot weather). Products include:
Bentyl Capsules 724
Bentyl Injection 724
Bentyl Syrup 724

Bentyl Tablets 724

Dobutamine Hydrochloride (Effects of concurrent use not specified; careful adjustment of dosage and close supervision are required).
No products indexed under this heading.

Dopamine Hydrochloride (Effects of concurrent use not specified; careful adjustment of dosage and close supervision are required).
No products indexed under this heading.

Doxepin Hydrochloride (Co-administration with cytochrome P4502D6 inhibitors, such as antidepressants, may make normal metabolizer resemble poor metabolizer leading to higher than expected plasma concentration of TCA with resultant toxicity; lower than usual doses of either drug may be required).
No products indexed under this heading.

Droperidol (Co-administration results in enhanced response to CNS depressants).
No products indexed under this heading.

Enflurane (Co-administration results in enhanced response to CNS depressants).
No products indexed under this heading.

Ephedrine Hydrochloride (Effects of concurrent use not specified; careful adjustment of dosage and close supervision are required). Products include:
Primatene Tablets 749

Ephedrine Sulfate (Effects of concurrent use not specified; careful adjustment of dosage and close supervision are required).
No products indexed under this heading.

Ephedrine Tannate (Effects of concurrent use not specified; careful adjustment of dosage and close supervision are required).
No products indexed under this heading.

Epinephrine (Effects of concurrent use not specified; careful adjustment of dosage and close supervision are required). Products include:
EpiPen 1061
Primatene Mist 749

Epinephrine Bitartrate (Effects of concurrent use not specified; careful adjustment of dosage and close supervision are required).
No products indexed under this heading.

Epinephrine Hydrochloride (Effects of concurrent use not specified; careful adjustment of dosage and close supervision are required).
No products indexed under this heading.

Estazolam (Co-administration results in enhanced response to CNS depressants). Products include:
ProSom Tablets 512

Ethanol (Co-administration results in enhanced response to CNS depressants).
No products indexed under this heading.

Ethchlorvynol (Co-administration results in enhanced response to CNS depressants).
No products indexed under this heading.

Ethinamate (Co-administration results in enhanced response to CNS depressants).
No products indexed under this heading.

Ethyl Alcohol (Co-administration results in enhanced response to CNS depressants).
No products indexed under this heading.

Fentanyl (Co-administration results in enhanced response to CNS depressants). Products include:
Duragesic Transdermal System 2448

Fentanyl Citrate (Co-administration results in enhanced response to CNS depressants). Products include:
Actiq 993

Flecainide Acetate (Co-administration with cytochrome P4502D6 inhibitors, such as flecainide, may make normal metabolizer resemble poor metabolizer leading to higher than expected plasma concentration of TCA with resultant toxicity; lower than usual doses of either drug may be required). Products include:
Tambocor Tablets 1824

Fluoxetine Hydrochloride (Co-administration with cytochrome P4502D6 inhibitors, such as antidepressants, may make normal metabolizer resemble poor metabolizer leading to higher than expected plasma concentration of TCA with resultant toxicity; due to variation in the extent of inhibition of P4502D6 and long half-life of fluoxetine, sufficient time, at least 5 weeks, should elapse in switching to TCA). Products include:
Prozac Pulvules and Liquid 1771
Symbyax Capsules 1788

Fluphenazine Decanoate (Co-administration with cytochrome P4502D6 inhibitors, such as phenothiazines, may make normal metabolizer resemble poor metabolizer leading to higher than expected plasma concentration of TCA with resultant toxicity; lower than usual doses of either drug may be required; co-administration results in enhanced response to CNS depressants).
No products indexed under this heading.

Fluphenazine Enanthate (Co-administration with cytochrome P4502D6 inhibitors, such as phenothiazines, may make normal metabolizer resemble poor metabolizer leading to higher than expected plasma concentration of TCA with resultant toxicity; lower than usual doses of either drug may be required; co-administration results in enhanced response to CNS depressants).
No products indexed under this heading.

Fluphenazine Hydrochloride (Co-administration with cytochrome P4502D6 inhibitors, such as phenothiazines, may make normal metabolizer resemble poor metabolizer leading to higher than expected plasma concentration of TCA with resultant toxicity; lower than usual doses of either drug may be required; co-administration results in enhanced response to CNS depressants).
No products indexed under this heading.

Flurazepam Hydrochloride (Co-administration results in enhanced response to CNS depressants). Products include:
Dalmane Capsules 3343

Fluvoxamine Maleate (Co-administration with cytochrome P4502D6 inhibitors, such as antidepressants, may make normal metabolizer resemble poor metabolizer leading to higher than expected plasma concentration of TCA with resultant toxicity; due to variation in the extent of inhibition of P4502D6, sufficient time should elapse in switching from one class to the other).
No products indexed under this heading.

Glutethimide (Co-administration results in enhanced response to CNS depressants).
No products indexed under this heading.

Glycopyrrolate (Co-administration may result in hyperpyrexia, particularly during hot weather).
No products indexed under this heading.

Guanadrel Sulfate (Protriptyline may block the antihypertensive action of guanadrel).
No products indexed under this heading.

Guanethidine Monosulfate (Protriptyline may block the antihypertensive action of guanethidine).
No products indexed under this heading.

Haloperidol (Co-administration results in enhanced response to CNS depressants).
No products indexed under this heading.

Haloperidol Decanoate (Co-administration results in enhanced response to CNS depressants).
No products indexed under this heading.

Hydrocodone Bitartrate (Co-administration results in enhanced response to CNS depressants). Products include:
Hycodan 1104
Hycomine Compound Tablets 1105
Hycotuss Expectorant Syrup 1106
Lortab 3315
Lortab Elixir 3312
Vicodin Tablets 530
Vicodin ES Tablets 531
Vicodin HP Tablets 532
Vicoprofen Tablets 533
Zydone Tablets 1118

Hydrocodone Polistirex (Co-administration results in enhanced response to CNS depressants). Products include:
Tussionex Pennkinetic Extended-Release Suspension 3322

Hydromorphone Hydrochloride (Co-administration results in enhanced response to CNS depressants). Products include:
Dilaudid 439
Dilaudid Oral Liquid 443
Dilaudid Non-Sterile Powder 439
Dilaudid Rectal Suppositories 439
Dilaudid Tablets 439
Dilaudid Tablets - 8 mg 443
Dilaudid-HP 441

Hydroxyzine Hydrochloride (Co-administration results in enhanced response to CNS depressants).
No products indexed under this heading.

Hyoscyamine (Co-administration may result in hyperpyrexia, particularly during hot weather).
No products indexed under this heading.

Hyoscyamine Sulfate (Co-administration may result in hyperpyrexia, particularly during hot weather).
No products indexed under this heading.

Imipramine Hydrochloride (Co-administration with cytochrome P4502D6 inhibitors, such as antidepressants, may make normal metabolizer resemble poor metabolizer leading to higher than expected plasma concentration of TCA with resultant toxicity; lower than usual doses of either drug may be required).
No products indexed under this heading.

Imipramine Pamoate (Co-administration with cytochrome P4502D6 inhibitors, such as antidepressants, may make normal metabolizer resemble poor metabolizer leading to higher than expected plasma concentration of TCA with resultant toxicity; lower than usual doses of either drug may be required).
No products indexed under this heading.

Ipratropium Bromide (Co-administration may result in hyperpyrexia, particularly during hot weather). Products include:
Atrovent HFA Inhalation Aerosol 872
Atrovent Inhalation Solution 868
Atrovent Nasal Spray 0.03% 869
Atrovent Nasal Spray 0.06% 870
Combivent Inhalation Aerosol 878
DuoNeb Inhalation Solution 1058

Isocarboxazid (Co-administration of tricyclic antidepressants and MAO inhibitors has resulted in hyperpyretic crises, severe convulsions, and deaths; concurrent and/or sequential use is contraindicated).
No products indexed under this heading.

Isoflurane (Co-administration results in enhanced response to CNS depressants).
No products indexed under this heading.

Isoproterenol Hydrochloride (Effects of concurrent use not specified; careful adjustment of dosage and close supervision are required).
No products indexed under this heading.

Isoproterenol Sulfate (Effects of concurrent use not specified; careful adjustment of dosage and close supervision are required).
No products indexed under this heading.

Ketamine Hydrochloride (Co-administration results in enhanced response to CNS depressants).
No products indexed under this heading.

Levalbuterol Hydrochloride (Effects of concurrent use not specified; careful adjustment of dosage and close supervision are required). Products include:
Xopenex Inhalation Solution 3143
Xopenex Inhalation Solution Concentrate 3147

Levomethadyl Acetate Hydrochloride (Co-administration results in enhanced response to CNS depressants).
No products indexed under this heading.

Levorphanol Tartrate (Co-administration results in enhanced response to CNS depressants).
No products indexed under this heading.

Levothyroxine Sodium (On rare occasions, concurrent use may result in arrhythmias). Products include:
- Levothroid Tablets 1189
- Levoxyl Tablets 1680
- Synthroid Tablets 515
- Unithroid Tablets 3521

Liothyronine Sodium (On rare occasions, concurrent use may result in arrhythmias). Products include:
- Cytomel Tablets 1678

Liotrix (On rare occasions, concurrent use may result in arrhythmias). Products include:
- Thyrolar 1203

Lorazepam (Co-administration results in enhanced response to CNS depressants).
No products indexed under this heading.

Loxapine Hydrochloride (Co-administration results in enhanced response to CNS depressants).
No products indexed under this heading.

Loxapine Succinate (Co-administration results in enhanced response to CNS depressants).
No products indexed under this heading.

Maprotiline Hydrochloride (Co-administration with cytochrome P4502D6 inhibitors, such as antidepressants, may make normal metabolizer resemble poor metabolizer leading to higher than expected plasma concentration of TCA with resultant toxicity; lower than usual doses of either drug may be required).
No products indexed under this heading.

Mepenzolate Bromide (Co-administration may result in hyperpyrexia, particularly during hot weather).
No products indexed under this heading.

Meperidine Hydrochloride (Co-administration results in enhanced response to CNS depressants).
No products indexed under this heading.

Mephobarbital (Co-administration results in enhanced response to CNS depressants). Products include:
- Mebaral Tablets, USP 2483

Meprobamate (Co-administration results in enhanced response to CNS depressants).
No products indexed under this heading.

Mesoridazine Besylate (Co-administration with cytochrome P4502D6 inhibitors, such as phenothiazines, may make normal metabolizer resemble poor metabolizer leading to higher than expected plasma concentration of TCA with resultant toxicity; lower than usual doses of either drug may be required; co-administration results in enhanced response to CNS depressants).
No products indexed under this heading.

Metaproterenol Sulfate (Effects of concurrent use not specified; careful adjustment of dosage and close supervision are required). Products include:
- Alupent Inhalation Aerosol 858

Metaraminol Bitartrate (Effects of concurrent use not specified; careful adjustment of dosage and close supervision are required). Products include:
- Aramine Injection 1889

Methadone Hydrochloride (Co-administration results in enhanced response to CNS depressants).
No products indexed under this heading.

Methohexital Sodium (Co-administration results in enhanced response to CNS depressants).
No products indexed under this heading.

Methotrimeprazine (Co-administration with cytochrome P4502D6 inhibitors, such as phenothiazines, may make normal metabolizer resemble poor metabolizer leading to higher than expected plasma concentration of TCA with resultant toxicity; lower than usual doses of either drug may be required; co-administration results in enhanced response to CNS depressants).
No products indexed under this heading.

Methoxamine Hydrochloride (Effects of concurrent use not specified; careful adjustment of dosage and close supervision are required).
No products indexed under this heading.

Methoxyflurane (Co-administration results in enhanced response to CNS depressants).
No products indexed under this heading.

Midazolam Hydrochloride (Co-administration results in enhanced response to CNS depressants).
No products indexed under this heading.

Mirtazapine (Co-administration with cytochrome P4502D6 inhibitors, such as antidepressants, may make normal metabolizer resemble poor metabolizer leading to higher than expected plasma concentration of TCA with resultant toxicity; lower than usual doses of either drug may be required).
No products indexed under this heading.

Moclobemide (Co-administration of tricyclic antidepressants and MAO inhibitors has resulted in hyperpyretic crises, severe convulsions, and deaths; concurrent and/or sequential use is contraindicated).
No products indexed under this heading.

Molindone Hydrochloride (Co-administration results in enhanced response to CNS depressants). Products include:
- Moban Tablets 1108

Morphine Sulfate (Co-administration results in enhanced response to CNS depressants). Products include:
- Avinza Capsules 1714
- Kadian Capsules 572
- MS Contin Tablets 2703

Nefazodone Hydrochloride (Co-administration with cytochrome P4502D6 inhibitors, such as antidepressants, may make normal metabolizer resemble poor metabolizer leading to higher than expected plasma concentration of TCA with resultant toxicity; lower than usual doses of either drug may be required).
No products indexed under this heading.

Norepinephrine Bitartrate (Effects of concurrent use not specified; careful adjustment of dosage and close supervision are required).
No products indexed under this heading.

Nortriptyline Hydrochloride (Co-administration with cytochrome P4502D6 inhibitors, such as antidepressants, may make normal metabolizer resemble poor metabolizer leading to higher than expected plasma concentration of TCA with resultant toxicity; lower than usual doses of either drug may be required).
No products indexed under this heading.

Olanzapine (Co-administration results in enhanced response to CNS depressants). Products include:
- Symbyax Capsules 1788
- Zyprexa Tablets 1798
- Zyprexa IntraMuscular 1798
- Zyprexa ZYDIS Orally Disintegrating Tablets 1798

Oxazepam (Co-administration results in enhanced response to CNS depressants).
No products indexed under this heading.

Oxybutynin Chloride (Co-administration may result in hyperpyrexia, particularly during hot weather). Products include:
- Ditropan XL Extended Release Tablets 2391

Oxycodone Hydrochloride (Co-administration results in enhanced response to CNS depressants). Products include:
- Combunox Tablets 1183
- OxyContin Tablets 2699
- OxyFast Oral Concentrate Solution 2704
- OxyIR Capsules 2704
- Percocet Tablets 1114
- Percodan Tablets 1115

Pargyline Hydrochloride (Co-administration of tricyclic antidepressants and MAO inhibitors has resulted in hyperpyretic crises, severe convulsions, and deaths; concurrent and/or sequential use is contraindicated).
No products indexed under this heading.

Paroxetine Hydrochloride (Co-administration with cytochrome P4502D6 inhibitors, such as antidepressants, may make normal metabolizer resemble poor metabolizer leading to higher than expected plasma concentration of TCA with resultant toxicity; lower than usual doses of either drug may be required). Products include:
- Paxil CR Controlled-Release Tablets 1509
- Paxil 1501

Pentobarbital Sodium (Co-administration results in enhanced response to CNS depressants). Products include:
- Nembutal Sodium Solution, USP 2484

Perphenazine (Co-administration with cytochrome P4502D6 inhibitors, such as phenothiazines, may make normal metabolizer resemble poor metabolizer leading to higher than expected plasma concentration of TCA with resultant toxicity; lower than usual doses of either drug may be required; co-administration results in enhanced response to CNS depressants).
No products indexed under this heading.

Phenelzine Sulfate (Co-administration of tricyclic antidepressants and MAO inhibitors has resulted in hyperpyretic crises, severe convulsions, and deaths; concurrent and/or sequential use is contraindicated).
No products indexed under this heading.

Phenobarbital (Co-administration results in enhanced response to CNS depressants).
No products indexed under this heading.

Phenylephrine Bitartrate (Effects of concurrent use not specified; careful adjustment of dosage and close supervision are required).
No products indexed under this heading.

Phenylephrine Hydrochloride (Effects of concurrent use not specified; careful adjustment of dosage and close supervision are required). Products include:
- Alacol DM Syrup 739
- Hycomine Compound Tablets 1105
- Preparation H Maximum Strength Cream .... ▣747
- Preparation H Cooling Gel .... ▣747
- Preparation H .... ▣747
- Sudafed PE Tablets .... ▣711
- Vicks Sinex Nasal Spray and Ultra Fine Mist for Sinus Relief 2677
- Zicam Concentrated Cough Mist for Kids Plus D Cool Cherry .... ▣643
- Zicam Concentrated Cough Mist Plus D Cool Cherry .... ▣642

Phenylephrine Tannate (Effects of concurrent use not specified; careful adjustment of dosage and close supervision are required).
No products indexed under this heading.

Phenylpropanolamine Hydrochloride (Effects of concurrent use not specified; careful adjustment of dosage and close supervision are required).
No products indexed under this heading.

Pirbuterol Acetate (Effects of concurrent use not specified; careful adjustment of dosage and close supervision are required). Products include:
- Maxair Autohaler 1820

Prazepam (Co-administration results in enhanced response to CNS depressants).
No products indexed under this heading.

Procarbazine Hydrochloride (Co-administration of tricyclic antidepressants and MAO inhibitors has resulted in hyperpyretic crises, severe convulsions, and deaths; concurrent and/or sequential use is contraindicated). Products include:
- Matulane Capsules 3188

Prochlorperazine (Co-administration with cytochrome P4502D6 inhibitors, such as phenothiazines, may make normal metabolizer resemble poor metabolizer leading to higher than expected plasma concentration of TCA with resultant toxicity; lower than usual doses of either drug may be required; co-administration results in enhanced response to CNS depressants).
No products indexed under this heading.

Procyclidine Hydrochloride (Co-administration may result in hyperpyrexia, particularly during hot weather).
No products indexed under this heading.

Promethazine Hydrochloride (Co-administration with cytochrome P4502D6 inhibitors, such as phenothiazines, may make normal metabolizer resemble poor metabolizer leading to higher than expected plasma concentration of TCA with resultant toxicity; lower than usual doses of either drug may be required; co-administration results in enhanced response to CNS depressants). Products include:
Phenergan 3438

Propafenone Hydrochloride (Co-administration with cytochrome P4502D6 inhibitors, such as propafenone, may make normal metabolizer resemble poor metabolizer leading to higher than expected plasma concentration of TCA with resultant toxicity; lower than usual doses of either drug may be required). Products include:
Rythmol SR Capsules 2736

Propantheline Bromide (Co-administration may result in hyperpyrexia, particularly during hot weather).
No products indexed under this heading.

Propofol (Co-administration results in enhanced response to CNS depressants). Products include:
Diprivan Injectable Emulsion 676

Propoxyphene Hydrochloride (Co-administration results in enhanced response to CNS depressants).
No products indexed under this heading.

Propoxyphene Napsylate (Co-administration results in enhanced response to CNS depressants). Products include:
Darvocet A 500 Tablets 3497

Pseudoephedrine Hydrochloride (Effects of concurrent use not specified; careful adjustment of dosage and close supervision are required). Products include:
Advil Allergy Sinus Caplets 737
Advil Cold & Sinus 739
Advil Flu & Body Ache Caplets 739
Children's Advil Cold Suspension ... 741
Advil Multi-Symptom Cold Caplets 738
Allegra-D 12 Hour Extended-Release Tablets 2860
Allegra-D 24 Hour Extended-Release Tablets 2862
Balamine DM 739
BC Cold Powder 612
Benadryl Allergy & Cold Tablets 692
Benadryl Allergy & Sinus Headache Caplets & Gelcaps 693
Children's Benadryl Allergy & Cold Fastmelt Tablets 695
Benadryl Maximum Strength Severe Allergy & Sinus Headache Caplets 694
Children's Benadryl D Allergy & Sinus Fastmelt Tablets 694
Children's Benadryl D Liquid Medication 693
Benadryl D Tablets 694
Contac Non-Drowsy 12 Hour Cold Caplets 614
Contac Non-Drowsy Timed Release 12 Hour Cold Caplets 615
Contac Severe Cold and Flu Caplets Maximum Strength 615
Contac Severe Cold and Flu Caplets Non-Drowsy 615
Children's Dimetapp Cold & Allergy Elixir 745
Children's Dimetapp DM Cold & Cough Elixir 745
Children's Dimetapp Long Acting Cough Plus Cold Syrup 746
Dimetapp Infant Drops Decongestant Plus Cough 746
Children's Motrin Cold Non-Staining Dye-Free Oral Suspension 1838
Children's Motrin Cold Oral Suspension 1838
Motrin Cold & Sinus Caplets 1836
PediaCare Decongestant & Cough Infant Drops 705
PediaCare Decongestant Infants' Drops 705
PediaCare Long-Acting Cough Plus Cold Liquid 704
PediaCare Multi-Symptom Cold Liquid 704
PediaCare NightRest Cough & Cold Liquid 704
Robitussin Allergy & Cough Syrup .. 750
Robitussin CF Liquid 755
Robitussin Cough & Cold Liquid-filled Capsules 750
Robitussin Cough, Cold & Flu Liquid-filled Capsules 750
Robitussin Cough & Cold Infant Drops 755
Robitussin Flu Liquid 752
Robitussin Maximum Strength Cough & Cold Liquid 754
Robitussin PE Syrup 753
Robitussin Pediatric Cough & Cold Liquid 754
Robitussin PM Cough & Cold Liquid 752
Robitussin Severe Congestion Liquid-filled Capsules 751
Simply Stuffy Liquid 1841
Singlet Caplets 636
Sudafed 12 Hour Caplets 708
Sudafed 24 Hour Tablets 709
Sudafed Nasal Decongestant Tablets 709
Sudafed Severe Cold 710
Sudafed Non-Drying Sinus Liquid Caps 709
Sudafed Sinus & Allergy Tablets 710
Sudafed Sinus Headache 711
TheraFlu Cold & Cough Hot Liquid 680
TheraFlu Cold & Sore Throat Hot Liquid 680
TheraFlu Flu & Chest Congestion Non-Drowsy Hot Liquid 681
TheraFlu Flu & Sore Throat Hot Liquid 681
TheraFlu Severe Cold Non-Drowsy Hot Liquid 683
TheraFlu Severe Cold & Cough Hot Liquid 683
TheraFlu Severe Cold Caplets 679
TheraFlu Severe Cold Hot Liquid 682
TheraFlu Severe Cold Non-Drowsy Caplets 679
Triaminic Chest & Nasal Congestion Liquid 685
Triaminic Cold & Allergy Liquid 685
Triaminic Cold & Cough Liquid 685
Triaminic Cough Liquid 687
Triaminic Cough & Nasal Congestion Liquid 687
Triaminic Cough & Sore Throat Liquid 687
Triaminic Flu, Cough & Fever Liquid 685
Triaminic Night Time Cough & Cold Liquid 685
Triaminic Allergy Runny Nose & Congestion Softchews 688
Triaminic Cold & Cough Softchews 688
Triaminic Cough & Sore Throat Softchews 689
Tylenol Sinus NightTime Caplets 663
Children's Tylenol Plus Cold & Allergy Suspension Liquid 1850
Children's Tylenol Plus Cold NightTime Suspension Liquid 1851
Children's Tylenol Plus Cold & Cough Suspension Liquid and Chewable Tablets 1851
Children's Tylenol Plus Cold Chewable Tablets 1851
Children's Tylenol Plus Cold Daytime Non-Drowsy Suspension Liquid 1851
Children's Tylenol Plus Flu Suspension Liquid 1853
Concentrated Tylenol Infants' Drops Plus Cold 1851
Concentrated Tylenol Infants' Drops Plus Cold and Cough 1851
Tylenol Cold & Flu Severe Daytime Liquid with Cool Burst 1846
Tylenol Cold & Flu Severe NightTime Liquid with Cool Burst 1846
Tylenol Cold Severe Congestion Non-Drowsy Caplets with Cool Burst 1846
Tylenol Allergy Complete Night Time Caplets 1844
Tylenol Allergy Complete Multi-Symptom Caplets and Gelcaps with Cool Burst 1844
Tylenol Flu NightTime Gelcaps 1846
Tylenol Flu Day Non-Drowsy Gelcaps 1846
Concentrated Tylenol Infants' Drops Plus Cold Nasal Congestant, Fever Reducer & Pain Reliever 668
Concentrated Tylenol Infants' Drops Plus Cold & Cough Nasal Decongestant, Fever Reducer & Pain Reliever 668
Multi-Symptom Tylenol Cold Night Time Caplets 1845
Multi-Symptom Tylenol Cold Day Non-Drowsy Caplets and Gelcaps 1845
Tylenol Sinus Day Non-Drowsy 1848
Tylenol Sinus Night Time Caplets 1848
Tylenol Sinus Severe Congestion Caplets with Cool Burst 1848
Vicks 44D Cough & Head Congestion Relief 2676
Vicks 44D Cough & Head Congestion Relief Liquid 721
Vicks 44M Cough, Cold & Flu Relief 2676
Pediatric Vicks 44m Cough & Cold Relief 2673
Vicks DayQuil LiquiCaps/Liquid Multi-Symptom Cold/Flu Relief 723
Vicks DayQuil Multi-Symptom Cold/Flu Relief LiquiCaps 2675
Vicks DayQuil Multi-Symptom Cold/Flu Relief Liquid 2675
Children's Vicks NyQuil Cold/Cough Relief 2671
Vicks NyQuil LiquiCaps 2677
Vicks NyQuil LiquiCaps/Liquid Multi-Symptom Cold/Flu Relief 725
Vicks NyQuil Liquid 2677
Zyrtec-D 12 Hour Extended Release Tablets 2591

Pseudoephedrine Sulfate (Effects of concurrent use not specified; careful adjustment of dosage and close supervision are required). Products include:
Alavert Allergy & Sinus D-12 Hour Tablets 743
Clarinex-D 24-Hour Extended-Release Tablets 3012
Claritin-D Non-Drowsy 12 Hour Tablets 731
Claritin-D Non-Drowsy 24 Hour Tablets 731

Quazepam (Co-administration results in enhanced response to CNS depressants).
No products indexed under this heading.

Quetiapine Fumarate (Co-administration results in enhanced response to CNS depressants). Products include:
Seroquel Tablets 691

Quinidine (Co-administration with cytochrome P4502D6 inhibitors, such as quinidine, may make normal metabolizer resemble poor metabolizer leading to higher than expected plasma concentration of TCA with resultant toxicity; lower than usual doses of either drug may be required).
No products indexed under this heading.

Quinidine Gluconate (Co-administration with cytochrome P4502D6 inhibitors, such as quinidine, may make normal metabolizer resemble poor metabolizer leading to higher than expected plasma concentration of TCA with resultant toxicity; lower than usual doses of either drug may be required).
No products indexed under this heading.

Quinidine Hydrochloride (Co-administration with cytochrome P4502D6 inhibitors, such as quinidine, may make normal metabolizer resemble poor metabolizer leading to higher than expected plasma concentration of TCA with resultant toxicity; lower than usual doses of either drug may be required).
No products indexed under this heading.

Quinidine Polygalacturonate (Co-administration with cytochrome P4502D6 inhibitors, such as quinidine, may make normal metabolizer resemble poor metabolizer leading to higher than expected plasma concentration of TCA with resultant toxicity; lower than usual doses of either drug may be required).
No products indexed under this heading.

Quinidine Sulfate (Co-administration with cytochrome P4502D6 inhibitors, such as quinidine, may make normal metabolizer resemble poor metabolizer leading to higher than expected plasma concentration of TCA with resultant toxicity; lower than usual doses of either drug may be required).
No products indexed under this heading.

Remifentanil Hydrochloride (Co-administration results in enhanced response to CNS depressants).
No products indexed under this heading.

Risperidone (Co-administration results in enhanced response to CNS depressants). Products include:
Risperdal Consta Long-Acting Injection 1664
Risperdal M-Tab Orally Disintegrating Tablets 1658
Risperdal 1658

Salmeterol Xinafoate (Effects of concurrent use not specified; careful adjustment of dosage and close supervision are required). Products include:
Advair Diskus 100/50 1291
Advair Diskus 250/50 1291
Advair Diskus 500/50 1291
Serevent Diskus 1540

Scopolamine (Co-administration may result in hyperpyrexia, particularly during hot weather). Products include:
Transderm Scōp Transdermal Therapeutic System **2166**

Scopolamine Hydrobromide (Co-administration may result in hyperpyrexia, particularly during hot weather).
No products indexed under this heading.

Secobarbital Sodium (Co-administration results in enhanced response to CNS depressants).
No products indexed under this heading.

Selegiline Hydrochloride (Co-administration of tricyclic antidepressants and MAO inhibitors has resulted in hyperpyretic crises, severe convulsions, and deaths; concurrent and/or sequential use is contraindicated). Products include:
Eldepryl Capsules **3209**

Sertraline Hydrochloride (Co-administration with cytochrome P4502D6 inhibitors, such as antidepressants, may make normal metabolizer resemble poor metabolizer leading to higher than expected plasma concentration of TCA with resultant toxicity; lower than usual doses of either drug may be required). Products include:
Zoloft **2581**

Sevoflurane (Co-administration results in enhanced response to CNS depressants). Products include:
Ultane Liquid for Inhalation **526**

Sufentanil Citrate (Co-administration results in enhanced response to CNS depressants).
No products indexed under this heading.

Temazepam (Co-administration results in enhanced response to CNS depressants).
No products indexed under this heading.

Terbutaline Sulfate (Effects of concurrent use not specified; careful adjustment of dosage and close supervision are required).
No products indexed under this heading.

Thiamylal Sodium (Co-administration results in enhanced response to CNS depressants).
No products indexed under this heading.

Thioridazine Hydrochloride (Co-administration with cytochrome P4502D6 inhibitors, such as phenothiazines, may make normal metabolizer resemble poor metabolizer leading to higher than expected plasma concentration of TCA with resultant toxicity; lower than usual doses of either drug may be required; co-administration results in enhanced response to CNS depressants). Products include:
Thioridazine Hydrochloride Tablets **2122**

Thiothixene (Co-administration results in enhanced response to CNS depressants). Products include:
Thiothixene Capsules **2124**

Thyroglobulin (On rare occasions, concurrent use may result in arrhythmias).
No products indexed under this heading.

Thyroid (On rare occasions, concurrent use may result in arrhythmias).
No products indexed under this heading.

Thyroxine (On rare occasions, concurrent use may result in arrhythmias).
No products indexed under this heading.

Thyroxine Sodium (On rare occasions, concurrent use may result in arrhythmias).
No products indexed under this heading.

Tolterodine Tartrate (Co-administration may result in hyperpyrexia, particularly during hot weather). Products include:
Detrol Tablets **2626**
Detrol LA Capsules **2629**

Tramadol Hydrochloride (Tricyclic antidepressants may enhance the seizure risk in patients taking tramadol). Products include:
Ultracet Tablets **2462**

Tranylcypromine Sulfate (Co-administration of tricyclic antidepressants and MAO inhibitors has resulted in hyperpyretic crises, severe convulsions, and deaths; concurrent and/or sequential use is contraindicated). Products include:
Parnate Tablets **1499**

Trazodone Hydrochloride (Co-administration with cytochrome P4502D6 inhibitors, such as antidepressants, may make normal metabolizer resemble poor metabolizer leading to higher than expected plasma concentration of TCA with resultant toxicity; lower than usual doses of either drug may be required).
No products indexed under this heading.

Triazolam (Co-administration results in enhanced response to CNS depressants).
No products indexed under this heading.

Tridihexethyl Chloride (Co-administration may result in hyperpyrexia, particularly during hot weather).
No products indexed under this heading.

Trifluoperazine Hydrochloride (Co-administration with cytochrome P4502D6 inhibitors, such as phenothiazines, may make normal metabolizer resemble poor metabolizer leading to higher than expected plasma concentration of TCA with resultant toxicity; lower than usual doses of either drug may be required; co-administration results in enhanced response to CNS depressants).
No products indexed under this heading.

Trihexyphenidyl Hydrochloride (Co-administration may result in hyperpyrexia, particularly during hot weather).
No products indexed under this heading.

Trimipramine Maleate (Co-administration with cytochrome P4502D6 inhibitors, such as antidepressants, may make normal metabolizer resemble poor metabolizer leading to higher than expected plasma concentration of TCA with resultant toxicity; lower than usual doses of either drug may be required). Products include:
Surmontil Capsules **2347**

Venlafaxine Hydrochloride (Co-administration with cytochrome P4502D6 inhibitors, such as antidepressants, may make normal metabolizer resemble poor metabolizer leading to higher than expected plasma concentration of TCA with resultant toxicity; lower than usual doses of either drug may be required). Products include:
Effexor Tablets **3405**
Effexor XR Capsules **3411**

Zaleplon (Co-administration results in enhanced response to CNS depressants). Products include:
Sonata Capsules **1686**

Ziprasidone Hydrochloride (Co-administration results in enhanced response to CNS depressants). Products include:
Geodon Capsules **2514**

Zolpidem Tartrate (Co-administration results in enhanced response to CNS depressants). Products include:
Ambien Tablets **2867**

Food Interactions

Alcohol (Co-administration results in enhanced response to alcohol).

VIVARIN CAPLETS

(Caffeine) .... ◘**639**
May interact with:

Beverages, containing medications (Concurrent use may cause nervousness, irritability, sleeplessness, and occasionally, rapid heartbeat).
No products indexed under this heading.

Caffeine-containing medications (Concurrent use may cause nervousness, irritability, sleeplessness, and occasionally, rapid heartbeat).
No products indexed under this heading.

Food, containing medications (Concurrent use may cause nervousness, irritability, sleeplessness, and occasionally, rapid heartbeat).
No products indexed under this heading.

VIVARIN TABLETS

(Caffeine) .... ◘**639**
See Vivarin Caplets

VIVELLE TRANSDERMAL SYSTEM

(Estradiol) **2288**
May interact with erythromycin, thyroid preparations, and certain other agents. Compounds in these categories include:

Carbamazepine (Co-administration of estrogens with inducers of CYP3A4, such as carbamazepine, may reduce plasma concentrations of estrogens, possibly resulting in a decrease in therapeutic effects and/or changes in the uterine bleeding profile). Products include:
Carbatrol Capsules **3174**
Equetro Extended-Release Capsules **3178**
Tegretol/Tegretol-XR **2278**

Clarithromycin (Co-administration of estrogens with inhibitors of CYP3A4, such as clarithromycin, may increase plasma concentrations of estrogens and may result in side effects). Products include:
Biaxin/Biaxin XL **402**
PREVPAC **3281**

Erythromycin (Co-administration of estrogens with inhibitors of CYP3A4, such as erythromycin, may reduce plasma concentrations of estrogens and may result in side effects). Products include:
Erygel Topical Gel **2096**
Ery-Tab Tablets **447**
Erythromycin Base Filmtab Tablets **454**
Erythromycin Delayed-Release Capsules, USP **456**
PCE Dispertab Tablets **510**

Erythromycin Estolate (Co-administration of estrogens with inhibitors of CYP3A4, such as erythromycin, may reduce plasma concentrations of estrogens and may result in side effects).
No products indexed under this heading.

Erythromycin Ethylsuccinate (Co-administration of estrogens with inhibitors of CYP3A4, such as erythromycin, may reduce plasma concentrations of estrogens and may result in side effects). Products include:
E.E.S. **449**
EryPed **445**

Erythromycin Gluceptate (Co-administration of estrogens with inhibitors of CYP3A4, such as erythromycin, may reduce plasma concentrations of estrogens and may result in side effects).
No products indexed under this heading.

Erythromycin Lactobionate (Co-administration of estrogens with inhibitors of CYP3A4, such as erythromycin, may reduce plasma concentrations of estrogens and may result in side effects).
No products indexed under this heading.

Erythromycin Stearate (Co-administration of estrogens with inhibitors of CYP3A4, such as erythromycin, may reduce plasma concentrations of estrogens and may result in side effects). Products include:
Erythrocin Stearate Filmtab Tablets **452**

Hypericum (Co-administration of estrogens with inducers of CYP3A4, such as St. John's Wort, may reduce plasma concentrations of estrogens, possibly resulting in a decrease in therapeutic effects and/or changes in the uterine bleeding profile).
No products indexed under this heading.

Itraconazole (Co-administration of estrogens with inhibitors of CYP3A4, such as itraconazole, may increase plasma concentrations of estrogens and may result in side effects).
No products indexed under this heading.

Ketoconazole (Co-administration of estrogens with inhibitors of CYP3A4, such as ketoconazole, may increase plasma concentrations of estrogens and may result in side effects). Products include:
Nizoral A-D Shampoo, 1% **1839**
Nizoral 2% Shampoo **1838**

Levothyroxine Sodium (Patients on thyroid replacement therapy may require higher doses of thyroid hormone). Products include:
Levothroid Tablets **1189**
Levoxyl Tablets **1680**
Synthroid Tablets **515**
Unithroid Tablets **3521**

Liothyronine Sodium (Patients on thyroid replacement therapy may require higher doses of thyroid hormone). Products include:
- Cytomel Tablets 1678

Liotrix (Patients on thyroid replacement therapy may require higher doses of thyroid hormone). Products include:
- Thyrolar 1203

Phenobarbital (Co-administration of estrogens with inducers of CYP3A4, such as phenobarbital, may reduce plasma concentrations of estrogens, possibly resulting in a decrease in therapeutic effects and/or changes in the uterine bleeding profile).
No products indexed under this heading.

Phenobarbital Sodium (Co-administration of estrogens with inducers of CYP3A4, such as phenobarbital, may reduce plasma concentrations of estrogens, possibly resulting in a decrease in therapeutic effects and/or changes in the uterine bleeding profile).
No products indexed under this heading.

Rifampin (Co-administration of estrogens with inducers of CYP3A4, such as rifampin, may reduce plasma concentrations of estrogens, possibly resulting in a decrease in therapeutic effects and/or changes in the uterine bleeding profile).
No products indexed under this heading.

Ritonavir (Co-administration of estrogens with inhibitors of CYP3A4, such as ritonavir, may increase plasma concentrations of estrogens and may result in side effects). Products include:
- Kaletra 474
- Norvir 499

Thyroglobulin (Patients on thyroid replacement therapy may require higher doses of thyroid hormone).
No products indexed under this heading.

Thyroid (Patients on thyroid replacement therapy may require higher doses of thyroid hormone).
No products indexed under this heading.

Thyroxine (Patients on thyroid replacement therapy may require higher doses of thyroid hormone).
No products indexed under this heading.

Thyroxine Sodium (Patients on thyroid replacement therapy may require higher doses of thyroid hormone).
No products indexed under this heading.

Food Interactions

Grapefruit Juice (Co-administration of estrogens with inhibitors of CYP3A4, such as grapefruit juice, may increase plasma concentrations of estrogens and may result in side effects).

VIVELLE-DOT TRANSDERMAL SYSTEM

(Estradiol) 2293

See Vivelle Transdermal System

VIVOTIF

(Typhoid Vaccine Live Oral TY21a) 834

May interact with:

Chloroquine Phosphate (Several antimalarials, such as chloroquine, possess antibacterial activity which may interfere with the immune response rate; in one study, concomitant treatment did not result in significant reduction in the immune response, therefore, these drugs can be administered together).
No products indexed under this heading.

Mefloquine Hydrochloride (Several antimalarials, such as mefloquine, possess antibacterial activity which may interfere with the immune response rate; in one study, concomitant treatment did not result in significant reduction in the immune response, therefore, these drugs can be administered together). Products include:
- Lariam Tablets 2790

Proguanil (The simultaneous administration of proguanil results in a significant decrease in the immune response rate).
No products indexed under this heading.

VOLTAREN OPHTHALMIC SOLUTION

(Diclofenac Sodium) 2300

None cited in PDR database.

VOLTAREN TABLETS

(Diclofenac Sodium) 2298

May interact with ACE inhibitors, lithium preparations, thiazides, and certain other agents. Compounds in these categories include:

Aspirin (When diclofenac is administered with aspirin, its protein binding is reduced; the clinical significance of this interaction is not known). Products include:
- Aggrenox Capsules 855
- Bayer, Aspirin Regimen 606
- Bayer Aspirin Tablets 3515
- BC Powder 612
- BC Allergy Sinus Cold Powder 612
- Arthritis Strength BC Powder 612
- BC Sinus Cold Powder 612
- Ecotrin Enteric Coated Aspirin Low, Regular and Maximum Strength Tablets 1627
- Goody's Body Pain Formula Powder 621
- Goody's Extra Strength Headache Powder 621
- Goody's Extra Strength Pain Relief Tablets 621
- Percodan Tablets 1115
- St. Joseph 81 mg Aspirin Chewable and Enteric Coated Tablets 1841

Benazepril Hydrochloride (Reports suggest that NSAIDs may diminish the antihypertensive effect of ACE inhibitors; this interaction should be given consideration in patients taking NSAIDs concomitantly with ACE inhibitors). Products include:
- Lotensin Tablets 2232
- Lotensin HCT Tablets 2235
- Lotrel Capsules 2238

Bendroflumethiazide (Studies have shown that diclofenac can reduce the natriuretic effect of furosemide and thiazides in some patients; during concomitant therapy with NSAIDs, the patient should be observed closely for signs of renal failure, as well as to assure diuretic efficacy).
No products indexed under this heading.

Captopril (Reports suggest that NSAIDs may diminish the antihypertensive effect of ACE inhibitors; this interaction should be given consideration in patients taking NSAIDs concomitantly with ACE inhibitors). Products include:
- Captopril Tablets 2114

Chlorothiazide (Studies have shown that diclofenac can reduce the natriuretic effect of furosemide and thiazides in some patients; during concomitant therapy with NSAIDs, the patient should be observed closely for signs of renal failure, as well as to assure diuretic efficacy). Products include:
- Aldoclor Tablets 1881
- Diuril Oral 1936

Chlorothiazide Sodium (Studies have shown that diclofenac can reduce the natriuretic effect of furosemide and thiazides in some patients; during concomitant therapy with NSAIDs, the patient should be observed closely for signs of renal failure, as well as to assure diuretic efficacy). Products include:
- Diuril Sodium Intravenous 1934

Cyclosporine (Diclofenac may affect renal prostaglandins and increase the toxicity of certain drugs; concomitant therapy with diclofenac may increase cyclosporine's nephrotoxicity; caution should be used when administered concomitantly with cyclosporine). Products include:
- Gengraf Capsules 458
- Neoral Soft Gelatin Capsules 2247
- Neoral Oral Solution 2247
- Restasis Ophthalmic Emulsion 570
- Sandimmune 2259

Enalapril Maleate (Reports suggest that NSAIDs may diminish the antihypertensive effect of ACE inhibitors; this interaction should be given consideration in patients taking NSAIDs concomitantly with ACE inhibitors). Products include:
- Vaseretic Tablets 2073
- Vasotec I.V. Injection 2076

Enalaprilat (Reports suggest that NSAIDs may diminish the antihypertensive effect of ACE inhibitors; this interaction should be given consideration in patients taking NSAIDs concomitantly with ACE inhibitors).
No products indexed under this heading.

Fosinopril Sodium (Reports suggest that NSAIDs may diminish the antihypertensive effect of ACE inhibitors; this interaction should be given consideration in patients taking NSAIDs concomitantly with ACE inhibitors).
No products indexed under this heading.

Furosemide (Studies have shown that diclofenac can reduce the natriuretic effect of furosemide and thiazides in some patients; during concomitant therapy with NSAIDs, the patient should be observed closely for signs of renal failure, as well as to assure diuretic efficacy). Products include:
- Furosemide Tablets 2117

Hydrochlorothiazide (Studies have shown that diclofenac can reduce the natriuretic effect of furosemide and thiazides in some patients; during concomitant therapy with NSAIDs, the patient should be observed closely for signs of renal failure, as well as to assure diuretic efficacy). Products include:
- Aldoril Tablets 1884
- Atacand HCT 637
- Avalide Tablets 2889
- Avalide Tablets 922
- Benicar HCT Tablets 2852
- Diovan HCT Tablets 2195
- Dyazide Capsules 1389
- Hyzaar 1964
- Lotensin HCT Tablets 2235
- Maxzide 2150
- Micardis HCT Tablets 886
- Moduretic Tablets 2003
- Prinzide Tablets 2033
- Teveten HCT Tablets 1710
- Timolide Tablets 2056
- Uniretic Tablets 3114
- Vaseretic Tablets 2073
- Zestoretic Tablets 701

Hydroflumethiazide (Studies have shown that diclofenac can reduce the natriuretic effect of furosemide and thiazides in some patients; during concomitant therapy with NSAIDs, the patient should be observed closely for signs of renal failure, as well as to assure diuretic efficacy).
No products indexed under this heading.

Lisinopril (Reports suggest that NSAIDs may diminish the antihypertensive effect of ACE inhibitors; this interaction should be given consideration in patients taking NSAIDs concomitantly with ACE inhibitors). Products include:
- Prinivil Tablets 2029
- Prinzide Tablets 2033
- Zestoretic Tablets 701
- Zestril Tablets 704

Lithium (NSAIDs have produced an elevation of plasma lithium levels and a reduction in renal lithium clearance; these effects have been attributed to inhibition of renal prostaglandin synthesis by the NSAID; monitor for signs of lithium toxicity).
No products indexed under this heading.

Lithium Carbonate (NSAIDs have produced an elevation of plasma lithium levels and a reduction in renal lithium clearance; these effects have been attributed to inhibition of renal prostaglandin synthesis by the NSAID; monitor for signs of lithium toxicity). Products include:
- Eskalith 1406
- Lithobid Tablets 1670

Lithium Citrate (NSAIDs have produced an elevation of plasma lithium levels and a reduction in renal lithium clearance; these effects have been attributed to inhibition of renal prostaglandin synthesis by the NSAID; monitor for signs of lithium toxicity).
No products indexed under this heading.

Methotrexate Sodium (NSAIDs have been reported to competitively inhibit methotrexate accumulation in animal studies; this may indicate that they could enhance the toxicity of methotrexate; caution should be given when NSAIDs are administered concomitantly with methotrexate).
No products indexed under this heading.

Methyclothiazide (Studies have shown that diclofenac can reduce the natriuretic effect of furosemide and thiazides in some patients; during concomitant therapy with NSAIDs, the patient should be observed closely for signs of renal failure, as well as to assure diuretic efficacy).
No products indexed under this heading.

Moexipril Hydrochloride (Reports suggest that NSAIDs may diminish the antihypertensive effect of ACE inhibitors; this interaction should be given consideration in patients taking NSAIDs concomitantly with ACE inhibitors). Products include:
Uniretic Tablets 3114
Univasc Tablets 3118

Perindopril Erbumine (Reports suggest that NSAIDs may diminish the antihypertensive effect of ACE inhibitors; this interaction should be given consideration in patients taking NSAIDs concomitantly with ACE inhibitors). Products include:
Aceon Tablets (2 mg, 4 mg, 8 mg) 3191

Polythiazide (Studies have shown that diclofenac can reduce the natriuretic effect of furosemide and thiazides in some patients; during concomitant therapy with NSAIDs, the patient should be observed closely for signs of renal failure, as well as to assure diuretic efficacy).
No products indexed under this heading.

Quinapril Hydrochloride (Reports suggest that NSAIDs may diminish the antihypertensive effect of ACE inhibitors; this interaction should be given consideration in patients taking NSAIDs concomitantly with ACE inhibitors).
No products indexed under this heading.

Ramipril (Reports suggest that NSAIDs may diminish the antihypertensive effect of ACE inhibitors; this interaction should be given consideration in patients taking NSAIDs concomitantly with ACE inhibitors). Products include:
Altace Capsules 1673

Spirapril Hydrochloride (Reports suggest that NSAIDs may diminish the antihypertensive effect of ACE inhibitors; this interaction should be given consideration in patients taking NSAIDs concomitantly with ACE inhibitors).
No products indexed under this heading.

Trandolapril (Reports suggest that NSAIDs may diminish the antihypertensive effect of ACE inhibitors; this interaction should be given consideration in patients taking NSAIDs concomitantly with ACE inhibitors). Products include:
Mavik Tablets 482
Tarka Tablets 519

Warfarin Sodium (The effects of warfarin and NSAIDs on GI bleeding are synergistic, such that users of both drugs together have a risk of serious GI bleeding higher than users of either drug alone). Products include:
Coumadin for Injection 932
Coumadin Tablets 932

VOLTAREN-XR TABLETS

(Diclofenac Sodium) 2301
See Voltaren Tablets

VOSPIRE EXTENDED-RELEASE TABLETS

(Albuterol Sulfate) 2352
May interact with beta blockers, monoamine oxidase inhibitors, non-potassium-sparing diuretics, oral sympathomimetics, tricyclic antidepressants, and certain other agents. Compounds in these categories include:

Acebutolol Hydrochloride (Co-administration of albuterol with beta-blockers not only blocks the pulmonary effect of beta-agonists, but may produce severe bronchospasm in asthmatic patients).
No products indexed under this heading.

Amitriptyline Hydrochloride (Administer albuterol with extreme caution to patients being treated with tricyclics, or within 2 weeks of discontinuing such agents, because action on vascular system may be potentiated).
No products indexed under this heading.

Amoxapine (Administer albuterol with extreme caution to patients being treated with tricyclics, or within 2 weeks of discontinuing such agents, because action on vascular system may be potentiated).
No products indexed under this heading.

Atenolol (Co-administration of albuterol with beta-blockers not only blocks the pulmonary effect of beta-agonists, but may produce severe bronchospasm in asthmatic patients). Products include:
Tenormin I.V. Injection 698
Tenormin Tablets 695

Bendroflumethiazide (Caution is advised in the co-administration of beta-agonists with non-potassium sparing diuretics, since the ECG changes and/or hypokalemia that may result from the administration of non-potassium sparing diuretics can be acutely worsened by beta-agonists, especially when the recommended dose of the beta-agonist is exceeded; clinical significance not known).
No products indexed under this heading.

Betaxolol Hydrochloride (Co-administration of albuterol with beta-blockers not only blocks the pulmonary effect of beta-agonists, but may produce severe bronchospasm in asthmatic patients). Products include:
Betoptic S Ophthalmic Suspension 554

Bisoprolol Fumarate (Co-administration of albuterol with beta-blockers not only blocks the pulmonary effect of beta-agonists, but may produce severe bronchospasm in asthmatic patients).
No products indexed under this heading.

Bumetanide (Caution is advised in the co-administration of beta-agonists with non-potassium sparing diuretics, since the ECG changes and/or hypokalemia that may result from the administration of non-potassium sparing diuretics can be acutely worsened by beta-agonists, especially when the recommended dose of the beta-agonist is exceeded; clinical significance not known).
No products indexed under this heading.

Carteolol Hydrochloride (Co-administration of albuterol with beta-blockers not only blocks the pulmonary effect of beta-agonists, but may produce severe bronchospasm in asthmatic patients). Products include:
Carteolol Hydrochloride Ophthalmic Solution USP, 1% .... ⊙246

Chlorothiazide (Caution is advised in the co-administration of beta-agonists with non-potassium sparing diuretics, since the ECG changes and/or hypokalemia that may result from the administration of non-potassium sparing diuretics can be acutely worsened by beta-agonists, especially when the recommended dose of the beta-agonist is exceeded; clinical significance not known). Products include:
Aldoclor Tablets 1881
Diuril Oral 1936

Chlorothiazide Sodium (Caution is advised in the co-administration of beta-agonists with non-potassium sparing diuretics, since the ECG changes and/or hypokalemia that may result from the administration of non-potassium sparing diuretics can be acutely worsened by beta-agonists, especially when the recommended dose of the beta-agonist is exceeded; clinical significance not known). Products include:
Diuril Sodium Intravenous 1934

Clomipramine Hydrochloride (Administer albuterol with extreme caution to patients being treated with tricyclics, or within 2 weeks of discontinuing such agents, because action on vascular system may be potentiated).
No products indexed under this heading.

Desipramine Hydrochloride (Administer albuterol with extreme caution to patients being treated with tricyclics, or within 2 weeks of discontinuing such agents, because action on vascular system may be potentiated).
No products indexed under this heading.

Digoxin (Monitor serum digoxin levels in patients receiving digoxin and albuterol, since co-administration may decrease serum digoxin levels; clinical significance on chronic therapy is unclear). Products include:
Digitek Tablets 2146
Lanoxicaps Capsules 1458
Lanoxin Injection 1462
Lanoxin Tablets 1468
Lanoxin Injection Pediatric 1465

Doxepin Hydrochloride (Administer albuterol with extreme caution to patients being treated with tricyclics, or within 2 weeks of discontinuing such agents, because action on vascular system may be potentiated).
No products indexed under this heading.

Ephedrine Hydrochloride (Concomitant use of albuterol and other oral sympathomimetic agents is not recommended since combined use may lead to deleterious cardiovascular effects). Products include:
Primatene Tablets .... ■749

Ephedrine Sulfate (Concomitant use of albuterol and other oral sympathomimetic agents is not recommended since combined use may lead to deleterious cardiovascular effects).
No products indexed under this heading.

Ephedrine Tannate (Concomitant use of albuterol and other oral sympathomimetic agents is not recommended since combined use may lead to deleterious cardiovascular effects).
No products indexed under this heading.

Esmolol Hydrochloride (Co-administration of albuterol with beta-blockers not only blocks the pulmonary effect of beta-agonists, but may produce severe bronchospasm in asthmatic patients). Products include:
Brevibloc Concentrate 766
Brevibloc Injection 766
Brevibloc Double Strength Injection 766
Brevibloc Premixed Injection 766
Brevibloc Double Strength Premixed Injection 766

Ethacrynic Acid (Caution is advised in the co-administration of beta-agonists with non-potassium sparing diuretics, since the ECG changes and/or hypokalemia that may result from the administration of non-potassium sparing diuretics can be acutely worsened by beta-agonists, especially when the recommended dose of the beta-agonist is exceeded; clinical significance not known). Products include:
Edecrin Tablets 1941

Furosemide (Caution is advised in the co-administration of beta-agonists with non-potassium sparing diuretics, since the ECG changes and/or hypokalemia that may result from the administration of non-potassium sparing diuretics can be acutely worsened by beta-agonists, especially when the recommended dose of the beta-agonist is exceeded; clinical significance not known). Products include:
Furosemide Tablets 2117

Hydrochlorothiazide (Caution is advised in the co-administration of beta-agonists with non-potassium sparing diuretics, since the ECG changes and/or hypokalemia that may result from the administration of non-potassium sparing diuretics can be acutely worsened by beta-agonists, especially when the recommended dose of the beta-agonist is exceeded; clinical significance not known). Products include:
Aldoril Tablets 1884
Atacand HCT 637
Avalide Tablets 2889
Avalide Tablets 922
Benicar HCT Tablets 2852
Diovan HCT Tablets 2195
Dyazide Capsules 1389
Hyzaar 1964
Lotensin HCT Tablets 2235
Maxzide 2150
Micardis HCT Tablets 886
Moduretic Tablets 2003
Prinzide Tablets 2033
Teveten HCT Tablets 1710

Timolide Tablets 2056
Uniretic Tablets 3114
Vaseretic Tablets 2073
Zestoretic Tablets 701

Hydroflumethiazide (Caution is advised in the co-administration of beta-agonists with non-potassium sparing diuretics, since the ECG changes and/or hypokalemia that may result from the administration of non-potassium sparing diuretics can be acutely worsened by beta-agonists, especially when the recommended dose of the beta-agonist is exceeded; clinical significance not known).
No products indexed under this heading.

Imipramine Hydrochloride (Administer albuterol with extreme caution to patients being treated with tricyclics, or within 2 weeks of discontinuing such agents, because action on vascular system may be potentiated).
No products indexed under this heading.

Imipramine Pamoate (Administer albuterol with extreme caution to patients being treated with tricyclics, or within 2 weeks of discontinuing such agents, because action on vascular system may be potentiated).
No products indexed under this heading.

Isocarboxazid (Administer albuterol with extreme caution to patients being treated with MAO inhibitors, or within 2 weeks of discontinuing such agents, because action on vascular system may be potentiated).
No products indexed under this heading.

Labetalol Hydrochloride (Co-administration of albuterol with beta-blockers not only blocks the pulmonary effect of beta-agonists, but may produce severe bronchospasm in asthmatic patients).
No products indexed under this heading.

Levobunolol Hydrochloride (Co-administration of albuterol with beta-blockers not only blocks the pulmonary effect of beta-agonists, but may produce severe bronchospasm in asthmatic patients). Products include:
Betagan Ophthalmic Solution, USP.. ⊙217

Maprotiline Hydrochloride (Administer albuterol with extreme caution to patients being treated with tricyclics, or within 2 weeks of discontinuing such agents, because action on vascular system may be potentiated).
No products indexed under this heading.

Metaproterenol Sulfate (Concomitant use of albuterol and other oral sympathomimetic agents is not recommended since combined use may lead to deleterious cardiovascular effects). Products include:
Alupent Inhalation Aerosol 858

Methyclothiazide (Caution is advised in the co-administration of beta-agonists with non-potassium sparing diuretics, since the ECG changes and/or hypokalemia that may result from the administration of non-potassium sparing diuretics can be acutely worsened by beta-agonists, especially when the recommended dose of the beta-agonist is exceeded; clinical significance not known).
No products indexed under this heading.

Metipranolol Hydrochloride (Co-administration of albuterol with beta-blockers not only blocks the pulmonary effect of beta-agonists, but may produce severe bronchospasm in asthmatic patients).
No products indexed under this heading.

Metoprolol Succinate (Co-administration of albuterol with beta-blockers not only blocks the pulmonary effect of beta-agonists, but may produce severe bronchospasm in asthmatic patients). Products include:
Toprol-XL Tablets 660

Metoprolol Tartrate (Co-administration of albuterol with beta-blockers not only blocks the pulmonary effect of beta-agonists, but may produce severe bronchospasm in asthmatic patients).
No products indexed under this heading.

Moclobemide (Administer albuterol with extreme caution to patients being treated with MAO inhibitors, or within 2 weeks of discontinuing such agents, because action on vascular system may be potentiated).
No products indexed under this heading.

Nadolol (Co-administration of albuterol with beta-blockers not only blocks the pulmonary effect of beta-agonists, but may produce severe bronchospasm in asthmatic patients). Products include:
Nadolol Tablets 2121

Nortriptyline Hydrochloride (Administer albuterol with extreme caution to patients being treated with tricyclics, or within 2 weeks of discontinuing such agents, because action on vascular system may be potentiated).
No products indexed under this heading.

Pargyline Hydrochloride (Administer albuterol with extreme caution to patients being treated with MAO inhibitors, or within 2 weeks of discontinuing such agents, because action on vascular system may be potentiated).
No products indexed under this heading.

Penbutolol Sulfate (Co-administration of albuterol with beta-blockers not only blocks the pulmonary effect of beta-agonists, but may produce severe bronchospasm in asthmatic patients).
No products indexed under this heading.

Phenelzine Sulfate (Administer albuterol with extreme caution to patients being treated with MAO inhibitors, or within 2 weeks of discontinuing such agents, because action on vascular system may be potentiated).
No products indexed under this heading.

Phenylephrine Hydrochloride (Concomitant use of albuterol and other oral sympathomimetic agents is not recommended since combined use may lead to deleterious cardiovascular effects). Products include:
Alacol DM Syrup 739
Hycomine Compound Tablets 1105
Preparation H Maximum Strength Cream 747
Preparation H Cooling Gel 747
Preparation H 747
Sudafed PE Tablets 711
Vicks Sinex Nasal Spray and Ultra Fine Mist for Sinus Relief.............. 2677
Zicam Concentrated Cough Mist for Kids Plus D Cool Cherry......... 643
Zicam Concentrated Cough Mist Plus D Cool Cherry..................... 642

Phenylephrine Tannate (Concomitant use of albuterol and other oral sympathomimetic agents is not recommended since combined use may lead to deleterious cardiovascular effects).
No products indexed under this heading.

Phenylpropanolamine Hydrochloride (Concomitant use of albuterol and other oral sympathomimetic agents is not recommended since combined use may lead to deleterious cardiovascular effects).
No products indexed under this heading.

Pindolol (Co-administration of albuterol with beta-blockers not only blocks the pulmonary effect of beta-agonists, but may produce severe bronchospasm in asthmatic patients).
No products indexed under this heading.

Polythiazide (Caution is advised in the co-administration of beta-agonists with non-potassium sparing diuretics, since the ECG changes and/or hypokalemia that may result from the administration of non-potassium sparing diuretics can be acutely worsened by beta-agonists, especially when the recommended dose of the beta-agonist is exceeded; clinical significance not known).
No products indexed under this heading.

Procarbazine Hydrochloride (Administer albuterol with extreme caution to patients being treated with MAO inhibitors, or within 2 weeks of discontinuing such agents, because action on vascular system may be potentiated). Products include:
Matulane Capsules 3188

Propranolol Hydrochloride (Co-administration of albuterol with beta-blockers not only blocks the pulmonary effect of beta-agonists, but may produce severe bronchospasm in asthmatic patients). Products include:
Inderal LA Long-Acting Capsules 3421
InnoPran XL Capsules 2728

Protriptyline Hydrochloride (Administer albuterol with extreme caution to patients being treated with tricyclics, or within 2 weeks of discontinuing such agents, because action on vascular system may be potentiated). Products include:
Vivactil Tablets 2350

Pseudoephedrine Hydrochloride (Concomitant use of albuterol and other oral sympathomimetic agents is not recommended since combined use may lead to deleterious cardiovascular effects). Products include:
Advil Allergy Sinus Caplets 737
Advil Cold & Sinus 739
Advil Flu & Body Ache Caplets 739
Children's Advil Cold Suspension ... 741
Advil Multi-Symptom Cold Caplets.............................. 738
Allegra-D 12 Hour Extended-Release Tablets............ 2860
Allegra-D 24 Hour Extended-Release Tablets............ 2862
Balamine DM 739
BC Cold Powder 612
Benadryl Allergy & Cold Tablets 692
Benadryl Allergy & Sinus Headache Caplets & Gelcaps...... 693
Children's Benadryl Allergy & Cold Fastmelt Tablets................ 695
Benadryl Maximum Strength Severe Allergy & Sinus Headache Caplets...................... 694
Children's Benadryl D Allergy & Sinus Fastmelt Tablets............... 694
Children's Benadryl D Liquid Medication.............................. 693
Benadryl D Tablets 694
Contac Non-Drowsy 12 Hour Cold Caplets.............................. 614
Contac Non-Drowsy Timed Release 12 Hour Cold Caplets 615
Contac Severe Cold and Flu Caplets Maximum Strength......... 615
Contac Severe Cold and Flu Caplets Non-Drowsy................. 615
Children's Dimetapp Cold & Allergy Elixir.............................. 745
Children's Dimetapp DM Cold & Cough Elixir 745
Children's Dimetapp Long Acting Cough Plus Cold Syrup.............. 746
Dimetapp Infant Drops Decongestant Plus Cough.......... 746
Children's Motrin Cold Non-Staining Dye-Free Oral Suspension.............................. 1838
Children's Motrin Cold Oral Suspension.............................. 1838
Motrin Cold & Sinus Caplets 1836
PediaCare Decongestant & Cough Infant Drops....................... 705
PediaCare Decongestant Infants' Drops.............................. 705
PediaCare Long-Acting Cough Plus Cold Liquid....................... 704
PediaCare Multi-Symptom Cold Liquid.............................. 704
PediaCare NightRest Cough & Cold Liquid.............................. 704
Robitussin Allergy & Cough Syrup .. 750
Robitussin CF Liquid 755
Robitussin Cough & Cold Liquid-filled Capsules.................. 750
Robitussin Cough, Cold & Flu Liquid-filled Capsules.................. 750
Robitussin Cough & Cold Infant Drops.............................. 755
Robitussin Flu Liquid 752
Robitussin Maximum Strength Cough & Cold Liquid 754
Robitussin PE Syrup 753
Robitussin Pediatric Cough & Cold Liquid.............................. 754
Robitussin PM Cough & Cold Liquid.............................. 752
Robitussin Severe Congestion Liquid-filled Capsules.................. 751
Simply Stuffy Liquid 1841
Singlet Caplets 636
Sudafed 12 Hour Caplets 708
Sudafed 24 Hour Tablets 709
Sudafed Nasal Decongestant Tablets.............................. 709
Sudafed Severe Cold 710
Sudafed Non-Drying Sinus Liquid Caps.............................. 709
Sudafed Sinus & Allergy Tablets 710
Sudafed Sinus Headache 711

TheraFlu Cold & Cough Hot Liquid ■ 680
TheraFlu Cold & Sore Throat Hot Liquid ■ 680
TheraFlu Flu & Chest Congestion Non-Drowsy Hot Liquid ■ 681
TheraFlu Flu & Sore Throat Hot Liquid ■ 681
TheraFlu Severe Cold Non-Drowsy Hot Liquid ■ 683
TheraFlu Severe Cold & Cough Hot Liquid ■ 683
TheraFlu Severe Cold Caplets ■ 679
TheraFlu Severe Cold Hot Liquid ■ 682
TheraFlu Severe Cold Non-Drowsy Caplets ■ 679
Triaminic Chest & Nasal Congestion Liquid ■ 685
Triaminic Cold & Allergy Liquid ■ 685
Triaminic Cold & Cough Liquid ■ 685
Triaminic Cough Liquid ■ 687
Triaminic Cough & Nasal Congestion Liquid ■ 687
Triaminic Cough & Sore Throat Liquid ■ 687
Triaminic Flu, Cough & Fever Liquid ■ 685
Triaminic Night Time Cough & Cold Liquid ■ 685
Triaminic Allergy Runny Nose & Congestion Softchews ■ 688
Triaminic Cold & Cough Softchews ■ 688
Triaminic Cough & Sore Throat Softchews ■ 689
Tylenol Sinus NightTime Caplets ■ 663
Children's Tylenol Plus Cold & Allergy Suspension Liquid 1850
Children's Tylenol Plus Cold NightTime Suspension Liquid 1851
Children's Tylenol Plus Cold & Cough Suspension Liquid and Chewable Tablets 1851
Children's Tylenol Plus Cold Chewable Tablets 1851
Children's Tylenol Plus Cold Daytime Non-Drowsy Suspension Liquid 1851
Children's Tylenol Plus Flu Suspension Liquid 1853
Concentrated Tylenol Infants' Drops Plus Cold 1851
Concentrated Tylenol Infants' Drops Plus Cold and Cough 1851
Tylenol Cold & Flu Severe Daytime Liquid with Cool Bust 1846
Tylenol Cold & Flu Severe NightTime Liquid with Cool Burst 1846
Tylenol Cold Severe Congestion Non-Drowsy Caplets with Cool Burst 1846
Tylenol Allergy Complete Night Time Caplets 1844
Tylenol Allergy Complete Multi-Symptom Caplets and Gelcaps with Cool Burst 1844
Tylenol Flu NightTime Gelcaps 1846
Tylenol Flu Day Non-Drowsy Gelcaps 1846
Concentrated Tylenol Infants' Drops Plus Cold Nasal Congestant, Fever Reducer & Pain Reliever ■ 668
Concentrated Tylenol Infants' Drops Plus Cold & Cough Nasal Decongestant, Fever Reducer & Pain Reliever ■ 668
Multi-Symptom Tylenol Cold Night Time Caplets 1845
Multi-Symptom Tylenol Cold Day Non-Drowsy Caplets and Gelcaps 1845
Tylenol Sinus Day Non-Drowsy 1848
Tylenol Sinus Night Time Caplets 1848
Tylenol Sinus Severe Congestion Caplets with Cool Burst 1848
Vicks 44D Cough & Head Congestion Relief 2676
Vicks 44D Cough & Head Congestion Relief Liquid ■ 721
Vicks 44M Cough, Cold & Flu Relief 2676
Pediatric Vicks 44m Cough & Cold Relief 2673
Vicks DayQuil LiquiCaps/Liquid Multi-Symptom Cold/Flu Relief ■ 723
Vicks DayQuil Multi-Symptom Cold/Flu Relief LiquiCaps 2675
Vicks DayQuil Multi-Symptom Cold/Flu Relief Liquid 2675
Children's Vicks NyQuil Cold/Cough Relief 2671
Vicks NyQuil LiquiCaps 2677
Vicks NyQuil LiquiCaps/Liquid Multi-Symptom Cold/Flu Relief ■ 725
Vicks NyQuil Liquid 2677
Zyrtec-D 12 Hour Extended Release Tablets 2591

Pseudoephedrine Sulfate (Concomitant use of albuterol and other oral sympathomimetic agents is not recommended since combined use may lead to deleterious cardiovascular effects). Products include:
Alavert Allergy & Sinus D-12 Hour Tablets ■ 743
Clarinex-D 24-Hour Extended-Release Tablets 3012
Claritin-D Non-Drowsy 12 Hour Tablets ■ 731
Claritin-D Non-Drowsy 24 Hour Tablets ■ 731

Selegiline Hydrochloride (Administer albuterol with extreme caution to patients being treated with MAO inhibitors, or within 2 weeks of discontinuing such agents, because action on vascular system may be potentiated). Products include:
Eldepryl Capsules 3209

Sotalol Hydrochloride (Co-administration of albuterol with beta-blockers not only blocks the pulmonary effect of beta-agonists, but may produce severe bronchospasm in asthmatic patients).
No products indexed under this heading.

Terbutaline Sulfate (Concomitant use of albuterol and other oral sympathomimetic agents is not recommended since combined use may lead to deleterious cardiovascular effects).
No products indexed under this heading.

Timolol Hemihydrate (Co-administration of albuterol with beta-blockers not only blocks the pulmonary effect of beta-agonists, but may produce severe bronchospasm in asthmatic patients). Products include:
Betimol Ophthalmic Solution 3371
Betimol Ophthalmic Solution ⊙ 283

Timolol Maleate (Co-administration of albuterol with beta-blockers not only blocks the pulmonary effect of beta-agonists, but may produce severe bronchospasm in asthmatic patients). Products include:
Blocadren Tablets 1891
Cosopt Sterile Ophthalmic Solution 1910
Timolide Tablets 2056
Timoptic in Ocudose 2061
Timoptic Sterile Ophthalmic Solution 2058
Timoptic-XE Sterile Ophthalmic Gel Forming Solution 2062

Torsemide (Caution is advised in the co-administration of beta-agonists with non-potassium sparing diuretics, since the ECG changes and/or hypokalemia that may result from the administration of non-potassium sparing diuretics can be acutely worsened by beta-agonists, especially when the recommended dose of the beta-agonist is exceeded; clinical significance not known).
No products indexed under this heading.

Tranylcypromine Sulfate (Administer albuterol with extreme caution to patients being treated with MAO inhibitors, or within 2 weeks of discontinuing such agents, because action on vascular system may be potentiated). Products include:
Parnate Tablets 1499

Trimipramine Maleate (Administer albuterol with extreme caution to patients being treated with tricyclics, or within 2 weeks of discontinuing such agents, because action on vascular system may be potentiated). Products include:
Surmontil Capsules 2347

VYTORIN 10/10 TABLETS

(Ezetimibe, Simvastatin) 2084
May interact with oral anticoagulants, erythromycin, fibrates, protease inhibitors, and certain other agents. Compounds in these categories include:

Amiodarone Hydrochloride (Co-administration increases the risk of myopathy/rhabdomyolysis; caution should be exercised and the dose of ezetimibe/simvastatin should not exceed 10/20 mg). Products include:
Pacerone Tablets 3337

Amprenavir (Co-administration with potent CYP3A4 inhibitors, such as HIV protease inhibitors, increases the risk of myopathy/rhabdomyolysis; concurrent use should be avoided). Products include:
Agenerase Capsules 1299
Agenerase Oral Solution 1304

Anisindione (Simvastatin modestly potentiated the effect of coumarin anticoagulants; monitor prothrombin time during co-administration). Products include:
Miradon Tablets 3056

Cholestyramine (Co-administration decreased the mean AUC of total ezetimibe by approximately 55%; therefore, the incremental LDL-C reduction due to adding ezetimibe/simvastatin to cholestyramine may be reduced).
No products indexed under this heading.

Clarithromycin (Co-administration with potent CYP3A4 inhibitors, such as clarithromycin, increases the risk of myopathy/rhabdomyolysis; the dose of ezetimibe/simvastatin should not exceed 10/10 mg). Products include:
Biaxin/Biaxin XL 402
PREVPAC 3281

Clofibrate (Co-administration with other lipid-lowering drugs that can cause myopathy when given alone, such as fibrates, increases the risk of myopathy/rhabdomyolysis; concurrent use should be avoided).
No products indexed under this heading.

Cyclosporine (Caution should be exercised when using Vytorin and cyclosporine concomitantly due to increased exposure to both ezetimibe and cyclosporine. Cyclosporine concentrations should be monitored in patients receiving Vytorin and cyclosporine). Products include:
Gengraf Capsules 458
Neoral Soft Gelatin Capsules 2247
Neoral Oral Solution 2247
Restasis Ophthalmic Emulsion 570
Sandimmune 2259

Dicumarol (Simvastatin modestly potentiated the effect of coumarin anticoagulants; monitor prothrombin time during co-administration).
No products indexed under this heading.

Digoxin (Co-administration resulted in a slight elevation (less than 0.3 ng/mL) in plasma digoxin concentrations). Products include:
Digitek Tablets 2146
Lanoxicaps Capsules 1458
Lanoxin Injection 1462
Lanoxin Tablets 1468
Lanoxin Injection Pediatric 1465

Erythromycin (Co-administration with potent CYP3A4 inhibitors, such as erythromycin, increases the risk of myopathy/rhabdomyolysis; concurrent use should be avoided). Products include:
Erygel Topical Gel 2096
Ery-Tab Tablets 447
Erythromycin Base Filmtab Tablets 454
Erythromycin Delayed-Release Capsules, USP 456
PCE Dispertab Tablets 510

Erythromycin Estolate (Co-administration with potent CYP3A4 inhibitors, such as erythromycin, increases the risk of myopathy/rhabdomyolysis; concurrent use should be avoided).
No products indexed under this heading.

Erythromycin Ethylsuccinate (Co-administration with potent CYP3A4 inhibitors, such as erythromycin, increases the risk of myopathy/rhabdomyolysis; concurrent use should be avoided). Products include:
E.E.S. 449
EryPed 445

Erythromycin Gluceptate (Co-administration with potent CYP3A4 inhibitors, such as erythromycin, increases the risk of myopathy/rhabdomyolysis; concurrent use should be avoided).
No products indexed under this heading.

Erythromycin Lactobionate (Co-administration with potent CYP3A4 inhibitors, such as erythromycin, increases the risk of myopathy/rhabdomyolysis; concurrent use should be avoided).
No products indexed under this heading.

Erythromycin Stearate (Co-administration with potent CYP3A4 inhibitors, such as erythromycin, increases the risk of myopathy/rhabdomyolysis; concurrent use should be avoided). Products include:
Erythrocin Stearate Filmtab Tablets 452

Fenofibrate (Co-administration with fibrates increases the risk of myopathy/rhabdomyolysis; concurrent use should be avoided. In a pharmacokinetic study, fenofibrate increased total ezetimibe concentrations by 1.5-fold). Products include:
Antara Capsules 2723
Lofibra Capsules 1217
Tricor Tablets 523
Triglide Tablets 1165

Gemfibrozil (Co-administration with gemfibrozil increases the risk of myopathy/rhabdomyolysis. In a pharmacokinetic study, gemfibrozil increased total ezetimibe concentrations by 1.7-fold).
No products indexed under this heading.

Indinavir Sulfate (Co-administration with potent CYP3A4 inhibitors, such as HIV protease inhibitors, increases the risk of myopathy/rhabdomyolysis; concurrent use should be avoided). Products include:
Crixivan Capsules **1918**

Itraconazole (Co-administration with potent CYP3A4 inhibitors, such as itraconazole, increases the risk of myopathy/rhabdomyolysis; concurrent use should be avoided).
No products indexed under this heading.

Ketoconazole (Co-administration with potent CYP3A4 inhibitors, such as ketoconazole, increases the risk of myopathy/rhabdomyolysis; concurrent use should be avoided). Products include:
Nizoral A-D Shampoo, 1% **1839**
Nizoral 2% Shampoo **1838**

Lopinavir (Co-administration with potent CYP3A4 inhibitors, such as HIV protease inhibitors, increases the risk of myopathy/rhabdomyolysis; concurrent use should be avoided). Products include:
Kaletra **474**

Nefazodone Hydrochloride (Co-administration with potent CYP3A4 inhibitors, such as nefazodone, increases the risk of myopathy/rhabdomyolysis; concurrent use should be avoided).
No products indexed under this heading.

Nelfinavir Mesylate (Co-administration with potent CYP3A4 inhibitors, such as HIV protease inhibitors, increases the risk of myopathy/rhabdomyolysis; concurrent use should be avoided). Products include:
Viracept **2556**

Niacin (Caution with greater than or equal to 1 gram per day of niacin with ezetimibe/simvastatin as niacin can cause myopathy when given alone). Products include:
Advicor Tablets **1694**
Niaspan Extended-Release Tablets **1703**

Ritonavir (Co-administration with potent CYP3A4 inhibitors, such as HIV protease inhibitors, increases the risk of myopathy/rhabdomyolysis; concurrent use should be avoided). Products include:
Kaletra **474**
Norvir **499**

Saquinavir (Co-administration with potent CYP3A4 inhibitors, such as HIV protease inhibitors, increases the risk of myopathy/rhabdomyolysis; concurrent use should be avoided).
No products indexed under this heading.

Saquinavir Mesylate (Co-administration with potent CYP3A4 inhibitors, such as HIV protease inhibitors, increases the risk of myopathy/rhabdomyolysis; concurrent use should be avoided). Products include:
Invirase **2776**

Verapamil Hydrochloride (Co-administration increases the risk of myopathy/rhabdomyolysis; caution should be exercised and the dose of ezetimibe/simvastatin should not exceed 10/20 mg). Products include:
Covera-HS Tablets **3135**
Tarka Tablets **519**
Verelan PM Capsules **3120**

Warfarin Sodium (Simvastatin modestly potentiated the effect of coumarin anticoagulants; monitor prothrombin time during co-administration). Products include:
Coumadin for Injection **932**
Coumadin Tablets **932**

Food Interactions

Grapefruit Juice (Co-administration with potent CYP3A4 inhibitors, such as large quantities of grapefruit juice (greater than 1 quart daily), increases the risk of myopathy/rhabdomyolysis; concurrent use should be avoided).

VYTORIN 10/10 TABLETS

(Ezetimibe, Simvastatin) **3092**
May interact with oral anticoagulants, erythromycin, fibrates, protease inhibitors, and certain other agents. Compounds in these categories include:

Amiodarone Hydrochloride (Co-administration increases the risk of myopathy/rhabdomyolysis; caution should be exercised and the dose of ezetimibe/simvastatin should not exceed 10/20 mg). Products include:
Pacerone Tablets **3337**

Amprenavir (Co-administration with potent CYP3A4 inhibitors, such as HIV protease inhibitors, increases the risk of myopathy/rhabdomyolysis; concurrent use should be avoided). Products include:
Agenerase Capsules **1299**
Agenerase Oral Solution **1304**

Anisindione (Simvastatin modestly potentiated the effect of coumarin anticoagulants). Products include:
Miradon Tablets **3056**

Cholestyramine (Co-administration decreased the mean AUC of total ezetimibe by approximately 55%; therefore, the incremental LDL-C reduction due to adding ezetimibe/simvastatin to cholestyramine may be reduced).
No products indexed under this heading.

Clarithromycin (Co-administration with potent CYP3A4 inhibitors, such as clarithromycin, increases the risk of myopathy/rhabdomyolysis; the dose of ezetimibe/simvastatin should not exceed 10/10 mg). Products include:
Biaxin/Biaxin XL **402**
PREVPAC **3281**

Clofibrate (Co-administration with other lipid-lowering drugs that can cause myopathy when given alone, such as fibrates, increases the risk of myopathy/rhabdomyolysis; concurrent use should be avoided).
No products indexed under this heading.

Cyclosporine (Co-administration with potent CYP3A4 inhibitors, such as cyclosporine, increases the risk of myopathy/rhabdomyolysis; the dose of ezetimibe/simvastatin should not exceed 10/10 mg). Products include:
Gengraf Capsules **458**
Neoral Soft Gelatin Capsules **2247**
Neoral Oral Solution **2247**
Restasis Ophthalmic Emulsion **570**
Sandimmune **2259**

Dicumarol (Simvastatin modestly potentiated the effect of coumarin anticoagulants).
No products indexed under this heading.

Digoxin (Co-administration resulted in a slight elevation (less than 0.3 ng/mL) in plasma digoxin concentrations). Products include:
Digitek Tablets **2146**
Lanoxicaps Capsules **1458**
Lanoxin Injection **1462**
Lanoxin Tablets **1468**
Lanoxin Injection Pediatric **1465**

Erythromycin (Co-administration with potent CYP3A4 inhibitors, such as erythromycin, increases the risk of myopathy/rhabdomyolysis; concurrent use should be avoided). Products include:
Erygel Topical Gel **2096**
Ery-Tab Tablets **447**
Erythromycin Base Filmtab Tablets **454**
Erythromycin Delayed-Release Capsules, USP **456**
PCE Dispertab Tablets **510**

Erythromycin Estolate (Co-administration with potent CYP3A4 inhibitors, such as erythromycin, increases the risk of myopathy/rhabdomyolysis; concurrent use should be avoided).
No products indexed under this heading.

Erythromycin Ethylsuccinate (Co-administration with potent CYP3A4 inhibitors, such as erythromycin, increases the risk of myopathy/rhabdomyolysis; concurrent use should be avoided). Products include:
E.E.S. **449**
EryPed **445**

Erythromycin Gluceptate (Co-administration with potent CYP3A4 inhibitors, such as erythromycin, increases the risk of myopathy/rhabdomyolysis; concurrent use should be avoided).
No products indexed under this heading.

Erythromycin Lactobionate (Co-administration with potent CYP3A4 inhibitors, such as erythromycin, increases the risk of myopathy/rhabdomyolysis; concurrent use should be avoided).
No products indexed under this heading.

Erythromycin Stearate (Co-administration with potent CYP3A4 inhibitors, such as erythromycin, increases the risk of myopathy/rhabdomyolysis; concurrent use should be avoided). Products include:
Erythrocin Stearate Filmtab Tablets **452**

Fenofibrate (Co-administration with fibrates increases the risk of myopathy/rhabdomyolysis; concurrent use should be avoided. In a pharmacokinetic study, fenofibrate increased total ezetimibe concentrations by 1.5-fold). Products include:
Antara Capsules **2723**
Lofibra Capsules **1217**
Tricor Tablets **523**
Triglide Tablets **1165**

Gemfibrozil (Co-administration with gemfibrozil increases the risk of myopathy/rhabdomyolysis. In a pharmacokinetic study, gemfibrozil increased total ezetimibe concentrations by 1.7-fold).
No products indexed under this heading.

Indinavir Sulfate (Co-administration with potent CYP3A4 inhibitors, such as HIV protease inhibitors, increases the risk of myopathy/rhabdomyolysis; concurrent use should be avoided). Products include:
Crixivan Capsules **1918**

Itraconazole (Co-administration with potent CYP3A4 inhibitors, such as itraconazole, increases the risk of myopathy/rhabdomyolysis; concurrent use should be avoided).
No products indexed under this heading.

Ketoconazole (Co-administration with potent CYP3A4 inhibitors, such as ketoconazole, increases the risk of myopathy/rhabdomyolysis; concurrent use should be avoided). Products include:
Nizoral A-D Shampoo, 1% **1839**
Nizoral 2% Shampoo **1838**

Lopinavir (Co-administration with potent CYP3A4 inhibitors, such as HIV protease inhibitors, increases the risk of myopathy/rhabdomyolysis; concurrent use should be avoided). Products include:
Kaletra **474**

Nefazodone Hydrochloride (Co-administration with potent CYP3A4 inhibitors, such as nefazodone, increases the risk of myopathy/rhabdomyolysis; concurrent use should be avoided).
No products indexed under this heading.

Nelfinavir Mesylate (Co-administration with potent CYP3A4 inhibitors, such as HIV protease inhibitors, increases the risk of myopathy/rhabdomyolysis; concurrent use should be avoided). Products include:
Viracept **2556**

Niacin (Caution with greater than or equal to 1 gram per day of niacin with ezetimibe/simvastatin as niacin can cause myopathy when given alone). Products include:
Advicor Tablets **1694**
Niaspan Extended-Release Tablets **1703**

Ritonavir (Co-administration with potent CYP3A4 inhibitors, such as HIV protease inhibitors, increases the risk of myopathy/rhabdomyolysis; concurrent use should be avoided). Products include:
Kaletra **474**
Norvir **499**

Saquinavir (Co-administration with potent CYP3A4 inhibitors, such as HIV protease inhibitors, increases the risk of myopathy/rhabdomyolysis; concurrent use should be avoided).
No products indexed under this heading.

Saquinavir Mesylate (Co-administration with potent CYP3A4 inhibitors, such as HIV protease inhibitors, increases the risk of myopathy/rhabdomyolysis; concurrent use should be avoided). Products include:

Invirase 2776

Verapamil Hydrochloride (Co-administration increases the risk of myopathy/rhabdomyolysis; caution should be exercised and the dose of ezetimibe/simvastatin should not exceed 10/20 mg). Products include:

Covera-HS Tablets 3135
Tarka Tablets 519
Verelan PM Capsules 3120

Warfarin Sodium (Simvastatin modestly potentiated the effect of coumarin anticoagulants). Products include:

Coumadin for Injection 932
Coumadin Tablets 932

Food Interactions

Grapefruit Juice (Co-administration with potent CYP3A4 inhibitors, such as large quantities of grapefruit juice (greater than 1 quart daily), increases the risk of myopathy/rhabdomyolysis; concurrent use should be avoided).

VYTORIN 10/20 TABLETS
(Ezetimibe, Simvastatin) 2084
See Vytorin 10/10 Tablets

VYTORIN 10/20 TABLETS
(Ezetimibe, Simvastatin) 3092
See Vytorin 10/10 Tablets

VYTORIN 10/40 TABLETS
(Ezetimibe, Simvastatin) 3092
See Vytorin 10/10 Tablets

VYTORIN 10/40 TABLETS
(Ezetimibe, Simvastatin) 2084
See Vytorin 10/10 Tablets

VYTORIN 10/80 TABLETS
(Ezetimibe, Simvastatin) 3092
See Vytorin 10/10 Tablets

VYTORIN 10/80 TABLETS
(Ezetimibe, Simvastatin) 2084
See Vytorin 10/10 Tablets

WELCHOL TABLETS
(Colesevelam Hydrochloride) 2855
May interact with:

Verapamil Hydrochloride (Co-administration of sustained-release verapamil with colesevelam results in decreased Cmax and AUC of sustained-release verapamil by approximately 31% and 11%, respectively; because of high variability in the bioavailability of verapamil, the clinical significance of this finding is unclear). Products include:

Covera-HS Tablets 3135
Tarka Tablets 519
Verelan PM Capsules 3120

WELLBUTRIN TABLETS
(Bupropion Hydrochloride) 1579
See Wellbutrin SR Sustained-Release Tablets

WELLBUTRIN SR SUSTAINED-RELEASE TABLETS
(Bupropion Hydrochloride) 1583
May interact with benzodiazepines, corticosteroids, cytochrome p450 2d6 substrates (selected), antidepressant drugs, monoamine oxidase inhibitors, antipsychotic agents, phenytoin, drugs which lower seizure threshold, xanthines, and certain other agents. Compounds in these categories include:

Alprazolam (Bupropion is associated with a dose-related risk of seizures; excessive use of benzodiazepine sedatives is associated with increased risk of seizures; bupropion is contraindicated in patients undergoing abrupt discontinuation of benzodiazepine sedatives). Products include:

Niravam Orally Disintegrating Tablets 3106
Xanax XR Tablets 2655

Amantadine Hydrochloride (Limited clinical data suggest higher incidence of adverse experiences with co-administration; use small initial dose and gradually increase doses). Products include:

Symmetrel 1115

Aminophylline (Bupropion is associated with a dose-related risk of seizures; co-administration with drugs that lower seizure threshold may increase the risk of seizures with bupropion; concurrent use should be undertaken with extreme caution).

No products indexed under this heading.

Amitriptyline Hydrochloride (Bupropion is associated with a dose-related risk of seizures; co-administration with drugs that lower seizure threshold may increase the risk of seizure with bupropion; concurrent use should be undertaken with extreme caution).

No products indexed under this heading.

Amoxapine (Bupropion is associated with a dose-related risk of seizures; co-administration with drugs that lower seizure threshold may increase the risk of seizure with bupropion; concurrent use should be undertaken with extreme caution).

No products indexed under this heading.

Amphetamine Aspartate (Co-administration of bupropion with drugs that are metabolized by the CYP2D6 isoenzyme should be approached with caution and should be initiated at the lower end of the dose range of the concomitant medication. If bupropion is added to the treatment regimen of a patient already receiving a drug metabolized by CYP2D6, the need to decrease the dose of the original medication should be considered, particularly for those concomitant medications with a narrow therapeutic index). Products include:

Adderall Tablets 3168
Adderall XR Capsules 3169

Amphetamine Aspartate Monohydrate (Co-administration of bupropion with drugs that are metabolized by the CYP2D6 isoenzyme should be approached with caution and should be initiated at the lower end of the dose range of the concomitant medication. If bupropion is added to the treatment regimen of a patient already receiving a drug metabolized by CYP2D6, the need to decrease the dose of the original medication should be considered, particularly for those concomitant medications with a narrow therapeutic index).

No products indexed under this heading.

Amphetamine Sulfate (Co-administration of bupropion with drugs that are metabolized by the CYP2D6 isoenzyme should be approached with caution and should be initiated at the lower end of the dose range of the concomitant medication. If bupropion is added to the treatment regimen of a patient already receiving a drug metabolized by CYP2D6, the need to decrease the dose of the original medication should be considered, particularly for those concomitant medications with a narrow therapeutic index). Products include:

Adderall Tablets 3168
Adderall XR Capsules 3169

Aripiprazole (Concurrent administration of bupropion and agents that lower seizure threshold (e.g., antipsychotics) should be undertaken only with extreme caution. Low initial dosing and gradual dose increases should be employed). Products include:

Abilify Tablets 2472
Abilify Tablets 916

Atomoxetine Hydrochloride (Co-administration of bupropion with drugs that are metabolized by the CYP2D6 isoenzyme should be approached with caution and should be initiated at the lower end of the dose range of the concomitant medication. If bupropion is added to the treatment regimen of a patient already receiving a drug metabolized by CYP2D6, the need to decrease the dose of the original medication should be considered, particularly for those concomitant medications with a narrow therapeutic index). Products include:

Strattera Capsules 1784

Betamethasone Acetate (Bupropion is associated with a dose-related risk of seizures; co-administration with drugs that lower seizure threshold, such as systemic steroids, may increase the risk of seizure with bupropion).

No products indexed under this heading.

Betamethasone Sodium Phosphate (Bupropion is associated with a dose-related risk of seizures; co-administration with drugs that lower seizure threshold, such as systemic steroids, may increase the risk of seizure with bupropion).

No products indexed under this heading.

Bisoprolol Fumarate (Co-administration of bupropion with drugs that are metabolized by the CYP2D6 isoenzyme should be approached with caution and should be initiated at the lower end of the dose range of the concomitant medication. If bupropion is added to the treatment regimen of a patient already receiving a drug metabolized by CYP2D6, the need to decrease the dose of the original medication should be considered, particularly for those concomitant medications with a narrow therapeutic index).

No products indexed under this heading.

Bupropion (Patients should be made aware that both formulations of Wellbutrin contain the same active moiety found in Zyban, an aid to smoking cessation; combination is contraindicated).

No products indexed under this heading.

Captopril (Co-administration of bupropion with drugs that are metabolized by the CYP2D6 isoenzyme should be approached with caution and should be initiated at the lower end of the dose range of the concomitant medication. If bupropion is added to the treatment regimen of a patient already receiving a drug metabolized by CYP2D6, the need to decrease the dose of the original medication should be considered, particularly for those concomitant medications with a narrow therapeutic index). Products include:

Captopril Tablets 2114

Carbamazepine (May induce the metabolism of bupropion). Products include:

Carbatrol Capsules 3174
Equetro Extended-Release Capsules 3178
Tegretol/Tegretol-XR 2278

Carvedilol (Co-administration of bupropion with drugs that are metabolized by the CYP2D6 isoenzyme should be approached with caution and should be initiated at the lower end of the dose range of the concomitant medication. If bupropion is added to the treatment regimen of a patient already receiving a drug metabolized by CYP2D6, the need to decrease the dose of the original medication should be considered, particularly for those concomitant medications with a narrow therapeutic index). Products include:

Coreg Tablets 1376

Cevimeline Hydrochloride (Co-administration of bupropion with drugs that are metabolized by the CYP2D6 isoenzyme should be approached with caution and should be initiated at the lower end of the dose range of the concomitant medication. If bupropion is added to the treatment regimen of a patient already receiving a drug metabolized by CYP2D6, the need to decrease the dose of the original medication should be considered, particularly for those concomitant medications with a narrow therapeutic index). Products include:

Evoxac Capsules 1042

Chlordiazepoxide (Bupropion is associated with a dose-related risk of seizures; excessive use of benzodiazepine sedatives is associated with increased risk of seizures; bupropion is contraindicated in patients undergoing abrupt discontinuation of benzodiazepine sedatives).

No products indexed under this heading.

Chlordiazepoxide Hydrochloride (Bupropion is associated with a dose-related risk of seizures; excessive use of benzodiazepine sedatives is associated with increased risk of seizures; bupropion is contraindicated in patients undergoing abrupt discontinuation of benzodiazepine sedatives). Products include:

Librium Capsules 3349

Chlorpromazine (Bupropion is associated with a dose-related risk of seizures; co-administration with drugs that lower seizure threshold may increase the risk of seizure with bupropion; concurrent use should be undertaken with extreme caution).

No products indexed under this heading.

Chlorpromazine Hydrochloride (Bupropion is associated with a dose-related risk of seizures; co-administration with drugs that lower seizure threshold may increase the risk of seizure with bupropion; concurrent use should be undertaken with extreme caution).

No products indexed under this heading.

Chlorpropamide (Co-administration of bupropion with drugs that are metabolized by the CYP2D6 isoenzyme should be approached with caution and should be initiated at the lower end of the dose range of the concomitant medication. If bupropion is added to the treatment regimen of a patient already receiving a drug metabolized by CYP2D6, the need to decrease the dose of the original medication should be considered, particularly for those concomitant medications with a narrow therapeutic index).
No products indexed under this heading.

Chlorprothixene (Concurrent administration of bupropion and agents that lower seizure threshold (e.g., antipsychotics) should be undertaken only with extreme caution. Low initial dosing and gradual dose increases should be employed).
No products indexed under this heading.

Chlorprothixene Hydrochloride (Concurrent administration of bupropion and agents that lower seizure threshold (e.g., antipsychotics) should be undertaken only with extreme caution. Low initial dosing and gradual dose increases should be employed).
No products indexed under this heading.

Cimetidine (May inhibit the metabolism of bupropion). Products include:
Tagamet HB 200 Tablets 637
Tagamet Tablets 1547

Cimetidine Hydrochloride (May induce the metabolism of bupropion).
No products indexed under this heading.

Citalopram Hydrobromide (Concurrent administration of bupropion and agents that lower seizure threshold (e.g., other antidepressants) should be undertaken only with extreme caution. Low initial dosing and gradual dose increases should be employed). Products include:
Celexa 1177

Clomipramine Hydrochloride (Co-administration of bupropion with drugs that are metabolized by the CYP2D6 isoenzyme should be approached with caution and should be initiated at the lower end of the dose range of the concomitant medication. If bupropion is added to the treatment regimen of a patient already receiving a drug metabolized by CYP2D6, the need to decrease the dose of the original medication should be considered, particularly for those concomitant medications with a narrow therapeutic index).
No products indexed under this heading.

Clorazepate Dipotassium (Bupropion is associated with a dose-related risk of seizures; excessive use of benzodiazepine sedatives is associated with increased risk of seizures; bupropion is contraindicated in patients undergoing abrupt discontinuation of benzodiazepine sedatives). Products include:
Tranxene 2488

Clozapine (Co-administration of bupropion with drugs that are metabolized by the CYP2D6 isoenzyme should be approached with caution and should be initiated at the lower end of the dose range of the concomitant medication. If bupropion is added to the treatment regimen of a patient already receiving a drug metabolized by CYP2D6, the need to decrease the dose of the original medication should be considered, particularly for those concomitant medications with a narrow therapeutic index). Products include:
Clozapine Tablets 2141
Clozaril Tablets 2174
FazaClo Orally Disintegrating Tablets 547

Codeine Phosphate (Co-administration of bupropion with drugs that are metabolized by the CYP2D6 isoenzyme should be approached with caution and should be initiated at the lower end of the dose range of the concomitant medication. If bupropion is added to the treatment regimen of a patient already receiving a drug metabolized by CYP2D6, the need to decrease the dose of the original medication should be considered, particularly for those concomitant medications with a narrow therapeutic index). Products include:
Tylenol with Codeine 2461

Codeine Sulfate (Co-administration of bupropion with drugs that are metabolized by the CYP2D6 isoenzyme should be approached with caution and should be initiated at the lower end of the dose range of the concomitant medication. If bupropion is added to the treatment regimen of a patient already receiving a drug metabolized by CYP2D6, the need to decrease the dose of the original medication should be considered, particularly for those concomitant medications with a narrow therapeutic index).
No products indexed under this heading.

Cortisone Acetate (Bupropion is associated with a dose-related risk of seizures; co-administration with drugs that lower seizure threshold, such as systemic steroids, may increase the risk of seizure with bupropion).
No products indexed under this heading.

Cyclobenzaprine Hydrochloride (Co-administration of bupropion with drugs that are metabolized by the CYP2D6 isoenzyme should be approached with caution and should be initiated at the lower end of the dose range of the concomitant medication. If bupropion is added to the treatment regimen of a patient already receiving a drug metabolized by CYP2D6, the need to decrease the dose of the original medication should be considered, particularly for those concomitant medications with a narrow therapeutic index). Products include:
Flexeril Tablets 1832

Cyclophosphamide (Bupropion is primarily metabolized, based on in vitro studies, to the morpholinol metabolite by cytochrome P450IIB6 isoenzyme; therefore, the potential exists for a drug interaction with agents that affect the cytochrome P450IIB6 metabolism, such as cyclophosphamide).
No products indexed under this heading.

Desipramine Hydrochloride (Co-administration of bupropion with drugs that are metabolized by the CYP2D6 isoenzyme, including desipramine, should be approached with caution and should be initiated at the lower end of the dose range of the concomitant medication. If bupropion is added to the treatment regimen of a patient already receiving a drug metabolized by CYP2D6, the need to decrease the dose of the original medication should be considered, particularly for those concomitant medications with a narrow therapeutic index).
No products indexed under this heading.

Dexamethasone (Bupropion is associated with a dose-related risk of seizures; co-administration with drugs that lower seizure threshold, such as systemic steroids, may increase the risk of seizure with bupropion). Products include:
Ciprodex Otic Suspension 555
Decadron Tablets 1929
TobraDex Ophthalmic Ointment 558
TobraDex Ophthalmic Suspension ... 558

Dexamethasone Acetate (Bupropion is associated with a dose-related risk of seizures; co-administration with drugs that lower seizure threshold, such as systemic steroids, may increase the risk of seizure with bupropion).
No products indexed under this heading.

Dexamethasone Sodium Phosphate (Bupropion is associated with a dose-related risk of seizures; co-administration with drugs that lower seizure threshold, such as systemic steroids, may increase the risk of seizure with bupropion). Products include:
Decadron Phosphate Injection 1931

Dexfenfluramine Hydrochloride (Co-administration of bupropion with drugs that are metabolized by the CYP2D6 isoenzyme should be approached with caution and should be initiated at the lower end of the dose range of the concomitant medication. If bupropion is added to the treatment regimen of a patient already receiving a drug metabolized by CYP2D6, the need to decrease the dose of the original medication should be considered, particularly for those concomitant medications with a narrow therapeutic index).
No products indexed under this heading.

Dextromethorphan Hydrobromide (Co-administration of bupropion with drugs that are metabolized by the CYP2D6 isoenzyme should be approached with caution and should be initiated at the lower end of the dose range of the concomitant medication. If bupropion is added to the treatment regimen of a patient already receiving a drug metabolized by CYP2D6, the need to decrease the dose of the original medication should be considered, particularly for those concomitant medications with a narrow therapeutic index). Products include:
Alacol DM Syrup 739
Balamine DM 739
Contac Severe Cold and Flu Caplets Maximum Strength 615
Contac Severe Cold and Flu Caplets Non-Drowsy 615
Children's Dimetapp DM Cold & Cough Elixir 745
Children's Dimetapp Long Acting Cough Plus Cold Syrup 746
Dimetapp Infant Drops Decongestant Plus Cough 746
Mucinex DM Tablets 602
PediaCare Decongestant & Cough Infant Drops 705
PediaCare Freezer Pops Long-Acting Cough-Glacier Grape and Polar Berry Blue 706
PediaCare Long-Acting Cough Infant Drops 705
PediaCare Long-Acting Cough Plus Cold Liquid 704
PediaCare Multi-Symptom Cold Liquid 704
PediaCare NightRest Cough & Cold Liquid 704
Robitussin Allergy & Cough Syrup .. 750
Robitussin CF Liquid 755
Robitussin Cough & Cold Liquid-filled Capsules 750
Robitussin Cough, Cold & Flu Liquid-filled Capsules 750
Robitussin Cough & Cold Infant Drops 755
Robitussin DM Infant Drops 753
Robitussin DM Liquid 753
Robitussin Flu Liquid 752
Robitussin Maximum Strength Cough Liquid 754
Robitussin Maximum Strength Cough & Cold Liquid 754
Robitussin Pediatric Cough Liquid 754
Robitussin Pediatric Cough & Cold Liquid 754
Robitussin PM Cough & Cold Liquid 752
Robitussin Sugar Free Cough Liquid 753
Simply Cough Liquid 1840
Sudafed Severe Cold 710
TheraFlu Cold & Cough Hot Liquid 680
TheraFlu Flu & Chest Congestion Non-Drowsy Hot Liquid 681
TheraFlu Severe Cold Non-Drowsy Hot Liquid 683
TheraFlu Severe Cold & Cough Hot Liquid 683
TheraFlu Severe Cold Caplets 679
TheraFlu Severe Cold Hot Liquid 682
TheraFlu Severe Cold Non-Drowsy Caplets 679
TheraFlu Thin Strips Long Acting Cough 684
Triaminic Cold & Cough Liquid 685
Triaminic Cough Liquid 687
Triaminic Cough & Nasal Congestion Liquid 687
Triaminic Cough & Sore Throat Liquid 687
Triaminic Flu, Cough & Fever Liquid 685
Triaminic Night Time Cough & Cold Liquid 685
Triaminic Cold & Cough Softchews 688
Triaminic Cough & Sore Throat Softchews 689
Triaminic Thin Strips Long Acting Cough 689
Children's Tylenol Plus Cold & Cough Suspension Liquid and Chewable Tablets 1851
Children's Tylenol Plus Flu Suspension Liquid 1853
Concentrated Tylenol Infants' Drops Plus Cold and Cough 1851
Tylenol Cold & Flu Severe Daytime Liquid with Cool Bust 1846
Tylenol Cold & Flu Severe NightTime Liquid with Cool Burst 1846
Tylenol Cold Severe Congestion Non-Drowsy Caplets with Cool Burst 1846
Tylenol Cough & Sore Throat Daytime Liquid with Cool Burst 1849
Tylenol Cough & Sore Throat NightTime Liquid with Cool Burst 1849
Tylenol Flu Day Non-Drowsy Gelcaps 1846
Concentrated Tylenol Infants' Drops Plus Cold & Cough Nasal Decongestant, Fever Reducer & Pain Reliever 668
Multi-Symptom Tylenol Cold Night Time Caplets 1845

Multi-Symptom Tylenol Cold Day Non-Drowsy Caplets and Gelcaps **1845**
Vicks 44 Cough Relief **2675**
Vicks 44D Cough & Head Congestion Relief **2676**
Vicks 44D Cough & Head Congestion Relief Liquid .... ▣ **721**
Vicks 44E Cough & Chest Congestion Relief **2676**
Pediatric Vicks 44e Cough & Chest Congestion Relief Liquid **2673**
Vicks 44M Cough, Cold & Flu Relief **2676**
Pediatric Vicks 44m Cough & Cold Relief **2673**
Vicks DayQuil LiquiCaps/Liquid Multi-Symptom Cold/Flu Relief .... ▣ **723**
Vicks DayQuil Multi-Symptom Cold/Flu Relief LiquiCaps **2675**
Vicks DayQuil Multi-Symptom Cold/Flu Relief Liquid **2675**
Children's Vicks NyQuil Cold/Cough Relief **2671**
Vicks NyQuil Cough Liquid **2677**
Vicks NyQuil LiquiCaps **2677**
Vicks NyQuil LiquiCaps/Liquid Multi-Symptom Cold/Flu Relief .... ▣ **725**
Vicks NyQuil Liquid **2677**
Zicam Concentrated Cough Mist for Kids Cool Cherry .... ▣ **643**
Zicam Concentrated Cough Mist for Kids Plus D Cool Cherry .... ▣ **643**
Zicam Concentrated Cough Mist Nite-Cool Cherry .... ▣ **642**
Zicam Concentrated Cough Mist Plus D Cool Cherry .... ▣ **642**
Zicam Concentrated Cough Mist-Honey Lemon & Cool Cherry .... ▣ **642**

Dextromethorphan Polistirex (Co-administration of bupropion with drugs that are metabolized by the CYP2D6 isoenzyme should be approached with caution and should be initiated at the lower end of the dose range of the concomitant medication. If bupropion is added to the treatment regimen of a patient already receiving a drug metabolized by CYP2D6, the need to decrease the dose of the original medication should be considered, particularly for those concomitant medications with a narrow therapeutic index). Products include:
Delsym Extended-Release Suspension .... ▣ **611**
Delsym 12 Hour Cough Suppressant for Children .... ▣ **611**

Diazepam (Bupropion is associated with a dose-related risk of seizures; excessive use of benzodiazepine sedatives is associated with increased risk of seizures; bupropion is contraindicated in patients undergoing abrupt discontinuation of benzodiazepine sedatives). Products include:
Diastat Rectal Delivery System **3344**
Valium Tablets **2822**

Dolasetron Mesylate (Co-administration of bupropion with drugs that are metabolized by the CYP2D6 isoenzyme should be approached with caution and should be initiated at the lower end of the dose range of the concomitant medication. If bupropion is added to the treatment regimen of a patient already receiving a drug metabolized by CYP2D6, the need to decrease the dose of the original medication should be considered, particularly for those concomitant medications with a narrow therapeutic index). Products include:
Anzemet Injection **2871**
Anzemet Tablets **2874**

Donepezil Hydrochloride (Co-administration of bupropion with drugs that are metabolized by the CYP2D6 isoenzyme should be approached with caution and should be initiated at the lower end of the dose range of the concomitant medication. If bupropion is added to the treatment regimen of a patient already receiving a drug metabolized by CYP2D6, the need to decrease the dose of the original medication should be considered, particularly for those concomitant medications with a narrow therapeutic index). Products include:
Aricept Tablets **1086**
Aricept ODT Tablets **1086**

Doxepin Hydrochloride (Bupropion is associated with a dose-related risk of seizures; co-administration with drugs that lower seizure threshold may increase the risk of seizure with bupropion; concurrent use should be undertaken with extreme caution).
No products indexed under this heading.

Dyphylline (Bupropion is associated with a dose-related risk of seizures; co-administration with drugs that lower seizure threshold may increase the risk of seizures with bupropion; concurrent use should be undertaken with extreme caution).
No products indexed under this heading.

Encainide Hydrochloride (Co-administration of bupropion with drugs that are metabolized by the CYP2D6 isoenzyme should be approached with caution and should be initiated at the lower end of the dose range of the concomitant medication. If bupropion is added to the treatment regimen of a patient already receiving a drug metabolized by CYP2D6, the need to decrease the dose of the original medication should be considered, particularly for those concomitant medications with a narrow therapeutic index).
No products indexed under this heading.

Escitalopram Oxalate (Concurrent administration of bupropion and agents that lower seizure threshold (e.g., other antidepressants) should be undertaken only with extreme caution. Low initial dosing and gradual dose increases should be employed). Products include:
Lexapro Oral Solution **1193**
Lexapro Tablets **1193**

Estazolam (Bupropion is associated with a dose-related risk of seizures; excessive use of benzodiazepine sedatives is associated with increased risk of seizures; bupropion is contraindicated in patients undergoing abrupt discontinuation of benzodiazepine sedatives). Products include:
ProSom Tablets **512**

Fentanyl (Co-administration of bupropion with drugs that are metabolized by the CYP2D6 isoenzyme should be approached with caution and should be initiated at the lower end of the dose range of the concomitant medication. If bupropion is added to the treatment regimen of a patient already receiving a drug metabolized by CYP2D6, the need to decrease the dose of the original medication should be considered, particularly for those concomitant medications with a narrow therapeutic index). Products include:
Duragesic Transdermal System **2448**

Fentanyl Citrate (Co-administration of bupropion with drugs that are metabolized by the CYP2D6 isoenzyme should be approached with caution and should be initiated at the lower end of the dose range of the concomitant medication. If bupropion is added to the treatment regimen of a patient already receiving a drug metabolized by CYP2D6, the need to decrease the dose of the original medication should be considered, particularly for those concomitant medications with a narrow therapeutic index). Products include:
Actiq **993**

Flecainide Acetate (Co-administration of bupropion with drugs that are metabolized by the CYP2D6 isoenzyme, including flecainide, should be approached with caution and should be initiated at the lower end of the dose range of the concomitant medication. If bupropion is added to the treatment regimen of a patient already receiving a drug metabolized by CYP2D6, the need to decrease the dose of the original medication should be considered, particularly for those concomitant medications with a narrow therapeutic index). Products include:
Tambocor Tablets **1824**

Fludrocortisone Acetate (Bupropion is associated with a dose-related risk of seizures; co-administration with drugs that lower seizure threshold, such as systemic steroids, may increase the risk of seizure with bupropion).
No products indexed under this heading.

Fluoxetine (Co-administration of bupropion with drugs that are metabolized by the CYP2D6 isoenzyme, including fluoxetine, should be approached with caution and should be initiated at the lower end of the dose range of the concomitant medication. If bupropion is added to the treatment regimen of a patient already receiving a drug metabolized by CYP2D6, the need to decrease the dose of the original medication should be considered, particularly for those concomitant medications with a narrow therapeutic index).
No products indexed under this heading.

Fluoxetine Hydrochloride (Co-administration of bupropion with drugs that are metabolized by the CYP2D6 isoenzyme, including fluoxetine, should be approached with caution and should be initiated at the lower end of the dose range of the concomitant medication. If bupropion is added to the treatment regimen of a patient already receiving a drug metabolized by CYP2D6, the need to decrease the dose of the original medication should be considered, particularly for those concomitant medications with a narrow therapeutic index). Products include:
Prozac Pulvules and Liquid **1771**
Symbyax Capsules **1788**

Fluphenazine Decanoate (Bupropion is associated with a dose-related risk of seizures; co-administration with drugs that lower seizure threshold may increase the risk of seizure with bupropion; concurrent use should be undertaken with extreme caution).
No products indexed under this heading.

Fluphenazine Enanthate (Bupropion is associated with a dose-related risk of seizures; co-administration with drugs that lower seizure threshold may increase the risk of seizure with bupropion; concurrent use should be undertaken with extreme caution).
No products indexed under this heading.

Fluphenazine Hydrochloride (Bupropion is associated with a dose-related risk of seizures; co-administration with drugs that lower seizure threshold may increase the risk of seizure with bupropion; concurrent use should be undertaken with extreme caution).
No products indexed under this heading.

Flurazepam Hydrochloride (Bupropion is associated with a dose-related risk of seizures; excessive use of benzodiazepine sedatives is associated with increased risk of seizures; bupropion is contraindicated in patients undergoing abrupt discontinuation of benzodiazepine sedatives). Products include:
Dalmane Capsules **3343**

Fluvoxamine Maleate (Co-administration of bupropion with drugs that are metabolized by the CYP2D6 isoenzyme should be approached with caution and should be initiated at the lower end of the dose range of the concomitant medication. If bupropion is added to the treatment regimen of a patient already receiving a drug metabolized by CYP2D6, the need to decrease the dose of the original medication should be considered, particularly for those concomitant medications with a narrow therapeutic index).
No products indexed under this heading.

Formoterol Fumarate (Co-administration of bupropion with drugs that are metabolized by the CYP2D6 isoenzyme should be approached with caution and should be initiated at the lower end of the dose range of the concomitant medication. If bupropion is added to the treatment regimen of a patient already receiving a drug metabolized by CYP2D6, the need to decrease the dose of the original medication should be considered, particularly for those concomitant medications with a narrow therapeutic index). Products include:
Foradil Aerolizer **3024**

Fosphenytoin Sodium (May induce the metabolism of bupropion).
No products indexed under this heading.

Galantamine Hydrobromide (Co-administration of bupropion with drugs that are metabolized by the CYP2D6 isoenzyme should be approached with caution and should be initiated at the lower end of the dose range of the concomitant medication. If bupropion is added to the treatment regimen of a patient already receiving a drug metabolized by CYP2D6, the need to decrease the dose of the original medication should be considered, particularly for those concomitant medications with a narrow therapeutic index). Products include:
Razadyne ER Extended-Release Capsules **2434**
Razadyne **2434**

Halazepam (Bupropion is associated with a dose-related risk of seizures; excessive use of benzodiazepine sedatives is associated with increased risk of seizures; bupropion is contraindicated in patients undergoing abrupt discontinuation of benzodiazepine sedatives).
No products indexed under this heading.

Haloperidol (Co-administration of bupropion with drugs that are metabolized by the CYP2D6 isoenzyme, including haloperidol, should be approached with caution and should be initiated at the lower end of the dose range of the concomitant medication. If bupropion is added to the treatment regimen of a patient already receiving a drug metabolized by CYP2D6, the need to decrease the dose of the original medication should be considered, particularly for those concomitant medications with a narrow therapeutic index).
No products indexed under this heading.

Haloperidol Decanoate (Co-administration of bupropion with drugs that are metabolized by the CYP2D6 isoenzyme, including haloperidol, should be approached with caution and should be initiated at the lower end of the dose range of the concomitant medication. If bupropion is added to the treatment regimen of a patient already receiving a drug metabolized by CYP2D6, the need to decrease the dose of the original medication should be considered, particularly for those concomitant medications with a narrow therapeutic index).
No products indexed under this heading.

Haloperidol Lactate (Co-administration of bupropion with drugs that are metabolized by the CYP2D6 isoenzyme, including haloperidol, should be approached with caution and should be initiated at the lower end of the dose range of the concomitant medication. If bupropion is added to the treatment regimen of a patient already receiving a drug metabolized by CYP2D6, the need to decrease the dose of the original medication should be considered, particularly for those concomitant medications with a narrow therapeutic index).
No products indexed under this heading.

Hydrocodone Bitartrate (Co-administration of bupropion with drugs that are metabolized by the CYP2D6 isoenzyme should be approached with caution and should be initiated at the lower end of the dose range of the concomitant medication. If bupropion is added to the treatment regimen of a patient already receiving a drug metabolized by CYP2D6, the need to decrease the dose of the original medication should be considered, particularly for those concomitant medications with a narrow therapeutic index). Products include:

- Hycodan 1104
- Hycomine Compound Tablets 1105
- Hycotuss Expectorant Syrup 1106
- Lortab 3315
- Lortab Elixir 3312
- Vicodin Tablets 530
- Vicodin ES Tablets 531
- Vicodin HP Tablets 532
- Vicoprofen Tablets 533
- Zydone Tablets 1118

Hydrocortisone (Bupropion is associated with a dose-related risk of seizures; co-administration with drugs that lower seizure threshold, such as systemic steroids, may increase the risk of seizure with bupropion). Products include:

- Cortizone•5 Ointment 699
- Cortizone•10 Creme 699
- Cortizone•10 Ointment 699
- Cortizone•10 Plus Creme 700
- Cortizone•10 Maximum Strength Quick Shot Spray 700
- Hydrocortone Tablets 1963
- Preparation H Hydrocortisone Cream 748

Hydrocortisone Acetate (Bupropion is associated with a dose-related risk of seizures; co-administration with drugs that lower seizure threshold, such as systemic steroids, may increase the risk of seizure with bupropion). Products include:

- Analpram-HC 1136
- Pramosone 1139
- ProctoFoam-HC 3113
- Tucks Anti-Itch Ointment 712
- U-cort 1% Cream 3289

Hydrocortisone Sodium Phosphate (Bupropion is associated with a dose-related risk of seizures; co-administration with drugs that lower seizure threshold, such as systemic steroids, may increase the risk of seizure with bupropion).
No products indexed under this heading.

Hydrocortisone Sodium Succinate (Bupropion is associated with a dose-related risk of seizures; co-administration with drugs that lower seizure threshold, such as systemic steroids, may increase the risk of seizure with bupropion).
No products indexed under this heading.

Imipramine Hydrochloride (Co-administration of bupropion with drugs that are metabolized by the CYP2D6 isoenzyme, including imipramine, should be approached with caution and should be initiated at the lower end of the dose range of the concomitant medication. If bupropion is added to the treatment regimen of a patient already receiving a drug metabolized by CYP2D6, the need to decrease the dose of the original medication should be considered, particularly for those concomitant medications with a narrow therapeutic index).
No products indexed under this heading.

Imipramine Pamoate (Co-administration of bupropion with drugs that are metabolized by the CYP2D6 isoenzyme, including imipramine, should be approached with caution and should be initiated at the lower end of the dose range of the concomitant medication. If bupropion is added to the treatment regimen of a patient already receiving a drug metabolized by CYP2D6, the need to decrease the dose of the original medication should be considered, particularly for those concomitant medications with a narrow therapeutic index).
No products indexed under this heading.

Indoramin Hydrochloride (Co-administration of bupropion with drugs that are metabolized by the CYP2D6 isoenzyme should be approached with caution and should be initiated at the lower end of the dose range of the concomitant medication. If bupropion is added to the treatment regimen of a patient already receiving a drug metabolized by CYP2D6, the need to decrease the dose of the original medication should be considered, particularly for those concomitant medications with a narrow therapeutic index).
No products indexed under this heading.

Isocarboxazid (Concurrent and/or sequential use with MAO inhibitors is contraindicated).
No products indexed under this heading.

Labetalol Hydrochloride (Co-administration of bupropion with drugs that are metabolized by the CYP2D6 isoenzyme should be approached with caution and should be initiated at the lower end of the dose range of the concomitant medication. If bupropion is added to the treatment regimen of a patient already receiving a drug metabolized by CYP2D6, the need to decrease the dose of the original medication should be considered, particularly for those concomitant medications with a narrow therapeutic index).
No products indexed under this heading.

Levodopa (Limited clinical data suggest higher incidence of adverse experiences with co-administration; use small initial dose and gradually increase doses). Products include:

- Parcopa Orally Disintegrating Tablets 3111
- Stalevo Tablets 2270

Lidocaine (Co-administration of bupropion with drugs that are metabolized by the CYP2D6 isoenzyme should be approached with caution and should be initiated at the lower end of the dose range of the concomitant medication. If bupropion is added to the treatment regimen of a patient already receiving a drug metabolized by CYP2D6, the need to decrease the dose of the original medication should be considered, particularly for those concomitant medications with a narrow therapeutic index). Products include:

- Lidoderm Patch 1107

Lidocaine Hydrochloride (Co-administration of bupropion with drugs that are metabolized by the CYP2D6 isoenzyme should be approached with caution and should be initiated at the lower end of the dose range of the concomitant medication. If bupropion is added to the treatment regimen of a patient already receiving a drug metabolized by CYP2D6, the need to decrease the dose of the original medication should be considered, particularly for those concomitant medications with a narrow therapeutic index).
No products indexed under this heading.

Lithium Carbonate (Concurrent administration of bupropion and agents that lower seizure threshold (e.g., antipsychotics) should be undertaken only with extreme caution. Low initial dosing and gradual dose increases should be employed). Products include:

- Eskalith 1406
- Lithobid Tablets 1670

Lithium Citrate (Concurrent administration of bupropion and agents that lower seizure threshold (e.g., antipsychotics) should be undertaken only with extreme caution. Low initial dosing and gradual dose increases should be employed).
No products indexed under this heading.

Lorazepam (Bupropion is associated with a dose-related risk of seizures; excessive use of benzodiazepine sedatives is associated with increased risk of seizures; bupropion is contraindicated in patients undergoing abrupt discontinuation of benzodiazepine sedatives).
No products indexed under this heading.

Loxapine Hydrochloride (Concurrent administration of bupropion and agents that lower seizure threshold (e.g., antipsychotics) should be undertaken only with extreme caution. Low initial dosing and gradual dose increases should be employed).
No products indexed under this heading.

Loxapine Succinate (Concurrent administration of bupropion and agents that lower seizure threshold (e.g., antipsychotics) should be undertaken only with extreme caution. Low initial dosing and gradual dose increases should be employed).
No products indexed under this heading.

Maprotiline Hydrochloride (Bupropion is associated with a dose-related risk of seizures; co-administration with drugs that lower seizure threshold may increase the risk of seizure with bupropion; concurrent use should be undertaken with extreme caution).
No products indexed under this heading.

Meperidine Hydrochloride (Co-administration of bupropion with drugs that are metabolized by the CYP2D6 isoenzyme should be approached with caution and should be initiated at the lower end of the dose range of the concomitant medication. If bupropion is added to the treatment regimen of a patient already receiving a drug metabolized by CYP2D6, the need to decrease the dose of the original medication should be considered, particularly for those concomitant medications with a narrow therapeutic index).
No products indexed under this heading.

Mesoridazine Besylate (Bupropion is associated with a dose-related risk of seizures; co-administration with drugs that lower seizure threshold may increase the risk of seizure with bupropion; concurrent use should be undertaken with extreme caution).
No products indexed under this heading.

Methadone Hydrochloride (Co-administration of bupropion with drugs that are metabolized by the CYP2D6 isoenzyme should be approached with caution and should be initiated at the lower end of the dose range of the concomitant medication. If bupropion is added to the treatment regimen of a patient already receiving a drug metabolized by CYP2D6, the need to decrease

the dose of the original medication should be considered, particularly for those concomitant medications with a narrow therapeutic index).
No products indexed under this heading.

Methamphetamine Hydrochloride (Co-administration of bupropion with drugs that are metabolized by the CYP2D6 isoenzyme should be approached with caution and should be initiated at the lower end of the dose range of the concomitant medication. If bupropion is added to the treatment regimen of a patient already receiving a drug metabolized by CYP2D6, the need to decrease the dose of the original medication should be considered, particularly for those concomitant medications with a narrow therapeutic index). Products include:
Desoxyn Tablets, USP 2482

Methotrimeprazine (Concurrent administration of bupropion and agents that lower seizure threshold (e.g., antipsychotics) should be undertaken only with extreme caution. Low initial dosing and gradual dose increases should be employed).
No products indexed under this heading.

Methylprednisolone Acetate (Bupropion is associated with a dose-related risk of seizures; co-administration with drugs that lower seizure threshold, such as systemic steroids, may increase the risk of seizure with bupropion). Products include:
Depo-Medrol Injectable Suspension 2615
Depo-Medrol Single-Dose Vial 2617

Methylprednisolone Sodium Succinate (Bupropion is associated with a dose-related risk of seizures; co-administration with drugs that lower seizure threshold, such as systemic steroids, may increase the risk of seizure with bupropion).
No products indexed under this heading.

Metoprolol Succinate (Co-administration of bupropion with drugs that are metabolized by the CYP2D6 isoenzyme, including metoprolol, should be approached with caution and should be initiated at the lower end of the dose range of the concomitant medication. If bupropion is added to the treatment regimen of a patient already receiving a drug metabolized by CYP2D6, the need to decrease the dose of the original medication should be considered, particularly for those concomitant medications with a narrow therapeutic index). Products include:
Toprol-XL Tablets 660

Metoprolol Tartrate (Co-administration of bupropion with drugs that are metabolized by the CYP2D6 isoenzyme, including metoprolol, should be approached with caution and should be initiated at the lower end of the dose range of the concomitant medication. If bupropion is added to the treatment regimen of a patient already receiving a drug metabolized by CYP2D6, the need to decrease the dose of the original medication should be considered, particularly for those concomitant medications with a narrow therapeutic index).
No products indexed under this heading.

Mexiletine Hydrochloride (Co-administration of bupropion with drugs that are metabolized by the CYP2D6 isoenzyme should be approached with caution and should be initiated at the lower end of the dose range of the concomitant medication. If bupropion is added to the treatment regimen of a patient already receiving a drug metabolized by CYP2D6, the need to decrease the dose of the original medication should be considered, particularly for those concomitant medications with a narrow therapeutic index).
No products indexed under this heading.

Midazolam Hydrochloride (Bupropion is associated with a dose-related risk of seizures; excessive use of benzodiazepine sedatives is associated with increased risk of seizures; bupropion is contraindicated in patients undergoing abrupt discontinuation of benzodiazepine sedatives).
No products indexed under this heading.

Mirtazapine (Co-administration of bupropion with drugs that are metabolized by the CYP2D6 isoenzyme should be approached with caution and should be initiated at the lower end of the dose range of the concomitant medication. If bupropion is added to the treatment regimen of a patient already receiving a drug metabolized by CYP2D6, the need to decrease the dose of the original medication should be considered, particularly for those concomitant medications with a narrow therapeutic index).
No products indexed under this heading.

Moclobemide (Concurrent and/or sequential use with MAO inhibitors is contraindicated).
No products indexed under this heading.

Molindone Hydrochloride (Concurrent administration of bupropion and agents that lower seizure threshold (e.g., antipsychotics) should be undertaken only with extreme caution. Low initial dosing and gradual dose increases should be employed). Products include:
Moban Tablets 1108

Morphine Sulfate (Co-administration of bupropion with drugs that are metabolized by the CYP2D6 isoenzyme should be approached with caution and should be initiated at the lower end of the dose range of the concomitant medication. If bupropion is added to the treatment regimen of a patient already receiving a drug metabolized by CYP2D6, the need to decrease the dose of the original medication should be considered, particularly for those concomitant medications with a narrow therapeutic index). Products include:
Avinza Capsules 1714
Kadian Capsules 572
MS Contin Tablets 2703

Nefazodone Hydrochloride (Concurrent administration of bupropion and agents that lower seizure threshold (e.g., other antidepressants) should be undertaken only with extreme caution. Low initial dosing and gradual dose increases should be employed).
No products indexed under this heading.

Nelfinavir Mesylate (Co-administration of bupropion with drugs that are metabolized by the CYP2D6 isoenzyme should be approached with caution and should be initiated at the lower end of the dose range of the concomitant medication. If bupropion is added to the treatment regimen of a patient already receiving a drug metabolized by CYP2D6, the need to decrease the dose of the original medication should be considered, particularly for those concomitant medications with a narrow therapeutic index). Products include:
Viracept 2556

Nicotine (Co-administration has resulted in a higher incidence of treatment-emergent hypertension). Products include:
Nicoderm CQ Patch 1629
NicoDerm CQ Clear Patch .... ▣ 627
Nicotrol Inhaler 2594
Nicotrol NS 2596

Nortriptyline Hydrochloride (Co-administration of bupropion with drugs that are metabolized by the CYP2D6 isoenzyme, including nortriptyline, should be approached with caution and should be initiated at the lower end of the dose range of the concomitant medication. If bupropion is added to the treatment regimen of a patient already receiving a drug metabolized by CYP2D6, the need to decrease the dose of the original medication should be considered, particularly for those concomitant medications with a narrow therapeutic index).
No products indexed under this heading.

Olanzapine (Co-administration of bupropion with drugs that are metabolized by the CYP2D6 isoenzyme should be approached with caution and should be initiated at the lower end of the dose range of the concomitant medication. If bupropion is added to the treatment regimen of a patient already receiving a drug metabolized by CYP2D6, the need to decrease the dose of the original medication should be considered, particularly for those concomitant medications with a narrow therapeutic index). Products include:
Symbyax Capsules 1788
Zyprexa Tablets 1798
Zyprexa IntraMuscular 1798
Zyprexa ZYDIS Orally Disintegrating Tablets 1798

Omeprazole (Co-administration of bupropion with drugs that are metabolized by the CYP2D6 isoenzyme should be approached with caution and should be initiated at the lower end of the dose range of the concomitant medication. If bupropion is added to the treatment regimen of a patient already receiving a drug metabolized by CYP2D6, the need to decrease the dose of the original medication should be considered, particularly for those concomitant medications with a narrow therapeutic index). Products include:
Zegerid Powder for Oral Solution 2972

Ondansetron (Co-administration of bupropion with drugs that are metabolized by the CYP2D6 isoenzyme should be approached with caution and should be initiated at the lower end of the dose range of the concomitant medication. If bupropion is added to the treatment regimen of a patient already receiving a drug metabolized by CYP2D6, the need to decrease the dose of the original medication should be considered, particularly for those concomitant medications with a narrow therapeutic index). Products include:
Zofran ODT Orally Disintegrating Tablets 1613

Ondansetron Hydrochloride (Co-administration of bupropion with drugs that are metabolized by the CYP2D6 isoenzyme should be approached with caution and should be initiated at the lower end of the dose range of the concomitant medication. If bupropion is added to the treatment regimen of a patient already receiving a drug metabolized by CYP2D6, the need to decrease the dose of the original medication should be considered, particularly for those concomitant medications with a narrow therapeutic index). Products include:
Zofran Injection 1607
Zofran 1613

Orphenadrine Citrate (Bupropion is primarily metabolized, based on in vitro studies, to the morpholinol metabolite by cytochrome P450IIB6 isoenzyme; therefore, the potential exists for a drug interaction with agents that affect the cytochrome P450IIB6 metabolism, such as orphenadrine). Products include:
Norflex Injection 1824

Oxazepam (Bupropion is associated with a dose-related risk of seizures; excessive use of benzodiazepine sedatives is associated with increased risk of seizures; bupropion is contraindicated in patients undergoing abrupt discontinuation of benzodiazepine sedatives).
No products indexed under this heading.

Oxycodone Hydrochloride (Co-administration of bupropion with drugs that are metabolized by the CYP2D6 isoenzyme should be approached with caution and should be initiated at the lower end of the dose range of the concomitant medication. If bupropion is added to the treatment regimen of a patient already receiving a drug metabolized by CYP2D6, the need to decrease the dose of the original medication should be considered, particularly for those concomitant medications with a narrow therapeutic index). Products include:
Combunox Tablets 1183
OxyContin Tablets 2699
OxyFast Oral Concentrate Solution 2704
OxyIR Capsules 2704
Percocet Tablets 1114
Percodan Tablets 1115

Paclitaxel (Co-administration of bupropion with drugs that are metabolized by the CYP2D6 isoenzyme should be approached with caution and should be initiated at the lower end of the dose range of the concomitant medication. If bupropion is added to the treatment regimen of a patient already receiving a drug metabolized by CYP2D6, the need to decrease the dose of the original medication should be considered, particularly for those concomitant medications with a narrow therapeutic index).
No products indexed under this heading.

Pargyline Hydrochloride (Concurrent and/or sequential use with MAO inhibitors is contraindicated).
No products indexed under this heading.

Paroxetine Hydrochloride (Co-administration of bupropion with drugs that are metabolized by the CYP2D6 isoenzyme, including paroxetine, should be approached with caution and should be initiated at the lower end of the dose range of the concomitant medication. If bupropion is added to the treatment regimen of a patient already receiving a drug metabolized by CYP2D6, the need to decrease the dose of the original medication should be considered, particularly for those concomitant medications with a narrow therapeutic index). Products include:
Paxil CR Controlled-Release Tablets 1509
Paxil 1501

Perphenazine (Bupropion is associated with a dose-related risk of seizures; co-administration with drugs that lower seizure threshold may increase the risk of seizure with bupropion; concurrent use should be undertaken with extreme caution).
No products indexed under this heading.

Phenelzine Sulfate (Concurrent and/or sequential use with MAO inhibitors is contraindicated; acute toxicity of bupropion is enhanced by phenelzine in animal models).
No products indexed under this heading.

Phenobarbital (May induce the metabolism of bupropion).
No products indexed under this heading.

Phenytoin (May induce the metabolism of bupropion).
No products indexed under this heading.

Phenytoin Sodium (May induce the metabolism of bupropion). Products include:
Phenytek Capsules 2153

Pimozide (Concurrent administration of bupropion and agents that lower seizure threshold (e.g., antipsychotics) should be undertaken only with extreme caution. Low initial dosing and gradual dose increases should be employed). Products include:
Orap Tablets 1220

Pindolol (Co-administration of bupropion with drugs that are metabolized by the CYP2D6 isoenzyme should be approached with caution and should be initiated at the lower end of the dose range of the concomitant medication. If bupropion is added to the treatment regimen of a patient already receiving a drug metabolized by CYP2D6, the need to decrease the dose of the original medication should be considered, particularly for those concomitant medications with a narrow therapeutic index).
No products indexed under this heading.

Prazepam (Bupropion is associated with a dose-related risk of seizures; excessive use of benzodiazepine sedatives is associated with increased risk of seizures; bupropion is contraindicated in patients undergoing abrupt discontinuation of benzodiazepine sedatives).
No products indexed under this heading.

Prednisolone Acetate (Bupropion is associated with a dose-related risk of seizures; co-administration with drugs that lower seizure threshold, such as systemic steroids, may increase the risk of seizure with bupropion). Products include:
Blephamide Ophthalmic Ointment 563
Blephamide Ophthalmic Suspension 564
Poly-Pred Liquifilm Ophthalmic Suspension .... ⊙231
Pred Forte Ophthalmic Suspension .... ⊙233
Pred Mild Sterile Ophthalmic Suspension .... ⊙236
Pred-G Ophthalmic Suspension .... ⊙234
Pred-G Sterile Ophthalmic Ointment .... ⊙235

Prednisolone Sodium Phosphate (Bupropion is associated with a dose-related risk of seizures; co-administration with drugs that lower seizure threshold, such as systemic steroids, may increase the risk of seizure with bupropion). Products include:
Pediapred Oral Solution 3319

Prednisolone Tebutate (Bupropion is associated with a dose-related risk of seizures; co-administration with drugs that lower seizure threshold, such as systemic steroids, may increase the risk of seizure with bupropion).
No products indexed under this heading.

Prednisone (Bupropion is associated with a dose-related risk of seizures; co-administration with drugs that lower seizure threshold, such as systemic steroids, may increase the risk of seizure with bupropion).
No products indexed under this heading.

Procarbazine Hydrochloride (Concurrent and/or sequential use with MAO inhibitors is contraindicated). Products include:
Matulane Capsules 3188

Prochlorperazine (Bupropion is associated with a dose-related risk of seizures; co-administration with drugs that lower seizure threshold may increase the risk of seizure with bupropion; concurrent use should be undertaken with extreme caution).
No products indexed under this heading.

Promethazine Hydrochloride (Bupropion is associated with a dose-related risk of seizures; co-administration with drugs that lower seizure threshold may increase the risk of seizure with bupropion; concurrent use should be undertaken with extreme caution). Products include:
Phenergan 3438

Propafenone Hydrochloride (Co-administration of bupropion with drugs that are metabolized by the CYP2D6 isoenzyme, including propafenone, should be approached with caution and should be initiated at the lower end of the dose range of the concomitant medication. If bupropion is added to the treatment regimen of a patient already receiving a drug metabolized by CYP2D6, the need to decrease the dose of the original medication should be considered, particularly for those concomitant medications with a narrow therapeutic index). Products include:
Rythmol SR Capsules 2736

Propoxyphene Hydrochloride (Co-administration of bupropion with drugs that are metabolized by the CYP2D6 isoenzyme should be approached with caution and should be initiated at the lower end of the dose range of the concomitant medication. If bupropion is added to the treatment regimen of a patient already receiving a drug metabolized by CYP2D6, the need to decrease the dose of the original medication should be considered, particularly for those concomitant medications with a narrow therapeutic index).
No products indexed under this heading.

Propoxyphene Napsylate (Co-administration of bupropion with drugs that are metabolized by the CYP2D6 isoenzyme should be approached with caution and should be initiated at the lower end of the dose range of the concomitant medication. If bupropion is added to the treatment regimen of a patient already receiving a drug metabolized by CYP2D6, the need to decrease the dose of the original medication should be considered, particularly for those concomitant medications with a narrow therapeutic index). Products include:
Darvocet A 500 Tablets 3497

Propranolol Hydrochloride (Co-administration of bupropion with drugs that are metabolized by the CYP2D6 isoenzyme should be approached with caution and should be initiated at the lower end of the dose range of the concomitant medication. If bupropion is added to the treatment regimen of a patient already receiving a drug metabolized by CYP2D6, the need to decrease the dose of the original medication should be considered, particularly for those concomitant medications with a narrow therapeutic index). Products include:
Inderal LA Long-Acting Capsules 3421
InnoPran XL Capsules 2728

Protriptyline Hydrochloride (Bupropion is associated with a dose-related risk of seizures; co-administration with drugs that lower seizure threshold may increase the risk of seizure with bupropion; concurrent use should be undertaken with extreme caution). Products include:
Vivactil Tablets 2350

Quazepam (Bupropion is associated with a dose-related risk of seizures; excessive use of benzodiazepine sedatives is associated with increased risk of seizures; bupropion is contraindicated in patients undergoing abrupt discontinuation of benzodiazepine sedatives).
No products indexed under this heading.

Quetiapine Fumarate (Co-administration of bupropion with drugs that are metabolized by the CYP2D6 isoenzyme should be approached with caution and should be initiated at the lower end of the dose range of the concomitant medication. If bupropion is added to the treatment regimen of a patient already receiving a drug metabolized by CYP2D6, the need to decrease the dose of the original medication should be considered, particularly for those concomitant medications with a narrow therapeutic index). Products include:
Seroquel Tablets 691

Quinidine Gluconate (Co-administration of bupropion with drugs that are metabolized by the CYP2D6 isoenzyme should be approached with caution and should be initiated at the lower end of the dose range of the concomitant medication. If bupropion is added to the treatment regimen of a patient already receiving a drug metabolized by CYP2D6, the need to decrease the dose of the original medication should be considered, particularly for those concomitant medications with a narrow therapeutic index).
No products indexed under this heading.

Quinidine Hydrochloride (Co-administration of bupropion with drugs that are metabolized by the CYP2D6 isoenzyme should be approached with caution and should be initiated at the lower end of the dose range of the concomitant medication. If bupropion is added to the treatment regimen of a patient already receiving a drug metabolized by CYP2D6, the need to decrease the dose of the original medication should be considered, particularly for those concomitant medications with a narrow therapeutic index).
No products indexed under this heading.

Quinidine Polygalacturonate (Co-administration of bupropion with drugs that are metabolized by the CYP2D6 isoenzyme should be approached with caution and should be initiated at the lower end of the dose range of the concomitant medication. If bupropion is added to the treatment regimen of a patient already receiving a drug metabolized by CYP2D6, the need to decrease the dose of the original medication should be considered, particularly for those concomitant medications with a narrow therapeutic index).
No products indexed under this heading.

Quinidine Sulfate (Co-administration of bupropion with drugs that are metabolized by the CYP2D6 isoenzyme should be approached with caution and should be initiated at the lower end of the dose range of the concomitant medication. If bupropion is added to the treatment regimen of a patient already receiving a drug metabolized by CYP2D6, the need to decrease the dose of the original medication should be considered, particularly for those concomitant medications with a narrow therapeutic index).
No products indexed under this heading.

Risperidone (Co-administration of bupropion with drugs that are metabolized by the CYP2D6 isoenzyme, including risperidone, should be approached with caution and should be initiated at the lower end of the dose range of the concomitant medication. If bupropion is added to the treatment regimen of a patient already receiving a drug metabolized by CYP2D6, the need to decrease the dose of the original medication should be considered, particularly for those concomitant medications with a narrow therapeutic index). Products include:
Risperdal Consta Long-Acting Injection 1664
Risperdal M-Tab Orally Disintegrating Tablets 1658

Risperdal 1658

Ritonavir (Co-administration of bupropion with drugs that are metabolized by the CYP2D6 isoenzyme should be approached with caution and should be initiated at the lower end of the dose range of the concomitant medication. If bupropion is added to the treatment regimen of a patient already receiving a drug metabolized by CYP2D6, the need to decrease the dose of the original medication should be considered, particularly for those concomitant medications with a narrow therapeutic index). Products include:

Kaletra 474
Norvir 499

Selegiline Hydrochloride (Concurrent and/or sequential use with MAO inhibitors is contraindicated). Products include:

Eldepryl Capsules 3209

Sertraline Hydrochloride (Co-administration of bupropion with drugs that are metabolized by the CYP2D6 isoenzyme, including sertraline, should be approached with caution and should be initiated at the lower end of the dose range of the concomitant medication. If bupropion is added to the treatment regimen of a patient already receiving a drug metabolized by CYP2D6, the need to decrease the dose of the original medication should be considered, particularly for those concomitant medications with a narrow therapeutic index). Products include:

Zoloft 2581

Tamoxifen Citrate (Co-administration of bupropion with drugs that are metabolized by the CYP2D6 isoenzyme should be approached with caution and should be initiated at the lower end of the dose range of the concomitant medication. If bupropion is added to the treatment regimen of a patient already receiving a drug metabolized by CYP2D6, the need to decrease the dose of the original medication should be considered, particularly for those concomitant medications with a narrow therapeutic index).

No products indexed under this heading.

Temazepam (Bupropion is associated with a dose-related risk of seizures; excessive use of benzodiazepine sedatives is associated with increased risk of seizures; bupropion is contraindicated in patients undergoing abrupt discontinuation of benzodiazepine sedatives).

No products indexed under this heading.

Teniposide (Co-administration of bupropion with drugs that are metabolized by the CYP2D6 isoenzyme should be approached with caution and should be initiated at the lower end of the dose range of the concomitant medication. If bupropion is added to the treatment regimen of a patient already receiving a drug metabolized by CYP2D6, the need to decrease the dose of the original medication should be considered, particularly for those concomitant medications with a narrow therapeutic index).

No products indexed under this heading.

Testosterone (Co-administration of bupropion with drugs that are metabolized by the CYP2D6 isoenzyme should be approached with caution and should be initiated at the lower end of the dose range of the concomitant medication. If bupropion is added to the treatment regimen of a patient already receiving a drug metabolized by CYP2D6, the need to decrease the dose of the original medication should be considered, particularly for those concomitant medications with a narrow therapeutic index). Products include:

AndroGel 3330
Striant Mucoadhesive 1022
Testim 1% Gel 722

Testosterone Cypionate (Co-administration of bupropion with drugs that are metabolized by the CYP2D6 isoenzyme should be approached with caution and should be initiated at the lower end of the dose range of the concomitant medication. If bupropion is added to the treatment regimen of a patient already receiving a drug metabolized by CYP2D6, the need to decrease the dose of the original medication should be considered, particularly for those concomitant medications with a narrow therapeutic index).

No products indexed under this heading.

Testosterone Enanthate (Co-administration of bupropion with drugs that are metabolized by the CYP2D6 isoenzyme should be approached with caution and should be initiated at the lower end of the dose range of the concomitant medication. If bupropion is added to the treatment regimen of a patient already receiving a drug metabolized by CYP2D6, the need to decrease the dose of the original medication should be considered, particularly for those concomitant medications with a narrow therapeutic index). Products include:

Delatestryl Injection 2976

Testosterone Propionate (Co-administration of bupropion with drugs that are metabolized by the CYP2D6 isoenzyme should be approached with caution and should be initiated at the lower end of the dose range of the concomitant medication. If bupropion is added to the treatment regimen of a patient already receiving a drug metabolized by CYP2D6, the need to decrease the dose of the original medication should be considered, particularly for those concomitant medications with a narrow therapeutic index).

No products indexed under this heading.

Theophylline (Bupropion is associated with a dose-related risk of seizures; co-administration with drugs that lower seizure threshold may increase the risk of seizures with bupropion; concurrent use should be undertaken with extreme caution).

No products indexed under this heading.

Theophylline Anhydrous (Bupropion is associated with a dose-related risk of seizures; co-administration with drugs that lower seizure threshold may increase the risk of seizures with bupropion; concurrent use should be undertaken with extreme caution). Products include:

Uniphyl Tablets 2708

Theophylline Calcium Salicylate (Bupropion is associated with a dose-related risk of seizures; co-administration with drugs that lower seizure threshold may increase the risk of seizures with bupropion; concurrent use should be undertaken with extreme caution).

No products indexed under this heading.

Theophylline Dihydroxypropyl (Glyceryl) (Bupropion is associated with a dose-related risk of seizures; co-administration with drugs that lower seizure threshold may increase the risk of seizures with bupropion; concurrent use should be undertaken with extreme caution).

No products indexed under this heading.

Theophylline Ethylenediamine (Bupropion is associated with a dose-related risk of seizures; co-administration with drugs that lower seizure threshold may increase the risk of seizures with bupropion; concurrent use should be undertaken with extreme caution).

No products indexed under this heading.

Theophylline Sodium Glycinate (Bupropion is associated with a dose-related risk of seizures; co-administration with drugs that lower seizure threshold may increase the risk of seizures with bupropion; concurrent use should be undertaken with extreme caution).

No products indexed under this heading.

Thioridazine (Co-administration of bupropion with drugs that are metabolized by the CYP2D6 isoenzyme, including thioridazine, should be approached with caution and should be initiated at the lower end of the dose range of the concomitant medication. If bupropion is added to the treatment regimen of a patient already receiving a drug metabolized by CYP2D6, the need to decrease the dose of the original medication should be considered, particularly for those concomitant medications with a narrow therapeutic index).

No products indexed under this heading.

Thioridazine Hydrochloride (Co-administration of bupropion with drugs that are metabolized by the CYP2D6 isoenzyme, including thioridazine, should be approached with caution and should be initiated at the lower end of the dose range of the concomitant medication. If bupropion is added to the treatment regimen of a patient already receiving a drug metabolized by CYP2D6, the need to decrease the dose of the original medication should be considered, particularly for those concomitant medications with a narrow therapeutic index). Products include:

Thioridazine Hydrochloride Tablets 2122

Thiothixene (Concurrent administration of bupropion and agents that lower seizure threshold (e.g., antipsychotics) should be undertaken only with extreme caution. Low initial dosing and gradual dose increases should be employed). Products include:

Thiothixene Capsules 2124

Timolol Maleate (Co-administration of bupropion with drugs that are metabolized by the CYP2D6 isoenzyme should be approached with caution and should be initiated at the lower end of the dose range of the concomitant medication. If bupropion is added to the treatment regimen of a patient already receiving a drug metabolized by CYP2D6, the need to decrease the dose of the original medication should be considered, particularly for those concomitant medications with a narrow therapeutic index). Products include:

Blocadren Tablets 1891
Cosopt Sterile Ophthalmic Solution 1910
Timolide Tablets 2056
Timoptic in Ocudose 2061
Timoptic Sterile Ophthalmic Solution 2058
Timoptic-XE Sterile Ophthalmic Gel Forming Solution 2062

Tolterodine Tartrate (Co-administration of bupropion with drugs that are metabolized by the CYP2D6 isoenzyme should be approached with caution and should be initiated at the lower end of the dose range of the concomitant medication. If bupropion is added to the treatment regimen of a patient already receiving a drug metabolized by CYP2D6, the need to decrease the dose of the original medication should be considered, particularly for those concomitant medications with a narrow therapeutic index). Products include:

Detrol Tablets 2626
Detrol LA Capsules 2629

Tramadol Hydrochloride (Co-administration of bupropion with drugs that are metabolized by the CYP2D6 isoenzyme should be approached with caution and should be initiated at the lower end of the dose range of the concomitant medication. If bupropion is added to the treatment regimen of a patient already receiving a drug metabolized by CYP2D6, the need to decrease the dose of the original medication should be considered, particularly for those concomitant medications with a narrow therapeutic index). Products include:

Ultracet Tablets 2462

Tranylcypromine Sulfate (Concurrent and/or sequential use with MAO inhibitors is contraindicated). Products include:

Parnate Tablets 1499

Trazodone Hydrochloride (Bupropion is associated with a dose-related risk of seizures; co-administration with drugs that lower seizure threshold may increase the risk of seizure with bupropion; concurrent use should be undertaken with extreme caution).

No products indexed under this heading.

Triamcinolone (Bupropion is associated with a dose-related risk of seizures; co-administration with drugs that lower seizure threshold, such as systemic steroids, may increase the risk of seizure with bupropion).

No products indexed under this heading.

Triamcinolone Acetonide (Bupropion is associated with a dose-related risk of seizures; co-administration with drugs that lower seizure threshold, such as systemic steroids, may increase the risk of seizure with bupropion). Products include:

Azmacort Inhalation Aerosol 1701

Nasacort HFA Inhalation Aerosol 2939
Nasacort AQ Nasal Spray 2937

Triamcinolone Diacetate (Bupropion is associated with a dose-related risk of seizures; co-administration with drugs that lower seizure threshold, such as systemic steroids, may increase the risk of seizure with bupropion).
No products indexed under this heading.

Triamcinolone Hexacetonide (Bupropion is associated with a dose-related risk of seizures; co-administration with drugs that lower seizure threshold, such as systemic steroids, may increase the risk of seizure with bupropion).
No products indexed under this heading.

Triazolam (Bupropion is associated with a dose-related risk of seizures; excessive use of benzodiazepine sedatives is associated with increased risk of seizures; bupropion is contraindicated in patients undergoing abrupt discontinuation of benzodiazepine sedatives).
No products indexed under this heading.

Trifluoperazine Hydrochloride (Bupropion is associated with a dose-related risk of seizures; co-administration with drugs that lower seizure threshold may increase the risk of seizure with bupropion; concurrent use should be undertaken with extreme caution).
No products indexed under this heading.

Trimipramine Maleate (Bupropion is associated with a dose-related risk of seizures; co-administration with drugs that lower seizure threshold may increase the risk of seizure with bupropion; concurrent use should be undertaken with extreme caution). Products include:
Surmontil Capsules 2347

Venlafaxine Hydrochloride (Co-administration of bupropion with drugs that are metabolized by the CYP2D6 isoenzyme should be approached with caution and should be initiated at the lower end of the dose range of the concomitant medication. If bupropion is added to the treatment regimen of a patient already receiving a drug metabolized by CYP2D6, the need to decrease the dose of the original medication should be considered, particularly for those concomitant medications with a narrow therapeutic index). Products include:
Effexor Tablets 3405
Effexor XR Capsules 3411

Vinblastine Sulfate (Co-administration of bupropion with drugs that are metabolized by the CYP2D6 isoenzyme should be approached with caution and should be initiated at the lower end of the dose range of the concomitant medication. If bupropion is added to the treatment regimen of a patient already receiving a drug metabolized by CYP2D6, the need to decrease the dose of the original medication should be considered, particularly for those concomitant medications with a narrow therapeutic index).
No products indexed under this heading.

Warfarin Sodium (Altered PT and/or INR, infrequently associated with hemorrhagic or thrombotic complications, were observed when bupropion was co-administered with warfarin). Products include:
Coumadin for Injection 932
Coumadin Tablets 932

Ziprasidone Hydrochloride (Concurrent administration of bupropion and agents that lower seizure threshold (e.g., antipsychotics) should be undertaken only with extreme caution. Low initial dosing and gradual dose increases should be employed). Products include:
Geodon Capsules 2514

Zonisamide (Co-administration of bupropion with drugs that are metabolized by the CYP2D6 isoenzyme should be approached with caution and should be initiated at the lower end of the dose range of the concomitant medication. If bupropion is added to the treatment regimen of a patient already receiving a drug metabolized by CYP2D6, the need to decrease the dose of the original medication should be considered, particularly for those concomitant medications with a narrow therapeutic index). Products include:
Zonegran Capsules 1089

Food Interactions

Alcohol (Bupropion hydrochloride is contraindicated in patients undergoing abrupt discontinuation of alcohol. The consumption of alcohol during treatment with bupropion hydrochloride should be minimized or avoided).

Food, unspecified (Food increases Cmax and AUC of bupropion by 11% and 17%, respectively; no clinically significant food effect).

WELLBUTRIN XL EXTENDED-RELEASE TABLETS

(Bupropion Hydrochloride) 1588

See Wellbutrin SR Sustained-Release Tablets

WINRHO SDF

(Rh$_0$ (D) Immune Globulin (Human)) 763
May interact with vaccines, live. Compounds in these categories include:

BCG Vaccine (Other antibodies contained in WinRho SDF may interfere with the response to live virus vaccines such as measles, mumps, polio or rubella. Therefore, immunization with live vaccines should not be given within 3 months after WinRho SDF administration).
No products indexed under this heading.

Measles, Mumps & Rubella Virus Vaccine, Live (Other antibodies contained in WinRho SDF may interfere with the response to live virus vaccines such as measles, mumps, polio or rubella. Therefore, immunization with live vaccines should not be given within 3 months after WinRho SDF administration). Products include:
M-M-R II 1980

Measles & Rubella Virus Vaccine Live (Other antibodies contained in WinRho SDF may interfere with the response to live virus vaccines such as measles, mumps, polio or rubella. Therefore, immunization with live vaccines should not be given within 3 months after WinRho SDF administration).
No products indexed under this heading.

Measles Virus Vaccine Live (Other antibodies contained in WinRho SDF may interfere with the response to live virus vaccines such as measles, mumps, polio or rubella. Therefore, immunization with live vaccines should not be given within 3 months after WinRho SDF administration). Products include:
Attenuvax 1889

Mumps Virus Vaccine, Live (Other antibodies contained in WinRho SDF may interfere with the response to live virus vaccines such as measles, mumps, polio or rubella. Therefore, immunization with live vaccines should not be given within 3 months after WinRho SDF administration). Products include:
Mumpsvax 2005

Poliovirus Vaccine, Live, Oral, Trivalent, Types 1,2,3 (Sabin) (Other antibodies contained in WinRho SDF may interfere with the response to live virus vaccines such as measles, mumps, polio or rubella. Therefore, immunization with live vaccines should not be given within 3 months after WinRho SDF administration).
No products indexed under this heading.

Rotavirus Vaccine, Live, Oral, Tetravalent (Other antibodies contained in WinRho SDF may interfere with the response to live virus vaccines such as measles, mumps, polio or rubella. Therefore, immunization with live vaccines should not be given within 3 months after WinRho SDF administration).
No products indexed under this heading.

Rubella & Mumps Virus Vaccine Live (Other antibodies contained in WinRho SDF may interfere with the response to live virus vaccines such as measles, mumps, polio or rubella. Therefore, immunization with live vaccines should not be given within 3 months after WinRho SDF administration).
No products indexed under this heading.

Rubella Virus Vaccine Live (Other antibodies contained in WinRho SDF may interfere with the response to live virus vaccines such as measles, mumps, polio or rubella. Therefore, immunization with live vaccines should not be given within 3 months after WinRho SDF administration). Products include:
Meruvax II 1994

Smallpox Vaccine (Other antibodies contained in WinRho SDF may interfere with the response to live virus vaccines such as measles, mumps, polio or rubella. Therefore, immunization with live vaccines should not be given within 3 months after WinRho SDF administration).
No products indexed under this heading.

Typhoid Vaccine (Other antibodies contained in WinRho SDF may interfere with the response to live virus vaccines such as measles, mumps, polio or rubella. Therefore, immunization with live vaccines should not be given within 3 months after WinRho SDF administration).
No products indexed under this heading.

Varicella Virus Vaccine Live (Other antibodies contained in WinRho SDF may interfere with the response to live virus vaccines such as measles, mumps, polio or rubella. Therefore, immunization with live vaccines should not be given within 3 months after WinRho SDF administration). Products include:
Varivax 2070

Yellow Fever Vaccine (Other antibodies contained in WinRho SDF may interfere with the response to live virus vaccines such as measles, mumps, polio or rubella. Therefore, immunization with live vaccines should not be given within 3 months after WinRho SDF administration).
No products indexed under this heading.

WOBENZYM TABLETS

(Dietary Supplement) 3525
May interact with oral anticoagulants. Compounds in these categories include:

Anisindione (The use of Wobenzym should be graduated when taken in conjunction with anticoagulants). Products include:
Miradon Tablets 3056

Dicumarol (The use of Wobenzym should be graduated when taken in conjunction with anticoagulants).
No products indexed under this heading.

Warfarin Sodium (The use of Wobenzym should be graduated when taken in conjunction with anticoagulants). Products include:
Coumadin for Injection 932
Coumadin Tablets 932

XALATAN STERILE OPHTHALMIC SOLUTION

(Latanoprost) 2654
May interact with:

Thimerosal (In vitro studies have shown that precipitation occurs when eye drops containing thimerosal are mixed with Xalatan; administer with an interval of at least five minutes between applications).
No products indexed under this heading.

XANAX XR TABLETS

(Alprazolam) 2655
May interact with antihistamines, azole antifungals, central nervous system depressants, cytochrome p450 3a4 inducers (selected), cytochrome p450 3a4 inhibitors (selected), anticonvulsants, macrolide antibiotics, oral contraceptives, and certain other agents. Compounds in these categories include:

Acetazolamide (Drugs that inhibit metabolism via cytochrome P4503A may have a profound effect on the clearance of alprazolam. Potent inhibitors of CYP3A would be expected to increase plasma alprazolam concentrations. Co-administration with very potent inhibitors of CYP3A should be avoided. Concurrent use of alprazolam with drugs inhibiting CYP3A to a lesser but still significant degree requires caution).
No products indexed under this heading.

Acrivastine (Additive CNS depressant effects).
No products indexed under this heading.

Alfentanil Hydrochloride (Additive CNS depressant effects).
No products indexed under this heading.

Allium sativum (CYP3A4 inducers would be expected to decrease alprazolam concentrations).
No products indexed under this heading.

Amiodarone Hydrochloride (Data from in vitro studies of benzodiazepines other than alprazolam suggest a possible interaction when co-administered; concurrent use requires caution). Products include:
Pacerone Tablets **3337**

Amprenavir (Drugs that inhibit metabolism via cytochrome P4503A may have a profound effect on the clearance of alprazolam. Potent inhibitors of CYP3A would be expected to increase plasma alprazolam concentrations. Co-administration with very potent inhibitors of CYP3A should be avoided. Concurrent use of alprazolam with drugs inhibiting CYP3A to a lesser but still significant degree requires caution). Products include:
Agenerase Capsules **1299**
Agenerase Oral Solution **1304**

Anastrozole (Drugs that inhibit metabolism via cytochrome P4503A may have a profound effect on the clearance of alprazolam. Potent inhibitors of CYP3A would be expected to increase plasma alprazolam concentrations. Co-administration with very potent inhibitors of CYP3A should be avoided. Concurrent use of alprazolam with drugs inhibiting CYP3A to a lesser but still significant degree requires caution). Products include:
Arimidex Tablets **665**

Aprepitant (Drugs that inhibit metabolism via cytochrome P4503A may have a profound effect on the clearance of alprazolam. Potent inhibitors of CYP3A would be expected to increase plasma alprazolam concentrations. Co-administration with very potent inhibitors of CYP3A should be avoided. Concurrent use of alprazolam with drugs inhibiting CYP3A to a lesser but still significant degree requires caution). Products include:
Emend Capsules **1944**

Aprobarbital (Additive CNS depressant effects).
No products indexed under this heading.

Astemizole (Additive CNS depressant effects).
No products indexed under this heading.

Azatadine Maleate (Additive CNS depressant effects).
No products indexed under this heading.

Azithromycin Dihydrate (Possible interaction based on the clinical studies involving other benzodiazepines metabolized similarly as alprazolam; co-administration requires caution). Products include:
Zithromax **2568**
Zithromax for IV Infusion **2573**
Zithromax for Oral Suspension, 300 mg, 600 mg, 900 mg, 1200 mg **2561**
Zithromax Tablets, 250 mg, 500 mg **2561**
Zithromax Tri-Pak **2561**
Zithromax Z-Pak **2568**

Betamethasone Acetate (CYP3A4 inducers would be expected to decrease alprazolam concentrations).
No products indexed under this heading.

Betamethasone Sodium Phosphate (CYP3A4 inducers would be expected to decrease alprazolam concentrations).
No products indexed under this heading.

Bromodiphenhydramine Hydrochloride (Additive CNS depressant effects).
No products indexed under this heading.

Brompheniramine Maleate (Additive CNS depressant effects). Products include:
Alacol DM Syrup **739**
Children's Dimetapp Cold & Allergy Elixir .... ▣**745**
Children's Dimetapp DM Cold & Cough Elixir .... ▣**745**
Robitussin Allergy & Cough Syrup .... ▣**750**

Buprenorphine Hydrochloride (Additive CNS depressant effects). Products include:
Buprenex Injectable **2718**
Suboxone Tablets **2719**
Subutex Tablets **2719**

Buspirone Hydrochloride (Additive CNS depressant effects).
No products indexed under this heading.

Butabarbital (Additive CNS depressant effects).
No products indexed under this heading.

Butalbital (Additive CNS depressant effects). Products include:
Sedapap Tablets 50 mg/650 mg **2098**

Carbamazepine (Co-administration of carbamazepine with alprazolam can increase alprazolam metabolism and therefore can decrease plasma levels of alprazolam). Products include:
Carbatrol Capsules **3174**
Equetro Extended-Release Capsules **3178**
Tegretol/Tegretol-XR **2278**

Cetirizine Hydrochloride (Additive CNS depressant effects). Products include:
Zyrtec Chewable Tablets **2589**
Zyrtec **2589**
Zyrtec-D 12 Hour Extended Release Tablets **2591**

Chlordiazepoxide (Additive CNS depressant effects).
No products indexed under this heading.

Chlordiazepoxide Hydrochloride (Additive CNS depressant effects). Products include:
Librium Capsules **3349**

Chlorpheniramine Maleate (Additive CNS depressant effects). Products include:
Advil Allergy Sinus Caplets .... ▣**737**
Advil Multi-Symptom Cold Caplets .... ▣**738**
BC Allergy Sinus Cold Powder .... ▣**612**
Contac Severe Cold and Flu Caplets Maximum Strength .... ▣**615**
Hycomine Compound Tablets **1105**
PediaCare Multi-Symptom Cold Liquid .... ▣**704**
PediaCare NightRest Cough & Cold Liquid .... ▣**704**
Robitussin Flu Liquid .... ▣**752**
Robitussin PM Cough & Cold Liquid .... ▣**752**
Singlet Caplets .... ▣**636**
Sudafed Sinus & Allergy Tablets .... ▣**710**
TheraFlu Cold & Cough Hot Liquid .... ▣**680**
TheraFlu Cold & Sore Throat Hot Liquid .... ▣**680**
TheraFlu Flu & Sore Throat Hot Liquid .... ▣**681**
TheraFlu Severe Cold & Cough Hot Liquid .... ▣**683**
TheraFlu Severe Cold Caplets .... ▣**679**
TheraFlu Severe Cold Hot Liquid .... ▣**682**
Triaminic Cold & Allergy Liquid .... ▣**685**
Triaminic Cold & Cough Liquid .... ▣**685**
Triaminic Flu, Cough & Fever Liquid .... ▣**685**
Triaminic Night Time Cough & Cold Liquid .... ▣**685**
Triaminic Allergy Runny Nose & Congestion Softchews .... ▣**688**
Triaminic Cold & Cough Softchews .... ▣**688**
Children's Tylenol Plus Cold NightTime Suspension Liquid **1851**
Children's Tylenol Plus Cold & Cough Suspension Liquid and Chewable Tablets **1851**
Children's Tylenol Plus Cold Chewable Tablets **1851**
Children's Tylenol Plus Flu Suspension Liquid **1853**
Tylenol Allergy Complete Multi-Symptom Caplets and Gelcaps with Cool Burst **1844**
Multi-Symptom Tylenol Cold Night Time Caplets **1845**
Vicks 44M Cough, Cold & Flu Relief **2676**
Pediatric Vicks 44m Cough & Cold Relief **2673**
Children's Vicks NyQuil Cold/Cough Relief **2671**

Chlorpheniramine Polistirex (Additive CNS depressant effects). Products include:
Tussionex Pennkinetic Extended-Release Suspension **3322**

Chlorpheniramine Tannate (Additive CNS depressant effects).
No products indexed under this heading.

Chlorpromazine (Additive CNS depressant effects).
No products indexed under this heading.

Chlorpromazine Hydrochloride (Additive CNS depressant effects).
No products indexed under this heading.

Chlorprothixene (Additive CNS depressant effects).
No products indexed under this heading.

Chlorprothixene Hydrochloride (Additive CNS depressant effects).
No products indexed under this heading.

Chlorprothixene Lactate (Additive CNS depressant effects).
No products indexed under this heading.

Cimetidine (Drugs that inhibit metabolism via cytochrome P4503A may have a profound effect on the clearance of alprazolam. Potent inhibitors of CYP3A would be expected to increase plasma alprazolam concentrations. Co-administration with very potent inhibitors of CYP3A should be avoided. Concurrent use of alprazolam with drugs inhibiting CYP3A to a lesser but still significant degree requires caution). Products include:
Tagamet HB 200 Tablets .... ▣**637**
Tagamet Tablets **1547**

Cimetidine Hydrochloride (Drugs that inhibit metabolism via cytochrome P4503A may have a profound effect on the clearance of alprazolam. Potent inhibitors of CYP3A would be expected to increase plasma alprazolam concentrations. Co-administration with very potent inhibitors of CYP3A should be avoided. Concurrent use of alprazolam with drugs inhibiting CYP3A to a lesser but still significant degree requires caution).
No products indexed under this heading.

Ciprofloxacin (Drugs that inhibit metabolism via cytochrome P4503A may have a profound effect on the clearance of alprazolam. Potent inhibitors of CYP3A would be expected to increase plasma alprazolam concentrations. Co-administration with very potent inhibitors of CYP3A should be avoided. Concurrent use of alprazolam with drugs inhibiting CYP3A to a lesser but still significant degree requires caution). Products include:
Cipro I.V. **2998**
Cipro I.V. Pharmacy Bulk Package **3509**
Cipro Oral Suspension **2991**
Cipro XR Tablets **3004**
Ciprodex Otic Suspension **555**

Ciprofloxacin Hydrochloride (CYP3A4 inducers would be expected to decrease alprazolam concentrations). Products include:
Ciloxan Ophthalmic Ointment **554**
Cipro Tablets **2991**

Cisplatin (CYP3A4 inducers would be expected to decrease alprazolam concentrations).
No products indexed under this heading.

Clarithromycin (Possible interaction based on the clinical studies involving other benzodiazepines metabolized similarly as alprazolam; co-administration requires caution). Products include:
Biaxin/Biaxin XL **402**
PREVPAC **3281**

Clemastine Fumarate (Additive CNS depressant effects).
No products indexed under this heading.

Clorazepate Dipotassium (Additive CNS depressant effects). Products include:
Tranxene **2488**

Clotrimazole (Azole-type antifungal agents are potent CYP3A inhibitors and have been shown to increase plasma alprazolam concentrations. Co-administration is not recommended). Products include:
Lotrimin **3053**
Lotrisone **3054**

Clozapine (Additive CNS depressant effects). Products include:
Clozapine Tablets **2141**
Clozaril Tablets **2174**
FazaClo Orally Disintegrating Tablets **547**

Codeine Phosphate (Additive CNS depressant effects). Products include:
Tylenol with Codeine **2461**

Cortisone Acetate (CYP3A4 inducers would be expected to decrease alprazolam concentrations).
No products indexed under this heading.

Cyclosporine (Data from in vitro studies of benzodiazepines other than alprazolam suggest a possible interaction when co-administered; concurrent use requires caution). Products include:
Gengraf Capsules **458**
Neoral Soft Gelatin Capsules **2247**
Neoral Oral Solution **2247**
Restasis Ophthalmic Emulsion **570**
Sandimmune **2259**

Cyproheptadine Hydrochloride (Additive CNS depressant effects).
No products indexed under this heading.

Dalfopristin (Drugs that inhibit metabolism via cytochrome P4503A may have a profound effect on the clearance of alprazolam. Potent inhibitors of CYP3A would be expected to increase plasma alprazolam concentrations. Co-administration with very potent inhibitors of CYP3A should be avoided. Concurrent use of alprazolam with drugs inhibiting CYP3A to a lesser but still significant degree requires caution). Products include:
Synercid I.V. 1690

Danazol (Drugs that inhibit metabolism via cytochrome P4503A may have a profound effect on the clearance of alprazolam. Potent inhibitors of CYP3A would be expected to increase plasma alprazolam concentrations. Co-administration with very potent inhibitors of CYP3A should be avoided. Concurrent use of alprazolam with drugs inhibiting CYP3A to a lesser but still significant degree requires caution).
No products indexed under this heading.

Delavirdine Mesylate (Drugs that inhibit metabolism via cytochrome P4503A may have a profound effect on the clearance of alprazolam. Potent inhibitors of CYP3A would be expected to increase plasma alprazolam concentrations. Co-administration with very potent inhibitors of CYP3A should be avoided. Concurrent use of alprazolam with drugs inhibiting CYP3A to a lesser but still significant degree requires caution). Products include:
Rescriptor Tablets 2535

Desflurane (Additive CNS depressant effects). Products include:
Suprane Liquid for Inhalation 770

Desipramine Hydrochloride (Concomitant administration of alprazolam and desipramine increased steady state plasma concentrations of desipramine by 20%).
No products indexed under this heading.

Desogestrel (Co-administration with oral contraceptives increased the maximum plasma concentration of alprazolam by 18%, decreased clearance by 22%, and increased half-life by 29%). Products include:
Ortho-Cept Tablets 2395

Dexamethasone (CYP3A4 inducers would be expected to decrease alprazolam concentrations). Products include:
Ciprodex Otic Suspension 555
Decadron Tablets 1929
TobraDex Ophthalmic Ointment 558
TobraDex Ophthalmic Suspension ... 558

Dexamethasone Acetate (CYP3A4 inducers would be expected to decrease alprazolam concentrations).
No products indexed under this heading.

Dexamethasone Sodium Phosphate (CYP3A4 inducers would be expected to decrease alprazolam concentrations). Products include:
Decadron Phosphate Injection 1931

Dexchlorpheniramine Maleate (Additive CNS depressant effects).
No products indexed under this heading.

Dezocine (Additive CNS depressant effects).
No products indexed under this heading.

Diazepam (Additive CNS depressant effects). Products include:
Diastat Rectal Delivery System 3344
Valium Tablets 2822

Diltiazem Hydrochloride (Possible interaction based on the clinical studies involving other benzodiazepines metabolized similarly as alprazolam; co-administration requires caution). Products include:
Cardizem LA Extended Release Tablets 1699
Tiazac Capsules 1204

Diltiazem Maleate (Drugs that inhibit metabolism via cytochrome P4503A may have a profound effect on the clearance of alprazolam. Potent inhibitors of CYP3A would be expected to increase plasma alprazolam concentrations. Co-administration with very potent inhibitors of CYP3A should be avoided. Concurrent use of alprazolam with drugs inhibiting CYP3A to a lesser but still significant degree requires caution).
No products indexed under this heading.

Diphenhydramine Citrate (Additive CNS depressant effects). Products include:
Children's Benadryl Allergy & Cold Fastmelt Tablets.................. 695
Children's Benadryl D Allergy & Sinus Fastmelt Tablets 694
Children's Benadryl Allergy Fastmelt Tablets 696
Goody's PM Powder 622

Diphenhydramine Hydrochloride (Additive CNS depressant effects). Products include:
Benadryl Allergy & Cold Tablets 692
Benadryl Allergy 691
Benadryl Allergy & Sinus Headache Caplets & Gelcaps...... 693
Children's Benadryl Allergy Liquid ... 695
Children's Benadryl Dye-Free Allergy Liquid 695
Benadryl Dye-Free Allergy Liqui-Gels Softgels 692
Benadryl Itch Relief Stick Extra Strength 696
Benadryl Itch Stopping Cream Extra Strength 697
Benadryl Itch Stopping Gel Extra Strength 697
Benadryl Itch Stopping Spray Extra Strength 697
Benadryl Maximum Strength Severe Allergy & Sinus Headache Caplets....................... 694
Children's Benadryl D Liquid Medication................................ 693
Benadryl D Tablets 694
Nytol QuickCaps Caplets 635
Maximum Strength Nytol QuickGels Softgels 635
Simply Sleep Caplets 1841
Sominex Original Formula Tablets .. 637
TheraFlu Thin Strips Multi Symptom.................................... 684
Triaminic Thin Strips Cough & Runny Nose 690
Children's Tylenol Plus Cold & Allergy Suspension Liquid 1850
Tylenol Allergy Complete Night Time Caplets 1844
Tylenol Severe Allergy Caplets 1844
Tylenol Flu NightTime Gelcaps 1846
Extra Strength Tylenol PM Caplets, Geltabs, Gelcaps and Liquid 1847
Unisom Maximum Strength SleepGels 712

Diphenylpyraline Hydrochloride (Additive CNS depressant effects).
No products indexed under this heading.

Dirithromycin (Possible interaction based on the clinical studies involving other benzodiazepines metabolized similarly as alprazolam; co-administration requires caution).
No products indexed under this heading.

Divalproex Sodium (Additive CNS depressant effects). Products include:
Depakote Sprinkle Capsules 422
Depakote Tablets 427
Depakote ER Tablets 433

Doxorubicin Hydrochloride (CYP3A4 inducers would be expected to decrease alprazolam concentrations). Products include:
Adriamycin for Injection, USP 786
Adriamycin Injection, USP 786

Droperidol (Additive CNS depressant effects).
No products indexed under this heading.

Efavirenz (Drugs that inhibit metabolism via cytochrome P4503A may have a profound effect on the clearance of alprazolam. Potent inhibitors of CYP3A would be expected to increase plasma alprazolam concentrations. Co-administration with very potent inhibitors of CYP3A should be avoided. Concurrent use of alprazolam with drugs inhibiting CYP3A to a lesser but still significant degree requires caution). Products include:
Sustiva Capsules 957

Enflurane (Additive CNS depressant effects).
No products indexed under this heading.

Ergotamine Tartrate (Data from in vitro studies of benzodiazepines other than alprazolam suggest a possible interaction when co-administered; concurrent use requires caution).
No products indexed under this heading.

Erythromycin (Possible interaction based on the clinical studies involving other benzodiazepines metabolized similarly as alprazolam; co-administration requires caution). Products include:
Erygel Topical Gel 2096
Ery-Tab Tablets 447
Erythromycin Base Filmtab Tablets 454
Erythromycin Delayed-Release Capsules, USP............................ 456
PCE Dispertab Tablets 510

Erythromycin Estolate (Possible interaction based on the clinical studies involving other benzodiazepines metabolized similarly as alprazolam; co-administration requires caution).
No products indexed under this heading.

Erythromycin Ethylsuccinate (Possible interaction based on the clinical studies involving other benzodiazepines metabolized similarly as alprazolam; co-administration requires caution). Products include:
E.E.S. 449
EryPed 445

Erythromycin Gluceptate (Possible interaction based on the clinical studies involving other benzodiazepines metabolized similarly as alprazolam; co-administration requires caution).
No products indexed under this heading.

Erythromycin Lactobionate (Drugs that inhibit metabolism via cytochrome P4503A may have a profound effect on the clearance of alprazolam. Potent inhibitors of CYP3A would be expected to increase plasma alprazolam concentrations. Co-administration with very potent inhibitors of CYP3A should be avoided. Concurrent use of alprazolam with drugs inhibiting CYP3A to a lesser but still significant degree requires caution).
No products indexed under this heading.

Erythromycin Stearate (Possible interaction based on the clinical studies involving other benzodiazepines metabolized similarly as alprazolam; co-administration requires caution). Products include:
Erythrocin Stearate Filmtab Tablets 452

Esomeprazole Magnesium (Drugs that inhibit metabolism via cytochrome P4503A may have a profound effect on the clearance of alprazolam. Potent inhibitors of CYP3A would be expected to increase plasma alprazolam concentrations. Co-administration with very potent inhibitors of CYP3A should be avoided. Concurrent use of alprazolam with drugs inhibiting CYP3A to a lesser but still significant degree requires caution). Products include:
Nexium Delayed-Release Capsules 645

Estazolam (Additive CNS depressant effects). Products include:
ProSom Tablets 512

Ethanol (Additive CNS depressant effects).
No products indexed under this heading.

Ethchlorvynol (Additive CNS depressant effects).
No products indexed under this heading.

Ethinamate (Additive CNS depressant effects).
No products indexed under this heading.

Ethinyl Estradiol (Co-administration with oral contraceptives increased the maximum plasma concentration of alprazolam by 18%, decreased clearance by 22%, and increased half-life by 29%). Products include:
Alesse-28 Tablets 3392
Lo/Ovral-28 Tablets 3423
NuvaRing 2357
Ortho-Cept Tablets 2395
Ortho-Cyclen/Ortho Tri-Cyclen 2414
Ortho Evra Transdermal System 2402
Ortho Tri-Cyclen Lo Tablets 2421
Seasonale Tablets 1073
Triphasil-28 Tablets 3483
Yasmin 28 Tablets 818

Ethosuximide (Additive CNS depressant effects).
No products indexed under this heading.

Ethotoin (Additive CNS depressant effects). Products include:
Peganone Tablets, USP 2487

Ethyl Alcohol (Additive CNS depressant effects).
No products indexed under this heading.

Ethynodiol Diacetate (Co-administration with oral contraceptives increased the maximum plasma concentration of alprazolam by 18%, decreased clearance by 22%, and increased half-life by 29%).
No products indexed under this heading.

Felbamate (Additive CNS depressant effects).
No products indexed under this heading.

Fentanyl (Additive CNS depressant effects). Products include:
Duragesic Transdermal System **2448**

Fentanyl Citrate (Additive CNS depressant effects). Products include:
Actiq **993**

Fexofenadine Hydrochloride (Additive CNS depressant effects). Products include:
Allegra **2857**
Allegra-D 12 Hour Extended-Release Tablets **2860**
Allegra-D 24 Hour Extended-Release Tablets **2862**

Fluconazole (Azole-type antifungal agents are potent CYP3A inhibitors and have been shown to increase plasma alprazolam concentrations. Co-administration is not recommended).
No products indexed under this heading.

Fludrocortisone Acetate (CYP3A4 inducers would be expected to decrease alprazolam concentrations).
No products indexed under this heading.

Fluoxetine Hydrochloride (Co-administration of fluoxetine with alprazolam increased the maximum plasma concentration of alprazolam by 46%, decreased clearance by 21%, increased half-life by 17%, and decreased measured psychomotor performance; concurrent use requires caution). Products include:
Prozac Pulvules and Liquid **1771**
Symbyax Capsules **1788**

Fluphenazine Decanoate (Additive CNS depressant effects).
No products indexed under this heading.

Fluphenazine Enanthate (Additive CNS depressant effects).
No products indexed under this heading.

Fluphenazine Hydrochloride (Additive CNS depressant effects).
No products indexed under this heading.

Flurazepam Hydrochloride (Additive CNS depressant effects). Products include:
Dalmane Capsules **3343**

Fluvoxamine Maleate (Co-administration of fluvoxamine and alprazolam approximately doubled the maximum plasma concentration of alprazolam, decreased clearance by 49%, increased half-life by 71%, and decreased measured psychomotor performance).
No products indexed under this heading.

Fosamprenavir Calcium (Drugs that inhibit metabolism via cytochrome P4503A may have a profound effect on the clearance of alprazolam. Potent inhibitors of CYP3A would be expected to increase plasma alprazolam concentrations. Co-administration with very potent inhibitors of CYP3A should be avoided. Concurrent use of alprazolam with drugs inhibiting CYP3A to a lesser but still significant degree requires caution). Products include:
Lexiva Tablets **1473**

Fosphenytoin (Additive CNS depressant effects).
No products indexed under this heading.

Fosphenytoin Sodium (Additive CNS depressant effects).
No products indexed under this heading.

Gabapentin (Additive CNS depressant effects). Products include:
Neurontin Capsules **2498**
Neurontin Oral Solution **2498**
Neurontin Tablets **2498**

Garlic Extract (CYP3A4 inducers would be expected to decrease alprazolam concentrations).
No products indexed under this heading.

Garlic Oil (CYP3A4 inducers would be expected to decrease alprazolam concentrations).
No products indexed under this heading.

Glutethimide (Additive CNS depressant effects).
No products indexed under this heading.

Haloperidol (Additive CNS depressant effects).
No products indexed under this heading.

Haloperidol Decanoate (Additive CNS depressant effects).
No products indexed under this heading.

Hydrocodone Bitartrate (Additive CNS depressant effects). Products include:
Hycodan **1104**
Hycomine Compound Tablets **1105**
Hycotuss Expectorant Syrup **1106**
Lortab **3315**
Lortab Elixir **3312**
Vicodin Tablets **530**
Vicodin ES Tablets **531**
Vicodin HP Tablets **532**
Vicoprofen Tablets **533**
Zydone Tablets **1118**

Hydrocodone Polistirex (Additive CNS depressant effects). Products include:
Tussionex Pennkinetic Extended-Release Suspension **3322**

Hydrocortisone (CYP3A4 inducers would be expected to decrease alprazolam concentrations). Products include:
Cortizone•5 Ointment .... ▣**699**
Cortizone•10 Creme .... ▣**699**
Cortizone•10 Ointment .... ▣**699**
Cortizone•10 Plus Creme .... ▣**700**
Cortizone•10 Maximum Strength Quick Shot Spray .... ▣**700**
Hydrocortone Tablets **1963**
Preparation H Hydrocortisone Cream .... ▣**748**

Hydrocortisone Acetate (CYP3A4 inducers would be expected to decrease alprazolam concentrations). Products include:
Analpram-HC **1136**
Pramosone **1139**
ProctoFoam-HC **3113**
Tucks Anti-Itch Ointment .... ▣**712**
U-cort 1% Cream **3289**

Hydrocortisone Butyrate (CYP3A4 inducers would be expected to decrease alprazolam concentrations). Products include:
Locoid **1138**
Locoid Lipocream Cream **1138**

Hydrocortisone Cypionate (CYP3A4 inducers would be expected to decrease alprazolam concentrations).
No products indexed under this heading.

Hydrocortisone Hemisuccinate (CYP3A4 inducers would be expected to decrease alprazolam concentrations).
No products indexed under this heading.

Hydrocortisone Probutate (CYP3A4 inducers would be expected to decrease alprazolam concentrations). Products include:
Pandel Cream, 0.1% **1017**

Hydrocortisone Sodium Phosphate (CYP3A4 inducers would be expected to decrease alprazolam concentrations).
No products indexed under this heading.

Hydrocortisone Sodium Succinate (CYP3A4 inducers would be expected to decrease alprazolam concentrations).
No products indexed under this heading.

Hydrocortisone Valerate (CYP3A4 inducers would be expected to decrease alprazolam concentrations).
No products indexed under this heading.

Hydromorphone Hydrochloride (Additive CNS depressant effects). Products include:
Dilaudid **439**
Dilaudid Oral Liquid **443**
Dilaudid Non-Sterile Powder **439**
Dilaudid Rectal Suppositories **439**
Dilaudid Tablets **439**
Dilaudid Tablets - 8 mg **443**
Dilaudid-HP **441**

Hydroxyzine Hydrochloride (Additive CNS depressant effects).
No products indexed under this heading.

Hypericum (CYP3A4 inducers would be expected to decrease alprazolam concentrations).
No products indexed under this heading.

Hypericum Perforatum (CYP3A4 inducers would be expected to decrease alprazolam concentrations).
No products indexed under this heading.

Imipramine Hydrochloride (Concomitant administration of alprazolam and imipramine increased steady state plasma concentrations of imipramine by 31%).
No products indexed under this heading.

Imipramine Pamoate (Concomitant administration of alprazolam and imipramine increased steady state plasma concentrations of imipramine by 31%).
No products indexed under this heading.

Indinavir Sulfate (Drugs that inhibit metabolism via cytochrome P4503A may have a profound effect on the clearance of alprazolam. Potent inhibitors of CYP3A would be expected to increase plasma alprazolam concentrations. Co-administration with very potent inhibitors of CYP3A should be avoided. Concurrent use of alprazolam with drugs inhibiting CYP3A to a lesser but still significant degree requires caution). Products include:
Crixivan Capsules **1918**

Isoflurane (Additive CNS depressant effects).
No products indexed under this heading.

Isoniazid (Possible interaction based on the clinical studies involving other benzodiazepines metabolized similarly as alprazolam; co-administration requires caution).
No products indexed under this heading.

Itraconazole (Azole-type antifungal agents are potent CYP3A inhibitors and have been shown to increase plasma alprazolam concentrations. Co-administration is not recommended).
No products indexed under this heading.

Ketamine Hydrochloride (Additive CNS depressant effects).
No products indexed under this heading.

Ketoconazole (Azole-type antifungal agents are potent CYP3A inhibitors and have been shown to increase plasma alprazolam concentrations. Co-administration is not recommended). Products include:
Nizoral A-D Shampoo, 1% **1839**
Nizoral 2% Shampoo **1838**

Lamotrigine (Additive CNS depressant effects). Products include:
Lamictal **1449**

Levetiracetam (Additive CNS depressant effects). Products include:
Keppra Oral Solution **3307**
Keppra Tablets **3307**

Levomethadyl Acetate Hydrochloride (Additive CNS depressant effects).
No products indexed under this heading.

Levonorgestrel (Co-administration with oral contraceptives increased the maximum plasma concentration of alprazolam by 18%, decreased clearance by 22%, and increased half-life by 29%). Products include:
Alesse-28 Tablets **3392**
Climara Pro Transdermal System **800**
Mirena Intrauterine System **810**
Plan B Tablets **1068**
Seasonale Tablets **1073**
Triphasil-28 Tablets **3483**

Levorphanol Tartrate (Additive CNS depressant effects).
No products indexed under this heading.

Lopinavir (Drugs that inhibit metabolism via cytochrome P4503A may have a profound effect on the clearance of alprazolam. Potent inhibitors of CYP3A would be expected to increase plasma alprazolam concentrations. Co-administration with very potent inhibitors of CYP3A should be avoided. Concurrent use of alprazolam with drugs inhibiting CYP3A to a lesser but still significant degree requires caution). Products include:
Kaletra **474**

Loratadine (Additive CNS depressant effects). Products include:
Alavert Allergy & Sinus D-12 Hour Tablets .... ▣**743**
Alavert .... ▣**743**
Children's Claritin 24 Hour Non-Drowsy Allergy Syrup .... ▣**732**
Claritin Non-Drowsy 24 Hour Tablets .... ▣**731**
Non-Drowsy Claritin Hives Relief Tablets .... ▣**733**
Claritin Reditabs 24 Hour Non-Drowsy Tablets .... ▣**732**
Claritin-D Non-Drowsy 12 Hour Tablets .... ▣**731**
Claritin-D Non-Drowsy 24 Hour Tablets .... ▣**731**
Children's Dimetapp ND Non-Drowsy Allergy Syrup .... ▣**746**

Triaminic Allerchews .... ▣ 684

Lorazepam (Additive CNS depressant effects).
No products indexed under this heading.

Loxapine Hydrochloride (Additive CNS depressant effects).
No products indexed under this heading.

Loxapine Succinate (Additive CNS depressant effects).
No products indexed under this heading.

Meperidine Hydrochloride (Additive CNS depressant effects).
No products indexed under this heading.

Mephenytoin (Additive CNS depressant effects).
No products indexed under this heading.

Mephobarbital (Additive CNS depressant effects). Products include:
Mebaral Tablets, USP 2483

Meprobamate (Additive CNS depressant effects).
No products indexed under this heading.

Mesoridazine Besylate (Additive CNS depressant effects).
No products indexed under this heading.

Mestranol (Co-administration with oral contraceptives increased the maximum plasma concentration of alprazolam by 18%, decreased clearance by 22%, and increased half-life by 29%).
No products indexed under this heading.

Methadone Hydrochloride (Additive CNS depressant effects).
No products indexed under this heading.

Methdilazine Hydrochloride (Additive CNS depressant effects).
No products indexed under this heading.

Methohexital Sodium (Additive CNS depressant effects).
No products indexed under this heading.

Methotrimeprazine (Additive CNS depressant effects).
No products indexed under this heading.

Methoxyflurane (Additive CNS depressant effects).
No products indexed under this heading.

Methsuximide (Additive CNS depressant effects).
No products indexed under this heading.

Methylprednisolone (CYP3A4 inducers would be expected to decrease alprazolam concentrations).
No products indexed under this heading.

Methylprednisolone Acetate (CYP3A4 inducers would be expected to decrease alprazolam concentrations). Products include:
Depo-Medrol Injectable Suspension 2615
Depo-Medrol Single-Dose Vial 2617

Methylprednisolone Sodium Succinate (CYP3A4 inducers would be expected to decrease alprazolam concentrations).
No products indexed under this heading.

Metronidazole (Drugs that inhibit metabolism via cytochrome P4503A may have a profound effect on the clearance of alprazolam. Potent inhibitors of CYP3A would be expected to increase plasma alprazolam concentrations. Co-administration with very potent inhibitors of CYP3A should be avoided. Concurrent use of alprazolam with drugs inhibiting CYP3A to a lesser but still significant degree requires caution). Products include:
Metrogel 1% 1212
MetroGel-Vaginal Gel 1822
Noritate Cream, 1% 1051

Metronidazole Benzoate (Drugs that inhibit metabolism via cytochrome P4503A may have a profound effect on the clearance of alprazolam. Potent inhibitors of CYP3A would be expected to increase plasma alprazolam concentrations. Co-administration with very potent inhibitors of CYP3A should be avoided. Concurrent use of alprazolam with drugs inhibiting CYP3A to a lesser but still significant degree requires caution).
No products indexed under this heading.

Metronidazole Hydrochloride (Drugs that inhibit metabolism via cytochrome P4503A may have a profound effect on the clearance of alprazolam. Potent inhibitors of CYP3A would be expected to increase plasma alprazolam concentrations. Co-administration with very potent inhibitors of CYP3A should be avoided. Concurrent use of alprazolam with drugs inhibiting CYP3A to a lesser but still significant degree requires caution).
No products indexed under this heading.

Miconazole (Azole-type antifungal agents are potent CYP3A inhibitors and have been shown to increase plasma alprazolam concentrations. Co-administration is not recommended).
No products indexed under this heading.

Miconazole Nitrate (Drugs that inhibit metabolism via cytochrome P4503A may have a profound effect on the clearance of alprazolam. Potent inhibitors of CYP3A would be expected to increase plasma alprazolam concentrations. Co-administration with very potent inhibitors of CYP3A should be avoided. Concurrent use of alprazolam with drugs inhibiting CYP3A to a lesser but still significant degree requires caution). Products include:
Desenex .... ▣ 674
Desenex Jock Itch Spray Powder ... ▣ 674

Midazolam Hydrochloride (Additive CNS depressant effects).
No products indexed under this heading.

Modafinil (CYP3A4 inducers would be expected to decrease alprazolam concentrations). Products include:
Provigil Tablets 1002

Molindone Hydrochloride (Additive CNS depressant effects). Products include:
Moban Tablets 1108

Morphine Sulfate (Additive CNS depressant effects). Products include:
Avinza Capsules 1714
Kadian Capsules 572
MS Contin Tablets 2703

Nefazodone Hydrochloride (Co-administration of nefazodone and alprazolam increased alprazolam concentration two-fold).
No products indexed under this heading.

Nelfinavir Mesylate (Drugs that inhibit metabolism via cytochrome P4503A may have a profound effect on the clearance of alprazolam. Potent inhibitors of CYP3A would be expected to increase plasma alprazolam concentrations. Co-administration with very potent inhibitors of CYP3A should be avoided. Concurrent use of alprazolam with drugs inhibiting CYP3A to a lesser but still significant degree requires caution). Products include:
Viracept 2556

Nevirapine (Drugs that inhibit metabolism via cytochrome P4503A may have a profound effect on the clearance of alprazolam. Potent inhibitors of CYP3A would be expected to increase plasma alprazolam concentrations. Co-administration with very potent inhibitors of CYP3A should be avoided. Concurrent use of alprazolam with drugs inhibiting CYP3A to a lesser but still significant degree requires caution). Products include:
Viramune Oral Suspension 903
Viramune Tablets 903

Niacinamide (Drugs that inhibit metabolism via cytochrome P4503A may have a profound effect on the clearance of alprazolam. Potent inhibitors of CYP3A would be expected to increase plasma alprazolam concentrations. Co-administration with very potent inhibitors of CYP3A should be avoided. Concurrent use of alprazolam with drugs inhibiting CYP3A to a lesser but still significant degree requires caution).
No products indexed under this heading.

Nicardipine Hydrochloride (Data from in vitro studies of benzodiazepines other than alprazolam suggest a possible interaction when co-administered; concurrent use requires caution). Products include:
Cardene I.V. 1129

Nicotinamide (Drugs that inhibit metabolism via cytochrome P4503A may have a profound effect on the clearance of alprazolam. Potent inhibitors of CYP3A would be expected to increase plasma alprazolam concentrations. Co-administration with very potent inhibitors of CYP3A should be avoided. Concurrent use of alprazolam with drugs inhibiting CYP3A to a lesser but still significant degree requires caution). Products include:
Nicomide Tablets 3190

Nifedipine (Data from in vitro studies of benzodiazepines other than alprazolam suggest a possible interaction when co-administered; concurrent use requires caution). Products include:
Adalat CC Tablets 2978

Norethindrone (Co-administration with oral contraceptives increased the maximum plasma concentration of alprazolam by 18%, decreased clearance by 22%, and increased half-life by 29%). Products include:
Ortho Micronor Tablets 2411

Norethynodrel (Co-administration with oral contraceptives increased the maximum plasma concentration of alprazolam by 18%, decreased clearance by 22%, and increased half-life by 29%).
No products indexed under this heading.

Norfloxacin (Drugs that inhibit metabolism via cytochrome P4503A may have a profound effect on the clearance of alprazolam. Potent inhibitors of CYP3A would be expected to increase plasma alprazolam concentrations. Co-administration with very potent inhibitors of CYP3A should be avoided. Concurrent use of alprazolam with drugs inhibiting CYP3A to a lesser but still significant degree requires caution). Products include:
Noroxin Tablets 2009

Norgestimate (Co-administration with oral contraceptives increased the maximum plasma concentration of alprazolam by 18%, decreased clearance by 22%, and increased half-life by 29%). Products include:
Ortho-Cyclen/Ortho Tri-Cyclen 2414
Ortho Tri-Cyclen Lo Tablets 2421
Prefest Tablets 1069

Norgestrel (Co-administration with oral contraceptives increased the maximum plasma concentration of alprazolam by 18%, decreased clearance by 22%, and increased half-life by 29%). Products include:
Lo/Ovral-28 Tablets 3423

Olanzapine (Additive CNS depressant effects). Products include:
Symbyax Capsules 1788
Zyprexa Tablets 1798
Zyprexa IntraMuscular 1798
Zyprexa ZYDIS Orally Disintegrating Tablets 1798

Omeprazole (Drugs that inhibit metabolism via cytochrome P4503A may have a profound effect on the clearance of alprazolam. Potent inhibitors of CYP3A would be expected to increase plasma alprazolam concentrations. Co-administration with very potent inhibitors of CYP3A should be avoided. Concurrent use of alprazolam with drugs inhibiting CYP3A to a lesser but still significant degree requires caution). Products include:
Zegerid Powder for Oral Solution 2972

Oxazepam (Additive CNS depressant effects).
No products indexed under this heading.

Oxcarbazepine (Additive CNS depressant effects). Products include:
Trileptal Oral Suspension 2281
Trileptal Tablets 2281

Oxiconazole Nitrate (Azole-type antifungal agents are potent CYP3A inhibitors and have been shown to increase plasma alprazolam concentrations. Co-administration is not recommended). Products include:
Oxistat 1498

Oxycodone Hydrochloride (Additive CNS depressant effects). Products include:
Combunox Tablets 1183
OxyContin Tablets 2699
OxyFast Oral Concentrate Solution 2704
OxyIR Capsules 2704
Percocet Tablets 1114
Percodan Tablets 1115

Paramethadione (Additive CNS depressant effects).
No products indexed under this heading.

Paroxetine Hydrochloride (Possible interaction based on the data from in vitro studies of alprazolam; concurrent use requires caution). Products include:
Paxil CR Controlled-Release Tablets 1509
Paxil 1501

Pentobarbital Sodium (Additive CNS depressant effects). Products include:
Nembutal Sodium Solution, USP 2484

Perphenazine (Additive CNS depressant effects).
No products indexed under this heading.

Phenacemide (Additive CNS depressant effects).
No products indexed under this heading.

Phenobarbital (Additive CNS depressant effects).
No products indexed under this heading.

Phenobarbital Sodium (CYP3A4 inducers would be expected to decrease alprazolam concentrations).
No products indexed under this heading.

Phensuximide (Additive CNS depressant effects).
No products indexed under this heading.

Phenytoin (Additive CNS depressant effects).
No products indexed under this heading.

Phenytoin Sodium (Additive CNS depressant effects). Products include:
Phenytek Capsules 2153

Prazepam (Additive CNS depressant effects).
No products indexed under this heading.

Prednisolone Acetate (CYP3A4 inducers would be expected to decrease alprazolam concentrations). Products include:
Blephamide Ophthalmic Ointment 563
Blephamide Ophthalmic Suspension 564
Poly-Pred Liquifilm Ophthalmic Suspension .... ⊙ 231
Pred Forte Ophthalmic Suspension .... ⊙ 233
Pred Mild Sterile Ophthalmic Suspension .... ⊙ 236
Pred-G Ophthalmic Suspension ...... ⊙ 234
Pred-G Sterile Ophthalmic Ointment .... ⊙ 235

Prednisolone Sodium Phosphate (CYP3A4 inducers would be expected to decrease alprazolam concentrations). Products include:
Pediapred Oral Solution 3319

Prednisolone Tebutate (CYP3A4 inducers would be expected to decrease alprazolam concentrations).
No products indexed under this heading.

Prednisone (CYP3A4 inducers would be expected to decrease alprazolam concentrations).
No products indexed under this heading.

Primidone (Additive CNS depressant effects).
No products indexed under this heading.

Prochlorperazine (Additive CNS depressant effects).
No products indexed under this heading.

Promethazine Hydrochloride (Additive CNS depressant effects). Products include:
Phenergan 3438

Propofol (Additive CNS depressant effects). Products include:
Diprivan Injectable Emulsion 676

Propoxyphene Hydrochloride (Co-administration of propoxyphene with alprazolam decreased the maximum plasma concentration of alprazolam by 6%, decreased clearance by 38%, and increased half-life by 58%; concurrent use requires caution).
No products indexed under this heading.

Propoxyphene Napsylate (Co-administration of propoxyphene with alprazolam decreased the maximum plasma concentration of alprazolam by 6%, decreased clearance by 38%, and increased half-life by 58%; concurrent use requires caution). Products include:
Darvocet A 500 Tablets 3497

Pyrilamine Maleate (Additive CNS depressant effects).
No products indexed under this heading.

Pyrilamine Tannate (Additive CNS depressant effects).
No products indexed under this heading.

Quazepam (Additive CNS depressant effects).
No products indexed under this heading.

Quetiapine Fumarate (Additive CNS depressant effects). Products include:
Seroquel Tablets 691

Quinidine (Drugs that inhibit metabolism via cytochrome P4503A may have a profound effect on the clearance of alprazolam. Potent inhibitors of CYP3A would be expected to increase plasma alprazolam concentrations. Co-administration with very potent inhibitors of CYP3A should be avoided. Concurrent use of alprazolam with drugs inhibiting CYP3A to a lesser but still significant degree requires caution).
No products indexed under this heading.

Quinidine Hydrochloride (Drugs that inhibit metabolism via cytochrome P4503A may have a profound effect on the clearance of alprazolam. Potent inhibitors of CYP3A would be expected to increase plasma alprazolam concentrations. Co-administration with very potent inhibitors of CYP3A should be avoided. Concurrent use of alprazolam with drugs inhibiting CYP3A to a lesser but still significant degree requires caution).
No products indexed under this heading.

Quinidine Polygalacturonate (Drugs that inhibit metabolism via cytochrome P4503A may have a profound effect on the clearance of alprazolam. Potent inhibitors of CYP3A would be expected to increase plasma alprazolam concentrations. Co-administration with very potent inhibitors of CYP3A should be avoided. Concurrent use of alprazolam with drugs inhibiting CYP3A to a lesser but still significant degree requires caution).
No products indexed under this heading.

Quinidine Sulfate (Drugs that inhibit metabolism via cytochrome P4503A may have a profound effect on the clearance of alprazolam. Potent inhibitors of CYP3A would be expected to increase plasma alprazolam concentrations. Co-administration with very potent inhibitors of CYP3A should be avoided. Concurrent use of alprazolam with drugs inhibiting CYP3A to a lesser but still significant degree requires caution).
No products indexed under this heading.

Quinine (Drugs that inhibit metabolism via cytochrome P4503A may have a profound effect on the clearance of alprazolam. Potent inhibitors of CYP3A would be expected to increase plasma alprazolam concentrations. Co-administration with very potent inhibitors of CYP3A should be avoided. Concurrent use of alprazolam with drugs inhibiting CYP3A to a lesser but still significant degree requires caution).
No products indexed under this heading.

Quinine Sulfate (Drugs that inhibit metabolism via cytochrome P4503A may have a profound effect on the clearance of alprazolam. Potent inhibitors of CYP3A would be expected to increase plasma alprazolam concentrations. Co-administration with very potent inhibitors of CYP3A should be avoided. Concurrent use of alprazolam with drugs inhibiting CYP3A to a lesser but still significant degree requires caution).
No products indexed under this heading.

Quinupristin (Drugs that inhibit metabolism via cytochrome P4503A may have a profound effect on the clearance of alprazolam. Potent inhibitors of CYP3A would be expected to increase plasma alprazolam concentrations. Co-administration with very potent inhibitors of CYP3A should be avoided. Concurrent use of alprazolam with drugs inhibiting CYP3A to a lesser but still significant degree requires caution). Products include:
Synercid I.V. 1690

Ranitidine Bismuth Citrate (Drugs that inhibit metabolism via cytochrome P4503A may have a profound effect on the clearance of alprazolam. Potent inhibitors of CYP3A would be expected to increase plasma alprazolam concentrations. Co-administration with very potent inhibitors of CYP3A should be avoided. Concurrent use of alprazolam with drugs inhibiting CYP3A to a lesser but still significant degree requires caution).
No products indexed under this heading.

Ranitidine Hydrochloride (Drugs that inhibit metabolism via cytochrome P4503A may have a profound effect on the clearance of alprazolam. Potent inhibitors of CYP3A would be expected to increase plasma alprazolam concentrations. Co-administration with very potent inhibitors of CYP3A should be avoided. Concurrent use of alprazolam with drugs inhibiting CYP3A to a lesser but still significant degree requires caution). Products include:
Zantac 1597
Zantac Injection 1593
Zantac 75 Tablets .... ▣ 715
Zantac 150 Maximum Strength Tablets .... ▣ 715
Zantac Injection Pharmacy Bulk Package 1595

Remifentanil Hydrochloride (Additive CNS depressant effects).
No products indexed under this heading.

Rifabutin (CYP3A4 inducers would be expected to decrease alprazolam concentrations).
No products indexed under this heading.

Rifampicin (CYP3A4 inducers would be expected to decrease alprazolam concentrations).
No products indexed under this heading.

Rifampin (CYP3A4 inducers would be expected to decrease alprazolam concentrations).
No products indexed under this heading.

Rifapentine (CYP3A4 inducers would be expected to decrease alprazolam concentrations).
No products indexed under this heading.

Risperidone (Additive CNS depressant effects). Products include:
Risperdal Consta Long-Acting Injection 1664
Risperdal M-Tab Orally Disintegrating Tablets 1658
Risperdal 1658

Ritonavir (Drugs that inhibit metabolism via cytochrome P4503A may have a profound effect on the clearance of alprazolam. Potent inhibitors of CYP3A would be expected to increase plasma alprazolam concentrations. Co-administration with very potent inhibitors of CYP3A should be avoided. Concurrent use of alprazolam with drugs inhibiting CYP3A to a lesser but still significant degree requires caution). Products include:
Kaletra 474
Norvir 499

Saquinavir (Drugs that inhibit metabolism via cytochrome P4503A may have a profound effect on the clearance of alprazolam. Potent inhibitors of CYP3A would be expected to increase plasma alprazolam concentrations. Co-administration with very potent inhibitors of CYP3A should be avoided. Concurrent use of alprazolam with drugs inhibiting CYP3A to a lesser but still significant degree requires caution).
No products indexed under this heading.

Saquinavir Mesylate (Drugs that inhibit metabolism via cytochrome P4503A may have a profound effect on the clearance of alprazolam. Potent inhibitors of CYP3A would be expected to increase plasma alprazolam concentrations. Co-administration with very potent inhibitors of CYP3A should be avoided. Concurrent use of alprazolam with drugs inhibiting CYP3A to a lesser but still significant degree requires caution). Products include:
Invirase 2776

Secobarbital Sodium (Additive CNS depressant effects).
No products indexed under this heading.

Sertraline Hydrochloride (Possible interaction based on the data from in vitro studies of alprazolam; concurrent use requires caution). Products include:
- Zoloft ... **2581**

Sevoflurane (Additive CNS depressant effects). Products include:
- Ultane Liquid for Inhalation ... **526**

Sodium Oxybate (Additive CNS depressant effects).
- No products indexed under this heading.

Sufentanil Citrate (Additive CNS depressant effects).
- No products indexed under this heading.

Sulfinpyrazone (CYP3A4 inducers would be expected to decrease alprazolam concentrations).
- No products indexed under this heading.

Telithromycin (Drugs that inhibit metabolism via cytochrome P4503A may have a profound effect on the clearance of alprazolam. Potent inhibitors of CYP3A would be expected to increase plasma alprazolam concentrations. Co-administration with very potent inhibitors of CYP3A should be avoided. Concurrent use of alprazolam with drugs inhibiting CYP3A to a lesser but still significant degree requires caution). Products include:
- Ketek Tablets ... **2920**

Temazepam (Additive CNS depressant effects).
- No products indexed under this heading.

Terconazole (Azole-type antifungal agents are potent CYP3A inhibitors and have been shown to increase plasma alprazolam concentrations. Co-administration is not recommended).
- No products indexed under this heading.

Terfenadine (Additive CNS depressant effects).
- No products indexed under this heading.

Theophylline (CYP3A4 inducers would be expected to decrease alprazolam concentrations).
- No products indexed under this heading.

Thiamylal Sodium (Additive CNS depressant effects).
- No products indexed under this heading.

Thioridazine Hydrochloride (Additive CNS depressant effects). Products include:
- Thioridazine Hydrochloride Tablets ... **2122**

Thiothixene (Additive CNS depressant effects). Products include:
- Thiothixene Capsules ... **2124**

Tiagabine Hydrochloride (Additive CNS depressant effects). Products include:
- Gabitril Tablets ... **998**

Topiramate (Additive CNS depressant effects). Products include:
- Topamax Sprinkle Capsules ... **2438**
- Topamax Tablets ... **2438**

Triamcinolone (CYP3A4 inducers would be expected to decrease alprazolam concentrations).
- No products indexed under this heading.

Triamcinolone Acetonide (CYP3A4 inducers would be expected to decrease alprazolam concentrations). Products include:
- Azmacort Inhalation Aerosol ... **1701**
- Nasacort HFA Inhalation Aerosol ... **2939**
- Nasacort AQ Nasal Spray ... **2937**

Triamcinolone Diacetate (CYP3A4 inducers would be expected to decrease alprazolam concentrations).
- No products indexed under this heading.

Triamcinolone Hexacetonide (CYP3A4 inducers would be expected to decrease alprazolam concentrations).
- No products indexed under this heading.

Triazolam (Additive CNS depressant effects).
- No products indexed under this heading.

Trifluoperazine Hydrochloride (Additive CNS depressant effects).
- No products indexed under this heading.

Trimeprazine Tartrate (Additive CNS depressant effects).
- No products indexed under this heading.

Trimethadione (Additive CNS depressant effects).
- No products indexed under this heading.

Tripelennamine Hydrochloride (Additive CNS depressant effects).
- No products indexed under this heading.

Triprolidine Hydrochloride (Additive CNS depressant effects).
- No products indexed under this heading.

Troglitazone (Drugs that inhibit metabolism via cytochrome P4503A may have a profound effect on the clearance of alprazolam. Potent inhibitors of CYP3A would be expected to increase plasma alprazolam concentrations. Co-administration with very potent inhibitors of CYP3A should be avoided. Concurrent use of alprazolam with drugs inhibiting CYP3A to a lesser but still significant degree requires caution).
- No products indexed under this heading.

Troleandomycin (Possible interaction based on the clinical studies involving other benzodiazepines metabolized similarly as alprazolam; co-administration requires caution).
- No products indexed under this heading.

Valproate Sodium (Additive CNS depressant effects). Products include:
- Depacon Injection ... **412**

Valproic Acid (Additive CNS depressant effects). Products include:
- Depakene ... **417**

Verapamil Hydrochloride (Drugs that inhibit metabolism via cytochrome P4503A may have a profound effect on the clearance of alprazolam. Potent inhibitors of CYP3A would be expected to increase plasma alprazolam concentrations. Co-administration with very potent inhibitors of CYP3A should be avoided. Concurrent use of alprazolam with drugs inhibiting CYP3A to a lesser but still significant degree requires caution). Products include:
- Covera-HS Tablets ... **3135**
- Tarka Tablets ... **519**
- Verelan PM Capsules ... **3120**

Voriconazole (Drugs that inhibit metabolism via cytochrome P4503A may have a profound effect on the clearance of alprazolam. Potent inhibitors of CYP3A would be expected to increase plasma alprazolam concentrations. Co-administration with very potent inhibitors of CYP3A should be avoided. Concurrent use of alprazolam with drugs inhibiting CYP3A to a lesser but still significant degree requires caution). Products include:
- VFEND I.V. ... **2543**
- VFEND Oral Suspension ... **2543**
- VFEND Tablets ... **2543**

Zafirlukast (Drugs that inhibit metabolism via cytochrome P4503A may have a profound effect on the clearance of alprazolam. Potent inhibitors of CYP3A would be expected to increase plasma alprazolam concentrations. Co-administration with very potent inhibitors of CYP3A should be avoided. Concurrent use of alprazolam with drugs inhibiting CYP3A to a lesser but still significant degree requires caution). Products include:
- Accolate Tablets ... **663**

Zaleplon (Additive CNS depressant effects). Products include:
- Sonata Capsules ... **1686**

Zileuton (Drugs that inhibit metabolism via cytochrome P4503A may have a profound effect on the clearance of alprazolam. Potent inhibitors of CYP3A would be expected to increase plasma alprazolam concentrations. Co-administration with very potent inhibitors of CYP3A should be avoided. Concurrent use of alprazolam with drugs inhibiting CYP3A to a lesser but still significant degree requires caution).
- No products indexed under this heading.

Ziprasidone Hydrochloride (Additive CNS depressant effects). Products include:
- Geodon Capsules ... **2514**

Zolpidem Tartrate (Additive CNS depressant effects). Products include:
- Ambien Tablets ... **2867**

Zonisamide (Additive CNS depressant effects). Products include:
- Zonegran Capsules ... **1089**

Food Interactions

Alcohol (Additive CNS depressant effects).

Food, unspecified (Food has a significant influence on the bioavailability of Xanax XR. A high fat meal given up to 2 hours before dosing with Xanax XR increased the mean Cmax and the effect of this meal on Tmax depended on the timing of this meal).

Grapefruit (Drugs that inhibit metabolism via cytochrome P4503A may have a profound effect on the clearance of alprazolam. Potent inhibitors of CYP3A would be expected to increase plasma alprazolam concentrations. Co-administration with very potent inhibitors of CYP3A should be avoided. Concurrent use of alprazolam with drugs inhibiting CYP3A to a lesser but still significant degree requires caution).

Grapefruit Juice (Possible interaction based on the clinical studies involving other benzodiazepines metabolized similarly as alprazolam; concurrent use requires caution).

XELODA TABLETS

(Capecitabine) ... **2825**

May interact with oral anticoagulants, phenytoin, and certain other agents. Compounds in these categories include:

Aluminum Hydroxide (Co-administration of capecitabine with aluminum hydroxide- and magnesium hydroxide-containing antacids has resulted in a small increase in plasma concentrations of capecitabine and one metabolite (5'DFCR)). Products include:
- Gaviscon Regular Strength Liquid ... **620**
- Gaviscon Regular Strength Tablets ... **619**
- Gaviscon Extra Strength Liquid ... **620**
- Gaviscon Extra Strength Tablets ... **619**
- Maalox Max Maximum Strength Antacid/Anti-Gas Liquid ... **2165**
- Maalox Regular Strength Antacid/Antigas Liquid ... **2164**

Anisindione (Co-administration has resulted in altered coagulation parameters and/or bleeding). Products include:
- Miradon Tablets ... **3056**

Dicumarol (Co-administration has resulted in altered coagulation parameters and/or bleeding).
- No products indexed under this heading.

Fosphenytoin Sodium (Co-administration has resulted in toxicity associated with elevated phenytoin levels).
- No products indexed under this heading.

Leucovorin Calcium (The concentrations of 5-fluorouracil, capecitabine is a prodrug and it is converted to 5-FU, is increased and its toxicity may be enhanced by leucovorin; deaths from severe enterocolitis, diarrhea, and dehydration have been reported in elderly patients receiving fluorouracil and leucovorin).
- No products indexed under this heading.

Magnesium Hydroxide (Co-administration of capecitabine with aluminum hydroxide- and magnesium hydroxide-containing antacids has resulted in a small increase in plasma concentrations of capecitabine and one metabolite (5'DFCR)). Products include:
- Maalox Max Maximum Strength Antacid/Anti-Gas Liquid ... **2165**
- Maalox Regular Strength Antacid/Antigas Liquid ... **2164**
- Pepcid Complete Chewable Tablets ... **1672**
- Rolaids Tablets ... **707**
- Extra Strength Rolaids Tablets ... **707**
- Rolaids Multi-Symptom Antacid & Antigas Tablets ... **708**

Phenytoin (Co-administration has resulted in toxicity associated with elevated phenytoin levels).
- No products indexed under this heading.

Phenytoin Sodium (Co-administration has resulted in toxicity associated with elevated phenytoin levels). Products include:
- Phenytek Capsules ... **2153**

Warfarin Sodium (Co-administration has resulted in altered coagulation parameters and/or bleeding). Products include:
- Coumadin for Injection ... **932**
- Coumadin Tablets ... **932**

Food Interactions

Food, unspecified (Reduces both rate and extent of absorption of capecitabine and delays Tmax of both parent and 5-FU).

XENADERM OINTMENT

(Balsam Peru, Castor Oil, Trypsin) **1638**
None cited in PDR database.

XENICAL CAPSULES

(Orlistat) **2834**
May interact with:

Beta-Carotene (Orlistat has been shown to reduce the absorption of some fat soluble vitamins; the vitamin supplement should be taken once a day at least 2 hours before or after the administration of orlistat).
No products indexed under this heading.

Cyclosporine (Co-administration has resulted in reduction in cyclosporine plasma levels; concurrent use is not recommended; if used concurrently, cyclosporine should be taken at least 2 hours before or after Xenical). Products include:
Gengraf Capsules **458**
Neoral Soft Gelatin Capsules **2247**
Neoral Oral Solution **2247**
Restasis Ophthalmic Emulsion **570**
Sandimmune **2259**

Pravastatin Sodium (Co-administration results in additive lipid lowering effect of pravastatin; modest increases in pravastatin plasma concentrations were observed during co-administration). Products include:
Pravachol Tablets **943**

Vitamin A (Orlistat has been shown to reduce the absorption of some fat soluble vitamins; the vitamin supplement should be taken once a day at least 2 hours before or after the administration of orlistat). Products include:
Visutein Capsules **3328**

Vitamin D (Orlistat has been shown to reduce the absorption of some fat soluble vitamins; the vitamin supplement should be taken once a day at least 2 hours before or after the administration of orlistat). Products include:
Active Calcium Tablets **3342**
Caltrate 600 PLUS Chewables .... ▣ **779**
Caltrate 600 PLUS Tablets .... ▣ **779**
Caltrate 600 + D Tablets .... ▣ **779**
Os-Cal 250 + D Tablets .... ▣ **765**
Os-Cal 500 + D Tablets .... ▣ **766**

Vitamin E (Orlistat has been shown to reduce the absorption of some fat soluble vitamins; the vitamin supplement should be taken once a day at least 2 hours before or after the administration of orlistat). Products include:
MarineOmega Softgel Capsules **2669**
Unique E Vitamin E Concentrate Capsules .... ▣ **602**

Vitamin K_1 (Absorption of vitamin K may be decreased). Products include:
AquaMEPHYTON Injection **1887**
Mephyton Tablets **1993**

Warfarin Sodium (Vitamin K absorption may be decreased with orlistat; patients on chronic stable doses of warfarin who are prescribed orlistat should be monitored closely for changes in coagulation parameters). Products include:
Coumadin for Injection **932**
Coumadin Tablets **932**

Food Interactions

Food, unspecified (Gastrointestinal events may increase when orlistat is taken with a diet high in fat).

XERAC AC SOLUTION

(Aluminum Chloride) **2507**
None cited in PDR database.

XIFAXAN TABLETS

(Rifaximin) **2847**
None cited in PDR database.

XIGRIS POWDER FOR INTRAVENOUS INFUSION

(Drotrecogin alfa (activated)) **1796**
May interact with oral anticoagulants, glycoprotein (GP) IIb/IIIa inhibitors, platelet inhibitors, thrombolytics, and certain other agents. Compounds in these categories include:

Abciximab (Bleeding is the most common serious adverse effect associated with drotrecogin alfa therapy; recent administration (within 7 days) of glycoprotein IIb/IIIa therapy increases the risk of bleeding). Products include:
ReoPro Vials **1779**

Alteplase (Bleeding is the most common serious adverse effect associated with drotrecogin alfa therapy; recent administration (within 3 days) of thrombolytic therapy increases the risk of bleeding). Products include:
Activase I.V. **1225**
Cathflo Activase **1232**

Anisindione (Bleeding is the most common serious adverse effect associated with drotrecogin alfa therapy; recent administration (within 7 days) of oral anticoagulant therapy increases the risk of bleeding). Products include:
Miradon Tablets **3056**

Anistreplase (Bleeding is the most common serious adverse effect associated with drotrecogin alfa therapy; recent administration (within 3 days) of thrombolytic therapy increases the risk of bleeding).
No products indexed under this heading.

Aspirin (Bleeding is the most common serious adverse effect associated with drotrecogin alfa therapy; recent administration (within 7 days) of more than 650mg per day of aspirin or other platelet inhibitors increases the risk of bleeding). Products include:
Aggrenox Capsules **855**
Bayer, Aspirin Regimen .... ▣ **606**
Bayer Aspirin Tablets **3515**
BC Powder .... ▣ **612**
BC Allergy Sinus Cold Powder .... ▣ **612**
Arthritis Strength BC Powder .... ▣ **612**
BC Sinus Cold Powder .... ▣ **612**
Ecotrin Enteric Coated Aspirin Low, Regular and Maximum Strength Tablets **1627**
Goody's Body Pain Formula Powder .... ▣ **621**
Goody's Extra Strength Headache Powder .... ▣ **621**
Goody's Extra Strength Pain Relief Tablets .... ▣ **621**
Percodan Tablets **1115**
St. Joseph 81 mg Aspirin Chewable and Enteric Coated Tablets **1841**

Aspirin, Enteric Coated (Bleeding is the most common serious adverse effect associated with drotrecogin alfa therapy; recent administration (within 7 days) of more than 650mg per day of aspirin or other platelet inhibitors increases the risk of bleeding).
No products indexed under this heading.

Aspirin Buffered (Bleeding is the most common serious adverse effect associated with drotrecogin alfa therapy; recent administration (within 7 days) of more than 650mg per day of aspirin or other platelet inhibitors increases the risk of bleeding).
No products indexed under this heading.

Azlocillin Sodium (Bleeding is the most common serious adverse effect associated with drotrecogin alfa therapy; recent administration (within 7 days) of more than 650mg per day of aspirin or other platelet inhibitors increases the risk of bleeding).
No products indexed under this heading.

Carbenicillin Indanyl Sodium (Bleeding is the most common serious adverse effect associated with drotrecogin alfa therapy; recent administration (within 7 days) of more than 650mg per day of aspirin or other platelet inhibitors increases the risk of bleeding).
No products indexed under this heading.

Choline Magnesium Trisalicylate (Bleeding is the most common serious adverse effect associated with drotrecogin alfa therapy; recent administration (within 7 days) of more than 650mg per day of aspirin or other platelet inhibitors increases the risk of bleeding).
No products indexed under this heading.

Clopidogrel Bisulfate (Bleeding is the most common serious adverse effect associated with drotrecogin alfa therapy; recent administration (within 7 days) of more than 650mg per day of aspirin or other platelet inhibitors increases the risk of bleeding). Products include:
Plavix Tablets **940**
Plavix Tablets **2942**

Diclofenac Potassium (Bleeding is the most common serious adverse effect associated with drotrecogin alfa therapy; recent administration (within 7 days) of more than 650mg per day of aspirin or other platelet inhibitors increases the risk of bleeding). Products include:
Cataflam Tablets **2173**

Diclofenac Sodium (Bleeding is the most common serious adverse effect associated with drotrecogin alfa therapy; recent administration (within 7 days) of more than 650mg per day of aspirin or other platelet inhibitors increases the risk of bleeding). Products include:
Arthrotec Tablets **3126**
Voltaren Ophthalmic Solution **2300**
Voltaren Tablets **2298**
Voltaren-XR Tablets **2301**

Dicumarol (Bleeding is the most common serious adverse effect associated with drotrecogin alfa therapy; recent administration (within 7 days) of oral anticoagulant therapy increases the risk of bleeding).
No products indexed under this heading.

Diflunisal (Bleeding is the most common serious adverse effect associated with drotrecogin alfa therapy; recent administration (within 7 days) of more than 650mg per day of aspirin or other platelet inhibitors increases the risk of bleeding). Products include:
Dolobid Tablets **1937**

Dipyridamole (Bleeding is the most common serious adverse effect associated with drotrecogin alfa therapy; recent administration (within 7 days) of more than 650mg per day of aspirin or other platelet inhibitors increases the risk of bleeding). Products include:
Aggrenox Capsules **855**
Persantine Tablets **898**

Eptifibatide (Bleeding is the most common serious adverse effect associated with drotrecogin alfa therapy; recent administration (within 7 days) of glycoprotein IIb/IIIa therapy increases the risk of bleeding). Products include:
Integrilin Injection **3034**

Fenoprofen Calcium (Bleeding is the most common serious adverse effect associated with drotrecogin alfa therapy; recent administration (within 7 days) of more than 650mg per day of aspirin or other platelet inhibitors increases the risk of bleeding). Products include:
Nalfon Capsules **2504**

Flurbiprofen (Bleeding is the most common serious adverse effect associated with drotrecogin alfa therapy; recent administration (within 7 days) of more than 650mg per day of aspirin or other platelet inhibitors increases the risk of bleeding).
No products indexed under this heading.

Heparin Sodium (Bleeding is the most common serious adverse effect associated with drotrecogin alfa therapy; concurrent therapeutic dosing of heparin used to treat an active thrombotic or embolic event increases the risk of bleeding; low dose heparin does not appear to affect safety).
No products indexed under this heading.

Ibuprofen (Bleeding is the most common serious adverse effect associated with drotrecogin alfa therapy; recent administration (within 7 days) of more than 650mg per day of aspirin or other platelet inhibitors increases the risk of bleeding). Products include:
Advil Allergy Sinus Caplets .... ▣ **737**
Advil .... ▣ **737**
Children's Advil Suspension .... ▣ **742**
Children's Advil Chewable Tablets .. ▣ **741**
Advil Cold & Sinus .... ▣ **739**
Advil Flu & Body Ache Caplets .... ▣ **739**
Children's Advil Cold Suspension ... ▣ **741**
Infants' Advil Concentrated Drops .. ▣ **743**
Junior Strength Advil Swallow Tablets .... ▣ **740**
Advil Migraine Liquigels .... ▣ **740**
Advil Multi-Symptom Cold Caplets .... ▣ **738**
Combunox Tablets **1183**
Children's Motrin Oral Suspension and Chewable Tablets **1837**

Children's Motrin Cold Non-Staining Dye-Free Oral Suspension 1838
Children's Motrin Cold Oral Suspension 1838
Children's Motrin Non-Staining Dye-Free Oral Suspension 1837
Motrin Cold & Sinus Caplets 1836
Motrin IB Tablets and Caplets 1836
Infants' Motrin Concentrated Drops 1837
Infants' Motrin Non-Staining Dye-Free Drops 1837
Junior Strength Motrin Caplets and Chewable Tablets 1837
Vicoprofen Tablets 533

Indomethacin (Bleeding is the most common serious adverse effect associated with drotrecogin alfa therapy; recent administration (within 7 days) of more than 650mg per day of aspirin or other platelet inhibitors increases the risk of bleeding). Products include:
Indocin 1968

Indomethacin Sodium Trihydrate (Bleeding is the most common serious adverse effect associated with drotrecogin alfa therapy; recent administration (within 7 days) of more than 650mg per day of aspirin or other platelet inhibitors increases the risk of bleeding). Products include:
Indocin I.V. 1973

Ketoprofen (Bleeding is the most common serious adverse effect associated with drotrecogin alfa therapy; recent administration (within 7 days) of more than 650mg per day of aspirin or other platelet inhibitors increases the risk of bleeding).
No products indexed under this heading.

Magnesium Salicylate (Bleeding is the most common serious adverse effect associated with drotrecogin alfa therapy; recent administration (within 7 days) of more than 650mg per day of aspirin or other platelet inhibitors increases the risk of bleeding).
No products indexed under this heading.

Meclofenamate Sodium (Bleeding is the most common serious adverse effect associated with drotrecogin alfa therapy; recent administration (within 7 days) of more than 650mg per day of aspirin or other platelet inhibitors increases the risk of bleeding).
No products indexed under this heading.

Mefenamic Acid (Bleeding is the most common serious adverse effect associated with drotrecogin alfa therapy; recent administration (within 7 days) of more than 650mg per day of aspirin or other platelet inhibitors increases the risk of bleeding).
No products indexed under this heading.

Mezlocillin Sodium (Bleeding is the most common serious adverse effect associated with drotrecogin alfa therapy; recent administration (within 7 days) of more than 650mg per day of aspirin or other platelet inhibitors increases the risk of bleeding).
No products indexed under this heading.

Nafcillin Sodium (Bleeding is the most common serious adverse effect associated with drotrecogin alfa therapy; recent administration (within 7 days) of more than 650mg per day of aspirin or other platelet inhibitors increases the risk of bleeding).
No products indexed under this heading.

Naproxen (Bleeding is the most common serious adverse effect associated with drotrecogin alfa therapy; recent administration (within 7 days) of more than 650mg per day of aspirin or other platelet inhibitors increases the risk of bleeding). Products include:
EC-Naprosyn Delayed-Release Tablets 2769
Naprosyn Suspension 2769
Naprosyn Tablets 2769
Prevacid NapraPAC 3277

Naproxen Sodium (Bleeding is the most common serious adverse effect associated with drotrecogin alfa therapy; recent administration (within 7 days) of more than 650mg per day of aspirin or other platelet inhibitors increases the risk of bleeding). Products include:
Aleve Tablets, Caplets and Gelcaps 605
Anaprox Tablets 2769
Anaprox DS Tablets 2769

Penicillin G Benzathine (Bleeding is the most common serious adverse effect associated with drotrecogin alfa therapy; recent administration (within 7 days) of more than 650mg per day of aspirin or other platelet inhibitors increases the risk of bleeding).
No products indexed under this heading.

Penicillin G Procaine (Bleeding is the most common serious adverse effect associated with drotrecogin alfa therapy; recent administration (within 7 days) of more than 650mg per day of aspirin or other platelet inhibitors increases the risk of bleeding).
No products indexed under this heading.

Phenylbutazone (Bleeding is the most common serious adverse effect associated with drotrecogin alfa therapy; recent administration (within 7 days) of more than 650mg per day of aspirin or other platelet inhibitors increases the risk of bleeding).
No products indexed under this heading.

Piroxicam (Bleeding is the most common serious adverse effect associated with drotrecogin alfa therapy; recent administration (within 7 days) of more than 650mg per day of aspirin or other platelet inhibitors increases the risk of bleeding).
No products indexed under this heading.

Reteplase (Bleeding is the most common serious adverse effect associated with drotrecogin alfa therapy; recent administration (within 3 days) of thrombolytic therapy increases the risk of bleeding). Products include:
Retavase 1131

Salsalate (Bleeding is the most common serious adverse effect associated with drotrecogin alfa therapy; recent administration (within 7 days) of more than 650mg per day of aspirin or other platelet inhibitors increases the risk of bleeding).
No products indexed under this heading.

Streptokinase (Bleeding is the most common serious adverse effect associated with drotrecogin alfa therapy; recent administration (within 3 days) of thrombolytic therapy increases the risk of bleeding).
No products indexed under this heading.

Sulindac (Bleeding is the most common serious adverse effect associated with drotrecogin alfa therapy; recent administration (within 7 days) of more than 650mg per day of aspirin or other platelet inhibitors increases the risk of bleeding). Products include:
Clinoril Tablets 1899

Ticarcillin Disodium (Bleeding is the most common serious adverse effect associated with drotrecogin alfa therapy; recent administration (within 7 days) of more than 650mg per day of aspirin or other platelet inhibitors increases the risk of bleeding). Products include:
Timentin ADD-Vantage 1556
Timentin Injection Galaxy Container 1559
Timentin IV Infusion 1553
Timentin Pharmacy Bulk Package 1562

Ticlopidine Hydrochloride (Bleeding is the most common serious adverse effect associated with drotrecogin alfa therapy; recent administration (within 7 days) of more than 650mg per day of aspirin or other platelet inhibitors increases the risk of bleeding). Products include:
Ticlid Tablets 2813

Tirofiban Hydrochloride (Bleeding is the most common serious adverse effect associated with drotrecogin alfa therapy; recent administration (within 7 days) of glycoprotein IIb/IIIa therapy increases the risk of bleeding). Products include:
Aggrastat 1878

Tolmetin Sodium (Bleeding is the most common serious adverse effect associated with drotrecogin alfa therapy; recent administration (within 7 days) of more than 650mg per day of aspirin or other platelet inhibitors increases the risk of bleeding).
No products indexed under this heading.

Urokinase (Bleeding is the most common serious adverse effect associated with drotrecogin alfa therapy; recent administration (within 3 days) of thrombolytic therapy increases the risk of bleeding).
No products indexed under this heading.

Warfarin Sodium (Bleeding is the most common serious adverse effect associated with drotrecogin alfa therapy; recent administration (within 7 days) of oral anticoagulant therapy increases the risk of bleeding). Products include:
Coumadin for Injection 932
Coumadin Tablets 932

XOLAIR
(Omalizumab) 1259
None cited in PDR database.

XOPENEX HFA INHALATION AEROSOL
(Levalbuterol Tartrate) 3151
See Xopenex Inhalation Solution

XOPENEX INHALATION SOLUTION
(Levalbuterol Hydrochloride) 3143
May interact with beta blockers, monoamine oxidase inhibitors, potassium-depleting diuretics, sympathomimetic aerosol bronchodilators, tricyclic antidepressants, and certain other agents. Compounds in these categories include:

Acebutolol Hydrochloride (Beta-adrenergic receptor blocking agents block the pulmonary effect of beta agonist and may produce severe bronchospasm in asthmatic patients).
No products indexed under this heading.

Albuterol (Potential for deleterious cardiovascular effects with concomitant use). Products include:
Proventil Inhalation Aerosol 3067

Amitriptyline Hydrochloride (Action of levalbuterol on the vascular system may be potentiated).
No products indexed under this heading.

Amoxapine (Action of levalbuterol on the vascular system may be potentiated).
No products indexed under this heading.

Atenolol (Beta-adrenergic receptor blocking agents block the pulmonary effect of beta agonist and may produce severe bronchospasm in asthmatic patients). Products include:
Tenormin I.V. Injection 698
Tenormin Tablets 695

Bendroflumethiazide (The ECG changes and/or hypokalemia that may result from the administration of non-potassium sparing diuretics can be acutely worsened by beta-agonists).
No products indexed under this heading.

Betaxolol Hydrochloride (Beta-adrenergic receptor blocking agents block the pulmonary effect of beta agonist and may produce severe bronchospasm in asthmatic patients). Products include:
Betoptic S Ophthalmic Suspension 554

Bisoprolol Fumarate (Beta-adrenergic receptor blocking agents block the pulmonary effect of beta agonist and may produce severe bronchospasm in asthmatic patients).
No products indexed under this heading.

Bitolterol Mesylate (Potential for deleterious cardiovascular effects with concomitant use).
No products indexed under this heading.

Bumetanide (The ECG changes and/or hypokalemia that may result from the administration of non-potassium sparing diuretics can be acutely worsened by beta-agonists).
No products indexed under this heading.

Carteolol Hydrochloride (Beta-adrenergic receptor blocking agents block the pulmonary effect of beta

agonist and may produce severe bronchospasm in asthmatic patients). Products include:

Carteolol Hydrochloride Ophthalmic Solution USP, 1%....... ⊙ 246

Chlorothiazide (The ECG changes and/or hypokalemia that may result from the administration of non-potassium sparing diuretics can be acutely worsened by beta-agonists). Products include:

Aldoclor Tablets 1881
Diuril Oral 1936

Chlorothiazide Sodium (The ECG changes and/or hypokalemia that may result from the administration of non-potassium sparing diuretics can be acutely worsened by beta-agonists). Products include:

Diuril Sodium Intravenous 1934

Clomipramine Hydrochloride (Action of levalbuterol on the vascular system may be potentiated).

No products indexed under this heading.

Desipramine Hydrochloride (Action of levalbuterol on the vascular system may be potentiated).

No products indexed under this heading.

Digoxin (Mean decreases of 16% and 22% in serum digoxin levels were demonstrated after the single-dose intravenous and oral administration of racemic albuterol, respectively; clinical significance of this finding is unclear). Products include:

Digitek Tablets 2146
Lanoxicaps Capsules 1458
Lanoxin Injection 1462
Lanoxin Tablets 1468
Lanoxin Injection Pediatric 1465

Doxepin Hydrochloride (Action of levalbuterol on the vascular system may be potentiated).

No products indexed under this heading.

Esmolol Hydrochloride (Beta-adrenergic receptor blocking agents block the pulmonary effect of beta agonist and may produce severe bronchospasm in asthmatic patients). Products include:

Brevibloc Concentrate 766
Brevibloc Injection 766
Brevibloc Double Strength Injection 766
Brevibloc Premixed Injection 766
Brevibloc Double Strength Premixed Injection 766

Ethacrynic Acid (The ECG changes and/or hypokalemia that may result from the administration of non-potassium sparing diuretics can be acutely worsened by beta-agonists). Products include:

Edecrin Tablets 1941

Furosemide (The ECG changes and/or hypokalemia that may result from the administration of non-potassium sparing diuretics can be acutely worsened by beta-agonists). Products include:

Furosemide Tablets 2117

Hydrochlorothiazide (The ECG changes and/or hypokalemia that may result from the administration of non-potassium sparing diuretics can be acutely worsened by beta-agonists). Products include:

Aldoril Tablets 1884
Atacand HCT 637
Avalide Tablets 2889
Avalide Tablets 922
Benicar HCT Tablets 2852
Diovan HCT Tablets 2195
Dyazide Capsules 1389
Hyzaar 1964
Lotensin HCT Tablets 2235
Maxzide 2150
Micardis HCT Tablets 886
Moduretic Tablets 2003
Prinzide Tablets 2033
Teveten HCT Tablets 1710
Timolide Tablets 2056
Uniretic Tablets 3114
Vaseretic Tablets 2073
Zestoretic Tablets 701

Hydroflumethiazide (The ECG changes and/or hypokalemia that may result from the administration of non-potassium sparing diuretics can be acutely worsened by beta-agonists).

No products indexed under this heading.

Imipramine Hydrochloride (Action of levalbuterol on the vascular system may be potentiated).

No products indexed under this heading.

Imipramine Pamoate (Action of levalbuterol on the vascular system may be potentiated).

No products indexed under this heading.

Isocarboxazid (Action of levalbuterol on the vascular system may be potentiated).

No products indexed under this heading.

Isoetharine (Potential for deleterious cardiovascular effects with concomitant use).

No products indexed under this heading.

Isoproterenol Hydrochloride (Potential for deleterious cardiovascular effects with concomitant use).

No products indexed under this heading.

Labetalol Hydrochloride (Beta-adrenergic receptor blocking agents block the pulmonary effect of beta agonist and may produce severe bronchospasm in asthmatic patients).

No products indexed under this heading.

Levobunolol Hydrochloride (Beta-adrenergic receptor blocking agents block the pulmonary effect of beta agonist and may produce severe bronchospasm in asthmatic patients). Products include:

Betagan Ophthalmic Solution, USP.......... ⊙ 217

Maprotiline Hydrochloride (Action of levalbuterol on the vascular system may be potentiated).

No products indexed under this heading.

Metaproterenol Sulfate (Potential for deleterious cardiovascular effects with concomitant use). Products include:

Alupent Inhalation Aerosol 858

Methyclothiazide (The ECG changes and/or hypokalemia that may result from the administration of non-potassium sparing diuretics can be acutely worsened by beta-agonists).

No products indexed under this heading.

Metipranolol Hydrochloride (Beta-adrenergic receptor blocking agents block the pulmonary effect of beta agonist and may produce severe bronchospasm in asthmatic patients).

No products indexed under this heading.

Metoprolol Succinate (Beta-adrenergic receptor blocking agents block the pulmonary effect of beta agonist and may produce severe bronchospasm in asthmatic patients). Products include:

Toprol-XL Tablets 660

Metoprolol Tartrate (Beta-adrenergic receptor blocking agents block the pulmonary effect of beta agonist and may produce severe bronchospasm in asthmatic patients).

No products indexed under this heading.

Moclobemide (Action of levalbuterol on the vascular system may be potentiated).

No products indexed under this heading.

Nadolol (Beta-adrenergic receptor blocking agents block the pulmonary effect of beta agonist and may produce severe bronchospasm in asthmatic patients). Products include:

Nadolol Tablets 2121

Nortriptyline Hydrochloride (Action of levalbuterol on the vascular system may be potentiated).

No products indexed under this heading.

Pargyline Hydrochloride (Action of levalbuterol on the vascular system may be potentiated).

No products indexed under this heading.

Penbutolol Sulfate (Beta-adrenergic receptor blocking agents block the pulmonary effect of beta agonist and may produce severe bronchospasm in asthmatic patients).

No products indexed under this heading.

Phenelzine Sulfate (Action of levalbuterol on the vascular system may be potentiated).

No products indexed under this heading.

Pindolol (Beta-adrenergic receptor blocking agents block the pulmonary effect of beta agonist and may produce severe bronchospasm in asthmatic patients).

No products indexed under this heading.

Pirbuterol Acetate (Potential for deleterious cardiovascular effects with concomitant use). Products include:

Maxair Autohaler 1820

Polythiazide (The ECG changes and/or hypokalemia that may result from the administration of non-potassium sparing diuretics can be acutely worsened by beta-agonists).

No products indexed under this heading.

Procarbazine Hydrochloride (Action of levalbuterol on the vascular system may be potentiated). Products include:

Matulane Capsules 3188

Propranolol Hydrochloride (Beta-adrenergic receptor blocking agents block the pulmonary effect of beta agonist and may produce severe bronchospasm in asthmatic patients). Products include:

Inderal LA Long-Acting Capsules 3421
InnoPran XL Capsules 2728

Protriptyline Hydrochloride (Action of levalbuterol on the vascular system may be potentiated). Products include:

Vivactil Tablets 2350

Salmeterol Xinafoate (Potential for deleterious cardiovascular effects with concomitant use). Products include:

Advair Diskus 100/50 1291
Advair Diskus 250/50 1291
Advair Diskus 500/50 1291
Serevent Diskus 1540

Selegiline Hydrochloride (Action of levalbuterol on the vascular system may be potentiated). Products include:

Eldepryl Capsules 3209

Sotalol Hydrochloride (Beta-adrenergic receptor blocking agents block the pulmonary effect of beta agonist and may produce severe bronchospasm in asthmatic patients).

No products indexed under this heading.

Terbutaline Sulfate (Potential for deleterious cardiovascular effects with concomitant use).

No products indexed under this heading.

Timolol Hemihydrate (Beta-adrenergic receptor blocking agents block the pulmonary effect of beta agonist and may produce severe bronchospasm in asthmatic patients). Products include:

Betimol Ophthalmic Solution 3371
Betimol Ophthalmic Solution .... ⊙ 283

Timolol Maleate (Beta-adrenergic receptor blocking agents block the pulmonary effect of beta agonist and may produce severe bronchospasm in asthmatic patients). Products include:

Blocadren Tablets 1891
Cosopt Sterile Ophthalmic Solution 1910
Timolide Tablets 2056
Timoptic in Ocudose 2061
Timoptic Sterile Ophthalmic Solution 2058
Timoptic-XE Sterile Ophthalmic Gel Forming Solution 2062

Torsemide (The ECG changes and/or hypokalemia that may result from the administration of non-potassium sparing diuretics can be acutely worsened by beta-agonists).

No products indexed under this heading.

Tranylcypromine Sulfate (Action of levalbuterol on the vascular system may be potentiated). Products include:

Parnate Tablets 1499

Trimipramine Maleate (Action of levalbuterol on the vascular system may be potentiated). Products include:

Surmontil Capsules 2347

XOPENEX INHALATION SOLUTION CONCENTRATE

(Levalbuterol Hydrochloride) 3147

See Xopenex Inhalation Solution

YASMIN 28 TABLETS

(Drospirenone, Ethinyl Estradiol) 818

May interact with ACE inhibitors, aldosterone-inhibiting diuretic agents, angiotensin-II receptor antagonists, non-steroidal anti-inflammatory agents, phenytoin, prednisolone, potassium sparing diuretics, tetracyclines, xanthines, and certain other agents. Compounds in these categories include:

Acetaminophen (May increase plasma levels of ethinyl estradiol possibly by inhibition of conjugation; co-administration may decrease plasma concentrations of acetaminophen). Products include:

Benadryl Allergy & Cold Tablets .... ▣ 692
Benadryl Allergy & Sinus Headache Caplets & Gelcaps .... ▣ 693

Benadryl Maximum Strength Severe Allergy & Sinus Headache Caplets ... 694
Contac Severe Cold and Flu Caplets Maximum Strength ... 615
Contac Severe Cold and Flu Caplets Non-Drowsy ... 615
Darvocet A 500 Tablets ... 3497
Goody's Body Pain Formula Powder ... 621
Goody's Extra Strength Headache Powder ... 621
Goody's Extra Strength Pain Relief Tablets ... 621
Goody's PM Powder ... 622
Hycomine Compound Tablets ... 1105
Lortab ... 3315
Lortab Elixir ... 3312
Percocet Tablets ... 1114
Robitussin Cough, Cold & Flu Liquid-filled Capsules ... 750
Robitussin Flu Liquid ... 752
Sedapap Tablets 50 mg/650 mg ... 2098
Singlet Caplets ... 636
Sudafed Severe Cold ... 710
Sudafed Sinus Headache ... 711
TheraFlu Cold & Cough Hot Liquid ... 680
TheraFlu Cold & Sore Throat Hot Liquid ... 680
TheraFlu Flu & Chest Congestion Non-Drowsy Hot Liquid ... 681
TheraFlu Flu & Sore Throat Hot Liquid ... 681
TheraFlu Severe Cold Non-Drowsy Hot Liquid ... 683
TheraFlu Severe Cold & Cough Hot Liquid ... 683
TheraFlu Severe Cold Caplets ... 679
TheraFlu Severe Cold Hot Liquid ... 682
TheraFlu Severe Cold Non-Drowsy Caplets ... 679
Triaminic Cough & Sore Throat Liquid ... 687
Triaminic Flu, Cough & Fever Liquid ... 685
Triaminic Cough & Sore Throat Softchews ... 689
Tylenol 8 Hour Extended Release Geltabs and Caplets ... 1843
Tylenol Sinus NightTime Caplets ... 663
Children's Tylenol Suspension Liquid and Meltaways ... 1850
Children's Tylenol Plus Cold & Allergy Suspension Liquid ... 1850
Children's Tylenol Plus Cold NightTime Suspension Liquid ... 1851
Children's Tylenol Plus Cold & Cough Suspension Liquid and Chewable Tablets ... 1851
Children's Tylenol Plus Cold Chewable Tablets ... 1851
Children's Tylenol Plus Cold Daytime Non-Drowsy Suspension Liquid ... 1851
Children's Tylenol Plus Flu Suspension Liquid ... 1853
Concentrated Tylenol Infants' Drops Plus Cold ... 1851
Concentrated Tylenol Infants' Drops Plus Cold and Cough ... 1851
Concentrated Tylenol Infants' Drops ... 1850
Junior Tylenol Meltaways ... 1850
Tylenol Cold & Flu Severe Daytime Liquid with Cool Bust ... 1846
Tylenol Cold & Flu Severe NightTime Liquid with Cool Burst ... 1846
Tylenol Cold Severe Congestion Non-Drowsy Caplets with Cool Burst ... 1846
Tylenol Cough & Sore Throat Daytime Liquid with Cool Burst ... 1849
Tylenol Cough & Sore Throat NightTime Liquid with Cool Burst ... 1849
Tylenol ... 1843
Extra Strength Tylenol Rapid Release Gels ... 1843
Tylenol ... 1843
Tylenol Allergy Complete Night Time Caplets ... 1844
Tylenol Allergy Complete Multi-Symptom Caplets and Gelcaps with Cool Burst ... 1844
Tylenol Severe Allergy Caplets ... 1844
Tylenol Flu NightTime Gelcaps ... 1846
Tylenol Flu Day Non-Drowsy Gelcaps ... 1846
Concentrated Tylenol Infants' Drops Plus Cold Nasal Congestant, Fever Reducer & Pain Reliever ... 668
Concentrated Tylenol Infants' Drops Plus Cold & Cough Nasal Decongestant, Fever Reducer & Pain Reliever ... 668
Multi-Symptom Tylenol Cold Night Time Caplets ... 1845
Multi-Symptom Tylenol Cold Day Non-Drowsy Caplets and Gelcaps ... 1845
Extra Strength Tylenol PM Caplets, Geltabs, Gelcaps and Liquid ... 1847
Tylenol Sinus Day Non-Drowsy ... 1848
Tylenol Sinus Night Time Caplets ... 1848
Tylenol Sinus Severe Congestion Caplets with Cool Burst ... 1848
Tylenol Sore Throat Daytime Liquid with Cool Burst ... 1849
Tylenol Sore Throat NightTime Liquid with Cool Burst ... 1849
Tylenol with Codeine ... 2461
Women's Tylenol Menstrual Relief Caplets ... 1849
Ultracet Tablets ... 2462
Vicks 44M Cough, Cold & Flu Relief ... 2676
Vicks DayQuil LiquiCaps/Liquid Multi-Symptom Cold/Flu Relief ... 723
Vicks DayQuil Multi-Symptom Cold/Flu Relief LiquiCaps ... 2675
Vicks DayQuil Multi-Symptom Cold/Flu Relief Liquid ... 2675
Vicks NyQuil LiquiCaps ... 2677
Vicks NyQuil LiquiCaps/Liquid Multi-Symptom Cold/Flu Relief ... 725
Vicks NyQuil Liquid ... 2677
Vicodin Tablets ... 530
Vicodin ES Tablets ... 531
Vicodin HP Tablets ... 532
Zydone Tablets ... 1118

Amiloride Hydrochloride (Yasmin has the potential to cause hyperkalemia in high-risk patients; co-administration with other drugs that have the potential to increase serum potassium, such as potassium-sparing diuretics, may increase this risk further). Products include:
Midamor Tablets ... 2000
Moduretic Tablets ... 2003

Aminophylline (Co-administration of products containing ethinyl estradiol may inhibit the metabolism of other compounds, such as theophylline, resulting in increased plasma concentrations of theophylline).
No products indexed under this heading.

Ampicillin (Pregnancy while taking oral contraceptives has been reported when oral contraceptives were administered with ampicillin; clinical pharmacokinetic studies have not demonstrated any consistent effect of antibiotics (other than rifampin) on plasma concentrations of synthetic steroids).
No products indexed under this heading.

Ampicillin Sodium (Pregnancy while taking oral contraceptives has been reported when oral contraceptives were administered with ampicillin; clinical pharmacokinetic studies have not demonstrated any consistent effect of antibiotics (other than rifampin) on plasma concentrations of synthetic steroids).
No products indexed under this heading.

Atorvastatin Calcium (Co-administration of atorvastatin and an oral contraceptive increased AUC values for ethinyl estradiol by approximately 20%). Products include:
Caduet Tablets ... 2507
Lipitor Tablets ... 2495

Benazepril Hydrochloride (Yasmin has the potential to cause hyperkalemia in high-risk patients; co-administration with other drugs that have the potential to increase serum potassium, such as ACE inhibitors, may increase this risk further). Products include:
Lotensin Tablets ... 2232
Lotensin HCT Tablets ... 2235
Lotrel Capsules ... 2238

Candesartan Cilexetil (Yasmin has the potential to cause hyperkalemia in high-risk patients; co-administration with other drugs that have the potential to increase serum potassium, such as angiotensin-II receptor antagonists, may increase this risk further). Products include:
Atacand Tablets ... 634
Atacand HCT ... 637

Captopril (Yasmin has the potential to cause hyperkalemia in high-risk patients; co-administration with other drugs that have the potential to increase serum potassium, such as ACE inhibitors, may increase this risk further). Products include:
Captopril Tablets ... 2114

Carbamazepine (Co-administration results in increased metabolism of ethinyl estradiol and/or some progestins which could result in a reduction of contraceptive effectiveness). Products include:
Carbatrol Capsules ... 3174
Equetro Extended-Release Capsules ... 3178
Tegretol/Tegretol-XR ... 2278

Celecoxib (Yasmin has the potential to cause hyperkalemia in high-risk patients; co-administration with other drugs that have the potential to increase serum potassium, such as NSAIDs, may increase this risk further). Products include:
Celebrex Capsules ... 3130

Clofibrate (Co-administration of products containing ethinyl estradiol may increase clearance of clofibric acid).
No products indexed under this heading.

Cyclosporine (Co-administration of products containing ethinyl estradiol may inhibit the metabolism of other compounds, such as cyclosporine, resulting in increased plasma concentrations of cyclosporine).
Products include:
Gengraf Capsules ... 458
Neoral Soft Gelatin Capsules ... 2247
Neoral Oral Solution ... 2247
Restasis Ophthalmic Emulsion ... 570
Sandimmune ... 2259

Demeclocycline Hydrochloride (Pregnancy while taking oral contraceptives has been reported when oral contraceptives were administered with tetracyclines; clinical pharmacokinetic studies have not demonstrated any consistent effect of antibiotics (other than rifampin) on plasma concentrations of synthetic steroids).
No products indexed under this heading.

Diclofenac Potassium (Yasmin has the potential to cause hyperkalemia in high-risk patients; co-administration with other drugs that have the potential to increase serum potassium, such as NSAIDs, may increase this risk further). Products include:
Cataflam Tablets ... 2173

Diclofenac Sodium (Yasmin has the potential to cause hyperkalemia in high-risk patients; co-administration with other drugs that have the potential to increase serum potassium, such as NSAIDs, may increase this risk further). Products include:
Arthrotec Tablets ... 3126
Voltaren Ophthalmic Solution ... 2300
Voltaren Tablets ... 2298
Voltaren-XR Tablets ... 2301

Doxycycline Calcium (Pregnancy while taking oral contraceptives has been reported when oral contraceptives were administered with tetracyclines; clinical pharmacokinetic studies have not demonstrated any consistent effect of antibiotics (other than rifampin) on plasma concentrations of synthetic steroids).
No products indexed under this heading.

Doxycycline Hyclate (Pregnancy while taking oral contraceptives has been reported when oral contraceptives were administered with tetracyclines; clinical pharmacokinetic studies have not demonstrated any consistent effect of antibiotics (other than rifampin) on plasma concentrations of synthetic steroids).
No products indexed under this heading.

Doxycycline Monohydrate (Pregnancy while taking oral contraceptives has been reported when oral contraceptives were administered with tetracyclines; clinical pharmacokinetic studies have not demonstrated any consistent effect of antibiotics (other than rifampin) on plasma concentrations of synthetic steroids).
No products indexed under this heading.

Dyphylline (Co-administration of products containing ethinyl estradiol may inhibit the metabolism of other compounds, such as theophylline, resulting in increased plasma concentrations of theophylline).
No products indexed under this heading.

Enalapril Maleate (Yasmin has the potential to cause hyperkalemia in high-risk patients; co-administration with other drugs that have the potential to increase serum potassium, such as ACE inhibitors, may increase this risk further). Products include:
Vaseretic Tablets ... 2073
Vasotec I.V. Injection ... 2076

Enalaprilat (Yasmin has the potential to cause hyperkalemia in high-risk patients; co-administration with other drugs that have the potential to increase serum potassium, such as ACE inhibitors, may increase this risk further).
No products indexed under this heading.

Eprosartan Mesylate (Yasmin has the potential to cause hyperkalemia in high-risk patients; co-administration with other drugs that have the potential to increase serum potassium, such as angiotensin-II receptor antagonists, may increase this risk further). Products include:
Teveten Tablets ... 1707
Teveten HCT Tablets ... 1710

Etodolac (Yasmin has the potential to cause hyperkalemia in high-risk patients; co-administration with other drugs that have the potential to increase serum potassium, such as NSAIDs, may increase this risk further).
No products indexed under this heading.

Fenoprofen Calcium (Yasmin has the potential to cause hyperkalemia in high-risk patients; co-administration with other drugs that have the potential to increase serum potassium, such as NSAIDs, may increase this risk further). Products include:
Nalfon Capsules 2504

Flurbiprofen (Yasmin has the potential to cause hyperkalemia in high-risk patients; co-administration with other drugs that have the potential to increase serum potassium, such as NSAIDs, may increase this risk further).
No products indexed under this heading.

Fosinopril Sodium (Yasmin has the potential to cause hyperkalemia in high-risk patients; co-administration with other drugs that have the potential to increase serum potassium, such as ACE inhibitors, may increase this risk further).
No products indexed under this heading.

Fosphenytoin Sodium (Co-administration results in increased metabolism of ethinyl estradiol and/or some progestins which could result in a reduction of contraceptive effectiveness).
No products indexed under this heading.

Griseofulvin (Pregnancy while taking oral contraceptives has been reported when oral contraceptives were administered with griseofulvin; clinical pharmacokinetic studies have not demonstrated any consistent effect of antibiotics (other than rifampin) on plasma concentrations of synthetic steroids). Products include:
Grifulvin V Tablets Microsize and Oral Suspension Microsize 2384
Gris-PEG Tablets 2504

Heparin Sodium (Yasmin has the potential to cause hyperkalemia in high-risk patients; co-administration with other drugs that have the potential to increase serum potassium, such as heparin, may increase this risk further).
No products indexed under this heading.

Hypericum (Herbal products containing St. John's Wort may induce hepatic enzyme and p-glycoprotein transport and may reduce the effectiveness of oral contraceptives and emergency contraceptive pills; potential for breakthrough bleeding).
No products indexed under this heading.

Ibuprofen (Yasmin has the potential to cause hyperkalemia in high-risk patients; co-administration with other drugs that have the potential to increase serum potassium, such as NSAIDs, may increase this risk further). Products include:
Advil Allergy Sinus Caplets .... ▣737
Advil .... ▣737
Children's Advil Suspension .... ▣742
Children's Advil Chewable Tablets .... ▣741
Advil Cold & Sinus .... ▣739
Advil Flu & Body Ache Caplets .... ▣739
Children's Advil Cold Suspension .... ▣741
Infants' Advil Concentrated Drops .... ▣743
Junior Strength Advil Swallow Tablets .... ▣740
Advil Migraine Liquigels .... ▣740
Advil Multi-Symptom Cold Caplets .... ▣738
Combunox Tablets 1183
Children's Motrin Oral Suspension and Chewable Tablets 1837
Children's Motrin Cold Non-Staining Dye-Free Oral Suspension 1838
Children's Motrin Cold Oral Suspension 1838
Children's Motrin Non-Staining Dye-Free Oral Suspension 1837
Motrin Cold & Sinus Caplets 1836
Motrin IB Tablets and Caplets 1836
Infants' Motrin Concentrated Drops 1837
Infants' Motrin Non-Staining Dye-Free Drops 1837
Junior Strength Motrin Caplets and Chewable Tablets 1837
Vicoprofen Tablets 533

Indomethacin (Yasmin has the potential to cause hyperkalemia in high-risk patients; co-administration with other drugs that have the potential to increase serum potassium, such as NSAIDs, may increase this risk further). Products include:
Indocin 1968

Indomethacin Sodium Trihydrate (Yasmin has the potential to cause hyperkalemia in high-risk patients; co-administration with other drugs that have the potential to increase serum potassium, such as NSAIDs, may increase this risk further). Products include:
Indocin I.V. 1973

Irbesartan (Yasmin has the potential to cause hyperkalemia in high-risk patients; co-administration with other drugs that have the potential to increase serum potassium, such as angiotensin-II receptor antagonists, may increase this risk further). Products include:
Avalide Tablets 922
Avalide Tablets 2889
Avapro Tablets 925
Avapro Tablets 2886

Ketoprofen (Yasmin has the potential to cause hyperkalemia in high-risk patients; co-administration with other drugs that have the potential to increase serum potassium, such as NSAIDs, may increase this risk further).
No products indexed under this heading.

Ketorolac Tromethamine (Yasmin has the potential to cause hyperkalemia in high-risk patients; co-administration with other drugs that have the potential to increase serum potassium, such as NSAIDs, may increase this risk further). Products include:
Acular Ophthalmic Solution 561
Acular LS Ophthalmic Solution 562

Lisinopril (Yasmin has the potential to cause hyperkalemia in high-risk patients; co-administration with other drugs that have the potential to increase serum potassium, such as ACE inhibitors, may increase this risk further). Products include:
Prinivil Tablets 2029
Prinzide Tablets 2033
Zestoretic Tablets 701
Zestril Tablets 704

Losartan Potassium (Yasmin has the potential to cause hyperkalemia in high-risk patients; co-administration with other drugs that have the potential to increase serum potassium, such as angiotensin-II receptor antagonists, may increase this risk further). Products include:
Cozaar Tablets 1913
Hyzaar 1964

Meclofenamate Sodium (Yasmin has the potential to cause hyperkalemia in high-risk patients; co-administration with other drugs that have the potential to increase serum potassium, such as NSAIDs, may increase this risk further).
No products indexed under this heading.

Mefenamic Acid (Yasmin has the potential to cause hyperkalemia in high-risk patients; co-administration with other drugs that have the potential to increase serum potassium, such as NSAIDs, may increase this risk further).
No products indexed under this heading.

Meloxicam (Yasmin has the potential to cause hyperkalemia in high-risk patients; co-administration with other drugs that have the potential to increase serum potassium, such as NSAIDs, may increase this risk further). Products include:
Mobic Oral Suspension 893
Mobic Tablets 893

Methacycline Hydrochloride (Pregnancy while taking oral contraceptives has been reported when oral contraceptives were administered with tetracyclines; clinical pharmacokinetic studies have not demonstrated any consistent effect of antibiotics (other than rifampin) on plasma concentrations of synthetic steroids).
No products indexed under this heading.

Minocycline Hydrochloride (Pregnancy while taking oral contraceptives has been reported when oral contraceptives were administered with tetracyclines; clinical pharmacokinetic studies have not demonstrated any consistent effect of antibiotics (other than rifampin) on plasma concentrations of synthetic steroids). Products include:
Dynacin Tablets 1859

Moexipril Hydrochloride (Yasmin has the potential to cause hyperkalemia in high-risk patients; co-administration with other drugs that have the potential to increase serum potassium, such as ACE inhibitors, may increase this risk further). Products include:
Uniretic Tablets 3114
Univasc Tablets 3118

Morphine Sulfate (Co-administration of products containing ethinyl estradiol may increase clearance of morphine). Products include:
Avinza Capsules 1714
Kadian Capsules 572
MS Contin Tablets 2703

Nabumetone (Yasmin has the potential to cause hyperkalemia in high-risk patients; co-administration with other drugs that have the potential to increase serum potassium, such as NSAIDs, may increase this risk further). Products include:
Relafen Tablets 1523

Naproxen (Yasmin has the potential to cause hyperkalemia in high-risk patients; co-administration with other drugs that have the potential to increase serum potassium, such as NSAIDs, may increase this risk further). Products include:
EC-Naprosyn Delayed-Release Tablets 2769
Naprosyn Suspension 2769
Naprosyn Tablets 2769
Prevacid NapraPAC 3277

Naproxen Sodium (Yasmin has the potential to cause hyperkalemia in high-risk patients; co-administration with other drugs that have the potential to increase serum potassium, such as NSAIDs, may increase this risk further). Products include:
Aleve Tablets, Caplets and Gelcaps .... ▣605
Anaprox Tablets 2769
Anaprox DS Tablets 2769

Oxaprozin (Yasmin has the potential to cause hyperkalemia in high-risk patients; co-administration with other drugs that have the potential to increase serum potassium, such as NSAIDs, may increase this risk further).
No products indexed under this heading.

Oxytetracycline Hydrochloride (Pregnancy while taking oral contraceptives has been reported when oral contraceptives were administered with tetracyclines; clinical pharmacokinetic studies have not demonstrated any consistent effect of antibiotics (other than rifampin) on plasma concentrations of synthetic steroids).
No products indexed under this heading.

Perindopril Erbumine (Yasmin has the potential to cause hyperkalemia in high-risk patients; co-administration with other drugs that have the potential to increase serum potassium, such as ACE inhibitors, may increase this risk further). Products include:
Aceon Tablets (2 mg, 4 mg, 8 mg) 3191

Phenobarbital (Co-administration results in increased metabolism of ethinyl estradiol and/or some progestins which could result in a reduction of contraceptive effectiveness).
No products indexed under this heading.

Phenylbutazone (A reduction in contraceptive effectiveness and an increased incidence of menstrual irregularities has been suggested with phenylbutazone).
No products indexed under this heading.

Phenytoin (Co-administration results in increased metabolism of ethinyl estradiol and/or some progestins which could result in a reduction of contraceptive effectiveness).
No products indexed under this heading.

Phenytoin Sodium (Co-administration results in increased metabolism of ethinyl estradiol and/or some progestins which could result in a reduction of contraceptive effectiveness). Products include:
Phenytek Capsules 2153

Piroxicam (Yasmin has the potential to cause hyperkalemia in high-risk patients; co-administration with other drugs that have the potential to increase serum potassium, such as NSAIDs, may increase this risk further).
No products indexed under this heading.

Prednisolone (Co-administration of products containing ethinyl estradiol may inhibit the metabolism of other compounds, such as prednisolone, resulting in increased plasma concentrations of prednisolone).
No products indexed under this heading.

Prednisolone Acetate (Co-administration of products containing ethinyl estradiol may inhibit the metabolism of other compounds, such as prednisolone, resulting in increased plasma concentrations of prednisolone). Products include:
Blephamide Ophthalmic Ointment 563
Blephamide Ophthalmic Suspension 564
Poly-Pred Liquifilm Ophthalmic Suspension .... ⊙231
Pred Forte Ophthalmic Suspension .... ⊙233
Pred Mild Sterile Ophthalmic Suspension .... ⊙236
Pred-G Ophthalmic Suspension ...... ⊙234
Pred-G Sterile Ophthalmic Ointment .... ⊙235

Prednisolone Sodium Phosphate (Co-administration of products containing ethinyl estradiol may inhibit the metabolism of other compounds, such as prednisolone, resulting in increased plasma concentrations of prednisolone). Products include:
Pediapred Oral Solution 3319

Prednisolone Tebutate (Co-administration of products containing ethinyl estradiol may inhibit the metabolism of other compounds, such as prednisolone, resulting in increased plasma concentrations of prednisolone).
No products indexed under this heading.

Quinapril Hydrochloride (Yasmin has the potential to cause hyperkalemia in high-risk patients; co-administration with other drugs that have the potential to increase serum potassium, such as ACE inhibitors, may increase this risk further).
No products indexed under this heading.

Ramipril (Yasmin has the potential to cause hyperkalemia in high-risk patients; co-administration with other drugs that have the potential to increase serum potassium, such as ACE inhibitors, may increase this risk further). Products include:
Altace Capsules 1673

Rifampin (Co-administration results in increased metabolism of ethinyl estradiol precipitating a reduction in contraceptive effectiveness and an increase in menstrual irregularities).
No products indexed under this heading.

Rofecoxib (Yasmin has the potential to cause hyperkalemia in high-risk patients; co-administration with other drugs that have the potential to increase serum potassium, such as NSAIDs, may increase this risk further).
No products indexed under this heading.

Salicylic Acid (Co-administration of products containing ethinyl estradiol may increase clearance of salicylic acid).
No products indexed under this heading.

Spirapril Hydrochloride (Yasmin has the potential to cause hyperkalemia in high-risk patients; co-administration with other drugs that have the potential to increase serum potassium, such as ACE inhibitors, may increase this risk further).
No products indexed under this heading.

Spironolactone (Yasmin has the potential to cause hyperkalemia in high-risk patients; co-administration with other drugs that have the potential to increase serum potassium, such as potassium-sparing diuretics, may increase this risk further).
No products indexed under this heading.

Sulindac (Yasmin has the potential to cause hyperkalemia in high-risk patients; co-administration with other drugs that have the potential to increase serum potassium, such as NSAIDs, may increase this risk further). Products include:
Clinoril Tablets 1899

Telmisartan (Yasmin has the potential to cause hyperkalemia in high-risk patients; co-administration with other drugs that have the potential to increase serum potassium, such as angiotensin-II receptor antagonists, may increase this risk further). Products include:
Micardis Tablets 884
Micardis HCT Tablets 886

Temazepam (Co-administration of products containing ethinyl estradiol may increase clearance of temazepam).
No products indexed under this heading.

Tetracycline Hydrochloride (Pregnancy while taking oral contraceptives has been reported when oral contraceptives were administered with tetracyclines; clinical pharmacokinetic studies have not demonstrated any consistent effect of antibiotics (other than rifampin) on plasma concentrations of synthetic steroids).
No products indexed under this heading.

Theophylline (Co-administration of products containing ethinyl estradiol may inhibit the metabolism of other compounds, such as theophylline, resulting in increased plasma concentrations of theophylline).
No products indexed under this heading.

Theophylline Anhydrous (Co-administration of products containing ethinyl estradiol may inhibit the metabolism of other compounds, such as theophylline, resulting in increased plasma concentrations of theophylline). Products include:
Uniphyl Tablets 2708

Theophylline Calcium Salicylate (Co-administration of products containing ethinyl estradiol may inhibit the metabolism of other compounds, such as theophylline, resulting in increased plasma concentrations of theophylline).
No products indexed under this heading.

Theophylline Dihydroxypropyl (Glyceryl) (Co-administration of products containing ethinyl estradiol may inhibit the metabolism of other compounds, such as theophylline, resulting in increased plasma concentrations of theophylline).
No products indexed under this heading.

Theophylline Ethylenediamine (Co-administration of products containing ethinyl estradiol may inhibit the metabolism of other compounds, such as theophylline, resulting in increased plasma concentrations of theophylline).
No products indexed under this heading.

Theophylline Sodium Glycinate (Co-administration of products containing ethinyl estradiol may inhibit the metabolism of other compounds, such as theophylline, resulting in increased plasma concentrations of theophylline).
No products indexed under this heading.

Tolmetin Sodium (Yasmin has the potential to cause hyperkalemia in high-risk patients; co-administration with other drugs that have the potential to increase serum potassium, such as NSAIDs, may increase this risk further).
No products indexed under this heading.

Trandolapril (Yasmin has the potential to cause hyperkalemia in high-risk patients; co-administration with other drugs that have the potential to increase serum potassium, such as ACE inhibitors, may increase this risk further). Products include:
Mavik Tablets 482
Tarka Tablets 519

Triamterene (Yasmin has the potential to cause hyperkalemia in high-risk patients; co-administration with other drugs that have the potential to increase serum potassium, such as potassium-sparing diuretics, may increase this risk further). Products include:
Dyazide Capsules 1389
Dyrenium Capsules 3390
Maxzide 2150

Valdecoxib (Yasmin has the potential to cause hyperkalemia in high-risk patients; co-administration with other drugs that have the potential to increase serum potassium, such as NSAIDs, may increase this risk further).
No products indexed under this heading.

Valsartan (Yasmin has the potential to cause hyperkalemia in high-risk patients; co-administration with other drugs that have the potential to increase serum potassium, such as angiotensin-II receptor antagonists, may increase this risk further). Products include:
Diovan HCT Tablets 2195
Diovan Tablets 2191

Vitamin C (May increase plasma levels of ethinyl estradiol possibly by inhibition of conjugation). Products include:
Chromagen Forte Soft Gelatin Capsules 3296
Halls Defense Sugarfree Vitamin C Drops .... ▣611
Niferex-150 Forte Capsules 3299
Peridin-C Tablets .... ▣761
Repliva 21/7 Tablets 3301

ZADITOR OPHTHALMIC SOLUTION
(Ketotifen Fumarate) 2302
None cited in PDR database.

ZANTAC 150 TABLETS
(Ranitidine Hydrochloride) 1597
May interact with:

Triazolam (Ranitidine, similar to other agents that lower gastric acidity, has been shown to increase the absorption of triazolam resulting in increased plasma concentrations on average 14% to 28%; the clinical significance of this finding is unknown).
No products indexed under this heading.

Warfarin Sodium (Potential for increased or decreased prothrombin time; doses of ranitidine up to 400 mg per day had no effect on prothrombin time or warfarin clearance). Products include:
Coumadin for Injection 932
Coumadin Tablets 932

ZANTAC 300 TABLETS
(Ranitidine Hydrochloride) 1597
See Zantac 150 Tablets

ZANTAC 25 EFFERDOSE TABLETS
(Ranitidine Hydrochloride) 1597
See Zantac 150 Tablets

ZANTAC 150 EFFERDOSE TABLETS
(Ranitidine Hydrochloride) 1597
See Zantac 150 Tablets

ZANTAC INJECTION
(Ranitidine Hydrochloride) 1593
See Zantac 150 Tablets

ZANTAC INJECTION PREMIXED
(Ranitidine Hydrochloride) 1593
See Zantac 150 Tablets

ZANTAC 75 TABLETS
(Ranitidine Hydrochloride) .... ▣715
None cited in PDR database.

ZANTAC 150 MAXIMUM STRENGTH TABLETS
(Ranitidine Hydrochloride) .... ▣715
None cited in PDR database.

ZANTAC INJECTION PHARMACY BULK PACKAGE
(Ranitidine Hydrochloride) 1595
May interact with:

Triazolam (Ranitidine, similar to other agents that lower gastric acidity, has been shown to increase the absorption of triazolam resulting in increased plasma concentrations on average 14% to 28%; the clinical significance of this finding is unknown).
No products indexed under this heading.

Warfarin Sodium (Potential for increased or decreased prothrombin time; doses of ranitidine up to 400 mg per day had no effect on prothrombin time or warfarin clearance). Products include:
Coumadin for Injection 932
Coumadin Tablets 932

ZANTAC SYRUP
(Ranitidine Hydrochloride) 1597
See Zantac 150 Tablets

ZAVESCA CAPSULES
(Miglustat) 543
May interact with:

Imiglucerase (Miglustat appeared to increase the clearance of imiglucerase by 70%; combination therapy is not indicated). Products include:
- Cerezyme for Injection 1263

ZEEL SOLUTION
(Arnica montana, Herbals, Multiple, Sulfur).. 1639
None cited in PDR database.

ZEGERID POWDER FOR ORAL SOLUTION
(Omeprazole) 2972
May interact with benzodiazepines, iron containing oral preparations, phenytoin, and certain other agents. Compounds in these categories include:

Alprazolam (Potential for metabolism interaction via cytochrome P450 system). Products include:
- Niravam Orally Disintegrating Tablets 3106
- Xanax XR Tablets 2655

Bacampicillin Hydrochloride (Omeprazole may interfere with gastric absorption of drugs, such as ampicillin esters, where gastric pH is an important determinant of their bioavailability).
- No products indexed under this heading.

Chlordiazepoxide (Potential for metabolism interaction via cytochrome P450 system).
- No products indexed under this heading.

Chlordiazepoxide Hydrochloride (Potential for metabolism interaction via cytochrome P450 system). Products include:
- Librium Capsules 3349

Clarithromycin (Co-administration may result in increases in plasma levels of omeprazole, clarithromycin, and 14-hydroxy-clarithromycin). Products include:
- Biaxin/Biaxin XL 402
- PREVPAC 3281

Clorazepate Dipotassium (Potential for metabolism interaction via cytochrome P450 system). Products include:
- Tranxene 2488

Cyclosporine (Potential for metabolism interaction via cytochrome P450 system). Products include:
- Gengraf Capsules 458
- Neoral Soft Gelatin Capsules 2247
- Neoral Oral Solution 2247
- Restasis Ophthalmic Emulsion 570
- Sandimmune 2259

Diazepam (Potential for metabolism interaction via cytochrome P450 system; prolonged elimination of diazepam). Products include:
- Diastat Rectal Delivery System 3344
- Valium Tablets 2822

Disulfiram (Potential for metabolism interaction via cytochrome P450 system). Products include:
- Antabuse Tablets 2343

Estazolam (Potential for metabolism interaction via cytochrome P450 system). Products include:
- ProSom Tablets 512

Ferrous Fumarate (Omeprazole may interfere with gastric absorption of drugs, such as iron salts, where gastric pH is an important determinant of their bioavailability). Products include:
- Chromagen Forte Soft Gelatin Capsules 3296
- Ferretts Tablets .... ■ 773
- Repliva 21/7 Tablets 3301

Ferrous Gluconate (Omeprazole may interfere with gastric absorption of drugs, such as iron salts, where gastric pH is an important determinant of their bioavailability).
- No products indexed under this heading.

Ferrous Sulfate (Omeprazole may interfere with gastric absorption of drugs, such as iron salts, where gastric pH is an important determinant of their bioavailability). Products include:
- Feosol Tablets 1629
- Slow Fe Iron Tablets .... ■ 772
- Slow Fe with Folic Acid Tablets .... ■ 773

Flurazepam Hydrochloride (Potential for metabolism interaction via cytochrome P450 system). Products include:
- Dalmane Capsules 3343

Fosphenytoin Sodium (Prolonged elimination of phenytoin).
- No products indexed under this heading.

Halazepam (Potential for metabolism interaction via cytochrome P450 system).
- No products indexed under this heading.

Iron (Omeprazole may interfere with gastric absorption of drugs, such as iron salts, where gastric pH is an important determinant of their bioavailability). Products include:
- Chromagen Forte Soft Gelatin Capsules 3296
- Ferretts IPS Liquid .... ■ 773
- OptiNate 1162
- Repliva 21/7 Tablets 3301

Ketoconazole (Omeprazole may interfere with gastric absorption of drugs, such as ketoconazole, where gastric pH is an important determinant of their bioavailability). Products include:
- Nizoral A-D Shampoo, 1% 1839
- Nizoral 2% Shampoo 1838

Lorazepam (Potential for metabolism interaction via cytochrome P450 system).
- No products indexed under this heading.

Midazolam Hydrochloride (Potential for metabolism interaction via cytochrome P450 system).
- No products indexed under this heading.

Oxazepam (Potential for metabolism interaction via cytochrome P450 system).
- No products indexed under this heading.

Phenytoin (Prolonged elimination of phenytoin).
- No products indexed under this heading.

Phenytoin Sodium (Prolonged elimination of phenytoin). Products include:
- Phenytek Capsules 2153

Polysaccharide Iron Complex (Omeprazole may interfere with gastric absorption of drugs, such as iron salts, where gastric pH is an important determinant of their bioavailability). Products include:
- Niferex-150 Forte Capsules 3299
- Nu-Iron 150 Capsules 2098

Prazepam (Potential for metabolism interaction via cytochrome P450 system).
- No products indexed under this heading.

Quazepam (Potential for metabolism interaction via cytochrome P450 system).
- No products indexed under this heading.

Temazepam (Potential for metabolism interaction via cytochrome P450 system).
- No products indexed under this heading.

Triazolam (Potential for metabolism interaction via cytochrome P450 system).
- No products indexed under this heading.

Warfarin Sodium (Prolonged elimination of warfarin, and reports of increased INR and prothrombin time with concurrent use). Products include:
- Coumadin for Injection 932
- Coumadin Tablets 932

ZELNORM TABLETS
(Tegaserod maleate) 2303
May interact with:

Digoxin (Reduced peak plasma concentrations of digoxin by approximately 15%; this reduction in bioavailability is not considered clinically relevant). Products include:
- Digitek Tablets 2146
- Lanoxicaps Capsules 1458
- Lanoxin Injection 1462
- Lanoxin Tablets 1468
- Lanoxin Injection Pediatric 1465

Food Interactions

Food, unspecified (Reduces the bioavailability of tegaserod; Zelnorm should be taken before meals).

ZEMAIRA
(Alpha$_1$-Proteinase Inhibitor (Human)).. 3506
None cited in PDR database.

ZEMPLAR CAPSULES
(Paricalcitol) 535
May interact with cytochrome p450 3a4 inhibitors, potent and certain other agents. Compounds in these categories include:

Amprenavir (A study has demonstrated that ketoconazole approximately doubled paricalcitol AUC. Since paricalcitol is partially metabolized by CYP3A and ketoconazole is known to be a strong inhibitor of cytochrome P450 3A enzyme, care should be taken while dosing paricalcitol with ketoconazole and other strong P450 3A inhibitors. Dose adjustment of paricalcitol capsules may be required and iPTH and serum calcium concentrations should be closely monitored if a patient initiates or discontinues therapy with a strong CYP3A4 inhibitor, such as ketoconazole). Products include:
- Agenerase Capsules 1299
- Agenerase Oral Solution 1304

Atazanavir (A study has demonstrated that ketoconazole approximately doubled paricalcitol AUC. Since paricalcitol is partially metabolized by CYP3A and ketoconazole is known to be a strong inhibitor of cytochrome P450 3A enzyme, care should be taken while dosing paricalcitol with ketoconazole and other strong P450 3A inhibitors. Dose adjustment of paricalcitol capsules may be required and iPTH and serum calcium concentrations should be closely monitored if a patient initiates or discontinues therapy with a strong CYP3A4 inhibitor, such as ketoconazole).
- No products indexed under this heading.

Atazanavir sulfate (A study has demonstrated that ketoconazole approximately doubled paricalcitol AUC. Since paricalcitol is partially metabolized by CYP3A and ketoconazole is known to be a strong inhibitor of cytochrome P450 3A enzyme, care should be taken while dosing paricalcitol with ketoconazole and other strong P450 3A inhibitors. Dose adjustment of paricalcitol capsules may be required and iPTH and serum calcium concentrations should be closely monitored if a patient initiates or discontinues therapy with a strong CYP3A4 inhibitor, such as ketoconazole). Products include:
- Reyataz Capsules 948

Cholestyramine (Drugs that impair intestinal absorption of fat-soluble vitamins, such as cholestyramine, may interfere with the absorption of paricalcitol).
- No products indexed under this heading.

Clarithromycin (A study has demonstrated that ketoconazole approximately doubled paricalcitol AUC. Since paricalcitol is partially metabolized by CYP3A and ketoconazole is known to be a strong inhibitor of cytochrome P450 3A enzyme, care should be taken while dosing paricalcitol with ketoconazole and other strong P450 3A inhibitors. Dose adjustment of paricalcitol capsules may be required and iPTH and serum calcium concentrations should be closely monitored if a patient initiates or discontinues therapy with a strong CYP3A4 inhibitor, such as ketoconazole). Products include:
- Biaxin/Biaxin XL 402
- PREVPAC 3281

Fosamprenavir Calcium (A study has demonstrated that ketoconazole approximately doubled paricalcitol AUC. Since paricalcitol is partially metabolized by CYP3A and ketoconazole is known to be a strong inhibitor of cytochrome P450 3A enzyme, care should be taken while dosing paricalcitol with ketoconazole and other strong P450 3A inhibitors. Dose adjustment of paricalcitol capsules may be required and iPTH and serum calcium concentrations should be closely monitored if a patient initiates or discontinues therapy with a strong CYP3A4 inhibitor, such as ketoconazole). Products include:
- Lexiva Tablets 1473

Indinavir Sulfate (A study has demonstrated that ketoconazole approximately doubled paricalcitol AUC. Since paricalcitol is partially metabolized by CYP3A and ketoconazole is known to be a strong inhibitor of cytochrome P450 3A enzyme, care should be taken while dosing paricalcitol with ketoconazole and other strong P450 3A inhibitors. Dose adjustment of paricalcitol capsules may be required and iPTH and serum calcium concentrations should be

closely monitored if a patient initiates or discontinues therapy with a strong CYP3A4 inhibitor, such as ketoconazole). Products include:

Crixivan Capsules 1918

Itraconazole (A study has demonstrated that ketoconazole approximately doubled paricalcitol AUC. Since paricalcitol is partially metabolized by CYP3A and ketoconazole is known to be a strong inhibitor of cytochrome P450 3A enzyme, care should be taken while dosing paricalcitol with ketoconazole and other strong P450 3A inhibitors. Dose adjustment of paricalcitol capsules may be required and iPTH and serum calcium concentrations should be closely monitored if a patient initiates or discontinues therapy with a strong CYP3A4 inhibitor, such as ketoconazole).

No products indexed under this heading.

Ketoconazole (A study has demonstrated that ketoconazole approximately doubled paricalcitol AUC. Since paricalcitol is partially metabolized by CYP3A and ketoconazole is known to be a strong inhibitor of cytochrome P450 3A enzyme, care should be taken while dosing paricalcitol with ketoconazole and other strong P450 3A inhibitors. Dose adjustment of paricalcitol capsules may be required and iPTH and serum calcium concentrations should be closely monitored if a patient initiates or discontinues therapy with a strong CYP3A4 inhibitor, such as ketoconazole). Products include:

Nizoral A-D Shampoo, 1% 1839
Nizoral 2% Shampoo 1838

Lopinavir (A study has demonstrated that ketoconazole approximately doubled paricalcitol AUC. Since paricalcitol is partially metabolized by CYP3A and ketoconazole is known to be a strong inhibitor of cytochrome P450 3A enzyme, care should be taken while dosing paricalcitol with ketoconazole and other strong P450 3A inhibitors. Dose adjustment of paricalcitol capsules may be required and iPTH and serum calcium concentrations should be closely monitored if a patient initiates or discontinues therapy with a strong CYP3A4 inhibitor, such as ketoconazole). Products include:

Kaletra 474

Nefazodone Hydrochloride (A study has demonstrated that ketoconazole approximately doubled paricalcitol AUC. Since paricalcitol is partially metabolized by CYP3A and ketoconazole is known to be a strong inhibitor of cytochrome P450 3A enzyme, care should be taken while dosing paricalcitol with ketoconazole and other strong P450 3A inhibitors. Dose adjustment of paricalcitol capsules may be required and iPTH and serum calcium concentrations should be closely monitored if a patient initiates or discontinues therapy with a strong CYP3A4 inhibitor, such as ketoconazole).

No products indexed under this heading.

Nelfinavir Mesylate (A study has demonstrated that ketoconazole approximately doubled paricalcitol AUC. Since paricalcitol is partially metabolized by CYP3A and ketoconazole is known to be a strong inhibitor of cytochrome P450 3A enzyme, care should be taken while dosing paricalcitol with ketoconazole and other strong P450 3A inhibitors. Dose adjustment of paricalcitol capsules may be required and iPTH and serum calcium concentrations should be closely monitored if a patient initiates or discontinues therapy with a strong CYP3A4 inhibitor, such as ketoconazole). Products include:

Viracept 2556

Ritonavir (A study has demonstrated that ketoconazole approximately doubled paricalcitol AUC. Since paricalcitol is partially metabolized by CYP3A and ketoconazole is known to be a strong inhibitor of cytochrome P450 3A enzyme, care should be taken while dosing paricalcitol with ketoconazole and other strong P450 3A inhibitors. Dose adjustment of paricalcitol capsules may be required and iPTH and serum calcium concentrations should be closely monitored if a patient initiates or discontinues therapy with a strong CYP3A4 inhibitor, such as ketoconazole). Products include:

Kaletra 474
Norvir 499

Saquinavir (A study has demonstrated that ketoconazole approximately doubled paricalcitol AUC. Since paricalcitol is partially metabolized by CYP3A and ketoconazole is known to be a strong inhibitor of cytochrome P450 3A enzyme, care should be taken while dosing paricalcitol with ketoconazole and other strong P450 3A inhibitors. Dose adjustment of paricalcitol capsules may be required and iPTH and serum calcium concentrations should be closely monitored if a patient initiates or discontinues therapy with a strong CYP3A4 inhibitor, such as ketoconazole).

No products indexed under this heading.

Saquinavir Mesylate (A study has demonstrated that ketoconazole approximately doubled paricalcitol AUC. Since paricalcitol is partially metabolized by CYP3A and ketoconazole is known to be a strong inhibitor of cytochrome P450 3A enzyme, care should be taken while dosing paricalcitol with ketoconazole and other strong P450 3A inhibitors. Dose adjustment of paricalcitol capsules may be required and iPTH and serum calcium concentrations should be closely monitored if a patient initiates or discontinues therapy with a strong CYP3A4 inhibitor, such as ketoconazole). Products include:

Invirase 2776

Telithromycin (A study has demonstrated that ketoconazole approximately doubled paricalcitol AUC. Since paricalcitol is partially metabolized by CYP3A and ketoconazole is known to be a strong inhibitor of cytochrome P450 3A enzyme, care should be taken while dosing paricalcitol with ketoconazole and other strong P450 3A inhibitors. Dose adjustment of paricalcitol capsules may be required and iPTH and serum calcium concentrations should be closely monitored if a patient initiates or discontinues therapy with a strong CYP3A4 inhibitor, such as ketoconazole). Products include:

Ketek Tablets 2920

Troleandomycin (A study has demonstrated that ketoconazole approximately doubled paricalcitol AUC. Since paricalcitol is partially metabolized by CYP3A and ketoconazole is known to be a strong inhibitor of cytochrome P450 3A enzyme, care should be taken while dosing paricalcitol with ketoconazole and other strong P450 3A inhibitors. Dose adjustment of paricalcitol capsules may be required and iPTH and serum calcium concentrations should be closely monitored if a patient initiates or discontinues therapy with a strong CYP3A4 inhibitor, such as ketoconazole).

No products indexed under this heading.

Voriconazole (A study has demonstrated that ketoconazole approximately doubled paricalcitol AUC. Since paricalcitol is partially metabolized by CYP3A and ketoconazole is known to be a strong inhibitor of cytochrome P450 3A enzyme, care should be taken while dosing paricalcitol with ketoconazole and other strong P450 3A inhibitors. Dose adjustment of paricalcitol capsules may be required and iPTH and serum calcium concentrations should be closely monitored if a patient initiates or discontinues therapy with a strong CYP3A4 inhibitor, such as ketoconazole). Products include:

VFEND I.V. 2543
VFEND Oral Suspension 2543
VFEND Tablets 2543

ZEMPLAR INJECTION

(Paricalcitol) 538

May interact with cardiac glycosides and certain other agents. Compounds in these categories include:

Calcitriol (Vitamin D-related compounds should not be taken concomitantly with paricalcitol). Products include:

Calcijex Injection 411

Deslanoside (Digitalis toxicity is potentiated by hypercalcemia of any cause, so caution should be applied when digitalis compounds are prescribed concomitantly with paricalcitol).

No products indexed under this heading.

Digitalis Glycoside Preparations (Digitalis toxicity is potentiated by hypercalcemia of any cause, so caution should be applied when digitalis compounds are prescribed concomitantly with paricalcitol).

No products indexed under this heading.

Digitoxin (Digitalis toxicity is potentiated by hypercalcemia of any cause, so caution should be applied when digitalis compounds are prescribed concomitantly with paricalcitol).

No products indexed under this heading.

Digoxin (Digitalis toxicity is potentiated by hypercalcemia of any cause, so caution should be applied when digitalis compounds are prescribed concomitantly with paricalcitol). Products include:

Digitek Tablets 2146
Lanoxicaps Capsules 1458
Lanoxin Injection 1462
Lanoxin Tablets 1468
Lanoxin Injection Pediatric 1465

Potassium Acid Phosphate (Phosphate compounds should not be taken concomitantly with paricalcitol). Products include:

K-Phos Original (Sodium Free) Tablets 785

Potassium Phosphate (Phosphate compounds should not be taken concomitantly with paricalcitol). Products include:

K-Phos Neutral Tablets 785

ZEMURON INJECTION

(Rocuronium Bromide) 2363

May interact with aminoglycosides, anticonvulsants, inhalant anesthetics, tetracyclines, and certain other agents. Compounds in these categories include:

Amikacin Sulfate (Possible prolongation of neuromuscular blockade).

No products indexed under this heading.

Bacitracin (Possible prolongation of neuromuscular blockade). Products include:

Neosporin Ointment 702
Neosporin + Pain Relief Maximum Strength Ointment....... 703
Polysporin Ointment 706

Carbamazepine (Potential for apparent resistance to the effects of rocuronium in the form of diminished magnitude of neuromuscular blockade). Products include:

Carbatrol Capsules 3174
Equetro Extended-Release Capsules 3178
Tegretol/Tegretol-XR 2278

Colistimethate Sodium (Possible prolongation of neuromuscular blockade).

No products indexed under this heading.

Colistin Sulfate (Possible prolongation of neuromuscular blockade).

No products indexed under this heading.

Demeclocycline Hydrochloride (Possible prolongation of neuromuscular blockade).

No products indexed under this heading.

Desflurane (Possible enhanced activity of neuromuscular blocking agent). Products include:

Suprane Liquid for Inhalation 770

Divalproex Sodium (Potential for apparent resistance to the effects of rocuronium in the form of diminished magnitude of neuromuscular blockade). Products include:

Depakote Sprinkle Capsules 422
Depakote Tablets 427
Depakote ER Tablets 433

Doxycycline Calcium (Possible prolongation of neuromuscular blockade).

No products indexed under this heading.

Doxycycline Hyclate (Possible prolongation of neuromuscular blockade).

No products indexed under this heading.

Doxycycline Monohydrate (Possible prolongation of neuromuscular blockade).

No products indexed under this heading.

Enflurane (Possible enhanced activity of neuromuscular blocking agent; may prolong the duration of action).

No products indexed under this heading.

Ethosuximide (Potential for apparent resistance to the effects of rocuronium in the form of diminished magnitude of neuromuscular blockade).

No products indexed under this heading.

Ethotoin (Potential for apparent resistance to the effects of rocuronium in the form of diminished magnitude of neuromuscular blockade). Products include:
- Peganone Tablets, USP 2487

Felbamate (Potential for apparent resistance to the effects of rocuronium in the form of diminished magnitude of neuromuscular blockade).
- No products indexed under this heading.

Fosphenytoin (Potential for apparent resistance to the effects of rocuronium in the form of diminished magnitude of neuromuscular blockade).
- No products indexed under this heading.

Fosphenytoin Sodium (Potential for apparent resistance to the effects of rocuronium in the form of diminished magnitude of neuromuscular blockade).
- No products indexed under this heading.

Gabapentin (Potential for apparent resistance to the effects of rocuronium in the form of diminished magnitude of neuromuscular blockade). Products include:
- Neurontin Capsules 2498
- Neurontin Oral Solution 2498
- Neurontin Tablets 2498

Gentamicin Sulfate (Possible prolongation of neuromuscular blockade). Products include:
- Garamycin Injectable 3028
- Genoptic Sterile Ophthalmic Solution .... ⊙ 227
- Pred-G Ophthalmic Suspension .... ⊙ 234
- Pred-G Sterile Ophthalmic Ointment .... ⊙ 235

Halothane (Possible enhanced activity of neuromuscular blocking agent).
- No products indexed under this heading.

Isoflurane (Possible enhanced activity of neuromuscular blocking agent; may prolong the duration of action).
- No products indexed under this heading.

Kanamycin Sulfate (Possible prolongation of neuromuscular blockade).
- No products indexed under this heading.

Lamotrigine (Potential for apparent resistance to the effects of rocuronium in the form of diminished magnitude of neuromuscular blockade). Products include:
- Lamictal 1449

Levetiracetam (Potential for apparent resistance to the effects of rocuronium in the form of diminished magnitude of neuromuscular blockade). Products include:
- Keppra Oral Solution 3307
- Keppra Tablets 3307

Lithium Carbonate (May increase the duration of neuromuscular block). Products include:
- Eskalith 1406
- Lithobid Tablets 1670

Lithium Citrate (May increase the duration of neuromuscular block).
- No products indexed under this heading.

Magnesium Sulfate Injection (May enhance the neuromuscular blockade).
- No products indexed under this heading.

Mephenytoin (Potential for apparent resistance to the effects of rocuronium in the form of diminished magnitude of neuromuscular blockade).
- No products indexed under this heading.

Methacycline Hydrochloride (Possible prolongation of neuromuscular blockade).
- No products indexed under this heading.

Methoxyflurane (Possible enhanced activity of neuromuscular blocking agent).
- No products indexed under this heading.

Methsuximide (Potential for apparent resistance to the effects of rocuronium in the form of diminished magnitude of neuromuscular blockade).
- No products indexed under this heading.

Minocycline Hydrochloride (Possible prolongation of neuromuscular blockade). Products include:
- Dynacin Tablets 1859

Oxcarbazepine (Potential for apparent resistance to the effects of rocuronium in the form of diminished magnitude of neuromuscular blockade). Products include:
- Trileptal Oral Suspension 2281
- Trileptal Tablets 2281

Oxytetracycline Hydrochloride (Possible prolongation of neuromuscular blockade).
- No products indexed under this heading.

Paramethadione (Potential for apparent resistance to the effects of rocuronium in the form of diminished magnitude of neuromuscular blockade).
- No products indexed under this heading.

Phenacemide (Potential for apparent resistance to the effects of rocuronium in the form of diminished magnitude of neuromuscular blockade).
- No products indexed under this heading.

Phenobarbital (Potential for apparent resistance to the effects of rocuronium in the form of diminished magnitude of neuromuscular blockade).
- No products indexed under this heading.

Phensuximide (Potential for apparent resistance to the effects of rocuronium in the form of diminished magnitude of neuromuscular blockade).
- No products indexed under this heading.

Phenytoin (Potential for apparent resistance to the effects of rocuronium in the form of diminished magnitude of neuromuscular blockade).
- No products indexed under this heading.

Phenytoin Sodium (Potential for apparent resistance to the effects of rocuronium in the form of diminished magnitude of neuromuscular blockade). Products include:
- Phenytek Capsules 2153

Polymyxin B Sulfate (Possible prolongation of neuromuscular blockade). Products include:
- Neosporin Ointment .... ▣ 702
- Neosporin + Pain Relief Maximum Strength Cream .... ▣ 703
- Neosporin + Pain Relief Maximum Strength Ointment .... ▣ 703
- Poly-Pred Liquifilm Ophthalmic Suspension .... ⊙ 231
- Polysporin Ointment .... ▣ 706
- Polytrim Ophthalmic Solution 570

Primidone (Potential for apparent resistance to the effects of rocuronium in the form of diminished magnitude of neuromuscular blockade).
- No products indexed under this heading.

Procainamide Hydrochloride (May increase the duration of neuromuscular block).
- No products indexed under this heading.

Quinidine Gluconate (Possible recurrent paralysis; increased duration of neuromusclar block).
- No products indexed under this heading.

Quinidine Polygalacturonate (Possible recurrent paralysis; increased duration of neuromusclar block).
- No products indexed under this heading.

Quinidine Sulfate (Possible recurrent paralysis; increased duration of neuromusclar block).
- No products indexed under this heading.

Streptomycin Sulfate (Possible prolongation of neuromuscular blockade).
- No products indexed under this heading.

Succinylcholine Chloride (Rocuronium should not be given until recovery from succinylcholine has been observed).
- No products indexed under this heading.

Tetracycline Hydrochloride (Possible prolongation of neuromuscular blockade).
- No products indexed under this heading.

Tiagabine Hydrochloride (Potential for apparent resistance to the effects of rocuronium in the form of diminished magnitude of neuromuscular blockade). Products include:
- Gabitril Tablets 998

Tobramycin (Possible prolongation of neuromuscular blockade). Products include:
- TOBI Solution for Inhalation 1015
- TobraDex Ophthalmic Ointment 558
- TobraDex Ophthalmic Suspension 558
- Zylet Ophthalmic Suspension 3508

Tobramycin Sulfate (Possible prolongation of neuromuscular blockade).
- No products indexed under this heading.

Topiramate (Potential for apparent resistance to the effects of rocuronium in the form of diminished magnitude of neuromuscular blockade). Products include:
- Topamax Sprinkle Capsules 2438
- Topamax Tablets 2438

Trimethadione (Potential for apparent resistance to the effects of rocuronium in the form of diminished magnitude of neuromuscular blockade).
- No products indexed under this heading.

Valproate Sodium (Potential for apparent resistance to the effects of rocuronium in the form of diminished magnitude of neuromuscular blockade). Products include:
- Depacon Injection 412

Valproic Acid (Potential for apparent resistance to the effects of rocuronium in the form of diminished magnitude of neuromuscular blockade). Products include:
- Depakene 417

Vancomycin Hydrochloride (Possible prolongation of neuromuscular blockade). Products include:
- Vancocin HCl Capsules, USP 3370

Zonisamide (Potential for apparent resistance to the effects of rocuronium in the form of diminished magnitude of neuromuscular blockade). Products include:
- Zonegran Capsules 1089

ZENAPAX FOR INJECTION

(Daclizumab) 2838

None cited in PDR database.

ZERIT CAPSULES

(Stavudine) 971

May interact with drugs that may exacerbate peripheral neuropathy (selected) and certain other agents. Compounds in these categories include:

Carboplatin (Concurrent use may exacerbate peripheral neuropathy).
- No products indexed under this heading.

Didanosine (Co-administration of stavudine and didanosine with other antiretroviral agents has resulted in fatal lactic acidosis in pregnant women; pancreatitis, peripheral neuropathy and liver function abnormalities occur more frequently with concurrent use).
- No products indexed under this heading.

Doxorubicin Hydrochloride (Co-administration may inhibit the phosporylation of stavudine at certain concentrations; administer with caution). Products include:
- Adriamycin for Injection, USP 786
- Adriamycin Injection, USP 786

Doxorubicin Hydrochloride Liposome (Co-administration may inhibit the phosporylation of stavudine at certain concentrations; administer with caution). Products include:
- Doxil Injection 3302

Isoniazid (Concurrent use may exacerbate peripheral neuropathy).
- No products indexed under this heading.

Paclitaxel (Concurrent use may exacerbate peripheral neuropathy).
- No products indexed under this heading.

Ribavirin (Co-administration may inhibit the phosporylation of stavudine at certain concentrations; administer with caution). Products include:
- Copegus Tablets 2759
- Rebetol 3073
- Rebetron Combination Therapy 3078
- Ribavirin, USP Capsules 3083
- Virazole for Inhalation Solution 3365

Zalcitabine (Concurrent use may exacerbate peripheral neuropathy).
- No products indexed under this heading.

Zidovudine (May competitively inhibit the intracellular phosphorylation of stavudine; concurrent use is not recommended). Products include:
- Combivir Tablets 1373
- Retrovir 1533
- Retrovir IV Infusion 1537

Trizivir Tablets 1565

Food Interactions

Meal, unspecified (Co-administration with food decreases Cmax by approximately 45%; however, the systemic availability (AUC) is unchanged; Zerit Capsules can be taken without regard to meals).

ZERIT FOR ORAL SOLUTION

(Stavudine) 971
See Zerit Capsules

ZESTORETIC TABLETS

(Hydrochlorothiazide, Lisinopril) 701
May interact with antihypertensives, barbiturates, corticosteroids, diuretics, cardiac glycosides, oral hypoglycemic agents, insulin, lithium preparations, narcotic analgesics, nondepolarizing neuromuscular blocking agents, non-steroidal anti-inflammatory agents, potassium preparations, potassium sparing diuretics, and certain other agents. Compounds in these categories include:

Acarbose (Hydrochlorothiazide produces hyperglycemia; dosage adjustment of the antidiabetic agent may be required). Products include:
Precose Tablets 776

Acebutolol Hydrochloride (Co-administration with other antihypertensive drugs may result in additive effect or potentiation).
No products indexed under this heading.

ACTH (Intensifies electrolyte depletion particularly hypokalemia).
No products indexed under this heading.

Alfentanil Hydrochloride (Potentiation of orthostatic hypotension may occur).
No products indexed under this heading.

Amiloride Hydrochloride (Concurrent use with potassium sparing diuretic may result in increased risk of hyperkalemia; co-administration with other antihypertensive drugs may result in additive effect or potentiation). Products include:
Midamor Tablets 2000
Moduretic Tablets 2003

Amlodipine Besylate (Co-administration with other antihypertensive drugs may result in additive effect or potentiation). Products include:
Caduet Tablets 2507
Lotrel Capsules 2238
Norvasc Tablets 2529

Aprobarbital (Potentiation of orthostatic hypotension may occur).
No products indexed under this heading.

Atenolol (Co-administration with other antihypertensive drugs may result in additive effect or potentiation). Products include:
Tenormin I.V. Injection 698
Tenormin Tablets 695

Atracurium Besylate (Possible increased responsiveness to the muscle relaxant).
No products indexed under this heading.

Benazepril Hydrochloride (Co-administration with other antihypertensive drugs may result in additive effect or potentiation). Products include:
Lotensin Tablets 2232
Lotensin HCT Tablets 2235
Lotrel Capsules 2238

Bendroflumethiazide (Possible excessive reduction of blood pressure after initiation of lisinopril; co-administration with other antihypertensive drugs may result in additive effect or potentiation).
No products indexed under this heading.

Betamethasone Acetate (Corticosteroids intensify electrolyte depletion particularly hypokalemia).
No products indexed under this heading.

Betamethasone Sodium Phosphate (Corticosteroids intensify electrolyte depletion particularly hypokalemia).
No products indexed under this heading.

Betaxolol Hydrochloride (Co-administration with other antihypertensive drugs may result in additive effect or potentiation). Products include:
Betoptic S Ophthalmic Suspension........................ 554

Bisoprolol Fumarate (Co-administration with other antihypertensive drugs may result in additive effect or potentiation).
No products indexed under this heading.

Bumetanide (Possible excessive reduction of blood pressure after initiation of lisinopril; co-administration with other antihypertensive drugs may result in additive effect or potentiation).
No products indexed under this heading.

Buprenorphine Hydrochloride (Potentiation of orthostatic hypotension may occur). Products include:
Buprenex Injectable 2718
Suboxone Tablets 2719
Subutex Tablets 2719

Butabarbital (Potentiation of orthostatic hypotension may occur).
No products indexed under this heading.

Butalbital (Potentiation of orthostatic hypotension may occur). Products include:
Sedapap Tablets 50 mg/650 mg 2098

Candesartan Cilexetil (Co-administration with other antihypertensive drugs may result in additive effect or potentiation). Products include:
Atacand Tablets 634
Atacand HCT 637

Captopril (Co-administration with other antihypertensive drugs may result in additive effect or potentiation). Products include:
Captopril Tablets 2114

Carteolol Hydrochloride (Co-administration with other antihypertensive drugs may result in additive effect or potentiation). Products include:
Carteolol Hydrochloride Ophthalmic Solution USP, 1%....... ⊙246

Celecoxib (Co-administration of non-steroidal anti-inflammatory agents can reduce the diuretic, natriuretic, and antihypertensive effects; possible further deterioration of renal function). Products include:
Celebrex Capsules 3130

Chlorothiazide (Possible excessive reduction of blood pressure after initiation of lisinopril; co-administration with other antihypertensive drugs may result in additive effect or potentiation). Products include:
Aldoclor Tablets 1881
Diuril Oral 1936

Chlorothiazide Sodium (Possible excessive reduction of blood pressure after initiation of lisinopril; co-administration with other antihypertensive drugs may result in additive effect or potentiation). Products include:
Diuril Sodium Intravenous 1934

Chlorpropamide (Hydrochlorothiazide produces hyperglycemia; dosage adjustment of the antidiabetic agent may be required).
No products indexed under this heading.

Chlorthalidone (Possible excessive reduction of blood pressure after initiation of lisinopril; co-administration with other antihypertensive drugs may result in additive effect or potentiation). Products include:
Clorpres Tablets 2139

Cholestyramine (Impairs the absorption of hydrochlorothiazide by binding in the GI tract and reducing the absorption by 85%).
No products indexed under this heading.

Cisatracurium Besylate (Possible increased responsiveness to the muscle relaxant). Products include:
Nimbex Injection 494

Clonidine (Co-administration with other antihypertensive drugs may result in additive effect or potentiation). Products include:
Catapres-TTS 875

Clonidine Hydrochloride (Co-administration with other antihypertensive drugs may result in additive effect or potentiation). Products include:
Catapres Tablets 874
Clorpres Tablets 2139

Codeine Phosphate (Potentiation of orthostatic hypotension may occur). Products include:
Tylenol with Codeine 2461

Colestipol Hydrochloride (Impairs the absorption of hydrochlorothiazide by binding in the GI tract and reducing the absorption by 43%).
No products indexed under this heading.

Cortisone Acetate (Corticosteroids intensify electrolyte depletion particularly hypokalemia).
No products indexed under this heading.

Deserpidine (Co-administration with other antihypertensive drugs may result in additive effect or potentiation).
No products indexed under this heading.

Deslanoside (Hypokalemia may develop during thiazide therapy and may sensitize or exaggerate the response of the heart to the toxic effects of digitalis, such as increased ventricular irritability).
No products indexed under this heading.

Dexamethasone (Corticosteroids intensify electrolyte depletion particularly hypokalemia). Products include:
Ciprodex Otic Suspension 555
Decadron Tablets 1929
TobraDex Ophthalmic Ointment 558
TobraDex Ophthalmic Suspension ... 558

Dexamethasone Acetate (Corticosteroids intensify electrolyte depletion particularly hypokalemia).
No products indexed under this heading.

Dexamethasone Sodium Phosphate (Corticosteroids intensify electrolyte depletion particularly hypokalemia). Products include:
Decadron Phosphate Injection 1931

Dezocine (Potentiation of orthostatic hypotension may occur).
No products indexed under this heading.

Diazoxide (Co-administration with other antihypertensive drugs may result in additive effect or potentiation). Products include:
Hyperstat I.V. Injection 3031

Diclofenac Potassium (Co-administration of non-steroidal anti-inflammatory agents can reduce the diuretic, natriuretic, and antihypertensive effects; possible further deterioration of renal function). Products include:
Cataflam Tablets 2173

Diclofenac Sodium (Co-administration of non-steroidal anti-inflammatory agents can reduce the diuretic, natriuretic, and antihypertensive effects; possible further deterioration of renal function). Products include:
Arthrotec Tablets 3126
Voltaren Ophthalmic Solution 2300
Voltaren Tablets 2298
Voltaren-XR Tablets 2301

Digitalis Glycoside Preparations (Hypokalemia may develop during thiazide therapy and may sensitize or exaggerate the response of the heart to the toxic effects of digitalis, such as increased ventricular irritability).
No products indexed under this heading.

Digitoxin (Hypokalemia may develop during thiazide therapy and may sensitize or exaggerate the response of the heart to the toxic effects of digitalis, such as increased ventricular irritability).
No products indexed under this heading.

Digoxin (Hypokalemia may develop during thiazide therapy and may sensitize or exaggerate the response of the heart to the toxic effects of digitalis, such as increased ventricular irritability). Products include:
Digitek Tablets 2146
Lanoxicaps Capsules 1458
Lanoxin Injection 1462
Lanoxin Tablets 1468
Lanoxin Injection Pediatric 1465

Diltiazem Hydrochloride (Co-administration with other antihypertensive drugs may result in additive effect or potentiation). Products include:
Cardizem LA Extended Release Tablets 1699
Tiazac Capsules 1204

Doxazosin Mesylate (Co-administration with other antihypertensive drugs may result in additive effect or potentiation).
No products indexed under this heading.

Enalapril Maleate (Co-administration with other antihypertensive drugs may result in additive effect or potentiation). Products include:
Vaseretic Tablets 2073
Vasotec I.V. Injection 2076

Enalaprilat (Co-administration with other antihypertensive drugs may result in additive effect or potentiation).
No products indexed under this heading.

Eprosartan Mesylate (Co-administration with other antihypertensive drugs may result in additive effect or potentiation). Products include:
Teveten Tablets 1707
Teveten HCT Tablets 1710

Esmolol Hydrochloride (Co-administration with other antihypertensive drugs may result in additive effect or potentiation). Products include:
Brevibloc Concentrate 766
Brevibloc Injection 766
Brevibloc Double Strength Injection.. 766
Brevibloc Premixed Injection 766
Brevibloc Double Strength Premixed Injection 766

Ethacrynic Acid (Possible excessive reduction of blood pressure after initiation of lisinopril; co-administration with other antihypertensive drugs may result in additive effect or potentiation). Products include:
Edecrin Tablets 1941

Etodolac (Co-administration of non-steroidal anti-inflammatory agents can reduce the diuretic, natriuretic, and antihypertensive effects; possible further deterioration of renal function).
No products indexed under this heading.

Felodipine (Co-administration with other antihypertensive drugs may result in additive effect or potentiation). Products include:
Plendil Extended-Release Tablets 651

Fenoprofen Calcium (Co-administration of non-steroidal anti-inflammatory agents can reduce the diuretic, natriuretic, and antihypertensive effects; possible further deterioration of renal function). Products include:
Nalfon Capsules 2504

Fentanyl (Potentiation of orthostatic hypotension may occur). Products include:
Duragesic Transdermal System 2448

Fentanyl Citrate (Potentiation of orthostatic hypotension may occur). Products include:
Actiq 993

Fludrocortisone Acetate (Corticosteroids intensify electrolyte depletion particularly hypokalemia).
No products indexed under this heading.

Flurbiprofen (Co-administration of non-steroidal anti-inflammatory agents can reduce the diuretic, natriuretic, and antihypertensive effects; possible further deterioration of renal function).
No products indexed under this heading.

Fosinopril Sodium (Co-administration with other antihypertensive drugs may result in additive effect or potentiation).
No products indexed under this heading.

Furosemide (Possible excessive reduction of blood pressure after initiation of lisinopril; co-administration with other antihypertensive drugs may result in additive effect or potentiation). Products include:
Furosemide Tablets 2117

Glimepiride (Hydrochlorothiazide produces hyperglycemia; dosage adjustment of the antidiabetic agent may be required). Products include:
Amaryl Tablets 2864

Glipizide (Hydrochlorothiazide produces hyperglycemia; dosage adjustment of the antidiabetic agent may be required).
No products indexed under this heading.

Glyburide (Hydrochlorothiazide produces hyperglycemia; dosage adjustment of the antidiabetic agent may be required).
No products indexed under this heading.

Guanabenz Acetate (Co-administration with other antihypertensive drugs may result in additive effect or potentiation).
No products indexed under this heading.

Guanethidine Monosulfate (Co-administration with other antihypertensive drugs may result in additive effect or potentiation).
No products indexed under this heading.

Hydralazine Hydrochloride (Co-administration with other antihypertensive drugs may result in additive effect or potentiation). Products include:
BiDil Tablets 2161

Hydrocodone Bitartrate (Potentiation of orthostatic hypotension may occur). Products include:
Hycodan 1104
Hycomine Compound Tablets 1105
Hycotuss Expectorant Syrup 1106
Lortab 3315
Lortab Elixir 3312
Vicodin Tablets 530
Vicodin ES Tablets 531
Vicodin HP Tablets 532
Vicoprofen Tablets 533
Zydone Tablets 1118

Hydrocodone Polistirex (Potentiation of orthostatic hypotension may occur). Products include:
Tussionex Pennkinetic Extended-Release Suspension...... 3322

Hydrocortisone (Corticosteroids intensify electrolyte depletion particularly hypokalemia). Products include:
Cortizone•5 Ointment .... ▣699
Cortizone•10 Creme .... ▣699
Cortizone•10 Ointment .... ▣699
Cortizone•10 Plus Creme .... ▣700
Cortizone•10 Maximum Strength Quick Shot Spray.......................... ▣700
Hydrocortone Tablets 1963
Preparation H Hydrocortisone Cream .... ▣748

Hydrocortisone Acetate (Corticosteroids intensify electrolyte depletion particularly hypokalemia). Products include:
Analpram-HC 1136
Pramosone 1139
ProctoFoam-HC 3113
Tucks Anti-Itch Ointment .... ▣712
U-cort 1% Cream 3289

Hydrocortisone Sodium Phosphate (Corticosteroids intensify electrolyte depletion particularly hypokalemia).
No products indexed under this heading.

Hydrocortisone Sodium Succinate (Corticosteroids intensify electrolyte depletion particularly hypokalemia).
No products indexed under this heading.

Hydroflumethiazide (Possible excessive reduction of blood pressure after initiation of lisinopril; co-administration with other antihypertensive drugs may result in additive effect or potentiation).
No products indexed under this heading.

Hydromorphone Hydrochloride (Potentiation of orthostatic hypotension may occur). Products include:
Dilaudid 439
Dilaudid Oral Liquid 443
Dilaudid Non-Sterile Powder 439
Dilaudid Rectal Suppositories 439
Dilaudid Tablets 439
Dilaudid Tablets - 8 mg 443
Dilaudid-HP 441

Ibuprofen (Co-administration of non-steroidal anti-inflammatory agents can reduce the diuretic, natriuretic, and antihypertensive effects; possible further deterioration of renal function). Products include:
Advil Allergy Sinus Caplets .... ▣737
Advil .... ▣737
Children's Advil Suspension .... ▣742
Children's Advil Chewable Tablets .. ▣741
Advil Cold & Sinus .... ▣739
Advil Flu & Body Ache Caplets .... ▣739
Children's Advil Cold Suspension ... ▣741
Infants' Advil Concentrated Drops .. ▣743
Junior Strength Advil Swallow Tablets.. ▣740
Advil Migraine Liquigels .... ▣740
Advil Multi-Symptom Cold Caplets .... ▣738
Combunox Tablets 1183
Children's Motrin Oral Suspension and Chewable Tablets.................. 1837
Children's Motrin Cold Non-Staining Dye-Free Oral Suspension 1838
Children's Motrin Cold Oral Suspension 1838
Children's Motrin Non-Staining Dye-Free Oral Suspension............. 1837
Motrin Cold & Sinus Caplets 1836
Motrin IB Tablets and Caplets 1836
Infants' Motrin Concentrated Drops... 1837
Infants' Motrin Non-Staining Dye-Free Drops............................. 1837
Junior Strength Motrin Caplets and Chewable Tablets.................. 1837
Vicoprofen Tablets 533

Indapamide (Possible excessive reduction of blood pressure after initiation of lisinopril; co-administration with other antihypertensive drugs may result in additive effect or potentiation). Products include:
Indapamide Tablets 2119

Indomethacin (Co-administration of non-steroidal anti-inflammatory agents can reduce the diuretic, natriuretic, and antihypertensive effects; possible further deterioration of renal function). Products include:
Indocin 1968

Indomethacin Sodium Trihydrate (Co-administration of non-steroidal anti-inflammatory agents can reduce the diuretic, natriuretic, and antihypertensive effects; possible further deterioration of renal function). Products include:
Indocin I.V. 1973

Insulin, Human, Zinc Suspension (Hydrochlorothiazide produces hyperglycemia; dosage adjustment of the insulin agent may be required). Products include:
Humulin L, 100 Units 1763
Humulin U, 100 Units 1770

Insulin, Human NPH (Hydrochlorothiazide produces hyperglycemia; dosage adjustment of the insulin agent may be required). Products include:
Humulin N, 100 Units 1764
Humulin N Pen 1765
Novolin N Human Insulin 10 ml Vials 2322
Novolin N InnoLet 2322
Novolin N PenFill 3 ml Cartridges 2325
Novolin R InnoLet 2322

Insulin, Human Regular (Hydrochlorothiazide produces hyperglycemia; dosage adjustment of the insulin agent may be required). Products include:
Humulin R (U-500) 1768
Humulin R, 100 Units 1767
Novolin R Human Insulin 10 ml Vials 2322
Novolin R PenFill 2325

Insulin, Human Regular and Human NPH Mixture (Hydrochlorothiazide produces hyperglycemia; dosage adjustment of the insulin agent may be required). Products include:
Humulin 50/50, 100 Units 1760
Humulin 70/30 Pen 1761
Novolin 70/30 Human Insulin 10 ml Vials 2321
Novolin 70/30 InnoLet 2322
Novolin 70/30 PenFill 3 ml Cartridges.. 2325

Insulin, NPH (Hydrochlorothiazide produces hyperglycemia; dosage adjustment of the insulin agent may be required).
No products indexed under this heading.

Insulin, Regular (Hydrochlorothiazide produces hyperglycemia; dosage adjustment of the insulin agent may be required).
No products indexed under this heading.

Insulin, Zinc Crystals (Hydrochlorothiazide produces hyperglycemia; dosage adjustment of the insulin agent may be required).
No products indexed under this heading.

Insulin, Zinc Suspension (Hydrochlorothiazide produces hyperglycemia; dosage adjustment of the insulin agent may be required).
No products indexed under this heading.

Insulin Aspart, Human Regular (Hydrochlorothiazide produces hyperglycemia; dosage adjustment of the insulin agent may be required). Products include:
NovoLog Injection 2326

Insulin glargine (Hydrochlorothiazide produces hyperglycemia; dosage adjustment of the insulin agent may be required). Products include:
Lantus Injection 2925

Insulin Lispro, Human (Hydrochlorothiazide produces hyperglycemia; dosage adjustment of the insulin agent may be required). Products include:
Humalog-Pen 1751
Humalog Mix 75/25-Pen 1754

Insulin Lispro Protamine, Human (Hydrochlorothiazide produces hyperglycemia; dosage adjustment of the insulin agent may be required). Products include:
Humalog Mix 75/25-Pen 1754

Irbesartan (Co-administration with other antihypertensive drugs may result in additive effect or potentiation). Products include:
Avalide Tablets 922
Avalide Tablets 2889
Avapro Tablets 925

Avapro Tablets 2886

Isradipine (Co-administration with other antihypertensive drugs may result in additive effect or potentiation). Products include:
DynaCirc CR Tablets 2726

Ketoprofen (Co-administration of non-steroidal anti-inflammatory agents can reduce the diuretic, natriuretic, and antihypertensive effects; possible further deterioration of renal function).
No products indexed under this heading.

Ketorolac Tromethamine (Co-administration of non-steroidal anti-inflammatory agents can reduce the diuretic, natriuretic, and antihypertensive effects; possible further deterioration of renal function). Products include:
Acular Ophthalmic Solution 561
Acular LS Ophthalmic Solution 562

Labetalol Hydrochloride (Co-administration with other antihypertensive drugs may result in additive effect or potentiation).
No products indexed under this heading.

Levorphanol Tartrate (Potentiation of orthostatic hypotension may occur).
No products indexed under this heading.

Lithium (Diuretics reduce the renal clearance and add a high risk of lithium toxicity; lithium toxicity has been reported in patients receiving drugs which cause sodium elimination, including ACE inhibitors).
No products indexed under this heading.

Lithium Carbonate (Diuretics reduce the renal clearance and add a high risk of lithium toxicity; lithium toxicity has been reported in patients receiving drugs which cause sodium elimination, including ACE inhibitors). Products include:
Eskalith 1406
Lithobid Tablets 1670

Lithium Citrate (Diuretics reduce the renal clearance and add a high risk of lithium toxicity; lithium toxicity has been reported in patients receiving drugs which cause sodium elimination, including ACE inhibitors).
No products indexed under this heading.

Losartan Potassium (Co-administration with other antihypertensive drugs may result in additive effect or potentiation). Products include:
Cozaar Tablets 1913
Hyzaar 1964

Mecamylamine Hydrochloride (Co-administration with other antihypertensive drugs may result in additive effect or potentiation). Products include:
Inversine Tablets 3286

Meclofenamate Sodium (Co-administration of non-steroidal anti-inflammatory agents can reduce the diuretic, natriuretic, and antihypertensive effects; possible further deterioration of renal function).
No products indexed under this heading.

Mefenamic Acid (Co-administration of non-steroidal anti-inflammatory agents can reduce the diuretic, natriuretic, and antihypertensive effects; possible further deterioration of renal function).
No products indexed under this heading.

Meloxicam (Co-administration of non-steroidal anti-inflammatory agents can reduce the diuretic, natriuretic, and antihypertensive effects; possible further deterioration of renal function). Products include:
Mobic Oral Suspension 893
Mobic Tablets 893

Meperidine Hydrochloride (Potentiation of orthostatic hypotension may occur).
No products indexed under this heading.

Mephobarbital (Potentiation of orthostatic hypotension may occur). Products include:
Mebaral Tablets, USP 2483

Metformin Hydrochloride (Hydrochlorothiazide produces hyperglycemia; dosage adjustment of the antidiabetic agent may be required). Products include:
ActoPlus Met Tablets 3219
Avandamet Tablets 1343
Fortamet Extended-Release Tablets 1156

Methadone Hydrochloride (Potentiation of orthostatic hypotension may occur).
No products indexed under this heading.

Methyclothiazide (Possible excessive reduction of blood pressure after initiation of lisinopril; co-administration with other antihypertensive drugs may result in additive effect or potentiation).
No products indexed under this heading.

Methyldopa (Co-administration with other antihypertensive drugs may result in additive effect or potentiation). Products include:
Aldoclor Tablets 1881
Aldoril Tablets 1884

Methyldopate Hydrochloride (Co-administration with other antihypertensive drugs may result in additive effect or potentiation).
No products indexed under this heading.

Methylprednisolone Acetate (Corticosteroids intensify electrolyte depletion particularly hypokalemia). Products include:
Depo-Medrol Injectable Suspension 2615
Depo-Medrol Single-Dose Vial 2617

Methylprednisolone Sodium Succinate (Corticosteroids intensify electrolyte depletion particularly hypokalemia).
No products indexed under this heading.

Metocurine Iodide (Possible increased responsiveness to the muscle relaxant).
No products indexed under this heading.

Metolazone (Possible excessive reduction of blood pressure after initiation of lisinopril; co-administration with other antihypertensive drugs may result in additive effect or potentiation).
No products indexed under this heading.

Metoprolol Succinate (Co-administration with other antihypertensive drugs may result in additive effect or potentiation). Products include:
Toprol-XL Tablets 660

Metoprolol Tartrate (Co-administration with other antihypertensive drugs may result in additive effect or potentiation).
No products indexed under this heading.

Metyrosine (Co-administration with other antihypertensive drugs may result in additive effect or potentiation). Products include:
Demser Capsules 1933

Mibefradil Dihydrochloride (Co-administration with other antihypertensive drugs may result in additive effect or potentiation).
No products indexed under this heading.

Miglitol (Hydrochlorothiazide produces hyperglycemia; dosage adjustment of the antidiabetic agent may be required).
No products indexed under this heading.

Minoxidil (Co-administration with other antihypertensive drugs may result in additive effect or potentiation). Products include:
Men's Rogaine Extra Strength Topical Solution, Ocean Rush Scent and Original Unscented 706
Women's Rogaine Topical Solution, Spring Bloom Scent and Original Unscented 707

Mivacurium Chloride (Possible increased responsiveness to the muscle relaxant). Products include:
Mivacron Injection 489

Moexipril Hydrochloride (Co-administration with other antihypertensive drugs may result in additive effect or potentiation). Products include:
Uniretic Tablets 3114
Univasc Tablets 3118

Morphine Sulfate (Potentiation of orthostatic hypotension may occur). Products include:
Avinza Capsules 1714
Kadian Capsules 572
MS Contin Tablets 2703

Nabumetone (Co-administration of non-steroidal anti-inflammatory agents can reduce the diuretic, natriuretic, and antihypertensive effects; possible further deterioration of renal function). Products include:
Relafen Tablets 1523

Nadolol (Co-administration with other antihypertensive drugs may result in additive effect or potentiation). Products include:
Nadolol Tablets 2121

Naproxen (Co-administration of non-steroidal anti-inflammatory agents can reduce the diuretic, natriuretic, and antihypertensive effects; possible further deterioration of renal function). Products include:
EC-Naprosyn Delayed-Release Tablets 2769
Naprosyn Suspension 2769
Naprosyn Tablets 2769
Prevacid NapraPAC 3277

Naproxen Sodium (Co-administration of non-steroidal anti-inflammatory agents can reduce the diuretic, natriuretic, and antihypertensive effects; possible further deterioration of renal function). Products include:
Aleve Tablets, Caplets and Gelcaps 605
Anaprox Tablets 2769
Anaprox DS Tablets 2769

Nicardipine Hydrochloride (Co-administration with other antihypertensive drugs may result in additive effect or potentiation). Products include:
Cardene I.V. 1129

Nifedipine (Co-administration with other antihypertensive drugs may result in additive effect or potentiation). Products include:
Adalat CC Tablets 2978

Nisoldipine (Co-administration with other antihypertensive drugs may result in additive effect or potentiation). Products include:
Sular Tablets 1163

Nitroglycerin (Co-administration with other antihypertensive drugs may result in additive effect or potentiation). Products include:
Nitro-Dur Transdermal Infusion System 3060
Nitrolingual Pumpspray 1161

Norepinephrine Bitartrate (Possible decreased response to pressor amines).
No products indexed under this heading.

Oxaprozin (Co-administration of non-steroidal anti-inflammatory agents can reduce the diuretic, natriuretic, and antihypertensive effects; possible further deterioration of renal function).
No products indexed under this heading.

Oxycodone Hydrochloride (Potentiation of orthostatic hypotension may occur). Products include:
Combunox Tablets 1183
OxyContin Tablets 2699
OxyFast Oral Concentrate Solution 2704
OxyIR Capsules 2704
Percocet Tablets 1114
Percodan Tablets 1115

Pancuronium Bromide (Possible increased responsiveness to the muscle relaxant).
No products indexed under this heading.

Penbutolol Sulfate (Co-administration with other antihypertensive drugs may result in additive effect or potentiation).
No products indexed under this heading.

Pentobarbital Sodium (Potentiation of orthostatic hypotension may occur). Products include:
Nembutal Sodium Solution, USP 2484

Perindopril Erbumine (Co-administration with other antihypertensive drugs may result in additive effect or potentiation). Products include:
Aceon Tablets (2 mg, 4 mg, 8 mg) 3191

Phenobarbital (Potentiation of orthostatic hypotension may occur).
No products indexed under this heading.

Phenoxybenzamine Hydrochloride (Co-administration with other antihypertensive drugs may result in additive effect or potentiation). Products include:
Dibenzyline Capsules 3390

Phentolamine Mesylate (Co-administration with other antihypertensive drugs may result in additive effect or potentiation).
No products indexed under this heading.

Phenylbutazone (Co-administration of non-steroidal anti-inflammatory agents can reduce the diuretic, natriuretic, and antihypertensive effects; possible further deterioration of renal function).
No products indexed under this heading.

Pindolol (Co-administration with other antihypertensive drugs may result in additive effect or potentiation).
No products indexed under this heading.

Pioglitazone Hydrochloride (Hydrochlorothiazide produces hyperglycemia; dosage adjustment of the antidiabetic agent may be required). Products include:
ActoPlus Met Tablets 3219
Actos Tablets 3224

Piroxicam (Co-administration of non-steroidal anti-inflammatory agents can reduce the diuretic, natriuretic, and antihypertensive effects; possible further deterioration of renal function).
No products indexed under this heading.

Polythiazide (Possible excessive reduction of blood pressure after initiation of lisinopril; co-administration with other antihypertensive drugs may result in additive effect or potentiation).
No products indexed under this heading.

Potassium Acid Phosphate (Concurrent use with potassium sparing diuretic may result in increased risk of hyperkalemia). Products include:
K-Phos Original (Sodium Free) Tablets 785

Potassium Bicarbonate (Concurrent use with potassium sparing diuretic may result in increased risk of hyperkalemia).
No products indexed under this heading.

Potassium Chloride (Concurrent use with potassium sparing diuretic may result in increased risk of hyperkalemia). Products include:
Colyte with Flavor Packs for Oral Solution 3102
HalfLytely and Bisacodyl Tablets Bowel Prep Kit with Flavors Packs 915
K-Dur Extended-Relase Tablets 3047
K-Lor Powder Packets 472
K-Tab Filmtab Tablets 473
TriLyte with Flavor Packs for Oral Solution 3114

Potassium Citrate (Concurrent use with potassium sparing diuretic may result in increased risk of hyperkalemia). Products include:
Urocit-K Tablets 2109

Potassium Gluconate (Concurrent use with potassium sparing diuretic may result in increased risk of hyperkalemia).
No products indexed under this heading.

Potassium Phosphate (Concurrent use with potassium sparing diuretic may result in increased risk of hyperkalemia). Products include:
K-Phos Neutral Tablets 785

Prazosin Hydrochloride (Co-administration with other antihypertensive drugs may result in additive effect or potentiation).
No products indexed under this heading.

Prednisolone Acetate (Corticosteroids intensify electrolyte depletion particularly hypokalemia). Products include:
Blephamide Ophthalmic Ointment 563
Blephamide Ophthalmic Suspension 564
Poly-Pred Liquifilm Ophthalmic Suspension .... ⊙ 231
Pred Forte Ophthalmic Suspension .... ⊙ 233
Pred Mild Sterile Ophthalmic Suspension .... ⊙ 236
Pred-G Ophthalmic Suspension .... ⊙ 234
Pred-G Sterile Ophthalmic Ointment .... ⊙ 235

Prednisolone Sodium Phosphate (Corticosteroids intensify electrolyte depletion particularly hypokalemia). Products include:
Pediapred Oral Solution 3319

Prednisolone Tebutate (Corticosteroids intensify electrolyte depletion particularly hypokalemia).
No products indexed under this heading.

Prednisone (Corticosteroids intensify electrolyte depletion particularly hypokalemia).
No products indexed under this heading.

Propoxyphene Hydrochloride (Potentiation of orthostatic hypotension may occur).
No products indexed under this heading.

Propoxyphene Napsylate (Potentiation of orthostatic hypotension may occur). Products include:
Darvocet A 500 Tablets 3497

Propranolol Hydrochloride (Co-administration with other antihypertensive drugs may result in additive effect or potentiation). Products include:
Inderal LA Long-Acting Capsules 3421
InnoPran XL Capsules 2728

Quinapril Hydrochloride (Co-administration with other antihypertensive drugs may result in additive effect or potentiation).
No products indexed under this heading.

Ramipril (Co-administration with other antihypertensive drugs may result in additive effect or potentiation). Products include:
Altace Capsules 1673

Rapacuronium Bromide (Possible increased responsiveness to the muscle relaxant).
No products indexed under this heading.

Rauwolfia Serpentina (Co-administration with other antihypertensive drugs may result in additive effect or potentiation).
No products indexed under this heading.

Remifentanil Hydrochloride (Potentiation of orthostatic hypotension may occur).
No products indexed under this heading.

Repaglinide (Hydrochlorothiazide produces hyperglycemia; dosage adjustment of the antidiabetic agent may be required). Products include:
Prandin Tablets (0.5, 1, and 2 mg) 2337

Rescinnamine (Co-administration with other antihypertensive drugs may result in additive effect or potentiation).
No products indexed under this heading.

Reserpine (Co-administration with other antihypertensive drugs may result in additive effect or potentiation).
No products indexed under this heading.

Rocuronium Bromide (Possible increased responsiveness to the muscle relaxant). Products include:
Zemuron Injection 2363

Rofecoxib (Co-administration of non-steroidal anti-inflammatory agents can reduce the diuretic, natriuretic, and antihypertensive effects; possible further deterioration of renal function).
No products indexed under this heading.

Rosiglitazone Maleate (Hydrochlorothiazide produces hyperglycemia; dosage adjustment of the antidiabetic agent may be required). Products include:
Avandamet Tablets 1343
Avandia Tablets 1348

Secobarbital Sodium (Potentiation of orthostatic hypotension may occur).
No products indexed under this heading.

Sodium Nitroprusside (Co-administration with other antihypertensive drugs may result in additive effect or potentiation).
No products indexed under this heading.

Sotalol Hydrochloride (Co-administration with other antihypertensive drugs may result in additive effect or potentiation).
No products indexed under this heading.

Spirapril Hydrochloride (Co-administration with other antihypertensive drugs may result in additive effect or potentiation).
No products indexed under this heading.

Spironolactone (Concurrent use with potassium sparing diuretic may result in increased risk of hyperkalemia; co-administration with other antihypertensive drugs may result in additive effect or potentiation).
No products indexed under this heading.

Sufentanil Citrate (Potentiation of orthostatic hypotension may occur).
No products indexed under this heading.

Sulindac (Co-administration of non-steroidal anti-inflammatory agents can reduce the diuretic, natriuretic, and antihypertensive effects; possible further deterioration of renal function). Products include:
Clinoril Tablets 1899

Telmisartan (Co-administration with other antihypertensive drugs may result in additive effect or potentiation). Products include:
Micardis Tablets 884
Micardis HCT Tablets 886

Terazosin Hydrochloride (Co-administration with other antihypertensive drugs may result in additive effect or potentiation). Products include:
Hytrin Capsules 469

Thiamylal Sodium (Potentiation of orthostatic hypotension may occur).
No products indexed under this heading.

Timolol Maleate (Co-administration with other antihypertensive drugs may result in additive effect or potentiation). Products include:
Blocadren Tablets 1891
Cosopt Sterile Ophthalmic Solution 1910
Timolide Tablets 2056
Timoptic in Ocudose 2061
Timoptic Sterile Ophthalmic Solution 2058
Timoptic-XE Sterile Ophthalmic Gel Forming Solution 2062

Tolazamide (Hydrochlorothiazide produces hyperglycemia; dosage adjustment of the antidiabetic agent may be required).
No products indexed under this heading.

Tolbutamide (Hydrochlorothiazide produces hyperglycemia; dosage adjustment of the antidiabetic agent may be required).
No products indexed under this heading.

Tolmetin Sodium (Co-administration of non-steroidal anti-inflammatory agents can reduce the diuretic, natriuretic, and antihypertensive effects; possible further deterioration of renal function).
No products indexed under this heading.

Torsemide (Possible excessive reduction of blood pressure after initiation of lisinopril; co-administration with other antihypertensive drugs may result in additive effect or potentiation).
No products indexed under this heading.

Trandolapril (Co-administration with other antihypertensive drugs may result in additive effect or potentiation). Products include:
Mavik Tablets 482
Tarka Tablets 519

Triamcinolone (Corticosteroids intensify electrolyte depletion particularly hypokalemia).
No products indexed under this heading.

Triamcinolone Acetonide (Corticosteroids intensify electrolyte depletion particularly hypokalemia). Products include:
Azmacort Inhalation Aerosol 1701
Nasacort HFA Inhalation Aerosol 2939
Nasacort AQ Nasal Spray 2937

Triamcinolone Diacetate (Corticosteroids intensify electrolyte depletion particularly hypokalemia).
No products indexed under this heading.

Triamcinolone Hexacetonide (Corticosteroids intensify electrolyte depletion particularly hypokalemia).
No products indexed under this heading.

Triamterene (Concurrent use with potassium sparing diuretic may result in increased risk of hyperkalemia; co-administration with other antihypertensive drugs may result in additive effect or potentiation). Products include:
Dyazide Capsules 1389
Dyrenium Capsules 3390
Maxzide 2150

Trimethaphan Camsylate (Co-administration with other antihypertensive drugs may result in additive effect or potentiation).
No products indexed under this heading.

Troglitazone (Hydrochlorothiazide produces hyperglycemia; dosage adjustment of the antidiabetic agent may be required).
No products indexed under this heading.

Tubocurarine Chloride (Possible increased responsiveness to the muscle relaxant).
No products indexed under this heading.

Valdecoxib (Co-administration of non-steroidal anti-inflammatory agents can reduce the diuretic, natriuretic, and antihypertensive effects; possible further deterioration of renal function).
No products indexed under this heading.

Valsartan (Co-administration with other antihypertensive drugs may result in additive effect or potentiation). Products include:
Diovan HCT Tablets ... 2195
Diovan Tablets ... 2191

Vecuronium Bromide (Possible increased responsiveness to the muscle relaxant).
No products indexed under this heading.

Verapamil Hydrochloride (Co-administration with other antihypertensive drugs may result in additive effect or potentiation). Products include:
Covera-HS Tablets ... 3135
Tarka Tablets ... 519
Verelan PM Capsules ... 3120

Food Interactions

Alcohol (Potentiation of orthostatic hypotension may occur).

ZESTRIL TABLETS

(Lisinopril) ... 704
May interact with diuretics, lithium preparations, non-steroidal anti-inflammatory agents, potassium preparations, potassium sparing diuretics, thiazides, and certain other agents. Compounds in these categories include:

Amiloride Hydrochloride (Potential for significant hyperkalemia; possibility of excessive reduction in blood pressure). Products include:
Midamor Tablets ... 2000
Moduretic Tablets ... 2003

Bendroflumethiazide (Thiazide-induced potassium loss attenuated; possibility of excessive reduction in blood pressure).
No products indexed under this heading.

Bumetanide (Possibility of excessive reduction in blood pressure).
No products indexed under this heading.

Celecoxib (In some patients with compromised renal function who are being treated with non-steroidal anti-inflammatory drugs, the co-administration of lisinopril may result in further deterioration of renal function; these effects are usually reversible). Products include:
Celebrex Capsules ... 3130

Chlorothiazide (Thiazide-induced potassium loss attenuated; possibility of excessive reduction in blood pressure). Products include:
Aldoclor Tablets ... 1881
Diuril Oral ... 1936

Chlorothiazide Sodium (Thiazide-induced potassium loss attenuated; possibility of excessive reduction in blood pressure). Products include:
Diuril Sodium Intravenous ... 1934

Chlorthalidone (Possibility of excessive reduction in blood pressure). Products include:
Clorpres Tablets ... 2139

Diclofenac Potassium (In some patients with compromised renal function who are being treated with non-steroidal anti-inflammatory drugs, the co-administration of lisinopril may result in further deterioration of renal function; these effects are usually reversible). Products include:
Cataflam Tablets ... 2173

Diclofenac Sodium (In some patients with compromised renal function who are being treated with non-steroidal anti-inflammatory drugs, the co-administration of lisinopril may result in further deterioration of renal function; these effects are usually reversible). Products include:
Arthrotec Tablets ... 3126
Voltaren Ophthalmic Solution ... 2300
Voltaren Tablets ... 2298
Voltaren-XR Tablets ... 2301

Ethacrynic Acid (Possibility of excessive reduction in blood pressure). Products include:
Edecrin Tablets ... 1941

Etodolac (In some patients with compromised renal function who are being treated with non-steroidal anti-inflammatory drugs, the co-administration of lisinopril may result in further deterioration of renal function; these effects are usually reversible).
No products indexed under this heading.

Fenoprofen Calcium (In some patients with compromised renal function who are being treated with non-steroidal anti-inflammatory drugs, the co-administration of lisinopril may result in further deterioration of renal function; these effects are usually reversible). Products include:
Nalfon Capsules ... 2504

Flurbiprofen (In some patients with compromised renal function who are being treated with non-steroidal anti-inflammatory drugs, the co-administration of lisinopril may result in further deterioration of renal function; these effects are usually reversible).
No products indexed under this heading.

Furosemide (Possibility of excessive reduction in blood pressure). Products include:
Furosemide Tablets ... 2117

Hydrochlorothiazide (Thiazide-induced potassium loss attenuated; possibility of excessive reduction in blood pressure). Products include:
Aldoril Tablets ... 1884
Atacand HCT ... 637
Avalide Tablets ... 2889
Avalide Tablets ... 922
Benicar HCT Tablets ... 2852
Diovan HCT Tablets ... 2195
Dyazide Capsules ... 1389
Hyzaar ... 1964
Lotensin HCT Tablets ... 2235
Maxzide ... 2150
Micardis HCT Tablets ... 886
Moduretic Tablets ... 2003
Prinzide Tablets ... 2033
Teveten HCT Tablets ... 1710
Timolide Tablets ... 2056
Uniretic Tablets ... 3114
Vaseretic Tablets ... 2073
Zestoretic Tablets ... 701

Hydroflumethiazide (Thiazide-induced potassium loss attenuated; possibility of excessive reduction in blood pressure).
No products indexed under this heading.

Ibuprofen (In some patients with compromised renal function who are being treated with non-steroidal anti-inflammatory drugs, the co-administration of lisinopril may result in further deterioration of renal function; these effects are usually reversible). Products include:
Advil Allergy Sinus Caplets ... 737
Advil ... 737
Children's Advil Suspension ... 742
Children's Advil Chewable Tablets ... 741
Advil Cold & Sinus ... 739
Advil Flu & Body Ache Caplets ... 739
Children's Advil Cold Suspension ... 741
Infants' Advil Concentrated Drops ... 743
Junior Strength Advil Swallow Tablets ... 740
Advil Migraine Liquigels ... 740
Advil Multi-Symptom Cold Caplets ... 738
Combunox Tablets ... 1183
Children's Motrin Oral Suspension and Chewable Tablets ... 1837
Children's Motrin Cold Non-Staining Dye-Free Oral Suspension ... 1838
Children's Motrin Cold Oral Suspension ... 1838
Children's Motrin Non-Staining Dye-Free Oral Suspension ... 1837
Motrin Cold & Sinus Caplets ... 1836
Motrin IB Tablets and Caplets ... 1836
Infants' Motrin Concentrated Drops ... 1837
Infants' Motrin Non-Staining Dye-Free Drops ... 1837
Junior Strength Motrin Caplets and Chewable Tablets ... 1837
Vicoprofen Tablets ... 533

Indapamide (Possibility of excessive reduction in blood pressure). Products include:
Indapamide Tablets ... 2119

Indomethacin (Reduces antihypertensive effect). Products include:
Indocin ... 1968

Indomethacin Sodium Trihydrate (Reduces antihypertensive effect). Products include:
Indocin I.V. ... 1973

Ketoprofen (In some patients with compromised renal function who are being treated with non-steroidal anti-inflammatory drugs, the co-administration of lisinopril may result in further deterioration of renal function; these effects are usually reversible).
No products indexed under this heading.

Ketorolac Tromethamine (In some patients with compromised renal function who are being treated with non-steroidal anti-inflammatory drugs, the co-administration of lisinopril may result in further deterioration of renal function; these effects are usually reversible). Products include:
Acular Ophthalmic Solution ... 561
Acular LS Ophthalmic Solution ... 562

Lithium (Possibility of lithium toxicity–serum lithium levels should be monitored frequently).
No products indexed under this heading.

Lithium Carbonate (Possibility of lithium toxicity–serum lithium levels should be monitored frequently). Products include:
Eskalith ... 1406
Lithobid Tablets ... 1670

Lithium Citrate (Possibility of lithium toxicity–serum lithium levels should be monitored frequently).
No products indexed under this heading.

Meclofenamate Sodium (In some patients with compromised renal function who are being treated with non-steroidal anti-inflammatory drugs, the co-administration of lisinopril may result in further deterioration of renal function; these effects are usually reversible).
No products indexed under this heading.

Mefenamic Acid (In some patients with compromised renal function who are being treated with non-steroidal anti-inflammatory drugs, the co-administration of lisinopril may result in further deterioration of renal function; these effects are usually reversible).
No products indexed under this heading.

Meloxicam (In some patients with compromised renal function who are being treated with non-steroidal anti-inflammatory drugs, the co-administration of lisinopril may result in further deterioration of renal function; these effects are usually reversible). Products include:
Mobic Oral Suspension ... 893
Mobic Tablets ... 893

Methyclothiazide (Thiazide-induced potassium loss attenuated; possibility of excessive reduction in blood pressure).
No products indexed under this heading.

Metolazone (Possibility of excessive reduction in blood pressure).
No products indexed under this heading.

Nabumetone (In some patients with compromised renal function who are being treated with non-steroidal anti-inflammatory drugs, the co-administration of lisinopril may result in further deterioration of renal function; these effects are usually reversible). Products include:
Relafen Tablets ... 1523

Naproxen (In some patients with compromised renal function who are being treated with non-steroidal anti-inflammatory drugs, the co-administration of lisinopril may result in further deterioration of renal function; these effects are usually reversible). Products include:
EC-Naprosyn Delayed-Release Tablets ... 2769
Naprosyn Suspension ... 2769
Naprosyn Tablets ... 2769
Prevacid NapraPAC ... 3277

Naproxen Sodium (In some patients with compromised renal function who are being treated with non-steroidal anti-inflammatory drugs, the co-administration of lisinopril may result in further deterioration of renal function; these effects are usually reversible). Products include:
Aleve Tablets, Caplets and Gelcaps ... 605
Anaprox Tablets ... 2769
Anaprox DS Tablets ... 2769

Oxaprozin (In some patients with compromised renal function who are being treated with non-steroidal anti-inflammatory drugs, the co-administration of lisinopril may result in further deterioration of renal function; these effects are usually reversible).
No products indexed under this heading.

Phenylbutazone (In some patients with compromised renal function who are being treated with non-steroidal anti-inflammatory drugs, the co-administration of lisinopril may result in further deterioration of renal function; these effects are usually reversible).
No products indexed under this heading.

Piroxicam (In some patients with compromised renal function who are being treated with non-steroidal anti-inflammatory drugs, the co-administration of lisinopril may result in further deterioration of renal function; these effects are usually reversible).
No products indexed under this heading.

Polythiazide (Thiazide-induced potassium loss attenuated; possibility of excessive reduction in blood pressure).
No products indexed under this heading.

Potassium Acid Phosphate (Potential for significant hyperkalemia). Products include:
K-Phos Original (Sodium Free) Tablets 785

Potassium Bicarbonate (Potential for significant hyperkalemia).
No products indexed under this heading.

Potassium Chloride (Potential for significant hyperkalemia). Products include:
Colyte with Flavor Packs for Oral Solution 3102
HalfLytely and Bisacodyl Tablets Bowel Prep Kit with Flavors Packs 915
K-Dur Extended-Relase Tablets 3047
K-Lor Powder Packets 472
K-Tab Filmtab Tablets 473
TriLyte with Flavor Packs for Oral Solution 3114

Potassium Citrate (Potential for significant hyperkalemia). Products include:
Urocit-K Tablets 2109

Potassium Gluconate (Potential for significant hyperkalemia).
No products indexed under this heading.

Potassium Phosphate (Potential for significant hyperkalemia). Products include:
K-Phos Neutral Tablets 785

Rofecoxib (In some patients with compromised renal function who are being treated with non-steroidal anti-inflammatory drugs, the co-administration of lisinopril may result in further deterioration of renal function; these effects are usually reversible).
No products indexed under this heading.

Spironolactone (Potential for significant hyperkalemia; possibility of excessive reduction in blood pressure).
No products indexed under this heading.

Sulindac (In some patients with compromised renal function who are being treated with non-steroidal anti-inflammatory drugs, the co-administration of lisinopril may result in further deterioration of renal function; these effects are usually reversible). Products include:
Clinoril Tablets 1899

Tolmetin Sodium (In some patients with compromised renal function who are being treated with non-steroidal anti-inflammatory drugs, the co-administration of lisinopril may result in further deterioration of renal function; these effects are usually reversible).
No products indexed under this heading.

Torsemide (Possibility of excessive reduction in blood pressure).
No products indexed under this heading.

Triamterene (Potential for significant hyperkalemia; possibility of excessive reduction in blood pressure). Products include:
Dyazide Capsules 1389
Dyrenium Capsules 3390
Maxzide 2150

Valdecoxib (In some patients with compromised renal function who are being treated with non-steroidal anti-inflammatory drugs, the co-administration of lisinopril may result in further deterioration of renal function; these effects are usually reversible).
No products indexed under this heading.

ZETIA TABLETS

(Ezetimibe) 2090
May interact with fibrates and certain other agents. Compounds in these categories include:

Cholestyramine (Co-administration decreased the mean AUC of total ezetimibe by approximately 55%. Incremental LDL-C reduction may be reduced).
No products indexed under this heading.

Clofibrate (Concurrent use is not recommended).
No products indexed under this heading.

Cyclosporine (Caution should be exercised when initiating ezetimibe in patients treated with cyclosporine due to increased exposure to ezetimibe. This exposure may be greater in patients with severe renal insufficiency). Products include:
Gengraf Capsules 458
Neoral Soft Gelatin Capsules 2247
Neoral Oral Solution 2247
Restasis Ophthalmic Emulsion 570
Sandimmune 2259

Fenofibrate (Co-administration increased total ezetimibe by approximately 1.5-fold. Concurrent use of fibrates is not recommended). Products include:
Antara Capsules 2723
Lofibra Capsules 1217
Tricor Tablets 523
Triglide Tablets 1165

Gemfibrozil (Co-administration increased total ezetimibe by approximately 1.7-fold).
No products indexed under this heading.

Warfarin Sodium (There have been post-marketing reports of increased INR in patients who had ezetimibe added to warfarin. Most of these patients were also on other medications). Products include:
Coumadin for Injection 932
Coumadin Tablets 932

ZETIA TABLETS

(Ezetimibe) 3098
May interact with fibrates, HMG-CoA reductase inhibitors, and certain other agents. Compounds in these categories include:

Atorvastatin Calcium (In controlled clinical studies of ezetimbe initiated concurrently with an HMG-CoA reductase inhibitor, the incidence of consecutive elevations (greater than or equal to 3 x ULN) in serum transaminases was 1.3% for patients treated with ezetimbe administered with HMG-CoA reductase inhibitors and 0.4% for patients treated with HMG-CoA reductase inhibitors alone. When ezetimbe is co-administered with an HMG-CoA reductase inhibitor, liver function tests should be performed at initiation of therapy and according to the recommendations of the HMG-CoA reductase inhibitor. The combination of ezetimbe with a HMG-CoA inhibitor is contraindicated in patients with active liver disease or unexplained persistent elevations in serum transaminases). Products include:
Caduet Tablets 2507
Lipitor Tablets 2495

Cerivastatin Sodium (In controlled clinical studies of ezetimbe initiated concurrently with an HMG-CoA reductase inhibitor, the incidence of consecutive elevations (greater than or equal to 3 x ULN) in serum transaminases was 1.3% for patients treated with ezetimbe administered with HMG-CoA reductase inhibitors and 0.4% for patients treated with HMG-CoA reductase inhibitors alone. When ezetimbe is co-administered with an HMG-CoA reductase inhibitor, liver function tests should be performed at initiation of therapy and according to the recommendations of the HMG-CoA reductase inhibitor. The combination of ezetimbe with a HMG-CoA inhibitor is contraindicated in patients with active liver disease or unexplained persistent elevations in serum transaminases).
No products indexed under this heading.

Cholestyramine (Co-administration decreased the mean AUC of total ezetimibe by approximately 55%. Incremental LDL-C reduction may be reduced).
No products indexed under this heading.

Clofibrate (The safety and effectiveness of ezetimbe administration with fibrates has not been established. Co-administration of ezetimbe with fibrates is not recommended until use in patients is studied).
No products indexed under this heading.

Cyclosporine (Caution should be exercised when initiating ezetimibe in patients treated with cyclosporine due to increased exposure to ezetimibe. This exposure may be greater in patients with severe renal insufficiency). Products include:
Gengraf Capsules 458
Neoral Soft Gelatin Capsules 2247
Neoral Oral Solution 2247
Restasis Ophthalmic Emulsion 570
Sandimmune 2259

Fenofibrate (Co-administration increased total ezetimibe concentrations by approximately 1.5-fold. Concurrent use of fibrates is not recommended). Products include:
Antara Capsules 2723
Lofibra Capsules 1217
Tricor Tablets 523
Triglide Tablets 1165

Fluvastatin Sodium (In controlled clinical studies of ezetimbe initiated concurrently with an HMG-CoA reductase inhibitor, the incidence of consecutive elevations (greater than or equal to 3 x ULN) in serum transaminases was 1.3% for patients treated with ezetimbe administered with HMG-CoA reductase inhibitors and 0.4% for patients treated with HMG-CoA reductase inhibitors alone. When ezetimbe is co-administered with an HMG-CoA reductase inhibitor, liver function tests should be performed at initiation of therapy and according to the recommendations of the HMG-CoA reductase inhibitor. The combination of ezetimbe with a HMG-CoA inhibitor is contraindicated in patients with active liver disease or unexplained persistent elevations in serum transaminases). Products include:
Lescol Capsules 2227
Lescol 2730
Lescol XL Tablets 2227

Gemfibrozil (Co-administration increased total ezetimbe concentrations by approximately 1.7-fold).
No products indexed under this heading.

Lovastatin (In controlled clinical studies of ezetimbe initiated concurrently with an HMG-CoA reductase inhibitor, the incidence of consecutive elevations (greater than or equal to 3 x ULN) in serum transaminases was 1.3% for patients treated with ezetimbe administered with HMG-CoA reductase inhibitors and 0.4% for patients treated with HMG-CoA reductase inhibitors alone. When ezetimbe is co-administered with an HMG-CoA reductase inhibitor, liver function tests should be performed at initiation of therapy and according to the recommendations of the HMG-CoA reductase inhibitor. The combination of ezetimbe with a HMG-CoA inhibitor is contraindicated in patients with active liver disease or unexplained persistent elevations in serum transaminases). Products include:
Advicor Tablets 1694
Altoprev Extended-Release Tablets 1151
Mevacor Tablets 1996

Pravastatin Sodium (In controlled clinical studies of ezetimbe initiated concurrently with an HMG-CoA reductase inhibitor, the incidence of consecutive elevations (greater than or equal to 3 x ULN) in serum transaminases was 1.3% for patients treated with ezetimbe administered with HMG-CoA reductase inhibitors and 0.4% for patients treated with HMG-CoA reductase inhibitors alone. When ezetimbe is co-administered with an HMG-CoA reductase inhibitor, liver function tests should be performed at initiation of therapy and according to the recommendations of the HMG-CoA reductase inhibitor. The combination of ezetimbe with a HMG-CoA inhibitor is contraindicated in patients with active liver disease or unexplained persistent elevations in serum transaminases). Products include:

Pravachol Tablets 943

Simvastatin (In controlled clinical studies of ezetimbe initiated concurrently with an HMG-CoA reductase inhibitor, the incidence of consecutive elevations (greater than or equal to 3 x ULN) in serum transaminases was 1.3% for patients treated with ezetimbe administered with HMG-CoA reductase inhibitors and 0.4% for patients treated with HMG-CoA reductase inhibitors alone. When ezetimbe is co-administered with an HMG-CoA reductase inhibitor, liver function tests should be performed at initiation of therapy and according to the recommendations of the HMG-CoA reductase inhibitor. The combination of ezetimbe with a HMG-CoA inhibitor is contraindicated in patients with active liver disease or unexplained persistent elevations in serum transaminases). Products include:

Vytorin 10/10 Tablets 2084
Vytorin 10/10 Tablets 3092
Vytorin 10/20 Tablets 2084
Vytorin 10/20 Tablets 3092
Vytorin 10/40 Tablets 3092
Vytorin 10/40 Tablets 2084
Vytorin 10/80 Tablets 2084
Vytorin 10/80 Tablets 3092
Zocor Tablets 2078

ZEVALIN INJECTION

(Ibritumomab Tiuxetan) 848
None cited in PDR database.

ZIAGEN ORAL SOLUTION

(Abacavir Sulfate) 1600
See Ziagen Tablets

ZIAGEN TABLETS

(Abacavir Sulfate) 1600
May interact with:

Methadone Hydrochloride (Co-administration in patients on methadone-maintenance therapy has resulted in increased methadone clearance by 22%; this alteration will not result in a methadone dose modification in the majority of patients; however, an increased methadone dose may be required in a small number of patients).
No products indexed under this heading.

Food Interactions

Alcohol (Decreases the elimination of abacavir causing an increase in overall exposure).

ZICAM ALLERGY RELIEF NASAL PUMP

(Galphimia Glauca, Histanium Hydrochloricum, Luffa operculata, Sulfur)...
None cited in PDR database.

ZICAM COLD REMEDY CHEWABLES

(Zincum Aceticum, Zincum Gluconicum)...
None cited in PDR database.

ZICAM COLD REMEDY NASAL PUMP

(Zincum Gluconicum) ....
None cited in PDR database.

ZICAM COLD REMEDY ORAL MIST

(Zincum Aceticum, Zincum Gluconicum)...
None cited in PDR database.

ZICAM COLD REMEDY RAPIDMELTS

(Zincum Aceticum, Zincum Gluconicum)...
None cited in PDR database.

ZICAM COLD REMEDY SWABS

(Zincum Gluconicum) ....
None cited in PDR database.

ZICAM COLD REMEDY SWABS KIDS SIZE

(Zincum Gluconicum) ....
None cited in PDR database.

ZICAM CONCENTRATED COUGH MIST FOR KIDS COOL CHERRY

(Dextromethorphan Hydrobromide)............................... 643
May interact with monoamine oxidase inhibitors. Compounds in these categories include:

Isocarboxazid (Do not use with, or for two weeks after stopping, MAOI drugs).
No products indexed under this heading.

Moclobemide (Do not use with, or for two weeks after stopping, MAOI drugs).
No products indexed under this heading.

Pargyline Hydrochloride (Do not use with, or for two weeks after stopping, MAOI drugs).
No products indexed under this heading.

Phenelzine Sulfate (Do not use with, or for two weeks after stopping, MAOI drugs).
No products indexed under this heading.

Procarbazine Hydrochloride (Do not use with, or for two weeks after stopping, MAOI drugs). Products include:
Matulane Capsules 3188

Selegiline Hydrochloride (Do not use with, or for two weeks after stopping, MAOI drugs). Products include:
Eldepryl Capsules 3209

Tranylcypromine Sulfate (Do not use with, or for two weeks after stopping, MAOI drugs). Products include:
Parnate Tablets 1499

ZICAM CONCENTRATED COUGH MIST FOR KIDS PLUS D COOL CHERRY

(Dextromethorphan Hydrobromide, Phenylephrine Hydrochloride)................................ 643
May interact with monoamine oxidase inhibitors. Compounds in these categories include:

Isocarboxazid (Do not use with, or for two weeks after stopping, MAOI drugs).
No products indexed under this heading.

Moclobemide (Do not use with, or for two weeks after stopping, MAOI drugs).
No products indexed under this heading.

Pargyline Hydrochloride (Do not use with, or for two weeks after stopping, MAOI drugs).
No products indexed under this heading.

Phenelzine Sulfate (Do not use with, or for two weeks after stopping, MAOI drugs).
No products indexed under this heading.

Procarbazine Hydrochloride (Do not use with, or for two weeks after stopping, MAOI drugs). Products include:
Matulane Capsules 3188

Selegiline Hydrochloride (Do not use with, or for two weeks after stopping, MAOI drugs). Products include:
Eldepryl Capsules 3209

Tranylcypromine Sulfate (Do not use with, or for two weeks after stopping, MAOI drugs). Products include:
Parnate Tablets 1499

ZICAM CONCENTRATED COUGH MIST NITE-COOL CHERRY

(Dextromethorphan Hydrobromide)................................ 642
May interact with monoamine oxidase inhibitors. Compounds in these categories include:

Isocarboxazid (Do not use with, or for two weeks after stopping, MAOI drugs).
No products indexed under this heading.

Moclobemide (Do not use with, or for two weeks after stopping, MAOI drugs).
No products indexed under this heading.

Pargyline Hydrochloride (Do not use with, or for two weeks after stopping, MAOI drugs).
No products indexed under this heading.

Phenelzine Sulfate (Do not use with, or for two weeks after stopping, MAOI drugs).
No products indexed under this heading.

Procarbazine Hydrochloride (Do not use with, or for two weeks after stopping, MAOI drugs). Products include:
Matulane Capsules 3188

Selegiline Hydrochloride (Do not use with, or for two weeks after stopping, MAOI drugs). Products include:
Eldepryl Capsules 3209

Tranylcypromine Sulfate (Do not use with, or for two weeks after stopping, MAOI drugs). Products include:
Parnate Tablets 1499

ZICAM CONCENTRATED COUGH MIST PLUS D COOL CHERRY

(Dextromethorphan Hydrobromide, Phenylephrine Hydrochloride)................................ 642
May interact with monoamine oxidase inhibitors. Compounds in these categories include:

Isocarboxazid (Do not use with, or for two weeks after stopping, MAOI drugs).
No products indexed under this heading.

Moclobemide (Do not use with, or for two weeks after stopping, MAOI drugs).
No products indexed under this heading.

Pargyline Hydrochloride (Do not use with, or for two weeks after stopping, MAOI drugs).
No products indexed under this heading.

Phenelzine Sulfate (Do not use with, or for two weeks after stopping, MAOI drugs).
No products indexed under this heading.

Procarbazine Hydrochloride (Do not use with, or for two weeks after stopping, MAOI drugs). Products include:
Matulane Capsules 3188

Selegiline Hydrochloride (Do not use with, or for two weeks after stopping, MAOI drugs). Products include:
Eldepryl Capsules 3209

Tranylcypromine Sulfate (Do not use with, or for two weeks after stopping, MAOI drugs). Products include:
Parnate Tablets 1499

ZICAM CONCENTRATED COUGH MIST-HONEY LEMON & COOL CHERRY

(Dextromethorphan Hydrobromide)................................ 642
May interact with monoamine oxidase inhibitors. Compounds in these categories include:

Isocarboxazid (Do not use with, or for two weeks after stopping, MAOI drugs).
No products indexed under this heading.

Moclobemide (Do not use with, or for two weeks after stopping, MAOI drugs).
No products indexed under this heading.

Pargyline Hydrochloride (Do not use with, or for two weeks after stopping, MAOI drugs).
No products indexed under this heading.

Phenelzine Sulfate (Do not use with, or for two weeks after stopping, MAOI drugs).
No products indexed under this heading.

Procarbazine Hydrochloride (Do not use with, or for two weeks after stopping, MAOI drugs). Products include:
Matulane Capsules 3188

Selegiline Hydrochloride (Do not use with, or for two weeks after stopping, MAOI drugs). Products include:
Eldepryl Capsules 3209

Tranylcypromine Sulfate (Do not use with, or for two weeks after stopping, MAOI drugs). Products include:
Parnate Tablets 1499

ZICAM EXTREME CONGESTION RELIEF NASAL PUMP

(Oxymetazoline Hydrochloride) ....
None cited in PDR database.

ZICAM NO-DRIP LIQUID NASAL MOISTURIZER

(Glycerin) 643
None cited in PDR database.

ZICAM SINUS RELIEF NASAL PUMP

(Oxymetazoline Hydrochloride) ....
None cited in PDR database.

ZINACEF INJECTION
(Cefuroxime) 1604
May interact with aminoglycosides, oral anticoagulants, and certain other agents. Compounds in these categories include:

Amikacin Sulfate (Concomitant administration may produce nephrotoxicity).
No products indexed under this heading.

Anisindione (Cephalosporins may be associated with a fall in prothrombin activity; those at risk include patients stabilized on anticoagulants). Products include:
Miradon Tablets 3056

Dicumarol (Cephalosporins may be associated with a fall in prothrombin activity; those at risk include patients stabilized on anticoagulants).
No products indexed under this heading.

Gentamicin Sulfate (Concomitant administration may produce nephrotoxicity). Products include:
Garamycin Injectable 3028
Genoptic Sterile Ophthalmic Solution.. ⊙227
Pred-G Ophthalmic Suspension ...... ⊙234
Pred-G Sterile Ophthalmic Ointment.. ⊙235

Kanamycin Sulfate (Concomitant administration may produce nephrotoxicity).
No products indexed under this heading.

Probenecid (Concurrent administration of probenecid decreases renal clearance and increases peak serum levels of cefuroxime).
No products indexed under this heading.

Streptomycin Sulfate (Concomitant administration may produce nephrotoxicity).
No products indexed under this heading.

Tobramycin (Concomitant administration may produce nephrotoxicity). Products include:
TOBI Solution for Inhalation 1015
TobraDex Ophthalmic Ointment 558
TobraDex Ophthalmic Suspension ... 558
Zylet Ophthalmic Suspension 3508

Tobramycin Sulfate (Concomitant administration may produce nephrotoxicity).
No products indexed under this heading.

Warfarin Sodium (Cephalosporins may be associated with a fall in prothrombin activity; those at risk include patients stabilized on anticoagulants). Products include:
Coumadin for Injection 932
Coumadin Tablets 932

ZINACEF FOR INJECTION
(Cefuroxime) 1604
See Zinacef Injection

ZINC-220 CAPSULES
(Zinc Sulfate) 576
None cited in PDR database.

ZINECARD FOR INJECTION
(Dexrazoxane) 2659
May interact with antineoplastics and certain other agents. Compounds in these categories include:

Altretamine (Dexrazoxane may add to the myelosuppression caused by chemotherapeutic agents). Products include:
Hexalen Capsules 2101

Anastrozole (Dexrazoxane may add to the myelosuppression caused by chemotherapeutic agents). Products include:
Arimidex Tablets 665

Asparaginase (Dexrazoxane may add to the myelosuppression caused by chemotherapeutic agents). Products include:
Elspar for Injection 1943

Bicalutamide (Dexrazoxane may add to the myelosuppression caused by chemotherapeutic agents). Products include:
Casodex Tablets 670

Bleomycin Sulfate (Dexrazoxane may add to the myelosuppression caused by chemotherapeutic agents).
No products indexed under this heading.

Busulfan (Dexrazoxane may add to the myelosuppression caused by chemotherapeutic agents). Products include:
I.V. Busulfex 1125
Myleran Tablets 1492

Carboplatin (Dexrazoxane may add to the myelosuppression caused by chemotherapeutic agents).
No products indexed under this heading.

Carmustine (BCNU) (Dexrazoxane may add to the myelosuppression caused by chemotherapeutic agents).
No products indexed under this heading.

Chlorambucil (Dexrazoxane may add to the myelosuppression caused by chemotherapeutic agents). Products include:
Leukeran Tablets 1472

Cisplatin (Dexrazoxane may add to the myelosuppression caused by chemotherapeutic agents).
No products indexed under this heading.

Cyclophosphamide (Use of dexrazoxane concurrently with the initiation of fluorouracil, doxorubicin and cyclophosphamide (FAC) therapy may interfere with the antitumor efficacy of the regimen).
No products indexed under this heading.

Dacarbazine (Dexrazoxane may add to the myelosuppression caused by chemotherapeutic agents).
No products indexed under this heading.

Daunorubicin Citrate (Use of dexrazoxane concurrently with the initiation of fluorouracil, doxorubicin and cyclophosphamide (FAC) therapy may interfere with the antitumor efficacy of the regimen).
No products indexed under this heading.

Daunorubicin Hydrochloride (Dexrazoxane may add to the myelosuppression caused by chemotherapeutic agents). Products include:
Cerubidine for Injection 788

Denileukin Diftitox (Dexrazoxane may add to the myelosuppression caused by chemotherapeutic agents). Products include:
Ontak Vials 1717

Docetaxel (Dexrazoxane may add to the myelosuppression caused by chemotherapeutic agents). Products include:
Taxotere Injection Concentrate 2947

Doxorubicin Hydrochloride (Use of dexrazoxane concurrently with the initiation of fluorouracil, doxorubicin and cyclophosphamide (FAC) therapy may interfere with the antitumor efficacy of the regimen). Products include:
Adriamycin for Injection, USP 786
Adriamycin Injection, USP 786

Epirubicin Hydrochloride (Dexrazoxane may add to the myelosuppression caused by chemotherapeutic agents). Products include:
Ellence Injection 2632

Estramustine Phosphate Sodium (Dexrazoxane may add to the myelosuppression caused by chemotherapeutic agents). Products include:
Emcyt Capsules 3137

Etoposide (Dexrazoxane may add to the myelosuppression caused by chemotherapeutic agents).
No products indexed under this heading.

Exemestane (Dexrazoxane may add to the myelosuppression caused by chemotherapeutic agents). Products include:
Aromasin Tablets 2600

Floxuridine (Dexrazoxane may add to the myelosuppression caused by chemotherapeutic agents).
No products indexed under this heading.

Fluorouracil (Use of dexrazoxane concurrently with the initiation of fluorouracil, doxorubicin and cyclophosphamide (FAC) therapy may interfere with the antitumor efficacy of the regimen). Products include:
Carac Cream, 0.5% 1048
Efudex 3348

Flutamide (Dexrazoxane may add to the myelosuppression caused by chemotherapeutic agents). Products include:
Eulexin Capsules 3023

Gemcitabine Hydrochloride (Dexrazoxane may add to the myelosuppression caused by chemotherapeutic agents). Products include:
Gemzar for Injection 1743

Hydroxyurea (Dexrazoxane may add to the myelosuppression caused by chemotherapeutic agents).
No products indexed under this heading.

Idarubicin Hydrochloride (Dexrazoxane may add to the myelosuppression caused by chemotherapeutic agents). Products include:
Idamycin PFS Injection 2645

Ifosfamide (Dexrazoxane may add to the myelosuppression caused by chemotherapeutic agents).
No products indexed under this heading.

Interferon alfa-2a, Recombinant (Dexrazoxane may add to the myelosuppression caused by chemotherapeutic agents). Products include:
Roferon-A Injection 2805

Interferon alfa-2b, Recombinant (Dexrazoxane may add to the myelosuppression caused by chemotherapeutic agents). Products include:
Intron A for Injection 3038
Rebetron Combination Therapy 3078

Irinotecan Hydrochloride (Dexrazoxane may add to the myelosuppression caused by chemotherapeutic agents). Products include:
Camptosar Injection 2602

Levamisole Hydrochloride (Dexrazoxane may add to the myelosuppression caused by chemotherapeutic agents).
No products indexed under this heading.

Lomustine (CCNU) (Dexrazoxane may add to the myelosuppression caused by chemotherapeutic agents).
No products indexed under this heading.

Mechlorethamine Hydrochloride (Dexrazoxane may add to the myelosuppression caused by chemotherapeutic agents). Products include:
Mustargen for Injection 2007

Megestrol Acetate (Dexrazoxane may add to the myelosuppression caused by chemotherapeutic agents). Products include:
Megace ES Oral Suspension 2492

Melphalan (Dexrazoxane may add to the myelosuppression caused by chemotherapeutic agents). Products include:
Alkeran Tablets 977

Mercaptopurine (Dexrazoxane may add to the myelosuppression caused by chemotherapeutic agents). Products include:
Purinethol Tablets 1222

Methotrexate Sodium (Dexrazoxane may add to the myelosuppression caused by chemotherapeutic agents).
No products indexed under this heading.

Mitomycin (Mitomycin-C) (Dexrazoxane may add to the myelosuppression caused by chemotherapeutic agents).
No products indexed under this heading.

Mitotane (Dexrazoxane may add to the myelosuppression caused by chemotherapeutic agents).
No products indexed under this heading.

Mitoxantrone Hydrochloride (Dexrazoxane may add to the myelosuppression caused by chemotherapeutic agents). Products include:
Novantrone for Injection Concentrate 3158

Paclitaxel (Dexrazoxane may add to the myelosuppression caused by chemotherapeutic agents).
No products indexed under this heading.

Procarbazine Hydrochloride (Dexrazoxane may add to the myelosuppression caused by chemotherapeutic agents). Products include:
Matulane Capsules 3188

Streptozocin (Dexrazoxane may add to the myelosuppression caused by chemotherapeutic agents).
No products indexed under this heading.

Tamoxifen Citrate (Dexrazoxane may add to the myelosuppression caused by chemotherapeutic agents).
No products indexed under this heading.

Teniposide (Dexrazoxane may add to the myelosuppression caused by chemotherapeutic agents).
No products indexed under this heading.

Thioguanine (Dexrazoxane may add to the myelosuppression caused by chemotherapeutic agents). Products include:

Tabloid Tablets 1545

Thiotepa (Dexrazoxane may add to the myelosuppression caused by chemotherapeutic agents).
No products indexed under this heading.

Topotecan Hydrochloride (Dexrazoxane may add to the myelosuppression caused by chemotherapeutic agents). Products include:
Hycamtin for Injection 1427

Toremifene Citrate (Dexrazoxane may add to the myelosuppression caused by chemotherapeutic agents).
No products indexed under this heading.

Valrubicin (Dexrazoxane may add to the myelosuppression caused by chemotherapeutic agents).
No products indexed under this heading.

Vincristine Sulfate (Dexrazoxane may add to the myelosuppression caused by chemotherapeutic agents).
No products indexed under this heading.

Vinorelbine Tartrate (Dexrazoxane may add to the myelosuppression caused by chemotherapeutic agents). Products include:
Navelbine Injection 1494

ZITHROMAX CAPSULES, 250 MG

(Azithromycin Dihydrate) 2568

May interact with antacids containing aluminum, calcium and magnesium, oral anticoagulants, phenytoin, xanthines, and certain other agents. Compounds in these categories include:

Aluminum Carbonate (Aluminum- and magnesium-containing antacids reduce the peak serum levels (rate) but not the AUC (extent) of azithromycin absorption; simultaneous administration should be avoided).
No products indexed under this heading.

Aluminum Hydroxide (Aluminum- and magnesium-containing antacids reduce the peak serum levels (rate) but not the AUC (extent) of azithromycin absorption; simultaneous administration should be avoided). Products include:
Gaviscon Regular Strength Liquid .. 620
Gaviscon Regular Strength Tablets....................................... 619
Gaviscon Extra Strength Liquid 620
Gaviscon Extra Strength Tablets 619
Maalox Max Maximum Strength Antacid/Anti-Gas Liquid................. 2165
Maalox Regular Strength Antacid/Antigas Liquid.................. 2164

Aminophylline (Concurrent use of macrolides and theophylline has been associated with increases in the serum concentrations of theophylline; the effect of azithromycin on the plasma levels of theophylline administered in multiple doses is not known).
No products indexed under this heading.

Anisindione (Concurrent use of macrolides and warfarin in clinical practice has been associated with increased anticoagulant effects). Products include:
Miradon Tablets 3056

Carbamazepine (Caution is advised since co-administration of drugs metabolized by cytochrome P450 system and macrolide antibiotics is associated with elevation in carbamazepine serum levels). Products include:
Carbatrol Capsules 3174
Equetro Extended-Release Capsules.................................... 3178
Tegretol/Tegretol-XR 2278

Cyclosporine (Caution is advised since co-administration of drugs metabolized by cytochrome P450 system and macrolide antibiotics is associated with elevation in cyclosporine serum levels). Products include:
Gengraf Capsules 458
Neoral Soft Gelatin Capsules 2247
Neoral Oral Solution 2247
Restasis Ophthalmic Emulsion 570
Sandimmune 2259

Dicumarol (Concurrent use of macrolides and warfarin in clinical practice has been associated with increased anticoagulant effects).
No products indexed under this heading.

Digoxin (Caution is advised since macrolide antibiotics elevate digoxin serum levels). Products include:
Digitek Tablets 2146
Lanoxicaps Capsules 1458
Lanoxin Injection 1462
Lanoxin Tablets 1468
Lanoxin Injection Pediatric 1465

Dihydroergotamine Mesylate (Caution is advised since macrolide antibiotics and ergotamine co-administration is associated with acute ergot toxicity). Products include:
Migranal Nasal Spray 3350

Dyphylline (Concurrent use of macrolides and theophylline has been associated with increases in the serum concentrations of theophylline; the effect of azithromycin on the plasma levels of theophylline administered in multiple doses is not known).
No products indexed under this heading.

Efavirenz (Co-administration produced a 22% increase in the Cmax of azithromycin). Products include:
Sustiva Capsules 957

Ergotamine Tartrate (Caution is advised since macrolide antibiotics and ergotamine co-administration is associated with acute ergot toxicity).
No products indexed under this heading.

Fosphenytoin Sodium (Caution is advised since co-administration of drugs metabolized by cytochrome P450 system and macrolide antibiotics is associated with elevation in phenytoin serum levels).
No products indexed under this heading.

Hexobarbital (Caution is advised since co-administration of drugs metabolized by cytochrome P450 system and macrolide antibiotics is associated with elevation in hexobarbital serum levels).
No products indexed under this heading.

Magaldrate (Aluminum- and magnesium-containing antacids reduce the peak serum levels (rate) but not the AUC (extent) of azithromycin absorption; simultaneous administration should be avoided).
No products indexed under this heading.

Magnesium Hydroxide (Aluminum- and magnesium-containing antacids reduce the peak serum levels (rate) but not the AUC (extent) of azithromycin absorption; simultaneous administration should be avoided). Products include:
Maalox Max Maximum Strength Antacid/Anti-Gas Liquid................ 2165
Maalox Regular Strength Antacid/Antigas Liquid................. 2164
Pepcid Complete Chewable Tablets.. 1672
Rolaids Tablets 707
Extra Strength Rolaids Tablets 707
Rolaids Multi-Symptom Antacid & Antigas Tablets 708

Magnesium Oxide (Aluminum- and magnesium-containing antacids reduce the peak serum levels (rate) but not the AUC (extent) of azithromycin absorption; simultaneous administration should be avoided). Products include:
Beelith Tablets 784
PremCal Light, Regular, and Extra Strength Tablets................ 762

Nelfinavir Mesylate (Co-administration produced a decrease of approximately 15% in mean AUC of nelfinavir and its M8 metabolite; no dosage adjustment is necessary). Products include:
Viracept 2556

Phenytoin (Caution is advised since co-administration of drugs metabolized by cytochrome P450 system and macrolide antibiotics is associated with elevation in phenytoin serum levels).
No products indexed under this heading.

Phenytoin Sodium (Caution is advised since co-administration of drugs metabolized by cytochrome P450 system and macrolide antibiotics is associated with elevation in phenytoin serum levels). Products include:
Phenytek Capsules 2153

Terfenadine (Caution is advised since co-administration of drugs metabolized by cytochrome P450 system and macrolide antibiotics is associated with elevation in terfenadine serum levels).
No products indexed under this heading.

Theophylline (Concurrent use of macrolides and theophylline has been associated with increases in the serum concentrations of theophylline; the effect of azithromycin on the plasma levels of theophylline administered in multiple doses is not known).
No products indexed under this heading.

Theophylline Anhydrous (Concurrent use of macrolides and theophylline has been associated with increases in the serum concentrations of theophylline; the effect of azithromycin on the plasma levels of theophylline administered in multiple doses is not known). Products include:
Uniphyl Tablets 2708

Theophylline Calcium Salicylate (Concurrent use of macrolides and theophylline has been associated with increases in the serum concentrations of theophylline; the effect of azithromycin on the plasma levels of theophylline administered in multiple doses is not known).
No products indexed under this heading.

Theophylline Dihydroxypropyl (Glyceryl) (Concurrent use of macrolides and theophylline has been associated with increases in the serum concentrations of theophylline; the effect of azithromycin on the plasma levels of theophylline administered in multiple doses is not known).
No products indexed under this heading.

Theophylline Ethylenediamine (Concurrent use of macrolides and theophylline has been associated with increases in the serum concentrations of theophylline; the effect of azithromycin on the plasma levels of theophylline administered in multiple doses is not known).
No products indexed under this heading.

Theophylline Sodium Glycinate (Concurrent use of macrolides and theophylline has been associated with increases in the serum concentrations of theophylline; the effect of azithromycin on the plasma levels of theophylline administered in multiple doses is not known).
No products indexed under this heading.

Triazolam (Caution is advised since macrolide antibiotics decrease the clearance of triazolam and thereby increasing the pharmacologic effect of triazolam).
No products indexed under this heading.

Warfarin Sodium (Concurrent use of macrolides and warfarin in clinical practice has been associated with increased anticoagulant effects). Products include:
Coumadin for Injection 932
Coumadin Tablets 932

Food Interactions

Food, unspecified (Zithromax should not be taken with food; reduces the rate of absorption (Cmax) of azithromycin capsules by 52% and the extent of absorption (AUC) by 43%; when oral suspension of azithromycin was administered with food the Cmax increased by 56% and the AUC was unchanged).

ZITHROMAX FOR IV INFUSION

(Azithromycin Dihydrate) 2573

May interact with oral anticoagulants, phenytoin, and certain other agents. Compounds in these categories include:

Anisindione (Concurrent use of macrolides and warfarin in clinical practice has been associated with increased anticoagulant effects). Products include:
Miradon Tablets 3056

Carbamazepine (Caution is advised since co-administration of drugs metabolized by cytochrome P450 system and macrolide antibiotics is associated with elevation in carbamazepine serum levels). Products include:
Carbatrol Capsules 3174
Equetro Extended-Release Capsules.................................... 3178
Tegretol/Tegretol-XR 2278

Cyclosporine (Caution is advised since co-administration of drugs metabolized by cytochrome P450 system and macrolide antibiotics is associated with elevation in cyclosporine serum levels). Products include:

Gengraf Capsules 458
Neoral Soft Gelatin Capsules 2247
Neoral Oral Solution 2247
Restasis Ophthalmic Emulsion 570
Sandimmune 2259

Dicumarol (Concurrent use of macrolides and warfarin in clinical practice has been associated with increased anticoagulant effects).
No products indexed under this heading.

Digoxin (Caution is advised since macrolide antibiotics elevate digoxin serum levels). Products include:
Digitek Tablets 2146
Lanoxicaps Capsules 1458
Lanoxin Injection 1462
Lanoxin Tablets 1468
Lanoxin Injection Pediatric 1465

Dihydroergotamine Mesylate (Caution is advised since macrolide antibiotics and ergotamine co-administration is associated with acute ergot toxicity). Products include:
Migranal Nasal Spray 3350

Efavirenz (Co-administration produced a 22% increase in the Cmax of azithromycin). Products include:
Sustiva Capsules 957

Ergotamine Tartrate (Caution is advised since macrolide antibiotics and ergotamine co-administration is associated with acute ergot toxicity).
No products indexed under this heading.

Fosphenytoin Sodium (Caution is advised since co-administration of drugs metabolized by cytochrome P450 system and macrolide antibiotics is associated with elevation in phenytoin serum levels).
No products indexed under this heading.

Hexobarbital (Caution is advised since co-administration of drugs metabolized by cytochrome P450 system and macrolide antibiotics is associated with elevation in hexobarbital serum levels).
No products indexed under this heading.

Nelfinavir Mesylate (Co-administration of nelfinavir at steady-state with a single oral dose of azithromycin resulted in increased azithromycin serum concentrations. Although a dose adjustment of azithromycin is not recommended when administered in combination with nelfinavir, close monitoring for known side effects of azithromycin is warranted). Products include:
Viracept 2556

Phenytoin (Caution is advised since co-administration of drugs metabolized by cytochrome P450 system and macrolide antibiotics is associated with elevation in phenytoin serum levels).
No products indexed under this heading.

Phenytoin Sodium (Caution is advised since co-administration of drugs metabolized by cytochrome P450 system and macrolide antibiotics is associated with elevation in phenytoin serum levels). Products include:
Phenytek Capsules 2153

Terfenadine (Caution is advised since co-administration of drugs metabolized by cytochrome P450 system and macrolide antibiotics is associated with elevation in terfenadine serum levels).
No products indexed under this heading.

Warfarin Sodium (Concurrent use of macrolides and warfarin in clinical practice has been associated with increased anticoagulant effects). Products include:
Coumadin for Injection 932
Coumadin Tablets 932

Food Interactions

Food, unspecified (Zithromax should not be taken with food; reduces the rate of absorption (Cmax) of azithromycin capsules by 52% and the extent of absorption (AUC) by 43%; when oral suspension of azithromycin was administered with food the Cmax increased by 56% and the AUC was unchanged).

ZITHROMAX FOR ORAL SUSPENSION, 1 G

(Azithromycin Dihydrate) 2568
See Zithromax Capsules, 250 mg

ZITHROMAX FOR ORAL SUSPENSION, 300 MG, 600 MG, 900 MG, 1200 MG

(Azithromycin Dihydrate) 2561
See Zithromax Capsules, 250 mg

ZITHROMAX TABLETS, 250 MG, 500 MG

(Azithromycin Dihydrate) 2561
See Zithromax Capsules, 250 mg

ZITHROMAX TABLETS, 600 MG

(Azithromycin Dihydrate) 2568
See Zithromax Capsules, 250 mg

ZITHROMAX TRI-PAK

(Azithromycin Dihydrate) 2561
See Zithromax Capsules, 250 mg

ZITHROMAX Z-PAK

(Azithromycin Dihydrate) 2568
See Zithromax Capsules, 250 mg

ZMAX FOR ORAL SUSPENSION

(Azithromycin) 2577
May interact with phenytoin and certain other agents. Compounds in these categories include:

Cyclosporine (Carefully monitor cyclosporine concentrations when used concomitantly with azithromycin). Products include:
Gengraf Capsules 458
Neoral Soft Gelatin Capsules 2247
Neoral Oral Solution 2247
Restasis Ophthalmic Emulsion 570
Sandimmune 2259

Digoxin (Caution is advised since macrolide antibiotics elevate digoxin serum levels). Products include:
Digitek Tablets 2146
Lanoxicaps Capsules 1458
Lanoxin Injection 1462
Lanoxin Tablets 1468
Lanoxin Injection Pediatric 1465

Dihydroergotamine Mesylate (Carefully monitor patients taking dihydroergotamine and azithromycin concomitantly, due to acute ergot toxicity characterized by severe peripheral vasospams and dysesthesia). Products include:
Migranal Nasal Spray 3350

Ergotamine Tartrate (Carefully monitor patients taking ergotamine and azithromycin concomitantly, due to acute ergot toxicity characterized by severe peripheral vasospams and dysesthesia).
No products indexed under this heading.

Fosphenytoin Sodium (Carefully monitor phenytoin concentrations when used concomitantly with azithromycin).
No products indexed under this heading.

Hexobarbital (Carefully monitor hexobarbital concentrations when used concomitantly with azithromycin).
No products indexed under this heading.

Nelfinavir Mesylate (Co-administration of nelfinavir at steady-state with a single dose of azithromycin (2 x 600 mg tablets) results in increased azithromycin serum concentrations. Although a dose adjustment of azithromycin is not recommended when administered in combination with nelfinavir, close monitoring for known side effects of azithromycin, such as liver enzyme abnormalties and hearing impairment, is warranted). Products include:
Viracept 2556

Phenytoin (Carefully monitor phenytoin concentrations when used concomitantly with azithromycin).
No products indexed under this heading.

Phenytoin Sodium (Carefully monitor phenytoin concentrations when used concomitantly with azithromycin). Products include:
Phenytek Capsules 2153

Warfarin Sodium (Azithromycin did not affect the prothrombin time response to a single dose of warfarin. However, prudent medical practice dictates careful monitoring of prothrombin time in all patients treated with azithromycin and warfarin concomitantly. Concurrent use of macrolides and warfarin in clinical practice has been associated with increased anticoagulant effects). Products include:
Coumadin for Injection 932
Coumadin Tablets 932

ZOCOR TABLETS

(Simvastatin) 2078
May interact with azole antifungals, oral anticoagulants, erythromycin, fibrates, protease inhibitors, and certain other agents. Compounds in these categories include:

Amiodarone Hydrochloride (Co-administration has resulted in myopathy, especially in patients on a higher dose of simvastatin; the dose of simvastatin should not exceed 20 mg daily in patients on concomitant amiodarone). Products include:
Pacerone Tablets 3337

Amprenavir (Simvastatin is metabolized by CYP3A4; co-administration with potent inhibitors of CYP3A4, such as protease inhibitors, increases the risk of myopathy by reducing the elimination of simvastatin; concurrent use should be avoided). Products include:
Agenerase Capsules 1299
Agenerase Oral Solution 1304

Anisindione (Simvastatin modestly potentiates the effect of coumarin anticoagulants; the prothrombin time is increased from baseline). Products include:
Miradon Tablets 3056

Clarithromycin (Simvastatin is metabolized by CYP3A4; co-administration with potent inhibitors of CYP3A4, such as clarithromycin increases the risk of myopathy by reducing the elimination of simvastatin; concurrent use should be avoided). Products include:
Biaxin/Biaxin XL 402
PREVPAC 3281

Clofibrate (The incidence and severity of myopathy are increased by co-administration of HMG-CoA reductase inhibitors with drugs that cause myopathy when given alone, such as fibrates. In patients on concomitant fibrates, the dose of simvastatin should generally not exceed 10 mg/day).
No products indexed under this heading.

Clotrimazole (The risk of myopathy appears to be increased by high levels of HMG-CoA reductase inhibitory activity and the drugs that share the same metabolic pathways as simvastatin, such as antifungal azoles, can raise the plasma levels of simvastatin and may increase the risk of myopathy). Products include:
Lotrimin 3053
Lotrisone 3054

Cyclosporine (The risk of myopathy appears to be increased by high levels of HMG-CoA reductase inhibitory activity and the drugs that share the same metabolic pathways as simvastatin, such as cyclosporine, can raise the plasma levels of simvastatin and may increase the risk of myopathy; in patients on concomitant cyclosporine, the dose of simvastatin should begin with 5 mg/day and not exceed 10 mg/day). Products include:
Gengraf Capsules 458
Neoral Soft Gelatin Capsules 2247
Neoral Oral Solution 2247
Restasis Ophthalmic Emulsion 570
Sandimmune 2259

Danazol (The risk of myopathy/rhabdomyolysis is increased by concomitant administration of danazol, particularly with higher doses of simvastatin. The does of simvastatin should not exceed 10 mg daily in patients receiving concomitant medication with danazol).
No products indexed under this heading.

Dicumarol (Simvastatin modestly potentiates the effect of coumarin anticoagulants; the prothrombin time is increased from baseline).
No products indexed under this heading.

Digoxin (Slight elevation in digoxin plasma levels; patients taking digoxin should be monitored appropriately when simvastatin is initiated). Products include:
Digitek Tablets 2146
Lanoxicaps Capsules 1458
Lanoxin Injection 1462
Lanoxin Tablets 1468
Lanoxin Injection Pediatric 1465

Erythromycin (Simvastatin is metabolized by CYP3A4; co-administration with potent inhibitors of CYP3A4, such as erythromycin, increases the risk of myopathy by reducing the elimination of simvastatin; concurrent use should be avoided). Products include:

Erygel Topical Gel 2096
Ery-Tab Tablets 447
Erythromycin Base Filmtab Tablets 454
Erythromycin Delayed-Release Capsules, USP 456
PCE Dispertab Tablets 510

Erythromycin Estolate (Simvastatin is metabolized by CYP3A4; co-administration with potent inhibitors of CYP3A4, such as erythromycin, increases the risk of myopathy by reducing the elimination of simvastatin; concurrent use should be avoided).
No products indexed under this heading.

Erythromycin Ethylsuccinate (Simvastatin is metabolized by CYP3A4; co-administration with potent inhibitors of CYP3A4, such as erythromycin, increases the risk of myopathy by reducing the elimination of simvastatin; concurrent use should be avoided). Products include:
E.E.S. 449
EryPed 445

Erythromycin Gluceptate (Simvastatin is metabolized by CYP3A4; co-administration with potent inhibitors of CYP3A4, such as erythromycin, increases the risk of myopathy by reducing the elimination of simvastatin; concurrent use should be avoided).
No products indexed under this heading.

Erythromycin Lactobionate (Simvastatin is metabolized by CYP3A4; co-administration with potent inhibitors of CYP3A4, such as erythromycin, increases the risk of myopathy by reducing the elimination of simvastatin; concurrent use should be avoided).
No products indexed under this heading.

Erythromycin Stearate (Simvastatin is metabolized by CYP3A4; co-administration with potent inhibitors of CYP3A4, such as erythromycin, increases the risk of myopathy by reducing the elimination of simvastatin; concurrent use should be avoided). Products include:
Erythrocin Stearate Filmtab Tablets 452

Fenofibrate (The incidence and severity of myopathy are increased by co-administration of HMG-CoA reductase inhibitors with drugs that cause myopathy when given alone, such as fibrates. In patients on concomitant fibrates, the dose of simvastatin should generally not exceed 10 mg/day). Products include:
Antara Capsules 2723
Lofibra Capsules 1217
Tricor Tablets 523
Triglide Tablets 1165

Fluconazole (The risk of myopathy appears to be increased by high levels of HMG-CoA reductase inhibitory activity and the drugs that share the same metabolic pathways as simvastatin, such as antifungal azoles, can raise the plasma levels of simvastatin and may increase the risk of myopathy).
No products indexed under this heading.

Gemfibrozil (The incidence and severity of myopathy are increased by co-administration of HMG-CoA reductase inhibitors with drugs that cause myopathy when given alone, such as fibrates. In patients on concomitant fibrates, the dose of simvastatin should generally not exceed 10 mg/day).
No products indexed under this heading.

Indinavir Sulfate (Simvastatin is metabolized by CYP3A4; co-administration with potent inhibitors of CYP3A4, such as protease inhibitors, increases the risk of myopathy by reducing the elimination of simvastatin; concurrent use should be avoided). Products include:
Crixivan Capsules 1918

Itraconazole (Simvastatin is metabolized by CYP3A4; co-administration with potent inhibitors of CYP3A4, such as itraconazole, increases the risk of myopathy by reducing the elimination of simvastatin; concurrent use should be avoided).
No products indexed under this heading.

Ketoconazole (Simvastatin is metabolized by CYP3A4; co-administration with potent inhibitors of CYP3A4, such as ketoconazole, increases the risk of myopathy by reducing the elimination of simvastatin; concurrent use should be avoided). Products include:
Nizoral A-D Shampoo, 1% 1839
Nizoral 2% Shampoo 1838

Lopinavir (Simvastatin is metabolized by CYP3A4; co-administration with potent inhibitors of CYP3A4, such as protease inhibitors, increases the risk of myopathy by reducing the elimination of simvastatin; concurrent use should be avoided). Products include:
Kaletra 474

Miconazole (The risk of myopathy appears to be increased by high levels of HMG-CoA reductase inhibitory activity and the drugs that share the same metabolic pathways as simvastatin, such as antifungal azoles, can raise the plasma levels of simvastatin and may increase the risk of myopathy).
No products indexed under this heading.

Nefazodone Hydrochloride (Simvastatin is metabolized by CYP3A4; co-administration with potent inhibitors of CYP3A4, such as nefazodone, increases the risk of myopathy by reducing the elimination of simvastatin; concurrent use should be avoided).
No products indexed under this heading.

Nelfinavir Mesylate (Simvastatin is metabolized by CYP3A4; co-administration with potent inhibitors of CYP3A4, such as protease inhibitors, increases the risk of myopathy by reducing the elimination of simvastatin; concurrent use should be avoided). Products include:
Viracept 2556

Niacin (The incidence and severity of myopathy are increased by co-administration of HMG-CoA reductase inhibitors with drugs that cause myopathy when given alone, such as lipid-lowering doses of niacin (greater than or equal to 1g/day); in patients on concomitant niacin, the dose of simvastatin should generally not exceed 10 mg). Products include:
Advicor Tablets 1694
Niaspan Extended-Release Tablets 1703

Oxiconazole Nitrate (The risk of myopathy appears to be increased by high levels of HMG-CoA reductase inhibitory activity and the drugs that share the same metabolic pathways as simvastatin, such as antifungal azoles, can raise the plasma levels of simvastatin and may increase the risk of myopathy). Products include:
Oxistat 1498

Propranolol Hydrochloride (Significant decreases in mean Cmax, but no change in AUC). Products include:
Inderal LA Long-Acting Capsules 3421
InnoPran XL Capsules 2728

Ritonavir (Simvastatin is metabolized by CYP3A4; co-administration with potent inhibitors of CYP3A4, such as protease inhibitors, increases the risk of myopathy by reducing the elimination of simvastatin; concurrent use should be avoided). Products include:
Kaletra 474
Norvir 499

Saquinavir (Simvastatin is metabolized by CYP3A4; co-administration with potent inhibitors of CYP3A4, such as protease inhibitors, increases the risk of myopathy by reducing the elimination of simvastatin; concurrent use should be avoided).
No products indexed under this heading.

Saquinavir Mesylate (Simvastatin is metabolized by CYP3A4; co-administration with potent inhibitors of CYP3A4, such as protease inhibitors, increases the risk of myopathy by reducing the elimination of simvastatin; concurrent use should be avoided). Products include:
Invirase 2776

Telithromycin (Simvastatin is metabolized by CYP3A4; co-administration with potent inhibitors of CYP3A4, such as telithromycin, increases the risk of myopathy by reducing the elimination of simvastatin; concurrent use should be avoided). Products include:
Ketek Tablets 2920

Terconazole (The risk of myopathy appears to be increased by high levels of HMG-CoA reductase inhibitory activity and the drugs that share the same metabolic pathways as simvastatin, such as antifungal azoles, can raise the plasma levels of simvastatin and may increase the risk of myopathy).
No products indexed under this heading.

Verapamil Hydrochloride (Co-administration has resulted in myopathy, especially in patients on a higher dose of simvastatin; the dose of simvastatin should not exceed 20 mg daily in patients on concomitant verapamil). Products include:
Covera-HS Tablets 3135
Tarka Tablets 519
Verelan PM Capsules 3120

Warfarin Sodium (Simvastatin modestly potentiates the effect of coumarin anticoagulants; the prothrombin time is increased from baseline). Products include:
Coumadin for Injection 932
Coumadin Tablets 932

Food Interactions

Alcohol (Simvastatin causes persistent increases in serum transaminase in 1% of patients; therefore, it should be used with caution in patients who consume substantial quantities of alcohol).

Grapefruit Juice (Simvastatin is a substrate for CYP4503A4 and grapefruit juice contains one or more components that inhibit CYP3A4; co-administration with grapefruit juice can increase the plasma concentrations of simvastatin and its B-hydroxyacid metabolite; large quantities of grapefruit juice (>1 quart daily) significantly increase the serum concentrations and should be avoided).

ZOFRAN INJECTION
(Ondansetron Hydrochloride) 1607
See Zofran Tablets

ZOFRAN INJECTION PREMIXED
(Ondansetron Hydrochloride) 1607
See Zofran Tablets

ZOFRAN ORAL SOLUTION
(Ondansetron Hydrochloride) 1613
See Zofran Tablets

ZOFRAN TABLETS
(Ondansetron Hydrochloride) 1613
May interact with phenytoin and certain other agents. Compounds in these categories include:

Carbamazepine (Co-administration with potent inducers of CYP3A4, such as carbamazepine, may increase the clearance and decrease ondansetron blood concentrations; based on available data, no dosage adjustment is recommended). Products include:
Carbatrol Capsules 3174
Equetro Extended-Release Capsules 3178
Tegretol/Tegretol-XR 2278

Fosphenytoin Sodium (Co-administration with potent inducers of CYP3A4, such as phenytoin, may increase the clearance and decrease ondansetron blood concentrations; based on the available data, no dosage adjustment is recommended).
No products indexed under this heading.

Phenytoin (Co-administration with potent inducers of CYP3A4, such as phenytoin, may increase the clearance and decrease ondansetron blood concentrations; based on the available data, no dosage adjustment is recommended).
No products indexed under this heading.

Phenytoin Sodium (Co-administration with potent inducers of CYP3A4, such as phenytoin, may increase the clearance and decrease ondansetron blood concentrations; based on the available data, no dosage adjustment is recommended). Products include:
Phenytek Capsules 2153

Rifampin (Co-administration with potent inducers of CYP3A4, such as rifampin, may increase the clearance and decrease ondansetron blood concentrations; based on available data, no dosage adjustment is recommended).
No products indexed under this heading.

Tramadol Hydrochloride (Ondansetron may be associated

with an increase in patient-controlled administration of tramadol). Products include:

Ultracet Tablets 2462

Food Interactions

Food, unspecified (Bioavailability slightly enhanced by food).

ZOFRAN ODT ORALLY DISINTEGRATING TABLETS

(Ondansetron) 1613

See Zofran Tablets

ZOLADEX

(Goserelin Acetate) 709

None cited in PDR database.

ZOLADEX 3-MONTH

(Goserelin Acetate) 712

None cited in PDR database.

ZOLOFT ORAL CONCENTRATE

(Sertraline Hydrochloride) 2581

May interact with anticoagulants, cytochrome p450 2d6 substrates (selected), antidepressant drugs, lithium preparations, monoamine oxidase inhibitors, non-steroidal anti-inflammatory agents, highly protein bound drugs (selected), tricyclic antidepressants, and certain other agents. Compounds in these categories include:

Amiodarone Hydrochloride (Co-administration with drugs that are highly protein bound may cause a shift in plasma concentrations, potentially resulting in an adverse effect). Products include:

Pacerone Tablets 3337

Amitriptyline Hydrochloride (Concurrent use of drugs that inhibit the biochemical activity of P450IID6, such as tricyclic antidepressants, may increase plasma concentrations of co-administered drugs that are metabolized by P450IID6; changes in the dosage may be required; the duration of an appropriate washout period which should intervene before switching has not been established).

No products indexed under this heading.

Amoxapine (Concurrent use of drugs that inhibit the biochemical activity of P450IID6, such as tricyclic antidepressants, may increase plasma concentrations of co-administered drugs that are metabolized by P450IID6; changes in the dosage may be required; the duration of an appropriate washout period which should intervene before switching has not been established).

No products indexed under this heading.

Amphetamine Aspartate (Many drugs effective in the treatment of major depressive disorder, eg, the SSRIs, including sertraline, and most tricyclic antidepressant drugs effective in the treatment of major depressive disorder inhibit the biochemical activity of the drug metabolizing isoenzyme cytochrome P450 2D6, and, thus, may increase the plasma concentrations of co-administered drugs that are metabolized by CYP2D6. The drugs for which this potential interaction is of greatest concern are those metabolized by CYP2D6 and which have a narrow therapeutic index). Products include:

Adderall Tablets 3168

Adderall XR Capsules 3169

Amphetamine Aspartate Monohydrate (Many drugs effective in the treatment of major depressive disorder, eg, the SSRIs, including sertraline, and most tricyclic antidepressant drugs effective in the treatment of major depressive disorder inhibit the biochemical activity of the drug metabolizing isoenzyme cytochrome P450 2D6, and, thus, may increase the plasma concentrations of co-administered drugs that are metabolized by CYP2D6. The drugs for which this potential interaction is of greatest concern are those metabolized by CYP2D6 and which have a narrow therapeutic index).

No products indexed under this heading.

Amphetamine Sulfate (Many drugs effective in the treatment of major depressive disorder, eg, the SSRIs, including sertraline, and most tricyclic antidepressant drugs effective in the treatment of major depressive disorder inhibit the biochemical activity of the drug metabolizing isoenzyme cytochrome P450 2D6, and, thus, may increase the plasma concentrations of co-administered drugs that are metabolized by CYP2D6. The drugs for which this potential interaction is of greatest concern are those metabolized by CYP2D6 and which have a narrow therapeutic index). Products include:

Adderall Tablets 3168

Adderall XR Capsules 3169

Anisindione (Patients should be cautioned about the concomitant use of sertraline hydrochloride and drugs that affect coagulation since the combined use of psychotropic drugs that interfere with serotonin reuptake and these agents has been associated with an increased risk of bleeding). Products include:

Miradon Tablets 3056

Ardeparin Sodium (Patients should be cautioned about the concomitant use of sertraline hydrochloride and drugs that affect coagulation since the combined use of psychotropic drugs that interfere with serotonin reuptake and these agents has been associated with an increased risk of bleeding).

No products indexed under this heading.

Aspirin (Patients should be cautioned about the concomitant use of sertraline hydrochloride and aspirin since the combined use of psychotropic drugs that interfere with serotonin reuptake and these agents has been associated with an increased risk of bleeding). Products include:

Aggrenox Capsules 855

Bayer, Aspirin Regimen .... ▣ 606

Bayer Aspirin Tablets 3515

BC Powder .... ▣ 612

BC Allergy Sinus Cold Powder .... ▣ 612

Arthritis Strength BC Powder .... ▣ 612

BC Sinus Cold Powder .... ▣ 612

Ecotrin Enteric Coated Aspirin Low, Regular and Maximum Strength Tablets 1627

Goody's Body Pain Formula Powder .... ▣ 621

Goody's Extra Strength Headache Powder .... ▣ 621

Goody's Extra Strength Pain Relief Tablets .... ▣ 621

Percodan Tablets 1115

St. Joseph 81 mg Aspirin Chewable and Enteric Coated Tablets 1841

Aspirin, Enteric Coated (Patients should be cautioned about the concomitant use of sertraline hydrochloride and aspirin since the combined use of psychotropic drugs that interfere with serotonin reuptake and these agents has been associated with an increased risk of bleeding).

No products indexed under this heading.

Aspirin Buffered (Patients should be cautioned about the concomitant use of sertraline hydrochloride and aspirin since the combined use of psychotropic drugs that interfere with serotonin reuptake and these agents has been associated with an increased risk of bleeding).

No products indexed under this heading.

Astemizole (Sertraline has been shown to have some inhibition of P4503A4 *in vitro*, astemizole is metabolized by P4503A4 isoenzyme and inhibition of this enzyme system may result in increased serum levels of astemizole; co-administration requires caution).

No products indexed under this heading.

Atomoxetine Hydrochloride (Many drugs effective in the treatment of major depressive disorder, eg, the SSRIs, including sertraline, and most tricyclic antidepressant drugs effective in the treatment of major depressive disorder inhibit the biochemical activity of the drug metabolizing isoenzyme cytochrome P450 2D6, and, thus, may increase the plasma concentrations of co-administered drugs that are metabolized by CYP2D6. The drugs for which this potential interaction is of greatest concern are those metabolized by CYP2D6 and which have a narrow therapeutic index). Products include:

Strattera Capsules 1784

Atovaquone (Co-administration with drugs that are highly protein bound may cause a shift in plasma concentrations, potentially resulting in an adverse effect). Products include:

Malarone Tablets 1484

Malarone Pediatric Tablets 1484

Mepron Suspension 1487

Bisoprolol Fumarate (Many drugs effective in the treatment of major depressive disorder, eg, the SSRIs, including sertraline, and most tricyclic antidepressant drugs effective in the treatment of major depressive disorder inhibit the biochemical activity of the drug metabolizing isoenzyme cytochrome P450 2D6, and, thus, may increase the plasma concentrations of co-administered drugs that are metabolized by CYP2D6. The drugs for which this potential interaction is of greatest concern are those metabolized by CYP2D6 and which have a narrow therapeutic index).

No products indexed under this heading.

Bupropion Hydrochloride (Concurrent use of drugs that inhibit the biochemical activity of P450IID6, such as tricyclic antidepressants, may increase plasma concentrations of co-administered drugs that are metabolized by P450IID6; changes in the dosage may be required; the duration of an appropriate washout period which should intervene before switching has not been established). Products include:

Wellbutrin Tablets 1579

Wellbutrin SR Sustained-Release Tablets 1583

Wellbutrin XL Extended-Release Tablets 1588

Zyban Sustained-Release Tablets 1620

Captopril (Many drugs effective in the treatment of major depressive disorder, eg, the SSRIs, including sertraline, and most tricyclic antidepressant drugs effective in the treatment of major depressive disorder inhibit the biochemical activity of the drug metabolizing isoenzyme cytochrome P450 2D6, and, thus, may increase the plasma concentrations of co-administered drugs that are metabolized by CYP2D6. The drugs for which this potential interaction is of greatest concern are those metabolized by CYP2D6 and which have a narrow therapeutic index). Products include:

Captopril Tablets 2114

Carvedilol (Many drugs effective in the treatment of major depressive disorder, eg, the SSRIs, including sertraline, and most tricyclic antidepressant drugs effective in the treatment of major depressive disorder inhibit the biochemical activity of the drug metabolizing isoenzyme cytochrome P450 2D6, and, thus, may increase the plasma concentrations of co-administered drugs that are metabolized by CYP2D6. The drugs for which this potential interaction is of greatest concern are those metabolized by CYP2D6 and which have a narrow therapeutic index). Products include:

Coreg Tablets 1376

Cefonicid Sodium (Co-administration with drugs that are highly protein bound may cause a shift in plasma concentrations, potentially resulting in an adverse effect).

No products indexed under this heading.

Celecoxib (Co-administration with drugs that are highly protein bound may cause a shift in plasma concentrations, potentially resulting in an adverse effect). Products include:

Celebrex Capsules 3130

Cevimeline Hydrochloride (Many drugs effective in the treatment of major depressive disorder, eg, the SSRIs, including sertraline, and most tricyclic antidepressant drugs effective in the treatment of major depressive disorder inhibit the biochemical activity of the drug metabolizing isoenzyme cytochrome P450 2D6, and, thus, may increase the plasma concentrations of co-administered drugs that are metabolized by CYP2D6. The drugs for which this potential interaction is of greatest concern are those metabolized by CYP2D6 and which have a narrow therapeutic index). Products include:

Evoxac Capsules 1042

Chlordiazepoxide (Co-administration with drugs that are highly protein bound may cause a shift in plasma concentrations, potentially resulting in an adverse effect).

No products indexed under this heading.

Chlordiazepoxide Hydrochloride (Co-administration with drugs that are highly protein bound may cause a shift in plasma concentrations, potentially resulting in an adverse effect). Products include:

Librium Capsules 3349

Chlorpromazine (Co-administration with drugs that are highly protein bound may cause a shift in plasma concentrations, potentially resulting in an adverse effect).

No products indexed under this heading.

Chlorpromazine Hydrochloride (Co-administration with drugs that are highly protein bound may cause a shift in plasma concentrations, potentially resulting in an adverse effect).

No products indexed under this heading.

Chlorpropamide (Many drugs effective in the treatment of major depressive disorder, eg, the SSRIs, including sertraline, and most tricyclic antidepressant drugs effective in the treatment of major depressive disorder inhibit the biochemical activity of the drug metabolizing isoenzyme cytochrome P450 2D6, and, thus, may increase the plasma concentrations of co-administered drugs that are metabolized by CYP2D6. The drugs for which this potential interaction is of greatest concern are those metabolized by CYP2D6 and which have a narrow therapeutic index).

No products indexed under this heading.

Cimetidine (Potential for increase in Zoloft mean AUC (50%), Cmax (24%) and half-life (26%); clinical significance is unknown). Products include:

Tagamet HB 200 Tablets 637
Tagamet Tablets 1547

Cimetidine Hydrochloride (Potential for increase in Zoloft mean AUC (50%), Cmax (24%) and half-life (26%); clinical significance is unknown).

No products indexed under this heading.

Cisapride (Sertraline induces the metabolism of cisapride (cisapride AUC and Cmax were reduced by about 35%)).

No products indexed under this heading.

Citalopram Hydrobromide (Concurrent use of drugs that inhibit the biochemical activity of P450IID6, such as tricyclic antidepressants, may increase plasma concentrations of co-administered drugs that are metabolized by P450IID6; changes in the dosage may be required; the duration of an appropriate washout period which should intervene before switching has not been established). Products include:

Celexa 1177

Clomipramine Hydrochloride (Concurrent use of drugs that inhibit the biochemical activity of P450IID6, such as tricyclic antidepressants, may increase plasma concentrations of co-administered drugs that are metabolized by P450IID6; changes in the dosage may be required; the duration of an appropriate washout period which should intervene before switching has not been established).

No products indexed under this heading.

Clozapine (Co-administration with drugs that are highly protein bound may cause a shift in plasma concentrations, potentially resulting in an adverse effect). Products include:

Clozapine Tablets 2141
Clozaril Tablets 2174
FazaClo Orally Disintegrating Tablets 547

CNS-Active Drugs, unspecified (Caution is advised if Zoloft is co-administered with other CNS-active drugs).

No products indexed under this heading.

Codeine Phosphate (Many drugs effective in the treatment of major depressive disorder, eg, the SSRIs, including sertraline, and most tricyclic antidepressant drugs effective in the treatment of major depressive disorder inhibit the biochemical activity of the drug metabolizing isoenzyme cytochrome P450 2D6, and, thus, may increase the plasma concentrations of co-administered drugs that are metabolized by CYP2D6. The drugs for which this potential interaction is of greatest concern are those metabolized by CYP2D6 and which have a narrow therapeutic index). Products include:

Tylenol with Codeine 2461

Codeine Sulfate (Many drugs effective in the treatment of major depressive disorder, eg, the SSRIs, including sertraline, and most tricyclic antidepressant drugs effective in the treatment of major depressive disorder inhibit the biochemical activity of the drug metabolizing isoenzyme cytochrome P450 2D6, and, thus, may increase the plasma concentrations of co-administered drugs that are metabolized by CYP2D6. The drugs for which this potential interaction is of greatest concern are those metabolized by CYP2D6 and which have a narrow therapeutic index).

No products indexed under this heading.

Cyclobenzaprine Hydrochloride (Many drugs effective in the treatment of major depressive disorder, eg, the SSRIs, including sertraline, and most tricyclic antidepressant drugs effective in the treatment of major depressive disorder inhibit the biochemical activity of the drug metabolizing isoenzyme cytochrome P450 2D6, and, thus, may increase the plasma concentrations of co-administered drugs that are metabolized by CYP2D6. The drugs for which this potential interaction is of greatest concern are those metabolized by CYP2D6 and which have a narrow therapeutic index). Products include:

Flexeril Tablets 1832

Cyclosporine (Co-administration with drugs that are highly protein bound may cause a shift in plasma concentrations, potentially resulting in an adverse effect). Products include:

Gengraf Capsules 458
Neoral Soft Gelatin Capsules 2247
Neoral Oral Solution 2247
Restasis Ophthalmic Emulsion 570
Sandimmune 2259

Dalteparin Sodium (Patients should be cautioned about the concomitant use of sertraline hydrochloride and drugs that affect coagulation since the combined use of psychotropic drugs that interfere with serotonin reuptake and these agents has been associated with an increased risk of bleeding). Products include:

Fragmin Injection 2638

Danaparoid Sodium (Patients should be cautioned about the concomitant use of sertraline hydrochloride and drugs that affect coagulation since the combined use of psychotropic drugs that interfere with serotonin reuptake and these agents has been associated with an increased risk of bleeding).

No products indexed under this heading.

Desipramine Hydrochloride (Concurrent use of drugs that inhibit the biochemical activity of P450IID6, such as tricyclic antidepressants, may increase plasma concentrations of co-administered drugs that are metabolized by P450IID6; changes in the dosage may be required; the duration of an appropriate washout period which should intervene before switching has not been established).

No products indexed under this heading.

Dexfenfluramine Hydrochloride (Many drugs effective in the treatment of major depressive disorder, eg, the SSRIs, including sertraline, and most tricyclic antidepressant drugs effective in the treatment of major depressive disorder inhibit the biochemical activity of the drug metabolizing isoenzyme cytochrome P450 2D6, and, thus, may increase the plasma concentrations of co-administered drugs that are metabolized by CYP2D6. The drugs for which this potential interaction is of greatest concern are those metabolized by CYP2D6 and which have a narrow therapeutic index).

No products indexed under this heading.

Dextromethorphan Hydrobromide (Many drugs effective in the treatment of major depressive disorder, eg, the SSRIs, including sertraline, and most tricyclic antidepressant drugs effective in the treatment of major depressive disorder inhibit the biochemical activity of the drug metabolizing isoenzyme cytochrome P450 2D6, and, thus, may increase the plasma concentrations of co-administered drugs that are metabolized by CYP2D6. The drugs for which this potential interaction is of greatest concern are those metabolized by CYP2D6 and which have a narrow therapeutic index). Products include:

Alacol DM Syrup 739
Balamine DM 739
Contac Severe Cold and Flu Caplets Maximum Strength 615
Contac Severe Cold and Flu Caplets Non-Drowsy 615
Children's Dimetapp DM Cold & Cough Elixir 745
Children's Dimetapp Long Acting Cough Plus Cold Syrup 746
Dimetapp Infant Drops Decongestant Plus Cough 746
Mucinex DM Tablets 602
PediaCare Decongestant & Cough Infant Drops 705
PediaCare Freezer Pops Long-Acting Cough-Glacier Grape and Polar Berry Blue 706
PediaCare Long-Acting Cough Infant Drops 705
PediaCare Long-Acting Cough Plus Cold Liquid 704
PediaCare Multi-Symptom Cold Liquid 704
PediaCare NightRest Cough & Cold Liquid 704
Robitussin Allergy & Cough Syrup .. 750
Robitussin CF Liquid 755
Robitussin Cough & Cold Liquid-filled Capsules 750
Robitussin Cough, Cold & Flu Liquid-filled Capsules 750
Robitussin Cough & Cold Infant Drops 755
Robitussin DM Infant Drops 753
Robitussin DM Liquid 753
Robitussin Flu Liquid 752
Robitussin Maximum Strength Cough Liquid 754
Robitussin Maximum Strength Cough & Cold Liquid 754
Robitussin Pediatric Cough Liquid 754
Robitussin Pediatric Cough & Cold Liquid 754
Robitussin PM Cough & Cold Liquid 752
Robitussin Sugar Free Cough Liquid 753
Simply Cough Liquid 1840
Sudafed Severe Cold 710
TheraFlu Cold & Cough Hot Liquid 680
TheraFlu Flu & Chest Congestion Non-Drowsy Hot Liquid 681
TheraFlu Severe Cold Non-Drowsy Hot Liquid 683
TheraFlu Severe Cold & Cough Hot Liquid 683
TheraFlu Severe Cold Caplets 679
TheraFlu Severe Cold Hot Liquid 682
TheraFlu Severe Cold Non-Drowsy Caplets 679
TheraFlu Thin Strips Long Acting Cough 684
Triaminic Cold & Cough Liquid 685
Triaminic Cough Liquid 687
Triaminic Cough & Nasal Congestion Liquid 687
Triaminic Cough & Sore Throat Liquid 687
Triaminic Flu, Cough & Fever Liquid 685
Triaminic Night Time Cough & Cold Liquid 685
Triaminic Cold & Cough Softchews 688
Triaminic Cough & Sore Throat Softchews 689
Triaminic Thin Strips Long Acting Cough 689
Children's Tylenol Plus Cold & Cough Suspension Liquid and Chewable Tablets 1851
Children's Tylenol Plus Flu Suspension Liquid 1853
Concentrated Tylenol Infants' Drops Plus Cold and Cough 1851
Tylenol Cold & Flu Severe Daytime Liquid with Cool Bust 1846
Tylenol Cold & Flu Severe NightTime Liquid with Cool Burst 1846
Tylenol Cold Severe Congestion Non-Drowsy Caplets with Cool Burst 1846
Tylenol Cough & Sore Throat Daytime Liquid with Cool Burst 1849
Tylenol Cough & Sore Throat NightTime Liquid with Cool Burst 1849
Tylenol Flu Day Non-Drowsy Gelcaps 1846
Concentrated Tylenol Infants' Drops Plus Cold & Cough Nasal Decongestant, Fever Reducer & Pain Reliever 668
Multi-Symptom Tylenol Cold Night Time Caplets 1845
Multi-Symptom Tylenol Cold Day Non-Drowsy Caplets and Gelcaps 1845
Vicks 44 Cough Relief 2675
Vicks 44D Cough & Head Congestion Relief 2676
Vicks 44D Cough & Head Congestion Relief Liquid 721
Vicks 44E Cough & Chest Congestion Relief 2676
Pediatric Vicks 44e Cough & Chest Congestion Relief Liquid 2673
Vicks 44M Cough, Cold & Flu Relief 2676
Pediatric Vicks 44m Cough & Cold Relief 2673

Vicks DayQuil LiquiCaps/Liquid Multi-Symptom Cold/Flu Relief..... ▣ 723
Vicks DayQuil Multi-Symptom Cold/Flu Relief LiquiCaps..... 2675
Vicks DayQuil Multi-Symptom Cold/Flu Relief Liquid..... 2675
Children's Vicks NyQuil Cold/Cough Relief..... 2671
Vicks NyQuil Cough Liquid..... 2677
Vicks NyQuil LiquiCaps..... 2677
Vicks NyQuil LiquiCaps/Liquid Multi-Symptom Cold/Flu Relief..... ▣ 725
Vicks NyQuil Liquid..... 2677
Zicam Concentrated Cough Mist for Kids Cool Cherry..... ▣ 643
Zicam Concentrated Cough Mist for Kids Plus D Cool Cherry..... ▣ 643
Zicam Concentrated Cough Mist Nite-Cool Cherry..... ▣ 642
Zicam Concentrated Cough Mist Plus D Cool Cherry..... ▣ 642
Zicam Concentrated Cough Mist-Honey Lemon & Cool Cherry..... ▣ 642

Dextromethorphan Polistirex (Many drugs effective in the treatment of major depressive disorder, eg, the SSRIs, including sertraline, and most tricyclic antidepressant drugs effective in the treatment of major depressive disorder inhibit the biochemical activity of the drug metabolizing isoenzyme cytochrome P450 2D6, and, thus, may increase the plasma concentrations of co-administered drugs that are metabolized by CYP2D6. The drugs for which this potential interaction is of greatest concern are those metabolized by CYP2D6 and which have a narrow therapeutic index). Products include:
Delsym Extended-Release Suspension..... ▣ 611
Delsym 12 Hour Cough Suppressant for Children..... ▣ 611

Diazepam (Co-administration with intravenous diazepam has resulted in decrease in relative to baseline diazepam clearance and increase in Tmax for desmethyldiazepam; the clinical significance is unknown). Products include:
Diastat Rectal Delivery System..... 3344
Valium Tablets..... 2822

Diclofenac Potassium (Co-administration with drugs that are highly protein bound may cause a shift in plasma concentrations, potentially resulting in an adverse effect). Products include:
Cataflam Tablets..... 2173

Diclofenac Sodium (Co-administration with drugs that are highly protein bound may cause a shift in plasma concentrations, potentially resulting in an adverse effect). Products include:
Arthrotec Tablets..... 3126
Voltaren Ophthalmic Solution..... 2300
Voltaren Tablets..... 2298
Voltaren-XR Tablets..... 2301

Dicumarol (Patients should be cautioned about the concomitant use of sertraline hydrochloride and drugs that affect coagulation since the combined use of psychotropic drugs that interfere with serotonin reuptake and these agents has been associated with an increased risk of bleeding).
No products indexed under this heading.

Digitoxin (Co-administration with drugs that are highly protein bound, such as digitoxin, may cause a shift in plasma concentrations, potentially resulting in an adverse effect).
No products indexed under this heading.

Dipyridamole (Co-administration with drugs that are highly protein bound may cause a shift in plasma concentrations, potentially resulting in an adverse effect). Products include:
Aggrenox Capsules..... 855
Persantine Tablets..... 898

Disulfiram (Zoloft Oral Concentrate contains 12% alcohol; concurrent use with disulfiram may result in Antabuse-Alcohol reaction; co-administration of Zoloft Oral Concentrate and disulfiram is contraindicated). Products include:
Antabuse Tablets..... 2343

Dolasetron Mesylate (Many drugs effective in the treatment of major depressive disorder, eg, the SSRIs, including sertraline, and most tricyclic antidepressant drugs effective in the treatment of major depressive disorder inhibit the biochemical activity of the drug metabolizing isoenzyme cytochrome P450 2D6, and, thus, may increase the plasma concentrations of co-administered drugs that are metabolized by CYP2D6. The drugs for which this potential interaction is of greatest concern are those metabolized by CYP2D6 and which have a narrow therapeutic index). Products include:
Anzemet Injection..... 2871
Anzemet Tablets..... 2874

Donepezil Hydrochloride (Many drugs effective in the treatment of major depressive disorder, eg, the SSRIs, including sertraline, and most tricyclic antidepressant drugs effective in the treatment of major depressive disorder inhibit the biochemical activity of the drug metabolizing isoenzyme cytochrome P450 2D6, and, thus, may increase the plasma concentrations of co-administered drugs that are metabolized by CYP2D6. The drugs for which this potential interaction is of greatest concern are those metabolized by CYP2D6 and which have a narrow therapeutic index). Products include:
Aricept Tablets..... 1086
Aricept ODT Tablets..... 1086

Doxepin Hydrochloride (Concurrent use of drugs that inhibit the biochemical activity of P450IID6, such as tricyclic antidepressants, may increase plasma concentrations of co-administered drugs that are metabolized by P450IID6; changes in the dosage may be required; the duration of an appropriate washout period which should intervene before switching has not been established).
No products indexed under this heading.

Encainide Hydrochloride (Many drugs effective in the treatment of major depressive disorder, eg, the SSRIs, including sertraline, and most tricyclic antidepressant drugs effective in the treatment of major depressive disorder inhibit the biochemical activity of the drug metabolizing isoenzyme cytochrome P450 2D6, and, thus, may increase the plasma concentrations of co-administered drugs that are metabolized by CYP2D6. The drugs for which this potential interaction is of greatest concern are those metabolized by CYP2D6 and which have a narrow therapeutic index).
No products indexed under this heading.

Enoxaparin Sodium (Patients should be cautioned about the concomitant use of sertraline hydrochloride and drugs that affect coagulation since the combined use of psychotropic drugs that interfere with serotonin reuptake and these agents has been associated with an increased risk of bleeding). Products include:
Lovenox Injection..... 2931

Escitalopram Oxalate (Concurrent use of drugs that inhibit the biochemical activity of P450IID6, such as tricyclic antidepressants, may increase plasma concentrations of co-administered drugs that are metabolized by P450IID6; changes in the dosage may be required; the duration of an appropriate washout period which should intervene before switching has not been established). Products include:
Lexapro Oral Solution..... 1193
Lexapro Tablets..... 1193

Ethanol (Patients should be told that although sertraline hydrochloride has not been shown in experiments with normal subjects to increase the mental and motor skill impairments caused by alcohol, the concomitant use of sertraline hydrochloride and alcohol is not advised).
No products indexed under this heading.

Etodolac (Patients should be cautioned about the concomitant use of sertraline hydrochloride and non-selective NSAIDs (eg, NSAIDs that inhibit both cyclooxygenase isoenzymes, COX 1 and 2), since the combined use of psychotropic drugs that interfere with serotonin reuptake and these agents has been associated with an increased risk of bleeding).
No products indexed under this heading.

Fenoprofen Calcium (Co-administration with drugs that are highly protein bound may cause a shift in plasma concentrations, potentially resulting in an adverse effect). Products include:
Nalfon Capsules..... 2504

Fentanyl (Many drugs effective in the treatment of major depressive disorder, eg, the SSRIs, including sertraline, and most tricyclic antidepressant drugs effective in the treatment of major depressive disorder inhibit the biochemical activity of the drug metabolizing isoenzyme cytochrome P450 2D6, and, thus, may increase the plasma concentrations of co-administered drugs that are metabolized by CYP2D6. The drugs for which this potential interaction is of greatest concern are those metabolized by CYP2D6 and which have a narrow therapeutic index). Products include:
Duragesic Transdermal System..... 2448

Fentanyl Citrate (Many drugs effective in the treatment of major depressive disorder, eg, the SSRIs, including sertraline, and most tricyclic antidepressant drugs effective in the treatment of major depressive disorder inhibit the biochemical activity of the drug metabolizing isoenzyme cytochrome P450 2D6, and, thus, may increase the plasma concentrations of co-administered drugs that are metabolized by CYP2D6. The drugs for which this potential interaction is of greatest concern are those metabolized by CYP2D6 and which have a narrow therapeutic index). Products include:
Actiq..... 993

Flecainide Acetate (Concurrent use of drugs that inhibit the biochemical activity of P450IID6, such as flecainide, may increase plasma concentrations of co-administered drugs that are metabolized by P450IID6; changes in the dosage may be required). Products include:
Tambocor Tablets..... 1824

Fluoxetine (Many drugs effective in the treatment of major depressive disorder, eg, the SSRIs, including sertraline, and most tricyclic antidepressant drugs effective in the treatment of major depressive disorder inhibit the biochemical activity of the drug metabolizing isoenzyme cytochrome P450 2D6, and, thus, may increase the plasma concentrations of co-administered drugs that are metabolized by CYP2D6. The drugs for which this potential interaction is of greatest concern are those metabolized by CYP2D6 and which have a narrow therapeutic index).
No products indexed under this heading.

Fluoxetine Hydrochloride (Concurrent use of drugs that inhibit the biochemical activity of P450IID6, such as SSRIs, may increase plasma concentrations of co-administered drugs that are metabolized by P450IID6; changes in the dosage may be required; the duration of an appropriate washout period, which should intervene before switching, has not been established). Products include:
Prozac Pulvules and Liquid..... 1771
Symbyax Capsules..... 1788

Fluphenazine Decanoate (Many drugs effective in the treatment of major depressive disorder, eg, the SSRIs, including sertraline, and most tricyclic antidepressant drugs effective in the treatment of major depressive disorder inhibit the biochemical activity of the drug metabolizing isoenzyme cytochrome P450 2D6, and, thus, may increase the plasma concentrations of co-administered drugs that are metabolized by CYP2D6. The drugs for which this potential interaction is of greatest concern are those metabolized by CYP2D6 and which have a narrow therapeutic index).
No products indexed under this heading.

Fluphenazine Enanthate (Many drugs effective in the treatment of major depressive disorder, eg, the SSRIs, including sertraline, and most tricyclic antidepressant drugs effective in the treatment of major depressive disorder inhibit the biochemical activity of the drug metabolizing isoenzyme cytochrome P450 2D6, and, thus, may increase the plasma concentrations of co-administered drugs that are metabolized by CYP2D6. The drugs for which this potential interaction is of greatest concern are those metabolized by CYP2D6 and which have a narrow therapeutic index).
No products indexed under this heading.

Fluphenazine Hydrochloride (Many drugs effective in the treatment of major depressive disorder, eg, the SSRIs, including sertraline, and most tricyclic antidepressant drugs effective in the treatment of major depressive disorder inhibit the biochemical activity of the drug

metabolizing isoenzyme cytochrome P450 2D6, and, thus, may increase the plasma concentrations of co-administered drugs that are metabolized by CYP2D6. The drugs for which this potential interaction is of greatest concern are those metabolized by CYP2D6 and which have a narrow therapeutic index).
No products indexed under this heading.

Flurazepam Hydrochloride (Co-administration with drugs that are highly protein bound may cause a shift in plasma concentrations, potentially resulting in an adverse effect). Products include:
Dalmane Capsules … **3343**

Flurbiprofen (Co-administration with drugs that are highly protein bound may cause a shift in plasma concentrations, potentially resulting in an adverse effect).
No products indexed under this heading.

Fluvoxamine Maleate (Concurrent use of drugs that inhibit the biochemical activity of P450IID6, such as SSRIs, may increase plasma concentrations of co-administered drugs that are metabolized by P450IID6; changes in the dosage may be required; the duration of an appropriate washout period, which should intervene before switching, has not been established).
No products indexed under this heading.

Fondaparinux Sodium (Patients should be cautioned about the concomitant use of sertraline hydrochloride and drugs that affect coagulation since the combined use of psychotropic drugs that interfere with serotonin reuptake and these agents has been associated with an increased risk of bleeding). Products include:
Arixtra Injection … **1325**

Formoterol Fumarate (Many drugs effective in the treatment of major depressive disorder, eg, the SSRIs, including sertraline, and most tricyclic antidepressant drugs effective in the treatment of major depressive disorder inhibit the biochemical activity of the drug metabolizing isoenzyme cytochrome P450 2D6, and, thus, may increase the plasma concentrations of co-administered drugs that are metabolized by CYP2D6. The drugs for which this potential interaction is of greatest concern are those metabolized by CYP2D6 and which have a narrow therapeutic index). Products include:
Foradil Aerolizer … **3024**

Galantamine Hydrobromide (Many drugs effective in the treatment of major depressive disorder, eg, the SSRIs, including sertraline, and most tricyclic antidepressant drugs effective in the treatment of major depressive disorder inhibit the biochemical activity of the drug metabolizing isoenzyme cytochrome P450 2D6, and, thus, may increase the plasma concentrations of co-administered drugs that are metabolized by CYP2D6. The drugs for which this potential interaction is of greatest concern are those metabolized by CYP2D6 and which have a narrow therapeutic index). Products include:
Razadyne ER Extended-Release Capsules … **2434**
Razadyne … **2434**

Glipizide (Co-administration with drugs that are highly protein bound may cause a shift in plasma concentrations, potentially resulting in an adverse effect).
No products indexed under this heading.

Haloperidol (Many drugs effective in the treatment of major depressive disorder, eg, the SSRIs, including sertraline, and most tricyclic antidepressant drugs effective in the treatment of major depressive disorder inhibit the biochemical activity of the drug metabolizing isoenzyme cytochrome P450 2D6, and, thus, may increase the plasma concentrations of co-administered drugs that are metabolized by CYP2D6. The drugs for which this potential interaction is of greatest concern are those metabolized by CYP2D6 and which have a narrow therapeutic index).
No products indexed under this heading.

Haloperidol Decanoate (Many drugs effective in the treatment of major depressive disorder, eg, the SSRIs, including sertraline, and most tricyclic antidepressant drugs effective in the treatment of major depressive disorder inhibit the biochemical activity of the drug metabolizing isoenzyme cytochrome P450 2D6, and, thus, may increase the plasma concentrations of co-administered drugs that are metabolized by CYP2D6. The drugs for which this potential interaction is of greatest concern are those metabolized by CYP2D6 and which have a narrow therapeutic index).
No products indexed under this heading.

Heparin Calcium (Patients should be cautioned about the concomitant use of sertraline hydrochloride and drugs that affect coagulation since the combined use of psychotropic drugs that interfere with serotonin reuptake and these agents has been associated with an increased risk of bleeding).
No products indexed under this heading.

Heparin Sodium (Patients should be cautioned about the concomitant use of sertraline hydrochloride and drugs that affect coagulation since the combined use of psychotropic drugs that interfere with serotonin reuptake and these agents has been associated with an increased risk of bleeding).
No products indexed under this heading.

Hydrocodone Bitartrate (Many drugs effective in the treatment of major depressive disorder, eg, the SSRIs, including sertraline, and most tricyclic antidepressant drugs effective in the treatment of major depressive disorder inhibit the biochemical activity of the drug metabolizing isoenzyme cytochrome P450 2D6, and, thus, may increase the plasma concentrations of co-administered drugs that are metabolized by CYP2D6. The drugs for which this potential interaction is of greatest concern are those metabolized by CYP2D6 and which have a narrow therapeutic index). Products include:
Hycodan … **1104**
Hycomine Compound Tablets … **1105**
Hycotuss Expectorant Syrup … **1106**
Lortab … **3315**
Lortab Elixir … **3312**
Vicodin Tablets … **530**
Vicodin ES Tablets … **531**
Vicodin HP Tablets … **532**
Vicoprofen Tablets … **533**
Zydone Tablets … **1118**

Ibuprofen (Co-administration with drugs that are highly protein bound may cause a shift in plasma concentrations, potentially resulting in an adverse effect). Products include:
Advil Allergy Sinus Caplets … ▣ **737**
Advil … ▣ **737**
Children's Advil Suspension … ▣ **742**
Children's Advil Chewable Tablets … ▣ **741**
Advil Cold & Sinus … ▣ **739**
Advil Flu & Body Ache Caplets … ▣ **739**
Children's Advil Cold Suspension … ▣ **741**
Infants' Advil Concentrated Drops … ▣ **743**
Junior Strength Advil Swallow Tablets … ▣ **740**
Advil Migraine Liquigels … ▣ **740**
Advil Multi-Symptom Cold Caplets … ▣ **738**
Combunox Tablets … **1183**
Children's Motrin Oral Suspension and Chewable Tablets … **1837**
Children's Motrin Cold Non-Staining Dye-Free Oral Suspension … **1838**
Children's Motrin Cold Oral Suspension … **1838**
Children's Motrin Non-Staining Dye-Free Oral Suspension … **1837**
Motrin Cold & Sinus Caplets … **1836**
Motrin IB Tablets and Caplets … **1836**
Infants' Motrin Concentrated Drops … **1837**
Infants' Motrin Non-Staining Dye-Free Drops … **1837**
Junior Strength Motrin Caplets and Chewable Tablets … **1837**
Vicoprofen Tablets … **533**

Imipramine Hydrochloride (Concurrent use of drugs that inhibit the biochemical activity of P450IID6, such as tricyclic antidepressants, may increase plasma concentrations of co-administered drugs that are metabolized by P450IID6; changes in the dosage may be required; the duration of an appropriate washout period which should intervene before switching has not been established).
No products indexed under this heading.

Imipramine Pamoate (Concurrent use of drugs that inhibit the biochemical activity of P450IID6, such as tricyclic antidepressants, may increase plasma concentrations of co-administered drugs that are metabolized by P450IID6; changes in the dosage may be required; the duration of an appropriate washout period which should intervene before switching has not been established).
No products indexed under this heading.

Indomethacin (Co-administration with drugs that are highly protein bound may cause a shift in plasma concentrations, potentially resulting in an adverse effect). Products include:
Indocin … **1968**

Indomethacin Sodium Trihydrate (Co-administration with drugs that are highly protein bound may cause a shift in plasma concentrations, potentially resulting in an adverse effect). Products include:
Indocin I.V. … **1973**

Indoramin Hydrochloride (Many drugs effective in the treatment of major depressive disorder, eg, the SSRIs, including sertraline, and most tricyclic antidepressant drugs effective in the treatment of major depressive disorder inhibit the biochemical activity of the drug metabolizing isoenzyme cytochrome P450 2D6, and, thus, may increase the plasma concentrations of co-administered drugs that are metabolized by CYP2D6. The drugs for which this potential interaction is of greatest concern are those metabolized by CYP2D6 and which have a narrow therapeutic index).
No products indexed under this heading.

Isocarboxazid (Co-administration has resulted in serious, sometimes fatal, reactions including hyperthermia, rigidity, myoclonus, autonomic instability, extreme agitation progressing to delirium and coma; concurrent and/or sequential use is contraindicated).
No products indexed under this heading.

Ketoprofen (Co-administration with drugs that are highly protein bound may cause a shift in plasma concentrations, potentially resulting in an adverse effect).
No products indexed under this heading.

Ketorolac Tromethamine (Co-administration with drugs that are highly protein bound may cause a shift in plasma concentrations, potentially resulting in an adverse effect). Products include:
Acular Ophthalmic Solution … **561**
Acular LS Ophthalmic Solution … **562**

Labetalol Hydrochloride (Many drugs effective in the treatment of major depressive disorder, eg, the SSRIs, including sertraline, and most tricyclic antidepressant drugs effective in the treatment of major depressive disorder inhibit the biochemical activity of the drug metabolizing isoenzyme cytochrome P450 2D6, and, thus, may increase the plasma concentrations of co-administered drugs that are metabolized by CYP2D6. The drugs for which this potential interaction is of greatest concern are those metabolized by CYP2D6 and which have a narrow therapeutic index).
No products indexed under this heading.

Lidocaine (Many drugs effective in the treatment of major depressive disorder, eg, the SSRIs, including sertraline, and most tricyclic antidepressant drugs effective in the treatment of major depressive disorder inhibit the biochemical activity of the drug metabolizing isoenzyme cytochrome P450 2D6, and, thus, may increase the plasma concentrations of co-administered drugs that are metabolized by CYP2D6. The drugs for which this potential interaction is of greatest concern are those metabolized by CYP2D6 and which have a narrow therapeutic index). Products include:
Lidoderm Patch … **1107**

Lidocaine Hydrochloride (Many drugs effective in the treatment of major depressive disorder, eg, the SSRIs, including sertraline, and most tricyclic antidepressant drugs effective in the treatment of major depressive disorder inhibit the biochemical activity of the drug metabolizing isoenzyme cytochrome P450 2D6, and, thus, may increase the plasma concentrations of co-administered drugs that are metabolized by CYP2D6. The drugs for which this potential interaction is of greatest

concern are those metabolized by CYP2D6 and which have a narrow therapeutic index).
No products indexed under this heading.

Lithium (No significant alteration in plasma lithium levels or renal clearance; nonetheless, plasma lithium levels should be monitored).
No products indexed under this heading.

Lithium Carbonate (No significant alteration in plasma lithium levels or renal clearance; nonetheless, plasma lithium levels should be monitored). Products include:
Eskalith 1406
Lithobid Tablets 1670

Lithium Citrate (No significant alteration in plasma lithium levels or renal clearance; nonetheless, plasma lithium levels should be monitored).
No products indexed under this heading.

Low Molecular Weight Heparins (Patients should be cautioned about the concomitant use of sertraline hydrochloride and drugs that affect coagulation since the combined use of psychotropic drugs that interfere with serotonin reuptake and these agents has been associated with an increased risk of bleeding).
No products indexed under this heading.

Maprotiline Hydrochloride (Concurrent use of drugs that inhibit the biochemical activity of P450IID6, such as tricyclic antidepressants, may increase plasma concentrations of co-administered drugs that are metabolized by P450IID6; changes in the dosage may be required; the duration of an appropriate washout period which should intervene before switching has not been established).
No products indexed under this heading.

Meclofenamate Sodium (Co-administration with drugs that are highly protein bound may cause a shift in plasma concentrations, potentially resulting in an adverse effect).
No products indexed under this heading.

Mefenamic Acid (Co-administration with drugs that are highly protein bound may cause a shift in plasma concentrations, potentially resulting in an adverse effect).
No products indexed under this heading.

Meloxicam (Patients should be cautioned about the concomitant use of sertraline hydrochloride and non-selective NSAIDs (eg, NSAIDs that inhibit both cyclooxygenase isoenzymes, COX 1 and 2), since the combined use of psychotropic drugs that interfere with serotonin reuptake and these agents has been associated with an increased risk of bleeding). Products include:
Mobic Oral Suspension 893
Mobic Tablets 893

Meperidine Hydrochloride (Many drugs effective in the treatment of major depressive disorder, eg, the SSRIs, including sertraline, and most tricyclic antidepressant drugs effective in the treatment of major depressive disorder inhibit the biochemical activity of the drug metabolizing isoenzyme cytochrome P450 2D6, and, thus, may increase the plasma concentrations of co-administered drugs that are metabolized by CYP2D6. The drugs for which this potential interaction is of greatest concern are those metabolized by CYP2D6 and which have a narrow therapeutic index).
No products indexed under this heading.

Methadone Hydrochloride (Many drugs effective in the treatment of major depressive disorder, eg, the SSRIs, including sertraline, and most tricyclic antidepressant drugs effective in the treatment of major depressive disorder inhibit the biochemical activity of the drug metabolizing isoenzyme cytochrome P450 2D6, and, thus, may increase the plasma concentrations of co-administered drugs that are metabolized by CYP2D6. The drugs for which this potential interaction is of greatest concern are those metabolized by CYP2D6 and which have a narrow therapeutic index).
No products indexed under this heading.

Methamphetamine Hydrochloride (Many drugs effective in the treatment of major depressive disorder, eg, the SSRIs, including sertraline, and most tricyclic antidepressant drugs effective in the treatment of major depressive disorder inhibit the biochemical activity of the drug metabolizing isoenzyme cytochrome P450 2D6, and, thus, may increase the plasma concentrations of co-administered drugs that are metabolized by CYP2D6. The drugs for which this potential interaction is of greatest concern are those metabolized by CYP2D6 and which have a narrow therapeutic index). Products include:
Desoxyn Tablets, USP 2482

Metoprolol Succinate (Many drugs effective in the treatment of major depressive disorder, eg, the SSRIs, including sertraline, and most tricyclic antidepressant drugs effective in the treatment of major depressive disorder inhibit the biochemical activity of the drug metabolizing isoenzyme cytochrome P450 2D6, and, thus, may increase the plasma concentrations of co-administered drugs that are metabolized by CYP2D6. The drugs for which this potential interaction is of greatest concern are those metabolized by CYP2D6 and which have a narrow therapeutic index). Products include:
Toprol-XL Tablets 660

Metoprolol Tartrate (Many drugs effective in the treatment of major depressive disorder, eg, the SSRIs, including sertraline, and most tricyclic antidepressant drugs effective in the treatment of major depressive disorder inhibit the biochemical activity of the drug metabolizing isoenzyme cytochrome P450 2D6, and, thus, may increase the plasma concentrations of co-administered drugs that are metabolized by CYP2D6. The drugs for which this potential interaction is of greatest concern are those metabolized by CYP2D6 and which have a narrow therapeutic index).
No products indexed under this heading.

Mexiletine Hydrochloride (Many drugs effective in the treatment of major depressive disorder, eg, the SSRIs, including sertraline, and most tricyclic antidepressant drugs effective in the treatment of major depressive disorder inhibit the biochemical activity of the drug metabolizing isoenzyme cytochrome P450 2D6, and, thus, may increase the plasma concentrations of co-administered drugs that are metabolized by CYP2D6. The drugs for which this potential interaction is of greatest concern are those metabolized by CYP2D6 and which have a narrow therapeutic index).
No products indexed under this heading.

Midazolam Hydrochloride (Co-administration with drugs that are highly protein bound may cause a shift in plasma concentrations, potentially resulting in an adverse effect).
No products indexed under this heading.

Mirtazapine (Concurrent use of drugs that inhibit the biochemical activity of P450IID6, such as tricyclic antidepressants, may increase plasma concentrations of co-administered drugs that are metabolized by P450IID6; changes in the dosage may be required; the duration of an appropriate washout period which should intervene before switching has not been established).
No products indexed under this heading.

Moclobemide (Concomitant use in patients taking MAO inhibitors and SSRIs, such as sertraline, has resulted in cases of serious fatal reactions including hyperthermia, rigidity, myoclonus, autonomic instability, delirium and coma; concurrent and/or sequential use is contraindicated).
No products indexed under this heading.

Morphine Sulfate (Many drugs effective in the treatment of major depressive disorder, eg, the SSRIs, including sertraline, and most tricyclic antidepressant drugs effective in the treatment of major depressive disorder inhibit the biochemical activity of the drug metabolizing isoenzyme cytochrome P450 2D6, and, thus, may increase the plasma concentrations of co-administered drugs that are metabolized by CYP2D6. The drugs for which this potential interaction is of greatest concern are those metabolized by CYP2D6 and which have a narrow therapeutic index). Products include:
Avinza Capsules 1714
Kadian Capsules 572
MS Contin Tablets 2703

Nabumetone (Patients should be cautioned about the concomitant use of sertraline hydrochloride and non-selective NSAIDs (eg, NSAIDs that inhibit both cyclooxygenase isoenzymes, COX 1 and 2), since the combined use of psychotropic drugs that interfere with serotonin reuptake and these agents has been associated with an increased risk of bleeding). Products include:
Relafen Tablets 1523

Naproxen (Co-administration with drugs that are highly protein bound may cause a shift in plasma concentrations, potentially resulting in an adverse effect). Products include:
EC-Naprosyn Delayed-Release Tablets 2769
Naprosyn Suspension 2769
Naprosyn Tablets 2769
Prevacid NapraPAC 3277

Naproxen Sodium (Co-administration with drugs that are highly protein bound may cause a shift in plasma concentrations, potentially resulting in an adverse effect). Products include:
Aleve Tablets, Caplets and Gelcaps .... ▣ 605
Anaprox Tablets 2769
Anaprox DS Tablets 2769

Nefazodone Hydrochloride (Care and prudent medical judgment should be exercised regarding the optimal timing of switching from another antidepressant to Zoloft; the duration of an appropriate washout period, which should intervene before switching, has not been established).
No products indexed under this heading.

Nelfinavir Mesylate (Many drugs effective in the treatment of major depressive disorder, eg, the SSRIs, including sertraline, and most tricyclic antidepressant drugs effective in the treatment of major depressive disorder inhibit the biochemical activity of the drug metabolizing isoenzyme cytochrome P450 2D6, and, thus, may increase the plasma concentrations of co-administered drugs that are metabolized by CYP2D6. The drugs for which this potential interaction is of greatest concern are those metabolized by CYP2D6 and which have a narrow therapeutic index). Products include:
Viracept 2556

Nortriptyline Hydrochloride (Concurrent use of drugs that inhibit the biochemical activity of P450IID6, such as tricyclic antidepressants, may increase plasma concentrations of co-administered drugs that are metabolized by P450IID6; changes in the dosage may be required; the duration of an appropriate washout period which should intervene before switching has not been established).
No products indexed under this heading.

Olanzapine (Many drugs effective in the treatment of major depressive disorder, eg, the SSRIs, including sertraline, and most tricyclic antidepressant drugs effective in the treatment of major depressive disorder inhibit the biochemical activity of the drug metabolizing isoenzyme cytochrome P450 2D6, and, thus, may increase the plasma concentrations of co-administered drugs that are metabolized by CYP2D6. The drugs for which this potential interaction is of greatest concern are those metabolized by CYP2D6 and which have a narrow therapeutic index). Products include:
Symbyax Capsules 1788
Zyprexa Tablets 1798
Zyprexa IntraMuscular 1798
Zyprexa ZYDIS Orally Disintegrating Tablets 1798

Omeprazole (Many drugs effective in the treatment of major depressive disorder, eg, the SSRIs, including sertraline, and most tricyclic antidepressant drugs effective in the treatment of major depressive disorder inhibit the biochemical activity of the drug metabolizing isoenzyme cytochrome P450 2D6, and, thus, may increase the plasma concentrations of co-administered drugs that are metabolized by CYP2D6. The drugs for which this potential interaction is

and which have a narrow therapeutic index).
No products indexed under this heading.

Risperidone (Many drugs effective in the treatment of major depressive disorder, eg, the SSRIs, including sertraline, and most tricyclic antidepressant drugs effective in the treatment of major depressive disorder inhibit the biochemical activity of the drug metabolizing isoenzyme cytochrome P450 2D6, and, thus, may increase the plasma concentrations of co-administered drugs that are metabolized by CYP2D6. The drugs for which this potential interaction is of greatest concern are those metabolized by CYP2D6 and which have a narrow therapeutic index). Products include:
Risperdal Consta Long-Acting Injection 1664
Risperdal M-Tab Orally Disintegrating Tablets 1658
Risperdal 1658

Ritonavir (Many drugs effective in the treatment of major depressive disorder, eg, the SSRIs, including sertraline, and most tricyclic antidepressant drugs effective in the treatment of major depressive disorder inhibit the biochemical activity of the drug metabolizing isoenzyme cytochrome P450 2D6, and, thus, may increase the plasma concentrations of co-administered drugs that are metabolized by CYP2D6. The drugs for which this potential interaction is of greatest concern are those metabolized by CYP2D6 and which have a narrow therapeutic index). Products include:
Kaletra 474
Norvir 499

Rofecoxib (Patients should be cautioned about the concomitant use of sertraline hydrochloride and nonselective NSAIDs (eg, NSAIDs that inhibit both cyclooxygenase isoenzymes, COX 1 and 2), since the combined use of psychotropic drugs that interfere with serotonin reuptake and these agents has been associated with an increased risk of bleeding).
No products indexed under this heading.

Selegiline Hydrochloride (Concomitant use in patients taking MAO inhibitors and SSRIs, such as sertraline, has resulted in cases of serious fatal reactions including hyperthermia, rigidity, myoclonus, autonomic instability, delirium and coma; concurrent and/or sequential use is contraindicated). Products include:
Eldepryl Capsules 3209

Sulindac (Co-administration with drugs that are highly protein bound may cause a shift in plasma concentrations, potentially resulting in an adverse effect). Products include:
Clinoril Tablets 1899

Sumatriptan (Co-administration of SSRIs and sumatriptan has resulted in rare reports of weakness, hyperreflexia, and incoordination). Products include:
Imitrex Nasal Spray 1435

Sumatriptan Succinate (Co-administration of SSRIs and sumatriptan has resulted in rare reports of weakness, hyperreflexia, and incoordination). Products include:
Imitrex Injection 1431
Imitrex Tablets 1440

Tamoxifen Citrate (Many drugs effective in the treatment of major depressive disorder, eg, the SSRIs, including sertraline, and most tricyclic antidepressant drugs effective in the treatment of major depressive disorder inhibit the biochemical activity of the drug metabolizing isoenzyme cytochrome P450 2D6, and, thus, may increase the plasma concentrations of co-administered drugs that are metabolized by CYP2D6. The drugs for which this potential interaction is of greatest concern are those metabolized by CYP2D6 and which have a narrow therapeutic index).
No products indexed under this heading.

Temazepam (Co-administration with drugs that are highly protein bound may cause a shift in plasma concentrations, potentially resulting in an adverse effect).
No products indexed under this heading.

Teniposide (Many drugs effective in the treatment of major depressive disorder, eg, the SSRIs, including sertraline, and most tricyclic antidepressant drugs effective in the treatment of major depressive disorder inhibit the biochemical activity of the drug metabolizing isoenzyme cytochrome P450 2D6, and, thus, may increase the plasma concentrations of co-administered drugs that are metabolized by CYP2D6. The drugs for which this potential interaction is of greatest concern are those metabolized by CYP2D6 and which have a narrow therapeutic index).
No products indexed under this heading.

Testosterone (Many drugs effective in the treatment of major depressive disorder, eg, the SSRIs, including sertraline, and most tricyclic antidepressant drugs effective in the treatment of major depressive disorder inhibit the biochemical activity of the drug metabolizing isoenzyme cytochrome P450 2D6, and, thus, may increase the plasma concentrations of co-administered drugs that are metabolized by CYP2D6. The drugs for which this potential interaction is of greatest concern are those metabolized by CYP2D6 and which have a narrow therapeutic index). Products include:
AndroGel 3330
Striant Mucoadhesive 1022
Testim 1% Gel 722

Testosterone Cypionate (Many drugs effective in the treatment of major depressive disorder, eg, the SSRIs, including sertraline, and most tricyclic antidepressant drugs effective in the treatment of major depressive disorder inhibit the biochemical activity of the drug metabolizing isoenzyme cytochrome P450 2D6, and, thus, may increase the plasma concentrations of co-administered drugs that are metabolized by CYP2D6. The drugs for which this potential interaction is of greatest concern are those metabolized by CYP2D6 and which have a narrow therapeutic index).
No products indexed under this heading.

Testosterone Enanthate (Many drugs effective in the treatment of major depressive disorder, eg, the SSRIs, including sertraline, and most tricyclic antidepressant drugs effective in the treatment of major depressive disorder inhibit the biochemical activity of the drug metabolizing isoenzyme cytochrome P450 2D6, and, thus, may increase the plasma concentrations of co-administered drugs that are metabolized by CYP2D6. The drugs for which this potential interaction is of greatest concern are those metabolized by CYP2D6 and which have a narrow therapeutic index). Products include:
Delatestryl Injection 2976

Testosterone Propionate (Many drugs effective in the treatment of major depressive disorder, eg, the SSRIs, including sertraline, and most tricyclic antidepressant drugs effective in the treatment of major depressive disorder inhibit the biochemical activity of the drug metabolizing isoenzyme cytochrome P450 2D6, and, thus, may increase the plasma concentrations of co-administered drugs that are metabolized by CYP2D6. The drugs for which this potential interaction is of greatest concern are those metabolized by CYP2D6 and which have a narrow therapeutic index).
No products indexed under this heading.

Thioridazine (Many drugs effective in the treatment of major depressive disorder, eg, the SSRIs, including sertraline, and most tricyclic antidepressant drugs effective in the treatment of major depressive disorder inhibit the biochemical activity of the drug metabolizing isoenzyme cytochrome P450 2D6, and, thus, may increase the plasma concentrations of co-administered drugs that are metabolized by CYP2D6. The drugs for which this potential interaction is of greatest concern are those metabolized by CYP2D6 and which have a narrow therapeutic index).
No products indexed under this heading.

Thioridazine Hydrochloride (Many drugs effective in the treatment of major depressive disorder, eg, the SSRIs, including sertraline, and most tricyclic antidepressant drugs effective in the treatment of major depressive disorder inhibit the biochemical activity of the drug metabolizing isoenzyme cytochrome P450 2D6, and, thus, may increase the plasma concentrations of co-administered drugs that are metabolized by CYP2D6. The drugs for which this potential interaction is of greatest concern are those metabolized by CYP2D6 and which have a narrow therapeutic index). Products include:
Thioridazine Hydrochloride Tablets 2122

Timolol Maleate (Many drugs effective in the treatment of major depressive disorder, eg, the SSRIs, including sertraline, and most tricyclic antidepressant drugs effective in the treatment of major depressive disorder inhibit the biochemical activity of the drug metabolizing isoenzyme cytochrome P450 2D6, and, thus, may increase the plasma concentrations of co-administered drugs that are metabolized by CYP2D6. The drugs for which this potential interaction is of greatest concern are those metabolized by CYP2D6 and which have a narrow therapeutic index). Products include:
Blocadren Tablets 1891
Cosopt Sterile Ophthalmic Solution 1910
Timolide Tablets 2056
Timoptic in Ocudose 2061
Timoptic Sterile Ophthalmic Solution 2058
Timoptic-XE Sterile Ophthalmic Gel Forming Solution 2062

Tinzaparin Sodium (Patients should be cautioned about the concomitant use of sertraline hydrochloride and drugs that affect coagulation since the combined use of psychotropic drugs that interfere with serotonin reuptake and these agents has been associated with an increased risk of bleeding).
No products indexed under this heading.

Tolbutamide (Co-administration has caused a statistically significant 16% decrease from baseline in the clearance of tolbutamide; the clinical significance of this finding is unknown).
No products indexed under this heading.

Tolmetin Sodium (Co-administration with drugs that are highly protein bound may cause a shift in plasma concentrations, potentially resulting in an adverse effect).
No products indexed under this heading.

Tolterodine Tartrate (Many drugs effective in the treatment of major depressive disorder, eg, the SSRIs, including sertraline, and most tricyclic antidepressant drugs effective in the treatment of major depressive disorder inhibit the biochemical activity of the drug metabolizing isoenzyme cytochrome P450 2D6, and, thus, may increase the plasma concentrations of co-administered drugs that are metabolized by CYP2D6. The drugs for which this potential interaction is of greatest concern are those metabolized by CYP2D6 and which have a narrow therapeutic index). Products include:
Detrol Tablets 2626
Detrol LA Capsules 2629

Tramadol Hydrochloride (Many drugs effective in the treatment of major depressive disorder, eg, the SSRIs, including sertraline, and most tricyclic antidepressant drugs effective in the treatment of major depressive disorder inhibit the biochemical activity of the drug metabolizing isoenzyme cytochrome P450 2D6, and, thus, may increase the plasma concentrations of co-administered drugs that are metabolized by CYP2D6. The drugs for which this potential interaction is of greatest concern are those metabolized by CYP2D6 and which have a narrow therapeutic index). Products include:
Ultracet Tablets 2462

Tranylcypromine Sulfate (Concomitant use in patients taking MAO inhibitors and SSRIs, such as sertraline, has resulted in cases of serious fatal reactions including hyperthermia, rigidity, myoclonus, autonomic instability, delirium and coma; concurrent and/or sequential use is contraindicated). Products include:
Parnate Tablets 1499

Trazodone Hydrochloride (Concurrent use of drugs that inhibit the biochemical activity of P450IID6, such as tricyclic antidepressants, may increase plasma concentrations of co-administered drugs that are metabolized by P450IID6; changes in the dosage may be required; the duration of an appropriate washout period which should intervene before switching has not been established).
No products indexed under this heading.

Triazolam (Many drugs effective in the treatment of major depressive disorder, eg, the SSRIs, including sertraline, and most tricyclic antidepressant drugs effective in the treatment of major depressive disorder inhibit the biochemical activity of the drug metabolizing isoenzyme cytochrome P450 2D6, and, thus, may increase the plasma concentrations of co-administered drugs that are metabolized by CYP2D6. The drugs for which this potential interaction is of greatest concern are those metabolized by CYP2D6 and which have a narrow therapeutic index).
No products indexed under this heading.

Trimipramine Maleate (Concurrent use of drugs that inhibit the biochemical activity of P450IID6, such as tricyclic antidepressants, may increase plasma concentrations of co-administered drugs that are metabolized by P450IID6; changes in the dosage may be required; the duration of an appropriate washout period which should intervene before switching has not been established). Products include:
Surmontil Capsules 2347

Valdecoxib (Patients should be cautioned about the concomitant use of sertraline hydrochloride and non-selective NSAIDs (eg, NSAIDs that inhibit both cyclooxygenase isoenzymes, COX 1 and 2), since the combined use of psychotropic drugs that interfere with serotonin reuptake and these agents has been associated with an increased risk of bleeding).
No products indexed under this heading.

Venlafaxine Hydrochloride (Concurrent use of drugs that inhibit the biochemical activity of P450IID6, such as SSRIs, may increase plasma concentrations of co-administered drugs that are metabolized by P450IID6; changes in the dosage may be required; the duration of an appropriate washout period, which should intervene before switching, has not been established). Products include:
Effexor Tablets 3405
Effexor XR Capsules 3411

Vinblastine Sulfate (Many drugs effective in the treatment of major depressive disorder, eg, the SSRIs, including sertraline, and most tricyclic antidepressant drugs effective in the treatment of major depressive disorder inhibit the biochemical activity of the drug metabolizing isoenzyme cytochrome P450 2D6, and, thus, may increase the plasma concentrations of co-administered drugs that are metabolized by CYP2D6. The drugs for which this potential interaction is of greatest concern are those metabolized by CYP2D6 and which have a narrow therapeutic index).
No products indexed under this heading.

Warfarin Sodium (Co-administration has resulted in a mean increase in prothrombin time of 8% relative to baseline for sertraline; the clinical significance of this change is not known). Products include:
Coumadin for Injection 932
Coumadin Tablets 932

Zonisamide (Many drugs effective in the treatment of major depressive disorder, eg, the SSRIs, including sertraline, and most tricyclic antidepressant drugs effective in the treatment of major depressive disorder inhibit the biochemical activity of the drug metabolizing isoenzyme cytochrome P450 2D6, and, thus, may increase the plasma concentrations of co-administered drugs that are metabolized by CYP2D6. The drugs for which this potential interaction is of greatest concern are those metabolized by CYP2D6 and which have a narrow therapeutic index). Products include:
Zonegran Capsules 1089

Food Interactions

Alcohol (Patients should be told that although sertraline hydrochloride has not been shown in experiments with normal subjects to increase the mental and motor skill impairments caused by alcohol, the concomitant use of sertraline hydrochloride and alcohol is not advised).

Food, unspecified (Co-administration of Zoloft Tablets with food slightly increased AUC but the Cmax was 25% greater, while time to reach peak plasma concentration (Tmax) decreased from 8 hours to 5.5 hours; for oral concentrate, Tmax was slightly prolonged from 5.9 hours to 7 hours with food).

ZOLOFT TABLETS

(Sertraline Hydrochloride) 2581
See Zoloft Oral Concentrate

ZOMETA FOR INTRAVENOUS INFUSION

(Zoledronic acid) 2306
May interact with aminoglycosides and loop diuretics. Compounds in these categories include:

Amikacin Sulfate (Co-administration with aminoglycosides may have an additive effect to lower serum calcium for prolonged period).
No products indexed under this heading.

Bumetanide (Increased risk of hypocalcemia).
No products indexed under this heading.

Ethacrynic Acid (Increased risk of hypocalcemia). Products include:
Edecrin Tablets 1941

Furosemide (Increased risk of hypocalcemia). Products include:
Furosemide Tablets 2117

Gentamicin Sulfate (Co-administration with aminoglycosides may have an additive effect to lower serum calcium for prolonged period). Products include:
Garamycin Injectable 3028
Genoptic Sterile Ophthalmic Solution .... ⊙ 227
Pred-G Ophthalmic Suspension ...... ⊙ 234
Pred-G Sterile Ophthalmic Ointment .... ⊙ 235

Kanamycin Sulfate (Co-administration with aminoglycosides may have an additive effect to lower serum calcium for prolonged period).
No products indexed under this heading.

Streptomycin Sulfate (Co-administration with aminoglycosides may have an additive effect to lower serum calcium for prolonged period).
No products indexed under this heading.

Tobramycin (Co-administration with aminoglycosides may have an additive effect to lower serum calcium for prolonged period). Products include:
TOBI Solution for Inhalation 1015
TobraDex Ophthalmic Ointment 558
TobraDex Ophthalmic Suspension ... 558
Zylet Ophthalmic Suspension 3508

Tobramycin Sulfate (Co-administration with aminoglycosides may have an additive effect to lower serum calcium for prolonged period).
No products indexed under this heading.

Torsemide (Increased risk of hypocalcemia).
No products indexed under this heading.

ZOMIG NASAL SPRAY

(Zolmitriptan) 718
May interact with 5HT1-receptor agonists, ergot-containing drugs, monoamine oxidase inhibitors, oral contraceptives, selective serotonin reuptake inhibitors, and certain other agents. Compounds in these categories include:

Acetaminophen (Zolmitriptan delayed the Tmax of acetaminophen by one hour in a single dose study). Products include:
Benadryl Allergy & Cold Tablets 692
Benadryl Allergy & Sinus Headache Caplets & Gelcaps 693
Benadryl Maximum Strength Severe Allergy & Sinus Headache Caplets 694
Contac Severe Cold and Flu Caplets Maximum Strength 615
Contac Severe Cold and Flu Caplets Non-Drowsy 615
Darvocet A 500 Tablets 3497
Goody's Body Pain Formula Powder 621
Goody's Extra Strength Headache Powder 621
Goody's Extra Strength Pain Relief Tablets 621
Goody's PM Powder 622
Hycomine Compound Tablets 1105
Lortab 3315
Lortab Elixir 3312
Percocet Tablets 1114
Robitussin Cough, Cold & Flu Liquid-filled Capsules 750
Robitussin Flu Liquid 752
Sedapap Tablets 50 mg/650 mg 2098
Singlet Caplets 636
Sudafed Severe Cold 710
Sudafed Sinus Headache 711
TheraFlu Cold & Cough Hot Liquid 680
TheraFlu Cold & Sore Throat Hot Liquid 680
TheraFlu Flu & Chest Congestion Non-Drowsy Hot Liquid 681
TheraFlu Flu & Sore Throat Hot Liquid 681
TheraFlu Severe Cold Non-Drowsy Hot Liquid 683
TheraFlu Severe Cold & Cough Hot Liquid 683
TheraFlu Severe Cold Caplets 679
TheraFlu Severe Cold Hot Liquid 682
TheraFlu Severe Cold Non-Drowsy Caplets 679
Triaminic Cough & Sore Throat Liquid 687
Triaminic Flu, Cough & Fever Liquid 685
Triaminic Cough & Sore Throat Softchews 689
Tylenol 8 Hour Extended Release Geltabs and Caplets 1843
Tylenol Sinus NightTime Caplets 663
Children's Tylenol Suspension Liquid and Meltaways 1850
Children's Tylenol Plus Cold & Allergy Suspension Liquid 1850
Children's Tylenol Plus Cold NightTime Suspension Liquid 1851
Children's Tylenol Plus Cold & Cough Suspension Liquid and Chewable Tablets 1851
Children's Tylenol Plus Cold Chewable Tablets 1851
Children's Tylenol Plus Cold Daytime Non-Drowsy Suspension Liquid 1851
Children's Tylenol Plus Flu Suspension Liquid 1853
Concentrated Tylenol Infants' Drops Plus Cold 1851
Concentrated Tylenol Infants' Drops Plus Cold and Cough 1851
Concentrated Tylenol Infants' Drops 1850
Junior Tylenol Meltaways 1850
Tylenol Cold & Flu Severe Daytime Liquid with Cool Burst....... 1846
Tylenol Cold & Flu Severe NightTime Liquid with Cool Burst 1846
Tylenol Cold Severe Congestion Non-Drowsy Caplets with Cool Burst 1846
Tylenol Cough & Sore Throat Daytime Liquid with Cool Burst...... 1849
Tylenol Cough & Sore Throat NightTime Liquid with Cool Burst 1849
Tylenol 1843
Extra Strength Tylenol Rapid Release Gels 1843
Tylenol 1843
Tylenol Allergy Complete Night Time Caplets 1844
Tylenol Allergy Complete Multi-Symptom Caplets and Gelcaps with Cool Burst............... 1844
Tylenol Severe Allergy Caplets 1844
Tylenol Flu NightTime Gelcaps 1846
Tylenol Flu Day Non-Drowsy Gelcaps 1846
Concentrated Tylenol Infants' Drops Plus Cold Nasal Congestant, Fever Reducer & Pain Reliever 668
Concentrated Tylenol Infants' Drops Plus Cold & Cough Nasal Decongestant, Fever Reducer & Pain Reliever 668
Multi-Symptom Tylenol Cold Night Time Caplets 1845
Multi-Symptom Tylenol Cold Day Non-Drowsy Caplets and Gelcaps 1845
Extra Strength Tylenol PM Caplets, Geltabs, Gelcaps and Liquid 1847
Tylenol Sinus Day Non-Drowsy 1848
Tylenol Sinus Night Time Caplets 1848
Tylenol Sinus Severe Congestion Caplets with Cool Burst 1848
Tylenol Sore Throat Daytime Liquid with Cool Burst 1849
Tylenol Sore Throat NightTime Liquid with Cool Burst 1849
Tylenol with Codeine 2461
Women's Tylenol Menstrual Relief Caplets... 1849
Ultracet Tablets 2462
Vicks 44M Cough, Cold & Flu Relief 2676
Vicks DayQuil LiquiCaps/Liquid Multi-Symptom Cold/Flu Relief..... 723
Vicks DayQuil Multi-Symptom Cold/Flu Relief LiquiCaps............. 2675
Vicks DayQuil Multi-Symptom Cold/Flu Relief Liquid..................... 2675

- Vicks NyQuil LiquiCaps **2677**
- Vicks NyQuil LiquiCaps/Liquid Multi-Symptom Cold/Flu Relief..... ▣ **725**
- Vicks NyQuil Liquid **2677**
- Vicodin Tablets **530**
- Vicodin ES Tablets **531**
- Vicodin HP Tablets **532**
- Zydone Tablets **1118**

Cimetidine (Following administration of cimetidine, the half-life and AUC of zolmitriptan and its active metabolites were approximately doubled). Products include:

- Tagamet HB 200 Tablets .... ▣ **637**
- Tagamet Tablets **1547**

Cimetidine Hydrochloride (Following administration of cimetidine, the half-life and AUC of zolmitriptan and its active metabolites were approximately doubled).

No products indexed under this heading.

Citalopram Hydrobromide (Co-administration of 5-HT1 agonists with selective serotonin reuptake inhibitors has resulted, rarely, in hyperreflexia, weakness and incoordination). Products include:

- Celexa **1177**

Desogestrel (Retrospective analysis of pharmacokinetic data indicates the mean plasma concentrations, Cmax and AUC, of zolmitriptan were generally higher in females taking oral contraceptives, Tmax was delayed by one-half hour in these females). Products include:

- Ortho-Cept Tablets **2395**

Dihydroergotamine Mesylate (Ergot-containing drugs have been reported to cause prolonged vasospastic reactions; because there is a theoretical basis that these effects may be additive, use of ergot-type agents and zolmitriptan within 24 hours is contraindicated). Products include:

- Migranal Nasal Spray **3350**

3-Diphenylacrylate (Co-administration with other 5-HT1 agonists within 24 hours of each other is contraindicated).

No products indexed under this heading.

Ergonovine Maleate (Ergot-containing drugs have been reported to cause prolonged vasospastic reactions; because there is a theoretical basis that these effects may be additive, use of ergot-type agents and zolmitriptan within 24 hours is contraindicated).

No products indexed under this heading.

Ergotamine Tartrate (Ergot-containing drugs have been reported to cause prolonged vasospastic reactions; because there is a theoretical basis that these effects may be additive, use of ergot-type agents and zolmitriptan within 24 hours is contraindicated).

No products indexed under this heading.

Escitalopram Oxalate (Co-administration of 5-HT1 agonists with selective serotonin reuptake inhibitors has resulted, rarely, in hyperreflexia, weakness and incoordination). Products include:

- Lexapro Oral Solution **1193**
- Lexapro Tablets **1193**

Ethinyl Estradiol (Retrospective analysis of pharmacokinetic data indicates the mean plasma concentrations, Cmax and AUC, of zolmitriptan were generally higher in females taking oral contraceptives, Tmax was delayed by one-half hour in these females). Products include:

- Alesse-28 Tablets **3392**
- Lo/Ovral-28 Tablets **3423**
- NuvaRing **2357**
- Ortho-Cept Tablets **2395**
- Ortho-Cyclen/Ortho Tri-Cyclen **2414**
- Ortho Evra Transdermal System **2402**
- Ortho Tri-Cyclen Lo Tablets **2421**
- Seasonale Tablets **1073**
- Triphasil-28 Tablets **3483**
- Yasmin 28 Tablets **818**

Ethynodiol Diacetate (Retrospective analysis of pharmacokinetic data indicates the mean plasma concentrations, Cmax and AUC, of zolmitriptan were generally higher in females taking oral contraceptives, Tmax was delayed by one-half hour in these females).

No products indexed under this heading.

Fluoxetine Hydrochloride (Co-administration of 5-HT1 agonists with selective serotonin reuptake inhibitors has resulted, rarely, in hyperreflexia, weakness and incoordination). Products include:

- Prozac Pulvules and Liquid **1771**
- Symbyax Capsules **1788**

Fluvoxamine Maleate (Co-administration of 5-HT1 agonists with selective serotonin reuptake inhibitors has resulted, rarely, in hyperreflexia, weakness and incoordination).

No products indexed under this heading.

Isocarboxazid (MAO-A inhibitors increase the systemic exposure of zolmitriptan; concurrent and/or sequential use is contraindicated).

No products indexed under this heading.

Levonorgestrel (Retrospective analysis of pharmacokinetic data indicates the mean plasma concentrations, Cmax and AUC, of zolmitriptan were generally higher in females taking oral contraceptives, Tmax was delayed by one-half hour in these females). Products include:

- Alesse-28 Tablets **3392**
- Climara Pro Transdermal System **800**
- Mirena Intrauterine System **810**
- Plan B Tablets **1068**
- Seasonale Tablets **1073**
- Triphasil-28 Tablets **3483**

Mestranol (Retrospective analysis of pharmacokinetic data indicates the mean plasma concentrations, Cmax and AUC, of zolmitriptan were generally higher in females taking oral contraceptives, Tmax was delayed by one-half hour in these females).

No products indexed under this heading.

Methylergonovine Maleate (Ergot-containing drugs have been reported to cause prolonged vasospastic reactions; because there is a theoretical basis that these effects may be additive, use of ergot-type agents and zolmitriptan within 24 hours is contraindicated).

No products indexed under this heading.

Methysergide Maleate (Ergot-containing drugs have been reported to cause prolonged vasospastic reactions; because there is a theoretical basis that these effects may be additive, use of ergot-type agents and zolmitriptan within 24 hours is contraindicated).

No products indexed under this heading.

Moclobemide (MAO-A inhibitors increase the systemic exposure of zolmitriptan; concurrent and/or sequential use is contraindicated).

No products indexed under this heading.

Naratriptan Hydrochloride (Co-administration with other 5-HT1 agonists within 24 hours of each other is contraindicated). Products include:

- Amerge Tablets **1312**

Norethindrone (Retrospective analysis of pharmacokinetic data indicates the mean plasma concentrations, Cmax and AUC, of zolmitriptan were generally higher in females taking oral contraceptives, Tmax was delayed by one-half hour in these females). Products include:

- Ortho Micronor Tablets **2411**

Norethynodrel (Retrospective analysis of pharmacokinetic data indicates the mean plasma concentrations, Cmax and AUC, of zolmitriptan were generally higher in females taking oral contraceptives, Tmax was delayed by one-half hour in these females).

No products indexed under this heading.

Norgestimate (Retrospective analysis of pharmacokinetic data indicates the mean plasma concentrations, Cmax and AUC, of zolmitriptan were generally higher in females taking oral contraceptives, Tmax was delayed by one-half hour in these females). Products include:

- Ortho-Cyclen/Ortho Tri-Cyclen **2414**
- Ortho Tri-Cyclen Lo Tablets **2421**
- Prefest Tablets **1069**

Norgestrel (Retrospective analysis of pharmacokinetic data indicates the mean plasma concentrations, Cmax and AUC, of zolmitriptan were generally higher in females taking oral contraceptives, Tmax was delayed by one-half hour in these females). Products include:

- Lo/Ovral-28 Tablets **3423**

Pargyline Hydrochloride (MAO-A inhibitors increase the systemic exposure of zolmitriptan; concurrent and/or sequential use is contraindicated).

No products indexed under this heading.

Paroxetine Hydrochloride (Co-administration of 5-HT1 agonists with selective serotonin reuptake inhibitors has resulted, rarely, in hyperreflexia, weakness and incoordination). Products include:

- Paxil CR Controlled-Release Tablets **1509**
- Paxil **1501**

Phenelzine Sulfate (MAO-A inhibitors increase the systemic exposure of zolmitriptan; concurrent and/or sequential use is contraindicated).

No products indexed under this heading.

Procarbazine Hydrochloride (MAO-A inhibitors increase the systemic exposure of zolmitriptan; concurrent and/or sequential use is contraindicated). Products include:

- Matulane Capsules **3188**

Propanolol (Cmax and AUC of zolmitriptan increased after one week of dosing with propanolol; Cmax and AUC of N-desmethyl metabolite was reduced).

No products indexed under this heading.

Rizatriptan Benzoate (Co-administration with other 5-HT1 agonists within 24 hours of each other is contraindicated). Products include:

- Maxalt Tablets **1983**
- Maxalt-MLT Orally Disintegrating Tablets **1983**

Selegiline Hydrochloride (MAO-A inhibitors increase the systemic exposure of zolmitriptan; concurrent and/or sequential use is contraindicated). Products include:

- Eldepryl Capsules **3209**

Sertraline Hydrochloride (Co-administration of 5-HT1 agonists with selective serotonin reuptake inhibitors has resulted, rarely, in hyperreflexia, weakness and incoordination). Products include:

- Zoloft **2581**

Sumatriptan (Co-administration with other 5-HT1 agonists within 24 hours of each other is contraindicated). Products include:

- Imitrex Nasal Spray **1435**

Sumatriptan Succinate (Co-administration with other 5-HT1 agonists within 24 hours of each other is contraindicated). Products include:

- Imitrex Injection **1431**
- Imitrex Tablets **1440**

Tranylcypromine Sulfate (MAO-A inhibitors increase the systemic exposure of zolmitriptan; concurrent and/or sequential use is contraindicated). Products include:

- Parnate Tablets **1499**

ZOMIG TABLETS

(Zolmitriptan) **714**

May interact with 5HT1-receptor agonists, ergot-containing drugs, monoamine oxidase inhibitors, oral contraceptives, selective serotonin reuptake inhibitors, and certain other agents. Compounds in these categories include:

Acetaminophen (Zolmitriptan delayed the Tmax of acetaminophen by 1 hour in a single dose study). Products include:

- Benadryl Allergy & Cold Tablets .... ▣ **692**
- Benadryl Allergy & Sinus Headache Caplets & Gelcaps .... ▣ **693**
- Benadryl Maximum Strength Severe Allergy & Sinus Headache Caplets .... ▣ **694**
- Contac Severe Cold and Flu Caplets Maximum Strength .... ▣ **615**
- Contac Severe Cold and Flu Caplets Non-Drowsy .... ▣ **615**
- Darvocet A 500 Tablets **3497**
- Goody's Body Pain Formula Powder .... ▣ **621**
- Goody's Extra Strength Headache Powder .... ▣ **621**
- Goody's Extra Strength Pain Relief Tablets .... ▣ **621**
- Goody's PM Powder .... ▣ **622**
- Hycomine Compound Tablets **1105**
- Lortab **3315**
- Lortab Elixir **3312**
- Percocet Tablets **1114**
- Robitussin Cough, Cold & Flu Liquid-filled Capsules .... ▣ **750**
- Robitussin Flu Liquid .... ▣ **752**
- Sedapap Tablets 50 mg/650 mg **2098**
- Singlet Caplets .... ▣ **636**
- Sudafed Severe Cold .... ▣ **710**
- Sudafed Sinus Headache .... ▣ **711**
- TheraFlu Cold & Cough Hot Liquid .... ▣ **680**
- TheraFlu Cold & Sore Throat Hot Liquid .... ▣ **680**
- TheraFlu Flu & Chest Congestion Non-Drowsy Hot Liquid .... ▣ **681**
- TheraFlu Flu & Sore Throat Hot Liquid .... ▣ **681**
- TheraFlu Severe Cold Non-Drowsy Hot Liquid .... ▣ **683**

TheraFlu Severe Cold & Cough Hot Liquid 683
TheraFlu Severe Cold Caplets 679
TheraFlu Severe Cold Hot Liquid 682
TheraFlu Severe Cold Non-Drowsy Caplets 679
Triaminic Cough & Sore Throat Liquid 687
Triaminic Flu, Cough & Fever Liquid 685
Triaminic Cough & Sore Throat Softchews 689
Tylenol 8 Hour Extended Release Geltabs and Caplets 1843
Tylenol Sinus NightTime Caplets 663
Children's Tylenol Suspension Liquid and Meltaways 1850
Children's Tylenol Plus Cold & Allergy Suspension Liquid 1850
Children's Tylenol Plus Cold NightTime Suspension Liquid 1851
Children's Tylenol Plus Cold & Cough Suspension Liquid and Chewable Tablets 1851
Children's Tylenol Plus Cold Chewable Tablets 1851
Children's Tylenol Plus Cold Daytime Non-Drowsy Suspension Liquid 1851
Children's Tylenol Plus Flu Suspension Liquid 1853
Concentrated Tylenol Infants' Drops Plus Cold 1851
Concentrated Tylenol Infants' Drops Plus Cold and Cough 1851
Concentrated Tylenol Infants' Drops 1850
Junior Tylenol Meltaways 1850
Tylenol Cold & Flu Severe Daytime Liquid with Cool Bust 1846
Tylenol Cold & Flu Severe NightTime Liquid with Cool Burst 1846
Tylenol Cold Severe Congestion Non-Drowsy Caplets with Cool Burst 1846
Tylenol Cough & Sore Throat Daytime Liquid with Cool Burst 1849
Tylenol Cough & Sore Throat NightTime Liquid with Cool Burst 1849
Tylenol 1843
Extra Strength Tylenol Rapid Release Gels 1843
Tylenol 1843
Tylenol Allergy Complete Night Time Caplets 1844
Tylenol Allergy Complete Multi-Symptom Caplets and Gelcaps with Cool Burst 1844
Tylenol Severe Allergy Caplets 1844
Tylenol Flu NightTime Gelcaps 1846
Tylenol Flu Day Non-Drowsy Gelcaps 1846
Concentrated Tylenol Infants' Drops Plus Cold Nasal Congestant, Fever Reducer & Pain Reliever 668
Concentrated Tylenol Infants' Drops Plus Cold & Cough Nasal Decongestant, Fever Reducer & Pain Reliever 668
Multi-Symptom Tylenol Cold Night Time Caplets 1845
Multi-Symptom Tylenol Cold Day Non-Drowsy Caplets and Gelcaps 1845
Extra Strength Tylenol PM Caplets, Geltabs, Gelcaps and Liquid 1847
Tylenol Sinus Day Non-Drowsy 1848
Tylenol Sinus Night Time Caplets 1848
Tylenol Sinus Severe Congestion Caplets with Cool Burst 1848
Tylenol Sore Throat Daytime Liquid with Cool Burst 1849
Tylenol Sore Throat NightTime Liquid with Cool Burst 1849
Tylenol with Codeine 2461
Women's Tylenol Menstrual Relief Caplets 1849
Ultracet Tablets 2462
Vicks 44M Cough, Cold & Flu Relief 2676
Vicks DayQuil LiquiCaps/Liquid Multi-Symptom Cold/Flu Relief 723
Vicks DayQuil Multi-Symptom Cold/Flu Relief LiquiCaps 2675
Vicks DayQuil Multi-Symptom Cold/Flu Relief Liquid 2675
Vicks NyQuil LiquiCaps 2677
Vicks NyQuil LiquiCaps/Liquid Multi-Symptom Cold/Flu Relief 725
Vicks NyQuil Liquid 2677
Vicodin Tablets 530
Vicodin ES Tablets 531
Vicodin HP Tablets 532
Zydone Tablets 1118

Cimetidine (Following the administration of cimetidine, the half-life and AUC of a 5 mg dose of zolmitriptan and its active metabolite were approximately doubled). Products include:
Tagamet HB 200 Tablets 637
Tagamet Tablets 1547

Cimetidine Hydrochloride (Following the administration of cimetidine, the half-life and AUC of a 5 mg dose of zolmitriptan and its active metabolite were approximately doubled).
No products indexed under this heading.

Citalopram Hydrobromide (Co-administration of 5-HT1 agonists with selective serotonin reuptake inhibitors (SSRIs) has resulted, rarely, in hyperreflexia, weakness, and incoordination). Products include:
Celexa 1177

Desogestrel (Retrospective analysis of pharmacokinetic data indicates that mean plasma concentrations, Cmax and AUC, of zolmitriptan were generally higher in females taking oral contraceptives; Tmax was delayed by one-half hour in these females). Products include:
Ortho-Cept Tablets 2395

Dihydroergotamine Mesylate (Ergot-containing drugs have been reported to cause prolonged vasospastic reactions; because there is a theoretical basis that these effects may be additive, use of ergot-type agents and zolmitriptan within 24 hours is contraindicated). Products include:
Migranal Nasal Spray 3350

3-Diphenylacrylate (Co-administration with other 5-HT1 agonists within 24 hours of each other is contraindicated because the vasospastic effects may be additive).
No products indexed under this heading.

Ergonovine Maleate (Ergot-containing drugs have been reported to cause prolonged vasospastic reactions; because there is a theoretical basis that these effects may be additive, use of ergot-type agents and zolmitriptan within 24 hours is contraindicated).
No products indexed under this heading.

Ergotamine Tartrate (Ergot-containing drugs have been reported to cause prolonged vasospastic reactions; because there is a theoretical basis that these effects may be additive, use of ergot-type agents and zolmitriptan within 24 hours is contraindicated).
No products indexed under this heading.

Escitalopram Oxalate (Co-administration of 5-HT1 agonists with selective serotonin reuptake inhibitors (SSRIs) has resulted, rarely, in hyperreflexia, weakness, and incoordination). Products include:
Lexapro Oral Solution 1193
Lexapro Tablets 1193

Ethinyl Estradiol (Retrospective analysis of pharmacokinetic data indicates that mean plasma concentrations, Cmax and AUC, of zolmitriptan were generally higher in females taking oral contraceptives; Tmax was delayed by one-half hour in these females). Products include:
Alesse-28 Tablets 3392
Lo/Ovral-28 Tablets 3423
NuvaRing 2357
Ortho-Cept Tablets 2395
Ortho-Cyclen/Ortho Tri-Cyclen 2414
Ortho Evra Transdermal System 2402
Ortho Tri-Cyclen Lo Tablets 2421
Seasonale Tablets 1073
Triphasil-28 Tablets 3483
Yasmin 28 Tablets 818

Ethynodiol Diacetate (Retrospective analysis of pharmacokinetic data indicates that mean plasma concentrations, Cmax and AUC, of zolmitriptan were generally higher in females taking oral contraceptives; Tmax was delayed by one-half hour in these females).
No products indexed under this heading.

Fluoxetine Hydrochloride (Co-administration of 5-HT1 agonists with selective serotonin reuptake inhibitors (SSRIs) has resulted, rarely, in hyperreflexia, weakness, and incoordination). Products include:
Prozac Pulvules and Liquid 1771
Symbyax Capsules 1788

Fluvoxamine Maleate (Co-administration of 5-HT1 agonists with selective serotonin reuptake inhibitors (SSRIs) has resulted, rarely, in hyperreflexia, weakness, and incoordination).
No products indexed under this heading.

Isocarboxazid (MAO-A inhibitors increase the systemic exposure of zolmitriptan; concurrent and/or sequential use is contraindicated).
No products indexed under this heading.

Levonorgestrel (Retrospective analysis of pharmacokinetic data indicates that mean plasma concentrations, Cmax and AUC, of zolmitriptan were generally higher in females taking oral contraceptives; Tmax was delayed by one-half hour in these females). Products include:
Alesse-28 Tablets 3392
Climara Pro Transdermal System 800
Mirena Intrauterine System 810
Plan B Tablets 1068
Seasonale Tablets 1073
Triphasil-28 Tablets 3483

Mestranol (Retrospective analysis of pharmacokinetic data indicates that mean plasma concentrations, Cmax and AUC, of zolmitriptan were generally higher in females taking oral contraceptives; Tmax was delayed by one-half hour in these females).
No products indexed under this heading.

Methylergonovine Maleate (Ergot-containing drugs have been reported to cause prolonged vasospastic reactions; because there is a theoretical basis that these effects may be additive, use of ergot-type agents and zolmitriptan within 24 hours is contraindicated).
No products indexed under this heading.

Methysergide Maleate (Ergot-containing drugs have been reported to cause prolonged vasospastic reactions; because there is a theoretical basis that these effects may be additive, use of ergot-type agents and zolmitriptan within 24 hours is contraindicated).
No products indexed under this heading.

Moclobemide (MAO-A inhibitors increase the systemic exposure of zolmitriptan; concurrent and/or sequential use is contraindicated).
No products indexed under this heading.

Naratriptan Hydrochloride (Co-administration with other 5-HT1 agonists within 24 hours of each other is contraindicated because the vasospastic effects may be additive). Products include:
Amerge Tablets 1312

Norethindrone (Retrospective analysis of pharmacokinetic data indicates that mean plasma concentrations, Cmax and AUC, of zolmitriptan were generally higher in females taking oral contraceptives; Tmax was delayed by one-half hour in these females). Products include:
Ortho Micronor Tablets 2411

Norethynodrel (Retrospective analysis of pharmacokinetic data indicates that mean plasma concentrations, Cmax and AUC, of zolmitriptan were generally higher in females taking oral contraceptives; Tmax was delayed by one-half hour in these females).
No products indexed under this heading.

Norgestimate (Retrospective analysis of pharmacokinetic data indicates that mean plasma concentrations, Cmax and AUC, of zolmitriptan were generally higher in females taking oral contraceptives; Tmax was delayed by one-half hour in these females). Products include:
Ortho-Cyclen/Ortho Tri-Cyclen 2414
Ortho Tri-Cyclen Lo Tablets 2421
Prefest Tablets 1069

Norgestrel (Retrospective analysis of pharmacokinetic data indicates that mean plasma concentrations, Cmax and AUC, of zolmitriptan were generally higher in females taking oral contraceptives; Tmax was delayed by one-half hour in these females). Products include:
Lo/Ovral-28 Tablets 3423

Pargyline Hydrochloride (MAO-A inhibitors increase the systemic exposure of zolmitriptan; concurrent and/or sequential use is contraindicated).
No products indexed under this heading.

Paroxetine Hydrochloride (Co-administration of 5-HT1 agonists with selective serotonin reuptake inhibitors (SSRIs) has resulted, rarely, in hyperreflexia, weakness, and incoordination). Products include:
Paxil CR Controlled-Release Tablets 1509
Paxil 1501

Phenelzine Sulfate (MAO-A inhibitors increase the systemic exposure of zolmitriptan; concurrent and/or sequential use is contraindicated).
No products indexed under this heading.

Procarbazine Hydrochloride (MAO-A inhibitors increase the sys-

temic exposure of zolmitriptan; concurrent and/or sequential use is contraindicated). Products include:

Matulane Capsules 3188

Propranolol Hydrochloride (Co-administration has resulted in increased (1.5-fold) Cmax and AUC of zolmitriptan after one week of propranolol dosing). Products include:

Inderal LA Long-Acting Capsules 3421
InnoPran XL Capsules 2728

Rizatriptan Benzoate (Co-administration with other 5-HT1 agonists within 24 hours of each other is contraindicated because the vasospastic effects may be additive). Products include:

Maxalt Tablets 1983
Maxalt-MLT Orally Disintegrating Tablets 1983

Selegiline Hydrochloride (MAO-A inhibitors increase the systemic exposure of zolmitriptan; concurrent and/or sequential use is contraindicated). Products include:

Eldepryl Capsules 3209

Sertraline Hydrochloride (Co-administration of 5-HT1 agonists with selective serotonin reuptake inhibitors (SSRIs) has resulted, rarely, in hyperreflexia, weakness, and incoordination). Products include:

Zoloft 2581

Sumatriptan (Co-administration with other 5-HT1 agonists within 24 hours of each other is contraindicated because the vasospastic effects may be additive). Products include:

Imitrex Nasal Spray 1435

Sumatriptan Succinate (Co-administration with other 5-HT1 agonists within 24 hours of each other is contraindicated because the vasospastic effects may be additive). Products include:

Imitrex Injection 1431
Imitrex Tablets 1440

Tranylcypromine Sulfate (MAO-A inhibitors increase the systemic exposure of zolmitriptan; concurrent and/or sequential use is contraindicated). Products include:

Parnate Tablets 1499

ZOMIG-ZMT TABLETS

(Zolmitriptan) 714
See Zomig Tablets

ZONEGRAN CAPSULES

(Zonisamide) 1089
May interact with phenytoin, valproate, and certain other agents. Compounds in these categories include:

Carbamazepine (Co-administration with drugs that induce liver enzymes increases the metabolism and clearance of zonisamide and decreases the half-life to 38 hours). Products include:

Carbatrol Capsules 3174
Equetro Extended-Release Capsules 3178
Tegretol/Tegretol-XR 2278

Divalproex Sodium (The half-life of zonisamide in patients concurrently on the non-enzyme inducing AED, valproate, was 46 hours). Products include:

Depakote Sprinkle Capsules 422
Depakote Tablets 427
Depakote ER Tablets 433

Fosphenytoin Sodium (Co-administration with drugs that induce liver enzymes increases the metabolism and clearance of zonisamide and decreases the half-life to 27 hours).

No products indexed under this heading.

Phenobarbital (Co-administration with drugs that induce liver enzymes increases the metabolism and clearance of zonisamide and decreases the half-life to 38 hours).

No products indexed under this heading.

Phenytoin (Co-administration with drugs that induce liver enzymes increases the metabolism and clearance of zonisamide and decreases the half-life to 27 hours).

No products indexed under this heading.

Phenytoin Sodium (Co-administration with drugs that induce liver enzymes increases the metabolism and clearance of zonisamide and decreases the half-life to 27 hours). Products include:

Phenytek Capsules 2153

Valproate Sodium (The half-life of zonisamide in patients concurrently on the non-enzyme inducing AED, valproate, was 46 hours). Products include:

Depacon Injection 412

Valproic Acid (The half-life of zonisamide in patients concurrently on the non-enzyme inducing AED, valproate, was 46 hours). Products include:

Depakene 417

ZOSYN

(Piperacillin Sodium, Tazobactam Sodium)... 3492
May interact with aminoglycosides, anticoagulants, nondepolarizing neuromuscular blocking agents, and certain other agents. Compounds in these categories include:

Amikacin Sulfate (The mixing of Zosyn with an aminoglycoside *in vitro* can result in substantial inactivation due to penicillin-aminoglycoside complex; this complex is microbiologically inactive and of unknown toxicity).

No products indexed under this heading.

Anisindione (Coagulation parameters should be tested more frequently and monitored regularly during simultaneous administration; effect of concurrent use is not specified). Products include:

Miradon Tablets 3056

Ardeparin Sodium (Coagulation parameters should be tested more frequently and monitored regularly during simultaneous administration; effect of concurrent use is not specified).

No products indexed under this heading.

Atracurium Besylate (Due to similar mechanism of action as vecuronium, it is expected that the neuromuscular blockade produced by other non-depolarizing muscle relaxants could be prolonged in the presence of piperacillin).

No products indexed under this heading.

Cisatracurium Besylate (Due to similar mechanism of action as vecuronium, it is expected that the neuromuscular blockade produced by other non-depolarizing muscle relaxants could be prolonged in the presence of piperacillin). Products include:

Nimbex Injection 494

Dalteparin Sodium (Coagulation parameters should be tested more frequently and monitored regularly during simultaneous administration; effect of concurrent use is not specified). Products include:

Fragmin Injection 2638

Danaparoid Sodium (Coagulation parameters should be tested more frequently and monitored regularly during simultaneous administration; effect of concurrent use is not specified).

No products indexed under this heading.

Dicumarol (Coagulation parameters should be tested more frequently and monitored regularly during simultaneous administration; effect of concurrent use is not specified).

No products indexed under this heading.

Enoxaparin Sodium (Coagulation parameters should be tested more frequently and monitored regularly during simultaneous administration; effect of concurrent use is not specified). Products include:

Lovenox Injection 2931

Fondaparinux Sodium (Coagulation parameters should be tested more frequently and monitored regularly during simultaneous administration; effect of concurrent use is not specified). Products include:

Arixtra Injection 1325

Gentamicin Sulfate (The mixing of Zosyn with an aminoglycoside *in vitro* can result in substantial inactivation due to penicillin-aminoglycoside complex; this complex is microbiologically inactive and of unknown toxicity). Products include:

Garamycin Injectable 3028
Genoptic Sterile Ophthalmic Solution.. ⊙ 227
Pred-G Ophthalmic Suspension ...... ⊙ 234
Pred-G Sterile Ophthalmic Ointment .... ⊙ 235

Heparin Calcium (Coagulation parameters should be tested more frequently and monitored regularly during simultaneous administration; effect of concurrent use is not specified).

No products indexed under this heading.

Heparin Sodium (Coagulation parameters should be tested more frequently and monitored regularly during simultaneous administration; effect of concurrent use is not specified).

No products indexed under this heading.

Kanamycin Sulfate (The mixing of Zosyn with an aminoglycoside *in vitro* can result in substantial inactivation due to penicillin-aminoglycoside complex; this complex is microbiologically inactive and of unknown toxicity).

No products indexed under this heading.

Low Molecular Weight Heparins (Coagulation parameters should be tested more frequently and monitored regularly during simultaneous administration; effect of concurrent use is not specified).

No products indexed under this heading.

Methotrexate (Limited data suggests that co-administration of methotrexate and piperacillin may reduce the clearance of methotrexate due to competition for renal excretion).

No products indexed under this heading.

Metocurine Iodide (Due to similar mechanism of action as vecuronium, it is expected that the neuromuscular blockade produced by other non-depolarizing muscle relaxants could be prolonged in the presence of piperacillin).

No products indexed under this heading.

Mivacurium Chloride (Due to similar mechanism of action as vecuronium, it is expected that the neuromuscular blockade produced by other non-depolarizing muscle relaxants could be prolonged in the presence of piperacillin). Products include:

Mivacron Injection 489

Pancuronium Bromide (Due to similar mechanism of action as vecuronium, it is expected that the neuromuscular blockade produced by other non-depolarizing muscle relaxants could be prolonged in the presence of piperacillin).

No products indexed under this heading.

Probenecid (Concomitant administration prolongs half-life of piperacillin by 21% and of tazobactam by 71%).

No products indexed under this heading.

Rapacuronium Bromide (Due to similar mechanism of action as vecuronium, it is expected that the neuromuscular blockade produced by other non-depolarizing muscle relaxants could be prolonged in the presence of piperacillin).

No products indexed under this heading.

Rocuronium Bromide (Due to similar mechanism of action as vecuronium, it is expected that the neuromuscular blockade produced by other non-depolarizing muscle relaxants could be prolonged in the presence of piperacillin). Products include:

Zemuron Injection 2363

Streptomycin Sulfate (The mixing of Zosyn with an aminoglycoside *in vitro* can result in substantial inactivation due to penicillin-aminoglycoside complex; this complex is microbiologically inactive and of unknown toxicity).

No products indexed under this heading.

Tinzaparin Sodium (Coagulation parameters should be tested more frequently and monitored regularly during simultaneous administration; effect of concurrent use is not specified).

No products indexed under this heading.

Tobramycin (The mixing of Zosyn with an aminoglycoside *in vitro* can result in substantial inactivation due to penicillin-aminoglycoside complex; this complex is microbiologically inactive and of unknown toxicity). Products include:

TOBI Solution for Inhalation 1015
TobraDex Ophthalmic Ointment 558
TobraDex Ophthalmic Suspension ... 558
Zylet Ophthalmic Suspension 3508

Tobramycin Sulfate (Co-administration has resulted in the alteration of tobramycin pharmacokinetics which may be due to *in vitro* and *in vivo* inactivation of tobramycin).
No products indexed under this heading.

Vecuronium Bromide (Co-administration of piperacillin and vecuronium has been implicated in the prolongation of the neuromuscular blockade).
No products indexed under this heading.

Warfarin Sodium (Coagulation parameters should be tested more frequently and monitored regularly during simultaneous administration; effect of concurrent use is not specified). Products include:
Coumadin for Injection 932
Coumadin Tablets 932

ZOSYN IN GALAXY CONTAINERS

(Piperacillin Sodium, Tazobactam Sodium).. 3492
See Zosyn

ZOVIRAX CAPSULES

(Acyclovir) 1616
May interact with:

Nephrotoxic Drugs (Increased risk of renal dysfunction).
No products indexed under this heading.

Probenecid (Co-administration of probenecid with intravenous acyclovir has been shown to increase acyclovir half-life and systemic exposure; urinary excretion and renal clearance were correspondingly reduced).
No products indexed under this heading.

ZOVIRAX CREAM

(Acyclovir) 853
None cited in PDR database.

ZOVIRAX FOR INJECTION

(Acyclovir Sodium) 1618
See Zovirax Capsules

ZOVIRAX OINTMENT

(Acyclovir) 854
None cited in PDR database.

ZOVIRAX SUSPENSION

(Acyclovir) 1616
See Zovirax Capsules

ZOVIRAX TABLETS

(Acyclovir) 1616
See Zovirax Capsules

ZYBAN SUSTAINED-RELEASE TABLETS

(Bupropion Hydrochloride) 1620
May interact with benzodiazepines, corticosteroids, antidepressant drugs, hypnotics and sedatives, monoamine oxidase inhibitors, antipsychotic agents, phenytoin, drugs which lower seizure threshold, xanthines, and certain other agents. Compounds in these categories include:

Alprazolam (Bupropion is associated with a dose-related risk of seizures; excessive use of benzodiazepine sedatives is associated with increased risk of seizures; bupropion is contraindicated in patients undergoing abrupt discontinuation of benzodiazepine sedatives). Products include:
Niravam Orally Disintegrating Tablets 3106
Xanax XR Tablets 2655

Amantadine Hydrochloride (Limited clinical data suggests higher incidence of adverse experiences with co-administration; use small initial dose and gradually increase doses). Products include:
Symmetrel 1115

Aminophylline (Bupropion is associated with a dose-related risk of seizures; co-administration with drugs that lower seizure threshold may increase the risk of seizures with bupropion; concurrent use should be undertaken with extreme caution).
No products indexed under this heading.

Amitriptyline Hydrochloride (Bupropion is associated with dose-dependent risk of seizures; co-administration with drugs that lower seizure threshold may increase the risk of seizure with bupropion).
No products indexed under this heading.

Amoxapine (Bupropion is associated with dose-dependent risk of seizures; co-administration with drugs that lower seizure threshold may increase the risk of seizure with bupropion).
No products indexed under this heading.

Aripiprazole (Bupropion is associated with dose-dependent risk of seizures; co-administration with drugs that lower seizure threshold, such as antipsychotics, may increase the risk of seizure with bupropion). Products include:
Abilify Tablets 2472
Abilify Tablets 916

Betamethasone Acetate (Concurrent administration of bupropion hydrochloride and agents that lower seizure threshold, such as systemic steroids, should be undertaken only with extreme caution).
No products indexed under this heading.

Betamethasone Sodium Phosphate (Concurrent administration of bupropion hydrochloride and agents that lower seizure threshold, such as systemic steroids, should be undertaken only with extreme caution).
No products indexed under this heading.

Bupropion (Zyban should not be used in combination with any other medications containing bupropion, such as Wellbutrin or Wellbutrin SR).
No products indexed under this heading.

Carbamazepine (May induce the metabolism of bupropion). Products include:
Carbatrol Capsules 3174
Equetro Extended-Release Capsules 3178
Tegretol/Tegretol-XR 2278

Chlordiazepoxide (Bupropion is associated with a dose-related risk of seizures; excessive use of benzodiazepine sedatives is associated with increased risk of seizures; bupropion is contraindicated in patients undergoing abrupt discontinuation of benzodiazepine sedatives).
No products indexed under this heading.

Chlordiazepoxide Hydrochloride (Bupropion is associated with a dose-related risk of seizures; excessive use of benzodiazepine sedatives is associated with increased risk of seizures; bupropion is contraindicated in patients undergoing abrupt discontinuation of benzodiazepine sedatives). Products include:
Librium Capsules 3349

Chlorpromazine (Bupropion is associated with dose-dependent risk of seizures; co-administration with drugs that lower seizure threshold, such as antipsychotics, may increase the risk of seizure with bupropion).
No products indexed under this heading.

Chlorpromazine Hydrochloride (Bupropion is associated with dose-dependent risk of seizures; co-administration with drugs that lower seizure threshold, such as antipsychotics, may increase the risk of seizure with bupropion).
No products indexed under this heading.

Chlorprothixene (Bupropion is associated with dose-dependent risk of seizures; co-administration with drugs that lower seizure threshold, such as antipsychotics, may increase the risk of seizure with bupropion).
No products indexed under this heading.

Chlorprothixene Hydrochloride (Bupropion is associated with dose-dependent risk of seizures; co-administration with drugs that lower seizure threshold, such as antipsychotics, may increase the risk of seizure with bupropion).
No products indexed under this heading.

Cimetidine (May inhibit the metabolism of bupropion). Products include:
Tagamet HB 200 Tablets 637
Tagamet Tablets 1547

Cimetidine Hydrochloride (May inhibit the metabolism of bupropion).
No products indexed under this heading.

Citalopram Hydrobromide (Bupropion is associated with dose-dependent risk of seizures; co-administration with drugs that lower seizure threshold, such as antidepressants, may increase the risk of seizure with bupropion). Products include:
Celexa 1177

Clorazepate Dipotassium (Bupropion is associated with a dose-related risk of seizures; excessive use of benzodiazepine sedatives is associated with increased risk of seizures; bupropion is contraindicated in patients undergoing abrupt discontinuation of benzodiazepine sedatives). Products include:
Tranxene 2488

Clozapine (Bupropion is associated with dose-dependent risk of seizures; co-administration with drugs that lower seizure threshold, such as antipsychotics, may increase the risk of seizure with bupropion). Products include:
Clozapine Tablets 2141
Clozaril Tablets 2174
FazaClo Orally Disintegrating Tablets 547

Cortisone Acetate (Concurrent administration of bupropion hydrochloride and agents that lower seizure threshold, such as systemic steroids, should be undertaken only with extreme caution).
No products indexed under this heading.

Cyclophosphamide (Bupropion is primarily metabolized, based on in vitro studies, to hydroxybupropion by the CYP2B6 isoenzyme, therefore the potential exists for a drug interaction with agents that affect the CYP2B6 isoenzyme metabolism, such as cyclophosphamide).
No products indexed under this heading.

Desipramine Hydrochloride (Co-administration in male subjects who were extensive metabolizers of the CYP2D6 isoenzyme with daily doses of bupropion followed by a single dose of desipramine increased the Cmax, AUC and t1/2 of desipramine by an average of approximately two-, five-, and two-fold respectively; co-administration should be initiated at the lower end of the dose range of desipramine; potential for increased risk of seizures).
No products indexed under this heading.

Dexamethasone (Concurrent administration of bupropion hydrochloride and agents that lower seizure threshold, such as systemic steroids, should be undertaken only with extreme caution). Products include:
Ciprodex Otic Suspension 555
Decadron Tablets 1929
TobraDex Ophthalmic Ointment 558
TobraDex Ophthalmic Suspension ... 558

Dexamethasone Acetate (Concurrent administration of bupropion hydrochloride and agents that lower seizure threshold, such as systemic steroids, should be undertaken only with extreme caution).
No products indexed under this heading.

Dexamethasone Sodium Phosphate (Concurrent administration of bupropion hydrochloride and agents that lower seizure threshold, such as systemic steroids, should be undertaken only with extreme caution). Products include:
Decadron Phosphate Injection 1931

Diazepam (Bupropion is associated with a dose-related risk of seizures; excessive use of benzodiazepine sedatives is associated with increased risk of seizures; bupropion is contraindicated in patients undergoing abrupt discontinuation of benzodiazepine sedatives). Products include:
Diastat Rectal Delivery System 3344
Valium Tablets 2822

Doxepin Hydrochloride (Bupropion is associated with dose-dependent risk of seizures; co-administration with drugs that lower seizure threshold may increase the risk of seizure with bupropion).
No products indexed under this heading.

Dyphylline (Bupropion is associated with a dose-related risk of seizures; co-administration with drugs that lower seizure threshold may increase the risk of seizures with bupropion; concurrent use should be undertaken with extreme caution).
No products indexed under this heading.

Escitalopram Oxalate (Bupropion is associated with dose-dependent risk of seizures; co-administration with drugs that lower seizure threshold, such as antidepressants, may increase the risk of seizure with bupropion). Products include:
Lexapro Oral Solution 1193
Lexapro Tablets 1193

Estazolam (Bupropion is associated with a dose-related risk of seizures; excessive use of benzodiazepine sedatives is associated with increased risk of seizures; bupropion is contraindicated in patients undergoing abrupt discontinuation of benzodiazepine sedatives). Products include:
ProSom Tablets 512

Ethchlorvynol (Bupropion hydrochloride is contraindicated in patients undergoing abrupt discontinuation of sedatives).
No products indexed under this heading.

Ethinamate (Bupropion hydrochloride is contraindicated in patients undergoing abrupt discontinuation of sedatives).
No products indexed under this heading.

Flecainide Acetate (Co-administration of bupropion with drugs that are metabolized by CYP2D6 isoenzyme, such as flecainide, may result in, based on data with desipramine, increased Cmax, AUC and t1/2; co-administration should be initiated at the lower end of the dose range of flecainide). Products include:
Tambocor Tablets 1824

Fludrocortisone Acetate (Concurrent administration of bupropion hydrochloride and agents that lower seizure threshold, such as systemic steroids, should be undertaken only with extreme caution).
No products indexed under this heading.

Fluoxetine Hydrochloride (Co-administration of bupropion with drugs that are metabolized by CYP2D6 isoenzyme, such as fluoxetine, may result in, based on data with desipramine, increased Cmax, AUC and t1/2; co-administration should be initiated at the lower end of the dose range of fluoxetine). Products include:
Prozac Pulvules and Liquid 1771
Symbyax Capsules 1788

Fluphenazine Decanoate (Bupropion is associated with dose-dependent risk of seizures; co-administration with drugs that lower seizure threshold, such as antipsychotics, may increase the risk of seizure with bupropion).
No products indexed under this heading.

Fluphenazine Enanthate (Bupropion is associated with dose-dependent risk of seizures; co-administration with drugs that lower seizure threshold, such as antipsychotics, may increase the risk of seizure with bupropion).
No products indexed under this heading.

Fluphenazine Hydrochloride (Bupropion is associated with dose-dependent risk of seizures; co-administration with drugs that lower seizure threshold, such as antipsychotics, may increase the risk of seizure with bupropion).
No products indexed under this heading.

Flurazepam Hydrochloride (Bupropion is associated with a dose-related risk of seizures; excessive use of benzodiazepine sedatives is associated with increased risk of seizures; bupropion is contraindicated in patients undergoing abrupt discontinuation of benzodiazepine sedatives). Products include:
Dalmane Capsules 3343

Fosphenytoin Sodium (May induce the metabolism of bupropion).
No products indexed under this heading.

Glutethimide (Bupropion hydrochloride is contraindicated in patients undergoing abrupt discontinuation of sedatives).
No products indexed under this heading.

Halazepam (Bupropion is associated with a dose-related risk of seizures; excessive use of benzodiazepine sedatives is associated with increased risk of seizures; bupropion is contraindicated in patients undergoing abrupt discontinuation of benzodiazepine sedatives).
No products indexed under this heading.

Haloperidol (Co-administration of bupropion with drugs that are metabolized by CYP2D6 isoenzyme, such as haloperidol, may result in, based on data with desipramine, increased Cmax, AUC and t1/2; co-administration should be initiated at the lower end of the dose range of haloperidol; potential for increased risk of seizures).
No products indexed under this heading.

Haloperidol Decanoate (Co-administration of bupropion with drugs that are metabolized by CYP2D6 isoenzyme, such as haloperidol, may result in, based on data with desipramine, increased Cmax, AUC and t1/2; co-administration should be initiated at the lower end of the dose range of haloperidol; potential for increased risk of seizures).
No products indexed under this heading.

Hydrocortisone (Concurrent administration of bupropion hydrochloride and agents that lower seizure threshold, such as systemic steroids, should be undertaken only with extreme caution). Products include:
Cortizone•5 Ointment ..... ▣699
Cortizone•10 Creme ..... ▣699
Cortizone•10 Ointment ..... ▣699
Cortizone•10 Plus Creme ..... ▣700
Cortizone•10 Maximum Strength Quick Shot Spray ..... ▣700
Hydrocortone Tablets 1963
Preparation H Hydrocortisone Cream ..... ▣748

Hydrocortisone Acetate (Concurrent administration of bupropion hydrochloride and agents that lower seizure threshold, such as systemic steroids, should be undertaken only with extreme caution). Products include:
Analpram-HC 1136
Pramosone 1139
ProctoFoam-HC 3113
Tucks Anti-Itch Ointment ..... ▣712
U-cort 1% Cream 3289

Hydrocortisone Sodium Phosphate (Concurrent administration of bupropion hydrochloride and agents that lower seizure threshold, such as systemic steroids, should be undertaken only with extreme caution).
No products indexed under this heading.

Hydrocortisone Sodium Succinate (Concurrent administration of bupropion hydrochloride and agents that lower seizure threshold, such as systemic steroids, should be undertaken only with extreme caution).
No products indexed under this heading.

Imipramine Hydrochloride (Co-administration of bupropion with drugs that are metabolized by CYP2D6 isoenzyme, such as imipramine, may result in, based on data with desipramine, increased Cmax, AUC and t1/2; co-administration should be initiated at the lower end of the dose range of imipramine; potential for increased risk of seizures).
No products indexed under this heading.

Imipramine Pamoate (Co-administration of bupropion with drugs that are metabolized by CYP2D6 isoenzyme, such as imipramine, may result in, based on data with desipramine, increased Cmax, AUC and t1/2; co-administration should be initiated at the lower end of the dose range of imipramine; potential for increased risk of seizures).
No products indexed under this heading.

Isocarboxazid (Concurrent and/or sequential use with MAO inhibitors is contraindicated).
No products indexed under this heading.

Levodopa (Limited clinical data suggests higher incidence of adverse experiences with co-administration; use small initial dose and gradually increase doses). Products include:
Parcopa Orally Disintegrating Tablets 3111
Stalevo Tablets 2270

Lithium Carbonate (Bupropion is associated with dose-dependent risk of seizures; co-administration with drugs that lower seizure threshold, such as antipsychotics, may increase the risk of seizure with bupropion). Products include:
Eskalith 1406
Lithobid Tablets 1670

Lithium Citrate (Bupropion is associated with dose-dependent risk of seizures; co-administration with drugs that lower seizure threshold, such as antipsychotics, may increase the risk of seizure with bupropion).
No products indexed under this heading.

Lorazepam (Bupropion is associated with a dose-related risk of seizures; excessive use of benzodiazepine sedatives is associated with increased risk of seizures; bupropion is contraindicated in patients undergoing abrupt discontinuation of benzodiazepine sedatives).
No products indexed under this heading.

Loxapine Hydrochloride (Bupropion is associated with dose-dependent risk of seizures; co-administration with drugs that lower seizure threshold, such as antipsychotics, may increase the risk of seizure with bupropion).
No products indexed under this heading.

Loxapine Succinate (Bupropion is associated with dose-dependent risk of seizures; co-administration with drugs that lower seizure threshold, such as antipsychotics, may increase the risk of seizure with bupropion).
No products indexed under this heading.

Maprotiline Hydrochloride (Bupropion is associated with dose-dependent risk of seizures; co-administration with drugs that lower seizure threshold may increase the risk of seizure with bupropion).
No products indexed under this heading.

Mesoridazine Besylate (Bupropion is associated with dose-dependent risk of seizures; co-administration with drugs that lower seizure threshold, such as antipsychotics, may increase the risk of seizure with bupropion).
No products indexed under this heading.

Methotrimeprazine (Bupropion is associated with dose-dependent risk of seizures; co-administration with drugs that lower seizure threshold, such as antipsychotics, may increase the risk of seizure with bupropion).
No products indexed under this heading.

Methylprednisolone Acetate (Concurrent administration of bupropion hydrochloride and agents that lower seizure threshold, such as systemic steroids, should be undertaken only with extreme caution). Products include:
Depo-Medrol Injectable Suspension 2615
Depo-Medrol Single-Dose Vial 2617

Methylprednisolone Sodium Succinate (Concurrent administration of bupropion hydrochloride and agents that lower seizure threshold, such as systemic steroids, should be undertaken only with extreme caution).
No products indexed under this heading.

Metoprolol Succinate (Co-administration of bupropion with drugs that are metabolized by CYP2D6 isoenzyme, such as metoprolol, may result in, based on data with desipramine, increased Cmax, AUC and t1/2; co-administration should be initiated at the lower end of the dose range of metoprolol). Products include:
Toprol-XL Tablets 660

Metoprolol Tartrate (Co-administration of bupropion with drugs that are metabolized by CYP2D6 isoenzyme, such as metoprolol, may result in, based on data with desipramine, increased Cmax, AUC and t1/2; co-administration should be initiated at the lower end of the dose range of metoprolol).
No products indexed under this heading.

Midazolam Hydrochloride (Bupropion is associated with a dose-related risk of seizures; excessive use of benzodiazepine sedatives is associated with increased risk of seizures; bupropion is contraindicated in patients undergoing abrupt discontinuation of benzodiazepine sedatives).
No products indexed under this heading.

Mirtazapine (Bupropion is associated with dose-dependent risk of seizures; co-administration with drugs that lower seizure threshold, such as antidepressants, may increase the risk of seizure with bupropion).
No products indexed under this heading.

Moclobemide (Concurrent and/or sequential use with MAO inhibitors is contraindicated).
No products indexed under this heading.

Molindone Hydrochloride (Bupropion is associated with dose-dependent risk of seizures; co-administration with drugs that lower seizure threshold, such as antipsychotics, may increase the risk of seizure with bupropion). Products include:
Moban Tablets **1108**

Nefazodone Hydrochloride (Bupropion is associated with dose-dependent risk of seizures; co-administration with drugs that lower seizure threshold, such as antidepressants, may increase the risk of seizure with bupropion).
No products indexed under this heading.

Nicotine (Co-administration of bupropion and nicotine transdermal system has resulted in a higher incidence of treatment-emergent hypertension). Products include:
Nicoderm CQ Patch **1629**
NicoDerm CQ Clear Patch .... ▣**627**
Nicotrol Inhaler **2594**
Nicotrol NS **2596**

Nortriptyline Hydrochloride (Co-administration of bupropion with drugs that are metabolized by CYP2D6 isoenzyme, such as nortriptyline, may result in, based on data with desipramine, increased Cmax, AUC and t1/2; co-administration should be initiated at the lower end of the dose range of nortriptyline; potential for increased risk of seizures).
No products indexed under this heading.

Olanzapine (Bupropion is associated with dose-dependent risk of seizures; co-administration with drugs that lower seizure threshold, such as antipsychotics, may increase the risk of seizure with bupropion). Products include:
Symbyax Capsules **1788**
Zyprexa Tablets **1798**
Zyprexa IntraMuscular **1798**
Zyprexa ZYDIS Orally Disintegrating Tablets **1798**

Orphenadrine Citrate (Bupropion is primarily metabolized, based on in vitro studies, to hydroxybupropion by the CYP2B6 isoenzyme, therefore the potential exists for a drug interaction with agents that affect the CYP2B6 isoenzyme metabolism, such as orphenadrine). Products include:
Norflex Injection **1824**

Oxazepam (Bupropion is associated with a dose-related risk of seizures; excessive use of benzodiazepine sedatives is associated with increased risk of seizures; bupropion is contraindicated in patients undergoing abrupt discontinuation of benzodiazepine sedatives).
No products indexed under this heading.

Pargyline Hydrochloride (Concurrent and/or sequential use with MAO inhibitors is contraindicated).
No products indexed under this heading.

Paroxetine Hydrochloride (Co-administration of bupropion with drugs that are metabolized by CYP2D6 isoenzyme, such as paroxetine, may result in, based on data with desipramine, increased Cmax, AUC and t1/2; co-administration should be initiated at the lower end of the dose range of paroxetine). Products include:
Paxil CR Controlled-Release Tablets **1509**
Paxil **1501**

Perphenazine (Bupropion is associated with dose-dependent risk of seizures; co-administration with drugs that lower seizure threshold, such as antipsychotics, may increase the risk of seizure with bupropion).
No products indexed under this heading.

Phenelzine Sulfate (Concurrent and/or sequential use with MAO inhibitors is contraindicated; acute toxicity of bupropion is enhanced by phenelzine in animal models).
No products indexed under this heading.

Phenobarbital (May induce the metabolism of bupropion).
No products indexed under this heading.

Phenytoin (May induce the metabolism of bupropion).
No products indexed under this heading.

Phenytoin Sodium (May induce the metabolism of bupropion). Products include:
Phenytek Capsules **2153**

Pimozide (Bupropion is associated with dose-dependent risk of seizures; co-administration with drugs that lower seizure threshold, such as antipsychotics, may increase the risk of seizure with bupropion). Products include:
Orap Tablets **1220**

Prazepam (Bupropion is associated with a dose-related risk of seizures; excessive use of benzodiazepine sedatives is associated with increased risk of seizures; bupropion is contraindicated in patients undergoing abrupt discontinuation of benzodiazepine sedatives).
No products indexed under this heading.

Prednisolone Acetate (Concurrent administration of bupropion hydrochloride and agents that lower seizure threshold, such as systemic steroids, should be undertaken only with extreme caution). Products include:
Blephamide Ophthalmic Ointment **563**
Blephamide Ophthalmic Suspension **564**
Poly-Pred Liquifilm Ophthalmic Suspension .... ⊙**231**
Pred Forte Ophthalmic Suspension .... ⊙**233**
Pred Mild Sterile Ophthalmic Suspension .... ⊙**236**
Pred-G Ophthalmic Suspension .... ⊙**234**
Pred-G Sterile Ophthalmic Ointment .... ⊙**235**

Prednisolone Sodium Phosphate (Concurrent administration of bupropion hydrochloride and agents that lower seizure threshold, such as systemic steroids, should be undertaken only with extreme caution). Products include:
Pediapred Oral Solution **3319**

Prednisolone Tebutate (Concurrent administration of bupropion hydrochloride and agents that lower seizure threshold, such as systemic steroids, should be undertaken only with extreme caution).
No products indexed under this heading.

Prednisone (Concurrent administration of bupropion hydrochloride and agents that lower seizure threshold, such as systemic steroids, should be undertaken only with extreme caution).
No products indexed under this heading.

Procarbazine Hydrochloride (Concurrent and/or sequential use with MAO inhibitors is contraindicated). Products include:
Matulane Capsules **3188**

Prochlorperazine (Bupropion is associated with dose-dependent risk of seizures; co-administration with drugs that lower seizure threshold, such as antipsychotics, may increase the risk of seizure with bupropion).
No products indexed under this heading.

Promethazine Hydrochloride (Bupropion is associated with dose-dependent risk of seizures; co-administration with drugs that lower seizure threshold, such as antipsychotics, may increase the risk of seizure with bupropion). Products include:
Phenergan **3438**

Propafenone Hydrochloride (Co-administration of bupropion with drugs that are metabolized by CYP2D6 isoenzyme, such as propafenone, may result in, based on data with desipramine, increased Cmax, AUC and t1/2; co-administration should be initiated at the lower end of the dose range of propafenone). Products include:
Rythmol SR Capsules **2736**

Propofol (Bupropion hydrochloride is contraindicated in patients undergoing abrupt discontinuation of sedatives). Products include:
Diprivan Injectable Emulsion **676**

Protriptyline Hydrochloride (Bupropion is associated with dose-dependent risk of seizures; co-administration with drugs that lower seizure threshold may increase the risk of seizure with bupropion). Products include:
Vivactil Tablets **2350**

Quazepam (Bupropion is associated with a dose-related risk of seizures; excessive use of benzodiazepine sedatives is associated with increased risk of seizures; bupropion is contraindicated in patients undergoing abrupt discontinuation of benzodiazepine sedatives).
No products indexed under this heading.

Quetiapine Fumarate (Bupropion is associated with dose-dependent risk of seizures; co-administration with drugs that lower seizure threshold, such as antipsychotics, may increase the risk of seizure with bupropion). Products include:
Seroquel Tablets **691**

Risperidone (Co-administration of bupropion with drugs that are metabolized by CYP2D6 isoenzyme, such as risperidone, may result in, based on data with desipramine, increased Cmax, AUC and t1/2; co-administration should be initiated at the lower end of the dose range of risperidone; potential for increased risk of seizures). Products include:
Risperdal Consta Long-Acting Injection **1664**
Risperdal M-Tab Orally Disintegrating Tablets **1658**
Risperdal **1658**

Secobarbital Sodium (Bupropion hydrochloride is contraindicated in patients undergoing abrupt discontinuation of sedatives).
No products indexed under this heading.

Selegiline Hydrochloride (Concurrent and/or sequential use with MAO inhibitors is contraindicated). Products include:
Eldepryl Capsules **3209**

Sertraline Hydrochloride (Co-administration of bupropion with drugs that are metabolized by CYP2D6 isoenzyme, such as sertraline, may result in, based on data with desipramine, increased Cmax, AUC and t1/2; co-administration should be initiated at the lower end of the dose range of sertraline). Products include:
Zoloft **2581**

Temazepam (Bupropion is associated with a dose-related risk of seizures; excessive use of benzodiazepine sedatives is associated with increased risk of seizures; bupropion is contraindicated in patients undergoing abrupt discontinuation of benzodiazepine sedatives).
No products indexed under this heading.

Theophylline (Bupropion is associated with a dose-related risk of seizures; co-administration with drugs that lower seizure threshold may increase the risk of seizures with bupropion; concurrent use should be undertaken with extreme caution).
No products indexed under this heading.

Theophylline Anhydrous (Bupropion is associated with a dose-related risk of seizures; co-administration with drugs that lower seizure threshold may increase the risk of seizures with bupropion; concurrent use should be undertaken with extreme caution). Products include:
Uniphyl Tablets **2708**

Theophylline Calcium Salicylate (Bupropion is associated with a dose-related risk of seizures; co-administration with drugs that lower seizure threshold may increase the risk of seizures with bupropion; concurrent use should be undertaken with extreme caution).
No products indexed under this heading.

Theophylline Dihydroxypropyl (Glyceryl) (Bupropion is associated with a dose-related risk of seizures; co-administration with drugs that lower seizure threshold may increase the risk of seizures with bupropion; concurrent use should be undertaken with extreme caution).
No products indexed under this heading.

Theophylline Ethylenediamine (Bupropion is associated with a dose-related risk of seizures; co-administration with drugs that lower seizure threshold may increase the risk of seizures with bupropion; concurrent use should be undertaken with extreme caution).
No products indexed under this heading.

Theophylline Sodium Glycinate (Bupropion is associated with a dose-related risk of seizures; co-administration with drugs that lower seizure threshold may increase the risk of seizures with bupropion; concurrent use should be undertaken with extreme caution).
No products indexed under this heading.

Thioridazine Hydrochloride (Co-administration of bupropion with drugs that are metabolized by CYP2D6 isoenzyme, such as thioridazine, may result in, based on data with desipramine, increased Cmax, AUC and t1/2; co-administration should be initiated at the lower end of the dose range of thioridazine; potential for increased risk of seizures). Products include:
Thioridazine Hydrochloride Tablets 2122

Thiothixene (Bupropion is associated with dose-dependent risk of seizures; co-administration with drugs that lower seizure threshold, such as antipsychotics, may increase the risk of seizure with bupropion). Products include:
Thiothixene Capsules 2124

Tranylcypromine Sulfate (Concurrent and/or sequential use with MAO inhibitors is contraindicated). Products include:
Parnate Tablets 1499

Trazodone Hydrochloride (Bupropion is associated with dose-dependent risk of seizures; co-administration with drugs that lower seizure threshold may increase the risk of seizure with bupropion).
No products indexed under this heading.

Triamcinolone (Concurrent administration of bupropion hydrochloride and agents that lower seizure threshold, such as systemic steroids, should be undertaken only with extreme caution).
No products indexed under this heading.

Triamcinolone Acetonide (Concurrent administration of bupropion hydrochloride and agents that lower seizure threshold, such as systemic steroids, should be undertaken only with extreme caution). Products include:
Azmacort Inhalation Aerosol 1701
Nasacort HFA Inhalation Aerosol 2939
Nasacort AQ Nasal Spray 2937

Triamcinolone Diacetate (Concurrent administration of bupropion hydrochloride and agents that lower seizure threshold, such as systemic steroids, should be undertaken only with extreme caution).
No products indexed under this heading.

Triamcinolone Hexacetonide (Concurrent administration of bupropion hydrochloride and agents that lower seizure threshold, such as systemic steroids, should be undertaken only with extreme caution).
No products indexed under this heading.

Triazolam (Bupropion is associated with a dose-related risk of seizures; excessive use of benzodiazepine sedatives is associated with increased risk of seizures; bupropion is contraindicated in patients undergoing abrupt discontinuation of benzodiazepine sedatives).
No products indexed under this heading.

Trifluoperazine Hydrochloride (Bupropion is associated with dose-dependent risk of seizures; co-administration with drugs that lower seizure threshold, such as antipsychotics, may increase the risk of seizure with bupropion).
No products indexed under this heading.

Trimipramine Maleate (Bupropion is associated with dose-dependent risk of seizures; co-administration with drugs that lower seizure threshold may increase the risk of seizure with bupropion). Products include:
Surmontil Capsules 2347

Venlafaxine Hydrochloride (Bupropion is associated with dose-dependent risk of seizures; co-administration with drugs that lower seizure threshold, such as antidepressants, may increase the risk of seizure with bupropion). Products include:
Effexor Tablets 3405
Effexor XR Capsules 3411

Warfarin Sodium (Altered PT and/or INR infrequently associated with hemorrhagic or thrombotic complications were observed when bupropion was co-administered with warfarin). Products include:
Coumadin for Injection 932
Coumadin Tablets 932

Zaleplon (Bupropion hydrochloride is contraindicated in patients undergoing abrupt discontinuation of sedatives). Products include:
Sonata Capsules 1686

Ziprasidone Hydrochloride (Bupropion is associated with dose-dependent risk of seizures; co-administration with drugs that lower seizure threshold, such as antipsychotics, may increase the risk of seizure with bupropion). Products include:
Geodon Capsules 2514

Zolpidem Tartrate (Bupropion hydrochloride is contraindicated in patients undergoing abrupt discontinuation of sedatives). Products include:
Ambien Tablets 2867

Food Interactions

Alcohol (Bupropion hydrochloride is contraindicated in patients undergoing abrupt discontinuation of alcohol. The consumption of alcohol during treatment with bupropion hydrochloride should be minimized or avoided).

Food, unspecified (Food increases Cmax and AUC of bupropion by 11% and 17% respectively; the mean time to peak concentration Tmax was prolonged by 1 hour; this effect was of no clinical significance).

ZYDONE TABLETS
(Acetaminophen, Hydrocodone Bitartrate) 1118
May interact with anticholinergics, central nervous system depressants, monoamine oxidase inhibitors, narcotic analgesics, tricyclic antidepressants, and certain other agents. Compounds in these categories include:

Alfentanil Hydrochloride (Co-administration may exhibit additive CNS depression).
No products indexed under this heading.

Alprazolam (Co-administration may exhibit additive CNS depression). Products include:
Niravam Orally Disintegrating Tablets 3106
Xanax XR Tablets 2655

Amitriptyline Hydrochloride (Co-administration of tricyclic antidepressants with hydrocodone may increase the effect of either hydrocodone or antidepressant).
No products indexed under this heading.

Amoxapine (Co-administration of tricyclic antidepressants with hydrocodone may increase the effect of either hydrocodone or antidepressant).
No products indexed under this heading.

Aprobarbital (Co-administration may exhibit additive CNS depression).
No products indexed under this heading.

Atropine Sulfate (Co-administration may produce paralytic ileus).
No products indexed under this heading.

Belladonna Alkaloids (Co-administration may produce paralytic ileus). Products include:
Hyland's Teething Tablets .... ▣736

Benztropine Mesylate (Co-administration may produce paralytic ileus). Products include:
Cogentin Injection 1903

Biperiden Hydrochloride (Co-administration may produce paralytic ileus).
No products indexed under this heading.

Buprenorphine Hydrochloride (Co-administration may exhibit additive CNS depression). Products include:
Buprenex Injectable 2718
Suboxone Tablets 2719
Subutex Tablets 2719

Buspirone Hydrochloride (Co-administration may exhibit additive CNS depression).
No products indexed under this heading.

Butabarbital (Co-administration may exhibit additive CNS depression).
No products indexed under this heading.

Butalbital (Co-administration may exhibit additive CNS depression). Products include:
Sedapap Tablets 50 mg/650 mg 2098

Chlordiazepoxide (Co-administration may exhibit additive CNS depression).
No products indexed under this heading.

Chlordiazepoxide Hydrochloride (Co-administration may exhibit additive CNS depression). Products include:
Librium Capsules 3349

Chlorpromazine (Co-administration may exhibit additive CNS depression).
No products indexed under this heading.

Chlorpromazine Hydrochloride (Co-administration may exhibit additive CNS depression).
No products indexed under this heading.

Chlorprothixene (Co-administration may exhibit additive CNS depression).
No products indexed under this heading.

Chlorprothixene Hydrochloride (Co-administration may exhibit additive CNS depression).
No products indexed under this heading.

Chlorprothixene Lactate (Co-administration may exhibit additive CNS depression).
No products indexed under this heading.

Clidinium Bromide (Co-administration may produce paralytic ileus).
No products indexed under this heading.

Clomipramine Hydrochloride (Co-administration of tricyclic antidepressants with hydrocodone may increase the effect of either hydrocodone or antidepressant).
No products indexed under this heading.

Clorazepate Dipotassium (Co-administration may exhibit additive CNS depression). Products include:
Tranxene 2488

Clozapine (Co-administration may exhibit additive CNS depression). Products include:
Clozapine Tablets 2141
Clozaril Tablets 2174
FazaClo Orally Disintegrating Tablets 547

Codeine Phosphate (Co-administration may exhibit additive CNS depression). Products include:
Tylenol with Codeine 2461

Desflurane (Co-administration may exhibit additive CNS depression). Products include:
Suprane Liquid for Inhalation 770

Desipramine Hydrochloride (Co-administration of tricyclic antidepressants with hydrocodone may increase the effect of either hydrocodone or antidepressant).
No products indexed under this heading.

Dezocine (Co-administration may exhibit additive CNS depression).
No products indexed under this heading.

Diazepam (Co-administration may exhibit additive CNS depression). Products include:
Diastat Rectal Delivery System 3344
Valium Tablets 2822

Dicyclomine Hydrochloride (Co-administration may produce paralytic ileus). Products include:

Bentyl Capsules 724
Bentyl Injection 724
Bentyl Syrup 724
Bentyl Tablets 724

Doxepin Hydrochloride (Co-administration of tricyclic antidepressants with hydrocodone may increase the effect of either hydrocodone or antidepressant).
No products indexed under this heading.

Droperidol (Co-administration may exhibit additive CNS depression).
No products indexed under this heading.

Enflurane (Co-administration may exhibit additive CNS depression).
No products indexed under this heading.

Estazolam (Co-administration may exhibit additive CNS depression). Products include:
ProSom Tablets 512

Ethanol (Co-administration may exhibit additive CNS depression).
No products indexed under this heading.

Ethchlorvynol (Co-administration may exhibit additive CNS depression).
No products indexed under this heading.

Ethinamate (Co-administration may exhibit additive CNS depression).
No products indexed under this heading.

Ethyl Alcohol (Co-administration may exhibit additive CNS depression).
No products indexed under this heading.

Fentanyl (Co-administration may exhibit additive CNS depression). Products include:
Duragesic Transdermal System 2448

Fentanyl Citrate (Co-administration may exhibit additive CNS depression). Products include:
Actiq 993

Fluphenazine Decanoate (Co-administration may exhibit additive CNS depression).
No products indexed under this heading.

Fluphenazine Enanthate (Co-administration may exhibit additive CNS depression).
No products indexed under this heading.

Fluphenazine Hydrochloride (Co-administration may exhibit additive CNS depression).
No products indexed under this heading.

Flurazepam Hydrochloride (Co-administration may exhibit additive CNS depression). Products include:
Dalmane Capsules 3343

Glutethimide (Co-administration may exhibit additive CNS depression).
No products indexed under this heading.

Glycopyrrolate (Co-administration may produce paralytic ileus).
No products indexed under this heading.

Haloperidol (Co-administration may exhibit additive CNS depression).
No products indexed under this heading.

Haloperidol Decanoate (Co-administration may exhibit additive CNS depression).
No products indexed under this heading.

Hydrocodone Polistirex (Co-administration may exhibit additive CNS depression). Products include:
Tussionex Pennkinetic Extended-Release Suspension 3322

Hydromorphone Hydrochloride (Co-administration may exhibit additive CNS depression). Products include:
Dilaudid 439
Dilaudid Oral Liquid 443
Dilaudid Non-Sterile Powder 439
Dilaudid Rectal Suppositories 439
Dilaudid Tablets 439
Dilaudid Tablets - 8 mg 443
Dilaudid-HP 441

Hydroxyzine Hydrochloride (Co-administration may exhibit additive CNS depression).
No products indexed under this heading.

Hyoscyamine (Co-administration may produce paralytic ileus).
No products indexed under this heading.

Hyoscyamine Sulfate (Co-administration may produce paralytic ileus).
No products indexed under this heading.

Imipramine Hydrochloride (Co-administration of tricyclic antidepressants with hydrocodone may increase the effect of either hydrocodone or antidepressant).
No products indexed under this heading.

Imipramine Pamoate (Co-administration of tricyclic antidepressants with hydrocodone may increase the effect of either hydrocodone or antidepressant).
No products indexed under this heading.

Ipratropium Bromide (Co-administration may produce paralytic ileus). Products include:
Atrovent HFA Inhalation Aerosol 872
Atrovent Inhalation Solution 868
Atrovent Nasal Spray 0.03% 869
Atrovent Nasal Spray 0.06% 870
Combivent Inhalation Aerosol 878
DuoNeb Inhalation Solution 1058

Isocarboxazid (Co-administration of MAO inhibitors with hydrocodone may increase the effect of either hydrocodone or MAO inhibitor).
No products indexed under this heading.

Isoflurane (Co-administration may exhibit additive CNS depression).
No products indexed under this heading.

Ketamine Hydrochloride (Co-administration may exhibit additive CNS depression).
No products indexed under this heading.

Levomethadyl Acetate Hydrochloride (Co-administration may exhibit additive CNS depression).
No products indexed under this heading.

Levorphanol Tartrate (Co-administration may exhibit additive CNS depression).
No products indexed under this heading.

Lorazepam (Co-administration may exhibit additive CNS depression).
No products indexed under this heading.

Loxapine Hydrochloride (Co-administration may exhibit additive CNS depression).
No products indexed under this heading.

Loxapine Succinate (Co-administration may exhibit additive CNS depression).
No products indexed under this heading.

Maprotiline Hydrochloride (Co-administration of tricyclic antidepressants with hydrocodone may increase the effect of either hydrocodone or antidepressant).
No products indexed under this heading.

Mepenzolate Bromide (Co-administration may produce paralytic ileus).
No products indexed under this heading.

Meperidine Hydrochloride (Co-administration may exhibit additive CNS depression).
No products indexed under this heading.

Mephobarbital (Co-administration may exhibit additive CNS depression). Products include:
Mebaral Tablets, USP 2483

Meprobamate (Co-administration may exhibit additive CNS depression).
No products indexed under this heading.

Mesoridazine Besylate (Co-administration may exhibit additive CNS depression).
No products indexed under this heading.

Methadone Hydrochloride (Co-administration may exhibit additive CNS depression).
No products indexed under this heading.

Methohexital Sodium (Co-administration may exhibit additive CNS depression).
No products indexed under this heading.

Methotrimeprazine (Co-administration may exhibit additive CNS depression).
No products indexed under this heading.

Methoxyflurane (Co-administration may exhibit additive CNS depression).
No products indexed under this heading.

Midazolam Hydrochloride (Co-administration may exhibit additive CNS depression).
No products indexed under this heading.

Moclobemide (Co-administration of MAO inhibitors with hydrocodone may increase the effect of either hydrocodone or MAO inhibitor).
No products indexed under this heading.

Molindone Hydrochloride (Co-administration may exhibit additive CNS depression). Products include:
Moban Tablets 1108

Morphine Sulfate (Co-administration may exhibit additive CNS depression). Products include:
Avinza Capsules 1714
Kadian Capsules 572
MS Contin Tablets 2703

Nortriptyline Hydrochloride (Co-administration of tricyclic antidepressants with hydrocodone may increase the effect of either hydrocodone or antidepressant).
No products indexed under this heading.

Olanzapine (Co-administration may exhibit additive CNS depression). Products include:
Symbyax Capsules 1788
Zyprexa Tablets 1798
Zyprexa IntraMuscular 1798
Zyprexa ZYDIS Orally Disintegrating Tablets 1798

Oxazepam (Co-administration may exhibit additive CNS depression).
No products indexed under this heading.

Oxybutynin Chloride (Co-administration may produce paralytic ileus). Products include:
Ditropan XL Extended Release Tablets 2391

Oxycodone Hydrochloride (Co-administration may exhibit additive CNS depression). Products include:
Combunox Tablets 1183
OxyContin Tablets 2699
OxyFast Oral Concentrate Solution 2704
OxyIR Capsules 2704
Percocet Tablets 1114
Percodan Tablets 1115

Pargyline Hydrochloride (Co-administration of MAO inhibitors with hydrocodone may increase the effect of either hydrocodone or MAO inhibitor).
No products indexed under this heading.

Pentobarbital Sodium (Co-administration may exhibit additive CNS depression). Products include:
Nembutal Sodium Solution, USP 2484

Perphenazine (Co-administration may exhibit additive CNS depression).
No products indexed under this heading.

Phenelzine Sulfate (Co-administration of MAO inhibitors with hydrocodone may increase the effect of either hydrocodone or MAO inhibitor).
No products indexed under this heading.

Phenobarbital (Co-administration may exhibit additive CNS depression).
No products indexed under this heading.

Prazepam (Co-administration may exhibit additive CNS depression).
No products indexed under this heading.

Procarbazine Hydrochloride (Co-administration of MAO inhibitors with hydrocodone may increase the effect of either hydrocodone or MAO inhibitor). Products include:
Matulane Capsules 3188

Prochlorperazine (Co-administration may exhibit additive CNS depression).
No products indexed under this heading.

Procyclidine Hydrochloride (Co-administration may produce paralytic ileus).
No products indexed under this heading.

Promethazine Hydrochloride (Co-administration may exhibit additive CNS depression). Products include:
Phenergan 3438

Propantheline Bromide (Co-administration may produce paralytic ileus).
No products indexed under this heading.

Propofol (Co-administration may exhibit additive CNS depression). Products include:
Diprivan Injectable Emulsion 676

Propoxyphene Hydrochloride (Co-administration may exhibit additive CNS depression).
No products indexed under this heading.

Propoxyphene Napsylate (Co-administration may exhibit additive CNS depression). Products include:
Darvocet A 500 Tablets 3497

Protriptyline Hydrochloride (Co-administration of tricyclic antidepressants with hydrocodone may increase the effect of either hydrocodone or antidepressant). Products include:
Vivactil Tablets 2350

Quazepam (Co-administration may exhibit additive CNS depression).
No products indexed under this heading.

Quetiapine Fumarate (Co-administration may exhibit additive CNS depression). Products include:
Seroquel Tablets 691

Remifentanil Hydrochloride (Co-administration may exhibit additive CNS depression).
No products indexed under this heading.

Risperidone (Co-administration may exhibit additive CNS depression). Products include:
Risperdal Consta Long-Acting Injection 1664
Risperdal M-Tab Orally Disintegrating Tablets 1658
Risperdal 1658

Scopolamine (Co-administration may produce paralytic ileus). Products include:
Transderm Scōp Transdermal Therapeutic System 2166

Scopolamine Hydrobromide (Co-administration may produce paralytic ileus).
No products indexed under this heading.

Secobarbital Sodium (Co-administration may exhibit additive CNS depression).
No products indexed under this heading.

Selegiline Hydrochloride (Co-administration of MAO inhibitors with hydrocodone may increase the effect of either hydrocodone or MAO inhibitor). Products include:
Eldepryl Capsules 3209

Sevoflurane (Co-administration may exhibit additive CNS depression). Products include:
Ultane Liquid for Inhalation 526

Sodium Oxybate (Co-administration may exhibit additive CNS depression).
No products indexed under this heading.

Sufentanil Citrate (Co-administration may exhibit additive CNS depression).
No products indexed under this heading.

Temazepam (Co-administration may exhibit additive CNS depression).
No products indexed under this heading.

Thiamylal Sodium (Co-administration may exhibit additive CNS depression).
No products indexed under this heading.

Thioridazine Hydrochloride (Co-administration may exhibit additive CNS depression). Products include:
Thioridazine Hydrochloride Tablets 2122

Thiothixene (Co-administration may exhibit additive CNS depression). Products include:
Thiothixene Capsules 2124

Tolterodine Tartrate (Co-administration may produce paralytic ileus). Products include:
Detrol Tablets 2626
Detrol LA Capsules 2629

Tranylcypromine Sulfate (Co-administration of MAO inhibitors with hydrocodone may increase the effect of either hydrocodone or MAO inhibitor). Products include:
Parnate Tablets 1499

Triazolam (Co-administration may exhibit additive CNS depression).
No products indexed under this heading.

Tridihexethyl Chloride (Co-administration may produce paralytic ileus).
No products indexed under this heading.

Trifluoperazine Hydrochloride (Co-administration may exhibit additive CNS depression).
No products indexed under this heading.

Trihexyphenidyl Hydrochloride (Co-administration may produce paralytic ileus).
No products indexed under this heading.

Trimipramine Maleate (Co-administration of tricyclic antidepressants with hydrocodone may increase the effect of either hydrocodone or antidepressant). Products include:
Surmontil Capsules 2347

Zaleplon (Co-administration may exhibit additive CNS depression). Products include:
Sonata Capsules 1686

Ziprasidone Hydrochloride (Co-administration may exhibit additive CNS depression). Products include:
Geodon Capsules 2514

Zolpidem Tartrate (Co-administration may exhibit additive CNS depression). Products include:
Ambien Tablets 2867

Food Interactions

Alcohol (Co-administration may exhibit additive CNS depression).

ZYLET OPHTHALMIC SUSPENSION
(Loteprednol Etabonate, Tobramycin)............ 3508
None cited in PDR database.

ZYMAR OPHTHALMIC SOLUTION
(Gatifloxacin) 571
None cited in PDR database.

ZYPREXA TABLETS
(Olanzapine) 1798
May interact with antihypertensives, benzodiazepines, central nervous system depressants, cytochrome p450 1a2 inducers (selected), cytochrome p450 1a2 inhibitors (selected), dopamine agonists, drugs that elevate levels of glucuronosyl transferase, and certain other agents. Compounds in these categories include:

Acebutolol Hydrochloride (Olanzapine, because of its potential for inducing hypotension, may enhance the effects of certain antihypertensive agents).
No products indexed under this heading.

Alatrofloxacin Mesylate (Can potentially inhibit olanzapine clearance; therefore, a dosage decrease might be considered).
No products indexed under this heading.

Alfentanil Hydrochloride (Given the primary CNS effects of olanzapine, caution should be used when olanzapine is taken in combination with other centrally-acting drugs).
No products indexed under this heading.

Alprazolam (Given the primary CNS effects of olanzapine, caution should be used when olanzapine is taken in combination with other centrally-acting drugs). Products include:
Niravam Orally Disintegrating Tablets 3106
Xanax XR Tablets 2655

Amiodarone Hydrochloride (Can potentially inhibit olanzapine clearance; therefore, a dosage decrease might be considered). Products include:
Pacerone Tablets 3337

Amlodipine Besylate (Olanzapine, because of its potential for inducing hypotension, may enhance the effects of certain antihypertensive agents). Products include:
Caduet Tablets 2507
Lotrel Capsules 2238
Norvasc Tablets 2529

Anastrozole (Can potentially inhibit olanzapine clearance; therefore, a dosage decrease might be considered). Products include:
Arimidex Tablets 665

Aprobarbital (Given the primary CNS effects of olanzapine, caution should be used when olanzapine is taken in combination with other centrally-acting drugs).
No products indexed under this heading.

Atenolol (Olanzapine, because of its potential for inducing hypotension, may enhance the effects of certain antihypertensive agents). Products include:
Tenormin I.V. Injection 698
Tenormin Tablets 695

Benazepril Hydrochloride (Olanzapine, because of its potential for inducing hypotension, may enhance the effects of certain antihypertensive agents). Products include:
Lotensin Tablets 2232
Lotensin HCT Tablets 2235
Lotrel Capsules 2238

Bendroflumethiazide (Olanzapine, because of its potential for inducing hypotension, may enhance the effects of certain antihypertensive agents).
No products indexed under this heading.

Betaxolol Hydrochloride (Olanzapine, because of its potential for inducing hypotension, may enhance the effects of certain antihypertensive agents). Products include:
Betoptic S Ophthalmic Suspension............ 554

Bisoprolol Fumarate (Olanzapine, because of its potential for inducing hypotension, may enhance the effects of certain antihypertensive agents).
No products indexed under this heading.

Bromocriptine Mesylate (Olanzapine may antagonize the effects of dopamine agonists).
No products indexed under this heading.

Buprenorphine Hydrochloride (Given the primary CNS effects of olanzapine, caution should be used when olanzapine is taken in combination with other centrally-acting drugs). Products include:
Buprenex Injectable 2718
Suboxone Tablets 2719
Subutex Tablets 2719

Buspirone Hydrochloride (Given the primary CNS effects of olanzapine, caution should be used when olanzapine is taken in combination with other centrally-acting drugs).
No products indexed under this heading.

Butabarbital (Given the primary CNS effects of olanzapine, caution should be used when olanzapine is taken in combination with other centrally-acting drugs).
No products indexed under this heading.

Butalbital (Given the primary CNS effects of olanzapine, caution should be used when olanzapine is taken in combination with other centrally-acting drugs). Products include:
Sedapap Tablets 50 mg/650 mg 2098

Candesartan Cilexetil (Olanzapine, because of its potential for inducing hypotension, may enhance the effects of certain antihypertensive agents). Products include:
Atacand Tablets 634
Atacand HCT 637

Captopril (Olanzapine, because of its potential for inducing hypotension, may enhance the effects of certain antihypertensive agents). Products include:
Captopril Tablets 2114

Carbamazepine (Causes an approximately 50% increase in the clearance of olanzapine at 400 mg daily; higher daily doses of carbamazepine may cause an even greater increase in olanzapine clearance). Products include:
Carbatrol Capsules 3174
Equetro Extended-Release Capsules............ 3178
Tegretol/Tegretol-XR 2278

Carteolol Hydrochloride (Olanzapine, because of its potential for inducing hypotension, may enhance the effects of certain antihypertensive agents). Products include:
Carteolol Hydrochloride Ophthalmic Solution USP, 1%....... ⊙246

Charcoal, Activated (Co-administration with activated charcoal reduces the Cmax and AUC of olanzapine by about 60%).
No products indexed under this heading.

Chlordiazepoxide (Given the primary CNS effects of olanzapine, caution should be used when olanzapine is taken in combination with other centrally-acting drugs).
No products indexed under this heading.

Chlordiazepoxide Hydrochloride (Given the primary CNS effects of olanzapine, caution should be used when olanzapine is taken in combination with other centrally-acting drugs). Products include:
Librium Capsules 3349

Chlorothiazide (Olanzapine, because of its potential for inducing hypotension, may enhance the effects of certain antihypertensive agents). Products include:
Aldoclor Tablets 1881
Diuril Oral 1936

Chlorothiazide Sodium (Olanzapine, because of its potential for inducing hypotension, may enhance the effects of certain antihypertensive agents). Products include:
Diuril Sodium Intravenous 1934

Chlorpromazine (Given the primary CNS effects of olanzapine, caution should be used when olanzapine is taken in combination with other centrally-acting drugs).
No products indexed under this heading.

Chlorpromazine Hydrochloride (Given the primary CNS effects of olanzapine, caution should be used when olanzapine is taken in combination with other centrally-acting drugs).
No products indexed under this heading.

Chlorprothixene (Given the primary CNS effects of olanzapine, caution should be used when olanzapine is taken in combination with other centrally-acting drugs).
No products indexed under this heading.

Chlorprothixene Hydrochloride (Given the primary CNS effects of olanzapine, caution should be used when olanzapine is taken in combination with other centrally-acting drugs).
No products indexed under this heading.

Chlorprothixene Lactate (Given the primary CNS effects of olanzapine, caution should be used when olanzapine is taken in combination with other centrally-acting drugs).
No products indexed under this heading.

Chlorthalidone (Olanzapine, because of its potential for inducing hypotension, may enhance the effects of certain antihypertensive agents). Products include:
Clorpres Tablets 2139

Cimetidine (Can potentially inhibit olanzapine clearance; therefore, a dosage decrease might be considered). Products include:
Tagamet HB 200 Tablets .... ▣637
Tagamet Tablets 1547

Cimetidine Hydrochloride (Can potentially inhibit olanzapine clearance; therefore, a dosage decrease might be considered).
No products indexed under this heading.

Ciprofloxacin (Can potentially inhibit olanzapine clearance; therefore, a dosage decrease might be considered). Products include:
Cipro I.V. 2998
Cipro I.V. Pharmacy Bulk Package 3509
Cipro Oral Suspension 2991
Cipro XR Tablets 3004
Ciprodex Otic Suspension 555

Ciprofloxacin Hydrochloride (Can potentially inhibit olanzapine clearance; therefore, a dosage decrease might be considered). Products include:
Ciloxan Ophthalmic Ointment 554
Cipro Tablets 2991

Citalopram Hydrobromide (May cause an increase in olanzapine clearance; therefore, a dosage increase might be considered). Products include:
Celexa 1177

Clarithromycin (Can potentially inhibit olanzapine clearance; therefore, a dosage decrease might be considered). Products include:
Biaxin/Biaxin XL 402
PREVPAC 3281

Clonidine (Olanzapine, because of its potential for inducing hypotension, may enhance the effects of certain antihypertensive agents). Products include:
Catapres-TTS 875

Clonidine Hydrochloride (Olanzapine, because of its potential for inducing hypotension, may enhance the effects of certain antihypertensive agents). Products include:
Catapres Tablets 874
Clorpres Tablets 2139

Clorazepate Dipotassium (Given the primary CNS effects of olanzapine, caution should be used when olanzapine is taken in combination with other centrally-acting drugs). Products include:
Tranxene 2488

Clozapine (Given the primary CNS effects of olanzapine, caution should be used when olanzapine is taken in combination with other centrally-acting drugs). Products include:
Clozapine Tablets 2141
Clozaril Tablets 2174
FazaClo Orally Disintegrating Tablets 547

Codeine Phosphate (Given the primary CNS effects of olanzapine, caution should be used when olanzapine is taken in combination with other centrally-acting drugs). Products include:
Tylenol with Codeine 2461

Deserpidine (Olanzapine, because of its potential for inducing hypotension, may enhance the effects of certain antihypertensive agents).
No products indexed under this heading.

Desflurane (Given the primary CNS effects of olanzapine, caution should be used when olanzapine is taken in combination with other centrally-acting drugs). Products include:
Suprane Liquid for Inhalation 770

Desogestrel (Can potentially inhibit olanzapine clearance; therefore, a dosage decrease might be considered). Products include:
Ortho-Cept Tablets 2395

Dezocine (Given the primary CNS effects of olanzapine, caution should be used when olanzapine is taken in combination with other centrally-acting drugs).
No products indexed under this heading.

Diazepam (Co-administration of diazepam with olanzapine may potentiate orthostatic hypotension. Concomitant administration of intramuscular olanzapine and parenteral benzodiazepine has not been studied and is therefore not recommended. If use of intramuscular olanzapine in combination with parenteral benzodiazepines is considered, careful evaluation of clinical status for excessive sedation and cardiorespiratory depression is recommended). Products include:
Diastat Rectal Delivery System 3344
Valium Tablets 2822

Diazoxide (Olanzapine, because of its potential for inducing hypotension, may enhance the effects of certain antihypertensive agents). Products include:
Hyperstat I.V. Injection 3031

Diltiazem Hydrochloride (Olanzapine, because of its potential for inducing hypotension, may enhance the effects of certain antihypertensive agents). Products include:
Cardizem LA Extended Release Tablets 1699
Tiazac Capsules 1204

Diltiazem Maleate (May cause an increase in olanzapine clearance; therefore, a dosage increase might be considered).
No products indexed under this heading.

Dopamine Hydrochloride (Olanzapine may antagonize the effects of dopamine agonists).
No products indexed under this heading.

Doxazosin Mesylate (Olanzapine, because of its potential for inducing hypotension, may enhance the effects of certain antihypertensive agents).
No products indexed under this heading.

Droperidol (Given the primary CNS effects of olanzapine, caution should be used when olanzapine is taken in combination with other centrally-acting drugs).
No products indexed under this heading.

Enalapril Maleate (Olanzapine, because of its potential for inducing hypotension, may enhance the effects of certain antihypertensive agents). Products include:
Vaseretic Tablets 2073
Vasotec I.V. Injection 2076

Enalaprilat (Olanzapine, because of its potential for inducing hypotension, may enhance the effects of certain antihypertensive agents).
No products indexed under this heading.

Enflurane (Given the primary CNS effects of olanzapine, caution should be used when olanzapine is taken in combination with other centrally-acting drugs).
No products indexed under this heading.

Enoxacin (Can potentially inhibit olanzapine clearance; therefore, a dosage decrease might be considered).
No products indexed under this heading.

Eprosartan Mesylate (Olanzapine, because of its potential for inducing hypotension, may enhance the effects of certain antihypertensive agents). Products include:
Teveten Tablets 1707
Teveten HCT Tablets 1710

Erythromycin (May cause an increase in olanzapine clearance; therefore, a dosage increase might be considered). Products include:
Erygel Topical Gel 2096
Ery-Tab Tablets 447
Erythromycin Base Filmtab Tablets 454
Erythromycin Delayed-Release Capsules, USP 456
PCE Dispertab Tablets 510

Erythromycin Estolate (May cause an increase in olanzapine clearance; therefore, a dosage increase might be considered).
No products indexed under this heading.

Erythromycin Ethylsuccinate (May cause an increase in olanzapine clearance; therefore, a dosage increase might be considered). Products include:
E.E.S. 449
EryPed 445

Erythromycin Gluceptate (May cause an increase in olanzapine clearance; therefore, a dosage increase might be considered).
No products indexed under this heading.

Erythromycin Lactobionate (May cause an increase in olanzapine clearance; therefore, a dosage increase might be considered).
No products indexed under this heading.

Erythromycin Stearate (May cause an increase in olanzapine clearance; therefore, a dosage increase might be considered). Products include:
Erythrocin Stearate Filmtab Tablets 452

Esmolol Hydrochloride (Olanzapine, because of its potential for inducing hypotension, may enhance the effects of certain antihypertensive agents). Products include:
Brevibloc Concentrate 766
Brevibloc Injection 766
Brevibloc Double Strength Injection 766
Brevibloc Premixed Injection 766
Brevibloc Double Strength Premixed Injection 766

Estazolam (Given the primary CNS effects of olanzapine, caution should be used when olanzapine is taken in combination with other centrally-acting drugs). Products include:
ProSom Tablets 512

Ethanol (Given the primary CNS effects of olanzapine, caution should be used when olanzapine is taken in combination with other centrally-acting drugs).
No products indexed under this heading.

Ethchlorvynol (Given the primary CNS effects of olanzapine, caution should be used when olanzapine is taken in combination with other centrally-acting drugs).
No products indexed under this heading.

IMPORTANT NOTE: Always consult each drug listing in the patient's regimen for possible interactions.

Ethinamate (Given the primary CNS effects of olanzapine, caution should be used when olanzapine is taken in combination with other centrally-acting drugs).
No products indexed under this heading.

Ethinyl Estradiol (Can potentially inhibit olanzapine clearance; therefore, a dosage decrease might be considered). Products include:
Alesse-28 Tablets 3392
Lo/Ovral-28 Tablets 3423
NuvaRing 2357
Ortho-Cept Tablets 2395
Ortho-Cyclen/Ortho Tri-Cyclen 2414
Ortho Evra Transdermal System 2402
Ortho Tri-Cyclen Lo Tablets 2421
Seasonale Tablets 1073
Triphasil-28 Tablets 3483
Yasmin 28 Tablets 818

Ethyl Alcohol (Given the primary CNS effects of olanzapine, caution should be used when olanzapine is taken in combination with other centrally-acting drugs).
No products indexed under this heading.

Felodipine (Olanzapine, because of its potential for inducing hypotension, may enhance the effects of certain antihypertensive agents). Products include:
Plendil Extended-Release Tablets 651

Fentanyl (Given the primary CNS effects of olanzapine, caution should be used when olanzapine is taken in combination with other centrally-acting drugs). Products include:
Duragesic Transdermal System 2448

Fentanyl Citrate (Given the primary CNS effects of olanzapine, caution should be used when olanzapine is taken in combination with other centrally-acting drugs). Products include:
Actiq 993

Fluoxetine Hydrochloride (Co-administration causes a small increase in the maximum concentration of olanzapine and a small decrease in olanzapine clearance; the magnitude of the impact of this factor is small in comparison to the overall variability between individuals and, therefore, dose modification is not routinely recommended). Products include:
Prozac Pulvules and Liquid 1771
Symbyax Capsules 1788

Fluphenazine Decanoate (Given the primary CNS effects of olanzapine, caution should be used when olanzapine is taken in combination with other centrally-acting drugs).
No products indexed under this heading.

Fluphenazine Enanthate (Given the primary CNS effects of olanzapine, caution should be used when olanzapine is taken in combination with other centrally-acting drugs).
No products indexed under this heading.

Fluphenazine Hydrochloride (Given the primary CNS effects of olanzapine, caution should be used when olanzapine is taken in combination with other centrally-acting drugs).
No products indexed under this heading.

Flurazepam Hydrochloride (Given the primary CNS effects of olanzapine, caution should be used when olanzapine is taken in combination with other centrally-acting drugs). Products include:
Dalmane Capsules 3343

Fluvoxamine (Can potentially inhibit olanzapine clearance; therefore, a dosage decrease might be considered).
No products indexed under this heading.

Fluvoxamine Maleate (Decreases the clearance of olanzapine leading to a mean increase in olanzapine Cmax and AUC; lower doses of olanzapine should be considered or co-administered).
No products indexed under this heading.

Fosinopril Sodium (Olanzapine, because of its potential for inducing hypotension, may enhance the effects of certain antihypertensive agents).
No products indexed under this heading.

Furosemide (Olanzapine, because of its potential for inducing hypotension, may enhance the effects of certain antihypertensive agents). Products include:
Furosemide Tablets 2117

Gatifloxacin (Can potentially inhibit olanzapine clearance; therefore, a dosage decrease might be considered). Products include:
Tequin Injection 964
Tequin Tablets 964
Zymar Ophthalmic Solution 571

Gemifloxacin Mesylate (Can potentially inhibit olanzapine clearance; therefore, a dosage decrease might be considered). Products include:
Factive Tablets 2464

Glutethimide (Given the primary CNS effects of olanzapine, caution should be used when olanzapine is taken in combination with other centrally-acting drugs).
No products indexed under this heading.

Grepafloxacin Hydrochloride (Can potentially inhibit olanzapine clearance; therefore, a dosage decrease might be considered).
No products indexed under this heading.

Guanabenz Acetate (Olanzapine, because of its potential for inducing hypotension, may enhance the effects of certain antihypertensive agents).
No products indexed under this heading.

Guanethidine Monosulfate (Olanzapine, because of its potential for inducing hypotension, may enhance the effects of certain antihypertensive agents).
No products indexed under this heading.

Halazepam (Concomitant administration of intramuscular olanzapine and parenteral benzodiazepine has not been studied and is therefore not recommended. If use of intramuscular olanzapine in combination with parenteral benzodiazepines is considered, careful evaluation of clinical status for excessive sedation and cardiorespiratory depression is recommended).
No products indexed under this heading.

Haloperidol (Given the primary CNS effects of olanzapine, caution should be used when olanzapine is taken in combination with other centrally-acting drugs).
No products indexed under this heading.

Haloperidol Decanoate (Given the primary CNS effects of olanzapine, caution should be used when olanzapine is taken in combination with other centrally-acting drugs).
No products indexed under this heading.

Hydralazine Hydrochloride (Olanzapine, because of its potential for inducing hypotension, may enhance the effects of certain antihypertensive agents). Products include:
BiDil Tablets 2161

Hydrochlorothiazide (Olanzapine, because of its potential for inducing hypotension, may enhance the effects of certain antihypertensive agents). Products include:
Aldoril Tablets 1884
Atacand HCT 637
Avalide Tablets 2889
Avalide Tablets 922
Benicar HCT Tablets 2852
Diovan HCT Tablets 2195
Dyazide Capsules 1389
Hyzaar 1964
Lotensin HCT Tablets 2235
Maxzide 2150
Micardis HCT Tablets 886
Moduretic Tablets 2003
Prinzide Tablets 2033
Teveten HCT Tablets 1710
Timolide Tablets 2056
Uniretic Tablets 3114
Vaseretic Tablets 2073
Zestoretic Tablets 701

Hydrocodone Bitartrate (Given the primary CNS effects of olanzapine, caution should be used when olanzapine is taken in combination with other centrally-acting drugs). Products include:
Hycodan 1104
Hycomine Compound Tablets 1105
Hycotuss Expectorant Syrup 1106
Lortab 3315
Lortab Elixir 3312
Vicodin Tablets 530
Vicodin ES Tablets 531
Vicodin HP Tablets 532
Vicoprofen Tablets 533
Zydone Tablets 1118

Hydrocodone Polistirex (Given the primary CNS effects of olanzapine, caution should be used when olanzapine is taken in combination with other centrally-acting drugs). Products include:
Tussionex Pennkinetic Extended-Release Suspension 3322

Hydroflumethiazide (Olanzapine, because of its potential for inducing hypotension, may enhance the effects of certain antihypertensive agents).
No products indexed under this heading.

Hydromorphone Hydrochloride (Given the primary CNS effects of olanzapine, caution should be used when olanzapine is taken in combination with other centrally-acting drugs). Products include:
Dilaudid 439
Dilaudid Oral Liquid 443
Dilaudid Non-Sterile Powder 439
Dilaudid Rectal Suppositories 439
Dilaudid Tablets 439
Dilaudid Tablets - 8 mg 443
Dilaudid-HP 441

Hydroxyzine Hydrochloride (Given the primary CNS effects of olanzapine, caution should be used when olanzapine is taken in combination with other centrally-acting drugs).
No products indexed under this heading.

Hypericum (May cause an increase in olanzapine clearance; therefore, a dosage increase might be considered).
No products indexed under this heading.

Indapamide (Olanzapine, because of its potential for inducing hypotension, may enhance the effects of certain antihypertensive agents). Products include:
Indapamide Tablets 2119

Insulin (May cause an increase in olanzapine clearance; therefore, a dosage increase might be considered).
No products indexed under this heading.

Irbesartan (Olanzapine, because of its potential for inducing hypotension, may enhance the effects of certain antihypertensive agents). Products include:
Avalide Tablets 922
Avalide Tablets 2889
Avapro Tablets 925
Avapro Tablets 2886

Isoflurane (Given the primary CNS effects of olanzapine, caution should be used when olanzapine is taken in combination with other centrally-acting drugs).
No products indexed under this heading.

Isoniazid (Can potentially inhibit olanzapine clearance; therefore, a dosage decrease might be considered).
No products indexed under this heading.

Isradipine (Olanzapine, because of its potential for inducing hypotension, may enhance the effects of certain antihypertensive agents). Products include:
DynaCirc CR Tablets 2726

Ketamine Hydrochloride (Given the primary CNS effects of olanzapine, caution should be used when olanzapine is taken in combination with other centrally-acting drugs).
No products indexed under this heading.

Ketoconazole (Can potentially inhibit olanzapine clearance; therefore, a dosage decrease might be considered). Products include:
Nizoral A-D Shampoo, 1% 1839
Nizoral 2% Shampoo 1838

Labetalol Hydrochloride (Olanzapine, because of its potential for inducing hypotension, may enhance the effects of certain antihypertensive agents).
No products indexed under this heading.

Lansoprazole (May cause an increase in olanzapine clearance; therefore, a dosage increase might be considered). Products include:
Prevacid Delayed-Release Capsules 3268
Prevacid for Delayed-Release Oral Suspension 3268
Prevacid I.V. for Injection 3274
Prevacid NapraPAC 3277
Prevacid SoluTab Delayed-Release Orally Disintegrating Tablets 3268
PREVPAC 3281

Levodopa (Olanzapine may antagonize the effects of levodopa). Products include:
- Parcopa Orally Disintegrating Tablets 3111
- Stalevo Tablets 2270

Levofloxacin (Can potentially inhibit olanzapine clearance; therefore, a dosage decrease might be considered). Products include:
- Levaquin in 5% Dextrose Injection 2453
- Levaquin 2453
- Quixin Ophthalmic Solution 3373

Levomethadyl Acetate Hydrochloride (Given the primary CNS effects of olanzapine, caution should be used when olanzapine is taken in combination with other centrally-acting drugs).
- No products indexed under this heading.

Levonorgestrel (Can potentially inhibit olanzapine clearance; therefore, a dosage decrease might be considered). Products include:
- Alesse-28 Tablets 3392
- Climara Pro Transdermal System 800
- Mirena Intrauterine System 810
- Plan B Tablets 1068
- Seasonale Tablets 1073
- Triphasil-28 Tablets 3483

Levorphanol Tartrate (Given the primary CNS effects of olanzapine, caution should be used when olanzapine is taken in combination with other centrally-acting drugs).
- No products indexed under this heading.

Lisinopril (Olanzapine, because of its potential for inducing hypotension, may enhance the effects of certain antihypertensive agents). Products include:
- Prinivil Tablets 2029
- Prinzide Tablets 2033
- Zestoretic Tablets 701
- Zestril Tablets 704

Lomefloxacin Hydrochloride (Can potentially inhibit olanzapine clearance; therefore, a dosage decrease might be considered).
- No products indexed under this heading.

Lorazepam (Given the primary CNS effects of olanzapine, caution should be used when olanzapine is taken in combination with other centrally-acting drugs).
- No products indexed under this heading.

Losartan Potassium (Olanzapine, because of its potential for inducing hypotension, may enhance the effects of certain antihypertensive agents). Products include:
- Cozaar Tablets 1913
- Hyzaar 1964

Loxapine Hydrochloride (Given the primary CNS effects of olanzapine, caution should be used when olanzapine is taken in combination with other centrally-acting drugs).
- No products indexed under this heading.

Loxapine Succinate (Given the primary CNS effects of olanzapine, caution should be used when olanzapine is taken in combination with other centrally-acting drugs).
- No products indexed under this heading.

Mecamylamine Hydrochloride (Olanzapine, because of its potential for inducing hypotension, may enhance the effects of certain antihypertensive agents). Products include:
- Inversine Tablets 3286

Meperidine Hydrochloride (Given the primary CNS effects of olanzapine, caution should be used when olanzapine is taken in combination with other centrally-acting drugs).
- No products indexed under this heading.

Mephobarbital (Given the primary CNS effects of olanzapine, caution should be used when olanzapine is taken in combination with other centrally-acting drugs). Products include:
- Mebaral Tablets, USP 2483

Meprobamate (Given the primary CNS effects of olanzapine, caution should be used when olanzapine is taken in combination with other centrally-acting drugs).
- No products indexed under this heading.

Mesoridazine Besylate (Given the primary CNS effects of olanzapine, caution should be used when olanzapine is taken in combination with other centrally-acting drugs).
- No products indexed under this heading.

Mestranol (Can potentially inhibit olanzapine clearance; therefore, a dosage decrease might be considered).
- No products indexed under this heading.

Methadone Hydrochloride (Given the primary CNS effects of olanzapine, caution should be used when olanzapine is taken in combination with other centrally-acting drugs).
- No products indexed under this heading.

Methohexital Sodium (Given the primary CNS effects of olanzapine, caution should be used when olanzapine is taken in combination with other centrally-acting drugs).
- No products indexed under this heading.

Methotrimeprazine (Given the primary CNS effects of olanzapine, caution should be used when olanzapine is taken in combination with other centrally-acting drugs).
- No products indexed under this heading.

Methoxsalen (Can potentially inhibit olanzapine clearance; therefore, a dosage decrease might be considered). Products include:
- Oxsoralen Lotion 1% 3354
- Oxsoralen-Ultra Capsules 3354

Methoxyflurane (Given the primary CNS effects of olanzapine, caution should be used when olanzapine is taken in combination with other centrally-acting drugs).
- No products indexed under this heading.

Methyclothiazide (Olanzapine, because of its potential for inducing hypotension, may enhance the effects of certain antihypertensive agents).
- No products indexed under this heading.

Methyldopa (Olanzapine, because of its potential for inducing hypotension, may enhance the effects of certain antihypertensive agents). Products include:
- Aldoclor Tablets 1881
- Aldoril Tablets 1884

Methyldopate Hydrochloride (Olanzapine, because of its potential for inducing hypotension, may enhance the effects of certain antihypertensive agents).
- No products indexed under this heading.

Metolazone (Olanzapine, because of its potential for inducing hypotension, may enhance the effects of certain antihypertensive agents).
- No products indexed under this heading.

Metoprolol Succinate (Olanzapine, because of its potential for inducing hypotension, may enhance the effects of certain antihypertensive agents). Products include:
- Toprol-XL Tablets 660

Metoprolol Tartrate (Olanzapine, because of its potential for inducing hypotension, may enhance the effects of certain antihypertensive agents).
- No products indexed under this heading.

Metyrosine (Olanzapine, because of its potential for inducing hypotension, may enhance the effects of certain antihypertensive agents). Products include:
- Demser Capsules 1933

Mexiletine Hydrochloride (Can potentially inhibit olanzapine clearance; therefore, a dosage decrease might be considered).
- No products indexed under this heading.

Mibefradil Dihydrochloride (Olanzapine, because of its potential for inducing hypotension, may enhance the effects of certain antihypertensive agents).
- No products indexed under this heading.

Midazolam Hydrochloride (Given the primary CNS effects of olanzapine, caution should be used when olanzapine is taken in combination with other centrally-acting drugs).
- No products indexed under this heading.

Minoxidil (Olanzapine, because of its potential for inducing hypotension, may enhance the effects of certain antihypertensive agents). Products include:
- Men's Rogaine Extra Strength Topical Solution, Ocean Rush Scent and Original Unscented 706
- Women's Rogaine Topical Solution, Spring Bloom Scent and Original Unscented 707

Moexipril Hydrochloride (Olanzapine, because of its potential for inducing hypotension, may enhance the effects of certain antihypertensive agents). Products include:
- Uniretic Tablets 3114
- Univasc Tablets 3118

Molindone Hydrochloride (Given the primary CNS effects of olanzapine, caution should be used when olanzapine is taken in combination with other centrally-acting drugs). Products include:
- Moban Tablets 1108

Morphine Sulfate (Given the primary CNS effects of olanzapine, caution should be used when olanzapine is taken in combination with other centrally-acting drugs). Products include:
- Avinza Capsules 1714
- Kadian Capsules 572
- MS Contin Tablets 2703

Moxifloxacin Hydrochloride (Can potentially inhibit olanzapine clearance; therefore, a dosage decrease might be considered). Products include:
- Avelox 2984
- Vigamox Ophthalmic Solution 560

Nadolol (Olanzapine, because of its potential for inducing hypotension, may enhance the effects of certain antihypertensive agents). Products include:
- Nadolol Tablets 2121

Nafcillin Sodium (May cause an increase in olanzapine clearance; therefore, a dosage increase might be considered).
- No products indexed under this heading.

Nalidixic Acid (Can potentially inhibit olanzapine clearance; therefore, a dosage decrease might be considered).
- No products indexed under this heading.

Nicardipine Hydrochloride (Olanzapine, because of its potential for inducing hypotension, may enhance the effects of certain antihypertensive agents). Products include:
- Cardene I.V. 1129

Nicotine (May cause an increase in olanzapine clearance; therefore, a dosage increase might be considered). Products include:
- Nicoderm CQ Patch 1629
- NicoDerm CQ Clear Patch 627
- Nicotrol Inhaler 2594
- Nicotrol NS 2596

Nicotine Polacrilex (May cause an increase in olanzapine clearance; therefore, a dosage increase might be considered). Products include:
- Commit Lozenges 1625
- Nicorette Gum 1632

Nicotine Salicylate (May cause an increase in olanzapine clearance; therefore, a dosage increase might be considered).
- No products indexed under this heading.

Nicotine Sulfate (May cause an increase in olanzapine clearance; therefore, a dosage increase might be considered).
- No products indexed under this heading.

Nifedipine (Olanzapine, because of its potential for inducing hypotension, may enhance the effects of certain antihypertensive agents). Products include:
- Adalat CC Tablets 2978

Nisoldipine (Olanzapine, because of its potential for inducing hypotension, may enhance the effects of certain antihypertensive agents). Products include:
- Sular Tablets 1163

Nitroglycerin (Olanzapine, because of its potential for inducing hypotension, may enhance the effects of certain antihypertensive agents). Products include:
- Nitro-Dur Transdermal Infusion System 3060
- Nitrolingual Pumpspray 1161

Norethindrone (Can potentially inhibit olanzapine clearance; therefore, a dosage decrease might be considered). Products include:
- Ortho Micronor Tablets 2411

Norfloxacin (Can potentially inhibit olanzapine clearance; therefore, a dosage decrease might be considered). Products include:

IMPORTANT NOTE: Always consult each drug listing in the patient's regimen for possible interactions.

Noroxin Tablets 2009

Norgestrel (Can potentially inhibit olanzapine clearance; therefore, a dosage decrease might be considered). Products include:

Lo/Ovral-28 Tablets 3423

Ofloxacin (Can potentially inhibit olanzapine clearance; therefore, a dosage decrease might be considered). Products include:

Floxin Otic Singles 1045
Floxin Otic Solution 1043

Omeprazole (May cause an increase in olanzapine clearance by inducing CYP1A2 or glucuronyl transferase clearance). Products include:

Zegerid Powder for Oral Solution 2972

Oxazepam (Given the primary CNS effects of olanzapine, caution should be used when olanzapine is taken in combination with other centrally-acting drugs).

No products indexed under this heading.

Oxycodone Hydrochloride (Given the primary CNS effects of olanzapine, caution should be used when olanzapine is taken in combination with other centrally-acting drugs). Products include:

Combunox Tablets 1183
OxyContin Tablets 2699
OxyFast Oral Concentrate Solution 2704
OxyIR Capsules 2704
Percocet Tablets 1114
Percodan Tablets 1115

Paroxetine Hydrochloride (Can potentially inhibit olanzapine clearance; therefore, a dosage decrease might be considered). Products include:

Paxil CR Controlled-Release Tablets 1509
Paxil 1501

Penbutolol Sulfate (Olanzapine, because of its potential for inducing hypotension, may enhance the effects of certain antihypertensive agents).

No products indexed under this heading.

Pentobarbital Sodium (Given the primary CNS effects of olanzapine, caution should be used when olanzapine is taken in combination with other centrally-acting drugs). Products include:

Nembutal Sodium Solution, USP 2484

Pergolide Mesylate (Olanzapine may antagonize the effects of dopamine agonists). Products include:

Permax Tablets 3357

Perindopril Erbumine (Olanzapine, because of its potential for inducing hypotension, may enhance the effects of certain antihypertensive agents). Products include:

Aceon Tablets (2 mg, 4 mg, 8 mg) 3191

Perphenazine (Given the primary CNS effects of olanzapine, caution should be used when olanzapine is taken in combination with other centrally-acting drugs).

No products indexed under this heading.

Phenobarbital (Given the primary CNS effects of olanzapine, caution should be used when olanzapine is taken in combination with other centrally-acting drugs).

No products indexed under this heading.

Phenoxybenzamine Hydrochloride (Olanzapine, because of its potential for inducing hypotension, may enhance the effects of certain antihypertensive agents). Products include:

Dibenzyline Capsules 3390

Phentolamine Mesylate (Olanzapine, because of its potential for inducing hypotension, may enhance the effects of certain antihypertensive agents).

No products indexed under this heading.

Phenytoin (May cause an increase in olanzapine clearance; therefore, a dosage increase might be considered).

No products indexed under this heading.

Phenytoin Sodium (May cause an increase in olanzapine clearance; therefore, a dosage increase might be considered). Products include:

Phenytek Capsules 2153

Pindolol (Olanzapine, because of its potential for inducing hypotension, may enhance the effects of certain antihypertensive agents).

No products indexed under this heading.

Polythiazide (Olanzapine, because of its potential for inducing hypotension, may enhance the effects of certain antihypertensive agents).

No products indexed under this heading.

Pramipexole Dihydrochloride (Olanzapine may antagonize the effects of dopamine agonists). Products include:

Mirapex Tablets 889

Prazepam (Given the primary CNS effects of olanzapine, caution should be used when olanzapine is taken in combination with other centrally-acting drugs).

No products indexed under this heading.

Prazosin Hydrochloride (Olanzapine, because of its potential for inducing hypotension, may enhance the effects of certain antihypertensive agents).

No products indexed under this heading.

Primidone (May cause an increase in olanzapine clearance; therefore, a dosage increase might be considered).

No products indexed under this heading.

Prochlorperazine (Given the primary CNS effects of olanzapine, caution should be used when olanzapine is taken in combination with other centrally-acting drugs).

No products indexed under this heading.

Promethazine Hydrochloride (Given the primary CNS effects of olanzapine, caution should be used when olanzapine is taken in combination with other centrally-acting drugs). Products include:

Phenergan 3438

Propofol (Given the primary CNS effects of olanzapine, caution should be used when olanzapine is taken in combination with other centrally-acting drugs). Products include:

Diprivan Injectable Emulsion 676

Propoxyphene Hydrochloride (Given the primary CNS effects of olanzapine, caution should be used when olanzapine is taken in combination with other centrally-acting drugs).

No products indexed under this heading.

Propoxyphene Napsylate (Given the primary CNS effects of olanzapine, caution should be used when olanzapine is taken in combination with other centrally-acting drugs). Products include:

Darvocet A 500 Tablets 3497

Propranolol Hydrochloride (Olanzapine, because of its potential for inducing hypotension, may enhance the effects of certain antihypertensive agents). Products include:

Inderal LA Long-Acting Capsules 3421
InnoPran XL Capsules 2728

Quazepam (Given the primary CNS effects of olanzapine, caution should be used when olanzapine is taken in combination with other centrally-acting drugs).

No products indexed under this heading.

Quetiapine Fumarate (Given the primary CNS effects of olanzapine, caution should be used when olanzapine is taken in combination with other centrally-acting drugs). Products include:

Seroquel Tablets 691

Quinapril Hydrochloride (Olanzapine, because of its potential for inducing hypotension, may enhance the effects of certain antihypertensive agents).

No products indexed under this heading.

Ramipril (Olanzapine, because of its potential for inducing hypotension, may enhance the effects of certain antihypertensive agents). Products include:

Altace Capsules 1673

Ranitidine Hydrochloride (Can potentially inhibit olanzapine clearance; therefore, a dosage decrease might be considered). Products include:

Zantac 1597
Zantac Injection 1593
Zantac 75 Tablets .... ▣715
Zantac 150 Maximum Strength Tablets .... ▣715
Zantac Injection Pharmacy Bulk Package 1595

Rauwolfia Serpentina (Olanzapine, because of its potential for inducing hypotension, may enhance the effects of certain antihypertensive agents).

No products indexed under this heading.

Remifentanil Hydrochloride (Given the primary CNS effects of olanzapine, caution should be used when olanzapine is taken in combination with other centrally-acting drugs).

No products indexed under this heading.

Rescinnamine (Olanzapine, because of its potential for inducing hypotension, may enhance the effects of certain antihypertensive agents).

No products indexed under this heading.

Reserpine (Olanzapine, because of its potential for inducing hypotension, may enhance the effects of certain antihypertensive agents).

No products indexed under this heading.

Rifampicin (May cause an increase in olanzapine clearance; therefore, a dosage increase might be considered).

No products indexed under this heading.

Rifampin (May cause an increase in olanzapine clearance by inducing CYP1A2 or glucuronyl tranferase clearance).

No products indexed under this heading.

Risperidone (Given the primary CNS effects of olanzapine, caution should be used when olanzapine is taken in combination with other centrally-acting drugs). Products include:

Risperdal Consta Long-Acting Injection 1664
Risperdal M-Tab Orally Disintegrating Tablets 1658
Risperdal 1658

Ritonavir (May cause an increase in olanzapine clearance; therefore, a dosage increase might be considered). Products include:

Kaletra 474
Norvir 499

Ropinirole Hydrochloride (Olanzapine may antagonize the effects of dopamine agonists). Products include:

Requip Tablets 1528

Secobarbital Sodium (Given the primary CNS effects of olanzapine, caution should be used when olanzapine is taken in combination with other centrally-acting drugs).

No products indexed under this heading.

Sevoflurane (Given the primary CNS effects of olanzapine, caution should be used when olanzapine is taken in combination with other centrally-acting drugs). Products include:

Ultane Liquid for Inhalation 526

Sodium Nitroprusside (Olanzapine, because of its potential for inducing hypotension, may enhance the effects of certain antihypertensive agents).

No products indexed under this heading.

Sodium Oxybate (Given the primary CNS effects of olanzapine, caution should be used when olanzapine is taken in combination with other centrally-acting drugs).

No products indexed under this heading.

Sotalol Hydrochloride (Olanzapine, because of its potential for inducing hypotension, may enhance the effects of certain antihypertensive agents).

No products indexed under this heading.

Sparfloxacin (Can potentially inhibit olanzapine clearance; therefore, a dosage decrease might be considered).

No products indexed under this heading.

Spirapril Hydrochloride (Olanzapine, because of its potential for inducing hypotension, may enhance the effects of certain antihypertensive agents).

No products indexed under this heading.

Sufentanil Citrate (Given the primary CNS effects of olanzapine, caution should be used when olanzapine is taken in combination with other centrally-acting drugs).
No products indexed under this heading.

Tacrine Hydrochloride (Can potentially inhibit olanzapine clearance; therefore, a dosage decrease might be considered).
No products indexed under this heading.

Telmisartan (Olanzapine, because of its potential for inducing hypotension, may enhance the effects of certain antihypertensive agents). Products include:
Micardis Tablets 884
Micardis HCT Tablets 886

Temazepam (Given the primary CNS effects of olanzapine, caution should be used when olanzapine is taken in combination with other centrally-acting drugs).
No products indexed under this heading.

Terazosin Hydrochloride (Olanzapine, because of its potential for inducing hypotension, may enhance the effects of certain antihypertensive agents). Products include:
Hytrin Capsules 469

Thiamylal Sodium (Given the primary CNS effects of olanzapine, caution should be used when olanzapine is taken in combination with other centrally-acting drugs).
No products indexed under this heading.

Thioridazine Hydrochloride (Given the primary CNS effects of olanzapine, caution should be used when olanzapine is taken in combination with other centrally-acting drugs). Products include:
Thioridazine Hydrochloride Tablets 2122

Thiothixene (Given the primary CNS effects of olanzapine, caution should be used when olanzapine is taken in combination with other centrally-acting drugs). Products include:
Thiothixene Capsules 2124

Ticlopidine Hydrochloride (Can potentially inhibit olanzapine clearance; therefore, a dosage decrease might be considered). Products include:
Ticlid Tablets 2813

Timolol Maleate (Olanzapine, because of its potential for inducing hypotension, may enhance the effects of certain antihypertensive agents). Products include:
Blocadren Tablets 1891
Cosopt Sterile Ophthalmic Solution 1910
Timolide Tablets 2056
Timoptic in Ocudose 2061
Timoptic Sterile Ophthalmic Solution 2058
Timoptic-XE Sterile Ophthalmic Gel Forming Solution 2062

Tobacco (May cause an increase in olanzapine clearance; therefore, a dosage increase might be considered).
No products indexed under this heading.

Torsemide (Olanzapine, because of its potential for inducing hypotension, may enhance the effects of certain antihypertensive agents).
No products indexed under this heading.

Trandolapril (Olanzapine, because of its potential for inducing hypotension, may enhance the effects of certain antihypertensive agents). Products include:
Mavik Tablets 482
Tarka Tablets 519

Triazolam (Given the primary CNS effects of olanzapine, caution should be used when olanzapine is taken in combination with other centrally-acting drugs).
No products indexed under this heading.

Trifluoperazine Hydrochloride (Given the primary CNS effects of olanzapine, caution should be used when olanzapine is taken in combination with other centrally-acting drugs).
No products indexed under this heading.

Trimethaphan Camsylate (Olanzapine, because of its potential for inducing hypotension, may enhance the effects of certain antihypertensive agents).
No products indexed under this heading.

Troleandomycin (Can potentially inhibit olanzapine clearance; therefore, a dosage decrease might be considered).
No products indexed under this heading.

Trovafloxacin Mesylate (Can potentially inhibit olanzapine clearance; therefore, a dosage decrease might be considered).
No products indexed under this heading.

Valsartan (Olanzapine, because of its potential for inducing hypotension, may enhance the effects of certain antihypertensive agents). Products include:
Diovan HCT Tablets 2195
Diovan Tablets 2191

Verapamil Hydrochloride (Olanzapine, because of its potential for inducing hypotension, may enhance the effects of certain antihypertensive agents). Products include:
Covera-HS Tablets 3135
Tarka Tablets 519
Verelan PM Capsules 3120

Zaleplon (Given the primary CNS effects of olanzapine, caution should be used when olanzapine is taken in combination with other centrally-acting drugs). Products include:
Sonata Capsules 1686

Zileuton (Can potentially inhibit olanzapine clearance; therefore, a dosage decrease might be considered).
No products indexed under this heading.

Ziprasidone Hydrochloride (Given the primary CNS effects of olanzapine, caution should be used when olanzapine is taken in combination with other centrally-acting drugs). Products include:
Geodon Capsules 2514

Zolpidem Tartrate (Given the primary CNS effects of olanzapine, caution should be used when olanzapine is taken in combination with other centrally-acting drugs). Products include:
Ambien Tablets 2867

Food Interactions

Alcohol (Co-administration of alcohol with olanzapine potentiates orthostatic hypotension; concurrent use should be avoided).

Broccoli (May cause an increase in olanzapine clearance; therefore, a dosage increase might be considered).

Brussel Sprouts (May cause an increase in olanzapine clearance; therefore, a dosage increase might be considered).

Charbroiled Food (May cause an increase in olanzapine clearance; therefore, a dosage increase might be considered).

Grapefruit Juice (Can potentially inhibit olanzapine clearance; therefore, a dosage decrease might be considered).

ZYPREXA INTRAMUSCULAR

(Olanzapine) 1798
May interact with antihypertensives, benzodiazepines, central nervous system depressants, cytochrome p450 1a2 inducers (selected), cytochrome p450 1a2 inhibitors (selected), dopamine agonists, drugs that elevate levels of glucuronosyl transferase, and certain other agents. Compounds in these categories include:

Acebutolol Hydrochloride (Olanzapine, because of its potential for inducing hypotension, may enhance the effects of certain antihypertensive agents).
No products indexed under this heading.

Alatrofloxacin Mesylate (Can potentially inhibit olanzapine clearance; therefore, a dosage decrease might be considered).
No products indexed under this heading.

Alfentanil Hydrochloride (Given the primary CNS effects of olanzapine, caution should be used when olanzapine is taken in combination with other centrally-acting drugs).
No products indexed under this heading.

Alprazolam (Given the primary CNS effects of olanzapine, caution should be used when olanzapine is taken in combination with other centrally-acting drugs). Products include:
Niravam Orally Disintegrating Tablets 3106
Xanax XR Tablets 2655

Amiodarone Hydrochloride (Can potentially inhibit olanzapine clearance; therefore, a dosage decrease might be considered). Products include:
Pacerone Tablets 3337

Amlodipine Besylate (Olanzapine, because of its potential for inducing hypotension, may enhance the effects of certain antihypertensive agents). Products include:
Caduet Tablets 2507
Lotrel Capsules 2238
Norvasc Tablets 2529

Anastrozole (Can potentially inhibit olanzapine clearance; therefore, a dosage decrease might be considered). Products include:
Arimidex Tablets 665

Aprobarbital (Given the primary CNS effects of olanzapine, caution should be used when olanzapine is taken in combination with other centrally-acting drugs).
No products indexed under this heading.

Atenolol (Olanzapine, because of its potential for inducing hypotension, may enhance the effects of certain antihypertensive agents). Products include:
Tenormin I.V. Injection 698
Tenormin Tablets 695

Benazepril Hydrochloride (Olanzapine, because of its potential for inducing hypotension, may enhance the effects of certain antihypertensive agents). Products include:
Lotensin Tablets 2232
Lotensin HCT Tablets 2235
Lotrel Capsules 2238

Bendroflumethiazide (Olanzapine, because of its potential for inducing hypotension, may enhance the effects of certain antihypertensive agents).
No products indexed under this heading.

Betaxolol Hydrochloride (Olanzapine, because of its potential for inducing hypotension, may enhance the effects of certain antihypertensive agents). Products include:
Betoptic S Ophthalmic Suspension 554

Bisoprolol Fumarate (Olanzapine, because of its potential for inducing hypotension, may enhance the effects of certain antihypertensive agents).
No products indexed under this heading.

Bromocriptine Mesylate (Olanzapine may antagonize the effects of dopamine agonists).
No products indexed under this heading.

Buprenorphine Hydrochloride (Given the primary CNS effects of olanzapine, caution should be used when olanzapine is taken in combination with other centrally-acting drugs). Products include:
Buprenex Injectable 2718
Suboxone Tablets 2719
Subutex Tablets 2719

Buspirone Hydrochloride (Given the primary CNS effects of olanzapine, caution should be used when olanzapine is taken in combination with other centrally-acting drugs).
No products indexed under this heading.

Butabarbital (Given the primary CNS effects of olanzapine, caution should be used when olanzapine is taken in combination with other centrally-acting drugs).
No products indexed under this heading.

Butalbital (Given the primary CNS effects of olanzapine, caution should be used when olanzapine is taken in combination with other centrally-acting drugs). Products include:
Sedapap Tablets 50 mg/650 mg 2098

Candesartan Cilexetil (Olanzapine, because of its potential for inducing hypotension, may enhance the effects of certain antihypertensive agents). Products include:
Atacand Tablets 634
Atacand HCT 637

Captopril (Olanzapine, because of its potential for inducing hypotension, may enhance the effects of certain antihypertensive agents). Products include:
Captopril Tablets 2114

Carbamazepine (Causes an approximately 50% increase in the clearance of olanzapine at 400 mg daily; higher daily doses of carbamazepine may cause an even greater increase in olanzapine clearance). Products include:
Carbatrol Capsules 3174

Equetro Extended-Release Capsules 3178
Tegretol/Tegretol-XR 2278

Carteolol Hydrochloride (Olanzapine, because of its potential for inducing hypotension, may enhance the effects of certain antihypertensive agents). Products include:
Carteolol Hydrochloride Ophthalmic Solution USP, 1% .... ⊙ 246

Chlordiazepoxide (Given the primary CNS effects of olanzapine, caution should be used when olanzapine is taken in combination with other centrally-acting drugs).
No products indexed under this heading.

Chlordiazepoxide Hydrochloride (Given the primary CNS effects of olanzapine, caution should be used when olanzapine is taken in combination with other centrally-acting drugs). Products include:
Librium Capsules 3349

Chlorothiazide (Olanzapine, because of its potential for inducing hypotension, may enhance the effects of certain antihypertensive agents). Products include:
Aldoclor Tablets 1881
Diuril Oral 1936

Chlorothiazide Sodium (Olanzapine, because of its potential for inducing hypotension, may enhance the effects of certain antihypertensive agents). Products include:
Diuril Sodium Intravenous 1934

Chlorpromazine (Given the primary CNS effects of olanzapine, caution should be used when olanzapine is taken in combination with other centrally-acting drugs).
No products indexed under this heading.

Chlorpromazine Hydrochloride (Given the primary CNS effects of olanzapine, caution should be used when olanzapine is taken in combination with other centrally-acting drugs).
No products indexed under this heading.

Chlorprothixene (Given the primary CNS effects of olanzapine, caution should be used when olanzapine is taken in combination with other centrally-acting drugs).
No products indexed under this heading.

Chlorprothixene Hydrochloride (Given the primary CNS effects of olanzapine, caution should be used when olanzapine is taken in combination with other centrally-acting drugs).
No products indexed under this heading.

Chlorprothixene Lactate (Given the primary CNS effects of olanzapine, caution should be used when olanzapine is taken in combination with other centrally-acting drugs).
No products indexed under this heading.

Chlorthalidone (Olanzapine, because of its potential for inducing hypotension, may enhance the effects of certain antihypertensive agents). Products include:
Clorpres Tablets 2139

Cimetidine (Can potentially inhibit olanzapine clearance; therefore, a dosage decrease might be considered). Products include:
Tagamet HB 200 Tablets .... ▣ 637
Tagamet Tablets 1547

Cimetidine Hydrochloride (Can potentially inhibit olanzapine clearance; therefore, a dosage decrease might be considered).
No products indexed under this heading.

Ciprofloxacin (Can potentially inhibit olanzapine clearance; therefore, a dosage decrease might be considered). Products include:
Cipro I.V. 2998
Cipro I.V. Pharmacy Bulk Package ... 3509
Cipro Oral Suspension 2991
Cipro XR Tablets 3004
Ciprodex Otic Suspension 555

Ciprofloxacin Hydrochloride (Can potentially inhibit olanzapine clearance; therefore, a dosage decrease might be considered). Products include:
Ciloxan Ophthalmic Ointment 554
Cipro Tablets 2991

Citalopram Hydrobromide (May cause an increase in olanzapine clearance; therefore, a dosage increase might be considered). Products include:
Celexa 1177

Clarithromycin (Can potentially inhibit olanzapine clearance; therefore, a dosage decrease might be considered). Products include:
Biaxin/Biaxin XL 402
PREVPAC 3281

Clonidine (Olanzapine, because of its potential for inducing hypotension, may enhance the effects of certain antihypertensive agents). Products include:
Catapres-TTS 875

Clonidine Hydrochloride (Olanzapine, because of its potential for inducing hypotension, may enhance the effects of certain antihypertensive agents). Products include:
Catapres Tablets 874
Clorpres Tablets 2139

Clorazepate Dipotassium (Given the primary CNS effects of olanzapine, caution should be used when olanzapine is taken in combination with other centrally-acting drugs). Products include:
Tranxene 2488

Clozapine (Given the primary CNS effects of olanzapine, caution should be used when olanzapine is taken in combination with other centrally-acting drugs). Products include:
Clozapine Tablets 2141
Clozaril Tablets 2174
FazaClo Orally Disintegrating Tablets 547

Codeine Phosphate (Given the primary CNS effects of olanzapine, caution should be used when olanzapine is taken in combination with other centrally-acting drugs). Products include:
Tylenol with Codeine 2461

Deserpidine (Olanzapine, because of its potential for inducing hypotension, may enhance the effects of certain antihypertensive agents).
No products indexed under this heading.

Desflurane (Given the primary CNS effects of olanzapine, caution should be used when olanzapine is taken in combination with other centrally-acting drugs). Products include:
Suprane Liquid for Inhalation 770

Desogestrel (Can potentially inhibit olanzapine clearance; therefore, a dosage decrease might be considered). Products include:
Ortho-Cept Tablets 2395

Dezocine (Given the primary CNS effects of olanzapine, caution should be used when olanzapine is taken in combination with other centrally-acting drugs).
No products indexed under this heading.

Diazepam (Co-administration of diazepam with olanzapine may potentiate orthostatic hypotension. Concomitant administration of intramuscular olanzapine and parenteral benzodiazepine has not been studied and is therefore not recommended. If use of intramuscular olanzapine in combination with parenteral benzodiazepines is considered, careful evaluation of clinical status for excessive sedation and cardiorespiratory depression is recommended). Products include:
Diastat Rectal Delivery System 3344
Valium Tablets 2822

Diazoxide (Olanzapine, because of its potential for inducing hypotension, may enhance the effects of certain antihypertensive agents). Products include:
Hyperstat I.V. Injection 3031

Diltiazem Hydrochloride (Olanzapine, because of its potential for inducing hypotension, may enhance the effects of certain antihypertensive agents). Products include:
Cardizem LA Extended Release Tablets 1699
Tiazac Capsules 1204

Diltiazem Maleate (May cause an increase in olanzapine clearance; therefore, a dosage increase might be considered).
No products indexed under this heading.

Dopamine Hydrochloride (Olanzapine may antagonize the effects of dopamine agonists).
No products indexed under this heading.

Doxazosin Mesylate (Olanzapine, because of its potential for inducing hypotension, may enhance the effects of certain antihypertensive agents).
No products indexed under this heading.

Droperidol (Given the primary CNS effects of olanzapine, caution should be used when olanzapine is taken in combination with other centrally-acting drugs).
No products indexed under this heading.

Enalapril Maleate (Olanzapine, because of its potential for inducing hypotension, may enhance the effects of certain antihypertensive agents). Products include:
Vaseretic Tablets 2073
Vasotec I.V. Injection 2076

Enalaprilat (Olanzapine, because of its potential for inducing hypotension, may enhance the effects of certain antihypertensive agents).
No products indexed under this heading.

Enflurane (Given the primary CNS effects of olanzapine, caution should be used when olanzapine is taken in combination with other centrally-acting drugs).
No products indexed under this heading.

Enoxacin (Can potentially inhibit olanzapine clearance; therefore, a dosage decrease might be considered).
No products indexed under this heading.

Eprosartan Mesylate (Olanzapine, because of its potential for inducing hypotension, may enhance the effects of certain antihypertensive agents). Products include:
Teveten Tablets 1707
Teveten HCT Tablets 1710

Erythromycin (May cause an increase in olanzapine clearance; therefore, a dosage increase might be considered). Products include:
Erygel Topical Gel 2096
Ery-Tab Tablets 447
Erythromycin Base Filmtab Tablets 454
Erythromycin Delayed-Release Capsules, USP 456
PCE Dispertab Tablets 510

Erythromycin Estolate (May cause an increase in olanzapine clearance; therefore, a dosage increase might be considered).
No products indexed under this heading.

Erythromycin Ethylsuccinate (May cause an increase in olanzapine clearance; therefore, a dosage increase might be considered). Products include:
E.E.S. 449
EryPed 445

Erythromycin Gluceptate (May cause an increase in olanzapine clearance; therefore, a dosage increase might be considered).
No products indexed under this heading.

Erythromycin Lactobionate (May cause an increase in olanzapine clearance; therefore, a dosage increase might be considered).
No products indexed under this heading.

Erythromycin Stearate (May cause an increase in olanzapine clearance; therefore, a dosage increase might be considered). Products include:
Erythrocin Stearate Filmtab Tablets 452

Esmolol Hydrochloride (Olanzapine, because of its potential for inducing hypotension, may enhance the effects of certain antihypertensive agents). Products include:
Brevibloc Concentrate 766
Brevibloc Injection 766
Brevibloc Double Strength Injection 766
Brevibloc Premixed Injection 766
Brevibloc Double Strength Premixed Injection 766

Estazolam (Given the primary CNS effects of olanzapine, caution should be used when olanzapine is taken in combination with other centrally-acting drugs). Products include:
ProSom Tablets 512

Ethanol (Given the primary CNS effects of olanzapine, caution should be used when olanzapine is taken in combination with other centrally-acting drugs).
No products indexed under this heading.

Ethchlorvynol (Given the primary CNS effects of olanzapine, caution should be used when olanzapine is taken in combination with other centrally-acting drugs).
No products indexed under this heading.

Levodopa (Olanzapine may antagonize the effects of levodopa). Products include:
Parcopa Orally Disintegrating Tablets ... 3111
Stalevo Tablets ... 2270

Levofloxacin (Can potentially inhibit olanzapine clearance; therefore, a dosage decrease might be considered). Products include:
Levaquin in 5% Dextrose Injection ... 2453
Levaquin ... 2453
Quixin Ophthalmic Solution ... 3373

Levomethadyl Acetate Hydrochloride (Given the primary CNS effects of olanzapine, caution should be used when olanzapine is taken in combination with other centrally-acting drugs).
No products indexed under this heading.

Levonorgestrel (Can potentially inhibit olanzapine clearance; therefore, a dosage decrease might be considered). Products include:
Alesse-28 Tablets ... 3392
Climara Pro Transdermal System ... 800
Mirena Intrauterine System ... 810
Plan B Tablets ... 1068
Seasonale Tablets ... 1073
Triphasil-28 Tablets ... 3483

Levorphanol Tartrate (Given the primary CNS effects of olanzapine, caution should be used when olanzapine is taken in combination with other centrally-acting drugs).
No products indexed under this heading.

Lisinopril (Olanzapine, because of its potential for inducing hypotension, may enhance the effects of certain antihypertensive agents). Products include:
Prinivil Tablets ... 2029
Prinzide Tablets ... 2033
Zestoretic Tablets ... 701
Zestril Tablets ... 704

Lomefloxacin Hydrochloride (Can potentially inhibit olanzapine clearance; therefore, a dosage decrease might be considered).
No products indexed under this heading.

Lorazepam (Co-administration added to the somnolence observed with either intramuscular drug alone).
No products indexed under this heading.

Losartan Potassium (Olanzapine, because of its potential for inducing hypotension, may enhance the effects of certain antihypertensive agents). Products include:
Cozaar Tablets ... 1913
Hyzaar ... 1964

Loxapine Hydrochloride (Given the primary CNS effects of olanzapine, caution should be used when olanzapine is taken in combination with other centrally-acting drugs).
No products indexed under this heading.

Loxapine Succinate (Given the primary CNS effects of olanzapine, caution should be used when olanzapine is taken in combination with other centrally-acting drugs).
No products indexed under this heading.

Mecamylamine Hydrochloride (Olanzapine, because of its potential for inducing hypotension, may enhance the effects of certain antihypertensive agents). Products include:
Inversine Tablets ... 3286

Meperidine Hydrochloride (Given the primary CNS effects of olanzapine, caution should be used when olanzapine is taken in combination with other centrally-acting drugs).
No products indexed under this heading.

Mephobarbital (Given the primary CNS effects of olanzapine, caution should be used when olanzapine is taken in combination with other centrally-acting drugs). Products include:
Mebaral Tablets, USP ... 2483

Meprobamate (Given the primary CNS effects of olanzapine, caution should be used when olanzapine is taken in combination with other centrally-acting drugs).
No products indexed under this heading.

Mesoridazine Besylate (Given the primary CNS effects of olanzapine, caution should be used when olanzapine is taken in combination with other centrally-acting drugs).
No products indexed under this heading.

Mestranol (Can potentially inhibit olanzapine clearance; therefore, a dosage decrease might be considered).
No products indexed under this heading.

Methadone Hydrochloride (Given the primary CNS effects of olanzapine, caution should be used when olanzapine is taken in combination with other centrally-acting drugs).
No products indexed under this heading.

Methohexital Sodium (Given the primary CNS effects of olanzapine, caution should be used when olanzapine is taken in combination with other centrally-acting drugs).
No products indexed under this heading.

Methotrimeprazine (Given the primary CNS effects of olanzapine, caution should be used when olanzapine is taken in combination with other centrally-acting drugs).
No products indexed under this heading.

Methoxsalen (Can potentially inhibit olanzapine clearance; therefore, a dosage decrease might be considered). Products include:
Oxsoralen Lotion 1% ... 3354
Oxsoralen-Ultra Capsules ... 3354

Methoxyflurane (Given the primary CNS effects of olanzapine, caution should be used when olanzapine is taken in combination with other centrally-acting drugs).
No products indexed under this heading.

Methyclothiazide (Olanzapine, because of its potential for inducing hypotension, may enhance the effects of certain antihypertensive agents).
No products indexed under this heading.

Methyldopa (Olanzapine, because of its potential for inducing hypotension, may enhance the effects of certain antihypertensive agents). Products include:
Aldoclor Tablets ... 1881
Aldoril Tablets ... 1884

Methyldopate Hydrochloride (Olanzapine, because of its potential for inducing hypotension, may enhance the effects of certain antihypertensive agents).
No products indexed under this heading.

Metolazone (Olanzapine, because of its potential for inducing hypotension, may enhance the effects of certain antihypertensive agents).
No products indexed under this heading.

Metoprolol Succinate (Olanzapine, because of its potential for inducing hypotension, may enhance the effects of certain antihypertensive agents). Products include:
Toprol-XL Tablets ... 660

Metoprolol Tartrate (Olanzapine, because of its potential for inducing hypotension, may enhance the effects of certain antihypertensive agents).
No products indexed under this heading.

Metyrosine (Olanzapine, because of its potential for inducing hypotension, may enhance the effects of certain antihypertensive agents). Products include:
Demser Capsules ... 1933

Mexiletine Hydrochloride (Can potentially inhibit olanzapine clearance; therefore, a dosage decrease might be considered).
No products indexed under this heading.

Mibefradil Dihydrochloride (Olanzapine, because of its potential for inducing hypotension, may enhance the effects of certain antihypertensive agents).
No products indexed under this heading.

Midazolam Hydrochloride (Given the primary CNS effects of olanzapine, caution should be used when olanzapine is taken in combination with other centrally-acting drugs).
No products indexed under this heading.

Minoxidil (Olanzapine, because of its potential for inducing hypotension, may enhance the effects of certain antihypertensive agents). Products include:
Men's Rogaine Extra Strength Topical Solution, Ocean Rush Scent and Original Unscented ... ▣ 706
Women's Rogaine Topical Solution, Spring Bloom Scent and Original Unscented ... ▣ 707

Moexipril Hydrochloride (Olanzapine, because of its potential for inducing hypotension, may enhance the effects of certain antihypertensive agents). Products include:
Uniretic Tablets ... 3114
Univasc Tablets ... 3118

Molindone Hydrochloride (Given the primary CNS effects of olanzapine, caution should be used when olanzapine is taken in combination with other centrally-acting drugs). Products include:
Moban Tablets ... 1108

Morphine Sulfate (Given the primary CNS effects of olanzapine, caution should be used when olanzapine is taken in combination with other centrally-acting drugs). Products include:
Avinza Capsules ... 1714
Kadian Capsules ... 572
MS Contin Tablets ... 2703

Moxifloxacin Hydrochloride (Can potentially inhibit olanzapine clearance; therefore, a dosage decrease might be considered). Products include:
Avelox ... 2984
Vigamox Ophthalmic Solution ... ⊙ 560

Nadolol (Olanzapine, because of its potential for inducing hypotension, may enhance the effects of certain antihypertensive agents). Products include:
Nadolol Tablets ... 2121

Nafcillin Sodium (May cause an increase in olanzapine clearance; therefore, a dosage increase might be considered).
No products indexed under this heading.

Nalidixic Acid (Can potentially inhibit olanzapine clearance; therefore, a dosage decrease might be considered).
No products indexed under this heading.

Nicardipine Hydrochloride (Olanzapine, because of its potential for inducing hypotension, may enhance the effects of certain antihypertensive agents). Products include:
Cardene I.V. ... 1129

Nicotine (May cause an increase in olanzapine clearance; therefore, a dosage increase might be considered). Products include:
Nicoderm CQ Patch ... 1629
NicoDerm CQ Clear Patch ... ▣ 627
Nicotrol Inhaler ... 2594
Nicotrol NS ... 2596

Nicotine Polacrilex (May cause an increase in olanzapine clearance; therefore, a dosage increase might be considered). Products include:
Commit Lozenges ... 1625
Nicorette Gum ... 1632

Nicotine Salicylate (May cause an increase in olanzapine clearance; therefore, a dosage increase might be considered).
No products indexed under this heading.

Nicotine Sulfate (May cause an increase in olanzapine clearance; therefore, a dosage increase might be considered).
No products indexed under this heading.

Nifedipine (Olanzapine, because of its potential for inducing hypotension, may enhance the effects of certain antihypertensive agents). Products include:
Adalat CC Tablets ... 2978

Nisoldipine (Olanzapine, because of its potential for inducing hypotension, may enhance the effects of certain antihypertensive agents). Products include:
Sular Tablets ... 1163

Nitroglycerin (Olanzapine, because of its potential for inducing hypotension, may enhance the effects of certain antihypertensive agents). Products include:
Nitro-Dur Transdermal Infusion System ... 3060
Nitrolingual Pumpspray ... 1161

Norethindrone (Can potentially inhibit olanzapine clearance; therefore, a dosage decrease might be considered). Products include:
Ortho Micronor Tablets ... 2411

Norfloxacin (Can potentially inhibit olanzapine clearance; therefore, a dosage decrease might be considered). Products include:

Noroxin Tablets 2009

Norgestrel (Can potentially inhibit olanzapine clearance; therefore, a dosage decrease might be considered). Products include:
Lo/Ovral-28 Tablets 3423

Ofloxacin (Can potentially inhibit olanzapine clearance; therefore, a dosage decrease might be considered). Products include:
Floxin Otic Singles 1045
Floxin Otic Solution 1043

Omeprazole (May cause an increase in olanzapine clearance by inducing CYP1A2 or glucuronyl transferase clearance). Products include:
Zegerid Powder for Oral Solution 2972

Oxazepam (Given the primary CNS effects of olanzapine, caution should be used when olanzapine is taken in combination with other centrally-acting drugs).
No products indexed under this heading.

Oxycodone Hydrochloride (Given the primary CNS effects of olanzapine, caution should be used when olanzapine is taken in combination with other centrally-acting drugs). Products include:
Combunox Tablets 1183
OxyContin Tablets 2699
OxyFast Oral Concentrate Solution 2704
OxyIR Capsules 2704
Percocet Tablets 1114
Percodan Tablets 1115

Paroxetine Hydrochloride (Can potentially inhibit olanzapine clearance; therefore, a dosage decrease might be considered). Products include:
Paxil CR Controlled-Release Tablets 1509
Paxil 1501

Penbutolol Sulfate (Olanzapine, because of its potential for inducing hypotension, may enhance the effects of certain antihypertensive agents).
No products indexed under this heading.

Pentobarbital Sodium (Given the primary CNS effects of olanzapine, caution should be used when olanzapine is taken in combination with other centrally-acting drugs). Products include:
Nembutal Sodium Solution, USP 2484

Pergolide Mesylate (Olanzapine may antagonize the effects of dopamine agonists). Products include:
Permax Tablets 3357

Perindopril Erbumine (Olanzapine, because of its potential for inducing hypotension, may enhance the effects of certain antihypertensive agents). Products include:
Aceon Tablets (2 mg, 4 mg, 8 mg) 3191

Perphenazine (Given the primary CNS effects of olanzapine, caution should be used when olanzapine is taken in combination with other centrally-acting drugs).
No products indexed under this heading.

Phenobarbital (Given the primary CNS effects of olanzapine, caution should be used when olanzapine is taken in combination with other centrally-acting drugs).
No products indexed under this heading.

Phenoxybenzamine Hydrochloride (Olanzapine, because of its potential for inducing hypotension, may enhance the effects of certain antihypertensive agents). Products include:
Dibenzyline Capsules 3390

Phentolamine Mesylate (Olanzapine, because of its potential for inducing hypotension, may enhance the effects of certain antihypertensive agents).
No products indexed under this heading.

Phenytoin (May cause an increase in olanzapine clearance; therefore, a dosage increase might be considered).
No products indexed under this heading.

Phenytoin Sodium (May cause an increase in olanzapine clearance; therefore, a dosage increase might be considered). Products include:
Phenytek Capsules 2153

Pindolol (Olanzapine, because of its potential for inducing hypotension, may enhance the effects of certain antihypertensive agents).
No products indexed under this heading.

Polythiazide (Olanzapine, because of its potential for inducing hypotension, may enhance the effects of certain antihypertensive agents).
No products indexed under this heading.

Pramipexole Dihydrochloride (Olanzapine may antagonize the effects of dopamine agonists). Products include:
Mirapex Tablets 889

Prazepam (Given the primary CNS effects of olanzapine, caution should be used when olanzapine is taken in combination with other centrally-acting drugs).
No products indexed under this heading.

Prazosin Hydrochloride (Olanzapine, because of its potential for inducing hypotension, may enhance the effects of certain antihypertensive agents).
No products indexed under this heading.

Primidone (May cause an increase in olanzapine clearance; therefore, a dosage increase might be considered).
No products indexed under this heading.

Prochlorperazine (Given the primary CNS effects of olanzapine, caution should be used when olanzapine is taken in combination with other centrally-acting drugs).
No products indexed under this heading.

Promethazine Hydrochloride (Given the primary CNS effects of olanzapine, caution should be used when olanzapine is taken in combination with other centrally-acting drugs). Products include:
Phenergan 3438

Propofol (Given the primary CNS effects of olanzapine, caution should be used when olanzapine is taken in combination with other centrally-acting drugs). Products include:
Diprivan Injectable Emulsion 676

Propoxyphene Hydrochloride (Given the primary CNS effects of olanzapine, caution should be used when olanzapine is taken in combination with other centrally-acting drugs).
No products indexed under this heading.

Propoxyphene Napsylate (Given the primary CNS effects of olanzapine, caution should be used when olanzapine is taken in combination with other centrally-acting drugs). Products include:
Darvocet A 500 Tablets 3497

Propranolol Hydrochloride (Olanzapine, because of its potential for inducing hypotension, may enhance the effects of certain antihypertensive agents). Products include:
Inderal LA Long-Acting Capsules 3421
InnoPran XL Capsules 2728

Quazepam (Given the primary CNS effects of olanzapine, caution should be used when olanzapine is taken in combination with other centrally-acting drugs).
No products indexed under this heading.

Quetiapine Fumarate (Given the primary CNS effects of olanzapine, caution should be used when olanzapine is taken in combination with other centrally-acting drugs). Products include:
Seroquel Tablets 691

Quinapril Hydrochloride (Olanzapine, because of its potential for inducing hypotension, may enhance the effects of certain antihypertensive agents).
No products indexed under this heading.

Ramipril (Olanzapine, because of its potential for inducing hypotension, may enhance the effects of certain antihypertensive agents). Products include:
Altace Capsules 1673

Ranitidine Hydrochloride (Can potentially inhibit olanzapine clearance; therefore, a dosage decrease might be considered). Products include:
Zantac 1597
Zantac Injection 1593
Zantac 75 Tablets 715
Zantac 150 Maximum Strength Tablets 715
Zantac Injection Pharmacy Bulk Package 1595

Rauwolfia Serpentina (Olanzapine, because of its potential for inducing hypotension, may enhance the effects of certain antihypertensive agents).
No products indexed under this heading.

Remifentanil Hydrochloride (Given the primary CNS effects of olanzapine, caution should be used when olanzapine is taken in combination with other centrally-acting drugs).
No products indexed under this heading.

Rescinnamine (Olanzapine, because of its potential for inducing hypotension, may enhance the effects of certain antihypertensive agents).
No products indexed under this heading.

Reserpine (Olanzapine, because of its potential for inducing hypotension, may enhance the effects of certain antihypertensive agents).
No products indexed under this heading.

Rifampicin (May cause an increase in olanzapine clearance; therefore, a dosage increase might be considered).
No products indexed under this heading.

Rifampin (May cause an increase in olanzapine clearance by inducing CYP1A2 or glucuronyl tranferase clearance).
No products indexed under this heading.

Risperidone (Given the primary CNS effects of olanzapine, caution should be used when olanzapine is taken in combination with other centrally-acting drugs). Products include:
Risperdal Consta Long-Acting Injection 1664
Risperdal M-Tab Orally Disintegrating Tablets 1658
Risperdal 1658

Ritonavir (May cause an increase in olanzapine clearance; therefore, a dosage increase might be considered). Products include:
Kaletra 474
Norvir 499

Ropinirole Hydrochloride (Olanzapine may antagonize the effects of dopamine agonists). Products include:
Requip Tablets 1528

Secobarbital Sodium (Given the primary CNS effects of olanzapine, caution should be used when olanzapine is taken in combination with other centrally-acting drugs).
No products indexed under this heading.

Sevoflurane (Given the primary CNS effects of olanzapine, caution should be used when olanzapine is taken in combination with other centrally-acting drugs). Products include:
Ultane Liquid for Inhalation 526

Sodium Nitroprusside (Olanzapine, because of its potential for inducing hypotension, may enhance the effects of certain antihypertensive agents).
No products indexed under this heading.

Sodium Oxybate (Given the primary CNS effects of olanzapine, caution should be used when olanzapine is taken in combination with other centrally-acting drugs).
No products indexed under this heading.

Sotalol Hydrochloride (Olanzapine, because of its potential for inducing hypotension, may enhance the effects of certain antihypertensive agents).
No products indexed under this heading.

Sparfloxacin (Can potentially inhibit olanzapine clearance; therefore, a dosage decrease might be considered).
No products indexed under this heading.

Spirapril Hydrochloride (Olanzapine, because of its potential for inducing hypotension, may enhance the effects of certain antihypertensive agents).
No products indexed under this heading.

Sufentanil Citrate (Given the primary CNS effects of olanzapine, caution should be used when olanzapine is taken in combination with other centrally-acting drugs).
No products indexed under this heading.

Tacrine Hydrochloride (Can potentially inhibit olanzapine clearance; therefore, a dosage decrease might be considered).
No products indexed under this heading.

Telmisartan (Olanzapine, because of its potential for inducing hypotension, may enhance the effects of certain antihypertensive agents). Products include:
Micardis Tablets 884
Micardis HCT Tablets 886

Temazepam (Given the primary CNS effects of olanzapine, caution should be used when olanzapine is taken in combination with other centrally-acting drugs).
No products indexed under this heading.

Terazosin Hydrochloride (Olanzapine, because of its potential for inducing hypotension, may enhance the effects of certain antihypertensive agents). Products include:
Hytrin Capsules 469

Thiamylal Sodium (Given the primary CNS effects of olanzapine, caution should be used when olanzapine is taken in combination with other centrally-acting drugs).
No products indexed under this heading.

Thioridazine Hydrochloride (Given the primary CNS effects of olanzapine, caution should be used when olanzapine is taken in combination with other centrally-acting drugs). Products include:
Thioridazine Hydrochloride Tablets 2122

Thiothixene (Given the primary CNS effects of olanzapine, caution should be used when olanzapine is taken in combination with other centrally-acting drugs). Products include:
Thiothixene Capsules 2124

Ticlopidine Hydrochloride (Can potentially inhibit olanzapine clearance; therefore, a dosage decrease might be considered). Products include:
Ticlid Tablets 2813

Timolol Maleate (Olanzapine, because of its potential for inducing hypotension, may enhance the effects of certain antihypertensive agents). Products include:
Blocadren Tablets 1891
Cosopt Sterile Ophthalmic Solution 1910
Timolide Tablets 2056
Timoptic in Ocudose 2061
Timoptic Sterile Ophthalmic Solution 2058
Timoptic-XE Sterile Ophthalmic Gel Forming Solution 2062

Tobacco (May cause an increase in olanzapine clearance; therefore, a dosage increase might be considered).
No products indexed under this heading.

Torsemide (Olanzapine, because of its potential for inducing hypotension, may enhance the effects of certain antihypertensive agents).
No products indexed under this heading.

Trandolapril (Olanzapine, because of its potential for inducing hypotension, may enhance the effects of certain antihypertensive agents). Products include:
Mavik Tablets 482
Tarka Tablets 519

Triazolam (Given the primary CNS effects of olanzapine, caution should be used when olanzapine is taken in combination with other centrally-acting drugs).
No products indexed under this heading.

Trifluoperazine Hydrochloride (Given the primary CNS effects of olanzapine, caution should be used when olanzapine is taken in combination with other centrally-acting drugs).
No products indexed under this heading.

Trimethaphan Camsylate (Olanzapine, because of its potential for inducing hypotension, may enhance the effects of certain antihypertensive agents).
No products indexed under this heading.

Troleandomycin (Can potentially inhibit olanzapine clearance; therefore, a dosage decrease might be considered).
No products indexed under this heading.

Trovafloxacin Mesylate (Can potentially inhibit olanzapine clearance; therefore, a dosage decrease might be considered).
No products indexed under this heading.

Valsartan (Olanzapine, because of its potential for inducing hypotension, may enhance the effects of certain antihypertensive agents). Products include:
Diovan HCT Tablets 2195
Diovan Tablets 2191

Verapamil Hydrochloride (Olanzapine, because of its potential for inducing hypotension, may enhance the effects of certain antihypertensive agents). Products include:
Covera-HS Tablets 3135
Tarka Tablets 519
Verelan PM Capsules 3120

Zaleplon (Given the primary CNS effects of olanzapine, caution should be used when olanzapine is taken in combination with other centrally-acting drugs). Products include:
Sonata Capsules 1686

Zileuton (Can potentially inhibit olanzapine clearance; therefore, a dosage decrease might be considered).
No products indexed under this heading.

Ziprasidone Hydrochloride (Given the primary CNS effects of olanzapine, caution should be used when olanzapine is taken in combination with other centrally-acting drugs). Products include:
Geodon Capsules 2514

Zolpidem Tartrate (Given the primary CNS effects of olanzapine, caution should be used when olanzapine is taken in combination with other centrally-acting drugs). Products include:
Ambien Tablets 2867

Food Interactions

Alcohol (Co-administration of alcohol with olanzapine potentiates orthostatic hypotension; concurrent use should be avoided).

Broccoli (May cause an increase in olanzapine clearance; therefore, a dosage increase might be considered).

Brussel Sprouts (May cause an increase in olanzapine clearance; therefore, a dosage increase might be considered).

Charbroiled Food (May cause an increase in olanzapine clearance; therefore, a dosage increase might be considered).

Grapefruit Juice (Can potentially inhibit olanzapine clearance; therefore, a dosage decrease might be considered).

ZYPREXA ZYDIS ORALLY DISINTEGRATING TABLETS

(Olanzapine) 1798
See Zyprexa Tablets

ZYRTEC CHEWABLE TABLETS

(Cetirizine Hydrochloride) 2589
See Zyrtec Tablets

ZYRTEC SYRUP

(Cetirizine Hydrochloride) 2589
See Zyrtec Tablets

ZYRTEC TABLETS

(Cetirizine Hydrochloride) 2589
May interact with central nervous system depressants, xanthines, and certain other agents. Compounds in these categories include:

Alfentanil Hydrochloride (Concurrent use may result in additional impairment of CNS performance and reduction in mental alertness).
No products indexed under this heading.

Alprazolam (Concurrent use may result in additional impairment of CNS performance and reduction in mental alertness). Products include:
Niravam Orally Disintegrating Tablets 3106
Xanax XR Tablets 2655

Aminophylline (Small decrease in the clearance of cetirizine caused by a larger dose, e.g., 400 mg dose of theophylline).
No products indexed under this heading.

Aprobarbital (Concurrent use may result in additional impairment of CNS performance and reduction in mental alertness).
No products indexed under this heading.

Buprenorphine Hydrochloride (Concurrent use may result in additional impairment of CNS performance and reduction in mental alertness). Products include:
Buprenex Injectable 2718
Suboxone Tablets 2719
Subutex Tablets 2719

Buspirone Hydrochloride (Concurrent use may result in additional impairment of CNS performance and reduction in mental alertness).
No products indexed under this heading.

Butabarbital (Concurrent use may result in additional impairment of CNS performance and reduction in mental alertness).
No products indexed under this heading.

Butalbital (Concurrent use may result in additional impairment of CNS performance and reduction in mental alertness). Products include:
Sedapap Tablets 50 mg/650 mg 2098

Chlordiazepoxide (Concurrent use may result in additional impairment of CNS performance and reduction in mental alertness).
No products indexed under this heading.

Chlordiazepoxide Hydrochloride (Concurrent use may result in additional impairment of CNS performance and reduction in mental alertness). Products include:
Librium Capsules 3349

Chlorpromazine (Concurrent use may result in additional impairment of CNS performance and reduction in mental alertness).
No products indexed under this heading.

Chlorpromazine Hydrochloride (Concurrent use may result in additional impairment of CNS performance and reduction in mental alertness).
No products indexed under this heading.

Chlorprothixene (Concurrent use may result in additional impairment of CNS performance and reduction in mental alertness).
No products indexed under this heading.

Chlorprothixene Hydrochloride (Concurrent use may result in additional impairment of CNS performance and reduction in mental alertness).
No products indexed under this heading.

Chlorprothixene Lactate (Concurrent use may result in additional impairment of CNS performance and reduction in mental alertness).
No products indexed under this heading.

Clorazepate Dipotassium (Concurrent use may result in additional impairment of CNS performance and reduction in mental alertness). Products include:
Tranxene 2488

Clozapine (Concurrent use may result in additional impairment of CNS performance and reduction in mental alertness). Products include:
Clozapine Tablets 2141
Clozaril Tablets 2174
FazaClo Orally Disintegrating Tablets 547

Codeine Phosphate (Concurrent use may result in additional impairment of CNS performance and reduction in mental alertness). Products include:
Tylenol with Codeine 2461

Desflurane (Concurrent use may result in additional impairment of CNS performance and reduction in mental alertness). Products include:
Suprane Liquid for Inhalation 770

Dezocine (Concurrent use may result in additional impairment of CNS performance and reduction in mental alertness).
No products indexed under this heading.

Diazepam (Concurrent use may result in additional impairment of CNS performance and reduction in mental alertness). Products include:
Diastat Rectal Delivery System 3344
Valium Tablets 2822

Droperidol (Concurrent use may result in additional impairment of CNS performance and reduction in mental alertness).
No products indexed under this heading.

Dyphylline (Small decrease in the clearance of cetirizine caused by a larger dose, e.g., 400 mg dose of theophylline).
No products indexed under this heading.

Enflurane (Concurrent use may result in additional impairment of CNS performance and reduction in mental alertness).
No products indexed under this heading.

Estazolam (Concurrent use may result in additional impairment of CNS performance and reduction in mental alertness). Products include:
ProSom Tablets **512**

Ethanol (Concurrent use may result in additional impairment of CNS performance and reduction in mental alertness).
No products indexed under this heading.

Ethchlorvynol (Concurrent use may result in additional impairment of CNS performance and reduction in mental alertness).
No products indexed under this heading.

Ethinamate (Concurrent use may result in additional impairment of CNS performance and reduction in mental alertness).
No products indexed under this heading.

Ethyl Alcohol (Concurrent use may result in additional impairment of CNS performance and reduction in mental alertness).
No products indexed under this heading.

Fentanyl (Concurrent use may result in additional impairment of CNS performance and reduction in mental alertness). Products include:
Duragesic Transdermal System **2448**

Fentanyl Citrate (Concurrent use may result in additional impairment of CNS performance and reduction in mental alertness). Products include:
Actiq **993**

Fluphenazine Decanoate (Concurrent use may result in additional impairment of CNS performance and reduction in mental alertness).
No products indexed under this heading.

Fluphenazine Enanthate (Concurrent use may result in additional impairment of CNS performance and reduction in mental alertness).
No products indexed under this heading.

Fluphenazine Hydrochloride (Concurrent use may result in additional impairment of CNS performance and reduction in mental alertness).
No products indexed under this heading.

Flurazepam Hydrochloride (Concurrent use may result in additional impairment of CNS performance and reduction in mental alertness). Products include:
Dalmane Capsules **3343**

Glutethimide (Concurrent use may result in additional impairment of CNS performance and reduction in mental alertness).
No products indexed under this heading.

Haloperidol (Concurrent use may result in additional impairment of CNS performance and reduction in mental alertness).
No products indexed under this heading.

Haloperidol Decanoate (Concurrent use may result in additional impairment of CNS performance and reduction in mental alertness).
No products indexed under this heading.

Hydrocodone Bitartrate (Concurrent use may result in additional impairment of CNS performance and reduction in mental alertness). Products include:
Hycodan **1104**
Hycomine Compound Tablets **1105**
Hycotuss Expectorant Syrup **1106**
Lortab **3315**
Lortab Elixir **3312**
Vicodin Tablets **530**
Vicodin ES Tablets **531**
Vicodin HP Tablets **532**
Vicoprofen Tablets **533**
Zydone Tablets **1118**

Hydrocodone Polistirex (Concurrent use may result in additional impairment of CNS performance and reduction in mental alertness). Products include:
Tussionex Pennkinetic Extended-Release Suspension **3322**

Hydromorphone Hydrochloride (Concurrent use may result in additional impairment of CNS performance and reduction in mental alertness). Products include:
Dilaudid **439**
Dilaudid Oral Liquid **443**
Dilaudid Non-Sterile Powder **439**
Dilaudid Rectal Suppositories **439**
Dilaudid Tablets **439**
Dilaudid Tablets - 8 mg **443**
Dilaudid-HP **441**

Hydroxyzine Hydrochloride (Concurrent use may result in additional impairment of CNS performance and reduction in mental alertness).
No products indexed under this heading.

Isoflurane (Concurrent use may result in additional impairment of CNS performance and reduction in mental alertness).
No products indexed under this heading.

Ketamine Hydrochloride (Concurrent use may result in additional impairment of CNS performance and reduction in mental alertness).
No products indexed under this heading.

Levomethadyl Acetate Hydrochloride (Concurrent use may result in additional impairment of CNS performance and reduction in mental alertness).
No products indexed under this heading.

Levorphanol Tartrate (Concurrent use may result in additional impairment of CNS performance and reduction in mental alertness).
No products indexed under this heading.

Lorazepam (Concurrent use may result in additional impairment of CNS performance and reduction in mental alertness).
No products indexed under this heading.

Loxapine Hydrochloride (Concurrent use may result in additional impairment of CNS performance and reduction in mental alertness).
No products indexed under this heading.

Loxapine Succinate (Concurrent use may result in additional impairment of CNS performance and reduction in mental alertness).
No products indexed under this heading.

Meperidine Hydrochloride (Concurrent use may result in additional impairment of CNS performance and reduction in mental alertness).
No products indexed under this heading.

Mephobarbital (Concurrent use may result in additional impairment of CNS performance and reduction in mental alertness). Products include:
Mebaral Tablets, USP **2483**

Meprobamate (Concurrent use may result in additional impairment of CNS performance and reduction in mental alertness).
No products indexed under this heading.

Mesoridazine Besylate (Concurrent use may result in additional impairment of CNS performance and reduction in mental alertness).
No products indexed under this heading.

Methadone Hydrochloride (Concurrent use may result in additional impairment of CNS performance and reduction in mental alertness).
No products indexed under this heading.

Methohexital Sodium (Concurrent use may result in additional impairment of CNS performance and reduction in mental alertness).
No products indexed under this heading.

Methotrimeprazine (Concurrent use may result in additional impairment of CNS performance and reduction in mental alertness).
No products indexed under this heading.

Methoxyflurane (Concurrent use may result in additional impairment of CNS performance and reduction in mental alertness).
No products indexed under this heading.

Midazolam Hydrochloride (Concurrent use may result in additional impairment of CNS performance and reduction in mental alertness).
No products indexed under this heading.

Molindone Hydrochloride (Concurrent use may result in additional impairment of CNS performance and reduction in mental alertness). Products include:
Moban Tablets **1108**

Morphine Sulfate (Concurrent use may result in additional impairment of CNS performance and reduction in mental alertness). Products include:
Avinza Capsules **1714**
Kadian Capsules **572**
MS Contin Tablets **2703**

Olanzapine (Concurrent use may result in additional impairment of CNS performance and reduction in mental alertness). Products include:
Symbyax Capsules **1788**
Zyprexa Tablets **1798**
Zyprexa IntraMuscular **1798**
Zyprexa ZYDIS Orally Disintegrating Tablets **1798**

Oxazepam (Concurrent use may result in additional impairment of CNS performance and reduction in mental alertness).
No products indexed under this heading.

Oxycodone Hydrochloride (Concurrent use may result in additional impairment of CNS performance and reduction in mental alertness). Products include:
Combunox Tablets **1183**
OxyContin Tablets **2699**
OxyFast Oral Concentrate Solution **2704**
OxyIR Capsules **2704**
Percocet Tablets **1114**
Percodan Tablets **1115**

Pentobarbital Sodium (Concurrent use may result in additional impairment of CNS performance and reduction in mental alertness). Products include:
Nembutal Sodium Solution, USP **2484**

Perphenazine (Concurrent use may result in additional impairment of CNS performance and reduction in mental alertness).
No products indexed under this heading.

Phenobarbital (Concurrent use may result in additional impairment of CNS performance and reduction in mental alertness).
No products indexed under this heading.

Prazepam (Concurrent use may result in additional impairment of CNS performance and reduction in mental alertness).
No products indexed under this heading.

Prochlorperazine (Concurrent use may result in additional impairment of CNS performance and reduction in mental alertness).
No products indexed under this heading.

Promethazine Hydrochloride (Concurrent use may result in additional impairment of CNS performance and reduction in mental alertness). Products include:
Phenergan **3438**

Propofol (Concurrent use may result in additional impairment of CNS performance and reduction in mental alertness). Products include:
Diprivan Injectable Emulsion **676**

Propoxyphene Hydrochloride (Concurrent use may result in additional impairment of CNS performance and reduction in mental alertness).
No products indexed under this heading.

Propoxyphene Napsylate (Concurrent use may result in additional impairment of CNS performance and reduction in mental alertness). Products include:
Darvocet A 500 Tablets **3497**

Quazepam (Concurrent use may result in additional impairment of CNS performance and reduction in mental alertness).
No products indexed under this heading.

Quetiapine Fumarate (Concurrent use may result in additional impairment of CNS performance and reduction in mental alertness). Products include:
- Seroquel Tablets 691

Remifentanil Hydrochloride (Concurrent use may result in additional impairment of CNS performance and reduction in mental alertness).
- No products indexed under this heading.

Risperidone (Concurrent use may result in additional impairment of CNS performance and reduction in mental alertness). Products include:
- Risperdal Consta Long-Acting Injection 1664
- Risperdal M-Tab Orally Disintegrating Tablets.................... 1658
- Risperdal 1658

Secobarbital Sodium (Concurrent use may result in additional impairment of CNS performance and reduction in mental alertness).
- No products indexed under this heading.

Sevoflurane (Concurrent use may result in additional impairment of CNS performance and reduction in mental alertness). Products include:
- Ultane Liquid for Inhalation 526

Sodium Oxybate (Concurrent use may result in additional impairment of CNS performance and reduction in mental alertness).
- No products indexed under this heading.

Sufentanil Citrate (Concurrent use may result in additional impairment of CNS performance and reduction in mental alertness).
- No products indexed under this heading.

Temazepam (Concurrent use may result in additional impairment of CNS performance and reduction in mental alertness).
- No products indexed under this heading.

Theophylline (Small decrease in the clearance of cetirizine caused by a larger dose, e.g., 400 mg dose of theophylline).
- No products indexed under this heading.

Theophylline Anhydrous (Small decrease in the clearance of cetirizine caused by a larger dose, e.g., 400 mg dose of theophylline). Products include:
- Uniphyl Tablets 2708

Theophylline Calcium Salicylate (Small decrease in the clearance of cetirizine caused by a larger dose, e.g., 400 mg dose of theophylline).
- No products indexed under this heading.

Theophylline Dihydroxypropyl (Glyceryl) (Small decrease in the clearance of cetirizine caused by a larger dose, e.g., 400 mg dose of theophylline).
- No products indexed under this heading.

Theophylline Ethylenediamine (Small decrease in the clearance of cetirizine caused by a larger dose, e.g., 400 mg dose of theophylline).
- No products indexed under this heading.

Theophylline Sodium Glycinate (Small decrease in the clearance of cetirizine caused by a larger dose, e.g., 400 mg dose of theophylline).
- No products indexed under this heading.

Thiamylal Sodium (Concurrent use may result in additional impairment of CNS performance and reduction in mental alertness).
- No products indexed under this heading.

Thioridazine Hydrochloride (Concurrent use may result in additional impairment of CNS performance and reduction in mental alertness). Products include:
- Thioridazine Hydrochloride Tablets.. 2122

Thiothixene (Concurrent use may result in additional impairment of CNS performance and reduction in mental alertness). Products include:
- Thiothixene Capsules 2124

Triazolam (Concurrent use may result in additional impairment of CNS performance and reduction in mental alertness).
- No products indexed under this heading.

Trifluoperazine Hydrochloride (Concurrent use may result in additional impairment of CNS performance and reduction in mental alertness).
- No products indexed under this heading.

Zaleplon (Concurrent use may result in additional impairment of CNS performance and reduction in mental alertness). Products include:
- Sonata Capsules 1686

Ziprasidone Hydrochloride (Concurrent use may result in additional impairment of CNS performance and reduction in mental alertness). Products include:
- Geodon Capsules 2514

Zolpidem Tartrate (Concurrent use may result in additional impairment of CNS performance and reduction in mental alertness). Products include:
- Ambien Tablets 2867

Food Interactions

Alcohol (Concurrent use may result in additional impairment of CNS performance and reduction in mental alertness).

Food, unspecified (Food has no effect on the extent of cetirizine absorption, but Tmax may be delayed and Cmax may be decreased in the presence of food).

ZYRTEC-D 12 HOUR EXTENDED RELEASE TABLETS

(Cetirizine Hydrochloride, Pseudoephedrine Hydrochloride)........ 2591

May interact with central nervous system depressants, cardiac glycosides, histamine H_2-receptor antagonists, monoamine oxidase inhibitors, proton pump inhibitor, sympathomimetics, xanthines, and certain other agents. Compounds in these categories include:

Albuterol (Co-administration with other sympathomimetic agents may result in harmful cardiovascular effects). Products include:
- Proventil Inhalation Aerosol 3067

Albuterol Sulfate (Co-administration with other sympathomimetic agents may result in harmful cardiovascular effects). Products include:
- AccuNeb Inhalation Solution 1055
- Combivent Inhalation Aerosol 878
- DuoNeb Inhalation Solution 1058
- Proventil Inhalation Solution 0.083%... 3069
- Proventil HFA Inhalation Aerosol 3071
- Ventolin HFA Inhalation Aerosol 1576
- VoSpire Extended-Release Tablets ... 2352

Alfentanil Hydrochloride (Concurrent use may result in additional reduction in alertness impairment of CNS performance).
- No products indexed under this heading.

Alprazolam (Concurrent use may result in additional reduction in alertness impairment of CNS performance). Products include:
- Niravam Orally Disintegrating Tablets.. 3106
- Xanax XR Tablets 2655

Aminophylline (Small decrease in the clearance of cetirizine caused by a 400 mg dose of theophylline; it is possible that larger theophylline doses could have a greater effect).
- No products indexed under this heading.

Aprobarbital (Concurrent use may result in additional reduction in alertness impairment of CNS performance).
- No products indexed under this heading.

Buprenorphine Hydrochloride (Concurrent use may result in additional reduction in alertness impairment of CNS performance). Products include:
- Buprenex Injectable 2718
- Suboxone Tablets 2719
- Subutex Tablets 2719

Buspirone Hydrochloride (Concurrent use may result in additional reduction in alertness impairment of CNS performance).
- No products indexed under this heading.

Butabarbital (Concurrent use may result in additional reduction in alertness impairment of CNS performance).
- No products indexed under this heading.

Butalbital (Concurrent use may result in additional reduction in alertness impairment of CNS performance). Products include:
- Sedapap Tablets 50 mg/650 mg 2098

Chlordiazepoxide (Concurrent use may result in additional reduction in alertness impairment of CNS performance).
- No products indexed under this heading.

Chlordiazepoxide Hydrochloride (Concurrent use may result in additional reduction in alertness impairment of CNS performance). Products include:
- Librium Capsules 3349

Chlorpromazine (Concurrent use may result in additional reduction in alertness impairment of CNS performance).
- No products indexed under this heading.

Chlorpromazine Hydrochloride (Concurrent use may result in additional reduction in alertness impairment of CNS performance).
- No products indexed under this heading.

Chlorprothixene (Concurrent use may result in additional reduction in alertness impairment of CNS performance).
- No products indexed under this heading.

Chlorprothixene Hydrochloride (Concurrent use may result in additional reduction in alertness impairment of CNS performance).
- No products indexed under this heading.

Chlorprothixene Lactate (Concurrent use may result in additional reduction in alertness impairment of CNS performance).
- No products indexed under this heading.

Cimetidine (H2 antagonists increase gastric pH and may reduce the absorption of delavirdine; chronic use of these drugs with delavirdine is not recommended). Products include:
- Tagamet HB 200 Tablets .... ■637
- Tagamet Tablets 1547

Cimetidine Hydrochloride (H2 antagonists increase gastric pH and may reduce the absorption of delavirdine; chronic use of these drugs with delavirdine is not recommended).
- No products indexed under this heading.

Clorazepate Dipotassium (Concurrent use may result in additional reduction in alertness impairment of CNS performance). Products include:
- Tranxene 2488

Clozapine (Concurrent use may result in additional reduction in alertness impairment of CNS performance). Products include:
- Clozapine Tablets 2141
- Clozaril Tablets 2174
- FazaClo Orally Disintegrating Tablets... 547

Codeine Phosphate (Concurrent use may result in additional reduction in alertness impairment of CNS performance). Products include:
- Tylenol with Codeine 2461

Desflurane (Concurrent use may result in additional reduction in alertness impairment of CNS performance). Products include:
- Suprane Liquid for Inhalation 770

Deslanoside (Co-administration of pseudoephedrine may increase ectopic pacemaker activity).
- No products indexed under this heading.

Dezocine (Concurrent use may result in additional reduction in alertness impairment of CNS performance).
- No products indexed under this heading.

Diazepam (Concurrent use may result in additional reduction in alertness impairment of CNS performance). Products include:
- Diastat Rectal Delivery System 3344
- Valium Tablets 2822

Digitalis Glycoside Preparations (Co-administration of pseudoephedrine may increase ectopic pacemaker activity).
- No products indexed under this heading.

Digitoxin (Co-administration of pseudoephedrine may increase ectopic pacemaker activity).
- No products indexed under this heading.

Digoxin (Co-administration of pseudoephedrine may increase ectopic pacemaker activity). Products include:
- Digitek Tablets 2146
- Lanoxicaps Capsules 1458

Lanoxin Injection **1462**
Lanoxin Tablets **1468**
Lanoxin Injection Pediatric **1465**

Dobutamine Hydrochloride (Co-administration with other sympathomimetic agents may result in harmful cardiovascular effects).
No products indexed under this heading.

Dopamine Hydrochloride (Co-administration with other sympathomimetic agents may result in harmful cardiovascular effects).
No products indexed under this heading.

Droperidol (Concurrent use may result in additional reduction in alertness impairment of CNS performance).
No products indexed under this heading.

Dyphylline (Small decrease in the clearance of cetirizine caused by a 400 mg dose of theophylline; it is possible that larger theophylline doses could have a greater effect).
No products indexed under this heading.

Enflurane (Concurrent use may result in additional reduction in alertness impairment of CNS performance).
No products indexed under this heading.

Ephedrine Hydrochloride (Co-administration with other sympathomimetic agents may result in harmful cardiovascular effects). Products include:
Primatene Tablets **749**

Ephedrine Sulfate (Co-administration with other sympathomimetic agents may result in harmful cardiovascular effects).
No products indexed under this heading.

Ephedrine Tannate (Co-administration with other sympathomimetic agents may result in harmful cardiovascular effects).
No products indexed under this heading.

Epinephrine (Co-administration with other sympathomimetic agents may result in harmful cardiovascular effects). Products include:
EpiPen **1061**
Primatene Mist **749**

Epinephrine Bitartrate (Co-administration with other sympathomimetic agents may result in harmful cardiovascular effects).
No products indexed under this heading.

Epinephrine Hydrochloride (Co-administration with other sympathomimetic agents may result in harmful cardiovascular effects).
No products indexed under this heading.

Esomeprazole Magnesium (Proton pump inhibitors increase gastric pH and may reduce the absorption of delavirdine chronic use of these drugs with delavirdine is not recommended). Products include:
Nexium Delayed-Release Capsules **645**

Estazolam (Concurrent use may result in additional reduction in alertness impairment of CNS performance). Products include:
ProSom Tablets **512**

Ethanol (Concurrent use may result in additional reduction in alertness impairment of CNS performance).
No products indexed under this heading.

Ethchlorvynol (Concurrent use may result in additional reduction in alertness impairment of CNS performance).
No products indexed under this heading.

Ethinamate (Concurrent use may result in additional reduction in alertness impairment of CNS performance).
No products indexed under this heading.

Ethyl Alcohol (Concurrent use may result in additional reduction in alertness impairment of CNS performance).
No products indexed under this heading.

Famotidine (H2 antagonists increase gastric pH and may reduce the absorption of delavirdine; chronic use of these drugs with delavirdine is not recommended). Products include:
Pepcid AC Chewable Tablets **1672**
Pepcid AC Gelcaps **1672**
Pepcid AC Tablets **1672**
Maximum Strength Pepcid AC Tablets **1672**
Pepcid Complete Chewable Tablets **1672**
Pepcid Injection **2017**
Pepcid **2014**

Fentanyl (Concurrent use may result in additional reduction in alertness impairment of CNS performance). Products include:
Duragesic Transdermal System **2448**

Fentanyl Citrate (Concurrent use may result in additional reduction in alertness impairment of CNS performance). Products include:
Actiq **993**

Fluphenazine Decanoate (Concurrent use may result in additional reduction in alertness impairment of CNS performance).
No products indexed under this heading.

Fluphenazine Enanthate (Concurrent use may result in additional reduction in alertness impairment of CNS performance).
No products indexed under this heading.

Fluphenazine Hydrochloride (Concurrent use may result in additional reduction in alertness impairment of CNS performance).
No products indexed under this heading.

Flurazepam Hydrochloride (Concurrent use may result in additional reduction in alertness impairment of CNS performance). Products include:
Dalmane Capsules **3343**

Glutethimide (Concurrent use may result in additional reduction in alertness impairment of CNS performance).
No products indexed under this heading.

Haloperidol (Concurrent use may result in additional reduction in alertness impairment of CNS performance).
No products indexed under this heading.

Haloperidol Decanoate (Concurrent use may result in additional reduction in alertness impairment of CNS performance).
No products indexed under this heading.

Hydrocodone Bitartrate (Concurrent use may result in additional reduction in alertness impairment of CNS performance). Products include:
Hycodan **1104**
Hycomine Compound Tablets **1105**
Hycotuss Expectorant Syrup **1106**
Lortab **3315**
Lortab Elixir **3312**
Vicodin Tablets **530**
Vicodin ES Tablets **531**
Vicodin HP Tablets **532**
Vicoprofen Tablets **533**
Zydone Tablets **1118**

Hydrocodone Polistirex (Concurrent use may result in additional reduction in alertness impairment of CNS performance). Products include:
Tussionex Pennkinetic Extended-Release Suspension **3322**

Hydromorphone Hydrochloride (Concurrent use may result in additional reduction in alertness impairment of CNS performance). Products include:
Dilaudid **439**
Dilaudid Oral Liquid **443**
Dilaudid Non-Sterile Powder **439**
Dilaudid Rectal Suppositories **439**
Dilaudid Tablets **439**
Dilaudid Tablets - 8 mg **443**
Dilaudid-HP **441**

Hydroxyzine Hydrochloride (Concurrent use may result in additional reduction in alertness impairment of CNS performance).
No products indexed under this heading.

Isocarboxazid (Concurrent and/or sequential use with MAO inhibitors is contraindicated).
No products indexed under this heading.

Isoflurane (Concurrent use may result in additional reduction in alertness impairment of CNS performance).
No products indexed under this heading.

Isoproterenol Hydrochloride (Co-administration with other sympathomimetic agents may result in harmful cardiovascular effects).
No products indexed under this heading.

Isoproterenol Sulfate (Co-administration with other sympathomimetic agents may result in harmful cardiovascular effects).
No products indexed under this heading.

Ketamine Hydrochloride (Concurrent use may result in additional reduction in alertness impairment of CNS performance).
No products indexed under this heading.

Lansoprazole (Proton pump inhibitors increase gastric pH and may reduce the absorption of delavirdine chronic use of these drugs with delavirdine is not recommended). Products include:
Prevacid Delayed-Release Capsules **3268**
Prevacid for Delayed-Release Oral Suspension **3268**
Prevacid I.V. for Injection **3274**
Prevacid NapraPAC **3277**
Prevacid SoluTab Delayed-Release Orally Disintegrating Tablets **3268**
PREVPAC **3281**

Levalbuterol Hydrochloride (Co-administration with other sympathomimetic agents may result in harmful cardiovascular effects). Products include:
Xopenex Inhalation Solution **3143**
Xopenex Inhalation Solution Concentrate **3147**

Levomethadyl Acetate Hydrochloride (Concurrent use may result in additional reduction in alertness impairment of CNS performance).
No products indexed under this heading.

Levorphanol Tartrate (Concurrent use may result in additional reduction in alertness impairment of CNS performance).
No products indexed under this heading.

Lorazepam (Concurrent use may result in additional reduction in alertness impairment of CNS performance).
No products indexed under this heading.

Loxapine Hydrochloride (Concurrent use may result in additional reduction in alertness impairment of CNS performance).
No products indexed under this heading.

Loxapine Succinate (Concurrent use may result in additional reduction in alertness impairment of CNS performance).
No products indexed under this heading.

Mecamylamine Hydrochloride (Pseudoephedrine may reduce the antihypertensive effect). Products include:
Inversine Tablets **3286**

Meperidine Hydrochloride (Concurrent use may result in additional reduction in alertness impairment of CNS performance).
No products indexed under this heading.

Mephobarbital (Concurrent use may result in additional reduction in alertness impairment of CNS performance). Products include:
Mebaral Tablets, USP **2483**

Meprobamate (Concurrent use may result in additional reduction in alertness impairment of CNS performance).
No products indexed under this heading.

Mesoridazine Besylate (Concurrent use may result in additional reduction in alertness impairment of CNS performance).
No products indexed under this heading.

Metaproterenol Sulfate (Co-administration with other sympathomimetic agents may result in harmful cardiovascular effects). Products include:
Alupent Inhalation Aerosol **858**

Metaraminol Bitartrate (Co-administration with other sympathomimetic agents may result in harmful cardiovascular effects). Products include:
Aramine Injection **1889**

IMPORTANT NOTE: Always consult each drug listing in the patient's regimen for possible interactions.

Methadone Hydrochloride (Concurrent use may result in additional reduction in alertness impairment of CNS performance).
No products indexed under this heading.

Methohexital Sodium (Concurrent use may result in additional reduction in alertness impairment of CNS performance).
No products indexed under this heading.

Methotrimeprazine (Concurrent use may result in additional reduction in alertness impairment of CNS performance).
No products indexed under this heading.

Methoxamine Hydrochloride (Co-administration with other sympathomimetic agents may result in harmful cardiovascular effects).
No products indexed under this heading.

Methoxyflurane (Concurrent use may result in additional reduction in alertness impairment of CNS performance).
No products indexed under this heading.

Methyldopa (Pseudoephedrine may reduce the antihypertensive effect). Products include:
Aldoclor Tablets 1881
Aldoril Tablets 1884

Methyldopate Hydrochloride (Pseudoephedrine may reduce the antihypertensive effect).
No products indexed under this heading.

Midazolam Hydrochloride (Concurrent use may result in additional reduction in alertness impairment of CNS performance).
No products indexed under this heading.

Moclobemide (Concurrent and/or sequential use with MAO inhibitors is contraindicated).
No products indexed under this heading.

Molindone Hydrochloride (Concurrent use may result in additional reduction in alertness impairment of CNS performance). Products include:
Moban Tablets 1108

Morphine Sulfate (Concurrent use may result in additional reduction in alertness impairment of CNS performance). Products include:
Avinza Capsules 1714
Kadian Capsules 572
MS Contin Tablets 2703

Nizatidine (H2 antagonists increase gastric pH and may reduce the absorption of delavirdine; chronic use of these drugs with delavirdine is not recommended). Products include:
Axid Oral Solution 913

Norepinephrine Bitartrate (Co-administration with other sympathomimetic agents may result in harmful cardiovascular effects).
No products indexed under this heading.

Olanzapine (Concurrent use may result in additional reduction in alertness impairment of CNS performance). Products include:
Symbyax Capsules 1788
Zyprexa Tablets 1798
Zyprexa IntraMuscular 1798
Zyprexa ZYDIS Orally Disintegrating Tablets 1798

Omeprazole (Proton pump inhibitors increase gastric pH and may reduce the absorption of delavirdine chronic use of these drugs with delavirdine is not recommended). Products include:
Zegerid Powder for Oral Solution 2972

Oxazepam (Concurrent use may result in additional reduction in alertness impairment of CNS performance).
No products indexed under this heading.

Oxycodone Hydrochloride (Concurrent use may result in additional reduction in alertness impairment of CNS performance). Products include:
Combunox Tablets 1183
OxyContin Tablets 2699
OxyFast Oral Concentrate Solution 2704
OxyIR Capsules 2704
Percocet Tablets 1114
Percodan Tablets 1115

Pantoprazole Sodium (Proton pump inhibitors increase gastric pH and may reduce the absorption of delavirdine chronic use of these drugs with delavirdine is not recommended). Products include:
Protonix I.V. 3468
Protonix Tablets 3465

Pargyline Hydrochloride (Concurrent and/or sequential use with MAO inhibitors is contraindicated).
No products indexed under this heading.

Pentobarbital Sodium (Concurrent use may result in additional reduction in alertness impairment of CNS performance). Products include:
Nembutal Sodium Solution, USP 2484

Perphenazine (Concurrent use may result in additional reduction in alertness impairment of CNS performance).
No products indexed under this heading.

Phenelzine Sulfate (Concurrent and/or sequential use with MAO inhibitors is contraindicated).
No products indexed under this heading.

Phenobarbital (Concurrent use may result in additional reduction in alertness impairment of CNS performance).
No products indexed under this heading.

Phenylephrine Bitartrate (Co-administration with other sympathomimetic agents may result in harmful cardiovascular effects).
No products indexed under this heading.

Phenylephrine Hydrochloride (Co-administration with other sympathomimetic agents may result in harmful cardiovascular effects). Products include:
Alacol DM Syrup 739
Hycomine Compound Tablets 1105
Preparation H Maximum Strength Cream .... ▣747
Preparation H Cooling Gel .... ▣747
Preparation H .... ▣747
Sudafed PE Tablets .... ▣711
Vicks Sinex Nasal Spray and Ultra Fine Mist for Sinus Relief 2677
Zicam Concentrated Cough Mist for Kids Plus D Cool Cherry .... ▣643
Zicam Concentrated Cough Mist Plus D Cool Cherry .... ▣642

Phenylephrine Tannate (Co-administration with other sympathomimetic agents may result in harmful cardiovascular effects).
No products indexed under this heading.

Phenylpropanolamine Hydrochloride (Co-administration with other sympathomimetic agents may result in harmful cardiovascular effects).
No products indexed under this heading.

Pirbuterol Acetate (Co-administration with other sympathomimetic agents may result in harmful cardiovascular effects). Products include:
Maxair Autohaler 1820

Prazepam (Concurrent use may result in additional reduction in alertness impairment of CNS performance).
No products indexed under this heading.

Procarbazine Hydrochloride (Concurrent and/or sequential use with MAO inhibitors is contraindicated). Products include:
Matulane Capsules 3188

Prochlorperazine (Concurrent use may result in additional reduction in alertness impairment of CNS performance).
No products indexed under this heading.

Promethazine Hydrochloride (Concurrent use may result in additional reduction in alertness impairment of CNS performance). Products include:
Phenergan 3438

Propofol (Concurrent use may result in additional reduction in alertness impairment of CNS performance). Products include:
Diprivan Injectable Emulsion 676

Propoxyphene Hydrochloride (Concurrent use may result in additional reduction in alertness impairment of CNS performance).
No products indexed under this heading.

Propoxyphene Napsylate (Concurrent use may result in additional reduction in alertness impairment of CNS performance). Products include:
Darvocet A 500 Tablets 3497

Pseudoephedrine Sulfate (Co-administration with other sympathomimetic agents may result in harmful cardiovascular effects). Products include:
Alavert Allergy & Sinus D-12 Hour Tablets .... ▣743
Clarinex-D 24-Hour Extended-Release Tablets 3012
Claritin-D Non-Drowsy 12 Hour Tablets .... ▣731
Claritin-D Non-Drowsy 24 Hour Tablets .... ▣731

Quazepam (Concurrent use may result in additional reduction in alertness impairment of CNS performance).
No products indexed under this heading.

Quetiapine Fumarate (Concurrent use may result in additional reduction in alertness impairment of CNS performance). Products include:
Seroquel Tablets 691

Rabeprazole Sodium (Proton pump inhibitors increase gastric pH and may reduce the absorption of delavirdine chronic use of these drugs with delavirdine is not recommended). Products include:
Aciphex Tablets 1081

Ranitidine Bismuth Citrate (H2 antagonists increase gastric pH and may reduce the absorption of delavirdine; chronic use of these drugs with delavirdine is not recommended).
No products indexed under this heading.

Ranitidine Hydrochloride (H2 antagonists increase gastric pH and may reduce the absorption of delavirdine; chronic use of these drugs with delavirdine is not recommended). Products include:
Zantac 1597
Zantac Injection 1593
Zantac 75 Tablets .... ▣715
Zantac 150 Maximum Strength Tablets .... ▣715
Zantac Injection Pharmacy Bulk Package 1595

Remifentanil Hydrochloride (Concurrent use may result in additional reduction in alertness impairment of CNS performance).
No products indexed under this heading.

Reserpine (Pseudoephedrine may reduce the antihypertensive effect).
No products indexed under this heading.

Risperidone (Concurrent use may result in additional reduction in alertness impairment of CNS performance). Products include:
Risperdal Consta Long-Acting Injection 1664
Risperdal M-Tab Orally Disintegrating Tablets 1658
Risperdal 1658

Salmeterol Xinafoate (Co-administration with other sympathomimetic agents may result in harmful cardiovascular effects). Products include:
Advair Diskus 100/50 1291
Advair Diskus 250/50 1291
Advair Diskus 500/50 1291
Serevent Diskus 1540

Secobarbital Sodium (Concurrent use may result in additional reduction in alertness impairment of CNS performance).
No products indexed under this heading.

Selegiline Hydrochloride (Concurrent and/or sequential use with MAO inhibitors is contraindicated). Products include:
Eldepryl Capsules 3209

Sevoflurane (Concurrent use may result in additional reduction in alertness impairment of CNS performance). Products include:
Ultane Liquid for Inhalation 526

Sufentanil Citrate (Concurrent use may result in additional reduction in alertness impairment of CNS performance).
No products indexed under this heading.

Temazepam (Concurrent use may result in additional reduction in alertness impairment of CNS performance).
No products indexed under this heading.

Terbutaline Sulfate (Co-administration with other sympathomimetic agents may result in harmful cardiovascular effects).
No products indexed under this heading.

Theophylline (Small decrease in the clearance of cetirizine caused by a 400 mg dose of theophylline; it is possible that larger theophylline doses could have a greater effect).
No products indexed under this heading.

Theophylline Anhydrous (Small decrease in the clearance of cetirizine caused by a 400 mg dose of theophylline; it is possible that larger theophylline doses could have a greater effect). Products include:
Uniphyl Tablets 2708

Theophylline Calcium Salicylate (Small decrease in the clearance of cetirizine caused by a 400 mg dose of theophylline; it is possible that larger theophylline doses could have a greater effect).
No products indexed under this heading.

Theophylline Dihydroxypropyl (Glyceryl) (Small decrease in the clearance of cetirizine caused by a 400 mg dose of theophylline; it is possible that larger theophylline doses could have a greater effect).
No products indexed under this heading.

Theophylline Ethylenediamine (Small decrease in the clearance of cetirizine caused by a 400 mg dose of theophylline; it is possible that larger theophylline doses could have a greater effect).
No products indexed under this heading.

Theophylline Sodium Glycinate (Small decrease in the clearance of cetirizine caused by a 400 mg dose of theophylline; it is possible that larger theophylline doses could have a greater effect).
No products indexed under this heading.

Thiamylal Sodium (Concurrent use may result in additional reduction in alertness impairment of CNS performance).
No products indexed under this heading.

Thioridazine Hydrochloride (Concurrent use may result in additional reduction in alertness impairment of CNS performance). Products include:
Thioridazine Hydrochloride Tablets 2122

Thiothixene (Concurrent use may result in additional reduction in alertness impairment of CNS performance). Products include:
Thiothixene Capsules 2124

Tranylcypromine Sulfate (Concurrent and/or sequential use with MAO inhibitors is contraindicated). Products include:
Parnate Tablets 1499

Triazolam (Concurrent use may result in additional reduction in alertness impairment of CNS performance).
No products indexed under this heading.

Trifluoperazine Hydrochloride (Concurrent use may result in additional reduction in alertness impairment of CNS performance).
No products indexed under this heading.

Zaleplon (Concurrent use may result in additional reduction in alertness impairment of CNS performance). Products include:
Sonata Capsules 1686

Ziprasidone Hydrochloride (Concurrent use may result in additional reduction in alertness impairment of CNS performance). Products include:
Geodon Capsules 2514

Zolpidem Tartrate (Concurrent use may result in additional reduction in alertness impairment of CNS performance). Products include:
Ambien Tablets 2867

Food Interactions

Alcohol (Concurrent use may result in additional reduction in alertness impairment of CNS performance).

ZYVOX INJECTION

(Linezolid) 2661
See Zyvox Tablets

ZYVOX FOR ORAL SUSPENSION

(Linezolid) 2661
See Zyvox Tablets

ZYVOX TABLETS

(Linezolid) 2661
May interact with serotoninergic agents, sympathomimetics, and certain other agents. Compounds in these categories include:

Albuterol (Linezolid is a reversible nonselective inhibitor of MAO; therefore, linezolid has the potential for interaction with adrenergic agents). Products include:
Proventil Inhalation Aerosol 3067

Albuterol Sulfate (Linezolid is a reversible nonselective inhibitor of MAO; therefore, linezolid has the potential for interaction with adrenergic agents). Products include:
AccuNeb Inhalation Solution 1055
Combivent Inhalation Aerosol 878
DuoNeb Inhalation Solution 1058
Proventil Inhalation Solution 0.083% 3069
Proventil HFA Inhalation Aerosol 3071
Ventolin HFA Inhalation Aerosol 1576
VoSpire Extended-Release Tablets ... 2352

Citalopram Hydrobromide (Linezolid is a reversible nonselective inhibitor of monoamine oxidase. Therefore, linezolid has the potential for interaction with serotonergic agents. Spontaneous reports of serotonin syndrome associated with co-administration of linezolid and serotinergic agents, including antidepressants such as selective serotonin reuptake inhibitors (SSRIs), have been reported. Patients who are treated with linezolid and concomitant serotinergic agents should be closely observed for signs and symptoms of serotonin syndrome (e.g., cognitive dysfunction, hyperpyrexia, hyperreflexia, incoordination). If any signs or symptoms occur, physicians should consider discontinuation of either one or both agents (linezolid or concomitant serotinergic agents)). Products include:
Celexa 1177

Dobutamine Hydrochloride (Linezolid is a reversible nonselective inhibitor of MAO; therefore, linezolid has the potential for interaction with adrenergic agents).
No products indexed under this heading.

Dopamine Hydrochloride (Some patients receiving Zyvox with dopaminergic agents may experience a reversible enhancement of pressor response; initial dose of dopamine should be reduced and titrated to achieve the desired response).
No products indexed under this heading.

Ephedrine Hydrochloride (Linezolid is a reversible nonselective inhibitor of MAO; therefore, linezolid has the potential for interaction with adrenergic agents). Products include:
Primatene Tablets 749

Ephedrine Sulfate (Linezolid is a reversible nonselective inhibitor of MAO; therefore, linezolid has the potential for interaction with adrenergic agents).
No products indexed under this heading.

Ephedrine Tannate (Linezolid is a reversible nonselective inhibitor of MAO; therefore, linezolid has the potential for interaction with adrenergic agents).
No products indexed under this heading.

Epinephrine (Linezolid is a reversible nonselective inhibitor of MAO; therefore, linezolid has the potential for interaction with adrenergic agents). Products include:
EpiPen 1061
Primatene Mist 749

Epinephrine Bitartrate (Linezolid is a reversible nonselective inhibitor of MAO; therefore, linezolid has the potential for interaction with adrenergic agents).
No products indexed under this heading.

Epinephrine Hydrochloride (Some patients receiving Zyvox with vasopressors may experience a reversible enhancement of pressor response; initial dose of epinephrine should be reduced and titrated to achieve the desired response).
No products indexed under this heading.

Escitalopram Oxalate (Linezolid is a reversible nonselective inhibitor of monoamine oxidase. Therefore, linezolid has the potential for interaction with serotonergic agents. Spontaneous reports of serotonin syndrome associated with co-administration of linezolid and serotinergic agents, including antidepressants such as selective serotonin reuptake inhibitors (SSRIs), have been reported. Patients who are treated with linezolid and concomitant serotinergic agents should be closely observed for signs and symptoms of serotonin syndrome (e.g., cognitive dysfunction, hyperpyrexia, hyperreflexia, incoordination). If any signs or symptoms occur, physicians should consider discontinuation of either one or both agents (linezolid or concomitant serotinergic agents)). Products include:
Lexapro Oral Solution 1193
Lexapro Tablets 1193

Fluoxetine Hydrochloride (Linezolid is a reversible nonselective inhibitor of monoamine oxidase. Therefore, linezolid has the potential for interaction with serotonergic agents. Spontaneous reports of serotonin syndrome associated with co-administration of linezolid and serotinergic agents, including antidepressants such as selective serotonin reuptake inhibitors (SSRIs), have been reported. Patients who are treated with linezolid and concomitant serotinergic agents should be closely observed for signs and symptoms of serotonin syndrome (e.g., cognitive dysfunction, hyperpyrexia, hyperreflexia, incoordination). If any signs or symptoms occur, physicians should consider discontinuation of either one or both agents (linezolid or concomitant serotinergic agents)). Products include:
Prozac Pulvules and Liquid 1771
Symbyax Capsules 1788

Fluvoxamine Maleate (Linezolid is a reversible nonselective inhibitor of monoamine oxidase. Therefore, linezolid has the potential for interaction with serotonergic agents. Spontaneous reports of serotonin syndrome associated with co-administration of linezolid and serotinergic agents, including antidepressants such as selective serotonin reuptake inhibitors (SSRIs), have been reported. Patients who are treated with linezolid and concomitant serotinergic agents should be closely observed for signs and symptoms of serotonin syndrome (e.g., cognitive dysfunction, hyperpyrexia, hyperreflexia, incoordination). If any signs or symptoms occur, physicians should consider discontinuation of either one or both agents (linezolid or concomitant serotinergic agents)).
No products indexed under this heading.

Isoproterenol Hydrochloride (Linezolid is a reversible nonselective inhibitor of MAO; therefore, linezolid has the potential for interaction with adrenergic agents).
No products indexed under this heading.

Isoproterenol Sulfate (Linezolid is a reversible nonselective inhibitor of MAO; therefore, linezolid has the potential for interaction with adrenergic agents).
No products indexed under this heading.

Levalbuterol Hydrochloride (Linezolid is a reversible nonselective inhibitor of MAO; therefore, linezolid has the potential for interaction with adrenergic agents). Products include:
Xopenex Inhalation Solution 3143
Xopenex Inhalation Solution Concentrate 3147

Metaproterenol Sulfate (Linezolid is a reversible nonselective inhibitor of MAO; therefore, linezolid has the potential for interaction with adrenergic agents). Products include:
Alupent Inhalation Aerosol 858

Metaraminol Bitartrate (Linezolid is a reversible nonselective inhibitor of MAO; therefore, linezolid has the potential for interaction with adrenergic agents). Products include:
Aramine Injection 1889

Methoxamine Hydrochloride (Linezolid is a reversible nonselective inhibitor of MAO; therefore, linezolid has the potential for interaction with adrenergic agents).
No products indexed under this heading.

Norepinephrine Bitartrate (Linezolid is a reversible nonselective inhibitor of MAO; therefore, linezolid has the potential for interaction with adrenergic agents).
No products indexed under this heading.

Paroxetine Hydrochloride (Linezolid is a reversible nonselective inhibitor of monoamine oxidase. Therefore, linezolid has the potential for interaction with serotonergic agents. Spontaneous reports of serotonin syndrome associated with co-administration of linezolid and serotinergic agents, including antidepressants such as selective serotonin reuptake inhibitors (SSRIs), have been reported. Patients who are treated with linezolid and concomitant serotinergic agents should be closely observed for signs and symptoms of serotonin syndrome (e.g., cognitive dysfunction, hyperpyrexia, hyperreflexia, incoordination). If any signs or symptoms occur, physicians should consider discontinuation of either one or both agents (linezolid or concomitant serotinergic agents)). Products include:

Paxil CR Controlled-Release Tablets ... 1509
Paxil ... 1501

Phenylephrine Bitartrate (Linezolid is a reversible nonselective inhibitor of MAO; therefore, linezolid has the potential for interaction with adrenergic agents).

No products indexed under this heading.

Phenylephrine Hydrochloride (Linezolid is a reversible nonselective inhibitor of MAO; therefore, linezolid has the potential for interaction with adrenergic agents). Products include:

Alacol DM Syrup ... 739
Hycomine Compound Tablets ... 1105
Preparation H Maximum Strength Cream ... ■ 747
Preparation H Cooling Gel ... ■ 747
Preparation H ... ■ 747
Sudafed PE Tablets ... ■ 711
Vicks Sinex Nasal Spray and Ultra Fine Mist for Sinus Relief ... 2677
Zicam Concentrated Cough Mist for Kids Plus D Cool Cherry ... ■ 643
Zicam Concentrated Cough Mist Plus D Cool Cherry ... ■ 642

Phenylephrine Tannate (Linezolid is a reversible nonselective inhibitor of MAO; therefore, linezolid has the potential for interaction with adrenergic agents).

No products indexed under this heading.

Phenylpropanolamine Hydrochloride (Co-administration has resulted in a reversible enhancement of pressor response of phenylpropanolamine).

No products indexed under this heading.

Pirbuterol Acetate (Linezolid is a reversible nonselective inhibitor of MAO; therefore, linezolid has the potential for interaction with adrenergic agents). Products include:

Maxair Autohaler ... 1820

Pseudoephedrine Hydrochloride (Co-administration has resulted in a reversible enhancement of pressor response of pseudoephedrine). Products include:

Advil Allergy Sinus Caplets ... ■ 737
Advil Cold & Sinus ... ■ 739
Advil Flu & Body Ache Caplets ... ■ 739
Children's Advil Cold Suspension ... ■ 741
Advil Multi-Symptom Cold Caplets ... ■ 738
Allegra-D 12 Hour Extended-Release Tablets ... 2860
Allegra-D 24 Hour Extended-Release Tablets ... 2862
Balamine DM ... 739
BC Cold Powder ... ■ 612
Benadryl Allergy & Cold Tablets ... ■ 692
Benadryl Allergy & Sinus Headache Caplets & Gelcaps ... ■ 693
Children's Benadryl Allergy & Cold Fastmelt Tablets ... ■ 695
Benadryl Maximum Strength Severe Allergy & Sinus Headache Caplets ... ■ 694
Children's Benadryl D Allergy & Sinus Fastmelt Tablets ... ■ 694
Children's Benadryl D Liquid Medication ... ■ 693
Benadryl D Tablets ... ■ 694
Contac Non-Drowsy 12 Hour Cold Caplets ... ■ 614
Contac Non-Drowsy Timed Release 12 Hour Cold Caplets ... ■ 615
Contac Severe Cold and Flu Caplets Maximum Strength ... ■ 615
Contac Severe Cold and Flu Caplets Non-Drowsy ... ■ 615
Children's Dimetapp Cold & Allergy Elixir ... ■ 745
Children's Dimetapp DM Cold & Cough Elixir ... ■ 745
Children's Dimetapp Long Acting Cough Plus Cold Syrup ... ■ 746
Dimetapp Infant Drops Decongestant Plus Cough ... ■ 746
Children's Motrin Cold Non-Staining Dye-Free Oral Suspension ... 1838
Children's Motrin Cold Oral Suspension ... 1838
Motrin Cold & Sinus Caplets ... 1836
PediaCare Decongestant & Cough Infant Drops ... ■ 705
PediaCare Decongestant Infants' Drops ... ■ 705
PediaCare Long-Acting Cough Plus Cold Liquid ... ■ 704
PediaCare Multi-Symptom Cold Liquid ... ■ 704
PediaCare NightRest Cough & Cold Liquid ... ■ 704
Robitussin Allergy & Cough Syrup ... ■ 750
Robitussin CF Liquid ... ■ 755
Robitussin Cough & Cold Liquid-filled Capsules ... ■ 750
Robitussin Cough, Cold & Flu Liquid-filled Capsules ... ■ 750
Robitussin Cough & Cold Infant Drops ... ■ 755
Robitussin Flu Liquid ... ■ 752
Robitussin Maximum Strength Cough & Cold Liquid ... ■ 754
Robitussin PE Syrup ... ■ 753
Robitussin Pediatric Cough & Cold Liquid ... ■ 754
Robitussin PM Cough & Cold Liquid ... ■ 752
Robitussin Severe Congestion Liquid-filled Capsules ... ■ 751
Simply Stuffy Liquid ... 1841
Singlet Caplets ... ■ 636
Sudafed 12 Hour Caplets ... ■ 708
Sudafed 24 Hour Tablets ... ■ 709
Sudafed Nasal Decongestant Tablets ... ■ 709
Sudafed Severe Cold ... ■ 710
Sudafed Non-Drying Sinus Liquid Caps ... ■ 709
Sudafed Sinus & Allergy Tablets ... ■ 710
Sudafed Sinus Headache ... ■ 711
TheraFlu Cold & Cough Hot Liquid ... ■ 680
TheraFlu Cold & Sore Throat Hot Liquid ... ■ 680
TheraFlu Flu & Chest Congestion Non-Drowsy Hot Liquid ... ■ 681
TheraFlu Flu & Sore Throat Hot Liquid ... ■ 681
TheraFlu Severe Cold Non-Drowsy Hot Liquid ... ■ 683
TheraFlu Severe Cold & Cough Hot Liquid ... ■ 683
TheraFlu Severe Cold Caplets ... ■ 679
TheraFlu Severe Cold Hot Liquid ... ■ 682
TheraFlu Severe Cold Non-Drowsy Caplets ... ■ 679
Triaminic Chest & Nasal Congestion Liquid ... ■ 685
Triaminic Cold & Allergy Liquid ... ■ 685
Triaminic Cold & Cough Liquid ... ■ 685
Triaminic Cough Liquid ... ■ 687
Triaminic Cough & Nasal Congestion Liquid ... ■ 687
Triaminic Cough & Sore Throat Liquid ... ■ 687
Triaminic Flu, Cough & Fever Liquid ... ■ 685
Triaminic Night Time Cough & Cold Liquid ... ■ 685
Triaminic Allergy Runny Nose & Congestion Softchews ... ■ 688
Triaminic Cold & Cough Softchews ... ■ 688
Triaminic Cough & Sore Throat Softchews ... ■ 689
Tylenol Sinus NightTime Caplets ... ■ 663
Children's Tylenol Plus Cold & Allergy Suspension Liquid ... 1850
Children's Tylenol Plus Cold NightTime Suspension Liquid ... 1851
Children's Tylenol Plus Cold & Cough Suspension Liquid and Chewable Tablets ... 1851
Children's Tylenol Plus Cold Chewable Tablets ... 1851
Children's Tylenol Plus Cold Daytime Non-Drowsy Suspension Liquid ... 1851
Children's Tylenol Plus Flu Suspension Liquid ... 1853
Concentrated Tylenol Infants' Drops Plus Cold ... 1851
Concentrated Tylenol Infants' Drops Plus Cold and Cough ... 1851
Tylenol Cold & Flu Severe Daytime Liquid with Cool Bust ... 1846
Tylenol Cold & Flu Severe NightTime Liquid with Cool Burst ... 1846
Tylenol Cold Severe Congestion Non-Drowsy Caplets with Cool Burst ... 1846
Tylenol Allergy Complete Night Time Caplets ... 1844
Tylenol Allergy Complete Multi-Symptom Caplets and Gelcaps with Cool Burst ... 1844
Tylenol Flu NightTime Gelcaps ... 1846
Tylenol Flu Day Non-Drowsy Gelcaps ... 1846
Concentrated Tylenol Infants' Drops Plus Cold Nasal Congestant, Fever Reducer & Pain Reliever ... ■ 668
Concentrated Tylenol Infants' Drops Plus Cold & Cough Nasal Decongestant, Fever Reducer & Pain Reliever ... ■ 668
Multi-Symptom Tylenol Cold Night Time Caplets ... 1845
Multi-Symptom Tylenol Cold Day Non-Drowsy Caplets and Gelcaps ... 1845
Tylenol Sinus Day Non-Drowsy ... 1848
Tylenol Sinus Night Time Caplets ... 1848
Tylenol Sinus Severe Congestion Caplets with Cool Burst ... 1848
Vicks 44D Cough & Head Congestion Relief ... 2676
Vicks 44D Cough & Head Congestion Relief Liquid ... ■ 721
Vicks 44M Cough, Cold & Flu Relief ... 2676
Pediatric Vicks 44m Cough & Cold Relief ... 2673
Vicks DayQuil LiquiCaps/Liquid Multi-Symptom Cold/Flu Relief ... ■ 723
Vicks DayQuil Multi-Symptom Cold/Flu Relief LiquiCaps ... 2675
Vicks DayQuil Multi-Symptom Cold/Flu Relief Liquid ... 2675
Children's Vicks NyQuil Cold/Cough Relief ... 2671
Vicks NyQuil LiquiCaps ... 2677
Vicks NyQuil LiquiCaps/Liquid Multi-Symptom Cold/Flu Relief ... ■ 725
Vicks NyQuil Liquid ... 2677
Zyrtec-D 12 Hour Extended Release Tablets ... 2591

Pseudoephedrine Sulfate (Linezolid is a reversible nonselective inhibitor of MAO; therefore, linezolid has the potential for interaction with adrenergic agents). Products include:

Alavert Allergy & Sinus D-12 Hour Tablets ... ■ 743
Clarinex-D 24-Hour Extended-Release Tablets ... 3012
Claritin-D Non-Drowsy 12 Hour Tablets ... ■ 731
Claritin-D Non-Drowsy 24 Hour Tablets ... ■ 731

Salmeterol Xinafoate (Linezolid is a reversible nonselective inhibitor of MAO; therefore, linezolid has the potential for interaction with adrenergic agents). Products include:

Advair Diskus 100/50 ... 1291
Advair Diskus 250/50 ... 1291
Advair Diskus 500/50 ... 1291
Serevent Diskus ... 1540

Sertraline Hydrochloride (Linezolid is a reversible nonselective inhibitor of monoamine oxidase. Therefore, linezolid has the potential for interaction with serotonergic agents. Spontaneous reports of serotonin syndrome associated with co-administration of linezolid and serotinergic agents, including antidepressants such as selective serotonin reuptake inhibitors (SSRIs), have been reported. Patients who are treated with linezolid and concomitant serotinergic agents should be closely observed for signs and symptoms of serotonin syndrome (e.g., cognitive dysfunction, hyperpyrexia, hyperreflexia, incoordination). If any signs or symptoms occur, physicians should consider discontinuation of either one or both agents (linezolid or concomitant serotinergic agents)). Products include:

Zoloft ... 2581

Terbutaline Sulfate (Linezolid is a reversible nonselective inhibitor of MAO; therefore, linezolid has the potential for interaction with adrenergic agents).

No products indexed under this heading.

Tyramine (Co-administration has resulted in a significant pressor response).

No products indexed under this heading.

Venlafaxine Hydrochloride (Linezolid is a reversible nonselective inhibitor of monoamine oxidase. Therefore, linezolid has the potential for interaction with serotonergic agents. Spontaneous reports of serotonin syndrome associated with co-administration of linezolid and serotinergic agents, including antidepressants such as selective serotonin reuptake inhibitors (SSRIs), have been reported. Patients who are treated with linezolid and concomitant serotinergic agents should be closely observed for signs and symptoms of serotonin syndrome (e.g., cognitive dysfunction, hyperpyrexia, hyperreflexia, incoordination). If any signs or symptoms occur, physicians should consider discontinuation of either one or both agents (linezolid or concomitant serotinergic agents)). Products include:

Effexor Tablets ... 3405
Effexor XR Capsules ... 3411

Food Interactions

Beverages with high tyramine (Co-administration has resulted in a significant pressor response; patients receiving linezolid should avoid consuming large amounts of beverages containing tyramine).

Food, unspecified (The time to reach maximum concentration is delayed from 1.5 hours to 2.2 hours and Cmax is decreased by about 17% when linezolid is co-administered with high fat food; linezolid may be administered without regard to the timing of meals).

Food high in tyramine (Co-administration has resulted in a significant pressor response; patients receiving linezolid should avoid consuming large amounts of food containing tyramine).

SECTION 2

FOOD INTERACTIONS CROSS-REFERENCE

In this section, drug/food and drug/alcohol interactions listed in the preceding index are cross-referenced by dietary item. Under each entry is an alphabetical list, by brand name, of drugs said to interact with the item. A brief description of the interaction follows each brand, along with the page number of the underlying text. Page numbers refer to the 2006 editions of *PDR®* and *PDR for Ophthalmic Medicines™* and the 2005 edition of *PDR for Nonprescription Drugs and Dietary Supplements™*, which is published later each year. A key to the symbols denoting the companion volumes appears in the bottom margin.

Entries in this section are limited to drug/food and drug/alcohol interactions listed in official prescribing information as published by *PDR®*.

Alcohol

Actiq (Concurrent use with alcoholic beverages may result in increased depressant effects; hypoventilation, hypotension, and profound sedation may occur)........................ 993

ActoPlus Met Tablets (Alcohol is known to potentiate the effect of metformin on lactate metabolism. Patients, therefore, should be warned against excessive alcohol intake, acute or chronic, while receiving Actoplus Met)..................3219

Adipex-P Tablets (May result in adverse drug interaction) 1216

Advicor Tablets (Concomitant alcohol may increase the flushing and its use should be avoided around the time of Advicor administration)...................1694

Advil Allergy Sinus Caplets (Avoid alcohol; concurrent use may increase drowsiness. Heavy alcohol users, three or more drinks per day, should consult their physician for advice on when and how they should take pain relievers/fever reducers, including ibuprofen.)....................▣ 737

Advil Multi-Symptom Cold Caplets (Avoid alcohol; concurrent use may increase drowsiness. Heavy alcohol users, three or more drinks per day, should consult their physician for advice on when and how they should take pain relievers/fever reducers, including ibuprofen.)....................▣ 738

Agenerase Oral Solution (Concurrent use of Agenerase Oral Solution with alcoholic beverages is not recommended).....1304

Aggrenox Capsules (Patients who consume three or more alcoholic drinks every day should be counseled about the bleeding risks involved with chronic, heavy alcohol use while taking aspirin)................................ 855

Alacol DM Syrup (Antihistamines have additive effects with alcohol) 739

Aldoclor Tablets (Aggravates orthostatic hypotension) 1881

Aldoril Tablets (Aggravates orthostatic hypotension) 1884

Aleve Tablets, Caplets and Gelcaps (Individuals consuming 3 or more alcohol-containing drinks per day should consult their physicians for advice on when and how they should take this product).....................................▣ 605

Alphagan P Ophthalmic Solution (Possible additive or potentiating effect with CNS depressants) 563

Ambien Tablets (Co-administration produces additive effects on psychomotor performance) 2867

Antabuse Tablets (Disulfiram plus alcohol, even small amounts, produce flushing, throbbing in head and neck, throbbing headache, respiratory difficulty, nausea, vomiting, and confusion; concurrent use with alcohol-containing preparations, such as cough syrups, tonics, sauces, vinegars, and even aftershave lotion and back rubs should be avoided).........................2343

Apidra Injection (Alcohol may either potentiate or weaken the blood glucose-lowering effect of insulin) 2876

Apokyn Injection (The effects of apomorphine on blood pressure may be increased by the concomitant use of alcohol; concurrent use should be avoided) 2132

Astelin Nasal Spray (Concurrent use may result in additional reduction in alertness and impairment of CNS performance; alcohol intake should be avoided).........................1876

Atacand HCT 16-12.5 Tablets (May aggravate orthostatic hypotension produced by hydrochlorothiazide)....................... 637

Avalide Tablets (Potentiation of orthostatic hypotension) 2889

Avalide Tablets (Potentiation of orthostatic hypotension) 922

Avandamet Tablets (Alcohol potentiates the effect of metformin on lactate metabolism; patients should be warned against excessive alcohol intake, acute or chronic).....1343

Avinza Capsules (Concurrent use increases the risk of respiratory depression, hypotension, profound sedation, or coma) 1714

Balamine DM Oral Drops (Antihistamines have additive effects with alcohol)....................... 739

Aspirin Regimen Bayer Adult Low Strength 81 mg Tablets (Chronic heavy alcohol users, 3 or more drinks per day, should consult their physicians for advice on when and how they should take pain relievers/fever reducers including aspirin)..........................▣ 606

BC Allergy Sinus Cold Powder (Individuals consuming 3 or more alcohol-containing drinks per day should consult their physician for advice on when and how they should take this product; increases drowsiness; avoid concurrent use)...................▣ 612

Benadryl Allergy & Cold Tablets (Concurrent use may increase drowsiness) ....▣ 692

Benadryl Allergy Kapseal Capsules (May increase drowsiness effect) ....▣ 691

Children's Benadryl Allergy & Cold Fastmelt Tablets (May increase drowsiness effect; avoid concurrent use)...................▣ 695

Children's Benadryl Dye-Free Allergy Liquid (May increase the drowsiness effect)...................▣ 695

Benadryl D Tablets (Increases drowsiness effect; avoid concomitant use) ....▣ 694

Benicar HCT Tablets (Concurrent administration could cause potentiation of orthostatic hypotension)..................................2852

BiDil Tablets (The effects of BiDil on vasodilators, including alcohol, may be additive)................2161

Buprenex Injectable (Increased CNS depression)...........................2718

Captopril Tablets (Drugs having vasodilator activity should, if possible, be discontinued before starting captopril)................2114

Catapres Tablets (Clonidine may potentiate the CNS-depressive effects) 874

(▣ Described in PDR For Nonprescription Drugs)

(⊙ Described in PDR For Ophthalmic Medicines™)

Catapres-TTS (Clonidine may potentiate the CNS-depressive effects) 875

Celexa Tablets (Although citalopram did not potentiate cognitive and motor effects of alcohol, concurrent use is not recommended) 1177

Children's Benadryl Allergy Fastmelt Tablets (Alcohol may increase drowsiness. Avoid alcoholic drinks) .... ▣696

Cialis Tablets (Both tadalafil and alcohol act as mild vasodilators. When mild vasodilators are taken in combination, blood-pressure lowering effects of each individual compound may be increased. Substantial consumption of alcohol in combination with tadalafil may increase the potential for orthostatic signs and symptoms, including increase in heart rate, decrease in standing blood pressure, dizziness, and headache) 1806

Clorpres Tablets (Clonidine may enhance the CNS-depressive effects of alcohol; orthostatic hypotension may be aggravated by alcohol) 2139

Clozapine Tablets (Clozapine induces drowsiness and sedation in a significant number of patients; caution is advised with concomitant use) 2141

Clozaril Tablets (Given the primary CNS effect of clozapine, caution is advised in using it concomitantly with alcohol) 2174

Combunox Tablets (Patients receiving other CNS depressants (including alcohol) concomitantly with oxycodone may exhibit an additive CNS depression. Interactive effects resulting in respiratory depression, hypotension, profound sedation, or coma may result if these drugs are taken in combination with the usual dosage of oxycodone. When such combined therapy is contemplated, the dose of one or both agents should be reduced) 1183

Comtan Tablets (Possible additive sedative effects) 2186

Contac Severe Cold and Flu Caplets Maximum Strength (May increase drowsiness effect; concurrent use should be avoided) .... ▣615

Coumadin Tablets (Decreased or increased prothrombin time response) 932

Covera-HS Tablets (Verapamil may increase blood alcohol concentrations and prolong its effect) 3135

Cymbalta Delayed-Release Capsules (Use of duloxetine concomitantly with heavy alcohol intake may be associated with severe liver injury; therefore, duloxetine should ordinarily not be prescribed for patients with substantial alcohol use) 1729

Dantrium Capsules (Co-administration may result in increased drowsiness; caution should be exercised) 2690

Darvocet A 500 Tablets (Additive CNS depressant effects) 3497

Demser Capsules (Additive sedative effects) 1933

Depacon Injection (Co-administration may result in additive CNS depression) 412

Depakene Capsules (Valproate produces CNS depression, especially when combined with another CNS depressant, such as alcohol) 417

Depakote Tablets (Valproate produces CNS depression, especially when combined with another CNS depressant, such as alcohol) 427

DepoDur Extended-Release Injection (The concurrent use of other central nervous system (CNS) depressants, including alcohol, increases the risk of respiratory depression, hypotension, profound sedation or coma. Use with caution and with vigilant monitoring in patients taking these agents) 1098

Diastat Rectal Delivery System (Potential for synergistic CNS-depressant effect) 3344

Dilaudid Ampules (Additive CNS depression) 439

Dilaudid Oral Liquid (May exhibit an additive CNS depression) 443

Children's Dimetapp Cold & Allergy Elixir (May increase drowsiness effect) .... ▣745

Children's Dimetapp DM Cold & Cough Elixir (Increases drowsiness effect; avoid concurrent use) .... ▣745

Diovan HCT Tablets (Co-administration of thiazide diuretics and alcohol may result in potentiation of orthostatic hypotension) 2195

Ditropan XL Extended Release Tablets (Enhances the drowsiness effect caused by anticholinergic agents such as oxybutynin) 2391

Diuril Oral Suspension (Potentiation of orthostatic hypotension may occur) 1936

Diuril Sodium Intravenous (Potentiation of orthostatic hypotension may occur) 1934

Duragesic Transdermal System (The concomitant use of fentanyl with other CNS depressants, including alcohol, may cause repiratory depression, hypotension, and profound sedation or potentially result in coma. When such combined therapy is contemplated, the dose of one or both agents should be significantly reduced) 2448

Ecotrin Enteric Coated Aspirin Low, Regular and Maximum Strength Tablets (Chronic heavy alcohol users, 3 or more drinks per day, in combination with analgesic/antipyretic drug products containing aspirin increases the risk of adverse GI events, including stomach bleeding) 1627

Effexor XR Capsules (Co-administration of venlafaxine as a stable regimen did not exaggerate the psychomotor and psychometric effects of alcohol; however, patients should be advised to avoid alcohol while taking venlafaxine) 3411

Equetro Extended-Release Capsules (Because of its primary CNS effect, caution should be used when carbamazepine is taken with alcohol) 3178

FazaClo Orally Disintegrating Tablets (Given the primary CNS effect of clozapine, caution is advised in using it concomitantly with alcohol) 547

Flexeril Tablets (Concurrent use results in enhanced effects) 1832

Flolan for Injection (Additional reductions in blood pressure may occur) 1408

Fortamet Extended-Release Tablets (Alcohol is known to potentiate the effect of metformin on lactate metabolism; therefore, patients should be warned against excessive acute or chronic intake) 1156

Furosemide Tablets (Aggravates orthostatic hypotension) 2117

Gabitril Tablets (Possible additive depressive effects) 998

Geodon Capsules (Somnolence was a commonly reported adverse event in patients treated with ziprasidone; concurrent use with alcohol or other CNS active drugs, such as depressants, should be undertaken with caution) 2514

Goody's Extra Strength Pain Relief Tablets (Individuals consuming 3 or more alcohol-containing drinks per day should consult their physicians for advice on when and how they should take this product) .... ▣621

Goody's PM Powder (Individuals consuming 3 or more alcohol-containing drinks per day should consult their physicians for advice on when and how they should take this product; avoid alcoholic beverages since diphenhydramine causes drowsiness) .... ▣622

Gris-PEG Tablets (The effects of alcohol may be potentiated by griseofulvin, producing such effects as tachycardia and flushing) 2504

Humalog-Pen (Co-administration with drugs with hypoglycemic activity may result in decreased insulin requirements) 1751

Hycodan Tablets (Exhibits an additive CNS depression) 1104

Hycomine Compound Tablets (Exhibits an additive CNS depression) 1105

Hycotuss Expectorant Syrup (Exhibits an additive CNS depression) 1106

Hyzaar 50-12.5 Tablets (Potentiation of orthostatic hypotension) 1964

Imdur Tablets (Additive vasodilating effects) 3032

Indapamide Tablets (Aggravates orthostatic hypotension) 2119

Inderal LA Long-Acting Capsules (Slows the rate of absorption of propranolol) 3421

Inversine Tablets (The action of mecamylamine may be potentiated by alcohol) 3286

Kadian Capsules (Co-administration may increase the risk of respiratory depression, hypotension and profound sedation and coma) 572

Klonopin Tablets (Potentiates CNS-depressant action) 2782

Lantus Injection (May either potentiate or weaken the blood-glucose-lowering effect of insulin) 2925

Lexapro Tablets (Given the primary CNS effects of escitalopram, concurrent use is not recommended) 1193

Lortab 10/500 Tablets (Co-administration may exhibit additive CNS-depression; concurrent use should be avoided) 3315

Lotensin HCT Tablets (Orthostatic hypotension produced by thiazides may be potentiated by alcohol) 2235

Lunesta Tablets (An additive effect on psychomotor performance was seen with co-administration of eszopiclone and alcohol 0.70 g/kg for up to 4 hours after alcohol consumption) 3139

Marinol Capsules (Co-administration results in additive drowsiness and CNS depression) 3334

Matulane Capsules (Concurrent use may produce an Antabuse-like reaction; concomitant use should be avoided) 3188

Maxzide Tablets (May aggravate orthostatic hypotension) 2150

Meridia Capsules (Concurrent use has not resulted in psychomotor reactions of clinical significance, however, concomitant use with excessive alcohol is not recommended) 485

MetroGel-Vaginal Gel (Possibility of a disulfiram-like reaction) 1822

Mevacor Tablets (Lovastatin should be used with caution in patients who have consumed substantial quantity of alcohol and have a past history of liver disease; active liver disease and unexplained elevation in transaminase are contraindications to the use of lovastatin) 1996

Micardis HCT Tablets (Potentiation of orthostatic hypotension) 886

Miradon Tablets (Has been reported to diminish and/or increase oral anticoagulant response, i.e., decreased prothrombin time response significantly) 3056

Moduretic Tablets (Potentiation of orthostatic hypotension) 2003

Motrin Cold & Sinus Caplets (Chronic heavy alcohol users, three or more drinks per day, should consult their physicians for advice on when and how they should take pain relievers/fever reducers including ibuprofen) 1836

MS Contin Tablets (Respiratory depression, hypotension and profound sedation or coma may result) 2703

Nembutal Sodium Solution, USP (Concomitant use of other CNS depressants may produce additive depressant effects) 2484

Niaspan Extended-Release Tablets (Concomitant alcohol may increase the side effects of flushing and pruritus and should be avoided around the time of Niaspan ingestion) 1703

Nitro-Dur Transdermal Infusion System (Enhances sensitivity to the hypotensive effects) 3060

Nitrolingual Pumpspray (Enhanced sensitivity to hypotensive effects) 1161

NovoLog Injection (May either potentiate or weaken the blood-glucose-lowering effect of insulin) 2326

Nubain Injection (Additive CNS depression) 1111

Numorphan Injection (Concomitant use may produce additive CNS depressant effects) 1112

Maximum Strength Nytol QuickGels Softgels (Concurrent use will heighten the depressant effect of Nytol; avoid alcoholic beverages while taking this product) .... ▣635

Orap Tablets (Pimozide may be capable of potentiating CNS depressants, including alcohol) 1220

OxyContin Tablets (Concurrent use with the usual dose of OxyContin may result in respiratory depression, profound sedation or coma) 2699

OxyIR Capsules (Concomitant use may exhibit an additive CNS depression) 2704

Oxytrol Transdermal System (May enhance drowsiness caused by anticholinergic agents such as oxybutynin) 3383

Parnate Tablets (Concurrent use is contraindicated; a marked potentiating effect on alcohol has been reported) **1499**

Paxil Tablets (Concurrent use should be avoided) **1501**

Percocet Tablets (Additive CNS depression) **1114**

Percodan Tablets (Additive CNS depression) **1115**

Permax Tablets (Pergolide may cause somnolence; concurrent use with alcohol may result in additive sedative effects) **3357**

Phenergan Suppositories (Promethazine may increase, prolong, or intensify the sedative action of other CNS depressants, such as alcohol) **3438**

Phenytek Capsules (Acute alcohol intake may increase phenytoin serum levels; chronic alcohol abuse may decrease phenytoin serum levels) **2153**

Photofrin for Injection (Compounds that quench active oxygen species or scavenge radicals, such as ethanol, would be expected to decrease photodynamic therapy; no human data available to support or rebut this possibility) **729**

Prinzide Tablets (Co-administration of thiazide and alcohol may potentiate orthostatic hypotension) **2033**

ProSom Tablets (Co-administration may result in increased CNS depression) **512**

Provigil Tablets (The use of modafinil in combination with alcohol has not been studied. It is advisable to avoid alcohol while taking modafinil) **1002**

Prozac Pulvules and Liquid (Concurrent use with CNS active agents, such as alcohol, requires caution) **1771**

Renova 0.05% Cream (Topical products with high concentration of alcohol may increase the irritation when used concurrently) **2387**

Requip Tablets (Possible additive sedative effects) **1528**

Rilutek Tablets (Alcohol may increase the risk of hepatotoxicity; patients on riluzole should be discouraged from drinking excessive amounts of alcohol) **2945**

Risperdal Tablets (Given the primary CNS effects of risperidone, caution should be taken if used with alcohol) **1658**

Robitussin Allergy & Cough Syrup (May increase drowsiness effect) .... ▣ **750**

Robitussin Cough, Cold & Flu Liquid-filled Capsules (Chronic heavy alcohol users, 3 or more drinks per day, should consult their physicians for advice on when and how they should take pain relievers/fever reducers including acetaminophen) .... ▣ **750**

Robitussin Flu Liquid (Chronic heavy alcohol users, 3 or more drinks per day, should consult their physicians for advice on when and how they should take pain relievers/fever reducers including acetaminophen; increases drowsiness effect) .... ▣ **752**

Robitussin PM Cough & Cold Liquid (Chronic heavy alcohol users, 3 or more drinks per day, should consult their physician for advice on when and how they should take pain relievers/fever reducers including acetaminophen; increases drowsiness effect; avoid alcoholic beverages) .... ▣ **752**

Rozerem Tablets (With single-dose, daytime co-administration of ramelteon 32 mg and alcohol (0.6 g/kg), there were no clinically meaningful or statistically significant effects on peak or total exposure to ramelteon. However, an additive effect was seen on some measures of psychomotor performance (ie. the Digit Symbol Substitution Test, the Psychomotor Vigilance Task Test, and a Visual Analog Scale of sedation) at some post-dose time points. No additive effect was seen on the Delayed Word Recognition Test. Because alcohol by itself impairs performance, and the intended effect of ramelteon is to promote sleep, patients should be cautioned not to consume alcohol when using ramelteon) **3228**

Sedapap Tablets 50 mg/650 mg (Additive CNS depression) **2098**

Seromycin Capsules (Concurrent use increases the possibility and risk of epileptic episodes) **1783**

Seroquel Tablets (The cognitive and motor effect of alcohol is potentiated; alcohol use should be avoided) **691**

Simply Sleep Caplets (Diphenhydramine is an antihistamine with sedative properties; concurrent use with alcoholic beverages should be avoided) **1841**

Singlet Caplets (Chronic heavy alcohol users, 3 or more drinks per day, should consult their physicians for advice on when and how they should take pain relievers/fever reducers including acetaminophen; increases drowsiness effect) .... ▣ **636**

Skelaxin Tablets (Skelaxin may enhance the effects of alcohol, barbiturates and other CNS depressants) **1685**

Solage Topical Solution (Concomitant topical products with a strong skin drying effect, such as products with high concentrations of alcohol, should be used with caution in patients being treated with Solage because they may increase irritation when used with Solage) **740**

Sominex Original Formula Tablets (Concurrent use of alcoholic beverages is not recommended) .... ▣ **637**

Sonata Capsules (Concurrent use may produce additive CNS depressant effects) **1686**

Soriatane Capsules (Clinical evidence has shown that etretinate can be formed with concurrent ingestion of acitretin and ethanol) **1028**

St. Joseph 81 mg Aspirin Chewable and Enteric Coated Tablets (Chronic heavy alcohol users, 3 or more drinks per day, in combination with analgesic/antipyretic drug products containing aspirin increases the risk of adverse GI events, including stomach bleeding) **1841**

Sudafed Non-Drowsy Severe Cold Caplets (Chronic heavy alcohol users, 3 or more drinks per day, should consult their physicians for advice on when and how they should take pain relievers/fever reducers including acetaminophen) .... ▣ **710**

Sudafed Sinus & Allergy Tablets (May increase drowsiness effect) .... ▣ **710**

Surmontil Capsules (Concurrent use is associated with exaggerated effects) **2347**

Sustiva Capsules (Potential for additive central nervous system effects when Sustiva is used concomitantly with alcohol) **957**

Symbyax Capsules (Alcohol may potentiate the orthostatic effect of olanzapine, increasing the risk of orthostatic hypotension. Therefore, patients should be advised to avoid alcohol while taking Symbyax) **1788**

Symmetrel Tablets (May increase the potential for CNS effects such as dizziness, confusion, light-headedness and orthostatic hypotension; avoid excessive alcohol usage) **1115**

Tasmar Tablets (Possible additive sedative effects when used in combination with CNS depressants, such as alcohol) **3360**

Teveten HCT Tablets (May potentiate orthostatic hypotension) **1710**

Thalomid Capsules (Thalidomide has been reported to enhance the sedative activity of alcohol) **979**

TheraFlu Cold & Cough Hot Liquid (Concurrent use may increase drowsiness; avoid alcoholic drinks) .... ▣ **680**

TheraFlu Cold & Sore Throat Hot Liquid (Concurrent use may increase drowsiness; avoid alcoholic drinks) .... ▣ **680**

TheraFlu Flu & Chest Congestion Non-Drowsy Hot Liquid (Concurrent use may increase drowsiness; avoid alcoholic drinks) .... ▣ **681**

TheraFlu Flu & Sore Throat Hot Liquid (Concurrent use may increase drowsiness; avoid alcoholic drinks) .... ▣ **681**

TheraFlu Severe Cold Non-Drowsy Hot Liquid (Chronic heavy alcohol users, 3 or more drinks per day, should consult their physicians for advice on when and how they should take pain relievers/fever reducers, including acetaminophen; may increase the drowsiness effect) .... ▣ **683**

TheraFlu Severe Cold & Cough Hot Liquid (Concurrent use may increase drowsiness; avoid alcoholic drinks) .... ▣ **683**

TheraFlu Severe Cold Caplets (Concurrent use may increase drowsiness; avoid alcoholic drinks) .... ▣ **679**

TheraFlu Severe Cold Hot Liquid (Concurrent use may increase drowsiness; avoid alcoholic drinks) .... ▣ **682**

TheraFlu Thin Strips Multi Symptom (Co-administration with alcohol may increase drowsiness) .... ▣ **684**

Thioridazine Hydrochloride Tablets (Thioridazine is capable of potentiating CNS depressants) **2122**

Thiothixene Capsules (Possible additive effects which may include hypotension) **2124**

Tindamax (Alcoholic beverages should be avoided during tinidazole therapy and for three days afterward because abdominal cramps, nausea, vomiting, headaches and flushing may occur) **2670**

Topamax Tablets (Potential for increased CNS depression) **2438**

Transderm Scōp Transdermal Therapeutic System (Scopolamine is an anticholinergic agent and causes certain CNS effects, such as drowsiness and dizziness, and hence it should be used with care in patients on concomitant therapy) **2166**

Tranxene T-TAB Tablets (Actions of benzodiazepines may be potentiated; prolonged sleeping time) **2488**

Trecator Tablets (Excessive ethanol ingestion should be avoided because a psychotic reaction has been reported) **3482**

Triaminic Cold & Cough Softchews (May increase drowsiness effect) .... ▣ **688**

Trileptal Tablets (Oxcarbazepine causes dizziness and somnolence, concurrent use with alcohol could result in possible additive sedative effect) **2281**

Tri-Luma Cream (Patients should avoid topical products containing high alcohol concentrations) **1213**

Trizivir Tablets (Concurrent use decreases the elimination of abacavir causing an increase in overall exposure) **1565**

Tussionex Pennkinetic Extended-Release Suspension (Combined use may result in additive CNS depression) **3322**

Tylenol 8-Hour Extended Release Geltabs/Caplets (Chronic heavy alcohol users, 3 or more drinks per day, should consult their physicians for advice on when and how they should take pain relievers including acetaminophen) .... ▣ **655**

Tylenol Cough & Sore Throat NightTime Liquid with Cool Burst (Co-administration with alcohol may increase drowsiness; avoid concurrent alcohol use) .... ▣ **664**

Tylenol Cold Severe Congestion Non-Drowsy Caplets with Cool Burst (Chronic heavy alcohol abusers, 3 or more drinks per day, may be at increased risk of liver toxicity from acetaminophen use) **1846**

Tylenol Cough & Sore Throat NightTime Liquid with Cool Burst (Co-administration with alcohol may increase drowsiness; avoid concurrent alcohol use) **1849**

Regular Strength Tylenol Tablets (Chronic heavy alcohol users, 3 or more drinks per day, should consult their physicians for advice on when and how they should take pain relievers including acetaminophen) **1843**

Tylenol Allergy Complete Night Time Caplets (Concurrent use may increase drowsiness effect; chronic heavy alcohol abusers, 3 or more drinks per day, may be at increased risk of liver toxicity from excessive acetaminophen use) **1844**

Tylenol Flu NightTime Gelcaps (Concurrent use may increase drowsiness effect; chronic heavy alcohol abusers, 3 or more drinks per day, may be at increased risk of liver toxicity from excessive acetaminophen use) **1846**

Extra Strength Tylenol PM Caplets, Geltabs, Gelcaps and Liquid (Avoid concurrent use; chronic heavy alcohol abusers, 3 or more drinks per day, may be at increased risk of liver toxicity from acetaminophen use) **1847**

Tylenol Sinus Night Time Caplets (May increase drowsiness effect) **1848**

Tylenol with Codeine Elixir (Concurrent use with other CNS depressants may exhibit an additive CNS depression) **2461**

Women's Tylenol Menstrual Relief Caplets (Chronic heavy alcohol users, 3 or more drinks per day, should consult their physicians for advice on when and how they should take pain relievers, including acetaminophen) **1849**

Ultracet Tablets (Tramadol increases the risk of CNS and respiratory depression with concurrent use; alcohol consumption with Ultracet is not recommended) **2462**

Uniphyl Tablets (Concurrent use with a single dose of alcohol (3mL/kg of whiskey) decreases theophylline clearance for up to 24 hours)....2708
Uniretic Tablets (Co-administration of alcohol with thiazide diuretics may result in potentiation of orthostatic hypotension)....3114
Unisom SleepTabs (Use Unisom cautiously)....■ 713
Unisom Maximum Strength SleepGels (Concurrent use with alcoholic beverages should be avoided)....■ 712
Valium Tablets (May potentiate the actions of diazepam)....2822
Vaseretic Tablets (Co-administration of thiazide and alcohol may potentiate orthostatic hypotension)....2073
Ventavis Inhalation Solution (Iloprost has the potential to increase the hypotensive effect of vasodilators and antihypertensive agents)....1036
Verelan PM Capsules (Verapamil has been found to significantly inhibit ethanol elimination resulting in elevated blood ethanol concentration that may prolong the intoxicating effects of alcohol)....3120
Vicks 44M Cough, Cold & Flu Relief (May increase drowsiness effect; patients consuming 3 or more alcoholic drinks per day should consult their physician for advice on when and how they should take this medication)....2676
Pediatric Vicks 44m Cough & Cold Relief (May increase drowsiness effect)....2673
Vicks DayQuil Multi-Symptom Cold/Flu Relief Liquid (Patients consuming 3 or more alcoholic drinks per day should consult their physician for advice on when and how they should take this medication)....2675
Children's Vicks NyQuil Cold/Cough Relief (May increase drowsiness effect)....2671
Vicks NyQuil LiquiCaps (May increase drowsiness effect; patients consuming 3 or more alcoholic drinks per day should consult their physician for advice on when and how they should take this medication)....2677
Vicks NyQuil LiquiCaps/Liquid Multi-Symptom Cold/Flu Relief (Chronic heavy alcohol users, 3 or more drinks per day, are at increased risk of liver toxicity from excessive acetaminophen use; alcohol increases drowsiness effect and concurrent use of alcoholic beverages should be avoided)....■ 725
Vicodin Tablets (May exhibit an additive CNS depression).... 530
Vicodin ES Tablets (Additive CNS depression).... 531
Vicodin HP Tablets (Concurrent use results in an additive CNS depression).... 532
Vicoprofen Tablets (May exhibit additive CNS depression).... 533
Visudyne for Injection (Co-administration with compounds that quench active oxygen species or scavenge radicals, such as ethanol, would be expected to decrease verteporfin activity)....2286
Vivactil Tablets (Co-administration results in enhanced response to alcohol)....2350
Wellbutrin SR Sustained-Release Tablets (Bupropion hydrochloride is contraindicated in patients undergoing abrupt discontinuation of alcohol. The consumption of alcohol during treatment with bupropion hydrochloride should be minimized or avoided)....1583
Xanax XR Tablets (Additive CNS depressant effects)....2655
Zestoretic Tablets (Potentiation of orthostatic hypotension may occur).... 701
Ziagen Tablets (Decreases the elimination of abacavir causing an increase in overall exposure)....1600
Zocor Tablets (Simvastatin causes persistent increases in serum transaminase in 1% of patients; therefore, it should be used with caution in patients who consume substantial quantities of alcohol)....2078
Zoloft Oral Concentrate (Patients should be told that although sertraline hydrochloride has not been shown in experiments with normal subjects to increase the mental and motor skill impairments caused by alcohol, the concomitant use of sertraline hydrochloride and alcohol is not advised)....2581
Zyban Sustained-Release Tablets (Bupropion hydrochloride is contraindicated in patients undergoing abrupt discontinuation of alcohol. The consumption of alcohol during treatment with bupropion hydrochloride should be minimized or avoided)....1620
Zydone Tablets (Co-administration may exhibit additive CNS depression)....1118
Zyprexa Tablets (Co-administration of alcohol with olanzapine potentiates orthostatic hypotension; concurrent use should be avoided)....1798
Zyprexa IntraMuscular (Co-administration of alcohol with olanzapine potentiates orthostatic hypotension; concurrent use should be avoided)....1798
Zyrtec Tablets (Concurrent use may result in additional impairment of CNS performance and reduction in mental alertness)....2589
Zyrtec-D 12 Hour Extended Release Tablets (Concurrent use may result in additional reduction in alertness impairment of CNS performance)....2591

Anchovies
Parnate Tablets (Potential for hypertensive crisis; concurrent use is contraindicated)....1499

Avocados
Parnate Tablets (Potential for hypertensive crisis; concurrent use is contraindicated)....1499

Bananas
Matulane Capsules (Procarbazine exhibits some MAO inhibitory activity: concurrent use should be avoided)....3188
Parnate Tablets (Potential for hypertensive crisis; concurrent use is contraindicated)....1499

Beans, broad
Parnate Tablets (Potential for hypertensive crisis; concurrent use is contraindicated)....1499

Beans, Fava
Parnate Tablets (Potential for hypertensive crisis; concurrent use is contraindicated)....1499

Beer, alcohol-free
Parnate Tablets (Potential for hypertensive crisis; concurrent use is contraindicated)....1499

Beer, unspecified
Parnate Tablets (Potential for hypertensive crisis; concurrent use is contraindicated)....1499

Beverages, caffeine-containing
Fosamax Tablets (Concomitant administration of alendronate with coffee reduces bioavailability by approximately 60%)....1949
Fosamax Plus D Tablets (Concomitant administration of alendronate with coffee reduces bioavailability by approximately 60%)....1956
Parnate Tablets (Potential for hypertensive crisis; concurrent use is contraindicated)....1499

Beverages with high tyramine
Zyvox Tablets (Co-administration has resulted in a significant pressor response; patients receiving linezolid should avoid consuming large amounts of beverages containing tyramine)....2661

Broccoli
Biltricide Tablets (Concomitant administration of drugs that increase the activity of drug metabolizing liver enzymes (Cytochrome P450) may reduce plasma levels of praziquantel)....2990
Cafcit Injection (Caffeine has the potential to interact with drugs that induce CYP1A2)....1854
Rozerem Tablets (Efficacy may be reduced when ramelteon is used in combination with strong CYP enzyme inducers such as rifampin)....3228
Symbyax Capsules (Agents that induce CYP1A2 or glucuronyl transferase enzymes may cause an increase in olanzapine concentration)....1788
Zyprexa Tablets (May cause an increase in olanzapine clearance; therefore, a dosage increase might be considered)....1798
Zyprexa IntraMuscular (May cause an increase in olanzapine clearance; therefore, a dosage increase might be considered)....1798

Brussel Sprouts
Biltricide Tablets (Concomitant administration of drugs that increase the activity of drug metabolizing liver enzymes (Cytochrome P450) may reduce plasma levels of praziquantel)....2990
Cafcit Injection (Caffeine has the potential to interact with drugs that induce CYP1A2)....1854
Rozerem Tablets (Efficacy may be reduced when ramelteon is used in combination with strong CYP enzyme inducers such as rifampin)....3228
Symbyax Capsules (Agents that induce CYP1A2 or glucuronyl transferase enzymes may cause an increase in olanzapine concentration)....1788
Zyprexa Tablets (May cause an increase in olanzapine clearance; therefore, a dosage increase might be considered)....1798
Zyprexa IntraMuscular (May cause an increase in olanzapine clearance; therefore, a dosage increase might be considered)....1798

Caviar
Parnate Tablets (Potential for hypertensive crisis; concurrent use is contraindicated)....1499

Charbroiled Food
Biltricide Tablets (Concomitant administration of drugs that increase the activity of drug metabolizing liver enzymes (Cytochrome P450) may reduce plasma levels of praziquantel)....2990
Cafcit Injection (Caffeine has the potential to interact with drugs that induce CYP1A2)....1854
Rozerem Tablets (Efficacy may be reduced when ramelteon is used in combination with strong CYP enzyme inducers such as rifampin)....3228
Symbyax Capsules (Agents that induce CYP1A2 or glucuronyl transferase enzymes may cause an increase in olanzapine concentration)....1788
Zyprexa Tablets (May cause an increase in olanzapine clearance; therefore, a dosage increase might be considered)....1798
Zyprexa IntraMuscular (May cause an increase in olanzapine clearance; therefore, a dosage increase might be considered)....1798

Cheese, aged
Matulane Capsules (Procarbazine exhibits some MAO inhibitory activity: concurrent use should be avoided)....3188
Parnate Tablets (Potential for hypertensive crisis; concurrent use is contraindicated)....1499

Cheese, strong, unpasteurized
Parnate Tablets (Potential for hypertensive crisis; concurrent use is contraindicated)....1499

Cheese, unspecified
Parnate Tablets (Potential for hypertensive crisis; concurrent use is contraindicated)....1499

Chocolate
Parnate Tablets (Potential for hypertensive crisis; concurrent use is contraindicated)....1499

Cotton seed meal
Levoxyl Tablets (Concurrent use of cotton seed meal may bind and decrease the absorption of levothyroxine sodium from GI tract)....1680
Unithroid Tablets (Concurrent use of cotton seed meal may bind and decrease the absorption of levothyroxine sodium from GI tract)....3521

Cream, sour
Parnate Tablets (Potential for hypertensive crisis; concurrent use is contraindicated)....1499

Dairy products
Cipro I.V. (Oral ciprofloxacin should not be taken concurrently with milk or yogurt alone, since absorption of ciprofloxacin may be significantly reduced; dietary calcium as part of a meal; however, does not significantly affect ciprofloxacin absorption)....2998
Cipro Tablets (Oral ciprofloxacin should not be taken concurrently with milk or yogurt alone, since absorption of ciprofloxacin may be significantly reduced; dietary calcium as part of a meal, however, does not significantly affect ciprofloxacin absorption)....2991
Cipro XR Tablets (Concurrent administration of ciprofloxacin with dairy products should be avoided since decreased absorption of ciprofloxacin is possible)....3004
Cuprimine Capsules (In all patients receiving penicillamine, it is important that penicillamine be given at least one hour apart from milk. This permits maximim absorption and reduces the likelihood of inactivation by metal binding in the gastrointestinal tract)....1925
Dulcolax Tablets (Dulcolax should not be taken within one hour of taking milk)....■ 607
Emcyt Capsules (Calcium-rich foods may impair the absorption of estramustine)....3137
Fleet Phospho-soda ACCU-PREP (Concurrent use within one hour should be avoided)....1171
Fleet Prep Kits (Concurrent use within one hour should be avoided)....1172

Noroxin Tablets (Avoid simultaneous ingestion; administer norfloxacin at least one hour before or two hours after ingestion of milk and/or other dairy products) 2009
Relafen Tablets (Potential for more rapid absorption; however, the total amount of GMNA in the plasma is unchanged) 1523
Tambocor Tablets (Milk may inhibit absorption in infants; a reduction in Tambocor dosage should be considered when milk is removed from the diet of infants) 1824

Diet, high-lipid

Adalat CC Tablets (High-fat meal increases peak plasma nifedipine concentrations by 60%, a prolongation in the time to peak concentration, but no significant change in the AUC; administer on an empty stomach) 2978
Albenza Tablets (Oral bioavailability appears to be enhanced when albendazole is co-administered with a fatty meal) 1310
Allegra-D 12 Hour Extended-Release Tablets (Co-administration with a high-fat meal decreased fexofenadine plasma concentrations Cmax and AUC, and Tmax was delayed by 50%; the rate of extent of pseudoephedrine absorption was not affected by food; administration of Allegra-D with food should be avoided) 2860
Gengraf Capsules (A high fat meal within one-half hour before cyclosporine administration decreases the AUC by 13% and Cmax by 33%) 458
Neoral Soft Gelatin Capsules (A high-fat meal consumed within one-half hour before Neoral administration decreased the AUC by 13% and Cmax by 33%) 2247
Rilutek Tablets (Co-administration with high-fat meal decreases absorption, reduces AUC by about 20% and peak blood levels by about 45%) 2945
Sular Tablets (Food with a high fat content has a pronounced effect on the release of nisoldipine resulting in a significant increase in peak concentration (Cmax) by up to 300%; concomitant intake of high-fat meal should be avoided) 1163
Uniphyl Tablets (Co-administration with a standardized high-fat meal results in increased peak plasma concentration and bioavailability; however, a precipitous increase in the rate and extent of absorption was not evident; the dosing should be ideally administered consistently either with or without food) 2708

Diet, potassium-rich

Maxzide Tablets (Concurrent use is contraindicated) 2150
Midamor Tablets (Potential for rapid increases in serum potassium levels) 2000
Moduretic Tablets (Potential for rapid increases in serum potassium levels) 2003

Diet high in vitamin K

Coumadin Tablets (Decreased prothrombin time) 932
Miradon Tablets (Has been reported to diminish oral anticoagulant response, i.e., decreased prothrombin time response significantly) 3056

Dietary Fiber

Levoxyl Tablets (Concurrent use of dietary fiber may bind and decrease the absorption of levothyroxine sodium from GI tract) 1680
Unithroid Tablets (Concurrent use of dietary fiber may bind and decrease the absorption of levothyroxine sodium from GI tract) 3521

Drinks, hot, unspecified

Advicor Tablets (Concomitant hot drinks may increase the flushing and its use should be avoided around the time of Advicor administration) 1694
Niaspan Extended-Release Tablets (Concomitant hot drinks may increase the side effects of flushing and pruritus and should be avoided around the time of Niaspan ingestion) 1703

Figs, canned

Parnate Tablets (Potential for hypertensive crisis; concurrent use is contraindicated) 1499

Food, calcium-rich

Cipro XR Tablets (Concurrent administration of ciprofloxacin with calcium-fortified juices should be avoided since decreased absorption of ciprofloxacin is possible) 3004
Emcyt Capsules (Calcium-rich foods may impair the absorption of estramustine) 3137

Food, charcoal-broiled

Rilutek Tablets (Potential inducers of CYP1A2, such as charcoal-broiled food, could increase the rate of riluzole elimination) 2945

Food, unspecified

Accolate Tablets (Co-administration with food reduces mean bioavailability by approximately 40%; patients should be instructed to take Accolate at least 1 hour before or 2 hours after meals) 663
Aceon Tablets (2 mg, 4 mg, 8 mg) (The presence of food in the GI tract does not affect the rate or extent of absorption of perindopril but reduces bioavailability of perindoprilat by about 35%; in clinical trials, perindopril was generally administered in a non-fasting state) 3191
Actonel Tablets (Mean oral bioavailability is decreased when risedronate is administered with food; risedronate sodium is effective when administered at least 30 minutes before breakfast) 2679
Actonel with Calcium Tablets (Mean oral bioavailability is decreased when risedronate is administered with food; risedronate sodium is effective when administered at least 30 minutes before breakfast) 2684
Adderall XR Capsules (Concurrent use with food prolongs T_{max} by 2.5 hours, however, food does not affect the extent of absorption) 3169
Agenerase Oral Solution (High-fat meals may decrease the absorption of Agenerase and should be avoided; Agenerase may be taken with meals of normal fat content) 1304
Altace Capsules (The rate of absorption is reduced, not the extent of absorption) 1673
Altoprev Extended-Release Tablets (Decreases the bioavailability of Altoprev) 1151
Aromasin Tablets (Exemestane plasma levels increased approximately 40% after high-fat breakfast) 2600
Avandamet Tablets (Food decreases the extent and slightly delays the absorption of metformin) 1343
Biaxin Filmtab Tablets (Food slightly delays both the onset of absorption and the formation of the active metabolite, but does not affect the extent of bioavailability; Biaxin may be administered without regard to food) 402
Captopril Tablets (Reduces absorption by about 30% to 40%; should be given one hour before meals) 2114
Carbatrol Capsules (A high fat meal increased the rat of absorption of a single 400 mg dose but not the AUC; elimination half-life remains unchanged between fasting and fed states) 3174
Ceftin Tablets (Absorption is greater when taken after food) 1369
Celebrex Capsules (Co-administration with a high-fat meal delayed peak plasma levels for about 1 to 2 hours with an increase in total absorption (AUC) of 10% to 20%; Celebrex can be administered without regard to the timing of meals) 3130
CellCept Capsules (Food has no effect on MPA AUC, but has been shown to decrease MPA Cmax by 40%; it is recommended that CellCept be administered on an empty stomach) 2751
Cipro I.V. (Delays the oral absorption of the drug resulting in peak concentrations that are closer to two hours after dosing) 2998
Cipro Tablets (Delays the oral absorption of the drug resulting in peak concentrations that are closer to two hours after dosing) 2991
Clinoril Tablets (The peak plasma concentrations of biologically active sulfide metabolite is delayed slightly in the presence of food) 1899
Coreg Tablets (When carvedilol is administered with food, the rate of absorption is slowed, as evidenced by a delay in the time to reach peak plasma levels, with no significant difference in extent of bioavailability; patients should be instructed to take Coreg with food in order to minimize the risk of hypotension) 1376
Crixivan Capsules (Co-administration with a meal high in calories, fat, and protein has resulted in a 77% ± 8% reduction in AUC and an 84% ± 7% reduction in Cmax; administer without food 1 hour before or 2 hours after a meal) 1918
Cuprimine Capsules (Food reduces the absorption of penicillamine. In all patients receiving penicillamine, it is important that penicillamine be given on an empty stomach, at least one hour before meals or two hours after meals. This permits maximum absorption and reduces the likelihood of inactivation by metal binding in the gastrointestinal tract) 1925
Diovan Tablets (Decreases the exposure (as measured by AUC) to valsartan about 40% and peak plasma concentration by about 50%) 2191
EC-Naprosyn Delayed-Release Tablets (The presence of food prolonged the time the EC-Naprosyn remained in the stomach, time to first detectable serum naproxen levels, and time to maximal naproxen levels (Tmax), but did not affect peak naproxen levels (Cmax)) 2769
Eldepryl Capsules (The bioavailability of selegiline is increased 3 to 4 fold when it is taken with food) 3209
Epivir Tablets (Absorption of lamivudine was slower in the fed state compared with fasted state; there was no significant difference in systemic exposure in the fed state and fasted states; Epivir may be given with or without food) 1394
Erythromycin Delayed-Release Capsules, USP (Lowers the blood levels of systemically available erythromycin) 456
Evista Tablets (Administration of raloxifene with a standardized, high fat meal increases the absorption of raloxifene, but does not lead to clinically meaningful changes in systemic exposure; Evista can be administered without regard to meals) 1735
Evoxac Capsules (Co-administration with food decreases the rate of absorption, with a fasting Tmax of 1.53 hours and a Tmax of 2.86 hours after a meal; the peak concentration is reduced by 17.3%) 1042
Exelon Capsules (Co-administration with food delays absorption (tmax) by 90 minutes, lowers Cmax by approximately 30% and increases AUC by approximately 30%) 2204
Flomax Capsules (Tmax is reached by 4 to 5 hours under fasting conditions and by 6 to 7 hours when tamsulosin is administered with food; taking tamsulosin under fasted conditions results in a 30% increase in AUC and 40% to 70% increase in Cmax compared to fed conditions; Flomax should be taken approximately 30 minutes following the meal) 881
Gabitril Tablets (A high fat meal decreases the rate (mean Tmax was prolonged to 2.5 hours, and Cmax was reduced by about 40%) but not the extent (AUC) of tiagabine) 998
Gengraf Capsules (The administration of food with Gengraf decreases the cyclosporine AUC and Cmax) 458
Hytrin Capsules (Delays the time to peak concentration by about 40 minutes; minimal effect on the extent of absorption) 469
Imdur Tablets (May decrease the rate (increase in Tmax) but not the extent (AUC) of absorption) 3032
Imitrex Tablets (Delays the Tmax slightly by about 0.5 hour with no significant effect on the bioavailability) 1440
Invirase Capsules (Saquinavir 24-hour AUC and Cmax following the administration of a high calorie meal were an average two times higher than after a lower calorie, lower fat meal; the effect of food has been shown to persist for up to 2 hours) 2776
Kadian Capsules (Slows the rate of absorption of Kadian, the extent of absorption is not affected and Kadian can be administered without regard to meals; the pellets in Kadian should not be dissolved) 572
Kaletra Capsules (Co-administration with moderate fat meal was associated with a mean increase in AUC and Cmax; to enhance bioavailability Kaletra should be taken with food) 474
Keppra Tablets (Decreases Cmax by 20% and delays Tmax by 1.5 hours; does not affect the extent of absorption) 3307

Kytril Tablets (When oral granisetron was administered with food, AUC was decreased by 5% and Cmax increased by 30% in non-fasted individuals) 2788

Lamisil Tablets (Co-administration has resulted in an increase in the AUC of terbinafine of less than 20%) 2226

Lescol Capsules (Administration of regular formulation of fluvastatin with food reduces the rate but not the extent of absorption; administration with evening meal results in a two-fold decrease in Cmax and more than a two-fold increase in tmax as compared to administration 4 hours after the evening meal; administration of Lescol XL with a high fat meal delayed the absorption and increased the bioavailability by 50%) 2227

Lescol Capsules (Administration of regular formulation of fluvastatin with food reduces the rate but not the extent of absorption; administration with evening meal results in a two-fold decrease in Cmax and more than a two-fold increase in tmax as compared to administration 4 hours after the evening meal; administration of Lescol XL with a high fat meal delayed the absorption and increased the bioavailability by 50%) 2730

Levaquin Tablets (Co-administration slightly prolongs the time to peak concentration by approximately 1 hour and slightly decreases the peak concentration by approximately 14%; levofloxacin can be administered without regard to food) 2453

Lofibra Capsules (The absorption of fenofibrate is increased when administered with food; Lofibra should be given with meals) 1217

Lotronex Tablets (Alosetron absorption is decreased by approximately 25% by co-administration with food with a mean delay in time to peak concentration of 15 minutes; Lotronex can be taken with or without food) 1479

Malarone Tablets (Dietary fat intake with atovaquone increases the rate and extent of absorption; Malarone should be taken with food or milky drink) 1484

Mavik Tablets (Slows absorption of trandolapril but does not affect AUC or Cmax) 482

Maxalt Tablets (Delays the time to reach peak concentration by an hour; no significant effect on the bioavailability) 1983

Mepron Suspension (Food enhances absorption by approximately two-fold) 1487

Meridia Capsules (Co-administration with a standard breakfast has resulted in reduced peak M1 and M2 amine concentrations and delayed the time to peak by approximately three hours; the AUCs of M1 and M2 were not significantly altered) 485

Micardis Tablets (Slightly reduces the bioavailability of telmisartan; Micardis tablets may be administered with or without food) 884

Micardis HCT Tablets (Slightly reduces the bioavailability of telmisartan with reduction in AUC of about 6%) 886

Mirapex Tablets (Food does not affect the extent of pramipexole absorption, although the time of maximum plasma concentration is increased by about 1 hour when the drug is taken with a meal) 889

Mobic Tablets (Co-administration with a high-fat breakfast did not affect extent of absorption of meloxicam capsules but led to 22% higher Cmax values; mean Cmax values were achieved between 5 to 6 hours; Mobic tablets can be administered without regard to timing of meals) 893

Neoral Soft Gelatin Capsules (Administration of food with Neoral decreases the AUC and Cmax) 2247

Noroxin Tablets (Co-administration may decrease the absorption of norfloxacin; administer at least one hour before or two hours after a meal) 2009

Omnicef Capsules (Although Cmax and AUC of cefdinir absorption from capsules are reduced by 44% and 33%, respectively, when given with a high-fat meal, the magnitude of these reductions is not likely to be clinically significant; therefore, cefdinir may be taken without regard to food) 506

Paxil Tablets (Co-administration with food resulted in slight increase (6%) in AUC, but Cmax was 29% greater; time to reach peak plasma concentration decreased from 6.4 hours post-dosing to 4.9 hours) 1501

Pepcid for Oral Suspension (Bioavailability may be slightly increased by antacids) 2014

Plendil Extended-Release Tablets (When Plendil is administered either with a high fat or carbohydrate diet, Cmax is increased by approximately 60%, AUC is unchanged; Plendil should regularly be taken either without food or with a light meal) 651

Pletal Tablets (Co-administration with a high-fat meal increases absorption, with an approximately 90% increase in Cmax and a 25% increase in AUC; patients should be advised to take Pletal at least one hour before or two hours after breakfast and dinner) 2478

Prandin Tablets (0.5, 1, and 2 mg) (When repaglinide was given with food the mean Cmax and AUC were decreased 20% and 12.4%, respectively; Tmax was unchanged) 2337

Premphase Tablets (Administration with a high fat breakfast decreased total estrone Cmax and increased total equilin Cmax compared to fasting state, no other effect on rate or extent of absorption; administration with food doubles MPA Cmax and increases MPA AUC) 3452

Prempro Tablets (Administration with food decreased Cmax of total estrone compared to fasting state, no other effect on rate or extent of absorption; administration with food doubles MPA Cmax and increases MPA AUC) 3452

Prevacid Delayed-Release Capsules (Cmax and AUC are diminished by about 50% if the drug is given 30 minutes after food as opposed to the fasting condition; Prevacid should be taken before eating) 3268

PREVPAC (Both Cmax and AUC are diminished by about 50% if the lansoprazole is given 30 minutes after food as opposed to the fasting condition) 3281

Prilosec OTC Tablets (Absorption begins only after the granules leave the stomach; Prilosec should be taken before eating) 2674

Prograf Capsules and Injection (The presence and composition of food has decreased both the rate and extent of tacrolimus absorption; this effect was most pronounced with a high-fat meal; the rate and extent of tacrolimus absorption were greatest under fasted conditions) 624

Prometrium Capsules (100 mg, 200 mg) (Concomitant food ingestion increases the bioavailability of Prometrium Capsules relative to the fasting state) 3205

Provigil Tablets (Delays the absorption (tmax) by approximately one hour; no effect on overall bioavailability) 1002

Prozac Pulvules and Liquid (May delay absorption of fluoxetine inconsequentially; Prozac may be administered with or without food) 1771

Rapamune Oral Solution and Tablets (A high-fat meal altered the bioavailability characteristics of sirolimus compared to fasting; 34% decrease in the peak blood sirolimus concentration, a 3.5-fold increase in the time-to-peak concentration and 35% increase in total exposure; to minimize variability, Rapamune should be taken consistently with or without food) 3472

Rebetron Combination Therapy (Both AUC and Cmax increased by 70% when Rebetron was administered with a high-fat meal in a single-dose pharmacokinetic study; there are insufficient data to address the clinical relevance of these results) 3078

Relafen Tablets (Potential for more rapid absorption; however, the total amount of GMNA in the plasma is unchanged) 1523

Requip Tablets (Food does not affect the extent of absorption of ropinirole, although Tmax is increased by 2.5 hours and Cmax is decreased by 25% when taken with a high fat meal) 1528

Ritalin LA Capsules (When Ritalin LA was administered with a high fat breakfast to adults, Ritalin LA had a longer lag time until absorption began and variable delays in the time until the peak concentration, the time until the interpeak minimum, and the time until the second peak; administration times relative to meals and meal composition may need to be individually titrated) 2255

Rythmol SR Capsules (Increased peak blood level and bioavailability in a single dose study) 2736

Seroquel Tablets (The bioavailability of quetiapine is marginally affected by administration with food, with Cmax and AUC values increased by 25% and 15%, respectively) 691

Sonata Capsules (A high-fat/heavy meal prolongs the absorption of zaleplon compared to fasting state, delays tmax by approximately 2 hours and reduces Cmax approximately 35%; the effect of Sonata on sleep onset may be reduced if it is taken with or immediately after a high-fat/heavy meal) 1686

Starlix Tablets (Administration of nateglinide with liquid meal significantly reduces peak plasma levels) 2276

Suprax (Increases time to maximal absorption approximately 0.8 hour) 1811

Sustiva Capsules (High fat meal may increase the absorption of Sustiva and should be avoided; it can be taken with or without meals of normal composition) 957

Targretin Capsules (Co-administration with a fat-containing meal has resulted in higher plasma bexarotene AUC and Cmax values; because safety and efficacy data are based upon administration with food, it is recommended that Targretin capsules be administered with or immediately following a meal) 1719

Tarka Tablets (Co-administration with food decreases verapamil bioavailability and the time to peak plasma concentration is delayed; bioavailability of trandolapril is not altered; Tarka should be administered with food) 519

Tasmar Tablets (Food given within 1 hour before and 2 hours after dosing of tolcapone decreases the relative bioavailability by 10% to 20%; Tasmar may be taken with or without food) 3360

Temodar Capsules (Co-administration with a modified high-fat breakfast has resulted in decrease in mean plasma concentration and AUC by 32% and 9%, respectively, and 2-fold increase in Tmax) 3088

Teveten Tablets (Co-administration with food delays absorption and causes variable changes in Cmax and AUC values which do not appear clinically important) 1707

Thalomid Capsules (Co-administration of Thalomid with a high fat meal causes minor changes in the observed AUC and Cmax values; however, it causes an increase in Tmax to approximately 6 hours) 979

Tricor Tablets (The absorption of fenofibrate is increased when administered with food; Tricor should be given with meals) 523

Uniretic Tablets (Bioavailability varies with formulation and food intake which reduces Cmax and AUC of moexiprilat by about 70% and 40% respectively after ingestion of low-fat breakfast or by 80% and 50% respectively after the ingestion of a high-fat breakfast; patients should be advised to take Uniretic one hour before a meal) 3114

Univasc Tablets (Food reduces Cmax and AUC by about 70% and 40% respectively after ingestion of a low-fat breakfast or by 80% and 50% respectively after the ingestion of high-fat breakfast) 3118

Valcyte Tablets (Co-administration with high fat meals has resulted in increased steady-state ganciclovir AUC and Cmax without any prolongation in time to peak plasma concentrations; Valcyte should be administered with food) 2816

Vantin Tablets and Oral Suspension (The extent of absorption and the mean peak plasma concentration increased when film-coated tablets were administered with food) 2650

Vesanoid Capsules (The absorption of retinoids as a class has been shown to be enhanced when taken with food) 2823

VFEND Tablets (When multiple doses of voriconazole are administered with high fat meals, the mean Cmax and AUC are reduced; VFEND tablets should be taken at least one hour before or one hour following a meal) ... 2543
Viagra Tablets (When Viagra is taken with a high fat meal, the rate of absorption is reduced with a mean delay in Tmax of 60 minutes and a mean reduction in Cmax of 29%) ... 2552
Viracept Tablets (Maximum plasma concentrations and AUC were 2- to 3-fold higher under fed conditions compared to fasting; Viracept should be taken with a meal or light snack) ... 2556
Viread Tablets (Increases the bioavailability and delays the time to tenofovir Cmax; Viread should be taken with a meal) ... 1284
Wellbutrin SR Sustained-Release Tablets (Food increases Cmax and AUC of bupropion by 11% and 17%, respectively; no clinically significant food effect) ... 1583
Xanax XR Tablets (Food has a significant influence on the bioavailability of Xanax XR. A high fat meal given up to 2 hours before dosing with Xanax XR increased the mean Cmax and the effect of this meal on Tmax depended on the timing of this meal) ... 2655
Xeloda Tablets (Reduces both rate and extent of absorption of capecitabine and delays Tmax of both parent and 5-FU) ... 2825
Xenical Capsules (Gastrointestinal events may increase when orlistat is taken with a diet high in fat) ... 2834
Zelnorm Tablets (Reduces the bioavailability of tegaserod; Zelnorm should be taken before meals) ... 2303
Zithromax Capsules, 250 mg (Zithromax should not be taken with food; reduces the rate of absorption (Cmax) of azithromycin capsules by 52% and the extent of absorption (AUC) by 43%; when oral suspension of azithromycin was administered with food the Cmax increased by 56% and the AUC was unchanged) ... 2568
Zithromax for IV Infusion (Zithromax should not be taken with food; reduces the rate of absorption (Cmax) of azithromycin capsules by 52% and the extent of absorption (AUC) by 43%; when oral suspension of azithromycin was administered with food the Cmax increased by 56% and the AUC was unchanged) ... 2573
Zofran Tablets (Bioavailability slightly enhanced by food) ... 1613
Zoloft Oral Concentrate (Co-administration of Zoloft Tablets with food slightly increased AUC but the Cmax was 25% greater, while time to reach peak plasma concentration (Tmax) decreased from 8 hours to 5.5 hours; for oral concentrate, Tmax was slightly prolonged from 5.9 hours to 7 hours with food) ... 2581
Zyban Sustained-Release Tablets (Food increases Cmax and AUC of bupropion by 11% and 17% respectively; the mean time to peak concentration Tmax was prolonged by 1 hour; this effect was of no clinical significance) ... 1620
Zyrtec Tablets (Food has no effect on the extent of cetirizine absorption, but Tmax may be delayed and Cmax may be decreased in the presence of food) ... 2589
Zyvox Tablets (The time to reach maximum concentration is delayed from 1.5 hours to 2.2 hours and Cmax is decreased by about 17% when linezolid is co-administered with high fat food; linezolid may be administered without regard to the timing of meals) ... 2661

Food having a pH greater than 5.5

Creon 5 Capsules (Can dissolve the protective coating resulting in early release of enzymes, irritation of oral mucosa, and/or loss of enzyme activity) ... 3195
Ultrase Capsules (Can dissolve the protective coating resulting in early release of enzymes, irritation of oral mucosa, and/or loss of enzyme activity) ... 735
Ultrase MT Capsules (Can dissolve the protective enteric shell) ... 736

Food high in tyramine

Zyvox Tablets (Co-administration has resulted in a significant pressor response; patients receiving linezolid should avoid consuming large amounts of food containing tyramine) ... 2661

Food with high concentration of tyramine

Matulane Capsules (Procarbazine exhibits some MAO inhibitory activity: concurrent use should be avoided) ... 3188
Parnate Tablets (Potential for hypertensive crisis; concurrent use is contraindicated) ... 1499

Fruit juices, unspecified

Dexedrine Spansule Capsules (Lowers absorption of amphetamines) ... 1386
DextroStat Tablets (Lowers absorption of amphetamines by acting as gastrointestinal acidifying agent) ... 3177

Fruits, dried

Parnate Tablets (Potential for hypertensive crisis; concurrent use is contraindicated) ... 1499

Fruits, overripe

Parnate Tablets (Potential for hypertensive crisis; concurrent use is contraindicated) ... 1499

Grapefruit

Abilify Tablets (Inhibitors of CYP3A4 or CYP2D6 can inhibit aripiprazole elimination and cause increased blood levels) ... 2472
Abilify Tablets (Inhibitors of CYP3A4 or CYP2D6 can inhibit aripiprazole elimination and cause increased blood levels) ... 916
Adalat CC Tablets (Nifedipine is mainly eliminated by metabolism and is a substrate of CYP3A4. Inhibitors of CYP3A4 can impact the exposure to nifedipine and consequently its desirable and undesirable effects) ... 2978
Alesse-28 Tablets (Co-administration may increase plasma hormone levels) ... 3392
Avodart Soft Gelatin Capsules (Blood concentrations of dutasteride may increase in the presence of CYP3A4 inhibitors) ... 1353
Biltricide Tablets (Grapefruit juice was reported to produce a 1.6-fold increase in the Cmax and a 1.9-fold increase in the AUC of praziquantel) ... 2990
Buprenex Injectable (Buprenorphine is metabolized by the CYP3A4 isoenzyme; co-administration with inhibitors of CYP3A4 may cause decrease in clearance of buprenorphine) ... 2718
Carbatrol Capsules (Carbamazepine is metabolized mainly by cytochrome P450 (CYP) 3A4 to the active carbamazepine 10,11 -epoxide, which is further metabolized to the trans-diol by epoxide hydrolase. Therefore, the potential exists for interaction between carbamazepine and any agent that inhibits CYP3A4 and/or epoxide hydrolase) ... 3174
Cenestin Tablets, 0.45mg, 0.625mg, 0.9mg, 1.25mg (Co-administration of estrogens with CYP3A4 inhibitors may increase plasma concentrations of estrogens and may result in side effects) ... 1063
Cialis Tablets (Tadalafil is metabolized predominantly by CYP3A4 in the liver. The dose of tadalafil should be limited to 10 mg no more than once every 72 hours in patients taking potent inhibitors of CYP3A4) ... 1806
Climara Pro Transdermal System (Inhibitors of CYP3A4 such as erythromycin, clarithromycin, ketoconazole, itraconazole, ritonavir and grapefruit juice may increase plasma concentrations of estrogens and may result in side effects) ... 800
CombiPatch Transdermal System (Studies have shown that estrogens are metabolized partially by cytochrome P4503A. Inhibitors of CYP3A4 may increase concentrations of estrogens and in side effects) ... 2180
Covera-HS Tablets (Clinically significant interactions have been reported with inhibitors of CYP3A4 causing elevation of plasma levels of verapamil while inducers of CYP3A4 have caused a lowering of plasma levels of verapamil) ... 3135
Decadron Tablets (Drugs which inhibit cytochrome P450 3A4 enzyme activity have the potential to result in increased plasma concentrations of corticosteroids) ... 1929
Diastat Rectal Delivery System (Studies suggest that CYP2C19 and CYP3A4 are the principal enzymes involved in the initial oxidative metabolism of diazepam. Therefore, potential interactions may occur when diazepam is given concurrently with agents that affect CYP2C19 and CYP3A4 activity. Potential inhibitors of CYP3A4 could decrease the rate of diazepam elimination) ... 3344
Duragesic Transdermal System (The concurrent use of CYP3A4 inhibitors with transdermal fentanyl may result in an increase in fentanyl plasma concentrations, which could increase or prolong adverse drug effects and may cause serious respiratory depression. In this situation, special patient care and observation are appropriate) ... 2448
Emend Capsules (Co-administration of EMEND with drugs that inhibit CYP3A4 activity may result in increased plasma concentrations of aprepitant and should be approached with caution) ... 1944
Entocort EC Capsules (Concurrent use with extensive intake of grapefruit juice has caused rise in systemic exposure of budesonide by two-fold; ingestion of grapefruit should be avoided) ... 2694
Equetro Extended-Release Capsules (Carbamazepine is metabolized mainly by CYP3A4 the active carbamazepine 10,11-epoxide, which is futher metabolized to the trans-diol by epoxide hydrolase. Therefore, the potential exists for interaction between carbamazepine and any agent that inhibits CYP3A4 and/or epoxide hydrolase. Agents that are CYP3A4 inhibitors may increase the plasma levels of carbamazepine. Thus, if a patient has been titrated to a stable dosage of carbamazepine, and then begins a course of treatment with a CYP3A4 or epoxide hydrolase inhibitor, it is reasonable to expect that a dose reduction for carbamazepine may be necessary) ... 3178
Estratest H.S. Tablets (Co-administration with inhibitors of CYP3A4 may increase plasma concentrations of estrogens and may result in side effects) ... 3196
Evoxac Capsules (Drugs which inhibit CYP3A3/4 also inhibit the metabolism of cevimeline) ... 1042
Flonase Nasal Spray (Caution should be exercised when potent cytochrome P450 3A4 inhibitors are co-administered with fluticasone propionate) ... 1412
Gengraf Capsules (Affects the metabolism of cyclosporine by increasing blood concentration of cyclosporine; concurrent use should be avoided) ... 458
Gleevec Tablets (Caution is recommended when administering Gleevec with inhibitors of the CYP3A4 family. Substances that inhibit CYP3A4 activity may decrease metabolism and increase imatinib concentrations. There is a significant increase in exposure to imatinib when Gleevec is co-administered with ketoconazole) ... 2221
Hectorol Capsules (Cytochrome P450 inhibitors may inhibit the 25-hydroxylation of doxercalciferol. Hence, formation of the active doxercalciferol moiety may be hindered) ... 909
Inspra Tablets (Eplerenone should not be used with strong inhibitors of CYP450 3A4. Potent inhibitors of CYP3A4 caused increased exposure of about 5-fold, while less potent CYP3A4 inhibitors (e.g., erythromycin, saquinavir, verapamil, fluconazole) gave approximately 2-fold increases in exposure. Grapefruit juice caused only a small increase (about 25%) in exposure) ... 2520
Levitra Tablets (Concomitant use with moderate/strong CYP 3A4 inhibitors results in significant increases in plasma levels of vardenafil) ... 3048
Lexiva Tablets (Amprenavir, the active metabolite of fosamprenavir, is metabolized in the liver by the cytochrome P450 enzyme system. Amprenavir may inhibit or induce CYP3A4. Caution should be used when co-administering medications that are substrates, inhibitors, or inducers of CYP3A4, or potentially toxic medications that are metabolized by CYP3A4) ... 1473
Mevacor Tablets (The risk of myopathy/rhabdomyolysis is increased by concomitant use of lovastatin with potent inhibitors of CYP3A4, particularly with higher doses of lovastatin; concomitant use should be avoided unless the benefits of combined therapy outweigh the increased risk) ... 1996

Migranal Nasal Spray (Co-administration of dihydroergotamin with potent CYP3A4 inhibitors results in vasospasm that can lead to cerebral ischemia and/or ischemia of the extremities, therefore it is contraindicated)........3350
Navelbine Injection (Co-administration of vinorelbine with an inhibitor of CYP3A metabolic pathway may cause an earlier onset and/or an increased severity of side effects) 1494
Neoral Soft Gelatin Capsules (Affects the metabolism of cyclosporine and should be avoided) 2247
Niravam Orally Disintegrating Tablets (Available data from clinical studies of benzodiazepines, other than alprazolam, suggest a possible drug interaction with alprazolam and grapefruit juice; caution is recommended during co-administration).........................3106
Pacerone Tablets (Grapefruit juice given to healthy volunteers increased amiodarone AUC by 50% and Cmax by 84%. Grapefruit juice inhibits CYP3A4-mediated metabolism of oral amiodarone in the intestinal mucosa, resulting in increased plasma levels of amiodarone; therefore, grapefruit juice should not be taken during treatment with oral amiodarone. This information should be considered when changing from intravenous amiodarone to oral amiodarone).....3337
Pletal Tablets (A reduced dose of cilostazol should be considered when taken concomitantly with CYP3A4 inhibitors).........................2478
Prefest Tablets (Inhibitors of CYP3A4 may increase plasma concentrations of estrogens and may result in side effects) 1069
Premarin Tablets (Co-administration of inhibitors of CYP3A4 with estrogens may affect estrogen drug metabolism. Inhibitors of CYP3A4 may increase plasma concentrations of estrogens and may result in side effects) 3443
Premphase Tablets (Co-administration of estrogens with inhibitors of CYP3A4 may increase plasma concentrations of estrogens and may result in side effects) 3452
Prempro Tablets (Co-administration of estrogens with inhibitors of CYP3A4 may increase plasma concentrations of estrogens and may result in side effects) 3452
Prograf Capsules and Injection (Since tacrolimus is metabolized mainly by the CYP3A enzyme systems, substances known to inhibit these enzymes may decrease the metabolism or increase bioavailability of tacrolimus as indicated by increased whole blood or plasma concentrations. Monitoringof blood concentrations and appropriate dosage adjustments are essential when such drugs are used concomitantly) 624
Provigil Tablets (Co-administration of potent inhibitors of CYP3A4 could alter the plasma levels of modafinil) 1002
Pulmicort Respules (Concomitant administration of budesonide with known inhibitors of CYP3A4 may inhibit the metabolism of, and increase the systemic exposure to, budesonide; care should be exercised)...................... 654
Rapamune Oral Solution and Tablets (Sirolimus is extensively metabolized by the CYP3A4 isoenzyme in the gut wall and liver. Co-administration with inhibitors of CYP3A4 may decrease the metabolism of sirolimus and increase sirolimus levels. Co-administration with strong inducers of CYP3A4 is not recommended) 3472
Relpax Tablets (Eletriptan should not be used within 72 hours of drugs that have demonstrated potent CYP3A4 inhibition) 2531
Revatio Tablets (Sildenafil metabolism is principally mediated by the CYP3A4 (major route) and CYP2C9 (minor route) cytochrome P450 isoforms. Therefore, inhibitors of these isoenzymes may reduce sildenafil clearance)............2541
Reyataz Capsules (Co-administration of atazanavir sulfate and other drugs that inhibit CYP3A may increase atazanavir sulfate plasma concentrations)............................. 948
Rhinocort Aqua Nasal Spray (Co-administration with inhibitors of CYP4503A4 may inhibit the metabolism of, and increase the systemic exposure to budesonide)............................. 658
Rozerem Tablets (Ramelteon should be administered with caution in subjects taking strong CYP2C9 inhibitors such as fluconazole)..............................3228
Rythmol SR Capsules (Drugs that inhibit CYP3A4 might lead to increased plasma levels of propafenone; patients should be closely monitored and the propafenone dose adjusted accordingly) 2736
Sandimmune I.V. Ampuls for Infusion (Co-administration results in increased blood concentrations of cyclosporine; concurrent use should be avoided)..2259
Seasonale Tablets (CYP 3A4 inhibitors may increase plasma ethinyl estradiol levels) 1073
Sensipar Tablets (Since cinacalcet hydrochloride is metabolized in part by CYP3A4, dose adjustment of cinacalcet hydrochloride may be required and PTH and serum calcium concentrations closely monitored if a patient initiates or discontinues therapy with a strong CYP3A4 inhibitor) 603
Seroquel Tablets (Co-administration with an inhibitor of CYP4503A may reduce oral clearance of quetiapine, resulting in an increase in maximum plasma concentration of quetiapine; dose adjustment of quetiapine will be necessary) 691
Sonata Capsules (CYP3A4 inhibitors may decrease zaleplon's clearance, possibly increasing its concentration) 1686
Suboxone Tablets (Buprenorphine is metabolized to norbuprenorphine by cytochrome CYP3A4. Because CYP3A4 inhibitors may increase plasma concentrations of buprenorphine, patients already on CYP3A4 inhibitors should have their dose of Subutex or Subuxone adjusted.) 2719
Subutex Tablets (Buprenorphine is metabolized to norbuprenorphine by cytochrome CYP3A4. Because CYP3A4 inhibitors may increase plasma concentrations of buprenorphine, patients already on CYP3A4 inhibitors should have their dose of Subutex or Subuxone adjusted.) 2719
Tarceva Tablets (Caution when administering or taking erlotinib with strong CYP3A4 inhibitors such as atazanavir, clarithromycin, indinavir, itraconazole, nefazodone, nelfinavir, ritonavir, saquinavir, telithromycin, troleandomycin, and voriconazole).........................1254
Tarceva Tablets (Caution when administering or taking erlotinib with strong CYP3A4 inhibitors such as atazanavir, clarithromycin, indinavir, itraconazole, nefazodone, nelfinavir, ritonavir, saquinavir, telithromycin, troleandomycin, and voriconazole)..........................2470
Taxotere Injection Concentrate (Metabolism of docetaxel may be inhibited by co-administration with CYP3A4 inhibitors, thereby leading to substantial increases in docetaxel blood concentrations).....2947
Uroxatral Tablets (Uroxatral should not be co-administered with potent CYP3A4 inhibitors such as ketoconazole, itraconazole, and ritonavir, since alfuzosin blood levels are increased) 2957
Velcade for Injection (Patients who are concomitantly receiving Velcade and drugs that are inhibitors or inducers of cytochrome P450 3A4 should be closely monitored for either toxicities or reduced efficacy) 2102
Verelan PM Capsules (Grapefruit juice may significantly increase concentrations of verapamil) 3120
Vesanoid Capsules (Tretinoin is metabolized by the hepatic P450 system; therefore, there is a potential for alteration of pharmacokinetic parameters in patients administered concomitant medications that are also inducers of this system. To date, there is no data to suggestthat co-use with these medications increases or decreases either efficacy or toxicity of tretinoin) 2823
VFEND Tablets (CYP3A4 inhibitors may increase voriconazole systemic exposure (plasma concentrations))............................2543
Viracept Tablets (Nelfinavir is metabolized by CYP3A and CYP2C19; co-administration of Viracept and drugs that inhibit CYP3A or CYP2C19 may increase nelfinavir plasma concentrations)............................2556
Xanax XR Tablets (Drugs that inhibit metabolism via cytochrome P4503A may have a profound effect on the clearance of alprazolam. Potent inhibitors of CYP3A would be expected to increase plasma alprazolam concentrations. Co-administration with very potent inhibitors of CYP3A should be avoided. Concurrent use of alprazolam with drugs inhibiting CYP3A to a lesser but still significant degree requires caution) 2655

Grapefruit Juice

Abilify Tablets (Inhibitors of CYP3A4 or CYP2D6 can inhibit aripiprazole elimination and cause increased blood levels) 2472
Abilify Tablets (Inhibitors of CYP3A4 or CYP2D6 can inhibit aripiprazole elimination and cause increased blood levels) 916
Adalat CC Tablets (Co-administration of nifedipine with grapefruit juice results in up to a 2-fold increase in AUC and Cmax, due to inhibition of CYP3A4-related first-pass metabolism. This effect of grapefruit juice may last for at least 3 days; co-administration should beavoided)..........................2978
Advicor Tablets (Inhibits CYP3A4 and can increase the plasma concentration of lovastatin; concurrent use should be avoided) 1694
Agrylin Capsules (Anagrelide is metabolized at least in part by CYP1A2. Therefore, CYP1A2 inhibitors could theoretically adversely influence the clearance of anagrelide)................3172
Alesse-28 Tablets (Co-administration may increase plasma hormone levels)................3392
Allegra-D 12 Hour Extended-Release Tablets (Co-administration with grapefruit, orange or apple juice will reduce the bioavailability and exposure or fexofenadine) 2860
Altoprev Extended-Release Tablets (Co-administration with potent CYP3A4 inhibitors, such as large quantities of grapefruit juice (greater than 1 quart daily), increases the risk of myopathy/rhabdomyolysis; concurrent use should be avoided) 1151
Avodart Soft Gelatin Capsules (Blood concentrations of dutasteride may increase in the presence of CYP3A4 inhibitors) 1353
Biltricide Tablets (Grapefruit juice was reported to produce a 1.6-fold increase in the Cmax and a 1.9-fold increase in the AUC of praziquantel).......................2990
Buprenex Injectable (Buprenorphine is metabolized by the CYP3A4 isoenzyme; co-administration with inhibitors of CYP3A4 may cause decrease in clearance of buprenorphine) 2718
Cafcit Injection (Caffeine has the potential to interact with drugs that inhibit CYP1A2).......................1854
Carbatrol Capsules (Carbamazepine is metabolized mainly by cytochrome P450 (CYP) 3A4 to the active carbamazepine 10,11 -epoxide, which is further metabolized to the trans-diol by epoxide hydrolase. Therefore, the potential exists for interaction between carbamazepine and any agent that inhibits CYP3A4 and/or epoxide hydrolase) 3174
Cenestin Tablets, 0.45mg, 0.625mg, 0.9mg, 1.25mg (Co-administration of estrogens with CYP3A4 inhibitors, such as grapefruit juice, may increase plasma concentrations of estrogens and may result in side effects) 1063
Cialis Tablets (YP3A4 inhibitors such as grapefruit juice may likely increase tadalafil exposure) 1806
Climara Transdermal System (Inducers of CYP3A4, such as grapefruit juice, may increase plasma concentrations of estrogens and may result in side effects) 795
Climara Pro Transdermal System (Inhibitors of CYP3A4 such as erythromycin, clarithromycin, ketoconazole, itraconazole, ritonavir and grapefruit juice may increase plasma concentrations of estrogens and may result in side effects) 800
CombiPatch Transdermal System (Studies have shown that estrogens are metabolized partially by cytochrome P4503A. Inhibitors of CYP3A4 may increase concentrations of estrogens and in side effects) 2180

Covera-HS Tablets (Grapefruit juice may significantly increase concentrations of verapamil) 3135

Crixivan Capsules (Potential for decrease in indinavir AUC) 1918

Cymbalta Delayed-Release Capsules (Concomitant use of duloxetine with fluvoxamine, an inhibitor of CYP1A2, results in approximately a 6-fold increase in AUC and about a 2.5-fold increase in Cmax of duloxetine. Since duloxetine is metabolized in part by CYP1A2, concomitant use of duloxetine with other inhibitors of CYP1A2, would be expected to have the same effects; these combinations should be avoided) 1729

Decadron Tablets (Drugs which inhibit cytochrome P450 3A4 enzyme activity have the potential to result in increased plasma concentrations of corticosteroids) 1929

Diastat Rectal Delivery System (Studies suggest that CYP2C19 and CYP3A4 are the principal enzymes involved in the initial oxidative metabolism of diazepam. Therefore, potential interactions may occur when diazepam is given concurrently with agents that affect CYP2C19 and CYP3A4 activity. Potential inhibitors of CYP3A4 could decrease the rate of diazepam elimination) 3344

Duragesic Transdermal System (The concurrent use of CYP3A4 inhibitors with transdermal fentanyl may result in an increase in fentanyl plasma concentrations, which could increase or prolong adverse drug effects and may cause serious respiratory depression. In this situation, special patient care and observation are appropriate) 2448

Emend Capsules (Co-administration of EMEND with drugs that inhibit CYP3A4 activity may result in increased plasma concentrations of aprepitant and should be approached with caution) 1944

Entocort EC Capsules (Concurrent use with extensive intake of grapefruit juice has caused rise in systemic exposure of budesonide by two-fold; ingestion of grapefruit juice should be avoided) 2694

Equetro Extended-Release Capsules (Carbamazepine is metabolized mainly by CYP3A4 the active carbamazepine 10,11-epoxide, which is futher metabolized to the trans-diol by epoxide hydrolase. Therefore, the potential exists for interaction between carbamazepine and any agent that inhibits CYP3A4 and/or epoxide hydrolase. Agents that are CYP3A4 inhibitors may increase the plasma levels of carbamazepine. Thus, if a patient has been titrated to a stable dosage of carbamazepine, and then begins a course of treatment with a CYP3A4 or epoxide hydrolase inhibitor, it is reasonable to expect that a dose reduction for carbamazepine may be necessary) 3178

Estratest H.S. Tablets (Co-administration with inhibitors of CYP3A4 may increase plasma concentrations of estrogens and may result in side effects) 3196

Estrogel 0.06% (Inhibitors of CYP3A4, such as grapefruit juice, may increase plasma concentrations of estrogens and may result in side effects) 3200

Evoxac Capsules (Co-administration with drugs which inhibit CYP3A3/4, such as grapefruit juice, may inhibit the metabolism of cevimeline resulting in a higher risk of adverse events) 1042

Flonase Nasal Spray (Caution should be exercised when potent cytochrome P450 3A4 inhibitors are co-administered with fluticasone propionate) 1412

Gengraf Capsules (Affects the metabolism of cyclosporine by increasing blood concentration of cyclosporine; concurrent use should be avoided) 458

Gleevec Tablets (Caution is recommended when administering Gleevec with inhibitors of the CYP3A4 family. Substances that inhibit CYP3A4 activity may decrease metabolism and increase imatinib concentrations. There is a significant increase in exposure to imatinib when Gleevec is co-administered with ketoconazole) 2221

Hectorol Capsules (Cytochrome P450 inhibitors may inhibit the 25-hydroxylation of doxercalciferol. Hence, formation of the active doxercalciferol moiety may be hindered) 909

InnoPran XL Capsules (Blood levels and/or toxicity of propranolol may be increased by administration of propranolol hydrochloride extended-release capsules with inhibitors of CYP1A2) 2728

Inspra Tablets (Eplerenone should not be used with strong inhibitors of CYP450 3A4. Potent inhibitors of CYP3A4 caused increased exposure of about 5-fold, while less potent CYP3A4 inhibitors (e.g., erythromycin, saquinavir, verapamil, fluconazole) gave approximately 2-fold increases in exposure. Grapefruit juice caused only a small increase (about 25%) in exposure) 2520

Levitra Tablets (Concomitant use with moderate/strong CYP 3A4 inhibitors results in significant increases in plasma levels of vardenafil) 3048

Lexiva Tablets (Amprenavir, the active metabolite of fosamprenavir, is metabolized in the liver by the cytochrome P450 enzyme system. Amprenavir may inhibit or induce CYP3A4. Caution should be used when co-administering medications that are substrates, inhibitors, or inducers of CYP3A4, or potentially toxic medications that are metabolized by CYP3A4) 1473

Lotronex Tablets (Concomitant administration of alosetron and moderate CYP1A2 inhibitors, including quinolone antibiotics and cimetidine, has not been evaluated, but should be avoided unless clinically necessary because of potential drug interactions) 1479

Menostar Transdermal System (Inhibitors of CYP3A4, such as grapefruit juice, may increase plasma concentrations of estrogens and may result in side effects) 805

Mevacor Tablets (The risk of myopathy/rhabdomyolysis is increased by concomitant use of lovastatin with potent inhibitors of CYP3A4, particularly with higher doses of lovastatin; concomitant use should be avoided unless the benefits of combined therapy outweigh the increased risk) 1996

Migranal Nasal Spray (Co-administration of dihydroergotamin with potent CYP3A4 inhibitors results in vasospasm that can lead to cerebral ischemia and/or ischemia of the extremities, therefore it is contraindicated) 3350

Navelbine Injection (Co-administration of vinorelbine with an inhibitor of CYP3A metabolic pathway may cause an earlier onset and/or an increased severity of side effects) 1494

Neoral Soft Gelatin Capsules (Affects the metabolism of cyclosporine and should be avoided) 2247

Niravam Orally Disintegrating Tablets (Available data from clinical studies of benzodiazepines, other than alprazolam, suggest a possible drug interaction with alprazolam and grapefruit juice; caution is recommended during co-administration) 3106

Pacerone Tablets (Grapefruit juice given to healthy volunteers increased amiodarone AUC by 50% and Cmax by 84%. Grapefruit juice inhibits CYP3A4-mediated metabolism of oral amiodarone in the intestinal mucosa, resulting in increased plasma levels of amiodarone; therefore, grapefruit juice should not be taken during treatment with oral amiodarone. This information should be considered when changing from intravenous amiodarone to oral amiodarone) 3337

Plendil Extended-Release Tablets (The bioavailability of felodipine is increased more than two-fold when taken with doubly concentrated grapefruit juice) 651

Pletal Tablets (Co-administration of cilostazol with inhibitors of CYP3A4, such as grapefruit juice, increase cilostazol plasma concentration by 50%; concurrent consumption of grapefruit juice should be avoided) 2478

Prefest Tablets (Inhibitors of CYP3A4 may increase plasma concentrations of estrogens and may result in side effects) 1069

Premarin Tablets (Co-administration of grapefruit juice with estrogens may increase plasma concentrations of estrogens and may result in side effects) 3443

Premphase Tablets (Co-administration of estrogens with inhibitors of CYP3A4, such as grapefruit juice, may increase plasma concentrations of estrogens and may result in side effects) 3452

Prempro Tablets (Co-administration of estrogens with inhibitors of CYP3A4, such as grapefruit juice, may increase plasma concentrations of estrogens and may result in side effects) 3452

Prograf Capsules and Injection (Co-administered grapefruit juice has been reported to increase tacrolimus blood trough concentrations in liver transplant patients; grapefruit juice should be avoided) 624

Provigil Tablets (Co-administration of potent inhibitors of CYP3A4 could alter the plasma levels of modafinil) 1002

Pulmicort Respules (Concomitant administration of budesonide with known inhibitors of CYP3A4 may inhibit the metabolism of, and increase the systemic exposure to, budesonide; care should be exercised) 654

Rapamune Oral Solution and Tablets (Induces CYP3A4-mediated metabolism of sirolimus; Rapamune must not be administered or diluted with grapefruit juice) 3472

Relpax Tablets (Eletriptan should not be used within 72 hours of drugs that have demonstrated potent CYP3A4 inhibition) 2531

Requip Tablets (If therapy with a drug known to be a potent inhibitor of CYP1A2 is stopped or started during treatment with ropinirole hydrochloride, adjustment of the dose of ropinirole hydrocholoride may be required) 1528

Revatio Tablets (Sildenafil metabolism is principally mediated by the CYP3A4 (major route) and CYP2C9 (minor route) cytochrome P450 isoforms. Therefore, inhibitors of these isoenzymes may reduce sildenafil clearance) 2541

Rhinocort Aqua Nasal Spray (Co-administration with inhibitors of CYP4503A4 may inhibit the metabolism of, and increase the systemic exposure to budesonide) 658

Rozerem Tablets (Ramelteon should be administered with caution in subjects taking strong CYP2C9 inhibitors such as fluconazole) 3228

Rythmol SR Capsules (Drugs that inhibit CYP1A2 might lead to increased plasma levels of propafenone; patients should be closely monitored and the propafenone dose adjusted accordingly) 2736

Sandimmune I.V. Ampuls for Infusion (Co-administration results in increased blood concentrations of cyclosporine; concurrent use should be avoided) 2259

Seasonale Tablets (CYP 3A4 inhibitors may increase plasma ethinyl estradiol levels) 1073

Seroquel Tablets (Co-administration with an inhibitor of CYP4503A may reduce oral clearance of quetiapine, resulting in an increase in maximum plasma concentration of quetiapine; dose adjustment of quetiapine will be necessary) 691

Sonata Capsules (CYP3A4 inhibitors may decrease zaleplon's clearance, possibly increasing its concentration) 1686

Suboxone Tablets (Buprenorphine is metabolized to norbuprenorphine by cytochrome CYP3A4. Because CYP3A4 inhibitors may increase plasma concentrations of buprenorphine, patients already on CYP3A4 inhibitors should have their dose of Subutex or Subuxone adjusted.) 2719

Subutex Tablets (Buprenorphine is metabolized to norbuprenorphine by cytochrome CYP3A4. Because CYP3A4 inhibitors may increase plasma concentrations of buprenorphine, patients already on CYP3A4 inhibitors should have their dose of Subutex or Subuxone adjusted.) 2719

Tarceva Tablets (Caution when administering or taking erlotinib with strong CYP3A4 inhibitors such as atazanavir, clarithromycin, indinavir, itraconazole, nefazodone, nelfinavir, ritonavir, saquinavir, telithromycin, troleandomycin, and voriconazole) 1254

Tarceva Tablets (Caution when administering or taking erlotinib with strong CYP3A4 inhibitors such as atazanavir, clarithromycin, indinavir, itraconazole, nefazodone, nelfinavir, ritonavir, saquinavir, telithromycin, troleandomycin, and voriconazole) 2470

Targretin Capsules (Bexarotene is metabolized by CYP403A4; co-administration with inhibitors of CYP4503A4, such as grapefruit juice, would be expected to lead to an increase in plasma bexarotene concentrations) 1719

Taxotere Injection Concentrate (Metabolism of docetaxel may be inhibited by co-administration with CYP3A4 inhibitors, thereby leading to substantial increases in docetaxel blood concentrations) 2947

Uroxatral Tablets (Uroxatral should not be co-administered with potent CYP3A4 inhibitors such as ketoconazole, itraconazole, and ritonavir, since alfuzosin blood levels are increased) 2957

Velcade for Injection (Patients who are concomitantly receiving Velcade and drugs that are inhibitors or inducers of cytochrome P450 3A4 should be closely monitored for either toxicities or reduced efficacy) 2102

Verelan PM Capsules (Grapefruit juice may significantly increase concentrations of verapamil) 3120

Vesanoid Capsules (Tretinoin is metabolized by the hepatic P450 system; therefore, there is a potential for alteration of pharmacokinetic parameters in patients administered concomitant medications that are also inducers of this system. To date, there is no data to suggestthat co-use with these medications increases or decreases either efficacy or toxicity of tretinoin) 2823

VFEND Tablets (CYP3A4 inhibitors may increase voriconazole systemic exposure (plasma concentrations)) 2543

Vivelle Transdermal System (Co-administration of estrogens with inhibitors of CYP3A4, such as grapefruit juice, may increase plasma concentrations of estrogens and may result in side effects) 2288

Vytorin 10/10 Tablets (Co-administration with potent CYP3A4 inhibitors, such as large quantities of grapefruit juice (greater than 1 quart daily), increases the risk of myopathy/rhabdomyolysis; concurrent use should be avoided) 2084

Vytorin 10/10 Tablets (Co-administration with potent CYP3A4 inhibitors, such as large quantities of grapefruit juice (greater than 1 quart daily), increases the risk of myopathy/rhabdomyolysis; concurrent use should be avoided) 3092

Xanax XR Tablets (Possible interaction based on the clinical studies involving other benzodiazepines metabolized similarly as alprazolam; concurrent use requires caution) 2655

Zocor Tablets (Simvastatin is a substrate for CYP4503A4 and grapefruit juice contains one or more components that inhibit CYP3A4; co-administration with grapefruit juice can increase the plasma concentrations of simvastatin and its B-hydroxyacid metabolite; large quantities of grapefruit juice (>1 quart daily) significantly increase the serum concentrations and should be avoided) 2078

Zyprexa Tablets (Can potentially inhibit olanzapine clearance; therefore, a dosage decrease might be considered) 1798

Zyprexa IntraMuscular (Can potentially inhibit olanzapine clearance; therefore, a dosage decrease might be considered) 1798

Herring, pickled

Parnate Tablets (Potential for hypertensive crisis; concurrent use is contraindicated) 1499

Liqueurs

Parnate Tablets (Potential for hypertensive crisis; concurrent use is contraindicated) 1499

Liver

Parnate Tablets (Potential for hypertensive crisis; concurrent use is contraindicated) 1499

Meal, high in bran fiber

Digitek Tablets (The amount of digoxin from an oral dose may be reduced when taken with meal high in bran fiber) 2146

Lanoxin Tablets (The amount of digoxin from an oral dose may be reduced) 1468

Meal, unspecified

Amaryl Tablets (When glimepiride is given with meals the mean Tmax is slightly increased (12%) and mean Cmax and AUC are slightly decreased) 2864

Ambien Tablets (Mean AUC and Cmax decreased by 15% and 25% respectively, while Tmax was prolonged by 60%; for faster sleep onset, Ambien should not be administered with or immediately after meal) 2867

Cozaar Tablets (Meal slows absorption and decreases Cmax, but has minor effects on losartan AUC or on the AUC of the metabolite) 1913

Cytovene Capsules (Meal containing 46.5% fat increases the steady-state AUC of oral Cytovene by 22% ± 22% and significant prolongation of time Tmax and a higher Cmax; patients should take Cytovene Capsules with food to maximize bioavailability) 2763

Digitek Tablets (Slows the rate of absorption) 2146

Famvir Tablets (Penciclovir Cmax decreased approximately 50% and Tmax was delayed by 1.5 hours when a capsule formulation of famciclovir was administered with food; there is no effect on the extent of availability (AUC) of penciclovir) 2207

Fosamax Tablets (Standardized breakfast decreases bioavailability by approximately 40% when alendronate is administered either one-half or 1 hour before breakfast) 1949

Fosamax Plus D Tablets (Bioavailability was decreased (by approximately 40%) when 10 mg alendronate was administered either 0.5 or 1 hour before a standardized breakfast, when compared to dosing 2 hours before eating) 1956

Hyzaar 50-12.5 Tablets (Meal slows absorption and decreases Cmax but has minor effects on losartan AUC or on the AUC of the metabolite) 1964

Lanoxin Tablets (Slows the rate of absorption) 1468

Mevacor Tablets (When lovastatin was given under fasting conditions, plasma concentrations of total inhibitors were on average about two-thirds those found when lovastatin was administered immediately after a standard meal) 1996

Nimotop Capsules (Administration of nimodipine capsules following a standard breakfast resulted in 68% lower peak plasma concentration and 38% lower bioavailability) 774

Norvir Soft Gelatin Capsules (Relative to fasting conditions, the extent of absorption of ritonavir from capsule formulation was 15% higher when administered with a meal; decreased peak ritonavir concentrations when oral solution was given under non-fasting condition) 499

PCE Dispertab Tablets (Presence of food results in lower blood levels; optimal blood levels are obtained when PCE is given in the fasting state (at least ½ hour and preferably 2 hours before meals)) 510

Ticlid Tablets (Administration after meals results in a 20% increase in the AUC of ticlopidine) 2813

Zerit Capsules (Co-administration with food decreases Cmax by approximately 45%; however, the systemic availability (AUC) is unchanged; Zerit Capsules can be taken without regard to meals) 971

Meat extracts

Parnate Tablets (Potential for hypertensive crisis; concurrent use is contraindicated) 1499

Meat prepared with tenderizers

Parnate Tablets (Potential for hypertensive crisis; concurrent use is contraindicated) 1499

Milk, low fat

Dyazide Capsules (Concurrent use of low-salt milk with triamterene may result in hyperkalemia, especially in patients with renal insufficiency) 1389

Milk, low salt

Dyrenium Capsules (Co-administration may promote serum potassium accumulation and possibly result in hyperkalemia) 3390

Orange Juice

Allegra-D 12 Hour Extended-Release Tablets (Co-administration with grapefruit, orange or apple juice will reduce the bioavailability and exposure or fexofenadine) 2860

Fosamax Tablets (Concomitant administration of alendronate with orange juice reduces bioavailability by approximately 60%) 1949

Fosamax Plus D Tablets (Concomitant administration of alendronate with orange juice reduces bioavailability by approximately 60%) 1956

Prunes

Parnate Tablets (Potential for hypertensive crisis; concurrent use is contraindicated) 1499

Raisins

Parnate Tablets (Potential for hypertensive crisis; concurrent use is contraindicated) 1499

Raspberries

Parnate Tablets (Potential for hypertensive crisis; concurrent use is contraindicated) 1499

Salt Substitutes, Potassium-Containing

Altace Capsules (Increases risk of hyperkalemia) 1673

Inspra Tablets (Eplerenone is contraindicated in patients treated concomitantly with salt substitutes containing potassium) 2520

Sauerkraut

Parnate Tablets (Potential for hypertensive crisis; concurrent use is contraindicated) 1499

Sherry

Parnate Tablets (Potential for hypertensive crisis; concurrent use is contraindicated) 1499

Soy Sauce

Parnate Tablets (Potential for hypertensive crisis; concurrent use is contraindicated) 1499

Soybean Formula, Children's

Levoxyl Tablets (Concurrent use of soybean flour may bind and decrease the absorption of levothyroxine sodium from GI tract) 1680

Synthroid Tablets (Binds and decreases absorption of levothyroxine sodium from the gastrointestinal tract) 515

Unithroid Tablets (Concurrent use of soybean flour may bind and decrease the absorption of levothyroxine sodium from GI tract) 3521

Vegetables, green leafy

Coumadin Tablets (Large amounts of green leafy vegetables may affect warfarin therapy) 932

Walnuts

Levoxyl Tablets (Concurrent use of walnuts may bind and decrease the absorption of levothyroxine sodium from GI tract) 1680

Unithroid Tablets (Concurrent use of walnuts may bind and decrease the absorption of levothyroxine sodium from GI tract) 3521

Wine, Chianti

Parnate Tablets (Potential for hypertensive crisis; concurrent use is contraindicated) 1499

Wine, unspecified

Matulane Capsules (Procarbazine exhibits some MAO inhibitory activity: concurrent use should be avoided) 3188

Yeast Extract

Parnate Tablets (Potential for hypertensive crisis; concurrent use is contraindicated) 1499

Yogurt

Matulane Capsules (Procarbazine exhibits some MAO inhibitory activity: concurrent use should be avoided) 3188

Parnate Tablets (Potential for hypertensive crisis; concurrent use is contraindicated) 1499

SECTION 3

SIDE EFFECTS INDEX

Presented in this section is an alphabetical list of every side effect reported in the "Adverse Reactions" section of the product descriptions in *PDR*® and its companion volumes. Under each side effect is an alphabetical list of brands associated with the reaction.

If noted in the underlying text, incidence is shown in parentheses immediately after the brand name. Products reporting an incidence rate of 3% or more are marked with a ▲ symbol at their left. Because incidence data are sometimes drawn from controlled clinical trials, the rates seen in actual clinical practice may vary from those found in the published reports.

This index lists only side effects noted in official prescribing information as published by *PDR*®. To alert you to the full range of possibilities, the entries include adverse effects shared by an entire class of drugs, but not necessarily reported for the specific drug in question. The index is restricted to reactions that may be expected to occur at recommended dosages in the general patient population. Precautions to be taken under special circumstances are not listed, nor are the effects of overdosage.

The page numbers shown for the products refer to the 2006 editions of *PDR*® and *PDR for Ophthalmic Medicines™*, and the 2005 edition of *PDR for Nonprescription Drugs and Dietary Supplements™*, which is published later in the year. A key to the symbols denoting the companion volumes appears in the bottom margin.

A

Abdomen, enlarged
Abilify Tablets (Infrequent) ... 916
Abilify Tablets (Infrequent) ... 2472
▲ Bravelle for Intramuscular or Subcutaneous Injection (2.7% to 6.7%) ... 1140
Campral Tablets (Rare) ... 1175
▲ Camptosar Injection (0% to 10%) ... 2602
Combunox Tablets (Less than 1%) ... 1183
▲ Follistim AQ Cartridge (8%) ... 2354
▲ Gonal-f RFF Pen for Injection (Greater than 10%) ... 3155
▲ I.V. Busulfex (23%) ... 1125
Menopur for Subcutaneous Injection (2.4%) ... 1145
Omacor Capsules ... 2735
Prevacid NapraPAC (Less than 1%) .. 3277
Relpax Tablets (Rare) ... 2531
Reyataz Capsules (Less than 3%) ... 948

Abdomen, redistribution/accumulation of body fat
Kaletra ... 474
Retrovir ... 1533

Abdominal bloating
Abilify Tablets (Infrequent) ... 916
Abilify Tablets (Infrequent) ... 2472
Aciphex Tablets (Rare) ... 1081
Activella Tablets ... 2311
Actonel with Calcium Tablets ... 2684
Aerobid/Aerobid-M (Less than 1%) ... 1172
Alesse-28 Tablets ... 3392
Aralast (Greater than or equal to 0.2%) ... 745
Aricept Tablets (Frequent) ... 1086
Aricept ODT Tablets (Frequent) ... 1086
Asacol Delayed-Release Tablets (2% or greater) ... 2688
Bentyl Capsules ... 724
Bentyl Injection ... 724
Bentyl Syrup ... 724
Bentyl Tablets ... 724
Cenestin Tablets, 0.45mg, 0.625mg, 0.9mg, 1.25mg ... 1063
Cenestin Tablets, 0.3mg ... 1063
Climara Transdermal System ... 795
Climara Pro Transdermal System ... 800
Colazal Capsules ... 2845
▲ Colyte with Flavor Packs for Oral Solution (Up to 50%) ... 3102
Coumadin for Injection (Infrequent) ... 932
Coumadin Tablets (Infrequent) ... 932
▲ Creon 5 Capsules (Among most frequent) ... 3195
▲ Creon 10 Capsules (Among most frequent) ... 3195
▲ Creon 20 Capsules (Among most frequent) ... 3196
▲ Depo-Provera Contraceptive Injection (1% to 5%) ... 2619
Estratest Tablets ... 3196
Estratest H.S. Tablets ... 3196
Estrogel 0.06% ... 3200
▲ HalfLytely and Bisacodyl Tablets Bowel Prep Kit with Flavors Packs (22.3% to 50%) ... 915
Imitrex Nasal Spray ... 1435
Indocin Capsules (Less than 1%) ... 1968
Indocin I.V. (Less than 1%) ... 1973
Indocin (Less than 1%) ... 1968
Lexapro Oral Solution (Infrequent) ... 1193
Lexapro Tablets (Infrequent) ... 1193
Lo/Ovral-28 Tablets ... 3423
Menostar Transdermal System ... 805
MetroGel-Vaginal Gel (Less than 1%) ... 1822
Midamor Tablets (Less than or equal to 1%) ... 2000
Moduretic Tablets (Less than or equal to 1%) ... 2003
Nadolol Tablets (1 to 5 of 1000 patients) ... 2121
Noroxin Tablets (Less frequent) ... 2009
Norvir (Less than 2%) ... 499
Ortho-Cept Tablets ... 2395
Ortho-Cyclen Tablets ... 2414
Ortho Evra Transdermal System ... 2402
Ortho Tri-Cyclen Tablets ... 2414
Ortho Tri-Cyclen Lo Tablets ... 2421
Prefest Tablets ... 1069
Premarin Intravenous ... 3440
Premarin Tablets ... 3443
Premarin Vaginal Cream ... 3449
Premphase Tablets ... 3452
Prempro Tablets ... 3452
Prilosec OTC Tablets (Less than 1%) ... 2674
▲ Prochieve 4% Gel (7%) ... 1018
▲ Prochieve 8% Gel (7%) ... 1018
▲ Prometrium Capsules (100 mg, 200 mg) (12%) ... 3205
ProNutra Protein Supplement ... 1643
Reishimax Capsules ... 2669
Repronex for Intramuscular and Subcutaneous Injection ... 1148
Roferon-A Injection (Infrequent) ... 2805
Senokot Wheat Bran ... 2717
▲ Thrombate III (1 of 17) ... 3254
Ticlid Tablets (0.5% to 1.0%) ... 2813
▲ TriLyte with Flavor Packs for Oral Solution (Up to 50%) ... 3114
Triphasil-28 Tablets ... 3483
Vivelle Transdermal System ... 2288
Vivelle-Dot Transdermal System ... 2293
Yasmin 28 Tablets ... 818
▲ Zavesca Capsules (6%) ... 543
Zegerid Powder for Oral Solution (Less than 1%) ... 2972

Abdominal discomfort
(*see also under* Distress, abdominal; Distress, gastrointestinal)
Biaxin/Biaxin XL (2%) ... 402
Brevibloc Concentrate (Less than 1%) ... 766
Brevibloc Injection (Less than 1%) ... 766
Brevibloc Double Strength Injection (Less than 1%) ... 766
Brevibloc Premixed Injection (Less than 1%) ... 766
Brevibloc Double Strength Premixed Injection (Less than 1%) ... 766
Carafate Tablets (Less than 0.5%) ... 728
Cipro I.V. (1.7%) ... 2998
Cipro I.V. Pharmacy Bulk Package (1.7%) ... 3509
Cipro (Less than 1%) ... 2991
Cipro XR Tablets (Less than 1%) ... 3004
▲ Clozapine Tablets (4%) ... 2141
▲ Clozaril Tablets (4%) ... 2174
▲ Depo-Provera Contraceptive Injection (Greater than 5%) ... 2619
Desferal Vials ... 2190
Dulcolax Suppositories ... ▣ 608
Dulcolax Tablets ... ▣ 607
DynaCirc CR Tablets (1.3% to 5.1%) ... 2726
▲ Epivir-HBV (16%) ... 1398
▲ FazaClo Orally Disintegrating Tablets (4%) ... 547
Fleet Bisacodyl Laxatives ... 1169
Fleet Prep Kits ... 1172
▲ Flovent Diskus 50 mcg (3%) ... 1415
▲ Gengraf Capsules (Up to 7%) ... 458
Hyperstat I.V. Injection ... 3031
Imitrex Nasal Spray (Infrequent) ... 1435
Imitrex Tablets ... 1440
Imodium Capsules ... 1834
K-Dur Extended-Relase Tablets ... 3047
Klonopin (Infrequent) ... 2782
Lexapro Oral Solution (Infrequent) ... 1193
Lexapro Tablets (Infrequent) ... 1193
Lithobid Tablets ... 1670
▲ Lotronex Tablets (7%) ... 1479
Children's Motrin Oral Suspension and Chewable Tablets ... ▣ 647
Children's Motrin Non-Staining Dye-Free Oral Suspension ... ▣ 647
Children's Motrin Oral Suspension and Chewable Tablets ... 1837
Children's Motrin Non-Staining Dye-Free Oral Suspension ... 1837
Infants' Motrin Concentrated Drops ... 1837
Infants' Motrin Non-Staining Dye-Free Drops ... 1837

Junior Strength Motrin Caplets and Chewable Tablets ... 1837
Nadolol Tablets (1 to 5 of 1000 patients) ... 2121
▲ Neoral Soft Gelatin Capsules (Up to 7%) ... 2247
▲ Neoral Oral Solution (Up to 7%) ... 2247
▲ Niravam Orally Disintegrating Tablets (18.3%) ... 3106
Pepcid Injection (Infrequent) ... 2017
Pepcid (Infrequent) ... 2014
Relpax Tablets (1% to 2%) ... 2531
▲ Sandimmune (Less than 1% to 7%) ... 2259
▲ Sandostatin Injection (34% to 61%) ... 2263
▲ Trisenox Injection (8%) ... 983
Urecholine Tablets ... 2349
Urocit-K Tablets (Some patients) ... 2109
Vantas (Less than 2%) ... 3367
▲ Xenical Capsules (25.5%) ... 2834
Zelnorm Tablets ... 2303

Abdominal distention

Actiq (1% or greater) ... 993
Aldoclor Tablets ... 1881
Aldoril Tablets ... 1884
Aloprim for Injection (Less than 1%) ... 2156
AmBisome for Injection (Less common) ... 615
Ammonul Injection ... 3323
Aptivus Capsules (Less than 2%) ... 859
Avalide Tablets ... 922
Avalide Tablets ... 2889
Avapro Tablets (Less than 1%) ... 925
Avapro Tablets (Less than 1%) ... 2886
▲ CellCept Capsules (3% to less than 20%) ... 2751
▲ CellCept Intravenous (3% to less than 20%) ... 2751
▲ CellCept Oral Suspension (3% to less than 20%) ... 2751
▲ CellCept Tablets (3% to less than 20%) ... 2751
Clozapine Tablets (Less than 1%) ... 2141
Clozaril Tablets (Less than 1%) ... 2174
Crixivan Capsules ... 1918
Cubicin for Injection (Less than 1%) ... 1038
Cytovene (At least 3 subjects) ... 2763
Decadron Phosphate Injection ... 1931
Decadron Tablets ... 1929
▲ DepoDur Extended-Release Injection (2% to 5%) ... 1098
Depo-Medrol Injectable Suspension ... 2615
Depo-Medrol Single-Dose Vial ... 2617
▲ depo-subQ provera 104 Injectable Suspension (1% to less than 5%) ... 2622
▲ Doxil Injection (1% to 10%) ... 3302
Duragesic Transdermal System (Less than 1%) ... 2448
DynaCirc CR Tablets (1.2%) ... 2726
Effexor Tablets (Infrequent) ... 3405
▲ Eloxatin for Injection (2% to 5%) ... 2908
Evoxac Capsules ... 1042
FazaClo Orally Disintegrating Tablets (Less than 1%) ... 547
▲ Flolan for Injection (4%) ... 1408
Follistim AQ Cartridge ... 2354
Fosamax (Up to 1.4%) ... 1949
Fosamax Plus D Tablets (0% to 1.4%) ... 1956
Gengraf Capsules (1% to less than 3%) ... 458
Gleevec Tablets (Less common) ... 2221
Hydrocortone Tablets ... 1963
Imitrex Nasal Spray ... 1435
Imodium Capsules ... 1834
Indocin I.V. (1% to 3%) ... 1973
▲ Intron A for Injection (Less than 5%) ... 3038
Invanz for Injection (Greater than 0.1%) ... 1974
Kaletra (Less than 2%) ... 474
Ketek Tablets (Greater than or equal to 0.2% to less than 2%) ... 2920
Lamictal (Rare) ... 1449
▲ Leukine (4%) ... 829
Lotronex Tablets (2%) ... 1479
Mavik Tablets (0.3% to 1.0%) ... 482
Merrem I.V. (Greater than 0.1% to 1%) ... 687
Mirapex Tablets (Less than 1%) ... 889
▲ Myfortic Tablets (3% to less than 20%) ... 2244
Neoral Soft Gelatin Capsules (1% to less than 3%) ... 2247
Neoral Oral Solution (1% to less than 3%) ... 2247
Nexium Delayed-Release Capsules (Less than 1%) ... 645
Nexium I.V. (Less than 1%) ... 649
Pediapred Oral Solution ... 3319
Pentasa Capsules (Less than 1%) ... 3182
Permax Tablets (Infrequent) ... 3357
Prevacid Delayed-Release Capsules (Less than 1%) ... 3268
Prevacid for Delayed-Release Oral Suspension (Less than 1%) ... 3268
Prevacid SoluTab Delayed-Release Orally Disintegrating Tablets (Less than 1%) ... 3268
PREVPAC (Less than 1%) ... 3281
▲ Prograf Capsules and Injection (3% to 15%) ... 624
▲ Proleukin for Injection (10%) ... 1007
▲ Prometrium Capsules (100 mg, 200 mg) (6% to 8%) ... 3205
▲ Rapamune Oral Solution and Tablets (3% to 20%) ... 3472
ReoPro Vials (0.1%) ... 1779
▲ Repronex for Intramuscular and Subcutaneous Injection (2.1% to 6%) ... 1148
Requip Tablets (Infrequent) ... 1528
Rescriptor Tablets ... 2535
Rilutek Tablets (Infrequent) ... 2945
Risperdal M-Tab Orally Disintegrating Tablets (Rare) ... 1658
Risperdal (Rare) ... 1658
▲ Rituxan for Infusion (1% to 5%) ... 845
Rythmol SR Capsules ... 2736
Sanctura Tablets (Greater than or equal to 0.5%) ... 1133
▲ Sandostatin Injection (Less than 10% to 35%) ... 2263
Sandostatin LAR Depot (Rare) ... 2264
Seroquel Tablets (Rare) ... 691
▲ Simulect for Injection (3% to 10%) ... 2268
▲ Taxotere Injection Concentrate (6%) ... 2947
Thalomid Capsules ... 979
Tiazac Capsules (2%) ... 1204
Topamax Sprinkle Capsules (Infrequent) ... 2438
Topamax Tablets (Infrequent) ... 2438
▲ Trisenox Injection (8%) ... 983
▲ Valcyte Tablets (Less than 5%) ... 2816
Vantin Tablets and Oral Suspension (Less than 1%) ... 2650
▲ Vesanoid Capsules (11%) ... 2823
VFEND I.V. (Less than 2%) ... 2543
VFEND Oral Suspension (Less than 2%) ... 2543
VFEND Tablets (Less than 2%) ... 2543
▲ Vivelle Transdermal System (1.5% to 3.8%) ... 2288
▲ Vivelle-Dot Transdermal System (1.5% to 3.8%) ... 2293
▲ Xeloda Tablets (Less than 5%) ... 2825
Xifaxan Tablets (Less than 2%) ... 2847
▲ Zavesca Capsules (8%) ... 543
▲ Zelnorm Tablets (3% to 4%) ... 2303
▲ Zenapax for Injection (Greater than 5%) ... 2838
▲ Zevalin Injection (5%) ... 848
Zyprexa Tablets (Rare) ... 1798
Zyprexa ZYDIS Orally Disintegrating Tablets (Rare) ... 1798
Zyrtec Chewable Tablets (Less than 2%) ... 2589
Zyrtec (Less than 2%) ... 2589
Zyrtec-D 12 Hour Extended Release Tablets (Less than 2%) ... 2591

Abdominal guarding

Sandostatin LAR Depot (Rare) ... 2264

Abdominal mass

Estratest Tablets ... 3196
Estratest H.S. Tablets ... 3196

Abdominal pain, gynecological

▲ Follistim AQ Cartridge (25%) ... 2354

Abdominal pain/cramps

▲ Abelcet Injection (4%) ... 1119
Abilify Tablets ... 916
Abilify Tablets ... 2472
Accolate Tablets (1.8% to 2.8%) ... 663
Aceon Tablets (2 mg, 4 mg, 8 mg) (2.7%) ... 3191
Aciphex Tablets ... 1081
▲ Actimmune (8%) ... 1646
Actiq (1% or greater) ... 993
Activella Tablets ... 2311
▲ Actonel Tablets (7.3% to 11.6%) ... 2679
▲ Actonel with Calcium Tablets (7.3% to 11.6%) ... 2684
Adalat CC Tablets (Less than 1%) ... 2978
▲ Adderall XR Capsules (11% to 14%) ... 3169
Advair Diskus 100/50 ... 1291
Advair Diskus 250/50 ... 1291
Advair Diskus 500/50 ... 1291
Advate Injection (0.6%) ... 742
▲ Advicor Tablets (4%) ... 1694
▲ Aerobid/Aerobid-M (3% to 9%) ... 1172
▲ Agenerase Capsules (14%) ... 1299
Agenerase Oral Solution ... 1304
▲ Aggrenox Capsules (17.5%) ... 855
▲ Agrylin Capsules (16.4%) ... 3172
▲ Albenza Tablets (Up to 6.0%) ... 1310
Aldoclor Tablets ... 1881
Aldoril Tablets ... 1884
Alesse-28 Tablets ... 3392
▲ Alinia for Oral Suspension (7.8%) ... 2840
▲ Alinia Tablets (7.8%) ... 2840
Allegra-D 12 Hour Extended-Release Tablets (1.4%) ... 2860
Allegra-D 24 Hour Extended-Release Tablets (1.4%) ... 2862
Aloxi Injection (Less than 1%) ... 2099
Altace Capsules (Less than 1%) ... 1673
Altoprev Extended-Release Tablets (2% to 2.5%) ... 1151
Ambien Tablets (2%) ... 2867
▲ AmBisome for Injection (9.9% to 19.8%) ... 615
Amerge Tablets (Infrequent) ... 1312
Aminohippurate Sodium "PAH" Injection ... 1886
▲ Anaprox Tablets (3% to 9%) ... 2769
▲ Anaprox DS Tablets (3% to 9%) ... 2769
Ancef for Injection ... 1318
▲ Angiomax for Injection (5%) ... 1856
▲ Antara Capsules (4.6%) ... 2723
▲ Anzemet Injection (3.2%) ... 2871
Anzemet Tablets (Rare) ... 2874
Aptivus Capsules (2.8%) ... 859
▲ Aranesp for Injection (12%) ... 576
▲ Arava Tablets (6%) ... 2881
▲ Aredia for Injection (22.6%) ... 2168
▲ Argatroban Injection (2.6% to 3.6%) ... 1321
Aricept Tablets ... 1086
Aricept ODT Tablets ... 1086
▲ Arimidex Tablets (6% to 8%) ... 665
Arixtra Injection (1.4%) ... 1325
▲ Aromasin Tablets (6%) ... 2600
▲ Arthrotec Tablets (21%) ... 3126
▲ Asacol Delayed-Release Tablets (18%) ... 2688
▲ Asmanex Twisthaler (2% to 3%) ... 2981
Astelin Nasal Spray (Infrequent) ... 1876
Atacand Tablets (More than 1%) ... 634
Atacand HCT (0.5% or greater) ... 637
Augmentin XR Extended-Release Tablets (1.6%) ... 1340
Avalide Tablets (2%) ... 922
Avalide Tablets (2%) ... 2889
Avapro Tablets (1% or greater) ... 925
Avapro Tablets (1% or greater) ... 2886
▲ Avastin IV (8% to 61%) ... 1229
Avelox (0.1% to less than 2%) ... 2984
▲ Avinza Capsules (5% to 10%) ... 1714
▲ Avonex (8%) ... 839
Axert Tablets (Infrequent) ... 2430
▲ Axid Oral Solution (7.5%) ... 913
Azasan Tablets (Rare) ... 2844
▲ Azmacort Inhalation Aerosol (1% to 3%) ... 1701
Bactroban Cream (Less than 1%) ... 1356
Beano ... ▣ 764
Benicar Tablets (Greater than 0.5%) ... 2850
Benicar HCT Tablets (Greater than 1%) ... 2852
Bentyl Capsules ... 724
Bentyl Injection ... 724
Bentyl Syrup ... 724
Bentyl Tablets ... 724
▲ Betaseron for SC Injection (19%) ... 791
▲ Bexxar (3% to 15%) ... 1360
Biaxin/Biaxin XL (2% to 3%) ... 402
Biltricide Tablets ... 2990
Blocadren Tablets ... 1891
▲ Boniva Tablets (5.3% to 7.8%) ... 2747
▲ Boostrix (3% to 26%) ... 1366
▲ Bravelle for Intramuscular or Subcutaneous Injection (2.9% to 14%) ... 1140
Buphenyl Powder (Less than or equal to 2%) ... 3327
Buphenyl Tablets (Less than or equal to 2%) ... 3327
▲ Caduet Tablets (1.6% to 3.8%) ... 2507
▲ Campath Ampules (2% to 11%) ... 826
Campral Tablets (Frequent) ... 1175
▲ Camptosar Injection (9% to 67.7%) ... 2602
▲ Canasa Rectal Suppositories (5.2%) ... 726
▲ Cancidas for Injection (0% to 3.6%) ... 1894
Captopril Tablets (About 0.5% to 2%) ... 2114
Carbatrol Capsules ... 3174
Cardene I.V. (0.7%) ... 1129
Carimune NF ... 3501
▲ Carnitor Injection (5% to 21%) ... 3185
Carnitor Tablets and Oral Solution ... 3187
▲ Casodex Tablets (8%) ... 670
▲ Cataflam Tablets (1% to 10%) ... 2173
Catapres Tablets (Rare) ... 874
Ceftin (0.1% to 1%) ... 1369
▲ Celebrex Capsules (4.1%) ... 3130
▲ Celexa (3%) ... 1177
▲ CellCept Capsules (24.7% to 62.5%) ... 2751
▲ CellCept Intravenous (24.7% to 62.5%) ... 2751
▲ CellCept Oral Suspension (24.7% to 62.5%) ... 2751
▲ CellCept Tablets (24.7% to 62.5%) ... 2751
▲ Cenestin Tablets, 0.45mg, 0.625mg, 0.9mg, 1.25mg (9.4% to 28%) ... 1063
Cenestin Tablets, 0.3mg ... 1063
▲ Cerezyme for Injection (Approximately 6.5%) ... 1263
Cervidil Vaginal Insert (Less than 1%) ... 1182
▲ Chemet Capsules (5.2% to 15.7%) ... 2480
Chromagen Soft Gelatin Capsules ... 3296
Chromagen Forte Soft Gelatin Capsules ... 3296
Cialis Tablets (Less than 2%) ... 1806
▲ Cipro I.V. (1% or less to 3.3%) ... 2998
▲ Cipro I.V. Pharmacy Bulk Package (1% or less to 3.3%) ... 3509
▲ Cipro (Less than 1% to 3.3%) ... 2991
Cipro XR Tablets (Less than 1%) ... 3004
Cleocin Vaginal Ovules (Less than 1%) ... 2613
▲ Climara Transdermal System (11% to 16%) ... 795
▲ Climara Pro Transdermal System (4.2%) ... 800
Clindagel ... 1207
Clindesse Vaginal Cream (Rare) ... 3296
▲ Clinoril Tablets (10%) ... 1899
▲ Clolar for Intravenous Infusion (36%) ... 1264
▲ Colazal Capsules (6%) ... 2845
Colyte with Flavor Packs for Oral Solution (Less frequent) ... 3102
▲ CombiPatch Transdermal System (12% to 14%) ... 2180
▲ Combivir Tablets (6% to 9%) ... 1373
Combunox Tablets (Less than 1%) ... 1183
▲ Comtan Tablets (8%) ... 2186
▲ Concerta Extended-Release Tablets (0.7% to 7%) ... 1828
Copaxone for Injection (At least 2%) ... 3292
▲ Copegus Tablets (8%) ... 2759
Cosmegen for Injection ... 1907
Cosopt Sterile Ophthalmic Solution (1% to 5%) ... 1910
Coumadin for Injection (Infrequent) ... 932
Coumadin Tablets (Infrequent) ... 932
Cozaar Tablets (1% or greater) ... 1913
▲ Creon 5 Capsules (Among most frequent) ... 3195
▲ Creon 10 Capsules (Among most frequent) ... 3195
▲ Creon 20 Capsules (Among most frequent) ... 3196
Crestor Tablets (Greater than or equal to 2%) ... 672
▲ Crixivan Capsules (16.6%) ... 1918
Cubicin for Injection (1% to 2%) ... 1038
Cymbalta Delayed-Release Capsules (Infrequent) ... 1729
Cytovene (At least 3 subjects) ... 2763
Dalmane Capsules ... 3343
Dantrium Capsules (Less frequent) ... 2690
Dapsone Tablets USP ... 1656
Darvocet A 500 Tablets ... 3497
DDAVP Injection 4 mcg/mL (Infrequent) ... 2893
DDAVP Nasal Spray (2%) ... 2894
DDAVP Tablets ... 2895
Demser Capsules (Infrequent) ... 1933
▲ Depacon Injection (1.1% to 23%) ... 412
▲ Depakene (12% to 23%) ... 417
▲ Depakote Sprinkle Capsules (9% to 23%) ... 422
▲ Depakote Tablets (9% to 23%) ... 427
▲ Depakote ER Tablets (7% to 23%) ... 433
▲ Depo-Provera Contraceptive Injection (Greater than 5%) ... 2619
▲ depo-subQ provera 104 Injectable Suspension (1% to less than 5%) ... 2622
Desmopressin Acetate Injection (Infrequent) ... 1143
Desmopressin Acetate Rhinal Tube (2%) ... 1144
▲ Detrol Tablets (7.6%) ... 2626
▲ Detrol LA Capsules (4%) ... 2629
Diastat Rectal Delivery System (1% or more) ... 3344
Digitek Tablets ... 2146

Dilaudid-HP (Less frequent) 441
Diovan HCT Tablets (Greater than 0.2%) 2195
Diovan Tablets (2%) 2191
Diprivan Injectable Emulsion (Less than 1%) 676
▲ Ditropan XL Extended Release Tablets (2% to less than 5%) 2391
Diuril Sodium Intravenous 1934
▲ Dostinex Tablets (5%) 2631
▲ Doxil Injection (1% to 33.5%) 3302
Duac Topical Gel 3214
▲ Duragesic Transdermal System (3% to 10%) 2448
Dyazide Capsules 1389
▲ EC-Naprosyn Delayed-Release Tablets (3% to 9%) 2769
Edecrin 1941
▲ E.E.S. (Among most frequent) 449
▲ Effexor Tablets (2.2% to 8.0%) 3405
▲ Effexor XR Capsules (4%) 3411
▲ Eldepryl Capsules (4 of 49 patients) 3209
▲ Elitek (20%) 2906
Elmiron Capsules (2%) 2393
▲ Eloxatin for Injection (1% to 33%) 2908
Elspar for Injection 1943
▲ Emend Capsules (4.6%) 1944
▲ Emtriva Capsules (8% to 14%) 1272
▲ Enablex Extended-Release Tablets (2.4% to 3.9%) 2201
▲ Enbrel for Injection (5% to 19%) 580
Engerix-B Vaccine (Less than 1%) 1391
▲ Entocort EC Capsules (6%) 2694
▲ Epivir (6% to 9%) 1394
▲ Epivir-HBV (16%) 1398
Epogen for Injection 586
▲ Epzicom Tablets (4% to 5%) 1402
Equetro Extended-Release Capsules 3178
▲ Erbitux (25%) 937
▲ EryPed (Among most frequent) 445
▲ Ery-Tab Tablets (Among most frequent) 447
▲ Erythrocin Stearate Filmtab Tablets (Among most frequent) 452
▲ Erythromycin Base Filmtab Tablets (Among most frequent) 454
▲ Erythromycin Delayed-Release Capsules, USP (Among most frequent) 456
Eskalith 1406
Estratest Tablets 3196
Estratest H.S. Tablets 3196
▲ Estrogel 0.06% (7.7%) 3200
▲ Evista Tablets (6.6%) 1735
Evoclin Foam, 1% 1025
▲ Evoxac Capsules (7.6%) 1042
▲ Exelon Capsules (13%) 2204
Factive Tablets (0.9%) 2464
▲ Famvir Tablets (1.1% to 7.9%) 2207
▲ Faslodex Injection (11.8%) 682
▲ Femara Tablets (4% to 6%) 2210
▲ Ferrlecit Injection (3% to 15%) 3379
Fleet Bisacodyl Laxatives 1169
Fleet Prep Kits 1172
▲ Flolan for Injection (5% to 27%) 1408
▲ Flonase Nasal Spray (1% to 3%) 1412
▲ Flovent Diskus 50 mcg (3%) 1415
Floxin Otic Singles (Reported in a single subject) 1045
Floxin Otic Solution (Single report) 1043
Flumadine (1.4%) 1186
▲ Flumist Vaccine (3.7%) 1872
▲ Focalin Tablets (15%) 2214
Focalin XR Capsules 2217
▲ Follistim AQ Cartridge (5% to 28%) 2354
▲ Fortamet Extended-Release Tablets (3.3%) 1156
Fortaz (1 in 416) 1422
▲ Fortical Nasal Spray (1% to 3%) 3336
▲ Fosamax (0.9% to 6.6%) 1949
▲ Fosamax Plus D Tablets (0.9% to 6.6%) 1956
▲ Fosrenol Chewable Tablets (5% to 17%) 3180
Frova Tablets (Frequent) 1101
Furosemide Tablets 2117
▲ Fuzeon Injection (3.9%) 2772
▲ Gabitril Tablets (5% to 7%) 998
Gammagard Liquid 751
Gammagard S/D 754
▲ Gamunex Immune Globulin I.V., 10% (4%) 3232
▲ Gengraf Capsules (2.7% to 15%) 458
Geodon (Frequent) 2514
▲ Gleevec Tablets (23.4% to 37%) 2221
▲ Gonal-f RFF Pen for Injection (Greater than 12%) 3155
Guanidine Hydrochloride Tablets 3030
▲ Gynazole-1 Vaginal Cream (5.7%) 3298
▲ HalfLytely and Bisacodyl Tablets Bowel Prep Kit with Flavors Packs (9.1% to 50%) 915
Havrix Vaccine (Less than 1%) 1425
▲ Hepsera Tablets (2% to 9%) 1275
▲ Herceptin I.V. (22%) 1234
▲ Humira Injection (7%) 464
▲ Hycamtin for Injection (Less than 1% to 33%) 1427
Hytrin Capsules (At least 1%) 469
Hyzaar (1.2%) 1964
▲ Idamycin PFS Injection (73%) 2645
▲ Imdur Tablets (Less than or equal to 5%) 3032
Imitrex Injection 1431
Imitrex Nasal Spray 1435
Imitrex Tablets 1440
Imodium Capsules 1834
Indapamide Tablets (Less than 5%) 2119
Inderal LA Long-Acting Capsules 3421
Indocin (Greater than 1%) 1968
Infed Injection 3381
▲ Infergen (24% to 41%) 1647
InnoPran XL Capsules 2728
Inspra Tablets (1%) 2520
▲ Intron A for Injection (1% to 21%) 3038
▲ Invanz for Injection (3.6% to 4.7%) 1974
▲ Invirase (0.3% to 6.1%) 2776
▲ I.V. Busulfex (3% to 72%) 1125
Iveegam EN 759
Kadian Capsules (Less than 3%) 572
▲ Kaletra (4% to 10%) 474
K-Dur Extended-Relase Tablets 3047
Keppra Oral Solution (1% to 2%) 3307
Keppra Tablets (1% to 2%) 3307
Ketek Tablets (Greater than or equal to 0.2% to less than 2%) 2920
▲ Kineret Injection (5%) 594
Klonopin (1%) 2782
▲ K-Lor Powder Packets (Among most common) 472
Kristalose for Oral Solution 2149
▲ Kytril Tablets (4% to 6%) 2788
▲ Lamictal (5% to 10%) 1449
Lamisil Tablets (2.4%) 2226
Lanoxicaps Capsules (Rare) 1458
Lanoxin Injection (Rare) 1462
Lanoxin Tablets (Rare) 1468
Lanoxin Injection Pediatric (Rare) 1465
▲ Lariam Tablets (Among most frequent) 2790
▲ Lescol Capsules (4.9%) 2227
▲ Lescol Capsules (4.9%) 2730
▲ Lescol XL Tablets (3.7%) 2227
▲ Lescol XL Tablets (3.7%) 2730
▲ Leukine (38%) 829
▲ Leustatin Injection (6%) 2368
Levaquin in 5% Dextrose Injection (0.4% to 2.5%) 2453
Levaquin (0.4% to 2.5%) 2453
Levitra Tablets (Less than 2%) 3048
Levothroid Tablets 1189
Levoxyl Tablets 1680
Lexapro Oral Solution (2%) 1193
Lexapro Tablets (2%) 1193
▲ Lexiva Tablets (Less than 1% to 11%) 1473
▲ Lipitor Tablets (Up to 3.8%) 2495
Lithobid Tablets 1670
▲ Lofibra Capsules (4.6%) 1217
Lo/Ovral-28 Tablets 3423
Lotensin HCT Tablets (0.3% to 1%) 2235
Lotrel Capsules 2238
▲ Lotronex Tablets (7%) 1479
Lunesta Tablets 3139
Lyrica Capsules (Greather than or equal to 1%) 2524
▲ Malarone Tablets (2% to 31%) 1484
▲ Malarone Pediatric Tablets (2% to 31%) 1484
▲ Marinol Capsules (3% to 10%) 3334
Matulane Capsules 3188
Mavik Tablets (0.3% to 1.0%) 482
Maxair Autohaler 1820
Mefoxin for Injection 1987
Mefoxin Premixed Intravenous Solution 1990
▲ Megace ES Oral Suspension (1% to 3%) 2492
▲ Menopur for Subcutaneous Injection (6% to 17.6%) 1145
▲ Menostar Transdermal System (46%) 805
▲ Mepron Suspension (4% to 21%) 1487
▲ Meridia Capsules (4.5%) 485
Merrem I.V. (Greater than 0.1% to 1%) 687
▲ Metadate CD Capsules (7%) 3316
▲ Mevacor Tablets (2.0% to 5.7%) 1996
Miacalcin Injection 2241
Miacalcin Nasal Spray (1% to 3%) 2242
Micardis Tablets (1%) 884
Micardis HCT Tablets (Less than 2%) 886
▲ Midamor Tablets (Between 1% and 3%) 2000
Migranal Nasal Spray (Rare) 3350
Mintezol 2002
Miradon Tablets 3056
Mirapex Tablets (1% or more) 889
▲ Mirena Intrauterine System (5% or more) 810
▲ Mobic Oral Suspension (1.9% to 4.7%) 893
▲ Mobic Tablets (1.9% to 4.7%) 893
Moduretic Tablets (Greater than 1%, less than 3%) 2003
MS Contin Tablets (Less frequent) 2703
Mycamine for Injection (0.5% to 1.9%) 620
▲ Myfortic Tablets (3% to less than 20%) 2244
▲ Mylotarg for Injection (26% to 39%) 3429
Nabi-HB 2159
Nalfon Capsules (2%) 2504
▲ Naprosyn Suspension (3% to 9%) 2769
▲ Naprosyn Tablets (3% to 9%) 2769
▲ Natrecor for Injection (1% to 3%) 3123
Navelbine Injection 1494
▲ Neoral Soft Gelatin Capsules (2.7% to 15%) 2247
▲ Neoral Oral Solution (2.7% to 15%) 2247
▲ Neulasta Injection (15% to 72%) 596
▲ Neumega for Injection (Greater than or equal to 10%) 3433
Neupogen for Injection (Infrequent) 598
Neurontin Capsules (2.7%) 2498
Neurontin Oral Solution (2.7%) 2498
Neurontin Tablets (2.7%) 2498
▲ Nexium Delayed-Release Capsules (Greater than or equal to 1% to 3.8%) 645
▲ Nexium I.V. (Greater than or equal to 1% to 3.8%) 649
▲ Niaspan Extended-Release Tablets (2% to 5%) 1703
▲ Nicotrol NS (3%) 2596
Niferex-150 Forte Capsules 3299
▲ Nipent for Injection (4% to 16%) 3216
Noroxin Tablets (0.3% to 1.6%) 2009
Norvasc Tablets (1.6%) 2529
▲ Norvir (6% to 8.3%) 499
Nubain Injection (1% or less) 1111
Numorphan 1112
Omnicef Capsules (1%) 506
Omnicef for Oral Suspension (0.8%) 506
▲ Oncaspar (Greater than 1% but less than 5%) 1123
Ortho-Cept Tablets 2395
Ortho-Cyclen Tablets 2414
▲ Ortho Evra Transdermal System (9% to 22%) 2402
Ortho Tri-Cyclen Tablets 2414
Ortho Tri-Cyclen Lo Tablets 2421
Orthoclone OKT3 Sterile Solution 2370
▲ OxyContin Tablets (Between 1% and 5%) 2699
▲ Oxytrol Transdermal System (Greater than 1%) 3383
▲ Pacerone Tablets (1% to 3%) 3337
▲ Pancrease MT Capsules (Among most frequent) 1839
Parcopa Orally Disintegrating Tablets 3111
Parnate Tablets 1499
▲ Paser Granules (Among most common) 1657
▲ Paxil CR Controlled-Release Tablets (4%) 1509
▲ Paxil (4%) 1501
▲ PCE Dispertab Tablets (Among most frequent) 510
Pediarix Vaccine 1518
▲ Pegasys (15%) 2793
▲ PEG-Intron Powder for Injection (15%) 3062
Pentasa Capsules (1.1% to 1.7%) 3182
Peri-Colace Tablets 2716
▲ Permax Tablets (5.8%) 3357
▲ Photofrin for Injection (12% to 20%) 729
▲ Plan B Tablets (17.6%) 1068
▲ Plavix Tablets (5.6%) 940
▲ Plavix Tablets (5.6%) 2942
Plendil Extended-Release Tablets (0.5% to 1.5%) 651
▲ Pletal Tablets (4% to 5%) 2478
▲ Pravachol Tablets (2.0% to 5.4%) 943
▲ Precose Tablets (19%) 776
▲ Prefest Tablets (Up to 12%) 1069
Premarin Intravenous 3440
▲ Premarin Tablets (15% to 17%) 3443
Premarin Vaginal Cream 3449
▲ Premphase Tablets (13% to 23%) 3452
▲ Prempro Tablets (13% to 23%) 3452
▲ Prevacid Delayed-Release Capsules (2.1% to 5%) 3268
▲ Prevacid for Delayed-Release Oral Suspension (2.1% to 5%) 3268
Prevacid I.V. for Injection (Less than 1%) 3274
▲ Prevacid NapraPAC (2.1% to 9%) 3277
▲ Prevacid SoluTab Delayed-Release Orally Disintegrating Tablets (2.1% to 5%) 3268
▲ PREVPAC (1.8% to 3%) 3281
▲ Prilosec OTC Tablets (2.4% to 5.2%) 2674
Primaxin I.M. 2022
Primaxin I.V. (Less than 0.2%) 2024
▲ Prinivil Tablets (0.3% to 4.0%) 2029
Prinzide Tablets (0.3% to 1%) 2033
▲ Prochieve 4% Gel (12% to 15%) 1018
▲ Prochieve 8% Gel (12% to 15%) 1018
▲ Prograf Capsules and Injection (29% to 59%) 624
▲ Proleukin for Injection (11%) 1007
▲ Prometrium Capsules (100 mg, 200 mg) (10% to 20%) 3205
ProNutra Protein Supplement 1643
ProSom Tablets (1%) 512
▲ Protonix I.V. (12%) 3468
▲ Protonix Tablets (1% to 4%) 3465
Protopic Ointment (1% to 5%) 629
Provigil Tablets (At least 1%) 1002
Prozac Pulvules and Liquid 1771
Pulmicort Respules (2% to 3%) 654
Pulmozyme Inhalation Solution 1245
▲ Rapamune Oral Solution and Tablets (28% to 36%) 3472
▲ Razadyne ER Extended-Release Capsules (5%) 2434
▲ Razadyne (5%) 2434
▲ Rebetol (13%) 3073
▲ Rebif Prefilled Syringe for Injection (20% to 22%) 3163
Recombivax HB (Less than 1%) 2045
ReFacto Vials 3479
▲ Relafen Tablets (12%) 1523
Relenza Rotadisk (Less than 1.5%) 1525
Relpax Tablets (1% to 2%) 2531
▲ Remicade for IV Injection (12%) 987
Renagel Tablets 1268
Repliva 21/7 Tablets 3301
▲ Repronex for Intramuscular and Subcutaneous Injection (5.2% to 6.9%) 1148
▲ Requip Tablets (3% to 9%) 1528
▲ Rescriptor Tablets (2.4% to 5%) 2535
▲ Retrovir Capsules (3.2%) 1533
▲ Retrovir IV Infusion (4%) 1537
▲ Retrovir (3.2%) 1533
▲ Reyataz Capsules (5% to 10%) 948
▲ Ribavirin, USP Capsules (13%) 3083
▲ Rilutek Tablets (6.8% to 7.8%) 2945
Risperdal Consta Long-Acting Injection (Frequent) 1664
▲ Risperdal M-Tab Orally Disintegrating Tablets (1% to 4%) 1658
▲ Risperdal (1% to 4%) 1658
Ritalin Hydrochloride Tablets 2254
Ritalin LA Capsules 2255
Ritalin-SR Tablets 2254
▲ Rituxan for Infusion (1% to 6%) 845
▲ Rituxan I.V. (14%) 1251
Rocephin Injectable Vials, ADD-Vantage, Galaxy, Bulk (Rare) 2801
▲ Roferon-A Injection (12%) 2805
Rythmol SR Capsules 2736
Sanctura Tablets (1.5%) 1133
▲ Sandostatin LAR Depot (29.1%) 2264
▲ Sedapap Tablets 50 mg/650 mg (Among the most frequent) 2098
▲ Seroquel Tablets (4%) 691
▲ Simulect for Injection (Greater than or equal to 10%) 2268
Singulair (Greater than or equal to 2% to 2.9%) 2047
▲ Sonata Capsules (6%) 1686
▲ Soriatane Capsules (1% to 10%) 1028
Spectracef Tablets (2%) 2706
▲ Spiriva HandiHaler (5% to 6%) 899
▲ Stalevo Tablets (5% to 8%) 2270
▲ Strattera Capsules (2% to 20%) 1784
Striant Mucoadhesive 1022
Stromectol Tablets (0.9%) 2053
▲ Suboxone Tablets (11.20%) 2719
▲ Subutex Tablets (11.7%) 2719
▲ Suprax (3%) 1811
Surmontil Capsules 2347
Sustiva Capsules (1% to 3%) 957
Synercid I.V. (Less than 1%) 1690
▲ Tambocor Tablets (3.3%) 1824
▲ Tamiflu Capsules (2% to 4.7%) 2810
▲ Tamiflu Oral Suspension (2% to 4.7%) 2810
▲ Tarceva Tablets (Less than 1% to 11%) 1254
▲ Tarceva Tablets (Less than 1% to 11%) 2470
▲ Targretin Capsules (3.8% to 10.7%) 1719

▲ Tasmar Tablets (5% to 6%) ... 3360
Taxotere Injection Concentrate ... 2947
Tegretol/Tegretol-XR ... 2278
▲ Temodar Capsules (5% to 9%) ... 3088
▲ Tequin Injection (0.1% to 3%) ... 964
▲ Tequin Tablets (0.1% to 3%) ... 964
Teveten Tablets (2%) ... 1707
Teveten HCT Tablets (Less than 1%) ... 1710
▲ Thalomid Capsules (4.2%) ... 979
▲ Thymoglobulin for Injection (37.8%) ... 2848
Tindamax ... 2670
▲ TOBI Solution for Inhalation (12.8%) ... 1015
▲ Topamax Sprinkle Capsules (5% to 7%) ... 2438
▲ Topamax Tablets (5% to 7%) ... 2438
Toprol-XL Tablets (Greater than 1%) ... 660
Tracleer Tablets ... 539
Trecator Tablets ... 3482
Trelstar LA Suspension (1.1%) ... 3387
▲ Tricor Tablets (4.6%) ... 523
▲ Triglide Tablets (4.6%) ... 1165
▲ Trileptal Oral Suspension (3% to 13%) ... 2281
▲ Trileptal Tablets (3% to 13%) ... 2281
TriLyte with Flavor Packs for Oral Solution ... 3114
Triphasil-28 Tablets (Occasional) ... 3483
▲ Trisenox Injection (58%) ... 983
▲ Trizivir Tablets (6% to 9%) ... 1565
▲ Truvada Tablets (Greater than 5%) ... 1279
Twinrix Vaccine (Less than 1%) ... 1571
▲ Tygacil for Injection (6.8%) ... 3489
Tylenol with Codeine ... 2461
Ultracet Tablets (At least 1%) ... 2462
Ultrase Capsules ... 735
▲ Ultrase MT Capsules (5.7%) ... 736
Uniretic Tablets (More than 1%) ... 3114
Unithroid Tablets ... 3521
Univasc Tablets (Less than 1%) ... 3118
Urecholine Tablets ... 2349
Uroxatral Tablets (1% to 2%) ... 2957
▲ Vagifem Tablets (7%) ... 2340
▲ Valcyte Tablets (15%) ... 2816
▲ Valtrex Caplets (1% to 11%) ... 1573
Vantin Tablets and Oral Suspension (Less than 1% to 1.6%) ... 2650
Vaqta (1.1% to 1.6%) ... 2067
Varivax (Greater than or equal to 1%) ... 2070
Vaseretic Tablets (0.5% to 2.0%) ... 2073
Vasotec I.V. Injection (1.6%) ... 2076
▲ Velcade for Injection (16%) ... 2102
Vermox Chewable Tablets ... 1853
▲ Vesanoid Capsules (31%) ... 2823
VESIcare Tablets (1.2% to 1.9%) ... 631
VFEND I.V. (Less than 2%) ... 2543
VFEND Oral Suspension (Less than 2%) ... 2543
VFEND Tablets (Less than 2%) ... 2543
Viadur Implant (Less than 2%) ... 782
Viagra Tablets (Less than 2%) ... 2552
▲ Vicoprofen Tablets (3% to 9%) ... 533
Viracept (Less than 2%) ... 2556
Viramune Oral Suspension (1%) ... 903
Viramune Tablets (1%) ... 903
▲ Viread Tablets (4% to 7%) ... 1284
Vivactil Tablets ... 2350
▲ Vivelle Transdermal System (1.9% to 3.8%) ... 2288
▲ Vivelle-Dot Transdermal System (1.9% to 3.8%) ... 2293
Vivotif ... 834
▲ Voltaren Ophthalmic Solution (Less than or equal to 3%) ... 2300
▲ Voltaren Tablets (1% to 10%) ... 2298
▲ Voltaren-XR Tablets (1% to 10%) ... 2301
Vytorin 10/10 Tablets ... 2084
Vytorin 10/10 Tablets ... 3092
Vytorin 10/20 Tablets ... 2084
Vytorin 10/20 Tablets ... 3092
Vytorin 10/40 Tablets ... 2084
Vytorin 10/40 Tablets ... 3092
Vytorin 10/80 Tablets ... 2084
Vytorin 10/80 Tablets ... 3092
▲ WelChol Tablets (5%) ... 2855
▲ Wellbutrin SR Sustained-Release Tablets (3% to 9%) ... 1583
▲ Wellbutrin XL Extended-Release Tablets (3% to 9%) ... 1588
WinRho SDF ... 763
Xanax XR Tablets (Frequent) ... 2655
▲ Xeloda Tablets (9% to 35%) ... 2825
▲ Xenical Capsules (25.5%) ... 2834
▲ Xifaxan Tablets (7.2%) ... 2847
Xopenex HFA Inhalation Aerosol (1.5%) ... 3151
Xopenex Inhalation Solution (1.5%) ... 3143
Xopenex Inhalation Solution Concentrate (1.5%) ... 3147
Yasmin 28 Tablets (Greater than 1%) ... 818
Zantac ... 1597
Zantac Injection ... 1593
Zantac Injection Pharmacy Bulk Package (Frequent) ... 1595
Zantac Syrup ... 1597
▲ Zavesca Capsules (18% to 67%) ... 543
▲ Zegerid Powder for Oral Solution (2.4% to 5.2%) ... 2972
▲ Zelnorm Tablets (2% to 12%) ... 2303
Zemaira (0.2% to 0.4%) ... 3506
▲ Zenapax for Injection (Greater than 5%) ... 2838
▲ Zerit (34%) ... 971
Zestoretic Tablets (0.3% to 1.0%) ... 701
Zestril Tablets (0.3% to 2.2%) ... 704
▲ Zetia Tablets (2.7% to 3%) ... 2090
▲ Zetia Tablets (2.7% to 3%) ... 3098
▲ Zevalin Injection (16%) ... 848
▲ Ziagen (6%) ... 1600
Zinacef Injection ... 1604
Zinacef for Injection ... 1604
▲ Zithromax Capsules, 250 mg (2% to 7%) ... 2568
▲ Zithromax for IV Infusion (1.9% to 3.7%) ... 2573
▲ Zithromax for Oral Suspension, 1 g (3% to 5%) ... 2568
▲ Zithromax for Oral Suspension, 300 mg, 600 mg, 900 mg, 1200 mg (2% to 7%) ... 2561
▲ Zithromax Tablets, 250 mg, 500 mg (2% to 7%) ... 2561
▲ Zithromax Tablets, 600 mg (3% to 5%) ... 2568
▲ Zithromax Tri-Pak (2% to 7%) ... 2561
▲ Zithromax Z-Pak (3% to 5%) ... 2568
Zmax for Oral Suspension (2.7%) ... 2577
▲ Zocor Tablets (3.2%) ... 2078
Zofran Injection (2%) ... 1607
Zofran (1% to 3%) ... 1613
Zofran ODT Orally Disintegrating Tablets (1% to 3%) ... 1613
▲ Zoladex (7% to 11%) ... 709
Zoladex 3-month (1% to 5%) ... 712
▲ Zoloft (2% to 7%) ... 2581
▲ Zometa for Intravenous Infusion (14% to 16.3%) ... 2306
Zomig Nasal Spray (Very rare to less than 2%) ... 718
Zomig Tablets (Very rare) ... 714
▲ Zonegran Capsules (6%) ... 1089
Zosyn (1.3%) ... 3492
Zovirax for Injection (Less than 1%) ... 1618
▲ Zyban Sustained-Release Tablets (3%) ... 1620
▲ Zyprexa Tablets (4%) ... 1798
Zyprexa IntraMuscular (Infrequent) ... 1798
▲ Zyprexa ZYDIS Orally Disintegrating Tablets (4%) ... 1798
▲ Zyrtec Chewable Tablets (4.4% to 5.6%) ... 2589
▲ Zyrtec (4.4% to 5.6%) ... 2589
▲ Zyrtec-D 12 Hour Extended Release Tablets (4.4% to 5.6%) ... 2591
Zyvox (0% to 2.4%) ... 2661

Abdominal surgeries, increased risk of

Zelnorm Tablets (0.3%) ... 2303

Abdominal symptom complex, acute

Permax Tablets (Rare) ... 3357
Prozac Pulvules and Liquid (Rare) ... 1771

Abdominal symptoms, unspecified

▲ Agenerase Oral Solution (14%) ... 1304

Abortion

Copaxone for Injection (Infrequent) .. 3292
Effexor Tablets (Rare) ... 3405
Effexor XR Capsules (Rare) ... 3411
Gabitril Tablets (Infrequent) ... 998
Imitrex Injection ... 1431
Imitrex Nasal Spray ... 1435
Imitrex Tablets (Rare) ... 1440
Paxil CR Controlled-Release Tablets (Infrequent) ... 1509
Paxil (Infrequent) ... 1501
Permax Tablets (Infrequent) ... 3357
Prozac Pulvules and Liquid (Infrequent) ... 1771

Abortion, spontaneous

Bravelle for Intramuscular or Subcutaneous Injection ... 1140
Celexa ... 1177
Gonal-f RFF Pen for Injection ... 3155
Lexapro Oral Solution ... 1193
Lexapro Tablets ... 1193
Lupron Depot-PED 7.5 mg, 11.25 mg and 15 mg (Possible) ... 3266
Rebif Prefilled Syringe for Injection ... 3163

Abrasion

Neurontin Oral Solution (1.3%) ... 2498

Abscess

Actiq (Less than 1%) ... 993
Aldurazyme for Intravenous Infusion (2%) ... 1261
Ambien Tablets (Rare) ... 2867
Aramine Injection ... 1889
▲ Aranesp for Injection (27%) ... 576
▲ Arava Tablets (1% to 3%) ... 2881
Aricept Tablets (Infrequent) ... 1086
Aricept ODT Tablets (Infrequent) ... 1086
Campath Ampules ... 826
Campral Tablets (Infrequent) ... 1175
Capastat Sulfate for Injection ... 1728
▲ CellCept Capsules (3% to less than 20%) ... 2751
▲ CellCept Intravenous (3% to less than 20%) ... 2751
▲ CellCept Oral Suspension (3% to less than 20%) ... 2751
▲ CellCept Tablets (3% to less than 20%) ... 2751
Colazal Capsules ... 2845
Decadron Phosphate Injection ... 1931
Depo-Medrol Single-Dose Vial ... 2617
Doxil Injection (Less than 1%) ... 3302
▲ Evoxac Capsules (1% to 3%) ... 1042
Ferrlecit Injection ... 3379
Gabitril Tablets (Infrequent) ... 998
▲ Gengraf Capsules (4.4%) ... 458
▲ Hectorol Capsules (3.3%) ... 909
▲ Hectorol Injection (3.3%) ... 911
Infed Injection ... 3381
▲ Intron A for Injection (Less than 5%) ... 3038
Invirase (Less than 2%) ... 2776
Lamictal (Rare) ... 1449
Levaquin in 5% Dextrose Injection (0.1% to 0.9%) ... 2453
Levaquin (0.1% to 0.9%) ... 2453
▲ Lupron Depot-PED 7.5 mg, 11.25 mg and 15 mg (5%) ... 3266
Lyrica Capsules (0.1% to 1%) ... 2524
Micardis Tablets (More than 0.3%) ... 884
Micardis HCT Tablets ... 886
▲ Neoral Soft Gelatin Capsules (1% to 4.4%) ... 2247
Neurontin Capsules (Infrequent) ... 2498
Neurontin Oral Solution (Infrequent) ... 2498
Neurontin Tablets (Infrequent) ... 2498
Nipent for Injection (2%) ... 3216
Paxil CR Controlled-Release Tablets (Rare) ... 1509
Paxil (Rare) ... 1501
PEG-Intron Powder for Injection (Less than or equal to 1%) ... 3062
Permax Tablets (Infrequent) ... 3357
▲ Prograf Capsules and Injection (3% to 15%) ... 624
Prometrium Capsules (100 mg, 200 mg) (Less than 5%) ... 3205
Protonix I.V. (Less than 1%) ... 3468
Protonix Tablets (Less than 1%) ... 3465
▲ Rapamune Oral Solution and Tablets (3% to 20%) ... 3472
Raptiva for Injection ... 1247
Relpax Tablets (Rare) ... 2531
▲ Remicade for IV Injection (15%) ... 987
ReoPro Vials (0.2%) ... 1779
Requip Tablets (Infrequent) ... 1528
Rescriptor Tablets ... 2535
Rilutek Tablets (Infrequent) ... 2945
Risperdal Consta Long-Acting Injection (Infrequent) ... 1664
▲ Sandimmune (4.4% to 5.3%) ... 2259
Suboxone Tablets (2%) ... 2719
Subutex Tablets (2%) ... 2719
Tasmar Tablets (Infrequent) ... 3360
▲ Tygacil for Injection (3.2%) ... 3489
Uniretic Tablets (Less than 1%) ... 3114
Vantin Tablets and Oral Suspension (Less than 1%) ... 2650

Abscess, abdominal

Enbrel for Injection ... 580
Invanz for Injection (1%) ... 1974

Abscess, dental

Clindesse Vaginal Cream (Less than 1%) ... 3296

Abscess, foot

Enbrel for Injection ... 580

Abscess, periodontal

Abilify Tablets (Infrequent) ... 916
Abilify Tablets (Infrequent) ... 2472
Actiq (1% or greater) ... 993
Aricept Tablets (Infrequent) ... 1086
Aricept ODT Tablets (Infrequent) ... 1086
▲ Casodex Tablets (2% to 5%) ... 670
Copaxone for Injection (At least 2%) ... 3292
Crestor Tablets (Greater than or equal to 1%) ... 672
▲ Depacon Injection (1% to 5%) ... 412
▲ Depakene (1% to 5%) ... 417
▲ Depakote Sprinkle Capsules (1% to 5%) ... 422
▲ Depakote Tablets (1% to 5%) ... 427
Depakote ER Tablets (Greater than 1%) ... 433
Doxil Injection (Less than 1%) ... 3302
Gabitril Tablets (Infrequent) ... 998
Neurontin Capsules (Infrequent) ... 2498
Neurontin Oral Solution (Infrequent) ... 2498
Neurontin Tablets (Infrequent) ... 2498
Norvir (Less than 2%) ... 499
Permax Tablets (Infrequent) ... 3357
Pletal Tablets (Less than 2%) ... 2478
Protonix I.V. (Less than 1%) ... 3468
Protonix Tablets (Less than 1%) ... 3465
Protopic Ointment (Up to 3%) ... 629
Provigil Tablets (Greater than or equal to 1%) ... 1002
Rescriptor Tablets ... 2535
Symbyax Capsules (Infrequent) ... 1788
Uniretic Tablets (Less than 1%) ... 3114
Zyprexa Tablets (Infrequent) ... 1798
Zyprexa ZYDIS Orally Disintegrating Tablets (Infrequent) ... 1798

Abscess, peritonsillar

Amevive ... 836
Tamiflu Capsules (Less than 1%) ... 2810
Tamiflu Oral Suspension (Less than 1%) ... 2810

Abscess, renal

Gengraf Capsules (1% to less than 3%) ... 458
Neoral Oral Solution (1% to less than 3%) ... 2247
Sandostatin LAR Depot (1% to 4%) .. 2264

Abscess at injection site

Adacel Vaccine (Very rare) ... 2959
Avonex (Rare) ... 839
Cerezyme for Injection (Less than 1%) ... 1263
Copaxone for Injection (Frequent) ... 3292
Cytovene-IV ... 2763
Lupron Depot 3.75 mg ... 3257
Lupron Depot 7.5 mg ... 3261
Lupron Depot–3 Month 11.25 mg ... 3262
Lupron Injection Pediatric ... 3256
Liquid PedvaxHIB ... 2012

Abuse

Ambien Tablets (Rare) ... 2867
Prozac Pulvules and Liquid ... 1771
Sonata Capsules ... 1686

Acanthosis nigricans

Advicor Tablets ... 1694
Niaspan Extended-Release Tablets ... 1703

Accommodation, impaired

Amaryl Tablets ... 2864
Ambien Tablets (Rare) ... 2867
Blephamide Ophthalmic Ointment (Occasional) ... 563
Blephamide Ophthalmic Suspension ... 564
Caduet Tablets (Less than or equal to 0.1%) ... 2507
Celexa (Frequent) ... 1177
Concerta Extended-Release Tablets ... 1828
▲ Detrol Tablets (4.7%) ... 2626
▲ Effexor Tablets (5.6% to 9.1%) ... 3405
Effexor XR Capsules (Frequent) ... 3411
FML Ophthalmic Ointment (Occasional) ... ⊙ 225
FML Ophthalmic Suspension (Occasional) ... ⊙ 224
FML Forte Ophthalmic Suspension (Occasional) ... ⊙ 223
Focalin Tablets ... 2214
HMS Sterile Ophthalmic Suspension ... ⊙ 228
Imitrex Nasal Spray ... 1435
Lamictal (Infrequent) ... 1449
Lyrica Capsules (0.1% to 1%) ... 2524
Metadate CD Capsules ... 3316
▲ Mirapex Tablets (Greater than 1% to 4%) ... 889
Neurontin Capsules (Rare) ... 2498
Neurontin Oral Solution (Rare) ... 2498
Neurontin Tablets (Rare) ... 2498
Norvasc Tablets (Less than or equal to 0.1%) ... 2529

▲ Orap Tablets (4 of 20 patients) 1220
Paxil CR Controlled-Release Tablets (Infrequent) 1509
Paxil (Infrequent) 1501
Pred Forte Ophthalmic Suspension (Occasional) ⊙ 233
Pred Mild Sterile Ophthalmic Suspension (Occasional) ⊙ 236
Relpax Tablets (Rare) 2531
Requip Tablets (Infrequent) 1528
Risperdal Consta Long-Acting Injection (Infrequent) 1664
Risperdal M-Tab Orally Disintegrating Tablets (Infrequent) 1658
Risperdal (Infrequent) 1658
Ritalin Hydrochloride Tablets 2254
Ritalin LA Capsules 2255
Ritalin-SR Tablets 2254
Seroquel Tablets (Rare) 691
Sonata Capsules (Rare) 1686
Surmontil Capsules 2347
Symbyax Capsules (Infrequent) 1788
Topamax Sprinkle Capsules (Greater than 1%) 2438
Topamax Tablets (Greater than 1%) 2438
Transderm Scōp Transdermal Therapeutic System 2166
Trileptal Oral Suspension (Up to 2%) 2281
Trileptal Tablets (Up to 2%) 2281
VFEND I.V. (Less than 2%) 2543
VFEND Oral Suspension (Less than 2%) 2543
VFEND Tablets (Less than 2%) 2543
Vivactil Tablets 2350
Wellbutrin SR Sustained-Release Tablets (Infrequent) 1583
Wellbutrin XL Extended-Release Tablets (Infrequent) 1588
Zantac (Rare) 1597
Zantac Injection (Rare) 1593
Zantac Syrup (Rare) 1597
Zofran Injection 1607
Zoloft (Infrequent) 2581
Zyban Sustained-Release Tablets (Infrequent) 1620
Zyprexa Tablets (Rare) 1798
Zyprexa ZYDIS Orally Disintegrating Tablets (Rare) 1798
Zyrtec Chewable Tablets (Less than 2%) 2589
Zyrtec (Less than 2%) 2589
Zyrtec-D 12 Hour Extended Release Tablets (Less than 2%) 2591

Accommodation paresis
DAPTACEL 2964
Miradon Tablets 3056

Aches
▲ Adacel Vaccine (1.2% to 30.4%) 2959
Asacol Delayed-Release Tablets 2688
Cipro I.V. (1% or less) 2998
Cipro I.V. Pharmacy Bulk Package (1% or less) 3509
Cipro (Less than 1%) 2991
Cipro XR Tablets 3004
Cosopt Sterile Ophthalmic Solution 1910
Eldepryl Capsules (1 of 49 patients) 3209
▲ Flonase Nasal Spray (1% to 3%) 1412
Inderal LA Long-Acting Capsules 3421
Midamor Tablets (Less than or equal to 1%) 2000
▲ Nabi-HB (3%) 2159
Nadolol Tablets 2121
Navelbine Injection 1494
Orthoclone OKT3 Sterile Solution 2370
Recombivax HB (Less than 1%) 2045
Repronex for Intramuscular and Subcutaneous Injection 1148
Serevent Diskus (1% to 3%) 1540
Tenormin I.V. Injection 698
Tenormin Tablets 695
Timoptic in Ocudose 2061
Timoptic Sterile Ophthalmic Solution 2058
Timoptic-XE Sterile Ophthalmic Gel Forming Solution 2062
Toprol-XL Tablets 660

Aches, joints
(*see under* Arthralgia)

Acholia
Reyataz Capsules (Less than 3%) 948

Acidosis
▲ Abelcet Injection (3%) 1119
Actiq (Less than 1%) 993
AmBisome for Injection (Less common) 615
▲ Ammonul Injection (3%) 3323
Cafcit (2.2%) 1854
Campath Ampules 826
▲ CellCept Capsules (3% to less than 20%) 2751
▲ CellCept Intravenous (3% to less than 20%) 2751
▲ CellCept Oral Suspension (3% to less than 20%) 2751
▲ CellCept Tablets (3% to less than 20%) 2751
Cipro I.V. (1% or less) 2998
Cipro I.V. Pharmacy Bulk Package (1% or less) 3509
Cipro (Less than 1%) 2991
Cipro XR Tablets 3004
Cytovene 2763
Dyazide Capsules 1389
Fleet Enema 1169
Fleet Phospho-soda 1170
Fleet Phospho-soda ACCU-PREP 1171
Fleet Prep Kits 1172
Indocin I.V. (Less than 3%) 1973
Mycamine for Injection 620
Permax Tablets (Rare) 3357
▲ Prograf Capsules and Injection (3% to 15%) 624
▲ Proleukin for Injection (12%) 1007
▲ Rapamune Oral Solution and Tablets (3% to 20%) 3472
Requip Tablets (Infrequent) 1528
▲ Simulect for Injection (3% to 10%) 2268
Symbyax Capsules (Rare) 1788
Topamax Sprinkle Capsules (Infrequent) 2438
Topamax Tablets (Infrequent) 2438
Trasylol Injection (1% to 2%) 779
▲ Trisenox Injection (5%) 983
Tygacil for Injection 3489
Ultane Liquid for Inhalation (Less than 1%) 526
▲ Vesanoid Capsules (3%) 2823
Zyprexa Tablets (Frequent) 1798
Zyprexa ZYDIS Orally Disintegrating Tablets (Frequent) 1798

Acidosis, hypochloremic metabolic
Gengraf Capsules 458
Sandimmune (Occasional) 2259
▲ Topamax Sprinkle Capsules (2% to 67%) 2438
▲ Topamax Tablets (2% to 67%) 2438

Acidosis, metabolic
Aggrenox Capsules 855
Aloprim for Injection (Less than 1%) 2156
Aloxi Injection (Less than 1%) 2099
▲ Ammonul Injection (4%) 3323
Bayer Aspirin Tablets 3515
▲ Buphenyl Powder (14%) 3327
▲ Buphenyl Tablets (14%) 3327
Daranide Tablets 1928
Diprivan Injectable Emulsion (Less than 1%) 676
Ecotrin Enteric Coated Aspirin Low, Regular and Maximum Strength Tablets 1627
Eloxatin for Injection 2908
Foradil Aerolizer 3024
Oncaspar 1123
St. Joseph 81 mg Aspirin Chewable and Enteric Coated Tablets 1841
Sulfamylon Cream 2154
Sulfamylon for 5% Topical Solution 2155
Topamax Sprinkle Capsules 2438
Topamax Tablets 2438
Viracept 2556

Acidosis, renal tubular
Abelcet Injection 1119
Buphenyl Powder (Less than or equal to 2%) 3327
Buphenyl Tablets (Less than or equal to 2%) 3327
Topamax Sprinkle Capsules 2438
Topamax Tablets 2438

Acidosis, respiratory
Ammonul Injection 3323
▲ CellCept Capsules (3% to less than 20%) 2751
▲ CellCept Intravenous (3% to less than 20%) 2751
▲ CellCept Oral Suspension (3% to less than 20%) 2751
▲ CellCept Tablets (3% to less than 20%) 2751
▲ Diprivan Injectable Emulsion (3% to 10%) 676
Rilutek Tablets (Infrequent) 2945

Acne
(*see under* Acneiform eruptions)

Acne, cystic, flare-up
Parnate Tablets 1499

Acne, flare-up of
Differin Cream (Less than 1%) 1210
Noritate Cream, 1% (One patient) 1051

Acne, transient exacerbation of
Oxandrin Tablets 2977

Acne fulminaris
Accutane Capsules 2740
Amnesteem Capsules 2126

Acneiform eruptions
Abilify Tablets (Infrequent) 916
Abilify Tablets (Infrequent) 2472
Aclovate (Infrequent) 1290
Activella Tablets 2311
Aerobid/Aerobid-M (1% to 3%) 1172
Alesse-28 Tablets 3392
Ambien Tablets (Rare) 2867
Amerge Tablets (Rare) 1312
Anadrol-50 Tablets 3329
Analpram-HC 1136
▲ AndroGel (1% to 8%) 3330
Antabuse Tablets 2343
Antara Capsules 2723
▲ Arava Tablets (1% to 3%) 2881
Arthrotec Tablets (Rare) 3126
Asacol Delayed-Release Tablets (1% to 2%) 2688
Aygestin Tablets 1062
Bravelle for Intramuscular or Subcutaneous Injection (2.9%) 1140
Caduet Tablets (Less than 2%) 2507
Campral Tablets (Infrequent) 1175
Canasa Rectal Suppositories (1.2%) 726
Celexa (Infrequent) 1177
▲ CellCept Capsules (3% to less than 20%) 2751
▲ CellCept Intravenous (3% to less than 20%) 2751
▲ CellCept Oral Suspension (3% to less than 20%) 2751
▲ CellCept Tablets (3% to less than 20%) 2751
Clobevate Gel 3213
Clobex Shampoo 1209
Clobex Lotion 1208
▲ CombiPatch Transdermal System (4% to 5%) 2180
Copaxone for Injection (At least 2%) 3292
Cosmegen for Injection 1907
Cutivate Cream (Infrequent) 1381
Cutivate Ointment (Infrequent to more frequent) 1384
Cymbalta Delayed-Release Capsules (Infrequent) 1729
Dantrium Capsules (Less frequent) 2690
Decadron Tablets 1929
Delatestryl Injection 2976
▲ Depo-Provera Contraceptive Injection (1% to 5%) 2619
▲ depo-subQ provera 104 Injectable Suspension (1% to less than 5%) 2622
Diprolene Gel 0.05% 3015
Diprolene Lotion 0.05% (1%) 3016
Diprolene Ointment 0.05% (Infrequent) 3017
Diprolene AF Cream 0.05% (Infrequent) 3014
Diprosone Cream, USP 0.05% 3018
▲ Dostinex Tablets (1% to less than 10%) 2631
▲ Doxil Injection (1% to 10%) 3302
Effexor Tablets (Infrequent) 3405
Effexor XR Capsules (Infrequent) 3411
Elidel Cream 1% (0.9% to 1.8%) 2198
Elocon Cream 0.1% (Infrequent) 3019
Elocon Lotion 0.1% (Infrequent) 3020
Elocon Ointment 0.1% (Infrequent) 3021
▲ Entocort EC Capsules (15%) 2694
Eskalith 1406
Estratest Tablets 3196
Estratest H.S. Tablets 3196
Evoxac Capsules (Less than 1%) 1042
Finacea Gel (1% or less) 1644
▲ Flovent Diskus 50 mcg (1% to 3%) 1415
Gabitril Tablets (1% or more) 998
▲ Gengraf Capsules (1% to 6%) 458
▲ Gonal-f RFF Pen for Injection (3.6%) 3155
Herceptin I.V. (2%) 1234
Humatrope Vials and Cartridges (Up to 5.8%) 1756
▲ Imdur Tablets (Less than or equal to 5%) 3032
▲ Intron A for Injection (Less than 5%) 3038
Invirase (Less than 2%) 2776
▲ Iressa Tablets (25% to 37%) 684
Kaletra (Less than 2%) 474
Lamictal (1.3%) 1449
Lexapro Oral Solution (Infrequent) 1193
Lexapro Tablets (Infrequent) 1193
Lipitor Tablets (Less than 2%) 2495
Lithobid Tablets 1670
Locoid Lipocream Cream (Infrequent) 1138
Lofibra Capsules 1217
Lo/Ovral-28 Tablets 3423
Loprox Gel 1861
Lotrisone 3054
Lotronex Tablets (Rare) 1479
Lunesta Tablets (Infrequent) 3139
▲ Lupron Depot–3 Month 11.25 mg (Up to 10%) 3262
Lupron Depot-PED 7.5 mg, 11.25 mg and 15 mg (2%) 3266
Lupron Injection Pediatric 3256
Luxíq Foam (One patient) 1026
Maxalt Tablets (Rare) 1983
Maxalt-MLT Orally Disintegrating Tablets (Rare) 1983
Meridia Capsules (1%) 485
▲ Mirena Intrauterine System (5% or more) 810
▲ Myfortic Tablets (3% to less than 20%) 2244
Namenda (More than one patient) 1199
▲ Neoral Soft Gelatin Capsules (1% to 6%) 2247
▲ Neoral Oral Solution (1% to 6%) 2247
Neurontin Capsules 2498
Neurontin Oral Solution 2498
Neurontin Tablets 2498
Nexium Delayed-Release Capsules (Less than 1%) 645
Nexium I.V. (Less than 1%) 649
▲ Nicotrol NS (3%) 2596
Nimotop Capsules (Up to 1.4%) 774
Nipent for Injection (Less than 3%) 3216
Noritate Cream, 1% (One patient) 1051
Norvir (Less than 2%) 499
Olux Foam 1027
Ortho-Cept Tablets 2395
Ortho-Cyclen Tablets 2414
Ortho Evra Transdermal System 2402
Ortho Micronor Tablets (Rare) 2411
Ortho Tri-Cyclen Tablets 2414
Ortho Tri-Cyclen Lo Tablets 2421
Oxandrin Tablets 2977
Pandel Cream, 0.1% 1017
Paxil CR Controlled-Release Tablets (Infrequent) 1509
Paxil (Infrequent) 1501
Pentasa Capsules (0.2%) 3182
Pepcid Injection (Infrequent) 2017
Pepcid (Infrequent) 2014
Permax Tablets (Infrequent) 3357
Pramosone 1139
Premphase Tablets 3452
Prempro Tablets 3452
Prevacid Delayed-Release Capsules (Less than 1%) 3268
Prevacid for Delayed-Release Oral Suspension (Less than 1%) 3268
Prevacid NapraPAC (Less than 1%) 3277
Prevacid SoluTab Delayed-Release Orally Disintegrating Tablets (Less than 1%) 3268
PREVPAC (Less than 1%) 3281
Prochieve 4% Gel 1018
Prochieve 8% Gel 1018
ProctoFoam-HC 3113
▲ Prograf Capsules and Injection (3% to 15%) 624
Prometrium Capsules (100 mg, 200 mg) (Less than 5%) 3205
ProSom Tablets (Rare) 512
Protonix I.V. (Less than 1%) 3468
Protonix Tablets (Less than 1%) 3465
▲ Protopic Ointment (2% to 7%) 629
Prozac Pulvules and Liquid (Infrequent) 1771
▲ Rapamune Oral Solution and Tablets (20% to 31%) 3472
▲ Raptiva for Injection (4%) 1247
ReFacto Vials 3479
Relafen Tablets (Less than 1%) 1523
Retrovir Capsules 1533
Retrovir IV Infusion 1537
Retrovir 1533
Risperdal Consta Long-Acting Injection (2%) 1664

Risperdal M-Tab Orally Disintegrating Tablets (Infrequent to 2%) 1658
Risperdal (Infrequent to 2%) 1658
▲ Sandimmune (1% to 6%) 2259
Sandostatin LAR Depot (1% to 4%) 2264
Seasonale Tablets 1073
Seroquel Tablets (Infrequent) 691
▲ Simulect for Injection (Greater than or equal to 10%) 2268
Sonata Capsules (Infrequent) 1686
Soriatane Capsules (Less than 1%) 1028
Striant Mucoadhesive 1022
Sular Tablets (Less than or equal to 1%) 1163
Symbyax Capsules (Infrequent) 1788
Targretin Capsules 1719
Temovate Cream 1549
Temovate Gel (Infrequent) 1550
Temovate Ointment 1549
Temovate Scalp Application (Infrequent) 1551
Temovate E Emollient (Infrequent) 1552
Testim 1% Gel (Less than 1%) 722
▲ Thalomid Capsules (3.1% to 11.1%) 979
▲ Topamax Sprinkle Capsules (2% to 3%) 2438
▲ Topamax Tablets (2% to 3%) 2438
Topicort .05% Gel 3288
Topicort .25% Cream 3288
Topicort .25% Ointment 3288
Topicort LP .05% Cream 3288
Trecator Tablets 3482
Tricor Tablets 523
Trileptal Oral Suspension (1% to 2%) 2281
Trileptal Tablets (1% to 2%) 2281
▲ Tri-Luma Cream (5%) 1213
Triphasil-28 Tablets 3483
U-cort 1% Cream 3289
Uniretic Tablets (Less than 1%) 3114
▲ Valcyte Tablets (Less than 5%) 2816
Vanos Cream 1864
Vantin Tablets and Oral Suspension (Less than 1%) 2650
Vivelle Transdermal System (2.3%) 2288
Vivelle-Dot Transdermal System (2.3%) 2293
Wellbutrin Tablets (Rare) 1579
Wellbutrin SR Sustained-Release Tablets (At least 1%) 1583
Wellbutrin XL Extended-Release Tablets (At least 1%) 1588
Yasmin 28 Tablets (Greater than 1%) 818
▲ Zenapax for Injection (Greater than 5%) 2838
▲ Zoladex (42%) 709
Zoladex 3-month 712
Zoloft (Infrequent) 2581
Zonegran Capsules (Infrequent) 1089
Zyban Sustained-Release Tablets (Infrequent) 1620
Zyrtec Chewable Tablets (Less than 2%) 2589
Zyrtec (Less than 2%) 2589
Zyrtec-D 12 Hour Extended Release Tablets (Less than 2%) 2591

Acneiform reactions

Cutivate Lotion 0.05% (Rare) 1383
Elocon Lotion 0.1% (2 in 209 patients) 3020
▲ Erbitux (90%) 937
▲ I.V. Busulfex (7%) 1125

Acrocyanosis, exacerbation

R-Gene 10 for Intravenous Use (One patient) 2647

Addiction

Lyrica Capsules (Rare) 2524

Adenitis

Clinoril Tablets 1899
Dolobid Tablets (Less than 1 in 100) 1937
Pneumovax 23 (Rare) 2020
Surmontil Capsules 2347
Vivactil Tablets (Rare) 2350

Adenoma, unspecified

▲ Humira Injection (Less than 5%) 464

Adenomas, endocrine system

Permax Tablets (Infrequent) 3357

Adenopathy

Carbatrol Capsules 3174
Enbrel for Injection 580
Equetro Extended-Release Capsules 3178
Kogenate FS 3517
Rescriptor Tablets 2535
Tegretol/Tegretol-XR 2278

ADH syndrome, inappropriate

Amaryl Tablets 2864
Carbatrol Capsules 3174
Celexa (Several cases) 1177
Cytovene 2763
Depacon Injection 412
Depakene 417
Depakote Sprinkle Capsules 422
Depakote Tablets 427
Depakote ER Tablets 433
Effexor Tablets 3405
Effexor XR Capsules 3411
Equetro Extended-Release Capsules 3178
Flexeril Tablets (Rare) 1832
Kadian Capsules (Less than 3%) 572
Lexapro Oral Solution 1193
Lexapro Tablets 1193
Navelbine Injection (Less than 1%) 1494
OxyContin Tablets (Less than 1%) 2699
Parnate Tablets 1499
Paxil CR Controlled-Release Tablets 1509
Paxil 1501
Permax Tablets (Infrequent) 3357
Requip Tablets (Rare) 1528
Seroquel Tablets 691
Surmontil Capsules 2347
Tegretol/Tegretol-XR 2278
Thalomid Capsules 979
Vivactil Tablets 2350
Wellbutrin Tablets 1579
Wellbutrin SR Sustained-Release Tablets 1583
Wellbutrin XL Extended-Release Tablets 1588
Zyban Sustained-Release Tablets 1620

Adnexal torsion, ovarian

Bravelle for Intramuscular or Subcutaneous Injection 1140
Follistim AQ Cartridge 2354
Gonal-f RFF Pen for Injection 3155
Repronex for Intramuscular and Subcutaneous Injection 1148

Adrenal crisis

Advair Diskus 100/50 1291
Advair Diskus 250/50 1291
Advair Diskus 500/50 1291

Adrenal insufficiency

Azmacort Inhalation Aerosol 1701
Beconase AQ Nasal Spray 1359
Cutivate Ointment 1384
Pulmicort Respules (Less than 1%) 654
VFEND I.V. (Less than 2%) 2543
VFEND Oral Suspension (Less than 2%) 2543
VFEND Tablets (Less than 2%) 2543

Adrenal suppression

(*see under* HPA axis suppression)

Adrenergic syndrome, unspecified

Paxil CR Controlled-Release Tablets (Rare) 1509
Paxil (Rare) 1501

Adrenocortical unresponsiveness, secondary

Decadron Phosphate Injection 1931
Decadron Tablets 1929
Depo-Medrol Injectable Suspension 2615
Depo-Medrol Single-Dose Vial 2617
Hydrocortone Tablets 1963
Pediapred Oral Solution 3319

Affect, blunted

Abilify Tablets (Rare) 916
Abilify Tablets (Rare) 2472

Afibrinogenemia

Depacon Injection (One infant) 412
Depakene (One infant) 417
Depakote Tablets (One infant) 427
Depakote ER Tablets (One infant) 433

Aftertaste

▲ Nasarel Nasal Spray (8% to 17%) 1652

Ageusia

▲ Aerobid/Aerobid-M (3% to 9%) 1172
Aggrenox Capsules (Less than 1%) 855
Arthrotec Tablets (Rare) 3126
Astelin Nasal Spray (Infrequent) 1876
Beconase AQ Nasal Spray (Rare) 1359
Bentyl Capsules 724
Bentyl Injection 724
Bentyl Syrup 724
Bentyl Tablets 724
Caduet Tablets (Less than 2%) 2507
Campath Ampules 826
Captopril Tablets (Approximately 2 to 4 of 100 patients) 2114
Celexa (Rare) 1177
Cipro I.V. 2998
Cipro I.V. Pharmacy Bulk Package 3509
Cipro 2991
Cipro XR Tablets 3004
Clinoril Tablets (Less than 1 in 100) 1899
Copaxone for Injection (Infrequent) 3292
Doxil Injection (Less than 1%) 3302
Effexor Tablets (Infrequent) 3405
Effexor XR Capsules (Infrequent) 3411
Exelon Capsules (Infrequent) 2204
Flexeril Tablets (Less than 1%) 1832
Flonase Nasal Spray 1412
Flumadine (Less than 0.3%) 1186
Gabitril Tablets (Infrequent) 998
▲ Intron A for Injection (Less than 5%) 3038
Klonopin (Infrequent) 2782
Lamictal (Rare) 1449
Lamisil Tablets (Uncommon) 2226
Lipitor Tablets (Less than 2%) 2495
Lyrica Capsules (0.1% to 1%) 2524
Neurontin Capsules (Infrequent) 2498
Neurontin Oral Solution (Infrequent) 2498
Neurontin Tablets (Infrequent) 2498
Nexium Delayed-Release Capsules (Less than 1%) 645
Nexium I.V. (Less than 1%) 649
Norvir (Less than 2%) 499
Paxil CR Controlled-Release Tablets (Infrequent) 1509
Paxil (Infrequent) 1501
Prevacid Delayed-Release Capsules (Less than 1%) 3268
Prevacid for Delayed-Release Oral Suspension (Less than 1%) 3268
Prevacid NapraPAC (Less than 1%) 3277
Prevacid SoluTab Delayed-Release Orally Disintegrating Tablets (Less than 1%) 3268
PREVPAC (Less than 1%) 3281
Prozac Pulvules and Liquid (Rare) 1771
Rilutek Tablets (Rare) 2945
Sonata Capsules (Rare) 1686
Soriatane Capsules (Less than 1%) 1028
Tequin Injection (Less than 0.1%) 964
Tequin Tablets (Less than 0.1%) 964
Topamax Sprinkle Capsules (1% to 2%) 2438
Topamax Tablets (1% to 2%) 2438
Vantin Tablets and Oral Suspension (Less than 1%) 2650
VFEND I.V. (Less than 2%) 2543
VFEND Oral Suspension (Less than 2%) 2543
VFEND Tablets (Less than 2%) 2543
▲ Xeloda Tablets (Less than 5%) 2825
Xifaxan Tablets (Less than 2%) 2847
Zyrtec Chewable Tablets (Less than 2%) 2589
Zyrtec (Less than 2%) 2589
Zyrtec-D 12 Hour Extended Release Tablets (Less than 2%) 2591

Aggression

Accutane Capsules 2740
Advair Diskus 100/50 1291
Advair Diskus 250/50 1291
Advair Diskus 500/50 1291
Ambien Tablets (Rare) 2867
Amerge Tablets (Rare) 1312
Ammonul Injection 3323
Amnesteem Capsules (Rare) 2126
Aricept Tablets (Frequent) 1086
Aricept ODT Tablets (Frequent) 1086
Celexa (Infrequent) 1177
Copegus Tablets (Less than 1%) 2759
Depacon Injection 412
Depakene 417
Depakote Sprinkle Capsules 422
Depakote Tablets 427
Depakote ER Tablets 433
Effexor Tablets 3405
Effexor XR Capsules 3411
Evoxac Capsules 1042
▲ Exelon Capsules (3%) 2204
Flexeril Tablets 1832
Flovent Diskus 50 mcg 1415
Flovent HFA 1418
Genotropin Lyophilized Powder 2642
Imitrex Injection 1431
Imitrex Tablets (Rare) 1440
▲ Intron A for Injection (Less than 5%) 3038
Klonopin (Infrequent) 2782
Levaquin in 5% Dextrose Injection (0.1% to 0.9%) 2453
Levaquin (0.1% to 0.9%) 2453
Lexapro Oral Solution (Infrequent) 1193
Lexapro Tablets (Infrequent) 1193
Neurontin Capsules 2498
Neurontin Oral Solution 2498
Neurontin Tablets 2498
Niravam Orally Disintegrating Tablets (Rare) 3106
Paxil CR Controlled-Release Tablets 1509
Paxil 1501
Pegasys (Less than 1%) 2793
PEG-Intron Powder for Injection (Less than or equal to 1%) 3062
Prilosec OTC Tablets (Less than 1%) 2674
Prochieve 4% Gel 1018
Prochieve 8% Gel 1018
Prozac Pulvules and Liquid 1771
Pulmicort Respules (Less than 1%) 654
Razadyne ER Extended-Release Capsules 2434
Razadyne 2434
Requip Tablets (Infrequent) 1528
▲ Risperdal M-Tab Orally Disintegrating Tablets (1% to 3%) 1658
▲ Risperdal (1% to 3%) 1658
Seromycin Capsules 1783
Singulair 2047
Soriatane Capsules 1028
Strattera Capsules (0.50%) 1784
Surmontil Capsules 2347
Sustiva Capsules (0.4%) 957
Symbyax Capsules 1788
Symmetrel 1115
▲ Topamax Sprinkle Capsules (2% to 9%) 2438
▲ Topamax Tablets (2% to 9%) 2438
Trileptal Oral Suspension 2281
Trileptal Tablets 2281
Vivactil Tablets 2350
Xanax XR Tablets (Rare to infrequent) 2655
Zegerid Powder for Oral Solution (Less than 1%) 2972
Zoloft (Infrequent to 2%) 2581

Aggressive reaction

Namenda (Frequent) 1199
Zmax for Oral Suspension 2577
Zyrtec Chewable Tablets (Rare) 2589
Zyrtec (Rare) 2589
Zyrtec-D 12 Hour Extended Release Tablets (Rare) 2591

Agitation

▲ Abilify Tablets (25%) 916
▲ Abilify Tablets (25%) 2472
Aciphex Tablets (Rare) 1081
Actiq (Less than 1%) 993
▲ Adderall XR Capsules (8%) 3169
Advair Diskus 100/50 1291
Advair Diskus 250/50 1291
Advair Diskus 500/50 1291
Aggrenox Capsules (Less than 1%) 855
Aldara Cream, 5% 1814
Allegra-D 12 Hour Extended-Release Tablets (1.9%) 2860
Allegra-D 24 Hour Extended-Release Tablets (1.9%) 2862
Aloprim for Injection (Less than 1%) 2156
Ambien Tablets (Infrequent) 2867
AmBisome for Injection (Less common) 615
Amerge Tablets (Rare) 1312
▲ Ammonul Injection (3%) 3323
Amoxil Capsules (Rare) 1315
Amoxil Chewable Tablets (Rare) 1315
Amoxil Pediatric Drops for Oral Suspension (Rare) 1315
Amoxil Powder for Oral Suspension (Rare) 1315
Amoxil Tablets (Rare) 1315
Anzemet Injection (Infrequently) 2871
Anzemet Tablets (Infrequently) 2874
Apokyn Injection 2132
Aricept Tablets 1086
Aricept ODT Tablets 1086
Augmentin (Rare) 1331
Augmentin Tablets (Rare) 1334
Augmentin XR Extended-Release Tablets (Rare) 1340
Augmentin ES-600 Powder for Oral Suspension (Rare) 1337
Avelox (Less than 0.1%) 2984

Avinza Capsules (Less than 5%) 1714
Bayer Aspirin Tablets 3515
Brevibloc Concentrate (About 2%) 766
Brevibloc Injection (About 2%) 766
Brevibloc Double Strength Injection (About 2%) 766
Brevibloc Premixed Injection (About 2%) 766
Brevibloc Double Strength Premixed Injection (About 2%) 766
Buprenex Injectable (Rare) 2718
Caduet Tablets (Less than or equal to 0.1%) 2507
Campral Tablets (Infrequent) 1175
Carbatrol Capsules 3174
Catapres Tablets (About 3 in 100 patients) 874
Catapres-TTS (0.5% or less) 875
▲ Celexa (3%) 1177
▲ CellCept Capsules (3% to less than 20%) 2751
▲ CellCept Intravenous (3% to less than 20%) 2751
▲ CellCept Oral Suspension (3% to less than 20%) 2751
▲ CellCept Tablets (3% to less than 20%) 2751
Cipro I.V. 2998
Cipro I.V. Pharmacy Bulk Package 3509
Cipro 2991
Cipro XR Tablets 3004
Clorpres Tablets (About 3%) 2139
▲ Clozapine Tablets (4%) 2141
▲ Clozaril Tablets (4%) 2174
Comtan Tablets (1%) 2186
Comvax 1904
▲ Copaxone for Injection (4%) 3292
Cuprimine Capsules 1925
Depacon Injection (1% or more) 412
Depakene (1% or more) 417
Depakote Sprinkle Capsules 422
▲ Depakote Tablets (1% to 5%) 427
Depakote ER Tablets (Greater than 1%) 433
Dexedrine 1386
Diastat Rectal Delivery System (Greater than or equal to 1%) 3344
Dilaudid 439
Dilaudid Oral Liquid (Less frequent) 443
Dilaudid Non-Sterile Powder 439
Dilaudid Rectal Suppositories 439
Dilaudid Tablets 439
Dilaudid Tablets - 8 mg (Less frequent) 443
Dilaudid-HP (Less frequent) 441
Diprivan Injectable Emulsion (Less than 1%) 676
▲ Doxil Injection (1% to 10%) 3302
Duragesic Transdermal System (1% or greater) 2448
Ecotrin Enteric Coated Aspirin Low, Regular and Maximum Strength Tablets 1627
▲ Effexor Tablets (2% to 4.5%) 3405
▲ Effexor XR Capsules (4%) 3411
Eldepryl Capsules 3209
Elspar for Injection 1943
Engerix-B Vaccine (Less than 1%) 1391
▲ Entocort EC Capsules (Less than 5%) 2694
Equetro Extended-Release Capsules 3178
Evoxac Capsules (Less than 1%) 1042
Exelon Capsules (2% or more) 2204
▲ FazaClo Orally Disintegrating Tablets (4%) 547
Ferrlecit Injection 3379
Flexeril Tablets (Less than 1%) 1832
▲ Flolan for Injection (11%) 1408
Flovent Diskus 50 mcg 1415
Flovent HFA 1418
Flumadine (0.3% to 1%) 1186
Fortical Nasal Spray (Less than 1%) 3336
Frova Tablets (Infrequent) 1101
Gabitril Tablets (1%) 998
Geodon Capsules (Frequent) 2514
Imitrex Injection (Infrequent) 1431
Imitrex Nasal Spray (Infrequent) 1435
Imitrex Tablets (Up to 2%) 1440
▲ Indapamide Tablets (Greater than or equal to 5%) 2119
▲ Infergen (4% to 6%) 1647
▲ Intron A for Injection (Less than 5%) 3038
▲ Invanz for Injection (3.3% to 5.1%) 1974
Invirase (Less than 2%) 2776
I.V. Busulfex (2%) 1125
Kadian Capsules (Less than 3%) 572
Kaletra (Less than 2%) 474
▲ Keppra Oral Solution (6%) 3307
▲ Keppra Tablets (6%) 3307
Klonopin 2782
Kytril Injection (Less than 2%) 2785
Lamictal (Infrequent) 1449
Lariam Tablets (Occasional) 2790
Leukeran Tablets (Rare) 1472
Levaquin in 5% Dextrose Injection (0.1% to 0.9%) 2453
Levaquin (0.1% to 0.9%) 2453
Lexapro Oral Solution (Infrequent) 1193
Lexapro Tablets (Infrequent) 1193
Lunesta Tablets (Infrequent) 3139
Lupron Depot 7.5 mg (Less than 5%) 3261
Lupron Depot–3 Month 11.25 mg 3262
Lyrica Capsules (0.1% to 1%) 2524
Maxalt Tablets (Infrequent) 1983
Maxalt-MLT Orally Disintegrating Tablets (Infrequent) 1983
Mebaral Tablets, USP (Less than 1 in 100 patients) 2483
Meridia Capsules (Greater than or equal to 1%) 485
Merrem I.V. (Greater than 0.1% to 1%) 687
Miacalcin Nasal Spray (Less than 1%) 2242
Mirapex Tablets (Less than 1%) 889
MS Contin Tablets (Less frequent) 2703
Namenda (Greater than or equal to 2%) 1199
Narcan Injection 1109
Naropin Injection (Less than 1%) 640
Nembutal Sodium Solution, USP (Less than 1%) 2484
Neurontin Capsules (Infrequent) 2498
Neurontin Oral Solution (Infrequent) 2498
Neurontin Tablets (Infrequent) 2498
Niravam Orally Disintegrating Tablets (2.9%) 3106
Norflex Injection 1824
Norvasc Tablets (Less than or equal to 0.1%) 2529
Norvir (Less than 2%) 499
Nubain Injection 1111
Orthoclone OKT3 Sterile Solution 2370
OxyContin Tablets (Less than 1%) 2699
Parcopa Orally Disintegrating Tablets 3111
Parnate Tablets 1499
▲ Paxil CR Controlled-Release Tablets (1.1% to 5%) 1509
▲ Paxil (1.1% to 5%) 1501
PEG-Intron Powder for Injection (2%) 3062
Pepcid Injection (Infrequent) 2017
Pepcid (Infrequent) 2014
Permax Tablets (Infrequent) 3357
Phenergan 3438
Prevacid Delayed-Release Capsules (Less than 1%) 3268
Prevacid for Delayed-Release Oral Suspension (Less than 1%) 3268
Prevacid NapraPAC (Less than 1%) 3277
Prevacid SoluTab Delayed-Release Orally Disintegrating Tablets (Less than 1%) 3268
PREVPAC (Less than 1%) 3281
▲ Prograf Capsules and Injection (3% to 15%) 624
Proleukin for Injection 1007
ProSom Tablets (Infrequent) 512
Provigil Tablets (1%) 1002
Prozac Pulvules and Liquid (At least 2%) 1771
Razadyne ER Extended-Release Capsules (Greater than or equal to 2%) 2434
Razadyne (Greater than or equal to 2%) 2434
▲ Rebetol (5% to 8%) 3073
Recombivax HB 2045
Relafen Tablets (1%) 1523
Relpax Tablets (Infrequent) 2531
ReoPro Vials (0.7%) 1779
Requip Tablets (Infrequent) 1528
Rescriptor Tablets 2535
Reyataz Capsules (Less than 3%) 948
▲ Ribavirin, USP Capsules (5% to 8%) 3083
Rilutek Tablets (Frequent) 2945
Risperdal Consta Long-Acting Injection (Frequent) 1664
▲ Risperdal M-Tab Orally Disintegrating Tablets (8% to 26%) 1658
▲ Risperdal (8% to 26%) 1658
▲ Rituxan for Infusion (1% to 5%) 845
▲ Rituxan I.V. (1% to 5%) 1251
Roferon-A Injection 2805
Sedapap Tablets 50 mg/650 mg (Infrequent) 2098
▲ Seroquel Tablets (4%) 691
▲ Simulect for Injection (3% to 10%) 2268
Singulair 2047
Sonata Capsules (Infrequent) 1686
St. Joseph 81 mg Aspirin Chewable and Enteric Coated Tablets 1841
Stalevo Tablets (1%) 2270
Suprane Liquid for Inhalation (Less than 1%) 770
Surmontil Capsules 2347
Sustiva Capsules (Less than 2%) 957
Symbyax Capsules 1788
Symmetrel (1% to 5%) 1115
Tagamet Tablets 1547
Targretin Capsules 1719
Tasmar Tablets (1%) 3360
Tegretol/Tegretol-XR 2278
Tequin Injection (Less than 0.1%) 964
Tequin Tablets (Less than 0.1%) 964
Thalomid Capsules 979
Thioridazine Hydrochloride Tablets 2122
Thiothixene Capsules 2124
▲ Topamax Sprinkle Capsules (1% to 3%) 2438
▲ Topamax Tablets (1% to 3%) 2438
Trasylol Injection (1% to 2%) 779
Trileptal Oral Suspension (1% to 2%) 2281
Trileptal Tablets (1% to 2%) 2281
▲ Trisenox Injection (5%) 983
Twinrix Vaccine (Less than 1%) 1571
▲ Ultane Liquid for Inhalation (7% to 15%) 526
▲ Valcyte Tablets (Less than 5%) 2816
Valtrex Caplets 1573
▲ Vesanoid Capsules (9%) 2823
VFEND I.V. (Less than 2%) 2543
VFEND Oral Suspension (Less than 2%) 2543
VFEND Tablets (Less than 2%) 2543
Vicoprofen Tablets (Less than 1%) 533
Vivactil Tablets 2350
▲ Wellbutrin Tablets (31.9%) 1579
▲ Wellbutrin SR Sustained-Release Tablets (3% to 9%) 1583
▲ Wellbutrin XL Extended-Release Tablets (3% to 9%) 1588
Xanax XR Tablets (Rare to frequent) 2655
Zantac (Rare) 1597
Zantac Injection 1593
Zantac Injection Pharmacy Bulk Package (Rare) 1595
Zantac Syrup (Rare) 1597
Zithromax Capsules, 250 mg (1% or less) 2568
Zithromax for Oral Suspension, 300 mg, 600 mg, 900 mg, 1200 mg (1% or less) 2561
Zithromax Tablets, 250 mg, 500 mg (1% or less) 2561
Zithromax Tri-Pak (1% or less) 2561
Zmax for Oral Suspension 2577
▲ Zofran Injection (2% to 6%) 1607
▲ Zofran (6%) 1613
▲ Zofran ODT Orally Disintegrating Tablets (6%) 1613
▲ Zoloft (1% to 6%) 2581
▲ Zometa for Intravenous Infusion (12.8%) 2306
Zomig Nasal Spray (Infrequent to less than 2%) 718
Zomig Tablets (Infrequent) 714
Zomig-ZMT Tablets (Infrequent) 714
▲ Zonegran Capsules (9%) 1089
▲ Zosyn (2.1% to 7.1%) 3492
Zovirax Capsules 1616
Zovirax for Injection (Approximately 1%) 1618
Zovirax 1616
Zyban Sustained-Release Tablets (Frequent) 1620
▲ Zyprexa Tablets (23%) 1798
▲ Zyprexa ZYDIS Orally Disintegrating Tablets (23%) 1798
Zyrtec Chewable Tablets (Less than 2%) 2589
Zyrtec (Less than 2%) 2589
Zyrtec-D 12 Hour Extended Release Tablets (Less than 2%) 2591

Agnosia

▲ Vesanoid Capsules (3%) 2823

Agranulocytosis

Accolate Tablets 663
Accutane Capsules 2740
Aceon Tablets (2 mg, 4 mg, 8 mg) 3191
Aciphex Tablets 1081
Alacol DM Syrup 739
Albenza Tablets (Rare) 1310
Aldoclor Tablets 1881
Aldoril Tablets 1884
Altace Capsules (Rare) 1673
Amaryl Tablets 2864
AmBisome for Injection (Infrequent) 615
Amnesteem Capsules (Rare) 2126
Amoxil Capsules 1315
Amoxil Chewable Tablets 1315
Amoxil Pediatric Drops for Oral Suspension 1315
Amoxil Powder for Oral Suspension 1315
Amoxil Tablets 1315
Anaprox Tablets (Less than 1%) 2769
Anaprox DS Tablets (Less than 1%) 2769
Antara Capsules 2723
Arava Tablets (Rare) 2881
Arthrotec Tablets (Rare) 3126
Asacol Delayed-Release Tablets (Rare) 2688
Atacand Tablets (Very rare) 634
Atacand HCT 637
Augmentin 1331
Augmentin Tablets 1334
Augmentin XR Extended-Release Tablets 1340
Augmentin ES-600 Powder for Oral Suspension 1337
Avalide Tablets 922
Avalide Tablets 2889
BiDil Tablets 2161
▲ Blephamide Ophthalmic Ointment (Among most often) 563
Blephamide Ophthalmic Suspension 564
Blocadren Tablets 1891
Campath Ampules 826
Captopril Tablets 2114
Carbatrol Capsules 3174
Cataflam Tablets (Rarely) 2173
Ceftin 1369
Cipro I.V. (1% or less) 2998
Cipro I.V. Pharmacy Bulk Package (1% or less) 3509
Cipro 2991
Cipro XR Tablets 3004
Cleocin Vaginal Ovules 2613
Clindesse Vaginal Cream (Rare) 3296
Clinoril Tablets (Less than 1%) 1899
Clorpres Tablets 2139
▲ Clozapine Tablets (1% to 13%) 2141
Clozaril Tablets (1% to 1.3%) 2174
Cosmegen for Injection 1907
Cosopt Sterile Ophthalmic Solution 1910
Cuprimine Capsules 1925
Dapsone Tablets USP 1656
Daranide Tablets 1928
Didronel Tablets (Rare) 2693
Diovan HCT Tablets 2195
Diuril Oral 1936
Diuril Sodium Intravenous 1934
Dolobid Tablets (Less than 1 in 100) 1937
Dyazide Capsules 1389
EC-Naprosyn Delayed-Release Tablets (Less than 1%) 2769
Edecrin 1941
Effexor Tablets 3405
Effexor XR Capsules 3411
Equetro Extended-Release Capsules 3178
FazaClo Orally Disintegrating Tablets (1%) 547
FML-S Liquifilm Sterile Ophthalmic Suspension ⊙226
Fortaz (Very rare) 1422
Furosemide Tablets 2117
Garamycin Injectable 3028
▲ Humira Injection (Less than 5%) 464
Hyzaar 1964
Indapamide Tablets 2119
Inderal LA Long-Acting Capsules 3421
Indocin Capsules (Less than 1%) 1968
Indocin I.V. (Less than 1%) 1973
Indocin (Less than 1%) 1968
InnoPran XL Capsules 2728
Lamictal 1449
Lamisil Tablets (Rare) 2226
▲ Leukine (6%) 829
Levaquin in 5% Dextrose Injection (0.1% to 0.9%) 2453
Levaquin (0.1% to 0.9%) 2453
Lofibra Capsules (Rare) 1217
Lortab 3315
Lortab Elixir 3312
Lotensin HCT Tablets 2235
Lotrel Capsules 2238
Mavik Tablets (Rare) 482
Maxipime for Injection 1093
Maxzide 2150

Mefoxin for Injection 1987
Mefoxin Premixed Intravenous Solution 1990
Micardis HCT Tablets 886
Miradon Tablets 3056
Mobic Oral Suspension (Less than 0.1%) 893
Mobic Tablets (Less than 0.1%) 893
Moduretic Tablets 2003
Mustargen for Injection (Relatively infrequent) 2007
Nadolol Tablets 2121
Nalfon Capsules (Less than 1%) 2504
Naprosyn Suspension (Less than 1%) 2769
Naprosyn Tablets (Less than 1%) 2769
▲ Nipent for Injection (3% to 10%) 3216
Noroxin Tablets 2009
Omnicef Capsules 506
Omnicef for Oral Suspension 506
Oncaspar 1123
Parcopa Orally Disintegrating Tablets 3111
Parnate Tablets 1499
Paser Granules 1657
Paxil CR Controlled-Release Tablets 1509
Paxil 1501
Pentasa Capsules 3182
Pepcid Injection (Rare) 2017
Pepcid (Rare) 2014
Phenergan 3438
Phenytek Capsules (Occasional) 2153
Plavix Tablets (Less than 1%) 940
Plavix Tablets (Less than 1%) 2942
Pletal Tablets (Very rare) 2478
Prevacid Delayed-Release Capsules (Less than 1%) 3268
Prevacid for Delayed-Release Oral Suspension (Less than 1%) 3268
Prevacid NapraPAC (Less than 1%) .. 3277
Prevacid SoluTab Delayed-Release Orally Disintegrating Tablets (Less than 1%) 3268
PREVPAC 3281
Prilosec OTC Tablets (Rare) 2674
Primaxin I.M. 2022
Primaxin I.V. 2024
Prinivil Tablets (Rare to frequent) 2029
Prinzide Tablets (Rare) 2033
ProSom Tablets (Rare) 512
Provigil Tablets 1002
Rocephin Injectable Vials, ADD-Vantage, Galaxy, Bulk 2801
Sedapap Tablets 50 mg/650 mg 2098
Seroquel Tablets 691
Stalevo Tablets 2270
Suprax 1811
Surmontil Capsules 2347
Tagamet Tablets (Approximately 3 per 1,000,000) 1547
Tegretol/Tegretol-XR (Very low incidence) 2278
Tenormin I.V. Injection 698
Tenormin Tablets 695
Teveten HCT Tablets 1710
Thioridazine Hydrochloride Tablets (Infrequent) 2122
Thiothixene Capsules 2124
Ticlid Tablets (Rare) 2813
Timolide Tablets 2056
Timoptic in Ocudose 2061
Timoptic Sterile Ophthalmic Solution 2058
Timoptic-XE Sterile Ophthalmic Gel Forming Solution 2062
Toprol-XL Tablets (Rare) 660
Tricor Tablets (Rare) 523
Trusopt Sterile Ophthalmic Solution (Rare) 2065
Uniretic Tablets (More than 1%) 3114
Vantin Tablets and Oral Suspension 2650
Vaseretic Tablets (Rare) 2073
Vasotec I.V. Injection (Several cases) 2076
Vermox Chewable Tablets 1853
VFEND I.V. (Less than 2%) 2543
VFEND Oral Suspension (Less than 2%) 2543
VFEND Tablets (Less than 2%) 2543
Vicodin Tablets 530
Vicodin ES Tablets 531
Vicodin HP Tablets 532
Vivactil Tablets 2350
Voltaren Tablets (Rarely) 2298
Voltaren-XR Tablets (Rarely) 2301
▲ Xeloda Tablets (Less than 5%) 2825
Zantac (Rare) 1597
Zantac Injection (Rare) 1593
Zantac Injection Pharmacy Bulk Package (Rare) 1595
Zantac Syrup (Rare) 1597
Zegerid Powder for Oral Solution (Rare) 2972
Zestoretic Tablets 701
Zestril Tablets 704
Zinacef Injection 1604
Zinacef for Injection 1604
Zoloft 2581
Zonegran Capsules (Rare) 1089
Zosyn (1% or less) 3492

Airway constriction

Amerge Tablets (Rare) 1312

Airway obstruction

Altace Capsules 1673
Amerge Tablets (Rare) 1312
Captopril Tablets 2114
Diprivan Injectable Emulsion (Less than 1%) 676
▲ Infasurf Intratracheal Suspension (39%) 1188
Levaquin in 5% Dextrose Injection (0.1% to 0.9%) 2453
Levaquin (0.1% to 0.9%) 2453
Orthoclone OKT3 Sterile Solution 2370
Prinivil Tablets 2029
Prinzide Tablets 2033
▲ Ultane Liquid for Inhalation (8%) 526
Vaseretic Tablets 2073
Vasotec I.V. Injection 2076
Zestoretic Tablets 701
Zestril Tablets 704

Akathisia

▲ Abilify Tablets (12% to 17%) 916
▲ Abilify Tablets (12% to 17%) 2472
Celexa 1177
▲ Clozapine Tablets (3%) 2141
▲ Clozaril Tablets (3%) 2174
Effexor Tablets (Infrequent) 3405
Effexor XR Capsules (Infrequent) 3411
▲ FazaClo Orally Disintegrating Tablets (3%) 547
▲ Geodon (8% to 10%) 2514
Lamictal (Infrequent) 1449
Lexapro Oral Solution 1193
Lexapro Tablets 1193
▲ Mirapex Tablets (2% to 3%) 889
Moban Tablets 1108
▲ Niravam Orally Disintegrating Tablets (1.6% to 3%) 3106
▲ Orap Tablets (8 of 20 patients) 1220
Paxil CR Controlled-Release Tablets 1509
Paxil 1501
Permax Tablets (1.6%) 3357
Prozac Pulvules and Liquid (Infrequent) 1771
▲ Risperdal Consta Long-Acting Injection (2% to 9%) 1664
▲ Risperdal M-Tab Orally Disintegrating Tablets (16% to 34%) 1658
▲ Risperdal (16% to 34%) 1658
Surmontil Capsules 2347
Symbyax Capsules 1788
Thioridazine Hydrochloride Tablets .. 2122
Thiothixene Capsules 2124
VFEND I.V. (Less than 2%) 2543
VFEND Oral Suspension (Less than 2%) 2543
VFEND Tablets (Less than 2%) 2543
Vivactil Tablets 2350
Wellbutrin Tablets (1.5%) 1579
Zoloft 2581
Zomig Tablets (Rare) 714
Zomig-ZMT Tablets (Rare) 714
▲ Zyprexa Tablets (5% to 27%) 1798
▲ Zyprexa IntraMuscular (2% to 5%) ... 1798
▲ Zyprexa ZYDIS Orally Disintegrating Tablets (5% to 27%) 1798

Akinesia

Abilify Tablets (Infrequent) 916
Abilify Tablets (Infrequent) 2472
▲ Clozapine Tablets (4%) 2141
▲ Clozaril Tablets (4%) 2174
Effexor Tablets (Rare) 3405
Effexor XR Capsules (Rare) 3411
▲ FazaClo Orally Disintegrating Tablets (4%) 547
Geodon Capsules (Frequent) 2514
Maxalt Tablets (Rare) 1983
Maxalt-MLT Orally Disintegrating Tablets (Rare) 1983
Moban Tablets 1108
▲ Orap Tablets (8 of 20 patients) 1220
Parnate Tablets 1499
Paxil CR Controlled-Release Tablets (Infrequent) 1509
Paxil (Infrequent) 1501
Permax Tablets (1.1%) 3357
Thioridazine Hydrochloride Tablets... 2122
▲ Wellbutrin Tablets (8.0%) 1579
Wellbutrin SR Sustained-Release Tablets 1583
Wellbutrin XL Extended-Release Tablets 1588
Zyban Sustained-Release Tablets 1620
Zyprexa Tablets (Infrequent) 1798
▲ Zyprexa ZYDIS Orally Disintegrating Tablets (8% to 20%) 1798

Alanine aminotransferase levels, changes in

Parcopa Orally Disintegrating Tablets 3111
Prozac Pulvules and Liquid (Infrequent) 1771
▲ Zyvox (0% to 10.1%) 2661

Alanine aminotransferase levels, elevation of

Abelcet Injection 1119
Abilify Tablets (Infrequent) 916
Abilify Tablets (Infrequent) 2472
Accolate Tablets (1.5%) 663
Accutane Capsules 2740
Aceon Tablets (2 mg, 4 mg, 8 mg) (1.6% to 1.7%) 3191
Aciphex Tablets (0.2%) 1081
Actos Tablets (0.3%) 3224
Adalat CC Tablets (Rare) 2978
▲ Alimta for Injection (1% to 10%) 1722
Alinia for Oral Suspension (Less than 1.1%) 2840
Alinia Tablets (Less than 1.1%) 2840
Aloxi Injection (Less than 1%) 2099
Altoprev Extended-Release Tablets .. 1151
Ambien Tablets (Infrequent) 2867
▲ AmBisome for Injection (14.6%) 615
Amnesteem Capsules 2126
Amoxil Capsules 1315
Amoxil Chewable Tablets 1315
Amoxil Pediatric Drops for Oral Suspension 1315
Amoxil Powder for Oral Suspension 1315
Amoxil Tablets 1315
Anaprox Tablets (Less than 1%) 2769
Anaprox DS Tablets (Less than 1%) .. 2769
Ancef for Injection 1318
▲ Antara Capsules (3%) 2723
Anzemet Injection 2871
Anzemet Tablets 2874
▲ Aptivus Capsules (2.7% to 17.5%) .. 859
▲ Aralast (11.1%) 745
▲ Arava Tablets (1.5% to 4.4%) 2881
▲ Arimidex Tablets (2% to 5%) 665
Arixtra Injection (0.3% to 2.6%) 1325
Asacol Delayed-Release Tablets 2688
Astelin Nasal Spray (Infrequent) 1876
Augmentin (Infrequent) 1331
Augmentin Tablets (Infrequent) 1334
Augmentin XR Extended-Release Tablets (Infrequent) 1340
Augmentin ES-600 Powder for Oral Suspension 1337
Avandamet Tablets (0.2%) 1343
Avandia Tablets (0.2%) 1348
Axid Oral Solution (Less common) 913
Aygestin Tablets 1062
▲ Baraclude (2% to 12%) 928
BeneFix for Injection (1.6%) 3402
Benicar HCT Tablets (Greater than 1%) 2852
▲ Betaseron for SC Injection (10%) 791
Biaxin/Biaxin XL 402
Calcijex Injection 411
Calcium Disodium Versenate Injection 1819
Campral Tablets (Infrequent) 1175
▲ Cancidas for Injection (3.7% to 10.8%) 1894
Cardizem LA Extended Release Tablets (Less than 2%) 1699
▲ Casodex Tablets (2% to 5%) 670
Ceftin (0.1% to 1%) 1369
Celebrex Capsules (0.1% to 1.9%) ... 3130
▲ CellCept Capsules (3% to less than 20%) 2751
▲ CellCept Intravenous (3% to less than 20%) 2751
▲ CellCept Oral Suspension (3% to less than 20%) 2751
▲ CellCept Tablets (3% to less than 20%) 2751
▲ Chemet Capsules (4.2% to 10.4%) 2480
▲ Cipro I.V. (Among most frequent) 2998
▲ Cipro I.V. Pharmacy Bulk Package (Among most frequent) 3509
Cipro (1.9%) 2991
▲ Clolar for Intravenous Infusion (44%) 1264
Colazal Capsules 2845
Combivir Tablets 1373
▲ Coreg Tablets (Greater than 1% to 3%) 1376
Covera-HS Tablets (1.4%) 3135
▲ Crixivan Capsules (4.9%) 1918
Cutivate Lotion 0.05% (Rare) 1383
Cymbalta Delayed-Release Capsules 1729
Cytovene (At least 3 subjects) 2763
Dalmane Capsules (Rare) 3343
▲ Depacon Injection (1% to 5%) 412
Depakene (Frequent) 417
▲ Depakote Sprinkle Capsules (1% to 5%) 422
▲ Depakote Tablets (Frequent) 427
Depakote ER Tablets (Greater than 1%) 433
Depo-Medrol Single-Dose Vial 2617
Dolobid Tablets 1937
▲ Doxil Injection (1% to 5%) 3302
EC-Naprosyn Delayed-Release Tablets (Less than 1%) 2769
Effexor Tablets (Infrequent) 3405
Effexor XR Capsules (Rare) 3411
▲ Eloxatin for Injection (0% to 36%) 2908
Elspar for Injection 1943
▲ Emend Capsules (6%) 1944
▲ Emtriva Capsules (2% to 5%) 1272
▲ Epivir (3.7% to 4%) 1394
▲ Epivir-HBV (11%) 1398
Eulexin Capsules 3023
Evoxac Capsules (Less than 1%) 1042
Factive Tablets (1.5%) 2464
▲ Famvir Tablets (3.2%) 2207
Femara Tablets 2210
▲ Fortaz (1 in 15) 1422
Fuzeon Injection 2772
▲ Gamunex Immune Globulin I.V., 10% (7% to 18%) 3232
Garamycin Injectable 3028
▲ Gemzar for Injection (38% to 72%) 1743
▲ Gleevec Tablets (Up to 4%) 2221
Hectorol Capsules 909
▲ Hepsera Tablets (2% to 20%) 1275
▲ Humatrope Vials and Cartridges (6.25% to 6.67%) 1756
▲ Hycamtin for Injection (Less than 1% to 5%) 1427
▲ Imdur Tablets (Less than or equal to 5%) 3032
Increlex Injection 3290
Inspra Tablets (15 patients) 2520
▲ Intron A for Injection (Up to 15% of patients) 3038
▲ Invanz for Injection (8.3% to 8.8%) 1974
▲ Invirase (Less than 1% to 4%) 2776
▲ I.V. Busulfex (7% to 31%) 1125
▲ Kaletra (4% to 10%) 474
▲ Kytril Injection (3.3%) 2785
▲ Kytril Tablets (6%) 2788
▲ Leukine (13%) 829
▲ Lexiva Tablets (6%) 1473
▲ Lofibra Capsules (Up to 3.4%) 1217
Lotronex Tablets (1%) 1479
▲ Lovenox Injection (Up to 5.5%) 2931
Malarone Tablets 1484
Malarone Pediatric Tablets 1484
Marinol Capsules (Less than 1%) 3334
Mavik Tablets (0.3% to 1.0%) 482
Maxipime for Injection (2.8%) 1093
Mefoxin for Injection 1987
Mefoxin Premixed Intravenous Solution 1990
▲ Mepron Suspension (6%) 1487
Meridia Capsules (1.6%) 485
Merrem I.V. (Greater than 0.2%) 687
Mevacor Tablets 1996
Mobic Oral Suspension (Less than 2%) 893
Mobic Tablets (Less than 2%) 893
Mycamine for Injection (0.4% to 2.6%) 620
▲ Mylotarg for Injection (9%) 3429
Naprosyn Suspension (Less than 1%) 2769
Naprosyn Tablets (Less than 1%) 2769
Nexium Delayed-Release Capsules (Less than 1%) 645
Nexium I.V. (Less than 1%) 649
Niaspan Extended-Release Tablets ... 1703
Nimotop Capsules (0.2%; rare) 774
Noroxin Tablets (1.4%) 2009
▲ Norvir (7.8% to 8.5%) 499
▲ Novantrone for Injection Concentrate (8% to 9%) 3158
Omacor Capsules 2735
Omnicef Capsules (0.7%) 506
Omnicef for Oral Suspension (0.4%) 506
▲ Oncaspar (Greater than 5%) 1123

Orthoclone OKT3 Sterile Solution 2370
Oxandrin Tablets 2977
Pacerone Tablets 3337
Paxil CR Controlled-Release Tablets (Infrequent) 1509
Paxil (Infrequent) 1501
Pegasys (Less than 1%) 2793
▲ PEG-Intron Powder for Injection (10%) 3062
Pentasa Capsules (Less than 1%) 3182
Plendil Extended-Release Tablets (0.5% to 1.5%) 651
Pravachol Tablets 943
Precose Tablets 776
Prevacid Delayed-Release Capsules 3268
Prevacid for Delayed-Release Oral Suspension 3268
Prevacid NapraPAC 3277
Prevacid SoluTab Delayed-Release Orally Disintegrating Tablets 3268
PREVPAC (Less than 1%) 3281
Prilosec OTC Tablets (Rare) 2674
Primaxin I.M. 2022
Primaxin I.V. 2024
▲ Prograf Capsules and Injection (3% to 15%) 624
Protonix I.V. (Greater than or equal to 1%) 3468
Protonix Tablets (Greater than or equal to 1%) 3465
Protopic Ointment (Greater than or equal to 1%) 629
Prozac Pulvules and Liquid (Rare) 1771
▲ Rapamune Oral Solution and Tablets (3% to 20%) 3472
▲ Rebif Prefilled Syringe for Injection (20% to 27%) 3163
▲ Rescriptor Tablets (4.1% to 5.1%) 2535
Risperdal Consta Long-Acting Injection (Infrequent) 1664
Risperdal M-Tab Orally Disintegrating Tablets (Infrequent) 1658
Risperdal (Infrequent) 1658
▲ Rocephin Injectable Vials, ADD-Vantage, Galaxy, Bulk (3.3%) 2801
Rythmol SR Capsules 2736
▲ Seroquel Tablets (5%) 691
Singulair (1% to 2.1%) 2047
Somavert Injection (0.8% to 1.2%) 2648
Sonata Capsules (Rare) 1686
▲ Soriatane Capsules (Approximately 1 in 3 patients) 1028
Stromectol Tablets (2%) 2053
Suprax (Less than 2%) 1811
Sustiva Capsules (2%) 957
Symmetrel 1115
Synagis (More than 1%) 1868
Tarceva Tablets 1254
Tarceva Tablets 2470
Targretin Capsules 1719
Tarka Tablets 519
Tasmar Tablets (1% to 5%) 3360
▲ Taxotere Injection Concentrate (4.3%) 2947
Tequin Injection (Less than 0.1%) 964
Tequin Tablets (Less than 0.1%) 964
Teveten Tablets (Less than 1%) 1707
Teveten HCT Tablets (Less than 1%) 1710
Thalomid Capsules 979
Tiazac Capsules (Less than 2%) 1204
Ticlid Tablets (Rare) 2813
Timentin ADD-Vantage 1556
Timentin Injection Galaxy Container 1559
Timentin IV Infusion 1553
Timentin Pharmacy Bulk Package 1562
Topamax Sprinkle Capsules (Infrequent) 2438
Topamax Tablets (Infrequent) 2438
▲ Tracleer Tablets (11%) 539
Trasylol Injection 779
Trecator Tablets 3482
▲ Tricor Tablets (3.0%) 523
▲ Triglide Tablets (3%) 1165
▲ Trisenox Injection (20%) 983
▲ Trizivir Tablets (3.7%) 1565
▲ Truvada Tablets (1% to 12%) 1279
▲ Tygacil for Injection (5.6%) 3489
Ultane Liquid for Inhalation (Less than 1%) 526
Uniretic Tablets (More than 1%) 3114
▲ Valtrex Caplets (14%) 1573
Vantin Tablets and Oral Suspension 2650
Verelan PM Capsules 3120
Vermox Chewable Tablets (Rare) 1853
▲ VFEND I.V. (1.8% to 18.9%) 2543
▲ VFEND Oral Suspension (1.8% to 18.9%) 2543
▲ VFEND Tablets (1.8% to 18.9%) 2543
Viracept (Less than 2%) 2556
▲ Viramune Oral Suspension (3.4%) 903
▲ Viramune Tablets (3.4%) 903
▲ Viread Tablets (2% to 4%) 1284
Xeloda Tablets (1.6%) 2825
Zantac 1597
Zantac Injection 1593
Zantac Syrup 1597
Zegerid Powder for Oral Solution (Rare) 2972
▲ Zerit (13%) 971
▲ Ziagen (6%) 1600
▲ Zinacef Injection (1 in 25 patients) 1604
▲ Zinacef for Injection (1 in 25 patients) 1604
Zithromax Capsules, 250 mg (1% to 2%) 2568
▲ Zithromax for IV Infusion (4% to 6%) 2573
Zithromax for Oral Suspension, 1 g (1% to 2%) 2568
Zithromax for Oral Suspension, 300 mg, 600 mg, 900 mg, 1200 mg (1% to 2%) 2561
Zithromax Tablets, 250 mg, 500 mg (1% to 2%) 2561
Zithromax Tablets, 600 mg (1% to 2%) 2568
Zithromax Tri-Pak (1% to 2%) 2561
Zithromax Z-Pak (1% to 2%) 2568
Zmax for Oral Suspension (Less then 1%) 2577
Zocor Tablets 2078
▲ Zofran Injection (Approximately 5% of patients) 1607
Zofran (Approximately 1% to 2%) 1613
Zofran ODT Orally Disintegrating Tablets (Approximately 1% to 2%) 1613
Zoladex (Less than 1%) 709
Zoladex 3-month 712
Zoloft (Infrequent) 2581
Zonegran Capsules (Rare) 1089
Zosyn 3492
Zyprexa Tablets (2%) 1798
Zyprexa ZYDIS Orally Disintegrating Tablets (2%) 1798

Albuminuria

Abilify Tablets (Infrequent) 916
Abilify Tablets (Infrequent) 2472
Aciphex Tablets 1081
▲ Arava Tablets (1% to 3%) 2881
Astelin Nasal Spray (Infrequent) 1876
Atacand Tablets (More than 1%) 634
Atacand HCT 637
Caduet Tablets (Less than 2%) 2507
Calcijex Injection 411
Carbatrol Capsules 3174
Cardizem LA Extended Release Tablets (Less than 2%) 1699
▲ CellCept Capsules (3% to less than 20%) 2751
▲ CellCept Intravenous (3% to less than 20%) 2751
▲ CellCept Oral Suspension (3% to less than 20%) 2751
▲ CellCept Tablets (3% to less than 20%) 2751
Cipro I.V. 2998
Cipro I.V. Pharmacy Bulk Package 3509
Cipro 2991
▲ Coreg Tablets (Greater than 1% to 3%) 1376
Dapsone Tablets USP 1656
▲ Doxil Injection (1% to 5%) 3302
Effexor Tablets (Infrequent) 3405
Effexor XR Capsules (Infrequent) 3411
Equetro Extended-Release Capsules 3178
Eskalith 1406
Evoxac Capsules (Less than 1%) 1042
Exelon Capsules (Infrequent) 2204
Geodon Capsules (Infrequent) 2514
Hectorol Capsules 909
Hectorol Injection 911
Inspra Tablets (1%) 2520
▲ Intron A for Injection (Less than 5%) 3038
▲ Keppra Oral Solution (4%) 3307
▲ Keppra Tablets (4%) 3307
Lipitor Tablets (Less than 2%) 2495
Lithobid Tablets 1670
Lyrica Capsules (0.1% to 1%) 2524
▲ Megace ES Oral Suspension (1% to 3%) 2492
Miradon Tablets 3056
Mobic Oral Suspension (Less than 2%) 893
Mobic Tablets (Less than 2%) 893
Nexium Delayed-Release Capsules (Less than 1%) 645
Nexium I.V. (Less than 1%) 649
Noroxin Tablets 2009
▲ Ontak Vials (10%) 1717
Pentasa Capsules (Less than 1%) 3182
Pletal Tablets (Less than 2%) 2478
Prevacid Delayed-Release Capsules (Less than 1%) 3268
Prevacid for Delayed-Release Oral Suspension 3268
Prevacid NapraPAC 3277
Prevacid SoluTab Delayed-Release Orally Disintegrating Tablets (Less than 1%) 3268
PREVPAC (Less than 1%) 3281
▲ Prograf Capsules and Injection (3% to 15%) 624
Protonix I.V. (Less than 1%) 3468
Protonix Tablets (Less than 1%) 3465
Provigil Tablets (1%) 1002
Prozac Pulvules and Liquid (Infrequent) 1771
▲ Rapamune Oral Solution and Tablets (3% to 20%) 3472
Relafen Tablets (Less than 1%) 1523
Requip Tablets (Infrequent) 1528
Sandostatin LAR Depot (1% to 4%) 2264
▲ Simulect for Injection (3% to 10%) 2268
Sonata Capsules (Rare) 1686
Targretin Capsules 1719
Tegretol/Tegretol-XR 2278
Teveten Tablets (Less than 1%) 1707
Teveten HCT Tablets (Less than 1%) 1710
▲ Thalomid Capsules (3.1% to 8.3%) 979
Topamax Sprinkle Capsules (Infrequent) 2438
Topamax Tablets (Infrequent) 2438
Ultane Liquid for Inhalation (Less than 1%) 526
Ultracet Tablets (Less than 1%) 2462
Uniretic Tablets (Less than 1%) 3114
Uroqid-Acid No. 2 Tablets 785
VFEND I.V. (Less than 2%) 2543
VFEND Oral Suspension (Less than 2%) 2543
VFEND Tablets (Less than 2%) 2543
▲ Visudyne for Injection (1% to 10%) 2286
Zonegran Capsules (Rare) 1089
Zyprexa Tablets (Rare) 1798
Zyprexa ZYDIS Orally Disintegrating Tablets (Rare) 1798

Alcohol, increased sensitivity to

Catapres Tablets 874
Celexa (Infrequent) 1177
Clorpres Tablets 2139
Copaxone for Injection (Infrequent) 3292
Effexor Tablets (Rare) 3405
Effexor XR Capsules (Rare) 3411
Lamictal (Rare) 1449
Neurontin Capsules (Rare) 2498
Neurontin Oral Solution (Rare) 2498
Neurontin Tablets (Rare) 2498
▲ Protopic Ointment (Up to 7%) 629
Prozac Pulvules and Liquid (Rare) 1771
Rescriptor Tablets 2535
Seroquel Tablets (Infrequent) 691
Soriatane Capsules (Less than 1%) 1028
Symbyax Capsules (Infrequent) 1788
Tequin Injection (Less than 0.1%) 964
Tequin Tablets (Less than 0.1%) 964
Teveten Tablets (Less than 1%) 1707
Teveten HCT Tablets (Less than 1%) 1710
Topamax Sprinkle Capsules (Rare) 2438
Topamax Tablets (Rare) 2438

Alcohol abuse

Effexor Tablets (Rare) 3405
Effexor XR Capsules (Rare) 3411
Paxil CR Controlled-Release Tablets (Infrequent) 1509
Paxil (Infrequent) 1501
Zyprexa Tablets (Infrequent) 1798
Zyprexa ZYDIS Orally Disintegrating Tablets (Infrequent) 1798

Alcohol craving

Campral Tablets (Rare) 1175

Alkalosis

Ammonul Injection 3323
▲ Buphenyl Powder (7%) 3327
▲ Buphenyl Tablets (7%) 3327
▲ CellCept Capsules (3% to less than 20%) 2751
▲ CellCept Intravenous (3% to less than 20%) 2751
▲ CellCept Oral Suspension (3% to less than 20%) 2751
▲ CellCept Tablets (3% to less than 20%) 2751
▲ Prograf Capsules and Injection (3% to 15%) 624
▲ Proleukin for Injection (4%) 1007

Alkalosis, metabolic

Indocin I.V. (Less than 3%) 1973

Alkalosis, respiratory

Ammonul Injection 3323
Bayer Aspirin Tablets 3515

Allergic reactions

Abelcet Injection 1119
Abilify Tablets (Rare) 916
Abilify Tablets (Rare) 2472
AccuNeb Inhalation Solution (0.9% to 3.4%) 1055
Accutane Capsules 2740
Aceon Tablets (2 mg, 4 mg, 8 mg) (2.0%) 3191
Aciphex Tablets 1081
Actiq (Less than 1%) 993
Activase I.V. (Very rare) 1225
Activella Tablets 2311
Actonel Tablets (1.9% to 2.5%) 2679
Actonel with Calcium Tablets (1.9% to 2.5%) 2684
▲ Acular Ophthalmic Solution (Approximately 1% to 10%) 561
▲ Acular LS Ophthalmic Solution (1% to 10%) 562
Adacel Vaccine 2959
Adalat CC Tablets (Less than 1%) 2978
Adipex-P 1216
▲ Advair Diskus 100/50 (1% to 3%) 1291
▲ Advair Diskus 250/50 (1% to 3%) 1291
▲ Advair Diskus 500/50 (1% to 3%) 1291
Advil ■ 737
Children's Advil Suspension ■ 742
Children's Advil Chewable Tablets ■ 741
Advil Cold & Sinus ■ 739
Advil Flu & Body Ache Caplets ■ 739
Children's Advil Cold Suspension ■ 741
Infants' Advil Concentrated Drops ■ 743
Advil Migraine Liquigels ■ 740
Aggrastat 1878
Aggrenox Capsules (Less than 1%) 855
Alamast Ophthalmic Solution (Less than 5%) 3371
Albenza Tablets (Rare) 1310
▲ Alimta for Injection (Up to 8%) 1722
Alinia for Oral Suspension (Less than 1%) 2840
Alinia Tablets (Less than 1%) 2840
Alkeran for Injection 976
Alkeran Tablets 977
Alphagan P Ophthalmic Solution (1% to 4%) 563
Amaryl Tablets (Less than 1%) 2864
Ambien Tablets (Rare) 2867
AmBisome for Injection (Less common) 615
Amerge Tablets (Rare) 1312
Amnesteem Capsules 2126
Amoxil Capsules 1315
Amoxil Chewable Tablets 1315
Amoxil Pediatric Drops for Oral Suspension 1315
Amoxil Powder for Oral Suspension 1315
Amoxil Tablets 1315
Ancef for Injection 1318
Antara Capsules 2723
Antivenin (Micrurus fulvius) 3401
Antivenin Polyvalent 3399
Apidra Injection 2876
Apokyn Injection 2132
Aquacel AG with Hydrofiber 1035
AquaMEPHYTON Injection 1887
Aranesp for Injection (Rare) 576
Arava Tablets (2%) 2881
Aredia for Injection (Rare) 2168
Argatroban Injection 1321
Arimidex Tablets (Very rare) 665
Arthrotec Tablets (0.1%) 3126
Astelin Nasal Spray (Infrequent) 1876
Atrovent HFA Inhalation Aerosol 872
Attenuvax (Rare) 1889
Augmentin 1331
Augmentin Tablets 1334
Avelox (0.1% to less than 2%) 2984
Azopt Ophthalmic Suspension (Less than 1%) 553
Beano (Rare) ■ 764
BeneFix for Injection (1.5%) 3402
Bentyl Capsules 724
Bentyl Injection 724
Bentyl Syrup 724
Bentyl Tablets 724
Betasept Surgical Scrub 2715
Betimol Ophthalmic Solution (1% to 5%) ⊙ 283
Betimol Ophthalmic Solution (1% to 5%) 3371

Betoptic S Ophthalmic Suspension .. 554
Bexxar 1360
Biaxin/Biaxin XL 402
BiDil Tablets (1% to less than 2%) 2161
Biltricide Tablets 2990
Boniva Tablets (2.5%) 2747
▲ Brimonidine Tartrate Ophthalmic Solution 0.2% (10% to 30%) .... ⊙245
Caduet Tablets (Greater than 0.1% to 2.8%) 2507
Campath Ampules 826
Campral Tablets (Infrequent) 1175
Carac Cream, 0.5% (1.2%) 1048
Cardizem LA Extended Release Tablets (Less than 2%) 1699
▲ Carnitor Injection (2% to 6%) 3185
Catapres Tablets 874
Ceftin 1369
Celebrex Capsules (0.1% to 1.9%) ... 3130
Celexa 1177
Cetacaine Topical Anesthetic 1007
Ciloxan Ophthalmic Ointment (Less than 1%) 554
Cipro I.V. (1% or less) 2998
Cipro I.V. Pharmacy Bulk Package (1% or less) 3509
Cipro (Less than 1%) 2991
Cipro XR Tablets 3004
Cogentin Injection 1903
Colyte with Flavor Packs for Oral Solution (Isolated cases) 3102
Copaxone for Injection (Rare) 3292
▲ Coreg Tablets (Greater than 1% to 3%) 1376
Cosopt Sterile Ophthalmic Solution 1910
Coumadin for Injection (Infrequent) ... 932
Coumadin Tablets (Infrequent) 932
Creon 5 Capsules (Less frequent) 3195
Creon 10 Capsules (Less frequent) .. 3195
Creon 20 Capsules (Less frequent) .. 3196
Cutivate Lotion 0.05% (Less than 1%) 1383
CytoGam Intravenous (Rare) 1866
Cytomel Tablets (Rare) 1678
Cytovene 2763
DDAVP Injection 4 mcg/mL (Rare) 2893
DDAVP Nasal Spray 2894
DDAVP Tablets (Rare) 2895
Depacon Injection 412
Depakene 417
Depakote Sprinkle Capsules 422
▲ Depakote Tablets (1% to 5%) 427
Depakote ER Tablets 433
Depo-Medrol Single-Dose Vial 2617
Depo-Provera Contraceptive Injection (Less than 1%) 2619
depo-subQ provera 104 Injectable Suspension 2622
Desmopressin Acetate Injection (Rare) 1143
Digibind for Injection (Rare) 1388
Dilaudid Oral Liquid 443
Dilaudid Tablets - 8 mg 443
Diovan HCT Tablets (Greater than 0.2%) 2195
Diovan Tablets 2191
▲ Doxil Injection (1% to 5%) 3302
Duragesic Transdermal System (1% or greater) 2448
E.E.S. 449
Effexor Tablets (Infrequent) 3405
Effexor XR Capsules (Infrequent) 3411
Elitek 2906
Elmiron Capsules (Less than or equal to 1%) 2393
▲ Eloxatin for Injection (3% to 10%) 2908
Elspar for Injection 1943
Emcyt Capsules 3137
Enbrel for Injection (Less than 0.5%) 580
Epogen for Injection (Rare) 586
▲ Equetro Extended-Release Capsules (Less than 5%) 3178
EryPed 445
Ery-Tab Tablets 447
Erythrocin Stearate Filmtab Tablets 452
Erythromycin Delayed-Release Capsules, USP 456
Ethyol for Injection 1869
▲ Evoxac Capsules (1% to 3%) 1042
Exelon Capsules (Frequent) 2204
Feiba VH 749
Ferrlecit Injection (0.5%) 3379
Flomax Capsules 881
FML Ophthalmic Suspension .... ⊙224
Focalin Tablets 2214
▲ Fortaz (Among most common) 1422
Fortical Nasal Spray 3336
Fragmin Injection (Rare) 2638
Gabitril Tablets (Frequent) 998
Gengraf Capsules (1% to less than 3%) 458
Genoptic Sterile Ophthalmic Solution (Rare) .... ⊙227
Geodon 2514
GlucaGen for Injection 790
Glucagon for Injection Vials and Emergency Kit 1749
Hemofil M (Extremely rare) 757
▲ Herceptin I.V. (3%) 1234
HMS Sterile Ophthalmic Suspension .... ⊙228
Humalog-Pen (Less common) 1751
Humalog Mix 75/25-Pen 1754
Humulin 50/50, 100 Units (Less common to occasional) 1760
Humulin 70/30 Pen 1761
Humulin L, 100 Units 1763
Humulin R (U-500) 1768
Humulin N Pen 1765
Hurricaine Topical Anesthetic Gel, 1 oz. Fresh Mint, Wild Cherry, Pina Colada, Watermelon, 1/6 oz. Wild Cherry (Rare) .... ▣607
Hurricaine Topical Anesthetic Liquid, 1 oz. Wild Cherry, Pina Colada, .25 ml Swab Applicator Wild Cherry (Rare) .... ▣607
Hurricaine Topical Anesthetic Spray Extension Tubes (200) (Rare) .... ▣607
Hurricaine Topical Anesthetic Spray Kit, 2 oz. Wild Cherry (Rare) .... ▣607
Hurricaine Topical Anesthetic Spray, 2 oz. Wild Cherry (Rare) ... ▣607
Hyalgan Solution (Three cases) 2917
Hycamtin for Injection (Infrequent) 1427
Hytrin Capsules (Rare) 469
Imodium Capsules (Extremely rare) 1834
Increlex Injection 3290
Infanrix Vaccine 1444
▲ Infergen (3% to 7%) 1647
Integrilin Injection 3034
Invirase (Less than 2%) 2776
Iressa Tablets (Very rare) 684
▲ I.V. Busulfex (2% to 26%) 1125
Kaletra (Less than 2%) 474
Keppra Oral Solution (2%) 3307
Keppra Tablets (2%) 3307
Ketek Tablets (Rare) 2920
Klonopin (2%) 2782
Koāte-DVI 3247
Kogenate FS 3517
Kytril Injection (Rare) 2785
Lamictal (Infrequent) 1449
Lamisil Tablets (Rare) 2226
Lantus Injection 2925
Lescol Capsules (2.3%) 2227
Lescol Capsules (2.3%) 2730
Lescol XL Tablets (1%) 2227
Lescol XL Tablets (1%) 2730
Leukeran Tablets 1472
▲ Leukine (12%) 829
Levaquin in 5% Dextrose Injection (0.1% to 0.9%) 2453
Levaquin (0.1% to 0.9%) 2453
Lexapro Oral Solution (Frequent) 1193
Lexapro Tablets (Frequent) 1193
Lidoderm Patch (Rare) 1107
Lipitor Tablets (Up to 2.8%) 2495
Lofibra Capsules 1217
Lortab 3315
Lortab Elixir 3312
Lotronex Tablets (Rare) 1479
Lovenox Injection 2931
Lunesta Tablets (Infrequent) 3139
Lyrica Capsules (Greater than or equal to 1%) 2524
Matulane Capsules 3188
Mefoxin for Injection 1987
Mefoxin Premixed Intravenous Solution 1990
Mepron Suspension (0.8% to 1.1%) 1487
Meridia Capsules (1.5%) 485
Merrem I.V. 687
Metamucil 2672
Miacalcin Injection (A few cases) 2241
Miacalcin Nasal Spray (Less than 1%) 2242
Micardis Tablets (More than 0.3%) ... 884
Micardis HCT Tablets 886
Mirapex Tablets (1% or more) 889
Mivacron Injection 489
Mobic Oral Suspension (Less than 2%) 893
Mobic Tablets (Less than 2%) 893
Children's Motrin Oral Suspension and Chewable Tablets .... ▣647
Children's Motrin Non-Staining Dye-Free Oral Suspension .... ▣647
Children's Motrin Oral Suspension and Chewable Tablets 1837
Children's Motrin Cold Non-Staining Dye-Free Oral Suspension 1838
Children's Motrin Cold Oral Suspension 1838
Children's Motrin Non-Staining Dye-Free Oral Suspension 1837
Motrin Cold & Sinus Caplets 1836
Motrin IB Tablets and Caplets 1836
Infants' Motrin Concentrated Drops 1837
Infants' Motrin Non-Staining Dye-Free Drops 1837
Junior Strength Motrin Caplets and Chewable Tablets 1837
Mumpsvax (Extremely rare) 2005
Namenda (Infrequent) 1199
Naropin Injection (Rare) 640
Nasacort HFA Inhalation Aerosol 2939
Natacyn Antifungal Ophthalmic Suspension (One case) .... ⊙207
Navelbine Injection 1494
Neoral Soft Gelatin Capsules (1% to less than 3%) 2247
Neoral Oral Solution (1% to less than 3%) 2247
Neosporin Scar Solution .... ▣702
Neulasta Injection 596
Neumega for Injection 3433
Neupogen for Injection (Less than 1 in 4000) 598
Neurontin Capsules (Infrequent) 2498
Neurontin Oral Solution 2498
Neurontin Tablets (Infrequent) 2498
Nexium Delayed-Release Capsules (Less than 1%) 645
Nexium I.V. (Less than 1%) 649
▲ Nicotrol Inhaler (Greater than 3%) ... 2594
Nicotrol NS (Less than1%) 2596
▲ Nipent for Injection (2% to 11%) 3216
Nitro-Dur Transdermal Infusion System (Uncommon) 3060
Noritate Cream, 1% (Uncommon) 1051
Noroxin Tablets (Less frequent) 2009
Norvasc Tablets (More than 0.1% to 1%) 2529
Norvir (Less than 2%) 499
Novolin 70/30 PenFill 3 ml Cartridges (Rare) 2325
Novolin N PenFill 3 ml Cartridges (Rare) 2325
Novolin R PenFill (Rare) 2325
NovoLog Injection 2326
NovoLog Mix 70/30 2331
NovoSeven (1%) 2335
Nubain Injection (1% or less) 1111
Numorphan 1112
Nutropin for Injection 1238
Nutropin AQ Injection 1241
Nutropin AQ Pen 1241
Nutropin AQ Pen Cartridge 1241
Nystatin Vaginal Tablets, USP (Rare) 2347
Omnicef Capsules 506
Omnicef for Oral Suspension 506
▲ Oncaspar (Greater than 5%) 1123
OptiPranolol Metipranolol Ophthalmic Solution 0.3% (A small number of patients) .... ⊙254
Paxil CR Controlled-Release Tablets (Infrequent) 1509
Paxil (Infrequent) 1501
PCE Dispertab Tablets 510
Pentasa Capsules 3182
PhosLo GelCaps 2158
Plasbumin-5 (Rare) 3249
Plasbumin-20 (Rare) 3249
Plasbumin-25 (Rare) 3251
Plavix Tablets (Less than 1%) 940
Plavix Tablets (Less than 1%) 2942
Prandin Tablets (0.5, 1, and 2 mg) (1% to 2%) 2337
Pred Forte Ophthalmic Suspension .... ⊙233
Pred Mild Sterile Ophthalmic Suspension .... ⊙236
Prevacid Delayed-Release Capsules (Less than 1%) 3268
Prevacid for Delayed-Release Oral Suspension (Less than 1%) 3268
Prevacid NapraPAC (Less than 1%) .. 3277
Prevacid SoluTab Delayed-Release Orally Disintegrating Tablets (Less than 1%) 3268
PREVPAC 3281
Prilosec OTC Tablets 2674
Primaxin I.M. 2022
Prochieve 4% Gel 1018
Prochieve 8% Gel 1018
Procrit for Injection (Rare) 2374
▲ Prograf Capsules and Injection (3% to 15%) 624
Prolastin (Occasional) 3252
Proleukin for Injection (1%) 1007
Propine Ophthalmic Solution .... ⊙237
ProSom Tablets (Infrequent) 512
Protonix I.V. (Less than 1%) 3468
Protonix Tablets (Less than 1%) 3465
▲ Protopic Ointment (6% to 22%) 629
▲ Proventil HFA Inhalation Aerosol (6%) 3071
Provigil Tablets (At least 1%) 1002
Psoriatec Cream (Very few instances) 3191
Pulmicort Respules (1% to 3%) 654
Quixin Ophthalmic Solution (Less than 1%) 3373
Rabies Vaccine RabAvert (Rare) 1011
Recombinate (Extremely rare) 762
ReFacto Vials 3479
▲ Refludan for Injection (3.5%) 815
Relpax Tablets (Rare) 2531
Remicade for IV Injection (Greater than or equal to 0.2%) 987
ReoPro Vials 1779
Repronex for Intramuscular and Subcutaneous Injection 1148
Rescriptor Tablets 2535
Retavase (3 patients) 1131
Reyataz Capsules (Less than 3%) 948
R-Gene 10 for Intravenous Use (One patient) 2647
Rhophylac (Rare) 3504
Risperdal M-Tab Orally Disintegrating Tablets (Rare) 1658
Risperdal (Rare) 1658
Sandimmune (2% or less) 2259
Sandostatin Injection (Less than 1%) 2263
▲ Sandostatin LAR Depot (5% to 15%) 2264
Sedapap Tablets 50 mg/650 mg (Infrequent) 2098
Seromycin Capsules 1783
Sonata Capsules 1686
Spectracef Tablets (0.1% to 1%) 2706
▲ Spiriva HandiHaler (1% to 3%) 899
Suprax 1811
Sustiva Capsules 957
▲ Symlin Injection (Less than 1% to 6%) 608
Symmetrel 1115
Synercid I.V. (Less than 1%) 1690
Tagamet Tablets (Rare) 1547
Tasmar Tablets (Infrequent) 3360
▲ Temodar Capsules (3%) 3088
▲ Tequin Injection (0.1% to 3%) 964
▲ Tequin Tablets (0.1% to 3%) 964
Thalomid Capsules 979
Thiothixene Capsules 2124
Thrombin-JMI 1693
Tiazac Capsules (1%) 1204
Ticlid Tablets 2813
Timoptic in Ocudose 2061
Timoptic Sterile Ophthalmic Solution 2058
Timoptic-XE Sterile Ophthalmic Gel Forming Solution 2062
TNKase I.V. (Rare) 1256
▲ Topamax Sprinkle Capsules (Less than 1% to 3%) 2438
▲ Topamax Tablets (Less than 1% to 3%) 2438
Trasylol Injection (0.3%) 779
Traumeel Injection Solution (Rare) 1638
Tricor Tablets 523
Trileptal Oral Suspension (Up to 2%) 2281
Trileptal Tablets (Up to 2%) 2281
Trusopt Sterile Ophthalmic Solution 2065
▲ Truvada Tablets (Greater than 5%) 1279
Twinrix Vaccine 1571
Tygacil for Injection (0.2% to less than 2%) 3489
Tylenol with Codeine 2461
Ultane Liquid for Inhalation (Less than 1%) 526
Ultracet Tablets 2462
Ultrase Capsules (Less frequent) 735
Ultrase MT Capsules (Less frequent) 736
Uniretic Tablets (Less than 1%) 3114
▲ Vagifem Tablets (3% to 5%) 2340
Vantin Tablets and Oral Suspension 2650
Varivax (Greater than or equal to 1%) 2070
VFEND I.V. (Less than 2%) 2543

VFEND Oral Suspension (Less than 2%) 2543
VFEND Tablets (Less than 2%) 2543
Viagra Tablets (Less than 2%) 2552
Vicodin Tablets 530
Vicodin ES Tablets 531
Vicodin HP Tablets 532
Vicoprofen Tablets (Less than 1%) 533
Viracept (Less than 2%) 2556
Viramune Oral Suspension 903
Viramune Tablets 903
Wellbutrin Tablets 1579
Wellbutrin SR Sustained-Release Tablets 1583
Wellbutrin XL Extended-Release Tablets 1588
Yasmin 28 Tablets 818
Zaditor Ophthalmic Solution (Less than 5%) 2302
Zeel Solution 1639
Zegerid Powder for Oral Solution 2972
Zelnorm Tablets 2303
Zemplar Capsules (Rare) 535
Zemplar Injection (Rare) 538
Zemuron Injection (Rare) 2363
▲ Zerit (9%) 971
Zevalin Injection (2%) 848
Zinacef Injection 1604
Zinacef for Injection 1604
Zithromax Capsules, 250 mg (Rare) 2568
Zithromax for IV Infusion (Rare) 2573
Zithromax for Oral Suspension, 1 g (Rare) 2568
Zithromax for Oral Suspension, 300 mg, 600 mg, 900 mg, 1200 mg (Rare) 2561
Zithromax Tablets, 250 mg, 500 mg (1% or less) 2561
Zithromax Tablets, 600 mg (Rare) 2568
Zithromax Tri-Pak (1% or less) 2561
Zithromax Z-Pak (Rare) 2568
Zoladex (1% or greater) 709
Zoladex 3-month 712
Zoloft (Rare) 2581
Zomig Nasal Spray (Infrequent) 718
Zomig Tablets (Infrequent) 714
Zomig-ZMT Tablets (Infrequent) 714
Zonegran Capsules (Infrequent) 1089
Zosyn 3492
Zyban Sustained-Release Tablets (1%) 1620

Allergic sensitization

▲ Alferon N Injection (1% to 18%) 1640
▲ Blephamide Ophthalmic Ointment (Among most often) 563
▲ Blephamide Ophthalmic Suspension (Most often) 564
▲ Catapres-TTS (5 of 101 patients) 875
Chromagen Forte Soft Gelatin Capsules 3296
Citracal Prenatal Rx Tablets 2108
Encora Capsules 3298
Encora AM Tablets 3298
Encora PM Tablets 3298
▲ FML-S Liquifilm Sterile Ophthalmic Suspension (Among most often) ⊙ 226
Metamucil Capsules 2672
Niferex-150 Forte Capsules 3299
OptiNate 1162
▲ Poly-Pred Liquifilm Ophthalmic Suspension (Most often) ⊙ 231
PreCare Chewables Tablets 3300
PreCare Prenatal Caplets 3300
▲ Pred-G Ophthalmic Suspension (Most often) ⊙ 234
Pred-G Sterile Ophthalmic Ointment ⊙ 235
PremesisRx Tablets 3300
Prenate Elite Tablets 1163
PrimaCare AM Capsules 3300
PrimaCare One Capsules 3301
PrimaCare PM Tablets 3300

Allergy

(*see under* Allergic reactions)

Alopecia

Abilify Tablets (Infrequent) 916
Abilify Tablets (Infrequent) 2472
Accutane Capsules 2740
Aciphex Tablets 1081
Actiq (Less than 1%) 993
Activella Tablets 2311
Adalat CC Tablets (Rare) 2978
▲ Adriamycin for Injection, USP (Most cases) 786
▲ Adriamycin Injection, USP (Most cases) 786
Advicor Tablets 1694
Aggrenox Capsules 855
Agrylin Capsules (1% to 5%) 3172
Albenza Tablets (Less than 1.0% to 1.6%) 1310
Aldara Cream, 5% (1.4%) 1814
Aldoclor Tablets 1881
Aldoril Tablets 1884
Alesse-28 Tablets 3392
▲ Alimta for Injection (11%) 1722
Alkeran for Injection 976
Alkeran Tablets 977
Aloprim for Injection (Less than 1%) 2156
Altoprev Extended-Release Tablets 1151
AmBisome for Injection (Less common) 615
Amerge Tablets (Rare) 1312
Ammonul Injection 3323
Amnesteem Capsules 2126
Anadrol-50 Tablets 3329
Anaprox Tablets (Less than 1%) 2769
Anaprox DS Tablets (Less than 1%) 2769
AndroGel (1%) 3330
Antara Capsules 2723
▲ Arava Tablets (10%) 2881
Aricept Tablets (Infrequent) 1086
Aricept ODT Tablets (Infrequent) 1086
▲ Aromasin Tablets (2% to 5%) 2600
Arthrotec Tablets (Rare) 3126
Asacol Delayed-Release Tablets 2688
Atacand HCT 637
▲ Avastin IV (6% to 32%) 1229
▲ Avonex (4%) 839
Azasan Tablets (Less than 1%) 2844
Azopt Ophthalmic Suspension (Less than 1%) 553
Benicar Tablets 2850
Benicar HCT Tablets (Rare) 2852
Betagan Ophthalmic Solution, USP ⊙ 217
▲ Betaseron for SC Injection (4%) 791
▲ Betimol Ophthalmic Solution (More than 5%) ⊙ 283
▲ Betimol Ophthalmic Solution (More than 5%) 3371
Betoptic S Ophthalmic Suspension (Rare) 554
BiDil Tablets (1% to less than 2%) 2161
Blocadren Tablets (Less than 1%) 1891
Caduet Tablets (Less than 2%) 2507
Campral Tablets (Infrequent) 1175
▲ Camptosar Injection (60%) 2602
Canasa Rectal Suppositories 726
Captopril Tablets (About 0.5% to 2%) 2114
Carbatrol Capsules 3174
Cardizem LA Extended Release Tablets (Infrequent) 1699
▲ Casodex Tablets (2% to 5%) 670
Cataflam Tablets (Occasionally) 2173
Catapres Tablets 874
Catapres-TTS 875
Celebrex Capsules (0.1% to 1.9%) 3130
Celexa (Infrequent) 1177
▲ CellCept Capsules (3% to less than 20%) 2751
▲ CellCept Intravenous (3% to less than 20%) 2751
▲ CellCept Oral Suspension (3% to less than 20%) 2751
▲ CellCept Tablets (3% to less than 20%) 2751
Cenestin Tablets, 0.3mg 1063
▲ Cerubidine for Injection (In most patients) 788
Climara Transdermal System 795
Climara Pro Transdermal System 800
Clinoril Tablets (Less than 1%) 1899
Clobex Shampoo 1209
Clorpres Tablets (About 2 in 1,000) 2139
Colazal Capsules 2845
Combivent Inhalation Aerosol 878
Combivir Tablets 1373
Comvax 1904
Concerta Extended-Release Tablets 1828
Copaxone for Injection (At least 2%) 3292
▲ Copegus Tablets (28%) 2759
Coreg Tablets (Less than or equal to 0.1%) 1376
Cosmegen for Injection 1907
Cosopt Sterile Ophthalmic Solution 1910
Coumadin for Injection (Infrequent) 932
Coumadin Tablets (Infrequent) 932
Covera-HS Tablets (Less than 2%) 3135
Cozaar Tablets (Less than 1%) 1913
Crixivan Capsules 1918
Cuprimine Capsules (Rare) 1925
Cymbalta Delayed-Release Capsules (Infrequent) 1729
Cytovene (At least 3 subjects) 2763
Delatestryl Injection 2976
▲ Depacon Injection (6% to 24%) 412
▲ Depakene (6% to 24%) 417
▲ Depakote Sprinkle Capsules (6% to 24%) 422
▲ Depakote Tablets (1% to 24%) 427
▲ Depakote ER Tablets (6% to 24%) 433
▲ Depo-Provera Contraceptive Injection (1% to 5%) 2619
Didronel Tablets 2693
Diovan HCT Tablets 2195
Diovan Tablets 2191
Diuril Oral 1936
Diuril Sodium Intravenous 1934
▲ Doxil Injection (8.9% to 19.2%) 3302
EC-Naprosyn Delayed-Release Tablets (Less than 1%) 2769
Effexor Tablets (Infrequent) 3405
Effexor XR Capsules (Infrequent) 3411
Efudex 3348
Eldepryl Capsules 3209
Eligard 7.5 mg (Less than 2%) 2896
Eligard 30 mg (2.2%) 2901
▲ Ellence Injection (19.3% to 95.5%) 2632
▲ Elmiron Capsules (4%) 2393
▲ Eloxatin for Injection (3% to 30%) 2908
Emcyt Capsules (1%) 3137
Emend Capsules (Greater than 0.5%) 1944
▲ Enbrel for Injection (1% to 6%) 580
Engerix-B Vaccine 1391
▲ Entocort EC Capsules (Less than 5%) 2694
Epivir 1394
Epivir-HBV 1398
Epzicom Tablets 1402
▲ Equetro Extended-Release Capsules (Less than 5%) 3178
▲ Erbitux (5%) 937
Eskalith 1406
Estratest Tablets 3196
Estratest H.S. Tablets 3196
Estrogel 0.06% 3200
Evoxac Capsules (Less than 1%) 1042
Exelon Capsules (Infrequent) 2204
▲ Femara Tablets (5%) 2210
Flexeril Tablets (Rare) 1832
Focalin Tablets 2214
Focalin XR Capsules 2217
Follistim AQ Cartridge 2354
Fortical Nasal Spray (Less than 1%) 3336
Gabitril Tablets (Frequent) 998
Garamycin Injectable 3028
▲ Gemzar for Injection (15% to 18%) 1743
▲ Gengraf Capsules (4%) 458
Genotropin Lyophilized Powder 2642
Geodon Capsules (Infrequent) 2514
Gleevec Tablets (Less common) 2221
Hexalen Capsules (Less than 1%) 2101
▲ Hycamtin for Injection (42% to 62%) 1427
Hyzaar 1964
▲ Idamycin PFS Injection (77%) 2645
Inderal LA Long-Acting Capsules (Rare) 3421
Indocin Capsules (Less than 1%) 1968
Indocin I.V. (Less than 1%) 1973
Indocin (Less than 1%) 1968
▲ Infergen (10% to 14%) 1647
InnoPran XL Capsules (Rare) 2728
▲ Intron A for Injection (Up to 38%) 3038
Invirase (Less than 2%) 2776
▲ I.V. Busulfex (2% to 15%) 1125
Kaletra (Less than 2%) 474
Keppra Oral Solution (1% to 2%) 3307
Keppra Tablets (1% to 2%) 3307
Klonopin (Infrequent) 2782
▲ Kytril Tablets (3%) 2788
Lamictal (1.3%) 1449
Lamisil Tablets 2226
Lariam Tablets (Less than 1%) 2790
Lescol Capsules 2227
Lescol Capsules 2730
Lescol XL Tablets 2227
Lescol XL Tablets 2730
▲ Leukine (37% to 73%) 829
Levaquin in 5% Dextrose Injection (0.1% to 0.9%) 2453
Levaquin (0.1% to 0.9%) 2453
Levothroid Tablets 1189
Levoxyl Tablets 1680
Lexapro Oral Solution (Infrequent) 1193
Lexapro Tablets (Infrequent) 1193
Lipitor Tablets (Less than 2%) 2495
Lithobid Tablets 1670
Lofibra Capsules (Less than 1%) 1217
Lo/Ovral-28 Tablets 3423
Loprox Gel 1861
Lotensin Tablets (Less than 1%) 2232
Lotensin HCT Tablets (0.3% or more) 2235
Lotrel Capsules (Infrequent) 2238
Lotronex Tablets (Rare) 1479
Lunesta Tablets (Infrequent) 3139
▲ Lupron Depot 3.75 mg (Among most frequent) 3257
Lupron Depot–3 Month 11.25 mg (Less than 5%) 3262
Lupron Depot-PED 7.5 mg, 11.25 mg and 15 mg (Less than 2%) 3266
Lupron Injection Pediatric (Less than 2%) 3256
Luxíq Foam (One patient) 1026
Lyrica Capsules (0.1% to 1%) 2524
Matulane Capsules 3188
Maxair Autohaler 1820
▲ Megace ES Oral Suspension (1% to 3%) 2492
Menostar Transdermal System 805
Meridia Capsules 485
Metadate CD Capsules 3316
Mevacor Tablets (0.5% to 1.0%) 1996
Miacalcin Nasal Spray (Less than 1%) 2242
Midamor Tablets (Less than or equal to 1%) 2000
Miradon Tablets 3056
Mobic Oral Suspension (Less than 2%) 893
Mobic Tablets (Less than 2%) 893
Moduretic Tablets 2003
Mustargen for Injection (Infrequent) 2007
Myleran Tablets (Rare) 1492
Nadolol Tablets (Infrequent) 2121
Nalfon Capsules (Less than 1%) 2504
Namenda (Infrequent) 1199
Naprosyn Suspension (Less than 1%) 2769
Naprosyn Tablets (Less than 1%) 2769
▲ Navelbine Injection (Up to 34%) 1494
▲ Neoral Soft Gelatin Capsules (4%) 2247
▲ Neoral Oral Solution (4%) 2247
▲ Neulasta Injection (15% to 72%) 596
▲ Neumega for Injection (Greater than or equal to 10%) 3433
▲ Neupogen for Injection (18%) 598
Neurontin Capsules (Infrequent) 2498
Neurontin Oral Solution (Infrequent) 2498
Neurontin Tablets (Infrequent) 2498
Nipent for Injection (Less than 3%) 3216
Nizoral 2% Shampoo (Less than 1%) 1838
Norvasc Tablets (Less than or equal to 0.1%) 2529
▲ Novantrone for Injection Concentrate (38% to 61%) 3158
Omacor Capsules 2735
Oncaspar 1123
Ortho-Cept Tablets 2395
Ortho-Cyclen Tablets 2414
Ortho Evra Transdermal System 2402
Ortho Tri-Cyclen Tablets 2414
Ortho Tri-Cyclen Lo Tablets 2421
Pacerone Tablets (Less than 1%) 3337
Parcopa Orally Disintegrating Tablets 3111
Parnate Tablets 1499
Paxil CR Controlled-Release Tablets (Infrequent) 1509
Paxil (Infrequent) 1501
Pediarix Vaccine 1518
▲ Pegasys (23%) 2793
▲ PEG-Intron Powder for Injection (22%) 3062
Pentasa Capsules (Less than 1%) 3182
Pepcid Injection (Infrequent) 2017
Pepcid (Infrequent) 2014
Permax Tablets (Infrequent) 3357
Persantine Tablets (Rare) 898
Prandin Tablets (0.5, 1, and 2 mg) (Rare) 2337
Pravachol Tablets 943
Prefest Tablets 1069
Premarin Intravenous 3440
Premarin Tablets 3443
Premarin Vaginal Cream 3449
Premphase Tablets 3452
Prempro Tablets 3452
Prevacid Delayed-Release Capsules (Less than 1%) 3268
Prevacid for Delayed-Release Oral Suspension (Less than 1%) 3268
Prevacid NapraPAC (Less than 1%) 3277
Prevacid SoluTab Delayed-Release Orally Disintegrating Tablets (Less than 1%) 3268
PREVPAC (Less than 1%) 3281
Prilosec OTC Tablets (Less than 1%) 2674
Prinivil Tablets (0.3% to 1.0%) 2029
Prinzide Tablets 2033

▲ Prograf Capsules and Injection (3% to 15%) 624
Proleukin for Injection (1%) 1007
Protonix I.V. (Less than 1%) 3468
Protonix Tablets (Less than 1%) 3465
Prozac Pulvules and Liquid (Infrequent) 1771
Purinethol Tablets 1222
▲ Rebetol (23% to 36%) 3073
▲ Rebetron Combination Therapy (27% to 32%) 3078
Relafen Tablets (Less than 1%) 1523
Relpax Tablets (Rare) 2531
Requip Tablets (Infrequent) 1528
Rescriptor Tablets 2535
Reyataz Capsules (Less than 3%) 948
▲ Ribavirin, USP Capsules (23% to 36%) 3083
Rilutek Tablets (Up to 1.2%) 2945
Risperdal Consta Long-Acting Injection (Infrequent) 1664
Risperdal M-Tab Orally Disintegrating Tablets (Infrequent) 1658
Risperdal (Infrequent) 1658
Ritalin Hydrochloride Tablets (A few instances) 2254
Ritalin LA Capsules 2255
Ritalin-SR Tablets (A few instances) 2254
▲ Roferon-A Injection (17% to 22%) 2805
Rythmol SR Capsules 2736
▲ Sandostatin Injection (1% to 4%) 2263
Sandostatin LAR Depot (1% to 4%) 2264
Seasonale Tablets 1073
Sonata Capsules (Infrequent) 1686
▲ Soriatane Capsules (50% to 75%) 1028
Stalevo Tablets 2270
Sular Tablets (Less than or equal to 1%) 1163
Surmontil Capsules 2347
Sustiva Capsules (Less than 2%) 957
Symbyax Capsules (Infrequent) 1788
Synthroid Tablets 515
Tagamet Tablets (Very rare) 1547
Tambocor Tablets (Less than 1%) 1824
▲ Targretin Capsules (3.6% to 11.3%) 1719
Tarka Tablets 519
Tasmar Tablets (1%) 3360
▲ Taxotere Injection Concentrate (Less than 1% to 75.8%) 2947
Tegretol/Tegretol-XR 2278
▲ Temodar Capsules (55%) 3088
Temovate Scalp Application (1 of 294 patients) 1551
Tenormin I.V. Injection 698
Tenormin Tablets 695
Teveten HCT Tablets 1710
Thalomid Capsules 979
Thyrolar 1203
Tiazac Capsules (Infrequent) 1204
Timolide Tablets 2056
Timoptic in Ocudose (Less frequent) 2061
Timoptic Sterile Ophthalmic Solution (Less frequent) 2058
Timoptic-XE Sterile Ophthalmic Gel Forming Solution 2062
▲ Topamax Sprinkle Capsules (Greater than 1% to 5%) 2438
▲ Topamax Tablets (Greater than 1% to 5%) 2438
Toprol-XL Tablets (Rare) 660
Tricor Tablets 523
Trileptal Oral Suspension 2281
Trileptal Tablets 2281
Triphasil-28 Tablets 3483
Trizivir Tablets 1565
Twinrix Vaccine 1571
Uniretic Tablets (Less than 1%) 3114
Unithroid Tablets 3521
Univasc Tablets (Less than 1%) 3118
Valtrex Caplets 1573
Vantin Tablets and Oral Suspension (Less than 1%) 2650
Vaseretic Tablets 2073
Vasotec I.V. Injection (0.5% to 1.0%) 2076
Verelan PM Capsules (2% or less) 3120
▲ Vesanoid Capsules (14%) 2823
VFEND I.V. (Less than 2%) 2543
VFEND Oral Suspension (Less than 2%) 2543
VFEND Tablets (Less than 2%) 2543
Viadur Implant (2.3%) 782
Vivactil Tablets 2350
Vivelle Transdermal System 2288
Vivelle-Dot Transdermal System 2293
Voltaren Tablets (Occasionally) 2298
Voltaren-XR Tablets (Occasionally) 2301
Vytorin 10/10 Tablets 2084
Vytorin 10/10 Tablets 3092
Vytorin 10/20 Tablets 2084
Vytorin 10/20 Tablets 3092
Vytorin 10/40 Tablets 2084
Vytorin 10/40 Tablets 3092
Vytorin 10/80 Tablets 2084
Vytorin 10/80 Tablets 3092
Wellbutrin Tablets (Infrequent) 1579
Wellbutrin SR Sustained-Release Tablets 1583
Wellbutrin XL Extended-Release Tablets 1588
Yasmin 28 Tablets 818
Zantac (Rare) 1597
Zantac Injection (Rare) 1593
Zantac Injection Pharmacy Bulk Package (Rare) 1595
Zantac Syrup (Rare) 1597
Zegerid Powder for Oral Solution (Less than 1%) 2972
Zestoretic Tablets 701
Zestril Tablets (0.3% to 1.0%) 704
▲ Zinecard for Injection (94% to 100%) 2659
Zocor Tablets 2078
Zoladex (1% or greater) 709
Zoladex 3-month 712
Zoloft (Infrequent) 2581
▲ Zometa for Intravenous Infusion (12%) 2306
Zonegran Capsules (Infrequent) 1089
Zovirax Capsules 1616
Zovirax for Injection 1618
Zovirax 1616
Zyprexa Tablets (Infrequent) 1798
Zyprexa ZYDIS Orally Disintegrating Tablets (Infrequent) 1798
Zyrtec Chewable Tablets (Less than 2%) 2589
Zyrtec (Less than 2%) 2589
Zyrtec-D 12 Hour Extended Release Tablets (Less than 2%) 2591

Alopecia hereditaria
Anadrol-50 Tablets 3329
Estratest Tablets 3196
Estratest H.S. Tablets 3196
Oxandrin Tablets 2977

Alpha-glutamyl transferase, elevation
Eulexin Capsules 3023

ALT elevation
(*see under* Alanine aminotransferase levels, elevation of)

Alveolitis
Cuprimine Capsules 1925
Pacerone Tablets 3337

Alveolitis, allergic
Paxil CR Controlled-Release Tablets 1509
Paxil 1501
Relafen Tablets (Less than 1%) 1523
Tricor Tablets 523

Alveolitis, fibrosing
Canasa Rectal Suppositories 726

Amaurosis
Zofran Injection (One patient) 1607

Amblyopia
Abilify Tablets (Rare) 916
Abilify Tablets (Rare) 2472
Aciphex Tablets 1081
▲ Actonel Tablets (3.3%) 2679
Adalat CC Tablets (Less than 1%) 2978
Advicor Tablets 1694
Agrylin Capsules (1% to 5%) 3172
Aloxi Injection (Less than 1%) 2099
Antara Capsules 2723
Arthrotec Tablets (Rare) 3126
Avelox (Less then 0.1%) 2984
Avinza Capsules (Less than 5%) 1714
Axid Oral Solution (1.0%) 913
▲ BiDil Tablets (3%) 2161
Buprenex Injectable (Infrequent) 2718
Caduet Tablets (Less than 2%) 2507
Campral Tablets (Infrequent) 1175
Cardizem LA Extended Release Tablets (Less than 2%) 1699
▲ Carnitor Injection (3% to 6%) 3185
▲ CellCept Capsules (3% to less than 20%) 2751
▲ CellCept Intravenous (3% to less than 20%) 2751
▲ CellCept Oral Suspension (3% to less than 20%) 2751
▲ CellCept Tablets (3% to less than 20%) 2751
Combunox Tablets (Less than 2%) 1183
Copaxone for Injection (At least 2%) 3292
▲ Depacon Injection (4% to 12%) 412
▲ Depakene (8% to 12%) 417
▲ Depakote Sprinkle Capsules (4% to 12%) 422
▲ Depakote Tablets (1% to 12%) 427
▲ Depakote ER Tablets (4% to 12%) 433
Diprivan Injectable Emulsion (Less than 1%) 676
Doxil Injection (Less than 1%) 3302
Duragesic Transdermal System (Less than 1%) 2448
Elmiron Capsules (Less than or equal to 1%) 2393
▲ Equetro Extended-Release Capsules (6%) 3178
▲ Flolan for Injection (8%) 1408
Flomax Capsules (0.2% to 2.0%) 881
▲ Gabitril Tablets (1% to 9%) 998
Herceptin I.V. (At least one of the 958 patients) 1234
Hytrin Capsules (0.6% to 1.3%) 469
Iressa Tablets (2%) 684
Kadian Capsules (Less than 3%) 572
Keppra Oral Solution (1% or 2%) 3307
Keppra Tablets (1% or 2%) 3307
Lipitor Tablets (Less than 2%) 2495
Lofibra Capsules 1217
▲ Megace ES Oral Suspension (1% to 3%) 2492
Meridia Capsules (Greater than or equal to 1%) 485
Natrecor for Injection (Greater than or equal to 1%) 3123
Neumega for Injection 3433
▲ Neurontin Capsules (2.7% to 4.2%) 2498
▲ Neurontin Oral Solution (2.7% to 4.2%) 2498
▲ Neurontin Tablets (2.7% to 4.2%) 2498
Niaspan Extended-Release Tablets 1703
Nipent for Injection (Less than 3%) 3216
Norvir (Less than 2%) 499
Paxil CR Controlled-Release Tablets (Rare) 1509
Paxil (Rare) 1501
Pletal Tablets (Less than 2%) 2478
Prevacid Delayed-Release Capsules (Less than 1%) 3268
Prevacid for Delayed-Release Oral Suspension (Less than 1%) 3268
Prevacid SoluTab Delayed-Release Orally Disintegrating Tablets (Less than 1%) 3268
PREVPAC (Less than 1%) 3281
▲ Prograf Capsules and Injection (3% to 15%) 624
Protonix I.V. (Less than 1%) 3468
Protonix Tablets (Less than 1%) 3465
Provigil Tablets (1%) 1002
Retrovir Capsules 1533
Retrovir IV Infusion 1537
Retrovir 1533
Rilutek Tablets (Infrequent) 2945
Seroquel Tablets (2%) 691
Sular Tablets (Less than or equal to 1%) 1163
Thalomid Capsules 979
Tiazac Capsules (Less than 2%) 1204
Tricor Tablets 523
Ultane Liquid for Inhalation (Less than 1%) 526
▲ Wellbutrin SR Sustained-Release Tablets (2% to 3%) 1583
▲ Wellbutrin XL Extended-Release Tablets (2% to 3%) 1588
Zoladex (1% or greater) 709
Zoladex 3-month 712
Zomig Nasal Spray (Infrequent) 718
Zonegran Capsules (Frequent) 1089
Zyban Sustained-Release Tablets (Frequent) 1620
▲ Zyprexa Tablets (5%) 1798
▲ Zyprexa ZYDIS Orally Disintegrating Tablets (5%) 1798

Ambylopia
▲ Symbyax Capsules (4% to 5%) 1788

Amelia
Thalomid Capsules 979

Amenorrhea
Abilify Tablets (Infrequent) 916
Abilify Tablets (Infrequent) 2472
Aldoclor Tablets 1881
Aldoril Tablets 1884
Alesse-28 Tablets 3392
Alinia for Oral Suspension (Less than 1%) 2840
Alinia Tablets (Less than 1%) 2840
Alkeran for Injection 976
Alkeran Tablets (A significant number of patients) 977
Astelin Nasal Spray (Infrequent) 1876
Aygestin Tablets 1062
▲ Buphenyl Powder (23%) 3327
▲ Buphenyl Tablets (23%) 3327
Celexa (Frequent) 1177
▲ Delatestryl Injection (Among most frequent) 2976
▲ Depacon Injection (1% to 5%) 412
▲ Depakene (1% to 5%) 417
▲ Depakote Sprinkle Capsules (1% to 5%) 422
▲ Depakote Tablets (1% to 5%) 427
▲ Depakote ER Tablets (1% to 5%) 433
▲ depo-subQ provera 104 Injectable Suspension (6%) 2622
Effexor Tablets (Infrequent) 3405
Effexor XR Capsules (Infrequent) 3411
▲ Ellence Injection (0% to 71.8%) 2632
▲ Estratest Tablets (Among most common) 3196
▲ Estratest H.S. Tablets (Among most common) 3196
Evoxac Capsules (Less than 1%) 1042
Gabitril Tablets (Infrequent) 998
Geodon Capsules (Infrequent) 2514
▲ Intron A for Injection (Less than 5%) 3038
I.V. Busulfex 1125
Kadian Capsules (Less than 3%) 572
Lamictal (1.9%) 1449
Leukeran Tablets 1472
Lo/Ovral-28 Tablets 3423
Lunesta Tablets (Infrequent) 3139
Lyrica Capsules (0.1% to 1%) 2524
▲ Mirena Intrauterine System (20%) 810
Moban Tablets (Infrequent) 1108
Mustargen for Injection 2007
Neurontin Capsules (Infrequent) 2498
Neurontin Oral Solution (Infrequent) 2498
Neurontin Tablets (Infrequent) 2498
Nipent for Injection (Less than 3%) 3216
▲ Novantrone for Injection Concentrate (28% to 43%) 3158
Ortho-Cept Tablets 2395
Ortho-Cyclen Tablets 2414
Ortho Evra Transdermal System 2402
Ortho Micronor Tablets 2411
Ortho Tri-Cyclen Tablets 2414
Ortho Tri-Cyclen Lo Tablets 2421
OxyContin Tablets 2699
Paxil CR Controlled-Release Tablets (Infrequent) 1509
Paxil (Infrequent) 1501
Pentasa Capsules (Less than 1%) 3182
Permax Tablets (Rare) 3357
Premarin Intravenous 3440
Premarin Vaginal Cream 3449
Premphase Tablets 3452
Prempro Tablets 3452
Prometrium Capsules (100 mg, 200 mg) 3205
Prozac Pulvules and Liquid (Infrequent) 1771
Requip Tablets (Infrequent) 1528
Rescriptor Tablets 2535
Reyataz Capsules (Less than 3%) 948
Rilutek Tablets (Rare) 2945
Risperdal Consta Long-Acting Injection (Frequent) 1664
Risperdal M-Tab Orally Disintegrating Tablets (Infrequent) 1658
Risperdal (Infrequent) 1658
Sandostatin Injection (Less than 1%) 2263
Seasonale Tablets 1073
Seroquel Tablets (Infrequent) 691
Symbyax Capsules (Infrequent) 1788
Thalomid Capsules 979
Thioridazine Hydrochloride Tablets 2122
Thiothixene Capsules 2124
Topamax Sprinkle Capsules (2%) 2438
Topamax Tablets (2%) 2438
Triphasil-28 Tablets 3483
Yasmin 28 Tablets 818
Zoladex (Rare) 709
Zoloft (Infrequent) 2581
Zonegran Capsules (Infrequent) 1089
Zyprexa Tablets (Infrequent) 1798
Zyprexa ZYDIS Orally Disintegrating Tablets (Infrequent) 1798

Amentia
Clozapine Tablets (Less than 1%) 2141
Clozaril Tablets (Less than 1%) 2174
FazaClo Orally Disintegrating Tablets (Less than 1%) 547

Amnesia

Abilify Tablets (Infrequent) 916
Abilify Tablets (Infrequent) 2472
Aceon Tablets (2 mg, 4 mg, 8 mg) (0.3% to 1%) 3191
Aciphex Tablets (Rare) 1081
Actiq (Less than 1%) 993
Aggrenox Capsules (2.4%) 855
Agrylin Capsules (1% to 5%) 3172
Altace Capsules (Less than 1%) 1673
Ambien Tablets (1%) 2867
AndroGel (Fewer than 1%) 3330
Avelox (Less than 0.1%) 2984
Avinza Capsules (Less than 5%) 1714
Caduet Tablets (Less than 2%) 2507
Campral Tablets (Frequent) 1175
Cardizem LA Extended Release Tablets (Less than 2%) 1699
Celexa (Frequent) 1177
Clozapine Tablets (Less than 1%) 2141
Clozaril Tablets (Less than 1%) 2174
Copaxone for Injection (At least 2%) 3292
Coreg Tablets (Less than or equal to 0.1%) 1376
▲ Depacon Injection (4% to 7%) 412
▲ Depakene (5% to 7%) 417
▲ Depakote Sprinkle Capsules (4% to 7%) 422
▲ Depakote Tablets (1% to 7%) 427
▲ Depakote ER Tablets (4% to 7%) 433
Didronel Tablets 2693
Duragesic Transdermal System (1% or greater) 2448
Effexor Tablets 3405
Effexor XR Capsules (Frequent) 3411
▲ Equetro Extended-Release Capsules (8%) 3178
Evoxac Capsules 1042
Exelon Capsules (Infrequent) 2204
FazaClo Orally Disintegrating Tablets (Less than 1%) 547
Frova Tablets (Infrequent) 1101
Geodon Capsules (Frequent) 2514
▲ Infergen (2% to 10%) 1647
▲ Intron A for Injection (Up to 14%) 3038
Invirase (Less than 2%) 2776
Kadian Capsules (Less than 3%) 572
Kaletra (Less than 2%) 474
Keppra Oral Solution (2%) 3307
Keppra Tablets (2%) 3307
Klonopin 2782
Lamictal (Frequent) 1449
Lexapro Oral Solution (Infrequent) 1193
Lexapro Tablets (Infrequent) 1193
Lipitor Tablets (Less than 2%) 2495
▲ Lyrica Capsules (1% to 6%) 2524
Marinol Capsules (Greater than 1%) 3334
Meridia Capsules 485
▲ Mirapex Tablets (4% to 6%) 889
Namenda (Infrequent) 1199
Naropin Injection (Less than 1%) 640
Neurontin Capsules (1.2% to 2.2%) 2498
Neurontin Oral Solution (1.2% to 2.2%) 2498
Neurontin Tablets (1.2% to 2.2%) 2498
Nicotrol NS (Less than 1%) 2596
Niravam Orally Disintegrating Tablets 3106
Norvasc Tablets (Less than or equal to 0.1%) 2529
Norvir (Less than 2%) 499
OxyContin Tablets (Less than 1%) 2699
Paxil CR Controlled-Release Tablets (2%) 1509
Paxil (2%) 1501
Permax Tablets (Frequent) 3357
Prevacid Delayed-Release Capsules (Less than 1%) 3268
Prevacid for Delayed-Release Oral Suspension (Less than 1%) 3268
Prevacid NapraPAC (Less than 1%) 3277
Prevacid SoluTab Delayed-Release Orally Disintegrating Tablets (Less than 1%) 3268
PREVPAC (Less than 1%) 3281
▲ Prograf Capsules and Injection (3% to 15%) 624
ProSom Tablets (Infrequent) 512
Provigil Tablets (1%) 1002
Prozac Pulvules and Liquid (Frequent) 1771
Relpax Tablets (Rare) 2531
▲ Requip Tablets (3%) 1528
Rescriptor Tablets 2535
Reyataz Capsules (Less than 3%) 948
Rilutek Tablets (Infrequent) 2945
Risperdal Consta Long-Acting Injection (Infrequent) 1664
Risperdal M-Tab Orally Disintegrating Tablets (Infrequent) 1658
Risperdal (Infrequent) 1658
Roferon-A Injection (Less than 3%) 2805
Sandostatin Injection (Less than 1%) 2263
Seroquel Tablets (Infrequent) 691
▲ Sonata Capsules (2% to 4%) 1686
Sular Tablets (Less than or equal to 1%) 1163
Sustiva Capsules (Less than 2%) 957
▲ Symbyax Capsules (1% to 3%) 1788
Symmetrel (0.1% to 1%) 1115
Tambocor Tablets (Less than 1%) 1824
Tasmar Tablets (Infrequent) 3360
▲ Temodar Capsules (10%) 3088
Thalomid Capsules 979
Tiazac Capsules (Less than 2%) 1204
▲ Trileptal Oral Suspension (1% to 5%) 2281
▲ Trileptal Tablets (1% to 5%) 2281
Ultracet Tablets (Less than 1%) 2462
Uniretic Tablets (Less than 1%) 3114
VFEND I.V. (Less than 2%) 2543
VFEND Oral Suspension (Less than 2%) 2543
VFEND Tablets (Less than 2%) 2543
Viadur Implant (Less than 2%) 782
Vytorin 10/10 Tablets 2084
Vytorin 10/10 Tablets 3092
Vytorin 10/20 Tablets 2084
Vytorin 10/20 Tablets 3092
Vytorin 10/40 Tablets 2084
Vytorin 10/40 Tablets 3092
Vytorin 10/80 Tablets 2084
Vytorin 10/80 Tablets 3092
Wellbutrin SR Sustained-Release Tablets (Rare) 1583
Wellbutrin XL Extended-Release Tablets (Rare) 1588
Xanax XR Tablets (Infrequent) 2655
Zoloft (Infrequent) 2581
Zomig Nasal Spray (Infrequent) 718
Zomig Tablets (Rare) 714
Zomig-ZMT Tablets (Rare) 714
Zyban Sustained-Release Tablets (Rare) 1620
Zyprexa Tablets (Frequent) 1798
Zyprexa ZYDIS Orally Disintegrating Tablets (2%) 1798
Zyrtec Chewable Tablets (Less than 2%) 2589
Zyrtec (Less than 2%) 2589
Zyrtec-D 12 Hour Extended Release Tablets (Less than 2%) 2591

Amyloidosis

Thalomid Capsules 979

ANA, positive

Aceon Tablets (2 mg, 4 mg, 8 mg) 3191
Adalat CC Tablets (Rare) 2978
Advicor Tablets 1694
Aldoclor Tablets 1881
Aldoril Tablets 1884
Altace Capsules (Less than 1%) 1673
Altoprev Extended-Release Tablets (Rare) 1151
Captopril Tablets 2114
▲ Enbrel for Injection (11%) 580
Lescol Capsules (Rare) 2227
Lescol Capsules (Rare) 2730
Lescol XL Tablets 2227
Lescol XL Tablets 2730
Mevacor Tablets (Rare) 1996
Pravachol Tablets (Rare) 943
Prinivil Tablets (0.3% to 1.0%) 2029
Prinzide Tablets 2033
Tenormin I.V. Injection 698
Tenormin Tablets 695
Ticlid Tablets (Rare) 2813
Vaseretic Tablets 2073
Vasotec I.V. Injection (0.5% to 1.0%) 2076
Vytorin 10/10 Tablets 2084
Vytorin 10/10 Tablets 3092
Vytorin 10/20 Tablets 2084
Vytorin 10/20 Tablets 3092
Vytorin 10/40 Tablets 2084
Vytorin 10/40 Tablets 3092
Vytorin 10/80 Tablets 2084
Vytorin 10/80 Tablets 3092
Zestoretic Tablets 701
Zestril Tablets (0.3% to 1.0%) 704
Zocor Tablets (Rare) 2078

Analgesia, reversal

Narcan Injection 1109

Anaphylactic reactions

Abilify Tablets (Rare) 916
Abilify Tablets (Rare) 2472
Aceon Tablets (2 mg, 4 mg, 8 mg) (0.3% to 1%) 3191
Adacel Vaccine 2959
Adalat CC Tablets (Rare) 2978
Advair Diskus 100/50 (Very rare) 1291
Advair Diskus 250/50 (Very rare) 1291
Advair Diskus 500/50 (Very rare) 1291
Aggrastat 1878
Aldoclor Tablets 1881
Aldoril Tablets 1884
Alesse-28 Tablets 3392
Amoxil Capsules 1315
Amoxil Chewable Tablets 1315
Amoxil Pediatric Drops for Oral Suspension 1315
Amoxil Powder for Oral Suspension 1315
Amoxil Tablets 1315
Ancef for Injection 1318
Antivenin (Black Widow Spider Antivenin) 1887
Anzemet Injection (Rare) 2871
Anzemet Tablets (Rare) 2874
Apokyn Injection 2132
AquaMEPHYTON Injection 1887
Arava Tablets (One case) 2881
Atacand HCT 637
Atrovent HFA Inhalation Aerosol 872
Atrovent Nasal Spray 0.06% 870
Augmentin 1331
Augmentin Tablets 1334
Augmentin ES-600 Powder for Oral Suspension 1337
Avalide Tablets 922
Avalide Tablets 2889
Avelox 2984
Aygestin Tablets 1062
Beconase AQ Nasal Spray 1359
Bexxar 1360
Boostrix (Rarely) 1366
Camptosar Injection 2602
Cataflam Tablets (Rarely) 2173
Celebrex Capsules (Less than 0.1%) 3130
Cipro I.V. (1% or less) 2998
Cipro I.V. Pharmacy Bulk Package (1% or less) 3509
Cipro 2991
Cipro XR Tablets (Rare) 3004
Climara Transdermal System 795
Climara Pro Transdermal System 800
Clindesse Vaginal Cream (Rare) 3296
Combivent Inhalation Aerosol (Less than 2%) 878
Cozaar Tablets 1913
Cytovene 2763
depo-subQ provera 104 Injectable Suspension (Infrequent) 2622
Desferal Vials 2190
Digibind for Injection 1388
Dilaudid Oral Liquid 443
Dilaudid Tablets - 8 mg 443
Diuril Oral 1936
Diuril Sodium Intravenous 1934
Dolobid Tablets (Less than 1 in 100) 1937
Eligard 22.5 mg 2899
Eligard 30 mg 2901
Elspar for Injection 1943
Estrogel 0.06% 3200
Flovent HFA (Very rare) 1418
Foradil Aerolizer (Rare) 3024
Fortaz 1422
GamaSTAN 3231
Gammagard Liquid 751
Gammagard S/D (A remote possibility) 754
Gamunex Immune Globulin I.V., 10% 3232
HalfLytely and Bisacodyl Tablets Bowel Prep Kit with Flavors Packs (Rare) 915
HibTITER 3419
Humalog-Pen (Less common) 1751
Humalog Mix 75/25-Pen 1754
HyperHep B S/D (Rare) 3237
Hyzaar 1964
Indapamide Tablets 2119
Inderal LA Long-Acting Capsules 3421
Infanrix Vaccine 1444
Infed Injection 3381
Kogenate FS 3517
Levitra Tablets (Less than 2%) 3048
Lo/Ovral-28 Tablets 3423
Lotensin HCT Tablets 2235
Lupron Depot 7.5 mg (One report) 3261
Lupron Injection Pediatric (Infrequent) 3256
Mefoxin Premixed Intravenous Solution 1990
Menostar Transdermal System 805
Meruvax II 1994
Micardis HCT Tablets 886
Mintezol 2002
Mivacron Injection 489
Moduretic Tablets 2003
Nabi-HB (Rare) 2159
Nexium Delayed-Release Capsules (Rare) 645
Nexium I.V. (Rare) 649
Nimbex Injection 494
Norflex Injection (Rare) 1824
Noroxin Tablets (Occasional) 2009
Nubain Injection (1% or less) 1111
▲ Oncaspar (Greater than 1% but less than 5%) 1123
Orthoclone OKT3 Sterile Solution 2370
OxyContin Tablets (Less than 1%) 2699
Pediarix Vaccine (Rare) 1518
Pegasys 2793
Pred Mild Sterile Ophthalmic Suspension ⊙236
Prefest Tablets 1069
Premarin Vaginal Cream 3449
Prevnar for Injection 3460
PREVPAC 3281
Primaxin I.M. 2022
Primaxin I.V. 2024
Prinzide Tablets 2033
Prograf Capsules and Injection (A few patients) 624
Rabies Vaccine RabAvert 1011
Rapamune Oral Solution and Tablets 3472
Refludan for Injection 815
Repronex for Intramuscular and Subcutaneous Injection (Some patients) 1148
Rhophylac (Rare) 3504
Risperdal M-Tab Orally Disintegrating Tablets 1658
Risperdal 1658
Roferon-A Injection (Rare) 2805
Sanctura Tablets 1133
Sandimmune I.V. Ampuls for Infusion (Rare) 2259
Sonata Capsules 1686
Symmetrel 1115
Tequin Injection 964
Tequin Tablets 964
Teveten HCT Tablets 1710
Timentin ADD-Vantage 1556
Timentin Injection Galaxy Container 1559
Timentin IV Infusion 1553
Timentin Pharmacy Bulk Package 1562
Timolide Tablets 2056
Trasylol Injection (Less than 0.5%) 779
Triphasil-28 Tablets 3483
Vaseretic Tablets 2073
Vivelle Transdermal System 2288
Vivelle-Dot Transdermal System 2293
Voltaren Tablets (Rarely) 2298
Voltaren-XR Tablets (Rarely) 2301
Zeel Solution 1639
Zemuron Injection (Rare) 2363
Zestoretic Tablets 701
Zoladex 3-month (One report) 712
Zosyn (Occasional) 3492

Anaphylactic shock

Ambien Tablets (Rare) 2867
Aredia for Injection (Very rare) 2168
Avelox 2984
CytoGam Intravenous (A possibility) 1866
Eloxatin for Injection 2908
Fortical Nasal Spray (1 patient) 3336
GlucaGen for Injection (Rare) 790
HyperRAB (Rare) 3239
HyperTET (Few isolated cases) 3245
Imodium Capsules (Extremely rare) 1834
Levaquin in 5% Dextrose Injection 2453
Levaquin 2453
Maxipime for Injection 1093
Meridia Capsules 485
Miacalcin Injection (A few cases) 2241
Orthoclone OKT3 Sterile Solution 2370
Protonix I.V. 3468
Protonix Tablets 3465
Rabies Vaccine RabAvert 1011
Sandostatin Injection 2263
Sandostatin LAR Depot (Rare) 2264
Trasylol Injection 779
Vantin Tablets and Oral Suspension (Less than 1%) 2650
Wellbutrin Tablets (Rare) 1579
Wellbutrin SR Sustained-Release Tablets (Rare) 1583
Wellbutrin XL Extended-Release Tablets (Rare) 1588
Zosyn (1% or less) 3492

Zyban Sustained-Release Tablets (Rare) ... 1620

Anaphylactoid reactions

Abelcet Injection ... 1119
Activase I.V. (Very rare) ... 1225
Alesse-28 Tablets ... 3392
Altace Capsules (Less than 1%) ... 1673
Amerge Tablets ... 1312
Amoxil Capsules (Occasional) ... 1315
Amoxil Chewable Tablets (Occasional) ... 1315
Amoxil Pediatric Drops for Oral Suspension (Occasional) ... 1315
Amoxil Powder for Oral Suspension (Occasional) ... 1315
Amoxil Tablets (Occasional) ... 1315
Anaprox Tablets (Less than 1%) ... 2769
Anaprox DS Tablets (Less than 1%) .. 2769
Arthrotec Tablets ... 3126
Astelin Nasal Spray ... 1876
Attenuvax ... 1889
Aygestin Tablets ... 1062
Beconase AQ Nasal Spray ... 1359
Campath Ampules ... 826
Camptosar Injection ... 2602
Captopril Tablets ... 2114
Carimune NF ... 3501
Cenestin Tablets, 0.45mg, 0.625mg, 0.9mg, 1.25mg ... 1063
Cenestin Tablets, 0.3mg ... 1063
Cerezyme for Injection ... 1263
Cerubidine for Injection (Rare) ... 788
Cleocin Vaginal Ovules (A few cases) ... 2613
Climara Transdermal System ... 795
Climara Pro Transdermal System ... 800
Copaxone for Injection (Rare) ... 3292
Crixivan Capsules ... 1918
Decadron Phosphate Injection ... 1931
Decadron Tablets ... 1929
Delatestryl Injection (Rare) ... 2976
Depo-Provera Contraceptive Injection ... 2619
Detrol Tablets ... 2626
Detrol LA Capsules ... 2629
Digibind for Injection ... 1388
Diprivan Injectable Emulsion (Less than 1%) ... 676
Dolobid Tablets ... 1937
Doxil Injection (Less than 1%) ... 3302
EC-Naprosyn Delayed-Release Tablets (Less than 1%) ... 2769
Engerix-B Vaccine ... 1391
Epogen for Injection ... 586
Estratest Tablets (Rare) ... 3196
Estratest H.S. Tablets (Rare) ... 3196
Estrogel 0.06% ... 3200
Ethyol for Injection (Rare) ... 1869
Feiba VH ... 749
Flonase Nasal Spray ... 1412
Fortaz ... 1422
Fragmin Injection (A few cases) ... 2638
Garamycin Injectable ... 3028
Gemzar for Injection (Rare) ... 1743
Gonal-f RFF Pen for Injection ... 3155
Havrix Vaccine (Rare) ... 1425
Herceptin I.V. (At least one of the 958 patients) ... 1234
HibTITER ... 3419
Hyalgan Solution ... 2917
Hycamtin for Injection (Rare) ... 1427
Imitrex Injection (Rare) ... 1431
Imitrex Nasal Spray ... 1435
Imitrex Tablets (Rare) ... 1440
Inderal LA Long-Acting Capsules ... 3421
Invanz for Injection (Very rare) ... 1974
Kytril Injection (Rare) ... 2785
Levaquin in 5% Dextrose Injection ... 2453
Levaquin ... 2453
Lidoderm Patch (Rare) ... 1107
Lo/Ovral-28 Tablets ... 3423
Lotrel Capsules ... 2238
Lovenox Injection ... 2931
Lupron Depot 3.75 mg (Rare) ... 3257
Lupron Depot 7.5 mg (Rare) ... 3261
Lupron Depot–3 Month 11.25 mg ... 3262
Lupron Depot-PED 7.5 mg, 11.25 mg and 15 mg ... 3266
Lyrica Capsules (Rare) ... 2524
Mavik Tablets ... 482
Menostar Transdermal System ... 805
Mephyton Tablets ... 1993
Meridia Capsules ... 485
Meruvax II ... 1994
Mivacron Injection ... 489
M-M-R II ... 1980
Mobic Oral Suspension (Less than 0.1%) ... 893
Mobic Tablets (Less than 0.1%) ... 893
Mumpsvax ... 2005
Naprosyn Suspension (Less than 1%) ... 2769
Naprosyn Tablets (Less than 1%) ... 2769
Naropin Injection ... 640
Nimbex Injection ... 494
Nitro-Dur Transdermal Infusion System (A few reports) ... 3060
Noroxin Tablets (Occasional) ... 2009
Nubain Injection (1% or less) ... 1111
Orthoclone OKT3 Sterile Solution ... 2370
OxyContin Tablets (Less than 1%) ... 2699
Plavix Tablets (Very rare) ... 940
Plavix Tablets (Very rare) ... 2942
Pneumovax 23 (Rare) ... 2020
Prandin Tablets (0.5, 1, and 2 mg) (One patient) ... 2337
Prefest Tablets ... 1069
Premarin Vaginal Cream ... 3449
Premphase Tablets ... 3452
Prempro Tablets ... 3452
Prevacid Delayed-Release Capsules ... 3268
Prevacid for Delayed-Release Oral Suspension ... 3268
Prevacid NapraPAC (Less than 1%) .. 3277
Prevacid SoluTab Delayed-Release Orally Disintegrating Tablets ... 3268
Prevnar for Injection ... 3460
PREVPAC ... 3281
Prinivil Tablets (0.3% to 1.0%) ... 2029
Prinzide Tablets ... 2033
Procrit for Injection ... 2374
Prometrium Capsules (100 mg, 200 mg) ... 3205
Protopic Ointment (Greater than or equal to 1%) ... 629
Rapamune Oral Solution and Tablets ... 3472
Relafen Tablets (Less than 1%) ... 1523
Retavase (2 patients) ... 1131
Sandostatin Injection ... 2263
Sandostatin LAR Depot (Rare) ... 2264
Seasonale Tablets ... 1073
Skelaxin Tablets (Rare) ... 1685
Suprax ... 1811
Trasylol Injection ... 779
TriLyte with Flavor Packs for Oral Solution (Rare) ... 3114
Triphasil-28 Tablets ... 3483
Twinrix Vaccine ... 1571
Ultane Liquid for Inhalation (Less than 1%) ... 526
Uniretic Tablets (More than 1%) ... 3114
Vaseretic Tablets ... 2073
Vasotec I.V. Injection (0.5% to 1.0%) ... 2076
VFEND I.V. (Less than 2%) ... 2543
VFEND Oral Suspension (Less than 2%) ... 2543
VFEND Tablets (Less than 2%) ... 2543
Vivelle Transdermal System ... 2288
Vivelle-Dot Transdermal System ... 2293
Wellbutrin Tablets ... 1579
Wellbutrin SR Sustained-Release Tablets ... 1583
Wellbutrin XL Extended-Release Tablets ... 1588
Zemuron Injection (Rare) ... 2363
Zestoretic Tablets ... 701
Zestril Tablets (0.3% to 1.0%) ... 704
Zofran Injection ... 1607
Zofran ... 1613
Zofran ODT Orally Disintegrating Tablets ... 1613
Zoloft ... 2581
Zomig Nasal Spray (Very rare) ... 718
Zomig Tablets (Very rare) ... 714
Zosyn ... 3492
Zyban Sustained-Release Tablets ... 1620
Zyprexa Tablets ... 1798
Zyprexa ZYDIS Orally Disintegrating Tablets ... 1798

Anaphylaxis

Abelcet Injection (Less than 0.1%) ... 1119
Aciphex Tablets ... 1081
Adriamycin for Injection, USP ... 786
Adriamycin Injection, USP ... 786
Advicor Tablets (Rare) ... 1694
Aggrastat ... 1878
Aldurazyme for Intravenous Infusion ... 1261
Alferon N Injection ... 1640
Alkeran for Injection (2.4%) ... 976
Alkeran Tablets (Rare) ... 977
Allegra (Rare) ... 2857
Allegra-D 12 Hour Extended-Release Tablets (Rare) ... 2860
Allegra-D 24 Hour Extended-Release Tablets (Rare) ... 2862
Altoprev Extended-Release Tablets (Rare) ... 1151
Amerge Tablets ... 1312
Aminohippurate Sodium "PAH" Injection ... 1886
Amoxil Capsules ... 1315
Amoxil Chewable Tablets ... 1315
Amoxil Pediatric Drops for Oral Suspension ... 1315
Amoxil Powder for Oral Suspension ... 1315
Amoxil Tablets ... 1315
Ancef for Injection ... 1318
Antivenin (Black Widow Spider Antivenin) ... 1887
Antivenin (Micrurus fulvius) ... 3401
Antivenin Polyvalent ... 3399
AquaMEPHYTON Injection ... 1887
Arimidex Tablets (Very rare) ... 665
Atrovent HFA Inhalation Aerosol ... 872
Atrovent Inhalation Solution (A single case) ... 868
Attenuvax ... 1889
Avonex (Rare) ... 839
Axid Oral Solution (Rare) ... 913
Azmacort Inhalation Aerosol ... 1701
Bayer Aspirin Tablets ... 3515
BeneFix for Injection ... 3402
Bentyl Capsules ... 724
Bentyl Injection ... 724
Bentyl Syrup ... 724
Bentyl Tablets ... 724
Betaseron for SC Injection ... 791
Bexxar ... 1360
Biaxin/Biaxin XL (Rare) ... 402
Blocadren Tablets ... 1891
Caduet Tablets ... 2507
Cancidas for Injection (0%) ... 1894
Ceftin ... 1369
Celexa ... 1177
Clarinex Syrup (Rare) ... 3009
Clarinex Tablets (Rare) ... 3009
Clarinex Reditabs Tablets (Rare) ... 3009
Clarinex-D 24-Hour Extended-Release Tablets ... 3012
Clinoril Tablets ... 1899
Colyte with Flavor Packs for Oral Solution (Rare) ... 3102
Combivent Inhalation Aerosol (Rare) ... 878
Combivir Tablets ... 1373
Comvax ... 1904
Coreg Tablets (Less than or equal to 0.1%) ... 1376
Cosopt Sterile Ophthalmic Solution ... 1910
CytoGam Intravenous ... 1866
Dantrium Capsules (Less frequent) .. 2690
Dantrium Intravenous (One case) ... 2691
Daraprim Tablets ... 1385
DDAVP Injection 4 mcg/mL (Rare) ... 2893
DDAVP Nasal Spray (Rare) ... 2894
Decadron Tablets ... 1929
Depakene ... 417
Depakote Sprinkle Capsules ... 422
Depakote Tablets ... 427
Depakote ER Tablets ... 433
Depo-Medrol Single-Dose Vial ... 2617
Depo-Provera Contraceptive Injection ... 2619
depo-subQ provera 104 Injectable Suspension (Infrequent) ... 2622
Desmopressin Acetate Injection (Rare) ... 1143
Digibind for Injection ... 1388
Diovan HCT Tablets (Greater than 0.2%) ... 2195
Diprivan Injectable Emulsion (Rare) .. 676
Dyazide Capsules ... 1389
Dynacin Tablets ... 1859
Dyrenium Capsules ... 3390
Ecotrin Enteric Coated Aspirin Low, Regular and Maximum Strength Tablets ... 1627
E.E.S. ... 449
Effexor Tablets ... 3405
Effexor XR Capsules ... 3411
Elitek (Less than 1%) ... 2906
Ellence Injection ... 2632
Elspar for Injection ... 1943
Engerix-B Vaccine ... 1391
Epivir ... 1394
Epivir-HBV ... 1398
Epzicom Tablets ... 1402
EryPed ... 445
Ery-Tab Tablets ... 447
Erythrocin Stearate Filmtab Tablets ... 452
Erythromycin Base Filmtab Tablets .. 454
Erythromycin Delayed-Release Capsules, USP ... 456
Flexeril Tablets ... 1832
Flonase Nasal Spray ... 1412
Flumist Vaccine ... 1872
Fluorescite Injection ... ⊙207
Fortaz (Very rare) ... 1422
GamaSTAN (Rare) ... 3231
Gammagard S/D ... 754
Havrix Vaccine (Rare) ... 1425
Herceptin I.V. ... 1234
Humira Injection ... 464
Hytrin Capsules (Rare) ... 469
Imitrex Injection (Rare) ... 1431
Imitrex Nasal Spray ... 1435
Imitrex Tablets (Rare) ... 1440
Imodium Capsules (Extremely rare) ... 1834
Indocin Capsules (Less than 1%) ... 1968
Indocin I.V. (Less than 1%) ... 1973
Indocin (Less than 1%) ... 1968
Infed Injection ... 3381
Integrilin Injection (One patient) ... 3034
Intron A for Injection (Rare) ... 3038
Invanz for Injection (Very rare) ... 1974
Ketek Tablets (Rare) ... 2920
Kytril Injection (Rare) ... 2785
Kytril Tablets (Rare) ... 2788
Lamisil Tablets (Rare) ... 2226
Lescol Capsules (Rare) ... 2227
Lescol Capsules (Rare) ... 2730
Lescol XL Tablets ... 2227
Lescol XL Tablets ... 2730
Lexapro Oral Solution (Infrequent) ... 1193
Lexapro Tablets (Infrequent) ... 1193
Lipitor Tablets ... 2495
Malarone Tablets (One case) ... 1484
Malarone Pediatric Tablets (One case) ... 1484
Maxipime for Injection ... 1093
Maxzide ... 2150
Mefoxin for Injection ... 1987
Mefoxin Premixed Intravenous Solution ... 1990
Meruvax II ... 1994
Mevacor Tablets (Rare) ... 1996
Miacalcin Injection (One case) ... 2241
Miacalcin Nasal Spray (One case) ... 2242
Mintezol ... 2002
M-M-R II ... 1980
MS Contin Tablets (Extremely rare) .. 2703
Mumpsvax ... 2005
Mustargen for Injection ... 2007
Mylotarg for Injection ... 3429
Nalfon Capsules (Less than 1%) ... 2504
Nasonex Nasal Spray ... 3058
Navelbine Injection ... 1494
Neulasta Injection ... 596
Neumega for Injection ... 3433
Norvir (Rare) ... 499
Novantrone for Injection Concentrate (Rare) ... 3158
Omnicef Capsules ... 506
Omnicef for Oral Suspension ... 506
Oncaspar ... 1123
Orthoclone OKT3 Sterile Solution ... 2370
Paxil CR Controlled-Release Tablets ... 1509
Paxil ... 1501
PCE Dispertab Tablets ... 510
Pepcid Injection (Infrequent) ... 2017
Pepcid (Infrequent) ... 2014
Poly-Pred Liquifilm Ophthalmic Suspension ... ⊙231
Pravachol Tablets (Rare) ... 943
Premarin Tablets ... 3443
Premphase Tablets ... 3452
Prempro Tablets ... 3452
PREVPAC (Rare) ... 3281
Prilosec OTC Tablets (Rare) ... 2674
Prograf Capsules and Injection (A small percentage of patients) ... 624
Proleukin for Injection ... 1007
Prometrium Capsules (100 mg, 200 mg) ... 3205
Protonix I.V. ... 3468
Protonix Tablets ... 3465
Rebetron Combination Therapy ... 3078
Recombivax HB (Less than 1%) ... 2045
ReFacto Vials ... 3479
Relafen Tablets (Less than 1%) ... 1523
Remicade for IV Injection (Less than 1%) ... 987
ReoPro Vials ... 1779
Retrovir Capsules (One patient) ... 1533
Retrovir IV Infusion (One patient) ... 1537
Retrovir (One patient) ... 1533
Rocephin Injectable Vials, ADD-Vantage, Galaxy, Bulk (Rare) ... 2801
Serevent Diskus ... 1540
Seroquel Tablets ... 691
Simulect for Injection ... 2268
Singulair ... 2047

St. Joseph 81 mg Aspirin Chewable and Enteric Coated Tablets 1841
Suprax 1811
Synagis (Less than 1 case per 100,000 patients) 1868
Tagamet Tablets (Rare) 1547
Temodar Capsules (Rare) 3088
Thiothixene Capsules (Rare) 2124
Ticlid Tablets 2813
Timoptic in Ocudose 2061
Timoptic Sterile Ophthalmic Solution 2058
Timoptic-XE Sterile Ophthalmic Gel Forming Solution 2062
TNKase I.V. (Rare) 1256
Trasylol Injection 779
Trizivir Tablets 1565
Twinrix Vaccine 1571
Ultracet Tablets 2462
Valtrex Caplets 1573
Vancocin HCl Capsules, USP 3370
Varivax 2070
Viramune Oral Suspension 903
Viramune Tablets 903
Vivelle Transdermal System (Isolated reports) 2288
Vytorin 10/10 Tablets 2084
Vytorin 10/10 Tablets 3092
Vytorin 10/20 Tablets 2084
Vytorin 10/20 Tablets 3092
Vytorin 10/40 Tablets 2084
Vytorin 10/40 Tablets 3092
Vytorin 10/80 Tablets 2084
Vytorin 10/80 Tablets 3092
Xenical Capsules 2834
Xolair 1259
Xopenex HFA Inhalation Aerosol 3151
Xopenex Inhalation Solution 3143
Xopenex Inhalation Solution Concentrate 3147
Zantac (Rare) 1597
Zantac Injection (Rare) 1593
Zantac Injection Pharmacy Bulk Package (Rare) 1595
Zantac Syrup (Rare) 1597
Zegerid Powder for Oral Solution (Rare) 2972
Zenapax for Injection 2838
Ziagen 1600
Zinacef Injection (Rare) 1604
Zinacef for Injection (Rare) 1604
Zithromax Capsules, 250 mg (Rare) 2568
Zithromax for IV Infusion (Rare) 2573
Zithromax for Oral Suspension, 1 g (Rare) 2568
Zithromax for Oral Suspension, 300 mg, 600 mg, 900 mg, 1200 mg (Rare) 2561
Zithromax Tablets, 250 mg, 500 mg (Rare) 2561
Zithromax Tablets, 600 mg (Rare) 2568
Zithromax Tri-Pak (Rare) 2561
Zithromax Z-Pak (Rare) 2568
Zmax for Oral Suspension 2577
Zocor Tablets (Rare) 2078
Zofran Injection (Rare) 1607
Zofran (Rare) 1613
Zofran ODT Orally Disintegrating Tablets (Rare) 1613
Zoladex (Rare) 709
Zoladex 3-month (Rare) 712
Zomig Nasal Spray (Very rare) 718
Zomig Tablets (Very rare) 714
Zosyn (1.0% or less) 3492
Zovirax Capsules (Rare) 1616
Zovirax Cream 853
Zovirax for Injection (Rare) 1618
Zovirax (Rare) 1616
Zyrtec Chewable Tablets (Rare) 2589
Zyrtec (Rare) 2589
Zyrtec-D 12 Hour Extended Release Tablets (Rare) 2591

Anasarca

▲ Gleevec Tablets (2% to 16%) 2221

Anastomotic disruption

Avastin IV (Rare) 1229
Rapamune Oral Solution and Tablets 3472

Androgen excess, signs or symptoms of

Lupron Depot 3.75 mg (Less than 5%) 3257
Lupron Depot–3 Month 11.25 mg (Less than 5%) 3262

Anemia

▲ Abelcet Injection (4%) 1119
Abilify Tablets (Frequent) 916
Abilify Tablets (Frequent) 2472
Accutane Capsules 2740
Aceon Tablets (2 mg, 4 mg, 8 mg) 3191
Aciphex Tablets 1081
Actiq (Less than 1%) 993
Actonel Tablets (2.4%) 2679
Actonel with Calcium Tablets (2.4%) 2684
Actos Tablets (Less than or equal to 2%) 3224
Adalat CC Tablets (Rare) 2978
Aggrenox Capsules (1.6%) 855
Agrylin Capsules (1% to 5%) 3172
▲ Alimta for Injection (1% to 33%) 1722
Alinia for Oral Suspension (Less than 1%) 2840
Alinia Tablets (Less than 1%) 2840
Alkeran for Injection 976
Alkeran Tablets 977
Aloprim for Injection (Less than 1%) 2156
Ambien Tablets (Rare) 2867
AmBisome for Injection (Less common) 615
Amerge Tablets (Rare) 1312
▲ Ammonul Injection (4%) 3323
Amnesteem Capsules 2126
Amoxil Capsules 1315
Amoxil Chewable Tablets 1315
Amoxil Pediatric Drops for Oral Suspension 1315
Amoxil Powder for Oral Suspension 1315
Amoxil Tablets 1315
Anaprox Tablets (Less than 1%) 2769
Anaprox DS Tablets (Less than 1%) 2769
Antara Capsules 2723
Anzemet Injection (Infrequently) 2871
Anzemet Tablets (Infrequently) 2874
Aptivus Capsules (Less than 2%) 859
▲ Arava Tablets (1% to 3%) 2881
▲ Aredia for Injection (42.5%) 2168
Aricept Tablets (Infrequent) 1086
Aricept ODT Tablets (Infrequent) 1086
▲ Arimidex Tablets (2% to 5%) 665
▲ Arixtra Injection (1.5% to 19.6%) 1325
Arthrotec Tablets (Rare) 3126
Asacol Delayed-Release Tablets 2688
Atacand Tablets 634
Augmentin 1331
Augmentin Tablets 1334
Augmentin XR Extended-Release Tablets 1340
Augmentin ES-600 Powder for Oral Suspension 1337
▲ Avandamet Tablets (7.1%) 1343
Avandia Tablets (1.9%) 1348
Avelox (0.1% to less than 2%) 2984
Avinza Capsules (Less than 5%) 1714
▲ Avonex (4%) 839
Axid Oral Solution (More frequent) 913
Betaseron for SC Injection 791
Bexxar 1360
▲ Buphenyl Powder (9%) 3327
▲ Buphenyl Tablets (9%) 3327
Caduet Tablets (Less than 2%) 2507
Calcium Disodium Versenate Injection 1819
▲ Campath Ampules (38% to 80%) 826
Campral Tablets (Infrequent) 1175
▲ Camptosar Injection (4.5% to 96.9%) 2602
▲ Cancidas for Injection (0% to 3.8%) 1894
Captopril Tablets 2114
▲ Carnitor Injection (3% to 12%) 3185
▲ Casodex Tablets (7%) 670
▲ Cataflam Tablets (1% to 10%) 2173
Celebrex Capsules (0.1% to 1.9%) 3130
▲ Celexa (Infrequent) 1177
▲ CellCept Capsules (25.6% to 43%) 2751
▲ CellCept Intravenous (25.6% to 43%) 2751
▲ CellCept Oral Suspension (25.6% to 43%) 2751
▲ CellCept Tablets (25.6% to 43%) 2751
Cipro (Less than 0.1%) 2991
Cipro XR Tablets 3004
Clinoril Tablets (Less than 1%) 1899
Clolar for Intravenous Infusion 1264
Clozapine Tablets (Less than 1%) 2141
Clozaril Tablets (Less than 1%) 2174
Colazal Capsules 2845
Combivir Tablets (2.9%) 1373
Combunox Tablets (Less than 1%) 1183
Concerta Extended-Release Tablets 1828
▲ Copegus Tablets (11% to 22%) 2759
▲ Coreg Tablets (Greater than 0.1% to greater than 3%) 1376
Cosmegen for Injection 1907
▲ Cozaar Tablets (Less than 1% to 14%) 1913
Crestor Tablets (Greater than or equal to 1%) 672
Crixivan Capsules (0.6%) 1918
Cubicin for Injection (2.1%) 1038
▲ Cytovene (1% to 19%) 2763
Demser Capsules (Rare) 1933
Depacon Injection 412
Depakene 417
Depakote Sprinkle Capsules 422
Depakote Tablets 427
Depakote ER Tablets (Greater than 1%) 433
DepoCyt Injection (1%) 1121
▲ DepoDur Extended-Release Injection (Greater than 10%) 1098
Depo-Provera Contraceptive Injection (Less than 1%) 2619
depo-subQ provera 104 Injectable Suspension 2622
Diastat Rectal Delivery System (Less than 1%) 3344
Dolobid Tablets 1937
▲ Doxil Injection (5.8% to 52.6%) 3302
EC-Naprosyn Delayed-Release Tablets (Less than 1%) 2769
Effexor Tablets (Infrequent) 3405
Effexor XR Capsules (Infrequent) 3411
Eldepryl Capsules 3209
▲ Ellence Injection (0% to 72.2%) 2632
Elmiron Capsules (Less than or equal to 1%) 2393
▲ Eloxatin for Injection (1% to 81%) 2908
Emend Capsules (Greater than 0.5%) 1944
Enbrel for Injection 580
Epivir 1394
Epivir-HBV 1398
Epzicom Tablets 1402
▲ Erbitux (10%) 937
▲ Eulexin Capsules (6%) 3023
▲ Evoxac Capsules (1% to 3%) 1042
Exelon Capsules (Frequent) 2204
Factive Tablets (Less than or equal to 0.1%) 2464
Famvir Tablets (0.1%) 2207
▲ Faslodex Injection (4.5%) 682
FazaClo Orally Disintegrating Tablets (Less than 1%) 547
Ferrlecit Injection 3379
Flolan for Injection 1408
Focalin Tablets 2214
Focalin XR Capsules 2217
Fortical Nasal Spray (Less than 1%) 3336
Furosemide Tablets 2117
Gabitril Tablets (Infrequent) 998
Garamycin Injectable 3028
▲ Gemzar for Injection (45% to 73%) 1743
Gengraf Capsules (1% to less than 3%) 458
Geodon Capsules (Infrequent) 2514
▲ Gleevec Tablets (Up to 41%) 2221
Guanidine Hydrochloride Tablets 3030
▲ Hectorol Capsules (Greater than or equal to 5%) 909
▲ Herceptin I.V. (4%) 1234
▲ Hycamtin for Injection (40% to 95%) 1427
Hyzaar 1964
Imitrex Injection 1431
Imitrex Nasal Spray 1435
Imitrex Tablets (Rare) 1440
Indocin Capsules (Less than 1%) 1968
Indocin I.V. (Less than 1%) 1973
Indocin (Less than 1%) 1968
▲ Intron A for Injection (Less than 5% to 22%) 3038
Invirase (Less than or equal to 2%) 2776
I.V. Busulfex (100%) 1125
Kadian Capsules (Less than 3%) 572
Kaletra (Less than 2%) 474
Klonopin 2782
Kogenate FS 3517
▲ Kytril Tablets (4%) 2788
Lamictal (Infrequent) 1449
▲ Leustatin Injection (37%) 2368
Levaquin in 5% Dextrose Injection (0.1% to 0.9%) 2453
Levaquin (0.1% to 0.9%) 2453
Lexapro Oral Solution (Infrequent) 1193
Lexapro Tablets (Infrequent) 1193
Lipitor Tablets (Less than 2%) 2495
Lofibra Capsules 1217
▲ Lovenox Injection (2% to 16%) 2931
Lunesta Tablets (Infrequent) 3139
Lyrica Capsules (0.1% to 1%) 2524
Matulane Capsules (Frequent) 3188
Mefoxin for Injection 1987
Mefoxin Premixed Intravenous Solution 1990
▲ Megace ES Oral Suspension (0% to 5%) 2492
▲ Mepron Suspension (4% to 6%) 1487
Meridia Capsules 485
▲ Merrem I.V. (Greater than 1% to 5.5%) 687
Metadate CD Capsules 3316
Miacalcin Nasal Spray (Less than 1%) 2242
Miradon Tablets 3056
▲ Mobic Oral Suspension (0% to 4.1%) 893
▲ Mobic Tablets (0% to 4.1%) 893
Mycamine for Injection (0.8% to 1.2%) 620
▲ Myfortic Tablets (3% to 21.6%) 2244
Myleran Tablets 1492
▲ Mylotarg for Injection (22%) 3429
Namenda (Frequent) 1199
Naprosyn Suspension (Less than 1%) 2769
Naprosyn Tablets (Less than 1%) 2769
▲ Naropin Injection (1% to 5%) 640
Natrecor for Injection (Greater than or equal to 1%) 3123
▲ Navelbine Injection (3% to 88%) 1494
Neoral Soft Gelatin Capsules (1% to less than 3%) 2247
Neoral Oral Solution (1% to less than 3%) 2247
▲ Neupogen for Injection (Approximately 10%) 598
Neurontin Capsules (Infrequent) 2498
Neurontin Oral Solution (Infrequent) 2498
Neurontin Tablets (Infrequent) 2498
Nexium Delayed-Release Capsules (Less than 1%) 645
Nexium I.V. (Less than 1%) 649
Nimotop Capsules (Less than 1%) 774
▲ Nipent for Injection (8% to 35%) 3216
Norvir (Less than 2%) 499
▲ Novantrone for Injection Concentrate (6% to 9%) 3158
Oncaspar 1123
▲ Ontak Vials (18%) 1717
Parnate Tablets 1499
Paxil CR Controlled-Release Tablets (Infrequent) 1509
Paxil (Infrequent) 1501
Pegasys (2%) 2793
PEG-Intron Powder for Injection 3062
Pentasa Capsules 3182
Permax Tablets (1.1%) 3357
▲ Photofrin for Injection (32%) 729
Plavix Tablets (1% to 2.5%) 940
Plavix Tablets (1% to 2.5%) 2942
Plendil Extended-Release Tablets (0.5% to 1.5%) 651
Pletal Tablets (Less than 2%) 2478
Pravachol Tablets 943
Prefest Tablets 1069
Prevacid Delayed-Release Capsules (Less than 1%) 3268
Prevacid for Delayed-Release Oral Suspension (Less than 1%) 3268
Prevacid NapraPAC (Less than 1%) 3277
Prevacid SoluTab Delayed-Release Orally Disintegrating Tablets (Less than 1%) 3268
PREVPAC (Less than 1%) 3281
Prilosec OTC Tablets (Rare) 2674
Prinivil Tablets 2029
Prochieve 4% Gel 1018
Prochieve 8% Gel 1018
▲ Prograf Capsules and Injection (5% to 47%) 624
▲ Proleukin for Injection (29%) 1007
Protonix I.V. (Less than 1%) 3468
Protonix Tablets (Less than 1%) 3465
Provigil Tablets (At least 1%) 1002
Prozac Pulvules and Liquid (Infrequent) 1771
Purinethol Tablets (Frequent) 1222
▲ Rapamune Oral Solution and Tablets (23% to 37%) 3472
Raptiva for Injection 1247
▲ Razadyne ER Extended-Release Capsules (3%) 2434
▲ Razadyne (3%) 2434
▲ Rebetol (12% to 17%) 3073
▲ Rebetron Combination Therapy (10%) 3078
▲ Rebif Prefilled Syringe for Injection (3% to 5%) 3163
▲ Refludan for Injection (12.4%) 815
Relafen Tablets (Less than 1%) 1523
Relpax Tablets (Rare) 2531
Remicade for IV Injection (Greater than or equal to 0.2%) 987
ReoPro Vials (1.2%) 1779
Requip Tablets (1% or more) 1528
Rescriptor Tablets (0.7% to 1.0%) 2535
Retavase (0.9% to 2.6%) 1131

▲ Retrovir Capsules (1.1% to 29%) 1533
▲ Retrovir IV Infusion (1.1% to 29%) ... 1537
▲ Retrovir (1.1% to 29%) 1533
▲ Ribavirin, USP Capsules (12% to 17%) 3083
Rilutek Tablets (Infrequent) 2945
Risperdal Consta Long-Acting Injection (Frequent) 1664
Risperdal M-Tab Orally Disintegrating Tablets (Infrequent) 1658
Risperdal (Infrequent) 1658
Ritalin Hydrochloride Tablets 2254
Ritalin LA Capsules 2255
Ritalin-SR Tablets 2254
Rituxan for Infusion (1%) 845
▲ Rituxan I.V. (8%) 1251
Rocephin Injectable Vials, ADD-Vantage, Galaxy, Bulk (Less than 1%) 2801
▲ Roferon-A Injection (4% to 31%) 2805
Rythmol SR Capsules 2736
Sandimmune (2% or less) 2259
Sandostatin Injection (Less than 1%) 2263
▲ Sandostatin LAR Depot (5% to 15%) 2264
Seroquel Tablets (Infrequent) 691
▲ Simulect for Injection (Greater than or equal to 10%) 2268
Sonata Capsules (Infrequent) 1686
Stromectol Tablets (One patient) 2053
Sular Tablets (Less than or equal to 1%) 1163
Symbyax Capsules (Infrequent) 1788
Synagis (More than 1%) 1868
Tabloid Tablets 1545
Tamiflu Capsules (Less than 1%) 2810
Tamiflu Oral Suspension (Less than 1%) 2810
▲ Targretin Capsules (6% to 24.5%) ... 1719
Tasmar Tablets (Infrequent) 3360
▲ Taxotere Injection Concentrate (7.7% to 93.6%) 2947
Temodar Capsules 3088
Teveten Tablets (Less than 1%) 1707
Teveten HCT Tablets (Less than 1%) 1710
▲ Thalomid Capsules (5.6% to 12.5%) 979
Thioridazine Hydrochloride Tablets .. 2122
Ticlid Tablets 2813
Topamax Sprinkle Capsules (1% to 2%) 2438
Topamax Tablets (1% to 2%) 2438
▲ Tracleer Tablets (3%) 539
Trasylol Injection (2%) 779
Trelstar Depot (1.4%) 3385
Tricor Tablets 523
Triglide Tablets 1165
▲ Trisenox Injection (20%) 983
Trizivir Tablets (2.9%) 1565
▲ Tygacil for Injection (4.2%) 3489
Ultracet Tablets (Less than 1%) 2462
Uniretic Tablets (Less than 1%) 3114
▲ Valcyte Tablets (8% to 26%) 2816
Valtrex Caplets (Up to 0.8%) 1573
Vantas (Less than 2%) 3367
Vantin Tablets and Oral Suspension (Less than 1%) 2650
Vaseretic Tablets 2073
Vasotec I.V. Injection 2076
▲ Velcade for Injection (26%) 2102
VFEND I.V. (0.1%) 2543
VFEND Oral Suspension (0.1%) 2543
VFEND Tablets (0.1%) 2543
Viadur Implant (2.3%) 782
Viagra Tablets (Less than 2%) 2552
Viracept (Less than 2%) 2556
Viramune Oral Suspension 903
Viramune Tablets 903
Virazole for Inhalation Solution 3365
▲ Visudyne for Injection (1% to 10%) .. 2286
▲ Voltaren Tablets (1% to 10%) 2298
▲ Voltaren-XR Tablets (1% to 10%) 2301
Wellbutrin Tablets (Rare) 1579
Wellbutrin SR Sustained-Release Tablets 1583
Wellbutrin XL Extended-Release Tablets 1588
▲ Xeloda Tablets (1% to 80%) 2825
▲ Zegerid Powder for Oral Solution (7.9%) 2972
Zerit (Fewer than 1%) 971
Zestoretic Tablets 701
▲ Zevalin Injection (61%) 848
Ziagen (<1%) 1600
Zoladex (1% to 5%) 709
Zoladex 3-month (1% to 5%) 712
Zoloft (Rare) 2581
▲ Zometa for Intravenous Infusion (22.1% to 33%) 2306
Zonegran Capsules (Infrequent) 1089
Zosyn (1% or less) 3492
Zovirax Capsules 1616
Zovirax for Injection (Less than 1%) 1618
Zovirax 1616
Zyban Sustained-Release Tablets 1620
Zyprexa Tablets (Infrequent) 1798
Zyprexa IntraMuscular (Infrequent) ... 1798
Zyprexa ZYDIS Orally Disintegrating Tablets (Infrequent) 1798
▲ Zyvox (0% to 5.6%) 2661

Anemia, aplastic

Aceon Tablets (2 mg, 4 mg, 8 mg) ... 3191
Aggrenox Capsules 855
Aldoclor Tablets 1881
Aldoril Tablets 1884
Amaryl Tablets 2864
Anaprox Tablets (Less than 1%) 2769
Anaprox DS Tablets (Less than 1%) .. 2769
Arthrotec Tablets (Rare) 3126
Asacol Delayed-Release Tablets (Rare) 2688
Atacand HCT 637
Avalide Tablets 922
Avalide Tablets 2889
▲ Blephamide Ophthalmic Ointment (Among most often) 563
Blephamide Ophthalmic Suspension 564
Buphenyl Powder (One patient) 3327
Buphenyl Tablets (One patient) 3327
Carbatrol Capsules 3174
Cataflam Tablets (Rarely) 2173
Ceftin 1369
Clinoril Tablets (Less than 1 in 100) 1899
Clorpres Tablets 2139
Copegus Tablets (Less than 1%) 2759
Coreg Tablets (Rare) 1376
Cosmegen for Injection 1907
Cuprimine Capsules 1925
Dantrium Capsules (Less frequent) .. 2690
Dantrium Intravenous 2691
Dapsone Tablets USP 1656
Depacon Injection 412
Depakene 417
Depakote Sprinkle Capsules 422
Depakote Tablets 427
Depakote ER Tablets 433
Diovan HCT Tablets 2195
Diuril Oral 1936
Diuril Sodium Intravenous 1934
Dyazide Capsules 1389
EC-Naprosyn Delayed-Release Tablets (Less than 1%) 2769
Effexor Tablets 3405
Effexor XR Capsules 3411
Enbrel for Injection 580
Epzicom Tablets 1402
Equetro Extended-Release Capsules 3178
FML-S Liquifilm Sterile Ophthalmic Suspension ..... ⊙ 226
Fortaz 1422
Furosemide Tablets 2117
Gleevec Tablets (Rare) 2221
▲ Hexalen Capsules (13% to 33%) 2101
Humira Injection 464
Hyzaar 1964
Indapamide Tablets 2119
Indocin Capsules (Less than 1%) 1968
Indocin I.V. (Less than 1%) 1973
Indocin (Less than 1%) 1968
Intron A for Injection (Very rare) 3038
Lamictal (Rare) 1449
Leustatin Injection (Some reports) ... 2368
Levaquin in 5% Dextrose Injection (Rare) 2453
Levaquin (Rare) 2453
Lotensin HCT Tablets 2235
Maxipime for Injection 1093
Maxzide 2150
Mefoxin for Injection 1987
Mefoxin Premixed Intravenous Solution 1990
Micardis HCT Tablets 886
Midamor Tablets (Rare) 2000
Moduretic Tablets 2003
Myleran Tablets 1492
Nalfon Capsules (Less than 1%) 2504
Naprosyn Suspension (Less than 1%) 2769
Naprosyn Tablets (Less than 1%) 2769
Nipent for Injection (Less than 3%) ... 3216
Norflex Injection (Very rare) 1824
Omnicef Capsules 506
Omnicef for Oral Suspension 506
Orthoclone OKT3 Sterile Solution 2370
Paxil CR Controlled-Release Tablets 1509
Paxil 1501
Pentasa Capsules 3182
Plavix Tablets (Less than 1%) 940
Plavix Tablets (Less than 1%) 2942
Prevacid Delayed-Release Capsules (Less than 1%) 3268
Prevacid for Delayed-Release Oral Suspension (Less than 1%) 3268
Prevacid NapraPAC (Less than 1%) .. 3277
Prevacid SoluTab Delayed-Release Orally Disintegrating Tablets (Less than 1%) 3268
PREVPAC 3281
Prinzide Tablets 2033
Prozac Pulvules and Liquid 1771
Rebetron Combination Therapy (Very rare) 3078
Retrovir Capsules 1533
Retrovir IV Infusion 1537
Retrovir 1533
Rilutek Tablets (Rare) 2945
Rituxan for Infusion (One case) 845
Roferon-A Injection (Rare) 2805
Suprax 1811
Tagamet Tablets (Very rare) 1547
Tegretol/Tegretol-XR (Very low incidence) 2278
Teveten HCT Tablets 1710
Thalomid Capsules 979
Thioridazine Hydrochloride Tablets .. 2122
Ticlid Tablets (Rare) 2813
Timolide Tablets 2056
Trizivir Tablets 1565
Trusopt Sterile Ophthalmic Solution (Rare) 2065
▲ Valcyte Tablets (Less than 5%) 2816
Valtrex Caplets 1573
Vantin Tablets and Oral Suspension 2650
Vaseretic Tablets 2073
VFEND I.V. (Less than 2%) 2543
VFEND Oral Suspension (Less than 2%) 2543
VFEND Tablets (Less than 2%) 2543
Voltaren Tablets (Rarely) 2298
Voltaren-XR Tablets (Rarely) 2301
Zantac (Rare) 1597
Zantac Injection (Rare) 1593
Zantac Injection Pharmacy Bulk Package (Rare) 1595
Zantac Syrup (Rare) 1597
Zestoretic Tablets 701
Zinacef Injection 1604
Zinacef for Injection 1604
Zoloft 2581
Zonegran Capsules (Rare) 1089

Anemia, dilutional

Neumega for Injection 3433
Prolastin 3252

Anemia, hemolytic

Aceon Tablets (2 mg, 4 mg, 8 mg) ... 3191
Aciphex Tablets 1081
Advicor Tablets 1694
Agenerase Capsules 1299
Agenerase Oral Solution 1304
Alacol DM Syrup 739
Aldoclor Tablets 1881
Aldoril Tablets 1884
Alkeran for Injection 976
Alkeran Tablets 977
Altace Capsules (Less than 1%) 1673
Altoprev Extended-Release Tablets (Rare) 1151
Amaryl Tablets 2864
Amoxil Capsules 1315
Amoxil Chewable Tablets 1315
Amoxil Pediatric Drops for Oral Suspension 1315
Amoxil Powder for Oral Suspension 1315
Amoxil Tablets 1315
Anaprox Tablets (Less than 1%) 2769
Anaprox DS Tablets (Less than 1%) .. 2769
Aricept Tablets (Rare) 1086
Aricept ODT Tablets (Rare) 1086
Arthrotec Tablets (Rare) 3126
Atacand HCT 637
Augmentin 1331
Augmentin Tablets 1334
Augmentin XR Extended-Release Tablets 1340
Augmentin ES-600 Powder for Oral Suspension 1337
Avalide Tablets 922
Avalide Tablets 2889
Campath Ampules 826
Captopril Tablets 2114
Cardizem LA Extended Release Tablets (Infrequent) 1699
Cataflam Tablets (Rarely) 2173
Ceftin 1369
Celexa 1177
Cipro I.V. (Rare) 2998
Cipro I.V. Pharmacy Bulk Package (Rare) 3509
Cipro 2991
Cipro XR Tablets 3004
Clinoril Tablets (Less than 1 in 100) 1899
Crixivan Capsules 1918
Cuprimine Capsules 1925
Cytovene 2763
Diovan HCT Tablets 2195
Diuril Oral 1936
Diuril Sodium Intravenous 1934
Dolobid Tablets (Less than 1 in 100) 1937
Dyazide Capsules 1389
Dynacin Tablets 1859
EC-Naprosyn Delayed-Release Tablets (Less than 1%) 2769
Eloxatin for Injection 2908
Eulexin Capsules 3023
Fortaz (Rare) 1422
Furosemide Tablets 2117
Gamunex Immune Globulin I.V., 10% (Very rare) 3232
Gengraf Capsules 458
Hyzaar 1964
Imitrex Injection 1431
Imitrex Tablets 1440
Indocin Capsules (Less than 1%) 1968
Indocin I.V. (Less than 1%) 1973
Indocin (Less than 1%) 1968
▲ Intron A for Injection (Less than 5%) 3038
Invirase (Rare) 2776
Lamictal 1449
Lescol Capsules (Rare) 2227
Lescol Capsules (Rare) 2730
Lescol XL Tablets 2227
Lescol XL Tablets 2730
Leustatin Injection (Some reports) ... 2368
Levaquin in 5% Dextrose Injection (Rare) 2453
Levaquin (Rare) 2453
Lexapro Oral Solution 1193
Lexapro Tablets 1193
Lotensin Tablets (Less than 1%) 2232
Lotensin HCT Tablets (Rare) 2235
Lotrel Capsules (Rare) 2238
Matulane Capsules 3188
Maxipime for Injection 1093
Maxzide 2150
Mefoxin for Injection 1987
Mefoxin Premixed Intravenous Solution 1990
Mevacor Tablets (Rare) 1996
Micardis HCT Tablets 886
Moduretic Tablets 2003
Mustargen for Injection (Rare) 2007
Mycamine for Injection 620
Nalfon Capsules (Less than 1 %) 2504
Naprosyn Suspension (Less than 1%) 2769
Naprosyn Tablets (Less than 1%) 2769
Neoral Soft Gelatin Capsules 2247
Neoral Oral Solution 2247
Nipent for Injection (Less than 3%) ... 3216
Noroxin Tablets (Rare) 2009
Omnicef Capsules 506
Omnicef for Oral Suspension 506
Oncaspar (Greater than 1% but less than 5%) 1123
Orap Tablets 1220
Orthoclone OKT3 Sterile Solution 2370
Parcopa Orally Disintegrating Tablets 3111
Paser Granules 1657
Paxil CR Controlled-Release Tablets 1509
Paxil 1501
PEG-Intron Powder for Injection 3062
Pneumovax 23 (Rare) 2020
Prandin Tablets (0.5, 1, and 2 mg) (Rare) 2337
Pravachol Tablets (Rare) 943
Prevacid Delayed-Release Capsules (Less than 1%) 3268
Prevacid for Delayed-Release Oral Suspension (Less than 1%) 3268
Prevacid NapraPAC (Less than 1%) .. 3277
Prevacid SoluTab Delayed-Release Orally Disintegrating Tablets (Less than 1%) 3268
PREVPAC 3281
Prilosec OTC Tablets (Rare) 2674
Primaxin I.M. 2022
Primaxin I.V. 2024
Prinivil Tablets (Rare) 2029
Prinzide Tablets 2033

Prograf Capsules and Injection ... 624
Raptiva for Injection ... 1247
▲ Rebetol (10%) ... 3073
▲ Rebetron Combination Therapy (10%) ... 3078
Remicade for IV Injection (Greater than or equal to 0.2%) ... 987
ReoPro Vials (0.3%) ... 1779
Rescriptor Tablets ... 2535
Retrovir Capsules ... 1533
Retrovir IV Infusion ... 1537
Retrovir ... 1533
Rituxan for Infusion (Two cases) ... 845
Rocephin Injectable Vials, ADD-Vantage, Galaxy, Bulk (Less than 1%) ... 2801
Roferon-A Injection (Rare) ... 2805
Skelaxin Tablets ... 1685
Stalevo Tablets ... 2270
Sulfamylon Cream ... 2154
Sulfamylon for 5% Topical Solution ... 2155
Suprax ... 1811
Teveten HCT Tablets ... 1710
Thiothixene Capsules ... 2124
Tiazac Capsules (Infrequent) ... 1204
Ticlid Tablets (Rare) ... 2813
Timolide Tablets ... 2056
Uniretic Tablets (Less than 1%) ... 3114
Univasc Tablets (Less than 1%) ... 3118
Vantin Tablets and Oral Suspension ... 2650
Vaseretic Tablets ... 2073
Vasotec I.V. Injection ... 2076
VFEND I.V. (Less than 2%) ... 2543
VFEND Oral Suspension (Less than 2%) ... 2543
VFEND Tablets (Less than 2%) ... 2543
Virazole for Inhalation Solution ... 3365
Voltaren Tablets (Rarely) ... 2298
Voltaren-XR Tablets (Rarely) ... 2301
Vytorin 10/10 Tablets ... 2084
Vytorin 10/10 Tablets ... 3092
Vytorin 10/20 Tablets ... 2084
Vytorin 10/20 Tablets ... 3092
Vytorin 10/40 Tablets ... 2084
Vytorin 10/40 Tablets ... 3092
Vytorin 10/80 Tablets ... 2084
Vytorin 10/80 Tablets ... 3092
Zegerid Powder for Oral Solution (Rare) ... 2972
Zestoretic Tablets ... 701
Zestril Tablets (Rare) ... 704
Zinacef Injection ... 1604
Zinacef for Injection ... 1604
Zocor Tablets (Rare) ... 2078
Zosyn ... 3492
Zyrtec Chewable Tablets (Rare) ... 2589
Zyrtec (Rare) ... 2589
Zyrtec-D 12 Hour Extended Release Tablets (Rare) ... 2591

Anemia, hemolytic, immune
Campath Ampules ... 826
Prozac Pulvules and Liquid ... 1771
Tagamet Tablets (Extremely rare) ... 1547
Zantac (Exceedingly rare) ... 1597
Zantac Injection (Exceedingly rare) ... 1593
Zantac Injection Pharmacy Bulk Package (Rare) ... 1595
Zantac Syrup (Exceedingly rare) ... 1597

Anemia, hypochromic
Abilify Tablets (Infrequent) ... 916
Abilify Tablets (Infrequent) ... 2472
Aciphex Tablets ... 1081
▲ Casodex Tablets (7%) ... 670
Celexa (Rare) ... 1177
▲ CellCept Capsules (24.6%) ... 2751
▲ CellCept Intravenous (24.6%) ... 2751
▲ CellCept Oral Suspension (24.6%) ... 2751
▲ CellCept Tablets (24.6%) ... 2751
▲ Doxil Injection (5.2% to 9.8%) ... 3302
Evoxac Capsules (Less than 1%) ... 1042
Exelon Capsules (Infrequent) ... 2204
Geodon Capsules (Rare) ... 2514
▲ Imdur Tablets (Less than or equal to 5%) ... 3032
Lovenox Injection (2%) ... 2931
Lyrica Capsules (0.1% to 1%) ... 2524
Merrem I.V. (Greater than 0.1% to 1%) ... 687
Nexium Delayed-Release Capsules (Less than 1%) ... 645
Nexium I.V. (Less than 1%) ... 649
Paxil CR Controlled-Release Tablets (Rare) ... 1509
Paxil (Rare) ... 1501
Plavix Tablets (Less than 1%) ... 940
Plavix Tablets (Less than 1%) ... 2942
▲ Prograf Capsules and Injection (3% to 15%) ... 624
Protonix I.V. (Less than 1%) ... 3468
Protonix Tablets (Less than 1%) ... 3465
Prozac Pulvules and Liquid (Rare) ... 1771
Requip Tablets (Infrequent) ... 1528
Rilutek Tablets (Rare) ... 2945
Risperdal M-Tab Orally Disintegrating Tablets (Infrequent) ... 1658
Risperdal (Infrequent) ... 1658
Seroquel Tablets (Infrequent) ... 691
▲ Targretin Capsules (3.6% to 13.2%) ... 1719
Thalomid Capsules ... 979
Uniretic Tablets (Less than 1%) ... 3114

Anemia, iron deficiency
Abilify Tablets (Infrequent) ... 916
Abilify Tablets (Infrequent) ... 2472
Anadrol-50 Tablets ... 3329
▲ Arava Tablets (1% to 3%) ... 2881
▲ Casodex Tablets (7%) ... 670
Lamictal (Rare) ... 1449
Paxil CR Controlled-Release Tablets (Rare) ... 1509
Paxil (Rare) ... 1501
Permax Tablets (Infrequent) ... 3357
Pletal Tablets (Less than 2%) ... 2478
Protonix I.V. (Less than 1%) ... 3468
Protonix Tablets (Less than 1%) ... 3465
Rilutek Tablets (Rare) ... 2945
Viadur Implant (Less than 2%) ... 782

Anemia, macrocytic
Abilify Tablets (Infrequent) ... 916
Abilify Tablets (Infrequent) ... 2472
Ambien Tablets (Rare) ... 2867
Azasan Tablets ... 2844
Depacon Injection ... 412
Depakene ... 417
Depakote Tablets ... 427
Depakote ER Tablets ... 433
Eulexin Capsules ... 3023
Lamictal (Rare) ... 1449
Thalomid Capsules ... 979
VFEND I.V. (Less than 2%) ... 2543
VFEND Oral Suspension (Less than 2%) ... 2543
VFEND Tablets (Less than 2%) ... 2543

Anemia, megaloblastic
Daraprim Tablets ... 1385
Dyazide Capsules ... 1389
Dyrenium Capsules (Rare) ... 3390
Mebaral Tablets, USP (Less than 1 in 100 patients) ... 2483
Nembutal Sodium Solution, USP ... 2484
Peganone Tablets, USP ... 2487
Permax Tablets (Infrequent) ... 3357
Phenytek Capsules ... 2153
Thalomid Capsules ... 979
VFEND I.V. (Less than 2%) ... 2543
VFEND Oral Suspension (Less than 2%) ... 2543
VFEND Tablets (Less than 2%) ... 2543
Zovirax for Injection (Less than 1%) ... 1618

Anemia, microangiopathic hemolytic
Gengraf Capsules ... 458
Plavix Tablets ... 940
Plavix Tablets ... 2942
Sandimmune (Occasional) ... 2259

Anemia, microcytic
Paxil CR Controlled-Release Tablets (Rare) ... 1509
Paxil (Rare) ... 1501
Thalomid Capsules ... 979
VFEND I.V. (Less than 2%) ... 2543
VFEND Oral Suspension (Less than 2%) ... 2543
VFEND Tablets (Less than 2%) ... 2543
Zonegran Capsules (Rare) ... 1089

Anemia, nonhemolytic
Parcopa Orally Disintegrating Tablets ... 3111
Stalevo Tablets ... 2270

Anemia, normocytic
Paxil CR Controlled-Release Tablets (Rare) ... 1509
Paxil (Rare) ... 1501
Risperdal M-Tab Orally Disintegrating Tablets (Rare) ... 1658
Risperdal (Rare) ... 1658
VFEND I.V. (Less than 2%) ... 2543
VFEND Oral Suspension (Less than 2%) ... 2543
VFEND Tablets (Less than 2%) ... 2543
Zyprexa Tablets (Infrequent) ... 1798
Zyprexa ZYDIS Orally Disintegrating Tablets (Infrequent) ... 1798

Anemia, sideroblastic
Cuprimine Capsules ... 1925

Anesthesia, local
Denavir Cream (0.9%) ... 2163
Migranal Nasal Spray (Infrequent) ... 3350

Anesthesia, persistent
Naropin Injection ... 640

Anesthetic effect
Lithobid Tablets ... 1670

Anetoderma
Cuprimine Capsules (Rare) ... 1925

Aneurysm
Requip Tablets (Infrequent) ... 1528
Sandostatin LAR Depot (Rare) ... 2264

Aneurysm, aortic
Effexor Tablets (Rare) ... 3405
Effexor XR Capsules (Rare) ... 3411
Imitrex Nasal Spray (Rare) ... 1435

Anger
Meridia Capsules ... 485
Xanax XR Tablets (Infrequent) ... 2655

Angiectases, cutaneous
Adalat CC Tablets (Less than 1%) ... 2978

Angiitis
Indocin Capsules (Less than 1%) ... 1968
Indocin I.V. (Less than 1%) ... 1973
Indocin (Less than 1%) ... 1968
Timolide Tablets ... 2056

Angina
Amerge Tablets ... 1312
▲ Apokyn Injection (4% to 15%) ... 2132
Caduet Tablets ... 2507
Cardizem LA Extended Release Tablets (Less than 2%) ... 1699
Clozapine Tablets (1%) ... 2141
Clozaril Tablets (1%) ... 2174
Combivent Inhalation Aerosol (Less than 2%) ... 878
Concerta Extended-Release Tablets ... 1828
Copegus Tablets (Less than 1%) ... 2759
FazaClo Orally Disintegrating Tablets (1%) ... 547
Femara Tablets (Less than or equal to 2%) ... 2210
Focalin Tablets ... 2214
Focalin XR Capsules ... 2217
Foradil Aerolizer ... 3024
Hyperstat I.V. Injection ... 3031
Imitrex Nasal Spray ... 1435
Imitrex Tablets (Rare) ... 1440
▲ Intron A for Injection (Less than 5%) ... 3038
Levothroid Tablets ... 1189
Levoxyl Tablets ... 1680
Lofibra Capsules ... 1217
Lupron Depot 7.5 mg (Less than 5%) ... 3261
Metadate CD Capsules ... 3316
Migranal Nasal Spray (Rare) ... 3350
OptiPranolol Metipranolol Ophthalmic Solution 0.3% (A small number of patients) ... ⊙ 254
Orthoclone OKT3 Sterile Solution (Less than 1%) ... 2370
PEG-Intron Powder for Injection (Less than or equal to 1%) ... 3062
Prandin Tablets (0.5, 1, and 2 mg) (1.8%) ... 2337
▲ Pravachol Tablets (0.1% to 4.0%) ... 943
Prevacid Delayed-Release Capsules (Less than 1%) ... 3268
Prevacid for Delayed-Release Oral Suspension (Less than 1%) ... 3268
Prevacid NapraPAC (Less than 1%) ... 3277
Prevacid SoluTab Delayed-Release Orally Disintegrating Tablets (Less than 1%) ... 3268
PREVPAC (Less than 1%) ... 3281
Prilosec OTC Tablets (Less than 1%) ... 2674
Proleukin for Injection ... 1007
Proventil Inhalation Aerosol ... 3067
Proventil HFA Inhalation Aerosol ... 3071
Relafen Tablets (Less than 1%) ... 1523
Ritalin Hydrochloride Tablets ... 2254
Ritalin LA Capsules ... 2255
Ritalin-SR Tablets ... 2254
Rituxan for Infusion (One patient) ... 845
Rituxan I.V. ... 1251
Tamiflu Capsules (Less than 1%) ... 2810
Tamiflu Oral Suspension (Less than 1%) ... 2810
Tarka Tablets (0.3% or more) ... 519
Taxotere Injection Concentrate (Rare) ... 2947
Tiazac Capsules (Less than 2%) ... 1204
Tricor Tablets ... 523
Triglide Tablets ... 1165
Unithroid Tablets ... 3521
Univasc Tablets (Less than 1%) ... 3118
Ventolin HFA Inhalation Aerosol ... 1576
VoSpire Extended-Release Tablets ... 2352
Zegerid Powder for Oral Solution (Less than 1%) ... 2972
Zofran Injection (Rare) ... 1607
Zofran (Rare) ... 1613
Zofran ODT Orally Disintegrating Tablets (Rare) ... 1613

Angina, crescendo
BiDil Tablets ... 2161
Nitro-Dur Transdermal Infusion System (Uncommon) ... 3060

Angina, increased
Lotrel Capsules (Rare) ... 2238
Nitro-Dur Transdermal Infusion System (2%) ... 3060
Norvasc Tablets (Rare) ... 2529

Angina, Prinzmetal's, episodes of
Imitrex Injection ... 1431
Imitrex Nasal Spray ... 1435

Angina pectoris
Abilify Tablets (Infrequent) ... 916
Abilify Tablets (Infrequent) ... 2472
Aciphex Tablets ... 1081
Actiq (Less than 1%) ... 993
Actonel Tablets (2.5%) ... 2679
Actonel with Calcium Tablets (2.5%) ... 2684
Aggrenox Capsules ... 855
Agrylin Capsules (1% to 5%) ... 3172
▲ Altace Capsules (3%) ... 1673
Ambien Tablets (Rare) ... 2867
▲ Angiomax for Injection (5.3%) ... 1856
Antara Capsules ... 2723
▲ Aranesp for Injection (8%) ... 576
▲ Arava Tablets (1% to 3%) ... 2881
Argatroban Injection (1.8%) ... 1321
Aricept Tablets (Infrequent) ... 1086
Aricept ODT Tablets (Infrequent) ... 1086
Arimidex Tablets (1.7%) ... 665
Atacand Tablets (Less frequently) ... 634
Atacand HCT (Less than 0.5%) ... 637
Avalide Tablets ... 922
Avalide Tablets ... 2889
Avapro Tablets (Less than 1%) ... 925
Avapro Tablets (Less than 1%) ... 2886
Caduet Tablets (Less than 2%) ... 2507
Campath Ampules ... 826
Campral Tablets (Infrequent) ... 1175
Camptosar Injection ... 2602
Captopril Tablets (2 to 3 of 1000 patients) ... 2114
Cardene I.V. (Rare) ... 1129
▲ Casodex Tablets (2% to 5%) ... 670
Celebrex Capsules (0.1% to 1.9%) ... 3130
Celexa (Infrequent) ... 1177
▲ CellCept Capsules (3% to less than 20%) ... 2751
▲ CellCept Intravenous (3% to less than 20%) ... 2751
▲ CellCept Oral Suspension (3% to less than 20%) ... 2751
▲ CellCept Tablets (3% to less than 20%) ... 2751
Cialis Tablets (Less than 2%) ... 1806
Cipro I.V. (1% or less) ... 2998
Cipro I.V. Pharmacy Bulk Package (1% or less) ... 3509
Cipro (Less than 1%) ... 2991
Cipro XR Tablets ... 3004
▲ Coreg Tablets (2% to 6%) ... 1376
Cosopt Sterile Ophthalmic Solution ... 1910
Covera-HS Tablets (2% or less) ... 3135
Cozaar Tablets (Less than 1%) ... 1913
Crestor Tablets (Greater than or equal to 1%) ... 672
Crixivan Capsules ... 1918
Doxil Injection (Less than 1%) ... 3302
Effexor Tablets (Infrequent) ... 3405
Effexor XR Capsules (Infrequent) ... 3411
Eldepryl Capsules ... 3209
Evoxac Capsules (Less than 1%) ... 1042
Exelon Capsules (Frequent) ... 2204
Ferrlecit Injection ... 3379
▲ Flolan for Injection (19%) ... 1408
Forteo for Injection (2.5%) ... 1739
▲ Fortical Nasal Spray (1% to 3%) ... 3336
Fuzeon Injection ... 2772

Gabitril Tablets (Infrequent) 998
Geodon Capsules (Infrequent) 2514
Hyzaar 1964
Imitrex Injection 1431
Imitrex Tablets 1440
Inspra Tablets 2520
Kytril Tablets (Rare) 2788
Lamictal (Rare) 1449
Levaquin in 5% Dextrose Injection (0.1% to 0.9%) 2453
Levaquin (0.1% to 0.9%) 2453
Levitra Tablets (Less than 2%) 3048
Lipitor Tablets (Less than 2%) 2495
Lofibra Capsules 1217
Maxalt Tablets (Rare) 1983
Maxalt-MLT Orally Disintegrating Tablets (Rare) 1983
Meridia Capsules 485
Miacalcin Nasal Spray (1% to 3%) 2242
Micardis Tablets (More than 0.3%) 884
Micardis HCT Tablets 886
Midamor Tablets (Less than or equal to 1%) 2000
Mirapex Tablets (Less than 1%) 889
Mobic Oral Suspension (Less than 2%) 893
Mobic Tablets (Less than 2%) 893
Moduretic Tablets (Less than or equal to 1%) 2003
Namenda (Infrequent) 1199
▲ Natrecor for Injection (2% to 6%) 3123
Neurontin Capsules (Infrequent) 2498
Neurontin Oral Solution (Infrequent) 2498
Neurontin Tablets (Infrequent) 2498
Nipent for Injection (Less than 3%) 3216
Omacor Capsules (1.3%) 2735
Ortho-Cyclen/Ortho Tri-Cyclen 2414
Ortho Tri-Cyclen Lo Tablets 2421
Paxil CR Controlled-Release Tablets (Rare) 1509
Paxil (Rare) 1501
Permax Tablets (Infrequent) 3357
Persantine Tablets (Rare) 898
Photofrin for Injection 729
Plendil Extended-Release Tablets (0.5% to 1.5%) 651
Pletal Tablets (2% or greater) 2478
Prinivil Tablets (Greater than 1%) 2029
Prinzide Tablets 2033
▲ Prograf Capsules and Injection (3% to 15%) 624
Prometrium Capsules (100 mg, 200 mg) (Less than 5%) 3205
Protonix I.V. (Less than 1%) 3468
Protonix Tablets (Less than 1%) 3465
Protopic Ointment (Greater than or equal to 1%) 629
Prozac Pulvules and Liquid (Infrequent) 1771
ReFacto Vials 3479
Relpax Tablets (Rare) 2531
Requip Tablets (Infrequent) 1528
Rilutek Tablets (Infrequent) 2945
Risperdal Consta Long-Acting Injection (Infrequent) 1664
Risperdal M-Tab Orally Disintegrating Tablets (Rare) 1658
Risperdal (Rare) 1658
Rythmol SR Capsules (2%) 2736
Seroquel Tablets (Infrequent) 691
▲ Simulect for Injection (3% to 10%) 2268
Sonata Capsules (Infrequent) 1686
▲ Spiriva HandiHaler (1% to 3%) 899
Symbyax Capsules (Rare) 1788
Tambocor Tablets (Less than 1%) 1824
Targretin Capsules 1719
Tasmar Tablets (Infrequent) 3360
Teveten Tablets (Less than 1%) 1707
Teveten HCT Tablets (Less than 1%) 1710
Thalomid Capsules 979
Timolide Tablets 2056
Topamax Sprinkle Capsules (Infrequent) 2438
Topamax Tablets (Infrequent) 2438
Travatan Ophthalmic Solution (1% to 5%) 559
Tricor Tablets 523
Triglide Tablets 1165
Vaseretic Tablets 2073
Vasotec I.V. Injection (1.5%) 2076
Verelan PM Capsules (2% or less) 3120
Viagra Tablets (Less than 2%) 2552
Xalatan Sterile Ophthalmic Solution (1% to 2%) 2654
Zelnorm Tablets 2303
Zestoretic Tablets 701
Zestril Tablets (Greater than 1%) 704
Zoladex 3-month (1% to 5%) 712
Zomig Nasal Spray (Rare) 718
Zomig Tablets 714
Zomig-ZMT Tablets 714

Angina pectoris, aggravation
Aldoclor Tablets 1881
Aldoril Tablets 1884
Blocadren Tablets (Less than 1%) 1891
▲ Coreg Tablets (Greater than 1% to 3%) 1376
Eldepryl Capsules 3209
▲ Imdur Tablets (Less than or equal to 5%) 3032
Sandostatin LAR Depot (Rare) 2264
▲ Spiriva HandiHaler (1% to 3%) 899
Timoptic in Ocudose (Less frequent) 2061
Timoptic Sterile Ophthalmic Solution (Less frequent) 2058
Timoptic-XE Sterile Ophthalmic Gel Forming Solution 2062

Angina pectoris, exacerbation of, post-abrupt discontinuation
Inderal LA Long-Acting Capsules 3421
Tenormin I.V. Injection 698
Tenormin Tablets 695
Toprol-XL Tablets 660

Angina tonsillaris
Invirase (Less than 2%) 2776

Angina, unstable
Rythmol SR Capsules 2736

Angioedema
(*see also under* Edema, angioneurotic)
Abilify Tablets (Rare) 916
Abilify Tablets (Rare) 2472
Aceon Tablets (2 mg, 4 mg, 8 mg) (0.1%) 3191
Aciphex Tablets 1081
Actonel with Calcium Tablets 2684
Advicor Tablets (Rare) 1694
Aldara Cream, 5% 1814
Aldurazyme for Intravenous Infusion 1261
Alesse-28 Tablets 3392
Allegra (Rare) 2857
Allegra-D 12 Hour Extended-Release Tablets (Rare) 2860
Allegra-D 24 Hour Extended-Release Tablets (Rare) 2862
AmBisome for Injection (Infrequent) 615
Amevive 836
Aminohippurate Sodium "PAH" Injection 1886
Aredia for Injection (Rare) 2168
Arimidex Tablets (Very rare) 665
Arthrotec Tablets (Rare) 3126
Atacand Tablets (Less frequently) 634
Atacand HCT (Less than 0.5%) 637
Atrovent HFA Inhalation Aerosol 872
Avalide Tablets (Rare) 922
Avalide Tablets (Rare) 2889
Avapro Tablets (Rare) 925
Avapro Tablets (Rare) 2886
Avelox 2984
Bayer Aspirin Tablets 3515
Beconase AQ Nasal Spray (Rare) 1359
BeneFix for Injection 3402
Benicar Tablets 2850
Benicar HCT Tablets (Rare) 2852
BiDil Tablets (1% to less than 2%) 2161
Caduet Tablets (Greater than 0.1% to less than or equal to 1%) 2507
Campath Ampules 826
Captopril Tablets (Approximately 1 in 1000 patients) 2114
Cardizem LA Extended Release Tablets (Infrequent) 1699
Cataflam Tablets (Rarely) 2173
Catapres Tablets 874
Ceftin 1369
Celebrex Capsules (Less than 0.1%) 3130
Celexa 1177
Cenestin Tablets, 0.45mg, 0.625mg, 0.9mg, 1.25mg 1063
Cenestin Tablets, 0.3mg 1063
▲ Cerezyme for Injection (Approximately 6.6%) 1263
Cipro I.V. (1% or less) 2998
Cipro I.V. Pharmacy Bulk Package (1% or less) 3509
Cipro (Less than 1%) 2991
Colazal Capsules 2845
CombiPatch Transdermal System 2180
Comvax 1904
Copaxone for Injection (Infrequent) 3292
Cosopt Sterile Ophthalmic Solution 1910
Cozaar Tablets (Rare) 1913
Crestor Tablets (Less than 1%) 672
Decadron Tablets 1929
depo-subQ provera 104 Injectable Suspension 2622
Detrol LA Capsules 2629
Didronel Tablets 2693
Diovan HCT Tablets (Rare) 2195
Diovan Tablets (Rare) 2191
Ecotrin Enteric Coated Aspirin Low, Regular and Maximum Strength Tablets 1627
Eloxatin for Injection 2908
Emcyt Capsules 3137
Emend Capsules (One patient) 1944
Enbrel for Injection 580
Eskalith 1406
Estratest Tablets 3196
Estratest H.S. Tablets 3196
Faslodex Injection (Less than 1%) 682
Flovent Diskus 50 mcg (Rare) 1415
Flovent HFA 1418
Foradil Aerolizer (Rare) 3024
Fortaz (Very rare) 1422
Fosamax (Rare) 1949
Fosamax Plus D Tablets (Rarely) 1956
GamaSTAN 3231
Gleevec Tablets (Rare) 2221
Herceptin I.V. 1234
Hycamtin for Injection (Rare) 1427
Hyzaar (Rare) 1964
Indocin (Less than 1%) 1968
Ketek Tablets (Rare) 2920
Lamisil Tablets (Rare) 2226
Levaquin in 5% Dextrose Injection 2453
Levaquin 2453
Levothroid Tablets 1189
Levoxyl Tablets 1680
Lexapro Oral Solution 1193
Lexapro Tablets 1193
Lidoderm Patch (Rare) 1107
Lithobid Tablets 1670
Lo/Ovral-28 Tablets 3423
Lotensin Tablets (Less than 1%) 2232
Lotensin HCT Tablets (0.3%) 2235
Lotrel Capsules (About 0.5%) 2238
Lyrica Capsules (Rare) 2524
Maxalt Tablets 1983
Maxalt-MLT Orally Disintegrating Tablets 1983
Menostar Transdermal System 805
Merrem I.V. 687
Micardis Tablets (Single case) 884
Micardis HCT Tablets 886
Mintezol 2002
Mobic Oral Suspension (Less than 2%) 893
Mobic Tablets (Less than 2%) 893
Nalfon Capsules (Less than 1%) 2504
Nasonex Nasal Spray 3058
Navelbine Injection 1494
Nembutal Sodium Solution, USP 2484
Neurontin Capsules 2498
Neurontin Oral Solution 2498
Neurontin Tablets 2498
Nexium Delayed-Release Capsules (Less than 1%) 645
Nexium I.V. (Less than 1%) 649
Noroxin Tablets 2009
Norvasc Tablets (More than 0.1% to 1%) 2529
Novarel for Injection 1147
Parcopa Orally Disintegrating Tablets 3111
Pediarix Vaccine 1518
Persantine Tablets (Rare) 898
Plavix Tablets 940
Plavix Tablets 2942
Plendil Extended-Release Tablets 651
Pravachol Tablets 943
Prefest Tablets 1069
Premarin Intravenous 3440
Premarin Tablets 3443
Premphase Tablets 3452
Prempro Tablets 3452
Prinivil Tablets (0.1% to 1.0%) 2029
Protonix I.V. 3468
Protonix Tablets 3465
Protopic Ointment (Greater than or equal to 1%) 629
Proventil Inhalation Aerosol 3067
Qvar Inhalation Aerosol (Rare) 1654
Rebetron Combination Therapy 3078
Recombivax HB (Less than 1%) 2045
Reyataz Capsules (Less than 3%) 948
Rhinocort Aqua Nasal Spray (Rare) 658
▲ Rituxan for Infusion (0.3% to 13%) 845
▲ Rituxan I.V. (0.3% to 13%) 1251
Seasonale Tablets 1073
Singulair 2047
Spiriva HandiHaler (Less than 1%) 899
St. Joseph 81 mg Aspirin Chewable and Enteric Coated Tablets 1841
Stalevo Tablets 2270
Suprax 1811
Thalomid Capsules 979
Timoptic in Ocudose 2061
Timoptic Sterile Ophthalmic Solution 2058
Timoptic-XE Sterile Ophthalmic Gel Forming Solution 2062
Tindamax 2670
TNKase I.V. (Rare) 1256
Triphasil-28 Tablets 3483
Trusopt Sterile Ophthalmic Solution 2065
Twinrix Vaccine 1571
Uniretic Tablets (Less than 0.5% to more than 1%) 3114
Unithroid Tablets 3521
Univasc Tablets (Less than 1%) 3118
Valtrex Caplets 1573
Vaseretic Tablets (0.6%) 2073
Vasotec I.V. Injection 2076
Ventolin HFA Inhalation Aerosol 1576
VFEND I.V. (Less than 2%) 2543
VFEND Oral Suspension (Less than 2%) 2543
VFEND Tablets (Less than 2%) 2543
Viramune Oral Suspension 903
Viramune Tablets 903
Voltaren Tablets (Rarely) 2298
Voltaren-XR Tablets (Rarely) 2301
Vytorin 10/40 Tablets 2084
Xenical Capsules 2834
Xopenex HFA Inhalation Aerosol 3151
Xopenex Inhalation Solution 3143
Xopenex Inhalation Solution Concentrate 3147
Zestril Tablets (0.1%) 704
Zetia Tablets 2090
Zetia Tablets 3098
▲ Zevalin Injection (5%) 848
Zinacef Injection 1604
Zinacef for Injection 1604
Zithromax Capsules, 250 mg (1% or less; rare) 2568
Zithromax for IV Infusion (Rare) 2573
Zithromax for Oral Suspension, 1 g (1% or less) 2568
Zithromax for Oral Suspension, 300 mg, 600 mg, 900 mg, 1200 mg (1% or less; rare) 2561
Zithromax Tablets, 250 mg, 500 mg (1% or less; rare) 2561
Zithromax Tablets, 600 mg (1% or less) 2568
Zithromax Tri-Pak (1% or less; rare) 2561
Zithromax Z-Pak (1% or less) 2568
Zmax for Oral Suspension 2577
Zofran Injection 1607
Zofran 1613
Zofran ODT Orally Disintegrating Tablets 1613
Zoloft 2581
Zomig Tablets (Rare) 714
Zovirax for Injection 1618
Zyprexa Tablets 1798
Zyprexa ZYDIS Orally Disintegrating Tablets 1798

Angioedema, extremities
Aceon Tablets (2 mg, 4 mg, 8 mg) (0.1%) 3191
Altace Capsules 1673
Captopril Tablets (Approximately 1 in 1000 patients) 2114
Lotensin Tablets 2232
Lotrel Capsules 2238
Mavik Tablets 482
Pegasys 2793
Prinivil Tablets (0.1%) 2029
Prinzide Tablets (Rare) 2033
Uniretic Tablets 3114
Vaseretic Tablets 2073
Vasotec I.V. Injection 2076
Zestoretic Tablets (Rare) 701
Zestril Tablets 704

Angioedema, eyes
Altace Capsules 1673
Captopril Tablets 2114
Uniretic Tablets 3114
Zestoretic Tablets 701
Zestril Tablets 704

Angioedema, face
Aceon Tablets (2 mg, 4 mg, 8 mg) (0.3% to 1%) 3191
Altace Capsules 1673
Atrovent HFA Inhalation Aerosol 872
Atrovent Nasal Spray 0.06% 870

Avalide Tablets (Rare) 922
Avalide Tablets (Rare) 2889
Avapro Tablets (Rare) 925
Avapro Tablets (Rare) 2886
Captopril Tablets (Approximately 1 in 1000 patients) 2114
Catapres-TTS (2 of 3,539 patients) 875
Cozaar Tablets (Rare) 1913
Crestor Tablets (Less than 1%) 672
Flomax Capsules 881
Hyzaar (Rare) 1964
Lotensin Tablets 2232
Lotrel Capsules (About 0.5%) 2238
Mavik Tablets (0.13%) 482
Prinivil Tablets 2029
Prinzide Tablets (Rare) 2033
Uniretic Tablets (Less than 0.5%) 3114
Vaseretic Tablets 2073
Vasotec I.V. Injection 2076
Zestoretic Tablets (Rare) 701
Zestril Tablets 704

Angioedema, glottis
Aceon Tablets (2 mg, 4 mg, 8 mg) (0.1%) 3191
Altace Capsules 1673
Captopril Tablets (Approximately 1 in 1000 patients) 2114
Cozaar Tablets 1913
Hyzaar 1964
Lotensin Tablets 2232
Lotrel Capsules (About 0.5%) 2238
Mavik Tablets (0.3% to 1.0%) 482
Prinivil Tablets 2029
Prinzide Tablets (Rare) 2033
Tarka Tablets 519
Uniretic Tablets 3114
Vaseretic Tablets 2073
Vasotec I.V. Injection 2076
Zestoretic Tablets (Rare) 701
Zestril Tablets 704

Angioedema, intestinal
Aceon Tablets (2 mg, 4 mg, 8 mg) 3191
Altace Capsules 1673
Captopril Tablets 2114
Lotensin Tablets 2232
Mavik Tablets 482
Prinivil Tablets (Rare) 2029
Prinzide Tablets (Rare) 2033
Zestoretic Tablets 701
Zestril Tablets (Very rare) 704

Angioedema, larynx
Aceon Tablets (2 mg, 4 mg, 8 mg) (0.1%) 3191
Activase I.V. 1225
Altace Capsules 1673
Captopril Tablets (Approximately 1 in 1000 patients) 2114
Levaquin in 5% Dextrose Injection 2453
Levaquin 2453
Lotensin Tablets 2232
Mavik Tablets 482
Prinivil Tablets 2029
Prinzide Tablets (Rare) 2033
Uniretic Tablets 3114
Vaseretic Tablets 2073
Vasotec I.V. Injection 2076
Zestoretic Tablets (Rare) 701
Zestril Tablets 704

Angioedema, lips
Aceon Tablets (2 mg, 4 mg, 8 mg) (0.1%) 3191
Altace Capsules 1673
Atrovent HFA Inhalation Aerosol 872
Atrovent Nasal Spray 0.06% 870
Avalide Tablets (Rare) 922
Avalide Tablets (Rare) 2889
Avapro Tablets (Rare) 925
Avapro Tablets (Rare) 2886
Captopril Tablets (Approximately 1 in 1000 patients) 2114
Cozaar Tablets (Rare) 1913
Flomax Capsules 881
Hyzaar (Rare) 1964
Lotensin Tablets 2232
Lotrel Capsules 2238
Mavik Tablets 482
Prinivil Tablets 2029
Prinzide Tablets (Rare) 2033
Uniretic Tablets 3114
Vaseretic Tablets 2073
Vasotec I.V. Injection 2076
Zestoretic Tablets (Rare) 701
Zestril Tablets 704

Angioedema, mucous membranes of the mouth
Activase I.V. 1225
Captopril Tablets 2114

Angioedema, oropharyngeal
Avalide Tablets (Rare) 922
Avalide Tablets (Rare) 2889
Avapro Tablets (Rare) 925
Avapro Tablets (Rare) 2886
Cozaar Tablets (Rare) 1913
Hyzaar (Rare) 1964

Angioedema, throat
Levaquin in 5% Dextrose Injection 2453
Levaquin 2453

Angioedema of tongue
Aceon Tablets (2 mg, 4 mg, 8 mg) (0.1%) 3191
Altace Capsules 1673
Atrovent HFA Inhalation Aerosol 872
Atrovent Nasal Spray 0.06% 870
Avalide Tablets (Rare) 922
Avalide Tablets (Rare) 2889
Avapro Tablets (Rare) 925
Avapro Tablets (Rare) 2886
Captopril Tablets (Approximately 1 in 1000 patients) 2114
Catapres-TTS (One case) 875
Cozaar Tablets (Rare) 1913
Flomax Capsules 881
Hyzaar (Rare) 1964
Levaquin in 5% Dextrose Injection 2453
Levaquin 2453
Lotensin Tablets 2232
Lotrel Capsules (About 0.5%) 2238
Mavik Tablets 482
Prinivil Tablets 2029
Prinzide Tablets (Rare) 2033
Uniretic Tablets 3114
Vaseretic Tablets 2073
Vasotec I.V. Injection 2076
Zestoretic Tablets (Rare) 701
Zestril Tablets 704

Anhidrosis
Cogentin Injection 1903

Anisocoria
Betoptic S Ophthalmic Suspension 554
Lyrica Capsules (Rare) 2524
Paxil CR Controlled-Release Tablets (Rare) 1509
Paxil (Rare) 1501

Anophthalmos
Thalomid Capsules 979

Anorexia
Abelcet Injection 1119
Abilify Tablets 916
Abilify Tablets 2472
Aciphex Tablets 1081
▲ Actimmune (3%) 1646
Actiq (Less than 1%) 993
Adderall Tablets 3168
▲ Adderall XR Capsules (2.9% to 33%) 3169
Adriamycin for Injection, USP (Occasional) 786
Adriamycin Injection, USP (Occasional) 786
Advicor Tablets 1694
Aggrenox Capsules (1.2%) 855
▲ Agrylin Capsules (7.7%) 3172
Alacol DM Syrup 739
Aldoclor Tablets 1881
Aldoril Tablets 1884
▲ Alferon N Injection (1% to 68%) 1640
▲ Alimta for Injection (1% to 62%) 1722
Alinia for Oral Suspension (Less than 1%) 2840
Alinia Tablets (Less than 1%) 2840
Aloxi Injection (Less than 1%) 2099
Altace Capsules (Less than 1%) 1673
Altoprev Extended-Release Tablets (Rare) 1151
Ambien Tablets (1%) 2867
AmBisome for Injection (Less common) 615
Ancef for Injection 1318
Antara Capsules 2723
Anzemet Injection (Rare) 2871
Anzemet Tablets (Rare) 2874
Aptivus Capsules (Less than 2%) 859
▲ Arava Tablets (3%) 2881
▲ Aredia for Injection (1% to 20.8%) 2168
▲ Aricept Tablets (3% to 7%) 1086
▲ Aricept ODT Tablets (3% to 7%) 1086
▲ Arimidex Tablets (5% to 8%) 665
▲ Aromasin Tablets (6%) 2600
Arthrotec Tablets (Rare) 3126
Asacol Delayed-Release Tablets 2688
Asmanex Twisthaler (1% to less than 3%) 2981
Atacand HCT 637
Avalide Tablets 922
Avalide Tablets 2889
▲ Avastin IV (35% to 43%) 1229
Avelox (0.1% to less than 2%) 2984
▲ Avinza Capsules (5% to 10%) 1714
Axid Oral Solution (1.2%) 913
Balamine DM 739
Bentyl Capsules 724
Bentyl Injection 724
Bentyl Syrup 724
Bentyl Tablets 724
▲ Bexxar (0% to 14%) 1360
Biaxin/Biaxin XL 402
Biltricide Tablets 2990
Brevibloc Concentrate (Less than 1%) 766
Brevibloc Injection (Less than 1%) 766
Brevibloc Double Strength Injection (Less than 1%) 766
Brevibloc Premixed Injection (Less than 1%) 766
Brevibloc Double Strength Premixed Injection (Less than 1%) 766
Buprenex Injectable (Rare) 2718
Caduet Tablets (Greater than 0.1% to less than 2%) 2507
Calcijex Injection 411
Calcium Disodium Versenate Injection 1819
▲ Campath Ampules (20%) 826
▲ Campral Tablets (2% to 5%) 1175
▲ Camptosar Injection (5% to 55%%) 2602
Cancidas for Injection (0% to 1.3%) 1894
Captopril Tablets (About 0.5% to 2%) 2114
Carbatrol Capsules 3174
Cardizem LA Extended Release Tablets (Less than 2%) 1699
▲ Carnitor Injection (3% to 6%) 3185
▲ Casodex Tablets (5%) 670
Catapres Tablets (About 1 in 100 patients) 874
Catapres-TTS (0.5% or less) 875
Ceftin Tablets (0.1% to 1%) 1369
Celebrex Capsules (0.1% to 1.9%) 3130
▲ Celexa (4%) 1177
▲ CellCept Capsules (3% to 25.3%) 2751
▲ CellCept Intravenous (3% to 25.3%) 2751
▲ CellCept Oral Suspension (3% to 25.3%) 2751
▲ CellCept Tablets (3% to 25.3%) 2751
Cipro I.V. (1% or less) 2998
Cipro I.V. Pharmacy Bulk Package (1% or less) 3509
Cipro (Less than 1%) 2991
Cipro XR Tablets (Less than 1%) 3004
▲ Clarinex Syrup (4.5%) 3009
Clarinex-D 24-Hour Extended-Release Tablets (2%) 3012
Clinoril Tablets (Greater than 1%) 1899
▲ Clolar for Intravenous Infusion (31%) 1264
Clorpres Tablets (About 1%) 2139
Clozapine Tablets (1%) 2141
Clozaril Tablets (1%) 2174
Colazal Capsules (2%) 2845
▲ Combivir Tablets (10%) 1373
Comvax (0.8% to 3.9%) 1904
▲ Concerta Extended-Release Tablets (0.7% to 4%) 1828
▲ Copaxone for Injection (8%) 3292
▲ Copegus Tablets (24%) 2759
Cosmegen for Injection 1907
Cosopt Sterile Ophthalmic Solution 1910
Cozaar Tablets (Less than 1%) 1913
Crixivan Capsules (2.7%) 1918
Cuprimine Capsules 1925
▲ Cymbalta Delayed-Release Capsules (3% to 5%) 1729
▲ Cytovene (15%) 2763
Dalmane Capsules (Rare) 3343
Dantrium Capsules (Rare) 2690
▲ DAPTACEL (9% to 17.6%) 2964
▲ Daranide Tablets (Among the most common effects) 1928
Daraprim Tablets 1385
▲ Depacon Injection (4% to 12%) 412
▲ Depakene (11% to 12%) 417
▲ Depakote Sprinkle Capsules (4% to 12%) 422
▲ Depakote Tablets (1% to 12%) 427
▲ Depakote ER Tablets (11% to 12%) 433
Dexedrine 1386
DextroStat Tablets 3177
Diastat Rectal Delivery System (Less than 1%) 3344
Digitek Tablets (1%) 2146
Dilaudid 439
Dilaudid Oral Liquid 443
Dilaudid Non-Sterile Powder 439
Dilaudid Rectal Suppositories 439
Dilaudid Tablets 439
Dilaudid Tablets - 8 mg 443
Dilaudid-HP (Less frequent) 441
Diovan HCT Tablets (Less frequent) 2195
Diovan Tablets (Less frequent) 2191
Diuril Oral 1936
Diuril Sodium Intravenous 1934
Dolobid Tablets (Less than 1 in 100) 1937
▲ Dostinex Tablets (1% to less than 10%) 2631
▲ Doxil Injection (1% to 20.1%) 3302
▲ Duragesic Transdermal System (3% to 10%) 2448
Dynacin Tablets 1859
Edecrin 1941
▲ E.E.S. (Among most frequent) 449
▲ Effexor Tablets (11% to 17.0%) 3405
▲ Effexor XR Capsules (5% to 20%) 3411
Eldepryl Capsules 3209
Ellence Injection (0% to 2.9%) 2632
Elmiron Capsules (Less than or equal to 1%) 2393
▲ Eloxatin for Injection (1% to 29%) 2908
Elspar for Injection 1943
▲ Emcyt Capsules (4%) 3137
▲ Emend Capsules (10.1%) 1944
Enbrel for Injection 580
Engerix-B Vaccine (Less than 1%) 1391
▲ Epivir (10%) 1394
Equetro Extended-Release Capsules 3178
▲ Erbitux (25%) 937
▲ EryPed (Among most frequent) 445
▲ Ery-Tab Tablets (Among most frequent) 447
▲ Erythrocin Stearate Filmtab Tablets (Among most frequent) 452
▲ Erythromycin Base Filmtab Tablets (Among most frequent) 454
▲ Erythromycin Delayed-Release Capsules, USP (Among most frequent) 456
Eskalith 1406
▲ Eulexin Capsules (4%) 3023
▲ Evoxac Capsules (1% to 3%) 1042
▲ Exelon Capsules (17%) 2204
Factive Tablets (0.1% to 1%) 2464
Famvir Tablets (1.1% to 2.6%) 2207
▲ Faslodex Injection (9%) 682
FazaClo Orally Disintegrating Tablets (1%) 547
▲ Femara Tablets (3% to 5%) 2210
Ferrlecit Injection 3379
Flexeril Tablets (Less than 1%) 1832
▲ Flolan for Injection (25% to 66%) 1408
Flumadine (1.6%) 1186
▲ Focalin Tablets (6%) 2214
Focalin XR Capsules 2217
Fortical Nasal Spray (Less than 1%) 3336
Frova Tablets (Infrequent) 1101
Furosemide Tablets 2117
Fuzeon Injection (2.3%) 2772
Gabitril Tablets (1% or more) 998
Gemzar for Injection (Common) 1743
▲ Gengraf Capsules (Less than 2% to 3%) 458
Geodon (2% to frequent) 2514
▲ Gleevec Tablets (7% to 17%) 2221
Guanidine Hydrochloride Tablets 3030
▲ Havrix Vaccine (1% to 10%) 1425
▲ Hectorol Capsules (4.9%) 909
▲ Hectorol Injection (4.9%) 911
▲ Herceptin I.V. (14%) 1234
Hexalen Capsules (1%) 2101
HibTITER 3419
▲ Hycamtin for Injection (Up to 19%) 1427
Hyperstat I.V. Injection 3031
Hyzaar 1964
Indapamide Tablets (Less than 5%) 2119
Indocin (Less than 1%) 1968
▲ Infergen (21% to 24%) 1647
▲ Intron A for Injection (1% to 69%) 3038
Invanz for Injection (Greater than 0.1%) 1974
Inversine Tablets 3286
Invirase (Less than 2%) 2776
▲ Iressa Tablets (7% to 11%) 684
▲ I.V. Busulfex (21% to 85%) 1125
Kadian Capsules (Less than 3%) 572
Kaletra (Up to 2%) 474
▲ Keppra Oral Solution (3% to 13%) 3307
▲ Keppra Tablets (3% to 13%) 3307
Ketek Tablets (Greater than or equal to 0.2% to less than 2%) 2920
Klonopin 2782
Lamictal (2%) 1449
Lamisil Tablets 2226
Lanoxicaps Capsules (Common) 1458
Lanoxin Injection (Common) 1462
Lanoxin Tablets 1468

Lanoxin Injection Pediatric 1465
▲ Lariam Tablets (Among most frequent)............................... 2790
Lescol Capsules.............................. 2227
Lescol Capsules.............................. 2730
Lescol XL Tablets 2227
Lescol XL Tablets 2730
▲ Leukine (13% to 54%) 829
Levaquin in 5% Dextrose Injection (0.1% to 0.9%).............................. 2453
Levaquin (0.1% to 0.9%)................... 2453
Lexapro Oral Solution 1193
Lexapro Tablets.............................. 1193
Lipitor Tablets (Less than 2%).......... 2495
Lithobid Tablets 1670
Lofibra Capsules 1217
Lotensin HCT Tablets (0.3% to 1%).. 2235
Lunesta Tablets (Infrequent)............ 3139
Lupron Depot 7.5 mg (Less than 5%)... 3261
▲ Malarone Tablets (5%) 1484
▲ Malarone Pediatric Tablets (5%) 1484
Marinol Capsules (Less than 1%)...... 3334
Matulane Capsules 3188
Maxair Autohaler............................. 1820
Maxalt Tablets (Rare)....................... 1983
Maxalt-MLT Orally Disintegrating Tablets (Rare)............................. 1983
Maxzide.. 2150
▲ Menactra Vaccine (0.3% to 11.8%)... 2968
▲ Mepron Suspension (7%) 1487
▲ Meridia Capsules (13%) 485
Merrem I.V. (Greater than 0.1% to 1%)... 687
▲ Metadate CD Capsules (9%) 3316
Mevacor Tablets (Rare)..................... 1996
Miacalcin Nasal Spray (Less than 1%)... 2242
▲ Midamor Tablets (3% to 8%) 2000
Migranal Nasal Spray (Rare)............. 3350
Mintezol... 2002
Miradon Tablets.............................. 3056
▲ Mirapex Tablets (Greater than or equal to 1% to 4%)..................... 889
▲ Moduretic Tablets (3% to 8%) 2003
MS Contin Tablets (Less frequent).... 2703
Mustargen for Injection.................... 2007
Mycamine for Injection..................... 620
Myleran Tablets 1492
▲ Mylotarg for Injection (22% to 27%).. 3429
Nadolol Tablets (1 to 5 of 1000 patients)...................................... 2121
Nalfon Capsules (Less than 1%)....... 2504
Namenda (Greater than or equal to 2%)... 1199
▲ Navelbine Injection (Less than 46%).. 1494
Neoral Soft Gelatin Capsules (2% or less to 3%)............................. 2247
Neoral Oral Solution (2% or less to 3%)... 2247
▲ Neulasta Injection (15% to 72%) 596
▲ Neumega for Injection (Greater than or equal to 10%).................. 3433
▲ Neupogen for Injection (9%) 598
Neurontin Capsules (Frequent).......... 2498
Neurontin Oral Solution (More than 2%)... 2498
Neurontin Tablets (Frequent)............ 2498
Nexium Delayed-Release Capsules (Less than 1%)............................ 645
Nexium I.V. (Less than 1%).............. 649
▲ Nipent for Injection (13% to 16%) 3216
Niravam Orally Disintegrating Tablets 3106
Noroxin Tablets (Less frequent)........ 2009
Norvasc Tablets (More than 0.1% to 1%).. 2529
▲ Norvir (1.7% to 7.8%) 499
Omacor Capsules............................ 2735
Omnicef Capsules (0.3%).................. 506
Omnicef for Oral Suspension (0.3%).. 506
▲ Oncaspar (Greater than 1% but less than 5%).............................. 1123
▲ Ontak Vials (36%) 1717
Orap Tablets.................................. 1220
Ortho-Cyclen/Ortho Tri-Cyclen 2414
Ortho Tri-Cyclen Lo Tablets............... 2421
Orthoclone OKT3 Sterile Solution (Less than 1%)............................ 2370
▲ OxyContin Tablets (Between 1% and 5%)....................................... 2699
▲ Pacerone Tablets (4% to 9%) 3337
Parcopa Orally Disintegrating Tablets 3111
Parnate Tablets 1499
Paser Granules (Less frequent)........ 1657
▲ PCE Dispertab Tablets (Among most frequent)............................. 510
Pediarix Vaccine 1518
▲ Pegasys (17%) 2793
▲ PEG-Intron Powder for Injection (20%) 3062
Pentasa Capsules (Less than 1% to 1.1%)....................................... 3182
Pepcid Injection (Infrequent)............. 2017
Pepcid (Infrequent).......................... 2014
▲ Permax Tablets (4.8%) 3357
PhosLo GelCaps.............................. 2158
▲ Photofrin for Injection (4% to 8%) 729
Pletal Tablets (Less than 2%)........... 2478
Potaba (Infrequent).......................... 1634
Pravachol Tablets (Rare).................. 943
Prevacid Delayed-Release Capsules (Less than 1%).............. 3268
Prevacid for Delayed-Release Oral Suspension (Less than 1%)........... 3268
Prevacid NapraPAC (Less than 1%).. 3277
Prevacid SoluTab Delayed-Release Orally Disintegrating Tablets (Less than 1%)............................ 3268
PREVPAC (Less than 1%)................. 3281
Prilosec OTC Tablets (Less than 1%) 2674
Prinivil Tablets (Greater than 1%) 2029
Prinzide Tablets 2033
▲ Prograf Capsules and Injection (3% to 34%) 624
▲ Proleukin for Injection (20%) 1007
Prometrium Capsules (100 mg, 200 mg) 3205
Protonix I.V. (Less than 1%) 3468
Protonix Tablets (Less than 1%) 3465
Protopic Ointment (Greater than or equal to 1%) 629
▲ Provigil Tablets (4%) 1002
▲ Prozac Pulvules and Liquid (8% to 17%).. 1771
Pulmicort Respules (1% to 3%) 654
Purinethol Tablets (Uncommon) 1222
▲ Rapamune Oral Solution and Tablets (3% to 20%)..................... 3472
▲ Razadyne ER Extended-Release Capsules (7% to 9%) 2434
▲ Razadyne (7% to 9%) 2434
▲ Rebetol (21% to 51%) 3073
▲ Rebetron Combination Therapy (21% to 27%)............................. 3078
ReFacto Vials 3479
Relafen Tablets (Less than 1%) 1523
Relpax Tablets (Infrequent) 2531
▲ Requip Tablets (4%) 1528
Rescriptor Tablets 2535
▲ Retrovir Capsules (11% to 20.1%) .. 1533
▲ Retrovir IV Infusion (11% to 20.1%)..................................... 1537
▲ Retrovir (11% to 20.1%) 1533
Reyataz Capsules (Less than 3%) 948
▲ Ribavirin, USP Capsules (21% to 51%).. 3083
▲ Rilutek Tablets (3.8% to 8.6%) 2945
Risperdal Consta Long-Acting Injection (Infrequent) 1664
Risperdal M-Tab Orally Disintegrating Tablets (Frequent) ... 1658
Risperdal (Frequent) 1658
Ritalin Hydrochloride Tablets 2254
▲ Ritalin LA Capsules (3.1%) 2255
Ritalin-SR Tablets 2254
▲ Rituxan for Infusion (Among most frequent) 845
▲ Rituxan I.V. (1% to 5%) 1251
▲ Roferon-A Injection (14% to 48%) 2805
Rythmol SR Capsules 2736
Sandimmune (2% or less) 2259
▲ Sandostatin LAR Depot (5% to 15%) 2264
▲ Sensipar Tablets (6%) 603
Seroquel Tablets (Frequent) 691
Sonata Capsules (Less than 1% to 2%) 1686
▲ Soriatane Capsules (1% to 10%) 1028
Spectracef Tablets (0.1% to 1%) 2706
Stalevo Tablets 2270
Strattera Capsules 1784
Stromectol Tablets (0.9%) 2053
Sular Tablets (Less than or equal to 1%) 1163
Surmontil Capsules 2347
Sustiva Capsules (Less than 1% to 2%) 957
▲ Symlin Injection (0% to 17%) 608
Symmetrel (1% to 5%) 1115
Tabloid Tablets (Less frequent) 1545
Tambocor Tablets (1% to 3%) 1824
▲ Tarceva Tablets (1% to 52%) 1254
▲ Tarceva Tablets (1% to 52%) 2470
▲ Targretin Capsules (2.4% to 22.6%)....................................... 1719
▲ Tasmar Tablets (19% to 23%) 3360
▲ Taxotere Injection Concentrate (5% to 42%) 2947
Tegretol/Tegretol-XR 2278
▲ Temodar Capsules (9% to 27%) 3088
Tequin Injection (Less than 0.1%) 964
Tequin Tablets (Less than 0.1%)....... 964
Teveten Tablets (Less than 1%)........ 1707
Teveten HCT Tablets (Less than 1%)... 1710
▲ Thalomid Capsules (2.8% to 9.4%)... 979
Thioridazine Hydrochloride Tablets... 2122
Thiothixene Capsules....................... 2124
Tiazac Capsules (Less than 2%)....... 1204
Ticlid Tablets (1.0%)........................ 2813
Timolide Tablets 2056
Timoptic in Ocudose (Less frequent)...................................... 2061
Timoptic Sterile Ophthalmic Solution (Less frequent)............... 2058
Timoptic-XE Sterile Ophthalmic Gel Forming Solution 2062
Tindamax (1.5% to 2.5%)................. 2670
▲ TOBI Solution for Inhalation (18.6%)...................................... 1015
▲ Topamax Sprinkle Capsules (4% to 24%) 2438
▲ Topamax Tablets (4% to 24%) 2438
Trecator Tablets 3482
Trelstar LA Suspension (1.7%) 3387
Tricor Tablets 523
Triglide Tablets 1165
▲ Trileptal Oral Suspension (3% to 5%) 2281
▲ Trileptal Tablets (3% to 5%) 2281
▲ Trisenox Injection (23%) 983
▲ Trizivir Tablets (15%) 1565
Truvada Tablets 1279
Twinrix Vaccine (Less than 1%) 1571
Tygacil for Injection (0.2% to less than 2%) 3489
▲ Ultracet Tablets (3%) 2462
Uniretic Tablets (Less than 1%) 3114
Valtrex Caplets (Less than 1% to 2%) 1573
Vantin Tablets and Oral Suspension (Less than 1%) 2650
Vaqta (1.2%) 2067
Vaseretic Tablets 2073
Vasotec I.V. Injection (0.5% to 1.0%)... 2076
▲ Velcade for Injection (34%) 2102
▲ Vesanoid Capsules (17%) 2823
VFEND I.V. (Less than 2%) 2543
VFEND Oral Suspension (Less than 2%) 2543
VFEND Tablets (Less than 2%) 2543
Vicoprofen Tablets (Less than 3%) ... 533
Viracept (Less than 2%) 2556
▲ Viread Tablets (3% to 4%) 1284
Vivactil Tablets 2350
Vytorin 10/10 Tablets 2084
Vytorin 10/10 Tablets 3092
Vytorin 10/20 Tablets 2084
Vytorin 10/20 Tablets 3092
Vytorin 10/40 Tablets 2084
Vytorin 10/40 Tablets 3092
Vytorin 10/80 Tablets 2084
Vytorin 10/80 Tablets 3092
▲ Wellbutrin Tablets (18.3%) 1579
▲ Wellbutrin SR Sustained-Release Tablets (3% to greater than or equal to 5%) 1583
▲ Wellbutrin XL Extended-Release Tablets (3% to greater than or equal to 5%) 1588
Xanax XR Tablets (1.5%) 2655
▲ Xeloda Tablets (1% to 13%) 2825
Xifaxan Tablets (Less than 2%) 2847
▲ Zavesca Capsules (7%) 543
Zegerid Powder for Oral Solution (Less than 1%) 2972
▲ Zerit (19%) 971
Zestoretic Tablets 701
Zestril Tablets (Greater than 1%) 704
▲ Zevalin Injection (8%) 848
▲ Zinecard for Injection (27% to 42%) 2659
Zithromax Capsules, 250 mg (1% or less) 2568
Zithromax for IV Infusion (1.9%) 2573
Zithromax for Oral Suspension, 300 mg, 600 mg, 900 mg, 1200 mg (1% or less) 2561
Zithromax Tablets, 250 mg, 500 mg (1% or less) 2561
Zithromax Tri-Pak (1% or less) 2561
Zmax for Oral Suspension 2577
Zocor Tablets 2078
Zoladex (1% to 5%) 709
Zoladex 3-month 712
▲ Zoloft (3% to 11%) 2581
▲ Zometa for Intravenous Infusion (9.3% to 22%) 2306
Zomig Tablets (Rare) 714
Zomig-ZMT Tablets (Rare) 714
▲ Zonegran Capsules (13%) 1089
Zovirax for Injection (Less than 1%) 1618
▲ Zyban Sustained-Release Tablets (1% to 3%)................................ 1620
Zyprexa Tablets 1798
Zyprexa ZYDIS Orally Disintegrating Tablets 1798
Zyrtec Chewable Tablets (Less than 2%)...................................... 2589
Zyrtec (Less than 2%)...................... 2589
Zyrtec-D 12 Hour Extended Release Tablets (Less than 2%)..... 2591

Anorgasmia

Abilify Tablets (Rare)........................ 916
Abilify Tablets (Rare) 2472
▲ Depo-Provera Contraceptive Injection (1% to 5%)...................... 2619
▲ Duragesic Transdermal System (4%)... 2448
Effexor Tablets 3405
▲ Effexor XR Capsules (3% to 17%) 3411
Eldepryl Capsules 3209
Geodon Capsules (Infrequent).......... 2514
Lamictal (Rare)............................... 1449
▲ Lexapro Oral Solution (2% to 6%) 1193
▲ Lexapro Tablets (2% to 6%) 1193
Lyrica Capsules (Greater than or equal to 1%) 2524
Neurontin Capsules (Infrequent)....... 2498
Neurontin Oral Solution (Infrequent)................................... 2498
Neurontin Tablets (Infrequent).......... 2498
▲ Paxil CR Controlled-Release Tablets (2% to 10.0%).................. 1509
▲ Paxil (2% to 10.0%) 1501
Prozac Pulvules and Liquid (Infrequent)................................... 1771
Risperdal M-Tab Orally Disintegrating Tablets (Frequent)... 1658
Risperdal (Frequent)......................... 1658
▲ Symbyax Capsules (1% to 3%) 1788
Viagra Tablets (Less than 2%).......... 2552

Anosmia

▲ Aerobid/Aerobid-M (3% to 9%) 1172
Beconase AQ Nasal Spray (Rare)..... 1359
Cipro I.V. (1% or less)..................... 2998
Cipro I.V. Pharmacy Bulk Package (1% or less)................................ 3509
Cipro... 2991
Cipro XR Tablets 3004
Cytovene.. 2763
Flonase Nasal Spray....................... 1412
Rhinocort Aqua Nasal Spray (Rare)... 658
Vaseretic Tablets 2073
Vasotec I.V. Injection (0.5% to 1.0%)... 2076

Anotia

Thalomid Capsules.......................... 979

Anotia, fetal

Accutane Capsules.......................... 2740

Anovulation, prolonged

depo-subQ provera 104 Injectable Suspension 2622

Antibodies, development of

NovoLog Injection........................... 2326

Anticholinergic syndrome

Clozapine Tablets 2141
Clozaril Tablets 2174
Diprivan Injectable Emulsion (Less than 1%).................................. 676

Antidiuretic effect

Dilaudid... 439
Dilaudid Non-Sterile Powder............. 439
Dilaudid Rectal Suppositories........... 439
Dilaudid Tablets.............................. 439
Dilaudid-HP (Less frequent).............. 441
MS Contin Tablets (Less frequent).... 2703
Risperdal M-Tab Orally Disintegrating Tablets (Rare)......... 1658
Risperdal (Rare).............................. 1658

Antisocial reaction

Prozac Pulvules and Liquid (Rare)..... 1771
Zyprexa Tablets (Infrequent)............. 1798
Zyprexa ZYDIS Orally Disintegrating Tablets (Infrequent).................................. 1798

Antithrombin, decrease

Estratest Tablets 3196
Estratest H.S. Tablets...................... 3196
Oncaspar 1123
Ortho-Cyclen/Ortho Tri-Cyclen 2414
Premarin Tablets............................. 3443

Anuria

Abelcet Injection............................. 1119
Ammonul Injection.......................... 3323

Campath Ampules ... 826
Carimune NF ... 3501
CytoGam Intravenous ... 1866
Effexor Tablets (Rare) ... 3405
Effexor XR Capsules (Rare) ... 3411
Gammagard S/D (Some patients) ... 754
Invanz for Injection (Greater than 0.1%) ... 1974
Iveegam EN (0.3% to 0.8%) ... 759
Miradon Tablets ... 3056
Mycamine for Injection ... 620
Nalfon Capsules (Less than 1%) ... 2504
Neurontin Capsules (Rare) ... 2498
Neurontin Oral Solution (Rare) ... 2498
Neurontin Tablets (Rare) ... 2498
Orthoclone OKT3 Sterile Solution (Less than 1%) ... 2370
Primaxin I.M. ... 2022
Primaxin I.V. (2.2%) ... 2024
Prinivil Tablets (0.3% to 1.0%) ... 2029
Prinzide Tablets ... 2033
▲ Proleukin for Injection (5%) ... 1007
VFEND I.V. (Less than 2%) ... 2543
VFEND Oral Suspension (Less than 2%) ... 2543
VFEND Tablets (Less than 2%) ... 2543
Zestoretic Tablets ... 701
Zestril Tablets (0.3% to 1.0%) ... 704
Zovirax for Injection (Less than 1%) ... 1618

Anuria, neonatal

Aceon Tablets (2 mg, 4 mg, 8 mg) ... 3191
Altace Capsules ... 1673
Avapro Tablets ... 925
Avapro Tablets ... 2886
Captopril Tablets ... 2114
Cozaar Tablets ... 1913
Hyzaar ... 1964
Lotrel Capsules ... 2238
Prinivil Tablets ... 2029
Prinzide Tablets ... 2033
Vaseretic Tablets ... 2073
Vasotec I.V. Injection ... 2076
Zestoretic Tablets ... 701
Zestril Tablets ... 704

Anxiety

▲ Abilify Tablets (20%) ... 916
▲ Abilify Tablets (20%) ... 2472
Aceon Tablets (2 mg, 4 mg, 8 mg) (0.3% to 1%) ... 3191
Aciphex Tablets ... 1081
▲ Actonel Tablets (0.6% to 4.3%) ... 2679
▲ Actonel with Calcium Tablets (0.6% to 4.7%) ... 2684
Adalat CC Tablets (Less than 1%) ... 2978
▲ Adderall XR Capsules (8%) ... 3169
Advicor Tablets ... 1694
Aerobid/Aerobid-M (1% to 3%) ... 1172
Allegra-D 12 Hour Extended-Release Tablets (1.4%) ... 2860
Allegra-D 24 Hour Extended-Release Tablets (1.4%) ... 2862
Aloxi Injection (1%) ... 2099
Altace Capsules (Less than 1%) ... 1673
Altoprev Extended-Release Tablets ... 1151
Ambien Tablets (1%) ... 2867
▲ AmBisome for Injection (7.4% to 13.7%) ... 615
Amerge Tablets (Infrequent) ... 1312
Amoxil Capsules (Rare) ... 1315
Amoxil Chewable Tablets (Rare) ... 1315
Amoxil Pediatric Drops for Oral Suspension (Rare) ... 1315
Amoxil Powder for Oral Suspension (Rare) ... 1315
Amoxil Tablets (Rare) ... 1315
Anaprox Tablets (Less than 1%) ... 2769
Anaprox DS Tablets (Less than 1%) ... 2769
AndroGel (Fewer than 1%) ... 3330
▲ Angiomax for Injection (6%) ... 1856
Antara Capsules ... 2723
Anzemet Injection (Infrequently) ... 2871
Anzemet Tablets (Infrequently) ... 2874
▲ Apokyn Injection (At least 5%) ... 2132
▲ Arava Tablets (1% to 3%) ... 2881
▲ Aredia for Injection (14.3%) ... 2168
▲ Arimidex Tablets (2% to 5%) ... 665
Arixtra Injection (0.8%) ... 1325
▲ Aromasin Tablets (10%) ... 2600
Arthrotec Tablets (Rare) ... 3126
Asacol Delayed-Release Tablets (2% or greater) ... 2688
Astelin Nasal Spray (Infrequent) ... 1876
Atacand Tablets (0.5% or greater) ... 634
Atacand HCT (0.5% or greater) ... 637
Augmentin (Rare) ... 1331
Augmentin Tablets (Rare) ... 1334
Augmentin XR Extended-Release Tablets (Rare) ... 1340
Augmentin ES-600 Powder for Oral Suspension (Rare) ... 1337
Avalide Tablets (1% or greater) ... 922
Avalide Tablets (1% or greater) ... 2889
Avapro Tablets (Less than 1%) ... 925
Avapro Tablets (Less than 1%) ... 2886
Avelox (0.1% to less than 2%) ... 2984
Avinza Capsules (Less than 5%) ... 1714
Axert Tablets (Infrequent) ... 2430
Axid Oral Solution (1.8%) ... 913
▲ Betaseron for SC Injection (10%) ... 791
Biaxin/Biaxin XL ... 402
▲ Botox Purified Neurotoxin Complex (3% to 10%) ... 565
Brevibloc Concentrate (Less than 1%) ... 766
Brevibloc Injection (Less than 1%) ... 766
Brevibloc Double Strength Injection (Less than 1%) ... 766
Brevibloc Premixed Injection (Less than 1%) ... 766
Brevibloc Double Strength Premixed Injection (Less than 1%) ... 766
Brimonidine Tartrate Ophthalmic Solution 0.2% (Less than 3%) ... ⊙ 245
Caduet Tablets (Greater than 0.1% to less than or equal to 1%) ... 2507
Campral Tablets (5% to 8%) ... 1175
Carnitor Injection (1% to 2%) ... 3185
▲ Casodex Tablets (2% to 5%) ... 670
Cataflam Tablets (Occasionally) ... 2173
Catapres Tablets ... 874
Catapres-TTS (0.5% or less) ... 875
Celebrex Capsules (0.1% to 1.9%) ... 3130
▲ Celexa (4%) ... 1177
▲ CellCept Capsules (3% to 28.4%) ... 2751
▲ CellCept Intravenous (3% to 28.4%) ... 2751
▲ CellCept Oral Suspension (3% to 28.4%) ... 2751
▲ CellCept Tablets (3% to 28.4%) ... 2751
▲ Cenestin Tablets, 0.45mg, 0.625mg, 0.9mg, 1.25mg (5.7%) ... 1063
Cipro I.V. (1% or less) ... 2998
Cipro I.V. Pharmacy Bulk Package (1% or less) ... 3509
Cipro ... 2991
Cipro XR Tablets ... 3004
Clindesse Vaginal Cream (Less than 1%) ... 3296
▲ Clolar for Intravenous Infusion (22%) ... 1264
Clorpres Tablets ... 2139
Clozapine Tablets (1%) ... 2141
Clozaril Tablets (1%) ... 2174
Colazal Capsules ... 2845
Combunox Tablets (Less than 2%) ... 1183
Comtan Tablets (2%) ... 2186
▲ Copaxone for Injection (23%) ... 3292
▲ Copegus Tablets (33%) ... 2759
Cosopt Sterile Ophthalmic Solution ... 1910
Cozaar Tablets (Less than 1%) ... 1913
Crestor Tablets (Greater than or equal to 1%) ... 672
Crixivan Capsules (Less than 2%) ... 1918
Cubicin for Injection (1% to 2%) ... 1038
Cuprimine Capsules ... 1925
▲ Cymbalta Delayed-Release Capsules (3%) ... 1729
Cytovene (At least 3 subjects) ... 2763
▲ DAPTACEL (23.6% to 39.6%) ... 2964
Delatestryl Injection ... 2976
Demser Capsules ... 1933
▲ Depacon Injection (1% to 5%) ... 412
▲ Depakene (1% to 5%) ... 417
▲ Depakote Sprinkle Capsules (1% to 5%) ... 422
▲ Depakote Tablets (1% to 5%) ... 427
▲ Depakote ER Tablets (1% to 5%) ... 433
▲ DepoDur Extended-Release Injection (2% to 5%) ... 1098
▲ depo-subQ provera 104 Injectable Suspension (1% to less than 5%) ... 2622
Detrol LA Capsules (1%) ... 2629
Digitek Tablets ... 2146
Dilaudid ... 439
Dilaudid Non-Sterile Powder ... 439
Dilaudid Rectal Suppositories ... 439
Dilaudid Tablets ... 439
Diovan HCT Tablets (Greater than 0.2%) ... 2195
Diovan Tablets ... 2191
Diprivan Injectable Emulsion (Less than 1%) ... 676
▲ Dostinex Tablets (1% to less than 10%) ... 2631
▲ Doxil Injection (Less than 1% to 10%) ... 3302
▲ Duragesic Transdermal System (3% to 10%) ... 2448
EC-Naprosyn Delayed-Release Tablets (Less than 1%) ... 2769
▲ Effexor Tablets (2% to 11.2%) ... 3405
Effexor XR Capsules (1%) ... 3411
Eldepryl Capsules (1 of 49 patients) ... 3209
▲ Eloxatin for Injection (2% to 5%) ... 2908
Emcyt Capsules (1%) ... 3137
Emend Capsules (Greater than 0.5%) ... 1944
EpiPen ... 1061
▲ Epogen for Injection (2% to 7%) ... 586
▲ Epzicom Tablets (3% to 5%) ... 1402
▲ Equetro Extended-Release Capsules (7%) ... 3178
Estratest Tablets ... 3196
Estratest H.S. Tablets ... 3196
Estrogel 0.06% (1.8%) ... 3200
Eulexin Capsules (1%) ... 3023
Evoxac Capsules (1.3%) ... 1042
▲ Exelon Capsules (5%) ... 2204
▲ Fabrazyme for Intravenous Infusion (8%) ... 1267
▲ Faslodex Injection (5%) ... 682
FazaClo Orally Disintegrating Tablets (1%) ... 547
Femara Tablets (Less frequent) ... 2210
Flexeril Tablets (Less than 1%) ... 1832
▲ Flolan for Injection (7% to 21%) ... 1408
▲ Focalin XR Capsules (5% to 11%) ... 2217
Foradil Aerolizer (1.5%) ... 3024
Fortical Nasal Spray (Less than 1%) ... 3336
Frova Tablets (Frequent) ... 1101
Fuzeon Injection ... 2772
Gabitril Tablets (1% or more) ... 998
Gengraf Capsules (1% to less than 3%) ... 458
▲ Geodon (5%) ... 2514
▲ Gleevec Tablets (8% to 12%) ... 2221
Hycodan ... 1104
Hycomine Compound Tablets ... 1105
Hycotuss Expectorant Syrup ... 1106
Hyperstat I.V. Injection ... 3031
Hytrin Capsules (At least 1%) ... 469
Hyzaar ... 1964
▲ Imdur Tablets (Less than or equal to 5%) ... 3032
Imitrex Injection (1.1%) ... 1431
Imitrex Nasal Spray (Infrequent) ... 1435
Imitrex Tablets ... 1440
▲ Indapamide Tablets (Greater than or equal to 5%) ... 2119
Indocin (Less than 1%) ... 1968
▲ Infanrix Vaccine (3.3% to 9.2%) ... 1444
▲ Infergen (10% to 19%) ... 1647
▲ Intron A for Injection (Up to 5%) ... 3038
Invanz for Injection (0.8% to 1.1%) ... 1974
Invirase (Greater than or equal to 2%) ... 2776
▲ I.V. Busulfex (72% to 75%) ... 1125
▲ Kadian Capsules (Less than 3% to 6%) ... 572
Kaletra (Less than 2%) ... 474
Keppra Oral Solution (2%) ... 3307
Keppra Tablets (2%) ... 3307
Ketek Tablets (Less than 0.2%) ... 2920
Klonopin (Infrequent) ... 2782
Kytril Injection (Less than 2%) ... 2785
Kytril Tablets (2%) ... 2788
▲ Lamictal (3.8%) ... 1449
Lanoxicaps Capsules ... 1458
Lanoxin Injection ... 1462
Lanoxin Tablets ... 1468
Lanoxin Injection Pediatric ... 1465
Lariam Tablets (Occasional) ... 2790
Lescol Capsules ... 2227
Lescol Capsules ... 2730
Lescol XL Tablets ... 2227
Lescol XL Tablets ... 2730
▲ Leukine (11%) ... 829
Levaquin in 5% Dextrose Injection (1.2%) ... 2453
Levaquin (1.2%) ... 2453
Levothroid Tablets ... 1189
Levoxyl Tablets ... 1680
Lexapro Oral Solution (At least 2%) ... 1193
Lexapro Tablets (At least 2%) ... 1193
Lofibra Capsules ... 1217
Lortab ... 3315
Lortab Elixir ... 3312
Lotensin Tablets (Less than 1%) ... 2232
Lotrel Capsules ... 2238
Lotronex Tablets (Infrequent) ... 1479
Lunesta Tablets (Infrequent) ... 3139
▲ Lupron Depot 3.75 mg (3%) ... 3257
▲ Lupron Depot–3 Month 11.25 mg (3%) ... 3262
Lyrica Capsules (Greater than or equal to 1%) ... 2524
Malarone Tablets (Less than 1%) ... 1484
Malarone Pediatric Tablets (Less than 1%) ... 1484
Marinol Capsules (Greater than 1%) ... 3334
Mavik Tablets (0.3% to 1.0%) ... 482
Maxair Autohaler ... 1820
Maxalt Tablets (Infrequent) ... 1983
Maxalt-MLT Orally Disintegrating Tablets (Infrequent) ... 1983
Maxzide ... 2150
Mebaral Tablets, USP (Less than 1 in 100 patients) ... 2483
▲ Mepron Suspension (7%) ... 1487
▲ Meridia Capsules (4.5%) ... 485
Merrem I.V. (Greater than 0.1% to 1%) ... 687
Mevacor Tablets (0.5% to 1.0%) ... 1996
Miacalcin Nasal Spray (Less than 1%) ... 2242
Micardis Tablets (More than 0.3%) ... 884
Micardis HCT Tablets ... 886
Migranal Nasal Spray (Rare) ... 3350
Mirapex Tablets (1% or more) ... 889
Mobic Oral Suspension (Less than 2%) ... 893
Mobic Tablets (Less than 2%) ... 893
▲ Myfortic Tablets (3% to less than 20%) ... 2244
▲ Mylotarg for Injection (7% to 10%) ... 3429
Namenda (Greater than or equal to 2%) ... 1199
Naprosyn Suspension (Less than 1%) ... 2769
Naprosyn Tablets (Less than 1%) ... 2769
▲ Naropin Injection (1% to 5%) ... 640
▲ Natrecor for Injection (2% to 3%) ... 3123
Nembutal Sodium Solution, USP (Less than 1%) ... 2484
Neoral Soft Gelatin Capsules (1% to less than 3%) ... 2247
Neoral Oral Solution (1% to less than 3%) ... 2247
Neurontin Capsules (Frequent) ... 2498
Neurontin Oral Solution (Frequent) ... 2498
Neurontin Tablets (Frequent) ... 2498
▲ Nicotrol Inhaler (Greater than 3%) ... 2594
▲ Nicotrol NS (Greater than 5%) ... 2596
▲ Nipent for Injection (3% to 10%) ... 3216
▲ Niravam Orally Disintegrating Tablets (16.6% to 19.2%) ... 3106
Noroxin Tablets (Less frequent) ... 2009
Norvasc Tablets (More than 0.1% to 1%) ... 2529
Norvir (0 to 1.7%) ... 499
OptiPranolol Metipranolol Ophthalmic Solution 0.3% (A small number of patients) ... ⊙ 254
▲ OxyContin Tablets (Between 1% and 5%) ... 2699
Parcopa Orally Disintegrating Tablets ... 3111
Parnate Tablets ... 1499
▲ Paxil CR Controlled-Release Tablets (1% to 5.9%) ... 1509
▲ Paxil (1% to 5.9%) ... 1501
▲ Pegasys (19%) ... 2793
▲ PEG-Intron Powder for Injection (28%) ... 3062
Pepcid Injection (Infrequent) ... 2017
Pepcid (Infrequent) ... 2014
▲ Permax Tablets (6.4%) ... 3357
▲ Photofrin for Injection (3% to 7%) ... 729
Plavix Tablets (1% to 2.5%) ... 940
Plavix Tablets (1% to 2.5%) ... 2942
Plendil Extended-Release Tablets (0.5% to 1.5%) ... 651
Pletal Tablets (Less than 2%) ... 2478
Pravachol Tablets ... 943
▲ Premphase Tablets (2% to 5%) ... 3452
▲ Prempro Tablets (2% to 5%) ... 3452
Prevacid Delayed-Release Capsules (Less than 1%) ... 3268
Prevacid for Delayed-Release Oral Suspension (Less than 1%) ... 3268
Prevacid NapraPAC (Less than 1%) ... 3277
Prevacid SoluTab Delayed-Release Orally Disintegrating Tablets (Less than 1%) ... 3268
PREVPAC (Less than 1%) ... 3281
Prilosec OTC Tablets (Less than 1%) ... 2674
ProAmatine Tablets (Less frequent) ... 3183
▲ Procrit for Injection (2% to 11%) ... 2374
▲ Prograf Capsules and Injection (3% to 15%) ... 624
▲ Proleukin for Injection (12%) ... 1007
Prometrium Capsules (100 mg, 200 mg) (Less than 5%) ... 3205
ProSom Tablets (Frequent) ... 512
Protonix I.V. (Greater than or equal to 1%) ... 3468
Protonix Tablets (Greater than or equal to 1%) ... 3465
Proventil HFA Inhalation Aerosol (Less than 3%) ... 3071
▲ Provigil Tablets (5%) ... 1002

▲ Prozac Pulvules and Liquid (4% to 17%) ... 1771
Pulmicort Respules (Less than 1%) ... 654
▲ Rapamune Oral Solution and Tablets (3% to 20%) ... 3472
Razadyne ER Extended-Release Capsules (Greater than or equal to 2%) ... 2434
Razadyne (Greater than or equal to 2%) ... 2434
▲ Rebetol (47%) ... 3073
Relafen Tablets (Less than 1%) ... 1523
Relpax Tablets (Infrequent) ... 2531
ReoPro Vials (1.7%) ... 1779
Requip Tablets (1% or more) ... 1528
▲ Rescriptor Tablets (2.4% to 6.7%) ... 2535
Retrovir Capsules ... 1533
Retrovir IV Infusion ... 1537
Retrovir ... 1533
Reyataz Capsules (Less than 3%) ... 948
▲ Ribavirin, USP Capsules (47%) ... 3083
Risperdal Consta Long-Acting Injection (Frequent) ... 1664
▲ Risperdal M-Tab Orally Disintegrating Tablets (4% to 20%) ... 1658
▲ Risperdal (4% to 20%) ... 1658
▲ Rituxan I.V. (5%) ... 1251
▲ Roferon-A Injection (5% to 6%) ... 2805
▲ Rythmol SR Capsules (10% to 13%) ... 2736
Sandimmune (Rare) ... 2259
Sandostatin Injection (Less than 1%) ... 2263
▲ Sandostatin LAR Depot (5% to 15%) ... 2264
Serevent Diskus (1% to 3%) ... 1540
▲ Seroquel Tablets (4%) ... 691
▲ Simulect for Injection (3% to 10%) ... 2268
Sonata Capsules (Frequent) ... 1686
Soriatane Capsules (Less than 1%) ... 1028
Stalevo Tablets (2%) ... 2270
Striant Mucoadhesive ... 1022
▲ Suboxone Tablets (12%) ... 2719
▲ Subutex Tablets (12%) ... 2719
Sular Tablets (Less than or equal to 1%) ... 1163
Surmontil Capsules ... 2347
▲ Sustiva Capsules (2% to 13%) ... 957
Symbyax Capsules ... 1788
Symmetrel (1% to 5%) ... 1115
Synercid I.V. (Less than 1%) ... 1690
Tagamet Tablets ... 1547
Tambocor Tablets (1% to 3%) ... 1824
Tarka Tablets (0.3% or more) ... 519
Tasmar Tablets (1% or more) ... 3360
▲ Temodar Capsules (7%) ... 3088
Tequin Injection (Less than 0.1%) ... 964
Tequin Tablets (Less than 0.1%) ... 964
Teveten Tablets (Less than 1%) ... 1707
Teveten HCT Tablets (Less than 1%) ... 1710
Thalomid Capsules ... 979
Thyrolar ... 1203
Timoptic in Ocudose (Less frequent) ... 2061
Timoptic Sterile Ophthalmic Solution (Less frequent) ... 2058
Timoptic-XE Sterile Ophthalmic Gel Forming Solution ... 2062
▲ Topamax Sprinkle Capsules (4% to 24%) ... 2438
▲ Topamax Tablets (4% to 24%) ... 2438
Toprol-XL Tablets ... 660
Trasylol Injection (1% to 2%) ... 779
Travatan Ophthalmic Solution (1% to 5%) ... 559
Tricor Tablets ... 523
▲ Trileptal Oral Suspension (5% to 7%) ... 2281
▲ Trileptal Tablets (5% to 7%) ... 2281
▲ Trisenox Injection (30%) ... 983
Tussionex Pennkinetic Extended-Release Suspension ... 3322
Ultracet Tablets (At least 1%) ... 2462
Uniretic Tablets (Less than 1%) ... 3114
Unithroid Tablets ... 3521
Univasc Tablets (Less than 1%) ... 3118
Vantin Tablets and Oral Suspension (Less than 1%) ... 2650
▲ Velcade for Injection (14%) ... 2102
▲ Vesanoid Capsules (17%) ... 2823
VFEND I.V. (Less than 2%) ... 2543
VFEND Oral Suspension (Less than 2%) ... 2543
VFEND Tablets (Less than 2%) ... 2543
Viadur Implant (Less than 2%) ... 782
Viagra Tablets ... 2552
Vicodin Tablets ... 530
Vicodin ES Tablets ... 531
Vicodin HP Tablets ... 532
▲ Vicoprofen Tablets (3% to 9%) ... 533
Viracept (Less than 2%) ... 2556
Vivactil Tablets ... 2350
Vivelle-Dot Transdermal System ... 2293
Voltaren Tablets (Occasionally) ... 2298
Voltaren-XR Tablets (Occasionally) ... 2301
Vytorin 10/10 Tablets ... 2084
Vytorin 10/10 Tablets ... 3092
Vytorin 10/20 Tablets ... 2084
Vytorin 10/20 Tablets ... 3092
Vytorin 10/40 Tablets ... 2084
Vytorin 10/40 Tablets ... 3092
Vytorin 10/80 Tablets ... 2084
Vytorin 10/80 Tablets ... 3092
▲ Wellbutrin Tablets (3.1%) ... 1579
▲ Wellbutrin SR Sustained-Release Tablets (5% to 6%) ... 1583
▲ Wellbutrin XL Extended-Release Tablets (5% to 6%) ... 1588
▲ Xanax XR Tablets (1.1% to 7.8%) ... 2655
▲ Xenical Capsules (2.8% to 4.4%) ... 2834
Xopenex HFA Inhalation Aerosol (2.7%) ... 3151
Xopenex Inhalation Solution (2.7%) ... 3143
Xopenex Inhalation Solution Concentrate (2.7%) ... 3147
Zegerid Powder for Oral Solution (Less than 1%) ... 2972
▲ Zenapax for Injection (2% to 5%) ... 2838
▲ Zevalin Injection (4%) ... 848
▲ Ziagen (5%) ... 1600
Zmax for Oral Suspension ... 2577
Zocor Tablets ... 2078
▲ Zofran Injection (2% to 6%) ... 1607
▲ Zofran (6%) ... 1613
▲ Zofran ODT Orally Disintegrating Tablets (6%) ... 1613
Zoladex (1% to 5%) ... 709
Zoladex 3-month ... 712
▲ Zoloft (4%) ... 2581
▲ Zometa for Intravenous Infusion (11% to 14%) ... 2306
Zomig Nasal Spray (Infrequent) ... 718
Zomig Tablets (Infrequent) ... 714
Zomig-ZMT Tablets (Infrequent) ... 714
▲ Zonegran Capsules (3%) ... 1089
▲ Zosyn (1.2% to 3.2%) ... 3492
▲ Zyban Sustained-Release Tablets (8%) ... 1620
Zydone Tablets ... 1118
▲ Zyprexa Tablets (9%) ... 1798
▲ Zyprexa ZYDIS Orally Disintegrating Tablets (9%) ... 1798
Zyrtec Chewable Tablets (Less than 2%) ... 2589
Zyrtec (Less than 2%) ... 2589
Zyrtec-D 12 Hour Extended Release Tablets (Less than 2%) ... 2591

Anxiety, paradoxical

Diastat Rectal Delivery System ... 3344
Valium Tablets ... 2822
Vivactil Tablets ... 2350

Apathy

Abilify Tablets (Infrequent) ... 916
Abilify Tablets (Infrequent) ... 2472
Ambien Tablets (Rare) ... 2867
Caduet Tablets (Less than or equal to 0.1%) ... 2507
Campath Ampules ... 826
Campral Tablets (Infrequent) ... 1175
Celexa (Infrequent) ... 1177
Digitek Tablets ... 2146
Effexor Tablets (Infrequent) ... 3405
Effexor XR Capsules (Infrequent) ... 3411
Eldepryl Capsules ... 3209
Evoxac Capsules ... 1042
Exelon Capsules (Infrequent) ... 2204
Gabitril Tablets (Infrequent) ... 998
Hectorol Capsules ... 909
Hectorol Injection ... 911
Imitrex Injection ... 1431
Imitrex Nasal Spray (Rare) ... 1435
Imitrex Tablets (Rare) ... 1440
▲ Intron A for Injection (Less than 5%) ... 3038
Kadian Capsules (Less than 3%) ... 572
Keppra Oral Solution ... 3307
Keppra Tablets ... 3307
Klonopin (Infrequent) ... 2782
Lamictal (Infrequent) ... 1449
Lanoxicaps Capsules ... 1458
Lanoxin Injection ... 1462
Lanoxin Tablets ... 1468
Lanoxin Injection Pediatric ... 1465
Lexapro Oral Solution (Infrequent) ... 1193
Lexapro Tablets (Infrequent) ... 1193
Lunesta Tablets ... 3139
Lyrica Capsules (0.1% to 1%) ... 2524
Mirapex Tablets (1% or more) ... 889
Namenda (Infrequent) ... 1199
Neurontin Capsules (Infrequent) ... 2498
Neurontin Oral Solution (Infrequent) ... 2498
Neurontin Tablets (Infrequent) ... 2498
Nexium Delayed-Release Capsules (Less than 1%) ... 645
Nexium I.V. (Less than 1%) ... 649
▲ Nicotrol NS (Less than 5%) ... 2596
Norvasc Tablets (Less than or equal to 0.1%) ... 2529
Permax Tablets (Infrequent) ... 3357
Prevacid Delayed-Release Capsules (Less than 1%) ... 3268
Prevacid for Delayed-Release Oral Suspension (Less than 1%) ... 3268
Prevacid NapraPAC (Less than 1%) ... 3277
Prevacid SoluTab Delayed-Release Orally Disintegrating Tablets (Less than 1%) ... 3268
PREVPAC (Less than 1%) ... 3281
Prilosec OTC Tablets (Less than 1%) ... 2674
ProSom Tablets (Infrequent) ... 512
Prozac Pulvules and Liquid (Infrequent) ... 1771
Razadyne ER Extended-Release Capsules (Infrequent) ... 2434
Razadyne (Infrequent) ... 2434
Relpax Tablets (Infrequent) ... 2531
Requip Tablets (Infrequent) ... 1528
Rilutek Tablets (Infrequent) ... 2945
Risperdal Consta Long-Acting Injection (Frequent) ... 1664
Risperdal M-Tab Orally Disintegrating Tablets (Infrequent) ... 1658
Risperdal (Infrequent) ... 1658
Roferon-A Injection (Infrequent) ... 2805
Seroquel Tablets (Infrequent) ... 691
Sonata Capsules (Frequent) ... 1686
Sustiva Capsules (Less than 2%) ... 957
Tambocor Tablets (Less than 1%) ... 1824
Tasmar Tablets (Infrequent) ... 3360
▲ Topamax Sprinkle Capsules (1% to 3%) ... 2438
▲ Topamax Tablets (1% to 3%) ... 2438
Trileptal Oral Suspension ... 2281
Trileptal Tablets ... 2281
Xanax XR Tablets (Infrequent) ... 2655
Zegerid Powder for Oral Solution (Less than 1%) ... 2972
Zoloft (Infrequent) ... 2581
Zomig Nasal Spray (Rare) ... 718
Zomig Tablets (Rare) ... 714
Zomig-ZMT Tablets (Rare) ... 714
Zyprexa Tablets ... 1798
Zyprexa ZYDIS Orally Disintegrating Tablets ... 1798

Aphasia

Amerge Tablets (Rare) ... 1312
Aricept Tablets (Frequent) ... 1086
Aricept ODT Tablets (Frequent) ... 1086
Avelox (Less than 0.1%) ... 2984
Campath Ampules ... 826
Colazal Capsules ... 2845
Duragesic Transdermal System (Less than 1%) ... 2448
Effexor Tablets (Rare) ... 3405
Effexor XR Capsules (Rare) ... 3411
Evoxac Capsules ... 1042
Exelon Capsules (Infrequent) ... 2204
▲ Intron A for Injection (Less than 5%) ... 3038
Lamictal (Infrequent) ... 1449
Lyrica Capsules (0.1% to 1%) ... 2524
Namenda (Infrequent) ... 1199
Neurontin Capsules (Infrequent) ... 2498
Neurontin Oral Solution (Infrequent) ... 2498
Neurontin Tablets (Infrequent) ... 2498
Nicotrol NS (Less than 1%) ... 2596
Norvir (Less than 2%) ... 499
Orthoclone OKT3 Sterile Solution (Less than 1%) ... 2370
Paxil CR Controlled-Release Tablets (Rare) ... 1509
Paxil (Rare) ... 1501
Razadyne ER Extended-Release Capsules (Infrequent) ... 2434
Razadyne (Infrequent) ... 2434
Relpax Tablets (Rare) ... 2531
Requip Tablets (Infrequent) ... 1528
Risperdal M-Tab Orally Disintegrating Tablets (Rare) ... 1658
Risperdal (Rare) ... 1658
Roferon-A Injection (Infrequent) ... 2805
Sandostatin LAR Depot (Rare) ... 2264
Seroquel Tablets (Rare) ... 691
Symbyax Capsules (Rare) ... 1788
Trileptal Oral Suspension ... 2281
Trileptal Tablets ... 2281
▲ Vesanoid Capsules (3%) ... 2823
Wellbutrin Tablets (Rare) ... 1579
Wellbutrin SR Sustained-Release Tablets ... 1583
Wellbutrin XL Extended-Release Tablets ... 1588
Zyban Sustained-Release Tablets ... 1620

Aphonia

Advair Diskus 100/50 ... 1291
Advair Diskus 250/50 ... 1291
Advair Diskus 500/50 ... 1291
Flovent Diskus 50 mcg ... 1415
Flovent HFA ... 1418
Klonopin ... 2782
Migranal Nasal Spray (Rare) ... 3350
Roferon-A Injection (Infrequent) ... 2805

Aphthous stomatitis

(*see under* Stomatitis, ulcerative)

APL differentiation syndrome

Trisenox Injection ... 983

Aplasia, bone marrow

Paxil CR Controlled-Release Tablets ... 1509
Paxil ... 1501

Aplasia, red cell

Combivir Tablets ... 1373
Cuprimine Capsules ... 1925
Epivir ... 1394
Epivir-HBV ... 1398
Epogen for Injection ... 586
Lamictal (Rare) ... 1449
Miradon Tablets ... 3056
Retrovir Capsules ... 1533
Retrovir IV Infusion ... 1537
Retrovir ... 1533
Trizivir Tablets ... 1565

Aplasia, unspecified

Campath Ampules ... 826

Aplastic anemia

(*see under* Anemia, aplastic)

Apnea

Abilify Tablets (Rare) ... 916
Abilify Tablets (Rare) ... 2472
Aciphex Tablets (Rare) ... 1081
Actiq ... 993
Aloprim for Injection (Less than 1%) ... 2156
Alphagan P Ophthalmic Solution ... 563
Aricept Tablets (Infrequent) ... 1086
Aricept ODT Tablets (Infrequent) ... 1086
Bentyl Capsules ... 724
Bentyl Injection ... 724
Bentyl Syrup ... 724
Bentyl Tablets ... 724
Brimonidine Tartrate Ophthalmic Solution 0.2% ... ⊙ 245
Buprenex Injectable (Infrequent) ... 2718
Carimune NF ... 3501
▲ CellCept Capsules (3% to less than 20%) ... 2751
▲ CellCept Intravenous (3% to less than 20%) ... 2751
▲ CellCept Oral Suspension (3% to less than 20%) ... 2751
▲ CellCept Tablets (3% to less than 20%) ... 2751
Dilaudid Oral Liquid ... 443
Dilaudid Tablets - 8 mg ... 443
Dilaudid-HP ... 441
Diprivan Injectable Emulsion (1% to 3%) ... 676
▲ Doxil Injection (1% to 10%) ... 3302
▲ Duragesic Transdermal System (3% to 10%) ... 2448
Effexor XR Capsules (Rare) ... 3411
Ethyol for Injection ... 1869
Evoxac Capsules ... 1042
Exelon Capsules (Infrequent) ... 2204
Gabitril Tablets (Infrequent) ... 998
Gammagard Liquid ... 751
Gammagard S/D (Rare) ... 754
Gamunex Immune Globulin I.V., 10% (Rare) ... 3232
Herceptin I.V. (At least one of the 958 patients) ... 1234
HibTITER ... 3419
Indocin I.V. (Less than 3%) ... 1973
▲ Infasurf Intratracheal Suspension (61% to 76%) ... 1188
Iveegam EN (Rare) ... 759
Lamictal ... 1449
Lyrica Capsules (Rare) ... 2524
Mebaral Tablets, USP (Less than 1 in 100 patients) ... 2483
Merrem I.V. (1.3%) ... 687
MS Contin Tablets ... 2703
Mycamine for Injection ... 620
Namenda (Infrequent) ... 1199

Natrecor for Injection (Greater than or equal to 1%) 3123
Nembutal Sodium Solution, USP (Less than 1%) 2484
Neurontin Capsules (Infrequent) 2498
Neurontin Oral Solution (Infrequent) 2498
Neurontin Tablets (Infrequent) 2498
Orthoclone OKT3 Sterile Solution (Less than 1%) 2370
OxyContin Tablets 2699
Permax Tablets (Infrequent) 3357
Phenergan 3438
Proleukin for Injection (1%) 1007
Prozac Pulvules and Liquid (Rare) 1771
Pulmozyme Inhalation Solution 1245
Rilutek Tablets (More than 2%) 2945
Risperdal M-Tab Orally Disintegrating Tablets 1658
Risperdal 1658
Sonata Capsules (Rare) 1686
Striant Mucoadhesive 1022
▲ Suprane Liquid for Inhalation (3% to 15%) 770
Symbyax Capsules (Infrequent) 1788
Synagis (More than 1%) 1868
Tasmar Tablets (Rare) 3360
Thalomid Capsules 979
▲ Trasylol Injection (3%) 779
Ultane Liquid for Inhalation (Less than 1% to 2%) 526
Virazole for Inhalation Solution 3365
Xanax XR Tablets (Infrequent) 2655
Zevalin Injection (1%) 848
Zomig Tablets (Rare) 714
Zomig-ZMT Tablets (Rare) 714
Zonegran Capsules (Rare) 1089
Zyprexa Tablets (Infrequent) 1798
Zyprexa ZYDIS Orally Disintegrating Tablets (Infrequent) 1798
Zyvox (0% to 2.3%) 2661

Appendicitis
▲ Advair Diskus 100/50 (1% to 3%) 1291
▲ Advair Diskus 250/50 (1% to 3%) 1291
▲ Advair Diskus 500/50 (1% to 3%) 1291
Amevive 836
Effexor Tablets (Rare) 3405
Effexor XR Capsules (Rare) 3411
Enbrel for Injection 580
Evoxac Capsules (Less than 1%) 1042
Sandostatin Injection (Less than 1%) 2263
Sandostatin LAR Depot (Rare) 2264

Appetite, changes
Activella Tablets 2311
Alesse-28 Tablets 3392
Anaprox Tablets (Less than 1%) 2769
Anaprox DS Tablets (Less than 1%) 2769
Arthrotec Tablets (Rare) 3126
Cataflam Tablets (Rarely) 2173
Decadron Phosphate Injection 1931
Decadron Tablets 1929
Depo-Provera Contraceptive Injection (Less than 1%) 2619
EC-Naprosyn Delayed-Release Tablets (Less than 1%) 2769
▲ Effexor Tablets (1% to 6%) 3405
▲ Effexor XR Capsules (1% to 6%) 3411
Eldepryl Capsules 3209
Gleevec Tablets (Infrequent) 2221
Hydrocortone Tablets 1963
Invirase (Greater than or equal to 2%) 2776
Lo/Ovral-28 Tablets 3423
Lupron Depot 3.75 mg (2%) 3257
Lupron Depot–3 Month 11.25 mg (Less than 5%) 3262
Maxzide 2150
▲ Midamor Tablets (Between 1% and 3%) 2000
Moduretic Tablets (Less than or equal to 1%) 2003
Naprosyn Suspension (Less than 1%) 2769
Naprosyn Tablets (Less than 1%) 2769
Ortho-Cept Tablets 2395
Ortho-Cyclen Tablets 2414
Ortho Evra Transdermal System 2402
Ortho Tri-Cyclen Tablets 2414
Ortho Tri-Cyclen Lo Tablets 2421
Premphase Tablets 3452
Prempro Tablets 3452
Seasonale Tablets 1073
Triphasil-28 Tablets 3483
Univasc Tablets (Less than 1%) 3118
Voltaren Tablets (Rarely) 2298
Voltaren-XR Tablets (Rarely) 2301
▲ Wellbutrin Tablets (3.7%) 1579
Yasmin 28 Tablets 818

Appetite, decreased
▲ Adderall XR Capsules (36%) 3169
▲ Aerobid/Aerobid-M (3% to 9%) 1172
Aloxi Injection (Less than 1%) 2099
Aptivus Capsules (Less than 2%) 859
▲ Buphenyl Powder (4%) 3327
▲ Buphenyl Tablets (4%) 3327
▲ Byetta Injection (Greater than or equal to 1% to less than 5%) 605
▲ Clolar for Intravenous Infusion (11%) 1264
▲ Combivir Tablets (10%) 1373
Cubicin for Injection (1% to 2%) 1038
▲ Cymbalta Delayed-Release Capsules (3% to 11%) 1729
DynaCirc CR Tablets (0.5% to 1%) 2726
Emend Capsules (Greater than 0.5%) 1944
▲ Epivir (10%) 1394
▲ Femara Tablets (4%) 2210
▲ Focalin XR Capsules (30%) 2217
▲ Fuzeon Injection (3.2%) 2772
Garamycin Injectable 3028
Imitrex Injection (Rare) 1431
Imitrex Nasal Spray (Rare) 1435
Imitrex Tablets (Rare) 1440
Invirase (Greater than or equal to 2%) 2776
Klonopin (1%) 2782
▲ Kytril Tablets (5%) 2788
▲ Leustatin Injection (17%) 2368
▲ Lexapro Oral Solution (3%) 1193
▲ Lexapro Tablets (3%) 1193
MetroGel-Vaginal Gel (1%) 1822
Mycamine for Injection (0.7%) 620
▲ Niravam Orally Disintegrating Tablets (12.8% to 27.8%) 3106
Oncaspar 1123
▲ Paxil CR Controlled-Release Tablets (2.0% to 9%) 1509
▲ Paxil (2.0% to 9%) 1501
▲ Prevnar for Injection (0% to 30%) 3460
Prochieve 4% Gel 1018
Prochieve 8% Gel 1018
ProSom Tablets (Infrequent) 512
Recombivax HB (Greater than 1%) 2045
Rescriptor Tablets 2535
Ritalin LA Capsules 2255
▲ Strattera Capsules (5% to 23%) 1784
▲ Trisenox Injection (15%) 983
▲ Valcyte Tablets (Less than 5%) 2816
Vantin Tablets and Oral Suspension (Less than 1%) 2650
▲ Velcade for Injection (43%) 2102
▲ Xanax XR Tablets (7.3% to 9.5%) 2655
▲ Zometa for Intravenous Infusion (13%) 2306

Appetite, increased
Abilify Tablets (Infrequent) 916
Abilify Tablets (Infrequent) 2472
Aceon Tablets (2 mg, 4 mg, 8 mg) (0.3% to 1%) 3191
Aciphex Tablets 1081
Aerobid/Aerobid-M (1% to 3%) 1172
Alinia for Oral Suspension (Less than 1%) 2840
Alinia Tablets (Less than 1%) 2840
Ambien Tablets (Rare) 2867
Antara Capsules 2723
Aricept Tablets (Infrequent) 1086
Aricept ODT Tablets (Infrequent) 1086
▲ Aromasin Tablets (3%) 2600
Asacol Delayed-Release Tablets 2688
Astelin Nasal Spray (Infrequent) 1876
Caduet Tablets (Less than 2%) 2507
Campral Tablets (Frequent) 1175
Celebrex Capsules (0.1% to 1.9%) 3130
Celexa (Frequent) 1177
▲ Clarinex Syrup (3.1%) 3009
Clozapine Tablets (Less than 1%) 2141
Clozaril Tablets (Less than 1%) 2174
Copaxone for Injection (Infrequent) 3292
Crixivan Capsules (2.1%) 1918
Cymbalta Delayed-Release Capsules (Frequent) 1729
Decadron Tablets 1929
▲ Depacon Injection (1% to 5%) 412
▲ Depakene (1% to 5%) 417
▲ Depakote Sprinkle Capsules (1% to 5%) 422
▲ Depakote Tablets (1% to 6%) 427
▲ Depakote ER Tablets (6%) 433
Diovan HCT Tablets (Greater than 0.2%) 2195
Doxil Injection (Less than 1%) 3302
DynaCirc CR Tablets (0.5% to 1%) 2726
▲ Entocort EC Capsules (Less than 5%) 2694
Evoxac Capsules (Less than 1%) 1042
FazaClo Orally Disintegrating Tablets (Less than 1%) 547
Fortical Nasal Spray (Less than 1%) 3336
Gabitril Tablets (2%) 998
Gengraf Capsules (1% to less than 3%) 458
▲ Intron A for Injection (Less than 5%) 3038
Kaletra (Less than 2%) 474
Klonopin (Infrequent) 2782
Lamictal (Infrequent) 1449
Levothroid Tablets 1189
Levoxyl Tablets 1680
Lexapro Oral Solution (Frequent) 1193
Lexapro Tablets (Frequent) 1193
Lipitor Tablets (Less than 2%) 2495
Lofibra Capsules 1217
Lunesta Tablets (Infrequent) 3139
▲ Lyrica Capsules (1% to 6%) 2524
Maxalt Tablets (Rare) 1983
Maxalt-MLT Orally Disintegrating Tablets (Rare) 1983
▲ Meridia Capsules (8.7%) 485
Miacalcin Nasal Spray (Less than 1%) 2242
Namenda (Infrequent) 1199
Neoral Soft Gelatin Capsules (1% to less than 3%) 2247
Neoral Oral Solution (1% to less than 3%) 2247
Neurontin Capsules (1.1%) 2498
Neurontin Oral Solution (1.1%) 2498
Neurontin Tablets (1.1%) 2498
Nexium Delayed-Release Capsules (Less than 1%) 645
Nexium I.V. (Less than 1%) 649
▲ Nicotrol NS (Less than 5%) 2596
▲ Niravam Orally Disintegrating Tablets (32.7%) 3106
Norvasc Tablets (Less than or equal to 0.1%) 2529
Omacor Capsules 2735
Oncaspar (Less than 1%) 1123
▲ Orap Tablets (1 of 20 patients) 1220
OxyContin Tablets (Less than 1%) 2699
▲ Paxil CR Controlled-Release Tablets (4%) 1509
▲ Paxil (4%) 1501
Permax Tablets (Infrequent) 3357
Prevacid Delayed-Release Capsules (Less than 1%) 3268
Prevacid for Delayed-Release Oral Suspension (Less than 1%) 3268
Prevacid NapraPAC (Less than 1%) 3277
Prevacid SoluTab Delayed-Release Orally Disintegrating Tablets (Less than 1%) 3268
PREVPAC (Less than 1%) 3281
Prochieve 4% Gel 1018
Prochieve 8% Gel 1018
▲ Prograf Capsules and Injection (3% to 15%) 624
Prometrium Capsules (100 mg, 200 mg) 3205
ProSom Tablets (Infrequent) 512
Protonix I.V. (Less than 1%) 3468
Protonix Tablets (Less than 1%) 3465
Provigil Tablets (At least 1%) 1002
Prozac Pulvules and Liquid (Frequent) 1771
Relafen Tablets (Less than 1%) 1523
Relpax Tablets (Rare) 2531
Rescriptor Tablets 2535
Reyataz Capsules (Less than 3%) 948
Rilutek Tablets (Infrequent) 2945
Risperdal Consta Long-Acting Injection (Infrequent) 1664
Risperdal M-Tab Orally Disintegrating Tablets (Infrequent) 1658
Risperdal (Infrequent) 1658
Seroquel Tablets (Infrequent) 691
Sonata Capsules (Infrequent) 1686
▲ Soriatane Capsules (1% to 10%) 1028
Spectracef Tablets (0.1% to 1%) 2706
Sular Tablets (Less than or equal to 1%) 1163
▲ Symbyax Capsules (Greater than or equal to 5% to 16%) 1788
Testim 1% Gel (Less than 1%) 722
Thalomid Capsules 979
Thiothixene Capsules 2124
Topamax Sprinkle Capsules (1%) 2438
Topamax Tablets (1%) 2438
Tricor Tablets 523
Triglide Tablets 1165
Trileptal Oral Suspension 2281
Trileptal Tablets 2281
Uniretic Tablets (Less than 1%) 3114
Unithroid Tablets 3521
Vantas (Less than 2%) 3367
Wellbutrin SR Sustained-Release Tablets (At least 1%) 1583
Wellbutrin XL Extended-Release Tablets (At least 1%) 1588
▲ Xanax XR Tablets (7%) 2655
Zelnorm Tablets 2303
Zoladex (2%) 709
Zoladex 3-month 712
Zoloft (Frequent) 2581
Zomig Nasal Spray (Rare) 718
Zomig Tablets (Infrequent) 714
Zomig-ZMT Tablets (Infrequent) 714
Zyban Sustained-Release Tablets (2%) 1620
Zyprexa Tablets (2%) 1798
Zyprexa ZYDIS Orally Disintegrating Tablets (2%) 1798
Zyrtec Chewable Tablets (Less than 2%) 2589
Zyrtec (Less than 2%) 2589
Zyrtec-D 12 Hour Extended Release Tablets (Less than 2%) 2591

Appetite, loss of
(*see also under* Anorexia)
▲ Chemet Capsules (12.0% to 20.9%) 2480
▲ Concerta Extended-Release Tablets (4%) 1828
▲ Focalin Tablets (Among more frequent) 2214
Focalin XR Capsules 2217
HibTITER (23 of 1,118 vaccinations) 3419
▲ Infanrix Vaccine (6.0% to 27.8%) 1444
Metadate CD Capsules 3316
Miacalcin Injection 2241
Numorphan 1112
▲ Pediarix Vaccine (21.6% or less) 1518
Tasmar Tablets 3360
Varivax (Greater than or equal to 1%) 2070
Ziagen 1600

Application site macules
Oxytrol Transdermal System (2.5%) 3383

Application site rash
▲ Aldara Cream, 5% (20.5%) 1814
▲ Oxytrol Transdermal System (3.3%) 3383
ThermaCare Heat Wraps 2674

Application site reaction, unspecified
▲ Aldara Cream, 5% (33%) 1814
Centany Ointment, 2% (1%) 2382
▲ Climara Pro Transdermal System (40.6%) 800
▲ CombiPatch Transdermal System (20% to 23%) 2180
▲ Duragesic Transdermal System (3% to 10%) 2448
Ertaczo Cream, 2% 2383
Estrogel 0.06% (0.6%) 3200
Evoclin Foam, 1% (1%) 1025
Floxin Otic Singles (0.6% to 16.8%) 1045
Loprox Shampoo 1862
▲ Menostar Transdermal System (9%) 805
▲ Tri-Luma Cream (5.45%) 1213
Vanos Cream (0.4% to 1.4%) 1864

Apprehension
Adenocard Injection (Less than 1%) 612
Dalmane Capsules 3343
Dilaudid Oral Liquid (Less frequent) 443
Dilaudid Tablets - 8 mg (Less frequent) 443
Dilaudid-HP (Less frequent) 441
Edecrin 1941
EpiPen 1061
Hyperstat I.V. Injection 3031
Lidoderm Patch 1107
Matulane Capsules 3188
Maxalt Tablets (Rare) 1983
Maxalt-MLT Orally Disintegrating Tablets (Rare) 1983
MS Contin Tablets (Less frequent) 2703

Apraxia
Eldepryl Capsules 3209
Exelon Capsules (Infrequent) 2204
Neurontin Capsules (Rare) 2498
Neurontin Oral Solution (Rare) 2498
Neurontin Tablets (Rare) 2498
Razadyne ER Extended-Release Capsules (Infrequent) 2434
Razadyne (Infrequent) 2434
Risperdal Consta Long-Acting Injection (Infrequent) 1664
Topamax Sprinkle Capsules (Infrequent) 2438
Topamax Tablets (Infrequent) 2438

Arachnoiditis
Depo-Medrol Single-Dose Vial 2617

Areflexia
Ammonul Injection ... 3323
Neurontin Capsules (Frequent) ... 2498
Neurontin Oral Solution ... 2498
Neurontin Tablets (Frequent) ... 2498

Arm, stiffness of
Engerix-B Vaccine (Less than 1%) ... 1391

Arrhythmia, exacerbation of
Pacerone Tablets ... 3337
Toprol-XL Tablets (Greater than 1%) ... 660

Arrhythmia, nodal
Pletal Tablets (Less than 2%) ... 2478
ReoPro Vials (0.2%) ... 1779
Rythmol SR Capsules ... 2736
VFEND I.V. (Less than 2%) ... 2543
VFEND Oral Suspension (Less than 2%) ... 2543
VFEND Tablets (Less than 2%) ... 2543

Arrhythmias
Abelcet Injection (Rare) ... 1119
Activase I.V. ... 1225
Adenocard Injection ... 612
Adenoscan (1%) ... 613
Adriamycin for Injection, USP ... 786
Adriamycin Injection, USP ... 786
Advair Diskus 100/50 ... 1291
Advair Diskus 250/50 ... 1291
Advair Diskus 500/50 ... 1291
Advicor Tablets ... 1694
Aggrenox Capsules (Less than 1%) ... 855
Agrylin Capsules (1% to 5%) ... 3172
Alacol DM Syrup ... 739
Aldara Cream, 5% ... 1814
Allegra-D 12 Hour Extended-Release Tablets ... 2860
Allegra-D 24 Hour Extended-Release Tablets ... 2862
Ambien Tablets (Rare) ... 2867
AmBisome for Injection (Less common) ... 615
Anaprox Tablets (Less than 1%) ... 2769
Anaprox DS Tablets (Less than 1%) ... 2769
Antara Capsules ... 2723
Aramine Injection ... 1889
▲ Aranesp for Injection (10%) ... 576
Arthrotec Tablets (Rare) ... 3126
Avalide Tablets ... 922
Avalide Tablets ... 2889
Avapro Tablets (Less than 1%) ... 925
Avapro Tablets (Less than 1%) ... 2886
Avonex ... 839
Balamine DM ... 739
Bayer Aspirin Tablets ... 3515
Betagan Ophthalmic Solution, USP ... ⊙ 217
Betimol Ophthalmic Solution ... ⊙ 283
Betimol Ophthalmic Solution ... 3371
Biltricide Tablets ... 2990
Blocadren Tablets (Greater than 1.1%) ... 1891
Brimonidine Tartrate Ophthalmic Solution 0.2% (Less than 3%) ... ⊙ 245
Buphenyl Powder (One patient) ... 3327
Buphenyl Tablets (One patient) ... 3327
Caduet Tablets (Greater than 0.1% to less than 2%) ... 2507
Calcijex Injection ... 411
Campath Ampules ... 826
Carbatrol Capsules ... 3174
Cardizem LA Extended Release Tablets (Less than 2%) ... 1699
Carnitor Injection (2% to 3%) ... 3185
Carteolol Hydrochloride Ophthalmic Solution USP, 1% (Occasional) ... ⊙ 246
Cataflam Tablets (Rarely) ... 2173
Catapres Tablets (Rare) ... 874
Catapres-TTS (0.5% or less) ... 875
▲ CellCept Capsules (3% to less than 20%) ... 2751
▲ CellCept Intravenous (3% to less than 20%) ... 2751
▲ CellCept Oral Suspension (3% to less than 20%) ... 2751
▲ CellCept Tablets (3% to less than 20%) ... 2751
Chemet Capsules (Up to 1.8%) ... 2480
Cipro I.V. (1% or less) ... 2998
Cipro I.V. Pharmacy Bulk Package (1% or less) ... 3509
Cipro XR Tablets ... 3004
Clinoril Tablets (Rare) ... 1899
Clorpres Tablets (Rare) ... 2139
Clozapine Tablets (Several patients) ... 2141
Clozaril Tablets (Several patients) ... 2174
Combivent Inhalation Aerosol (Less than 2%) ... 878
Concerta Extended-Release Tablets ... 1828
Copaxone for Injection ... 3292
Copegus Tablets (Less than 1%) ... 2759
Cosopt Sterile Ophthalmic Solution ... 1910
Cozaar Tablets (Less than 1%) ... 1913
Crestor Tablets (Less than 1%) ... 672
Decadron Tablets ... 1929
Depakote ER Tablets (Greater than 1%) ... 433
Diprivan Injectable Emulsion (1.2%) ... 676
Ditropan XL Extended Release Tablets (Rare) ... 2391
Doxil Injection (Less than 1%) ... 3302
Duragesic Transdermal System (1% or greater) ... 2448
Dyazide Capsules ... 1389
EC-Naprosyn Delayed-Release Tablets (Less than 1%) ... 2769
Effexor Tablets (Infrequent) ... 3405
Effexor XR Capsules (Infrequent) ... 3411
Eldepryl Capsules ... 3209
Elitek (Less than or equal to 1%) ... 2906
EpiPen ... 1061
Equetro Extended-Release Capsules ... 3178
Ery-Tab Tablets (Occasional reports) ... 447
Erythrocin Stearate Filmtab Tablets (Occasional reports) ... 452
Erythromycin Base Filmtab Tablets (Occasional reports) ... 454
Erythromycin Delayed-Release Capsules, USP (Occasional reports) ... 456
Eskalith ... 1406
Ethyol for Injection (Rare) ... 1869
Evoxac Capsules (Less than 1%) ... 1042
Fabrazyme for Intravenous Infusion ... 1267
Flexeril Tablets (Less than 1%) ... 1832
▲ Flolan for Injection (27%) ... 1408
Focalin Tablets ... 2214
Focalin XR Capsules ... 2217
Foradil Aerolizer ... 3024
Furosemide Tablets ... 2117
Gemzar for Injection (2%) ... 1743
Gengraf Capsules (2%) ... 458
Hectorol Capsules ... 909
Hectorol Injection ... 911
Herceptin I.V. (At least one of the 958 patients) ... 1234
▲ Humira Injection (Less than 5%) ... 464
Hytrin Capsules (At least 1%) ... 469
Hyzaar ... 1964
Idamycin PFS Injection ... 2645
▲ Imdur Tablets (Less than or equal to 5%) ... 3032
Imitrex Injection (Rare) ... 1431
Imitrex Nasal Spray (Infrequent) ... 1435
Imitrex Tablets (Rare to infrequent) ... 1440
Indocin Capsules (Less than 1%) ... 1968
Indocin I.V. (Less than 1%) ... 1973
Indocin (Less than 1%) ... 1968
Infed Injection ... 3381
▲ Intron A for Injection (Less than 5%) ... 3038
Invanz for Injection (Greater than 0.1%) ... 1974
▲ I.V. Busulfex (5%) ... 1125
Kytril Injection (Rare) ... 2785
Lanoxicaps Capsules ... 1458
Lanoxin Injection ... 1462
Lanoxin Injection Pediatric ... 1465
Leukine ... 829
Levaquin in 5% Dextrose Injection (0.1% to 0.9%) ... 2453
Levaquin (0.1% to 0.9%) ... 2453
Levothroid Tablets ... 1189
Levoxyl Tablets ... 1680
Lipitor Tablets (Less than 2%) ... 2495
Lithobid Tablets ... 1670
Lofibra Capsules ... 1217
Lotronex Tablets (Rare) ... 1479
Lupron Depot 7.5 mg (Less than 5%) ... 3261
Maxalt Tablets (Infrequent) ... 1983
Maxalt-MLT Orally Disintegrating Tablets (Infrequent) ... 1983
Metadate CD Capsules ... 3316
Midamor Tablets (Less than or equal to 1%) ... 2000
Mirapex Tablets (Less than 1%) ... 889
Mivacron Injection (Less than 1%) ... 489
Moban Tablets ... 1108
Mobic Oral Suspension (Less than 2%) ... 893
Mobic Tablets (Less than 2%) ... 893
Moduretic Tablets (Greater than 1%, less than 3%) ... 2003
Mycamine for Injection ... 620
Naprosyn Suspension (Less than 1%) ... 2769
Naprosyn Tablets (Less than 1%) ... 2769
Naropin Injection (Less than 1%) ... 640
Neoral Soft Gelatin Capsules (2%) ... 2247
Neoral Oral Solution (2%) ... 2247
▲ Neupogen for Injection (11 of 375 cancer patients) ... 598
Niaspan Extended-Release Tablets ... 1703
Nipent for Injection (Less than 3%) ... 3216
Norvasc Tablets (More than 0.1% to 1%) ... 2529
▲ Novantrone for Injection Concentrate (6% to 18%) ... 3158
Omacor Capsules ... 2735
▲ Ontak Vials (6%) ... 1717
Orap Tablets ... 1220
Orthoclone OKT3 Sterile Solution (Less than 1%) ... 2370
▲ Pacerone Tablets (1% to 3%) ... 3337
Paxil CR Controlled-Release Tablets (Rare) ... 1509
Paxil (Rare) ... 1501
Pepcid Injection (Infrequent) ... 2017
Pepcid (Infrequent) ... 2014
Permax Tablets (1.1%) ... 3357
Phenergan ... 3438
Plendil Extended-Release Tablets (0.5% to 1.5%) ... 651
Prandin Tablets (0.5, 1, and 2 mg) (Less than or equal to 1%) ... 2337
Prevacid Delayed-Release Capsules (Less than 1%) ... 3268
Prevacid for Delayed-Release Oral Suspension (Less than 1%) ... 3268
Prevacid NapraPAC (Less than 1%) ... 3277
Prevacid SoluTab Delayed-Release Orally Disintegrating Tablets (Less than 1%) ... 3268
PREVPAC (Less than 1%) ... 3281
Prinivil Tablets (0.3% to 1.0%) ... 2029
Prinzide Tablets ... 2033
Prograf Capsules and Injection ... 624
▲ Proleukin for Injection (10%) ... 1007
Propine Ophthalmic Solution ... ⊙ 237
ProSom Tablets (Rare) ... 512
Protonix I.V. (Less than 1%) ... 3468
Protonix Tablets (Less than 1%) ... 3465
Protopic Ointment (Greater than or equal to 1%) ... 629
Proventil Inhalation Aerosol ... 3067
Provigil Tablets (1%) ... 1002
Prozac Pulvules and Liquid (Infrequent) ... 1771
Relafen Tablets (Less than 1%) ... 1523
Relpax Tablets (Rare) ... 2531
Remicade for IV Injection (Greater than or equal to 0.2%) ... 987
Rescriptor Tablets ... 2535
Retavase ... 1131
Risperdal M-Tab Orally Disintegrating Tablets ... 1658
Risperdal ... 1658
Ritalin Hydrochloride Tablets ... 2254
Ritalin LA Capsules ... 2255
Ritalin-SR Tablets ... 2254
Rituxan for Infusion (Four patients) ... 845
Rituxan I.V. ... 1251
Roferon-A Injection (1% to 3%) ... 2805
Rythmol SR Capsules ... 2736
▲ Sandostatin Injection (9%) ... 2263
Serevent Diskus ... 1540
Seroquel Tablets ... 691
Suprane Liquid for Inhalation (Less than 1%) ... 770
Surmontil Capsules ... 2347
Symbyax Capsules (Infrequent) ... 1788
Symmetrel ... 1115
Tamiflu Capsules ... 2810
Tamiflu Oral Suspension ... 2810
Tasmar Tablets (Infrequent) ... 3360
Tegretol/Tegretol-XR ... 2278
Thalomid Capsules ... 979
Timolide Tablets (Less than 1%) ... 2056
Timoptic in Ocudose (Less frequent) ... 2061
Timoptic Sterile Ophthalmic Solution (Less frequent) ... 2058
Timoptic-XE Sterile Ophthalmic Gel Forming Solution ... 2062
TNKase I.V. ... 1256
▲ Trasylol Injection (4%) ... 779
Tricor Tablets ... 523
Triglide Tablets ... 1165
Ultane Liquid for Inhalation (Less than 1%) ... 526
Uniphyl Tablets ... 2708
Uniretic Tablets (Less than 1%) ... 3114
Unithroid Tablets ... 3521
Vaseretic Tablets ... 2073
Vasotec I.V. Injection (0.5% to 1.0%) ... 2076
Ventolin HFA Inhalation Aerosol ... 1576
▲ Vesanoid Capsules (23%) ... 2823
Vicoprofen Tablets (Less than 1%) ... 533
Vivactil Tablets ... 2350
Voltaren Tablets (Rarely) ... 2298
Voltaren-XR Tablets (Rarely) ... 2301
▲ Wellbutrin Tablets (5.3%) ... 1579
Xopenex HFA Inhalation Aerosol ... 3151
Xopenex Inhalation Solution ... 3143
Xopenex Inhalation Solution Concentrate ... 3147
Zantac (Rare) ... 1597
Zantac Injection (Rare) ... 1593
Zantac Injection Pharmacy Bulk Package (Rare) ... 1595
Zantac Syrup (Rare) ... 1597
Zemuron Injection (Less than 1%) ... 2363
Zestoretic Tablets ... 701
Zestril Tablets (0.3% to 1.0%) ... 704
Zithromax Capsules, 250 mg ... 2568
Zithromax for IV Infusion ... 2573
Zithromax for Oral Suspension, 300 mg, 600 mg, 900 mg, 1200 mg ... 2561
Zithromax Tablets, 250 mg, 500 mg ... 2561
Zithromax Tri-Pak ... 2561
Zofran Injection ... 1607
Zoladex (1% to 5%) ... 709
Zoladex 3-month ... 712
Zomig Nasal Spray (Infrequent) ... 718
Zomig Tablets (Infrequent) ... 714
Zomig-ZMT Tablets (Infrequent) ... 714
Zosyn (1.0% or less) ... 3492
Zyrtec-D 12 Hour Extended Release Tablets ... 2591

Arrhythmias, junctional
Proleukin for Injection (1%) ... 1007

Arrhythmias, malignant
Symmetrel ... 1115

Arrhythmias, sinus
Aloxi Injection (Less than 1%) ... 2099
Anzemet Injection ... 2871
Anzemet Tablets ... 2874
Imitrex Injection (Infrequent) ... 1431
Imitrex Nasal Spray ... 1435
Imitrex Tablets ... 1440
Rythmol SR Capsules ... 2736

Arrhythmias, supraventricular
Cubicin for Injection (Less than 1%) ... 1038
Intron A for Injection (Rare) ... 3038
Leukine (Occasional) ... 829
Pegasys (Less than 1%) ... 2793
PEG-Intron Powder for Injection (Less than or equal to 1%) ... 3062
▲ Proleukin for Injection (5%) ... 1007
Rituxan for Infusion (Four patients) ... 845
Rituxan I.V. ... 1251
Sanctura Tablets ... 1133

Arterial carbon dioxide, decrease
Sulfamylon Cream ... 2154

Arterial insufficiency
Blocadren Tablets ... 1891
Cosopt Sterile Ophthalmic Solution ... 1910
Inderal LA Long-Acting Capsules ... 3421
InnoPran XL Capsules ... 2728
Timolide Tablets ... 2056
Timoptic in Ocudose ... 2061
Timoptic Sterile Ophthalmic Solution ... 2058
Timoptic-XE Sterile Ophthalmic Gel Forming Solution ... 2062
Toprol-XL Tablets (About 1 of 100 patients) ... 660

Arteriosclerosis
Tasmar Tablets (Rare) ... 3360

Arteriospasm
Fortaz ... 1422
Tasmar Tablets (Infrequent) ... 3360

Arteritis
Ambien Tablets (Rare) ... 2867
Aricept Tablets (Infrequent) ... 1086
Aricept ODT Tablets (Infrequent) ... 1086
Effexor Tablets (Rare) ... 3405
Effexor XR Capsules (Rare) ... 3411
Zyprexa Tablets (Rare) ... 1798

Zyprexa ZYDIS Orally Disintegrating Tablets (Rare) 1798

Arteritis, temporal

Imitrex Nasal Spray 1435
Imitrex Tablets 1440
Orthoclone OKT3 Sterile Solution (Less than 1%) 2370

Arthralgia

Abelcet Injection 1119
Abilify Tablets (Infrequent) 916
Abilify Tablets (Infrequent) 2472
Accutane Capsules 2740
Aceon Tablets (2 mg, 4 mg, 8 mg) (0.3% to 1.1%) 3191
Actimmune (2%) 1646
Actiq (1% or greater) 993
Activella Tablets 2311
▲ Actonel Tablets (11.5% to 32.8%) 2679
▲ Actonel with Calcium Tablets (11.5% to 23.7%) 2684
▲ Adacel Vaccine (0.3% to 14%) 2959
Adalat CC Tablets (Less than 1%) 2978
▲ Advair Diskus 100/50 (1% to 3%) 1291
▲ Advair Diskus 250/50 (1% to 3%) 1291
▲ Advair Diskus 500/50 (1% to 3%) 1291
▲ Advate Injection (23.3%) 742
Advicor Tablets 1694
▲ Aggrenox Capsules (5.5%) 855
Agrylin Capsules (1% to 5%) 3172
Aldara Cream, 5% (0.9%) 1814
Aldoclor Tablets 1881
Aldoril Tablets 1884
▲ Alferon N Injection (3% to 10%) 1640
▲ Alimta for Injection (Up to 8%) 1722
Aloprim for Injection (Less than 1%) 2156
Aloxi Injection (Less than 1%) 2099
Altace Capsules (Less than 1%) 1673
▲ Altoprev Extended-Release Tablets (5%) 1151
▲ Ambien Tablets (4%) 2867
AmBisome for Injection (Less common) 615
Amerge Tablets (Infrequent) 1312
Antara Capsules 2723
Anzemet Injection (Rare) 2871
Anzemet Tablets (Rare) 2874
▲ Apokyn Injection (At least 5%) 2132
▲ Aranesp for Injection (11% to 13%) 576
Arava Tablets (1%) 2881
▲ Aredia for Injection (11.5% to 26%) 2168
▲ Arimidex Tablets (2% to 13%) 665
▲ Aromasin Tablets (2% to 5%) 2600
Arthrotec Tablets (Rare) 3126
▲ Asacol Delayed-Release Tablets (5%) 2688
▲ Asmanex Twisthaler (13%) 2981
Atacand Tablets (More than 1%) 634
Atacand HCT (0.5% or greater) 637
Augmentin 1331
Augmentin Tablets 1334
Augmentin XR Extended-Release Tablets 1340
Augmentin ES-600 Powder for Oral Suspension 1337
Avalide Tablets 922
Avalide Tablets 2889
▲ Avandamet Tablets (5%) 1343
Avapro Tablets (Less than 1%) 925
Avapro Tablets (Less than 1%) 2886
Avelox (0.1% to less than 2%) 2984
▲ Avonex (9%) 839
Axert Tablets (Rare) 2430
Azasan Tablets (Less than 1%) 2844
Azmacort Inhalation Aerosol 1701
Beconase AQ Nasal Spray 1359
Benicar Tablets (Greater than 0.5%) 2850
Benicar HCT Tablets (Greater than 1%) 2852
▲ Betaseron for SC Injection (31%) 791
▲ Bexxar (1% to 10%) 1360
BiDil Tablets (1% to less than 2%) 2161
Blocadren Tablets (Less than 1%) 1891
▲ Boniva Tablets (3.5% to 5.6%) 2747
Boostrix 1366
▲ Caduet Tablets (Greater than 0.1% to 5.1%) 2507
Calcium Disodium Versenate Injection 1819
Campral Tablets (Frequent) 1175
▲ Captopril Tablets (About 4 to 7 of 100 patients) 2114
Carbatrol Capsules 3174
Catapres Tablets (About 6 in 1,000 patients) 874
Catapres-TTS (0.5% or less) 875
Ceftin for Oral Suspension (0.1% to 1%) 1369
Celebrex Capsules (0.1% to 1.9%) 3130
Celexa (2%) 1177
▲ CellCept Capsules (3% to less than 20%) 2751
▲ CellCept Intravenous (3% to less than 20%) 2751
▲ CellCept Oral Suspension (3% to less than 20%) 2751
▲ CellCept Tablets (3% to less than 20%) 2751
▲ Cenestin Tablets, 0.45mg, 0.625mg, 0.9mg, 1.25mg (9.4% to 25%) 1063
Cenestin Tablets, 0.3mg 1063
Cialis Tablets (Less than 2%) 1806
Cipro I.V. (1% or less) 2998
Cipro I.V. Pharmacy Bulk Package (1% or less) 3509
Cipro (Less than 1%) 2991
Cipro XR Tablets 3004
Climara Transdermal System (1% to 5%) 795
▲ Climara Pro Transdermal System (4.2%) 800
Clindesse Vaginal Cream (Less than 1%) 3296
Clinoril Tablets (Less than 1 in 100) 1899
▲ Clolar for Intravenous Infusion (11%) 1264
Clorpres Tablets (About 6 in 1,000) 2139
Clozapine Tablets (Less than 1%) 2141
Clozaril Tablets (Less than 1%) 2174
▲ Colazal Capsules (4%) 2845
▲ CombiPatch Transdermal System (6%) 2180
Combivent Inhalation Aerosol (Less than 2%) 878
▲ Combivir Tablets (5%) 1373
Comvax 1904
Concerta Extended-Release Tablets 1828
▲ Copaxone for Injection (24%) 3292
▲ Copegus Tablets (22%) 2759
▲ Coreg Tablets (1% to 6%) 1376
Cosopt Sterile Ophthalmic Solution 1910
Coumadin for Injection 932
Coumadin Tablets 932
Covera-HS Tablets (Less than 2%) 3135
Cozaar Tablets (Less than 1%) 1913
Crestor Tablets (Greater than or equal to 2%) 672
Crixivan Capsules 1918
Cubicin for Injection (0.9%) 1038
Cuprimine Capsules 1925
CytoGam Intravenous (Less than 5.0%) 1866
Cytovene (At least 3 subjects) 2763
Dalmane Capsules 3343
▲ Depacon Injection (1% to 5%) 412
▲ Depakene (1% to 5%) 417
▲ Depakote Sprinkle Capsules (1% to 5%) 422
▲ Depakote Tablets (1% to 5%) 427
Depakote ER Tablets (Greater than 1%) 433
▲ Depo-Provera Contraceptive Injection (1% to 5%) 2619
▲ depo-subQ provera 104 Injectable Suspension (1% to less than 5%) 2622
Desferal Vials 2190
Detrol Tablets (2.3%) 2626
Didronel Tablets (Infrequent) 2693
Diovan HCT Tablets (Greater than 0.2%) 2195
▲ Diovan Tablets (1% to 3%) 2191
Dolobid Tablets (Less than 1 in 100) 1937
Dostinex Tablets (1%) 2631
▲ Doxil Injection (1% to 10%) 3302
DynaCirc CR Tablets (0.5% to 1%) 2726
Effexor Tablets 3405
Effexor XR Capsules (Frequent) 3411
Elidel Cream 1% (Up to 1.5%) 2198
Eligard 7.5 mg (Less than 2%) 2896
▲ Eligard 22.5 mg (3.4%) 2899
▲ Eloxatin for Injection (7% to 10%) 2908
Elspar for Injection 1943
▲ Emtriva Capsules (3% to 5%) 1272
Enablex Extended-Release Tablets (Greater than or equal to 1%) 2201
Enbrel for Injection 580
Engerix-B Vaccine (Less than 1%) 1391
▲ Epivir (5%) 1394
▲ Epivir-HBV (7%) 1398
Epogen for Injection (Rare) 586
Equetro Extended-Release Capsules 3178
Eskalith 1406
Estratest Tablets 3196
Estratest H.S. Tablets 3196
Estrogel 0.06% 3200
▲ Evista Tablets (10.7% to 15.5%) 1735
▲ Evoxac Capsules (3.7%) 1042
Exelon Capsules (2% or more) 2204
Factive Tablets (0.1% to 1%) 2464
Famvir Tablets (1.3% to 1.5%) 2207
FazaClo Orally Disintegrating Tablets (Less than 1%) 547
▲ Femara Tablets (1% to 22%) 2210
Ferrlecit Injection 3379
▲ Flolan for Injection (6% to 84%) 1408
▲ Flovent Diskus 50 mcg (1% to 17%) 1415
Focalin XR Capsules 2217
Follistim AQ Cartridge 2354
▲ Forteo for Injection (10.1%) 1739
▲ Fortical Nasal Spray (3.8%) 3336
▲ Fosamax (0.4% to approximately 6%) 1949
▲ Fosamax Plus D Tablets (0.4% to 4.1%) 1956
Frova Tablets (Infrequent) 1101
▲ Gamunex Immune Globulin I.V., 10% (4%) 3232
Garamycin Injectable 3028
▲ Gengraf Capsules (1% to 6%) 458
Genotropin Lyophilized Powder 2642
Geodon Capsules 2514
▲ Gleevec Tablets (25% to 40%) 2221
Havrix Vaccine (Less than 1%) 1425
▲ Hectorol Capsules (4.9%) 909
▲ Hectorol Injection (4.9%) 911
▲ Herceptin I.V. (6%) 1234
▲ Humatrope Vials and Cartridges (10.8% to 17.3%) 1756
Hycamtin for Injection (0.2% to 0.9%) 1427
Hytrin Capsules (At least 1%) 469
Hyzaar 1964
▲ Imdur Tablets (Less than or equal to 5%) 3032
Imitrex Injection (Infrequent) 1431
▲ Increlex Injection (Greater than or equal to 5%) 3290
Infed Injection 3381
▲ Infergen (43% to 51%) 1647
▲ Intron A for Injection (Up to 19%) 3038
Invanz for Injection (Greater than 0.5%) 1974
Invirase (Less than 2%) 2776
▲ I.V. Busulfex (13%) 1125
Kadian Capsules (Less than 3%) 572
Kaletra (Less than 2%) 474
▲ Kepivance (10%) 592
Keppra Oral Solution (1% or more) 3307
Keppra Tablets (1% or more) 3307
▲ Kineret Injection (6%) 594
Klonopin (Infrequent) 2782
K-Phos Neutral Tablets 785
K-Phos Original (Sodium Free) Tablets (Less frequent) 785
Lamictal (2.0%) 1449
Lamisil Tablets 2226
Lariam Tablets (Infrequent) 2790
▲ Lescol Capsules (4.0%) 2227
Lescol XL Tablets (1.3%) 2227
▲ Leukine (11% to 21%) 829
▲ Leustatin Injection (5%) 2368
Levaquin in 5% Dextrose Injection (0.1% to 0.9%) 2453
Levaquin (0.1% to 0.9%) 2453
Levitra Tablets (Less than 2%) 3048
Levothroid Tablets 1189
Levoxyl Tablets 1680
Lexapro Oral Solution (Frequent) 1193
Lexapro Tablets (Frequent) 1193
▲ Lipitor Tablets (Up to 5.1%) 2495
Lithobid Tablets 1670
Lofibra Capsules 1217
Lotensin Tablets (Less than 1%) 2232
Lotensin HCT Tablets (0.3% to 1%) 2235
Lunesta Tablets (Infrequent) 3139
Lupron Depot–3 Month 11.25 mg 3262
Lyrica Capsules (Greather than or equal to 1%) 2524
Matulane Capsules 3188
Maxalt Tablets (Infrequent) 1983
Maxalt-MLT Orally Disintegrating Tablets (Infrequent) 1983
▲ Menactra Vaccine (0.3% to 19.8%) 2968
▲ Menostar Transdermal System (12%) 805
▲ Meridia Capsules (5.9%) 485
Meruvax II 1994
Metadate CD Capsules 3316
Mevacor Tablets (0.5% to 1.0%) 1996
▲ Miacalcin Nasal Spray (3.8%) 2242
Micardis Tablets (More than 0.3%) 884
Micardis HCT Tablets 886
Midamor Tablets (Less than or equal to 1%) 2000
Migranal Nasal Spray (Rare) 3350
Mirapex Tablets (Greater than or equal to 1%) 889
M-M-R II 1980
▲ Mobic Oral Suspension (0% to 5.3%) 893
▲ Mobic Tablets (0% to 5.3%) 893
Moduretic Tablets (Less than or equal to 1%) 2003
Mycamine for Injection 620
▲ Myfortic Tablets (3% to less than 20%) 2244
Namenda (Greater than or equal to 2%) 1199
Nasonex Nasal Spray (Greater than or equal to 2%) 3058
▲ Navelbine Injection (Up to 12%) 1494
▲ Neoral Soft Gelatin Capsules (1% to 6%) 2247
▲ Neoral Oral Solution (1% to 6%) 2247
▲ Neulasta Injection (15% to 72%) 596
Neupogen for Injection (Infrequent) 598
Neurontin Capsules (Frequent) 2498
Neurontin Oral Solution (Frequent) 2498
Neurontin Tablets (Frequent) 2498
Nexium Delayed-Release Capsules (Less than 1%) 645
Nexium I.V. (Less than 1%) 649
▲ Nicotrol NS (5%) 2596
▲ Nipent for Injection (3% to 10%) 3216
▲ Norditropin Cartridges (19%) 2318
Noroxin Tablets 2009
Norvasc Tablets (More than 0.1% to 1%) 2529
Norvir (0 to1.7%) 499
Nutropin for Injection 1238
Nutropin AQ Injection 1241
Nutropin AQ Pen 1241
Nutropin AQ Pen Cartridge 1241
Omacor Capsules 2735
▲ Oncaspar (Greater than 1% but less than 5%) 1123
▲ Ontak Vials (8%) 1717
Orthoclone OKT3 Sterile Solution (Less than 1%) 2370
▲ Orthovisc Injection (12.6%) 3518
Paxil CR Controlled-Release Tablets (Frequent) 1509
Paxil (Frequent) 1501
Pediarix Vaccine 1518
▲ Pegasys (28%) 2793
▲ PEG-Intron Powder for Injection (23%) 3062
Pentasa Capsules (Less than 1%) 3182
Pepcid Injection (Infrequent) 2017
Pepcid (Infrequent) 2014
Permax Tablets (1.6%) 3357
Phenytek Capsules 2153
▲ Photofrin for Injection (31%) 729
▲ Plavix Tablets (6.3%) 940
▲ Plavix Tablets (6.3%) 2942
Plendil Extended-Release Tablets (0.5% to 1.5%) 651
Pletal Tablets (Less than 2%) 2478
Pneumovax 23 (Rare) 2020
▲ Prandin Tablets (0.5, 1, and 2 mg) (3% to 6%) 2337
Pravachol Tablets (Rare) 943
▲ Prefest Tablets (9%) 1069
▲ Premarin Tablets (7% to 14%) 3443
Premarin Vaginal Cream 3449
▲ Premphase Tablets (7% to 13%) 3452
▲ Prempro Tablets (7% to 13%) 3452
Prevacid Delayed-Release Capsules (Less than 1%) 3268
Prevacid for Delayed-Release Oral Suspension (Less than 1%) 3268
Prevacid NapraPAC (Less than 1%) 3277
Prevacid SoluTab Delayed-Release Orally Disintegrating Tablets (Less than 1%) 3268
PREVPAC (Less than 1%) 3281
Prilosec OTC Tablets (Less than 1%) 2674
Prinivil Tablets (0.3% to 1.0%) 2029
Prinzide Tablets 2033
▲ Prochieve 4% Gel (8%) 1018
▲ Prochieve 8% Gel (8%) 1018
▲ Procrit for Injection (Rare to 11%) 2374
▲ Prograf Capsules and Injection (3% to 15%) 624
▲ Proleukin for Injection (6%) 1007
▲ Prometrium Capsules (100 mg, 200 mg) (20%) 3205
ProSom Tablets (Rare) 512
Protonix I.V. (Greater than or equal to 1%) 3468
Protonix Tablets (Greater than or equal to 1%) 3465
Protopic Ointment (Greater than or equal to 1%) 629
Provigil Tablets (At least 1%) 1002
Prozac Pulvules and Liquid 1771
Rabies Vaccine RabAvert (Common) 1011

▲ Rapamune Oral Solution and Tablets (25% to 31%) 3472
Raptiva for Injection 1247
▲ Rebetol (15% to 34%) 3073
▲ Rebetron Combination Therapy (29% to 33%) 3078
Recombivax HB (Less than 1%) 2045
Relenza Rotadisk (Less than 1.5%) 1525
Relpax Tablets (Infrequent) 2531
▲ Remicade for IV Injection (8%) 987
▲ Renagel Tablets (12.1%) 1268
Repronex for Intramuscular and Subcutaneous Injection 1148
▲ Requip Tablets (4% to 7%) 1528
Rescriptor Tablets 2535
▲ Retisert Implant (5% to 15%) ⊙ 256
Retrovir Capsules 1533
Retrovir IV Infusion 1537
Retrovir 1533
▲ Reyataz Capsules (Less than 1% to 4%) 948
▲ Ribavirin, USP Capsules (15% to 33%) 3083
▲ Rilutek Tablets (1.6% to 5.1%) 2945
Risperdal Consta Long-Acting Injection (Frequent) 1664
▲ Risperdal M-Tab Orally Disintegrating Tablets (2% to 3%) 1658
Risperdal (2% to 3%) 1658
Ritalin Hydrochloride Tablets 2254
Ritalin LA Capsules 2255
Ritalin-SR Tablets 2254
Rituxan for Infusion (0.3%) 845
▲ Rituxan I.V. (10%) 1251
▲ Roferon-A Injection (47% to 51%) 2805
Rozerem Tablets (2%) 3228
Sandimmune (Rare) 2259
▲ Sandostatin Injection (1% to 4%) 2263
▲ Sandostatin LAR Depot (5% to 15%) 2264
Serevent Diskus (1% to 3%) 1540
Seroquel Tablets (Infrequent) 691
▲ Simulect for Injection (3% to 10%) 2268
Singulair 2047
Sonata Capsules (Frequent) 1686
▲ Soriatane Capsules (10% to 25%) 1028
▲ Strattera Capsules (2% or greater) 1784
▲ Stromectol Tablets (9.3%) 2053
Sular Tablets (Less than or equal to 1%) 1163
Sustiva Capsules (Less than 2%) 957
▲ Symbyax Capsules (3% to 5%) 1788
▲ Symlin Injection (2% to 7%) 608
Synercid I.V. (Less than 1%) 1690
Tagamet Tablets (Rare) 1547
Tambocor Tablets (Less than 1%) 1824
Targretin Capsules 1719
Tarka Tablets (0.3% to 1.7%) 519
Tasmar Tablets (1% or more) 3360
▲ Taxotere Injection Concentrate (3.4% to 9.2%) 2947
Tegretol/Tegretol-XR 2278
▲ Temodar Capsules (6%) 3088
Tequin Injection (Less than 0.1%) 964
Tequin Tablets (Less than 0.1%) 964
Teveten Tablets (2%) 1707
Teveten HCT Tablets (Less than 1%) 1710
Thalomid Capsules 979
Thyrolar 1203
Timentin ADD-Vantage 1556
Timentin Injection Galaxy Container 1559
Timentin IV Infusion 1553
Timentin Pharmacy Bulk Package 1562
Timolide Tablets 2056
Timoptic in Ocudose 2061
Timoptic Sterile Ophthalmic Solution 2058
Timoptic-XE Sterile Ophthalmic Gel Forming Solution 2062
Tindamax 2670
▲ Topamax Sprinkle Capsules (1% to 7%) 2438
▲ Topamax Tablets (1% to 7%) 2438
Toprol-XL Tablets 660
Trasylol Injection (1% to 2%) 779
Trelstar LA Suspension (2.3%) 3387
Tricor Tablets 523
Trileptal Oral Suspension 2281
Trileptal Tablets 2281
▲ Trisenox Injection (33%) 983
▲ Trizivir Tablets (5%) 1565
Truvada Tablets 1279
Twinrix Vaccine (Less than 1%) 1571
Uniretic Tablets (Less than 1%) 3114
Unithroid Tablets 3521
Univasc Tablets (Less than 1%) 3118
Uroqid-Acid No. 2 Tablets 785
▲ Valcyte Tablets (Less than 5%) 2816
▲ Valtrex Caplets (Less than 1% to 6%) 1573
Vantas (Less than 2%) 3367
Varivax (Greater than or equal to 1%) 2070
Vaseretic Tablets (0.5% to 2.0%) 2073
Vasotec I.V. Injection (0.5% to 1.0%) 2076
▲ Velcade for Injection (14%) 2102
Verelan PM Capsules (2% or less) 3120
VFEND I.V. (Less than 2%) 2543
VFEND Oral Suspension (Less than 2%) 2543
VFEND Tablets (Less than 2%) 2543
Viagra Tablets (Greater than 2%) 2552
Vicoprofen Tablets (Less than 1%) 533
Viracept (Less than 2%) 2556
▲ Viramune Oral Suspension (2% to 6%) 903
▲ Viramune Tablets (2% to 6%) 903
▲ Visudyne for Injection (1% to 10%) 2286
Vivelle Transdermal System 2288
Vivelle-Dot Transdermal System 2293
Vytorin 10/10 Tablets 2084
Vytorin 10/10 Tablets 3092
Vytorin 10/20 Tablets 2084
Vytorin 10/20 Tablets 3092
Vytorin 10/40 Tablets 2084
Vytorin 10/40 Tablets 3092
Vytorin 10/80 Tablets 2084
Vytorin 10/80 Tablets 3092
Wellbutrin Tablets 1579
Wellbutrin SR Sustained-Release Tablets (1% to 4%) 1583
Wellbutrin XL Extended-Release Tablets (1% to 4%) 1588
WinRho SDF 763
Xalatan Sterile Ophthalmic Solution (1% to 2%) 2654
Xanax XR Tablets (2.4%) 2655
Xifaxan Tablets (Less than 2%) 2847
▲ Xolair (8%) 1259
Zantac (Rare) 1597
Zantac Injection (Rare) 1593
Zantac Injection Pharmacy Bulk Package (Rare) 1595
Zantac Syrup (Rare) 1597
Zegerid Powder for Oral Solution (Less than 1%) 2972
▲ Zenapax for Injection (2% to 5%) 2838
Zestoretic Tablets 701
Zestril Tablets (0.3% to 1.0%) 704
▲ Zetia Tablets (3.8%) 2090
▲ Zetia Tablets (3.8%) 3098
▲ Zevalin Injection (7%) 848
Ziagen 1600
Zithromax Capsules, 250 mg 2568
Zithromax for IV Infusion 2573
Zithromax for Oral Suspension, 300 mg, 600 mg, 900 mg, 1200 mg 2561
Zithromax Tablets, 250 mg, 500 mg 2561
Zithromax Tri-Pak 2561
Zmax for Oral Suspension 2577
Zocor Tablets 2078
Zofran Injection (2%) 1607
Zoladex (1% or greater) 709
Zoladex 3-month 712
Zoloft (Infrequent) 2581
▲ Zometa for Intravenous Infusion (5% to 21%) 2306
Zomig Nasal Spray (Infrequent) 718
Zonegran Capsules (Infrequent) 1089
Zosyn (1.0% or less) 3492
▲ Zyban Sustained-Release Tablets (4% to 5%) 1620
▲ Zyprexa Tablets (5%) 1798
▲ Zyprexa ZYDIS Orally Disintegrating Tablets (5%) 1798
Zyrtec Chewable Tablets (Less than 2%) 2589
Zyrtec (Less than 2%) 2589
Zyrtec-D 12 Hour Extended Release Tablets (Less than 2%) 2591

Arthralgia, monoarticular

Recombivax HB (Less than 1%) 2045

Arthritis

Abilify Tablets (Infrequent) 916
Abilify Tablets (Infrequent) 2472
Accutane Capsules 2740
Aceon Tablets (2 mg, 4 mg, 8 mg) (1.0%) 3191
Aciphex Tablets 1081
Actiq (Less than 1%) 993
▲ Actonel Tablets (4.1% to 4.8%) 2679
▲ Actonel with Calcium Tablets (4.1% to 4.8%) 2684
Adalat CC Tablets (Less than 1%) 2978
Advicor Tablets 1694
Aggrenox Capsules (2.1%) 855
Aldara Cream, 5% (0.9%) 1814
Altace Capsules (Less than 1%) 1673
Altoprev Extended-Release Tablets (Rare) 1151
Ambien Tablets (Infrequent) 2867
Amnesteem Capsules 2126
Antara Capsules 2723
Aricept Tablets (2%) 1086
Aricept ODT Tablets (2%) 1086
▲ Arimidex Tablets (12% to 14%) 665
Asacol Delayed-Release Tablets (1% to 2%) 2688
Atacand HCT (0.5% or greater) 637
Atrovent Inhalation Solution (0.9%) 868
Augmentin 1331
Augmentin Tablets 1334
Augmentin XR Extended-Release Tablets 1340
Augmentin ES-600 Powder for Oral Suspension 1337
Avalide Tablets 922
Avalide Tablets 2889
Avapro Tablets (Less than 1%) 925
Avapro Tablets (Less than 1%) 2886
Avelox (Less than 0.1%) 2984
Axert Tablets (Rare) 2430
Benicar Tablets (Greater than 0.5%) 2850
Benicar HCT Tablets (Greater than 1%) 2852
▲ Boniva Tablets (3.2%) 2747
Caduet Tablets (Greater than or equal to 2%) 2507
Campath Ampules 826
▲ Casodex Tablets (5%) 670
Celexa (Infrequent) 1177
Clinoril Tablets (Less than 1 in 100) 1899
Colazal Capsules 2845
Combunox Tablets (Less than 2%) 1183
Comvax 1904
Copaxone for Injection (Infrequent) 3292
▲ Coreg Tablets (Greater than 1% to 3%) 1376
Cozaar Tablets (Less than 1%) 1913
Crestor Tablets (Greater than or equal to 2%) 672
Cytovene 2763
Didronel Tablets 2693
▲ Ditropan XL Extended Release Tablets (2% to less than 5%) 2391
Dolobid Tablets (Less than 1 in 100) 1937
Effexor Tablets (Infrequent) 3405
Effexor XR Capsules (Infrequent) 3411
Engerix-B Vaccine (Less than 1%) 1391
Evoxac Capsules (Less than 1%) 1042
Exelon Capsules (Frequent) 2204
Faslodex Injection (2.8%) 682
▲ Femara Tablets (0.4% to 6.7%) 2210
▲ Flolan for Injection (52%) 1408
Fortical Nasal Spray (Less than 1%) 3336
Gabitril Tablets (Infrequent) 998
▲ Humira Injection (Less than 5%) 464
Hytrin Capsules (At least 1%) 469
Hyzaar 1964
Imitrex Nasal Spray (Infrequent) 1435
Imitrex Tablets 1440
Infed Injection 3381
▲ Intron A for Injection (Less than 5%) 3038
Invirase (Less than 2%) 2776
Lamictal (Rare) 1449
Lescol Capsules (Rare) 2227
Lescol Capsules (Rare) 2730
Lescol XL Tablets (1.3%) 2227
Lescol XL Tablets (1.3%) 2730
Levaquin in 5% Dextrose Injection (0.1% to 0.9%) 2453
Levaquin (0.1% to 0.9%) 2453
Lexapro Oral Solution (Infrequent) 1193
Lexapro Tablets (Infrequent) 1193
Lipitor Tablets (Greater than or equal to 2%) 2495
Lofibra Capsules 1217
Lotensin Tablets (Less than 1%) 2232
Lotensin HCT Tablets (0.3% or more) 2235
Lunesta Tablets (Infrequent) 3139
▲ Menostar Transdermal System (5%) 805
Meridia Capsules (Greater than or equal to 1%) 485
Meruvax II (Rare) 1994
Mevacor Tablets (Rare) 1996
Miacalcin Nasal Spray (Less than 1%) 2242
Micardis Tablets (More than 0.3%) 884
Micardis HCT Tablets 886
▲ Mirapex Tablets (3%) 889
M-M-R II 1980
Neurontin Capsules (Infrequent) 2498
Neurontin Oral Solution (Infrequent) 2498
Neurontin Tablets (Infrequent) 2498
Nipent for Injection (Less than 3%) 3216
Noroxin Tablets 2009
Omacor Capsules 2735
OptiPranolol Metipranolol Ophthalmic Solution 0.3% (A small number of patients) ⊙ 254
Orthoclone OKT3 Sterile Solution (Less than 1%) 2370
Orthovisc Injection (0.7%) 3518
Paxil CR Controlled-Release Tablets (Infrequent) 1509
Paxil (Infrequent) 1501
Permax Tablets (Infrequent) 3357
Persantine Tablets (Rare) 898
Plavix Tablets (1% to 2.5%) 940
Plavix Tablets (1% to 2.5%) 2942
Pletal Tablets (2% or greater) 2478
Pneumovax 23 2020
Pravachol Tablets (Rare) 943
Prevacid Delayed-Release Capsules (Less than 1%) 3268
Prevacid for Delayed-Release Oral Suspension (Less than 1%) 3268
Prevacid NapraPAC (Less than 1%) 3277
Prevacid SoluTab Delayed-Release Orally Disintegrating Tablets (Less than 1%) 3268
PREVPAC (Less than 1%) 3281
Prinivil Tablets (0.3% to 1.0%) 2029
Prinzide Tablets 2033
Proleukin for Injection (1%) 1007
Prometrium Capsules (100 mg, 200 mg) (Less than 5%) 3205
ProSom Tablets (Infrequent) 512
Protonix I.V. (Less than 1%) 3468
Protonix Tablets (Less than 1%) 3465
Protopic Ointment (Greater than or equal to 1%) 629
Provigil Tablets (At least 1%) 1002
Prozac Pulvules and Liquid (Infrequent) 1771
Rabies Vaccine RabAvert (Rare) 1011
Raptiva for Injection 1247
Recombivax HB (Greater than 1%) 2045
Relpax Tablets (Infrequent) 2531
Requip Tablets (1% or more) 1528
Rescriptor Tablets 2535
Risperdal Consta Long-Acting Injection (Infrequent) 1664
Risperdal M-Tab Orally Disintegrating Tablets (Rare) 1658
Risperdal (Rare) 1658
▲ Roferon-A Injection (5%) 2805
Rythmol SR Capsules 2736
Sandostatin Injection (Less than 1%) 2263
Sandostatin LAR Depot (Rare) 2264
Seroquel Tablets (Infrequent) 691
Sonata Capsules (Frequent) 1686
▲ Soriatane Capsules (1% to 10%) 1028
▲ Spiriva HandiHaler (Greater than or equal to 3%) 899
Sular Tablets (Less than or equal to 1%) 1163
Symbyax Capsules (Infrequent) 1788
Tasmar Tablets (1% to 2%) 3360
Teveten Tablets (Less than 1%) 1707
Teveten HCT Tablets (Less than 1%) 1710
Thalomid Capsules 979
Tindamax 2670
Travatan Ophthalmic Solution (1% to 5%) 559
Tricor Tablets 523
Twinrix Vaccine 1571
Uniretic Tablets (Less than 1%) 3114
Vaseretic Tablets 2073
Vasotec I.V. Injection (0.5% to 1.0%) 2076
VFEND I.V. (Less than 2%) 2543
VFEND Oral Suspension (Less than 2%) 2543
VFEND Tablets (Less than 2%) 2543
Viadur Implant (Less than 2%) 782
Viagra Tablets (Less than 2%) 2552
Viracept (Less than 2%) 2556
Vivelle Transdermal System 2288
Vivelle-Dot Transdermal System 2293
Vytorin 10/10 Tablets 2084
Vytorin 10/10 Tablets 3092
Vytorin 10/20 Tablets 2084
Vytorin 10/20 Tablets 3092
Vytorin 10/40 Tablets 2084
Vytorin 10/40 Tablets 3092
Vytorin 10/80 Tablets 2084
Vytorin 10/80 Tablets 3092
▲ Wellbutrin Tablets (3.1%) 1579
Wellbutrin SR Sustained-Release Tablets (Up to 2%) 1583

Wellbutrin XL Extended-Release Tablets (Up to 2%) 1588
▲ Xeloda Tablets (Less than 5%) 2825
▲ Xenical Capsules (5.4%) 2834
Zestoretic Tablets 701
Zestril Tablets (0.3% to 1.0%) 704
Zevalin Injection (Less than 1%) 848
Zocor Tablets (Rare) 2078
Zomig Tablets (Rare) 714
Zomig-ZMT Tablets (Rare) 714
Zonegran Capsules (Infrequent) 1089
Zyban Sustained-Release Tablets 1620
Zyprexa Tablets (Infrequent) 1798
Zyprexa ZYDIS Orally Disintegrating Tablets (Infrequent) 1798
Zyrtec Chewable Tablets (Less than 2%) 2589
Zyrtec (Less than 2%) 2589
Zyrtec-D 12 Hour Extended Release Tablets (Less than 2%) 2591

Arthritis, exacerbation of
Campath Ampules 826
▲ Entocort EC Capsules (Less than 5%) 2694
Evoxac Capsules (Less than 1%) 1042
Nexium Delayed-Release Capsules (Less than 1%) 645
Nexium I.V. (Less than 1%) 649
Teveten Tablets (Less than 1%) 1707
Teveten HCT Tablets (Less than 1%) 1710

Arthritis, inflammatory
Raptiva for Injection (0.4%) 1247

Arthritis, polyarticular
Rituxan for Infusion (Less than 0.1%) 845
▲ Rituxan I.V. (1% to 5%) 1251

Arthritis, psoriatic
Raptiva for Injection 1247

Arthritis, pyogenic
▲ Humira Injection (Less than 5%) 464

Arthritis, septic
Humira Injection 464
Raptiva for Injection 1247

Arthritis, tuberculous
Enbrel 580

Arthropathy, Charcot-like
Decadron Phosphate Injection 1931
Depo-Medrol Single-Dose Vial 2617

Arthropathy, unspecified
Campath Ampules 826
Colazal Capsules 2845
Didronel Tablets 2693
Evoxac Capsules (Less than 1%) 1042
▲ Gengraf Capsules (4%) 458
▲ Lescol XL Tablets (3.2%) 2227
▲ Lescol XL Tablets (3.2%) 2730
Lexapro Oral Solution (Infrequent) 1193
Lexapro Tablets (Infrequent) 1193
▲ Neoral Soft Gelatin Capsules (4%) 2247
▲ Neoral Oral Solution (4%) 2247
Nexium Delayed-Release Capsules (Less than 1%) 645
Nexium I.V. (Less than 1%) 649
Orthovisc Injection (0.9%) 3518
Risperdal Consta Long-Acting Injection (Infrequent) 1664
▲ Simulect for Injection (3% to 10%) 2268
▲ Starlix Tablets (3.3%) 2276
Ticlid Tablets (Rare) 2813
Zelnorm Tablets 2303

Arthroplasty, knee
Orthovisc Injection (0.5%) 3518

Arthrosis
Abilify Tablets (Infrequent) 916
Abilify Tablets (Infrequent) 2472
Aciphex Tablets 1081
Aggrenox Capsules (1.1%) 855
Ambien Tablets (Rare) 2867
Antara Capsules 2723
▲ Arava Tablets (1% to 3%) 2881
▲ Aredia for Injection (At least 10%) 2168
▲ Arimidex Tablets (4% to 6%) 665
Atacand HCT (0.5% or greater) 637
Caduet Tablets (Greater than 0.1% to less than or equal to 1%) 2507
Celebrex Capsules (0.1% to 1.9%) 3130
Depacon Injection (1% or more) 412
Depakene (1% or more) 417
Depakote Sprinkle Capsules 422
▲ Depakote Tablets (1% to 5%) 427
Depakote ER Tablets (Greater than 1%) 433
Effexor Tablets (Infrequent) 3405
Effexor XR Capsules (Infrequent) 3411
▲ Fabrazyme for Intravenous Infusion (3%) 1267
▲ Fortical Nasal Spray (1% to 3%) 3336
Frova Tablets (Infrequent) 1101
Gabitril Tablets (Infrequent) 998
▲ Humatrope Vials and Cartridges (10.8%) 1756
▲ Intron A for Injection (Less than 5%) 3038
Kaletra (Less than 2%) 474
Levaquin in 5% Dextrose Injection (0.1% to 0.9%) 2453
Levaquin (0.1% to 0.9%) 2453
Lofibra Capsules 1217
Lunesta Tablets (Rare) 3139
Lyrica Capsules (0.1% to 1%) 2524
Meridia Capsules 485
Miacalcin Nasal Spray (1% to 3%) 2242
Neurontin Capsules (Infrequent) 2498
Neurontin Oral Solution (Infrequent) 2498
Neurontin Tablets (Infrequent) 2498
Norvasc Tablets (More than 0.1% to 1%) 2529
Norvir (Less than 2%) 499
NovoSeven (1%) 2335
Paxil CR Controlled-Release Tablets (Rare) 1509
Paxil (Rare) 1501
Plavix Tablets (1% to 2.5%) 940
Plavix Tablets (1% to 2.5%) 2942
Protonix I.V. (Less than 1%) 3468
Protonix Tablets (Less than 1%) 3465
Prozac Pulvules and Liquid (Rare) 1771
▲ Rapamune Oral Solution and Tablets (3% to 20%) 3472
Relpax Tablets (Infrequent) 2531
Requip Tablets (1% or more) 1528
Rilutek Tablets (Infrequent) 2945
Risperdal Consta Long-Acting Injection (Infrequent) 1664
Risperdal M-Tab Orally Disintegrating Tablets (Rare) 1658
Risperdal (Rare) 1658
Sonata Capsules (Infrequent) 1686
▲ Soriatane Capsules (1% to 10%) 1028
Symbyax Capsules (Rare) 1788
Targretin Capsules 1719
Tasmar Tablets (Infrequent) 3360
Teveten Tablets (Less than 1%) 1707
Teveten HCT Tablets (Less than 1%) 1710
Topamax Sprinkle Capsules (Infrequent) 2438
Topamax Tablets (Infrequent) 2438
Tricor Tablets 523
Uniretic Tablets (Less than 1%) 3114
Viagra Tablets (Less than 2%) 2552
▲ Visudyne for Injection (1% to 10%) 2286
Zoloft (Infrequent) 2581
Zyprexa Tablets (Infrequent) 1798
Zyprexa ZYDIS Orally Disintegrating Tablets (Infrequent) 1798
Zyrtec Chewable Tablets (Less than 2%) 2589
Zyrtec (Less than 2%) 2589
Zyrtec-D 12 Hour Extended Release Tablets (Less than 2%) 2591

Ascaris, appearance in mouth and nose
Mintezol 2002

Ascites
Actiq (1% or greater) 993
Campath Ampules 826
Campral Tablets (Rare) 1175
▲ Camptosar Injection (9%) 2602
▲ CellCept Capsules (24.2%) 2751
▲ CellCept Intravenous (24.2%) 2751
▲ CellCept Oral Suspension (24.2%) 2751
▲ CellCept Tablets (24.2%) 2751
Cosmegen for Injection 1907
▲ Doxil Injection (1% to 10%) 3302
Ellence Injection 2632
▲ Eloxatin for Injection (2% to 5%) 2908
▲ Flolan for Injection (12% to 23%) 1408
Follistim AQ Cartridge 2354
▲ Gleevec Tablets (2% to 16%) 2221
Herceptin I.V. (At least one of the 958 patients) 1234
▲ Intron A for Injection (Less than 5%) 3038
Invirase (Rare) 2776
Levaquin in 5% Dextrose Injection (0.1% to 0.9%) 2453
Levaquin (0.1% to 0.9%) 2453
Lyrica Capsules (Rare) 2524
Mylotarg for Injection (Observed in 8 out of 274 patients) 3429
Oncaspar 1123
▲ Prograf Capsules and Injection (7% to 27%) 624
▲ Proleukin for Injection (4%) 1007
▲ Rapamune Oral Solution and Tablets (3% to 20%) 3472
Requip Tablets (Rare) 1528
Risperdal M-Tab Orally Disintegrating Tablets (Rare) 1658
Risperdal (Rare) 1658
Sandostatin LAR Depot (1% to 4%) 2264
Tabloid Tablets 1545
Taxotere Injection Concentrate (Less frequent) 2947
Thalomid Capsules 979
▲ Valcyte Tablets (Less than 5%) 2816
▲ Vesanoid Capsules (3%) 2823
VFEND I.V. (Less than 2%) 2543
VFEND Oral Suspension (Less than 2%) 2543
VFEND Tablets (Less than 2%) 2543
▲ Xeloda Tablets (Less than 5%) 2825

Aseptic meningitis syndrome
Carimune NF 3501
Clinoril Tablets (Less than 1 in 100) 1899
CytoGam Intravenous (Infrequent) 1866
Gammagard Liquid (Infrequent) 751
Orthoclone OKT3 Sterile Solution (Less than 1%) 2370

Aseptic necrosis of femoral/humeral heads
Decadron Phosphate Injection 1931
Decadron Tablets 1929
Depo-Medrol Injectable Suspension 2615
Depo-Medrol Single-Dose Vial 2617
Hydrocortone Tablets 1963
Pediapred Oral Solution 3319

Aspartate aminotransferase levels, changes in
Abilify Tablets (Infrequent) 916
Abilify Tablets (Infrequent) 2472
▲ Emcyt Capsules (2% to 34%) 3137
Parcopa Orally Disintegrating Tablets 3111
Prozac Pulvules and Liquid (Infrequent) 1771
▲ Roferon-A Injection (1% to 9%) 2805
▲ Zyvox (1.7% to 5%) 2661

Aspartate aminotransferase levels, elevation of
Abelcet Injection 1119
Accutane Capsules 2740
Aceon Tablets (2 mg, 4 mg, 8 mg) (0.3% to 1%) 3191
Aciphex Tablets (0.2%) 1081
Adalat CC Tablets (Rare) 2978
▲ Alimta for Injection (Less than 1% to 8%) 1722
Aloxi Injection (Less than 1%) 2099
Altoprev Extended-Release Tablets 1151
Ambien Tablets (Rare) 2867
▲ AmBisome for Injection (12.8%) 615
Amnesteem Capsules 2126
Amoxil Capsules 1315
Amoxil Chewable Tablets 1315
Amoxil Pediatric Drops for Oral Suspension 1315
Amoxil Powder for Oral Suspension 1315
Amoxil Tablets 1315
Anadrol-50 Tablets 3329
Anaprox Tablets (Less than 1%) 2769
Anaprox DS Tablets (Less than 1%) 2769
Ancef for Injection 1318
▲ Antara Capsules (3.4%) 2723
Anzemet Injection 2871
Anzemet Tablets 2874
▲ Aptivus Capsules (0.7% to 17.5%) 859
▲ Aralast (11.1%) 745
Arava Tablets (1.5% to 2.2%) 2881
▲ Arimidex Tablets (2% to 5%) 665
Arixtra Injection (0.2% to 2.6%) 1325
Asacol Delayed-Release Tablets 2688
Augmentin (Infrequent) 1331
Augmentin Tablets (Infrequent) 1334
Augmentin XR Extended-Release Tablets (Infrequent) 1340
Augmentin ES-600 Powder for Oral Suspension 1337
Axid Oral Solution (Less common) 913
Aygestin Tablets 1062
▲ Baraclude (5%) 928
BeneFix for Injection (1.6%) 3402
Benicar HCT Tablets (Greater than 1%) 2852
▲ Betaseron for SC Injection (3%) 791
Biaxin/Biaxin XL (Less than 1%) 402
Calcijex Injection 411
Calcium Disodium Versenate Injection 1819
Campral Tablets (Infrequent) 1175
▲ Camptosar Injection (1% to 10%) 2602
▲ Cancidas for Injection (1.9% to 13%) 1894
Cardizem LA Extended Release Tablets (Less than 2%) 1699
▲ Casodex Tablets (2% to 5%) 670
Ceftin (0.1% to 1%) 1369
Celebrex Capsules (0.1% to 1.9%) 3130
▲ CellCept Capsules (3% to less than 20%) 2751
▲ CellCept Intravenous (3% to less than 20%) 2751
▲ CellCept Oral Suspension (3% to less than 20%) 2751
▲ CellCept Tablets (3% to less than 20%) 2751
▲ Chemet Capsules (4.2% to 10.4%) 2480
▲ Cipro I.V. (Among most frequent) 2998
▲ Cipro I.V. Pharmacy Bulk Package (Among most frequent) 3509
Cipro (1.7%) 2991
▲ Clolar for Intravenous Infusion (38%) 1264
Colazal Capsules 2845
Combivir Tablets 1373
▲ Coreg Tablets (Greater than 1% to 3%) 1376
Covera-HS Tablets (1.4%) 3135
▲ Crixivan Capsules (3.7%) 1918
Cutivate Lotion 0.05% (Rare) 1383
Cymbalta Delayed-Release Capsules 1729
Cytovene (At least 3 subjects) 2763
Dalmane Capsules (Rare) 3343
DDAVP Tablets 2895
Demser Capsules (Rare) 1933
▲ Depacon Injection (1% to 5%) 412
Depakene (Frequent) 417
▲ Depakote Sprinkle Capsules (1% to 5%) 422
Depakote Tablets (Frequent) 427
Depakote ER Tablets (Greater than 1%) 433
Depo-Medrol Single-Dose Vial 2617
Dolobid Tablets 1937
EC-Naprosyn Delayed-Release Tablets (Less than 1%) 2769
Effexor Tablets (Infrequent) 3405
Effexor XR Capsules (Infrequent) 3411
▲ Eloxatin for Injection (0% to 54%) 2908
Elspar for Injection 1943
▲ Emend Capsules (3%) 1944
▲ Emtriva Capsules (3% to 6%) 1272
Epivir (Up to 1.7%) 1394
Eulexin Capsules 3023
Evoxac Capsules (Less than 1%) 1042
Factive Tablets (1.1%) 2464
Famvir Tablets (2.3%) 2207
Femara Tablets 2210
▲ Fortaz (1 in 16) 1422
Fuzeon Injection 2772
Gamunex Immune Globulin I.V., 10% 3232
Garamycin Injectable 3028
▲ Gemzar for Injection (52% to 78%) 1743
▲ Gleevec Tablets (Up to 3%) 2221
Hectorol Capsules 909
Hectorol Injection 911
▲ Hepsera Tablets (2% to 8%) 1275
▲ Humatrope Vials and Cartridges (6.67% to 12.50%) 1756
▲ Hycamtin for Injection (Less than 1% to 5%) 1427
▲ Imdur Tablets (Less than or equal to 5%) 3032
Increlex Injection 3290
▲ Intron A for Injection (Up to 63% of patients) 3038
▲ Invanz for Injection (7.1% to 8.4%) 1974
▲ Invirase (Less than 1% to 4%) 2776
▲ Kaletra (2% to 10%) 474
Kytril Injection (2.8%) 2785
▲ Kytril Tablets (5%) 2788
▲ Lexiva Tablets (6%) 1473
▲ Lofibra Capsules (Up to 3%) 1217
Lotronex Tablets 1479
▲ Lovenox Injection (Up to 3.9%) 2931
Lupron Depot 3.75 mg (One patient) 3257
Lupron Depot 7.5 mg (Greater than or equal to 5%) 3261
Malarone Tablets 1484
Malarone Pediatric Tablets 1484
Marinol Capsules (Less than 1%) 3334
Maxipime for Injection (2.4%) 1093
Mefoxin for Injection 1987
Mefoxin Premixed Intravenous Solution 1990
▲ Mepron Suspension (4%) 1487

Meridia Capsules (1.6%) 485
Merrem I.V. (Greater than 0.2%) 687
Mevacor Tablets 1996
Mobic Oral Suspension (Less than 2%) 893
Mobic Tablets (Less than 2%) 893
Mycamine for Injection (0.7% to 2.7%) 620
▲ Mylotarg for Injection (18%) 3429
Nabi-HB (2%) 2159
Nalfon Capsules (Less than 1%) 2504
Naprosyn Suspension (Less than 1%) 2769
Naprosyn Tablets (Less than 1%) 2769
▲ Navelbine Injection (1% to 54%) 1494
Nexium Delayed-Release Capsules (Less than 1%) 645
Nexium I.V. (Less than 1%) 649
Niaspan Extended-Release Tablets 1703
Noroxin Tablets (1.4% to 1.6%) 2009
▲ Norvir (6.4% to 9.5%) 499
▲ Novantrone for Injection Concentrate (5% to 6%) 3158
Omacor Capsules 2735
Omnicef Capsules (0.4%) 506
Omnicef for Oral Suspension (0.2%) 506
Oncaspar (Greater than 1% but less than 5%) 1123
Orthoclone OKT3 Sterile Solution (Less than 1%) 2370
Oxandrin Tablets 2977
Pacerone Tablets 3337
Paxil CR Controlled-Release Tablets (Infrequent) 1509
Paxil (Infrequent) 1501
Pentasa Capsules (Less than 1%) 3182
Pravachol Tablets 943
Precose Tablets 776
Prevacid Delayed-Release Capsules 3268
Prevacid for Delayed-Release Oral Suspension 3268
Prevacid NapraPAC 3277
Prevacid SoluTab Delayed-Release Orally Disintegrating Tablets 3268
PREVPAC (Less than 1%) 3281
Prilosec OTC Tablets (Rare) 2674
Primaxin I.M. 2022
Primaxin I.V. 2024
▲ Prograf Capsules and Injection (3% to 15%) 624
▲ Proleukin for Injection (23%) 1007
ProSom Tablets (Rare) 512
Protonix I.V. (Greater than or equal to 1%) 3468
Protonix Tablets (Less than 1%) 3465
Protopic Ointment (Greater than or equal to 1%) 629
Provigil Tablets (At least 1%) 1002
▲ Rapamune Oral Solution and Tablets (3% to 20%) 3472
▲ Rebif Prefilled Syringe for Injection (10% to 17%) 3163
▲ Rescriptor Tablets (2.3% to 3.4%) 2535
Risperdal Consta Long-Acting Injection (Rare) 1664
Risperdal M-Tab Orally Disintegrating Tablets (Infrequent) 1658
Risperdal (Infrequent) 1658
▲ Rocephin Injectable Vials, ADD-Vantage, Galaxy, Bulk (3.1%) 2801
Rythmol SR Capsules 2736
▲ Seroquel Tablets (3%) 691
Singulair (1.6%) 2047
Somavert Injection (0.8%) 2648
Sonata Capsules (Rare) 1686
▲ Soriatane Capsules (Approximately 1 in 3 patients) 1028
Stromectol Tablets (2%) 2053
Suprax (Less than 2%) 1811
Sustiva Capsules (2%) 957
Symmetrel 1115
▲ Synagis (3.0%) 1868
Tarceva Tablets 1254
Tarceva Tablets 2470
Targretin Capsules 1719
Tarka Tablets 519
Tasmar Tablets (1% to 5%) 3360
▲ Taxotere Injection Concentrate (4.3%) 2947
Tequin Injection (Less than 0.1%) 964
Tequin Tablets (Less than 0.1%) 964
Teveten Tablets (Less than 1%) 1707
Teveten HCT Tablets (Less than 1%) 1710
▲ Thalomid Capsules (2.8% to 12.5%) 979
Tiazac Capsules (Less than 2%) 1204
Ticlid Tablets (Rare) 2813
Timentin ADD-Vantage 1556
Timentin Injection Galaxy Container 1559
Timentin IV Infusion 1553
Timentin Pharmacy Bulk Package 1562
Topamax Sprinkle Capsules (Infrequent) 2438
Topamax Tablets (Infrequent) 2438
▲ Tracleer Tablets (11%) 539
Trecator Tablets 3482
▲ Tricor Tablets (3.4%) 523
▲ Triglide Tablets (3.4%) 1165
▲ Trisenox Injection (13%) 983
Trizivir Tablets (1.7%) 1565
▲ Truvada Tablets (1% to 12%) 1279
▲ Tygacil for Injection (4.3%) 3489
Ultane Liquid for Inhalation (Less than 1%) 526
Uniretic Tablets (Less than 1%) 3114
▲ Valtrex Caplets (1% to 16%) 1573
Vantas (Less than 2%) 3367
Vantin Tablets and Oral Suspension 2650
Verelan PM Capsules 3120
Vermox Chewable Tablets (Rare) 1853
▲ VFEND I.V. (1.9% to 20.3%) 2543
▲ VFEND Oral Suspension (1.9% to 20.3%) 2543
▲ VFEND Tablets (1.9% to 20.3%) 2543
Viracept (Less than 2%) 2556
Viramune Oral Suspension (2.0%) 903
Viramune Tablets (2.0%) 903
▲ Viread Tablets (3% to 4%) 1284
Xifaxan Tablets (Less than 2%) 2847
Zegerid Powder for Oral Solution (Rare) 2972
▲ Zerit (11%) 971
▲ Ziagen (6%) 1600
▲ Zinacef Injection (1 in 25 patients) 1604
▲ Zinacef for Injection (1 in 25 patients) 1604
Zithromax Capsules, 250 mg (1% to 2%) 2568
▲ Zithromax for IV Infusion (4% to 6%) 2573
Zithromax for Oral Suspension, 1 g (1% to 2%) 2568
Zithromax for Oral Suspension, 300 mg, 600 mg, 900 mg, 1200 mg (1% to 2%) 2561
Zithromax Tablets, 250 mg, 500 mg (1% to 2%) 2561
Zithromax Tablets, 600 mg (1% to 2%) 2568
Zithromax Tri-Pak (1% to 2%) 2561
Zithromax Z-Pak (1% to 2%) 2568
Zmax for Oral Suspension (Less then 1%) 2577
Zocor Tablets 2078
▲ Zofran Injection (Approximately 5% of patients) 1607
Zofran (Approximately 1% to 2%) 1613
Zofran ODT Orally Disintegrating Tablets (Approximately 1% to 2%) 1613
Zoladex (Less than 1%) 709
Zoladex 3-month 712
Zoloft (Infrequent) 2581
Zonegran Capsules (Rare) 1089
Zosyn 3492

Asphyxia

Bentyl Capsules 724
Bentyl Injection 724
Bentyl Syrup 724
Bentyl Tablets 724

Aspiration

Clozapine Tablets 2141
Clozaril Tablets 2174
FazaClo Orally Disintegrating Tablets 547
Levaquin in 5% Dextrose Injection (0.1% to 0.9%) 2453
Levaquin (0.1% to 0.9%) 2453
Risperdal M-Tab Orally Disintegrating Tablets (Rare) 1658
Risperdal (Rare) 1658
Seroquel Tablets 691

AST elevation

(*see under* Aspartate aminotransferase levels, elevation of)

Asterixis

Depacon Injection 412
Depakene 417
Depakote Sprinkle Capsules 422
Depakote Tablets 427
Depakote ER Tablets 433
Fortaz 1422
Orthoclone OKT3 Sterile Solution (Less than 1%) 2370
Phenytek Capsules (Rare) 2153
▲ Vesanoid Capsules (3%) 2823

Asthenia

▲ Abilify Tablets (Infrequent to 8%) 916
▲ Abilify Tablets (Infrequent to 8%) 2472
Accolate Tablets (1.8%) 663
Accutane Capsules 2740
▲ Aceon Tablets (2 mg, 4 mg, 8 mg) (7.9%) 3191
Aciphex Tablets 1081
▲ Actiq (4% to 38%) 993
▲ Actonel Tablets (3.5% to 5.1%) 2679
▲ Actonel with Calcium Tablets (3.5% to 5.4%) 2684
▲ Adacel Vaccine (1.2% to 30.4%) 2959
Adalat CC Tablets (Less than 1%) 2978
▲ Adderall XR Capsules (2% to 6%) 3169
Adenoscan (Less than 1%) 613
▲ Advicor Tablets (5%) 1694
Aerobid/Aerobid-M (1% to 3%) 1172
Aggrenox Capsules (1.8%) 855
▲ Agrylin Capsules (23.1%) 3172
Alacol DM Syrup 739
Albalon Ophthalmic Solution .... ⊙216
Aldoclor Tablets 1881
Aldoril Tablets 1884
Alinia for Oral Suspension (Less than 1%) 2840
Alinia Tablets (Less than 1%) 2840
Allegra-D 12 Hour Extended-Release Tablets 2860
Allegra-D 24 Hour Extended-Release Tablets 2862
Aloxi Injection (1%) 2099
Alphagan P Ophthalmic Solution (1% to 4%) 563
Altace Capsules (0.3% to 2.0%) 1673
▲ Altoprev Extended-Release Tablets (3%) 1151
Amaryl Tablets (1.6%) 2864
Ambien Tablets (Frequent) 2867
▲ AmBisome for Injection (6.2% to 13.1%) 615
Ammonul Injection 3323
Amnesteem Capsules 2126
AndroGel (0% to 3%) 3330
Antara Capsules (2.1%) 2723
▲ Apokyn Injection (At least 5%) 2132
Aptivus Capsules (1.5%) 859
▲ Aranesp for Injection (5%) 576
▲ Arava Tablets (3%) 2881
▲ Aredia for Injection (22.2%) 2168
▲ Arimidex Tablets (13% to 17%) 665
Aromasin Tablets (Less frequent) 2600
Arthrotec Tablets (Rare) 3126
▲ Asacol Delayed-Release Tablets (7%) 2688
Atacand Tablets (0.5% or greater) 634
Atacand HCT (0.5% or greater) 637
Avalide Tablets 922
Avalide Tablets 2889
Avapro Tablets (1% or greater) 925
Avapro Tablets (1% or greater) 2886
▲ Avastin IV (10% to 74%) 1229
Avelox (0.1% to less than 2%) 2984
▲ Avinza Capsules (5% to 10%) 1714
▲ Avonex (24%) 839
Axert Tablets (Infrequent) 2430
▲ Axid Oral Solution (3.1%) 913
Balamine DM 739
Benicar Tablets 2850
Benicar HCT Tablets (Rare) 2852
▲ Bentyl Capsules (7%) 724
▲ Bentyl Injection (7%) 724
▲ Bentyl Syrup (7%) 724
▲ Bentyl Tablets (7%) 724
Betagan Ophthalmic Solution, USP .... ⊙217
▲ Betaseron for SC Injection (61%) 791
Betimol Ophthalmic Solution (1% to 5%) .... ⊙283
Betimol Ophthalmic Solution (1% to 5%) 3371
▲ Bexxar (2% to 46%) 1360
▲ BiDil Tablets (14%) 2161
Biltricide Tablets 2990
Blocadren Tablets (0.6%) 1891
▲ Boniva Tablets (3.5%) 2747
▲ Botox Purified Neurotoxin Complex (2% to 10%) 565
Brevibloc Concentrate (Less than 1%) 766
Brevibloc Injection (Less than 1%) 766
Brevibloc Double Strength Injection (Less than 1%) 766
Brevibloc Premixed Injection (Less than 1%) 766
Brevibloc Double Strength Premixed Injection (Less than 1%) 766
▲ Brimonidine Tartrate Ophthalmic Solution 0.2% (3% to 9%) .... ⊙245
▲ Byetta Injection (Greater than or equal to 1% to less than 5%) 605
▲ Caduet Tablets (Less than 1% to 3.8%) 2507
Calcijex Injection 411
▲ Campath Ampules (4% to 13%) 826
▲ Campral Tablets (5% to 7%) 1175
▲ Camptosar Injection (12% to 76%) 2602
Cancidas for Injection (0%) 1894
Captopril Tablets 2114
Cardene I.V. (0.7%) 1129
Cardizem LA Extended Release Tablets (2.6%) 1699
▲ Carnitor Injection (8% to 12%) 3185
Carteolol Hydrochloride Ophthalmic Solution USP, 1% (Occasional) .... ⊙246
▲ Casodex Tablets (15%) 670
Cataflam Tablets (Occasionally) 2173
▲ Catapres Tablets (About 10 in 100 patients) 874
Catapres-TTS (0.5% or less) 875
Cathflo Activase (2%) 1232
Caverject Impulse Injection (Less than 1%) 2610
Celebrex Capsules (0.1% to 1.9%) 3130
Celexa (At least 2%) 1177
▲ CellCept Capsules (35.4% to 43.3%) 2751
▲ CellCept Intravenous (35.4% to 43.3%) 2751
▲ CellCept Oral Suspension (35.4% to 43.3%) 2751
▲ CellCept Tablets (35.4% to 43.3%) 2751
▲ Cenestin Tablets, 0.45mg, 0.625mg, 0.9mg, 1.25mg (11.3% to 33%) 1063
Cialis Tablets (Less than 2%) 1806
Cipro I.V. (1% or less) 2998
Cipro I.V. Pharmacy Bulk Package (1% or less) 3509
Cipro (Less than 1%) 2991
Cipro XR Tablets (Less than 1%) 3004
Clinoril Tablets (Less than 1 in 100) 1899
▲ Clorpres Tablets (About 10%) 2139
Clozapine Tablets (1%) 2141
Clozaril Tablets (1%) 2174
Cogentin Injection 1903
Colazal Capsules 2845
▲ CombiPatch Transdermal System (10% to 13%) 2180
Combivent Inhalation Aerosol 878
Combivir Tablets 1373
▲ Combunox Tablets (Less than 1% to 3.3%) 1183
Comtan Tablets (2%) 2186
▲ Copaxone for Injection (41%) 3292
▲ Copegus Tablets (65%) 2759
▲ Coreg Tablets (7% to 11%) 1376
Cosopt Sterile Ophthalmic Solution 1910
Coumadin for Injection (Infrequent) 932
Coumadin Tablets (Infrequent) 932
Cozaar Tablets (1% or greater) 1913
Crestor Tablets (2.7%) 672
Crixivan Capsules (2.1%) 1918
Cubicin for Injection (Less than 1%) 1038
▲ Cymbalta Delayed-Release Capsules (2% to 8%) 1729
Cytovene (At least 3 subjects) 2763
Dalmane Capsules 3343
▲ Dantrium Capsules (Among most frequent) 2690
Dapsone Tablets USP 1656
Daranide Tablets 1928
Darvocet A 500 Tablets 3497
DDAVP Nasal Spray (Up to 2%) 2894
Decadron Tablets 1929
▲ Depacon Injection (10% to 27%) 412
▲ Depakene (21% to 27%) 417
▲ Depakote Sprinkle Capsules (10% to 27%) 422
▲ Depakote Tablets (10% to 27%) 427
▲ Depakote ER Tablets (20% to 27%) 433
▲ DepoCyt Injection (5% to 19%) 1121
▲ Depo-Provera Contraceptive Injection (Greater than 5%) 2619
depo-subQ provera 104 Injectable Suspension 2622
Desmopressin Acetate Rhinal Tube (Up to 2%) 1144
Diastat Rectal Delivery System (At least 1%) 3344
Digitek Tablets 2146
Dilaudid 439
Dilaudid Oral Liquid (Less frequent) 443
Dilaudid Non-Sterile Powder 439
Dilaudid Rectal Suppositories 439
Dilaudid Tablets 439

Dilaudid Tablets - 8 mg (Less frequent) 443
Dilaudid-HP (Less frequent) 441
Diovan HCT Tablets (Greater than 0.2%) 2195
Diovan Tablets 2191
Diprivan Injectable Emulsion (Less than 1%) 676
▲ Ditropan XL Extended Release Tablets (3% to 7%) 2391
Diuril Oral 1936
Diuril Sodium Intravenous 1934
Dolobid Tablets (Less than 1 in 100) 1937
▲ Dostinex Tablets (6% to 9%) 2631
▲ Doxil Injection (6.5% to 40.2%) 3302
▲ Duragesic Transdermal System (10% or more) 2448
Dyazide Capsules 1389
DynaCirc CR Tablets 2726
Dyrenium Capsules (Rare) 3390
▲ Effexor Tablets (2% to 16.9%) 3405
▲ Effexor XR Capsules (1% to 17%) 3411
Eldepryl Capsules 3209
Eligard 22.5 mg (Less than 2%) 2899
▲ Eligard 45 mg (3.6%) 2904
▲ Emend Capsules (17.8%) 1944
▲ Emtriva Capsules (12% to 16%) 1272
Enablex Extended-Release Tablets (1.5% to 2.7%) 2201
▲ Enbrel for Injection (5% to 11%) 580
Engerix-B Vaccine (Less than 1%) 1391
▲ Entocort EC Capsules (Less than 5%) 2694
EpiPen 1061
Epivir 1394
Epivir-HBV 1398
▲ Epogen for Injection (7% to 13%) 586
Epzicom Tablets 1402
▲ Equetro Extended-Release Capsules (8%) 3178
▲ Erbitux (49%) 937
Eskalith 1406
▲ Estrogel 0.06% (4.8%) 3200
Evoxac Capsules (0.5%) 1042
▲ Exelon Capsules (6%) 2204
Factive Tablets (Less than or equal to 0.1%) 2464
▲ Faslodex Injection (22.7%) 682
FazaClo Orally Disintegrating Tablets (1%) 547
▲ Femara Tablets (0.6% to 33.6%) 2210
▲ Ferrlecit Injection (7%) 3379
▲ Flexeril Tablets (1% to 3%) 1832
▲ Flolan for Injection (87% to 100%) 1408
▲ Flomax Capsules (7.8% to 8.5%) 881
Flumadine (1.4%) 1186
▲ Flumist Vaccine (25.7%) 1872
▲ Forteo for Injection (8.7%) 1739
Frova Tablets (Infrequent) 1101
Furosemide Tablets 2117
Fuzeon Injection 2772
▲ Gabitril Tablets (18% to 23%) 998
▲ Gamunex Immune Globulin I.V., 10% (4% to 10%) 3232
Gemzar for Injection (Common) 1743
Gengraf Capsules (Rare) 458
▲ Geodon (5% to 6%) 2514
▲ Gleevec Tablets (15% to 21%) 2221
Hectorol Capsules 909
Hectorol Injection 911
▲ Hepsera Tablets (2% to 13%) 1275
▲ Herceptin I.V. (42%) 1234
▲ Humatrope Vials and Cartridges (3.33% to 6.25%) 1756
▲ Hycamtin for Injection (Less than 1% to 21%) 1427
Hyperstat I.V. Injection (2%) 3031
▲ Hytrin Capsules (1.6% to 11.3%) 469
Hyzaar (1% or greater) 1964
▲ Imdur Tablets (Less than or equal to 5%) 3032
▲ Imitrex Injection (4.9%) 1431
Imitrex Nasal Spray (Infrequent) 1435
Imitrex Tablets (Less than 1% to 2%) 1440
Indapamide Tablets (Less than 5%) 2119
Inderal LA Long-Acting Capsules 3421
Infed Injection 3381
▲ Infergen (9% to 10%) 1647
InnoPran XL Capsules 2728
▲ Intron A for Injection (Up to 40%) 3038
Invanz for Injection (1.2%) 1974
Inversine Tablets 3286
▲ Invirase (0.3% to 9.2%) 2776
▲ Iressa Tablets (5% to 6%) 684
▲ I.V. Busulfex (2% to 51%) 1125
Kadian Capsules (Less than 3%) 572
▲ Kaletra (3% to 9%) 474
▲ Keppra Oral Solution (8.9% to 15%) 3307
▲ Keppra Tablets (8.9% to 15%) 3307
K-Phos Neutral Tablets 785
▲ Kytril Injection (5%) 2785
▲ Kytril Tablets (5% to 14%) 2788
▲ Lamictal (2% to 8%) 1449
Lanoxicaps Capsules 1458
Lanoxin Injection 1462
Lanoxin Tablets 1468
Lanoxin Injection Pediatric 1465
Lariam Tablets (Less than 1%) 2790
Lescol Capsules (Rare) 2227
Lescol Capsules (Rare) 2730
Lescol XL Tablets 2227
Lescol XL Tablets 2730
▲ Leukine (17% to 66%) 829
▲ Leustatin Injection (9%) 2368
Levaquin in 5% Dextrose Injection (0.1% to 0.9%) 2453
Levaquin (0.1% to 0.9%) 2453
Levitra Tablets (Less than 2%) 3048
Levothroid Tablets 1189
Lexapro Oral Solution (Infrequent) 1193
Lexapro Tablets (Infrequent) 1193
Lidoderm Patch 1107
▲ Lipitor Tablets (Up to 3.8%) 2495
Lofibra Capsules (2.1%) 1217
Lotensin Tablets (Less than 1%) 2232
Lotensin HCT Tablets (0.3% to1%) 2235
Lotrel Capsules 2238
▲ Lumigan Ophthalmic Solution (1% to 5%) 569
Lunesta Tablets 3139
▲ Lupron Depot 3.75 mg (9%) 3257
Lupron Depot 7.5 mg (Less than 5%) 3261
▲ Lupron Depot–3 Month 11.25 mg (9%) 3262
▲ Lyrica Capsules (2% to 7%) 2524
▲ Malarone Tablets (3% to 8%) 1484
▲ Malarone Pediatric Tablets (3% to 8%) 1484
Marinol Capsules (Greater than 1%) 3334
Matulane Capsules 3188
▲ Mavik Tablets (3.3%) 482
Maxair Autohaler 1820
▲ Maxalt Tablets (4% to 7%) 1983
▲ Maxalt-MLT Orally Disintegrating Tablets (4% to 7%) 1983
Maxzide 2150
▲ Megace ES Oral Suspension (2% to 6%) 2492
▲ Mepron Suspension (8% to 31%) 1487
▲ Meridia Capsules (5.9%) 485
Mevacor Tablets (1.2% to 1.7%) 1996
Micardis Tablets 884
Micardis HCT Tablets 886
▲ Midamor Tablets (Between 1% and 3%) 2000
Migranal Nasal Spray (1%) 3350
Mintezol 2002
▲ Mirapex Tablets (10% to 14%) 889
▲ Moduretic Tablets (3% to 8%) 2003
MS Contin Tablets (Less frequent) 2703
Mustargen for Injection 2007
Myleran Tablets 1492
▲ Mylotarg for Injection (37%) 3429
▲ Nalfon Capsules (5.4%) 2504
Narcan Injection 1109
Naropin Injection (Less than 1%) 640
▲ Navelbine Injection (Up to 27%) 1494
Neoral Soft Gelatin Capsules (Rare) 2247
Neoral Oral Solution (Rare) 2247
▲ Neulasta Injection (15% to 72%) 596
▲ Neumega for Injection (14%) 3433
▲ Neupogen for Injection (4%) 598
▲ Neurontin Capsules (5.7%) 2498
▲ Neurontin Oral Solution (5.7%) 2498
▲ Neurontin Tablets (5.7%) 2498
Nexium Delayed-Release Capsules (Less than 1%) 645
Nexium I.V. (Less than 1%) 649
Niaspan Extended-Release Tablets 1703
▲ Nipent for Injection (10% to 13%) 3216
▲ Niravam Orally Disintegrating Tablets (5.8% to 7.1%) 3106
Nitrolingual Pumpspray 1161
Norditropin Cartridges 2318
Norflex Injection 1824
Noroxin Tablets (Less frequent) 2009
Norvasc Tablets (Less than 1% to 2%) 2529
▲ Norvir (10.3% to 15.3%) 499
Nubain Injection (1% or less) 1111
Numorphan 1112
Omacor Capsules 2735
Omnicef Capsules (0.2%) 506
Omnicef for Oral Suspension (0.2%) 506
▲ Ontak Vials (66%) 1717
OptiPranolol Metipranolol Ophthalmic Solution 0.3% (A small number of patients) ⊙254
▲ Orap Tablets (25.0%) 1220
Ortho-Cyclen/Ortho Tri-Cyclen 2414
Ortho Tri-Cyclen Lo Tablets 2421
Orthoclone OKT3 Sterile Solution (Less than 1%) 2370
▲ OxyContin Tablets (6%) 2699
Parcopa Orally Disintegrating Tablets 3111
Parnate Tablets 1499
Patanol Ophthalmic Solution (Less than 5%) 557
▲ Paxil CR Controlled-Release Tablets (1.6% to 22%) 1509
▲ Paxil (1.6% to 22%) 1501
Pediarix Vaccine 1518
▲ Pegasys (56%) 2793
▲ PEG-Intron Powder for Injection (52%) 3062
Pentasa Capsules (Less than 1%) 3182
Pepcid Injection (Infrequent) 2017
Pepcid (Infrequent) 2014
▲ Permax Tablets (4.2%) 3357
▲ Photofrin for Injection (6%) 729
Plavix Tablets (1% to 2.5%) 940
Plavix Tablets (1% to 2.5%) 2942
▲ Plendil Extended-Release Tablets (2.2% to 3.9%) 651
Pletal Tablets (2% or greater) 2478
Pneumovax 23 2020
Pravachol Tablets (Rare) 943
▲ Premarin Tablets (7% to 8%) 3443
▲ Premphase Tablets (6% to 10%) 3452
▲ Prempro Tablets (6% to 10%) 3452
Prevacid Delayed-Release Capsules (Less than 1%) 3268
Prevacid for Delayed-Release Oral Suspension (Less than 1%) 3268
Prevacid NapraPAC (Less than 1%) 3277
Prevacid SoluTab Delayed-Release Orally Disintegrating Tablets (Less than 1%) 3268
PREVPAC (Less than 1%) 3281
Prilosec OTC Tablets (1.1% to 1.3%) 2674
Primaxin I.M. 2022
Primaxin I.V. (Less than 0.2%) 2024
Prinivil Tablets (Greater than 1%) 2029
Prinzide Tablets (1.8%) 2033
ProAmatine Tablets (Rare) 3183
Prochieve 4% Gel 1018
Prochieve 8% Gel 1018
▲ Procrit for Injection (7% to 13%) 2374
▲ Prograf Capsules and Injection (11% to 52%) 624
▲ Proleukin for Injection (23%) 1007
Prometrium Capsules (100 mg, 200 mg) 3205
▲ ProSom Tablets (11%) 512
Protonix I.V. (Greater than or equal to 1%) 3468
Protonix Tablets (Greater than or equal to 1%) 3465
Protopic Ointment (1% to 3%) 629
Provigil Tablets (At least 1%) 1002
▲ Prozac Pulvules and Liquid (7% to 21%) 1771
Pulmozyme Inhalation Solution 1245
Rabies Vaccine RabAvert (Common) 1011
▲ Rapamune Oral Solution and Tablets (22% to 40%) 3472
Raptiva for Injection 1247
Razadyne ER Extended-Release Capsules (Greater than or equal to 2%) 2434
Razadyne (Frequent) 2434
▲ Rebetol (5% to 66%) 3073
▲ Rebetron Combination Therapy (4% to 9%) 3078
Recombivax HB (Equal to or greater than 1%) 2045
ReFacto Vials 3479
Relafen Tablets (Less than 1%) 1523
▲ Relpax Tablets (4% to 10%) 2531
ReoPro Vials (0.7%) 1779
Requip Tablets (Infrequent) 1528
▲ Rescriptor Tablets (5.3% to 16%) 2535
▲ Retrovir Capsules (8.6% to 69%) 1533
▲ Retrovir IV Infusion (8.6% to 69%) 1537
▲ Retrovir (8.6% to 69%) 1533
Reyataz Capsules (Less than 3%) 948
▲ Ribavirin, USP Capsules (5% to 10%) 3083
▲ Rilutek Tablets (14.8% to 20.1%) 2945
Risperdal Consta Long-Acting Injection (Frequent) 1664
Risperdal M-Tab Orally Disintegrating Tablets 1658
Risperdal 1658
▲ Rituxan for Infusion (16%) 845
▲ Rituxan I.V. (26%) 1251
▲ Roferon-A Injection (Less than 0.5% to 88%) 2805
▲ Rythmol SR Capsules (3% to 4%) 2736
Sandimmune (Rare) 2259
▲ Sandostatin Injection (1% to 4%) 2263
▲ Sandostatin LAR Depot (5% to 15%) 2264
▲ Sensipar Tablets (7%) 603
▲ Seroquel Tablets (5%) 691
▲ Simulect for Injection (3% to 10%) 2268
Singulair (1.8%) 2047
▲ Sonata Capsules (5% to 7%) 1686
Spectracef Tablets (0.1% to 1%) 2706
Stalevo Tablets (2%) 2270
Stromectol Tablets (0.9%) 2053
▲ Suboxone Tablets (6.5% to 14%) 2719
▲ Subutex Tablets (4.9% to 14%) 2719
Surmontil Capsules 2347
Sustiva Capsules (Less than 2%) 957
▲ Symbyax Capsules (Up to 15%) 1788
Symmetrel (0.1% to 1%) 1115
▲ Tambocor Tablets (Less than 1% to 4.9%) 1824
▲ Targretin Capsules (20.2% to 45.3%) 1719
Tarka Tablets (0.3% or more) 519
Tasmar Tablets (1% or more) 3360
▲ Taxotere Injection Concentrate (12.8% to 74%) 2947
▲ Temodar Capsules (7% to 13%) 3088
Tequin Injection (Less than 0.1%) 964
Tequin Tablets (Less than 0.1%) 964
Teveten Tablets (Less than 1%) 1707
Teveten HCT Tablets (Less than 1%) 1710
▲ Thalomid Capsules (8.3%) 979
Thiothixene Capsules 2124
▲ Thymoglobulin for Injection (26.8%) 2848
▲ Thyrogen for Injection (3.4%) 1270
Thyrolar 1203
Tiazac Capsules (1% to 4%) 1204
Ticlid Tablets (0.5% to 1.0%) 2813
Timolide Tablets (1.9%) 2056
Timoptic in Ocudose (Less frequent) 2061
Timoptic Sterile Ophthalmic Solution (Less frequent) 2058
Timoptic-XE Sterile Ophthalmic Gel Forming Solution 2062
Tindamax (1.1% to 2.1%) 2670
▲ TOBI Solution for Inhalation (35.7%) 1015
▲ Topamax Sprinkle Capsules (Less than 1% to 6%) 2438
▲ Topamax Tablets (Less than 1% to 6%) 2438
Trasylol Injection (2%) 779
Trelstar LA Suspension (1.1%) 3387
Tricor Tablets (2.1%) 523
Triglide Tablets (2.1%) 1165
▲ Trileptal Oral Suspension (3% to 6%) 2281
▲ Trileptal Tablets (3% to 6%) 2281
▲ Trisenox Injection (10%) 983
Trizivir Tablets 1565
Trusopt Sterile Ophthalmic Solution (Infrequent) 2065
▲ Truvada Tablets (Greater than 5%) 1279
Twinrix Vaccine (Less than 1%) 1571
Tygacil for Injection (2.5%) 3489
Ultane Liquid for Inhalation (Less than 1%) 526
Ultracet Tablets (At least 1%) 2462
Uniretic Tablets (Less than 1%) 3114
Uroqid-Acid No. 2 Tablets 785
▲ Urso 250 Tablets (11.7%) 737
▲ Urso Forte Tablets (11.7%) 737
▲ Valcyte Tablets (Less than 5%) 2816
▲ Valtrex Caplets (1% to 4%) 1573
Vantas (Less than 2%) 3367
Vantin Tablets and Oral Suspension (Less than 1%) 2650
▲ Vaqta (3.9%) 2067
Vaseretic Tablets (2.4%) 2073
Vasotec I.V. Injection (1.1% to 1.6%) 2076
Verelan PM Capsules (2%) 3120
Vesanoid Capsules 2823
VFEND I.V. (Less than 2%) 2543
VFEND Oral Suspension (Less than 2%) 2543
VFEND Tablets (Less than 2%) 2543
▲ Viadur Implant (7.6%) 782
Viagra Tablets (Less than 2%) 2552
▲ Vicoprofen Tablets (3% to 9%) 533
Viracept (Less than 2%) 2556
Virazole for Inhalation Solution 3365
▲ Viread Tablets (7% to 11%) 1284
▲ Visudyne for Injection (1% to 10%) 2286
Vivactil Tablets 2350
▲ Voltaren Ophthalmic Solution (Less than or equal to 3%) 2300
Voltaren Tablets (Occasionally) 2298
Voltaren-XR Tablets (Occasionally) 2301
VoSpire Extended-Release Tablets (Less frequent) 2352
Vytorin 10/10 Tablets 2084
Vytorin 10/10 Tablets 3092

Vytorin 10/20 Tablets 2084
Vytorin 10/20 Tablets 3092
Vytorin 10/40 Tablets 2084
Vytorin 10/40 Tablets 3092
Vytorin 10/80 Tablets 2084
Vytorin 10/80 Tablets 3092
▲ WelChol Tablets (4%) 2855
▲ Wellbutrin SR Sustained-Release Tablets (2% to 4%) 1583
▲ Wellbutrin XL Extended-Release Tablets (2% to 4%) 1588
WinRho SDF 763
Xanax XR Tablets (Frequent) 2655
▲ Xeloda Tablets (Less than 1% to 26%) 2825
Xifaxan Tablets (Less than 2%) 2847
▲ Xopenex HFA Inhalation Aerosol (3%) 3151
▲ Xopenex Inhalation Solution (3%) 3143
▲ Xopenex Inhalation Solution Concentrate (3%) 3147
Yasmin 28 Tablets (Greater than 1%) 818
▲ Zavesca Capsules (17%) 543
Zegerid Powder for Oral Solution (1.1% to 1.3%) 2972
Zemaira (0.6%) 3506
▲ Zemplar Capsules (3%) 535
▲ Zemplar Injection (3%) 538
▲ Zenapax for Injection (2% to 5%) 2838
Zestoretic Tablets (1.8%) 701
Zestril Tablets (Greater than 1% to 1.3%) 704
▲ Zevalin Injection (43%) 848
Zithromax Capsules, 250 mg 2568
Zithromax for IV Infusion 2573
Zithromax for Oral Suspension, 1 g 2568
Zithromax for Oral Suspension, 300 mg, 600 mg, 900 mg, 1200 mg 2561
Zithromax Tablets, 250 mg, 500 mg 2561
Zithromax Tablets, 600 mg 2568
Zithromax Tri-Pak 2561
Zithromax Z-Pak 2568
Zmax for Oral Suspension (Less then 1%) 2577
Zocor Tablets (1.6%) 2078
Zofran (Up to 2%) 1613
Zofran ODT Orally Disintegrating Tablets (Up to 2%) 1613
▲ Zoladex (11%) 709
Zoloft (Frequent) 2581
▲ Zometa for Intravenous Infusion (5% to 24%) 2306
▲ Zomig Nasal Spray (0% to 3%) 718
▲ Zomig Tablets (3% to 9%) 714
▲ Zomig-ZMT Tablets (3% to 9%) 714
Zonegran Capsules (Frequent) 1089
Zyban Sustained-Release Tablets (Frequent) 1620
▲ Zyprexa Tablets (8% to 20%) 1798
Zyprexa IntraMuscular (2%) 1798
▲ Zyprexa ZYDIS Orally Disintegrating Tablets (8% to 20%) 1798
Zyrtec Chewable Tablets (Less than 2%) 2589
Zyrtec (Less than 2%) 2589
Zyrtec-D 12 Hour Extended Release Tablets (Less than 2%) 2591

Asthenopia

▲ Lumigan Ophthalmic Solution (1% to 3%) 569

Asthma, allergic

Abelcet Injection 1119

Asthma, bronchial

Agrylin Capsules (1% to 5%) 3172
Aralast (Greater than or equal to 0.2%) 745
BeneFix for Injection (1.6%) 3402
Caduet Tablets (Less than 2%) 2507
Cataflam Tablets (Occasionally) 2173
Cipro I.V. (1.8%) 2998
Cipro I.V. Pharmacy Bulk Package (1.8%) 3509
Coreg Tablets (Greater than 0.1% to 1%) 1376
Cuprimine Capsules 1925
Cytovene-IV (One report) 2763
Doxil Injection (Less than 1%) 3302
▲ Gamunex Immune Globulin I.V., 10% (3% to 29%) 3232
▲ I.V. Busulfex (8%) 1125
Kadian Capsules (Less than 3%) 572
Kaletra (Less than 2%) 474
Levaquin in 5% Dextrose Injection (0.1% to 0.9%) 2453
Levaquin (0.1% to 0.9%) 2453
Lipitor Tablets (Less than 2%) 2495
Norvir (Less than 2%) 499
Nubain Injection (1% or less) 1111
Omacor Capsules 2735
Permax Tablets (Infrequent) 3357
Prevacid Delayed-Release Capsules (Less than 1%) 3268
Prevacid for Delayed-Release Oral Suspension (Less than 1%) 3268
Prevacid NapraPAC (Less than 1%) 3277
Prevacid SoluTab Delayed-Release Orally Disintegrating Tablets (Less than 1%) 3268
PREVPAC (Less than 1%) 3281
Prinivil Tablets (0.3% to 1.0%) 2029
Prochieve 4% Gel 1018
Prochieve 8% Gel 1018
Prozac Pulvules and Liquid (Infrequent) 1771
Relafen Tablets (Less than 1%) 1523
Tasmar Tablets (Infrequent) 3360
Uniretic Tablets (Less than 1%) 3114
Vaqta (Less than 1%) 2067
Vaseretic Tablets 2073
Vasotec I.V. Injection (0.5% to 1.0%) 2076
▲ Vesanoid Capsules (3%) 2823
Vicoprofen Tablets (Less than 1%) 533
Voltaren Tablets (Occasionally) 2298
Voltaren-XR Tablets (Occasionally) 2301
Zestoretic Tablets 701

Asthma, worsening of

▲ AccuNeb Inhalation Solution (1.3% to 11.1%) 1055
▲ Asacol Delayed-Release Tablets (5% or greater) 2688
Cenestin Tablets, 0.45mg, 0.625mg, 0.9mg, 1.25mg 1063
Cenestin Tablets, 0.3mg 1063
Climara Transdermal System 795
Climara Pro Transdermal System 800
CombiPatch Transdermal System 2180
Elidel Cream 1% (Up to 3.9%) 2198
Estratest Tablets 3196
Estratest H.S. Tablets 3196
Estrogel 0.06% 3200
Finacea Gel (Rare) 1644
Flovent Diskus 50 mcg 1415
Flovent HFA 1418
Foradil Aerolizer 3024
Menostar Transdermal System 805
Nexium Delayed-Release Capsules (Less than 1%) 645
Nexium I.V. (Less than 1%) 649
Premarin Intravenous 3440
Premarin Tablets 3443
Premarin Vaginal Cream 3449
Premphase Tablets 3452
Prempro Tablets 3452
Qvar Inhalation Aerosol (Up to 4%) 1654
Striant Mucoadhesive 1022
Stromectol Tablets 2053
▲ Tamiflu Capsules (3.5%) 2810
▲ Tamiflu Oral Suspension (3.5%) 2810
Vaqta 2067
Vivelle Transdermal System 2288
Vivelle-Dot Transdermal System 2293
Xalatan Sterile Ophthalmic Solution 2654
▲ Xopenex HFA Inhalation Aerosol (9%) 3151
▲ Xopenex Inhalation Solution (9%) 3143
▲ Xopenex Inhalation Solution Concentrate (9%) 3147

Asthmatic episodes

Abilify Tablets (Frequent) 916
Abilify Tablets (Frequent) 2472
Aciphex Tablets 1081
Actiq (Less than 1%) 993
Aggrenox Capsules (Less than 1%) 855
Alupent Inhalation Aerosol (1 to 4%) 858
AmBisome for Injection (Less common) 615
Amerge Tablets (Rare) 1312
Antara Capsules 2723
Apokyn Injection 2132
▲ Arava Tablets (1% to 3%) 2881
Arthrotec Tablets (Rare) 3126
Avelox (Less than 1%) 2984
Bayer Aspirin Tablets 3515
Betoptic S Ophthalmic Suspension (Rare) 554
Campath Ampules 826
Campral Tablets (Infrequent) 1175
▲ Casodex Tablets (2% to 5%) 670
Celexa (Rare) 1177
▲ CellCept Capsules (3% to less than 20%) 2751
▲ CellCept Intravenous (3% to less than 20%) 2751
▲ CellCept Oral Suspension (3% to less than 20%) 2751
▲ CellCept Tablets (3% to less than 20%) 2751
Cipro (1.8%) 2991
Copaxone for Injection (Infrequent) 3292
Crestor Tablets (Greater than or equal to 1%) 672
depo-subQ provera 104 Injectable Suspension 2622
Desferal Vials 2190
Diastat Rectal Delivery System (2%) 3344
Dilaudid Oral Liquid 443
Dilaudid Tablets - 8 mg 443
Doxil Injection (Less than 1%) 3302
Duragesic Transdermal System (Less than 1%) 2448
Ecotrin Enteric Coated Aspirin Low, Regular and Maximum Strength Tablets 1627
Effexor Tablets (Infrequent) 3405
Effexor XR Capsules (Infrequent) 3411
Eldepryl Capsules 3209
Elidel Cream 1% (0.7% to 3.3%) 2198
Engerix-B Vaccine 1391
Evoxac Capsules (Less than 1%) 1042
▲ Flonase Nasal Spray (3.3% to 7.2%) 1412
Flumist Vaccine 1872
Gabitril Tablets (Infrequent) 998
Gengraf Capsules (1% to less than 3%) 458
Herceptin I.V. (At least one of the 958 patients) 1234
▲ Humira Injection (Less than 5%) 464
Imitrex Injection 1431
Imitrex Nasal Spray (Rare) 1435
Imitrex Tablets (Infrequent) 1440
Indocin Capsules (Less than 1%) 1968
Indocin I.V. (Less than 1%) 1973
Indocin (Less than 1%) 1968
Invanz for Injection (Greater than 0.1%) 1974
Keppra Oral Solution (2%) 3307
Keppra Tablets (2%) 3307
Klonopin (Infrequent) 2782
Levaquin in 5% Dextrose Injection (0.1% to 0.9%) 2453
Levaquin (0.1% to 0.9%) 2453
Lexapro Oral Solution (Infrequent) 1193
Lexapro Tablets (Infrequent) 1193
Lofibra Capsules 1217
Lotensin Tablets (Less than 1%) 2232
Lunesta Tablets (Infrequent) 3139
Lupron Depot 3.75 mg (Rare) 3257
Lupron Depot 7.5 mg (Rare) 3261
Lupron Depot–3 Month 11.25 mg 3262
Lupron Depot-PED 7.5 mg, 11.25 mg and 15 mg 3266
Merrem I.V. (Greater than 0.1% to 1%) 687
Micardis Tablets (More than 0.3%) 884
Micardis HCT Tablets 886
Mobic Oral Suspension (Less than 2%) 893
Mobic Tablets (Less than 2%) 893
Children's Motrin Oral Suspension and Chewable Tablets ▣ 647
Children's Motrin Non-Staining Dye-Free Oral Suspension ▣ 647
Children's Motrin Oral Suspension and Chewable Tablets 1837
Children's Motrin Cold Non-Staining Dye-Free Oral Suspension 1838
Children's Motrin Cold Oral Suspension 1838
Children's Motrin Non-Staining Dye-Free Oral Suspension 1837
Motrin Cold & Sinus Caplets 1836
Motrin IB Tablets and Caplets 1836
Infants' Motrin Concentrated Drops 1837
Infants' Motrin Non-Staining Dye-Free Drops 1837
Junior Strength Motrin Caplets and Chewable Tablets 1837
Namenda (Infrequent) 1199
Nasacort AQ Nasal Spray 2937
Nasonex Nasal Spray (Greater than or equal to 2%) 3058
Neurontin Capsules (Infrequent) 2498
Neurontin Oral Solution (Infrequent) 2498
Neurontin Tablets (Infrequent) 2498
▲ Nipent for Injection (3% to 10%) 3216
Omnicef Capsules 506
Omnicef for Oral Suspension 506
▲ Optivar Ophthalmic Solution (1% to 10%) 1877
Paxil CR Controlled-Release Tablets (Infrequent) 1509
Paxil (Infrequent) 1501
Phenergan 3438
Pletal Tablets (Less than 2%) 2478
Pred Mild Sterile Ophthalmic Suspension ⊙ 236
Prefest Tablets 1069
Prevnar for Injection 3460
Prinzide Tablets 2033
▲ Prograf Capsules and Injection (3% to 15%) 624
Proleukin for Injection 1007
ProSom Tablets (Infrequent) 512
Protonix I.V. (Less than 1%) 3468
Protonix Tablets (Less than 1%) 3465
▲ Protopic Ointment (4% to 16%) 629
Provigil Tablets (1%) 1002
▲ Rapamune Oral Solution and Tablets (3% to 20%) 3472
Raptiva for Injection 1247
Relenza Rotadisk (Less than 1%) 1525
Relpax Tablets (Infrequent) 2531
Requip Tablets (Infrequent) 1528
Rilutek Tablets (Infrequent) 2945
Risperdal M-Tab Orally Disintegrating Tablets (Rare) 1658
Risperdal (Rare) 1658
Rituxan for Infusion (0.3%) 845
▲ Serevent Diskus (3% to 4%) 1540
Seroquel Tablets (Rare) 691
Sonata Capsules (Infrequent) 1686
St. Joseph 81 mg Aspirin Chewable and Enteric Coated Tablets 1841
Sular Tablets (Less than or equal to 1%) 1163
Suprane Liquid for Inhalation (Less than 1%) 770
Sustiva Capsules (Less than 2%) 957
Symbyax Capsules (Infrequent) 1788
Synagis (More than 1%) 1868
▲ Tamiflu Capsules (3.5%) 2810
▲ Tamiflu Oral Suspension (3.5%) 2810
Tequin Injection (Less than 0.1%) 964
Tequin Tablets (Less than 0.1%) 964
Teveten Tablets (Less than 1%) 1707
Teveten HCT Tablets (Less than 1%) 1710
Thioridazine Hydrochloride Tablets 2122
▲ TOBI Solution for Inhalation (15.9%) 1015
Topamax Sprinkle Capsules (Greater than 1%) 2438
Topamax Tablets (Greater than 1%) 2438
Trasylol Injection (2%) 779
Tricor Tablets 523
Trileptal Oral Suspension 2281
Trileptal Tablets 2281
Twinrix Vaccine 1571
Urecholine Tablets 2349
Vantin Tablets and Oral Suspension (Less than 1%) 2650
Vaqta 2067
Viagra Tablets (Less than 2%) 2552
Viokase 738
Xalatan Sterile Ophthalmic Solution 2654
▲ Xeloda Tablets (Less than 5%) 2825
Zemuron Injection (Less than 1%) 2363
Zestril Tablets (0.3% to 1.0%) 704
Zyprexa Tablets (Infrequent) 1798
Zyprexa ZYDIS Orally Disintegrating Tablets (Infrequent) 1798

Asystole

Acthrel for Injection (One patient) 3528
Adenocard Injection 612
Brevibloc Concentrate (2 Patients) 766
Brevibloc Injection (2 Patients) 766
Brevibloc Double Strength Injection (2 Patients) 766
Brevibloc Premixed Injection (2 Patients) 766
Brevibloc Double Strength Premixed Injection (2 Patients) 766
Cardizem LA Extended Release Tablets (Infrequent) 1699
Digitek Tablets 2146
Diprivan Injectable Emulsion 676
Invanz for Injection (Greater than 0.1%) 1974
Lanoxicaps Capsules 1458
Lanoxin Injection 1462
Lanoxin Tablets 1468
Lanoxin Injection Pediatric 1465
TriLyte with Flavor Packs for Oral Solution 3114
Zantac Injection (Rare) 1593
Zantac Injection Pharmacy Bulk Package (Rare) 1595

Ataxia

Abilify Tablets (Rare to Infrequent) 916

Abilify Tablets (Rare to Infrequent).... 2472
Actiq (Less than 1%)........ 993
Ambien Tablets (Frequent)........ 2867
Ammonul Injection........ 3323
Anzemet Injection (Rare)........ 2871
Anzemet Tablets (Rare)........ 2874
Aricept Tablets (Frequent)........ 1086
Aricept ODT Tablets (Frequent)........ 1086
Attenuvax (Rare)........ 1889
Avinza Capsules (Less than 5%)....... 1714
Axert Tablets (Rare)........ 2430
Betagan Ophthalmic Solution, USP (Rare)........ ⊙ 217
▲ Betaseron for SC Injection (21%) 791
Buprenex Injectable (Rare)........ 2718
Caduet Tablets (Less than 2%)........ 2507
Captopril Tablets........ 2114
Celebrex Capsules (Less than 0.1%)........ 3130
Celexa (Infrequent)........ 1177
Cipro I.V. (1% or less)........ 2998
Cipro I.V. Pharmacy Bulk Package (1% or less)........ 3509
Cipro (Less than 1%)........ 2991
Cipro XR Tablets (Less than 1%)........ 3004
Clozapine Tablets (1%)........ 2141
Clozaril Tablets (1%)........ 2174
Copaxone for Injection (At least 2%)........ 3292
Cozaar Tablets (Less than 1%)........ 1913
Cymbalta Delayed-Release Capsules (Infrequent)........ 1729
Dalmane Capsules........ 3343
Daranide Tablets........ 1928
▲ Depacon Injection (8%)........ 412
▲ Depakene (8%)........ 417
▲ Depakote Sprinkle Capsules (1% to 8%)........ 422
▲ Depakote Tablets (1% to 8%)........ 427
▲ Depakote ER Tablets (8%)........ 433
▲ Diastat Rectal Delivery System (3%)........ 3344
Doxil Injection (Less than 1%)........ 3302
Effexor Tablets (Infrequent)........ 3405
Effexor XR Capsules (Infrequent)........ 3411
▲ Eloxatin for Injection (2% to 5%)........ 2908
▲ Equetro Extended-Release Capsules (5% to 15%)........ 3178
Eskalith........ 1406
Exelon Capsules (Frequent)........ 2204
Fabrazyme for Intravenous Infusion........ 1267
FazaClo Orally Disintegrating Tablets (1%)........ 547
Flexeril Tablets (Less than 1%)........ 1832
Flumadine (0.3% to 1%)........ 1186
Frova Tablets (Infrequent)........ 1101
▲ Gabitril Tablets (5%)........ 998
Garamycin Injectable........ 3028
Geodon Capsules (Frequent)........ 2514
Guanidine Hydrochloride Tablets........ 3030
Herceptin I.V. (At least one of the 958 patients)........ 1234
Hexalen Capsules........ 2101
Hyzaar........ 1964
Imitrex Tablets (Infrequent)........ 1440
▲ Intron A for Injection (Less than 5%)........ 3038
Invirase (Less than 2%)........ 2776
Kadian Capsules (Less than 3%)........ 572
Kaletra (Less than 2%)........ 474
▲ Keppra Oral Solution (2% to 3%)........ 3307
▲ Keppra Tablets (2% to 3%)........ 3307
▲ Klonopin (30%)........ 2782
▲ Lamictal (5% to 28%)........ 1449
Lariam Tablets (Occasional)........ 2790
Leukeran Tablets (Rare)........ 1472
Levaquin in 5% Dextrose Injection (0.1% to 0.9%)........ 2453
Levaquin (0.1% to 0.9%)........ 2453
Librium Capsules........ 3349
Lithobid Tablets........ 1670
Lunesta Tablets (Infrequent)........ 3139
▲ Lyrica Capsules (1% to 20%)........ 2524
Marinol Capsules (Greater than 1%)........ 3334
Matulane Capsules........ 3188
Maxalt Tablets (Infrequent)........ 1983
Maxalt-MLT Orally Disintegrating Tablets (Infrequent)........ 1983
Mebaral Tablets, USP (Less than 1 in 100 patients)........ 2483
Mintezol........ 2002
Mirapex Tablets (1% or more)........ 889
M-M-R II (Rare)........ 1980
Namenda (Frequent)........ 1199
Nembutal Sodium Solution, USP (Less than 1%)........ 2484
▲ Neurontin Capsules (3.3% to 12.5%)........ 2498
▲ Neurontin Oral Solution (3.3% to 12.5%)........ 2498
▲ Neurontin Tablets (3.3% to 12.5%)........ 2498
▲ Nicotrol NS (Less than 5%)........ 2596
Nipent for Injection (Less than 3%)... 3216
Niravam Orally Disintegrating Tablets........ 3106
Noroxin Tablets........ 2009
Norvasc Tablets (Less than or equal to 0.1%)........ 2529
Norvir (Less than 2%)........ 499
▲ Pacerone Tablets (4% to 9%)........ 3337
Parcopa Orally Disintegrating Tablets........ 3111
Parnate Tablets........ 1499
Paxil CR Controlled-Release Tablets (Rare to infrequent)........ 1509
Paxil (Rare to infrequent)........ 1501
Peganone Tablets, USP (Rare)........ 2487
Permax Tablets (1.6%)........ 3357
Phenergan........ 3438
▲ Phenytek Capsules (Among most common)........ 2153
Prinivil Tablets (0.3% to 1.0%)........ 2029
Prinzide Tablets........ 2033
▲ Prograf Capsules and Injection (3% to 15%)........ 624
ProSom Tablets (Rare)........ 512
Proventil HFA Inhalation Aerosol (Less than 3%)........ 3071
Provigil Tablets (1%)........ 1002
Prozac Pulvules and Liquid (Infrequent)........ 1771
Razadyne ER Extended-Release Capsules (Infrequent)........ 2434
Razadyne (Infrequent)........ 2434
Relpax Tablets (Infrequent)........ 2531
Rilutek Tablets (Infrequent)........ 2945
Risperdal Consta Long-Acting Injection (Infrequent)........ 1664
▲ Risperdal M-Tab Orally Disintegrating Tablets (17% to 34%)........ 1658
▲ Risperdal (17% to 34%)........ 1658
Rythmol SR Capsules........ 2736
Seroquel Tablets (Infrequent)........ 691
Sonata Capsules (Infrequent)........ 1686
Stalevo Tablets........ 2270
Sular Tablets (Less than or equal to 1%)........ 1163
Surmontil Capsules........ 2347
Sustiva Capsules........ 957
Symbyax Capsules (Infrequent)........ 1788
Symmetrel (1% to 5%)........ 1115
Tambocor Tablets (1% to 3%)........ 1824
Targretin Capsules........ 1719
▲ Temodar Capsules (8%)........ 3088
▲ Tequin Injection (Less than 0.1%)........ 964
▲ Tequin Tablets (Less than 0.1%)........ 964
Teveten Tablets (Less than 1%)........ 1707
Teveten HCT Tablets (Less than 1%)........ 1710
Thalomid Capsules........ 979
Tindamax........ 2670
▲ Topamax Sprinkle Capsules (1% to 16%)........ 2438
▲ Topamax Tablets (1% to 16%)........ 2438
Tranxene........ 2488
▲ Trileptal Oral Suspension (5% to 31%)........ 2281
▲ Trileptal Tablets (5% to 31%)........ 2281
Ultracet Tablets (Less than 1%)........ 2462
Uniretic Tablets (Less than 1%)........ 3114
Valcyte Tablets........ 2816
▲ Valium Tablets (Among most common)........ 2822
Valtrex Caplets........ 1573
Varivax........ 2070
Vaseretic Tablets........ 2073
Vasotec I.V. Injection (0.5% to 1.0%)........ 2076
VFEND I.V. (Less than 2%)........ 2543
VFEND Oral Suspension (Less than 2%)........ 2543
VFEND Tablets (Less than 2%)........ 2543
Viagra Tablets (Less than 2%)........ 2552
Vivactil Tablets........ 2350
Wellbutrin Tablets (Frequent)........ 1579
Wellbutrin SR Sustained-Release Tablets (Rare)........ 1583
Wellbutrin XL Extended-Release Tablets (Rare)........ 1588
▲ Xanax XR Tablets (7.2%)........ 2655
▲ Xeloda Tablets (Less than 5%)........ 2825
Zestoretic Tablets........ 701
Zestril Tablets (0.3% to 1.0%)........ 704
Zoloft (Infrequent)........ 2581
Zomig Nasal Spray (Infrequent)........ 718
Zomig Tablets (Rare)........ 714
Zomig-ZMT Tablets (Rare)........ 714
▲ Zonegran Capsules (6%)........ 1089
Zovirax........ 1616
Zyban Sustained-Release Tablets (Rare)........ 1620
Zyprexa Tablets (Infrequent)........ 1798
Zyprexa ZYDIS Orally Disintegrating Tablets (Infrequent)........ 1798
Zyrtec Chewable Tablets (Less than 2%)........ 2589
Zyrtec (Less than 2%)........ 2589
Zyrtec-D 12 Hour Extended Release Tablets (Less than 2%)........ 2591

Ataxia, cerebellar

Vaqta (Very rare)........ 2067

Atelectasis

AmBisome for Injection (Less common)........ 615
Bravelle for Intramuscular or Subcutaneous Injection........ 1140
▲ CellCept Capsules (3% to less than 20%)........ 2751
▲ CellCept Intravenous (3% to less than 20%)........ 2751
▲ CellCept Oral Suspension (3% to less than 20%)........ 2751
▲ CellCept Tablets (3% to less than 20%)........ 2751
Effexor Tablets (Rare)........ 3405
Effexor XR Capsules (Rare)........ 3411
Evoxac Capsules........ 1042
I.V. Busulfex (2%)........ 1125
Kadian Capsules (Less than 3%)........ 572
Lyrica Capsules (Rare)........ 2524
Numorphan........ 1112
▲ Prograf Capsules and Injection (5% to 28%)........ 624
Prozac Pulvules and Liquid (Rare)........ 1771
▲ Rapamune Oral Solution and Tablets (3% to 20%)........ 3472
Repronex for Intramuscular and Subcutaneous Injection........ 1148
Rythmol SR Capsules........ 2736
▲ Trasylol Injection (5%)........ 779
Virazole for Inhalation Solution (Infrequent)........ 3365
▲ Zenapax for Injection (2% to 5%)........ 2838
Zyprexa Tablets (Rare)........ 1798
Zyprexa ZYDIS Orally Disintegrating Tablets (Infrequent)........ 1798

Atherosclerosis

Imitrex Injection........ 1431
Imitrex Nasal Spray........ 1435

Atrial arrhythmias

Diprivan Injectable Emulsion (Less than 1%)........ 676
Hyperstat I.V. Injection........ 3031
▲ Imdur Tablets (Less than or equal to 5%)........ 3032
Ketek Tablets........ 2920
Mirapex Tablets (Less than 1%)........ 889
▲ Neumega for Injection (15%)........ 3433
Proleukin for Injection (Less than 1%)........ 1007
Razadyne (Infrequent)........ 2434
Symbyax Capsules (Rare)........ 1788
▲ Trasylol Injection (3%)........ 779
Ultane Liquid for Inhalation (Less than 1%)........ 526
VFEND I.V. (Less than 2%)........ 2543
VFEND Oral Suspension (Less than 2%)........ 2543
VFEND Tablets (Less than 2%)........ 2543
Zoloft........ 2581

Atrial contractions, premature

Adenocard Injection........ 612
Diprivan Injectable Emulsion (Less than 1%)........ 676
Neurontin Capsules (Rare)........ 2498
Neurontin Oral Solution (Rare)........ 2498
Neurontin Tablets (Rare)........ 2498
▲ Proleukin for Injection (4%)........ 1007
Risperdal M-Tab Orally Disintegrating Tablets (Rare)........ 1658
Risperdal (Rare)........ 1658

Atrial fibrillations

Abilify Tablets (Infrequent)........ 916
Abilify Tablets (Infrequent)........ 2472
Adalat CC Tablets (Less than 1%)........ 2978
Advair Diskus 100/50........ 1291
Advair Diskus 250/50........ 1291
Advair Diskus 500/50........ 1291
Advicor Tablets........ 1694
Agrylin Capsules........ 3172
Aldara Cream, 5% (1.4%)........ 1814
AmBisome for Injection (Less common)........ 615
Amerge Tablets (Infrequent)........ 1312
Antara Capsules........ 2723
Anzemet Injection........ 2871
Anzemet Tablets........ 2874
Aredia for Injection (Up to 6%)........ 2168
▲ Argatroban Injection (3%)........ 1321
Aricept Tablets (Frequent)........ 1086
Aricept ODT Tablets (Frequent)........ 1086
Arthrotec Tablets (Rare)........ 3126
Atrovent HFA Inhalation Aerosol........ 872
Avelox (Less than 0.1%)........ 2984
Caduet Tablets (Greater than 0.1% to less than or equal to 1%)........ 2507
Campath Ampules........ 826
▲ Carnitor Injection (2% to 6%)........ 3185
Celexa (Rare)........ 1177
▲ CellCept Capsules (3% to less than 20%)........ 2751
▲ CellCept Intravenous (3% to less than 20%)........ 2751
▲ CellCept Oral Suspension (3% to less than 20%)........ 2751
▲ CellCept Tablets (3% to less than 20%)........ 2751
Clozapine Tablets........ 2141
Clozaril Tablets........ 2174
Copaxone for Injection (Infrequent) .. 3292
Cozaar Tablets (Less than 1%)........ 1913
Cymbalta Delayed-Release Capsules (Infrequent)........ 1729
Diprivan Injectable Emulsion (Less than 1%)........ 676
DynaCirc CR Tablets (0.5% to 1%)........ 2726
Effexor Tablets........ 3405
Effexor XR Capsules........ 3411
Ethyol for Injection (Rare)........ 1869
Exelon Capsules (Frequent)........ 2204
FazaClo Orally Disintegrating Tablets........ 547
Geodon Capsules (Infrequent)........ 2514
Guanidine Hydrochloride Tablets........ 3030
▲ Humira Injection (Less than 5%)........ 464
Hyzaar........ 1964
Idamycin PFS Injection........ 2645
▲ Imdur Tablets (Less than or equal to 5%)........ 3032
Imitrex Injection (Extremely rare)........ 1431
Imitrex Nasal Spray........ 1435
Imitrex Tablets (Rare)........ 1440
▲ Intron A for Injection (Less than 5%)........ 3038
Invanz for Injection (Greater than 0.1%)........ 1974
I.V. Busulfex (2%)........ 1125
Kadian Capsules (Less than 3%)........ 572
Kaletra (Less than 2%)........ 474
Kytril Injection (Rare)........ 2785
Kytril Tablets (Rare)........ 2788
Lamictal (Rare)........ 1449
Levaquin in 5% Dextrose Injection (0.1% to 0.9%)........ 2453
Levaquin (0.1% to 0.9%)........ 2453
Lexapro Oral Solution........ 1193
Lexapro Tablets........ 1193
Lofibra Capsules........ 1217
Lovenox Injection (0.7%)........ 2931
Meridia Capsules........ 485
Micardis Tablets........ 884
Micardis HCT Tablets........ 886
Mirapex Tablets (Less than 1%)........ 889
Nalfon Capsules (Less than 1%)........ 2504
Namenda (Infrequent)........ 1199
Naropin Injection (Less than 1%)........ 640
Natrecor for Injection (Greater than or equal to 1%)........ 3123
▲ Neumega for Injection (12%)........ 3433
Neurontin Capsules (Rare)........ 2498
Neurontin Oral Solution (Rare)........ 2498
Neurontin Tablets (Rare)........ 2498
Niaspan Extended-Release Tablets ... 1703
Norvasc Tablets (More than 0.1% to 1%)........ 2529
OptiPranolol Metipranolol Ophthalmic Solution 0.3% (A small number of patients)........ ⊙ 254
Paxil CR Controlled-Release Tablets (Rare)........ 1509
Paxil (Rare)........ 1501
Permax Tablets (Infrequent)........ 3357
▲ Photofrin for Injection (10%)........ 729
Plavix Tablets (1% to 2.5%)........ 940
Plavix Tablets (1% to 2.5%)........ 2942
Pletal Tablets (Less than 2%)........ 2478
Prinivil Tablets (0.3% to 1.0%)........ 2029
Prinzide Tablets........ 2033
Protonix I.V.........3468
Protonix Tablets (Less than 1%)........ 3465
Proventil Inhalation Aerosol........ 3067
Prozac Pulvules and Liquid (Rare)........ 1771
▲ Rapamune Oral Solution and Tablets (3% to 20%)........ 3472
Razadyne ER Extended-Release Capsules (Infrequent)........ 2434
Razadyne (Infrequent)........ 2434
Relpax Tablets (Rare)........ 2531
▲ ReoPro Vials (3.5%)........ 1779
Requip Tablets (2%)........ 1528
Rilutek Tablets (Infrequent)........ 2945

- Risperdal M-Tab Orally Disintegrating Tablets 1658
- Risperdal 1658
- Sandostatin LAR Depot (Rare) 2264
- Serevent Diskus 1540
- Seroquel Tablets (Rare) 691
- ▲ Simulect for Injection (3% to 10%) 2268
- Spiriva HandiHaler (Less than 1%) 899
- Sular Tablets (Less than or equal to 1%) 1163
- Symbyax Capsules (Rare) 1788
- Tasmar Tablets (Infrequent) 3360
- Taxotere Injection Concentrate 2947
- ▲ Tenormin I.V. Injection (5%) 698
- ▲ Tenormin Tablets (5%) 695
- Teveten Tablets (Less than 1%) 1707
- Teveten HCT Tablets (Less than 1%) 1710
- Thalomid Capsules 979
- ▲ Trasylol Injection (21%) 779
- Tricor Tablets 523
- Triglide Tablets 1165
- Ultane Liquid for Inhalation (Less than 1%) 526
- Uniretic Tablets (Less than 1%) 3114
- Vaseretic Tablets 2073
- Vasotec I.V. Injection (0.5% to 1.0%) 2076
- Ventolin HFA Inhalation Aerosol 1576
- VFEND I.V. (Less than 2%) 2543
- VFEND Oral Suspension (Less than 2%) 2543
- VFEND Tablets (Less than 2%) 2543
- ▲ Visudyne for Injection (1% to 10%) 2286
- ▲ Xeloda Tablets (Less than 5%) 2825
- Xopenex HFA Inhalation Aerosol 3151
- Xopenex Inhalation Solution 3143
- Xopenex Inhalation Solution Concentrate 3147
- ▲ Zegerid Powder for Oral Solution (6.2%) 2972
- Zestril Tablets (0.3% to 1.0%) 704
- Zofran Injection 1607
- Zomig Nasal Spray (Rare) 718
- Zonegran Capsules (Rare) 1089
- Zosyn (1.0% or less) 3492
- Zyprexa Tablets (Infrequent) 1798
- Zyprexa ZYDIS Orally Disintegrating Tablets 1798

Atrial flutter
- Abilify Tablets (Rare) 916
- Abilify Tablets (Rare) 2472
- Amerge Tablets (Infrequent) 1312
- Anzemet Injection 2871
- Anzemet Tablets 2874
- Aredia for Injection (Up to 1%) 2168
- ▲ CellCept Capsules (3% to less than 20%) 2751
- ▲ CellCept Intravenous (3% to less than 20%) 2751
- ▲ CellCept Oral Suspension (3% to less than 20%) 2751
- ▲ CellCept Tablets (3% to less than 20%) 2751
- Cipro I.V. (1% or less) 2998
- Cipro I.V. Pharmacy Bulk Package (1% or less) 3509
- Cipro (Less than 1%) 2991
- Cipro XR Tablets 3004
- Ethyol for Injection (Rare) 1869
- ▲ Neumega for Injection (12%) 3433
- Pletal Tablets (Less than 2%) 2478
- Protonix I.V. 3468
- Protonix Tablets (Less than 1%) 3465
- ▲ ReoPro Vials (3.5%) 1779
- Rythmol SR Capsules 2736
- Taxotere Injection Concentrate (Rare) 2947
- Tenormin I.V. Injection (1.6%) 698
- Tenormin Tablets (1.6%) 695
- ▲ Trasylol Injection (6%) 779
- Uniphyl Tablets 2708

Atrial hypertrophy
- Rythmol SR Capsules 2736

Atrial rupture
- Ammonul Injection 3323

Atrial tachycardia
- Digitek Tablets 2146
- Lanoxicaps Capsules 1458
- Lanoxin Injection 1462
- Lanoxin Tablets 1468
- Lanoxin Injection Pediatric 1465
- Prinivil Tablets (0.3% to 1.0%) 2029
- Prinzide Tablets 2033
- Uniphyl Tablets 2708
- Vaseretic Tablets 2073
- Vasotec I.V. Injection (0.5% to 1.0%) 2076
- Zestril Tablets (0.3% to 1.0%) 704

Atrioventricular dissociation
- Covera-HS Tablets (Less than 2%) 3135
- Digitek Tablets 2146
- Lanoxicaps Capsules (Common) 1458
- Lanoxin Injection (Common) 1462
- Lanoxin Tablets (Common) 1468
- Tarka Tablets 519
- Verelan PM Capsules (2% or less) 3120

Atrophy
- Cuprimine Capsules 1925

Atrophy, cutaneous
- Decadron Phosphate Injection 1931
- Depo-Medrol Single-Dose Vial 2617

Atrophy, subcutaneous
- Decadron Phosphate Injection 1931
- Depo-Medrol Single-Dose Vial 2617
- Garamycin Injectable (Rare) 3028

Atrophy, testicular
- ▲ Eligard 45 mg (7.2%) 2904
- ▲ Vantas (5.3%) 3367

Attention, disturbance in
- ▲ Topamax Sprinkle Capsules (3% to 14%) 2438
- ▲ Topamax Tablets (3% to 14%) 2438
- ▲ Xanax XR Tablets (3.2%) 2655

Atypical measles
- Attenuvax 1889

Auditory acuity, decrease
- ▲ Capastat Sulfate for Injection (Approximately 11%) 1728
- Desferal Vials 2190

Auditory canals, small or absent, fetal
- Accutane Capsules 2740

Auditory disturbances
- Navelbine Injection 1494
- ▲ Wellbutrin Tablets (5.3%) 1579

Aura disappeared
- Neurontin Capsules 2498
- Neurontin Oral Solution 2498
- Neurontin Tablets 2498

Autoimmune disorders
- Avonex 839

Autoimmune disorders, life-threatening, aggravation of
- Copegus Tablets (Less than 1%) 2759
- Roferon-A Injection 2805

Autonomic deficit, persistent
- Symmetrel (Uncommon) 1115

A-V block
- Abilify Tablets (Infrequent) 916
- Abilify Tablets (Infrequent) 2472
- Activase I.V. 1225
- Adenocard Injection 612
- Anzemet Injection 2871
- Anzemet Tablets 2874
- Biltricide Tablets 2990
- Blocadren Tablets (Less than 1%) 1891
- Carbatrol Capsules 3174
- Cardene I.V. (Rare) 1129
- Catapres Tablets (Rare) 874
- Catapres-TTS (0.5% or less) 875
- Clorpres Tablets (Rare) 2139
- ▲ Coreg Tablets (Greater than 1% to 3%) 1376
- Covera-HS Tablets (0.8% to 2%) 3135
- Digitek Tablets 2146
- Diprivan Injectable Emulsion (Less than 1%) 676
- Ellence Injection 2632
- Equetro Extended-Release Capsules 3178
- Exelon Capsules (Infrequent) 2204
- Kytril Injection (Rare) 2785
- Lanoxicaps Capsules 1458
- Lanoxin Injection 1462
- Lanoxin Tablets 1468
- Lanoxin Injection Pediatric (Common) 1465
- Lariam Tablets (Infrequent) 2790
- Namenda 1199
- Nipent for Injection (Less than 3%) 3216
- Pepcid Injection (Infrequent) 2017
- Pepcid (Infrequent) 2014
- Permax Tablets (Infrequent) 3357
- Razadyne ER Extended-Release Capsules (Infrequent) 2434
- Razadyne (Infrequent) 2434
- ReoPro Vials (1.3%) 1779
- Retavase 1131
- Risperdal Consta Long-Acting Injection (Infrequent) 1664
- Risperdal M-Tab Orally Disintegrating Tablets (Infrequent) 1658
- Risperdal (Infrequent) 1658
- Rythmol SR Capsules 2736
- Tagamet Tablets (Rare) 1547
- Tambocor Tablets 1824
- Tegretol/Tegretol-XR 2278
- ▲ Tiazac Capsules (4%) 1204
- Timolide Tablets 2056
- TNKase I.V. 1256
- Topamax Sprinkle Capsules (Infrequent) 2438
- Topamax Tablets (Infrequent) 2438
- Ultane Liquid for Inhalation (Less than 1%) 526
- Verelan PM Capsules (0.8% to 1.2%) 3120
- VFEND I.V. (Less than 2%) 2543
- VFEND Oral Suspension (Less than 2%) 2543
- VFEND Tablets (Less than 2%) 2543
- Viagra Tablets (Less than 2%) 2552
- Wellbutrin SR Sustained-Release Tablets 1583
- Wellbutrin XL Extended-Release Tablets 1588
- Zantac (Rare) 1597
- Zantac Injection (Rare) 1593
- Zantac Injection Pharmacy Bulk Package (Rare) 1595
- Zantac Syrup (Rare) 1597
- Zoloft 2581
- Zyban Sustained-Release Tablets 1620
- Zyprexa IntraMuscular (Infrequent) 1798

A-V block, first-degree
- Adenocard Injection 612
- Adenoscan (2.9% to 3%) 613
- Aricept Tablets (Infrequent) 1086
- Aricept ODT Tablets (Infrequent) 1086
- ▲ Cardizem LA Extended Release Tablets (2.4% to 3.2%) 1699
- Cathflo Activase (1.2%) 1232
- Covera-HS Tablets (1.2% to 1.7%) 3135
- Digitek Tablets 2146
- Effexor Tablets (Rare) 3405
- Effexor XR Capsules (Rare) 3411
- Geodon Capsules (Rare) 2514
- Lanoxicaps Capsules 1458
- Lanoxin Injection 1462
- Lanoxin Tablets 1468
- Lanoxin Injection Pediatric 1465
- Mavik Tablets (0.3% to 1.0%) 482
- ▲ Rythmol SR Capsules (2% to 3%) 2736
- Seroquel Tablets (Infrequent) 691
- Sular Tablets (Less than or equal to 1%) 1163
- ▲ Tarka Tablets (3.9%) 519
- Uniretic Tablets (Less than 1%) 3114
- Verelan PM Capsules (1.2%) 3120

A-V block, intensification of
- Blocadren Tablets 1891
- Inderal LA Long-Acting Capsules 3421
- InnoPran XL Capsules 2728
- Nadolol Tablets (Single instance) 2121
- Toprol-XL Tablets 660

A-V block, second-degree
- Adenocard Injection 612
- Adenoscan (2.6% to 3%) 613
- Blocadren Tablets (Less than 1%) 1891
- Cardizem LA Extended Release Tablets (Less than 2%) 1699
- Covera-HS Tablets (0.8% to 2%) 3135
- Cozaar Tablets (Less than 1%) 1913
- Digitek Tablets 2146
- Hyzaar 1964
- Lanoxicaps Capsules 1458
- Lanoxin Injection 1462
- Lanoxin Tablets 1468
- Lanoxin Injection Pediatric 1465
- Proleukin for Injection (Less than 1%) 1007
- Reyataz Capsules (Rare) 948
- Tambocor Tablets (Less than 1%) 1824
- Tarka Tablets (Less frequent) 519
- Ultane Liquid for Inhalation (Less than 1%) 526
- Verelan PM Capsules (0.8% to 1.2%) 3120

A-V block, third-degree
- Adenocard Injection 612
- Adenoscan (0.8%; less than 1%) 613
- Blocadren Tablets (Less than 1%) 1891
- Cardizem LA Extended Release Tablets (Less than 2%) 1699
- Coreg Tablets (Less than or equal to 0.1%) 1376
- Covera-HS Tablets (0.8% to 2%) 3135
- Digitek Tablets 2146
- Lanoxicaps Capsules 1458
- Lanoxin Injection 1462
- Lanoxin Tablets 1468
- Lanoxin Injection Pediatric 1465
- Tambocor Tablets (Less than 1%) 1824
- Tarka Tablets 519
- Verelan PM Capsules (0.8% to 1.2%) 3120
- Wellbutrin Tablets 1579

A-V conduction, prolongation
- Timolide Tablets 2056

A-V conduction changes, unspecified
- Natrecor for Injection (Greater than or equal to 1%) 3123
- Nimotop Capsules 774

A-V shunt, thrombosis of
(*see under* Thrombosis of vascular access)

Avitaminosis
- Campral Tablets (Infrequent) 1175
- Kaletra (Less than 2%) 474
- Norvir (Less than 2%) 499
- Thalomid Capsules 979

Awareness, altered
- Diprivan Injectable Emulsion (Less than 1%) 676

Awareness, heightened
- Demser Capsules 1933
- Imitrex Tablets (Rare) 1440
- ▲ Marinol Capsules (8% to 24%) 3334

Azoospermia
- Mustargen for Injection 2007

Azotemia
- Altace Capsules 1673
- Aredia for Injection (Up to 4%) 2168
- Avalide Tablets 922
- Avalide Tablets 2889
- Carbatrol Capsules 3174
- Cleocin Vaginal Ovules (Rare) 2613
- Clindesse Vaginal Cream (Rare) 3296
- Diuril Sodium Intravenous 1934
- Dyrenium Capsules (Rare) 3390
- Effexor Tablets (Rare) 3405
- Effexor XR Capsules (Rare) 3411
- Elspar for Injection (Frequent) 1943
- Equetro Extended-Release Capsules 3178
- Furosemide Tablets 2117
- Guanidine Hydrochloride Tablets 3030
- Hyzaar 1964
- ▲ Indocin I.V. (41% of infants) 1973
- Lotrel Capsules 2238
- Nalfon Capsules (Less than 1%) 2504
- Prinivil Tablets (0.3% to 1.0%) 2029
- Prinzide Tablets 2033
- Relafen Tablets (Less than 1%) 1523
- Requip Tablets (Rare) 1528
- Tegretol/Tegretol-XR 2278
- Teveten HCT Tablets 1710
- Tygacil for Injection 3489
- Vancocin HCl Capsules, USP 3370
- Vaseretic Tablets 2073
- Vasotec I.V. Injection 2076
- VFEND I.V. (Less than 2%) 2543
- VFEND Oral Suspension (Less than 2%) 2543
- VFEND Tablets (Less than 2%) 2543
- Zestoretic Tablets 701
- Zestril Tablets (0.3% to 1.0%) 704

B

Babinski's phenomenon, bilateral
- Neurontin Capsules (Infrequent) 2498
- Neurontin Oral Solution (Infrequent) 2498
- Neurontin Tablets (Infrequent) 2498

Back strain
- Prinzide Tablets (0.3% to 1%) 2033
- Zestoretic Tablets (0.3% to 1.0%) 701

Backache
- Abilify Tablets 916
- Abilify Tablets 2472
- Accolate Tablets (1.5%) 663
- ▲ Aceon Tablets (2 mg, 4 mg, 8 mg) (Up to 5.8%) 3191
- Actimmune (2%) 1646
- Actiq (1% or greater) 993
- ▲ Activella Tablets (3% to 6%) 2311

▲ Actonel Tablets (8.7% to 26.1%) 2679
▲ Actonel with Calcium Tablets (8.7% to 26.1%) 2684
Adenocard Injection (Less than 1%) 612
Adenoscan (Less than 1%) 613
Advair Diskus 100/50 1291
Advair Diskus 250/50 1291
Advair Diskus 500/50 1291
▲ Advicor Tablets (5%) 1694
▲ Aggrenox Capsules (4.6%) 855
▲ Agrylin Capsules (5.9%) 3172
Alamast Ophthalmic Solution (Less than 5%) 3371
Aldara Cream, 5% (1.4%) 1814
Alferon N Injection (Up to 4%) 1640
Allegra (2.2% to 2.8%) 2857
Allegra-D 12 Hour Extended-Release Tablets (1.9%) 2860
Allegra-D 24 Hour Extended-Release Tablets (1.9%) 2862
▲ Altoprev Extended-Release Tablets (5%) 1151
▲ Ambien Tablets (3%) 2867
▲ AmBisome for Injection (12%) 615
▲ Angiomax for Injection (9.2% to 42%) 1856
▲ Antara Capsules (3.4%) 2723
▲ Apokyn Injection (At least 5%) 2132
Aralast (Greater than or equal to 0.2%) 745
▲ Aranesp for Injection (8%) 576
▲ Arava Tablets (5%) 2881
▲ Aredia for Injection (At least 5%) 2168
▲ Argatroban Injection (8%) 1321
▲ Arimidex Tablets (8% to 12%) 665
Arixtra Injection (1.3%) 1325
▲ Aromasin Tablets (2% to 5%) 2600
▲ Asacol Delayed-Release Tablets (7%) 2688
▲ Asmanex Twisthaler (3% to 6%) 2981
Astelin Nasal Spray (Infrequent) 1876
▲ Atacand Tablets (3%) 634
▲ Atacand HCT (3.3%) 637
▲ Atrovent HFA Inhalation Aerosol (2% to 7%) 872
▲ Atrovent Inhalation Solution (3.2%) 868
▲ Avandamet Tablets (5%) 1343
▲ Avandia Tablets (4%) 1348
Avelox (Less than 0.1%) 2984
▲ Avinza Capsules (5% to 10%) 1714
Axert Tablets (Infrequent) 2430
Axid Oral Solution (2.4%) 913
▲ Azmacort Inhalation Aerosol (2% to 4%) 1701
Benicar HCT Tablets (Greater than 1%) 2852
▲ Bexxar (1% to 8%) 1360
▲ Boniva Tablets (4.3% to 13.5%) 2747
Boostrix 1366
▲ Botox Purified Neurotoxin Complex (2% to 10%) 565
▲ Caduet Tablets (Greater than 0.1% to 3.8%) 2507
▲ Campath Ampules (3% to 10%) 826
Campral Tablets (Frequent) 1175
▲ Camptosar Injection (2% to 14%) 2602
Cancidas for Injection (0% to 0.7%) 1894
Carafate Suspension (Less than 0.5%) 727
Carafate Tablets (Less than 0.5%) 728
Carimune NF 3501
▲ Carnitor Injection (6% to 9%) 3185
▲ Casodex Tablets (15%) 670
Caverject Impulse Injection (1%) 2610
Celebrex Capsules (2.8%) 3130
Celexa (At least 2%) 1177
▲ CellCept Capsules (34.6% to 46.6%) 2751
▲ CellCept Intravenous (34.6% to 46.6%) 2751
▲ CellCept Oral Suspension (34.6% to 46.6%) 2751
▲ CellCept Tablets (34.6% to 46.6%) 2751
▲ Cenestin Tablets, 0.45mg, 0.625mg, 0.9mg, 1.25mg (14%) 1063
▲ Cerezyme for Injection (Approximately 6.5%) 1263
▲ Chemet Capsules (5.2% to 15.7%) 2480
▲ Cialis Tablets (3% to 6%) 1806
Cipro I.V. (1% or less) 2998
Cipro I.V. Pharmacy Bulk Package (1% or less) 3509
Cipro (Less than 1%) 2991
Cipro XR Tablets 3004
▲ Climara Transdermal System (4% to 9%) 795
▲ Climara Pro Transdermal System (6.1%) 800
Clindesse Vaginal Cream (1.6%) 3296
▲ Clolar for Intravenous Infusion (13%) 1264
Clozapine Tablets (1%) 2141
Clozaril Tablets (1%) 2174
Colazal Capsules (2%) 2845
▲ CombiPatch Transdermal System (14% to 15%) 2180
Combunox Tablets (Less than 2%) 1183
Comtan Tablets (2%) 2186
▲ Copaxone for Injection (16%) 3292
▲ Copegus Tablets (5%) 2759
Cosopt Sterile Ophthalmic Solution (1% to 5%) 1910
▲ Cozaar Tablets (2% to 12%) 1913
Crestor Tablets (2.6%) 672
▲ Crixivan Capsules (8.4%) 1918
Cubicin for Injection (1% to 2%) 1038
CytoGam Intravenous (Less than 5.0%) 1866
Dantrium Capsules (Less frequent) 2690
▲ Depacon Injection (1% to 5%) 412
▲ Depakene (1% to 5%) 417
▲ Depakote Sprinkle Capsules (1% to 5%) 422
▲ Depakote Tablets (1% to 8%) 427
▲ Depakote ER Tablets (8%) 433
▲ DepoCyt Injection (7%) 1121
▲ DepoDur Extended-Release Injection (2% to 5%) 1098
▲ Depo-Provera Contraceptive Injection (1% to 5%) 2619
▲ depo-subQ provera 104 Injectable Suspension (1% to less than 5%) 2622
Detrol Tablets (2.7%) 2626
Diovan HCT Tablets (More than 2%) 2195
▲ Diovan Tablets (3%) 2191
▲ Ditropan XL Extended Release Tablets (2% to less than 5%) 2391
▲ Doxil Injection (6.8% to 11.7%) 3302
DuoNeb Inhalation Solution 1058
Duragesic Transdermal System (Greater than or equal to 1%) 2448
DynaCirc CR Tablets (0.5% to 1%) 2726
Edex Injection (2%) 3103
Effexor Tablets 3405
Effexor XR Capsules 3411
Eldepryl Capsules (1 of 49 patients) 3209
Elidel Cream 1% (0.3% to 1.8%) 2198
Eligard 7.5 mg (Less than 2%) 2896
▲ Eloxatin for Injection (11% to 19%) 2908
Enablex Extended-Release Tablets (Greater than or equal to 1%) 2201
Engerix-B Vaccine (Less than 1%) 1391
▲ Entocort EC Capsules (7%) 2694
▲ Equetro Extended-Release Capsules (5%) 3178
▲ Erbitux (11%) 937
▲ Estrogel 0.06% (4.8%) 3200
▲ Evoxac Capsules (4.5%) 1042
Exelon Capsules (2% or more) 2204
Factive Tablets (Less than or equal to 0.1%) 2464
Famvir Tablets (1.5% to 1.9%) 2207
▲ Faslodex Injection (14.4%) 682
FazaClo Orally Disintegrating Tablets (1%) 547
▲ Femara Tablets (0.3% to 22%) 2210
Ferrlecit Injection (0.4%) 3379
▲ Flolan for Injection (2% to 13%) 1408
▲ Flomax Capsules (7.0% to 8.3%) 881
▲ Follistim AQ Cartridge (7%) 2354
▲ Foradil Aerolizer (4.2%) 3024
▲ Fortical Nasal Spray (5%) 3336
Frova Tablets (Infrequent) 1101
Gabitril Tablets (1% or more) 998
Gammagard Liquid 751
Gammagard S/D (Occasional) 754
▲ Gamunex Immune Globulin I.V., 10% (6%) 3232
Geodon for Injection (Up to 1%) 2514
▲ Gleevec Tablets (1% to 11%) 2221
▲ Gonal-f RFF Pen for Injection (3.6%) 3155
▲ Herceptin I.V. (22%) 1234
▲ Humatrope Vials and Cartridges (9.1% to 9.6%) 1756
▲ Humira Injection (6%) 464
Hycamtin for Injection (2%) 1427
Hyperstat I.V. Injection 3031
Hytrin Capsules (2.4%) 469
Hyzaar (2.1%) 1964
▲ Imdur Tablets (Less than or equal to 5%) 3032
Imitrex Injection (Rare) 1431
Imitrex Nasal Spray (Infrequent) 1435
▲ Indapamide Tablets (Greater than or equal to 5%) 2119
Infed Injection 3381
▲ Infergen (29% to 42%) 1647
▲ Intron A for Injection (Up to 19%) 3038
Invirase (Less than or equal to 2%) 2776
▲ I.V. Busulfex (23%) 1125
Iveegam EN 759
Kadian Capsules (Less than 3%) 572
Kaletra (Less than 2%) 474
Keppra Oral Solution (1% or more) 3307
Keppra Tablets (1% or more) 3307
Klonopin (Infrequent) 2782
▲ Lamictal (8%) 1449
▲ Lescol Capsules (5.7%) 2227
▲ Lescol XL Tablets (4.7%) 2227
▲ Leukine (9%) 829
Levaquin in 5% Dextrose Injection (1.2%) 2453
Levaquin (1.2%) 2453
Levitra Tablets (Less than or equal to 2%) 3048
Lexapro Oral Solution (At least 2%) 1193
Lexapro Tablets (At least 2%) 1193
▲ Lipitor Tablets (Up to 3.8%) 2495
▲ Lofibra Capsules (3.4%) 1217
Lotensin HCT Tablets (More than 1%) 2235
Lotrel Capsules 2238
Lunesta Tablets 3139
Lyrica Capsules (1% to 2%) 2524
▲ Menopur for Subcutaneous Injection (3.2%) 1145
▲ Meridia Capsules (8.2%) 485
Merrem I.V. (Greater than 0.1% to 1%) 687
Metrogel 1% (0.5%) 1212
▲ Miacalcin Nasal Spray (5.0%) 2242
▲ Micardis Tablets (3%) 884
Micardis HCT Tablets (Less than 2%) 886
Midamor Tablets (Less than or equal to 1%) 2000
Mirapex Tablets (Greater than or equal to 1%) 889
▲ Mirena Intrauterine System (5% or more) 810
▲ Mobic Oral Suspension (0.4% to 3%) 893
▲ Mobic Tablets (0.4% to 3%) 893
Moduretic Tablets (Less than or equal to 1%) 2003
▲ Myfortic Tablets (3% to less than 20%) 2244
▲ Mylotarg for Injection (12% to 16%) 3429
▲ Namenda (3%) 1199
▲ Naropin Injection (More than 5% to 16.4%) 640
▲ Natrecor for Injection (1% to 4%) 3123
Navelbine Injection 1494
Neurontin Capsules (1% to 1.8%) 2498
Neurontin Oral Solution (1% to 1.8%) 2498
Neurontin Tablets (1% to 1.8%) 2498
Nexium Delayed-Release Capsules (Less than 1%) 645
Nexium I.V. (Less than 1%) 649
▲ Nicotrol Inhaler (Greater than 3%) 2594
▲ Nicotrol NS (6%) 2596
Noroxin Tablets (0.3% to 1.0%) 2009
Norvasc Tablets (More than 0.1% to 1%) 2529
Norvir (Less than 2%) 499
▲ Novantrone for Injection Concentrate (6% to 8%) 3158
Omacor Capsules (2.2%) 2735
▲ Orthovisc Injection (6.9%) 3518
▲ Oxytrol Transdermal System (Greater than 1%) 3383
Parcopa Orally Disintegrating Tablets 3111
▲ Paxil CR Controlled-Release Tablets (3%) 1509
▲ Paxil (3%) 1501
▲ Pegasys (9%) 2793
Permax Tablets (1.6%) 3357
▲ Photofrin for Injection (5% to 11%) 729
Plasmanate (Occasional) 3252
▲ Plavix Tablets (5.8%) 940
▲ Plavix Tablets (5.8%) 2942
Plendil Extended-Release Tablets (0.5% to 1.5%) 651
▲ Pletal Tablets (6% to 7%) 2478
▲ Prandin Tablets (0.5, 1, and 2 mg) (5% to 6%) 2337
▲ Prefest Tablets (12%) 1069
▲ Premarin Tablets (13% to 14%) 3443
▲ Premphase Tablets (13% to 16%) 3452
▲ Prempro Tablets (13% to 16%) 3452
Prevacid Delayed-Release Capsules (Less than 1%) 3268
Prevacid for Delayed-Release Oral Suspension (Less than 1%) 3268
Prevacid NapraPAC (Less than 1%) 3277
Prevacid SoluTab Delayed-Release Orally Disintegrating Tablets (Less than 1%) 3268
PREVPAC (Less than 1%) 3281
Prilosec OTC Tablets (1.1%) 2674
Prinivil Tablets (0.3% to greater than 1.0%) 2029
Prinzide Tablets (0.3% to 1%) 2033
ProAmatine Tablets (Rare) 3183
Prochieve 4% Gel 1018
Prochieve 8% Gel 1018
▲ Prograf Capsules and Injection (17% to 30%) 624
▲ Proleukin for Injection (9%) 1007
▲ Prometrium Capsules (100 mg, 200 mg) (8%) 3205
ProSom Tablets (2%) 512
Protonix I.V. (Greater than or equal to 1%) 3468
Protonix Tablets (Greater than or equal to 1%) 3465
Protopic Ointment (1% to 3%) 629
▲ Proventil HFA Inhalation Aerosol (4%) 3071
▲ Provigil Tablets (6%) 1002
Prozac Pulvules and Liquid 1771
Qvar Inhalation Aerosol (Less than 1% to 4%) 1654
▲ Rapamune Oral Solution and Tablets (16% to 26%) 3472
▲ Raptiva for Injection (4%) 1247
Razadyne ER Extended-Release Capsules (Greater than or equal to 2%) 2434
Razadyne (Greater than or equal to 2%) 2434
▲ Rebif Prefilled Syringe for Injection (23% to 25%) 3163
Recombivax HB (Less than 1%) 2045
Relpax Tablets (Frequent) 2531
▲ Remicade for IV Injection (8%) 987
▲ Renagel Tablets (4%) 1268
Requip Tablets (1% or more) 1528
▲ Retisert Implant (5% to 15%) ⊙256
Retrovir Capsules 1533
Retrovir IV Infusion 1537
Retrovir 1533
▲ Reyataz Capsules (2% to 6%) 948
▲ Rilutek Tablets (1.7% to 4.1%) 2945
Risperdal Consta Long-Acting Injection (Frequent) 1664
Risperdal M-Tab Orally Disintegrating Tablets (Up to 2%) 1658
Risperdal (Up to 2%) 1658
▲ Rituxan for Infusion (1% to 5%) 845
▲ Rituxan I.V. (10%) 1251
▲ Roferon-A Injection (16%) 2805
▲ Sandostatin Injection (1% to 4%) 2263
▲ Seroquel Tablets (3%) 691
▲ Simulect for Injection (3% to 10%) 2268
▲ Somavert Injection (4% to 8%) 2648
Sonata Capsules (Frequent) 1686
▲ Soriatane Capsules (1% to 10%) 1028
▲ Stalevo Tablets (2% to 4%) 2270
▲ Starlix Tablets (4%) 2276
▲ Strattera Capsules (2% or greater) 1784
Stromectol Tablets 2053
▲ Suboxone Tablets (3.7% to 14%) 2719
▲ Subutex Tablets (7.8% to 14%) 2719
▲ Targretin Capsules (2.4% to 11.3%) 1719
Tarka Tablets (2.2%) 519
Taxotere Injection Concentrate 2947
▲ Temodar Capsules (8%) 3088
▲ Tequin Injection (0.1% to 3%) 964
▲ Tequin Tablets (0.1% to 3%) 964
Teveten Tablets (Less than 1%) 1707
Teveten HCT Tablets (2.6%) 1710
Thalomid Capsules (4.2%) 979
▲ TOBI Solution for Inhalation (7%) 1015
▲ Topamax Sprinkle Capsules (1% to 5%) 2438
▲ Topamax Tablets (1% to 5%) 2438
Travatan Ophthalmic Solution (1% to 5%) 559
Trelstar LA Suspension (2.9%) 3387
▲ Tricor Tablets (3.4%) 523
▲ Triglide Tablets (3.4%) 1165
▲ Trileptal Oral Suspension (2% to 4%) 2281
▲ Trileptal Tablets (2% to 4%) 2281
▲ Trisenox Injection (18%) 983
Truvada Tablets 1279
Twinrix Vaccine (Less than 1%) 1571
Tygacil for Injection (1.2%) 3489
Uniretic Tablets (More than 1%) 3114
▲ Vagifem Tablets (7%) 2340
▲ Valcyte Tablets (Less than 5%) 2816
Vancocin HCl Capsules, USP 3370
Vantas (Less than 2%) 3367
Vantin Tablets and Oral Suspension (Less than 1%) 2650
Vaqta (1.1%) 2067
Vaseretic Tablets (0.5% to 2.0%) 2073
▲ Velcade for Injection (14%) 2102
▲ Ventavis Inhalation Solution (7%) 1036
VFEND I.V. (Less than 2%) 2543
VFEND Oral Suspension (Less than 2%) 2543

VFEND Tablets (Less than 2%).......... 2543
Viagra Tablets (Greater than 2%)...... 2552
Viracept (Less than 2%)................. 2556
▲ Viread Tablets (3% to 4%) 1284
▲ Visudyne for Injection (1% to 10%) .. 2286
Vivelle Transdermal System.............. 2288
Vivelle-Dot Transdermal System....... 2293
Vytorin 10/10 Tablets...................... 2084
Vytorin 10/10 Tablets...................... 3092
Vytorin 10/20 Tablets...................... 2084
Vytorin 10/20 Tablets...................... 3092
Vytorin 10/40 Tablets...................... 2084
Vytorin 10/40 Tablets...................... 3092
Vytorin 10/80 Tablets...................... 2084
Vytorin 10/80 Tablets...................... 3092
▲ WelChol Tablets (3%) 2855
Wellbutrin SR Sustained-Release Tablets (At least 1%)................. 1583
Wellbutrin XL Extended-Release Tablets (At least 1%)................. 1588
WinRho SDF.................................... 763
Xalatan Sterile Ophthalmic Solution (1% to 2%) 2654
Xanax XR Tablets (Frequent) 2655
▲ Xeloda Tablets (Less than 1% to 12%) 2825
▲ Xenical Capsules (13.90%) 2834
Yasmin 28 Tablets (Greater than 1%) 818
▲ Zavesca Capsules (8%) 543
Zegerid Powder for Oral Solution (1.1%) 2972
▲ Zelnorm Tablets (2% to 5%) 2303
Zemaira (0.2% to 0.4%) 3506
▲ Zenapax for Injection (Greater than 5%).. 2838
Zestoretic Tablets (0.3% to 1%) 701
Zestril Tablets (0.3% to 1.0%) 704
▲ Zetia Tablets (3.4% to 4.1%) 2090
▲ Zetia Tablets (3.4% to 4.1%) 3098
▲ Zevalin Injection (8%) 848
▲ Zoladex (4% to 7%) 709
Zoladex 3-month (1% to 5%) 712
Zoloft (Frequent) 2581
▲ Zometa for Intravenous Infusion (15%)... 2306
Zomig Nasal Spray (Infrequent) 718
Zomig Tablets (Infrequent) 714
Zomig-ZMT Tablets (Infrequent) 714
Zosyn (1.0% or less) 3492
Zyban Sustained-Release Tablets (Infrequent) 1620
▲ Zyprexa Tablets (4%) 1798
▲ Zyprexa ZYDIS Orally Disintegrating Tablets (4%) 1798
Zyrtec Chewable Tablets (Less than 2%) 2589
Zyrtec (Less than 2%) 2589
Zyrtec-D 12 Hour Extended Release Tablets (Less than 2%) 2591

Bacteremia
▲ Aranesp for Injection (27%) 576
Bexxar 1360
▲ Clolar for Intravenous Infusion (10%)... 1264
Crixivan Capsules 1918
Effexor Tablets (Rare) 3405
Enbrel for Injection 580
Retrovir Capsules (1.6%) 1533
Retrovir IV Infusion (2%) 1537
Retrovir (1.6%) 1533
Zenapax for Injection 2838

Bacteriuria
Primaxin I.M. 2022

Bad breath
(*see under* Halitosis)

Balance, loss of
(*see also under* Equilibrium dysfunction)
Dalmane Capsules 3343
Eldepryl Capsules 3209
Rythmol SR Capsules 2736
Tarka Tablets (Less frequent) 519
Tasmar Tablets (2% to 3%) 3360
▲ Xanax XR Tablets (3.2%) 2655

Balanitis
Doxil Injection (Less than 1%) 3302
Dynacin Tablets 1859
Effexor XR Capsules (Rare) 3411
Lupron Depot 7.5 mg (Less than 5%)... 3261
Lyrica Capsules (Rare) 2524
Protonix I.V. (Less than 1%) 3468
Protonix Tablets (Less than 1%) 3465

Balanoposthitis
Requip Tablets (Infrequent) 1528
Zoloft (Rare) 2581

Baldness, male pattern
(*see under* Alopecia hereditaria)

Barrett's esophagus
Nexium Delayed-Release Capsules (Less than 1%)........................... 645
Nexium I.V. (Less than 1%)............... 649

Bartter's syndrome
Capastat Sulfate for Injection (1 patient).. 1728

Basophils, increase
Effexor Tablets (Rare)....................... 3405
Effexor XR Capsules (Rare)............... 3411
Geodon Capsules (Rare)................... 2514
Paxil CR Controlled-Release Tablets (Rare)............................... 1509
Paxil (Rare).................................... 1501
Primaxin I.M.................................... 2022
Primaxin I.V..................................... 2024
Rocephin Injectable Vials, ADD-Vantage, Galaxy, Bulk (Rare)... 2801
Vantin Tablets and Oral Suspension 2650
Vesanoid Capsules (Isolated cases).. 2823
Zithromax for Oral Suspension, 300 mg, 600 mg, 900 mg, 1200 mg (Less than 1%) 2561
Zithromax Tablets, 250 mg, 500 mg (Less than 1%) 2561
Zithromax Tri-Pak (Less than 1%) 2561

BBB + Major Axis Deviation
▲ Tenormin I.V. Injection (6.6%) 698
▲ Tenormin Tablets (6.6%) 695

Behavior, hostile
Niravam Orally Disintegrating Tablets (Rare) 3106

Behavior, inappropriate
Apokyn Injection (Rare) 2132
Diprivan Injectable Emulsion (Less than 1%) 676
Phenergan 3438
ProSom Tablets 512
Ritalin Hydrochloride Tablets 2254
Ritalin LA Capsules 2255
Ritalin-SR Tablets 2254
Symmetrel 1115
Tessalon Capsules (Isolated instances) 1202
Tessalon Perles (Isolated instances) 1202
Zovirax for Injection 1618

Behavior, schizophrenic
Zonegran Capsules (2%) 1089

Behavior, violent
Accutane Capsules 2740
Amnesteem Capsules 2126
Invanz for Injection (Greater than 0.1%)... 1974
Prozac Pulvules and Liquid 1771
Zovirax 1616

Behavioral changes
Ambien Tablets 2867
Amoxil Capsules (Rare) 1315
Amoxil Chewable Tablets (Rare) 1315
Amoxil Pediatric Drops for Oral Suspension (Rare) 1315
Amoxil Powder for Oral Suspension (Rare) 1315
Amoxil Tablets (Rare) 1315
Augmentin (Rare) 1331
Augmentin Tablets (Rare) 1334
Augmentin XR Extended-Release Tablets (Rare) 1340
Augmentin ES-600 Powder for Oral Suspension (Rare) 1337
Biaxin/Biaxin XL 402
Catapres Tablets 874
Catapres-TTS (0.5% or less) 875
Clorpres Tablets 2139
Cosopt Sterile Ophthalmic Solution 1910
Effexor Tablets 3405
Effexor XR Capsules 3411
Eldepryl Capsules 3209
▲ Keppra Oral Solution (38%) 3307
▲ Keppra Tablets (38%) 3307
▲ Klonopin (5% to 25%) 2782
Nadolol Tablets (6 of 1000 patients)....................................... 2121
Neurontin Capsules 2498
Neurontin Oral Solution 2498
Neurontin Tablets 2498
▲ Orap Tablets (27.7%) 1220
Paxil CR Controlled-Release Tablets 1509
Paxil 1501
PREVPAC 3281
▲ Roferon-A Injection (3%) 2805
Surmontil Capsules 2347
Thioridazine Hydrochloride Tablets... 2122
Timoptic in Ocudose (Less frequent)..................................... 2061
Timoptic Sterile Ophthalmic Solution (Less frequent)............... 2058
Timoptic-XE Sterile Ophthalmic Gel Forming Solution 2062
Uniphyl Tablets 2708
Valtrex Caplets 1573
Zoloft 2581
Zyprexa Tablets 1798
Zyprexa ZYDIS Orally Disintegrating Tablets 1798

Behavioral deterioration
Depacon Injection 412
Depakene 417
Depakote Sprinkle Capsules 422
Depakote Tablets 427
Depakote ER Tablets 433

Behavioral disturbances, exacerbation of
Focalin XR Capsules 2217

BEI, increase
Aygestin Tablets 1062

Belching
▲ Actonel Tablets (3.3%) 2679
Lexapro Oral Solution (Infrequent) 1193
Lexapro Tablets (Infrequent) 1193
Urecholine Tablets 2349

Bell's palsy
Aldoclor Tablets 1881
Aldoril Tablets 1884
▲ Altoprev Extended-Release Tablets (0.5% to 1%) 1151
Comvax 1904
Cytovene 2763
Depo-Provera Contraceptive Injection (Less than 1%) 2619
Engerix-B Vaccine 1391
Flexeril Tablets (Rare) 1832
▲ Intron A for Injection (Less than 5%)... 3038
Mevacor Tablets (0.5% to 1.0%) 1996
Permax Tablets (Rare) 3357
Pravachol Tablets 943
Recombivax HB 2045
Sandostatin Injection (Less than 1%)... 2263
Sandostatin LAR Depot (Rare) 2264
Soriatane Capsules (Less than 5%) .. 1028
Thalomid Capsules 979
Twinrix Vaccine 1571
Varivax 2070
Zocor Tablets 2078

Benzyl alcohol, sensitivity to
AquaMEPHYTON Injection 1887
Depo-Medrol Injectable Suspension 2615
Epogen for Injection 586
Fragmin Injection 2638
Herceptin I.V. 1234
Leukine 829
Leustatin Injection 2368
Lupron Injection Pediatric 3256
Mivacron Injection 489
Nimbex Injection 494
Norditropin Cartridges 2318
Nutropin for Injection 1238
Nutropin AQ Pen 1241
Nutropin AQ Pen Cartridge 1241
Procrit for Injection 2374
Roferon-A Injection 2805

Bezoar
Carafate Suspension 727
Carafate Tablets 728
Ecotrin Enteric Coated Aspirin Low, Regular and Maximum Strength Tablets 1627
Prevacid Delayed-Release Capsules (Less than 1%) 3268
Prevacid for Delayed-Release Oral Suspension (Less than 1%) 3268
Prevacid NapraPAC (Less than 1%) .. 3277
Prevacid SoluTab Delayed-Release Orally Disintegrating Tablets (Less than 1%) 3268
PREVPAC (Less than 1%) 3281
St. Joseph 81 mg Aspirin Chewable and Enteric Coated Tablets 1841

Bigeminy
Digitek Tablets 2146
Diprivan Injectable Emulsion (Less than 1%)............................. 676
Effexor Tablets (Rare)...................... 3405
Effexor XR Capsules (Rare).............. 3411
Lanoxicaps Capsules....................... 1458
Lanoxin Injection............................ 1462
Lanoxin Tablets.............................. 1468
Lanoxin Injection Pediatric 1465
Sonata Capsules (Rare) 1686
Suprane Liquid for Inhalation (Less than 1%) 770
Ultane Liquid for Inhalation (Less than 1%)............................... 526
Uniretic Tablets (Less than 1%) 3114
VFEND I.V. (Less than 2%)............... 2543
VFEND Oral Suspension (Less than 2%).. 2543
VFEND Tablets (Less than 2%).......... 2543
Virazole for Inhalation Solution (Infrequent) 3365

Bile duct obstruction
Thalomid Capsules 979
Zelnorm Tablets 2303

Bile duct sludge, presence of metabolites
Clinoril Tablets (Rare) 1899

Biliary lithiasis
Rocephin 2801

Biliary sludge
Sandostatin Injection (Frequent) 2263

Biliary stasis
Thioridazine Hydrochloride Tablets .. 2122

Bilirubin, total, decrease
▲ Avastin IV (1% to 6%) 1229

Bilirubin, total, increase
Aloxi Injection (Less than 1%) 2099
▲ Baraclude (2% to 3%) 928
Epzicom Tablets 1402
Maxipime for Injection (Greater than 0.1% to less than 1%) 1093
▲ Truvada Tablets (1% to 12%) 1279

Bilirubinemia
▲ Abelcet Injection (4%) 1119
Abilify Tablets (Infrequent) 916
Abilify Tablets (Infrequent) 2472
Aldurazyme for Intravenous Infusion (2%)................................ 1261
Ambien Tablets (Rare) 2867
▲ AmBisome for Injection (11.1% to 18.1%).. 615
Arthrotec Tablets (Rare) 3126
Asacol Delayed-Release Tablets 2688
Campral Tablets (Infrequent) 1175
▲ Cancidas for Injection (0% to 3.8%)... 1894
Celexa (Rare) 1177
▲ CellCept Capsules (3% to less than 20%)....................................... 2751
▲ CellCept Intravenous (3% to less than 20%)....................................... 2751
▲ CellCept Oral Suspension (3% to less than 20%).............................. 2751
▲ CellCept Tablets (3% to less than 20%).. 2751
Coreg Tablets (Greater than 0.1% to 1%) 1376
Doxil Injection (Less than 1%) 3302
Effexor Tablets (Rare) 3405
Effexor XR Capsules (Rare) 3411
▲ Eloxatin for Injection (1% to 20%) 2908
Factive Tablets (Less than or equal to 0.1%) 2464
Gengraf Capsules (1% to less than 3%).. 458
▲ Intron A for Injection (Less than 5%)... 3038
Lamictal (Rare) 1449
Lexapro Oral Solution 1193
Lexapro Tablets 1193
Lotronex Tablets (Rare) 1479
Mefoxin for Injection 1987
Mefoxin Premixed Intravenous Solution 1990
Mobic Oral Suspension (Less than 2%).. 893
Mobic Tablets (Less than 2%) 893
▲ Mylotarg for Injection (11% to 13%).. 3429
Neoral Soft Gelatin Capsules (1% to less than 3%)........................ 2247
Neoral Oral Solution (1% to less than 3%) 2247
Nexium Delayed-Release Capsules (Less than 1%) 645
Nexium I.V. (Less than 1%) 649

Niaspan Extended-Release Tablets... 1703
Oncaspar (Greater than 1% but less than 5%)... 1123
Paxil CR Controlled-Release Tablets (Rare)... 1509
Paxil (Rare)... 1501
Plavix Tablets (Less than 1%)... 940
Plavix Tablets (Less than 1%)... 2942
Prevacid Delayed-Release Capsules... 3268
Prevacid for Delayed-Release Oral Suspension... 3268
Prevacid NapraPAC... 3277
Prevacid SoluTab Delayed-Release Orally Disintegrating Tablets... 3268
PREVPAC... 3281
▲ Prograf Capsules and Injection (3% to 15%)... 624
▲ Proleukin for Injection (40%)... 1007
Protonix I.V. (Less than 1%)... 3468
Protonix Tablets (Less than 1%)... 3465
Protopic Ointment (Greater than or equal to 1%)... 629
▲ Rebif Prefilled Syringe for Injection (2% to 3%)... 3163
ReFacto Vials... 3479
Relpax Tablets (Rare)... 2531
Requip Tablets (Infrequent)... 1528
Rescriptor Tablets... 2535
Risperdal Consta Long-Acting Injection (Rare)... 1664
Sonata Capsules (Rare)... 1686
Symbyax Capsules (Rare)... 1788
Thalomid Capsules... 979
Tygacil for Injection (2.3%)... 3489
Ultane Liquid for Inhalation (Less than 1%)... 526
Uniretic Tablets (Less than 1%)... 3114
VFEND I.V. (0.5% to 1.1%)... 2543
VFEND Oral Suspension (0.5% to 1.1%)... 2543
VFEND Tablets (0.5% to 1.1%)... 2543
Viracept... 2556
Zyprexa Tablets (Infrequent)... 1798
Zyprexa ZYDIS Orally Disintegrating Tablets (Infrequent)... 1798

Bilirubinuria
Primaxin I.M.... 2022
Primaxin I.V.... 2024
Relafen Tablets (Less than 1%)... 1523

Birth, premature
Accutane Capsules... 2740
Paxil CR Controlled-Release Tablets... 1509
Sandimmune... 2259

Birth defects, increased risk of
Activella Tablets... 2311
Arava Tablets... 2881
Aygestin Tablets... 1062
Coumadin for Injection... 932
Coumadin Tablets... 932
Cuprimine Capsules... 1925
Depacon Injection (Multiple reports)... 412
Depakene (Multiple reports)... 417
Depakote Tablets (Multiple reports)... 427
Depakote ER Tablets (Multiple reports)... 433
Efudex... 3348
Klonopin... 2782
Lo/Ovral-28 Tablets... 3423
Phenytek Capsules... 2153
Premarin Intravenous... 3440
Premarin Vaginal Cream... 3449
Premphase Tablets... 3452
Prempro Tablets... 3452
Rebetol... 3073
Rebetron Combination Therapy... 3078
Repronex for Intramuscular and Subcutaneous Injection (1.7%)... 1148
Soriatane Capsules... 1028
Thalomid Capsules... 979
Tracleer Tablets... 539
Triphasil-28 Tablets... 3483
Vivelle Transdermal System... 2288
Vivelle-Dot Transdermal System... 2293

Birth weight, low
Adderall Tablets... 3168
Adderall XR Capsules... 3169
Aggrenox Capsules... 855
Bayer Aspirin Tablets... 3515
Dexedrine... 1386
Ecotrin Enteric Coated Aspirin Low, Regular and Maximum Strength Tablets... 1627
Sandimmune... 2259
St. Joseph 81 mg Aspirin Chewable and Enteric Coated Tablets... 1841

Births, multiple
▲ Repronex for Intramuscular and Subcutaneous Injection (20%)... 1148

Black stools
Chromagen Soft Gelatin Capsules... 3296
Chromagen Forte Soft Gelatin Capsules... 3296

Blackout spells
Eskalith... 1406
Lithobid Tablets... 1670

Bladder, irritability
Anadrol-50 Tablets... 3329
Oxandrin Tablets... 2977

Bladder, spasms
Clindesse Vaginal Cream (Less than 1%)... 3296
▲ DepoDur Extended-Release Injection (2% to 5%)... 1098
Furosemide Tablets... 2117
Midamor Tablets (Less than or equal to 1%)... 2000
Moduretic Tablets... 2003
▲ Myfortic Tablets (3% to less than 20%)... 2244

Bladder dysfunction
Aricept Tablets (Infrequent)... 1086
Aricept ODT Tablets (Infrequent)... 1086
DepoCyt Injection... 1121
Depo-Medrol Single-Dose Vial... 2617
Invanz for Injection (Greater than 0.1%)... 1974

Blanching
Catapres-TTS (1 of 101 patients)... 875

Blebs, filtering (ocular)
Blephamide Ophthalmic Ointment (Increased incidence)... 563
FML Ophthalmic Ointment... ⊙ 225
FML Ophthalmic Suspension... ⊙ 224
FML Forte Ophthalmic Suspension... ⊙ 223
HMS Sterile Ophthalmic Suspension... ⊙ 228
Pred Forte Ophthalmic Suspension... ⊙ 233
Pred Mild Sterile Ophthalmic Suspension... ⊙ 236

Bleeding
Abilify Tablets (Infrequent)... 916
Abilify Tablets (Infrequent)... 2472
Accolate Tablets... 663
▲ Activase I.V. (Most common complication)... 1225
Adriamycin for Injection, USP... 786
Adriamycin Injection, USP... 786
▲ Aggrastat (Among most common)... 1878
▲ Aggrenox Capsules (3.2%)... 855
Agrylin Capsules (1% to 5%)... 3172
Aldara Cream, 5% (More than 1%)... 1814
Alkeran for Injection... 976
Alkeran Tablets... 977
Aloprim for Injection (Less than 1%)... 2156
AmBisome for Injection (Less common)... 615
Ammonul Injection... 3323
▲ Angiomax for Injection (0.6% to 3%)... 1856
Aquacel AG with Hydrofiber... 1035
▲ Arixtra Injection (0% to 3.4%)... 1325
Azasan Tablets... 2844
Bexxar... 1360
Cafcit (2.2%)... 1854
▲ Camptosar Injection (1% to 5%)... 2602
▲ Carnitor Injection (2% to 9%)... 3185
▲ Cathflo Activase (Among most frequent)... 1232
Ceftin... 1369
▲ CellCept Capsules (3% to less than 20%)... 2751
▲ CellCept Intravenous (3% to less than 20%)... 2751
▲ CellCept Oral Suspension (3% to less than 20%)... 2751
▲ CellCept Tablets (3% to less than 20%)... 2751
Colazal Capsules... 2845
Coumadin for Injection... 932
Coumadin Tablets... 932
Crixivan Capsules... 1918
Cytovene-IV (1% or less)... 2763
Depacon Injection... 412
Depakene... 417
Depakote Sprinkle Capsules... 422
Depakote Tablets... 427
Depakote ER Tablets... 433
Diprivan Injectable Emulsion (Less than 1%)... 676
▲ Doxil Injection (1% to 5%)... 3302
Effexor Tablets... 3405
Effexor XR Capsules... 3411
Elitek (Less than or equal to 1%)... 2906
Elspar for Injection... 1943
Ferrlecit Injection (Two or more patients)... 3379
▲ Flolan for Injection (11%)... 1408
Fortaz... 1422
Fragmin Injection... 2638
Gabitril Tablets (Infrequent)... 998
▲ Gamunex Immune Globulin I.V., 10% (29%)... 3232
▲ Gemzar for Injection (Up to 17%)... 1743
▲ Gleevec Tablets (18.9% to 53%)... 2221
Herceptin I.V. (At least one of the 958 patients)... 1234
Hycamtin for Injection (Rare)... 1427
▲ Idamycin PFS Injection (63%)... 2645
▲ Integrilin Injection (10.5% to 14.2%)... 3034
▲ Intron A for Injection (8%)... 3038
Invanz for Injection (Greater than 0.1%)... 1974
Iressa Tablets... 684
I.V. Busulfex... 1125
Lamictal (2%)... 1449
Leukeran Tablets... 1472
▲ Leukine (23% to 29%)... 829
Lotronex Tablets (Rare)... 1479
▲ Lovenox Injection (1% to 13%)... 2931
Maxipime for Injection... 1093
Mefoxin for Injection... 1987
Mefoxin Premixed Intravenous Solution... 1990
Meridia Capsules... 485
Miradon Tablets... 3056
Mustargen for Injection... 2007
▲ Mylotarg for Injection (9% to 13%)... 3429
Nalfon Capsules (Less than 1%)... 2504
▲ Nipent for Injection (3% to 10%)... 3216
Norvir (Less than 2%)... 499
NovoSeven (Greater than or equal to 2%)... 2335
Omnicef Capsules... 506
Omnicef for Oral Suspension... 506
Oncaspar... 1123
Pletal Tablets (Less than 2%)... 2478
▲ Prograf Capsules and Injection (3% to 15%)... 624
Proleukin for Injection (Less than 1%)... 1007
Protonix I.V. (Less than 1%)... 3468
Protonix Tablets (Less than 1%)... 3465
Prozac Pulvules and Liquid (Frequent)... 1771
▲ Rapamune Oral Solution and Tablets (3% to 20%)... 3472
ReFacto Vials... 3479
▲ ReoPro Vials (10.6% to 16.8%)... 1779
▲ Retavase (21.1%)... 1131
Rilutek Tablets (Rare)... 2945
Risperdal M-Tab Orally Disintegrating Tablets (Rare)... 1658
Risperdal (Rare)... 1658
Rythmol SR Capsules... 2736
▲ Simulect for Injection (3% to 10%)... 2268
Soriatane Capsules (Less than 1%)... 1028
Suprane Liquid for Inhalation (Less than 1%)... 770
Suprax... 1811
Targretin Capsules... 1719
Tasmar Tablets (1%)... 3360
Taxotere Injection Concentrate... 2947
Thrombin-JMI... 1693
Ticlid Tablets... 2813
▲ TNKase I.V. (4.7% to 21.8%)... 1256
Trasylol Injection (1% to 2%)... 779
▲ Trisenox Injection (8%)... 983
Ultane Liquid for Inhalation (Less than 1%)... 526
Uniretic Tablets (Less than 1%)... 3114
▲ Valcyte Tablets (Less than 5%)... 2816
Vantin Tablets and Oral Suspension... 2650
▲ Vesanoid Capsules (60%)... 2823
▲ Xeloda Tablets (Less than 5%)... 2825
▲ Xigris Powder for Intravenous Infusion (Most common)... 1796
Zemaira (0.2% to 0.4%)... 3506
▲ Zenapax for Injection (Greater than 5%)... 2838
Zinacef Injection... 1604
Zinacef for Injection... 1604
Zinecard for Injection (2% to 3%)... 2659
Zoladex (1% or greater)... 709
Zoladex 3-month... 712
Zoloft... 2581
Zosyn (1.0% or less)... 3492
Zyprexa Tablets (Infrequent)... 1798
Zyprexa ZYDIS Orally Disintegrating Tablets (Infrequent)... 1798

Bleeding, antepartum
Aggrenox Capsules... 855
Bayer Aspirin Tablets... 3515
Ecotrin Enteric Coated Aspirin Low, Regular and Maximum Strength Tablets... 1627
St. Joseph 81 mg Aspirin Chewable and Enteric Coated Tablets... 1841

Bleeding, at site of administration
▲ Aldara Cream, 5% (3.3%)... 1814
▲ Aranesp for Injection (6%)... 576
Avonex... 839
▲ Copaxone for Injection (5%)... 3292
Doxil Injection (Less than 1%)... 3302
Enbrel for Injection... 580
▲ Flolan for Injection (11%)... 1408
Genotropin Lyophilized Powder (Infrequent)... 2642
▲ Intron A for Injection (Less than 5%)... 3038
ReoPro Vials (1 to 50 events)... 1779

Bleeding, breakthrough
Activella Tablets... 2311
Alesse-28 Tablets... 3392
Aygestin Tablets... 1062
Cenestin Tablets, 0.45mg, 0.625mg, 0.9mg, 1.25mg... 1063
Cenestin Tablets, 0.3mg... 1063
Climara Transdermal System... 795
Climara Pro Transdermal System... 800
Estratest Tablets... 3196
Estratest H.S. Tablets... 3196
Estrogel 0.06%... 3200
Lo/Ovral-28 Tablets... 3423
Menostar Transdermal System... 805
Ortho-Cept Tablets... 2395
Ortho-Cyclen Tablets... 2414
Ortho Evra Transdermal System... 2402
Ortho Tri-Cyclen Tablets... 2414
Ortho Tri-Cyclen Lo Tablets... 2421
Prefest Tablets... 1069
Premarin Intravenous... 3440
Premarin Tablets... 3443
Premarin Vaginal Cream... 3449
Premphase Tablets... 3452
Prempro Tablets... 3452
Prometrium Capsules (100 mg, 200 mg)... 3205
Seasonale Tablets... 1073
Triphasil-28 Tablets... 3483
Vivelle Transdermal System... 2288
Vivelle-Dot Transdermal System... 2293
Yasmin 28 Tablets... 818

Bleeding, dental
Abilify Tablets (Rare)... 916
Abilify Tablets (Rare)... 2472
Accutane Capsules... 2740
Actiq (Less than 1%)... 993
Activase I.V. (Less than 1%)... 1225
Aggrenox Capsules (Less than 1%)... 855
AmBisome for Injection (Less common)... 615
▲ Avastin IV (6%)... 1229
Celexa (Rare)... 1177
▲ Clolar for Intravenous Infusion (15%)... 1264
Copaxone for Injection (Infrequent)... 3292
Coumadin for Injection... 932
Coumadin Tablets... 932
Crixivan Capsules (Less than 2%)... 1918
Depakote ER Tablets (Greater than 1%)... 433
Doxil Injection (Less than 1%)... 3302
Effexor Tablets (Rare)... 3405
Effexor XR Capsules (Rare)... 3411
Elmiron Capsules (Less than or equal to 1%)... 2393
Gengraf Capsules (1% to less than 3%)... 458
Geodon Capsules (Rare)... 2514
▲ Intron A for Injection (Less than 5%)... 3038
Lamictal (Rare)... 1449
Lipitor Tablets (Less than 2%)... 2495
Mustargen for Injection... 2007
Neoral Soft Gelatin Capsules (1% to less than 3%)... 2247
Neoral Oral Solution (1% to less than 3%)... 2247
Neurontin Capsules (Infrequent)... 2498
Neurontin Oral Solution (Infrequent)... 2498
Neurontin Tablets (Infrequent)... 2498

Pletal Tablets (Less than 2%)........... 2478
Prevacid Delayed-Release Capsules (Less than 1%).............. 3268
Prevacid for Delayed-Release Oral Suspension (Less than 1%)........... 3268
Prevacid SoluTab Delayed-Release Orally Disintegrating Tablets (Less than 1%)........................... 3268
PREVPAC (Less than 1%)................ 3281
Prozac Pulvules and Liquid (Infrequent)................................. 1771
Rescriptor Tablets 2535
Retrovir Capsules 1533
Retrovir IV Infusion.......................... 1537
Retrovir.. 1533
Rilutek Tablets (Infrequent)............. 2945
Roferon-A Injection (2%).................. 2805
Rythmol SR Capsules...................... 2736
Seroquel Tablets (Infrequent)........... 691
Sonata Capsules (Rare) 1686
▲ Soriatane Capsules (1% to 10%) 1028
Topamax Sprinkle Capsules (Infrequent)................................ 2438
Topamax Tablets (Infrequent) 2438
Trileptal Oral Suspension 2281
Trileptal Tablets 2281
VFEND I.V. (Less than 2%) 2543
VFEND Oral Suspension (Less than 2%) 2543
VFEND Tablets (Less than 2%) 2543
Wellbutrin SR Sustained-Release Tablets 1583
Wellbutrin XL Extended-Release Tablets 1588
Zonegran Capsules (Infrequent) 1089
Zyban Sustained-Release Tablets 1620

Bleeding, duodenal ulcer

Emend Capsules (Isolated cases) 1944

Bleeding, gastrointestinal

▲ Abelcet Injection (4%) 1119
Abilify Tablets (Infrequent) 916
Abilify Tablets (Infrequent) 2472
Aciphex Tablets (Rare) 1081
Actimmune (Rare) 1646
Actiq (1% or greater) 993
▲ Activase I.V. (5%) 1225
Adalat CC Tablets (Less than 1%) 2978
Advil Allergy Sinus Caplets .... ▣ 737
Advil .... ▣ 737
Advil Cold & Sinus .... ▣ 739
Advil Flu & Body Ache Caplets .... ▣ 739
Advil Migraine Liquigels .... ▣ 740
Advil Multi-Symptom Cold Caplets .. ▣ 738
Aggrastat (0.1%) 1878
Aggrenox Capsules (1.2%) 855
Agrylin Capsules (1% to 5%) 3172
Aleve Tablets, Caplets and Gelcaps .... ▣ 605
Aloprim for Injection (Less than 1%) 2156
▲ AmBisome for Injection (9.9%) 615
Ammonul Injection 3323
Anaprox Tablets (Less than 1%) 2769
Anaprox DS Tablets (Less than 1%) .. 2769
▲ Aredia for Injection (Up to 6%) 2168
▲ Argatroban Injection (2.3% to 14.4%) 1321
Aricept Tablets (Frequent) 1086
Aricept ODT Tablets (Frequent) 1086
Arthrotec Tablets (Rare) 3126
Asacol Delayed-Release Tablets (2% to 5%) 2688
▲ Avastin IV (19% to 24%) 1229
Bayer, Aspirin Regimen .... ▣ 606
Bayer Aspirin 3515
BC Powder .... ▣ 612
BC Allergy Sinus Cold Powder .... ▣ 612
Arthritis Strength BC Powder .... ▣ 612
BC Sinus Cold Powder .... ▣ 612
Cafcit (2.2%) 1854
Campath Ampules 826
Campral Tablets (Infrequent) 1175
Cataflam Tablets (Occasionally) 2173
Cathflo Activase 1232
Celebrex Capsules (Less than 0.1%) 3130
Celexa 1177
▲ CellCept Capsules (1.7% to less than 20%) 2751
▲ CellCept Intravenous (1.7% to less than 20%) 2751
▲ CellCept Oral Suspension (1.7% to less than 20%) 2751
▲ CellCept Tablets (1.7% to less than 20%) 2751
Cipro I.V. (Less than 1%) 2998
Cipro I.V. Pharmacy Bulk Package (Less than 1%) 3509
Cipro (Less than 1%) 2991
Cipro XR Tablets 3004
Clinoril Tablets (Less than 1%) 1899
Combunox Tablets........................... 1183
Copegus Tablets (Less than 1%)...... 2759
Coreg Tablets (Less than or equal to 0.1%) 1376
Dantrium Capsules (Rare) 2690
Dolobid Tablets (Less than 1 in 100) 1937
Doxil Injection (Less than 1%).......... 3302
EC-Naprosyn Delayed-Release Tablets (Less than 1%)................ 2769
Ecotrin Enteric Coated Aspirin Low, Regular and Maximum Strength Tablets 1627
Edecrin 1941
Effexor Tablets (Rare) 3405
Effexor XR Capsules (Rare) 3411
Eldepryl Capsules............................ 3209
Emcyt Capsules (1%)....................... 3137
Enbrel for Injection (Infrequent)......... 580
Evoxac Capsules (Less than 1%)..... 1042
Exelon Capsules (Infrequent)............ 2204
Fosamax (Occasional) 1949
Gabitril Tablets (Infrequent) 998
Gengraf Capsules (1% to less than 3%) 458
▲ Gleevec Tablets (2% to 8%) 2221
Goody's Body Pain Formula Powder .... ▣ 621
Goody's Extra Strength Headache Powder .... ▣ 621
Goody's Extra Strength Pain Relief Tablets .... ▣ 621
▲ Humira Injection (Less than 5%) 464
Imitrex Injection 1431
Imitrex Nasal Spray (Rare) 1435
Imitrex Tablets (Rare) 1440
Indocin Capsules (Less than 1%) 1968
▲ Indocin I.V. (3% to 9%) 1973
Indocin (Less than 1%) 1968
Integrilin Injection 3034
▲ Intron A for Injection (Less than 5%) 3038
Invanz for Injection (Greater than 0.1%) 1974
K-Dur Extended-Relase Tablets 3047
K-Tab Filmtab Tablets 473
Lamictal (Rare) 1449
▲ Leukine (11% to 27%) 829
Levaquin in 5% Dextrose Injection (0.1% to 0.9%) 2453
Levaquin (0.1% to 0.9%) 2453
Lexapro Oral Solution 1193
Lexapro Tablets 1193
Lyrica Capsules (0.1% to 1%) 2524
Meridia Capsules 485
Merrem I.V. (0.5%) 687
Midamor Tablets (Less than or equal to 1%) 2000
Mobic Oral Suspension (Less than 2%) 893
Mobic Tablets (Less than 2%) 893
Moduretic Tablets (Less than or equal to 1%) 2003
Children's Motrin Oral Suspension and Chewable Tablets 1837
Children's Motrin Cold Non-Staining Dye-Free Oral Suspension 1838
Children's Motrin Cold Oral Suspension 1838
Children's Motrin Non-Staining Dye-Free Oral Suspension 1837
Motrin Cold & Sinus Caplets 1836
Motrin IB Tablets and Caplets 1836
Infants' Motrin Concentrated Drops 1837
Infants' Motrin Non-Staining Dye-Free Drops 1837
Junior Strength Motrin Caplets and Chewable Tablets 1837
Mustargen for Injection 2007
Myfortic Tablets 2244
Mylotarg for Injection 3429
Nalfon Capsules (Less than 1%) 2504
Namenda (Infrequent) 1199
Naprosyn Suspension (Less than 1%) 2769
Naprosyn Tablets (Less than 1%) 2769
Neoral Soft Gelatin Capsules (1% to less than 3%) 2247
Neoral Oral Solution (1% to less than 3%) 2247
Nexium Delayed-Release Capsules (Less than 1%) 645
Nexium I.V. (Less than 1%) 649
Nimotop Capsules (Less than 1%) 774
Norvir (Less than 2%) 499
NovoSeven 2335
Omnicef Capsules 506
Omnicef for Oral Suspension 506
Orthoclone OKT3 Sterile Solution (Less than 1%) 2370
Parcopa Orally Disintegrating Tablets 3111
Pegasys (Less than 1%).................. 2793
Pentasa Capsules (Less than 1%).... 3182
Plavix Tablets (1% to 2.5%)............. 940
Plavix Tablets (1% to 2.5%)............. 2942
Pletal Tablets (Very rare)................. 2478
Prevacid Delayed-Release Capsules (Less than 1%).............. 3268
Prevacid for Delayed-Release Oral Suspension (Less than 1%)........... 3268
Prevacid NapraPAC (Less than 1%).. 3277
Prevacid SoluTab Delayed-Release Orally Disintegrating Tablets (Less than 1%)............................. 3268
PREVPAC (Less than 1%) 3281
▲ Prograf Capsules and Injection (3% to 15%)................................ 624
▲ Proleukin for Injection (13%) 1007
Protonix I.V. (Less than 1%).............. 3468
Protonix Tablets (Less than 1%) 3465
Prozac Pulvules and Liquid (Rare) 1771
Razadyne ER Extended-Release Capsules 2434
Razadyne 2434
▲ Refludan for Injection (5.3%) 815
Relafen Tablets (Less than 1%) 1523
Remicade for IV Injection (Greater than or equal to 0.2%) 987
ReoPro Vials (11 events) 1779
Requip Tablets (Infrequent) 1528
Rescriptor Tablets 2535
▲ Retavase (1.8% to 9%) 1131
Rilutek Tablets (Infrequent) 2945
Risperdal M-Tab Orally Disintegrating Tablets (Rare) 1658
Risperdal (Rare) 1658
Roferon-A Injection (Infrequent) 2805
Sandimmune (Rare) 2259
Sandostatin Injection (Less than 1%) 2263
Sandostatin LAR Depot (Rare) 2264
▲ Simulect for Injection (3% to 10%) ... 2268
St. Joseph 81 mg Aspirin Chewable and Enteric Coated Tablets 1841
Stalevo Tablets 2270
Sular Tablets (Less than or equal to 1%) 1163
Symbyax Capsules (Rare) 1788
Tarceva Tablets 1254
Tarceva Tablets 2470
Tasmar Tablets (Infrequent) 3360
Taxotere Injection Concentrate (One patient) 2947
Tequin Injection (Less than 0.1%) 964
Tequin Tablets (Less than 0.1%) 964
Thalomid Capsules 979
Ticlid Tablets 2813
TNKase I.V. (1%) 1256
Trasylol Injection (1% to 2%) 779
TriLyte with Flavor Packs for Oral Solution 3114
▲ Trisenox Injection (8%) 983
Ultracet Tablets 2462
Uniretic Tablets (Less than 1%) 3114
▲ Vesanoid Capsules (34%) 2823
VFEND I.V. (Less than 2%) 2543
VFEND Oral Suspension (Less than 2%) 2543
VFEND Tablets (Less than 2%) 2543
Viracept (Less than 2%) 2556
Voltaren Tablets (Occasionally) 2298
Voltaren-XR Tablets (Occasionally) 2301
Wellbutrin Tablets (Rare) 1579
Wellbutrin SR Sustained-Release Tablets 1583
Wellbutrin XL Extended-Release Tablets 1588
▲ Xeloda Tablets (1% to 6%) 2825
▲ Xigris Powder for Intravenous Infusion (5%) 1796
▲ Zemplar Capsules (5%) 535
▲ Zemplar Injection (5%) 538
Zevalin Injection (1%) 848
Zyban Sustained-Release Tablets 1620
Zyvox (0% to 2.3%) 2661

Bleeding, genitourinary tract

▲ Activase I.V. (4%) 1225
Activella Tablets 2311
Aggrastat (0.1%) 1878
Argatroban Injection (1.8%) 1321
Premphase Tablets 3452
Prempro Tablets 3452
ReoPro Vials (5 to 8 events) 1779
▲ Retavase (0.9% to 9.5%) 1131
Xigris Powder for Intravenous Infusion (2%) 1796

Bleeding, gingival

(*see under* Bleeding, dental)

Bleeding, gums

Adalat CC Tablets (Less than 1%)..... 2978
Caduet Tablets (Less than 2%)......... 2507
▲ Mylotarg for Injection (5% to 14%) ... 3429
Prevacid NapraPAC (Less than 1%).. 3277
Raptiva for Injection 1247
Symbyax Capsules (Rare) 1788

Bleeding, intermenstrual

Arthrotec Tablets (Rare).................. 3126
Clindesse Vaginal Cream (Less than 1%) 3296
▲ depo-subQ provera 104 Injectable Suspension (7%)........... 2622
▲ Entocort EC Capsules (Less than 5%)... 2694
Evoxac Capsules (Less than 1%)..... 1042
▲ Gonal-f RFF Pen for Injection (3.8%).. 3155
Imitrex Injection 1431
Imitrex Nasal Spray 1435
Imitrex Tablets (Infrequent)............... 1440
Risperdal M-Tab Orally Disintegrating Tablets (Infrequent) 1658
Risperdal (Infrequent) 1658
Topamax Sprinkle Capsules (Greater than 1%) 2438
Topamax Tablets (Greater than 1%) 2438
Trileptal Oral Suspension 2281
Trileptal Tablets 2281
▲ Trisenox Injection (8%) 983
Yasmin 28 Tablets (Greater than 1%) 818
Zoloft (Infrequent) 2581
Zyrtec Chewable Tablets (Less than 2%) 2589
Zyrtec (Less than 2%) 2589
Zyrtec-D 12 Hour Extended Release Tablets (Less than 2%) 2591

Bleeding, internal

Activase I.V. 1225

Bleeding, intra-abdominal

Xigris Powder for Intravenous Infusion (2%) 1796

Bleeding, intracerebral

▲ Gleevec Tablets (0.9% to 7%) 2221
Revatio Tablets 2541
Ticlid Tablets (Rare) 2813
Viagra Tablets 2552

Bleeding, intracranial

Abilify Tablets (Rare) 916
Abilify Tablets (Rare) 2472
Activase I.V. (0.4% to 1.3%) 1225
Aggrastat (0.1%) 1878
Aggrenox Capsules (Less than 1%) .. 855
Angiomax for Injection (Less than 0.1%) 1856
▲ Argatroban Injection (1% to 4.3%) ... 1321
Aricept Tablets (Infrequent) 1086
Aricept ODT Tablets (Infrequent) 1086
Bayer Aspirin Tablets 3515
Campath Ampules 826
Cardene I.V. (0.7%) 1129
Ecotrin Enteric Coated Aspirin Low, Regular and Maximum Strength Tablets 1627
Elspar for Injection 1943
Exelon Capsules (Infrequent) 2204
▲ Indocin I.V. (3% to 9%) 1973
▲ Infasurf Intratracheal Suspension (29% to 36%) 1188
Integrilin Injection (Rare) 3034
Invirase (Rare) 2776
Lovenox Injection 2931
Mylotarg for Injection (1%) 3429
Namenda 1199
Neurontin Capsules (Infrequent) 2498
Neurontin Oral Solution (Infrequent) 2498
Neurontin Tablets (Infrequent) 2498
Plavix Tablets (Less than 1%) 940
Plavix Tablets (Less than 1%) 2942
Pletal Tablets (Very rare) 2478
Refludan for Injection 815
ReoPro Vials (1 to 3 events) 1779
Retavase (0.8%) 1131
Sandostatin LAR Depot (Rare) 2264
St. Joseph 81 mg Aspirin Chewable and Enteric Coated Tablets 1841
Xigris (2%) 1796

Bleeding, lip

Neurontin Capsules (Rare) 2498
Neurontin Oral Solution (Rare) 2498

Neurontin Tablets (Rare) 2498

Bleeding, menstrual, heavy
depo-subQ provera 104 2622

Bleeding, mouth
Evoxac Capsules (Less than 1%) 1042
▲ Intron A for Injection (Less than 5%) 3038
ReoPro Vials (4 events) 1779

Bleeding, mucosal
Effexor Tablets (Rare) 3405

Bleeding, nasal
(*see under* Epistaxis)

Bleeding, oropharyngeal
Integrilin Injection 3034

Bleeding, otic
Relenza Rotadisk (Less than 1%) 1525
ReoPro Vials (9 to 11 events) 1779

Bleeding, pericardial
Activase I.V. 1225

Bleeding, perioperative
Ticlid Tablets 2813

Bleeding, pharyngeal
▲ TNKase I.V. (3.1%) 1256

Bleeding, postmenopausal
▲ Activella Tablets (5% to 11%) 2311

Bleeding, postoperative
▲ Arixtra Injection (4.3%) 1325
Persantine Tablets (Rare) 898

Bleeding, puncture site
Capastat Sulfate for Injection 1728
TNKase I.V. (Less than 1%) 1256

Bleeding, renal-pelvic
Cipro I.V. (1% or less) 2998
Cipro I.V. Pharmacy Bulk Package (1% or less) 3509

Bleeding, respiratory tract
TNKase I.V. (Less than 1%) 1256

Bleeding, retroperitoneal
Activase I.V. (Less than 1%) 1225
Aggrastat (0.6%) 1878
Angiomax for Injection (0.2%) 1856
Argatroban Injection (0.9%) 1321
Integrilin Injection 3034
Lovenox Injection 2931
Plavix Tablets (Less than 1%) 940
Plavix Tablets (Less than 1%) 2942
Pletal Tablets (Less than 2%) 2478
Proleukin for Injection 1007
ReoPro Vials (2 to 12 events) 1779
TNKase I.V. (Less than 1%) 1256
▲ Xigris (3%) 1796

Bleeding, subcutaneous
Imitrex Injection 1431

Bleeding, subdural
Bayer Aspirin Tablets 3515

Bleeding, superficial
Activase I.V. 1225

Bleeding, upper GI
(*see under* Bleeding, gastrointestinal)

Bleeding, urethral
Ceftin Tablets (0.1% to 1%) 1369
Cipro (Less than 1%) 2991
Cipro XR Tablets 3004
Klonopin (Infrequent) 2782

Bleeding, urinary tract
Amerge Tablets (Rare) 1312
Eligard 22.5 mg (Less than 2%) 2899
Lotronex Tablets 1479
TNKase I.V. (Less than 1% to 3.7%) 1256
▲ Zenapax for Injection (2% to 5%) 2838

Bleeding, uterine
Abilify Tablets (Rare) 916
Abilify Tablets (Rare) 2472
Activella Tablets 2311
Aggrenox Capsules (Less than 1%) 855
Caduet Tablets (Less than 2%) 2507
Climara Transdermal System 795
Clindesse Vaginal Cream (Less than 1%) 3296
▲ depo-subQ provera 104 Injectable Suspension (1% to less than 5%) 2622
Effexor Tablets (Rare) 3405
Effexor XR Capsules (Infrequent) 3411
Estratest Tablets 3196
Estratest H.S. Tablets 3196
Evoxac Capsules (Less than 1%) 1042
Gengraf Capsules (1% to less than 3%) 458
Geodon Capsules (Rare) 2514
Gonal-f RFF Pen for Injection (2.4%) 3155
▲ Intron A for Injection (Less than 5%) 3038
Lipitor Tablets (Less than 2%) 2495
Lunesta Tablets 3139
Neoral Soft Gelatin Capsules (1% to less than 3%) 2247
Neoral Oral Solution (1% to less than 3%) 2247
Permax Tablets (Infrequent) 3357
Prefest Tablets 1069
Premarin Intravenous 3440
Premarin Vaginal Cream 3449
Premphase Tablets 3452
Prempro Tablets 3452
Prozac Pulvules and Liquid (Rare) 1771
Requip Tablets (Rare) 1528
Rilutek Tablets (Rare) 2945
Tasmar Tablets (Rare) 3360
VFEND I.V. (Less than 2%) 2543
VFEND Oral Suspension (Less than 2%) 2543
VFEND Tablets (Less than 2%) 2543
▲ Zoladex (6%) 709

Bleeding, uterine, irregularities
depo-subQ provera 104 Injectable Suspension 2622

Bleeding, vaginal
Abilify Tablets (Infrequent) 916
Abilify Tablets (Infrequent) 2472
Actiq (Less than 1%) 993
Activella Tablets 2311
AmBisome for Injection (Less common) 615
▲ Arimidex Tablets (1% to 5%) 665
Arthrotec Tablets (Rare) 3126
▲ Avastin IV (6%) 1229
Caduet Tablets (Less than 2%) 2507
Celebrex Capsules (0.1% to 1.9%) 3130
Celexa (Infrequent) 1177
Climara Transdermal System 795
▲ Climara Pro Transdermal System (36.8%) 800
Clinoril Tablets (Less than 1%) 1899
▲ CombiPatch Transdermal System (3% to 6%) 2180
Coumadin for Injection 932
Coumadin Tablets 932
Depacon Injection (1% or more) 412
Depakene (1% or more) 417
Depakote Sprinkle Capsules 422
▲ Depakote Tablets (1% to 5%) 427
Depakote ER Tablets (1% or more) 433
▲ depo-subQ provera 104 Injectable Suspension (1% to less than 5%) 2622
▲ Doxil Injection (1% to 10%) 3302
Effexor Tablets (Infrequent) 3405
Effexor XR Capsules (Infrequent) 3411
▲ Eloxatin for Injection (2% to 5%) 2908
Estratest Tablets 3196
Estratest H.S. Tablets 3196
Estrogel 0.06% (1.2%) 3200
▲ Evista Tablets (2.5% to 6.2%) 1735
Evoxac Capsules (Less than 1%) 1042
Faslodex Injection (Less than 1%) 682
Gabitril Tablets (Infrequent) 998
Geodon Capsules (Rare) 2514
▲ Gonal-f RFF Pen for Injection (6%) 3155
Indocin Capsules (Less than 1%) 1968
Indocin I.V. (Less than 1%) 1973
Indocin (Less than 1%) 1968
Inspra Tablets (0.4%) 2520
Lipitor Tablets (Less than 2%) 2495
Lo/Ovral-28 Tablets 3423
Lunesta Tablets (Infrequent) 3139
Lupron Depot-PED 7.5 mg, 11.25 mg and 15 mg (2%) 3266
Lupron Injection Pediatric 3256
Menostar Transdermal System 805
▲ Mylotarg for Injection (4% to 13%) 3429
Neurontin Capsules (Infrequent) 2498
Neurontin Oral Solution (Infrequent) 2498
Neurontin Tablets (Infrequent) 2498
Ortho-Cyclen/Ortho Tri-Cyclen 2414
Ortho Tri-Cyclen Lo Tablets 2421
Paxil CR Controlled-Release Tablets (Rare) 1509
Paxil (Rare) 1501
Permax Tablets (Infrequent) 3357
Pletal Tablets (Less than 2%) 2478
▲ Prefest Tablets (9%) 1069
▲ Premarin Tablets (2% to 14%) 3443
▲ Premphase Tablets (1% to 6%) 3452
▲ Prempro Tablets (1% to 6%) 3452
Prozac Pulvules and Liquid (Infrequent) 1771
Refludan for Injection (1.8%) 815
Relafen Tablets (Less than 1%) 1523
▲ Repronex for Intramuscular and Subcutaneous Injection (3.1% to 7.9%) 1148
Requip Tablets (Infrequent) 1528
Risperdal M-Tab Orally Disintegrating Tablets (Infrequent) 1658
Risperdal (Infrequent) 1658
Seroquel Tablets (Infrequent) 691
Sonata Capsules (Rare) 1686
Sular Tablets (Less than or equal to 1%) 1163
Symbyax Capsules (Infrequent) 1788
▲ Topamax Sprinkle Capsules (0% to 3%) 2438
▲ Topamax Tablets (0% to 3%) 2438
Triphasil-28 Tablets 3483
▲ Trisenox Injection (13%) 983
Uniretic Tablets (Less than 1%) 3114
VFEND I.V. (Less than 2%) 2543
VFEND Oral Suspension (Less than 2%) 2543
VFEND Tablets (Less than 2%) 2543
Vivelle Transdermal System 2288
Vivelle-Dot Transdermal System 2293
Wellbutrin SR Sustained-Release Tablets (Up to 2%) 1583
Wellbutrin XL Extended-Release Tablets (Up to 2%) 1588
Zevalin Injection (Less than 1%) 848
Zoladex (1% or greater) 709
Zoloft (Infrequent) 2581

Bleeding at injection site
▲ Amevive (4%) 836
Ammonul Injection 3323
Angiomax for Injection (0.9%) 1856
▲ Botox Purified Neurotoxin Complex (3% to 10%) 565
▲ Edex Injection (6% to 15%) 3103
▲ Humira Injection (20%) 464
▲ Lovenox Injection (3% to 5%) 2931
▲ Retavase (4.6% to 48.6%) 1131
Zemaira (0.9%) 3506

Bleeding diathesis
Cipro I.V. (Rare) 2998
Cipro I.V. Pharmacy Bulk Package (Rare) 3509
Cipro (Less than 0.1%) 2991
Cipro XR Tablets 3004

Bleeding irregularities
Activella Tablets 2311
Climara Transdermal System 795
Climara Pro Transdermal System 800
Menostar Transdermal System 805
Mirena Intrauterine System 810
Ortho Micronor Tablets 2411
Plavix Tablets (1% to 2.5%) 940
Plavix Tablets (1% to 2.5%) 2942
Premphase Tablets 3452
Prempro Tablets 3452

Bleeding secondary to eczema
Bactroban Cream (One report) 1356

Bleeding tendency, increased
Pletal Tablets (Very rare) 2478
Singulair 2047

Bleeding time, prolongation
Actiq (Less than 1%) 993
Acular LS Ophthalmic Solution 562
Advate Injection (0.6%) 742
▲ Anaprox Tablets (1% to 10%) 2769
▲ Anaprox DS Tablets (1% to 10%) 2769
Cardizem LA Extended Release Tablets (Infrequent) 1699
▲ Cataflam Tablets (1% to 10%) 2173
Depakote ER Tablets (Greater than 1%) 433
Dolobid Tablets 1937
▲ EC-Naprosyn Delayed-Release Tablets (1% to 10%) 2769
Elmiron Capsules 2393
▲ Naprosyn Suspension (1% to 10%) 2769
▲ Naprosyn Tablets (1% to 10%) 2769
Neurontin Capsules (Rare) 2498
Neurontin Oral Solution (Rare) 2498
Neurontin Tablets (Rare) 2498
Paxil CR Controlled-Release Tablets (Rare) 1509
Paxil (Rare) 1501
Soriatane Capsules (Less than 1%) 1028
Tiazac Capsules (Infrequent) 1204
Timentin ADD-Vantage 1556
Timentin Injection Galaxy Container 1559
Timentin IV Infusion 1553
Timentin Pharmacy Bulk Package 1562
VFEND I.V. (Less than 2%) 2543
VFEND Oral Suspension (Less than 2%) 2543
VFEND Tablets (Less than 2%) 2543
▲ Voltaren Tablets (1% to 10%) 2298
▲ Voltaren-XR Tablets (1% to 10%) 2301
Zosyn 3492

Blepharitis
Abilify Tablets (Infrequent) 916
Abilify Tablets (Infrequent) 2472
Alphagan P Ophthalmic Solution (1% to 4%) 563
Aricept Tablets (Infrequent) 1086
Aricept ODT Tablets (Infrequent) 1086
Azopt Ophthalmic Suspension (1% to 5%) 553
Bactroban Nasal (Less than 1%) 1357
Betimol Ophthalmic Solution (1% to 5%) ⊙ 283
Betimol Ophthalmic Solution (1% to 5%) 3371
▲ Brimonidine Tartrate Ophthalmic Solution 0.2% (3% to 9%) ⊙ 245
Cosopt Sterile Ophthalmic Solution (1% to 5%) 1910
Doxil Injection (Less than 1%) 3302
Effexor Tablets (Rare) 3405
Effexor XR Capsules (Rare) 3411
Evoxac Capsules (Less than 1%) 1042
Exelon Capsules (Infrequent) 2204
Gabitril Tablets (Infrequent) 998
Geodon Capsules (Infrequent) 2514
Invirase (Less than 2%) 2776
▲ Lumigan Ophthalmic Solution (3% to 10%) 569
Lyrica Capsules (0.1% to 1%) 2524
Namenda (Infrequent) 1199
Norvir (Less than 2%) 499
OptiPranolol Metipranolol Ophthalmic Solution 0.3% (A small number of patients) ⊙ 254
Paxil CR Controlled-Release Tablets (Rare) 1509
Paxil (Rare) 1501
Prozac Pulvules and Liquid (Rare) 1771
Requip Tablets (Infrequent) 1528
Rescriptor Tablets 2535
▲ Retisert Implant (5% to 9%) ⊙ 256
Rilutek Tablets (Rare) 2945
Risperdal M-Tab Orally Disintegrating Tablets (Rare) 1658
Risperdal (Rare) 1658
Seroquel Tablets (Infrequent) 691
Sonata Capsules (Rare) 1686
Soriatane Capsules (Less than 5%) 1028
Sular Tablets (Less than or equal to 1%) 1163
Targretin Capsules 1719
Timoptic in Ocudose (Less frequent) 2061
Timoptic Sterile Ophthalmic Solution (Less frequent) 2058
Timoptic-XE Sterile Ophthalmic Gel Forming Solution 2062
Travatan Ophthalmic Solution (1% to 4%) 559
VFEND I.V. (Less than 2%) 2543
VFEND Oral Suspension (Less than 2%) 2543
VFEND Tablets (Less than 2%) 2543
▲ Visudyne for Injection (1% to 10%) 2286
Zyprexa Tablets (Infrequent) 1798
Zyprexa ZYDIS Orally Disintegrating Tablets (2%) 1798

Blepharoconjunctivitis
▲ Betagan Ophthalmic Solution, USP (About 1 in 20 patients) ⊙ 217
Carteolol Hydrochloride Ophthalmic Solution USP, 1% (Occasional) ⊙ 246
▲ Flovent Diskus 50 mcg (1% to 3%) 1415

Blepharoptosis
(*see also under* Ptosis, eyelids)
Betagan Ophthalmic Solution, USP ⊙ 217
Betimol Ophthalmic Solution ⊙ 283
Betimol Ophthalmic Solution 3371

Blepharospasm
Eldepryl Capsules 3209
Parcopa Orally Disintegrating Tablets 3111
Requip Tablets (Infrequent) 1528
Stalevo Tablets 2270

Blind spot, enlargement
Eskalith 1406

Blindness
Ammonul Injection 3323
Decadron Phosphate Injection (Rare) 1931
DepoCyt Injection 1121
Doxil Injection (Less than 1%) 3302
Eskalith 1406
Gabitril Tablets (Infrequent) 998
Imitrex Nasal Spray 1435
Imitrex Tablets 1440
Lithobid Tablets 1670
Lyrica Capsules (Rare) 2524
Neoral Soft Gelatin Capsules 2247
Neoral Oral Solution 2247
Neurontin Capsules (Rare) 2498
Neurontin Oral Solution (Rare) 2498
Neurontin Tablets (Rare) 2498
Ortho-Cyclen/Ortho Tri-Cyclen (Rare) 2414
Orthoclone OKT3 Sterile Solution (Less than 1%) 2370
Pacerone Tablets 3337
PEG-Intron Powder for Injection (Less than or equal to 1%) 3062
Permax Tablets (Rare) 3357
Pletal Tablets (Less than 2%) 2478
Proleukin for Injection (Less than 1%) 1007
Sandimmune 2259
Zofran (Rare) 1613
Zofran ODT Orally Disintegrating Tablets (Rare) 1613
Zoloft 2581
Zyrtec Chewable Tablets (Less than 2%) 2589
Zyrtec (Less than 2%) 2589
Zyrtec-D 12 Hour Extended Release Tablets (Less than 2%) 2591

Blindness, color
VFEND I.V. (Less than 2%) 2543
VFEND Oral Suspension (Less than 2%) 2543
VFEND Tablets (Less than 2%) 2543

Blindness, night
(*see under* Nyctalopia)

Blindness, transient
Adalat CC Tablets (Rare) 2978
Imitrex Tablets 1440
Proleukin for Injection (Less than 1%) 1007
Zofran Injection 1607
Zofran 1613
Zofran ODT Orally Disintegrating Tablets 1613

Blistering
Accolate Tablets 663
Ammonul Injection 3323
Avita Cream 2136
Avita Gel 2138
Cutivate Cream (0.8%) 1381
Efudex (Infrequent) 3348
Lotrimin 3053
Lotrisone 3054
Children's Motrin Oral Suspension and Chewable Tablets 1837
Children's Motrin Cold Non-Staining Dye-Free Oral Suspension 1838
Children's Motrin Cold Oral Suspension 1838
Children's Motrin Non-Staining Dye-Free Oral Suspension 1837
Motrin Cold & Sinus Caplets 1836
Motrin IB Tablets and Caplets 1836
Infants' Motrin Concentrated Drops 1837
Infants' Motrin Non-Staining Dye-Free Drops 1837
Junior Strength Motrin Caplets and Chewable Tablets 1837
Navelbine Injection 1494
Retin-A Micro 0.1%/0.04% 2388
Somavert Injection 2648
Striant Mucoadhesive 1022
Sulfamylon Cream 2154
Sulfamylon for 5% Topical Solution 2155
▲ Trisenox Injection (8%) 983
Viramune Oral Suspension 903
Viramune Tablets 903

Blistering, nasal
Nicotrol NS 2596

Blisters at application site
Lidoderm Patch 1107

Bloating
(*see under* Abdominal bloating)

Blood carbon dioxide, changes
Ammonul Injection 3323

Blood clotting, mechanisms, disorders of
Plavix Tablets (Less than 1%) 940
Plavix Tablets (Less than 1%) 2942

Blood counts, peripheral, decreased
Avonex 839

Blood disorders, unspecified
▲ Ammonul Injection (11%) 3323

Blood dyscrasias
Abelcet Injection 1119
Asacol Delayed-Release Tablets 2688
BiDil Tablets 2161
▲ Blephamide Ophthalmic Ointment (Among most often) 563
Blephamide Ophthalmic Suspension 564
Campath Ampules 826
Dapsone Tablets USP 1656
Depo-Provera Contraceptive Injection (Less than 1%) 2619
depo-subQ provera 104 Injectable Suspension 2622
Furosemide Tablets 2117
▲ Leukine (25%) 829
Librium Capsules 3349
Peganone Tablets, USP 2487
Prozac Pulvules and Liquid (Rare) 1771
Tambocor Tablets (Extremely rare) 1824
Trusopt Sterile Ophthalmic Solution (Rare) 2065
Zonegran Capsules (Rare) 1089

Blood glucose, elevation
(*see under* Hyperglycinemia)

Blood glucose, reduction
(*see under* Hypoglycemia)

Blood loss, increase
(*see under* Bleeding)

Blood pH, increased
Ammonul Injection 3323

Blood pressure, changes
Activella Tablets 2311
Clozapine Tablets 2141
Clozaril Tablets 2174
Dantrium Capsules (Less frequent) 2690
DDAVP Injection 4 mcg/mL (Infrequent) 2893
Desmopressin Acetate Injection (Infrequent) 1143
Desoxyn Tablets, USP 2482
Evoxac Capsules 1042
Focalin XR Capsules 2217
Gammagard Liquid 751
Moban Tablets 1108
Orap Tablets 1220
Plasbumin-5 (Rare) 3249
Plasbumin-20 (Rare) 3249
Plasbumin-25 (Rare) 3251
Premphase Tablets 3452
Prempro Tablets (Occasional) 3452
Risperdal M-Tab Orally Disintegrating Tablets 1658
Risperdal 1658
Ritalin Hydrochloride Tablets 2254
Ritalin LA Capsules 2255
Ritalin-SR Tablets 2254
Rythmol SR Capsules 2736
Sandimmune 2259
Zemuron Injection 2363

Blood pressure, elevation
(*see under* Hypertension)

Blood pressure, reduction
(*see under* Hypotension)

Blood urea levels, increase
Cancidas for Injection (0% to 1.9%) 1894
Fortaz (Occasional) 1422
Roferon-A Injection 2805
Rythmol SR Capsules 2736

Blood urea nitrogen levels, increase
(*see under* BUN levels, elevation)

Blurred vision
(*see under* Vision, blurred)

Body fat accumulation
Truvada Tablets 1279

Body odor
▲ Buphenyl Powder (3%) 3327
▲ Buphenyl Tablets (3%) 3327
Carnitor Injection (Less frequent) 3185
Carnitor Tablets and Oral Solution 3187
Depo-Provera Contraceptive Injection (Less than 1%) 2619
depo-subQ provera 104 Injectable Suspension 2622
Effexor Tablets (Rare) 3405
Lupron Depot 3.75 mg (Less than 5%) 3257
Lupron Depot-PED 7.5 mg, 11.25 mg and 15 mg (Less than 2%) 3266
Lupron Injection Pediatric (Less than 2%) 3256
Neurontin Capsules (Rare) 2498
Neurontin Oral Solution (Rare) 2498
Neurontin Tablets (Rare) 2498
Omacor Capsules 2735
Retrovir Capsules 1533
Retrovir IV Infusion 1537
Retrovir 1533
Topamax Sprinkle Capsules (1%) 2438
Topamax Tablets (1%) 2438
Wellbutrin Tablets (Rare) 1579

Bone density, changes
Advair Diskus 100/50 1291
Advair Diskus 250/50 1291
Advair Diskus 500/50 1291
Lupron Depot 3.75 mg 3257
Lupron Depot–3 Month 11.25 mg 3262
Viadur Implant (Less than 2%) 782
▲ Zoladex (4.3% decrease) 709

Bone density, decreased
Amnesteem Capsules 2126
Arimidex Tablets 665
Depo-Provera Contraceptive Injection 2619
Eligard 7.5 mg (Less than 2%) 2896
Eligard 22.5 mg 2899
Eligard 30 mg 2901
Eligard 45 mg 2904
Truvada Tablets 1279
Vantas 3367
Viread Tablets 1284

Bone disorders
Accutane Capsules 2740
▲ Actonel Tablets (4%) 2679
▲ Actonel with Calcium Tablets (4%) 2684
▲ Advair Diskus 100/50 (1% to 3%) 1291
▲ Advair Diskus 250/50 (1% to 3%) 1291
▲ Advair Diskus 500/50 (1% to 3%) 1291
Amnesteem Capsules 2126
Celebrex Capsules (0.1% to 1.9%) 3130
Desferal Vials 2190
Effexor Tablets (Infrequent) 3405
Evoxac Capsules (Less than 1%) 1042
▲ Humatrope Vials and Cartridges (9.6%) 1756
▲ Humira Injection (Less than 5%) 464
Prevacid Delayed-Release Capsules (Less than 1%) 3268
Prevacid for Delayed-Release Oral Suspension (Less than 1%) 3268
Prevacid NapraPAC (Less than 1%) 3277
Prevacid SoluTab Delayed-Release Orally Disintegrating Tablets (Less than 1%) 3268
PREVPAC (Less than 1%) 3281
Protonix I.V. (Less than 1%) 3468
Protonix Tablets (Less than 1%) 3465
Rescriptor Tablets 2535
Risperdal M-Tab Orally Disintegrating Tablets (Rare) 1658
Risperdal (Rare) 1658
Soriatane Capsules (Less than 1%) 1028
Symbyax Capsules (Infrequent) 1788
Thalomid Capsules 979
▲ Vesanoid Capsules (3%) 2823

Bone fractures
▲ Actonel Tablets (5% to 6.4%) 2679
▲ Actonel with Calcium Tablets (5% to 6.4%) 2684
Alinia for Oral Suspension (Less than 1%) 2840
Alinia Tablets (Less than 1%) 2840
Aricept Tablets (Frequent) 1086
Aricept ODT Tablets (Frequent) 1086
▲ Arimidex Tablets (3% to 7%) 665
Campath Ampules 826
Didronel Tablets 2693
Gengraf Capsules (1% to less than 3%) 458
▲ Humira Injection (Less than 5%) 464
Namenda (More than one patient) 1199
Neoral Soft Gelatin Capsules (1% to less than 3%) 2247
Neoral Oral Solution (1% to less than 3%) 2247
Zoladex 3-month 712

Bone marrow depression
Adriamycin for Injection, USP (High incidence) 786
Adriamycin Injection, USP (High incidence) 786
Aldoclor Tablets 1881
Aldoril Tablets 1884
Altace Capsules (Rare) 1673
Azasan Tablets 2844
Calcium Disodium Versenate Injection 1819
Campath Ampules 826
Carbatrol Capsules 3174
Cipro I.V. 2998
Cipro I.V. Pharmacy Bulk Package 3509
Cipro 2991
Cipro XR Tablets 3004
Clinoril Tablets (Less than 1%) 1899
Cuprimine Capsules 1925
Doxil Injection 3302
Elspar for Injection (Rare) 1943
Equetro Extended-Release Capsules 3178
Flexeril Tablets (Rare) 1832
FML-S Liquifilm Sterile Ophthalmic Suspension ⊙ 226
Indocin Capsules (Less than 1%) 1968
Indocin I.V. (Less than 1%) 1973
Indocin (Less than 1%) 1968
Lotrel Capsules 2238
Mavik Tablets (Rare) 482
Mefoxin for Injection 1987
Mefoxin Premixed Intravenous Solution 1990
Primaxin I.M. 2022
Primaxin I.V. 2024
Prinivil Tablets (Rare) 2029
Prinzide Tablets (Rare) 2033
Sulfamylon Cream (A single case) 2154
Sulfamylon for 5% Topical Solution 2155
Surmontil Capsules 2347
Tegretol/Tegretol-XR 2278
Ticlid Tablets 2813
Topamax Sprinkle Capsules (Rare) 2438
Topamax Tablets (Rare) 2438
▲ Valcyte Tablets (Less than 5%) 2816
Vaseretic Tablets (Rare) 2073
Vasotec I.V. Injection (Rare) 2076
VFEND I.V. (Less than 2%) 2543
VFEND Oral Suspension (Less than 2%) 2543
VFEND Tablets (Less than 2%) 2543
Vivactil Tablets 2350
Zestoretic Tablets (Rare) 701
Zestril Tablets (Rare) 704

Bone marrow hypoplasia
Campath Ampules 826
Captopril Tablets 2114
Retrovir Capsules 1533
Retrovir IV Infusion 1537
Retrovir 1533
Rituxan for Infusion 845
Rituxan I.V. 1251
Zantac (Rare) 1597
Zantac Injection (Sometimes) 1593
Zantac Injection Pharmacy Bulk Package (Rare) 1595
Zantac Syrup (Rare) 1597

Bone marrow suppression
▲ Alkeran for Injection (Most common) 976
▲ Alkeran Tablets (Most common) 977
Aloprim for Injection (Less than 1%) 2156
▲ Cerubidine for Injection (All patients) 788
Clozapine Tablets 2141
Clozaril Tablets 2174
Depacon Injection 412
Depakene 417
Depakote Sprinkle Capsules 422
Depakote Tablets 427
Depakote ER Tablets 433
Doxil Injection 3302
Hycamtin for Injection 1427
Leukeran Tablets (Frequent) 1472

Leustatin Injection (Common) 2368
Phenytek Capsules 2153
Purinethol Tablets (Frequent) 1222
Tabloid Tablets 1545
Taxotere Injection Concentrate 2947

Bone mineral density, decreased
Accutane Capsules 2740
depo-subQ provera 104 Injectable Suspension 2622
Levothroid Tablets 1189
Zoladex 3-month 712

Borborygmi
Urecholine Tablets 2349

Bowel, gangrenous
Zelnorm Tablets 2303

Bowel disease, inflammatory, exacerbation of
Accutane Capsules 2740
Amnesteem Capsules 2126
Asacol Delayed-Release Tablets 2688

Bowel dysfunction
DepoCyt Injection 1121
Depo-Medrol Single-Dose Vial 2617

Bowel frequency, increase
Invirase (Less than 2%) 2776
Klonopin (Infrequent) 2782

Bowel habits, changes
Colace Capsules 50 mg 2715
Colace Capsules 100 mg 2715
Colace Glycerin Suppositories, USP 1.2 grams - Infants and Children 2715
Colace Glycerin Suppositories, USP 2.1 grams - Adults and Children 2716
Colace Liquid 1% Solution 2716
Colace Syrup ▣729
Evoxac Capsules 1042
Frova Tablets (Rare) 1101
Mineral Oil 2716
Nexium Delayed-Release Capsules (Less than 1%) 645
Nexium I.V. (Less than 1%) 649
Peri-Colace Tablets 2716

Bowel infarction
Activase I.V. 1225
Orthoclone OKT3 Sterile Solution (Less than 1%) 2370
Proleukin for Injection 1007

Bowel strictures, fibrotic
Pancrease MT Capsules 1839

Bowel syndrome, irritable
Cymbalta Delayed-Release Capsules (Infrequent) 1729
Evoxac Capsules (Less than 1%) 1042
Neurontin Capsules (Rare) 2498
Neurontin Oral Solution (Rare) 2498
Neurontin Tablets (Rare) 2498
Risperdal Consta Long-Acting Injection (Infrequent) 1664
Zelnorm Tablets 2303

Bowel urgency
Copaxone for Injection (Frequent) 3292

Bowels, perforation
Decadron Phosphate Injection 1931
Decadron Tablets 1929
Hydrocortone Tablets 1963
Indocin I.V. (1% to 3%) 1973
Proleukin for Injection 1007

Brachial plexus neuropathies
Botox Purified Neurotoxin Complex 565
DAPTACEL 2964

Bradycardia
Abilify Tablets (Frequent) 916
Abilify Tablets (Frequent) 2472
Aciphex Tablets (Rare) 1081
Adalat CC Tablets (Less than 1%) 2978
Adenoscan (Less than 1%) 613
▲ Aggrastat (4%) 1878
Aldoclor Tablets 1881
Aldoril Tablets 1884
Aloprim for Injection (Less than 1%) 2156
Aloxi Injection (1%) 2099
Alphagan P Ophthalmic Solution 563
AmBisome for Injection (Less common) 615
Amerge Tablets (Rare) 1312
Ammonul Injection 3323
▲ Angiomax for Injection (5%) 1856
▲ Anzemet Injection (5.1%) 2871
▲ Anzemet Tablets (5.1%) 2874
▲ Argatroban Injection (4.5%) 1321
Aricept Tablets (Infrequent) 1086
Aricept ODT Tablets (Infrequent) 1086
Atacand HCT (0.5% or greater) 637
Avinza Capsules (Less than 5%) 1714
Betagan Ophthalmic Solution, USP ⊙217
Betimol Ophthalmic Solution ⊙283
Betimol Ophthalmic Solution 3371
Betoptic S Ophthalmic Suspension (Rare) 554
Biltricide Tablets 2990
▲ Blocadren Tablets (5% to 9.1%) 1891
Brevibloc Concentrate (Less than 1%) 766
Brevibloc Injection (Less than 1%) 766
Brevibloc Double Strength Injection (Less than 1%) 766
Brevibloc Premixed Injection (Less than 1%) 766
Brevibloc Double Strength Premixed Injection (Less than 1%) 766
Brimonidine Tartrate Ophthalmic Solution 0.2% ⊙245
Buprenex Injectable (Less than 1%) 2718
Caduet Tablets (Greater than 0.1% to less than or equal to 1%) 2507
Camptosar Injection 2602
▲ Cardizem LA Extended Release Tablets (1.7% to 3.6%) 1699
Carteolol Hydrochloride Ophthalmic Solution USP, 1% ⊙246
Catapres Tablets (About 5 in 1,000 patients) 874
Catapres-TTS (0.5% or less) 875
Celexa (Infrequent) 1177
▲ CellCept Capsules (3% to less than 20%) 2751
▲ CellCept Intravenous (3% to less than 20%) 2751
▲ CellCept Oral Suspension (3% to less than 20%) 2751
▲ CellCept Tablets (3% to less than 20%) 2751
Cipro XR Tablets (Less than 1%) 3004
Clorpres Tablets (About 5 in 1,000) 2139
Clozapine Tablets (Less than 1%) 2141
Clozaril Tablets (Less than 1%) 2174
Colazal Capsules 2845
Copaxone for Injection (Infrequent) 3292
▲ Coreg Tablets (2% to 10%) 1376
Cosopt Sterile Ophthalmic Solution (Less than 1%) 1910
Covera-HS Tablets (1.4%) 3135
Curosurf Intratracheal Suspension 1057
Decadron Tablets 1929
Depacon Injection 412
Depakene 417
Depakote Sprinkle Capsules 422
Depakote Tablets 427
Depakote ER Tablets 433
▲ DepoDur Extended-Release Injection (2% to 5%) 1098
Diastat Rectal Delivery System (Infrequent) 3344
Dilaudid 439
Dilaudid Oral Liquid 443
Dilaudid Non-Sterile Powder 439
Dilaudid Rectal Suppositories 439
Dilaudid Tablets 439
Dilaudid Tablets - 8 mg 443
Dilaudid-HP (Less frequent) 441
Diprivan Injectable Emulsion (1% to 3%) 676
Doxil Injection (Less than 1%) 3302
Duragesic Transdermal System (Less than 1%) 2448
Effexor Tablets (Rare) 3405
Effexor XR Capsules (Rare) 3411
Ellence Injection 2632
Emend Capsules (Isolated cases) 1944
Eskalith 1406
Ethyol for Injection 1869
Exelon Capsules (Frequent) 2204
Fabrazyme for Intravenous Infusion 1267
FazaClo Orally Disintegrating Tablets (Less than 1%) 547
Ferrlecit Injection 3379
▲ Flolan for Injection (5% to 15%) 1408
Frova Tablets (Rare) 1101
Geodon Capsules (Infrequent) 2514
▲ Hectorol Capsules (6.6%) 909
▲ Hectorol Injection (6.6%) 911
Hyperstat I.V. Injection 3031
▲ Imdur Tablets (Less than or equal to 5%) 3032
Imitrex Injection (Infrequent) 1431
Imitrex Nasal Spray (Rare) 1435
Imitrex Tablets (Rare) 1440
Inderal LA Long-Acting Capsules 3421
Indocin I.V. (Less than 3%) 1973
▲ Infasurf Intratracheal Suspension (34%) 1188
Infed Injection 3381
InnoPran XL Capsules 2728
▲ Intron A for Injection (Less than 5%) 3038
Invanz for Injection (Greater than 0.1%) 1974
Kadian Capsules (Less than 3%) 572
Kaletra 474
Ketek Tablets (Less than 0.2%) 2920
Lariam Tablets (Less than 1%) 2790
Levaquin in 5% Dextrose Injection (0.1% to 0.9%) 2453
Levaquin (0.1% to 0.9%) 2453
Lexapro Oral Solution (Infrequent) 1193
Lexapro Tablets (Infrequent) 1193
Lidoderm Patch 1107
Lithobid Tablets 1670
▲ Mavik Tablets (0.3% to 4.7%) 482
Maxalt Tablets (Infrequent) 1983
Maxalt-MLT Orally Disintegrating Tablets (Infrequent) 1983
Mebaral Tablets, USP (Less than 1 in 100 patients) 2483
Merrem I.V. (Greater than 0.1% to 1%) 687
Midamor Tablets 2000
Mirena Intrauterine System 810
Mivacron Injection (Less than 1%) 489
MS Contin Tablets (Less frequent) 2703
Nadolol Tablets (Common) 2121
Namenda (Infrequent) 1199
▲ Naropin Injection (More than 5% to 19.5%) 640
▲ Natrecor for Injection (1% to 5%) 3123
Nembutal Sodium Solution, USP (Less than 1%) 2484
Neurontin Capsules (Rare) 2498
Neurontin Oral Solution (Rare) 2498
Neurontin Tablets (Rare) 2498
Nimbex Injection (0.4%) 494
Nimotop Capsules (Up to 1.0%) 774
Nipent for Injection (Less than 3%) 3216
Norvasc Tablets (More than 0.1% to 1%) 2529
NovoSeven (1%) 2335
Nubain Injection (1% or less) 1111
Numorphan 1112
OptiPranolol Metipranolol Ophthalmic Solution 0.3% (A small number of patients) ⊙254
Orthoclone OKT3 Sterile Solution (Less than 1%) 2370
Pacerone Tablets (Uncommon) 3337
Paxil CR Controlled-Release Tablets (Infrequent) 1509
Paxil (Infrequent) 1501
Permax Tablets (Infrequent) 3357
Phenergan 3438
Photofrin for Injection 729
Prevacid Delayed-Release Capsules (Less than 1%) 3268
Prevacid for Delayed-Release Oral Suspension (Less than 1%) 3268
Prevacid NapraPAC (Less than 1%) 3277
Prevacid SoluTab Delayed-Release Orally Disintegrating Tablets (Less than 1%) 3268
PREVPAC (Less than 1%) 3281
Prilosec OTC Tablets (Less than 1%) 2674
Prinivil Tablets (0.3% to 1.0%) 2029
Prinzide Tablets 2033
▲ Proleukin for Injection (7%) 1007
Provigil Tablets (At least 1%) 1002
Prozac Pulvules and Liquid (Rare) 1771
Razadyne ER Extended-Release Capsules (2%) 2434
Razadyne (2%) 2434
Relpax Tablets (Rare) 2531
Remicade for IV Injection (Greater than or equal to 0.2%) 987
▲ ReoPro Vials (5.2%) 1779
Requip Tablets (Infrequent) 1528
Rilutek Tablets (Rare) 2945
Risperdal Consta Long-Acting Injection (Infrequent) 1664
Risperdal M-Tab Orally Disintegrating Tablets 1658
Risperdal 1658
▲ Rituxan for Infusion (1% to 5%) 845
▲ Rituxan I.V. (1% to 5%) 1251
▲ Rythmol SR Capsules (3% to 4%) 2736
Seroquel Tablets (Infrequent) 691
Suprane Liquid for Inhalation (Greater than 1%) 770
Symbyax Capsules (Infrequent) 1788
Tagamet Tablets (Rare) 1547
Tambocor Tablets (Less than 1%) 1824
Tarka Tablets (1.8%) 519
Tasmar Tablets (Infrequent) 3360
▲ Tenormin I.V. Injection (3% to 18%) 698
▲ Tenormin Tablets (3% to 18%) 695
Tequin Injection (Less than 0.1%) 964
Tequin Tablets (Less than 0.1%) 964
Teveten Tablets (Less than 1%) 1707
Teveten HCT Tablets (Less than 1%) 1710
Thalomid Capsules 979
Timolide Tablets (1.2%) 2056
Timoptic in Ocudose (Less frequent) 2061
Timoptic Sterile Ophthalmic Solution (Less frequent) 2058
Timoptic-XE Sterile Ophthalmic Gel Forming Solution 2062
Topamax Sprinkle Capsules (1%) 2438
Topamax Tablets (1%) 2438
Toprol-XL Tablets (1.5% to approximately 3 of 100 patients) 660
Trasylol Injection (1% to 2%) 779
Travatan Ophthalmic Solution (1% to 5%) 559
Trileptal Oral Suspension 2281
Trileptal Tablets 2281
Tygacil for Injection (0.2% to less than 2%) 3489
▲ Ultane Liquid for Inhalation (5%) 526
Uniretic Tablets (Less than 1%) 3114
Vaseretic Tablets 2073
Vasotec I.V. Injection (0.5% to 1.0%) 2076
Verelan PM Capsules (1.4%) 3120
VFEND I.V. (Less than 2%) 2543
VFEND Oral Suspension (Less than 2%) 2543
VFEND Tablets (Less than 2%) 2543
Virazole for Inhalation Solution (Infrequent) 3365
▲ Xeloda Tablets (Less than 5%) 2825
Zantac (Rare) 1597
Zantac Injection (Rare) 1593
Zantac Injection Pharmacy Bulk Package (Rare) 1595
Zantac Syrup (Rare) 1597
▲ Zegerid Powder for Oral Solution (3.9%) 2972
Zestril Tablets (0.3% to 1.0%) 704
Zofran Injection (Rare) 1607
▲ Zofran (6%) 1613
▲ Zofran ODT Orally Disintegrating Tablets (6%) 1613
Zoloft 2581
Zomig Nasal Spray (Rare) 718
Zomig Tablets (Rare) 714
Zomig-ZMT Tablets (Rare) 714
Zonegran Capsules (Infrequent) 1089
Zosyn (1.0% or less) 3492
Zyprexa Tablets (Infrequent) 1798
Zyprexa IntraMuscular 1798
Zyprexa ZYDIS Orally Disintegrating Tablets (Infrequent) 1798

Bradycardia, fetal
▲ Naropin Injection (More than 5% to 17.2%) 640

Bradycardia, neonatal
Tenormin I.V. Injection 698
Tenormin Tablets 695

Bradycardia, severe
Brevibloc Concentrate 766
Brevibloc Injection 766
Brevibloc Double Strength Injection 766
Brevibloc Premixed Injection 766
Brevibloc Double Strength Premixed Injection 766
Eskalith 1406

Bradycardia, symptomatic
Nadolol Tablets (2 of 100 patients) 2121

Bradycardia, transient
Covera-HS Tablets (1.4%) 3135

Bradykinesia
Abilify Tablets (Infrequent) 916
Abilify Tablets (Infrequent) 2472
Effexor Tablets (Rare) 3405
Effexor XR Capsules (Rare) 3411
Eldepryl Capsules 3209
Maxalt Tablets (Rare) 1983
Maxalt-MLT Orally Disintegrating Tablets (Rare) 1983

Paxil CR Controlled-Release Tablets ... 1509
Paxil ... 1501
Risperdal Consta Long-Acting Injection (Infrequent) ... 1664
▲ Wellbutrin Tablets (8.0%) ... 1579

Bradykinetic episodes
Parcopa Orally Disintegrating Tablets ... 3111
Stalevo Tablets ... 2270

Bradylogia
Imitrex Tablets (Rare) ... 1440

Bradypnea
Zoloft (Rare) ... 2581

Brain damage
Rythmol SR Capsules ... 2736

Brain death
Ammonul Injection ... 3323

Brain syndrome, acute
Actiq (Less than 1%) ... 993
Doxil Injection (Less than 1%) ... 3302
Permax Tablets (Infrequent) ... 3357
Prozac Pulvules and Liquid (Infrequent) ... 1771
Rilutek Tablets (Rare) ... 2945
Symbyax Capsules (Rare) ... 1788
VFEND I.V. (Less than 2%) ... 2543
VFEND Oral Suspension (Less than 2%) ... 2543
VFEND Tablets (Less than 2%) ... 2543
Virazole for Inhalation Solution ... 3365

Brain syndrome, organic, acute
Garamycin Injectable ... 3028

Breast, redistribution/ accumulation of body fat
Retrovir ... 1533

Breast abscess
Lamictal (Rare) ... 1449
Rilutek Tablets (Rare) ... 2945

Breast atrophy
Paxil CR Controlled-Release Tablets (Rare) ... 1509
Paxil (Rare) ... 1501
▲ Zoladex (33%) ... 709

Breast changes, unspecified
▲ Emcyt Capsules (Up to 66%) ... 3137
Lo/Ovral-28 Tablets ... 3423
▲ Lupron Depot 3.75 mg (3%) ... 3257
▲ Lupron Depot–3 Month 11.25 mg (3%) ... 3262
Lupron Depot-PED 7.5 mg, 11.25 mg and 15 mg (Less than 2%) ... 3266
Lupron Injection Pediatric (Less than 2%) ... 3256
Ortho-Cept Tablets ... 2395
Ortho-Cyclen Tablets ... 2414
▲ Ortho Evra Transdermal System (9% to 22%) ... 2402
Ortho Tri-Cyclen Tablets ... 2414
Ortho Tri-Cyclen Lo Tablets ... 2421
Premphase Tablets ... 3452
Prempro Tablets ... 3452
Seasonale Tablets ... 1073
Triphasil-28 Tablets ... 3483

Breast discharge
Cenestin Tablets, 0.45mg, 0.625mg, 0.9mg, 1.25mg ... 1063
Cenestin Tablets, 0.3mg ... 1063
Climara Transdermal System ... 795
Climara Pro Transdermal System ... 800
Effexor Tablets (Rare) ... 3405
Effexor XR Capsules (Rare) ... 3411
Estrogel 0.06% ... 3200
Menostar Transdermal System ... 805
Premarin Tablets ... 3443
Premphase Tablets ... 3452
Prempro Tablets ... 3452
Vivelle Transdermal System ... 2288
Vivelle-Dot Transdermal System ... 2293

Breast engorgement
Adalat CC Tablets (Less than 1%) ... 2978
Copaxone for Injection (Infrequent) ... 3292
Effexor Tablets (Rare) ... 3405
Effexor XR Capsules (Rare) ... 3411
Permax Tablets (Rare) ... 3357
Prozac Pulvules and Liquid (Rare) ... 1771
Symbyax Capsules (Rare) ... 1788
Thioridazine Hydrochloride Tablets ... 2122
Zoladex (1% to 5%) ... 709

Breast enlargement
Aciphex Tablets (Rare) ... 1081
Activella Tablets ... 2311
Aldoclor Tablets ... 1881
Aldoril Tablets ... 1884
Alesse-28 Tablets ... 3392
Aptivus Capsules ... 859
Aygestin Tablets ... 1062
Caduet Tablets (Less than 2%) ... 2507
Catapres-TTS (0.5% or less) ... 875
Celexa (Infrequent) ... 1177
Cenestin Tablets, 0.45mg, 0.625mg, 0.9mg, 1.25mg ... 1063
Cenestin Tablets, 0.3mg ... 1063
Climara Transdermal System ... 795
Climara Pro Transdermal System ... 800
▲ CombiPatch Transdermal System (2% to 7%) ... 2180
Combivir Tablets ... 1373
Copaxone for Injection (Infrequent) ... 3292
Crixivan Capsules ... 1918
Demser Capsules (Infrequent) ... 1933
Depacon Injection ... 412
Depakene ... 417
Depakote Sprinkle Capsules ... 422
Depakote Tablets ... 427
Depakote ER Tablets ... 433
Effexor Tablets (Rare) ... 3405
Effexor XR Capsules (Rare) ... 3411
Eligard 30 mg (1.1%) ... 2901
▲ Emcyt Capsules (60%) ... 3137
Estratest Tablets ... 3196
Estratest H.S. Tablets ... 3196
Estrogel 0.06% ... 3200
Flexeril Tablets (Rare) ... 1832
Gabitril Tablets (Infrequent) ... 998
Gleevec Tablets (Infrequent) ... 2221
Imitrex Nasal Spray ... 1435
Indocin Capsules (Less than 1%) ... 1968
Indocin I.V. (Less than 1%) ... 1973
Indocin (Less than 1%) ... 1968
Invirase ... 2776
Lipitor Tablets (Less than 2%) ... 2495
Lunesta Tablets (Infrequent) ... 3139
Lupron Depot 7.5 mg (Less than 5%) ... 3261
Menostar Transdermal System ... 805
Norvir ... 499
Ortho-Cept Tablets ... 2395
Ortho-Cyclen Tablets ... 2414
Ortho Evra Transdermal System ... 2402
Ortho Tri-Cyclen Tablets ... 2414
Ortho Tri-Cyclen Lo Tablets ... 2421
Paxil CR Controlled-Release Tablets (Rare) ... 1509
Paxil (Rare) ... 1501
Prefest Tablets ... 1069
Premarin Intravenous ... 3440
Premarin Tablets ... 3443
Premarin Vaginal Cream ... 3449
▲ Premphase Tablets (2% to 5%) ... 3452
▲ Prempro Tablets (2% to 5%) ... 3452
Prevacid Delayed-Release Capsules (Less than 1%) ... 3268
Prevacid for Delayed-Release Oral Suspension (Less than 1%) ... 3268
Prevacid NapraPAC (Less than 1%) ... 3277
Prevacid SoluTab Delayed-Release Orally Disintegrating Tablets (Less than 1%) ... 3268
PREVPAC (Less than 1%) ... 3281
▲ Prochieve 4% Gel (40%) ... 1018
▲ Prochieve 8% Gel (40%) ... 1018
Prometrium Capsules (100 mg, 200 mg) ... 3205
Propecia Tablets (0.5% to 1.8%) ... 2036
Proscar Tablets (0.5% to 1.8%) ... 2040
ProSom Tablets (Rare) ... 512
Prozac Pulvules and Liquid (Infrequent) ... 1771
Requip Tablets (Rare) ... 1528
Rescriptor Tablets ... 2535
Seasonale Tablets ... 1073
Striant Mucoadhesive ... 1022
Surmontil Capsules ... 2347
Symbyax Capsules (Infrequent) ... 1788
Thiothixene Capsules ... 2124
Triphasil-28 Tablets ... 3483
Trizivir Tablets ... 1565
Truvada Tablets ... 1279
Uniretic Tablets (Less than 1%) ... 3114
▲ Viadur Implant (6.9%) ... 782
Viagra Tablets (Less than 2%) ... 2552
Viracept ... 2556
Viramune Oral Suspension ... 903
Viramune Tablets ... 903
Viread Tablets ... 1284
Vivactil Tablets ... 2350
Vivelle Transdermal System ... 2288
Vivelle-Dot Transdermal System ... 2293
Yasmin 28 Tablets ... 818
Zerit ... 971
Ziagen ... 1600
▲ Zoladex (18%) ... 709
Zoloft (Rare) ... 2581
Zyprexa Tablets (Rare) ... 1798

Breast fibroadenosis
Ambien Tablets (Rare) ... 2867
Aricept Tablets (Infrequent) ... 1086
Aricept ODT Tablets (Infrequent) ... 1086
Celebrex Capsules (0.1% to 1.9%) ... 3130
Gengraf Capsules (1% to less than 3%) ... 458
Neoral Soft Gelatin Capsules (1% to less than 3%) ... 2247
Neoral Oral Solution (1% to less than 3%) ... 2247

Breast fibrocystic
Aricept Tablets (Infrequent) ... 1086
Aricept ODT Tablets (Infrequent) ... 1086
Caduet Tablets (Less than 2%) ... 2507
Cenestin Tablets, 0.45mg, 0.625mg, 0.9mg, 1.25mg ... 1063
Cenestin Tablets, 0.3mg ... 1063
Climara Transdermal System ... 795
Climara Pro Transdermal System ... 800
CombiPatch Transdermal System ... 2180
Copaxone for Injection (Infrequent) .. 3292
Effexor Tablets (Rare) ... 3405
Effexor XR Capsules (Rare) ... 3411
Estratest Tablets ... 3196
Estratest H.S. Tablets ... 3196
Estrogel 0.06% ... 3200
Gabitril Tablets (Infrequent) ... 998
Lipitor Tablets (Less than 2%) ... 2495
Menostar Transdermal System ... 805
Ortho-Cyclen/Ortho Tri-Cyclen ... 2414
Ortho Tri-Cyclen Lo Tablets ... 2421
Paxil CR Controlled-Release Tablets (Rare) ... 1509
Paxil (Rare) ... 1501
Permax Tablets (Infrequent) ... 3357
Prefest Tablets ... 1069
Premarin Tablets ... 3443
Premarin Vaginal Cream ... 3449
Premphase Tablets ... 3452
Prempro Tablets ... 3452
Prozac Pulvules and Liquid (Infrequent) ... 1771
Symbyax Capsules (Infrequent) ... 1788
Vivelle Transdermal System ... 2288
Vivelle-Dot Transdermal System ... 2293
Zomig Nasal Spray (Rare) ... 718

Breast lumps
Amerge Tablets (Rare) ... 1312
Depo-Provera Contraceptive Injection (Less than 1%) ... 2619
depo-subQ provera 104 Injectable Suspension ... 2622
Imitrex Nasal Spray ... 1435
Nipent for Injection (Less than 3%) ... 3216
Ortho-Cyclen/Ortho Tri-Cyclen ... 2414
Ortho Tri-Cyclen Lo Tablets ... 2421

Breast milk, maternal, excreted in
Accolate Tablets ... 663
Activella Tablets ... 2311
Adalat CC Tablets ... 2978
Adderall Tablets ... 3168
Adderall XR Capsules ... 3169
Advicor Tablets ... 1694
Aggrenox Capsules ... 855
Aldoclor Tablets ... 1881
Aldoril Tablets ... 1884
Alesse-28 Tablets ... 3392
Aloprim for Injection ... 2156
Altace Capsules ... 1673
Ambien Tablets ... 2867
Anaprox Tablets ... 2769
Anaprox DS Tablets ... 2769
Arthrotec Tablets ... 3126
Asacol Delayed-Release Tablets ... 2688
Augmentin ... 1331
Augmentin Tablets ... 1334
Augmentin XR Extended-Release Tablets ... 1340
Augmentin ES-600 Powder for Oral Suspension ... 1337
Avalide Tablets ... 922
Avalide Tablets ... 2889
Avinza Capsules ... 1714
Axid Oral Solution ... 913
Biltricide Tablets ... 2990
Blocadren Tablets ... 1891
Captopril Tablets ... 2114
Carbatrol Capsules ... 3174
Catapres Tablets ... 874
Catapres-TTS ... 875
Ceftin Tablets ... 1369
Celexa ... 1177
Cipro I.V. ... 2998
Cipro I.V. Pharmacy Bulk Package ... 3509
Cipro ... 2991
Cipro XR Tablets ... 3004
Clarinex Tablets ... 3009
Clarinex Reditabs Tablets ... 3009
Cleocin Vaginal Ovules ... 2613
Clorpres Tablets ... 2139
Clozapine Tablets ... 2141
Clozaril Tablets ... 2174
CombiPatch Transdermal System ... 2180
Cosopt Sterile Ophthalmic Solution ... 1910
Coumadin for Injection ... 932
Covera-HS Tablets ... 3135
Dapsone Tablets USP ... 1656
Daraprim Tablets ... 1385
Decadron Phosphate Injection ... 1931
Decadron Tablets ... 1929
Depacon Injection ... 412
Depakene ... 417
Depakote Sprinkle Capsules ... 422
Depakote Tablets ... 427
Depakote ER Tablets ... 433
Desoxyn Tablets, USP ... 2482
Dexedrine ... 1386
DextroStat Tablets ... 3177
Diastat Rectal Delivery System ... 3344
Digitek Tablets ... 2146
Dilaudid Oral Liquid ... 443
Dilaudid Tablets - 8 mg ... 443
Dilaudid-HP ... 441
Diovan HCT Tablets ... 2195
Diprivan Injectable Emulsion ... 676
Diuril Oral ... 1936
Diuril Sodium Intravenous ... 1934
Dolobid Tablets ... 1937
Duragesic Transdermal System ... 2448
Dyazide Capsules ... 1389
Dyrenium Capsules ... 3390
EC-Naprosyn Delayed-Release Tablets ... 2769
Ecotrin Enteric Coated Aspirin Low, Regular and Maximum Strength Tablets ... 1627
E.E.S. ... 449
Effexor Tablets ... 3405
Effexor XR Capsules ... 3411
EryPed ... 445
Ery-Tab Tablets ... 447
Erythrocin Stearate Filmtab Tablets ... 452
Eskalith ... 1406
Fluorescite Injection ... ⊙ 207
Fortaz ... 1422
Furosemide Tablets ... 2117
Gengraf Capsules ... 458
Hydrocortone Tablets ... 1963
Imitrex Injection ... 1431
Imitrex Nasal Spray ... 1435
Imitrex Tablets ... 1440
Inderal LA Long-Acting Capsules ... 3421
Indocin ... 1968
Infed Injection ... 3381
Invanz for Injection ... 1974
Inversine Tablets ... 3286
Kadian Capsules ... 572
Lamictal ... 1449
Lamisil Tablets ... 2226
Lanoxicaps Capsules ... 1458
Lanoxin Injection ... 1462
Lanoxin Tablets ... 1468
Lanoxin Injection Pediatric ... 1465
Lariam Tablets ... 2790
Lescol Capsules ... 2227
Lescol Capsules ... 2730
Lescol XL Tablets ... 2227
Lescol XL Tablets ... 2730
Levoxyl Tablets ... 1680
Lexapro Oral Solution ... 1193
Lexapro Tablets ... 1193
Lo/Ovral-28 Tablets ... 3423
Lortab ... 3315
Lortab Elixir ... 3312
Lotensin Tablets ... 2232
Lotensin HCT Tablets ... 2235
Lotrel Capsules ... 2238
Marinol Capsules ... 3334
Maxzide ... 2150
Mefoxin for Injection ... 1987
Mefoxin Premixed Intravenous Solution ... 1990
Meruvax II ... 1994
Midamor Tablets ... 2000
Migranal Nasal Spray ... 3350
Moduretic Tablets ... 2003
MS Contin Tablets ... 2703
Naprosyn Suspension ... 2769
Naprosyn Tablets ... 2769
Nembutal Sodium Solution, USP ... 2484
Neoral Soft Gelatin Capsules ... 2247
Neoral Oral Solution ... 2247

Neurontin Capsules 2498
Neurontin Oral Solution 2498
Neurontin Tablets 2498
Niaspan Extended-Release Tablets 1703
Noritate Cream, 1% 1051
Nubain Injection 1111
Ortho-Cept Tablets 2395
Ortho-Cyclen Tablets 2414
Ortho Evra Transdermal System 2402
Ortho Micronor Tablets 2411
Ortho Tri-Cyclen Tablets 2414
Ortho Tri-Cyclen Lo Tablets 2421
Oxistat 1498
OxyContin Tablets 2699
OxyFast Oral Concentrate Solution 2704
OxyIR Capsules 2704
Pacerone Tablets 3337
Paxil CR Controlled-Release Tablets 1509
Paxil 1501
PCE Dispertab Tablets 510
Pediapred Oral Solution 3319
Pentasa Capsules 3182
Pepcid Injection 2017
Pepcid 2014
Persantine Tablets 898
Phenytek Capsules 2153
Pravachol Tablets 943
Premphase Tablets 3452
Prempro Tablets 3452
Prevacid Delayed-Release Capsules 3268
Prevacid for Delayed-Release Oral Suspension 3268
Prevacid SoluTab Delayed-Release Orally Disintegrating Tablets 3268
PREVPAC 3281
Prinzide Tablets 2033
Prograf Capsules and Injection 624
Protopic Ointment 629
Pulmicort Respules 654
Qvar Inhalation Aerosol 1654
Retrovir Capsules 1533
Retrovir IV Infusion 1537
Retrovir 1533
Rocephin Injectable Vials, ADD-Vantage, Galaxy, Bulk 2801
Sandimmune 2259
Sedapap Tablets 50 mg/650 mg 2098
Sonata Capsules 1686
St. Joseph 81 mg Aspirin Chewable and Enteric Coated Tablets 1841
Stromectol Tablets 2053
Symmetrel 1115
Synthroid Tablets 515
Tagamet Tablets 1547
Tambocor Tablets 1824
Tarka Tablets 519
Tegretol/Tegretol-XR 2278
Tenormin I.V. Injection 698
Tenormin Tablets 695
Tiazac Capsules 1204
Timolide Tablets 2056
Timoptic in Ocudose 2061
Timoptic Sterile Ophthalmic Solution 2058
Timoptic-XE Sterile Ophthalmic Gel Forming Solution 2062
Toprol-XL Tablets 660
Tranxene 2488
Trileptal Oral Suspension 2281
Trileptal Tablets 2281
Triphasil-28 Tablets 3483
Trisenox Injection 983
Trizivir Tablets 1565
Tylenol with Codeine 2461
Ultracet Tablets 2462
Uniphyl Tablets 2708
Uniretic Tablets 3114
Unithroid Tablets 3521
Uroqid-Acid No. 2 Tablets 785
Vancocin HCl Capsules, USP 3370
Vantin Tablets and Oral Suspension 2650
Vaseretic Tablets 2073
Vasotec I.V. Injection 2076
Verelan PM Capsules 3120
Vicodin Tablets 530
Vicodin ES Tablets 531
Vicodin HP Tablets 532
Viramune Oral Suspension 903
Viramune Tablets 903
Wellbutrin SR Sustained-Release Tablets 1583
Wellbutrin XL Extended-Release Tablets 1588
Xanax XR Tablets 2655
Yasmin 28 Tablets 818
Zantac 1597
Zantac Injection 1593
Zantac Syrup 1597
Zestoretic Tablets 701
Zinacef Injection 1604
Zinacef for Injection 1604
Zosyn 3492
Zovirax Capsules 1616
Zovirax for Injection 1618
Zovirax 1616
Zyban Sustained-Release Tablets 1620
Zyrtec Chewable Tablets 2589
Zyrtec 2589
Zyrtec-D 12 Hour Extended Release Tablets 2591

Breast nipple bleeding

Depo-Provera Contraceptive Injection (Less than 1%) 2619
depo-subQ provera 104 Injectable Suspension 2622

Breast pain

Abilify Tablets (Infrequent) 916
Abilify Tablets (Infrequent) 2472
Actiq (1% or greater) 993
▲ Activella Tablets (17% to 24%) 2311
Ambien Tablets (Rare) 2867
AndroGel (1% to 3%) 3330
Arthrotec Tablets (Rare) 3126
Astelin Nasal Spray (Infrequent) 1876
▲ Casodex Tablets (6%) 670
Celebrex Capsules (0.1% to 1.9%) 3130
Celexa (Infrequent) 1177
▲ Cenestin Tablets, 0.45mg, 0.625mg, 0.9mg, 1.25mg (29%) 1063
Cenestin Tablets, 0.3mg 1063
Cipro I.V. (1% or less) 2998
Cipro I.V. Pharmacy Bulk Package (1% or less) 3509
Cipro (0.3% to 1%) 2991
Cipro XR Tablets 3004
▲ Climara Transdermal System (5% to 29%) 795
▲ Climara Pro Transdermal System (18.9%) 800
Clozapine Tablets (Less than 1%) 2141
Clozaril Tablets (Less than 1%) 2174
▲ CombiPatch Transdermal System (34% to 48%) 2180
Copaxone for Injection (At least 2%) 3292
▲ Depo-Provera Contraceptive Injection (1% to 5%) 2619
▲ depo-subQ provera 104 Injectable Suspension (1% to less than 5%) 2622
Dostinex Tablets (1% to 2%) 2631
Doxil Injection (Less than 1%) 3302
Effexor Tablets (Infrequent) 3405
Effexor XR Capsules (Infrequent) 3411
Estratest Tablets 3196
Estratest H.S. Tablets 3196
▲ Estrogel 0.06% (12.5%) 3200
▲ Evista Tablets (4.4%) 1735
Evoxac Capsules (Less than 1%) 1042
Exelon Capsules (Infrequent) 2204
FazaClo Orally Disintegrating Tablets (Less than 1%) 547
▲ Femara Tablets (7%) 2210
▲ Follistim AQ Cartridge (15%) 2354
Gabitril Tablets (Infrequent) 998
Gengraf Capsules (1% to less than 3%) 458
▲ Gonal-f RFF Pen for Injection (6%) 3155
▲ Imdur Tablets (Less than or equal to 5%) 3032
Infergen (2%) 1647
Klonopin (Infrequent) 2782
Lamictal (Infrequent) 1449
Lo/Ovral-28 Tablets 3423
Lunesta Tablets (Infrequent) 3139
▲ Lupron Depot 3.75 mg (3%) 3257
▲ Lupron Depot–3 Month 11.25 mg (3%) 3262
▲ Menostar Transdermal System (5%) 805
▲ Mirena Intrauterine System (5% or more) 810
Neoral Soft Gelatin Capsules (1% to less than 3%) 2247
Neoral Oral Solution (1% to less than 3%) 2247
Neurontin Capsules (Rare) 2498
Neurontin Oral Solution (Rare) 2498
Neurontin Tablets (Rare) 2498
Paxil CR Controlled-Release Tablets (Infrequent) 1509
Paxil (Infrequent) 1501
Pentasa Capsules (Less than 1%) 3182
Permax Tablets (Infrequent) 3357
▲ Prefest Tablets (16%) 1069
▲ Premarin Tablets (7% to 12%) 3443
▲ Premphase Tablets (13% to 38%) 3452
▲ Prempro Tablets (13% to 38%) 3452
Prevacid Delayed-Release Capsules (Less than 1%) 3268
Prevacid for Delayed-Release Oral Suspension (Less than 1%) 3268
Prevacid NapraPAC (Less than 1%) 3277
Prevacid SoluTab Delayed-Release Orally Disintegrating Tablets (Less than 1%) 3268
PREVPAC (Less than 1%) 3281
Prinivil Tablets (0.3% to 1.0%) 2029
Prinzide Tablets 2033
▲ Prochieve 4% Gel (13%) 1018
▲ Prochieve 8% Gel (13%) 1018
▲ Prometrium Capsules (100 mg, 200 mg) (6% to 16%) 3205
Protonix I.V. (Less than 1%) 3468
Protonix Tablets (Less than 1%) 3465
Protopic Ointment (Greater than or equal to 1%) 629
Prozac Pulvules and Liquid (Infrequent) 1771
Relpax Tablets (Rare) 2531
Rilutek Tablets (Rare) 2945
Risperdal Consta Long-Acting Injection (Infrequent) 1664
Risperdal M-Tab Orally Disintegrating Tablets (Rare to infrequent) 1658
Risperdal (Rare to infrequent) 1658
Rythmol SR Capsules 2736
Sandostatin LAR Depot (1% to 4%) 2264
Sonata Capsules (Infrequent) 1686
Soriatane Capsules (Less than 1%) 1028
Striant Mucoadhesive 1022
Symbyax Capsules (Frequent) 1788
Targretin Capsules 1719
▲ Temodar Capsules (6%) 3088
▲ Topamax Sprinkle Capsules (4%) 2438
▲ Topamax Tablets (4%) 2438
Trelstar LA Suspension (2.3%) 3387
Triphasil-28 Tablets 3483
Uniretic Tablets (Less than 1%) 3114
Vantas (Less than 2%) 3367
▲ Viadur Implant (3.1%) 782
Vivelle Transdermal System 2288
Vivelle-Dot Transdermal System 2293
Yasmin 28 Tablets (Greater than 1%) 818
Zestril Tablets (0.3% to 1.0%) 704
▲ Zoladex (7%) 709
Zoladex 3-month (1% to 5%) 712
Zoloft (Rare) 2581
Zyprexa Tablets (Infrequent) 1798
Zyprexa ZYDIS Orally Disintegrating Tablets (Infrequent) 1798
Zyrtec Chewable Tablets (Less than 2%) 2589
Zyrtec (Less than 2%) 2589
Zyrtec-D 12 Hour Extended Release Tablets (Less than 2%) 2591

Breast secretion

Alesse-28 Tablets 3392
Amerge Tablets (Rare) 1312
Estratest Tablets 3196
Estratest H.S. Tablets 3196
Imitrex Nasal Spray 1435
Imitrex Tablets (Rare) 1440
Ortho-Cept Tablets 2395
Ortho-Cyclen Tablets 2414
Ortho Evra Transdermal System 2402
Ortho Tri-Cyclen Tablets 2414
Ortho Tri-Cyclen Lo Tablets 2421
Premarin Intravenous 3440
Premarin Vaginal Cream 3449
Seasonale Tablets 1073
Topamax Sprinkle Capsules (Infrequent) 2438
Topamax Tablets (Infrequent) 2438
Yasmin 28 Tablets 818

Breast size, changes

Depo-Provera Contraceptive Injection (Less than 1%) 2619

Breast tenderness

Activella Tablets 2311
Alesse-28 Tablets 3392
Aygestin Tablets 1062
Bravelle for Intramuscular or Subcutaneous Injection (2%) 1140
Cenestin Tablets, 0.45mg, 0.625mg, 0.9mg, 1.25mg 1063
Cenestin Tablets, 0.3mg 1063
Climara Transdermal System 795
Climara Pro Transdermal System 800
▲ depo-subQ provera 104 Injectable Suspension (1% to less than 5%) 2622
Eligard 22.5 mg (Less than 2%) 2899
▲ Emcyt Capsules (66%) 3137
Estratest Tablets 3196
Estratest H.S. Tablets 3196
Estrogel 0.06% 3200
Follistim AQ Cartridge 2354
Imitrex Nasal Spray 1435
Imitrex Tablets (Infrequent) 1440
Indocin Capsules (Less than 1%) 1968
Indocin I.V. (Less than 1%) 1973
Indocin (Less than 1%) 1968
Lo/Ovral-28 Tablets 3423
▲ Lupron Depot 3.75 mg (3%) 3257
▲ Lupron Depot–3 Month 11.25 mg (3%) 3262
Menopur for Subcutaneous Injection (1.8% to 2.6%) 1145
Menostar Transdermal System 805
Ortho-Cept Tablets 2395
Ortho-Cyclen Tablets 2414
Ortho Evra Transdermal System 2402
Ortho Micronor Tablets 2411
Ortho Tri-Cyclen Tablets 2414
Ortho Tri-Cyclen Lo Tablets 2421
▲ Plan B Tablets (10.7%) 1068
Prefest Tablets 1069
Premarin Intravenous 3440
Premarin Tablets 3443
Premarin Vaginal Cream 3449
Premphase Tablets 3452
Prempro Tablets 3452
Prevacid Delayed-Release Capsules (Less than 1%) 3268
Prevacid for Delayed-Release Oral Suspension (Less than 1%) 3268
Prevacid NapraPAC (Less than 1%) 3277
Prevacid SoluTab Delayed-Release Orally Disintegrating Tablets (Less than 1%) 3268
PREVPAC (Less than 1%) 3281
▲ Prometrium Capsules (100 mg, 200 mg) (27%) 3205
Propecia Tablets (0.4% to 0.7%) 2036
Proscar Tablets (0.4% to 0.7%) 2040
Repronex for Intramuscular and Subcutaneous Injection (2%) 1148
Seasonale Tablets 1073
Triphasil-28 Tablets 3483
Vantas (Less than 2%) 3367
▲ Vivelle Transdermal System (6.5% to 17%) 2288
▲ Vivelle-Dot Transdermal System (6.5% to 17%) 2293
Yasmin 28 Tablets 818
Zoladex (1% to 5%) 709
Zoladex 3-month 712

Breath sounds, abnormal

Epivir 1394
Epivir-HBV 1398
▲ Trisenox Injection (10%) 983
Trizivir Tablets 1565
▲ Zenapax for Injection (2% to 5%) 2838

Breathholding

▲ Suprane Liquid for Inhalation (30% to 68%) 770
▲ Ultane Liquid for Inhalation (2% to 5%) 526

Breathing, difficult

(*see under* Dyspnea)

Breathing, irregular

Dilaudid 439
Dilaudid Non-Sterile Powder 439
Dilaudid Rectal Suppositories 439
Dilaudid Tablets 439
Dilaudid-HP 441
Imitrex Nasal Spray 1435
Lortab 3315
Lortab Elixir 3312
Lotronex Tablets (Infrequent) 1479
Parcopa Orally Disintegrating Tablets 3111
Stalevo Tablets 2270
Vicodin Tablets 530
Vicodin ES Tablets 531
Vicoprofen Tablets 533
Zydone Tablets 1118

Breathing, labored

(*see under* Dyspnea)

Breathing, shallow

(*see under* Hypopnea)

Breathing, stertorous

Duragesic Transdermal System (Less than 1%) 2448
Neurontin Capsules (Rare) 2498
Neurontin Oral Solution (3.4%) 2498
Neurontin Tablets (Rare) 2498

Breathing sound, abnormal

Combivir Tablets 1373
Epzicom Tablets 1402

Bromsulphalein retention, increase
(*see under* BSP retention, increase)

Bronchial anastomotic dehiscence
Rapamune Oral Solution and Tablets 3472

Bronchial constriction
Vaqta (Less than 1%) 2067

Bronchial obstruction
Blocadren Tablets 1891
Cosopt Sterile Ophthalmic Solution 1910
Timoptic in Ocudose 2061
Timoptic Sterile Ophthalmic Solution 2058
Timoptic-XE Sterile Ophthalmic Gel Forming Solution 2062

Bronchial secretions, thickening
▲ Alacol DM Syrup (Among most frequent) 739
Betoptic S Ophthalmic Suspension (Rare) 554

Bronchiectasis
Pulmozyme Inhalation Solution 1245

Bronchiolitis
Comvax (Two vaccinees) 1904
Cuprimine Capsules 1925
Flumist Vaccine 1872
Lyrica Capsules (Rare) 2524
Prevnar for Injection 3460
Synagis (More than 1%) 1868
Vaqta 2067

Bronchiolitis, obliterative
PEG-Intron Powder for Injection 3062
Pentasa Capsules (One case) 3182
Rituxan for Infusion (0.3%) 845
Rituxan I.V. (0.3%) 1251
Tarceva Tablets 1254
Tarceva Tablets 2470

Bronchiolitis obliterans
Pegasys 2793
Raptiva for Injection (1 case) 1247

Bronchiolitis obliterans organizing pneumonia
Pacerone Tablets 3337
Rapamune Oral Solution and Tablets (Infrequent) 3472

Bronchitis
AccuNeb Inhalation Solution (0.9% to 1.7%) 1055
Aceon Tablets (2 mg, 4 mg, 8 mg) (0.3% to 1%) 3191
Actiq (1% or greater) 993
▲ Actonel Tablets (2.3% to 4.9%) 2679
▲ Actonel with Calcium Tablets (2.3% to 4.9%) 2684
Advair Diskus 100/50 (2%) 1291
▲ Advair Diskus 250/50 (8%) 1291
▲ Advair Diskus 500/50 (2% to 8%) 1291
Aerobid/Aerobid-M (1% to 3%) 1172
Agrylin Capsules (1% to 5%) 3172
Alamast Ophthalmic Solution (Less than 5%) 3371
Aldara Cream, 5% (0.9%) 1814
Alphagan P Ophthalmic Solution (1% to 4%) 563
Ambien Tablets (Infrequent) 2867
Amerge Tablets (Infrequent) 1312
Antara Capsules 2723
Aptivus Capsules (2.9%) 859
Aralast (Greater than or equal to 0.2%) 745
▲ Aranesp for Injection (6%) 576
Arava Tablets (7%) 2881
Aricept Tablets (Frequent) 1086
Aricept ODT Tablets (Frequent) 1086
▲ Arimidex Tablets (2% to 5%) 665
Aromasin Tablets (Less frequent) 2600
Asacol Delayed-Release Tablets (2% or greater) 2688
Atacand Tablets (More than 1%) 634
Atacand HCT (0.5% or greater) 637
▲ Atrovent HFA Inhalation Aerosol (10% to 23%) 872
▲ Atrovent Inhalation Solution (14.6%) 868
▲ Avonex (8%) 839
Axert Tablets (Infrequent) 2430
Bexxar 1360
▲ BiDil Tablets (8%) 2161
▲ Boniva Tablets (2.5% to 10%) 2747
Caduet Tablets (Greater than or equal to 2%) 2507
▲ Campath Ampules (13% to 21%) 826
Campral Tablets (Frequent) 1175
▲ Carnitor Injection (3% to 5%) 3185
▲ Casodex Tablets (6%) 670
Celebrex Capsules (0.1% to 1.9%) 3130
Celexa (Infrequent) 1177
▲ CellCept Capsules (3% to less than 20%) 2751
▲ CellCept Intravenous (3% to less than 20%) 2751
▲ CellCept Oral Suspension (3% to less than 20%) 2751
▲ CellCept Tablets (3% to less than 20%) 2751
▲ Clarinex Syrup (6.1%) 3009
▲ Climara Pro Transdermal System (4.2%) 800
Clozapine Tablets (Less than 1%) 2141
Clozaril Tablets (Less than 1%) 2174
▲ CombiPatch Transdermal System (3% to 5%) 2180
▲ Combivent Inhalation Aerosol (12.3%) 878
▲ Copaxone for Injection (9%) 3292
▲ Coreg Tablets (5%) 1376
Cosopt Sterile Ophthalmic Solution (1% to 5%) 1910
▲ Cozaar Tablets (Less than 1% to 10%) 1913
Crestor Tablets (Greater than or equal to 2%) 672
▲ Depacon Injection (5%) 412
▲ Depakene (5%) 417
▲ Depakote Sprinkle Capsules (5%) 422
▲ Depakote Tablets (5%) 427
▲ Depakote ER Tablets (5%) 433
▲ depo-subQ provera 104 Injectable Suspension (1% to less than 5%) 2622
Detrol Tablets (2.1%) 2626
▲ Ditropan XL Extended Release Tablets (2% to less than 5%) 2391
Doxil Injection (Less than 1%) 3302
DuoNeb Inhalation Solution (1.7%) 1058
Duragesic Transdermal System (Greater than or equal to 1%) 2448
Effexor Tablets (Frequent) 3405
▲ Elidel Cream 1% (0.4% to 10.7%) 2198
Enablex Extended-Release Tablets (Greater than or equal to 1%) 2201
Enbrel for Injection 580
▲ Entocort EC Capsules (Less than 5%) 2694
▲ Epivir-HBV (Among most common) 1398
▲ Equetro Extended-Release Capsules (Less than 5%) 3178
▲ Evoxac Capsules (4.1%) 1042
Exelon Capsules (2% or more) 2204
▲ Fabrazyme for Intravenous Infusion (3%) 1267
FazaClo Orally Disintegrating Tablets (Less than 1%) 547
▲ Flonase Nasal Spray (1% to 3%) 1412
▲ Flovent Diskus 50 mcg (3%) 1415
Flovent HFA (2%) 1418
Flumist Vaccine 1872
▲ Foradil Aerolizer (4.6%) 3024
Fortical Nasal Spray (Less than 1%) 3336
▲ Fosrenol Chewable Tablets (5%) 3180
Gabitril Tablets (Frequent) 998
Gengraf Capsules (1%) 458
Humira Injection 464
Hytrin Capsules (At least 1%) 469
Hyzaar (1% or greater) 1964
▲ Imdur Tablets (Less than or equal to 5%) 3032
Imitrex Nasal Spray 1435
▲ Infergen (2% to 6%) 1647
Intron A for Injection (Less than or equal to 5%) 3038
Invirase (Less than 2% to 2.7%) 2776
Kaletra (Up to 2%) 474
Keppra Oral Solution (1% or more) 3307
Keppra Tablets (1% or more) 3307
Klonopin (1%) 2782
▲ Lamictal (2% to 7%) 1449
Lescol Capsules (1.8%) 2227
Lescol Capsules (1.8%) 2730
Lescol XL Tablets (2.6%) 2227
Lescol XL Tablets (2.6%) 2730
Levaquin in 5% Dextrose Injection (0.1% to 0.9%) 2453
Levaquin (0.1% to 0.9%) 2453
Lexapro Oral Solution (Frequent) 1193
Lexapro Tablets (Frequent) 1193
Lipitor Tablets (Greater than or equal to 2%) 2495
Lofibra Capsules 1217
Lotensin Tablets (Less than 1%) 2232
Lotensin HCT Tablets (0.3% or more) 2235
Lunesta Tablets (Infrequent) 3139
▲ Lyrica Capsules (1% to 3%) 2524
▲ Menostar Transdermal System (6%) 805
Meridia Capsules (Greater than or equal to 1%) 485
Metrogel 1% (1.1%) 1212
Miacalcin Nasal Spray (Less than 1%) 2242
Micardis Tablets (More than 0.3%) 884
Micardis HCT Tablets (Less than 2%) 886
Migranal Nasal Spray (Rare) 3350
Namenda (Greater than or equal to 2%) 1199
Nasonex Nasal Spray (Greater than or equal to 2%) 3058
Neoral Soft Gelatin Capsules (1%) 2247
Neoral Oral Solution (1%) 2247
▲ Neurontin Oral Solution (3.4%) 2498
▲ Nicotrol Inhaler (Greater than 3%) 2594
Nicotrol NS (Less than 1%) 2596
▲ Nipent for Injection (3%) 3216
▲ Norditropin Cartridges (9%) 2318
Omacor Capsules 2735
OptiPranolol Metipranolol Ophthalmic Solution 0.3% (A small number of patients) ⊙254
Paxil CR Controlled-Release Tablets (Infrequent) 1509
Paxil (Infrequent) 1501
Permax Tablets (Infrequent) 3357
▲ Photofrin for Injection (4%) 729
▲ Plavix Tablets (3.7%) 940
▲ Plavix Tablets (3.7%) 2942
Plendil Extended-Release Tablets (0.5% to 1.5%) 651
Pletal Tablets (2% or greater) 2478
▲ Prandin Tablets (0.5, 1, and 2 mg) (2% to 6%) 2337
Prevacid Delayed-Release Capsules (Less than 1%) 3268
Prevacid for Delayed-Release Oral Suspension (Less than 1%) 3268
Prevacid NapraPAC (Less than 1%) 3277
Prevacid SoluTab Delayed-Release Orally Disintegrating Tablets (Less than 1%) 3268
PREVPAC (Less than 1%) 3281
Prinivil Tablets (0.3% to 1.0%) 2029
Prinzide Tablets (0.3% to 1%) 2033
▲ Prograf Capsules and Injection (3% to 15%) 624
Prometrium Capsules (100 mg, 200 mg) (Less than 5%) 3205
Protonix I.V. (Greater than or equal to 1%) 3468
Protonix Tablets (Greater than or equal to 1%) 3465
▲ Protopic Ointment (2% to 6%) 629
Proventil Inhalation Solution 0.083% (1.5% to 4%) 3069
Provigil Tablets (At least 1%) 1002
Pulmozyme Inhalation Solution 1245
▲ Rapamune Oral Solution and Tablets (3% to 20%) 3472
Raptiva for Injection 1247
Razadyne ER Extended-Release Capsules (Greater than or equal to 2%) 2434
Razadyne (Greater than or equal to 2%) 2434
Relenza Rotadisk (2%) 1525
Relpax Tablets (Rare) 2531
▲ Remicade for IV Injection (10%) 987
▲ Renagel Tablets (11.1%) 1268
ReoPro Vials (0.3%) 1779
▲ Requip Tablets (3%) 1528
▲ Rescriptor Tablets (3.5% to 6.7%) 2535
Rilutek Tablets (More than 2%) 2945
▲ Rituxan for Infusion (1% to 5%) 845
▲ Rituxan I.V. (1% to 5%) 1251
Sandostatin LAR Depot (1% to 4%) 2264
▲ Serevent Diskus (4% to 7%) 1540
▲ Simulect for Injection (3% to 10%) 2268
Singulair (Greater than or equal to 2%) 2047
Sonata Capsules (Frequent) 1686
Starlix Tablets (2.7%) 2276
Symbyax Capsules (Frequent) 1788
Synagis (More than 1%) 1868
Tamiflu Capsules (0.7% to 2.3%) 2810
Tamiflu Oral Suspension (0.7% to 2.3%) 2810
Targretin Capsules 1719
Tarka Tablets (1.5%) 519
Tasmar Tablets (Frequent) 3360
Teveten Tablets (1% or greater) 1707
Teveten HCT Tablets (Less than 1%) 1710
Tiazac Capsules (1% to 4%) 1204
▲ Topamax Sprinkle Capsules (2% to 7%) 2438
▲ Topamax Tablets (2% to 7%) 2438
Travatan Ophthalmic Solution (1% to 5%) 559
Tricor Tablets 523
▲ Trileptal Oral Suspension (Up to 3%) 2281
▲ Trileptal Tablets (Up to 3%) 2281
Uniretic Tablets (More than 1%) 3114
Uroxatral Tablets (1% to 2%) 2957
▲ Vagifem Tablets (3% to 5%) 2340
Vantin Tablets and Oral Suspension (Less than 1%) 2650
Vaseretic Tablets 2073
Vasotec I.V. Injection (0.5% to 1.0%) 2076
Viagra Tablets (Less than 2%) 2552
Vicoprofen Tablets (Less than 1%) 533
Vivelle Transdermal System (1.5% to 2.3%) 2288
Vivelle-Dot Transdermal System (1.5% to 2.3%) 2293
Wellbutrin Tablets (Infrequent) 1579
Wellbutrin SR Sustained-Release Tablets (At least 1%) 1583
Wellbutrin XL Extended-Release Tablets (At least 1%) 1588
▲ Xeloda Tablets (Less than 5%) 2825
Yasmin 28 Tablets (Greater than 1%) 818
Zemaira (0.8%) 3506
Zestoretic Tablets (0.3% to 1%) 701
Zestril Tablets (0.3% to 1.0%) 704
▲ Ziagen (4%) 1600
Zoladex (1% or greater) 709
Zoladex 3-month 712
Zoloft (Rare) 2581
Zomig Nasal Spray (Infrequent) 718
Zomig Tablets (Infrequent) 714
Zomig-ZMT Tablets (Infrequent) 714
Zyban Sustained-Release Tablets (2%) 1620
Zyrtec Chewable Tablets (Less than 2%) 2589
Zyrtec (Less than 2%) 2589
Zyrtec-D 12 Hour Extended Release Tablets (Less than 2%) 2591

Bronchoconstriction
Intron A for Injection (Rare) 3038
Invanz for Injection (Greater than 0.1%) 1974
Pegasys 2793
Rebetron Combination Therapy 3078
Urecholine Tablets 2349

Bronchopneumonia
▲ Xeloda Tablets (Less than 5%) 2825

Bronchopulmonary dysplasia
I.V. Busulfex (Rare) 1125
Myleran Tablets 1492

Bronchospasm
Abelcet Injection (Rare) 1119
Accutane Capsules 2740
Actimmune (Rare) 1646
Adenocard Injection 612
Advair Diskus 100/50 1291
Advair Diskus 250/50 1291
Advair Diskus 500/50 1291
Aggrenox Capsules (Less than 1%) 855
Aldurazyme for Intravenous Infusion 1261
Alkeran for Injection (In some patients) 976
Ambien Tablets (Rare) 2867
Amnesteem Capsules 2126
Anzemet Injection (Rare) 2871
Anzemet Tablets (Rare) 2874
Astelin Nasal Spray (Infrequent) 1876
Atrovent HFA Inhalation Aerosol 872
Atrovent Inhalation Solution (2.3%) 868
Atrovent Nasal Spray 0.06% (Rare) 870
Attenuvax 1889
Axid Oral Solution (Rare) 913
Bayer Aspirin Tablets 3515
Beconase AQ Nasal Spray (Rare) 1359
Betagan Ophthalmic Solution, USP ⊙217
Betaseron for SC Injection 791
▲ Betimol Ophthalmic Solution (More than 5%) ⊙283
▲ Betimol Ophthalmic Solution (More than 5%) 3371
Betoptic S Ophthalmic Suspension (Rare) 554
Bexxar 1360
Blocadren Tablets (0.6%) 1891

Brevibloc Concentrate (Less than 1%) 766
Brevibloc Injection (Less than 1%) 766
Brevibloc Double Strength Injection (Less than 1%) 766
Brevibloc Premixed Injection (Less than 1%) 766
Brevibloc Double Strength Premixed Injection (Less than 1%) 766
▲ Campath Ampules (2% to 9%) 826
Captopril Tablets 2114
Carimune NF 3501
Carteolol Hydrochloride Ophthalmic Solution USP, 1% ⊙246
Celebrex Capsules (0.1% to 1.9%) 3130
Celexa (Rare) 1177
Cipro I.V. (1% or less) 2998
Cipro I.V. Pharmacy Bulk Package (1% or less) 3509
Cipro (Less than 1%) 2991
Cipro XR Tablets 3004
Clinoril Tablets (Less than 1 in 100) 1899
Colazal Capsules 2845
Combivent Inhalation Aerosol (0.3%; rare) 878
Coreg Tablets (Less than or equal to 0.1%) 1376
Cosopt Sterile Ophthalmic Solution 1910
Cytovene 2763
Dilaudid 439
Dilaudid Oral Liquid 443
Dilaudid Non-Sterile Powder 439
Dilaudid Rectal Suppositories 439
Dilaudid Tablets 439
Dilaudid Tablets - 8 mg 443
Dilaudid-HP (Less frequent) 441
Diovan HCT Tablets (Greater than 0.2%) 2195
Diprivan Injectable Emulsion (Rare) 676
Dolobid Tablets (Less than 1 in 100) 1937
Ecotrin Enteric Coated Aspirin Low, Regular and Maximum Strength Tablets 1627
Elitek 2906
Eloxatin for Injection (Rare) 2908
Engerix-B Vaccine 1391
Evoxac Capsules (Less than 1%) 1042
Exelon Capsules (Infrequent) 2204
Fabrazyme for Intravenous Infusion (2%) 1267
Flonase Nasal Spray 1412
Flovent HFA 1418
Flumadine (Less than 0.3%) 1186
Fluorescite Injection ⊙207
Fortaz (Very rare) 1422
▲ Fortical Nasal Spray (1% to 3%) 3336
Gammagard Liquid 751
Gammagard S/D 754
Gamunex Immune Globulin I.V., 10% 3232
Gemzar for Injection (Less than 2%) 1743
▲ Gengraf Capsules (1% to 5%) 458
Herceptin I.V. 1234
▲ Humira Injection (Less than 5%) 464
▲ Imdur Tablets (Less than or equal to 5%) 3032
Imitrex Injection 1431
Imitrex Nasal Spray 1435
Inderal LA Long-Acting Capsules 3421
Infed Injection 3381
InnoPran XL Capsules 2728
▲ Intron A for Injection (Less than or equal to 5%) 3038
Iveegam EN 759
Lamictal (2%) 1449
Levaquin in 5% Dextrose Injection (0.1% to 0.9%) 2453
Levaquin (0.1% to 0.9%) 2453
Lidoderm Patch (Rare) 1107
Meruvax II 1994
Miacalcin Injection (A few cases) 2241
Miacalcin Nasal Spray (1% to 3%) 2242
Migranal Nasal Spray (Rare) 3350
Mivacron Injection (Less than 1%) 489
M-M-R II 1980
Mobic Oral Suspension (Less than 2%) 893
Mobic Tablets (Less than 2%) 893
Mumpsvax 2005
Nadolol Tablets (1 of 1000 patients) 2121
Naropin Injection (Less than 1%) 640
Navelbine Injection (Infrequent) 1494
▲ Neoral Soft Gelatin Capsules (1% to 5%) 2247
▲ Neoral Oral Solution (1% to 5%) 2247
Neurontin Capsules (Rare) 2498
Neurontin Oral Solution (Rare) 2498
Neurontin Tablets (Rare) 2498
Nicotrol NS (Less than 1%) 2596
Nimbex Injection (0.2%) 494
Nipent for Injection (Less than 3%) 3216
Norvir 499
Nubain Injection (1% or less) 1111
Numorphan 1112
▲ Oncaspar (Less than 1% to greater than 5%) 1123
Orthoclone OKT3 Sterile Solution (Less than 1%) 2370
Pepcid Injection (Infrequent) 2017
Pepcid (Infrequent) 2014
Persantine Tablets (Rare) 898
Photofrin for Injection 729
Plavix Tablets (Very rare) 940
Plavix Tablets (Very rare) 2942
Prevnar for Injection 3460
Prinivil Tablets (0.3% to 1.0%) 2029
Prinzide Tablets 2033
Proventil Inhalation Aerosol 3067
▲ Proventil Inhalation Solution 0.083% (8% to 15.4%) 3069
Proventil HFA Inhalation Aerosol (Rare) 3071
Pulmicort Respules (Less than 1%) 654
Qvar Inhalation Aerosol (Rare) 1654
Rabies Vaccine RabAvert 1011
Recombivax HB (Less than 1%) 2045
Refludan for Injection (Common) 815
Relenza Rotadisk (Less than 1%) 1525
Remicade for IV Injection 987
ReoPro Vials (0.3%) 1779
Rhinocort Aqua Nasal Spray (2%) 658
Risperdal M-Tab Orally Disintegrating Tablets (Infrequent) 1658
Risperdal (Infrequent) 1658
▲ Rituxan for Infusion (1% to 8%) 845
▲ Rituxan I.V. (1% to 8%) 1251
Rocephin Injectable Vials, ADD-Vantage, Galaxy, Bulk (Rare) 2801
Roferon-A Injection (Rare to infrequent) 2805
▲ Simulect for Injection (3% to 10%) 2268
St. Joseph 81 mg Aspirin Chewable and Enteric Coated Tablets 1841
▲ Suprane Liquid for Inhalation (3% to 10%) 770
Tambocor Tablets (Less than 1%) 1824
Taxotere Injection Concentrate (0.9%) 2947
Tenormin I.V. Injection (1.2%) 698
Tenormin Tablets (1.2%) 695
Tequin Injection (Less than 0.1%) 964
Tequin Tablets (Less than 0.1%) 964
Tessalon Capsules 1202
Tessalon Perles 1202
Timolide Tablets (1.6%) 2056
Timoptic in Ocudose (Less frequent) 2061
Timoptic Sterile Ophthalmic Solution (Less frequent) 2058
Timoptic-XE Sterile Ophthalmic Gel Forming Solution 2062
Tindamax (Rare) 2670
TOBI Solution for Inhalation 1015
Toprol-XL Tablets (About 1 of 100 patients) 660
Trusopt Sterile Ophthalmic Solution 2065
Twinrix Vaccine 1571
Ultane Liquid for Inhalation (Less than 1%) 526
Univasc Tablets (Less than 1%) 3118
Vaseretic Tablets 2073
Vasotec I.V. Injection (0.5% to 1.0%) 2076
Ventolin HFA Inhalation Aerosol 1576
Viracept 2556
Virazole for Inhalation Solution (Infrequent) 3365
VoSpire Extended-Release Tablets (Rare) 2352
Wellbutrin SR Sustained-Release Tablets (Rare) 1583
Wellbutrin XL Extended-Release Tablets (Rare) 1588
Zantac (Rare) 1597
Zantac Injection 1593
Zantac Injection Pharmacy Bulk Package (Rare) 1595
Zantac Syrup (Rare) 1597
Zemaira (0.5%) 3506
Zemuron Injection (Less than 1%) 2363
Zestoretic Tablets 701
Zestril Tablets (0.3% to 1.0%) 704
▲ Zevalin Injection (5%) 848
Zithromax for IV Infusion (1% or less) 2573
Zofran Injection (Rare to less than 1%) 1607
Zofran (Rare) 1613
Zofran ODT Orally Disintegrating Tablets (Rare) 1613
Zoloft (Infrequent) 2581
Zomig Tablets (Infrequent) 714
Zomig-ZMT Tablets (Infrequent) 714
Zosyn (1.0% or less) 3492
Zyban Sustained-Release Tablets (Rare) 1620
▲ Zyrtec Chewable Tablets (1.9% to 3.1%) 2589
▲ Zyrtec (1.9% to 3.1%) 2589
▲ Zyrtec-D 12 Hour Extended Release Tablets (1.9% to 3.1%) 2591

Bronchospasm, exacerbation of
AccuNeb Inhalation Solution 1055
Celebrex Capsules (0.1% to 1.9%) 3130
Didronel Tablets (Rare) 2693
Serevent Diskus 1540

Bronchospasm, paradoxical
AccuNeb Inhalation Solution 1055
Advair Diskus 100/50 1291
Advair Diskus 250/50 1291
Advair Diskus 500/50 1291
Alupent Inhalation Aerosol 858
Combivent Inhalation Aerosol (Less than 2%) 878
DuoNeb Inhalation Solution 1058
Flovent Diskus 50 mcg 1415
Flovent HFA 1418
Proventil HFA Inhalation Aerosol 3071
Serevent Diskus 1540
Ventolin HFA Inhalation Aerosol 1576
Xopenex HFA Inhalation Aerosol 3151
Xopenex Inhalation Solution 3143
Xopenex Inhalation Solution Concentrate 3147

Browache
OptiPranolol Metipranolol Ophthalmic Solution 0.3% (A small number of patients) ⊙254
▲ Rēv-Eyes Ophthalmic Eyedrops 0.5% (10% to 40%) ⊙256

Bruising
Accolate Tablets 663
Accutane Capsules 2740
Amnesteem Capsules 2126
▲ Apokyn Injection (16%) 2132
Arixtra Injection (1%) 1325
Arthrotec Tablets (Rare) 3126
Azmacort Inhalation Aerosol 1701
Carbatrol Capsules 3174
Clindesse Vaginal Cream (Less than 1%) 3296
Clozapine Tablets (Less than 1%) 2141
Clozaril Tablets (Less than 1%) 2174
Coumadin for Injection 932
Coumadin Tablets 932
Covera-HS Tablets (Less than 2%) 3135
Cymbalta Delayed-Release Capsules (Infrequent) 1729
Depacon Injection 412
Depakene 417
Depakote Sprinkle Capsules 422
Depakote Tablets 427
Depakote ER Tablets 433
▲ Eligard 22.5 mg (3.4%) 2899
Elocon Cream 0.1% (1 in 97 patients) 3019
▲ Emcyt Capsules (3%) 3137
Enbrel for Injection 580
▲ Entocort EC Capsules (15%) 2694
FazaClo Orally Disintegrating Tablets (Less than 1%) 547
Hycamtin for Injection 1427
Imitrex Injection 1431
▲ Increlex Injection (Greater than or equal to 5%) 3290
Lexapro Oral Solution (Infrequent) 1193
Lexapro Tablets (Infrequent) 1193
Maxair Autohaler (0.6%) 1820
Nalfon Capsules (Less than 1%) 2504
Neurontin Capsules (Frequent) 2498
Neurontin Oral Solution (Frequent) 2498
Neurontin Tablets (Frequent) 2498
Oncaspar 1123
Plendil Extended-Release Tablets (0.5% to 1.5%) 651
Raptiva for Injection 1247
ReFacto Vials 3479
Rescriptor Tablets 2535
Roferon-A Injection (Less than 4%) 2805
▲ Sandostatin Injection (1% to 4%) 2263
Singulair 2047
Tarka Tablets 519
Tegretol/Tegretol-XR 2278
Trileptal Oral Suspension 2281
Trileptal Tablets 2281
Verelan PM Capsules (2% or less) 3120
Xolair 1259

Bruising at application site
Lidoderm Patch 1107

Bruising at injection site
Adacel Vaccine (Very rare) 2959
Eligard 45 mg (Less than 1% to 2.3%) 2904
▲ Gonal-f RFF Pen for Injection (9.7%) 3155
▲ Vantas (7.2%) 3367

Bruxism
Effexor Tablets (Infrequent) 3405
Effexor XR Capsules (Infrequent) 3411
Eldepryl Capsules 3209
Lexapro Oral Solution (Infrequent) 1193
Lexapro Tablets (Infrequent) 1193
Parcopa Orally Disintegrating Tablets 3111
Paxil CR Controlled-Release Tablets (Infrequent) 1509
Paxil (Infrequent) 1501
Seroquel Tablets (Infrequent) 691
Sonata Capsules (Rare) 1686
Stalevo Tablets 2270
Wellbutrin Tablets (Infrequent) 1579
Wellbutrin SR Sustained-Release Tablets (Infrequent) 1583
Wellbutrin XL Extended-Release Tablets (Infrequent) 1588
Zyban Sustained-Release Tablets (Infrequent) 1620

BSP retention
Capastat Sulfate for Injection 1728

BSP retention, increase
Anadrol-50 Tablets 3329
Estratest Tablets 3196
Estratest H.S. Tablets 3196
Oxandrin Tablets 2977

Buccoglossal syndrome
Abilify Tablets (Rare) 916
Abilify Tablets (Rare) 2472
Effexor Tablets (Rare) 3405
Effexor XR Capsules (Rare) 3411
Geodon Capsules (Frequent) 2514
Prozac Pulvules and Liquid (Infrequent) 1771
Seroquel Tablets (Rare) 691
Symbyax Capsules (Infrequent) 1788
Zyprexa Tablets (Up to 2%) 1798
Zyprexa ZYDIS Orally Disintegrating Tablets (Up to 2%) 1798

Bucking
Diprivan Injectable Emulsion (Less than 1%) 676

Budd-Chiari syndrome
Alesse-28 Tablets 3392
Lo/Ovral-28 Tablets 3423
Ortho-Cept Tablets 2395
Ortho-Cyclen Tablets 2414
Ortho Evra Transdermal System 2402
Ortho Tri-Cyclen Tablets 2414
Ortho Tri-Cyclen Lo Tablets 2421
Seasonale Tablets 1073
Triphasil-28 Tablets 3483
Yasmin 28 Tablets 818

Buffalo hump

(*see under* Dorsocervical fat enlargement)

Bulbus oculi, perforation
Alrex Ophthalmic Suspension 0.2% ⊙243
Blephamide Ophthalmic Ointment 563
Blephamide Ophthalmic Suspension 564
FML Ophthalmic Ointment ⊙225
FML Ophthalmic Suspension ⊙224
FML Forte Ophthalmic Suspension ⊙223
FML-S Liquifilm Sterile Ophthalmic Suspension ⊙226
Lotemax Ophthalmic Suspension 0.5% ⊙249
Poly-Pred Liquifilm Ophthalmic Suspension ⊙231
Pred Forte Ophthalmic Suspension ⊙233

Pred Mild Sterile Ophthalmic Suspension ⊙ 236
Retisert Implant ⊙ 256
TobraDex Ophthalmic Ointment 558
TobraDex Ophthalmic Suspension 558
Zylet Ophthalmic Suspension 3508

Bulimia
Paxil CR Controlled-Release Tablets (Rare) 1509
Paxil (Rare) 1501

BUN levels, abnormal
Zyvox (0.2% to 2.1%) 2661

BUN levels, changes
Azasan Tablets (Less than 1%) 2844
Decadron Phosphate Injection 1931
Decadron Tablets 1929
Depo-Medrol Injectable Suspension 2615
Depo-Medrol Single-Dose Vial 2617
▲ Intron A for Injection (Up to 12%) 3038
Moban Tablets 1108
Neurontin Capsules (Rare) 2498
Neurontin Oral Solution (Rare) 2498
Neurontin Tablets (Rare) 2498
Parcopa Orally Disintegrating Tablets 3111
Pediapred Oral Solution 3319
▲ Vasotec I.V. Injection (About 0.2% to 20%) 2076

BUN levels, decrease
Cipro I.V. (Infrequent) 2998
Cipro I.V. Pharmacy Bulk Package (Infrequent) 3509

BUN levels, elevation
Abilify Tablets (Infrequent) 916
Abilify Tablets (Infrequent) 2472
Aceon Tablets (2 mg, 4 mg, 8 mg) 3191
Aldoclor Tablets 1881
Aldoril Tablets 1884
▲ Altace Capsules (0.5% to 3%) 1673
Ambien Tablets (Rare) 2867
▲ AmBisome for Injection (21%) 615
Ancef for Injection (Very rare) 1318
Aredia for Injection 2168
Arthrotec Tablets (Rare) 3126
Asacol Delayed-Release Tablets 2688
Atacand Tablets (Infrequent) 634
Atacand HCT (0.5% or greater) 637
Avalide Tablets 922
Avalide Tablets 2889
Avapro Tablets (Less than 0.7%) 925
Avapro Tablets (Less than 0.7%) 2886
Bayer Aspirin Tablets 3515
Benicar HCT Tablets (1.3%) 2852
▲ Biaxin/Biaxin XL (4%) 402
Blocadren Tablets 1891
Calcijex Injection 411
▲ Capastat Sulfate for Injection (36%) 1728
Captopril Tablets 2114
Carbatrol Capsules 3174
Carimune NF 3501
▲ Casodex Tablets (2% to 5%) 670
Ceftin 1369
Celebrex Capsules (0.1% to 1.9%) 3130
▲ CellCept Capsules (34.6%) 2751
▲ CellCept Intravenous (34.6%) 2751
▲ CellCept Oral Suspension (34.6%) 2751
▲ CellCept Tablets (34.6%) 2751
Cipro I.V. 2998
Cipro I.V. Pharmacy Bulk Package 3509
Cipro (0.9%) 2991
▲ Coreg Tablets (Less than or equal to 1% to 6%) 1376
Cozaar Tablets (Less than 0.1%) 1913
CytoGam Intravenous 1866
▲ Diovan Tablets (16.6%) 2191
Diprivan Injectable Emulsion (Less than 1%) 676
Doxil Injection (Less than 1%) 3302
Dyazide Capsules 1389
Dynacin Tablets 1859
Dyrenium Capsules (Rare) 3390
Ecotrin Enteric Coated Aspirin Low, Regular and Maximum Strength Tablets 1627
Effexor Tablets (Rare) 3405
Effexor XR Capsules (Rare) 3411
▲ Emend Capsules (4.7%) 1944
Equetro Extended-Release Capsules 3178
Eulexin Capsules 3023
Evoxac Capsules (Less than 1%) 1042
Fortaz (Occasional) 1422
Gammagard S/D 754
Garamycin Injectable 3028
▲ Gemzar for Injection (8% to 16%) 1743
Gengraf Capsules (1% to less than 3%) 458
Geodon Capsules (Rare) 2514
Hectorol Capsules 909
Hectorol Injection 911
▲ Hexalen Capsules (1% to 9%) 2101
Hyzaar (0.6%) 1964
Indapamide Tablets (Less than 5%) 2119
Indocin Capsules (Less than 1%) 1968
▲ Indocin I.V. (41% of infants) 1973
Indocin (Less than 1%) 1968
Inspra Tablets (0.5%) 2520
▲ Intron A for Injection (Less than 5%) 3038
Invanz for Injection (0.1% to 1%) 1974
▲ I.V. Busulfex (2% to 3%) 1125
Iveegam EN (0.3% to 0.8%) 759
▲ Leukine (23%) 829
Lotensin HCT Tablets 2235
Lotrel Capsules 2238
Lupron Depot 7.5 mg (Greater than or equal to 5%) 3261
▲ Mavik Tablets (0.6% to 9%) 482
Maxipime for Injection (Greater than 0.1% to less than 1%) 1093
Maxzide 2150
Mefoxin for Injection 1987
Mefoxin Premixed Intravenous Solution 1990
Mepron Suspension (1%) 1487
Merrem I.V. (Greater than 0.2%) 687
Micardis HCT Tablets 886
Mobic Oral Suspension (Less than 2%) 893
Mobic Tablets (Less than 2%) 893
Mycamine for Injection (0.5%) 620
Neoral Soft Gelatin Capsules (1% to less than 3%) 2247
Neoral Oral Solution (1% to less than 3%) 2247
Noroxin Tablets (Less frequent) 2009
Omnicef Capsules (0.3%) 506
Omnicef for Oral Suspension (0.2%) 506
Paxil CR Controlled-Release Tablets (Rare) 1509
Paxil (Rare) 1501
Pletal Tablets (Very rare) 2478
▲ PREVPAC (4%) 3281
Primaxin I.M. 2022
Primaxin I.V. 2024
▲ Prinivil Tablets (2.0% to 11.6%) 2029
Prinzide Tablets 2033
▲ Prograf Capsules and Injection (3% to 15%) 624
▲ Proleukin for Injection (63%) 1007
Prozac Pulvules and Liquid (Rare) 1771
▲ Rapamune Oral Solution and Tablets (3% to 20%) 3472
Requip Tablets (Frequent) 1528
Rocephin Injectable Vials, ADD-Vantage, Galaxy, Bulk (1.2%) 2801
Sandimmune 2259
St. Joseph 81 mg Aspirin Chewable and Enteric Coated Tablets 1841
Sular Tablets (Less than or equal to 1%) 1163
Suprax (Less than 2%) 1811
Symmetrel 1115
Tegretol/Tegretol-XR 2278
Teveten Tablets (0.6%) 1707
Teveten HCT Tablets (1.3%) 1710
Thalomid Capsules 979
Timentin ADD-Vantage 1556
Timentin Injection Galaxy Container 1559
Timentin IV Infusion 1553
Timentin Pharmacy Bulk Package 1562
Tygacil for Injection (2.1%) 3489
Ultane Liquid for Inhalation (Less than 1%) 526
Uniretic Tablets (Less than 1%) 3114
Univasc Tablets (1%) 3118
Vancocin HCl Capsules, USP (Rare) 3370
Vantin Tablets and Oral Suspension 2650
▲ Vaseretic Tablets (About 0.6% to 20%) 2073
VFEND I.V. (Less than 2%) 2543
VFEND Oral Suspension (Less than 2%) 2543
VFEND Tablets (Less than 2%) 2543
Zestoretic Tablets 701
Zestril Tablets (About 2.0%) 704
Zinacef Injection 1604
Zinacef for Injection 1604
Zithromax (Less than 1%) 2568
Zithromax for Oral Suspension, 300 mg, 600 mg, 900 mg, 1200 mg (Less than 1%) 2561
Zithromax Tablets, 250 mg, 500 mg (Less than 1%) 2561
Zithromax Tablets, 600 mg (Less than 1%) 2568
Zithromax Tri-Pak (Less than 1%) 2561
Zithromax Z-Pak (Less than 1%) 2568
Zmax for Oral Suspension (Less then 1%) 2577
Zonegran Capsules 1089
Zosyn 3492
Zovirax Capsules 1616
▲ Zovirax for Injection (5% to 10%) 1618
Zovirax 1616

Bundle branch block
Abilify Tablets (Rare) 916
Abilify Tablets (Rare) 2472
Aciphex Tablets 1081
Anzemet Injection 2871
Anzemet Tablets 2874
Cardizem LA Extended Release Tablets (Less than 2%) 1699
Celexa (Rare) 1177
Coreg Tablets (Less than or equal to 0.1%) 1376
Cymbalta Delayed-Release Capsules (Infrequent) 1729
Diprivan Injectable Emulsion (Less than 1%) 676
Doxil Injection (Less than 1%) 3302
Effexor Tablets (Rare) 3405
Effexor XR Capsules (Infrequent) 3411
Ellence Injection 2632
Evoxac Capsules 1042
Exelon Capsules (Infrequent) 2204
Fortical Nasal Spray (Less than 1%) 3336
Geodon Capsules (Rare) 2514
▲ Imdur Tablets (Less than or equal to 5%) 3032
Lexapro Oral Solution 1193
Lexapro Tablets 1193
Miacalcin Nasal Spray (Less than 1%) 2242
Paxil CR Controlled-Release Tablets (Rare) 1509
Paxil (Rare) 1501
Razadyne ER Extended-Release Capsules (Infrequent) 2434
Razadyne (Infrequent) 2434
Rilutek Tablets (Infrequent) 2945
Risperdal Consta Long-Acting Injection (Infrequent) 1664
Rythmol SR Capsules (Greater than or equal to 2%) 2736
Seroquel Tablets (Infrequent) 691
Sonata Capsules (Infrequent) 1686
Symbyax Capsules (Rare) 1788
Tarka Tablets (Less frequent) 519
▲ Tenormin I.V. Injection (6.6%) 698
▲ Tenormin Tablets (6.6%) 695
Tiazac Capsules (Less than 2%) 1204
Trasylol Injection (1% to 2%) 779
Uniretic Tablets (Less than 1%) 3114
VFEND I.V. (Less than 2%) 2543
VFEND Oral Suspension (Less than 2%) 2543
VFEND Tablets (Less than 2%) 2543

Burn wound infection
Amevive 836

Burning
Aclovate (Approximately 2%) 1290
▲ Acular Ophthalmic Solution (Up to 40%) 561
▲ Acular LS Ophthalmic Solution (20% to 40%) 562
Analpram-HC 1136
Bactroban Nasal (2%) 1357
Bactroban Ointment (1.5%) 1358
▲ Brimonidine Tartrate Ophthalmic Solution 0.2% (10% to 30%) ⊙ 245
Catapres-TTS (3 of 101 patients) 875
Clobevate Gel (Less than 2%) 3213
Clobex Shampoo 1209
Cutivate Cream (0.6% to 1.6%) 1381
Cutivate Lotion 0.05% (2%) 1383
Cutivate Ointment (Less than 1%) 1384
Decadron Phosphate Injection 1931
Elocon Cream 0.1% (1.6%) 3019
Elocon Lotion 0.1% (4 in 209 patients) 3020
▲ Elocon Ointment 0.1% (4.8%) 3021
Evoxac Capsules (Less than 1%) 1042
▲ Finacea Gel (4% to 20%) 1644
Fleet Bisacodyl Laxatives 1169
Fleet Prep Kits 1172
Garamycin Injectable 3028
Locoid (Infrequent) 1138
Lotrimin 3053
▲ Metrogel 1% (1.3% to 7.2%) 1212
▲ Naftin Gel (5.0%) 2097
Olux Foam (Less than 2%) 1027
Ophthetic Ophthalmic Solution (Occasional) ⊙ 230
Panafil Ointment (Occasional) 1637
Panafil Spray (Occasional) 1637
Pandel Cream, 0.1% (1.8%) 1017
Pramosone 1139
Pred-G Ophthalmic Suspension ⊙ 234
▲ Renova 0.02% Cream (Almost all subjects) 2384
▲ Renova 0.05% Cream (Almost all subjects) 2387
▲ Rēv-Eyes Ophthalmic Eyedrops 0.5% (Approximately 50%) ⊙ 256
▲ Solage Topical Solution (21.9% to 26%) 740
▲ Spectazole Cream (3%) 2390
Tasmar Tablets (1% to 2%) 3360
Temovate Cream (1%) 1549
▲ Temovate Gel (Among most frequent) 1550
Temovate Scalp Application (Infrequent) 1551
▲ Temovate E Emollient (5%) 1552
Tindamax 2670
U-Kera Cream 3290
Vanos Cream 1864
Zantac Injection 1593
Zantac Injection Pharmacy Bulk Package (Frequent) 1595
▲ Zovirax Ointment (28.3%) 854

Burning, extremities
Zerit 971

Burning, local
Acticin Cream 2125
▲ Aldara Cream, 5% (More than 1% to 26%) 1814
▲ Alphagan P Ophthalmic Solution (Approximately 5% to 9%) 563
Bactroban Cream (Less than 1% to 3.6%) 1356
▲ Dovonex Scalp Solution 0.005% (Approximately 23%) 3375
▲ Efudex (Among most frequent) 3348
▲ Elidel Cream 1% (1.5% to 25.9%) 2198
Klaron Lotion 10% 1050
Locoid Lipocream Cream (Infrequent) 1138
Mentax Cream (Approximately 1%) 2152
Mumpsvax 2005
▲ Naftin Cream (6%) 2097
Spectazole Cream 2390
Sulfamylon for 5% Topical Solution 2155
Topicort .05% Gel 3288
Topicort .25% Cream 3288
Topicort .25% Ointment 3288
Topicort LP .05% Cream 3288
U-cort 1% Cream 3289
▲ Zylet Ophthalmic Suspension (9%) 3508

Burning, vaginal
(*see under* Vaginal burning)

Burning, vulvovaginal
(*see under* Vaginal burning)

Burning at application site
▲ Aldara Cream, 5% (5.6%) 1814
▲ Cutivate Lotion 0.05% (5%) 1383
▲ Evoclin Foam, 1% (6%) 1025
Lidoderm Patch 1107
▲ Oxytrol Transdermal System (Greater than 1%) 3383
Premarin Vaginal Cream 3449
Ultralytic 2 Cream 20% 1651
Ultralytic 2 Foam 20% 1652
▲ Vanos Cream (1.8% to 6.6%) 1864

Burning at injection site
Anzemet Injection 2871
Attenuvax 1889
Brevibloc Concentrate (Less than 1%) 766
Brevibloc Injection (Less than 1%) 766
Brevibloc Double Strength Injection (Less than 1%) 766
Brevibloc Premixed Injection (Less than 1%) 766
Brevibloc Double Strength Premixed Injection (Less than 1%) 766
Cerezyme for Injection (Less than 1%) 1263
Cipro I.V. (1% or less) 2998
Cipro I.V. Pharmacy Bulk Package (1% or less) 3509
DDAVP Injection 4 mcg/mL (Occasional) 2893
Desferal Vials 2190
Desmopressin Acetate Injection (Occasional) 1143
▲ Diprivan Injectable Emulsion (10% to 17.6%) 676
▲ Eligard 22.5 mg (21.7%) 2899

▲ Eligard 30 mg (20%) 2901
▲ Eligard 45 mg (16%) 2904
Genotropin Lyophilized Powder (Infrequent).......... 2642
▲ Intron A for Injection (Less than 5%).......... 3038
Invanz for Injection (1.3%).......... 1974
Meruvax II.......... 1994
M-M-R II.......... 1980
Mumpsvax.......... 2005
Nubain Injection.......... 1111
ThermaCare Heat Wraps 2674
Timentin ADD-Vantage 1556
Timentin Injection Galaxy Container 1559
Timentin IV Infusion.......... 1553
Timentin Pharmacy Bulk Package 1562
Xolair.......... 1259
▲ Zofran Injection (4%) 1607

Burning sensation
Accuzyme Debriding Ointment (A small percentage) 1636
Accuzyme Spray (A small percentage) 1637
Adenocard Injection (Less than 1%) 612
Adriamycin for Injection, USP 786
Adriamycin Injection, USP 786
Amerge Tablets (Infrequent) 1312
BeneFix for Injection (1.5%) 3402
Clobevate Gel (1.8%) 3213
Copaxone for Injection (Infrequent) .. 3292
Doxil Injection 3302
Fleet Glycerin Laxatives 1168
Idamycin PFS Injection 2645
▲ Imitrex Injection (7.5%) 1431
Imitrex Nasal Spray (0.4% to 1.4%) 1435
Imitrex Tablets (Frequent) 1440
▲ Olux Foam (10%) 1027
Reyataz Capsules (Less than 3%) 948
▲ Sulfamylon Cream (One of two most frequent) 2154
Temovate Cream (1%) 1549
Temovate Gel (1.8%) 1550
Temovate Ointment (0.5%) 1549
▲ Temovate Scalp Application (29 of 294 patients) 1551

Bursitis
Abilify Tablets (Infrequent) 916
Abilify Tablets (Infrequent) 2472
Aciphex Tablets 1081
▲ Actonel Tablets (1.3% to 3%) 2679
▲ Actonel with Calcium Tablets (1.3% to 3%) 2684
Antara Capsules 2723
▲ Arava Tablets (1% to 3%) 2881
Avalide Tablets 922
Avalide Tablets 2889
Avapro Tablets (Less than 1%) 925
Avapro Tablets (Less than 1%) 2886
▲ Azmacort Inhalation Aerosol (1% to 3%) 1701
Caduet Tablets (Less than 2%) 2507
Celexa (Rare) 1177
Copaxone for Injection (Infrequent) .. 3292
Effexor Tablets (Infrequent) 3405
Effexor XR Capsules (Infrequent) 3411
Enbrel for Injection (Infrequent) 580
Evoxac Capsules (Less than 1%) 1042
Gabitril Tablets (Infrequent) 998
Gengraf Capsules (1% to less than 3%) 458
Lamictal (Rare) 1449
Lipitor Tablets (Less than 2%) 2495
Lofibra Capsules 1217
Lunesta Tablets (Infrequent) 3139
Meridia Capsules 485
Mirapex Tablets (2%) 889
Neoral Soft Gelatin Capsules (1% to less than 3%) 2247
Neoral Oral Solution (1% to less than 3%) 2247
Neurontin Capsules (Rare) 2498
Neurontin Oral Solution (Rare) 2498
Neurontin Tablets (Rare) 2498
Noroxin Tablets (Less frequent) 2009
Orthovisc Injection (1.1%) 3518
Paxil CR Controlled-Release Tablets (Rare) 1509
Paxil (Rare) 1501
Permax Tablets (1.6%) 3357
Pletal Tablets (Less than 2%) 2478
Protonix I.V. (Less than 1%) 3468
Protonix Tablets (Less than 1%) 3465
Prozac Pulvules and Liquid (Infrequent) 1771
Requip Tablets (Infrequent) 1528
Risperdal M-Tab Orally Disintegrating Tablets (Rare) 1658
Risperdal (Rare) 1658
Rythmol SR Capsules.......... 2736
Sonata Capsules (Infrequent).......... 1686
Symbyax Capsules (Rare).......... 1788
Tricor Tablets.......... 523
Uniretic Tablets (Less than 1%).......... 3114
Zyprexa Tablets (Rare).......... 1798
Zyprexa ZYDIS Orally Disintegrating Tablets (Infrequent).......... 1798

C

Cachexia
Actiq (1% or greater).......... 993
Cytovene-IV (One report).......... 2763
▲ Doxil Injection (1% to 10%) 3302
Exelon Capsules (Infrequent).......... 2204
▲ Intron A for Injection (Less than or equal to 5%).......... 3038
Norvir (Less than 2%).......... 499
Permax Tablets (Rare).......... 3357
Risperdal M-Tab Orally Disintegrating Tablets (Rare).......... 1658
Risperdal (Rare).......... 1658
Sandostatin LAR Depot (1% to 4%)... 2264
▲ Xeloda Tablets (Less than 5%) 2825

Calcification, ectopic
Calcijex Injection.......... 411
Hectorol Capsules.......... 909
Hectorol Injection.......... 911

Calcium, metabolism, disorders of
Lotronex Tablets (Rare).......... 1479

Calcium retention
Estratest Tablets 3196
Estratest H.S. Tablets.......... 3196
Oxandrin Tablets.......... 2977

Calf muscles, need to flex
Imitrex Injection (Rare).......... 1431

Callus formation, post bone fracture
Miradon Tablets.......... 3056

Calming
Nicotrol NS.......... 2596

Cancer, breast
Cenestin Tablets, 0.45mg, 0.625mg, 0.9mg, 1.25mg.......... 1063
Cenestin Tablets, 0.3mg.......... 1063
Climara Pro Transdermal System.......... 800
Depo-Provera Contraceptive Injection (Less than 1%).......... 2619
depo-subQ provera 104 Injectable Suspension 2622
Estrogel 0.06%.......... 3200
Menostar Transdermal System.......... 805
Neurontin Capsules (Infrequent).......... 2498
Neurontin Oral Solution (Infrequent).......... 2498
Neurontin Tablets (Infrequent).......... 2498
Premarin Tablets.......... 3443
Premarin Vaginal Cream.......... 3449
Propecia Tablets (Four cases).......... 2036
Proscar Tablets (Four cases).......... 2040

Cancer, cervical
Depo-Provera Contraceptive Injection (Less than 1%).......... 2619
depo-subQ provera 104 Injectable Suspension 2622
Estratest Tablets 3196
Estratest H.S. Tablets.......... 3196
Ortho-Cyclen/Ortho Tri-Cyclen.......... 2414
Ortho Tri-Cyclen Lo Tablets.......... 2421
Permax Tablets (Infrequent).......... 3357
Premarin Intravenous.......... 3440
Premarin Vaginal Cream.......... 3449

Cancer, skin, non-melanoma
Myfortic Tablets (0.9% to 1.8%).......... 2244
Raptiva for Injection.......... 1247

Cancer, vaginal
Estratest Tablets 3196
Estratest H.S. Tablets.......... 3196
Premarin Intravenous.......... 3440
Premarin Vaginal Cream.......... 3449
Vivelle Transdermal System.......... 2288
Vivelle-Dot Transdermal System.......... 2293

Candidiasis
Abilify Tablets (Rare).......... 916
Abilify Tablets (Rare).......... 2472
▲ Advair Diskus 100/50 (3%) 1291
▲ Advair Diskus 250/50 (1% to 3%) ... 1291
Advair Diskus 500/50 (Up to 3%)..... 1291
▲ Aerobid/Aerobid-M (3% to 9%) 1172
Aredia for Injection (Up to 6%).......... 2168
Augmentin.......... 1331
Augmentin Tablets 1334
Augmentin XR Extended-Release Tablets 1340
Augmentin ES-600 Powder for Oral Suspension (1.4%).......... 1337
Avelox (0.1% to less than 2%).......... 2984
Biaxin/Biaxin XL.......... 402
▲ Campath Ampules (1% to 8%) 826
Ceftin for Oral Suspension (0.1% to 1%).......... 1369
Celebrex Capsules (0.1% to 1.9%)... 3130
▲ CellCept Capsules (17% to 22.4%).......... 2751
▲ CellCept Intravenous (17% to 22.4%).......... 2751
▲ CellCept Oral Suspension (17% to 22.4%).......... 2751
▲ CellCept Tablets (17% to 22.4%) 2751
▲ Chemet Capsules (5.2% to 15.7%).......... 2480
Cipro I.V. (1% or less) 2998
Cipro I.V. Pharmacy Bulk Package (1% or less) 3509
Cipro (Less than 1%) 2991
Cipro XR Tablets 3004
Cleocin Vaginal Ovules (Less than 1%) 2613
Colazal Capsules 2845
▲ Doxil Injection (23.5%) 3302
Effexor Tablets (Infrequent) 3405
Elocon Cream 0.1% (1 in 182 patients) 3019
▲ Evoxac Capsules (1% to 3%) 1042
Factive Tablets (0.1% to 1%) 2464
Fortaz (Less than 1%) 1422
▲ Imdur Tablets (Less than or equal to 5%).......... 3032
▲ Intron A for Injection (Up to 17%) 3038
Invanz for Injection (Greater than 0.1%) 1974
Invirase (Less than 2%) 2776
Klonopin (Infrequent) 2782
Levaquin in 5% Dextrose Injection (0.1% to 0.9%) 2453
Levaquin (0.1% to 0.9%) 2453
▲ Megace ES Oral Suspension (1% to 3%) 2492
Merrem I.V. (0.1% to 2.0%) 687
▲ Myfortic Tablets (Less than or equal to 5.6%) 2244
Nipent for Injection (2%) 3216
Norvir (Less than 2%) 499
Omnicef Capsules (0.2%) 506
Omnicef for Oral Suspension (1%) 506
Paxil CR Controlled-Release Tablets (Infrequent) 1509
Paxil (Infrequent) 1501
Pentasa Capsules (Less than 1%) 3182
Permax Tablets (Infrequent) 3357
▲ Photofrin for Injection (9%) 729
Prevacid Delayed-Release Capsules (Less than 1%) 3268
Prevacid for Delayed-Release Oral Suspension (Less than 1%) 3268
Prevacid NapraPAC (Less than 1%) .. 3277
Prevacid SoluTab Delayed-Release Orally Disintegrating Tablets (Less than 1%) 3268
PREVPAC (Less than 1%) 3281
Primaxin I.M. 2022
Primaxin I.V. (Less than 0.2%) 2024
Protonix I.V. (Less than 1%) 3468
Protonix Tablets (Less than 1%) 3465
▲ Pulmicort Respules (3% to 4%) 654
Relpax Tablets (Rare) 2531
▲ Remicade for IV Injection (5%) 987
Rilutek Tablets (0.4% to 1.2%) 2945
Sandostatin LAR Depot (1% to 4%) .. 2264
Seasonale Tablets 1073
Seroquel Tablets (Infrequent) 691
▲ Simulect for Injection (3% to 10%) ... 2268
Soriatane Capsules (Less than 1%) .. 1028
▲ Spiriva HandiHaler (3% to 4%) 899
Suprax (Less than 2%) 1811
Symbyax Capsules (Infrequent) 1788
Targretin Capsules 1719
Thalomid Capsules 979
Uniretic Tablets (Less than 1%) 3114
Vantin Tablets and Oral Suspension (Less than 1%) 2650
Vivelle Transdermal System 2288
Vivelle-Dot Transdermal System 2293
▲ Xeloda Tablets (Less than 5%) 2825
Zithromax for IV Infusion (1% or less) 2573
▲ Zometa for Intravenous Infusion (11.6%) 2306
Zosyn (1.6%) 3492
Zyprexa Tablets (Infrequent) 1798
Zyprexa ZYDIS Orally Disintegrating Tablets (Infrequent) 1798

Candidiasis, cutaneous
Cipro XR Tablets.......... 3004
Omnicef for Oral Suspension (0.9%).......... 506

Candidiasis, esophageal
Prilosec OTC Tablets (Less than 1%).......... 2674
▲ Zegerid Powder for Oral Solution (3.9%).......... 2972

Candidiasis, gastrointestinal
▲ CellCept Capsules (3% to less than 20%).......... 2751
▲ CellCept Intravenous (3% to less than 20%).......... 2751
▲ CellCept Oral Suspension (3% to less than 20%).......... 2751
▲ CellCept Tablets (3% to less than 20%).......... 2751
Cipro.......... 2991
Protonix I.V. (Less than 1%).......... 3468
Protonix Tablets (Less than 1%).......... 3465
▲ Thymoglobulin for Injection (4.9%) .. 2848
Zyrtec-D 12 Hour Extended Release Tablets.......... 2591

Candidiasis, genital
(*see also under* Vaginal candidiasis)
Activella Tablets (0% to 6%).......... 2311
▲ Azmacort Inhalation Aerosol (1% to 3%).......... 1701
Celebrex Capsules (0.1% to 1.9%)... 3130
Effexor Tablets (Infrequent).......... 3405
Effexor XR Capsules.......... 3411
Evoxac Capsules (Less than 1%).......... 1042
Factive Tablets (0.1% to 1%).......... 2464
Infergen (2%).......... 1647
Lamictal (Infrequent).......... 1449
Levaquin in 5% Dextrose Injection (0.2%).......... 2453
Levaquin (0.2%).......... 2453
Mefoxin for Injection 1987
Mefoxin Premixed Intravenous Solution.......... 1990
Nexium Delayed-Release Capsules (Less than 1%).......... 645
Nexium I.V. (Less than 1%).......... 649
Paxil CR Controlled-Release Tablets (Rare) 1509
Paxil (Rare).......... 1501
PREVPAC (Less than 3%).......... 3281
▲ Prochieve 4% Gel (5%) 1018
▲ Prochieve 8% Gel (5%) 1018
Requip Tablets (Infrequent).......... 1528
Rilutek Tablets (Rare).......... 2945
Rocephin Injectable Vials, ADD-Vantage, Galaxy, Bulk (Occasional).......... 2801
▲ Vagifem Tablets (5%) 2340

Candidiasis, mouth
(*see under* Candidiasis, oral)

Candidiasis, nasal
Nasonex Nasal Spray (Rare).......... 3058

Candidiasis, oral
Abilify Tablets (Infrequent).......... 916
Abilify Tablets (Infrequent).......... 2472
Actiq (Less than 1%).......... 993
▲ Advair Diskus 100/50 (1% to 4%) ... 1291
▲ Advair Diskus 250/50 (1% to 4%) ... 1291
▲ Advair Diskus 500/50 (1% to 4%) ... 1291
Ancef for Injection.......... 1318
▲ Arava Tablets (1% to 3%) 2881
▲ Asmanex Twisthaler (4% to 22%) ... 2981
Augmentin ES-600 Powder for Oral Suspension.......... 1337
Avelox (0.1% to less than 2%).......... 2984
Azmacort Inhalation Aerosol (A few cases).......... 1701
▲ CellCept Capsules (3% to less than 20%).......... 2751
▲ CellCept Intravenous (3% to less than 20%).......... 2751
▲ CellCept Oral Suspension (3% to less than 20%).......... 2751
▲ CellCept Tablets (3% to less than 20%).......... 2751
Cipro I.V. (1% or less).......... 2998
Cipro I.V. Pharmacy Bulk Package (1% or less).......... 3509
Cipro (Less than 1%).......... 2991
Cipro XR Tablets.......... 3004
▲ Clolar for Intravenous Infusion (13%).......... 1264
Comvax (0.2% to 0.8%).......... 1904
Copaxone for Injection (Frequent)..... 3292
▲ Doxil Injection (1% to 10%) 3302
Effexor Tablets (Infrequent).......... 3405
Effexor XR Capsules (Infrequent)...... 3411

▲ Flovent Diskus 50 mcg (9% to 31%) ... 1415
▲ Flovent HFA (4%) ... 1418
Fortaz (Less than 1%) ... 1422
Grifulvin V Tablets Microsize and Oral Suspension Microsize (Occasional) ... 2384
Gris-PEG Tablets (Occasional) ... 2504
Invanz for Injection (0.1% to 1%) ... 1974
Ketek Tablets (Greater than or equal to 0.2% to less than 2%) ... 2920
Maxipime for Injection (Greater than 0.1% to less than 1%) ... 1093
▲ Megace ES Oral Suspension (1% to 3%) ... 2492
▲ Mepron Suspension (5% to 10%) ... 1487
Merrem I.V. (Greater than 0.1% to 1%) ... 687
▲ Myfortic Tablets (3% to less than 20%) ... 2244
Nasonex Nasal Spray (Rare) ... 3058
▲ Neumega for Injection (14%) ... 3433
Neurontin Capsules (Infrequent) ... 2498
Neurontin Oral Solution (Infrequent) ... 2498
Neurontin Tablets (Infrequent) ... 2498
Prevacid Delayed-Release Capsules (Less than 1%) ... 3268
Prevacid for Delayed-Release Oral Suspension (Less than 1%) ... 3268
Prevacid NapraPAC (Less than 1%) ... 3277
Prevacid SoluTab Delayed-Release Orally Disintegrating Tablets (Less than 1%) ... 3268
Prevnar for Injection ... 3460
PREVPAC (Less than 1%) ... 3281
▲ Prograf Capsules and Injection (3% to 15%) ... 624
Protonix I.V. (Less than 1%) ... 3468
Protonix Tablets (Less than 1%) ... 3465
▲ Rapamune Oral Solution and Tablets (3% to 20%) ... 3472
Rescriptor Tablets ... 2535
Serevent Diskus (1% to 3%) ... 1540
Spectracef Tablets (0.1% to 1%) ... 2706
Synagis (More than 1%) ... 1868
Synercid I.V. (Less than 1%) ... 1690
▲ Tequin Injection (0.1% to 3%) ... 964
▲ Tequin Tablets (0.1% to 3%) ... 964
▲ Thalomid Capsules (4.2%) ... 979
▲ Thymoglobulin for Injection (3.7%) ... 2848
Tindamax ... 2670
▲ Trisenox Injection (5%) ... 983
Vantin Tablets and Oral Suspension (Less than 1%) ... 2650
▲ Xeloda Tablets (Less than 1% to 7%) ... 2825
Zithromax (1% or less) ... 2568
Zithromax for Oral Suspension, 300 mg, 600 mg, 900 mg, 1200 mg (1% or less) ... 2561
Zithromax Tablets, 250 mg, 500 mg (1% or less) ... 2561
Zithromax Tablets, 600 mg ... 2568
Zithromax Tri-Pak (1% or less) ... 2561
Zithromax Z-Pak ... 2568
Zmax for Oral Suspension (Less then 1%) ... 2577
▲ Zosyn (3.9%) ... 3492
Zyprexa Tablets (Infrequent) ... 1798
Zyprexa ZYDIS Orally Disintegrating Tablets (Infrequent) ... 1798
Zyvox (0% to 1.1%) ... 2661

Candidiasis, pharynx
Azmacort Inhalation Aerosol ... 1701
Serevent Diskus (1% to 3%) ... 1540

Candidiasis, urinary tract
Nexium Delayed-Release Capsules (Less than 1%) ... 645
Nexium I.V. (Less than 1%) ... 649

Candidiasis, vaginal
Avelox (0.1% to less than 2%) ... 2984
▲ Doxil Injection (1% to 10%) ... 3302

Candiduria
Cipro I.V. ... 2998
Cipro I.V. Pharmacy Bulk Package ... 3509
Cipro ... 2991
Cipro XR Tablets ... 3004
Noroxin Tablets ... 2009
Zosyn (1.0% or less) ... 3492

Capillary fragility
Aerobid/Aerobid-M (1% to 3%) ... 1172
Campath Ampules ... 826
Neurontin Capsules (Rare) ... 2498
Neurontin Oral Solution (Rare) ... 2498
Neurontin Tablets (Rare) ... 2498

Capillary leak syndrome
Aldara Cream, 5% ... 1814
Betaseron for SC Injection ... 791
Clolar for Intravenous Infusion ... 1264
I.V. Busulfex ... 1125
Leukine ... 829
Neumega for Injection ... 3433
Neupogen for Injection (One event) .. 598
Orthoclone OKT3 Sterile Solution (Less than 1%) ... 2370
Proleukin for Injection ... 1007
Simulect for Injection ... 2268

Carbohydrate craving
Lexapro Oral Solution (Infrequent) ... 1193
Lexapro Tablets (Infrequent) ... 1193

Carbohydrate tolerance, decrease
Activella Tablets ... 2311
Alesse-28 Tablets ... 3392
Cenestin Tablets, 0.45mg, 0.625mg, 0.9mg, 1.25mg ... 1063
Cenestin Tablets, 0.3mg ... 1063
Climara Transdermal System ... 795
Climara Pro Transdermal System ... 800
Decadron Phosphate Injection ... 1931
Decadron Tablets ... 1929
Depo-Medrol Injectable Suspension ... 2615
Depo-Medrol Single-Dose Vial ... 2617
Estratest Tablets ... 3196
Estratest H.S. Tablets ... 3196
Estrogel 0.06% ... 3200
Hydrocortone Tablets ... 1963
Lo/Ovral-28 Tablets ... 3423
Menostar Transdermal System ... 805
Ortho-Cept Tablets ... 2395
Ortho-Cyclen Tablets ... 2414
Ortho Evra Transdermal System ... 2402
Ortho Tri-Cyclen Tablets ... 2414
Ortho Tri-Cyclen Lo Tablets ... 2421
Premarin Intravenous ... 3440
Premarin Vaginal Cream ... 3449
Premphase Tablets ... 3452
Prempro Tablets ... 3452
Triphasil-28 Tablets ... 3483
Vivelle Transdermal System ... 2288
Vivelle-Dot Transdermal System ... 2293
Yasmin 28 Tablets ... 818

Carbohydrate tolerance, reduced
Prefest Tablets ... 1069

Carbon dioxide, changes
Ammonul Injection ... 3323

Carcinogenic

Carcinoma, basal cell
Aldara Cream, 5% (2.3%) ... 1814
Amevive (Less than 0.1%) ... 836
Evoxac Capsules (Less than 1%) ... 1042
Metrogel 1% (0.2%) ... 1212
Neoral Soft Gelatin Capsules (0.4%) ... 2247
Neoral Oral Solution (0.4%) ... 2247
▲ Rapamune Oral Solution and Tablets (0.7% to 4.7%) ... 3472
Remicade for IV Injection (Greater than or equal to 0.2%) ... 987
Requip Tablets (1% or more) ... 1528
Sandostatin Injection (Less than 1%) ... 2263
Sandostatin LAR Depot (Rare) ... 2264

Carcinoma, bile duct
▲ Humira Injection (Less than 5%) ... 464

Carcinoma, bladder
Bexxar ... 1360
Requip Tablets (Infrequent) ... 1528
Zoladex 3-month (1% to 5%) ... 712

Carcinoma, breast
Actiq (1% or greater) ... 993
Activella Tablets ... 2311
Ambien Tablets (Rare) ... 2867
Bexxar ... 1360
Celebrex Capsules (0.1% to 1.9%) ... 3130
Climara Transdermal System ... 795
CombiPatch Transdermal System ... 2180
Estratest Tablets ... 3196
Estratest H.S. Tablets ... 3196
Eulexin Capsules (Two reports) ... 3023
▲ Humira Injection (Less than 5%) ... 464
Imitrex Nasal Spray ... 1435
Lamictal (Rare) ... 1449
Lo/Ovral-28 Tablets ... 3423
Ortho-Cyclen/Ortho Tri-Cyclen ... 2414
Ortho Tri-Cyclen Lo Tablets ... 2421
Paxil CR Controlled-Release Tablets (Rare) ... 1509
Paxil (Rare) ... 1501
Permax Tablets (Infrequent) ... 3357
Prefest Tablets ... 1069
Premphase Tablets ... 3452
Prempro Tablets ... 3452
Prometrium Capsules (100 mg, 200 mg) (2%) ... 3205
Remicade for IV Injection (Greater than or equal to 0.2%) ... 987
Requip Tablets (Infrequent) ... 1528
Sandostatin LAR Depot (Rare) ... 2264
Symbyax Capsules (Rare) ... 1788
Tasmar Tablets (Infrequent) ... 3360
Uniretic Tablets (Less than 1%) ... 3114
Vivelle Transdermal System (1.29%) ... 2288
Vivelle-Dot Transdermal System ... 2293
Zelnorm Tablets ... 2303
Zomig Nasal Spray (Rare) ... 718

Carcinoma, cervix
Copaxone for Injection (Infrequent) ... 3292
▲ Humira (Less than 5%) ... 464

Carcinoma, colorectal
Bexxar ... 1360

Carcinoma, endometrial
Activella Tablets ... 2311
Arimidex Tablets (0.1%) ... 665
Cenestin Tablets, 0.45mg, 0.625mg, 0.9mg, 1.25mg ... 1063
Cenestin Tablets, 0.3mg ... 1063
Climara Transdermal System ... 795
Climara Pro Transdermal System ... 800
CombiPatch Transdermal System ... 2180
Estratest Tablets ... 3196
Estratest H.S. Tablets ... 3196
Estrogel 0.06% ... 3200
Menostar Transdermal System ... 805
Omacor Capsules ... 2735
Prefest Tablets ... 1069
Premarin Intravenous ... 3440
Premarin Tablets ... 3443
Premarin Vaginal Cream ... 3449
Premphase Tablets ... 3452
Prempro Tablets ... 3452
Vivelle Transdermal System ... 2288
Vivelle-Dot Transdermal System ... 2293

Carcinoma, esophageal
Requip Tablets (Infrequent) ... 1528

Carcinoma, gallbladder
▲ Humira Injection (Less than 5%) ... 464

Carcinoma, gastric
Bexxar ... 1360

Carcinoma, gastrointestinal
▲ Casodex Tablets (2% to 5%) ... 670
Copaxone for Injection (Infrequent) .. 3292
Protonix I.V. (Less than 1%) ... 3468
Protonix Tablets (Less than 1%) ... 3465
Tasmar Tablets (Rare) ... 3360
▲ Visudyne for Injection (1% to 10%) .. 2286
Zomig Nasal Spray (Rare) ... 718

Carcinoma, head and neck
Bexxar ... 1360

Carcinoma, hepatocellular
Anadrol-50 Tablets (Rare) ... 3329
Delatestryl Injection ... 2976
Ortho-Cyclen/Ortho Tri-Cyclen (Rare) ... 2414
Ortho Tri-Cyclen Lo Tablets ... 2421
Testim 1% Gel ... 722

Carcinoma, laryngeal
Prevacid Delayed-Release Capsules (Less than 1%) ... 3268
Prevacid for Delayed-Release Oral Suspension (Less than 1%) ... 3268
Prevacid NapraPAC (Less than 1%) .. 3277
Prevacid SoluTab Delayed-Release Orally Disintegrating Tablets (Less than 1%) ... 3268
PREVPAC (Less than 1%) ... 3281

Carcinoma, liver
Campral Tablets (Rare) ... 1175

Carcinoma, lung
Bexxar ... 1360
Matulane Capsules ... 3188
Permax Tablets (Rare) ... 3357
Prinivil Tablets (0.3% to 1.0%) ... 2029
Rilutek Tablets (Infrequent) ... 2945
Uniretic Tablets (Less than 1%) ... 3114

Carcinoma, lung, non-small cell
Emend Capsules (Greater than 0.5%) ... 1944

Carcinoma, ovarian
Cenestin Tablets, 0.45mg, 0.625mg, 0.9mg, 1.25mg ... 1063
Cenestin Tablets, 0.3mg ... 1063
Climara Transdermal System ... 795
Climara Pro Transdermal System ... 800
CombiPatch Transdermal System ... 2180
Estratest Tablets ... 3196
Estratest H.S. Tablets ... 3196
Estrogel 0.06% ... 3200
Menostar Transdermal System ... 805
Prefest Tablets ... 1069
Premarin Tablets ... 3443
Premarin Vaginal Cream ... 3449
Premphase Tablets ... 3452
Prempro Tablets ... 3452
Repronex for Intramuscular and Subcutaneous Injection (Infrequent) ... 1148
Tasmar Tablets (Rare) ... 3360
Vivelle Transdermal System ... 2288
Vivelle-Dot Transdermal System ... 2293

Carcinoma, prostate
Campath Ampules ... 826
▲ Humira Injection (Less than 5%) ... 464
Mirapex Tablets (Less than 1%) ... 889
Paxil CR Controlled-Release Tablets (Rare) ... 1509
Paxil (Rare) ... 1501
▲ Propecia Tablets (6.4%) ... 2036
▲ Proscar Tablets (6.4%) ... 2040
Rilutek Tablets (Infrequent) ... 2945
Striant Mucoadhesive ... 1022
Tasmar Tablets (Infrequent) ... 3360
Testim 1% Gel ... 722

Carcinoma, prostate, increased risk of

Carcinoma, rectal
▲ Humira Injection (Less than 5%) ... 464
Requip Tablets (Infrequent) ... 1528

Carcinoma, reproductive organs
Lo/Ovral-28 Tablets ... 3423

Carcinoma, skin
Actonel Tablets (2%) ... 2679
Actonel with Calcium Tablets (2%) ... 2684
Bexxar ... 1360
▲ Casodex Tablets (2% to 5%) ... 670
▲ CellCept Capsules (1.6% to less than 20%) ... 2751
▲ CellCept Intravenous (1.6% to less than 20%) ... 2751
▲ CellCept Oral Suspension (1.6% to less than 20%) ... 2751
▲ CellCept Tablets (1.6% to less than 20%) ... 2751
Copaxone for Injection (Infrequent) .. 3292
Gabitril Tablets (Infrequent) ... 998
Neurontin Capsules (Rare) ... 2498
Neurontin Oral Solution (Rare) ... 2498
Neurontin Tablets (Rare) ... 2498
Orthoclone OKT3 Sterile Solution ... 2370
Permax Tablets (Infrequent) ... 3357
Prevacid Delayed-Release Capsules (Less than 1%) ... 3268
Prevacid for Delayed-Release Oral Suspension (Less than 1%) ... 3268
Prevacid NapraPAC (Less than 1%) .. 3277
Prevacid SoluTab Delayed-Release Orally Disintegrating Tablets (Less than 1%) ... 3268
PREVPAC (Less than 1%) ... 3281
▲ Prograf Capsules and Injection (One of the two most common forms) ... 624
▲ Rapamune Oral Solution and Tablets (1.1% to 6.5%) ... 3472
Sandimmune ... 2259
Uniretic Tablets (Less than 1%) ... 3114

Carcinoma, skin, benign
▲ CellCept Capsules (3% to less than 20%) ... 2751
▲ CellCept Intravenous (3% to less than 20%) ... 2751
▲ CellCept Oral Suspension (3% to less than 20%) ... 2751
▲ CellCept Tablets (3% to less than 20%) ... 2751
Copaxone for Injection (Infrequent) .. 3292
Gabitril Tablets (Infrequent) ... 998
Kaletra (Less than 2%) ... 474
Permax Tablets (Rare) ... 3357
Protopic Ointment (1% to 3%) ... 629
Thalomid Capsules ... 979
Virazole for Inhalation Solution ... 3365

Carcinoma, squamous
▲ Aldara Cream, 5% (3.7%) ... 1814
Amevive (Less than 0.1%) ... 836

Campath Ampules 826
Evoxac Capsules (Less than 1%) 1042
Rapamune Oral Solution and Tablets (0.4% to 2.7%) 3472

Carcinoma, testicular
Campath Ampules 826

Carcinoma, unspecified
▲ Actonel Tablets (0.8% to 3.3%) 2679
▲ Actonel with Calcium Tablets (0.8% to 3.3%) 2684
Aggrenox Capsules (1.7%) 855
Azasan Tablets (2.8%) 2844
▲ Casodex Tablets (2% to 5%) 670
▲ CellCept Capsules (3% to less than 20%) 2751
▲ CellCept Intravenous (3% to less than 20%) 2751
▲ CellCept Oral Suspension (3% to less than 20%) 2751
▲ CellCept Tablets (3% to less than 20%) 2751
Colazal Capsules 2845
Effexor Tablets (Rare) 3405
Effexor XR Capsules (Rare) 3411
Ferrlecit Injection 3379
Gabitril Tablets (Infrequent) 998
Gengraf Capsules 458
▲ Humira Injection (Less than 5%) 464
Levaquin in 5% Dextrose Injection (0.1% to 0.9%) 2453
Levaquin (0.1% to 0.9%) 2453
Lupron Depot 7.5 mg (Less than 5%) 3261
Neoral Soft Gelatin Capsules (1% to less than 3%) 2247
Neoral Oral Solution (1% to less than 3%) 2247
Nipent for Injection (Less than 3%) 3216
Omacor Capsules 2735
Paxil CR Controlled-Release Tablets (Infrequent) 1509
Paxil (Infrequent) 1501
Permax Tablets (Infrequent) 3357
Prevacid Delayed-Release Capsules (Less than 1%) 3268
Prevacid for Delayed-Release Oral Suspension (Less than 1%) 3268
Prevacid NapraPAC (Less than 1%) 3277
Prevacid SoluTab Delayed-Release Orally Disintegrating Tablets (Less than 1%) 3268
PREVPAC (Less than 1%) 3281
Protonix I.V. (Less than 1%) 3468
Protonix Tablets (Less than 1%) 3465
Rilutek Tablets (Infrequent) 2945
Tasmar Tablets (Infrequent) 3360
Zomig Nasal Spray (Rare to infrequent) 718

Carcinoma, uterine
▲ Humira Injection (Less than 5%) 464
Requip Tablets (Rare) 1528

Cardiac abnormalities
Accolate Tablets (Rare) 663
Albalon Ophthalmic Solution ⊙ 216
Clozapine Tablets (1%) 2141
Clozaril Tablets (1%) 2174
FazaClo Orally Disintegrating Tablets (1%) 547
Flovent Diskus 50 mcg 1415
▲ Leukine (23%) 829
Pacerone Tablets (Infrequent) 3337
Parcopa Orally Disintegrating Tablets 3111
Rythmol SR Capsules 2736

Cardiac anomalies
Eskalith 1406
Repronex for Intramuscular and Subcutaneous Injection (One report) 1148
Stalevo Tablets 2270

Cardiac arrest
▲ Abelcet Injection (6%) 1119
Abilify Tablets (Infrequent) 916
Abilify Tablets (Infrequent) 2472
Aceon Tablets (2 mg, 4 mg, 8 mg) 3191
Activase I.V. 1225
Adalat CC Tablets (Less than 1%) 2978
Adenoscan 613
AmBisome for Injection (Less common) 615
Ammonul Injection 3323
Antivenin Polyvalent (Isolated cases) 3399
▲ Apokyn Injection (4%) 2132
AquaMEPHYTON Injection 1887
▲ Aranesp for Injection (10%) 576
▲ Argatroban Injection (5.8%) 1321
Avelox (Very rare) 2984
Betagan Ophthalmic Solution, USP ⊙ 217
Betimol Ophthalmic Solution ⊙ 283
Betimol Ophthalmic Solution 3371
Blocadren Tablets (Less than 1%) 1891
Campath Ampules 826
Camptosar Injection 2602
Captopril Tablets 2114
Carimune NF 3501
▲ Casodex Tablets (2% to 5%) 670
Celexa (Rare) 1177
▲ CellCept Capsules (3% to less than 20%) 2751
▲ CellCept Intravenous (3% to less than 20%) 2751
▲ CellCept Oral Suspension (3% to less than 20%) 2751
▲ CellCept Tablets (3% to less than 20%) 2751
Clozapine Tablets (Rare) 2141
Clozaril Tablets (Rare) 2174
Cosopt Sterile Ophthalmic Solution 1910
Cytovene 2763
Decadron Tablets 1929
Digitek Tablets (1%) 2146
Dilaudid 439
Dilaudid Oral Liquid 443
Dilaudid Tablets - 8 mg 443
Dilaudid-HP 441
Diprivan Injectable Emulsion (Rare to very rare) 676
▲ Doxil Injection (1% to 10%) 3302
Effexor Tablets (Rare) 3405
Effexor XR Capsules (Rare) 3411
Elitek (Less than or equal to 1%) 2906
Ethyol for Injection (Rare) 1869
Exelon Capsules (Infrequent) 2204
Fabrazyme for Intravenous Infusion 1267
Fluorescite Injection ⊙ 207
Gammagard Liquid 751
Gammagard S/D (Rare) 754
Gamunex Immune Globulin I.V., 10% (Rare) 3232
Herceptin I.V. (At least one of the 958 patients) 1234
▲ Humira Injection (Less than 5%) 464
Imitrex Injection 1431
Imitrex Tablets 1440
Infed Injection 3381
Invanz for Injection (Greater than 0.1%) 1974
Iveegam EN (Rare) 759
Kadian Capsules 572
K-Lor Powder Packets 472
K-Tab Filmtab Tablets 473
Lanoxicaps Capsules 1458
Lanoxin Injection 1462
Lanoxin Tablets 1468
Lanoxin Injection Pediatric 1465
Levaquin in 5% Dextrose Injection (0.1% to 0.9%) 2453
Levaquin (0.1% to 0.9%) 2453
Levothroid Tablets 1189
Levoxyl Tablets 1680
Lexapro Oral Solution 1193
Lexapro Tablets 1193
Lidoderm Patch 1107
Meridia Capsules 485
Merrem I.V. (Greater than 0.1% to 1%) 687
MS Contin Tablets 2703
Mycamine for Injection 620
Namenda (Infrequent) 1199
Narcan Injection 1109
Naropin Injection 640
Neumega for Injection 3433
Nipent for Injection (Less than 3%) 3216
Nubain Injection (1% or less) 1111
Omacor Capsules 2735
Orthoclone OKT3 Sterile Solution (Less than 1%) 2370
Permax Tablets (Infrequent) 3357
Pletal Tablets (Less than 2%) 2478
Prinivil Tablets (0.3% to 1.0%) 2029
Prinzide Tablets 2033
Proleukin for Injection (Less than 1% to 2%) 1007
Proventil Inhalation Aerosol 3067
Prozac Pulvules and Liquid (Rare) 1771
Pulmozyme Inhalation Solution 1245
Remicade for IV Injection (Greater than or equal to 0.2%) 987
Requip Tablets (Infrequent) 1528
Retavase 1131
Reyataz Capsules (Less than 3%) 948
Rilutek Tablets (More than 2%) 2945
Rythmol SR Capsules 2736
Sandostatin LAR Depot (Rare) 2264
Symmetrel 1115
▲ Tambocor Tablets (5.1%) 1824
Tasmar Tablets (Infrequent) 3360
Tenormin I.V. Injection (1.6%) 698
Tenormin Tablets (1.6%) 695
Thalomid Capsules 979
Thioridazine Hydrochloride Tablets 2122
Timolide Tablets 2056
Timoptic in Ocudose (Less frequent) 2061
Timoptic Sterile Ophthalmic Solution (Less frequent) 2058
Timoptic-XE Sterile Ophthalmic Gel Forming Solution 2062
TNKase I.V. 1256
Trasylol Injection (1% to 2%) 779
Uniretic Tablets (Less than 1%) 3114
Unithroid Tablets 3521
Vaseretic Tablets 2073
Vasotec I.V. Injection (0.5% to 1.0%) 2076
▲ Vesanoid Capsules (3%) 2823
VFEND I.V. (Less than 2%) 2543
VFEND Oral Suspension (Less than 2%) 2543
VFEND Tablets (Less than 2%) 2543
Viagra Tablets (Less than 2%) 2552
Virazole for Inhalation Solution 3365
Zestoretic Tablets 701
Zestril Tablets (0.3% to 1.0%) 704
Zosyn (1.0% or less) 3492
Zyprexa Tablets (Rare) 1798
Zyprexa ZYDIS Orally Disintegrating Tablets (Rare) 1798

Cardiac arrhythmias
(*see under* Arrhythmias)

Cardiac asystole
(*see under* Asystole)

Cardiac collapse
Botox Purified Neurotoxin Complex (2 patients) 565

Cardiac death
Cialis Tablets 1806
Revatio Tablets 2541
Viagra Tablets 2552

Cardiac disorders, unspecified
▲ Ammonul Injection (9%) 3323

Cardiac dysrhythmias
(*see under* Arrhythmias)

Cardiac enlargement
Decadron Tablets 1929

Cardiac failure
(*see under* Heart failure)

Cardiac insufficiency
Rescriptor Tablets 2535

Cardiac murmur
Aceon Tablets (2 mg, 4 mg, 8 mg) (0.3% to 1%) 3191
Amerge Tablets (Rare) 1312
Avalide Tablets 922
Avalide Tablets 2889
Avapro Tablets (Less than 1%) 925
Avapro Tablets (Less than 1%) 2886
Cipro I.V. (1% or less) 2998
Cipro I.V. Pharmacy Bulk Package (1% or less) 3509
Cipro XR Tablets 3004
Copaxone for Injection (Infrequent) 3292
Evoxac Capsules (Less than 1%) 1042
▲ Imdur Tablets (Less than or equal to 5%) 3032
▲ Increlex Injection (Greater than or equal to 5%) 3290
Invanz for Injection (Greater than 0.1%) 1974
Invirase (Less than 2%) 2776
Neurontin Capsules (Infrequent) 2498
Neurontin Oral Solution (Infrequent) 2498
Neurontin Tablets (Infrequent) 2498
▲ Roferon-A Injection (Less than 5%) 2805
▲ Rythmol SR Capsules (2% to 4%) 2736
Thalomid Capsules 979
▲ Vesanoid Capsules (3%) 2823

Cardiac output, decrease
Ammonul Injection 3323
Digibind for Injection (Few instances) 1388
Diprivan Injectable Emulsion (1% to 3%) 676
Fabrazyme for Intravenous Infusion 1267
Naropin Injection 640
Paxil CR Controlled-Release Tablets (Rare) 1509
Paxil (Rare) 1501

Cardiac rhythms, disturbances
Calcium Disodium Versenate Injection 1819
Captopril Tablets 2114
Daraprim Tablets 1385
Digitek Tablets 2146
Lanoxicaps Capsules 1458
Lanoxin Injection 1462
Lanoxin Tablets 1468
Lanoxin Injection Pediatric 1465
Nadolol Tablets (1 of 100 patients) 2121
Prinzide Tablets 2033
Rescriptor Tablets 2535
Univasc Tablets (Less than 1%) 3118
Vaseretic Tablets 2073
Vasotec I.V. Injection (0.5% to 1.0%) 2076
Zestoretic Tablets 701

Cardiac rhythms, ectopic
Biltricide Tablets 2990

Cardiac tamponade
Activase I.V. 1225
I.V. Busulfex 1125
Myleran Tablets (A small number of patients) 1492
Retavase 1131
▲ Taxotere Injection Concentrate (6%) 2947
TNKase I.V. 1256
Zovirax for Injection (Less than 1%) 1618

Cardiac toxicity, unspecified
Adriamycin for Injection, USP 786
Adriamycin Injection, USP 786
Cerubidine for Injection 788
Digitek Tablets 2146
Doxil Injection 3302
Ellence Injection (1.4% to 1.8%) 2632
▲ Idamycin PFS Injection (16%) 2645
Lanoxicaps Capsules 1458
Lanoxin Injection 1462
Lanoxin Tablets 1468
Lanoxin Injection Pediatric 1465

Cardiac valve disorder, unspecified
Adipex-P 1216
Apokyn Injection 2132
Permax Tablets 3357

Cardialgia
(*see under* Heartburn)

Cardiodynia
(*see under* Heartburn)

Cardiogenic shock
Activase I.V. 1225
Ammonul Injection 3323
▲ Mavik Tablets (3.8%) 482
Retavase 1131
Rituxan for Infusion 845
Rituxan I.V. 1251
Tenormin I.V. Injection (0.4%) 698
Tenormin Tablets (0.4%) 695
TNKase I.V. 1256

Cardiomegaly
Abilify Tablets (Rare) 916
Abilify Tablets (Rare) 2472
Agrylin Capsules 3172
AmBisome for Injection (Less common) 615
Doxil Injection (Less than 1%) 3302
Evoxac Capsules 1042
▲ Fabrazyme for Intravenous Infusion (3%) 1267
Geodon Capsules (Rare) 2514
▲ I.V. Busulfex (5%) 1125
▲ Neumega for Injection (21%) 3433
Requip Tablets (Infrequent) 1528
VFEND I.V. (Less than 2%) 2543
VFEND Oral Suspension (Less than 2%) 2543
VFEND Tablets (Less than 2%) 2543

Cardiomyopathy
Abelcet Injection 1119
Adderall Tablets (Isolated reports) 3168
Adderall XR Capsules (Isolated cases) 3169
Adriamycin for Injection, USP 786
Adriamycin Injection, USP 786
Agrylin Capsules 3172
Aldara Cream, 5% 1814
Ammonul Injection 3323
Avonex (Rare) 839
Betaseron for SC Injection 791
Campral Tablets (Rare) 1175

Clozapine Tablets 2141
Clozaril Tablets 2174
Combivir Tablets 1373
Dexedrine (Isolated reports) 1386
DextroStat Tablets (Isolated reports) 3177
▲ Doxil Injection (1% to 5%) 3302
Ellence Injection 2632
Herceptin I.V. 1234
Idamycin PFS Injection 2645
Imitrex Injection 1431
Imitrex Nasal Spray 1435
Imitrex Tablets 1440
▲ Intron A for Injection (Less than 5%) 3038
▲ Megace ES Oral Suspension (1% to 3%) 2492
PEG-Intron Powder for Injection (Less than or equal to 1%) 3062
Proleukin for Injection 1007
Rescriptor Tablets 2535
Retrovir Capsules (0.8%) 1533
Retrovir IV Infusion (1%) 1537
Retrovir (0.8%) 1533
Roferon-A Injection (Rare to infrequent) 2805
Trizivir Tablets 1565
VFEND I.V. (Less than 2%) 2543
VFEND Oral Suspension (Less than 2%) 2543
VFEND Tablets (Less than 2%) 2543
Viagra Tablets (Less than 2%) 2552

Cardiomyopathy, hypertrophic
Decadron Phosphate Injection 1931

Cardiomyopathy, hypertrophic, premature infants
Decadron Tablets 1929

Cardiopulmonary arrest
Abilify Tablets (Infrequent to Rare) 916
Abilify Tablets (Infrequent to Rare) 2472
Ammonul Injection 3323
Cipro I.V. (1% or less) 2998
Cipro I.V. Pharmacy Bulk Package (1% or less) 3509
Cipro (Less than 1%) 2991
Cipro XR Tablets 3004
Fortaz 1422
Lariam Tablets (One patient) 2790
Pulmozyme Inhalation Solution 1245
Risperdal M-Tab Orally Disintegrating Tablets 1658
Risperdal 1658
Zofran Injection 1607
Zofran 1613
Zofran ODT Orally Disintegrating Tablets 1613

Cardiorespiratory arrest
Aloprim for Injection (Less than 1%) 2156
Avalide Tablets 922
Avalide Tablets 2889
Avapro Tablets (Less than 1%) 925
Avapro Tablets (Less than 1%) 2886
Orthoclone OKT3 Sterile Solution 2370

Cardiospasm
Paxil CR Controlled-Release Tablets (Rare) 1509
Paxil (Rare) 1501
Prevacid Delayed-Release Capsules (Less than 1%) 3268
Prevacid for Delayed-Release Oral Suspension (Less than 1%) 3268
Prevacid NapraPAC (Less than 1%) 3277
Prevacid SoluTab Delayed-Release Orally Disintegrating Tablets (Less than 1%) 3268
PREVPAC (Less than 1%) 3281
Protonix I.V. (Less than 1%) 3468
Protonix Tablets (Less than 1%) 3465
Sonata Capsules (Rare) 1686

Cardiotoxicity
Novantrone for Injection Concentrate 3158

Cardiovascular abnormalities, fetal
Accutane Capsules 2740
Clinoril Tablets 1899
Dolobid Tablets 1937

Cardiovascular collapse
Allegra-D 12 Hour Extended-Release Tablets 2860
Allegra-D 24 Hour Extended-Release Tablets 2862
Carbatrol Capsules 3174
Cipro I.V. (1% or less) 2998
Cipro I.V. Pharmacy Bulk Package (1% or less) 3509
Cipro 2991
Cipro XR Tablets 3004
Clarinex-D 24-Hour Extended-Release Tablets 3012
Diastat Rectal Delivery System (Infrequent) 3344
Equetro Extended-Release Capsules 3178
Infed Injection 3381
Levaquin in 5% Dextrose Injection 2453
Levaquin 2453
Lidoderm Patch 1107
Noroxin Tablets 2009
Orthoclone OKT3 Sterile Solution 2370
Tegretol/Tegretol-XR 2278
Tessalon Capsules 1202
Tessalon Perles 1202
Zyrtec-D 12 Hour Extended Release Tablets 2591

Cardiovascular disorders
Actonel Tablets (2.5%) 2679
Actonel with Calcium Tablets (2.5%) 2684
Agrylin Capsules (1% to 5%) 3172
Allegra-D 12 Hour Extended-Release Tablets (Rare) 2860
Allegra-D 24 Hour Extended-Release Tablets (Rare) 2862
Aloprim for Injection (Less than 1%) 2156
Antara Capsules 2723
Argatroban Injection (2.3%) 1321
Avonex 839
▲ Carnitor Injection (3% to 6%) 3185
▲ CellCept Capsules (3% to 25.6%) 2751
▲ CellCept Intravenous (3% to 25.6%) 2751
▲ CellCept Oral Suspension (3% to 25.6%) 2751
▲ CellCept Tablets (3% to 25.6%) 2751
▲ Clozapine Tablets (Greater than 5%) 2141
▲ Clozaril Tablets (Greater than 5%) 2174
Crixivan Capsules 1918
Evoxac Capsules (Less than 1%) 1042
▲ Humira Injection (Less than 5%) 464
Lofibra Capsules 1217
Menostar Transdermal System (10%) 805
▲ Neoral Soft Gelatin Capsules (28.0%) 2247
▲ Neoral Oral Solution (28.0%) 2247
Neumega for Injection 3433
Protonix I.V. (Less than 1%) 3468
Protonix Tablets (Less than 1%) 3465
Risperdal Consta Long-Acting Injection 1664
Risperdal M-Tab Orally Disintegrating Tablets 1658
Risperdal 1658
Singulair 2047
Tasmar Tablets (Rare) 3360
Tricor Tablets 523
Zomig Tablets 714
Zyban Sustained-Release Tablets 1620

Cardiovascular events
CombiPatch Transdermal System 2180

Carnitine concentrations, decreased
Depacon Injection 412
Depakene 417
Depakote Sprinkle Capsules 422
Depakote Tablets 427
Depakote ER Tablets 433

Carotid bruit
Rythmol SR Capsules 2736

Carotid sinus hypersensitivity
Aldoclor Tablets 1881
Aldoril Tablets 1884

Carpal tunnel syndrome
Evoxac Capsules (Less than 1%) 1042
Humatrope Vials and Cartridges (Rare) 1756
▲ Intron A for Injection (Less than 5%) 3038
Lexapro Oral Solution (Infrequent) 1193
Lexapro Tablets (Infrequent) 1193
Namenda (More than one patient) 1199
Nutropin for Injection (Rare) 1238
Nutropin AQ Injection (Rare) 1241
Nutropin AQ Pen (Rare) 1241
Nutropin AQ Pen Cartridge (Rare) 1241
Prozac Pulvules and Liquid 1771
Thalomid Capsules 979
Vivelle Transdermal System 2288
Vivelle-Dot Transdermal System 2293

Cataplexy
Clozapine Tablets 2141
Clozaril Tablets 2174
FazaClo Orally Disintegrating Tablets 547
Provigil Tablets (Greater than or equal to 1%) 1002

Cataracts
Abilify Tablets (Infrequent) 916
Abilify Tablets (Infrequent) 2472
Accutane Capsules 2740
Aciphex Tablets 1081
▲ Actonel Tablets (1.9% to 5.9%) 2679
▲ Actonel with Calcium Tablets (1.9% to 5.9%) 2684
Advair Diskus 100/50 1291
Advair Diskus 250/50 1291
Advair Diskus 500/50 1291
Alesse-28 Tablets 3392
Altoprev Extended-Release Tablets 1151
Amnesteem Capsules 2126
Antara Capsules 2723
▲ Arava Tablets (1% to 3%) 2881
Aricept Tablets (Frequent) 1086
Aricept ODT Tablets (Frequent) 1086
▲ Arimidex Tablets (4%) 665
Azmacort Inhalation Aerosol (Rare) 1701
Beconase AQ Nasal Spray (Rare) 1359
Betimol Ophthalmic Solution (1% to 5%) ⊙283
Betimol Ophthalmic Solution (1% to 5%) 3371
▲ Casodex Tablets (2% to 5%) 670
Celebrex Capsules (0.1% to 1.9%) 3130
Celexa (Rare) 1177
▲ CellCept Capsules (3% to less than 20%) 2751
▲ CellCept Intravenous (3% to less than 20%) 2751
▲ CellCept Oral Suspension (3% to less than 20%) 2751
▲ CellCept Tablets (3% to less than 20%) 2751
Copaxone for Injection (Infrequent) 3292
▲ Cozaar Tablets (7%) 1913
Cytovene 2763
Desferal Vials 2190
Effexor Tablets (Infrequent) 3405
Effexor XR Capsules (Infrequent) 3411
Evoxac Capsules (Less than 1%) 1042
Exelon Capsules (Frequent) 2204
Flonase Nasal Spray 1412
Flovent Diskus 50 mcg 1415
Flovent HFA 1418
Gengraf Capsules (1% to less than 3%) 458
Geodon Capsules (Infrequent) 2514
▲ Humira Injection (Less than 5%) 464
Hyperstat I.V. Injection 3031
Lescol Capsules 2227
Lescol Capsules 2730
Lescol XL Tablets 2227
Lescol XL Tablets 2730
Levaquin in 5% Dextrose Injection 2453
Levaquin 2453
Lofibra Capsules 1217
Lo/Ovral-28 Tablets 3423
▲ Lumigan Ophthalmic Solution (3% to 10%) 569
Mirapex Tablets (Less than 1%) 889
Myleran Tablets (Rare) 1492
Namenda (Frequent) 1199
Nasacort HFA Inhalation Aerosol 2939
Neoral Soft Gelatin Capsules (1% to less than 3%) 2247
Neoral Oral Solution (1% to less than 3%) 2247
Neurontin Capsules (Infrequent) 2498
Neurontin Oral Solution (Infrequent) 2498
Neurontin Tablets (Infrequent) 2498
Omacor Capsules 2735
Orap Tablets 1220
Ortho-Cept Tablets 2395
Ortho-Cyclen Tablets 2414
Ortho Evra Transdermal System 2402
Ortho Tri-Cyclen Tablets 2414
Ortho Tri-Cyclen Lo Tablets 2421
Paxil CR Controlled-Release Tablets (Rare) 1509
Paxil (Rare) 1501
Permax Tablets (Rare) 3357
Photofrin for Injection 729
Plavix Tablets (1% to 2.5%) 940
Plavix Tablets (1% to 2.5%) 2942
Pravachol Tablets 943
Protonix I.V. (Less than 1%) 3468
Protonix Tablets (Less than 1%) 3465
Prozac Pulvules and Liquid 1771
Pulmicort Respules (Rare) 654
▲ Rapamune Oral Solution and Tablets (3% to 20%) 3472
▲ Retisert Implant (50% to 90%) ⊙256
Rilutek Tablets (Rare) 2945
Seasonale Tablets 1073
Sonata Capsules (Rare) 1686
▲ Spiriva HandiHaler (1% to 3%) 899
Tasmar Tablets (Rare) 3360
Travatan Ophthalmic Solution (1% to 4%) 559
Tricor Tablets 523
Trileptal Oral Suspension 2281
Trileptal Tablets 2281
Triphasil-28 Tablets 3483
Uniretic Tablets (Less than 1%) 3114
Viagra Tablets (Less than 2%) 2552
▲ Visudyne for Injection (1% to 10%) 2286
Vytorin 10/10 Tablets 2084
Vytorin 10/10 Tablets 3092
Vytorin 10/20 Tablets 2084
Vytorin 10/20 Tablets 3092
Vytorin 10/40 Tablets 2084
Vytorin 10/40 Tablets 3092
Vytorin 10/80 Tablets 2084
Vytorin 10/80 Tablets 3092
Yasmin 28 Tablets 818
Zoloft 2581
Zyprexa Tablets (Infrequent) 1798
Zyprexa ZYDIS Orally Disintegrating Tablets (Infrequent) 1798

Cataracts, posterior subcapsular
Alrex Ophthalmic Suspension 0.2% ⊙243
Blephamide Ophthalmic Ointment (Infrequent) 563
Blephamide Ophthalmic Suspension 564
Cosopt Sterile Ophthalmic Solution (1% to 5%) 1910
Decadron Phosphate Injection 1931
Decadron Tablets 1929
Depo-Medrol Injectable Suspension 2615
Depo-Medrol Single-Dose Vial 2617
FML Ophthalmic Ointment (Infrequent) ⊙225
FML Ophthalmic Suspension ⊙224
FML Forte Ophthalmic Suspension (Infrequent) ⊙223
FML-S Liquifilm Sterile Ophthalmic Suspension ⊙226
HMS Sterile Ophthalmic Suspension (Rare) ⊙228
Hydrocortone Tablets 1963
Lotemax Ophthalmic Suspension 0.5% ⊙249
Pediapred Oral Solution 3319
Poly-Pred Liquifilm Ophthalmic Suspension ⊙231
Pred Forte Ophthalmic Suspension ⊙233
Pred Mild Sterile Ophthalmic Suspension (Infrequent) ⊙236
Pred-G Ophthalmic Suspension ⊙234
Pred-G Sterile Ophthalmic Ointment ⊙235
Retisert Implant ⊙256
▲ Soriatane Capsules (1% to 5%) 1028
TobraDex Ophthalmic Ointment 558
TobraDex Ophthalmic Suspension 558
Zylet Ophthalmic Suspension 3508

Catatonia
Blocadren Tablets 1891
Celexa (Rare) 1177
Cosopt Sterile Ophthalmic Solution 1910
Depacon Injection (1% or more) 412
Depakene (1% or more) 417
Depakote Sprinkle Capsules 422
▲ Depakote Tablets (1% to 5%) 427
Depakote ER Tablets (Greater than 1%) 433
Effexor Tablets 3405
Effexor XR Capsules 3411
Inderal LA Long-Acting Capsules 3421
InnoPran XL Capsules 2728
Nadolol Tablets 2121
Phenergan 3438
Relpax Tablets (Rare) 2531
Risperdal M-Tab Orally Disintegrating Tablets (Infrequent) 1658
Risperdal (Infrequent) 1658
Seroquel Tablets (Infrequent) 691
Tenormin I.V. Injection 698
Tenormin Tablets 695

Timolide Tablets ... 2056
Timoptic in Ocudose ... 2061
Timoptic Sterile Ophthalmic Solution ... 2058
Timoptic-XE Sterile Ophthalmic Gel Forming Solution ... 2062
Toprol-XL Tablets ... 660

Causalgia

Thalomid ... 979

Cellulitis

Actiq (1% or greater) ... 993
Adalat CC Tablets (Less than 1%) ... 2978
Adriamycin for Injection, USP ... 786
Adriamycin Injection, USP ... 786
Aloprim for Injection (Less than 1%) ... 2156
AmBisome for Injection (Less common) ... 615
Aricept Tablets (Infrequent) ... 1086
Aricept ODT Tablets (Infrequent) ... 1086
Bactroban Cream (Less than 1%) ... 1356
BeneFix for Injection (1.5%) ... 3402
Campath Ampules ... 826
Celebrex Capsules (0.1% to 1.9%) ... 3130
Celexa (Rare) ... 1177
▲ CellCept Capsules (3% to less than 20%) ... 2751
▲ CellCept Intravenous (3% to less than 20%) ... 2751
▲ CellCept Oral Suspension (3% to less than 20%) ... 2751
▲ CellCept Tablets (3% to less than 20%) ... 2751
▲ Clolar for Intravenous Infusion (11%) ... 1264
Copaxone for Injection (Infrequent) .. 3292
▲ Cozaar Tablets (7%) ... 1913
Cubicin for Injection (1% to 2%) ... 1038
Doxil Injection (Less than 1%) ... 3302
Effexor Tablets (Rare) ... 3405
Effexor XR Capsules (Rare) ... 3411
Elitek (Less than or equal to 1%) ... 2906
Enbrel for Injection ... 580
Evoxac Capsules (Less than 1%) ... 1042
Exelon Capsules (Infrequent) ... 2204
Gabitril Tablets (Infrequent) ... 998
Gemzar for Injection (Rare) ... 1743
Gengraf Capsules (1% to less than 3%) ... 458
Herceptin I.V. (At least one of the 958 patients) ... 1234
▲ Humira Injection (Less than 5%) ... 464
Hyperstat I.V. Injection ... 3031
Infanrix Vaccine ... 1444
▲ Intron A for Injection (Less than 5%) ... 3038
Invirase (Less than 2%) ... 2776
Kineret Injection ... 594
Klonopin (Infrequent) ... 2782
Lunesta Tablets (Infrequent) ... 3139
Lupron Depot 7.5 mg (Less than 5%) ... 3261
Lyrica Capsules (0.1% to 1%) ... 2524
Namenda (Infrequent) ... 1199
Neoral Soft Gelatin Capsules (1% to less than 3%) ... 2247
Neoral Oral Solution (1% to less than 3%) ... 2247
Neurontin Capsules (Infrequent) ... 2498
Neurontin Oral Solution (Infrequent) ... 2498
Neurontin Tablets (Infrequent) ... 2498
▲ Nipent for Injection (6%) ... 3216
Paxil CR Controlled-Release Tablets (Rare) ... 1509
Paxil (Rare) ... 1501
Pediarix Vaccine ... 1518
PEG-Intron Powder for Injection (Less than or equal to 1%) ... 3062
Permax Tablets (Infrequent) ... 3357
▲ Prograf Capsules and Injection (3% to 15%) ... 624
Proleukin for Injection ... 1007
Protopic Ointment (Greater than or equal to 1%) ... 629
▲ Rapamune Oral Solution and Tablets (3% to 20%) ... 3472
Raptiva for Injection ... 1247
Remicade for IV Injection (Greater than or equal to 0.2%) ... 987
ReoPro Vials (0.3%) ... 1779
Requip Tablets (Infrequent) ... 1528
Reyataz Capsules (Less than 3%) ... 948
Rilutek Tablets (Infrequent) ... 2945
Sandostatin Injection (Less than 1%) ... 2263
Sandostatin LAR Depot (1% to 4%) .. 2264
Sular Tablets (Less than or equal to 1%) ... 1163
Symbyax Capsules (Infrequent) ... 1788
Targretin Capsules ... 1719
Tasmar Tablets (Infrequent) ... 3360
Thalomid Capsules ... 979
Uniretic Tablets (Less than 1%) ... 3114
Varivax ... 2070
▲ Vesanoid Capsules (8%) ... 2823
VFEND I.V. (Less than 2%) ... 2543
VFEND Oral Suspension (Less than 2%) ... 2543
VFEND Tablets (Less than 2%) ... 2543
Zevalin Injection ... 848
Zomig Nasal Spray (Rare) ... 718

Cellulitis, at injection site

Avonex (Rare) ... 839
Infed Injection ... 3381

Cellulitis, pre-septal

Amevive ... 836

Cellulitis-like reactions

Pneumovax 23 (Rare) ... 2020

Central nervous system demyelinating disorders

Adacel Vaccine ... 2959

Centrilobular sinusoidal fibrosis

Myleran Tablets ... 1492

Cephalin flocculation test, positive

Cuprimine Capsules ... 1925

Cerebellar dysfunction

▲ Idamycin PFS Injection (4%) ... 2645
Neurontin Capsules (Infrequent) ... 2498
Neurontin Oral Solution (Infrequent) ... 2498
Neurontin Tablets (Infrequent) ... 2498

Cerebellar malformation, fetal

Accutane Capsules ... 2740

Cerebellar syndrome, acute

Lamictal (Rare) ... 1449
Lyrica Capsules (Rare) ... 2524
Topamax Sprinkle Capsules (Rare) ... 2438
Topamax Tablets (Rare) ... 2438

Cerebral abnormalities, fetal

Accutane Capsules ... 2740

Cerebral arterial insufficiency, symptoms

Carbatrol Capsules ... 3174
Equetro Extended-Release Capsules ... 3178
Tegretol/Tegretol-XR ... 2278

Cerebral arteritis

Concerta Extended-Release Tablets (Isolated cases) ... 1828
Focalin Tablets ... 2214
Focalin XR Capsules ... 2217
Metadate CD Capsules (Isolated cases) ... 3316
Ritalin Hydrochloride Tablets (Isolated cases) ... 2254
Ritalin LA Capsules ... 2255
Ritalin-SR Tablets (Isolated cases) ... 2254

Cerebral atrophy

Ammonul Injection ... 3323
Depacon Injection (Several cases) ... 412
Depakene (Several reports) ... 417
Depakote Sprinkle Capsules (Several reports) ... 422
Depakote Tablets (Several reports) ... 427
Depakote ER Tablets (Several reports) ... 433

Cerebral bleeding

(*see under* Cerebral hemorrhage)

Cerebral embolism

Aygestin Tablets ... 1062
Prozac Pulvules and Liquid (Rare) ... 1771
Rilutek Tablets (Rare) ... 2945
Trasylol Injection (1% to 2%) ... 779

Cerebral hemorrhage

Alesse-28 Tablets ... 3392
Ammonul Injection ... 3323
Cafcit (2.2%) ... 1854
Campath Ampules ... 826
Copegus Tablets (Less than 1%) ... 2759
Imitrex Injection ... 1431
Imitrex Tablets ... 1440
I.V. Busulfex (One patient) ... 1125
Kaletra (Less than 2%) ... 474
Lo/Ovral-28 Tablets ... 3423
Mylotarg for Injection (2%) ... 3429
Namenda (Infrequent) ... 1199
Ortho-Cept Tablets ... 2395
Ortho-Cyclen Tablets ... 2414
Ortho Evra Transdermal System ... 2402
Ortho Tri-Cyclen Tablets ... 2414
Ortho Tri-Cyclen Lo Tablets ... 2421
Pegasys (Less than 1%) ... 2793
Permax Tablets (Rare) ... 3357
Pletal Tablets (Very rare) ... 2478
Proleukin for Injection ... 1007
Rilutek Tablets (Infrequent) ... 2945
Seasonale Tablets ... 1073
Tasmar Tablets (Infrequent) ... 3360
Trileptal Oral Suspension ... 2281
Trileptal Tablets ... 2281
Triphasil-28 Tablets ... 3483
▲ Vesanoid Capsules (9%) ... 2823
VFEND I.V. (Less than 2%) ... 2543
VFEND Oral Suspension (Less than 2%) ... 2543
VFEND Tablets (Less than 2%) ... 2543
Yasmin 28 Tablets ... 818
Zomig Tablets ... 714
Zomig-ZMT Tablets ... 714

Cerebral herniation

Activase I.V. ... 1225
Ammonul Injection ... 3323

Cerebral infarction

Activase I.V. ... 1225
Aloprim for Injection (Less than 1%) ... 2156
Amerge Tablets ... 1312
Ammonul Injection ... 3323
Camptosar Injection ... 2602
Geodon Capsules (Rare) ... 2514
Hyperstat I.V. Injection ... 3031
Namenda ... 1199
Pletal Tablets (Less than 2%) ... 2478
Prevacid Delayed-Release Capsules (Less than 1%) ... 3268
Prevacid for Delayed-Release Oral Suspension (Less than 1%) ... 3268
Prevacid NapraPAC (Less than 1%) .. 3277
Prevacid SoluTab Delayed-Release Orally Disintegrating Tablets (Less than 1%) ... 3268
PREVPAC (Less than 1%) ... 3281
Remicade for IV Injection (Greater than or equal to 0.2%) ... 987
Uniretic Tablets (Less than 1%) ... 3114

Cerebral ischemia

(*see under* Ischemia, cerebral)

Cerebral lesions

Proleukin for Injection ... 1007

Cerebral occlusion

Concerta Extended-Release Tablets (Isolated cases) ... 1828
Focalin Tablets ... 2214
Focalin XR Capsules ... 2217
Metadate CD Capsules (Isolated cases) ... 3316
Ritalin Hydrochloride Tablets (Isolated cases) ... 2254
Ritalin LA Capsules ... 2255
Ritalin-SR Tablets (Isolated cases) ... 2254

Cerebral thrombosis

Activella Tablets ... 2311
Alesse-28 Tablets ... 3392
Aygestin Tablets ... 1062
Cipro I.V. (1% or less) ... 2998
Cipro I.V. Pharmacy Bulk Package (1% or less) ... 3509
Cipro (Less than 1%) ... 2991
Cipro XR Tablets ... 3004
DDAVP Injection 4 mcg/mL (Rare) ... 2893
Desmopressin Acetate Injection (Rare) ... 1143
Lamictal (Rare) ... 1449
Lo/Ovral-28 Tablets ... 3423
Ortho-Cept Tablets ... 2395
Ortho-Cyclen Tablets ... 2414
Ortho Evra Transdermal System ... 2402
Ortho Tri-Cyclen Tablets ... 2414
Ortho Tri-Cyclen Lo Tablets ... 2421
Seasonale Tablets ... 1073
Trasylol Injection (0.5%) ... 779
Triphasil-28 Tablets ... 3483
Viagra Tablets (Less than 2%) ... 2552
Yasmin 28 Tablets ... 818

Cerebrospinal fluid proteins, changes

Thiothixene Capsules ... 2124

Cerebrovascular accident

Abelcet Injection ... 1119
Abilify Tablets (Infrequent) ... 916
Abilify Tablets (Infrequent) ... 2472
Aceon Tablets (2 mg, 4 mg, 8 mg) (0.2%) ... 3191
Agrylin Capsules (1% to 5%) ... 3172
Aldara Cream, 5% ... 1814
Amerge Tablets ... 1312
Aricept Tablets (Infrequent) ... 1086
Aricept ODT Tablets (Infrequent) ... 1086
Arimidex Tablets (1%) ... 665
Avalide Tablets ... 922
Avalide Tablets ... 2889
Avapro Tablets (Less than 1%) ... 925
Avapro Tablets (Less than 1%) ... 2886
Betagan Ophthalmic Solution, USP ... ⊙ 217
Betimol Ophthalmic Solution ... ⊙ 283
Betimol Ophthalmic Solution ... 3371
Blocadren Tablets (Less than 1%) ... 1891
Camptosar Injection ... 2602
Captopril Tablets ... 2114
Carteolol Hydrochloride Ophthalmic Solution USP, 1% ... ⊙ 246
Catapres-TTS (0.5% or less) ... 875
Celebrex Capsules (Less than 0.1%) ... 3130
Celexa (Infrequent) ... 1177
▲ Coreg Tablets (Greater than 1% to 3%) ... 1376
Cosopt Sterile Ophthalmic Solution (Less than 1%) ... 1910
Covera-HS Tablets (Less than 2%) ... 3135
Cozaar Tablets (Less than 1%) ... 1913
Effexor Tablets (Rare) ... 3405
Effexor XR Capsules (Rare) ... 3411
Emcyt Capsules (2%) ... 3137
Epogen for Injection (0.4%) ... 586
▲ Flolan for Injection (4%) ... 1408
Fortical Nasal Spray (Less than 1%) ... 3336
Gammagard S/D ... 754
Gemzar for Injection (2%) ... 1743
Geodon Capsules (Rare) ... 2514
Hyzaar ... 1964
Imitrex Injection ... 1431
Imitrex Nasal Spray ... 1435
Imitrex Tablets ... 1440
Lamictal (Rare) ... 1449
Maxalt Tablets (Very rare) ... 1983
Maxalt-MLT Orally Disintegrating Tablets (Very rare) ... 1983
Meridia Capsules ... 485
Miacalcin Nasal Spray (Less than 1%) ... 2242
Namenda (Frequent) ... 1199
Neurontin Capsules (Rare) ... 2498
Neurontin Oral Solution (Rare) ... 2498
Neurontin Tablets (Rare) ... 2498
Orthoclone OKT3 Sterile Solution ... 2370
Paxil CR Controlled-Release Tablets (Rare) ... 1509
Paxil (Rare) ... 1501
Permax Tablets (Infrequent) ... 3357
Pletal Tablets (Very rare) ... 2478
Prefest Tablets ... 1069
Prevacid Delayed-Release Capsules (Less than 1%) ... 3268
Prevacid for Delayed-Release Oral Suspension (Less than 1%) ... 3268
Prevacid NapraPAC (Less than 1%) .. 3277
Prevacid SoluTab Delayed-Release Orally Disintegrating Tablets (Less than 1%) ... 3268
PREVPAC (Less than 1%) ... 3281
Prinivil Tablets (0.3% to 1.0%) ... 2029
Prinzide Tablets ... 2033
▲ Procrit for Injection (0.4% to 3.2%) ... 2374
Protopic Ointment (Greater than or equal to 1%) ... 629
Prozac Pulvules and Liquid (Rare) ... 1771
Razadyne (Infrequent) ... 2434
Risperdal M-Tab Orally Disintegrating Tablets ... 1658
Risperdal ... 1658
Rythmol SR Capsules ... 2736
Seroquel Tablets (Infrequent) ... 691
Sular Tablets (Less than or equal to 1%) ... 1163
Targretin Capsules ... 1719
Tarka Tablets ... 519
Tasmar Tablets (Infrequent) ... 3360
Thalomid Capsules ... 979
Timolide Tablets ... 2056
Timoptic in Ocudose (Less frequent) ... 2061
Timoptic Sterile Ophthalmic Solution (Less frequent) ... 2058
Timoptic-XE Sterile Ophthalmic Gel Forming Solution ... 2062
Trasylol Injection (1% to 2%) ... 779
Univasc Tablets (Less than 1%) ... 3118

Varivax ... 2070
Vaseretic Tablets ... 2073
Vasotec I.V. Injection (0.5% to 1.0%) ... 2076
Verelan PM Capsules (2% or less) ... 3120
Vesanoid Capsules ... 2823
VFEND I.V. (Less than 2%) ... 2543
VFEND Oral Suspension (Less than 2%) ... 2543
VFEND Tablets (Less than 2%) ... 2543
Zestoretic Tablets ... 701
Zestril Tablets (0.3% to 1.0%) ... 704
Zoladex (1% to 5%) ... 709
Zoladex 3-month (1% to 5%) ... 712
Zonegran Capsules (Infrequent) ... 1089
Zosyn (1.0% or less) ... 3492
Zyprexa Tablets (Infrequent) ... 1798
Zyprexa ZYDIS Orally Disintegrating Tablets (Infrequent) ... 1798

Cerebrovascular disorders
Abilify Tablets ... 916
Abilify Tablets ... 2472
Activella Tablets ... 2311
Aldoclor Tablets ... 1881
Aldoril Tablets ... 1884
Ambien Tablets (Infrequent) ... 2867
Campath Ampules ... 826
Coreg Tablets (Less than or equal to 0.1%) ... 1376
Crixivan Capsules ... 1918
Elitek (Less than or equal to 1%) ... 2906
Flumadine (Less than 0.3%) ... 1186
Levaquin in 5% Dextrose Injection (0.1% to 0.9%) ... 2453
Levaquin (0.1% to 0.9%) ... 2453
Lo/Ovral-28 Tablets ... 3423
Micardis Tablets (More than 0.3%) ... 884
Micardis HCT Tablets (More than 0.3%) ... 886
Ortho-Cyclen/Ortho Tri-Cyclen ... 2414
Ortho Tri-Cyclen Lo Tablets ... 2421
Relpax Tablets (Rare) ... 2531
Risperdal M-Tab Orally Disintegrating Tablets ... 1658
Risperdal ... 1658
Toprol-XL Tablets (Greater than 1%) ... 660
Triphasil-28 Tablets ... 3483
Zoloft (Rare) ... 2581
Zomig Tablets ... 714
Zomig-ZMT Tablets ... 714

Cerebrovascular insufficiency
Captopril Tablets ... 2114

Cerumen, increased
Norvir (Less than 2%) ... 499

Cervical disorders
(*see under* Cervical irregularities)

Cervical dysplasia
Campath Ampules ... 826
Clindesse Vaginal Cream (Less than 1%) ... 3296

Cervical ectropion, changes
(*see also under* Cervical erosion, changes)
Cenestin Tablets, 0.45mg, 0.625mg, 0.9mg, 1.25mg ... 1063
Cenestin Tablets, 0.3mg ... 1063
Climara Transdermal System ... 795
Climara Pro Transdermal System ... 800
Estrogel 0.06% ... 3200
Menostar Transdermal System ... 805
Premarin Tablets ... 3443
Seasonale Tablets ... 1073
Vivelle Transdermal System ... 2288
Vivelle-Dot Transdermal System ... 2293

Cervical erosion, changes
(*see also under* Cervical ectropion, changes)
Activella Tablets ... 2311
Alesse-28 Tablets ... 3392
Aygestin Tablets ... 1062
Estratest Tablets ... 3196
Estratest H.S. Tablets ... 3196
Lo/Ovral-28 Tablets ... 3423
Ortho-Cept Tablets ... 2395
Ortho-Cyclen/Ortho Tri-Cyclen ... 2414
Ortho Tri-Cyclen Lo Tablets ... 2421
Prefest Tablets ... 1069
Premarin Intravenous ... 3440
Premarin Vaginal Cream ... 3449
Premphase Tablets ... 3452
Prempro Tablets ... 3452
Triphasil-28 Tablets ... 3483
Yasmin 28 Tablets ... 818

Cervical eversion, changes in
(*see under* Cervical ectropion, changes; Cervical erosion, changes)

Cervical irregularities
Bravelle for Intramuscular or Subcutaneous Injection (2.9%) ... 1140
Clindesse Vaginal Cream (Less than 1%) ... 3296
Lupron Depot-PED 7.5 mg, 11.25 mg and 15 mg (Less than 2%) ... 3266
Lupron Injection Pediatric (Less than 2%) ... 3256
▲ Premphase Tablets (4% to 5%) ... 3452
▲ Prempro Tablets (4% to 5%) ... 3452

Cervical secretion, changes
Activella Tablets ... 2311
Alesse-28 Tablets ... 3392
Aygestin Tablets ... 1062
Cenestin Tablets, 0.45mg, 0.625mg, 0.9mg, 1.25mg ... 1063
Cenestin Tablets, 0.3mg ... 1063
Climara Transdermal System ... 795
Climara Pro Transdermal System ... 800
Estratest Tablets ... 3196
Estratest H.S. Tablets ... 3196
Estrogel 0.06% ... 3200
Lo/Ovral-28 Tablets ... 3423
Menostar Transdermal System ... 805
Ortho-Cept Tablets ... 2395
Ortho-Cyclen/Ortho Tri-Cyclen ... 2414
Ortho Tri-Cyclen Lo Tablets ... 2421
Prefest Tablets ... 1069
Premarin Intravenous ... 3440
Premarin Tablets ... 3443
Premarin Vaginal Cream ... 3449
Premphase Tablets ... 3452
Prempro Tablets ... 3452
Prometrium Capsules (100 mg, 200 mg) ... 3205
Seasonale Tablets ... 1073
Triphasil-28 Tablets ... 3483
Vivelle Transdermal System ... 2288
Vivelle-Dot Transdermal System ... 2293
Yasmin 28 Tablets ... 818

Cervical smear test, abnormal
▲ Estrogel 0.06% (5.4%) ... 3200
Zomig Nasal Spray (Rare) ... 718

Cervical smear test, positive
Evoxac Capsules (Less than 1%) ... 1042

Cervicitis
Abilify Tablets (Rare) ... 916
Abilify Tablets (Rare) ... 2472
Effexor Tablets (Rare) ... 3405
Effexor XR Capsules (Rare) ... 3411
Lyrica Capsules (Rare) ... 2524

Chalazion
Invirase (Less than 2%) ... 2776
Soriatane Capsules (Less than 1%) ... 1028

Changes in blood glucose levels
Ammonul Injection ... 3323
Amnesteem Capsules ... 2126
Neurontin Capsules ... 2498
Neurontin Oral Solution ... 2498
Neurontin Tablets ... 2498
Ortho-Cyclen/Ortho Tri-Cyclen ... 2414

Character changes
Seromycin Capsules ... 1783

Charcot's syndrome
▲ Imdur Tablets (Less than or equal to 5%) ... 3032
▲ Mavik Tablets (3.8%) ... 482
ReoPro Vials (0.4%) ... 1779
Risperdal Consta Long-Acting Injection (Rare) ... 1664
Soriatane Capsules (Less than 1%) ... 1028
Timolide Tablets ... 2056

Cheek puffing
Moban Tablets ... 1108
Orap Tablets ... 1220
Thiothixene Capsules ... 2124

Cheilitis
Accutane Capsules ... 2740
Actiq (Less than 1%) ... 993
Amnesteem Capsules ... 2126
Caduet Tablets (Less than 2%) ... 2507
Cosmegen for Injection ... 1907
Effexor Tablets (Rare) ... 3405
Effexor XR Capsules (Rare) ... 3411
Frova Tablets (Rare) ... 1101
Invirase (Less than 2%) ... 2776
Lipitor Tablets (Less than 2%) ... 2495
Norvir (Less than 2%) ... 499
Protopic Ointment (Greater than or equal to 1%) ... 629
Rilutek Tablets (Rare) ... 2945
Sonata Capsules (Rare) ... 1686
▲ Soriatane Capsules (More than 75%) ... 1028
Targretin Capsules ... 1719
Tequin Injection (Less than 0.1%) ... 964
Tequin Tablets (Less than 0.1%) ... 964
Uniretic Tablets (Less than 1%) ... 3114
VFEND I.V. (Less than 2%) ... 2543
VFEND Oral Suspension (Less than 2%) ... 2543
VFEND Tablets (Less than 2%) ... 2543

Cheilosis
Calcium Disodium Versenate Injection ... 1819
Cuprimine Capsules (Rare) ... 1925

Chemosis
▲ Alrex Ophthalmic Suspension 0.2% (5% to 15%) ... ⊙243
▲ Lotemax Ophthalmic Suspension 0.5% (5% to 15%) ... ⊙249
▲ Rēv-Eyes Ophthalmic Eyedrops 0.5% (10% to 40%) ... ⊙256
▲ Zymar Ophthalmic Solution (1% to 4%) ... 571

Chest congestion
Advair Diskus 100/50 ... 1291
Advair Diskus 250/50 ... 1291
Advair Diskus 500/50 ... 1291
Aerobid/Aerobid-M (3% to 9%) ... 1172
▲ Azmacort Inhalation Aerosol (1% to 3%) ... 1701
Effexor Tablets (Infrequent) ... 3405
Effexor XR Capsules (Infrequent) ... 3411
Klonopin ... 2782
Rescriptor Tablets ... 2535

Chest numbness
Tessalon Capsules ... 1202
Tessalon Perles ... 1202

Chest pain
▲ Abelcet Injection (3%) ... 1119
Abilify Tablets (Frequent) ... 916
Abilify Tablets (Frequent) ... 2472
AccuNeb Inhalation Solution (0.9% to 1.7%) ... 1055
Accutane Capsules (Less frequent) ... 2740
Aceon Tablets (2 mg, 4 mg, 8 mg) (2.4%) ... 3191
Actiq (1% or greater) ... 993
▲ Actonel Tablets (2.3% to 6.6%) ... 2679
▲ Actonel with Calcium Tablets (2.3% to 5%) ... 2684
▲ Adalat CC Tablets (3% or less) ... 2978
Adenocard Injection (Less than 1%) ... 612
Advate Injection (0.6%) ... 742
Advicor Tablets ... 1694
▲ Aerobid/Aerobid-M (3% to 9%) ... 1172
Aggrenox Capsules ... 855
▲ Agrylin Capsules (7.8%) ... 3172
Aldara Cream, 5% (0.5%) ... 1814
Aldurazyme for Intravenous Infusion (2%) ... 1261
Alesse-28 Tablets ... 3392
▲ Alferon N Injection (6% to 10%) ... 1640
▲ Alimta for Injection (Less than 1% to 40%) ... 1722
Altace Capsules (1.1%) ... 1673
Altoprev Extended-Release Tablets (0.5% to 1%) ... 1151
Ambien Tablets (1%) ... 2867
▲ AmBisome for Injection (8.2% to 12%) ... 615
Ammonul Injection ... 3323
Amnesteem Capsules ... 2126
Angiomax for Injection (2.3%) ... 1856
Antara Capsules ... 2723
Anzemet Injection (Rare) ... 2871
Anzemet Tablets (Rare) ... 2874
▲ Apokyn Injection (15%) ... 2132
Aralast (0.1%) ... 745
▲ Aranesp for Injection (6%) ... 576
Arava Tablets (2%) ... 2881
▲ Argatroban Injection (15.2%) ... 1321
Aricept Tablets (Frequent) ... 1086
Aricept ODT Tablets (Frequent) ... 1086
▲ Arimidex Tablets (5% to 7%) ... 665
Arixtra Injection (1.4%) ... 1325
▲ Aromasin Tablets (2% to 5%) ... 2600
▲ Asacol Delayed-Release Tablets (3%) ... 2688
Astelin Nasal Spray ... 1876
Atacand Tablets (More than 1%) ... 634
Atacand HCT (0.5% or greater) ... 637
▲ Atrovent Inhalation Solution (3.2%) ... 868
Avalide Tablets (2%) ... 922
Avalide Tablets (2%) ... 2889
Avapro Tablets (1% or greater) ... 925
Avapro Tablets (1% or greater) ... 2886
Avelox (Less than 0.1%) ... 2984
▲ Avonex (5%) ... 839
Axert Tablets (Infrequent) ... 2430
Axid Oral Solution (2.3%) ... 913
Azopt Ophthalmic Suspension (Less than 1%) ... 553
Benicar Tablets (Greater than 0.5%) ... 2850
Benicar HCT Tablets (Greater than 1%) ... 2852
Betagan Ophthalmic Solution, USP ... ⊙217
▲ Betaseron for SC Injection (11%) ... 791
Betimol Ophthalmic Solution ... ⊙283
Betimol Ophthalmic Solution ... 3371
▲ Bexxar (0% to 7%) ... 1360
▲ BiDil Tablets (16%) ... 2161
Blocadren Tablets (0.6%) ... 1891
Brevibloc Concentrate (Less than 1%) ... 766
Brevibloc Injection (Less than 1%) ... 766
Brevibloc Double Strength Injection (Less than 1%) ... 766
Brevibloc Premixed Injection (Less than 1%) ... 766
Brevibloc Double Strength Premixed Injection (Less than 1%) ... 766
Caduet Tablets (Greater than 0.1%) ... 2507
▲ Campath Ampules (1% to 10%) ... 826
Campral Tablets (Frequent) ... 1175
Captopril Tablets (Approximately 1 in 100 patients) ... 2114
Cardene I.V. (0.7%) ... 1129
▲ Carnitor Injection (6% to 15%) ... 3185
▲ Casodex Tablets (6%) ... 670
Catapres-TTS (0.5% or less) ... 875
Ceftin Tablets (0.1% to 1%) ... 1369
Celebrex Capsules (0.1% to 1.9%) ... 3130
Celexa ... 1177
▲ CellCept Capsules (26.3%) ... 2751
▲ CellCept Intravenous (26.3%) ... 2751
▲ CellCept Oral Suspension (26.3%) ... 2751
▲ CellCept Tablets (26.3%) ... 2751
Cialis Tablets (Less than 2%) ... 1806
Cipro I.V. (1% or less) ... 2998
Cipro I.V. Pharmacy Bulk Package (1% or less) ... 3509
Cipro (Less than 1%) ... 2991
Cipro XR Tablets ... 3004
Clinoril Tablets (Less than 1 in 100) ... 1899
Clozapine Tablets (1%) ... 2141
Clozaril Tablets (1%) ... 2174
Colazal Capsules ... 2845
Combivent Inhalation Aerosol (0.3%) ... 878
Combunox Tablets (Less than 1%) ... 1183
▲ Copaxone for Injection (21%) ... 3292
Coreg Tablets ... 1376
Cosopt Sterile Ophthalmic Solution (Less than 1%) ... 1910
Coumadin for Injection ... 932
Coumadin Tablets ... 932
Covera-HS Tablets (Less than 2%) ... 3135
Cozaar Tablets (1% or greater) ... 1913
Crestor Tablets (Greater than or equal to 2%) ... 672
Cubicin for Injection (1% to 2%) ... 1038
Cytovene (At least 3 subjects) ... 2763
Dalmane Capsules ... 3343
▲ Depacon Injection (1% to 5%) ... 412
▲ Depakene (1% to 5%) ... 417
▲ Depakote Sprinkle Capsules (1% to 5%) ... 422
▲ Depakote Tablets (1% to 5%) ... 427
▲ Depakote ER Tablets (1% to 5%) ... 433
Depo-Provera Contraceptive Injection (Less than 1%) ... 2619
depo-subQ provera 104 Injectable Suspension ... 2622
▲ Detrol Tablets (3.4%) ... 2626
Diovan HCT Tablets (More than 2%) ... 2195
Diovan Tablets (Less frequent) ... 2191
Diprivan Injectable Emulsion (Less than 1%) ... 676
Dolobid Tablets (Rare) ... 1937
▲ Doxil Injection (1% to 5%) ... 3302
DuoNeb Inhalation Solution (2.6%) ... 1058
Duragesic Transdermal System (1% or greater) ... 2448
DynaCirc CR Tablets (0.5% to 1%) ... 2726
Effexor Tablets (2%) ... 3405
Effexor XR Capsules (Frequent) ... 3411
Elitek (Less than or equal to 1%) ... 2906

▲ Eloxatin for Injection (5% to 8%) 2908
Emcyt Capsules (1%)...................... 3137
Enbrel for Injection........................... 580
▲ Entocort EC Capsules (Less than 5%)... 2694
▲ Epogen for Injection (7%) 586
▲ Equetro Extended-Release Capsules (5%)........................... 3178
Ery-Tab Tablets (Isolated reports)..... 447
Erythrocin Stearate Filmtab Tablets (Isolated reports)............ 452
Erythromycin Base Filmtab Tablets (Isolated reports)........................ 454
Erythromycin Delayed-Release Capsules, USP (Isolated reports)... 456
Ethyol for Injection......................... 1869
▲ Evista Tablets (4%) 1735
▲ Evoxac Capsules (1% to 3%) 1042
Exelon Capsules (2% or more)......... 2204
▲ Fabrazyme for Intravenous Infusion (5%)........................... 1267
▲ Faslodex Injection (7.1%) 682
FazaClo Orally Disintegrating Tablets (1%) 547
▲ Femara Tablets (3% to 8%) 2210
▲ Ferrlecit Injection (0.5% to 10%) 3379
Flexeril Tablets (Rare) 1832
▲ Flolan for Injection (11% to 67%) 1408
▲ Flomax Capsules (4.0% to 4.1%) 881
▲ Foradil Aerolizer (3.2%) 3024
Frova Tablets (2%) 1101
Gabitril Tablets (1% or more) 998
Gammagard Liquid 751
▲ Gengraf Capsules (6%) 458
▲ Geodon Capsules (3%) 2514
▲ Gleevec Tablets (7% to 11%) 2221
▲ Hectorol Capsules (Greater than or equal to 5%) 909
▲ Humira Injection (Less than 5%) 464
Hytrin Capsules (At least 1%) 469
Hyzaar 1964
Idamycin PFS Injection 2645
▲ Imdur Tablets (Less than or equal to 5%) 3032
Imitrex Injection 1431
Imitrex Nasal Spray 1435
Imitrex Tablets (Frequent) 1440
Indapamide Tablets (Less than 5%) .. 2119
Indocin (Less than 1%) 1968
Infed Injection 3381
▲ Infergen (5% to 13%) 1647
▲ Intron A for Injection (Up to 28%) 3038
Invanz for Injection (1% to 1.5%) 1974
Invirase (Greater than or equal to 2%) 2776
▲ I.V. Busulfex (26%) 1125
Kadian Capsules (Less than 3%) 572
Kaletra (Less than 2%) 474
Keppra Oral Solution (1% or more) ... 3307
Keppra Tablets (1% or more) 3307
Klonopin (Infrequent) 2782
Lamictal (More than 1%) 1449
Lariam Tablets (Infrequent) 2790
▲ Leukine (15%) 829
Levaquin in 5% Dextrose Injection (1.2%) 2453
Levaquin (1.2%) 2453
Levitra Tablets (Less than 2%) 3048
Lexapro Oral Solution (Frequent) 1193
Lexapro Tablets (Frequent) 1193
Lipitor Tablets (Greater than or equal to 2%) 2495
Lofibra Capsules 1217
Lotensin HCT Tablets (0.3% to 1%) .. 2235
Lotrel Capsules (Infrequent) 2238
Lunesta Tablets (Frequent) 3139
▲ Lyrica Capsules (1% to 4%) 2524
Mavik Tablets (0.3% to 1.0%) 482
Maxair Autohaler (1.3%) 1820
Maxalt Tablets (Less than 2% to 3%) 1983
Maxalt-MLT Orally Disintegrating Tablets (Less than 2% to 3%) 1983
Maxzide 2150
▲ Megace ES Oral Suspension (1% to 3%) 2492
▲ Meridia Capsules (1.8%) 485
Merrem I.V. (Greater than 0.1% to 1%) 687
Mevacor Tablets (0.5% to 1.0%) 1996
Micardis Tablets (1%) 884
Micardis HCT Tablets 886
Midamor Tablets (Less than or equal to 1%) 2000
▲ Mirapex Tablets (Greater than or equal to 1% to 3%) 889
Moduretic Tablets (Less than or equal to 1%) 2003
▲ Myfortic Tablets (3% to less than 20%) 2244
Namenda 1199
▲ Naropin Injection (1% to 5%) 640
Nasonex Nasal Spray (Greater than or equal to 2%) 3058
▲ Navelbine Injection (5%) 1494
▲ Neoral Soft Gelatin Capsules (6%) ... 2247
▲ Neoral Oral Solution (6%) 2247
Neumega for Injection 3433
▲ Neupogen for Injection (5%) 598
Neurontin Capsules (Infrequent)....... 2498
Neurontin Oral Solution (Infrequent)................................. 2498
Neurontin Tablets (Infrequent) 2498
▲ Nipent for Injection (3% to 10%) 3216
▲ Niravam Orally Disintegrating Tablets (10.6%) 3106
Noroxin Tablets (Less frequent)........ 2009
Norvasc Tablets (More than 0.1% to 1%) 2529
Norvir (Less than 2%) 499
Omacor Capsules........................... 2735
Omnicef Capsules........................... 506
Omnicef for Oral Suspension 506
Oncaspar (Less than 1%)................. 1123
▲ Ontak Vials (24%) 1717
Orap Tablets 1220
Ortho-Cyclen/Ortho Tri-Cyclen 2414
Ortho Tri-Cyclen Lo Tablets 2421
▲ Orthoclone OKT3 Sterile Solution (14%) 2370
OxyContin Tablets (Less than 1%) 2699
Parcopa Orally Disintegrating Tablets 3111
▲ Paxil CR Controlled-Release Tablets (3%) 1509
▲ Paxil (3%) 1501
Peganone Tablets, USP 2487
Pegasys 2793
▲ PEG-Intron Powder for Injection (6%) 3062
Pentasa Capsules (Infrequent) 3182
▲ Permax Tablets (3.7%) 3357
▲ Photofrin for Injection (22% to 35%) 729
▲ Plavix Tablets (8.3%) 940
▲ Plavix Tablets (8.3%) 2942
Plendil Extended-Release Tablets (0.5% to 1.5%) 651
Pletal Tablets (Very rare) 2478
▲ Prandin Tablets (0.5, 1, and 2 mg) (1.8% to 3%) 2337
▲ Pravachol Tablets (0.3% to 3.7%) 943
Prevacid Delayed-Release Capsules (Less than 1%) 3268
Prevacid for Delayed-Release Oral Suspension (Less than 1%) 3268
Prevacid NapraPAC (Less than 1%) .. 3277
Prevacid SoluTab Delayed-Release Orally Disintegrating Tablets (Less than 1%) 3268
PREVPAC (Less than 1%) 3281
Prilosec OTC Tablets (Less than 1%) 2674
▲ Prinivil Tablets (3.4%) 2029
Prinzide Tablets (0.3% to 1%) 2033
▲ Procrit for Injection (7%) 2374
▲ Prograf Capsules and Injection (3% to 19%) 624
▲ Proleukin for Injection (12%) 1007
▲ Prometrium Capsules (100 mg, 200 mg) (5% to 7%) 3205
ProSom Tablets (1%) 512
▲ Protonix I.V. (6%) 3468
Protonix Tablets (Greater than or equal to 1%) 3465
Proventil HFA Inhalation Aerosol (Less than 3%) 3071
▲ Provigil Tablets (3%) 1002
Prozac Pulvules and Liquid (Frequent) 1771
Pulmicort Respules (1% to 3%) 654
▲ Pulmozyme Inhalation Solution (18% to 25%) 1245
▲ Rapamune Oral Solution and Tablets (16% to 24%) 3472
Razadyne ER Extended-Release Capsules (Frequent) 2434
Razadyne (Frequent) 2434
▲ Rebetol (5% to 9%) 3073
▲ Rebetron Combination Therapy (5% to 9%) 3078
▲ Rebif Prefilled Syringe for Injection (6% to 8%) 3163
▲ Relpax Tablets (1% to 4%) 2531
Remicade for IV Injection (1%) 987
▲ Requip Tablets (4%) 1528
Retrovir Capsules 1533
Retrovir IV Infusion 1537
Retrovir 1533
Reyataz Capsules (Less than 3%) 948
▲ Ribavirin, USP Capsules (5% to 9%) 3083
Risperdal Consta Long-Acting Injection (Frequent) 1664
▲ Risperdal M-Tab Orally Disintegrating Tablets (2% to 3%) 1658
▲ Risperdal (2% to 3%) 1658
▲ Rituxan for Infusion (1% to 5%) 845
▲ Rituxan I.V. (1% to 5%) 1251
▲ Roferon-A Injection (Less than 4% to 11%) 2805
Men's Rogaine Extra Strength Topical Solution, Ocean Rush Scent and Original Unscented ..... ▣ 706
Women's Rogaine Topical Solution, Spring Bloom Scent and Original Unscented.............. ▣ 707
Rythmol SR Capsules..................... 2736
Sanctura Tablets............................ 1133
Sandimmune (Rare)........................ 2259
Sandostatin Injection (Less than 1%).. 2263
▲ Sensipar Tablets (6%) 603
▲ Simulect for Injection (3% to 10%) ... 2268
▲ Somavert Injection (4% to 8%) 2648
Sonata Capsules (Frequent)............. 1686
Soriatane Capsules (Less than 1%).. 1028
▲ Spiriva HandiHaler (5% to 7%) 899
Stalevo Tablets 2270
Strattera Capsules (0.70%) 1784
Sular Tablets (2%) 1163
Symbyax Capsules (Up to 1%) 1788
Synercid I.V. (Less than 1%) 1690
▲ Tambocor Tablets (5.4%) 1824
Targretin Capsules 1719
Tarka Tablets (0.3% to 2.2%) 519
Tasmar Tablets (1% to 3%) 3360
Taxotere Injection Concentrate 2947
▲ Tequin Injection (0.1% to 3%) 964
▲ Tequin Tablets (0.1% to 3%) 964
Teveten Tablets (1% or greater) 1707
Teveten HCT Tablets (Less than 1%) 1710
Thalomid Capsules 979
▲ Thrombate III (1 of 17) 3254
Thyrolar 1203
Timolide Tablets (Less than 1%) 2056
Timoptic in Ocudose (Less frequent) 2061
Timoptic Sterile Ophthalmic Solution (Less frequent) 2058
Timoptic-XE Sterile Ophthalmic Gel Forming Solution 2062
▲ TOBI Solution for Inhalation (26%) ... 1015
▲ Topamax Sprinkle Capsules (Greater than 1% to 4%) 2438
▲ Topamax Tablets (Greater than 1% to 4%) 2438
Toprol-XL Tablets (Greater than 1%) 660
Trasylol Injection (2%) 779
Travatan Ophthalmic Solution (1% to 5%) 559
Trelstar LA Suspension (1.7%) 3387
Tricor Tablets 523
Triglide Tablets 1165
Trileptal Oral Suspension (Up to 2%) 2281
Trileptal Tablets (Up to 2%) 2281
▲ Trisenox Injection (25%) 983
Truvada Tablets 1279
Ultracet Tablets (Less than 1%) 2462
Uniretic Tablets (More than 1%) 3114
Univasc Tablets (Greater than 1%) ... 3118
Uroxatral Tablets 2957
▲ Urso 250 Tablets (5%) 737
▲ Urso Forte Tablets (5%) 737
Vancocin HCl Capsules, USP 3370
Vantin Tablets and Oral Suspension (Less than 1%) 2650
Vaseretic Tablets (0.5% to 2.0%) 2073
Vasotec I.V. Injection (0.5% to 2.1%) 2076
Ventavis Inhalation Solution 1036
Verelan PM Capsules (2% or less) 3120
VFEND I.V. (Less than 2%) 2543
VFEND Oral Suspension (Less than 2%) 2543
VFEND Tablets (Less than 2%) 2543
Viagra Tablets (Less than 2%) 2552
Virazole for Inhalation Solution 3365
▲ Viread Tablets (3%) 1284
Visudyne for Injection (Less than 1%) 2286
Vivelle Transdermal System (1.5%) .. 2288
Vivelle-Dot Transdermal System (1.5%) 2293
Wellbutrin Tablets (Infrequent) 1579
▲ Wellbutrin SR Sustained-Release Tablets (3% to 4%) 1583
▲ Wellbutrin XL Extended-Release Tablets (3% to 4%) 1588
Xalatan Sterile Ophthalmic Solution (1% to 2%) 2654
Xanax XR Tablets (Frequent) 2655
▲ Xeloda Tablets (Less than 5%) 2825
Xifaxan Tablets (Less than 2%) 2847
Xopenex HFA Inhalation Aerosol 3151
Xopenex Inhalation Solution 3143
Xopenex Inhalation Solution Concentrate 3147
Zegerid Powder for Oral Solution (Less than 1%)............................ 2972
Zelnorm Tablets............................. 2303
Zemaira (0.5%).............................. 3506
▲ Zenapax for Injection (Greater than 5%)...................................... 2838
Zestoretic Tablets (0.3% to 1.0%).... 701
▲ Zestril Tablets (3.4%) 704
▲ Zetia Tablets (3.4%) 2090
▲ Zetia Tablets (3.4%) 3098
Zithromax (1% or less).................... 2568
Zithromax for Oral Suspension, 300 mg, 600 mg, 900 mg, 1200 mg (1% or less).................. 2561
Zithromax Tablets, 250 mg, 500 mg (1% or less)..................... 2561
Zithromax Tablets, 600 mg (1% or less).. 2568
Zithromax Tri-Pak (1% or less)......... 2561
Zithromax Z-Pak (1% or less)........... 2568
Zmax for Oral Suspension (Less then 1%) 2577
Zofran Injection (Rare) 1607
Zofran (Rare) 1613
Zofran ODT Orally Disintegrating Tablets (Rare) 1613
Zoladex (1% or greater) 709
Zoladex 3-month 712
Zoloft (Frequent) 2581
▲ Zometa for Intravenous Infusion (5% to 10%) 2306
Zomig Nasal Spray (Infrequent) 718
▲ Zomig Tablets (2% to 4%) 714
▲ Zomig-ZMT Tablets (2% to 4%) 714
Zonegran Capsules (Infrequent) 1089
Zovirax for Injection (Less than 1%) 1618
Zyban Sustained-Release Tablets (Less than 1%) 1620
▲ Zyprexa Tablets (4%) 1798
▲ Zyprexa ZYDIS Orally Disintegrating Tablets (4%) 1798
Zyrtec Chewable Tablets (Less than 2%) 2589
Zyrtec (Less than 2%) 2589
Zyrtec-D 12 Hour Extended Release Tablets (Less than 2%) 2591

Chest pain, musculoskeletal

▲ Trelstar LA Suspension (13.2%) 3387
Wellbutrin SR Sustained-Release Tablets (Infrequent) 1583
Wellbutrin XL Extended-Release Tablets (Infrequent) 1588

Chest pain, substernal

Aciphex Tablets 1081
Adalat CC Tablets (Less than 1%) 2978
Effexor Tablets (Frequent) 3405
Effexor XR Capsules (Frequent) 3411
▲ Intron A for Injection (Less than 5%) 3038
Kaletra (Less than 2%) 474
Nexium Delayed-Release Capsules (Less than 1%) 645
Nexium I.V. (Less than 1%) 649
Norvir (Less than 2%) 499
▲ Photofrin for Injection (5%) 729
Protonix I.V. (Less than 1%) 3468
Protonix Tablets (Less than 1%) 3465
Reyataz Capsules (Less than 3%) 948
Tequin Injection (Less than 0.1%) 964
Tequin Tablets (Less than 0.1%) 964
VFEND I.V. (Less than 2%) 2543
VFEND Oral Suspension (Less than 2%) 2543
VFEND Tablets (Less than 2%) 2543
Zoloft (Rare) 2581

Chest sound, abnormalities

Gengraf Capsules (1% to less than 3%) 458
▲ Imdur Tablets (Less than or equal to 5%) 3032
▲ Leustatin Injection (9%) 2368
Neoral Soft Gelatin Capsules (1% to less than 3%) 2247
Neoral Oral Solution (1% to less than 3%) 2247
Orthoclone OKT3 Sterile Solution 2370
Prinivil Tablets (Greater than 1%) 2029
Prinzide Tablets 2033
▲ Simulect for Injection (3% to 10%) ... 2268
Zestoretic Tablets 701
Zestril Tablets (Greater than 1%) 704

Chest tightness

Abilify Tablets (Infrequent) 916
Abilify Tablets (Infrequent) 2472
Acthrel for Injection 3528
▲ Adenocard Injection (7%) 612
Advair Diskus 100/50 1291
Advair Diskus 250/50 1291
Advair Diskus 500/50 1291

Aerobid/Aerobid-M (1% to 3%) ... 1172
Alacol DM Syrup ... 739
Alferon N Injection ... 1640
Allegra (Rare) ... 2857
Allegra-D 12 Hour Extended-Release Tablets (Rare) ... 2860
Allegra-D 24 Hour Extended-Release Tablets (Rare) ... 2862
▲ Apokyn Injection (15%) ... 2132
BeneFix for Injection (1.5%) ... 3402
Carimune NF ... 3501
Ceftin Tablets (0.1% to 1%) ... 1369
▲ Doxil Injection (Approximately 6.8%) ... 3302
Elitek ... 2906
Eskalith ... 1406
Ethyol for Injection (Rare) ... 1869
Flovent Diskus 50 mcg ... 1415
Flovent HFA ... 1418
Gammagard Liquid ... 751
Hyperstat I.V. Injection ... 3031
Imitrex Injection (2.7%) ... 1431
Imitrex Nasal Spray (Infrequent) ... 1435
Imitrex Tablets (Frequent) ... 1440
Infed Injection ... 3381
Lexapro Oral Solution (Infrequent) ... 1193
Lexapro Tablets (Infrequent) ... 1193
Lithobid Tablets ... 1670
Maxair Autohaler (1.3%) ... 1820
Maxalt Tablets (Less than 2% to 3%) ... 1983
Maxalt-MLT Orally Disintegrating Tablets (Less than 2% to 3%) ... 1983
Meridia Capsules ... 485
Nicotrol NS ... 2596
Ortho-Cyclen/Ortho Tri-Cyclen ... 2414
Ortho Tri-Cyclen Lo Tablets ... 2421
Orthoclone OKT3 Sterile Solution ... 2370
▲ Relpax Tablets (1% to 4%) ... 2531
Sular Tablets (Very rare) ... 1163
Taxotere Injection Concentrate ... 2947
▲ Thrombate III (3 of 17) ... 3254
Tussionex Pennkinetic Extended-Release Suspension (Occasional) ... 3322
Ventavis Inhalation Solution ... 1036
Xanax XR Tablets (Infrequent) ... 2655
Zomig Nasal Spray (1% to less than 2%) ... 718
▲ Zomig Tablets (2% to 4%) ... 714
▲ Zomig-ZMT Tablets (2% to 4%) ... 714

Chewing movements

Moban Tablets ... 1108
Orap Tablets ... 1220
Thioridazine Hydrochloride Tablets ... 2122
Thiothixene Capsules ... 2124

CHF

(*see under* Congestive heart failure)

Chills

▲ Abelcet Injection (18%) ... 1119
Abilify Tablets (Infrequent) ... 916
Abilify Tablets (Infrequent) ... 2472
Aceon Tablets (2 mg, 4 mg, 8 mg) (0.3% to 1%) ... 3191
Aciphex Tablets ... 1081
▲ Actimmune (14%) ... 1646
Actiq (1% or greater) ... 993
▲ Adacel Vaccine (0.5% to 15.1%) ... 2959
Adalat CC Tablets (Less than 1%) ... 2978
Adriamycin for Injection, USP (Occasional) ... 786
Adriamycin Injection, USP (Occasional) ... 786
Advicor Tablets ... 1694
Aerobid/Aerobid-M (1% to 3%) ... 1172
Aggrastat ... 1878
▲ Agrylin Capsules (1% to 5%) ... 3172
▲ Alferon N Injection (14% to 87%) ... 1640
Alinia for Oral Suspension (Less than 1%) ... 2840
Alinia Tablets (Less than 1%) ... 2840
Aloprim for Injection (Less than 1%) ... 2156
Altoprev Extended-Release Tablets (Rare) ... 1151
▲ AmBisome for Injection (40% to 48.1%) ... 615
Amerge Tablets (Infrequent) ... 1312
▲ Amevive (6%) ... 836
Anadrol-50 Tablets ... 3329
Anaprox Tablets (Less than 1%) ... 2769
Anaprox DS Tablets (Less than 1%) ... 2769
Anzemet Injection (2%) ... 2871
Anzemet Tablets (1.3%) ... 2874
Aralast (0.1%) ... 745
Aricept Tablets (Infrequent) ... 1086
Aricept ODT Tablets (Infrequent) ... 1086
▲ Asacol Delayed-Release Tablets (3%) ... 2688
Avalide Tablets (2%) ... 922
Avalide Tablets (2%) ... 2889
Avapro Tablets (Less than 1%) ... 925
Avapro Tablets (Less than 1%) ... 2886
▲ Avonex (19%) ... 839
Axert Tablets (Infrequent) ... 2430
BeneFix for Injection (1.6%) ... 3402
▲ Betaseron for SC Injection (25%) ... 791
▲ Bexxar (1% to 18%) ... 1360
Buminate 5% Solution, USP (Occasional) ... 747
Buminate 25% Solution, USP (Occasional) ... 748
Buprenex Injectable (Less than 1%) ... 2718
Calcium Disodium Versenate Injection ... 1819
Campral Tablets (Frequent) ... 1175
▲ Camptosar Injection (0% to 14%) ... 2602
▲ Cancidas for Injection (0% to 13.8%) ... 1894
Carbatrol Capsules ... 3174
Carimune NF ... 3501
▲ Casodex Tablets (2% to 5%) ... 670
Ceftin Tablets (0.1% to 1%) ... 1369
▲ CellCept Capsules (3% to less than 20%) ... 2751
▲ CellCept Intravenous (3% to less than 20%) ... 2751
▲ CellCept Oral Suspension (3% to less than 20%) ... 2751
▲ CellCept Tablets (3% to less than 20%) ... 2751
▲ Cerezyme for Injection (Approximately 6.5%) ... 1263
Cerubidine for Injection (Rare) ... 788
▲ Chemet Capsules (5.2% to 15.7%) ... 2480
Cipro I.V. (1% or less) ... 2998
Cipro I.V. Pharmacy Bulk Package (1% or less) ... 3509
Cipro (Less than 1%) ... 2991
Cipro XR Tablets ... 3004
Clinoril Tablets (Less than 1 in 100) ... 1899
Clozapine Tablets (Less than 1%) ... 2141
Clozaril Tablets (Less than 1%) ... 2174
Colazal Capsules ... 2845
▲ Combivir Tablets (10%) ... 1373
Combunox Tablets (Less than 2%) ... 1183
▲ Copaxone for Injection (4%) ... 3292
Coumadin for Injection (Infrequent) ... 932
Coumadin Tablets (Infrequent) ... 932
CytoGam Intravenous (Less than 5.0%) ... 1866
▲ Cytovene (7%) ... 2763
Dantrium Capsules (Less frequent) ... 2690
DDAVP Nasal Spray (Up to 2%) ... 2894
Depacon Injection (1% or more) ... 412
Depakene (1% or more) ... 417
Depakote Sprinkle Capsules ... 422
▲ Depakote Tablets (1% to 5%) ... 427
Depakote ER Tablets (Greater than 1%) ... 433
Depo-Provera Contraceptive Injection (Less than 1%) ... 2619
Desmopressin Acetate Rhinal Tube (Up to 2%) ... 1144
Dilaudid ... 439
Dilaudid Oral Liquid ... 443
Dilaudid Non-Sterile Powder ... 439
Dilaudid Rectal Suppositories ... 439
Dilaudid Tablets ... 439
Dilaudid Tablets - 8 mg ... 443
Dilaudid-HP (Less frequent) ... 441
Diprivan Injectable Emulsion (Less than 1%) ... 676
Dolobid Tablets (Less than 1 in 100) ... 1937
▲ Doxil Injection (1% to 5%) ... 3302
EC-Naprosyn Delayed-Release Tablets (Less than 1%) ... 2769
Edecrin ... 1941
▲ Effexor Tablets (2.2% to 6.8%) ... 3405
Effexor XR Capsules (Frequent) ... 3411
Eldepryl Capsules ... 3209
Ellence Injection ... 2632
Elspar for Injection ... 1943
Engerix-B Vaccine (Less than 1%) ... 1391
▲ Epivir (10%) ... 1394
▲ Epivir-HBV (7%) ... 1398
Equetro Extended-Release Capsules ... 3178
Ethyol for Injection ... 1869
FazaClo Orally Disintegrating Tablets (Less than 1%) ... 547
Ferrlecit Injection ... 3379
▲ Flolan for Injection (13% to 25%) ... 1408
▲ Flumist Vaccine (2.5% to 8.6%) ... 1872
Follistim AQ Cartridge ... 2354
Gabitril Tablets (Frequent) ... 998
▲ Gammagard Liquid (1.69% to 13.1%) ... 751
Gammagard S/D (Occasional) ... 754
Gemzar for Injection (Common) ... 1743
Geodon Capsules (Frequent) ... 2514
Hemofil M (Extremely rare) ... 757
▲ Herceptin I.V. (32%) ... 1234
Imitrex Injection (Infrequent) ... 1431
Imitrex Nasal Spray (Infrequent) ... 1435
Imitrex Tablets ... 1440
Infed Injection ... 3381
▲ Intron A for Injection (Up to 54%) ... 3038
Invanz for Injection (Greater than 0.1%) ... 1974
▲ I.V. Busulfex (46%) ... 1125
Kadian Capsules (Less than 3%) ... 572
Kaletra (Up to 2%) ... 474
Lamictal (1.3%) ... 1449
▲ Lariam Tablets (Among most frequent) ... 2790
Lescol Capsules (Rare) ... 2227
Lescol Capsules (Rare) ... 2730
Lescol XL Tablets ... 2227
Lescol XL Tablets ... 2730
▲ Leukine (19% to 25%) ... 829
▲ Leustatin Injection (9%) ... 2368
Lexapro Oral Solution (Infrequent) ... 1193
Lexapro Tablets (Infrequent) ... 1193
Lotensin HCT Tablets (0.3% or more) ... 2235
Lupron Depot 7.5 mg (Less than 5%) ... 3261
Lyrica Capsules (0.1% to 1%) ... 2524
Marinol Capsules (Less than 1%) ... 3334
Matulane Capsules ... 3188
Maxalt Tablets (Infrequent) ... 1983
Maxalt-MLT Orally Disintegrating Tablets (Infrequent) ... 1983
▲ Menactra Vaccine (0.2% to 9.7%) ... 2968
Merrem I.V. (Greater than 0.1% to 1%) ... 687
Mevacor Tablets (Rare) ... 1996
Mintezol ... 2002
MS Contin Tablets (Less frequent) ... 2703
▲ Mylotarg for Injection (64% to 68%) ... 3429
Nabi-HB ... 2159
Naprosyn Suspension (Less than 1%) ... 2769
Naprosyn Tablets (Less than 1%) ... 2769
▲ Naropin Injection (2.2% to 4.4%) ... 640
Navelbine Injection ... 1494
▲ Neumega for Injection (Greater than or equal to 10%) ... 3433
Neurontin Capsules (Infrequent) ... 2498
Neurontin Oral Solution (Infrequent) ... 2498
Neurontin Tablets (Infrequent) ... 2498
Niaspan Extended-Release Tablets ... 1703
▲ Nipent for Injection (11% to 19%) ... 3216
Noroxin Tablets (Less frequent) ... 2009
Norvir (Less than 2%) ... 499
Omacor Capsules ... 2735
▲ Oncaspar (Greater than 5%) ... 1123
▲ Ontak Vials (81%) ... 1717
▲ Orthoclone OKT3 Sterile Solution (59%) ... 2370
▲ OxyContin Tablets (Between 1% and 5%) ... 2699
Parnate Tablets ... 1499
Paxil CR Controlled-Release Tablets (2%) ... 1509
Paxil (2%) ... 1501
Permax Tablets (1.1%) ... 3357
Plasbumin-5 (Rare) ... 3249
Plasbumin-20 (Rare) ... 3249
Plasbumin-25 (Rare) ... 3251
Pletal Tablets (Less than 2%) ... 2478
Pravachol Tablets (Rare) ... 943
Prevacid Delayed-Release Capsules (Less than 1%) ... 3268
Prevacid for Delayed-Release Oral Suspension (Less than 1%) ... 3268
Prevacid NapraPAC (Less than 1%) ... 3277
Prevacid SoluTab Delayed-Release Orally Disintegrating Tablets (Less than 1%) ... 3268
PREVPAC (Less than 1%) ... 3281
Prinivil Tablets (0.3% to 1.0%) ... 2029
Prinzide Tablets ... 2033
▲ ProAmatine Tablets (4.9%) ... 3183
▲ Prograf Capsules and Injection (3% to 15%) ... 624
Prolastin (Occasional) ... 3252
▲ Proleukin for Injection (52%) ... 1007
ProSom Tablets (Infrequent) ... 512
Protonix I.V. (Less than 1%) ... 3468
Protonix Tablets (Less than 1%) ... 3465
Protopic Ointment (Greater than or equal to 1%) ... 629
Provigil Tablets (1%) ... 1002
Prozac Pulvules and Liquid (Frequent) ... 1771
Rabies Vaccine RabAvert (Rare) ... 1011
▲ Rapamune Oral Solution and Tablets (3% to 20%) ... 3472
▲ Raptiva for Injection (13%) ... 1247
Recombinate (Extremely rare) ... 762
Recombivax HB (Less than 1%) ... 2045
ReFacto Vials ... 3479
Refludan for Injection (Uncommon) ... 815
Relafen Tablets (Less than 1%) ... 1523
Relpax Tablets (Frequent) ... 2531
Repronex for Intramuscular and Subcutaneous Injection ... 1148
Rescriptor Tablets ... 2535
Retrovir Capsules ... 1533
Retrovir IV Infusion ... 1537
Retrovir ... 1533
Rhophylac (Occasionally) ... 3504
Rilutek Tablets (Infrequent) ... 2945
▲ Rituxan for Infusion (32%) ... 845
▲ Rituxan I.V. (33%) ... 1251
Rocephin Injectable Vials, ADD-Vantage, Galaxy, Bulk (Less than 1%) ... 2801
▲ Roferon-A Injection (23% to 64%) ... 2805
Seroquel Tablets (Infrequent) ... 691
Sonata Capsules (Infrequent) ... 1686
▲ Suboxone Tablets (6% to 7.5%) ... 2719
▲ Subutex Tablets (6% to 7.8%) ... 2719
Sular Tablets (Less than or equal to 1%) ... 1163
Symbyax Capsules (Frequent) ... 1788
▲ Targretin Capsules (9.5% to 13.2%) ... 1719
Tasmar Tablets (Infrequent) ... 3360
Taxotere Injection Concentrate ... 2947
Tegretol/Tegretol-XR ... 2278
▲ Tequin Injection (0.1% to 3%) ... 964
▲ Tequin Tablets (0.1% to 3%) ... 964
Tessalon Capsules ... 1202
Tessalon Perles ... 1202
▲ Thalomid Capsules (4.2%) ... 979
▲ Thrombate III (2 of 17) ... 3254
▲ Thymoglobulin for Injection (57.3%) ... 2848
Thyrogen for Injection (1%) ... 1270
Ticlid Tablets ... 2813
Timentin ADD-Vantage ... 1556
Timentin Injection Galaxy Container ... 1559
Timentin IV Infusion ... 1553
Timentin Pharmacy Bulk Package ... 1562
▲ Trizivir Tablets (20%) ... 1565
Tygacil for Injection (0.2% to less than 2%) ... 3489
Uniretic Tablets (Less than 1%) ... 3114
Vancocin HCl Capsules, USP (Infrequent) ... 3370
Vantin Tablets and Oral Suspension (Less than 1%) ... 2650
Varivax (Greater than or equal to 1%) ... 2070
▲ VFEND I.V. (0.2% to 3.7%) ... 2543
▲ VFEND Oral Suspension (0.2% to 3.7%) ... 2543
▲ VFEND Tablets (0.2% to 3.7%) ... 2543
Viadur Implant (Less than 2%) ... 782
Viagra Tablets (Less than 2%) ... 2552
Vytorin 10/10 Tablets ... 2084
Vytorin 10/10 Tablets ... 3092
Vytorin 10/20 Tablets ... 2084
Vytorin 10/20 Tablets ... 3092
Vytorin 10/40 Tablets ... 2084
Vytorin 10/40 Tablets ... 3092
Vytorin 10/80 Tablets ... 2084
Vytorin 10/80 Tablets ... 3092
Wellbutrin Tablets (1.2%) ... 1579
Wellbutrin SR Sustained-Release Tablets (Infrequent) ... 1583
Wellbutrin XL Extended-Release Tablets (Infrequent) ... 1588
WinRho SDF (Less than 2%) ... 763
Xopenex HFA Inhalation Aerosol (Less than 2%) ... 3151
Xopenex Inhalation Solution (Less than 2%) ... 3143
Xopenex Inhalation Solution Concentrate (Less than 2%) ... 3147
▲ Zemplar Capsules (5%) ... 535
▲ Zemplar Injection (5%) ... 538
▲ Zerit (50%) ... 971
Zestoretic Tablets ... 701
Zestril Tablets (0.3% to 1.0%) ... 704
▲ Zevalin Injection (24%) ... 848
▲ Ziagen (6% to 9 %) ... 1600
Zocor Tablets (Rare) ... 2078
Zoladex (1% to 5%) ... 709
Zoladex 3-month ... 712
Zometa for Intravenous Infusion ... 2306
Zomig Nasal Spray (Infrequent) ... 718
Zomig Tablets (Infrequent) ... 714
Zomig-ZMT Tablets (Infrequent) ... 714
Zyban Sustained-Release Tablets (Infrequent) ... 1620
Zyprexa Tablets (Rare) ... 1798

Zyprexa ZYDIS Orally Disintegrating Tablets (Infrequent) ... 1798

Chloasma
Activella Tablets ... 2311
Alesse-28 Tablets ... 3392
Aygestin Tablets ... 1062
Climara Transdermal System ... 795
Climara Pro Transdermal System ... 800
Depo-Provera Contraceptive Injection (Less than 1%) ... 2619
depo-subQ provera 104 Injectable Suspension ... 2622
Estratest Tablets ... 3196
Estratest H.S. Tablets ... 3196
Lo/Ovral-28 Tablets ... 3423
Menostar Transdermal System ... 805
Ortho-Cept Tablets ... 2395
Ortho-Cyclen Tablets ... 2414
Ortho Evra Transdermal System ... 2402
Ortho Tri-Cyclen Tablets ... 2414
Ortho Tri-Cyclen Lo Tablets ... 2421
Prefest Tablets ... 1069
Premarin Intravenous ... 3440
Premarin Vaginal Cream ... 3449
Premphase Tablets ... 3452
Prempro Tablets ... 3452
Prometrium Capsules (100 mg, 200 mg) ... 3205
Seasonale Tablets ... 1073
Topamax Sprinkle Capsules (Rare) ... 2438
Topamax Tablets (Rare) ... 2438
Triphasil-28 Tablets ... 3483
Vivelle Transdermal System ... 2288
Vivelle-Dot Transdermal System ... 2293

Chloasma, possibly persistent
Cenestin Tablets, 0.45mg, 0.625mg, 0.9mg, 1.25mg ... 1063
Cenestin Tablets, 0.3mg ... 1063
Estrogel 0.06% ... 3200

Chloride retention
Estratest Tablets ... 3196
Estratest H.S. Tablets ... 3196
Oxandrin Tablets ... 2977

Choking sensation
Advair Diskus 100/50 ... 1291
Advair Diskus 250/50 ... 1291
Advair Diskus 500/50 ... 1291
Dantrium Intravenous ... 2691
Evoxac Capsules (Less than 1%) ... 1042
Hyperstat I.V. Injection ... 3031
Relpax Tablets (Rare) ... 2531
Risperdal Consta Long-Acting Injection (Infrequent) ... 1664
Serevent Diskus (Rare) ... 1540
Xanax XR Tablets (Infrequent) ... 2655

Cholangitis
Abelcet Injection ... 1119
Aciphex Tablets (Rare) ... 1081
▲ CellCept Capsules (3% to less than 20%) ... 2751
▲ CellCept Intravenous (3% to less than 20%) ... 2751
▲ CellCept Oral Suspension (3% to less than 20%) ... 2751
▲ CellCept Tablets (3% to less than 20%) ... 2751
Copegus Tablets (Less than 1%) ... 2759
Kaletra (Less than 2%) ... 474
Norvir (Less than 2%) ... 499
Pegasys (Less than 1%) ... 2793
▲ Prograf Capsules and Injection (3% to 15%) ... 624
Thalomid Capsules ... 979
Zevalin Injection (2%) ... 848
Zonegran Capsules (Rare) ... 1089

Cholangitis, sclerosing
Doxil Injection (Less than 1%) ... 3302

Cholecystectomy
Prometrium Capsules (100 mg, 200 mg) (2%) ... 3205

Cholecystitis
Abelcet Injection ... 1119
Abilify Tablets (Infrequent) ... 916
Abilify Tablets (Infrequent) ... 2472
Aciphex Tablets ... 1081
Amevive ... 836
Antara Capsules ... 2723
Aricept Tablets ... 1086
Aricept ODT Tablets ... 1086
Asacol Delayed-Release Tablets ... 2688
BiDil Tablets (1% to less than 2%) ... 2161
Campral Tablets (Rare) ... 1175
Celexa (Rare) ... 1177
Copaxone for Injection (Infrequent) ... 3292
Effexor Tablets (Rare) ... 3405
Effexor XR Capsules (Rare) ... 3411
Enbrel for Injection (Infrequent) ... 580
Evoxac Capsules ... 1042
Exelon Capsules (Infrequent) ... 2204
▲ Flovent Diskus 50 mcg (1% to 3%) ... 1415
Gabitril Tablets (Infrequent) ... 998
▲ Humira Injection (Less than 5%) ... 464
Kaletra (Less than 2%) ... 474
Lofibra Capsules ... 1217
Lotronex Tablets (Rare) ... 1479
Lyrica Capsules (0.1% to 1%) ... 2524
Meridia Capsules ... 485
Neurontin Capsules (Rare) ... 2498
Neurontin Oral Solution (Rare) ... 2498
Neurontin Tablets (Rare) ... 2498
Permax Tablets (Rare) ... 3357
Proleukin for Injection ... 1007
Protonix I.V. (Less than 1%) ... 3468
Protonix Tablets (Less than 1%) ... 3465
Prozac Pulvules and Liquid (Rare) ... 1771
Remicade for IV Injection (Greater than or equal to 0.2%) ... 987
Requip Tablets (Infrequent) ... 1528
Rilutek Tablets (Rare) ... 2945
Risperdal M-Tab Orally Disintegrating Tablets (Rare) ... 1658
Risperdal (Rare) ... 1658
Tasmar Tablets (Rare) ... 3360
Tricor Tablets ... 523
Triglide Tablets ... 1165
VFEND I.V. (Less than 2%) ... 2543
VFEND Oral Suspension (Less than 2%) ... 2543
VFEND Tablets (Less than 2%) ... 2543
Vytorin 10/10 Tablets ... 2084
Vytorin 10/10 Tablets ... 3092
Vytorin 10/20 Tablets ... 2084
Vytorin 10/20 Tablets ... 3092
Vytorin 10/40 Tablets ... 2084
Vytorin 10/40 Tablets ... 3092
Vytorin 10/80 Tablets ... 2084
Vytorin 10/80 Tablets ... 3092
Zelnorm Tablets ... 2303
Zetia Tablets ... 2090
Zetia Tablets ... 3098
Zonegran Capsules (Rare) ... 1089

Cholelithiasis
Abilify Tablets (Infrequent) ... 916
Abilify Tablets (Infrequent) ... 2472
Aciphex Tablets ... 1081
Aggrenox Capsules (Less than 1%) ... 855
Antara Capsules ... 2723
▲ Arava Tablets (1% to 3%) ... 2881
Aricept Tablets (Infrequent) ... 1086
Aricept ODT Tablets (Infrequent) ... 1086
Celebrex Capsules (Less than 0.1%) ... 3130
Celexa (Rare) ... 1177
Cytovene ... 2763
Effexor Tablets (Rare) ... 3405
Effexor XR Capsules (Rare) ... 3411
Evoxac Capsules (Less than 1%) ... 1042
Fortical Nasal Spray (Less than 1%) ... 3336
Gabitril Tablets (Infrequent) ... 998
▲ Humira Injection (Less than 5%) ... 464
Invanz for Injection (Greater than 0.1%) ... 1974
Levaquin in 5% Dextrose Injection (0.1% to 0.9%) ... 2453
Levaquin (0.1% to 0.9%) ... 2453
Lofibra Capsules ... 1217
Lunesta Tablets (Infrequent) ... 3139
Lyrica Capsules (0.1% to 1%) ... 2524
Meridia Capsules ... 485
Miacalcin Nasal Spray (Less than 1%) ... 2242
Neurontin Capsules (Rare) ... 2498
Neurontin Oral Solution (Rare) ... 2498
Neurontin Tablets (Rare) ... 2498
Paxil CR Controlled-Release Tablets (Rare) ... 1509
Paxil (Rare) ... 1501
Permax Tablets (Infrequent) ... 3357
Persantine Tablets (Rare) ... 898
Pletal Tablets (Less than 2%) ... 2478
Prevacid Delayed-Release Capsules (Less than 1%) ... 3268
Prevacid for Delayed-Release Oral Suspension (Less than 1%) ... 3268
Prevacid NapraPAC (Less than 1%) ... 3277
Prevacid SoluTab Delayed-Release Orally Disintegrating Tablets (Less than 1%) ... 3268
PREVPAC (Less than 1%) ... 3281
Protonix I.V. (Less than 1%) ... 3468
Protonix Tablets (Less than 1%) ... 3465
Prozac Pulvules and Liquid (Infrequent) ... 1771
Remicade for IV Injection (Greater than or equal to 0.2%) ... 987
Requip Tablets (Infrequent) ... 1528
Risperdal M-Tab Orally Disintegrating Tablets (Rare) ... 1658
Risperdal (Rare) ... 1658
Sonata Capsules (Rare) ... 1686
Symbyax Capsules (Infrequent) ... 1788
Tasmar Tablets (Infrequent) ... 3360
Tricor Tablets ... 523
Triglide Tablets ... 1165
Trileptal Oral Suspension ... 2281
Trileptal Tablets ... 2281
Uniretic Tablets (Less than 1%) ... 3114
VFEND I.V. (Less than 2%) ... 2543
VFEND Oral Suspension (Less than 2%) ... 2543
VFEND Tablets (Less than 2%) ... 2543
Vytorin 10/10 Tablets ... 2084
Vytorin 10/10 Tablets ... 3092
Vytorin 10/20 Tablets ... 2084
Vytorin 10/20 Tablets ... 3092
Vytorin 10/40 Tablets ... 2084
Vytorin 10/40 Tablets ... 3092
Vytorin 10/80 Tablets ... 2084
Vytorin 10/80 Tablets ... 3092
Zelnorm Tablets ... 2303
Zetia Tablets ... 2090
Zetia Tablets ... 3098
Zonegran Capsules (Infrequent) ... 1089

Cholestasis
Amaryl Tablets (Isolated cases) ... 2864
Ammonul Injection ... 3323
Arava Tablets (Rare) ... 2881
Captopril Tablets (Rare) ... 2114
Ceftin ... 1369
Clinoril Tablets (Less than 1%) ... 1899
Clozapine Tablets ... 2141
Clozaril Tablets ... 2174
Cytovene ... 2763
Dolobid Tablets (Less than 1 in 100) ... 1937
FazaClo Orally Disintegrating Tablets ... 547
Flexeril Tablets (Less than 1%) ... 1832
Fortaz ... 1422
Maxipime for Injection ... 1093
Mefoxin for Injection ... 1987
Mefoxin Premixed Intravenous Solution ... 1990
Mintezol ... 2002
Norvasc Tablets ... 2529
Omnicef Capsules ... 506
Omnicef for Oral Suspension ... 506
Suprax ... 1811
Tagamet Tablets (Rare) ... 1547
Tambocor Tablets (Rare) ... 1824
Ticlid Tablets ... 2813
Vantin Tablets and Oral Suspension ... 2650
Zinacef Injection ... 1604
Zinacef for Injection ... 1604
Zyrtec Chewable Tablets (Rare) ... 2589
Zyrtec (Rare) ... 2589
Zyrtec-D 12 Hour Extended Release Tablets (Rare) ... 2591

Cholestasis, intrahepatic
Amoxil Capsules ... 1315
Amoxil Chewable Tablets ... 1315
Amoxil Pediatric Drops for Oral Suspension ... 1315
Amoxil Powder for Oral Suspension ... 1315
Amoxil Tablets ... 1315
Cuprimine Capsules (Rare) ... 1925

Cholestatic hepatic injury
Axid Oral Solution (Rare) ... 913
Coumadin for Injection (Infrequent) ... 932
Coumadin Tablets (Infrequent) ... 932

Cholesterol, systemic, microembolism
Coumadin for Injection (Infrequent) ... 932
Coumadin Tablets (Infrequent) ... 932

Cholinergic reactions
Camptosar Injection ... 2602
Evoxac Capsules ... 1042
Risperdal M-Tab Orally Disintegrating Tablets (Rare) ... 1658
Risperdal (Rare) ... 1658

Choluria
Xifaxan Tablets (Less than 2%) ... 2847

Chondrodystrophy
Prozac Pulvules and Liquid (Rare) ... 1771

Chorea
Activella Tablets ... 2311
Cenestin Tablets, 0.45mg, 0.625mg, 0.9mg, 1.25mg ... 1063
Cenestin Tablets, 0.3mg ... 1063
Climara Transdermal System ... 795
Climara Pro Transdermal System ... 800
CombiPatch Transdermal System ... 2180
Dilaudid-HP ... 441
Eldepryl Capsules ... 3209
Estratest Tablets ... 3196
Estratest H.S. Tablets ... 3196
Estrogel 0.06% ... 3200
Inversine Tablets ... 3286
Klonopin ... 2782
Lo/Ovral-28 Tablets ... 3423
Menostar Transdermal System ... 805
Phenytek Capsules (Rare) ... 2153
Prefest Tablets ... 1069
Premarin Intravenous ... 3440
Premarin Tablets ... 3443
Premarin Vaginal Cream ... 3449
Premphase Tablets ... 3452
Prempro Tablets ... 3452
Triphasil-28 Tablets ... 3483
Vivelle Transdermal System ... 2288
Vivelle-Dot Transdermal System ... 2293

Chorea, exacerbation of
Seasonale Tablets ... 1073

Choreiform
Parcopa Orally Disintegrating Tablets (Common) ... 3111

Choreoathetosis
Celexa ... 1177
Gabitril Tablets (Infrequent) ... 998
Geodon Capsules (Frequent) ... 2514
Lexapro Oral Solution ... 1193
Lexapro Tablets ... 1193
Neurontin Capsules (Rare) ... 2498
Neurontin Oral Solution (Rare) ... 2498
Neurontin Tablets (Rare) ... 2498
Requip Tablets (Infrequent) ... 1528
Seroquel Tablets (Rare) ... 691

Choreoathetotic movements
Aldoclor Tablets ... 1881
Aldoril Tablets ... 1884
Eskalith ... 1406
Lamictal (Rare) ... 1449
Lithobid Tablets ... 1670
Neurontin Capsules (Rare) ... 2498
Neurontin Oral Solution (Rare) ... 2498
Neurontin Tablets (Rare) ... 2498
Paxil CR Controlled-Release Tablets (Rare) ... 1509
Paxil (Rare) ... 1501
Permax Tablets (Frequent) ... 3357
Risperdal M-Tab Orally Disintegrating Tablets (Rare) ... 1658
Risperdal (Rare) ... 1658
Tasmar Tablets (Infrequent) ... 3360
Thioridazine Hydrochloride Tablets ... 2122
Zoloft (Rare) ... 2581
Zyprexa Tablets (Up to 2%) ... 1798
Zyprexa ZYDIS Orally Disintegrating Tablets (Up to 2%) ... 1798

Chorioretinitis
Neurontin Capsules (Rare) ... 2498
Neurontin Oral Solution (Rare) ... 2498
Neurontin Tablets (Rare) ... 2498
Stromectol Tablets ... 2053

Choroidal detachment
▲ Retisert Implant (5% to 9%) ... ⊙ 256

Choroidal detachment, post-filtration procedures
Cosopt Sterile Ophthalmic Solution ... 1910
Timoptic in Ocudose ... 2061
Timoptic Sterile Ophthalmic Solution ... 2058
Timoptic-XE Sterile Ophthalmic Gel Forming Solution ... 2062
Trusopt Sterile Ophthalmic Solution ... 2065

Choroiditis
Stromectol Tablets ... 2053

Chromatopsia
Cipro I.V. (1% or less) ... 2998
Cipro I.V. Pharmacy Bulk Package (1% or less) ... 3509
Cipro (Less than 1%) ... 2991
Cipro XR Tablets ... 3004
Effexor Tablets (Rare) ... 3405
Effexor XR Capsules (Rare) ... 3411
Levitra Tablets (Less than 2%) ... 3048
VFEND I.V. (0.4% to 1.2%) ... 2543

VFEND Oral Suspension (0.4% to 1.2%) 2543
VFEND Tablets (0.4% to 1.2%) 2543

Chromaturia
Rescriptor Tablets 2535

Chromosomal abnormalities
Mustargen for Injection 2007
Roferon-A Injection (One case) 2805

Churg-Strauss syndrome
Accolate Tablets (Rare) 663
Advair Diskus 100/50 (Rare) 1291
Advair Diskus 250/50 (Rare) 1291
Advair Diskus 500/50 (Rare) 1291
Flovent Diskus 50 mcg (Rare) 1415
Flovent HFA (Rare) 1418
Singulair 2047

Circulatory collapse
Amerge Tablets 1312
Decadron Tablets 1929
Furosemide Tablets 2117

Circulatory collapse, peripheral
Eskalith 1406
▲ Intron A for Injection (Less than or equal to 5%) 3038
Lithobid Tablets 1670
Tenormin I.V. Injection 698
Tenormin Tablets 695

Circulatory depression
Actiq 993
Dilaudid 439
Dilaudid Oral Liquid 443
Dilaudid Tablets - 8 mg 443
Dilaudid-HP 441
MS Contin Tablets 2703
OxyContin Tablets 2699

Circulatory failure
Ambien Tablets (Rare) 2867
Dilaudid 439
Levaquin in 5% Dextrose Injection (0.1% to 0.9%) 2453
Levaquin (0.1% to 0.9%) 2453
Prevacid Delayed-Release Capsules (Less than 1%) 3268
Prevacid for Delayed-Release Oral Suspension (Less than 1%) 3268
Prevacid NapraPAC (Less than 1%) 3277
Prevacid SoluTab Delayed-Release Orally Disintegrating Tablets (Less than 1%) 3268
PREVPAC (Less than 1%) 3281
Remicade for IV Injection (Greater than or equal to 0.2%) 987
Trasylol Injection 779
Zosyn (1.0% or less) 3492

Cirrhosis, hepatic
(*see under* Cirrhosis of liver)

Cirrhosis of liver
Advicor Tablets (Rare) 1694
Altoprev Extended-Release Tablets 1151
Campral Tablets (Infrequent) 1175
Colazal Capsules 2845
Lescol Capsules (Rare) 2227
Lescol Capsules (Rare) 2730
Lescol XL Tablets (Rare) 2227
Lescol XL Tablets (Rare) 2730
Mevacor Tablets (Rare) 1996
Pacerone Tablets (Rare) 3337
Pentasa Capsules 3182
Pravachol Tablets (Rare) 943
Vytorin 10/10 Tablets (Rare) 2084
Vytorin 10/10 Tablets (Rare) 3092
Vytorin 10/20 Tablets (Rare) 2084
Vytorin 10/20 Tablets (Rare) 3092
Vytorin 10/40 Tablets (Rare) 2084
Vytorin 10/40 Tablets (Rare) 3092
Vytorin 10/80 Tablets (Rare) 2084
Vytorin 10/80 Tablets (Rare) 3092
Zocor Tablets (Rare) 2078

Clamminess
Eligard 22.5 mg (Less than 2%) 2899
▲ Eligard 30 mg (4.4%) 2901
Evoxac Capsules (Less than 1%) 1042
Exelon Capsules (Infrequent) 2204
▲ Intron A for Injection (Less than 5%) 3038
Migranal Nasal Spray (Infrequent) 3350
Norvasc Tablets (Less than or equal to 0.1%) 2529
▲ Nubain Injection (9%) 1111
Xanax XR Tablets (Infrequent) 2655
Xifaxan Tablets (Less than 2%) 2847
Zoloft (Infrequent) 2581

Claudication
Blocadren Tablets 1891
Cosopt Sterile Ophthalmic Solution 1910
Covera-HS Tablets (Less than 2%) 3135
Namenda (More than one patient) 1199
Tarka Tablets 519
Timolide Tablets 2056
Timoptic in Ocudose 2061
Timoptic Sterile Ophthalmic Solution 2058
Timoptic-XE Sterile Ophthalmic Gel Forming Solution 2062
Verelan PM Capsules (2% or less) 3120

Claudication, intermittent
(*see under* Charcot's syndrome)

Claustrophobia
Roferon-A Injection (Infrequent) 2805

Cleft palate, neonatal
Accutane Capsules 2740
Proventil Inhalation Aerosol 3067
Proventil Inhalation Solution 0.083% 3069

Clitoris, enlargement
(*see under* Clitoromegaly)

Clitoromegaly
Anadrol-50 Tablets 3329
▲ Delatestryl Injection (Among most frequent) 2976
Estratest Tablets 3196
Estratest H.S. Tablets 3196
Oxandrin Tablets 2977

Clonic movements of whole limbs
Diprivan Injectable Emulsion (Less than 1%) 676
Eskalith 1406

Clonus
Ammonul Injection 3323

Clotting disorder, intravascular
Cosmegen for Injection 1907

Clotting time, prolongation
Anadrol-50 Tablets 3329
Oncaspar (Less than 1%) 1123
Testim 1% Gel (Less than 1%) 722
Zosyn 3492

CNS, unresponsiveness, unspecified
Cipro I.V. 2998
Cipro I.V. Pharmacy Bulk Package 3509
Cipro XR Tablets 3004

CNS abnormalities, fetal
Accutane Capsules 2740

CNS depression
Anaprox Tablets (Less than 1%) 2769
Anaprox DS Tablets (Less than 1%) 2769
Depacon Injection 412
Depakene 417
Depakote Tablets 427
Depakote ER Tablets 433
Diastat Rectal Delivery System 3344
EC-Naprosyn Delayed-Release Tablets (Less than 1%) 2769
▲ Klonopin (Most frequent) 2782
Lamictal (Infrequent) 1449
Mebaral Tablets, USP (Less than 1 in 100 patients) 2483
Naprosyn Suspension (Less than 1%) 2769
Naprosyn Tablets (Less than 1%) 2769
Nembutal Sodium Solution, USP (Less than 1%) 2484
Neurontin Capsules 2498
Neurontin Oral Solution 2498
Neurontin Tablets 2498
Prozac Pulvules and Liquid (Infrequent) 1771
Rilutek Tablets (Rare) 2945
▲ Vesanoid Capsules (3%) 2823
Xanax XR Tablets 2655

CNS reactions
Attenuvax 1889
Clozapine Tablets 2141
Clozaril Tablets 2174
Digitek Tablets 2146
Hexalen Capsules 2101
▲ Intron A for Injection (Less than 5%) 3038
Lanoxicaps Capsules (Rare) 1458
Lanoxin Injection 1462
Lanoxin Tablets 1468
Lanoxin Injection Pediatric 1465
Lariam Tablets 2790
▲ Leukine (11%) 829
▲ Nipent for Injection (1% to 11%) 3216
Noroxin Tablets 2009
Orap Tablets 1220
Orthoclone OKT3 Sterile Solution 2370
Roferon-A Injection (Less than 5%) 2805
Stalevo Tablets 2270

CNS stimulation
Adipex-P 1216
Avelox 2984
Axert Tablets (Infrequent) 2430
Balamine DM 739
Cafcit 1854
Cipro I.V. 2998
Cipro I.V. Pharmacy Bulk Package 3509
Cipro 2991
Cipro XR Tablets 3004
Clarinex-D 24-Hour Extended-Release Tablets 3012
Combivent Inhalation Aerosol 878
Effexor Tablets (Infrequent) 3405
Effexor XR Capsules (Infrequent) 3411
Kytril Injection (Less than 2%) 2785
Lamictal (Rare) 1449
Lidoderm Patch 1107
Meridia Capsules (1.5%) 485
Mirapex Tablets (Less than 1%) 889
Noroxin Tablets 2009
Paxil CR Controlled-Release Tablets (Frequent) 1509
Paxil (Frequent) 1501
Proventil Inhalation Aerosol 3067
Proventil HFA Inhalation Aerosol 3071
Prozac Pulvules and Liquid (Infrequent) 1771
Tequin Injection 964
Tequin Tablets 964
Ventolin HFA Inhalation Aerosol 1576
VoSpire Extended-Release Tablets 2352
Wellbutrin SR Sustained-Release Tablets (1% to 2%) 1583
Wellbutrin XL Extended-Release Tablets (1% to 2%) 1588
Zyban Sustained-Release Tablets (Infrequent) 1620
Zyprexa Tablets (Infrequent) 1798
Zyprexa ZYDIS Orally Disintegrating Tablets (Infrequent) 1798
Zyrtec-D 12 Hour Extended Release Tablets 2591

CNS stimulation, paradoxical
Diastat Rectal Delivery System 3344
Niravam Orally Disintegrating Tablets (Rare) 3106
Numorphan 1112

CNS toxicity
DepoCyt Injection 1121
▲ Nipent for Injection (1% to 11%) 3216

Coagulation defects, neonatal
Phenytek Capsules 2153

Coagulation dysfunction
Abelcet Injection 1119
AmBisome for Injection (Less common) 615
Campath Ampules 826
Celexa (Rare) 1177
▲ CellCept Capsules (3% to less than 20%) 2751
▲ CellCept Intravenous (3% to less than 20%) 2751
▲ CellCept Oral Suspension (3% to less than 20%) 2751
▲ CellCept Tablets (3% to less than 20%) 2751
Depacon Injection 412
Depakene 417
Depakote Tablets 427
Depakote ER Tablets 433
Diprivan Injectable Emulsion (Less than 1%) 676
Elspar for Injection 1943
Estratest Tablets 3196
Estratest H.S. Tablets 3196
Herceptin I.V. (At least one of the 958 patients) 1234
▲ Leukine (19%) 829
Lo/Ovral-28 Tablets 3423
Neurontin Capsules 2498
Neurontin Oral Solution 2498
Neurontin Tablets 2498
Nimotop Capsules (Less than 1%) 774
NovoSeven (1%) 2335
Omnicef Capsules 506
Omnicef for Oral Suspension 506
Oncaspar (Less than 1%) 1123
Orthoclone OKT3 Sterile Solution 2370
▲ Pacerone Tablets (1% to 3%) 3337
Plavix Tablets (1% to 2.5%) 940
Plavix Tablets (1% to 2.5%) 2942
Premarin Intravenous 3440
Premarin Vaginal Cream 3449
▲ Prograf Capsules and Injection (3% to 15%) 624
▲ Proleukin for Injection (10%) 1007
Rituxan for Infusion (0.3%) 845
Roferon-A Injection (Less than 4%) 2805
Symbyax Capsules (Rare) 1788
▲ Xeloda Tablets (Less than 5%) 2825

Coagulation tests, altered results
Zosyn 3492

Coagulation time, increase in
Arthrotec Tablets (Rare) 3126
Spectracef Tablets (0.1% to 1%) 2706
Zoloft 2581

Coagulopathy
Aggrenox Capsules 855
Ammonul Injection (Less than 3%) 3323
Bayer Aspirin Tablets 3515
Ecotrin Enteric Coated Aspirin Low, Regular and Maximum Strength Tablets 1627
Enbrel for Injection 580
Mycamine for Injection 620
St. Joseph 81 mg Aspirin Chewable and Enteric Coated Tablets 1841

Coccidioidomycosis, disseminated
Remicade for IV Injection 987

Cochlear lesion
DAPTACEL 2964

Cognitive dysfunction
Ambien Tablets (Infrequent) 2867
Amerge Tablets (Infrequent) 1312
Anaprox Tablets (Rare) 2769
Anaprox DS Tablets (Rare) 2769
EC-Naprosyn Delayed-Release Tablets (Rare) 2769
Naprosyn Suspension (Rare) 2769
Naprosyn Tablets (Rare) 2769
▲ Niravam Orally Disintegrating Tablets (10.3% to 28.8%) 3106
Orthoclone OKT3 Sterile Solution 2370
Prevacid NapraPAC (Less than 1%) 3277
Rescriptor Tablets 2535
Risperdal M-Tab Orally Disintegrating Tablets 1658
Risperdal 1658
▲ Topamax Sprinkle Capsules (0% to 7%) 2438
▲ Topamax Tablets (0% to 7%) 2438
Ultracet Tablets 2462

Cogwheel rigidity
Abilify Tablets (Infrequent) 916
Abilify Tablets (Infrequent) 2472
Eskalith 1406
Geodon (Frequent) 2514
Lithobid Tablets 1670
Lyrica Capsules (Rare) 2524
Paxil CR Controlled-Release Tablets 1509
Paxil 1501
Symbyax Capsules (Infrequent) 1788
Thioridazine Hydrochloride Tablets 2122
Thiothixene Capsules 2124
▲ Zyprexa Tablets (8% to 20%) 1798
▲ Zyprexa ZYDIS Orally Disintegrating Tablets (8% to 20%) 1798

Cold, reduced tolerance
Coumadin for Injection (Infrequent) 932
Coumadin Tablets (Infrequent) 932

Cold sensations
Aceon Tablets (2 mg, 4 mg, 8 mg) (0.3% to 1%) 3191
Aricept Tablets (Infrequent) 1086
Aricept ODT Tablets (Infrequent) 1086
Buprenex Injectable (Less than 1%) 2718
Coumadin for Injection (Infrequent) 932
Coumadin Tablets (Infrequent) 932

Ethyol for Injection 1869
▲ Frova Tablets (3%) 1101
Guanidine Hydrochloride Tablets 3030
Imitrex Injection (1.1%) 1431
Imitrex Nasal Spray (Rare) 1435
Imitrex Tablets (Rare) 1440
Migranal Nasal Spray (Infrequent) 3350
Roferon-A Injection (Infrequent) 2805
Zofran Injection (2%) 1607
▲ Zomig Tablets (5% to 7%) 714
▲ Zomig-ZMT Tablets (5% to 7%) 714

Cold sore, non-herpetic
▲ Intron A for Injection (Less than 5%) 3038
Varivax (Greater than or equal to 1%) 2070

Cold symptoms, unspecified
AccuNeb Inhalation Solution (Up to 3.4%) 1055
▲ Aerobid/Aerobid-M (15%) 1172
▲ Alamast Ophthalmic Solution (10% to 25%) 3371
Carac Cream, 0.5% (2.3%) 1048
▲ Cutivate Lotion 0.05% (4%) 1383
▲ Elestat Ophthalmic Solution (Approximately 10%) 1643
▲ Geodon Capsules (8%) 2514
Patanol Ophthalmic Solution (Less than 5%) 557
Paxil CR Controlled-Release Tablets 1509
Paxil 1501
Prinivil Tablets (1.1%) 2029
▲ ProSom Tablets (3%) 512
▲ Sandostatin Injection (1% to 4%) 2263
Somavert Injection 2648
▲ Xalatan Sterile Ophthalmic Solution (Approximately 4%) 2654
Zestril Tablets (1.1%) 704

Coldness of extremities
▲ Blocadren Tablets (8%) 1891
Cosopt Sterile Ophthalmic Solution 1910
Effexor Tablets (Infrequent) 3405
Effexor XR Capsules (Infrequent) 3411
Eskalith (A few reports) 1406
Gleevec Tablets (Infrequent) 2221
Lithobid Tablets 1670
Maxalt Tablets (Infrequent) 1983
Maxalt-MLT Orally Disintegrating Tablets (Infrequent) 1983
ReoPro Vials (0.2%) 1779
Rythmol SR Capsules 2736
Strattera Capsules 1784
▲ Tenormin I.V. Injection (Up to 12%) 698
▲ Tenormin Tablets (Up to 12%) 695
Timolide Tablets 2056
Timoptic in Ocudose 2061
Timoptic Sterile Ophthalmic Solution 2058
Timoptic-XE Sterile Ophthalmic Gel Forming Solution 2062
Toprol-XL Tablets (About 1 of 100 patients) 660

Colds, susceptibility
Betimol Ophthalmic Solution (1% to 5%) ⊙ 283
Betimol Ophthalmic Solution (1% to 5%) 3371
Hytrin Capsules (At least 1%) 469
▲ Pravachol Tablets (Up to 7.0%) 943
Prinzide Tablets (0.3% to 1%) 2033
Zestoretic Tablets (0.3% to 1%) 701

Colic
Invirase (Less than 2%) 2776
Prevnar for Injection 3460
Urecholine Tablets 2349

Colic, biliary
Kadian Capsules (Less than 3%) 572

Colitis
Abilify Tablets (Frequent) 916
Abilify Tablets (Frequent) 2472
Accutane Capsules 2740
Aciphex Tablets 1081
▲ Actonel Tablets (0.8% to 3.3%) 2679
▲ Actonel with Calcium Tablets (0.8% to 2.5%) 2684
Aldoclor Tablets 1881
Aldoril Tablets 1884
Alesse-28 Tablets 3392
Amnesteem Capsules 2126
Anaprox Tablets (Less than 1%) 2769
Anaprox DS Tablets (Less than 1%) 2769
Ancef for Injection 1318
Antara Capsules 2723
▲ Arava Tablets (1% to 3%) 2881
▲ Avastin IV (1% to 6%) 1229
Benzaclin Topical Gel 1046
Caduet Tablets (Less than 2%) 2507
Campath Ampules 826
Campral Tablets (Rare) 1175
Camptosar Injection (Rare) 2602
Canasa Rectal Suppositories (1.2%) 726
Cataflam Tablets (Rarely) 2173
Celebrex Capsules (Less than 0.1%) 3130
Celexa (Rare) 1177
CellCept Capsules 2751
CellCept Intravenous 2751
CellCept Oral Suspension 2751
CellCept Tablets 2751
Cleocin Vaginal Ovules 2613
Clindagel 1207
Clinoril Tablets (Less than 1%) 1899
Copaxone for Injection (Infrequent) 3292
Copegus Tablets (Less than 1%) 2759
Doxil Injection (Less than 1%) 3302
Duac Topical Gel 3214
EC-Naprosyn Delayed-Release Tablets (Less than 1%) 2769
Effexor Tablets (Infrequent) 3405
Effexor XR Capsules (Infrequent) 3411
Eligard 7.5 mg (2.5%) 2896
Elmiron Capsules (Less than or equal to 1%) 2393
Eloxatin for Injection 2908
Evoclin Foam, 1% (Rarely) 1025
Exelon Capsules (Infrequent) 2204
Fortaz 1422
Gleevec Tablets (Rare) 2221
Herceptin I.V. (At least one of the 958 patients) 1234
Imitrex Nasal Spray (Rare) 1435
Imitrex Tablets 1440
Lipitor Tablets (Less than 2%) 2495
Lofibra Capsules 1217
Lo/Ovral-28 Tablets 3423
Lotronex Tablets (Rare) 1479
Lunesta Tablets (Rare) 3139
Lyrica Capsules (0.1% to 1%) 2524
Maxipime for Injection (Greater than 0.1% to less than 1%) 1093
Mefoxin for Injection 1987
Mefoxin Premixed Intravenous Solution 1990
Mobic Oral Suspension (Less than 2%) 893
Mobic Tablets (Less than 2%) 893
Myfortic Tablets 2244
Namenda 1199
Naprosyn Suspension (Less than 1%) 2769
Naprosyn Tablets (Less than 1%) 2769
Neurontin Capsules (Rare) 2498
Neurontin Oral Solution (Rare) 2498
Neurontin Tablets (Rare) 2498
Norvir (Less than 2%) 499
Omacor Capsules 2735
Oncaspar 1123
Ortho-Cept Tablets 2395
Ortho-Cyclen Tablets 2414
Ortho Evra Transdermal System 2402
Ortho Tri-Cyclen Tablets 2414
Ortho Tri-Cyclen Lo Tablets 2421
Paxil CR Controlled-Release Tablets (Rare) 1509
Paxil (Rare) 1501
Permax Tablets (Rare) 3357
Plavix Tablets 940
Plavix Tablets 2942
Pletal Tablets (Less than 2%) 2478
Prevacid Delayed-Release Capsules (Less than 1%) 3268
Prevacid for Delayed-Release Oral Suspension (Less than 1%) 3268
Prevacid NapraPAC (Less than 1%) 3277
Prevacid SoluTab Delayed-Release Orally Disintegrating Tablets (Less than 1%) 3268
Prevnar for Injection 3460
PREVPAC (Less than 1%) 3281
Proleukin for Injection 1007
Protonix I.V. (Less than 1%) 3468
Protonix Tablets (Less than 1%) 3465
Prozac Pulvules and Liquid (Infrequent) 1771
Requip Tablets (Infrequent) 1528
Rescriptor Tablets 2535
Reyataz Capsules (Less than 3%) 948
Risperdal Consta Long-Acting Injection (Infrequent) 1664
Rocephin Injectable Vials, ADD-Vantage, Galaxy, Bulk (Rare) 2801
Roferon-A Injection (Infrequent) 2805
Sandostatin LAR Depot (1% to 4%) 2264
Seasonale Tablets 1073
Sonata Capsules (Less than 1%) 1686
Sular Tablets (Less than or equal to 1%) 1163
Suprax 1811
Symbyax Capsules (Infrequent) 1788
Targretin Capsules 1719
Tasmar Tablets (Infrequent) 3360
Tequin Injection (Less than 0.1%) 964
Tequin Tablets (Less than 0.1%) 964
Thalomid Capsules 979
Ticlid Tablets 2813
Tricor Tablets 523
Triglide Tablets 1165
Trileptal Oral Suspension 2281
Trileptal Tablets 2281
Triphasil-28 Tablets 3483
Uniretic Tablets (Less than 1%) 3114
Voltaren Tablets (Rarely) 2298
Voltaren-XR Tablets (Rarely) 2301
Wellbutrin Tablets (Rare) 1579
Wellbutrin SR Sustained-Release Tablets 1583
Wellbutrin XL Extended-Release Tablets 1588
Yasmin 28 Tablets 818
Zevalin Injection 848
Zinacef Injection 1604
Zinacef for Injection 1604
Zoloft (Rare) 2581
Zomig Nasal Spray (Rare) 718
Zonegran Capsules (Rare) 1089
Zyban Sustained-Release Tablets 1620

Colitis, hemorrhagic
Augmentin ES-600 Powder for Oral Suspension 1337
Pegasys (Less than 1%) 2793
PEG-Intron Powder for Injection 3062
Roferon-A Injection 2805

Colitis, ischemic
Blocadren Tablets 1891
Cosopt Sterile Ophthalmic Solution 1910
Imitrex Injection 1431
Imitrex Nasal Spray 1435
Imitrex Tablets 1440
InnoPran XL Capsules 2728
Lotronex Tablets (Infrequent) 1479
Nadolol Tablets 2121
Pegasys (Less than 1%) 2793
PEG-Intron Powder for Injection 3062
Roferon-A Injection 2805
Tenormin I.V. Injection 698
Tenormin Tablets 695
Timoptic-XE Sterile Ophthalmic Gel Forming Solution 2062
Zelnorm Tablets 2303
Zomig Nasal Spray (Very rare) 718
Zomig Tablets (Very rare) 714

Colitis, lymphocytic
Plavix Tablets 940
Plavix Tablets 2942

Colitis, necrotizing
Adriamycin for Injection, USP 786
Adriamycin Injection, USP 786

Colitis, pseudomembranous
(*see under* Pseudomembranous colitis)

Colitis, ulcerative
Camptosar Injection 2602
Evoxac Capsules (Less than 1%) 1042
Indocin (Less than 1%) 1968
Lotronex Tablets (Rare) 1479
Pegasys (Less than 1%) 2793
Plavix Tablets 940
Plavix Tablets 2942
Prevacid Delayed-Release Capsules (Less than 1%) 3268
Prevacid for Delayed-Release Oral Suspension (Less than 1%) 3268
Prevacid NapraPAC (Less than 1%) 3277
Prevacid SoluTab Delayed-Release Orally Disintegrating Tablets (Less than 1%) 3268
PREVPAC (Less than 1%) 3281
Protonix I.V. (Less than 1%) 3468
Protonix Tablets (Less than 1%) 3465
Vantin Tablets and Oral Suspension 2650

Colitis, ulcerative, worsening of
▲ Asacol Delayed-Release Tablets (3%) 2688
Colazal Capsules 2845
Pentasa Capsules (0.4%) 3182

Collagen disease, unspecified
▲ Flolan for Injection (82%) 1408
Rythmol SR Capsules 2736

Collapse
Carbatrol Capsules 3174
Clozapine Tablets (Rare) 2141
Clozaril Tablets (Rare) 2174
Mintezol 2002
Nitrolingual Pumpspray 1161
Tegretol/Tegretol-XR 2278
▲ Xeloda Tablets (Less than 5%) 2825

Colon, irritable
Aricept Tablets (Infrequent) 1086
Aricept ODT Tablets (Infrequent) 1086
Prilosec OTC Tablets (Less than 1%) 2674
Zegerid Powder for Oral Solution (Less than 1%) 2972

Colon obstruction
VESIcare Tablets 631

Colonic strictures
Creon 5 Capsules 3195
Creon 10 Capsules 3195
Creon 20 Capsules 3196
Ultrase Capsules 735
Ultrase MT Capsules 736

Color perception, disturbed
Amnesteem Capsules 2126
Cialis Tablets (Less than 2%) 1806
Cipro (Less than 1%) 2991
Cipro XR Tablets 3004

Color vision, changes
Levitra Tablets (Less than 2%) 3048
▲ VFEND I.V. (Approximately 21%) 2543
▲ VFEND Oral Suspension (Approximately 21%) 2543
▲ VFEND Tablets (Approximately 21%) 2543

Coma
Aciphex Tablets 1081
Aggrenox Capsules (Less than 1%) 855
Aloprim for Injection (Less than 1%) 2156
AmBisome for Injection (Less common) 615
▲ Ammonul Injection (3%) 3323
Anaprox Tablets (Less than 1%) 2769
Anaprox DS Tablets (Less than 1%) 2769
Arthrotec Tablets (Rare) 3126
Avinza Capsules (Less than 5%) 1714
Bayer Aspirin Tablets 3515
Buprenex Injectable (Infrequent) 2718
Campath Ampules 826
Carimune NF 3501
Cataflam Tablets (Rarely) 2173
Copaxone for Injection (Infrequent) 3292
Copegus Tablets (Less than 1%) 2759
Dalmane Capsules 3343
DDAVP Injection 4 mcg/mL (Rare) 2893
DDAVP Nasal Spray (Rare) 2894
Depacon Injection (Rare) 412
▲ Depakene (Rare) 417
Depakote Sprinkle Capsules (Rare) 422
Depakote Tablets (Rare) 427
Depakote ER Tablets (Rare) 433
Desmopressin Acetate Injection (Rare) 1143
EC-Naprosyn Delayed-Release Tablets (Less than 1%) 2769
Ecotrin Enteric Coated Aspirin Low, Regular and Maximum Strength Tablets 1627
Elspar for Injection 1943
Eskalith 1406
Evoxac Capsules (Less than 1%) 1042
Fortaz 1422
Gabitril Tablets (Infrequent) 998
Gammagard Liquid 751
Gammagard S/D (Rare) 754
Gamunex Immune Globulin I.V., 10% (Rare) 3232
Indocin Capsules (Less than 1%) 1968
Indocin I.V. (Less than 1%) 1973
Indocin (Less than 1%) 1968
▲ Intron A for Injection (Less than 5%) 3038
I.V. Busulfex (One patient) 1125
Iveegam EN (Rare) 759
Klonopin 2782
Levaquin in 5% Dextrose Injection (0.1% to 0.9%) 2453
Levaquin (0.1% to 0.9%) 2453
Lithobid Tablets 1670
Lyrica Capsules (Rare) 2524
Matulane Capsules 3188
Maxipime for Injection 1093
Naprosyn Suspension (Less than 1%) 2769
Naprosyn Tablets (Less than 1%) 2769

Naropin Injection (Less than 1%) 640
Oncaspar 1123
Orthoclone OKT3 Sterile Solution 2370
Pegasys (Less than 1%) 2793
Permax Tablets (Infrequent) 3357
PhosLo GelCaps 2158
Prograf Capsules and Injection 624
Proleukin for Injection (1%) 1007
Prozac Pulvules and Liquid (Rare) 1771
ReoPro Vials (0.4%) 1779
Requip Tablets (Infrequent) 1528
Rilutek Tablets (Infrequent) 2945
Risperdal M-Tab Orally Disintegrating Tablets (Rare) 1658
Risperdal (Rare) 1658
Roferon-A Injection (Rare to infrequent) 2805
Seromycin Capsules 1783
St. Joseph 81 mg Aspirin Chewable and Enteric Coated Tablets 1841
Stromectol Tablets 2053
Symbyax Capsules (Infrequent) 1788
Symmetrel 1115
Tindamax (Rare) 2670
▲ Trisenox Injection (5%) 983
Valtrex Caplets 1573
▲ Vesanoid Capsules (3%) 2823
VFEND I.V. (Less than 2%) 2543
VFEND Oral Suspension (Less than 2%) 2543
VFEND Tablets (Less than 2%) 2543
Voltaren Tablets (Rarely) 2298
Voltaren-XR Tablets (Rarely) 2301
Wellbutrin Tablets 1579
Wellbutrin SR Sustained-Release Tablets 1583
Wellbutrin XL Extended-Release Tablets 1588
Zoloft (Rare) 2581
Zovirax Capsules 1616
Zovirax for Injection (Approximately 1%) 1618
Zovirax 1616
Zyban Sustained-Release Tablets 1620
Zyprexa Tablets (Rare) 1798
Zyprexa ZYDIS Orally Disintegrating Tablets (Infrequent) 1798

Coma, hyperosmolar
FazaClo Orally Disintegrating Tablets 547

Coma, hepatic
(*see under* Hepatic coma)

Coma, hyperosmolar non-ketonic
Hyperstat I.V. Injection 3031

Combativeness
Diprivan Injectable Emulsion (Less than 1%) 676
Orthoclone OKT3 Sterile Solution 2370
Zosyn (1.0% or less) 3492

Complement activation
Visudyne for Injection (Less than 1%) 2286

Condition aggravated
Denavir Cream 2163
Levaquin in 5% Dextrose Injection (0.1% to 0.9%) 2453
Levaquin (0.1% to 0.9%) 2453

Conduction disturbances
Aceon Tablets (2 mg, 4 mg, 8 mg) (0.3% to 1%) 3191
Avalide Tablets 922
Avalide Tablets 2889
Avapro Tablets (Less than 1%) 925
Avapro Tablets (Less than 1%) 2886
Blocadren Tablets 1891
Catapres-TTS 875
Clorpres Tablets (Rare) 2139
Cytovene 2763
Digitek Tablets 2146
▲ Lanoxicaps Capsules (Among most common) 1458
▲ Lanoxin Injection (Among most common) 1462
▲ Lanoxin Tablets (Among most common) 1468
▲ Lanoxin Injection Pediatric (Among most common) 1465
Lariam Tablets (Infrequent) 2790
Nadolol Tablets (1 of 100 patients) 2121
Paxil CR Controlled-Release Tablets (Infrequent) 1509
Paxil (Infrequent) 1501
Reyataz Capsules (Rare) 948
Rythmol SR Capsules (Greater than or equal to 2%) 2736

Confusion
Abilify Tablets (Frequent) 916
Abilify Tablets (Frequent) 2472
Aciphex Tablets (Rare) 1081
Actimmune (Rare) 1646
▲ Actiq (1% to 6%) 993
Adalat CC Tablets (Less than 1%) 2978
Aggrenox Capsules (1.1%) 855
Agrylin Capsules (1% to 5%) 3172
Aldoclor Tablets 1881
Aldoril Tablets 1884
Alferon N Injection (One patient to 3%) 1640
Ambien Tablets (Frequent) 2867
▲ AmBisome for Injection (8.6% to 12.9%) 615
Amerge Tablets (Rare) 1312
Ammonul Injection 3323
Amoxil Capsules (Rare) 1315
Amoxil Chewable Tablets (Rare) 1315
Amoxil Pediatric Drops for Oral Suspension (Rare) 1315
Amoxil Powder for Oral Suspension (Rare) 1315
Amoxil Tablets (Rare) 1315
Anaprox Tablets (Less than 1%) 2769
Anaprox DS Tablets (Less than 1%) 2769
Angiomax for Injection (Rare) 1856
Anzemet Injection (Infrequently) 2871
Anzemet Tablets (Infrequently) 2874
▲ Apokyn Injection (5% to 10%) 2132
Aricept Tablets 1086
Aricept ODT Tablets 1086
▲ Arimidex Tablets (2% to 5%) 665
▲ Arixtra Injection (1.2% to 3.1%) 1325
▲ Aromasin Tablets (2% to 5%) 2600
Arthrotec Tablets (Rare) 3126
Asacol Delayed-Release Tablets 2688
Astelin Nasal Spray 1876
Augmentin (Rare) 1331
Augmentin Tablets (Rare) 1334
Augmentin XR Extended-Release Tablets (Rare) 1340
Augmentin ES-600 Powder for Oral Suspension (Rare) 1337
Avalide Tablets 922
Avalide Tablets 2889
▲ Avastin IV (1% to 6%) 1229
Avelox (Less than 0.1%) 2984
Avinza Capsules (Less than 5%) 1714
Axid Oral Solution (Rare) 913
Bayer Aspirin Tablets 3515
Bentyl Capsules 724
Bentyl Injection 724
Bentyl Syrup 724
Bentyl Tablets 724
Betagan Ophthalmic Solution, USP ⊙ 217
Betaseron for SC Injection 791
Biaxin/Biaxin XL 402
Brevibloc Concentrate (About 2%) 766
Brevibloc Injection (About 2%) 766
Brevibloc Double Strength Injection (About 2%) 766
Brevibloc Premixed Injection (About 2%) 766
Brevibloc Double Strength Premixed Injection (About 2%) 766
Campath Ampules 826
Campral Tablets (Infrequent) 1175
Camptosar Injection (0% to 2.7%) 2602
Captopril Tablets 2114
Carbatrol Capsules 3174
Cardene I.V. (Rare) 1129
▲ Casodex Tablets (2% to 5%) 670
Cataflam Tablets (Occasionally) 2173
Celexa (Frequent) 1177
▲ CellCept Capsules (3% to less than 20%) 2751
▲ CellCept Intravenous (3% to less than 20%) 2751
▲ CellCept Oral Suspension (3% to less than 20%) 2751
▲ CellCept Tablets (3% to less than 20%) 2751
Cipro I.V. (1% or less) 2998
Cipro I.V. Pharmacy Bulk Package (1% or less) 3509
Cipro 2991
Cipro XR Tablets 3004
▲ Clozapine Tablets (3%) 2141
▲ Clozaril Tablets (3%) 2174
Cogentin Injection 1903
Copaxone for Injection (2%) 3292
Cosopt Sterile Ophthalmic Solution 1910
Covera-HS Tablets (Less than 2%) 3135
Cozaar Tablets (Less than 1%) 1913
Cubicin for Injection (1% to 2%) 1038
Cytovene (At least 3 subjects) 2763
Dalmane Capsules (Rare) 3343
Dantrium Capsules (Less frequent) 2690
Daranide Tablets 1928
Demser Capsules 1933
▲ Depacon Injection (1% to 5%) 412
▲ Depakene (1% to 5%) 417
▲ Depakote Sprinkle Capsules (1% to 5%) 422
▲ Depakote Tablets (1% to 5%) 427
▲ Depakote ER Tablets (1% to 5%) 433
▲ DepoCyt Injection (4% to 14%) 1121
Diastat Rectal Delivery System (Greater than or equal to 1%) 3344
Didronel Tablets 2693
Digitek Tablets 2146
Diovan HCT Tablets 2195
Diprivan Injectable Emulsion (Less than 1%) 676
▲ Ditropan XL Extended Release Tablets (2% to less than 5%) 2391
Diuril Oral 1936
Diuril Sodium Intravenous 1934
Dolobid Tablets (Less than 1 in 100) 1937
Dostinex Tablets 2631
▲ Doxil Injection (1% to 10%) 3302
▲ Duragesic Transdermal System (10% or more) 2448
Dyazide Capsules 1389
EC-Naprosyn Delayed-Release Tablets (Less than 1%) 2769
Ecotrin Enteric Coated Aspirin Low, Regular and Maximum Strength Tablets 1627
Edecrin 1941
Effexor Tablets (2%) 3405
Effexor XR Capsules (Frequent) 3411
▲ Eldepryl Capsules (3 of 49 patients) 3209
Elspar for Injection 1943
Emend Capsules (Greater than 0.5%) 1944
▲ Entocort EC Capsules (Less than 5%) 2694
Equetro Extended-Release Capsules 3178
Ery-Tab Tablets (Isolated reports) 447
Erythrocin Stearate Filmtab Tablets (Isolated reports) 452
Erythromycin Base Filmtab Tablets (Isolated reports) 454
Erythromycin Delayed-Release Capsules, USP (Isolated reports) 456
Eskalith 1406
Eulexin Capsules (1%) 3023
Evoxac Capsules (Less than 1%) 1042
▲ Exelon Capsules (8%) 2204
Famvir Tablets (Infrequent) 2207
▲ FazaClo Orally Disintegrating Tablets (3%) 547
▲ Flexeril Tablets (1% to 3%) 1832
▲ Flolan for Injection (6%) 1408
Flovent HFA 1418
Flumadine (Less than 0.3%) 1186
Frova Tablets (Infrequent) 1101
▲ Gabitril Tablets (5%) 998
Garamycin Injectable 3028
Gengraf Capsules (1% to less than 3%) 458
Geodon Capsules (Frequent) 2514
Gleevec Tablets (Rare) 2221
Grifulvin V Tablets Microsize and Oral Suspension Microsize (Occasional) 2384
Gris-PEG Tablets (Occasional) 2504
Guanidine Hydrochloride Tablets 3030
Herceptin I.V. (At least one of the 958 patients) 1234
▲ Humira Injection (Less than 5%) 464
Hyperstat I.V. Injection 3031
Hyzaar 1964
▲ Imdur Tablets (Less than or equal to 5%) 3032
Imitrex Injection (Infrequent) 1431
Imitrex Nasal Spray (Infrequent) 1435
Imitrex Tablets (Infrequent) 1440
Indocin (Less than 1%) 1968
▲ Infergen (4%) 1647
▲ Intron A for Injection (Up to 12%) 3038
▲ Invanz for Injection (3.3% to 5.1%) 1974
Invirase (Less than 2%) 2776
▲ I.V. Busulfex (11%) 1125
Kadian Capsules (Less than 3%) 572
Kaletra (Less than 2%) 474
Keppra Oral Solution (1% to 2%) 3307
Keppra Tablets (1% to 2%) 3307
Klonopin (1%) 2782
K-Phos Neutral Tablets 785
K-Phos Original (Sodium Free) Tablets (Less frequent) 785
Lamictal (1.8%) 1449
Lanoxicaps Capsules 1458
Lanoxin Injection 1462
Lanoxin Tablets 1468
Lanoxin Injection Pediatric 1465
Lariam Tablets (Occasional) 2790
Leukeran Tablets (Rare) 1472
Levaquin in 5% Dextrose Injection (0.1% to 0.9%) 2453
Levaquin (0.1% to 0.9%) 2453
Lexapro Oral Solution (Infrequent) 1193
Lexapro Tablets (Infrequent) 1193
Librium Capsules 3349
Lidoderm Patch 1107
Lithobid Tablets 1670
Lotronex Tablets (Rare) 1479
Lovenox Injection (2.2%) 2931
▲ Lunesta Tablets (0% to 3%) 3139
Lupron Depot 3.75 mg 3257
▲ Lyrica Capsules (1% to 7%) 2524
Marinol Capsules (Greater than 1%) 3334
Matulane Capsules 3188
Maxair Autohaler 1820
Maxalt Tablets (Infrequent) 1983
Maxalt-MLT Orally Disintegrating Tablets (Infrequent) 1983
Maxipime for Injection 1093
Mebaral Tablets, USP (Less than 1 in 100 patients) 2483
▲ Megace ES Oral Suspension (1% to 3%) 2492
Meridia Capsules 485
Merrem I.V. (Greater than 0.1% to 1%) 687
Midamor Tablets (Less than or equal to 1%) 2000
Migranal Nasal Spray (Infrequent) 3350
Mintezol 2002
▲ Mirapex Tablets (4% to 10%) 889
Mobic Oral Suspension (Less than 2%) 893
Mobic Tablets (Less than 2%) 893
Moduretic Tablets (Less than or equal to 1%) 2003
Nalfon Capsules (1.4%) 2504
▲ Namenda (6%) 1199
Naprosyn Suspension (Less than 1%) 2769
Naprosyn Tablets (Less than 1%) 2769
Naropin Injection (Less than 1%) 640
Natrecor for Injection (Greater than or equal to 1%) 3123
Nembutal Sodium Solution, USP (Less than 1%) 2484
Neoral Soft Gelatin Capsules (1% to less than 3%) 2247
Neoral Oral Solution (1% to less than 3%) 2247
Neumega for Injection 3433
Neurontin Capsules 2498
Neurontin Oral Solution 2498
Neurontin Tablets 2498
Nexium Delayed-Release Capsules (Less than 1%) 645
Nexium I.V. (Less than 1%) 649
▲ Nicotrol NS (Less than 5%) 2596
▲ Niravam Orally Disintegrating Tablets (5% to 10.4%) 3106
Norflex Injection (Infrequent) 1824
Noroxin Tablets 2009
Norvir (0.6% to 0.9%) 499
Nubain Injection (1% or less) 1111
Numorphan 1112
Oncaspar (Less than 1%) 1123
▲ Ontak Vials (8%) 1717
Orthoclone OKT3 Sterile Solution 2370
▲ OxyContin Tablets (Between 1% and 5%) 2699
Parcopa Orally Disintegrating Tablets 3111
Parnate Tablets 1499
Paxil CR Controlled-Release Tablets (1%) 1509
Paxil (1%) 1501
Pepcid Injection (Infrequent) 2017
Pepcid (Infrequent) 2014
▲ Permax Tablets (11.1%) 3357
Phenergan Suppositories 3438
▲ Phenytek Capsules (Among most common) 2153
PhosLo GelCaps 2158
▲ Photofrin for Injection (8%) 729
Plavix Tablets 940
Plavix Tablets 2942
Prevacid Delayed-Release Capsules (Less than 1%) 3268
Prevacid for Delayed-Release Oral Suspension (Less than 1%) 3268
Prevacid NapraPAC (Less than 1%) 3277
Prevacid SoluTab Delayed-Release Orally Disintegrating Tablets (Less than 1%) 3268
▲ PREVPAC (Less than 1% to 3%) 3281

Prilosec OTC Tablets (Less than 1%) 2674
Primaxin I.M. 2022
Primaxin I.V. (Less than 0.2%) 2024
Prinivil Tablets (0.3% to 1.0%) 2029
Prinzide Tablets 2033
ProAmatine Tablets (Less frequent) 3183
▲ Prograf Capsules and Injection (3% to 15%) 624
▲ Proleukin for Injection (34%) 1007
Prometrium Capsules (100 mg, 200 mg) (Less than 5%) 3205
ProSom Tablets (2%) 512
Protonix I.V. (Less than 1%) 3468
Protonix Tablets (Less than 1%) 3465
Provigil Tablets (1%) 1002
Prozac Pulvules and Liquid (Frequent) 1771
▲ Rapamune Oral Solution and Tablets (3% to 20%) 3472
Razadyne ER Extended-Release Capsules (Greater than or equal to 2%) 2434
Razadyne (Greater than or equal to 2%) 2434
Relafen Tablets (Less than 1%) 1523
Relpax Tablets (Infrequent) 2531
Remicade for IV Injection (Greater than or equal to 0.2%) 987
ReoPro Vials (0.6%) 1779
▲ Requip Tablets (5%) 1528
Rescriptor Tablets 2535
Retrovir Capsules 1533
Retrovir IV Infusion 1537
Retrovir 1533
Reyataz Capsules (Less than 3%) 948
Rilutek Tablets (Infrequent) 2945
Risperdal Consta Long-Acting Injection (Infrequent) 1664
Risperdal M-Tab Orally Disintegrating Tablets (Infrequent) 1658
Risperdal (Infrequent) 1658
▲ Roferon-A Injection (Less than 4% to 7%) 2805
Sandimmune (2% or less) 2259
▲ Sandostatin LAR Depot (5% to 15%) 2264
Sedapap Tablets 50 mg/650 mg (Infrequent) 2098
Seromycin Capsules 1783
Seroquel Tablets (Infrequent) 691
Sonata Capsules (1% or less) 1686
St. Joseph 81 mg Aspirin Chewable and Enteric Coated Tablets 1841
Stalevo Tablets 2270
Stromectol Tablets 2053
Sular Tablets (Less than or equal to 1%) 1163
Surmontil Capsules 2347
Sustiva Capsules (Less than 2%) 957
Symbyax Capsules (Infrequent) 1788
Symmetrel (0.1% to 5%) 1115
Synercid I.V. (Less than 1%) 1690
Tagamet Tablets (Occasional) 1547
Tambocor Tablets (Less than 1%) 1824
Tamiflu Capsules 2810
Tamiflu Oral Suspension 2810
Targretin Capsules 1719
Tarka Tablets 519
▲ Tasmar Tablets (10% to 11%) 3360
Taxotere Injection Concentrate 2947
Tegretol/Tegretol-XR 2278
▲ Temodar Capsules (5%) 3088
Tequin Injection (Less than 0.1%) 964
Tequin Tablets (Less than 0.1%) 964
Tessalon Capsules 1202
Tessalon Perles 1202
Thalomid Capsules 979
Timolide Tablets (Less than 1%) 2056
Timoptic in Ocudose (Less frequent) 2061
Timoptic Sterile Ophthalmic Solution (Less frequent) 2058
Timoptic-XE Sterile Ophthalmic Gel Forming Solution 2062
Tindamax (Rare) 2670
▲ Topamax Sprinkle Capsules (2% to 14%) 2438
▲ Topamax Tablets (2% to 14%) 2438
Toprol-XL Tablets 660
Transderm Scōp Transdermal Therapeutic System (Infrequent) 2166
Tranxene (Less common) 2488
▲ Trasylol Injection (4%) 779
Tricor Tablets 523
Trileptal Oral Suspension (1% to 2%) 2281
Trileptal Tablets (1% to 2%) 2281
▲ Trisenox Injection (5%) 983
Ultane Liquid for Inhalation (Less than 1%) 526
Ultracet Tablets (At least 1%) 2462
Uroqid-Acid No. 2 Tablets 785
▲ Valcyte Tablets (Less than 5%) 2816
Valium Tablets (Infrequent) 2822
Valtrex Caplets 1573
Vantin Tablets and Oral Suspension (Less than 1%) 2650
Vaseretic Tablets 2073
Vasotec I.V. Injection (0.5% to 1%) 2076
Verelan PM Capsules (2% or less) 3120
▲ Vesanoid Capsules (14%) 2823
VFEND I.V. (Less than 2%) 2543
VFEND Oral Suspension (Less than 2%) 2543
VFEND Tablets (Less than 2%) 2543
Vicoprofen Tablets (Less than 3%) 533
Vivactil Tablets 2350
Voltaren Tablets (Occasionally) 2298
Voltaren-XR Tablets (Occasionally) 2301
▲ Wellbutrin Tablets (8.4%) 1579
Wellbutrin SR Sustained-Release Tablets 1583
Wellbutrin XL Extended-Release Tablets 1588
Xanax XR Tablets (1.5%) 2655
▲ Xeloda Tablets (Less than 5%) 2825
Zantac (Rare) 1597
Zantac Injection (Rare) 1593
Zantac Injection Pharmacy Bulk Package (Rare) 1595
Zantac Syrup (Rare) 1597
Zegerid Powder for Oral Solution (Less than 1%) 2972
Zestoretic Tablets 701
Zestril Tablets (0.3% to 1.0%) 704
Zoloft (Infrequent) 2581
▲ Zometa for Intravenous Infusion (7% to 12.8%) 2306
Zomig Nasal Spray (Infrequent) 718
▲ Zonegran Capsules (6%) 1089
Zosyn (1.0% or less) 3492
Zovirax Capsules 1616
Zovirax for Injection (Approximately 1%) 1618
Zovirax 1616
Zyban Sustained-Release Tablets (Infrequent) 1620
Zyprexa Tablets 1798
Zyprexa IntraMuscular (Infrequent) 1798
Zyprexa ZYDIS Orally Disintegrating Tablets 1798
Zyrtec Chewable Tablets (Less than 2%) 2589
Zyrtec (Less than 2%) 2589
Zyrtec-D 12 Hour Extended Release Tablets (Less than 2%) 2591

Confusion, mental
(*see under* Confusion)

Confusion, nocturnal
Thioridazine Hydrochloride Tablets (Extremely rare) 2122

Confusional state
(*see under* Confusion)

Congelation
Eldepryl Capsules 3209

Congenital anomalies
Altoprev Extended-Release Tablets (Rare) 1151
Arthrotec Tablets 3126
Aygestin Tablets 1062
Bravelle for Intramuscular or Subcutaneous Injection 1140
Cytovene 2763
Depacon Injection 412
Depakene 417
Depakote Tablets 427
Depakote ER Tablets 433
Effexor Tablets 3405
Effexor XR Capsules 3411
Havrix Vaccine (Rare) 1425
Lescol Capsules (Rare) 2227
Lescol Capsules (Rare) 2730
Lescol XL Tablets 2227
Lescol XL Tablets 2730
Lo/Ovral-28 Tablets 3423
Mevacor Tablets (Rare) 1996
Permax Tablets 3357
Premarin Intravenous 3440
Proventil Inhalation Aerosol 3067
Proventil Inhalation Solution 0.083% 3069
Repronex for Intramuscular and Subcutaneous Injection 1148
Retrovir Capsules 1533
Retrovir IV Infusion 1537
Retrovir 1533
Triphasil-28 Tablets 3483
Twinrix Vaccine 1571
Vivelle Transdermal System 2288
Vivelle-Dot Transdermal System 2293

Congenital malformation
Activella Tablets 2311
Carbatrol Capsules 3174
Diastat Rectal Delivery System 3344
Follistim AQ Cartridge 2354
Phenytek Capsules 2153
Pravachol Tablets (One case) 943
Tegretol/Tegretol-XR 2278
Tranxene 2488
Valium Tablets 2822

Congestion
▲ Advair Diskus 100/50 (1% to 3%) 1291
▲ Advair Diskus 250/50 (1% to 3%) 1291
▲ Advair Diskus 500/50 (1% to 3%) 1291
Avalide Tablets 922
Avalide Tablets 2889
Avapro Tablets (Less than 1%) 925
Avapro Tablets (Less than 1%) 2886
▲ Infergen (5% to 12%) 1647
Tricor Tablets 523
▲ Zenapax for Injection (2% to 5%) 2838

Congestion, nasal
(*see under* Nasal congestion)

Congestive heart failure
Actos Tablets (1.1%) 3224
Adriamycin for Injection, USP 786
Adriamycin Injection, USP 786
Agrylin Capsules 3172
Aldoclor Tablets 1881
Aldoril Tablets 1884
Aminohippurate Sodium "PAH" Injection 1886
Anaprox Tablets (Less than 1%) 2769
Anaprox DS Tablets (Less than 1%) 2769
▲ Apokyn Injection (5%) 2132
▲ Aranesp for Injection (6%) 576
Aricept Tablets (Infrequent) 1086
Aricept ODT Tablets (Infrequent) 1086
Arthrotec Tablets (Rare) 3126
Avastin IV 1229
Avonex (Rare) 839
Betagan Ophthalmic Solution, USP ⊙ 217
Betoptic S Ophthalmic Suspension (Rare) 554
Captopril Tablets (2 to 3 of 1000 patients) 2114
Carbatrol Capsules 3174
Cardizem LA Extended Release Tablets (Less than 2%) 1699
Carteolol Hydrochloride Ophthalmic Solution USP, 1% ⊙ 246
▲ Casodex Tablets (2% to 5%) 670
Cataflam Tablets (Occasionally) 2173
Catapres Tablets (Rare) 874
Catapres-TTS (0.5% or less) 875
Celebrex Capsules (Less than 0.1%) 3130
▲ CellCept Capsules (3% to less than 20%) 2751
▲ CellCept Intravenous (3% to less than 20%) 2751
▲ CellCept Oral Suspension (3% to less than 20%) 2751
▲ CellCept Tablets (3% to less than 20%) 2751
Cerubidine for Injection 788
Clinoril Tablets (Less than 1%) 1899
Clorpres Tablets (Rare) 2139
Clozapine Tablets 2141
Clozaril Tablets 2174
Covera-HS Tablets (1.8% to 2%) 3135
Cymbalta Delayed-Release Capsules (Infrequent) 1729
Decadron Phosphate Injection 1931
Decadron Tablets 1929
Depo-Medrol Injectable Suspension 2615
Depo-Medrol Single-Dose Vial 2617
Digibind for Injection (Few instances) 1388
Dolobid Tablets 1937
▲ Doxil Injection (1% to 5%) 3302
EC-Naprosyn Delayed-Release Tablets (Less than 1%) 2769
Effexor Tablets (Rare) 3405
Effexor XR Capsules (Infrequent) 3411
Ellence Injection (0.4% to 1.5%) 2632
▲ Emcyt Capsules (3%) 3137
Enbrel for Injection 580
Equetro Extended-Release Capsules 3178
Gemzar for Injection (Very rare) 1743
▲ Herceptin I.V. (7%) 1234
▲ Humira Injection (Less than 5%) 464
Hydrocortone Tablets 1963
Idamycin PFS Injection 2645
Inderal LA Long-Acting Capsules 3421
Indocin Capsules (Less than 1%) 1968
Indocin I.V. (Less than 1%) 1973
Indocin (Less than 1%) 1968
InnoPran XL Capsules 2728
Iveegam EN 759
Lupron Depot 7.5 mg (Less than 5%) 3261
Meridia Capsules 485
Micardis Tablets 884
Micardis HCT Tablets 886
Naprosyn Suspension (Less than 1%) 2769
Naprosyn Tablets (Less than 1%) 2769
Neumega for Injection 3433
Neurontin Capsules (Infrequent) 2498
Neurontin Oral Solution (Infrequent) 2498
Neurontin Tablets (Infrequent) 2498
Nimotop Capsules (Less than 1%) 774
Novantrone for Injection Concentrate 3158
▲ Pacerone Tablets (1% to 3%) 3337
Paxil CR Controlled-Release Tablets (Rare) 1509
Paxil (Rare) 1501
Pediapred Oral Solution 3319
Permax Tablets (Frequent) 3357
Pletal Tablets (Less than 2%) 2478
Prevacid NapraPAC (Less than 1%) 3277
Prevnar for Injection 3460
Proleukin for Injection (1%) 1007
Protonix I.V. (Less than 1%) 3468
Protonix Tablets (Less than 1%) 3465
Prozac Pulvules and Liquid (Infrequent) 1771
▲ Rapamune Oral Solution and Tablets (3% to 20%) 3472
Remicade for IV Injection 987
Retrovir Capsules (0.8%) 1533
Retrovir IV Infusion (1%) 1537
Retrovir (0.8%) 1533
Rilutek Tablets (Infrequent) 2945
Roferon-A Injection (Infrequent) 2805
Rythmol SR Capsules (1% to 2%) 2736
Sandostatin Injection (Less than 1%) 2263
Seromycin Capsules 1783
Seroquel Tablets (Infrequent) 691
Sular Tablets (Less than or equal to 1%) 1163
Symbyax Capsules (Rare) 1788
Symmetrel (0.1% to 1%) 1115
Tambocor Tablets 1824
Tarka Tablets 519
Tegretol/Tegretol-XR 2278
Thalomid Capsules 979
Tiazac Capsules (Less than 2%) 1204
Toprol-XL Tablets (About 1 of 100 patients) 660
Trasylol Injection (1% to 2%) 779
Vantin Tablets and Oral Suspension (Less than 1%) 2650
▲ Velcade for Injection (5%) 2102
Ventavis Inhalation Solution 1036
Verelan PM Capsules (1.8%) 3120
VFEND I.V. (Less than 2%) 2543
VFEND Oral Suspension (Less than 2%) 2543
VFEND Tablets (Less than 2%) 2543
Voltaren Tablets (Occasionally) 2298
Voltaren-XR Tablets (Occasionally) 2301
▲ Zoladex (5%) 709
Zoladex 3-month (1% to 5%) 712
Zyprexa Tablets (Infrequent) 1798
Zyprexa ZYDIS Orally Disintegrating Tablets (Infrequent) 1798

Conjunctiva, suffusion
Brimonidine Tartrate Ophthalmic Solution 0.2% (Less than 3%) ⊙ 245

Conjunctival blanching
▲ Brimonidine Tartrate Ophthalmic Solution 0.2% (3% to 9%) ⊙ 245

Conjunctival chemosis
Natacyn Antifungal Ophthalmic Suspension (One case) ⊙ 207
▲ Retisert Implant (5% to 9%) ⊙ 256

Conjunctival deposits
Propine Ophthalmic Solution ⊙ 237

Conjunctival epithelial defects, unspecified
▲ Genoptic Sterile Ophthalmic Solution (Among most frequent) ⊙ 227

Conjunctival erythema

Poly-Pred Liquifilm Ophthalmic Suspension ⊙231
▲ Zylet Ophthalmic Suspension (Less than 4%) 3508

Conjunctival follicles

▲ Brimonidine Tartrate Ophthalmic Solution 0.2% (10% to 30%) ⊙245
Cosopt Sterile Ophthalmic Solution (1% to 5%) 1910

Conjunctival hyperemia

▲ Lumigan Ophthalmic Solution (15% to 45%) 569
Poly-Pred Liquifilm Ophthalmic Suspension ⊙231
▲ Retisert Implant (10% to 35%) ⊙256

Conjunctival injection

▲ Betimol Ophthalmic Solution (More than 5%) ⊙283
▲ Betimol Ophthalmic Solution (More than 5%) 3371
Cosopt Sterile Ophthalmic Solution (1% to 5%) 1910
Crolom Cromolyn Sodium Sterile Ophthalmic Solution USP 4% (Infrequent) ⊙248
Mintezol 2002
▲ Neumega for Injection (19% to 58%) 3433
Pepcid Injection (Infrequent) 2017
Pepcid (Infrequent) 2014
▲ Rēv-Eyes Ophthalmic Eyedrops 0.5% (80%) ⊙256
▲ Visudyne for Injection (1% to 10%) 2286
▲ Zaditor Ophthalmic Solution (10% to 25%) 2302

Conjunctival irritation

▲ Brimonidine Tartrate Ophthalmic Solution 0.2% (3% to 9%) ⊙245
Efudex (Infrequent) 3348
▲ Zymar Ophthalmic Solution (5% to 10%) 571

Conjunctival microhemorrhage

Brimonidine Tartrate Ophthalmic Solution 0.2% (Less than 3%) ⊙245

Conjunctivitis

Abilify Tablets (Frequent) 916
Abilify Tablets (Frequent) 2472
Accutane Capsules 2740
Aceon Tablets (2 mg, 4 mg, 8 mg) (0.3% to 1%) 3191
Actiq (1% or greater) 993
▲ Actonel Tablets (3.1%) 2679
▲ Actonel with Calcium Tablets (3.1%) 2684
Adalat CC Tablets (Less than 1%) 2978
Adriamycin for Injection, USP (Rare) 786
Adriamycin Injection, USP (Rare) 786
▲ Advair Diskus 100/50 (1% to 3%) 1291
▲ Advair Diskus 250/50 (1% to 3%) 1291
▲ Advair Diskus 500/50 (1% to 3%) 1291
Aldara Cream, 5% (0.5%) 1814
Alphagan P Ophthalmic Solution (1% to 4%) 563
Alrex Ophthalmic Suspension 0.2% (Less than 5%) ⊙243
Ambien Tablets (Rare) 2867
AmBisome for Injection (Less common) 615
Amnesteem Capsules 2126
Anaprox Tablets (Less than 1%) 2769
Anaprox DS Tablets (Less than 1%) 2769
Antara Capsules 2723
▲ Arava Tablets (1% to 3%) 2881
Arthrotec Tablets (Rare) 3126
Asacol Delayed-Release Tablets (1% to 2%) 2688
Astelin Nasal Spray (Infrequent) 1876
Atacand HCT (0.5% or greater) 637
Atrovent Nasal Spray 0.03% (Less than 2%) 869
Atrovent Nasal Spray 0.06% (Less than 1%) 870
Attenuvax 1889
Avalide Tablets 922
Avalide Tablets 2889
Avapro Tablets (Less than 1%) 925
Avapro Tablets (Less than 1%) 2886
Axert Tablets (Rare) 2430
Azopt Ophthalmic Suspension (Less than 1%) 553
Betimol Ophthalmic Solution ⊙283
Betimol Ophthalmic Solution 3371
BiDil Tablets 2161
Buprenex Injectable (Less than 1%) 2718
Caduet Tablets (Greater than 0.1% to less than or equal to 1%) 2507
Carbatrol Capsules 3174
Cardene I.V. (Rare) 1129
Cataflam Tablets (Rarely) 2173
Celebrex Capsules (0.1% to 1.9%) 3130
Celexa (Infrequent) 1177
▲ CellCept Capsules (3% to less than 20%) 2751
▲ CellCept Intravenous (3% to less than 20%) 2751
▲ CellCept Oral Suspension (3% to less than 20%) 2751
▲ CellCept Tablets (3% to less than 20%) 2751
Cialis Tablets (Less than 2%) 1806
Clinoril Tablets (Less than 1 in 100) 1899
Colazal Capsules 2845
Comvax 1904
Copaxone for Injection (At least 2%) 3292
Cosopt Sterile Ophthalmic Solution (1% to 5%) 1910
Cozaar Tablets (Less than 1%) 1913
DDAVP Nasal Spray (Up to 2%) 2894
Depacon Injection (1% or more) 412
Depakene (1% or more) 417
Depakote Sprinkle Capsules 422
▲ Depakote Tablets (1% to 5%) 427
Depakote ER Tablets (Greater than 1%) 433
Desmopressin Acetate Rhinal Tube (Up to 2%) 1144
Differin Cream (Less than 1%) 1210
▲ Doxil Injection (1% to 10%) 3302
EC-Naprosyn Delayed-Release Tablets (Less than 1%) 2769
Effexor Tablets (Infrequent) 3405
Effexor XR Capsules (Infrequent) 3411
Ellence Injection (0% to 14.8%) 2632
Elmiron Capsules (Less than or equal to 1%) 2393
▲ Eloxatin for Injection (2% to 9%) 2908
Engerix-B Vaccine 1391
Equetro Extended-Release Capsules 3178
▲ Erbitux (7%) 937
▲ Evoxac Capsules (4.3%) 1042
Ferrlecit Injection 3379
Flonase Nasal Spray 1412
▲ Flovent Diskus 50 mcg (1% to 3%) 1415
Flumist Vaccine 1872
FML Ophthalmic Ointment (Occasional) ⊙225
FML Ophthalmic Suspension (Occasional) ⊙224
FML Forte Ophthalmic Suspension (Occasional) ⊙223
FML-S Liquifilm Sterile Ophthalmic Suspension ⊙226
▲ Fortical Nasal Spray (1% to 3%) 3336
Frova Tablets (Infrequent) 1101
Fuzeon Injection (2%) 2772
Gabitril Tablets (1% or more) 998
Gengraf Capsules (1% to less than 3%) 458
▲ Genoptic Sterile Ophthalmic Solution (Among most frequent) ⊙227
Geodon Capsules (Infrequent) 2514
Gleevec Tablets (Less common) 2221
Hectorol Capsules 909
Hectorol Injection 911
HMS Sterile Ophthalmic Suspension ⊙228
Hytrin Capsules (At least 1%) 469
Hyzaar 1964
▲ Imdur Tablets (Less than or equal to 5%) 3032
Imitrex Injection 1431
Imitrex Nasal Spray 1435
Indapamide Tablets (Less than 5%) 2119
▲ Infergen (4% to 8%) 1647
▲ Intron A for Injection (Less than 5%) 3038
Iressa Tablets (2%) 684
Kadian Capsules (Less than 3%) 572
Lamictal (Infrequent) 1449
Levaquin in 5% Dextrose Injection (0.1% to 0.9%) 2453
Levaquin (0.1% to 0.9%) 2453
Levitra Tablets (Less than 2%) 3048
Lexapro Oral Solution (Infrequent) 1193
Lexapro Tablets (Infrequent) 1193
Lofibra Capsules 1217
Lotemax Ophthalmic Suspension 0.5% (Less than 5%) ⊙249
Lotensin HCT Tablets (0.3% or more) 2235
Lunesta Tablets (Infrequent) 3139
Lupron Depot 3.75 mg (Less than 5%) 3257
Lupron Depot–3 Month 11.25 mg (Less than 5%) 3262
Luxíq Foam (One patient) 1026
Lyrica Capsules (Greater than or equal to 1%) 2524
Marinol Capsules (0.3% to 1%) 3334
Meruvax II 1994
Miacalcin Nasal Spray (1% to 3%) 2242
Micardis Tablets (More than 0.3%) 884
Micardis HCT Tablets 886
Migranal Nasal Spray (Infrequent) 3350
Mirapex Tablets (1% or more) 889
M-M-R II 1980
Mobic Oral Suspension (Less than 2%) 893
Mobic Tablets (Less than 2%) 893
Mumpsvax 2005
Namenda (Frequent) 1199
Naprosyn Suspension (Less than 1%) 2769
Naprosyn Tablets (Less than 1%) 2769
Nasonex Nasal Spray (Greater than or equal to 2%) 3058
Neoral Soft Gelatin Capsules (1% to less than 3%) 2247
Neoral Oral Solution (1% to less than 3%) 2247
Neurontin Capsules (1.2%) 2498
Neurontin Oral Solution (1.2%) 2498
Neurontin Tablets (1.2%) 2498
Nexium Delayed-Release Capsules (Less than 1%) 645
Nexium I.V. (Less than 1%) 649
▲ Nipent for Injection (4%) 3216
Norvasc Tablets (More than 0.1% to 1%) 2529
Omnicef Capsules 506
Omnicef for Oral Suspension 506
OptiPranolol Metipranolol Ophthalmic Solution 0.3% (A small number of patients) ⊙254
▲ Optivar Ophthalmic Solution (1% to 10%) 1877
Orthoclone OKT3 Sterile Solution 2370
Ovide .5% Lotion 3287
Paxil CR Controlled-Release Tablets (Infrequent) 1509
Paxil (Infrequent) 1501
▲ PEG-Intron Powder for Injection (4%) 3062
Pentasa Capsules (Less than 1%) 3182
Permax Tablets (Infrequent) 3357
Plavix Tablets (1% to 2.5%) 940
Plavix Tablets (1% to 2.5%) 2942
Pletal Tablets (Less than 2%) 2478
Poly-Pred Liquifilm Ophthalmic Suspension ⊙231
Pred Forte Ophthalmic Suspension (Occasional) ⊙233
Pred Mild Sterile Ophthalmic Suspension (Occasional) ⊙236
Prevacid Delayed-Release Capsules (Less than 1%) 3268
Prevacid for Delayed-Release Oral Suspension (Less than 1%) 3268
Prevacid NapraPAC (Less than 1%) 3277
Prevacid SoluTab Delayed-Release Orally Disintegrating Tablets (Less than 1%) 3268
Prevnar for Injection 3460
PREVPAC (Less than 1%) 3281
Prochieve 4% Gel 1018
Prochieve 8% Gel 1018
▲ Proleukin for Injection (4%) 1007
Protopic Ointment (2% to 4%) 629
Provigil Tablets (Greater than or equal to 1%) 1002
Prozac Pulvules and Liquid (Infrequent) 1771
Pulmicort Respules (Less than 1% to 4%) 654
Pulmozyme Inhalation Solution (1% to 5%) 1245
▲ Rapamune Oral Solution and Tablets (3% to 20%) 3472
▲ Rebetol (4% to 5%) 3073
Recombivax HB 2045
Relpax Tablets (Infrequent) 2531
Requip Tablets (Infrequent) 1528
Rescriptor Tablets 2535
▲ Ribavirin, USP Capsules (4% to 5%) 3083
Risperdal Consta Long-Acting Injection (Infrequent) 1664
▲ Rituxan for Infusion (1% to 5%) 845
▲ Rituxan I.V. (1% to 5%) 1251
▲ Roferon-A Injection (4%) 2805
Sandimmune (2% or less) 2259
Serevent Diskus (1% to 3%) 1540
Seroquel Tablets (Infrequent) 691
▲ Simulect for Injection (3% to 10%) 2268
Singulair (Greater than or equal to 2%) 2047
Sonata Capsules (Frequent) 1686
▲ Soriatane Capsules (1% to 10%) 1028
Stromectol Tablets 2053
Sular Tablets (Less than or equal to 1%) 1163
Suprane Liquid for Inhalation (Greater than 1%) 770
Symbyax Capsules (Infrequent) 1788
Synagis (More than 1%) 1868
Tamiflu Capsules (1%) 2810
Tamiflu Oral Suspension (1%) 2810
▲ Tarceva Tablets (0% to 12%) 1254
▲ Tarceva Tablets (0% to 12%) 2470
Targretin Capsules 1719
Taxotere Injection Concentrate 2947
Tegretol/Tegretol-XR 2278
Teveten Tablets (Less than 1%) 1707
Teveten HCT Tablets (Less than 1%) 1710
Tiazac Capsules (2%) 1204
Timoptic in Ocudose (Less frequent) 2061
Timoptic Sterile Ophthalmic Solution (Less frequent) 2058
Timoptic-XE Sterile Ophthalmic Gel Forming Solution (1% to 5%) 2062
Topamax Sprinkle Capsules (1% to 2%) 2438
Topamax Tablets (1% to 2%) 2438
Travatan Ophthalmic Solution (1% to 4%) 559
Trelstar LA Suspension (1.1%) 3387
Tricor Tablets 523
Trizivir Tablets 1565
Trusopt Sterile Ophthalmic Solution (Approximately 1% to 5%) 2065
Twinrix Vaccine 1571
Ultane Liquid for Inhalation (Less than 1%) 526
Uniretic Tablets (Less than 1%) 3114
Vaqta (1.3%) 2067
Vaseretic Tablets 2073
Vasotec I.V. Injection (0.5% to 1.0%) 2076
VFEND I.V. (Less than 2%) 2543
VFEND Oral Suspension (Less than 2%) 2543
VFEND Tablets (Less than 2%) 2543
Viagra Tablets (Less than 2%) 2552
▲ Vigamox Ophthalmic Solution (1% to 6%) 560
Viramune Oral Suspension 903
Viramune Tablets 903
Virazole for Inhalation Solution 3365
▲ Visudyne for Injection (1% to 10%) 2286
▲ Voltaren Ophthalmic Solution (Less than or equal to 5%) 2300
Voltaren Tablets (Rarely) 2298
Voltaren-XR Tablets (Rarely) 2301
Xalatan Sterile Ophthalmic Solution (Less than 1%) 2654
▲ Xeloda Tablets (Less than 5%) 2825
Zaditor Ophthalmic Solution (Less than 5%) 2302
Ziagen 1600
Zithromax Capsules, 250 mg (1% or less) 2568
Zithromax for Oral Suspension, 300 mg, 600 mg, 900 mg, 1200 mg (1% or less) 2561
Zithromax Tablets, 250 mg, 500 mg (1% or less) 2561
Zithromax Tri-Pak (1% or less) 2561
Zoloft (Infrequent) 2581
Zomig Nasal Spray (Rare) 718
Zonegran Capsules (Infrequent) 1089
▲ Zymar Ophthalmic Solution (5% to 10%) 571
Zyprexa Tablets 1798
Zyprexa ZYDIS Orally Disintegrating Tablets 1798
Zyrtec Chewable Tablets (Less than 2%) 2589
Zyrtec (Less than 2%) 2589
Zyrtec-D 12 Hour Extended Release Tablets (Less than 2%) 2591

Conjunctivitis, allergic

▲ Alphagan P Ophthalmic Solution (Approximately 10% to 20%) 563
▲ Lumigan Ophthalmic Solution (1% to 3%) 569

Conjunctivitis, calcific

Calcijex Injection 411

Conjunctivitis, follicular

▲ Alphagan P Ophthalmic Solution (Approximately 5% to 9%) 563
Propine Ophthalmic Solution ⊙237

Conjunctivitis, hemorrhagic
Alphagan P Ophthalmic Solution (1% to 4%) 563

Conjunctivitis, nonspecific
▲ Keppra Oral Solution (3%) 3307
▲ Keppra Tablets (3%) 3307

Conjunctivitis sicca
Cymbalta Delayed-Release Capsules (Infrequent) 1729
Thyrolar 1203

Consciousness, decreased
Abilify Tablets (Infrequent) 916
Abilify Tablets (Infrequent) 2472
Ammonul Injection 3323
Xanax XR Tablets (Infrequent) 2655

Consciousness, disorders of
Amerge Tablets (Rare) 1312
Comtan Tablets 2186
Hexalen Capsules 2101
▲ Intron A for Injection (Less than 5%) 3038
Neoral Soft Gelatin Capsules 2247
Neoral Oral Solution 2247
Permax Tablets 3357
Sandimmune 2259
Symmetrel (Uncommon) 1115
Tasmar Tablets (Four cases) 3360
Valtrex Caplets 1573
Zovirax 1616

Consciousness, loss of
Acthrel for Injection (Two patients) 3528
Carimune NF 3501
Cipro I.V. (1% or less) 2998
Cipro I.V. Pharmacy Bulk Package (1% or less) 3509
Cipro 2991
Cipro XR Tablets 3004
Effexor Tablets (Rare) 3405
Effexor XR Capsules (Rare) 3411
Ferrlecit Injection 3379
Gammagard Liquid 751
Gammagard S/D (Rare) 754
Gamunex Immune Globulin I.V., 10% (Rare) 3232
Hyperstat I.V. Injection 3031
Infed Injection 3381
Invirase (Less than 2%) 2776
Iveegam EN (Rare) 759
Levaquin in 5% Dextrose Injection 2453
Levaquin 2453
Lidoderm Patch 1107
Naropin Injection 640
Neumega for Injection 3433
Noroxin Tablets 2009
Omnicef Capsules 506
Omnicef for Oral Suspension 506
Orthoclone OKT3 Sterile Solution 2370
PEG-Intron Powder for Injection (Less than or equal to 1%) 3062
Taxotere Injection Concentrate 2947
▲ Vesanoid Capsules (3%) 2823
▲ Xeloda Tablets (Less than 5%) 2825

Constipation
▲ Abilify Tablets (11% to 13%) 916
▲ Abilify Tablets (11% to 13%) 2472
Aceon Tablets (2 mg, 4 mg, 8 mg) (0.3% to 1%) 3191
Aciphex Tablets 1081
Actiq (1% to 4%) 993
▲ Actonel Tablets (6.6% to 12.2%) 2679
▲ Actonel with Calcium Tablets (12.2% to 12.5%) 2684
▲ Adalat CC Tablets (1% to 3%) 2978
Adderall Tablets 3168
▲ Adderall XR Capsules (2% to 4%) 3169
Adipex-P 1216
▲ Advair Diskus 100/50 (1% to 3%) 1291
▲ Advair Diskus 250/50 (1% to 3%) 1291
▲ Advair Diskus 500/50 (1% to 3%) 1291
Advicor Tablets 1694
Aerobid/Aerobid-M (1% to 3%) 1172
Agrylin Capsules (1% to 5%) 3172
Alacol DM Syrup 739
Aldoclor Tablets 1881
Aldoril Tablets 1884
Alferon N Injection (One patient) 1640
▲ Alimta for Injection (Up to 44%) 1722
Alinia for Oral Suspension (Less than 1%) 2840
Alinia Tablets (Less than 1%) 2840
Aloprim for Injection (Less than 1%) 2156
▲ Aloxi Injection (5%) 2099
Altace Capsules (Less than 1%) 1673
▲ Altoprev Extended-Release Tablets (2% to 3.5%) 1151
Ambien Tablets (Infrequent) 2867
AmBisome for Injection (Less common) 615
Amerge Tablets (Infrequent) 1312
▲ Anaprox Tablets (3% to 9%) 2769
▲ Anaprox DS Tablets (3% to 9%) 2769
Antara Capsules (2.1%) 2723
Anzemet Injection (Rare) 2871
Anzemet Tablets (Rare) 2874
▲ Apokyn Injection (At least 5%) 2132
▲ Aranesp for Injection (5% to 18%) 576
▲ Arava Tablets (1% to 3%) 2881
▲ Aredia for Injection (33.2%) 2168
▲ Arimidex Tablets (7% to 9%) 665
▲ Arixtra Injection (1.8% to 8.5%) 1325
▲ Aromasin Tablets (5%) 2600
Arthrotec Tablets (Rare) 3126
▲ Asacol Delayed-Release Tablets (5%) 2688
Astelin Nasal Spray (Infrequent) 1876
Atacand HCT 637
Atrovent HFA Inhalation Aerosol 872
Atrovent Inhalation Solution (0.9%) 868
Atrovent Nasal Spray 0.03% 869
Atrovent Nasal Spray 0.06% 870
Avalide Tablets 922
Avalide Tablets 2889
Avapro Tablets (Less than 1%) 925
Avapro Tablets (Less than 1%) 2886
▲ Avastin IV (4%) 1229
Avelox (Less than 0.1%) 2984
▲ Avinza Capsules (Greater than 10%) 1714
Axid Oral Solution (2.5%) 913
Bentyl Capsules 724
Bentyl Injection 724
Bentyl Syrup 724
Bentyl Tablets 724
▲ Betaseron for SC Injection (20%) 791
▲ Bexxar (1% to 6%) 1360
▲ Boniva Tablets (2.5% to 4%) 2747
Bravelle for Intramuscular or Subcutaneous Injection (2% to 2.7%) 1140
Brevibloc Concentrate (Less than 1%) 766
Brevibloc Injection (Less than 1%) 766
Brevibloc Double Strength Injection (Less than 1%) 766
Brevibloc Premixed Injection (Less than 1%) 766
Brevibloc Double Strength Premixed Injection (Less than 1%) 766
Buphenyl Powder (One patient) 3327
Buphenyl Tablets (One patient) 3327
Buprenex Injectable (Less than 1%) 2718
Caduet Tablets (Greater than 0.1% to 2.5%) 2507
Calcijex Injection 411
▲ Campath Ampules (1% to 9%) 826
Campral Tablets (Frequent) 1175
▲ Camptosar Injection (0.4% to 32.3%) 2602
Captopril Tablets (About 0.5% to 2%) 2114
Carafate Suspension (2%) 727
Carafate Tablets (2%) 728
Carbatrol Capsules 3174
Cardizem LA Extended Release Tablets (Less than 2%) 1699
▲ Carnitor Injection (3%) 3185
▲ Casodex Tablets (17%) 670
▲ Cataflam Tablets (1% to 10%) 2173
▲ Catapres Tablets (About 10 in 100 patients) 874
Catapres-TTS (1 of 101 patients) 875
Celebrex Capsules (0.1% to 1.9%) 3130
Celexa (At least 2%) 1177
▲ CellCept Capsules (18.5% to 41.2%) 2751
▲ CellCept Intravenous (18.5% to 41.2%) 2751
▲ CellCept Oral Suspension (18.5% to 41.2%) 2751
▲ CellCept Tablets (18.5% to 41.2%) 2751
▲ Cenestin Tablets, 0.45mg, 0.625mg, 0.9mg, 1.25mg (6%) 1063
Chromagen Soft Gelatin Capsules 3296
Chromagen Forte Soft Gelatin Capsules 3296
Cipro I.V. (1% or less) 2998
Cipro I.V. Pharmacy Bulk Package (1% or less) 3509
Cipro 2991
Cipro XR Tablets (Less than 1%) 3004
Clindesse Vaginal Cream (1.1%) 3296
▲ Clinoril Tablets (3% to 9%) 1899
▲ Clolar for Intravenous Infusion (21%) 1264
▲ Clorpres Tablets (About 10%) 2139
▲ Clozapine Tablets (More than 5% to 14%) 2141
▲ Clozaril Tablets (More than 5% to 25%) 2174
Cogentin Injection 1903
Colazal Capsules (1%) 2845
▲ CombiPatch Transdermal System (2% to 5%) 2180
Combivent Inhalation Aerosol 878
▲ Combunox Tablets (Less than 1% to 4.5%) 1183
▲ Comtan Tablets (6%) 2186
Copaxone for Injection (At least 2%) 3292
▲ Covera-HS Tablets (7.2% to 11.7%) 3135
Cozaar Tablets (Less than 1%) 1913
▲ Creon 5 Capsules (Among most frequent) 3195
▲ Creon 10 Capsules (Among most frequent) 3195
▲ Creon 20 Capsules (Among most frequent) 3196
Crestor Tablets (Greater than or equal to 2%) 672
▲ Cubicin for Injection (6.2%) 1038
▲ Cymbalta Delayed-Release Capsules (11%) 1729
Cytovene (At least 3 subjects) 2763
Dalmane Capsules 3343
Dantrium Capsules (Less frequent) 2690
Daranide Tablets 1928
Darvocet A 500 Tablets 3497
▲ Depacon Injection (Up to 5%) 412
▲ Depakene (5%) 417
▲ Depakote Sprinkle Capsules (5%) 422
▲ Depakote Tablets (1% to 5%) 427
▲ Depakote ER Tablets (5%) 433
▲ DepoCyt Injection (7%) 1121
▲ DepoDur Extended-Release Injection (Greater than 10%) 1098
Desoxyn Tablets, USP 2482
▲ Detrol Tablets (6.5%) 2626
▲ Detrol LA Capsules (6%) 2629
Dexedrine 1386
DextroStat Tablets 3177
Diastat Rectal Delivery System (Infrequent) 3344
Dilaudid 439
Dilaudid Oral Liquid 443
Dilaudid Non-Sterile Powder 439
Dilaudid Rectal Suppositories 439
Dilaudid Tablets 439
Dilaudid Tablets - 8 mg 443
Dilaudid-HP (Less frequent) 441
Diovan HCT Tablets (Greater than 0.2%) 2195
Diovan Tablets 2191
▲ Ditropan XL Extended Release Tablets (7% to 13%) 2391
Diuril Oral 1936
Diuril Sodium Intravenous 1934
Dolobid Tablets (Greater than 1 in 100) 1937
▲ Dostinex Tablets (7% to 10%) 2631
▲ Doxil Injection (1% to 30.1%) 3302
DuoNeb Inhalation Solution (More than 1%) 1058
▲ Duragesic Transdermal System (10% or more) 2448
Dyazide Capsules 1389
DynaCirc CR Tablets (1.2% to 3.8%) 2726
▲ EC-Naprosyn Delayed-Release Tablets (3% to 9%) 2769
▲ Effexor Tablets (15%) 3405
▲ Effexor XR Capsules (5% to 10%) 3411
Eldepryl Capsules 3209
Elidel Cream 1% (0.4% to 3.4%) 2198
Eligard 7.5 mg (Less than 2%) 2896
▲ Elitek (20%) 2906
Elmiron Capsules (Less than or equal to 1%) 2393
▲ Eloxatin for Injection (22% to 32%) 2908
▲ Emend Capsules (10.3%) 1944
▲ Enablex Extended-Release Tablets (14.8% to 21.3%) 2201
Engerix-B Vaccine (Less than 1%) 1391
▲ Epogen for Injection (42% to 43%) 586
▲ Equetro Extended-Release Capsules (5%) 3178
▲ Erbitux (28%) 937
Estrogel 0.06% 3200
▲ Evoxac Capsules (1% to 3%) 1042
▲ Exelon Capsules (5%) 2204
Factive Tablets (0.1% to 1%) 2464
▲ Famvir Tablets (1.4% to 4.4%) 2207
▲ Faslodex Injection (12%) 682
▲ FazaClo Orally Disintegrating Tablets (Greater than 5% to 14%) 547
▲ Femara Tablets (0.2% to 11.3%) 2210
Feosol Caplets (Occasional) 1629
Feosol Tablets (Occasional) 1629
▲ Flexeril Tablets (1% to 3%) 1832
▲ Flolan for Injection (4% to 6%) 1408
Flomax Capsules (Infrequent) 881
Flumadine 1186
▲ Follistim AQ Cartridge (5%) 2354
▲ Forteo for Injection (5.4%) 1739
▲ Fortical Nasal Spray (1% to 3%) 3336
▲ Fosamax (Up to 3.1%) 1949
▲ Fosamax Plus D Tablets (0% to 3.1%) 1956
▲ Fosrenol Chewable Tablets (6% to 14%) 3180
Frova Tablets (Infrequent) 1101
Furosemide Tablets 2117
▲ Fuzeon Injection (3.9%) 2772
Gabitril Tablets (1% or more) 998
▲ Gemzar for Injection (10% to 31%) 1743
Gengraf Capsules (1% to less than 3%) 458
▲ Geodon (9%) 2514
▲ Gleevec Tablets (9% to 16%) 2221
Gonal-f RFF Pen for Injection (2.4%) 3155
▲ Hectorol Capsules (3.3% to greater than or equal to 5%) 909
▲ Hectorol Injection (3.3%) 911
▲ Hycamtin for Injection (Less than 1% to 39%) 1427
Hycodan 1104
Hyperstat I.V. Injection 3031
Hytrin Capsules (At least 1%) 469
Hyzaar 1964
▲ Imdur Tablets (Less than or equal to 5%) 3032
Imitrex Nasal Spray (Infrequent) 1435
Imitrex Tablets (Infrequent) 1440
Imodium Capsules 1834
Indapamide Tablets (Less than 5%) 2119
Inderal LA Long-Acting Capsules 3421
Indocin Capsules (Greater than 1%) 1968
Indocin I.V. (1% to 3%) 1973
Indocin (Greater than 1%) 1968
▲ Infergen (5% to 9%) 1647
▲ InnoPran XL Capsules (1% to 3%) 2728
▲ Intron A for Injection (Up to 10%) 3038
▲ Invanz for Injection (2.3% to 4%) 1974
Inversine Tablets 3286
Invirase (Greater than or equal to 2%) 2776
▲ I.V. Busulfex (35% to 38%) 1125
▲ Kadian Capsules (Virtually all patients) 572
Kaletra (Less than 2%) 474
▲ Keppra Oral Solution (1% to 3%) 3307
▲ Keppra Tablets (1% to 3%) 3307
Ketek Tablets (Greater than or equal to 0.2% to less than 2%) 2920
Klonopin (2%) 2782
Kogenate FS 3517
▲ Kytril Injection (3%) 2785
▲ Kytril Tablets (3% to 18%) 2788
▲ Lamictal (4%) 1449
▲ Lescol Capsules (3.1%) 2227
Lescol XL Tablets (2.3%) 2227
▲ Leukine (8%) 829
▲ Leustatin Injection (9%) 2368
▲ Levaquin in 5% Dextrose Injection (0.1% to 3.1%) 2453
▲ Levaquin (0.1% to 3.1%) 2453
▲ Lexapro Oral Solution (3% to 6%) 1193
▲ Lexapro Tablets (3% to 6%) 1193
Librium Capsules 3349
Lipitor Tablets (Up to 2.5%) 2495
Lofibra Capsules (2.1%) 1217
Lortab 3315
Lortab Elixir 3312
Lotensin Tablets (Less than 1%) 2232
Lotensin HCT Tablets (0.3% to 1%) 2235
Lotrel Capsules 2238
▲ Lotronex Tablets (29%) 1479
▲ Lyrica Capsules (1% to 7%) 2524
Matulane Capsules 3188
Mavik Tablets (0.3% to 1.0%) 482
Maxalt Tablets (Infrequent) 1983
Maxalt-MLT Orally Disintegrating Tablets (Infrequent) 1983
Maxzide 2150
Mebaral Tablets, USP (Less than 1 in 100 patients) 2483
▲ Megace ES Oral Suspension (1% to 3%) 2492
Menopur for Subcutaneous Injection (1.6%) 1145
▲ Menostar Transdermal System (5%) 805
▲ Mepron Suspension (3%) 1487
▲ Meridia Capsules (11.5%) 485
▲ Merrem I.V. (1.4% to 7%) 687
▲ Mevacor Tablets (2.0% to 4.9%) 1996
Miacalcin Nasal Spray (1% to 3%) 2242
Micardis Tablets (More than 0.3%) 884
Micardis HCT Tablets 886
▲ Midamor Tablets (Between 1% and 3%) 2000
▲ Mirapex Tablets (10% to 14%) 889
Moban Tablets 1108

Mobic Oral Suspension (0.8% to 1.8%) 893
Mobic Tablets (0.8% to 1.8%) 893
Moduretic Tablets (Less than or equal to 1%) 2003
▲ MS Contin Tablets (Less frequent to among most frequent) 2703
Mycamine for Injection (0.2%) 620
▲ Myfortic Tablets (3% to 38%) 2244
▲ Mylotarg for Injection (23%) 3429
Nadolol Tablets (1 to 5 of 1000 patients) 2121
▲ Nalfon Capsules (7%) 2504
▲ Namenda (5%) 1199
▲ Naprosyn Suspension (3% to 9%) 2769
▲ Naprosyn Tablets (3% to 9%) 2769
▲ Navelbine Injection (Up to 35%) 1494
Nembutal Sodium Solution, USP (Less than 1%) 2484
Neoral Soft Gelatin Capsules (1% to less than 3%) 2247
Neoral Oral Solution (1% to less than 3%) 2247
▲ Neulasta Injection (15% to 72%) 596
▲ Neumega for Injection (Greater than or equal to 10%) 3433
▲ Neupogen for Injection (5%) 598
Neurontin Capsules (1.5% to 3.9%) 2498
Neurontin Oral Solution (1.5% to 3.9%) 2498
Neurontin Tablets (1.5% to 3.9%) 2498
Nexium Delayed-Release Capsules (Greater than or equal to 1%) 645
Nexium I.V. (Greater than or equal to 1%) 649
Nicotrol NS 2596
Niferex-150 Forte Capsules 3299
Nipent for Injection (Less than 3%) 3216
▲ Niravam Orally Disintegrating Tablets (10.4% to 26.2%) 3106
Norflex Injection 1824
Noroxin Tablets (0.3% to 1.0%) 2009
Norvasc Tablets (More than 0.1% to 1%) 2529
Norvir (0% to 0.7%) 499
▲ Novantrone for Injection Concentrate (10% to 14%) 3158
Numorphan 1112
Omacor Capsules 2735
Omnicef Capsules (0.3%) 506
Omnicef for Oral Suspension (0.3%) 506
Oncaspar (Less than 1%) 1123
▲ Ontak Vials (9%) 1717
▲ Orap Tablets (4 of 20 patients) 1220
▲ OxyContin Tablets (23%) 2699
OxyFast Oral Concentrate Solution 2704
OxyIR Capsules 2704
▲ Oxytrol Transdermal System (3.3%) 3383
▲ Pacerone Tablets (4% to 9%) 3337
▲ Pancrease MT Capsules (Among most frequent) 1839
Parcopa Orally Disintegrating Tablets 3111
Parnate Tablets 1499
▲ Paxil CR Controlled-Release Tablets (1.1% to 16%) 1509
▲ Paxil (1.1% to 16%) 1501
PEG-Intron Powder for Injection (1%) 3062
Pentasa Capsules (Less than 1%) 3182
Pepcid Injection (1.2%) 2017
Pepcid (1.2%) 2014
Percocet Tablets 1114
Percodan Tablets 1115
▲ Permax Tablets (10.6%; frequent) 3357
Phenytek Capsules 2153
PhosLo GelCaps 2158
▲ Photofrin for Injection (17% to 24%) 729
Plavix Tablets (1% to 2.5%) 940
Plavix Tablets (1% to 2.5%) 2942
Plendil Extended-Release Tablets (0.3% to 1.5%) 651
▲ Prandin Tablets (0.5, 1, and 2 mg) (2% to 3%) 2337
▲ Pravachol Tablets (2.4% to 4.0%) 943
Prevacid Delayed-Release Capsules (1%) 3268
Prevacid for Delayed-Release Oral Suspension (1%) 3268
▲ Prevacid NapraPAC (1% to 9%) 3277
Prevacid SoluTab Delayed-Release Orally Disintegrating Tablets (1%) 3268
PREVPAC (1%) 3281
Prilosec OTC Tablets (1.1% to 1.5%) 2674
Prinivil Tablets (0.3% to 1.0%) 2029
Prinzide Tablets (0.3% to 1%) 2033
▲ Prochieve 4% Gel (27%) 1018
▲ Prochieve 8% Gel (27%) 1018
▲ Procrit for Injection (42% to 53%) 2374
▲ Prograf Capsules and Injection (23% to 35%) 624
▲ Proleukin for Injection (5%) 1007
Prometrium Capsules (100 mg, 200 mg) (Less than 5%) 3205
ProSom Tablets (Frequent) 512
Protonix I.V. (Greater than or equal to 1%) 3468
Protonix Tablets (Greater than or equal to 1%) 3465
Protopic Ointment (Greater than or equal to 1%) 629
Provigil Tablets (2%) 1002
▲ Prozac Pulvules and Liquid (5%) 1771
▲ Rapamune Oral Solution and Tablets (28% to 38%) 3472
Razadyne ER Extended-Release Capsules (Greater than or equal to 2%) 2434
Razadyne (Greater than or equal to 2%) 2434
▲ Rebetol (5%) 3073
Recombivax HB 2045
ReFacto Vials 3479
▲ Relafen Tablets (3% to 9%) 1523
Relpax Tablets (Infrequent) 2531
Remicade for IV Injection (Greater than or equal to 0.2%) 987
▲ Renagel Tablets (2% to 8.1%) 1268
ReoPro Vials (0.3%) 1779
Repliva 21/7 Tablets 3301
▲ Requip Tablets (6%) 1528
Rescriptor Tablets 2535
▲ Retrovir Capsules (6.4%) 1533
▲ Retrovir IV Infusion (6.4%) 1537
▲ Retrovir (6.4%) 1533
Reyataz Capsules (Less than 3%) 948
▲ Ribavirin, USP Capsules (5%) 3083
Rilutek Tablets (More than 2%) 2945
▲ Risperdal Consta Long-Acting Injection (5% to 7%) 1664
▲ Risperdal M-Tab Orally Disintegrating Tablets (7% to 13%) 1658
▲ Risperdal (7% to 13%) 1658
▲ Rythmol SR Capsules (8% to 14%) 2736
▲ Sanctura Tablets (9.6%) 1133
Sandimmune (Rare) 2259
▲ Sandostatin Injection (Less than 10%) 2263
▲ Sandostatin LAR Depot (18.8%) 2264
Sedapap Tablets 50 mg/650 mg (Infrequent) 2098
▲ Seroquel Tablets (8%) 691
▲ Simulect for Injection (Greater than or equal to 10%) 2268
Sonata Capsules (Frequent) 1686
Soriatane Capsules (Less than 1%) 1028
Spectracef Tablets (0.1% to 1%) 2706
▲ Spiriva HandiHaler (1% to 4%) 899
▲ Stalevo Tablets (6%) 2270
▲ Strattera Capsules (Less than 1% to 10%) 1784
Stromectol Tablets (0.9%) 2053
▲ Suboxone Tablets (11% to 12.1%) 2719
▲ Subutex Tablets (7.8% to 11%) 2719
Surmontil Capsules 2347
Sustiva Capsules 957
Symmetrel (1% to 5%) 1115
Synercid I.V. (Less than 1%) 1690
▲ Tambocor Tablets (4.4%) 1824
Targretin Capsules 1719
▲ Tarka Tablets (3.3%) 519
▲ Tasmar Tablets (6% to 8%) 3360
Taxotere Injection Concentrate 2947
Tegretol/Tegretol-XR 2278
▲ Temodar Capsules (22% to 33%) 3088
▲ Tequin Injection (0.1% to 3%) 964
▲ Tequin Tablets (0.1% to 3%) 964
Tessalon Capsules 1202
Tessalon Perles 1202
Teveten Tablets (Less than 1%) 1707
Teveten HCT Tablets (Less than 1%) 1710
▲ Thalomid Capsules (4.2%) 979
Thioridazine Hydrochloride Tablets 2122
Thiothixene Capsules (Infrequently) 2124
Tiazac Capsules (Less than 2%) 1204
Timolide Tablets (Less than 1%) 2056
Tindamax (0.4% to 1.4%) 2670
▲ Topamax Sprinkle Capsules (Greater than 1% to 5%) 2438
▲ Topamax Tablets (Greater than 1% to 5%) 2438
Toprol-XL Tablets (About 1 of 100 patients) 660
▲ Trasylol Injection (4%) 779
Trelstar LA Suspension (1.7%) 3387
Tricor Tablets (2.1%) 523
Triglide Tablets (2.1%) 1165
▲ Trileptal Oral Suspension (2% to 6%) 2281
▲ Trileptal Tablets (2% to 6%) 2281
▲ Trisenox Injection (28%) 983
Tussionex Pennkinetic Extended-Release Suspension 3322
Twinrix Vaccine (Less than 1%) 1571
Tygacil for Injection (2.8%) 3489
Tylenol with Codeine 2461
▲ Ultracet Tablets (6%) 2462
Uniretic Tablets (Less than 1%) 3114
Univasc Tablets (Less than 1%) 3118
Uroxatral Tablets (1% to 2%) 2957
▲ Valcyte Tablets (Less than 5%) 2816
Valium Tablets (Infrequent) 2822
▲ Valtrex Caplets (Less than 1% to 4%) 1573
▲ Vantas (3.5%) 3367
Varivax (Greater than or equal to 1%) 2070
Vaseretic Tablets (0.5% to 2.0%) 2073
Vasotec I.V. Injection (0.5% to 1.0%) 2076
▲ Velcade for Injection (42%) 2102
▲ Verelan PM Capsules (7.3% to 8.8%) 3120
▲ Vesanoid Capsules (17%) 2823
▲ VESIcare Tablets (5.4% to 13.4%) 631
VFEND I.V. (Less than 2%) 2543
VFEND Oral Suspension (Less than 2%) 2543
VFEND Tablets (Less than 2%) 2543
Viadur Implant (Less than 2%) 782
Vicodin Tablets 530
Vicodin ES Tablets 531
Vicodin HP Tablets 532
▲ Vicoprofen Tablets (22%) 533
▲ Visudyne for Injection (1% to 10%) 2286
Vivactil Tablets 2350
▲ Vivelle Transdermal System (1.5% to 6.5%) 2288
▲ Vivelle-Dot Transdermal System (1.5% to 6.5%) 2293
▲ Voltaren Tablets (1% to 10%) 2298
▲ Voltaren-XR Tablets (1% to 10%) 2301
Vytorin 10/10 Tablets 2084
Vytorin 10/10 Tablets 3092
Vytorin 10/20 Tablets 2084
Vytorin 10/20 Tablets 3092
Vytorin 10/40 Tablets 2084
Vytorin 10/40 Tablets 3092
Vytorin 10/80 Tablets 2084
Vytorin 10/80 Tablets 3092
▲ WelChol Tablets (11%) 2855
▲ Wellbutrin Tablets (26.0%) 1579
▲ Wellbutrin SR Sustained-Release Tablets (5% to 10%) 1583
▲ Wellbutrin XL Extended-Release Tablets (5% to 10%) 1588
▲ Xanax XR Tablets (8.1%) 2655
▲ Xeloda Tablets (1% to 14%) 2825
▲ Xifaxan Tablets (3.8%) 2847
Zantac 1597
Zantac Injection 1593
Zantac Injection Pharmacy Bulk Package (Frequency) 1595
Zantac Syrup 1597
▲ Zavesca Capsules (8%) 543
▲ Zegerid Powder for Oral Solution (1.1% to 4.5%) 2972
▲ Zenapax for Injection (Greater than 5%) 2838
Zestoretic Tablets (0.3% to 1%) 701
Zestril Tablets (0.3% to 1.0%) 704
▲ Zevalin Injection (5%) 848
Zithromax Capsules, 250 mg (1% or less) 2568
Zithromax for IV Infusion 2573
Zithromax for Oral Suspension, 300 mg, 600 mg, 900 mg, 1200 mg (1% or less) 2561
Zithromax Tablets, 250 mg, 500 mg (1% or less) 2561
Zithromax Tri-Pak (1% or less) 2561
Zmax for Oral Suspension (Less then 1%) 2577
Zocor Tablets (2.3%) 2078
▲ Zofran Injection (11%) 1607
▲ Zofran (6% to 9%) 1613
▲ Zofran ODT Orally Disintegrating Tablets (6% to 9%) 1613
Zoladex (1% to 5%) 709
Zoladex 3-month 712
▲ Zoloft (1% to 8%) 2581
▲ Zometa for Intravenous Infusion (26.7% to 31%) 2306
Zomig Nasal Spray (Rare) 718
Zomig Tablets (Rare) 714
Zomig-ZMT Tablets (Rare) 714
Zonegran Capsules (2%) 1089
▲ Zosyn (7.7% to 8.4%) 3492
▲ Zyban Sustained-Release Tablets (8%) 1620
Zydone Tablets 1118
▲ Zyprexa Tablets (9% to 11%) 1798
▲ Zyprexa ZYDIS Orally Disintegrating Tablets (9% to 11%) 1798
Zyrtec Chewable Tablets (Less than 2%) 2589
Zyrtec (Less than 2%) 2589
Zyrtec-D 12 Hour Extended Release Tablets (Less than 2%) 2591
Zyvox (2.2%) 2661

Constipation, aggravation of

Nexium Delayed-Release Capsules (Less than 1%) 645
Nexium I.V. (Less than 1%) 649
Sanctura Tablets (1.4%) 1133

Constitutional symptoms, unspecified

▲ Alimta for Injection (1% to 11%) 1722

Constriction, pupillary

(*see under* Miosis)

Constriction, pupils

(*see under* Miosis)

Contact lenses, intolerance

Accutane Capsules 2740
Activella Tablets 2311
Alesse-28 Tablets 3392
Cenestin Tablets, 0.45mg, 0.625mg, 0.9mg, 1.25mg 1063
Cenestin Tablets, 0.3mg 1063
Climara Transdermal System 795
Climara Pro Transdermal System 800
Estratest Tablets 3196
Estratest H.S. Tablets 3196
Estrogel 0.06% 3200
Lo/Ovral-28 Tablets 3423
Menostar Transdermal System 805
Ortho-Cept Tablets 2395
Ortho-Cyclen Tablets 2414
Ortho Evra Transdermal System 2402
Ortho Tri-Cyclen Tablets 2414
Ortho Tri-Cyclen Lo Tablets 2421
Prefest Tablets 1069
Premarin Intravenous 3440
Premarin Tablets 3443
Premarin Vaginal Cream 3449
Premphase Tablets 3452
Prempro Tablets 3452
Seasonale Tablets 1073
Vivelle Transdermal System 2288
Vivelle-Dot Transdermal System 2293
Yasmin 28 Tablets 818

Contusions

▲ Advair Diskus 100/50 (1% to 3%) 1291
▲ Advair Diskus 250/50 (1% to 3%) 1291
▲ Advair Diskus 500/50 (1% to 3%) 1291
▲ Clolar for Intravenous Infusion (11%) 1264
▲ Flovent Diskus 50 mcg (1% to 3%) 1415
Lotronex Tablets (Rare) 1479
▲ Myfortic Tablets (3% to less than 20%) 2244
Vantas (Less than 2%) 3367

Convulsions

Abelcet Injection 1119
Aciphex Tablets 1081
Aggrenox Capsules (1.7%) 855
Alacol DM Syrup 739
Aldara Cream, 5% 1814
Aldoclor Tablets 1881
Aldoril Tablets 1884
Altace Capsules (Less than 1%) 1673
Ambien Tablets 2867
AmBisome for Injection (Less common) 615
Amerge Tablets (Rare) 1312
▲ Ammonul Injection (6%) 3323
Anaprox Tablets (Less than 1%) 2769
Anaprox DS Tablets (Less than 1%) 2769
Aricept Tablets 1086
Aricept ODT Tablets 1086
Arthrotec Tablets (Rare) 3126
Attenuvax (Rare) 1889
Augmentin (Rare) 1331
Augmentin Tablets (Rare) 1334
Augmentin XR Extended-Release Tablets (Rare) 1340
Augmentin ES-600 Powder for Oral Suspension (Rare) 1337
Avelox 2984
Avinza Capsules (Less than 5%) 1714
Balamine DM 739
Betaseron for SC Injection 791
Biaxin/Biaxin XL 402
Biltricide Tablets 2990
Boostrix 1366
Brevibloc Concentrate (Less than 1%) 766
Brevibloc Injection (Less than 1%) 766

Brevibloc Double Strength Injection (Less than 1%) 766
Brevibloc Premixed Injection (Less than 1%) 766
Brevibloc Double Strength Premixed Injection (Less than 1%) 766
Buprenex Injectable (Rare) 2718
Campral Tablets (Infrequent) 1175
Cataflam Tablets (Rarely) 2173
Ceftin for Oral Suspension 1369
▲ CellCept Capsules (3% to less than 20%) 2751
▲ CellCept Intravenous (3% to less than 20%) 2751
▲ CellCept Oral Suspension (3% to less than 20%) 2751
▲ CellCept Tablets (3% to less than 20%) 2751
Cipro I.V. 2998
Cipro I.V. Pharmacy Bulk Package 3509
Cipro 2991
Cipro XR Tablets 3004
Clarinex-D 24-Hour Extended-Release Tablets 3012
Clinoril Tablets (Less than 1%) 1899
▲ Clozapine Tablets (3%) 2141
▲ Clozaril Tablets (3%) 2174
Coreg Tablets (Less than or equal to 0.1%) 1376
Cytovene (At least 3 subjects) 2763
Decadron Phosphate Injection 1931
Decadron Tablets 1929
Depo-Medrol Injectable Suspension 2615
Depo-Medrol Single-Dose Vial 2617
Depo-Provera Contraceptive Injection (Less than 1%) 2619
depo-subQ provera 104 Injectable Suspension 2622
Diastat Rectal Delivery System (Greater than or equal to 1%) 3344
Diprivan Injectable Emulsion (Rare) 676
Ditropan XL Extended Release Tablets (Rare) 2391
Diuril Oral 1936
Diuril Sodium Intravenous 1934
Doxil Injection (Less than 1%) 3302
Duragesic Transdermal System (1% or greater) 2448
EC-Naprosyn Delayed-Release Tablets (Less than 1%) 2769
E.E.S. 449
Effexor Tablets (Infrequent) 3405
Effexor XR Capsules (Infrequent) 3411
Elitek (Less than or equal to 1%) 2906
Epzicom Tablets 1402
Erythrocin Stearate Filmtab Tablets (Rare) 452
Erythromycin Delayed-Release Capsules, USP (Rare) 456
Ethyol for Injection 1869
Evoxac Capsules 1042
Exelon Capsules (Frequent) 2204
▲ FazaClo Orally Disintegrating Tablets (3%) 547
Ferrlecit Injection 3379
Flexeril Tablets (Less than 1%) 1832
▲ Flolan for Injection (4%) 1408
Flumadine (Less than 0.3%) 1186
Fluorescite Injection ⊙207
Gabitril Tablets 998
Garamycin Injectable 3028
Gengraf Capsules 458
Gleevec Tablets (Rare) 2221
Havrix Vaccine (Rare) 1425
Herceptin I.V. (At least one of the 958 patients) 1234
HibTITER 3419
Hydrocortone Tablets 1963
Hyperstat I.V. Injection 3031
Imitrex Injection (Rare) 1431
Imitrex Tablets (Rare) 1440
▲ Increlex Injection (Greater than or equal to 5%) 3290
Indocin Capsules (Less than 1%) 1968
Indocin I.V. (Less than 1%) 1973
Indocin (Less than 1%) 1968
Infanrix Vaccine 1444
Infed Injection 3381
▲ Intron A for Injection (Less than 5%) 3038
Inversine Tablets 3286
Invirase (Less than 2%) 2776
Kaletra (Less than 2%) 474
Keppra Oral Solution (1% to 2%) 3307
Keppra Tablets (1% to 2%) 3307
▲ Lamictal (2% to 3%) 1449
Lariam Tablets (Occasional) 2790
Levaquin in 5% Dextrose Injection (0.1% to 0.9%) 2453
Levaquin (0.1% to 0.9%) 2453
Lexapro Oral Solution 1193
Lexapro Tablets 1193
Lidoderm Patch 1107
Matulane Capsules 3188
▲ Megace ES Oral Suspension (1% to 3%) 2492
Meridia Capsules (0.1%) 485
Mintezol 2002
Mirapex Tablets (Less than 1%) 889
Mobic Oral Suspension (Less than 2%) 893
Mobic Tablets (Less than 2%) 893
Mycamine for Injection 620
Namenda (Infrequent) 1199
Naprosyn Suspension (Less than 1%) 2769
Naprosyn Tablets (Less than 1%) 2769
Narcan Injection 1109
Naropin Injection (Less than 1%) 640
▲ Neoral Soft Gelatin Capsules (1% to 5%) 2247
▲ Neoral Oral Solution (1% to 5%) 2247
Neurontin Capsules (More than 1%) 2498
Neurontin Oral Solution 2498
Neurontin Tablets (More than 1%) 2498
Nipent for Injection (Less than 3%) 3216
Noroxin Tablets 2009
Norvir (Less than 2%) 499
Oncaspar (Greater than 1% but less than 5%) 1123
Parcopa Orally Disintegrating Tablets 3111
Paxil CR Controlled-Release Tablets (0.1%) 1509
Paxil (0.1%) 1501
PCE Dispertab Tablets (Rare) 510
Pediapred Oral Solution 3319
Pediarix Vaccine 1518
Permax Tablets (Infrequent) 3357
Prevacid Delayed-Release Capsules (Less than 1%) 3268
Prevacid for Delayed-Release Oral Suspension (Less than 1%) 3268
Prevacid NapraPAC (Less than 1%) 3277
Prevacid SoluTab Delayed-Release Orally Disintegrating Tablets (Less than 1%) 3268
PREVPAC (Less than 1%) 3281
▲ Primaxin I.V. (5.9%) 2024
▲ Prograf Capsules and Injection (3% to 15%) 624
Protonix I.V. (Less than 1%) 3468
Protonix Tablets (Less than 1%) 3465
Prozac Pulvules and Liquid (0.1% to 0.2%) 1771
Razadyne ER Extended-Release Capsules (Infrequent) 2434
Razadyne (Infrequent) 2434
▲ Rebif Prefilled Syringe for Injection (4% to 5%) 3163
Remicade for IV Injection (Less than 1%) 987
Requip Tablets (Infrequent) 1528
Reyataz Capsules (Less than 3%) 948
Rilutek Tablets (Infrequent) 2945
Risperdal Consta Long-Acting Injection (Infrequent) 1664
▲ Sandimmune (1% to 5%) 2259
Sandostatin LAR Depot (Rare) 2264
Sedapap Tablets 50 mg/650 mg (Infrequent) 2098
Seromycin Capsules 1783
Stalevo Tablets 2270
Sustiva Capsules (Less than 2%) 957
Symmetrel (Less than 0.1%) 1115
Tambocor Tablets (Less than 1%) 1824
▲ Temodar Capsules (6% to 23%) 3088
Tequin Injection (Less than 0.1%) 964
Tequin Tablets (Less than 0.1%) 964
Timolide Tablets 2056
Tindamax 2670
Trasylol Injection (1% to 2%) 779
▲ Trisenox Injection (8%) 983
Twinrix Vaccine 1571
Ultracet Tablets (Less than 1%) 2462
▲ Valcyte Tablets (Less than 5%) 2816
Valtrex Caplets 1573
Vantin Tablets and Oral Suspension 2650
Vermox Chewable Tablets (Very rare) 1853
▲ Vesanoid Capsules (3%) 2823
VFEND I.V. (Less than 2%) 2543
VFEND Oral Suspension (Less than 2%) 2543
VFEND Tablets (Less than 2%) 2543
Virazole for Inhalation Solution 3365
Voltaren Tablets (Rarely) 2298
Voltaren-XR Tablets (Rarely) 2301
Zestoretic Tablets 701
Zithromax Capsules, 250 mg 2568
Zithromax for IV Infusion 2573
Zithromax for Oral Suspension, 300 mg, 600 mg, 900 mg, 1200 mg 2561
Zithromax Tablets, 250 mg, 500 mg 2561
Zithromax Tri-Pak 2561
Zmax for Oral Suspension 2577
Zoloft 2581
Zomig Nasal Spray (Rare) 718
Zonegran Capsules (Frequent) 1089
Zosyn (1.0% or less) 3492
Zovirax for Injection 1618
Zyrtec Chewable Tablets (Rare) 2589
Zyrtec (Rare) 2589
Zyrtec-D 12 Hour Extended Release Tablets (Rare) 2591
Zyvox (0% to 2.8%) 2661

Convulsions, aggravated
Topamax Sprinkle Capsules (More than 1%) 2438
Topamax Tablets (More than 1%) 2438
Trileptal Oral Suspension (1% to 2%) 2281
Trileptal Tablets (1% to 2%) 2281

Convulsions, clonic
Seromycin Capsules 1783
Uniphyl Tablets (A few isolated reports) 2708

Convulsions, grand mal
Campath Ampules 826
Celexa 1177
Cipro (Less than 1%) 2991
Diastat Rectal Delivery System (Fewer than 1%) 3344
Keppra Oral Solution (1% or more) 3307
Keppra Tablets (1% or more) 3307
Lamictal (Rare) 1449
Lexapro Oral Solution 1193
Lexapro Tablets 1193
Namenda 1199
Narcan Injection 1109
Norvir (Less than 2%) 499
Paxil CR Controlled-Release Tablets (Rare) 1509
Paxil (Rare) 1501
Requip Tablets (Rare) 1528
Topamax Sprinkle Capsules (1%) 2438
Topamax Tablets (1%) 2438
VFEND I.V. (Less than 2%) 2543
VFEND Oral Suspension (Less than 2%) 2543
VFEND Tablets (Less than 2%) 2543

Convulsions, local
▲ Temodar Capsules (6%) 3088

Convulsions, major
Seromycin Capsules 1783

Convulsions, tonic generalized
Uniphyl Tablets (A few isolated reports) 2708

Coombs' test, positive
Adalat CC Tablets 2978
Aldoclor Tablets 1881
Aldoril Tablets 1884
Carimune NF 3501
Catapres Tablets 874
Ceftin (0.1% to 1%) 1369
Clorpres Tablets 2139
▲ Fortaz (1 in 23) 1422
Gammagard Liquid 751
Gamunex Immune Globulin I.V., 10% 3232
Iveegam EN 759
▲ Maxipime for Injection (16.2%) 1093
Mefoxin for Injection 1987
Mefoxin Premixed Intravenous Solution 1990
Merrem I.V. (Greater than 0.2%) 687
Paser Granules 1657
Primaxin I.M. 2022
Primaxin I.V. 2024
Rilutek Tablets (Infrequent) 2945
Roferon-A Injection (Rare) 2805
Suprax 1811
Vantin Tablets and Oral Suspension (Occasional) 2650
Zinacef Injection (Fewer than 1 in 250 patients) 1604
Zinacef for Injection (Fewer than 1 in 250 patients) 1604
Zosyn 3492

Coordination, disturbed
(*see under* Coordination, impaired)

Coordination, impaired
Alacol DM Syrup 739
Amerge Tablets (Rare) 1312
Arthrotec Tablets (Rare) 3126
Avelox (Less than 0.1%) 2984
Carbatrol Capsules 3174
Celexa (Rare) 1177
Cipro XR Tablets (Less than 1%) 3004
Clozapine Tablets (Less than 1%) 2141
Clozaril Tablets (Less than 1%) 2174
Combivent Inhalation Aerosol 878
▲ Depacon Injection (1% to 5%) 412
▲ Diastat Rectal Delivery System (3%) 3344
Duragesic Transdermal System (1% or greater) 2448
Equetro Extended-Release Capsules 3178
Evoxac Capsules (Less than 1%) 1042
FazaClo Orally Disintegrating Tablets (Less than 1%) 547
▲ Intron A for Injection (Less than 5%) 3038
▲ Klonopin (6%) 2782
▲ Lamictal (6.0%) 1449
Levaquin in 5% Dextrose Injection (0.1% to 0.9%) 2453
Levaquin (0.1% to 0.9%) 2453
Lexapro Oral Solution (Infrequent) 1193
Lexapro Tablets (Infrequent) 1193
Marinol Capsules 3334
Namenda (Infrequent) 1199
Neurontin Capsules (1.1%) 2498
Neurontin Oral Solution (1.1%) 2498
Neurontin Tablets (1.1%) 2498
▲ Niravam Orally Disintegrating Tablets (6.6% to 40.1%) 3106
▲ Pacerone Tablets (4% to 9%) 3337
▲ Phenytek Capsules (Among most common) 2153
▲ ProSom Tablets (4%) 512
▲ Rebif Prefilled Syringe for Injection (4% to 5%) 3163
Requip Tablets (Infrequent) 1528
Rescriptor Tablets 2535
Rilutek Tablets (Infrequent) 2945
Roferon-A Injection (Less than 0.5%) 2805
Tegretol/Tegretol-XR 2278
▲ Temodar Capsules (11%) 3088
▲ Topamax Sprinkle Capsules (4%) 2438
▲ Topamax Tablets (4%) 2438
▲ Trileptal Oral Suspension (1% to 3%) 2281
▲ Trileptal Tablets (1% to 3%) 2281
Wellbutrin SR Sustained-Release Tablets (Infrequent) 1583
Wellbutrin XL Extended-Release Tablets (Infrequent) 1588
▲ Xanax XR Tablets (9.4%) 2655
Zoloft (Infrequent) 2581
Zomig Nasal Spray (Infrequent) 718
Zyban Sustained-Release Tablets (Infrequent) 1620
Zyrtec Chewable Tablets (Less than 2%) 2589
Zyrtec (Less than 2%) 2589
Zyrtec-D 12 Hour Extended Release Tablets (Less than 2%) 2591

Coordination, lack of
(*see under* Ataxia)

Coordination difficulty
(*see under* Coordination, impaired)

Cor pulmonale
Pulmozyme Inhalation Solution 1245

Cornea, discoloration
Xalatan Sterile Ophthalmic Solution 2654

Cornea, gray, ground-glass appearance
Ophthetic Ophthalmic Solution ⊙230

Cornea, opacities
Accutane Capsules 2740
Amnesteem Capsules 2126
Imitrex Injection 1431
Imitrex Tablets 1440
Symmetrel (0.1% to 1%) 1115

Cornea, white crystalline precipitates, presence of
▲ Ciloxan Ophthalmic Ointment (Approximately 17%) 554

Corneal changes
Efudex (Infrequent) 3348
Neurontin Capsules (Rare) 2498
Neurontin Oral Solution (Rare) 2498
Neurontin Tablets (Rare) 2498

Corneal clouding
▲ Chemet Capsules (1.0% to 3.7%) 2480

Corneal curvature, steepening
Activella Tablets.............................. 2311
Alesse-28 Tablets.............................. 3392
Climara Transdermal System........... 795
Climara Pro Transdermal System..... 800
Estratest Tablets.............................. 3196
Estratest H.S. Tablets...................... 3196
Lo/Ovral-28 Tablets......................... 3423
Ortho-Cept Tablets.......................... 2395
Ortho-Cyclen Tablets....................... 2414
Ortho Evra Transdermal System...... 2402
Ortho Tri-Cyclen Tablets.................. 2414
Ortho Tri-Cyclen Lo Tablets............. 2421
Premarin Vaginal Cream.................. 3449
Premphase Tablets........................... 3452
Prempro Tablets............................... 3452
Seasonale Tablets............................ 1073
Triphasil-28 Tablets......................... 3483
Vivelle Transdermal System............ 2288
Vivelle-Dot Transdermal System....... 2293
Yasmin 28 Tablets........................... 818

Corneal decompensation
Amvisc Plus..................................... ⊙289
Cytovene-IV (One report)................. 2763
Ocucoat.. ⊙290

Corneal degeneration
Pacerone Tablets.............................. 3337

Corneal deposits
Indocin (Less than 1%)..................... 1968
▲ Pacerone Tablets (Majority of adults)... 3337
Propine Ophthalmic Solution........... ⊙237
Thioridazine Hydrochloride Tablets... 2122
▲ Voltaren Ophthalmic Solution (Less than or equal to 5%)............. 2300
▲ Zylet Ophthalmic Suspension (Less than 4%).................................. 3508

Corneal epithelial breakdown
Acular Ophthalmic Solution.............. 561
Acular LS Ophthalmic Solution......... 562
Iressa Tablets (Very rare)................. 684
Voltaren Ophthalmic Solution........... 2300

Corneal erosion
Acular Ophthalmic Solution.............. 561
Acular LS Ophthalmic Solution......... 562
▲ Brimonidine Tartrate Ophthalmic Solution 0.2% (3% to 9%)............. ⊙245
Iressa Tablets.................................. 684
Sonata Capsules (Rare).................... 1686
Voltaren Ophthalmic Solution........... 2300
Xalatan Sterile Ophthalmic Solution.. 2654

Corneal infiltrate
Acular Ophthalmic Solution (Rare).... 561
▲ Acular LS Ophthalmic Solution (1% to 5%).. 562
Ciloxan Ophthalmic Ointment (Less than 1%).................................. 554
Voltaren Ophthalmic Solution........... 2300

Corneal opacity
Aciphex Tablets................................ 1081
Aldurazyme for Intravenous Infusion (2%)..................................... 1261
Evoxac Capsules (Less than 1%)...... 1042
Namenda (Infrequent)...................... 1199
VFEND I.V. (Less than 2%)............... 2543
VFEND Oral Suspension (Less than 2%)... 2543
VFEND Tablets (Less than 2%).......... 2543
▲ Voltaren Ophthalmic Solution (Less than or equal to 5%)............. 2300

Corneal perforation
Acular Ophthalmic Solution.............. 561
Acular LS Ophthalmic Solution......... 562
HMS Sterile Ophthalmic Suspension.................................... ⊙228
Voltaren Ophthalmic Solution........... 2300

Corneal punctate, defects
Symmetrel (0.1% to 1%).................... 1115

Corneal punctate keratitis
Betoptic S Ophthalmic Suspension (Small number of patients)............ 554
Voltaren Ophthalmic Solution........... 2300

Corneal sensitivity, decrease
Betagan Ophthalmic Solution, USP (A small number of patients)....................................... ⊙217
Betimol Ophthalmic Solution............ ⊙283
Betimol Ophthalmic Solution............ 3371
Betoptic S Ophthalmic Suspension.. 554
Cosopt Sterile Ophthalmic Solution.. 1910
Timoptic in Ocudose (Less frequent).. 2061
Timoptic Sterile Ophthalmic Solution (Less frequent)............... 2058
Timoptic-XE Sterile Ophthalmic Gel Forming Solution........................ 2062

Corneal sensitivity, unspecified
Carteolol Hydrochloride Ophthalmic Solution USP, 1% (Occasional).................................. ⊙246

Corneal staining
Betimol Ophthalmic Solution (1% to 5%).. ⊙283
Betimol Ophthalmic Solution (1% to 5%).. 3371
▲ Brimonidine Tartrate Ophthalmic Solution 0.2% (3% to 9%)............ ⊙245
Carteolol Hydrochloride Ophthalmic Solution USP, 1% (Occasional).................................. ⊙246
Ciloxan Ophthalmic Ointment (Less than 1%).................................. 554

Corneal thinning
Acular Ophthalmic Solution 561
Acular LS Ophthalmic Solution 562
HMS Sterile Ophthalmic Suspension .... ⊙228
Myleran Tablets 1492
Pred-G Sterile Ophthalmic Ointment .... ⊙235
Voltaren Ophthalmic Solution 2300

Corneal ulceration
Acular Ophthalmic Solution (Rare) 561
Ambien Tablets (Rare) 2867
Botox Purified Neurotoxin Complex 565
Copegus Tablets (Less than 1%) 2759
Evoxac Capsules (Less than 1%) 1042
Paxil CR Controlled-Release Tablets (Rare) 1509
Paxil (Rare) 1501
Pegasys (Less than 1%) 2793
Pred Forte Ophthalmic Suspension (Occasional) .... ⊙233
Pred Mild Sterile Ophthalmic Suspension (Occasional) .... ⊙236
Soriatane Capsules (Less than 1%) .. 1028
Tarceva Tablets 1254
Tarceva Tablets 2470
Voltaren Ophthalmic Solution 2300

Coronary artery disease, aggravation
Carbatrol Capsules 3174
Equetro Extended-Release Capsules 3178
Tegretol/Tegretol-XR 2278

Coronary artery disease, unspecified
Amevive (Less than 1%) 836
Antara Capsules 2723
Campath Ampules 826
▲ Casodex Tablets (2% to 5%) 670
Celebrex Capsules (0.1% to 1.9%) ... 3130
Cymbalta Delayed-Release Capsules (Infrequent) 1729
Effexor Tablets (Rare) 3405
Effexor XR Capsules (Rare) 3411
▲ Humira Injection (Less than 5%) 464
▲ Intron A for Injection (Less than 5%) 3038
Lofibra Capsules 1217
Proleukin for Injection (Less than 1%) 1007
Rythmol SR Capsules 2736
Tasmar Tablets (Infrequent) 3360
Testim 1% Gel 722
Toprol-XL Tablets (Greater than 1%) 660
Tricor Tablets 523
Triglide Tablets 1165

Coronary heart disease
Premarin Tablets 3443

Coronary occlusion
Omacor Capsules 2735
Trasylol Injection (1% to 2%) 779

Coronary thrombosis
Levaquin in 5% Dextrose Injection (0.1% to 0.9%) 2453
Levaquin (0.1% to 0.9%) 2453
Lo/Ovral-28 Tablets 3423
Triphasil-28 Tablets 3483

Corpuscular volume, mean, elevation
Thalomid Capsules 979

Cortical lens opacities, scattered punctate
Carbatrol Capsules 3174
Equetro Extended-Release Capsules 3178
Tegretol/Tegretol-XR 2278

Corticosteroid binding globulin, elevated
Premphase Tablets 3452
Prempro Tablets 3452

Costochondritis
Evoxac Capsules (Less than 1%) 1042
Neurontin Capsules (Rare) 2498
Neurontin Oral Solution (Rare) 2498
Neurontin Tablets (Rare) 2498
Rythmol SR Capsules 2736

Cough
▲ Abilify Tablets (3%) 916
▲ Abilify Tablets (3%) 2472
▲ Aceon Tablets (2 mg, 4 mg, 8 mg) (6.0% to 12.0%) 3191
Actiq (1% or greater) 993
▲ Actonel Tablets (2.5% to 3.1%) 2679
▲ Actonel with Calcium Tablets (2.5% to 3.1%) 2684
Adalat CC Tablets (Less than 1%) 2978
Adenoscan (Less than 1%) 613
▲ Advair Diskus 100/50 (3%) 1291
▲ Advair Diskus 250/50 (6%) 1291
▲ Advair Diskus 500/50 (3% to 6%) ... 1291
▲ Advate Injection (15.3%) 742
▲ Aerobid/Aerobid-M (3% to 9%) 1172
Aggrenox Capsules (1.5%) 855
▲ Agrylin Capsules (6.3%) 3172
Alamast Ophthalmic Solution (Less than 5%) 3371
Aldara Cream, 5% (2.8%) 1814
Aldurazyme for Intravenous Infusion 1261
Alferon N Injection (One patient to 1%) 1640
Alkeran for Injection 976
Alkeran Tablets 977
▲ Allegra (3.8%) 2857
Alphagan P Ophthalmic Solution (1% to 4%) 563
▲ Altace Capsules (7.6% to 12%) 1673
▲ Alupent Inhalation Aerosol (3.3%) ... 858
Ambien Tablets (Infrequent) 2867
▲ AmBisome for Injection (17.8%) 615
Amerge Tablets (Infrequent) 1312
Amevive (Common) 836
Aptivus Capsules (0.8%) 859
▲ Aranesp for Injection (10%) 576
▲ Arava Tablets (3%) 2881
▲ Aredia for Injection (25.7%) 2168
Argatroban Injection (2.8%) 1321
▲ Arimidex Tablets (7% to 11%) 665
Arixtra Injection (2.1%) 1325
▲ Aromasin Tablets (6%) 2600
Arthrotec Tablets (Rare) 3126
Asacol Delayed-Release Tablets (1% to 2%) 2688
Astelin Nasal Spray (Infrequent) 1876
Atacand Tablets (More than 1%) 634
Atacand HCT (0.5% or greater) 637
▲ Atrovent HFA Inhalation Aerosol (3% to 5%) 872
▲ Atrovent Inhalation Solution (4.6%) 868
Atrovent Nasal Spray 0.03% (Less than 2%) 869
Atrovent Nasal Spray 0.06% (Less than 1%) 870
Attenuvax 1889
Avalide Tablets (1% or greater) 922
Avalide Tablets (1% or greater) 2889
Avapro Tablets (2.8%) 925
Avapro Tablets (2.8%) 2886
Axid Oral Solution (2.0%) 913
Azmacort Inhalation Aerosol 1701
Bactroban Nasal (2%) 1357
BeneFix for Injection (1.5%) 3402
Benicar HCT Tablets (Greater than 1%) 2852
Blocadren Tablets 1891
▲ Botox Purified Neurotoxin Complex (2% to 10%) 565
Caduet Tablets (Less than or equal to 0.1%) 2507
▲ Campath Ampules (2% to 25%) 826
▲ Camptosar Injection (0% to 20.2%) 2602
Captopril Tablets (0.5% to 2%) 2114
Cardizem LA Extended Release Tablets (2%) 1699
▲ Carnitor Injection (9% to 18%) 3185
▲ Casodex Tablets (2% to 5%) 670
Caverject Impulse Injection (1%) 2610
Ceftin for Oral Suspension (0.1% to 1%) 1369
Celebrex Capsules (0.1% to 1.9%)... 3130
Celexa (Frequent)............................. 1177
▲ Cenestin Tablets, 0.45mg, 0.625mg, 0.9mg, 1.25mg (6%)... 1063
▲ Cerezyme for Injection (Approximately 6.6%)................... 1263
▲ Chemet Capsules (0.7% to 3.7%) 2480
▲ Clarinex Syrup (10.6% to 10.8%) 3009
Clindesse Vaginal Cream (Less than 1%)...................................... 3296
▲ Clolar for Intravenous Infusion (19%)... 1264
Clozapine Tablets (Less than 1%)..... 2141
Clozaril Tablets (Less than 1%)......... 2174
Colazal Capsules (2%)..................... 2845
▲ Combivent Inhalation Aerosol (4.2%)... 878
▲ Combivir Tablets (18%) 1373
Comvax (0.2% to 0.9%).................... 1904
▲ Concerta Extended-Release Tablets (4%).................................. 1828
Copaxone for Injection (At least 2%)... 3292
▲ Copegus Tablets (10%) 2759
▲ Coreg Tablets (5% to 8%) 1376
Cosopt Sterile Ophthalmic Solution (1% to 5%)...................... 1910
Cozaar Tablets (1% or greater)......... 1913
Crixivan Capsules (1.5%).................. 1918
Cubicin for Injection (1% to 2%)....... 1038
▲ Cutivate Lotion 0.05% (3%) 1383
▲ Cymbalta Delayed-Release Capsules (3% to 6%)...................... 1729
Cytovene (At least 3 subjects).......... 2763
DDAVP Nasal Spray......................... 2894
▲ Depacon Injection (1% to 5%) 412
▲ Depakene (1% to 5%) 417
▲ Depakote Sprinkle Capsules (1% to 5%)... 422
▲ Depakote Tablets (1% to 5%) 427
▲ Depakote ER Tablets (1% to 5%) 433
Desmopressin Acetate Rhinal Tube.. 1144
Detrol Tablets (2.1%)........................ 2626
Diastat Rectal Delivery System (Less than 1%).............................. 3344
▲ Diovan HCT Tablets (3%) 2195
Diovan Tablets (0.6% to 2.6%).......... 2191
Diprivan Injectable Emulsion (Less than 1%)...................................... 676
▲ Ditropan XL Extended Release Tablets (2% to less than 5%)......... 2391
▲ Doxil Injection (Less than 1% to 9.6%)... 3302
Duragesic Transdermal System (1% or greater)............................... 2448
DynaCirc CR Tablets (0.5% to 1%).... 2726
Effexor Tablets................................. 3405
▲ Effexor XR Capsules (3%) 3411
▲ Elidel Cream 1% (2.4% to 15.8%) 2198
▲ Eloxatin for Injection (11% to 19%)... 2908
Emend Capsules (Greater than 0.5%)... 1944
▲ Enbrel for Injection (5% to 6%) 580
▲ Epivir (18%) 1394
▲ Epivir-HBV (Among most common).. 1398
▲ Epogen for Injection (18%) 586
▲ Erbitux (10%) 937
▲ Evista Tablets (6% to 9.3%) 1735
▲ Evoxac Capsules (6.1%) 1042
Exelon Capsules (2% or more).......... 2204
▲ Faslodex Injection (10.4%) 682
FazaClo Orally Disintegrating Tablets (Less than 1%).................. 547
▲ Femara Tablets (5% to 13%) 2210
▲ Ferrlecit Injection (6%) 3379
▲ Flolan for Injection (38% to 82%) 1408
▲ Flomax Capsules (3.4% to 4.5%) 881
▲ Flonase Nasal Spray (3.6% to 3.8%)... 1412
▲ Flovent Diskus 50 mcg (5% to 9%)... 1415
▲ Flovent HFA (4%) 1418
Floxin Otic Singles (Reported in a single subject)............................. 1045
Floxin Otic Solution (Single report)... 1043
Flumadine (Less than 0.3%)............. 1186
▲ Flumist Vaccine (13.9% to 38.5%) ... 1872
▲ Forteo for Injection (6.4%) 1739
Fortical Nasal Spray (Less than 1%)... 3336
▲ Fuzeon Injection (3.9%) 2772
▲ Gabitril Tablets (4%) 998
▲ Gammagard Liquid (0.61% to 8.2%)... 751
Gemzar for Injection (Common)........ 1743
▲ Gengraf Capsules (4% to 5%) 458
▲ Gleevec Tablets (12.5% to 27%) 2221
Gonal-f RFF Pen for Injection (2.4%)... 3155
Hepsera Tablets (2% or greater)....... 1275
▲ Herceptin I.V. (26%) 1234

▲ Humatrope Vials and Cartridges (Up to 6.25%) 1756
Hycamtin for Injection (1%) 1427
Hyperstat I.V. Injection 3031
Hytrin Capsules (At least 1%) 469
Hyzaar (2.6%) 1964
▲ Imdur Tablets (Less than or equal to 5%) 3032
Imitrex Nasal Spray (Infrequent) 1435
Imitrex Tablets (Infrequent) 1440
Indapamide Tablets (Less than 5%) 2119
Inspra Tablets (2%) 2520
▲ Intron A for Injection (Up to 31%) 3038
▲ Invanz for Injection (1.3% to 4.4%) 1974
Invirase (Less than 2%) 2776
▲ I.V. Busulfex (28%) 1125
Iveegam EN 759
▲ Keppra Oral Solution (2% to 11%) 3307
▲ Keppra Tablets (2% to 11%) 3307
Klonopin (2%) 2782
▲ Lamictal (7% to 8%) 1449
Lescol Capsules (2.4%) 2227
Lescol XL Tablets (1.9%) 2227
Leukeran Tablets 1472
▲ Leustatin Injection (7% to 10%) 2368
Levaquin in 5% Dextrose Injection (0.1% to 0.9%) 2453
Levaquin (0.1% to 0.9%) 2453
Lexapro Oral Solution (Frequent) 1193
Lexapro Tablets (Frequent) 1193
Lofibra Capsules 1217
Lotensin Tablets (1.2%) 2232
Lotensin HCT Tablets (2.1%) 2235
▲ Lotrel Capsules (3.3%) 2238
Lotronex Tablets (Rare) 1479
▲ Malarone Tablets (Less than 1% to 10%) 1484
▲ Malarone Pediatric Tablets (Less than 1% to 10%) 1484
Marinol Capsules (Less than 1%) 3334
Matulane Capsules 3188
▲ Mavik Tablets (0.3% to 35%) 482
Maxair Autohaler (1.2%) 1820
Maxalt Tablets (Rare) 1983
Maxalt-MLT Orally Disintegrating Tablets (Rare) 1983
▲ Megace ES Oral Suspension (1% to 3%) 2492
Menopur for Subcutaneous Injection (1.6% to 2.6%) 1145
▲ Mepron Suspension (25%) 1487
▲ Meridia Capsules (3.8%) 485
Meruvax II 1994
Miacalcin Nasal Spray (Less than 1%) 2242
Micardis Tablets (1%) 884
Micardis HCT Tablets (2% or greater) 886
▲ Midamor Tablets (Between 1% and 3%) 2000
Mirapex Tablets (1% or more) 889
M-M-R II 1980
Mobic Oral Suspension (0.2% to 2.4%) 893
Mobic Tablets (0.2% to 2.4%) 893
Moduretic Tablets 2003
Mumpsvax 2005
▲ Myfortic Tablets (3% to less than 20%) 2244
▲ Mylotarg for Injection (16% to 18%) 3429
Nadolol Tablets (1 to 5 of 1000 patients) 2121
▲ Namenda (4%) 1199
Naropin Injection (Less than 1%) 640
Nasacort HFA Inhalation Aerosol 2939
Nasacort AQ Nasal Spray (2.1%) 2937
Nasarel Nasal Spray (Greater than 1%) 1652
▲ Nasonex Nasal Spray (7% to 13%) 3058
Navelbine Injection 1494
▲ Neoral Soft Gelatin Capsules (4% to 5%) 2247
▲ Neoral Oral Solution (4% to 5%) 2247
▲ Neumega for Injection (29%) 3433
▲ Neupogen for Injection (6%) 598
Neurontin Capsules (1.8%) 2498
Neurontin Oral Solution (1.8%) 2498
Neurontin Tablets (1.8%) 2498
Nexium Delayed-Release Capsules (Less than 1%) 645
Nexium I.V. (Less than 1%) 649
▲ Nicotrol Inhaler (32%) 2594
Nicotrol NS 2596
▲ Nipent for Injection (17% to 20%) 3216
Norvasc Tablets (Less than or equal to 0.1%) 2529
Norvir (Less than 2%) 499
Omacor Capsules 2735
Oncaspar (Less than 1%) 1123
▲ Ontak Vials (26%) 1717
OptiPranolol Metipranolol Ophthalmic Solution 0.3% (A small number of patients) ⊙ 254
OxyContin Tablets (Less than 1%) 2699
▲ Pacerone Tablets (2% to 7%) 3337
Parcopa Orally Disintegrating Tablets 3111
Paxil CR Controlled-Release Tablets (Frequent) 1509
Paxil (Frequent) 1501
▲ Pegasys (4%) 2793
▲ PEG-Intron Powder for Injection (8%) 3062
▲ Photofrin for Injection (7% to 9%) 729
▲ Plavix Tablets (3.1%) 940
▲ Plavix Tablets (3.1%) 2942
Plendil Extended-Release Tablets (0.8% to 1.7%) 651
▲ Pletal Tablets (3% to 4%) 2478
Pravachol Tablets (0.1% to 2.6%) 943
▲ Prefest Tablets (5%) 1069
Prevacid Delayed-Release Capsules (Less than 1%) 3268
Prevacid for Delayed-Release Oral Suspension (Less than 1%) 3268
Prevacid SoluTab Delayed-Release Orally Disintegrating Tablets (Less than 1%) 3268
PREVPAC (Less than 1%) 3281
Prilosec OTC Tablets (1.1%) 2674
▲ Prinivil Tablets (1% to 3.5%) 2029
▲ Prinzide Tablets (3.9%) 2033
▲ Procrit for Injection (18%) 2374
▲ Prograf Capsules and Injection (3% to 18%) 624
▲ Proleukin for Injection (11%) 1007
▲ Prometrium Capsules (100 mg, 200 mg) (8%) 3205
ProSom Tablets (Infrequent) 512
Protonix I.V. (Greater than or equal to 1%) 3468
Protonix Tablets (Greater than or equal to 1%) 3465
▲ Protopic Ointment (1% to 15%) 629
▲ Proventil Inhalation Solution 0.083% (3.1% to 4%) 3069
Provigil Tablets (At least 1%) 1002
Prozac Pulvules and Liquid 1771
▲ Pulmicort Respules (5% to 9%) 654
Pulmozyme Inhalation Solution 1245
▲ Rapamune Oral Solution and Tablets (3% to 20%) 3472
Razadyne ER Extended-Release Capsules (Greater than or equal to 2%) 2434
Razadyne (Greater than or equal to 2%) 2434
▲ Rebetol (16% to 23%) 3073
Recombivax HB (Less than 1%) 2045
ReFacto Vials 3479
Refludan for Injection (Common) 815
Relafen Tablets (Less than 1%) 1523
Relenza Rotadisk (Less than 2%) 1525
Relpax Tablets (Rare) 2531
▲ Remicade for IV Injection (12%) 987
▲ Renagel Tablets (7.1%) 1268
▲ Requip Tablets (1% to 3%) 1528
▲ Rescriptor Tablets (3.5% to 5%) 2535
▲ Retisert Implant (5% to 15%) ⊙ 256
Retrovir Capsules 1533
Retrovir IV Infusion 1537
Retrovir 1533
Rhinocort Aqua Nasal Spray (2%) 658
▲ Ribavirin, USP Capsules (16% to 23%) 3083
▲ Rilutek Tablets (2.1% to 3.7%) 2945
▲ Risperdal Consta Long-Acting Injection (2% to 5%) 1664
▲ Risperdal M-Tab Orally Disintegrating Tablets (2% to 3%) 1658
▲ Risperdal (2% to 3%) 1658
Rituxan for Infusion (0.3%) 845
▲ Rituxan I.V. (13%) 1251
▲ Roferon-A Injection (1% to 19%) 2805
Rythmol SR Capsules 2736
▲ Serevent Diskus (Greater than 3%) 1540
Seroquel Tablets (Infrequent) 691
▲ Simulect for Injection (Greater than or equal to 10%) 2268
Singulair (1% to 2.7%) 2047
Soriatane Capsules (Less than 1%) 1028
▲ Spiriva HandiHaler (Greater than or equal to 3%) 899
Stalevo Tablets 2270
Starlix Tablets (2.4%) 2276
▲ Strattera Capsules (2% to 11%) 1784
▲ Suboxone Tablets (4%) 2719
▲ Subutex Tablets (4%) 2719
Sular Tablets (Less than or equal to 1%) 1163
▲ Suprane Liquid for Inhalation (34% to 72%) 770
▲ Sustiva Capsules (25%) 957
Synagis (More than 1%) 1868
▲ Tamiflu Capsules (1.2% to 5.6%) 2810
▲ Tamiflu Oral Suspension (1.2% to 5.6%) 2810
▲ Tarceva Tablets (0% to 33%) 1254
▲ Tarceva Tablets (0% to 33%) 2470
Targretin Capsules 1719
▲ Tarka Tablets (4.6%) 519
Tasmar Tablets (Infrequent) 3360
▲ Temodar Capsules (5% to 8%) 3088
▲ Teveten Tablets (4%) 1707
Teveten HCT Tablets (Less than 1%) 1710
Thalomid Capsules 979
Tiazac Capsules (1% to 2%) 1204
Timolide Tablets 2056
Timoptic in Ocudose (Less frequent) 2061
Timoptic Sterile Ophthalmic Solution (Less frequent) 2058
Timoptic-XE Sterile Ophthalmic Gel Forming Solution 2062
▲ TOBI Solution for Inhalation (46.1%) 1015
▲ Topamax Sprinkle Capsules (2% to 4%) 2438
▲ Topamax Tablets (2% to 4%) 2438
Trelstar LA Suspension (1.7%) 3387
▲ Trileptal Oral Suspension (Up to 5%) 2281
▲ Trileptal Tablets (Up to 5%) 2281
▲ Trisenox Injection (65%) 983
▲ Trizivir Tablets (18%) 1565
Truvada Tablets 1279
Uniretic Tablets (Less than 1% to 3%) 3114
▲ Valcyte Tablets (Less than 5%) 2816
Vantin Tablets and Oral Suspension (Less than 1%) 2650
▲ Vaqta (1% to 5.1%) 2067
Varivax (Greater than or equal to 1%) 2070
▲ Vaseretic Tablets (3.5%) 2073
Vasotec I.V. Injection (1.3% to 2.2%) 2076
▲ Velcade for Injection (21%) 2102
▲ Ventolin HFA Inhalation Aerosol (5%) 1576
VESIcare Tablets (0.2% to 1.1%) 631
VFEND I.V. (Less than 2%) 2543
VFEND Oral Suspension (Less than 2%) 2543
VFEND Tablets (Less than 2%) 2543
Viagra Tablets (Less than 2%) 2552
Vicoprofen Tablets (Less than 1%) 533
▲ Vigamox Ophthalmic Solution (1% to 4%) ⊙ 212
▲ Visudyne for Injection (1% to 10%) 2286
Vivelle Transdermal System 2288
Vivelle-Dot Transdermal System 2293
Vytorin 10/10 Tablets 2084
Vytorin 10/10 Tablets 3092
Vytorin 10/20 Tablets 2084
Vytorin 10/20 Tablets 3092
Vytorin 10/40 Tablets 2084
Vytorin 10/40 Tablets 3092
Vytorin 10/80 Tablets 2084
Vytorin 10/80 Tablets 3092
WelChol Tablets (2%) 2855
Wellbutrin SR Sustained-Release Tablets (1% to 2%) 1583
Wellbutrin XL Extended-Release Tablets (1% to 2%) 1588
▲ Xeloda Tablets (Less than 5%) 2825
▲ Xopenex HFA Inhalation Aerosol (1.4% to 4.1%) 3151
▲ Xopenex Inhalation Solution (1.4% to 4.1%) 3143
▲ Xopenex Inhalation Solution Concentrate (1.4% to 4.1%) 3147
Zegerid Powder for Oral Solution (1.1%) 2972
▲ Zenapax for Injection (Greater than 5%) 2838
▲ Zestoretic Tablets (3.9%) 701
▲ Zestril Tablets (Greater than 1% to 3.5%) 704
Zetia Tablets (2.3%) 2090
Zetia Tablets (2.3%) 3098
▲ Zevalin Injection (10%) 848
Ziagen 1600
Zithromax for Oral Suspension, 300 mg, 600 mg, 900 mg, 1200 mg (1% or less) 2561
Zithromax Tablets, 250 mg, 500 mg (1% or less) 2561
Zithromax Tri-Pak (1% or less) 2561
Zoladex (1% or greater) 709
Zoladex 3-month (1% to 5%) 712
Zoloft (Infrequent) 2581
▲ Zometa for Intravenous Infusion (11.6% to 22%) 2306
Zosyn (1.0% or less) 3492
▲ Zyban Sustained-Release Tablets (3%) 1620
▲ Zyprexa Tablets (5%) 1798
▲ Zyprexa ZYDIS Orally Disintegrating Tablets (5%) 1798
▲ Zyrtec Chewable Tablets (2.8% to 4.4%) 2589
▲ Zyrtec (2.8% to 4.4%) 2589
Zyrtec-D 12 Hour Extended Release Tablets (2.8% to 4.4%) 2591
Zyvox 2661

Cough, increased

Antara Capsules 2723
Aralast (0.1% to 0.6%) 745
▲ Bexxar (1% to 21%) 1360
Campral Tablets (Frequent) 1175
▲ CellCept Capsules (31.1%) 2751
▲ CellCept Intravenous (31.1%) 2751
▲ CellCept Oral Suspension (31.1%) 2751
▲ CellCept Tablets (31.1%) 2751
Crestor Tablets (Greater than or equal to 2%) 672
▲ Elestat Ophthalmic Solution (1% to 3%) 1643
▲ Emtriva Capsules (14%) 1272
▲ Gamunex Immune Globulin I.V., 10% (1.7% to 54%) 3232
▲ Geodon Capsules (3%) 2514
▲ Hectorol Capsules (Greater than or equal to 5%) 909
Merrem I.V. (Greater than 0.1% to 1%) 687
Natrecor for Injection (Greater than or equal to 1%) 3123
▲ Premarin Tablets (4% to 7%) 3443
▲ Premphase Tablets (5% to 8%) 3452
▲ Prempro Tablets (5% to 8%) 3452
Prevacid NapraPAC (Less than 1%) 3277
▲ Reyataz Capsules (1% to 5%) 948
Tricor Tablets 523
▲ Tygacil for Injection (3.7%) 3489
▲ Ultane Liquid for Inhalation (5% to 11%) 526
▲ Univasc Tablets (6.1%) 3118
▲ Ventavis Inhalation Solution (39%) 1036
▲ Vigamox Ophthalmic Solution (1% to 4%) 560
Zemaira (0.4%) 3506
Zomig Nasal Spray (Infrequent) 718

Cough, productive

Permax Tablets (Frequent) 3357

Cough reflex, depression

Kadian Capsules (Less than 3%) 572
Prozac Pulvules and Liquid (Rare) 1771

CPK, elevation

(*see under* Creatine kinase, increase)

Cramping

Advair Diskus 100/50 1291
Advair Diskus 250/50 1291
Advair Diskus 500/50 1291
Aldoclor Tablets 1881
Aldoril Tablets 1884
Alferon N Injection (One patient) 1640
Aminohippurate Sodium "PAH" Injection 1886
Asacol Delayed-Release Tablets 2688
Atacand HCT 637
Avalide Tablets 922
Avalide Tablets 2889
Clinoril Tablets (Greater than 1%) 1899
Clorpres Tablets 2139
Colazal Capsules (1%) 2845
Coumadin for Injection (Infrequent) 932
Coumadin Tablets (Infrequent) 932
Dilaudid 439
Dilaudid Oral Liquid 443
Dilaudid Non-Sterile Powder 439
Dilaudid Rectal Suppositories 439
Dilaudid Tablets 439
Dilaudid Tablets - 8 mg 443
Diovan HCT Tablets 2195
Diuril Oral 1936
Diuril Sodium Intravenous 1934
Exelon Capsules (Infrequent) 2204
▲ Ferrlecit Injection (25%) 3379
▲ Gengraf Capsules (1% to 4%) 458
Hyzaar 1964
Lotensin HCT Tablets 2235
Maxzide 2150
MetroGel-Vaginal Gel (1%) 1822
Moduretic Tablets 2003
▲ Neoral Soft Gelatin Capsules (1% to 4%) 2247
Neoral Oral Solution (1% to 4%) 2247
Nexium Delayed-Release Capsules (Less than 1%) 645
Nexium I.V. (Less than 1%) 649
Prinzide Tablets 2033
▲ Sandimmune (Up to 4%) 2259

Teveten HCT Tablets 1710
▲ Thrombate III (2 of 17) 3254
Timolide Tablets 2056
Tindamax (1.4% to 1.8%) 2670
Uniretic Tablets 3114
Vaseretic Tablets 2073
▲ Zavesca Capsules (11%) 543
Zestoretic Tablets (0.3% to 1%) 701

Cramping, abdominal
(*see under* Abdominal pain/cramps)

Cramping, muscular
Abilify Tablets (Frequent) 916
Abilify Tablets (Frequent) 2472
Adalat CC Tablets (Rare) 2978
▲ Advair Diskus 250/50 (3%) 1291
Advicor Tablets 1694
Alferon N Injection (1%) 1640
Altoprev Extended-Release Tablets (0.6% to 1.1%) 1151
Amerge Tablets (Infrequent) 1312
Anadrol-50 Tablets 3329
Antivenin (Black Widow Spider Antivenin) 1887
Aptivus Capsules (Less than 2%) 859
▲ Arava Tablets (1% to 3%) 2881
▲ Aricept Tablets (3% to 8%) 1086
▲ Aricept ODT Tablets (3% to 8%) 1086
Asacol Delayed-Release Tablets 2688
Avalide Tablets (1% or greater) 922
Avalide Tablets (1% or greater) 2889
Avapro Tablets (Less than 1%) 925
Avapro Tablets (Less than 1%) 2886
BiDil Tablets 2161
Boniva Tablets (1.8% to 2%) 2747
Caduet Tablets (Less than 1% to 2%) 2507
Cardizem LA Extended Release Tablets (Less than 2%) 1699
Ceftin Tablets (0.1% to 1%) 1369
Climara Transdermal System 795
▲ Coreg Tablets (Greater than 1% to 3%) 1376
Covera-HS Tablets (Less than 2%) 3135
Cozaar Tablets (1%) 1913
Cubicin for Injection (Less than 1%) 1038
▲ Cymbalta Delayed-Release Capsules (4% to 5%) 1729
CytoGam Intravenous (Less than 5.0%) 1866
Diovan HCT Tablets (Greater than 0.2%) 2195
Diovan Tablets 2191
Diuril Sodium Intravenous 1934
Dolobid Tablets (Rare) 1937
Dyazide Capsules 1389
Eldepryl Capsules 3209
▲ Entocort EC Capsules (Less than 5%) 2694
Foradil Aerolizer 3024
▲ Fosamax (Up to approximately 6%) 1949
Fosamax Plus D Tablets (0% to 1.1%) 1956
Furosemide Tablets 2117
Gammagard Liquid 751
▲ Gleevec Tablets (28% to 62%) 2221
▲ Humira Injection (Less than 5%) 464
Hyzaar 1964
Imitrex Injection (1.1%) 1431
Imitrex Nasal Spray (Rare) 1435
Imitrex Tablets (Infrequent) 1440
▲ Indapamide Tablets (Greater than or equal to 5%) 2119
Invirase (Less than 2%) 2776
Ketek Tablets 2920
Klonopin (Infrequent) 2782
K-Phos Neutral Tablets 785
K-Phos Original (Sodium Free) Tablets (Less frequent) 785
Lariam Tablets (Infrequent) 2790
Lescol Capsules 2227
Lescol Capsules 2730
Lescol XL Tablets 2227
Lescol XL Tablets 2730
Lexapro Oral Solution (Infrequent) 1193
Lexapro Tablets (Infrequent) 1193
Lotrel Capsules 2238
Mavik Tablets (0.3% to 1.0%) 482
Maxalt Tablets (Infrequent) 1983
Maxalt-MLT Orally Disintegrating Tablets (Infrequent) 1983
Maxzide 2150
Mevacor Tablets (0.6% to 1.1%) 1996
Micardis Tablets 884
Micardis HCT Tablets 886
▲ Midamor Tablets (Between 1% and 3%) 2000
Migranal Nasal Spray (Infrequent) 3350
Moduretic Tablets (Less than or equal to 1%) 2003
▲ Myfortic Tablets (3% to less than 20%) 2244
Naropin Injection (Less than 1%) 640
Nimotop Capsules (Up to 1.4%) 774
Niravam Orally Disintegrating Tablets (2.4%) 3106
Norvasc Tablets (Less than 1% to 2%) 2529
Norvir (Less than 2%) 499
Oncaspar 1123
Parcopa Orally Disintegrating Tablets 3111
Pepcid Injection (Infrequent) 2017
Pepcid (Infrequent) 2014
Plendil Extended-Release Tablets (0.5% to 1.5%) 651
Prilosec OTC Tablets (Less than 1%) 2674
Prinivil Tablets (Greater than 1%) 2029
Prinzide Tablets (2%) 2033
▲ Prograf Capsules and Injection (3% to 15%) 624
Prozac Pulvules and Liquid (Infrequent) 1771
▲ Requip Tablets (3%) 1528
Rescriptor Tablets 2535
Roferon-A Injection (Infrequent) 2805
Rythmol SR Capsules 2736
▲ Simulect for Injection (3% to 10%) 2268
Singulair 2047
Stalevo Tablets 2270
▲ Tasmar Tablets (17% to 18%) 3360
Teveten Tablets (Less than 1%) 1707
Tiazac Capsules (Less than 2%) 1204
Timolide Tablets 2056
Uroqid-Acid No. 2 Tablets 785
▲ Valcyte Tablets (Less than 5%) 2816
Vaseretic Tablets (2.7%) 2073
Vasotec I.V. Injection (0.5% to 1.0%) 2076
▲ Velcade for Injection (12%) 2102
▲ Ventavis Inhalation Solution (6%) 1036
Verelan PM Capsules (2% or less) 3120
Viracept (Less than 2%) 2556
▲ VoSpire Extended-Release Tablets (1.2% to 6.9%) 2352
Vytorin 10/10 Tablets 2084
Vytorin 10/10 Tablets 3092
Vytorin 10/20 Tablets 2084
Vytorin 10/20 Tablets 3092
Vytorin 10/40 Tablets 2084
Vytorin 10/40 Tablets 3092
Vytorin 10/80 Tablets 2084
Vytorin 10/80 Tablets 3092
Xanax XR Tablets (Frequent) 2655
Zegerid Powder for Oral Solution (Less than 1%) 2972
Zestoretic Tablets (2.0%) 701
Zestril Tablets (0.5% to greater than 1%) 704
Zocor Tablets 2078
Zoloft (Infrequent) 2581

Cramps, abdominal
(*see under* Abdominal pain/cramps)

Cramps, lower limbs
Aciphex Tablets 1081
Actiq (1% or greater) 993
▲ Actonel Tablets (3.3% to 3.5%) 2679
▲ Adalat CC Tablets (3% or less) 2978
Agrylin Capsules (1% to 5%) 3172
Alinia for Oral Suspension (Less than 1%) 2840
Alinia Tablets (Less than 1%) 2840
Ambien Tablets (Infrequent) 2867
Antara Capsules 2723
Arava Tablets (1%) 2881
Atacand HCT (0.5% or greater) 637
▲ Betaseron for SC Injection (4%) 791
Caduet Tablets (Less than 2%) 2507
Campral Tablets (Frequent) 1175
Carbatrol Capsules 3174
▲ Carnitor Injection (4% to 8%) 3185
▲ Casodex Tablets (2% to 5%) 670
Catapres Tablets (About 3 in 1,000) 874
Catapres-TTS (0.5% or less) 875
Caverject Impulse Injection (Less than 1%) 2610
Celebrex Capsules (0.1% to 1.9%) 3130
Celexa (Infrequent) 1177
▲ CellCept Capsules (3% to less than 20%) 2751
▲ CellCept Intravenous (3% to less than 20%) 2751
▲ CellCept Oral Suspension (3% to less than 20%) 2751
▲ CellCept Tablets (3% to less than 20%) 2751
▲ Cenestin Tablets, 0.45mg, 0.625mg, 0.9mg, 1.25mg (10%) 1063
Cenestin Tablets, 0.3mg 1063
Climara Transdermal System 795
Climara Pro Transdermal System 800
Clorpres Tablets (About 3 in 1,000) 2139
Cytovene (At least 3 subjects) 2763
▲ Depacon Injection (1% to 5%) 412
▲ Depakene (1% to 5%) 417
▲ Depakote Sprinkle Capsules (1% to 5%) 422
▲ Depakote Tablets (1% to 5%) 427
▲ Depakote ER Tablets (1% to 5%) 433
▲ Depo-Provera Contraceptive Injection (1% to 5%) 2619
Desferal Vials 2190
Didronel Tablets 2693
DuoNeb Inhalation Solution (1.4%) 1058
DynaCirc CR Tablets (0.5% to 1%) 2726
Effexor Tablets (Infrequent) 3405
Effexor XR Capsules (Infrequent) 3411
▲ Emcyt Capsules (8%) 3137
Equetro Extended-Release Capsules 3178
Estratest H.S. Tablets 3196
Estrogel 0.06% 3200
▲ Evista Tablets (5.9% to 7%) 1735
▲ Evoxac Capsules (1% to 3%) 1042
Exelon Capsules (Frequent) 2204
Factive Tablets (Less than or equal to 0.1%) 2464
▲ Ferrlecit Injection (10%) 3379
Foradil Aerolizer (1.7%) 3024
Forteo for Injection (2.6%) 1739
Frova Tablets (Infrequent) 1101
Gabitril Tablets (Infrequent) 998
Gammagard S/D (Occasional) 754
▲ Gengraf Capsules (12%) 458
▲ Intron A for Injection (Less than 5%) 3038
Invirase (Less than 2%) 2776
Klonopin (Infrequent) 2782
Lamictal (Rare) 1449
Levaquin in 5% Dextrose Injection (0.1% to 0.9%) 2453
Levaquin (0.1% to 0.9%) 2453
Lipitor Tablets (Less than 2%) 2495
Lofibra Capsules 1217
Lunesta Tablets (Infrequent) 3139
Lyrica Capsules (Grather than or equal to 1%) 2524
Menostar Transdermal System 805
Meridia Capsules (Greater than or equal to 1%) 485
Micardis Tablets (More than 0.3%) 884
Micardis HCT Tablets 886
Mirapex Tablets (1% or more) 889
Natrecor for Injection (Greater than or equal to 1%) 3123
▲ Neoral Soft Gelatin Capsules (12%) 2247
▲ Neoral Oral Solution (12%) 2247
Neurontin Capsules (Infrequent) 2498
Neurontin Oral Solution (Infrequent) 2498
Neurontin Tablets (Infrequent) 2498
Oxsoralen-Ultra Capsules 3354
Pentasa Capsules (Less than 1%) 3182
Plavix Tablets (1% to 2.5%) 940
Plavix Tablets (1% to 2.5%) 2942
Pletal Tablets (2% or greater) 2478
Prefest Tablets 1069
▲ Premarin Tablets (3% to 7%) 3443
Premarin Vaginal Cream 3449
▲ Premphase Tablets (3% to 7%) 3452
▲ Prempro Tablets (3% to 7%) 3452
Prevacid Delayed-Release Capsules (Less than 1%) 3268
Prevacid for Delayed-Release Oral Suspension (Less than 1%) 3268
Prevacid NapraPAC (Less than 1%) 3277
Prevacid SoluTab Delayed-Release Orally Disintegrating Tablets (Less than 1%) 3268
PREVPAC (Less than 1%) 3281
ProAmatine Tablets (Rare) 3183
Prochieve 4% Gel 1018
Prochieve 8% Gel 1018
▲ Prograf Capsules and Injection (3% to 15%) 624
Prometrium Capsules (100 mg, 200 mg) (Less than 5%) 3205
Protonix I.V. (Less than 1%) 3468
Protonix Tablets (Less than 1%) 3465
Proventil HFA Inhalation Aerosol (Less than 3%) 3071
Provigil Tablets (At least 1%) 1002
Prozac Pulvules and Liquid (Infrequent) 1771
▲ Rapamune Oral Solution and Tablets (3% to 20%) 3472
Razadyne (Infrequent) 2434
Requip Tablets (1% or more) 1528
Rilutek Tablets (Infrequent) 2945
Risperdal Consta Long-Acting Injection (Infrequent) 1664
Risperdal M-Tab Orally Disintegrating Tablets (Rare) 1658
Risperdal (Rare) 1658
▲ Roferon-A Injection (3%) 2805
▲ Sandostatin LAR Depot (5% to 15%) 2264
Seroquel Tablets (Infrequent) 691
Sular Tablets (Less than or equal to 1%) 1163
Symbyax Capsules (Infrequent) 1788
Synercid I.V. (Less than 1%) 1690
Tegretol/Tegretol-XR 2278
Tequin Injection (Less than 0.1%) 964
Tequin Tablets (Less than 0.1%) 964
Teveten HCT Tablets (Less than 1%) 1710
Thalomid Capsules 979
Topamax Sprinkle Capsules (2%) 2438
Topamax Tablets (2%) 2438
Tricor Tablets 523
VFEND I.V. (Less than 2%) 2543
VFEND Oral Suspension (Less than 2%) 2543
VFEND Tablets (Less than 2%) 2543
Vivelle Transdermal System 2288
Vivelle-Dot Transdermal System 2293
Wellbutrin SR Sustained-Release Tablets (Infrequent) 1583
Wellbutrin XL Extended-Release Tablets (Infrequent) 1588
Xopenex HFA Inhalation Aerosol (2.7%) 3151
Xopenex Inhalation Solution (2.7%) 3143
Xopenex Inhalation Solution Concentrate (2.7%) 3147
▲ Zavesca Capsules (4% to 11%) 543
▲ Zenapax for Injection (2% to 5%) 2838
Zoladex (2%) 709
Zoladex 3-month 712
Zoloft (Infrequent) 2581
Zomig Tablets (Infrequent) 714
Zomig-ZMT Tablets (Infrequent) 714
Zonegran Capsules (Infrequent) 1089
Zyban Sustained-Release Tablets (Infrequent) 1620
Zyprexa Tablets (Infrequent) 1798
Zyprexa ZYDIS Orally Disintegrating Tablets (Infrequent) 1798
Zyrtec Chewable Tablets (Less than 2%) 2589
Zyrtec (Less than 2%) 2589
Zyrtec-D 12 Hour Extended Release Tablets (Less than 2%) 2591

Cramps, pelvic
▲ Menopur for Subcutaneous Injection (3.9%) 1145

Cranial nerve, dysfunction
Advicor Tablets 1694
Garamycin Injectable 3028
Lescol Capsules 2227
Lescol Capsules 2730
Lescol XL Tablets 2227
Lescol XL Tablets 2730
Pravachol Tablets 943
Zocor Tablets 2078

Cranial nerve, paralysis of
Amerge Tablets (Rare) 1312
Eloxatin for Injection 2908

Cranial nerve deficit, fetal
Accutane Capsules 2740

Craniofacial deformities
Altace Capsules 1673
Captopril Tablets 2114
Cozaar Tablets 1913
Hyzaar 1964
Lotrel Capsules 2238
Prinivil Tablets 2029
Prinzide Tablets 2033
Vaseretic Tablets 2073
Vasotec I.V. Injection 2076
Zestoretic Tablets 701
Zestril Tablets 704

Craniosynostosis
Synthroid Tablets 515

Cravings, unspecified
▲ Nicotrol NS (Greater than 5%) 2596

Creatine kinase, increase
Accutane Capsules 2740
Aciphex Tablets 1081
Actos Tablets 3224

Adalat CC Tablets (Rare)........ 2978
Advicor Tablets........ 1694
▲ Altoprev Extended-Release Tablets (11%)........ 1151
Amnesteem Capsules........ 2126
Anadrol-50 Tablets........ 3329
▲ Arava Tablets (1% to 3%)........ 2881
Atacand Tablets (0.5% or greater)........ 634
Atacand HCT (0.5% or greater)........ 637
Axert Tablets (Infrequent)........ 2430
Cardizem LA Extended Release Tablets (Less than 2%)........ 1699
Clozapine Tablets........ 2141
Clozaril Tablets........ 2174
Colazal Capsules........ 2845
Combivir Tablets........ 1373
Comtan Tablets........ 2186
Cubicin for Injection (2.8%)........ 1038
Effexor Tablets........ 3405
Effexor XR Capsules........ 3411
▲ Emtriva Capsules (11% to 12%)........ 1272
Epivir........ 1394
▲ Epivir-HBV (9%)........ 1398
Evoxac Capsules........ 1042
Factive Tablets (0.8%)........ 2464
Gleevec Tablets (up to 1.5%)........ 2221
▲ Hepsera Tablets (7%)........ 1275
Levitra Tablets (2%)........ 3048
▲ Lofibra Capsules (3%)........ 1217
▲ Mevacor Tablets (11%)........ 1996
Noroxin Tablets (Rare)........ 2009
Orap Tablets........ 1220
Oxandrin Tablets........ 2977
Paxil CR Controlled-Release Tablets (Rare)........ 1509
Paxil (Rare)........ 1501
Pravachol Tablets (Rare)........ 943
▲ Rapamune Oral Solution and Tablets (3% to 20%)........ 3472
ReFacto Vials........ 3479
Retrovir IV Infusion........ 1537
Sandostatin Injection (Less than 1%)........ 2263
Sandostatin LAR Depot (Rare)........ 2264
Seroquel Tablets........ 691
Symmetrel........ 1115
Tasmar Tablets (Three cases)........ 3360
Teveten Tablets (Less than 1%)........ 1707
Teveten HCT Tablets (Less than 1%)........ 1710
Tiazac Capsules (Less than 2%)........ 1204
▲ Tricor Tablets (3%)........ 523
Trizivir Tablets........ 1565
▲ Truvada Tablets (1% to 12%)........ 1279
Twinrix Vaccine........ 1571
Uniretic Tablets (Less than 1%)........ 3114
▲ Viread Tablets (7% to 12%)........ 1284
Ziagen........ 1600
Zmax for Oral Suspension (Less then 1%)........ 2577
Zocor Tablets........ 2078

Creatine phosphokinase, increase

Vytorin 10/40 Tablets........ 2084
Zetia Tablets........ 2090
Zetia Tablets........ 3098

Creatinine, increase

(*see under* Serum creatinine, elevation)

Creatinine clearance, decrease

▲ Alimta for Injection (Up to 5%)........ 1722
Cytovene (At least 3 subjects)........ 2763
Eskalith........ 1406
Lithobid Tablets........ 1670
▲ Valcyte Tablets (Less than 5%)........ 2816
Vantas (Less than 2%)........ 3367
VFEND I.V. (Less than 2%)........ 2543
VFEND Oral Suspension (Less than 2%)........ 2543
VFEND Tablets (Less than 2%)........ 2543
Zinacef Injection........ 1604
Zinacef for Injection........ 1604

Crepitations

▲ Trisenox Injection (10%)........ 983

Crohn's disease, exacerbation

▲ Entocort EC Capsules (Less than 5%)........ 2694
Proleukin for Injection (Two patients)........ 1007

Croup

(*see under* Laryngotracheobronchitis)

Crusting

Solage Topical Solution (2.4%)........ 740

Crying

Ambien Tablets........ 2867
Aricept Tablets (Frequent)........ 1086
Aricept ODT Tablets (Frequent)........ 1086
▲ Comvax (0.2% to 10.6%)........ 1904
DAPTACEL (1% to 2.5%)........ 2964
HibTITER (38 of 1,118 vaccinations)........ 3419
▲ Infanrix Vaccine (2.2% to 3.9%)........ 1444
Lexapro Oral Solution (Infrequent)........ 1193
Lexapro Tablets (Infrequent)........ 1193
Namenda (Infrequent)........ 1199
Nubain Injection (1% or less)........ 1111
Paxil CR Controlled-Release Tablets........ 1509
Paxil........ 1501
▲ Pediarix Vaccine (1.4% to 24.9%)........ 1518
Prochieve 4% Gel........ 1018
Prochieve 8% Gel........ 1018
Recombivax HB (Greater than 1%)........ 2045
Strattera Capsules (2%)........ 1784
Ultane Liquid for Inhalation (Less than 1%)........ 526
Vaqta (1.8%)........ 2067

Cryptococcosis

▲ CellCept Capsules (Less than 4%)........ 2751
▲ CellCept Intravenous (Less than 4%)........ 2751
▲ CellCept Oral Suspension (Less than 4%)........ 2751
▲ CellCept Tablets (Less than 4%)........ 2751
Doxil Injection (Less than 1%)........ 3302

Crystalluria

Amoxil Capsules........ 1315
Amoxil Chewable Tablets........ 1315
Amoxil Pediatric Drops for Oral Suspension........ 1315
Amoxil Powder for Oral Suspension........ 1315
Amoxil Tablets........ 1315
Augmentin........ 1331
Augmentin Tablets........ 1334
Augmentin XR Extended-Release Tablets........ 1340
Cardizem LA Extended Release Tablets (Less than 2%)........ 1699
Cipro I.V. (1% or less)........ 2998
Cipro I.V. Pharmacy Bulk Package (1% or less)........ 3509
Cipro (Rare)........ 2991
Cipro XR Tablets........ 3004
Clinoril Tablets (Less than 1 in 100)........ 1899
Crixivan Capsules........ 1918
Dantrium Capsules (Less frequent)........ 2690
Demser Capsules (A few patients)........ 1933
Effexor Tablets (Rare)........ 3405
Effexor XR Capsules (Rare)........ 3411
Levaquin in 5% Dextrose Injection........ 2453
Levaquin........ 2453
Lyrica Capsules (Rare)........ 2524
Mintezol........ 2002
Noroxin Tablets........ 2009
Paser Granules........ 1657
Reyataz Capsules (Less than 3%)........ 948
Uniretic Tablets (Less than 1%)........ 3114

Cushingoid appearance

Advair Diskus 100/50........ 1291
Advair Diskus 250/50........ 1291
Advair Diskus 500/50........ 1291
Aptivus Capsules........ 859
Crixivan Capsules........ 1918
Retrovir........ 1533
Truvada Tablets........ 1279

Cushingoid state

(*see under* Cushing's syndrome)

Cushing's syndrome

Aclovate........ 1290
Advair Diskus 100/50........ 1291
Advair Diskus 250/50........ 1291
Advair Diskus 500/50........ 1291
▲ CellCept Capsules (3% to less than 20%)........ 2751
▲ CellCept Intravenous (3% to less than 20%)........ 2751
▲ CellCept Oral Suspension (3% to less than 20%)........ 2751
▲ CellCept Tablets (3% to less than 20%)........ 2751
Clobevate Gel........ 3213
Clobex Shampoo........ 1209
Copaxone for Injection (Infrequent)........ 3292
Cutivate Cream........ 1381
Cutivate Lotion 0.05% (Rare)........ 1383
Cutivate Ointment........ 1384
Decadron Phosphate Injection........ 1931
Decadron Tablets........ 1929
Depo-Medrol Injectable Suspension........ 2615
Depo-Medrol Single-Dose Vial........ 2617
Diprolene Gel 0.05%........ 3015
Diprolene Lotion 0.05%........ 3016
Diprolene Ointment 0.05% (Some patients)........ 3017
Diprolene AF Cream 0.05% (Some patients)........ 3014
Diprosone Cream, USP 0.05%........ 3018
Elocon Cream 0.1%........ 3019
Elocon Lotion 0.1%........ 3020
Elocon Ointment 0.1%........ 3021
Flovent Diskus 50 mcg........ 1415
Flovent HFA........ 1418
Hydrocortone Tablets........ 1963
Kaletra (Less than 2%)........ 474
Lotrisone........ 3054
▲ Myfortic Tablets (3% to less than 20%)........ 2244
Nasacort HFA Inhalation Aerosol........ 2939
Neurontin Capsules (Rare)........ 2498
Neurontin Oral Solution (Rare)........ 2498
Neurontin Tablets (Rare)........ 2498
Olux Foam........ 1027
Pediapred Oral Solution........ 3319
▲ Prograf Capsules and Injection (3% to 15%)........ 624
▲ Rapamune Oral Solution and Tablets (3% to 20%)........ 3472
Temovate Cream........ 1549
Temovate Gel........ 1550
Temovate Ointment........ 1549
Temovate Scalp Application........ 1551
Temovate E Emollient........ 1552
Vanos Cream........ 1864

Cutaneous reactions, severe

Celexa (Rare)........ 1177

Cutaneous reactions, unspecified

Ertaczo Cream, 2% (2%)........ 2383
Lotrisone Cream........ 3054
Malarone Tablets........ 1484
Malarone Pediatric Tablets........ 1484

Cutaneous tenderness

Oxsoralen-Ultra Capsules........ 3354

Cyanosis

Abilify Tablets (Infrequent)........ 916
Abilify Tablets (Infrequent)........ 2472
AmBisome for Injection (Infrequent)........ 615
AquaMEPHYTON Injection........ 1887
BeneFix for Injection........ 3402
Buprenex Injectable (Less than 1%)........ 2718
Campath Ampules........ 826
Carimune NF........ 3501
▲ Cerezyme for Injection (Approximately 6.6%)........ 1263
Clozapine Tablets (Less than 1%)........ 2141
Clozaril Tablets (Less than 1%)........ 2174
Copaxone for Injection (Infrequent)........ 3292
Cytovene-IV (One report)........ 2763
Effexor Tablets (Rare)........ 3405
Effexor XR Capsules (Rare)........ 3411
Elitek (Less than or equal to 1%)........ 2906
FazaClo Orally Disintegrating Tablets (Less than 1%)........ 547
▲ Flolan for Injection (31% to 54%)........ 1408
Gammagard Liquid........ 751
Gammagard S/D........ 754
Gamunex Immune Globulin I.V., 10%........ 3232
Imitrex Injection........ 1431
Imitrex Nasal Spray........ 1435
Imitrex Tablets........ 1440
Infanrix Vaccine........ 1444
▲ Infasurf Intratracheal Suspension (65%)........ 1188
Infed Injection........ 3381
▲ Intron A for Injection (Less than or equal to 5%)........ 3038
Invirase (Less than 2%)........ 2776
Iveegam EN........ 759
Mephyton Tablets (Rare)........ 1993
Mycamine for Injection........ 620
Pediarix Vaccine........ 1518
Permax Tablets (Infrequent)........ 3357
Primaxin I.M........ 2022
Primaxin I.V. (Less than 0.2%)........ 2024
Relpax Tablets (Rare)........ 2531
Rilutek Tablets (Rare)........ 2945
Seroquel Tablets (Rare)........ 691
Sonata Capsules (Rare)........ 1686
Soriatane Capsules (Less than 1%)........ 1028
Tequin Injection (Less than 0.1%)........ 964
Tequin Tablets (Less than 0.1%)........ 964
Thalomid Capsules........ 979
VFEND I.V. (Less than 2%)........ 2543
VFEND Oral Suspension (Less than 2%)........ 2543
VFEND Tablets (Less than 2%)........ 2543
Virazole for Inhalation Solution (Infrequent)........ 3365
Zomig Nasal Spray (Infrequent)........ 718
Zomig Tablets (Rare)........ 714
Zomig-ZMT Tablets (Rare)........ 714
Zyprexa Tablets (Infrequent)........ 1798
Zyprexa ZYDIS Orally Disintegrating Tablets (Infrequent)........ 1798

Cyanosis, hand

▲ Intron A for Injection (Less than 5%)........ 3038

Cycloplegia

Bentyl Capsules........ 724
Bentyl Injection........ 724
Bentyl Syrup........ 724
Bentyl Tablets........ 724
Ditropan XL Extended Release Tablets........ 2391

Cylindruria

Cipro I.V. (1% or less)........ 2998
Cipro I.V. Pharmacy Bulk Package (1% or less)........ 3509
Cipro........ 2991
Levaquin in 5% Dextrose Injection........ 2453
Levaquin........ 2453
Noroxin Tablets........ 2009

Cyst, Baker's

Orthovisc Injection (0.4%)........ 3518

Cyst, sebaceous

Rescriptor Tablets........ 2535

Cyst, synovial

Gengraf Capsules (1% to less than 3%)........ 458
Neoral Soft Gelatin Capsules (1% to less than 3%)........ 2247
Neoral Oral Solution (1% to less than 3%)........ 2247

Cyst, unspecified

Actiq (Less than 1%)........ 993
Antara Capsules........ 2723
▲ Arava Tablets (1% to 3%)........ 2881
▲ Casodex Tablets (2% to 5%)........ 670
▲ CellCept Capsules (3% to less than 20%)........ 2751
▲ CellCept Intravenous (3% to less than 20%)........ 2751
▲ CellCept Oral Suspension (3% to less than 20%)........ 2751
▲ CellCept Tablets (3% to less than 20%)........ 2751
Copaxone for Injection (2%)........ 3292
Gabitril Tablets (Frequent)........ 998
Imitrex Injection........ 1431
Lofibra Capsules........ 1217
Neurontin Capsules (Rare)........ 2498
Neurontin Oral Solution (Rare)........ 2498
Neurontin Tablets (Rare)........ 2498
Prochieve 4% Gel........ 1018
Prochieve 8% Gel........ 1018
Protonix I.V. (Less than 1%)........ 3468
Protonix Tablets (Less than 1%)........ 3465
Protopic Ointment (Up to 3%)........ 629
▲ Simulect for Injection (3% to 10%)........ 2268
Soriatane Capsules (Less than 1%)........ 1028
Symbyax Capsules (Infrequent)........ 1788
Thalomid Capsules........ 979
Tricor Tablets........ 523
Uniretic Tablets (Less than 1%)........ 3114
Zomig Nasal Spray (Infrequent)........ 718

Cystitis

Abilify Tablets (Infrequent)........ 916
Abilify Tablets (Infrequent)........ 2472
Aciphex Tablets........ 1081
Activella Tablets........ 2311
▲ Actonel Tablets (4.1%)........ 2679
▲ Actonel with Calcium Tablets (4.1%)........ 2684
Alesse-28 Tablets........ 3392
Ambien Tablets (Infrequent)........ 2867
Anaprox Tablets (Less than 1%)........ 2769
Anaprox DS Tablets (Less than 1%)........ 2769
Antara Capsules........ 2723
▲ Arava Tablets (1% to 3%)........ 2881
Aricept Tablets (Infrequent)........ 1086
Aricept ODT Tablets (Infrequent)........ 1086
Atacand HCT (0.5% or greater)........ 637
▲ Azmacort Inhalation Aerosol (1% to 3%)........ 1701
Caduet Tablets (Less than 2%)........ 2507
Cataflam Tablets (Occasionally)........ 2173
Copaxone for Injection (At least 2%)........ 3292
Depacon Injection (1% or more)........ 412
Depakene (1% or more)........ 417
Depakote Sprinkle Capsules........ 422
▲ Depakote Tablets (1% to 5%)........ 427

Depakote ER Tablets (Greater than 1%) 433
▲ Ditropan XL Extended Release Tablets (2% to less than 5%) 2391
▲ Doxil Injection (Less than 1% to 10%) 3302
EC-Naprosyn Delayed-Release Tablets (Less than 1%) 2769
Effexor Tablets (Infrequent) 3405
Effexor XR Capsules (Infrequent) 3411
Estratest Tablets 3196
Estratest H.S. Tablets 3196
▲ Eulexin Capsules (16%) 3023
▲ Evista Tablets (3.3% to 4.6%) 1735
▲ Evoxac Capsules (1% to 3%) 1042
Exelon Capsules (Infrequent) 2204
▲ Fortical Nasal Spray (1% to 3%) 3336
Gabitril Tablets (Infrequent) 998
Gonal-f RFF Pen for Injection (2.4%) 3155
▲ Humira Injection (Less than 5%) 464
▲ Intron A for Injection (Less than 5%) 3038
Klonopin (Infrequent) 2782
Lamictal (Rare) 1449
Leukeran Tablets 1472
Lipitor Tablets (Less than 2%) 2495
Lofibra Capsules 1217
Lo/Ovral-28 Tablets 3423
Lunesta Tablets (Infrequent) 3139
Miacalcin Nasal Spray (1% to 3%) 2242
Micardis Tablets (More than 0.3%) 884
Micardis HCT Tablets 886
Migranal Nasal Spray (Infrequent) 3350
Nalfon Capsules (Less than 1%) 2504
Naprosyn Suspension (Less than 1%) 2769
Naprosyn Tablets (Less than 1%) 2769
Neurontin Capsules (Infrequent) 2498
Neurontin Oral Solution (Infrequent) 2498
Neurontin Tablets (Infrequent) 2498
Nexium Delayed-Release Capsules (Less than 1%) 645
Nexium I.V. (Less than 1%) 649
Ortho-Cept Tablets 2395
Ortho-Cyclen Tablets 2414
Ortho Evra Transdermal System 2402
Ortho Tri-Cyclen Tablets 2414
Ortho Tri-Cyclen Lo Tablets 2421
Paxil CR Controlled-Release Tablets (Infrequent) 1509
Paxil (Infrequent) 1501
Permax Tablets (Infrequent) 3357
Plavix Tablets (1% to 2.5%) 940
Plavix Tablets (1% to 2.5%) 2942
Pletal Tablets (Less than 2%) 2478
Premarin Intravenous 3440
Premarin Vaginal Cream 3449
Premphase Tablets 3452
Prempro Tablets 3452
Prochieve 4% Gel 1018
Prochieve 8% Gel 1018
▲ Prograf Capsules and Injection (3% to 15%) 624
Protonix I.V. (Less than 1%) 3468
Protonix Tablets (Less than 1%) 3465
Provigil Tablets (At least 1%) 1002
Prozac Pulvules and Liquid (Infrequent) 1771
Razadyne ER Extended-Release Capsules (Infrequent) 2434
Razadyne (Infrequent) 2434
Risperdal M-Tab Orally Disintegrating Tablets (Rare) 1658
Risperdal (Rare) 1658
Seasonale Tablets 1073
Seroquel Tablets (Infrequent) 691
Sonata Capsules (Infrequent) 1686
Symbyax Capsules (Infrequent) 1788
Teveten Tablets (Less than 1%) 1707
Teveten HCT Tablets (Less than 1%) 1710
▲ Topamax Sprinkle Capsules (1% to 3%) 2438
▲ Topamax Tablets (1% to 3%) 2438
Tricor Tablets 523
Triglide Tablets 1165
Triphasil-28 Tablets 3483
Uniretic Tablets (Less than 1%) 3114
Viagra Tablets (Less than 2%) 2552
Vicoprofen Tablets (Less than 1%) 533
Voltaren Tablets (Occasionally) 2298
Voltaren-XR Tablets (Occasionally) 2301
Wellbutrin Tablets (Rare) 1579
Wellbutrin SR Sustained-Release Tablets 1583
Wellbutrin XL Extended-Release Tablets 1588
Yasmin 28 Tablets (Greater than 1%) 818
▲ Zoladex (16%) 709
▲ Zoladex 3-month (16%) 712
Zoloft (Rare) 2581
Zomig Tablets (Infrequent) 714
Zomig-ZMT Tablets (Infrequent) 714
Zyban Sustained-Release Tablets 1620
Zyprexa Tablets (Infrequent) 1798
Zyprexa ZYDIS Orally Disintegrating Tablets (Infrequent) 1798
Zyrtec Chewable Tablets (Less than 2%) 2589
Zyrtec (Less than 2%) 2589
Zyrtec-D 12 Hour Extended Release Tablets (Less than 2%) 2591

Cystitis, hemorrhagic
Adriamycin for Injection, USP 786
Adriamycin Injection, USP 786
AmBisome for Injection (Infrequent) 615
Cipro I.V. (1% or less) 2998
Cipro I.V. Pharmacy Bulk Package (1% or less) 3509
Cipro XR Tablets 3004
Herceptin I.V. (At least one of the 958 patients) 1234
▲ I.V. Busulfex (7%) 1125
Navelbine Injection (Less than 1%) 1494
Oncaspar 1123
VFEND I.V. (Less than 2%) 2543
VFEND Oral Suspension (Less than 2%) 2543
VFEND Tablets (Less than 2%) 2543

Cystitis, viral
Retrovir Capsules (0.8%) 1533
Retrovir IV Infusion (1%) 1537
Retrovir (0.8%) 1533

Cysts, epidermal
Rescriptor Tablets 2535

Cysts, vaginal
Depo-Provera Contraceptive Injection (Less than 1%) 2619
depo-subQ provera 104 Injectable Suspension 2622

Cysts at injection site
▲ Fuzeon Injection (80%) 2772

Cytokine Released Syndrome
Orthoclone OKT3 Sterile Solution (Occasional) 2370
Simulect for Injection 2268

Cytopenia, unspecified
Bexxar 1360
Pegasys 2793

D

Deafness
Abelcet Injection 1119
Abilify Tablets (Infrequent) 916
Abilify Tablets (Infrequent) 2472
Aciphex Tablets 1081
Actiq (Less than 1%) 993
Aggrenox Capsules (Less than 1%) 855
Betasept Surgical Scrub 2715
Caduet Tablets (Less than 2%) 2507
Campral Tablets (Infrequent) 1175
Celebrex Capsules (0.1% to 1.9%) 3130
▲ CellCept Capsules (3% to less than 20%) 2751
▲ CellCept Intravenous (3% to less than 20%) 2751
▲ CellCept Oral Suspension (3% to less than 20%) 2751
▲ CellCept Tablets (3% to less than 20%) 2751
Copaxone for Injection (At least 2%) 3292
▲ Depacon Injection (1% to 5%) 412
▲ Depakene (1% to 5%) 417
▲ Depakote Sprinkle Capsules (1% to 5%) 422
▲ Depakote Tablets (1% to 5%) 427
Depakote ER Tablets (Greater than 1%) 433
DepoCyt Injection 1121
Edecrin 1941
Effexor Tablets (Rare) 3405
Effexor XR Capsules (Rare) 3411
Eloxatin for Injection 2908
Evoxac Capsules (Less than 1%) 1042
Gabitril Tablets (Infrequent) 998
Gengraf Capsules (1% to less than 3%) 458
Herceptin I.V. (At least one of the 958 patients) 1234
Imitrex Injection 1431
Imitrex Nasal Spray 1435
Imitrex Tablets 1440
Indocin Capsules (Less than 1%) 1968
Indocin I.V. (Less than 1%) 1973
Indocin (Less than 1%) 1968
Lamictal (Rare) 1449
Lipitor Tablets (Less than 2%) 2495
Neoral Soft Gelatin Capsules (1% to less than 3%) 2247
Neoral Oral Solution (1% to less than 3%) 2247
Neurontin Capsules (Infrequent) 2498
Neurontin Oral Solution (Infrequent) 2498
Neurontin Tablets (Infrequent) 2498
Nipent for Injection (Less than 3%) 3216
Paxil CR Controlled-Release Tablets (Rare) 1509
Paxil (Rare) 1501
Permax Tablets (Infrequent) 3357
Prevacid Delayed-Release Capsules (Less than 1%) 3268
Prevacid for Delayed-Release Oral Suspension (Less than 1%) 3268
Prevacid NapraPAC (Less than 1%) 3277
Prevacid SoluTab Delayed-Release Orally Disintegrating Tablets (Less than 1%) 3268
PREVPAC (Less than 1%) 3281
Prograf Capsules and Injection 624
Protonix I.V. (Less than 1%) 3468
Protonix Tablets (Less than 1%) 3465
▲ Rapamune Oral Solution and Tablets (3% to 20%) 3472
Rilutek Tablets (Rare) 2945
Risperdal Consta Long-Acting Injection (Infrequent) 1664
Sandostatin LAR Depot (Rare) 2264
Seroquel Tablets (Infrequent) 691
Sonata Capsules (Rare) 1686
Soriatane Capsules (Less than 1%) 1028
Symbyax Capsules (Infrequent) 1788
Uniretic Tablets (Less than 1%) 3114
VFEND I.V. (Less than 2%) 2543
VFEND Oral Suspension (Less than 2%) 2543
VFEND Tablets (Less than 2%) 2543
Viagra Tablets (Less than 2%) 2552
Wellbutrin SR Sustained-Release Tablets 1583
Wellbutrin XL Extended-Release Tablets 1588
Zithromax Capsules, 250 mg 2568
Zithromax for IV Infusion 2573
Zithromax for Oral Suspension, 300 mg, 600 mg, 900 mg, 1200 mg 2561
Zithromax Tablets, 250 mg, 500 mg 2561
Zithromax Tri-Pak 2561
Zmax for Oral Suspension 2577
Zonegran Capsules (Infrequent) 1089
Zyban Sustained-Release Tablets 1620
Zyprexa Tablets (Infrequent) 1798
Zyprexa ZYDIS Orally Disintegrating Tablets (Infrequent) 1798
Zyrtec Chewable Tablets (Less than 2%) 2589
Zyrtec (Less than 2%) 2589
Zyrtec-D 12 Hour Extended Release Tablets (Less than 2%) 2591

Deafness, transient
Actiq (Less than 1%) 993

Death
Abilify Tablets 916
Abilify Tablets 2472
Anaprox Tablets (Less than 1%) 2769
Anaprox DS Tablets (Less than 1%) 2769
▲ Aranesp for Injection (7%) 576
Cataflam Tablets (Rarely) 2173
EC-Naprosyn Delayed-Release Tablets (Less than 1%) 2769
Gemzar for Injection (Rare) 1743
Mephyton Tablets 1993
Naprosyn Suspension (Less than 1%) 2769
Naprosyn Tablets (Less than 1%) 2769
Rapamune Oral Solution and Tablets (0.8% to 1.7%) 3472
Razadyne ER Extended-Release Capsules 2434
Razadyne 2434
Symbyax Capsules (Rare) 1788
Voltaren Tablets (Rarely) 2298
Voltaren-XR Tablets (Rarely) 2301

Death, fetal
Aceon Tablets (2 mg, 4 mg, 8 mg) 3191
Altace Capsules 1673
Arthrotec Tablets 3126
Atacand Tablets 634
Atacand HCT 637
Avalide Tablets 922
Avalide Tablets 2889
Avapro Tablets 925
Avapro Tablets 2886
Captopril Tablets 2114
Cozaar Tablets 1913
Hyzaar 1964
Lotrel Capsules 2238
Prinivil Tablets 2029
Prinzide Tablets 2033
Prometrium Capsules (100 mg, 200 mg) (Rare) 3205
Thalomid Capsules 979
Uniretic Tablets (More than 1%) 3114
Vaseretic Tablets 2073
Vasotec I.V. Injection 2076
Zestoretic Tablets 701
Zestril Tablets 704
Zyrtec Chewable Tablets (Rare) 2589
Zyrtec (Rare) 2589

Death, infants
Virazole for Inhalation Solution (20 cases) 3365

Death, sudden
Aciphex Tablets 1081
Adderall Tablets 3168
Adderall XR Capsules 3169
▲ Apokyn Injection (4%) 2132
Campral Tablets (Rare) 1175
Camptosar Injection 2602
Celebrex Capsules (Less than 0.1%) 3130
Clozapine Tablets (Rare) 2141
Clozaril Tablets (Rare) 2174
Gabitril Tablets (Infrequent) 998
Imitrex Tablets 1440
Meridia Capsules 485
Namenda 1199
Orap Tablets 1220
Phenergan 3438
Prozac Pulvules and Liquid 1771
Risperdal M-Tab Orally Disintegrating Tablets (Rare) 1658
Risperdal (Rare) 1658
Thioridazine Hydrochloride Tablets 2122
Topamax Sprinkle Capsules (Rare) 2438
Topamax Tablets (Rare) 2438
Zyprexa Tablets (Rare) 1798
Zyprexa ZYDIS Orally Disintegrating Tablets (Rare) 1798

Deep tendon reflexes, loss
Eloxatin for Injection 2908

Defecate, desire to
Aminohippurate Sodium "PAH" Injection 1886

Defecation, increased
▲ Xenical Capsules (2.8% to 10.8%) 2834

Defecation, painful
Invirase (Less than 2%) 2776

Dehydration
Abilify Tablets (Frequent) 916
Abilify Tablets (Frequent) 2472
Aciphex Tablets 1081
Actiq (1% or greater) 993
Aggrenox Capsules 855
Agrylin Capsules (1% to 5%) 3172
▲ Alimta for Injection (Up to 9%) 1722
Amerge Tablets (Infrequent) 1312
Ammonul Injection 3323
▲ Apokyn Injection (At least 5%) 2132
Aptivus Capsules (Less than 2%) 859
▲ Aranesp for Injection (5%) 576
Aricept Tablets (Frequent) 1086
Aricept ODT Tablets (Frequent) 1086
Arthrotec Tablets (Rare) 3126
Bayer Aspirin Tablets 3515
Bexxar 1360
Bravelle for Intramuscular or Subcutaneous Injection (2.7%) 1140
Campath Ampules 826
▲ Camptosar Injection (4% to 15%) 2602
Captopril Tablets 2114
▲ Casodex Tablets (2% to 5%) 670
Celexa (Rare) 1177
▲ CellCept Capsules (3% to less than 20%) 2751
▲ CellCept Intravenous (3% to less than 20%) 2751
▲ CellCept Oral Suspension (3% to less than 20%) 2751
▲ CellCept Tablets (3% to less than 20%) 2751
Cymbalta Delayed-Release Capsules (Infrequent) 1729
Diovan HCT Tablets (Greater than 0.2%) 2195

Diprivan Injectable Emulsion (Less than 1%) 676
▲ Doxil Injection (1% to 10%) 3302
Ecotrin Enteric Coated Aspirin Low, Regular and Maximum Strength Tablets 1627
Effexor Tablets (Rare) 3405
Effexor XR Capsules (Rare) 3411
Elitek (Less than or equal to 1%) 2906
Ellence Injection 2632
▲ Eloxatin for Injection (5% to 8%) 2908
▲ Emend Capsules (5.9%) 1944
Epivir 1394
▲ Erbitux (2% to 9%) 937
Eskalith 1406
Evoxac Capsules (Less than 1%) 1042
Exelon Capsules (Frequent) 2204
Fleet Enema 1169
Frova Tablets (Infrequent) 1101
Furosemide Tablets 2117
Gabitril Tablets (Infrequent) 998
Garamycin Injectable 3028
Geodon Capsules (Infrequent) 2514
Gleevec Tablets (Infrequent) 2221
▲ Hectorol Capsules (Greater than or equal to 5%) 909
Hectorol Injection 911
▲ Humira Injection (Less than 5%) 464
Imitrex Injection (Rare) 1431
Imitrex Nasal Spray 1435
Imitrex Tablets 1440
▲ Intron A for Injection (Less than or equal to 5%) 3038
Invanz for Injection (Greater than 0.1%) 1974
Invirase (Less than 2%) 2776
Kaletra (Less than 2%) 474
Keppra Oral Solution (2%) 3307
Keppra Tablets (2%) 3307
Klonopin 2782
Levaquin in 5% Dextrose Injection (0.1% to 0.9%) 2453
Levaquin (0.1% to 0.9%) 2453
Lithobid Tablets 1670
Lunesta Tablets (Rare) 3139
Maxalt Tablets (Infrequent) 1983
Maxalt-MLT Orally Disintegrating Tablets (Infrequent) 1983
Mobic Oral Suspension (Less than 2%) 893
Mobic Tablets (Less than 2%) 893
Moduretic Tablets (Less than or equal to 1%) 2003
▲ Myfortic Tablets (3% to less than 20%) 2244
Namenda (Infrequent) 1199
Neumega for Injection 3433
Neurontin Capsules 2498
Neurontin Oral Solution 2498
Neurontin Tablets 2498
Norvir (Less than 2%) 499
▲ Ontak Vials (9%) 1717
OxyContin Tablets (Less than 1%) 2699
Paxil CR Controlled-Release Tablets (Rare) 1509
Paxil (Rare) 1501
Permax Tablets (Infrequent) 3357
▲ Photofrin for Injection (7% to 10%) 729
Prevacid Delayed-Release Capsules (Less than 1%) 3268
Prevacid for Delayed-Release Oral Suspension (Less than 1%) 3268
Prevacid NapraPAC (Less than 1%) 3277
Prevacid SoluTab Delayed-Release Orally Disintegrating Tablets (Less than 1%) 3268
PREVPAC (Less than 1%) 3281
Prinivil Tablets (0.3% to 1.0%) 2029
Prinzide Tablets 2033
▲ Prograf Capsules and Injection (3% to 15%) 624
Protonix I.V. 3468
Protonix Tablets 3465
Protopic Ointment (Greater than or equal to 1%) 629
Prozac Pulvules and Liquid (Infrequent) 1771
▲ Rapamune Oral Solution and Tablets (3% to 20%) 3472
Razadyne ER Extended-Release Capsules 2434
Razadyne 2434
Remicade for IV Injection (Greater than or equal to 0.2%) 987
Requip Tablets (Infrequent) 1528
Reyataz Capsules (Less than 3%) 948
Risperdal Consta Long-Acting Injection (Infrequent) 1664
Risperdal M-Tab Orally Disintegrating Tablets (Rare) 1658
Risperdal (Rare) 1658
Rythmol SR Capsules 2736
▲ Sandostatin LAR Depot (5% to 15%) 2264
Seroquel Tablets (Infrequent) 691
▲ Simulect for Injection (3% to 10%) 2268
St. Joseph 81 mg Aspirin Chewable and Enteric Coated Tablets 1841
Symbyax Capsules (Infrequent) 1788
Tasmar Tablets (Infrequent) 3360
Taxotere Injection Concentrate (Rare) 2947
Thalomid Capsules 979
Topamax Sprinkle Capsules (Infrequent) 2438
Topamax Tablets (Infrequent) 2438
Uniretic Tablets (Less than 1%) 3114
▲ Valcyte Tablets (Less than 5%) 2816
Vantin Tablets and Oral Suspension (Less than 1%) 2650
Vaqta 2067
Vaseretic Tablets 2073
Vasotec I.V. Injection 2076
▲ Velcade for Injection (18%) 2102
Viracept (Less than 2%) 2556
▲ Xeloda Tablets (2% to 10%) 2825
Xifaxan Tablets (Less than 2%) 2847
▲ Zenapax for Injection (2% to 5%) 2838
Zestoretic Tablets 701
Zestril Tablets (0.3% to 1.0%) 704
Zithromax Capsules, 250 mg (Rare) 2568
Zithromax for IV Infusion (Rare) 2573
Zithromax for Oral Suspension, 300 mg, 600 mg, 900 mg, 1200 mg (Rare) 2561
Zithromax Tablets, 250 mg, 500 mg (Rare) 2561
Zithromax Tri-Pak (Rare) 2561
Zmax for Oral Suspension 2577
Zoloft (Rare) 2581
▲ Zometa for Intravenous Infusion (5% to 14%) 2306
Zomig Nasal Spray (Rare) 718
Zonegran Capsules (Infrequent) 1089
Zyprexa Tablets (Infrequent) 1798
Zyprexa IntraMuscular (Infrequent) 1798
Zyprexa ZYDIS Orally Disintegrating Tablets (Infrequent) 1798
Zyrtec Chewable Tablets (Less than 2%) 2589
Zyrtec (Less than 2%) 2589
Zyrtec-D 12 Hour Extended Release Tablets (Less than 2%) 2591

Delirium

Abilify Tablets (Infrequent) 916
Abilify Tablets (Infrequent) 2472
Aciphex Tablets 1081
Avinza Capsules (Less than 5%) 1714
Catapres Tablets 874
Catapres-TTS (0.5% or less) 875
Celexa 1177
▲ CellCept Capsules (3% to less than 20%) 2751
▲ CellCept Intravenous (3% to less than 20%) 2751
▲ CellCept Oral Suspension (3% to less than 20%) 2751
▲ CellCept Tablets (3% to less than 20%) 2751
Cipro I.V. 2998
Cipro I.V. Pharmacy Bulk Package 3509
Cipro 2991
Cipro XR Tablets 3004
Clorpres Tablets 2139
Clozapine Tablets 2141
Clozaril Tablets 2174
Digitek Tablets 2146
Diprivan Injectable Emulsion (Less than 1%) 676
Effexor Tablets 3405
Effexor XR Capsules 3411
Evoxac Capsules 1042
Exelon Capsules (Infrequent) 2204
Famvir Tablets (Infrequent) 2207
FazaClo Orally Disintegrating Tablets 547
Geodon Capsules (Frequent) 2514
I.V. Busulfex (2%) 1125
Lamictal (Rare) 1449
Lanoxicaps Capsules 1458
Lanoxin Injection 1462
Lanoxin Tablets 1468
Lanoxin Injection Pediatric 1465
Levaquin in 5% Dextrose Injection (0.1% to 0.9%) 2453
Levaquin (0.1% to 0.9%) 2453
Lexapro Oral Solution 1193
Lexapro Tablets 1193
Lyrica Capsules (Rare) 2524
Merrem I.V. (Greater than 0.1% to 1%) 687
Mycamine for Injection (0.8%) 620
Namenda (Infrequent) 1199
Orthoclone OKT3 Sterile Solution (Less than 1%) 2370
Paxil CR Controlled-Release Tablets (Rare) 1509
Paxil (Rare) 1501
Phenergan 3438
PhosLo GelCaps 2158
Prograf Capsules and Injection 624
Razadyne ER Extended-Release Capsules (Infrequent) 2434
Razadyne (Infrequent) 2434
Requip Tablets (Infrequent) 1528
Rilutek Tablets (Infrequent) 2945
Risperdal Consta Long-Acting Injection (Infrequent) 1664
Risperdal M-Tab Orally Disintegrating Tablets (Rare) 1658
Risperdal (Rare) 1658
Sanctura Tablets 1133
Seroquel Tablets (Rare) 691
Symmetrel 1115
Tasmar Tablets (Rare) 3360
Topamax Sprinkle Capsules (Infrequent) 2438
Topamax Tablets (Infrequent) 2438
Trileptal Oral Suspension 2281
Trileptal Tablets 2281
VFEND I.V. (Less than 2%) 2543
VFEND Oral Suspension (Less than 2%) 2543
VFEND Tablets (Less than 2%) 2543
Wellbutrin Tablets 1579
Wellbutrin SR Sustained-Release Tablets 1583
Wellbutrin XL Extended-Release Tablets 1588
Zovirax Capsules 1616
Zovirax for Injection 1618
Zovirax 1616
Zyban Sustained-Release Tablets 1620
Zyprexa Tablets (Infrequent) 1798
Zyprexa ZYDIS Orally Disintegrating Tablets (Infrequent) 1798

Delivery complications, unspecified

Advil ◘ 737
Advil Cold & Sinus ◘ 739
Advil Flu & Body Ache Caplets ◘ 739
Advil Migraine Liquigels ◘ 740
Aleve Tablets, Caplets and Gelcaps ◘ 605
Bayer, Aspirin Regimen ◘ 606
Bayer Aspirin Tablets 3515
BC Powder ◘ 612
BC Allergy Sinus Cold Powder ◘ 612
Arthritis Strength BC Powder ◘ 612
BC Sinus Cold Powder ◘ 612
Ecotrin Enteric Coated Aspirin Low, Regular and Maximum Strength Tablets 1627
Epivir 1394
Goody's Body Pain Formula Powder ◘ 621
Goody's Extra Strength Headache Powder ◘ 621
Goody's Extra Strength Pain Relief Tablets ◘ 621
Motrin Cold & Sinus Caplets 1836
Motrin IB Tablets and Caplets 1836
St. Joseph 81 mg Aspirin Chewable and Enteric Coated Tablets 1841

Delusions

Abilify Tablets (Frequent) 916
Abilify Tablets (Frequent) 2472
Ambien Tablets (Rare) 2867
Aricept Tablets (Frequent) 1086
Aricept ODT Tablets (Frequent) 1086
Celexa (Rare) 1177
Clozapine Tablets (Less than 1%) 2141
Clozaril Tablets (Less than 1%) 2174
Effexor Tablets (Rare) 3405
Effexor XR Capsules (Rare) 3411
Eldepryl Capsules 3209
Evoxac Capsules 1042
Exelon Capsules (2% or more) 2204
FazaClo Orally Disintegrating Tablets (Less than 1%) 547
Flexeril Tablets (Rare) 1832
Gabitril Tablets (Infrequent) 998
Lamictal (Rare) 1449
▲ Lupron Depot 3.75 mg (Among most frequent) 3257
Lupron Depot–3 Month 11.25 mg (Less than 5%) 3262
Lyrica Capsules (Rare) 2524
Mirapex Tablets (1%) 889
Namenda (Infrequent) 1199
Nubain Injection (1% or less) 1111
Parcopa Orally Disintegrating Tablets 3111
Paxil CR Controlled-Release Tablets (Rare) 1509
Paxil (Rare) 1501
Permax Tablets (Infrequent) 3357
Prozac Pulvules and Liquid (Rare) 1771
Requip Tablets (Infrequent) 1528
Rilutek Tablets (Infrequent) 2945
Risperdal Consta Long-Acting Injection (Frequent) 1664
Seroquel Tablets (Infrequent) 691
Sonata Capsules (Rare) 1686
Stalevo Tablets 2270
Surmontil Capsules 2347
Sustiva Capsules 957
Symmetrel 1115
Tasmar Tablets (Infrequent) 3360
Topamax Sprinkle Capsules (Infrequent) 2438
Topamax Tablets (Infrequent) 2438
Trileptal Oral Suspension 2281
Trileptal Tablets 2281
Vivactil Tablets 2350
Wellbutrin Tablets (1.2%) 1579
Wellbutrin SR Sustained-Release Tablets 1583
Wellbutrin XL Extended-Release Tablets 1588
Zoloft (Infrequent) 2581
Zyban Sustained-Release Tablets 1620
Zyprexa Tablets (Frequent) 1798

Dementia

Ambien Tablets (Rare) 2867
Cenestin Tablets, 0.45mg, 0.625mg, 0.9mg, 1.25mg 1063
Cenestin Tablets, 0.3mg 1063
CombiPatch Transdermal System 2180
Depacon Injection (Several reports) 412
Depakene (Several reports) 417
Depakote Sprinkle Capsules (Several reports) 422
Depakote Tablets (Several reports) 427
Depakote ER Tablets (Several reports) 433
Effexor Tablets (Rare) 3405
Effexor XR Capsules (Rare) 3411
Estratest Tablets (1.8%) 3196
Estratest H.S. Tablets (1.8%) 3196
Evoxac Capsules 1042
Exelon Capsules (Infrequent) 2204
Menostar Transdermal System 805
Parcopa Orally Disintegrating Tablets 3111
Prefest Tablets 1069
Premarin Intravenous 3440
Premarin Tablets 3443
Premarin Vaginal Cream 3449
Premphase Tablets 3452
Prempro Tablets 3452
Relpax Tablets (Rare) 2531
Requip Tablets (Infrequent) 1528
Rilutek Tablets (Rare) 2945
Risperdal Consta Long-Acting Injection (Infrequent) 1664
Rythmol SR Capsules 2736
Stalevo Tablets 2270
▲ Vesanoid Capsules (3%) 2823
VFEND I.V. (Less than 2%) 2543
VFEND Oral Suspension (Less than 2%) 2543
VFEND Tablets (Less than 2%) 2543
Vivelle Transdermal System (1.8%) 2288
Vivelle-Dot Transdermal System 2293
Zyprexa Tablets (Infrequent) 1798

Demyelination

Infanrix Vaccine 1444
Proleukin for Injection 1007
Remicade for IV Injection 987

Dental caries

Abilify Tablets (Infrequent) 916
Abilify Tablets (Infrequent) 2472
Actiq (Less than 1%) 993
Ambien Tablets (Rare) 2867
Copaxone for Injection (Frequent) 3292
Eskalith 1406
Gabitril Tablets (Infrequent) 998
Lithobid Tablets 1670
Paxil CR Controlled-Release Tablets (Rare) 1509
Paxil (Rare) 1501
Permax Tablets (Infrequent) 3357
Seroquel Tablets (Infrequent) 691
Symbyax Capsules (Infrequent) 1788
Uniretic Tablets (Less than 1%) 3114
Zoloft (Infrequent) 2581

Dependence, drug
Actiq 993
Adderall Tablets 3168
Adderall XR Capsules 3169
Adipex-P 1216
Ambien Tablets (Rare) 2867
Avinza Capsules 1714
▲ Carnitor Injection (2% to 6%) 3185
Celexa (Infrequent) 1177
Darvocet A 500 Tablets 3497
Dexedrine 1386
DextroStat Tablets 3177
Dilaudid 439
Dilaudid Oral Liquid 443
Dilaudid Non-Sterile Powder 439
Dilaudid Rectal Suppositories 439
Dilaudid Tablets 439
Dilaudid Tablets - 8 mg 443
Duragesic Transdermal System 2448
Lortab 3315
Lortab Elixir 3312
MS Contin Tablets 2703
Nembutal Sodium Solution, USP 2484
▲ Nicotrol Inhaler (Greater than 3%) 2594
Nicotrol NS 2596
OxyFast Oral Concentrate Solution 2704
OxyIR Capsules 2704
Paxil CR Controlled-Release Tablets (Rare) 1509
Paxil (Rare) 1501
Percocet Tablets 1114
Percodan Tablets 1115
Peri-Colace Tablets 2716
Ritalin Hydrochloride Tablets 2254
Ritalin LA Capsules 2255
Ritalin-SR Tablets 2254
Sonata Capsules 1686
Tranxene 2488
Tylenol with Codeine 2461
Valium Tablets 2822
Vicoprofen Tablets 533

Dependence, physical
Dexedrine 1386
Dilaudid Ampules 439
Dilaudid Oral Liquid 443
Dilaudid Non-Sterile Powder 439
Dilaudid Rectal Suppositories 439
Dilaudid Tablets 439
Dilaudid Tablets - 8 mg 443
Duragesic Transdermal System 2448
Hycodan 1104
Hycomine Compound Tablets 1105
Hycotuss Expectorant Syrup 1106
Klonopin 2782
Lortab 3315
Lortab Elixir 3312
Marinol Capsules (Uncommon) 3334
MS Contin Tablets 2703
OxyContin Tablets 2699
Percocet Tablets 1114
Percodan Tablets 1115
ProSom Tablets 512
Sedapap Tablets 50 mg/650 mg 2098
Tranxene 2488
Tylenol with Codeine 2461
Vicodin HP Tablets 532
Vicoprofen Tablets 533
Xanax XR Tablets 2655

Dependence, psychic
(*see under* Dependence, psychological)

Dependence, psychological
Adderall Tablets 3168
Adderall XR Capsules 3169
Avinza Capsules 1714
Darvocet A 500 Tablets 3497
Desoxyn Tablets, USP 2482
Dexedrine 1386
DextroStat Tablets 3177
Dilaudid 439
Dilaudid Oral Liquid 443
Dilaudid Non-Sterile Powder 439
Dilaudid Rectal Suppositories 439
Dilaudid Tablets 439
Dilaudid Tablets - 8 mg 443
Duragesic Transdermal System 2448
Hycodan 1104
Hycomine Compound Tablets 1105
Hycotuss Expectorant Syrup 1106
Kadian Capsules (Very rare) 572
Klonopin 2782
Lortab 3315
Lortab Elixir 3312
Marinol Capsules (Uncommon) 3334
MS Contin Tablets (Very rare) 2703
Nembutal Sodium Solution, USP 2484
Numorphan 1112
OxyContin Tablets 2699
OxyFast Oral Concentrate Solution 2704
OxyIR Capsules 2704
Percocet Tablets 1114
Percodan Tablets 1115
ProSom Tablets 512
Ritalin Hydrochloride Tablets 2254
Ritalin LA Capsules 2255
Ritalin-SR Tablets 2254
Sedapap Tablets 50 mg/650 mg 2098
Tranxene 2488
Tussionex Pennkinetic Extended-Release Suspension 3322
Tylenol with Codeine 2461
Vicodin Tablets 530
Vicodin ES Tablets 531
Vicodin HP Tablets 532
Vicoprofen Tablets 533
Xanax XR Tablets 2655
Zydone Tablets 1118

Depersonalization
Abilify Tablets (Infrequent) 916
Abilify Tablets (Infrequent) 2472
Ambien Tablets (Rare) 2867
Anzemet Injection (Infrequently) 2871
Anzemet Tablets (Infrequently) 2874
Astelin Nasal Spray (Infrequent) 1876
Avelox (Less than 0.1%) 2984
Betaseron for SC Injection 791
Biaxin/Biaxin XL 402
Buprenex Injectable (Infrequent) 2718
Caduet Tablets (Greater than 0.1% to less than or equal to 1%) 2507
Campral Tablets (Rare) 1175
Celexa (Infrequent) 1177
Cipro I.V. (1% or less) 2998
Cipro I.V. Pharmacy Bulk Package (1% or less) 3509
Cipro (Less than 1%) 2991
Cipro XR Tablets (Less than 1%) 3004
Copaxone for Injection (Infrequent) 3292
Duragesic Transdermal System (Less than 1%) 2448
Effexor Tablets (1%) 3405
Effexor XR Capsules (Frequent) 3411
▲ Equetro Extended-Release Capsules (Less than 5%) 3178
Evoxac Capsules (Less than 1%) 1042
Exelon Capsules (Infrequent) 2204
Frova Tablets (Infrequent) 1101
Gabitril Tablets (Frequent) 998
Indocin (Less than 1%) 1968
Keppra Oral Solution 3307
Keppra Tablets 3307
Klonopin (Infrequent) 2782
Kogenate FS 3517
Lamictal (Infrequent) 1449
Lexapro Oral Solution (Infrequent) 1193
Lexapro Tablets (Infrequent) 1193
Lyrica Capsules (Greather than or equal to 1%) 2524
Marinol Capsules (Greater than 1%) 3334
Maxalt Tablets (Rare) 1983
Maxalt-MLT Orally Disintegrating Tablets (Rare) 1983
Namenda (Infrequent) 1199
Neurontin Capsules (Infrequent) 2498
Neurontin Oral Solution (Infrequent) 2498
Neurontin Tablets (Infrequent) 2498
Niravam Orally Disintegrating Tablets 3106
Norvasc Tablets (More than 0.1% to 1%) 2529
Nubain Injection (1% or less) 1111
OxyContin Tablets (Less than 1%) 2699
Paxil CR Controlled-Release Tablets (Infrequent) 1509
Paxil (Infrequent) 1501
Prevacid Delayed-Release Capsules (Less than 1%) 3268
Prevacid for Delayed-Release Oral Suspension (Less than 1%) 3268
Prevacid NapraPAC (Less than 1%) 3277
Prevacid SoluTab Delayed-Release Orally Disintegrating Tablets (Less than 1%) 3268
PREVPAC 3281
Prozac Pulvules and Liquid (Infrequent) 1771
Relpax Tablets (Infrequent) 2531
Requip Tablets (Infrequent) 1528
Rilutek Tablets (Infrequent) 2945
Risperdal Consta Long-Acting Injection (Infrequent) 1664
Seroquel Tablets (Infrequent) 691
Sonata Capsules (Less than 1% to 2%) 1686
Symbyax Capsules (Infrequent) 1788
Tambocor Tablets (Less than 1%) 1824
Tequin Injection (Less than 0.1%) 964
Tequin Tablets (Less than 0.1%) 964
Topamax Sprinkle Capsules (1% to 2%) 2438
Topamax Tablets (1% to 2%) 2438
Ultracet Tablets (Less than 1%) 2462
VFEND I.V. (Less than 2%) 2543
VFEND Oral Suspension (Less than 2%) 2543
VFEND Tablets (Less than 2%) 2543
Wellbutrin Tablets (Infrequent) 1579
Wellbutrin SR Sustained-Release Tablets (Infrequent) 1583
Wellbutrin XL Extended-Release Tablets (Infrequent) 1588
▲ Xanax XR Tablets (5.7%) 2655
Zoloft (Infrequent) 2581
Zomig Nasal Spray (Infrequent) 718
Zyban Sustained-Release Tablets (Infrequent) 1620
Zyprexa Tablets (Infrequent) 1798
Zyprexa ZYDIS Orally Disintegrating Tablets (Infrequent) 1798
Zyrtec Chewable Tablets (Less than 2%) 2589
Zyrtec (Less than 2%) 2589
Zyrtec-D 12 Hour Extended Release Tablets (Less than 2%) 2591

Depigmentation
Finacea Gel (Rare) 1644
▲ Intron A for Injection (Less than 5%) 3038

Depigmentation at application site
Lidoderm Patch 1107

Depression
Abilify Tablets (Frequent) 916
Abilify Tablets (Frequent) 2472
Accutane Capsules 2740
Aceon Tablets (2 mg, 4 mg, 8 mg) (2.0%) 3191
Aciphex Tablets 1081
▲ Actimmune (3%) 1646
Activella Tablets 2311
▲ Actonel Tablets (2.3% to 6.8%) 2679
▲ Actonel with Calcium Tablets (2.3% to 6.8%) 2684
Adalat CC Tablets (Less than 1%) 2978
Adderall Tablets 3168
Adderall XR Capsules (0.7%) 3169
Advair Diskus 100/50 1291
Advair Diskus 250/50 1291
Advair Diskus 500/50 1291
Aerobid/Aerobid-M (1% to 3%) 1172
▲ Agenerase Capsules (4% to 16%) 1299
▲ Agenerase Oral Solution (4% to 16%) 1304
Agrylin Capsules (1% to 5%) 3172
Aldara Cream, 5% 1814
Aldoclor Tablets 1881
Aldoril Tablets 1884
Alesse-28 Tablets 3392
Alferon N Injection (One patient to 3%) 1640
▲ Alimta for Injection (Up to 14%) 1722
Altace Capsules (Less than 1%) 1673
Altoprev Extended-Release Tablets 1151
Ambien Tablets (2%) 2867
AmBisome for Injection (Less common) 615
Amerge Tablets (Infrequent) 1312
Amnesteem Capsules 2126
AndroGel (Up to 1%) 3330
Antara Capsules 2723
▲ Apokyn Injection (At least 5%) 2132
Aptivus Capsules (2%) 859
▲ Arava Tablets (1% to 3%) 2881
▲ Aricept Tablets (3%) 1086
▲ Aricept ODT Tablets (3%) 1086
▲ Arimidex Tablets (2% to 11%) 665
▲ Aromasin Tablets (13%) 2600
Arthrotec Tablets (Rare) 3126
Asacol Delayed-Release Tablets 2688
▲ Asmanex Twisthaler (11%) 2981
Astelin Nasal Spray (Infrequent) 1876
Atacand Tablets (0.5% or greater) 634
Atacand HCT (0.5% or greater) 637
Avalide Tablets 922
Avalide Tablets 2889
Avapro Tablets (Less than 1%) 925
Avapro Tablets (Less than 1%) 2886
Avelox 2984
▲ Avonex (18% to 20%) 839
Axert Tablets (Rare) 2430
Aygestin Tablets 1062
Azmacort Inhalation Aerosol 1701
Beconase AQ Nasal Spray 1359
Betagan Ophthalmic Solution, USP ⊙217
▲ Betaseron for SC Injection (34%) 791
Betimol Ophthalmic Solution ⊙283
Betimol Ophthalmic Solution 3371
Betoptic S Ophthalmic Suspension (Rare) 554
Blocadren Tablets 1891
Bravelle for Intramuscular or Subcutaneous Injection (2.7%) 1140
Brevibloc Concentrate (Less than 1%) 766
Brevibloc Injection (Less than 1%) 766
Brevibloc Double Strength Injection (Less than 1%) 766
Brevibloc Premixed Injection (Less than 1%) 766
Brevibloc Double Strength Premixed Injection (Less than 1%) 766
Brimonidine Tartrate Ophthalmic Solution 0.2% (Less than 3%) ⊙245
Buphenyl Powder (Less than or equal to 2%) 3327
Buphenyl Tablets (Less than or equal to 2%) 3327
Caduet Tablets (Greater than 0.1% to less than 2%) 2507
▲ Campath Ampules (1% to 7%) 826
▲ Campral Tablets (4% to 8%) 1175
Captopril Tablets 2114
Carbatrol Capsules 3174
Cardizem LA Extended Release Tablets (Less than 2%) 1699
▲ Carnitor Injection (5% to 6%) 3185
Carteolol Hydrochloride Ophthalmic Solution USP, 1% ⊙246
▲ Casodex Tablets (4%) 670
Cataflam Tablets (Occasionally) 2173
Catapres Tablets (About 1 in 100 patients) 874
Catapres-TTS (0.5% or less) 875
Celebrex Capsules (0.1% to 1.9%) 3130
Celexa (Frequent) 1177
▲ CellCept Capsules (3% to less than 20%) 2751
▲ CellCept Intravenous (3% to less than 20%) 2751
▲ CellCept Oral Suspension (3% to less than 20%) 2751
▲ CellCept Tablets (3% to less than 20%) 2751
▲ Cenestin Tablets, 0.45mg, 0.625mg, 0.9mg, 1.25mg (3.8% to 28%) 1063
Cenestin Tablets, 0.3mg 1063
Cipro I.V. (1% or less) 2998
Cipro I.V. Pharmacy Bulk Package (1% or less) 3509
Cipro (Less than 1%) 2991
Cipro XR Tablets (Less than 1%) 3004
▲ Climara Transdermal System (1% to 8%) 795
▲ Climara Pro Transdermal System (5.7%) 800
Clinoril Tablets (Less than 1%) 1899
▲ Clolar for Intravenous Infusion (11%) 1264
Clorpres Tablets (About 1%) 2139
Clozapine Tablets (1%) 2141
Clozaril Tablets (1%) 2174
Cogentin Injection 1903
Colazal Capsules 2845
▲ CombiPatch Transdermal System (8% to 9%) 2180
Concerta Extended-Release Tablets 1828
Copaxone for Injection (At least 2%) 3292
▲ Copegus Tablets (20%) 2759
▲ Coreg Tablets (Greater than 1% to 3%) 1376
Cosopt Sterile Ophthalmic Solution (Less than 1%) 1910
Cozaar Tablets (Less than 1%) 1913
Crestor Tablets (Greater than or equal to 2%) 672
Crixivan Capsules 1918
Cytovene (At least 3 subjects) 2763
Dalmane Capsules (Rare) 3343
Dantrium Capsules (Less frequent) 2690
Daranide Tablets 1928
DDAVP Nasal Spray 2894
Decadron Phosphate Injection 1931
Decadron Tablets 1929
Delatestryl Injection 2976
Demser Capsules 1933
▲ Depacon Injection (4% to 5%) 412
▲ Depakene (5%) 417
▲ Depakote Sprinkle Capsules (4% to 5%) 422
▲ Depakote Tablets (1% to 5%) 427
▲ Depakote ER Tablets (4% to 5%) 433
▲ Depo-Provera Contraceptive Injection (1% to 5%) 2619
▲ depo-subQ provera 104 Injectable Suspension (1% to less than 5%) 2622
Desmopressin Acetate Rhinal Tube 1144

Diastat Rectal Delivery System (Infrequent) ... 3344
Didronel Tablets ... 2693
Digitek Tablets ... 2146
Dilaudid Oral Liquid (Less frequent) ... 443
Dilaudid Tablets - 8 mg (Less frequent) ... 443
Dilaudid-HP (Less frequent) ... 441
Diovan HCT Tablets (Greater than 0.2%) ... 2195
Diprivan Injectable Emulsion (Less than 1%) ... 676
Dolobid Tablets (Less than 1 in 100) ... 1937
▲ Dostinex Tablets (3%) ... 2631
▲ Doxil Injection (Less than 1% to 10%) ... 3302
▲ Duragesic Transdermal System (3% to 10%) ... 2448
DynaCirc CR Tablets (0.5% to 1%) ... 2726
Effexor Tablets (1%) ... 3405
▲ Effexor XR Capsules (3%) ... 3411
Eldepryl Capsules ... 3209
Eligard 7.5 mg (Less than 2%) ... 2896
Eligard 30 mg (1.1%) ... 2901
Elmiron Capsules ... 2393
▲ Eloxatin for Injection (2% to 5%) ... 2908
Elspar for Injection ... 1943
Emend Capsules (Greater than 0.5%) ... 1944
▲ Emtriva Capsules (6% to 9%) ... 1272
Enbrel for Injection (Infrequent) ... 580
▲ Epzicom Tablets (7%) ... 1402
▲ Equetro Extended-Release Capsules (7%) ... 3178
▲ Erbitux (9%) ... 937
Estratest Tablets ... 3196
Estratest H.S. Tablets ... 3196
▲ Estrogel 0.06% (3%) ... 3200
Eulexin Capsules (1%) ... 3023
▲ Evista Tablets (6.4%) ... 1735
▲ Evoxac Capsules (1% to 3%) ... 1042
▲ Exelon Capsules (6%) ... 2204
▲ Fabrazyme for Intravenous Infusion (3%) ... 1267
▲ Faslodex Injection (5.7%) ... 682
FazaClo Orally Disintegrating Tablets (1%) ... 547
Femara Tablets (Less frequent) ... 2210
Flexeril Tablets (Less than 1%) ... 1832
▲ Flolan for Injection (13% to 37%) ... 1408
Flovent Diskus 50 mcg ... 1415
Flovent HFA ... 1418
Flumadine (0.3% to 1%) ... 1186
Focalin Tablets ... 2214
Focalin XR Capsules ... 2217
▲ Forteo for Injection (4.1%) ... 1739
▲ Fortical Nasal Spray (1% to 3%) ... 3336
Frova Tablets (Infrequent) ... 1101
Fuzeon Injection ... 2772
▲ Gabitril Tablets (3%) ... 998
Garamycin Injectable ... 3028
Gengraf Capsules (Rare) ... 458
Geodon Capsules ... 2514
Gleevec Tablets (Infrequent) ... 2221
▲ Hectorol Capsules (Greater than or equal to 5%) ... 909
▲ Herceptin I.V. (6%) ... 1234
Hydrocortone Tablets ... 1963
Hytrin Capsules (0.3%) ... 469
Hyzaar ... 1964
▲ Imdur Tablets (Less than or equal to 5%) ... 3032
Imitrex Injection (Rare) ... 1431
Imitrex Nasal Spray (Infrequent) ... 1435
Imitrex Tablets (Infrequent) ... 1440
Indapamide Tablets (Less than 5%) ... 2119
Inderal LA Long-Acting Capsules ... 3421
Indocin (Greater than 1%) ... 1968
▲ Infergen (18% to 26%) ... 1647
InnoPran XL Capsules ... 2728
▲ Intron A for Injection (2% to 40%) ... 3038
Invanz for Injection (Greater than 0.1%) ... 1974
Invirase (Greater than or equal to 2%) ... 2776
▲ I.V. Busulfex (23%) ... 1125
Kadian Capsules (Less than 3%) ... 572
Kaletra (Up to 2%) ... 474
▲ Keppra Oral Solution (3% to 4%) ... 3307
▲ Keppra Tablets (3% to 4%) ... 3307
▲ Klonopin (4% to 7%) ... 2782
▲ Lamictal (4.2%) ... 1449
Lanoxicaps Capsules ... 1458
Lanoxin Injection ... 1462
Lanoxin Tablets ... 1468
Lanoxin Injection Pediatric ... 1465
Lariam Tablets (Occasional) ... 2790
Lescol Capsules ... 2227
Lescol Capsules ... 2730
Lescol XL Tablets ... 2227
Lescol XL Tablets ... 2730
Levaquin in 5% Dextrose Injection (0.1% to 0.9%) ... 2453
Levaquin (0.1% to 0.9%) ... 2453
Lexapro Oral Solution (Infrequent) ... 1193
Lexapro Tablets (Infrequent) ... 1193
▲ Lexiva Tablets (Less than 1% to 11%) ... 1473
Lidoderm Patch ... 1107
Lipitor Tablets (Less than 2%) ... 2495
Lofibra Capsules ... 1217
Lo/Ovral-28 Tablets ... 3423
Lotronex Tablets (2%) ... 1479
▲ Lunesta Tablets (1% to 4%) ... 3139
▲ Lupron Depot 3.75 mg (16%) ... 3257
▲ Lupron Depot–3 Month 11.25 mg (16%) ... 3262
Malarone Tablets (Less than 1%) ... 1484
Malarone Pediatric Tablets (Less than 1%) ... 1484
Marinol Capsules (Less than 1%) ... 3334
Matulane Capsules ... 3188
Maxair Autohaler ... 1820
Maxalt Tablets (Infrequent) ... 1983
Maxalt-MLT Orally Disintegrating Tablets (Infrequent) ... 1983
Maxzide ... 2150
▲ Megace ES Oral Suspension (1% to 3%) ... 2492
Menostar Transdermal System ... 805
▲ Meridia Capsules (4.3%) ... 485
Merrem I.V. (Greater than 0.1% to 1%) ... 687
Metadate CD Capsules ... 3316
MetroGel-Vaginal Gel (Less than 1%) ... 1822
Mevacor Tablets (0.5% to 1.0%) ... 1996
Miacalcin Nasal Spray (1% to 3%) ... 2242
Micardis Tablets (More than 0.3%) ... 884
Micardis HCT Tablets ... 886
Midamor Tablets (Less than or equal to 1%) ... 2000
Migranal Nasal Spray (Rare) ... 3350
Mintezol ... 2002
Mirapex Tablets (1% or more) ... 889
▲ Mirena Intrauterine System (5% or more) ... 810
Moban Tablets (Less frequent) ... 1108
Mobic Oral Suspension (Less than 2%) ... 893
Mobic Tablets (Less than 2%) ... 893
Moduretic Tablets (Less than or equal to 1%) ... 2003
MS Contin Tablets (Less frequent) ... 2703
▲ Myfortic Tablets (3% to less than 20%) ... 2244
▲ Mylotarg for Injection (8% to 10%) ... 3429
Nadolol Tablets ... 2121
Nalfon Capsules (Less than 1%) ... 2504
Namenda (Greater than or equal to 2%) ... 1199
Naropin Injection ... 640
Neoral Soft Gelatin Capsules (1%) ... 2247
Neoral Oral Solution (1%) ... 2247
Neurontin Capsules (1.8%) ... 2498
Neurontin Oral Solution (1.8%) ... 2498
Neurontin Tablets (1.8%) ... 2498
▲ Nicotrol Inhaler (Greater than 3%) ... 2594
Nicotrol NS (Greater than 5%) ... 2596
Nimotop Capsules (Up to 1.4%) ... 774
▲ Nipent for Injection (3% to 10%) ... 3216
▲ Niravam Orally Disintegrating Tablets (5.1% to 13.9%) ... 3106
Noroxin Tablets (Less frequent) ... 2009
Norvasc Tablets (More than 0.1% to 1%) ... 2529
Norvir (1.7%) ... 499
Novarel for Injection ... 1147
Nubain Injection (1% or less) ... 1111
Numorphan ... 1112
Omacor Capsules ... 2735
OptiPranolol Metipranolol Ophthalmic Solution 0.3% (A small number of patients) ... ⊙254
▲ Orap Tablets (2 of 20 patients) ... 1220
Ortho-Cept Tablets ... 2395
Ortho-Cyclen Tablets ... 2414
Ortho Evra Transdermal System ... 2402
Ortho Tri-Cyclen Tablets ... 2414
Ortho Tri-Cyclen Lo Tablets ... 2421
Oxandrin Tablets ... 2977
Oxsoralen-Ultra Capsules ... 3354
OxyContin Tablets (Less than 1%) ... 2699
Parcopa Orally Disintegrating Tablets ... 3111
Paxil CR Controlled-Release Tablets (Frequent) ... 1509
Paxil (Frequent) ... 1501
▲ Pegasys (18%) ... 2793
▲ PEG-Intron Powder for Injection (29%) ... 3062
Pentasa Capsules (Less than 1%) ... 3182
Pepcid Injection (Infrequent) ... 2017
Pepcid (Infrequent) ... 2014
▲ Permax Tablets (3.2%) ... 3357
▲ Plavix Tablets (3.6%) ... 940
▲ Plavix Tablets (3.6%) ... 2942
Plendil Extended-Release Tablets (0.5% to 1.5%) ... 651
Pravachol Tablets ... 943
▲ Prefest Tablets (5%) ... 1069
Premarin Intravenous ... 3440
▲ Premarin Tablets (5% to 8%) ... 3443
Premarin Vaginal Cream ... 3449
▲ Premphase Tablets (6% to 11%) ... 3452
▲ Prempro Tablets (6% to 11%) ... 3452
Prevacid Delayed-Release Capsules (Less than 1%) ... 3268
Prevacid for Delayed-Release Oral Suspension (Less than 1%) ... 3268
Prevacid NapraPAC (Less than 1%) ... 3277
Prevacid SoluTab Delayed-Release Orally Disintegrating Tablets (Less than 1%) ... 3268
PREVPAC (Less than 1%) ... 3281
Prilosec OTC Tablets (Less than 1%) ... 2674
Prinivil Tablets (Greater than 1%) ... 2029
Prinzide Tablets (0.3% to 1%) ... 2033
▲ Prochieve 4% Gel (8% to 11%) ... 1018
▲ Prochieve 8% Gel (8% to 11%) ... 1018
▲ Prograf Capsules and Injection (3% to 15%) ... 624
Proleukin for Injection (Less than 1%) ... 1007
▲ Prometrium Capsules (100 mg, 200 mg) (5% to 19%) ... 3205
ProSom Tablets (2%) ... 512
Protonix I.V. (Less than 1%) ... 3468
Protonix Tablets (Less than 1%) ... 3465
Protopic Ointment (Greater than or equal to 1%) ... 629
Proventil HFA Inhalation Aerosol (Less than 3%) ... 3071
Provigil Tablets (2%) ... 1002
Prozac Pulvules and Liquid ... 1771
Pulmicort Respules (Less than 1%) ... 654
▲ Rapamune Oral Solution and Tablets (3% to 20%) ... 3472
▲ Razadyne ER Extended-Release Capsules (7%) ... 2434
▲ Razadyne (7%) ... 2434
▲ Rebetol (13% to 36%) ... 3073
▲ Rebetron Combination Therapy (23% to 36%) ... 3078
▲ Rebif Prefilled Syringe for Injection (25%) ... 3163
Relafen Tablets (Less than 1%) ... 1523
Relpax Tablets (Infrequent) ... 2531
Requip Tablets (1% or more) ... 1528
Retrovir Capsules ... 1533
Retrovir IV Infusion ... 1537
Retrovir ... 1533
▲ Reyataz Capsules (3% to 8%) ... 948
▲ Ribavirin, USP Capsules (13% to 36%) ... 3083
▲ Rilutek Tablets (4.2% to 6.1%) ... 2945
Risperdal Consta Long-Acting Injection (Frequent) ... 1664
Risperdal M-Tab Orally Disintegrating Tablets (Infrequent) ... 1658
Risperdal (Infrequent) ... 1658
Ritalin Hydrochloride Tablets ... 2254
Ritalin LA Capsules ... 2255
Ritalin-SR Tablets ... 2254
▲ Rituxan for Infusion (Among most frequent) ... 845
▲ Rituxan I.V. (1% to 5%) ... 1251
▲ Roferon-A Injection (16% to 28%) ... 2805
Rozerem Tablets (2%) ... 3228
▲ Rythmol SR Capsules (1% to 3%) ... 2736
Sandimmune (Rare) ... 2259
▲ Sandostatin Injection (1% to 4%) ... 2263
▲ Sandostatin LAR Depot (5% to 15%) ... 2264
Seasonale Tablets ... 1073
Sedapap Tablets 50 mg/650 mg (Infrequent) ... 2098
▲ Simulect for Injection (3% to 10%) ... 2268
Sonata Capsules (Frequent) ... 1686
▲ Soriatane Capsules (1% to 10%) ... 1028
▲ Spiriva HandiHaler (1% to 3%) ... 899
Stalevo Tablets ... 2270
▲ Strattera Capsules (2% to 6%) ... 1784
Striant Mucoadhesive ... 1022
▲ Suboxone Tablets (11%) ... 2719
▲ Subutex Tablets (11%) ... 2719
Sular Tablets (Less than or equal to 1%) ... 1163
▲ Sustiva Capsules (2% to 19%) ... 957
Symmetrel (1% to 5%) ... 1115
Tagamet Tablets ... 1547
Tambocor Tablets (1% to 3%) ... 1824
Targretin Capsules ... 1719
Tasmar Tablets (Frequent) ... 3360
Tegretol/Tegretol-XR ... 2278
▲ Temodar Capsules (6%) ... 3088
▲ Tenormin I.V. Injection (0.6% to 12%) ... 698
▲ Tenormin Tablets (0.6% to 12%) ... 695
Tequin Injection (Less than 0.1%) ... 964
Tequin Tablets (Less than 0.1%) ... 964
Testim 1% Gel ... 722
Teveten Tablets (1%) ... 1707
Teveten HCT Tablets (Less than 1%) ... 1710
Thalomid Capsules ... 979
Thyrolar ... 1203
Tiazac Capsules (Less than 2%) ... 1204
Timolide Tablets ... 2056
Timoptic in Ocudose (Less frequent) ... 2061
Timoptic Sterile Ophthalmic Solution (Less frequent) ... 2058
Timoptic-XE Sterile Ophthalmic Gel Forming Solution ... 2062
Tindamax (Rare) ... 2670
▲ Topamax Sprinkle Capsules (1% to 13%) ... 2438
▲ Topamax Tablets (1% to 13%) ... 2438
▲ Toprol-XL Tablets (About 5 of 100 patients) ... 660
Tranxene ... 2488
Travatan Ophthalmic Solution (1% to 5%) ... 559
Trecator Tablets ... 3482
Tricor Tablets ... 523
Triphasil-28 Tablets ... 3483
▲ Trisenox Injection (20%) ... 983
▲ Trizivir Tablets (9%) ... 1565
▲ Truvada Tablets (Greater than 5%) ... 1279
Ultracet Tablets (Less than 1%) ... 2462
Uniretic Tablets (Less than 1%) ... 3114
▲ Valcyte Tablets (Less than 5%) ... 2816
Valium Tablets (Infrequent) ... 2822
▲ Valtrex Caplets (Less than 1% to 7%) ... 1573
Vantas (Less than 2%) ... 3367
Vaseretic Tablets ... 2073
Vasotec I.V. Injection (0.5% to 1%) ... 2076
▲ Vesanoid Capsules (14%) ... 2823
VESIcare Tablets (0.8% to 1.2%) ... 631
VFEND I.V. (Less than 2%) ... 2543
VFEND Oral Suspension (Less than 2%) ... 2543
VFEND Tablets (Less than 2%) ... 2543
▲ Viadur Implant (5.3%) ... 782
Viagra Tablets (Less than 2%) ... 2552
Vicoprofen Tablets (Less than 1%) ... 533
Viracept (Less than 2%) ... 2556
▲ Viread Tablets (4% to 8%) ... 1284
▲ Vivelle Transdermal System (3% to 10.6%) ... 2288
▲ Vivelle-Dot Transdermal System (3% to 10.6%) ... 2293
Voltaren Tablets (Occasionally) ... 2298
Voltaren-XR Tablets (Occasionally) ... 2301
Vytorin 10/10 Tablets ... 2084
Vytorin 10/10 Tablets ... 3092
Vytorin 10/20 Tablets ... 2084
Vytorin 10/20 Tablets ... 3092
Vytorin 10/40 Tablets ... 2084
Vytorin 10/40 Tablets ... 3092
Vytorin 10/80 Tablets ... 2084
Vytorin 10/80 Tablets ... 3092
Wellbutrin Tablets (Frequent) ... 1579
▲ Xanax XR Tablets (1.3% to 12.1%) ... 2655
▲ Xeloda Tablets (Less than 5%) ... 2825
▲ Xenical Capsules (3.4%) ... 2834
Yasmin 28 Tablets (Greater than 1%) ... 818
Zantac (Rare) ... 1597
Zantac Injection (Rare) ... 1593
Zantac Injection Pharmacy Bulk Package (Rare) ... 1595
Zantac Syrup (Rare) ... 1597
Zegerid Powder for Oral Solution (Less than 1%) ... 2972
Zelnorm Tablets ... 2303
▲ Zenapax for Injection (2% to 5%) ... 2838
Zestoretic Tablets (0.3% to 1%) ... 701
Zestril Tablets (Greater than 1%) ... 704
Zocor Tablets ... 2078
▲ Zoladex (1% to 54%) ... 709
Zoladex 3-month ... 712
Zoloft (Infrequent) ... 2581
▲ Zometa for Intravenous Infusion (14%) ... 2306
Zomig Nasal Spray (Infrequent) ... 718
Zomig Tablets (Infrequent) ... 714
Zomig-ZMT Tablets (Infrequent) ... 714
▲ Zonegran Capsules (6%) ... 1089
Zosyn (1.0% or less) ... 3492
Zyban Sustained-Release Tablets (Frequent) ... 1620
Zyprexa Tablets ... 1798
Zyprexa ZYDIS Orally Disintegrating Tablets ... 1798
Zyrtec Chewable Tablets (Less than 2%) ... 2589

Zyrtec (Less than 2%) 2589
Zyrtec-D 12 Hour Extended Release Tablets (Less than 2%) 2591

Depression, aggravation of
Celexa (Frequent) 1177
Coreg Tablets (Greater than 0.1% to 1%) 1376
Evoxac Capsules (Less than 1%) 1042
Frova Tablets (Rare) 1101
▲ Intron A for Injection (Less than 5%) 3038
Lexapro Oral Solution (Infrequent) 1193
Lexapro Tablets (Infrequent) 1193
Lupron Depot 3.75 mg 3257
Lupron Depot–3 Month 11.25 mg (Possible) 3262
Meridia Capsules 485
Nexium Delayed-Release Capsules (Less than 1%) 645
Nexium I.V. (Less than 1%) 649
Sustiva Capsules (Less than 2%) 957
Tegretol-XR Tablets 2278
Ziagen (5 patients) 1600
Zoloft (Infrequent) 2581

Depression, circulatory
Kadian Capsules 572

Depression, mood
(*see under* Depression)

Depression, psychotic
Celexa (Infrequent) 1177
Copaxone for Injection (Infrequent) 3292
Effexor Tablets (Rare) 3405
Effexor XR Capsules (Infrequent) 3411
Lyrica Capsules (Rare) 2524
Paxil CR Controlled-Release Tablets (Rare) 1509
Paxil (Rare) 1501
Relpax Tablets (Rare) 2531
Rilutek Tablets (Rare) 2945
Risperdal Consta Long-Acting Injection (Infrequent) 1664

Depression, respiratory, neonatal
Dilaudid 439
Dilaudid Non-Sterile Powder 439
Dilaudid Rectal Suppositories 439
Dilaudid Tablets 439
Kadian Capsules 572
Lortab 3315
Lortab Elixir 3312
MS Contin Tablets 2703
Percocet Tablets 1114
Tussionex Pennkinetic Extended-Release Suspension 3322
Tylenol with Codeine 2461
Vicodin Tablets 530
Vicodin ES Tablets 531

Depression, worsening
Paxil CR Controlled-Release Tablets 1509
Paxil 1501
Symbyax Capsules 1788

Depressive reactions
▲ Combivir Tablets (9%) 1373
▲ Epivir (9%) 1394
▲ Rescriptor Tablets (4.9% to 12.6%) 2535
Truvada Tablets 1279
▲ Ziagen (6%) 1600

Derealization
Abilify Tablets (Rare) 916
Abilify Tablets (Rare) 2472
Niravam Orally Disintegrating Tablets (1.9%) 3106
Wellbutrin SR Sustained-Release Tablets (Rare) 1583
Wellbutrin XL Extended-Release Tablets (Rare) 1588
▲ Xanax XR Tablets (8%) 2655

Dermatitis
Aldara Cream, 5% (1.4%) 1814
Ambien Tablets (Rare) 2867
Amerge Tablets (Rare) 1312
Aricept Tablets (Infrequent) 1086
Aricept ODT Tablets (Infrequent) 1086
Atacand HCT (0.5% or greater) 637
Avalide Tablets 922
Avalide Tablets 2889
Avapro Tablets (Less than 1%) 925
Avapro Tablets (Less than 1%) 2886
Axert Tablets (Rare) 2430
Azopt Ophthalmic Suspension (1% to 5%) 553
Bactroban Cream (Less than 1%) 1356
Caduet Tablets (Less than or equal to 0.1%) 2507
Celebrex Capsules (0.1% to 1.9%) 3130
Celexa (Infrequent) 1177
Ciloxan Ophthalmic Ointment (Less than 1%) 554
Clindagel 1207
Clindesse Vaginal Cream (Less than 1%) 3296
▲ Clolar for Intravenous Infusion (41%) 1264
Clozapine Tablets (Less than 1%) 2141
Clozaril Tablets (Less than 1%) 2174
Colazal Capsules 2845
Colyte with Flavor Packs for Oral Solution (Isolated cases) 3102
Copaxone for Injection (Infrequent) 3292
▲ Copegus Tablets (16%) 2759
Cosopt Sterile Ophthalmic Solution 1910
Coumadin for Injection (Infrequent) 932
Coumadin Tablets (Infrequent) 932
Cozaar Tablets (Less than 1%) 1913
Differin Cream (Less than 1%) 1210
▲ Dovonex Cream 0.005% (1% to 10%) 3374
▲ Dovonex Ointment 0.005% (1% to 10%) 3375
▲ Entocort EC Capsules (Less than 5%) 2694
Evoxac Capsules (Less than 1%) 1042
Factive Tablets (0.1% to 1%) 2464
FazaClo Orally Disintegrating Tablets (Less than 1%) 547
▲ Flovent Diskus 50 mcg (1% to 3%) 1415
Floxin Otic Singles 1045
Floxin Otic Solution (Single report) 1043
Gengraf Capsules (1% to less than 3%) 458
HalfLytely and Bisacodyl Tablets Bowel Prep Kit with Flavors Packs 915
Hycamtin for Injection (Rare) 1427
Hyzaar 1964
▲ Intron A for Injection (Up to 8%) 3038
Invanz for Injection (1%) 1974
Invirase (Less than 2%) 2776
Lexapro Oral Solution (Infrequent) 1193
Lexapro Tablets (Infrequent) 1193
Lidoderm Patch 1107
Lotensin Tablets (Less than 1%) 2232
Lotrel Capsules 2238
Lotronex Tablets (Rare) 1479
Lupron Depot 7.5 mg (Less than 5%) 3261
Maxair Autohaler 1820
Meridia Capsules 485
Micardis Tablets (More than 0.3%) 884
Micardis HCT Tablets 886
Miradon Tablets 3056
Namenda (Infrequent) 1199
Neoral Soft Gelatin Capsules (1% to less than 3%) 2247
Neoral Oral Solution (1% to less than 3%) 2247
Nexium Delayed-Release Capsules (Less than 1%) 645
Nexium I.V. (Less than 1%) 649
Norvasc Tablets (Less than or equal to 0.1%) 2529
Pancrease MT Capsules (Frequent) 1839
▲ Pegasys (8%) 2793
Phenergan 3438
Phenytek Capsules (Rare) 2153
Prevnar for Injection 3460
Prilosec OTC Tablets 2674
Prinzide Tablets (0.3% to 1%) 2033
Requip Tablets (Infrequent) 1528
Rescriptor Tablets 2535
Risperdal Consta Long-Acting Injection (Infrequent) 1664
Rythmol SR Capsules 2736
Singulair (Greater than or equal to 2%) 2047
Solage Topical Solution (2%) 740
▲ Soriatane Capsules (1% to 10%) 1028
▲ Strattera Capsules (2% to 4%) 1784
Tamiflu Capsules (1%) 2810
Tamiflu Oral Suspension (1%) 2810
Temovate Scalp Application (1 of 294 patients) 1551
Thioridazine Hydrochloride Tablets (Infrequent) 2122
Topamax Sprinkle Capsules (2%) 2438
Topamax Tablets (2%) 2438
TriLyte with Flavor Packs for Oral Solution 3114
▲ Trisenox Injection (43%) 983
▲ Valcyte Tablets (Less than 5%) 2816
Vaqta (Less than 1%) 2067
Varivax (Greater than or equal to 1%) 2070
VFEND I.V. (Less than 2%) 2543
VFEND Oral Suspension (Less than 2%) 2543
VFEND Tablets (Less than 2%) 2543
Viracept (Less than 2%) 2556
▲ Xeloda Tablets (1% to 37%) 2825
Xolair (2%) 1259
Zegerid Powder for Oral Solution 2972
Zoloft (Rare) 2581
▲ Zometa for Intravenous Infusion (11%) 2306
Zyrtec Chewable Tablets (Less than 2%) 2589
Zyrtec (Less than 2%) 2589
Zyrtec-D 12 Hour Extended Release Tablets (Less than 2%) 2591

Dermatitis, allergic
Aloxi Injection (Less than 1%) 2099
Antabuse Tablets 2343
Decadron Phosphate Injection 1931
Decadron Tablets 1929
Hydrocortone Tablets 1963
▲ Niravam Orally Disintegrating Tablets (3.8%) 3106
ProctoFoam-HC 3113
Xifaxan Tablets 2847

Dermatitis, allergic contact
Aclovate (Infrequent) 1290
Analpram-HC 1136
▲ Catapres-TTS (About 19 in 100) 875
Clinac BPO 7 Gel USP 1137
Clobevate Gel 3213
Clobex Shampoo (Infrequent) 1209
Clobex Lotion 1208
Cutivate Cream (Infrequent) 1381
Cutivate Ointment (Infrequent to more frequent) 1384
Diprolene Gel 0.05% 3015
Diprolene Lotion 0.05% (Infrequent) 3016
Diprolene Ointment 0.05% (Infrequent) 3017
Diprolene AF Cream 0.05% (Infrequent) 3014
Diprosone Cream, USP 0.05% 3018
▲ Efudex (Among most frequent) 3348
Elocon Cream 0.1% (Infrequent) 3019
Elocon Lotion 0.1% (Infrequent) 3020
Elocon Ointment 0.1% (Infrequent) 3021
Locoid Cream (Infrequent) 1138
Locoid Lipocream Cream (Infrequent) 1138
Locoid (Infrequent) 1138
Lotrisone 3054
Luxiq Foam 1026
Olux Foam 1027
Ophthetic Ophthalmic Solution ⊙ 230
Oxistat Cream 1498
Pandel Cream, 0.1% 1017
Pramosone 1139
Retin-A Micro 0.1%/0.04% (Rare) 2388
Temovate Cream 1549
Temovate Gel (Infrequent) 1550
Temovate Ointment 1549
Temovate Scalp Application (Infrequent) 1551
Temovate E Emollient (Infrequent) 1552
Topicort .05% Gel 3288
Topicort .25% Cream 3288
Topicort .25% Ointment 3288
Topicort LP .05% Cream 3288
Triaz 1864
Triaz Pads 1864
Tri-Luma Cream 1213
U-cort 1% Cream 3289
Vanos Cream 1864

Dermatitis, application site
Lidoderm Patch 1107

Dermatitis, atopic
Cutivate Cream (0.8%) 1381
Cutivate Lotion 0.05% (Less than 1%) 1383
Invanz for Injection (Greater than 0.5%) 1974

Dermatitis, bullous
Carimune NF 3501
Gammagard Liquid 751
Gammagard S/D (Rare) 754
Gamunex Immune Globulin I.V., 10% (Rare) 3232
Iveegam EN (Rare) 759
Phenytek Capsules 2153
Zevalin Injection 848

Dermatitis, contact
Advair Diskus 100/50 1291
Advair Diskus 250/50 1291
Advair Diskus 500/50 1291
Antara Capsules 2723
▲ Arava Tablets (1% to 3%) 2881
Astelin Nasal Spray (Infrequent) 1876
▲ Augmentin ES-600 Powder for Oral Suspension (3.5%) 1337
Bactroban Ointment (Less than 1%) 1358
Caduet Tablets (Less than 2%) 2507
▲ Catapres-TTS (About 8 to 34 in 100 patients) 875
Celebrex Capsules (0.1% to 1.9%) 3130
Centany Ointment, 2% (0.7%) 2382
Claripel Cream 3212
Clindagel 1207
Copaxone for Injection (Infrequent) 3292
Cosopt Sterile Ophthalmic Solution 1910
Cutivate Lotion 0.05% (Less than 1%) 1383
Doxil Injection (Less than 1%) 3302
Effexor Tablets (Infrequent) 3405
Effexor XR Capsules (Infrequent) 3411
Ertaczo Cream, 2% 2383
Evoxac Capsules (Less than 1%) 1042
Exelon Capsules (Infrequent) 2204
Finacea Gel (1% or less) 1644
Gabitril Tablets (Infrequent) 998
Geodon Capsules (Infrequent) 2514
Klonopin (Infrequent) 2782
▲ Lamictal (2% to 5%) 1449
Lipitor Tablets (Less than 2%) 2495
Lofibra Capsules 1217
Loprox Gel (1% to 5%) 1861
Lunesta Tablets (Infrequent) 3139
Lustra Cream 3287
Lustra-AF Cream 3287
Lustra-Ultra Cream 3287
Mentax Cream (Less than 2%) 2152
Metrogel 1% (1.3%) 1212
Nitro-Dur Transdermal Infusion System (Uncommon) 3060
Norvir (Less than 2%) 499
Paxil CR Controlled-Release Tablets (Rare) 1509
Paxil (Rare) 1501
Prevacid Delayed-Release Capsules (Less than 1%) 3268
Prevacid for Delayed-Release Oral Suspension (Less than 1%) 3268
Prevacid NapraPAC (Less than 1%) 3277
Prevacid SoluTab Delayed-Release Orally Disintegrating Tablets (Less than 1%) 3268
PREVPAC (Less than 1%) 3281
Protonix I.V. (Less than 1%) 3468
Protonix Tablets (Less than 1%) 3465
Protopic Ointment (1% to 3%) 629
Prozac Pulvules and Liquid (Infrequent) 1771
Pulmicort Respules (1% to 3%) 654
Rilutek Tablets (Rare) 2945
Serevent Diskus (1% to 3%) 1540
Seroquel Tablets (Infrequent) 691
Sonata Capsules (Infrequent) 1686
Symbyax Capsules (Infrequent) 1788
Thioridazine Hydrochloride Tablets 2122
Thiothixene Capsules 2124
Tricor Tablets 523
Trileptal Oral Suspension 2281
Trileptal Tablets 2281
Trusopt Sterile Ophthalmic Solution 2065
Uniretic Tablets (Less than 1%) 3114
Varivax (Greater than or equal to 1%) 2070
VFEND I.V. (Less than 2%) 2543
VFEND Oral Suspension (Less than 2%) 2543
VFEND Tablets (Less than 2%) 2543
Viagra Tablets (Less than 2%) 2552
Zoloft (Rare) 2581
Zovirax Cream 853
Zyprexa Tablets (Infrequent) 1798
Zyprexa ZYDIS Orally Disintegrating Tablets (Infrequent) 1798

Dermatitis, eczematoid
Symmetrel (Less than 0.1%) 1115

Dermatitis, exfoliative
Abelcet Injection 1119
Abilify Tablets (Infrequent) 916
Abilify Tablets (Infrequent) 2472
Aceon Tablets (2 mg, 4 mg, 8 mg) 3191
Actiq (Less than 1%) 993
Adalat CC Tablets (Rare) 2978
Aldara Cream, 5% 1814
Aldoclor Tablets 1881
Aldoril Tablets 1884
Amoxil Capsules 1315

Amoxil Chewable Tablets 1315
Amoxil Pediatric Drops for Oral Suspension 1315
Amoxil Powder for Oral Suspension 1315
Amoxil Tablets 1315
Anaprox Tablets (Less than 1%) 2769
Anaprox DS Tablets (Less than 1%) 2769
Arthrotec Tablets (Rare) 3126
Atacand HCT 637
Augmentin (Occasional case) 1331
Augmentin Tablets (Occasional) 1334
Augmentin XR Extended-Release Tablets (Occasional) 1340
Augmentin ES-600 Powder for Oral Suspension (Occasional) 1337
Avalide Tablets 922
Avalide Tablets 2889
▲ Avastin IV (3% to 19%) 1229
Axid Oral Solution 913
Bravelle for Intramuscular or Subcutaneous Injection (2.7%) 1140
Campral Tablets (Infrequent) 1175
Camptosar Injection (Up to 0.9%) 2602
Captopril Tablets 2114
Carbatrol Capsules 3174
Cardizem LA Extended Release Tablets (Infrequent) 1699
Cataflam Tablets (Rarely) 2173
Celebrex Capsules (Less than 0.1%) 3130
Centany Ointment, 2% (0.3%) 2382
Cialis Tablets 1806
Cipro I.V. (1% or less) 2998
Cipro I.V. Pharmacy Bulk Package (1% or less) 3509
Cipro 2991
Cipro XR Tablets 3004
Clinoril Tablets 1899
Concerta Extended-Release Tablets 1828
Coreg Tablets (Less than or equal to 0.1%) 1376
Cuprimine Capsules 1925
Cymbalta Delayed-Release Capsules (Infrequent) 1729
Cytovene 2763
Diovan HCT Tablets 2195
Diuril Oral 1936
Diuril Sodium Intravenous 1934
Dolobid Tablets (Less than 1 in 100) 1937
▲ Doxil Injection (Less than 1% to 10%) 3302
Duragesic Transdermal System (Less than 1%) 2448
Dynacin Tablets (Uncommon) 1859
EC-Naprosyn Delayed-Release Tablets (Less than 1%) 2769
Effexor Tablets (Rare) 3405
Effexor XR Capsules (Rare) 3411
Equetro Extended-Release Capsules 3178
Focalin Tablets 2214
Focalin XR Capsules 2217
Furosemide Tablets 2117
Gabitril Tablets (Infrequent) 998
Geodon Capsules (Infrequent) 2514
Gleevec Tablets (Infrequent) 2221
Hyzaar 1964
Imitrex Tablets (Rare) 1440
Inderal LA Long-Acting Capsules 3421
Indocin Capsules (Less than 1%) 1968
Indocin I.V. (Less than 1%) 1973
Indocin (Less than 1%) 1968
▲ I.V. Busulfex (5%) 1125
Kaletra (Less than 2%) 474
Lamictal (Rare) 1449
Lyrica Capsules (Rare) 2524
Mefoxin for Injection 1987
Mefoxin Premixed Intravenous Solution 1990
Metadate CD Capsules 3316
Micardis HCT Tablets 886
Miradon Tablets 3056
Mobic Oral Suspension 893
Mobic Tablets 893
Moduretic Tablets 2003
Nalfon Capsules (Less than 1%) 2504
Naprosyn Suspension (Less than 1%) 2769
Naprosyn Tablets (Less than 1%) 2769
Nembutal Sodium Solution, USP 2484
Neumega for Injection 3433
Nitrolingual Pumpspray 1161
Noroxin Tablets 2009
Omnicef Capsules 506
Omnicef for Oral Suspension 506
OxyContin Tablets (Less than 1%) 2699
Paser Granules 1657
Paxil CR Controlled-Release Tablets (Rare) 1509
Paxil (Rare) 1501
Phenytek Capsules 2153
Prinzide Tablets 2033
▲ Prograf Capsules and Injection (3% to 15%) 624
▲ Proleukin for Injection (18%) 1007
Protopic Ointment (Up to 3%) 629
Prozac Pulvules and Liquid 1771
Relpax Tablets (Rare) 2531
Rilutek Tablets (Up to 1.2%) 2945
Risperdal M-Tab Orally Disintegrating Tablets (Infrequent) 1658
Risperdal (Infrequent) 1658
Ritalin Hydrochloride Tablets 2254
Ritalin LA Capsules 2255
Ritalin-SR Tablets 2254
Seroquel Tablets (Rare) 691
Sular Tablets (Less than or equal to 1%) 1163
▲ Sustiva Capsules (Up to 3.5%) 957
Symbyax Capsules (Rare) 1788
Tagamet Tablets (Very rare) 1547
Tambocor Tablets (Less than 1%) 1824
▲ Targretin Capsules (9.5% to 28.3%) 1719
Tegretol/Tegretol-XR 2278
Teveten HCT Tablets 1710
Thalomid Capsules 979
Thioridazine Hydrochloride Tablets 2122
Thiothixene Capsules 2124
Tiazac Capsules (Infrequent) 1204
Ticlid Tablets (Rare) 2813
Timolide Tablets 2056
Vancocin HCl Capsules, USP (Infrequent) 3370
Vantin Tablets and Oral Suspension (Less than 1%) 2650
Vaseretic Tablets 2073
Vasotec I.V. Injection (0.5% to 1.0%) 2076
VFEND I.V. (Less than 2%) 2543
VFEND Oral Suspension (Less than 2%) 2543
VFEND Tablets (Less than 2%) 2543
Viagra Tablets (Less than 2%) 2552
Voltaren Tablets (Rarely) 2298
Voltaren-XR Tablets (Rarely) 2301
Wellbutrin Tablets 1579
Wellbutrin SR Sustained-Release Tablets 1583
Wellbutrin XL Extended-Release Tablets 1588
Zestoretic Tablets 701
Zevalin Injection 848
Zyban Sustained-Release Tablets 1620

Dermatitis, eyelid
OptiPranolol Metipranolol Ophthalmic Solution 0.3% (A small number of patients) ⊙254
Vantin Tablets and Oral Suspension 2650

Dermatitis, fungal
Antara Capsules 2723
▲ Arava Tablets (1% to 3%) 2881
Aricept Tablets (Infrequent) 1086
Aricept ODT Tablets (Infrequent) 1086
▲ CellCept Capsules (3% to less than 20%) 2751
▲ CellCept Intravenous (3% to less than 20%) 2751
▲ CellCept Oral Suspension (3% to less than 20%) 2751
▲ CellCept Tablets (3% to less than 20%) 2751
Clindagel 1207
Copaxone for Injection (Infrequent) 3292
▲ Doxil Injection (1% to 10%) 3302
Effexor Tablets (Rare) 3405
Geodon Capsules (2%) 2514
Lamictal (Rare) 1449
Lofibra Capsules 1217
Neurontin Capsules (Infrequent) 2498
Neurontin Oral Solution (Infrequent) 2498
Neurontin Tablets (Infrequent) 2498
Paxil CR Controlled-Release Tablets (Rare) 1509
Paxil (Rare) 1501
Permax Tablets (Infrequent) 3357
▲ Prograf Capsules and Injection (3% to 15%) 624
Protonix I.V. (Less than 1%) 3468
Protonix Tablets (Less than 1%) 3465
▲ Protopic Ointment (1% to 6%) 629
▲ Rapamune Oral Solution and Tablets (3% to 20%) 3472
Requip Tablets (Infrequent) 1528
Rescriptor Tablets 2535
Rilutek Tablets (Infrequent) 2945
Sular Tablets (Less than or equal to 1%) 1163
Synagis (More than 1%) 1868
▲ Thalomid Capsules (4.2%) 979
Tricor Tablets 523
Uniretic Tablets (Less than 1%) 3114
Vantin Tablets and Oral Suspension (Less than 1%) 2650
Viracept (Less than 2%) 2556
Zithromax for Oral Suspension, 300 mg, 600 mg, 900 mg, 1200 mg (1% or less) 2561
Zithromax Tablets, 250 mg, 500 mg (1% or less) 2561
Zithromax Tri-Pak (1% or less) 2561

Dermatitis, herpes simplex
Elidel Cream 1% (0.3% to 1.5%) 2198
▲ Mylotarg for Injection (21%) 3429

Dermatitis, irritant
Clobex Shampoo 1209

Dermatitis, lichenoides
Effexor Tablets (Rare) 3405
Effexor XR Capsules (Rare) 3411
Evoxac Capsules (Less than 1%) 1042
▲ Intron A for Injection (Less than 5%) 3038
Lyrica Capsules (Rare) 2524
Permax Tablets (Rare) 3357
Protonix I.V. (Less than 1%) 3468
Protonix Tablets (Less than 1%) 3465
Risperdal M-Tab Orally Disintegrating Tablets (Rare) 1658
Risperdal (Rare) 1658

Dermatitis, perioral
Aclovate (Infrequent) 1290
Analpram-HC 1136
Clobevate Gel 3213
Clobex Shampoo (Infrequent) 1209
Clobex Lotion 1208
Cutivate Cream (Infrequent) 1381
Cutivate Lotion 0.05% (Rare) 1383
Cutivate Ointment (Infrequent to more frequent) 1384
Diprolene Gel 0.05% 3015
Diprolene Lotion 0.05% (Infrequent) 3016
Diprolene Ointment 0.05% (Infrequent) 3017
Diprolene AF Cream 0.05% (Infrequent) 3014
Diprosone Cream, USP 0.05% 3018
Elocon Cream 0.1% (Infrequent) 3019
Elocon Lotion 0.1% (Infrequent) 3020
Elocon Ointment 0.1% (Infrequent) 3021
Locoid Cream (Infrequent) 1138
Locoid Lipocream Cream (Infrequent) 1138
Locoid (Infrequent) 1138
Lotrisone 3054
Luxiq Foam 1026
Olux Foam 1027
Pandel Cream, 0.1% 1017
Pramosone 1139
ProctoFoam-HC 3113
Temovate Cream 1549
Temovate Gel (Infrequent) 1550
Temovate Ointment 1549
Temovate Scalp Application (Infrequent) 1551
Temovate E Emollient (Infrequent) 1552
Topicort .05% Gel 3288
Topicort .25% Cream 3288
Topicort .25% Ointment 3288
Topicort LP .05% Cream 3288
Tri-Luma Cream 1213
U-cort 1% Cream 3289
Vanos Cream 1864

Dermatitis, photosensitive
Advair Diskus 100/50 1291
Advair Diskus 250/50 1291
Advair Diskus 500/50 1291
Amerge Tablets (Rare) 1312
Anaprox Tablets (Less than 1%) 2769
Anaprox DS Tablets (Less than 1%) 2769
EC-Naprosyn Delayed-Release Tablets (Less than 1%) 2769
▲ Flovent Diskus 50 mcg (1% to 3%) 1415
Naprosyn Suspension (Less than 1%) 2769
Naprosyn Tablets (Less than 1%) 2769
▲ Pacerone Tablets (4% to 9%) 3337
Prevacid NapraPAC (Less than 1%) 3277

Dermatitis, purpuric
Phenytek Capsules 2153

Dermatitis, radiation recall
Navelbine Injection 1494

Dermatitis, vesicular bullous
(*see under* Dermatitis, bullous)

Dermatitis seborrhic
Imitrex Injection 1431
Imitrex Nasal Spray 1435

Dermatologic reactions, unspecified
Aceon Tablets (2 mg, 4 mg, 8 mg) 3191
Altace Capsules (Less than 1%) 1673
Captopril Tablets 2114
Clinoril Tablets (Less than 1 in 100) 1899
Erbitux (1%) 937
Follistim AQ Cartridge 2354
▲ Idamycin PFS Injection (46%) 2645
Nexium Delayed-Release Capsules (Rare) 645
Nexium I.V. (Rare) 649
Norflex Injection (Rare) 1824
Prinivil Tablets (0.3% to 1.0%) 2029
Prinzide Tablets 2033
Protonix I.V. 3468
Protonix Tablets 3465
Sedapap Tablets 50 mg/650 mg (Several cases) 2098
Tasmar Tablets (Infrequent) 3360
Vaseretic Tablets 2073
Vasotec I.V. Injection (0.5% to 1.0%) 2076
Zestoretic Tablets 701
Zestril Tablets (0.3% to 1.0%) 704
Zithromax Capsules, 250 mg (Rare) 2568
Zithromax for IV Infusion (Rare) 2573
Zithromax for Oral Suspension, 300 mg, 600 mg, 900 mg, 1200 mg (Rare) 2561
Zithromax Tablets, 250 mg, 500 mg (Rare) 2561
Zithromax Tri-Pak (Rare) 2561

Dermatomyositis
Altoprev Extended-Release Tablets 1151
Cuprimine Capsules (Rare) 1925
Mevacor Tablets 1996
Pravachol Tablets (Rare) 943
Vytorin 10/10 Tablets 2084
Vytorin 10/10 Tablets 3092
Vytorin 10/20 Tablets 2084
Vytorin 10/20 Tablets 3092
Vytorin 10/40 Tablets 2084
Vytorin 10/40 Tablets 3092
Vytorin 10/80 Tablets 2084
Vytorin 10/80 Tablets 3092
Zocor Tablets 2078

Dermatomyositis, exacerbation of
Actimmune (Rare) 1646

Dermatosis
Amerge Tablets (Rare) 1312
▲ Flovent Diskus 50 mcg (1% to 3%) 1415
Lotronex Tablets (Rare) 1479

Descemetitis
Ophthetic Ophthalmic Solution ⊙230

Desquamation
▲ Alimta for Injection (Up to 22%) 1722
Doxil Injection (Some patients) 3302
Ertaczo Cream, 2% 2383
Invanz for Injection (Greater than 0.1%) 1974
Neurontin Capsules (Rare) 2498
Neurontin Oral Solution (Rare) 2498
Neurontin Tablets (Rare) 2498
Oxistat Lotion (0.4%) 1498
Rescriptor Tablets 2535
▲ Solage Topical Solution (12.6% to 14%) 740
▲ Sustiva Capsules (16.7% to 24.5%) 957
▲ Taxotere Injection Concentrate (5.6%) 2947
▲ Tri-Luma Cream (25.48% to 38%) 1213
Vantin Tablets and Oral Suspension (Less than 1%) 2650
Xeloda Tablets 2825
Zovirax Cream (Less than 1%) 853

Diabetes
(*see under* Diabetes mellitus)

Diabetes, aggravation of
▲ ActoPlus Met Tablets (5.1%) 3219
Campath Ampules 826
CombiPatch Transdermal System 2180
Geodon 2514

Namenda (Infrequent) 1199
Prefest Tablets 1069
Premphase Tablets 3452
Prempro Tablets 3452
Tamiflu Capsules 2810
Tamiflu Oral Suspension 2810

Diabetes, unstable

Viagra Tablets (Less than 2%) 2552

Diabetes insipidus

Sandostatin LAR Depot (Rare) 2264
VFEND I.V. (Less than 2%) 2543
VFEND Oral Suspension (Less than 2%) 2543
VFEND Tablets (Less than 2%) 2543

Diabetes insipidus, nephrogenic

Eskalith (Some reports) 1406
Viread Tablets 1284

Diabetes mellitus

Abilify Tablets (Infrequent) 916
Abilify Tablets (Infrequent) 2472
Accutane Capsules 2740
Antara Capsules 2723
Aptivus Capsules (Less than 2%) 859
▲ Arava Tablets (1% to 3%) 2881
Aricept Tablets (Infrequent) 1086
Aricept ODT Tablets (Infrequent) 1086
Boostrix 1366
Campral Tablets (Infrequent) 1175
Celebrex Capsules (0.1% to 1.9%) 3130
▲ CellCept Capsules (3% to less than 20%) 2751
▲ CellCept Intravenous (3% to less than 20%) 2751
▲ CellCept Oral Suspension (3% to less than 20%) 2751
▲ CellCept Tablets (3% to less than 20%) 2751
Copegus Tablets (Less than 1%) 2759
▲ Coreg Tablets (Greater than 1% to 3%) 1376
Crestor Tablets (Greater than or equal to 1%) 672
Crixivan Capsules 1918
Doxil Injection (Less than 1%) 3302
Dyazide Capsules 1389
Effexor Tablets (Rare) 3405
Effexor XR Capsules (Infrequent) 3411
Emend Capsules (Greater than 0.5%) 1944
Evoxac Capsules (Less than 1%) 1042
Exelon Capsules (Infrequent) 2204
Gengraf Capsules (1% to less than 3%) 458
Geodon 2514
Invirase (2.7%) 2776
Kaletra (Less than 2%) 474
Lofibra Capsules 1217
Lupron Depot 7.5 mg (Less than 5%) 3261
Maxzide 2150
Micardis Tablets (More than 0.3%) 884
Micardis HCT Tablets 886
M-M-R II 1980
Mumpsvax 2005
▲ Myfortic Tablets (3% to less than 20%) 2244
Neoral Soft Gelatin Capsules (1% to less than 3%) 2247
Neoral Oral Solution (1% to less than 3%) 2247
Neurontin Capsules (Infrequent) 2498
Neurontin Oral Solution (Infrequent) 2498
Neurontin Tablets (Infrequent) 2498
▲ Norditropin Cartridges (5%) 2318
Norvir (Less than 2%) 499
Paxil CR Controlled-Release Tablets (Rare) 1509
Paxil (Rare) 1501
Pegasys (Less than 1%) 2793
Permax Tablets (Infrequent) 3357
Pletal Tablets (Less than 2%) 2478
Prevacid Delayed-Release Capsules (Less than 1%) 3268
Prevacid for Delayed-Release Oral Suspension (Less than 1%) 3268
Prevacid NapraPAC (Less than 1%) 3277
Prevacid SoluTab Delayed-Release Orally Disintegrating Tablets (Less than 1%) 3268
PREVPAC (Less than 1%) 3281
Prinivil Tablets (0.3% to 1.0%) 2029
Prinzide Tablets 2033
▲ Prograf Capsules and Injection (3% to 24%) 624
Protonix I.V. (Less than 1%) 3468
Protonix Tablets (Less than 1%) 3465
Proventil HFA Inhalation Aerosol (Less than 3%) 3071
Prozac Pulvules and Liquid (Rare) 1771
Pulmozyme Inhalation Solution 1245
▲ Rapamune Oral Solution and Tablets (3% to 20%) 3472
Rebetron Combination Therapy 3078
ReoPro Vials (0.1%) 1779
Requip Tablets (Infrequent) 1528
Reyataz Capsules (Less than 3%) 948
Rilutek Tablets (Infrequent) 2945
Risperdal Consta Long-Acting Injection (Infrequent) 1664
Risperdal M-Tab Orally Disintegrating Tablets (Infrequent) 1658
Risperdal (Infrequent) 1658
Roferon-A Injection (Infrequent) 2805
Rythmol SR Capsules 2736
Sandostatin Injection (Less than 1%) 2263
Sandostatin LAR Depot (Rare) 2264
Seroquel Tablets (Infrequent) 691
▲ Simulect for Injection (3% to 10%) 2268
Sonata Capsules (Rare) 1686
Sular Tablets (Less than or equal to 1%) 1163
Tasmar Tablets (Infrequent) 3360
Tequin Injection (Less than 0.1%) 964
Tequin Tablets (Less than 0.1%) 964
Teveten Tablets (Less than 1%) 1707
Teveten HCT Tablets (Less than 1%) 1710
Thalomid Capsules 979
Topamax Sprinkle Capsules (Infrequent) 2438
Topamax Tablets (Infrequent) 2438
Toprol-XL Tablets (Greater than 1%) 660
Tricor Tablets 523
Triglide Tablets 1165
Uniretic Tablets (Less than 1%) 3114
Viracept 2556
▲ Zenapax for Injection (2% to 5%) 2838
Zestoretic Tablets 701
Zestril Tablets (0.3% to 1.0%) 704
Zoladex 3-month (1% to 5%) 712
Zyprexa Tablets (Infrequent) 1798
Zyprexa ZYDIS Orally Disintegrating Tablets (Infrequent) 1798
Zyrtec Chewable Tablets (Less than 2%) 2589
Zyrtec (Less than 2%) 2589
Zyrtec-D 12 Hour Extended Release Tablets (Less than 2%) 2591

Diabetes mellitus, increase

▲ Actos Tablets (5.1%) 3224
Agenerase Capsules 1299
Agenerase Oral Solution 1304
Levaquin in 5% Dextrose Injection (0.1% to 0.9%) 2453
Levaquin (0.1% to 0.9%) 2453
Toprol-XL Tablets (Greater than 1%) 660

Diabetes mellitus, insulin-dependent, post-transplant

▲ Prograf Capsules and Injection (20%) 624

Diabetes mellitus, precipitation of latent

Decadron Phosphate Injection 1931
Decadron Tablets 1929
Depo-Medrol Injectable Suspension 2615
Depo-Medrol Single-Dose Vial 2617
Furosemide Tablets 2117
Hydrocortone Tablets 1963
▲ Intron A for Injection (Less than 5%) 3038
Levaquin in 5% Dextrose Injection (0.1% to 0.9%) 2453
Levaquin (0.1% to 0.9%) 2453
Maxzide 2150
Pediapred Oral Solution 3319
Prinzide Tablets 2033
Risperdal M-Tab Orally Disintegrating Tablets 1658
Risperdal 1658
Vaseretic Tablets 2073
Viracept 2556
Zestoretic Tablets 701

Diabetes mellitus, type I

Enbrel for Injection 580

Diabetes mellitus de novo

Agenerase Capsules (2 patients) 1299
Agenerase Oral Solution (Two patients) 1304

Diabetic acidosis

Prozac Pulvules and Liquid (Rare) 1771
Zyprexa Tablets (Rare) 1798
Zyprexa ZYDIS Orally Disintegrating Tablets (Rare) 1798

Diabetic ketoacidosis

Agenerase Capsules 1299
Agenerase Oral Solution 1304
Aptivus Capsules 859
Neurontin Capsules (Rare) 2498
Neurontin Oral Solution (Rare) 2498
Neurontin Tablets (Rare) 2498
Risperdal M-Tab Orally Disintegrating Tablets 1658
Risperdal 1658
Viracept (Some cases) 2556

Diabetic retinopathy

Neurontin Capsules (Rare) 2498
Neurontin Oral Solution (Rare) 2498
Neurontin Tablets (Rare) 2498

Dialysis encephalopathy

Maalox Regular Strength Antacid/Anti-Gas Liquid .... ▣ 677
Maalox Max Maximum Strength Antacid/Anti-Gas Liquid 2165
Maalox Regular Strength Antacid/Antigas Liquid 2164

Dialysis graft complication

▲ Fosrenol (3% to 26%) 3180

Dialysis osteomalacia, results in, or worsening of

Maalox Regular Strength Antacid/Anti-Gas Liquid .... ▣ 677
Maalox Max Maximum Strength Antacid/Anti-Gas Liquid 2165
Maalox Regular Strength Antacid/Antigas Liquid 2164

Diaphoresis

Abilify Tablets (Frequent) 916
Abilify Tablets (Frequent) 2472
Accutane Capsules 2740
Aceon Tablets (2 mg, 4 mg, 8 mg) (0.3% to 1%) 3191
Aciphex Tablets 1081
Actiq (1% to 2%) 993
Adalat CC Tablets (Less than 1%) 2978
▲ Adderall XR Capsules (2% to 4%) 3169
Adenocard Injection (Less than 1%) 612
Adenoscan (Less than 1%) 613
▲ Advair Diskus 100/50 (1% to 3%) 1291
▲ Advair Diskus 250/50 (1% to 3%) 1291
▲ Advair Diskus 500/50 (1% to 3%) 1291
Advicor Tablets 1694
Aerobid/Aerobid-M (1% to 3%) 1172
Aggrastat (2%) 1878
Albalon Ophthalmic Solution .... ⊙ 216
Alferon N Injection (One patient to 3%) 1640
Alinia for Oral Suspension (Less than 1%) 2840
Alinia Tablets (Less than 1%) 2840
Aloprim for Injection (Less than 1%) 2156
Altace Capsules (Less than 1%) 1673
Ambien Tablets (Infrequent) 2867
▲ AmBisome for Injection (7%) 615
Amerge Tablets (Infrequent) 1312
Amnesteem Capsules 2126
Anaprox Tablets (Less than 3%) 2769
Anaprox DS Tablets (Less than 3%) 2769
AndroGel (Fewer than 1%) 3330
Antara Capsules 2723
Anzemet Injection (Rare) 2871
Anzemet Tablets (Rare) 2874
AquaMEPHYTON Injection 1887
▲ Arava Tablets (1% to 3%) 2881
Aredia for Injection 2168
Aricept Tablets (Frequent) 1086
Aricept ODT Tablets (Frequent) 1086
▲ Arimidex Tablets (1% to 5%) 665
▲ Aromasin Tablets (6%) 2600
Arthrotec Tablets (Rare) 3126
▲ Asacol Delayed-Release Tablets (3%) 2688
Atacand Tablets (0.5% or greater) 634
Atacand HCT (0.5% or greater) 637
Avelox (0.1% to less than 2%) 2984
▲ Avinza Capsules (5% to 10%) 1714
Axert Tablets (Rare) 2430
Axid Oral Solution (More frequent) 913
▲ Betaseron for SC Injection (8%) 791
▲ Bexxar (Less than 1% to 8%) 1360
BiDil Tablets (1% to less than 2%) 2161
Blocadren Tablets (Less than 1%) 1891
▲ Brevibloc Concentrate (12%) 766
▲ Brevibloc Injection (12%) 766
▲ Brevibloc Double Strength Injection (12%) 766
▲ Brevibloc Premixed Injection (12%) 766
▲ Brevibloc Double Strength Premixed Injection (12%) 766
▲ Buprenex Injectable (1% to 5%) 2718
Caduet Tablets (Less than 2%) 2507
▲ Campath Ampules (1% to 19%) 826
▲ Campral Tablets (2% to 3%) 1175
▲ Camptosar Injection (0% to 16%) 2602
Cancidas for Injection (0% to 2.8%) 1894
Captopril Tablets 2114
Carbatrol Capsules 3174
Cardene I.V. (1.4%) 1129
Carimune NF 3501
▲ Casodex Tablets (5%) 670
Caverject Impulse Injection (Less than 1%) 2610
Celebrex Capsules (0.1% to 1.9%) 3130
▲ Celexa (11%) 1177
▲ CellCept Capsules (3% to less than 20%) 2751
▲ CellCept Intravenous (3% to less than 20%) 2751
▲ CellCept Oral Suspension (3% to less than 20%) 2751
▲ CellCept Tablets (3% to less than 20%) 2751
Cialis Tablets (Less than 2%) 1806
Cipro I.V. (1% or less) 2998
Cipro I.V. Pharmacy Bulk Package (1% or less) 3509
Cipro (Less than 1%) 2991
Cipro XR Tablets 3004
Clinoril Tablets (Less than 1 in 100) 1899
▲ Clozapine Tablets (More than 5% to 6%) 2141
▲ Clozaril Tablets (More than 5% to 6%) 2174
Combunox Tablets (1.6%) 1183
Comtan Tablets (2%) 2186
▲ Copaxone for Injection (15%) 3292
Coreg Tablets (Greater than 0.1% to 1%) 1376
Cosopt Sterile Ophthalmic Solution 1910
Covera-HS Tablets (Less than 2%) 3135
Cozaar Tablets (Less than 1%) 1913
▲ Cytovene (11%) 2763
Dalmane Capsules (Rare) 3343
Dantrium Capsules (Less frequent) 2690
Decadron Phosphate Injection 1931
Decadron Tablets 1929
Depacon Injection (0.9%) 412
Depakote ER Tablets (Greater than 1%) 433
Depo-Medrol Injectable Suspension 2615
Depo-Medrol Single-Dose Vial 2617
Diastat Rectal Delivery System (Less than 1%) 3344
Dilaudid 439
Dilaudid Oral Liquid 443
Dilaudid Non-Sterile Powder 439
Dilaudid Rectal Suppositories 439
Dilaudid Tablets 439
Dilaudid Tablets - 8 mg 443
▲ Dilaudid-HP (Among most frequent) 441
Diovan HCT Tablets (Greater than 0.2%) 2195
Diprivan Injectable Emulsion (Less than 1%) 676
Dolobid Tablets (Less than 1 in 100) 1937
▲ Doxil Injection (1% to 10%) 3302
▲ Duragesic Transdermal System (10% or more) 2448
Dyazide Capsules 1389
EC-Naprosyn Delayed-Release Tablets (Less than 3%) 2769
▲ Effexor Tablets (2% to 19.3%) 3405
▲ Effexor XR Capsules (1% to 14%) 3411
Eldepryl Capsules 3209
▲ Eligard 7.5 mg (25% to 56.7%) 2896
▲ Eligard 22.5 mg (56.4%) 2899
▲ Eloxatin for Injection (2% to 5%) 2908
Emend Capsules (Greater than 0.5%) 1944
Engerix-B Vaccine (Less than 1%) 1391
▲ Entocort EC Capsules (Less than 5%) 2694
Equetro Extended-Release Capsules 3178
Evista Tablets (2.5% to 3.1%) 1735
▲ Evoxac Capsules (18.7%) 1042
▲ Exelon Capsules (4%) 2204
▲ Faslodex Injection (5%) 682
▲ FazaClo Orally Disintegrating Tablets (Greater than 5% to 6%) 547

▲ Femara Tablets (Less than 0.1% to 24.2%) 2210
Ferrlecit Injection 3379
Flexeril Tablets (Less than 1%) 1832
▲ Flolan for Injection (1% to 41%) 1408
Flumadine 1186
▲ Forteo for Injection (4.2%) 1739
Fortical Nasal Spray (Less than 1%) 3336
Frova Tablets (Frequent) 1101
Gabitril Tablets (Frequent) 998
Gemzar for Injection (Infrequent) 1743
Gengraf Capsules (1% to less than 3%) 458
Geodon for Injection (Up to 2%) 2514
Guanidine Hydrochloride Tablets 3030
Humalog-Pen (Less common) 1751
Humalog Mix 75/25-Pen (Less common) 1754
Humulin 50/50, 100 Units 1760
Humulin 70/30 Pen 1761
Humulin L, 100 Units (Less common) 1763
Humulin R (U-500) (Less common) 1768
Humulin N Pen 1765
Hydrocortone Tablets 1963
Hyperstat I.V. Injection 3031
Hytrin Capsules (At least 1%) 469
Hyzaar 1964
▲ Imdur Tablets (Less than or equal to 5%) 3032
Imitrex Injection (1.6%) 1431
Imitrex Nasal Spray (Infrequent) 1435
Imitrex Tablets (Infrequent) 1440
Indocin (Less than 1%) 1968
Infed Injection 3381
▲ Infergen (12% to 13%) 1647
▲ Intron A for Injection (1% to 21%) 3038
Invanz for Injection (Greater than 0.1%) 1974
Invirase (Less than 2%) 2776
Kadian Capsules (Less than 3%) 572
Kaletra (Less than 2%) 474
▲ Lamictal (2% to 5%) 1449
Lariam Tablets 2790
▲ Leukine (6%) 829
▲ Leustatin Injection (9%) 2368
Levaquin in 5% Dextrose Injection (0.1% to 0.9%) 2453
Levaquin (0.1% to 0.9%) 2453
Levitra Tablets (Less than 2%) 3048
Levoxyl Tablets 1680
▲ Lexapro Oral Solution (3% to 8%) 1193
▲ Lexapro Tablets (3% to 8%) 1193
Lipitor Tablets (Less than 2%) 2495
Lofibra Capsules 1217
Lotensin Tablets (Less than 1%) 2232
Lotensin HCT Tablets (0.3% to 1%) 2235
Lotronex Tablets (Infrequent) 1479
Lunesta Tablets 3139
▲ Lupron Depot 3.75 mg (50%) 3257
▲ Lupron Depot 7.5 mg (57.1%) 3261
▲ Lupron Depot–3 Month 11.25 mg (50%) 3262
Marinol Capsules (Less than 1%) 3334
Matulane Capsules 3188
Maxalt Tablets (Infrequent) 1983
Maxalt-MLT Orally Disintegrating Tablets (Infrequent) 1983
▲ Megace ES Oral Suspension (1% to 3%) 2492
Mephyton Tablets (Rare) 1993
▲ Mepron Suspension (10%) 1487
Meridia Capsules (2.5%) 485
Merrem I.V. (Greater than 0.1% to 1%) 687
Micardis Tablets (More than 0.3%) 884
Micardis HCT Tablets 886
Migranal Nasal Spray (Infrequent) 3350
Mirapex Tablets (1% or more) 889
Moban Tablets 1108
Mobic Oral Suspension (Less than 2%) 893
Mobic Tablets (Less than 2%) 893
Moduretic Tablets (Less than or equal to 1%) 2003
▲ MS Contin Tablets (Less frequent to among most frequent) 2703
Nadolol Tablets (1 to 5 of 1000 patients) 2121
Naprosyn Suspension (Less than 3%) 2769
Naprosyn Tablets (Less than 3%) 2769
Narcan Injection 1109
Naropin Injection 640
Natrecor for Injection (Greater than or equal to 1%) 3123
Neoral Soft Gelatin Capsules (1% to less than 3%) 2247
Neoral Oral Solution (1% to less than 3%) 2247
Neurontin Capsules (Infrequent) 2498
Neurontin Oral Solution (Infrequent) 2498
Neurontin Tablets (Infrequent) 2498
Nexium Delayed-Release Capsules (Less than 1%) 645
Nexium I.V. (Less than 1%) 649
Niaspan Extended-Release Tablets 1703
Nimotop Capsules (Less than 1%) 774
▲ Nipent for Injection (8% to 10%) 3216
▲ Niravam Orally Disintegrating Tablets (14.4% to 15.1%) 3106
Nitrolingual Pumpspray 1161
Norvasc Tablets (More than 0.1% to 1%) 2529
Norvir (1.7% to 2.6%) 499
Novolin 70/30 PenFill 3 ml Cartridges (Rare) 2325
Novolin N PenFill 3 ml Cartridges (Rare) 2325
Novolin R PenFill (Rare) 2325
▲ Nubain Injection (9%) 1111
Numorphan 1112
Omacor Capsules 2735
▲ Ontak Vials (10%) 1717
Orap Tablets 1220
Orthoclone OKT3 Sterile Solution (Less than 1%) 2370
▲ OxyContin Tablets (5%) 2699
▲ Paxil CR Controlled-Release Tablets (1.1% to 19.2%) 1509
▲ Paxil (1.1% to 19.2%) 1501
Pediapred Oral Solution 3319
▲ Pegasys (6%) 2793
▲ PEG-Intron Powder for Injection (6%) 3062
Pentasa Capsules (Less than 1%) 3182
Permax Tablets (2.1%) 3357
Phenergan 3438
Prevacid Delayed-Release Capsules (Less than 1%) 3268
Prevacid for Delayed-Release Oral Suspension (Less than 1%) 3268
Prevacid NapraPAC (Less than 3%) 3277
Prevacid SoluTab Delayed-Release Orally Disintegrating Tablets (Less than 1%) 3268
PREVPAC (Less than 1%) 3281
Prinivil Tablets (0.3% to 1.0%) 2029
Prinzide Tablets (0.3% to 1%) 2033
▲ Prograf Capsules and Injection (3% to 15%) 624
Prometrium Capsules (100 mg, 200 mg) 3205
ProSom Tablets (Infrequent) 512
Protonix I.V. (Less than 1%) 3468
Protonix Tablets (Less than 1%) 3465
Protopic Ointment (Greater than or equal to 1%) 629
Proventil HFA Inhalation Aerosol (Less than 3%) 3071
Provigil Tablets (1%) 1002
▲ Prozac Pulvules and Liquid (2% to 8%) 1771
Rabies Vaccine RabAvert (Rare) 1011
▲ Rapamune Oral Solution and Tablets (3% to 20%) 3472
▲ Rebetol (7% to 11%) 3073
Recombivax HB (Less than 1%) 2045
ReFacto Vials 3479
Reishimax Capsules 2669
Relafen Tablets (1% to 3%) 1523
Relpax Tablets (Frequent) 2531
Remicade for IV Injection (Greater than or equal to 0.2%) 987
ReoPro Vials (1%) 1779
▲ Requip Tablets (6% to 7%) 1528
Rescriptor Tablets 2535
▲ Retrovir Capsules (5%) 1533
▲ Retrovir IV Infusion (5%) 1537
▲ Retrovir (5%) 1533
Reyataz Capsules (Less than 3%) 948
▲ Ribavirin, USP Capsules (7%) 3083
Risperdal M-Tab Orally Disintegrating Tablets (Infrequent) 1658
Risperdal (Infrequent) 1658
Rocephin Injectable Vials, ADD-Vantage, Galaxy, Bulk (Occasional) 2801
▲ Roferon-A Injection (More than 1% to 22%) 2805
▲ Sandostatin LAR Depot (5% to 15%) 2264
Seroquel Tablets (Frequent) 691
Sonata Capsules (Infrequent) 1686
▲ Soriatane Capsules (1% to 10%) 1028
Spectracef Tablets (0.1% to 1%) 2706
▲ Suboxone Tablets (12% to 14%) 2719
▲ Subutex Tablets (12% to 12.6%) 2719
Sular Tablets (Less than or equal to 1%) 1163
Surmontil Capsules 2347
Sustiva Capsules (1% to 2%) 957
Symmetrel 1115
Synercid I.V. (Less than 1%) 1690
Tambocor Tablets (1% to 3%) 1824
Tarka Tablets 519
▲ Tasmar Tablets (4% to 7%) 3360
Tegretol/Tegretol-XR 2278
▲ Tequin Injection (0.1% to 3%) 964
▲ Tequin Tablets (0.1% to 3%) 964
Teveten Tablets (Less than 1%) 1707
Teveten HCT Tablets (Less than 1%) 1710
Thalomid Capsules 979
Thiothixene Capsules (Infrequently) 2124
Timolide Tablets 2056
Timoptic in Ocudose 2061
Timoptic Sterile Ophthalmic Solution 2058
Timoptic-XE Sterile Ophthalmic Gel Forming Solution 2062
Tindamax 2670
Topamax Sprinkle Capsules (2%) 2438
Topamax Tablets (2%) 2438
Tricor Tablets 523
▲ Trileptal Oral Suspension (Up to 3%) 2281
▲ Trileptal Tablets (Up to 3%) 2281
▲ Trisenox Injection (13%) 983
Truvada Tablets 1279
Twinrix Vaccine (Less than 1%) 1571
Tygacil for Injection (2.3%) 3489
▲ Ultracet Tablets (4%) 2462
Uniretic Tablets (Less than 1%) 3114
Unithroid Tablets 3521
Univasc Tablets (Less than 1%) 3118
Urecholine Tablets 2349
Vaseretic Tablets (0.5% to 2.0%) 2073
Vasotec I.V. Injection (0.5% to 1.0%) 2076
Verelan PM Capsules (2% or less) 3120
▲ Vesanoid Capsules (20%) 2823
VFEND I.V. (Less than 2%) 2543
VFEND Oral Suspension (Less than 2%) 2543
VFEND Tablets (Less than 2%) 2543
▲ Viadur Implant (5.3%) 782
Viagra Tablets (Less than 2%) 2552
▲ Vicoprofen Tablets (3% to 9%) 533
Viracept (Less than 2%) 2556
▲ Viread Tablets (3%) 1284
Vivactil Tablets 2350
▲ Wellbutrin Tablets (22.3%) 1579
▲ Wellbutrin SR Sustained-Release Tablets (5% to 6%) 1583
▲ Wellbutrin XL Extended-Release Tablets (5% to 6%) 1588
WinRho SDF 763
▲ Xeloda Tablets (Less than 5%) 2825
Xopenex HFA Inhalation Aerosol 3151
Xopenex Inhalation Solution 3143
Xopenex Inhalation Solution Concentrate 3147
▲ Zenapax for Injection (2% to 5%) 2838
Zestoretic Tablets (0.3% to 1%) 701
Zestril Tablets (0.3% to 1.0%) 704
▲ Zevalin Injection (4%) 848
Zithromax for Oral Suspension, 300 mg, 600 mg, 900 mg, 1200 mg (1% or less) 2561
Zithromax Tablets, 250 mg, 500 mg (1% or less) 2561
Zithromax Tri-Pak (1% or less) 2561
▲ Zoladex (6% to 45%) 709
Zoladex 3-month 712
▲ Zoloft (5% to 8%) 2581
Zomig Nasal Spray (Infrequent) 718
Zomig Tablets (2% to 3%) 714
▲ Zomig-ZMT Tablets (2% to 3%) 714
Zonegran Capsules (Infrequent) 1089
Zosyn (1.0% or less) 3492
Zovirax for Injection (Less than 1%) 1618
Zyban Sustained-Release Tablets (Frequent) 1620
Zyprexa Tablets 1798
Zyprexa IntraMuscular (Infrequent) 1798
Zyprexa ZYDIS Orally Disintegrating Tablets 1798
Zyrtec Chewable Tablets (Less than 2%) 2589
Zyrtec (Less than 2%) 2589
Zyrtec-D 12 Hour Extended Release Tablets (Less than 2%) 2591

Diaphoresis, nocturnal

Sandimmune (Rare) 2259

Diaphragmatic hernia

(*see under* Hernia, hiatal)

Diarrhea

▲ Abelcet Injection (6%) 1119
Abilify Tablets 916
Abilify Tablets 2472
Accolate Tablets (2.8%) 663
Accutane Capsules 2740
▲ Aceon Tablets (2 mg, 4 mg, 8 mg) (4.3%) 3191
Aciphex Tablets 1081
▲ Actimmune (14%) 1646
Actiq (1% or greater) 993
▲ Actonel Tablets (4.9% to 19.7%) 2679
▲ Actonel with Calcium Tablets (4.9% to 10.6%) 2684
▲ ActoPlus Met Tablets (4.6% to 5.8%) 3219
▲ Adacel Vaccine (0.3% to 10.3%) 2959
Adalat CC Tablets (Less than 1%) 2978
Adderall Tablets 3168
▲ Adderall XR Capsules (2% to 6%) 3169
Adipex-P 1216
Adriamycin for Injection, USP (Occasional) 786
Adriamycin Injection, USP (Occasional) 786
▲ Advair Diskus 100/50 (4%) 1291
Advair Diskus 250/50 (2%) 1291
▲ Advair Diskus 500/50 (2% to 4%) 1291
Advate Injection (0.6%) 742
▲ Advicor Tablets (6%) 1694
▲ Aerobid/Aerobid-M (10%) 1172
▲ Agenerase Capsules (28% to 60%) 1299
▲ Agenerase Oral Solution (28% to 60%) 1304
▲ Aggrenox Capsules (12.7%) 855
▲ Agrylin Capsules (25.7%) 3172
Alacol DM Syrup 739
Aldara Cream, 5% (More than 1%) 1814
Aldoclor Tablets 1881
Aldoril Tablets 1884
▲ Alferon N Injection (2% to 6%) 1640
▲ Alimta for Injection (Up to 26%) 1722
Alinia for Oral Suspension (2.1%) 2840
Alinia Tablets (2.1%) 2840
Alkeran for Injection (Infrequent) 976
Alkeran Tablets (Infrequent) 977
Aloprim for Injection (Less than 1%) 2156
Aloxi Injection (1%) 2099
Altace Capsules (Less than 1% to 1.1%) 1673
▲ Altoprev Extended-Release Tablets (3%) 1151
Amaryl Tablets (Less than 1%) 2864
Ambien Tablets (1% to 3%) 2867
▲ AmBisome for Injection (15.3% to 30.3%) 615
Amerge Tablets (Infrequent) 1312
▲ Ammonul Injection (3%) 3323
▲ Amoxil Capsules (8%) 1315
▲ Amoxil Chewable Tablets (8%) 1315
▲ Amoxil Pediatric Drops for Oral Suspension (8%) 1315
▲ Amoxil Powder for Oral Suspension (8%) 1315
▲ Amoxil Tablets (8%) 1315
Anadrol-50 Tablets 3329
Anaprox Tablets (Less than 3%) 2769
Anaprox DS Tablets (Less than 3%) 2769
Ancef for Injection 1318
Antara Capsules (2.3%) 2723
▲ Anzemet Injection (12.4%) 2871
Anzemet Tablets (2.1%) 2874
▲ Apokyn Injection (At least 5%) 2132
▲ Aptivus Capsules (10.9%) 859
▲ Aranesp for Injection (16% to 22%) 576
▲ Arava Tablets (17%) 2881
▲ Aredia for Injection (28.5%) 2168
▲ Argatroban Injection (6.2%) 1321
▲ Aricept Tablets (8% to 15%) 1086
▲ Aricept ODT Tablets (8% to 15%) 1086
▲ Arimidex Tablets (6% to 8%) 665
Arixtra Injection (1.9% to 2.5%) 1325
▲ Aromasin Tablets (4%) 2600
▲ Arthrotec Tablets (19%) 3126
▲ Asacol Delayed-Release Tablets (7%) 2688
Astelin Nasal Spray 1876
Atacand Tablets (More than 1%) 634
Atacand HCT (0.5% or greater) 637
Attenuvax (Rare) 1889
▲ Augmentin (9%) 1331
▲ Augmentin Tablets (9%) 1334
▲ Augmentin XR Extended-Release Tablets (15.6%) 1340
Augmentin ES-600 Powder for Oral Suspension (2.9%) 1337
Avalide Tablets (1% or greater) 922
Avalide Tablets (1% or greater) 2889
▲ Avandamet Tablets (12.7%) 1343
Avandia Tablets (2.3%) 1348
▲ Avapro Tablets (3%) 925
▲ Avapro Tablets (3%) 2886
▲ Avastin IV (34%) 1229
▲ Avelox (5%) 2984
▲ Avinza Capsules (5% to 10%) 1714
Axert Tablets (Infrequent) 2430
▲ Axid Oral Solution (7.2%) 913
Azasan Tablets (Less than 1%) 2844

▲ Azmacort Inhalation Aerosol (1% to 3%) 1701
Azopt Ophthalmic Suspension (Less than 1%) 553
Bactroban Nasal (Less than 1%) 1357
Balamine DM 739
Baraclude (Less than or equal to 1%) 928
Beano ▣ 764
BeneFix for Injection (1.5% to 1.6%) 3402
Benicar HCT Tablets (Greater than 1%) 2852
Benzaclin Topical Gel 1046
Betagan Ophthalmic Solution, USP ⊙ 217
▲ Betaseron for SC Injection (19%) 791
Betimol Ophthalmic Solution ⊙ 283
Betimol Ophthalmic Solution 3371
▲ Bexxar (1% to 12%) 1360
▲ Biaxin/Biaxin XL (3% to 6%) 402
Blocadren Tablets (Less than 1%) 1891
▲ Boniva Tablets (4.1% to 6.8%) 2747
▲ Boostrix (3% to 26%) 1366
Bravelle for Intramuscular or Subcutaneous Injection (2.7%) 1140
Buprenex Injectable (Rare) 2718
▲ Byetta Injection (13%) 605
▲ Caduet Tablets (Greater than 0.1% to 5.3%) 2507
▲ Campath Ampules (1% to 22%) 826
▲ Campral Tablets (10% to 17%) 1175
▲ Camptosar Injection (6.7% to 88%) 2602
▲ Canasa Rectal Suppositories (3.1%) 726
▲ Cancidas for Injection (1.3% to 3.6%) 1894
Captopril Tablets (About 0.5% to 2%) 2114
Carafate Suspension (Less than 0.5%) 727
Carafate Tablets (Less than 0.5%) 728
Carbatrol Capsules 3174
Cardizem LA Extended Release Tablets (Less than 2%) 1699
▲ Carnitor Injection (9% to 35%) 3185
Carnitor Tablets and Oral Solution 3187
▲ Casodex Tablets (10%) 670
▲ Cataflam Tablets (1% to 10%) 2173
▲ Ceftin (8.6%) 1369
▲ Celebrex Capsules (5.6%) 3130
▲ Celexa (8%) 1177
▲ CellCept Capsules (31% to 51.3%) 2751
▲ CellCept Intravenous (31% to 51.3%) 2751
▲ CellCept Oral Suspension (31% to 51.3%) 2751
▲ CellCept Tablets (31% to 51.3%) 2751
▲ Cenestin Tablets, 0.45mg, 0.625mg, 0.9mg, 1.25mg (6%) 1063
▲ Cerezyme for Injection (Approximately 6.5%) 1263
Cerubidine for Injection (Occasional) 788
Cervidil Vaginal Insert (Less than 1%) 1182
▲ Chemet Capsules (12.0% to 20.9%) 2480
Chromagen Soft Gelatin Capsules 3296
Chromagen Forte Soft Gelatin Capsules 3296
Cialis Tablets (Less than 2%) 1806
▲ Cipro I.V. (Greater than 1% to 4.8%) 2998
▲ Cipro I.V. Pharmacy Bulk Package (Greater than 1% to 4.8%) 3509
▲ Cipro (1.6% to 4.8%) 2991
Cipro XR Tablets (2%) 3004
▲ Clarinex Syrup (15.4% to 19.7%) 3009
Cleocin Vaginal Ovules (Less than 1%) 2613
Clindagel 1207
Clindesse Vaginal Cream (Less than 1%) 3296
▲ Clinoril Tablets (3% to 9%) 1899
▲ Clolar for Intravenous Infusion (53%) 1264
Clorpres Tablets 2139
Clozapine Tablets (2%) 2141
Clozaril Tablets (2%) 2174
▲ Colazal Capsules (5%) 2845
▲ CombiPatch Transdermal System (9% to 14%) 2180
Combivent Inhalation Aerosol (Less than 2%) 878
▲ Combivir Tablets (18%) 1373
Combunox Tablets (2.1%) 1183
▲ Comtan Tablets (10%) 2186
Comvax (0.8% to 2.2%) 1904
Concerta Extended-Release Tablets (2%) 1828
▲ Copaxone for Injection (12%) 3292
▲ Copegus Tablets (11%) 2759
▲ Coreg Tablets (2% to 12%) 1376
Cosmegen for Injection 1907
Cosopt Sterile Ophthalmic Solution (Less than 1%) 1910
Coumadin for Injection (Infrequent) 932
Coumadin Tablets (Infrequent) 932
Covera-HS Tablets (Less than 2%) 3135
Cozaar Tablets (1% or greater) 1913
▲ Creon 5 Capsules (Among most frequent) 3195
▲ Creon 10 Capsules (Among most frequent) 3195
▲ Creon 20 Capsules (Among most frequent) 3196
▲ Crestor Tablets (3.4%) 672
▲ Crixivan Capsules (3.3%) 1918
▲ Cubicin for Injection (5.2%) 1038
Cuprimine Capsules 1925
Cutivate Lotion 0.05% (1%) 1383
▲ Cymbalta Delayed-Release Capsules (7% to 13%) 1729
▲ Cytovene (41%) 2763
Dalmane Capsules 3343
▲ Dantrium Capsules (Among most frequent) 2690
DDAVP Tablets 2895
▲ Demser Capsules (10%) 1933
▲ Depacon Injection (0.9% to 23%) 412
▲ Depakene (13% to 23%) 417
▲ Depakote Sprinkle Capsules (13% to 23%) 422
▲ Depakote Tablets (12% to 23%) 427
▲ Depakote ER Tablets (7% to 23%) 433
▲ depo-subQ provera 104 Injectable Suspension (1% to less than 5%) 2622
Desferal Vials 2190
Desoxyn Tablets, USP 2482
▲ Detrol Tablets (4%) 2626
Dexedrine 1386
DextroStat Tablets 3177
▲ Diastat Rectal Delivery System (4%) 3344
▲ Didronel Tablets (About 1 patient in 15; possibly 2 or 3 in 10) 2693
▲ Digitek Tablets (4%) 2146
Dilaudid 439
Dilaudid Oral Liquid 443
Dilaudid Non-Sterile Powder 439
Dilaudid Rectal Suppositories 439
Dilaudid Tablets 439
Dilaudid Tablets - 8 mg 443
Dilaudid-HP (Less frequent) 441
▲ Diovan HCT Tablets (3%) 2195
▲ Diovan Tablets (1% to 5%) 2191
Diprivan Injectable Emulsion (Less than 1%) 676
▲ Ditropan XL Extended Release Tablets (7% to 9%) 2391
Diuril Oral 1936
Diuril Sodium Intravenous 1934
▲ Dolobid Tablets (3% to 9%) 1937
▲ Dostinex Tablets (2% to less than 10%) 2631
▲ Doxil Injection (5.2% to 20.9%) 3302
Duac Topical Gel 3214
DuoNeb Inhalation Solution (1.8%) 1058
▲ Duragesic Transdermal System (3% to 10%) 2448
Dyazide Capsules 1389
Dynacin Tablets (Infrequent) 1859
DynaCirc CR Tablets (0.5% to 1%) 2726
Dyrenium Capsules (Rare) 3390
EC-Naprosyn Delayed-Release Tablets (Less than 3%) 2769
Edecrin 1941
▲ E.E.S. (Among most frequent) 449
▲ Effexor Tablets (8%) 3405
▲ Effexor XR Capsules (6%) 3411
Eldepryl Capsules (1 of 49 patients) 3209
Elidel Cream 1% (0.6% to 7.7%) 2198
▲ Elitek (20%) 2906
▲ Ellence Injection (0% to 24.8%) 2632
▲ Elmiron Capsules (4%) 2393
▲ Eloxatin for Injection (11% to 67%) 2908
▲ Emcyt Capsules (12%) 3137
▲ Emend Capsules (10.3%) 1944
▲ Emtriva Capsules (23%) 1272
Enablex Extended-Release Tablets (0.9% to 2.1%) 2201
Enbrel for Injection 580
Engerix-B Vaccine (Less than 1%) 1391
▲ Epivir (18%) 1394
▲ Epivir-HBV (14%) 1398
▲ Epogen for Injection (0.11% to 21%) 586
▲ Epzicom Tablets (5% to 6%) 1402
▲ Equetro Extended-Release Capsules (10%) 3178
▲ Erbitux (28%) 937
▲ EryPed (Among most frequent) 445
▲ Ery-Tab Tablets (Among most frequent) 447
▲ Erythrocin Stearate Filmtab Tablets (Among most frequent) 452
▲ Erythromycin Base Filmtab Tablets (Among most frequent) 454
▲ Erythromycin Delayed-Release Capsules, USP (Among most frequent) 456
Eskalith 1406
▲ Estrogel 0.06% (4.2%) 3200
▲ Eulexin Capsules (12% to 40%) 3023
Evoclin Foam, 1% (Rarely) 1025
▲ Evoxac Capsules (10.3%) 1042
▲ Exelon Capsules (19%) 2204
▲ Factive Tablets (4.6%) 2464
▲ Famvir Tablets (4.5% to 9%) 2207
▲ Faslodex Injection (12.3%) 682
FazaClo Orally Disintegrating Tablets (2%) 547
▲ Femara Tablets (0.5% to 8%) 2210
Feosol Caplets (Occasional) 1629
Feosol Tablets (Occasional) 1629
▲ Ferrlecit Injection (2% to 35%) 3379
▲ Flexeril Tablets (1% to 3%) 1832
▲ Flolan for Injection (37% to 50%) 1408
▲ Flomax Capsules (4.3% to 6.2%) 881
▲ Flonase Nasal Spray (1% to 3%) 1412
▲ Flovent Diskus 50 mcg (1% to 3%) 1415
▲ Flovent HFA (1% to 3%) 1418
Floxin Otic Singles (0.6%) 1045
Floxin Otic Solution (0.6%) 1043
Flumadine (0.3% to 1%) 1186
▲ Flumist Vaccine (3.7%) 1872
Follistim AQ Cartridge 2354
▲ Fortamet Extended-Release Tablets (16.7%) 1156
Fortaz (1 in 78 patients) 1422
▲ Forteo for Injection (5.1%) 1739
▲ Fortical Nasal Spray (1% to 3%) 3336
▲ Fosamax (0.6% to 3.1%) 1949
▲ Fosamax Plus D Tablets (0% to 3.1%) 1956
▲ Fosrenol Chewable Tablets (13% to 23%) 3180
Frova Tablets (Frequent) 1101
Furosemide Tablets 2117
▲ Fuzeon Injection (31.7%) 2772
▲ Gabitril Tablets (2% to 10%) 998
▲ Gammagard Liquid (0.85% to 8.2%) 751
▲ Gamunex Immune Globulin I.V., 10% (28%) 3232
▲ Gemzar for Injection (19% to 31%) 1743
▲ Gengraf Capsules (3% to 13%) 458
▲ Geodon (5%) 2514
▲ Gleevec Tablets (30.3% to 60%) 2221
▲ Gonal-f RFF Pen for Injection (3.6%) 3155
Grifulvin V Tablets Microsize and Oral Suspension Microsize (Occasional) 2384
Gris-PEG Tablets (Occasional) 2504
Guanidine Hydrochloride Tablets 3030
Havrix Vaccine (Less than 1%) 1425
▲ Hepsera Tablets (2% to 3%) 1275
▲ Herceptin I.V. (25%) 1234
HibTITER (2 of 1,118 vaccinations) 3419
▲ Hycamtin for Injection (Less than 1% to 42%) 1427
Hyperstat I.V. Injection 3031
Hytrin Capsules (At least 1%) 469
Hyzaar (1% or greater) 1964
▲ Idamycin PFS Injection (73%) 2645
▲ Imdur Tablets (Less than or equal to 5%) 3032
Imitrex Injection (Infrequent) 1431
Imitrex Nasal Spray (Infrequent) 1435
Imitrex Tablets (Frequent) 1440
Indapamide Tablets (Less than 5%) 2119
Inderal LA Long-Acting Capsules 3421
Indocin Capsules (Greater than 1%) 1968
Indocin I.V. (1% to 3%) 1973
Indocin (Greater than 1%) 1968
▲ Infanrix Vaccine (3.8% to 4.3%) 1444
Infed Injection 3381
▲ Infergen (24% to 29%) 1647
InnoPran XL Capsules 2728
Inspra Tablets (2%) 2520
▲ Intron A for Injection (2% to 45%) 3038
▲ Invanz for Injection (9.2% to 11.7%) 1974
▲ Invirase (1% to 8.1%) 2776
▲ Iressa Tablets (49% to 76%) 684
▲ I.V. Busulfex (5% to 84%) 1125
Kadian Capsules (Less than 3%) 572
▲ Kaletra (7% to 27%) 474
K-Dur Extended-Relase Tablets 3047
▲ Keppra Oral Solution (1% to 8%) 3307
▲ Keppra Tablets (1% to 8%) 3307
▲ Ketek Tablets (10% to 10.8%) 2920
▲ Kineret Injection (7%) 594
Klonopin 2782
▲ K-Lor Powder Packets (Among most common) 472
K-Phos Neutral Tablets 785
K-Phos Original (Sodium Free) Tablets 785
Kristalose for Oral Solution 2149
▲ K-Tab Filmtab Tablets (Most common) 473
▲ Kytril Injection (4%) 2785
▲ Kytril Tablets (4% to 9%) 2788
▲ Lamictal (5% to 11%) 1449
▲ Lamisil Tablets (5.6%) 2226
Lanoxicaps Capsules (Less common) 1458
Lanoxin Injection (Less common) 1462
Lanoxin Tablets (Less common) 1468
Lanoxin Injection Pediatric 1465
▲ Lariam Tablets (Among most frequent) 2790
▲ Lescol Capsules (4.9%) 2227
▲ Lescol Capsules (4.9%) 2730
▲ Lescol XL Tablets (3.3%) 2227
▲ Lescol XL Tablets (3.3%) 2730
Leukeran Tablets (Infrequent) 1472
▲ Leukine (52% to 89%) 829
▲ Leustatin Injection (10%) 2368
▲ Levaquin in 5% Dextrose Injection (1.2% to 5.4%) 2453
▲ Levaquin (1.2% to 5.4%) 2453
Levitra Tablets (Less than 2%) 3048
Levothroid Tablets 1189
Levoxyl Tablets 1680
▲ Lexapro Oral Solution (6% to 14%) 1193
▲ Lexapro Tablets (6% to 14%) 1193
▲ Lexiva Tablets (5% to 52%) 1473
▲ Lipitor Tablets (Up to 5.3%) 2495
Lithobid Tablets 1670
Lofibra Capsules (2.3%) 1217
Lotensin HCT Tablets (0.3% to 1%) 2235
Lotrel Capsules 2238
Lovenox Injection (2.2%) 2931
▲ Lunesta Tablets (2% to 4%) 3139
Lupron Depot 7.5 mg (Less than 5%) 3261
▲ Malarone Tablets (1% to 8%) 1484
▲ Malarone Pediatric Tablets (1% to 8%) 1484
Marinol Capsules (0.3% to 1%) 3334
Matulane Capsules 3188
Mavik Tablets (0.3% to 1.0%) 482
Maxair Autohaler (1.3%) 1820
Maxalt Tablets (Frequent) 1983
Maxalt-MLT Orally Disintegrating Tablets (Frequent) 1983
▲ Maxipime for Injection (Greater than 0.1% to 3%) 1093
Maxzide 2150
Mefoxin for Injection 1987
Mefoxin Premixed Intravenous Solution 1990
▲ Megace ES Oral Suspension (6% to 13%) 2492
▲ Menactra Vaccine (0.3% to 16%) 2968
Menopur for Subcutaneous Injection (2.6% to 2.8%) 1145
▲ Mepron Suspension (2.1% to 42%) 1487
Meridia Capsules (Greater than or equal to 1%) 485
▲ Merrem I.V. (3.5% to 7%) 687
Meruvax II 1994
MetroGel-Vaginal Gel (1%) 1822
▲ Mevacor Tablets (2.2% to 5.5%) 1996
Miacalcin Nasal Spray (1% to 3%) 2242
▲ Micardis Tablets (3%) 884
▲ Micardis HCT Tablets (3%) 886
▲ Midamor Tablets (3% to 8%) 2000
Migranal Nasal Spray (2%) 3350
Mintezol 2002
Miradon Tablets 3056
Mirapex Tablets (Greater than or equal to 1%) 889
M-M-R II 1980
▲ Mobic Oral Suspension (1.9% to 7.8%) 893
▲ Mobic Tablets (1.9% to 7.8%) 893
Moduretic Tablets (Greater than 1%, less than 3%) 2003
MS Contin Tablets (Less frequent) 2703
Mumpsvax 2005
Mustargen for Injection 2007
Mycamine for Injection (1.6% to 2.1%) 620
▲ Myfortic Tablets (21.4% to 23.5%) 2244
▲ Mylotarg for Injection (30% to 36%) 3429
▲ Nabi-HB (3%) 2159
Nadolol Tablets (1 to 5 of 1000 patients) 2121
Nalfon Capsules (1.8%) 2504
Namenda (Greater than or equal to 2%) 1199

Naprosyn Suspension (Less than 3%) 2769
Naprosyn Tablets (Less than 3%) 2769
Narcan Injection 1109
Nasonex Nasal Spray (Greater than or equal to 2%) 3058
▲ Navelbine Injection (Up to 17%) 1494
▲ Neoral Soft Gelatin Capsules (3% to 13%) 2247
▲ Neoral Oral Solution (3% to 13%) 2247
▲ Neulasta Injection (15% to 72%) 596
▲ Neumega for Injection (43%) 3433
▲ Neupogen for Injection (14%) 598
▲ Neurontin Capsules (5.7%) 2498
▲ Neurontin Oral Solution (5.7%) 2498
▲ Neurontin Tablets (5.7%) 2498
▲ Nexium Delayed-Release Capsules (Greater than or equal to 1% to 9.2%) 645
▲ Nexium I.V. (Greater than or equal to 1% to 9.2%) 649
▲ Niaspan Extended-Release Tablets (6% to 8%) 1703
Nicomide Tablets 3190
▲ Nicotrol Inhaler (Greater than 3%) 2594
Nicotrol NS (Less than 1%) 2596
Niferex-150 Forte Capsules 3299
▲ Nimotop Capsules (Up to 4.2%) 774
▲ Nipent for Injection (15% to 17%) 3216
▲ Niravam Orally Disintegrating Tablets (10.1% to 20.6%) 3106
Noroxin Tablets (0.3% to 1.0%) 2009
Norvasc Tablets (More than 0.1% to 1%) 2529
▲ Norvir (15.4% to 23.3%) 499
▲ Novantrone for Injection Concentrate (16% to 25%) 3158
▲ Omnicef Capsules (15%) 506
▲ Omnicef for Oral Suspension (8%) 506
▲ Oncaspar (Greater than 1% but less than 5%) 1123
▲ Ontak Vials (29%) 1717
▲ Orap Tablets (1 of 20 patients) 1220
▲ Orthoclone OKT3 Sterile Solution (14%) 2370
▲ OxyContin Tablets (Between 1% and 5%) 2699
▲ Oxytrol Transdermal System (3.2%) 3383
▲ Pancrease MT Capsules (Among most frequent) 1839
Parcopa Orally Disintegrating Tablets 3111
Parnate Tablets 1499
▲ Paser Granules (Among most common) 1657
▲ Paxil CR Controlled-Release Tablets (1.0% to 12%) 1509
▲ Paxil (1.0% to 12%) 1501
▲ PCE Dispertab Tablets (Among most frequent) 510
Pediarix Vaccine 1518
Liquid PedvaxHIB (One case) 2012
Peganone Tablets, USP 2487
▲ Pegasys (16%) 2793
▲ PEG-Intron Powder for Injection (18%) 3062
▲ Pentasa Capsules (3.4% to 3.5%) 3182
Pepcid Injection (1.7%) 2017
Pepcid (1.7%) 2014
▲ Permax Tablets (6.4%) 3357
Persantine Tablets 898
▲ Photofrin for Injection (5% to 9%) 729
▲ Plan B Tablets (5%) 1068
▲ Plavix Tablets (4.5%) 940
▲ Plavix Tablets (4.5%) 2942
Plendil Extended-Release Tablets (0.5% to 1.5%) 651
▲ Pletal Tablets (12% to 19%) 2478
▲ Prandin Tablets (0.5, 1, and 2 mg) (4% to 5%) 2337
▲ Pravachol Tablets (2.0% to 6.2%) 943
▲ Precose Tablets (31%) 776
▲ Premarin Tablets (6% to 7%) 3443
▲ Premphase Tablets (5% to 7%) 3452
▲ Prempro Tablets (5% to 7%) 3452
▲ Prevacid Delayed-Release Capsules (1.4% to 7.4%) 3268
▲ Prevacid for Delayed-Release Oral Suspension (1.4% to 7.4%) 3268
Prevacid I.V. for Injection (Less than 1%) 3274
▲ Prevacid NapraPAC (Less than 1% to 5%) 3277
▲ Prevacid SoluTab Delayed-Release Orally Disintegrating Tablets (1.4% to 7.4%) 3268
▲ Prevnar for Injection (8.3% to 13.7%) 3460
▲ PREVPAC (3% to 7.4%) 3281
▲ Prilosec OTC Tablets (3.0% to 14%) 2674
Primaxin I.M. (0.6%) 2022
Primaxin I.V. (1.8% to 3.9%) 2024
▲ Prinivil Tablets (3.7%) 2029
Prinzide Tablets (2.5%) 2033
▲ Prochieve 4% Gel (8%) 1018
▲ Prochieve 8% Gel (8%) 1018
▲ Procrit for Injection (0.11% to 21%) 2374
▲ Prograf Capsules and Injection (37% to 72%) 624
▲ Proleukin for Injection (67%) 1007
▲ Prometrium Capsules (100 mg, 200 mg) (7%) 3205
Protonix I.V. (Greater than 1%) 3468
▲ Protonix Tablets (4% to 6%) 3465
▲ Protopic Ointment (3% to 6%) 629
▲ Provigil Tablets (6%) 1002
▲ Prozac Pulvules and Liquid (8% to 18%) 1771
Pulmicort Respules (2% to 4%) 654
Purinethol Tablets (Occasional) 1222
▲ Rapamune Oral Solution and Tablets (25% to 42%) 3472
▲ Razadyne ER Extended-Release Capsules (6% to 12%) 2434
▲ Razadyne (6% to 12%) 2434
▲ Rebetol (17% to 22%) 3073
Recombivax HB (Greater than 1%) 2045
ReFacto Vials 3479
▲ Relafen Tablets (14%) 1523
▲ Relenza Rotadisk (2% to 3%) 1525
Relpax Tablets (Infrequent) 2531
▲ Remicade for IV Injection (12%) 987
▲ Renagel Tablets (4% to 19.2%) 1268
ReoPro Vials (1.1%) 1779
Repliva 21/7 Tablets 3301
Repronex for Intramuscular and Subcutaneous Injection (Up to 2.1%) 1148
▲ Requip Tablets (1% to 5%) 1528
▲ Rescriptor Tablets (2.4% to 5.9%) 2535
▲ Retrovir Capsules (0.8% to 12%) 1533
▲ Retrovir IV Infusion (1% to 12%) 1537
▲ Retrovir (0.8% to 12%) 1533
▲ Revatio Tablets (9%) 2541
▲ Reyataz Capsules (6% to 25%) 948
▲ Ribavirin, USP Capsules (17% to 22%) 3083
▲ Rilutek Tablets (5.5% to 9.0%) 2945
▲ Risperdal Consta Long-Acting Injection (1% to 5%) 1664
Risperdal M-Tab Orally Disintegrating Tablets (Infrequent) 1658
Risperdal (Infrequent) 1658
▲ Rituxan for Infusion (1% to 5%) 845
▲ Rituxan I.V. (10%) 1251
Rocephin Injectable Vials, ADD-Vantage, Galaxy, Bulk (2.7%) 2801
▲ Roferon-A Injection (20% to 37%) 2805
Rozerem Tablets (2%) 3228
▲ Rythmol SR Capsules (2% to 4%) 2736
▲ Sandimmune (3% to 8%) 2259
▲ Sandostatin Injection (22% to 61%) 2263
▲ Sandostatin LAR Depot (36%) 2264
▲ Sensipar Tablets (21%) 603
▲ Simulect for Injection (Greater than or equal to 10%) 2268
Singulair (Greater than or equal to 2%) 2047
▲ Somavert Injection (4% to 14%) 2648
▲ Soriatane Capsules (1% to 10%) 1028
▲ Spectracef Tablets (11% to 15%) 2706
▲ Stalevo Tablets (5% to 10%) 2270
▲ Starlix Tablets (3.2%) 2276
▲ Strattera Capsules (2% to 4%) 1784
Stromectol Tablets (1.8%) 2053
▲ Suboxone Tablets (3.7% to 5%) 2719
▲ Subutex Tablets (4.9% to 5%) 2719
Sular Tablets (Less than or equal to 1%) 1163
▲ Suprax (16%) 1811
Surmontil Capsules 2347
▲ Sustiva Capsules (2% to 39%) 957
▲ Symbyax Capsules (8% to 19%) 1788
Symmetrel (1% to 5%) 1115
Synagis (More than 1%) 1868
Synercid I.V. (2.7%) 1690
Tagamet Tablets (Approximately 1 in 100) 1547
Tambocor Tablets (1% to 3%) 1824
▲ Tamiflu Capsules (3.2% to 9.5%) 2810
▲ Tamiflu Oral Suspension (3.2% to 9.5%) 2810
▲ Tarceva Tablets (Less than 1% to 54%) 1254
▲ Tarceva Tablets (Less than 1% to 54%) 2470
▲ Targretin Capsules (7.1% to 41.5%) 1719
Tarka Tablets (1.5%) 519
▲ Tasmar Tablets (16% to 18%) 3360
▲ Taxotere Injection Concentrate (2.8% to 55%) 2947
Tegretol/Tegretol-XR 2278
▲ Temodar Capsules (10% to 16%) 3088
Tenormin I.V. Injection (2% to 3%) 698
Tenormin Tablets (2% to 3%) 695
▲ Tequin Injection (4%) 964
▲ Tequin Tablets (4%) 964
Teveten Tablets (1% or greater) 1707
Teveten HCT Tablets (Less than 1%) 1710
▲ Thalomid Capsules (4.2%) 979
Thioridazine Hydrochloride Tablets 2122
Thiothixene Capsules 2124
▲ Thymoglobulin for Injection (36.6%) 2848
Tiazac Capsules (Less than 2%) 1204
▲ Ticlid Tablets (12.5%) 2813
Timentin ADD-Vantage 1556
Timentin Injection Galaxy Container 1559
Timentin IV Infusion 1553
Timentin Pharmacy Bulk Package 1562
Timolide Tablets (Less than 1%) 2056
Timoptic in Ocudose (Less frequent) 2061
Timoptic Sterile Ophthalmic Solution (Less frequent) 2058
Timoptic-XE Sterile Ophthalmic Gel Forming Solution 2062
Tindamax 2670
▲ TOBI Solution for Inhalation (6.2%) 1015
▲ Topamax Sprinkle Capsules (2% to 11%) 2438
▲ Topamax Tablets (2% to 11%) 2438
▲ Toprol-XL Tablets (About 5 of 100 patients) 660
▲ Trasylol Injection (3%) 779
Trecator Tablets 3482
Trelstar Depot (1.4%) 3385
Trelstar LA Suspension (1.1%) 3387
Tricor Tablets (2.3%) 523
Triglide Tablets (2.3%) 1165
▲ Trileptal Oral Suspension (5% to 7%) 2281
▲ Trileptal Tablets (5% to 7%) 2281
▲ Trisenox Injection (53%) 983
▲ Trizivir Tablets (12% to 26%) 1565
▲ Truvada Tablets (Greater than 5%) 1279
▲ Twinrix Vaccine (4% to 6%) 1571
▲ Tygacil for Injection (12.7%) 3489
▲ Ultracet Tablets (3%) 2462
Ultrase Capsules 735
▲ Ultrase MT Capsules (0.2% to 3.6%) 736
Uniphyl Tablets 2708
Uniretic Tablets (More than 1%) 3114
Unithroid Tablets 3521
▲ Univasc Tablets (3.1%) 3118
Urecholine Tablets 2349
Urocit-K Tablets (Some patients) 2109
Uroqid-Acid No. 2 Tablets 785
Urso 250 Tablets (1%) 737
Urso Forte Tablets (1%) 737
▲ Valcyte Tablets (16% to 41%) 2816
Valtrex Caplets 1573
▲ Vantin Tablets and Oral Suspension (1.2% to 7.2%) 2650
▲ Vaqta (1% to 5.9%) 2067
Varivax (Greater than or equal to 1%) 2070
Vaseretic Tablets (2.1%) 2073
Vasotec I.V. Injection (1.4% to 2.1%) 2076
▲ Velcade for Injection (57%) 2102
Ventolin HFA Inhalation Aerosol (Less than 3%) 1576
Verelan PM Capsules (2.4%) 3120
Vermox Chewable Tablets 1853
▲ Vesanoid Capsules (23%) 2823
VFEND I.V. (Less than 2%) 2543
VFEND Oral Suspension (Less than 2%) 2543
VFEND Tablets (Less than 2%) 2543
Viadur Implant (2.3%) 782
▲ Viagra Tablets (3%) 2552
▲ Vicoprofen Tablets (3% to 9%) 533
Viokase 738
▲ Viracept (14% to 20%) 2556
Viramune Oral Suspension (2%) 903
Viramune Tablets (2%) 903
▲ Viread Tablets (11% to 16%) 1284
Vivactil Tablets 2350
▲ Vivelle Transdermal System (1.9% to 4.3%) 2288
Vivelle-Dot Transdermal System (1.9% to 4.3%) 2293
Vivotif 834
▲ Voltaren Tablets (1% to 10%) 2298
▲ Voltaren-XR Tablets (1% to 10%) 2301
Vytorin 10/10 Tablets 2084
Vytorin 10/10 Tablets 3092
Vytorin 10/20 Tablets 2084
Vytorin 10/20 Tablets 3092
Vytorin 10/40 Tablets 2084
Vytorin 10/40 Tablets 3092
Vytorin 10/80 Tablets 2084
Vytorin 10/80 Tablets 3092
▲ WelChol Tablets (5%) 2855
▲ Wellbutrin Tablets (6.8%) 1579
▲ Wellbutrin SR Sustained-Release Tablets (5% to 7%) 1583
▲ Wellbutrin XL Extended-Release Tablets (5% to 7%) 1588
WinRho SDF 763
▲ Xanax XR Tablets (12.1%) 2655
▲ Xeloda Tablets (2% to 55%) 2825
Xifaxan Tablets (Less than 2%) 2847
▲ Xopenex HFA Inhalation Aerosol (6%) 3151
▲ Xopenex Inhalation Solution (6%) 3143
▲ Xopenex Inhalation Solution Concentrate (1.5% to 6%) 3147
Zantac 1597
Zantac Injection 1593
Zantac Injection Pharmacy Bulk Package (Frequent) 1595
Zantac Syrup 1597
▲ Zavesca Capsules (89% to 100%) 543
▲ Zegerid Powder for Oral Solution (3% to 7%) 2972
▲ Zelnorm Tablets (4% to 9%) 2303
Zemaira (0.2% to 0.4%) 3506
▲ Zenapax for Injection (Greater than 5%) 2838
▲ Zerit (34% to 50%) 971
Zestoretic Tablets (2.5%) 701
▲ Zestril Tablets (3.7%) 704
▲ Zetia Tablets (3.4% to 3.7%) 2090
▲ Zetia Tablets (3.4% to 3.7%) 3098
▲ Zevalin Injection (9%) 848
▲ Ziagen (0% to 7%) 1600
Zinacef Injection (1 in 220 patients) 1604
Zinacef for Injection (1 in 220 patients) 1604
▲ Zinecard for Injection (14% to 21%) 2659
▲ Zithromax Capsules, 250 mg (2% to 14%) 2568
▲ Zithromax for IV Infusion (Up to 8.5%) 2573
▲ Zithromax for Oral Suspension, 1 g (5% to 7%) 2568
▲ Zithromax for Oral Suspension, 300 mg, 600 mg, 900 mg, 1200 mg (2% to 14%) 2561
▲ Zithromax Tablets, 250 mg, 500 mg (2% to 14%) 2561
▲ Zithromax Tablets, 600 mg (5% to 7%) 2568
▲ Zithromax Tri-Pak (2% to 14%) 2561
▲ Zithromax Z-Pak (5% to 7%) 2568
Zmax for Oral Suspension (11.6%) 2577
Zocor Tablets (1.9%) 2078
▲ Zofran Injection (2% to 16%) 1607
▲ Zofran (4% to 6%) 1613
▲ Zofran ODT Orally Disintegrating Tablets (4% to 6%) 1613
▲ Zoladex (1% to 36%) 709
▲ Zoladex 3-month (1% to 40%) 712
▲ Zoloft (13% to 24%) 2581
▲ Zometa for Intravenous Infusion (17.4% to 24%) 2306
Zomig Nasal Spray (Infrequent) 718
▲ Zonegran Capsules (5%) 1089
▲ Zosyn (11.3% to 20%) 3492
Zovirax (2.4% to 3.2%) 1616
▲ Zyban Sustained-Release Tablets (4%) 1620
Zyprexa Tablets 1798
Zyprexa IntraMuscular (Infrequent) 1798
Zyprexa ZYDIS Orally Disintegrating Tablets 1798
▲ Zyrtec Chewable Tablets (1.9% to 3.1%) 2589
▲ Zyrtec (1.9% to 3.1%) 2589
▲ Zyrtec-D 12 Hour Extended Release Tablets (1.9% to 3.1%) 2591
▲ Zyvox (3.8% to 10.8%) 2661

Diarrhea, bloody

Aciphex Tablets (Rare) 1081
Asacol Delayed-Release Tablets 2688
Benzaclin Topical Gel 1046
Biltricide Tablets 2990
Canasa Rectal Suppositories 726
Cleocin Vaginal Ovules 2613
Clindagel 1207
Colazal Capsules 2845
Duac Topical Gel 3214
Evoclin Foam, 1% (Rarely) 1025
Imitrex Tablets 1440
Norvir (Less than 2%) 499
Omnicef Capsules 506
Omnicef for Oral Suspension 506
Paxil CR Controlled-Release Tablets (Rare) 1509
Paxil (Rare) 1501
Pentasa Capsules (0.9%) 3182
Proleukin for Injection (Less than 1%) 1007
Prozac Pulvules and Liquid (Rare) 1771
Ticlid Tablets 2813
Vantin Tablets and Oral Suspension 2650

Zomig Nasal Spray (Very rare) 718
Zomig Tablets (Very rare) 714

Diarrhea, C. difficile-associated
Cipro XR Tablets 3004
Invanz for Injection (Greater than 0.1%) 1974

Diarrhea, infectious
▲ Xenical Capsules (5.3%) 2834

Diastolic blood pressure, decreased
Agrylin Capsules 3172
Testim 1% Gel (1% or less) 722

Diastolic blood pressure changes
Focalin XR Capsules 2217

Digitalis toxicity
Lanoxicaps Capsules 1458
Virazole for Inhalation Solution 3365

Dim vision
Levitra Tablets (Less than 2%) 3048

Diplegia
Imitrex Injection (Rare) 1431
Imitrex Nasal Spray (Rare) 1435
Imitrex Tablets 1440

Diplopia
Abelcet Injection 1119
Abilify Tablets (Rare) 916
Abilify Tablets (Rare) 2472
Aciphex Tablets 1081
Adalat CC Tablets (Less than 1%) 2978
Agrylin Capsules (1% to 5%) 3172
Ambien Tablets (Frequent) 2867
Arthrotec Tablets (Rare) 3126
Axert Tablets (Rare) 2430
Azopt Ophthalmic Suspension (Less than 1%) 553
Balamine DM 739
Bentyl Capsules 724
Bentyl Injection 724
Bentyl Syrup 724
Bentyl Tablets 724
Betagan Ophthalmic Solution, USP .... ⊙ 217
Betimol Ophthalmic Solution .... ⊙ 283
Betimol Ophthalmic Solution 3371
Blocadren Tablets 1891
Botox Purified Neurotoxin Complex (Rare) 565
Buprenex Injectable (Less than 1%) 2718
Caduet Tablets (Greater than 0.1% to less than or equal to 1%) 2507
Campral Tablets (Rare) 1175
Carbatrol Capsules 3174
Carteolol Hydrochloride Ophthalmic Solution USP, 1% .... ⊙ 246
Celexa (Rare) 1177
Cipro I.V. (1% or less) 2998
Cipro I.V. Pharmacy Bulk Package (1% or less) 3509
Cipro (Less than 1%) 2991
Cipro XR Tablets (Less than 1%) 3004
Copaxone for Injection (At least 2%) 3292
Cosopt Sterile Ophthalmic Solution 1910
Cymbalta Delayed-Release Capsules (Infrequent) 1729
Dantrium Capsules (Less frequent) .. 2690
▲ Depacon Injection (16%) 412
▲ Depakene (16%) 417
▲ Depakote Sprinkle Capsules (16%) 422
▲ Depakote Tablets (1% to 16%) 427
▲ Depakote ER Tablets (16%) 433
Dilaudid 439
Dilaudid Oral Liquid (Less frequent) 443
Dilaudid Non-Sterile Powder 439
Dilaudid Rectal Suppositories 439
Dilaudid Tablets 439
Dilaudid Tablets - 8 mg (Less frequent) 443
Dilaudid-HP (Less frequent) 441
Diprivan Injectable Emulsion (Less than 1%) 676
Effexor Tablets (Infrequent) 3405
Effexor XR Capsules (Infrequent) 3411
Eldepryl Capsules 3209
▲ Equetro Extended-Release Capsules (Less than 5%) 3178
Evoxac Capsules (Less than 1%) 1042
Exelon Capsules (Infrequent) 2204
Flexeril Tablets (Less than 1%) 1832
Gabitril Tablets (1% or more) 998
Geodon Capsules (Frequent) 2514
Indocin (Less than 1%) 1968
▲ Intron A for Injection (Less than 5%) 3038
Kadian Capsules (Less than 3%) 572
Keppra Oral Solution (2%) 3307
Keppra Tablets (2%) 3307
Ketek Tablets (Greater than or equal to 0.2% to less than 2%) 2920
Klonopin (Infrequent) 2782
▲ Lamictal (5% to 49%) 1449
Levaquin in 5% Dextrose Injection (0.1% to 0.9%) 2453
Levaquin (0.1% to 0.9%) 2453
Lexapro Oral Solution 1193
Lexapro Tablets 1193
Lidoderm Patch 1107
▲ Lyrica Capsules (2% to 12%) 2524
Matulane Capsules 3188
Mirapex Tablets (1% or more) 889
MS Contin Tablets (Less frequent) 2703
Nalfon Capsules (Less than 1%) 2504
Namenda (Infrequent) 1199
▲ Neurontin Capsules (1.2% to 5.9%) 2498
▲ Neurontin Oral Solution (1.2 to 5.9%) 2498
▲ Neurontin Tablets (1.2% to 5.9%) 2498
Niravam Orally Disintegrating Tablets 3106
Noroxin Tablets 2009
Norvasc Tablets (More than 0.1% to 1%) 2529
Norvir (Less than 2%) 499
Numorphan 1112
Ortho-Cyclen/Ortho Tri-Cyclen (Rare) 2414
Ortho Tri-Cyclen Lo Tablets 2421
Orthoclone OKT3 Sterile Solution 2370
Parcopa Orally Disintegrating Tablets 3111
Paxil CR Controlled-Release Tablets (Rare) 1509
Paxil (Rare) 1501
Peganone Tablets, USP 2487
Permax Tablets (2.1%) 3357
Phenergan 3438
Photofrin for Injection 729
Pletal Tablets (Less than 2%) 2478
Premphase Tablets 3452
Prempro Tablets 3452
Prevacid Delayed-Release Capsules (Less than 1%) 3268
Prevacid for Delayed-Release Oral Suspension (Less than 1%) 3268
Prevacid NapraPAC (Less than 1%) .. 3277
Prevacid SoluTab Delayed-Release Orally Disintegrating Tablets (Less than 1%) 3268
PREVPAC (Less than 1%) 3281
Prilosec OTC Tablets (Less than 1%) 2674
Prinivil Tablets (0.3% to 1.0%) 2029
Prinzide Tablets 2033
ProSom Tablets (Rare) 512
Protonix I.V. (Less than 1%) 3468
Protonix Tablets (Less than 1%) 3465
Prozac Pulvules and Liquid (Rare) 1771
Relpax Tablets (Rare) 2531
ReoPro Vials (0.1%) 1779
Requip Tablets (2%) 1528
Rescriptor Tablets 2535
Rilutek Tablets (Rare) 2945
Risperdal M-Tab Orally Disintegrating Tablets (Rare) 1658
Risperdal (Rare) 1658
Sonata Capsules (Infrequent) 1686
▲ Soriatane Capsules (1% to 5%) 1028
Stalevo Tablets 2270
Sustiva Capsules (Less than 2%) 957
Symbyax Capsules (Infrequent) 1788
Tambocor Tablets (1% to 3%) 1824
Tasmar Tablets (Infrequent) 3360
Tegretol/Tegretol-XR 2278
▲ Temodar Capsules (5%) 3088
Thalomid Capsules 979
Timolide Tablets 2056
Timoptic in Ocudose (Less frequent) 2061
Timoptic Sterile Ophthalmic Solution (Less frequent) 2058
Timoptic-XE Sterile Ophthalmic Gel Forming Solution 2062
▲ Topamax Sprinkle Capsules (1% to 10%) 2438
▲ Topamax Tablets (1% to 10%) 2438
Tranxene 2488
Trecator Tablets 3482
▲ Trileptal Oral Suspension (5% to 40%) 2281
▲ Trileptal Tablets (5% to 40%) 2281
Valium Tablets (Infrequent) 2822
VFEND I.V. (Less than 2%) 2543
VFEND Oral Suspension (Less than 2%) 2543
VFEND Tablets (Less than 2%) 2543
Viagra Tablets 2552
▲ Visudyne for Injection (1% to 10%) .. 2286
Wellbutrin Tablets (Rare) 1579
Wellbutrin SR Sustained-Release Tablets 1583
Wellbutrin XL Extended-Release Tablets 1588
Xalatan Sterile Ophthalmic Solution (Less than 1%) 2654
Zegerid Powder for Oral Solution (Less than 1%) 2972
Zestoretic Tablets 701
Zestril Tablets (0.3% to 1.0%) 704
Zoloft (Rare) 2581
Zomig Tablets (Rare) 714
Zomig-ZMT Tablets (Rare) 714
▲ Zonegran Capsules (6%) 1089
Zyban Sustained-Release Tablets 1620
Zyprexa Tablets (Infrequent) 1798
Zyprexa ZYDIS Orally Disintegrating Tablets (Infrequent) 1798

Dipsesis
Abilify Tablets (Infrequent) 916
Abilify Tablets (Infrequent) 2472
Aciphex Tablets (Rare) 1081
Actiq (Less than 1%) 993
Aggrenox Capsules (Less than 1%) .. 855
Alferon N Injection (1%) 1640
Alinia for Oral Suspension (Less than 1%) 2840
Alinia Tablets (Less than 1%) 2840
Ambien Tablets (Infrequent) 2867
Amerge Tablets (Infrequent) 1312
Anaprox Tablets (Less than 3%) 2769
Anaprox DS Tablets (Less than 3%) .. 2769
Aricept Tablets (Infrequent) 1086
Aricept ODT Tablets (Infrequent) 1086
Atrovent Nasal Spray 0.06% (Less than 1%) 870
Avinza Capsules (Less than 5%) 1714
Axert Tablets (Rare) 2430
Bayer Aspirin Tablets 3515
Caduet Tablets (Greater than 0.1% to less than or equal to 1%) 2507
Calcium Disodium Versenate Injection 1819
Campral Tablets (Infrequent) 1175
Cardizem LA Extended Release Tablets (Less than 2%) 1699
Ceftin Tablets (0.1% to 1%) 1369
Celexa (Infrequent) 1177
▲ CellCept Capsules (3% to less than 20%) 2751
▲ CellCept Intravenous (3% to less than 20%) 2751
▲ CellCept Oral Suspension (3% to less than 20%) 2751
▲ CellCept Tablets (3% to less than 20%) 2751
Cipro XR Tablets (Less than 1%) 3004
Cymbalta Delayed-Release Capsules (Infrequent) 1729
Depo-Provera Contraceptive Injection (Less than 1%) 2619
depo-subQ provera 104 Injectable Suspension 2622
Dyazide Capsules 1389
EC-Naprosyn Delayed-Release Tablets (Less than 3%) 2769
Ecotrin Enteric Coated Aspirin Low, Regular and Maximum Strength Tablets 1627
Effexor Tablets (Infrequent) 3405
Effexor XR Capsules (Infrequent) 3411
Emcyt Capsules (1%) 3137
Eskalith 1406
Evoxac Capsules (Less than 1%) 1042
Exelon Capsules (Infrequent) 2204
Flexeril Tablets (Less than 1%) 1832
Fortical Nasal Spray (Less than 1%) 3336
Frova Tablets (Infrequent) 1101
Furosemide Tablets 2117
Gabitril Tablets (Infrequent) 998
Geodon Capsules (Infrequent) 2514
Imitrex Injection (Infrequent) 1431
Imitrex Nasal Spray (Infrequent) 1435
Imitrex Tablets (Infrequent) 1440
▲ Intron A for Injection (Less than or equal to 5%) 3038
Klonopin (Infrequent) 2782
K-Phos Neutral Tablets 785
Lamictal (Infrequent) 1449
Levaquin in 5% Dextrose Injection (0.1% to 0.9%) 2453
Levaquin (0.1% to 0.9%) 2453
Lexapro Oral Solution (Infrequent) 1193
Lexapro Tablets (Infrequent) 1193
Lithobid Tablets 1670
Lunesta Tablets (Infrequent) 3139
▲ Lupron Depot 3.75 mg (Among most frequent) 3257
Lupron Depot–3 Month 11.25 mg (Less than 5%) 3262
Maxalt Tablets (Infrequent) 1983
Maxalt-MLT Orally Disintegrating Tablets (Infrequent) 1983
Maxzide 2150
Meridia Capsules (1.7%) 485
MetroGel-Vaginal Gel (Less than 1%) 1822
Miacalcin Nasal Spray (Less than 1%) 2242
Midamor Tablets (Less than or equal to 1%) 2000
Mirapex Tablets (Less than 1%) 889
Moduretic Tablets (Less than or equal to 1%) 2003
Naprosyn Suspension (Less than 3%) 2769
Naprosyn Tablets (Less than 3%) 2769
Neurontin Capsules (Infrequent) 2498
Neurontin Oral Solution (Infrequent) 2498
Neurontin Tablets (Infrequent) 2498
Nexium Delayed-Release Capsules (Less than 1%) 645
Nexium I.V. (Less than 1%) 649
Norvasc Tablets (More than 0.1% to 1%) 2529
Norvir (Less than 2%) 499
Oncaspar (Less than 1%) 1123
▲ Orap Tablets (1 of 20 patients) 1220
OxyContin Tablets (Less than 1%) 2699
Paxil CR Controlled-Release Tablets (Infrequent) 1509
Paxil (Infrequent) 1501
Pentasa Capsules (Less than 1%) 3182
Permax Tablets (Infrequent) 3357
Prevacid Delayed-Release Capsules (Less than 1%) 3268
Prevacid for Delayed-Release Oral Suspension (Less than 1%) 3268
Prevacid NapraPAC (Less than 3%) .. 3277
Prevacid SoluTab Delayed-Release Orally Disintegrating Tablets (Less than 1%) 3268
▲ PREVPAC (Less than 1% to 3%) 3281
Prinzide Tablets 2033
Prochieve 4% Gel 1018
Prochieve 8% Gel 1018
ProSom Tablets (Infrequent) 512
Protonix I.V. (Less than 1%) 3468
Protonix Tablets (Less than 1%) 3465
Provigil Tablets (1%) 1002
Prozac Pulvules and Liquid (Infrequent to greater than or equal to 2%) 1771
Reishimax Capsules 2669
Relpax Tablets (Infrequent) 2531
Requip Tablets (Infrequent) 1528
Rescriptor Tablets 2535
Rilutek Tablets (Infrequent) 2945
Risperdal M-Tab Orally Disintegrating Tablets (Infrequent) 1658
Risperdal (Infrequent) 1658
Seroquel Tablets (Infrequent) 691
Sonata Capsules (Infrequent) 1686
▲ Soriatane Capsules (1% to 10%) 1028
Spectracef Tablets (0.1% to 1%) 2706
St. Joseph 81 mg Aspirin Chewable and Enteric Coated Tablets 1841
Symbyax Capsules (Frequent) 1788
Tasmar Tablets (Infrequent) 3360
Tequin Injection (Less than 0.1%) 964
Tequin Tablets (Less than 0.1%) 964
Tiazac Capsules (Less than 2%) 1204
Tindamax 2670
Topamax Sprinkle Capsules (1% to 2%) 2438
Topamax Tablets (1% to 2%) 2438
Trileptal Oral Suspension (Up to 2%) 2281
Trileptal Tablets (Up to 2%) 2281
Uniretic Tablets (Less than 1%) 3114
Uroqid-Acid No. 2 Tablets 785
Vantin Tablets and Oral Suspension (Less than 1%) 2650
Vaseretic Tablets 2073
Viagra Tablets (Less than 2%) 2552
Vicoprofen Tablets (Less than 3%) ... 533
Wellbutrin SR Sustained-Release Tablets (Infrequent) 1583
Wellbutrin XL Extended-Release Tablets (Infrequent) 1588
Xanax XR Tablets (Infrequent) 2655
▲ Xeloda Tablets (Less than 5%) 2825

Zestoretic Tablets 701
Zoloft (Infrequent) 2581
Zomig Nasal Spray (Infrequent) 718
Zomig Tablets (Infrequent) 714
Zomig-ZMT Tablets (Infrequent) 714
Zonegran Capsules (Infrequent) 1089
Zosyn (1.0% or less) 3492
Zovirax for Injection (Less than 1%) 1618
Zyban Sustained-Release Tablets (Less than 1%) 1620
Zyprexa Tablets (Frequent) 1798
Zyprexa ZYDIS Orally Disintegrating Tablets (Frequent) 1798
Zyrtec Chewable Tablets (Less than 2%) 2589
Zyrtec (Less than 2%) 2589
Zyrtec-D 12 Hour Extended Release Tablets (Less than 2%) 2591

Discharge, nipple
depo-subQ provera 104 Injectable Suspension 2622
Prefest Tablets 1069

Discoloration, application site
Lidoderm Patch 1107

Discoloration, injection site
Diprivan Injectable Emulsion (Less than 1%) 676
HibTITER 3419
▲ Navelbine Injection (Approximately 1/3 of patients) 1494
Neumega for Injection 3433

Discomfort, arm
▲ Adenoscan (4%) 613
Imitrex Injection 1431

Discomfort, chest
▲ Adenoscan (40%) 613
Amerge Tablets (Frequent) 1312
▲ Cerezyme for Injection (Approximately 6.6%) 1263
Imitrex Injection (Rare) 1431
Imitrex Nasal Spray (Infrequent) 1435
Imitrex Tablets (Frequent) 1440
▲ Nicotrol Inhaler (Greater than 3%) 2594
▲ Photofrin for Injection (11%) 729
Primaxin I.M. 2022
Primaxin I.V. (Less than 0.2%) 2024
Prinivil Tablets (0.3% to 1.0%) 2029
Prinzide Tablets (0.3% to 1%) 2033
Recombivax HB (Less than 1%) 2045
Tasmar Tablets (1% to 2%) 3360
Timentin ADD-Vantage 1556
Timentin Injection Galaxy Container 1559
Timentin IV Infusion 1553
Timentin Pharmacy Bulk Package 1562
Ventavis Inhalation Solution 1036
▲ Vesanoid Capsules (32%) 2823
VoSpire Extended-Release Tablets (Less frequent) 2352
Zestoretic Tablets (0.3% to 1.0%) 701
Zestril Tablets (0.3% to 1.0%) 704
Zomig Nasal Spray (Infrequent) 718

Discomfort, general
Coumadin for Injection 932
Coumadin Tablets 932
Cubicin for Injection (Less than 1%) 1038
Eskalith 1406
▲ HalfLytely and Bisacodyl Tablets Bowel Prep Kit with Flavors Packs (19.1%) 915
Zovirax Ointment 854

Discomfort, jaw
▲ Adenoscan (15%) 613
Imitrex Injection (1.8%) 1431
Zomig Nasal Spray (Rare) 718

Discomfort, local
Albalon Ophthalmic Solution ⊙ 216
▲ Betimol Ophthalmic Solution (More than 5%) ⊙ 283
▲ Betimol Ophthalmic Solution (More than 5%) 3371
▲ Ciloxan Ophthalmic Ointment (Among most frequent) 554
Efudex (Infrequent) 3348
OptiPranolol Metipranolol Ophthalmic Solution 0.3% (A small number of patients) ⊙ 254
ThermaCare Heat Wraps 2674

Discomfort, lower extremities
Adenoscan (Less than 1%) 613

Discomfort, nasal
Amerge Tablets (Frequent) 1312
Imitrex Injection (2.2%) 1431
Imitrex Nasal Spray (Infrequent) 1435
▲ Imitrex Tablets (5% to 7%) 1440
▲ Zomig Nasal Spray (1% to 3%) 718

Discomfort, nasal septum
▲ Nasacort HFA Inhalation Aerosol (Greater than or equal to 3% to 5.5%) 2939

Discomfort, vulvovaginal
Clindesse Vaginal Cream (Less than 1%) 3296

Discomfort at injection site
▲ Fuzeon Injection (96%) 2772
MICRhoGAM Ultra-Filtered 2429
Nutropin AQ Injection 1241
RhoGAM Ultra-Filtered 2429

Discontinuation syndrome
Catapres-TTS 875
Clorpres Tablets (About 1%) 2139

Disinhibition
Niravam Orally Disintegrating Tablets (2.7%) 3106

Disorientation
Aciphex Tablets 1081
Actimmune (Rare) 1646
Alferon N Injection (1%) 1640
Arthrotec Tablets (Rare) 3126
Asacol Delayed-Release Tablets 2688
Biaxin/Biaxin XL 402
BiDil Tablets 2161
Botox Purified Neurotoxin Complex 565
Buphenyl Powder 3327
Buphenyl Tablets 3327
Cosopt Sterile Ophthalmic Solution 1910
Dalmane Capsules 3343
Daranide Tablets 1928
Demser Capsules 1933
Dilaudid 439
Dilaudid Oral Liquid (Less frequent) 443
Dilaudid Non-Sterile Powder 439
Dilaudid Rectal Suppositories 439
Dilaudid Tablets 439
Dilaudid Tablets - 8 mg (Less frequent) 443
Dilaudid-HP (Less frequent) 441
Dolobid Tablets (Less than 1 in 100) 1937
Eldepryl Capsules 3209
Emend Capsules (Isolated cases) 1944
Famvir Tablets (Infrequent) 2207
Flexeril Tablets (Less than 1%) 1832
Infed Injection 3381
▲ Invanz for Injection (3.3% to 5.1%) 1974
Lexapro Oral Solution (Infrequent) 1193
Lexapro Tablets (Infrequent) 1193
Lidoderm Patch 1107
Maxalt Tablets (Infrequent) 1983
Maxalt-MLT Orally Disintegrating Tablets (Infrequent) 1983
MS Contin Tablets (Less frequent) 2703
Nalfon Capsules (Less than 1%) 2504
Oncaspar 1123
Orthoclone OKT3 Sterile Solution 2370
Parcopa Orally Disintegrating Tablets 3111
Parnate Tablets 1499
Phenergan Suppositories 3438
PREVPAC 3281
Rescriptor Tablets 2535
Seromycin Capsules 1783
Stalevo Tablets 2270
Surmontil Capsules 2347
Tagamet Tablets 1547
Timoptic in Ocudose (Less frequent) 2061
Timoptic Sterile Ophthalmic Solution (Less frequent) 2058
Timoptic-XE Sterile Ophthalmic Gel Forming Solution 2062
Transderm Scōp Transdermal Therapeutic System (Infrequent) 2166
Vivactil Tablets 2350
Xanax XR Tablets (1.5%) 2655

Disorientation, place
Blocadren Tablets 1891
Cosopt Sterile Ophthalmic Solution 1910
Inderal LA Long-Acting Capsules 3421
InnoPran XL Capsules 2728
Nadolol Tablets 2121
Tenormin I.V. Injection 698
Tenormin Tablets 695
Timolide Tablets 2056
Timoptic in Ocudose 2061
Timoptic Sterile Ophthalmic Solution 2058
Timoptic-XE Sterile Ophthalmic Gel Forming Solution 2062
Toprol-XL Tablets 660

Disorientation, time
Blocadren Tablets 1891
Cosopt Sterile Ophthalmic Solution 1910
Inderal LA Long-Acting Capsules 3421
InnoPran XL Capsules 2728
Nadolol Tablets 2121
Tenormin I.V. Injection 698
Tenormin Tablets 695
Timolide Tablets 2056
Timoptic in Ocudose 2061
Timoptic Sterile Ophthalmic Solution 2058
Timoptic-XE Sterile Ophthalmic Gel Forming Solution 2062
Toprol-XL Tablets 660

Distention, abdominal
(*see under* Abdominal distention)

Distress, abdominal
Ambien Tablets (Rare) 2867
Augmentin (Less frequent) 1331
Augmentin Tablets (Less frequent) 1334
Ery-Tab Tablets 447
Erythrocin Stearate Filmtab Tablets 452
Imitrex Injection (1.3%) 1431
Imitrex Tablets 1440
Indocin (Greater than 1%) 1968
Invirase (0.9% to greater than or equal to 2%) 2776
▲ K-Lor Powder Packets (Among most common) 472
▲ K-Tab Filmtab Tablets (Most common) 473
▲ Persantine Tablets (6.1%) 898
Stalevo Tablets 2270
▲ Ultrase MT Capsules (0.2%) 736
Zantac Injection 1593

Distress, epigastric
Abelcet Injection 1119
Alacol DM Syrup 739
Amaryl Tablets (Less than 1%) 2864
Aricept Tablets (Frequent) 1086
Aricept ODT Tablets (Frequent) 1086
Chromagen Forte Soft Gelatin Capsules 3296
Cipro I.V. (1% or less) 2998
Cipro I.V. Pharmacy Bulk Package (1% or less) 3509
Clorpres Tablets 2139
Colazal Capsules 2845
Cuprimine Capsules 1925
▲ Emend Capsules (4%) 1944
▲ Entocort EC Capsules (Less than 5%) 2694
Ferrlecit Injection 3379
Grifulvin V Tablets Microsize and Oral Suspension Microsize (Occasional) 2384
Gris-PEG Tablets (Occasional) 2504
Inderal LA Long-Acting Capsules 3421
▲ Indocin (3% to 9%) 1968
InnoPran XL Capsules 2728
▲ MetroGel-Vaginal Gel (7%) 1822
Mintezol 2002
Nexium Delayed-Release Capsules (Less than 1%) 645
Nexium I.V. (Less than 1%) 649
Oncaspar (Less than 1%) 1123
Sandostatin LAR Depot (Rare) 2264
Surmontil Capsules 2347
▲ Ticlid Tablets (3.7%) 2813
Timentin ADD-Vantage 1556
Timentin Injection Galaxy Container 1559
Timentin IV Infusion 1553
Timentin Pharmacy Bulk Package 1562
Tindamax (1.4% to 1.8%) 2670
Toprol-XL Tablets (About 1 of 100 patients) 660
Viracept (Less than 2%) 2556
Vivactil Tablets 2350
▲ Zavesca Capsules (6%) 543
▲ Zenapax for Injection (Greater than 5%) 2838

Distress, gastric
(*see under* Distress, gastrointestinal)

Distress, gastrointestinal
Advil Flu & Body Ache Caplets ▣ 739
Children's Advil Cold Suspension ▣ 741
Agrylin Capsules (1% to 5%) 3172
Alferon N Injection (One patient) 1640
Alupent Inhalation Aerosol (1 to 4%) 858
Appearex Tablets 2095
Biltricide Tablets 2990
Bios Life 2 Drink Mix 3328
Carafate Suspension (Less than 0.5%) 727
Carafate Tablets (Less than 0.5%) 728
Carbatrol Capsules 3174
Cardio Essentials Capsules 3328
▲ Clinoril Tablets (10%) 1899
CM Plex Softgels 3328
Colace Capsules 50 mg 2715
Colace Capsules 100 mg 2715
Colace Glycerin Suppositories, USP 1.2 grams - Infants and Children 2715
Colace Glycerin Suppositories, USP 2.1 grams - Adults and Children 2716
Colace Liquid 1% Solution 2716
Colace Syrup ▣ 729
Combivent Inhalation Aerosol 878
Covera-HS Tablets (Less than 2%) 3135
Cuprimine Capsules 1925
Depo-Provera Contraceptive Injection (Less than 1%) 2619
depo-subQ provera 104 Injectable Suspension 2622
▲ Dolobid Tablets (3% to 9%) 1937
▲ Emcyt Capsules (11%) 3137
Equetro Extended-Release Capsules 3178
Evoclin Foam, 1% 1025
Feosol Caplets 1629
Feosol Tablets (Occasional) 1629
Flexeril Tablets (Less than 1%) 1832
▲ Flovent HFA (1% to 3%) 1418
Fluorescite Injection ⊙ 207
Imitrex Tablets (Frequent) 1440
Kadian Capsules (Less than 3%) 572
K-Dur Extended-Relase Tablets 3047
▲ Lotronex Tablets (5%) 1479
▲ Lupron Depot–3 Month 11.25 mg (3% to 7%) 3262
Lupron Injection Pediatric 3256
▲ Midamor Tablets (Between 1% and 3%) 2000
Mineral Oil 2716
Moduretic Tablets (Greater than 1%, less than 3%) 2003
Orap Tablets 1220
Peri-Colace Tablets 2716
ProAmatine Tablets (Rare) 3183
Roferon-A Injection (Less than 1%) 2805
▲ Sandostatin LAR Depot (29.1%) 2264
Sedapap Tablets 50 mg/650 mg (Less frequent) 2098
Tegretol/Tegretol-XR 2278
Timolide Tablets (Less than 1%) 2056
Timoptic in Ocudose 2061
Timoptic Sterile Ophthalmic Solution 2058
Verelan PM Capsules (2% or less) 3120
Visutein Capsules 3328
Xifaxan Tablets (Less than 2%) 2847
Zovirax 1616

Distress, precordial
(*see under* Distress, epigastric)

Distress, stomach
(*see under* Distress, gastrointestinal)

Distress, upper GI
(*see under* Distress, epigastric)

Disturbances, emotional
(*see under* Emotional disturbances)

Disturbances, gastrointestinal
(*see under* Distress, gastrointestinal)

Disulfiram-like reactions
Amaryl Tablets 2864

Diuresis
Amerge Tablets (Infrequent) 1312
Lotronex Tablets (Rare) 1479
Sedapap Tablets 50 mg/650 mg (Infrequent) 2098

Diuresis, potentiation of
Uniphyl Tablets 2708

Diverticulitis
Aricept Tablets (Infrequent) 1086
Aricept ODT Tablets (Infrequent) 1086
Celebrex Capsules (0.1% to 1.9%) 3130
Celexa (Rare) 1177

Colazal Capsules 2845
Cymbalta Delayed-Release Capsules (Infrequent) 1729
Evoxac Capsules (Less than 1%) 1042
Humira Injection 464
Lotronex Tablets (Rare) 1479
Namenda (Infrequent) 1199
Razadyne ER Extended-Release Capsules (Infrequent) 2434
Razadyne (Infrequent) 2434
Requip Tablets (Infrequent) 1528
Rescriptor Tablets 2535
Risperdal M-Tab Orally Disintegrating Tablets (Rare) 1658
Risperdal (Rare) 1658
Sandostatin LAR Depot (1% to 4%) 2264
Zoloft (Rare) 2581

Dizziness

Accolate Tablets (1.6%) 663
Accutane Capsules 2740
Aciphex Tablets 1081
▲ Actiq (6% to 17%) 993
Activella Tablets 2311
▲ Actonel Tablets (4.9% to 6.6%) 2679
▲ Actonel with Calcium Tablets (4.9% to 6.4%) 2684
▲ ActoPlus Met Tablets (4.8% to 5.4%) 3219
▲ Adalat CC Tablets (4%) 2978
Adderall Tablets 3168
▲ Adderall XR Capsules (2% to 7%) 3169
Adenocard Injection (1%) 612
▲ Adenoscan (12%) 613
Adipex-P 1216
▲ Advair Diskus 250/50 (4%) 1291
Advate Injection (2%) 742
Advicor Tablets 1694
Advil Allergy Sinus Caplets ▣ 737
Advil Multi-Symptom Cold Caplets ▣ 738
▲ Aerobid/Aerobid-M (3% to 9%) 1172
▲ Aggrastat (3%) 1878
Aggrenox Capsules (Less than 1%) 855
▲ Agrylin Capsules (15.4%) 3172
▲ Alacol DM Syrup (Among most frequent) 739
Alavert Allergy & Sinus D-12 Hour Tablets ▣ 743
Albalon Ophthalmic Solution ⊙ 216
Albenza Tablets (Less than 1.0% to 1.2%) 1310
Aldara Cream, 5% (1.4%) 1814
Aldoclor Tablets 1881
Aldoril Tablets 1884
Alesse-28 Tablets 3392
▲ Alferon N Injection (9%) 1640
Alinia for Oral Suspension (Less than 1%) 2840
Alinia Tablets (Less than 1%) 2840
Allegra (2.2%) 2857
Allegra-D 12 Hour Extended-Release Tablets (1.9%) 2860
Allegra-D 24 Hour Extended-Release Tablets (1.9%) 2862
Aloxi Injection (1%) 2099
Alphagan P Ophthalmic Solution (1% to 4%) 563
▲ Altace Capsules (2.2% to 4.1%) 1673
Altoprev Extended-Release Tablets (2%) 1151
▲ Alupent Inhalation Aerosol (3.3%) 858
Amaryl Tablets (1.7%) 2864
Ambien Tablets (1% to 5%) 2867
AmBisome for Injection (Less common) 615
Amerge Tablets (1% to 2%) 1312
Amevive (Common) 836
Amnesteem Capsules 2126
Amoxil Capsules (Rare) 1315
Amoxil Chewable Tablets (Rare) 1315
Amoxil Pediatric Drops for Oral Suspension (Rare) 1315
Amoxil Powder for Oral Suspension (Rare) 1315
Amoxil Tablets (Rare) 1315
▲ Anaprox Tablets (3% to 9%) 2769
▲ Anaprox DS Tablets (3% to 9%) 2769
AndroGel (Fewer than 1%) 3330
Antara Capsules 2723
▲ Anzemet Injection (2.2% to 5.5%) 2871
Anzemet Tablets (1.3% to 4.4%) 2874
▲ Apokyn Injection (20%) 2132
Aptivus Capsules (Less than 2%) 859
AquaMEPHYTON Injection 1887
Aralast (Greater than or equal to 0.02% to 0.1%) 745
▲ Aranesp for Injection (8% to 14%) 576
▲ Arava Tablets (4%) 2881
Aredia for Injection 2168
▲ Aricept Tablets (8%) 1086
▲ Aricept ODT Tablets (8%) 1086
▲ Arimidex Tablets (5% to 6%) 665
▲ Arixtra Injection (0.6% to 3.6%) 1325
▲ Aromasin Tablets (8%) 2600
Arthrotec Tablets (Rare) 3126
▲ Asacol Delayed-Release Tablets (8%) 2688
Astelin Nasal Spray (2.0%) 1876
▲ Atacand Tablets (4%) 634
Atacand HCT (2.9%) 637
▲ Atrovent HFA Inhalation Aerosol (3%) 872
Atrovent Inhalation Solution (2.3%) 868
Atrovent Nasal Spray 0.03% (Less than 2%) 869
Atrovent Nasal Spray 0.06% (Less than 1%) 870
Attenuvax 1889
Augmentin (Rare) 1331
Augmentin Tablets (Rare) 1334
Augmentin XR Extended-Release Tablets (Rare) 1340
Augmentin ES-600 Powder for Oral Suspension 1337
▲ Avalide Tablets (8%) 922
▲ Avalide Tablets (8%) 2889
▲ Avapro Tablets (5.4% to 6%) 925
▲ Avapro Tablets (5.4% to 10.2%) 2886
▲ Avastin IV (19% to 26%) 1229
▲ Avelox (2%) 2984
▲ Avonex (14%) 839
Axert Tablets (Frequent) 2430
▲ Axid Oral Solution (4.6%) 913
Azopt Ophthalmic Suspension (Less than 1%) 553
Bactroban Cream (Less than 1%) 1356
Balamine DM 739
Baraclude (Less than 1%) 928
Bayer Aspirin Tablets 3515
▲ BeneFix for Injection (7.7%) 3402
▲ Benicar Tablets (3%) 2850
▲ Benicar HCT Tablets (9%) 2852
▲ Bentyl Capsules (29%) 724
▲ Bentyl Injection (29%) 724
▲ Bentyl Syrup (29%) 724
▲ Bentyl Tablets (29%) 724
Betagan Ophthalmic Solution, USP (Rare) ⊙ 217
▲ Betaseron for SC Injection (24%) 791
Betimol Ophthalmic Solution (1% to 5%) ⊙ 283
Betimol Ophthalmic Solution (1% to 5%) 3371
Betoptic S Ophthalmic Suspension (Rare) 554
▲ Bexxar (0% to 5%) 1360
Biaxin/Biaxin XL 402
▲ BiDil Tablets (32%) 2161
Biltricide Tablets 2990
Blocadren Tablets (2.3%) 1891
▲ Boniva Tablets (1% to 3.7%) 2747
▲ Botox Purified Neurotoxin Complex (2% to 10%) 565
▲ Brevibloc Concentrate (3% to 12%) 766
▲ Brevibloc Injection (3% to 12%) 766
▲ Brevibloc Double Strength Injection (3% to 12%) 766
▲ Brevibloc Premixed Injection (3% to 12%) 766
▲ Brevibloc Double Strength Premixed Injection (3% to 12%) 766
▲ Brimonidine Tartrate Ophthalmic Solution 0.2% (3% to 9%) ⊙ 245
▲ Buprenex Injectable (5% to 10%) 2718
▲ Byetta Injection (9%) 605
▲ Caduet Tablets (1.1% to 3.4%) 2507
▲ Campath Ampules (1% to 12%) 826
▲ Campral Tablets (3% to 4%) 1175
▲ Camptosar Injection (0% to 15%) 2602
▲ Canasa Rectal Suppositories (3%) 726
Cancidas for Injection (0% to 1.5%) 1894
Captopril Tablets (About 0.5% to 2%) 2114
Carafate Suspension (Less than 0.5%) 727
Carafate Tablets (Less than 0.5%) 728
▲ Carbatrol Capsules (Among most frequent) 3174
Cardene I.V. (1.4%) 1129
▲ Cardizem LA Extended Release Tablets (3.5% to 6.4%) 1699
Carimune NF 3501
▲ Carnitor Injection (5% to 6%) 3185
Carteolol Hydrochloride Ophthalmic Solution USP, 1% (Occasional) ⊙ 246
▲ Casodex Tablets (7%) 670
▲ Cataflam Tablets (1% to 10%) 2173
▲ Catapres Tablets (About 16 in 100 patients) 874
Catapres-TTS (2 of 101 patients) 875
Caverject Impulse Injection (1%) 2610
Ceftin Tablets (0.1% to 1%) 1369
Celebrex Capsules (2%) 3130
▲ Celexa (At least 2%) 1177
▲ CellCept Capsules (28.7%) 2751
▲ CellCept Intravenous (28.7%) 2751
▲ CellCept Oral Suspension (28.7%) 2751
▲ CellCept Tablets (28.7%) 2751
▲ Cenestin Tablets, 0.45mg, 0.625mg, 0.9mg, 1.25mg (11%) 1063
Cenestin Tablets, 0.3mg 1063
▲ Cerezyme for Injection (Approximately 6.5%) 1263
▲ Chemet Capsules (1.0% to 12.7%) 2480
Cialis Tablets (Less than 2%) 1806
Cipro I.V. (1% or less) 2998
Cipro I.V. Pharmacy Bulk Package (1% or less) 3509
Cipro (0.3% to 1%) 2991
Cipro XR Tablets (1% to 2%) 3004
▲ Clarinex Tablets (4%) 3009
▲ Clarinex Reditabs Tablets (4%) 3009
Clarinex-D 24-Hour Extended-Release Tablets (2%) 3012
Climara Transdermal System 795
Climara Pro Transdermal System 800
Clindesse Vaginal Cream (Less than 1%) 3296
▲ Clinoril Tablets (3% to 9%) 1899
▲ Clolar for Intravenous Infusion (16%) 1264
▲ Clorpres Tablets (About 16%) 2139
▲ Clozapine Tablets (More than 5% to 19%) 2141
▲ Clozaril Tablets (More than 5% to 27%) 2174
Colazal Capsules (1%) 2845
▲ CombiPatch Transdermal System (6% to 7%) 2180
Combivent Inhalation Aerosol (Less than 2%) 878
▲ Combivir Tablets (10%) 1373
▲ Combunox Tablets (5.1% to 19.2%) 1183
▲ Comtan Tablets (8%) 2186
Concerta Extended-Release Tablets (2%) 1828
Contac Non-Drowsy 12 Hour Cold Caplets ▣ 614
Contac Non-Drowsy Timed Release 12 Hour Cold Caplets ▣ 615
Contac Severe Cold and Flu Caplets Maximum Strength ▣ 615
Copaxone for Injection (At least 2%) 3292
▲ Copegus Tablets (14%) 2759
▲ Coreg Tablets (6% to 32%) 1376
Cosopt Sterile Ophthalmic Solution (1% to 5%) 1910
Coumadin for Injection (Infrequent) 932
Coumadin Tablets (Infrequent) 932
▲ Covera-HS Tablets (3.3% to 4.7%) 3135
▲ Cozaar Tablets (3%) 1913
Crestor Tablets (Greater than or equal to 2%) 672
▲ Crixivan Capsules (3%) 1918
Cubicin for Injection (2.2%) 1038
▲ Cymbalta Delayed-Release Capsules (6% to 17%) 1729
Cytovene (At least 3 subjects) 2763
Dalmane Capsules 3343
▲ Dantrium Capsules (Among most frequent) 2690
Daranide Tablets 1928
▲ Darvocet A 500 Tablets (Among most frequent) 3497
▲ DDAVP Nasal Spray (Up to 3%) 2894
▲ Depacon Injection (5.2% to 25%) 412
▲ Depakene (18% to 25%) 417
▲ Depakote Sprinkle Capsules (13% to 25%) 422
▲ Depakote Tablets (12% to 25%) 427
▲ Depakote ER Tablets (12% to 25%) 433
▲ DepoDur Extended-Release Injection (Greater than 10%) 1098
▲ Depo-Provera Contraceptive Injection (Greater than 5%) 2619
▲ depo-subQ provera 104 Injectable Suspension (1% to less than 5%) 2622
Desferal Vials 2190
Desmopressin Acetate Rhinal Tube (Up to 3%) 1144
Desoxyn Tablets, USP (Rare) 2482
▲ Detrol Tablets (8.6%) 2626
Detrol LA Capsules (2%) 2629
Dexedrine 1386
DextroStat Tablets 3177
▲ Diastat Rectal Delivery System (3%) 3344
▲ Digitek Tablets (6%) 2146
Dilaudid 439
Dilaudid Oral Liquid 443
Dilaudid Non-Sterile Powder 439
Dilaudid Rectal Suppositories 439
Dilaudid Tablets 439
Dilaudid Tablets - 8 mg 443
▲ Dilaudid-HP (Among most frequent) 441
Children's Dimetapp Long Acting Cough Plus Cold Syrup ▣ 746
▲ Diovan HCT Tablets (9%) 2195
▲ Diovan Tablets (1% to 17%) 2191
Diprivan Injectable Emulsion (Less than 1%) 676
▲ Ditropan XL Extended Release Tablets (4% to 6%) 2391
Diuril Oral 1936
Diuril Sodium Intravenous 1934
Dolobid Tablets (Greater than 1 in 100) 1937
▲ Dostinex Tablets (15% to 17%) 2631
▲ Doxil Injection (1% to 10%) 3302
▲ Duragesic Transdermal System (3% to 10%) 2448
Dyazide Capsules 1389
Dynacin Tablets 1859
▲ DynaCirc CR Tablets (3.7% to 6.4%) 2726
Dyrenium Capsules (Rare) 3390
▲ EC-Naprosyn Delayed-Release Tablets (3% to 9%) 2769
Ecotrin Enteric Coated Aspirin Low, Regular and Maximum Strength Tablets 1627
Edex Injection (Less than 1%) 3103
▲ Effexor Tablets (3% to 23.9%) 3405
▲ Effexor XR Capsules (2% to 20%) 3411
▲ Eldepryl Capsules (7 of 49 patients) 3209
▲ Eligard 7.5 mg (3.3%) 2896
▲ Eligard 30 mg (4.4%) 2901
Elmiron Capsules (1%) 2393
▲ Eloxatin for Injection (7% to 13%) 2908
▲ Emend Capsules (6.6%) 1944
▲ Emtriva Capsules (4% to 25%) 1272
Enablex Extended-Release Tablets (0.9% to 2.1%) 2201
▲ Enbrel for Injection (7% to 8%) 580
▲ Engerix-B Vaccine (1% to 10%) 1391
▲ Entocort EC Capsules (7%) 2694
EpiPen 1061
▲ Epivir (10%) 1394
▲ Epogen for Injection (5% to 12%) 586
▲ Epzicom Tablets (6%) 1402
▲ Equetro Extended-Release Capsules (16% to 44%) 3178
Ery-Tab Tablets (Isolated reports) 447
Erythrocin Stearate Filmtab Tablets (Isolated reports) 452
Erythromycin Base Filmtab Tablets (Isolated reports) 454
Erythromycin Delayed-Release Capsules, USP (Isolated reports) 456
Eskalith 1406
Estratest Tablets 3196
Estratest H.S. Tablets 3196
Estrogel 0.06% 3200
Ethyol for Injection 1869
▲ Evoxac Capsules (4.1%) 1042
▲ Exelon Capsules (21%) 2204
▲ Fabrazyme for Intravenous Infusion (4%) 1267
Factive Tablets (0.8%) 2464
▲ Famvir Tablets (3.3% to 5.5%) 2207
▲ Faslodex Injection (6.9%) 682
▲ FazaClo Orally Disintegrating Tablets (More than 5% to 19%) 547
▲ Femara Tablets (0.4% to 14.2%) 2210
▲ Ferrlecit Injection (13%) 3379
▲ Flexeril Tablets (3% to 11%) 1832
▲ Flolan for Injection (8% to 83%) 1408
▲ Flomax Capsules (14.9% to 17.1%) 881
▲ Flonase Nasal Spray (1% to 3%) 1412
▲ Flovent Diskus 50 mcg (1% to 3%) 1415
▲ Flovent HFA (1% to 3%) 1418
Floxin Otic Singles (0.6% to 1%) 1045
Floxin Otic Solution (0.6% to 1%) 1043
Flumadine (0.7% to 1.9%) 1186
Focalin Tablets 2214
▲ Focalin XR Capsules (6%) 2217
Follistim AQ Cartridge 2354
Foradil Aerolizer (1.6%) 3024
Fortaz (Less than 1%) 1422
▲ Forteo for Injection (8%) 1739
▲ Fortical Nasal Spray (1% to 3%) 3336
▲ Frova Tablets (8%) 1101
Furosemide Tablets 2117
▲ Gabitril Tablets (27% to 31%) 998
▲ Gammagard Liquid (0.85% to 9.8%) 751
Gamunex Immune Globulin I.V., 10% (2%) 3232
Garamycin Injectable 3028
▲ Gengraf Capsules (1% to 8%) 458
▲ Geodon (8% to 16%) 2514
▲ Gleevec Tablets (12% to 16%) 2221

Gonal-f RFF Pen for Injection (2.1% to 2.4%) ... 3155
Grifulvin V Tablets Microsize and Oral Suspension Microsize (Occasional) ... 2384
Gris-PEG Tablets (Occasional) ... 2504
Havrix Vaccine (Rare) ... 1425
▲ Hectorol Capsules (11.5%) ... 909
▲ Hectorol Injection (11.5%) ... 911
▲ Herceptin I.V. (13%) ... 1234
Hexalen Capsules ... 2101
Hycodan ... 1104
Hycomine Compound Tablets ... 1105
Hycotuss Expectorant Syrup ... 1106
Hyperstat I.V. Injection (2%) ... 3031
▲ Hytrin Capsules (2.0% to 28%) ... 469
▲ Hyzaar (5.7%) ... 1964
▲ Imdur Tablets (8% to 11%) ... 3032
▲ Imitrex Injection (11.9%) ... 1431
Imitrex Nasal Spray (1% to 1.7%) ... 1435
Imitrex Tablets ... 1440
Imodium Capsules ... 1834
Imodium A-D Liquid and Caplets ... 1835
Imodium Advanced Caplets and Chewable Tablets ... ▣ 644
▲ Increlex Injection (Greater than or equal to 5%) ... 3290
▲ Indapamide Tablets (Greater than or equal to 5%) ... 2119
▲ Indocin (3% to 9%) ... 1968
Infed Injection ... 3381
▲ Infergen (18% to 22%) ... 1647
▲ InnoPran XL Capsules (4% to 7%) ... 2728
▲ Inspra Tablets (3%) ... 2520
▲ Intron A for Injection (7% to 24%) ... 3038
▲ Invanz for Injection (1.5% to 2.1%) ... 1974
Inversine Tablets ... 3286
Invirase (0.3% to greater than or equal to 2%) ... 2776
▲ I.V. Busulfex (30%) ... 1125
▲ Kadian Capsules (Among most frequent) ... 572
Kaletra (Less than 2%) ... 474
▲ Keppra Oral Solution (7% to 9%) ... 3307
▲ Keppra Tablets (7% to 9%) ... 3307
▲ Ketek Tablets (2.8% to 3.7%) ... 2920
▲ Klonopin (1% to 8%) ... 2782
Kogenate FS ... 3517
K-Phos Neutral Tablets ... 785
K-Phos Original (Sodium Free) Tablets (Less frequent) ... 785
▲ Kytril Tablets (3% to 5%) ... 2788
▲ Lamictal (5% to 54%) ... 1449
Lanoxicaps Capsules ... 1458
Lanoxin Injection ... 1462
Lanoxin Tablets ... 1468
Lanoxin Injection Pediatric ... 1465
▲ Lariam Tablets (Among most frequent) ... 2790
Lescol Capsules (2.2%) ... 2227
Lescol XL Tablets (1.9%) ... 2227
▲ Leustatin Injection (9%) ... 2368
Levaquin in 5% Dextrose Injection (0.3% to 2.4%) ... 2453
Levaquin (0.3% to 2.4%) ... 2453
Levitra Tablets (2%) ... 3048
▲ Lexapro Oral Solution (4% to 7%) ... 1193
▲ Lexapro Tablets (4% to 7%) ... 1193
Lidoderm Patch ... 1107
Lithobid Tablets ... 1670
Lofibra Capsules ... 1217
Lo/Ovral-28 Tablets ... 3423
▲ Lortab (Among most frequent) ... 3315
▲ Lortab Elixir (Among most frequent) ... 3312
▲ Lotensin Tablets (3.6%) ... 2232
▲ Lotensin HCT Tablets (6.3%) ... 2235
Lotrel Capsules (1.3%) ... 2238
▲ Lunesta Tablets (1% to 7%) ... 3139
▲ Lupron Depot 3.75 mg (8%) ... 3257
▲ Lupron Depot–3 Month 11.25 mg (8%) ... 3262
▲ Lyrica Capsules (8% to 38%) ... 2524
▲ Malarone Tablets (2% to 5%) ... 1484
▲ Malarone Pediatric Tablets (2% to 5%) ... 1484
▲ Marinol Capsules (3% to 10%) ... 3334
Matulane Capsules ... 3188
▲ Mavik Tablets (1.3% to 23%) ... 482
Maxair Autohaler (0.6% to 1.2%) ... 1820
▲ Maxalt Tablets (4% to 9%) ... 1983
▲ Maxalt-MLT Orally Disintegrating Tablets (4% to 9%) ... 1983
Maxzide ... 2150
Mebaral Tablets, USP (Less than 1 in 100 patients) ... 2483
Menopur for Subcutaneous Injection (2.6%) ... 1145
▲ Menostar Transdermal System (5%) ... 805
Mephyton Tablets (Rare) ... 1993
▲ Mepron Suspension (3% to 8%) ... 1487
▲ Meridia Capsules (7%) ... 485
Merrem I.V. (Greater than 0.1% to 1%) ... 687
Meruvax II ... 1994
Metadate CD Capsules ... 3316
MetroGel-Vaginal Gel (2%) ... 1822
Mevacor Tablets (0.5% to 2.0%) ... 1996
Miacalcin Nasal Spray (1% to 3%) ... 2242
Micardis Tablets (1%) ... 884
▲ Micardis HCT Tablets (4% to 7%) ... 886
▲ Midamor Tablets (Between 1% and 3%) ... 2000
▲ Migranal Nasal Spray (4%) ... 3350
Mintezol ... 2002
▲ Mirapex Tablets (25% to 26%) ... 889
Mivacron Injection (Less than 1%) ... 489
M-M-R II ... 1980
▲ Mobic Oral Suspension (0.4% to 3.8%) ... 893
▲ Mobic Tablets (0.4% to 3.8%) ... 893
▲ Moduretic Tablets (3% to 8%) ... 2003
Motrin Cold & Sinus Caplets ... 1836
▲ MS Contin Tablets (Among most frequent) ... 2703
Mycamine for Injection (0.4% to 0.7%) ... 620
▲ Myfortic Tablets (3% to less than 20%) ... 2244
▲ Mylotarg for Injection (10% to 15%) ... 3429
Nadolol Tablets (2 of 100 patients) ... 2121
▲ Nalfon Capsules (6.5%) ... 2504
▲ Namenda (7%) ... 1199
▲ Naprosyn Suspension (3% to 9%) ... 2769
▲ Naprosyn Tablets (3% to 9%) ... 2769
▲ Naropin Injection (1% to 5%) ... 640
Nasacort HFA Inhalation Aerosol ... 2939
▲ Natrecor for Injection (3% to 6%) ... 3123
Nembutal Sodium Solution, USP (Less than 1%) ... 2484
▲ Neoral Soft Gelatin Capsules (1% to 8%) ... 2247
▲ Neoral Oral Solution (1% to 8%) ... 2247
▲ Neulasta Injection (15% to 72%) ... 596
▲ Neumega for Injection (38%) ... 3433
▲ Neurontin Capsules (17.1% to 28%) ... 2498
▲ Neurontin Oral Solution (17.1% to 28%) ... 2498
▲ Neurontin Tablets (17.1% to 28%) ... 2498
Nexium Delayed-Release Capsules (Less than 1%) ... 645
Nexium I.V. (Less than 1%) ... 649
Niaspan Extended-Release Tablets ... 1703
Nicomide Tablets ... 3190
▲ Nicotrol Inhaler (Greater than 3%) ... 2594
▲ Nicotrol NS (Greater than 5%) ... 2596
Nimotop Capsules (Less than 1%) ... 774
▲ Nipent for Injection (3% to 10%) ... 3216
▲ Niravam Orally Disintegrating Tablets (1.8% to 29.8%) ... 3106
Nitrolingual Pumpspray (Occasional) ... 1161
Norflex Injection ... 1824
Noroxin Tablets (1.7% to 2.6%) ... 2009
Norvasc Tablets (0.1% to 3.4%) ... 2529
▲ Norvir (2.6% to 3.9%) ... 499
▲ Nubain Injection (5%) ... 1111
Omacor Capsules ... 2735
Omnicef Capsules (0.3%) ... 506
Omnicef for Oral Suspension (0.2%) ... 506
Oncaspar (Less than 1%) ... 1123
▲ Ontak Vials (22%) ... 1717
OptiPranolol Metipranolol Ophthalmic Solution 0.3% (A small number of patients) ... ⊙ 254
Orap Tablets ... 1220
Ortho-Cept Tablets ... 2395
Ortho-Cyclen Tablets ... 2414
Ortho Micronor Tablets ... 2411
Ortho Tri-Cyclen Tablets ... 2414
Ortho Tri-Cyclen Lo Tablets ... 2421
Orthoclone OKT3 Sterile Solution ... 2370
Oxsoralen-Ultra Capsules ... 3354
▲ OxyContin Tablets (13%) ... 2699
▲ OxyFast Oral Concentrate Solution (Among most frequent) ... 2704
▲ OxyIR Capsules (Among most frequent) ... 2704
▲ Pacerone Tablets (4% to 9%) ... 3337
Parcopa Orally Disintegrating Tablets ... 3111
Parnate Tablets ... 1499
▲ Paxil CR Controlled-Release Tablets (1% to 14%) ... 1509
▲ Paxil (1% to 14%) ... 1501
Peganone Tablets, USP ... 2487
▲ Pegasys (16%) ... 2793
▲ PEG-Intron Powder for Injection (12%) ... 3062
Pentasa Capsules (Less than 1%) ... 3182
Pepcid Injection (1.3%) ... 2017
Pepcid (1.3%) ... 2014
▲ Percocet Tablets (Among most frequent) ... 1114
▲ Percodan Tablets (Among most frequent) ... 1115
▲ Permax Tablets (19.1%) ... 3357
▲ Persantine Tablets (13.6%) ... 898
Phenergan ... 3438
Phenytek Capsules ... 2153
▲ Plan B Tablets (11.2%) ... 1068
▲ Plavix Tablets (6.2%) ... 940
▲ Plavix Tablets (6.2%) ... 2942
▲ Plendil Extended-Release Tablets (2.7% to 3.7%) ... 651
▲ Pletal Tablets (9% to 10%) ... 2478
▲ Pravachol Tablets (1.0% to 3.3%) ... 943
▲ Prefest Tablets (5%) ... 1069
Premarin Intravenous ... 3440
▲ Premarin Tablets (4% to 6%) ... 3443
Premarin Vaginal Cream ... 3449
▲ Premphase Tablets (3% to 5%) ... 3452
▲ Prempro Tablets (3% to 5%) ... 3452
Prevacid Delayed-Release Capsules (Less than 1%) ... 3268
Prevacid for Delayed-Release Oral Suspension (Less than 1%) ... 3268
Prevacid I.V. for Injection (Less than 1%) ... 3274
▲ Prevacid NapraPAC (Less than 1% to 9%) ... 3277
Prevacid SoluTab Delayed-Release Orally Disintegrating Tablets (Less than 1%) ... 3268
▲ PREVPAC (Less than 1% to 3%) ... 3281
Prilosec OTC Tablets (1.5%) ... 2674
Primaxin I.M. ... 2022
Primaxin I.V. (0.3%) ... 2024
▲ Prinivil Tablets (5.4% to 11.8%) ... 2029
▲ Prinzide Tablets (7.5%) ... 2033
ProAmatine Tablets (Rare) ... 3183
▲ Prochieve 4% Gel (5%) ... 1018
▲ Prochieve 8% Gel (5%) ... 1018
▲ Procrit for Injection (5% to 21%) ... 2374
▲ Prograf Capsules and Injection (3% to 19%) ... 624
Prolastin (0.19%) ... 3252
▲ Proleukin for Injection (11%) ... 1007
▲ Prometrium Capsules (100 mg, 200 mg) (15% to 24%) ... 3205
▲ ProSom Tablets (7%) ... 512
Protonix I.V. (Greater than 1%) ... 3468
Protonix Tablets (Greater than or equal to 1%) ... 3465
Protopic Ointment (Greater than or equal to 1%) ... 629
▲ Proventil Inhalation Aerosol (Less than 5%) ... 3067
▲ Proventil Inhalation Solution 0.083% (7%) ... 3069
Proventil HFA Inhalation Aerosol (Less than 3%) ... 3071
▲ Provigil Tablets (5%) ... 1002
▲ Prozac Pulvules and Liquid (9%) ... 1771
▲ Rabies Vaccine RabAvert (15%) ... 1011
▲ Rapamune Oral Solution and Tablets (3% to 20%) ... 3472
▲ Razadyne ER Extended-Release Capsules (9%) ... 2434
▲ Razadyne (9%) ... 2434
▲ Rebetol (7% to 26%) ... 3073
▲ Rebetron Combination Therapy (6% to 17%) ... 3078
ReFacto Vials ... 3479
▲ Relafen Tablets (3% to 9%) ... 1523
Relenza Rotadisk (1% to 2%) ... 1525
▲ Relpax Tablets (3% to 7%) ... 2531
Remicade for IV Injection (Greater than or equal to 0.2%) ... 987
ReoPro Vials (2.9%) ... 1779
Repronex for Intramuscular and Subcutaneous Injection ... 1148
▲ Requip Tablets (11% to 40%) ... 1528
Rescriptor Tablets ... 2535
▲ Retisert Implant (5% to 15%) ... ⊙ 256
▲ Retrovir Capsules (6% to 17.9%) ... 1533
▲ Retrovir IV Infusion (6% to 17.9%) ... 1537
▲ Retrovir (6% to 17.9%) ... 1533
▲ Reyataz Capsules (1% to 8%) ... 948
▲ Ribavirin, USP Capsules (17% to 26%) ... 3083
▲ Rilutek Tablets (5.1% to 12.7%) ... 2945
▲ Risperdal Consta Long-Acting Injection (8% to 11%) ... 1664
▲ Risperdal M-Tab Orally Disintegrating Tablets (4% to 11%) ... 1658
▲ Risperdal (4% to 11%) ... 1658
Ritalin Hydrochloride Tablets ... 2254
Ritalin LA Capsules ... 2255
Ritalin-SR Tablets ... 2254
▲ Rituxan for Infusion (7%) ... 845
▲ Rituxan I.V. (10%) ... 1251
Robitussin CF Liquid ... ▣ 755
Robitussin Maximum Strength Cough & Cold Liquid ... ▣ 754
Robitussin PE Syrup ... ▣ 753
Robitussin Pediatric Cough & Cold Liquid ... ▣ 754
Rocephin Injectable Vials, ADD-Vantage, Galaxy, Bulk (Occasional) ... 2801
▲ Roferon-A Injection (11% to 21%) ... 2805
Men's Rogaine Extra Strength Topical Solution, Ocean Rush Scent and Original Unscented ... ▣ 706
Women's Rogaine Topical Solution, Spring Bloom Scent and Original Unscented ... ▣ 707
▲ Rozerem Tablets (5%) ... 3228
▲ Rythmol SR Capsules (21% to 23%) ... 2736
▲ Sandostatin Injection (5%) ... 2263
Seasonale Tablets ... 1073
▲ Sedapap Tablets 50 mg/650 mg (Among the most frequent) ... 2098
▲ Sensipar Tablets (10%) ... 603
▲ Seroquel Tablets (11%) ... 691
▲ Simulect for Injection (Greater than or equal to 10%) ... 2268
Singulair (1.9%) ... 2047
▲ Skelaxin Tablets (Most frequent) ... 1685
▲ Somavert Injection (4% to 8%) ... 2648
▲ Sonata Capsules (7% to 9%) ... 1686
Soriatane Capsules (Less than 1%) ... 1028
Spectracef Tablets (0.1% to 1%) ... 2706
St. Joseph 81 mg Aspirin Chewable and Enteric Coated Tablets ... 1841
▲ Stalevo Tablets (8%) ... 2270
Starlix Tablets (2.2%) ... 2276
▲ Strattera Capsules (5% or greater) ... 1784
Stromectol Tablets (2.8%) ... 2053
▲ Suboxone Tablets (4%) ... 2719
▲ Subutex Tablets (4%) ... 2719
Sudafed 12 Hour Caplets ... ▣ 708
Sudafed 24 Hour Tablets ... ▣ 709
Sudafed Nasal Decongestant Tablets ... ▣ 709
▲ Sular Tablets (5%) ... 1163
Suprane Liquid for Inhalation (Less than 1%) ... 770
Suprax (Less than 2%) ... 1811
Surmontil Capsules ... 2347
▲ Sustiva Capsules (2% to 10%) ... 957
▲ Symlin Injection (2% to 5%) ... 608
▲ Symmetrel (5% to 10%) ... 1115
Synercid I.V. (Less than 1%) ... 1690
Tagamet Tablets (Approximately 1 in 100) ... 1547
▲ Tambocor Tablets (18.9%) ... 1824
▲ Tamiflu Capsules (1.6% to 2.1%) ... 2810
▲ Tamiflu Oral Suspension (1.6% to 2.1%) ... 2810
Targretin Capsules ... 1719
▲ Tarka Tablets (3.1%) ... 519
▲ Tasmar Tablets (6% to 13%) ... 3360
▲ Tegretol/Tegretol-XR (Among most frequent) ... 2278
▲ Temodar Capsules (5% to 12%) ... 3088
▲ Tenormin I.V. Injection (4% to 13%) ... 698
▲ Tenormin Tablets (4% to 13%) ... 695
▲ Tequin Injection (3%) ... 964
▲ Tequin Tablets (3%) ... 964
Tessalon Capsules ... 1202
Tessalon Perles ... 1202
Teveten Tablets (1% or greater) ... 1707
▲ Teveten HCT Tablets (4.1%) ... 1710
▲ Thalomid Capsules (4.2%) ... 979
TheraFlu Cold & Cough Hot Liquid ... ▣ 680
TheraFlu Cold & Sore Throat Hot Liquid ... ▣ 680
TheraFlu Flu & Chest Congestion Non-Drowsy Hot Liquid ... ▣ 681
TheraFlu Flu & Sore Throat Hot Liquid ... ▣ 681
TheraFlu Severe Cold Non-Drowsy Hot Liquid ... ▣ 683
TheraFlu Severe Cold & Cough Hot Liquid ... ▣ 683
TheraFlu Severe Cold Caplets ... ▣ 679
TheraFlu Severe Cold Hot Liquid ... ▣ 682
TheraFlu Severe Cold Non-Drowsy Caplets ... ▣ 679
▲ Thrombate III (7 of 17) ... 3254
▲ Thymoglobulin for Injection (8.5%) ... 2848
Thyrogen for Injection (1.6%) ... 1270
▲ Tiazac Capsules (5%) ... 1204
Ticlid Tablets (1.1%) ... 2813
Timentin ADD-Vantage ... 1556
Timentin Injection Galaxy Container ... 1559
Timentin IV Infusion ... 1553
Timentin Pharmacy Bulk Package ... 1562
Timolide Tablets (1.2%) ... 2056
Timoptic in Ocudose (Less frequent) ... 2061
Timoptic Sterile Ophthalmic Solution (Less frequent) ... 2058
Timoptic-XE Sterile Ophthalmic Gel Forming Solution (1% to 5%) ... 2062

(▣ Described in PDR For Nonprescription Drugs) Incidence data in parenthesis; ▲ 3% or more (⊙ Described in PDR For Ophthalmic Medicines™)

Tindamax (0.5% to 1.1%) 2670
▲ TOBI Solution for Inhalation (5.8%) 1015
▲ Topamax Sprinkle Capsules (4% to 32%) 2438
▲ Topamax Tablets (4% to 32%) 2438
▲ Toprol-XL Tablets (1.8% to about 10 of 100 patients) 660
Transderm Scōp Transdermal Therapeutic System (Infrequent) 2166
Tranxene (Less common) 2488
Trasylol Injection (1% to 2%) 779
Trecator Tablets 3482
Trelstar Depot (1.4%) 3385
Trelstar LA Suspension (2.9%) 3387
Triaminic Chest & Nasal Congestion Liquid ▣685
Triaminic Cold & Allergy Liquid ▣685
Triaminic Cold & Cough Liquid ▣685
Triaminic Cough Liquid ▣687
Triaminic Cough & Nasal Congestion Liquid ▣687
Triaminic Cough & Sore Throat Liquid ▣687
Triaminic Flu, Cough & Fever Liquid ▣685
Triaminic Night Time Cough & Cold Liquid ▣685
Triaminic Cough & Sore Throat Softchews ▣689
Tricor Tablets 523
▲ Trileptal Oral Suspension (8% to 49%) 2281
▲ Trileptal Tablets (8% to 49%) 2281
Triphasil-28 Tablets 3483
▲ Trisenox Injection (23%) 983
▲ Trizivir Tablets (10%) 1565
Trusopt Sterile Ophthalmic Solution 2065
▲ Truvada Tablets (Greater than 5%) 1279
Tussionex Pennkinetic Extended-Release Suspension 3322
Twinrix Vaccine (Less than 1%) 1571
▲ Tygacil for Injection (3.5%) 3489
Children's Tylenol Plus Cold NightTime Suspension Liquid 1851
Children's Tylenol Plus Cold Chewable Tablets 1851
Tylenol Cold & Flu Severe Daytime Liquid with Cool Bust 1846
Tylenol Cold & Flu Severe NightTime Liquid with Cool Burst 1846
Tylenol Flu NightTime Gelcaps 1846
Tylenol Flu Day Non-Drowsy Gelcaps 1846
Concentrated Tylenol Infants' Drops Plus Cold Nasal Congestant, Fever Reducer & Pain Reliever ▣668
Concentrated Tylenol Infants' Drops Plus Cold & Cough Nasal Decongestant, Fever Reducer & Pain Reliever ▣668
Multi-Symptom Tylenol Cold Night Time Caplets 1845
Multi-Symptom Tylenol Cold Day Non-Drowsy Caplets and Gelcaps 1845
▲ Tylenol with Codeine (Among most frequent) 2461
▲ Ultane Liquid for Inhalation (4%) 526
Ultracet Tablets (At least 1%) 2462
Uniretic Tablets (Less than 1% to 1.4%) 3114
▲ Univasc Tablets (4.3%) 3118
Uroqid-Acid No. 2 Tablets 785
▲ Uroxatral Tablets (5.7%) 2957
Valcyte Tablets 2816
▲ Valtrex Caplets (2% to 4%) 1573
Vancocin HCl Capsules, USP (Rare) 3370
Vantas (Less than 2%) 3367
Vantin Tablets and Oral Suspension (Less than 1%) 2650
Varivax 2070
▲ Vaseretic Tablets (8.6%) 2073
▲ Vasotec I.V. Injection (4.3% to 7.9%) 2076
▲ Velcade for Injection (14%) 2102
Ventavis Inhalation Solution 1036
Ventolin HFA Inhalation Aerosol (Less than 3%) 1576
▲ Verelan PM Capsules (3% to 3.3%) 3120
▲ Vesanoid Capsules (20%) 2823
VESIcare Tablets (1.8% to 1.9%) 631
VFEND I.V. (1.3% to 2.6%) 2543
VFEND Oral Suspension (1.3% to 2.6%) 2543
VFEND Tablets (1.3% to 2.6%) 2543
Viadur Implant (Less than 2%) 782
Viagra Tablets (2%) 2552
Vicks 44D Cough & Head Congestion Relief 2676
Vicks 44M Cough, Cold & Flu Relief 2676
Pediatric Vicks 44m Cough & Cold Relief 2673
Vicks DayQuil Multi-Symptom Cold/Flu Relief LiquiCaps 2675
Vicks DayQuil Multi-Symptom Cold/Flu Relief Liquid 2675
Children's Vicks NyQuil Cold/Cough Relief 2671
Vicks NyQuil LiquiCaps 2677
Vicks NyQuil Liquid 2677
Vicodin Tablets 530
▲ Vicodin ES Tablets (Among most frequent) 531
▲ Vicodin HP Tablets (Among most frequent) 532
▲ Vicoprofen Tablets (14%) 533
Viracept (Less than 2%) 2556
▲ Viread Tablets (1% to 3%) 1284
Vivactil Tablets 2350
Vivelle Transdermal System 2288
Vivelle-Dot Transdermal System 2293
▲ Voltaren Tablets (1% to 10%) 2298
▲ Voltaren-XR Tablets (1% to 10%) 2301
VoSpire Extended-Release Tablets (1.5%) 2352
Vytorin 10/10 Tablets 2084
Vytorin 10/10 Tablets 3092
Vytorin 10/20 Tablets 2084
Vytorin 10/20 Tablets 3092
Vytorin 10/40 Tablets 2084
Vytorin 10/40 Tablets 3092
Vytorin 10/80 Tablets 2084
Vytorin 10/80 Tablets 3092
▲ Wellbutrin Tablets (22.3%) 1579
▲ Wellbutrin SR Sustained-Release Tablets (5% to 11%) 1583
▲ Wellbutrin XL Extended-Release Tablets (5% to 11%) 1588
WinRho SDF 763
Xanax XR Tablets (Frequent) 2655
▲ Xeloda Tablets (1% to 12%) 2825
▲ Xenical Capsules (5.2%) 2834
Xifaxan Tablets (Less than 2%) 2847
▲ Xolair (3%) 1259
Xopenex HFA Inhalation Aerosol (1.4% to 2.7%) 3151
Xopenex Inhalation Solution (1.4% to 2.7%) 3143
Xopenex Inhalation Solution Concentrate (1.4% to 2.7%) 3147
Yasmin 28 Tablets (Greater than 1%) 818
Zantac (Rare) 1597
Zantac Injection (Rare) 1593
Zantac Injection Pharmacy Bulk Package (Rare) 1595
Zantac Syrup (Rare) 1597
▲ Zavesca Capsules (8% to 11%) 543
Zegerid Powder for Oral Solution (1.5%) 2972
▲ Zelnorm Tablets (4%) 2303
Zemaira (0.2% to 0.4%) 3506
▲ Zenapax for Injection (Greater than 5%) 2838
▲ Zestoretic Tablets (7.5%) 701
▲ Zestril Tablets (5.4% to 11.8%) 704
Zetia Tablets (2.7%) 2090
Zetia Tablets (2.7%) 3098
▲ Zevalin Injection (10%) 848
▲ Ziagen (6%) 1600
Zithromax Capsules, 250 mg (1% or less) 2568
Zithromax for IV Infusion (1.9%) 2573
Zithromax for Oral Suspension, 1 g (1% or less) 2568
Zithromax for Oral Suspension, 300 mg, 600 mg, 900 mg, 1200 mg (1% or less) 2561
Zithromax Tablets, 250 mg, 500 mg (1% or less) 2561
Zithromax Tablets, 600 mg (1% or less) 2568
Zithromax Tri-Pak (1% or less) 2561
Zithromax Z-Pak (1% or less) 2568
Zmax for Oral Suspension (Less then 1%) 2577
Zocor Tablets 2078
▲ Zofran Injection (12%) 1607
▲ Zofran (4% to 7%) 1613
▲ Zofran ODT Orally Disintegrating Tablets (4% to 7%) 1613
▲ Zoladex (5% to 6%) 709
Zoladex 3-month (1% to 5%) 712
▲ Zoloft (6% to 17%) 2581
▲ Zometa for Intravenous Infusion (18%) 2306
▲ Zomig Nasal Spray (2% to 6%) 718
▲ Zomig Tablets (6% to 10%) 714
▲ Zomig-ZMT Tablets (6% to 10%) 714
▲ Zonegran Capsules (13%) 1089
Zosyn (1.4%) 3492
Zovirax Capsules 1616
Zovirax for Injection 1618
Zovirax 1616
▲ Zyban Sustained-Release Tablets (8% to 10%) 1620
▲ Zydone Tablets (Among most frequent) 1118
▲ Zyprexa Tablets (11% to 18%) 1798
▲ Zyprexa IntraMuscular (4%) 1798
▲ Zyprexa ZYDIS Orally Disintegrating Tablets (11% to 18%) 1798
Zyrtec Chewable Tablets (2%) 2589
Zyrtec (2%) 2589
Zyrtec-D 12 Hour Extended Release Tablets (2%) 2591
Zyvox (2%) 2661

Dorsocervical fat enlargement

Agenerase Capsules (1 patient) 1299
Agenerase Oral Solution (1 patient) 1304
Aptivus Capsules 859
Combivir Tablets 1373
Crixivan Capsules 1918
Epivir 1394
Invirase 2776
Norvir 499
Retrovir 1533
Reyataz Capsules (Less than 3%) 948
Sustiva Capsules 957
Trizivir Tablets 1565
Truvada Tablets 1279
Viracept 2556
Viramune Oral Suspension 903
Viramune Tablets 903
Viread Tablets 1284
Zerit 971
Ziagen 1600

Down's syndrome

Repronex for Intramuscular and Subcutaneous Injection 1148

Dreaming

Amerge Tablets (Rare) 1312
Dilaudid Oral Liquid (Less frequent) 443
Dilaudid Tablets - 8 mg (Less frequent) 443
▲ Malarone Tablets (2% to 7%) 1484
▲ Malarone Pediatric Tablets (2% to 7%) 1484
MS Contin Tablets (Less frequent) 2703
▲ Nicotrol NS (Less than 5%) 2596
Tenormin I.V. Injection (Up to 3%) 698
Tenormin Tablets (Up to 3%) 695

Dreaming abnormalities

Abilify Tablets (Frequent) 916
Abilify Tablets (Frequent) 2472
Aciphex Tablets 1081
Actiq (Less than 1%) 993
Ambien Tablets (1%) 2867
Anaprox Tablets (Less than 1%) 2769
Anaprox DS Tablets (Less than 1%) 2769
Anzemet Injection (Infrequently) 2871
Anzemet Tablets (Infrequently) 2874
▲ Aricept Tablets (3%) 1086
▲ Aricept ODT Tablets (3%) 1086
Arthrotec Tablets (Rare) 3126
Avelox (Less than 0.1%) 2984
Avinza Capsules (Less than 5%) 1714
Axert Tablets (Rare) 2430
Axid Oral Solution (1.9%) 913
Blocadren Tablets (Less than 1%) 1891
Buprenex Injectable (Less than 1%) 2718
Caduet Tablets (Greater than 0.1% to less than 2%) 2507
Campral Tablets (Infrequent) 1175
Cardizem LA Extended Release Tablets (Less than 2%) 1699
Cataflam Tablets (Occasionally) 2173
Catapres Tablets 874
Catapres-TTS (0.5% or less) 875
Cipro XR Tablets (Less than 1%) 3004
Clorpres Tablets 2139
Copaxone for Injection (Frequent) 3292
Cozaar Tablets (Less than 1%) 1913
Cytovene (At least 3 subjects) 2763
▲ Depacon Injection (1% to 5%) 412
▲ Depakene (1% to 5%) 417
▲ Depakote Sprinkle Capsules (1% to 5%) 422
▲ Depakote Tablets (1% to 5%) 427
▲ Depakote ER Tablets (1% to 5%) 433
Dilaudid-HP (Less frequent) 441
Diprivan Injectable Emulsion (Less than 1%) 676
Duragesic Transdermal System (1% or greater) 2448
EC-Naprosyn Delayed-Release Tablets (Less than 1%) 2769
▲ Effexor Tablets (4%) 3405
▲ Effexor XR Capsules (3% to 7%) 3411
▲ Eldepryl Capsules (2 of 49 patients) 3209
▲ Emtriva Capsules (2% to 11%) 1272
▲ Epzicom Tablets (4% to 5%) 1402
Evoxac Capsules (Less than 1%) 1042
Exelon Capsules (Infrequent) 2204
Flexeril Tablets (Less than 1%) 1832
Frova Tablets (Rare) 1101
Gabitril Tablets (Infrequent) 998
Hyzaar 1964
Inderal LA Long-Acting Capsules 3421
▲ Intron A for Injection (Less than 5%) 3038
Invirase (Less than 2%) 2776
Kadian Capsules (Less than 3%) 572
Kaletra (Less than 2%) 474
Klonopin (Infrequent) 2782
Lamictal (Infrequent) 1449
▲ Lariam Tablets (Among most frequent) 2790
Levaquin in 5% Dextrose Injection (0.1% to 0.9%) 2453
Levaquin (0.1% to 0.9%) 2453
▲ Lexapro Oral Solution (3%) 1193
▲ Lexapro Tablets (3%) 1193
Lipitor Tablets (Less than 2%) 2495
Lotensin HCT Tablets (0.3% or more) 2235
Lotronex Tablets (Rare) 1479
▲ Lunesta Tablets (1% to 3%) 3139
Lyrica Capsules (0.1% to 1%) 2524
Maxalt Tablets (Infrequent) 1983
Maxalt-MLT Orally Disintegrating Tablets (Infrequent) 1983
Meridia Capsules 485
▲ Mirapex Tablets (Greater than or equal to 1% to 11%) 889
Naprosyn Suspension (Less than 1%) 2769
Naprosyn Tablets (Less than 1%) 2769
Neurontin Capsules (Infrequent) 2498
Neurontin Oral Solution (Infrequent) 2498
Neurontin Tablets (Infrequent) 2498
Nipent for Injection (Less than 3%) 3216
Niravam Orally Disintegrating Tablets (1.8%) 3106
Norvasc Tablets (More than 0.1% to 1%) 2529
Norvir (Less than 2%) 499
Nubain Injection (1% or less) 1111
Orap Tablets (2.7%) 1220
▲ OxyContin Tablets (Between 1% and 5%) 2699
Parcopa Orally Disintegrating Tablets 3111
▲ Paxil CR Controlled-Release Tablets (3% to 4%) 1509
▲ Paxil (3% to 4%) 1501
Permax Tablets (2.7%) 3357
Prevacid Delayed-Release Capsules (Less than 1%) 3268
Prevacid for Delayed-Release Oral Suspension (Less than 1%) 3268
Prevacid NapraPAC (Less than 1%) 3277
Prevacid SoluTab Delayed-Release Orally Disintegrating Tablets (Less than 1%) 3268
PREVPAC (Less than 1%) 3281
Prilosec OTC Tablets (Less than 1%) 2674
▲ Prograf Capsules and Injection (3% to 15%) 624
ProSom Tablets (2%) 512
Protonix I.V. (Less than 1%) 3468
Protonix Tablets (Less than 1%) 3465
▲ Prozac Pulvules and Liquid (1% to 5%) 1771
Relpax Tablets (Infrequent) 2531
▲ Requip Tablets (11%) 1528
Rescriptor Tablets 2535
Reyataz Capsules (Less than 3%) 948
Rilutek Tablets (Rare) 2945
Risperdal Consta Long-Acting Injection (Up to 2%) 1664
Risperdal M-Tab Orally Disintegrating Tablets (Frequent) 1658
Risperdal (Frequent) 1658
Seroquel Tablets (Infrequent) 691
Singulair (Very rare) 2047
Spectracef Tablets (0.1% to 1%) 2706
Stalevo Tablets 2270
▲ Strattera Capsules (4%) 1784
Sular Tablets (Less than or equal to 1%) 1163
Sustiva Capsules (1% to 4%) 957
Symmetrel (1% to 5%) 1115
Tambocor Tablets (Less than 1%) 1824
▲ Tasmar Tablets (16% to 21%) 3360
▲ Tequin Injection (0.1% to 3%) 964
▲ Tequin Tablets (0.1% to 3%) 964
Thioridazine Hydrochloride Tablets 2122
Tiazac Capsules (Less than 2%) 1204

Topamax Sprinkle Capsules (Infrequent) 2438
Topamax Tablets (Infrequent) 2438
Truvada Tablets 1279
Vantin Tablets and Oral Suspension (Less than 1%) 2650
Vaseretic Tablets 2073
Vasotec I.V. Injection (0.5% to 1.0%) 2076
VFEND I.V. (Less than 2%) 2543
VFEND Oral Suspension (Less than 2%) 2543
VFEND Tablets (Less than 2%) 2543
Viagra Tablets (Less than 2%) 2552
Vicoprofen Tablets (Less than 1%) 533
Voltaren Tablets (Occasionally) 2298
Voltaren-XR Tablets (Occasionally) 2301
Wellbutrin Tablets 1579
Wellbutrin SR Sustained-Release Tablets (At least 1%) 1583
Wellbutrin XL Extended-Release Tablets (At least 1%) 1588
Xanax XR Tablets (Infrequent) 2655
Xifaxan Tablets (Less than 2%) 2847
Zegerid Powder for Oral Solution (Less than 1%) 2972
Zoloft (Infrequent) 2581
Zomig Nasal Spray (Rare) 718
Zonegran Capsules (Infrequent) 1089
▲ Zyban Sustained-Release Tablets (5%) 1620
Zyprexa Tablets 1798
Zyprexa ZYDIS Orally Disintegrating Tablets 1798

Drooling

Aricept Tablets 1086
Aricept ODT Tablets 1086
Dantrium Capsules (Less frequent) 2690
Demser Capsules 1933
Thioridazine Hydrochloride Tablets 2122
Thiothixene Capsules 2124

Drowsiness

▲ Abilify Tablets (7% to 15%) 916
▲ Abilify Tablets (7% to 15%) 2472
Accutane Capsules 2740
Aceon Tablets (2 mg, 4 mg, 8 mg) (1.3%) 3191
Aciphex Tablets 1081
▲ Actiq (9% to 20%) 993
Adalat CC Tablets (Less than 1%) 2978
▲ Adderall XR Capsules (2% to 4%) 3169
Adenoscan (Less than 1%) 613
Advil Allergy Sinus Caplets ▣ 737
Advil Multi-Symptom Cold Caplets ▣ 738
Aggrenox Capsules (1.2%) 855
Agrylin Capsules (1% to 5%) 3172
Alavert Allergy & Sinus D-12 Hour Tablets ▣ 743
Albalon Ophthalmic Solution ⊙ 216
▲ Alferon N Injection (3% to 10%) 1640
Alinia for Oral Suspension (Less than 1%) 2840
Alinia Tablets (Less than 1%) 2840
Allegra (1.3% to 2.2%) 2857
Allegra-D 12 Hour Extended-Release Tablets 2860
Allegra-D 24 Hour Extended-Release Tablets 2862
Aloxi Injection (Less than 1%) 2099
Alphagan P Ophthalmic Solution (Less than 1%) 563
Altace Capsules (Less than 1%) 1673
▲ Ambien Tablets (2% to 8%) 2867
AmBisome for Injection (Less common) 615
Amerge Tablets (1% to 2%) 1312
Amnesteem Capsules 2126
▲ Anaprox Tablets (3% to 9%) 2769
▲ Anaprox DS Tablets (3% to 9%) 2769
Antabuse Tablets 2343
Antara Capsules 2723
Anzemet Injection (2.4%) 2871
▲ Apokyn Injection (35%) 2132
Aptivus Capsules (Less than 2%) 859
Aralast (Greater than or equal to 0.2% to 0.3%) 745
▲ Aredia for Injection (Up to 6%) 2168
Aricept Tablets (2%) 1086
Aricept ODT Tablets (2%) 1086
▲ Arimidex Tablets (2% to 5%) 665
Arthrotec Tablets (Rare) 3126
Asacol Delayed-Release Tablets 2688
▲ Astelin Nasal Spray (3.2%) 1876
Atacand Tablets (0.5% or greater) 634
Atacand HCT 637
Avalide Tablets 922
Avalide Tablets 2889
Avapro Tablets (Less than 1%) 925
Avapro Tablets (Less than 1%) 2886
Avelox (0.1% to less than 2%) 2984
▲ Avinza Capsules (Greater than 10%) 1714
Axert Tablets (Frequent) 2430
Axid Oral Solution (1.9%) 913
Baraclude (Less than 1%) 928
BC Allergy Sinus Cold Powder ▣ 612
Benadryl Allergy & Cold Tablets ▣ 692
Benadryl Allergy ▣ 691
Benadryl Allergy & Sinus Headache Caplets & Gelcaps ▣ 693
Children's Benadryl Allergy Liquid ▣ 695
Children's Benadryl Allergy & Cold Fastmelt Tablets ▣ 695
Children's Benadryl Dye-Free Allergy Liquid ▣ 695
Benadryl Dye-Free Allergy Liqui-Gels Softgels ▣ 692
Benadryl Maximum Strength Severe Allergy & Sinus Headache Caplets ▣ 694
Children's Benadryl D Allergy & Sinus Fastmelt Tablets ▣ 694
Children's Benadryl D Liquid Medication ▣ 693
Benadryl D Tablets ▣ 694
BeneFix for Injection (1.5%) 3402
▲ Bentyl Capsules (9%) 724
▲ Bentyl Injection (9%) 724
▲ Bentyl Syrup (9%) 724
▲ Bentyl Tablets (9%) 724
▲ Bexxar (0% to 5%) 1360
BiDil Tablets (1% to less than 2%) 2161
Biltricide Tablets 2990
Blocadren Tablets (Less than 1%) 1891
▲ Botox Purified Neurotoxin Complex (2% to 10%) 565
▲ Brevibloc Concentrate (3%) 766
▲ Brevibloc Injection (3%) 766
▲ Brevibloc Double Strength Injection (3%) 766
▲ Brevibloc Premixed Injection (3%) 766
▲ Brevibloc Double Strength Premixed Injection (3%) 766
▲ Brimonidine Tartrate Ophthalmic Solution 0.2% (10% to 30%) ⊙ 245
Buphenyl Powder 3327
Buphenyl Tablets 3327
Caduet Tablets (1.3% to less than 2%) 2507
Calcijex Injection 411
▲ Campath Ampules (1% to 5%) 826
Campral Tablets (Frequent) 1175
▲ Camptosar Injection (1.3% to 9.4%) 2602
Captopril Tablets 2114
Carafate Suspension (Less than 0.5%) 727
Carafate Tablets (Less than 0.5%) 728
▲ Carbatrol Capsules (Among most frequent) 3174
Cardizem LA Extended Release Tablets (Less than 2%) 1699
▲ Casodex Tablets (2% to 5%) 670
Cataflam Tablets (Occasionally) 2173
▲ Catapres Tablets (About 33 in 100 patients) 874
▲ Catapres-TTS (12 of 101 patients) 875
Ceftin Tablets (0.1% to 1%) 1369
Celebrex Capsules (0.1% to 1.9%) 3130
▲ Celexa (18%) 1177
▲ CellCept Capsules (3% to less than 20%) 2751
▲ CellCept Intravenous (3% to less than 20%) 2751
▲ CellCept Oral Suspension (3% to less than 20%) 2751
▲ CellCept Tablets (3% to less than 20%) 2751
▲ Chemet Capsules (1.0% to 12.7%) 2480
Children's Benadryl Allergy Fastmelt Tablets ▣ 696
Cialis Tablets (Less than 2%) 1806
Cipro I.V. (1% or less) 2998
Cipro I.V. Pharmacy Bulk Package (1% or less) 3509
Cipro (Less than 1%) 2991
Cipro XR Tablets (Less than 1%) 3004
▲ Clarinex Syrup (9.1%) 3009
Clarinex Tablets (2.1%) 3009
Clarinex Reditabs Tablets (2.1%) 3009
▲ Clarinex-D 24-Hour Extended-Release Tablets (3%) 3012
Clinoril Tablets (Less than 1%) 1899
▲ Clolar for Intravenous Infusion (10%) 1264
▲ Clorpres Tablets (About 33%) 2139
▲ Clozapine Tablets (More than 5% to 39%) 2141
▲ Clozaril Tablets (More than 5% to 46%) 2174
Colazal Capsules 2845
Combivent Inhalation Aerosol 878
▲ Combunox Tablets (17.4%) 1183
Comtan Tablets (2%) 2186
▲ Comvax (21.1% to 49.5%) 1904
Concerta Extended-Release Tablets 1828
Contac Severe Cold and Flu Caplets Maximum Strength ▣ 615
Copaxone for Injection (At least 2%) 3292
▲ Coreg Tablets (Greater than 1% to 3%) 1376
Covera-HS Tablets (Less than 2%) 3135
Cozaar Tablets (Less than 1%) 1913
Crixivan Capsules (2.4%) 1918
▲ Cymbalta Delayed-Release Capsules (7% to 21%) 1729
CytoGam Intravenous (Infrequent) 1866
Cytovene (At least 3 subjects) 2763
Dalmane Capsules 3343
▲ Dantrium Capsules (Among most frequent) 2690
▲ DAPTACEL (13.3% to 43.2%) 2964
▲ Daranide Tablets (Among the most common effects) 1928
▲ Depacon Injection (1.7% to 30%) 412
▲ Depakene (27% to 30%) 417
▲ Depakote Sprinkle Capsules (18% to 30%) 422
▲ Depakote Tablets (17% to 30%) 427
▲ Depakote ER Tablets (7% to 30%) 433
▲ DepoCyt Injection (4% to 12%) 1121
▲ DepoDur Extended-Release Injection (2% to 5%) 1098
Depo-Provera Contraceptive Injection (Less than 1%) 2619
depo-subQ provera 104 Injectable Suspension 2622
▲ Detrol Tablets (3%) 2626
▲ Detrol LA Capsules (3%) 2629
▲ Diastat Rectal Delivery System (23%) 3344
Dibenzyline Capsules 3390
Dilaudid 439
Dilaudid Non-Sterile Powder 439
Dilaudid Rectal Suppositories 439
Dilaudid Tablets 439
Children's Dimetapp Cold & Allergy Elixir ▣ 745
Diovan HCT Tablets (Greater than 0.2%) 2195
Diovan Tablets 2191
Diprivan Injectable Emulsion (Less than 1%) 676
▲ Ditropan XL Extended Release Tablets (2% to 12%) 2391
Diuril Sodium Intravenous 1934
Dolobid Tablets (Greater than 1 in 100) 1937
▲ Dostinex Tablets (2% to less than 10%) 2631
▲ Doxil Injection (1% to 10%) 3302
DuoNeb Inhalation Solution 1058
▲ Duragesic Transdermal System (10% or more) 2448
Dyazide Capsules 1389
DynaCirc CR Tablets (0.5% to 1%) 2726
▲ EC-Naprosyn Delayed-Release Tablets (3% to 9%) 2769
▲ Effexor Tablets (3% to 26.1%) 3405
▲ Effexor XR Capsules (2% to 17%) 3411
Eldepryl Capsules 3209
▲ Eloxatin for Injection (2% to 5%) 2908
Elspar for Injection 1943
Engerix-B Vaccine (Less than 1%) 1391
▲ Entocort EC Capsules (Less than 5%) 2694
▲ Equetro Extended-Release Capsules (12% to 32%) 3178
Eskalith 1406
Ethyol for Injection 1869
Eulexin Capsules (1%) 3023
Evoxac Capsules (Less than 1%) 1042
▲ Exelon Capsules (5%) 2204
Factive Tablets (0.1% to 1%) 2464
Famvir Tablets (1.6% to 2.6%) 2207
▲ FazaClo Orally Disintegrating Tablets (More than 5% to 39%) 547
▲ Femara Tablets (2% to 4%) 2210
Ferrlecit Injection 3379
▲ Flexeril Tablets (16% to 39%) 1832
▲ Flolan for Injection (4%) 1408
▲ Flomax Capsules (3.0% to 4.3%) 881
Flumadine (0.3% to 1%) 1186
Focalin Tablets 2214
Focalin XR Capsules 2217
Frova Tablets (Greater than or equal to 2%) 1101
Furosemide Tablets 2117
▲ Gabitril Tablets (18%) 998
▲ Gemzar for Injection (5% to 11%) 1743
Gengraf Capsules (1% to less than 3%) 458
▲ Geodon (14% to 31%) 2514
Gleevec Tablets (Infrequent) 2221
Goody's PM Powder ▣ 622
Havrix Vaccine (Rare) 1425
Hectorol Capsules 909
Hectorol Injection 911
HibTITER (91 of 1,118 vaccinations) 3419
Hycodan 1104
Hycomine Compound Tablets 1105
Hycotuss Expectorant Syrup 1106
Hyperstat I.V. Injection 3031
▲ Hytrin Capsules (0.6% to 5.4%) 469
Hyzaar 1964
▲ Imdur Tablets (Less than or equal to 5%) 3032
Imitrex Injection (2.7%) 1431
Imitrex Nasal Spray (Infrequent) 1435
Imitrex Tablets 1440
Imodium Capsules 1834
Imodium A-D Liquid and Caplets 1835
Imodium Advanced Caplets and Chewable Tablets ▣ 644
Indapamide Tablets (Less than 5%) 2119
Indocin (Less than 1%) 1968
▲ Infanrix Vaccine (6.6% to 54%) 1444
▲ Infergen (4% to 5%) 1647
▲ Intron A for Injection (Up to 14%) 3038
▲ Invanz for Injection (Greater than 0.5% to 5.1%) 1974
Invirase (Less than 2%) 2776
▲ Kadian Capsules (Among most frequent) 572
Kaletra (Less than 2%) 474
▲ Keppra Oral Solution (3% to 23%) 3307
▲ Keppra Tablets (3% to 23%) 3307
Ketek Tablets (Greater than or equal to 0.2% to less than 2%) 2920
▲ Klonopin (7% to 50%) 2782
▲ Kytril Injection (4%) 2785
Kytril Tablets (1% to 4%) 2788
▲ Lamictal (5% to 17%) 1449
▲ Lariam Tablets (Among most frequent) 2790
Levaquin in 5% Dextrose Injection (0.1% to 0.9%) 2453
Levaquin (0.1% to 0.9%) 2453
Levitra Tablets (Less than 2%) 3048
▲ Lexapro Oral Solution (4% to 13%) 1193
▲ Lexapro Tablets (4% to 13%) 1193
Librium Capsules 3349
Lidoderm Patch 1107
Lipitor Tablets (Less than 2%) 2495
Lithobid Tablets 1670
Lofibra Capsules 1217
Lortab 3315
Lortab Elixir 3312
Lotensin Tablets (1.6%) 2232
Lotensin HCT Tablets (1.2%) 2235
Lotrel Capsules (Up to 0.3%) 2238
▲ Lunesta Tablets (8% to 10%) 3139
Lupron Depot-PED 7.5 mg, 11.25 mg and 15 mg (Less than 2%) 3266
Lupron Injection Pediatric (Less than 2%) 3256
▲ Lyrica Capsules (4% to 28%) 2524
▲ Marinol Capsules (3% to 10%) 3334
Matulane Capsules 3188
Mavik Tablets (0.3% to 1.0%) 482
▲ Maxalt Tablets (4% to 8%) 1983
▲ Maxalt-MLT Orally Disintegrating Tablets (4% to 8%) 1983
Maxzide 2150
▲ Mebaral Tablets, USP (1 to 3 per 100 patients) 2483
Meridia Capsules (1.7%) 485
Merrem I.V. (Greater than 0.1% to 1%) 687
Metadate CD Capsules 3316
Micardis Tablets (More than 0.3%) 884
Micardis HCT Tablets 886
Midamor Tablets (Less than or equal to 1%) 2000
▲ Migranal Nasal Spray (3%) 3350
Mintezol 2002
▲ Mirapex Tablets (9% to 22%) 889
▲ Moban Tablets (Most frequent) 1108
Mobic Oral Suspension (Less than 2%) 893
Mobic Tablets (Less than 2%) 893
Moduretic Tablets (Less than or equal to 1%) 2003
Mycamine for Injection (0.4% to 0.5%) 620
▲ Nalfon Capsules (8.5%) 2504
▲ Namenda (3%) 1199
▲ Naprosyn Suspension (3% to 9%) 2769
▲ Naprosyn Tablets (3% to 9%) 2769
Naropin Injection (Less than 1%) 640
Natrecor for Injection (Greater than or equal to 1%) 3123
Nembutal Sodium Solution, USP (1% to 3%) 2484
Neoral Soft Gelatin Capsules (1% to less than 3%) 2247

Neoral Oral Solution (1% to less than 3%) ... 2247
Neumega for Injection ... 3433
▲ Neurontin Capsules (19.3% to 21.4%) ... 2498
▲ Neurontin Oral Solution (19.3% to 21.4%) ... 2498
▲ Neurontin Tablets (19.3% to 21.4%) ... 2498
Nexium Delayed-Release Capsules (Less than 1%) ... 645
Nexium I.V. (Less than 1%) ... 649
▲ Nicotrol NS (Greater than 5%) ... 2596
▲ Nipent for Injection (3% to 10%) ... 3216
▲ Niravam Orally Disintegrating Tablets (41% to 76.8%) ... 3106
Norflex Injection ... 1824
Noroxin Tablets (0.3% to 1.0%) ... 2009
Norvasc Tablets (1.3% to 1.6%) ... 2529
Norvir (2.4% to 2.6%) ... 499
Numorphan ... 1112
Maximum Strength Nytol QuickGels Softgels ... □ 635
Omnicef Capsules (0.2%) ... 506
Omnicef for Oral Suspension (0.2%) ... 506
Oncaspar (Less than 1%) ... 1123
OptiPranolol Metipranolol Ophthalmic Solution 0.3% (A small number of patients) ... ⊙ 254
▲ Orap Tablets (27.7%) ... 1220
▲ OxyContin Tablets (23%) ... 2699
▲ Oxytrol Transdermal System (Greater than 1%) ... 3383
Parcopa Orally Disintegrating Tablets ... 3111
Parnate Tablets ... 1499
▲ Paxil CR Controlled-Release Tablets (1.9% to 24%) ... 1509
▲ Paxil (1.9% to 24%) ... 1501
PediaCare Multi-Symptom Cold Liquid ... □ 704
PediaCare NightRest Cough & Cold Liquid ... □ 704
Pediarix Vaccine ... 1518
▲ Liquid PedvaxHIB (Among most frequent) ... 2012
Pentasa Capsules (Less than 1%) ... 3182
Pepcid Injection (Infrequent) ... 2017
Pepcid (Infrequent) ... 2014
▲ Permax Tablets (10.1%) ... 3357
Phenergan ... 3438
Plendil Extended-Release Tablets (0.5% to 1.5%) ... 651
Premphase Tablets ... 3452
Prempro Tablets ... 3452
Prevacid Delayed-Release Capsules (Less than 1%) ... 3268
Prevacid for Delayed-Release Oral Suspension (Less than 1%) ... 3268
▲ Prevacid NapraPAC (Less than 1% to 9%) ... 3277
Prevacid SoluTab Delayed-Release Orally Disintegrating Tablets (Less than 1%) ... 3268
▲ Prevnar for Injection (11% to 40.7%) ... 3460
PREVPAC (Less than 1%) ... 3281
Prilosec OTC Tablets (Less than 1%) ... 2674
Primaxin I.M. ... 2022
Primaxin I.V. (0.2%) ... 2024
Prinivil Tablets (0.3% to 1.0%) ... 2029
Prinzide Tablets (0.3% to 1%) ... 2033
ProAmatine Tablets (Rare) ... 3183
▲ Prochieve 4% Gel (27%) ... 1018
▲ Prochieve 8% Gel (27%) ... 1018
▲ Prograf Capsules and Injection (3% to 15%) ... 624
▲ Proleukin for Injection (22%) ... 1007
Prometrium Capsules (100 mg, 200 mg) (Less than 5%) ... 3205
▲ ProSom Tablets (42%) ... 512
Protonix I.V. (Less than 1%) ... 3468
Protonix Tablets (Less than 1%) ... 3465
Proventil HFA Inhalation Aerosol (Less than 3%) ... 3071
Provigil Tablets (2%) ... 1002
▲ Prozac Pulvules and Liquid (5% to 17%) ... 1771
▲ Rapamune Oral Solution and Tablets (3% to 20%) ... 3472
▲ Razadyne ER Extended-Release Capsules (4%) ... 2434
▲ Razadyne (4%) ... 2434
▲ Rebif Prefilled Syringe for Injection (4% to 5%) ... 3163
Recombivax HB ... 2045
ReFacto Vials ... 3479
Reishimax Capsules ... 2669
Relafen Tablets (1% to 3%) ... 1523
▲ Relpax Tablets (3% to 7%) ... 2531
▲ Requip Tablets (12% to 40%) ... 1528
Rescriptor Tablets ... 2535
▲ Retrovir Capsules (8%) ... 1533
▲ Retrovir IV Infusion (8%) ... 1537
▲ Retrovir (8%) ... 1533
Reyataz Capsules (Less than 3%) ... 948
▲ Rilutek Tablets (0.8% to 4.1%) ... 2945
▲ Risperdal Consta Long-Acting Injection (5% to 6%) ... 1664
▲ Risperdal M-Tab Orally Disintegrating Tablets (3% to 41%) ... 1658
▲ Risperdal (3% to 41%) ... 1658
Ritalin Hydrochloride Tablets ... 2254
Ritalin LA Capsules ... 2255
Ritalin-SR Tablets ... 2254
▲ Rituxan I.V. (1% to 5%) ... 1251
Robitussin Allergy & Cough Syrup ... □ 750
Robitussin Flu Liquid ... □ 752
Robitussin PM Cough & Cold Liquid ... □ 752
▲ Rozerem Tablets (5%) ... 3228
▲ Rythmol SR Capsules (1% to 3%) ... 2736
Sandostatin LAR Depot (1% to 4%) ... 2264
▲ Sedapap Tablets 50 mg/650 mg (Among the most frequent) ... 2098
Seromycin Capsules ... 1783
▲ Seroquel Tablets (18%) ... 691
Singlet Caplets ... □ 636
Singulair (Very rare) ... 2047
▲ Skelaxin Tablets (Most frequent) ... 1685
▲ Sonata Capsules (5%) ... 1686
▲ Soriatane Capsules (1% to 10%) ... 1028
Spectracef Tablets (0.1% to 1%) ... 2706
Stalevo Tablets (2%) ... 2270
▲ Strattera Capsules (0.5% to 7%) ... 1784
Stromectol Tablets (0.9%) ... 2053
▲ Suboxone Tablets (5%) ... 2719
▲ Subutex Tablets (5%) ... 2719
Sudafed Sinus & Allergy Tablets ... □ 710
Sular Tablets (Less than or equal to 1%) ... 1163
Surmontil Capsules ... 2347
Sustiva Capsules (2% to 3%) ... 957
▲ Symbyax Capsules (Up to 22%) ... 1788
Symmetrel (1% to 5%) ... 1115
Tagamet Tablets (Approximately 1 in 100) ... 1547
Tambocor Tablets (1% to 3%) ... 1824
Tarka Tablets (0.3% or more) ... 519
▲ Tasmar Tablets (14% to 18%) ... 3360
▲ Tegretol/Tegretol-XR (Among most frequent) ... 2278
▲ Temodar Capsules (9%) ... 3088
Tenormin I.V. Injection (0.6% to 2%) ... 698
Tenormin Tablets (0.6% to 2%) ... 695
Tequin Injection (Less than 0.1%) ... 964
Tequin Tablets (Less than 0.1%) ... 964
Teveten Tablets (Less than 1%) ... 1707
Teveten HCT Tablets (Less than 1%) ... 1710
▲ Thalomid Capsules (37.5%) ... 979
TheraFlu Cold & Cough Hot Liquid ... □ 680
TheraFlu Cold & Sore Throat Hot Liquid ... □ 680
TheraFlu Flu & Sore Throat Hot Liquid ... □ 681
TheraFlu Severe Cold & Cough Hot Liquid ... □ 683
TheraFlu Severe Cold Caplets ... □ 679
TheraFlu Severe Cold Hot Liquid ... □ 682
TheraFlu Thin Strips Multi Symptom ... □ 684
Thioridazine Hydrochloride Tablets (Occasional) ... 2122
Thiothixene Capsules ... 2124
Tiazac Capsules (Less than 2%) ... 1204
Timolide Tablets (Less than 1%) ... 2056
Timoptic in Ocudose (Less frequent) ... 2061
Timoptic Sterile Ophthalmic Solution (Less frequent) ... 2058
Timoptic-XE Sterile Ophthalmic Gel Forming Solution ... 2062
Tindamax ... 2670
▲ Topamax Sprinkle Capsules (7% to 29%) ... 2438
▲ Topamax Tablets (7% to 29%) ... 2438
Toprol-XL Tablets ... 660
▲ Transderm Scōp Transdermal Therapeutic System (Less than one-sixth) ... 2166
▲ Tranxene (Most frequent) ... 2488
Trecator Tablets ... 3482
Triaminic Allerchews ... □ 684
Triaminic Cold & Allergy Liquid ... □ 685
Triaminic Cold & Cough Liquid ... □ 685
Triaminic Flu, Cough & Fever Liquid ... □ 685
Triaminic Night Time Cough & Cold Liquid ... □ 685
Triaminic Allergy Runny Nose & Congestion Softchews ... □ 688
Triaminic Cold & Cough Softchews ... □ 688
Triaminic Thin Strips Cough & Runny Nose ... □ 690
Tricor Tablets ... 523
▲ Trileptal Oral Suspension (5% to 36%) ... 2281
▲ Trileptal Tablets (5% to 36%) ... 2281
▲ Trisenox Injection (8%) ... 983
Tussionex Pennkinetic Extended-Release Suspension ... 3322
Twinrix Vaccine (Less than 1%) ... 1571
Tygacil for Injection (0.2% to less than 2%) ... 3489
Tylenol Cough & Sore Throat NightTime Liquid with Cool Burst ... □ 664
Children's Tylenol Plus Cold & Allergy Suspension Liquid ... 1850
Children's Tylenol Plus Cold NightTime Suspension Liquid ... 1851
Children's Tylenol Plus Cold & Cough Suspension Liquid and Chewable Tablets ... 1851
Children's Tylenol Plus Cold Chewable Tablets ... 1851
Children's Tylenol Plus Flu Suspension Liquid ... 1853
Tylenol Cold & Flu Severe NightTime Liquid with Cool Burst .. 1846
Tylenol Cough & Sore Throat NightTime Liquid with Cool Burst .. 1849
Tylenol Allergy Complete Night Time Caplets ... 1844
Tylenol Allergy Complete Multi-Symptom Caplets and Gelcaps with Cool Burst ... 1844
Tylenol Severe Allergy Caplets ... 1844
Tylenol Flu NightTime Gelcaps ... 1846
Multi-Symptom Tylenol Cold Night Time Caplets ... 1845
Extra Strength Tylenol PM Caplets, Geltabs, Gelcaps and Liquid ... 1847
Tylenol Sinus Night Time Caplets ... 1848
Tylenol Sore Throat NightTime Liquid with Cool Burst ... 1849
▲ Ultane Liquid for Inhalation (9%) ... 526
▲ Ultracet Tablets (6%) ... 2462
Uniretic Tablets (Less than 1%) ... 3114
Unisom SleepTabs ... □ 713
Unisom Maximum Strength SleepGels ... □ 712
Univasc Tablets (Less than 1%) ... 3118
▲ Valium Tablets (Among most common) ... 2822
Vantin Tablets and Oral Suspension (Less than 1%) ... 2650
Vaseretic Tablets (0.5% to 2.0%) ... 2073
Vasotec I.V. Injection (0.5% to 1.0%) ... 2076
Verelan PM Capsules (2% or less) ... 3120
▲ Vesanoid Capsules (3%) ... 2823
VFEND I.V. (Less than 2%) ... 2543
VFEND Oral Suspension (Less than 2%) ... 2543
VFEND Tablets (Less than 2%) ... 2543
Viagra Tablets (Less than 2%) ... 2552
Vicks 44M Cough, Cold & Flu Relief ... 2676
Pediatric Vicks 44m Cough & Cold Relief ... 2673
Children's Vicks NyQuil Cold/Cough Relief ... 2671
Vicks NyQuil Cough Liquid ... 2677
Vicks NyQuil LiquiCaps ... 2677
Vicks NyQuil LiquiCaps/Liquid Multi-Symptom Cold/Flu Relief ... □ 725
Vicks NyQuil Liquid ... 2677
Vicodin Tablets ... 530
Vicodin ES Tablets ... 531
Vicodin HP Tablets ... 532
▲ Vicoprofen Tablets (22%) ... 533
Viracept (Less than 2%) ... 2556
▲ Viramune Oral Suspension (3% to 8%) ... 903
▲ Viramune Tablets (3% to 8%) ... 903
Vivactil Tablets ... 2350
Voltaren Tablets (Occasionally) ... 2298
Voltaren-XR Tablets (Occasionally) ... 2301
VoSpire Extended-Release Tablets (0.3%) ... 2352
▲ Wellbutrin SR Sustained-Release Tablets (2% to 3%) ... 1583
▲ Wellbutrin XL Extended-Release Tablets (2% to 3%) ... 1588
WinRho SDF ... 763
▲ Xanax XR Tablets (23%) ... 2655
Zantac (Rare) ... 1597
Zantac Injection ... 1593
Zantac Injection Pharmacy Bulk Package (Rare) ... 1595
Zantac Syrup (Rare) ... 1597
Zegerid Powder for Oral Solution (Less than 1%) ... 2972
Zestoretic Tablets (0.3% to 1%) ... 701
Zestril Tablets (0.3% to 1.0%) ... 704
Zithromax Capsules, 250 mg (1% or less) ... 2568
Zithromax for IV Infusion (1% or less) ... 2573
Zithromax for Oral Suspension, 1 g (1% or less) ... 2568
Zithromax for Oral Suspension, 300 mg, 600 mg, 900 mg, 1200 mg (1% or less) ... 2561
Zithromax Tablets, 250 mg, 500 mg (1% or less) ... 2561
Zithromax Tablets, 600 mg (1% or less) ... 2568
Zithromax Tri-Pak (1% or less) ... 2561
Zithromax Z-Pak (1% or less) ... 2568
Zmax for Oral Suspension ... 2577
▲ Zofran Injection (5% to 8%) ... 1607
▲ Zofran (20%) ... 1613
▲ Zofran ODT Orally Disintegrating Tablets (20%) ... 1613
Zoladex (1% or greater) ... 709
Zoladex 3-month ... 712
▲ Zoloft (2% to 15%) ... 2581
▲ Zometa for Intravenous Infusion (5% to 10%) ... 2306
▲ Zomig Nasal Spray (0% to 4%) ... 718
▲ Zomig Tablets (5% to 8%) ... 714
▲ Zomig-ZMT Tablets (5% to 8%) ... 714
▲ Zonegran Capsules (17%) ... 1089
Zovirax ... 1616
Zyban Sustained-Release Tablets (2%) ... 1620
Zydone Tablets ... 1118
▲ Zyprexa Tablets (20% to 39%) ... 1798
▲ Zyprexa IntraMuscular (6%) ... 1798
▲ Zyprexa ZYDIS Orally Disintegrating Tablets (20% to 39%) ... 1798
▲ Zyrtec Chewable Tablets (1.9% to 13.7%) ... 2589
▲ Zyrtec (1.9% to 13.7%) ... 2589
▲ Zyrtec-D 12 Hour Extended Release Tablets (1.9% to 13.7%) ... 2591

Drug abuse

Copegus Tablets (Less than 1%) ... 2759

Drug administration site reactions, unspecified

Abelcet Injection ... 1119
Aloprim for Injection (Less than 1%) ... 2156
▲ Ammonul Injection (14%) ... 3323
▲ AndroGel (3% to 5%) ... 3330
▲ Avonex (3%) ... 839
Cardene I.V. (1.4%) ... 1129
▲ CombiPatch Transdermal System (2% to 23%) ... 2180
▲ Cytovene-IV (22%) ... 2763
Denavir Cream (1.3%) ... 2163
Depacon Injection (2.4%) ... 412
Doxil Injection ... 3302
Duragesic Transdermal System (1% or greater) ... 2448
Engerix-B Vaccine ... 1391
▲ Epogen for Injection (7% to 25%) ... 586
▲ Floxin Otic Solution (0.6% to 16.8%) ... 1043
▲ Fortaz (Among most common) ... 1422
Fragmin Injection (Rare) ... 2638
▲ Imitrex Injection (58.7%) ... 1431
▲ Intron A for Injection (Less than 5%) ... 3038
Leukine ... 829
▲ Leustatin Injection (9% to 19%) ... 2368
Lupron Depot 3.75 mg (1%) ... 3257
Lupron Depot–3 Month 11.25 mg (1%) ... 3262
▲ Lupron Depot-PED 7.5 mg, 11.25 mg and 15 mg (5%) ... 3266
Lupron Injection Pediatric ... 3256
Merrem I.V. (1.1%) ... 687
▲ Migranal Nasal Spray (6%) ... 3350
▲ Navelbine Injection (Up to 38%) ... 1494
Neupogen for Injection (Infrequent) .. 598
Oncaspar (Greater than 1% but less than 5%) ... 1123
▲ Ontak Vials (8%) ... 1717
▲ Ortho Evra Transdermal System (9% to 22%) ... 2402
▲ Procrit for Injection (7% to 29%) ... 2374
▲ Proleukin for Injection (3%) ... 1007
Retrovir IV Infusion (Infrequent) ... 1537
Rilutek Tablets (Infrequent) ... 2945
▲ Rocephin Injectable Vials, ADD-Vantage, Galaxy, Bulk (5% to 17%) ... 2801
▲ Roferon-A Injection (29%) ... 2805
Taxotere Injection Concentrate ... 2947
▲ Testim 1% Gel (2% to 4%) ... 722
▲ Vesanoid Capsules (17%) ... 2823
Zithromax for IV Infusion (1.9%) ... 2573
▲ Zoladex (6%) ... 709
Zoladex 3-month ... 712

Zosyn (0.5%) 3492
▲ Zyban Sustained-Release Tablets (11%) 1620

Drug effect, unspecified, diminished
Mivacron Injection 489

Drug effect, unspecified, prolonged
Diprivan Injectable Emulsion (Less than 1%) 676
Mivacron Injection (Less than 1%) 489

Drug fever
Aldoclor Tablets 1881
Aldoril Tablets 1884
Ancef for Injection 1318
Clozapine Tablets 2141
Clozaril Tablets 2174
DynaCirc CR Tablets (0.5% to 1%) 2726
Invirase (Rare) 2776
Leukeran Tablets 1472
Orap Tablets 1220
Primaxin I.M. 2022
Primaxin I.V. (Less than 0.2%) 2024
Purinethol Tablets (Very rare) 1222
Suprax (Less than 2%) 1811
Taxotere Injection Concentrate 2947
Timentin ADD-Vantage 1556
Timentin Injection Galaxy Container 1559
Timentin IV Infusion 1553
Timentin Pharmacy Bulk Package 1562
Vancocin HCl Capsules, USP (Infrequent) 3370
Vivactil Tablets 2350
Zinacef Injection (Rare) 1604
Zinacef for Injection (Rare) 1604

Drug idiosyncrasies
(*see under* Allergic reactions)

Drug overdose
Campral Tablets (Infrequent) 1175
Copegus Tablets (Less than 1%) 2759
Lyrica Capsules (0.1% to 1%) 2524
Pegasys (Less than 1%) 2793
Prozac Pulvules and Liquid (Infrequent) 1771
Reyataz Capsules (Less than 3%) 948
Symbyax Capsules (Infrequent) 1788

Dry mouth
(*see under* Xerostomia)

Dry skin
(*see under* Xerosis cutis)

Dry sockets
Celebrex Capsules 3130

Dryness
Aclovate Cream (Approximately 2%) 1290
Analpram-HC 1136
Cutivate Cream (1.2%) 1381
Cutivate Ointment (Infrequent to more frequent) 1384
Elocon Lotion 0.1% (Infrequent) 3020
Locoid Cream (Infrequent) 1138
Locoid Lipocream Cream (Infrequent) 1138
Locoid (Infrequent) 1138
▲ Naftin Cream (3%) 2097
Olux Foam (Less than 1%) 1027
Ophthetic Ophthalmic Solution ⊙ 230
Pandel Cream, 0.1% 1017
Pramosone 1139
Temovate Cream 1549
Temovate Gel (Infrequent) 1550
Temovate Ointment 1549
Temovate Scalp Application (Infrequent) 1551
Temovate E Emollient (Infrequent) 1552
Topicort .05% Gel 3288
Topicort .25% Cream 3288
Topicort .25% Ointment 3288
Topicort LP .05% Cream 3288
U-cort 1% Cream 3289
Vanos Cream 1864

Dryness, mucous membrane
Advicor Tablets 1694
Dolobid Tablets (Less than 1 in 100) 1937
Mintezol Chewable Tablets 2002
Myleran Tablets (Rare) 1492
Pravachol Tablets 943
Timolide Tablets (Less than 1%) 2056
▲ Vesanoid Capsules (77%) 2823
Vytorin 10/10 Tablets 2084
Vytorin 10/10 Tablets 3092
Vytorin 10/20 Tablets 2084
Vytorin 10/20 Tablets 3092
Vytorin 10/40 Tablets 2084
Vytorin 10/40 Tablets 3092
Vytorin 10/80 Tablets 2084
Vytorin 10/80 Tablets 3092

Dryness, nose
(*see under* Xeromycteria)

Dryness, vaginal
Effexor Tablets (Rare) 3405
Effexor XR Capsules (Rare) 3411
▲ Femara Tablets (5.3%) 2210

Dryness, vulvovaginal
Clindesse Vaginal Cream (Less than 1%) 3296

Dryness at application site
Evoclin Foam, 1% (1%) 1025

Duodenitis
Aciphex Tablets (Rare) 1081
Actonel with Calcium Tablets (0.1% to 1%) 2684
Effexor Tablets (Rare) 3405
Effexor XR Capsules (Rare) 3411
Evoxac Capsules (Less than 1%) 1042
Invanz for Injection (Greater than 0.1%) 1974
Nexium Delayed-Release Capsules (Less than 1%) 645
Nexium I.V. (Less than 1%) 649
Paxil CR Controlled-Release Tablets (Rare) 1509
Paxil (Rare) 1501
Permax Tablets (Rare) 3357
Pletal Tablets (Less than 2%) 2478
Protonix I.V. (Less than 1%) 3468
Protonix Tablets (Less than 1%) 3465
Relafen Tablets (Less than 1%) 1523
Requip Tablets (Infrequent) 1528
Rythmol SR Capsules 2736
VFEND I.V. (Less than 2%) 2543
VFEND Oral Suspension (Less than 2%) 2543
VFEND Tablets (Less than 2%) 2543
Zonegran Capsules (Rare) 1089

Dupuytren's contracture
Requip Tablets (Rare) 1528

Dypnea
▲ Clolar for Intravenous Infusion (13%) 1264
▲ Ribavirin, USP Capsules (24%) 3083
Ultane Liquid for Inhalation (Less than 1%) 526

Dysarthria
Abilify Tablets (Infrequent) 916
Abilify Tablets (Infrequent) 2472
Ambien Tablets (Infrequent) 2867
Aricept Tablets (Infrequent) 1086
Aricept ODT Tablets (Infrequent) 1086
Clozapine Tablets (Less than 1%) 2141
Clozaril Tablets (Less than 1%) 2174
Cymbalta Delayed-Release Capsules (Infrequent) 1729
Depacon Injection 412
Depakene 417
Depakote Sprinkle Capsules 422
▲ Depakote Tablets (1% to 5%) 427
Depakote ER Tablets (Greater than 1%) 433
Diastat Rectal Delivery System (Greater than or equal to 1%) 3344
Eloxatin for Injection 2908
FazaClo Orally Disintegrating Tablets (Less than 1%) 547
Flexeril Tablets (Less than 1%) 1832
Gabitril Tablets (Frequent) 998
Geodon Capsules (Frequent) 2514
Imitrex Injection (Rare) 1431
Imitrex Nasal Spray (Infrequent) 1435
Imitrex Tablets (Infrequent) 1440
Indocin Capsules (Less than 1%) 1968
Indocin I.V. (Less than 1%) 1973
Indocin (Less than 1%) 1968
Invirase (Less than 2%) 2776
Klonopin (2%) 2782
Lamictal (1.0%) 1449
Lyrica Capsules (0.1% to 1%) 2524
Maxalt Tablets (Infrequent) 1983
Maxalt-MLT Orally Disintegrating Tablets (Infrequent) 1983
Neumega for Injection 3433
Neurontin Capsules (2.4%) 2498
Neurontin Oral Solution (2.4%) 2498
Neurontin Tablets (2.4%) 2498
Nipent for Injection (Less than 3%) 3216
▲ Niravam Orally Disintegrating Tablets (23.3%) 3106
Paxil CR Controlled-Release Tablets (Rare) 1509
Paxil (Rare) 1501
Protonix I.V. (Less than 1%) 3468
Protonix Tablets (Less than 1%) 3465
Prozac Pulvules and Liquid (Rare) 1771
Rilutek Tablets (Infrequent) 2945
Risperdal M-Tab Orally Disintegrating Tablets (Infrequent) 1658
Risperdal (Infrequent) 1658
Roferon-A Injection (Less than 0.5%) 2805
Seromycin Capsules 1783
Seroquel Tablets (Frequent) 691
Sonata Capsules (Rare) 1686
Symbyax Capsules (Infrequent) 1788
Valium Tablets (Infrequent) 2822
Valtrex Caplets 1573
▲ Vesanoid Capsules (3%) 2823
Wellbutrin Tablets (Infrequent) 1579
Wellbutrin SR Sustained-Release Tablets 1583
Wellbutrin XL Extended-Release Tablets 1588
▲ Xanax XR Tablets (10.9%) 2655
▲ Xeloda Tablets (Less than 5%) 2825
Zonegran Capsules (Infrequent) 1089
Zovirax Capsules 1616
Zovirax for Injection 1618
Zovirax 1616
Zyban Sustained-Release Tablets 1620
Zyprexa Tablets (Infrequent) 1798
Zyprexa ZYDIS Orally Disintegrating Tablets (Infrequent) 1798

Dysautonomia
Lyrica Capsules (Rare) 2524

Dyschromatopsia
Desferal Vials 2190

Dyscrasias, blood
(*see under* Blood dyscrasias)

Dysdiadochokinesia
Klonopin 2782

Dysentery
Xifaxan Tablets (Less than 2%) 2847

Dysesthesia
AmBisome for Injection (Less common) 615
▲ Astelin Nasal Spray (7.9%) 1876
Avelox 2984
Copaxone for Injection (At least 2%) 3292
Cytovene 2763
Evoxac Capsules (Less than 1%) 1042
Factive Tablets (Rare) 2464
Floxin Otic Singles (Reported in a single subject) 1045
Floxin Otic Solution (Single report) 1043
Frova Tablets (Frequent) 1101
Imitrex Injection (Rare) 1431
Imitrex Nasal Spray (Rare) 1435
Imitrex Tablets (Rare) 1440
Invirase (Less than 2%) 2776
▲ Kepivance (12%) 592
Maxalt Tablets (Rare) 1983
Maxalt-MLT Orally Disintegrating Tablets (Rare) 1983
Neurontin Capsules (Infrequent) 2498
Neurontin Oral Solution (Infrequent) 2498
Neurontin Tablets (Infrequent) 2498
Prinivil Tablets (0.3% to 1.0%) 2029
Prinzide Tablets 2033
▲ Taxotere Injection Concentrate (7 of 134 patients) 2947
Tequin Injection 964
Tequin Tablets 964
Thalomid Capsules 979
Vaseretic Tablets 2073
Vasotec I.V. Injection (0.5% to 1.0%) 2076
▲ Velcade for Injection (23%) 2102
Zestril Tablets (0.3% to 1.0%) 704

Dysesthesia, hemifacial
Prilosec OTC Tablets (Less than 1%) 2674
Zegerid Powder for Oral Solution (Less than 1%) 2972

Dysgeusia
Advate Injection (2.6%) 742
Altoprev Extended-Release Tablets 1151
Buphenyl Powder 3327
Buphenyl Tablets 3327
Captopril Tablets (Approximately 2 to 4 of 100 patients) 2114
Cardizem LA Extended Release Tablets (Less than 2%) 1699
Emend Capsules (Greater than 0.5%) 1944
Eskalith 1406
Ferrlecit Injection 3379
Havrix Vaccine (Less than 1%) 1425
Ketek Tablets (1.5% to 1.6%) 2920
Lithobid Tablets 1670
Maxalt Tablets 1983
Maxalt-MLT Orally Disintegrating Tablets 1983
Mevacor Tablets (0.8%) 1996
Mycamine for Injection (0.7%) 620
Noroxin Tablets 2009
Rocephin Injectable Vials, ADD-Vantage, Galaxy, Bulk (Less than 1%) 2801
Rozerem Tablets (2%) 3228
Sanctura Tablets (Greater than or equal to 0.5%) 1133
Tiazac Capsules (Less than 1%) 1204
Twinrix Vaccine (Less than 1%) 1571
▲ Velcade for Injection (13%) 2102

Dyskinesia
Abilify Tablets (Infrequent) 916
Abilify Tablets (Infrequent) 2472
Adderall Tablets 3168
Adderall XR Capsules 3169
▲ Apokyn Injection (24% to 35%) 2132
Bentyl Capsules 724
Bentyl Injection 724
Bentyl Syrup 724
Bentyl Tablets 724
Celexa 1177
▲ Comtan Tablets (25%) 2186
Concerta Extended-Release Tablets 1828
Dexedrine 1386
DextroStat Tablets 3177
Dostinex Tablets 2631
▲ Eldepryl Capsules (2 of 49 patients) 3209
Evoxac Capsules (Less than 1%) 1042
Focalin Tablets 2214
Focalin XR Capsules 2217
▲ Geodon Capsules (14%) 2514
Kaletra (Less than 2%) 474
Lamictal (Infrequent) 1449
Lexapro Oral Solution 1193
Lexapro Tablets 1193
Lyrica Capsules (Rare) 2524
Metadate CD Capsules 3316
▲ Mirapex Tablets (47%) 889
Namenda 1199
Naropin Injection (Less than 1%) 640
Neurontin Capsules 2498
Neurontin Oral Solution 2498
Neurontin Tablets 2498
Orap Tablets 1220
Parcopa Orally Disintegrating Tablets (Common) 3111
Paxil CR Controlled-Release Tablets (Rare) 1509
Paxil (Rare) 1501
▲ Permax Tablets (62.4%) 3357
Phenytek Capsules (Rare) 2153
Provigil Tablets (1%) 1002
Prozac Pulvules and Liquid 1771
Requip Tablets (1% or more) 1528
Risperdal Consta Long-Acting Injection (Infrequent) 1664
Ritalin Hydrochloride Tablets 2254
Ritalin LA Capsules 2255
Ritalin-SR Tablets 2254
Seroquel Tablets (Infrequent) 691
▲ Stalevo Tablets (5% to 25%) 2270
▲ Tasmar Tablets (42% to 51%) 3360
Thalomid Capsules 979
Topamax Sprinkle Capsules (Infrequent) 2438
Topamax Tablets (Infrequent) 2438
Wellbutrin Tablets (Frequent) 1579
Wellbutrin SR Sustained-Release Tablets 1583
Wellbutrin XL Extended-Release Tablets 1588
Xanax XR Tablets (1.7%) 2655
Zoloft (Rare) 2581
Zonegran Capsules 1089
Zyban Sustained-Release Tablets 1620
Zyprexa Tablets (Up to 2%) 1798
Zyprexa ZYDIS Orally Disintegrating Tablets (Up to 2%) 1798

Dyskinesia, orofacial
Neurontin Capsules (Rare) 2498
Neurontin Oral Solution (Rare) 2498
Neurontin Tablets (Rare) 2498
Provigil Tablets (At least 1%) 1002
Zyrtec Chewable Tablets (Rare) 2589
Zyrtec (Rare) 2589

Zyrtec-D 12 Hour Extended Release Tablets (Rare) 2591

Dyskinesia, tardive
(*see under* Tardive dyskinesia)

Dyskinesia, transient
Orap Tablets 1220

Dyslipidemia
Cymbalta Delayed-Release Capsules (Infrequent) 1729

Dysmenorrhea
Abilify Tablets 916
Abilify Tablets 2472
Aciphex Tablets 1081
▲ Adderall XR Capsules (2% to 4%) 3169
Advair Diskus 100/50 1291
Advair Diskus 250/50 1291
Advair Diskus 500/50 1291
Alamast Ophthalmic Solution (Less than 5%) 3371
Alesse-28 Tablets 3392
Allegra (1.5%) 2857
Arthrotec Tablets (Rare) 3126
▲ Asacol Delayed-Release Tablets (3%) 2688
▲ Asmanex Twisthaler (4% to 9%) 2981
Axert Tablets (Infrequent) 2430
▲ Betaseron for SC Injection (7%) 791
Celebrex Capsules (0.1% to 1.9%) 3130
▲ Celexa (3%) 1177
▲ Cenestin Tablets, 0.45mg, 0.625mg, 0.9mg, 1.25mg (6%) 1063
Cenestin Tablets, 0.3mg 1063
Cipro XR Tablets (Less than 1%) 3004
Clarinex Tablets (2.1%) 3009
Clarinex Reditabs Tablets (2.1%) 3009
Clindesse Vaginal Cream (Less than 1%) 3296
Clozapine Tablets (Less than 1%) 2141
Clozaril Tablets (Less than 1%) 2174
▲ CombiPatch Transdermal System (30% to 31%) 2180
▲ Concerta Extended-Release Tablets (3%) 1828
▲ Copaxone for Injection (6%) 3292
▲ Depacon Injection (1% to 5%) 412
▲ Depakene (1% to 5%) 417
▲ Depakote Sprinkle Capsules (1% to 5%) 422
▲ Depakote Tablets (1% to 5%) 427
Depakote ER Tablets (Greater than 1%) 433
Depo-Provera Contraceptive Injection (Less than 1%) 2619
▲ Dostinex Tablets (1% to less than 10%) 2631
Effexor Tablets 3405
▲ Effexor XR Capsules (6%) 3411
Elidel Cream 1% (1.1% to 1.5%) 2198
Estratest Tablets 3196
Estratest H.S. Tablets 3196
Estrogel 0.06% 3200
Evoxac Capsules (Less than 1%) 1042
▲ Famvir Tablets (2.2% to 7.6%) 2207
FazaClo Orally Disintegrating Tablets (Less than 1%) 547
Gabitril Tablets (Frequent) 998
Geodon for Injection (Up to 2%) 2514
Imitrex Injection (Rare) 1431
Imitrex Nasal Spray (Infrequent) 1435
Imitrex Tablets (Infrequent) 1440
▲ Infergen (2% to 9%) 1647
▲ Intron A for Injection (Less than 5%) 3038
▲ Klonopin (3%) 2782
▲ Lamictal (6.6%) 1449
Levaquin in 5% Dextrose Injection (0.1% to 0.9%) 2453
Levaquin (0.1% to 0.9%) 2453
Lo/Ovral-28 Tablets 3423
▲ Lunesta Tablets (0% to 3%) 3139
Lyrica Capsules (0.1% to 1%) 2524
Menostar Transdermal System 805
▲ Meridia Capsules (3.5%) 485
▲ Mirena Intrauterine System (5% or more) 810
▲ Nasonex Nasal Spray (1% to 5%) 3058
Neurontin Capsules (Infrequent) 2498
Neurontin Oral Solution (Infrequent) 2498
Neurontin Tablets (Infrequent) 2498
Nexium Delayed-Release Capsules (Less than 1%) 645
Nexium I.V. (Less than 1%) 649
▲ Nicotrol NS (3%) 2596
Noroxin Tablets (Less frequent) 2009
Paxil CR Controlled-Release Tablets (Infrequent) 1509
Paxil (Infrequent) 1501
Permax Tablets (Frequent) 3357
▲ Prefest Tablets (8%) 1069
Premarin Intravenous 3440
Premarin Tablets 3443
Premarin Vaginal Cream 3449
▲ Premphase Tablets (3% to 13%) 3452
▲ Prempro Tablets (3% to 13%) 3452
Prevacid Delayed-Release Capsules (Less than 1%) 3268
Prevacid for Delayed-Release Oral Suspension (Less than 1%) 3268
Prevacid NapraPAC (Less than 1%) 3277
Prevacid SoluTab Delayed-Release Orally Disintegrating Tablets (Less than 1%) 3268
PREVPAC (Less than 1%) 3281
Prochieve 4% Gel 1018
Prochieve 8% Gel 1018
Protonix I.V. (Less than 1%) 3468
Protonix Tablets (Less than 1%) 3465
Protopic Ointment (Up to 4%) 629
Provigil Tablets (At least 1%) 1002
Prozac Pulvules and Liquid 1771
Qvar Inhalation Aerosol (1% to 3%) 1654
Risperdal Consta Long-Acting Injection (Infrequent) 1664
Risperdal M-Tab Orally Disintegrating Tablets (Infrequent) 1658
Risperdal (Infrequent) 1658
Seasonale Tablets 1073
Seroquel Tablets (Infrequent) 691
▲ Sonata Capsules (3% to 4%) 1686
▲ Strattera Capsules (5% or greater) 1784
Topamax Sprinkle Capsules (More than 1%) 2438
Topamax Tablets (More than 1%) 2438
Triphasil-28 Tablets 3483
Uniretic Tablets (Less than 1%) 3114
▲ Valtrex Caplets (Less than 1% to 8%) 1573
VFEND I.V. (Less than 2%) 2543
VFEND Oral Suspension (Less than 2%) 2543
VFEND Tablets (Less than 2%) 2543
Vivelle Transdermal System 2288
Vivelle-Dot Transdermal System 2293
Wellbutrin SR Sustained-Release Tablets (At least 1%) 1583
Wellbutrin XL Extended-Release Tablets (At least 1%) 1588
▲ Xanax XR Tablets (3.6%) 2655
Yasmin 28 Tablets (Greater than 1%) 818
Zelnorm Tablets (1% to 2%) 2303
▲ Zoladex (1% to 7%) 709
Zoloft (Infrequent) 2581
Zomig Nasal Spray (Rare) 718
Zomig Tablets (Rare) 714
Zomig-ZMT Tablets (Rare) 714
Zyprexa Tablets 1798
Zyprexa ZYDIS Orally Disintegrating Tablets 1798
Zyrtec Chewable Tablets (Less than 2%) 2589
Zyrtec (Less than 2%) 2589
Zyrtec-D 12 Hour Extended Release Tablets (Less than 2%) 2591

Dysmetria
Trileptal Oral Suspension 2281
Trileptal Tablets 2281

Dyspareunia
Depo-Provera Contraceptive Injection (Less than 1%) 2619
Lyrica Capsules (Rare) 2524
▲ Prochieve 4% Gel (6%) 1018
▲ Prochieve 8% Gel (6%) 1018
Wellbutrin Tablets (Rare) 1579
Wellbutrin SR Sustained-Release Tablets 1583
Wellbutrin XL Extended-Release Tablets 1588
▲ Zoladex (14%) 709
Zyban Sustained-Release Tablets 1620

Dyspepsia
Abelcet Injection 1119
▲ Abilify Tablets (15%) 916
▲ Abilify Tablets (15%) 2472
Accolate Tablets (1.5%) 663
Aceon Tablets (2 mg, 4 mg, 8 mg) (0.3% to 1.9%) 3191
Aciphex Tablets 1081
Actiq (1% or greater) 993
▲ Actonel Tablets (6.9% to 7.6%) 2679
▲ Actonel with Calcium Tablets (6.9% to 7.6%) 2684
Adalat CC Tablets (Less than 1%) 2978
Adderall XR Capsules (2%) 3169
Advair Diskus 100/50 1291
Advair Diskus 250/50 1291
Advair Diskus 500/50 1291
▲ Advicor Tablets (3%) 1694
Aerobid/Aerobid-M (1% to 3%) 1172
▲ Aggrenox Capsules (18.4%) 855
▲ Agrylin Capsules (5.2%) 3172
Aldara Cream, 5% (2.8%) 1814
▲ Alferon N Injection (3%) 1640
Alinia for Oral Suspension (Less than 1%) 2840
Alinia Tablets (Less than 1%) 2840
Allegra (1.3%) 2857
Allegra-D 12 Hour Extended-Release Tablets (2.8%) 2860
Allegra-D 24 Hour Extended-Release Tablets (2.8%) 2862
Aloxi Injection (Less than 1%) 2099
Alphagan P Ophthalmic Solution (1% to 4%) 563
Altace Capsules (Less than 1%) 1673
Altoprev Extended-Release Tablets (1% to 1.6%) 1151
▲ Ambien Tablets (5%) 2867
AmBisome for Injection (Less common) 615
Amerge Tablets (Infrequent) 1312
Anaprox Tablets (Less than 3%) 2769
Anaprox DS Tablets (Less than 3%) 2769
▲ Angiomax for Injection (5%) 1856
Antara Capsules 2723
▲ Anzemet Injection (3%) 2871
▲ Anzemet Tablets (3%) 2874
Aptivus Capsules (Less than 2%) 859
▲ Arava Tablets (5%) 2881
▲ Aredia for Injection (22.6%) 2168
▲ Arimidex Tablets (5%) 665
Arixtra Injection (0.3% to 2.4%) 1325
▲ Aromasin Tablets (2% to 5%) 2600
▲ Arthrotec Tablets (14%) 3126
▲ Asacol Delayed-Release Tablets (6%) 2688
▲ Asmanex Twisthaler (3% to 5%) 2981
Atacand Tablets (0.5% or greater) 634
Atacand HCT (0.5% or greater) 637
▲ Atrovent HFA Inhalation Aerosol (1% to 5%) 872
Avalide Tablets (2%) 922
Avalide Tablets (2%) 2889
Avapro Tablets (2%) 925
Avapro Tablets (2%) 2886
▲ Avastin IV (17% to 24%) 1229
Avelox (0.1% to less than 2%) 2984
Avinza Capsules (Less than 5%) 1714
Axert Tablets (Infrequent) 2430
▲ Axid Oral Solution (3.6%) 913
Azopt Ophthalmic Suspension (Less than 1%) 553
Baraclude (Less than or equal to 1%) 928
Bayer Aspirin Tablets 3515
Benicar Tablets (Greater than 0.5%) 2850
Benicar HCT Tablets (Greater than 1%) 2852
▲ Betaseron for SC Injection (14%) 791
▲ Bexxar (Less than 1% to 6%) 1360
Biaxin/Biaxin XL (2%) 402
Blocadren Tablets (0.6%) 1891
▲ Boniva Tablets (5.6% to 11.9%) 2747
Brevibloc Concentrate (Less than 1%) 766
Brevibloc Injection (Less than 1%) 766
Brevibloc Double Strength Injection (Less than 1%) 766
Brevibloc Premixed Injection (Less than 1%) 766
Brevibloc Double Strength Premixed Injection (Less than 1%) 766
Buprenex Injectable (Infrequent) 2718
▲ Byetta Injection (6%) 605
Caduet Tablets (Less than 1% to 2.8%) 2507
▲ Campath Ampules (10%) 826
Campral Tablets (Frequent) 1175
▲ Camptosar Injection (0% to 10%) 2602
Captopril Tablets 2114
Cardene I.V. (Rare) 1129
▲ Carnitor Injection (5% to 9%) 3185
Casodex Tablets (2% to 5%) 670
▲ Cataflam Tablets (1% to 10%) 2173
Ceftin Tablets (0.1% to 1%) 1369
▲ Celebrex Capsules (8.8%) 3130
▲ Celexa (5%) 1177
▲ CellCept Capsules (22.4%) 2751
▲ CellCept Intravenous (22.4%) 2751
▲ CellCept Oral Suspension (22.4%) 2751
▲ CellCept Tablets (22.4%) 2751
▲ Cenestin Tablets, 0.45mg, 0.625mg, 0.9mg, 1.25mg (10%) 1063
▲ Cialis Tablets (4% to 10%) 1806
Cipro I.V. (2.7%) 2998
Cipro I.V. Pharmacy Bulk Package (2.7%) 3509
Cipro (2.7%) 2991
Cipro XR Tablets (1%) 3004
▲ Clarinex Tablets (3%) 3009
▲ Clarinex Reditabs Tablets (3%) 3009
Clindesse Vaginal Cream (Less than 1%) 3296
▲ Clinoril Tablets (3% to 9%) 1899
▲ Clozaril Tablets (14%) 2174
Colazal Capsules (2%) 2845
▲ CombiPatch Transdermal System (6% to 8%) 2180
Combivent Inhalation Aerosol (Less than 2%) 878
▲ Combivir Tablets (5%) 1373
Combunox Tablets (Less than 1% to 2.1%) 1183
Comtan Tablets (2%) 2186
Copaxone for Injection (At least 2%) 3292
▲ Copegus Tablets (6%) 2759
Cosopt Sterile Ophthalmic Solution (1% to 5%) 1910
Cozaar Tablets (1% or greater) 1913
▲ Crestor Tablets (3.4%) 672
Crixivan Capsules (1.5%) 1918
Cubicin for Injection (0.9%) 1038
▲ Cymbalta Delayed-Release Capsules (4%) 1729
Cytovene (At least 3 subjects) 2763
Dalmane Capsules 3343
▲ Depacon Injection (8% to 11%) 412
▲ Depakene (8% to 11%) 417
▲ Depakote Sprinkle Capsules (8% to 11%) 422
▲ Depakote Tablets (8% to 13%) 427
▲ Depakote ER Tablets (7% to 13%) 433
▲ DepoDur Extended-Release Injection (2% to 5%) 1098
▲ Detrol Tablets (5.9%) 2626
▲ Detrol LA Capsules (3%) 2629
Diovan HCT Tablets (Greater than 0.2%) 2195
Diovan Tablets 2191
▲ Ditropan XL Extended Release Tablets (5% to 7%) 2391
▲ Dolobid Tablets (3% to 9%) 1937
▲ Dostinex Tablets (2% to 5%) 2631
▲ Doxil Injection (Less than 1% to 12.1%) 3302
DuoNeb Inhalation Solution (1.3%) 1058
▲ Duragesic Transdermal System (3% to 10%) 2448
EC-Naprosyn Delayed-Release Tablets (Less than 3%) 2769
Ecotrin Enteric Coated Aspirin Low, Regular and Maximum Strength Tablets 1627
▲ Effexor Tablets (4.5% to 5%) 3405
Effexor XR Capsules (At least 2%) 3411
Eligard 22.5 mg (Less than 2%) 2899
Elmiron Capsules (2%) 2393
▲ Eloxatin for Injection (7% to 14%) 2908
Emend Capsules (Greater than 0.5%) 1944
▲ Emtriva Capsules (4% to 8%) 1272
▲ Enablex Extended-Release Tablets (2.7% to 8.4%) 2201
▲ Enbrel for Injection (4% to 11%) 580
Engerix-B Vaccine 1391
▲ Entocort EC Capsules (6%) 2694
▲ Epivir (5%) 1394
▲ Epogen for Injection (9% to 11%) 586
▲ Equetro Extended-Release Capsules (10%) 3178
▲ Erbitux (7%) 937
Estrogel 0.06% 3200
▲ Evista Tablets (5.9%) 1735
▲ Evoxac Capsules (7.8%) 1042
▲ Exelon Capsules (9%) 2204
▲ Fabrazyme for Intravenous Infusion (3%) 1267
Factive Tablets (0.1% to 1%) 2464
▲ Famvir Tablets (1.1% to 3.4%) 2207
▲ Femara Tablets (3% to 4%) 2210
Ferrlecit Injection 3379
▲ Flexeril Tablets (1% to 3%) 1832
Flolan for Injection (1%) 1408
Floxin Otic Singles 1045
Floxin Otic Solution (Single report) 1043
Flumadine (0.3% to 1%) 1186
▲ Focalin XR Capsules (5% to 9%) 2217
▲ Fortamet Extended-Release Tablets (4.2%) 1156
▲ Forteo for Injection (5.2%) 1739
▲ Fortical Nasal Spray (1% to 3%) 3336
▲ Fosamax (1.1% to 3.6%) 1949
▲ Fosamax Plus D Tablets (1.1% to 3.6%) 1956
Frova Tablets (2%) 1101
Gabitril Tablets (1% or more) 998
▲ Gengraf Capsules (2.2% to 8%) 458
▲ Geodon (8%) 2514
▲ Gleevec Tablets (12% to 27%) 2221
Gonal-f RFF Pen for Injection (2.4%) 3155
▲ Hectorol Capsules (4.9% to greater than or equal to 5%) 909
▲ Hectorol Injection (4.9%) 911
▲ Hepsera Tablets (3%) 1275

Hytrin Capsules (At least 1%) 469
Hyzaar 1964
▲ Imdur Tablets (Less than or equal to 5%) 3032
Imitrex Nasal Spray 1435
Indapamide Tablets (Less than 5%) 2119
▲ Indocin (3% to 9%) 1968
▲ Infergen (12% to 21%) 1647
▲ Intron A for Injection (Up to 8%) 3038
Invanz for Injection (1% to 1.1%) 1974
Invirase (0.9% to greater than or equal to 2%) 2776
▲ I.V. Busulfex (44%) 1125
Kadian Capsules (Less than 3%) 572
▲ Kaletra (1% to 5%) 474
Keppra Oral Solution (1% or more) 3307
Keppra Tablets (1% or more) 3307
Ketek Tablets (Greater than or equal to 0.2% to less than 2%) 2920
Klonopin (Infrequent) 2782
▲ Kytril Tablets (4% to 6%) 2788
▲ Lamictal (2% to 7%) 1449
▲ Lamisil Tablets (4.3%) 2226
Lariam Tablets 2790
▲ Lescol Capsules (7.9%) 2227
▲ Lescol Capsules (7.9%) 2730
▲ Lescol XL Tablets (3.5%) 2227
▲ Lescol XL Tablets (3.5%) 2730
▲ Leukine (17%) 829
Levaquin in 5% Dextrose Injection (0.2% to 2.3%) 2453
Levaquin (0.2% to 2.3%) 2453
▲ Levitra Tablets (4%) 3048
Lexapro Oral Solution (Infrequent) 1193
Lexapro Tablets (Infrequent) 1193
Lipitor Tablets (1.3% to 2.8%) 2495
Lofibra Capsules 1217
Lotensin HCT Tablets (0.3% to 1%) 2235
Lotrel Capsules 2238
Lotronex Tablets (Infrequent) 1479
▲ Lunesta Tablets (2% to 6%) 3139
▲ Malarone Tablets (1% to 3%) 1484
▲ Malarone Pediatric Tablets (1% to 3%) 1484
▲ Mavik Tablets (0.3% to 6.4%) 482
Maxalt Tablets (Infrequent) 1983
Maxalt-MLT Orally Disintegrating Tablets (Infrequent) 1983
▲ Megace ES Oral Suspension (0% to 4%) 2492
▲ Menostar Transdermal System (5%) 805
▲ Mepron Suspension (5%) 1487
▲ Meridia Capsules (5%) 485
Merrem I.V. (Greater than 0.1% to 1%) 687
▲ Mevacor Tablets (1.0% to 3.9%) 1996
Miacalcin Nasal Spray (1% to 3%) 2242
Micardis Tablets (1%) 884
Micardis HCT Tablets (Less than 2%) 886
▲ Midamor Tablets (Less than or equal to 1%) 2000
Migranal Nasal Spray (Infrequent) 3350
Mirapex Tablets (Greater than or equal to 1%) 889
▲ Mobic Oral Suspension (3.8% to 8.9%) 893
▲ Mobic Tablets (3.8% to 8.9%) 893
Moduretic Tablets 2003
▲ Myfortic Tablets (3% to 22.5%) 2244
▲ Mylotarg for Injection (8% to 27%) 3429
▲ Nalfon Capsules (10.3%) 2504
Naprosyn Suspension (Less than 3%) 2769
Naprosyn Tablets (Less than 3%) 2769
Nasonex Nasal Spray (Greater than or equal to 2%) 3058
▲ Neoral Soft Gelatin Capsules (2.2% to 8%) 2247
▲ Neoral Oral Solution (2.2% to 8%) 2247
▲ Neulasta Injection (15% to 72%) 596
▲ Neumega for Injection (Greater than or equal to 10%) 3433
Neurontin Capsules (1% to 2.2%) 2498
Neurontin Oral Solution (1% to 2.2%) 2498
Neurontin Tablets (1% to 2.2%) 2498
Nexium Delayed-Release Capsules (Less than 1%) 645
Nexium I.V. (Less than 1%) 649
▲ Nicotrol Inhaler (18%) 2594
Nicotrol NS 2596
▲ Nipent for Injection (3% to 10%) 3216
Noroxin Tablets (0.3% to 1.0%) 2009
Norvasc Tablets (Less than 1% to 2%) 2529
▲ Norvir (0% to 5.9%) 499
Nubain Injection (1% or less) 1111
▲ Omacor Capsules (3.1%) 2735
Omnicef Capsules (0.7%) 506
Omnicef for Oral Suspension (0.2%) 506
▲ Ontak Vials (7%) 1717
▲ OxyContin Tablets (Between 1% and 5%) 2699
Parcopa Orally Disintegrating Tablets 3111
▲ Paxil CR Controlled-Release Tablets (2% to 5%) 1509
▲ Paxil (2% to 5%) 1501
Pegasys (Less than 1%) 2793
▲ PEG-Intron Powder for Injection (6%) 3062
Pentasa Capsules (1.6%) 3182
▲ Permax Tablets (6.4%) 3357
Persantine Tablets (Rare) 898
▲ Photofrin for Injection (6%) 729
▲ Plavix Tablets (5.2%) 940
▲ Plavix Tablets (5.2%) 2942
▲ Plendil Extended-Release Tablets (0.5% to 3.9%) 651
▲ Pletal Tablets (6%) 2478
▲ Prandin Tablets (0.5, 1, and 2 mg) (2% to 3%) 2337
▲ Premarin Tablets (9% to 11%) 3443
▲ Premphase Tablets (5% to 8%) 3452
▲ Prempro Tablets (5% to 8%) 3452
Prevacid Delayed-Release Capsules (Less than 1%) 3268
Prevacid for Delayed-Release Oral Suspension (Less than 1%) 3268
Prevacid I.V. for Injection (Less than 1%) 3274
Prevacid NapraPAC (Less than 3%) 3277
Prevacid SoluTab Delayed-Release Orally Disintegrating Tablets (Less than 1%) 3268
▲ PREVPAC (Less than 1% to 3%) 3281
Prinivil Tablets (0.3% to 1.0%) 2029
Prinzide Tablets (1.3%) 2033
Prochieve 4% Gel 1018
Prochieve 8% Gel 1018
▲ Procrit for Injection (7% to 11%) 2374
▲ Prograf Capsules and Injection (3% to 28%) 624
▲ Proleukin for Injection (7%) 1007
Prometrium Capsules (100 mg, 200 mg) (Less than 5%) 3205
ProSom Tablets (2%) 512
Protonix I.V. (Greater than 1%) 3468
Protonix Tablets (Greater than or equal to 1%) 3465
Protopic Ointment (1% to 4%) 629
Proventil Inhalation Solution 0.083% (1% to 1.5%) 3069
▲ Provigil Tablets (5%) 1002
▲ Prozac Pulvules and Liquid (6% to 10%) 1771
▲ Pulmozyme Inhalation Solution (3%) 1245
▲ Rapamune Oral Solution and Tablets (17% to 25%) 3472
▲ Razadyne ER Extended-Release Capsules (5%) 2434
▲ Razadyne (5%) 2434
▲ Rebetol (Less than 1% to 16%) 3073
▲ Rebetron Combination Therapy (14% to 16%) 3078
Recombivax HB (Less than 1%) 2045
ReFacto Vials 3479
▲ Relafen Tablets (13%) 1523
▲ Relpax Tablets (1% to 2%) 2531
▲ Remicade for IV Injection (10%) 987
▲ Renagel Tablets (5% to 16.2%) 1268
ReoPro Vials (2.1%) 1779
▲ Requip Tablets (4% to 10%) 1528
Rescriptor Tablets 2535
▲ Retrovir Capsules (5% to 6%) 1533
▲ Retrovir IV Infusion (5% to 6%) 1537
▲ Retrovir (5% to 6%) 1533
▲ Revatio Tablets (13%) 2541
Reyataz Capsules (Less than 3%) 948
▲ Ribavirin, USP Capsules (Less than 1% to 16%) 3083
▲ Rilutek Tablets (2.5% to 6.1%) 2945
▲ Risperdal Consta Long-Acting Injection (7%) 1664
▲ Risperdal M-Tab Orally Disintegrating Tablets (5% to 11%) 1658
▲ Risperdal (5% to 11%) 1658
▲ Rituxan for Infusion (1% to 5%) 845
▲ Rituxan I.V. (1% to 5%) 1251
Rocephin Injectable Vials, ADD-Vantage, Galaxy, Bulk (Rare) 2801
Rythmol SR Capsules 2736
Sanctura Tablets (1.2%) 1133
▲ Sandostatin LAR Depot (5% to 15%) 2264
Serevent Diskus (1% to 3%) 1540
▲ Seroquel Tablets (5%) 691
▲ Simulect for Injection (Greater than or equal to 10%) 2268
Singulair (2.1%) 2047
Sonata Capsules (Frequent) 1686
Soriatane Capsules (Less than 1%) 1028
Spectracef Tablets (1% to 2%) 2706
▲ Spiriva HandiHaler (1% to 6%) 899
St. Joseph 81 mg Aspirin Chewable and Enteric Coated Tablets 1841
Stalevo Tablets (2%) 2270
▲ Strattera Capsules (4% to 8%) 1784
▲ Suboxone Tablets (3%) 2719
▲ Subutex Tablets (3%) 2719
Sular Tablets (Less than or equal to 1%) 1163
▲ Suprax (3%) 1811
Sustiva Capsules (1% to 4%) 957
Synercid I.V. (Less than 1%) 1690
Tambocor Tablets (1% to 3%) 1824
Targretin Capsules 1719
Tarka Tablets (0.3% or more) 519
▲ Tasmar Tablets (3% to 4%) 3360
▲ Tequin Injection (0.1% to 3%) 964
▲ Tequin Tablets (0.1% to 3%) 964
Teveten Tablets (1% or greater) 1707
Teveten HCT Tablets (Less than 1%) 1710
Thalomid Capsules 979
▲ Tiazac Capsules (4%) 1204
▲ Ticlid Tablets (7.0%) 2813
Timolide Tablets (Less than 1%) 2056
Timoptic in Ocudose (Less frequent) 2061
Timoptic Sterile Ophthalmic Solution 2058
Timoptic-XE Sterile Ophthalmic Gel Forming Solution 2062
Tindamax (1.4% to 1.8%) 2670
▲ Topamax Sprinkle Capsules (2% to 7%) 2438
▲ Topamax Tablets (2% to 7%) 2438
▲ Tracleer Tablets (4%) 539
Trasylol Injection (1% to 2%) 779
Travatan Ophthalmic Solution (1% to 5%) 559
Trelstar LA Suspension (1.7%) 3387
Tricor Tablets 523
Triglide Tablets 1165
▲ Trileptal Oral Suspension (2% to 6%) 2281
▲ Trileptal Tablets (2% to 6%) 2281
▲ Trisenox Injection (10%) 983
▲ Trizivir Tablets (5%) 1565
Truvada Tablets 1279
Twinrix Vaccine 1571
Tygacil for Injection (2.9%) 3489
Ultracet Tablets (At least 1%) 2462
Uniretic Tablets (More than 1%) 3114
Univasc Tablets (Greater than 1%) 3118
Uroxatral Tablets (1% to 2%) 2957
▲ Urso 250 Tablets (10%) 737
▲ Urso Forte Tablets (10%) 737
▲ Vagifem Tablets (3% to 5%) 2340
▲ Valcyte Tablets (Less than 5%) 2816
Vantin Tablets and Oral Suspension (Less than 1%) 2650
Vaseretic Tablets (0.5% to 2.0%) 2073
Vasotec I.V. Injection (0.5% to 1.0%) 2076
▲ Velcade for Injection (13%) 2102
Verelan PM Capsules (2.7%) 3120
▲ Vesanoid Capsules (14%) 2823
▲ VESIcare Tablets (1.4% to 3.9%) 631
VFEND I.V. (Less than 2%) 2543
VFEND Oral Suspension (Less than 2%) 2543
VFEND Tablets (Less than 2%) 2543
▲ Viagra Tablets (7%) 2552
▲ Vicoprofen Tablets (12%) 533
Viracept (Less than 2%) 2556
▲ Viread Tablets (3% to 4%) 1284
▲ Vivelle Transdermal System (Up to 9.2%) 2288
▲ Vivelle-Dot Transdermal System (Up to 9.2%) 2293
▲ Voltaren Tablets (1% to 10%) 2298
▲ Voltaren-XR Tablets (1% to 10%) 2301
Vytorin 10/10 Tablets 2084
Vytorin 10/10 Tablets 3092
Vytorin 10/20 Tablets 2084
Vytorin 10/20 Tablets 3092
Vytorin 10/40 Tablets 2084
Vytorin 10/40 Tablets 3092
Vytorin 10/80 Tablets 2084
Vytorin 10/80 Tablets 3092
▲ WelChol Tablets (8%) 2855
▲ Wellbutrin Tablets (3.1%) 1579
Wellbutrin SR Sustained-Release Tablets (At least 1%) 1583
Wellbutrin XL Extended-Release Tablets (At least 1%) 1588
Xanax XR Tablets (Frequent) 2655
Xopenex HFA Inhalation Aerosol (1.4% to 2.7%) 3151
Xopenex Inhalation Solution (1.4% to 2.7%) 3143
Xopenex Inhalation Solution Concentrate (1.4% to 2.7%) 3147
▲ Zavesca Capsules (7%) 543
Zelnorm Tablets 2303
Zemaira (0.2% to 0.4%) 3506
▲ Zenapax for Injection (Greater than 5%) 2838
Zestoretic Tablets (1.3%) 701
Zestril Tablets (0.3% to 1.0%) 704
▲ Zevalin Injection (4%) 848
Zithromax Capsules, 250 mg (1% or less) 2568
Zithromax for IV Infusion (1% or less) 2573
Zithromax for Oral Suspension, 1 g (1% or less to 1%) 2568
Zithromax for Oral Suspension, 300 mg, 600 mg, 900 mg, 1200 mg (1% or less) 2561
Zithromax Tablets, 250 mg, 500 mg (1% or less) 2561
Zithromax Tablets, 600 mg (1% or less to 1%) 2568
Zithromax Tri-Pak (1% or less) 2561
Zithromax Z-Pak (1% or less to 1%) 2568
Zmax for Oral Suspension (Less then 1%) 2577
Zocor Tablets (1.1%) 2078
Zoladex (1% or greater) 709
Zoladex 3-month 712
▲ Zoloft (6% to 13%) 2581
▲ Zometa for Intravenous Infusion (10%) 2306
Zomig Nasal Spray (Infrequent) 718
Zomig Tablets (1% to 3%) 714
▲ Zomig-ZMT Tablets (1% to 3%) 714
▲ Zonegran Capsules (3%) 1089
▲ Zosyn (1.9% to 3.3%) 3492
Zyban Sustained-Release Tablets (Frequent) 1620
▲ Zyprexa Tablets (11%) 1798
▲ Zyprexa ZYDIS Orally Disintegrating Tablets (11%) 1798
Zyrtec Chewable Tablets (Less than 2%) 2589
Zyrtec (Less than 2%) 2589
Zyrtec-D 12 Hour Extended Release Tablets (Less than 2%) 2591
Zyvox 2661

Dysphagia

Abilify Tablets (Infrequent) 916
Abilify Tablets (Infrequent) 2472
Aciphex Tablets 1081
Actiq (1% or greater) 993
Actonel Tablets 2679
Actonel with Calcium Tablets 2684
Adalat CC Tablets (Less than 1%) 2978
▲ Alimta for Injection (Up to 6%) 1722
Altace Capsules (Less than 1%) 1673
Ambien Tablets (Infrequent) 2867
AmBisome for Injection (Less common) 615
Arthrotec Tablets (Rare) 3126
Avelox (Less than 0.1%) 2984
Avinza Capsules (Less than 5%) 1714
▲ Botox Purified Neurotoxin Complex (19%) 565
Caduet Tablets (Greater than 0.1% to less than 2%) 2507
Campral Tablets (Infrequent) 1175
▲ Casodex Tablets (2% to 5%) 670
Celebrex Capsules (0.1% to 1.9%) 3130
Celexa (Infrequent) 1177
▲ CellCept Capsules (3% to less than 20%) 2751
▲ CellCept Intravenous (3% to less than 20%) 2751
▲ CellCept Oral Suspension (3% to less than 20%) 2751
▲ CellCept Tablets (3% to less than 20%) 2751
Cialis Tablets (Less than 2%) 1806
Cipro I.V. (1% or less) 2998
Cipro I.V. Pharmacy Bulk Package (1% or less) 3509
Cipro (Less than 1%) 2991
Cipro XR Tablets 3004
Clozapine Tablets 2141
Clozaril Tablets 2174
Copaxone for Injection (At least 2%) 3292
Cosmegen for Injection 1907
Cymbalta Delayed-Release Capsules (Infrequent) 1729
Depakote ER Tablets (Greater than 1%) 433
▲ Doxil Injection (1% to 10%) 3302
Edecrin 1941
Effexor Tablets (Infrequent) 3405
Effexor XR Capsules (Infrequent) 3411
Eldepryl Capsules 3209
Emend Capsules (Greater than 0.5%) 1944
Evoxac Capsules (Less than 1%) 1042
Exelon Capsules (Infrequent) 2204
FazaClo Orally Disintegrating Tablets 547

Flumadine 1186
Fosamax (0.1% to 1%) 1949
Fosamax Plus D Tablets (0.1% to 1%) 1956
Frova Tablets (Infrequent) 1101
Gabitril Tablets (Infrequent) 998
Gengraf Capsules (1% to less than 3%) 458
Geodon Capsules (2%) 2514
Imitrex Injection (1.1%) 1431
Imitrex Nasal Spray (Infrequent) 1435
Imitrex Tablets (Infrequent) 1440
▲ Intron A for Injection (Less than 5%) 3038
Invanz for Injection (Greater than 0.1%) 1974
Invirase (Less than 2%) 2776
Kadian Capsules (Less than 3%) 572
Kaletra (Up to 2%) 474
Lamictal (Infrequent) 1449
▲ Leukine (11%) 829
Levaquin in 5% Dextrose Injection (0.1% to 0.9%) 2453
Levaquin (0.1% to 0.9%) 2453
Levitra Tablets (Less than 2%) 3048
Lipitor Tablets (Less than 2%) 2495
Lunesta Tablets (Rare) 3139
Lupron Depot 7.5 mg (Less than 5%) 3261
Lupron Depot-PED 7.5 mg, 11.25 mg and 15 mg (Less than 2%) 3266
Lupron Injection Pediatric (Less than 2%) 3256
Lyrica Capsules (0.1% to 1%) 2524
Matulane Capsules 3188
Maxalt Tablets (Infrequent) 1983
Maxalt-MLT Orally Disintegrating Tablets (Infrequent) 1983
Migranal Nasal Spray (Infrequent) 3350
Mirapex Tablets (2%) 889
Namenda 1199
Navelbine Injection 1494
Neoral Soft Gelatin Capsules (1% to less than 3%) 2247
Neoral Oral Solution (1% to less than 3%) 2247
Neurontin Capsules (Rare) 2498
Neurontin Oral Solution (Rare) 2498
Neurontin Tablets (Rare) 2498
Nexium Delayed-Release Capsules (Less than 1%) 645
Nexium I.V. (Less than 1%) 649
Nipent for Injection (Less than 3%) 3216
Noroxin Tablets 2009
Norvasc Tablets (More than 0.1% to 1%) 2529
Norvir (Less than 2%) 499
Omacor Capsules 2735
▲ Ontak Vials (6%) 1717
Orap Tablets (2.7%) 1220
OxyContin Tablets (Less than 1%) 2699
Parcopa Orally Disintegrating Tablets 3111
Paxil CR Controlled-Release Tablets (Infrequent) 1509
Paxil (Infrequent) 1501
Pentasa Capsules (Less than 1%) 3182
Permax Tablets (Frequent) 3357
▲ Photofrin for Injection (10% to 24%) 729
Prevacid Delayed-Release Capsules (Less than 1%) 3268
Prevacid for Delayed-Release Oral Suspension (Less than 1%) 3268
Prevacid NapraPAC (Less than 1%) 3277
Prevacid SoluTab Delayed-Release Orally Disintegrating Tablets (Less than 1%) 3268
PREVPAC (Less than 1%) 3281
▲ Prograf Capsules and Injection (3% to 15%) 624
Protonix I.V. (Less than 1%) 3468
Protonix Tablets (Less than 1%) 3465
Prozac Pulvules and Liquid (Infrequent) 1771
▲ Rapamune Oral Solution and Tablets (3% to 20%) 3472
Razadyne ER Extended-Release Capsules (Infrequent) 2434
Razadyne (Infrequent) 2434
Relafen Tablets (Less than 1%) 1523
Relpax Tablets (1% to 2%) 2531
Remicade for IV Injection 987
Requip Tablets (Infrequent) 1528
Rescriptor Tablets 2535
Retrovir Capsules 1533
Retrovir IV Infusion 1537
Retrovir 1533
Rilutek Tablets (More than 2%) 2945
Risperdal Consta Long-Acting Injection (Infrequent) 1664
Risperdal M-Tab Orally Disintegrating Tablets (Infrequent) 1658
Risperdal (Infrequent) 1658
Rythmol SR Capsules 2736
Sandostatin LAR Depot (1% to 4%) 2264
Seroquel Tablets (Infrequent) 691
Sonata Capsules (Rare) 1686
Stalevo Tablets 2270
Sular Tablets (Less than or equal to 1%) 1163
Symmetrel 1115
Tasmar Tablets (Infrequent) 3360
Tequin Injection (Less than 0.1%) 964
Tequin Tablets (Less than 0.1%) 964
Thalomid Capsules 979
Topamax Sprinkle Capsules (1%) 2438
Topamax Tablets (1%) 2438
Trileptal Oral Suspension 2281
Trileptal Tablets 2281
Ultracet Tablets (Less than 1%) 2462
Uniretic Tablets (Less than 1%) 3114
VFEND I.V. (Less than 2%) 2543
VFEND Oral Suspension (Less than 2%) 2543
VFEND Tablets (Less than 2%) 2543
Viagra Tablets (Less than 2%) 2552
Vicoprofen Tablets (Less than 1%) 533
Wellbutrin Tablets (Infrequent) 1579
Wellbutrin SR Sustained-Release Tablets (Up to 2%) 1583
Wellbutrin XL Extended-Release Tablets (Up to 2%) 1588
Xanax XR Tablets (Infrequent) 2655
▲ Xeloda Tablets (Less than 5%) 2825
▲ Zinecard for Injection (Up to 8%) 2659
Zoloft (Infrequent) 2581
▲ Zometa for Intravenous Infusion (5% to 10%) 2306
Zomig Nasal Spray (1% to less than 2%) 718
Zomig Tablets (2%) 714
Zomig-ZMT Tablets (2%) 714
Zonegran Capsules (Infrequent) 1089
Zyban Sustained-Release Tablets (Infrequent) 1620
Zyprexa Tablets (Infrequent) 1798
Zyprexa ZYDIS Orally Disintegrating Tablets (Infrequent) 1798

Dysphasia

Ambien Tablets (Rare) 2867
Aricept Tablets (Infrequent) 1086
Aricept ODT Tablets (Infrequent) 1086
Cipro I.V. (1% or less) 2998
Cipro I.V. Pharmacy Bulk Package (1% or less) 3509
Cipro 2991
Cipro XR Tablets 3004
Cytovene 2763
Dynacin Tablets 1859
Imitrex Injection 1431
Imitrex Nasal Spray 1435
Roferon-A Injection (Infrequent) 2805
▲ Temodar Capsules (7%) 3088
▲ Xeloda Tablets (Less than 5%) 2825

Dysphonia

▲ Advair Diskus 100/50 (5%) 1291
Advair Diskus 250/50 (2% to 5%) 1291
▲ Advair Diskus 500/50 (2% to 5%) 1291
Colazal Capsules 2845
Combivent Inhalation Aerosol (Less than 2%) 878
Evoxac Capsules (Less than 1%) 1042
Exelon Capsules (Infrequent) 2204
▲ Flovent Diskus 50 mcg (1% to 9%) 1415
Flovent HFA (2%) 1418
Foradil Aerolizer (1%) 3024
▲ Intron A for Injection (Less than 5%) 3038
Proventil HFA Inhalation Aerosol (Less than 3%) 3071
Pulmicort Respules (1% to 3%) 654
Qvar Inhalation Aerosol (Up to 4%) 1654
ReoPro Vials (0.3%) 1779
Requip Tablets (Infrequent) 1528
Sandostatin LAR Depot (1% to 4%) 2264
Soriatane Capsules (Less than 1%) 1028
▲ Spiriva HandiHaler (1% to 3%) 899
Topamax Sprinkle Capsules (Infrequent) 2438
Topamax Tablets (Infrequent) 2438
Trileptal Oral Suspension 2281
Trileptal Tablets 2281
Xanax XR Tablets (Infrequent) 2655
Zoloft (Rare) 2581
Zyrtec Chewable Tablets (Less than 2%) 2589
Zyrtec (Less than 2%) 2589
Zyrtec-D 12 Hour Extended Release Tablets (Less than 2%) 2591

Dysphoria

Abilify Tablets (Infrequent) 916
Abilify Tablets (Infrequent) 2472
Actiq 993
Adderall Tablets 3168
Adderall XR Capsules 3169
Adipex-P 1216
Advair Diskus 100/50 1291
Advair Diskus 250/50 1291
Advair Diskus 500/50 1291
Alacol DM Syrup 739
Aldoclor Tablets 1881
Aldoril Tablets 1884
Allegra-D 12 Hour Extended-Release Tablets 2860
Allegra-D 24 Hour Extended-Release Tablets 2862
Ambien Tablets 2867
Amerge Tablets (Rare) 1312
Aricept Tablets (Infrequent) 1086
Aricept ODT Tablets (Infrequent) 1086
Atacand HCT 637
Avalide Tablets 922
Avalide Tablets 2889
Axert Tablets (Infrequent) 2430
Buprenex Injectable (Rare) 2718
Cafcit 1854
Catapres Tablets 874
Catapres-TTS (0.5% or less) 875
Cipro I.V. (Greater than 1%) 2998
Cipro I.V. Pharmacy Bulk Package (Greater than 1%) 3509
Cipro (Less than 1.1%) 2991
Cipro XR Tablets 3004
Clorpres Tablets 2139
▲ Clozapine Tablets (4%) 2141
▲ Clozaril Tablets (4%) 2174
Cymbalta Delayed-Release Capsules (Frequent) 1729
Dalmane Capsules (Rare) 3343
Darvocet A 500 Tablets 3497
Desoxyn Tablets, USP (Rare) 2482
Dexedrine 1386
DextroStat Tablets 3177
Dilaudid 439
Dilaudid Oral Liquid 443
Dilaudid Non-Sterile Powder 439
Dilaudid Rectal Suppositories 439
Dilaudid Tablets 439
Dilaudid Tablets - 8 mg 443
Dilaudid-HP (Less frequent) 441
Diovan HCT Tablets 2195
Diuril Oral 1936
Diuril Sodium Intravenous 1934
Eldepryl Capsules 3209
Eskalith 1406
▲ FazaClo Orally Disintegrating Tablets (4%) 547
Flovent Diskus 50 mcg 1415
Flovent HFA 1418
Furosemide Tablets 2117
Hycodan 1104
Hycomine Compound Tablets 1105
Hycotuss Expectorant Syrup 1106
Hyzaar 1964
▲ Infanrix Vaccine (8.6% to 15.9%) 1444
Lamictal (Infrequent) 1449
Lariam Tablets 2790
Levaquin in 5% Dextrose Injection 2453
Levaquin 2453
Lexapro Oral Solution (Infrequent) 1193
Lexapro Tablets (Infrequent) 1193
Lithobid Tablets 1670
Lortab 3315
Lortab Elixir 3312
Lotensin HCT Tablets 2235
Maxzide 2150
Micardis HCT Tablets 886
Moduretic Tablets 2003
▲ MS Contin Tablets (Among most frequent) 2703
Namenda 1199
Narcan Injection 1109
Naropin Injection 640
Nitrolingual Pumpspray 1161
Noroxin Tablets 2009
Novarel for Injection 1147
Nubain Injection (1% or less) 1111
Numorphan 1112
Oxsoralen-Ultra Capsules 3354
OxyFast Oral Concentrate Solution 2704
OxyIR Capsules 2704
Parnate Tablets 1499
Percocet Tablets 1114
Percodan Tablets 1115
Prinzide Tablets 2033
Rescriptor Tablets 2535
Singulair (Very rare) 2047
Surmontil Capsules 2347
Tequin Injection 964
Tequin Tablets 964
Teveten HCT Tablets 1710
Thioridazine Hydrochloride Tablets (Extremely rare) 2122
Thiothixene Capsules 2124
Timolide Tablets 2056
Transderm Scōp Transdermal Therapeutic System (Infrequent) 2166
Trecator Tablets 3482
Tussionex Pennkinetic Extended-Release Suspension 3322
Tylenol with Codeine 2461
Uniphyl Tablets 2708
Uniretic Tablets 3114
Vaseretic Tablets 2073
Vicodin Tablets 530
Vicodin ES Tablets 531
Vicodin HP Tablets 532
Vivactil Tablets 2350
VoSpire Extended-Release Tablets (Less frequent) 2352
Wellbutrin Tablets (Infrequent) 1579
Wellbutrin SR Sustained-Release Tablets (Infrequent) 1583
Wellbutrin XL Extended-Release Tablets (Infrequent) 1588
Xanax XR Tablets (Frequent) 2655
Zelnorm Tablets 2303
Zestoretic Tablets 701
Zyban Sustained-Release Tablets (Less than 1%) 1620
Zydone Tablets 1118

Dysplasia, cervical

Vivelle Transdermal System 2288
▲ Vivelle-Dot Transdermal System (1.9% to 4.3%) 2293

Dysplasia, gastrointestinal

Nexium Delayed-Release Capsules (Less than 1%) 645
Nexium I.V. (Less than 1%) 649

Dysplasia, unspecified

Reyataz Capsules (Less than 3%) 948

Dyspnea

▲ Abelcet Injection (7%) 1119
Abilify Tablets (Frequent) 916
Abilify Tablets (Frequent) 2472
Aceon Tablets (2 mg, 4 mg, 8 mg) (0.3% to 1%) 3191
Aciphex Tablets 1081
Acthrel for Injection 3528
▲ Actiq (2% to 6%) 993
▲ Actonel Tablets (3.8%) 2679
▲ Actonel with Calcium Tablets (3.8%) 2684
Actos Tablets 3224
Adacel Vaccine 2959
Adalat CC Tablets (Less than 1%) 2978
▲ Adderall XR Capsules (2% to 4%) 3169
▲ Adenocard Injection (12%) 612
▲ Adenoscan (Approximately 28%) 613
Advair Diskus 100/50 1291
Advair Diskus 250/50 1291
Advair Diskus 500/50 1291
Advate Injection (0.6%) 742
Advicor Tablets 1694
Aerobid/Aerobid-M (1% to 3%) 1172
Aggrenox Capsules 855
▲ Agrylin Capsules (11.9%) 3172
Aldara Cream, 5% 1814
Aldurazyme for Intravenous Infusion 1261
▲ Alimta for Injection (1% to 72%) 1722
Alkeran for Injection (In some patients) 976
Allegra (Rare) 2857
Allegra-D 12 Hour Extended-Release Tablets (Rare) 2860
Allegra-D 24 Hour Extended-Release Tablets (Rare) 2862
Alphagan P Ophthalmic Solution (1% to 4%) 563
Altace Capsules (Less than 1%) 1673
Altoprev Extended-Release Tablets (Rare) 1151
Ambien Tablets (Infrequent) 2867
▲ AmBisome for Injection (17.6% to 23%) 615
Amerge Tablets 1312
Ammonul Injection 3323
▲ Anaprox Tablets (3% to 9%) 2769
▲ Anaprox DS Tablets (3% to 9%) 2769
Antara Capsules 2723
Anzemet Injection (Rare) 2871
Anzemet Tablets (Rare) 2874
▲ Apokyn Injection (At least 5%) 2132
Aptivus Capsules (Less than 2%) 859
AquaMEPHYTON Injection 1887

Aralast (0.1%) 745
▲ Aranesp for Injection (12%) 576
▲ Arava Tablets (1% to 3%) 2881
▲ Aredia for Injection (Up to 23.3%) 2168
▲ Argatroban Injection (8.1%) 1321
Aricept Tablets (Frequent) 1086
Aricept ODT Tablets (Frequent) 1086
▲ Arimidex Tablets (6% to 11%) 665
▲ Aromasin Tablets (10%) 2600
Arthrotec Tablets (Rare) 3126
Astelin Nasal Spray 1876
Atacand Tablets (0.5% or greater) 634
Atacand HCT (0.5% or greater) 637
▲ Atrovent HFA Inhalation Aerosol (7% to 8%) 872
▲ Atrovent Inhalation Solution (9.6%) 868
Avalide Tablets 922
Avalide Tablets 2889
Avapro Tablets (Less than 1%) 925
Avapro Tablets (Less than 1%) 2886
▲ Avastin IV (25% to 26%) 1229
Avelox (0.1% to less than 2%) 2984
▲ Avinza Capsules (5% to 10%) 1714
Avonex 839
Axert Tablets (Infrequent) 2430
Azopt Ophthalmic Suspension (Less than 1%) 553
▲ BeneFix for Injection (3.2%) 3402
Bentyl Capsules 724
Bentyl Injection 724
Bentyl Syrup 724
Bentyl Tablets 724
Betagan Ophthalmic Solution, USP ⊙ 217
▲ Betaseron for SC Injection (7%) 791
Betimol Ophthalmic Solution ⊙ 283
Betimol Ophthalmic Solution 3371
Betoptic S Ophthalmic Suspension (Rare) 554
▲ Bexxar (3% to 11%) 1360
Blocadren Tablets (1.7%) 1891
Boostrix (Rarely) 1366
Botox Purified Neurotoxin Complex (Rare) 565
Bravelle for Intramuscular or Subcutaneous Injection 1140
Brevibloc Concentrate (Less than 1%) 766
Brevibloc Injection (Less than 1%) 766
Brevibloc Double Strength Injection (Less than 1%) 766
Brevibloc Premixed Injection (Less than 1%) 766
Brevibloc Double Strength Premixed Injection (Less than 1%) 766
Buprenex Injectable (Less than 1%) 2718
Caduet Tablets (Less than 1% to 2%) 2507
Cafcit (2.2%) 1854
▲ Campath Ampules (9% to 26%) 826
Campral Tablets (Frequent) 1175
▲ Camptosar Injection (2.2% to 22%) 2602
Cancidas for Injection (2%) 1894
Captopril Tablets (About 0.5% to 2%) 2114
Carbatrol Capsules 3174
Cardene I.V. (0.7%) 1129
Cardizem LA Extended Release Tablets (Less than 2%) 1699
Carimune NF 3501
▲ Carnitor Injection (3% to 11%) 3185
Carteolol Hydrochloride Ophthalmic Solution USP, 1% (Occasional) ⊙ 246
▲ Casodex Tablets (7%) 670
Cataflam Tablets (Occasionally) 2173
Celebrex Capsules (0.1% to 1.9%) 3130
Celexa (Infrequent) 1177
▲ CellCept Capsules (31% to 36.7%) 2751
▲ CellCept Intravenous (31% to 36.7%) 2751
▲ CellCept Oral Suspension (31% to 36.7%) 2751
▲ CellCept Tablets (31% to 36.7%) 2751
▲ Cerezyme for Injection (Approximately 6.6%) 1263
Cialis Tablets (Less than 2%) 1806
Cipro I.V. (1% or less) 2998
Cipro I.V. Pharmacy Bulk Package (1% or less) 3509
Cipro (Less than 1%) 2991
Clarinex Syrup (Rare) 3009
Clarinex Tablets (Rare) 3009
Clarinex Reditabs Tablets (Rare) 3009
Clarinex-D 24-Hour Extended-Release Tablets 3012
Clinoril Tablets (Less than 1%) 1899
Clozapine Tablets (1%) 2141
Clozaril Tablets (1%) 2174
Colazal Capsules 2845
▲ Combivent Inhalation Aerosol (4.5%) 878
▲ Comtan Tablets (3%) 2186
Comvax 1904
▲ Copaxone for Injection (19%) 3292
▲ Copegus Tablets (13%) 2759
▲ Coreg Tablets (Greater than 3%) 1376
Cosopt Sterile Ophthalmic Solution (Less than 1%) 1910
Coumadin for Injection 932
Coumadin Tablets 932
Covera-HS Tablets (1.4% to 2%) 3135
Cozaar Tablets (Less than 1%) 1913
Crestor Tablets (Greater than or equal to 1%) 672
Crixivan Capsules 1918
Crolom Cromolyn Sodium Sterile Ophthalmic Solution USP 4% ⊙ 248
Cubicin for Injection (2.1%) 1038
Cytovene (At least 3 subjects) 2763
▲ Depacon Injection (1% to 5%) 412
▲ Depakene (5%) 417
▲ Depakote Sprinkle Capsules (1% to 5%) 422
▲ Depakote Tablets (1% to 5%) 427
▲ Depakote ER Tablets (1% to 5%) 433
▲ DepoDur Extended-Release Injection (2% to 5%) 1098
Depo-Provera Contraceptive Injection (Less than 1%) 2619
depo-subQ provera 104 Injectable Suspension 2622
Diovan HCT Tablets (Greater than 0.2%) 2195
Diovan Tablets 2191
Diprivan Injectable Emulsion (Less than 1%) 676
Dolobid Tablets (Rare) 1937
▲ Doxil Injection (1% to 15.1%) 3302
▲ Duragesic Transdermal System (3% to 10%) 2448
DynaCirc CR Tablets (0.5% to 1%) 2726
▲ EC-Naprosyn Delayed-Release Tablets (3% to 9%) 2769
Effexor Tablets (Frequent) 3405
Effexor XR Capsules (Frequent) 3411
Elitek 2906
Ellence Injection 2632
Elmiron Capsules (Less than or equal to 1%) 2393
▲ Eloxatin for Injection (5% to 20%) 2908
▲ Emcyt Capsules (11%) 3137
Emend Capsules (Greater than 0.5%) 1944
Enbrel for Injection (Infrequent) 580
▲ Entocort EC Capsules (Less than 5%) 2694
Equetro Extended-Release Capsules 3178
▲ Erbitux (20%) 937
Ethyol for Injection 1869
Evoxac Capsules (Less than 1%) 1042
Fabrazyme for Intravenous Infusion 1267
Factive Tablets (Less than or equal to 0.1%) 2464
▲ Faslodex Injection (14.9%) 682
FazaClo Orally Disintegrating Tablets (1%) 547
▲ Femara Tablets (0.8% to 18%) 2210
▲ Ferrlecit Injection (11%) 3379
Flexeril Tablets (Rare) 1832
▲ Flolan for Injection (2% to 100%) 1408
▲ Flonase Nasal Spray (1% to 3%) 1412
Flovent Diskus 50 mcg 1415
Flovent HFA 1418
Flumadine (0.3% to 1%) 1186
Follistim AQ Cartridge 2354
Foradil Aerolizer (2.1%) 3024
▲ Forteo for Injection (3.6%) 1739
Fortical Nasal Spray (Less than 1%) 3336
Frova Tablets (Infrequent) 1101
Gabitril Tablets (Frequent) 998
Gammagard Liquid 751
Gammagard S/D 754
Gamunex Immune Globulin I.V., 10% 3232
▲ Gemzar for Injection (3% to 23%) 1743
▲ Gengraf Capsules (1% to 5%) 458
Geodon Capsules (2%) 2514
▲ Gleevec Tablets (12% to 21%) 2221
GlucaGen for Injection (Rare) 790
Havrix Vaccine (Rare) 1425
▲ Hectorol Capsules (Greater than or equal to 5% to 11.5%) 909
▲ Hectorol Injection (11.5%) 911
▲ Herceptin I.V. (22%) 1234
▲ Humira Injection (Less than 5%) 464
▲ Hycamtin for Injection (1.8% to 20%) 1427
Hyperstat I.V. Injection 3031
▲ Hytrin Capsules (0.5% to 3.1%) 469
Hyzaar 1964
▲ Imdur Tablets (Less than or equal to 5%) 3032
Imitrex Injection (Infrequent) 1431
Imitrex Nasal Spray (Infrequent) 1435
Imitrex Tablets (Frequent) 1440
Indocin Capsules (Less than 1%) 1968
Indocin I.V. (Less than 1%) 1973
Indocin (Less than 1%) 1968
Infanrix Vaccine 1444
Infed Injection 3381
▲ Infergen (7% to 8%) 1647
▲ Intron A for Injection (Up to 34%) 3038
Invanz for Injection (1% to 2.6%) 1974
Invirase (Less than 2%) 2776
Iressa Tablets (2%) 684
▲ I.V. Busulfex (2% to 25%) 1125
Iveegam EN 759
Kadian Capsules (Less than 3%) 572
Kaletra (Less than 2%) 474
Klonopin (Infrequent) 2782
K-Phos Neutral Tablets 785
K-Phos Original (Sodium Free) Tablets (Less frequent) 785
Lamictal (1.1%) 1449
Lariam Tablets 2790
Lescol Capsules (Rare) 2227
Lescol Capsules (Rare) 2730
Lescol XL Tablets 2227
Lescol XL Tablets 2730
▲ Leukine (15% to 28%) 829
▲ Leustatin Injection (11%) 2368
Levaquin in 5% Dextrose Injection (0.1% to 1.3%) 2453
Levaquin (0.1% to 1.3%) 2453
Levitra Tablets (Less than 2%) 3048
Levothroid Tablets 1189
Levoxyl Tablets 1680
Lidoderm Patch 1107
Lipitor Tablets (Less than 2%) 2495
Lofibra Capsules 1217
Lortab 3315
Lortab Elixir 3312
Lotensin Tablets (Less than 1%) 2232
▲ Lovenox Injection (3.3%) 2931
Lunesta Tablets (Infrequent) 3139
▲ Lupron Depot 7.5 mg (5.4%) 3261
▲ Lyrica Capsules (2% to 3%) 2524
Mavik Tablets (0.3% to 1.0%) 482
Maxalt Tablets (Frequent) 1983
Maxalt-MLT Orally Disintegrating Tablets (Frequent) 1983
Mefoxin for Injection 1987
Mefoxin Premixed Intravenous Solution 1990
▲ Megace ES Oral Suspension (1% to 3%) 2492
Mephyton Tablets (Rare) 1993
▲ Mepron Suspension (15% to 21%) 1487
Meridia Capsules (Greater than or equal to 1%) 485
Merrem I.V. (Greater than 0.1% to 1%) 687
Mevacor Tablets (Rare) 1996
Miacalcin Nasal Spray (Less than 1%) 2242
Micardis Tablets (More than 0.3%) 884
Micardis HCT Tablets 886
▲ Midamor Tablets (Between 1% and 3%) 2000
Migranal Nasal Spray (Infrequent) 3350
▲ Mirapex Tablets (Greater than or equal to 1% to 4%) 889
Mobic Oral Suspension (Less than 2%) 893
Mobic Tablets (Less than 2%) 893
Moduretic Tablets (Greater than 1%, less than 3%) 2003
Mycamine for Injection 620
▲ Myfortic Tablets (3% to less than 20%) 2244
▲ Mylotarg for Injection (26%) 3429
Nalfon Capsules (2.8%) 2504
Namenda (2%) 1199
▲ Naprosyn Suspension (3% to 9%) 2769
▲ Naprosyn Tablets (3% to 9%) 2769
Narcan Injection 1109
Naropin Injection (Less than 1%) 640
Nasacort HFA Inhalation Aerosol 2939
Navelbine Injection (Up to 3%) 1494
▲ Neoral Soft Gelatin Capsules (1% to 5%) 2247
▲ Neoral Oral Solution (1% to 5.0%) 2247
▲ Neumega for Injection (48%) 3433
▲ Neupogen for Injection (9%) 598
Neurontin Capsules (Infrequent) 2498
Neurontin Oral Solution (Infrequent) 2498
Neurontin Tablets (Infrequent) 2498
Nexium Delayed-Release Capsules (Less than 1%) 645
Nexium I.V. (Less than 1%) 649
Niaspan Extended-Release Tablets 1703
Nicotrol NS (5%) 2596
Nimotop Capsules (Up to 1.2%) 774
▲ Nipent for Injection (8% to 11%) 3216
Noroxin Tablets 2009
Norvasc Tablets (Less than 1% to 2%) 2529
Norvir (Less than 2%) 499
Novantrone for Injection Concentrate 3158
Novarel for Injection 1147
Nubain Injection (1% or less) 1111
Omacor Capsules 2735
▲ Oncaspar (Greater than 5%) 1123
▲ Ontak Vials (29%) 1717
OptiPranolol Metipranolol Ophthalmic Solution 0.3% (A small number of patients) ⊙ 254
▲ Optivar Ophthalmic Solution (1% to 10%) 1877
▲ Orthoclone OKT3 Sterile Solution (21%) 2370
▲ OxyContin Tablets (Between 1% and 5%) 2699
▲ Pacerone Tablets (2% to 7%) 3337
Parcopa Orally Disintegrating Tablets 3111
Paxil CR Controlled-Release Tablets (Infrequent) 1509
Paxil (Infrequent) 1501
Pediarix Vaccine (Rare) 1518
▲ Pegasys (Less than 1% to 4%) 2793
▲ PEG-Intron Powder for Injection (4%) 3062
Pentasa Capsules (One case) 3182
▲ Permax Tablets (4.8%) 3357
▲ Photofrin for Injection (6% to 20%) 729
▲ Plavix Tablets (4.5%) 940
▲ Plavix Tablets (4.5%) 2942
Plendil Extended-Release Tablets (0.5% to 1.5%) 651
Pletal Tablets (2% or greater) 2478
Pravachol Tablets (Rare) 943
Prevacid Delayed-Release Capsules (Less than 1%) 3268
Prevacid for Delayed-Release Oral Suspension (Less than 1%) 3268
▲ Prevacid NapraPAC (Less than 1% to 9%) 3277
Prevacid SoluTab Delayed-Release Orally Disintegrating Tablets (Less than 1%) 3268
PREVPAC (Less than 1%) 3281
Primaxin I.M. 2022
Primaxin I.V. (Less than 0.2%) 2024
Prinivil Tablets (Greater than 1%) 2029
Prinzide Tablets (0.3% to 1%) 2033
Prochieve 4% Gel 1018
Prochieve 8% Gel 1018
▲ Prograf Capsules and Injection (5% to 29%) 624
Prolastin (Occasional) 3252
▲ Proleukin for Injection (43%) 1007
ProSom Tablets (Infrequent) 512
Protonix I.V. (Greater than or equal to 1%) 3468
Protonix Tablets (Greater than or equal to 1%) 3465
Protopic Ointment (Greater than or equal to 1%) 629
Proventil Inhalation Solution 0.083% (1.5%) 3069
Provigil Tablets (Greater than or equal to 1%) 1002
▲ Pulmozyme Inhalation Solution (17%) 1245
▲ Rapamune Oral Solution and Tablets (22% to 30%) 3472
Raptiva for Injection 1247
▲ Rebetol (5% to 26%) 3073
▲ Rebetron Combination Therapy (17% to 19%) 3078
Recombivax HB (Less than 1%) 2045
ReFacto Vials 3479
Refludan for Injection (Common) 815
Relafen Tablets (1%) 1523
Relenza Rotadisk (Less than 1%) 1525
Relpax Tablets (Infrequent) 2531
Remicade for IV Injection (1%) 987
▲ Renagel Tablets (10.1%) 1268
Repronex for Intramuscular and Subcutaneous Injection (1% to 2.1%) 1148
▲ Requip Tablets (3%) 1528
Rescriptor Tablets 2535
▲ Retrovir Capsules (5%) 1533
▲ Retrovir IV Infusion (5%) 1537
▲ Retrovir (5%) 1533
Reyataz Capsules (Less than 3%) 948
Rhophylac (Rare) 3504
▲ Ribavirin, USP Capsules (5% to 26%) 3083

(▣ Described in PDR For Nonprescription Drugs)   Incidence data in parenthesis; ▲ 3% or more   (⊙ Described in PDR For Ophthalmic Medicines™)

Rilutek Tablets (More than 2%) 2945
Risperdal Consta Long-Acting Injection (Frequent) 1664
Risperdal M-Tab Orally Disintegrating Tablets (Up to 1%) .. 1658
Risperdal (Up to 1%) 1658
Rituxan for Infusion (0.3%) 845
▲ Rituxan I.V. (7%) 1251
▲ Roferon-A Injection (More than 1% to 12%) 2805
▲ Rythmol SR Capsules (13% to 17%) 2736
Sandimmune 2259
Seroquel Tablets (Infrequent) 691
▲ Simulect for Injection (Greater than or equal to 10%) 2268
Sonata Capsules (Infrequent) 1686
▲ Stalevo Tablets (3%) 2270
Striant Mucoadhesive 1022
Stromectol Tablets 2053
Sular Tablets (Less than or equal to 1%) 1163
Suprane Liquid for Inhalation (Less than 1%) 770
Sustiva Capsules 957
Symbyax Capsules (1% to 2%) 1788
Symmetrel (0.1% to 1%) 1115
Synagis (More than 1%) 1868
Synercid I.V. (Less than 1%) 1690
▲ Tambocor Tablets (10.3%) 1824
▲ Tarceva Tablets (11% to 41%) 1254
▲ Tarceva Tablets (11% to 41%) 2470
Targretin Capsules 1719
Tarka Tablets (1.3%) 519
▲ Tasmar Tablets (3%) 3360
▲ Taxotere Injection Concentrate (6%) 2947
Tegretol/Tegretol-XR 2278
▲ Temodar Capsules (5%) 3088
▲ Tenormin I.V. Injection (0.6% to 6%) 698
▲ Tenormin Tablets (0.6% to 6%) 695
▲ Tequin Injection (0.1% to 3%) 964
▲ Tequin Tablets (0.1% to 3%) 964
Thalomid Capsules 979
▲ Thymoglobulin for Injection (28%) ... 2848
Tiazac Capsules (Less than 2%) 1204
Timolide Tablets (1.2%) 2056
Timoptic in Ocudose (Less frequent) 2061
Timoptic Sterile Ophthalmic Solution (Less frequent) 2058
Timoptic-XE Sterile Ophthalmic Gel Forming Solution 2062
Tindamax (Rare) 2670
▲ TOBI Solution for Inhalation (33.7%) 1015
▲ Topamax Sprinkle Capsules (1% to 3%) 2438
▲ Topamax Tablets (1% to 3%) 2438
Toprol-XL Tablets (Greater than 1%) 660
▲ Trasylol Injection (4%) 779
Trelstar LA Suspension (1.1%) 3387
Tricor Tablets 523
TriLyte with Flavor Packs for Oral Solution 3114
▲ Trisenox Injection (53%) 983
Trizivir Tablets 1565
Trusopt Sterile Ophthalmic Solution 2065
Truvada Tablets 1279
Twinrix Vaccine 1571
Tygacil for Injection (2.9%) 3489
Ultracet Tablets (Less than 1%) 2462
Uniretic Tablets (Less than 1%) 3114
Unithroid Tablets 3521
Univasc Tablets (Less than 1%) 3118
Uroqid-Acid No. 2 Tablets 785
▲ Valcyte Tablets (Less than 5%) 2816
Valtrex Caplets 1573
Vancocin HCl Capsules, USP 3370
Vantin Tablets and Oral Suspension (Less than 1%) 2650
Vaseretic Tablets (0.5% to 2.0%) 2073
Vasotec I.V. Injection (0.5% to 1.3%) 2076
▲ Velcade for Injection (20%) 2102
Ventavis Inhalation Solution 1036
Verelan PM Capsules (2% or less) 3120
▲ Vesanoid Capsules (60%) 2823
VFEND I.V. (Less than 2%) 2543
VFEND Oral Suspension (Less than 2%) 2543
VFEND Tablets (Less than 2%) 2543
Viadur Implant (2.3%) 782
Viagra Tablets (Less than 2%) 2552
Vicoprofen Tablets (Less than 3%) ... 533
Viracept (Less than 2%) 2556
Virazole for Inhalation Solution 3365
Viread Tablets 1284
Voltaren Tablets (Occasionally) 2298
Voltaren-XR Tablets (Occasionally) 2301
Vytorin 10/10 Tablets 2084
Vytorin 10/10 Tablets 3092
Vytorin 10/20 Tablets 2084
Vytorin 10/20 Tablets 3092
Vytorin 10/40 Tablets 2084
Vytorin 10/40 Tablets 3092
Vytorin 10/80 Tablets 2084
Vytorin 10/80 Tablets 3092
Wellbutrin Tablets (Infrequent) 1579
Wellbutrin SR Sustained-Release Tablets 1583
Wellbutrin XL Extended-Release Tablets 1588
Xalatan Sterile Ophthalmic Solution 2654
Xanax XR Tablets (1.5%) 2655
▲ Xeloda Tablets (Less than 5%) 2825
Xifaxan Tablets (Less than 2%) 2847
Xopenex HFA Inhalation Aerosol 3151
Xopenex Inhalation Solution 3143
Xopenex Inhalation Solution Concentrate 3147
Zelnorm Tablets 2303
Zemaira (0.2% to 0.4%) 3506
▲ Zenapax for Injection (Greater than 5%) 2838
Zestoretic Tablets (0.3% to 1%) 701
Zestril Tablets (Greater than 1%) 704
▲ Zevalin Injection (14%) 848
Ziagen 1600
Zithromax for IV Infusion (1.9%) 2573
Zocor Tablets (Rare) 2078
▲ Zoladex 3-month (1% to 5%) 712
Zoloft (Infrequent) 2581
▲ Zometa for Intravenous Infusion (22.1% to 27%) 2306
Zomig Nasal Spray (Infrequent) 718
Zonegran Capsules (Infrequent) 1089
Zyban Sustained-Release Tablets (1%) 1620
Zyprexa Tablets (Frequent) 1798
Zyprexa ZYDIS Orally Disintegrating Tablets (Frequent) ... 1798
Zyrtec Chewable Tablets (Less than 2%) 2589
Zyrtec (Less than 2%) 2589
Zyrtec-D 12 Hour Extended Release Tablets (Less than 2%) 2591
Zyvox 2661

Dyspnea, aggravation of

▲ Revatio Tablets (7%) 2541
Toprol-XL Tablets (Greater than 1%) 660

Dyspnea, exertional

Clozaril Tablets 2174
▲ Copegus Tablets (4%) 2759
▲ Myfortic Tablets (3% to less than 20%) 2244
Neumega for Injection 3433
Pegasys (Less than 1%) 2793
Vantas (Less than 2%) 3367

Dyspnea, nocturnal

Prinivil Tablets (0.3% to 1.0%) 2029
Prinzide Tablets 2033
Zestoretic Tablets 701
Zestril Tablets (0.3% to 1.0%) 704

Dyspnea, nocturnal, paroxysmal

Clozaril Tablets 2174
Herceptin I.V. 1234

Dysrhythmia

Camptosar Injection 2602
Ecotrin Enteric Coated Aspirin Low, Regular and Maximum Strength Tablets 1627
▲ Roferon-A Injection (7%) 2805
St. Joseph 81 mg Aspirin Chewable and Enteric Coated Tablets 1841
Taxotere Injection Concentrate (Rare) 2947

Dysthesias

▲ Campath Ampules (15%) 826

Dystonia

Abilify Tablets (Infrequent) 916
Abilify Tablets (Infrequent) 2472
Aloprim for Injection (Less than 1%) 2156
AmBisome for Injection (Less common) 615
Celexa (Infrequent) 1177
Clozapine Tablets 2141
Clozaril Tablets 2174
Cuprimine Capsules 1925
Diprivan Injectable Emulsion (Less than 1%) 676
Effexor Tablets (Rare) 3405
Effexor XR Capsules (Rare) 3411
Eldepryl Capsules 3209
Eskalith (One report in a child) 1406
Gabitril Tablets (Infrequent) 998
▲ Geodon Capsules (4% to 14%) 2514
Imitrex Injection (Rare) 1431
Imitrex Tablets (Rare) 1440
Lamictal (Rare) 1449
Lexapro Oral Solution 1193
Lexapro Tablets 1193
Lyrica Capsules (Rare) 2524
Migranal Nasal Spray (Infrequent) 3350
▲ Mirapex Tablets (2% to 8%) 889
Moban Tablets (Infrequent) 1108
Neurontin Capsules (Infrequent) 2498
Neurontin Oral Solution (Infrequent) 2498
Neurontin Tablets (Infrequent) 2498
Niravam Orally Disintegrating Tablets 3106
Orap Tablets (Less frequent) 1220
Parcopa Orally Disintegrating Tablets (Common) 3111
Paxil CR Controlled-Release Tablets (Infrequent) 1509
Paxil (Infrequent) 1501
▲ Permax Tablets (11.6%) 3357
Phenytek Capsules (Rare) 2153
Prozac Pulvules and Liquid (Rare) 1771
Relpax Tablets (Rare) 2531
Requip Tablets (1% or more) 1528
Risperdal Consta Long-Acting Injection (Frequent) 1664
▲ Risperdal M-Tab Orally Disintegrating Tablets (17% to 34%) 1658
▲ Risperdal (17% to 34%) 1658
Symbyax Capsules (Rare) 1788
Syprine Capsules 2055
▲ Tasmar Tablets (19% to 22%) 3360
Thioridazine Hydrochloride Tablets .. 2122
Thiothixene Capsules 2124
Topamax Sprinkle Capsules (Infrequent) 2438
Topamax Tablets (Infrequent) 2438
Trileptal Oral Suspension 2281
Trileptal Tablets 2281
Wellbutrin Tablets (Frequent) 1579
Wellbutrin SR Sustained-Release Tablets 1583
Wellbutrin XL Extended-Release Tablets 1588
Zofran Injection 1607
Zofran 1613
Zofran ODT Orally Disintegrating Tablets 1613
Zoloft (Infrequent) 2581
Zomig Tablets (Rare) 714
Zomig-ZMT Tablets (Rare) 714
Zonegran Capsules (Rare) 1089
Zyban Sustained-Release Tablets 1620
▲ Zyprexa Tablets (2% to 3%) 1798
Zyprexa ZYDIS Orally Disintegrating Tablets (2% to 3%) 1798

Dystonia, tardive

Thioridazine Hydrochloride Tablets .. 2122
Thiothixene Capsules 2124

Dystonic reactions
(*see under* Dystonia)

Dysuria

Abelcet Injection 1119
Abilify Tablets (Infrequent) 916
Abilify Tablets (Infrequent) 2472
Aciphex Tablets 1081
Actiq (Less than 1%) 993
Adalat CC Tablets (Less than 1%) 2978
Agrylin Capsules (1% to 5%) 3172
Alferon N Injection (1%) 1640
Alinia for Oral Suspension (Less than 1%) 2840
Alinia Tablets (Less than 1%) 2840
Allegra-D 12 Hour Extended-Release Tablets 2860
Allegra-D 24 Hour Extended-Release Tablets 2862
Ambien Tablets (Rare) 2867
AmBisome for Injection (Less common) 615
Anaprox Tablets (Less than 1%) 2769
Anaprox DS Tablets (Less than 1%) .. 2769
Antara Capsules 2723
Anzemet Injection (Rare) 2871
Anzemet Tablets (Rare) 2874
Aricept Tablets (Infrequent) 1086
Aricept ODT Tablets (Infrequent) 1086
Arthrotec Tablets (Rare) 3126
Asacol Delayed-Release Tablets 2688
Avinza Capsules (Less than 5%) 1714
Balamine DM 739
Caduet Tablets (Less than 2%) 2507
▲ Casodex Tablets (2% to 5%) 670
Cataflam Tablets (Occasionally) 2173
Ceftin Tablets (0.1% to 1%) 1369
Celexa (Infrequent) 1177
▲ CellCept Capsules (3% to less than 20%) 2751
▲ CellCept Intravenous (3% to less than 20%) 2751
▲ CellCept Oral Suspension (3% to less than 20%) 2751
▲ CellCept Tablets (3% to less than 20%) 2751
Cleocin Vaginal Ovules (Less than 1%) 2613
Clinoril Tablets 1899
Clorpres Tablets (Rare) 2139
Cogentin Injection 1903
Combivent Inhalation Aerosol (Less than 2%) 878
Copaxone for Injection (At least 2%) 3292
Crixivan Capsules (1.5%) 1918
Cymbalta Delayed-Release Capsules (Frequent) 1729
Demser Capsules (A few patients) ... 1933
Depacon Injection (1% or more) 412
Depakene (1% or more) 417
Depakote Sprinkle Capsules 422
▲ Depakote Tablets (1% to 5%) 427
Depakote ER Tablets (1% or more) ... 433
Desferal Vials 2190
Detrol Tablets (2.5%) 2626
Detrol LA Capsules (1%) 2629
Diovan HCT Tablets (Greater than 0.2%) 2195
Dolobid Tablets (Less than 1 in 100) 1937
▲ Doxil Injection (1% to 10%) 3302
DynaCirc CR Tablets (0.5% to 1%) 2726
EC-Naprosyn Delayed-Release Tablets (Less than 1%) 2769
Effexor Tablets (Infrequent) 3405
▲ Eloxatin for Injection (1% to 6%) 2908
Emend Capsules (Greater than 0.5%) 1944
▲ Entocort EC Capsules (Less than 5%) 2694
Evoxac Capsules (Less than 1%) 1042
Exelon Capsules (Infrequent) 2204
Gabitril Tablets (Frequent) 998
Gengraf Capsules (1%) 458
Imitrex Injection (Rare) 1431
Imitrex Nasal Spray (Infrequent) 1435
Imitrex Tablets (Up to 2%) 1440
▲ Intron A for Injection (Less than 5%) 3038
▲ I.V. Busulfex (7%) 1125
Klonopin (Infrequent) 2782
Lamictal (Rare) 1449
Lexapro Oral Solution (Infrequent) 1193
Lexapro Tablets (Infrequent) 1193
Lipitor Tablets (Less than 2%) 2495
Lunesta Tablets (Infrequent) 3139
▲ Lupron Depot 3.75 mg (Among most frequent) 3257
Lupron Depot 7.5 mg (Less than 5%) 3261
Lupron Depot–3 Month 11.25 mg (Less than 5%) 3262
Lyrica Capsules (0.1% to 1%) 2524
Maxalt Tablets (Rare) 1983
Maxalt-MLT Orally Disintegrating Tablets (Rare) 1983
Merrem I.V. (Greater than 0.1% to 1%) 687
Midamor Tablets (Less than or equal to 1%) 2000
Mirapex Tablets (Less than 1%) 889
Moduretic Tablets (Less than or equal to 1%) 2003
▲ Myfortic Tablets (3% to less than 20%) 2244
Nalfon Capsules (Less than 1%) 2504
Namenda (Infrequent) 1199
Naprosyn Suspension (Less than 1%) 2769
Naprosyn Tablets (Less than 1%) 2769
Neoral Soft Gelatin Capsules (1%) ... 2247
Neoral Oral Solution (1%) 2247
Neurontin Capsules (Infrequent) 2498
Neurontin Oral Solution (Infrequent) 2498
Neurontin Tablets (Infrequent) 2498
Nexium Delayed-Release Capsules (Less than 1%) 645
Nexium I.V. (Less than 1%) 649
Norvasc Tablets (Less than or equal to 0.1%) 2529
Norvir (Less than 2%) 499
OxyContin Tablets (Less than 1%) 2699
Oxytrol Transdermal System (2.4%) 3383

Paxil CR Controlled-Release Tablets (Infrequent) 1509
Paxil (Infrequent) 1501
Permax Tablets (Infrequent) 3357
Plendil Extended-Release Tablets (0.5% to 1.5%) 651
Prevacid Delayed-Release Capsules (Less than 1%) 3268
Prevacid for Delayed-Release Oral Suspension (Less than 1%) 3268
Prevacid NapraPAC (Less than 1%) 3277
Prevacid SoluTab Delayed-Release Orally Disintegrating Tablets (Less than 1%) 3268
PREVPAC (Less than 1%) 3281
Prinivil Tablets (0.3% to 1.0%) 2029
Prinzide Tablets 2033
▲ ProAmatine Tablets (13.4%) 3183
Prochieve 4% Gel 1018
Prochieve 8% Gel 1018
▲ Prograf Capsules and Injection (3% to 15%) 624
▲ Proleukin for Injection (3%) 1007
Protonix I.V. (Less than 1%) 3468
Protonix Tablets (Less than 1%) 3465
Prozac Pulvules and Liquid (Infrequent) 1771
▲ Rapamune Oral Solution and Tablets (3% to 20%) 3472
Recombivax HB (Less than 1%) 2045
Relafen Tablets (Less than 1%) 1523
ReoPro Vials (0.4%) 1779
Requip Tablets (Infrequent) 1528
Retrovir Capsules 1533
Retrovir IV Infusion 1537
Retrovir 1533
Rilutek Tablets (Up to 1.2%) 2945
Risperdal M-Tab Orally Disintegrating Tablets (Infrequent) 1658
Risperdal (Infrequent) 1658
Rythmol SR Capsules 2736
Seroquel Tablets (Infrequent) 691
▲ Simulect for Injection (3% to 10%) 2268
Sonata Capsules (Infrequent) 1686
Soriatane Capsules (Less than 1%) 1028
Sular Tablets (Less than or equal to 1%) 1163
Symbyax Capsules (Infrequent) 1788
Tasmar Tablets (Infrequent) 3360
▲ Tequin Injection (0.1% to 3%) 964
▲ Tequin Tablets (0.1% to 3%) 964
Topamax Sprinkle Capsules (0% to 2%) 2438
Topamax Tablets (0% to 2%) 2438
▲ Trelstar LA Suspension (4.6%) 3387
Trileptal Oral Suspension 2281
Trileptal Tablets 2281
Uniretic Tablets (Less than 1%) 3114
Uroqid-Acid No. 2 Tablets (Occasional) 785
▲ Valcyte Tablets (Less than 5%) 2816
Vantas (Less than 2%) 3367
Vantin Tablets and Oral Suspension (Less than 1%) 2650
▲ Vesanoid Capsules (9%) 2823
VFEND I.V. (Less than 2%) 2543
VFEND Oral Suspension (Less than 2%) 2543
VFEND Tablets (Less than 2%) 2543
Viadur Implant (Less than 2%) 782
Voltaren Tablets (Occasionally) 2298
Voltaren-XR Tablets (Occasionally) 2301
Wellbutrin Tablets (Rare) 1579
Wellbutrin SR Sustained-Release Tablets 1583
Wellbutrin XL Extended-Release Tablets 1588
Xifaxan Tablets (Less than 2%) 2847
▲ Zenapax for Injection (Greater than 5%) 2838
Zestril Tablets (0.3% to 1.0%) 704
Zofran Injection (2%) 1607
Zoloft (Infrequent) 2581
Zonegran Capsules (Infrequent) 1089
Zosyn (1.0% or less) 3492
Zyban Sustained-Release Tablets 1620
Zyprexa Tablets (Infrequent) 1798
Zyprexa ZYDIS Orally Disintegrating Tablets (Infrequent) 1798
Zyrtec Chewable Tablets (Less than 2%) 2589
Zyrtec (Less than 2%) 2589
Zyrtec-D 12 Hour Extended Release Tablets (Less than 2%) 2591

Dyuria

Lofibra Capsules 1217
Targretin Capsules 1719
Tricor Tablets 523

E

Ear, discomfort

Aerobid/Aerobid-M (1% to 3%) 1172
▲ Ciprodex Otic Suspension (3%) 555
Invirase (Less than 2%) 2776
Levaquin in 5% Dextrose Injection (0.1% to 0.9%) 2453
Levaquin (0.1% to 0.9%) 2453

Ear, disorders of

Ciprodex Otic Suspension (1 patient) 555
FazaClo Orally Disintegrating Tablets (Less than 1%) 547
▲ I.V. Busulfex (3%) 1125
Levaquin in 5% Dextrose Injection (0.1% to 0.9%) 2453
Levaquin (0.1% to 0.9%) 2453
Prevacid NapraPAC (Less than 1%) 3277
Relpax Tablets (Rare) 2531
▲ Risperdal Consta Long-Acting Injection (Up to 3%) 1664

Ear, external abnormalities, fetal

Accutane Capsules 2740

Ear congestion

Ciprodex (0.4%) 555

Ear disease, unspecified

Actiq (1% or greater) 993
▲ Advair Diskus 100/50 (3%) 1291
Advair Diskus 250/50 1291
▲ Advair Diskus 500/50 (3%) 1291
Asacol Delayed-Release Tablets (2% or greater) 2688
Avapro Tablets (Less than 1%) 925
Avapro Tablets (Less than 1%) 2886
Cardene I.V. (Rare) 1129
Celebrex Capsules (0.1% to 1.9%) 3130
▲ CellCept Capsules (3% to less than 20%) 2751
▲ CellCept Intravenous (3% to less than 20%) 2751
▲ CellCept Oral Suspension (3% to less than 20%) 2751
▲ CellCept Tablets (3% to less than 20%) 2751
Clozapine Tablets (Less than 1%) 2141
Clozaril Tablets (Less than 1%) 2174
▲ Depakote Tablets (1% to 5%) 427
Ferrlecit Injection 3379
Gengraf Capsules (1%) 458
▲ Humatrope Vials and Cartridges (11.8%) 1756
Lamictal (2%) 1449
Lotronex Tablets (Rare) 1479
Neoral Soft Gelatin Capsules (1%) 2247
Neoral Oral Solution (1%) 2247
Prevacid Delayed-Release Capsules (Less than 1%) 3268
Prevacid for Delayed-Release Oral Suspension (Less than 1%) 3268
Prevacid SoluTab Delayed-Release Orally Disintegrating Tablets (Less than 1%) 3268
PREVPAC (Less than 1%) 3281
Provigil Tablets (At least 1%) 1002
Tamiflu Capsules (1.7%) 2810
Tamiflu Oral Suspension (1.7%) 2810
▲ Vesanoid Capsules (6%) 2823

Ear drum, perforated

Neurontin Capsules (Rare) 2498
Neurontin Oral Solution (Rare) 2498
Neurontin Tablets (Rare) 2498

Ear precipitate

Ciprodex Otic Suspension (0.5%) 555

Earache

Fortical Nasal Spray (Less than 1%) 3336
Nicotrol NS 2596

Ears, blocked

Asacol Delayed-Release Tablets 2688
▲ Chemet Capsules (1.0% to 3.7%) 2480
Neurontin Capsules (Infrequent) 2498
Neurontin Oral Solution (Infrequent) 2498
Neurontin Tablets (Infrequent) 2498
Orthoclone OKT3 Sterile Solution 2370

Ears, ringing

(*see under* Tinnitus)

Ears, roaring in

Garamycin Injectable 3028

Ebriety, feeling of

▲ Intron A for Injection (Less than 5%) 3038

Ebstein's anomaly

Eskalith 1406

Ecchymoses

Abilify Tablets (Frequent) 916
Abilify Tablets (Frequent) 2472
Aceon Tablets (2 mg, 4 mg, 8 mg) (0.3% to 1%) 3191
Aciphex Tablets 1081
Actiq (1% or greater) 993
Activase I.V. (Less than 1% to 1%) 1225
▲ Actonel Tablets (4.3%) 2679
▲ Actonel with Calcium Tablets (4.3%) 2684
Advair Diskus 100/50 1291
Advair Diskus 250/50 1291
Advair Diskus 500/50 1291
Agrylin Capsules (1% to 5%) 3172
Aloprim for Injection (Less than 1%) 2156
▲ Anaprox Tablets (3% to 9%) 2769
▲ Anaprox DS Tablets (3% to 9%) 2769
▲ Arava Tablets (1% to 3%) 2881
▲ Aricept Tablets (4%) 1086
▲ Aricept ODT Tablets (4%) 1086
Arthrotec Tablets (Rare) 3126
Avalide Tablets 922
Avalide Tablets 2889
Avapro Tablets (Less than 1%) 925
Avapro Tablets (Less than 1%) 2886
▲ Avonex (6%) 839
Buphenyl Powder (One patient) 3327
Buphenyl Tablets (One patient) 3327
Campral Tablets (Infrequent) 1175
Cardizem LA Extended Release Tablets (Less than 2%) 1699
Cataflam Tablets (Occasionally) 2173
Caverject Impulse Injection (2%) 2610
Celebrex Capsules (0.1% to 1.9%) 3130
Celexa 1177
▲ CellCept Capsules (3% to less than 20%) 2751
▲ CellCept Intravenous (3% to less than 20%) 2751
▲ CellCept Oral Suspension (3% to less than 20%) 2751
▲ CellCept Tablets (3% to less than 20%) 2751
Clinoril Tablets (Less than 1%) 1899
Combunox Tablets (Less than 2%) 1183
Comvax 1904
▲ Copaxone for Injection (8%) 3292
Covera-HS Tablets (Less than 2%) 3135
Cozaar Tablets (Less than 1%) 1913
Crestor Tablets (Greater than or equal to 1%) 672
Cymbalta Delayed-Release Capsules (Infrequent) 1729
Decadron Phosphate Injection 1931
Decadron Tablets 1929
▲ Depacon Injection (4% to 5%) 412
▲ Depakene (5%) 417
▲ Depakote Sprinkle Capsules (4% to 5%) 422
▲ Depakote Tablets (1% to 5%) 427
▲ Depakote ER Tablets (1% to 5%) 433
Depo-Medrol Injectable Suspension 2615
Depo-Medrol Single-Dose Vial 2617
▲ Doxil Injection (1% to 10%) 3302
▲ EC-Naprosyn Delayed-Release Tablets (3% to 9%) 2769
Effexor Tablets (Frequent) 3405
Effexor XR Capsules (Frequent) 3411
Elmiron Capsules (Less than or equal to 1%) 2393
Engerix-B Vaccine (Less than 1%) 1391
Flovent Diskus 50 mcg 1415
Flovent HFA 1418
▲ Gabitril Tablets (1% to 6%) 998
▲ Gamunex Immune Globulin I.V., 10% (40%) 3232
Geodon Capsules (Infrequent) 2514
▲ Gleevec Tablets (0.4% to 11%) 2221
Guanidine Hydrochloride Tablets 3030
▲ Hyalgan Solution (14%) 2917
Hydrocortone Tablets 1963
Hyzaar 1964
Indocin Capsules (Less than 1%) 1968
Indocin I.V. (Less than 1%) 1973
Indocin (Less than 1%) 1968
▲ Infergen (4% to 6%) 1647
▲ Keppra Oral Solution (1% to 4%) 3307
▲ Keppra Tablets (1% to 4%) 3307
Lamictal (Infrequent) 1449
Lexapro Oral Solution 1193
Lexapro Tablets 1193
Lipitor Tablets (Less than 2%) 2495
Lofibra Capsules 1217
▲ Lovenox Injection (Up to 3%) 2931
▲ Lupron Depot 3.75 mg (Among most frequent) 3257
Lupron Depot 7.5 mg (Less than 5%) 3261
Lupron Depot–3 Month 11.25 mg (Less than 5%) 3262
Meridia Capsules (0.7%) 485
▲ Mylotarg for Injection (9% to 11%) 3429
Nabi-HB (2%) 2159
▲ Naprosyn Suspension (3% to 9%) 2769
▲ Naprosyn Tablets (3% to 9%) 2769
▲ Neumega for Injection (Greater than or equal to 10%) 3433
Neurontin Capsules (Infrequent) 2498
Neurontin Oral Solution (Infrequent) 2498
Neurontin Tablets (Infrequent) 2498
Norvir (Less than 2%) 499
Oncaspar 1123
Pacerone Tablets (Less than 1%) 3337
Paxil CR Controlled-Release Tablets (Infrequent) 1509
Paxil (Infrequent) 1501
Pentasa Capsules (Less than 1%) 3182
Pletal Tablets (Less than 2%) 2478
▲ Prevacid NapraPAC (3% to 9%) 3277
▲ Prograf Capsules and Injection (3% to 15%) 624
Protonix I.V. (Less than 1%) 3468
Protonix Tablets (Less than 1%) 3465
Protopic Ointment (Greater than or equal to 1%) 629
Provigil Tablets (At least 1%) 1002
Prozac Pulvules and Liquid (Infrequent) 1771
▲ Rapamune Oral Solution and Tablets (3% to 20%) 3472
Reyataz Capsules (Less than 3%) 948
Rilutek Tablets (Infrequent) 2945
▲ Roferon-A Injection (Less than 5%) 2805
▲ Rythmol SR Capsules (2% to 4%) 2736
Seroquel Tablets (Infrequent) 691
Sonata Capsules (Infrequent) 1686
Sular Tablets (Less than or equal to 1%) 1163
Tarka Tablets 519
Tequin Injection (Less than 0.1%) 964
Tequin Tablets (Less than 0.1%) 964
Ticlid Tablets 2813
Tricor Tablets 523
Triglide Tablets 1165
▲ Trisenox Injection (20%) 983
Twinrix Vaccine (Less than 1%) 1571
Uniretic Tablets (Less than 1%) 3114
Vaqta (1%) 2067
Verelan PM Capsules (2% or less) 3120
VFEND I.V. (Less than 2%) 2543
VFEND Oral Suspension (Less than 2%) 2543
VFEND Tablets (Less than 2%) 2543
▲ Viadur Implant (4.6%) 782
Voltaren Tablets (Occasionally) 2298
Voltaren-XR Tablets (Occasionally) 2301
Wellbutrin Tablets 1579
Wellbutrin SR Sustained-Release Tablets (Infrequent) 1583
Wellbutrin XL Extended-Release Tablets (Infrequent) 1588
Zemaira (0.2% to 0.4%) 3506
▲ Zevalin Injection (7%) 848
Zoladex (1% or greater) 709
Zoladex 3-month 712
Zomig Nasal Spray (Rare) 718
Zomig Tablets (Infrequent) 714
Zomig-ZMT Tablets (Infrequent) 714
Zonegran Capsules (2%) 1089
Zyban Sustained-Release Tablets (Infrequent) 1620
Zyprexa Tablets 1798
Zyprexa ZYDIS Orally Disintegrating Tablets 1798

Ecchymosis, injection site

▲ Edex Injection (4%) 3103
▲ Fuzeon Injection (52%) 2772

Ecchymosis, soft eyelid tissue

Botox Purified Neurotoxin Complex 565

Ecchymosis, unspecified

Antara Capsules 2723
▲ Apokyn Injection (At least 5%) 2132
Caduet Tablets (Less than 2%) 2507
Lyrica Capsules (Greater than or equal to 1%) 2524
Symbyax Capsules (Frequent) 1788

ECG changes

(*see under* EKG changes)

Eclampsia

Paxil CR Controlled-Release Tablets 1509
Paxil 1501

Ectropion

Botox Purified Neurotoxin Complex (Less than 1%) 565
Soriatane Capsules (Less than 1%) 1028

Eczema

Abilify Tablets (Infrequent) 916
Abilify Tablets (Infrequent) 2472
Accutane Capsules 2740
▲ Aerobid/Aerobid-M (3% to 9%) 1172
Aldara Cream, 5% (1.9%) 1814
Antara Capsules 2723
Arava Tablets (2%) 2881
Arthrotec Tablets (Rare) 3126
Astelin Nasal Spray (Infrequent) 1876
Atacand HCT (0.5% or greater) 637
Caduet Tablets (Less than 2%) 2507
Celexa (Infrequent) 1177
Clozapine Tablets (Less than 1%) 2141
Clozaril Tablets (Less than 1%) 2174
Copaxone for Injection (Frequent) 3292
▲ Copegus Tablets (5%) 2759
Cubicin for Injection (Less than 1%) 1038
Cutivate Cream (0.8%) 1381
Cymbalta Delayed-Release Capsules (Infrequent) 1729
Dantrium Capsules (Less frequent) 2690
Differin Cream (Less than 1%) 1210
Effexor Tablets (Infrequent) 3405
Effexor XR Capsules (Infrequent) 3411
Engerix-B Vaccine 1391
▲ Entocort EC Capsules (Less than 5%) 2694
Evoxac Capsules (Less than 1%) 1042
Exelon Capsules (Frequent) 2204
Factive Tablets (Less than or equal to 0.1%) 2464
FazaClo Orally Disintegrating Tablets (Less than 1%) 547
▲ Flolan for Injection (25%) 1408
▲ Flovent Diskus 50 mcg (1% to 3%) 1415
Floxin Otic Singles 1045
Floxin Otic Solution (Single report) 1043
Fortical Nasal Spray (Less than 1%) 3336
Gabitril Tablets (Infrequent) 998
Gengraf Capsules (1% to less than 3%) 458
Geodon Capsules (Infrequent) 2514
Imitrex Injection 1431
Imitrex Nasal Spray 1435
▲ Intron A for Injection (Less than 5%) 3038
Invirase (Greater than or equal to 2%) 2776
Kaletra (Less than 2%) 474
Ketek Tablets (Less than 0.2%) 2920
Lamictal (2%) 1449
Levaquin in 5% Dextrose Injection (0.1% to 0.9%) 2453
Levaquin (0.1% to 0.9%) 2453
Lexapro Oral Solution (Infrequent) 1193
Lexapro Tablets (Infrequent) 1193
Lipitor Tablets (Less than 2%) 2495
Lofibra Capsules 1217
Lotronex Tablets (Rare) 1479
Lunesta Tablets (Infrequent) 3139
Lyrica Capsules (0.1% to 1%) 2524
Miacalcin Nasal Spray (Less than 1%) 2242
Micardis Tablets (More than 0.3%) 884
Micardis HCT Tablets 886
Namenda (Infrequent) 1199
Neoral Soft Gelatin Capsules (1% to less than 3%) 2247
Neoral Oral Solution (1% to less than 3%) 2247
Neurontin Capsules (Infrequent) 2498
Neurontin Oral Solution (Infrequent) 2498
Neurontin Tablets (Infrequent) 2498
Nipent for Injection (Less than 3%) 3216
Norvir (Less than 2%) 499
Olux Foam (One case) 1027
Omacor Capsules 2735
Paxil CR Controlled-Release Tablets (Infrequent) 1509
Paxil (Infrequent) 1501
Pegasys (1%) 2793
Pentasa Capsules (Less than 1%) 3182
Permax Tablets (Infrequent) 3357
Plavix Tablets (1% to 2.5%) 940
Plavix Tablets (1% to 2.5%) 2942
Protonix I.V. (Less than 1%) 3468
Protonix Tablets (Less than 1%) 3465
Protopic Ointment (Up to 3%) 629
Prozac Pulvules and Liquid (Infrequent) 1771
Pulmicort Respules (1% to 3%) 654
Relpax Tablets (Rare) 2531
Requip Tablets (Infrequent) 1528
Reyataz Capsules (Less than 3%) 948
Rilutek Tablets (0.8% to 1.6%) 2945
Risperdal Consta Long-Acting Injection (Infrequent) 1664
Roferon-A Injection (Less than 1%) 2805
Serevent Diskus (1% to 3%) 1540
Seroquel Tablets (Infrequent) 691
Singulair (Greater than or equal to 2%) 2047
Sonata Capsules (Infrequent) 1686
Soriatane Capsules (Less than 1%) 1028
Sustiva Capsules (Less than 2%) 957
Symbyax Capsules (Infrequent) 1788
Synagis (More than 1%) 1868
Tasmar Tablets (Infrequent) 3360
Teveten Tablets (Less than 1%) 1707
Teveten HCT Tablets (Less than 1%) 1710
Thalomid Capsules 979
Topamax Sprinkle Capsules (1%) 2438
Topamax Tablets (1%) 2438
Tricor Tablets 523
Uniretic Tablets (Less than 1%) 3114
Varivax (Greater than or equal to 1%) 2070
VFEND I.V. (Less than 2%) 2543
VFEND Oral Suspension (Less than 2%) 2543
VFEND Tablets (Less than 2%) 2543
▲ Visudyne for Injection (1% to 10%) 2286
Vytorin 10/10 Tablets 2084
Vytorin 10/10 Tablets 3092
Vytorin 10/20 Tablets 2084
Vytorin 10/20 Tablets 3092
Vytorin 10/40 Tablets 2084
Vytorin 10/40 Tablets 3092
Vytorin 10/80 Tablets 2084
Vytorin 10/80 Tablets 3092
Xopenex HFA Inhalation Aerosol 3151
Xopenex Inhalation Solution 3143
Xopenex Inhalation Solution Concentrate 3147
Zithromax for Oral Suspension, 300 mg, 600 mg, 900 mg, 1200 mg (1% or less) 2561
Zithromax Tablets, 250 mg, 500 mg (1% or less) 2561
Zithromax Tri-Pak (1% or less) 2561
Zoloft (Rare) 2581
Zomig Nasal Spray (Rare) 718
Zonegran Capsules (Infrequent) 1089
▲ Zosyn (4.2%) 3492
Zovirax Cream 853
Zyprexa Tablets (Infrequent) 1798
Zyprexa ZYDIS Orally Disintegrating Tablets (Infrequent) 1798
Zyrtec Chewable Tablets (Less than 2%) 2589
Zyrtec (Less than 2%) 2589
Zyrtec-D 12 Hour Extended Release Tablets (Less than 2%) 2591

Eczema, dyshidrotic

Oxistat Lotion (0.4%) 1498

Eczema, exacerbation of

Cutivate (0.8% to 3.0%) 1381

Eczema herpeticum

Cutivate Lotion 0.05% (Rare) 1383
Protopic Ointment (Up to 2%) 629

Eczematous reactions

(*see under* Eczema)

Edema

Abilify Tablets (Infrequent) 916
Abilify Tablets (Infrequent) 2472
Accolate Tablets 663
Accutane Capsules 2740
▲ Aceon Tablets (2 mg, 4 mg, 8 mg) (0.3% to 3.9%) 3191
Aciphex Tablets 1081
Actiq (Less than 1%) 993
Activella Tablets 2311
▲ ActoPlus Met Tablets (4.8% to 6%) 3219
▲ Actos Tablets (4.8% to 7.2%) 3224
▲ Advair Diskus 100/50 (1% to 3%) 1291
▲ Advair Diskus 250/50 (1% to 3%) 1291
▲ Advair Diskus 500/50 (1% to 3%) 1291
Advicor Tablets 1694
▲ Aerobid/Aerobid-M (3% to 9%) 1172
Aggrastat (2%) 1878
▲ Agrylin Capsules (20.6%) 3172
▲ Aldara Cream, 5% (Up to 18%) 1814
Aldoclor Tablets 1881
Aldoril Tablets 1884
Alesse-28 Tablets 3392
Alferon N Injection (One patient) 1640
▲ Alimta for Injection (Up to 19%) 1722
Alkeran for Injection 976
Aloprim for Injection (Less than 1%) 2156
Altace Capsules (Less than 1%) 1673
Ambien Tablets (Infrequent) 2867
▲ AmBisome for Injection (12.3% to 14.3%) 615
Amerge Tablets (Infrequent) 1312
Amevive (2%) 836
Ammonul Injection 3323
Anadrol-50 Tablets 3329
▲ Anaprox Tablets (3% to 9%) 2769
▲ Anaprox DS Tablets (3% to 9%) 2769
Antara Capsules 2723
Anzemet Injection (Rare) 2871
Anzemet Tablets (Rare) 2874
▲ Apokyn Injection (10%) 2132
▲ Aranesp for Injection (6% to 21%) 576
Aredia for Injection (Up to 1%) 2168
▲ Arimidex Tablets (7% to 11%) 665
▲ Arixtra Injection (0.9% to 8.7%) 1325
▲ Aromasin Tablets (7%) 2600
Arthrotec Tablets (Rare) 3126
Asacol Delayed-Release Tablets 2688
▲ Avalide Tablets (3%) 922
▲ Avalide Tablets (3%) 2889
▲ Avandamet Tablets (4.4%) 1343
▲ Avandia Tablets (4.8%) 1348
Avapro Tablets (1% or greater) 925
Avapro Tablets (1% or greater) 2886
Avinza Capsules (Less than 5%) 1714
Aygestin Tablets 1062
Blocadren Tablets (0.6%) 1891
Brevibloc Concentrate (Less than 1%) 766
Brevibloc Injection (Less than 1%) 766
Brevibloc Double Strength Injection (Less than 1%) 766
Brevibloc Premixed Injection (Less than 1%) 766
Brevibloc Double Strength Premixed Injection (Less than 1%) 766
Buphenyl Powder (One patient) 3327
Buphenyl Tablets (One patient) 3327
▲ Caduet Tablets (1.8% to 14.6%) 2507
▲ Campath Ampules (1% to 13%) 826
▲ Camptosar Injection (1% to 10%) 2602
Cancidas for Injection (0%) 1894
Captopril Tablets 2114
Carbatrol Capsules 3174
▲ Cardizem LA Extended Release Tablets (Up to 4.6%) 1699
▲ Casodex Tablets (2% to 5%) 670
▲ Cataflam Tablets (1% to 10%) 2173
Catapres-TTS (3 of 101 patients) 875
Celebrex Capsules (0.1% to 1.9%) 3130
▲ CellCept Capsules (3% to 28.2%) 2751
▲ CellCept Intravenous (3% to 28.2%) 2751
▲ CellCept Oral Suspension (3% to 28.2%) 2751
▲ CellCept Tablets (3% to 28.2%) 2751
▲ Cenestin Tablets, 0.45mg, 0.625mg, 0.9mg, 1.25mg (3%) 1063
Cenestin Tablets, 0.3mg 1063
Clarinex Syrup (Rare) 3009
Clarinex Tablets (Rare) 3009
Clarinex Reditabs Tablets (Rare) 3009
Clarinex-D 24-Hour Extended-Release Tablets 3012
▲ Climara Transdermal System (0.5% to 13%) 795
▲ Climara Pro Transdermal System (3.8%) 800
Clinac BPO 7 Gel USP 1137
Clinoril Tablets (Greater than 1%) 1899
Clobex Shampoo 1209
▲ Clolar for Intravenous Infusion (20%) 1264
Clozapine Tablets (Less than 1%) 2141
Clozaril Tablets (Less than 1%) 2174
Colazal Capsules 2845
Combivent Inhalation Aerosol (Less than 2%) 878
Combunox Tablets (Less than 1%) 1183
Comvax 1904
▲ Copaxone for Injection (3%) 3292
▲ Coreg Tablets (5% to 6%) 1376
Coumadin for Injection (Infrequent) 932
Coumadin Tablets (Infrequent) 932
▲ Covera-HS Tablets (1.9% to 3.0%) 3135
Cozaar Tablets (1% or greater) 1913
Crolom Cromolyn Sodium Sterile Ophthalmic Solution USP 4% ⊙ 248
Cubicin for Injection (1% to 2%) 1038
Cutivate Lotion 0.05% (Rare) 1383
Cymbalta Delayed-Release Capsules (Infrequent) 1729
Cytovene (At least 3 subjects) 2763
DDAVP Tablets 2895
Decadron Phosphate Injection 1931
Decadron Tablets 1929
Delatestryl Injection 2976
▲ Depakote Tablets (1% to 5%) 427
▲ Depakote ER Tablets (1% to 5%) 433
Depo-Medrol Injectable Suspension 2615
Depo-Medrol Single-Dose Vial 2617
▲ Depo-Provera Contraceptive Injection (1% to 5%) 2619
depo-subQ provera 104 Injectable Suspension 2622
Diovan Tablets (More than 1%) 2191
Diprivan Injectable Emulsion (Less than 1%) 676
Dolobid Tablets (Less than 1 in 100) 1937
▲ Doxil Injection (1% to 10%) 3302
Duragesic Transdermal System (1% or greater) 2448
▲ DynaCirc CR Tablets (8.9% to 35.9%) 2726
▲ EC-Naprosyn Delayed-Release Tablets (3% to 9%) 2769
Effexor Tablets (Infrequent) 3405
Effexor XR Capsules (Frequent) 3411
▲ Eloxatin for Injection (10% to 15%) 2908
▲ Emcyt Capsules (19%) 3137
Emend Capsules (Greater than 0.5%) 1944
▲ Epogen for Injection (6% to 17%) 586
▲ Equetro Extended-Release Capsules (Less than 5%) 3178
Estratest Tablets 3196
Estratest H.S. Tablets 3196
Estrogel 0.06% 3200
▲ Eulexin Capsules (4%) 3023
▲ Evoxac Capsules (1% to 3%) 1042
Exelon Capsules (Frequent) 2204
FazaClo Orally Disintegrating Tablets (Less than 1%) 547
▲ Femara Tablets (0.2% to 18.4%) 2210
▲ Ferrlecit Injection (5%) 3379
Finacea Gel (1% or less) 1644
Flexeril Tablets (Rare) 1832
▲ Flolan for Injection (60% to 79%) 1408
▲ Flovent Diskus 50 mcg (1% to 3%) 1415
Gabitril Tablets (Frequent) 998
▲ Gemzar for Injection (Less than 1% to 13%) 1743
▲ Gengraf Capsules (10%) 458
Genotropin Lyophilized Powder 2642
▲ Gleevec Tablets (0.9% to 76%) 2221
▲ Hectorol Capsules (34.4%) 909
▲ Hectorol Injection (34.4%) 911
▲ Herceptin I.V. (8%) 1234
▲ Humatrope Vials and Cartridges (2.5% to 21.2%) 1756
Hydrocortone Tablets 1963
Hytrin Capsules (0.9%) 469
Hyzaar (1.3%) 1964
▲ Imdur Tablets (Less than or equal to 5%) 3032
Imitrex Nasal Spray (Infrequent) 1435
Imitrex Tablets (Rare to infrequent) 1440
Indocin Capsules (Less than 1%) 1968
Indocin I.V. (Less than 1%) 1973
Indocin (Less than 1%) 1968
▲ Intron A for Injection (Less than or equal to 5%) 3038
▲ Invanz for Injection (2.9% to 3.4%) 1974
Invirase (Less than 2%) 2776
▲ I.V. Busulfex (28% to 79%) 1125
Iveegam EN 759
Kadian Capsules (Less than 3%) 572
Kaletra (Less than 2%) 474
▲ Kepivance (28%) 592
Klaron Lotion 10% (One of 105 patients) 1050
Klonopin (Infrequent) 2782
Lamictal (2%) 1449
Lariam Tablets 2790
▲ Leukine (13% to 34%) 829
▲ Leustatin Injection (6%) 2368
Levaquin in 5% Dextrose Injection (0.1% to 0.9%) 2453
Levaquin (0.1% to 0.9%) 2453
Librium Capsules 3349
Lipitor Tablets (Less than 2%) 2495
Lithobid Tablets 1670
Lofibra Capsules 1217
Lo/Ovral-28 Tablets 3423
Lotrel Capsules (0.6% to 3.2%) 2238
Lotrimin 3053
Lotrisone (Less than 1%) 3054
Lovenox Injection (2%) 2931
▲ Lupron Depot 3.75 mg (5.4%) 3257
▲ Lupron Depot 7.5 mg (14.3%) 3261
▲ Lupron Depot–3 Month 11.25 mg (5.4% to 7%) 3262
▲ Lyrica Capsules (2% to 4%) 2524
Matulane Capsules 3188

Mavik Tablets (0.3% to 1.0%) 482
Maxair Autohaler 1820
Maxalt Tablets (Rare) 1983
Maxalt-MLT Orally Disintegrating Tablets (Rare) 1983
▲ Megace ES Oral Suspension (1% to 3%) 2492
Menostar Transdermal System 805
Meridia Capsules (1.2%) 485
Micardis Tablets 884
Micardis HCT Tablets 886
Migranal Nasal Spray (Infrequent) 3350
▲ Mirapex Tablets (4% to 5%) 889
▲ Mobic Oral Suspension (0.6% to 4.5%) 893
▲ Mobic Tablets (0.6% to 4.5%) 893
MS Contin Tablets (Less frequent) 2703
▲ Myfortic Tablets (3% to less than 20%) 2244
▲ Naprosyn Suspension (3% to 9%) 2769
▲ Naprosyn Tablets (3% to 9%) 2769
▲ Neoral Soft Gelatin Capsules (2% to 10%) 2247
▲ Neoral Oral Solution (2% to 10%) 2247
▲ Neumega for Injection (59%) 3433
Neurontin Capsules (Infrequent) 2498
Neurontin Oral Solution (Infrequent) 2498
Neurontin Tablets (Infrequent) 2498
Nexium Delayed-Release Capsules (Less than 1%) 645
Nexium I.V. (Less than 1%) 649
Niaspan Extended-Release Tablets 1703
Nimotop Capsules (Up to 1.2%) 774
▲ Niravam Orally Disintegrating Tablets (4.9%) 3106
▲ Norditropin Cartridges (25%) 2318
Noroxin Tablets (Less frequent) 2009
▲ Norvasc Tablets (1.8% to 14.6%) 2529
Norvir (Less than 2%) 499
Novarel for Injection 1147
NovoSeven (1%) 2335
Nubain Injection (1% or less) 1111
▲ Nutropin for Injection (41%) 1238
▲ Nutropin AQ Injection (41%) 1241
▲ Nutropin AQ Pen (41%) 1241
▲ Nutropin AQ Pen Cartridge (41%) 1241
Omacor Capsules 2735
▲ Oncaspar (Greater than 5%) 1123
▲ Ontak Vials (47%) 1717
OptiPranolol Metipranolol Ophthalmic Solution 0.3% (A small number of patients) ⊙ 254
Ortho-Cept Tablets 2395
Ortho-Cyclen Tablets 2414
Ortho Evra Transdermal System 2402
Ortho Tri-Cyclen Tablets 2414
Ortho Tri-Cyclen Lo Tablets 2421
Oxandrin Tablets 2977
Oxsoralen-Ultra Capsules 3354
OxyContin Tablets (Less than 1%) 2699
▲ Pacerone Tablets (1% to 3%) 3337
Parcopa Orally Disintegrating Tablets 3111
Parnate Tablets 1499
Paxil CR Controlled-Release Tablets (Frequent) 1509
Paxil (Frequent) 1501
Pediapred Oral Solution 3319
Pediarix Vaccine 1518
Pentasa Capsules (Less than 1%) 3182
Permax Tablets (1.6%) 3357
▲ Photofrin for Injection (5% to 18%) 729
▲ Plavix Tablets (4.1%) 940
▲ Plavix Tablets (4.1%) 2942
Pletal Tablets (Less than 2%) 2478
Precose Tablets (Rare) 776
Prefest Tablets 1069
Premarin Intravenous 3440
Premarin Tablets 3443
Premarin Vaginal Cream 3449
Premphase Tablets 3452
Prempro Tablets 3452
Prevacid Delayed-Release Capsules (Less than 1%) 3268
Prevacid for Delayed-Release Oral Suspension (Less than 1%) 3268
▲ Prevacid NapraPAC (Less than 1% to 9%) 3277
Prevacid SoluTab Delayed-Release Orally Disintegrating Tablets (Less than 1%) 3268
PREVPAC (Less than 1%) 3281
Prinivil Tablets (0.3% to 1.0%) 2029
Prinzide Tablets 2033
Prochieve 4% Gel 1018
Prochieve 8% Gel 1018
▲ Procrit for Injection (6% to 17%) 2374
▲ Prograf Capsules and Injection (3% to 18%) 624
▲ Proleukin for Injection (15%) 1007
Prometrium Capsules (100 mg, 200 mg) (Less than 5%) 3205
ProSom Tablets (Rare) 512
Protonix I.V. (Less than 1%) 3468
Protonix Tablets (Less than 1%) 3465
Protopic Ointment (Greater than or equal to 1%) 629
Proventil HFA Inhalation Aerosol (Less than 3%) 3071
Provigil Tablets (1%) 1002
Prozac Pulvules and Liquid (Infrequent) 1771
Rabies Vaccine RabAvert 1011
▲ Rapamune Oral Solution and Tablets (16% to 24%) 3472
Recombivax HB (Less than 1%) 2045
▲ Relafen Tablets (3% to 9%) 1523
Relpax Tablets (Infrequent) 2531
Remicade for IV Injection (Greater than or equal to 0.2%) 987
ReoPro Vials (0.3%) 1779
▲ Requip Tablets (Infrequent) 1528
Rescriptor Tablets 2535
Retrovir Capsules (0.8%) 1533
Retrovir IV Infusion (1%) 1537
Retrovir (0.8%) 1533
Reyataz Capsules (Less than 3%) 948
Rilutek Tablets (Rare to frequent) 2945
Risperdal M-Tab Orally Disintegrating Tablets (Infrequent) 1658
Risperdal (Infrequent) 1658
▲ Rituxan I.V. (1% to 5%) 1251
▲ Roferon-A Injection (More than 1% to 11%) 2805
▲ Rythmol SR Capsules (5% to 13%) 2736
Sandimmune (2% or less) 2259
▲ Sandostatin Injection (1% to 4%) 2263
Sandostatin LAR Depot (Rare) 2264
Seasonale Tablets 1073
Serevent Diskus (1% to 3%) 1540
▲ Simulect for Injection (Greater than or equal to 10%) 2268
Singulair 2047
Sonata Capsules (Infrequent) 1686
▲ Soriatane Capsules (1% to 10%) 1028
Stalevo Tablets 2270
Striant Mucoadhesive 1022
▲ Symbyax Capsules (Greater than or equal to 5%) 1788
Symmetrel 1115
▲ Tambocor Tablets (3.5%) 1824
Tarka Tablets (0.3% to 1.3%) 519
Tasmar Tablets (Infrequent) 3360
▲ Taxotere Injection Concentrate (2.8% to 66.7%) 2947
Tegretol/Tegretol-XR 2278
Tequin Injection (Less than 0.1%) 964
Tequin Tablets (Less than 0.1%) 964
Thalomid Capsules 979
Thioridazine Hydrochloride Tablets 2122
Thyrogen for Injection (4 patients out of 55) 1270
Tiazac Capsules (2%) 1204
Timolide Tablets 2056
Timoptic in Ocudose 2061
Timoptic Sterile Ophthalmic Solution 2058
Timoptic-XE Sterile Ophthalmic Gel Forming Solution 2062
Topamax Sprinkle Capsules (1% to 2%) 2438
Topamax Tablets (1% to 2%) 2438
▲ Tracleer Tablets (4%) 539
Trelstar LA Suspension (2.3%) 3387
Tricor Tablets 523
Triglide Tablets 1165
Trileptal Oral Suspension (1% to 2%) 2281
Trileptal Tablets (1% to 2%) 2281
Triphasil-28 Tablets 3483
▲ Trisenox Injection (40%) 983
Trizivir Tablets 1565
Uniretic Tablets (Less than 1%) 3114
▲ Valcyte Tablets (Less than 5%) 2816
Vantas (Less than 2%) 3367
Vaqta (Less than 1%) 2067
▲ Velcade for Injection (11%) 2102
Verelan PM Capsules (1.7% to 1.9%) 3120
▲ Vesanoid Capsules (29% to 32%) 2823
VFEND I.V. (Less than 2%) 2543
VFEND Oral Suspension (Less than 2%) 2543
VFEND Tablets (Less than 2%) 2543
Viadur Implant (Less than 2%) 782
Viagra Tablets (Less than 2%) 2552
▲ Vicoprofen Tablets (3% to 9%) 533
Viracept 2556
Vivactil Tablets 2350
▲ Vivelle Transdermal System (3.1% to 6.5%) 2288
▲ Vivelle-Dot Transdermal System (3.1% to 6.5%) 2293
▲ Voltaren Tablets (1% to 10%) 2298
▲ Voltaren-XR Tablets (1% to 10%) 2301
Wellbutrin Tablets (Frequent) 1579
Wellbutrin SR Sustained-Release Tablets (Infrequent) 1583
Wellbutrin XL Extended-Release Tablets (Infrequent) 1588
Xanax XR Tablets (Infrequent) 2655
▲ Xeloda Tablets (1% to 9%) 2825
Yasmin 28 Tablets 818
▲ Zemplar Capsules (7%) 535
▲ Zemplar Injection (7%) 538
▲ Zenapax for Injection (Greater than 5%) 2838
Zestoretic Tablets 701
Zestril Tablets (0.3% to 1.0%) 704
Ziagen 1600
Zithromax Capsules, 250 mg 2568
Zithromax for IV Infusion 2573
Zithromax for Oral Suspension, 300 mg, 600 mg, 900 mg, 1200 mg 2561
Zithromax Tablets, 250 mg, 500 mg 2561
Zithromax Tri-Pak 2561
Zmax for Oral Suspension 2577
▲ Zoladex (1% to 7%) 709
Zoladex 3-month 712
Zoloft (Infrequent) 2581
Zomig Tablets (Infrequent) 714
Zomig-ZMT Tablets (Infrequent) 714
Zonegran Capsules (Infrequent) 1089
Zosyn (0.1% to 1.9%) 3492
Zovirax for Injection (Less than 1%) 1618
Zyban Sustained-Release Tablets (Infrequent) 1620
Zyrtec Chewable Tablets (Less than 2%) 2589
Zyrtec (Less than 2%) 2589
Zyrtec-D 12 Hour Extended Release Tablets (Less than 2%) 2591
Zyvox (0% to 2.3%) 2661

Edema, aggravated

▲ Gleevec Tablets (2% to 16%) 2221

Edema, angioneurotic

Accolate Tablets 663
Adalat CC Tablets (Less than 1%) 2978
Altace Capsules (0.3%) 1673
Altoprev Extended-Release Tablets (Rare) 1151
Anaprox Tablets (Less than 1%) 2769
Anaprox DS Tablets (Less than 1%) 2769
Arava Tablets (Rare) 2881
Atrovent Nasal Spray 0.06% (Rare) 870
Augmentin 1331
Augmentin Tablets 1334
Augmentin XR Extended-Release Tablets 1340
Bexxar 1360
Bravelle for Intramuscular or Subcutaneous Injection 1140
Caduet Tablets 2507
Carafate Suspension 727
Carafate Tablets 728
Catapres Tablets (About 5 in 1,000 patients) 874
Catapres-TTS (0.5% or less) 875
Ceftin 1369
Cipro XR Tablets 3004
Climara Transdermal System 795
Climara Pro Transdermal System 800
Clinoril Tablets (Less than 1 in 100) 1899
Clorpres Tablets (About 5 in 1,000) 2139
Colyte with Flavor Packs for Oral Solution (Rare) 3102
Combivent Inhalation Aerosol (Rare) 878
Comvax (Rare) 1904
Cozaar Tablets (Rare) 1913
CytoGam Intravenous (A possibility) 1866
Decadron Phosphate Injection 1931
Decadron Tablets 1929
Diovan HCT Tablets (Less frequent) 2195
Diovan Tablets (Less frequent) 2191
Diprivan Injectable Emulsion (Rare) 676
Dolobid Tablets (Less than 1 in 100) 1937
Dynacin Tablets 1859
EC-Naprosyn Delayed-Release Tablets (Less than 1%) 2769
Engerix-B Vaccine 1391
Flexeril Tablets (Less than 1%) 1832
Flonase Nasal Spray 1412
Gengraf Capsules (1% to less than 3%) 458
Grifulvin V Tablets Microsize and Oral Suspension Microsize (Rare) 2384
Gris-PEG Tablets (Rare) 2504
Havrix Vaccine (Rare) 1425
HibTITER 3419
Hydrocortone Tablets 1963
HyperHep B S/D 3237
HyperRAB (Rare) 3239
HyperTET (Few isolated cases) 3245
Imitrex Injection 1431
Imitrex Nasal Spray 1435
Imitrex Tablets 1440
Intron A for Injection (Rare) 3038
Lamictal (Rare) 1449
Lescol Capsules (Rare) 2227
Lescol Capsules (Rare) 2730
Lescol XL Tablets 2227
Lescol XL Tablets 2730
Leukeran Tablets 1472
Lipitor Tablets 2495
Malarone Tablets 1484
Malarone Pediatric Tablets 1484
Mavik Tablets (0.13%) 482
Mefoxin for Injection 1987
Mefoxin Premixed Intravenous Solution 1990
Meridia Capsules 485
Mevacor Tablets (Rare) 1996
Micardis Tablets 884
Micardis HCT Tablets 886
M-M-R II 1980
Naprosyn Suspension (Less than 1%) 2769
Naprosyn Tablets (Less than 1%) 2769
Naropin Injection 640
Navelbine Injection 1494
Neoral Soft Gelatin Capsules (1% to less than 3%) 2247
Neoral Oral Solution (1% to less than 3%) 2247
Niaspan Extended-Release Tablets 1703
Noroxin Tablets 2009
Norvir 499
Orthoclone OKT3 Sterile Solution 2370
Pacerone Tablets 3337
Paxil CR Controlled-Release Tablets (Rare) 1509
Paxil (Rare) 1501
Liquid PedvaxHIB (Rare) 2012
Pepcid Injection (Infrequent) 2017
Pepcid (Infrequent) 2014
Phenergan Tablets 3438
Pravachol Tablets (Rare) 943
Premarin Vaginal Cream 3449
Prevacid NapraPAC (Less than 1%) 3277
Prevnar for Injection 3460
Prilosec OTC Tablets (Less than 1%) 2674
Primaxin I.M. 2022
Primaxin I.V. (Less than 0.2%) 2024
Prinzide Tablets (Rare) 2033
Proventil Inhalation Solution 0.083% (Rare) 3069
Proventil HFA Inhalation Aerosol (Rare) 3071
Pulmicort Respules (Less than 1%) 654
Raptiva for Injection 1247
Relafen Tablets (1%) 1523
Repronex for Intramuscular and Subcutaneous Injection 1148
Rescriptor Tablets 2535
Retin-A Micro 0.1%/0.04% 2388
Rilutek Tablets (Rare) 2945
Risperdal M-Tab Orally Disintegrating Tablets 1658
Risperdal 1658
Sanctura Tablets (One event) 1133
▲ Stromectol Tablets (22.7%) 2053
Sular Tablets (Very rare) 1163
Tarka Tablets (0.15%) 519
Tequin Injection 964
Tequin Tablets 964
Thioridazine Hydrochloride Tablets 2122
Trusopt Sterile Ophthalmic Solution 2065
Vermox Chewable Tablets (Rare) 1853
VESIcare Tablets 631
Vivelle Transdermal System 2288
Vivelle-Dot Transdermal System 2293
Vytorin 10/10 Tablets 2084
Vytorin 10/10 Tablets 3092
Vytorin 10/20 Tablets 2084
Vytorin 10/20 Tablets 3092
Vytorin 10/40 Tablets 2084
Vytorin 10/40 Tablets 3092
Vytorin 10/80 Tablets 2084
Vytorin 10/80 Tablets 3092
Wellbutrin Tablets 1579
Wellbutrin SR Sustained-Release Tablets 1583

Wellbutrin XL Extended-Release Tablets 1588
Xifaxan Tablets 2847
Zantac (Rare) 1597
Zantac Injection (Rare) 1593
Zantac Injection Pharmacy Bulk Package (Rare) 1595
Zantac Syrup (Rare) 1597
Zegerid Powder for Oral Solution (Less than 1%) 2972
Zestoretic Tablets (Very rare) 701
Zetia Tablets 2090
Zocor Tablets (Rare) 2078
Zofran Injection (Rare) 1607
Zomig Nasal Spray (Rare) 718
Zovirax Cream 853
Zyban Sustained-Release Tablets 1620
Zyrtec Chewable Tablets (Less than 2%) 2589
Zyrtec (Less than 2%) 2589
Zyrtec-D 12 Hour Extended Release Tablets (Less than 2%) 2591

Edema, aphakic cystoid macular

Cosopt Sterile Ophthalmic Solution 1910
Timoptic in Ocudose (Less frequent) 2061
Timoptic Sterile Ophthalmic Solution (Less frequent) 2058
Timoptic-XE Sterile Ophthalmic Gel Forming Solution 2062

Edema, brain

▲ Ammonul Injection (5%) 3323

Edema, cerebral

Activase I.V. 1225
Aggrenox Capsules 855
Bayer Aspirin Tablets 3515
Ecotrin Enteric Coated Aspirin Low, Regular and Maximum Strength Tablets 1627
Gleevec Tablets (Rare) 2221
Orthoclone OKT3 Sterile Solution 2370
Permax Tablets (Rare) 3357
Proleukin for Injection (Less than 1%) 1007
St. Joseph 81 mg Aspirin Chewable and Enteric Coated Tablets 1841
Thiothixene Capsules 2124
▲ Vesanoid Capsules (3%) 2823
VFEND I.V. (Less than 2%) 2543
VFEND Oral Suspension (Less than 2%) 2543
VFEND Tablets (Less than 2%) 2543

Edema, conjunctival

Alphagan P Ophthalmic Solution (1% to 4%) 563
▲ Brimonidine Tartrate Ophthalmic Solution 0.2% (3% to 9%) .... ⊙ 245
Cipro 2991
Cipro XR Tablets 3004
Cosopt Sterile Ophthalmic Solution (1% to 5%) 1910
Differin Cream (Less than 1%) 1210
Effexor Tablets (Rare) 3405
Effexor XR Capsules (Rare) 3411
▲ Lumigan Ophthalmic Solution (1% to 3%) 569
Patanol Ophthalmic Solution (Less than 5%) 557
Paxil CR Controlled-Release Tablets (Rare) 1509
Paxil (Rare) 1501
▲ Retisert Implant (5% to 9%) .... ⊙ 256
Trileptal Oral Suspension 2281
Trileptal Tablets 2281

Edema, corneal

▲ Acular Ophthalmic Solution (1% to 10%) 561
▲ Acular LS Ophthalmic Solution (1% to 10%) 562
Amvisc Plus .... ⊙ 289
Ocucoat .... ⊙ 290
▲ Retisert Implant (5% to 9%) .... ⊙ 256
▲ Rēv-Eyes Ophthalmic Eyedrops 0.5% (10% to 40%) .... ⊙ 256
Symmetrel (0.1% to 1%) 1115
▲ Voltaren Ophthalmic Solution (Less than or equal to 5%) 2300
Xalatan Sterile Ophthalmic Solution 2654

Edema, cystoid macular

Advicor Tablets 1694
Lumigan Ophthalmic Solution 569
Niaspan Extended-Release Tablets 1703
Travatan Ophthalmic Solution 559
Xalatan Sterile Ophthalmic Solution 2654

Edema, dependent

Aldurazyme for Intravenous Infusion (2%) 1261
▲ Coreg Tablets (4%) 1376
Diovan HCT Tablets (Greater than 0.2%) 2195
Ellence Injection 2632
▲ Entocort EC Capsules (Less than 5%) 2694
▲ Fabrazyme for Intravenous Infusion (6%) 1267
Micardis Tablets (More than 0.3%) 884
Micardis HCT Tablets 886
▲ Mobic Oral Suspension (0.6% to 4.5%) 893
▲ Mobic Tablets (0.6% to 4.5%) 893
Razadyne ER Extended-Release Capsules (Infrequent) 2434
Razadyne (Infrequent) 2434
▲ Requip Tablets (6%) 1528
▲ Simulect for Injection (3% to 10%) 2268
▲ Spiriva HandiHaler (3% to 5%) 899
Teveten Tablets (1% or greater) 1707
Teveten HCT Tablets (Less than 1%) 1710
Zoloft (Infrequent) 2581

Edema, ear

Fabrazyme for Intravenous Infusion 1267

Edema, esophageal

▲ Photofrin for Injection (8%) 729

Edema, extremities

Celexa (Infrequent) 1177
Cipro I.V. (1% or less) 2998
Cipro I.V. Pharmacy Bulk Package (1% or less) 3509
Cipro (Less than 1%) 2991
Cipro XR Tablets 3004
Depacon Injection 412
Depakene 417
Depakote Sprinkle Capsules 422
Depakote Tablets 427
Depakote ER Tablets 433
Lexapro Oral Solution (Infrequent) 1193
Lexapro Tablets (Infrequent) 1193
Tarka Tablets 519
Taxotere Injection Concentrate 2947
▲ Zenapax for Injection (Greater than 5%) 2838

Edema, eyelid

▲ Retisert Implant (10% to 35%) .... ⊙ 256

Edema, facial

Abilify Tablets (Infrequent) 916
Abilify Tablets (Infrequent) 2472
Aciphex Tablets (Rare) 1081
Actiq (Less than 1%) 993
Adalat CC Tablets (Less than 1%) 2978
Advair Diskus 100/50 1291
Advair Diskus 250/50 1291
Advair Diskus 500/50 1291
▲ Aldurazyme for Intravenous Infusion (9%) 1261
Ambien Tablets (Rare) 2867
AmBisome for Injection (Less common) 615
Anzemet Injection (Rare) 2871
Anzemet Tablets (Rare) 2874
Aricept Tablets (Infrequent) 1086
Aricept ODT Tablets (Infrequent) 1086
Asacol Delayed-Release Tablets 2688
Astelin Nasal Spray 1876
Attenuvax 1889
Avalide Tablets 922
Avalide Tablets 2889
Avapro Tablets (Less than 1%) 925
Avapro Tablets (Less than 1%) 2886
Avelox (Less than 0.1%) 2984
▲ Azmacort Inhalation Aerosol (1% to 3%) 1701
Benicar Tablets (Five patients) 2850
Benicar HCT Tablets (2 out of 1,243 patients) 2852
Bexxar 1360
Bravelle for Intramuscular or Subcutaneous Injection 1140
Caduet Tablets (Less than 2%) 2507
Campath Ampules 826
Campral Tablets (Rare) 1175
▲ Cancidas for Injection (0% to 3.1%) 1894
▲ Carac Cream, 0.5% (35.4%) 1048
Celebrex Capsules (0.1% to 1.9%) 3130
Celexa (Rare) 1177
▲ CellCept Capsules (3% to less than 20%) 2751
▲ CellCept Intravenous (3% to less than 20%) 2751
▲ CellCept Oral Suspension (3% to less than 20%) 2751
▲ CellCept Tablets (3% to less than 20%) 2751
Cialis Tablets (Less than 2%) 1806
Cipro I.V. (1% or less) 2998
Cipro I.V. Pharmacy Bulk Package (1% or less) 3509
Cipro (Less than 1%) 2991
Cipro XR Tablets 3004
Colyte with Flavor Packs for Oral Solution (Rare) 3102
Combivent Inhalation Aerosol (Less than 2%) 878
▲ Copaxone for Injection (6%) 3292
Cozaar Tablets (Rare) 1913
Cymbalta Delayed-Release Capsules (Infrequent) 1729
Depacon Injection (1% or more) 412
Depakene (1% or more) 417
Depakote Sprinkle Capsules 422
▲ Depakote Tablets (1% to 5%) 427
Depakote ER Tablets (1% or more) 433
▲ Dostinex Tablets (Less than 10%) 2631
Doxil Injection (Less than 1%) 3302
Effexor Tablets (Infrequent) 3405
Effexor XR Capsules (Infrequent) 3411
▲ Entocort EC Capsules (Less than 5%) 2694
Evoxac Capsules (Less than 1%) 1042
Exelon Capsules (Infrequent) 2204
Flexeril Tablets (Less than 1%) 1832
Flonase Nasal Spray 1412
Flovent HFA 1418
Flumist Vaccine 1872
Gabitril Tablets (Infrequent) 998
Geodon Capsules (Frequent) 2514
HibTITER 3419
Hytrin Capsules (At least 1%) 469
Imitrex Nasal Spray 1435
Imitrex Tablets 1440
▲ Intron A for Injection (Up to 10%) 3038
Invanz for Injection (Greater than 0.1%) 1974
Kaletra (Less than 2%) 474
Keppra Oral Solution (2%) 3307
Keppra Tablets (2%) 3307
Ketek Tablets 2920
Klonopin 2782
Lamictal (2%) 1449
Levaquin in 5% Dextrose Injection (0.1% to 0.9%) 2453
Levaquin (0.1% to 0.9%) 2453
Levitra Tablets (Less than 2%) 3048
Lipitor Tablets (Less than 2%) 2495
Lofibra Capsules (Less than 1%) 1217
Loprox Gel 1861
Lunesta Tablets (Infrequent) 3139
Lupron Depot–3 Month 11.25 mg 3262
▲ Lyrica Capsules (1% to 3%) 2524
Maxalt Tablets (Infrequent) 1983
Maxalt-MLT Orally Disintegrating Tablets (Infrequent) 1983
Meridia Capsules 485
Meruvax II 1994
Micardis Tablets 884
Micardis HCT Tablets 886
M-M-R II 1980
Mobic Oral Suspension (Less than 2%) 893
Mobic Tablets (Less than 2%) 893
Mumpsvax 2005
Neumega for Injection 3433
Neupogen for Injection 598
Neurontin Capsules (Frequent) 2498
Neurontin Oral Solution (Frequent) 2498
Neurontin Tablets (Frequent) 2498
Nexium Delayed-Release Capsules (Less than 1%) 645
Nexium I.V. (Less than 1%) 649
▲ Nipent for Injection (3% to 10%) 3216
Noroxin Tablets 2009
Norvir (Less than 2%) 499
Numorphan 1112
Omnicef Capsules 506
Omnicef for Oral Suspension 506
Oncaspar (Less than 1%) 1123
OxyContin Tablets (Less than 1%) 2699
Paxil CR Controlled-Release Tablets (Infrequent) 1509
Paxil (Infrequent) 1501
Pepcid Injection (Infrequent) 2017
Pepcid (Infrequent) 2014
Permax Tablets (1.1%) 3357
Plendil Extended-Release Tablets (0.5% to 1.5%) 651
Pletal Tablets (Less than 2%) 2478
Prevnar for Injection 3460
Primaxin I.V. (Less than 0.2%) 2024
Prinivil Tablets (0.3% to 1.0%) 2029
Prinzide Tablets 2033
Prochieve 4% Gel 1018
Prochieve 8% Gel 1018
Propecia Tablets 2036
Protonix I.V. (Less than 1%) 3468
Protonix Tablets (Less than 1%) 3465
Protopic Ointment (1% to 3%) 629
Prozac Pulvules and Liquid (Infrequent) 1771
▲ Rapamune Oral Solution and Tablets (3% to 20%) 3472
Relenza Rotadisk 1525
Relpax Tablets (Infrequent) 2531
Remicade for IV Injection 987
Repronex for Intramuscular and Subcutaneous Injection 1148
Rilutek Tablets (Infrequent) 2945
Sandostatin LAR Depot (Rare) 2264
Seroquel Tablets (Infrequent) 691
▲ Simulect for Injection (3% to 10%) 2268
Sonata Capsules (Infrequent) 1686
Spectracef Tablets (0.1% to 1%) 2706
Stromectol Tablets (1.2%) 2053
Sular Tablets (Less than or equal to 1%) 1163
Sulfamylon Cream 2154
Sulfamylon for 5% Topical Solution 2155
Suprax 1811
Surmontil Capsules 2347
Tarka Tablets 519
Tasmar Tablets (Infrequent) 3360
Tequin Injection (Less than 0.1%) 964
Tequin Tablets (Less than 0.1%) 964
Teveten HCT Tablets (Less than 1%) 1710
▲ Thalomid Capsules (4.2%) 979
Topamax Sprinkle Capsules (Infrequent) 2438
Topamax Tablets (Infrequent) 2438
Tricor Tablets 523
▲ Trisenox Injection (8%) 983
Valtrex Caplets 1573
Vantin Tablets and Oral Suspension (Less than 1%) 2650
▲ Vesanoid Capsules (6%) 2823
VFEND I.V. (Less than 2%) 2543
VFEND Oral Suspension (Less than 2%) 2543
VFEND Tablets (Less than 2%) 2543
Viagra Tablets (Less than 2%) 2552
Viramune Oral Suspension 903
Viramune Tablets 903
▲ Voltaren Ophthalmic Solution (Less than or equal to 3%) 2300
Wellbutrin SR Sustained-Release Tablets (Infrequent) 1583
Wellbutrin XL Extended-Release Tablets (Infrequent) 1588
Zestoretic Tablets 701
Zestril Tablets (0.3% to 1.0%) 704
Zithromax for Oral Suspension, 300 mg, 600 mg, 900 mg, 1200 mg (1% or less) 2561
Zithromax Tablets, 250 mg, 500 mg (1% or less) 2561
Zithromax Tri-Pak (1% or less) 2561
Zoloft (Infrequent) 2581
Zomig Nasal Spray (Infrequent) 718
Zomig Tablets (Infrequent) 714
Zomig-ZMT Tablets (Infrequent) 714
Zonegran Capsules (Infrequent) 1089
Zyban Sustained-Release Tablets (Less than 1%) 1620
Zyprexa Tablets (Infrequent) 1798
Zyprexa ZYDIS Orally Disintegrating Tablets (Infrequent) 1798
Zyrtec Chewable Tablets (Less than 2%) 2589
Zyrtec (Less than 2%) 2589
Zyrtec-D 12 Hour Extended Release Tablets (Less than 2%) 2591

Edema, generalized

Caduet Tablets (Less than 2%) 2507
Symbyax Capsules (Frequent) 1788

Edema, genital

Doxil Injection (Less than 1%) 3302
▲ Simulect for Injection (3% to 10%) 2268
Viagra Tablets (Less than 2%) 2552

Edema, hand

Cipro XR Tablets 3004
Remicade for IV Injection 987
Seroquel Tablets (Rare) 691

Edema, heart failure

(*see under* Congestive heart failure)

Edema, independent

Dostinex Tablets (1%) 2631

Edema, injection site

▲ Betaseron for SC Injection (3%) 791

Gonal-f RFF Pen for Injection (2.5%) ... 3155
Merrem I.V. (0.2%) ... 687
Orthovisc Injection (0.9%) ... 3518
Premarin Intravenous ... 3440
▲ Synercid I.V. (17.3%) ... 1690
Tygacil for Injection (0% to less than 2%) ... 3489

Edema, labia
Alinia for Oral Suspension (Less than 1%) ... 2840
Alinia Tablets (Less than 1%) ... 2840

Edema, laryngeal
Activase I.V. (Very rare) ... 1225
Arthrotec Tablets (Rare) ... 3126
Avelox ... 2984
Axid Oral Solution (Rare) ... 913
Bayer Aspirin Tablets ... 3515
BeneFix for Injection ... 3402
Bravelle for Intramuscular or Subcutaneous Injection ... 1140
Cipro I.V. (1% or less) ... 2998
Cipro I.V. Pharmacy Bulk Package (1% or less) ... 3509
Cipro (Less than 1%) ... 2991
Cipro XR Tablets ... 3004
Ecotrin Enteric Coated Aspirin Low, Regular and Maximum Strength Tablets ... 1627
Effexor XR Capsules (Rare) ... 3411
Ethyol for Injection (Rare) ... 1869
Fortaz ... 1422
Garamycin Injectable ... 3028
Levitra Tablets (Less than 2%) ... 3048
Lotrel Capsules (About 0.5%) ... 2238
Naropin Injection ... 640
Neumega for Injection ... 3433
Nexium Delayed-Release Capsules (Less than 1%) ... 645
Nexium I.V. (Less than 1%) ... 649
Nipent for Injection (Less than 3%) ... 3216
Nubain Injection (1% or less) ... 1111
Numorphan ... 1112
Omnicef Capsules ... 506
Omnicef for Oral Suspension ... 506
Orthoclone OKT3 Sterile Solution ... 2370
Permax Tablets (Rare) ... 3357
Persantine Tablets (Rare) ... 898
Prinivil Tablets (0.3% to 1.0%) ... 2029
Prinzide Tablets (Rare) ... 2033
Prozac Pulvules and Liquid (Rare) ... 1771
Remicade for IV Injection ... 987
Repronex for Intramuscular and Subcutaneous Injection ... 1148
St. Joseph 81 mg Aspirin Chewable and Enteric Coated Tablets ... 1841
Tarka Tablets ... 519
Thioridazine Hydrochloride Tablets .. 2122
Thyrogen for Injection (1 patient out of 55) ... 1270
TNKase I.V. (Rare) ... 1256
Vaseretic Tablets ... 2073
Vasotec I.V. Injection ... 2076
▲ Vesanoid Capsules (3%) ... 2823
Zestoretic Tablets ... 701
Zestril Tablets (0.3% to 1.0%) ... 704
Zofran Injection ... 1607
Zofran ... 1613
Zofran ODT Orally Disintegrating Tablets ... 1613
Zomig Nasal Spray (Infrequent) ... 718

Edema, laryngotracheal
Photofrin for Injection ... 729

Edema, legs
▲ Trelstar LA Suspension (6.3%) ... 3387

Edema, lesional
Oncaspar (Less than 1%) ... 1123

Edema, lips
Cipro I.V. (1% or less) ... 2998
Cipro I.V. Pharmacy Bulk Package (1% or less) ... 3509
Cipro (Less than 1%) ... 2991
Cipro XR Tablets ... 3004
Combivent Inhalation Aerosol (Less than 2%) ... 878
Cozaar Tablets (Rare) ... 1913
Fabrazyme for Intravenous Infusion ... 1267
Imitrex Tablets ... 1440
▲ Oncaspar (Greater than 1% but less than 5%) ... 1123
Orthoclone OKT3 Sterile Solution ... 2370
Propecia Tablets ... 2036
Remicade for IV Injection ... 987
Rescriptor Tablets ... 2535
Retrovir Capsules ... 1533
Retrovir IV Infusion ... 1537
Retrovir ... 1533
Tarka Tablets ... 519

Edema, local
Avita Gel ... 2138
Avodart Soft Gelatin Capsules ... 1353
Cleocin Vaginal Ovules (Less than 1%) ... 2613
Denavir Cream ... 2163
Desferal Vials ... 2190
Havrix Vaccine (Rare) ... 1425
Lidoderm Patch ... 1107
Oncaspar ... 1123
Rescriptor Tablets ... 2535
Striant Mucoadhesive (2.0%) ... 1022
Vantin Tablets and Oral Suspension (Less than 1%) ... 2650
Zovirax Ointment ... 854

Edema, lower extremities
▲ ActoPlus Met Tablets (2.9% to 11.3%) ... 3219
Advate Injection (0.6%) ... 742
▲ Aromasin Tablets (7%) ... 2600
▲ Cardizem LA Extended Release Tablets (5% to 8%) ... 1699
▲ Coreg Tablets (Greater than 1% to 3%) ... 1376
Eldepryl Capsules ... 3209
▲ Femara Tablets (5%) ... 2210
Ferrlecit Injection ... 3379
Miacalcin Injection ... 2241
Micardis Tablets (More than 0.3%) ... 884
Micardis HCT Tablets ... 886
▲ Mobic Oral Suspension (0.6% to 4.5%) ... 893
▲ Mobic Tablets (0.6% to 4.5%) ... 893
▲ Myfortic Tablets (3% to less than 20%) ... 2244
Nexium Delayed-Release Capsules (Less than 1%) ... 645
Nexium I.V. (Less than 1%) ... 649
▲ Norditropin Cartridges (15%) ... 2318
▲ Requip Tablets (6%) ... 1528
▲ Simulect for Injection (Greater than or equal to 10%) ... 2268
Taxotere Injection Concentrate ... 2947
▲ Tracleer Tablets (8%) ... 539
Trileptal Oral Suspension (1% to 2%) ... 2281
Trileptal Tablets (1% to 2%) ... 2281
VESIcare Tablets (0.3% to 1.1%) ... 631
Xenical Capsules (2.8%) ... 2834
▲ Zometa for Intravenous Infusion (5% to 21%) ... 2306
Zyprexa Tablets (1%) ... 1798
Zyprexa ZYDIS Orally Disintegrating Tablets (1%) ... 1798
Zyrtec Chewable Tablets (Less than 2%) ... 2589
Zyrtec (Less than 2%) ... 2589
Zyrtec-D 12 Hour Extended Release Tablets (Less than 2%) ... 2591

Edema, macular
Gleevec Tablets (Rare) ... 2221
Intron A for Injection ... 3038
Lumigan Ophthalmic Solution ... 569
Pegasys ... 2793
PEG-Intron Powder for Injection ... 3062
▲ Retisert Implant (5% to 9%) ... ⊙ 256
Retrovir Capsules (A single case) ... 1533
Retrovir IV Infusion (A single case) ... 1537
Retrovir (A single case) ... 1533
Travatan Ophthalmic Solution ... 559
Xalatan Sterile Ophthalmic Solution ... 2654

Edema, mouth
Campath Ampules ... 826
Evoxac Capsules (Less than 1%) ... 1042
Frova Tablets (Rare) ... 1101
Tequin Injection (Less than 0.1%) ... 964
Tequin Tablets (Less than 0.1%) ... 964

Edema, nasal
▲ Atrovent Nasal Spray 0.03% (3.1%) ... 869
Striant Mucoadhesive ... 1022

Edema, non-specific
(*see under* Edema)

Edema, oropharyngeal
Advair Diskus 100/50 ... 1291
Advair Diskus 250/50 ... 1291
Advair Diskus 500/50 ... 1291
Arthrotec Tablets (Rare) ... 3126
Atrovent HFA Inhalation Aerosol ... 872
Atrovent Nasal Spray 0.06% (Rare) .. 870
Cipro I.V. (1% or less) ... 2998
Cipro I.V. Pharmacy Bulk Package (1% or less) ... 3509
Cipro (Less than 1%) ... 2991
Cipro XR Tablets ... 3004
Combivent Inhalation Aerosol (Rare) ... 878
Denavir Cream ... 2163
Flovent HFA ... 1418
Proventil Inhalation Aerosol ... 3067
Proventil Inhalation Solution 0.083% (Rare) ... 3069
Proventil HFA Inhalation Aerosol (Rare) ... 3071
Relenza Rotadisk (Less than 1%) ... 1525
Ventolin HFA Inhalation Aerosol (Less than 3%) ... 1576
VoSpire Extended-Release Tablets (Rare) ... 2352

Edema, palpebral
Aredia for Injection (One patient) ... 2168
Betoptic S Ophthalmic Suspension .. 554
▲ Carteolol Hydrochloride Ophthalmic Solution USP, 1% (About 1 of 4 patients) ... ⊙ 246
Cipro I.V. (1% or less) ... 2998
Cipro I.V. Pharmacy Bulk Package (1% or less) ... 3509
Crolom Cromolyn Sodium Sterile Ophthalmic Solution USP 4% (Infrequent) ... ⊙ 248
DDAVP Nasal Spray (Up to 2%) ... 2894
Desmopressin Acetate Rhinal Tube (Up to 2%) ... 1144
Imitrex Nasal Spray ... 1435
Imitrex Tablets ... 1440
Maxalt Tablets (Infrequent) ... 1983
Maxalt-MLT Orally Disintegrating Tablets (Infrequent) ... 1983
Orthoclone OKT3 Sterile Solution ... 2370
Prinzide Tablets ... 2033
ProSom Tablets (Infrequent) ... 512
Vaseretic Tablets ... 2073
Vasotec I.V. Injection ... 2076
Viagra Tablets ... 2552
▲ Zymar Ophthalmic Solution (1% to 4%) ... 571

Edema, paramacular
Viagra Tablets ... 2552

Edema, penile
Caverject Impulse Injection (1%) ... 2610

Edema, periorbital
(*see under* Edema, peripheral)

Edema, peripheral
Abilify Tablets (2%) ... 916
Abilify Tablets (2%) ... 2472
Aciphex Tablets ... 1081
Actiq (1% or greater) ... 993
▲ Actonel Tablets (1.6% to 8.2%) ... 2679
▲ Actonel with Calcium Tablets (1.6% to 4.2%) ... 2684
▲ ActoPlus Met Tablets (6%) ... 3219
▲ Adalat CC Tablets (18% to 29%) ... 2978
Aerobid/Aerobid-M (1% to 3%) ... 1172
▲ Agrylin Capsules (8.9%) ... 3172
Ambien Tablets (Rare) ... 2867
▲ AmBisome for Injection (14.6%) ... 615
Anaprox Tablets (Some patients) ... 2769
Anaprox DS Tablets (Some patients) ... 2769
AndroGel (Fewer than 1%) ... 3330
Antara Capsules ... 2723
Anzemet Injection (Rare) ... 2871
Anzemet Tablets (Rare) ... 2874
Aralast (Greater than or equal to 0.2%) ... 745
▲ Aranesp for Injection (11%) ... 576
▲ Arava Tablets (1% to 3%) ... 2881
Aricept Tablets (Infrequent) ... 1086
Aricept ODT Tablets (Infrequent) ... 1086
▲ Arimidex Tablets (5% to 10%) ... 665
▲ Aromasin Tablets (7%) ... 2600
Arthrotec Tablets (Rare) ... 3126
▲ Asacol Delayed-Release Tablets (3%) ... 2688
Atacand HCT (0.5% or greater) ... 637
Attenuvax ... 1889
Avelox (0.1%) ... 2984
▲ Avinza Capsules (5% to 10%) ... 1714
Benicar Tablets (Greater than 0.5%) ... 2850
Benicar HCT Tablets (Greater than 1%) ... 2852
▲ Betaseron for SC Injection (15%) ... 791
Betimol Ophthalmic Solution (1% to 5%) ... ⊙ 283
Betimol Ophthalmic Solution (1% to 5%) ... 3371
▲ Bexxar (0% to 9%) ... 1360
Caduet Tablets (Greater than or equal to 2%) ... 2507
▲ Campath Ampules (1% to 13%) ... 826
Campral Tablets (Frequent) ... 1175
Cardene I.V. (Rare) ... 1129
▲ Carnitor Injection (3% to 6%) ... 3185
▲ Casodex Tablets (8%) ... 670
Celebrex Capsules (2.1%) ... 3130
▲ CellCept Capsules (27.0% to 64%) ... 2751
▲ CellCept Intravenous (27.0% to 64%) ... 2751
▲ CellCept Oral Suspension (27.0% to 64%) ... 2751
▲ CellCept Tablets (27.0% to 64%) ... 2751
▲ Cenestin Tablets, 0.45mg, 0.625mg, 0.9mg, 1.25mg (10%) ... 1063
Cerezyme for Injection ... 1263
Clozapine Tablets ... 2141
Clozaril Tablets ... 2174
▲ CombiPatch Transdermal System (6%) ... 2180
▲ Copaxone for Injection (7%) ... 3292
▲ Coreg Tablets (2% to 7%) ... 1376
Crestor Tablets (Greater than or equal to 2%) ... 672
Cymbalta Delayed-Release Capsules (Infrequent) ... 1729
Demser Capsules (Rare) ... 1933
▲ Depacon Injection (3% to 8%) ... 412
▲ Depakene (8%) ... 417
▲ Depakote Sprinkle Capsules (3% to 8%) ... 422
▲ Depakote Tablets (1% to 8%) ... 427
▲ Depakote ER Tablets (1% to 8%) ... 433
▲ DepoCyt Injection (7%) ... 1121
Detrol Tablets ... 2626
Detrol LA Capsules ... 2629
Ditropan XL Extended Release Tablets (Rare) ... 2391
Dostinex Tablets (1%) ... 2631
▲ Doxil Injection (1% to 11.3%) ... 3302
EC-Naprosyn Delayed-Release Tablets (Some patients) ... 2769
Effexor Tablets (Frequent) ... 3405
Eldepryl Capsules ... 3209
▲ Eloxatin for Injection (5% to 10%) ... 2908
Emcyt Capsules ... 3137
Enablex Extended-Release Tablets (Greater than or equal to 1%) ... 2201
▲ Enbrel for Injection (2% to 8%) ... 580
▲ Equetro Extended-Release Capsules (Less than 5%) ... 3178
▲ Erbitux (10%) ... 937
▲ Evista Tablets (3.3% to 5.2%) ... 1735
▲ Evoxac Capsules (Less than 1% to 3%) ... 1042
Exelon Capsules (2% or more) ... 2204
▲ Faslodex Injection (9%) ... 682
FazaClo Orally Disintegrating Tablets ... 547
▲ Femara Tablets (5%) ... 2210
Ferrlecit Injection ... 3379
▲ Flolan for Injection (79%) ... 1408
Fortical Nasal Spray (Less than 1%) ... 3336
Gabitril Tablets (Frequent) ... 998
▲ Gemzar for Injection (20%) ... 1743
Geodon Capsules (Infrequent) ... 2514
▲ Herceptin I.V. (10%) ... 1234
▲ Humatrope Vials and Cartridges (11.5% to 18.2%) ... 1756
▲ Humira Injection (Less than 5%) ... 464
▲ Hytrin Capsules (0.6% to 5.5%) ... 469
Imitrex Nasal Spray ... 1435
Imitrex Tablets ... 1440
Indapamide Tablets (Less than 5%) .. 2119
▲ Infergen (4% to 9%) ... 1647
▲ Intron A for Injection (Less than or equal to 5%) ... 3038
Iressa Tablets (2%) ... 684
Kadian Capsules (Less than 3%) ... 572
Kaletra (Less than 2%) ... 474
Klonopin (Infrequent) ... 2782
Lamictal (Infrequent) ... 1449
▲ Leukine (11% to 15%) ... 829
Levaquin in 5% Dextrose Injection (0.1% to 0.9%) ... 2453
Levaquin (0.1% to 0.9%) ... 2453
Lipitor Tablets (Greater than or equal to 2%) ... 2495
Lofibra Capsules ... 1217
▲ Lovenox Injection (3% to 6%) ... 2931
Lunesta Tablets (Frequent) ... 3139
Lupron Depot-PED 7.5 mg, 11.25 mg and 15 mg (Less than 2%) ... 3266
Lupron Injection Pediatric (Less than 2%) ... 3256
▲ Lyrica Capsules (3% to 12%) ... 2524
▲ Megace ES Oral Suspension (1% to 3%) ... 2492
Meridia Capsules (Greater than or equal to 1%) ... 485
Merrem I.V. (Greater than 0.1% to 1%) ... 687
Meruvax II ... 1994
Miacalcin Nasal Spray (Less than 1%) ... 2242

Micardis Tablets (1%) 884
Micardis HCT Tablets (1%) 886
Migranal Nasal Spray (Rare) 3350
▲ Mirapex Tablets (2% to 5%) 889
M-M-R II 1980
▲ Mobic Oral Suspension (0.6% to 4.5%) 893
▲ Mobic Tablets (0.6% to 4.5%) 893
Mumpsvax 2005
▲ Myfortic Tablets (3% to less than 20%) 2244
▲ Mylotarg for Injection (8% to 19%) ... 3429
▲ Nalfon Capsules (5%) 2504
Namenda (Greater than or equal to 2%) 1199
Naprosyn Suspension (Some patients) 2769
Naprosyn Tablets (Some patients) 2769
▲ Neulasta Injection (15% to 72%) 596
Neumega for Injection 3433
▲ Neurontin Capsules (1.7% to 8.3%) 2498
▲ Neurontin Oral Solution (1.7% to 8.3%) 2498
▲ Neurontin Tablets (1.7% to 8.3%) 2498
Nexium Delayed-Release Capsules (Less than 1%) 645
Nexium I.V. (Less than 1%) 649
Niaspan Extended-Release Tablets ... 1703
Nicotrol NS (Less than 1%) 2596
▲ Nipent for Injection (3% to 10%) 3216
▲ Norditropin Cartridges (42%) 2318
Norvir (Less than 2%) 499
▲ Nutropin for Injection (41%) 1238
▲ Nutropin AQ Injection (41%) 1241
▲ Nutropin AQ Pen (41%) 1241
▲ Nutropin AQ Pen Cartridge (41%) 1241
▲ Oncaspar (Greater than 1% but less than 5%) 1123
Orap Tablets 1220
OxyContin Tablets (Less than 1%) 2699
Paxil CR Controlled-Release Tablets (Infrequent) 1509
Paxil (Infrequent) 1501
Pepcid Injection (Infrequent) 2017
Pepcid (Infrequent) 2014
▲ Permax Tablets (7.4%) 3357
▲ Photofrin for Injection (7%) 729
▲ Plendil Extended-Release Tablets (2.0% to 17.4%) 651
▲ Pletal Tablets (7% to 9%) 2478
▲ Premphase Tablets (3% to 4%) 3452
▲ Prempro Tablets (3% to 4%) 3452
Prevacid Delayed-Release Capsules (Less than 1%) 3268
Prevacid for Delayed-Release Oral Suspension (Less than 1%) 3268
Prevacid NapraPAC (Less than 1%) .. 3277
Prevacid SoluTab Delayed-Release Orally Disintegrating Tablets (Less than 1%) 3268
PREVPAC (Less than 1%) 3281
Prilosec OTC Tablets (Less than 1%) 2674
Prinivil Tablets (0.3% to 1.0%) 2029
Prinzide Tablets 2033
▲ Prograf Capsules and Injection (12% to 36%) 624
▲ Proleukin for Injection (28%) 1007
Prometrium Capsules (100 mg, 200 mg) (Less than 5%) 3205
Protonix I.V. (Less than 1%) 3468
Protonix Tablets (Less than 1%) 3465
Protopic Ointment (1% to 4%) 629
Provigil Tablets (At least 1%) 1002
Prozac Pulvules and Liquid (Infrequent) 1771
▲ Rapamune Oral Solution and Tablets (54% to 64%) 3472
Raptiva for Injection 1247
Razadyne ER Extended-Release Capsules (Greater than or equal to 2%) 2434
Razadyne (Greater than or equal to 2%) 2434
Relpax Tablets (Infrequent) 2531
ReoPro Vials (1.6%) 1779
Requip Tablets (Infrequent) 1528
Reyataz Capsules (Less than 3%) 948
▲ Rilutek Tablets (3.3% to 4.2%) 2945
▲ Risperdal Consta Long-Acting Injection (2% to 3%) 1664
▲ Rituxan for Infusion (Among most frequent) 845
▲ Rituxan I.V. (8%) 1251
▲ Sandostatin LAR Depot (5% to 15%) 2264
Seroquel Tablets (Infrequent) 691
▲ Simulect for Injection (Greater than or equal to 10%) 2268
▲ Somavert Injection (4% to 8%) 2648
Sonata Capsules (Less than 1%) 1686
Spectracef Tablets (0.1% to 1%) 2706
▲ Stromectol Tablets (3.2%) 2053
▲ Sular Tablets (22%) 1163
Sustiva Capsules (Less than 2%) 957
▲ Symbyax Capsules (5% to 8%) 1788
Symmetrel (1% to 5%) 1115
Synercid I.V. (Less than 1%) 1690
▲ Targretin Capsules (4.8% to 11.3%) 1719
Tasmar Tablets (1% or more) 3360
▲ Taxotere Injection Concentrate (6% to 39%) 2947
▲ Temodar Capsules (11%) 3088
▲ Tequin Injection (0.1% to 3%) 964
▲ Tequin Tablets (0.1% to 3%) 964
Teveten Tablets (Less than 1%) 1707
Teveten HCT Tablets (Less than 1%) 1710
▲ Thalomid Capsules (4.2%) 979
Thioridazine Hydrochloride Tablets... 2122
Thiothixene Capsules 2124
▲ Thymoglobulin for Injection (34.1%) 2848
▲ Tiazac Capsules (3% to 5%) 1204
Toprol-XL Tablets (About 1 of 100 patients) 660
▲ Trasylol Injection (5%) 779
Trelstar LA Suspension (1.1%) 3387
Tricor Tablets 523
Triglide Tablets 1165
▲ Tygacil for Injection (3.3%) 3489
Uniretic Tablets (More than 1%) 3114
Univasc Tablets (Greater than 1%) ... 3118
▲ Urso 250 Tablets (8.3%) 737
▲ Urso Forte Tablets (8.3%) 737
▲ Valcyte Tablets (Less than 5%) 2816
Vantas (Less than 2%) 3367
Vantin Tablets and Oral Suspension (Less than 1%) 2650
Ventavis Inhalation Solution 1036
▲ Verelan PM Capsules (3.7%) 3120
▲ Vesanoid Capsules (52%) 2823
▲ VFEND I.V. (Less than 2%) 2543
▲ VFEND Oral Suspension (Less than 2%) 2543
▲ VFEND Tablets (Less than 2%) 2543
▲ Viadur Implant (3.1%) 782
Viagra Tablets (Less than 2%) 2552
▲ Vivelle Transdermal System (1.5% to 4.3%) 2288
▲ Vivelle-Dot Transdermal System (1.5% to 4.3%) 2293
Wellbutrin SR Sustained-Release Tablets (Infrequent) 1583
Wellbutrin XL Extended-Release Tablets (Infrequent) 1588
Zegerid Powder for Oral Solution (Less than 1%) 2972
Zelnorm Tablets 2303
Zestoretic Tablets 701
Zestril Tablets (0.3% to 1.0%) 704
▲ Zevalin Injection (8%) 848
▲ Zoladex (21%) 709
Zoladex 3-month (1% to 5%) 712
Zoloft (Infrequent) 2581
Zomig Nasal Spray (Rare) 718
Zonegran Capsules (Infrequent) 1089
Zovirax Capsules 1616
Zovirax for Injection 1618
Zovirax 1616
Zyban Sustained-Release Tablets (Infrequent) 1620
Zyprexa Tablets (2%) 1798
Zyprexa ZYDIS Orally Disintegrating Tablets (2%) 1798
Zyrtec Chewable Tablets (Less than 2%) 2589
Zyrtec (Less than 2%) 2589
Zyrtec-D 12 Hour Extended Release Tablets (Less than 2%) 2591

Edema, pharyngeal

Atacand Tablets (More than 1%) 634
Avelox (Less than 0.1%) 2984
Cipro 2991
Cipro XR Tablets 3004
Cozaar Tablets (Rare) 1913
Maxalt Tablets (Rare) 1983
Maxalt-MLT Orally Disintegrating Tablets (Rare) 1983
Noroxin Tablets 2009
Remicade for IV Injection 987
Xolair 1259

Edema, pulmonary

Abelcet Injection 1119
Abilify Tablets (Rare) 916
Abilify Tablets (Rare) 2472
Activase I.V. 1225
Aggrenox Capsules (Less than 1%) .. 855
Aldara Cream, 5% 1814
Aldoclor Tablets 1881
Aldoril Tablets 1884
Ambien Tablets (Rare) 2867
AmBisome for Injection (Less common) 615
Ammonul Injection 3323
Angiomax for Injection (Rare) 1856
Argatroban Injection (0.9%) 1321
Atacand HCT 637
Avalide Tablets 922
Avalide Tablets 2889
Bayer Aspirin Tablets 3515
Blocadren Tablets 1891
Brevibloc Concentrate (Less than 1%) 766
Brevibloc Injection (Less than 1%) 766
Brevibloc Double Strength Injection (Less than 1%) 766
Brevibloc Premixed Injection (Less than 1%) 766
Brevibloc Double Strength Premixed Injection (Less than 1%) 766
Cafcit (2.2%) 1854
Campath Ampules 826
Carimune NF 3501
▲ CellCept Capsules (3% to less than 20%) 2751
▲ CellCept Intravenous (3% to less than 20%) 2751
▲ CellCept Oral Suspension (3% to less than 20%) 2751
▲ CellCept Tablets (3% to less than 20%) 2751
Cipro I.V. (1% or less) 2998
Cipro I.V. Pharmacy Bulk Package (1% or less) 3509
Cipro (Less than 1%) 2991
Cipro XR Tablets 3004
Clolar for Intravenous Infusion 1264
▲ Coreg Tablets (Less than or equal to 0.1% to greater than 3%) 1376
Cosopt Sterile Ophthalmic Solution 1910
Covera-HS Tablets (1.8% to 2%) 3135
Dantrium Intravenous (Rare) 2691
Decadron Tablets 1929
Diovan HCT Tablets 2195
Diprivan Injectable Emulsion (Rare) .. 676
Diuril Oral 1936
Diuril Sodium Intravenous 1934
Dyazide Capsules 1389
Elitek (Less than or equal to 1%) 2906
Ellence Injection 2632
Ferrlecit Injection 3379
▲ Flolan for Injection (4%) 1408
Gammagard Liquid 751
Gammagard S/D 754
Gamunex Immune Globulin I.V., 10% 3232
▲ Gleevec Tablets (2% to 16%) 2221
Herceptin I.V. 1234
Hyzaar 1964
Indocin Capsules (Less than 1%) 1968
Indocin I.V. (Less than 1%) 1973
Indocin (Less than 1%) 1968
Inversine Tablets 3286
Iveegam EN 759
Kaletra (Less than 2%) 474
Levaquin in 5% Dextrose Injection (0.1% to 0.9%) 2453
Levaquin (0.1% to 0.9%) 2453
Lotensin HCT Tablets 2235
Lovenox Injection (0.7%) 2931
Lupron Depot 7.5 mg (Less than 5%) 3261
Lyrica Capsules (Rare) 2524
Micardis HCT Tablets 886
Moduretic Tablets 2003
Nalfon Capsules (Less than 1%) 2504
Namenda (Infrequent) 1199
Narcan Injection 1109
Navelbine Injection 1494
Neumega for Injection 3433
Neurontin Capsules (Rare) 2498
Neurontin Oral Solution (Rare) 2498
Neurontin Tablets (Rare) 2498
Nubain Injection 1111
Orthoclone OKT3 Sterile Solution (Less than 2%) 2370
Paxil CR Controlled-Release Tablets (Rare) 1509
Paxil (Rare) 1501
Permax Tablets (Infrequent) 3357
Photofrin for Injection 729
Prinivil Tablets (Greater than 1%) 2029
Prinzide Tablets 2033
▲ Prograf Capsules and Injection (3% to 15%) 624
▲ Proleukin for Injection (Less than 1% to 10%) 1007
Prozac Pulvules and Liquid (Rare) 1771
▲ Rapamune Oral Solution and Tablets (3% to 20%) 3472
Remicade for IV Injection (Greater than or equal to 0.2%) 987
ReoPro Vials (1.5%) 1779
Requip Tablets (Infrequent) 1528
Retavase 1131
Rilutek Tablets (Infrequent) 2945
Risperdal Consta Long-Acting Injection (Rare) 1664
▲ Roferon-A Injection (9%) 2805
▲ Simulect for Injection (3% to 10%) ... 2268
Symmetrel 1115
Targretin Capsules 1719
Tarka Tablets 519
Tasmar Tablets (Rare) 3360
Taxotere Injection Concentrate (Rare) 2947
Teveten HCT Tablets 1710
Thalomid Capsules 979
Timolide Tablets 2056
Timoptic in Ocudose (Less frequent) 2061
Timoptic Sterile Ophthalmic Solution (Less frequent) 2058
Timoptic-XE Sterile Ophthalmic Gel Forming Solution 2062
TNKase I.V. 1256
Trasylol Injection (1.2%) 779
TriLyte with Flavor Packs for Oral Solution 3114
Ultracet Tablets 2462
Uniretic Tablets 3114
Vaseretic Tablets 2073
Vasotec I.V. Injection (0.5% to 1.0%) 2076
Verelan PM Capsules (1.8%) 3120
▲ Vesanoid Capsules (3%) 2823
VFEND I.V. (Less than 2%) 2543
VFEND Oral Suspension (Less than 2%) 2543
VFEND Tablets (Less than 2%) 2543
Virazole for Inhalation Solution (Infrequent) 3365
▲ Zenapax for Injection (Greater than 5%) 2838
Zestoretic Tablets 701
Zestril Tablets (Greater than 1%) 704
Zevalin Injection (Less than 1%) 848
Zosyn (1.0% or less) 3492
Zovirax for Injection (Less than 1%) 1618

Edema, pulmonary, non-cardiogenic

Kadian Capsules (Less than 3%) 572

Edema, retinal

Lyrica Capsules (0.1% to 1%) 2524

Edema, scrotal

Actiq (1% or greater) 993
Caverject Impulse Injection (Less than 1%) 2610
▲ CellCept Capsules (3% to less than 20%) 2751
▲ CellCept Intravenous (3% to less than 20%) 2751
▲ CellCept Oral Suspension (3% to less than 20%) 2751
▲ CellCept Tablets (3% to less than 20%) 2751
▲ Intron A for Injection (Less than or equal to 5%) 3038
Protonix I.V. (Less than 1%) 3468
Protonix Tablets (Less than 1%) 3465
▲ Rapamune Oral Solution and Tablets (3% to 20%) 3472
Uniretic Tablets (Less than 1%) 3114
VFEND I.V. (Less than 2%) 2543
VFEND Oral Suspension (Less than 2%) 2543
VFEND Tablets (Less than 2%) 2543

Edema, skin

(*see under* Edema, angioneurotic)

Edema, superficial

▲ Gleevec Tablets (57.5% to 76%) 2221

Edema, tongue

Abilify Tablets (Infrequent) 916
Abilify Tablets (Infrequent) 2472
Aricept Tablets (Infrequent) 1086
Aricept ODT Tablets (Infrequent) 1086
Avonex 839
Betaseron for SC Injection 791
Colyte with Flavor Packs for Oral Solution (Rare) 3102
Combivent Inhalation Aerosol (Less than 2%) 878
Cozaar Tablets (Rare) 1913
Effexor Tablets (Infrequent) 3405
Effexor XR Capsules (Infrequent) 3411
▲ Entocort EC Capsules (Less than 5%) 2694
Flexeril Tablets (Less than 1%) 1832
Flonase Nasal Spray 1412

▲ Geodon Capsules (3%) 2514
Lamictal (Rare) 1449
Levaquin in 5% Dextrose Injection (0.1% to 0.9%) 2453
Levaquin (0.1% to 0.9%) 2453
Lunesta Tablets (Rare) 3139
Lyrica Capsules (0.1% to 1%) 2524
Maxalt Tablets (Infrequent) 1983
Maxalt-MLT Orally Disintegrating Tablets (Infrequent) 1983
Meridia Capsules 485
Neumega for Injection 3433
Nexium Delayed-Release Capsules (Less than 1%) 645
Nexium I.V. (Less than 1%) 649
Paxil CR Controlled-Release Tablets (Rare) 1509
Paxil (Rare) 1501
Pletal Tablets (Less than 2%) 2478
Prozac Pulvules and Liquid (Rare) 1771
Relpax Tablets (Rare) 2531
Requip Tablets (Infrequent) 1528
Retrovir Capsules 1533
Retrovir IV Infusion 1537
Retrovir 1533
Risperdal M-Tab Orally Disintegrating Tablets (Rare) 1658
Risperdal (Rare) 1658
Seroquel Tablets (Infrequent) 691
Sonata Capsules (Rare) 1686
Surmontil Capsules 2347
Tarka Tablets 519
Tequin Injection (Less than 0.1%) 964
Tequin Tablets (Less than 0.1%) 964
Topamax Sprinkle Capsules (Rare) 2438
Topamax Tablets (Rare) 2438
Ultracet Tablets (Less than 1%) 2462
Uniretic Tablets (Less than 1%) 3114
VFEND I.V. (Less than 2%) 2543
VFEND Oral Suspension (Less than 2%) 2543
VFEND Tablets (Less than 2%) 2543
Wellbutrin SR Sustained-Release Tablets (Rare) 1583
Wellbutrin XL Extended-Release Tablets (Rare) 1588
Xolair 1259
Zoloft (Rare) 2581
Zomig Nasal Spray (Infrequent) 718
Zomig Tablets (Infrequent) 714
Zomig-ZMT Tablets (Infrequent) 714
Zyban Sustained-Release Tablets (Rare) 1620
Zyprexa Tablets (Infrequent) 1798
Zyprexa ZYDIS Orally Disintegrating Tablets (Infrequent) 1798
Zyrtec Chewable Tablets (Less than 2%) 2589
Zyrtec (Less than 2%) 2589
Zyrtec-D 12 Hour Extended Release Tablets (Less than 2%) 2591

Edema, turbinate

Xopenex HFA Inhalation Aerosol (1.4% to 2.8%) 3151
Xopenex Inhalation Solution (1.4% to 2.8%) 3143
Xopenex Inhalation Solution Concentrate (1.4% to 2.8%) 3147

Edema, upper extremities

Avalide Tablets 922
Avalide Tablets 2889
Avapro Tablets (Less than 1%) 925
Avapro Tablets (Less than 1%) 2886
Zyprexa Tablets (Infrequent) 1798
Zyprexa ZYDIS Orally Disintegrating Tablets (Infrequent) 1798

EEG changes

Adacel Vaccine 2959
Clozapine Tablets 2141
Clozaril Tablets 2174
DAPTACEL 2964
Eskalith 1406
FazaClo Orally Disintegrating Tablets 547
Flexeril Tablets (Rare) 1832
Gabitril Tablets 998
Levaquin in 5% Dextrose Injection 2453
Levaquin 2453
Librium Capsules 3349
Paxil CR Controlled-Release Tablets (Rare) 1509
Paxil (Rare) 1501
ProSom Tablets 512
Prozac Pulvules and Liquid (Rare) 1771
Surmontil Capsules 2347
Topamax Sprinkle Capsules (Infrequent) 2438
Topamax Tablets (Infrequent) 2438
Trileptal Oral Suspension (Up to 2%) 2281
Trileptal Tablets (Up to 2%) 2281
Valium Tablets (Infrequent) 2822
Vivactil Tablets 2350
Wellbutrin Tablets (Rare) 1579
Wellbutrin SR Sustained-Release Tablets 1583
Wellbutrin XL Extended-Release Tablets 1588
Zyban Sustained-Release Tablets 1620

Efficacy, lack of

Neoral Soft Gelatin Capsules (1.4%) 2247
Neoral Oral Solution (1.4%) 2247

Ejaculate volume, decreased

▲ Proscar Tablets (1.5% to 3.7%) 2040

Ejaculation, delayed

▲ Cymbalta Delayed-Release Capsules (3%) 1729
▲ Effexor XR Capsules (17%) 3411
▲ Lexapro Oral Solution (9%) 1193
▲ Lexapro Tablets (9%) 1193
▲ Zoloft (14%) 2581

Ejaculation, inhibition

Demser Capsules (Infrequent) 1933
Dibenzyline Capsules 3390
Parnate Tablets 1499
▲ Paxil CR Controlled-Release Tablets (3.7% to 10.0%) 1509
▲ Paxil (3.7% to 10.0%) 1501
Wellbutrin Tablets (Infrequent) 1579

Ejaculation, retrograde

Flomax 881

Ejaculation disturbances

Abilify Tablets (Infrequent) 916
Abilify Tablets (Infrequent) 2472
Avinza Capsules (Less than 5%) 1714
Avodart Soft Gelatin Capsules (0.1% to 1.4%) 1353
Caduet Tablets (Less than 2%) 2507
Campral Tablets (Rare) 1175
▲ Celexa (6%) 1177
Clozapine Tablets (1%) 2141
Clozaril Tablets (1%) 2174
▲ Cymbalta Delayed-Release Capsules (3%) 1729
▲ Duragesic Transdermal System (4%) 2448
▲ Effexor Tablets (3% to 12.5%) 3405
▲ Effexor XR Capsules (5% to 16%) 3411
FazaClo Orally Disintegrating Tablets (1%) 547
▲ Flomax Capsules (8.4% to 18.1%) 881
Geodon Capsules (Infrequent) 2514
Kaletra (Less than 2%) 474
Klonopin (1%) 2782
Lamictal (Rare) 1449
Levitra Tablets (Less than 2%) 3048
▲ Lexapro Oral Solution (5% to 14%) 1193
▲ Lexapro Tablets (5% to 14%) 1193
Lipitor Tablets (Less than 2%) 2495
Lyrica Capsules (0.1% to 1%) 2524
Meridia Capsules 485
Mirapex Tablets (Less than 1%) 889
Neurontin Capsules (Infrequent) 2498
Neurontin Oral Solution (Infrequent) 2498
Neurontin Tablets (Infrequent) 2498
▲ Paxil CR Controlled-Release Tablets (1.6% to 25%) 1509
▲ Paxil (1.6% to 25%) 1501
▲ Propecia Tablets (0.2% to 3.7%) 2036
Proscar Tablets (0.2% to 0.8%) 2040
Provigil Tablets (1%) 1002
Prozac Pulvules and Liquid (Less than 1%) 1771
Requip Tablets (Rare) 1528
Risperdal M-Tab Orally Disintegrating Tablets (Infrequent) 1658
Risperdal (Infrequent) 1658
Seroquel Tablets (Infrequent) 691
▲ Strattera Capsules (5% or greater) 1784
Surmontil Capsules 2347
▲ Symbyax Capsules (2% to 7%) 1788
Thioridazine Hydrochloride Tablets 2122
▲ Topamax Sprinkle Capsules (Up to 3%) 2438
▲ Topamax Tablets (Up to 3%) 2438
Viagra Tablets (Less than 2%) 2552
Wellbutrin Tablets (Rare) 1579
Wellbutrin SR Sustained-Release Tablets 1583
Wellbutrin XL Extended-Release Tablets 1588
▲ Zoloft (7% to 19%) 2581
Zyban Sustained-Release Tablets 1620
Zyprexa Tablets (Infrequent) 1798
Zyprexa ZYDIS Orally Disintegrating Tablets (Infrequent) 1798

Ejaculation failure

Flomax Capsules 881
Levaquin in 5% Dextrose Injection (0.1% to 0.9%) 2453
Levaquin (0.1% to 0.9%) 2453
Risperdal Consta Long-Acting Injection (Infrequent) 1664
▲ Strattera Capsules (5%) 1784

Ejection fraction reduction

Adriamycin for Injection, USP 786
Adriamycin Injection, USP 786
Herceptin I.V. 1234

EKG changes

Aceon Tablets (2 mg, 4 mg, 8 mg) (1.8%) 3191
Aciphex Tablets 1081
Aloprim for Injection (Less than 1%) 2156
Amerge Tablets (Infrequent) 1312
Anzemet Injection (Rare) 2871
Anzemet Tablets (Rare) 2874
Atacand HCT (0.5% or greater) 637
Avelox (Less than 0.1%) 2984
Cardene I.V. (1.4%) 1129
Cardizem LA Extended Release Tablets (Less than 2%) 1699
▲ Carnitor Injection (2% to 6%) 3185
Catapres Tablets (Rare) 874
Catapres-TTS (0.5% or less) 875
Clorpres Tablets (Rare) 2139
Clozapine Tablets (1%) 2141
Clozaril Tablets (1%) 2174
Digitek Tablets 2146
Diprivan Injectable Emulsion (Less than 1%) 676
Effexor Tablets 3405
Effexor XR Capsules 3411
Eskalith 1406
Evoxac Capsules (Less than 1%) 1042
FazaClo Orally Disintegrating Tablets (1%) 547
Frova Tablets (Infrequent) 1101
Gabitril Tablets (Infrequent) 998
Hyperstat I.V. Injection 3031
Imitrex Nasal Spray (Infrequent) 1435
Imitrex Tablets (Infreqent) 1440
I.V. Busulfex (2%) 1125
Kytril Injection (Rare) 2785
Lamictal (Rare) 1449
Lanoxicaps Capsules 1458
Lanoxin Injection 1462
Lanoxin Tablets 1468
Lanoxin Injection Pediatric 1465
Lexapro Oral Solution (Infrequent) 1193
Lexapro Tablets (Infrequent) 1193
Lofibra Capsules 1217
Lotensin HCT Tablets 2235
Micardis Tablets (More than 0.3%) 884
Micardis HCT Tablets 886
Midamor Tablets 2000
Nalfon Capsules (Less than 1%) 2504
Naropin Injection (Less than 1%) 640
Nimotop Capsules (Up to 1.4%) 774
▲ Novantrone for Injection Concentrate (5% to 11%) 3158
Orap Tablets (2.7%) 1220
Paxil CR Controlled-Release Tablets (Infrequent) 1509
Paxil (Infrequent) 1501
Permax Tablets (Infrequent) 3357
Prandin Tablets (0.5, 1, and 2 mg) (Less than or equal to 1%) 2337
▲ Prograf Capsules and Injection (3% to 15%) 624
Protonix I.V. (Less than 1%) 3468
Protonix Tablets (Less than 1%) 3465
Retrovir Capsules (2.4%) 1533
▲ Retrovir IV Infusion (3%) 1537
Retrovir (2.4%) 1533
Seroquel Tablets (Rare) 691
Suprane Liquid for Inhalation (Less than 1%) 770
Taxotere Injection Concentrate 2947
Teveten Tablets (Less than 1%) 1707
Teveten HCT Tablets (Less than 1%) 1710
Thioridazine Hydrochloride Tablets 2122
Tiazac Capsules (Less than 2%) 1204
Tricor Tablets 523
Triglide Tablets 1165
Uniretic Tablets (More than 1%) 3114
Verelan PM Capsules (2%) 3120
Viagra Tablets (Less than 2%) 2552
Wellbutrin Tablets (Infrequent) 1579
Xopenex HFA Inhalation Aerosol 3151
Xopenex Inhalation Solution 3143
Xopenex Inhalation Solution Concentrate 3147
Zemuron Injection (Less than 1%) 2363
Zofran Injection (Rare) 1607
Zofran (Rare) 1613
Zofran ODT Orally Disintegrating Tablets (Rare) 1613
Zomig Tablets (Rare) 714
Zomig-ZMT Tablets (Rare) 714

EKG changes, PR prolongation

Amerge Tablets (Infrequent) 1312
Digitek Tablets 2146
Imitrex Injection (Infrequent) 1431
Imitrex Tablets 1440
Lanoxicaps Capsules 1458
Lanoxin Injection 1462
Lanoxin Tablets 1468
Lanoxin Injection Pediatric 1465

EKG changes, Q wave disturbances

▲ Imdur Tablets (Less than or equal to 5%) 3032

EKG changes, QRS interval prolonged

Seroquel Tablets (Infrequent) 691

EKG changes, QT interval prolonged

Abilify Tablets (Infrequent) 916
Abilify Tablets (Infrequent) 2472
Aciphex Tablets (Rare) 1081
Aloxi Injection (Less than 1%) 2099
Amerge Tablets (Infrequent) 1312
Apokyn Injection 2132
Avelox (0.1% to less than 2%) 2984
Celexa 1177
E.E.S. 449
Effexor Tablets (Rare) 3405
Effexor XR Capsules (Rare) 3411
Erythrocin Stearate Filmtab Tablets (Rare) 452
Erythromycin Base Filmtab Tablets (Rare) 454
Erythromycin Delayed-Release Capsules, USP 456
Factive Tablets 2464
Geodon Capsules 2514
Imitrex Injection (Infrequent) 1431
Levaquin in 5% Dextrose Injection 2453
Levaquin 2453
Lexapro Oral Solution 1193
Lexapro Tablets 1193
Namenda 1199
Noroxin Tablets (Rare) 2009
Orap Tablets 1220
PCE Dispertab Tablets 510
Pletal Tablets (Very rare) 2478
Prograf Capsules and Injection 624
Prozac Pulvules and Liquid 1771
Razadyne ER Extended-Release Capsules (Infrequent) 2434
Razadyne (Infrequent) 2434
Rythmol SR Capsules 2736
Seroquel Tablets (Infrequent) 691
Symbyax Capsules (Infrequent) 1788
Tequin Injection 964
Tequin Tablets 964
Thioridazine Hydrochloride Tablets 2122
▲ Trisenox Injection (8%) 983
Uniretic Tablets (Less than 1%) 3114
VFEND I.V. (Less than 2%) 2543
VFEND Oral Suspension (Less than 2%) 2543
VFEND Tablets (Less than 2%) 2543
Viracept 2556
Zithromax Capsules, 250 mg (Rare) 2568
Zithromax for IV Infusion 2573
Zithromax for Oral Suspension, 300 mg, 600 mg, 900 mg, 1200 mg (Rare) 2561
Zithromax Tablets, 250 mg, 500 mg (Rare) 2561
Zithromax Tri-Pak (Rare) 2561
Zoloft 2581
Zomig Tablets (Rare) 714
Zomig-ZMT Tablets (Rare) 714

EKG changes, reversible flattening

Eskalith 1406

EKG changes, sinus pause

Tambocor Tablets (1% to 3%) 1824

EKG changes, ST section

AccuNeb Inhalation Solution (One case) 1055
▲ Adenoscan (3%) 613
Amerge Tablets (Infrequent) 1312

Anzemet Injection 2871
Anzemet Tablets 2874
Cardene I.V. (Rare) 1129
Clozapine Tablets 2141
Clozaril Tablets 2174
Digitek Tablets 2146
Diprivan Injectable Emulsion (Less than 1%) 676
Ellence Injection 2632
Imitrex Injection (Infrequent) 1431
Imitrex Tablets 1440
Lanoxicaps Capsules 1458
Lanoxin Injection 1462
Lanoxin Tablets 1468
Lanoxin Injection Pediatric 1465
Naropin Injection (Less than 1%) 640
OxyContin Tablets (Less than 1%) 2699
Risperdal M-Tab Orally Disintegrating Tablets (Rare) 1658
Risperdal (Rare) 1658
Seroquel Tablets (Rare) 691
Tarka Tablets (0.3% or more) 519

EKG changes, T-wave
Adenoscan (Less than 1%) 613
Amerge Tablets (Infrequent) 1312
Anzemet Injection 2871
Anzemet Tablets 2874
Cardene I.V. (Rare) 1129
Clozapine Tablets 2141
Clozaril Tablets 2174
Eskalith 1406
Evoxac Capsules (Less than 1%) 1042
Imitrex Injection (Infrequent) 1431
Imitrex Tablets 1440
Lithobid Tablets (Rare) 1670
Moban Tablets (Rare) 1108
Orap Tablets 1220
Pentasa Capsules (Infrequent) 3182
Razadyne ER Extended-Release Capsules (Infrequent) 2434
Razadyne (Infrequent) 2434
Risperdal Consta Long-Acting Injection (Rare) 1664
Risperdal M-Tab Orally Disintegrating Tablets (Rare) 1658
Risperdal (Rare) 1658
Sular Tablets (Less than or equal to 1%) 1163
Symbyax Capsules (Rare) 1788
Tarka Tablets (0.3% or more) 519
Uniretic Tablets (less than 1%) 3114

Elastosis perforans, serpiginosa
Cuprimine Capsules (Rare) 1925

Elation
▲ Marinol Capsules (8% to 24%) 3334

Electrocardiogram, abnormal
Antara Capsules 2723
Edex Injection 3103
Provigil Tablets (Greater than or equal to 1%) 1002
Rythmol SR Capsules 2736
Symbyax Capsules (Infrequent) 1788

Electrocardiographic changes
(*see under* EKG changes)

Electroencephalographic changes
(*see under* EEG changes)

Electrolyte disturbances
(*see under* Electrolyte imbalance)

Electrolyte imbalance
Aldoclor Tablets 1881
Aldoril Tablets 1884
Aloprim for Injection (Less than 1%) 2156
Aloxi Injection (Less than 1%) 2099
Anadrol-50 Tablets 3329
Avalide Tablets 922
Avalide Tablets 2889
Benicar HCT Tablets 2852
Camptosar Injection 2602
Capastat Sulfate for Injection (1 patient) 1728
Cubicin for Injection (Less than 1%) 1038
Daranide Tablets 1928
Decadron Phosphate Injection 1931
Diovan HCT Tablets 2195
Diuril Oral 1936
Diuril Sodium Intravenous 1934
Dyazide Capsules 1389
Epivir 1394
Follistim AQ Cartridge 2354
Indapamide Tablets 2119
Levaquin in 5% Dextrose Injection (0.1% to 0.9%) 2453
Levaquin (0.1% to 0.9%) 2453
Maxzide 2150
Moduretic Tablets 2003
Navelbine Injection 1494
Permax Tablets (Rare) 3357
Pravachol Tablets 943
Prevacid Delayed-Release Capsules 3268
Prevacid for Delayed-Release Oral Suspension 3268
Prevacid NapraPAC 3277
Prevacid SoluTab Delayed-Release Orally Disintegrating Tablets 3268
PREVPAC 3281
Prinzide Tablets 2033
Risperdal M-Tab Orally Disintegrating Tablets 1658
Risperdal 1658
Tequin Injection (Less than 0.1%) 964
Tequin Tablets (Less than 0.1%) 964
Teveten HCT Tablets 1710
Thalomid Capsules 979
Timolide Tablets 2056
Uniretic Tablets (More than 1%) 3114
Vaseretic Tablets 2073
Zelnorm Tablets 2303
Zestoretic Tablets 701
Zosyn 3492

Electromechanical dissociation
Retavase 1131

Electro-oculogram, abnormal
Norvir (Less than 2%) 499

Elevated bilirubin levels
(*see under* Hyperbilirubinemia)

Embolism
Activase I.V. 1225
Activella Tablets 2311
▲ Alimta for Injection (1% to 7%) 1722
Aygestin Tablets 1062
Decadron Tablets 1929
Furosemide Tablets 2117
Gleevec Tablets (Rare) 2221
Levaquin in 5% Dextrose Injection (0.1% to 0.9%) 2453
Levaquin (0.1% to 0.9%) 2453
Navelbine Injection (Up to 10%) 1494
Ortho-Cept Tablets 2395
Ortho-Cyclen/Ortho Tri-Cyclen 2414
Ortho Tri-Cyclen Lo Tablets 2421
TNKase I.V. 1256
Trasylol Injection (1% to 2%) 779
Zosyn (1.0% or less) 3492

Embolism, arterial
Rythmol SR Capsules 2736

Embolism, cholesterol
Activase I.V. (Rare) 1225
TNKase I.V. 1256

Embolism, limb
ReoPro Vials (0.3%) 1779
Requip Tablets (Rare) 1528

Embolism, lower extremities
Camptosar Injection 2602
Rilutek Tablets (Infrequent) 2945

Embolism, pulmonary
Abelcet Injection 1119
Abilify Tablets (Rare) 916
Abilify Tablets (Rare) 2472
Aciphex Tablets (Rare) 1081
Actimmune (Rare) 1646
Activella Tablets 2311
Alesse-28 Tablets 3392
Aloprim for Injection (Less than 1%) 2156
Ambien Tablets (Rare) 2867
Apokyn Injection 2132
Aranesp for Injection (1.3%) 576
Arthrotec Tablets (Rare) 3126
▲ Avastin IV (16%) 1229
Aygestin Tablets 1062
Betaseron for SC Injection 791
Campath Ampules 826
Campral Tablets (Rare) 1175
Camptosar Injection 2602
Cathflo Activase 1232
Celebrex Capsules (Less than 0.1%) 3130
Celexa (Rare) 1177
Cenestin Tablets, 0.45mg, 0.625mg, 0.9mg, 1.25mg 1063
Cenestin Tablets, 0.3mg 1063
Cipro I.V. (1% or less) 2998
Cipro I.V. Pharmacy Bulk Package (1% or less) 3509
Cipro (Less than 1%) 2991
Cipro XR Tablets 3004
Climara Transdermal System 795
Climara Pro Transdermal System 800
Clozapine Tablets 2141
Clozaril Tablets 2174
CombiPatch Transdermal System 2180
Copegus Tablets (Less than 1%) 2759
Depo-Provera Contraceptive Injection (Less than 1%) 2619
depo-subQ provera 104 Injectable Suspension 2622
Effexor Tablets (Rare) 3405
Effexor XR Capsules (Rare) 3411
Emcyt Capsules (2%) 3137
Emend Capsules (Greater than 0.5%) 1944
Enbrel for Injection (Infrequent) 580
Epogen for Injection (Rare) 586
Erbitux (1%) 937
Estratest Tablets 3196
Estratest H.S. Tablets 3196
Estrogel 0.06% 3200
Evoxac Capsules (Less than 1%) 1042
Exelon Capsules (Infrequent) 2204
FazaClo Orally Disintegrating Tablets 547
Femara Tablets (Less than or equal to 2%) 2210
Gammagard S/D 754
Geodon Capsules (Rare) 2514
Imitrex Nasal Spray 1435
Imitrex Tablets 1440
Levaquin in 5% Dextrose Injection (0.1% to 0.9%) 2453
Levaquin (0.1% to 0.9%) 2453
Lexapro Oral Solution 1193
Lexapro Tablets 1193
Lo/Ovral-28 Tablets 3423
Lupron Depot–3 Month 11.25 mg 3262
Lupron Injection Pediatric 3256
Megace ES Oral Suspension 2492
Menostar Transdermal System 805
Merrem I.V. (Greater than 0.1% to 1%) 687
Mirapex Tablets (Less than 1%) 889
Mycamine for Injection 620
Namenda (Infrequent) 1199
Naropin Injection (Less than 1%) 640
Navelbine Injection 1494
Neurontin Capsules (Rare) 2498
Neurontin Oral Solution (Rare) 2498
Neurontin Tablets (Rare) 2498
Nipent for Injection (Less than 3%) 3216
Ortho-Cept Tablets 2395
Ortho-Cyclen Tablets 2414
Ortho Evra Transdermal System 2402
Ortho Tri-Cyclen Tablets 2414
Ortho Tri-Cyclen Lo Tablets 2421
Paxil CR Controlled-Release Tablets (Rare) 1509
Paxil (Rare) 1501
Pegasys (Less than 1%) 2793
Permax Tablets (Infrequent) 3357
Prefest Tablets 1069
Premarin Intravenous 3440
Premarin Tablets 3443
Premarin Vaginal Cream 3449
Premphase Tablets (1.3%) 3452
Prempro Tablets (1.3%) 3452
Prinivil Tablets (0.3% to 1.0%) 2029
Prinzide Tablets 2033
▲ Procrit for Injection (3.2%) 2374
Proleukin for Injection (Less than 1%) 1007
Prozac Pulvules and Liquid 1771
Remicade for IV Injection (Greater than or equal to 0.2%) 987
ReoPro Vials (0.3%) 1779
Requip Tablets (Rare) 1528
Risperdal Consta Long-Acting Injection (Rare) 1664
Risperdal M-Tab Orally Disintegrating Tablets 1658
Risperdal 1658
Sandostatin LAR Depot (1% to 4%) 2264
Seasonale Tablets 1073
Sonata Capsules (Rare) 1686
Tasmar Tablets (Infrequent) 3360
Taxotere Injection Concentrate 2947
Tenormin I.V. Injection (1.2%) 698
Tenormin Tablets (1.2%) 695
Thalomid Capsules 979
Topamax Sprinkle Capsules (Infrequent) 2438
Topamax Tablets (Infrequent) 2438
Trasylol Injection (1% to 2%) 779
Triphasil-28 Tablets 3483
Vaseretic Tablets 2073
Vasotec I.V. Injection (0.5% to 1.0%) 2076
VFEND I.V. (Less than 2%) 2543
VFEND Oral Suspension (Less than 2%) 2543
VFEND Tablets (Less than 2%) 2543
Vivelle Transdermal System 2288
Vivelle-Dot Transdermal System 2293
Wellbutrin Tablets (Rare) 1579
Wellbutrin SR Sustained-Release Tablets 1583
Wellbutrin XL Extended-Release Tablets 1588
▲ Xeloda Tablets (Less than 5%) 2825
Yasmin 28 Tablets 818
Zestoretic Tablets 701
Zestril Tablets (0.3% to 1.0%) 704
Zevalin Injection (Less than 1%) 848
Zoladex 3-month (1% to 5%) 712
Zonegran Capsules (Rare) 1089
Zosyn (1.0% or less) 3492
Zyban Sustained-Release Tablets 1620
Zyprexa Tablets 1798
Zyprexa ZYDIS Orally Disintegrating Tablets 1798

Embolism, retinal artery
Xalatan Sterile Ophthalmic Solution (Extremely rare) 2654

Embolism, venous
Retavase 1131

Emesis
(*see under* Vomiting)

Emotional disturbances
Accutane Capsules 2740
Avalide Tablets 922
Avalide Tablets 2889
Avapro Tablets (Less than 1%) 925
Avapro Tablets (Less than 1%) 2886
Decadron Tablets 1929
Depacon Injection 412
Depakene 417
Depakote Sprinkle Capsules 422
Depakote Tablets 427
Depakote ER Tablets 433
Efudex (Infrequent) 3348
Imitrex Nasal Spray (Rare) 1435
Lariam Tablets (Less than 1%) 2790
Paxil CR Controlled-Release Tablets (Infrequent) 1509
Paxil (Infrequent) 1501
Rythmol SR Capsules 2736

Emotional lability
Abilify Tablets (Infrequent) 916
Abilify Tablets (Infrequent) 2472
Accutane Capsules 2740
Actiq (Less than 1%) 993
Activella Tablets (0% to 6%) 2311
▲ Adderall XR Capsules (1% to 9%) 3169
Adenoscan (Less than 1%) 613
Ambien Tablets (Infrequent) 2867
Amnesteem Capsules 2126
AndroGel (Up to 3%) 3330
Aricept Tablets (Infrequent) 1086
Aricept ODT Tablets (Infrequent) 1086
Asacol Delayed-Release Tablets 2688
Avelox (Less than 0.1%) 2984
Betaseron for SC Injection 791
Blocadren Tablets 1891
Bravelle for Intramuscular or Subcutaneous Injection (2% to 2.7%) 1140
Caduet Tablets (Less than 2%) 2507
Celexa (Infrequent) 1177
▲ CellCept Capsules (3% to less than 20%) 2751
▲ CellCept Intravenous (3% to less than 20%) 2751
▲ CellCept Oral Suspension (3% to less than 20%) 2751
▲ CellCept Tablets (3% to less than 20%) 2751
▲ Clarinex Syrup (3.1%) 3009
Concerta Extended-Release Tablets (0.7%) 1828
Copaxone for Injection (At least 2%) 3292
Coreg Tablets (Greater than 0.1% to 1%) 1376
Cosopt Sterile Ophthalmic Solution 1910
▲ Depacon Injection (6%) 412
▲ Depakene (6%) 417
▲ Depakote Sprinkle Capsules (6%) 422
▲ Depakote Tablets (1% to 6%) 427
▲ Depakote ER Tablets (6%) 433

Diastat Rectal Delivery System (Greater than or equal to 1%) 3344
Diprivan Injectable Emulsion (Less than 1%) 676
▲ Doxil Injection (1% to 5%) 3302
Effexor Tablets (Infrequent) 3405
Effexor XR Capsules (Infrequent) 3411
Elmiron Capsules 2393
Emcyt Capsules (2%) 3137
Evoxac Capsules (Less than 1%) 1042
Exelon Capsules (Infrequent) 2204
Frova Tablets (Infrequent) 1101
▲ Gabitril Tablets (3%) 998
Gengraf Capsules (1% to less than 3%) 458
Guanidine Hydrochloride Tablets 3030
Inderal LA Long-Acting Capsules 3421
▲ Infergen (6% to 12%) 1647
InnoPran XL Capsules 2728
▲ Intron A for Injection (Less than 5%) 3038
Kaletra (Less than 2%) 474
▲ Keppra Oral Solution (2% to 6%) 3307
▲ Keppra Tablets (2% to 6%) 3307
Klonopin (1%) 2782
▲ Lamictal (4%) 1449
Levaquin in 5% Dextrose Injection (0.1% to 0.9%) 2453
Levaquin (0.1% to 0.9%) 2453
Levothroid Tablets 1189
Levoxyl Tablets 1680
Lexapro Oral Solution (Infrequent) 1193
Lexapro Tablets (Infrequent) 1193
Lipitor Tablets (Less than 2%) 2495
Lunesta Tablets (Infrequent) 3139
▲ Lupron Depot 3.75 mg (16%) 3257
▲ Lupron Depot–3 Month 11.25 mg (16%) 3262
Lupron Depot-PED 7.5 mg, 11.25 mg and 15 mg (Less than 2%) 3266
Lupron Injection Pediatric (Less than 2%) 3256
Meridia Capsules (1.3%) 485
Nadolol Tablets 2121
Namenda (Infrequent) 1199
Naropin Injection (Less than 1%) 640
Neoral Soft Gelatin Capsules (1% to less than 3%) 2247
Neoral Oral Solution (1% to less than 3%) 2247
▲ Neurontin Capsules (4.2% to 6%) 2498
▲ Neurontin Oral Solution (4.2% to 6%) 2498
▲ Neurontin Tablets (4.2% to 6%) 2498
▲ Nicotrol NS (Greater than 5%) 2596
Nipent for Injection (Less than 3%) 3216
Norvir (Less than 2%) 499
Omacor Capsules 2735
Oncaspar (Less than 1%) 1123
OxyContin Tablets (Less than 1%) 2699
Paxil CR Controlled-Release Tablets (Frequent) 1509
Paxil (Frequent) 1501
Pediapred Oral Solution 3319
▲ PEG-Intron Powder for Injection (28%) 3062
Permax Tablets (Infrequent) 3357
Prevacid Delayed-Release Capsules (Less than 1%) 3268
Prevacid for Delayed-Release Oral Suspension (Less than 1%) 3268
Prevacid NapraPAC (Less than 1%) 3277
Prevacid SoluTab Delayed-Release Orally Disintegrating Tablets (Less than 1%) 3268
PREVPAC (Less than 1%) 3281
Prochieve 4% Gel 1018
Prochieve 8% Gel 1018
▲ Prograf Capsules and Injection (3% to 15%) 624
▲ Prometrium Capsules (100 mg, 200 mg) (6%) 3205
ProSom Tablets (Infrequent) 512
Protonix I.V. (Less than 1%) 3468
Protonix Tablets (Less than 1%) 3465
Provigil Tablets (1%) 1002
Prozac Pulvules and Liquid (Frequent) 1771
Pulmicort Respules (1% to 3%) 654
▲ Rapamune Oral Solution and Tablets (3% to 20%) 3472
▲ Rebetol (7% to 47%) 3073
▲ Rebetron Combination Therapy (7% to 12%) 3078
Relpax Tablets (Infrequent) 2531
Requip Tablets (Infrequent) 1528
Rescriptor Tablets 2535
Retrovir Capsules 1533
Retrovir IV Infusion 1537
Retrovir 1533
Reyataz Capsules (Less than 3%) 948
▲ Ribavirin, USP Capsules (7% to 47%) 3083
Rilutek Tablets (Infrequent) 2945
Risperdal Consta Long-Acting Injection (Infrequent) 1664
Risperdal M-Tab Orally Disintegrating Tablets (Rare) 1658
Risperdal (Rare) 1658
Seroquel Tablets (Rare) 691
Sonata Capsules (Frequent) 1686
Striant Mucoadhesive 1022
Sustiva Capsules (Less than 2%) 957
Symbyax Capsules (Infrequent) 1788
Tasmar Tablets (Frequent) 3360
Tenormin I.V. Injection 698
Tenormin Tablets 695
Thalomid Capsules 979
Timolide Tablets 2056
Timoptic in Ocudose 2061
Timoptic Sterile Ophthalmic Solution 2058
Timoptic-XE Sterile Ophthalmic Gel Forming Solution 2062
▲ Topamax Sprinkle Capsules (3%) 2438
▲ Topamax Tablets (3%) 2438
Toprol-XL Tablets 660
Trelstar Depot (1.4%) 3385
▲ Trileptal Oral Suspension (2% to 3%) 2281
▲ Trileptal Tablets (2% to 3%) 2281
Ultracet Tablets (Less than 1%) 2462
Uniretic Tablets (Less than 1%) 3114
Unithroid Tablets 3521
Viracept (Less than 2%) 2556
Wellbutrin SR Sustained-Release Tablets (Infrequent) 1583
Wellbutrin XL Extended-Release Tablets (Infrequent) 1588
Yasmin 28 Tablets 818
▲ Zoladex (60%) 709
Zoladex 3-month 712
Zoloft (Infrequent) 2581
Zomig Tablets (Infrequent) 714
Zomig-ZMT Tablets (Infrequent) 714
Zyban Sustained-Release Tablets (Infrequent) 1620
Zyprexa Tablets 1798
Zyprexa IntraMuscular (Infrequent) 1798
Zyprexa ZYDIS Orally Disintegrating Tablets 1798
Zyrtec Chewable Tablets (Less than 2%) 2589
Zyrtec (Less than 2%) 2589
Zyrtec-D 12 Hour Extended Release Tablets (Less than 2%) 2591

Emphysema
Levaquin in 5% Dextrose Injection (0.1% to 0.9%) 2453
Levaquin (0.1% to 0.9%) 2453
Lupron Depot 7.5 mg (Less than 5%) 3261
Paxil CR Controlled-Release Tablets (Rare) 1509
Paxil (Rare) 1501
Permax Tablets (Infrequent) 3357
Prozac Pulvules and Liquid (Rare) 1771
Symbyax Capsules (Rare) 1788
Thalomid Capsules 979

Empyema
Zevalin Injection (2%) 848

Enanthema
Gengraf Capsules (1% to less than 3%) 458
Neoral Soft Gelatin Capsules (1% to less than 3%) 2247
Neoral Oral Solution (1% to less than 3%) 2247

Encephalitis
Attenuvax 1889
Boostrix 1366
M-M-R II (Very rare) 1980
Mumpsvax (Very rare) 2005
Nipent for Injection (Less than 3%) 3216
Orthoclone OKT3 Sterile Solution (Less than 1%) 2370
Rabies Vaccine RabAvert 1011
Recombivax HB 2045
Vaqta (Very rare) 2067
Varivax 2070
VFEND I.V. (Less than 2%) 2543
VFEND Oral Suspension (Less than 2%) 2543
VFEND Tablets (Less than 2%) 2543

Encephalitis, measles inclusion body
Attenuvax 1889
M-M-R II 1980

Encephalopathy
Abelcet Injection 1119
Adacel Vaccine 2959
Ammonul Injection 3323
Attenuvax 1889
Campral Tablets (Rare) 1175
Cytovene 2763
DAPTACEL 2964
Depacon Injection (Rare) 412
Depakene (Rare instances) 417
Depakote Sprinkle Capsules (Rare) 422
Depakote Tablets (Rare instances) 427
Depakote ER Tablets (Rare instances) 433
Fortaz 1422
Gabitril Tablets (Infrequent) 998
Garamycin Injectable 3028
Gengraf Capsules 458
Havrix Vaccine (Rare) 1425
Infanrix Vaccine 1444
I.V. Busulfex (2%) 1125
Kaletra (Less than 2%) 474
Lariam Tablets 2790
Levaquin in 5% Dextrose Injection (0.1% to 0.9%) 2453
Levaquin (0.1% to 0.9%) 2453
Lyrica Capsules (Rare) 2524
Maxipime for Injection 1093
▲ Midamor Tablets (Between 1% and 3%) 2000
M-M-R II (Very rare) 1980
Moduretic Tablets 2003
Mycamine for Injection 620
Neoral Soft Gelatin Capsules 2247
Neoral Oral Solution 2247
Neurontin Capsules (Rare) 2498
Neurontin Oral Solution (Rare) 2498
Neurontin Tablets (Rare) 2498
Orthoclone OKT3 Sterile Solution (Less than 1%) 2370
Paser Granules 1657
Pediarix Vaccine 1518
Primaxin I.M. 2022
Primaxin I.V. (Less than 0.2%) 2024
▲ Prograf Capsules and Injection (3% to 15%) 624
Proleukin for Injection 1007
Roferon-A Injection (Infrequent) 2805
Sandimmune 2259
Stromectol Tablets 2053
Tasmar Tablets (Rare) 3360
Topamax Sprinkle Capsules (Infrequent) 2438
Topamax Tablets (Infrequent) 2438
Twinrix Vaccine 1571
Valtrex Caplets 1573
▲ Vesanoid Capsules (3%) 2823
VFEND I.V. (Less than 2%) 2543
VFEND Oral Suspension (Less than 2%) 2543
VFEND Tablets (Less than 2%) 2543
▲ Xeloda Tablets (Less than 5%) 2825
Zevalin Injection (Less than 1%) 848
Zonegran Capsules (Rare) 1089
Zovirax Capsules 1616
Zovirax for Injection (Approximately 1%) 1618
Zovirax 1616
Zyprexa Tablets (Rare) 1798
Zyprexa ZYDIS Orally Disintegrating Tablets (Rare) 1798

Encephalopathy, hepatic
Aciphex Tablets (Rare) 1081
Eulexin Capsules 3023
Intron A for Injection (Very rare) 3038
Prilosec OTC Tablets (Rare) 2674
Zegerid Powder for Oral Solution (Rare) 2972

Encephalopathy, hypertensive
Catapres-TTS (Rare) 875
Clorpres Tablets 2139
Epogen for Injection (On occasion) 586
Humira Injection 464
Procrit for Injection (Occasional) 2374

Endocardial fibrosis
Myleran Tablets (One case) 1492

Endocarditis
▲ Copegus Tablets (3%) 2759
Oncaspar (Less than 1%) 1123
▲ Pegasys (3% to 5%) 2793
Proleukin for Injection (1%) 1007
VFEND I.V. (Less than 2%) 2543
VFEND Oral Suspension (Less than 2%) 2543
VFEND Tablets (Less than 2%) 2543

Endocarditis, infectious
CellCept Capsules (Occasional) 2751
CellCept Intravenous (Occasional) 2751
CellCept Oral Suspension (Occasional) 2751
CellCept Tablets (Occasional) 2751
Myfortic Tablets (Occasionally) 2244

Endocrine disturbances
Elocon Lotion 0.1% (1 in 65 patients) 3020
Imitrex Nasal Spray 1435
Permax Tablets (Rare) 3357
Pravachol Tablets 943

Endometrial carcinoma
(*see under* Carcinoma, endometrial)

Endometrial disorder, unspecified
▲ Estrogel 0.06% (1.8%) 3200
Evista Tablets 1735
Evoxac Capsules (Less than 1%) 1042
Symbyax Capsules (Rare) 1788

Endometrial hyperplasia
▲ Cenestin Tablets, 0.45mg, 0.625mg, 0.9mg, 1.25mg (18.9%) 1063
Cenestin Tablets, 0.3mg 1063
Climara Transdermal System 795
Climara Pro Transdermal System 800
Estratest Tablets 3196
Estratest H.S. Tablets 3196
Estrogel 0.06% 3200
Menostar Transdermal System 805
Prefest Tablets 1069
Premarin Tablets 3443
Premarin Vaginal Cream 3449
Premphase Tablets 3452
Prempro Tablets 3452
Vivelle Transdermal System 2288
Vivelle-Dot Transdermal System 2293

Endometriosis
Cenestin Tablets, 0.45mg, 0.625mg, 0.9mg, 1.25mg 1063
Effexor XR Capsules (Rare) 3411
Imitrex Injection 1431
Imitrex Nasal Spray (Rare) 1435
Imitrex Tablets 1440
Tarka Tablets (Less frequent) 519

Endometriosis, exacerbation of
CombiPatch Transdermal System 2180
Prefest Tablets 1069
Vivelle-Dot Transdermal System 2293

Endometrium disorders, unspecified
Amerge Tablets (Rare) 1312

Endophthalmitis
Campath Ampules 826

Endotracheal tube, reflux into
▲ Infasurf Intratracheal Suspension (21%) 1188

Endotracheal tube occlusion
Curosurf Intratracheal Suspension 1057

Energy, high
Eldepryl Capsules 3209
Sedapap Tablets 50 mg/650 mg (Infrequent) 2098
Xanax XR Tablets (Infrequent) 2655

Energy, loss of
▲ Gabitril Tablets (20%) 998
Ortho-Cyclen/Ortho Tri-Cyclen 2414
Ortho Tri-Cyclen Lo Tablets 2421

Enteritis
Ambien Tablets (Rare) 2867
Arthrotec Tablets (Rare) 3126
Caduet Tablets (Less than 2%) 2507
▲ Entocort EC Capsules (Less than 5%) 2694
Kaletra (Less than 2%) 474
Lipitor Tablets (Less than 2%) 2495
Micardis HCT Tablets 886
Paxil CR Controlled-Release Tablets (Rare) 1509
Paxil (Rare) 1501
Prevacid Delayed-Release Capsules (Less than 1%) 3268
Prevacid for Delayed-Release Oral Suspension (Less than 1%) 3268
Prevacid NapraPAC (Less than 1%) 3277
Prevacid SoluTab Delayed-Release Orally Disintegrating Tablets (Less than 1%) 3268
PREVPAC (Less than 1%) 3281
Protonix I.V. (Less than 1%) 3468
Protonix Tablets (Less than 1%) 3465
Prozac Pulvules and Liquid (Rare) 1771
Rescriptor Tablets 2535
Sonata Capsules (Rare) 1686

Trileptal Oral Suspension 2281
Trileptal Tablets 2281
Uniretic Tablets (Less than 1%) 3114
Zithromax for Oral Suspension, 300 mg, 600 mg, 900 mg, 1200 mg (1% or less) 2561
Zithromax Tablets, 250 mg, 500 mg (1% or less) 2561
Zithromax Tri-Pak (1% or less) 2561
Zyprexa Tablets (Rare) 1798
Zyprexa ZYDIS Orally Disintegrating Tablets (Rare) 1798

Enterocolitis
Augmentin 1331
Augmentin Tablets 1334
Augmentin XR Extended-Release Tablets 1340
Augmentin ES-600 Powder for Oral Suspension 1337
Dynacin Tablets 1859
Evoxac Capsules (Less than 1%) 1042
Indocin I.V. (Less than 3%) 1973
Kaletra (Less than 2%) 474
Omnicef Capsules 506
Omnicef for Oral Suspension 506
ProSom Tablets (Rare) 512

Enterocolitis, necrotizing
▲ Cafcit (4.3%) 1854
Indocin I.V. 1973
▲ Infasurf Intratracheal Suspension (5% to 17%) 1188
▲ Xeloda Tablets (Less than 5%) 2825

Enterocolitis, neutropenic
Taxotere Injection Concentrate 2947

Enterocolitis with perforation
Idamycin PFS Injection (Rare) 2645

Entropion
Botox Purified Neurotoxin Complex (Less than 1%) 565

Enuresis
Aricept Tablets 1086
Aricept ODT Tablets 1086
Depacon Injection 412
Depakene 417
Depakote Sprinkle Capsules 422
Depakote Tablets 427
Depakote ER Tablets 433
Klonopin (Infrequent) 2782
Mintezol 2002
Thalomid Capsules 979
Wellbutrin Tablets (Rare) 1579
Zonegran Capsules (Rare) 1089

Eosinophilia
Abelcet Injection 1119
Abilify Tablets (Rare to infrequent) 916
Abilify Tablets (Rare to infrequent) 2472
Accolate Tablets (Rare) 663
Aceon Tablets (2 mg, 4 mg, 8 mg) 3191
Adalat CC Tablets (Less than 1%) 2978
Advair Diskus 100/50 (Rare) 1291
Advair Diskus 250/50 (Rare) 1291
Advair Diskus 500/50 (Rare) 1291
Advicor Tablets 1694
Aldoclor Tablets 1881
Aldoril Tablets 1884
Aloprim for Injection (Less than 1%) 2156
Altace Capsules (Less than 1%) 1673
Altoprev Extended-Release Tablets 1151
Amoxil Capsules 1315
Amoxil Chewable Tablets 1315
Amoxil Pediatric Drops for Oral Suspension 1315
Amoxil Powder for Oral Suspension 1315
Amoxil Tablets 1315
Anaprox Tablets (Less than 1%) 2769
Anaprox DS Tablets (Less than 1%) 2769
Ancef for Injection 1318
Antara Capsules 2723
Arava Tablets (Rare) 2881
Aricept Tablets (Infrequent) 1086
Aricept ODT Tablets (Infrequent) 1086
Arthrotec Tablets (Rare) 3126
Asacol Delayed-Release Tablets 2688
Augmentin 1331
Augmentin Tablets 1334
Augmentin XR Extended-Release Tablets 1340
Augmentin ES-600 Powder for Oral Suspension 1337
Avelox (0.1% to less than 2%) 2984
Axid Oral Solution (Rare) 913
BiDil Tablets 2161
Campral Tablets (Infrequent) 1175
▲ Cancidas for Injection (3.1% to 3.2%) 1894
Capastat Sulfate for Injection (Majority of patients) 1728
▲ Captopril Tablets (About 4 to 7 of 100 patients) 2114
Carbatrol Capsules 3174
Cataflam Tablets (Occasionally) 2173
Ceftin (0.1% to 1%) 1369
Chemet Capsules (0.5% to 1.5%) 2480
Cipro I.V. (Greater than 1%) 2998
Cipro I.V. Pharmacy Bulk Package (Greater than 1%) 3509
Cipro (0.6%) 2991
Cipro XR Tablets (Rare) 3004
Cleocin Vaginal Ovules 2613
Clindesse Vaginal Cream (Rare) 3296
Clinoril Tablets (Less than 1 in 100) 1899
Clozapine Tablets (1%) 2141
Clozaril Tablets (1%) 2174
Colazal Capsules 2845
Copaxone for Injection (Infrequent) 3292
Cubicin for Injection (Less than 1%) 1038
Cuprimine Capsules 1925
Demser Capsules (Rare) 1933
Depacon Injection 412
Depakene 417
Depakote Sprinkle Capsules 422
Depakote Tablets 427
Depakote ER Tablets 433
Dolobid Tablets (Less than 1 in 100) 1937
Doxil Injection (Less than 1%) 3302
Dynacin Tablets 1859
EC-Naprosyn Delayed-Release Tablets (Less than 1%) 2769
Effexor Tablets (Rare) 3405
Effexor XR Capsules (Rare) 3411
Efudex 3348
Equetro Extended-Release Capsules 3178
Evoxac Capsules (Less than 1%) 1042
Factive Tablets (Less than or equal to 0.1%) 2464
FazaClo Orally Disintegrating Tablets (1%) 547
Flexeril Tablets (Rare) 1832
Flovent Diskus 50 mcg 1415
▲ Fortaz (1 in 13) 1422
▲ Fuzeon Injection (1.8% to 8.3%) 2772
Garamycin Injectable 3028
Geodon Capsules (Infrequent) 2514
Invanz for Injection (1.1% to 2.1%) 1974
Kineret Injection 594
Klonopin 2782
Lamictal (Infrequent) 1449
Lescol Capsules (Rare) 2227
Lescol Capsules (Rare) 2730
Lescol XL Tablets 2227
Lescol XL Tablets 2730
Leukine 829
Levaquin in 5% Dextrose Injection 2453
Levaquin 2453
Lofibra Capsules 1217
Lotensin HCT Tablets 2235
Lyrica Capsules (0.1% to 1%) 2524
Matulane Capsules 3188
Mefoxin for Injection 1987
Mefoxin Premixed Intravenous Solution 1990
Merrem I.V. (Greater than 0.2%) 687
Mevacor Tablets 1996
Miradon Tablets 3056
Naprosyn Suspension (Less than 1%) 2769
Naprosyn Tablets (Less than 1%) 2769
Noroxin Tablets (0.6% to 1.5%) 2009
Omnicef Capsules (0.7%) 506
Omnicef for Oral Suspension (1%) 506
Orthoclone OKT3 Sterile Solution (Less than 1%) 2370
▲ Paser Granules (55% of 38 patients with drug-induced hepatitis) 1657
Paxil CR Controlled-Release Tablets (Rare) 1509
Paxil (Rare) 1501
Pentasa Capsules 3182
Permax Tablets (Rare) 3357
Phenytek Capsules 2153
Pravachol Tablets (Rare) 943
Prevacid Delayed-Release Capsules (Less than 1%) 3268
Prevacid for Delayed-Release Oral Suspension (Less than 1%) 3268
Prevacid NapraPAC (Less than 1%) 3277
Prevacid SoluTab Delayed-Release Orally Disintegrating Tablets (Less than 1%) 3268
PREVPAC (Less than 1%) 3281
Primaxin I.M. 2022
Primaxin I.V. 2024
Prinivil Tablets (0.3% to 1.0%) 2029
Prinzide Tablets 2033
▲ Proleukin for Injection (6%) 1007
Protonix I.V. (Less than 1%) 3468
Protonix Tablets (Less than 1%) 3465
Provigil Tablets (1%) 1002
Requip Tablets (Infrequent) 1528
Rescriptor Tablets 2535
▲ Rocephin Injectable Vials, ADD-Vantage, Galaxy, Bulk (6%) 2801
Rythmol SR Capsules 2736
Seroquel Tablets (Infrequent) 691
Singulair (Rare) 2047
Sonata Capsules (Rare) 1686
▲ Stromectol Tablets (3%) 2053
Sulfamylon Cream 2154
Sulfamylon for 5% Topical Solution 2155
Suprax (Less than 2%) 1811
Surmontil Capsules 2347
Targretin Capsules 1719
Tegretol/Tegretol-XR 2278
Thalomid Capsules 979
Thioridazine Hydrochloride Tablets 2122
Thiothixene Capsules 2124
Ticlid Tablets 2813
Timentin ADD-Vantage 1556
Timentin Injection Galaxy Container 1559
Timentin IV Infusion 1553
Timentin Pharmacy Bulk Package 1562
Topamax Sprinkle Capsules (Infrequent) 2438
Topamax Tablets (Infrequent) 2438
Tricor Tablets 523
Triglide Tablets 1165
Trileptal Oral Suspension 2281
Trileptal Tablets 2281
Tygacil for Injection (0% to less than 2%) 3489
Uniretic Tablets (Less than 1%) 3114
Vancocin HCl Capsules, USP (Infrequent) 3370
Vantin Tablets and Oral Suspension 2650
Vaqta (Isolated reports) 2067
Vaseretic Tablets 2073
Vasotec I.V. Injection (0.5% to 1.0%) 2076
VFEND I.V. (Less than 2%) 2543
VFEND Oral Suspension (Less than 2%) 2543
VFEND Tablets (Less than 2%) 2543
Viramune Oral Suspension 903
Viramune Tablets 903
Vivactil Tablets 2350
Voltaren Tablets (Occasionally) 2298
Voltaren-XR Tablets (Occasionally) 2301
Vytorin 10/10 Tablets 2084
Vytorin 10/10 Tablets 3092
Vytorin 10/20 Tablets 2084
Vytorin 10/20 Tablets 3092
Vytorin 10/40 Tablets 2084
Vytorin 10/40 Tablets 3092
Vytorin 10/80 Tablets 2084
Vytorin 10/80 Tablets 3092
Zantac (Rare) 1597
Zantac Injection 1593
Zantac Injection Pharmacy Bulk Package (Rare) 1595
Zantac Syrup (Rare) 1597
Zestoretic Tablets 701
Zestril Tablets (0.3% to 1.0%) 704
▲ Zinacef Injection (1 in 14 patients) 1604
▲ Zinacef for Injection (1 in 14 patients) 1604
Zocor Tablets 2078
Zomig Tablets (Rare) 714
Zomig-ZMT Tablets (Rare) 714
Zosyn 3492
Zyvox (0.4% to 1.4%) 2661

Eosinophilia, myoclonus
Carbatrol Capsules (One case) 3174
Tegretol/Tegretol-XR (One case) 2278

Eosinophilia, peripheral
Carbatrol Capsules (One case) 3174
Tegretol/Tegretol-XR (One case) 2278

Eosinophilia, pulmonary
Dapsone Tablets USP 1656
Daraprim Tablets (Rare) 1385
Effexor Tablets 3405
Effexor XR Capsules 3411

Eosinophilic pneumonitis
(*see under* Pneumonitis, eosinophilic)

Epidermal necrolysis
(*see under* Necrolysis, epidermal, toxic)

Epidermal shedding
Plavix Tablets 2942

Epidermolysis
Carimune NF 3501
Gammagard Liquid 751
Gamunex Immune Globulin I.V., 10% (Rare) 3232
Iveegam EN (Rare) 759

Epidermolysis bullosa
Anaprox Tablets (Less than 1%) 2769
Anaprox DS Tablets (Less than 1%) 2769
EC-Naprosyn Delayed-Release Tablets (Less than 1%) 2769
Gammagard S/D (Rare) 754
Naprosyn Suspension (Less than 1%) 2769
Naprosyn Tablets (Less than 1%) 2769
Prevacid NapraPAC (Less than 1%) 3277

Epididymitis
Anadrol-50 Tablets 3329
Asacol Delayed-Release Tablets 2688
Caduet Tablets (Less than 2%) 2507
Evoxac Capsules (Less than 1%) 1042
Lamictal (Rare) 1449
Lipitor Tablets (Less than 2%) 2495
Lyrica Capsules (Rare) 2524
Neurontin Capsules (Rare) 2498
Neurontin Oral Solution (Rare) 2498
Neurontin Tablets (Rare) 2498
Omacor Capsules 2735
Oxandrin Tablets 2977
Pacerone Tablets (Rare) 3337
Paxil CR Controlled-Release Tablets (Rare) 1509
Paxil (Rare) 1501
Permax Tablets (Rare) 3357
Protonix I.V. (Less than 1%) 3468
Protonix Tablets (Less than 1%) 3465
Requip Tablets (Infrequent) 1528
Rescriptor Tablets 2535
VFEND I.V. (Less than 2%) 2543
VFEND Oral Suspension (Less than 2%) 2543
VFEND Tablets (Less than 2%) 2543

Epigastric pain
(*see under* Distress, epigastric)

Epilepsy, aggravation
Cenestin Tablets, 0.45mg, 0.625mg, 0.9mg, 1.25mg 1063
Cenestin Tablets, 0.3mg 1063
Climara Transdermal System 795
Climara Pro Transdermal System 800
CombiPatch Transdermal System 2180
Estratest Tablets 3196
Estratest H.S. Tablets 3196
Estrogel 0.06% 3200
Indocin Capsules (Less than 1%) 1968
Indocin I.V. (Less than 1%) 1973
Indocin (Less than 1%) 1968
Menostar Transdermal System 805
Prefest Tablets 1069
Premarin Intravenous 3440
Premarin Tablets 3443
Premarin Vaginal Cream 3449
Premphase Tablets 3452
Prempro Tablets 3452
Vivelle Transdermal System 2288
Vivelle-Dot Transdermal System 2293

Epileptic ictal phenomenon
Trileptal Oral Suspension 2281
Trileptal Tablets 2281

Epileptiform movements, unspecified
Clozapine Tablets (1%) 2141
Clozaril Tablets (1%) 2174
FazaClo Orally Disintegrating Tablets (1%) 547

Epiphora
Alphagan P Ophthalmic Solution (1% to 4%) 563
▲ Alrex Ophthalmic Suspension 0.2% (5% to 15%) ⊙243
Betimol Ophthalmic Solution (1% to 5%) ⊙283

Betimol Ophthalmic Solution (1% to 5%) ... 3371
▲ Lotemax Ophthalmic Suspension 0.5% (5% to 15%) ... ⊙ 249
▲ Restasis Ophthalmic Emulsion (1% to 5%) ... 570

Epiphyseal closure, premature

Accutane Capsules ... 2740
Amnesteem Capsules ... 2126
Anadrol-50 Tablets ... 3329
Estratest Tablets ... 3196
Estratest H.S. Tablets ... 3196
Oxandrin Tablets ... 2977

Episcleritis

Aredia for Injection (Rare) ... 2168
Fosamax ... 1949
Fosamax Plus D Tablets (Rarely) ... 1956

Epistaxis

Abilify Tablets (Infrequent) ... 916
Abilify Tablets (Infrequent) ... 2472
Accutane Capsules ... 2740
Aceon Tablets (2 mg, 4 mg, 8 mg) (0.3% to 1%) ... 3191
Aciphex Tablets ... 1081
Actiq (1% or greater) ... 993
Activase I.V. (Less than 1%) ... 1225
▲ Adalat CC Tablets (3% or less) ... 2978
▲ Advair Diskus 100/50 (1% to 4%) ... 1291
▲ Advair Diskus 250/50 (1% to 4%) ... 1291
▲ Advair Diskus 500/50 (1% to 4%) ... 1291
Aerobid/Aerobid-M (1% to 3%) ... 1172
Aggrenox Capsules (2.4%) ... 855
Agrylin Capsules (1% to 5%) ... 3172
Alferon N Injection (1%) ... 1640
Alinia for Oral Suspension (Less than 1%) ... 2840
Alinia Tablets (Less than 1%) ... 2840
Altace Capsules (Less than 1%) ... 1673
Ambien Tablets (Rare) ... 2867
▲ AmBisome for Injection (8.6% to 14.9%) ... 615
Amerge Tablets (Rare) ... 1312
Amnesteem Capsules ... 2126
Anzemet Injection (Rare) ... 2871
Anzemet Tablets (Rare) ... 2874
▲ Arava Tablets (1% to 3%) ... 2881
Aricept Tablets (Infrequent) ... 1086
Aricept ODT Tablets (Infrequent) ... 1086
Arixtra Injection (1.3%) ... 1325
Arthrotec Tablets (Rare) ... 3126
Asmanex Twisthaler (1% to less than 3%) ... 2981
Astelin Nasal Spray (2.0% to 3.2%) .. 1876
Atacand Tablets (0.5% or greater) ... 634
Atacand HCT (0.5% or greater) ... 637
▲ Atrovent Nasal Spray 0.03% (7.0% to 9.0%) ... 869
▲ Atrovent Nasal Spray 0.06% (8.2%) ... 870
Avalide Tablets ... 922
Avalide Tablets ... 2889
Avapro Tablets (Less than 1%) ... 925
Avapro Tablets (Less than 1%) ... 2886
▲ Avastin IV (32% to 35%) ... 1229
Axert Tablets (Infrequent) ... 2430
Bactroban Nasal (Less than 1%) ... 1357
Beconase AQ Nasal Spray (Fewer than 3 per 100 patients) ... 1359
Caduet Tablets (Greater than 0.1% to less than 2%) ... 2507
▲ Campath Ampules (1% to 7%) ... 826
Campral Tablets (Infrequent) ... 1175
Cardizem LA Extended Release Tablets (Less than 2%) ... 1699
▲ Casodex Tablets (2% to 5%) ... 670
Celebrex Capsules (0.1% to 1.9%) ... 3130
Celexa (Infrequent) ... 1177
▲ CellCept Capsules (3% to less than 20%) ... 2751
▲ CellCept Intravenous (3% to less than 20%) ... 2751
▲ CellCept Oral Suspension (3% to less than 20%) ... 2751
▲ CellCept Tablets (3% to less than 20%) ... 2751
Cialis Tablets (Less than 2%) ... 1806
Cipro I.V. (1% or less) ... 2998
Cipro I.V. Pharmacy Bulk Package (1% or less) ... 3509
Cipro (Less than 1%) ... 2991
Cipro XR Tablets ... 3004
▲ Clarinex Syrup (3.1%) ... 3009
Clindesse Vaginal Cream (Less than 1%) ... 3296
Clinoril Tablets (Less than 1%) ... 1899
▲ Clolar for Intravenous Infusion (31%) ... 1264
Clozapine Tablets (Less than 1%) ... 2141
Clozaril Tablets (Less than 1%) ... 2174
Colazal Capsules ... 2845
Copaxone for Injection (Infrequent) .. 3292
Cosopt Sterile Ophthalmic Solution ... 1910
Coumadin for Injection ... 932
Coumadin Tablets ... 932
Cozaar Tablets (Less than 1%) ... 1913
▲ DDAVP Nasal Spray (Up to 3%) ... 2894
▲ Depacon Injection (1% to 5%) ... 412
▲ Depakene (1% to 5%) ... 417
▲ Depakote Sprinkle Capsules (1% to 5%) ... 422
▲ Depakote Tablets (1% to 5%) ... 427
▲ Depakote ER Tablets (1% to 5%) ... 433
Desmopressin Acetate Rhinal Tube (Up to 3%) ... 1144
Diovan HCT Tablets (Greater than 0.2%) ... 2195
▲ Dostinex Tablets (Less than 10%) ... 2631
▲ Doxil Injection (1% to 10%) ... 3302
DynaCirc CR Tablets (0.5% to 1%) ... 2726
Effexor Tablets (Infrequent) ... 3405
Effexor XR Capsules (Infrequent) ... 3411
Elidel Cream 1% (Up to 3.3%) ... 2198
Elmiron Capsules (Less than or equal to 1%) ... 2393
▲ Eloxatin for Injection (2% to 16%) ... 2908
▲ Evoxac Capsules (1% to 3%) ... 1042
Exelon Capsules (Frequent) ... 2204
FazaClo Orally Disintegrating Tablets (Less than 1%) ... 547
▲ Flolan for Injection (4% to 9%) ... 1408
▲ Flonase Nasal Spray (6% to 6.9%) ... 1412
▲ Flovent Diskus 50 mcg (1% to 3%) ... 1415
Flumist Vaccine ... 1872
▲ Fortical Nasal Spray (3.5% to 10.6%) ... 3336
Frova Tablets (Infrequent) ... 1101
Gabitril Tablets (Frequent) ... 998
▲ Gamunex Immune Globulin I.V., 10% (23%) ... 3232
Gengraf Capsules (1% to less than 3%) ... 458
Geodon Capsules (Infrequent) ... 2514
▲ Gleevec Tablets (3% to 12%) ... 2221
Hytrin Capsules (At least 1%) ... 469
Hyzaar ... 1964
Imitrex Nasal Spray ... 1435
Indocin Capsules (Less than 1%) ... 1968
Indocin I.V. (Less than 1%) ... 1973
Indocin (Less than 1%) ... 1968
▲ Infergen (6% to 8%) ... 1647
▲ Intron A for Injection (Less than or equal to 5%) ... 3038
Invanz for Injection (Greater than 0.1%) ... 1974
Invirase (Less than 2%) ... 2776
Iressa Tablets ... 684
▲ I.V. Busulfex (25%) ... 1125
Keppra Oral Solution (2%) ... 3307
Keppra Tablets (2%) ... 3307
Klonopin (Infrequent) ... 2782
Lamictal (Infrequent) ... 1449
▲ Leukine (17%) ... 829
▲ Leustatin Injection (5%) ... 2368
Levaquin in 5% Dextrose Injection (0.1% to 0.9%) ... 2453
Levaquin (0.1% to 0.9%) ... 2453
Levitra Tablets (Less than 2%) ... 3048
Lexapro Oral Solution (Infrequent) ... 1193
Lexapro Tablets (Infrequent) ... 1193
Lipitor Tablets (Less than 2%) ... 2495
Lofibra Capsules (Less than 1%) ... 1217
Lotensin HCT Tablets (0.3% or more) ... 2235
Lunesta Tablets (Infrequent) ... 3139
Lupron Depot-PED 7.5 mg, 11.25 mg and 15 mg (Less than 2%) ... 3266
Lupron Injection Pediatric (Less than 2%) ... 3256
Matulane Capsules ... 3188
Mavik Tablets (0.3% to 1.0%) ... 482
Maxalt Tablets (Infrequent) ... 1983
Maxalt-MLT Orally Disintegrating Tablets (Infrequent) ... 1983
Meridia Capsules ... 485
Merrem I.V. (0.2%) ... 687
▲ Miacalcin Nasal Spray (3.5%) ... 2242
Micardis Tablets (More than 0.3%) ... 884
Micardis HCT Tablets ... 886
Migranal Nasal Spray (Rare) ... 3350
▲ Mylotarg for Injection (3% to 34%) ... 3429
▲ Nasacort HFA Inhalation Aerosol (Greater than or equal to 3%) ... 2939
Nasacort AQ Nasal Spray (2.7%) ... 2937
▲ Nasarel Nasal Spray (3% to 9%) ... 1652
▲ Nasonex Nasal Spray (8% to 11%) ... 3058
Neoral Soft Gelatin Capsules (1% to less than 3%) ... 2247
Neoral Oral Solution (1% to less than 3%) ... 2247
▲ Neupogen for Injection (9% to 15%) ... 598
Neurontin Capsules (Infrequent) ... 2498
Neurontin Oral Solution (Infrequent) ... 2498
Neurontin Tablets (Infrequent) ... 2498
Nexium Delayed-Release Capsules (Less than 1%) ... 645
Nexium I.V. (Less than 1%) ... 649
Nicotrol NS ... 2596
Norvasc Tablets (More than 0.1% to 1%) ... 2529
Norvir (Less than 2%) ... 499
Omacor Capsules ... 2735
Oncaspar (Less than 1%) ... 1123
OptiPranolol Metipranolol Ophthalmic Solution 0.3% (A small number of patients) ... ⊙ 254
Paxil CR Controlled-Release Tablets (Infrequent) ... 1509
Paxil (Infrequent) ... 1501
Permax Tablets (1.6%) ... 3357
Plavix Tablets (2.9%) ... 940
Plavix Tablets (2.9%) ... 2942
Plendil Extended-Release Tablets (0.5% to 1.5%) ... 651
Pletal Tablets (Less than 2%) ... 2478
Prevacid Delayed-Release Capsules (Less than 1%) ... 3268
Prevacid for Delayed-Release Oral Suspension (Less than 1%) ... 3268
Prevacid NapraPAC (Less than 1%) .. 3277
Prevacid SoluTab Delayed-Release Orally Disintegrating Tablets (Less than 1%) ... 3268
PREVPAC (Less than 1%) ... 3281
Prilosec OTC Tablets (Less than 1%) ... 2674
Prinivil Tablets (0.3% to 1.0%) ... 2029
Prinzide Tablets ... 2033
ProSom Tablets (Rare) ... 512
Protonix I.V. (Less than 1%) ... 3468
Protonix Tablets (Less than 1%) ... 3465
Protopic Ointment (Greater than or equal to 1%) ... 629
Provigil Tablets (1%) ... 1002
Prozac Pulvules and Liquid (Infrequent to greater than or equal to 2%) ... 1771
Pulmicort Respules (2% to 4%) ... 654
▲ Rapamune Oral Solution and Tablets (3% to 20%) ... 3472
Razadyne ER Extended-Release Capsules (Infrequent) ... 2434
Razadyne (Infrequent) ... 2434
Recombinate ... 762
▲ Refludan for Injection (4.4%) ... 815
Relenza Rotadisk (Less than 1%) ... 1525
Relpax Tablets (Rare) ... 2531
ReoPro Vials (9 to 11 events) ... 1779
Requip Tablets (Infrequent) ... 1528
Rescriptor Tablets ... 2535
Retrovir Capsules ... 1533
Retrovir IV Infusion ... 1537
Retrovir ... 1533
▲ Revatio Tablets (9%) ... 2541
▲ Rhinocort Aqua Nasal Spray (8%) ... 658
Rilutek Tablets (Infrequent) ... 2945
Risperdal Consta Long-Acting Injection (Infrequent) ... 1664
Risperdal M-Tab Orally Disintegrating Tablets (Infrequent) ... 1658
Risperdal (Infrequent) ... 1658
Rocephin Injectable Vials, ADD-Vantage, Galaxy, Bulk (Rare) ... 2801
▲ Roferon-A Injection (Less than 5%) .. 2805
Rythmol SR Capsules ... 2736
Sandostatin Injection (Less than 1%) ... 2263
Sandostatin LAR Depot (1% to 4%) .. 2264
Seroquel Tablets (Infrequent) ... 691
Singulair (Greater than or equal to 1%) ... 2047
Sonata Capsules (Less than 1%) ... 1686
▲ Spiriva HandiHaler (1% to 4%) ... 899
Sular Tablets (Less than or equal to 1%) ... 1163
Symbyax Capsules (Infrequent) ... 1788
▲ Tamiflu Capsules (3.1%) ... 2810
▲ Tamiflu Oral Suspension (3.1%) ... 2810
Tarka Tablets (Less frequent) ... 519
Tasmar Tablets (Infrequent) ... 3360
Tequin Injection (Less than 0.1%) ... 964
Tequin Tablets (Less than 0.1%) ... 964
Teveten Tablets (Less than 1%) ... 1707
Teveten HCT Tablets (Less than 1%) ... 1710
Thalomid Capsules ... 979
Tiazac Capsules (Less than 2%) ... 1204
Ticlid Tablets (0.5% to 1.0%) ... 2813
TNKase I.V. (1.5%) ... 1256
▲ TOBI Solution for Inhalation (7%) ... 1015
▲ Topamax Sprinkle Capsules (1% to 4%) ... 2438
▲ Topamax Tablets (1% to 4%) ... 2438
Tricor Tablets ... 523
▲ Trileptal Oral Suspension (2% to 4%) ... 2281
▲ Trileptal Tablets (2% to 4%) ... 2281
▲ Trisenox Injection (25%) ... 983
Trusopt Sterile Ophthalmic Solution ... 2065
Uniretic Tablets (Less than 1%) ... 3114
Vantin Tablets and Oral Suspension (Less than 1%) ... 2650
VFEND I.V. (Less than 2%) ... 2543
VFEND Oral Suspension (Less than 2%) ... 2543
VFEND Tablets (Less than 2%) ... 2543
Viagra Tablets ... 2552
Wellbutrin Tablets (Rare) ... 1579
Xanax XR Tablets (Infrequent) ... 2655
▲ Xeloda Tablets (Less than 5%) ... 2825
Zegerid Powder for Oral Solution (Less than 1%) ... 2972
Zestoretic Tablets ... 701
Zestril Tablets (0.3% to 1.0%) ... 704
▲ Zevalin Injection (3%) ... 848
Zoladex (1% or greater) ... 709
Zoladex 3-month ... 712
Zoloft (Infrequent to 2%) ... 2581
Zomig Nasal Spray (Infrequent) ... 718
Zomig Tablets (Infrequent) ... 714
Zomig-ZMT Tablets (Infrequent) ... 714
Zosyn (1.0% or less) ... 3492
Zyban Sustained-Release Tablets (2%) ... 1620
Zyprexa Tablets (Infrequent) ... 1798
Zyprexa ZYDIS Orally Disintegrating Tablets (Infrequent) ... 1798
▲ Zyrtec Chewable Tablets (1.9% to 3.7%) ... 2589
▲ Zyrtec (1.9% to 3.7%) ... 2589
▲ Zyrtec-D 12 Hour Extended Release Tablets (1.9% to 3.7%) ... 2591

Epitheliopathy

Ciloxan Ophthalmic Ointment (Less than 1%) ... 554

Equilibrium dysfunction

Amerge Tablets (Infrequent) ... 1312
Covera-HS Tablets (Less than 2%) ... 3135
Lariam Tablets ... 2790
Lexapro Oral Solution (Infrequent) ... 1193
Lexapro Tablets (Infrequent) ... 1193
Transderm Scōp Transdermal Therapeutic System (Few patients) ... 2166
Verelan PM Capsules (2% or less) ... 3120
▲ Xeloda Tablets (Less than 5%) ... 2825

Erection disturbances, unspecified

(*see also under* Impotence)

Advicor Tablets ... 1694
Altoprev Extended-Release Tablets ... 1151
Anadrol-50 Tablets ... 3329
▲ Cymbalta Delayed-Release Capsules (Up to 4%) ... 1729
Dantrium Capsules (Less frequent) .. 2690
Effexor Tablets (Rare) ... 3405
Effexor XR Capsules (Rare) ... 3411
Eligard 30 mg (1.1%) ... 2901
Lescol Capsules ... 2227
Lescol Capsules ... 2730
Lescol XL Tablets ... 2227
Lescol XL Tablets ... 2730
Mevacor Tablets (0.5% to 1.0%) ... 1996
Micardis Tablets ... 884
▲ Paxil CR Controlled-Release Tablets (3.7% to 10.0%) ... 1509
▲ Paxil (3.7% to 10.0%) ... 1501
Pravachol Tablets ... 943
Propecia Tablets (1.3%) ... 2036
Risperdal M-Tab Orally Disintegrating Tablets (Frequent) ... 1658
Risperdal (Frequent) ... 1658
▲ Vantas (3.5%) ... 3367
Wellbutrin Tablets (Infrequent) ... 1579
Wellbutrin SR Sustained-Release Tablets ... 1583
Wellbutrin XL Extended-Release Tablets ... 1588
Zocor Tablets ... 2078
▲ Zoladex (18%) ... 709
Zoladex 3-month ... 712
Zyban Sustained-Release Tablets ... 1620

Erosion, genital

▲ Aldara (1% to 31%) ... 1814

Eructation

Abilify Tablets (Infrequent) ... 916

Abilify Tablets (Infrequent) ... 2472
Aciphex Tablets ... 1081
Actiq (Less than 1%) ... 993
Adalat CC Tablets (Less than 1%) ... 2978
Agrylin Capsules (1% to 5%) ... 3172
Ambien Tablets (Rare) ... 2867
AmBisome for Injection (Less common) ... 615
Anaprox Tablets (Less than 1%) ... 2769
Anaprox DS Tablets (Less than 1%) ... 2769
Antara Capsules ... 2723
Aricept Tablets (Infrequent) ... 1086
Aricept ODT Tablets (Infrequent) ... 1086
Arthrotec Tablets (Rare) ... 3126
▲ Asacol Delayed-Release Tablets (16%) ... 2688
Caduet Tablets (Less than 2%) ... 2507
Campral Tablets (Infrequent) ... 1175
Cataflam Tablets (Rarely) ... 2173
Celebrex Capsules (0.1% to 1.9%) ... 3130
Celexa (Infrequent) ... 1177
Clozapine Tablets (Less than 1%) ... 2141
Clozaril Tablets (Less than 1%) ... 2174
Colazal Capsules ... 2845
Combunox Tablets (Less than 1%) ... 1183
Cytovene (At least 3 subjects) ... 2763
▲ Depacon Injection (1% to 5%) ... 412
▲ Depakene (1% to 5%) ... 417
▲ Depakote Sprinkle Capsules (1% to 5%) ... 422
▲ Depakote Tablets (1% to 5%) ... 427
Depakote ER Tablets (Greater than 1%) ... 433
Dolobid Tablets (Less than 1 in 100) ... 1937
Doxil Injection (Less than 1%) ... 3302
EC-Naprosyn Delayed-Release Tablets (Less than 1%) ... 2769
Effexor Tablets (Frequent) ... 3405
Effexor XR Capsules (2%) ... 3411
▲ Evoxac Capsules (1% to 3%) ... 1042
Exelon Capsules (2%) ... 2204
FazaClo Orally Disintegrating Tablets (Less than 1%) ... 547
Ferrlecit Injection ... 3379
Frova Tablets (Rare) ... 1101
Gabitril Tablets (Infrequent) ... 998
Gengraf Capsules (1% to less than 3%) ... 458
Imitrex Injection (Rare) ... 1431
Imitrex Nasal Spray (Rare) ... 1435
Imitrex Tablets ... 1440
▲ Intron A for Injection (Less than 5%) ... 3038
Invirase (Less than 2%) ... 2776
Kaletra (Less than 2%) ... 474
Lamictal (Rare) ... 1449
Lipitor Tablets (Less than 2%) ... 2495
Lofibra Capsules ... 1217
Lupron Depot 7.5 mg (Less than 5%) ... 3261
Maxalt Tablets (Rare) ... 1983
Maxalt-MLT Orally Disintegrating Tablets (Rare) ... 1983
Meridia Capsules ... 485
Mobic Oral Suspension (Less than 2%) ... 893
Mobic Tablets (Less than 2%) ... 893
Naprosyn Suspension (Less than 1%) ... 2769
Naprosyn Tablets (Less than 1%) ... 2769
Neoral Soft Gelatin Capsules (1% to less than 3%) ... 2247
Neoral Oral Solution (1% to less than 3%) ... 2247
Neurontin Capsules (Rare) ... 2498
Neurontin Oral Solution (Rare) ... 2498
Neurontin Tablets (Rare) ... 2498
Nexium Delayed-Release Capsules (Less than 1%) ... 645
Nexium I.V. (Less than 1%) ... 649
Niaspan Extended-Release Tablets ... 1703
Norvir (Less than 2%) ... 499
▲ Omacor Capsules (4.9%) ... 2735
Orap Tablets ... 1220
OxyContin Tablets (Less than 1%) ... 2699
Paxil CR Controlled-Release Tablets (Infrequent) ... 1509
Paxil (Infrequent) ... 1501
Pentasa Capsules (Less than 1%) ... 3182
Permax Tablets (Infrequent) ... 3357
▲ Photofrin for Injection (5%) ... 729
Prevacid Delayed-Release Capsules (Less than 1%) ... 3268
Prevacid for Delayed-Release Oral Suspension (Less than 1%) ... 3268
Prevacid NapraPAC (Less than 1%) ... 3277
Prevacid SoluTab Delayed-Release Orally Disintegrating Tablets (Less than 1%) ... 3268
PREVPAC (Less than 1%) ... 3281
Prochieve 4% Gel ... 1018
Prochieve 8% Gel ... 1018
Protonix I.V. (Greater than or equal to 1%) ... 3468
Protonix Tablets (1%) ... 3465
Proventil HFA Inhalation Aerosol (Less than 3%) ... 3071
Prozac Pulvules and Liquid (Infrequent) ... 1771
▲ Rapamune Oral Solution and Tablets (3% to 20%) ... 3472
Relafen Tablets (Less than 1%) ... 1523
Relpax Tablets (Infrequent) ... 2531
Requip Tablets (Infrequent) ... 1528
Rescriptor Tablets ... 2535
Retrovir Capsules ... 1533
Retrovir IV Infusion ... 1537
Retrovir ... 1533
Risperdal M-Tab Orally Disintegrating Tablets (Rare) ... 1658
Risperdal (Rare) ... 1658
Rythmol SR Capsules ... 2736
Sonata Capsules (Infrequent) ... 1686
Spectracef Tablets (0.1% to 1%) ... 2706
Symbyax Capsules (Infrequent) ... 1788
Thalomid Capsules ... 979
Tricor Tablets ... 523
Triglide Tablets ... 1165
Trileptal Oral Suspension ... 2281
Trileptal Tablets ... 2281
Uniretic Tablets (Less than 1%) ... 3114
Vantin Tablets and Oral Suspension (Less than 1%) ... 2650
Voltaren Tablets (Rarely) ... 2298
Voltaren-XR Tablets (Rarely) ... 2301
Zoloft (Infrequent) ... 2581
Zomig Nasal Spray (Rare) ... 718
Zyprexa Tablets (Rare) ... 1798
Zyprexa ZYDIS Orally Disintegrating Tablets (Infrequent) ... 1798
Zyrtec Chewable Tablets (Less than 2%) ... 2589
Zyrtec (Less than 2%) ... 2589
Zyrtec-D 12 Hour Extended Release Tablets (Less than 2%) ... 2591

Eruptions
Cuprimine Capsules ... 1925
Meridia Capsules ... 485
Raptiva for Injection ... 1247

Eruptions, acneiform
(*see under* Acneiform eruptions)

Eruptions, bullous
Aciphex Tablets ... 1081
Ambien Tablets (Rare) ... 2867
▲ Argatroban Injection (1% to 10%) ... 1321
▲ Arixtra Injection (0% to 3.1%) ... 1325
Campath Ampules ... 826
Coumadin for Injection (Infrequent) ... 932
Coumadin Tablets (Infrequent) ... 932
Eulexin Capsules ... 3023
Evoxac Capsules (Less than 1%) ... 1042
Fragmin Injection (Rare) ... 2638
Frova Tablets (Infrequent) ... 1101
Gengraf Capsules (1%) ... 458
Gleevec Tablets (Infrequent) ... 2221
Hycamtin for Injection (Less than 1%) ... 1427
Indapamide Tablets ... 2119
Invirase (Rare) ... 2776
Levaquin in 5% Dextrose Injection (0.1% to 0.9%) ... 2453
Levaquin (0.1% to 0.9%) ... 2453
Mobic Oral Suspension (Less than 2%) ... 893
Mobic Tablets (Less than 2%) ... 893
Neoral Soft Gelatin Capsules (1%) ... 2247
Neoral Oral Solution (1%) ... 2247
Plavix Tablets (Less than 1%) ... 940
Plavix Tablets (Less than 1%) ... 2942
Relafen Tablets (Less than 1%) ... 1523
ReoPro Vials (0.1%) ... 1779
Risperdal M-Tab Orally Disintegrating Tablets (Rare) ... 1658
Risperdal (Rare) ... 1658
▲ Soriatane Capsules (1% to 10%) ... 1028
Taxotere Injection Concentrate (Rare) ... 2947
Viramune Oral Suspension ... 903
Viramune Tablets ... 903
Zoloft (Rare) ... 2581
Zyrtec Chewable Tablets (Less than 2%) ... 2589
Zyrtec (Less than 2%) ... 2589
Zyrtec-D 12 Hour Extended Release Tablets (Less than 2%) ... 2591

Eruptions, cutaneous
Rhophylac (Occasionally) ... 3504
Roferon-A Injection (Less than 1%) ... 2805
Taxotere Injection Concentrate ... 2947

Eruptions, eczematoid
(*see under* Eczema)

Eruptions, fixed drug
Cipro I.V. ... 2998
Cipro I.V. Pharmacy Bulk Package ... 3509
Cipro ... 2991
Cipro XR Tablets ... 3004
Dynacin Tablets (Rarely reported) ... 1859
Nitro-Dur Transdermal Infusion System (Uncommon) ... 3060
Prevacid Delayed-Release Capsules (Less than 1%) ... 3268
Prevacid for Delayed-Release Oral Suspension (Less than 1%) ... 3268
Prevacid NapraPAC (Less than 1%) ... 3277
Prevacid SoluTab Delayed-Release Orally Disintegrating Tablets (Less than 1%) ... 3268
PREVPAC (Less than 1%) ... 3281
VFEND I.V. (Less than 2%) ... 2543
VFEND Oral Suspension (Less than 2%) ... 2543
VFEND Tablets (Less than 2%) ... 2543

Eruptions, hemorrhagic
Activella Tablets ... 2311
Alesse-28 Tablets ... 3392
Cenestin Tablets, 0.45mg, 0.625mg, 0.9mg, 1.25mg ... 1063
Cenestin Tablets, 0.3mg ... 1063
Climara Transdermal System ... 795
Climara Pro Transdermal System ... 800
CombiPatch Transdermal System ... 2180
Estratest Tablets ... 3196
Estratest H.S. Tablets ... 3196
Estrogel 0.06% ... 3200
Lo/Ovral-28 Tablets ... 3423
Menostar Transdermal System ... 805
Ortho-Cept Tablets ... 2395
Ortho-Cyclen Tablets ... 2414
Ortho Evra Transdermal System ... 2402
Ortho Tri-Cyclen Tablets ... 2414
Ortho Tri-Cyclen Lo Tablets ... 2421
Prefest Tablets ... 1069
Premarin Intravenous ... 3440
Premarin Tablets ... 3443
Premarin Vaginal Cream ... 3449
Premphase Tablets ... 3452
Prempro Tablets ... 3452
Seasonale Tablets ... 1073
Triphasil-28 Tablets ... 3483
Vivelle Transdermal System ... 2288
Vivelle-Dot Transdermal System ... 2293
Yasmin 28 Tablets ... 818

Eruptions, herpetic
▲ Chemet Capsules (2.6% to 11.2%) ... 2480

Eruptions, maculopapular
Amaryl Tablets (Less than 1%) ... 2864
Mustargen for Injection (Occasional) ... 2007
▲ Reyataz Capsules (21%) ... 948

Eruptions, morbilliform
Amaryl Tablets (Less than 1%) ... 2864

Eruptions, mucocutaneous
▲ Chemet Capsules (2.6% to 11.2%) ... 2480

Erysipelas
▲ Humira Injection (Less than 5%) ... 464

Erythema
Accutane Capsules ... 2740
Aceon Tablets (2 mg, 4 mg, 8 mg) (0.3% to 1%) ... 3191
Aclovate (Approximately 2%) ... 1290
Acticin Cream (1% to 2%) ... 2125
▲ Aldara Cream, 5% (1% to 65%) ... 1814
Alphagan P Ophthalmic Solution ... 563
Amaryl Tablets (Less than 1%) ... 2864
AmBisome for Injection (Infrequent) ... 615
Amerge Tablets (Infrequent) ... 1312
Aquacel AG with Hydrofiber ... 1035
Aricept Tablets (Infrequent) ... 1086
Aricept ODT Tablets (Infrequent) ... 1086
Avita Cream ... 2136
Avita Gel ... 2138
Axert Tablets (Rare) ... 2430
Bactroban Ointment (Less than 1%) ... 1358
Benzaclin Topical Gel (2%) ... 1046
Betoptic S Ophthalmic Suspension (Small number of patients) ... 554
Brevibloc Concentrate (Less than 1%) ... 766
Brevibloc Injection (Less than 1%) ... 766
Brevibloc Double Strength Injection (Less than 1%) ... 766
Brevibloc Premixed Injection (Less than 1%) ... 766
Brevibloc Double Strength Premixed Injection (Less than 1%) ... 766
Brevoxyl-4 Creamy Wash ... 3212
Brevoxyl-4 Gel ... 3211
Brevoxyl-8 Creamy Wash ... 3212
Brevoxyl-8 Gel ... 3211
Brimonidine Tartrate Ophthalmic Solution 0.2% ... ⊙245
Cancidas for Injection (1.2% to 1.5%) ... 1894
▲ Carac Cream, 0.5% (93.4%) ... 1048
▲ Catapres-TTS (26 of 101 patients) ... 875
Ceftin Tablets (0.1% to 1%) ... 1369
Cipro I.V. (1% or less) ... 2998
Cipro I.V. Pharmacy Bulk Package (1% or less) ... 3509
Ciprodex Otic Suspension (0.4%) ... 555
▲ Clarinex Syrup (3%) ... 3009
Climara Transdermal System ... 795
Clinac BPO 7 Gel USP ... 1137
▲ Clindets Pledgets (7% to 16%) ... 3212
Clobevate Gel (Less than 2%) ... 3213
Clobex Lotion ... 1208
▲ Clolar for Intravenous Infusion (18%) ... 1264
Clozapine Tablets (Less than 1%) ... 2141
Clozaril Tablets (Less than 1%) ... 2174
▲ Copaxone for Injection (4%) ... 3292
Cosmegen for Injection ... 1907
Cozaar Tablets (Less than 1%) ... 1913
Cutivate Cream (1.6%) ... 1381
Cutivate Ointment (Less than 1%) ... 1384
Cymbalta Delayed-Release Capsules (Infrequent) ... 1729
Dantrium Intravenous (Rare) ... 2691
Decadron Phosphate Injection ... 1931
Decadron Tablets ... 1929
Desferal Vials ... 2190
Detrol Tablets (1.9%) ... 2626
▲ Differin Cream (Less than 1% to 38%) ... 1210
▲ Differin Gel (10% to 40%) ... 1211
Digibind for Injection (One patient) ... 1388
Diprivan Injectable Emulsion (Rare) ... 676
Diprolene Gel 0.05% ... 3015
Diprolene Ointment 0.05% (3 per 767 patients) ... 3017
▲ Dovonex Ointment 0.005% (1% to 10%) ... 3375
▲ Doxil Injection (3.4%) ... 3302
Duac Topical Gel (2%) ... 3214
Duragesic Transdermal System (1% or greater) ... 2448
▲ Efudex (Among most frequent) ... 3348
Elidel Cream 1% (Up to 2.2%) ... 2198
Eligard 22.5 mg (1.7%) ... 2899
Eligard 30 mg (2.2%) ... 2901
Eloxatin for Injection (Less than 1%) ... 2908
Engerix-B Vaccine (Less than 1%) ... 1391
Ertaczo Cream, 2% ... 2383
Erygel Topical Gel ... 2096
Eulexin Capsules ... 3023
FazaClo Orally Disintegrating Tablets (Less than 1%) ... 547
Finacea Gel (2% or less) ... 1644
Follistim AQ Cartridge ... 2354
Fosamax (Rare) ... 1949
Hycamtin for Injection ... 1427
Hydrocortone Tablets ... 1963
Hyzaar ... 1964
Imitrex Injection (Infrequent) ... 1431
Imitrex Nasal Spray ... 1435
Imitrex Tablets (Infrequent) ... 1440
Infanrix Vaccine ... 1444
▲ Infergen (6%) ... 1647
▲ Intron A for Injection (Less than 5%) ... 3038
Invanz for Injection (1.2% to 1.6%) ... 1974
Invirase (Less than 2%) ... 2776
▲ Kepivance (32%) ... 592
Klaron Lotion 10% (One of 105 patients) ... 1050
Lamictal (Infrequent) ... 1449
▲ Leustatin Injection (6%) ... 2368
Lidoderm Patch ... 1107
Lotrimin ... 3053
Lotrisone ... 3054
Lovenox Injection ... 2931
Maxalt Tablets (Infrequent) ... 1983
Maxalt-MLT Orally Disintegrating Tablets (Infrequent) ... 1983
Mentax Cream (Less than 2%) ... 2152
Meruvax II ... 1994
▲ Miacalcin Nasal Spray (10.6%) ... 2242
Micardis Tablets ... 884
Miradon Tablets ... 3056

Mivacron Injection (less than1%) 489
M-M-R II ... 1980
▲ Nabi-HB (12%) ... 2159
Naftin Cream (2%) ... 2097
Naftin Gel (0.5%) ... 2097
Naropin Injection ... 640
Noroxin Tablets (Less frequent) ... 2009
Novarel for Injection ... 1147
Olux Foam (Less than 2%) ... 1027
▲ Oncaspar (Greater than 5%) ... 1123
Orthoclone OKT3 Sterile Solution (Less than 1%) ... 2370
Oxistat Cream (0.2%) ... 1498
Oxsoralen-Ultra Capsules ... 3354
▲ Pediarix Vaccine (0.6% to 41.9%) ... 1518
▲ Photofrin for Injection (Approximately 20%) ... 729
Plendil Extended-Release Tablets (0.5% to 1.5%) ... 651
▲ Prevnar for Injection (0% to 48.3%) ... 3460
Prinivil Tablets (0.3% to 1.0%) ... 2029
Prinzide Tablets ... 2033
▲ Proleukin for Injection (41%) ... 1007
▲ Protopic Ointment (9% to 28%) ... 629
Prozac Pulvules and Liquid ... 1771
Recombivax HB (Equal to or greater than 1%) ... 2045
▲ Renova 0.02% Cream (Almost all subjects) ... 2384
▲ Renova 0.05% Cream (Almost all subjects) ... 2387
Rescriptor Tablets ... 2535
Retin-A Micro 0.1%/0.04% ... 2388
▲ Revatio Tablets (6%) ... 2541
Rythmol SR Capsules ... 2736
▲ Solage Topical Solution (44.6% to 49%) ... 740
▲ Spectazole Cream (3%) ... 2390
Sulfamylon Cream ... 2154
Sulfamylon for 5% Topical Solution ... 2155
▲ Sustiva Capsules (8.8% to 9.9%) ... 957
Taxotere Injection Concentrate (0.9%) ... 2947
Temodar Capsules (1%) ... 3088
▲ Temovate Gel (Among most frequent) ... 1550
Temovate Ointment (Less frequent) ... 1549
Temovate E Emollient (Less than 2%) ... 1552
Thioridazine Hydrochloride Tablets ... 2122
Transderm Scōp Transdermal Therapeutic System (Infrequent) ... 2166
▲ Tri-Luma Cream (29.17% to 41%) ... 1213
▲ Trisenox Injection (13%) ... 983
Twinrix Vaccine (Less than 1%) ... 1571
Vaqta (Less than 1%) ... 2067
▲ Vivelle Transdermal System (One of the two most common) ... 2288
Vivelle-Dot Transdermal System (One of the two most common) ... 2293
Xeloda Tablets ... 2825
Zestoretic Tablets ... 701
Zestril Tablets (0.3% to 1.0%) ... 704
▲ Zinecard for Injection (4% to 5%) ... 2659
Zomig Nasal Spray (Rare) ... 718

Erythema, application site
▲ Humira Injection (20%) ... 464
Metrogel 1% ... 1212
▲ Oxytrol Transdermal System (5.6% to 8.3%) ... 3383
Vivelle Transdermal System (1.5% to 2.3%) ... 2288
Vivelle-Dot Transdermal System (1.5% to 2.3%) ... 2293

Erythema, conjunctival
▲ Rēv-Eyes Ophthalmic Eyedrops 0.5% (10% to 40%) ... ⊙ 256
TobraDex Ophthalmic Ointment (Less than 4%) ... 558
TobraDex Ophthalmic Suspension (Less than 4%) ... 558

Erythema, facial
Avalide Tablets ... 922
Avalide Tablets ... 2889
Avapro Tablets (Less than 1%) ... 925
Avapro Tablets (Less than 1%) ... 2886
▲ Carac Cream, 0.5% (89.4% to 96.5%) ... 1048
Depo-Medrol Injectable Suspension ... 2615
Depo-Medrol Single-Dose Vial ... 2617
Pediapred Oral Solution ... 3319

Erythema, hemorrhagic exudative
(*see under* Henoch-Schönlein purpura)

Erythema, insertion site
Vantas (2.8%) ... 3367

Erythema, nasal
▲ Fortical Nasal Spray (10.6%) ... 3336

Erythema, oral
▲ Advair Diskus 100/50 (1% to 3%) ... 1291
▲ Advair Diskus 250/50 (1% to 3%) ... 1291
▲ Advair Diskus 500/50 (1% to 3%) ... 1291

Erythema, penile
▲ Caverject Impulse Injection (3%) ... 2610

Erythema, periungual
▲ Penlac (5%) ... 1051

Erythema, vulvar
Clindesse Vaginal Cream (Less than 1%) ... 3296

Erythema at injection site
▲ Actimmune (14%) ... 1646
▲ Adacel Vaccine (2.7% to 24.7%) ... 2959
Attenuvax ... 1889
▲ Comvax (22.4% to 27.2%) ... 1904
▲ DAPTACEL (12.1% to 19.7%) ... 2964
DDAVP Injection 4 mcg/mL (Occasional) ... 2893
Desmopressin Acetate Injection (Occasional) ... 1143
Edex Injection (2%) ... 3103
▲ Enbrel for Injection (37%) ... 580
▲ Engerix-B Vaccine (1% to 10%) ... 1391
▲ Fuzeon Injection (91%) ... 2772
HibTITER (Less than 1% to 2.0%) ... 3419
Humalog-Pen ... 1751
▲ Infergen (17% to 23%) ... 1647
▲ Invanz for Injection (3.9%) ... 1974
▲ Leustatin Injection (9%) ... 2368
▲ Navelbine Injection (Approximately 1/3 of patients) ... 1494
Orthovisc Injection (0.4%) ... 3518
Pediarix Vaccine ... 1518
Liquid PedvaxHIB (0.4% to 2.2%) ... 2012
Pneumovax 23 (Common) ... 2020
Primaxin I.V. (0.4%) ... 2024
Rabies Vaccine RabAvert (Common) ... 1011
Risperdal Consta Long-Acting Injection (1%) ... 1664
Taxotere Injection Concentrate ... 2947
▲ Vaqta (0.8% to 13.1%) ... 2067
▲ Varivax (19.3% to 32.5%) ... 2070

Erythema multiforme
Abelcet Injection ... 1119
Aciphex Tablets ... 1081
Activella Tablets ... 2311
Advicor Tablets ... 1694
Aldoclor Tablets ... 1881
Aldoril Tablets ... 1884
Alesse-28 Tablets ... 3392
Altace Capsules (Less than 1%) ... 1673
Altoprev Extended-Release Tablets (Rare) ... 1151
Amoxil Capsules ... 1315
Amoxil Chewable Tablets ... 1315
Amoxil Pediatric Drops for Oral Suspension ... 1315
Amoxil Powder for Oral Suspension ... 1315
Amoxil Tablets ... 1315
Anaprox Tablets (Less than 1%) ... 2769
Anaprox DS Tablets (Less than 1%) ... 2769
Arava Tablets (Rare) ... 2881
Arimidex Tablets (Very rare) ... 665
Arthrotec Tablets (Rare) ... 3126
Atacand HCT ... 637
Attenuvax (Rare) ... 1889
Augmentin ... 1331
Augmentin Tablets ... 1334
Augmentin XR Extended-Release Tablets ... 1340
Augmentin ES-600 Powder for Oral Suspension ... 1337
Avalide Tablets ... 922
Avalide Tablets ... 2889
Caduet Tablets (Greater than 0.1% to less than or equal to 1%) ... 2507
Captopril Tablets ... 2114
Carbatrol Capsules ... 3174
Cardizem LA Extended Release Tablets (Infrequent) ... 1699
Carimune NF ... 3501
Cataflam Tablets (Rarely) ... 2173
Ceftin ... 1369
Celebrex Capsules (Less than 0.1%) ... 3130
Celexa (At least 3 patients) ... 1177
Cenestin Tablets, 0.45mg, 0.625mg, 0.9mg, 1.25mg ... 1063
Cenestin Tablets, 0.3mg ... 1063
Cipro I.V. (1% or less) ... 2998
Cipro I.V. Pharmacy Bulk Package (1% or less) ... 3509
Cipro ... 2991
Cipro XR Tablets ... 3004
Cleocin Vaginal Ovules (Rare) ... 2613
Climara Transdermal System ... 795
Climara Pro Transdermal System ... 800
Clindesse Vaginal Cream (Rare) ... 3296
Clinoril Tablets (Less than 1%) ... 1899
Clozapine Tablets ... 2141
Clozaril Tablets ... 2174
CombiPatch Transdermal System ... 2180
Combivir Tablets ... 1373
Comvax ... 1904
Concerta Extended-Release Tablets ... 1828
Covera-HS Tablets (Less than 2%) ... 3135
Crixivan Capsules ... 1918
Daraprim Tablets ... 1385
Depacon Injection ... 412
Depakene ... 417
Depakote Sprinkle Capsules ... 422
Depakote Tablets ... 427
Depakote ER Tablets ... 433
Diovan HCT Tablets ... 2195
Diuril Oral ... 1936
Diuril Sodium Intravenous ... 1934
Dolobid Tablets (Less than 1 in 100) ... 1937
Doxil Injection (Less than 1%) ... 3302
Dynacin Tablets ... 1859
EC-Naprosyn Delayed-Release Tablets (Less than 1%) ... 2769
E.E.S. (Rare) ... 449
Effexor Tablets ... 3405
Effexor XR Capsules ... 3411
Engerix-B Vaccine (Less than 1%) ... 1391
Epzicom Tablets ... 1402
Equetro Extended-Release Capsules ... 3178
EryPed (Rare) ... 445
Erythromycin Delayed-Release Capsules, USP (Rare) ... 456
Estratest Tablets ... 3196
Estratest H.S. Tablets ... 3196
Estrogel 0.06% ... 3200
Ethyol for Injection ... 1869
FazaClo Orally Disintegrating Tablets ... 547
Focalin Tablets ... 2214
Focalin XR Capsules ... 2217
Fortaz ... 1422
Furosemide Tablets ... 2117
Gammagard Liquid ... 751
Gammagard S/D (Rare) ... 754
Gamunex Immune Globulin I.V., 10% (Rare) ... 3232
Gleevec Tablets ... 2221
Grifulvin V Tablets Microsize and Oral Suspension Microsize ... 2384
Gris-PEG Tablets (Occasional) ... 2504
Havrix Vaccine (Rare) ... 1425
HibTITER ... 3419
Hyzaar ... 1964
Inderal LA Long-Acting Capsules ... 3421
Indocin Capsules (Less than 1%) ... 1968
Indocin I.V. (Less than 1%) ... 1973
Indocin (Less than 1%) ... 1968
Iressa Tablets (Very rare) ... 684
Iveegam EN (Rare) ... 759
Ketek Tablets (Less than 0.2%) ... 2920
Lamictal ... 1449
Lariam Tablets ... 2790
Lescol Capsules (Rare) ... 2227
Lescol Capsules (Rare) ... 2730
Lescol XL Tablets ... 2227
Lescol XL Tablets ... 2730
Leukeran Tablets (Rare) ... 1472
Levaquin in 5% Dextrose Injection ... 2453
Levaquin ... 2453
Lexapro Oral Solution ... 1193
Lexapro Tablets ... 1193
Lipitor Tablets ... 2495
Lo/Ovral-28 Tablets ... 3423
Lunesta Tablets (Rare) ... 3139
Lupron Depot-PED 7.5 mg, 11.25 mg and 15 mg (2%) ... 3266
Lupron Injection Pediatric ... 3256
Malarone Tablets (Rare) ... 1484
Malarone Pediatric Tablets (Rare) ... 1484
Maxipime for Injection ... 1093
Mefoxin for Injection ... 1987
Mefoxin Premixed Intravenous Solution ... 1990
Menostar Transdermal System ... 805
Mepron Suspension ... 1487
Merrem I.V. ... 687
Meruvax II (Rare) ... 1994
Metadate CD Capsules ... 3316
Mevacor Tablets (Rare) ... 1996
Micardis HCT Tablets ... 886
Mintezol ... 2002
M-M-R II (Rare) ... 1980
Mobic Oral Suspension (Less than 0.1%) ... 893
Mobic Tablets (Less than 0.1%) ... 893
Moduretic Tablets ... 2003
Mumpsvax (Rare) ... 2005
Mustargen for Injection ... 2007
Mycamine for Injection ... 620
Myleran Tablets (Rare) ... 1492
Naprosyn Suspension (Less than 1%) ... 2769
Naprosyn Tablets (Less than 1%) ... 2769
Neurontin Capsules ... 2498
Neurontin Oral Solution ... 2498
Neurontin Tablets ... 2498
Nexium Delayed-Release Capsules ... 645
Nexium I.V. ... 649
Noroxin Tablets ... 2009
Norvasc Tablets (More than 0.1% to 1%) ... 2529
Omnicef Capsules ... 506
Omnicef for Oral Suspension ... 506
Ortho-Cept Tablets ... 2395
Ortho-Cyclen Tablets ... 2414
Ortho Evra Transdermal System ... 2402
Ortho Tri-Cyclen Tablets ... 2414
Ortho Tri-Cyclen Lo Tablets ... 2421
Paxil CR Controlled-Release Tablets (Rare) ... 1509
Paxil (Rare) ... 1501
PCE Dispertab Tablets (Rare) ... 510
Pediarix Vaccine ... 1518
PEG-Intron Powder for Injection ... 3062
Plavix Tablets ... 940
Plavix Tablets ... 2942
Pravachol Tablets (Rare) ... 943
Prefest Tablets ... 1069
Premarin Intravenous ... 3440
Premarin Tablets ... 3443
Premarin Vaginal Cream ... 3449
Premphase Tablets ... 3452
Prempro Tablets ... 3452
Prevacid NapraPAC (Less than 1%) ... 3277
Prevnar for Injection ... 3460
PREVPAC ... 3281
Prilosec OTC Tablets (Very rare) ... 2674
Primaxin I.M. ... 2022
Primaxin I.V. (Less than 0.2%) ... 2024
Prinzide Tablets ... 2033
ProAmatine Tablets (Rare) ... 3183
Protonix I.V. ... 3468
Protonix Tablets ... 3465
Provigil Tablets (Rare) ... 1002
Raptiva for Injection ... 1247
Relafen Tablets (Less than 1%) ... 1523
Rescriptor Tablets ... 2535
Reyataz Capsules ... 948
Rilutek Tablets (Rare) ... 2945
Ritalin Hydrochloride Tablets ... 2254
Ritalin LA Capsules ... 2255
Ritalin-SR Tablets ... 2254
Seasonale Tablets ... 1073
Sedapap Tablets 50 mg/650 mg (Several cases) ... 2098
Suprax (Less than 2%) ... 1811
Sustiva Capsules (Up to 3.3%) ... 957
Tagamet Tablets (Very rare) ... 1547
Tarka Tablets ... 519
Tasmar Tablets (Infrequent) ... 3360
Taxotere Injection Concentrate ... 2947
Tegretol/Tegretol-XR ... 2278
Temodar Capsules (Rare) ... 3088
Teveten HCT Tablets ... 1710
Tiazac Capsules (Infrequent) ... 1204
Ticlid Tablets (Rare) ... 2813
Timentin ADD-Vantage ... 1556
Timentin Injection Galaxy Container ... 1559
Timentin IV Infusion ... 1553
Timentin Pharmacy Bulk Package ... 1562
Timolide Tablets ... 2056
Topamax Sprinkle Capsules ... 2438
Topamax Tablets ... 2438
Trileptal Oral Suspension ... 2281
Trileptal Tablets ... 2281
Triphasil-28 Tablets ... 3483
Trizivir Tablets ... 1565
Twinrix Vaccine ... 1571
Valtrex Caplets ... 1573
Vantin Tablets and Oral Suspension ... 2650
Varivax ... 2070
Vaseretic Tablets ... 2073
Vasotec I.V. Injection (0.5% to 1.0%) ... 2076
Verelan PM Capsules (2% or less) ... 3120
VFEND I.V. (Rare) ... 2543
VFEND Oral Suspension (Rare) ... 2543
VFEND Tablets (Rare) ... 2543
Vivelle Transdermal System ... 2288
Vivelle-Dot Transdermal System ... 2293
Voltaren Tablets (Rarely) ... 2298
Voltaren-XR Tablets (Rarely) ... 2301
Vytorin 10/10 Tablets ... 2084

Vytorin 10/10 Tablets ... 3092
Vytorin 10/20 Tablets ... 2084
Vytorin 10/20 Tablets ... 3092
Vytorin 10/40 Tablets ... 2084
Vytorin 10/40 Tablets ... 3092
Vytorin 10/80 Tablets ... 2084
Vytorin 10/80 Tablets ... 3092
Wellbutrin Tablets (Rare) ... 1579
Wellbutrin SR Sustained-Release Tablets (Rare) ... 1583
Wellbutrin XL Extended-Release Tablets (Rare) ... 1588
Yasmin 28 Tablets ... 818
Zantac (Rare) ... 1597
Zantac Injection (Rare) ... 1593
Zantac Syrup (Rare) ... 1597
Zegerid Powder for Oral Solution (Very rare) ... 2972
Zestoretic Tablets ... 701
Zevalin Injection ... 848
Ziagen ... 1600
Zinacef Injection (Rare) ... 1604
Zinacef for Injection (Rare) ... 1604
Zithromax Capsules, 250 mg (Rare) ... 2568
Zithromax for IV Infusion (Rare) ... 2573
Zithromax for Oral Suspension, 300 mg, 600 mg, 900 mg, 1200 mg (Rare) ... 2561
Zithromax Tablets, 250 mg, 500 mg (Rare) ... 2561
Zithromax Tri-Pak (Rare) ... 2561
Zmax for Oral Suspension (Rare) ... 2577
Zocor Tablets (Rare) ... 2078
Zomig Nasal Spray (Rare) ... 718
Zosyn (Rare) ... 3492
Zovirax Capsules ... 1616
Zovirax for Injection ... 1618
Zovirax ... 1616
Zyban Sustained-Release Tablets (Rare) ... 1620

Erythema nodosum
Accutane Capsules ... 2740
Activella Tablets ... 2311
Alesse-28 Tablets ... 3392
Asacol Delayed-Release Tablets ... 2688
Carbatrol Capsules ... 3174
Cenestin Tablets, 0.45mg, 0.625mg, 0.9mg, 1.25mg ... 1063
Cenestin Tablets, 0.3mg ... 1063
Cipro I.V. (1% or less) ... 2998
Cipro I.V. Pharmacy Bulk Package (1% or less) ... 3509
Cipro (Less than 1%) ... 2991
Cipro XR Tablets ... 3004
Climara Transdermal System ... 795
Climara Pro Transdermal System ... 800
Colazal Capsules ... 2845
CombiPatch Transdermal System ... 2180
Copaxone for Injection (Infrequent) ... 3292
Depakote ER Tablets (Greater than 1%) ... 433
Doxil Injection (Less than 1%) ... 3302
Effexor Tablets (Rare) ... 3405
Effexor XR Capsules (Rare) ... 3411
Engerix-B Vaccine (Less than 1%) ... 1391
Estratest Tablets ... 3196
Estratest H.S. Tablets ... 3196
Estrogel 0.06% ... 3200
Indocin Capsules (Less than 1%) ... 1968
Indocin I.V. (Less than 1%) ... 1973
Indocin (Less than 1%) ... 1968
▲ Intron A for Injection (Less than 5%) ... 3038
I.V. Busulfex (2%) ... 1125
Lo/Ovral-28 Tablets ... 3423
Menostar Transdermal System ... 805
Myleran Tablets (Rare) ... 1492
Neupogen for Injection (One event) ... 598
Omnicef Capsules ... 506
Omnicef for Oral Suspension ... 506
Ortho-Cept Tablets ... 2395
Ortho-Cyclen/Ortho Tri-Cyclen ... 2414
Ortho Tri-Cyclen Lo Tablets ... 2421
Paxil CR Controlled-Release Tablets (Rare) ... 1509
Paxil (Rare) ... 1501
Pentasa Capsules (Less than 1%) ... 3182
Prefest Tablets ... 1069
Premarin Intravenous ... 3440
Premarin Tablets ... 3443
Premarin Vaginal Cream ... 3449
Premphase Tablets ... 3452
Prempro Tablets ... 3452
Recombivax HB (Less than 1%) ... 2045
Seasonale Tablets ... 1073
Tegretol/Tegretol-XR ... 2278
Thalomid Capsules ... 979
Triphasil-28 Tablets ... 3483
Twinrix Vaccine ... 1571
Uniretic Tablets (Less than 1%) ... 3114
Vesanoid Capsules (Isolated cases) ... 2823
Vivelle Transdermal System ... 2288
Vivelle-Dot Transdermal System ... 2293
Yasmin 28 Tablets ... 818

Erythema simplex
Oncaspar (Less than 1%) ... 1123

Erythematous streaking
Adriamycin for Injection, USP ... 786
Adriamycin Injection, USP ... 786
▲ Zinecard for Injection (4% to 5%) ... 2659

Erythrocytes, abnormal
▲ Ferrlecit Injection (11%) ... 3379
Gabitril Tablets (Infrequent) ... 998
Paxil CR Controlled-Release Tablets (Rare) ... 1509
Paxil (Rare) ... 1501
Uniretic Tablets (Less than 1%) ... 3114

Erythrocytosis
Moban Tablets ... 1108
Repronex for Intramuscular and Subcutaneous Injection (One patient) ... 1148

Erythrocyturia
Emend Capsules (Greater than 0.5%) ... 1944

Erythroderma, exfoliative
Tagamet Tablets ... 1547

Erythroleukemia
Thalomid Capsules ... 979

Erythromelalgia
Adalat CC Tablets (Rare) ... 2978
Gammagard S/D ... 754

Erythropenia
Accutane Capsules ... 2740
Amnesteem Capsules ... 2126
Aricept Tablets (Infrequent) ... 1086
Aricept ODT Tablets (Infrequent) ... 1086
Factive Tablets (0.1%) ... 2464
Moban Tablets ... 1108
Mustargen for Injection ... 2007
Primaxin I.M. ... 2022

Escharotic effect
Cetacaine Topical Anesthetic ... 1007

Esophageal disease, unspecified
Myleran Tablets ... 1492
Nexium Delayed-Release Capsules (Less than 1%) ... 645
Nexium I.V. (Less than 1%) ... 649

Esophageal erosions
Fosamax ... 1949
Fosamax Plus D Tablets ... 1956

Esophageal perforation
Celebrex Capsules (Less than 0.1%) ... 3130
Fosamax (Rare) ... 1949
Fosamax Plus D Tablets (Rarely) ... 1956
Razadyne ER Extended-Release Capsules (Rare) ... 2434
Razadyne (Rare) ... 2434
TriLyte with Flavor Packs for Oral Solution ... 3114

Esophageal rupture
Exelon Capsules (One case) ... 2204

Esophageal stenosis
Actiq (Less than 1%) ... 993
Cymbalta Delayed-Release Capsules (Infrequent) ... 1729
Prevacid NapraPAC (Less than 1%) ... 3277
Rilutek Tablets (Infrequent) ... 2945

Esophageal stricture
Evoxac Capsules (Less than 1%) ... 1042
Fosamax (Rare) ... 1949
Fosamax Plus D Tablets (Rarely) ... 1956
Nexium Delayed-Release Capsules (Less than 1%) ... 645
Nexium I.V. (Less than 1%) ... 649
▲ Photofrin for Injection (6% to 38%) ... 729
Prevacid Delayed-Release Capsules (Less than 1%) ... 3268
Prevacid for Delayed-Release Oral Suspension (Less than 1%) ... 3268
Prevacid SoluTab Delayed-Release Orally Disintegrating Tablets (Less than 1%) ... 3268
PREVPAC (Less than 1%) ... 3281

Esophageal ulceration
Accutane Capsules ... 2740
Actonel with Calcium Tablets ... 2684
Arthrotec Tablets (Rare) ... 3126
Dynacin Tablets (Rare) ... 1859
Fosamax Plus D Tablets (0.1% to 1.5%) ... 1956
Pediapred Oral Solution ... 3319
Prevacid Delayed-Release Capsules (Less than 1%) ... 3268
Prevacid for Delayed-Release Oral Suspension (Less than 1%) ... 3268
Prevacid SoluTab Delayed-Release Orally Disintegrating Tablets (Less than 1%) ... 3268
PREVPAC (Less than 1%) ... 3281

Esophagitis
Abilify Tablets (Rare) ... 916
Abilify Tablets (Rare) ... 2472
Accutane Capsules ... 2740
Aciphex Tablets ... 1081
Actiq (Less than 1%) ... 993
Actonel with Calcium Tablets ... 2684
Adalat CC Tablets (Less than 1%) ... 2978
Adriamycin for Injection, USP ... 786
Adriamycin Injection, USP ... 786
▲ Alimta for Injection (Up to 6%) ... 1722
Amerge Tablets (Rare) ... 1312
Anaprox Tablets (Less than 1%) ... 2769
Anaprox DS Tablets (Less than 1%) ... 2769
Antara Capsules ... 2723
▲ Arava Tablets (1% to 3%) ... 2881
Arthrotec Tablets (Rare) ... 3126
Caduet Tablets (Less than 2%) ... 2507
Campath Ampules ... 826
Campral Tablets (Infrequent) ... 1175
Cataflam Tablets (Occasionally) ... 2173
Celebrex Capsules (0.1% to 1.9%) ... 3130
Celexa (Infrequent) ... 1177
▲ CellCept Capsules (3% to less than 20%) ... 2751
▲ CellCept Intravenous (3% to less than 20%) ... 2751
▲ CellCept Oral Suspension (3% to less than 20%) ... 2751
▲ CellCept Tablets (3% to less than 20%) ... 2751
Cialis Tablets (Less than 2%) ... 1806
Clindesse Vaginal Cream (Rare) ... 3296
Copaxone for Injection (Infrequent) ... 3292
Cosmegen for Injection ... 1907
Didronel Tablets ... 2693
▲ Doxil Injection (1% to 10%) ... 3302
Dynacin Tablets (Rare) ... 1859
EC-Naprosyn Delayed-Release Tablets (Less than 1%) ... 2769
Effexor Tablets (Infrequent) ... 3405
Effexor XR Capsules (Infrequent) ... 3411
Elmiron Capsules (Less than or equal to 1%) ... 2393
Enbrel for Injection ... 580
Evoxac Capsules (Less than 1%) ... 1042
Exelon Capsules (Infrequent) ... 2204
Fosamax ... 1949
Fosamax Plus D Tablets ... 1956
Gabitril Tablets (Infrequent) ... 998
Gengraf Capsules (1% to less than 3%) ... 458
▲ Humira Injection (Less than 5%) ... 464
▲ Intron A for Injection (Less than 5%) ... 3038
Invanz for Injection (Greater than 0.1%) ... 1974
Invirase (Less than 2%) ... 2776
I.V. Busulfex (2%) ... 1125
Kaletra (Less than 2%) ... 474
Lamictal ... 1449
Levaquin in 5% Dextrose Injection (0.1% to 0.9%) ... 2453
Levaquin (0.1% to 0.9%) ... 2453
Levitra Tablets (Less than 2%) ... 3048
Lipitor Tablets (Less than 2%) ... 2495
Lofibra Capsules ... 1217
Lotrel Capsules ... 2238
Lyrica Capsules (0.1% to 1%) ... 2524
Mobic Oral Suspension (Less than 2%) ... 893
Mobic Tablets (Less than 2%) ... 893
Myfortic Tablets ... 2244
Naprosyn Suspension (Less than 1%) ... 2769
Naprosyn Tablets (Less than 1%) ... 2769
Navelbine Injection ... 1494
Neoral Soft Gelatin Capsules (1% to less than 3%) ... 2247
Neoral Oral Solution (1% to less than 3%) ... 2247
Neurontin Capsules (Rare) ... 2498
Neurontin Oral Solution (Rare) ... 2498
Neurontin Tablets (Rare) ... 2498
Nexium Delayed-Release Capsules (Less than 1%) ... 645
Nexium I.V. (Less than 1%) ... 649
Norvir (Less than 2%) ... 499
Paxil CR Controlled-Release Tablets (Rare) ... 1509
Paxil (Rare) ... 1501
Permax Tablets (Infrequent) ... 3357
▲ Photofrin for Injection (5%) ... 729
Pletal Tablets (Less than 2%) ... 2478
Prevacid Delayed-Release Capsules (Less than 1%) ... 3268
Prevacid for Delayed-Release Oral Suspension (Less than 1%) ... 3268
Prevacid NapraPAC (Less than 1%) ... 3277
Prevacid SoluTab Delayed-Release Orally Disintegrating Tablets (Less than 1%) ... 3268
PREVPAC (Less than 1%) ... 3281
▲ Prograf Capsules and Injection (3% to 15%) ... 624
Protonix I.V. (Less than 1%) ... 3468
Protonix Tablets (Less than 1%) ... 3465
Prozac Pulvules and Liquid (Infrequent) ... 1771
▲ Rapamune Oral Solution and Tablets (3% to 20%) ... 3472
Relpax Tablets (Infrequent) ... 2531
Requip Tablets (Infrequent) ... 1528
Reyataz Capsules (Less than 3%) ... 948
Risperdal M-Tab Orally Disintegrating Tablets (Rare) ... 1658
Risperdal (Rare) ... 1658
▲ Simulect for Injection (3% to 10%) ... 2268
Sonata Capsules (Infrequent) ... 1686
Soriatane Capsules (Less than 1%) ... 1028
Symbyax Capsules (Infrequent) ... 1788
Tasmar Tablets (Infrequent) ... 3360
Taxotere Injection Concentrate ... 2947
Teveten Tablets (Less than 1%) ... 1707
Teveten HCT Tablets (Less than 1%) ... 1710
Thalomid Capsules ... 979
Topamax Sprinkle Capsules (Infrequent) ... 2438
Topamax Tablets (Infrequent) ... 2438
Tricor Tablets ... 523
Triglide Tablets ... 1165
Trileptal Oral Suspension ... 2281
Trileptal Tablets ... 2281
Uniretic Tablets (Less than 1%) ... 3114
VFEND I.V. (Less than 2%) ... 2543
VFEND Oral Suspension (Less than 2%) ... 2543
VFEND Tablets (Less than 2%) ... 2543
Viagra Tablets (Less than 2%) ... 2552
Vicoprofen Tablets (Less than 1%) ... 533
Voltaren Tablets (Occasionally) ... 2298
Voltaren-XR Tablets (Occasionally) ... 2301
Wellbutrin Tablets ... 1579
Wellbutrin SR Sustained-Release Tablets ... 1583
Wellbutrin XL Extended-Release Tablets ... 1588
Xeloda Tablets ... 2825
▲ Zinecard for Injection (3% to 6%) ... 2659
Zoloft (Infrequent) ... 2581
Zomig Tablets (Infrequent) ... 714
Zomig-ZMT Tablets (Infrequent) ... 714
Zonegran Capsules (Rare) ... 1089
Zyban Sustained-Release Tablets ... 1620
Zyprexa Tablets (Infrequent) ... 1798
Zyprexa ZYDIS Orally Disintegrating Tablets (Infrequent) ... 1798

Esophagitis, ulcerative
Decadron Phosphate Injection ... 1931
Decadron Tablets ... 1929
Depo-Medrol Injectable Suspension ... 2615
Depo-Medrol Single-Dose Vial ... 2617
Hydrocortone Tablets ... 1963
Indocin I.V. (Less than 1%) ... 1973

Esophagospasm
Ambien Tablets (Rare) ... 2867
Effexor XR Capsules (Rare) ... 3411
Frova Tablets (Infrequent) ... 1101
Migranal Nasal Spray (Rare) ... 3350
Neurontin Capsules (Rare) ... 2498
Neurontin Oral Solution (Rare) ... 2498
Neurontin Tablets (Rare) ... 2498

Esosinophilia
Zelnorm Tablets ... 2303

ESR, elevation
Accutane Capsules ... 2740
Aceon Tablets (2 mg, 4 mg, 8 mg) ... 3191
Advicor Tablets ... 1694
Altace Capsules (Less than 1%) ... 1673
Altoprev Extended-Release Tablets (Rare) ... 1151
Ambien Tablets (Rare) ... 2867
Amnesteem Capsules ... 2126
Captopril Tablets ... 2114

Cipro I.V. (Rare) 2998
Cipro I.V. Pharmacy Bulk Package (Rare) 3509
Clozapine Tablets 2141
Clozaril Tablets 2174
Comvax 1904
FazaClo Orally Disintegrating Tablets 547
Lescol Capsules (Rare) 2227
Lescol Capsules (Rare) 2730
Lescol XL Tablets 2227
Lescol XL Tablets 2730
Mevacor Tablets (Rare) 1996
Pravachol Tablets (Rare) 943
Prinivil Tablets (0.3% to 1.0%) 2029
Prinzide Tablets 2033
Recombivax HB 2045
Vaseretic Tablets 2073
Vasotec I.V. Injection (0.5% to 1.0%) 2076
Vytorin 10/10 Tablets 2084
Vytorin 10/10 Tablets 3092
Vytorin 10/20 Tablets 2084
Vytorin 10/20 Tablets 3092
Vytorin 10/40 Tablets 2084
Vytorin 10/40 Tablets 3092
Vytorin 10/80 Tablets 2084
Vytorin 10/80 Tablets 3092
Zestoretic Tablets 701
Zestril Tablets (0.3% to 1.0%) 704
Zocor Tablets (Rare) 2078

ESR decrease
Thalomid Capsules 979

Estradiol, elevated
Menopur for Subcutaneous Injection (2.4%) 1145

Euphoria
Abilify Tablets (Rare) 916
Abilify Tablets (Rare) 2472
Actiq (Less than 1%) 993
Adderall Tablets 3168
Adderall XR Capsules 3169
Adipex-P 1216
Alacol DM Syrup 739
Ambien Tablets (Frequent) 2867
Avinza Capsules (Less than 5%) 1714
Axert Tablets (Rare) 2430
Celexa (Infrequent) 1177
Combunox Tablets (Less than 1%) 1183
Copaxone for Injection (At least 2%) 3292
Dalmane Capsules (Rare) 3343
Darvocet A 500 Tablets 3497
Decadron Phosphate Injection 1931
Decadron Tablets 1929
Depacon Injection (0.9%) 412
Desoxyn Tablets, USP 2482
Dexedrine 1386
DextroStat Tablets 3177
▲ Diastat Rectal Delivery System (3%) 3344
Dilaudid 439
Dilaudid Oral Liquid 443
Dilaudid Non-Sterile Powder 439
Dilaudid Rectal Suppositories 439
Dilaudid Tablets 439
Dilaudid Tablets - 8 mg 443
Dilaudid-HP (Less frequent) 441
Diprivan Injectable Emulsion (Less than 1%) 676
▲ Duragesic Transdermal System (3% to 10%) 2448
Effexor Tablets (Infrequent) 3405
Effexor XR Capsules (Infrequent) 3411
Eldepryl Capsules 3209
Flumadine (Less than 0.3%) 1186
Frova Tablets (Infrequent) 1101
Gabitril Tablets (Frequent) 998
Hydrocortone Tablets 1963
Hyperstat I.V. Injection 3031
Imitrex Injection (Infrequent) 1431
Imitrex Nasal Spray (Infrequent) 1435
Imitrex Tablets (Infrequent) 1440
Invirase (Less than 2%) 2776
Kadian Capsules (Less than 3%) 572
Lamictal (Infrequent) 1449
Lidoderm Patch 1107
Lunesta Tablets (Rare) 3139
▲ Lyrica Capsules (2% to 3%) 2524
▲ Marinol Capsules (3% to 10%) 3334
Maxalt Tablets (Frequent) 1983
Maxalt-MLT Orally Disintegrating Tablets (Frequent) 1983
Migranal Nasal Spray (Infrequent) 3350
Moban Tablets (Less frequent) 1108
▲ MS Contin Tablets (Among most frequent) 2703
Neurontin Capsules (Infrequent) 2498
Neurontin Oral Solution (Infrequent) 2498
Neurontin Tablets (Infrequent) 2498
Norvir (Less than 2%) 499
Nubain Injection (1% or less) 1111
Numorphan 1112
▲ OxyContin Tablets (Between 1% and 5%) 2699
OxyFast Oral Concentrate Solution 2704
OxyIR Capsules 2704
Parcopa Orally Disintegrating Tablets 3111
Paxil CR Controlled-Release Tablets (Rare) 1509
Paxil (Rare) 1501
Percocet Tablets 1114
Percodan Tablets 1115
Permax Tablets (Infrequent) 3357
Phenergan 3438
ProSom Tablets (Infrequent) 512
Prozac Pulvules and Liquid (Infrequent) 1771
Relpax Tablets (Infrequent) 2531
Requip Tablets (Infrequent) 1528
Rescriptor Tablets 2535
Rilutek Tablets (Rare) 2945
Risperdal Consta Long-Acting Injection (Infrequent) 1664
Risperdal M-Tab Orally Disintegrating Tablets (Infrequent) 1658
Risperdal (Infrequent) 1658
Sedapap Tablets 50 mg/650 mg (Infrequent) 2098
Seroquel Tablets (Rare) 691
Sonata Capsules (Frequent) 1686
Stalevo Tablets 2270
Sustiva Capsules (Less than 2%) 957
Symbyax Capsules (Infrequent) 1788
Symmetrel (0.1% to 1%) 1115
Tambocor Tablets (Less than 1%) 1824
Tasmar Tablets (1%) 3360
Tequin Injection (Less than 0.1%) 964
Tequin Tablets (Less than 0.1%) 964
Thalomid Capsules 979
Topamax Sprinkle Capsules (Infrequent) 2438
Topamax Tablets (Infrequent) 2438
Trileptal Oral Suspension 2281
Trileptal Tablets 2281
Tussionex Pennkinetic Extended-Release Suspension 3322
Tylenol with Codeine 2461
Ultracet Tablets (At least 1%) 2462
VFEND I.V. (Less than 2%) 2543
VFEND Oral Suspension (Less than 2%) 2543
VFEND Tablets (Less than 2%) 2543
Vicoprofen Tablets (Less than 1%) 533
Wellbutrin Tablets (1.2%) 1579
Wellbutrin SR Sustained-Release Tablets 1583
Wellbutrin XL Extended-Release Tablets 1588
Xanax XR Tablets (Infrequent) 2655
Zoloft (Infrequent) 2581
Zomig Nasal Spray (Rare) 718
Zomig Tablets (Rare) 714
Zomig-ZMT Tablets (Rare) 714
Zonegran Capsules (Infrequent) 1089
Zyban Sustained-Release Tablets 1620
Zyprexa Tablets (2%) 1798
Zyprexa ZYDIS Orally Disintegrating Tablets (2%) 1798
Zyrtec Chewable Tablets (Less than 2%) 2589
Zyrtec (Less than 2%) 2589
Zyrtec-D 12 Hour Extended Release Tablets (Less than 2%) 2591

Eustachian tube dysfunction
Neurontin Capsules (Rare) 2498
Neurontin Oral Solution (Rare) 2498
Neurontin Tablets (Rare) 2498

Exanthema
Aptivus Capsules (Less than 2%) 859
Boostrix 1366
Copaxone for Injection (Infrequent) 3292
Covera-HS Tablets (Less than 2%) 3135
Lariam Tablets (Infrequent) 2790
Tarka Tablets 519
Verelan PM Capsules (2% or less) 3120

Exanthema, viral
Vaqta (1%) 2067

Excitability
Anadrol-50 Tablets 3329
Balamine DM (Rare) 739
BC Allergy Sinus Cold Powder ▣612
Benadryl Allergy & Cold Tablets ▣692
Benadryl Allergy ▣691
Benadryl Allergy & Sinus Headache Caplets & Gelcaps ▣693
Children's Benadryl Allergy Liquid ▣695
Children's Benadryl Dye-Free Allergy Liquid ▣695
Benadryl Dye-Free Allergy Liqui-Gels Softgels ▣692
Benadryl Maximum Strength Severe Allergy & Sinus Headache Caplets ▣694
Children's Benadryl D Allergy & Sinus Fastmelt Tablets ▣694
Children's Benadryl D Liquid Medication ▣693
Benadryl D Tablets ▣694
Bentyl Capsules 724
Bentyl Injection 724
Bentyl Syrup 724
Bentyl Tablets 724
Children's Benadryl Allergy Fastmelt Tablets ▣696
Cogentin Injection 1903
Contac Severe Cold and Flu Caplets Maximum Strength ▣615
Children's Dimetapp Cold & Allergy Elixir ▣745
Flexeril Tablets (Less than 1%) 1832
Klonopin (Infrequent) 2782
Lexapro Oral Solution (Infrequent) 1193
Lexapro Tablets (Infrequent) 1193
Narcan Injection 1109
Naropin Injection 640
Orap Tablets 1220
Oxandrin Tablets 2977
PediaCare Multi-Symptom Cold Liquid ▣704
PediaCare NightRest Cough & Cold Liquid ▣704
Phenergan 3438
Robitussin PM Cough & Cold Liquid ▣752
Sedapap Tablets 50 mg/650 mg (Infrequent) 2098
Singlet Caplets ▣636
Sudafed Sinus & Allergy Tablets ▣710
TheraFlu Cold & Cough Hot Liquid ▣680
TheraFlu Cold & Sore Throat Hot Liquid ▣680
TheraFlu Flu & Sore Throat Hot Liquid ▣681
TheraFlu Severe Cold & Cough Hot Liquid ▣683
TheraFlu Severe Cold Caplets ▣679
TheraFlu Severe Cold Hot Liquid ▣682
TheraFlu Thin Strips Multi Symptom ▣684
Triaminic Cold & Cough Softchews ▣688
Triaminic Thin Strips Cough & Runny Nose ▣690
Tylenol Cough & Sore Throat NightTime Liquid with Cool Burst ▣664
Children's Tylenol Plus Cold NightTime Suspension Liquid 1851
Children's Tylenol Plus Cold & Cough Suspension Liquid and Chewable Tablets 1851
Children's Tylenol Plus Cold Chewable Tablets 1851
Tylenol Cold & Flu Severe Daytime Liquid with Cool Bust 1846
Tylenol Cold & Flu Severe NightTime Liquid with Cool Burst 1846
Tylenol Cough & Sore Throat NightTime Liquid with Cool Burst 1849
Tylenol Allergy Complete Multi-Symptom Caplets and Gelcaps with Cool Burst 1844
Tylenol Flu NightTime Gelcaps 1846
Tylenol Flu Day Non-Drowsy Gelcaps 1846
Multi-Symptom Tylenol Cold Night Time Caplets 1845
Tylenol Sinus Night Time Caplets 1848
Pediatric Vicks 44m Cough & Cold Relief 2673
Children's Vicks NyQuil Cold/Cough Relief 2671
Vicks NyQuil LiquiCaps 2677
Vicks NyQuil LiquiCaps/Liquid Multi-Symptom Cold/Flu Relief ▣725
Vicks NyQuil Liquid 2677
Zyrtec-D 12 Hour Extended Release Tablets 2591

Excitement, paradoxical
ProSom Tablets 512
Valium Tablets 2822

Excoriation
▲ Aldara Cream, 5% (Up to 25%) 1814
Catapres-TTS (3 of 101 patients) 875
Cutivate Lotion 0.05% (2%) 1383
Sulfamylon Cream (Rare) 2154

Exercise tolerance, decreased
Blocadren Tablets 1891
Cosopt Sterile Ophthalmic Solution 1910
Timoptic in Ocudose (Less frequent) 2061
Timoptic Sterile Ophthalmic Solution (Less frequent) 2058
Timoptic-XE Sterile Ophthalmic Gel Forming Solution 2062

Exophthalmos
Decadron Phosphate Injection 1931
Decadron Tablets 1929
Depo-Medrol Injectable Suspension 2615
Depo-Medrol Single-Dose Vial 2617
Effexor Tablets (Rare) 3405
Effexor XR Capsules (Rare) 3411
Eskalith 1406
Hydrocortone Tablets 1963
Lyrica Capsules (Rare) 2524
Paxil CR Controlled-Release Tablets (Rare) 1509
Paxil (Rare) 1501
Pediapred Oral Solution 3319
Prozac Pulvules and Liquid (Rare) 1771
Zoloft (Rare) 2581

Extraocular movement, impairment of
Lescol Capsules 2227
Lescol Capsules 2730
Lescol XL Tablets 2227
Lescol XL Tablets 2730
Vytorin 10/10 Tablets 2084
Vytorin 10/10 Tablets 3092
Vytorin 10/20 Tablets 2084
Vytorin 10/20 Tablets 3092
Vytorin 10/40 Tablets 2084
Vytorin 10/40 Tablets 3092
Vytorin 10/80 Tablets 2084
Vytorin 10/80 Tablets 3092

Extrapyramidal disorder
Lexapro Oral Solution 1193
Lexapro Tablets 1193
Namenda (Infrequent) 1199
Parcopa Orally Disintegrating Tablets 3111
Symbyax Capsules (Infrequent) 1788

Extrapyramidal symptoms
Abelcet Injection 1119
▲ Abilify Tablets (6% to 17%) 916
▲ Abilify Tablets (6% to 17%) 2472
Aciphex Tablets (Rare) 1081
Cardizem LA Extended Release Tablets (Infrequent) 1699
Celexa (Infrequent) 1177
Clozapine Tablets 2141
Clozaril Tablets 2174
Cytovene 2763
▲ Demser Capsules (10%) 1933
Effexor Tablets 3405
Effexor XR Capsules 3411
▲ Equetro Extended-Release Capsules (Less than 5%) 3178
Eskalith 1406
Flexeril Tablets (Rare) 1832
▲ Geodon (14% to 31%) 2514
▲ Intron A for Injection (Less than 5%) 3038
Kytril Injection (Rare) 2785
Kytril Tablets (One case) 2788
Lamictal (Rare) 1449
Librium Capsules 3349
▲ Mirapex Tablets (Greater than or equal to 1% to 28%) 889
Moban Tablets 1108
Orap Tablets (Frequent) 1220
Paxil CR Controlled-Release Tablets (Rare) 1509
Paxil (Rare) 1501
Permax Tablets (1.6%) 3357
Phenergan 3438
Proleukin for Injection 1007
Prozac Pulvules and Liquid (Rare) 1771
Requip Tablets (Infrequent) 1528
Rilutek Tablets (Infrequent) 2945
Risperdal Consta Long-Acting Injection 1664
▲ Risperdal M-Tab Orally Disintegrating Tablets (17% to 34%) 1658
▲ Risperdal (17% to 34%) 1658
Seroquel Tablets 691
Stalevo Tablets 2270

Surmontil Capsules 2347
Tasmar Tablets (Infrequent) 3360
Thioridazine Hydrochloride Tablets (Infrequent) 2122
Thiothixene Capsules 2124
Tiazac Capsules (Infrequent) 1204
Trileptal Oral Suspension 2281
Trileptal Tablets 2281
VFEND I.V. (Less than 2%) 2543
VFEND Oral Suspension (Less than 2%) 2543
VFEND Tablets (Less than 2%) 2543
Vivactil Tablets 2350
Wellbutrin SR Sustained-Release Tablets 1583
Wellbutrin XL Extended-Release Tablets 1588
Zofran Injection (Rare) 1607
Zofran (Rare) 1613
Zofran ODT Orally Disintegrating Tablets (Rare) 1613
Zoloft 2581
Zyban Sustained-Release Tablets 1620
▲ Zyprexa Tablets (8% to 32%) 1798
▲ Zyprexa IntraMuscular (2% to 4%) 1798
▲ Zyprexa ZYDIS Orally Disintegrating Tablets (8% to 32%) 1798

Extrapyramidal syndrome
Lyrica Capsules (Rare) 2524

Extrasystoles
Abilify Tablets (Infrequent) 916
Abilify Tablets (Infrequent) 2472
Adalat CC Tablets (Less than 1%) 2978
Advair Diskus 100/50 1291
Advair Diskus 250/50 1291
Advair Diskus 500/50 1291
Aloxi Injection (Less than 1%) 2099
Ambien Tablets (Rare) 2867
Antara Capsules 2723
Anzemet Injection 2871
Anzemet Tablets 2874
Atacand HCT (0.5% or greater) 637
Caduet Tablets (Less than or equal to 0.1%) 2507
Cardene I.V. (0.7%) 1129
Celexa (Infrequent) 1177
▲ CellCept Capsules (3% to less than 20%) 2751
▲ CellCept Intravenous (3% to less than 20%) 2751
▲ CellCept Oral Suspension (3% to less than 20%) 2751
▲ CellCept Tablets (3% to less than 20%) 2751
Diprivan Injectable Emulsion (Less than 1%) 676
Effexor Tablets (Infrequent) 3405
Effexor XR Capsules (Infrequent) 3411
Ethyol for Injection 1869
Evoxac Capsules (Less than 1%) 1042
Exelon Capsules (Infrequent) 2204
▲ Imdur Tablets (Less than or equal to 5%) 3032
▲ Intron A for Injection (Less than 5%) 3038
Lariam Tablets (Occasional) 2790
Lofibra Capsules 1217
Lotronex Tablets (Rare) 1479
Meridia Capsules 485
Naropin Injection (Less than 1%) 640
Norvasc Tablets (Less than or equal to 0.1%) 2529
Proventil Inhalation Aerosol 3067
Prozac Pulvules and Liquid (Rare) 1771
Requip Tablets (2%) 1528
Rythmol SR Capsules 2736
Serevent Diskus 1540
Teveten Tablets (Less than 1%) 1707
Teveten HCT Tablets (Less than 1%) 1710
Tiazac Capsules (2%) 1204
Tricor Tablets 523
Ventolin HFA Inhalation Aerosol (Less than 3%) 1576
VFEND I.V. (Less than 2%) 2543
VFEND Oral Suspension (Less than 2%) 2543
VFEND Tablets (Less than 2%) 2543
Wellbutrin SR Sustained-Release Tablets 1583
Wellbutrin XL Extended-Release Tablets 1588
▲ Xeloda Tablets (Less than 5%) 2825
Xopenex HFA Inhalation Aerosol 3151
Xopenex Inhalation Solution 3143
Xopenex Inhalation Solution Concentrate 3147
Zomig Tablets (Rare) 714
Zomig-ZMT Tablets (Rare) 714
Zyban Sustained-Release Tablets 1620

Extrasystoles, supraventricular
Aloxi Injection (Less than 1%) 2099
Caverject Impulse Injection (Less than 1%) 2610
▲ CellCept Capsules (3% to less than 20%) 2751
▲ CellCept Intravenous (3% to less than 20%) 2751
▲ CellCept Oral Suspension (3% to less than 20%) 2751
▲ CellCept Tablets (3% to less than 20%) 2751
Rythmol SR Capsules 2736
Ultane Liquid for Inhalation (Less than 1%) 526

Extravasation
Adriamycin for Injection, USP 786
Adriamycin Injection, USP 786
Ammonul Injection 3323
Brevibloc Concentrate (Less than 1%) 766
Brevibloc Injection (Less than 1%) 766
Brevibloc Double Strength Injection (Less than 1%) 766
Brevibloc Premixed Injection (Less than 1%) 766
Brevibloc Double Strength Premixed Injection (Less than 1%) 766
Cerubidine for Injection 788
Cosmegen for Injection 1907
Doxil Injection 3302
Fluorescite Injection .... ⊙ 207
Gemzar for Injection (Infrequent) 1743
Hyperstat I.V. Injection 3031
Idamycin PFS Injection 2645
Novantrone for Injection Concentrate 3158
Taxotere Injection Concentrate 2947
▲ Visudyne for Injection (10% to 30%) 2286
Zinecard for Injection (1% to 3%) 2659

Extremities, rigidity of
Abilify Tablets (Frequent) 916
Abilify Tablets (Frequent) 2472

Extroversion
Ambien Tablets 2867

Exudate, increased
Bactroban Ointment (Less than 1%) 1358
▲ Thrombate III (1 of 17) 3254
Xalatan Sterile Ophthalmic Solution (Less than 1%) 2654

Eye abnormalities, fetal
Accutane Capsules 2740

Eye abnormality, unspecified
Topamax Sprinkle Capsules (2%) 2438
Topamax Tablets (2%) 2438

Eye discharge
Retisert Implant (5% to 9%) .... ⊙ 256
▲ Zylet Ophthalmic Suspension (Less than 4%) 3508

Eye disorder, unspecified
Lyrica Capsules (1% to 2%) 2524
▲ Zylet Ophthalmic Suspension (Less than 4%) 3508

Eye globe, perforation
(*see under* Bulbus oculi, perforation)

Eye movements, abnormal
Klonopin 2782
Mevacor Tablets (0.5% to 1.0%) 1996
Zocor Tablets 2078

Eye swelling
Poly-Pred Liquifilm Ophthalmic Suspension .... ⊙ 231
▲ Retisert Implant (5% to 9%) .... ⊙ 256

Eyeball, perforation
(*see under* Bulbus oculi, perforation)

Eyelash changes
Xalatan Sterile Ophthalmic Solution 2654

Eyelash darkening
▲ Lumigan Ophthalmic Solution (3% to 10%) 569
▲ Travatan Ophthalmic Solution (Among most frequent) 559
Xalatan Sterile Ophthalmic Solution 2654

Eyelashes, increase in growth
Iressa Tablets 684
▲ Lumigan Ophthalmic Solution (15% to 45%) 569
▲ Travatan Ophthalmic Solution (Among most frequent) 559

Eyelashes, matting of
Betoptic S Ophthalmic Suspension (Small number of patients) 554
Lacrisert Sterile Ophthalmic Insert 1979

Eyelid, discomfort
▲ Xalatan (1% to 4%) 2654

Eyelid crusting
Brimonidine Tartrate Ophthalmic Solution 0.2% (Less than 3%) .... ⊙ 245
Cosopt Sterile Ophthalmic Solution 1910
Travatan Ophthalmic Solution (1% to 4%) 559
Trusopt Sterile Ophthalmic Solution 2065
▲ Xalatan Sterile Ophthalmic Solution (1% to 4%) 2654

Eyelid disorder, unspecified
▲ Zylet Ophthalmic Suspension (Less than 4%) 3508

Eyelid skin darkening
▲ Lumigan Ophthalmic Solution (3% to 10%) 569
▲ Travatan Ophthalmic Solution (Among most frequent) 559
Xalatan Sterile Ophthalmic Solution 2654

Eyelid swelling
▲ Acular LS Ophthalmic Solution (1% to 5%) 562
Cialis Tablets (Less than 2%) 1806
▲ Voltaren Ophthalmic Solution (Less than or equal to 5%) 2300
▲ Zylet Ophthalmic Suspension (Less than 4%) 3508

Eyelids, deposits in
Soriatane Capsules (Less than 5%) 1028
Xalatan Sterile Ophthalmic Solution (1% to 4%) 2654

Eyelids, edema of
Alphagan P Ophthalmic Solution (1% to 4%) 563
Amnesteem Capsules 2126
Botox Purified Neurotoxin Complex (2 cases) 565
▲ Brimonidine Tartrate Ophthalmic Solution 0.2% (3% to 9%) .... ⊙ 245
Ciloxan Ophthalmic Ointment (Less than 1%) 554
Hyzaar 1964
Lacrisert Sterile Ophthalmic Insert 1979
Polytrim Ophthalmic Solution (Multiple reports) 570
Quixin Ophthalmic Solution (Less than 1%) 3373
▲ Rēv-Eyes Ophthalmic Eyedrops 0.5% (10% to 40%) .... ⊙ 256
Stromectol Tablets 2053
▲ Trisenox Injection (5%) 983
Xalatan Sterile Ophthalmic Solution (1% to 4%) 2654

Eyelids, erythema
Alphagan P Ophthalmic Solution (1% to 4%) 563
Alrex Ophthalmic Suspension 0.2% (Less than 5%) .... ⊙ 243
▲ Betimol Ophthalmic Solution (More than 5%) .... ⊙ 283
▲ Betimol Ophthalmic Solution (More than 5%) 3371
▲ Brimonidine Tartrate Ophthalmic Solution 0.2% (3% to 9%) .... ⊙ 245
Lotemax Ophthalmic Suspension 0.5% (Less than 5%) .... ⊙ 249
▲ Lumigan Ophthalmic Solution (3% to 10%) 569
Xalatan Sterile Ophthalmic Solution (1% to 4%) 2654

Eyelids, heavy
Sedapap Tablets 50 mg/650 mg (Infrequent) 2098

Eyelids, pruritis
Brimonidine Tartrate Ophthalmic Solution 0.2% .... ⊙ 245
▲ Zylet Ophthalmic Suspension (Less than 4%) 3508

Eyes, burning of
Alamast Ophthalmic Solution (Less than 5%) 3371
▲ Alrex Ophthalmic Suspension 0.2% (5% to 15%) .... ⊙ 243
▲ Betagan Ophthalmic Solution, USP (About 1 in 3 patients) .... ⊙ 217
▲ Betimol Ophthalmic Solution (1 in 8 patients) .... ⊙ 283
▲ Betimol Ophthalmic Solution (1 in 8 patients) 3371
Bleph-10 Ophthalmic Solution 10% .... ⊙ 219
▲ Carac Cream, 0.5% (5.4%) 1048
▲ Carteolol Hydrochloride Ophthalmic Solution USP, 1% (About 1 of 4 patients) .... ⊙ 246
Catapres Tablets 874
Catapres-TTS (0.5% or less) 875
▲ Ciloxan Ophthalmic Ointment (Among most frequent) 554
Clorpres Tablets 2139
▲ Cosopt Sterile Ophthalmic Solution (Up to 30%) 1910
Cozaar Tablets (Less than 1%) 1913
Dalmane Capsules (Rare) 3343
▲ Elestat Ophthalmic Solution (1% to 10%) 1643
FML Ophthalmic Suspension .... ⊙ 224
FML Forte Ophthalmic Suspension .... ⊙ 223
▲ Genoptic Sterile Ophthalmic Solution (Among most frequent) .... ⊙ 227
HMS Sterile Ophthalmic Suspension .... ⊙ 228
Hyzaar 1964
▲ Lotemax Ophthalmic Suspension 0.5% (5% to 15%) .... ⊙ 249
▲ Lumigan Ophthalmic Solution (3% to 10%) 569
Maxalt Tablets (Infrequent) 1983
Maxalt-MLT Orally Disintegrating Tablets (Infrequent) 1983
Muro 128 Ophthalmic Ointment .... ⊙ 251
Muro 128 Ophthalmic Solution 2% and 5% .... ⊙ 251
Nicotrol NS 2596
Ocufen Ophthalmic Solution .... ⊙ 230
Ophthetic Ophthalmic Solution .... ⊙ 230
▲ Optivar Ophthalmic Solution (Approximately 30%) 1877
Patanol Ophthalmic Solution (Less than 5%) 557
▲ Polytrim Ophthalmic Solution (Among most frequent) 570
Pred Forte Ophthalmic Suspension .... ⊙ 233
Pred Mild Sterile Ophthalmic Suspension .... ⊙ 236
▲ Propine Ophthalmic Solution (6%) .... ⊙ 237
Quixin Ophthalmic Solution (1% to 3%) 3373
▲ Restasis Ophthalmic Emulsion (17%) 570
Tessalon Capsules 1202
Tessalon Perles 1202
▲ Timoptic in Ocudose (Approximately 1 in 8 patients) 2061
▲ Timoptic Sterile Ophthalmic Solution (Approximately 1 in 8 patients) 2058
▲ Timoptic-XE Sterile Ophthalmic Gel Forming Solution (1 in 8 patients) 2062
▲ Trusopt Sterile Ophthalmic Solution (Approximately one-third of patients) 2065
Viagra Tablets 2552
Visine For Contacts Rewetting Drops .... ⊙ 278
▲ Xalatan Sterile Ophthalmic Solution (5% to 15%) 2654
Zaditor Ophthalmic Solution (Less than 5%) 2302

Eyes, cotton wool spots
Intron A for Injection 3038
PEG-Intron Powder for Injection 3062

Eyes, dilatation of pupil
(*see under* Mydriasis)

Eyes, discoloration
Alinia for Oral Suspension (Less than 1%) 2840
Alinia Tablets (Less than 1%) 2840
FazaClo Orally Disintegrating Tablets (Less than 1%) 547

Eyes, disorders of
Adalat CC Tablets (Less than 1%) 2978
Aerobid/Aerobid-M (1% to 3%) 1172
Alphagan P Ophthalmic Solution (1% to 4%) 563
Antara Capsules 2723
▲ Arava Tablets (1% to 3%) 2881
Astelin Nasal Spray (Infrequent) 1876
Avapro Tablets (Less than 1%) 925
Avapro Tablets (Less than 1%) 2886
▲ Avonex (4%) 839

Carbatrol Capsules 3174
▲ Carnitor Injection (3% to 6%) 3185
Clinoril Tablets (Less than 1%) 1899
▲ Copaxone for Injection (4%) 3292
Depakote ER Tablets (Greater than 1%) 433
Desferal Vials 2190
Kaletra (Less than 2%) 474
Lofibra Capsules 1217
▲ Lupron Depot 3.75 mg (Among most frequent) 3257
Mintezol 2002
Mirapex Tablets (Less than 1%) 889
Neurontin Capsules (Rare) 2498
Neurontin Oral Solution (Rare) 2498
Neurontin Tablets (Rare) 2498
Pacerone Tablets 3337
Permax Tablets (1.1%) 3357
Protopic Ointment (Greater than or equal to 1%) 629
▲ Requip Tablets (3%) 1528
▲ Soriatane Capsules (1% to 10%) 1028
Stromectol Tablets 2053
Tambocor Tablets 1824
Tegretol/Tegretol-XR 2278
▲ Thrombate III (1 of 17) 3254
Travatan Ophthalmic Solution (1% to 4%) 559
Tricor Tablets 523
Varivax (Greater than or equal to 1%) 2070
▲ Vesanoid Capsules (17%) 2823
Viracept (Less than 2%) 2556

Eyes, dry
(*see under* Xerophthalmia)

Eyes, irritation of
▲ Acular Ophthalmic Solution (Approximately 1% to 10%) 561
▲ Acular LS Ophthalmic Solution (1% to 10%) 562
Advicor Tablets 1694
Albalon Ophthalmic Solution ⊙ 216
Aloxi Injection (Less than 1%) 2099
Alphagan P Ophthalmic Solution (1% to 4%) 563
Alrex Ophthalmic Suspension 0.2% (Less than 5%) ⊙ 243
Altoprev Extended-Release Tablets (0.5% to 1%) 1151
Ambien Tablets (Infrequent) 2867
Aricept Tablets (Frequent) 1086
Aricept ODT Tablets (Frequent) 1086
Atrovent Nasal Spray 0.03% (Less than 2%) 869
Bleph-10 Ophthalmic Solution 10% ⊙ 219
Blocadren Tablets (1.1%) 1891
▲ Botox Purified Neurotoxin Complex (10.0%) 565
▲ Brimonidine Tartrate Ophthalmic Solution 0.2% (3% to 9%) ⊙ 245
▲ Carac Cream, 0.5% (5.4%) 1048
Cardizem LA Extended Release Tablets (Less than 2%) 1699
▲ Carteolol Hydrochloride Ophthalmic Solution USP, 1% (About 1 of 4 patients) ⊙ 246
Crolom Cromolyn Sodium Sterile Ophthalmic Solution USP 4% (Infrequent) ⊙ 248
Cubicin for Injection (Less than 1%) 1038
Erygel Topical Gel 2096
Flonase Nasal Spray 1412
FML Ophthalmic Suspension ⊙ 224
FML Forte Ophthalmic Suspension ⊙ 223
▲ Genoptic Sterile Ophthalmic Solution (Among most frequent) ⊙ 227
Imitrex Injection (Infrequent) 1431
Imitrex Nasal Spray (Infrequent) 1435
Imitrex Tablets (Up to 2%) 1440
Invirase (Less than 2%) 2776
Klonopin (Infrequent) 2782
Lacrisert Sterile Ophthalmic Insert 1979
Lexapro Oral Solution (Infrequent) 1193
Lexapro Tablets (Infrequent) 1193
Lotemax Ophthalmic Suspension 0.5% (Less than 5%) ⊙ 249
▲ Lumigan Ophthalmic Solution (3% to 10%) 569
Maxalt Tablets (Infrequent) 1983
Maxalt-MLT Orally Disintegrating Tablets (Infrequent) 1983
Mevacor Tablets (0.5% to 1.0%) 1996
Muro 128 Ophthalmic Ointment ⊙ 251
Muro 128 Ophthalmic Solution 2% and 5% ⊙ 251
Nicotrol NS 2596
Noritate Cream, 1% (Uncommon) 1051
Ocufen Ophthalmic Solution ⊙ 230
▲ Polytrim Ophthalmic Solution (Among most frequent) 570
Pred Forte Ophthalmic Suspension ⊙ 233
Pred Mild Sterile Ophthalmic Suspension ⊙ 236
Prilosec OTC Tablets (Less than 1%) 2674
ProSom Tablets (Infrequent) 512
▲ Retisert Implant (10% to 35%) ⊙ 256
▲ Soriatane Capsules (1% to 10%) 1028
Tambocor Tablets (Less than 1%) 1824
Temovate Scalp Application (1 of 294 patients) 1551
Tiazac Capsules (Less than 2%) 1204
Timolide Tablets 2056
Timoptic in Ocudose (Less frequent) 2061
Timoptic Sterile Ophthalmic Solution (Less frequent) 2058
Timoptic-XE Sterile Ophthalmic Gel Forming Solution 2062
▲ Trisenox Injection (10%) 983
Vaqta (Less than 1%) 2067
▲ Voltaren Ophthalmic Solution (Less than or equal to 5%) 2300
▲ Xeloda Tablets (13%) 2825
Zaditor Ophthalmic Solution (Less than 5%) 2302
Zegerid Powder for Oral Solution (Less than 1%) 2972
▲ Zymar Ophthalmic Solution (1% to 4%) 571

Eyes, nonreactive
Nipent for Injection (Less than 3%) 3216

Eyes, redness of
▲ Advair Diskus 100/50 (1% to 3%) 1291
▲ Advair Diskus 250/50 (1% to 3%) 1291
▲ Advair Diskus 500/50 (1% to 3%) 1291
Albalon Ophthalmic Solution ⊙ 216
Clozapine Tablets (Less than 1%) 2141
Clozaril Tablets (Less than 1%) 2174
▲ Polytrim Ophthalmic Solution (Among most frequent) 570
Transderm Scōp Transdermal Therapeutic System (Infrequent) 2166
▲ Travatan Ophthalmic Solution (35% to 50%) 559
Trusopt Sterile Ophthalmic Solution 2065
Viagra Tablets 2552
Visine For Contacts Rewetting Drops ⊙ 278
▲ Zymar Ophthalmic Solution (1% to 4%) 571

Eyes, "spots" before the
Aricept Tablets (Infrequent) 1086
Aricept ODT Tablets (Infrequent) 1086
Depacon Injection 412
Depakene 417
Depakote Sprinkle Capsules 422
Depakote Tablets 427
Depakote ER Tablets 433
Tambocor Tablets 1824

Eyes, stinging
▲ Restasis Ophthalmic Emulsion (1% to 5%) 570
▲ Voltaren Ophthalmic Solution (15%) 2300
▲ Xalatan Sterile Ophthalmic Solution (5% to 15%) 2654
▲ Zylet Ophthalmic Suspension (9%) 3508

Eyes, tearing
Astelin Nasal Spray (Infrequent) 1876
Beconase AQ Nasal Spray (Fewer than 3 per 100 patients) 1359
Betoptic S Ophthalmic Suspension (Small number of patients) 554
▲ Brimonidine Tartrate Ophthalmic Solution 0.2% (3% to 9%) ⊙ 245
▲ Carac Cream, 0.5% (5.4%) 1048
▲ Carteolol Hydrochloride Ophthalmic Solution USP, 1% (About 1 of 4 patients) ⊙ 246
▲ Chemet Capsules (1.0% to 3.7%) 2480
Ciloxan Ophthalmic Ointment (Less than 1%) 554
Cosopt Sterile Ophthalmic Solution 1910
Dantrium Capsules (Less frequent) 2690
Emcyt Capsules (1%) 3137
Levitra Tablets (Less than 2%) 3048
▲ Lumigan Ophthalmic Solution (1% to 3%) 569
Nipent for Injection (Less than 3%) 3216
Polytrim Ophthalmic Solution (Multiple reports) 570
▲ Retisert Implant (10% to 35%) ⊙ 256
Rēv-Eyes Ophthalmic Eyedrops 0.5% (Less frequently) ⊙ 256
Sonata Capsules (Infrequent) 1686
Strattera Capsules 1784
▲ Suboxone Tablets (5%) 2719
▲ Subutex Tablets (5%) 2719
Taxotere Injection Concentrate 2947
Timoptic in Ocudose (Less frequent) 2061
Timoptic Sterile Ophthalmic Solution (Less frequent) 2058
Timoptic-XE Sterile Ophthalmic Gel Forming Solution (1% to 5%) 2062
Travatan Ophthalmic Solution (1% to 4%) 559
Visine For Contacts Rewetting Drops ⊙ 278
Xalatan Sterile Ophthalmic Solution (1% to 4%) 2654
▲ Zymar Ophthalmic Solution (1% to 4%) 571

Eyes, watering
Nicotrol NS 2596

F

Face, rhythmical involuntary movements
Moban Tablets 1108
Orap Tablets 1220
Thiothixene Capsules 2124

Facial dehiscence
Rapamune Oral Solution and Tablets 3472

Facial dysmorphia, fetal
Accutane Capsules 2740

Facial features, coarsening
Phenytek Capsules 2153

Facial paresis
(*see also under* Bell's palsy)
Vytorin 10/10 Tablets 2084
Vytorin 10/10 Tablets 3092
Vytorin 10/20 Tablets 2084
Vytorin 10/20 Tablets 3092
Vytorin 10/40 Tablets 2084
Vytorin 10/40 Tablets 3092
Vytorin 10/80 Tablets 2084
Vytorin 10/80 Tablets 3092

Facial swelling
Altace Capsules 1673
Carafate Suspension 727
Carafate Tablets 728
▲ Doxil Injection (Approximately 6.8%) 3302
▲ Entocort EC Capsules (11%) 2694
Imitrex Nasal Spray (Rare) 1435
Levaquin in 5% Dextrose Injection 2453
Levaquin 2453
Children's Motrin Oral Suspension and Chewable Tablets 1837
Children's Motrin Cold Non-Staining Dye-Free Oral Suspension 1838
Children's Motrin Cold Oral Suspension 1838
Children's Motrin Non-Staining Dye-Free Oral Suspension 1837
Motrin Cold & Sinus Caplets 1836
Motrin IB Tablets and Caplets 1836
Infants' Motrin Concentrated Drops 1837
Infants' Motrin Non-Staining Dye-Free Drops 1837
Junior Strength Motrin Caplets and Chewable Tablets 1837
Nadolol Tablets (1 to 5 of 1000 patients) 2121
Proscar Tablets 2040
Tamiflu Capsules 2810
Tamiflu Oral Suspension 2810

Facial wasting
Aptivus Capsules (Less than 2%) 859
Combivir Tablets 1373
Crixivan Capsules 1918
Invirase 2776
Norvir 499
Retrovir 1533
Reyataz Capsules (Less than 3%) 948
Truvada Tablets 1279
Viracept 2556
Viramune Oral Suspension 903
Viramune Tablets 903
Viread Tablets 1284
Zerit 971

Facies, mask-like
Thiothixene Capsules 2124
▲ Zyprexa Tablets (8% to 20%) 1798
▲ Zyprexa ZYDIS Orally Disintegrating Tablets (8% to 20%) 1798

Factor VIII decrease
Advate Injection (0.6%) 742

Factors II, V, VII, X, decrease
Anadrol-50 Tablets 3329
Estratest Tablets 3196
Estratest H.S. Tablets 3196
Oxandrin Tablets 2977

Factors VII, VIII, IX, X, increase
Aygestin Tablets 1062
Estratest Tablets 3196
Estratest H.S. Tablets 3196
Ortho-Cyclen/Ortho Tri-Cyclen 2414

Fainting
(*see under* Syncope)

Faintness
Fleet Prep Kits 1172
Parcopa Orally Disintegrating Tablets 3111

Falling
▲ Advate Injection (12.7%) 742
Ambien Tablets (Infrequent) 2867
▲ Apokyn Injection (At least 5%) 2132
Dalmane Capsules 3343
Detrol Tablets (1.5%) 2626
Eldepryl Capsules 3209
Evoxac Capsules (Less than 1%) 1042
Geodon Capsules (Frequent) 2514
Klonopin (Infrequent) 2782
Lexapro Oral Solution (Infrequent) 1193
Lexapro Tablets (Infrequent) 1193
Matulane Capsules 3188
Mobic Oral Suspension (0% to 2.6%) 893
Mobic Tablets (0% to 2.6%) 893
Namenda (Greater than or equal to 2%) 1199
Parcopa Orally Disintegrating Tablets 3111
Razadyne ER Extended-Release Capsules (Greater than or equal to 2%) 2434
Razadyne (Greater than or equal to 2%) 2434
Requip Tablets (1% or more) 1528
▲ Tasmar Tablets (4% to 6%) 3360
▲ Trileptal Oral Suspension (Up to 4%) 2281
▲ Trileptal Tablets (Up to 4%) 2281
Viagra Tablets (Less than 2%) 2552
Xanax XR Tablets (Infrequent) 2655

Fanconi syndrome
Depacon Injection (Rare) 412
Depakene (Rare) 417
Depakote Sprinkle Capsules (Rare) 422
Depakote Tablets (Rare) 427
Depakote ER Tablets (Rare) 433
Garamycin Injectable 3028
Truvada Tablets 1279
Viread Tablets 1284

Fasciculations
Amerge Tablets (Rare) 1312
Aricept Tablets (Infrequent) 1086
Aricept ODT Tablets (Infrequent) 1086
Clozapine Tablets (Less than 1%) 2141
Clozaril Tablets (Less than 1%) 2174
▲ Depakote Sprinkle Capsules (1% to 5%) 422
Dilaudid Oral Liquid (Less frequent) 443
Dilaudid Tablets - 8 mg (Less frequent) 443
Dilaudid-HP 441
Eldepryl Capsules 3209
Eloxatin for Injection 2908
Eskalith 1406
Flexeril Tablets (Less than 1%) 1832
Garamycin Injectable 3028
Leukeran Tablets (Rare) 1472
Migranal Nasal Spray (Rare) 3350
MS Contin Tablets (Less frequent) 2703
▲ Niravam Orally Disintegrating Tablets (6.9% to 7.9%) 3106
Parcopa Orally Disintegrating Tablets 3111
Parnate Tablets 1499
Paxil CR Controlled-Release Tablets (Rare) 1509
Paxil (Rare) 1501
ReoPro Vials (0.4%) 1779
Retrovir 1533
Stalevo Tablets 2270
Uniphyl Tablets 2708
▲ Xanax XR Tablets (7.4%) 2655

Fasciitis, necrotizing
Raptiva for Injection 1247

Fasciitis, necrotizing fulminant
Clinoril Tablets (Rare) 1899
Dolobid Tablets 1937
Indocin (Rare) 1968

Fat deposits, abnormal
Decadron Tablets 1929

Fat redistribution, unspecified
Agenerase Capsules (Nine patients) 1299
Agenerase Oral Solution (Nine patients) 1304
Aptivus Capsules 859
Crixivan Capsules (2.1%) 1918
Epzicom Tablets 1402
Rescriptor Tablets 2535
Truvada Tablets 1279
Viracept (Less than 2%) 2556

Fatality, hepatic related
Eulexin Capsules 3023

Fatigue
Accutane Capsules 2740
▲ Actimmune (14%) 1646
Activella Tablets 2311
▲ Adacel Vaccine (1.2% to 30.2%) 2959
▲ Adalat CC Tablets (4%) 2978
▲ Advair Diskus 250/50 (3%) 1291
Aerobid/Aerobid-M (1% to 3%) 1172
▲ Agenerase Capsules (7% to 14%) 1299
▲ Agenerase Oral Solution (7% to 14%) 1304
▲ Aggrenox Capsules (5.8%) 855
Agrylin Capsules 3172
Aldara Cream, 5% (More than 1%) 1814
▲ Alferon N Injection (6% to 14%) 1640
▲ Alimta for Injection (Up to 87%) 1722
Allegra (1.3%) 2857
Aloxi Injection (Less than 1%) 2099
Altace Capsules (2%) 1673
Ambien Tablets (1%) 2867
Amerge Tablets (2%) 1312
Antabuse Tablets 2343
▲ Anzemet Injection (3.6%) 2871
Anzemet Tablets (2.6%) 2874
▲ Apokyn Injection (At least 5%) 2132
▲ Aptivus Capsules (4%) 859
▲ Aranesp for Injection (9% to 33%) 576
▲ Aredia for Injection (37.2%) 2168
▲ Aricept Tablets (3% to 8%) 1086
▲ Aricept ODT Tablets (3% to 8%) 1086
▲ Aromasin Tablets (22%) 2600
Arthrotec Tablets (Rare) 3126
▲ Asmanex Twisthaler (1% to 13%) 2981
Astelin Nasal Spray (2.3%) 1876
Atacand Tablets (More than 1%) 634
Atacand HCT (0.5% or greater) 637
▲ Avalide Tablets (7%) 922
▲ Avalide Tablets (7%) 2889
▲ Avandamet Tablets (6.2%) 1343
Avandia Tablets (3.6%) 1348
▲ Avapro Tablets (4%) 925
▲ Avapro Tablets (4%) 2886
Avonex 839
Axert Tablets (Infrequent) 2430
Azmacort Inhalation Aerosol 1701
Azopt Ophthalmic Suspension (Less than 1%) 553
▲ Baraclude (1% to 3%) 928
Benicar Tablets (Greater than 0.5%) 2850
▲ Blocadren Tablets (3.4% to 5%) 1891
▲ Boostrix (3.7% to 37%) 1366
Brevibloc Concentrate (About 1%) 766
Brevibloc Injection (About 1%) 766
Brevibloc Double Strength Injection (About 1%) 766
Brevibloc Premixed Injection (About 1%) 766
Brevibloc Double Strength Premixed Injection (About 1%) 766
▲ Brimonidine Tartrate Ophthalmic Solution 0.2% (10% to 30%) ⊙ 245
Buphenyl Powder 3327
Buphenyl Tablets 3327
▲ Caduet Tablets (4.5%) 2507
Calcium Disodium Versenate Injection 1819
▲ Campath Ampules (5% to 34%) 826
Cancidas for Injection (0%) 1894
Captopril Tablets (About 0.5% to 2%) 2114
Carbatrol Capsules 3174
▲ Cardizem LA Extended Release Tablets (4.8%) 1699
Casodex Tablets 670
▲ Catapres Tablets (About 4 in 100 patients) 874
▲ Catapres-TTS (6 of 101 patients) 875
Celebrex Capsules (0.1% to 1.9%) 3130
▲ Celexa (5%) 1177
▲ Cerezyme for Injection (Approximately 6.5%) 1263
▲ Chemet Capsules (5.2% to 15.7%) 2480
Cialis Tablets (Less than 2%) 1806
Clarinex Tablets (2.1% to 5%) 3009
Clarinex Reditabs Tablets (2.1% to 5%) 3009
▲ Clarinex-D 24-Hour Extended-Release Tablets (3%) 3012
Clindesse Vaginal Cream (Less than 1%) 3296
Clinoril Tablets (Less than 1 in 100) 1899
▲ Clolar for Intravenous Infusion (36%) 1264
▲ Clorpres Tablets (About 4%) 2139
Clozapine Tablets (2%) 2141
Clozaril Tablets (2%) 2174
Colazal Capsules (2%) 2845
Combivent Inhalation Aerosol (Less than 2%) 878
▲ Combivir Tablets (10%) 1373
▲ Comtan Tablets (6%) 2186
▲ Copegus Tablets (65%) 2759
▲ Coreg Tablets (24%) 1376
Cosmegen for Injection 1907
Cosopt Sterile Ophthalmic Solution 1910
Coumadin for Injection (Infrequent) 932
Coumadin Tablets (Infrequent) 932
▲ Covera-HS Tablets (1.7% to 4.5%) 3135
Cozaar Tablets (1% or greater) 1913
Crixivan Capsules (2.7%) 1918
Cubicin for Injection (Less than 1%) 1038
▲ Cymbalta Delayed-Release Capsules (2% to 12%) 1729
▲ Dantrium Capsules (Among most frequent) 2690
▲ depo-subQ provera 104 Injectable Suspension (1% to less than 5%) 2622
▲ Detrol Tablets (6.8%) 2626
Detrol LA Capsules (2%) 2629
Dibenzyline Capsules 3390
▲ Diovan HCT Tablets (5%) 2195
▲ Diovan Tablets (2% to 3%) 2191
Diprivan Injectable Emulsion (Less than 1%) 676
Dolobid Tablets (Greater than 1 in 100) 1937
▲ Dostinex Tablets (5% to 7%) 2631
Doxil Injection 3302
▲ Duragesic Transdermal System (3% to 10%) 2448
Dyazide Capsules 1389
▲ DynaCirc CR Tablets (2.5% to 7.6%) 2726
Dyrenium Capsules (Rare) 3390
Edecrin 1941
Effexor XR Capsules 3411
Eldepryl Capsules 3209
▲ Eligard 7.5 mg (17.5%) 2896
▲ Eligard 22.5 mg (6%) 2899
▲ Eligard 30 mg (13.3%) 2901
▲ Eligard 45 mg (11.7%) 2904
▲ Eloxatin for Injection (4% to 68%) 2908
Elspar for Injection 1943
▲ Emend Capsules (17.8%) 1944
Enbrel for Injection 580
▲ Engerix-B Vaccine (14%) 1391
▲ Entocort EC Capsules (5%) 2694
▲ Epivir (27%) 1394
▲ Epivir-HBV (24%) 1398
▲ Epogen for Injection (9% to 25%) 586
▲ Epzicom Tablets (6% to 8%) 1402
Equetro Extended-Release Capsules 3178
Eskalith 1406
Eulexin Capsules 3023
▲ Evoxac Capsules (3.3%) 1042
▲ Exelon Capsules (9%) 2204
Factive Tablets (0.1% to 1%) 2464
▲ Famvir Tablets (4% to 6.3%) 2207
FazaClo Orally Disintegrating Tablets (2%) 547
▲ Femara Tablets (6% to 13%) 2210
▲ Ferrlecit Injection (6%) 3379
▲ Flexeril Tablets (1% to 6%) 1832
Flolan for Injection 1408
▲ Flovent Diskus 50 mcg (1% to 16%) 1415
Flumadine (1.0%) 1186
▲ Flumist Vaccine (25.7%) 1872
Foradil Aerolizer 3024
▲ Fortical Nasal Spray (1% to 3%) 3336
▲ Frova Tablets (5%) 1101
▲ Fuzeon Injection (20.2%) 2772
Gabitril Tablets 998
▲ Gammagard Liquid (2.18% to 16.4%) 751
Gammagard S/D (Occasional) 754
▲ Gengraf Capsules (3%) 458
▲ Gleevec Tablets (30% to 48%) 2221
Grifulvin V Tablets Microsize and Oral Suspension Microsize (Occasional) 2384
Gris-PEG Tablets 2504
▲ Havrix Vaccine (1% to 10%) 1425
Hexalen Capsules (1%) 2101
▲ Hycamtin for Injection (Up to 37%) 1427
▲ Hytrin Capsules (7.4% to 11.3%) 469
Hyzaar (1% or greater) 1964
▲ Imdur Tablets (Less than or equal to 5%) 3032
Imitrex Injection (1.1%) 1431
Imitrex Tablets 1440
Imodium Capsules 1834
Imodium A-D Liquid and Caplets 1835
Imodium Advanced Caplets and Chewable Tablets ⊡ 644
▲ Indapamide Tablets (Greater than or equal to 5%) 2119
Inderal LA Long-Acting Capsules 3421
Indocin (Greater than 1%) 1968
▲ Infergen (65% to 69%) 1647
▲ InnoPran XL Capsules (5% to 7%) 2728
Inspra Tablets (2%) 2520
▲ Intron A for Injection (4% to 96%) 3038
Invanz for Injection (1.2%) 1974
Inversine Tablets 3286
▲ Invirase (Less than 2% to 6.1%) 2776
I.V. Busulfex (2%) 1125
Keppra Oral Solution 3307
Keppra Tablets 3307
Ketek Tablets (Greater than or equal to 0.2% to less than 2%) 2920
▲ Klonopin (7%) 2782
K-Phos Neutral Tablets 785
K-Phos Original (Sodium Free) Tablets (Less frequent) 785
▲ Lamictal (8%) 1449
Lamisil Tablets 2226
▲ Lariam Tablets (Among most frequent) 2790
Lescol Capsules (2.7%) 2227
Lescol Capsules (2.7%) 2730
Lescol XL Tablets (1.6%) 2227
Lescol XL Tablets (1.6%) 2730
▲ Leustatin Injection (11% to 45%) 2368
Levaquin in 5% Dextrose Injection (1.2%) 2453
Levaquin (1.2%) 2453
Levothroid Tablets 1189
Levoxyl Tablets 1680
▲ Lexapro Oral Solution (2% to 8%) 1193
▲ Lexapro Tablets (2% to 8%) 1193
▲ Lexiva Tablets (Less than 1% to 18%) 1473
Lithobid Tablets 1670
Lotensin Tablets (2.4%) 2232
▲ Lotensin HCT Tablets (5.2%) 2235
Lotrel Capsules 2238
Lotronex Tablets (Rare) 1479
Mavik Tablets (More than 1%) 482
Maxair Autohaler 1820
▲ Maxalt Tablets (4% to 7%) 1983
▲ Maxalt-MLT Orally Disintegrating Tablets (4% to 7%) 1983
Maxzide 2150
▲ Menactra Vaccine (0.9% to 34.7%) 2968
MetroGel-Vaginal Gel (Less than 1%) 1822
Miacalcin Nasal Spray (1% to 3%) 2242
Micardis Tablets (1%) 884
▲ Micardis HCT Tablets (3%) 886
▲ Midamor Tablets (Between 1% and 3%) 2000
Migranal Nasal Spray (1%) 3350
Mintezol 2002
Mobic Oral Suspension (Less than 2%) 893
Mobic Tablets (Less than 2%) 893
Moduretic Tablets (Greater than 1%, less than 3%) 2003
▲ Myfortic Tablets (3% to less than 20%) 2244
Myleran Tablets 1492
Nabi-HB 2159
Nadolol Tablets (2 of 100 patients) 2121
Nalfon Capsules (1.7%) 2504
Namenda (2%) 1199
▲ Navelbine Injection (67%) 1494
▲ Neoral Soft Gelatin Capsules (3%) 2247
▲ Neoral Oral Solution (3%) 2247
▲ Neulasta Injection (15% to 72%) 596
▲ Neupogen for Injection (11%) 598
▲ Neurontin Capsules (11%) 2498
▲ Neurontin Oral Solution (3.4% to 11%) 2498
▲ Neurontin Tablets (11%) 2498
Nexium Delayed-Release Capsules (Less than 1%) 645
Nexium I.V. (Less than 1%) 649
▲ Nicotrol Inhaler (Greater than 3%) 2594
▲ Nicotrol NS (Greater than 5%) 2596
▲ Nipent for Injection (29% to 42%) 3216
▲ Niravam Orally Disintegrating Tablets (18.4% to 48.6%) 3106
▲ Norvasc Tablets (4.5%) 2529
Novarel for Injection 1147
Numorphan 1112
Oncaspar 1123
▲ Optivar Ophthalmic Solution (1% to 10%) 1877
Ortho-Cyclen/Ortho Tri-Cyclen 2414
Ortho Tri-Cyclen Lo Tablets 2421
Orthoclone OKT3 Sterile Solution 2370
▲ Oxytrol Transdermal System (Greater than 1%) 3383
▲ Pacerone Tablets (4% to 9%) 3337
Parcopa Orally Disintegrating Tablets 3111
Peganone Tablets, USP 2487
▲ Pegasys (56%) 2793
▲ PEG-Intron Powder for Injection (52%) 3062
Pepcid Injection (Infrequent) 2017
Pepcid (Infrequent) 2014
Persantine Tablets (Rare) 898
Phenergan 3438
▲ Photofrin for Injection (4%) 729
▲ Plan B Tablets (16.9%) 1068
▲ Plavix Tablets (3.3%) 940
▲ Plavix Tablets (3.3%) 2942
▲ Pravachol Tablets (1.9% to 3.8%) 943
▲ Prefest Tablets (6%) 1069
Premphase Tablets 3452
Prempro Tablets 3452
Prilosec OTC Tablets (Less than 1%) 2674
Prinivil Tablets (2.5%) 2029
▲ Prinzide Tablets (3.7%) 2033
Prochieve 4% Gel 1018
Prochieve 8% Gel 1018
▲ Procrit for Injection (9% to 25%) 2374
▲ Proleukin for Injection (53%) 1007
▲ Prometrium Capsules (100 mg, 200 mg) (8% to 9%) 3205
Pulmicort Respules (1% to 3%) 654
Rabies Vaccine RabAvert (Rare) 1011
▲ Razadyne ER Extended-Release Capsules (5%) 2434
▲ Razadyne (5%) 2434
▲ Rebetol (58% to 70%) 3073
▲ Rebetron Combination Therapy (62% to 70%) 3078
▲ Rebif Prefilled Syringe for Injection (33% to 41%) 3163
Recombinate 762
Recombivax HB (Greater than 1%) 2045
Relafen Tablets (1% to 3%) 1523
Relenza Rotadisk (Less than 1.5%) 1525
▲ Remicade for IV Injection (9%) 987
▲ Requip Tablets (8% to 11%) 1528
▲ Rescriptor Tablets (5.3% to 16%) 2535
▲ Reyataz Capsules (2% to 3%) 948
RhoGAM Ultra-Filtered 2429
▲ Ribavirin, USP Capsules (60% to 70%) 3083
▲ Risperdal Consta Long-Acting Injection (3% to 7%) 1664
▲ Risperdal M-Tab Orally Disintegrating Tablets (Frequent to 4%) 1658
▲ Risperdal (Frequent to 4%) 1658
▲ Roferon-A Injection (58% to 88%) 2805
▲ Rozerem Tablets (4%) 3228
▲ Rythmol SR Capsules (11% to 13%) 2736
Sanctura Tablets (1.9%) 1133
▲ Sandostatin Injection (1% to 4%) 2263
Sedapap Tablets 50 mg/650 mg (Infrequent) 2098
▲ Simulect for Injection (3% to 10%) 2268
Singulair (1.8%) 2047
▲ Soriatane Capsules (1% to 10%) 1028
▲ Stalevo Tablets (6%) 2270
▲ Strattera Capsules (3%) 1784
Striant Mucoadhesive 1022
Stromectol Tablets (0.9%) 2053
Surmontil Capsules 2347
▲ Sustiva Capsules (2% to 8%) 957
▲ Symlin Injection (4.5% to 7%) 608
Symmetrel (0.1% to 5%) 1115
▲ Tambocor Tablets (7.7%) 1824
▲ Tamiflu Capsules (1% to 7.9%) 2810
▲ Tamiflu Oral Suspension (1% to 7.9%) 2810
▲ Tarceva Tablets (4% to 52%) 1254
▲ Tarceva Tablets (4% to 52%) 2470
Tarka Tablets (2.8%) 519
▲ Tasmar Tablets (3% to 8%) 3360
Tegretol/Tegretol-XR 2278
▲ Temodar Capsules (13% to 61%) 3088
▲ Tenormin I.V. Injection (0.6% to 26%) 698
▲ Tenormin Tablets (0.6% to 26%) 695
Teveten Tablets (2%) 1707
Teveten HCT Tablets (1.9%) 1710

Thiothixene Capsules ... 2124
Thyrolar ... 1203
Timolide Tablets (1.9%) ... 2056
Timoptic in Ocudose (Less frequent) ... 2061
Timoptic Sterile Ophthalmic Solution (Less frequent) ... 2058
Timoptic-XE Sterile Ophthalmic Gel Forming Solution ... 2062
Tindamax (1.1% to 2.1%) ... 2670
▲ Topamax Sprinkle Capsules (9% to 30%) ... 2438
▲ Topamax Tablets (9% to 30%) ... 2438
▲ Toprol-XL Tablets (About 10 of 100 patients) ... 660
▲ Tracleer Tablets (4%) ... 539
Tranxene ... 2488
Trelstar Depot (2.1%) ... 3385
Trelstar LA Suspension (2.3%) ... 3387
▲ Tricor Tablets (5%) ... 523
▲ Trileptal Oral Suspension (7% to 21%) ... 2281
▲ Trileptal Tablets (7% to 21%) ... 2281
▲ Trisenox Injection (63%) ... 983
▲ Trizivir Tablets (44%) ... 1565
Trusopt Sterile Ophthalmic Solution (Infrequent) ... 2065
▲ Twinrix Vaccine (11% to 14%) ... 1571
Ultracet Tablets (At least 1%) ... 2462
Uniretic Tablets (1%) ... 3114
Unithroid Tablets ... 3521
Univasc Tablets (2.4%) ... 3118
Uroqid-Acid No. 2 Tablets ... 785
Uroxatral Tablets (2.7%) ... 2957
▲ Valcyte Tablets (Less than 5%) ... 2816
▲ Valium Tablets (Among most common) ... 2822
▲ Valtrex Caplets (8%) ... 1573
▲ Vantas (9.9%) ... 3367
Vantin Tablets and Oral Suspension (Less than 1%) ... 2650
▲ Vaqta (3.9%) ... 2067
Varivax (Greater than or equal to 1%) ... 2070
▲ Vaseretic Tablets (3.9%) ... 2073
Vasotec I.V. Injection (1.8% to 3.0%) ... 2076
▲ Velcade for Injection (65%) ... 2102
Verelan PM Capsules (1.7%) ... 3120
Vesanoid Capsules ... 2823
VESIcare Tablets (1% to 2.1%) ... 631
Viadur Implant (Rare) ... 782
▲ Viramune Oral Suspension (7% to 19%) ... 903
▲ Viramune Tablets (7% to 19%) ... 903
Vivactil Tablets ... 2350
▲ Vivelle Transdermal System (1.9% to 4.3%) ... 2288
▲ Vivelle-Dot Transdermal System (1.9% to 4.3%) ... 2293
Vytorin 10/10 Tablets ... 2084
Vytorin 10/10 Tablets ... 3092
Vytorin 10/20 Tablets ... 2084
Vytorin 10/20 Tablets ... 3092
Vytorin 10/40 Tablets ... 2084
Vytorin 10/40 Tablets ... 3092
Vytorin 10/80 Tablets ... 2084
Vytorin 10/80 Tablets ... 3092
▲ Wellbutrin Tablets (5.0%) ... 1579
▲ Xanax XR Tablets (13.9%) ... 2655
▲ Xeloda Tablets (4% to 42%) ... 2825
▲ Xenical Capsules (3.1% to 7.2%) ... 2834
Xifaxan Tablets (Less than 2%) ... 2847
▲ Xolair (3%) ... 1259
Zegerid Powder for Oral Solution (Less than 1%) ... 2972
Zelnorm Tablets (1%) ... 2303
▲ Zenapax for Injection (Greater than 5%) ... 2838
▲ Zestoretic Tablets (3.7%) ... 701
Zestril Tablets (2.5%) ... 704
Zetia Tablets (1.9%) ... 2090
Zetia Tablets (1.9%) ... 3098
▲ Ziagen (12%) ... 1600
▲ Zinecard for Injection (48% to 61%) ... 2659
Zithromax (1% or less) ... 2568
Zithromax for Oral Suspension, 300 mg, 600 mg, 900 mg, 1200 mg (1% or less) ... 2561
Zithromax Tablets, 250 mg, 500 mg (1% or less) ... 2561
Zithromax Tablets, 600 mg (1% or less) ... 2568
Zithromax Tri-Pak (1% or less) ... 2561
Zithromax Z-Pak (1% or less) ... 2568
Zmax for Oral Suspension ... 2577
▲ Zofran Injection (5%) ... 1607
▲ Zofran (9% to 13%) ... 1613
▲ Zofran ODT Orally Disintegrating Tablets (9% to 13%) ... 1613
▲ Zoladex (5%) ... 709
▲ Zoloft (10% to 16%) ... 2581
▲ Zometa for Intravenous Infusion (39%) ... 2306
▲ Zonegran Capsules (8%) ... 1089
Zovirax for Injection ... 1618
▲ Zyrtec Chewable Tablets (3.6% to 5.9%) ... 2589
▲ Zyrtec (3.6% to 5.9%) ... 2589
▲ Zyrtec-D 12 Hour Extended Release Tablets (3.6% to 5.9%) ... 2591

Fatigue, muscular
Dyazide Capsules ... 1389
Furosemide Tablets ... 2117
Imitrex Injection (Rare) ... 1431
Maxzide ... 2150
Prinzide Tablets ... 2033
Sedapap Tablets 50 mg/650 mg (Infrequent) ... 2098
▲ Tenormin I.V. Injection (3% to 6%) ... 698
▲ Tenormin Tablets (3% to 6%) ... 695
Vaseretic Tablets ... 2073
Zestoretic Tablets ... 701

Fear
Dilaudid ... 439
Dilaudid Non-Sterile Powder ... 439
Dilaudid Rectal Suppositories ... 439
Dilaudid Tablets ... 439
Hycodan ... 1104
Hycomine Compound Tablets ... 1105
Hycotuss Expectorant Syrup ... 1106
Lortab ... 3315
Lortab Elixir ... 3312
Niravam Orally Disintegrating Tablets (1.4%) ... 3106
Tussionex Pennkinetic Extended-Release Suspension ... 3322
Vicodin Tablets ... 530
Vicodin ES Tablets ... 531
Vicodin HP Tablets ... 532
Zydone Tablets ... 1118
Zyrtec-D 12 Hour Extended Release Tablets ... 2591

Febrile reactions
Bravelle for Intramuscular or Subcutaneous Injection ... 1140
Capastat Sulfate for Injection ... 1728
Digibind for Injection ... 1388
Follistim AQ Cartridge ... 2354
Infed Injection ... 3381
▲ Leustatin Injection (11%) ... 2368
Liquid PedvaxHIB ... 2012
Repronex for Intramuscular and Subcutaneous Injection ... 1148
Varivax (Less than 0.1%) ... 2070

Fecal fat, increase
(*see under* Steatorrhea)

Fecal impaction
Abilify Tablets (Infrequent) ... 916
Abilify Tablets (Infrequent) ... 2472
Actiq (Less than 1%) ... 993
Clozapine Tablets ... 2141
Clozaril Tablets ... 2174
Doxil Injection (Less than 1%) ... 3302
FazaClo Orally Disintegrating Tablets ... 547
Geodon Capsules (Rare) ... 2514
Paxil CR Controlled-Release Tablets (Rare) ... 1509
Paxil (Rare) ... 1501
Rilutek Tablets (Infrequent) ... 2945
VESIcare Tablets ... 631
Zyprexa Tablets (Infrequent) ... 1798
Zyprexa ZYDIS Orally Disintegrating Tablets (Infrequent) ... 1798

Fecal urgency
▲ Xenical Capsules (2.8% to 22.1%) ... 2834
▲ Xifaxan Tablets (5.9%) ... 2847

Feces, color change
Prilosec OTC Tablets (Less than 1%) ... 2674
Zegerid Powder for Oral Solution (Less than 1%) ... 2972

Feces, discoloration
Invirase (Less than 2%) ... 2776
Prevacid Delayed-Release Capsules (Less than 1%) ... 3268
Prevacid for Delayed-Release Oral Suspension (Less than 1%) ... 3268
Prevacid SoluTab Delayed-Release Orally Disintegrating Tablets (Less than 1%) ... 3268
PREVPAC (Less than 1%) ... 3281
Risperdal M-Tab Orally Disintegrating Tablets (Rare) ... 1658
Risperdal (Rare) ... 1658

Feces abnormal
Colazal Capsules ... 2845
Xifaxan Tablets (Less than 2%) ... 2847

Feeling, drugged
▲ Ambien Tablets (3%) ... 2867
Neurontin Capsules (Infrequent) ... 2498
Neurontin Oral Solution (Infrequent) ... 2498
Neurontin Tablets (Infrequent) ... 2498
Paxil CR Controlled-Release Tablets (2%) ... 1509
Paxil (2%) ... 1501

Feeling, high
Neurontin Capsules (Rare) ... 2498
Neurontin Oral Solution (Rare) ... 2498
Neurontin Tablets (Rare) ... 2498

Feeling, intoxicated
(*see also under* Inebriated feeling)
Ambien Tablets (Rare) ... 2867
Effexor XR Capsules (Rare) ... 3411
Imitrex Injection (Rare) ... 1431
▲ Sedapap Tablets 50 mg/650 mg (Among the most frequent) ... 2098
Trileptal Oral Suspension ... 2281
Trileptal Tablets ... 2281
Xanax XR Tablets (Infrequent) ... 2655

Feeling, shaky
Koāte-DVI (0.7%) ... 3247

Feeling, strange
Ambien Tablets (Rare) ... 2867
Amerge Tablets (Infrequent) ... 1312
Imitrex Injection (2.2%) ... 1431
Imitrex Nasal Spray (Infrequent) ... 1435
Imitrex Tablets ... 1440
Lexapro Oral Solution (Infrequent) ... 1193
Lexapro Tablets (Infrequent) ... 1193
MS Contin Tablets (Less frequent) ... 2703
Neurontin Capsules (Rare) ... 2498
Neurontin Oral Solution (Rare) ... 2498
Neurontin Tablets (Rare) ... 2498
Trileptal Oral Suspension (1% to 2%) ... 2281
Trileptal Tablets (1% to 2%) ... 2281

Fertility, impairment of
Intron A for Injection ... 3038
Levothroid Tablets ... 1189

Fertility, male, decrease
Lofibra Capsules (Less than 1%) ... 1217
Reyataz Capsules (Less than 3%) ... 948
Tricor Tablets ... 523

Festination
Eldepryl Capsules ... 3209

Fetal death
(*see under* Death, fetal)

Fetal defects
Accutane Capsules ... 2740
Climara Transdermal System ... 795
Lotrel Capsules ... 2238
▲ Naropin Injection (1% to 5%) ... 640
Nembutal Sodium Solution, USP ... 2484

Fetal harm
Accutane Capsules ... 2740
Activella Tablets ... 2311
Advicor Tablets ... 1694
Advil ... ■ 737
Advil Cold & Sinus ... ■ 739
Advil Flu & Body Ache Caplets ... ■ 739
Advil Migraine Liquigels ... ■ 740
Albenza Tablets ... 1310
Alkeran for Injection ... 976
Alkeran Tablets ... 977
Altoprev Extended-Release Tablets ... 1151
Arava Tablets ... 2881
Aredia for Injection ... 2168
Arimidex Tablets ... 665
Aromasin Tablets ... 2600
Arthrotec Tablets ... 3126
Atacand Tablets ... 634
Atacand HCT ... 637
Avalide Tablets ... 922
Avalide Tablets ... 2889
Avapro Tablets ... 925
Avapro Tablets ... 2886
Aygestin Tablets ... 1062
Bayer, Aspirin Regimen ... ■ 606
BC Powder ... ■ 612
BC Allergy Sinus Cold Powder ... ■ 612
Arthritis Strength BC Powder ... ■ 612
BC Sinus Cold Powder ... ■ 612
Benicar Tablets ... 2850
Bravelle for Intramuscular or Subcutaneous Injection ... 1140
Camptosar Injection ... 2602
Captopril Tablets ... 2114
Carac Cream, 0.5% ... 1048
Carbatrol Capsules ... 3174
Casodex Tablets ... 670
Cerubidine for Injection ... 788
CombiPatch Transdermal System ... 2180
Cosmegen for Injection ... 1907
Cozaar Tablets ... 1913
Efudex ... 3348
Eligard 7.5 mg ... 2896
Eligard 22.5 mg ... 2899
Eligard 30 mg ... 2901
Eskalith ... 1406
Estratest Tablets ... 3196
Estratest H.S. Tablets ... 3196
Eulexin Capsules ... 3023
Evista Tablets ... 1735
Faslodex Injection ... 682
Femara Tablets ... 2210
Garamycin Injectable ... 3028
Gemzar for Injection ... 1743
Goody's Body Pain Formula Powder ... ■ 621
Goody's Extra Strength Headache Powder ... ■ 621
Goody's Extra Strength Pain Relief Tablets ... ■ 621
Hycamtin for Injection ... 1427
Hyzaar ... 1964
Lescol Capsules ... 2227
Lescol Capsules ... 2730
Lescol XL Tablets ... 2227
Lescol XL Tablets ... 2730
Leukeran Tablets ... 1472
Lotensin Tablets ... 2232
Lotrel Capsules ... 2238
Lupron Depot 7.5 mg ... 3261
Mavik Tablets ... 482
Maxzide ... 2150
Mevacor Tablets ... 1996
Micardis Tablets ... 884
Micardis HCT Tablets ... 886
Migranal Nasal Spray ... 3350
Motrin Cold & Sinus Caplets ... 1836
Mustargen for Injection ... 2007
Myleran Tablets ... 1492
Mylotarg for Injection ... 3429
Navelbine Injection ... 1494
Nembutal Sodium Solution, USP ... 2484
Niravam Orally Disintegrating Tablets ... 3106
Pravachol Tablets ... 943
Premarin Intravenous ... 3440
Prinivil Tablets ... 2029
Prinzide Tablets ... 2033
ProSom Tablets ... 512
Pulmicort Respules (Remote) ... 654
Purinethol Tablets ... 1222
Rebetol ... 3073
ReoPro Vials ... 1779
Repronex for Intramuscular and Subcutaneous Injection ... 1148
Tabloid Tablets ... 1545
Targretin Capsules ... 1719
Taxotere Injection Concentrate ... 2947
Tegretol/Tegretol-XR ... 2278
Temodar Capsules ... 3088
Tenormin I.V. Injection ... 698
Tenormin Tablets ... 695
Teveten HCT Tablets ... 1710
Thalomid Capsules ... 979
TOBI Solution for Inhalation ... 1015
Tracleer Tablets ... 539
Trisenox Injection ... 983
Tygacil for Injection ... 3489
Vaseretic Tablets ... 2073
Vasotec I.V. Injection ... 2076
Vesanoid Capsules ... 2823
Viadur Implant ... 782
Virazole for Inhalation Solution ... 3365
Vivelle Transdermal System ... 2288
Vivelle-Dot Transdermal System ... 2293
Xanax XR Tablets ... 2655
Xeloda Tablets ... 2825
Zestoretic Tablets ... 701
Zestril Tablets ... 704
Zevalin Injection ... 848
Zocor Tablets ... 2078
Zoladex ... 709

Fetal hemorrhage
Coumadin for Injection ... 932
Coumadin Tablets ... 932

Fetal hydantoin syndrome
Phenytek Capsules ... 2153

Fetal problems, unspecified
Aleve Tablets, Caplets and Gelcaps ... ■ 605
Bayer Aspirin Tablets ... 3515
BC Powder ... ■ 612
Cipro I.V. ... 2998
Cipro I.V. Pharmacy Bulk Package ... 3509

(■ Described in PDR For Nonprescription Drugs) Incidence data in parenthesis; ▲ 3% or more (⊙ Described in PDR For Ophthalmic Medicines™)

Polytrim Ophthalmic Solution 570
Vaseretic Tablets 2073
Vasotec I.V. Injection 2076

Fever

▲ Abelcet Injection (14%) 1119
Abilify Tablets (Frequent) 916
Abilify Tablets (Frequent) 2472
Accolate Tablets (1.6%) 663
Aceon Tablets (2 mg, 4 mg, 8 mg) (0.3% to 1.5%) 3191
Aciphex Tablets 1081
▲ Actimmune (52%) 1646
Actiq (1% or greater) 993
Activase I.V. 1225
▲ Adacel Vaccine (0% to 5%) 2959
Adalat CC Tablets (Rare) 2978
▲ Adderall XR Capsules (5%) 3169
Adriamycin for Injection, USP (Occasional) 786
Adriamycin Injection, USP (Occasional) 786
▲ Advair Diskus 100/50 (5%) 1291
▲ Advair Diskus 250/50 (5%) 1291
▲ Advair Diskus 500/50 (5%) 1291
▲ Advate Injection (16.7%) 742
Advicor Tablets 1694
▲ Aerobid/Aerobid-M (3% to 9%) 1172
Aggrastat (Less than 1%) 1878
Aggrenox Capsules (Less than 1%) 855
▲ Agrylin Capsules (8.9%) 3172
Alamast Ophthalmic Solution (Less than 5%) 3371
Albenza Tablets (Up to 1.0%) 1310
Aldara Cream, 5% (More than 1%) 1814
Aldoril Tablets 1884
Aldurazyme for Intravenous Infusion 1261
▲ Alferon N Injection (18% to 81%) 1640
▲ Alimta for Injection (Up to 26%) 1722
Alinia for Oral Suspension (Less than 1%) 2840
Alinia Tablets (Less than 1%) 2840
Alkeran for Injection 976
Alkeran Tablets 977
Allegra (2.4%) 2857
Aloprim for Injection (Less than 1%) 2156
Aloxi Injection (Less than 1%) 2099
Altace Capsules (Less than 1%) 1673
Altoprev Extended-Release Tablets (Rare) 1151
Ambien Tablets (Infrequent) 2867
Amerge Tablets (Infrequent) 1312
▲ Ammonul Injection (5%) 3323
Anaprox Tablets (Less than 1%) 2769
Anaprox DS Tablets (Less than 1%) 2769
▲ Angiomax for Injection (5%) 1856
Antara Capsules 2723
▲ Anzemet Injection (4.3%) 2871
▲ Anzemet Tablets (3.5%) 2874
Apokyn Injection 2132
▲ Aptivus Capsules (Less than 2% to 4.6%) 859
Aralast (0.1%) 745
▲ Aranesp for Injection (7% to 19%) 576
▲ Arava Tablets (1% to 3%) 2881
▲ Aredia for Injection (38.5%) 2168
▲ Argatroban Injection (3.6% to 6.9%) 1321
Aricept Tablets (Infrequent) 1086
Aricept ODT Tablets (Infrequent) 1086
▲ Arimidex Tablets (2% to 5%) 665
▲ Arixtra Injection (0.3% to 13.6%) 1325
Aromasin Tablets (Less frequent) 2600
Arthrotec Tablets (Rare) 3126
▲ Asacol Delayed-Release Tablets (6%) 2688
Asmanex Twisthaler (1% to less than 3%) 2981
Atacand Tablets (0.5% or greater) 634
Attenuvax (Occasional) 1889
Augmentin (Frequent) 1331
Augmentin Tablets (Frequent) 1334
Augmentin XR Extended-Release Tablets (Frequent) 1340
Augmentin ES-600 Powder for Oral Suspension 1337
Avalide Tablets 922
Avalide Tablets 2889
Avapro Tablets (Less than 1%) 925
Avapro Tablets (Less than 1%) 2886
▲ Avinza Capsules (5% to 10%) 1714
▲ Avonex (20%) 839
Axert Tablets (Rare) 2430
Axid Oral Solution (1.6%) 913
Azasan Tablets (Less than 1%) 2844
Bayer Aspirin Tablets 3515
▲ BeneFix for Injection (3.1%) 3402
▲ Betaseron for SC Injection (36%) 791
▲ Bexxar (2% to 37%) 1360
Blocadren Tablets 1891
▲ Boostrix (1.4% to 13.5%) 1366
▲ Botox Purified Neurotoxin Complex (2% to 10%) 565
Bravelle for Intramuscular or Subcutaneous Injection (2.7%) 1140
Brevibloc Concentrate (Less than 1%) 766
Brevibloc Injection (Less than 1%) 766
Brevibloc Double Strength Injection (Less than 1%) 766
Brevibloc Premixed Injection (Less than 1%) 766
Brevibloc Double Strength Premixed Injection (Less than 1%) 766
Buminate 5% Solution, USP (Occasional) 747
Buminate 25% Solution, USP (Occasional) 748
Caduet Tablets (Less than 2%) 2507
Calcium Disodium Versenate Injection 1819
▲ Campath Ampules (19% to 86%) 826
Campral Tablets (Infrequent) 1175
▲ Camptosar Injection (0.4% to 45%) 2602
Canasa Rectal Suppositories (1.2%) 726
▲ Cancidas for Injection (2.9% to 26.2%) 1894
▲ Captopril Tablets (About 4 to 7 of 100) 2114
Carbatrol Capsules 3174
Cardene I.V. (Rare) 1129
Carimune NF 3501
▲ Carnitor Injection (5% to 12%) 3185
▲ Casodex Tablets (2% to 5%) 670
Cataflam Tablets (Occasionally) 2173
Catapres Tablets 874
Catapres-TTS (0.5% or less) 875
Cathflo Activase 1232
Ceftin for Oral Suspension (0.1% to 1%) 1369
Celebrex Capsules (0.1% to 1.9%) 3130
Celexa (2%) 1177
▲ CellCept Capsules (3% to 52.3%) 2751
▲ CellCept Intravenous (3% to 52.3%) 2751
▲ CellCept Oral Suspension (3% to 52.3%) 2751
▲ CellCept Tablets (3% to 52.3%) 2751
Cenestin Tablets, 0.45mg, 0.625mg, 0.9mg, 1.25mg (1%) 1063
▲ Cerezyme for Injection (Approximately 6.5%) 1263
Cerubidine for Injection (Rare) 788
Cervidil Vaginal Insert (Less than 1%) 1182
▲ Chemet Capsules (5.2% to 15.7%) 2480
Cipro I.V. (1% or less to 2.1%) 2998
Cipro I.V. Pharmacy Bulk Package (1% or less to 2.1%) 3509
Cipro (Less than 1% to 2.1%) 2991
Cipro XR Tablets 3004
▲ Clarinex Syrup (5.5% to 16.9%) 3009
Cleocin Vaginal Ovules (Less than 1%) 2613
Clindesse Vaginal Cream (Less than 1%) 3296
Clinoril Tablets (Less than 1%) 1899
▲ Clolar for Intravenous Infusion (41%) 1264
Clorpres Tablets 2139
▲ Clozapine Tablets (1% to 5% or more) 2141
▲ Clozaril Tablets (1% to 5% or more) 2174
Cogentin Injection 1903
Colazal Capsules (2%) 2845
▲ Combivir Tablets (10%) 1373
▲ Combunox Tablets (Greater than or equal to 1% to 3%) 1183
Comtan Tablets 2186
▲ Comvax (0.8% to 14.2%) 1904
▲ Concerta Extended-Release Tablets (3%) 1828
▲ Copaxone for Injection (8%) 3292
▲ Copegus Tablets (41%) 2759
▲ Coreg Tablets (Greater than 1% to 3%) 1376
Cosmegen for Injection 1907
Cosopt Sterile Ophthalmic Solution 1910
Coumadin for Injection (Infrequent) 932
Coumadin Tablets (Infrequent) 932
Cozaar Tablets (Less than 1%) 1913
Crixivan Capsules (1.5%) 1918
Cubicin for Injection (1.9%) 1038
Cuprimine Capsules (Rare) 1925
▲ Cutivate Lotion 0.05% (4%) 1383
▲ Cymbalta Delayed-Release Capsules (1% to 3%) 1729
CytoGam Intravenous (Less than 5.0%) 1866
▲ Cytovene (38%) 2763
Dantrium Capsules (Less frequent) 2690
Dapsone Tablets USP 1656
▲ DAPTACEL (9.9% to 11.9%) 2964
Daranide Tablets 1928
▲ Depacon Injection (Rare to 6%) 412
▲ Depakene (6%) 417
▲ Depakote Sprinkle Capsules (6%) 422
▲ Depakote Tablets (1% to 6%) 427
▲ Depakote ER Tablets (6%) 433
▲ DepoCyt Injection (4% to 11%) 1121
▲ DepoDur Extended-Release Injection (Greater than 10%) 1098
Depo-Provera Contraceptive Injection (Less than 1%) 2619
depo-subQ provera 104 Injectable Suspension 2622
Desferal Vials 2190
Diovan HCT Tablets 2195
Diprivan Injectable Emulsion (Less than 1%) 676
Diuril Oral 1936
Diuril Sodium Intravenous 1934
Dolobid Tablets (Less than 1 in 100) 1937
▲ Doxil Injection (6.9% to 21.3%) 3302
▲ Duragesic Transdermal System (35%) 2448
EC-Naprosyn Delayed-Release Tablets (Less than 1%) 2769
Ecotrin Enteric Coated Aspirin Low, Regular and Maximum Strength Tablets 1627
Edecrin 1941
Effexor Tablets 3405
Effexor XR Capsules (Frequent) 3411
▲ Elidel Cream 1% (1.2% to 12.5%) 2198
▲ Elitek (46%) 2906
▲ Ellence Injection (0% to 5.2%) 2632
▲ Eloxatin for Injection (1% to 29%) 2908
Elspar for Injection 1943
Emend Capsules (2.9%) 1944
Enbrel for Injection 580
▲ Engerix-B Vaccine (1% to 10%) 1391
▲ Epivir (10%) 1394
▲ Epivir-HBV (7%) 1398
▲ Epogen for Injection (29% to 51%) 586
▲ Epzicom Tablets (3% to 5%) 1402
Equetro Extended-Release Capsules 3178
▲ Erbitux (5% to 33%) 937
Eskalith 1406
Ethyol for Injection 1869
▲ Evista Tablets (3.1% to 3.9%) 1735
▲ Evoxac Capsules (1% to 3%) 1042
Exelon Capsules (Frequent) 2204
▲ Fabrazyme for Intravenous Infusion (14%) 1267
▲ Famvir Tablets (0.8% to 3.3%) 2207
▲ Faslodex Injection (6.4%) 682
▲ FazaClo Orally Disintegrating Tablets (Greater than 5%) 547
▲ Ferrlecit Injection (3% to 15%) 3379
▲ Flolan for Injection (13% to 25%) 1408
▲ Flonase Nasal Spray (1% to 3%) 1412
▲ Flovent Diskus 50 mcg (7%) 1415
▲ Flovent HFA (1% to 3%) 1418
Floxin Otic Singles (0.3%) 1045
Floxin Otic Solution (0.3%) 1043
Flumadine 1186
▲ Flumist Vaccine (0% to 10.3%) 1872
▲ Focalin Tablets (5%) 2214
Focalin XR Capsules 2217
Follistim AQ Cartridge 2354
Foradil Aerolizer (2.2%) 3024
Fortaz (2%) 1422
Fortical Nasal Spray (Less than 1%) 3336
Fosamax (Rare) 1949
Fosamax Plus D Tablets (Rarely) 1956
Fragmin Injection (Rare) 2638
Frova Tablets (Infrequent) 1101
Furosemide Tablets 2117
Fuzeon Injection 2772
Gabitril Tablets (1% or more) 998
▲ Gammagard Liquid (2.3% to 21.3%) 751
Gammagard S/D (Occasional) 754
▲ Gamunex Immune Globulin I.V., 10% (0.1% to 28%) 3232
Garamycin Injectable 3028
▲ Gemzar for Injection (16% to 41%) 1743
▲ Gengraf Capsules (3%) 458
Geodon Capsules (Frequent) 2514
▲ Gleevec Tablets (5% to 41%) 2221
Gonal-f RFF Pen for Injection (2.4%) 3155
Guanidine Hydrochloride Tablets 3030
▲ Havrix Vaccine (1% to 10%) 1425
Hemofil M (Extremely rare) 757
Hepsera Tablets (2% or greater) 1275
▲ Herceptin I.V. (36%) 1234
HibTITER (0.6% to 1.4%) 3419
▲ Humira Injection (Less than 5%) 464
Hyalgan Solution (Seven cases) 2917
▲ Hycamtin for Injection (Less than 1% to 34%) 1427
Hyperstat I.V. Injection 3031
Hytrin Capsules (0.5% to at least 1%) 469
Hyzaar 1964
▲ Idamycin PFS Injection (26%) 2645
▲ Imdur Tablets (Less than or equal to 5%) 3032
Imitrex Injection (Rare) 1431
Imitrex Nasal Spray (Infrequent) 1435
Imitrex Tablets (Infrequent) 1440
Indapamide Tablets 2119
Inderal LA Long-Acting Capsules 3421
▲ Infanrix Vaccine (Up to 19.8%) 1444
Infed Injection 3381
▲ Infergen (58% to 61%) 1647
InnoPran XL Capsules 2728
▲ Intron A for Injection (3% to 86%) 3038
▲ Invanz for Injection (2.3% to 5%) 1974
▲ Invirase (Less than 2% to 3.4%) 2776
▲ I.V. Busulfex (3% to 80%) 1125
Iveegam EN (0.3% to 0.8%) 759
Kadian Capsules (Less than 3%) 572
Kaletra (Less than 2%) 474
▲ Kepivance (39%) 592
Keppra Oral Solution (1% to 2%) 3307
Keppra Tablets (1% to 2%) 3307
Klonopin (Infrequent) 2782
▲ Kytril Injection (3%) 2785
▲ Kytril Tablets (5%) 2788
▲ Lamictal (2% to 15%) 1449
▲ Lariam Tablets (Among most frequent) 2790
Lescol Capsules (Rare) 2227
Lescol Capsules (Rare) 2730
Lescol XL Tablets 2227
Lescol XL Tablets 2730
Leukeran Tablets 1472
▲ Leukine (77% to 95%) 829
▲ Leustatin Injection (11% to 69%) 2368
Levaquin in 5% Dextrose Injection (0.1% to 0.9%) 2453
Levaquin (0.1% to 0.9%) 2453
Levothroid Tablets 1189
Levoxyl Tablets 1680
Lexapro Oral Solution (Frequent) 1193
Lexapro Tablets (Frequent) 1193
Lipitor Tablets (Less than 2%) 2495
Lithobid Tablets 1670
Lofibra Capsules 1217
Lotensin HCT Tablets (0.3% or more) 2235
▲ Lovenox Injection (8%) 2931
Lunesta Tablets (Infrequent) 3139
Lupron Depot 7.5 mg (Less than 5%) 3261
Lupron Depot-PED 7.5 mg, 11.25 mg and 15 mg (Less than 2%) 3266
Lupron Injection Pediatric (Less than 2%) 3256
Lyrica Capsules (Greater than or equal to 1%) 2524
▲ Malarone Tablets (Less than 1% to 6%) 1484
▲ Malarone Pediatric Tablets (Less than 1% to 6%) 1484
Matulane Capsules 3188
Maxalt Tablets (Rare) 1983
Maxalt-MLT Orally Disintegrating Tablets (Rare) 1983
Maxipime for Injection (Greater than 0.1% to 1%) 1093
Maxzide 2150
Mebaral Tablets, USP (Less than 1 in 100 patients) 2483
Mefoxin for Injection 1987
Mefoxin Premixed Intravenous Solution 1990
▲ Megace ES Oral Suspension (1% to 6%) 2492
▲ Menactra Vaccine (0% to 5.1%) 2968
▲ Mepron Suspension (0.6% to 40%) 1487
Meridia Capsules (Greater than or equal to 1%) 485
Merrem I.V. (Greater than 0.1% to 1%) 687
Meruvax II 1994
Metadate CD Capsules 3316
Mevacor Tablets (Rare) 1996
Miacalcin Nasal Spray (Less than 1%) 2242
Micardis Tablets (More than 0.3%) 884
Micardis HCT Tablets 886
Migranal Nasal Spray (Infrequent) 3350
Mintezol 2002
Miradon Tablets 3056
Mirapex Tablets (1% or more) 889

M-M-R II ... 1980
Moban Tablets ... 1108
Mobic Oral Suspension (Less than 2%) ... 893
Mobic Tablets (Less than 2%) ... 893
Moduretic Tablets ... 2003
Mumpsvax (Uncommon) ... 2005
Mycamine for Injection (0.9% to 1.9%) ... 620
▲ Myfortic Tablets (3% to less than 20%) ... 2244
▲ Mylotarg for Injection (78% to 88%) ... 3429
Nadolol Tablets ... 2121
Nalfon Capsules (Less than 1%) ... 2504
Naprosyn Suspension (Less than 1%) ... 2769
Naprosyn Tablets (Less than 1%) ... 2769
Narcan Injection ... 1109
▲ Naropin Injection (1% to 5%) ... 640
Natrecor for Injection (Greater than or equal to 1%) ... 3123
▲ Navelbine Injection (Up to 20%) ... 1494
Nembutal Sodium Solution, USP ... 2484
Neoral Soft Gelatin Capsules (1% to less than 3%) ... 2247
Neoral Oral Solution (1% to less than 3%) ... 2247
▲ Neulasta Injection (15% to 72%) ... 596
▲ Neumega for Injection (36%) ... 3433
▲ Neupogen for Injection (12%) ... 598
Neurontin Capsules (More than 1%) ... 2498
▲ Neurontin Oral Solution (10.1%) ... 2498
Neurontin Tablets (More than 1%) ... 2498
Nexium Delayed-Release Capsules (Less than 1%) ... 645
Nexium I.V. (Less than 1%) ... 649
▲ Nicotrol Inhaler (Greater than 3%) ... 2594
▲ Nipent for Injection (42% to 46%) ... 3216
Noroxin Tablets (0.3% to 1.0%) ... 2009
▲ Norvir (0.9% to 5%) ... 499
NovoSeven (Greater than or equal to 2%) ... 2335
Omacor Capsules ... 2735
Omnicef Capsules ... 506
Omnicef for Oral Suspension ... 506
▲ Oncaspar (Greater than 5%) ... 1123
▲ Ontak Vials (81%) ... 1717
Orap Tablets ... 1220
Ortho-Cyclen/Ortho Tri-Cyclen ... 2414
Ortho Tri-Cyclen Lo Tablets ... 2421
▲ Orthoclone OKT3 Sterile Solution (89% to 90%) ... 2370
▲ OxyContin Tablets (Between 1% and 5%) ... 2699
Panhematin for Injection ... 2487
Paser Granules ... 1657
Paxil CR Controlled-Release Tablets (2%) ... 1509
Paxil (2%) ... 1501
▲ Pediarix Vaccine (31.3% or less) ... 1518
▲ Liquid PedvaxHIB (0.5% to 18.1%) ... 2012
Peganone Tablets, USP ... 2487
▲ Pegasys (37%) ... 2793
▲ PEG-Intron Powder for Injection (22%) ... 3062
Pentasa Capsules (0.9%) ... 3182
Pepcid Injection (Infrequent) ... 2017
Pepcid (Infrequent) ... 2014
Permax Tablets (Frequent) ... 3357
Phenergan ... 3438
Phenytek Capsules ... 2153
▲ Photofrin for Injection (19% to 31%) ... 729
Plasbumin-5 (Rare) ... 3249
Plasbumin-20 (Rare) ... 3249
Plasbumin-25 (Rare) ... 3251
Plavix Tablets (1% to 2.5%) ... 940
Plavix Tablets (1% to 2.5%) ... 2942
Pletal Tablets (Less than 2%) ... 2478
Pneumovax 23 (Common) ... 2020
Potaba (Infrequent) ... 1634
Pravachol Tablets (Rare) ... 943
Premphase Tablets ... 3452
Prempro Tablets ... 3452
Prevacid Delayed-Release Capsules (Less than 1%) ... 3268
Prevacid for Delayed-Release Oral Suspension (Less than 1%) ... 3268
Prevacid NapraPAC (Less than 1%) ... 3277
Prevacid SoluTab Delayed-Release Orally Disintegrating Tablets (Less than 1%) ... 3268
▲ Prevnar for Injection (0% to 36.7%) ... 3460
PREVPAC (Less than 1%) ... 3281
Prilosec OTC Tablets (Less than 1%) ... 2674
Primaxin I.M. ... 2022
Primaxin I.V. (0.5%) ... 2024
Prinivil Tablets (0.3% to 1.1%) ... 2029
Prinzide Tablets (0.3% to 1%) ... 2033
Prochieve 4% Gel ... 1018
Prochieve 8% Gel ... 1018
▲ Procrit for Injection (29% to 51%) ... 2374
▲ Prograf Capsules and Injection (19% to 48%) ... 624
Prolastin (0.77%) ... 3252
▲ Proleukin for Injection (29%) ... 1007
Prometrium Capsules (100 mg, 200 mg) (Less than 5%) ... 3205
ProSom Tablets (Infrequent) ... 512
Protonix I.V. (Less than 1%) ... 3468
Protonix Tablets (Less than 1%) ... 3465
▲ Protopic Ointment (1% to 18%) ... 629
▲ Proventil HFA Inhalation Aerosol (6%) ... 3071
Provigil Tablets (At least 1%) ... 1002
Prozac Pulvules and Liquid (2%) ... 1771
▲ Pulmozyme Inhalation Solution (32%) ... 1245
Purinethol Tablets (Very rare) ... 1222
Quixin Ophthalmic Solution (1% to 3%) ... 3373
Rabies Vaccine RabAvert (Uncommon) ... 1011
▲ Rapamune Oral Solution and Tablets (27% to 34%) ... 3472
▲ Raptiva for Injection (7%) ... 1247
Razadyne (Frequent) ... 2434
▲ Rebetol (32% to 61%) ... 3073
▲ Rebetron Combination Therapy (35% to 41%) ... 3078
▲ Rebif Prefilled Syringe for Injection (25% to 28%) ... 3163
Recombinate (Extremely rare) ... 762
Recombivax HB (Greater than 1%) ... 2045
ReFacto Vials ... 3479
▲ Refludan for Injection (4.4%) ... 815
Relafen Tablets (Less than 1%) ... 1523
Relenza Rotadisk (Less than 1.5%) ... 1525
Relpax Tablets (Rare) ... 2531
▲ Remicade for IV Injection (3% to 7%) ... 987
▲ Renagel Tablets (5.1%) ... 1268
Repronex for Intramuscular and Subcutaneous Injection ... 1148
Requip Tablets (Infrequent) ... 1528
▲ Rescriptor Tablets (1.6% to 7.1%) ... 2535
Retavase ... 1131
▲ Retisert Implant (5% to 15%) ... ⊙256
▲ Retrovir Capsules (3.2% to 16%) ... 1533
▲ Retrovir IV Infusion (4% to 16%) ... 1537
▲ Retrovir (3.2% to 16%) ... 1533
▲ Revatio Tablets (6%) ... 2541
▲ Reyataz Capsules (4% to 6%) ... 948
RhoGAM Ultra-Filtered ... 2429
Rhophylac (Occasionally) ... 3504
▲ Ribavirin, USP Capsules (32% to 61%) ... 3083
Risperdal Consta Long-Acting Injection (1% to 2%) ... 1664
▲ Risperdal M-Tab Orally Disintegrating Tablets (2% to 3%) ... 1658
Risperdal (2% to 3%) ... 1658
Ritalin Hydrochloride Tablets ... 2254
Ritalin LA Capsules ... 2255
Ritalin-SR Tablets ... 2254
▲ Rituxan for Infusion (49%) ... 845
▲ Rituxan I.V. (53%) ... 1251
Rocephin Injectable Vials, ADD-Vantage, Galaxy, Bulk (Less than 1%) ... 2801
▲ Roferon-A Injection (28% to 92%) ... 2805
Rythmol SR Capsules ... 2736
Sandimmune (2% or less) ... 2259
Sedapap Tablets 50 mg/650 mg (Infrequent) ... 2098
Serevent Diskus (1% to 3%) ... 1540
Seroquel Tablets (2%) ... 691
Singulair (1.5% to greater than or equal to 2%) ... 2047
Sonata Capsules (Frequent) ... 1686
Soriatane Capsules (Less than 1%) ... 1028
Spectracef Tablets (0.1% to 1%) ... 2706
St. Joseph 81 mg Aspirin Chewable and Enteric Coated Tablets ... 1841
▲ Strattera Capsules (3%) ... 1784
▲ Stromectol Tablets (22.6%) ... 2053
▲ Suboxone Tablets (3%) ... 2719
▲ Subutex Tablets (3%) ... 2719
Sular Tablets (Less than or equal to 1%) ... 1163
Suprane Liquid for Inhalation (Less than 1%) ... 770
▲ Sustiva Capsules (21%) ... 957
▲ Symbyax Capsules (3% to 4%) ... 1788
Symmetrel ... 1115
▲ Synagis (27.1%) ... 1868
Synercid I.V. (Less than 1%) ... 1690
Tagamet Tablets (Rare) ... 1547
Tambocor Tablets (1% to 3%) ... 1824
Tamiflu Capsules (Less than 1%) ... 2810
Tamiflu Oral Suspension (Less than 1%) ... 2810
▲ Targretin Capsules (4.8% to 17%) ... 1719
Tarka Tablets (Several cases) ... 519
Tasmar Tablets (1%) ... 3360
▲ Taxotere Injection Concentrate (2.1% to 41%) ... 2947
Tegretol/Tegretol-XR ... 2278
▲ Temodar Capsules (13%) ... 3088
Tenormin I.V. Injection ... 698
Tenormin Tablets ... 695
▲ Tequin Injection (0.1% to 3%) ... 964
▲ Tequin Tablets (0.1% to 3%) ... 964
Teveten Tablets (Less than 1%) ... 1707
Teveten HCT Tablets (Less than 1%) ... 1710
▲ Thalomid Capsules (19.4% to 21.9%) ... 979
Thioridazine Hydrochloride Tablets ... 2122
Thiothixene Capsules ... 2124
▲ Thrombate III (1 of 17) ... 3254
▲ Thymoglobulin for Injection (63.4%) ... 2848
Thyrogen for Injection (1%) ... 1270
Ticlid Tablets ... 2813
Timolide Tablets ... 2056
Timoptic in Ocudose ... 2061
Timoptic Sterile Ophthalmic Solution ... 2058
Timoptic-XE Sterile Ophthalmic Gel Forming Solution ... 2062
Tindamax ... 2670
TNKase I.V. ... 1256
▲ TOBI Solution for Inhalation (32.9%) ... 1015
▲ Topamax Sprinkle Capsules (0% to 9%) ... 2438
▲ Topamax Tablets (0% to 9%) ... 2438
Toprol-XL Tablets ... 660
Tracleer Tablets ... 539
▲ Trasylol Injection (15%) ... 779
Tricor Tablets ... 523
Triglide Tablets ... 1165
▲ Trileptal Oral Suspension (Up to 3%) ... 2281
▲ Trileptal Tablets (Up to 3%) ... 2281
▲ Trisenox Injection (63%) ... 983
▲ Trizivir Tablets (20%) ... 1565
Truvada Tablets ... 1279
Twinrix Vaccine (2% to 4%) ... 1571
▲ Tygacil for Injection (7.1%) ... 3489
Ultane Liquid for Inhalation (1%) ... 526
Uniretic Tablets (More than 1%) ... 3114
Unithroid Tablets ... 3521
Urso 250 Tablets ... 737
Urso Forte Tablets ... 737
▲ Valcyte Tablets (31%) ... 2816
Vantin Tablets and Oral Suspension (Less than 1%) ... 2650
▲ Vaqta (2.7% to 11.3%) ... 2067
▲ Varivax (10.2% to 14.7%) ... 2070
Vaseretic Tablets ... 2073
Vasotec I.V. Injection (0.5% to 1.0%) ... 2076
▲ Velcade for Injection (35%) ... 2102
Verelan PM Capsules ... 3120
▲ Vesanoid Capsules (83%) ... 2823
▲ VFEND I.V. (0% to 5.7%) ... 2543
▲ VFEND Oral Suspension (0% to 5.7%) ... 2543
▲ VFEND Tablets (0% to 5.7%) ... 2543
Vicoprofen Tablets (Rare; less than 3%) ... 533
▲ Vigamox Ophthalmic Solution (1% to 4%) ... 560
Viracept (Less than 2%) ... 2556
▲ Viramune Oral Suspension (3%) ... 903
▲ Viramune Tablets (3%) ... 903
▲ Viread Tablets (2% to 4%) ... 1284
▲ Visudyne for Injection (1% to 10%) ... 2286
Vivactil Tablets ... 2350
Vivotif ... 834
▲ Voltaren Ophthalmic Solution (Less than or equal to 3%) ... 2300
Voltaren Tablets (Occasionally) ... 2298
Voltaren-XR Tablets (Occasionally) ... 2301
Vytorin 10/10 Tablets ... 2084
Vytorin 10/10 Tablets ... 3092
Vytorin 10/20 Tablets ... 2084
Vytorin 10/20 Tablets ... 3092
Vytorin 10/40 Tablets ... 2084
Vytorin 10/40 Tablets ... 3092
Vytorin 10/80 Tablets ... 2084
Vytorin 10/80 Tablets ... 3092
Wellbutrin Tablets (1.2%) ... 1579
Wellbutrin SR Sustained-Release Tablets (1% to 2%) ... 1583
Wellbutrin XL Extended-Release Tablets (1% to 2%) ... 1588
WinRho SDF (1%) ... 763
Xanax XR Tablets (Infrequent) ... 2655
▲ Xeloda Tablets (1% to 12%) ... 2825
▲ Xifaxan Tablets (3.1%) ... 2847
▲ Xopenex HFA Inhalation Aerosol (3%) ... 3151
▲ Xopenex Inhalation Solution (3%) ... 3143
▲ Xopenex Inhalation Solution Concentrate (3% to 9.1%) ... 3147
Zantac (Rare) ... 1597
Zantac Injection ... 1593
Zantac Injection Pharmacy Bulk Package (Rare) ... 1595
Zantac Syrup (Rare) ... 1597
Zegerid Powder for Oral Solution (Less than 1%) ... 2972
Zemaira (0.6%) ... 3506
▲ Zemplar Capsules (5%) ... 535
▲ Zemplar Injection (5%) ... 538
▲ Zenapax for Injection (Greater than 5%) ... 2838
▲ Zerit (50%) ... 971
Zestoretic Tablets (0.3% to 1%) ... 701
Zestril Tablets (0.3% to 1.0%) ... 704
▲ Zevalin Injection (17%) ... 848
▲ Ziagen (6% to 9%) ... 1600
▲ Zinecard for Injection (22% to 34%) ... 2659
Zithromax Capsules, 250 mg (1% or less) ... 2568
Zithromax for Oral Suspension, 300 mg, 600 mg, 900 mg, 1200 mg (1% or less) ... 2561
Zithromax Tablets, 250 mg, 500 mg (1% or less) ... 2561
Zithromax Tri-Pak (1% or less) ... 2561
Zocor Tablets (Rare) ... 2078
▲ Zofran Injection (2% to 8%) ... 1607
▲ Zofran (8%) ... 1613
▲ Zofran ODT Orally Disintegrating Tablets (8%) ... 1613
Zoladex (1% to 5%) ... 709
Zoladex 3-month ... 712
Zoloft (Infrequent to 2%) ... 2581
▲ Zometa for Intravenous Infusion (32% to 44.2%) ... 2306
Zomig Nasal Spray (Rare) ... 718
Zomig Tablets (Infrequent) ... 714
Zomig-ZMT Tablets (Infrequent) ... 714
▲ Zosyn (2.4% to 3.2%) ... 3492
Zovirax Capsules ... 1616
Zovirax for Injection (Less than 1%) ... 1618
Zovirax ... 1616
Zyban Sustained-Release Tablets (Frequent) ... 1620
▲ Zyprexa Tablets (Rare to 5%) ... 1798
Zyprexa IntraMuscular (Infrequent) ... 1798
▲ Zyprexa ZYDIS Orally Disintegrating Tablets (5%) ... 1798
Zyrtec Chewable Tablets (Less than 2%) ... 2589
Zyrtec (Less than 2%) ... 2589
Zyrtec-D 12 Hour Extended Release Tablets (Less than 2%) ... 2591
▲ Zyvox (0% to 14.1%) ... 2661

Fever, neutropenic

Campath Ampules ... 826
▲ Camptosar Injection (2% to 5.8%) ... 2602
▲ Mylotarg for Injection (15% to 19%) ... 3429
▲ Neulasta Injection (15% to 72%) ... 596
▲ Neumega for Injection (48%) ... 3433
▲ Neupogen for Injection (13%) ... 598
▲ Xeloda Tablets (3% to 16%) ... 2825

Fever, postpartum

Gonal-f RFF Pen for Injection ... 3155

Fibrillations

Tambocor Tablets ... 1824

Fibrinolysis increased

NovoSeven (1%) ... 2335

Fibromyalgia

Cozaar Tablets (Less than 1%) ... 1913
Hyzaar ... 1964
Lupron Depot 7.5 mg ... 3261
Lupron Depot–3 Month 11.25 mg ... 3262
Nexium Delayed-Release Capsules (Less than 1%) ... 645
Nexium I.V. (Less than 1%) ... 649

Fibrosing colonopathy

Creon 5 Capsules ... 3195
Creon 10 Capsules ... 3195
Creon 20 Capsules ... 3196
Ultrase Capsules ... 735
Ultrase MT Capsules ... 736

Fibrosis

Apokyn Injection ... 2132
Copaxone for Injection (Infrequent) ... 3292
Genotropin Lyophilized Powder (Infrequent) ... 2642
Inversine Tablets ... 3286
Ocufen Ophthalmic Solution ... ⊙230
Permax Tablets ... 3357

▲ Xeloda Tablets (Less than 5%) 2825

Fibrosis, cavernous body
Edex Injection (2%)........................ 3103

Fibrosis, hepatic
▲ Xeloda Tablets (Less than 5%) 2825

Fibrosis, interstitial pulmonary
(*see under* Pulmonary fibrosis)

Fibrosis, penile
▲ Caverject Impulse Injection (3%) 2610
▲ Edex Injection (5%) 3103

Fibrosis, periportal
Tagamet Tablets (A single case)....... 1547

Fibrosis, perisinusoidal
Eloxatin for Injection 2908

Fibrosis, pleural
▲ Intron A for Injection (Less than or equal to 5%)............................ 3038
Migranal Nasal Spray..................... 3350
Permax Tablets (Rare).................... 3357

Fibrosis, retroperitoneal
Lyrica Capsules (Rare)..................... 2524
Migranal Nasal Spray..................... 3350
Permax Tablets (Rare)..................... 3357
Tasmar Tablets 3360

Fingernails, brittle
Gengraf Capsules (2% or less)......... 458
Neoral Soft Gelatin Capsules (2% or less)..................................... 2247
Neoral Oral Solution (2% or less)...... 2247
Sandimmune (2% or less)................ 2259

Fingers, discoloration
Eskalith 1406

Fissuring, fingertips
Ophthetic Ophthalmic Solution........ ⊙230

Fissuring, unspecified
Clobevate Gel (Less than 2%)........... 3213
Olux Foam (Less than 2%)............... 1027
Oxistat Cream (0.1%)...................... 1498
▲ Soriatane Capsules (1% to 10%) 1028
Temovate Cream (1 of 421 patients)..................................... 1549
▲ Temovate Gel (Among most frequent)..................................... 1550
Temovate E Emollient (Less than 2%).. 1552

Fistula, arteriovenous
ReoPro Vials (0.4%)........................ 1779

Fistula, tracheo-esophageal
▲ Photofrin for Injection (6%) 729
Proleukin for Injection (Less than 1%).. 1007

Flare
Humira Injection (0.7%)................... 464
Travatan Ophthalmic Solution (1% to 4%)... 559

Flare, postinjection
Attenuvax (Rare)............................. 1889
Decadron Phosphate Injection 1931
Depo-Medrol Single-Dose Vial 2617
Dilaudid-HP (Less frequent)............. 441
Meruvax II...................................... 1994
M-M-R II... 1980
Mumpsvax (Rare)............................. 2005

Flatulence
Abilify Tablets (Infrequent)............... 916
Abilify Tablets (Infrequent)............... 2472
Aceon Tablets (2 mg, 4 mg, 8 mg) (1.0%)... 3191
Aciphex Tablets 1081
Actiq (1% or greater)....................... 993
Activella Tablets.............................. 2311
▲ Actonel Tablets (3.1% to 4.6%)......... 2679
▲ Actonel with Calcium Tablets (3.1% to 4.6%)............................. 2684
Adalat CC Tablets (Less than 1%)..... 2978
Advicor Tablets............................... 1694
Aerobid/Aerobid-M (1% to 3%)......... 1172
▲ Agrylin Capsules (10.2%) 3172
Aldoclor Tablets.............................. 1881
Aldoril Tablets................................ 1884
Alinia for Oral Suspension (Less than 1%)...................................... 2840
Alinia Tablets (Less than 1%)........... 2840
Aloprim for Injection (Less than 1%).. 2156
Aloxi Injection (Less than 1%).......... 2099
▲ Altoprev Extended-Release Tablets (3.7% to 4.5%)................. 1151
Ambien Tablets (Infrequent)............. 2867
AmBisome for Injection (Less common)...................................... 615
▲ Anaprox Tablets (1% to 10%) 2769
▲ Anaprox DS Tablets (1% to 10%) 2769
Antara Capsules............................. 2723
Aptivus Capsules (Less than 2%)...... 859
▲ Arava Tablets (1% to 3%) 2881
Aricept Tablets (Infrequent)............. 1086
Aricept ODT Tablets (Infrequent)...... 1086
▲ Arthrotec Tablets (9%) 3126
▲ Asacol Delayed-Release Tablets (3% to 5%)................................. 2688
Asmanex Twisthaler (1% to less than 3%)...................................... 2981
Augmentin (Less frequent)............... 1331
Augmentin Tablets (Less frequent).... 1334
Avalide Tablets............................... 922
Avalide Tablets............................... 2889
Avapro Tablets (Less than 1%)......... 925
Avapro Tablets (Less than 1%) 2886
▲ Avastin IV (11% to 19%) 1229
Avelox (0.1% to less than 2%) 2984
▲ Axid Oral Solution (4.9%) 913
Buprenex Injectable (Infrequent) 2718
Caduet Tablets (Greater than 0.1% to 2.8%) 2507
▲ Campral Tablets (1% to 4%) 1175
▲ Camptosar Injection (0% to 12%) 2602
▲ Canasa Rectal Suppositories (5.2%) 726
Carafate Suspension (Less than 0.5%) 727
Carafate Tablets (Less than 0.5%) 728
▲ Casodex Tablets (5%) 670
▲ Cataflam Tablets (1% to 10%) 2173
Ceftin (0.1% to 1%) 1369
Celebrex Capsules (2.2%) 3130
Celexa (Frequent) 1177
▲ CellCept Capsules (3% to less than 20%) 2751
▲ CellCept Intravenous (3% to less than 20%) 2751
▲ CellCept Oral Suspension (3% to less than 20%) 2751
▲ CellCept Tablets (3% to less than 20%) 2751
▲ Cenestin Tablets, 0.45mg, 0.625mg, 0.9mg, 1.25mg (29%) 1063
Cipro I.V. (1% or less) 2998
Cipro I.V. Pharmacy Bulk Package (1% or less) 3509
Cipro 2991
Cipro XR Tablets (Less than 1%) 3004
▲ Climara Transdermal System (1% to 7%) 795
▲ Climara Pro Transdermal System (3.8%) 800
Clindesse Vaginal Cream (Less than 1%) 3296
▲ Clinoril Tablets (1% to 3%) 1899
Colazal Capsules (2%) 2845
▲ CombiPatch Transdermal System (5% to 7%) 2180
Combunox Tablets (1%) 1183
Comtan Tablets (2%) 2186
Copaxone for Injection (At least 2%) 3292
Coumadin for Injection (Infrequent) ... 932
Coumadin Tablets (Infrequent) 932
Cozaar Tablets (Less than 1%) 1913
Crestor Tablets (Greater than or equal to 1%) 672
Cubicin for Injection (Less than 1%) 1038
Cytovene 2763
▲ Depacon Injection (1% to 5%) 412
▲ Depakene (1% to 5%) 417
▲ Depakote Sprinkle Capsules (1% to 5%) 422
▲ Depakote Tablets (1% to 5%) 427
▲ Depakote ER Tablets (1% to 5%) 433
▲ DepoDur Extended-Release Injection (5% to 10%) 1098
Detrol Tablets (1.3%) 2626
Diovan HCT Tablets (Greater than 0.2%) 2195
Diovan Tablets 2191
▲ Ditropan XL Extended Release Tablets (2% to less than 5%) 2391
Dolobid Tablets (Greater than 1 in 100) 1937
▲ Dostinex Tablets (2% to less than 10%) 2631
▲ Doxil Injection (1% to 10%) 3302
Duragesic Transdermal System (1% or greater) 2448
▲ EC-Naprosyn Delayed-Release Tablets (1% to 10%) 2769
▲ Effexor Tablets (3%) 3405
▲ Effexor XR Capsules (4% to 5%) 3411
Eligard 7.5 mg (Less than 2%) 2896
Elmiron Capsules (Less than or equal to 1%) 2393
▲ Eloxatin for Injection (3% to 5%) 2908
Emcyt Capsules (2%) 3137
Emend Capsules (Greater than 0.5%) 1944
▲ Entocort EC Capsules (6%) 2694
Eskalith 1406
▲ Estrogel 0.06% (6.5%) 3200
▲ Evista Tablets (3.1%) 1735
▲ Evoxac Capsules (1% to 3%) 1042
▲ Exelon Capsules (4%) 2204
Factive Tablets (0.1% to 1%)............ 2464
Famvir Tablets (1.5% to 1.9%)......... 2207
Ferrlecit Injection........................... 3379
Flexeril Tablets (Less than 1%)......... 1832
▲ Flolan for Injection (5%) 1408
▲ Follistim AQ Cartridge (27%) 2354
▲ Fortamet Extended-Release Tablets (3.5%)............................ 1156
Fortical Nasal Spray (Less than 1%)... 3336
▲ Fosamax (Up to 4.1%) 1949
▲ Fosamax Plus D Tablets (0% to 4.1%) 1956
Frova Tablets (Infrequent) 1101
Gabitril Tablets (1% or more) 998
▲ Gengraf Capsules (4%) 458
▲ Gleevec Tablets (16% to 23%) 2221
▲ Gonal-f RFF Pen for Injection (3.6%) 3155
▲ Hepsera Tablets (2% to 4%) 1275
Hytrin Capsules (At least 1%) 469
Hyzaar 1964
▲ Imdur Tablets (Less than or equal to 5%) 3032
Imitrex Injection (Rare) 1431
Imitrex Nasal Spray (Rare) 1435
Imitrex Tablets 1440
Indocin Capsules (Less than 1%) 1968
Indocin I.V. (Less than 1%) 1973
Indocin (Less than 1%) 1968
▲ Infergen (6% to 8%) 1647
▲ Intron A for Injection (Less than 5%) 3038
Invanz for Injection (Greater than 0.1%) 1974
Invirase (Less than 2%) 2776
▲ Kaletra (1% to 4%) 474
K-Dur Extended-Relase Tablets 3047
Ketek Tablets (Greater than or equal to 0.2% to less than 2%) 2920
Klonopin (Infrequent) 2782
▲ K-Lor Powder Packets (Among most common) 472
Kristalose for Oral Solution 2149
▲ K-Tab Filmtab Tablets (Most common) 473
Lamictal (More than 1%) 1449
Lamisil Tablets (2.2%) 2226
Lescol Capsules (2.6%) 2227
Lescol Capsules (2.6%) 2730
Lescol XL Tablets (1.4%) 2227
Lescol XL Tablets (1.4%) 2730
Levaquin in 5% Dextrose Injection (0.2% to 1.2%) 2453
Levaquin (0.2% to 1.2%) 2453
Lexapro Oral Solution (2%) 1193
Lexapro Tablets (2%) 1193
Lipitor Tablets (1.1% to 2.8%) 2495
Lithobid Tablets 1670
Lofibra Capsules 1217
Lotensin HCT Tablets (0.3% or more) 2235
▲ Lotronex Tablets (3%) 1479
▲ Lyrica Capsules (1% to 3%) 2524
Maxalt Tablets (Infrequent) 1983
Maxalt-MLT Orally Disintegrating Tablets (Infrequent) 1983
▲ Megace ES Oral Suspension (0% to 10%) 2492
Meridia Capsules (Greater than or equal to 1%) 485
Merrem I.V. (Greater than 0.1% to 1%) 687
MetroGel-Vaginal Gel (Less than 1%) 1822
▲ Mevacor Tablets (3.7% to 6.4%) 1996
Miacalcin Nasal Spray (Less than 1%) 2242
Micardis Tablets (More than 0.3%) ... 884
Micardis HCT Tablets 886
Midamor Tablets (Less than or equal to 1%) 2000
Mirapex Tablets (Greater than or equal to 1%) 889
▲ Mobic Oral Suspension (0.4% to 3.2%) 893
▲ Mobic Tablets (0.4% to 3.2%) 893
Moduretic Tablets (Less than or equal to 1%) 2003
▲ Myfortic Tablets (3% to less than 20%) 2244
Nadolol Tablets (1 to 5 of 1000 patients) 2121
Nalfon Capsules (Less than 1%) 2504
▲ Naprosyn Suspension (1% to 10%) 2769
▲ Naprosyn Tablets (1% to 10%) 2769
▲ Neoral Soft Gelatin Capsules (4%) ... 2247
▲ Neoral Oral Solution (4%) 2247
Neurontin Capsules (2.1%).............. 2498
Neurontin Oral Solution (2.1%)......... 2498
Neurontin Tablets (2.1%)................. 2498
Nexium Delayed-Release Capsules (Greater than or equal to 1%) 645
Nexium I.V. (Greater than or equal to 1%)... 649
Niaspan Extended-Release Tablets... 1703
▲ Nicotrol Inhaler (Greater than 3%) 2594
▲ Nicotrol NS (4%) 2596
▲ Nipent for Injection (3% to 10%) 3216
Noroxin Tablets (0.3% to 1.0%)........ 2009
Norvasc Tablets (More than 0.1% to 1%)... 2529
Norvir (0.9% to 1.7%)..................... 499
Omnicef Capsules (0.7%)................. 506
Omnicef for Oral Suspension (0.6%) 506
Oncaspar (Less than 1%) 1123
OxyContin Tablets (Less than 1%) 2699
▲ Oxytrol Transdermal System (Greater than 1%) 3383
Parcopa Orally Disintegrating Tablets 3111
▲ Paxil CR Controlled-Release Tablets (4.0%) 1509
▲ Paxil (4.0%) 1501
Permax Tablets (Infrequent) 3357
Plendil Extended-Release Tablets (0.5% to 1.5%) 651
▲ Pletal Tablets (2% to 3%) 2478
▲ Pravachol Tablets (2.7% to 3.3%) 943
▲ Precose Tablets (74%) 776
▲ Prefest Tablets (5%) 1069
▲ Premarin Tablets (6% to 7%) 3443
▲ Premphase Tablets (5% to 9%) 3452
▲ Prempro Tablets (5% to 9%) 3452
Prevacid Delayed-Release Capsules (Less than 1%) 3268
Prevacid for Delayed-Release Oral Suspension (Less than 1%) 3268
Prevacid NapraPAC (Less than 1%) .. 3277
Prevacid SoluTab Delayed-Release Orally Disintegrating Tablets (Less than 1%) 3268
PREVPAC (Less than 1%) 3281
Prilosec OTC Tablets (Less than 1 to 2.7%) 2674
Prinivil Tablets (0.3% to 1.0%) 2029
Prinzide Tablets 2033
ProAmatine Tablets (Rare) 3183
Prochieve 4% Gel 1018
Prochieve 8% Gel 1018
▲ Prograf Capsules and Injection (3% to 15%) 624
ProSom Tablets (Infrequent) 512
Protonix I.V. (Greater than or equal to 1%) 3468
▲ Protonix Tablets (2% to 4%) 3465
Proventil HFA Inhalation Aerosol (Less than 3%) 3071
Provigil Tablets (1%) 1002
▲ Prozac Pulvules and Liquid (3%) 1771
▲ Rapamune Oral Solution and Tablets (3% to 20%) 3472
Razadyne ER Extended-Release Capsules (Frequent) 2434
Razadyne (Frequent) 2434
▲ Relafen Tablets (3% to 9%) 1523
Relpax Tablets (Infrequent) 2531
▲ Renagel Tablets (4%) 1268
Requip Tablets (2% to 3%) 1528
Rescriptor Tablets 2535
Retrovir Capsules 1533
Retrovir IV Infusion 1537
Retrovir 1533
Reyataz Capsules (Less than 3%) 948
Rilutek Tablets (2.0% to 2.5%) 2945
Risperdal Consta Long-Acting Injection (Infrequent) 1664
Risperdal M-Tab Orally Disintegrating Tablets (Infrequent) 1658
Risperdal (Infrequent) 1658
Rocephin Injectable Vials, ADD-Vantage, Galaxy, Bulk (Rare) 2801
▲ Roferon-A Injection (3%) 2805
Rythmol SR Capsules (1% to 2%) 2736
Sanctura Tablets (1.2%) 1133
▲ Sandostatin Injection (Less than 10%) 2263
▲ Sandostatin LAR Depot (25.7%) 2264
Sedapap Tablets 50 mg/650 mg (Infrequent) 2098
Seroquel Tablets (Infrequent) 691
▲ Simulect for Injection (3% to 10%) .. 2268
Sonata Capsules (Infrequent) 1686
Spectracef Tablets (0.1% to 1%) 2706

Stalevo Tablets (2%) 2270
Strattera Capsules (2%) 1784
Sular Tablets (Less than or equal to 1%) 1163
▲ Suprax (4%) 1811
Sustiva Capsules (1% to 2%) 957
Tambocor Tablets (Less than 1%) 1824
Targretin Capsules 1719
Tasmar Tablets (2% to 4%) 3360
Tequin Injection (Less than 0.1%) 964
Tequin Tablets (Less than 0.1%) 964
Teveten Tablets (Less than 1%) 1707
Teveten HCT Tablets (Less than 1%) 1710
▲ Thalomid Capsules (8.3%) 979
Ticlid Tablets (1.5%) 2813
Timentin ADD-Vantage 1556
Timentin Injection Galaxy Container 1559
Timentin IV Infusion 1553
Timentin Pharmacy Bulk Package 1562
Topamax Sprinkle Capsules (1% to frequent) 2438
Topamax Tablets (1% to frequent) 2438
Toprol-XL Tablets (About 1 of 100 patients) 660
▲ Tricor Tablets (3%) 523
Triglide Tablets 1165
Trileptal Oral Suspension 2281
Trileptal Tablets 2281
Truvada Tablets 1279
Ultracet Tablets (At least 1%) 2462
Ultrase MT Capsules (1.5%) 736
Uniretic Tablets (Less than 1%) 3114
Vantin Tablets and Oral Suspension (Less than 1%) 2650
Vaseretic Tablets (0.5% to 2.0%) 2073
VFEND I.V. (Less than 2%) 2543
VFEND Oral Suspension (Less than 2%) 2543
VFEND Tablets (Less than 2%) 2543
▲ Vicoprofen Tablets (3% to 9%) 533
▲ Viracept (1% to 5%) 2556
▲ Viread Tablets (3% to 4%) 1284
▲ Voltaren Tablets (1% to 10%) 2298
▲ Voltaren-XR Tablets (1% to 10%) 2301
Vytorin 10/10 Tablets 2084
Vytorin 10/10 Tablets 3092
Vytorin 10/20 Tablets 2084
Vytorin 10/20 Tablets 3092
Vytorin 10/40 Tablets 2084
Vytorin 10/40 Tablets 3092
Vytorin 10/80 Tablets 2084
Vytorin 10/80 Tablets 3092
▲ WelChol Tablets (12%) 2855
Wellbutrin SR Sustained-Release Tablets (At least 1%) 1583
Wellbutrin XL Extended-Release Tablets (At least 1%) 1588
▲ Xifaxan Tablets (11.3%) 2847
▲ Zavesca Capsules (29% to 50%) 543
▲ Zegerid Powder for Oral Solution (4.5% to 20.2%) 2972
▲ Zelnorm Tablets (6%) 2303
▲ Zenapax for Injection (2% to 5%) 2838
Zestoretic Tablets 701
Zestril Tablets (0.3% to 1.0%) 704
Zithromax Capsules, 250 mg (1% or less) 2568
Zithromax for IV Infusion (1% or less) 2573
Zithromax for Oral Suspension, 1 g (1% or less) 2568
Zithromax for Oral Suspension, 300 mg, 600 mg, 900 mg, 1200 mg (1% or less) 2561
Zithromax Tablets, 250 mg, 500 mg (1% or less) 2561
Zithromax Tablets, 600 mg (1% or less) 2568
Zithromax Tri-Pak (1% or less) 2561
Zithromax Z-Pak (1% or less) 2568
Zmax for Oral Suspension (Less then 1%) 2577
Zocor Tablets (1.9%) 2078
Zoladex (1% or greater) 709
Zoladex 3-month 712
▲ Zoloft (3%) 2581
Zonegran Capsules (Infrequent) 1089
Zosyn (1.0% or less to 1.3%) 3492
Zyban Sustained-Release Tablets (Frequent) 1620
Zyprexa Tablets (Frequent) 1798
Zyprexa ZYDIS Orally Disintegrating Tablets (Infrequent) 1798
Zyrtec Chewable Tablets (Less than 2%) 2589
Zyrtec (Less than 2%) 2589
Zyrtec-D 12 Hour Extended Release Tablets (Less than 2%) 2591

Flatus with discharge

▲ Xenical Capsules (2.1% to 23.9%) 2834

Floating feeling

Dilaudid Oral Liquid (Less frequent) 443
Dilaudid Tablets - 8 mg (Less frequent) 443
Dilaudid-HP (Less frequent) 441
Mintezol 2002
MS Contin Tablets (Less frequent) 2703
Nubain Injection (1% or less) 1111

Flu Syndrome

Abilify Tablets (Frequent) 916
Abilify Tablets (Frequent) 2472
▲ Actonel with Calcium Tablets (7.1% to 8.7%) 2684
Alinia for Oral Suspension (Less than 1%) 2840
Alinia Tablets (Less than 1%) 2840
Antara Capsules (2.1%) 2723
▲ Arimidex Tablets (2% to 7%) 665
▲ Caduet Tablets (2.2% to 3.2%) 2507
Campral Tablets (Frequent) 1175
▲ Climara Pro Transdermal System (4.7%) 800
Crestor Tablets (2.3%) 672
▲ Enablex Extended-Release Tablets (1% to 3%) 2201
▲ Estrogel 0.06% (5.4%) 3200
▲ Humira Injection (7%) 464
▲ Levitra Tablets (3%) 3048
Lunesta Tablets 3139
Menopur for Subcutaneous Injection (1.3% to 2.6%) 1145
Mirapex Tablets (Greater than or equal to 1%) 889
▲ Omacor Capsules (3.5%) 2735
▲ Premphase Tablets (8% to 13%) 3452
▲ Prempro Tablets (8% to 13%) 3452
Prevacid NapraPAC (Less than 1%) 3277
▲ Raptiva for Injection (7%) 1247
Relpax Tablets (Rare) 2531
▲ Somavert Injection (4% to 12%) 2648
Triglide Tablets (2.1%) 1165
▲ Univasc Tablets (3.1%) 3118
▲ Ventavis Inhalation Solution (14%) 1036
Zomig Nasal Spray (Infrequent) 718

Fluid depletion

Captopril Tablets 2114
Kristalose for Oral Solution 2149

Fluid imbalance

Benicar HCT Tablets 2852
Imitrex Nasal Spray 1435
Lotronex Tablets (Rare) 1479
Photofrin for Injection 729
Prinzide Tablets 2033
Vaseretic Tablets 2073
▲ Vesanoid Capsules (6%) 2823
Zestoretic Tablets 701

Fluid overload

AmBisome for Injection (Less common) 615
Ammonul Injection 3323
▲ Aredia for Injection (Up to at least 15%) 2168
Campath Ampules 826
▲ Coreg Tablets (Greater than 1% to 3%) 1376
Levaquin in 5% Dextrose Injection (0.1% to 0.9%) 2453
Levaquin (0.1% to 0.9%) 2453
▲ Myfortic Tablets (3% to less than 20%) 2244
Orthoclone OKT3 Sterile Solution 2370
Prinivil Tablets (0.3% to 1.0%) 2029
▲ Simulect for Injection (3% to 10%) 2268
Vivelle Transdermal System 2288
▲ Zegerid Powder for Oral Solution (5.1%) 2972
▲ Zenapax for Injection (2% to 5%) 2838
Zestoretic Tablets 701
Zestril Tablets (0.3% to 1.0%) 704
Zosyn (1.9%) 3492

Fluid retention

(see under Edema)

Flu-like symptoms

AccuNeb Inhalation Solution (2.6%) 1055
▲ Actimmune (Most common) 1646
Actiq (Less than 1%) 993
▲ Actonel Tablets (7.1% to 9.8%) 2679
Advair Diskus 100/50 1291
Advair Diskus 250/50 1291
Advair Diskus 500/50 1291
▲ Advicor Tablets (6%) 1694
▲ Aerobid/Aerobid-M (10%) 1172
Agrylin Capsules (1% to 5%) 3172
▲ Alamast Ophthalmic Solution (10% to 25%) 3371
▲ Aldara Cream, 5% (1% to 3%) 1814
▲ Alferon N Injection (30%) 1640
Allegra (2.5%) 2857
Aloxi Injection (Less than 1%) 2099
Alphagan P Ophthalmic Solution (1% to 4%) 563
Altace Capsules 1673
▲ Altoprev Extended-Release Tablets (5%) 1151
Ambien Tablets (2%) 2867
AmBisome for Injection (Less common) 615
Aptivus Capsules (Less than 2%) 859
▲ Aranesp for Injection (6%) 576
Arava Tablets (2%) 2881
Aricept Tablets (Frequent) 1086
Aricept ODT Tablets (Frequent) 1086
▲ Aromasin Tablets (6%) 2600
▲ Asacol Delayed-Release Tablets (3% to 5%) 2688
Asmanex Twisthaler (1% to less than 3%) 2981
Atacand HCT (2.5%) 637
▲ Atrovent HFA Inhalation Aerosol (4% to 8%) 872
▲ Atrovent Inhalation Solution (3.7%) 868
▲ Avalide Tablets (3%) 922
▲ Avalide Tablets (3%) 2889
Avapro Tablets (1% or greater) 925
Avapro Tablets (1% or greater) 2886
▲ Avinza Capsules (5% to 10%) 1714
▲ Avonex (49%) 839
▲ Azmacort Inhalation Aerosol (2% to 5%) 1701
▲ Betaseron for SC Injection (60%) 791
Bexxar 1360
▲ Boniva Tablets (0.8% to 3.3%) 2747
▲ Botox Purified Neurotoxin Complex (2% to 10%) 565
Campath Ampules 826
▲ Cancidas for Injection (0% to 3.1%) 1894
▲ Carnitor Injection (15% to 29%) 3185
▲ Casodex Tablets (4%) 670
Caverject Impulse Injection (2%) 2610
Celebrex Capsules (0.1% to 1.9%) 3130
Celexa (Infrequent) 1177
▲ CellCept Capsules (3% to less than 20%) 2751
▲ CellCept Intravenous (3% to less than 20%) 2751
▲ CellCept Oral Suspension (3% to less than 20%) 2751
▲ CellCept Tablets (3% to less than 20%) 2751
▲ Chemet Capsules (5.2% to 15.7%) 2480
Clozapine Tablets 2141
Clozaril Tablets 2174
Colazal Capsules (1%) 2845
▲ CombiPatch Transdermal System (10% to 14%) 2180
Combivent Inhalation Aerosol (1.4%) 878
▲ Copaxone for Injection (19%) 3292
▲ Coreg Tablets (Greater than 1% to 3%) 1376
▲ Cozaar Tablets (10%) 1913
Cymbalta Delayed-Release Capsules (Infrequent) 1729
▲ Depacon Injection (12%) 412
▲ Depakene (12%) 417
▲ Depakote Sprinkle Capsules (12%) 422
▲ Depakote Tablets (At least 5% to 12%) 427
▲ Depakote ER Tablets (12%) 433
▲ Detrol Tablets (4.4%) 2626
▲ Ditropan XL Extended Release Tablets (2% to less than 5%) 2391
▲ Dostinex Tablets (1% to less than 10%) 2631
Doxil Injection (Less than 1%) 3302
▲ Duragesic Transdermal System (3% to 10%) 2448
▲ Edex Injection (3%) 3103
Effexor Tablets 3405
▲ Effexor XR Capsules (6%) 3411
▲ Elidel Cream 1% (6.6% to 13.2%) 2198
Enbrel for Injection 580
Engerix-B Vaccine (Less than 1%) 1391
▲ Entocort EC Capsules (Less than 5%) 2694
Epogen for Injection (Rare) 586
Eulexin Capsules 3023
▲ Evista Tablets (13.5% to 14.6%) 1735
▲ Evoxac Capsules (1% to 3%) 1042
▲ Exelon Capsules (3%) 2204
▲ Faslodex Injection (7.1%) 682
▲ Femara Tablets (6%) 2210
Ferrlecit Injection 3379
▲ Flolan for Injection (13% to 25%) 1408
▲ Flonase Nasal Spray (1% to 3%) 1412
Follistim AQ Cartridge 2354
▲ Fortical Nasal Spray (1% to 3%) 3336
Fuzeon Injection (2.3%) 2772
▲ Gabitril Tablets (1% to 9%) 998
▲ Gemzar for Injection (19%) 1743
Gengraf Capsules (2%) 458
Geodon (Frequent) 2514
▲ Gleevec Tablets (0.8% to 11%) 2221
▲ Herceptin I.V. (10%) 1234
▲ Humatrope Vials and Cartridges (3.9% to 15.6%) 1756
Hytrin Capsules (At least 1% to 2.4%) 469
▲ Imdur Tablets (Less than or equal to 5%) 3032
Imitrex Injection (Rare) 1431
Imitrex Nasal Spray 1435
Imitrex Tablets 1440
Indapamide Tablets (Less than 5%) 2119
▲ Infergen (8% to 15%) 1647
Inspra Tablets (2%) 2520
▲ Intron A for Injection (Up to 79%) 3038
Invirase (Less than 2%) 2776
Kadian Capsules (Less than 3%) 572
Kaletra (Less than 2%) 474
▲ Keppra Oral Solution (1% to 3%) 3307
▲ Keppra Tablets (1% to 3%) 3307
▲ Kineret Injection (6%) 594
▲ Klonopin (4%) 2782
▲ Lamictal (5% to 7%) 1449
▲ Lescol Capsules (5.1%) 2227
▲ Lescol Capsules (5.1%) 2730
▲ Lescol XL Tablets (7.1%) 2227
▲ Lescol XL Tablets (7.1%) 2730
Levaquin in 5% Dextrose Injection (0.1% to 0.9%) 2453
Levaquin (0.1% to 0.9%) 2453
▲ Lexapro Oral Solution (5%) 1193
▲ Lexapro Tablets (5%) 1193
▲ Lipitor Tablets (Up to 3.2%) 2495
Lofibra Capsules (2.1%) 1217
Lotensin HCT Tablets (More than 1%) 2235
Lupron Depot 3.75 mg (Less than 5%) 3257
Lupron Depot–3 Month 11.25 mg (Less than 5%) 3262
Lyrica Capsules (1% to 2%) 2524
▲ Meridia Capsules (8.2%) 485
Miacalcin Nasal Spray (1% to 3%) 2242
Micardis Tablets (1%) 884
Micardis HCT Tablets (2%) 886
Migranal Nasal Spray (Rare) 3350
▲ Mobic Oral Suspension (2.3% to 5.8%) 893
▲ Mobic Tablets (2.3% to 5.8%) 893
Namenda (Greater than or equal to 2%) 1199
Nasonex Nasal Spray (Greater than or equal to 2%) 3058
▲ Neoral Soft Gelatin Capsules (3% to 9.9%) 2247
▲ Neoral Oral Solution (3% to 9.9%) 2247
Neumega for Injection 3433
Neurontin Capsules (More than 1%) 2498
Neurontin Oral Solution (More than 1%) 2498
Neurontin Tablets (More than 1%) 2498
Nexium Delayed-Release Capsules (Less than 1%) 645
Nexium I.V. (Less than 1%) 649
▲ Nicotrol Inhaler (Greater than 3%) 2594
Nipent for Injection (Less than 3%) 3216
▲ Norditropin Cartridges (8%) 2318
Norvir (Less than 2%) 499
▲ Ontak Vials (8%) 1717
▲ Optivar Ophthalmic Solution (1% to 10%) 1877
Orthoclone OKT3 Sterile Solution 2370
Paxil CR Controlled-Release Tablets (Infrequent) 1509
Paxil (Infrequent) 1501
▲ PEG-Intron Powder for Injection (46%) 3062
▲ Permax Tablets (3.2%) 3357
▲ Plavix Tablets (7.9%) 940
▲ Plavix Tablets (7.5%) 2942
Plendil Extended-Release Tablets (0.5% to 1.5%) 651
Pletal Tablets (2% or greater) 2478
Pravachol Tablets (Up to 2.4%) 943
▲ Prefest Tablets (11%) 1069
▲ Premarin Tablets (10% to 11%) 3443
Prevacid Delayed-Release Capsules (Less than 1%) 3268
Prevacid for Delayed-Release Oral Suspension (Less than 1%) 3268
Prevacid SoluTab Delayed-Release Orally Disintegrating Tablets (Less than 1%) 3268
Prevnar for Injection 3460
PREVPAC (Less than 1%) 3281
Prilosec OTC Tablets (1%) 2674
Prinivil Tablets (0.3%) 2029
Prinzide Tablets (0.3% to 1%) 2033

Prochieve 4% Gel................ 1018
Prochieve 8% Gel................ 1018
Procrit for Injection (Rare)................ 2374
▲ Prograf Capsules and Injection (3% to 15%)................ 624
Prolastin (Occasional)................ 3252
Protonix I.V. (Greater than or equal to 1%)................ 3468
Protonix Tablets (Greater than or equal to 1%)................ 3465
▲ Protopic Ointment (22% to 35%) 629
▲ Provigil Tablets (4%) 1002
▲ Prozac Pulvules and Liquid (3% to 10%)................ 1771
Pulmicort Respules (1% to 3%)......... 654
Pulmozyme Inhalation Solution......... 1245
Rabies Vaccine RabAvert (Common)................ 1011
▲ Rapamune Oral Solution and Tablets (3% to 20%)................ 3472
▲ Rebetol (13% to 31%) 3073
▲ Rebetron Combination Therapy (14% to 18%)................ 3078
▲ Rebif Prefilled Syringe for Injection (56% to 59%) 3163
Recombivax HB (Less than 1%) 2045
Repronex for Intramuscular and Subcutaneous Injection 1148
Requip Tablets (Infrequent) 1528
▲ Rescriptor Tablets (2.4% to 7.3%) ... 2535
Retrovir Capsules 1533
Retrovir IV Infusion 1537
Retrovir 1533
▲ Ribavirin, USP Capsules (13% to 31%) 3083
Rilutek Tablets (More than 2%) 2945
Risperdal M-Tab Orally Disintegrating Tablets (Infrequent) 1658
Risperdal (Infrequent) 1658
▲ Roferon-A Injection (16% to 33%) 2805
▲ Sandostatin Injection (1% to 4%) 2263
▲ Serevent Diskus (5%) 1540
Seroquel Tablets (Frequent) 691
Soriatane Capsules (Less than 1%) .. 1028
▲ Spiriva HandiHaler (Greater than or equal to 3%) 899
▲ Starlix Tablets (3.6%) 2276
▲ Suboxone Tablets (6%) 2719
▲ Subutex Tablets (6%) 2719
Sular Tablets (Less than or equal to 1%) 1163
Synagis (More than 1%) 1868
▲ Targretin Capsules (3.6% to 13.2%) 1719
▲ Tasmar Tablets (3% to 4%) 3360
Teveten Tablets (Less than 1%) 1707
Teveten HCT Tablets (Less than 1%) 1710
Thalomid Capsules 979
Thyrogen for Injection (1%) 1270
Tiazac Capsules (2%) 1204
▲ Topamax Sprinkle Capsules (Less than 1% to 4%) 2438
▲ Topamax Tablets (Less than 1% to 4%) 2438
Tricor Tablets (2.1%) 523
Twinrix Vaccine (Less than 1%) 1571
Uniretic Tablets (More than 1%) 3114
▲ Verelan PM Capsules (3.7%) 3120
VFEND I.V. (Less than 2%) 2543
VFEND Oral Suspension (Less than 2%) 2543
VFEND Tablets (Less than 2%) 2543
Viagra Tablets (Greater than 2%) 2552
Vicoprofen Tablets (Less than 3%) 533
▲ Visudyne for Injection (1% to 10%) .. 2286
▲ Vivelle Transdermal System (1.5% to 6.5%) 2288
▲ Vivelle-Dot Transdermal System (1.5% to 6.5%) 2293
▲ WelChol Tablets (3%) 2855
Wellbutrin Tablets (Frequent) 1579
Wellbutrin SR Sustained-Release Tablets (At least 1%) 1583
Wellbutrin XL Extended-Release Tablets (At least 1%) 1588
▲ Xalatan Sterile Ophthalmic Solution (Approximately 4%) 2654
▲ Xeloda Tablets (Less than 5%) 2825
▲ Xenical Capsules (39.7%) 2834
▲ Xopenex HFA Inhalation Aerosol (1.4% to 4.2%) 3151
▲ Xopenex Inhalation Solution (1.4% to 4.2%) 3143
▲ Xopenex Inhalation Solution Concentrate (1.4% to 4.2%) 3147
Yasmin 28 Tablets (Greater than 1%) 818
Zaditor Ophthalmic Solution (Less than 5%) 2302
Zegerid Powder for Oral Solution (1%) 2972
▲ Zemplar Capsules (5%) 535
▲ Zemplar Injection (5%) 538
Zestoretic Tablets (0.3% to 1%)....... 701
Zestril Tablets (0.3%)................ 704
▲ Zoladex (5%) 709
Zoladex 3-month (1% to 5%)............ 712
▲ Zometa for Intravenous Infusion (Less than 15%)................ 2306
▲ Zonegran Capsules (4%) 1089
Zyprexa Tablets (Frequent)................ 1798
Zyprexa ZYDIS Orally Disintegrating Tablets (Frequent)... 1798

Fluorosis

Ultane Liquid for Inhalation (Less than 1%)................ 526

Flushing

Accutane Capsules................ 2740
▲ Acthrel for Injection (16%) 3528
▲ Adalat CC Tablets (4%) 2978
▲ Adenoscan (44%) 613
▲ Advicor Tablets (71%) 1694
Aggrenox Capsules (Less than 1%).. 855
▲ Aldurazyme for Intravenous Infusion (5%) 1261
Allegra (Rare) 2857
Allegra-D 12 Hour Extended-Release Tablets (Rare) ... 2860
Allegra-D 24 Hour Extended-Release Tablets (Rare) ... 2862
Aloprim for Injection (Less than 1%) 2156
Altoprev Extended-Release Tablets (Rare) 1151
Ambien Tablets (Rare) 2867
AmBisome for Injection (Less common) 615
Aminohippurate Sodium "PAH" Injection 1886
Ammonul Injection 3323
Amnesteem Capsules 2126
Anzemet Injection (Infrequently) 2871
Anzemet Tablets (Infrequently) 2874
Apokyn Injection (Common) 2132
AquaMEPHYTON Injection 1887
Astelin Nasal Spray (Infrequent) 1876
Avalide Tablets 922
Avalide Tablets 2889
Avapro Tablets (Less than 1%) 925
Avapro Tablets (Less than 1%) 2886
▲ BeneFix for Injection (3.1%) 3402
BiDil Tablets 2161
Brevibloc Concentrate (Less than 1%) 766
Brevibloc Injection (Less than 1%) 766
Brevibloc Double Strength Injection (Less than 1%) 766
Brevibloc Premixed Injection (Less than 1%) 766
Brevibloc Double Strength Premixed Injection (Less than 1%) 766
Buprenex Injectable (Less than 1%) 2718
▲ Caduet Tablets (0.7% to 4.5%) 2507
Camptosar Injection 2602
Cancidas for Injection (1.8% to 2.9%) 1894
Captopril Tablets (2 to 5 of 1000 patients) 2114
Cardizem LA Extended Release Tablets (1.4%) 1699
Celexa (Infrequent) 1177
▲ Cerezyme for Injection (Approximately 6.6%) 1263
▲ Cialis Tablets (2% to 3%) 1806
Cipro I.V. (1% or less) 2998
Cipro I.V. Pharmacy Bulk Package (1% or less) 3509
Cipro (Less than 1%) 2991
Cipro XR Tablets 3004
Clinoril Tablets (Less than 1 in 100) 1899
▲ Clolar for Intravenous Infusion (18%) 1264
Combivent Inhalation Aerosol 878
Covera-HS Tablets (0.6% to 0.8%) ... 3135
Cozaar Tablets (Less than 1%) 1913
Cubicin for Injection (Less than 1%) 1038
CytoGam Intravenous (Less than 5.0%) 1866
Dalmane Capsules (Rare) 3343
DDAVP Nasal Spray (Occasional) 2894
DDAVP Tablets 2895
Desmopressin Acetate Rhinal Tube (Occasional) 1144
Dilaudid 439
Dilaudid Oral Liquid 443
Dilaudid Non-Sterile Powder 439
Dilaudid Rectal Suppositories 439
Dilaudid Tablets 439
Dilaudid Tablets - 8 mg 443
Diovan HCT Tablets (Greater than 0.2%) 2195
Diprivan Injectable Emulsion (Less than 1%) 676
Dolobid Tablets................ 1937
▲ Doxil Injection (Approximately 6.8%) 3302
DuoNeb Inhalation Solution................ 1058
Duragesic Transdermal System (1% or greater) 2448
DynaCirc CR Tablets (1.2% to 3.8%) 2726
Effexor Tablets 3405
▲ Eloxatin for Injection (3% to 10%) 2908
Emcyt Capsules (1%) 3137
Emend Capsules (Greater than 0.5%) 1944
Enbrel for Injection 580
Engerix-B Vaccine (Less than 1%)..... 1391
▲ Entocort EC Capsules (Less than 5%) 2694
Ethyol for Injection................ 1869
Evoxac Capsules (0.3%) 1042
Exelon Capsules (Infrequent) 2204
Factive Tablets (Less than or equal to 0.1%) 2464
▲ Femara Tablets (0.1% to 49.7%) 2210
Ferrlecit Injection (Two cases) 3379
▲ Flolan for Injection (23% to 58%) 1408
Floxin Otic Singles 1045
Floxin Otic Solution (Single report) ... 1043
Fortical Nasal Spray (Less than 1%) 3336
▲ Frova Tablets (4%) 1101
Gammagard Liquid 751
Gammagard S/D (Occasional) 754
▲ Gengraf Capsules (Less than 1% to 5%) 458
Gleevec Tablets (Infrequent) 2221
Gonal-f RFF Pen for Injection (2.4%) 3155
Hyperstat I.V. Injection 3031
Hyzaar 1964
▲ Imdur Tablets (Less than or equal to 5%) 3032
▲ Imitrex Injection (6.6%) 1431
Imitrex Nasal Spray (Infrequent) 1435
Imitrex Tablets (Up to 4%) 1440
Indapamide Tablets (Less than 5%) .. 2119
Indocin Capsules (Less than 1%) 1968
Indocin I.V. (Less than 1%) 1973
Indocin (Less than 1%) 1968
Infed Injection 3381
▲ Intron A for Injection (Less than 5%) 3038
Invanz for Injection (Greater than 0.1%) 1974
▲ I.V. Busulfex (25%) 1125
Iveegam EN (0.3% to 0.8%) 759
Ketek Tablets (Less than 0.2%) 2920
Klonopin (Infrequent) 2782
Lamictal (Infrequent) 1449
Lariam Tablets (Infrequent) 2790
Lescol Capsules (Rare) 2227
Lescol Capsules (Rare) 2730
Lescol XL Tablets 2227
Lescol XL Tablets 2730
Leukine 829
Levaquin in 5% Dextrose Injection (0.1% to 0.9%) 2453
Levaquin (0.1% to 0.9%) 2453
▲ Levitra Tablets (11%) 3048
Levothroid Tablets 1189
Levoxyl Tablets 1680
Lexapro Oral Solution (Infrequent) 1193
Lexapro Tablets (Infrequent) 1193
Lidoderm Patch 1107
Lotensin Tablets (Less than 1%) 2232
Lotensin HCT Tablets (0.3% to 1%) .. 2235
Lotrel Capsules (Up to 0.3%) 2238
Marinol Capsules (0.3% to 1%) 3334
Matulane Capsules 3188
Mavik Tablets (0.3% to 1.0%) 482
Maxair Autohaler 1820
Maxalt Tablets (Frequent) 1983
Maxalt-MLT Orally Disintegrating Tablets (Frequent) 1983
Mefoxin for Injection 1987
Mefoxin Premixed Intravenous Solution 1990
Menopur for Subcutaneous Injection (2.4%) 1145
Mephyton Tablets 1993
Mevacor Tablets (Rare) 1996
Miacalcin Nasal Spray (Less than 1%) 2242
Micardis Tablets (More than 0.3%) ... 884
Micardis HCT Tablets 886
▲ Mivacron Injection (16%) 489
Moduretic Tablets (Less than or equal to 1%) 2003
Mycamine for Injection (0.2% to 0.5%) 620
Narcan Injection................ 1109
Navelbine Injection................ 1494
▲ Neoral Soft Gelatin Capsules (1% to 5%)................ 2247
▲ Neoral Oral Solution (1% to 5%) 2247
Neumega for Injection 3433
Nexium Delayed-Release Capsules (Less than 1%)................ 645
Nexium I.V. (Less than 1%)................ 649
▲ Niaspan Extended-Release Tablets (Among most common).... 1703
Nicomide Tablets................ 3190
Nimbex Injection (0.2%)................ 494
Nimotop Capsules (Less than 1% to 2.1%)................ 774
Nitrolingual Pumpspray................ 1161
Norvasc Tablets (0.7% to 4.5%)....... 2529
Nubain Injection (1% or less)........... 1111
Numorphan 1112
Orthoclone OKT3 Sterile Solution..... 2370
▲ Oxytrol Transdermal System (Greater than 1%) 3383
▲ Pacerone Tablets (1% to 3%) 3337
Parcopa Orally Disintegrating Tablets 3111
▲ PEG-Intron Powder for Injection (6%) 3062
Pepcid Injection (Infrequent) 2017
Pepcid (Infrequent) 2014
Persantine Tablets 898
Plasmanate (Occasional) 3252
▲ Plendil Extended-Release Tablets (3.9% to 6.9%) 651
Pletal Tablets (Very rare) 2478
Pravachol Tablets (Rare) 943
Primaxin I.M. 2022
Primaxin I.V. (Less than 0.2%) 2024
Prinivil Tablets (0.3% to 1.0%) 2029
Prinzide Tablets (0.3% to 1%) 2033
ProSom Tablets (Infrequent) 512
Rabies Vaccine RabAvert 1011
▲ Rebetol (3% to 4%) 3073
Recombinate 762
Recombivax HB (Less than 1%) 2045
ReFacto Vials 3479
Refludan for Injection (Uncommon) ... 815
Remicade for IV Injection 987
▲ Requip Tablets (3%) 1528
▲ Revatio Tablets (10%) 2541
▲ R-Gene 10 for Intravenous Use (3%) 2647
▲ Ribavirin, USP Capsules (3% to 4%) 3083
Risperdal Consta Long-Acting Injection (Rare) 1664
Risperdal M-Tab Orally Disintegrating Tablets (Rare) 1658
Risperdal (Rare) 1658
▲ Rituxan for Infusion (Among most frequent) 845
▲ Rituxan I.V. (5%) 1251
Rocephin Injectable Vials, ADD-Vantage, Galaxy, Bulk (Occasional) 2801
Rythmol SR Capsules 2736
▲ Sandimmune (Less than 1% to 4%) 2259
▲ Sandostatin Injection (1% to 4%) 2263
▲ Soriatane Capsules (1% to 10%) 1028
Stalevo Tablets 2270
▲ Strattera Capsules (3%) 1784
Surmontil Capsules 2347
Sustiva Capsules (Less than 2%) 957
Tambocor Tablets (1% to 3%) 1824
Tarka Tablets (0.3% or more) 519
Taxotere Injection Concentrate 2947
Thyrogen for Injection 1270
Tindamax 2670
Topamax Sprinkle Capsules (Infrequent) 2438
Topamax Tablets (Infrequent) 2438
▲ Tracleer Tablets (9%) 539
Trileptal Oral Suspension 2281
Trileptal Tablets 2281
▲ Trisenox Injection (10%) 983
Twinrix Vaccine (Less than 1%) 1571
Uniretic Tablets (Less than 1%) 3114
Unithroid Tablets 3521
Univasc Tablets (1.6%) 3118
Vantas (Less than 2%) 3367
Vantin Tablets and Oral Suspension (Less than 1%) 2650
Vaseretic Tablets 2073
Vasotec I.V. Injection (0.5% to 1.0%) 2076
Verelan PM Capsules (0.6%) 3120
▲ Vesanoid Capsules (23%) 2823
▲ Viagra Tablets (10%) 2552
Vivactil Tablets 2350
VoSpire Extended-Release Tablets (Less frequent) 2352
Vytorin 10/10 Tablets 2084
Vytorin 10/10 Tablets 3092

Vytorin 10/20 Tablets 2084
Vytorin 10/20 Tablets 3092
Vytorin 10/40 Tablets 2084
Vytorin 10/40 Tablets 3092
Vytorin 10/80 Tablets 2084
Vytorin 10/80 Tablets 3092
Wellbutrin Tablets (Rare) 1579
▲ Wellbutrin SR Sustained-Release Tablets (1% to 4%) 1583
▲ Wellbutrin XL Extended-Release Tablets (1% to 4%) 1588
▲ Xeloda Tablets (5%) 2825
Zelnorm Tablets 2303
Zestoretic Tablets (0.3% to 1%) 701
Zestril Tablets (0.3% to 1.0%) 704
▲ Zevalin Injection (6%) 848
Zocor Tablets (Rare) 2078
Zofran Injection 1607
Zofran 1613
Zofran ODT Orally Disintegrating Tablets 1613
Zoloft (Infrequent) 2581
Zosyn (1.0% or less) 3492
Zyban Sustained-Release Tablets (Infrequent) 1620
Zyrtec Chewable Tablets (Less than 2%) 2589
Zyrtec (Less than 2%) 2589
Zyrtec-D 12 Hour Extended Release Tablets (Less than 2%) 2591

Flushing, cutaneous
Kadian Capsules (Less than 3%) 572
▲ Mivacron Injection (About 25%) 489
Nitrolingual Pumpspray 1161
Roferon-A Injection (Less than 0.5%) 2805

Flushing, facial
▲ Acthrel for Injection (16%) 3528
▲ Adenocard Injection (18%) 612
Adriamycin for Injection, USP 786
Adriamycin Injection, USP 786
Alferon N Injection (One patient) 1640
Carimune NF 3501
Chromagen Forte Soft Gelatin Capsules 3296
DDAVP Injection 4 mcg/mL (Occasional) 2893
Desmopressin Acetate Injection (Occasional) 1143
Dilaudid-HP (Less frequent) 441
Doxil Injection 3302
Ferrlecit Injection 3379
Imitrex Nasal Spray 1435
Imitrex Tablets 1440
Kadian Capsules (Less than 3%) 572
Marinol Capsules (Greater than 1%) 3334
Miacalcin Injection (About 2% to 5%) 2241
Mintezol 2002
MS Contin Tablets (Less frequent) 2703
Nicotrol NS 2596
ProAmatine Tablets (Less frequent) 3183
Relpax Tablets (2%) 2531
Sandimmune 2259
Urecholine Tablets 2349

Flushing, generalized
Chromagen Forte Soft Gelatin Capsules 3296

Flushing, hands
Miacalcin Injection (About 2% to 5%) 2241

Flushing, upper thorax
▲ Acthrel for Injection (16%) 3528
Sandimmune 2259

Folliculitis
Aclovate (Infrequent) 1290
Amerge Tablets (Rare) 1312
Analpram-HC 1136
Clindagel 1207
Clobevate Gel (Less than 2%) 3213
Clobex Shampoo 1209
Clobex Lotion 1208
Cutivate Cream (0.8%) 1381
Cutivate Lotion 0.05% (Less than 1%) 1383
Cutivate Ointment (Infrequent to more frequent) 1384
Didronel Tablets 2693
Diprolene Lotion 0.05% (2%) 3016
Diprolene Ointment 0.05% (2 per 767 patients) 3017
Diprolene AF Cream 0.05% (Infrequent) 3014
Diprosone Cream, USP 0.05% 3018
Dovonex Ointment 0.005% (Less than 1%) 3375
Dovonex Scalp Solution 0.005% 3375
Elidel Cream 1% (0.9% to 6.1%) 2198
Elocon Cream 0.1% (Infrequent) 3019
Elocon Lotion 0.1% (4 in 156 subjects) 3020
Elocon Ointment 0.1% (Infrequent) 3021
Eskalith 1406
Evoclin Foam, 1% 1025
▲ Flovent Diskus 50 mcg (1% to 3%) 1415
Fuzeon Injection (2.4%) 2772
Gengraf Capsules (1% to less than 3%) 458
Guanidine Hydrochloride Tablets 3030
▲ Intron A for Injection (Less than 5%) 3038
Invirase (Less than 2%) 2776
Lexapro Oral Solution (Infrequent) 1193
Lexapro Tablets (Infrequent) 1193
Lithobid Tablets 1670
Locoid Cream (Infrequent) 1138
Locoid Lipocream Cream (Infrequent) 1138
Locoid (Infrequent) 1138
Lotrisone 3054
Lotronex Tablets (Rare) 1479
Luxíq Foam 1026
Neoral Soft Gelatin Capsules (1% to less than 3%) 2247
Neoral Oral Solution (1% to less than 3%) 2247
Norvir (Less than 2%) 499
Olux Foam (Less than 2%) 1027
Oxistat Cream (0.3%) 1498
Oxsoralen-Ultra Capsules 3354
Pandel Cream, 0.1% 1017
Pramosone 1139
ProctoFoam-HC 3113
▲ Protopic Ointment (4% to 11%) 629
Rescriptor Tablets 2535
Sustiva Capsules (Less than 2%) 957
▲ Temovate Gel (Among most frequent) 1550
Temovate Ointment (Less frequent) 1549
Temovate Scalp Application (2 of 294 patients; infrequent) 1551
Temovate E Emollient (Less than 2%) 1552
Topicort .05% Gel 3288
Topicort .25% Cream 3288
Topicort .25% Ointment 3288
Topicort LP .05% Cream 3288
Tri-Luma Cream 1213
U-cort 1% Cream 3289
Vanos Cream 1864
Viracept (Less than 2%) 2556

Folliculosis
▲ Elestat Ophthalmic Solution (1% to 10%) 1643

Fontanels, bulging
Dynacin Tablets 1859

Food craving
Vantas (Less than 2%) 3367

Foot drop
Actiq (Less than 1%) 993
▲ Copaxone for Injection (3%) 3292
Kadian Capsules (Less than 3%) 572
Matulane Capsules 3188
Prozac Pulvules and Liquid (Rare) 1771
Thalomid Capsules 979

Forceps delivery, increased incidence
Naropin Injection 640

Foreign body reaction
Alamast Ophthalmic Solution (Less than 5%) 3371
Alphagan P Ophthalmic Solution (1% to 4%) 563
▲ Alrex Ophthalmic Suspension 0.2% (5% to 15%) ⊙243
▲ Ciloxan Ophthalmic Ointment (Less than 10%) 554
HMS Sterile Ophthalmic Suspension ⊙228
▲ Lotemax Ophthalmic Suspension 0.5% (5% to 15%) ⊙249
▲ Lumigan Ophthalmic Solution (3% to 10%) 569
▲ Travatan Ophthalmic Solution (5% to 10%) 559
▲ Xalatan Sterile Ophthalmic Solution (5% to 15%) 2654

Forgetfulness
Lariam Tablets (Occasional) 2790
Lexapro Oral Solution (Infrequent) 1193
Lexapro Tablets (Infrequent) 1193
Prochieve 4% Gel 1018
Prochieve 8% Gel 1018

Fracture, humerus
Tamiflu Capsules (Less than 1%) 2810
Tamiflu Oral Suspension (Less than 1%) 2810

Fracture, pathological
Actiq (Less than 1%) 993
▲ Arimidex Tablets (2% to 5%) 665
Aromasin Tablets (Less frequent) 2600
▲ Casodex Tablets (2% to 5%) 670
Depo-Medrol Injectable Suspension 2615
▲ Doxil Injection (1% to 10%) 3302
Effexor Tablets (Rare) 3405
Effexor XR Capsules (Rare) 3411
Herceptin I.V. (At least one of the 958 patients) 1234
Lamictal (Rare) 1449
Seroquel Tablets (Infrequent) 691

Fractures, long bones
Decadron Phosphate Injection 1931
Decadron Tablets 1929
Depo-Medrol Injectable Suspension 2615
Depo-Medrol Single-Dose Vial 2617
Hydrocortone Tablets 1963
Pediapred Oral Solution 3319

Fractures, osteoporotic
depo-subQ provera 104 Injectable Suspension (Rare) 2622

Fractures, unspecified
Celebrex Capsules (0.1% to 1.9%) 3130
Crestor Tablets (Greater than or equal to 1%) 672
Exelon Capsules (2% or more) 2204
Femara Tablets 2210
Klonopin (Infrequent) 2782
Levaquin in 5% Dextrose Injection (0.1% to 0.9%) 2453
Levaquin (0.1% to 0.9%) 2453
Neurontin Capsules (1.1%) 2498
Neurontin Oral Solution (1.1%) 2498
Neurontin Tablets (1.1%) 2498
Omacor Capsules 2735
Pulmicort Respules (1% to 3%) 654
▲ Simulect for Injection (3% to 10%) 2268
Tasmar Tablets (1% or more) 3360
Xolair (2%) 1259

Fractures, vertebral compression
Decadron Tablets 1929
Depo-Medrol Single-Dose Vial 2617
Hydrocortone Tablets 1963

Free T3 resin uptake, decrease
(*see under* T3, decrease)

Frequent blinking
Abilify Tablets (Rare) 916
Abilify Tablets (Rare) 2472

Fretfulness
(*see under* Anxiety)

Frigidity, unspecified
Wellbutrin Tablets (Infrequent) 1579

Fullness, abdominal
(*see under* Abdominal bloating)

Fundi with microhemorrhage, ocular
Neurontin Capsules (Rare) 2498
Neurontin Oral Solution (Rare) 2498
Neurontin Tablets (Rare) 2498

Fungal invasion
Blephamide Ophthalmic Ointment 563
Blephamide Ophthalmic Suspension 564
FML Ophthalmic Ointment (Possibility) ⊙225
FML Ophthalmic Suspension (Possibility) ⊙224
FML Forte Ophthalmic Suspension (Possibility) ⊙223
FML-S Liquifilm Sterile Ophthalmic Suspension ⊙226
Pred Mild Sterile Ophthalmic Suspension ⊙236
Pred-G Ophthalmic Suspension ⊙234
Pred-G Sterile Ophthalmic Ointment ⊙235
TobraDex Ophthalmic Ointment 558
TobraDex Ophthalmic Suspension 558

Furunculosis
Ambien Tablets (Rare) 2867
Astelin Nasal Spray (Infrequent) 1876
Centany Ointment, 2% (0.7%) 2382
Copaxone for Injection (Infrequent) 3292
Depacon Injection (1% or more) 412
Depakene (1% or more) 417
Depakote Sprinkle Capsules 422
▲ Depakote Tablets (1% to 5%) 427
Depakote ER Tablets (Greater than 1%) 433
▲ Doxil Injection (1% to 10%) 3302
Effexor Tablets (Rare) 3405
Effexor XR Capsules (Rare) 3411
▲ Elocon Cream 0.1% (Approximately 7%) 3019
▲ Elocon Ointment 0.1% (4.8% to approximately 7%) 3021
Evoxac Capsules (Less than 1%) 1042
Gabitril Tablets (Infrequent) 998
Geodon for Injection (Up to 2%) 2514
▲ Intron A for Injection (Less than 5%) 3038
Invirase (Less than 2%) 2776
Kaletra (Less than 2%) 474
Lexapro Oral Solution (Infrequent) 1193
Lexapro Tablets (Infrequent) 1193
Lunesta Tablets (Rare) 3139
Neurontin Capsules (Infrequent) 2498
Neurontin Oral Solution (Infrequent) 2498
Neurontin Tablets (Infrequent) 2498
▲ Nipent for Injection (4%) 3216
Paxil CR Controlled-Release Tablets (Infrequent) 1509
Paxil (Infrequent) 1501
Pletal Tablets (Less than 2%) 2478
Protopic Ointment (Greater than or equal to 1%) 629
Prozac Pulvules and Liquid (Rare) 1771
Requip Tablets (Infrequent) 1528
Rilutek Tablets (Rare) 2945
Risperdal M-Tab Orally Disintegrating Tablets (Rare) 1658
Risperdal (Rare) 1658
Soriatane Capsules (Less than 1%) 1028
Tasmar Tablets (Infrequent) 3360
Teveten Tablets (Less than 1%) 1707
Teveten HCT Tablets (Less than 1%) 1710
Uniretic Tablets (Less than 1%) 3114
VFEND I.V. (Less than 2%) 2543
VFEND Oral Suspension (Less than 2%) 2543
VFEND Tablets (Less than 2%) 2543
Zyrtec Chewable Tablets (Less than 2%) 2589
Zyrtec (Less than 2%) 2589
Zyrtec-D 12 Hour Extended Release Tablets (Less than 2%) 2591

Fussiness
▲ Prevnar for Injection (16.7% to 54.1%) 3460

G

Gagging
Lexapro Oral Solution (Infrequent) 1193
Lexapro Tablets (Infrequent) 1193

Gait, abnormal
Abilify Tablets (Frequent) 916
Abilify Tablets (Frequent) 2472
Actimmune (Rare) 1646
Actiq (1% to 4%) 993
Ambien Tablets (Rare) 2867
Aricept Tablets (Infrequent) 1086
Aricept ODT Tablets (Infrequent) 1086
▲ Avastin IV (1% to 5%) 1229
Avinza Capsules (Less than 5%) 1714
Campath Ampules 826
Cardizem LA Extended Release Tablets (Less than 2%) 1699
Celexa (Infrequent) 1177
Cipro I.V. (1% or less) 2998
Cipro I.V. Pharmacy Bulk Package (1% or less) 3509
Cipro (Less than 1%) 2991
Cipro XR Tablets 3004
Colazal Capsules 2845
Copaxone for Injection (At least 2%) 3292
▲ Depacon Injection (1% to 5%) 412
▲ Depakene (1% to 5%) 417
▲ Depakote Sprinkle Capsules (1% to 5%) 422
▲ Depakote Tablets (1% to 5%) 427
▲ Depakote ER Tablets (1% to 5%) 433
▲ DepoCyt Injection (1% to 4%) 1121
Duragesic Transdermal System (1% or greater) 2448
Effexor Tablets (Rare) 3405

Effexor XR Capsules (Rare) 3411
Evoxac Capsules 1042
Exelon Capsules (Frequent) 2204
Flexeril Tablets (Rare) 1832
Flumadine (Less than 0.3%) 1186
Frova Tablets (Infrequent) 1101
▲ Gabitril Tablets (3%) 998
Geodon Capsules (Frequent) 2514
▲ Intron A for Injection (Less than 5%) 3038
▲ Lamictal (4%) 1449
Levaquin in 5% Dextrose Injection (0.1% to 0.9%) 2453
Levaquin (0.1% to 0.9%) 2453
Lexapro Oral Solution 1193
Lexapro Tablets 1193
Lunesta Tablets (Rare) 3139
▲ Lyrica Capsules (1% to 8%) 2524
Maxalt Tablets (Infrequent) 1983
Maxalt-MLT Orally Disintegrating Tablets (Infrequent) 1983
Meridia Capsules 485
Migranal Nasal Spray (Rare) 3350
▲ Mirapex Tablets (Greater than or equal to 1% to 7%) 889
Namenda (Greater than or equal to 2%) 1199
Navelbine Injection 1494
Neurontin Capsules (1.5%) 2498
Neurontin Oral Solution (1.5%) 2498
Neurontin Tablets (1.5%) 2498
Norvir (Less than 2%) 499
OxyContin Tablets (Less than 1%) 2699
▲ Pacerone Tablets (4% to 9%) 3337
Parcopa Orally Disintegrating Tablets 3111
Paxil CR Controlled-Release Tablets (Rare) 1509
Paxil (Rare) 1501
Permax Tablets (1.6%) 3357
Prozac Pulvules and Liquid (Infrequent) 1771
Relpax Tablets (Rare) 2531
Requip Tablets (Infrequent) 1528
Reyataz Capsules (Less than 3%) 948
Rilutek Tablets (Infrequent) 2945
Risperdal Consta Long-Acting Injection (Infrequent) 1664
▲ Risperdal M-Tab Orally Disintegrating Tablets (17% to 34%) 1658
▲ Risperdal (17% to 34%) 1658
Roferon-A Injection (Infrequent) 2805
Rythmol SR Capsules 2736
Sandostatin LAR Depot (1% to 4%) 2264
Seroquel Tablets (Infrequent) 691
Sonata Capsules (Infrequent) 1686
Soriatane Capsules (Less than 1%) 1028
Stalevo Tablets 2270
Symbyax Capsules (Infrequent) 1788
Symmetrel 1115
Tasmar Tablets (1% or more) 3360
▲ Temodar Capsules (6%) 3088
Thalomid Capsules 979
Tiazac Capsules (Less than 2%) 1204
▲ Topamax Sprinkle Capsules (2% to 8%) 2438
▲ Topamax Tablets (2% to 8%) 2438
▲ Trileptal Oral Suspension (5% to 17%) 2281
▲ Trileptal Tablets (5% to 17%) 2281
▲ Vesanoid Capsules (3%) 2823
▲ Xeloda Tablets (Less than 5%) 2825
Zantac 150 Tablets 1597
Zantac Injection 1593
▲ Zavesca Capsules (8%) 543
Zoloft (Infrequent) 2581
Zonegran Capsules (Frequent) 1089
Zyprexa Tablets (Infrequent) 1798
Zyprexa IntraMuscular (Infrequent) 1798
Zyprexa ZYDIS Orally Disintegrating Tablets (Infrequent) 1798

Galactorrhea
Celexa (Infrequent) 1177
Cenestin Tablets, 0.45mg, 0.625mg, 0.9mg, 1.25mg 1063
Cenestin Tablets, 0.3mg 1063
Climara Transdermal System 795
Climara Pro Transdermal System 800
Covera-HS Tablets (Less than 2%) 3135
Demser Capsules (Infrequent) 1933
Depacon Injection 412
Depakene 417
Depakote Sprinkle Capsules 422
Depakote Tablets 427
Depakote ER Tablets 433
Depo-Provera Contraceptive Injection (Less than 1%) 2619
depo-subQ provera 104 Injectable Suspension 2622
Estratest Tablets 3196
Estratest H.S. Tablets 3196
Estrogel 0.06% 3200
Flexeril Tablets (Rare) 1832
Geodon 2514
Imitrex Injection 1431
Imitrex Nasal Spray (Rare) 1435
Imitrex Tablets (Rare) 1440
Menostar Transdermal System 805
Moban Tablets (Infrequent) 1108
Niravam Orally Disintegrating Tablets 3106
Paxil CR Controlled-Release Tablets 1509
Paxil 1501
Prefest Tablets 1069
Premarin Tablets 3443
Premphase Tablets 3452
Prempro Tablets 3452
Sandostatin Injection (Less than 1%) 2263
Sandostatin LAR Depot (Rare) 2264
Surmontil Capsules 2347
Tarka Tablets 519
Thalomid Capsules 979
Thioridazine Hydrochloride Tablets 2122
Verelan PM Capsules (2% or less) 3120
Vivactil Tablets 2350
Vivelle Transdermal System 2288
Vivelle-Dot Transdermal System 2293
Xanax XR Tablets 2655
Zoloft 2581

Gallbladder, sonographic abnormalities
Rocephin Injectable Vials, ADD-Vantage, Galaxy, Bulk 2801

Gallbladder disease
Activella Tablets 2311
Alesse-28 Tablets 3392
Cenestin Tablets, 0.45mg, 0.625mg, 0.9mg, 1.25mg 1063
Cenestin Tablets, 0.3mg 1063
Climara Transdermal System 795
Climara Pro Transdermal System 800
CombiPatch Transdermal System 2180
Estratest Tablets 3196
Estratest H.S. Tablets 3196
Estrogel 0.06% 3200
Lo/Ovral-28 Tablets 3423
Menostar Transdermal System 805
Ortho-Cept Tablets 2395
Ortho-Cyclen Tablets 2414
Ortho Evra Transdermal System 2402
Ortho Tri-Cyclen Tablets 2414
Ortho Tri-Cyclen Lo Tablets 2421
Prefest Tablets 1069
Premarin Intravenous 3440
Premarin Tablets 3443
Premarin Vaginal Cream 3449
Premphase Tablets 3452
Prempro Tablets 3452
Pulmozyme Inhalation Solution 1245
Rocephin Injectable Vials, ADD-Vantage, Galaxy, Bulk 2801
Sandostatin Injection (Frequent) 2263
Sandostatin LAR Depot (Rare) 2264
Seasonale Tablets 1073
Triphasil-28 Tablets 3483
Vivelle Transdermal System 2288
Vivelle-Dot Transdermal System 2293
Yasmin 28 Tablets 818

Gallstones
Imitrex Injection (Rare) 1431
Imitrex Nasal Spray 1435
Imitrex Tablets 1440
▲ Intron A for Injection (Less than 5%) 3038
Relafen Tablets (Less than 1%) 1523
Sandostatin Injection (Frequent) 2263

Gamma-glutamyl transferase, abnormal
Antara Capsules 2723
Vytorin 10/10 Tablets 2084
Vytorin 10/10 Tablets 3092
Vytorin 10/20 Tablets 2084
Vytorin 10/20 Tablets 3092
Vytorin 10/40 Tablets 2084
Vytorin 10/40 Tablets 3092
Vytorin 10/80 Tablets 2084
Vytorin 10/80 Tablets 3092

Gamma-glutamyl transferase, increase
Factive Tablets (0.5%) 2464
Zosyn 3492

Gamma-glutamyl transpeptidase, elevation
Accutane Capsules 2740
Adalat CC Tablets (Less than 1%) 2978
Advicor Tablets 1694
Altoprev Extended-Release Tablets 1151
Amnesteem Capsules 2126
▲ Arimidex Tablets (2% to 5%) 665
Asacol Delayed-Release Tablets 2688
Avelox (0.1% to less than 2%) 2984
Axert Tablets (Rare) 2430
Benicar HCT Tablets (Greater than 1%) 2852
Betaseron for SC Injection 791
Biaxin/Biaxin XL (Less than 1%) 402
▲ CellCept Capsules (3% to less than 20%) 2751
▲ CellCept Intravenous (3% to less than 20%) 2751
▲ CellCept Oral Suspension (3% to less than 20%) 2751
▲ CellCept Tablets (3% to less than 20%) 2751
Cialis Tablets (Less than 2%) 1806
Cipro I.V. (Infrequent) 2998
Cipro I.V. Pharmacy Bulk Package (Infrequent) 3509
Cipro (Less than 0.1%) 2991
▲ Coreg Tablets (Greater than 1% to 3%) 1376
Effexor Tablets 3405
Effexor XR Capsules 3411
Epzicom Tablets 1402
Evoxac Capsules (Less than 1%) 1042
Factive Tablets (Less than or equal to 0.1%) 2464
▲ Fortaz (1 in 19) 1422
Fuzeon Injection 2772
Geodon Capsules (Rare) 2514
Inspra Tablets 2520
▲ Kaletra (6% to 29%) 474
Lescol Capsules 2227
Lescol Capsules 2730
Lescol XL Tablets 2227
Lescol XL Tablets 2730
Levitra Tablets (Less than 2%) 3048
Lofibra Capsules 1217
Mevacor Tablets 1996
Mobic Oral Suspension (Less than 2%) 893
Mobic Tablets (Less than 2%) 893
Neurontin Capsules (Rare) 2498
Neurontin Oral Solution (Rare) 2498
Neurontin Tablets (Rare) 2498
▲ Novantrone for Injection Concentrate (3% to 15%) 3158
Omnicef Capsules (1%) 506
Oncaspar 1123
Pentasa Capsules (Less than 1%) 3182
Prevacid Delayed-Release Capsules 3268
Prevacid for Delayed-Release Oral Suspension 3268
Prevacid NapraPAC 3277
Prevacid SoluTab Delayed-Release Orally Disintegrating Tablets 3268
PREVPAC (Less than 1%) 3281
Prilosec OTC Tablets (Rare) 2674
▲ Prograf Capsules and Injection (3% to 15%) 624
Protonix I.V. (Less than 1%) 3468
Protonix Tablets (Less than 1%) 3465
Provigil Tablets (At least 1%) 1002
Rescriptor Tablets (Up to 1.8%) 2535
Rilutek Tablets (Infrequent) 2945
Risperdal Consta Long-Acting Injection (Rare) 1664
Rythmol SR Capsules 2736
Seroquel Tablets (Infrequent to 1%) 691
▲ Soriatane Capsules (Approximately 1 in 3 patients) 1028
Symmetrel 1115
Ticlid Tablets (Rare) 2813
▲ Topamax Sprinkle Capsules (1% to 3%) 2438
▲ Topamax Tablets (1% to 3%) 2438
Tricor Tablets 523
Trileptal Oral Suspension 2281
Trileptal Tablets 2281
Vantin Tablets and Oral Suspension 2650
▲ Ventavis Inhalation Solution (6%) 1036
Vermox Chewable Tablets (Rare) 1853
VFEND I.V. (Less than 2%) 2543
VFEND Oral Suspension (Less than 2%) 2543
VFEND Tablets (Less than 2%) 2543
Viracept (Less than 2%) 2556
Viramune Oral Suspension (2.4%) 903
Viramune Tablets (2.4%) 903
Zegerid Powder for Oral Solution (Rare) 2972
Ziagen 1600
Zithromax (1% to 2%) 2568
Zithromax for Oral Suspension, 300 mg, 600 mg, 900 mg, 1200 mg (1% to 2%) 2561
Zithromax Tablets, 250 mg, 500 mg (1% to 2%) 2561
Zithromax Tablets, 600 mg (1% to 2%) 2568
Zithromax Tri-Pak (1% to 2%) 2561
Zithromax Z-Pak (1% to 2%) 2568
Zocor Tablets 2078

Gangrene
Gemzar for Injection (Very rare) 1743
Levaquin in 5% Dextrose Injection (0.1% to 0.9%) 2453
Levaquin (0.1% to 0.9%) 2453
Proleukin for Injection (1%) 1007
Requip Tablets (Rare) 1528

Gangrene, cutaneous
Miradon Tablets 3056

Gangrene, peripheral
Celebrex Capsules (Less than 0.1%) 3130
Requip Tablets (Infrequent) 1528

Gasping syndrome
Novarel for Injection 1147

Gastric acid, regurgitation
Crixivan Capsules (2.7%) 1918
▲ Fosamax (Up to 4.1%) 1949
▲ Fosamax Plus D Tablets (0% to 4.2%) 1956
Prilosec OTC Tablets (1.9%) 2674
Zegerid Powder for Oral Solution (1.7%) 2972

Gastric discomfort
(*see under* Distress, gastrointestinal)

Gastric disorder
(*see under* Distress, gastrointestinal)

Gastric emptying, impaired
Cymbalta Delayed-Release Capsules (Infrequent) 1729

Gastric nodule
Prevacid NapraPAC (Less than 1%) 3277

Gastric regurgitation
Wellbutrin SR Sustained-Release Tablets (Infrequent) 1583
Wellbutrin XL Extended-Release Tablets (Infrequent) 1588

Gastritis
Abilify Tablets (Infrequent) 916
Abilify Tablets (Infrequent) 2472
Actonel Tablets (2.5%) 2679
Actonel with Calcium Tablets (2.5%) 2684
Aggrenox Capsules (Less than 1%) 855
Agrylin Capsules (1% to 5%) 3172
Ambien Tablets (Rare) 2867
Amerge Tablets (Rare) 1312
Anaprox Tablets (Less than 1%) 2769
Anaprox DS Tablets (Less than 1%) 2769
Antara Capsules 2723
▲ Arava Tablets (1% to 3%) 2881
Aricept Tablets (Infrequent) 1086
Aricept ODT Tablets (Infrequent) 1086
Arthrotec Tablets (Rare) 3126
Asacol Delayed-Release Tablets 2688
Atacand HCT (0.5% or greater) 637
Augmentin 1331
Augmentin Tablets 1334
Augmentin XR Extended-Release Tablets 1340
Augmentin ES-600 Powder for Oral Suspension 1337
Avelox (Less than 0.1%) 2984
Axert Tablets (Rare) 2430
Boniva Tablets (2.2%) 2747
Buphenyl Powder (Less than or equal to 2%) 3327
Buphenyl Tablets (Less than or equal to 2%) 3327
Caduet Tablets (Less than 2%) 2507
Cafcit (2.2%) 1854
Campral Tablets (Infrequent) 1175
Cancidas for Injection (0%) 1894
Carnitor Injection (Less frequent) 3185
Cataflam Tablets (Occasionally) 2173
Celebrex Capsules (0.1% to 1.9%) 3130
Celexa (Infrequent) 1177
▲ CellCept Capsules (3% to less than 20%) 2751
▲ CellCept Intravenous (3% to less than 20%) 2751

▲ CellCept Oral Suspension (3% to less than 20%) 2751
▲ CellCept Tablets (3% to less than 20%) 2751
Cialis Tablets (Less than 2%) 1806
Clinoril Tablets (Less than 1%) 1899
Comtan Tablets (1%) 2186
Copaxone for Injection (At least 2%) 3292
▲ Cozaar Tablets (Less than 1% to 5%) 1913
Crestor Tablets (Greater than or equal to 1%) 672
Cymbalta Delayed-Release Capsules (Frequent) 1729
Didronel Tablets 2693
Dolobid Tablets (Less than 1 in 100) 1937
Doxil Injection (Less than 1%) 3302
EC-Naprosyn Delayed-Release Tablets (Less than 1%) 2769
Effexor Tablets (Infrequent) 3405
Effexor XR Capsules (Infrequent) 3411
Elmiron Capsules (Less than or equal to 1%) 2393
▲ Emend Capsules (4.2%) 1944
Enbrel for Injection 580
Eskalith 1406
Evoxac Capsules (Less than 1%) 1042
Exelon Capsules (Frequent) 2204
Factive Tablets (0.1% to 1%) 2464
Flexeril Tablets (Less than 1%) 1832
▲ Flolan for Injection (61%) 1408
Fortical Nasal Spray (Less than 1%) 3336
Fosamax (0.2% to 1.1%) 1949
Fosamax Plus D Tablets (0.2% to 1.1%) 1956
Gabitril Tablets (Infrequent) 998
Gengraf Capsules (1% to less than 3%) 458
Gleevec Tablets (Infrequent) 2221
▲ Humatrope Vials and Cartridges (Up to 6.67%) 1756
Hyzaar 1964
▲ Imdur Tablets (Less than or equal to 5%) 3032
Imitrex Injection 1431
Imitrex Nasal Spray 1435
▲ Intron A for Injection (Less than 5%) 3038
Invanz for Injection (Greater than 0.1%) 1974
Invirase (Less than 2%) 2776
Kaletra (Less than 2%) 474
Ketek Tablets (Greater than or equal to 0.2% to less than 2%) 2920
Klonopin 2782
Lamictal (Rare) 1449
Levaquin in 5% Dextrose Injection (0.1% to 0.9%) 2453
Levaquin (0.1% to 0.9%) 2453
Levitra Tablets (Less than 2%) 3048
Lexapro Oral Solution (Infrequent) 1193
Lexapro Tablets (Infrequent) 1193
Lipitor Tablets (Less than 2%) 2495
Lithobid Tablets 1670
Lofibra Capsules 1217
Lotensin Tablets (Less than 1%) 2232
Lotronex Tablets (Rare) 1479
Lunesta Tablets (Rare) 3139
Lyrica Capsules (0.1% to 1%) 2524
▲ Malarone Tablets (2% to 3%) 1484
▲ Malarone Pediatric Tablets (2% to 3%) 1484
▲ Mavik Tablets (4.2%) 482
Maxalt Tablets (Rare) 1983
Maxalt-MLT Orally Disintegrating Tablets (Rare) 1983
Meridia Capsules (1.7%) 485
Miacalcin Nasal Spray (Less than 1%) 2242
Micardis Tablets (More than 0.3%) 884
Micardis HCT Tablets 886
Mobic Oral Suspension (Less than 2%) 893
Mobic Tablets (Less than 2%) 893
Nalfon Capsules (Less than 1%) 2504
Namenda 1199
Naprosyn Suspension (Less than 1%) 2769
Naprosyn Tablets (Less than 1%) 2769
Neoral Soft Gelatin Capsules (1% to less than 3%) 2247
Neoral Oral Solution (1% to less than 3%) 2247
Neurontin Capsules (Infrequent) 2498
Neurontin Oral Solution (Infrequent) 2498
Neurontin Tablets (Infrequent) 2498
Norvasc Tablets (Less than or equal to 0.1%) 2529
Norvir (Less than 2%) 499
Omacor Capsules 2735
▲ OxyContin Tablets (Between 1% and 5%) 2699
Permax Tablets (Infrequent) 3357
Pletal Tablets (Less than 2%) 2478
Prevacid Delayed-Release Capsules (Less than 1%) 3268
Prevacid for Delayed-Release Oral Suspension (Less than 1%) 3268
Prevacid NapraPAC (Less than 1%) 3277
Prevacid SoluTab Delayed-Release Orally Disintegrating Tablets (Less than 1%) 3268
PREVPAC (Less than 1%) 3281
Prinivil Tablets (0.3% to 1.0%) 2029
Prinzide Tablets 2033
Prochieve 4% Gel 1018
Prochieve 8% Gel 1018
▲ Prograf Capsules and Injection (3% to 15%) 624
Proleukin for Injection 1007
ProSom Tablets (Infrequent) 512
Protopic Ointment (Greater than or equal to 1%) 629
Prozac Pulvules and Liquid (Infrequent) 1771
▲ Rapamune Oral Solution and Tablets (3% to 20%) 3472
Razadyne ER Extended-Release Capsules (Infrequent) 2434
Razadyne (Infrequent) 2434
ReFacto Vials 3479
Relafen Tablets (1% to 3%) 1523
Relpax Tablets (Infrequent) 2531
Requip Tablets (Infrequent) 1528
▲ Revatio Tablets (3%) 2541
Reyataz Capsules (Less than 3%) 948
Rilutek Tablets (Infrequent) 2945
Risperdal Consta Long-Acting Injection (Infrequent) 1664
Risperdal M-Tab Orally Disintegrating Tablets (Infrequent) 1658
Risperdal (Infrequent) 1658
Rythmol SR Capsules 2736
Sanctura Tablets 1133
Sandimmune (2% or less) 2259
Sandostatin LAR Depot (1% to 4%) 2264
Seroquel Tablets (Infrequent) 691
Sonata Capsules (Infrequent) 1686
Soriatane Capsules (Less than 1%) 1028
Stalevo Tablets (1%) 2270
Sular Tablets (Less than or equal to 1%) 1163
Symbyax Capsules (Infrequent) 1788
Tequin Injection (Less than 0.1%) 964
Tequin Tablets (Less than 0.1%) 964
Teveten Tablets (Less than 1%) 1707
Teveten HCT Tablets (Less than 1%) 1710
Thymoglobulin for Injection (1.2%) 2848
▲ Topamax Sprinkle Capsules (0% to 3%) 2438
▲ Topamax Tablets (0% to 3%) 2438
Tricor Tablets 523
Triglide Tablets 1165
Trileptal Oral Suspension (1% to 2%) 2281
Trileptal Tablets (1% to 2%) 2281
Uniretic Tablets (Less than 1%) 3114
Vantin Tablets and Oral Suspension (Less than 1%) 2650
Viagra Tablets (Less than 2%) 2552
Vicoprofen Tablets (Less than 3%) 533
Voltaren Tablets (Occasionally) 2298
Voltaren-XR Tablets (Occasionally) 2301
Xeloda Tablets 2825
Zelnorm Tablets 2303
▲ Zenapax for Injection (2% to 5%) 2838
Zestoretic Tablets 701
Zestril Tablets (0.3% to 1.0%) 704
Zithromax Capsules, 250 mg (1% or less) 2568
Zithromax for IV Infusion (1% or less) 2573
Zithromax for Oral Suspension, 300 mg, 600 mg, 900 mg, 1200 mg (1% or less) 2561
Zithromax Tablets, 250 mg, 500 mg (1% or less) 2561
Zithromax Tri-Pak (1% or less) 2561
Zmax for Oral Suspension (Less then 1%) 2577
Zoloft (Rare) 2581
Zomig Nasal Spray (Rare) 718
Zomig Tablets (Rare) 714
Zomig-ZMT Tablets (Rare) 714
Zonegran Capsules (Infrequent) 1089
Zosyn (1.0% or less) 3492
Zyprexa Tablets (Infrequent) 1798
Zyprexa ZYDIS Orally Disintegrating Tablets (Infrequent) 1798
Zyrtec Chewable Tablets (Less than 2%) 2589
Zyrtec (Less than 2%) 2589
Zyrtec-D 12 Hour Extended Release Tablets (Less than 2%) 2591

Gastritis, hemorrhagic

Plavix Tablets (Less than 1%) 940
Plavix Tablets (Less than 1%) 2942
Requip Tablets (Rare) 1528

Gastroduodenitis

Lotronex Tablets (Rare) 1479

Gastroenteritis

Abilify Tablets (Infrequent) 916
Abilify Tablets (Infrequent) 2472
AccuNeb Inhalation Solution (0.9% to 3.4%) 1055
Aceon Tablets (2 mg, 4 mg, 8 mg) (0.3% to 1%) 3191
Aciphex Tablets 1081
Actiq (Less than 1%) 993
Activella Tablets (0% to 6%) 2311
▲ Actonel Tablets (3.5% to 3.8%) 2679
▲ Actonel with Calcium Tablets (3.5% to 3.8%) 2684
▲ Advair Diskus 100/50 (1% to 3%) 1291
▲ Advair Diskus 250/50 (1% to 3%) 1291
▲ Advair Diskus 500/50 (1% to 3%) 1291
Altace Capsules (Less than 1%) 1673
Ambien Tablets (Infrequent) 2867
Amerge Tablets (Infrequent) 1312
Amevive 836
Antara Capsules 2723
▲ Arava Tablets (3%) 2881
Aricept Tablets (Infrequent) 1086
Aricept ODT Tablets (Infrequent) 1086
Asacol Delayed-Release Tablets (2% or greater) 2688
Asmanex Twisthaler (1% to less than 3%) 2981
Astelin Nasal Spray (Infrequent) 1876
Atacand Tablets (0.5% or greater) 634
Atacand HCT (0.5% or greater) 637
Avalide Tablets 922
Avalide Tablets 2889
Avapro Tablets (Less than 1%) 925
Avapro Tablets (Less than 1%) 2886
Avinza Capsules (Less than 5%) 1714
Axert Tablets (Rare) 2430
Benicar Tablets (Greater than 0.5%) 2850
Benicar HCT Tablets (Greater than 1%) 2852
Caduet Tablets (Less than 2%) 2507
Campath Ampules 826
Campral Tablets (Infrequent) 1175
Celebrex Capsules (0.1% to 1.9%) 3130
Celexa (Infrequent) 1177
▲ CellCept Capsules (3% to less than 20%) 2751
▲ CellCept Intravenous (3% to less than 20%) 2751
▲ CellCept Oral Suspension (3% to less than 20%) 2751
▲ CellCept Tablets (3% to less than 20%) 2751
Clinoril Tablets (Less than 1%) 1899
Clozapine Tablets (Less than 1%) 2141
Clozaril Tablets (Less than 1%) 2174
Colazal Capsules 2845
▲ Copaxone for Injection (3%) 3292
Crestor Tablets (Greater than or equal to 2%) 672
Depacon Injection (1% or more) 412
Depakene (1% or more) 417
Depakote Sprinkle Capsules 422
▲ Depakote Tablets (1% to 5%) 427
Depakote ER Tablets (Greater than 1%) 433
Effexor Tablets (Infrequent) 3405
Effexor XR Capsules (Infrequent) 3411
▲ Elidel Cream 1% (1.8% to 7.4%) 2198
Eligard 7.5 mg (2.5%) 2896
Enbrel for Injection 580
Epivir 1394
Evista Tablets (2.6%) 1735
Evoxac Capsules (Less than 1%) 1042
Exelon Capsules (Infrequent) 2204
Factive Tablets (Less than or equal to 0.1%) 2464
FazaClo Orally Disintegrating Tablets (Less than 1%) 547
▲ Flovent Diskus 50 mcg (1% to 3%) 1415
Gabitril Tablets (1% or more) 998
Gengraf Capsules (1% to less than 3%) 458
Gleevec Tablets (Infrequent) 2221
Herceptin I.V. (At least one of the 958 patients) 1234
▲ Humira Injection (Less than 5%) 464
Imitrex Injection 1431
Imitrex Nasal Spray (Rare) 1435
Indocin Capsules (Less than 1%) 1968
Indocin I.V. (Less than 1%) 1973
Indocin (Less than 1%) 1968
▲ Intron A for Injection (Less than 5%) 3038
Invirase (Less than 2%) 2776
Kaletra (Less than 2%) 474
▲ Keppra Oral Solution (1% to 4%) 3307
▲ Keppra Tablets (1% to 4%) 3307
Ketek Tablets (Greater than or equal to 0.2% to less than 2%) 2920
Kogenate FS 3517
Levaquin in 5% Dextrose Injection (0.1% to 0.9%) 2453
Levaquin (0.1% to 0.9%) 2453
Lexapro Oral Solution (Frequent) 1193
Lexapro Tablets (Frequent) 1193
Lipitor Tablets (Less than 2%) 2495
Lofibra Capsules 1217
Lotensin HCT Tablets (0.3% or more) 2235
Lotronex Tablets (Rare) 1479
Lyrica Capsules (Greater than or equal to 1%) 2524
Meridia Capsules (Greater than or equal to 1%) 485
Micardis Tablets (More than 0.3%) 884
Micardis HCT Tablets 886
Namenda (Infrequent) 1199
Neoral Soft Gelatin Capsules (1% to less than 3%) 2247
Neoral Oral Solution (1% to less than 3%) 2247
Neurontin Capsules (Infrequent) 2498
Neurontin Oral Solution (Infrequent) 2498
Neurontin Tablets (Infrequent) 2498
Nexium Delayed-Release Capsules (Less than 1%) 645
Nexium I.V. (Less than 1%) 649
▲ Norditropin Cartridges (8%) 2318
Norvir (Less than 2%) 499
Omacor Capsules 2735
Paxil CR Controlled-Release Tablets (Rare) 1509
Paxil (Rare) 1501
PEG-Intron Powder for Injection (Less than or equal to 1%) 3062
Permax Tablets (Infrequent) 3357
Pletal Tablets (Less than 2%) 2478
Prevacid Delayed-Release Capsules (Less than 1%) 3268
Prevacid for Delayed-Release Oral Suspension (Less than 1%) 3268
Prevacid NapraPAC (Less than 1%) 3277
Prevacid SoluTab Delayed-Release Orally Disintegrating Tablets (Less than 1%) 3268
Prevnar for Injection 3460
PREVPAC (Less than 1%) 3281
Primaxin I.M. 2022
Primaxin I.V. (Less than 0.2%) 2024
Prograf Capsules and Injection 624
Prometrium Capsules (100 mg, 200 mg) (Less than 5%) 3205
Protonix I.V. (Greater than or equal to 1%) 3468
Protonix Tablets (Greater than or equal to 1%) 3465
Protopic Ointment (2% to 4%) 629
Provigil Tablets (At least 1%) 1002
Prozac Pulvules and Liquid (Infrequent) 1771
▲ Pulmicort Respules (5%) 654
▲ Rapamune Oral Solution and Tablets (3% to 20%) 3472
Raptiva for Injection 1247
Razadyne ER Extended-Release Capsules (Infrequent) 2434
Razadyne (Infrequent) 2434
ReFacto Vials 3479
Relafen Tablets (Less than 1%) 1523
Rescriptor Tablets 2535
Reyataz Capsules (Less than 3%) 948
Risperdal M-Tab Orally Disintegrating Tablets (Rare) 1658
Risperdal (Rare) 1658
Sandostatin LAR Depot (1% to 4%) 2264
Seroquel Tablets (Infrequent to 2%) 691
▲ Simulect for Injection (3% to 10%) 2268
Singulair (Greater than or equal to 2%) 2047
Sonata Capsules (Infrequent) 1686
Soriatane Capsules (Less than 1%) 1028
Symbyax Capsules (Infrequent) 1788

Synagis (More than 1%) 1868
Targretin Capsules 1719
Tasmar Tablets (Infrequent) 3360
Teveten Tablets (Less than 1%) 1707
Teveten HCT Tablets (Less than 1%) 1710
Thalomid Capsules 979
▲ Topamax Sprinkle Capsules (1% to 3%) 2438
▲ Topamax Tablets (1% to 3%) 2438
Tricor Tablets 523
Triglide Tablets 1165
Trizivir Tablets 1565
Uniretic Tablets (Less than 1%) 3114
Vaqta 2067
VFEND I.V. (Less than 2%) 2543
VFEND Oral Suspension (Less than 2%) 2543
VFEND Tablets (Less than 2%) 2543
Viagra Tablets (Less than 2%) 2552
Vicoprofen Tablets (Less than 1%) 533
▲ Xeloda Tablets (Less than 5%) 2825
Xopenex HFA Inhalation Aerosol 3151
Xopenex Inhalation Solution 3143
Xopenex Inhalation Solution Concentrate 3147
Yasmin 28 Tablets (Greater than 1%) 818
Zoloft (Infrequent) 2581
Zomig Tablets (Infrequent) 714
Zomig-ZMT Tablets (Infrequent) 714
Zonegran Capsules (Infrequent) 1089
Zyprexa Tablets (Infrequent) 1798
Zyprexa ZYDIS Orally Disintegrating Tablets (Infrequent) 1798

Gastroenteritis, infectious
Singulair (1.5%) 2047

Gastroenteritis, viral
▲ Flovent Diskus 50 mcg (3%) 1415
▲ Strattera Capsules (2% or greater) 1784

Gastroesophageal reflux
Abilify Tablets (Infrequent) 916
Abilify Tablets (Infrequent) 2472
Aldara Cream, 5% (1.4%) 1814
Amerge Tablets (Rare) 1312
Aptivus Capsules (Less than 2%) 859
Axert Tablets (Rare) 2430
▲ Byetta Injection (Greater than or equal to 1% to less than 5%) 605
Celebrex Capsules (0.1% to 1.9%) 3130
Celexa (Rare) 1177
Cialis Tablets (Less than 2%) 1806
▲ Ditropan XL Extended Release Tablets (2% to less than 5%) 2391
▲ Eloxatin for Injection (1% to 5%) 2908
Emend Capsules (Greater than 0.5%) 1944
▲ Evoxac Capsules (1% to 3%) 1042
Exelon Capsules (Infrequent) 2204
▲ Flolan for Injection (61%) 1408
Fosamax (0.7% to 2.8%) 1949
Fosamax Plus D Tablets (0.7% to 2.8%) 1956
Frova Tablets (Rare) 1101
Gleevec Tablets (Less common) 2221
Imitrex Injection (Infrequent) 1431
Imitrex Nasal Spray (Infrequent) 1435
Imitrex Tablets (Infrequent) 1440
Kadian Capsules (Less than 3%) 572
Levaquin in 5% Dextrose Injection (0.1% to 0.9%) 2453
Levaquin (0.1% to 0.9%) 2453
Levitra Tablets (Less than 2%) 3048
Lexapro Oral Solution (Frequent) 1193
Lexapro Tablets (Frequent) 1193
Micardis Tablets (More than 0.3%) 884
Micardis HCT Tablets 886
Mobic Oral Suspension (Less than 2%) 893
Mobic Tablets (Less than 2%) 893
▲ Myfortic Tablets (3% to less than 20%) 2244
Namenda 1199
ReoPro Vials (0.1%) 1779
Requip Tablets (Infrequent) 1528
Rescriptor Tablets 2535
Risperdal Consta Long-Acting Injection (Infrequent) 1664
Risperdal M-Tab Orally Disintegrating Tablets (Rare) 1658
Risperdal (Rare) 1658
Rythmol SR Capsules 2736
Seroquel Tablets (Infrequent) 691
▲ Spiriva HandiHaler (1% to 3%) 899
Topamax Sprinkle Capsules (Greater than 1%) 2438
Topamax Tablets (Greater than 1%) 2438
Zelnorm Tablets 2303

Gastrointestinal anomaly, unspecified
Prevacid Delayed-Release Capsules (Less than 1%) 3268
Prevacid for Delayed-Release Oral Suspension (Less than 1%) 3268
Prevacid NapraPAC (Less than 1%) 3277
Prevacid SoluTab Delayed-Release Orally Disintegrating Tablets (Less than 1%) 3268
PREVPAC (Less than 1%) 3281
Zomig Tablets 714

Gastrointestinal bleeding
(*see under* Bleeding, gastrointestinal)

Gastrointestinal disorders
Accutane Capsules 2740
Actonel Tablets (1.9% to 2.3%) 2679
Actonel with Calcium Tablets (1.9% to 2.5%) 2684
Adalat CC Tablets (Less than 1%) 2978
Adderall Tablets 3168
Adderall XR Capsules 3169
▲ Adenoscan (13%) 613
Adipex-P 1216
▲ Advair Diskus 100/50 (1% to 4%) 1291
Advair Diskus 250/50 (1%) 1291
▲ Advair Diskus 500/50 (1% to 4%) 1291
▲ Aerobid/Aerobid-M (1% to 10%) 1172
Aldoclor Tablets 1881
Alkeran for Injection (Infrequent) 976
Alkeran Tablets (Infrequent) 977
Amerge Tablets (Infrequent) 1312
▲ Ammonul Injection (13%) 3323
Amnesteem Capsules 2126
Anaprox Tablets 2769
Anaprox DS Tablets 2769
Antara Capsules 2723
Argatroban Injection (0.9%) 1321
▲ Arimidex Tablets (4% to 34%) 665
Avelox (Less than 0.1%) 2984
Axid Oral Solution (1.1%) 913
Balamine DM 739
▲ Boostrix (3% to 26%) 1366
Bravelle for Intramuscular or Subcutaneous Injection 1140
▲ Brimonidine Tartrate Ophthalmic Solution 0.2% (3% to 9%) ⊙245
Captopril Tablets 2114
▲ Carnitor Injection (2% to 6%) 3185
Carnitor Tablets and Oral Solution 3187
▲ CellCept Capsules (3% to less than 20%) 2751
▲ CellCept Intravenous (3% to less than 20%) 2751
▲ CellCept Oral Suspension (3% to less than 20%) 2751
▲ CellCept Tablets (3% to less than 20%) 2751
▲ Chemet Capsules (About 10%) 2480
Clindagel 1207
▲ Clinoril Tablets (3% to 9%) 1899
▲ Clozapine Tablets (Greater than 5%) 2141
▲ Clozaril Tablets (Greater than 5%) 2174
Comtan Tablets (1%) 2186
▲ Copaxone for Injection (5%) 3292
Cosopt Sterile Ophthalmic Solution 1910
▲ Creon 5 Capsules (Among most frequent) 3195
▲ Cuprimine Capsules (17%) 1925
▲ Daranide Tablets (Among the most common effects) 1928
DDAVP Nasal Spray (Up to 2%) 2894
Decadron Phosphate Injection 1931
Depacon Injection 412
Depakene 417
▲ Depakote Tablets (1% to 5%) 427
Depakote ER Tablets 433
Desmopressin Acetate Rhinal Tube (Up to 2%) 1144
Dexedrine 1386
DextroStat Tablets 3177
Didronel Tablets 2693
Dyazide Capsules 1389
EC-Naprosyn Delayed-Release Tablets 2769
Ecotrin Enteric Coated Aspirin Low, Regular and Maximum Strength Tablets 1627
▲ Eulexin Capsules (6%) 3023
▲ Evista Tablets (3.3%) 1735
Factive Tablets (Less than or equal to 0.1%) 2464
Ferrlecit Injection 3379
▲ Flovent Diskus 50 mcg (4%) 1415
▲ Flovent HFA (1% to 3%) 1418
▲ Fortaz (Among most common) 1422
Forteo for Injection (2.3%) 1739
Furosemide Tablets 2117
▲ Gengraf Capsules (4% to 19.8%) 458
▲ Humira Injection (Less than 5%) 464
▲ Hyalgan Solution (29%) 2917
Kaletra (Less than 2%) 474
K-Dur Extended-Relase Tablets 3047
Ketek Tablets (Greater than or equal to 0.2% to less than 2%) 2920
Klonopin (Infrequent) 2782
K-Phos Neutral Tablets 785
Lanoxicaps Capsules 1458
Leukeran Tablets (Infrequent) 1472
▲ Leukine (37%) 829
Lofibra Capsules 1217
Lupron Depot 3.75 mg (2%) 3257
▲ Lupron Depot 7.5 mg (14.3%) 3261
Lupron Depot–3 Month 11.25 mg (2%) 3262
Maxzide 2150
Micardis Tablets (More than 0.3%) 884
Micardis HCT Tablets 886
Midamor Tablets (Less than or equal to 1%) 2000
Moduretic Tablets (Less than or equal to 1%) 2003
Naprosyn Suspension 2769
Naprosyn Tablets 2769
▲ Neoral Soft Gelatin Capsules (4% to 19.8%) 2247
▲ Neoral Oral Solution (4% to 19.8%) 2247
Neurontin Capsules (Infrequent) 2498
Neurontin Oral Solution (Infrequent) 2498
Neurontin Tablets (Infrequent) 2498
Nexium Delayed-Release Capsules (Less than 1%) 645
Nexium I.V. (Less than 1%) 649
Nimotop Capsules (Up to 2.4%) 774
Nipent for Injection 3216
Norvir (Less than 2%) 499
Omacor Capsules 2735
Omnicef Capsules 506
Omnicef for Oral Suspension 506
Orap Tablets 1220
Ortho-Cyclen/Ortho Tri-Cyclen 2414
Ortho Tri-Cyclen Lo Tablets 2421
Oxsoralen-Ultra Capsules 3354
OxyContin Tablets (Less than 1%) 2699
▲ Pancrease MT Capsules (Among most frequent) 1839
▲ Plavix Tablets (About 27.1%) 940
▲ Plavix Tablets (About 27.1%) 2942
▲ Precose Tablets (Among most common) 776
Prevacid Delayed-Release Capsules (Less than 1%) 3268
Prevacid for Delayed-Release Oral Suspension (Less than 1%) 3268
Prevacid NapraPAC (Less than 1%) 3277
Prevacid SoluTab Delayed-Release Orally Disintegrating Tablets (Less than 1%) 3268
PREVPAC (Less than 1%) 3281
Prinzide Tablets (0.3% to 1%) 2033
Proleukin for Injection (Less than 1%) 1007
Protonix I.V. (Greater than or equal to 1%) 3468
Protonix Tablets (Greater than or equal to 1%) 3465
Provigil Tablets (At least 1%) 1002
Rabies Vaccine RabAvert (Uncommon) 1011
Relpax Tablets (Infrequent) 2531
Rescriptor Tablets 2535
▲ Retrovir Capsules (20%) 1533
▲ Retrovir IV Infusion (20%) 1537
▲ Retrovir (20%) 1533
Reyataz Capsules (Less than 3%) 948
Seasonale Tablets 1073
▲ Simulect for Injection (3% to 10%) 2268
▲ Skelaxin Tablets (Most frequent) 1685
Spectracef Tablets (0.1% to 1%) 2706
▲ Spiriva HandiHaler (1% to 3%) 899
St. Joseph 81 mg Aspirin Chewable and Enteric Coated Tablets 1841
Stalevo Tablets (1%) 2270
Striant Mucoadhesive 1022
▲ Suprax (30%) 1811
Taxotere Injection Concentrate 2947
Tessalon Capsules 1202
Tessalon Perles 1202
Thalomid Capsules 979
▲ Ticlid Tablets (30% to 40%) 2813
Timoptic-XE Sterile Ophthalmic Gel Forming Solution 2062
Topamax Sprinkle Capsules (1%) 2438
Topamax Tablets (1%) 2438
Toprol-XL Tablets 660
Tranxene (Less common) 2488
Travatan Ophthalmic Solution (1% to 5%) 559
Trecator Tablets 3482
Tricor Tablets 523
Triglide Tablets 1165
▲ Ultrase Capsules (Most frequent) 735
Uroqid-Acid No. 2 Tablets 785
▲ Urso 250 Tablets (5%) 737
▲ Urso Forte Tablets (5%) 737
Vantin Tablets and Oral Suspension 2650
Vaseretic Tablets 2073
▲ Vesanoid Capsules (26%) 2823
Viokase 738
▲ Xenical Capsules (Among most frequent) 2834
▲ Zenapax for Injection (Greater than 5%) 2838
Zestoretic Tablets (0.3% to 1.0%) 701
Zinacef Injection (1 in 150 patients) 1604
Zinacef for Injection (1 in 150 patients) 1604
Zomig Nasal Spray (Infrequent) 718
Zosyn 3492

Gastrointestinal disorders, unspecified
▲ Focalin XR Capsules (28% to 44%) 2217
Merrem I.V. (Greater than 1%) 687

Gastrointestinal fistula
▲ Entocort EC Capsules (Less than 5%) 2694

Gastrointestinal impaction
Lotronex Tablets 1479

Gastrointestinal infarction
Zomig Nasal Spray (Very rare) 718
Zomig Tablets (Very rare) 714

Gastrointestinal inflammation
Combunox Tablets 1183
Mobic Oral Suspension 893
Mobic Tablets 893

Gastrointestinal motility, decreased
Enablex Extended-Release Tablets 2201
Lotronex Tablets (Rare) 1479

Gastrointestinal neoplasm, benign
Arthrotec Tablets (Rare) 3126

Gastrointestinal obstruction
K-Dur Extended-Relase Tablets 3047
K-Tab Filmtab Tablets 473
Lotronex Tablets (Rare) 1479

Gastrointestinal perforation
Aggrenox Capsules (Less than 1%) 855
▲ Anaprox Tablets (Approximately 1% to 4%) 2769
▲ Anaprox DS Tablets (Approximately 1% to 4%) 2769
Avastin IV 1229
Bayer Aspirin Tablets 3515
▲ Cataflam Tablets (1% to 10%) 2173
CellCept Capsules (Rare) 2751
CellCept Intravenous (Rare) 2751
CellCept Oral Suspension (Rare) 2751
CellCept Tablets (Rare) 2751
Clinoril Tablets (Rare) 1899
Combunox Tablets 1183
Cytovene (At least 3 subjects) 2763
Dolobid Tablets (Less than 1 in 100) 1937
▲ EC-Naprosyn Delayed-Release Tablets (Approximately 1% to 4%) 2769
Ecotrin Enteric Coated Aspirin Low, Regular and Maximum Strength Tablets 1627
Indocin Capsules (Approximately 1%) 1968
Indocin I.V. 1973
Indocin (Approximately 1%) 1968
K-Dur Extended-Relase Tablets 3047
K-Tab Filmtab Tablets 473
Lotronex Tablets 1479
Mobic Oral Suspension 893
Mobic Tablets 893
▲ Naprosyn Suspension (Approximately 1% to 4%) 2769
▲ Naprosyn Tablets (Approximately 1% to 4%) 2769
Prevacid NapraPAC (Less than 1%) 3277
▲ Prograf Capsules and Injection (3%) 624
Relafen Tablets 1523

St. Joseph 81 mg Aspirin Chewable and Enteric Coated Tablets 1841
Taxotere Injection Concentrate 2947
▲ Voltaren Tablets (1% to 10%) 2298
▲ Voltaren-XR Tablets (1% to 10%) 2301

Gastrointestinal reactions
(*see under* Gastrointestinal disorders)

Gastrointestinal reflux
Arthrotec Tablets (Rare) 3126
Lotronex Tablets (Rare) 1479

Gastrointestinal symptoms
(*see under* Gastrointestinal disorders)

Gastrointestinal toxicity
Alkeran for Injection 976
Alkeran Tablets 977
Anaprox Tablets 2769
Anaprox DS Tablets 2769
EC-Naprosyn Delayed-Release Tablets 2769
I.V. Busulfex (Frequent) 1125
Naprosyn Suspension 2769
Naprosyn Tablets 2769

Gastrointestinal upset
(*see under* Gastrointestinal disorders)

Genital abnormalities
Vesanoid Capsules 2823

Genital malformation
Thalomid Capsules 979

Genital moniliasis
Ancef for Injection 1318
Augmentin XR Extended-Release Tablets (2.1%) 1340
Levaquin in 5% Dextrose Injection (0.1% to 0.9%) 2453
Levaquin (0.1% to 0.9%) 2453
Topamax Sprinkle Capsules (Greater than 1%) 2438
Topamax Tablets (Greater than 1%) 2438

Genitalia, male, external, abnormalities of
Propecia Tablets 2036
Proscar Tablets 2040

Genitourinary disturbances
Adalat CC Tablets (Less than 1%) 2978
Dalmane Capsules 3343
Eulexin Capsules (2%) 3023
▲ Leukine (50%) 829
▲ Nipent for Injection (Up to 15%) 3216
▲ Paxil CR Controlled-Release Tablets (3%) 1509
▲ Paxil (3%) 1501
Tranxene 2488

Germinal aplasia
Mustargen for Injection 2007

GGTP, elevation
(*see under* Gamma-glutamyl transpeptidase, elevation)

Giardiasis
Colazal Capsules 2845

Giddiness
(*see under* Dizziness)

Gingival disorder, unspecified
Adalat CC Tablets (Less than 1%) 2978
Xenical Capsules (2%) 2834
Xifaxan Tablets (Less than 2%) 2847

Gingival hyperplasia
Adalat CC Tablets (Rare) 2978
Caduet Tablets (Greater than 0.1% to less than or equal to 1%) 2507
Cardizem LA Extended Release Tablets (Infrequent) 1699
▲ CellCept Capsules (3% to less than 20%) 2751
▲ CellCept Intravenous (3% to less than 20%) 2751
▲ CellCept Oral Suspension (3% to less than 20%) 2751
▲ CellCept Tablets (3% to less than 20%) 2751
Covera-HS Tablets (Less than 2%) 3135
Evoxac Capsules 1042
Gabitril Tablets (Infrequent) 998
▲ Gengraf Capsules (4% to 16%) 458
▲ Intron A for Injection (Less than 5%) 3038
Lamictal (Infrequent) 1449
▲ Myfortic Tablets (3% to less than 20%) 2244
▲ Neoral Soft Gelatin Capsules (3.8% to 16%) 2247
▲ Neoral Oral Solution (3.8% to 16%) 2247
Norvasc Tablets (More than 0.1% to 1%) 2529
Orap Tablets (One patient) 1220
Phenytek Capsules 2153
Plendil Extended-Release Tablets (Less than 0.5%) 651
Rapamune Oral Solution and Tablets 3472
▲ Sandimmune (4% to 16%) 2259
▲ Simulect for Injection (3% to 10%) 2268
Soriatane Capsules (Less than 1%) 1028
Sular Tablets (Less than or equal to 1%) 1163
Tarka Tablets 519
Tiazac Capsules (Infrequent) 1204
Topamax Sprinkle Capsules (Infrequent to 1%) 2438
Topamax Tablets (Infrequent to 1%) 2438
Trileptal Oral Suspension 2281
Trileptal Tablets 2281
Verelan PM Capsules (2% or less) 3120
VFEND I.V. (Less than 2%) 2543
VFEND Oral Suspension (Less than 2%) 2543
VFEND Tablets (Less than 2%) 2543
Zoloft (Rare) 2581
Zonegran Capsules (Infrequent) 1089

Gingivitis
Abilify Tablets (Infrequent) 916
Abilify Tablets (Infrequent) 2472
Accutane Capsules 2740
Aciphex Tablets 1081
Actiq (1% or greater) 993
▲ Arava Tablets (1% to 3%) 2881
Aricept Tablets (Infrequent) 1086
Aricept ODT Tablets (Infrequent) 1086
Campath Ampules 826
Celexa (Infrequent) 1177
▲ CellCept Capsules (3% to less than 20%) 2751
▲ CellCept Intravenous (3% to less than 20%) 2751
▲ CellCept Oral Suspension (3% to less than 20%) 2751
▲ CellCept Tablets (3% to less than 20%) 2751
Copaxone for Injection (At least 2%) 3292
Cymbalta Delayed-Release Capsules (Infrequent) 1729
▲ Doxil Injection (1% to 10%) 3302
Effexor Tablets (Infrequent) 3405
Effexor XR Capsules (Infrequent) 3411
▲ Eloxatin for Injection (2% to 5%) 2908
Evoxac Capsules (Less than 1%) 1042
Exelon Capsules (Infrequent) 2204
Gabitril Tablets (Frequent) 998
Gengraf Capsules 458
▲ Intron A for Injection (Up to 14%) 3038
Invirase (Less than 2%) 2776
Keppra Oral Solution (1% or more) 3307
Keppra Tablets (1% or more) 3307
Klonopin 2782
Lamictal (Infrequent) 1449
Lupron Depot-PED 7.5 mg, 11.25 mg and 15 mg (Less than 2%) 3266
Lupron Injection Pediatric (Less than 2%) 3256
Neoral Soft Gelatin Capsules 2247
Neoral Oral Solution 2247
Neurontin Capsules (Frequent) 2498
Neurontin Oral Solution (Frequent) 2498
Neurontin Tablets (Frequent) 2498
▲ Nipent for Injection (3% to 10%) 3216
Norvir (Less than 2%) 499
Paxil CR Controlled-Release Tablets (Rare) 1509
Paxil (Rare) 1501
Permax Tablets (Infrequent) 3357
Protonix I.V. (Less than 1%) 3468
Protonix Tablets (Less than 1%) 3465
Provigil Tablets (1%) 1002
▲ Rapamune Oral Solution and Tablets (3% to 20%) 3472
Relafen Tablets (Less than 1%) 1523
Relpax Tablets (Rare) 2531
Requip Tablets (1% or more) 1528
Rescriptor Tablets 2535
Risperdal Consta Long-Acting Injection (Infrequent) 1664
Risperdal M-Tab Orally Disintegrating Tablets (Rare) 1658
Risperdal (Rare) 1658
Sandostatin LAR Depot (1% to 4%) 2264
Seroquel Tablets (Infrequent) 691
Sonata Capsules (Infrequent) 1686
▲ Soriatane Capsules (1% to 10%) 1028
Striant Mucoadhesive 1022
Symbyax Capsules (Infrequent) 1788
Targretin Capsules 1719
Tequin Injection (Less than 0.1%) 964
Tequin Tablets (Less than 0.1%) 964
Teveten Tablets (Less than 1%) 1707
Teveten HCT Tablets (Less than 1%) 1710
Topamax Sprinkle Capsules (1%) 2438
Topamax Tablets (1%) 2438
Uniretic Tablets (Less than 1%) 3114
VFEND I.V. (Less than 2%) 2543
VFEND Oral Suspension (Less than 2%) 2543
VFEND Tablets (Less than 2%) 2543
Viagra Tablets (Less than 2%) 2552
Wellbutrin SR Sustained-Release Tablets (Infrequent) 1583
Wellbutrin XL Extended-Release Tablets (Infrequent) 1588
Zomig Nasal Spray (Rare) 718
Zonegran Capsules (Infrequent) 1089
Zyban Sustained-Release Tablets (Infrequent) 1620
Zyprexa Tablets (Infrequent) 1798
Zyprexa ZYDIS Orally Disintegrating Tablets (Infrequent) 1798

Gingivostomatitis
Cuprimine Capsules (Rare) 1925

Glassy-eyed appearance
Klonopin 2782

Glaucoma
(*see also under* IOP, elevation of)
Aciphex Tablets 1081
Advair Diskus 100/50 1291
Advair Diskus 250/50 1291
Advair Diskus 500/50 1291
Ambien Tablets (Rare) 2867
Aricept Tablets (Infrequent) 1086
Aricept ODT Tablets (Infrequent) 1086
Arthrotec Tablets (Rare) 3126
Azmacort Inhalation Aerosol (Rare) 1701
Beconase AQ Nasal Spray (Rare) 1359
Blephamide Ophthalmic Ointment (A possibility) 563
Blephamide Ophthalmic Suspension 564
Celebrex Capsules (0.1% to 1.9%) 3130
Clozapine Tablets 2141
Clozaril Tablets 2174
Cymbalta Delayed-Release Capsules (Infrequent) 1729
Decadron Phosphate Injection 1931
Decadron Tablets 1929
Depo-Medrol Injectable Suspension 2615
Depo-Medrol Single-Dose Vial 2617
Effexor XR Capsules (Rare) 3411
Evoxac Capsules (Less than 1%) 1042
Exelon Capsules (Infrequent) 2204
Flonase Nasal Spray 1412
FML Forte Ophthalmic Suspension ⊙ 223
HMS Sterile Ophthalmic Suspension (Rare) ⊙ 228
Hydrocortone Tablets 1963
Levitra Tablets (Less than 2%) 3048
Lipitor Tablets (Less than 2%) 2495
Midamor Tablets (Less than or equal to 1%) 2000
Mirapex Tablets (Less than 1%) 889
Moduretic Tablets 2003
Namenda (Infrequent) 1199
Nasacort HFA Inhalation Aerosol 2939
Neurontin Capsules (Rare) 2498
Neurontin Oral Solution (Rare) 2498
Neurontin Tablets (Rare) 2498
Pediapred Oral Solution 3319
Poly-Pred Liquifilm Ophthalmic Suspension ⊙ 231
Pred-G Ophthalmic Suspension ⊙ 234
Pred-G Sterile Ophthalmic Ointment ⊙ 235
Protonix I.V. (Less than 1%) 3468
Protonix Tablets (Less than 1%) 3465
Prozac Pulvules and Liquid (Rare) 1771
Pulmicort Respules (Rare) 654
Requip Tablets (Infrequent) 1528
▲ Retisert Implant (50% to 90%) ⊙ 256
Rilutek Tablets (Rare) 2945
Sandostatin LAR Depot (Rare) 2264
Seroquel Tablets (Rare) 691
Sonata Capsules (Rare) 1686
Sular Tablets (Less than or equal to 1%) 1163
Tasmar Tablets (Rare) 3360
TobraDex Ophthalmic Ointment 558
TobraDex Ophthalmic Suspension 558
Uniretic Tablets (Less than 1%) 3114
Vivactil Tablets 2350
Zoloft (Rare) 2581
Zonegran Capsules (Infrequent) 1089
Zyprexa Tablets (Rare) 1798
Zyprexa ZYDIS Orally Disintegrating Tablets (Rare) 1798
Zyrtec Chewable Tablets (Less than 2%) 2589
Zyrtec (Less than 2%) 2589

Glaucoma, angle closure precipitation
Atrovent Nasal Spray 0.03% 869
Atrovent Nasal Spray 0.06% 870
Botox Purified Neurotoxin Complex (One report) 565
Combivent Inhalation Aerosol 878
DuoNeb Inhalation Solution 1058
Transderm Scōp Transdermal Therapeutic System (Infrequent) 2166

Glaucoma, corticosteroid-induced
Blephamide Ophthalmic Suspension 564
FML Ophthalmic Ointment ⊙ 225
FML Ophthalmic Suspension ⊙ 224
FML Forte Ophthalmic Suspension ⊙ 223
FML-S Liquifilm Sterile Ophthalmic Suspension ⊙ 226
HMS Sterile Ophthalmic Suspension ⊙ 228
Poly-Pred Liquifilm Ophthalmic Suspension ⊙ 231
Pred Forte Ophthalmic Suspension ⊙ 233
Pred Mild Sterile Ophthalmic Suspension ⊙ 236
Pred-G Ophthalmic Suspension ⊙ 234
TobraDex Ophthalmic Ointment 558
TobraDex Ophthalmic Suspension 558

Glaucoma, narrow-angle
Atrovent HFA Inhalation Aerosol 872
FazaClo Orally Disintegrating Tablets 547

Glaucoma, secondary
Topamax Sprinkle Capsules 2438
Topamax Tablets 2438

Glaucoma, worsening of narrow angle
Atrovent HFA Inhalation Aerosol 872
Atrovent Inhalation Solution 868
Atrovent Nasal Spray 0.03% 869
Atrovent Nasal Spray 0.06% 870
Combivent Inhalation Aerosol 878
DuoNeb Inhalation Solution 1058

Globus hystericus
Daranide Tablets 1928
Imitrex Injection (Rare) 1431

Glomerular filtration rate, decrease
Captopril Tablets 2114

Glomerulitis
Lyrica Capsules (Rare) 2524

Glomerulonephritis
Accutane Capsules 2740
Amnesteem Capsules 2126
Anaprox Tablets (Less than 1%) 2769
Anaprox DS Tablets (Less than 1%) 2769
Cuprimine Capsules 1925
EC-Naprosyn Delayed-Release Tablets (Less than 1%) 2769
Fuzeon Injection 2772
Naprosyn Suspension (Less than 1%) 2769
Naprosyn Tablets (Less than 1%) 2769
Orthoclone OKT3 Sterile Solution 2370
Prevacid NapraPAC (Less than 1%) 3277
Zyrtec Chewable Tablets (Rare) 2589
Zyrtec (Rare) 2589
Zyrtec-D 12 Hour Extended Release Tablets (Rare) 2591

Glomerulonephropathy, membranous
Enbrel for Injection (Infrequent) 580

Glomerulopathy
Herceptin I.V. (Rare) 1234
Plavix Tablets 940
Plavix Tablets 2942

Glossitis
Abilify Tablets (Rare) 916
Abilify Tablets (Rare) 2472
Aciphex Tablets 1081
Actiq (1% or greater) 993
Actonel with Calcium Tablets (0.1% to 1%) 2684
Aerobid/Aerobid-M (1% to 3%) 1172
Anaprox Tablets (Less than 1%) 2769
Anaprox DS Tablets (Less than 1%) 2769
Arthrotec Tablets (Rare) 3126
Astelin Nasal Spray (Infrequent) 1876
Augmentin 1331
Augmentin Tablets 1334
Augmentin XR Extended-Release Tablets 1340
Augmentin ES-600 Powder for Oral Suspension 1337
Avelox (0.1% to less than 2%) 2984
Betoptic S Ophthalmic Suspension (Rare) 554
Biaxin/Biaxin XL 402
Caduet Tablets (Less than 2%) 2507
Captopril Tablets 2114
Carbatrol Capsules 3174
Cataflam Tablets (Occasionally) 2173
Celexa (Rare) 1177
Clinoril Tablets (Less than 1%) 1899
Colazal Capsules 2845
Cuprimine Capsules 1925
Daraprim Tablets 1385
Depacon Injection (1% or more) 412
Depakene (1% or more) 417
Depakote Sprinkle Capsules 422
▲ Depakote Tablets (1% to 5%) 427
Depakote ER Tablets (Greater than 1%) 433
Didronel Tablets 2693
▲ Doxil Injection (1% to 5%) 3302
Dynacin Tablets 1859
EC-Naprosyn Delayed-Release Tablets (Less than 1%) 2769
Effexor Tablets (Infrequent) 3405
Effexor XR Capsules (Infrequent) 3411
▲ Entocort EC Capsules (Less than 5%) 2694
Equetro Extended-Release Capsules 3178
Evoxac Capsules (Less than 1%) 1042
Exelon Capsules (Infrequent) 2204
Gabitril Tablets (Infrequent) 998
Gengraf Capsules (1% to less than 3%) 458
▲ Imdur Tablets (Less than or equal to 5%) 3032
Inversine Tablets 3286
Invirase (Less than 2%) 2776
Ketek Tablets (Greater than or equal to 0.2% to less than 2%) 2920
Lamictal (Infrequent) 1449
Lipitor Tablets (Less than 2%) 2495
Lupron Depot 3.75 mg 3257
Lupron Depot–3 Month 11.25 mg 3262
Maxair Autohaler 1820
Merrem I.V. (1.0%) 687
Naprosyn Suspension (Less than 1%) 2769
Naprosyn Tablets (Less than 1%) 2769
Neoral Soft Gelatin Capsules (1% to less than 3%) 2247
Neoral Oral Solution (1% to less than 3%) 2247
Neurontin Capsules (Infrequent) 2498
Neurontin Oral Solution (Infrequent) 2498
Neurontin Tablets (Infrequent) 2498
Nipent for Injection (Less than 3%) 3216
Paxil CR Controlled-Release Tablets (Infrequent) 1509
Paxil (Infrequent) 1501
Permax Tablets (Rare) 3357
Prevacid Delayed-Release Capsules (Less than 1%) 3268
Prevacid for Delayed-Release Oral Suspension (Less than 1%) 3268
Prevacid NapraPAC (Less than 1%) 3277
Prevacid SoluTab Delayed-Release Orally Disintegrating Tablets (Less than 1%) 3268
PREVPAC (Less than 1%) 3281
Primaxin I.M. 2022
Primaxin I.V. (Less than 0.2%) 2024
Protonix I.V. (Less than 1%) 3468
Protonix Tablets (Less than 1%) 3465
Prozac Pulvules and Liquid (Infrequent) 1771
Relafen Tablets (Less than 1%) 1523
Relpax Tablets (Infrequent) 2531
Requip Tablets (Infrequent) 1528
Rilutek Tablets (Infrequent) 2945
Rythmol SR Capsules 2736
Sandostatin LAR Depot (1% to 4%) 2264
Seroquel Tablets (Infrequent) 691
Sonata Capsules (Infrequent) 1686
Soriatane Capsules (Less than 1%) 1028
Sular Tablets (Less than or equal to 1%) 1163
Tegretol/Tegretol-XR 2278
▲ Tequin Injection (0.1% to 3%) 964
▲ Tequin Tablets (0.1% to 3%) 964
Topamax Sprinkle Capsules (1%) 2438
Topamax Tablets (1%) 2438
Uniretic Tablets (Less than 1%) 3114
Vaseretic Tablets 2073
Vasotec I.V. Injection (0.5% to 1.0%) 2076
VFEND I.V. (Less than 2%) 2543
VFEND Oral Suspension (Less than 2%) 2543
VFEND Tablets (Less than 2%) 2543
Viagra Tablets (Less than 2%) 2552
Vicoprofen Tablets (Less than 1%) 533
Voltaren Tablets (Occasionally) 2298
Voltaren-XR Tablets (Occasionally) 2301
Wellbutrin Tablets (Rare) 1579
Wellbutrin SR Sustained-Release Tablets (Infrequent) 1583
Wellbutrin XL Extended-Release Tablets (Infrequent) 1588
Zoloft (Rare) 2581
Zonegran Capsules (Infrequent) 1089
Zyban Sustained-Release Tablets (Infrequent) 1620
Zyprexa Tablets (Infrequent) 1798
Zyprexa ZYDIS Orally Disintegrating Tablets (Infrequent) 1798

Glossodynia
Adenoscan (Less than 1%) 613
Aldoclor Tablets 1881
Aldoril Tablets 1884
Clozapine Tablets (1%) 2141
Clozaril Tablets (1%) 2174
▲ Imitrex Injection (4.9%) 1431
Imitrex Tablets 1440
Rythmol SR Capsules 2736

Glossoncus
Altace Capsules 1673
Ceftin Tablets (0.1% to 1%) 1369
Fortical Nasal Spray 3336
Maxalt Tablets 1983
Maxalt-MLT Orally Disintegrating Tablets 1983
Miacalcin Injection (A few cases) 2241
Miacalcin Nasal Spray (Few reports) 2242
Tambocor Tablets (Less than 1%) 1824
Tamiflu Capsules 2810
Tamiflu Oral Suspension 2810

Glossoplegia
Risperdal M-Tab Orally Disintegrating Tablets (Rare) 1658
Risperdal (Rare) 1658

Glossotrichia
Augmentin 1331
Augmentin Tablets 1334
Augmentin XR Extended-Release Tablets 1340
Augmentin ES-600 Powder for Oral Suspension 1337
Klonopin (Infrequent) 2782
PREVPAC 3281
Surmontil Capsules 2347
Vivactil Tablets 2350

Glucocorticoids, decreased
Elocon Cream 0.1% (2 in 182 subjects) 3019
▲ Elocon Lotion 0.1% (4 in 65 subjects) 3020
Elocon Ointment 0.1% (1 in 63 patients) 3021

Glucocorticoids, increased
Evoxac Capsules (Less than 1%) 1042
Prevacid NapraPAC 3277

Glucose tolerance, changes
Celexa (Infrequent) 1177
Estratest Tablets 3196
Estratest H.S. Tablets 3196
Furosemide Tablets 2117
Prefest Tablets 1069
Premarin Intravenous 3440

Glucose tolerance, decreased
Activella Tablets 2311
Anadrol-50 Tablets 3329
Decadron Tablets 1929
depo-subQ provera 104 Injectable Suspension 2622
Emcyt Capsules 3137
Kaletra (Less than 2%) 474
Lo/Ovral-28 Tablets 3423
Lyrica Capsules (Rare) 2524
Niaspan Extended-Release Tablets 1703
Nutropin for Injection 1238
Nutropin AQ Injection 1241
Nutropin AQ Pen 1241
Nutropin AQ Pen Cartridge 1241
Ortho-Cyclen/Ortho Tri-Cyclen 2414
Ortho Tri-Cyclen Lo Tablets 2421
Oxandrin Tablets 2977
Premarin Intravenous 3440
Premarin Vaginal Cream 3449
Triphasil-28 Tablets 3483
Uniretic Tablets (Less than 1%) 3114
VFEND I.V. (Less than 2%) 2543
VFEND Oral Suspension (Less than 2%) 2543
VFEND Tablets (Less than 2%) 2543
Vivelle Transdermal System 2288
Vivelle-Dot Transdermal System 2293

Glucose tolerance, impaired
Megace ES Oral Suspension 2492
▲ Norditropin Cartridges (6%) 2318
Premarin Tablets 3443
Premphase Tablets 3452
Prempro Tablets 3452

Glucosuria
Aclovate 1290
Clobex Shampoo 1209
Clobex Lotion 1208
Clorpres Tablets (Rare) 2139
Diprolene Gel 0.05% 3015
Diprolene Lotion 0.05% 3016
Diprolene Ointment 0.05% (Some patients) 3017
Diprolene AF Cream 0.05% (Some patients) 3014
Elspar for Injection (Low) 1943
Humatrope Vials and Cartridges (Infrequent) 1756
Lotrisone 3054
Norditropin Cartridges 2318
Olux Foam 1027
Temovate Cream 1549
Temovate Gel 1550
Temovate Ointment 1549
Temovate Scalp Application 1551
Vanos Cream 1864

Glycosuria
Abilify Tablets (Rare) 916
Abilify Tablets (Rare) 2472
Aldoclor Tablets 1881
Aldoril Tablets 1884
Aloprim for Injection (Less than 1%) 2156
Aloxi Injection (Less than 1%) 2099
Amerge Tablets (Rare) 1312
Arthrotec Tablets (Rare) 3126
Avalide Tablets 922
Avalide Tablets 2889
▲ Baraclude (4%) 928
Calcium Disodium Versenate Injection 1819
Carbatrol Capsules 3174
Clorpres Tablets 2139
▲ Coreg Tablets (Greater than 1% to 3%) 1376
Cutivate Lotion 0.05% (Rare) 1383
Decadron Tablets 1929
Diovan HCT Tablets 2195
Diprosone Cream, USP 0.05% 3018
Diuril Oral 1936
Diuril Sodium Intravenous 1934
Doxil Injection (Less than 1%) 3302
Dyazide Capsules 1389
Effexor Tablets (Rare) 3405
Effexor XR Capsules (Infrequent) 3411
Elocon Cream 0.1% 3019
Elocon Lotion 0.1% 3020
Elocon Ointment 0.1% 3021
Equetro Extended-Release Capsules 3178
Eskalith 1406
Evoxac Capsules 1042
Furosemide Tablets 2117
Geodon Capsules (Infrequent) 2514
Hepsera Tablets (1%) 1275
Hyzaar 1964
Indapamide Tablets (Less than 5%) 2119
Indocin Capsules (Less than 1%) 1968
Indocin I.V. (Less than 1%) 1973
Indocin (Less than 1%) 1968
Lithobid Tablets 1670
Lotensin HCT Tablets 2235
Maxzide 2150
Micardis HCT Tablets 886
Moduretic Tablets 2003
Neurontin Capsules (Rare) 2498
Neurontin Oral Solution (Rare) 2498
Neurontin Tablets (Rare) 2498
Nexium Delayed-Release Capsules (Less than 1%) 645
Nexium I.V. (Less than 1%) 649
Noroxin Tablets (Less frequent) 2009
Norvir (Less than 2%) 499
Prevacid Delayed-Release Capsules (Less than 1%) 3268
Prevacid for Delayed-Release Oral Suspension 3268
Prevacid NapraPAC 3277
Prevacid SoluTab Delayed-Release Orally Disintegrating Tablets (Less than 1%) 3268
PREVPAC (Less than 1%) 3281
Prilosec OTC Tablets (Less than 1%) 2674
Prograf Capsules and Injection 624
Protonix I.V. (Less than 1%) 3468
Protonix Tablets (Less than 1%) 3465
Prozac Pulvules and Liquid (Rare) 1771
▲ Rapamune Oral Solution and Tablets (3% to 20%) 3472
Requip Tablets (Infrequent) 1528
Risperdal Consta Long-Acting Injection (Infrequent) 1664
Rocephin Injectable Vials, ADD-Vantage, Galaxy, Bulk (Rare) 2801
Rythmol SR Capsules 2736
Seroquel Tablets (Infrequent) 691
Symbyax Capsules (Infrequent) 1788
Tegretol/Tegretol-XR 2278
Teveten Tablets (Less than 1%) 1707
Teveten HCT Tablets (Less than 1%) 1710
Thiothixene Capsules 2124
Timolide Tablets 2056
Ultane Liquid for Inhalation (Less than 1%) 526
Uniretic Tablets (Less than 1%) 3114
VFEND I.V. (Less than 2%) 2543
VFEND Oral Suspension (Less than 2%) 2543
VFEND Tablets (Less than 2%) 2543
Vicoprofen Tablets (Less than 1%) 533
Wellbutrin Tablets (Rare) 1579
Wellbutrin SR Sustained-Release Tablets 1583
Wellbutrin XL Extended-Release Tablets 1588
Zegerid Powder for Oral Solution (Less than 1%) 2972
Zyban Sustained-Release Tablets 1620

Goiter
Abilify Tablets (Rare) 916
Abilify Tablets (Rare) 2472
Aricept Tablets (Infrequent) 1086
Aricept ODT Tablets (Infrequent) 1086
Campral Tablets (Rare) 1175
Celexa (Rare) 1177
Copaxone for Injection (Infrequent) 3292
Effexor Tablets (Rare) 3405
Effexor XR Capsules (Rare) 3411
Evoxac Capsules (Less than 1%) 1042
Exelon Capsules (Infrequent) 2204
Fortical Nasal Spray (Less than 1%) 3336
Gabitril Tablets (Infrequent) 998
Gengraf Capsules (1% to less than 3%) 458
Lamictal (Rare) 1449
Meridia Capsules 485
Miacalcin Nasal Spray (Less than 1%) 2242
Neoral Soft Gelatin Capsules (1% to less than 3%) 2247
Neoral Oral Solution (1% to less than 3%) 2247
Neurontin Capsules (Rare) 2498
Neurontin Oral Solution (Rare) 2498
Neurontin Tablets (Rare) 2498
Nexium Delayed-Release Capsules (Less than 1%) 645
Nexium I.V. (Less than 1%) 649
Paxil CR Controlled-Release Tablets (Rare) 1509
Paxil (Rare) 1501
Prevacid Delayed-Release Capsules (Less than 1%) 3268
Prevacid for Delayed-Release Oral Suspension (Less than 1%) 3268
Prevacid NapraPAC (Less than 1%) 3277
Prevacid SoluTab Delayed-Release Orally Disintegrating Tablets (Less than 1%) 3268

- PREVPAC (Less than 1%) 3281
- Protonix I.V. (Less than 1%) 3468
- Protonix Tablets (Less than 1%) 3465
- Relpax Tablets (Rare) 2531
- ▲ Sandostatin Injection (6%) 2263
- ▲ Sandostatin LAR Depot (8%) 2264
- Sonata Capsules (Rare) 1686
- Uniretic Tablets (Less than 1%) 3114
- Zyprexa Tablets (Infrequent) 1798
- Zyprexa ZYDIS Orally Disintegrating Tablets (Infrequent) 1798

Goiter, euthyroid
- Eskalith 1406
- Lithobid Tablets 1670
- Zomig Nasal Spray (Rare) 718

Goiter production
(*see under* Goiter)

Gonadotropin secretion, inhibition
- ▲ Delatestryl Injection (Among most frequent) 2976
- ▲ Estratest Tablets (Among most common) 3196
- ▲ Estratest H.S. Tablets (Among most common) 3196
- Oxandrin Tablets 2977

Goodpasture's syndrome
- Campath Ampules 826
- Cuprimine Capsules 1925

Goosebumps
(*see under* Piloerection)

Gout
- Abilify Tablets (Rare) 916
- Abilify Tablets (Rare) 2472
- Aceon Tablets (2 mg, 4 mg, 8 mg) (0.3% to 1%) 3191
- Aciphex Tablets 1081
- Adalat CC Tablets (Less than 1%) 2978
- Advicor Tablets 1694
- Ambien Tablets (Rare) 2867
- Antara Capsules 2723
- Aricept Tablets (Infrequent) 1086
- Aricept ODT Tablets (Infrequent) 1086
- Arthrotec Tablets (Rare) 3126
- Asacol Delayed-Release Tablets 2688
- Avalide Tablets 922
- Avalide Tablets 2889
- Avapro Tablets (Less than 1%) 925
- Avapro Tablets (Less than 1%) 2886
- Caduet Tablets (Less than 2%) 2507
- Campral Tablets (Infrequent) 1175
- ▲ Casodex Tablets (2% to 5%) 670
- ▲ CellCept Capsules (3% to less than 20%) 2751
- ▲ CellCept Intravenous (3% to less than 20%) 2751
- ▲ CellCept Oral Suspension (3% to less than 20%) 2751
- ▲ CellCept Tablets (3% to less than 20%) 2751
- Cipro I.V. (1% or less) 2998
- Cipro I.V. Pharmacy Bulk Package (1% or less) 3509
- Cipro (Less than 1%) 2991
- Clorpres Tablets 2139
- Copaxone for Injection (Infrequent) .. 3292
- ▲ Coreg Tablets (Greater than 1% to 3%) 1376
- Cozaar Tablets (Less than 1%) 1913
- Diovan HCT Tablets (Greater than 0.2%) 2195
- Edecrin 1941
- Effexor Tablets (Rare) 3405
- Effexor XR Capsules (Rare) 3411
- Evoxac Capsules 1042
- Exelon Capsules (Infrequent) 2204
- Furosemide Tablets 2117
- Geodon Capsules (Rare) 2514
- Gleevec Tablets (Infrequent) 2221
- Hytrin Capsules (At least 1%) 469
- Hyzaar 1964
- Invanz for Injection (Greater than 0.1%) 1974
- Klonopin (Infrequent) 2782
- Levaquin in 5% Dextrose Injection (0.1% to 0.9%) 2453
- Levaquin (0.1% to 0.9%) 2453
- Lexapro Oral Solution (Infrequent) 1193
- Lexapro Tablets (Infrequent) 1193
- Lipitor Tablets (Less than 2%) 2495
- Lofibra Capsules 1217
- Lotensin HCT Tablets (0.3% to 1%) .. 2235
- Lotrel Capsules (Infrequent) 2238
- Lunesta Tablets (Rare) 3139
- Mavik Tablets (0.3% to 1.0%) 482
- Maxzide 2150
- Micardis Tablets (More than 0.3%) ... 884
- Micardis HCT Tablets 886
- Moduretic Tablets (Less than or equal to 1%) 2003
- Neurontin Capsules (Infrequent) 2498
- Neurontin Oral Solution (Infrequent) 2498
- Neurontin Tablets (Infrequent) 2498
- Niaspan Extended-Release Tablets... 1703
- Nipent for Injection (Less than 3%)... 3216
- Norvir (Less than 2%) 499
- Paxil CR Controlled-Release Tablets (Rare) 1509
- Paxil (Rare) 1501
- PEG-Intron Powder for Injection (Less than or equal to 1%) 3062
- Permax Tablets (Infrequent) 3357
- Plavix Tablets (1% to 2.5%) 940
- Plavix Tablets (1% to 2.5%) 2942
- Pletal Tablets (Less than 2%) 2478
- Prevacid Delayed-Release Capsules (Less than 1%) 3268
- Prevacid for Delayed-Release Oral Suspension (Less than 1%) 3268
- Prevacid NapraPAC (Less than 1%) .. 3277
- Prevacid SoluTab Delayed-Release Orally Disintegrating Tablets (Less than 1%) 3268
- PREVPAC (Less than 1%) 3281
- Prinivil Tablets (0.3% to 1.0%) 2029
- Prinzide Tablets 2033
- Protonix I.V. (Less than 1%) 3468
- Protonix Tablets (Less than 1%) 3465
- Prozac Pulvules and Liquid (Infrequent) 1771
- Requip Tablets (1% or more) 1528
- Reyataz Capsules (Less than 3%) 948
- Rilutek Tablets (Infrequent) 2945
- Rythmol SR Capsules 2736
- Sandostatin LAR Depot (1% to 4%) .. 2264
- Seroquel Tablets (Infrequent) 691
- Sonata Capsules (Infrequent) 1686
- Sular Tablets (Less than or equal to 1%) 1163
- Symbyax Capsules (Rare) 1788
- Synercid I.V. (Less than 1%) 1690
- Tarka Tablets (Less frequent) 519
- Teveten Tablets (Less than 1%) 1707
- Teveten HCT Tablets (Less than 1%) 1710
- Tiazac Capsules (1% to 2%) 1204
- Timolide Tablets 2056
- Tricor Tablets 523
- Triglide Tablets 1165
- Uniretic Tablets (Less than 1%) 3114
- Vantin Tablets and Oral Suspension (Less than 1%) 2650
- Vaseretic Tablets (0.5% to 2.0%) 2073
- Viagra Tablets (Less than 2%) 2552
- Zestoretic Tablets 701
- Zestril Tablets (0.3% to 1.0%) 704
- Zoladex (1% to 5%) 709
- Zoladex 3-month 712
- Zyprexa Tablets (Rare) 1798
- Zyprexa ZYDIS Orally Disintegrating Tablets (Rare) 1798

Gout, exacerbation of
- Cipro XR Tablets 3004

Graft loss
- ▲ Rapamune Oral Solution and Tablets (3.4% to 6.3%) 3472

Graft versus host reaction
- ▲ I.V. Busulfex (18%) 1125
- VFEND I.V. (Less than 2%) 2543
- VFEND Oral Suspension (Less than 2%) 2543
- VFEND Tablets (Less than 2%) 2543

Granulocytopenia
- Albenza Tablets (Rare) 1310
- Aldoclor Tablets 1881
- Aldoril Tablets 1884
- Anaprox Tablets (Less than 1%) 2769
- Anaprox DS Tablets (Less than 1%) .. 2769
- ▲ Aredia for Injection (19.8%) 2168
- Celexa (Rare) 1177
- Colazal Capsules 2845
- ▲ Cytovene (6%) 2763
- Dalmane Capsules (Rare) 3343
- EC-Naprosyn Delayed-Release Tablets (Less than 1%) 2769
- Evoxac Capsules (Less than 1%) 1042
- Factive Tablets (Less than or equal to 0.1%) 2464
- Garamycin Injectable 3028
- Grifulvin V Tablets Microsize and Oral Suspension Microsize 2384
- Gris-PEG Tablets 2504
- ▲ Humira Injection (Less than 5%) 464
- ▲ Infergen (23% to 42%) 1647
- ▲ Intron A for Injection (Less than 5%) 3038
- ▲ I.V. Busulfex (100%) 1125
- Levaquin in 5% Dextrose Injection (0.1% to 0.9%) 2453
- Levaquin (0.1% to 0.9%) 2453
- Mefoxin for Injection 1987
- Mefoxin Premixed Intravenous Solution 1990
- Mustargen for Injection 2007
- Naprosyn Suspension (Less than 1%) 2769
- Naprosyn Tablets (Less than 1%) 2769
- ▲ Navelbine Injection (20% to 89%) 1494
- ▲ Neulasta Injection (15% to 72%) 596
- ▲ Novantrone for Injection Concentrate (6%) 3158
- Omnicef Capsules 506
- Omnicef for Oral Suspension 506
- Phenytek Capsules (Occasional) 2153
- Plavix Tablets (Less than 1%) 940
- Plavix Tablets (Less than 1%) 2942
- Pletal Tablets (Very rare) 2478
- Prevacid NapraPAC (Less than 1%) .. 3277
- Relafen Tablets (Less than 1%) 1523
- ▲ Retrovir Capsules (1.8% to 47%) 1533
- ▲ Retrovir IV Infusion (1.8% to 47%) ... 1537
- ▲ Retrovir (1.8% to 47%) 1533
- Risperdal Consta Long-Acting Injection (Rare) 1664
- Thalomid Capsules 979
- Topamax Sprinkle Capsules (Infrequent) 2438
- Topamax Tablets (Infrequent) 2438
- Viramune Oral Suspension 903
- Viramune Tablets 903
- ▲ Xeloda Tablets (2% to 86%) 2825
- Zantac (A few patients) 1597
- Zantac Injection (Few patients) 1593
- Zantac Injection Pharmacy Bulk Package (Infrequent) 1595
- Zantac Syrup (A few patients) 1597
- Zinecard for Injection 2659
- ▲ Zometa for Intravenous Infusion (5% to 10%) 2306

Granulocytosis
- Rescriptor Tablets 2535
- Vantin Tablets and Oral Suspension 2650

Granuloma, unspecified
- Actiq (Less than 1%) 993
- ▲ Apokyn Injection (4%) 2132
- Fluorescite Injection .... ⊙ 207
- Lyrica Capsules (Rare) 2524
- VFEND I.V. (Less than 2%) 2543
- VFEND Oral Suspension (Less than 2%) 2543
- VFEND Tablets (Less than 2%) 2543

Granulomatosis, Wegener's
- Accutane Capsules 2740

Grave's Disease
- Campath Ampules 826

Groin pain
- Ferrlecit Injection 3379

Growth rate, decrease
- ▲ Sandostatin Injection (37%) 2263

Growth retardation
- Advair Diskus 100/50 1291
- Advair Diskus 250/50 1291
- Advair Diskus 500/50 1291
- Cosmegen for Injection 1907
- Desferal Vials 2190
- Elocon Cream 0.1% 3019
- Elocon Lotion 0.1% 3020
- Elocon Ointment 0.1% 3021
- Hectorol Capsules 909
- Hectorol Injection 911
- Herceptin I.V. (At least one of the 958 patients) 1234
- Lotrisone Cream 3054
- Phenytek Capsules 2153

Growth retardation, intrauterine
- Altace Capsules 1673
- Captopril Tablets 2114
- Cozaar Tablets 1913
- Hyzaar 1964
- Prinivil Tablets 2029
- Prinzide Tablets 2033
- Tenormin I.V. Injection 698
- Tenormin Tablets 695
- Vaseretic Tablets 2073
- Vasotec I.V. Injection 2076
- Zestoretic Tablets 701
- Zestril Tablets 704

Growth suppression
- Azmacort Inhalation Aerosol 1701
- Beconase AQ Nasal Spray 1359
- Decadron Phosphate Injection 1931
- Decadron Tablets 1929
- Depo-Medrol Injectable Suspension 2615
- Depo-Medrol Single-Dose Vial 2617
- Desoxyn Tablets, USP 2482
- Flonase Nasal Spray 1412
- Flovent Diskus 50 mcg 1415
- Flovent HFA 1418
- Focalin XR Capsules 2217
- Hydrocortone Tablets 1963
- Pediapred Oral Solution 3319
- Pulmicort Respules 654
- Rhinocort Aqua Nasal Spray 658

Guillain-Barré syndrome
- Adacel Vaccine 2959
- Asacol Delayed-Release Tablets (Rare) 2688
- Attenuvax (Rare) 1889
- Boostrix 1366
- Campath Ampules 826
- Comvax 1904
- Cuprimine Capsules 1925
- DAPTACEL 2964
- Effexor Tablets (Rare) 3405
- Effexor XR Capsules (Rare) 3411
- Engerix-B Vaccine (Less than 1%) 1391
- Flumist Vaccine 1872
- Fuzeon Injection 2772
- Havrix Vaccine (Rare) 1425
- HibTITER 3419
- Infanrix Vaccine 1444
- Lyrica Capsules (Rare) 2524
- Meruvax II (Isolated reports) 1994
- M-M-R II (Rare) 1980
- Mumpsvax 2005
- Noroxin Tablets 2009
- Paxil CR Controlled-Release Tablets 1509
- Paxil 1501
- Pediarix Vaccine 1518
- Liquid PedvaxHIB 2012
- Pneumovax 23 (Rare) 2020
- Rabies Vaccine RabAvert 1011
- Recombivax HB 2045
- Remicade for IV Injection 987
- Twinrix Vaccine 1571
- Vaqta (Very rare) 2067
- Varivax 2070
- VFEND I.V. (Less than 2%) 2543
- VFEND Oral Suspension (Less than 2%) 2543
- VFEND Tablets (Less than 2%) 2543

Gum problems, unspecified
- ▲ Nicotrol NS (4%) 2596

Gums, sore
- Rythmol SR Capsules 2736
- ▲ Striant Mucoadhesive (3.1%) 1022
- Wellbutrin (Infrequent) 1579

Gynecological disorders, unspecified
- ▲ Zofran (7%) 1613
- ▲ Zofran ODT Orally Disintegrating Tablets (7%) 1613

Gynecomastia
- Abilify Tablets (Infrequent) 916
- Abilify Tablets (Infrequent) 2472
- Adalat CC Tablets (Rare) 2978
- Advicor Tablets 1694
- Aldoclor Tablets 1881
- Aldoril Tablets 1884
- Altoprev Extended-Release Tablets 1151
- Anadrol-50 Tablets 3329
- AndroGel (Up to 3%) 3330
- Antara Capsules 2723
- Avodart Soft Gelatin Capsules (0.5% to 1.1%) 1353
- Axid Oral Solution (Rare) 913
- Caduet Tablets 2507
- Captopril Tablets 2114
- Cardizem LA Extended Release Tablets (Less than 2%) 1699
- ▲ Casodex Tablets (5%) 670
- Catapres Tablets (About 1 in 1,000 patients) 874
- Catapres-TTS (0.5% or less) 875
- Celexa (Rare) 1177
- Cipro I.V. (1% or less) 2998
- Cipro I.V. Pharmacy Bulk Package (1% or less) 3509
- Cipro XR Tablets 3004
- Clinoril Tablets (Rare) 1899
- Clorpres Tablets (About 1 in 1,000) 2139
- Covera-HS Tablets (Less than 2%) 3135
- Delatestryl Injection 2976
- Digitek Tablets (Occasional) 2146

Effexor Tablets (Rare) 3405
Effexor XR Capsules (Rare) 3411
Eligard 7.5 mg (Less than 2%) 2896
Eligard 22.5 mg (Less than 2%) 2899
Eligard 30 mg (2.2%) 2901
▲ Eligard 45 mg (3.6%) 2904
▲ Eulexin Capsules (9%) 3023
Flexeril Tablets (Rare) 1832
▲ Gengraf Capsules (Less than 1% to 4%) 458
Geodon Capsules (Rare) 2514
▲ Humatrope Vials and Cartridges (Rare to 5.4%) 1756
Indocin Capsules (Less than 1%) 1968
Indocin I.V. (Less than 1%) 1973
Indocin (Less than 1%) 1968
Inspra Tablets (0.4% to 1%) 2520
▲ Intron A for Injection (Less than 5%) 3038
Kadian Capsules (Less than 3%) 572
Kaletra (Less than 2%) 474
Lanoxicaps Capsules (Occasional) 1458
Lanoxin Injection (Occasional) 1462
Lanoxin Tablets (Occasional) 1468
Lanoxin Injection Pediatric (Occasional) 1465
Lescol Capsules 2227
Lescol Capsules 2730
Lescol XL Tablets 2227
Lescol XL Tablets 2730
Lofibra Capsules 1217
Lotrel Capsules 2238
▲ Lunesta Tablets (0% to 3%) 3139
Lupron Depot 7.5 mg (Less than 5%) 3261
Lupron Depot-PED 7.5 mg, 11.25 mg and 15 mg (Less than 2%) 3266
Lupron Injection Pediatric (Less than 2%) 3256
Matulane Capsules 3188
▲ Megace ES Oral Suspension (1% to 3%) 2492
Mevacor Tablets (0.5% to 1.0%) 1996
Midamor Tablets 2000
Moban Tablets (Infrequent) 1108
Moduretic Tablets 2003
Myleran Tablets (Rare) 1492
▲ Neoral Soft Gelatin Capsules (Less than 1% to 4%) 2247
Neoral Oral Solution (Less than 1% to 4%) 2247
Neurontin Capsules (Rare) 2498
Neurontin Oral Solution (Rare) 2498
Neurontin Tablets (Rare) 2498
Niravam Orally Disintegrating Tablets 3106
Norvasc Tablets (Infrequent) 2529
Novarel for Injection 1147
Nutropin for Injection (Rare) 1238
Nutropin AQ Injection (Rare) 1241
Nutropin AQ Pen (Rare) 1241
Nutropin AQ Pen Cartridge (Rare) 1241
Oxandrin Tablets 2977
Pepcid Injection (Rare) 2017
Pepcid (Rare) 2014
Plendil Extended-Release Tablets (0.5% to 1.5%) 651
Pravachol Tablets 943
Prevacid Delayed-Release Capsules (Less than 1%) 3268
Prevacid for Delayed-Release Oral Suspension (Less than 1%) 3268
Prevacid NapraPAC (Less than 1%) 3277
Prevacid SoluTab Delayed-Release Orally Disintegrating Tablets (Less than 1%) 3268
PREVPAC (Less than 1%) 3281
Prilosec OTC Tablets (Less than 1%) 2674
Prozac Pulvules and Liquid 1771
Repronex for Intramuscular and Subcutaneous Injection (Occasional) 1148
Requip Tablets (Infrequent) 1528
Retrovir Capsules 1533
Retrovir IV Infusion 1537
Retrovir 1533
Reyataz Capsules (Less than 3%) 948
Risperdal Consta Long-Acting Injection (Infrequent) 1664
Risperdal M-Tab Orally Disintegrating Tablets (Rare) 1658
Risperdal (Rare) 1658
▲ Sandimmune (Less than 1% to 4%) 2259
Sandostatin Injection (Less than 1%) 2263
Sandostatin LAR Depot (Rare) 2264
Seroquel Tablets (Rare) 691
Striant Mucoadhesive 1022
Sular Tablets 1163
Surmontil Capsules 2347
Sustiva Capsules 957
Symbyax Capsules (Rare) 1788
▲ Tagamet Tablets (4%; 0.3% to 1%) 1547
Tarka Tablets 519
Testim 1% Gel (1% or less) 722
Thalomid Capsules 979
Thioridazine Hydrochloride Tablets 2122
Thiothixene Capsules 2124
Tiazac Capsules (Less than 2%) 1204
Trecator Tablets 3482
Trelstar LA Suspension (1.7%) 3387
Tricor Tablets 523
Trizivir Tablets 1565
▲ Vantas (4.1%) 3367
Vaseretic Tablets 2073
Vasotec I.V. Injection (0.5% to 1.0%) 2076
Verelan PM Capsules (2% or less) 3120
▲ Viadur Implant (6.9%) 782
Vivactil Tablets 2350
Vytorin 10/10 Tablets 2084
Vytorin 10/10 Tablets 3092
Vytorin 10/20 Tablets 2084
Vytorin 10/20 Tablets 3092
Vytorin 10/40 Tablets 2084
Vytorin 10/40 Tablets 3092
Vytorin 10/80 Tablets 2084
Vytorin 10/80 Tablets 3092
Wellbutrin Tablets (Infrequent) 1579
Wellbutrin SR Sustained-Release Tablets 1583
Wellbutrin XL Extended-Release Tablets 1588
Xanax XR Tablets 2655
Zantac (Occasional) 1597
Zantac Injection 1593
Zantac Injection Pharmacy Bulk Package (Infrequent) 1595
Zantac Syrup (Occasional) 1597
Zegerid Powder for Oral Solution (Less than 1%) 2972
Zocor Tablets 2078
▲ Zoladex 3-month (8%) 712
Zoloft (Rare) 2581
Zonegran Capsules (Rare) 1089
Zyban Sustained-Release Tablets 1620
Zyprexa Tablets (Infrequent) 1798

Gynecomastia, aggravated

Vantas (Less than 2%) 3367

H

Haemophilus B disease

Liquid PedvaxHIB 2012

Hair, abnormal growth

(*see under* Hirsutism)

Hair, dry brittle

Eskalith 1406
Gengraf Capsules (Rare) 458
Lithobid Tablets 1670
Neoral Soft Gelatin Capsules (Rare) 2247
Neoral Oral Solution (Rare) 2247
Nizoral 2% Shampoo 1838
Sandimmune (Rare) 2259

Hair, oily

Nizoral 2% Shampoo 1838

Hair discoloration

▲ Arava Tablets (1% to 3%) 2881
Effexor Tablets (Rare) 3405
Effexor XR Capsules (Rare) 3411
Nizoral 2% Shampoo (Rare) 1838
Psoriatec Cream 3191
Men's Rogaine Extra Strength Topical Solution, Ocean Rush Scent and Original Unscented ▣ 706
Women's Rogaine Topical Solution, Spring Bloom Scent and Original Unscented ▣ 707
Soriatane Capsules (Less than 1%) 1028
Wellbutrin Tablets (Rare) 1579

Hair growth, unwanted

Lupron Injection Pediatric 3256
Men's Rogaine Extra Strength Topical Solution, Ocean Rush Scent and Original Unscented ▣ 706
Women's Rogaine Topical Solution, Spring Bloom Scent and Original Unscented ▣ 707

Hair loss

(*see under* Alopecia)

Hair problems, unspecified

Accutane Capsules 2740
Advicor Tablets 1694
Altoprev Extended-Release Tablets 1151
Amnesteem Capsules 2126
Emcyt Capsules (1%) 3137
Invirase (Less than 2%) 2776
Lescol Capsules 2227
Lescol Capsules 2730
Lescol XL Tablets 2227
Lescol XL Tablets 2730
▲ Lupron Depot 3.75 mg (Among most frequent) 3257
Lupron Depot 7.5 mg (Less than 5%) 3261
Lupron Depot–3 Month 11.25 mg (Less than 5%) 3262
Mevacor Tablets 1996
Neurontin Capsules (Rare) 2498
Neurontin Oral Solution (Rare) 2498
Neurontin Tablets (Rare) 2498
Pravachol Tablets 943
Prevacid Delayed-Release Capsules (Less than 1%) 3268
Prevacid for Delayed-Release Oral Suspension (Less than 1%) 3268
Prevacid NapraPAC (Less than 1%) 3277
Prevacid SoluTab Delayed-Release Orally Disintegrating Tablets (Less than 1%) 3268
PREVPAC (Less than 1%) 3281
Vytorin 10/10 Tablets 2084
Vytorin 10/10 Tablets 3092
Vytorin 10/20 Tablets 2084
Vytorin 10/20 Tablets 3092
Vytorin 10/40 Tablets 2084
Vytorin 10/40 Tablets 3092
Vytorin 10/80 Tablets 2084
Vytorin 10/80 Tablets 3092
Zocor Tablets 2078
▲ Zoladex (4%) 709
Zoladex 3-month 712
Zomig Nasal Spray (Rare) 718

Hair texture, abnormal

▲ Imdur Tablets (Less than or equal to 5%) 3032
▲ Intron A for Injection (Less than 5%) 3038
Nizoral 2% Shampoo (One occurrence in 41 patients) 1838
Men's Rogaine Extra Strength Topical Solution, Ocean Rush Scent and Original Unscented ▣ 706
Women's Rogaine Topical Solution, Spring Bloom Scent and Original Unscented ▣ 707
▲ Soriatane Capsules (1% to 10%) 1028
Topamax Sprinkle Capsules (Infrequent) 2438
Topamax Tablets (Infrequent) 2438
Zoloft (Rare) 2581

Hair thinning

Accutane Capsules 2740
▲ Arimidex Tablets (2% to 5%) 665
Clorpres Tablets 2139
Eskalith 1406
Intron A for Injection 3038
Lithobid Tablets 1670

Halitosis

Effexor Tablets (Rare) 3405
Exelon Capsules (Infrequent) 2204
Floxin Otic Singles (Reported in a single subject) 1045
Floxin Otic Solution (Single report) 1043
Gabitril Tablets (Infrequent) 998
▲ Intron A for Injection (Less than 5%) 3038
Lamictal (Infrequent) 1449
Lunesta Tablets (Infrequent) 3139
Prevacid Delayed-Release Capsules (Less than 1%) 3268
Prevacid for Delayed-Release Oral Suspension (Less than 1%) 3268
Prevacid NapraPAC (Less than 1%) 3277
Prevacid SoluTab Delayed-Release Orally Disintegrating Tablets (Less than 1%) 3268
PREVPAC (Less than 1%) 3281
Protonix I.V. (Less than 1%) 3468
Protonix Tablets (Less than 1%) 3465
Relpax Tablets (Rare) 2531
Rythmol SR Capsules 2736
Tequin Injection (Less than 0.1%) 964
Tequin Tablets (Less than 0.1%) 964

Hallucinations

Abilify Tablets (Infrequent to frequent) 916
Abilify Tablets (Infrequent to frequent) 2472
Actimmune (Rare) 1646
Actiq (1% to 2%) 993
Allegra-D 12 Hour Extended-Release Tablets 2860
Allegra-D 24 Hour Extended-Release Tablets 2862
Ambien Tablets (Infrequent) 2867
AmBisome for Injection (Less common) 615
Amerge Tablets (Rare) 1312
Ammonul Injection 3323
Anaprox Tablets (Less than 1%) 2769
Anaprox DS Tablets (Less than 1%) 2769
▲ Apokyn Injection (10% to 14%) 2132
Aricept Tablets 1086
Aricept ODT Tablets 1086
Arthrotec Tablets (Rare) 3126
Avelox (Less than 0.1%) 2984
Avinza Capsules (Less than 5%) 1714
Balamine DM 739
Biaxin/Biaxin XL 402
Blocadren Tablets (Less than 1%) 1891
Buprenex Injectable (Infrequent) 2718
Campath Ampules 826
Campral Tablets (Infrequent) 1175
Cardizem LA Extended Release Tablets (Less than 2%) 1699
Cataflam Tablets (Rarely) 2173
Catapres Tablets 874
Celexa (Infrequent) 1177
▲ CellCept Capsules (3% to less than 20%) 2751
▲ CellCept Intravenous (3% to less than 20%) 2751
▲ CellCept Oral Suspension (3% to less than 20%) 2751
▲ CellCept Tablets (3% to less than 20%) 2751
Cipro I.V. (1% or less) 2998
Cipro I.V. Pharmacy Bulk Package (1% or less) 3509
Cipro (Less than 1%) 2991
Cipro XR Tablets 3004
Clozapine Tablets (Less than 1%) 2141
Clozaril Tablets (Less than 1%) 2174
Cogentin Injection 1903
Comtan Tablets 2186
Copaxone for Injection (Infrequent) 3292
Cosopt Sterile Ophthalmic Solution 1910
Cytovene 2763
Dalmane Capsules (Rare) 3343
Darvocet A 500 Tablets 3497
Demser Capsules 1933
Depacon Injection 412
Depakene 417
Depakote Sprinkle Capsules 422
▲ Depakote Tablets (1% to 5%) 427
Depakote ER Tablets (Greater than 1%) 433
Detrol Tablets 2626
Didronel Tablets 2693
Digitek Tablets 2146
Dilaudid 439
Dilaudid Oral Liquid (Less frequent) 443
Dilaudid Non-Sterile Powder 439
Dilaudid Rectal Suppositories 439
Dilaudid Tablets 439
Dilaudid Tablets - 8 mg (Less frequent) 443
Dilaudid-HP (Less frequent) 441
Diprivan Injectable Emulsion (Less than 1%) 676
Ditropan XL Extended Release Tablets (Rare) 2391
Dolobid Tablets (Less than 1 in 100) 1937
Dostinex Tablets 2631
▲ Duragesic Transdermal System (3% to 10%) 2448
EC-Naprosyn Delayed-Release Tablets (Less than 1%) 2769
Effexor Tablets (Infrequent) 3405
Effexor XR Capsules (Infrequent) 3411
▲ Eldepryl Capsules (3 of 49 patients) 3209
Elspar for Injection 1943
Equetro Extended-Release Capsules 3178
Ery-Tab Tablets (Isolated reports) 447
Erythrocin Stearate Filmtab Tablets (Isolated reports) 452
Erythromycin Base Filmtab Tablets (Isolated reports) 454
Erythromycin Delayed-Release Capsules, USP (Isolated reports) 456
Eskalith 1406
Evoxac Capsules (Less than 1%) 1042
▲ Exelon Capsules (4%) 2204
Famvir Tablets (Infrequent) 2207
FazaClo Orally Disintegrating Tablets (Less than 1%) 547
Flexeril Tablets (Less than 1%) 1832

Flumadine (Less than 0.3%) 1186
Focalin Tablets 2214
Gabitril Tablets (Frequent) 998
Genoptic Sterile Ophthalmic Solution (Rare) ⊙ 227
Guanidine Hydrochloride Tablets 3030
Imitrex Injection 1431
Imitrex Tablets (Rare) 1440
Inderal LA Long-Acting Capsules 3421
InnoPran XL Capsules 2728
Invanz for Injection (Very rare) 1974
Invirase (Less than 2%) 2776
▲ I.V. Busulfex (5%) 1125
Kadian Capsules (Less than 3%) 572
Klonopin 2782
Lamictal (Infrequent) 1449
Lanoxicaps Capsules 1458
Lanoxin Injection 1462
Lanoxin Tablets 1468
Lanoxin Injection Pediatric 1465
Lariam Tablets (Occasional) 2790
Leukeran Tablets (Rare) 1472
Levaquin in 5% Dextrose Injection (0.1% to 0.9%) 2453
Levaquin (0.1% to 0.9%) 2453
Lithobid Tablets 1670
▲ Lunesta Tablets (1% to 3%) 3139
Lyrica Capsules (0.1% to 1%) 2524
Marinol Capsules (Greater than 1%) 3334
Matulane Capsules 3188
Maxipime for Injection 1093
Mebaral Tablets, USP (Less than 1 in 100 patients) 2483
Merrem I.V. (Greater than 0.1% to 1%) 687
▲ Mirapex Tablets (9% to 17%) 889
MS Contin Tablets (Less frequent) 2703
Nadolol Tablets 2121
Naprosyn Suspension (Less than 1%) 2769
Naprosyn Tablets (Less than 1%) 2769
Narcan Injection 1109
Naropin Injection (Less than 1%) 640
Nembutal Sodium Solution, USP (Less than 1%) 2484
Neurontin Capsules (Infrequent) 2498
Neurontin Oral Solution (Infrequent) 2498
Neurontin Tablets (Infrequent) 2498
Nipent for Injection (Less than 3%) 3216
Niravam Orally Disintegrating Tablets 3106
Norflex Injection 1824
Noroxin Tablets 2009
Norvir (Less than 2%) 499
Nubain Injection (1% or less) 1111
Numorphan 1112
OxyContin Tablets (Less than 1%) 2699
Parcopa Orally Disintegrating Tablets 3111
Paxil CR Controlled-Release Tablets (Infrequent) 1509
Paxil (Infrequent) 1501
Pepcid Injection (Infrequent) 2017
Pepcid (Infrequent) 2014
▲ Permax Tablets (13.8%) 3357
Phenergan 3438
Plavix Tablets 940
Plavix Tablets 2942
Prevacid Delayed-Release Capsules (Less than 1%) 3268
Prevacid for Delayed-Release Oral Suspension (Less than 1%) 3268
Prevacid NapraPAC (Less than 1%) 3277
Prevacid SoluTab Delayed-Release Orally Disintegrating Tablets (Less than 1%) 3268
PREVPAC (Less than 1%) 3281
Prilosec OTC Tablets (Less than 1%) 2674
Primaxin I.M. 2022
Primaxin I.V. 2024
▲ Prograf Capsules and Injection (3% to 15%) 624
ProSom Tablets (Rare) 512
Protonix I.V. (Less than 1%) 3468
Protonix Tablets (Less than 1%) 3465
Provigil Tablets (At least 1%) 1002
Prozac Pulvules and Liquid (Infrequent) 1771
Razadyne ER Extended-Release Capsules (Greater than or equal to 2%) 2434
Razadyne (Greater than or equal to 2%) 2434
Relpax Tablets (Rare) 2531
▲ Requip Tablets (5% to 10%) 1528
Rescriptor Tablets 2535
Reyataz Capsules (Less than 3%) 948
Rilutek Tablets (Infrequent) 2945
▲ Risperdal Consta Long-Acting Injection (6% to 7%) 1664
Roferon-A Injection (Infrequent) 2805
Sanctura Tablets 1133
Sandostatin LAR Depot (1% to 4%) 2264
Seroquel Tablets (Infrequent) 691
Singulair 2047
Sonata Capsules (Less than 1%) 1686
▲ Stalevo Tablets (4%) 2270
Surmontil Capsules 2347
Sustiva Capsules (Less than 2%) 957
Symmetrel (1% to 5%) 1115
Tagamet Tablets 1547
▲ Tasmar Tablets (8% to 10%) 3360
Tenormin I.V. Injection 698
Tenormin Tablets 695
Tequin Injection (Less than 0.1%) 964
Tequin Tablets (Less than 0.1%) 964
Tiazac Capsules (Less than 2%) 1204
Timolide Tablets 2056
Timoptic in Ocudose (Less frequent) 2061
Timoptic Sterile Ophthalmic Solution (Less frequent) 2058
Timoptic-XE Sterile Ophthalmic Gel Forming Solution 2062
Topamax Sprinkle Capsules (Frequent) 2438
Topamax Tablets (Frequent) 2438
Toprol-XL Tablets 660
Transderm Scōp Transdermal Therapeutic System (Infrequent) 2166
Ultracet Tablets (Less than 1%) 2462
▲ Valcyte Tablets (Less than 5%) 2816
Valium Tablets 2822
Vantin Tablets and Oral Suspension (Less than 1%) 2650
▲ Vesanoid Capsules (6%) 2823
VFEND I.V. (0% to 2.8%) 2543
VFEND Oral Suspension (0% to 2.8%) 2543
VFEND Tablets (0% to 2.8%) 2543
Vivactil Tablets 2350
Voltaren Tablets (Rarely) 2298
Voltaren-XR Tablets (Rarely) 2301
Wellbutrin Tablets (Frequent) 1579
Wellbutrin SR Sustained-Release Tablets 1583
Wellbutrin XL Extended-Release Tablets 1588
Xanax XR Tablets (Rare to infrequent) 2655
Zantac (Rare) 1597
Zantac Injection 1593
Zantac Injection Pharmacy Bulk Package (Rare) 1595
Zantac Syrup (Rare) 1597
Zegerid Powder for Oral Solution (Less than 1%) 2972
Zoloft (Infrequent) 2581
Zomig Tablets (Rare) 714
Zomig-ZMT Tablets (Rare) 714
Zosyn (1.0% or less) 3492
Zovirax Capsules 1616
Zovirax for Injection (Approximately 1%) 1618
Zovirax 1616
Zyban Sustained-Release Tablets 1620
Zyprexa Tablets 1798
Zyprexa ZYDIS Orally Disintegrating Tablets 1798
Zyrtec Chewable Tablets (Rare) 2589
Zyrtec (Rare) 2589
Zyrtec-D 12 Hour Extended Release Tablets 2591

Hallucinations, auditory
Catapres Tablets (Rare) 874
Catapres-TTS (0.5% or less) 875
Clorpres Tablets 2139
Lexapro Oral Solution (Infrequent) 1193
Lexapro Tablets (Infrequent) 1193
Orthoclone OKT3 Sterile Solution 2370
Valtrex Caplets 1573

Hallucinations, paradoxical
Diastat Rectal Delivery System 3344
Niravam Orally Disintegrating Tablets (Rare) 3106

Hallucinations, visual
Carbatrol Capsules 3174
Catapres Tablets (Rare) 874
Catapres-TTS (0.5% or less) 875
Clorpres Tablets 2139
Cogentin Injection 1903
Lexapro Oral Solution 1193
Lexapro Tablets 1193
Orthoclone OKT3 Sterile Solution 2370
Tegretol/Tegretol-XR 2278
Tessalon Capsules 1202
Tessalon Perles 1202
Valtrex Caplets 1573

Halos
Pacerone Tablets 3337

Hand-foot syndrome
(*see under* Palmar-plantar erythrodysesthesia syndrome)

Hangover
Aciphex Tablets (Rare) 1081
Effexor Tablets (Infrequent) 3405
Effexor XR Capsules (Infrequent) 3411
Lyrica Capsules (Rare) 2524
Maxalt Tablets (Infrequent) 1983
Maxalt-MLT Orally Disintegrating Tablets (Infrequent) 1983
Neurontin Capsules (Rare) 2498
Neurontin Oral Solution (Rare) 2498
Neurontin Tablets (Rare) 2498
Nipent for Injection (Less than 3%) 3216
▲ ProSom Tablets (3%) 512
Sonata Capsules (Infrequent) 1686
Thalomid Capsules 979
Xanax XR Tablets (Infrequent) 2655
Zyprexa Tablets (Infrequent) 1798
Zyprexa ZYDIS Orally Disintegrating Tablets (Infrequent) 1798

HDL, decrease
▲ Amnesteem Capsules (15%) 2126
Anadrol-50 Tablets 3329
▲ AndroGel (3% to 6%) 3330
Coreg Tablets (Less than or equal to 0.1%) 1376
Premphase Tablets 3452
Prempro Tablets 3452
Targretin Capsules 1719

HDL, increase
CombiPatch Transdermal System 2180
Equetro Extended-Release Capsules 3178
Premarin Tablets 3443
Premphase Tablets 3452
Prempro Tablets 3452

Head, tight feeling
Adenocard Injection (Less than 1%) 612
Aricept Tablets (Infrequent) 1086
Aricept ODT Tablets (Infrequent) 1086
Imitrex Injection (2.2%) 1431
Imitrex Tablets (Infrequent) 1440
Klonopin (Infrequent) 2782
ProAmatine Tablets (Less frequent) 3183

Headache
▲ Abelcet Injection (6%) 1119
▲ Abilify Tablets (31%) 916
▲ Abilify Tablets (31%) 2472
▲ Accolate Tablets (4.5% to 12.9%) 663
Accutane Capsules 2740
▲ Aceon Tablets (2 mg, 4 mg, 8 mg) (23.8%) 3191
Aciphex Tablets (2.4%) 1081
▲ Actimmune (33%) 1646
▲ Actiq (3% to 6%) 993
▲ Activella Tablets (11% to 16%) 2311
▲ Actonel Tablets (7.2% to 18%) 2679
▲ Actonel with Calcium Tablets (7.2% to 7.3%) 2684
▲ ActoPlus Met Tablets (4.6% to 6%) 3219
▲ Actos Tablets (9.1%) 3224
Acular Ophthalmic Solution (Rare) 561
▲ Acular LS Ophthalmic Solution (1% to 5%) 562
▲ Adacel Vaccine (2% to 44%) 2959
▲ Adalat CC Tablets (19%) 2978
Adderall Tablets 3168
▲ Adderall XR Capsules (26%) 3169
Adenocard Injection (2%) 612
▲ Adenoscan (18%) 613
Adipex-P 1216
▲ Advair Diskus 100/50 (12% to 20%) 1291
▲ Advair Diskus 250/50 (12% to 20%) 1291
▲ Advair Diskus 500/50 (12% to 20%) 1291
▲ Advate Injection (29.3%) 742
▲ Advicor Tablets (9%) 1694
▲ Aerobid/Aerobid-M (25%) 1172
▲ Agenerase Capsules (12% to 16%) 1299
▲ Agenerase Oral Solution (12% to 16%) 1304
Aggrastat (Less than 1%) 1878
▲ Aggrenox Capsules (39.2%) 855
▲ Agrylin Capsules (43.5%) 3172
Alacol DM Syrup 739
▲ Alamast Ophthalmic Solution (10% to 25%) 3371
Albalon Ophthalmic Solution ⊙ 216
▲ Albenza Tablets (1.3% to 11.0%) 1310
▲ Aldara Cream, 5% (More than 1% to 5%) 1814
Aldoclor Tablets 1881
Aldoril Tablets 1884
Aldurazyme for Intravenous Infusion 1261
Alesse-28 Tablets 3392
▲ Alferon N Injection (3% to 31%) 1640
Alinia for Oral Suspension (1.1%) 2840
Alinia Tablets (1.1%) 2840
▲ Allegra (7.2% to 10.6%) 2857
▲ Allegra-D 12 Hour Extended-Release Tablets (13.8%) 2860
▲ Allegra-D 24 Hour Extended-Release Tablets (13.8%) 2862
Aloprim for Injection (Less than 1%) 2156
▲ Aloxi Injection (9%) 2099
Alphagan P Ophthalmic Solution (1% to 4%) 563
▲ Altace Capsules (1.2% to 5.4%) 1673
▲ Altoprev Extended-Release Tablets (2.1% to 3.2%) 1151
▲ Alupent Inhalation Aerosol (3.3%) 858
Amaryl Tablets (1.5%) 2864
▲ Ambien Tablets (7% to 19%) 2867
▲ AmBisome for Injection (9.4% to 19.8%) 615
Amevive (0.20%) 836
Amnesteem Capsules 2126
▲ Amoxil Capsules (7%) 1315
▲ Amoxil Chewable Tablets (7%) 1315
▲ Amoxil Pediatric Drops for Oral Suspension (7%) 1315
▲ Amoxil Powder for Oral Suspension (7%) 1315
▲ Amoxil Tablets (7%) 1315
▲ Anaprox Tablets (3% to 9%) 2769
▲ Anaprox DS Tablets (3% to 9%) 2769
AndroGel (Up to 3%) 3330
▲ Angiomax for Injection (2.6% to 12%) 1856
Antabuse Tablets 2343
▲ Antara Capsules (3.2%) 2723
▲ Anzemet Injection (9.4% to 24.3%) 2871
▲ Anzemet Tablets (7% to 17.9%) 2874
▲ Apokyn Injection (At least 5%) 2132
▲ Aptivus Capsules (3.1%) 859
Aralast (0.3% to 0.7%) 745
▲ Aranesp for Injection (12% to 16%) 576
▲ Arava Tablets (7%) 2881
▲ Aredia for Injection (10% to 26.2%) 2168
▲ Argatroban Injection (5.4%) 1321
▲ Aricept Tablets (10%) 1086
▲ Aricept ODT Tablets (10%) 1086
▲ Arimidex Tablets (7% to 18%) 665
▲ Arixtra Injection (0% to 4.5%) 1325
▲ Aromasin Tablets (8%) 2600
Arthrotec Tablets (Rare) 3126
▲ Asacol Delayed-Release Tablets (35%) 2688
▲ Asmanex Twisthaler (17% to 22%) 2981
▲ Astelin Nasal Spray (7.9%) 1876
Atacand Tablets (More than 1%) 634
▲ Atrovent HFA Inhalation Aerosol (6% to 7%) 872
▲ Atrovent Inhalation Solution (6.4%) 868
▲ Atrovent Nasal Spray 0.03% (9.8%) 869
Attenuvax 1889
Augmentin (Less frequent) 1331
Augmentin Tablets (Less frequent) 1334
Augmentin XR Extended-Release Tablets (Rare) 1340
Avalide Tablets (1% or greater) 922
Avalide Tablets (1% or greater) 2889
▲ Avandamet Tablets (6.5%) 1343
▲ Avandia Tablets (5.9%) 1348
Avapro Tablets (1% or greater) 925
Avapro Tablets (1% or greater) 2886
▲ Avastin IV (26%) 1229
Avelox (2%) 2984
▲ Avinza Capsules (Greater than 10%) 1714
▲ Avonex (58%) 839
Axert Tablets (Frequent) 2430
▲ Axid Oral Solution (16.6%) 913
Aygestin Tablets 1062
▲ Azmacort Inhalation Aerosol (7% to 21%) 1701
Azopt Ophthalmic Suspension (1% to 5%) 553
Bactroban Cream (1.7% to 3.6%) 1356
▲ Bactroban Nasal (9%) 1357
Balamine DM 739
▲ Baraclude (2% to 5%) 928
Bayer Aspirin Tablets 3515
Beconase AQ Nasal Spray (Fewer than 5 per 100 patients) 1359
▲ BeneFix for Injection (10.8%) 3402

Benicar HCT Tablets (Greater than 2%) 2852
Bentyl Capsules 724
Bentyl Injection 724
Bentyl Syrup 724
Bentyl Tablets 724
Betagan Ophthalmic Solution, USP (Rare) ⊙ 217
▲ Betaseron for SC Injection (57%) 791
▲ Betimol Ophthalmic Solution (More than 5%) ⊙ 283
▲ Betimol Ophthalmic Solution (More than 5%) 3371
Betoptic S Ophthalmic Suspension (Rare) 554
▲ Bexxar (0% to 16%) 1360
Biaxin/Biaxin XL (2%) 402
▲ BiDil Tablets (50%) 2161
Biltricide Tablets 2990
Blocadren Tablets (Greater than 1%) 1891
▲ Boniva Tablets (3.3% to 6.5%) 2747
▲ Boostrix (3.7% to 43.1%) 1366
▲ Botox Purified Neurotoxin Complex (3% to 11%) 565
▲ Bravelle for Intramuscular or Subcutaneous Injection (8.1% to 12.7%) 1140
Brevibloc Concentrate (About 2%) 766
Brevibloc Injection (About 2%) 766
Brevibloc Double Strength Injection (About 2%) 766
Brevibloc Premixed Injection (About 2%) 766
Brevibloc Double Strength Premixed Injection (About 2%) 766
▲ Brimonidine Tartrate Ophthalmic Solution 0.2% (10% to 30%) ⊙ 245
Buphenyl Powder (Less than or equal to 2%) 3327
Buphenyl Tablets (Less than or equal to 2%) 3327
▲ Buprenex Injectable (1% to 5%) 2718
▲ Byetta Injection (9%) 605
▲ Caduet Tablets (2.5% to 16.7%) 2507
Calcijex Injection 411
Calcium Disodium Versenate Injection 1819
▲ Campath Ampules (1% to 24%) 826
Campral Tablets (Frequent) 1175
▲ Camptosar Injection (1% to 17%) 2602
▲ Canasa Rectal Suppositories (14.4%) 726
▲ Cancidas for Injection (4.3% to 11.3%) 1894
Captopril Tablets (About 0.5% to 2%) 2114
▲ Carac Cream, 0.5% (3.1%) 1048
Carafate Suspension (Less than 0.5%) 727
Carafate Tablets (Less than 0.5%) 728
Carbatrol Capsules 3174
▲ Cardene I.V. (14.6%) 1129
▲ Cardizem LA Extended Release Tablets (Up to 4.6%) 1699
Carimune NF 3501
▲ Carnitor Injection (3% to 37%) 3185
Carteolol Hydrochloride Ophthalmic Solution USP, 1% (Occasional) ⊙ 246
▲ Casodex Tablets (4%) 670
▲ Cataflam Tablets (1% to 10%) 2173
Catapres Tablets (About 1 in 100 patients) 874
▲ Catapres-TTS (5 of 101 patients) 875
Caverject Impulse Injection (2%) 2610
Ceftin Tablets (0.1% to 1%) 1369
▲ Celebrex Capsules (15.8%) 3130
Celexa (At least 2%) 1177
▲ CellCept Capsules (16.1% to 54.3%) 2751
▲ CellCept Intravenous (16.1% to 54.3%) 2751
▲ CellCept Oral Suspension (16.1% to 54.3%) 2751
▲ CellCept Tablets (16.1% to 54.3%) 2751
▲ Cenestin Tablets, 0.45mg, 0.625mg, 0.9mg, 1.25mg (11.3% to 68%) 1063
Cenestin Tablets, 0.3mg 1063
▲ Cerezyme for Injection (Approximately 6.5%) 1263
▲ Chemet Capsules (5.2% to 15.7%) 2480
▲ Cialis Tablets (11% to 15%) 1806
Cipro I.V. (Greater than 1%) 2998
Cipro I.V. Pharmacy Bulk Package (Greater than 1%) 3509
Cipro (Less than 1%) 2991
▲ Cipro XR Tablets (1% to 3%) 3004
▲ Clarinex Tablets (14%) 3009
▲ Clarinex Reditabs Tablets (14%) 3009
▲ Clarinex-D 24-Hour Extended-Release Tablets (6%) 3012
Cleocin Vaginal Ovules (Less than 1%) 2613
▲ Climara Transdermal System (5% to 18%) 795
▲ Climara Pro Transdermal System (5.2%) 800
Clindesse Vaginal Cream (2.7%) 3296
▲ Clinoril Tablets (3% to 9%) 1899
Clobex Shampoo (1.8%) 1209
▲ Clolar for Intravenous Infusion (46%) 1264
Clorpres Tablets (About 1 in 100) 2139
▲ Clozapine Tablets (More than 5% to 7%) 2141
▲ Clozaril Tablets (More than 5% to 7%) 2174
▲ Colazal Capsules (8%) 2845
▲ CombiPatch Transdermal System (17% to 25%) 2180
▲ Combivent Inhalation Aerosol (5.6%) 878
▲ Combivir Tablets (35%) 1373
▲ Combunox Tablets (Greater than or equal to 1% to 10.2%) 1183
▲ Concerta Extended-Release Tablets (9% to 14%) 1828
Copaxone for Injection (At least 2%) 3292
▲ Copegus Tablets (43%) 2759
▲ Coreg Tablets (5% to 8%) 1376
Cosopt Sterile Ophthalmic Solution (1% to 5%) 1910
Coumadin for Injection (Infrequent) 932
Coumadin Tablets (Infrequent) 932
▲ Covera-HS Tablets (2.2% to 6.6%) 3135
Cozaar Tablets (1% or greater) 1913
▲ Crestor Tablets (5.5%) 672
▲ Crixivan Capsules (5.4%) 1918
▲ Cubicin for Injection (5.4%) 1038
Cutivate Lotion 0.05% (2%) 1383
▲ Cymbalta Delayed-Release Capsules (13% to 15%) 1729
CytoGam Intravenous (Infrequent) 1866
Cytovene (At least 3 subjects) 2763
Dalmane Capsules 3343
Dantrium Capsules (Less frequent) 2690
Dapsone Tablets USP 1656
Daranide Tablets 1928
Darvocet A 500 Tablets 3497
DDAVP Injection 4 mcg/mL (Infrequent) 2893
▲ DDAVP Nasal Spray (2 to 5%) 2894
▲ DDAVP Tablets (4%) 2895
Decadron Phosphate Injection 1931
Decadron Tablets 1929
Delatestryl Injection 2976
Demser Capsules (Infrequent) 1933
Denavir Cream 2163
▲ Depacon Injection (4.3% to 31%) 412
▲ Depakene (31%) 417
▲ Depakote Sprinkle Capsules (31%) 422
▲ Depakote Tablets (31%) 427
▲ Depakote ER Tablets (31%) 433
▲ DepoCyt Injection (18% to 53%) 1121
▲ DepoDur Extended-Release Injection (Greater than 10%) 1098
Depo-Medrol Injectable Suspension 2615
Depo-Medrol Single-Dose Vial 2617
▲ Depo-Provera Contraceptive Injection (Greater than 5%) 2619
▲ depo-subQ provera 104 Injectable Suspension (9%) 2622
Desferal Vials 2190
▲ Desmopressin Acetate Rhinal Tube (2% to 5%) 1144
Desoxyn Tablets, USP 2482
▲ Detrol Tablets (11%) 2626
▲ Detrol LA Capsules (6%) 2629
Dexedrine 1386
DextroStat Tablets 3177
▲ Diastat Rectal Delivery System (5%) 3344
Didronel Tablets 2693
▲ Digitek Tablets (4%) 2146
Dilaudid 439
Dilaudid Oral Liquid (Less frequent) 443
Dilaudid Non-Sterile Powder 439
Dilaudid Rectal Suppositories 439
Dilaudid Tablets 439
Dilaudid Tablets - 8 mg (Less frequent) 443
Dilaudid-HP (Less frequent) 441
Diovan HCT Tablets (More than 2%) 2195
Diovan Tablets (More than 1%) 2191
Diprivan Injectable Emulsion (Less than 1%) 676
▲ Ditropan XL Extended Release Tablets (6% to 10%) 2391
Diuril Oral 1936
Diuril Sodium Intravenous 1934
▲ Dolobid Tablets (3% to 9%) 1937
▲ Dostinex Tablets (26%) 2631
▲ Doxil Injection (Approximately 5.3% to 10.5%) 3302
▲ Duragesic Transdermal System (3% to 10%) 2448
Dyazide Capsules 1389
Dynacin Tablets 1859
▲ DynaCirc CR Tablets (10.3% to 18.3%) 2726
Dyrenium Capsules (Rare) 3390
▲ EC-Naprosyn Delayed-Release Tablets (3% to 9%) 2769
Ecotrin Enteric Coated Aspirin Low, Regular and Maximum Strength Tablets 1627
Edecrin 1941
Edex Injection (2%) 3103
▲ Effexor Tablets (3% to 25%) 3405
▲ Effexor XR Capsules (2% to 34%) 3411
▲ Eldepryl Capsules (2 of 49 patients) 3209
▲ Elestat Ophthalmic Solution (1% to 3%) 1643
▲ Elidel Cream 1% (7% to 16%) 2198
▲ Elitek (26%) 2906
▲ Elmiron Capsules (3%) 2393
▲ Eloxatin for Injection (7% to 17%) 2908
Elspar for Injection 1943
Emcyt Capsules (1%) 3137
▲ Emend Capsules (8.5%) 1944
▲ Emtriva Capsules (13% to 22%) 1272
▲ Enablex Extended-Release Tablets (6.7%) 2201
▲ Enbrel for Injection (17% to 24%) 580
▲ Engerix-B Vaccine (1% to 10%) 1391
▲ Entocort EC Capsules (21%) 2694
EpiPen 1061
▲ Epivir (35%) 1394
▲ Epivir-HBV (21%) 1398
▲ Epogen for Injection (0.4% to 19%) 586
▲ Epzicom Tablets (6% to 7%) 1402
▲ Equetro Extended-Release Capsules (22%) 3178
▲ Erbitux (25%) 937
Eskalith 1406
Estratest Tablets 3196
Estratest H.S. Tablets 3196
▲ Estrogel 0.06% (20.2%) 3200
▲ Evoclin Foam, 1% (3%) 1025
▲ Evoxac Capsules (14.4%) 1042
▲ Exelon Capsules (17%) 2204
▲ Fabrazyme for Intravenous Infusion (13%) 1267
Factive Tablets (1.2%) 2464
▲ Famvir Tablets (16% to 39.3%) 2207
▲ Faslodex Injection (15.4%) 682
▲ FazaClo Orally Disintegrating Tablets (Greater than 5% to 7%) 547
▲ Femara Tablets (0.7% to 20%) 2210
▲ Ferrlecit Injection (7% to 29%) 3379
▲ Flexeril Tablets (1% to 5%) 1832
▲ Flolan for Injection (49% to 83%) 1408
▲ Flomax Capsules (19.3% to 21.1%) 881
▲ Flonase Nasal Spray (6.6% to 16.1%) 1412
▲ Flovent Diskus 50 mcg (12%) 1415
▲ Flovent HFA (11%) 1418
Floxin Otic Singles (0.3%) 1045
Floxin Otic Solution (0.2% to 0.3%) 1043
Flumadine (1.4%) 1186
▲ Flumist Vaccine (6.8% to 40.4%) 1872
Fluorescite Injection ⊙ 207
Focalin Tablets 2214
▲ Focalin XR Capsules (25% to 39%) 2217
▲ Follistim AQ Cartridge (5%) 2354
Foradil Aerolizer 3024
▲ Fortamet Extended-Release Tablets (4.7%) 1156
Fortaz (Less than 1%) 1422
▲ Forteo for Injection (7.5%) 1739
▲ Fortical Nasal Spray (3.2%) 3336
Fosamax (Up to 2.6%) 1949
Fosamax Plus D Tablets (0% to 2.6%) 1956
▲ Fosrenol Chewable Tablets (5% to 21%) 3180
▲ Frova Tablets (4%) 1101
Furosemide Tablets 2117
Gabitril Tablets (1% or more) 998
▲ Gammagard Liquid (6.9% to 36.1%) 751
Gammagard S/D (Occasional) 754
▲ Gamunex Immune Globulin I.V., 10% (0.8% to 58%) 3232
Garamycin Injectable 3028
Gemzar for Injection (Common) 1743
▲ Gengraf Capsules (2% to 25%) 458
Genotropin Lyophilized Powder 2642
▲ Geodon (18%) 2514
▲ Gleevec Tablets (25% to 35%) 2221
▲ Gonal-f RFF Pen for Injection (Greater than 10%) 3155
Grifulvin V Tablets Microsize and Oral Suspension Microsize (Occasional) 2384
Gris-PEG Tablets (Occasional) 2504
▲ Havrix Vaccine (9% to 14%) 1425
▲ Hectorol Capsules (27.9%) 909
▲ Hectorol Injection (27.9%) 911
▲ Hepsera Tablets (2% to 9%) 1275
▲ Herceptin I.V. (26%) 1234
HibTITER 3419
▲ Humatrope Vials and Cartridges (6.07% to 9.38%) 1756
▲ Humira Injection (12%) 464
▲ Hyalgan Solution (18%) 2917
▲ Hycamtin for Injection (0.2% to 21%) 1427
Hydrocortone Tablets 1963
Hyperstat I.V. Injection 3031
▲ Hytrin Capsules (1.1% to 16.2%) 469
Hyzaar (1% or greater) 1964
▲ Idamycin PFS Injection (20%) 2645
▲ Imdur Tablets (38% to 57%) 3032
Imitrex Injection (2.2%) 1431
Imitrex Tablets 1440
▲ Increlex Injection (Greater than or equal to 5%) 3290
▲ Indapamide Tablets (Greater than or equal to 5%) 2119
▲ Indocin (11.7%) 1968
Infed Injection 3381
▲ Infergen (78% to 82%) 1647
Inspra Tablets 2520
▲ Intron A for Injection (4% to 62%) 3038
▲ Invanz for Injection (4.4% to 6.8%) 1974
Invirase (Greater than or equal to 2%) 2776
▲ I.V. Busulfex (5% to 69%) 1125
Iveegam EN (0.3% to 0.8%) 759
Kadian Capsules (Less than 3%) 572
▲ Kaletra (2% to 7%) 474
▲ Keppra Oral Solution (2% to 14%) 3307
▲ Keppra Tablets (2% to 14%) 3307
▲ Ketek Tablets (2% to 5.5%) 2920
▲ Kineret Injection (12%) 594
Klonopin 2782
Koāte-DVI (0.7%) 3247
K-Phos Neutral Tablets 785
▲ Kytril Injection (14%) 2785
▲ Kytril Tablets (14% to 21%) 2788
▲ Lamictal (29.1%) 1449
▲ Lamisil Tablets (12.9%) 2226
Lanoxicaps Capsules 1458
Lanoxin Injection 1462
Lanoxin Tablets 1468
Lanoxin Injection Pediatric 1465
▲ Lariam Tablets (Among most frequent) 2790
▲ Lescol Capsules (8.9%) 2227
▲ Lescol Capsules (8.9%) 2730
▲ Lescol XL Tablets (4.7%) 2227
▲ Lescol XL Tablets (4.7%) 2730
▲ Leukine (26% to 36%) 829
▲ Leustatin Injection (7% to 22%) 2368
▲ Levaquin in 5% Dextrose Injection (0.1% to 5.8%) 2453
▲ Levaquin (0.1% to 5.8%) 2453
▲ Levitra Tablets (15%) 3048
Levothroid Tablets 1189
Levoxyl Tablets 1680
▲ Lexapro Oral Solution (24%) 1193
▲ Lexapro Tablets (24%) 1193
▲ Lexiva Tablets (2% to 27%) 1473
Lidoderm Patch 1107
▲ Lipitor Tablets (2.5% to 16.7%) 2495
Lithobid Tablets 1670
▲ Lofibra Capsules (3.2%) 1217
Lo/Ovral-28 Tablets 3423
Loprox Shampoo 1862
▲ Lotemax Ophthalmic Suspension 0.5% (Less than 15%) ⊙ 249
▲ Lotensin Tablets (6.2%) 2232
▲ Lotensin HCT Tablets (3.1%) 2235
Lotrel Capsules (2.2%) 2238
Lotronex Tablets 1479
▲ Lumigan Ophthalmic Solution (1% to 5%) 569
▲ Lunesta Tablets (13% to 21%) 3139
▲ Lupron Depot 3.75 mg (33%) 3257
Lupron Depot 7.5 mg (Less than 5%) 3261
▲ Lupron Depot–3 Month 11.25 mg (33%) 3262
Lupron Depot-PED 7.5 mg, 11.25 mg and 15 mg (Less than 2%) 3266
Lupron Injection Pediatric (Less than 2%) 3256
▲ Lyrica Capsules (5% to 8%) 2524
▲ Malarone Tablets (3% to 22%) 1484
▲ Malarone Pediatric Tablets (3% to 22%) 1484
Marinol Capsules (Less than 1%) 3334
Matulane Capsules 3188
Mavik Tablets (More than 1%) 482
Maxair Autohaler (1.3% to 2.0%) 1820

Maxalt Tablets (Less than 2%) 1983
Maxalt-MLT Orally Disintegrating Tablets (Less than 2%) 1983
Maxipime for Injection (Greater than 0.1% to 1%) 1093
Maxzide 2150
Mebaral Tablets, USP (Less than 1 in 100 patients) 2483
▲ Megace ES Oral Suspension (1% to 10%) 2492
▲ Menactra Vaccine (1.1% to 41.8%) 2968
▲ Menopur for Subcutaneous Injection (15.8% to 34.1%) 1145
Menostar Transdermal System 805
▲ Mepron Suspension (16% to 31%) 1487
▲ Meridia Capsules (30.3%) 485
▲ Merrem I.V. (2.3% to 7.8%) 687
Meruvax II 1994
▲ Metadate CD Capsules (12%) 3316
Metrogel 1% (2.2%) 1212
▲ MetroGel-Vaginal Gel (5%) 1822
▲ Mevacor Tablets (2.1% to 9.3%) 1996
▲ Miacalcin Nasal Spray (3.2%) 2242
Micardis Tablets (1%) 884
Micardis HCT Tablets (2% or greater) 886
▲ Midamor Tablets (3% to 8%) 2000
Mintezol 2002
Miradon Tablets 3056
Mirapex Tablets (1% or more) 889
▲ Mirena Intrauterine System (5% or more) 810
M-M-R II 1980
▲ Mobic Oral Suspension (2.4% to 8.3%) 893
▲ Mobic Tablets (2.4% to 8.3%) 893
▲ Moduretic Tablets (3% to 8%) 2003
MS Contin Tablets (Less frequent) 2703
Mycamine for Injection (0.9% to 2.7%) 620
▲ Myfortic Tablets (3% to less than 20%) 2244
▲ Mylotarg for Injection (27% to 50%) 3429
▲ Nabi-HB (14%) 2159
Nadolol Tablets (1 to 5 of 1000 patients) 2121
▲ Nalfon Capsules (8.7%) 2504
▲ Namenda (6%) 1199
▲ Naprosyn Suspension (3% to 9%) 2769
▲ Naprosyn Tablets (3% to 9%) 2769
▲ Naropin Injection (1% to 7.7%) 640
▲ Nasacort HFA Inhalation Aerosol (Greater than or equal to 3% to 10.3%) 2939
Nasacort AQ Nasal Spray (2% or greater) 2937
▲ Nasonex Nasal Spray (17% to 26%) 3058
▲ Natrecor for Injection (7% to 9%) 3123
Navelbine Injection 1494
Nembutal Sodium Solution, USP 2484
▲ Neoral Soft Gelatin Capsules (2% to 25%) 2247
▲ Neoral Oral Solution (2% to 25%) 2247
▲ Neulasta Injection (15% to 72%) 596
▲ Neumega for Injection (41%) 3433
▲ Neupogen for Injection (7%) 598
▲ Neurontin Capsules (3.3%) 2498
▲ Neurontin Oral Solution (3.3%) 2498
▲ Neurontin Tablets (3.3%) 2498
▲ Nexium Delayed-Release Capsules (3.8% to 5.5%) 645
▲ Nexium I.V. (3.8% to 5.5%) 649
▲ Niaspan Extended-Release Tablets (5% to 11%) 1703
Nicomide Tablets 3190
▲ Nicotrol Inhaler (26%) 2594
▲ Nicotrol NS (18%) 2596
Nimotop Capsules (Up to 4.1%) 774
▲ Nipent for Injection (13% to 17%) 3216
▲ Niravam Orally Disintegrating Tablets (12.9% to 29.2%) 3106
▲ Nitro-Dur Transdermal Infusion System (63%) 3060
▲ Nitrolingual Pumpspray (50%) 1161
▲ Norditropin Cartridges (Small number of patients -9%) 2318
Norflex Injection 1824
Noritate Cream, 1% (Uncommon) 1051
Noroxin Tablets (2.0% to 2.8%) 2009
▲ Norvasc Tablets (7.3%) 2529
▲ Norvir (6% to 6.5%) 499
▲ Novantrone for Injection Concentrate (6%) 3158
Novarel for Injection 1147
NovoSeven (1%) 2335
▲ Nubain Injection (3%) 1111
Numorphan 1112
Nutropin for Injection (A small number of patients) 1238
Nutropin AQ Injection (A small number of patients) 1241
Nutropin AQ Pen (A small number of patients) 1241
Nutropin AQ Pen Cartridge (A small number of patients) 1241
Omnicef Capsules (2%) 506
Omnicef for Oral Suspension (2%) 506
Oncaspar (Greater than 1% but less than 5%) 1123
▲ Ontak Vials (26%) 1717
OptiPranolol Metipranolol Ophthalmic Solution 0.3% (A small number of patients) .... ⊙254
▲ Optivar Ophthalmic Solution (Approximately 15%) 1877
▲ Orap Tablets (22.2%) 1220
Ortho-Cept Tablets 2395
Ortho-Cyclen Tablets 2414
▲ Ortho Evra Transdermal System (9% to 22%) 2402
Ortho Micronor Tablets 2411
Ortho Tri-Cyclen Tablets 2414
Ortho Tri-Cyclen Lo Tablets 2421
▲ Orthoclone OKT3 Sterile Solution (11% to 44%) 2370
▲ Orthovisc Injection (12.1%) 3518
Oxsoralen-Ultra Capsules 3354
▲ OxyContin Tablets (7%) 2699
▲ Oxytrol Transdermal System (Greater than 1%) 3383
▲ Pacerone Tablets (1% to 3%) 3337
Parcopa Orally Disintegrating Tablets 3111
Parnate Tablets 1499
▲ Patanol Ophthalmic Solution (7%) 557
▲ Paxil CR Controlled-Release Tablets (17% to 18%) 1509
▲ Paxil (17% to 18%) 1501
Pediapred Oral Solution 3319
Pediarix Vaccine 1518
Peganone Tablets, USP 2487
▲ Pegasys (54%) 2793
▲ PEG-Intron Powder for Injection (56%) 3062
Pentasa Capsules (2.0% to 2.2%) 3182
▲ Pepcid Injection (4.7%) 2017
▲ Pepcid (4.7%) 2014
▲ Permax Tablets (5.3%) 3357
Persantine Tablets (2.3%) 898
Phenytek Capsules 2153
▲ Photofrin for Injection (6%) 729
▲ Plan B Tablets (16.8%) 1068
Plasmanate (Occasional) 3252
▲ Plavix Tablets (7.6%) 940
▲ Plavix Tablets (7.6%) 2942
▲ Plendil Extended-Release Tablets (10.6% to 14.7%) 651
▲ Pletal Tablets (27% to 34%) 2478
Pneumovax 23 2020
▲ Prandin Tablets (0.5, 1, and 2 mg) (9% to 11%) 2337
▲ Pravachol Tablets (1.7% to 6.2%) 943
▲ Prefest Tablets (23%) 1069
Premarin Intravenous 3440
▲ Premarin Tablets (26% to 32%) 3443
Premarin Vaginal Cream 3449
▲ Premphase Tablets (28% to 37%) 3452
▲ Prempro Tablets (28% to 37%) 3452
▲ Prevacid Delayed-Release Capsules (Greater than 1% to 7%) 3268
▲ Prevacid for Delayed-Release Oral Suspension (Greater than 1% to 7%) 3268
Prevacid I.V. for Injection (1%) 3274
▲ Prevacid NapraPAC (3% to 9%) 3277
▲ Prevacid SoluTab Delayed-Release Orally Disintegrating Tablets (Greater than 1% to 7%) 3268
▲ PREVPAC (1% to 6%) 3281
▲ Prilosec OTC Tablets (2.9% to 7%) 2674
Primaxin I.M. 2022
Primaxin I.V. (Less than 0.2%) 2024
▲ Prinivil Tablets (4.4% to 5.7%) 2029
▲ Prinzide Tablets (5.2%) 2033
ProAmatine Tablets (Less frequent) 3183
▲ Prochieve 4% Gel (13%) 1018
▲ Prochieve 8% Gel (13%) 1018
▲ Procrit for Injection (0.40% to 19%) 2374
▲ Prograf Capsules and Injection (37% to 64%) 624
▲ Proleukin for Injection (12%) 1007
▲ Prometrium Capsules (100 mg, 200 mg) (10% to 31%) 3205
Propine Ophthalmic Solution .... ⊙237
▲ ProSom Tablets (16%) 512
Protonix I.V. (Greater than 1%) 3468
▲ Protonix Tablets (5% to 9%) 3465
▲ Protopic Ointment (10% to 20%) 629
Proventil Inhalation Aerosol 3067
▲ Proventil Inhalation Solution 0.083% (3% to 3.1%) 3069
Proventil HFA Inhalation Aerosol 3071
▲ Provigil Tablets (34%) 1002
▲ Prozac Pulvules and Liquid (21%) 1771
Quixin Ophthalmic Solution (1% to 3%) 3373
▲ Qvar Inhalation Aerosol (8% to 25%) 1654
▲ Rabies Vaccine RabAvert (10% to 52%) 1011
▲ Rapamune Oral Solution and Tablets (23% to 34%) 3472
▲ Raptiva for Injection (32%) 1247
▲ Razadyne ER Extended-Release Capsules (8%) 2434
▲ Razadyne (8%) 2434
▲ Rebetol (58% to 69%) 3073
▲ Rebetron Combination Therapy (63% to 67%) 3078
▲ Rebif Prefilled Syringe for Injection (65% to 70%) 3163
Recombivax HB (Greater than or equal to 1%) 2045
ReFacto Vials 3479
▲ Relafen Tablets (3% to 9%) 1523
Relenza Rotadisk (2%) 1525
▲ Relpax Tablets (3% to 4%) 2531
▲ Remicade for IV Injection (18%) 987
▲ Renagel Tablets (9.1%) 1268
▲ Repronex for Intramuscular and Subcutaneous Injection (5.2% to 6%) 1148
Requip Tablets (1% or more) 1528
▲ Rescriptor Tablets (11.2% to 16.8%) 2535
▲ Retisert Implant (31%) .... ⊙256
▲ Retrovir Capsules (1.6% to 62.5%) 1533
▲ Retrovir IV Infusion (2% to 62.5%) 1537
▲ Retrovir (1.6% to 62.5%) 1533
▲ Revatio Tablets (46%) 2541
▲ Rēv-Eyes Ophthalmic Eyedrops 0.5% (10% to 40%) .... ⊙256
▲ Reyataz Capsules (8% to 14%) 948
▲ R-Gene 10 for Intravenous Use (3%) 2647
Rhophylac (Occasionally) 3504
▲ Ribavirin, USP Capsules (58% to 69%) 3083
▲ Rilutek Tablets (7.0% to 8.0%) 2945
▲ Risperdal Consta Long-Acting Injection (15% to 22%) 1664
▲ Risperdal M-Tab Orally Disintegrating Tablets (12% to 14%) 1658
▲ Risperdal (12% to 14%) 1658
Ritalin Hydrochloride Tablets 2254
Ritalin LA Capsules 2255
Ritalin-SR Tablets 2254
▲ Rituxan for Infusion (14%) 845
▲ Rituxan I.V. (19%) 1251
Rocephin Injectable Vials, ADD-Vantage, Galaxy, Bulk (Occasional) 2801
▲ Roferon-A Injection (44% to 64%) 2805
▲ Rozerem Tablets (7%) 3228
▲ Rythmol SR Capsules (6% to 10%) 2736
▲ Sanctura Tablets (4.2%) 1133
▲ Sandimmune (2% to 15%) 2259
▲ Sandostatin Injection (6%) 2263
Sedapap Tablets 50 mg/650 mg (Infrequent) 2098
▲ Serevent Diskus (13% to 17%) 1540
Seromycin Capsules 1783
▲ Seroquel Tablets (21%) 691
▲ Simulect for Injection (Greater than or equal to 10%) 2268
▲ Singulair (1% to 18.4%) 2047
▲ Skelaxin Tablets (Most frequent) 1685
▲ Sonata Capsules (30% to 42%) 1686
▲ Soriatane Capsules (1% to 10%) 1028
▲ Spectracef Tablets (2% to 3%) 2706
St. Joseph 81 mg Aspirin Chewable and Enteric Coated Tablets 1841
Stalevo Tablets 2270
▲ Strattera Capsules (17% to 27%) 1784
▲ Striant Mucoadhesive (3.1%) 1022
Stromectol Tablets (0.2%) 2053
▲ Suboxone Tablets (30% to 36.4%) 2719
▲ Subutex Tablets (29.1% to 30%) 2719
▲ Sular Tablets (22%) 1163
Suprane Liquid for Inhalation (Greater than 1%) 770
Suprax (Less than 2%) 1811
Surmontil Capsules 2347
▲ Sustiva Capsules (5% to 11%) 957
Symmetrel (1% to 5%) 1115
Synercid I.V. (1.6%) 1690
Tagamet Tablets (2.1% to 3.5%) 1547
▲ Tambocor Tablets (9.6%) 1824
▲ Tamiflu Capsules (1.8% to 20.1%) 2810
▲ Tamiflu Oral Suspension (1.8% to 20.1%) 2810
▲ Targretin Capsules (29.8% to 41.5%) 1719
▲ Tarka Tablets (8.9%) 519
▲ Tasmar Tablets (10% to 11%) 3360
Tegretol/Tegretol-XR 2278
▲ Temodar Capsules (5% to 41%) 3088
Temovate Scalp Application (1 of 294 patients) 1551
Tenormin I.V. Injection 698
Tenormin Tablets 695
▲ Tequin Injection (3%) 964
▲ Tequin Tablets (3%) 964
Tessalon Capsules 1202
Tessalon Perles 1202
Testim 1% Gel (1%) 722
Teveten Tablets (1% or greater) 1707
▲ Teveten HCT Tablets (3.4%) 1710
Tev-Tropin for Injection (Infrequently) 1224
▲ Thalomid Capsules (12.5%) 979
Thioridazine Hydrochloride Tablets (Extremely rare) 2122
▲ Thymoglobulin for Injection (40.2%) 2848
▲ Thyrogen for Injection (7.3%) 1270
Thyrolar 1203
▲ Tiazac Capsules (8%) 1204
Ticlid Tablets (0.5% to 1.0%) 2813
Timentin ADD-Vantage 1556
Timentin Injection Galaxy Container 1559
Timentin IV Infusion 1553
Timentin Pharmacy Bulk Package 1562
Timolide Tablets (Less than 1%) 2056
Timoptic in Ocudose (Less frequent) 2061
Timoptic Sterile Ophthalmic Solution (Less frequent) 2058
Timoptic-XE Sterile Ophthalmic Gel Forming Solution (1% to 5%) 2062
Tindamax (0.7% to 1.3%) 2670
▲ TOBI Solution for Inhalation (26.7%) 1015
Topamax Sprinkle Capsules (More than 1%) 2438
Topamax Tablets (More than 1%) 2438
Toprol-XL Tablets 660
▲ Tracleer Tablets (22%) 539
Transderm Scōp Transdermal Therapeutic System (Few patients) 2166
Tranxene (Less common) 2488
Travatan Ophthalmic Solution (1% to 5%) 559
Trecator Tablets 3482
▲ Trelstar Depot (5%) 3385
▲ Trelstar LA Suspension (6.9%) 3387
▲ Tricor Tablets (3.2%) 523
▲ Triglide Tablets (3.2%) 1165
▲ Trileptal Oral Suspension (15% to 32%) 2281
▲ Trileptal Tablets (15% to 32%) 2281
Triphasil-28 Tablets 3483
▲ Trisenox Injection (60%) 983
▲ Trizivir Tablets (28%) 1565
Trusopt Sterile Ophthalmic Solution (Infrequent) 2065
▲ Truvada Tablets (Greater than 5%) 1279
▲ Twinrix Vaccine (13% to 22%) 1571
▲ Tygacil for Injection (5.9%) 3489
Tylenol Flu NightTime Gelcaps 1846
Ultane Liquid for Inhalation (1%) 526
Ultracet Tablets (At least 1%) 2462
Uniphyl Tablets 2708
Uniretic Tablets (More than 1%) 3114
Unithroid Tablets 3521
Univasc Tablets (Greater than 1%) 3118
Urecholine Tablets 2349
Uroqid-Acid No. 2 Tablets 785
▲ Uroxatral Tablets (3%) 2957
▲ Vagifem Tablets (9% to 10%) 2340
▲ Valcyte Tablets (9% to 22%) 2816
Valium Tablets (Infrequent) 2822
▲ Valtrex Caplets (13% to 38%) 1573
▲ Vanos Cream (2.8% to 4%) 1864
Vantas (2.9%) 3367
Vantin Tablets and Oral Suspension (Less than 1% to 1.1%) 2650
▲ Vaqta (0.4% to 16%) 2067
Varivax (Greater than or equal to 1%) 2070
▲ Vaseretic Tablets (5.5%) 2073
Vasotec I.V. Injection (1.8% to 5.2%) 2076
▲ Velcade for Injection (26%) 2102
▲ Ventavis Inhalation Solution (30%) 1036
Ventolin HFA Inhalation Aerosol 1576
▲ Verelan PM Capsules (2.2% to 12.1%) 3120
▲ Vesanoid Capsules (86%) 2823
▲ VFEND I.V. (0% to 3%) 2543
▲ VFEND Oral Suspension (0% to 3%) 2543
▲ VFEND Tablets (0% to 3%) 2543
▲ Viadur Implant (4.6%) 782
▲ Viagra Tablets (16%) 2552
▲ Vicoprofen Tablets (27%) 533
Viracept (Less than 2%) 2556
▲ Viramune Oral Suspension (3%) 903

▲ Viramune Tablets (3%) 903
▲ Viread Tablets (5% to 8%) 1284
Vivactil Tablets 2350
▲ Vivelle Transdermal System (14.9% to 50%) 2288
▲ Vivelle-Dot Transdermal System (14.9% to 50%) 2293
Vivotif 834
▲ Voltaren Ophthalmic Solution (Less than or equal to 3%) 2300
▲ Voltaren Tablets (1% to 10%) 2298
▲ Voltaren-XR Tablets (1% to 10%) 2301
▲ VoSpire Extended-Release Tablets (18.8%) 2352
▲ Vytorin 10/10 Tablets (6.8%) 2084
▲ Vytorin 10/10 Tablets (6.8%) 3092
▲ Vytorin 10/20 Tablets (6.8%) 2084
▲ Vytorin 10/20 Tablets (6.8%) 3092
▲ Vytorin 10/40 Tablets (6.8%) 2084
▲ Vytorin 10/40 Tablets (6.8%) 3092
▲ Vytorin 10/80 Tablets (6.8%) 2084
▲ Vytorin 10/80 Tablets (6.8%) 3092
▲ WelChol Tablets (6%) 2855
▲ Wellbutrin SR Sustained-Release Tablets (25% to 26%) 1583
▲ Wellbutrin XL Extended-Release Tablets (25% to 26%) 1588
WinRho SDF (2%) 763
▲ Xanax XR Tablets (26.5%) 2655
▲ Xeloda Tablets (1% to 9%) 2825
▲ Xenical Capsules (30.6%) 2834
▲ Xifaxan Tablets (9.7%) 2847
▲ Xolair (15%) 1259
▲ Xopenex HFA Inhalation Aerosol (11.9%) 3151
▲ Xopenex Inhalation Solution (11.9%) 3143
▲ Xopenex Inhalation Solution Concentrate (7.6% to 11.9%) 3147
Yasmin 28 Tablets (Greater than 1%) 818
▲ Zaditor Ophthalmic Solution (10% to 25%) 2302
Zantac 1597
Zantac Injection 1593
Zantac Injection Pharmacy Bulk Package (Frequent) 1595
Zantac Syrup 1597
▲ Zavesca Capsules (22%) 543
▲ Zegerid Powder for Oral Solution (2.9% to 7%) 2972
▲ Zelnorm Tablets (1% to 15%) 2303
Zemaira (2.5%) 3506
▲ Zenapax for Injection (Greater than 5%) 2838
▲ Zerit (25% to 54%) 971
▲ Zestoretic Tablets (5.2%) 701
▲ Zestril Tablets (4.4% to 5.7%) 704
▲ Zetia Tablets (8%) 2090
▲ Zetia Tablets (8%) 3098
▲ Zevalin Injection (12%) 848
▲ Ziagen (1% to 13%) 1600
Zithromax Capsules, 250 mg (1% or less) 2568
Zithromax for IV Infusion (1% or less) 2573
Zithromax for Oral Suspension, 1 g (1% or less) 2568
Zithromax for Oral Suspension, 300 mg, 600 mg, 900 mg, 1200 mg (1% or less) 2561
Zithromax Tablets, 250 mg, 500 mg (1% or less) 2561
Zithromax Tablets, 600 mg (1% or less) 2568
Zithromax Tri-Pak (1% or less) 2561
Zithromax Z-Pak (1% or less) 2568
Zmax for Oral Suspension (1.3%) 2577
▲ Zocor Tablets (3.5%) 2078
▲ Zofran Injection (17% to 25%) 1607
▲ Zofran (9% to 27%) 1613
▲ Zofran ODT Orally Disintegrating Tablets (9% to 27%) 1613
▲ Zoladex (1% to 75%) 709
Zoladex 3-month (1% to 5%) 712
▲ Zoloft (26%) 2581
▲ Zometa for Intravenous Infusion (5% to 19%) 2306
Zomig Nasal Spray (Rare to less than 2%) 718
Zomig Tablets (Rare) 714
▲ Zonegran Capsules (10%) 1089
▲ Zosyn (4.5% to 7.7%) 3492
Zovirax Capsules (2.2%) 1616
Zovirax for Injection (Less than 1%) 1618
Zovirax (2.2%) 1616
Zyban Sustained-Release Tablets (Frequent) 1620
▲ Zylet Ophthalmic Suspension (14%) 3508
▲ Zymar Ophthalmic Solution (1% to 4%) 571
▲ Zyprexa Tablets (17%) 1798
▲ Zyprexa ZYDIS Orally Disintegrating Tablets (17%) 1798
▲ Zyrtec Chewable Tablets (11.0% to 14.0%) 2589
▲ Zyrtec (11.0% to 14.0%) 2589
Zyrtec-D 12 Hour Extended Release Tablets 2591
▲ Zyvox (0% to 6.5%) 2661

Headache, migraine

(*see under* Migraine)

Headache, sinus

Lexapro Oral Solution (Frequent) 1193
Lexapro Tablets (Frequent) 1193
Serevent Diskus (1% to 3%) 1540
▲ Strattera Capsules (3%) 1784
▲ Vivelle Transdermal System (1.5% to 10.9%) 2288
▲ Vivelle-Dot Transdermal System (1.5% to 10.9%) 2293

Headache, throbbing

Hyperstat I.V. Injection 3031

Headache, transient

DDAVP Injection 4 mcg/mL (Infrequent) 2893
DDAVP Nasal Spray (Infrequent) 2894
Desmopressin Acetate Injection (Infrequent) 1143

Headache, vascular

Meridia Capsules 485
Paxil CR Controlled-Release Tablets 1509
Paxil 1501
Prozac Pulvules and Liquid (Infrequent) 1771

Healing, abnormal

Amnesteem Capsules 2126
Cafcit (2.2%) 1854
▲ CellCept Capsules (3% to less than 20%) 2751
▲ CellCept Intravenous (3% to less than 20%) 2751
▲ CellCept Oral Suspension (3% to less than 20%) 2751
▲ CellCept Tablets (3% to less than 20%) 2751
▲ Humira Injection (Less than 5%) 464
▲ Prograf Capsules and Injection (3% to 15%) 624
Soriatane Capsules (Less than 1%) 1028
▲ Tygacil for Injection (3.5%) 3489

Hearing, impaired

Accutane Capsules 2740
Amnesteem Capsules 2126
Anaprox Tablets (Less than 1%) 2769
Anaprox DS Tablets (Less than 1%) 2769
Arthrotec Tablets (Rare) 3126
Cataflam Tablets (Rarely) 2173
Desferal Vials 2190
EC-Naprosyn Delayed-Release Tablets (Less than 1%) 2769
Lariam Tablets 2790
Lortab 3315
Lortab Elixir 3312
Lupron Injection Pediatric 3256
Mustargen for Injection 2007
Naprosyn Suspension (Less than 1%) 2769
Naprosyn Tablets (Less than 1%) 2769
Naropin Injection (Less than 1%) 640
Norvir (Less than 2%) 499
Pegasys 2793
PEG-Intron Powder for Injection 3062
Prevacid NapraPAC (Less than 1%) 3277
Requip Tablets (Infrequent) 1528
Roferon-A Injection 2805
Rythmol SR Capsules 2736
Vesanoid Capsules (Less than 1%) 2823
Vicodin Tablets (Very rare) 530
Vicodin ES Tablets (Very rare) 531
Vicodin HP Tablets (Very rare) 532
Voltaren Tablets (Rarely) 2298
Voltaren-XR Tablets (Rarely) 2301

Hearing, loss of

Abelcet Injection 1119
Aggrenox Capsules 855
Altace Capsules (Less than 1%) 1673
Bayer Aspirin Tablets 3515
▲ Capastat Sulfate for Injection (3%) 1728
Cipro I.V. (1% or less) 2998
Cipro I.V. Pharmacy Bulk Package (1% or less) 3509
Cipro (Less than 1%) 2991
Cipro XR Tablets 3004
Coreg Tablets (Less than or equal to 0.1%) 1376
Depacon Injection 412
Depakene 417
Depakote Sprinkle Capsules 422
Depakote Tablets 427
Depakote ER Tablets 433
Desferal Vials 2190
Dolobid Tablets (Rare) 1937
Ecotrin Enteric Coated Aspirin Low, Regular and Maximum Strength Tablets 1627
Fabrazyme for Intravenous Infusion 1267
Floxin Otic Singles (Reported in a single subject) 1045
Floxin Otic Solution (Single report) 1043
Fortical Nasal Spray (Less than 1%) 3336
Furosemide Tablets 2117
Garamycin Injectable 3028
Gengraf Capsules (2% or less) 458
Imitrex Nasal Spray 1435
Kaopectate Anti-Diarrheal/Upset Stomach Reliever Liquid ▣701
Extra Strength Kaopectate Anti-Diarrheal Liquid ▣701
Lortab 3315
Lortab Elixir 3312
Maalox Maximum Strength Total Stomach Relief Peppermint Liquid ▣677
Maalox Maximum Strength Total Stomach Relief Strawberry Liquid ▣678
Matulane Capsules 3188
Miacalcin Nasal Spray (Less than 1%) 2242
Neoral Soft Gelatin Capsules (2% or less) 2247
Neoral Oral Solution (2% or less) 2247
Neurontin Capsules (Infrequent) 2498
Neurontin Oral Solution (Infrequent) 2498
Neurontin Tablets (Infrequent) 2498
Orthoclone OKT3 Sterile Solution 2370
Pegasys 2793
PEG-Intron Powder for Injection 3062
PREVPAC 3281
Primaxin I.M. 2022
Primaxin I.V. (Less than 0.2%) 2024
Prograf Capsules and Injection 624
Prozac Pulvules and Liquid (Rare) 1771
Raptiva for Injection (1 case) 1247
Retrovir Capsules 1533
Retrovir IV Infusion 1537
Retrovir 1533
Roferon-A Injection 2805
Sandimmune (2% or less) 2259
Sandostatin Injection (Less than 1%) 2263
St. Joseph 81 mg Aspirin Chewable and Enteric Coated Tablets 1841
TOBI Solution for Inhalation 1015
Vancocin HCl Capsules, USP (A few dozen cases) 3370
▲ Vesanoid Capsules (6%) 2823
Zinacef Injection (A few pediatric patients) 1604
Zinacef for Injection (A few pediatric patients) 1604
Zithromax Capsules, 250 mg 2568
Zithromax for IV Infusion 2573
Zithromax for Oral Suspension, 300 mg, 600 mg, 900 mg, 1200 mg 2561
Zithromax Tablets, 250 mg, 500 mg 2561
Zithromax Tri-Pak 2561
Zmax for Oral Suspension 2577

Hearing decreased

Aricept Tablets (Infrequent) 1086
Aricept ODT Tablets (Infrequent) 1086
Campath Ampules 826
Ciprodex Otic Suspension (1 patient) 555
Clinoril Tablets (Less than 1%) 1899
Dynacin Tablets (Rarely reported) 1859
Evoxac Capsules (Less than 1%) 1042
Invirase (Less than 2%) 2776
Nalfon Capsules (1.6%) 2504
Namenda (Infrequent) 1199
ProSom Tablets (Rare) 512
Risperdal Consta Long-Acting Injection (Infrequent) 1664
Risperdal M-Tab Orally Disintegrating Tablets (Rare) 1658
Risperdal (Rare) 1658
Topamax Sprinkle Capsules (1% to 2%) 2438
Topamax Tablets (1% to 2%) 2438
▲ Visudyne for Injection (1% to 10%) 2286

Hearing disturbances

Amerge Tablets (Infrequent) 1312
Anaprox Tablets (Less than 3%) 2769
Anaprox DS Tablets (Less than 3%) 2769
Avalide Tablets 922
Avalide Tablets 2889
Avapro Tablets (Less than 1%) 925
Avapro Tablets (Less than 1%) 2886
EC-Naprosyn Delayed-Release Tablets (Less than 3%) 2769
Imitrex Nasal Spray (Infrequent) 1435
Imitrex Tablets (Infrequent) 1440
Indocin Capsules (Less than 1%) 1968
Indocin I.V. (Less than 1%) 1973
Indocin (Less than 1%) 1968
▲ Intron A for Injection (Less than 5%) 3038
Naprosyn Suspension (Less than 3%) 2769
Naprosyn Tablets (Less than 3%) 2769
Prevacid NapraPAC (Less than 3%) 3277
Rebetol 3073
Ribavirin, USP Capsules 3083
▲ Roferon-A Injection (Less than 4%) 2805
Zithromax Capsules, 250 mg 2568
Zithromax for IV Infusion 2573
Zithromax for Oral Suspension, 300 mg, 600 mg, 900 mg, 1200 mg 2561
Zithromax Tablets, 250 mg, 500 mg 2561
Zithromax Tri-Pak 2561
Zmax for Oral Suspension 2577

Hearing loss, reversible

Depacon Injection 412
Depakene 417
Depakote Tablets 427
Depakote ER Tablets 433
E.E.S. (Isolated reports) 449
EryPed (Isolated reports) 445
Ery-Tab Tablets (Isolated reports) 447
Erythrocin Stearate Filmtab Tablets (Isolated reports) 452
Erythromycin Base Filmtab Tablets (Isolated reports) 454
Erythromycin Delayed-Release Capsules, USP (Isolated reports) 456
Hyperstat I.V. Injection 3031
PCE Dispertab Tablets (Isolated reports) 510

Heart beat, irregular

Adenocard Injection 612
Indapamide Tablets (Less than 5%) 2119
K-Phos Neutral Tablets 785
K-Phos Original (Sodium Free) Tablets (Less frequent) 785
Children's Motrin Oral Suspension and Chewable Tablets ▣647
Children's Motrin Non-Staining Dye-Free Oral Suspension ▣647
Children's Motrin Oral Suspension and Chewable Tablets 1837
Children's Motrin Non-Staining Dye-Free Oral Suspension 1837
Infants' Motrin Concentrated Drops 1837
Infants' Motrin Non-Staining Dye-Free Drops 1837
Junior Strength Motrin Caplets and Chewable Tablets 1837
Rythmol SR Capsules 2736
Uroqid-Acid No. 2 Tablets 785

Heart beats, ectopic

Imitrex Injection (Infrequent) 1431
Imitrex Nasal Spray 1435
Imitrex Tablets 1440

Heart beats, premature

Plendil Extended-Release Tablets (0.5% to 1.5%) 651

Heart block

(*see also under* Sinoatrial block)

Actimmune (Rare) 1646
Adenocard Injection 612
Agrylin Capsules 3172
Aricept Tablets 1086
Aricept ODT Tablets 1086
Betagan Ophthalmic Solution, USP ⊙217
Betimol Ophthalmic Solution ⊙283
Betimol Ophthalmic Solution 3371
Betoptic S Ophthalmic Suspension (Rare) 554
Brevibloc Concentrate (Less than 1%) 766
Brevibloc Injection (Less than 1%) 766
Brevibloc Double Strength Injection (Less than 1%) 766
Brevibloc Premixed Injection (Less than 1%) 766

Brevibloc Double Strength Premixed Injection (Less than 1%) 766
Carteolol Hydrochloride Ophthalmic Solution USP, 1% ⊙246
Digitek Tablets 2146
Diprivan Injectable Emulsion (Less than 1%) 676
Flexeril Tablets (Rare) 1832
Imitrex Nasal Spray 1435
Imitrex Tablets (Rare) 1440
Lanoxicaps Capsules 1458
Lanoxin Injection 1462
Lanoxin Tablets 1468
Lanoxin Injection Pediatric 1465
Levaquin in 5% Dextrose Injection (0.1% to 0.9%) 2453
Levaquin (0.1% to 0.9%) 2453
Naropin Injection 640
▲ Pacerone Tablets (2% to 5%) 3337
Paxil CR Controlled-Release Tablets (Rare) 1509
Paxil (Rare) 1501
Permax Tablets (Rare) 3357
Prozac Pulvules and Liquid (Rare) 1771
Relpax Tablets (Rare) 2531
Reyataz Capsules (Less than 3%) 948
Surmontil Capsules 2347
▲ Tenormin I.V. Injection (4.5%) 698
▲ Tenormin Tablets (4.5%) 695
Timoptic in Ocudose (Less frequent) 2061
Timoptic Sterile Ophthalmic Solution (Less frequent) 2058
Trasylol Injection (1% to 2%) 779
Vivactil Tablets 2350
Zyprexa IntraMuscular (Infrequent) 1798

Heart block, second degree
Toprol-XL Tablets 660
Zofran Injection (Rare) 1607

Heart block, third degree
I.V. Busulfex (2%) 1125
Nadolol Tablets (Single instance) 2121
Toprol-XL Tablets 660
Wellbutrin Tablets 1579

Heart defects, congenital
Thalomid Capsules 979

Heart disease
CombiPatch Transdermal System 2180

Heart failure
Abelcet Injection 1119
Abilify Tablets (Infrequent) 916
Abilify Tablets (Infrequent) 2472
Actimmune (Rare) 1646
Activase I.V. 1225
Aggrenox Capsules (1.6%) 855
Agrylin Capsules (1% to 5%) 3172
Aldara Cream, 5% 1814
Aloprim for Injection (Less than 1%) 2156
Altace Capsules (2%) 1673
Ammonul Injection 3323
Aredia for Injection (Up to 1%) 2168
Avalide Tablets 922
Avalide Tablets 2889
Avapro Tablets (Less than 1%) 925
Avapro Tablets (Less than 1%) 2886
Betimol Ophthalmic Solution ⊙283
Betimol Ophthalmic Solution 3371
Blocadren Tablets 1891
Brevibloc Concentrate 766
Brevibloc Injection 766
Brevibloc Double Strength Injection 766
Brevibloc Premixed Injection 766
Brevibloc Double Strength Premixed Injection 766
Caduet Tablets (Less than or equal to 0.1%) 2507
Campath Ampules 826
Campral Tablets (Rare) 1175
Carteolol Hydrochloride Ophthalmic Solution USP, 1% (In some cases) ⊙246
Celexa (Infrequent) 1177
▲ CellCept Capsules (3% to less than 20%) 2751
▲ CellCept Intravenous (3% to less than 20%) 2751
▲ CellCept Oral Suspension (3% to less than 20%) 2751
▲ CellCept Tablets (3% to less than 20%) 2751
Coreg Tablets 1376
Cosopt Sterile Ophthalmic Solution (Less than 1%) 1910
Cubicin for Injection (1% to 2%) 1038
Cymbalta Delayed-Release Capsules (Infrequent) 1729
Dantrium Capsules (Less frequent) 2690
Dantrium Intravenous 2691
Diprivan Injectable Emulsion (Less than 1%) 676
Dostinex Tablets (Rare) 2631
Doxil Injection (Less than 1%) 3302
DynaCirc CR Tablets (0.5% to 1%) 2726
Elitek (Less than or equal to 1%) 2906
Enbrel for Injection (Infrequent) 580
Exelon Capsules (Frequent) 2204
▲ Flolan for Injection (11%) 1408
Flumadine (Less than 0.3%) 1186
Gengraf Capsules (1% to less than 3%) 458
Gleevec Tablets (Infrequent) 2221
Herceptin I.V. 1234
▲ Imdur Tablets (Less than or equal to 5%) 3032
▲ Intron A for Injection (Less than 5%) 3038
Invanz for Injection (Greater than 0.1%) 1974
I.V. Busulfex (2%) 1125
Levothroid Tablets 1189
Levoxyl Tablets 1680
Lovenox Injection (0.95%) 2931
Lyrica Capsules (0.1% to 1%) 2524
Merrem I.V. (Greater than 0.1% to 1%) 687
Mirapex Tablets (Less than 1%) 889
Mobic Oral Suspension (Less than 2%) 893
Mobic Tablets (Less than 2%) 893
Nadolol Tablets (1 of 100 patients) 2121
Namenda (Frequent) 1199
Neoral Soft Gelatin Capsules (1% to less than 3%) 2247
Neoral Oral Solution (1% to less than 3%) 2247
Neurontin Capsules (Rare) 2498
Neurontin Oral Solution (Rare) 2498
Neurontin Tablets (Rare) 2498
Nipent for Injection (Less than 3%) 3216
Norvasc Tablets (Less than or equal to 0.1%) 2529
Omnicef Capsules 506
Omnicef for Oral Suspension 506
Orthoclone OKT3 Sterile Solution 2370
▲ Photofrin for Injection (7%) 729
Plavix Tablets (1% to 2.5%) 940
Plavix Tablets (1% to 2.5%) 2942
Pulmozyme Inhalation Solution 1245
Razadyne ER Extended-Release Capsules (Infrequent) 2434
Razadyne (Infrequent) 2434
▲ Refludan for Injection (3%) 815
Requip Tablets (Infrequent) 1528
Retavase 1131
Rilutek Tablets (Infrequent) 2945
Risperdal Consta Long-Acting Injection 1664
Risperdal M-Tab Orally Disintegrating Tablets 1658
Risperdal 1658
Rituxan for Infusion (Rare) 845
Rituxan I.V. (Rare) 1251
Sandostatin LAR Depot (1% to 4%) 2264
▲ Simulect for Injection (3% to 10%) 2268
Targretin Capsules 1719
Tasmar Tablets (Infrequent) 3360
Taxotere Injection Concentrate (Rare) 2947
▲ Tenormin I.V. Injection (19%) 698
▲ Tenormin Tablets (19%) 695
Thalomid Capsules 979
Timolide Tablets (Less than 1%) 2056
Timoptic in Ocudose (Less frequent) 2061
Timoptic Sterile Ophthalmic Solution (Less frequent) 2058
Timoptic-XE Sterile Ophthalmic Gel Forming Solution 2062
TNKase I.V. 1256
Toprol-XL Tablets 660
▲ Trasylol Injection (5%) 779
Trileptal Oral Suspension 2281
Trileptal Tablets 2281
Unithroid Tablets 3521
Verelan PM Capsules 3120
▲ Vesanoid Capsules (6%) 2823
Viagra Tablets (Less than 2%) 2552
Zonegran Capsules (Rare) 1089
Zosyn (1.0% or less) 3492
Zyprexa Tablets 1798
Zyprexa ZYDIS Orally Disintegrating Tablets 1798
Zyrtec Chewable Tablets (Less than 2%) 2589
Zyrtec (Less than 2%) 2589
Zyrtec-D 12 Hour Extended Release Tablets (Less than 2%) 2591

Heart failure, congestive
(*see under* Congestive heart failure)

Heart failure, worsening of
Avandia Tablets 1348
Prinivil Tablets (Greater than 1%) 2029
Prinzide Tablets 2033
Toprol-XL Tablets 660
Velcade for Injection 2102
Zestoretic Tablets 701
Zestril Tablets (Greater than 1%) 704

Heart rate, abnormal
Rescriptor Tablets 2535
Thyrolar 1203

Heart rate, changes
▲ Blocadren Tablets (5%) 1891
Invirase (Less than 2%) 2776
Zemuron Injection 2363
Zomig Tablets 714

Heart rate, decrease
Betagan Ophthalmic Solution, USP ⊙217
ProAmatine Tablets 3183

Heart rate, increased
Abilify Tablets 916
Abilify Tablets 2472
Balamine DM 739
DDAVP Injection 4 mcg/mL (Infrequent) 2893
Desmopressin Acetate Injection (Infrequent) 1143
Effexor Tablets 3405
Levaquin in 5% Dextrose Injection (0.1% to 0.9%) 2453
Levaquin (0.1% to 0.9%) 2453
Levothroid Tablets 1189
Meridia Capsules 485
Men's Rogaine Extra Strength Topical Solution, Ocean Rush Scent and Original Unscented ▣706
Women's Rogaine Topical Solution, Spring Bloom Scent and Original Unscented ▣707
Thyrolar 1203
▲ Xopenex HFA Inhalation Aerosol (0.8% to 6%) 3151
▲ Xopenex Inhalation Solution (0.8% to 6%) 3143
▲ Xopenex Inhalation Solution Concentrate (0.8% to 6%) 3147

Heart sounds, abnormal
Gengraf Capsules (1% to less than 3%) 458
Neoral Soft Gelatin Capsules (1% to less than 3%) 2247
Neoral Oral Solution (1% to less than 3%) 2247
Rythmol SR Capsules 2736
▲ Simulect for Injection (3% to 10%) 2268

Heart spasms
(*see under* Cardiospasm)

Heartburn
▲ Aerobid/Aerobid-M (3% to 9%) 1172
▲ Alferon N Injection (3%) 1640
Altoprev Extended-Release Tablets 1151
▲ Anaprox Tablets (3% to 9%) 2769
▲ Anaprox DS Tablets (3% to 9%) 2769
Arthrotec Tablets (Rare) 3126
Avalide Tablets (2%) 922
Avalide Tablets (2%) 2889
Avapro Tablets (2%) 925
Avapro Tablets (2%) 2886
Balamine DM 739
Bayer Aspirin Tablets 3515
▲ Cataflam Tablets (1% to 10%) 2173
▲ Clozapine Tablets (4%) 2141
▲ Clozaril Tablets (4%) 2174
Combivent Inhalation Aerosol 878
Dalmane Capsules 3343
▲ EC-Naprosyn Delayed-Release Tablets (3% to 9%) 2769
Ecotrin Enteric Coated Aspirin Low, Regular and Maximum Strength Tablets 1627
Eldepryl Capsules 3209
▲ Emend Capsules (5.3%) 1944
▲ FazaClo Orally Disintegrating Tablets (4%) 547
▲ Indocin (3% to 9%) 1968
Klonopin (Infrequent) 2782
Lexapro Oral Solution (Frequent) 1193
Lexapro Tablets (Frequent) 1193
Mevacor Tablets (1.6%) 1996
Midamor Tablets (Less than or equal to 1%) 2000
Moduretic Tablets 2003
▲ Naprosyn Suspension (3% to 9%) 2769
▲ Naprosyn Tablets (3% to 9%) 2769
Noroxin Tablets (0.3% to 1.0%) 2009
Parcopa Orally Disintegrating Tablets 3111
Pravachol Tablets (2.0% to 2.9%) 943
▲ Prevacid NapraPAC (3% to 9%) 3277
Primaxin I.M. 2022
Primaxin I.V. (Less than 0.2%) 2024
Prinivil Tablets (0.3% to 1.0%) 2029
Prinzide Tablets (0.3% to 1%) 2033
ProAmatine Tablets (Rare) 3183
▲ Proventil Inhalation Aerosol (Less than 5%) 3067
Sedapap Tablets 50 mg/650 mg (Infrequent) 2098
St. Joseph 81 mg Aspirin Chewable and Enteric Coated Tablets 1841
Stalevo Tablets 2270
Syprine Capsules 2055
Toprol-XL Tablets (About 1 of 100 patients) 660
▲ Voltaren Tablets (1% to 10%) 2298
▲ Voltaren-XR Tablets (1% to 10%) 2301
▲ Zenapax for Injection (Greater than 5%) 2838
Zestoretic Tablets (0.3% to 1%) 701
Zestril Tablets (0.3% to 1.0%) 704

Heat intolerance
Alferon N Injection (1%) 1640
Imitrex Tablets 1440
Levothroid Tablets 1189
Levoxyl Tablets 1680
Reyataz Capsules (Less than 3%) 948
Unithroid Tablets 3521

Heat stroke
Abilify Tablets (Rare) 916
Abilify Tablets (Rare) 2472
Clozapine Tablets 2141
Clozaril Tablets 2174
Cogentin Injection 1903
Evoxac Capsules (Less than 1%) 1042
Lunesta Tablets (Infrequent) 3139
Orap Tablets 1220
Protonix I.V. (Less than 1%) 3468
Protonix Tablets (Less than 1%) 3465

Heaviness, head
Abilify Tablets (Rare) 916
Abilify Tablets (Rare) 2472

Heavy sensation, arms
Adenocard Injection (Less than 1%) 612

Heavy sensation, legs
Eldepryl Capsules 3209
K-Phos Neutral Tablets 785
K-Phos Original (Sodium Free) Tablets (Less frequent) 785

Hemangioma, acquired
Ammonul Injection 3323

Hemarthrosis
Kaletra 474
NovoSeven (Greater than or equal to 2%) 2335

Hematemesis
Abilify Tablets (Rare) 916
Abilify Tablets (Rare) 2472
Aggrenox Capsules 855
AmBisome for Injection (Less common) 615
Anaprox Tablets (Less than 1%) 2769
Anaprox DS Tablets (Less than 1%) 2769
Argatroban Injection (2.6%) 1321
Arthrotec Tablets (Rare) 3126
Campath Ampules 826
Campral Tablets (Infrequent) 1175
Cataflam Tablets (Occasionally) 2173
Clozapine Tablets (Less than 1%) 2141
Clozaril Tablets (Less than 1%) 2174
Copaxone for Injection (Infrequent) 3292
▲ Depacon Injection (1% to 5%) 412
▲ Depakene (1% to 5%) 417
▲ Depakote Sprinkle Capsules (1% to 5%) 422
▲ Depakote Tablets (1% to 5%) 427
Depakote ER Tablets (Greater than 1%) 433
EC-Naprosyn Delayed-Release Tablets (Less than 1%) 2769
Effexor Tablets (Rare) 3405
Effexor XR Capsules (Rare) 3411
Exelon Capsules (Infrequent) 2204
FazaClo Orally Disintegrating Tablets (Less than 1%) 547
Geodon Capsules (Rare) 2514

Herceptin I.V. (At least one of the 958 patients) 1234
Imitrex Injection 1431
Imitrex Nasal Spray (Rare) 1435
Imitrex Tablets (Rare) 1440
I.V. Busulfex (2%) 1125
Lamictal 1449
▲ Leukine (13%) 829
Matulane Capsules 3188
Mobic Oral Suspension (Less than 2%) 893
Mobic Tablets (Less than 2%) 893
Naprosyn Suspension (Less than 1%) 2769
Naprosyn Tablets (Less than 1%) 2769
Neurontin Capsules (Rare) 2498
Neurontin Oral Solution (Rare) 2498
Neurontin Tablets (Rare) 2498
Paxil CR Controlled-Release Tablets (Rare) 1509
Paxil (Rare) 1501
Permax Tablets (Infrequent) 3357
▲ Photofrin for Injection (8%) 729
Pletal Tablets (Less than 2%) 2478
Prevacid Delayed-Release Capsules (Less than 1%) 3268
Prevacid for Delayed-Release Oral Suspension (Less than 1%) 3268
Prevacid NapraPAC (Less than 1%) 3277
Prevacid SoluTab Delayed-Release Orally Disintegrating Tablets (Less than 1%) 3268
PREVPAC (Less than 1%) 3281
Proleukin for Injection (Less than 1%) 1007
Protonix I.V. (Less than 1%) 3468
Protonix Tablets (Less than 1%) 3465
Prozac Pulvules and Liquid (Rare) 1771
Relpax Tablets (Rare) 2531
ReoPro Vials (5 to 11 events) 1779
Requip Tablets (Rare) 1528
Rilutek Tablets (Rare) 2945
Risperdal M-Tab Orally Disintegrating Tablets (Rare) 1658
Risperdal (Rare) 1658
Seroquel Tablets (Infrequent) 691
Tequin Injection (Less than 0.1%) 964
Tequin Tablets (Less than 0.1%) 964
Tricor Tablets 523
Trileptal Oral Suspension 2281
Trileptal Tablets 2281
VFEND I.V. (Less than 2%) 2543
VFEND Oral Suspension (Less than 2%) 2543
VFEND Tablets (Less than 2%) 2543
Voltaren Tablets (Occasionally) 2298
Voltaren-XR Tablets (Occasionally) 2301
Xeloda Tablets 2825
Zevalin Injection (Less than 1%) 848
Zoladex 3-month (1% to 5%) 712
Zomig Tablets (Rare) 714
Zomig-ZMT Tablets (Rare) 714
Zonegran Capsules (Rare) 1089

Hematochezia

Adriamycin for Injection, USP 786
Adriamycin Injection, USP 786
Camptosar Injection 2602
Coumadin for Injection 932
Cymbalta Delayed-Release Capsules (Infrequent) 1729
Invirase (Less than 2%) 2776
Nalfon Capsules (Less than 1%) 2504
Neurontin Capsules (Infrequent) 2498
Neurontin Oral Solution (Infrequent) 2498
Neurontin Tablets (Infrequent) 2498
Rescriptor Tablets 2535
Trileptal Oral Suspension 2281
Trileptal Tablets 2281
Xifaxan Tablets (Less than 2%) 2847

Hematocrit, decrease

Aceon Tablets (2 mg, 4 mg, 8 mg) 3191
ActoPlus Met Tablets 3219
Actos Tablets 3224
Advate Injection (0.6%) 742
Aggrastat (2.2%) 1878
Aggrenox Capsules 855
Altace Capsules (Rare) 1673
Antara Capsules 2723
▲ Argatroban Injection (10.4%) 1321
Atacand Tablets 634
Atacand HCT 637
Avandamet Tablets 1343
Avandia Tablets 1348
Benicar Tablets 2850
Benicar HCT Tablets (One patient) 2852
Blocadren Tablets 1891
▲ Cancidas for Injection (0.9% to 11.1%) 1894
▲ Cipro I.V. (Among most frequent) 2998
▲ Cipro I.V. Pharmacy Bulk Package (Among most frequent) 3509
▲ DepoDur Extended-Release Injection (2% to 5%) 1098
Diovan HCT Tablets 2195
Diovan Tablets (0.8%) 2191
Eligard 7.5 mg (Less than 2%) 2896
Hyzaar 1964
Infergen (1% or less) 1647
▲ Invanz for Injection (3% to 3.4%) 1974
▲ Lariam Tablets (Among most frequent) 2790
Lofibra Capsules 1217
Lupron Depot 7.5 mg (Greater than or equal to 5%) 3261
Maxipime for Injection (Greater than 0.1% to less than 1%) 1093
Merrem I.V. (Greater than 0.2%) 687
Micardis HCT Tablets (0.6%) 886
Neumega for Injection 3433
Noroxin Tablets (Less frequent) 2009
Omnicef for Oral Suspension (0.2%) 506
Panhematin for Injection 2487
Parcopa Orally Disintegrating Tablets 3111
Precose Tablets 776
Primaxin I.M. 2022
Primaxin I.V. 2024
Prinivil Tablets (Frequent) 2029
Prinzide Tablets (Frequent) 2033
ReoPro Vials (7 to 11 events) 1779
Teveten HCT Tablets (0.1%) 1710
Timentin ADD-Vantage 1556
Timentin Injection Galaxy Container 1559
Timentin IV Infusion 1553
Timentin Pharmacy Bulk Package 1562
Tracleer Tablets 539
Tranxene 2488
Vantin Tablets and Oral Suspension 2650
Vaseretic Tablets (0.5% to 2.0%) 2073
Vasotec I.V. Injection (Frequent) 2076
Zestoretic Tablets (Frequent) 701
Zestril Tablets (Frequent) 704
▲ Zinacef Injection (1 in 10 patients) 1604
▲ Zinacef for Injection (1 in 10 patients) 1604
Zithromax for Oral Suspension, 300 mg, 600 mg, 900 mg, 1200 mg (Greater than 1%) 2561
Zithromax Tablets, 250 mg, 500 mg (Greater than 1%) 2561
Zithromax Tri-Pak (Greater than 1%) 2561
Zosyn 3492

Hematocrit, increase

▲ AndroGel (3% to 6%) 3330
Clozapine Tablets 2141
Clozaril Tablets 2174
Epogen for Injection 586
Factive Tablets (0.1%) 2464
FazaClo Orally Disintegrating Tablets 547
Procrit for Injection 2374
Striant Mucoadhesive 1022
Testim 1% Gel (1% to 2%) 722

Hematologic reactions

Dapsone Tablets USP 1656
Daraprim Tablets 1385
Lamictal 1449
Rebif Prefilled Syringe for Injection 3163

Hematologic toxicity

Adriamycin for Injection, USP 786
Adriamycin Injection, USP 786
Bexxar 1360
Doxil Injection 3302
Retrovir IV Infusion 1537

Hematoma

Aceon Tablets (2 mg, 4 mg, 8 mg) (0.3% to 1%) 3191
▲ Advair Diskus 100/50 (1% to 3%) 1291
▲ Advair Diskus 250/50 (1% to 3%) 1291
▲ Advair Diskus 500/50 (1% to 3%) 1291
Advate Injection (0.6%) 742
Aggrenox Capsules (Less than 1%) 855
Anzemet Injection (Infrequently) 2871
Anzemet Tablets (Infrequently) 2874
▲ Arava Tablets (1% to 3%) 2881
▲ Argatroban Injection (3.6%) 1321
Arixtra Injection (2.1% to 2.8%) 1325
Campath Ampules 826
Caverject Impulse Injection 2610
Copaxone for Injection (Infrequent) 3292
Depacon Injection 412
Depakene 417
Depakote Sprinkle Capsules 422
Depakote Tablets 427
Depakote ER Tablets 433
Eldepryl Capsules 3209
Evoxac Capsules (Less than 1%) 1042
Exelon Capsules (Infrequent) 2204
▲ Flovent Diskus 50 mcg (1% to 3%) 1415
▲ Fragmin Injection (0.2% to 7.1%) 2638
Havrix Vaccine (Less than 1%) 1425
Imitrex Injection 1431
Imitrex Tablets (Rare) 1440
Invanz for Injection (Greater than 0.1%) 1974
Levaquin in 5% Dextrose Injection (0.1% to 0.9%) 2453
Levaquin (0.1% to 0.9%) 2453
Lexapro Oral Solution (Infrequent) 1193
Lexapro Tablets (Infrequent) 1193
Lotronex Tablets (Rare) 1479
Lovenox Injection 2931
Nimotop Capsules (Less than 1%) 774
Paxil CR Controlled-Release Tablets (Infrequent) 1509
Paxil (Infrequent) 1501
Plavix Tablets (1% to 2.5%) 940
Plavix Tablets (1% to 2.5%) 2942
ReFacto Vials 3479
▲ Refludan for Injection (10.6%) 815
ReoPro Vials 1779
Risperdal Consta Long-Acting Injection (Rare) 1664
Roferon-A Injection (1%) 2805
Rythmol SR Capsules 2736
▲ Sandostatin Injection (1% to 4%) 2263
Sandostatin LAR Depot (1% to 4%) 2264
▲ Simulect for Injection (3% to 10%) 2268
▲ Thrombate III (1 of 17) 3254
▲ TNKase I.V. (1.7% to 12.3%) 1256
Topamax Sprinkle Capsules (1%) 2438
Topamax Tablets (1%) 2438
Vantas (Less than 2%) 3367
Vantin Tablets and Oral Suspension (Less than 1%) 2650
▲ Varivax (24.4% to 32.5%) 2070

Hematoma, spinal-epidural

Aggrastat 1878

Hematoma, splenic

NovoSeven 2335

Hematoma, subdermal

Neurontin Oral Solution (Infrequent) 2498
Seroquel Tablets (Rare) 691

Hematoma, subdural

Actiq (Less than 1%) 993
Ammonul Injection 3323
▲ Humira Injection (Less than 5%) 464
Neurontin 2498
Pletal Tablets (Very rare) 2478
Rilutek Tablets (Infrequent) 2945
Zevalin Injection (Less than 1%) 848

Hematoma at injection site

▲ Edex Injection (5%) 3103

Hematopoietic depression

Cosmegen for Injection 1907
Mustargen for Injection (Occasional) 2007

Hematuria

Abilify Tablets (Infrequent) 916
Abilify Tablets (Infrequent) 2472
Accutane Capsules 2740
Aceon Tablets (2 mg, 4 mg, 8 mg) (0.3% to 1%) 3191
Aciphex Tablets (Rare) 1081
Actiq (Less than 1%) 993
Aggrenox Capsules (Less than 1%) 855
Agrylin Capsules (1% to 5%) 3172
Aloprim for Injection (Less than 1%) 2156
▲ AmBisome for Injection (14%) 615
Amnesteem Capsules 2126
Anaprox Tablets (Less than 1%) 2769
Anaprox DS Tablets (Less than 1%) 2769
Anzemet Injection (Rare) 2871
Anzemet Tablets (Rare) 2874
▲ Arava Tablets (1% to 3%) 2881
▲ Argatroban Injection (0.9% to 11.8%) 1321
Aricept Tablets (Infrequent) 1086
Aricept ODT Tablets (Infrequent) 1086
Arthrotec Tablets (Rare) 3126
Asacol Delayed-Release Tablets 2688
Astelin Nasal Spray (Infrequent) 1876
Atacand Tablets (0.5% or greater) 634
Atacand HCT (0.5% or greater) 637
Augmentin (Rare) 1331
Augmentin Tablets (Rare) 1334
Augmentin XR Extended-Release Tablets (Rare) 1340
Augmentin ES-600 Powder for Oral Suspension (Rare) 1337
▲ Baraclude (9%) 928
Benicar HCT Tablets (Greater than 1%) 2852
Caduet Tablets (Less than 2%) 2507
Campath Ampules 826
Campral Tablets (Rare) 1175
Cancidas for Injection (2.2%) 1894
Cardene I.V. (0.7%) 1129
▲ Casodex Tablets (7%) 670
Cataflam Tablets (Occasionally) 2173
Caverject Injection (Less than 1%) 2610
Celebrex Capsules (0.1% to 1.9%) 3130
Celexa (Rare) 1177
▲ CellCept Capsules (3% to less than 20%) 2751
▲ CellCept Intravenous (3% to less than 20%) 2751
▲ CellCept Oral Suspension (3% to less than 20%) 2751
▲ CellCept Tablets (3% to less than 20%) 2751
Cipro I.V. (1% or less) 2998
Cipro I.V. Pharmacy Bulk Package (1% or less) 3509
Cipro 2991
Cipro XR Tablets (Less than 1%) 3004
Clinoril Tablets (Less than 1%) 1899
▲ Clolar for Intravenous Infusion (17%) 1264
Colazal Capsules 2845
▲ Coreg Tablets (Greater than 1% to 3%) 1376
Coumadin for Injection 932
Coumadin Tablets 932
▲ Crixivan Capsules (Approximately 12.4%) 1918
Cuprimine Capsules 1925
Dantrium Capsules (Less frequent) 2690
Daraprim Tablets 1385
Demser Capsules (A few patients) 1933
Diuril Sodium Intravenous (1 case) 1934
Dolobid Tablets (Less than 1 in 100) 1937
▲ Doxil Injection (1% to 10%) 3302
EC-Naprosyn Delayed-Release Tablets (Less than 1%) 2769
Edecrin 1941
Effexor Tablets (Infrequent) 3405
Effexor XR Capsules (Infrequent) 3411
Eloxatin for Injection 2908
▲ Eulexin Capsules (7%) 3023
Evoxac Capsules (Less than 1%) 1042
Exelon Capsules (Frequent) 2204
▲ Flolan for Injection (5%) 1408
Fortical Nasal Spray (Less than 1%) 3336
Gabitril Tablets (Infrequent) 998
▲ Gemzar for Injection (Up to 35%) 1743
Gengraf Capsules (1% to less than 3%) 458
Genotropin Lyophilized Powder (Infrequent) 2642
Geodon Capsules (Infrequent) 2514
Gleevec Tablets (Infrequent) 2221
▲ Hepsera Tablets (11%) 1275
Herceptin I.V. (At least one of the 958 patients) 1234
▲ Humira Injection (5%) 464
Imitrex Nasal Spray 1435
Imitrex Tablets (Rare) 1440
Indocin Capsules (Less than 1%) 1968
Indocin I.V. (Less than 1%) 1973
Indocin (Less than 1%) 1968
Infed Injection 3381
▲ Intron A for Injection (Less than 5%) 3038
Invanz for Injection (Greater than 0.1%) 1974
Iressa Tablets 684
Lamictal (Infrequent) 1449
▲ Leukine (9%) 829
Levaquin in 5% Dextrose Injection (0.1% to 0.9%) 2453
Levaquin (0.1% to 0.9%) 2453
Lexapro Oral Solution (Infrequent) 1193
Lexapro Tablets (Infrequent) 1193
Lipitor Tablets (Less than 2%) 2495
Lovenox Injection (Less than 2%) 2931
Lunesta Tablets (Infrequent) 3139
Lupron Depot 7.5 mg (Less than 5%) 3261
Lyrica Capsules (0.1% to 1%) 2524
Matulane Capsules 3188
Meridia Capsules 485
Miacalcin Nasal Spray (Less than 1%) 2242
Mintezol 2002
Mirapex Tablets (Less than 1%) 889
Mobic Oral Suspension (Less than 2%) 893

Mobic Tablets (Less than 2%) 893
▲ Myfortic Tablets (3% to less than 20%) 2244
▲ Mylotarg for Injection (1% to 37%) 3429
Nalfon Capsules (Less than 1%) 2504
Namenda (Infrequent) 1199
Naprosyn Suspension (Less than 1%) 2769
Naprosyn Tablets (Less than 1%) 2769
Neoral Soft Gelatin Capsules (1% to less than 3%) 2247
Neoral Oral Solution (1% to less than 3%) 2247
Neupogen for Injection (Infrequent) 598
Neurontin Capsules (Infrequent) 2498
Neurontin Oral Solution (Infrequent) 2498
Neurontin Tablets (Infrequent) 2498
Nexium Delayed-Release Capsules (Less than 1%) 645
Nexium I.V. (Less than 1%) 649
Noroxin Tablets 2009
Norvir (Less than 2%) 499
Oncaspar (Less than 1%) 1123
▲ Ontak Vials (10%) 1717
OxyContin Tablets (Less than 1%) 2699
Parcopa Orally Disintegrating Tablets 3111
Paxil CR Controlled-Release Tablets (Infrequent) 1509
Paxil (Infrequent) 1501
Pentasa Capsules (Less than 1%) 3182
Permax Tablets (1.1%) 3357
Plavix Tablets (Less than 1%) 940
Plavix Tablets (Less than 1%) 2942
Pletal Tablets (2% or greater) 2478
Prevacid Delayed-Release Capsules (Less than 1%) 3268
Prevacid for Delayed-Release Oral Suspension 3268
Prevacid NapraPAC (Less than 1%) 3277
Prevacid SoluTab Delayed-Release Orally Disintegrating Tablets (Less than 1%) 3268
PREVPAC (Less than 1%) 3281
Prilosec OTC Tablets (Less than 1%) 2674
Primaxin I.M. 2022
Primaxin I.V. 2024
▲ Prograf Capsules and Injection (3% to 15%) 624
▲ Proleukin for Injection (9%) 1007
ProSom Tablets (Rare) 512
Protonix I.V. (Less than 1%) 3468
Protonix Tablets (Less than 1%) 3465
Provigil Tablets (1%) 1002
Prozac Pulvules and Liquid (Infrequent) 1771
▲ Rapamune Oral Solution and Tablets (3% to 20%) 3472
▲ Razadyne ER Extended-Release Capsules (3%) 2434
▲ Razadyne (3%) 2434
▲ Refludan for Injection (4.4%) 815
Relafen Tablets (Less than 1%) 1523
ReoPro Vials (4 events) 1779
Requip Tablets (Infrequent) 1528
Rescriptor Tablets 2535
Retrovir Capsules (0.8%) 1533
Retrovir IV Infusion (1%) 1537
Retrovir (0.8%) 1533
Reyataz Capsules (Less than 3%) 948
Rilutek Tablets (Infrequent) 2945
Risperdal Consta Long-Acting Injection (Infrequent) 1664
Risperdal M-Tab Orally Disintegrating Tablets (Infrequent) 1658
Risperdal (Infrequent) 1658
Rocephin Injectable Vials, ADD-Vantage, Galaxy, Bulk (Rare) 2801
▲ Rythmol SR Capsules (1% to 3%) 2736
Sandimmune (Rare) 2259
Sandostatin Injection (Less than 1%) 2263
Sandostatin LAR Depot (Rare) 2264
▲ Simulect for Injection (3% to 10%) 2268
Sonata Capsules (Infrequent) 1686
Sular Tablets (Less than or equal to 1%) 1163
Sustiva Capsules (Up to 1%) 957
Symbyax Capsules (Infrequent) 1788
Synercid I.V. (Less than 1%) 1690
Targretin Capsules 1719
Tarka Tablets (Less frequent) 519
Tasmar Tablets (Infrequent) 3360
▲ Tequin Injection (0.1% to 3%) 964
▲ Tequin Tablets (0.1% to 3%) 964
Teveten Tablets (Less than 1%) 1707
Teveten HCT Tablets (Less than 1%) 1710
Thalomid Capsules 979
Ticlid Tablets 2813
Topamax Sprinkle Capsules (Less than 1% to 2%) 2438
Topamax Tablets (Less than 1% to 2%) 2438
Trileptal Oral Suspension 2281
Trileptal Tablets 2281
▲ Truvada Tablets (2% to 12%) 1279
Uniretic Tablets (Less than 1%) 3114
Uroqid-Acid No. 2 Tablets (Rare) 785
▲ Vagifem Tablets (3% to 5%) 2340
Vantin Tablets and Oral Suspension (Less than 1%) 2650
VFEND I.V. (Less than 2%) 2543
VFEND Oral Suspension (Less than 2%) 2543
VFEND Tablets (Less than 2%) 2543
Viagra Tablets 2552
Voltaren Tablets (Occasionally) 2298
Voltaren-XR Tablets (Occasionally) 2301
Xifaxan Tablets (Less than 2%) 2847
Zegerid Powder for Oral Solution (Less than 1%) 2972
▲ Zoladex (7%) 709
▲ Zoladex 3-month (1% to 7%) 712
Zoloft (Rare) 2581
Zomig Tablets (Infrequent) 714
Zomig-ZMT Tablets (Infrequent) 714
Zonegran Capsules (Infrequent) 1089
Zosyn (1.0% or less) 3492
Zovirax Capsules 1616
Zovirax for Injection (Less than 1%) 1618
Zovirax 1616
Zyprexa Tablets (Infrequent) 1798
Zyprexa ZYDIS Orally Disintegrating Tablets (Frequent) 1798
Zyrtec Chewable Tablets (Less than 2%) 2589
Zyrtec (Less than 2%) 2589
Zyrtec-D 12 Hour Extended Release Tablets (Less than 2%) 2591

Hematuria, aggravated

Vantas (Less than 2%) 3367

Hematuria, microscopic

Calcium Disodium Versenate Injection 1819
▲ Crixivan Capsules (Approximately 12.4%) 1918
▲ Ontak Vials (Less than 5%) 1717

Hemianopsia

Trileptal Oral Suspension 2281
Trileptal Tablets 2281

Hemiparesis

Femara Tablets (Less than or equal to 2%) 2210
Klonopin 2782
Orthoclone OKT3 Sterile Solution 2370
Requip Tablets (Rare) 1528
Sandostatin LAR Depot (Rare) 2264
▲ Temodar Capsules (18%) 3088
Thyrogen for Injection (4 patients out of 55) 1270

Hemiplegia

Actiq (Less than 1%) 993
DepoCyt Injection 1121
Doxil Injection (Less than 1%) 3302
Gabitril Tablets (Infrequent) 998
Imitrex Injection (Rare) 1431
Imitrex Tablets 1440
Lamictal (Rare) 1449
Namenda (Infrequent) 1199
Neurontin Capsules (Infrequent) 2498
Neurontin Oral Solution (Infrequent) 2498
Neurontin Tablets (Infrequent) 2498
Orthoclone OKT3 Sterile Solution 2370
Permax Tablets (Rare) 3357
Prevacid Delayed-Release Capsules (Less than 1%) 3268
Prevacid for Delayed-Release Oral Suspension (Less than 1%) 3268
Prevacid NapraPAC (Less than 1%) 3277
Prevacid SoluTab Delayed-Release Orally Disintegrating Tablets (Less than 1%) 3268
PREVPAC (Less than 1%) 3281
Relpax Tablets (Rare) 2531
Requip Tablets (Rare) 1528
Rilutek Tablets (Infrequent) 2945
Seroquel Tablets (Infrequent) 691
Tasmar Tablets (Rare) 3360
Thyrogen for Injection (4 patients out of 55) 1270
Trileptal Oral Suspension 2281
Trileptal Tablets 2281
▲ Vesanoid Capsules (3%) 2823

Hemochromatosis

Effexor Tablets (Rare) 3405
Effexor XR Capsules (Rare) 3411

Hemoconcentration

Follistim AQ Cartridge 2354

Hemoglobin, decrease

Aceon Tablets (2 mg, 4 mg, 8 mg) 3191
ActoPlus Met Tablets 3219
Actos Tablets 3224
Aggrastat (2.1%) 1878
Aggrenox Capsules 855
Altace Capsules (Rare) 1673
Antara Capsules 2723
▲ Argatroban Injection (10.4%) 1321
Atacand Tablets 634
Atacand HCT 637
Avalide Tablets 922
Avalide Tablets 2889
Avandamet Tablets 1343
Avandia Tablets 1348
Avapro Tablets (Less than 0.2%) 925
Avapro Tablets (Less than 0.2%) 2886
Benicar Tablets 2850
Blocadren Tablets 1891
▲ Cancidas for Injection (0.9% to 12.3%) 1894
▲ Casodex Tablets (2% to 5%) 670
▲ Cipro I.V. (Among most frequent) 2998
▲ Cipro I.V. Pharmacy Bulk Package (Among most frequent) 3509
Cipro (Less than 0.1%) 2991
Crixivan Capsules (0.6%) 1918
▲ Dapsone Tablets USP (Almost all patients) 1656
Eligard 7.5 mg (Less than 2%) 2896
Factive Tablets (0.2%) 2464
Hyzaar 1964
Infergen (1% or less) 1647
▲ Invanz for Injection (4.5% to 4.9%) 1974
Invirase (Up to 1%) 2776
Lofibra Capsules 1217
Lupron Depot 7.5 mg (Greater than or equal to 5%) 3261
Merrem I.V. (Greater than 0.2%) 687
Micardis HCT Tablets (1.2%) 886
Mustargen for Injection 2007
▲ Myfortic Tablets (3% to less than 20%) 2244
Neumega for Injection 3433
Noroxin Tablets (0.6%) 2009
Omnicef Capsules (0.3%) 506
Omnicef for Oral Suspension (0.4%) 506
Parcopa Orally Disintegrating Tablets 3111
▲ Pegasys (17%) 2793
▲ PEG-Intron Powder for Injection (30%) 3062
Primaxin I.M. 2022
Primaxin I.V. 2024
Prinivil Tablets (Frequent) 2029
Prinzide Tablets (Frequent) 2033
Rebetol 3073
Rebetron Combination Therapy 3078
Refludan for Injection 815
ReoPro Vials (7 to 11 events) 1779
▲ Roferon-A Injection (Up to 31%) 2805
Rythmol SR Capsules 2736
▲ Temodar Capsules (51%) 3088
Teveten Tablets (0.1%) 1707
Teveten HCT Tablets (0.1%) 1710
Timentin ADD-Vantage 1556
Timentin Injection Galaxy Container 1559
Timentin IV Infusion 1553
Timentin Pharmacy Bulk Package 1562
Tracleer Tablets 539
Valtrex Caplets (Up to 0.8%) 1573
Vantin Tablets and Oral Suspension 2650
Vaseretic Tablets (0.5% to 2.0%) 2073
Vasotec I.V. Injection (Frequent) 2076
Viramune Oral Suspension (1.2%) 903
Viramune Tablets (1.2%) 903
WinRho SDF 763
Xeloda Tablets (1%) 2825
Zestoretic Tablets (Frequent) 701
Zestril Tablets (Frequent) 704
▲ Zinacef Injection (1 in 10 patients) 1604
▲ Zinacef for Injection (1 in 10 patients) 1604
Zithromax for Oral Suspension, 300 mg, 600 mg, 900 mg, 1200 mg (Greater than 1%) 2561
Zithromax Tablets, 250 mg, 500 mg (Greater than 1%) 2561
Zithromax Tri-Pak (Greater than 1%) 2561
Zosyn 3492

Hemoglobin, increase

Factive Tablets (0.1%) 2464
FazaClo Orally Disintegrating Tablets 547
Fuzeon Injection (0.6% to 1.5%) 2772
Testim 1% Gel (1% to 2%) 722

Hemoglobin content, deviation

Amerge Tablets (Rare) 1312
Diovan HCT Tablets (0.004%) 2195
Diovan Tablets (0.4%) 2191
▲ Intron A for Injection (Up to 32%) 3038
Lotronex Tablets (Rare) 1479

Hemoglobinemia

▲ AndroGel (3% to 6%) 3330
Clozapine Tablets 2141
Clozaril Tablets 2174
Stromectol Tablets (1%) 2053
Zovirax for Injection (Less than 1%) 1618

Hemoglobinuria

Mycamine for Injection 620
Raptiva for Injection 1247
WinRho SDF 763

Hemolysis

Campath Ampules 826
Carimune NF 3501
Cozaar Tablets 1913
▲ Dapsone Tablets USP (Most common) 1656
▲ Doxil Injection (1% to 5%) 3302
Elitek (Less than 1%) 2906
Gammagard Liquid 751
Gammagard S/D 754
Gamunex Immune Globulin I.V., 10% 3232
Hyzaar (One subject) 1964
Iveegam EN 759
Mycamine for Injection 620
Prevacid Delayed-Release Capsules (Less than 1%) 3268
Prevacid for Delayed-Release Oral Suspension (Less than 1%) 3268
Prevacid NapraPAC (Less than 1%) 3277
Prevacid SoluTab Delayed-Release Orally Disintegrating Tablets (Less than 1%) 3268
PREVPAC (Less than 1%) 3281
Rebetron Combination Therapy 3078
Seroquel Tablets (Rare) 691
Trasylol Injection (0.3%) 779
Uniretic Tablets (Less than 1%) 3114
Vaseretic Tablets (A few cases) 2073
Vasotec I.V. Injection (A few cases) 2076
Zovirax for Injection 1618

Hemolysis, neonatal

AquaMEPHYTON Injection 1887
Dapsone Tablets USP 1656
Mephyton Tablets 1993

Hemolytic icterus

(*see under* Jaundice)

Hemolytic-uremic syndrome

Alesse-28 Tablets 3392
Cytovene 2763
Eloxatin for Injection 2908
Gemzar for Injection (Rare) 1743
Gengraf Capsules 458
Lo/Ovral-28 Tablets 3423
Neoral Soft Gelatin Capsules 2247
Neoral Oral Solution 2247
Ortho-Cept Tablets 2395
Ortho-Cyclen Tablets 2414
Ortho Evra Transdermal System 2402
Ortho Tri-Cyclen Tablets 2414
Ortho Tri-Cyclen Lo Tablets 2421
▲ Rapamune Oral Solution and Tablets (3% to 20%) 3472
Seasonale Tablets 1073
Valtrex Caplets 1573
Yasmin 28 Tablets 818

Hemopericardium

Aggrastat 1878
Cardene I.V. (0.7%) 1129

Hemoperitoneum

Follistim AQ Cartridge 2354
Gonal-f RFF Pen for Injection 3155
Merrem I.V. (0.2%) 687
Repronex for Intramuscular and Subcutaneous Injection 1148
Trasylol Injection (1% to 2%) 779

Hemophilus

▲ Intron A for Injection (Less than 5%) 3038

Hemoptysis

Abelcet Injection 1119

Abilify Tablets (Rare) 916
Abilify Tablets (Rare) 2472
Actiq (Less than 1%) 993
Aggrenox Capsules (Less than 1%) 855
AmBisome for Injection (Less common) 615
Argatroban Injection (2.9%) 1321
Campath Ampules 826
▲ CellCept Capsules (3% to less than 20%) 2751
▲ CellCept Intravenous (3% to less than 20%) 2751
▲ CellCept Oral Suspension (3% to less than 20%) 2751
▲ CellCept Tablets (3% to less than 20%) 2751
Cipro I.V. (1% or less) 2998
Cipro I.V. Pharmacy Bulk Package (1% or less) 3509
Cipro (Less than 1%) 2991
Cipro XR Tablets 3004
Colazal Capsules 2845
Duragesic Transdermal System (1% or greater) 2448
Effexor Tablets (Rare) 3405
Effexor XR Capsules (Rare) 3411
▲ Eloxatin for Injection (2% to 5%) 2908
Evoxac Capsules (Less than 1%) 1042
Gabitril Tablets (Infrequent) 998
▲ Intron A for Injection (Less than or equal to 5%) 3038
Invanz for Injection (Greater than 0.1%) 1974
Invirase (Less than 2%) 2776
▲ I.V. Busulfex (3%) 1125
Levaquin in 5% Dextrose Injection (0.1% to 0.9%) 2453
Levaquin (0.1% to 0.9%) 2453
Lupron Depot 7.5 mg (Less than 5%) 3261
Matulane Capsules 3188
Namenda (Infrequent) 1199
Natrecor for Injection (Greater than or equal to 1%) 3123
Neurontin Capsules (Rare) 2498
Neurontin Oral Solution (Rare) 2498
Neurontin Tablets (Rare) 2498
Paxil CR Controlled-Release Tablets (Rare) 1509
Paxil (Rare) 1501
Permax Tablets (Infrequent) 3357
Photofrin for Injection (One patient) 729
Plavix Tablets (Less than 1%) 940
Plavix Tablets (Less than 1%) 2942
Pletal Tablets (Less than 2%) 2478
Prevacid Delayed-Release Capsules (Less than 1%) 3268
Prevacid for Delayed-Release Oral Suspension (Less than 1%) 3268
Prevacid NapraPAC (Less than 1%) 3277
Prevacid SoluTab Delayed-Release Orally Disintegrating Tablets (Less than 1%) 3268
PREVPAC (Less than 1%) 3281
Prinivil Tablets (0.3% to 1.0%) 2029
Prinzide Tablets 2033
Proleukin for Injection (1%) 1007
Prozac Pulvules and Liquid (Rare) 1771
Pulmozyme Inhalation Solution 1245
ReoPro Vials (9 to 11 events) 1779
Rilutek Tablets (Infrequent) 2945
Risperdal Consta Long-Acting Injection (Infrequent) 1664
Rythmol SR Capsules 2736
Symbyax Capsules (Rare) 1788
Targretin Capsules 1719
▲ TOBI Solution for Inhalation (19.4%) 1015
▲ Trisenox Injection (8%) 983
Uniretic Tablets (Less than 1%) 3114
▲ Ventavis Inhalation Solution (5%) 1036
VFEND I.V. (Less than 2%) 2543
VFEND Oral Suspension (Less than 2%) 2543
VFEND Tablets (Less than 2%) 2543
▲ Xeloda Tablets (Less than 5%) 2825
Zestoretic Tablets 701
Zestril Tablets (0.3% to 1.0%) 704
Zoloft (Rare) 2581
Zonegran Capsules (Rare) 1089
Zyprexa Tablets (Infrequent) 1798
Zyprexa ZYDIS Orally Disintegrating Tablets (Infrequent) 1798

Hemorrhage

(*see under* Bleeding)

Hemorrhage, cerebral

(*see under* Cerebral hemorrhage)

Hemorrhage, cerebrovascular

Mycamine for Injection 620
Revatio Tablets 2541
Viagra Tablets 2552

Hemorrhage, colon

Actiq (Less than 1%) 993
Prozac Pulvules and Liquid (Rare) 1771

Hemorrhage, conjunctival

Exelon Capsules (Infrequent) 2204
Gleevec Tablets (Infrequent) 2221
Namenda (Infrequent) 1199
Plavix Tablets 940
Plavix Tablets 2942
▲ Retisert Implant (10% to 35%) ⊙ 256
Stromectol Tablets 2053
Trileptal Oral Suspension 2281
Trileptal Tablets 2281
▲ Zymar Ophthalmic Solution (1% to 4%) 571

Hemorrhage, ear

Imitrex Nasal Spray 1435

Hemorrhage, esophageal

Pletal Tablets (Less than 2%) 2478
Protonix I.V. (Less than 1%) 3468
Protonix Tablets (Less than 1%) 3465

Hemorrhage, eye, anterior chamber

Evoxac Capsules (Less than 1%) 1042
Zoloft (Rare) 2581

Hemorrhage, eyes

Abilify Tablets (Infrequent) 916
Abilify Tablets (Infrequent) 2472
Actiq (Less than 1%) 993
Adalat CC Tablets (Less than 1%) 2978
AmBisome for Injection (Less common) 615
Amerge Tablets (Rare) 1312
Caduet Tablets (Less than 2%) 2507
▲ CellCept Capsules (3% to less than 20%) 2751
▲ CellCept Intravenous (3% to less than 20%) 2751
▲ CellCept Oral Suspension (3% to less than 20%) 2751
▲ CellCept Tablets (3% to less than 20%) 2751
Effexor Tablets 3405
Effexor XR Capsules 3411
Imitrex Nasal Spray 1435
Iressa Tablets (Very rare) 684
▲ Leukine (11%) 829
Lipitor Tablets (Less than 2%) 2495
Lyrica Capsules (0.1% to 1%) 2524
Neumega for Injection 3433
Neurontin Capsules (Infrequent) 2498
Neurontin Oral Solution (Infrequent) 2498
Neurontin Tablets (Infrequent) 2498
Ocufen Ophthalmic Solution ⊙ 230
Paxil CR Controlled-Release Tablets (Rare) 1509
Paxil (Rare) 1501
Permax Tablets (Infrequent) 3357
Plavix Tablets 940
Plavix Tablets 2942
Pletal Tablets (Less than 2%) 2478
Prozac Pulvules and Liquid (Rare) 1771
Relpax Tablets (Rare) 2531
ReoPro Vials (9 to 11 events) 1779
Rythmol SR Capsules 2736
Sonata Capsules (Rare) 1686
Soriatane Capsules (Less than 1%) 1028
Symbyax Capsules (Rare) 1788
Tasmar Tablets (Infrequent) 3360
Ticlid Tablets 2813
Uniretic Tablets (Less than 1%) 3114
VFEND I.V. (Less than 2%) 2543
VFEND Oral Suspension (Less than 2%) 2543
VFEND Tablets (Less than 2%) 2543
Viagra Tablets (Less than 2%) 2552
Zyprexa Tablets (Infrequent) 1798
Zyprexa ZYDIS Orally Disintegrating Tablets (Infrequent) 1798
Zyrtec Chewable Tablets (Less than 2%) 2589
Zyrtec (Less than 2%) 2589
Zyrtec-D 12 Hour Extended Release Tablets (Less than 2%) 2591

Hemorrhage, focal

Thyrogen for Injection (4 patients out of 55) 1270

Hemorrhage, gastrointestinal

(*see under* Bleeding, gastrointestinal)

Hemorrhage, intra-alveolar

▲ I.V. Busulfex (5%) 1125

Hemorrhage, intracerebral

(*see under* Bleeding, intracerebral)

Hemorrhage, postpartum

Aggrenox Capsules 855
Bayer Aspirin Tablets 3515
Ecotrin Enteric Coated Aspirin Low, Regular and Maximum Strength Tablets 1627
St. Joseph 81 mg Aspirin Chewable and Enteric Coated Tablets 1841

Hemorrhage, pulmonary

Aggrastat 1878
Ammonul Injection 3323
Mylotarg for Injection 3429
Photofrin for Injection 729
Plavix Tablets (Less than 1%) 940
Plavix Tablets (Less than 1%) 2942
Pletal Tablets (Very rare) 2478
ReoPro Vials (9 to 11 events) 1779
Revatio Tablets 2541
Viagra Tablets 2552

Hemorrhage, purpuric

Carbatrol Capsules 3174
Tegretol/Tegretol-XR 2278

Hemorrhage, rectal

Antara Capsules 2723
Caduet Tablets (Less than 2%) 2507
Campral Tablets (Infrequent) 1175
depo-subQ provera 104 Injectable Suspension 2622
Lyrica Capsules (0.1% to 1%) 2524
Prevacid NapraPAC (Less than 1%) 3277
Prozac Pulvules and Liquid (Rare) 1771
Risperdal Consta Long-Acting Injection (Infrequent) 1664
Tricor Tablets 523
Zelnorm Tablets 2303

Hemorrhage, retinal

Aricept Tablets (Infrequent) 1086
Aricept ODT Tablets (Infrequent) 1086
Effexor Tablets (Rare) 3405
Effexor XR Capsules (Rare) 3411
Elitek (Less than or equal to 1%) 2906
Elmiron Capsules (Less than or equal to 1%) 2393
Gleevec Tablets (Rare) 2221
Intron A for Injection (Rare) 3038
Matulane Capsules 3188
Namenda (Infrequent) 1199
Paxil CR Controlled-Release Tablets (Rare) 1509
Paxil (Rare) 1501
Pegasys 2793
PEG-Intron Powder for Injection 3062
Plavix Tablets 940
Plavix Tablets 2942
Pletal Tablets (Less than 2%) 2478
▲ Retisert Implant (5% to 9%) ⊙ 256
Revatio Tablets (1.4% to 1.9%) 2541
VFEND I.V. (Less than 2%) 2543
VFEND Oral Suspension (Less than 2%) 2543
VFEND Tablets (Less than 2%) 2543
Viagra Tablets 2552
▲ Visudyne for Injection (1% to 10%) 2286

Hemorrhage, subarachnoid

Aggrenox Capsules (Less than 1%) 855
Amerge Tablets 1312
Campath Ampules 826
Imitrex Injection 1431
Imitrex Nasal Spray 1435
Imitrex Tablets 1440
Orthoclone OKT3 Sterile Solution 2370
Requip Tablets (Rare) 1528
Revatio Tablets 2541
Rilutek Tablets (Rare) 2945
Symbyax Capsules (Rare) 1788
Viagra Tablets 2552
Zomig Tablets 714
Zomig-ZMT Tablets 714
Zyprexa Tablets (Rare) 1798
Zyprexa ZYDIS Orally Disintegrating Tablets (Rare) 1798

Hemorrhage, subconjunctival

Effexor Tablets (Rare) 3405
Effexor XR Capsules (Rare) 3411
Travatan Ophthalmic Solution (1% to 4%) 559
▲ Vigamox Ophthalmic Solution (1% to 6%) 560
▲ Visudyne for Injection (1% to 10%) 2286

Hemorrhage, subcutaneous

Mustargen for Injection 2007
Pletal Tablets (Very rare) 2478
Ticlid Tablets 2813

Hemorrhage, throat

Imitrex Nasal Spray 1435

Hemorrhage, uterine

Prozac Pulvules and Liquid (Rare) 1771

Hemorrhage, vitreous

Gleevec Tablets (Rare) 2221
▲ Retisert Implant (10% to 35%) ⊙ 256
▲ Visudyne for Injection (1% to 10%) 2286
Xalatan Sterile Ophthalmic Solution (Extremely rare) 2654

Hemorrhagic colitis

Amoxil Capsules 1315
Amoxil Chewable Tablets 1315
Amoxil Pediatric Drops for Oral Suspension 1315
Amoxil Powder for Oral Suspension 1315
Amoxil Tablets 1315
Augmentin 1331
Augmentin Tablets 1334
Augmentin XR Extended-Release Tablets 1340
Kaletra (Less than 2%) 474
Lamictal (Rare) 1449
Omnicef Capsules 506
Omnicef for Oral Suspension 506
Primaxin I.M. 2022
Primaxin I.V. (Less than 0.2%) 2024

Hemorrhagic complications

Coumadin for Injection 932
Coumadin Tablets 932
Fragmin Injection (Low incidence) 2638
Lovenox Injection (Low incidence) 2931

Hemorrhagic eruptions

(*see under* Eruptions, hemorrhagic)

Hemorrhagic tendency

Mustargen for Injection 2007

Hemorrhoids

Abilify Tablets (Infrequent) 916
Abilify Tablets (Infrequent) 2472
Aggrenox Capsules (1%) 855
Ambien Tablets (Rare) 2867
AmBisome for Injection (Less common) 615
Amerge Tablets (Rare) 1312
Aricept Tablets (Infrequent) 1086
Aricept ODT Tablets (Infrequent) 1086
Arthrotec Tablets (Rare) 3126
Campath Ampules 826
Celebrex Capsules (0.1% to 1.9%) 3130
Celexa (Infrequent) 1177
▲ Chemet Capsules (12.0% to 20.9%) 2480
Clindesse Vaginal Cream (Less than 1%) 3296
Colazal Capsules 2845
Effexor Tablets (Infrequent) 3405
Effexor XR Capsules (Infrequent) 3411
▲ Eloxatin for Injection (2% to 5%) 2908
▲ Entocort EC Capsules (Less than 5%) 2694
Evoxac Capsules (Less than 1%) 1042
Exelon Capsules (Infrequent) 2204
▲ Imdur Tablets (Less than or equal to 5%) 3032
▲ Infergen (1% to 6%) 1647
Invanz for Injection (Greater than 0.1%) 1974
Invirase (Less than 2%) 2776
Klonopin (Infrequent) 2782
Lexapro Oral Solution (Infrequent) 1193
Lexapro Tablets (Infrequent) 1193
Lotronex Tablets (2%) 1479
Micardis Tablets (More than 0.3%) 884
Micardis HCT Tablets 886
Neurontin Capsules (Infrequent) 2498
Neurontin Oral Solution (Infrequent) 2498
Neurontin Tablets (Infrequent) 2498
Requip Tablets (Infrequent) 1528
Risperdal Consta Long-Acting Injection (Infrequent) 1664

Risperdal M-Tab Orally Disintegrating Tablets (Infrequent) 1658
Risperdal (Infrequent) 1658
Sandostatin Injection (Less than 1%) 2263
▲ Sandostatin LAR Depot (5% to 15%) 2264
Seroquel Tablets (Infrequent) 691
Soriatane Capsules (Less than 1%) 1028
Topamax Sprinkle Capsules (Infrequent) 2438
Topamax Tablets (Infrequent) 2438
Trileptal Oral Suspension 2281
Trileptal Tablets 2281
Zelnorm Tablets 2303
▲ Zenapax for Injection (2% to 5%) 2838
Zyrtec Chewable Tablets (Less than 2%) 2589
Zyrtec (Less than 2%) 2589
Zyrtec-D 12 Hour Extended Release Tablets (Less than 2%) 2591

Hemospermia

Rescriptor Tablets 2535

Hemostasis, interference

Depacon Injection 412
Depakote Tablets 427

Hemothorax

Permax Tablets (Rare) 3357
Plavix Tablets (Less than 1%) 940
Plavix Tablets (Less than 1%) 2942
Refludan for Injection 815

Henoch-Schönlein purpura

Boostrix 1366
Cozaar Tablets 1913
Hyzaar 1964
Parcopa Orally Disintegrating Tablets 3111
Paxil CR Controlled-Release Tablets 1509
Paxil 1501
Stalevo Tablets 2270
Varivax 2070

Hepatic adenoma

Alesse-28 Tablets 3392
Estratest Tablets (Rare) 3196
Estratest H.S. Tablets (Rare) 3196
Lo/Ovral-28 Tablets 3423
Ortho-Cept Tablets 2395
Ortho-Cyclen Tablets 2414
Ortho Evra Transdermal System 2402
Ortho Tri-Cyclen Tablets 2414
Ortho Tri-Cyclen Lo Tablets 2421
Premarin Intravenous 3440
Premarin Vaginal Cream 3449
Seasonale Tablets 1073
Triphasil-28 Tablets 3483
Yasmin 28 Tablets 818

Hepatic coma

Concerta Extended-Release Tablets 1828
Focalin Tablets 2214
Focalin XR Capsules 2217
Levaquin in 5% Dextrose Injection (0.1% to 0.9%) 2453
Levaquin (0.1% to 0.9%) 2453
Maxzide 2150
Metadate CD Capsules 3316
Prinzide Tablets 2033
Ritalin Hydrochloride Tablets (Some instances) 2254
Ritalin LA Capsules 2255
Ritalin-SR Tablets (Some instances) 2254
Vaseretic Tablets 2073
VFEND I.V. (Less than 2%) 2543
VFEND Oral Suspension (Less than 2%) 2543
VFEND Tablets (Less than 2%) 2543
▲ Xeloda Tablets (Less than 5%) 2825
Zestoretic Tablets 701

Hepatic dysfunction

Accolate Tablets 663
Actimmune (Rare) 1646
▲ Advair Diskus 100/50 (1% to 3%) 1291
▲ Advair Diskus 250/50 (1% to 3%) 1291
▲ Advair Diskus 500/50 (1% to 3%) 1291
Advicor Tablets 1694
Aggrenox Capsules (Less than 1%) 855
▲ Albenza Tablets (Less than 1.0% to 15.6%) 1310
Aldara Cream, 5% 1814
Aldoclor Tablets 1881
Aldoril Tablets 1884
Alkeran for Injection 976
Alkeran Tablets 977
Altoprev Extended-Release Tablets 1151
Amaryl Tablets (Isolated cases) 2864
Ambien Tablets (Infrequent) 2867
AmBisome for Injection (Less common) 615
Amerge Tablets (Rare) 1312
Amoxil Capsules 1315
Amoxil Chewable Tablets 1315
Amoxil Pediatric Drops for Oral Suspension 1315
Amoxil Powder for Oral Suspension 1315
Amoxil Tablets 1315
Anadrol-50 Tablets 3329
Anaprox Tablets (Less than 1%) 2769
Anaprox DS Tablets (Less than 1%) 2769
▲ Anzemet Injection (3.6%) 2871
▲ Arava Tablets (5%) 2881
Arixtra Injection (0.4%) 1325
Arthrotec Tablets (Rare) 3126
Atacand Tablets 634
Atacand HCT 637
Augmentin (Infrequent) 1331
Augmentin Tablets (Infrequent) 1334
Augmentin XR Extended-Release Tablets (Infrequent) 1340
Augmentin ES-600 Powder for Oral Suspension (Infrequently) 1337
Avelox (1%) 2984
Avinza Capsules (Less than 5%) 1714
Avonex 839
Aygestin Tablets 1062
Biaxin/Biaxin XL (Infrequent) 402
Blocadren Tablets 1891
Capastat Sulfate for Injection 1728
Captopril Tablets 2114
Carbatrol Capsules 3174
Carimune NF 3501
Catapres Tablets 874
Ceftin 1369
Celebrex Capsules (0.1% to 1.9%) 3130
▲ CellCept Capsules (3% to less than 20%) 2751
▲ CellCept Intravenous (3% to less than 20%) 2751
▲ CellCept Oral Suspension (3% to less than 20%) 2751
▲ CellCept Tablets (3% to less than 20%) 2751
▲ Cipro I.V. (Among most frequent) 2998
▲ Cipro I.V. Pharmacy Bulk Package (Among most frequent) 3509
Cleocin Vaginal Ovules 2613
Clinoril Tablets (Less than 1 in 100) 1899
Concerta Extended-Release Tablets 1828
Copegus Tablets (Less than 1%) 2759
Cosmegen for Injection 1907
Crixivan Capsules 1918
Cuprimine Capsules 1925
Cytovene 2763
Dantrium Capsules 2690
Daranide Tablets 1928
Darvocet A 500 Tablets 3497
Delatestryl Injection 2976
Depacon Injection 412
Depakene 417
Depakote Sprinkle Capsules (Occasional) 422
Depakote Tablets 427
Depakote ER Tablets 433
Diovan Tablets (Occasional) 2191
Diprivan Injectable Emulsion (Less than 1%) 676
Dolobid Tablets (Less than 1 in 100) 1937
Dyazide Capsules 1389
EC-Naprosyn Delayed-Release Tablets (Less than 1%) 2769
Edecrin (Rare) 1941
E.E.S. 449
Effexor Tablets 3405
Effexor XR Capsules 3411
Elmiron Capsules (1%) 2393
Emcyt Capsules 3137
Engerix-B Vaccine 1391
Epivir 1394
EryPed 445
Ery-Tab Tablets 447
Erythrocin Stearate Filmtab Tablets 452
Erythromycin Base Filmtab Tablets 454
Erythromycin Delayed-Release Capsules, USP 456
Estratest Tablets 3196
Estratest H.S. Tablets 3196
Eulexin Capsules 3023
Evoxac Capsules (Less than 1%) 1042
Exelon Capsules (Infrequent) 2204
Flexeril Tablets (Less than 1%) 1832
Focalin Tablets 2214
Focalin XR Capsules 2217
Fortaz 1422
Gabitril Tablets (Infrequent) 998
Gammagard Liquid 751
Gammagard S/D 754
Gamunex Immune Globulin I.V., 10% 3232
Guanidine Hydrochloride Tablets 3030
Hepsera Tablets (2% or greater) 1275
Idamycin PFS Injection (Less than 5%) 2645
Imitrex Injection (Infrequent) 1431
Imitrex Nasal Spray 1435
Imitrex Tablets 1440
▲ Intron A for Injection (Less than 5%) 3038
Invirase (Rare) 2776
Iveegam EN 759
Kaletra 474
Ketek Tablets 2920
Lamictal (Infrequent) 1449
▲ Lamisil Tablets (3.3%) 2226
Leukine 829
Levaquin in 5% Dextrose Injection (0.1% to 0.9%) 2453
Levaquin (0.1% to 0.9%) 2453
Librium Capsules 3349
Lipitor Tablets (Less than 2%) 2495
▲ Lofibra Capsules (7.5%) 1217
▲ Lumigan Ophthalmic Solution (1% to 5%) 569
Lupron Injection Pediatric 3256
Matulane Capsules 3188
Maxipime for Injection 1093
Mefoxin for Injection 1987
Mefoxin Premixed Intravenous Solution 1990
Metadate CD Capsules 3316
Mevacor Tablets 1996
Midamor Tablets (Rare) 2000
Mintezol (Rare) 2002
Moban Tablets (Rare) 1108
Moduretic Tablets 2003
Mycamine for Injection 620
Naprosyn Suspension (Less than 1%) 2769
Naprosyn Tablets (Less than 1%) 2769
Neurontin Capsules 2498
Neurontin Oral Solution 2498
Neurontin Tablets 2498
Nexium Delayed-Release Capsules (Less than 1%) 645
Nexium I.V. (Less than 1%) 649
Niaspan Extended-Release Tablets 1703
Nimotop Capsules (Up to 1.2%) 774
▲ Nipent for Injection (2% to 19%) 3216
Norvir (Less than 2%) 499
Omnicef Capsules 506
Omnicef for Oral Suspension 506
Oncaspar (Greater than 1% but less than 5%) 1123
Oxandrin Tablets 2977
▲ Pacerone Tablets (4% to 9%) 3337
Paxil CR Controlled-Release Tablets 1509
Paxil 1501
PCE Dispertab Tablets 510
Pediarix Vaccine 1518
Pegasys (Less than 1%) 2793
Permax Tablets (Infrequent) 3357
Persantine Tablets (Rare) 898
Phenytek Capsules 2153
Plavix Tablets 940
Plavix Tablets 2942
Prandin Tablets (0.5, 1, and 2 mg) (Rare) 2337
Premarin Vaginal Cream 3449
Prevacid Delayed-Release Capsules 3268
Prevacid for Delayed-Release Oral Suspension 3268
Prevacid SoluTab Delayed-Release Orally Disintegrating Tablets 3268
PREVPAC (Infrequent) 3281
▲ Prograf Capsules and Injection (5% to 36%) 624
Proleukin for Injection 1007
Protopic Ointment (Greater than or equal to 1%) 629
▲ Provigil Tablets (2% to 3%) 1002
Prozac Pulvules and Liquid (Infrequent) 1771
▲ Rapamune Oral Solution and Tablets (3% to 20%) 3472
▲ Rebif Prefilled Syringe for Injection (4% to 18%) 3163
▲ Refludan for Injection (5.3%) 815
▲ Relafen Tablets (Up to 15%) 1523
Relpax Tablets (Infrequent) 2531
Remicade for IV Injection (Rare) 987
Repronex for Intramuscular and Subcutaneous Injection 1148
Rilutek Tablets (Infrequent) 2945
Ritalin Hydrochloride Tablets (Some instances) 2254
Ritalin LA Capsules 2255
Ritalin-SR Tablets (Some instances) 2254
▲ Somavert Injection (4% to 12%) 2648
Sonata Capsules (Rare) 1686
Soriatane Capsules (Less than 1%) 1028
Spectracef Tablets (0.1% to 1%) 2706
Strattera Capsules 1784
Striant Mucoadhesive 1022
Sular Tablets (Less than or equal to 1%) 1163
Suprax 1811
Surmontil Capsules 2347
Synagis (More than 1%) 1868
Tabloid Tablets (Occasional) 1545
Tambocor Tablets (Rare) 1824
Tamiflu Capsules 2810
Tamiflu Oral Suspension 2810
Tasmar Tablets 3360
Tegretol/Tegretol-XR 2278
Thalomid Capsules 979
Ticlid Tablets (1.0%) 2813
Timolide Tablets 2056
▲ Tracleer Tablets (8%) 539
Tranxene 2488
▲ Trasylol Injection (3%) 779
Trelstar LA Suspension (1.1%) 3387
Trileptal Oral Suspension 2281
Trileptal Tablets 2281
Ultane Liquid for Inhalation (Less than 1%) 526
Ultracet Tablets (Less than 1%) 2462
▲ Valcyte Tablets (Less than 5%) 2816
Valtrex Caplets 1573
Vantas (Less than 2%) 3367
Vantin Tablets and Oral Suspension 2650
Vaqta (Isolated reports) 2067
▲ Vesanoid Capsules (50% to 60%) 2823
VFEND I.V. (2.7%) 2543
VFEND Oral Suspension (2.7%) 2543
VFEND Tablets (2.7%) 2543
Viagra Tablets (Less than 2%) 2552
Viracept 2556
Viramune Oral Suspension 903
Viramune Tablets 903
Vivactil Tablets 2350
Vivelle Transdermal System (Rare) 2288
Vivelle-Dot Transdermal System (Rare) 2293
Wellbutrin SR Sustained-Release Tablets (Infrequent) 1583
Wellbutrin XL Extended-Release Tablets (Infrequent) 1588
Zestril Tablets (Rare) 704
Zinacef Injection 1604
Zinacef for Injection 1604
Zithromax Capsules, 250 mg 2568
Zithromax for IV Infusion 2573
Zithromax for Oral Suspension, 300 mg, 600 mg, 900 mg, 1200 mg 2561
Zithromax Tablets, 250 mg, 500 mg 2561
Zithromax Tri-Pak 2561
Zmax for Oral Suspension 2577
Zofran Injection 1607
Zofran 1613
Zofran ODT Orally Disintegrating Tablets 1613
Zoloft (Rare) 2581
Zomig Tablets (Infrequent) 714
Zomig-ZMT Tablets (Infrequent) 714
Zovirax Capsules 1616
Zovirax for Injection 1618
Zovirax 1616
Zyban Sustained-Release Tablets (Infrequent) 1620
Zyrtec Chewable Tablets (Less than 2%) 2589
Zyrtec (Less than 2%) 2589
Zyrtec-D 12 Hour Extended Release Tablets (Less than 2%) 2591
Zyvox (0.4% to 1.3%) 2661

Hepatic enzymes, elevation

(*see also under* Serum transaminase, elevation)

Accolate Tablets (Rare) 663
Accutane Capsules 2740
Agrylin Capsules (2 of 551 patients) 3172
Altace Capsules (Rare) 1673
Amaryl Tablets (Rare) 2864
▲ Anaprox Tablets (Up to 15%) 2769
▲ Anaprox DS Tablets (Up to 15%) 2769
Arixtra Injection (0.3%) 1325
Asacol Delayed-Release Tablets 2688
Atacand Tablets (Infrequent) 634
Atacand HCT 637

- Avandamet Tablets 1343
- Avandia Tablets 1348
- Avapro Tablets 925
- Avapro Tablets (Very rare) 2886
- Avonex 839
- Azasan Tablets 2844
- Benicar Tablets (Infrequently) 2850
- Betaseron for SC Injection 791
- Biaxin/Biaxin XL (Infrequent) 402
- Biltricide Tablets 2990
- Caduet Tablets 2507
- ▲ Camptosar Injection (Fewer than 10%) 2602
- Canasa Rectal Suppositories 726
- Captopril Tablets 2114
- ▲ Casodex Tablets (6%) 670
- ▲ Cataflam Tablets (1% to 10%) 2173
- Ceftin for Oral Suspension (0.1% to 1%) 1369
- Celexa (Infrequent) 1177
- Clarinex Syrup (Rare) 3009
- Clarinex Tablets (Rare) 3009
- Clarinex Reditabs Tablets (Rare) 3009
- Colazal Capsules 2845
- Comvax 1904
- Coreg Tablets (Greater than 0.1% to 1%) 1376
- Coumadin for Injection (Infrequent) 932
- Coumadin Tablets (Infrequent) 932
- Covera-HS Tablets (1.4%) 3135
- Dantrium Capsules 2690
- Depacon Injection 412
- Depakene 417
- Depakote Tablets 427
- Depakote ER Tablets 433
- Diovan HCT Tablets 2195
- Diovan Tablets 2191
- Dyazide Capsules 1389
- DynaCirc CR Tablets (0.5% to 1%) 2726
- Dyrenium Capsules (Rare) 3390
- ▲ EC-Naprosyn Delayed-Release Tablets (Up to 15%) 2769
- Ecotrin Enteric Coated Aspirin Low, Regular and Maximum Strength Tablets 1627
- EryPed 445
- Evoxac Capsules (Less than 1%) 1042
- Hycamtin for Injection (Less than 1%) 1427
- Hyzaar (Occasional) 1964
- Imitrex Nasal Spray 1435
- Imitrex Tablets 1440
- Ketek Tablets (Greater than or equal to 0.2% to less than 2%) 2920
- Lescol Capsules 2227
- Lescol Capsules 2730
- Lescol XL Tablets 2227
- Lescol XL Tablets 2730
- Lotrel Capsules (Scattered incidents) 2238
- Maxzide 2150
- Micardis HCT Tablets 886
- MS Contin Tablets 2703
- Nadolol Tablets 2121
- ▲ Naprosyn Suspension (Up to 15%) 2769
- ▲ Naprosyn Tablets (Up to 15%) 2769
- Navelbine Injection 1494
- Niaspan Extended-Release Tablets 1703
- Niravam Orally Disintegrating Tablets 3106
- Noroxin Tablets 2009
- Norvasc Tablets (Infrequent) 2529
- Paxil CR Controlled-Release Tablets 1509
- Paxil 1501
- Persantine Tablets 898
- Plavix Tablets (1% to 2.5%) 940
- Plavix Tablets (1% to 2.5%) 2942
- Prandin Tablets (0.5, 1, and 2 mg) (Less than 1%) 2337
- PREVPAC (Infrequent) 3281
- Prinivil Tablets (Rare) 2029
- Prinzide Tablets (Rare) 2033
- Provigil Tablets (At least 1%) 1002
- Rebif Prefilled Syringe for Injection 3163
- Recombivax HB 2045
- Relafen Tablets (Less than 1%) 1523
- Risperdal Consta Long-Acting Injection (Frequent) 1664
- Roferon-A Injection (Frequent) 2805
- Sandostatin Injection (Less than 1%) 2263
- Sandostatin LAR Depot (Rare) 2264
- St. Joseph 81 mg Aspirin Chewable and Enteric Coated Tablets 1841
- Sustiva Capsules 957
- Tabloid Tablets (Occasional) 1545
- Tarka Tablets (2.8%) 519
- Tasmar Tablets 3360
- Tegretol/Tegretol-XR 2278
- Tenormin I.V. Injection 698
- Tenormin Tablets 695
- Thalomid Capsules 979
- Trileptal Oral Suspension 2281
- Trileptal Tablets 2281
- Trizivir Tablets 1565
- Ultracet Tablets 2462
- Vaseretic Tablets (Rare) 2073
- Vasotec I.V. Injection 2076
- Verelan PM Capsules 3120
- Vermox Chewable Tablets (Rare) 1853
- VFEND I.V. (1.5% to 2.4%) 2543
- VFEND Oral Suspension (1.5% to 2.4%) 2543
- VFEND Tablets (1.5% to 2.4%) 2543
- ▲ Vicoprofen Tablets (Up to 15%) 533
- ▲ Visudyne for Injection (1% to 10%) 2286
- ▲ Voltaren Tablets (1% to 10%) 2298
- ▲ Voltaren-XR Tablets (1% to 10%) 2301
- Xanax XR Tablets 2655
- Zestoretic Tablets (Rare) 701
- Zestril Tablets (Rare) 704
- Zoloft (One or more patients) 2581
- Zovirax 1616

Hepatic enzymes, increased

- Aptivus Capsules (Less than 2%) 859
- Lexapro Oral Solution (Infrequent) 1193
- Lexapro Tablets (Infrequent) 1193
- MS Contin Tablets (Less frequent) 2703
- Nicomide Tablets 3190
- Univasc Tablets 3118

Hepatic eosinophilic infiltration

- Singulair (Very rare) 2047

Hepatic failure

- Abelcet Injection 1119
- Accolate Tablets (Rare) 663
- Aceon Tablets (2 mg, 4 mg, 8 mg) 3191
- Aloprim for Injection (Less than 1%) 2156
- Altace Capsules 1673
- Amaryl Tablets 2864
- Ammonul Injection 3323
- Anaprox Tablets (Less than 1%) 2769
- Anaprox DS Tablets (Less than 1%) 2769
- Antabuse Tablets 2343
- Aptivus Capsules (Less than 2%) 859
- Arava Tablets (Rare) 2881
- Arthrotec Tablets (Rare) 3126
- Asacol Delayed-Release Tablets (Rare) 2688
- Biaxin/Biaxin XL (Very rare) 402
- Campath Ampules 826
- Captopril Tablets (Rare) 2114
- Cataflam Tablets (Rarely) 2173
- Celebrex Capsules (Less than 0.1%) 3130
- Cipro I.V. 2998
- Cipro I.V. Pharmacy Bulk Package 3509
- Cipro 2991
- Cipro XR Tablets 3004
- Clinoril Tablets (Less than 1 in 100) 1899
- Colazal Capsules 2845
- Copegus Tablets (2%) 2759
- Cosmegen for Injection 1907
- Crixivan Capsules 1918
- Cytovene 2763
- Depacon Injection 412
- Depakene 417
- Depakote Sprinkle Capsules 422
- Depakote Tablets 427
- Depakote ER Tablets 433
- Dolobid Tablets 1937
- Doxil Injection (Less than 1%) 3302
- EC-Naprosyn Delayed-Release Tablets (Less than 1%) 2769
- Effexor Tablets 3405
- Effexor XR Capsules 3411
- Eulexin Capsules (Rare) 3023
- Flolan for Injection 1408
- Gemzar for Injection (Rare) 1743
- Hepsera Tablets (2% or greater) 1275
- Herceptin I.V. (At least one of the 958 patients) 1234
- Intron A for Injection (Very rare) 3038
- Lamisil Tablets (Rare) 2226
- Levaquin in 5% Dextrose Injection (0.1% to 0.9%) 2453
- Levaquin (0.1% to 0.9%) 2453
- Mavik Tablets (Rare) 482
- Merrem I.V. (Greater than 0.1% to 1%) 687
- Mintezol (Rare) 2002
- Mobic Oral Suspension (Less than 0.1%) 893
- Mobic Tablets (Less than 0.1%) 893
- Mycamine for Injection 620
- Mylotarg for Injection 3429
- Namenda 1199
- Naprosyn Suspension (Less than 1%) 2769
- Naprosyn Tablets (Less than 1%) 2769
- Niravam Orally Disintegrating Tablets 3106
- Omnicef Capsules 506
- Omnicef for Oral Suspension 506
- Oncaspar 1123
- Pentasa Capsules 3182
- Persantine Tablets 898
- Plavix Tablets 940
- PREVPAC (Very rare) 3281
- Prilosec OTC Tablets (Rare) 2674
- Prinivil Tablets (Rare) 2029
- Prinzide Tablets (Rare) 2033
- Proleukin for Injection (Less than 1%) 1007
- Protonix I.V. 3468
- Protonix Tablets 3465
- Prozac Pulvules and Liquid 1771
- Rebif Prefilled Syringe for Injection (Very rare) 3163
- Relafen Tablets (Less than 1%) 1523
- Rescriptor Tablets 2535
- Risperdal M-Tab Orally Disintegrating Tablets (Rare) 1658
- Risperdal (Rare) 1658
- Sustiva Capsules 957
- Tambocor Tablets (Rare) 1824
- Targretin Capsules 1719
- Tasmar Tablets 3360
- Tegretol/Tegretol-XR (Very rare) 2278
- Topamax Sprinkle Capsules 2438
- Topamax Tablets 2438
- Trasylol Injection (1% to 2%) 779
- Trizivir Tablets 1565
- Ultracet Tablets 2462
- Vaseretic Tablets (Rare) 2073
- Vasotec I.V. Injection (0.5% to 1.0%) 2076
- VFEND I.V. (Less than 2%) 2543
- VFEND Oral Suspension (Less than 2%) 2543
- VFEND Tablets (Less than 2%) 2543
- Viramune Oral Suspension 903
- Viramune Tablets 903
- Voltaren Tablets (Rarely) 2298
- Voltaren-XR Tablets (Rarely) 2301
- Xanax XR Tablets 2655
- ▲ Xeloda Tablets (Less than 5%) 2825
- Zantac (Rare) 1597
- Zantac Injection (Rare) 1593
- Zantac Injection Pharmacy Bulk Package (Rare) 1595
- Zantac Syrup (Rare) 1597
- Zegerid Powder for Oral Solution (Rare) 2972
- Zerit 971
- Zestoretic Tablets (Rare) 701
- Zestril Tablets (Rare) 704
- Ziagen 1600
- Zofran Injection 1607
- Zofran 1613
- Zofran ODT Orally Disintegrating Tablets 1613
- Zoloft (One or more patients) 2581

Hepatic failure, fulminant

- Tasmar Tablets (Three cases) 3360
- Zofran Injection Premixed 1607

Hepatic function tests, impaired

(*see under* Hepatic dysfunction)

Hepatic hemangioma, enlargement

- Cenestin Tablets, 0.45mg, 0.625mg, 0.9mg, 1.25mg 1063
- Cenestin Tablets, 0.3mg 1063
- Estrogel 0.06% 3200
- Menostar Transdermal System 805
- Prefest Tablets 1069
- Premarin Intravenous 3440
- Premarin Tablets 3443
- Premarin Vaginal Cream 3449
- Premphase Tablets 3452
- Prempro Tablets 3452
- Vivelle Transdermal System 2288
- Vivelle-Dot Transdermal System 2293

Hepatic necrosis

- Aceon Tablets (2 mg, 4 mg, 8 mg) (Rare) 3191
- Advicor Tablets 1694
- Altace Capsules (Rare) 1673
- Altoprev Extended-Release Tablets (Rare) 1151
- Arava Tablets (Rare) 2881
- Asacol Delayed-Release Tablets (Rare) 2688
- ▲ Blephamide Ophthalmic Ointment (Among most often) 563
- Blephamide Ophthalmic Suspension 564
- Captopril Tablets (Rare) 2114
- Celebrex Capsules (Rare) 3130
- Celexa 1177
- Cipro I.V. (1% or less) 2998
- Cipro I.V. Pharmacy Bulk Package (1% or less) 3509
- Cipro (Rare) 2991
- Cipro XR Tablets (Rare) 3004
- Colazal Capsules 2845
- Darvocet A 500 Tablets 3497
- Dolobid Tablets 1937
- Effexor Tablets 3405
- Effexor XR Capsules 3411
- Eulexin Capsules 3023
- FML-S Liquifilm Sterile Ophthalmic Suspension ⊙ 226
- ▲ Humira Injection (Less than 5%) 464
- Lescol Capsules (Rare) 2227
- Lescol Capsules (Rare) 2730
- Lescol XL Tablets 2227
- Lescol XL Tablets 2730
- Levaquin in 5% Dextrose Injection (Rare) 2453
- Levaquin (Rare) 2453
- Lexapro Oral Solution 1193
- Lexapro Tablets 1193
- Lotrel Capsules (Rare) 2238
- Mavik Tablets (Rare) 482
- Mevacor Tablets (Rare) 1996
- Myleran Tablets 1492
- Niaspan Extended-Release Tablets 1703
- Noroxin Tablets 2009
- Oxandrin Tablets (Rare) 2977
- Paxil CR Controlled-Release Tablets 1509
- Paxil 1501
- Pentasa Capsules 3182
- Pravachol Tablets (Rare) 943
- Prilosec OTC Tablets (Rare) 2674
- Prinivil Tablets (Rare) 2029
- Prinzide Tablets (Rare) 2033
- Rapamune Oral Solution and Tablets 3472
- Tabloid Tablets 1545
- Tarka Tablets (Rare) 519
- Ticlid Tablets (Rare) 2813
- Trusopt Sterile Ophthalmic Solution (Rare) 2065
- Uniretic Tablets (Rare) 3114
- Vaseretic Tablets (Rare) 2073
- Vasotec I.V. Injection (Rare) 2076
- Viramune Oral Suspension 903
- Viramune Tablets 903
- Vytorin 10/10 Tablets (Rare) 2084
- Vytorin 10/10 Tablets (Rare) 3092
- Vytorin 10/20 Tablets (Rare) 2084
- Vytorin 10/20 Tablets (Rare) 3092
- Vytorin 10/40 Tablets (Rare) 2084
- Vytorin 10/40 Tablets (Rare) 3092
- Vytorin 10/80 Tablets (Rare) 2084
- Vytorin 10/80 Tablets (Rare) 3092
- Zegerid Powder for Oral Solution (Rare) 2972
- Zestoretic Tablets (Rare) 701
- Zestril Tablets (Rare) 704
- Zocor Tablets (Rare) 2078
- Zonegran Capsules (Rare) 1089

Hepatic veno-occlusive disease

- Abelcet Injection 1119
- Alkeran for Injection 976
- AmBisome for Injection (Less common) 615
- Azasan Tablets 2844
- Cosmegen for Injection 1907
- ▲ I.V. Busulfex (8%) 1125
- Myleran Tablets 1492
- ▲ Mylotarg for Injection (5%) 3429
- Tabloid Tablets 1545

Hepatitis

- Abelcet Injection 1119
- Abilify Tablets (Rare) 916
- Abilify Tablets (Rare) 2472
- Accutane Capsules 2740
- Aciphex Tablets (Rare) 1081
- Advicor Tablets 1694
- Aldoclor Tablets 1881
- Aldoril Tablets 1884
- Alkeran for Injection 976
- Alkeran Tablets 977
- Altace Capsules (Less than 1%) 1673
- Altoprev Extended-Release Tablets 1151
- Amaryl Tablets (Isolated cases) 2864
- Amevive (1 case) 836
- Amnesteem Capsules 2126
- Anaprox Tablets (Less than 1%) 2769
- Anaprox DS Tablets (Less than 1%) 2769
- Ancef for Injection (Very rare) 1318

Antabuse Tablets 2343
Aptivus Capsules (Less than 2%) 859
Arava Tablets (Rare) 2881
Aricept Tablets 1086
Aricept ODT Tablets 1086
Arthrotec Tablets (Rare) 3126
Asacol Delayed-Release Tablets (Rare) 2688
Atacand Tablets 634
Atacand HCT 637
Augmentin (Rare) 1331
Augmentin Tablets (Rare) 1334
Avandamet Tablets 1343
Avandia Tablets 1348
Avelox 2984
Avonex 839
Axid Oral Solution 913
Bayer Aspirin Tablets 3515
Betaseron for SC Injection 791
BiDil Tablets 2161
Caduet Tablets (Less than 2%) 2507
Campral Tablets (Infrequent) 1175
Captopril Tablets 2114
Carbatrol Capsules 3174
Casodex Tablets 670
Cataflam Tablets (Occasionally) 2173
Catapres Tablets (Rare) 874
Ceftin 1369
Celebrex Capsules (Less than 0.1%) 3130
Celexa (Rare) 1177
▲ CellCept Capsules (3% to less than 20%) 2751
▲ CellCept Intravenous (3% to less than 20%) 2751
▲ CellCept Oral Suspension (3% to less than 20%) 2751
▲ CellCept Tablets (3% to less than 20%) 2751
Cipro I.V. (1% or less) 2998
Cipro I.V. Pharmacy Bulk Package (1% or less) 3509
Cipro (Less than 1%) 2991
Cipro XR Tablets 3004
Clarinex-D 24-Hour Extended-Release Tablets (Very rare) 3012
Clinoril Tablets (Less than 1%) 1899
Clorpres Tablets (Rare) 2139
Clozapine Tablets 2141
Clozaril Tablets 2174
Cosmegen for Injection 1907
Coumadin for Injection (Infrequent) 932
Coumadin Tablets (Infrequent) 932
Cozaar Tablets (Rare) 1913
Crestor Tablets (Less than 1%) 672
Crixivan Capsules 1918
Cytovene 2763
Dantrium Capsules (Less frequent) 2690
Diovan HCT Tablets (Very rare) 2195
Diovan Tablets (Very rare) 2191
Dolobid Tablets (Less than 1 in 100) 1937
Doxil Injection (Less than 1%) 3302
EC-Naprosyn Delayed-Release Tablets (Less than 1%) 2769
Ecotrin Enteric Coated Aspirin Low, Regular and Maximum Strength Tablets 1627
E.E.S. 449
Effexor Tablets (Rare) 3405
Effexor XR Capsules (Rare) 3411
Enbrel for Injection 580
Equetro Extended-Release Capsules 3178
EryPed 445
Erythromycin Delayed-Release Capsules, USP 456
Eulexin Capsules (Less than 1%) 3023
FazaClo Orally Disintegrating Tablets 547
Flexeril Tablets (Rare) 1832
Fortical Nasal Spray (Less than 1%) 3336
Havrix Vaccine (Rare) 1425
Herceptin I.V. (At least one of the 958 patients) 1234
Hyzaar (Rare) 1964
Invirase (Less than 2%) 2776
Ketek Tablets (Greater than or equal to 0.2% to less than 2%) 2920
Lamictal (Rare) 1449
Lescol Capsules 2227
Lescol Capsules 2730
Lescol XL Tablets 2227
Lescol XL Tablets 2730
Levaquin in 5% Dextrose Injection (Rare) 2453
Levaquin (Rare) 2453
Lexapro Oral Solution 1193
Lexapro Tablets 1193
Lipitor Tablets (Less than 2%) 2495
Lofibra Capsules 1217
Lotronex Tablets (A single case) 1479
Lunesta Tablets (Rare) 3139
Mevacor Tablets 1996
Miacalcin Nasal Spray (Less than 1%) 2242
Miradon Tablets 3056
Mobic Oral Suspension (Less than 2%) 893
Mobic Tablets (Less than 2%) 893
Naprosyn Suspension (Less than 1%) 2769
Naprosyn Tablets (Less than 1%) 2769
Neurontin Capsules 2498
Neurontin Oral Solution 2498
Neurontin Tablets 2498
Nexium Delayed-Release Capsules (Very rare) 645
Nexium I.V. (Very rare) 649
Nimotop Capsules (Less than 1%) 774
Niravam Orally Disintegrating Tablets 3106
Noroxin Tablets 2009
Norvasc Tablets (Less than or equal to 0.1%) 2529
Norvir (Less than 2%) 499
Omnicef Capsules 506
Omnicef for Oral Suspension 506
Orthoclone OKT3 Sterile Solution 2370
Pacerone Tablets 3337
Parnate Tablets (Rare) 1499
Paser Granules 1657
Paxil CR Controlled-Release Tablets (Rare) 1509
Paxil (Rare) 1501
PCE Dispertab Tablets 510
Pentasa Capsules (Infrequent) 3182
Permax Tablets (Infrequent) 3357
Persantine Tablets (Rare) 898
Plavix Tablets 940
Plavix Tablets 2942
Pravachol Tablets 943
Prilosec OTC Tablets (Rare) 2674
Primaxin I.M. 2022
Primaxin I.V. (Less than 0.2%) 2024
Prinivil Tablets (0.3% to 1.0%) 2029
Prinzide Tablets 2033
▲ Prograf Capsules and Injection (3% to 15%) 624
Proleukin for Injection 1007
Prometrium Capsules (100 mg, 200 mg) 3205
Protonix I.V. (Less than 1%) 3468
Protonix Tablets (Less than 1%) 3465
Prozac Pulvules and Liquid (Rare) 1771
Rebif Prefilled Syringe for Injection (Rare) 3163
Remicade for IV Injection (Greater than or equal to 0.2%) 987
Rescriptor Tablets 2535
Retrovir Capsules (Rare) 1533
Retrovir IV Infusion (Rare) 1537
Retrovir (Rare) 1533
Reyataz Capsules (Less than 3%) 948
Rilutek Tablets (Infrequent) 2945
Risperdal Consta Long-Acting Injection (Rare) 1664
Risperdal M-Tab Orally Disintegrating Tablets (Rare) 1658
Risperdal (Rare) 1658
Roferon-A Injection (Infrequent) 2805
Sandostatin Injection (Less than 1%) 2263
Sandostatin LAR Depot (Rare) 2264
Soriatane Capsules (Less than 1%) 1028
St. Joseph 81 mg Aspirin Chewable and Enteric Coated Tablets 1841
Suprane Liquid for Inhalation 770
Suprax 1811
Sustiva Capsules (Less than 2%) 957
Tamiflu Capsules 2810
Tamiflu Oral Suspension 2810
Taxotere Injection Concentrate (Rare) 2947
Tegretol/Tegretol-XR 2278
Tequin Injection 964
Tequin Tablets 964
Thalomid Capsules 979
Ticlid Tablets (Rare) 2813
Timentin ADD-Vantage (Rare) 1556
Timentin Injection Galaxy Container (Rare) 1559
Timentin IV Infusion (Rare) 1553
Timentin Pharmacy Bulk Package (Rare) 1562
Topamax Sprinkle Capsules 2438
Topamax Tablets 2438
Toprol-XL Tablets 660
Trecator Tablets 3482
Tricor Tablets 523
Twinrix Vaccine 1571
Ultane Liquid for Inhalation (Less than 1%) 526
Ultracet Tablets 2462
Univasc Tablets (Less than 1%) 3118
Valtrex Caplets 1573
Vaseretic Tablets 2073
Vasotec I.V. Injection (0.5% to 1.0%) 2076
Vermox Chewable Tablets (Rare) 1853
▲ Vesanoid Capsules (3%) 2823
VFEND I.V. (Less than 2%) 2543
VFEND Oral Suspension (Less than 2%) 2543
VFEND Tablets (Less than 2%) 2543
Viracept (Less than 2%) 2556
Viramune Oral Suspension (1%) 903
Viramune Tablets (1%) 903
Voltaren Tablets (Occasionally) 2298
Voltaren-XR Tablets (Occasionally) 2301
Vytorin 10/10 Tablets 2084
Vytorin 10/10 Tablets 3092
Vytorin 10/20 Tablets 2084
Vytorin 10/20 Tablets 3092
Vytorin 10/40 Tablets 2084
Vytorin 10/40 Tablets 3092
Vytorin 10/80 Tablets 2084
Vytorin 10/80 Tablets 3092
Wellbutrin Tablets 1579
Wellbutrin SR Sustained-Release Tablets 1583
Wellbutrin XL Extended-Release Tablets 1588
Xanax XR Tablets 2655
▲ Xeloda Tablets (Less than 5%) 2825
Zantac (Occasional) 1597
Zantac Injection 1593
Zantac Injection Pharmacy Bulk Package (Infrequent) 1595
Zantac Syrup (Occasional) 1597
Zegerid Powder for Oral Solution (Rare) 2972
Zerit 971
Zestoretic Tablets 701
Zestril Tablets (0.3% to 1.0%) 704
Zetia Tablets 2090
Zetia Tablets 3098
Zithromax Capsules, 250 mg 2568
Zithromax for IV Infusion 2573
Zithromax for Oral Suspension, 300 mg, 600 mg, 900 mg, 1200 mg 2561
Zithromax Tablets, 250 mg, 500 mg 2561
Zithromax Tri-Pak 2561
Zmax for Oral Suspension 2577
Zocor Tablets 2078
Zoloft (One or more patients) 2581
Zosyn 3492
Zovirax 1616
Zyban Sustained-Release Tablets 1620
Zyprexa Tablets (Infrequent) 1798
Zyprexa ZYDIS Orally Disintegrating Tablets (Infrequent) 1798
Zyrtec Chewable Tablets (Rare) 2589
Zyrtec (Rare) 2589
Zyrtec-D 12 Hour Extended Release Tablets (Rare) 2591

Hepatitis, allergic

Adalat CC Tablets (Rare) 2978

Hepatitis, autoimmune

Avonex (Rare) 839

Hepatitis, cholestatic

Anadrol-50 Tablets 3329
Antabuse Tablets 2343
Avelox 2984
Biaxin/Biaxin XL (Infrequent) 402
EryPed 445
Estratest Tablets 3196
Estratest H.S. Tablets 3196
Ketek Tablets 2920
Lamisil Tablets (Rare) 2226
Nalfon Capsules (Less than 1%) 2504
Oxandrin Tablets 2977
Pacerone Tablets (Rare) 3337
PREVPAC (Infrequent) 3281
Prilosec OTC Tablets (Rare) 2674
Risperdal M-Tab Orally Disintegrating Tablets (Rare) 1658
Risperdal (Rare) 1658
Singulair (Rare) 2047
Viramune Oral Suspension 903
Viramune Tablets 903
▲ Xeloda Tablets (Less than 5%) 2825
Zantac (Occasional) 1597
Zantac Injection (Occasional) 1593
Zantac Injection Pharmacy Bulk Package (Infrequent) 1595
Zantac Syrup (Occasional) 1597
Zegerid Powder for Oral Solution (Rare) 2972
Zosyn 3492

Hepatitis, cytolytic

Amoxil Capsules 1315
Amoxil Chewable Tablets 1315
Amoxil Pediatric Drops for Oral Suspension 1315
Amoxil Powder for Oral Suspension 1315
Amoxil Tablets 1315
PREVPAC 3281

Hepatitis, fulminant

Antabuse Tablets 2343
Celebrex Capsules (Less than 0.1%) 3130
Omnicef Capsules 506
Omnicef for Oral Suspension 506
Precose Tablets (Few cases) 776
Viramune Oral Suspension 903
Viramune Tablets 903

Hepatitis, hepatocellular

Ketek Tablets 2920

Hepatitis, idiopathic

Raptiva for Injection (1 case) 1247

Hepatitis, infectious

Plavix Tablets (Less than 1%) 940
Plavix Tablets (Less than 1%) 2942

Hepatitis, overt

Prilosec OTC Tablets (Rare) 2674
Zegerid Powder for Oral Solution (Rare) 2972

Hepatitis, post-treatment exacerbations of

Combivir Tablets 1373
Epivir 1394
Epivir-HBV 1398
Epzicom Tablets 1402
Trizivir Tablets 1565

Hepatitis, symptomatic

Accolate Tablets (Rare) 663

Hepatitis, toxic

Alkeran for Injection 976
Cuprimine Capsules (Rare) 1925
Dapsone Tablets USP 1656
Indocin Capsules (Less than 1%) 1968
Indocin I.V. (Less than 1%) 1973
Indocin (Less than 1%) 1968
Phenytek Capsules 2153

Hepatitis, viral

Evoxac Capsules (Less than 1%) 1042
Prolastin 3252
Zevalin Injection 848

Hepatobiliary dysfunction

Lamisil Tablets (Rare) 2226

Hepatocellular atrophy

Myleran Tablets 1492

Hepatocellular damage

Mycamine for Injection 620

Hepatomas

Aciphex Tablets (Rare) 1081
Advicor Tablets 1694
Altoprev Extended-Release Tablets (Rare) 1151
Lescol Capsules (Rare) 2227
Lescol Capsules (Rare) 2730
Lescol XL Tablets 2227
Lescol XL Tablets 2730
Mevacor Tablets (Rare) 1996
Pravachol Tablets (Rare) 943
Premarin Intravenous 3440
Premarin Vaginal Cream 3449
Seasonale Tablets 1073
Vytorin 10/10 Tablets (Rare) 2084
Vytorin 10/10 Tablets (Rare) 3092
Vytorin 10/20 Tablets (Rare) 2084
Vytorin 10/20 Tablets (Rare) 3092
Vytorin 10/40 Tablets (Rare) 2084
Vytorin 10/40 Tablets (Rare) 3092
Vytorin 10/80 Tablets (Rare) 2084
Vytorin 10/80 Tablets (Rare) 3092
Zocor Tablets (Rare) 2078

Hepatomas, benign

Lo/Ovral-28 Tablets 3423
Ortho-Cept Tablets 2395
Ortho-Cyclen/Ortho Tri-Cyclen (Rare) 2414
Ortho Tri-Cyclen Lo Tablets 2421

Triphasil-28 Tablets 3483

Hepatomegaly

Abelcet Injection 1119
Abilify Tablets (Rare) 916
Abilify Tablets (Rare) 2472
Aloprim for Injection (Less than 1%) 2156
AmBisome for Injection (Less common) 615
Blocadren Tablets 1891
Camptosar Injection 2602
▲ Clolar for Intravenous Infusion (15%) 1264
Combivir Tablets 1373
Copaxone for Injection (Infrequent) 3292
Cosmegen for Injection 1907
Cosopt Sterile Ophthalmic Solution 1910
Decadron Tablets 1929
Ellence Injection 2632
Epivir 1394
Epivir-HBV 1398
Epzicom Tablets 1402
Gabitril Tablets (Infrequent) 998
Garamycin Injectable 3028
Geodon Capsules (Rare) 2514
▲ Infergen (3% to 5%) 1647
Invirase (Less than 2%) 2776
▲ I.V. Busulfex (6%) 1125
Klonopin 2782
Lofibra Capsules (Less than 1%) 1217
Lunesta Tablets (Rare) 3139
▲ Megace ES Oral Suspension (1% to 3%) 2492
Mycamine for Injection 620
Neupogen for Injection (Infrequent) 598
Neurontin Capsules (Infrequent) 2498
Neurontin Oral Solution (Infrequent) 2498
Neurontin Tablets (Infrequent) 2498
Norvir (Less than 2%) 499
Oncaspar (Less than 1%) 1123
Orthoclone OKT3 Sterile Solution 2370
Paser Granules 1657
▲ PEG-Intron Powder for Injection (6%) 3062
Permax Tablets (Infrequent) 3357
Proleukin for Injection (1%) 1007
▲ Rebetol (4%) 3073
Rescriptor Tablets 2535
Retrovir Capsules (Rare) 1533
Retrovir IV Infusion (Rare) 1537
Retrovir (Rare) 1533
Reyataz Capsules (Less than 3%) 948
▲ Ribavirin, USP Capsules (4%) 3083
Risperdal Consta Long-Acting Injection (Infrequent) 1664
Rythmol SR Capsules 2736
Sular Tablets (Less than or equal to 1%) 1163
Symbyax Capsules (Infrequent) 1788
Tabloid Tablets 1545
Thalomid Capsules 979
Timolide Tablets 2056
Timoptic in Ocudose 2061
Timoptic Sterile Ophthalmic Solution 2058
Timoptic-XE Sterile Ophthalmic Gel Forming Solution 2062
Tricor Tablets 523
Trizivir Tablets 1565
Truvada Tablets 1279
Viread Tablets 1284
Zerit 971
Zoloft (One or more patients) 2581

Hepatorenal syndrome, unspecified

Actiq (Less than 1%) 993

Hepatosplenomegaly

Doxil Injection (Less than 1%) 3302
Invirase (Less than 2%) 2776
Mylotarg for Injection 3429
Proleukin for Injection 1007
Reyataz Capsules (Less than 3%) 948
Tegretol/Tegretol-XR 2278
▲ Vesanoid Capsules (9%) 2823

Hepatotoxicity

Accutane Capsules 2740
Adriamycin for Injection, USP 786
Adriamycin Injection, USP 786
Advicor Tablets 1694
Alkeran Tablets (Rare) 977
Ammonul Injection 3323
Amnesteem Capsules 2126
Anadrol-50 Tablets 3329
Antabuse Tablets 2343
Asacol Delayed-Release Tablets (Rare) 2688
Azasan Tablets 2844
Benadryl Allergy & Cold Tablets ▣ 692
Benadryl Allergy & Sinus Headache Caplets & Gelcaps ▣ 693
Benadryl Maximum Strength Severe Allergy & Sinus Headache Caplets ▣ 694
Campath Ampules 826
Carbatrol Capsules 3174
Casodex Tablets 670
▲ CellCept Capsules (3% to less than 20%) 2751
▲ CellCept Intravenous (3% to less than 20%) 2751
▲ CellCept Oral Suspension (3% to less than 20%) 2751
▲ CellCept Tablets (3% to less than 20%) 2751
Combivir Tablets 1373
Contac Severe Cold and Flu Caplets Maximum Strength ▣ 615
Contac Severe Cold and Flu Caplets Non-Drowsy ▣ 615
Cosmegen for Injection 1907
Dantrium Capsules 2690
Depacon Injection 412
Depakene 417
Depakote Sprinkle Capsules 422
Depakote Tablets 427
Depakote ER Tablets 433
Effexor Tablets 3405
Effexor XR Capsules 3411
Eloxatin for Injection 2908
Estratest Tablets 3196
Estratest H.S. Tablets 3196
Furosemide Tablets 2117
Gemzar for Injection (Rare) 1743
▲ Gengraf Capsules (Less than 1% to 7%) 458
▲ Gleevec Tablets (6% to 12%) 2221
Goody's Body Pain Formula Powder ▣ 621
Goody's Extra Strength Headache Powder ▣ 621
Goody's Extra Strength Pain Relief Tablets ▣ 621
Goody's PM Powder ▣ 622
Intron A for Injection (Rare) 3038
I.V. Busulfex 1125
Lamisil Tablets 2226
Leukeran Tablets 1472
▲ Leukine (13%) 829
Lunesta Tablets (Rare) 3139
Mebaral Tablets, USP (Less than 1 in 100 patients) 2483
Mintezol 2002
Miradon Tablets 3056
Mylotarg for Injection 3429
Nembutal Sodium Solution, USP 2484
▲ Neoral Soft Gelatin Capsules (Less than 1% to 7%) 2247
▲ Neoral Oral Solution (Less than 1% to 7%) 2247
Nicomide Tablets 3190
Norvir (Less than 2%) 499
Pentasa Capsules 3182
Phenytek Capsules 2153
Prevacid Delayed-Release Capsules 3268
Prevacid for Delayed-Release Oral Suspension 3268
Prevacid NapraPAC 3277
Prevacid SoluTab Delayed-Release Orally Disintegrating Tablets 3268
PREVPAC 3281
▲ Prograf Capsules and Injection (3% to 15%) 624
Purinethol Tablets (Frequent) 1222
Rapamune Oral Solution and Tablets 3472
Reyataz Capsules (Less than 3%) 948
Risperdal Consta Long-Acting Injection (Rare) 1664
Risperdal M-Tab Orally Disintegrating Tablets (Rare) 1658
Risperdal (Rare) 1658
Robitussin Cough, Cold & Flu Liquid-filled Capsules ▣ 750
Robitussin Flu Liquid ▣ 752
Roferon-A Injection (Unusual) 2805
▲ Sandimmune (Less than 1% to 7%) 2259
Singlet Caplets ▣ 636
Soriatane Capsules 1028
Sudafed Severe Cold ▣ 710
Sudafed Sinus Headache ▣ 711
Tegretol/Tegretol-XR 2278
TheraFlu Severe Cold Non-Drowsy Hot Liquid ▣ 683
TheraFlu Severe Cold Non-Drowsy Caplets ▣ 679
Trasylol Injection (0.5%) 779
Tylenol 8 Hour Extended Release Geltabs and Caplets 1843
Tylenol 8-Hour Extended Release Geltabs/Caplets ▣ 655
Tylenol Cough & Sore Throat Daytime Liquid with Cool Burst ▣ 664
Tylenol Cough & Sore Throat NightTime Liquid with Cool Burst ▣ 664
Tylenol Cold & Flu Severe Daytime Liquid with Cool Bust 1846
Tylenol Cold & Flu Severe NightTime Liquid with Cool Burst 1846
Tylenol Cough & Sore Throat Daytime Liquid with Cool Burst 1849
Tylenol Cough & Sore Throat NightTime Liquid with Cool Burst 1849
Tylenol 1843
Tylenol Flu Day Non-Drowsy Gelcaps 1846
Tylenol Sinus Day Non-Drowsy 1848
Tylenol Sinus Night Time Caplets 1848
Tylenol Sinus Severe Congestion Caplets with Cool Burst 1848
Tylenol Sore Throat Daytime Liquid with Cool Burst 1849
Tylenol Sore Throat NightTime Liquid with Cool Burst 1849
Women's Tylenol Menstrual Relief Caplets 1849
Vicks 44M Cough, Cold & Flu Relief 2676
Vicks DayQuil Multi-Symptom Cold/Flu Relief LiquiCaps 2675
Vicks DayQuil Multi-Symptom Cold/Flu Relief Liquid 2675
Vicks NyQuil LiquiCaps 2677
Vicks NyQuil Liquid 2677
Viramune Oral Suspension 903
Viramune Tablets 903
Wellbutrin Tablets (Infrequent) 1579
Wellbutrin SR Sustained-Release Tablets 1583
Wellbutrin XL Extended-Release Tablets 1588
▲ Xeloda Tablets (Less than 5%) 2825
Zerit 971
Zyban Sustained-Release Tablets 1620

Hernia, hiatal

Aricept Tablets (Infrequent) 1086
Aricept ODT Tablets (Infrequent) 1086
Celebrex Capsules (0.1% to 1.9%) 3130
Neurontin Capsules (Rare) 2498
Neurontin Oral Solution (Rare) 2498
Neurontin Tablets (Rare) 2498
Prometrium Capsules (100 mg, 200 mg) (Less than 5%) 3205
Remicade for IV Injection (Greater than or equal to 0.2%) 987
Triglide Tablets 1165

Hernia, inguinal

Edex Injection (1%) 3103
Prevnar for Injection 3460
Xifaxan Tablets (Less than 2%) 2847
Zyban Sustained-Release Tablets (Infrequent) 1620

Hernia, unspecified

Actonel Tablets (2.9%) 2679
Actonel with Calcium Tablets (2.9%) 2684
Antara Capsules 2723
▲ Arava Tablets (1% to 3%) 2881
Campral Tablets (Infrequent) 1175
▲ Casodex Tablets (2% to 5%) 670
▲ CellCept Capsules (3% to less than 20%) 2751
▲ CellCept Intravenous (3% to less than 20%) 2751
▲ CellCept Oral Suspension (3% to less than 20%) 2751
▲ CellCept Tablets (3% to less than 20%) 2751
Effexor XR Capsules 3411
Exelon Capsules (Infrequent) 2204
Gabitril Tablets (Infrequent) 998
Lofibra Capsules 1217
Lunesta Tablets (Infrequent) 3139
Neurontin Capsules (Rare) 2498
Neurontin Oral Solution (Rare) 2498
Neurontin Tablets (Rare) 2498
Nexium Delayed-Release Capsules (Less than 1%) 645
Nexium I.V. (Less than 1%) 649
Permax Tablets (Infrequent) 3357
Plavix Tablets (1% to 2.5%) 940
Plavix Tablets (1% to 2.5%) 2942
▲ Prograf Capsules and Injection (3% to 15%) 624
Protonix I.V. (Less than 1%) 3468
Protonix Tablets (Less than 1%) 3465
Protopic Ointment (Greater than or equal to 1%) 629
▲ Rapamune Oral Solution and Tablets (3% to 20%) 3472
Relpax Tablets (Rare) 2531
Rilutek Tablets (Infrequent) 2945
▲ Simulect for Injection (3% to 10%) 2268
Symbyax Capsules (Infrequent) 1788
▲ Synagis (4.1%) 1868
Tasmar Tablets (Infrequent) 3360
Thalomid Capsules 979
Tricor Tablets 523
Uniretic Tablets (Less than 1%) 3114

Herpes, precipitation

Oxsoralen-Ultra Capsules 3354

Herpes, unspecified

Bexxar 1360
Imitrex Nasal Spray (Rare) 1435
Matulane Capsules 3188
▲ Megace ES Oral Suspension (1% to 3%) 2492

Herpes labialis

Alferon N Injection (1%) 1640
Finacea Gel (Rare) 1644

Herpes simplex

Aceon Tablets (2 mg, 4 mg, 8 mg) (0.3% to 1%) 3191
Aldara Cream, 5% (1.9%) 1814
Alrex Ophthalmic Suspension 0.2% ⊙ 243
Ambien Tablets (Rare) 2867
AmBisome for Injection (Less common) 615
Amevive 836
Antara Capsules 2723
Aptivus Capsules (Less than 2%) 859
▲ Arava Tablets (1% to 3%) 2881
Aricept Tablets (Infrequent) 1086
Aricept ODT Tablets (Infrequent) 1086
Astelin Nasal Spray (Infrequent) 1876
Blephamide Ophthalmic Ointment 563
▲ Campath Ampules (1% to 11%) 826
Celebrex Capsules (0.1% to 1.9%) 3130
▲ CellCept Capsules (10.1% to 20.8%) 2751
▲ CellCept Intravenous (10.1% to 20.8%) 2751
▲ CellCept Oral Suspension (10.1% to 20.8%) 2751
▲ CellCept Tablets (10.1% to 20.8%) 2751
Clindesse Vaginal Cream (Less than 1%) 3296
▲ Clolar for Intravenous Infusion (11%) 1264
▲ Copaxone for Injection (4%) 3292
Cutivate Cream (0.8%) 1381
▲ Doxil Injection (1% to 10%) 3302
Effexor XR Capsules 3411
Efudex (Infrequent) 3348
Elidel Cream 1% (0.4% to 4%) 2198
Evoxac Capsules (Less than 1%) 1042
Exelon Capsules (Infrequent) 2204
FML Ophthalmic Ointment ⊙ 225
▲ Fuzeon Injection (3.5% to 4.1%) 2772
Gabitril Tablets (Infrequent) 998
Gengraf Capsules (1% to less than 3%) 458
Gleevec Tablets (Infrequent) 2221
Herceptin I.V. (2%) 1234
▲ Intron A for Injection (Up to 5%) 3038
Invanz for Injection (1%) 1974
Invirase (Less than 2%) 2776
Klonopin (Infrequent) 2782
Levaquin in 5% Dextrose Injection (0.1% to 0.9%) 2453
Levaquin (0.1% to 0.9%) 2453
Lofibra Capsules 1217
Lotemax Ophthalmic Suspension 0.5% ⊙ 249
Meridia Capsules (1.3%) 485
Migranal Nasal Spray (Rare) 3350
▲ Myfortic Tablets (1.3% to less than 20%) 2244
▲ Mylotarg for Injection (2% to 25%) 3429
Neoral Soft Gelatin Capsules (1% to less than 3%) 2247
Neoral Oral Solution (1% to less than 3%) 2247
Neurontin Capsules (Infrequent) 2498
Neurontin Oral Solution (Infrequent) 2498
Neurontin Tablets (Infrequent) 2498
▲ Nipent for Injection (4%) 3216
Oncaspar 1123
Paxil CR Controlled-Release Tablets (Rare) 1509
Paxil (Rare) 1501
Permax Tablets (Infrequent) 3357
▲ Prograf Capsules and Injection (3% to 15%) 624
Prometrium Capsules (100 mg, 200 mg) (Less than 5%) 3205

Protonix I.V. (Less than 1%) 3468
Protonix Tablets (Less than 1%) 3465
▲ Protopic Ointment (4% to 12%) 629
Provigil Tablets (1%) 1002
Pulmicort Respules (1% to 3%) 654
Requip Tablets (Infrequent) 1528
Rescriptor Tablets 2535
▲ Simulect for Injection (3% to 10%) 2268
Soriatane Capsules (Less than 1%) 1028
Sular Tablets (Less than or equal to 1%) 1163
Tasmar Tablets (Infrequent) 3360
Teveten Tablets (Less than 1%) 1707
Teveten HCT Tablets (Less than 1%) 1710
Thalomid Capsules 979
▲ Thymoglobulin for Injection (4.9%) 2848
Tricor Tablets 523
▲ Trisenox Injection (13%) 983
Uniretic Tablets (Less than 1%) 3114
VFEND I.V. (Less than 2%) 2543
VFEND Oral Suspension (Less than 2%) 2543
VFEND Tablets (Less than 2%) 2543
Viagra Tablets (Less than 2%) 2552
Vivelle Transdermal System 2288
Vivelle-Dot Transdermal System 2293
Zoladex 3-month (1% to 5%) 712

Herpes simplex, disseminated

Accutane Capsules 2740

Herpes zoster

Aciphex Tablets (Rare) 1081
Actiq (Less than 1%) 993
Ambien Tablets (Rare) 2867
Antara Capsules 2723
Aptivus Capsules (Less than 2%) 859
▲ Arava Tablets (1% to 3%) 2881
Aricept Tablets (Infrequent) 1086
Aricept ODT Tablets (Infrequent) 1086
Campath Ampules 826
▲ Casodex Tablets (2% to 5%) 670
Celebrex Capsules (0.1% to 1.9%) 3130
▲ CellCept Capsules (4% to 10.7%) 2751
▲ CellCept Intravenous (4% to 10.7%) 2751
▲ CellCept Oral Suspension (4% to 10.7%) 2751
▲ CellCept Tablets (4% to 10.7%) 2751
Copaxone for Injection (Frequent) 3292
▲ Doxil Injection (Less than 1% to 10%) 3302
Effexor XR Capsules 3411
Engerix-B Vaccine 1391
Evoxac Capsules (Less than 1%) 1042
Gabitril Tablets (Infrequent) 998
Gengraf Capsules (1% to less than 3%) 458
Gleevec Tablets (Infrequent) 2221
Herceptin I.V. (At least one of the 958 patients) 1234
▲ Humira Injection (Less than 5%) 464
▲ Intron A for Injection (Less than 5%) 3038
Invirase (Less than 2%) 2776
Lamictal (Rare) 1449
Leustatin Injection (8 episodes) 2368
Lofibra Capsules 1217
Lunesta Tablets (Rare) 3139
Mustargen for Injection 2007
▲ Myfortic Tablets (1.9% to less than 20%) 2244
Neoral Soft Gelatin Capsules (1% to less than 3%) 2247
Neoral Oral Solution (1% to less than 3%) 2247
Neurontin Capsules (Rare) 2498
Neurontin Oral Solution (Rare) 2498
Neurontin Tablets (Rare) 2498
▲ Nipent for Injection (8%) 3216
Paxil CR Controlled-Release Tablets (Rare) 1509
Paxil (Rare) 1501
Permax Tablets (Infrequent) 3357
Prinivil Tablets (0.3% to 1.0%) 2029
Prinzide Tablets 2033
Protonix I.V. (Less than 1%) 3468
Protonix Tablets (Less than 1%) 3465
Protopic Ointment (Up to 3%) 629
Prozac Pulvules and Liquid (Rare) 1771
▲ Rapamune Oral Solution and Tablets (3% to 20%) 3472
Recombivax HB 2045
Requip Tablets (Infrequent) 1528
Rescriptor Tablets 2535
▲ Simulect for Injection (3% to 10%) 2268
▲ Spiriva HandiHaler (1% to 3%) 899
Sular Tablets (Less than or equal to 1%) 1163
Tasmar Tablets (Infrequent) 3360
Tricor Tablets 523
▲ Trisenox Injection (8%) 983
Twinrix Vaccine 1571
Uniretic Tablets (Less than 1%) 3114
Varivax 2070
Vaseretic Tablets 2073
Vasotec I.V. Injection (0.5% to 1.0%) 2076
▲ Velcade for Injection (13%) 2102
Zestoretic Tablets 701
Zestril Tablets (0.3% to 1.0%) 704

Herxheimer's reaction

▲ Ceftin Tablets (5.6%) 1369

Hiccups

Abilify Tablets (Infrequent) 916
Abilify Tablets (Infrequent) 2472
Aciphex Tablets 1081
Actiq (Less than 1%) 993
Aloxi Injection (Less than 1%) 2099
Ambien Tablets (Frequent) 2867
AmBisome for Injection (Less common) 615
Avinza Capsules (Less than 5%) 1714
Celexa (Rare) 1177
▲ CellCept Capsules (3% to less than 20%) 2751
▲ CellCept Intravenous (3% to less than 20%) 2751
▲ CellCept Oral Suspension (3% to less than 20%) 2751
▲ CellCept Tablets (3% to less than 20%) 2751
Cipro I.V. (1% or less) 2998
Cipro I.V. Pharmacy Bulk Package (1% or less) 3509
Cipro (Less than 1%) 2991
Cipro XR Tablets 3004
Decadron Phosphate Injection 1931
Decadron Tablets 1929
Depakote ER Tablets (Greater than 1%) 433
Diastat Rectal Delivery System (Greater than or equal to 1%) 3344
Diprivan Injectable Emulsion (Less than 1%) 676
Doxil Injection (Less than 1%) 3302
Duragesic Transdermal System (1% or greater) 2448
▲ Eloxatin for Injection (2% to 5%) 2908
▲ Emend Capsules (10.8%) 1944
Ethyol for Injection 1869
▲ Evoxac Capsules (1% to 3%) 1042
Frova Tablets (Rare) 1101
Gabitril Tablets (Infrequent) 998
Gengraf Capsules (2% or less) 458
Imitrex Injection (Rare) 1431
Imitrex Nasal Spray 1435
Imitrex Tablets (Rare) 1440
Invanz for Injection (Greater than 0.1%) 1974
▲ I.V. Busulfex (18%) 1125
Kadian Capsules (Less than 3%) 572
Lamictal (Rare) 1449
Lunesta Tablets (Infrequent) 3139
Lyrica Capsules (Rare) 2524
Maxalt Tablets (Rare) 1983
Maxalt-MLT Orally Disintegrating Tablets (Rare) 1983
Migranal Nasal Spray (Infrequent) 3350
Moduretic Tablets (Less than or equal to 1%) 2003
Mycamine for Injection (0.2%) 620
Neoral Soft Gelatin Capsules (2% or less) 2247
Neoral Oral Solution (2% or less) 2247
Neurontin Capsules (Rare) 2498
Neurontin Oral Solution (Rare) 2498
Neurontin Tablets (Rare) 2498
Nexium Delayed-Release Capsules (Less than 1%) 645
Nexium I.V. (Less than 1%) 649
▲ Nicotrol Inhaler (Greater than 3%) 2594
Nicotrol NS (Less than 1%) 2596
Norvir (Less than 2%) 499
▲ OxyContin Tablets (Between 1% and 5%) 2699
Parcopa Orally Disintegrating Tablets 3111
Paxil CR Controlled-Release Tablets (Rare) 1509
Paxil (Rare) 1501
Permax Tablets (1.1%) 3357
▲ Photofrin for Injection (6%) 729
Prevacid Delayed-Release Capsules (Less than 1%) 3268
Prevacid for Delayed-Release Oral Suspension (Less than 1%) 3268
Prevacid NapraPAC (Less than 1%) 3277
Prevacid SoluTab Delayed-Release Orally Disintegrating Tablets (Less than 1%) 3268
PREVPAC (Less than 1%) 3281
Protonix I.V. (Less than 1%) 3468
Protonix Tablets (Less than 1%) 3465
Prozac Pulvules and Liquid (Infrequent) 1771
Razadyne ER Extended-Release Capsules (Infrequent) 2434
Razadyne (Infrequent) 2434
Relpax Tablets (Rare) 2531
Requip Tablets (Infrequent) 1528
Rescriptor Tablets 2535
Reyataz Capsules (Less than 3%) 948
Rilutek Tablets (Infrequent) 2945
Sandimmune (2% or less) 2259
Seroquel Tablets (Rare) 691
Sonata Capsules (Rare) 1686
Stalevo Tablets 2270
Symbyax Capsules (Infrequent) 1788
Tasmar Tablets (Infrequent) 3360
Trileptal Oral Suspension 2281
Trileptal Tablets 2281
Ultane Liquid for Inhalation (Less than 1%) 526
Vicoprofen Tablets (Less than 3%) 533
Zemuron Injection (Less than 1%) 2363
Zofran Injection 1607
Zofran 1613
Zofran ODT Orally Disintegrating Tablets 1613
Zoloft (Rare) 2581
Zomig Nasal Spray (Rare) 718
Zomig Tablets (Infrequent) 714
Zomig-ZMT Tablets (Infrequent) 714
Zosyn (1.0% or less to 2.6%) 3492
Zyprexa Tablets (Rare) 1798
Zyprexa ZYDIS Orally Disintegrating Tablets (Rare) 1798

Hirsutism

Accutane Capsules 2740
Activella Tablets 2311
Alesse-28 Tablets 3392
Amnesteem Capsules 2126
Anadrol-50 Tablets 3329
AndroGel (Fewer than 1%) 3330
Aricept Tablets (Infrequent) 1086
Aricept ODT Tablets (Infrequent) 1086
Carbatrol Capsules (Isolated cases) 3174
▲ CellCept Capsules (3% to less than 20%) 2751
▲ CellCept Intravenous (3% to less than 20%) 2751
▲ CellCept Oral Suspension (3% to less than 20%) 2751
▲ CellCept Tablets (3% to less than 20%) 2751
Cenestin Tablets, 0.45mg, 0.625mg, 0.9mg, 1.25mg 1063
Cenestin Tablets, 0.3mg 1063
Climara Transdermal System 795
Climara Pro Transdermal System 800
CombiPatch Transdermal System 2180
Dantrium Capsules (Less frequent) 2690
Decadron Phosphate Injection 1931
Decadron Tablets 1929
Delatestryl Injection 2976
Depo-Provera Contraceptive Injection (Less than 1%) 2619
Effexor Tablets (Rare) 3405
Effexor XR Capsules (Rare) 3411
Eldepryl Capsules 3209
▲ Entocort EC Capsules (5%) 2694
Equetro Extended-Release Capsules 3178
Estratest Tablets 3196
Estratest H.S. Tablets 3196
Estrogel 0.06% 3200
Gabitril Tablets (Infrequent) 998
▲ Gengraf Capsules (21% to 45%) 458
Hydrocortone Tablets 1963
Hyperstat I.V. Injection 3031
▲ Intron A for Injection (Less than 5%) 3038
Klonopin 2782
Lamictal (Infrequent) 1449
Lo/Ovral-28 Tablets 3423
▲ Lumigan Ophthalmic Solution (1% to 5%) 569
Lunesta Tablets (Rare) 3139
Lupron Depot 7.5 mg (Less than 5%) 3261
Lupron Depot–3 Month 11.25 mg (0.6% to 1%) 3262
Lyrica Capsules (0.1% to 1%) 2524
Menostar Transdermal System 805
▲ Myfortic Tablets (3% to less than 20%) 2244
▲ Neoral Soft Gelatin Capsules (21% to 45%) 2247
▲ Neoral Oral Solution (21% to 45%) 2247
Neurontin Capsules (Infrequent) 2498
Neurontin Oral Solution (Infrequent) 2498
Neurontin Tablets (Infrequent) 2498
Ortho-Cept Tablets 2395
Ortho-Cyclen Tablets 2414
Ortho Evra Transdermal System 2402
Ortho Micronor Tablets (Rare) 2411
Ortho Tri-Cyclen Tablets 2414
Ortho Tri-Cyclen Lo Tablets 2421
Oxandrin Tablets 2977
Paxil CR Controlled-Release Tablets (Rare) 1509
Paxil (Rare) 1501
Permax Tablets (Infrequent) 3357
Photofrin for Injection 729
Prefest Tablets 1069
Premarin Intravenous 3440
Premarin Tablets 3443
Premarin Vaginal Cream 3449
Premphase Tablets 3452
Prempro Tablets 3452
▲ Prograf Capsules and Injection (3% to 15%) 624
Prozac Pulvules and Liquid (Rare) 1771
▲ Rapamune Oral Solution and Tablets (3% to 20%) 3472
▲ Sandimmune (21% to 45%) 2259
Seasonale Tablets 1073
Tegretol/Tegretol-XR (Isolated cases) 2278
Triphasil-28 Tablets 3483
Viadur Implant (Less than 2%) 782
Vivelle Transdermal System 2288
Vivelle-Dot Transdermal System 2293
Wellbutrin Tablets (Rare) 1579
Wellbutrin SR Sustained-Release Tablets 1583
Wellbutrin XL Extended-Release Tablets 1588
Yasmin 28 Tablets 818
▲ Zenapax for Injection (2% to 5%) 2838
▲ Zoladex (7%) 709
Zonegran Capsules (Infrequent) 1089
Zyban Sustained-Release Tablets 1620
Zyprexa Tablets (Infrequent) 1798
Zyprexa ZYDIS Orally Disintegrating Tablets (Infrequent) 1798

Histoplasmosis

Remicade for IV Injection 987

Histrionic movements

FazaClo Orally Disintegrating Tablets (Less than 1%) 547

HIV viral load increase

Thalomid Capsules 979

Hives

(*see under* Urticaria)

Hives at injection site

Diprivan Injectable Emulsion (Less than 1%) 676
Idamycin PFS Injection 2645
Prevnar for Injection 3460
Xolair 1259

Hoarseness

Aceon Tablets (2 mg, 4 mg, 8 mg) (0.3% to 1%) 3191
▲ Advair Diskus 100/50 (5%) 1291
▲ Advair Diskus 250/50 (2% to 8%) 1291
▲ Advair Diskus 500/50 (2% to 5%) 1291
▲ Aerobid/Aerobid-M (3% to 9%) 1172
Atrovent Nasal Spray 0.03% (Less than 2%) 869
Atrovent Nasal Spray 0.06% (Less than 1%) 870
Azmacort Inhalation Aerosol 1701
Captopril Tablets 2114
Depo-Provera Contraceptive Injection (Less than 1%) 2619
depo-subQ provera 104 Injectable Suspension 2622
Emcyt Capsules (1%) 3137
Flonase Nasal Spray 1412
▲ Flovent Diskus 50 mcg (1% to 9%) 1415
Flovent HFA (2%) 1418
Klonopin (Infrequent) 2782
Levaquin in 5% Dextrose Injection 2453
Levaquin 2453
Matulane Capsules 3188
Maxalt Tablets (Rare) 1983
Maxalt-MLT Orally Disintegrating Tablets (Rare) 1983
Nasarel Nasal Spray (1% or less) 1652
Neurontin Capsules 2498
Neurontin Oral Solution 2498
Neurontin Tablets 2498
Nicotrol NS 2596
Oxandrin Tablets 2977

Parcopa Orally Disintegrating Tablets ... 3111
Proventil Inhalation Aerosol ... 3067
Retrovir Capsules ... 1533
Retrovir IV Infusion ... 1537
Retrovir ... 1533
Stalevo Tablets ... 2270
Vaseretic Tablets ... 2073
Vasotec I.V. Injection (0.5% to 1.0%) ... 2076
Ventolin HFA Inhalation Aerosol ... 1576
Vicoprofen Tablets (Less than 1%) ... 533
▲ Xeloda Tablets (Less than 5%) ... 2825

Hodgkin's disease
Phenytek Capsules ... 2153

Hodgkin's disease, nodular sclerosing
Thalomid Capsules ... 979

Homicidal ideation
Xanax XR Tablets (Infrequent) ... 2655

Hormonal imbalance
Norvir (Less than 2%) ... 499
Wellbutrin Tablets (Rare) ... 1579

Horner's syndrome
Naropin Injection (Less than 1%) ... 640
Parcopa Orally Disintegrating Tablets ... 3111
Stalevo Tablets ... 2270

Hostility
Abilify Tablets (Frequent) ... 916
Abilify Tablets (Frequent) ... 2472
Amerge Tablets (Rare) ... 1312
Aricept Tablets (Infrequent) ... 1086
Aricept ODT Tablets (Infrequent) ... 1086
Campral Tablets (Infrequent) ... 1175
Copaxone for Injection (Infrequent) .. 3292
Depacon Injection ... 412
Depakene ... 417
Depakote Sprinkle Capsules ... 422
Depakote Tablets ... 427
Depakote ER Tablets ... 433
Duragesic Transdermal System (Less than 1%) ... 2448
Effexor Tablets (Infrequent) ... 3405
Effexor XR Capsules (Infrequent) ... 3411
Gabitril Tablets (2%) ... 998
Geodon Capsules (Frequent) ... 2514
Keppra Oral Solution (12%) ... 3307
Keppra Tablets (12%) ... 3307
Klonopin ... 2782
Lamictal (Frequent) ... 1449
Lunesta Tablets (Infrequent) ... 3139
Lyrica Capsules (0.1% to 1%) ... 2524
▲ Neurontin Capsules (5.2% to 7.6%) ... 2498
▲ Neurontin Oral Solution (5.2% to 7.6%) ... 2498
▲ Neurontin Tablets (5.2% to 7.6%) ... 2498
Nipent for Injection (Less than 3%) ... 3216
Nubain Injection (1% or less) ... 1111
Paxil CR Controlled-Release Tablets (Infrequent) ... 1509
Paxil (Infrequent) ... 1501
Permax Tablets (Infrequent) ... 3357
Prevacid Delayed-Release Capsules (Less than 1%) ... 3268
Prevacid for Delayed-Release Oral Suspension (Less than 1%) ... 3268
Prevacid NapraPAC (Less than 1%) .. 3277
Prevacid SoluTab Delayed-Release Orally Disintegrating Tablets (Less than 1%) ... 3268
PREVPAC (Less than 1%) ... 3281
ProSom Tablets (Infrequent) ... 512
Prozac Pulvules and Liquid (Infrequent) ... 1771
Reyataz Capsules (Less than 3%) ... 948
Rilutek Tablets (Frequent) ... 2945
Sonata Capsules (Rare) ... 1686
Strattera Capsules ... 1784
Surmontil Capsules ... 2347
Symbyax Capsules (Infrequent) ... 1788
Tasmar Tablets (Infrequent) ... 3360
Tequin Injection (Less than 0.1%) ... 964
Tequin Tablets (Less than 0.1%) ... 964
Thalomid Capsules ... 979
Vivactil Tablets ... 2350
▲ Wellbutrin Tablets (5.6%) ... 1579
Wellbutrin SR Sustained-Release Tablets (Infrequent) ... 1583
Wellbutrin XL Extended-Release Tablets (Infrequent) ... 1588
Xanax XR Tablets (Rare) ... 2655
Zoloft ... 2581
Zyban Sustained-Release Tablets (Infrequent) ... 1620
▲ Zyprexa Tablets (15%) ... 1798
▲ Zyprexa ZYDIS Orally Disintegrating Tablets (15%) ... 1798

Hot flashes
Advate Injection (1.3%) ... 742
Alferon N Injection (1%) ... 1640
Aloxi Injection (Less than 1%) ... 2099
Ambien Tablets (Rare) ... 2867
Aricept Tablets (Frequent) ... 1086
Aricept ODT Tablets (Frequent) ... 1086
▲ Arimidex Tablets (11% to 35%) ... 665
▲ Aromasin Tablets (13%) ... 2600
▲ Bravelle for Intramuscular or Subcutaneous Injection (4% to 5.7%) ... 1140
Caduet Tablets (Greater than 0.1% to less than or equal to 1%) ... 2507
▲ Casodex Tablets (49%) ... 670
Celebrex Capsules (0.1% to 1.9%) ... 3130
Celexa (Infrequent) ... 1177
Clozapine Tablets (Less than 1%) ... 2141
Clozaril Tablets (Less than 1%) ... 2174
Colazal Capsules ... 2845
▲ Depo-Provera Contraceptive Injection (1% to 5%) ... 2619
Dostinex Tablets (1% to 3%) ... 2631
▲ Effexor XR Capsules (4%) ... 3411
▲ Eligard 7.5 mg (25% to 56.7%) ... 2896
▲ Eligard 22.5 mg (56.4%) ... 2899
▲ Eligard 30 mg (73.3%) ... 2901
▲ Eligard 45 mg (57.7%) ... 2904
Elitek (Less than or equal to 1%) ... 2906
▲ Ellence Injection (0% to 38.9%) ... 2632
▲ Eloxatin for Injection (2% to 5%) ... 2908
▲ Eulexin Capsules (46% to 61%) ... 3023
▲ Evista Tablets (9.7% to 24.6%) ... 1735
Evoxac Capsules (2.4%) ... 1042
Exelon Capsules (Frequent) ... 2204
Factive Tablets (Less than or equal to 0.1%) ... 2464
FazaClo Orally Disintegrating Tablets (Less than 1%) ... 547
▲ Femara Tablets (5% to 19%) ... 2210
Floxin Otic Singles ... 1045
Floxin Otic Solution (Single report) ... 1043
Frova Tablets (Infrequent) ... 1101
Gengraf Capsules (1% to less than 3%) ... 458
▲ Imdur Tablets (Less than or equal to 5%) ... 3032
▲ Infergen (7% to 13%) ... 1647
▲ Intron A for Injection (Less than 5%) ... 3038
Invirase (Less than 2%) ... 2776
▲ I.V. Busulfex (25%) ... 1125
Lamictal (1.3%) ... 1449
Levaquin in 5% Dextrose Injection (0.1% to 0.9%) ... 2453
Levaquin (0.1% to 0.9%) ... 2453
Lexapro Oral Solution (Frequent) ... 1193
Lexapro Tablets (Frequent) ... 1193
Lotrel Capsules ... 2238
▲ Lupron Depot 3.75 mg (50%) ... 3257
▲ Lupron Depot 7.5 mg (57.1%) ... 3261
▲ Lupron Depot–3 Month 11.25 mg (50%) ... 3262
Maxalt Tablets (Frequent) ... 1983
Maxalt-MLT Orally Disintegrating Tablets (Frequent) ... 1983
Menopur for Subcutaneous Injection (0.6% to 2.6%) ... 1145
Migranal Nasal Spray (1%) ... 3350
Mobic Oral Suspension (Less than 2%) ... 893
Mobic Tablets (Less than 2%) ... 893
Neoral Soft Gelatin Capsules (1% to less than 3%) ... 2247
Neoral Oral Solution (1% to less than 3%) ... 2247
Nexium Delayed-Release Capsules (Less than 1%) ... 645
Nexium I.V. (Less than 1%) ... 649
Norvasc Tablets (More than 0.1% to 1%) ... 2529
Parcopa Orally Disintegrating Tablets ... 3111
Prochieve 4% Gel ... 1018
Prochieve 8% Gel ... 1018
▲ Prometrium Capsules (100 mg, 200 mg) (11%) ... 3205
Requip Tablets (1% or more) ... 1528
Roferon-A Injection (Rare to infrequent) ... 2805
Sandostatin LAR Depot (1% to 4%) .. 2264
Sedapap Tablets 50 mg/650 mg (Infrequent) ... 2098
▲ Soriatane Capsules (1% to 10%) ... 1028
Stalevo Tablets ... 2270
Sustiva Capsules (Less than 2%) ... 957
Testim 1% Gel (1% or less) ... 722
Teveten Tablets (Less than 1%) ... 1707
Teveten HCT Tablets (Less than 1%) ... 1710
Topamax Sprinkle Capsules (1% to 2%) ... 2438
Topamax Tablets (1% to 2%) ... 2438
▲ Trelstar Depot (58.6%) ... 3385
▲ Trelstar LA Suspension (73%) ... 3387
Trileptal Oral Suspension (1% to 2%) ... 2281
Trileptal Tablets (1% to 2%) ... 2281
Ultracet Tablets (At least 1%) ... 2462
▲ Vagifem Tablets (3% to 5%) ... 2340
▲ Vantas (65.5%) ... 3367
Vivelle Transdermal System ... 2288
Vivelle-Dot Transdermal System ... 2293
▲ Wellbutrin SR Sustained-Release Tablets (1% to 3%) ... 1583
▲ Wellbutrin XL Extended-Release Tablets (1% to 3%) ... 1588
▲ Xanax XR Tablets (1.5% to 5.95%) .. 2655
▲ Xeloda Tablets (Less than 5%) ... 2825
Xifaxan Tablets (Less than 2%) ... 2847
▲ Zoladex (62% to 96%) ... 709
▲ Zoladex 3-month (46% to 64%) ... 712
Zoloft (2%) ... 2581
Zyban Sustained-Release Tablets (1%) ... 1620
Zyrtec Chewable Tablets (Less than 2%) ... 2589
Zyrtec (Less than 2%) ... 2589
Zyrtec-D 12 Hour Extended Release Tablets (Less than 2%) ... 2591

Hot flushes
Cymbalta Delayed-Release Capsules (2%) ... 1729
▲ depo-subQ provera 104 Injectable Suspension (1% to less than 5%) ... 2622

HPA axis suppression
Aclovate ... 1290
Advair Diskus 100/50 ... 1291
Advair Diskus 250/50 ... 1291
Advair Diskus 500/50 ... 1291
Clobex Shampoo ... 1209
Cutivate Cream ... 1381
Cutivate Ointment ... 1384
Diprolene Gel 0.05% ... 3015
Diprolene Lotion 0.05% ... 3016
Diprolene Ointment 0.05% (Some patients) ... 3017
Diprolene AF Cream 0.05% (Some patients) ... 3014
Diprosone Cream, USP 0.05% ... 3018
▲ Elocon Cream 0.1% (16%) ... 3019
Elocon Lotion 0.1% ... 3020
▲ Elocon Ointment 0.1% (27%) ... 3021
Lotrisone ... 3054
▲ Olux Foam (5 of 13 patients) ... 1027
Temovate Cream ... 1549
Temovate Gel ... 1550
Temovate Ointment ... 1549
Temovate Scalp Application ... 1551
Temovate E Emollient ... 1552
Vanos Cream ... 1864

HPA function suppression
Azmacort Inhalation Aerosol ... 1701

Hunger
Imitrex Injection (Rare) ... 1431
Imitrex Nasal Spray (Rare) ... 1435
Imitrex Tablets (Rare) ... 1440
Klonopin (Infrequent) ... 2782

Hydrocephalus
DepoCyt Injection ... 1121
Herceptin I.V. (At least one of the 958 patients) ... 1234
Repronex for Intramuscular and Subcutaneous Injection (One report) ... 1148

Hydrocephalus, fetal
Accutane Capsules ... 2740

Hydronephrosis
Actiq (1% or greater) ... 993
▲ Casodex Tablets (2% to 5%) ... 670
▲ CellCept Capsules (3% to less than 20%) ... 2751
▲ CellCept Intravenous (3% to less than 20%) ... 2751
▲ CellCept Oral Suspension (3% to less than 20%) ... 2751
▲ CellCept Tablets (3% to less than 20%) ... 2751
Crixivan Capsules (2.8%) ... 1918
Doxil Injection (Less than 1%) ... 3302
Herceptin I.V. (At least one of the 958 patients) ... 1234
▲ Myfortic Tablets (3% to less than 20%) ... 2244
▲ Prograf Capsules and Injection (3% to 15%) ... 624
▲ Rapamune Oral Solution and Tablets (3% to 20%) ... 3472
VFEND I.V. (Less than 2%) ... 2543
VFEND Oral Suspension (Less than 2%) ... 2543
VFEND Tablets (Less than 2%) ... 2543
▲ Zenapax for Injection (2% to 5%) ... 2838

Hydrothorax
Follistim AQ Cartridge ... 2354

Hypalgesia
Lyrica Capsules (Rare) ... 2524

Hyperacidity
Lotronex Tablets (Rare) ... 1479

Hyperactive deep tendon reflexes
Eskalith ... 1406
Lithobid Tablets ... 1670

Hyperactivity
Abilify Tablets (Infrequent) ... 916
Abilify Tablets (Infrequent) ... 2472
Aerobid/Aerobid-M (1% to 3%) ... 1172
Amerge Tablets (Rare) ... 1312
Amoxil Capsules (Rare) ... 1315
Amoxil Chewable Tablets (Rare) ... 1315
Amoxil Pediatric Drops for Oral Suspension (Rare) ... 1315
Amoxil Powder for Oral Suspension (Rare) ... 1315
Amoxil Tablets (Rare) ... 1315
Augmentin (Rare) ... 1331
Augmentin Tablets (Rare) ... 1334
Augmentin XR Extended-Release Tablets (Rare) ... 1340
Augmentin ES-600 Powder for Oral Suspension (Rare) ... 1337
Ceftin for Oral Suspension (0.1% to 1%) ... 1369
Clarinex-D 24-Hour Extended-Release Tablets (2%) ... 3012
Dalmane Capsules (Rare) ... 3343
Depacon Injection ... 412
Depakene ... 417
Depakote Sprinkle Capsules ... 422
Depakote Tablets ... 427
Depakote ER Tablets ... 433
Klonopin (Infrequent) ... 2782
Levothroid Tablets ... 1189
Levoxyl Tablets ... 1680
Moban Tablets (Less frequent) ... 1108
Neurontin Capsules ... 2498
Neurontin Oral Solution ... 2498
Neurontin Tablets ... 2498
PREVPAC ... 3281
Roferon-A Injection (Infrequent) ... 2805
Tasmar Tablets (1%) ... 3360
Thioridazine Hydrochloride Tablets (Extremely rare) ... 2122
Unithroid Tablets ... 3521
Zmax for Oral Suspension ... 2577

Hyperacusis
Axert Tablets (Infrequent) ... 2430
Carbatrol Capsules ... 3174
Effexor Tablets (Infrequent) ... 3405
Effexor XR Capsules (Infrequent) ... 3411
Equetro Extended-Release Capsules ... 3178
Frova Tablets (Infrequent) ... 1101
Gabitril Tablets (Infrequent) ... 998
Lunesta Tablets (Rare) ... 3139
Lyrica Capsules (0.1% to 1%) ... 2524
Maxalt Tablets (Rare) ... 1983
Maxalt-MLT Orally Disintegrating Tablets (Rare) ... 1983
Paxil CR Controlled-Release Tablets (Rare) ... 1509
Paxil (Rare) ... 1501
Prozac Pulvules and Liquid (Rare) ... 1771
Rilutek Tablets (Rare) ... 2945
Risperdal M-Tab Orally Disintegrating Tablets (Rare) ... 1658
Risperdal (Rare) ... 1658
Sonata Capsules (2%) ... 1686
Tegretol/Tegretol-XR ... 2278
Zoloft (Rare) ... 2581
Zomig Tablets (Infrequent) ... 714
Zomig-ZMT Tablets (Infrequent) ... 714

Hyperalgesia
Lamictal (Rare) ... 1449
Lyrica Capsules (0.1% to 1%) ... 2524
Paxil CR Controlled-Release Tablets (Rare) ... 1509
Paxil (Rare) ... 1501
Relpax Tablets (Rare) ... 2531
Retrovir Capsules ... 1533
Retrovir IV Infusion ... 1537
Retrovir ... 1533
Thalomid Capsules ... 979

Hyperammonemia
Aciphex Tablets ... 1081
▲ Ammonul Injection (5%) ... 3323
Depacon Injection ... 412
Depakene ... 417
Depakote Sprinkle Capsules ... 422
Depakote Tablets ... 427
Depakote ER Tablets ... 433
Oncaspar (Less than 1%) ... 1123

Hyperammonemic encephalopathy
Depacon Injection ... 412
Depakene ... 417
Depakote Sprinkle Capsules ... 422
Depakote Tablets ... 427
Depakote ER Tablets ... 433

Hyperamylasemia
Aptivus Capsules (Less than 2%) ... 859

Hyperbilirubinemia
Abelcet Injection ... 1119
Accolate Tablets (Rare) ... 663
Advicor Tablets ... 1694
Aloprim for Injection (Less than 1%) ... 2156
Altace Capsules ... 1673
Altoprev Extended-Release Tablets .. 1151
Anadrol-50 Tablets ... 3329
▲ AndroGel (3% to 6%) ... 3330
Anzemet Injection (Less than 1%) ... 2871
Anzemet Tablets (Less than 1%) ... 2874
AquaMEPHYTON Injection ... 1887
Atacand Tablets (Infrequent) ... 634
Atacand HCT ... 637
Augmentin (Infrequent) ... 1331
Augmentin Tablets (Infrequent) ... 1334
Augmentin XR Extended-Release Tablets (Infrequent) ... 1340
Augmentin ES-600 Powder for Oral Suspension (Infrequently) ... 1337
Avelox (Greater than or equal to 2%) ... 2984
Azasan Tablets ... 2844
Benicar Tablets (Infrequently) ... 2850
Biaxin/Biaxin XL (Less than 1%) ... 402
Buphenyl Powder (1%) ... 3327
Buphenyl Tablets (1%) ... 3327
Campath Ampules ... 826
▲ Camptosar Injection (7.2% to 83.9%) ... 2602
Captopril Tablets ... 2114
▲ Casodex Tablets (2% to 5%) ... 670
Ceftin ... 1369
▲ Cipro I.V. (Among most frequent) ... 2998
▲ Cipro I.V. Pharmacy Bulk Package (Among most frequent) ... 3509
Cipro (0.3%) ... 2991
Clarinex Tablets (Rare) ... 3009
Clarinex Reditabs Tablets (Rare) ... 3009
Clarinex-D 24-Hour Extended-Release Tablets ... 3012
▲ Clolar for Intravenous Infusion (15%) ... 1264
Colazal Capsules ... 2845
Covera-HS Tablets ... 3135
▲ Crixivan Capsules (11.9% to 14%) .. 1918
Dapsone Tablets USP ... 1656
Depacon Injection (Occasional) ... 412
Depakene ... 417
Depakote Sprinkle Capsules (Occasional) ... 422
Depakote Tablets (Occasional) ... 427
Depakote ER Tablets ... 433
▲ Doxil Injection (1% to 5%) ... 3302
▲ Eloxatin for Injection (13%) ... 2908
Elspar for Injection ... 1943
Emtriva Capsules (Less than 1%) ... 1272
Epivir (0.8%) ... 1394
Eulexin Capsules ... 3023
Factive Tablets (0.3%) ... 2464
Famvir Tablets (1.9%) ... 2207
Fortaz ... 1422
Garamycin Injectable ... 3028
▲ Gemzar for Injection (13% to 26%) ... 1743
Gengraf Capsules (1% to less than 3%) ... 458
▲ Gleevec Tablets (Up to 3.8%) ... 2221
Hycamtin for Injection (Less than 3%) ... 1427
HyperRho S/D Full Dose ... 3243
Hyperstat I.V. Injection ... 3031
Hyzaar (Occasional) ... 1964
Invanz for Injection (0.6% to 1.7%) ... 1974
▲ Invirase (Less than 1% to 4%) ... 2776
▲ I.V. Busulfex (30% to 49%) ... 1125
Kaletra (Up to 1%) ... 474
Ketek Tablets (Less than 0.2%) ... 2920
Lescol Capsules ... 2227
Lescol Capsules ... 2730
Lescol XL Tablets ... 2227
Lescol XL Tablets ... 2730
▲ Leukine (30%) ... 829
Leustatin Injection ... 2368
Levaquin in 5% Dextrose Injection (0.1% to 0.9%) ... 2453
Levaquin (0.1% to 0.9%) ... 2453
Lexapro Oral Solution (Infrequent) ... 1193
Lexapro Tablets (Infrequent) ... 1193
Lotrel Capsules (Rare) ... 2238
Lotronex Tablets ... 1479
Mavik Tablets (0.2% of patients) ... 482
Mephyton Tablets (Rare) ... 1993
Meridia Capsules (1.6%) ... 485
Merrem I.V. (Greater than 0.2%) ... 687
Mevacor Tablets ... 1996
Micardis HCT Tablets (Occasional) ... 886
Mycamine for Injection (1% to 2.8%) ... 620
Myleran Tablets ... 1492
▲ Mylotarg for Injection (29%) ... 3429
▲ Navelbine Injection (2% to 9%) ... 1494
Neoral Soft Gelatin Capsules (1% to less than 3%) ... 2247
Neoral Oral Solution (1% to less than 3%) ... 2247
Niravam Orally Disintegrating Tablets ... 3106
Omnicef Capsules (0.2%) ... 506
Omnicef for Oral Suspension (0.2%) ... 506
Oncaspar ... 1123
Oxandrin Tablets ... 2977
Pegasys ... 2793
▲ PEG-Intron Powder for Injection (10% to 14%) ... 3062
Pentasa Capsules ... 3182
Pravachol Tablets ... 943
PREVPAC (Less than 1%) ... 3281
Prilosec OTC Tablets (Rare) ... 2674
Primaxin I.M. ... 2022
Primaxin I.V. ... 2024
Prinivil Tablets (Rare) ... 2029
Prinzide Tablets (Rare) ... 2033
▲ Prograf Capsules and Injection (12% to 30%) ... 624
▲ Proleukin for Injection (64%) ... 1007
Protonix Tablets (Less than 1%) ... 3465
▲ Rebetol (10% to 14%) ... 3073
Rebetron Combination Therapy ... 3078
Rescriptor Tablets (0.5% to 1.0%) ... 2535
Retrovir Capsules (Rare) ... 1533
Retrovir IV Infusion (Rare) ... 1537
Retrovir (Rare) ... 1533
RhoGAM Ultra-Filtered ... 2429
Rocephin Injectable Vials, ADD-Vantage, Galaxy, Bulk (Less than 1%) ... 2801
Rythmol SR Capsules ... 2736
Strattera Capsules ... 1784
Suprax ... 1811
Symmetrel ... 1115
Tarceva Tablets ... 1254
Tarceva Tablets ... 2470
Tarka Tablets ... 519
Tenormin I.V. Injection ... 698
Tenormin Tablets ... 695
Tequin Injection (Less than 0.1%) ... 964
Tequin Tablets (Less than 0.1%) ... 964
Ticlid Tablets (Rare) ... 2813
Timentin ADD-Vantage ... 1556
Timentin Injection Galaxy Container ... 1559
Timentin IV Infusion ... 1553
Timentin Pharmacy Bulk Package ... 1562
Tracleer Tablets ... 539
Trecator Tablets ... 3482
Trizivir Tablets (0.8%) ... 1565
Vantin Tablets and Oral Suspension ... 2650
Vaseretic Tablets (Rare) ... 2073
Vasotec I.V. Injection ... 2076
Verelan PM Capsules ... 3120
▲ VFEND I.V. (4.3% to 19.4%) ... 2543
▲ VFEND Oral Suspension (4.3% to 19.4%) ... 2543
▲ VFEND Tablets (4.3% to 19.4%) ... 2543
Viramune Oral Suspension (0.4%) ... 903
Viramune Tablets (0.4%) ... 903
▲ Xeloda Tablets (2% to 22%) ... 2825
Zegerid Powder for Oral Solution (Rare) ... 2972
Zerit (2%) ... 971
Zestoretic Tablets (Rare) ... 701
Zestril Tablets (Rare) ... 704
Zinacef Injection (1 in 500 patients) ... 1604
Zinacef for Injection (1 in 500 patients) ... 1604
Zithromax Capsules, 250 mg (Less than 1%) ... 2568
▲ Zithromax for IV Infusion (1% to 3%) ... 2573
Zithromax for Oral Suspension, 1 g (Less than 1%) ... 2568
Zithromax for Oral Suspension, 300 mg, 600 mg, 900 mg, 1200 mg (Less than 1%) ... 2561
Zithromax Tablets, 250 mg, 500 mg (Less than 1%) ... 2561
Zithromax Tablets, 600 mg (Less than 1%) ... 2568
Zithromax Tri-Pak (Less than 1%) ... 2561
Zithromax Z-Pak (Less than 1%) ... 2568
Zmax for Oral Suspension (Less then 1%) ... 2577
Zocor Tablets ... 2078
Zoloft (One or more patients) ... 2581
Zosyn ... 3492
Zovirax Capsules ... 1616
Zovirax for Injection ... 1618
Zovirax ... 1616
Zyrtec Chewable Tablets (A single case) ... 2589
Zyrtec (A single case) ... 2589
Zyrtec-D 12 Hour Extended Release Tablets (A single case) ... 2591

Hypercalcemia
Abelcet Injection ... 1119
Actiq (Less than 1%) ... 993
Activella Tablets ... 2311
Aloprim for Injection (Less than 1%) ... 2156
Anadrol-50 Tablets ... 3329
Avelox (Greater than or equal to 2%) ... 2984
Benicar HCT Tablets ... 2852
Calcijex Injection ... 411
Calcium Disodium Versenate Injection ... 1819
▲ Carnitor Injection (6% to 15%) ... 3185
▲ CellCept Capsules (3% to less than 20%) ... 2751
▲ CellCept Intravenous (3% to less than 20%) ... 2751
▲ CellCept Oral Suspension (3% to less than 20%) ... 2751
▲ CellCept Tablets (3% to less than 20%) ... 2751
Cenestin Tablets, 0.45mg, 0.625mg, 0.9mg, 1.25mg ... 1063
Cenestin Tablets, 0.3mg ... 1063
Cipro I.V. (Infrequent) ... 2998
Cipro I.V. Pharmacy Bulk Package (Infrequent) ... 3509
Climara Transdermal System ... 795
CombiPatch Transdermal System ... 2180
Cytovene ... 2763
Delatestryl Injection ... 2976
Dovonex Ointment 0.005% (Less than 1%) ... 3375
Dovonex Scalp Solution 0.005% ... 3375
▲ Doxil Injection (1% to 10%) ... 3302
Eskalith ... 1406
Estratest Tablets ... 3196
Estratest H.S. Tablets ... 3196
Evoxac Capsules (Less than 1%) ... 1042
Factive Tablets (Less than 0.1%) ... 2464
Femara Tablets (Less frequent) ... 2210
▲ Flolan for Injection (48%) ... 1408
▲ Forteo for Injection (6% to 11.1%) ... 1739
▲ Fosrenol Chewable Tablets (0% to 4%) ... 3180
Hectorol Capsules ... 909
Hectorol Injection ... 911
Herceptin I.V. (At least one of the 958 patients) ... 1234
Hyzaar ... 1964
▲ Intron A for Injection (Less than or equal to 5%) ... 3038
▲ Invirase (Less than 1% to 4%) ... 2776
Lithobid Tablets ... 1670
Lupron Depot 7.5 mg (Less than 5%) ... 3261
Maxipime for Injection (Greater than 0.1% to less than 1%) ... 1093
Maxzide ... 2150
Micardis HCT Tablets ... 886
▲ Myfortic Tablets (3% to less than 20%) ... 2244
Nipent for Injection (Less than 3%) ... 3216
Oxandrin Tablets ... 2977
Paxil CR Controlled-Release Tablets (Rare) ... 1509
Paxil (Rare) ... 1501
PhosLo GelCaps ... 2158
Premarin Intravenous ... 3440
Premarin Vaginal Cream ... 3449
Premphase Tablets ... 3452
Prempro Tablets ... 3452
Prinzide Tablets ... 2033
▲ Prograf Capsules and Injection (3% to 15%) ... 624
Proleukin for Injection (1%) ... 1007
▲ Rapamune Oral Solution and Tablets (3% to 20%) ... 3472
Rilutek Tablets (Rare) ... 2945
▲ Simulect for Injection (3% to 10%) ... 2268
Timolide Tablets ... 2056
Uniretic Tablets (Less than 1%) ... 3114
Vantas (Less than 2%) ... 3367
Vaseretic Tablets ... 2073
Vesanoid Capsules (Isolated cases) ... 2823
VFEND I.V. (Less than 2%) ... 2543
VFEND Oral Suspension (Less than 2%) ... 2543
VFEND Tablets (Less than 2%) ... 2543
Vivelle Transdermal System ... 2288
Vivelle-Dot Transdermal System ... 2293
Xeloda Tablets (1.1%) ... 2825
Zemplar Capsules ... 535
Zemplar Injection ... 538
Zestoretic Tablets ... 701
Zoladex ... 709
Zoladex 3-month (Rare) ... 712
Zosyn ... 3492

Hypercalciuria
Calcijex Injection ... 411
Effexor XR Capsules (Rare) ... 3411
Hectorol Capsules ... 909

Hypercapnia
Ammonul Injection ... 3323
▲ DepoDur Extended-Release Injection (2% to 5%) ... 1098

Hyperchloremia
Anadrol-50 Tablets ... 3329
Avelox (Greater than or equal to 2%) ... 2984
▲ Buphenyl Powder (7%) ... 3327
▲ Buphenyl Tablets (7%) ... 3327
Daranide Tablets ... 1928
Delatestryl Injection ... 2976
Geodon Capsules (Rare) ... 2514
Primaxin I.M. ... 2022
Primaxin I.V. ... 2024
Sulfamylon Cream ... 2154
Sulfamylon for 5% Topical Solution .. 2155
Topamax Sprinkle Capsules (Infrequent) ... 2438
Topamax Tablets (Infrequent) ... 2438

Hyperchlorhydria
Effexor Tablets (Rare) ... 3405
Effexor XR Capsules (Rare) ... 3411
Prozac Pulvules and Liquid (Infrequent) ... 1771

Hypercholesterolemia
Abilify Tablets (Infrequent) ... 916
Abilify Tablets (Infrequent) ... 2472
Accutane Capsules ... 2740
Aceon Tablets (2 mg, 4 mg, 8 mg) (0.3% to 1%) ... 3191
Aciphex Tablets ... 1081
Agenerase Capsules ... 1299
Aldara Cream, 5% (1.9%) ... 1814
Ambien Tablets (Rare) ... 2867
Amerge Tablets (Rare) ... 1312
▲ Amnesteem Capsules (7%) ... 2126
▲ Aptivus Capsules (0.8% to 11.3%) .. 859
▲ Arimidex Tablets (2% to 7%) ... 665
Arthrotec Tablets (Rare) ... 3126
Axert Tablets (Rare) ... 2430
Benicar Tablets (Greater than 0.5%) ... 2850
Benicar HCT Tablets ... 2852
BiDil Tablets (1% to less than 2%) ... 2161
▲ Boniva Tablets (4.8%) ... 2747
Calcijex Injection ... 411
Carbatrol Capsules (Occasional) ... 3174
▲ Casodex Tablets (2% to 5%) ... 670
Celebrex Capsules (0.1% to 1.9%) ... 3130
▲ CellCept Capsules (3% to 41.2%) ... 2751
▲ CellCept Intravenous (3% to 41.2%) ... 2751
▲ CellCept Oral Suspension (3% to 41.2%) ... 2751
▲ CellCept Tablets (3% to 41.2%) ... 2751
▲ Chemet Capsules (4.2% to 10.4%) ... 2480
Cipro I.V. (Infrequent) ... 2998
Cipro I.V. Pharmacy Bulk Package (Infrequent) ... 3509
Cipro ... 2991
Clozaril Tablets (Rare) ... 2174
▲ Coreg Tablets (1% to 4%) ... 1376
Crixivan Capsules (0.9%) ... 1918
Cymbalta Delayed-Release Capsules (Infrequent) ... 1729
Delatestryl Injection ... 2976
Edex Injection (1%) ... 3103
▲ Effexor Tablets (5.3%) ... 3405
▲ Effexor XR Capsules (5.3%) ... 3411
Equetro Extended-Release Capsules ... 3178

Estratest Tablets 3196
Estratest H.S. Tablets 3196
Evoxac Capsules (Less than 1%) 1042
Exelon Capsules (Infrequent) 2204
▲ Femara Tablets (Less than 0.1% to 15.6%) 2210
Gabitril Tablets (Infrequent) 998
Gengraf Capsules (Less than 3%) 458
Geodon Capsules (Infrequent) 2514
Hectorol Capsules 909
Hectorol Injection 911
▲ Humira Injection (6%) 464
Hyzaar 1964
Inspra Tablets (0.3% to 1%) 2520
▲ Kaletra (9% to 39%) 474
▲ Leukine (17%) 829
Lexapro Oral Solution (Infrequent) 1193
Lexapro Tablets (Infrequent) 1193
Lunesta Tablets (Infrequent) 3139
▲ Lupron Depot 3.75 mg (7%) 3257
Lupron Depot 7.5 mg (Greater than or equal to 5%) 3261
Micardis Tablets (More than 0.3%) 884
Micardis HCT Tablets 886
▲ Myfortic Tablets (3% to less than 20%) 2244
Neoral Soft Gelatin Capsules (Less than 3%) 2247
Neoral Oral Solution (Less than 3%) 2247
Neurontin Capsules (Rare) 2498
Neurontin Oral Solution (Rare) 2498
Neurontin Tablets (Rare) 2498
Noroxin Tablets 2009
▲ Norvir (36.5% to 44.8%) 499
Oxandrin Tablets 2977
Paxil CR Controlled-Release Tablets (Rare) 1509
Paxil (Rare) 1501
Permax Tablets (Infrequent) 3357
▲ Plavix Tablets (4%) 940
▲ Plavix Tablets (4%) 2942
Prevacid Delayed-Release Capsules 3268
Prevacid for Delayed-Release Oral Suspension 3268
Prevacid NapraPAC 3277
Prevacid SoluTab Delayed-Release Orally Disintegrating Tablets 3268
PREVPAC 3281
Prinzide Tablets 2033
▲ Prograf Capsules and Injection (3% to 15%) 624
Prozac Pulvules and Liquid (Infrequent) 1771
▲ Rapamune Oral Solution and Tablets (38% to 46%) 3472
Requip Tablets (Infrequent) 1528
Rilutek Tablets (Rare) 2945
Risperdal Consta Long-Acting Injection (Infrequent) 1664
Rythmol SR Capsules 2736
Sonata Capsules (Infrequent) 1686
▲ Spiriva HandiHaler (1% to 3%) 899
Sustiva Capsules 957
▲ Targretin Capsules (32.1% to 62.3%) 1719
Tasmar Tablets (Infrequent) 3360
Tegretol/Tegretol-XR (Occasional) 2278
Teveten Tablets (Less than 1%) 1707
Teveten HCT Tablets (Less than 1%) 1710
Thalomid Capsules 979
Ticlid Tablets 2813
Timolide Tablets 2056
Travatan Ophthalmic Solution (1% to 5%) 559
Uniretic Tablets (Less than 1%) 3114
Vantas (Less than 2%) 3367
Vaseretic Tablets 2073
▲ Vesanoid Capsules (Up to 60%) 2823
VFEND I.V. (Less than 2%) 2543
VFEND Oral Suspension (Less than 2%) 2543
VFEND Tablets (Less than 2%) 2543
Zestoretic Tablets 701
Zoladex 709
Zoladex 3-month 712
▲ Zoloft (Approximately 3%) 2581
Zyprexa Tablets (Rare) 1798
Zyprexa ZYDIS Orally Disintegrating Tablets (Rare) 1798

Hypercorticism

Advair Diskus 100/50 1291
Advair Diskus 250/50 1291
Advair Diskus 500/50 1291
Beconase AQ Nasal Spray 1359
Blephamide Ophthalmic Ointment (Rare) 563
Blephamide Ophthalmic Suspension (Rare) 564
Entocort EC Capsules 2694
FML Ophthalmic Ointment (Rare) .... ⊙ 225
FML Ophthalmic Suspension (Rare) .... ⊙ 224
HMS Sterile Ophthalmic Suspension .... ⊙ 228
Nasacort HFA Inhalation Aerosol 2939
Pred Forte Ophthalmic Suspension (Rare) .... ⊙ 233
Pred Mild Sterile Ophthalmic Suspension (Rare) .... ⊙ 236
Pulmicort Respules (Less than 1%) 654

Hypercorticoidism

Poly-Pred Liquifilm Ophthalmic Suspension .... ⊙ 231

Hyperdipsia

(*see under* Dipsesis)

Hyperemia

Azopt Ophthalmic Suspension (1% to 5%) 553
▲ Elestat Ophthalmic Solution (1% to 10%) 1643
Lacrisert Sterile Ophthalmic Insert 1979
Patanol Ophthalmic Solution (Less than 5%) 557
Topamax Sprinkle Capsules 2438
Topamax Tablets 2438

Hyperemia, conjunctival

▲ Acular LS Ophthalmic Solution (1% to 5%) 562
▲ Alphagan P Ophthalmic Solution (Approximately 10% to 20%) 563
▲ Brimonidine Tartrate Ophthalmic Solution 0.2% (10% to 30%) .... ⊙ 245
▲ Carteolol Hydrochloride Ophthalmic Solution USP, 1% (About 1 of 4 patients) .... ⊙ 246
▲ Ciloxan Ophthalmic Ointment (Less than 10%) 554
▲ Cosopt Sterile Ophthalmic Solution (5% to 30%) 1910
Diprivan Injectable Emulsion (Less than 1%) 676
FML Ophthalmic Ointment (Occasional) .... ⊙ 225
FML Ophthalmic Suspension (Occasional) .... ⊙ 224
FML Forte Ophthalmic Suspension (Occasional) .... ⊙ 223
FML-S Liquifilm Sterile Ophthalmic Suspension .... ⊙ 226
▲ Genoptic Sterile Ophthalmic Solution (Among most frequent) .... ⊙ 227
HMS Sterile Ophthalmic Suspension .... ⊙ 228
▲ Lumigan Ophthalmic Solution (15% to 45%) 569
Natacyn Antifungal Ophthalmic Suspension (One case) .... ⊙ 207
Neurontin Capsules (Rare) 2498
Neurontin Oral Solution (Rare) 2498
Neurontin Tablets (Rare) 2498
Ophthetic Ophthalmic Solution .... ⊙ 230
Pred Forte Ophthalmic Suspension (Occasional) .... ⊙ 233
Pred Mild Sterile Ophthalmic Suspension (Occasional) .... ⊙ 236
▲ Restasis Ophthalmic Emulsion (1% to 5%) 570
Suprane Liquid for Inhalation (Greater than 1%) 770
▲ Travatan Ophthalmic Solution (15% to 45%) 559
▲ Vigamox Ophthalmic Solution (1% to 6%) 560
▲ Xalatan Sterile Ophthalmic Solution (5% to 15%) 2654

Hypereosinophilia

Ketek Tablets (Less than 0.2%) 2920
Leustatin Injection 2368
Maxipime for Injection (1.7%) 1093

Hyperesthesia

Abilify Tablets (Infrequent) 916
Abilify Tablets (Infrequent) 2472
Amerge Tablets (Rare) 1312
Arthrotec Tablets (Rare) 3126
Asacol Delayed-Release Tablets 2688
Axert Tablets (Infrequent) 2430
Celexa (Rare) 1177
Cipro I.V. 2998
Cipro I.V. Pharmacy Bulk Package 3509
Cipro 2991
Cipro XR Tablets 3004
Diprolene Lotion 0.05% (Less than 1%) 3016
Doxil Injection (Less than 1%) 3302
Effexor Tablets (Infrequent) 3405
Effexor XR Capsules (Frequent) 3411
Evoxac Capsules 1042
▲ Flolan for Injection (5% to 12%) 1408
Frova Tablets (Frequent) 1101
Gengraf Capsules 458
Imitrex Injection (Rare) 1431
Imitrex Tablets (Rare) 1440
▲ Intron A for Injection (Less than 5%) 3038
Invirase (Less than 2%) 2776
▲ Kepivance (12%) 592
Lamictal (Rare) 1449
Lidoderm Patch 1107
Lunesta Tablets (Rare) 3139
Lyrica Capsules (0.1% to 1%) 2524
Maxalt Tablets (Infrequent) 1983
Maxalt-MLT Orally Disintegrating Tablets (Infrequent) 1983
Neoral Soft Gelatin Capsules 2247
Neoral Oral Solution 2247
Neurontin Capsules (Rare) 2498
Neurontin Oral Solution (Rare) 2498
Neurontin Tablets (Rare) 2498
Norvir (Less than 2%) 499
Pletal Tablets (2% or greater) 2478
ProAmatine Tablets (Rare) 3183
▲ Protopic Ointment (Up to 7%) 629
Prozac Pulvules and Liquid (Rare) 1771
Relpax Tablets (Frequent) 2531
▲ Requip Tablets (4%) 1528
Rescriptor Tablets 2535
Sonata Capsules (Infrequent) 1686
▲ Soriatane Capsules (10% to 25%) 1028
Targretin Capsules 1719
Tequin Injection (Less than 0.1%) 964
Tequin Tablets (Less than 0.1%) 964
Thalomid Capsules 979
Topamax Sprinkle Capsules (Rare) 2438
Topamax Tablets (Rare) 2438
Tri-Luma Cream (2%) 1213
Zoloft (Infrequent) 2581
▲ Zomig Nasal Spray (0% to 5%) 718
Zomig Tablets (Infrequent) 714
Zomig-ZMT Tablets (Infrequent) 714
Zonegran Capsules (Rare) 1089
Zyrtec Chewable Tablets (Less than 2%) 2589
Zyrtec (Less than 2%) 2589
Zyrtec-D 12 Hour Extended Release Tablets (Less than 2%) 2591

Hyperesthesia, tongue

Alferon N Injection (1%) 1640

Hyperexcitability

Phenergan 3438

Hyperexcitability, paradoxical

Diastat Rectal Delivery System 3344

Hyperfibrinogenemia

Colazal Capsules 2845
Neumega for Injection 3433
Premarin Tablets 3443
Premphase Tablets 3452
Prempro Tablets 3452

Hypergammaglobulinemia

Prevacid Delayed-Release Capsules 3268
Prevacid for Delayed-Release Oral Suspension 3268
Prevacid SoluTab Delayed-Release Orally Disintegrating Tablets 3268
PREVPAC 3281

Hyperglycemia

Abelcet Injection 1119
Abilify Tablets (Infrequent) 916
Abilify Tablets (Infrequent) 2472
Accutane Capsules 2740
Aceon Tablets (2 mg, 4 mg, 8 mg) (0.3% to 1%) 3191
Aciphex Tablets 1081
Aclovate 1290
Actimmune (Rare) 1646
Actiq (1% or greater) 993
Adalat CC Tablets (Rare) 2978
Advair Diskus 100/50 1291
Advair Diskus 250/50 1291
Advair Diskus 500/50 1291
▲ Advicor Tablets (4%) 1694
▲ Agenerase Capsules (2% to 3%) 1299
Agenerase Oral Solution (2.3%) 1304
Aggrenox Capsules (Less than 1%) 855
Albalon Ophthalmic Solution .... ⊙ 216
Aldoclor Tablets 1881
Aldoril Tablets 1884
Aloprim for Injection (Less than 1%) 2156
Aloxi Injection (Less than 1%) 2099
Altace Capsules 1673
Ambien Tablets (Infrequent) 2867
▲ AmBisome for Injection (8.2% to 23%) 615
Amerge Tablets (Rare) 1312
▲ Ammonul Injection (7%) 3323
Anaprox Tablets (Less than 1%) 2769
Anaprox DS Tablets (Less than 1%) 2769
▲ AndroGel (3% to 6%) 3330
Aptivus Capsules (Less than 2%) 859
▲ Arava Tablets (1% to 3%) 2881
Aricept Tablets (Infrequent) 1086
Aricept ODT Tablets (Infrequent) 1086
Arthrotec Tablets (Rare) 3126
Atacand Tablets (0.5% or greater) 634
Atacand HCT (0.5% or greater) 637
Avalide Tablets 922
Avalide Tablets 2889
▲ Avandamet Tablets (5.9%) 1343
▲ Avandia Tablets (3.9%) 1348
Avelox (Less than 0.1%) 2984
Axert Tablets (Infrequent) 2430
Aygestin Tablets 1062
Baraclude (2%) 928
Bayer Aspirin Tablets 3515
Benicar HCT Tablets (Greater than 1%) 2852
▲ BiDil Tablets (4%) 2161
Blocadren Tablets 1891
Caduet Tablets (Greater than 0.1% to less than 2%) 2507
Cafcit 1854
Campath Ampules 826
Campral Tablets (Infrequent) 1175
Camptosar Injection 2602
Cardizem LA Extended Release Tablets (Less than 2%) 1699
▲ Casodex Tablets (6%) 670
Cataflam Tablets (Rarley) 2173
Catapres Tablets (Rare) 874
Celebrex Capsules (0.1% to 1.9%) 3130
▲ CellCept Capsules (43.7% to 46.7%) 2751
▲ CellCept Intravenous (43.7% to 46.7%) 2751
▲ CellCept Oral Suspension (43.7% to 46.7%) 2751
▲ CellCept Tablets (43.7% to 46.7%) 2751
▲ Cipro I.V. (Among most frequent) 2998
▲ Cipro I.V. Pharmacy Bulk Package (Among most frequent) 3509
Cipro 2991
Cipro XR Tablets (Less than 1%) 3004
Clinoril Tablets (Rare) 1899
Clobex Shampoo 1209
Clobex Lotion 1208
Clorpres Tablets 2139
Clozapine Tablets 2141
Clozaril Tablets 2174
Combivir Tablets 1373
▲ Coreg Tablets (5% to 12%) 1376
Cosopt Sterile Ophthalmic Solution 1910
Crixivan Capsules 1918
Cubicin for Injection (1% to 2%) 1038
Cutivate Lotion 0.05% (Rare) 1383
Decadron Phosphate Injection 1931
Decadron Tablets 1929
Diovan HCT Tablets 2195
Diprivan Injectable Emulsion (Less than 1%) 676
Diprolene Gel 0.05% 3015
Diprolene Lotion 0.05% 3016
Diprolene Ointment 0.05% (Some patients) 3017
Diprolene AF Cream 0.05% (Some patients) 3014
Diprosone Cream, USP 0.05% 3018
Diuril Oral 1936
Diuril Sodium Intravenous 1934
▲ Doxil Injection (1% to 10%) 3302
Dyazide Capsules 1389
EC-Naprosyn Delayed-Release Tablets (Less than 1%) 2769
Ecotrin Enteric Coated Aspirin Low, Regular and Maximum Strength Tablets 1627
Edecrin 1941
Edex Injection (1%) 3103
Effexor Tablets (Infrequent) 3405
Effexor XR Capsules (Infrequent) 3411
Elocon Cream 0.1% 3019
Elocon Lotion 0.1% 3020
Elocon Ointment 0.1% 3021
Elspar for Injection (Low) 1943
Emend Capsules (Greater than 0.5%) 1944
Epivir 1394
Epivir-HBV 1398
Epzicom Tablets 1402
Evoxac Capsules (Less than 1%) 1042
Exelon Capsules (Infrequent) 2204
Factive Tablets (0.1% to 1%) 2464
FazaClo Orally Disintegrating Tablets 547
Flexeril Tablets (Rare) 1832

Flovent Diskus 50 mcg ... 1415
Flovent HFA ... 1418
Foradil Aerolizer ... 3024
Furosemide Tablets ... 2117
Fuzeon Injection ... 2772
Gabitril Tablets (Infrequent) ... 998
Gengraf Capsules (2% or less) ... 458
Genotropin Lyophilized Powder (Infrequent) ... 2642
Geodon Capsules (Infrequent) ... 2514
Humatrope Vials and Cartridges (Infrequent) ... 1756
Hydrocortone Tablets ... 1963
Hyperstat I.V. Injection ... 3031
Hyzaar ... 1964
Imitrex Injection ... 1431
Imitrex Nasal Spray ... 1435
Imitrex Tablets (Rare) ... 1440
Indapamide Tablets (Less than 5%) .. 2119
Indocin Capsules (Less than 1%) ... 1968
Indocin I.V. (Less than 1%) ... 1973
Indocin (Less than 1%) ... 1968
▲ Intron A for Injection (Less than or equal to 5%) ... 3038
Invanz for Injection (1.2% to 1.7%) ... 1974
▲ Invirase (2.7% to less than or equal to 5%) ... 2776
▲ I.V. Busulfex (15% to 67%) ... 1125
▲ Kaletra (1% to 5%) ... 474
Lamictal (Rare) ... 1449
▲ Leukine (25% to 41%) ... 829
Levaquin in 5% Dextrose Injection (0.1% to 0.9%) ... 2453
Levaquin (0.1% to 0.9%) ... 2453
Lexapro Oral Solution (Infrequent) ... 1193
Lexapro Tablets (Infrequent) ... 1193
Lexiva Tablets (Less than 1%) ... 1473
Lipitor Tablets (Less than 2%) ... 2495
Lithobid Tablets ... 1670
Lo/Ovral-28 Tablets ... 3423
Lotensin HCT Tablets ... 2235
Lotrisone ... 3054
Lotronex Tablets (Rare) ... 1479
Lupron Depot 7.5 mg (Greater than or equal to 5%) ... 3261
Maxzide ... 2150
▲ Megace ES Oral Suspension (0% to 6%) ... 2492
▲ Mepron Suspension (9%) ... 1487
Meridia Capsules ... 485
Micardis HCT Tablets ... 886
Mintezol ... 2002
Moduretic Tablets ... 2003
▲ Myfortic Tablets (3% to less than 20%) ... 2244
▲ Mylotarg for Injection (10% to 11%) ... 3429
Naprosyn Suspension (Less than 1%) ... 2769
Naprosyn Tablets (Less than 1%) ... 2769
Neoral Soft Gelatin Capsules (2% or less) ... 2247
Neoral Oral Solution (2% or less) ... 2247
Neurontin Capsules (1.2%) ... 2498
Neurontin Oral Solution (1.2%) ... 2498
Neurontin Tablets (1.2%) ... 2498
Niaspan Extended-Release Tablets ... 1703
Nicomide Tablets ... 3190
Nimotop Capsules (0.8%; rare) ... 774
Norditropin Cartridges ... 2318
Noroxin Tablets ... 2009
Norvasc Tablets (More than 0.1% to 1%) ... 2529
Norvir ... 499
Olux Foam ... 1027
Omacor Capsules ... 2735
Omnicef Capsules (0.9%) ... 506
Omnicef for Oral Suspension (0.9%) ... 506
▲ Oncaspar (Greater than 1% but less than 5%) ... 1123
Paxil CR Controlled-Release Tablets (Infrequent) ... 1509
Paxil (Infrequent) ... 1501
Pegasys ... 2793
PEG-Intron Powder for Injection (Less than or equal to 1%) ... 3062
Permax Tablets (Infrequent) ... 3357
Phenytek Capsules ... 2153
Prevacid Delayed-Release Capsules (Less than 1%) ... 3268
Prevacid for Delayed-Release Oral Suspension (Less than 1%) ... 3268
Prevacid NapraPAC (Less than 1%) .. 3277
Prevacid SoluTab Delayed-Release Orally Disintegrating Tablets (Less than 1%) ... 3268
PREVPAC (Less than 1%) ... 3281
Prinzide Tablets ... 2033
▲ Prograf Capsules and Injection (Many patients; 13% to 47%) ... 624
Proleukin for Injection (2%) ... 1007
Protonix I.V. (Less than or equal to 1%) ... 3468
Protonix Tablets (Less than or equal to 1%) ... 3465
Protopic Ointment (Greater than or equal to 1%) ... 629
Provigil Tablets (Greater than or equal to 1%) ... 1002
▲ Rapamune Oral Solution and Tablets (3% to 20%) ... 3472
Razadyne ER Extended-Release Capsules (Infrequent) ... 2434
Razadyne (Infrequent) ... 2434
Rebetron Combination Therapy ... 3078
Relafen Tablets (Less than 1%) ... 1523
Relpax Tablets (Rare) ... 2531
Requip Tablets (1% or more) ... 1528
Rescriptor Tablets ... 2535
Risperdal Consta Long-Acting Injection (Infrequent) ... 1664
Risperdal M-Tab Orally Disintegrating Tablets ... 1658
Risperdal ... 1658
▲ Rituxan for Infusion (1% to 5%) ... 845
▲ Rituxan I.V. (9%) ... 1251
Roferon-A Injection (Rare) ... 2805
Rythmol SR Capsules ... 2736
Sandimmune (2% or less) ... 2259
▲ Sandostatin Injection (3% to 16%) ... 2263
▲ Sandostatin LAR Depot (15% to 27%) ... 2264
Serevent Diskus (1% to 3%) ... 1540
Seroquel Tablets (Infrequent) ... 691
▲ Simulect for Injection (Greater than or equal to 10%) ... 2268
Sonata Capsules (Rare) ... 1686
Spectracef Tablets (0.1% to 1%) ... 2706
▲ Spiriva HandiHaler (1% to 3%) ... 899
St. Joseph 81 mg Aspirin Chewable and Enteric Coated Tablets ... 1841
Suprane Liquid for Inhalation ... 770
Surmontil Capsules ... 2347
Targretin Capsules ... 1719
Temovate Cream ... 1549
Temovate Gel ... 1550
Temovate Ointment ... 1549
Temovate Scalp Application ... 1551
Tequin Injection (Less than 0.1%) ... 964
Tequin Tablets (Less than 0.1%) ... 964
Teveten Tablets (Less than 1%) ... 1707
Teveten HCT Tablets (Less than 1%) ... 1710
Thalomid Capsules ... 979
Thiothixene Capsules ... 2124
Tiazac Capsules (Less than 2%) ... 1204
Timolide Tablets ... 2056
Timoptic in Ocudose ... 2061
Timoptic Sterile Ophthalmic Solution ... 2058
Timoptic-XE Sterile Ophthalmic Gel Forming Solution ... 2062
Topamax Sprinkle Capsules (Infrequent) ... 2438
Topamax Tablets (Infrequent) ... 2438
Trasylol Injection (1% to 2%) ... 779
Trileptal Oral Suspension ... 2281
Trileptal Tablets ... 2281
Triphasil-28 Tablets ... 3483
▲ Trisenox Injection (45%) ... 983
Trizivir Tablets ... 1565
▲ Truvada Tablets (1% to 12%) ... 1279
Tygacil for Injection (1.8%) ... 3489
Ultane Liquid for Inhalation (Less than 1%) ... 526
Uniretic Tablets (More than 1%) ... 3114
Urso 250 Tablets (1%) ... 737
Urso Forte Tablets (1%) ... 737
▲ Valcyte Tablets (Less than 5%) ... 2816
Vanos Cream ... 1864
Vantas (Less than 2%) ... 3367
Vantin Tablets and Oral Suspension ... 2650
Vaseretic Tablets ... 2073
VFEND I.V. (Less than 2%) ... 2543
VFEND Oral Suspension (Less than 2%) ... 2543
VFEND Tablets (Less than 2%) ... 2543
Viagra Tablets (Less than 2%) ... 2552
Viracept (Less than 2%) ... 2556
▲ Viread Tablets (2% to 3%) ... 1284
Vivactil Tablets ... 2350
Voltaren Tablets (Rarely) ... 2298
Voltaren-XR Tablets (Rarely) ... 2301
Wellbutrin Tablets ... 1579
Wellbutrin SR Sustained-Release Tablets ... 1583
Wellbutrin XL Extended-Release Tablets ... 1588
▲ Xopenex HFA Inhalation Aerosol (2.6% to 5.2%) ... 3151
▲ Xopenex Inhalation Solution (2.6% to 5.2%) ... 3143
▲ Xopenex Inhalation Solution Concentrate (2.6% to 5.2%) ... 3147
Zegerid Powder for Oral Solution (0.7%) ... 2972
Zenapax for Injection ... 2838
Zestoretic Tablets ... 701
Ziagen ... 1600
Zithromax (Less than 1%) ... 2568
Zithromax for Oral Suspension, 300 mg, 600 mg, 900 mg, 1200 mg (Less than 1%) ... 2561
Zithromax Tablets, 250 mg, 500 mg (Less than 1%) ... 2561
Zithromax Tablets, 600 mg (Less than 1%) ... 2568
Zithromax Tri-Pak (Less than 1%) ... 2561
Zithromax Z-Pak (Less than 1%) ... 2568
Zoladex (1% to 5%) ... 709
Zoladex 3-month ... 712
Zoloft ... 2581
Zomig Tablets (Rare) ... 714
Zomig-ZMT Tablets (Rare) ... 714
Zosyn ... 3492
Zyprexa Tablets (Infrequent) ... 1798
Zyprexa ZYDIS Orally Disintegrating Tablets (Infrequent) ... 1798

Hyperglycemia, hyperosmolar nonketotic
Tequin Injection ... 964
Tequin Tablets ... 964

Hyperglycemia, transient
Eskalith ... 1406
▲ Rituxan for Infusion (1% to 5%) ... 845
▲ Rituxan I.V. (1% to 5%) ... 1251

Hyperglycinemia
Amnesteem Capsules ... 2126
Depacon Injection ... 412
Depakene ... 417
Depakote Sprinkle Capsules ... 422
Depakote Tablets ... 427
Depakote ER Tablets ... 433
▲ Emtriva Capsules (2% to 3%) ... 1272
Moban Tablets ... 1108
Parcopa Orally Disintegrating Tablets ... 3111
Pletal Tablets (Very rare) ... 2478
Rythmol SR Capsules ... 2736

Hypergranulation
Aquacel AG with Hydrofiber ... 1035

Hyperhemoglobinemia
Ambien Tablets (Rare) ... 2867
Evoxac Capsules ... 1042
Prevacid NapraPAC ... 3277

Hyperheparinemia
Mustargen for Injection (Rare) ... 2007

Hyperhidrosis
Accutane Capsules ... 2740
Byetta Injection (Greater than or equal to 1% to less than 5%) ... 605
▲ Cymbalta Delayed-Release Capsules (6% to 8%) ... 1729
DynaCirc CR Tablets (0.5% to 1%) ... 2726
Havrix Vaccine (Rare) ... 1425
Miacalcin Nasal Spray (Less than 1%) ... 2242
Noroxin Tablets (0.3% to 1.0%) ... 2009
Prilosec OTC Tablets (Less than 1%) ... 2674
Primaxin I.M. ... 2022
Primaxin I.V. (Less than 0.2%) ... 2024
Prinivil Tablets ... 2029
Prinzide Tablets (0.3% to 1%) ... 2033
▲ Requip Tablets (3%) ... 1528
Sedapap Tablets 50 mg/650 mg (Infrequent) ... 2098
Thyrolar ... 1203
Vaseretic Tablets ... 2073
Vasotec I.V. Injection ... 2076
Zegerid Powder for Oral Solution (Less than 1%) ... 2972
Zestoretic Tablets ... 701

Hyperhistaminemia
▲ Vesanoid Capsules (3%) ... 2823

Hyperirritability
Mintezol ... 2002
Seromycin Capsules ... 1783

Hyperirritability, muscle
Eskalith ... 1406
Lithobid Tablets ... 1670

Hyperirritability, neuromuscular
Timentin ADD-Vantage ... 1556
Timentin Injection Galaxy Container ... 1559
Timentin IV Infusion ... 1553
Timentin Pharmacy Bulk Package ... 1562

Hyperkalemia
Abelcet Injection ... 1119
Abilify Tablets (Infrequent) ... 916
Abilify Tablets (Infrequent) ... 2472
Aceon Tablets (2 mg, 4 mg, 8 mg) (1.4%) ... 3191
Aggrenox Capsules ... 855
Aloprim for Injection (Less than 1%) ... 2156
Aloxi Injection (1%) ... 2099
Altace Capsules (Approximately 1%) ... 1673
AmBisome for Injection (Less common) ... 615
Ammonul Injection ... 3323
Anadrol-50 Tablets ... 3329
Anaprox Tablets (Less than 1%) ... 2769
Anaprox DS Tablets (Less than 1%) .. 2769
Atacand Tablets ... 634
Atacand HCT (Very rare) ... 637
Avalide Tablets ... 922
Avalide Tablets ... 2889
▲ Avapro Tablets (18.6%) ... 925
▲ Avapro Tablets (18.6%) ... 2886
Bayer Aspirin Tablets ... 3515
Blocadren Tablets ... 1891
Campath Ampules ... 826
Cancidas for Injection (0% to 0.9%) ... 1894
Captopril Tablets ... 2114
▲ Carnitor Injection (6%) ... 3185
▲ CellCept Capsules (22%) ... 2751
▲ CellCept Intravenous (22%) ... 2751
▲ CellCept Oral Suspension (22%) ... 2751
▲ CellCept Tablets (22%) ... 2751
Cipro I.V. (Infrequent) ... 2998
Cipro I.V. Pharmacy Bulk Package (Infrequent) ... 3509
Cipro ... 2991
Clinoril Tablets (Less than 1 in 100) ... 1899
▲ Coreg Tablets (Greater than 1% to 3%) ... 1376
▲ Cozaar Tablets (7%) ... 1913
Delatestryl Injection ... 2976
Diovan HCT Tablets (0.3%) ... 2195
▲ Diovan Tablets (2% to 4.4%) ... 2191
Diprivan Injectable Emulsion (Less than 1%) ... 676
Doxil Injection (Less than 1%) ... 3302
Dyazide Capsules ... 1389
Dyrenium Capsules (Rare) ... 3390
EC-Naprosyn Delayed-Release Tablets (Less than 1%) ... 2769
Ecotrin Enteric Coated Aspirin Low, Regular and Maximum Strength Tablets ... 1627
Effexor Tablets (Rare) ... 3405
Effexor XR Capsules (Rare) ... 3411
Epogen for Injection (Approximately 0.11%) ... 586
Estratest Tablets ... 3196
Estratest H.S. Tablets ... 3196
Evoxac Capsules ... 1042
Factive Tablets (0.5%) ... 2464
▲ Ferrlecit Injection (6%) ... 3379
▲ Flolan for Injection (4%) ... 1408
Gengraf Capsules (1% to less than 3%) ... 458
Geodon Capsules (Rare) ... 2514
Gleevec Tablets (Rare) ... 2221
Hyzaar (0.4%) ... 1964
Indocin Capsules (Less than 1%) ... 1968
Indocin I.V. (Less than 1%) ... 1973
Indocin (Less than 1%) ... 1968
▲ Inspra Tablets (3.4% to 15.6%) ... 2520
Invanz for Injection (0.5% to 1.3%) ... 1974
▲ Invirase (Less than 1% to 4%) ... 2776
K-Dur Extended-Relase Tablets ... 3047
▲ K-Lor Powder Packets (Among most severe) ... 472
▲ K-Tab Filmtab Tablets (Most common) ... 473
Levaquin in 5% Dextrose Injection (0.1% to 0.9%) ... 2453
Levaquin (0.1% to 0.9%) ... 2453
Lotensin Tablets ... 2232
Lotrel Capsules (Approximately 1.5%) ... 2238
▲ Mavik Tablets (0.3% to 5.3%) ... 482
Maxipime for Injection (Greater than 0.1% to less than 1%) ... 1093
Maxzide ... 2150
Micardis Tablets ... 884
▲ Midamor Tablets (Between 1% and 3%) ... 2000
Moduretic Tablets (Greater than 1%, less than 3%) ... 2003

▲ Myfortic Tablets (3% to less than 20%) ... 2244
Naprosyn Suspension (Less than 1%) ... 2769
Naprosyn Tablets (Less than 1%) ... 2769
Neoral Soft Gelatin Capsules (1% to less than 3%) ... 2247
Neoral Oral Solution (1% to less than 3%) ... 2247
Noroxin Tablets ... 2009
Omnicef Capsules (0.2%) ... 506
Omnicef for Oral Suspension (0.2%) ... 506
Oxandrin Tablets ... 2977
Paxil CR Controlled-Release Tablets (Rare) ... 1509
Paxil (Rare) ... 1501
Prevacid NapraPAC (Less than 1%) .. 3277
Primaxin I.M. ... 2022
Primaxin I.V. ... 2024
▲ Prinivil Tablets (Approximately 2.2% to 4.8%) ... 2029
Prinzide Tablets (Approximately 1.4%) ... 2033
Procrit for Injection (0.11%) ... 2374
▲ Prograf Capsules and Injection (13% to 45%) ... 624
▲ Proleukin for Injection (4%) ... 1007
Prozac Pulvules and Liquid (Rare) ... 1771
▲ Rapamune Oral Solution and Tablets (12% to 17%) ... 3472
ReoPro Vials (0.1%) ... 1779
Requip Tablets (Infrequent) ... 1528
Rescriptor Tablets ... 2535
Rituxan for Infusion ... 845
Sandimmune (Occasional) ... 2259
▲ Simulect for Injection (Greater than or equal to 10%) ... 2268
St. Joseph 81 mg Aspirin Chewable and Enteric Coated Tablets ... 1841
Symbyax Capsules (Rare) ... 1788
Targretin Capsules ... 1719
Tarka Tablets ... 519
Teveten Tablets (Less than 1%) ... 1707
Teveten HCT Tablets (Less than 1%) ... 1710
Thalomid Capsules ... 979
▲ Thymoglobulin for Injection (26.8%) ... 2848
▲ Trisenox Injection (18%) ... 983
Uniretic Tablets (Less than 1%) ... 3114
Univasc Tablets ... 3118
▲ Valcyte Tablets (Less than 5%) ... 2816
Vaseretic Tablets ... 2073
Vasotec I.V. Injection (Approximately 1%) ... 2076
VFEND I.V. (Less than 2%) ... 2543
VFEND Oral Suspension (Less than 2%) ... 2543
VFEND Tablets (Less than 2%) ... 2543
Zegerid Powder for Oral Solution (2.2%) ... 2972
Zestoretic Tablets (Approximately 1.4%) ... 701
▲ Zestril Tablets (Approximately 2.2% to 4.8%) ... 704
Zithromax (1% to 2%) ... 2568
Zithromax for Oral Suspension, 300 mg, 600 mg, 900 mg, 1200 mg (1% to 2%) ... 2561
Zithromax Tablets, 250 mg, 500 mg (1% to 2%) ... 2561
Zithromax Tablets, 600 mg (1% to 2%) ... 2568
Zithromax Tri-Pak (1% to 2%) ... 2561
Zithromax Z-Pak (1% to 2%) ... 2568
Zmax for Oral Suspension (Less then 1%) ... 2577
Zosyn ... 3492
Zyprexa Tablets (Infrequent) ... 1798
Zyprexa IntraMuscular (Infrequent) ... 1798
Zyprexa ZYDIS Orally Disintegrating Tablets (Infrequent) ... 1798

Hyperkalemia, neonatal

Altace Capsules ... 1673
Prograf Capsules and Injection ... 624
Zestril Tablets ... 704

Hyperkeratosis

▲ Aldara Cream, 5% (8.8%) ... 1814
Aricept Tablets (Infrequent) ... 1086
Aricept ODT Tablets (Infrequent) ... 1086
Covera-HS Tablets (Less than 2%) ... 3135
Cymbalta Delayed-Release Capsules (Infrequent) ... 1729
Evoxac Capsules (Less than 1%) ... 1042
Requip Tablets (Infrequent) ... 1528
Risperdal M-Tab Orally Disintegrating Tablets (Infrequent) ... 1658
Risperdal (Infrequent) ... 1658
Soriatane Capsules (Less than 1%) .. 1028
Tarka Tablets ... 519
Zyrtec Chewable Tablets (Less than 2%) ... 2589
Zyrtec (Less than 2%) ... 2589
Zyrtec-D 12 Hour Extended Release Tablets (Less than 2%) ... 2591

Hyperkinesia

Abilify Tablets (Infrequent) ... 916
Abilify Tablets (Infrequent) ... 2472
Aciphex Tablets (Rare) ... 1081
AndroGel (One patient) ... 3330
Astelin Nasal Spray (Infrequent) ... 1876
Caduet Tablets (Less than 2%) ... 2507
Campral Tablets (Rare) ... 1175
Celexa (Infrequent) ... 1177
Clozapine Tablets (1%) ... 2141
Clozaril Tablets (1%) ... 2174
Combunox Tablets (Less than 2%) ... 1183
▲ Comtan Tablets (10%) ... 2186
Diastat Rectal Delivery System (Greater than or equal to 1%) ... 3344
Effexor Tablets (Infrequent) ... 3405
Effexor XR Capsules (Infrequent) ... 3411
▲ Entocort EC Capsules (Less than 5%) ... 2694
Evoxac Capsules (Less than 1%) ... 1042
Exelon Capsules (Infrequent) ... 2204
FazaClo Orally Disintegrating Tablets (1%) ... 547
▲ Flolan for Injection (7%) ... 1408
Floxin Otic Singles (Reported in a single subject) ... 1045
Floxin Otic Solution (Single report) ... 1043
Flumadine (Less than 0.3%) ... 1186
Gabitril Tablets (Frequent) ... 998
Geodon Capsules (Frequent) ... 2514
▲ Intron A for Injection (Less than 5%) ... 3038
Keppra Oral Solution (2%) ... 3307
Keppra Tablets (2%) ... 3307
Lamictal (Infrequent) ... 1449
Levaquin in 5% Dextrose Injection (0.1% to 0.9%) ... 2453
Levaquin (0.1% to 0.9%) ... 2453
Lipitor Tablets (Less than 2%) ... 2495
Lyrica Capsules (0.1% to 1%) ... 2524
Maxair Autohaler ... 1820
Maxalt Tablets (Rare) ... 1983
Maxalt-MLT Orally Disintegrating Tablets (Rare) ... 1983
Mebaral Tablets, USP (Less than 1 in 100 patients) ... 2483
Mirapex Tablets (Less than 1%) ... 889
Namenda (Infrequent) ... 1199
Nembutal Sodium Solution, USP (Less than 1%) ... 2484
▲ Neurontin Capsules (2.5% to 4.7%) ... 2498
▲ Neurontin Oral Solution (2.5% to 4.7%) ... 2498
▲ Neurontin Tablets (2.5% to 4.7%) ... 2498
Nipent for Injection (Less than 3%) ... 3216
Omnicef for Oral Suspension (0.2%) ... 506
▲ Orap Tablets (5.5%) ... 1220
OxyContin Tablets (Less than 1%) ... 2699
Paxil CR Controlled-Release Tablets (Infrequent) ... 1509
Paxil (Infrequent) ... 1501
Permax Tablets (Infrequent) ... 3357
Prevacid Delayed-Release Capsules (Less than 1%) ... 3268
Prevacid for Delayed-Release Oral Suspension (Less than 1%) ... 3268
Prevacid NapraPAC (Less than 1%) .. 3277
Prevacid SoluTab Delayed-Release Orally Disintegrating Tablets (Less than 1%) ... 3268
PREVPAC (Less than 1%) ... 3281
Protonix I.V. (Less than 1%) ... 3468
Protonix Tablets (Less than 1%) ... 3465
Proventil HFA Inhalation Aerosol (Less than 3%) ... 3071
Provigil Tablets (1%) ... 1002
Prozac Pulvules and Liquid (At least 2%) ... 1771
Pulmicort Respules (1% to 3%) ... 654
Razadyne ER Extended-Release Capsules (Infrequent) ... 2434
Razadyne (Infrequent) ... 2434
Relpax Tablets (Infrequent) ... 2531
Requip Tablets (2%) ... 1528
Reyataz Capsules (Less than 3%) ... 948
▲ Risperdal M-Tab Orally Disintegrating Tablets (17% to 34%) ... 1658
▲ Risperdal (17% to 34%) ... 1658
▲ Rituxan I.V. (1% to 5%) ... 1251
Sandostatin LAR Depot (1% to 4%) .. 2264
Seroquel Tablets (Infrequent) ... 691
Sonata Capsules (Infrequent) ... 1686
▲ Stalevo Tablets (5% to 10%) ... 2270
Symbyax Capsules (1% to 2%) ... 1788
Symmetrel (0.1% to 1%) ... 1115
Tasmar Tablets (2% to 3%) ... 3360
▲ Topamax Sprinkle Capsules (5%) ... 2438
▲ Topamax Tablets (5%) ... 2438
Trileptal Oral Suspension ... 2281
Trileptal Tablets ... 2281
Vantin Tablets and Oral Suspension (Less than 1%) ... 2650
Viracept (Less than 2%) ... 2556
Wellbutrin SR Sustained-Release Tablets (Infrequent) ... 1583
Wellbutrin XL Extended-Release Tablets (Infrequent) ... 1588
WinRho SDF ... 763
Zithromax Capsules, 250 mg (1% or less) ... 2568
Zithromax for Oral Suspension, 300 mg, 600 mg, 900 mg, 1200 mg (1% or less) ... 2561
Zithromax Tablets, 250 mg, 500 mg (1% or less) ... 2561
Zithromax Tri-Pak (1% or less) ... 2561
Zoloft (Infrequent to 2%) ... 2581
Zomig Tablets (Rare) ... 714
Zomig-ZMT Tablets (Rare) ... 714
Zonegran Capsules (Infrequent) ... 1089
Zyban Sustained-Release Tablets (Infrequent) ... 1620
▲ Zyprexa Tablets (5% to 11%) ... 1798
▲ Zyprexa ZYDIS Orally Disintegrating Tablets (5% to 11%) ... 1798
Zyrtec Chewable Tablets (Less than 2%) ... 2589
Zyrtec (Less than 2%) ... 2589
Zyrtec-D 12 Hour Extended Release Tablets (Less than 2%) ... 2591

Hyperlactemia

Zerit ... 971

Hyperlipemia

Abilify Tablets (Infrequent) ... 916
Abilify Tablets (Infrequent) ... 2472
Benicar HCT Tablets (Greater than 1%) ... 2852
Lunesta Tablets (Rare) ... 3139
Omacor Capsules ... 2735
Prevacid NapraPAC ... 3277
Prozac Pulvules and Liquid (Infrequent) ... 1771
Risperdal Consta Long-Acting Injection (Infrequent) ... 1664
Symbyax Capsules (Infrequent) ... 1788

Hyperlipidemia

Aciphex Tablets ... 1081
Ambien Tablets (Rare) ... 2867
Amerge Tablets (Rare) ... 1312
▲ Amnesteem Capsules (7%) ... 2126
▲ AndroGel (3% to 6%) ... 3330
▲ Arava Tablets (1% to 3%) ... 2881
Avelox (Less than 0.1%) ... 2984
Benicar Tablets (Greater than 0.5%) ... 2850
▲ BiDil Tablets (3%) ... 2161
▲ CellCept Capsules (3% to less than 20%) ... 2751
▲ CellCept Intravenous (3% to less than 20%) ... 2751
▲ CellCept Oral Suspension (3% to less than 20%) ... 2751
▲ CellCept Tablets (3% to less than 20%) ... 2751
Cymbalta Delayed-Release Capsules (Infrequent) ... 1729
▲ Diprivan Injectable Emulsion (Less than 1% to 10%) ... 676
Doxil Injection (Less than 1%) ... 3302
Effexor Tablets (Infrequent) ... 3405
Effexor XR Capsules (Infrequent) ... 3411
Evoxac Capsules (Less than 1%) ... 1042
Exelon Capsules (Infrequent) ... 2204
Gabitril Tablets (Infrequent) ... 998
Geodon Capsules (Rare) ... 2514
▲ Humatrope Vials and Cartridges (8.1%) ... 1756
▲ Humira Injection (7%) ... 464
Lovenox Injection (Rare) ... 2931
▲ Myfortic Tablets (3% to less than 20%) ... 2244
Namenda (More than one patient) ... 1199
Neurontin Capsules (Rare) ... 2498
Neurontin Oral Solution (Rare) ... 2498
Neurontin Tablets (Rare) ... 2498
▲ Norvir (1.7% to 4.1%) ... 499
Pletal Tablets (Less than 2%) ... 2478
Prevacid Delayed-Release Capsules ... 3268
Prevacid for Delayed-Release Oral Suspension ... 3268
Prevacid SoluTab Delayed-Release Orally Disintegrating Tablets ... 3268
PREVPAC ... 3281
▲ Prograf Capsules and Injection (3% to 15%) ... 624
Protonix I.V. (Greater than or equal to 1%) ... 3468
Protonix Tablets (Greater than or equal to 1%) ... 3465
▲ Rapamune Oral Solution and Tablets (38% to 57%) ... 3472
Rythmol SR Capsules ... 2736
Sandimmune ... 2259
Seroquel Tablets (Infrequent) ... 691
▲ Targretin Capsules (76.6% to 79.2%) ... 1719
▲ Thalomid Capsules (5.6% to 9.4%) ... 979
Topamax Sprinkle Capsules (Infrequent) ... 2438
Topamax Tablets (Infrequent) ... 2438
Uniretic Tablets (Less than 1%) ... 3114
Viracept (Less than 2%) ... 2556
Zyprexa Tablets (Rare) ... 1798
Zyprexa ZYDIS Orally Disintegrating Tablets (Rare) ... 1798

Hypermagnesemia

Doxil Injection (Less than 1%) ... 3302
VFEND I.V. (Less than 2%) ... 2543
VFEND Oral Suspension (Less than 2%) ... 2543
VFEND Tablets (Less than 2%) ... 2543
Zometa for Intravenous Infusion (2%) ... 2306

Hypermotility, gastrointestinal

Roferon-A Injection (Less than 1%) ... 2805

Hypernatremia

Abilify Tablets (Rare) ... 916
Abilify Tablets (Rare) ... 2472
Aloprim for Injection (Less than 1%) ... 2156
▲ AmBisome for Injection (4.1%) ... 615
Ammonul Injection ... 3323
Anadrol-50 Tablets ... 3329
Buphenyl Powder (1%) ... 3327
Buphenyl Tablets (1%) ... 3327
Doxil Injection (Less than 1%) ... 3302
Fleet Enema ... 1169
Fleet Phospho-soda ... 1170
Fleet Phospho-soda ACCU-PREP ... 1171
Fleet Prep Kits ... 1172
Invanz for Injection (0.1% to 1%) ... 1974
▲ Invirase (Less than 1% to 4%) ... 2776
Kristalose for Oral Solution ... 2149
Levaquin in 5% Dextrose Injection (0.1% to 0.9%) ... 2453
Levaquin (0.1% to 0.9%) ... 2453
Proleukin for Injection (1%) ... 1007
Timentin ADD-Vantage ... 1556
Timentin Injection Galaxy Container ... 1559
Timentin IV Infusion ... 1553
Timentin Pharmacy Bulk Package ... 1562
Topamax Sprinkle Capsules (Rare) ... 2438
Topamax Tablets (Rare) ... 2438
VFEND I.V. (Less than 2%) ... 2543
VFEND Oral Suspension (Less than 2%) ... 2543
VFEND Tablets (Less than 2%) ... 2543
Viagra Tablets (Less than 2%) ... 2552
Zegerid Powder for Oral Solution (1.7%) ... 2972
Zosyn ... 3492
Zyprexa Tablets (Rare) ... 1798
Zyprexa ZYDIS Orally Disintegrating Tablets (Rare) ... 1798

Hyperosmolarity

Diprivan Injectable Emulsion (Less than 1%) ... 676

Hyperostosis, skeletal

Accutane Capsules ... 2740
Amnesteem Capsules ... 2126
▲ Soriatane Capsules (Less than 1% to 25%) ... 1028

Hyperparathyroidism

Eskalith ... 1406
Lithobid Tablets ... 1670
Maxzide ... 2150
Prinzide Tablets ... 2033
Vaseretic Tablets ... 2073

Hyperperistalsis, intestinal

Camptosar Injection ... 2602

Hyperphenylalaninemia

Daraprim Tablets (Rare) ... 1385

Hyperphosphatemia

Aloprim for Injection (Less than 1%) ... 2156

AmBisome for Injection (Less common) 615
Anadrol-50 Tablets 3329
Buphenyl Powder (2%) 3327
Buphenyl Tablets (2%) 3327
Cancidas for Injection (0%) 1894
Delatestryl Injection 2976
Didronel Tablets 2693
Effexor Tablets (Rare) 3405
Effexor XR Capsules (Rare) 3411
Estratest Tablets 3196
Estratest H.S. Tablets 3196
Fleet Enema 1169
Fleet Phospho-soda 1170
Fleet Phospho-soda ACCU-PREP 1171
Fleet Prep Kits 1172
Hectorol Capsules 909
Hectorol Injection 911
▲ Myfortic Tablets (3% to less than 20%) 2244
Oxandrin Tablets 2977
Paxil CR Controlled-Release Tablets (Rare) 1509
Paxil (Rare) 1501
▲ Prograf Capsules and Injection (3% to 15%) 624
Proleukin for Injection (1%) 1007
▲ Rapamune Oral Solution and Tablets (3% to 20%) 3472
Requip Tablets (Infrequent) 1528
Risperdal M-Tab Orally Disintegrating Tablets (Rare) 1658
Risperdal (Rare) 1658
Rituxan for Infusion 845
▲ Roferon-A Injection (9%) 2805
Zithromax (Less than 1%) 2568
Zithromax for Oral Suspension, 300 mg, 600 mg, 900 mg, 1200 mg (Less than 1%) 2561
Zithromax Tablets, 250 mg, 500 mg (Less than 1%) 2561
Zithromax Tablets, 600 mg (Less than 1%) 2568
Zithromax Tri-Pak (Less than 1%) 2561
Zithromax Z-Pak (Less than 1%) 2568

Hyperpigmentation
Accutane Capsules 2740
Advicor Tablets 1694
Aldara Cream, 5% 1814
Amnesteem Capsules 2126
Avita Cream 2136
Avita Gel 2138
Blocadren Tablets 1891
▲ Catapres-TTS (5 of 101 patients) 875
Cipro I.V. (1% or less) 2998
Cipro I.V. Pharmacy Bulk Package (1% or less) 3509
Cipro (Less than 1%) 2991
Cipro XR Tablets 3004
Crixivan Capsules 1918
Decadron Phosphate Injection 1931
Depo-Medrol Single-Dose Vial 2617
Dovonex Ointment 0.005% (Less than 1%) 3375
Dovonex Scalp Solution 0.005% 3375
▲ Efudex (Among most frequent) 3348
Ellence Injection 2632
Ertaczo Cream, 2% 2383
Matulane Capsules 3188
▲ Myleran Tablets (5% to10%) 1492
Niaspan Extended-Release Tablets 1703
Purinethol Tablets 1222
Retin-A Micro 0.1%/0.04% 2388
Taxotere Injection Concentrate 2947
Tri-Luma Cream (18 occurrences in 27 patients) 1213
▲ Trisenox Injection (8%) 983

Hyperpigmentation, dermal creases
Adriamycin for Injection, USP (A few cases primarily in children) 786
Adriamycin Injection, USP (A few cases primarily in children) 786

Hyperpigmentation, nail beds
Adriamycin for Injection, USP (A few cases primarily in children) 786
Adriamycin Injection, USP (A few cases primarily in children) 786

Hyperplasia, endometrial
Premarin Tablets 3443

Hyperplasia, gingival
(*see under* Gingival hyperplasia)

Hyperplasia, mammary
Cuprimine Capsules (Rare) 1925

Hyperplasia, uterine
Depo-Provera Contraceptive Injection (Less than 1%) 2619
depo-subQ provera 104 Injectable Suspension 2622

Hyperpnea
Aggrenox Capsules (Less than 1%) 855
Bayer Aspirin Tablets 3515

Hyperprolactinemia
Aldoclor Tablets 1881
Aldoril Tablets 1884
Celexa 1177
Covera-HS Tablets (Less than 2%) 3135
Effexor Tablets 3405
Effexor XR Capsules 3411
Lexapro Oral Solution 1193
Lexapro Tablets 1193
Moban Tablets 1108
Niravam Orally Disintegrating Tablets 3106
Paxil CR Controlled-Release Tablets 1509
Paxil 1501
Prozac Pulvules and Liquid 1771
Risperdal Consta Long-Acting Injection (Infrequent) 1664
Risperdal M-Tab Orally Disintegrating Tablets 1658
Risperdal 1658
Rythmol SR Capsules 2736
Tarka Tablets 519
Verelan PM Capsules (2% or less) 3120
Xanax XR Tablets 2655
Zoloft 2581
Zyprexa Tablets 1798
Zyprexa ZYDIS Orally Disintegrating Tablets 1798

Hyperproteinemia
Evoxac Capsules 1042

Hyperprothrombinemia
AmBisome for Injection (Less common) 615
Avelox (Less than 0.1%) 2984
▲ Doxil Injection (1% to 10%) 3302
Estratest Tablets 3196
Estratest H.S. Tablets 3196
Rythmol SR Capsules 2736
Topamax Sprinkle Capsules (1%) 2438
Topamax Tablets (1%) 2438

Hyperpyrexia
(*see under* Fever)

Hyperreflexia
Abilify Tablets (Infrequent) 916
Abilify Tablets (Infrequent) 2472
▲ Aldurazyme for Intravenous Infusion (3%) 1261
Depacon Injection (1% or more) 412
Depakene (1% or more) 417
Depakote Sprinkle Capsules 422
▲ Depakote Tablets (1% to 5%) 427
Depakote ER Tablets (Greater than 1%) 433
Effexor Tablets (Rare) 3405
Effexor XR Capsules (Rare) 3411
Exelon Capsules (Infrequent) 2204
Gabitril Tablets (Infrequent) 998
Geodon Capsules (Rare) 2514
Invirase (Less than 2%) 2776
Keppra Oral Solution (2%) 3307
Keppra Tablets (2%) 3307
Lexapro Oral Solution (Infrequent) 1193
Lexapro Tablets (Infrequent) 1193
Neurontin Capsules (Frequent) 2498
Neurontin Oral Solution (Frequent) 2498
Neurontin Tablets (Frequent) 2498
Orap Tablets (Less frequent) 1220
Orthoclone OKT3 Sterile Solution 2370
Paxil CR Controlled-Release Tablets (Rare) 1509
Paxil (Rare) 1501
Prozac Pulvules and Liquid (Rare) 1771
Rescriptor Tablets 2535
Reyataz Capsules (Less than 3%) 948
Risperdal M-Tab Orally Disintegrating Tablets (Rare) 1658
Risperdal (Rare) 1658
Seromycin Capsules 1783
Sonata Capsules (Rare) 1686
Topamax Sprinkle Capsules (Infrequent) 2438
Topamax Tablets (Infrequent) 2438
Trileptal Oral Suspension 2281
Trileptal Tablets 2281
Zonegran Capsules (Infrequent) 1089

Hypersalivation
(*see under* Sialism)

Hypersecretion
Klonopin 2782

Hypersensitivity
▲ Alimta for Injection (Up to 8%) 1722
Alkeran for Injection 976
Amoxil Capsules 1315
Amoxil Chewable Tablets 1315
Amoxil Pediatric Drops for Oral Suspension 1315
Amoxil Powder for Oral Suspension 1315
Amoxil Tablets 1315
Aptivus Capsules (Less than 2%) 859
Betagan Ophthalmic Solution, USP .... ⊙217
Bleph-10 Ophthalmic Solution 10% .... ⊙219
Carteolol Hydrochloride Ophthalmic Solution USP, 1% .... ⊙246
Clindesse Vaginal Cream (Less than 1%) 3296
Clinoril Tablets (Less than 1%) 1899
Cubicin for Injection (Less than 1%) 1038
Daranide Tablets 1928
Decadron Phosphate Injection 1931
Demser Capsules (Rare) 1933
Dolobid Tablets (Less than 1 in 100) 1937
Elspar for Injection 1943
Estratest Tablets (Rare) 3196
Estratest H.S. Tablets (Rare) 3196
Flexeril Tablets 1832
Fluorescite Injection .... ⊙207
FML-S Liquifilm Sterile Ophthalmic Suspension .... ⊙226
Fortaz (Immediate in 1 in 285 patients) 1422
Hydrocortone Tablets 1963
Hyperstat I.V. Injection 3031
Imitrex Injection (Infrequent) 1431
Imitrex Nasal Spray (Rare) 1435
Imitrex Tablets (Frequent) 1440
Imodium Capsules 1834
Indocin (Less than 1%) 1968
Lacrisert Sterile Ophthalmic Insert 1979
Leukeran Tablets 1472
Micardis Tablets 884
Mustargen for Injection 2007
Nembutal Sodium Solution, USP 2484
Norflex Injection 1824
Noroxin Tablets (A few patients) 2009
Pediarix Vaccine 1518
Plavix Tablets 2942
Premarin Vaginal Cream 3449
PREVPAC 3281
Prinzide Tablets 2033
Rabies Vaccine RabAvert (Rare) 1011
Recombivax HB 2045
Ritalin Hydrochloride Tablets 2254
Ritalin LA Capsules 2255
Ritalin-SR Tablets 2254
Rocephin Injectable Vials, ADD-Vantage, Galaxy, Bulk 2801
Rosac Cream with Sunscreens (Rare) 3216
Seromycin Capsules 1783
Thyrolar 1203
Timoptic in Ocudose (Less frequent) 2061
Timoptic Sterile Ophthalmic Solution (Less frequent) 2058
TobraDex Ophthalmic Ointment (Less than 4%) 558
TobraDex Ophthalmic Suspension (Less than 4%) 558
Viramune Oral Suspension 903
Viramune Tablets 903
Zantac (Rare) 1597
Zantac Injection (Rare) 1593
Zantac Injection Pharmacy Bulk Package (Rare) 1595
Zantac Syrup (Rare) 1597
Zinacef Injection (Fewer than 1%) 1604
Zinacef for Injection (Fewer than 1%) 1604
▲ Zylet Ophthalmic Suspension (Less than 4%) 3508

Hypersensitivity at injection site
Amevive (Less than 1%) 836
▲ Betaseron for SC Injection (3%) 791
Bexxar 1360
HibTITER 3419

Hypersensitivity reactions, Arthus-type
Adacel Vaccine 2959
Boostrix 1366
Pediarix Vaccine 1518
Rabies Vaccine RabAvert 1011

Hypersensitivity reactions, general
Accolate Tablets 663
Advair Diskus 100/50 1291
Advair Diskus 250/50 1291
Advair Diskus 500/50 1291
Alferon N Injection 1640
Alkeran Tablets 977
Altace Capsules (Less than 1%) 1673
Altoprev Extended-Release Tablets (Rare) 1151
Aminohippurate Sodium "PAH" Injection 1886
Ancef for Injection 1318
Antara Capsules 2723
Antivenin (Black Widow Spider Antivenin) 1887
Asacol Delayed-Release Tablets (Some patients) 2688
Atrovent HFA Inhalation Aerosol 872
Augmentin 1331
Augmentin Tablets 1334
Augmentin XR Extended-Release Tablets 1340
Augmentin ES-600 Powder for Oral Suspension 1337
Axid Oral Solution (Rare) 913
Beconase AQ Nasal Spray (Rare) 1359
Benicar HCT Tablets 2852
▲ Betimol Ophthalmic Solution (More than 5%) .... ⊙283
▲ Betimol Ophthalmic Solution (More than 5%) 3371
Bexxar 1360
Carafate Suspension 727
Carafate Tablets 728
Carimune NF 3501
Ceftin 1369
Cialis Tablets 1806
Cipro 2991
Cipro XR Tablets (Rare) 3004
Clarinex Syrup (Rare) 3009
Clarinex-D 24-Hour Extended-Release Tablets 3012
Cleocin Vaginal Ovules 2613
Clozapine Tablets 2141
Clozaril Tablets 2174
Comvax 1904
Coumadin for Injection (Infrequent) 932
Coumadin Tablets (Infrequent) 932
Cozaar Tablets 1913
Crestor Tablets (Less than 1%) 672
Didronel Tablets 2693
Digibind for Injection 1388
Faslodex Injection (Less than 1%) 682
FazaClo Orally Disintegrating Tablets 547
Ferrlecit Injection 3379
Flovent HFA (Rare) 1418
Flumist Vaccine 1872
Focalin XR Capsules 2217
Fosamax 1949
Fosamax Plus D Tablets 1956
Furosemide Tablets 2117
Gammagard Liquid 751
Gonal-f RFF Pen for Injection 3155
Grifulvin V Tablets Microsize and Oral Suspension Microsize 2384
Humira Injection 464
Hyzaar 1964
Inderal LA Long-Acting Capsules 3421
Infanrix Vaccine 1444
Infed Injection 3381
Kytril Injection (Rare) 2785
Kytril Tablets (Rare) 2788
Lescol Capsules (Rare) 2227
Lescol Capsules (Rare) 2730
Lescol XL Tablets (Rare) 2227
Lescol XL Tablets (Rare) 2730
Levothroid Tablets 1189
Lidoderm Patch 1107
Maxzide 2150
Mebaral Tablets, USP (Less than 1 in 100 patients) 2483
Mephyton Tablets 1993
Mevacor Tablets (Rare) 1996
Mylotarg for Injection 3429
Neumega for Injection 3433
Nimbex Injection 494
Nubain Injection (1% or less) 1111
Oncaspar (Greater than 1% but less than 5%) 1123
Orthoclone OKT3 Sterile Solution 2370
Polytrim Ophthalmic Solution (Multiple reports) 570
Propecia Tablets 2036
Proscar Tablets 2040
Rapamune Oral Solution and Tablets 3472
▲ Raptiva for Injection (8%) 1247
Remicade for IV Injection 987

ReoPro Vials 1779
Repronex for Intramuscular and Subcutaneous Injection (Some patients) 1148
Singulair 2047
Skelaxin Tablets 1685
Sular Tablets (Very rare) 1163
Synagis (Rare) 1868
▲ Taxotere Injection Concentrate (Up to 33.3%) 2947
Tessalon Capsules 1202
Tessalon Perles 1202
Timoptic-XE Sterile Ophthalmic Gel Forming Solution 2062
Trasylol Injection 779
Trecator Tablets (Rare) 3482
Trileptal Oral Suspension 2281
Trileptal Tablets 2281
Trizivir Tablets 1565
Univasc Tablets (Less than 1%) 3118
▲ Valcyte Tablets (Less than 5%) 2816
Viracept 2556
Visudyne for Injection (Less than 1%) 2286
Vytorin 10/10 Tablets 2084
Vytorin 10/10 Tablets 3092
Vytorin 10/20 Tablets 2084
Vytorin 10/20 Tablets 3092
Vytorin 10/40 Tablets 2084
Vytorin 10/40 Tablets 3092
Vytorin 10/80 Tablets 2084
Vytorin 10/80 Tablets 3092
▲ Xeloda Tablets (Less than 5%) 2825
Xifaxan Tablets 2847
Zelnorm Tablets 2303
Zenapax for Injection 2838
Zetia Tablets 2090
Zetia Tablets 3098
▲ Ziagen (2% to 9%) 1600
Zocor Tablets (Rare) 2078
Zofran Injection (Rare) 1607
Zoladex (Rare) 709
Zoladex 3-month (Rare) 712
Zomig Nasal Spray (Rare) 718
Zomig Tablets (Rare) 714
Zosyn (1% or less) 3492

Hypersensitivity reactions, multi-organ

▲ Epzicom Tablets (2% to 9%) 1402
Tegretol/Tegretol-XR 2278

Hypersensitivity vasculitis

Aldoclor Tablets 1881
Aldoril Tablets 1884
Clinoril Tablets (Less than 1 in 100) 1899
Dolobid Tablets (Less than 1 in 100) 1937
Lovenox Injection (Rare) 2931
PREVPAC 3281
Tagamet Tablets (Rare) 1547

Hypersomnia

Abilify Tablets (Infrequent) 916
Abilify Tablets (Infrequent) 2472
Aloxi Injection (Less than 1%) 2099
Maxalt Tablets (Rare) 1983
Maxalt-MLT Orally Disintegrating Tablets (Rare) 1983
Permax Tablets 3357
Prinivil Tablets (0.3% to 1.0%) 2029
Prinzide Tablets 2033
Xanax XR Tablets (1.3%) 2655
Zestoretic Tablets 701
Zestril Tablets (0.3% to 1.0%) 704

Hypersplenism

Flolan for Injection 1408

Hypertension

▲ Abelcet Injection (5%) 1119
Abilify Tablets (2%) 916
Abilify Tablets (2%) 2472
Aciphex Tablets 1081
Actiq (Less than 1%) 993
Activase I.V. 1225
Activella Tablets 2311
▲ Actonel Tablets (4.9% to 5.8%) 2679
▲ Actonel with Calcium Tablets (4.9% to 10%) 2684
Adderall Tablets 3168
Adderall XR Capsules 3169
Adenocard Injection 612
Adenoscan (Less than 1%) 613
Adipex-P 1216
Aerobid/Aerobid-M (1% to 3%) 1172
Agrylin Capsules (1% to 5%) 3172
Alacol DM Syrup 739
Albalon Ophthalmic Solution ⊙216
Aldara Cream, 5% (1.4%) 1814
Alesse-28 Tablets 3392
▲ Alimta for Injection (3% to 11%) 1722
Alinia for Oral Suspension (Less than 1%) 2840
Alinia Tablets (Less than 1%) 2840
Aloprim for Injection (Less than 1%) 2156
Aloxi Injection (Less than 1%) 2099
▲ Alphagan P Ophthalmic Solution (Approximately 5% to 9%) 563
Alupent Inhalation Aerosol (Less frequent) 858
Ambien Tablets (Infrequent) 2867
▲ AmBisome for Injection (7.9% to 19.8%) 615
Amerge Tablets (Infrequent) 1312
Ammonul Injection 3323
Anaprox Tablets (Less than 1%) 2769
Anaprox DS Tablets (Less than 1%) 2769
▲ Angiomax for Injection (6%) 1856
Antara Capsules 2723
Anzemet Injection (2.9%) 2871
Anzemet Tablets (2.2%) 2874
▲ Aranesp for Injection (3.7% to 23%) 576
▲ Arava Tablets (10%) 2881
▲ Aredia for Injection (Up to at least 15%) 2168
Aricept Tablets (Frequent) 1086
Aricept ODT Tablets (Frequent) 1086
▲ Arimidex Tablets (2% to 9%) 665
Arixtra Injection (2.4%) 1325
▲ Aromasin Tablets (5%) 2600
Arthrotec Tablets (Rare) 3126
Astelin Nasal Spray (Infrequent) 1876
Atrovent Inhalation Solution (0.9%) 868
Avalide Tablets 922
Avalide Tablets 2889
Avapro Tablets (Less than 1%) 925
Avapro Tablets (Less than 1%) 2886
▲ Avastin IV (12% to 34%) 1229
Avelox (0.1% to less than 2%) 2984
Avinza Capsules (Less than 5%) 1714
Axert Tablets (Rare) 2430
Balamine DM 739
▲ Betaseron for SC Injection (7%) 791
Betimol Ophthalmic Solution (1% to 5%) ⊙283
Betimol Ophthalmic Solution (1% to 5%) 3371
▲ Boniva Tablets (6.3% to 7.3%) 2747
Bravelle for Intramuscular or Subcutaneous Injection (2.7%) 1140
Brimonidine Tartrate Ophthalmic Solution 0.2% (Less than 3%) ⊙245
Buprenex Injectable (Less than 1%) 2718
Caduet Tablets (Less than 2%) 2507
Calcijex Injection 411
▲ Campath Ampules (2% to 11%) 826
Campral Tablets (Frequent) 1175
Cancidas for Injection (1.1% to 1.8%) 1894
Carbatrol Capsules 3174
Cardene I.V. (0.7%) 1129
▲ Carnitor Injection (18% to 12%) 3185
▲ Casodex Tablets (5%) 670
Cataflam Tablets (Occasionally) 2173
Catapres-TTS (0.5% or less) 875
Caverject Impulse Injection (2%) 2610
Celexa (Infrequent) 1177
▲ CellCept Capsules (28.2% to 77.5%) 2751
▲ CellCept Intravenous (28.2% to 77.5%) 2751
▲ CellCept Oral Suspension (28.2% to 77.5%) 2751
▲ CellCept Tablets (28.2% to 77.5%) 2751
Cenestin Tablets, 0.3mg 1063
Cialis Tablets (Less than 2%) 1806
Cipro I.V. (1% or less) 2998
Cipro I.V. Pharmacy Bulk Package (1% or less) 3509
Cipro (Less than 1%) 2991
Cipro XR Tablets 3004
Climara Transdermal System 795
▲ Climara Pro Transdermal System (3.3%) 800
Clinoril Tablets (Less than 1%) 1899
▲ Clolar for Intravenous Infusion (11%) 1264
▲ Clozapine Tablets (4%) 2141
▲ Clozaril Tablets (4%) 2174
Colazal Capsules 2845
CombiPatch Transdermal System 2180
Combivent Inhalation Aerosol (Less than 2%) 878
Concerta Extended-Release Tablets 1828
Copaxone for Injection (Frequent) 3292
▲ Coreg Tablets (Greater than 1% to 3%) 1376
Cosopt Sterile Ophthalmic Solution (1% to 5%) 1910
Crestor Tablets (Greater than or equal to 2%) 672
Cubicin for Injection (1.1%) 1038
Cytovene (1% or less) 2763
DDAVP Injection 4 mcg/mL (Infrequent) 2893
Decadron Phosphate Injection 1931
Decadron Tablets 1929
▲ Depacon Injection (1% to 5%) 412
Depakene (1% or more) 417
▲ Depakote Sprinkle Capsules (1% to 5%) 422
▲ Depakote Tablets (1% to 5%) 427
Depakote ER Tablets (Greater than 1%) 433
▲ DepoDur Extended-Release Injection (2% to 5%) 1098
Depo-Medrol Injectable Suspension 2615
Depo-Medrol Single-Dose Vial 2617
Desmopressin Acetate Injection (Infrequent) 1143
Desmopressin Acetate Rhinal Tube (Infrequent) 1144
Desoxyn Tablets, USP 2482
Detrol Tablets (1.5%) 2626
Dexedrine 1386
DextroStat Tablets 3177
Dilaudid 439
Dilaudid Oral Liquid 443
Dilaudid Non-Sterile Powder 439
Dilaudid Rectal Suppositories 439
Dilaudid Tablets 439
Dilaudid Tablets - 8 mg 443
Dilaudid-HP (Less frequent) 441
▲ Diprivan Injectable Emulsion (Less than 1% to 8%) 676
▲ Ditropan XL Extended Release Tablets (2% to less than 5%) 2391
Dolobid Tablets 1937
Doxil Injection (Less than 1%) 3302
▲ Duragesic Transdermal System (1% to 3%) 2448
EC-Naprosyn Delayed-Release Tablets (Less than 1%) 2769
Ecotrin Enteric Coated Aspirin Low, Regular and Maximum Strength Tablets 1627
Edex Injection (2%) 3103
▲ Effexor Tablets (1.1% to 4.5%) 3405
▲ Effexor XR Capsules (4% to 5%) 3411
Eldepryl Capsules 3209
Eligard 22.5 mg (Less than 2%) 2899
Emcyt Capsules 3137
Emend Capsules (Greater than 0.5%) 1944
Enablex Extended-Release Tablets (Greater than or equal to 1%) 2201
Enbrel for Injection (Infrequent) 580
▲ Entocort EC Capsules (Less than 5%) 2694
▲ Epogen for Injection (0.75% to 24%) 586
Equetro Extended-Release Capsules 3178
Estratest Tablets (Common) 3196
Estratest H.S. Tablets (Common) 3196
Estrogel 0.06% 3200
Ethyol for Injection 1869
Eulexin Capsules (1%) 3023
Evoxac Capsules (Less than 1%) 1042
▲ Exelon Capsules (3%) 2204
▲ Fabrazyme for Intravenous Infusion (3%) 1267
▲ FazaClo Orally Disintegrating Tablets (4%) 547
▲ Femara Tablets (5% to 8%) 2210
▲ Ferrlecit Injection (0.6% to 23%) 3379
Flexeril Tablets (Rare) 1832
Floxin Otic Singles (Reported in a single subject) 1045
Floxin Otic Solution (Single report) 1043
Flumadine (Less than 0.3%) 1186
Focalin Tablets 2214
Focalin XR Capsules 2217
Foradil Aerolizer 3024
▲ Forteo for Injection (7.1%) 1739
▲ Fortical Nasal Spray (1% to 3%) 3336
Gabitril Tablets (Frequent) 998
Gammagard S/D (Occasional) 754
Garamycin Injectable 3028
Gemzar for Injection (2%) 1743
▲ Gengraf Capsules (25% to 50%) 458
▲ Geodon (3%) 2514
Gleevec Tablets (Infrequent) 2221
GlucaGen for Injection 790
Hectorol Capsules 909
Hectorol Injection 911
Herceptin I.V. 1234
▲ Humatrope Vials and Cartridges (2.7% to 7.7%) 1756
▲ Humira Injection (5%) 464
Hycomine Compound Tablets 1105
Hycotuss Expectorant Syrup 1106
Hydrocortone Tablets 1963
▲ Imdur Tablets (Less than or equal to 5%) 3032
Imitrex Injection (Infrequent) 1431
Imitrex Nasal Spray (Infrequent) 1435
Imitrex Tablets (Infrequent) 1440
Indocin Capsules (Less than 1%) 1968
Indocin I.V. (Less than 1%) 1973
Indocin (Less than 1%) 1968
Infed Injection 3381
▲ Infergen (2% to 5%) 1647
▲ Intron A for Injection (Less than 5% to 9%) 3038
Invanz for Injection (0.7% to 1.6%) 1974
Invirase (Less than 2%) 2776
▲ I.V. Busulfex (7% to 36%) 1125
Iveegam EN (0.3% to 0.8%) 759
Kadian Capsules (Less than 3%) 572
Kaletra (Less than 2%) 474
▲ Kepivance (7% to 14%) 592
Kogenate FS 3517
Kytril Injection (2%) 2785
Kytril Tablets (1%) 2788
Lamictal (Rare) 1449
Lariam Tablets (Infrequent) 2790
▲ Leukine (25% to 34%) 829
Levaquin in 5% Dextrose Injection (0.1% to 0.9%) 2453
Levaquin (0.1% to 0.9%) 2453
Levitra Tablets (Less than 2%) 3048
Levothroid Tablets 1189
Levoxyl Tablets 1680
Lexapro Oral Solution (Frequent) 1193
Lexapro Tablets (Frequent) 1193
Lipitor Tablets (Less than 2%) 2495
Lofibra Capsules 1217
Lo/Ovral-28 Tablets 3423
Lotronex Tablets (Rare) 1479
Lunesta Tablets (Frequent) 3139
Maxalt Tablets (Infrequent) 1983
Maxalt-MLT Orally Disintegrating Tablets (Infrequent) 1983
▲ Megace ES Oral Suspension (0% to 8%) 2492
Menostar Transdermal System 805
Meridia Capsules (2.1%) 485
Merrem I.V. (Greater than 0.1% to 1%) 687
Metadate CD Capsules 3316
Metrogel 1% (1.1%) 1212
Miacalcin Nasal Spray (1% to 3%) 2242
Micardis Tablets (1%) 884
Micardis HCT Tablets 886
Migranal Nasal Spray (Rare) 3350
Mirapex Tablets (1% or more) 889
▲ Mirena Intrauterine System (5% or more) 810
Mobic Oral Suspension (Less than 2%) 893
Mobic Tablets (Less than 2%) 893
MS Contin Tablets (Less frequent) 2703
Mycamine for Injection (0.6%) 620
▲ Myfortic Tablets (3% to less than 20%) 2244
▲ Mylotarg for Injection (13% to 17%) 3429
▲ Namenda (4%) 1199
Naprosyn Suspension (Less than 1%) 2769
Naprosyn Tablets (Less than 1%) 2769
Narcan Injection 1109
▲ Naropin Injection (1% to 5%) 640
Navelbine Injection 1494
▲ Neoral Soft Gelatin Capsules (25% to 50%) 2247
▲ Neoral Oral Solution (Approximately 25% to 50% most patients) 2247
▲ Neupogen for Injection (4%) 598
Neurontin Capsules (Frequent) 2498
Neurontin Oral Solution (Frequent) 2498
Neurontin Tablets (Frequent) 2498
Nexium Delayed-Release Capsules (Less than 1%) 645
Nexium I.V. (Less than 1%) 649
Nicoderm CQ Patch 1629
NicoDerm CQ Clear Patch ▣627
▲ Nicotrol Inhaler (Greater than 3%) 2594
Nimotop Capsules (Less than 1%) 774
Nipent for Injection (Less than 3%) 3216
▲ Norditropin Cartridges (8%) 2318
NovoSeven (Greater than or equal to 2%) 2335
Nubain Injection (1% or less) 1111
Omacor Capsules 2735
Omnicef Capsules 506
Omnicef for Oral Suspension 506
Oncaspar (Less than 1%) 1123
▲ Ontak Vials (6%) 1717
OptiPranolol Metipranolol Ophthalmic Solution 0.3% (A small number of patients) ⊙254
Orap Tablets 1220

Ortho-Cept Tablets 2395
Ortho-Cyclen Tablets 2414
Ortho Evra Transdermal System 2402
Ortho Tri-Cyclen Tablets 2414
Ortho Tri-Cyclen Lo Tablets 2421
▲ Orthoclone OKT3 Sterile Solution (8%) 2370
Parcopa Orally Disintegrating Tablets 3111
Paxil CR Controlled-Release Tablets (Frequent) 1509
Paxil (Frequent) 1501
Pediapred Oral Solution 3319
Pegasys 2793
Permax Tablets (1.6%) 3357
Phenergan 3438
▲ Photofrin for Injection (37% to 6%) 729
▲ Plavix Tablets (4.3%) 940
▲ Plavix Tablets (4.3%) 2942
Pletal Tablets (2% or greater) 2478
Prandin Tablets (0.5, 1, and 2 mg) (Less than or equal to 1%) 2337
Prefest Tablets 1069
Premarin Intravenous 3440
Premarin Tablets 3443
Premarin Vaginal Cream 3449
Premphase Tablets 3452
Prempro Tablets 3452
Prevacid Delayed-Release Capsules (Less than 1%) 3268
Prevacid for Delayed-Release Oral Suspension (Less than 1%) 3268
Prevacid NapraPAC (Less than 1%) 3277
Prevacid SoluTab Delayed-Release Orally Disintegrating Tablets (Less than 1%) 3268
PREVPAC (Less than 1%) 3281
Prilosec OTC Tablets (Less than 1%) 2674
▲ Procrit for Injection (0.75% to 24%) 2374
▲ Prograf Capsules and Injection (Common; 38% to 47%) 624
Prometrium Capsules (100 mg, 200 mg) (Less than 5%) 3205
Propine Ophthalmic Solution ⊙ 237
Protonix I.V. (Less than 1%) 3468
Protonix Tablets (Less than 1%) 3465
Protopic Ointment (Greater than or equal to 1%) 629
▲ Proventil Inhalation Aerosol (Less than 5%) 3067
Proventil Inhalation Solution 0.083% (1% to 3.1%) 3069
Proventil HFA Inhalation Aerosol 3071
▲ Provigil Tablets (3%) 1002
Prozac Pulvules and Liquid (Frequent) 1771
▲ Rapamune Oral Solution and Tablets (39% to 49%) 3472
Razadyne ER Extended-Release Capsules (Greater than or equal to 2%) 2434
Razadyne (Greater than or equal to 2%) 2434
Relafen Tablets (Less than 1%) 1523
Relpax Tablets (Infrequent) 2531
▲ Remicade for IV Injection (7%) 987
▲ Renagel Tablets (10.1%) 1268
▲ Requip Tablets (5%) 1528
Rescriptor Tablets 2535
Revatio Tablets 2541
Reyataz Capsules (Less than 3%) 948
▲ Rilutek Tablets (3.3% to 6.8%) 2945
▲ Risperdal Consta Long-Acting Injection (3%) 1664
▲ Risperdal M-Tab Orally Disintegrating Tablets (Infrequent to 3%) 1658
▲ Risperdal (Infrequent to 3%) 1658
Rituxan for Infusion (0.3%) 845
▲ Rituxan I.V. (6%) 1251
▲ Roferon-A Injection (11%) 2805
Rythmol SR Capsules 2736
▲ Sandimmune (13% to 53%) 2259
Sandostatin Injection (Less than 1%) 2263
▲ Sandostatin LAR Depot (5% to 15%) 2264
Seasonale Tablets 1073
▲ Sensipar Tablets (7%) 603
Serevent Diskus 1540
▲ Simulect for Injection (Greater than or equal to 10%) 2268
▲ Somavert Injection (8%) 2648
Sonata Capsules (Infrequent) 1686
St. Joseph 81 mg Aspirin Chewable and Enteric Coated Tablets 1841
Stalevo Tablets 2270
Strattera Capsules 1784
Striant Mucoadhesive 1022
Sular Tablets (Less than or equal to 1%) 1163
Suprane Liquid for Inhalation (Greater than 1%) 770
Surmontil Capsules 2347
Symbyax Capsules (2%) 1788
Symmetrel (0.1% to 1%) 1115
Tambocor Tablets (Less than 1%) 1824
Targretin Capsules 1719
Tasmar Tablets (Infrequent) 3360
Taxotere Injection Concentrate (Rare) 2947
Tegretol/Tegretol-XR 2278
Tequin Injection (Less than 0.1%) 964
Tequin Tablets (Less than 0.1%) 964
Testim 1% Gel (1%) 722
Thalomid Capsules 979
▲ Thymoglobulin for Injection (36.6%) 2848
Thyrolar 1203
Timoptic in Ocudose (Less frequent) 2061
Timoptic Sterile Ophthalmic Solution (Less frequent) 2058
Timoptic-XE Sterile Ophthalmic Gel Forming Solution 2062
Topamax Sprinkle Capsules (1% to 2%) 2438
Topamax Tablets (1% to 2%) 2438
▲ Trasylol Injection (4%) 779
Travatan Ophthalmic Solution (1% to 5%) 559
▲ Trelstar Depot (3.6%) 3385
▲ Trelstar LA Suspension (4%) 3387
Tricor Tablets 523
Triglide Tablets 1165
Trileptal Oral Suspension 2281
Trileptal Tablets 2281
Triphasil-28 Tablets 3483
▲ Trisenox Injection (10%) 983
▲ Tygacil for Injection (4.9%) 3489
Ultane Liquid for Inhalation (2%) 526
Ultracet Tablets (Less than 1%) 2462
Unithroid Tablets 3521
▲ Urso 250 Tablets (8.3%) 737
▲ Urso Forte Tablets (8.3%) 737
Valtrex Caplets 1573
Vantin Tablets and Oral Suspension (Less than 1%) 2650
Ventolin HFA Inhalation Aerosol 1576
Verelan PM Capsules (1.7%) 3120
▲ Vesanoid Capsules (11%) 2823
VESIcare Tablets (0.5% to 1.4%) 631
VFEND I.V. (Less than 2%) 2543
VFEND Oral Suspension (Less than 2%) 2543
VFEND Tablets (Less than 2%) 2543
Viadur Implant (Rare) 782
Viagra Tablets 2552
▲ Visudyne for Injection (1% to 10%) 2286
Vivactil Tablets 2350
Vivelle Transdermal System 2288
Vivelle-Dot Transdermal System 2293
Voltaren Tablets (Occasionally) 2298
Voltaren-XR Tablets (Occasionally) 2301
VoSpire Extended-Release Tablets 2352
▲ Wellbutrin Tablets (4.3%) 1579
Wellbutrin SR Sustained-Release Tablets (At least 1%) 1583
Wellbutrin XL Extended-Release Tablets (At least 1%) 1588
Xeloda Tablets 2825
Xopenex HFA Inhalation Aerosol 3151
Xopenex Inhalation Solution 3143
Xopenex Inhalation Solution Concentrate 3147
Yasmin 28 Tablets 818
▲ Zegerid Powder for Oral Solution (7.9%) 2972
Zemuron Injection (0.1%; 2%) 2363
▲ Zenapax for Injection (Greater than 5%) 2838
▲ Zestril Tablets (5.7%) 704
▲ Zoladex (Occasional) 709
Zoladex 3-month (Occasional) 712
Zoloft (Infrequent) 2581
Zomig Nasal Spray (Infrequent) 718
Zomig Tablets (Infrequent) 714
Zomig-ZMT Tablets (Infrequent) 714
Zonegran Capsules (Infrequent) 1089
Zosyn (1.3% to 1.6%) 3492
Zyban Sustained-Release Tablets (1% to 2.5%) 1620
Zyprexa Tablets 1798
Zyprexa ZYDIS Orally Disintegrating Tablets 1798
Zyrtec Chewable Tablets (Less than 2%) 2589
Zyrtec (Less than 2%) 2589
Zyrtec-D 12 Hour Extended Release Tablets (Less than 2%) 2591
Zyvox 2661

Hypertension, aggravation

Ambien Tablets (Rare) 2867
Atrovent Inhalation Solution (0.9%) 868
Brimonidine Tartrate Ophthalmic Solution 0.2% ⊙ 245
Carbatrol Capsules 3174
Celebrex Capsules (0.1% to 1.9%) 3130
Dolobid Tablets 1937
Equetro Extended-Release Capsules 3178
Ethyol for Injection 1869
Evoxac Capsules (Less than 1%) 1042
Micardis Tablets 884
▲ Myfortic Tablets (3% to less than 20%) 2244
Sandostatin LAR Depot (1% to 4%) 2264
Tegretol/Tegretol-XR 2278
Ultracet Tablets (Less than 1%) 2462
▲ Zenapax for Injection (Greater than 5%) 2838
Zoloft (Rare) 2581

Hypertension, intracranial

Aclovate 1290
Cutivate Cream 1381
Cutivate Ointment 1384
Cytovene 2763
Diprivan Injectable Emulsion (Less than 1%) 676
Diprolene Gel 0.05% 3015
Diprolene Lotion 0.05% 3016
Diprolene Ointment 0.05% (Some patients) 3017
Dynacin Tablets 1859
Elocon Cream 0.1% 3019
Elocon Ointment 0.1% 3021
Entocort EC Capsules (Three cases) 2694
Genotropin Lyophilized Powder (A small number of patients) 2642
Humatrope Vials and Cartridges 1756
Increlex Injection (3 subjects) 3290
Lithobid Tablets 1670
Lotrisone Cream 3054
Lyrica Capsules (Rare) 2524
Permax Tablets (Rare) 3357
▲ Vesanoid Capsules (9%) 2823
VFEND I.V. (Less than 2%) 2543
VFEND Oral Suspension (Less than 2%) 2543
VFEND Tablets (Less than 2%) 2543

Hypertension, portal

Invirase (Rare) 2776
Myleran Tablets 1492
Tabloid Tablets 1545

Hypertension, rebound

Nitro-Dur Transdermal Infusion System (Uncommon) 3060

Hypertension, supine

▲ ProAmatine Tablets (7.3%) 3183

Hypertensive crises

Avalide Tablets 922
Avalide Tablets 2889
Avapro Tablets (Less than 1%) 925
Avapro Tablets (Less than 1%) 2886
Avastin IV 1229
Imitrex Injection (Rare) 1431
Rythmol SR Capsules 2736
Sanctura Tablets 1133

Hyperthermia

Biltricide Tablets 2990
Calcijex Injection 411
Cogentin Injection 1903
Effexor Tablets 3405
Elspar for Injection 1943
Hectorol Capsules 909
Hectorol Injection 911
HyperRAB 3239
HyperRho S/D Full Dose 3243
HyperRho S/D Mini-Dose 3241
HyperTET 3245
MICRhoGAM Ultra-Filtered 2429
Risperdal M-Tab Orally Disintegrating Tablets 1658
Risperdal 1658

Hyperthyroidism

Abilify Tablets (Rare) 916
Abilify Tablets (Rare) 2472
Aciphex Tablets 1081
▲ Arava Tablets (1% to 3%) 2881
Avonex 839
Betaseron for SC Injection 791
Campath Ampules 826
Copaxone for Injection (Infrequent) 3292
Copegus Tablets (Less than 1%) 2759
Cytomel Tablets 1678
Effexor Tablets (Rare) 3405
Effexor XR Capsules (Rare) 3411
Eskalith (Rare) 1406
Flolan for Injection 1408
Fortical Nasal Spray (Less than 1%) 3336
▲ Intron A for Injection (Less than 5%) 3038
Levoxyl Tablets 1680
Lithobid Tablets 1670
Meridia Capsules 485
Miacalcin Nasal Spray (Less than 1%) 2242
Neurontin Capsules (Rare) 2498
Neurontin Oral Solution (Rare) 2498
Neurontin Tablets (Rare) 2498
▲ Ontak Vials (Less than 5%) 1717
▲ Pacerone Tablets (1% to 3%) 3337
Paxil CR Controlled-Release Tablets (Rare) 1509
Paxil (Rare) 1501
Pegasys (Less than 1%) 2793
PEG-Intron Powder for Injection (Less than or equal to 1%) 3062
Proleukin for Injection 1007
Requip Tablets (Infrequent) 1528
Roferon-A Injection (Infrequent) 2805
Seroquel Tablets (Rare) 691
Synthroid Tablets (Rare) 515
Tenormin I.V. Injection 698
Tenormin Tablets 695
Unithroid Tablets 3521
VFEND I.V. (Less than 2%) 2543
VFEND Oral Suspension (Less than 2%) 2543
VFEND Tablets (Less than 2%) 2543
Zomig Nasal Spray (Rare) 718

Hypertonia

Abilify Tablets 916
Abilify Tablets 2472
Aceon Tablets (2 mg, 4 mg, 8 mg) (0.2% to 2.7%) 3191
Aciphex Tablets 1081
Actonel Tablets (2.2%) 2679
Actonel with Calcium Tablets (2.2%) 2684
Adalat CC Tablets (Less than 1%) 2978
Antara Capsules 2723
Aricept Tablets (Infrequent) 1086
Aricept ODT Tablets (Infrequent) 1086
▲ Arimidex Tablets (3%) 665
Arthrotec Tablets (Rare) 3126
▲ Asacol Delayed-Release Tablets (5%) 2688
Avelox (Less than 0.1%) 2984
Avonex 839
Axert Tablets (Rare) 2430
Azopt Ophthalmic Suspension (Less than 1%) 553
▲ Betaseron for SC Injection (50%) 791
▲ Botox Purified Neurotoxin Complex (2% to 10%) 565
Caduet Tablets (Less than 2%) 2507
Cardene I.V. (Rare) 1129
Carnitor Injection (1% to 3%) 3185
▲ Casodex Tablets (2% to 5%) 670
Celebrex Capsules (0.1% to 1.9%) 3130
Celexa (Infrequent) 1177
▲ CellCept Capsules (3% to less than 20%) 2751
▲ CellCept Intravenous (3% to less than 20%) 2751
▲ CellCept Oral Suspension (3% to less than 20%) 2751
▲ CellCept Tablets (3% to less than 20%) 2751
▲ Cenestin Tablets, 0.45mg, 0.625mg, 0.9mg, 1.25mg (6%) 1063
Cipro I.V. 2998
Cipro I.V. Pharmacy Bulk Package 3509
Cipro 2991
Cipro XR Tablets 3004
Colazal Capsules 2845
Combunox Tablets (Less than 2%) 1183
▲ Copaxone for Injection (22%) 3292
Crestor Tablets (Greater than or equal to 2%) 672
▲ Depacon Injection (1% to 5%) 412
▲ Depakene (1% to 5%) 417
▲ Depakote Sprinkle Capsules (1% to 5%) 422
▲ Depakote Tablets (1% to 5%) 427
▲ Depakote ER Tablets (1% to 5%) 433
Diprivan Injectable Emulsion (Less than 1%) 676
▲ Doxil Injection (1% to 10%) 3302
Duragesic Transdermal System (Less than 1%) 2448
▲ Effexor Tablets (3%; Infrequent) 3405
Effexor XR Capsules (Infrequent) 3411
Eskalith 1406
▲ Evoxac Capsules (1% to 3%) 1042

Exelon Capsules (Infrequent) ... 2204
Ferrlecit Injection (Two or more patients) ... 3379
Flexeril Tablets (Less than 1%) ... 1832
Frova Tablets (Rare) ... 1101
Gabitril Tablets (Frequent) ... 998
▲ Geodon (3% to 14%) ... 2514
Havrix Vaccine (Less than 1%) ... 1425
▲ Hectorol Capsules (Greater than or equal to 5%) ... 909
Indapamide Tablets (Less than 5%) .. 2119
▲ Infergen (6% to 7%) ... 1647
▲ Intron A for Injection (Less than 5%) ... 3038
Kaletra (Less than 2%) ... 474
Klonopin (Infrequent) ... 2782
Lamictal (Rare) ... 1449
Levaquin in 5% Dextrose Injection (0.1% to 0.9%) ... 2453
Levaquin (0.1% to 0.9%) ... 2453
Levitra Tablets (Less than 2%) ... 3048
Lexapro Oral Solution (Infrequent) ... 1193
Lexapro Tablets (Infrequent) ... 1193
Lipitor Tablets (Less than 2%) ... 2495
Lithobid Tablets ... 1670
Lofibra Capsules ... 1217
Lotensin Tablets (Less than 1%) ... 2232
Lotensin HCT Tablets (1.5%) ... 2235
Lunesta Tablets (Infrequent) ... 3139
Lyrica Capsules (Greater than or equal to 1%) ... 2524
Meridia Capsules (Greater than or equal to 1%) ... 485
Mirapex Tablets (Greater than or equal to 1%) ... 889
Namenda (Infrequent) ... 1199
Neurontin Capsules (Rare) ... 2498
Neurontin Oral Solution (Rare) ... 2498
Neurontin Tablets (Rare) ... 2498
Nexium Delayed-Release Capsules (Less than 1%) ... 645
Nexium I.V. (Less than 1%) ... 649
Norvasc Tablets (Less than or equal to 0.1%) ... 2529
Paxil CR Controlled-Release Tablets (Infrequent) ... 1509
Paxil (Infrequent) ... 1501
▲ PEG-Intron Powder for Injection (5%) ... 3062
Permax Tablets (1.1%) ... 3357
▲ Premphase Tablets (3%) ... 3452
▲ Prempro Tablets (3% to 4%) ... 3452
Prevacid Delayed-Release Capsules (Less than 1%) ... 3268
Prevacid for Delayed-Release Oral Suspension (Less than 1%) ... 3268
Prevacid NapraPAC (Less than 1%) .. 3277
Prevacid SoluTab Delayed-Release Orally Disintegrating Tablets (Less than 1%) ... 3268
PREVPAC (Less than 1%) ... 3281
▲ Prograf Capsules and Injection (3% to 15%) ... 624
Prometrium Capsules (100 mg, 200 mg) (Less than 5%) ... 3205
Protonix I.V. (Greater than or equal to 1%) ... 3468
Protonix Tablets (Greater than or equal to 1%) ... 3465
Provigil Tablets (1%) ... 1002
Prozac Pulvules and Liquid (Infrequent) ... 1771
▲ Rapamune Oral Solution and Tablets (3% to 20%) ... 3472
Razadyne ER Extended-Release Capsules (Infrequent) ... 2434
Razadyne (Infrequent) ... 2434
▲ Rebif Prefilled Syringe for Injection (6% to 7%) ... 3163
Relpax Tablets (Frequent) ... 2531
ReoPro Vials (0.2%) ... 1779
Requip Tablets (Infrequent) ... 1528
Rescriptor Tablets ... 2535
▲ Rilutek Tablets (5.3% to 5.9%) ... 2945
Risperdal Consta Long-Acting Injection (Frequent) ... 1664
▲ Risperdal M-Tab Orally Disintegrating Tablets (17% to 34%) ... 1658
▲ Risperdal (17% to 34%) ... 1658
▲ Rituxan for Infusion (1% to 5%) ... 845
▲ Rituxan I.V. (1% to 5%) ... 1251
Rythmol SR Capsules ... 2736
Sandostatin LAR Depot (1% to 4%) .. 2264
Seroquel Tablets (Frequent) ... 691
Sonata Capsules (1%) ... 1686
▲ Soriatane Capsules (1% to 10%) ... 1028
Sular Tablets (Less than or equal to 1%) ... 1163
Symmetrel ... 1115
Synercid I.V. (Less than 1%) ... 1690
Tasmar Tablets (1%) ... 3360
Tequin Injection (Less than 0.1%) ... 964
Tequin Tablets (Less than 0.1%) ... 964
Thalomid Capsules ... 979
▲ Topamax Sprinkle Capsules (0% to 3%) ... 2438
▲ Topamax Tablets (0% to 3%) ... 2438
Tricor Tablets ... 523
Ultane Liquid for Inhalation (Less than 1%) ... 526
Ultracet Tablets (Less than 1%) ... 2462
Uniretic Tablets (More than 1%) ... 3114
VFEND I.V. (Less than 2%) ... 2543
VFEND Oral Suspension (Less than 2%) ... 2543
VFEND Tablets (Less than 2%) ... 2543
Viagra Tablets (Less than 2%) ... 2552
Vicoprofen Tablets (Less than 3%) ... 533
Wellbutrin SR Sustained-Release Tablets (Infrequent) ... 1583
Wellbutrin XL Extended-Release Tablets (Infrequent) ... 1588
Zoladex (1%) ... 709
Zoladex 3-month ... 712
Zoloft (Frequent) ... 2581
Zomig Nasal Spray (Rare to infrequent) ... 718
Zomig Tablets (Rare) ... 714
Zomig-ZMT Tablets (Rare) ... 714
Zonegran Capsules (Infrequent) ... 1089
Zyban Sustained-Release Tablets (Infrequent) ... 1620
▲ Zyprexa Tablets (4% to 20%) ... 1798
▲ Zyprexa ZYDIS Orally Disintegrating Tablets (4% to 20%) ... 1798
Zyrtec Chewable Tablets (Less than 2%) ... 2589
Zyrtec (Less than 2%) ... 2589
Zyrtec-D 12 Hour Extended Release Tablets (Less than 2%) ... 2591

Hypertrichosis

Analpram-HC ... 1136
Celexa (Rare) ... 1177
Clobevate Gel ... 3213
Cutivate Ointment (Less than 1%) ... 1384
Decadron Tablets ... 1929
Diprolene Lotion 0.05% (Infrequent) ... 3016
Diprolene Ointment 0.05% (Infrequent) ... 3017
Diprolene AF Cream 0.05% (Infrequent) ... 3014
Diprosone Cream, USP 0.05% ... 3018
Elocon Cream 0.1% (Infrequent) ... 3019
Elocon Lotion 0.1% (Infrequent) ... 3020
Elocon Ointment 0.1% (Infrequent) ... 3021
Finacea Gel (Rare) ... 1644
▲ Gengraf Capsules (6.6% to 15%) ... 458
Locoid Cream (Infrequent) ... 1138
Locoid Lipocream Cream (Infrequent) ... 1138
Locoid (Infrequent) ... 1138
Lotrisone ... 3054
▲ Neoral Soft Gelatin Capsules (6.6% to 15%) ... 2247
▲ Neoral Oral Solution (6.6% to 15%) ... 2247
Olux Foam ... 1027
Pandel Cream, 0.1% ... 1017
Phenytek Capsules ... 2153
Pramosone ... 1139
ProctoFoam-HC ... 3113
Risperdal M-Tab Orally Disintegrating Tablets (Rare) ... 1658
Risperdal (Rare) ... 1658
▲ Simulect for Injection (3% to 10%) ... 2268
Soriatane Capsules (Less than 1%) .. 1028
Temovate Gel (Infrequent) ... 1550
Temovate Scalp Application (Infrequent) ... 1551
Temovate E Emollient (Infrequent) ... 1552
Topamax Sprinkle Capsules (2%) ... 2438
Topamax Tablets (2%) ... 2438
Topicort .05% Gel ... 3288
Topicort .25% Cream ... 3288
Topicort .25% Ointment ... 3288
Topicort LP .05% Cream ... 3288
U-cort 1% Cream ... 3289
Vanos Cream ... 1864
Zoloft (Rare) ... 2581
Zyrtec Chewable Tablets (Less than 2%) ... 2589
Zyrtec (Less than 2%) ... 2589
Zyrtec-D 12 Hour Extended Release Tablets (Less than 2%) ... 2591

Hypertriglyceridemia

Accutane Capsules ... 2740
Aceon Tablets (2 mg, 4 mg, 8 mg) (1.3%) ... 3191
▲ Agenerase Capsules (8% to 13%) ... 1299
▲ Agenerase Oral Solution (8% to 13%) ... 1304
Alesse-28 Tablets ... 3392
▲ Amnesteem Capsules (25%) ... 2126
▲ AndroGel (3% to 6%) ... 3330
▲ Aptivus Capsules (6.1% to 26.2%) .. 859
Atacand Tablets (0.5% or greater) ... 634
Atacand HCT ... 637
Benicar HCT Tablets ... 2852
Betaseron for SC Injection ... 791
Blocadren Tablets ... 1891
Carbatrol Capsules (Occasional) ... 3174
Cenestin Tablets, 0.45mg, 0.625mg, 0.9mg, 1.25mg ... 1063
Cenestin Tablets, 0.3mg ... 1063
▲ Cipro I.V. (Among most frequent) ... 2998
▲ Cipro I.V. Pharmacy Bulk Package (Among most frequent) ... 3509
Cipro ... 2991
Climara Transdermal System ... 795
Climara Pro Transdermal System ... 800
Clozaril Tablets (Rare) ... 2174
CombiPatch Transdermal System ... 2180
Coreg Tablets (Greater than 0.1% to 1%) ... 1376
Crixivan Capsules ... 1918
Cymbalta Delayed-Release Capsules (Infrequent) ... 1729
Cytovene ... 2763
Edex Injection (2%) ... 3103
▲ Emtriva Capsules (9% to 10%) ... 1272
Epzicom Tablets ... 1402
Equetro Extended-Release Capsules ... 3178
Estratest Tablets ... 3196
Estratest H.S. Tablets ... 3196
Estrogel 0.06% ... 3200
Evoxac Capsules (Less than 1%) ... 1042
Fuzeon Injection ... 2772
▲ Gengraf Capsules (About 15%) ... 458
Hyzaar ... 1964
▲ Infergen (5% to 6%) ... 1647
▲ Inspra Tablets (1% to 15%) ... 2520
▲ Intron A for Injection (Less than 5%) ... 3038
▲ Kaletra (9% to 36%) ... 474
Lo/Ovral-28 Tablets ... 3423
Lovenox Injection ... 2931
▲ Lupron Depot 3.75 mg (12%) ... 3257
▲ Lupron Depot–3 Month 11.25 mg (32%) ... 3262
Menostar Transdermal System ... 805
▲ Neoral Soft Gelatin Capsules (About 15%) ... 2247
▲ Neoral Oral Solution (About 15%) ... 2247
Noroxin Tablets ... 2009
▲ Norvir (1.3% to 33.6%) ... 499
Ortho-Cyclen/Ortho Tri-Cyclen ... 2414
Ortho Tri-Cyclen Lo Tablets ... 2421
▲ Pegasys (20%) ... 2793
PEG-Intron Powder for Injection ... 3062
Prefest Tablets ... 1069
Premarin Tablets ... 3443
Premarin Vaginal Cream ... 3449
Premphase Tablets ... 3452
Prempro Tablets ... 3452
Prinzide Tablets ... 2033
Rapamune Oral Solution and Tablets ... 3472
Rebetron Combination Therapy ... 3078
Rescriptor Tablets ... 2535
Risperdal M-Tab Orally Disintegrating Tablets (Rare) ... 1658
Risperdal (Rare) ... 1658
Roferon-A Injection ... 2805
Rythmol SR Capsules ... 2736
▲ Simulect for Injection (3% to 10%) ... 2268
Soriatane Capsules (Less common) ... 1028
Sustiva Capsules ... 957
▲ Targretin Capsules (Approximately 70%) ... 1719
Tegretol/Tegretol-XR (Occasional) ... 2278
Teveten Tablets (1%) ... 1707
Teveten HCT Tablets (Less than 1%) ... 1710
Ticlid Tablets ... 2813
Timolide Tablets ... 2056
Triphasil-28 Tablets ... 3483
Trizivir Tablets ... 1565
▲ Truvada Tablets (1% to 12%) ... 1279
Vaseretic Tablets ... 2073
▲ Vesanoid Capsules (Up to 60%) ... 2823
▲ Viread Tablets (8% to 11%) ... 1284
Vivelle Transdermal System ... 2288
Vivelle-Dot Transdermal System ... 2293
WelChol Tablets ... 2855
▲ Xeloda Tablets (Less than 5%) ... 2825
Zestoretic Tablets ... 701
▲ Ziagen (6%) ... 1600
Zoladex ... 709
Zoladex 3-month ... 712
▲ Zoloft (Approximately 5%) ... 2581
Zyprexa Tablets (Rare) ... 1798
Zyprexa IntraMuscular (Rare) ... 1798
Zyprexa ZYDIS Orally Disintegrating Tablets (Rare) ... 1798

Hypertrophic papillae of the tongue

Primaxin I.M. ... 2022
Primaxin I.V. (Less than 0.2%) ... 2024

Hypertrophy, gum

Amnesteem Capsules ... 2126
Peganone Tablets, USP (Rare) ... 2487

Hypertrophy, thymus

▲ Increlex (Greater than or equal to 5%) ... 3290

Hypertrophy, unspecified

Kaletra (Less than 2%) ... 474

Hyperuricemia

Abelcet Injection ... 1119
Abilify Tablets (Infrequent) ... 916
Abilify Tablets (Infrequent) ... 2472
Accutane Capsules ... 2740
Aceon Tablets (2 mg, 4 mg, 8 mg) (0.3% to 1%) ... 3191
Advicor Tablets ... 1694
Aldoclor Tablets ... 1881
Aldoril Tablets ... 1884
Aloprim for Injection (Less than 1%) ... 2156
Altace Capsules ... 1673
Amnesteem Capsules ... 2126
Antara Capsules ... 2723
Arthrotec Tablets (Rare) ... 3126
Atacand Tablets (0.6%) ... 634
Atacand HCT (0.5% or greater) ... 637
Avalide Tablets ... 922
Avalide Tablets ... 2889
Avelox (Less than 0.1%) ... 2984
Axid Oral Solution ... 913
Benicar Tablets (Greater than 0.5%) ... 2850
▲ Benicar HCT Tablets (4%) ... 2852
Betaseron for SC Injection ... 791
Blocadren Tablets ... 1891
Buphenyl Powder (2%) ... 3327
Buphenyl Tablets (2%) ... 3327
Campral Tablets (Infrequent) ... 1175
Cardizem LA Extended Release Tablets (Less than 2%) ... 1699
▲ CellCept Capsules (3% to less than 20%) ... 2751
▲ CellCept Intravenous (3% to less than 20%) ... 2751
▲ CellCept Oral Suspension (3% to less than 20%) ... 2751
▲ CellCept Tablets (3% to less than 20%) ... 2751
Cerubidine for Injection ... 788
▲ Cipro I.V. (Among most frequent) ... 2998
▲ Cipro I.V. Pharmacy Bulk Package (Among most frequent) ... 3509
Cipro (Less than 0.1%) ... 2991
Clorpres Tablets ... 2139
Clozapine Tablets ... 2141
Clozaril Tablets ... 2174
▲ Coreg Tablets (Greater than 1% to 3%) ... 1376
Creon 5 Capsules ... 3195
Creon 10 Capsules ... 3195
Creon 20 Capsules ... 3196
Daranide Tablets ... 1928
Diovan HCT Tablets ... 2195
Diuril Oral ... 1936
Diuril Sodium Intravenous ... 1934
▲ Doxil Injection (1% to 5%) ... 3302
Dyazide Capsules ... 1389
Ecotrin Enteric Coated Aspirin Low, Regular and Maximum Strength Tablets ... 1627
Edecrin ... 1941
Effexor Tablets (Infrequent) ... 3405
Effexor XR Capsules (Infrequent) ... 3411
Ellence Injection ... 2632
Evoxac Capsules (Less than 1%) ... 1042
FazaClo Orally Disintegrating Tablets ... 547
Furosemide Tablets ... 2117
Gengraf Capsules (1% to less than 3%) ... 458
Geodon Capsules (Rare) ... 2514
Hyzaar ... 1964
▲ Imdur Tablets (Less than or equal to 5%) ... 3032
Indapamide Tablets (Less than 5%) .. 2119
Inspra Tablets (0.3%) ... 2520
▲ Kaletra (Up to 3%) ... 474
Lofibra Capsules ... 1217
Lotensin HCT Tablets ... 2235
Lotrel Capsules (Rare) ... 2238
Lupron Depot 7.5 mg (Greater than or equal to 5%) ... 3261
Lupron Injection Pediatric ... 3256

▲ Mavik Tablets (15%) 482
Maxzide 2150
Micardis HCT Tablets 886
Moduretic Tablets 2003
▲ Myfortic Tablets (3% to less than 20%) 2244
Myleran Tablets 1492
Neoral Soft Gelatin Capsules (1% to less than 3%) 2247
Neoral Oral Solution (1% to less than 3%) 2247
▲ Neulasta Injection (8%) 596
▲ Neupogen for Injection (27% to 58%) 598
Nexium Delayed-Release Capsules (Less than 1%) 645
Nexium I.V. (Less than 1%) 649
▲ Norvir (3.8%) 499
Oncaspar (Greater than 1% but less than 5%) 1123
Pancrease MT Capsules 1839
▲ PEG-Intron Powder for Injection (33% to 38%) 3062
Permax Tablets (Rare) 3357
Plavix Tablets (1% to 2.5%) 940
Plavix Tablets (1% to 2.5%) 2942
Pletal Tablets (Less than 2%) 2478
Prinzide Tablets 2033
▲ Prograf Capsules and Injection (3% to 15%) 624
▲ Proleukin for Injection (9%) 1007
Prozac Pulvules and Liquid (Rare) 1771
Purinethol Tablets 1222
Rapamune Oral Solution and Tablets 3472
▲ Rebetol (33% to 38%) 3073
Rebetron Combination Therapy 3078
Relafen Tablets (Less than 1%) 1523
Requip Tablets (Infrequent) 1528
Rescriptor Tablets 2535
Risperdal Consta Long-Acting Injection (Infrequent) 1664
Risperdal M-Tab Orally Disintegrating Tablets (Rare) 1658
Risperdal (Rare) 1658
Rituxan for Infusion 845
▲ Roferon-A Injection (10%) 2805
Rythmol SR Capsules 2736
Sandimmune (Occasional) 2259
▲ Simulect for Injection (Greater than or equal to 10%) 2268
Sonata Capsules (Rare) 1686
St. Joseph 81 mg Aspirin Chewable and Enteric Coated Tablets 1841
Starlix Tablets 2276
Tabloid Tablets (Frequent) 1545
Teveten HCT Tablets 1710
Thalomid Capsules 979
Tiazac Capsules (Less than 2%) 1204
Timolide Tablets 2056
Tricor Tablets 523
Triglide Tablets 1165
Ultrase Capsules 735
Ultrase MT Capsules 736
Uniretic Tablets (More than 1%) 3114
Univasc Tablets 3118
Vaseretic Tablets 2073
VFEND I.V. (Less than 2%) 2543
VFEND Oral Suspension (Less than 2%) 2543
VFEND Tablets (Less than 2%) 2543
Viagra Tablets (Less than 2%) 2552
Viokase 738
Viracept (Less than 2%) 2556
Zestoretic Tablets 701
Zyprexa Tablets (Infrequent) 1798
Zyprexa ZYDIS Orally Disintegrating Tablets (Infrequent) 1798

Hyperuricosuria
Creon 5 Capsules 3195
Creon 10 Capsules 3195
Creon 20 Capsules 3196
Myleran Tablets 1492
Pancrease MT Capsules 1839
Purinethol Tablets 1222
Ultrase Capsules 735
Ultrase MT Capsules 736

Hyperuricuria
Viokase 738

Hyperventilation
Aciphex Tablets 1081
Actiq (Less than 1%) 993
Adenocard Injection (Less than 1%) 612
AmBisome for Injection (Less common) 615
Ammonul Injection 3323
Aricept Tablets (Infrequent) 1086
Aricept ODT Tablets (Infrequent) 1086
Arthrotec Tablets (Rare) 3126
Axert Tablets (Rare) 2430
Clozapine Tablets (Less than 1%) 2141
Clozaril Tablets (Less than 1%) 2174
Copaxone for Injection (Frequent) 3292
Diprivan Injectable Emulsion (Less than 1%) 676
Doxil Injection (Less than 1%) 3302
Effexor Tablets (Infrequent) 3405
Effexor XR Capsules (Infrequent) 3411
FazaClo Orally Disintegrating Tablets (Less than 1%) 547
Frova Tablets (Infrequent) 1101
Gabitril Tablets (Infrequent) 998
▲ I.V. Busulfex (2% to 3%) 1125
Lamictal (Infrequent) 1449
Neurontin Capsules (Rare) 2498
Neurontin Oral Solution (Rare) 2498
Neurontin Tablets (Rare) 2498
▲ Niravam Orally Disintegrating Tablets (9.7%) 3106
Orthoclone OKT3 Sterile Solution 2370
Paxil CR Controlled-Release Tablets (Infrequent) 1509
Paxil (Infrequent) 1501
Permax Tablets (Infrequent) 3357
Primaxin I.M. 2022
Primaxin I.V. (Less than 0.2%) 2024
Prochieve 4% Gel 1018
Prochieve 8% Gel 1018
ProSom Tablets (Rare) 512
Prozac Pulvules and Liquid (Infrequent) 1771
Relpax Tablets (Rare) 2531
Rilutek Tablets (Infrequent) 2945
Risperdal M-Tab Orally Disintegrating Tablets (Infrequent) 1658
Risperdal (Infrequent) 1658
Seroquel Tablets (Rare) 691
Sonata Capsules (Rare) 1686
Sulfamylon Cream 2154
Sulfamylon for 5% Topical Solution 2155
Symbyax Capsules (Infrequent) 1788
Tasmar Tablets (Infrequent) 3360
Tequin Injection (Less than 0.1%) 964
Tequin Tablets (Less than 0.1%) 964
▲ TOBI Solution for Inhalation (5.4%) 1015
Ultane Liquid for Inhalation (Less than 1%) 526
▲ Xanax XR Tablets (8.5%) 2655
Zoloft (Rare) 2581
Zomig Nasal Spray (Rare) 718
Zyprexa Tablets (Infrequent) 1798
Zyprexa ZYDIS Orally Disintegrating Tablets (Infrequent) 1798
Zyrtec Chewable Tablets (Less than 2%) 2589
Zyrtec (Less than 2%) 2589
Zyrtec-D 12 Hour Extended Release Tablets (Less than 2%) 2591

Hypervolemia
Aloprim for Injection (Less than 1%) 2156
▲ AmBisome for Injection (8.2% to 12.2%) 615
▲ Carnitor Injection (3% to 12%) 3185
▲ CellCept Capsules (3% to less than 20%) 2751
▲ CellCept Intravenous (3% to less than 20%) 2751
▲ CellCept Oral Suspension (3% to less than 20%) 2751
▲ CellCept Tablets (3% to less than 20%) 2751
▲ Coreg Tablets (Greater than 1% to 3%) 1376
Ferrlecit Injection 3379
I.V. Busulfex 1125
Merrem I.V. (Greater than 0.1% to 1%) 687
▲ Prograf Capsules and Injection (3% to 15%) 624
▲ Rapamune Oral Solution and Tablets (3% to 20%) 3472
Trasylol Injection (1% to 2%) 779
VFEND I.V. (Less than 2%) 2543
VFEND Oral Suspension (Less than 2%) 2543
VFEND Tablets (Less than 2%) 2543

Hypesthesia
(*see under* Hypoesthesia)

Hypnagogic effects
▲ Advair Diskus 100/50 (1% to 3%) 1291
▲ Advair Diskus 250/50 (1% to 3%) 1291
▲ Advair Diskus 500/50 (1% to 3%) 1291
Lotronex Tablets (Infrequent) 1479

Hypoactivity
Aerobid/Aerobid-M (1% to 3%) 1172
▲ Flumist Vaccine (10.6 to 14%) 1872

Hypoacusis
Buphenyl Powder 3327
Buphenyl Tablets 3327
▲ Increlex Injection (Greater than or equal to 5%) 3290
VFEND I.V. (Less than 2%) 2543
VFEND Oral Suspension (Less than 2%) 2543
VFEND Tablets (Less than 2%) 2543

Hypoadrenalism
Sandostatin Injection (Less than 1%) 2263
Sandostatin LAR Depot (Rare) 2264

Hypoadrenalism, neonatal
Azmacort Inhalation Aerosol 1701
Decadron Phosphate Injection 1931
Decadron Tablets 1929
Hydrocortone Tablets 1963
Pulmicort Respules 654

Hypoalbuminemia
Baraclude (0% to less than 1%) 928
▲ Buphenyl Powder (11%) 3327
▲ Buphenyl Tablets (11%) 3327
Campath Ampules 826
▲ Cancidas for Injection (4.6% to 8.6%) 1894
Dapsone Tablets USP 1656
Evista Tablets 1735
▲ Leukine (27%) 829
Lupron Depot 7.5 mg (Greater than or equal to 5%) 3261
Oncaspar 1123
▲ Ontak Vials (83%) 1717
▲ Proleukin for Injection (8%) 1007
Vantin Tablets and Oral Suspension 2650
Zosyn 3492

Hypoalbuminuria
Elspar for Injection 1943
Invanz for Injection (0.9% to 1.7%) 1974

Hypocalcemia
Abelcet Injection 1119
Actiq (Less than 1%) 993
Actonel Tablets (0.8%) 2679
Actonel with Calcium Tablets (0.8%) 2684
Aloprim for Injection (Less than 1%) 2156
▲ AmBisome for Injection (4.9% to 18.4%) 615
▲ Ammonul Injection (3%) 3323
▲ Aredia for Injection (Up to 12%) 2168
Betaseron for SC Injection 791
Cancidas for Injection (0% to 1.9%) 1894
▲ CellCept Capsules (3% to 30%) 2751
▲ CellCept Intravenous (3% to 30%) 2751
▲ CellCept Oral Suspension (3% to 30%) 2751
▲ CellCept Tablets (3% to 30%) 2751
Cenestin Tablets, 0.45mg, 0.625mg, 0.9mg, 1.25mg 1063
Cenestin Tablets, 0.3mg 1063
Climara Transdermal System 795
Climara Pro Transdermal System 800
Colazal Capsules 2845
CombiPatch Transdermal System 2180
Cosmegen for Injection 1907
▲ Doxil Injection (1% to 5%) 3302
Equetro Extended-Release Capsules 3178
Estratest Tablets 3196
Estratest H.S. Tablets 3196
Estrogel 0.06% 3200
Ethyol for Injection (Rare) 1869
Evista Tablets 1735
Fleet Enema 1169
Fleet Phospho-soda 1170
Fleet Phospho-soda ACCU-PREP 1171
Fleet Prep Kits 1172
▲ Fosamax (Approximately 18%) 1949
▲ Fosamax Plus D Tablets (18%) 1956
Frova Tablets (Rare) 1101
Furosemide Tablets 2117
Garamycin Injectable 3028
Geodon Capsules (Rare) 2514
▲ Invirase (Less than 1% to 4%) 2776
▲ I.V. Busulfex (3% to 49%) 1125
Leukine (2%) 829
▲ Mavik Tablets (4.7%) 482
Maxipime for Injection (Greater than 0.1% to less than 1%) 1093
Menostar Transdermal System 805
Mycamine for Injection (1.2% to 1.9%) 620
▲ Myfortic Tablets (3% to less than 20%) 2244
▲ Mylotarg for Injection (10% to 12%) 3429
Omnicef for Oral Suspension (0.5%) 506
▲ Ontak Vials (17%) 1717
Paxil CR Controlled-Release Tablets (Rare) 1509
Paxil (Rare) 1501
Precose Tablets 776
Premarin Tablets 3443
Premarin Vaginal Cream 3449
Premphase Tablets 3452
Prempro Tablets 3452
▲ Prograf Capsules and Injection (3% to 15%) 624
▲ Proleukin for Injection (11%) 1007
Prozac Pulvules and Liquid (Rare) 1771
▲ Rapamune Oral Solution and Tablets (3% to 20%) 3472
Rescriptor Tablets 2535
Rituxan for Infusion 845
▲ Roferon-A Injection (28%) 2805
▲ Simulect for Injection (3% to 10%) 2268
Targretin Capsules 1719
Tegretol-XR Tablets 2278
Thalomid Capsules 979
Topamax Sprinkle Capsules (Infrequent) 2438
Topamax Tablets (Infrequent) 2438
Trileptal Oral Suspension 2281
Trileptal Tablets 2281
▲ Trisenox Injection (10%) 983
Tygacil for Injection (0% to less than 2%) 3489
Uniretic Tablets (Less than 1%) 3114
▲ Valcyte Tablets (Less than 5%) 2816
VFEND I.V. (Less than 2%) 2543
VFEND Oral Suspension (Less than 2%) 2543
VFEND Tablets (Less than 2%) 2543
Vivelle Transdermal System 2288
Vivelle-Dot Transdermal System 2293
Xeloda Tablets (2.3%) 2825
▲ Zometa for Intravenous Infusion (0.6% to less than 15%) 2306
Zosyn 3492

Hypochloremia
▲ CellCept Capsules (3% to less than 20%) 2751
▲ CellCept Intravenous (3% to less than 20%) 2751
▲ CellCept Oral Suspension (3% to less than 20%) 2751
▲ CellCept Tablets (3% to less than 20%) 2751
Doxil Injection (Less than 1%) 3302
Dyazide Capsules 1389
Geodon Capsules (Rare) 2514
Indapamide Tablets (Less than 5%) 2119
Maxzide 2150
Requip Tablets (Rare) 1528
Uniretic Tablets (Less than 1%) 3114

Hypochloremic alkalosis
Diuril Sodium Intravenous 1934
Furosemide Tablets 2117
Maxzide 2150
Prinzide Tablets 2033
Teveten HCT Tablets 1710
Vaseretic Tablets 2073
Zestoretic Tablets 701

Hypocholesterolemia
Evista Tablets 1735
Geodon Capsules (Rare) 2514
Prevacid Delayed-Release Capsules 3268
Prevacid for Delayed-Release Oral Suspension 3268
Prevacid NapraPAC 3277
Prevacid SoluTab Delayed-Release Orally Disintegrating Tablets 3268
PREVPAC 3281
Proleukin for Injection (1%) 1007
▲ Simulect for Injection (Greater than or equal to 10%) 2268
Topamax Sprinkle Capsules (Rare) 2438
Topamax Tablets (Rare) 2438

Hypoesthesia
Abilify Tablets (Infrequent) 916
Abilify Tablets (Infrequent) 2472
Actiq (1% or greater) 993
Adalat CC Tablets (Less than 1%) 2978
Alinia for Oral Suspension (Less than 1%) 2840
Alinia Tablets (Less than 1%) 2840
Ambien Tablets (Infrequent) 2867
Amerge Tablets (Rare) 1312
▲ Aromasin Tablets (2% to 5%) 2600
Arthrotec Tablets (Rare) 3126
Astelin Nasal Spray (Infrequent) 1876

Atacand HCT (0.5% or greater) 637
Avelox (Less than 0.1%) 2984
Caduet Tablets (Greater than 0.1% to less than 2%) 2507
Campral Tablets (Infrequent) 1175
Cardene I.V. (0.7%) 1129
Caverject Impulse Injection (Less than 1%) 2610
Celebrex Capsules (0.1% to 1.9%) 3130
Celexa (Infrequent) 1177
Cialis Tablets (Less than 2%) 1806
Cipro I.V. 2998
Cipro I.V. Pharmacy Bulk Package 3509
Cipro 2991
Cipro XR Tablets 3004
Clindesse Vaginal Cream (Less than 1%) 3296
Colazal Capsules 2845
Copaxone for Injection (At least 2%) 3292
▲ Coreg Tablets (Greater than 1% to 3%) 1376
▲ Cozaar Tablets (Less than 1% to 5%) 1913
Cymbalta Delayed-Release Capsules (Infrequent) 1729
Denavir Cream (0.9%) 2163
Depacon Injection (0.6%) 412
Depakene 417
Depakote Sprinkle Capsules 422
Depakote Tablets 427
Depakote ER Tablets 433
▲ DepoDur Extended-Release Injection (2% to 5%) 1098
Effexor Tablets 3405
Engerix-B Vaccine 1391
▲ Evoxac Capsules (1% to 3%) 1042
Exelon Capsules (Infrequent) 2204
Factive Tablets (Rare) 2464
Ferrlecit Injection 3379
▲ Flolan for Injection (1% to 12%) 1408
Floxin Otic Singles (Reported in a single subject) 1045
Floxin Otic Solution (Single report) 1043
Flumadine 1186
Frova Tablets (Infrequent) 1101
Gabitril Tablets (Frequent) 998
Gengraf Capsules (1% to less than 3%) 458
Geodon Capsules (2%) 2514
▲ Humatrope Vials and Cartridges (Up to 6.25%) 1756
Hyzaar 1964
▲ Imdur Tablets (Less than or equal to 5%) 3032
▲ Infergen (8% to 10%) 1647
▲ Intron A for Injection (Up to 10%) 3038
Invanz for Injection (Greater than 0.1%) 1974
Kadian Capsules (Less than 3%) 572
▲ Kepivance (12%) 592
Klonopin (Infrequent) 2782
Lamictal (Infrequent) 1449
Levaquin in 5% Dextrose Injection (0.1% to 0.9%) 2453
Levaquin (0.1% to 0.9%) 2453
Levitra Tablets (Less than 2%) 3048
Lidoderm Patch 1107
Lipitor Tablets (Less than 2%) 2495
Lotensin HCT Tablets (0.3% or more) 2235
Lotronex Tablets (Rare) 1479
Lunesta Tablets (Infrequent) 3139
Lupron Depot 3.75 mg 3257
Lupron Depot–3 Month 11.25 mg 3262
Lyrica Capsules (Greater than or equal to 1%) 2524
Maxalt Tablets (Frequent) 1983
Maxalt-MLT Orally Disintegrating Tablets (Frequent) 1983
▲ Megace ES Oral Suspension (1% to 3%) 2492
Meridia Capsules 485
Micardis Tablets (More than 0.3%) 884
Micardis HCT Tablets 886
Migranal Nasal Spray (Infrequent) 3350
▲ Mirapex Tablets (Greater than or equal to 1% to 3%) 889
Namenda (Infrequent) 1199
▲ Naropin Injection (1% to 5%) 640
▲ Navelbine Injection (Among most frequent) 1494
Neoral Soft Gelatin Capsules (1% to less than 3%) 2247
Neoral Oral Solution (1% to less than 3%) 2247
Neurontin Capsules (1.2%) 2498
Neurontin Oral Solution (1.2%) 2498
Neurontin Tablets (1.2%) 2498
Nexium Delayed-Release Capsules (Less than 1%) 645
Nexium I.V. (Less than 1%) 649
Norvasc Tablets (More than 0.1% to 1%) 2529
OxyContin Tablets (Less than 1%) 2699
Paxil CR Controlled-Release Tablets (Infrequent) 1509
Paxil (Infrequent) 1501
Plavix Tablets (1% to 2.5%) 940
Plavix Tablets (1% to 2.5%) 2942
Prevacid Delayed-Release Capsules (Less than 1%) 3268
Prevacid for Delayed-Release Oral Suspension (Less than 1%) 3268
Prevacid NapraPAC (Less than 1%) 3277
Prevacid SoluTab Delayed-Release Orally Disintegrating Tablets (Less than 1%) 3268
PREVPAC (Less than 1%) 3281
Protonix I.V. (Less than 1%) 3468
Protonix Tablets (Less than 1%) 3465
Prozac Pulvules and Liquid (Infrequent) 1771
▲ Rapamune Oral Solution and Tablets (3% to 20%) 3472
Recombivax HB 2045
ReoPro Vials (0.3%) 1779
Requip Tablets (Infrequent) 1528
Rescriptor Tablets 2535
Reyataz Capsules (Less than 3%) 948
Rilutek Tablets (Infrequent) 2945
Risperdal Consta Long-Acting Injection (Up to 2%) 1664
Risperdal M-Tab Orally Disintegrating Tablets (Rare to 2%) 1658
Risperdal (Rare to 2%) 1658
▲ Rituxan for Infusion (1% to 5%) 845
▲ Rituxan I.V. (1% to 5%) 1251
▲ Sandostatin LAR Depot (5% to 15%) 2264
▲ Simulect for Injection (3% to 10%) 2268
Singulair 2047
Sonata Capsules (Less than 1% to 2%) 1686
Soriatane Capsules (Less than 1%) 1028
Sular Tablets (Less than or equal to 1%) 1163
Sustiva Capsules (1% to 2%) 957
Symbyax Capsules (Infrequent) 1788
Tambocor Tablets (1% to 3%) 1824
Targretin Capsules 1719
Tarka Tablets (Less frequent) 519
Tasmar Tablets (Frequent) 3360
Tequin Injection 964
Tequin Tablets 964
▲ Topamax Sprinkle Capsules (1% to 8%) 2438
▲ Topamax Tablets (1% to 8%) 2438
▲ Trileptal Oral Suspension (1% to 3%) 2281
▲ Trileptal Tablets (1% to 3%) 2281
Uniretic Tablets (Less than 1%) 3114
VFEND I.V. (Less than 2%) 2543
VFEND Oral Suspension (Less than 2%) 2543
VFEND Tablets (Less than 2%) 2543
Viagra Tablets (Less than 2%) 2552
▲ Visudyne for Injection (1% to 10%) 2286
Vivelle Transdermal System 2288
Vivelle-Dot Transdermal System 2293
Wellbutrin SR Sustained-Release Tablets (Infrequent) 1583
Wellbutrin XL Extended-Release Tablets (Infrequent) 1588
▲ Xanax XR Tablets (1.3% to 7.8%) 2655
▲ Xeloda Tablets (Less than 1% to 4%) 2825
Xopenex HFA Inhalation Aerosol 3151
Xopenex Inhalation Solution 3143
Xopenex Inhalation Solution Concentrate 3147
Zoloft (Frequent) 2581
▲ Zometa for Intravenous Infusion (12%) 2306
Zomig Tablets (1% to 2%) 714
Zomig-ZMT Tablets (1% to 2%) 714
Zyban Sustained-Release Tablets (Infrequent) 1620
Zyprexa Tablets (Infrequent) 1798
Zyprexa ZYDIS Orally Disintegrating Tablets (Infrequent) 1798
Zyrtec Chewable Tablets (Less than 2%) 2589
Zyrtec (Less than 2%) 2589
Zyrtec-D 12 Hour Extended Release Tablets (Less than 2%) 2591

Hypoestrogeneism

▲ Lupron Depot 3.75 mg (Among most frequent) 3257
Lupron Depot–3 Month 11.25 mg 3262
Neurontin Capsules (Rare) 2498
Neurontin Oral Solution (Rare) 2498
Neurontin Tablets (Rare) 2498

Hypofibrinogenemia

Depacon Injection 412
Depakene 417
Depakote Sprinkle Capsules 422
Depakote Tablets 427
Depakote ER Tablets 433
Elspar for Injection 1943
Lamictal (Rare) 1449
NovoSeven (Greater than or equal to 2%) 2335
Oncaspar 1123
Panhematin for Injection 2487

Hypogeusia

Cuprimine Capsules (Some patients) 1925

Hypoglycemia

Abelcet Injection 1119
Abilify Tablets (Infrequent) 916
Abilify Tablets (Infrequent) 2472
Actiq (Less than 1%) 993
▲ Actos Tablets (8% to 15%) 3224
Aggrenox Capsules 855
Amaryl Tablets (0.9% to 1.7%) 2864
Ammonul Injection 3323
Anaprox Tablets (Less than 1%) 2769
Anaprox DS Tablets (Less than 1%) 2769
Antara Capsules 2723
Apidra Injection 2876
Arthrotec Tablets (Rare) 3126
▲ Avandamet Tablets (3%) 1343
Avandia Tablets (0.6%) 1348
Avelox (Greater than or equal to 2%) 2984
Aygestin Tablets 1062
Bayer Aspirin Tablets 3515
Biaxin/Biaxin XL (Rare) 402
Blocadren Tablets 1891
▲ Byetta Injection (3.3% to 35.7%) 605
Caduet Tablets (Less than 2%) 2507
Cafcit 1854
Campath Ampules 826
Celebrex Capsules (Less than 0.1%) 3130
Celexa (Rare) 1177
▲ CellCept Capsules (3% to less than 20%) 2751
▲ CellCept Intravenous (3% to less than 20%) 2751
▲ CellCept Oral Suspension (3% to less than 20%) 2751
▲ CellCept Tablets (3% to less than 20%) 2751
Cipro I.V. (Rare) 2998
Cipro I.V. Pharmacy Bulk Package (Rare) 3509
Cipro (Less than 0.1%) 2991
Cipro XR Tablets 3004
▲ Coreg Tablets (5% to 12%) 1376
Cosopt Sterile Ophthalmic Solution 1910
▲ Cozaar Tablets (14%) 1913
Cubicin for Injection (1% to 2%) 1038
Cuprimine Capsules 1925
Cymbalta Delayed-Release Capsules (Frequent) 1729
Doxil Injection (Less than 1%) 3302
EC-Naprosyn Delayed-Release Tablets (Less than 1%) 2769
Ecotrin Enteric Coated Aspirin Low, Regular and Maximum Strength Tablets 1627
Edecrin (In 2 uremic patients) 1941
Effexor Tablets (Infrequent) 3405
Effexor XR Capsules (Infrequent) 3411
Epivir 1394
Evoxac Capsules (Less than 1%) 1042
Exelon Capsules (Infrequent) 2204
Ferrlecit Injection 3379
Flexeril Tablets (Rare) 1832
Frova Tablets (Rare) 1101
Gabitril Tablets (Infrequent) 998
Gengraf Capsules (1% to less than 3%) 458
Geodon Capsules (Rare) 2514
Herceptin I.V. (At least one of the 958 patients) 1234
▲ Humalog-Pen (Most common) 1751
Humalog Mix 75/25-Pen 1754
Humulin 50/50, 100 Units 1760
Humulin 70/30 Pen 1761
Humulin L, 100 Units 1763
Humulin R (U-500) 1768
Humulin U, 100 Units 1770
Humulin N Pen 1765
Imitrex Nasal Spray 1435
Imitrex Tablets (Rare) 1440
▲ Increlex Injection (5% to 42%) 3290
Indocin I.V. (1% to 3%) 1973
▲ Invirase (Less than 1% to 4%) 2776
Lantus Injection 2925
Levaquin in 5% Dextrose Injection (0.1% to 0.9%) 2453
Levaquin (0.1% to 0.9%) 2453
Lipitor Tablets (Less than 2%) 2495
Lofibra Capsules 1217
Lotronex Tablets (Rare) 1479
▲ Lyrica Capsules (1% to 3%) 2524
Mepron Suspension (1%) 1487
Meridia Capsules 485
Merrem I.V. (Greater than 1%) 687
Moban Tablets 1108
Namenda 1199
Naprosyn Suspension (Less than 1%) 2769
Naprosyn Tablets (Less than 1%) 2769
Neoral Soft Gelatin Capsules (1% to less than 3%) 2247
Neoral Oral Solution (1% to less than 3%) 2247
Neurontin Capsules (Infrequent) 2498
Neurontin Oral Solution (Infrequent) 2498
Neurontin Tablets (Infrequent) 2498
Noroxin Tablets 2009
Novolin 70/30 InnoLet 2322
Novolin N InnoLet 2322
Novolin R InnoLet 2322
NovoLog Injection 2326
NovoLog Mix 70/30 2331
Omnicef Capsules (0.2%) 506
Omnicef for Oral Suspension (0.2%) 506
Oncaspar (Greater than 1% but less than 5%) 1123
Paser Granules 1657
Paxil CR Controlled-Release Tablets (Rare) 1509
Paxil (Rare) 1501
Pegasys (Less than 1%) 2793
Permax Tablets (Infrequent) 3357
▲ Prandin Tablets (0.5, 1, and 2 mg) (16% to 31%) 2337
Precose Tablets 776
Prevacid Delayed-Release Capsules (Less than 1%) 3268
Prevacid for Delayed-Release Oral Suspension (Less than 1%) 3268
Prevacid NapraPAC (Less than 1%) 3277
Prevacid SoluTab Delayed-Release Orally Disintegrating Tablets (Less than 1%) 3268
PREVPAC (Less than 1%) 3281
Prilosec OTC Tablets (Less than 1%) 2674
▲ Prograf Capsules and Injection (3% to 15%) 624
Proleukin for Injection (2%) 1007
Protopic Ointment (Greater than or equal to 1%) 629
Prozac Pulvules and Liquid 1771
▲ Rapamune Oral Solution and Tablets (3% to 20%) 3472
Requip Tablets (Infrequent) 1528
Risperdal M-Tab Orally Disintegrating Tablets (Rare) 1658
Risperdal (Rare) 1658
▲ Sandostatin Injection (3% to 16%) 2263
Sandostatin LAR Depot (2% to 4%) 2264
Seroquel Tablets (Infrequent) 691
Sonata Capsules (Rare) 1686
St. Joseph 81 mg Aspirin Chewable and Enteric Coated Tablets 1841
Starlix Tablets (2.4%) 2276
Surmontil Capsules 2347
Symbyax Capsules (Infrequent) 1788
▲ Symlin Injection (0.4% to 16.8%) 608
Tenormin I.V. Injection 698
Tenormin Tablets 695
Tequin Injection (Less than 0.1%) 964
Tequin Tablets (Less than 0.1%) 964
Thiothixene Capsules 2124
Timolide Tablets 2056
Timoptic-XE Sterile Ophthalmic Gel Forming Solution 2062
Topamax Sprinkle Capsules (1%) 2438
Topamax Tablets (1%) 2438
Trecator Tablets 3482
Tricor Tablets 523
Triglide Tablets 1165
Trileptal Oral Suspension 2281
Trileptal Tablets 2281
▲ Trisenox Injection (8%) 983
▲ Truvada Tablets (1% to 12%) 1279
Tygacil for Injection (0% to less than 2%) 3489
Vantin Tablets and Oral Suspension 2650
VFEND I.V. (Less than 2%) 2543
VFEND Oral Suspension (Less than 2%) 2543
VFEND Tablets (Less than 2%) 2543

Viagra Tablets (Less than 2%) 2552
Viracept (Less than 2%) 2556
Vivactil Tablets 2350
Wellbutrin Tablets 1579
Wellbutrin SR Sustained-Release Tablets 1583
Wellbutrin XL Extended-Release Tablets 1588
▲ Zegerid Powder for Oral Solution (3.4%) 2972
Zoloft (Rare) 2581
Zonegran Capsules (Rare) 1089
Zosyn (1.0% or less) 3492
Zyprexa Tablets (Infrequent) 1798
Zyprexa ZYDIS Orally Disintegrating Tablets (Infrequent) 1798

Hypoglycemia, masked symptoms of

Betagan Ophthalmic Solution, USP ⊙ 217
Betimol Ophthalmic Solution ⊙ 283
Betimol Ophthalmic Solution 3371
Timoptic in Ocudose (Less frequent) 2061
Timoptic-XE Sterile Ophthalmic Gel Forming Solution 2062

Hypoglycemic reactions

Abilify Tablets (Rare) 916
Abilify Tablets (Rare) 2472
Symbyax Capsules (Rare) 1788

Hypogonadism

Permax Tablets (Rare) 3357
Virazole for Inhalation Solution 3365

Hypogonadism, male

Kaletra (Up to 2%) 474

Hypohidrosis

Bentyl Capsules 724
Bentyl Injection 724
Bentyl Syrup 724
Bentyl Tablets 724
Celexa (Rare) 1177
Paxil CR Controlled-Release Tablets (Rare) 1509
Paxil (Rare) 1501
Risperdal M-Tab Orally Disintegrating Tablets (Infrequent) 1658
Risperdal (Infrequent) 1658
Zonegran Capsules 1089

Hypokalemia

▲ Abelcet Injection (5%) 1119
Abilify Tablets (Infrequent) 916
Abilify Tablets (Infrequent) 2472
Aceon Tablets (2 mg, 4 mg, 8 mg) (0.3% to 1%) 3191
Aciphex Tablets 1081
Actiq (1% or greater) 993
Aggrenox Capsules 855
Aldoclor Tablets 1881
Aldoril Tablets 1884
Aloprim for Injection (Less than 1%) 2156
▲ AmBisome for Injection (37.6% to 43.2%) 615
▲ Ammonul Injection (7%) 3323
▲ AndroGel (3% to 6%) 3330
Arava Tablets (1%) 2881
▲ Aredia for Injection (4% to 18%) 2168
Aricept Tablets (Infrequent) 1086
Aricept ODT Tablets (Infrequent) 1086
▲ Arixtra Injection (0% to 4.2%) 1325
Atacand HCT (0.5% or greater) 637
Avalide Tablets 922
Avalide Tablets 2889
▲ Avastin IV (12% to 16%) 1229
Benicar HCT Tablets 2852
Buphenyl Powder (1%) 3327
Buphenyl Tablets (1%) 3327
Campath Ampules 826
▲ Cancidas for Injection (0.9% to 10.8%) 1894
Capastat Sulfate for Injection 1728
Cardene I.V. (0.7%) 1129
Celebrex Capsules (0.1% to 1.9%) 3130
Celexa (Rare) 1177
▲ CellCept Capsules (31.8% to 37.2%) 2751
▲ CellCept Intravenous (31.8% to 37.2%) 2751
▲ CellCept Oral Suspension (31.8% to 37.2%) 2751
▲ CellCept Tablets (31.8% to 37.2%) 2751
Cipro I.V. (Infrequent) 2998
Cipro I.V. Pharmacy Bulk Package (Infrequent) 3509
Clorpres Tablets 2139
Colazal Capsules 2845
Combunox Tablets (Less than 2%) 1183
▲ Coreg Tablets (Greater than 1% to 3%) 1376
Cubicin for Injection (1% to 2%) 1038
▲ Cytovene (25%) 2763
Daranide Tablets 1928
Decadron Phosphate Injection 1931
Decadron Tablets 1929
▲ DepoDur Extended-Release Injection (2% to 5%) 1098
Depo-Medrol Injectable Suspension 2615
Depo-Medrol Single-Dose Vial 2617
Digibind for Injection 1388
▲ Diovan HCT Tablets (4.5%) 2195
Diuril Sodium Intravenous 1934
▲ Doxil Injection (1% to 10%) 3302
Dyazide Capsules (Uncommon) 1389
Dyrenium Capsules (Rare) 3390
Effexor Tablets (Infrequent) 3405
Effexor XR Capsules (Infrequent) 3411
▲ Eloxatin for Injection (3% to 9%) 2908
Emend Capsules (Greater than 0.5%) 1944
▲ Entocort EC Capsules (Less than 5%) 2694
Evoxac Capsules (Less than 1%) 1042
Exelon Capsules (Frequent) 2204
Ferrlecit Injection 3379
Fleet Enema for Children 1169
Fleet Phospho-soda 1170
Fleet Phospho-soda ACCU-PREP 1171
Fleet Prep Kits 1172
▲ Flolan for Injection (6%) 1408
Foradil Aerolizer 3024
Furosemide Tablets 2117
Gabitril Tablets (Infrequent) 998
Garamycin Injectable 3028
Geodon Capsules (Infrequent) 2514
▲ Gleevec Tablets (6% to 13%) 2221
Humalog-Pen 1751
Humalog Mix 75/25-Pen 1754
Hydrocortone Tablets 1963
▲ Hyzaar (6.7%) 1964
▲ Imdur Tablets (Less than or equal to 5%) 3032
▲ Indapamide Tablets (3% to 7%) 2119
▲ Inspra Tablets (0.6% to 8.4%) 2520
Invanz for Injection (1.7% to 1.8%) 1974
▲ Invirase (Less than 1% to 4%) 2776
▲ I.V. Busulfex (2% to 64%) 1125
Kristalose for Oral Solution 2149
Lanoxicaps Capsules 1458
Levaquin in 5% Dextrose Injection (0.1% to 0.9%) 2453
Levaquin (0.1% to 0.9%) 2453
Lotrel Capsules 2238
Lunesta Tablets (Rare) 3139
Maxzide 2150
Micardis HCT Tablets (Less than 2%) 886
Mycamine for Injection (0.9% to 1.1%) 620
▲ Myfortic Tablets (3% to less than 20%) 2244
▲ Mylotarg for Injection (24% to 29%) 3429
Naropin Injection (Less than 1%) 640
NovoLog Injection 2326
NovoLog Mix 70/30 2331
▲ Ontak Vials (6%) 1717
Parcopa Orally Disintegrating Tablets 3111
Paxil CR Controlled-Release Tablets (Rare) 1509
Paxil (Rare) 1501
Pediapred Oral Solution 3319
Permax Tablets (Infrequent) 3357
Prinzide Tablets 2033
▲ Prograf Capsules and Injection (13% to 29%) 624
▲ Proleukin for Injection (9%) 1007
Proventil HFA Inhalation Aerosol (Some patients) 3071
Prozac Pulvules and Liquid (Infrequent) 1771
▲ Rapamune Oral Solution and Tablets (11% to 21%) 3472
Razadyne ER Extended-Release Capsules 2434
Razadyne 2434
Relafen Tablets (Less than 1%) 1523
Requip Tablets (Infrequent) 1528
Rilutek Tablets (Infrequent) 2945
Risperdal Consta Long-Acting Injection (Infrequent) 1664
Risperdal M-Tab Orally Disintegrating Tablets (Rare) 1658
Risperdal (Rare) 1658
Rythmol SR Capsules 2736
Sandostatin LAR Depot (1% to 4%) 2264
Seroquel Tablets (Rare) 691
▲ Simulect for Injection (Greater than or equal to 10%) 2268
Sular Tablets (Less than or equal to 1%) 1163
Symbyax Capsules (Infrequent) 1788
Teveten Tablets (Less than 1%) 1707
Teveten HCT Tablets (Less than 1%) 1710
Timentin ADD-Vantage (Rare) 1556
Timentin Injection Galaxy Container 1559
Timentin IV Infusion (Rare) 1553
Timentin Pharmacy Bulk Package (Rare) 1562
Timolide Tablets 2056
Topamax Sprinkle Capsules (Infrequent) 2438
Topamax Tablets (Infrequent) 2438
Trasylol Injection (1% to 2%) 779
Trileptal Oral Suspension 2281
Trileptal Tablets 2281
▲ Trisenox Injection (50%) 983
Tygacil for Injection (2.1%) 3489
Uniretic Tablets (More than 1%) 3114
▲ Valcyte Tablets (Less than 5%) 2816
Vaseretic Tablets 2073
▲ VFEND I.V. (0% to 16.7%) 2543
▲ VFEND Oral Suspension (0% to 16.7%) 2543
▲ VFEND Tablets (0% to 16.7%) 2543
▲ Xeloda Tablets (Less than 5%) 2825
Xopenex HFA Inhalation Aerosol 3151
Xopenex Inhalation Solution 3143
Xopenex Inhalation Solution Concentrate 3147
Zestoretic Tablets 701
Zithromax for Oral Suspension, 300 mg, 600 mg, 900 mg, 1200 mg (Less than 1%) 2561
Zithromax Tablets, 250 mg, 500 mg (Less than 1%) 2561
Zithromax Tri-Pak (Less than 1%) 2561
Zofran Injection (Rare) 1607
Zofran (Rare) 1613
Zofran ODT Orally Disintegrating Tablets (Rare) 1613
▲ Zometa for Intravenous Infusion (Less than 15%) 2306
Zosyn 3492
Zovirax for Injection (Less than 1%) 1618
Zyprexa Tablets (Infrequent) 1798
Zyprexa ZYDIS Orally Disintegrating Tablets (Infrequent) 1798
Zyvox (0% to 2.8%) 2661

Hypokalemic alkalosis

Decadron Phosphate Injection 1931
Decadron Tablets 1929
Depo-Medrol Injectable Suspension 2615
Depo-Medrol Single-Dose Vial 2617
Hydrocortone Tablets 1963
Pediapred Oral Solution 3319

Hypokinesia

Abilify Tablets (Infrequent) 916
Abilify Tablets (Infrequent) 2472
Actiq (1% or greater) 993
Ambien Tablets (Rare) 2867
Aricept Tablets (Infrequent) 1086
Aricept ODT Tablets (Infrequent) 1086
Celexa (Infrequent) 1177
▲ Clozapine Tablets (4%) 2141
▲ Clozaril Tablets (4%) 2174
▲ Comtan Tablets (9%) 2186
Copaxone for Injection (Infrequent) 3292
Coreg Tablets (Greater than 0.1% to 1%) 1376
Depacon Injection (1% or more) 412
Depakene (1% or more) 417
Depakote Sprinkle Capsules 422
▲ Depakote Tablets (1% to 5%) 427
Depakote ER Tablets (Greater than 1%) 433
Doxil Injection (Less than 1%) 3302
Effexor Tablets (Rare) 3405
Effexor XR Capsules (Rare) 3411
Exelon Capsules (Infrequent) 2204
▲ FazaClo Orally Disintegrating Tablets (4%) 547
Gabitril Tablets (Frequent) 998
▲ Geodon Capsules (14%) 2514
▲ Intron A for Injection (Less than 5%) 3038
Lamictal (Rare) 1449
Lunesta Tablets (Rare) 3139
Lyrica Capsules (0.1% to 1%) 2524
Mirapex Tablets (1% or more) 889
Namenda (Frequent) 1199
Naropin Injection (Less than 1%) 640
Neurontin Capsules (Rare) 2498
Neurontin Oral Solution (Rare) 2498
Neurontin Tablets (Rare) 2498
Paxil CR Controlled-Release Tablets (Rare) 1509
Paxil (Rare) 1501
Permax Tablets (Infrequent) 3357
▲ ProSom Tablets (8%) 512
Protonix I.V. 3468
Razadyne ER Extended-Release Capsules (Infrequent) 2434
Razadyne (Infrequent) 2434
Relpax Tablets (Rare) 2531
Rilutek Tablets (Infrequent) 2945
Risperdal Consta Long-Acting Injection (Infrequent) 1664
▲ Risperdal M-Tab Orally Disintegrating Tablets (17% to 34%) 1658
▲ Risperdal (17% to 34%) 1658
Sonata Capsules (Rare) 1686
▲ Stalevo Tablets (9%) 2270
Symbyax Capsules (Infrequent) 1788
Symmetrel 1115
Tasmar Tablets (1% to 3%) 3360
Topamax Sprinkle Capsules (Frequent) 2438
Topamax Tablets (Frequent) 2438
Trileptal Oral Suspension 2281
Trileptal Tablets 2281
Uniretic Tablets (Less than 1%) 3114
Wellbutrin SR Sustained-Release Tablets 1583
Wellbutrin XL Extended-Release Tablets 1588
Zoloft (Infrequent) 2581
Zonegran Capsules (Rare) 1089
Zyban Sustained-Release Tablets 1620
▲ Zyprexa Tablets (8% to 20%) 1798
▲ Zyprexa ZYDIS Orally Disintegrating Tablets (8% to 20%) 1798

Hypomagnesemia

Abelcet Injection 1119
Actiq (1% or greater) 993
Aloprim for Injection (Less than 1%) 2156
▲ AmBisome for Injection (15.3% to 25.9%) 615
▲ Aredia for Injection (3.8% to at least 15%) 2168
Avalide Tablets 922
Avalide Tablets 2889
Benicar HCT Tablets 2852
Cancidas for Injection (2.3%) 1894
▲ CellCept Capsules (39%) 2751
▲ CellCept Intravenous (39%) 2751
▲ CellCept Oral Suspension (39%) 2751
▲ CellCept Tablets (39%) 2751
Cubicin for Injection (Less than 1%) 1038
Diovan HCT Tablets 2195
Diuril Sodium Intravenous 1934
Doxil Injection (Less than 1%) 3302
Furosemide Tablets 2117
Garamycin Injectable 3028
Gengraf Capsules 458
Geodon Capsules (Rare) 2514
Herceptin I.V. (At least one of the 958 patients) 1234
Hyzaar 1964
▲ I.V. Busulfex (77%) 1125
Lanoxicaps Capsules 1458
▲ Leukine (15%) 829
Levaquin in 5% Dextrose Injection (0.1% to 0.9%) 2453
Levaquin (0.1% to 0.9%) 2453
Maxzide 2150
Micardis HCT Tablets 886
Mycamine for Injection (1.1% to 1.2%) 620
▲ Myfortic Tablets (3% to less than 20%) 2244
▲ Mylotarg for Injection (3% to 10%) 3429
Naropin Injection (Less than 1%) 640
▲ Neoral Soft Gelatin Capsules (6%) 2247
▲ Neoral Oral Solution (6%) 2247
Prinzide Tablets 2033
▲ Prograf Capsules and Injection (16% to 48%) 624
▲ Proleukin for Injection (12%) 1007
▲ Rapamune Oral Solution and Tablets (3% to 20%) 3472
Sandimmune (In some patients) 2259
▲ Simulect for Injection (3% to 10%) 2268
Thalomid Capsules 979
Timolide Tablets 2056
▲ Trisenox Injection (45%) 983
Uniretic Tablets 3114
▲ Valcyte Tablets (Less than 5%) 2816
Vaseretic Tablets 2073
VFEND I.V. (Less than 2%) 2543
VFEND Oral Suspension (Less than 2%) 2543

VFEND Tablets (Less than 2%) 2543
▲ Xeloda Tablets (Less than 5%) 2825
Zegerid Powder for Oral Solution (0.1%) 2972
Zestoretic Tablets 701
Zometa for Intravenous Infusion (0.1% to 0.2%) 2306

Hypomania
Celexa 1177
Effexor Tablets (0.5%) 3405
Effexor XR Capsules (0.3%) 3411
Lamictal (Rare) 1449
Lexapro Oral Solution 1193
Paxil CR Controlled-Release Tablets (Approximately 1.0%) 1509
Paxil (Approximately 1.0%) 1501
Prozac Pulvules and Liquid (0.1% to 1.8%) 1771
Surmontil Capsules 2347
Symbyax Capsules 1788
Vivactil Tablets 2350
Wellbutrin Tablets (Frequent) 1579
Wellbutrin SR Sustained-Release Tablets (Rare) 1583
Wellbutrin XL Extended-Release Tablets (Rare) 1588
Xanax XR Tablets (Infrequent) 2655
Zoloft (Approximately 0.4%) 2581
Zyban Sustained-Release Tablets (Rare) 1620

Hypomenorrhea
Effexor Tablets (Rare) 3405
Effexor XR Capsules (Rare) 3411
Pentasa Capsules (Less than 1%) 3182
Prozac Pulvules and Liquid (Rare) 1771
Symbyax Capsules (Infrequent) 1788

Hyponatremia
Abilify Tablets (Infrequent) 916
Abilify Tablets (Infrequent) 2472
Aceon Tablets (2 mg, 4 mg, 8 mg) 3191
Aciphex Tablets 1081
Actimmune (Rare) 1646
Actiq (Less than 1%) 993
Aloprim for Injection (Less than 1%) 2156
Altace Capsules 1673
Amaryl Tablets 2864
AmBisome for Injection (Less common) 615
Aricept Tablets 1086
Aricept ODT Tablets 1086
Arthrotec Tablets (Rare) 3126
Atacand Tablets 634
Atacand HCT (Very rare) 637
Avastin IV (Rare) 1229
Benicar HCT Tablets 2852
Campath Ampules 826
Campral Tablets (Rare) 1175
Cancidas for Injection (1.5% to 1.9%) 1894
Captopril Tablets 2114
Carbatrol Capsules 3174
Celebrex Capsules (Less than 0.1%) 3130
Celexa (Several cases) 1177
▲ CellCept Capsules (3% to less than 20%) 2751
▲ CellCept Intravenous (3% to less than 20%) 2751
▲ CellCept Oral Suspension (3% to less than 20%) 2751
▲ CellCept Tablets (3% to less than 20%) 2751
Clozapine Tablets 2141
Clozaril Tablets 2174
Coreg Tablets (Greater than 1% to 3%) 1376
Cozaar Tablets 1913
Cytovene 2763
DDAVP Injection 4 mcg/mL 2893
DDAVP Nasal Spray 2894
DDAVP Tablets 2895
Depacon Injection 412
Depakene 417
Depakote Sprinkle Capsules 422
Depakote Tablets 427
Depakote ER Tablets 433
Desmopressin Acetate Injection 1143
Diuril Sodium Intravenous 1934
▲ Doxil Injection (1% to 10%) 3302
Dyazide Capsules 1389
Effexor Tablets (Rare) 3405
Effexor XR Capsules 3411
Emend Capsules (Greater than 0.5%) 1944
Equetro Extended-Release Capsules 3178
Evoxac Capsules (Less than 1%) 1042
Exelon Capsules (Infrequent) 2204
Factive Tablets (0.3%) 2464
FazaClo Orally Disintegrating Tablets 547
Furosemide Tablets 2117
Gabitril Tablets (Infrequent) 998
Garamycin Injectable 3028
Geodon Capsules (Rare) 2514
Gleevec Tablets (Rare) 2221
Herceptin I.V. (At least one of the 958 patients) 1234
Hyzaar 1964
Indapamide Tablets (Less than 5%) 2119
▲ Indocin I.V. (3% to 9%) 1973
Inspra Tablets (2.4%) 2520
▲ Invirase (Less than 1% to 4%) 2776
I.V. Busulfex (2%) 1125
Kadian Capsules (Less than 3%) 572
Lexapro Oral Solution (One case) 1193
Lexapro Tablets (One case) 1193
Lotensin HCT Tablets 2235
Mavik Tablets (0.3% to 1.0%) 482
Maxzide 2150
▲ Mepron Suspension (7% to 10%) 1487
Moduretic Tablets 2003
Mycamine for Injection 620
Namenda (Infrequent) 1199
Navelbine Injection 1494
Neurontin Capsules 2498
Neurontin Oral Solution 2498
Neurontin Tablets 2498
Nexium Delayed-Release Capsules (Less than 1%) 645
Nexium I.V. (Less than 1%) 649
Nimotop Capsules (Less than 1%) 774
Nipent for Injection (Less than 3%) 3216
Oncaspar (Less than 1%) 1123
Orap Tablets 1220
OxyContin Tablets (Less than 1%) 2699
Paxil CR Controlled-Release Tablets (Rare) 1509
Paxil (Rare) 1501
Prilosec OTC Tablets (Less than 1%) 2674
Primaxin I.M. 2022
Primaxin I.V. 2024
Prinivil Tablets 2029
Prinzide Tablets 2033
▲ Prograf Capsules and Injection (3% to 15%) 624
▲ Proleukin for Injection (4%) 1007
Prozac Pulvules and Liquid 1771
▲ Rapamune Oral Solution and Tablets (3% to 20%) 3472
Requip Tablets (Infrequent) 1528
Rescriptor Tablets 2535
Rilutek Tablets (Infrequent) 2945
Risperdal Consta Long-Acting Injection (Infrequent) 1664
Risperdal M-Tab Orally Disintegrating Tablets (Infrequent) 1658
Risperdal (Infrequent) 1658
Rythmol SR Capsules 2736
Seroquel Tablets 691
Tarka Tablets 519
Tegretol/Tegretol-XR 2278
Teveten Tablets (Less than 1%) 1707
Teveten HCT Tablets (Less than 1%) 1710
Ticlid Tablets (Rare) 2813
Topamax Sprinkle Capsules (Rare) 2438
Topamax Tablets (Rare) 2438
Trileptal Oral Suspension (2.5%) 2281
Trileptal Tablets (2.5%) 2281
Tygacil for Injection (0% to less than 2%) 3489
Uniretic Tablets (Less than 1%) 3114
Univasc Tablets 3118
Vaseretic Tablets 2073
Vasotec I.V. Injection 2076
VFEND I.V. (Less than 2%) 2543
VFEND Oral Suspension (Less than 2%) 2543
VFEND Tablets (Less than 2%) 2543
▲ Zegerid Powder for Oral Solution (3.9%) 2972
Zestoretic Tablets 701
Zestril Tablets 704
Zithromax for Oral Suspension, 300 mg, 600 mg, 900 mg, 1200 mg (Less than 1%) 2561
Zithromax Tablets, 250 mg, 500 mg (Less than 1%) 2561
Zithromax Tri-Pak (Less than 1%) 2561
Zoloft (Several cases) 2581
Zonegran Capsules (Rare) 1089
Zosyn 3492
Zyprexa Tablets (Infrequent) 1798
Zyprexa ZYDIS Orally Disintegrating Tablets (Infrequent) 1798

Hyponatremia, dilutional
Diuril Sodium Intravenous 1934
Hyzaar 1964
Maxzide 2150
Prinzide Tablets 2033
Vaseretic Tablets 2073
Zestoretic Tablets 701

Hypophosphatemia
Abelcet Injection 1119
Actonel Tablets (2.7%) 2679
Advicor Tablets 1694
AmBisome for Injection (Less common) 615
▲ Aredia for Injection (Up to 18%) 2168
▲ Buphenyl Powder (6%) 3327
▲ Buphenyl Tablets (6%) 3327
Cardene I.V. (Rare) 1129
▲ CellCept Capsules (3% to less than 20%) 2751
▲ CellCept Intravenous (3% to less than 20%) 2751
▲ CellCept Oral Suspension (3% to less than 20%) 2751
▲ CellCept Tablets (3% to less than 20%) 2751
Doxil Injection (Less than 1%) 3302
Effexor Tablets (Rare) 3405
Evista Tablets 1735
▲ Fosamax (Approximately 10%) 1949
▲ Fosamax Plus D Tablets (10%) 1956
Gleevec Tablets (Infrequent) 2221
▲ Invirase (Less than 1% to 4%) 2776
▲ I.V. Busulfex (17%) 1125
Levaquin in 5% Dextrose Injection (0.1% to 0.9%) 2453
Levaquin (0.1% to 0.9%) 2453
Maalox Regular Strength Antacid/Anti-Gas Liquid 677
Maalox Max Maximum Strength Antacid/Anti-Gas Liquid 2165
Maalox Regular Strength Antacid/Antigas Liquid 2164
Maxzide 2150
Mycamine for Injection (1.4%) 620
▲ Myfortic Tablets (3% to less than 20%) 2244
▲ Mylotarg for Injection (6% to 10%) 3429
Niaspan Extended-Release Tablets 1703
▲ Prograf Capsules and Injection (3% to 49%) 624
▲ Proleukin for Injection (11%) 1007
▲ Rapamune Oral Solution and Tablets (15% to 23%) 3472
Rescriptor Tablets 2535
▲ Roferon-A Injection (22%) 2805
▲ Simulect for Injection (Greater than or equal to 10%) 2268
Timolide Tablets 2056
Topamax Sprinkle Capsules (Rare) 2438
Topamax Tablets (Rare) 2438
Truvada Tablets 1279
Tygacil for Injection 3489
Ultane Liquid for Inhalation (Less than 1%) 526
▲ Valcyte Tablets (Less than 5%) 2816
VFEND I.V. (Less than 2%) 2543
VFEND Oral Suspension (Less than 2%) 2543
VFEND Tablets (Less than 2%) 2543
Viread Tablets 1284
▲ Zegerid Powder for Oral Solution (6.2%) 2972
▲ Zometa for Intravenous Infusion (0.5% to 11.8%) 2306

Hypopigmentation
Accutane Capsules 2740
Aclovate (Infrequent) 1290
Aldara Cream, 5% (More than 1%) 1814
Amnesteem Capsules 2126
Analpram-HC 1136
Avita Cream 2136
Avita Gel 2138
Catapres-TTS (0.5% or less) 875
Clobevate Gel 3213
Clobex Shampoo (Infrequent) 1209
Clobex Lotion 1208
Cutivate Cream (Infrequent) 1381
Cutivate Lotion 0.05% (Rare) 1383
Cutivate Ointment (Infrequent to more frequent) 1384
Decadron Phosphate Injection 1931
Depo-Medrol Single-Dose Vial 2617
Diprolene Gel 0.05% 3015
Diprolene Lotion 0.05% (Infrequent) 3016
Diprolene Ointment 0.05% (Infrequent) 3017
Diprolene AF Cream 0.05% (Infrequent) 3014
Diprosone Cream, USP 0.05% 3018
Elocon Cream 0.1% (Infrequent) 3019
Elocon Lotion 0.1% (Infrequent) 3020
Elocon Ointment 0.1% (Infrequent) 3021
Locoid Cream (Infrequent) 1138
Locoid Lipocream Cream (Infrequent) 1138
Locoid (Infrequent) 1138
Lotrisone 3054
Luxiq Foam 1026
Olux Foam 1027
Oxsoralen-Ultra Capsules 3354
Pandel Cream, 0.1% 1017
Pramosone 1139
ProctoFoam-HC 3113
Retin-A Micro 0.1%/0.04% 2388
▲ Solage Topical Solution (4.1% to 7%) 740
Taxotere Injection Concentrate 2947
Temovate Cream 1549
Temovate Gel (Infrequent) 1550
Temovate Ointment 1549
Temovate Scalp Application (Infrequent) 1551
Temovate E Emollient (Infrequent) 1552
Tri-Luma Cream (11 occurrences in 27 patients) 1213
U-cort 1% Cream 3289
Vanos Cream 1864

Hypoplasia, enamel
Dynacin Tablets 1859

Hypoplasia, erythroid
Captopril Tablets 2114

Hypoplasia, myeloid
(*see under* Bone marrow hypoplasia)

Hypoplastic anemia
(*see under* Anemia, hypoplastic)

Hypopnea
Vicoprofen Tablets (Less than 1%) 533

Hypoproteinemia
Actiq (Less than 1%) 993
AmBisome for Injection (Less common) 615
▲ Buphenyl Powder (3%) 3327
▲ Buphenyl Tablets (3%) 3327
▲ CellCept Capsules (3% to less than 20%) 2751
▲ CellCept Intravenous (3% to less than 20%) 2751
▲ CellCept Oral Suspension (3% to less than 20%) 2751
▲ CellCept Tablets (3% to less than 20%) 2751
Cipro I.V. 2998
Cipro I.V. Pharmacy Bulk Package 3509
Colazal Capsules 2845
Depakote ER Tablets (Greater than 1%) 433
Doxil Injection (Less than 1%) 3302
Effexor Tablets (Rare) 3405
Effexor XR Capsules (Rare) 3411
Evista Tablets 1735
Factive Tablets (0.1%) 2464
Geodon Capsules (Rare) 2514
Lupron Depot 7.5 mg (Greater than or equal to 5%) 3261
Oncaspar (Greater than 1% but less than 5%) 1123
▲ Prograf Capsules and Injection (3% to 15%) 624
▲ Proleukin for Injection (7%) 1007
Risperdal M-Tab Orally Disintegrating Tablets (Rare) 1658
Risperdal (Rare) 1658
Sandostatin LAR Depot (1% to 4%) 2264
▲ Simulect for Injection (3% to 10%) 2268
Targretin Capsules 1719
Thalomid Capsules 979
▲ Tygacil for Injection (4.5%) 3489
Uniretic Tablets (Less than 1%) 3114
Vantin Tablets and Oral Suspension 2650
Zosyn 3492
Zyprexa Tablets (Rare) 1798
Zyprexa ZYDIS Orally Disintegrating Tablets (Rare) 1798

Hypoprothrombinemia
AmBisome for Injection (Less common) 615
Arixtra Injection (1.3%) 1325
Celexa 1177
Cipro I.V. (Rare) 2998
Cipro I.V. Pharmacy Bulk Package (Rare) 3509
Cipro XR Tablets (Less than 1%) 3004
Colazal Capsules 2845
▲ Coreg Tablets (Greater than 1% to 3%) 1376
Dynacin Tablets 1859

Lexapro Oral Solution 1193
Lexapro Tablets 1193
Lyrica Capsules (Rare) 2524
Merrem I.V. (Greater than 0.2%) 687
Neurontin Capsules (Rare) 2498
Neurontin Oral Solution (Rare) 2498
Neurontin Tablets (Rare) 2498
NovoSeven (1%) 2335
Paser Granules 1657
▲ Prograf Capsules and Injection (3% to 15%) 624
Rocephin Injectable Vials, ADD-Vantage, Galaxy, Bulk (Rare) 2801
Rythmol SR Capsules 2736

Hypoptyalism

Amerge Tablets (Frequent) 1312
Demser Capsules 1933
▲ Flovent HFA (1% to 3%) 1418
Imitrex Injection 1431
Imitrex Nasal Spray 1435
▲ Infergen (4% to 6%) 1647
Lotronex Tablets (Infrequent) 1479
▲ Niravam Orally Disintegrating Tablets (10.6% to 32.8%) 3106
Risperdal M-Tab Orally Disintegrating Tablets (Frequent) 1658
Risperdal (Frequent) 1658
Serevent Diskus (1% to 3%) 1540
Vantin Tablets and Oral Suspension (Less than 1%) 2650

Hypopyon

Ocucoat (Rare) ⊙ 290

Hyporeflexia

Abilify Tablets (Rare) 916
Abilify Tablets (Rare) 2472
Axert Tablets (Rare) 2430
Effexor Tablets (Rare) 3405
▲ Evoxac Capsules (1% to 3%) 1042
Gabitril Tablets (Frequent) 998
Invirase (Less than 2%) 2776
Lunesta Tablets (Infrequent) 3139
Matulane Capsules 3188
Maxalt Tablets (Rare) 1983
Maxalt-MLT Orally Disintegrating Tablets (Rare) 1983
Navelbine Injection (Less than 5%) 1494
Neurontin Capsules (Frequent) 2498
Neurontin Oral Solution (Frequent) 2498
Neurontin Tablets (Frequent) 2498
Paxil CR Controlled-Release Tablets (Rare) 1509
Paxil (Rare) 1501
ProSom Tablets (Rare) 512
Protonix I.V. (Less than 1%) 3468
Protonix Tablets (Less than 1%) 3465
Prozac Pulvules and Liquid (Rare) 1771
▲ Retrovir Capsules (5.6%) 1533
▲ Retrovir IV Infusion (7%) 1537
▲ Retrovir (5.6%) 1533
▲ Risperdal M-Tab Orally Disintegrating Tablets (17% to 34%) 1658
▲ Risperdal (17% to 34%) 1658
Sonata Capsules (Rare) 1686
Thalomid Capsules 979
Thiothixene Capsules 2124
Topamax Sprinkle Capsules (2%) 2438
Topamax Tablets (2%) 2438
Trileptal Oral Suspension 2281
Trileptal Tablets 2281
▲ Vesanoid Capsules (3%) 2823
Viagra Tablets (Less than 2%) 2552
Zoloft (Rare) 2581

Hyporesponsive episode, unspecified

HibTITER (One case) 3419

Hyposalivation

(*see under* Hypoptyalism)

Hypospadias

Topamax Sprinkle Capsules 2438
Topamax Tablets 2438

Hypotaxia

▲ Vesanoid Capsules (3%) 2823

Hypotension

▲ Abelcet Injection (8%) 1119
Abilify Tablets (Frequent) 916
Abilify Tablets (Frequent) 2472
Aceon Tablets (2 mg, 4 mg, 8 mg) (0.3% to 1%) 3191
Acthrel for Injection 3528
Actimmune (Rare) 1646
Actiq (Less than 1%) 993
Activase I.V. 1225
Adacel Vaccine 2959
Adalat CC Tablets (Less than 1%) 2978
Adenocard Injection (Less than 1%) 612
Adenoscan (2%) 613
Advicor Tablets 1694
Aggrenox Capsules (Less than 1%) 855
Alacol DM Syrup 739
Aldoclor Tablets 1881
Aldoril Tablets 1884
Aldurazyme for Intravenous Infusion (2%) 1261
▲ Alferon N Injection (6%) 1640
Alkeran for Injection (In some patients) 976
Allegra-D 12 Hour Extended-Release Tablets 2860
Allegra-D 24 Hour Extended-Release Tablets 2862
Aloprim for Injection (Less than 1%) 2156
Aloxi Injection (1%) 2099
Alphagan P Ophthalmic Solution 563
▲ Altace Capsules (11%) 1673
Ambien Tablets (Rare) 2867
▲ AmBisome for Injection (7.4% to 14.3%) 615
Amerge Tablets (Infrequent) 1312
▲ Ammonul Injection (4%) 3323
Anaprox Tablets (Less than 1%) 2769
Anaprox DS Tablets (Less than 1%) 2769
▲ Angiomax for Injection (3.1% to 12%) 1856
Antara Capsules 2723
Anzemet Injection (Infrequently) 2871
▲ Anzemet Tablets (5.3%) 2874
▲ Apokyn Injection (11%) 2132
AquaMEPHYTON Injection 1887
▲ Aranesp for Injection (22%) 576
Aredia for Injection (Rare) 2168
▲ Argatroban Injection (7.2% to 10.7%) 1321
Aricept Tablets (Frequent) 1086
Aricept ODT Tablets (Frequent) 1086
▲ Arixtra Injection (0.3% to 3.5%) 1325
Arthrotec Tablets (Rare) 3126
Atacand HCT (Rare) 637
Atrovent HFA Inhalation Aerosol 872
Avalide Tablets 922
Avalide Tablets 2889
Avapro Tablets (0.4%) 925
Avapro Tablets (0.4%) 2886
▲ Avastin IV (7% to 15%) 1229
Avelox (Less than 0.1%) 2984
Avinza Capsules (Less than 5%) 1714
Azasan Tablets 2844
Bayer Aspirin Tablets 3515
BeneFix for Injection 3402
Benicar Tablets 2850
Betagan Ophthalmic Solution, USP ⊙ 217
Betimol Ophthalmic Solution ⊙ 283
Betimol Ophthalmic Solution 3371
▲ Bexxar (1% to 7%) 1360
▲ BiDil Tablets (8%) 2161
▲ Blocadren Tablets (3%) 1891
Boostrix (Rarely) 1366
▲ Brevibloc Concentrate (20% to 50%) 766
▲ Brevibloc Injection (20% to 50%) 766
▲ Brevibloc Double Strength Injection (20% to 50%) 766
▲ Brevibloc Premixed Injection (20% to 50%) 766
▲ Brevibloc Double Strength Premixed Injection (20% to 50%) 766
Brimonidine Tartrate Ophthalmic Solution 0.2% ⊙ 245
▲ Buprenex Injectable (1% to 5%) 2718
Caduet Tablets (Greater than 0.1% to less than or equal to 1%) 2507
Calcium Disodium Versenate Injection 1819
▲ Campath Ampules (5% to 32%) 826
Campral Tablets (Infrequent) 1175
▲ Camptosar Injection (1.7% to 5.8%) 2602
Cancidas for Injection (0.9%) 1894
Captopril Tablets (Rare) 2114
Carbatrol Capsules 3174
▲ Cardene I.V. (5.6%) 1129
Cardizem LA Extended Release Tablets (Less than 2%) 1699
Carimune NF 3501
▲ Carnitor Injection (3% to 19%) 3185
Carteolol Hydrochloride Ophthalmic Solution USP, 1% ⊙ 246
Cataflam Tablets (Rarely) 2173
Caverject Impulse Injection (Less than 1%) 2610
Celexa (Frequent) 1177
▲ CellCept Capsules (3% to 32.5%) 2751
▲ CellCept Intravenous (3% to 32.5%) 2751
▲ CellCept Oral Suspension (3% to 32.5%) 2751
▲ CellCept Tablets (3% to 32.5%) 2751
▲ Cerezyme for Injection (Approximately 6.6%) 1263
Cialis Tablets (Less than 2%) 1806
Cipro I.V. (1% or less) 2998
Cipro I.V. Pharmacy Bulk Package (1% or less) 3509
Cipro (Less than 1%) 2991
Cipro XR Tablets 3004
Clinoril Tablets (Less than 1 in 100) 1899
▲ Clolar for Intravenous Infusion (29%) 1264
▲ Clozapine Tablets (More than 5% to 9%) 2141
▲ Clozaril Tablets (More than 5% to 9%) 2174
Combivent Inhalation Aerosol 878
Combunox Tablets (Less than 1%) 1183
Comtan Tablets 2186
Comvax 1904
Concerta Extended-Release Tablets 1828
Copaxone for Injection (Infrequent) 3292
▲ Coreg Tablets (9% to 14%) 1376
Cosopt Sterile Ophthalmic Solution (Less than 1%) 1910
Coumadin for Injection 932
Coumadin Tablets 932
Covera-HS Tablets (0.7% to 2.5%) 3135
▲ Cozaar Tablets (Less than 1% to 7%) 1913
Cubicin for Injection (2.4%) 1038
Curosurf Intratracheal Suspension 1057
CytoGam Intravenous 1866
Dalmane Capsules (Rare) 3343
DDAVP Injection 4 mcg/mL (Infrequent) 2893
DDAVP Nasal Spray (Infrequent) 2894
Depacon Injection (1% or more) 412
Depakene (1% or more) 417
Depakote Sprinkle Capsules 422
▲ Depakote Tablets (1% to 5%) 427
Depakote ER Tablets (Greater than 1%) 433
▲ DepoDur Extended-Release Injection (Greater than 10%) 1098
Desferal Vials 2190
Desmopressin Acetate Injection (Infrequent) 1143
Diastat Rectal Delivery System (At least 1%) 3344
Dilaudid 439
Dilaudid Oral Liquid 443
Dilaudid Non-Sterile Powder 439
Dilaudid Rectal Suppositories 439
Dilaudid Tablets 439
Dilaudid Tablets - 8 mg 443
Dilaudid-HP (Less frequent) 441
Diovan HCT Tablets 2195
▲ Diovan Tablets (1.4% to 7%) 2191
Diprivan Injectable Emulsion (Rare) 676
Diuril Oral 1936
Diuril Sodium Intravenous 1934
▲ Dostinex Tablets (1% to less than 10%) 2631
▲ Doxil Injection (1% to 10%) 3302
▲ Duragesic Transdermal System (1% to 3%) 2448
Dyazide Capsules 1389
DynaCirc CR Tablets (0.5% to 1%) 2726
EC-Naprosyn Delayed-Release Tablets (Less than 1%) 2769
Ecotrin Enteric Coated Aspirin Low, Regular and Maximum Strength Tablets 1627
Edex Injection (Less than 1%) 3103
Effexor Tablets (Infrequent) 3405
Effexor XR Capsules (Infrequent) 3411
Eldepryl Capsules 3209
Eligard 22.5 mg (Less than 2%) 2899
Elitek 2906
Eloxatin for Injection (Rare) 2908
Emend Capsules (Greater than 0.5%) 1944
Enbrel for Injection (Infrequent) 580
Engerix-B Vaccine (Less than 1%) 1391
Equetro Extended-Release Capsules 3178
Eskalith 1406
▲ Ethyol for Injection (3% to 61%) 1869
Evoxac Capsules (Less than 1%) 1042
Exelon Capsules (Frequent) 2204
▲ Fabrazyme for Intravenous Infusion (4%) 1267
▲ FazaClo Orally Disintegrating Tablets (Greater than 5% to 9%) 547
▲ Ferrlecit Injection (1.3% to 41%) 3379
Flexeril Tablets (Less than 1%) 1832
▲ Flolan for Injection (13% to 27%) 1408
Fluorescite Injection ⊙ 207
Focalin Tablets 2214
Focalin XR Capsules 2217
Foradil Aerolizer (Rare) 3024
Fortaz (Very rare) 1422
▲ Fosrenol Chewable Tablets (8% to 16%) 3180
Furosemide Tablets 2117
Gabitril Tablets (Infrequent) 998
Gammagard Liquid 751
Gammagard S/D 754
Gamunex Immune Globulin I.V., 10% 3232
Garamycin Injectable 3028
Gleevec Tablets (Infrequent) 2221
GlucaGen for Injection (Rare) 790
Glucagon for Injection Vials and Emergency Kit 1749
Guanidine Hydrochloride Tablets 3030
Herceptin I.V. (At least one of the 958 patients) 1234
Humalog-Pen (Less common) 1751
Humalog Mix 75/25-Pen (Less common) 1754
Humulin 50/50, 100 Units 1760
Humulin 70/30 Pen (Less common) 1761
Humulin L, 100 Units (Less common) 1763
Humulin R (U-500) (Less common) 1768
Humulin N Pen (Less common) 1765
▲ Hyperstat I.V. Injection (7%) 3031
▲ Hytrin Capsules (0.6%; 21%) 469
Hyzaar 1964
▲ Imdur Tablets (Less than or equal to 5%) 3032
Imitrex Injection (Infrequent) 1431
Imitrex Nasal Spray (Rare) 1435
Imitrex Tablets (Infrequent) 1440
Inderal LA Long-Acting Capsules 3421
Indocin Capsules (Less than 1%) 1968
Indocin I.V. (Less than 1%) 1973
Indocin (Less than 1%) 1968
Infanrix Vaccine 1444
Infed Injection 3381
InnoPran XL Capsules 2728
▲ Integrilin Injection (7%) 3034
▲ Intron A for Injection (Less than 5%) 3038
Invanz for Injection (1% to 2%) 1974
Invirase (Less than 2%) 2776
▲ I.V. Busulfex (3% to 11%) 1125
Iveegam EN (0.36%) 759
Kadian Capsules (Less than 3%) 572
Ketek Tablets (Less than 0.2%) 2920
Kogenate FS (Very rare) 3517
Kytril Injection (Rare) 2785
Kytril Tablets (Rare) 2788
Lariam Tablets (Infrequent) 2790
▲ Leukine (13%) 829
Levaquin in 5% Dextrose Injection (0.1% to 0.9%) 2453
Levaquin (0.1% to 0.9%) 2453
Levitra Tablets (Less than 2%) 3048
Lexapro Oral Solution 1193
Lexapro Tablets 1193
Lidoderm Patch 1107
Lithobid Tablets 1670
Lofibra Capsules 1217
Lotensin HCT Tablets (0.6%) 2235
Lotrel Capsules (Rare) 2238
Lupron Depot 3.75 mg 3257
Lupron Depot 7.5 mg 3261
Lupron Depot–3 Month 11.25 mg 3262
Lupron Depot-PED 7.5 mg, 11.25 mg and 15 mg 3266
Lupron Injection Pediatric 3256
Lyrica Capsules (0.1% to 1%) 2524
Marinol Capsules (0.3 to 1%) 3334
Matulane Capsules 3188
▲ Mavik Tablets (0.3% to 11%) 482
Maxair Autohaler 1820
Maxzide 2150
Mebaral Tablets, USP (Less than 1 in 100 patients) 2483
Mefoxin for Injection 1987
Mefoxin Premixed Intravenous Solution 1990
Mephyton Tablets (Rare) 1993
Mepron Suspension (1%) 1487
Merrem I.V. (Greater than 0.1% to 1%) 687
Metadate CD Capsules 3316
Micardis Tablets 884
Migranal Nasal Spray (Rare) 3350
Mintezol 2002
Mirapex Tablets (Greater than or equal to 1%) 889
Mivacron Injection (Less than 1%) 489
Moban Tablets (Rare) 1108
Mobic Oral Suspension (Less than 2%) 893
Mobic Tablets (Less than 2%) 893

MS Contin Tablets (Less frequent).... 2703
Mycamine for Injection (0.2%).......... 620
▲ Myfortic Tablets (3% to less than 20%).. 2244
▲ Mylotarg for Injection (18% to 23%).. 3429
Nadolol Tablets (2 of 100 patients).. 2121
Namenda (Infrequent)........................ 1199
Naprosyn Suspension (Less than 1%).. 2769
Naprosyn Tablets (Less than 1%)..... 2769
Narcan Injection.............................. 1109
▲ Naropin Injection (More than 5% to 54.6%).. 640
▲ Natrecor for Injection (4% to 35%) .. 3123
Navelbine Injection........................ 1494
Nembutal Sodium Solution, USP (Less than 1%)............................... 2484
Neumega for Injection 3433
Neupogen for Injection (7 of 176 patients).. 598
Neurontin Capsules (Infrequent)....... 2498
Neurontin Oral Solution (Infrequent)...................................... 2498
Neurontin Tablets (Infrequent).......... 2498
Niaspan Extended-Release Tablets... 1703
Nimbex Injection (0.2%)................... 494
▲ Nimotop Capsules (1.2% to 50.0%).. 774
▲ Nipent for Injection (3% to 10%) 3216
▲ Niravam Orally Disintegrating Tablets (4.7%)................................ 3106
▲ Nitro-Dur Transdermal Infusion System (4%).................................. 3060
Nitrolingual Pumpspray.................... 1161
Norvasc Tablets (0.1% to 1%; rare).. 2529
Norvir (Less than 2%)..................... 499
Novantrone for Injection Concentrate..................................... 3158
Novolin 70/30 PenFill 3 ml Cartridges (Rare)........................... 2325
Novolin N PenFill 3 ml Cartridges (Rare).. 2325
Novolin R PenFill (Rare).................. 2325
NovoLog Injection............................ 2326
NovoSeven (1%)............................... 2335
Nubain Injection (1% or less)........... 1111
Numorphan...................................... 1112
Oncaspar (Greater than 1% but less than 5%)................................. 1123
▲ Ontak Vials (36%) 1717
Orap Tablets.................................... 1220
Orthoclone OKT3 Sterile Solution..... 2370
Oxsoralen-Ultra Capsules................. 3354
OxyContin Tablets............................ 2699
OxyFast Oral Concentrate Solution .. 2704
OxyIR Capsules................................ 2704
Pacerone Tablets (Less than 1%)..... 3337
Parcopa Orally Disintegrating Tablets.. 3111
Paxil CR Controlled-Release Tablets (Infrequent)...................... 1509
Paxil (Infrequent)............................ 1501
Pediarix Vaccine (Rare).................... 1518
Permax Tablets (2.1%)..................... 3357
Persantine Tablets (Rare)................ 898
Phenergan.. 3438
▲ Photofrin for Injection (7%) 729
Plasmanate....................................... 3252
Plavix Tablets.................................. 940
Plavix Tablets.................................. 2942
Plendil Extended-Release Tablets (0.5% to 1.5%)............................... 651
Pletal Tablets (Less than 2%)........... 2478
Pravachol Tablets............................ 943
Premarin Intravenous....................... 3440
Prevacid Delayed-Release Capsules (Less than 1%).............. 3268
Prevacid for Delayed-Release Oral Suspension (Less than 1%)......... 3268
Prevacid NapraPAC (Less than 1%).. 3277
Prevacid SoluTab Delayed-Release Orally Disintegrating Tablets (Less than 1%)............................... 3268
PREVPAC (Less than 1%)................. 3281
Primaxin I.M..................................... 2022
Primaxin I.V. (0.4%)......................... 2024
▲ Prinivil Tablets (0.3% to 4.4%; rare).. 2029
Prinzide Tablets (1.4%).................... 2033
▲ Prograf Capsules and Injection (3% to 15%)................................... 624
Prolastin (Rare)................................ 3252
▲ Proleukin for Injection (3% to 71%).. 1007
Prometrium Capsules (100 mg, 200 mg) (Rare)........................... 3205
Protonix I.V. (Less than 1%)............. 3468
Protonix Tablets (Less than 1%)....... 3465
Provigil Tablets (Greater than or equal to 1%)................................ 1002
Prozac Pulvules and Liquid (Infrequent).................................. 1771
▲ Rapamune Oral Solution and Tablets (3% to 20%)..................... 3472
Razadyne ER Extended-Release Capsules (Infrequent).................. 2434
Razadyne (Infrequent)...................... 2434
Recombivax HB (Less than 1%)........ 2045
ReFacto Vials................................... 3479
Refludan for Injection....................... 815
Relpax Tablets (Rare)...................... 2531
Remicade for IV Injection (Greater than or equal to 0.2%).................. 987
▲ Renagel Tablets (11%) 1268
▲ ReoPro Vials (21.1%) 1779
Requip Tablets (2%)......................... 1528
Retavase... 1131
Rhophylac (Rare).............................. 3504
Rilutek Tablets (Infrequent).............. 2945
Risperdal Consta Long-Acting Injection (Frequent)...................... 1664
Risperdal M-Tab Orally Disintegrating Tablets (Infrequent to 2%).......................... 1658
Risperdal (Infrequent to 2%) 1658
▲ Rituxan for Infusion (1% to 10%) 845
▲ Rituxan I.V. (1% to 10%) 1251
▲ Roferon-A Injection (Less than 4% to less than 5%).............................. 2805
Rythmol SR Capsules (Greater than or equal to 2%) 2736
▲ Simulect for Injection (3% to 10%) ... 2268
Sonata Capsules (Infrequent) 1686
St. Joseph 81 mg Aspirin Chewable and Enteric Coated Tablets 1841
Stalevo Tablets 2270
Sular Tablets (Less than or equal to 1%; very rare)......................... 1163
Surmontil Capsules 2347
Symbyax Capsules (Infrequent) 1788
Symmetrel 1115
Tambocor Tablets (Less than 1%) 1824
Tarka Tablets (0.3% to 0.6%) 519
Tasmar Tablets (2%)......................... 3360
▲ Taxotere Injection Concentrate (0.9% to 3.6%) 2947
Tegretol/Tegretol-XR 2278
▲ Tenormin I.V. Injection (25%) 698
▲ Tenormin Tablets (25%) 695
Tequin Injection 964
Tequin Tablets 964
Teveten Tablets (Less than 1%) 1707
Teveten HCT Tablets (Less than 1%).. 1710
Thalomid Capsules 979
Thioridazine Hydrochloride Tablets .. 2122
Thiothixene Capsules 2124
Tiazac Capsules (Less than 2%) 1204
Timolide Tablets (1.6%) 2056
Timoptic in Ocudose (Less frequent) 2061
Timoptic Sterile Ophthalmic Solution (Less frequent) 2058
Timoptic-XE Sterile Ophthalmic Gel Forming Solution 2062
TNKase I.V. 1256
Topamax Sprinkle Capsules (Infrequent) 2438
Topamax Tablets (Infrequent) 2438
Toprol-XL Tablets (About 1 of 100 patients) 660
▲ Tracleer Tablets (7%) 539
Tranxene 2488
▲ Trasylol Injection (8%) 779
Travatan Ophthalmic Solution (1% to 5%) 559
Tricor Tablets 523
Triglide Tablets 1165
Trileptal Oral Suspension (1% to 2%) 2281
Trileptal Tablets (1% to 2%) 2281
▲ Trisenox Injection (25%) 983
Trizivir Tablets 1565
Twinrix Vaccine (Less than 1%) 1571
Tygacil for Injection (2.3%) 3489
▲ Ultane Liquid for Inhalation (4% to 11%) 526
Ultracet Tablets (Less than 1%) 2462
Uniretic Tablets (More than 1%) 3114
Urecholine Tablets 2349
▲ Valcyte Tablets (Less than 5%) 2816
Valium Tablets (Infrequent) 2822
Vancocin HCl Capsules, USP 3370
Vantin Tablets and Oral Suspension (Less than 1%) 2650
Vaseretic Tablets (Rare; 0.9%) 2073
▲ Vasotec I.V. Injection (0.5% to 6.7%) 2076
▲ Velcade for Injection (11%-12%) 2102
▲ Ventavis Inhalation Solution (11%) ... 1036
Verelan PM Capsules (2.5%) 3120
▲ Vesanoid Capsules (14%; occasional)............................... 2823
VFEND I.V. (Less than 2%)............... 2543
VFEND Oral Suspension (Less than 2%).. 2543
VFEND Tablets (Less than 2%).......... 2543
Viagra Tablets (Less than 2%).......... 2552
Vicoprofen Tablets (Less than 1%).... 533
Virazole for Inhalation Solution......... 3365
Vivactil Tablets................................ 2350
Voltaren Tablets (Rarely).................. 2298
Voltaren-XR Tablets (Rarely)............. 2301
Wellbutrin Tablets (2.5%).................. 1579
Wellbutrin SR Sustained-Release Tablets 1583
Wellbutrin XL Extended-Release Tablets 1588
WinRho SDF..................................... 763
Xanax XR Tablets (Infrequent).......... 2655
Xeloda Tablets................................. 2825
Xopenex HFA Inhalation Aerosol...... 3151
Xopenex Inhalation Solution............. 3143
Xopenex Inhalation Solution Concentrate 3147
Zantac Injection 1593
▲ Zegerid Powder for Oral Solution (9.6%) 2972
Zelnorm Tablets (0.04%) 2303
Zemuron Injection (0.1%; 2%) 2363
▲ Zenapax for Injection (Greater than 5%) 2838
Zestoretic Tablets (1.4%; rare) 701
Zestril Tablets (Rare) 704
▲ Zevalin Injection (6%) 848
Ziagen 1600
Zithromax 2568
Zithromax for Oral Suspension, 300 mg, 600 mg, 900 mg, 1200 mg 2561
Zithromax Tablets, 250 mg, 500 mg 2561
Zithromax Tablets, 600 mg 2568
Zithromax Tri-Pak 2561
Zithromax Z-Pak 2568
Zmax for Oral Suspension 2577
Zofran Injection (Rare) 1607
▲ Zofran (5%) 1613
▲ Zofran ODT Orally Disintegrating Tablets (5%) 1613
Zoladex (Occasional) 709
Zoladex 3-month (Occasional) 712
Zoloft (Infrequent) 2581
▲ Zometa for Intravenous Infusion (10.5%) 2306
Zonegran Capsules (Infrequent) 1089
Zosyn (1.0% or less to 1.3%) 3492
Zovirax for Injection (Less than 1%) 1618
Zyban Sustained-Release Tablets 1620
Zyprexa Tablets (2%) 1798
Zyprexa IntraMuscular (2%) 1798
Zyprexa ZYDIS Orally Disintegrating Tablets (2%) 1798
Zyrtec Chewable Tablets (Rare) 2589
Zyrtec (Rare) 2589
Zyrtec-D 12 Hour Extended Release Tablets (Rare) 2591

Hypotension, asymptomatic

▲ Brevibloc Concentrate (About 25%) 766
▲ Brevibloc Injection (About 25%) 766
▲ Brevibloc Double Strength Injection (About 25%) 766
▲ Brevibloc Premixed Injection (About 25%) 766
▲ Brevibloc Double Strength Premixed Injection (About 25%) 766

Hypotension, neonatal

Aceon Tablets (2 mg, 4 mg, 8 mg) ... 3191
Altace Capsules 1673
Captopril Tablets 2114
Cozaar Tablets 1913
Hyzaar 1964
Lotrel Capsules 2238
Prinivil Tablets 2029
Prinzide Tablets 2033
Vaseretic Tablets 2073
Vasotec I.V. Injection 2076
Zestoretic Tablets 701
Zestril Tablets 704

Hypotension, orthostatic

Aceon Tablets (2 mg, 4 mg, 8 mg) (0.3% to 1%) 3191
Actiq (Less than 1%) 993
Adalat CC Tablets (Less than 1%) 2978
Advicor Tablets 1694
Agrylin Capsules (1% to 5%) 3172
Aldoclor Tablets 1881
Aldoril Tablets 1884
Altace Capsules (2%) 1673
Ambien Tablets (Infrequent) 2867
AmBisome for Injection (Less common)... 615
Anzemet Injection (Rare).................. 2871
Anzemet Tablets (Rare).................... 2874
▲ Apokyn Injection (11% to 20%) 2132
Aricept Tablets (Infrequent) 1086
Aricept ODT Tablets (Infrequent)....... 1086
Atacand HCT 637
Avalide Tablets................................ 922
Avalide Tablets 2889
▲ Avapro Tablets (5.4%) 925
▲ Avapro Tablets (5.4%) 2886
Caduet Tablets (Greater than 0.1% to less than 2%)............................ 2507
Campral Tablets (Infrequent)............ 1175
Camptosar Injection......................... 2602
Captopril Tablets 2114
Cardene I.V. (1.4%).......................... 1129
Catapres-TTS (0.5% or less) 875
Celexa (Frequent)............................. 1177
▲ CellCept Capsules (3% to less than 20%).................................... 2751
▲ CellCept Intravenous (3% to less than 20%).................................... 2751
▲ CellCept Oral Suspension (3% to less than 20%)........................... 2751
▲ CellCept Tablets (3% to less than 20%).. 2751
Cialis Tablets (Less than 2%)........... 1806
Cipro I.V. 2998
Cipro I.V. Pharmacy Bulk Package ... 3509
Cipro 2991
Cipro XR Tablets 3004
▲ Clorpres Tablets (About 3 in 100) 2139
Clozapine Tablets 2141
Clozaril Tablets................................ 2174
Comtan Tablets 2186
Copaxone for Injection (Infrequent)... 3292
▲ Coreg Tablets (1% to 3%) 1376
Covera-HS Tablets (0.4%)................. 3135
▲ Cozaar Tablets (4%) 1913
Depacon Injection (1% or more) 412
Depakene (1% or more).................... 417
Depakote Sprinkle Capsules 422
▲ Depakote Tablets (1% to 5%) 427
Depakote ER Tablets (Greater than 1%).. 433
Dibenzyline Capsules....................... 3390
Dilaudid Multiple Dose Vials............. 439
Diovan HCT Tablets.......................... 2195
Diovan Tablets (2%)......................... 2191
Diuril Oral 1936
Diuril Sodium Intravenous 1934
▲ Dostinex Tablets (4%) 2631
Doxil Injection (Less than 1%).......... 3302
Dyazide Capsules 1389
Effexor Tablets (1%)........................ 3405
Effexor XR Capsules (Frequent)....... 3411
Eldepryl Capsules 3209
Evoxac Capsules 1042
Exelon Capsules (Frequent).............. 2204
Flomax Capsules (0.2% to 0.4%)...... 881
Furosemide Tablets 2117
Gabitril Tablets (Infrequent) 998
Geodon (Frequent)........................... 2514
Hycomine Compound Tablets 1105
Hycotuss Expectorant Syrup 1106
Hyperstat I.V. Injection..................... 3031
Hytrin Capsules 469
Indapamide Tablets (Less than 5%).. 2119
▲ Intron A for Injection (Less than 5%).. 3038
Inversine Tablets 3286
Kadian Capsules 572
Kaletra (Less than 2%)..................... 474
Klonopin (Infrequent)........................ 2782
Lamictal (Infrequent)........................ 1449
Levaquin in 5% Dextrose Injection (0.1% to 0.9%)............................. 2453
Levaquin (0.1% to 0.9%).................. 2453
Levitra Tablets (Less than 2%)......... 3048
Lexapro Oral Solution 1193
Lexapro Tablets 1193
Lipitor Tablets (Less than 2%).......... 2495
Lotensin Tablets (0.4%).................... 2232
Lotensin HCT Tablets (0.3%)............ 2235
Lyrica Capsules (0.1% to 1%)........... 2524
Maxzide... 2150
Micardis Tablets............................... 884
Micardis HCT Tablets (Less than 2%).. 886
Midamor Tablets (Less than or equal to 1%)................................ 2000
▲ Mirapex Tablets (Greater than or equal to 1% to 53%).................... 889
Moduretic Tablets (Less than or equal to 1%)................................ 2003
MS Contin Tablets............................ 2703
Namenda (Infrequent)....................... 1199
Naropin Injection (Less than 1%)...... 640
Niaspan Extended-Release Tablets... 1703
Nitrolingual Pumpspray (Occasional)...................................... 1161

Noroxin Tablets.......... 2009
Norvasc Tablets (More than 0.1% to 1%).......... 2529
Norvir (Less than 2%).......... 499
Numorphan.......... 1112
Orap Tablets.......... 1220
▲ OxyContin Tablets (Between 1% and 5%).......... 2699
Parcopa Orally Disintegrating Tablets.......... 3111
Paxil CR Controlled-Release Tablets (1.2%).......... 1509
Paxil (1.2%).......... 1501
▲ Permax Tablets (9.0% to 10.0%).......... 3357
Pletal Tablets (Less than 2%).......... 2478
Prinivil Tablets (0.3% to 1.2%).......... 2029
Prinzide Tablets (0.5% to 1.0%).......... 2033
▲ Prograf Capsules and Injection (3% to 15%).......... 624
Prometrium Capsules (100 mg, 200 mg) (Rare).......... 3205
Prozac Pulvules and Liquid (Infrequent).......... 1771
▲ Rapamune Oral Solution and Tablets (3% to 20%).......... 3472
Razadyne ER Extended-Release Capsules (Infrequent).......... 2434
Razadyne (Infrequent).......... 2434
▲ Requip Tablets (6%).......... 1528
Rescriptor Tablets.......... 2535
Rilutek Tablets (0.8% to 1.6%).......... 2945
Risperdal Consta Long-Acting Injection (Infrequent to 2%).......... 1664
Risperdal M-Tab Orally Disintegrating Tablets.......... 1658
Risperdal.......... 1658
▲ Rituxan for Infusion (1% to 5%).......... 845
▲ Rituxan I.V. (1% to 5%).......... 1251
Sandostatin Injection (Less than 1%).......... 2263
Sandostatin LAR Depot (Rare).......... 2264
▲ Seroquel Tablets (4%).......... 691
Sonata Capsules (Rare).......... 1686
Stalevo Tablets.......... 2270
Stromectol Tablets (1.1%).......... 2053
Sular Tablets (Less than or equal to 1%).......... 1163
Symbyax Capsules.......... 1788
Symmetrel (1% to 5%).......... 1115
▲ Tasmar Tablets (13% to 14%).......... 3360
▲ Tenormin I.V. Injection (2% to 4%).......... 698
Tenormin Tablets (2% to 4%).......... 695
Teveten Tablets (Less than 1%).......... 1707
Teveten HCT Tablets (Less than 1%).......... 1710
Thalomid Capsules.......... 979
Timolide Tablets.......... 2056
Topamax Sprinkle Capsules (Infrequent).......... 2438
Topamax Tablets (Infrequent).......... 2438
Trecator Tablets.......... 3482
Trileptal Oral Suspension.......... 2281
Trileptal Tablets.......... 2281
Ultracet Tablets.......... 2462
Uniretic Tablets.......... 3114
Univasc Tablets (0.51%).......... 3118
Uroxatral Tablets (0.4%).......... 2957
Vaseretic Tablets (0.5% to 2.0%).......... 2073
Vasotec I.V. Injection (0.5% to 1.6%).......... 2076
▲ Velcade for Injection (12%).......... 2102
VFEND I.V. (Less than 2%).......... 2543
VFEND Oral Suspension (Less than 2%).......... 2543
VFEND Tablets (Less than 2%).......... 2543
Viagra Tablets (Less than 2%).......... 2552
Vivactil Tablets.......... 2350
Wellbutrin Tablets.......... 1579
Wellbutrin SR Sustained-Release Tablets (Infrequent).......... 1583
Wellbutrin XL Extended-Release Tablets (Infrequent).......... 1588
▲ Xeloda Tablets (Less than 5%).......... 2825
Zestoretic Tablets (0.3% to 1%).......... 701
Zestril Tablets (0.3% to 1.2%).......... 704
Zoloft (Infrequent).......... 2581
Zomig Tablets (Rare).......... 714
Zomig-ZMT Tablets (Rare).......... 714
Zyban Sustained-Release Tablets (Infrequent).......... 1620
Zyprexa Tablets.......... 1798
Zyprexa IntraMuscular (1%).......... 1798
Zyprexa ZYDIS Orally Disintegrating Tablets.......... 1798

Hypotension, postural
(*see under* Hypotension, orthostatic)

Hypotension, secondary to spinal block
Naropin Injection.......... 640

Hypotension, symptomatic
Aceon Tablets (2 mg, 4 mg, 8 mg).......... 3191
Altace Capsules (0.5%).......... 1673
Benicar HCT Tablets.......... 2852
▲ Brevibloc Concentrate (12%).......... 766
▲ Brevibloc Injection (12%).......... 766
▲ Brevibloc Double Strength Injection (12%).......... 766
▲ Brevibloc Premixed Injection (12%).......... 766
▲ Brevibloc Double Strength Premixed Injection (12%).......... 766
Covera-HS Tablets.......... 3135
Cozaar Tablets.......... 1913
Hyzaar.......... 1964
Lotensin Tablets (0.3%).......... 2232
Lotrel Capsules.......... 2238
Mavik Tablets (Rare; 0.6%).......... 482
Prinivil Tablets.......... 2029
Tarka Tablets.......... 519
Uniretic Tablets.......... 3114
Univasc Tablets (0.51%).......... 3118

Hypotensive crisis
Acthrel for Injection (One patient).......... 3528
Cymbalta Delayed-Release Capsules (Infrequent).......... 1729
Hyalgan Solution (One case).......... 2917

Hypothalamic-pituitary dysfunction
Lotronex Tablets (Rare).......... 1479

Hypothermia
Aggrenox Capsules.......... 855
Alphagan P Ophthalmic Solution.......... 563
Bayer Aspirin Tablets.......... 3515
Brimonidine Tartrate Ophthalmic Solution 0.2%.......... ⊙ 245
Clozapine Tablets (Less than 1%).......... 2141
Clozaril Tablets (Less than 1%).......... 2174
Depacon Injection.......... 412
Depakene.......... 417
Depakote Sprinkle Capsules.......... 422
Depakote Tablets.......... 427
Depakote ER Tablets.......... 433
Doxil Injection (Less than 1%).......... 3302
Ecotrin Enteric Coated Aspirin Low, Regular and Maximum Strength Tablets.......... 1627
Exelon Capsules (Infrequent).......... 2204
FazaClo Orally Disintegrating Tablets (Less than 1%).......... 547
Geodon Capsules (Frequent).......... 2514
Invanz for Injection (1.6%).......... 1974
Namenda (Infrequent).......... 1199
Naropin Injection (Less than 1%).......... 640
Norvir (Less than 2%).......... 499
Permax Tablets (Infrequent).......... 3357
Proleukin for Injection (Less than 1%).......... 1007
Provigil Tablets (At least 1%).......... 1002
Prozac Pulvules and Liquid (Rare).......... 1771
Relpax Tablets (Rare).......... 2531
Rilutek Tablets (Rare).......... 2945
Risperdal M-Tab Orally Disintegrating Tablets.......... 1658
Risperdal.......... 1658
St. Joseph 81 mg Aspirin Chewable and Enteric Coated Tablets.......... 1841
Ultane Liquid for Inhalation (1%).......... 526
▲ Vesanoid Capsules (3%).......... 2823

Hypothesia
Rythmol SR Capsules.......... 2736

Hypothyroidism
Abilify Tablets (Infrequent).......... 916
Abilify Tablets (Infrequent).......... 2472
Aciphex Tablets.......... 1081
▲ Advair Diskus 250/50 (1% to 3%).......... 1291
Amerge Tablets (Rare).......... 1312
▲ Aredia for Injection (Up to 6%).......... 2168
Avonex.......... 839
Betaseron for SC Injection.......... 791
▲ Bexxar (0% to 7%).......... 1360
Campral Tablets (Rare).......... 1175
Celexa (Rare).......... 1177
▲ CellCept Capsules (3% to less than 20%).......... 2751
▲ CellCept Intravenous (3% to less than 20%).......... 2751
▲ CellCept Oral Suspension (3% to less than 20%).......... 2751
▲ CellCept Tablets (3% to less than 20%).......... 2751
Cenestin Tablets, 0.45mg, 0.625mg, 0.9mg, 1.25mg.......... 1063
Cenestin Tablets, 0.3mg.......... 1063
Copaxone for Injection (Infrequent).......... 3292
▲ Copegus Tablets (Less than 1% to 4%).......... 2759
Effexor Tablets (Rare).......... 3405
Effexor XR Capsules (Rare).......... 3411
Eskalith.......... 1406
Evoxac Capsules (Less than 1%).......... 1042
Exelon Capsules (Infrequent).......... 2204
Gabitril Tablets (Infrequent).......... 998
Genotropin Lyophilized Powder (Infrequent).......... 2642
Herceptin I.V. (At least one of the 958 patients).......... 1234
▲ Humatrope Vials and Cartridges (11%).......... 1756
Imitrex Injection.......... 1431
Imitrex Nasal Spray (Rare).......... 1435
Imitrex Tablets (Rare).......... 1440
▲ Intron A for Injection (Less than 5%).......... 3038
Kaletra (Less than 2%).......... 474
Lamictal (Rare).......... 1449
Lithobid Tablets.......... 1670
Meridia Capsules.......... 485
Neurontin Capsules (Rare).......... 2498
Neurontin Oral Solution (Rare).......... 2498
Neurontin Tablets (Rare).......... 2498
▲ Ontak Vials (Less than 5%).......... 1717
▲ Pacerone Tablets (1% to 3%).......... 3337
Paxil CR Controlled-Release Tablets (Rare).......... 1509
Paxil (Rare).......... 1501
▲ Pegasys (3% to 4%).......... 2793
▲ PEG-Intron Powder for Injection (5%).......... 3062
Permax Tablets (Infrequent).......... 3357
Premarin Tablets.......... 3443
Prevacid Delayed-Release Capsules (Less than 1%).......... 3268
Prevacid for Delayed-Release Oral Suspension (Less than 1%).......... 3268
Prevacid NapraPAC (Less than 1%).......... 3277
Prevacid SoluTab Delayed-Release Orally Disintegrating Tablets (Less than 1%).......... 3268
PREVPAC (Less than 1%).......... 3281
Proleukin for Injection (Less than 1%).......... 1007
Prozac Pulvules and Liquid (Infrequent).......... 1771
▲ Rebetol (4% to 5%).......... 3073
Requip Tablets (Infrequent).......... 1528
▲ Ribavirin, USP Capsules (4% to 5%).......... 3083
Risperdal Consta Long-Acting Injection (Infrequent).......... 1664
Roferon-A Injection (Rare to infrequent).......... 2805
▲ Sandostatin Injection (12%).......... 2263
▲ Sandostatin LAR Depot (12%).......... 2264
Seroquel Tablets (Infrequent).......... 691
Sonata Capsules (Rare).......... 1686
Symbyax Capsules (Infrequent).......... 1788
▲ Targretin Capsules (28.6% to 52.8%).......... 1719
Thalomid Capsules.......... 979
Thyrolar.......... 1203
VFEND I.V. (Less than 2%).......... 2543
VFEND Oral Suspension (Less than 2%).......... 2543
VFEND Tablets (Less than 2%).......... 2543
Zoloft.......... 2581

Hypotonia
Abilify Tablets (Rare).......... 916
Abilify Tablets (Rare).......... 2472
Aloprim for Injection (Less than 1%).......... 2156
Alphagan P Ophthalmic Solution.......... 563
Ambien Tablets (Rare).......... 2867
Brimonidine Tartrate Ophthalmic Solution 0.2%.......... ⊙ 245
▲ Coreg Tablets (Greater than 1% to 3%).......... 1376
Diprivan Injectable Emulsion (Less than 1%).......... 676
Doxil Injection (Less than 1%).......... 3302
Duragesic Transdermal System (Less than 1%).......... 2448
Effexor Tablets (Infrequent).......... 3405
Effexor XR Capsules (Infrequent).......... 3411
Frova Tablets (Rare).......... 1101
Gabitril Tablets (Frequent).......... 998
Geodon Capsules (Frequent).......... 2514
HibTITER.......... 3419
Infanrix Vaccine.......... 1444
Klonopin.......... 2782
Lamictal (Rare).......... 1449
Lyrica Capsules (0.1% to 1%).......... 2524
Naropin Injection (Less than 1%).......... 640
Neurontin Capsules (Infrequent).......... 2498
Neurontin Oral Solution (Infrequent).......... 2498
Neurontin Tablets (Infrequent).......... 2498
Orthoclone OKT3 Sterile Solution (Less than 1%).......... 2370
OxyContin Tablets (Less than 1%).......... 2699
Pediarix Vaccine.......... 1518
Permax Tablets (Infrequent).......... 3357
▲ Rapamune Oral Solution and Tablets (3% to 20%).......... 3472
Requip Tablets (Infrequent).......... 1528
Rilutek Tablets (Rare).......... 2945
Risperdal M-Tab Orally Disintegrating Tablets (Rare).......... 1658
Risperdal (Rare).......... 1658
Sonata Capsules (Infrequent).......... 1686
Trileptal Oral Suspension.......... 2281
Trileptal Tablets.......... 2281
Xanax XR Tablets (Infrequent).......... 2655
Zoloft (Rare).......... 2581
Zomig Tablets (Rare).......... 714
Zomig-ZMT Tablets (Rare).......... 714
Zonegran Capsules (Infrequent).......... 1089
Zyprexa Tablets (Infrequent).......... 1798
Zyprexa ZYDIS Orally Disintegrating Tablets (Infrequent).......... 1798

Hypotonic-hyporesponsive episode
DAPTACEL (0.39%).......... 2964
Infanrix Vaccine.......... 1444

Hypotrichosis
Vantas (Less than 2%).......... 3367

Hypouresis
▲ Chemet Capsules (Up to 3.7%).......... 2480
Cymbalta Delayed-Release Capsules (Infrequent).......... 1729
Dilaudid-HP.......... 441
▲ Indocin I.V. (41% of infants).......... 1973
K-Phos Neutral Tablets.......... 785
Prograf Capsules and Injection.......... 624
Uroqid-Acid No. 2 Tablets.......... 785

Hypouricemia
Cipro I.V. (Infrequent).......... 2998
Cipro I.V. Pharmacy Bulk Package (Infrequent).......... 3509
Timentin ADD-Vantage.......... 1556
Timentin Injection Galaxy Container.......... 1559
Timentin IV Infusion.......... 1553
Timentin Pharmacy Bulk Package.......... 1562
Zoloft.......... 2581

Hypoventilation
Aciphex Tablets (Rare).......... 1081
Avinza Capsules (Less than 5%).......... 1714
▲ Buprenex Injectable (1% to 5%).......... 2718
Copaxone for Injection (Infrequent).......... 3292
Diastat Rectal Delivery System (Two patients).......... 3344
Diprivan Injectable Emulsion (Less than 1%).......... 676
▲ Duragesic Transdermal System (2% to 10%).......... 2448
Effexor XR Capsules (Rare).......... 3411
Mebaral Tablets, USP (Less than 1 in 100 patients).......... 2483
Nembutal Sodium Solution, USP (Less than 1%).......... 2484
Neurontin Capsules (Rare).......... 2498
Neurontin Oral Solution (Rare).......... 2498
Neurontin Tablets (Rare).......... 2498
Norvir (Less than 2%).......... 499
Permax Tablets (Rare).......... 3357
Prozac Pulvules and Liquid (Rare).......... 1771
Rilutek Tablets (Infrequent).......... 2945
Ultane Liquid for Inhalation (Less than 1%).......... 526
Virazole for Inhalation Solution (Infrequent).......... 3365
Zyprexa Tablets (Rare).......... 1798
Zyprexa ZYDIS Orally Disintegrating Tablets (Rare).......... 1798

Hypovolemia
Campath Ampules.......... 826
▲ CellCept Capsules (3% to less than 20%).......... 2751
▲ CellCept Intravenous (3% to less than 20%).......... 2751
▲ CellCept Oral Suspension (3% to less than 20%).......... 2751
▲ CellCept Tablets (3% to less than 20%).......... 2751
▲ Coreg Tablets (Greater than 1% to 3%).......... 1376
Estrastest Tablets.......... 3196
Estratest H.S. Tablets.......... 3196
Follistim AQ Cartridge.......... 2354
Zelnorm Tablets (0.04%).......... 2303

Hypoxemia
Carimune NF.......... 3501
Gammagard Liquid.......... 751
Gammagard S/D.......... 754
Gamunex Immune Globulin I.V., 10%.......... 3232

(▣ Described in PDR For Nonprescription Drugs) Incidence data in parenthesis; ▲ 3% or more (⊙ Described in PDR For Ophthalmic Medicines™)

Invanz for Injection (Greater than 0.1%) ... 1974
Iveegam EN ... 759
Mivacron Injection (Less than 1%) ... 489
Orthoclone OKT3 Sterile Solution ... 2370

Hypoxia
Abilify Tablets (Rare) ... 916
Abilify Tablets (Rare) ... 2472
Ambien Tablets (Rare) ... 2867
▲ AmBisome for Injection (6.2% to 7.5%) ... 615
Aricept Tablets (Infrequent) ... 1086
Aricept ODT Tablets (Infrequent) ... 1086
BeneFix for Injection (1.5%) ... 3402
Campath Ampules ... 826
Carbatrol Capsules ... 3174
▲ CellCept Capsules (3% to less than 20%) ... 2751
▲ CellCept Intravenous (3% to less than 20%) ... 2751
▲ CellCept Oral Suspension (3% to less than 20%) ... 2751
▲ CellCept Tablets (3% to less than 20%) ... 2751
Combunox Tablets (Less than 1%) ... 1183
▲ DepoDur Extended-Release Injection (5% to 10%) ... 1098
Diprivan Injectable Emulsion (Less than 1%) ... 676
Effexor Tablets (Rare) ... 3405
Effexor XR Capsules (Rare) ... 3411
Elitek ... 2906
Ethyol for Injection (Rare) ... 1869
▲ Flolan for Injection (55%) ... 1408
Herceptin I.V. (At least one of the 958 patients) ... 1234
I.V. Busulfex (2%) ... 1125
Kadian Capsules (Less than 3%) ... 572
Leukine ... 829
Levaquin in 5% Dextrose Injection (0.1% to 0.9%) ... 2453
Levaquin (0.1% to 0.9%) ... 2453
Merrem I.V. (Greater than 0.1% to 1%) ... 687
Mycamine for Injection ... 620
▲ Mylotarg for Injection (5%) ... 3429
Narcan Injection ... 1109
Neulasta Injection (Single case) ... 596
Orthoclone OKT3 Sterile Solution ... 2370
Permax Tablets (Rare) ... 3357
Protopic Ointment (Greater than or equal to 1%) ... 629
Prozac Pulvules and Liquid (Rare) ... 1771
Pulmozyme Inhalation Solution ... 1245
▲ Rapamune Oral Solution and Tablets (3% to 20%) ... 3472
Reyataz Capsules (Less than 3%) ... 948
Rilutek Tablets (Infrequent) ... 2945
Rituxan for Infusion (0.3%) ... 845
Rituxan I.V. (0.3%) ... 1251
Suprane Liquid for Inhalation (Less than 1%) ... 770
Targretin Capsules ... 1719
Tasmar Tablets (Rare) ... 3360
Tegretol/Tegretol-XR ... 2278
Trasylol Injection (2%) ... 779
▲ Trisenox Injection (23%) ... 983
Ultane Liquid for Inhalation (Less than 1%) ... 526
VFEND I.V. (Less than 2%) ... 2543
VFEND Oral Suspension (Less than 2%) ... 2543
VFEND Tablets (Less than 2%) ... 2543
▲ Zenapax for Injection (2% to 5%) ... 2838
▲ Zofran (9%) ... 1613
▲ Zofran ODT Orally Disintegrating Tablets (9%) ... 1613
Zyprexa Tablets (Infrequent) ... 1798
Zyprexa ZYDIS Orally Disintegrating Tablets (Rare) ... 1798

Hysteria
Ambien Tablets (Rare) ... 2867
Diprivan Injectable Emulsion (Less than 1%) ... 676
Imitrex Injection (Rare) ... 1431
Imitrex Tablets (Rare) ... 1440
Klonopin ... 2782
Neurontin Capsules (Rare) ... 2498
Neurontin Oral Solution (Rare) ... 2498
Neurontin Tablets (Rare) ... 2498
Paxil CR Controlled-Release Tablets (Rare) ... 1509
Paxil (Rare) ... 1501
Phenergan ... 3438
Relpax Tablets (Rare) ... 2531
Trileptal Oral Suspension ... 2281
Trileptal Tablets ... 2281

I

Ichthyosis
▲ Advair Diskus 100/50 (1% to 3%) ... 1291
▲ Advair Diskus 250/50 (1% to 3%) ... 1291
▲ Advair Diskus 500/50 (1% to 3%) ... 1291
Efudex (Infrequent) ... 3348
▲ Metrogel 1% (0.6% to 16.2%) ... 1212
Thalomid Capsules ... 979
Tricor Tablets ... 523

Icterus
(*see under* Jaundice)

Idiosyncrasy
Furosemide Tablets ... 2117

Idiosyncratic reactions
(*see under* Idiosyncrasy)

Idioventricular rhythm, accelerated
Retavase ... 1131

Idioventricular rhythms
Activase I.V. ... 1225

Ileitis, regional
Accutane Capsules ... 2740
Amnesteem Capsules ... 2126
Effexor XR Capsules (Rare) ... 3411
Indocin (Less than 1%) ... 1968
Norvir (Less than 2%) ... 499
Paxil CR Controlled-Release Tablets (Rare) ... 1509
Paxil (Rare) ... 1501

Ileus
Aricept Tablets (Infrequent) ... 1086
Aricept ODT Tablets (Infrequent) ... 1086
Camptosar Injection (Rare) ... 2602
Celebrex Capsules (Less than 0.1%) ... 3130
▲ CellCept Capsules (3% to less than 20%) ... 2751
▲ CellCept Intravenous (3% to less than 20%) ... 2751
▲ CellCept Oral Suspension (3% to less than 20%) ... 2751
▲ CellCept Tablets (3% to less than 20%) ... 2751
Cipro I.V. (1% or less) ... 2998
Cipro I.V. Pharmacy Bulk Package (1% or less) ... 3509
Cipro XR Tablets ... 3004
Cogentin Injection ... 1903
Combunox Tablets (Less than 1%) ... 1183
Dilaudid ... 439
Dilaudid Oral Liquid ... 443
Dilaudid Non-Sterile Powder ... 439
Dilaudid Rectal Suppositories ... 439
Dilaudid Tablets ... 439
Dilaudid Tablets - 8 mg ... 443
Diprivan Injectable Emulsion (Less than 1%) ... 676
▲ Doxil Injection (1% to 10%) ... 3302
Effexor Tablets (Rare) ... 3405
Effexor XR Capsules ... 3411
Elitek (Less than or equal to 1%) ... 2906
Eloxatin for Injection ... 2908
Evoxac Capsules (Less than 1%) ... 1042
Herceptin I.V. (At least one of the 958 patients) ... 1234
Hyperstat I.V. Injection ... 3031
Indocin I.V. (1% to 3%) ... 1973
Invanz for Injection (Greater than 0.1%) ... 1974
Inversine Tablets ... 3286
▲ I.V. Busulfex (2% to 8%) ... 1125
Lotronex Tablets (Rare) ... 1479
Merrem I.V. (Greater than 0.1% to 1%) ... 687
MS Contin Tablets (Less frequent) ... 2703
Myfortic Tablets ... 2244
Namenda ... 1199
Nimotop Capsules (Rare) ... 774
Nipent for Injection (Less than 3%) ... 3216
Omnicef Capsules ... 506
Omnicef for Oral Suspension ... 506
OxyContin Tablets (Less than 1%) ... 2699
Paxil CR Controlled-Release Tablets (Rare) ... 1509
Paxil (Rare) ... 1501
▲ Photofrin for Injection (Less than 5%) ... 729
▲ Prograf Capsules and Injection (3% to 15%) ... 624
Proleukin for Injection (2%) ... 1007
▲ Rapamune Oral Solution and Tablets (3% to 20%) ... 3472
Remicade for IV Injection (Greater than or equal to 0.2%) ... 987
ReoPro Vials (0.3%) ... 1779
Rilutek Tablets (Rare) ... 2945
Taxotere Injection Concentrate ... 2947
Vaseretic Tablets ... 2073
Vasotec I.V. Injection (0.5% to 1.0%) ... 2076
▲ Xeloda Tablets (1% to 6%) ... 2825
Zosyn (1.0% or less) ... 3492
Zyprexa Tablets (Rare) ... 1798
Zyprexa ZYDIS Orally Disintegrating Tablets (Rare) ... 1798

Ileus, adynamic
Thiothixene Capsules ... 2124

Ileus, paralytic
BiDil Tablets ... 2161
Campath Ampules ... 826
Clozapine Tablets ... 2141
Clozaril Tablets ... 2174
Cogentin Injection ... 1903
Covera-HS Tablets (Infrequent) ... 3135
▲ DepoDur Extended-Release Injection (5% to 10%) ... 1098
FazaClo Orally Disintegrating Tablets ... 547
Flexeril Tablets (Rare) ... 1832
Imodium Capsules (Rare) ... 1834
Navelbine Injection (1%) ... 1494
Numorphan ... 1112
Surmontil Capsules ... 2347
Tarka Tablets (Infrequent) ... 519
Thioridazine Hydrochloride Tablets ... 2122
Vivactil Tablets ... 2350

Illusion, unspecified
Ambien Tablets (Infrequent) ... 2867
Evoxac Capsules ... 1042
Klonopin (Infrequent) ... 2782
Zoloft (Rare) ... 2581

Immobility
Moban Tablets ... 1108

Immune reconstitution syndrome
Viread Tablets ... 1284

Immunogenicity
▲ Bexxar (1% to 7%) ... 1360
▲ Enbrel for Injection (6%) ... 580
Epogen for Injection ... 586
▲ Erbitux (5%) ... 937
Forteo for Injection (2.8%) ... 1739
Neumega for Injection (2%) ... 3433
NovoLog Injection ... 2326
PEG-Intron Powder for Injection ... 3062
Procrit for Injection ... 2374
▲ Raptiva for Injection (6.3%) ... 1247
Synagis ... 1868

Immunoglobulin, abnormalities
Phenytek Capsules ... 2153
Rilutek Tablets (Infrequent) ... 2945
Xolair ... 1259

Immunosuppression
Azasan Tablets ... 2844
Cutivate Lotion 0.05% (Rare) ... 1383
HMS Sterile Ophthalmic Suspension ... ⊙ 228
Purinethol Tablets ... 1222

Immunosuppression, progressive
Lamictal ... 1449

Impaired concentration
Abilify Tablets (Infrequent) ... 916
Abilify Tablets (Infrequent) ... 2472
▲ Copegus Tablets (10%) ... 2759
Coreg Tablets (Greater than 0.1% to 1%) ... 1376
▲ Imdur Tablets (Less than or equal to 5%) ... 3032
Levaquin in 5% Dextrose Injection (0.1% to 0.9%) ... 2453
Levaquin (0.1% to 0.9%) ... 2453
Lunesta Tablets (Infrequent) ... 3139
▲ Nicotrol NS (Greater than 5%) ... 2596
Niravam Orally Disintegrating Tablets ... 3106
▲ Pegasys (8%) ... 2793
▲ PEG-Intron Powder for Injection (10%) ... 3062
Prevacid NapraPAC (Less than 1%) ... 3277
▲ Rebetol (5% to 21%) ... 3073
Rescriptor Tablets ... 2535
▲ Ribavirin, USP Capsules (5% to 21%) ... 3083
Risperdal Consta Long-Acting Injection (Infrequent) ... 1664
Risperdal M-Tab Orally Disintegrating Tablets (2%) ... 1658
Risperdal (2%) ... 1658
▲ Topamax Sprinkle Capsules (3% to 14%) ... 2438
▲ Topamax Tablets (3% to 14%) ... 2438
Wellbutrin SR Sustained-Release Tablets ... 1583
Wellbutrin XL Extended-Release Tablets ... 1588

Impetigo
Cutivate Cream (0.8%) ... 1381
Elidel Cream 1% (1.9% to 4%) ... 2198
Varivax ... 2070

Impotence
(*see also under* Sexual dysfunction)
Abelcet Injection ... 1119
Abilify Tablets (Infrequent) ... 916
Abilify Tablets (Infrequent) ... 2472
Aciphex Tablets (Rare) ... 1081
▲ Adalat CC Tablets (3% or less) ... 2978
Adderall Tablets ... 3168
▲ Adderall XR Capsules (2% to 4%) ... 3169
Adipex-P ... 1216
Advicor Tablets ... 1694
Aldoclor Tablets ... 1881
Aldoril Tablets ... 1884
Altace Capsules (Less than 1%) ... 1673
Ambien Tablets (Rare) ... 2867
Anadrol-50 Tablets ... 3329
Antabuse Tablets ... 2343
Arthrotec Tablets (Rare) ... 3126
Atacand HCT ... 637
Avinza Capsules (Less than 5%) ... 1714
▲ Avodart Soft Gelatin Capsules (0.8% to 4.7%) ... 1353
Axid Oral Solution ... 913
Betagan Ophthalmic Solution, USP ... ⊙ 217
▲ Betaseron for SC Injection (9%) ... 791
Betimol Ophthalmic Solution ... ⊙ 283
Betimol Ophthalmic Solution ... 3371
Blocadren Tablets (Less than 1%) ... 1891
Caduet Tablets (Less than 2%) ... 2507
Campral Tablets (Frequent) ... 1175
Captopril Tablets ... 2114
Carbatrol Capsules ... 3174
Cardizem LA Extended Release Tablets (Less than 2%) ... 1699
▲ Casodex Tablets (5%) ... 670
▲ Catapres Tablets (About 3 in 100 patients) ... 874
Catapres-TTS (2 of 101 patients) ... 875
▲ Celexa (3%) ... 1177
▲ CellCept Capsules (3% to less than 20%) ... 2751
▲ CellCept Intravenous (3% to less than 20%) ... 2751
▲ CellCept Oral Suspension (3% to less than 20%) ... 2751
▲ CellCept Tablets (3% to less than 20%) ... 2751
▲ Clorpres Tablets (About 3%) ... 2139
Clozapine Tablets (Less than 1%) ... 2141
Clozaril Tablets (Less than 1%) ... 2174
▲ Coreg Tablets (Greater than 1% to 3%) ... 1376
Cosopt Sterile Ophthalmic Solution ... 1910
Covera-HS Tablets (Less than 2%) ... 3135
Cozaar Tablets (Less than 1%) ... 1913
Demser Capsules (Infrequent) ... 1933
Desoxyn Tablets, USP ... 2482
Dexedrine ... 1386
DextroStat Tablets ... 3177
Diovan HCT Tablets (Greater than 0.2%) ... 2195
Diovan Tablets ... 2191
Ditropan XL Extended Release Tablets (Rare) ... 2391
Diuril Oral ... 1936
Diuril Sodium Intravenous ... 1934
Dyazide Capsules ... 1389
DynaCirc CR Tablets (0.5% to 1%) ... 2726
▲ Effexor Tablets (2.1% to 6%) ... 3405
▲ Effexor XR Capsules (3% to 10%) ... 3411
Eligard 7.5 mg (Less than 2%) ... 2896
Eligard 22.5 mg (Less than 2%) ... 2899
Eligard 30 mg ... 2901
Equetro Extended-Release Capsules ... 3178
Eskalith ... 1406
▲ Eulexin Capsules (33%) ... 3023
Evoxac Capsules ... 1042
Exelon Capsules (Infrequent) ... 2204
FazaClo Orally Disintegrating Tablets (Less than 1%) ... 547
Flexeril Tablets (Rare) ... 1832
Gabitril Tablets (Infrequent) ... 998
Geodon Capsules (Infrequent) ... 2514
Hytrin Capsules (1.2% to 1.6%) ... 469
Hyzaar ... 1964
▲ Imdur Tablets (Less than or equal to 5%) ... 3032
Indapamide Tablets (Less than 5%) ... 2119
Inderal LA Long-Acting Capsules (Rare) ... 3421
InnoPran XL Capsules (Rare) ... 2728

▲ Intron A for Injection (Less than 5%) 3038
Inversine Tablets 3286
Invirase (Less than 2%) 2776
Klonopin (1%) 2782
▲ Lamictal (13%) 1449
Levaquin in 5% Dextrose Injection (0.1% to 0.9%) 2453
Levaquin (0.1% to 0.9%) 2453
▲ Lexapro Oral Solution (Less than 1% to 3%) 1193
▲ Lexapro Tablets (Less than 1% to 3%) 1193
Lipitor Tablets (Less than 2%) 2495
Lithobid Tablets 1670
Lotensin Tablets (Less than 1%) 2232
Lotensin HCT Tablets (1.2%) 2235
Lotrel Capsules 2238
▲ Lupron Depot 7.5 mg (5.4%) 3261
Lyrica Capsules (Greater than or equal to 1%) 2524
Mavik Tablets (0.3% to 1.0%) 482
▲ Megace ES Oral Suspension (4% to 14%) 2492
Meridia Capsules 485
Micardis Tablets (More than 0.3%) 884
Micardis HCT Tablets 886
▲ Midamor Tablets (Between 1% and 3%) 2000
Mirapex Tablets (2%) 889
Moduretic Tablets (Less than or equal to 1%) 2003
MS Contin Tablets (Less frequent) 2703
Nadolol Tablets (1 to 5 of 1000 patients) 2121
Namenda (More than one patient) 1199
Neurontin Capsules (1.5%) 2498
Neurontin Oral Solution (1.5%) 2498
Neurontin Tablets (1.5%) 2498
Nexium Delayed-Release Capsules (Less than 1%) 645
Nexium I.V. (Less than 1%) 649
Nipent for Injection (Less than 3%) 3216
Norvir (Less than 2%) 499
Omacor Capsules 2735
▲ Orap Tablets (3 of 20 patients) 1220
Oxandrin Tablets 2977
OxyContin Tablets (Less than 1%) 2699
Parnate Tablets 1499
▲ Paxil CR Controlled-Release Tablets (4% to 10.0%) 1509
▲ Paxil (4% to 10.0%) 1501
Pepcid Injection (Rare) 2017
Pepcid (Rare) 2014
Permax Tablets (Infrequent) 3357
Plendil Extended-Release Tablets (0.5% to 1.5%) 651
Prevacid Delayed-Release Capsules (Less than 1%) 3268
Prevacid for Delayed-Release Oral Suspension (Less than 1%) 3268
Prevacid NapraPAC (Less than 1%) 3277
Prevacid SoluTab Delayed-Release Orally Disintegrating Tablets (Less than 1%) 3268
PREVPAC (Less than 1%) 3281
Prinivil Tablets (1.0%) 2029
Prinzide Tablets (1.2%) 2033
▲ Propecia Tablets (5.1% to 8.1%) 2036
▲ Proscar Tablets (5.15 to 8.1%) 2040
Protonix I.V. (Less than 1%) 3468
Protonix Tablets (Less than 1%) 3465
Prozac Pulvules and Liquid (Less than 1%) 1771
▲ Rapamune Oral Solution and Tablets (3% to 20%) 3472
Relafen Tablets (Less than 1%) 1523
Relpax Tablets (Infrequent) 2531
▲ Requip Tablets (3%) 1528
Rescriptor Tablets 2535
Reyataz Capsules (Less than 3%) 948
Rilutek Tablets (Infrequent) 2945
Risperdal Consta Long-Acting Injection (Infrequent) 1664
▲ Roferon-A Injection (Less than 4%) 2805
Rythmol SR Capsules 2736
Sandostatin LAR Depot (1% to 4%) 2264
Seroquel Tablets (Infrequent) 691
▲ Simulect for Injection (3% to 10%) 2268
Sonata Capsules (Infrequent) 1686
Sular Tablets (Less than or equal to 1%) 1163
Surmontil Capsules 2347
▲ Symbyax Capsules (2% to 4%) 1788
Tagamet Tablets 1547
Tambocor Tablets (Less than 1%) 1824
Tarka Tablets (0.3% or more) 519
Tasmar Tablets (Frequent) 3360
Tegretol/Tegretol-XR 2278
Tenormin I.V. Injection 698
Tenormin Tablets 695
Teveten HCT Tablets 1710
▲ Thalomid Capsules (8.3%) 979
Thiothixene Capsules (Infrequently) 2124
Tiazac Capsules (Less than 2%) 1204
Timolide Tablets 2056
Timoptic in Ocudose (Less frequent) 2061
Timoptic Sterile Ophthalmic Solution (Less frequent) 2058
Timoptic-XE Sterile Ophthalmic Gel Forming Solution 2062
Topamax Sprinkle Capsules (Frequent) 2438
Topamax Tablets (Frequent) 2438
Toprol-XL Tablets 660
Trecator Tablets 3482
▲ Trelstar Depot (7.1%) 3385
Trelstar LA Suspension (2.3%) 3387
Ultracet Tablets (Less than 1%) 2462
Uniretic Tablets (More than 1%) 3114
Uroxatral Tablets (1% to 2%) 2957
Vaseretic Tablets (2.2%) 2073
Vasotec I.V. Injection (0.5% to 1.0%) 2076
Verelan PM Capsules (2% or less) 3120
VFEND I.V. (Less than 2%) 2543
VFEND Oral Suspension (Less than 2%) 2543
VFEND Tablets (Less than 2%) 2543
Viadur Implant (2.3%) 782
Vicoprofen Tablets (Less than 1%) 533
Vivactil Tablets 2350
Vytorin 10/10 Tablets 2084
Vytorin 10/10 Tablets 3092
Vytorin 10/20 Tablets 2084
Vytorin 10/20 Tablets 3092
Vytorin 10/40 Tablets 2084
Vytorin 10/40 Tablets 3092
Vytorin 10/80 Tablets 2084
Vytorin 10/80 Tablets 3092
▲ Wellbutrin Tablets (3.4%) 1579
Wellbutrin SR Sustained-Release Tablets (Infrequent) 1583
Wellbutrin XL Extended-Release Tablets (Infrequent) 1588
Zantac (Occasional) 1597
Zantac Injection 1593
Zantac Injection Pharmacy Bulk Package (Infrequent) 1595
Zantac Syrup (Occasional) 1597
Zestoretic Tablets (1.2%) 701
Zestril Tablets (1.0%) 704
Zoladex 3-month (1% to 5%) 712
Zoloft (Frequent) 2581
Zonegran Capsules (Infrequent) 1089
Zyban Sustained-Release Tablets (Infrequent) 1620
Zyprexa Tablets (Infrequent) 1798
Zyprexa ZYDIS Orally Disintegrating Tablets (Infrequent) 1798

Impulse control, impaired
Effexor Tablets (Rare) 3405
Paxil CR Controlled-Release Tablets 1509
Paxil 1501
Prozac Pulvules and Liquid 1771
Surmontil Capsules 2347
Symbyax Capsules 1788
Vivactil Tablets 2350
Xanax XR Tablets (Infrequent) 2655
Zoloft 2581

Incontinence
Moduretic Tablets (Less than or equal to 1%) 2003
Namenda (Greater than or equal to 2%) 1199
Niravam Orally Disintegrating Tablets (1.5%) 3106
Razadyne ER Extended-Release Capsules (Frequent) 2434
Razadyne (Frequent) 2434
Sandostatin LAR Depot (1% to 4%) 2264
Valium Tablets (Infrequent) 2822

Incontinence, fecal
Abilify Tablets 916
Abilify Tablets 2472
Actiq (Less than 1%) 993
AmBisome for Injection (Less common) 615
Aricept Tablets (Frequent) 1086
Aricept ODT Tablets (Frequent) 1086
Colazal Capsules 2845
Copaxone for Injection (At least 2%) 3292
Depacon Injection (1% or more) 412
Depakene (1% or more) 417
Depakote Sprinkle Capsules 422
▲ Depakote Tablets (1% to 5%) 427
Depakote ER Tablets (Greater than 1%) 433
Eskalith 1406
Exelon Capsules (Frequent) 2204
Gabitril Tablets (Infrequent) 998
Kaletra (Less than 2%) 474
Klonopin 2782
Lithobid Tablets 1670
Marinol Capsules (Less than 1%) 3334
Naropin Injection (Less than 1%) 640
Neurontin Capsules (Infrequent) 2498
Neurontin Oral Solution (Infrequent) 2498
Neurontin Tablets (Infrequent) 2498
Omacor Capsules 2735
Paxil CR Controlled-Release Tablets (Rare) 1509
Paxil (Rare) 1501
Pentasa Capsules (Less than 1%) 3182
Permax Tablets (Rare) 3357
Prozac Pulvules and Liquid (Rare) 1771
Requip Tablets (Infrequent) 1528
Rilutek Tablets (Infrequent) 2945
Risperdal Consta Long-Acting Injection (Infrequent) 1664
Risperdal M-Tab Orally Disintegrating Tablets (Rare) 1658
Risperdal (Rare) 1658
Seroquel Tablets (Infrequent) 691
Stromectol Tablets 2053
Symbyax Capsules (Rare) 1788
Topamax Sprinkle Capsules (Infrequent to 1%) 2438
Topamax Tablets (Infrequent to 1%) 2438
▲ Trisenox Injection (8%) 983
▲ Xenical Capsules (1.8% to 7.7%) 2834
Zelnorm Tablets 2303
Zoloft (Rare) 2581
Zonegran Capsules (Rare) 1089
Zyprexa Tablets (Infrequent) 1798
Zyprexa ZYDIS Orally Disintegrating Tablets (Infrequent) 1798

Incoordination
(*see under* Ataxia)

Indigestion
Asacol Delayed-Release Tablets 2688
Augmentin 1331
Augmentin Tablets 1334
Augmentin XR Extended-Release Tablets 1340
Augmentin ES-600 Powder for Oral Suspension 1337
Carafate Suspension (Less than 0.5%) 727
Carafate Tablets (Less than 0.5%) 728
Ceftin Tablets (0.1% to 1%) 1369
▲ Depacon Injection (Among most common) 412
Depakote Sprinkle Capsules 422
▲ Depakote Tablets (Among most common) 427
Depakote ER Tablets 433
Eskalith 1406
▲ Indocin (3% to 9%) 1968
▲ Lexapro Oral Solution (2% to 6%) 1193
▲ Lexapro Tablets (2% to 6%) 1193
Lithobid Tablets 1670
Nadolol Tablets (1 to 5 of 1000 patients) 2121
Oncaspar 1123
Roferon-A Injection (2%) 2805

Induration at injection site
Ancef for Injection 1318
▲ Aredia for Injection (Up to 41%) 2168
Boostrix 1366
▲ Brevibloc Concentrate (About 8%) 766
▲ Brevibloc Injection (About 8%) 766
▲ Brevibloc Double Strength Injection (About 8%) 766
▲ Brevibloc Premixed Injection (About 8%) 766
▲ Brevibloc Double Strength Premixed Injection (About 8%) 766
▲ Cancidas for Injection (0% to 3.1%) 1894
Capastat Sulfate for Injection 1728
▲ Comvax (27.2% to 27.6%) 1904
▲ Copaxone for Injection (13%) 3292
Desferal Vials 2190
▲ Engerix-B Vaccine (1% to 10 %) 1391
▲ Fuzeon Injection (90%) 2772
▲ Havrix Vaccine (1% to 10%) 1425
HibTITER 3419
Imitrex Injection 1431
Invanz for Injection (1%) 1974
Lupron Depot 3.75 mg 3257
Lupron Depot 7.5 mg 3261
Lupron Depot–3 Month 11.25 mg 3262
Lupron Depot-PED 7.5 mg, 11.25 mg and 15 mg 3266
Lupron Injection Pediatric 3256
▲ Menactra Vaccine (0.3% to 17.1%) 2968
Meruvax II 1994
M-M-R II 1980
Oncaspar 1123
Liquid PedvaxHIB 2012
Pneumovax 23 (Common) 2020
▲ Prevnar for Injection (0% to 48.3%) 3460
Primaxin I.V. (0.2%) 2024
Rabies Vaccine RabAvert (Common) 1011
Risperdal Consta Long-Acting Injection (1%) 1664
Rocephin Injectable Vials, ADD-Vantage, Galaxy, Bulk (1%) 2801
Timentin ADD-Vantage 1556
Timentin Injection Galaxy Container 1559
Timentin IV Infusion 1553
Timentin Pharmacy Bulk Package 1562
▲ Twinrix Vaccine (1% to 10%) 1571
▲ Varivax (19.35% to 32.5%) 2070
Xolair 1259

Inebriated feeling
Klonopin (Infrequent) 2782

Infection, access site
▲ Sensipar Tablets (5%) 603

Infection, acquired immunodeficiency syndrome
Thalomid Capsules 979

Infection, aspergillus
Myfortic Tablets (Rare) 2244

Infection, bacterial
Actiq (Less than 1%) 993
▲ Advair Diskus 100/50 (1% to 3%) 1291
▲ Advair Diskus 250/50 (1% to 3%) 1291
▲ Advair Diskus 500/50 (1% to 3%) 1291
Campath Ampules 826
Celebrex Capsules (0.1% to 1.9%) 3130
Comtan Tablets (1%) 2186
▲ Copaxone for Injection (5%) 3292
▲ Copegus Tablets (Less than 1% to 3%) 2759
Elidel Cream 1% (1.1% to 1.8%) 2198
Elocon Cream 0.1% (1 in 182 patients) 3019
Elocon Ointment 0.1% (1 in 63 patients) 3021
Enbrel for Injection 580
▲ Equetro Extended-Release Capsules (Less than 5%) 3178
Evoxac Capsules (Less than 1%) 1042
▲ Flovent Diskus 50 mcg (1% to 3%) 1415
Gengraf Capsules (1% to less than 3%) 458
▲ Humira Injection (Less than 5%) 464
▲ Imdur Tablets (Less than or equal to 5%) 3032
▲ Intron A for Injection (Less than 5%) 3038
Invirase (Less than 2%) 2776
Kaletra (Less than 2%) 474
▲ Leustatin Injection (42%) 2368
Levaquin in 5% Dextrose Injection (0.1% to 0.9%) 2453
Levaquin (0.1% to 0.9%) 2453
Neoral Soft Gelatin Capsules (1% to less than 3%) 2247
Neoral Oral Solution (1% to less than 3%) 2247
▲ Nipent for Injection (5%) 3216
Orthoclone OKT3 Sterile Solution 2370
Pegasys 2793
Remicade for IV Injection 987
Rituxan for Infusion 845
▲ Rituxan I.V. (19%) 1251
Sandostatin LAR Depot (1% to 4%) 2264
Stalevo Tablets (1%) 2270
▲ Targretin Capsules (1.2% to 13.2%) 1719
Tasmar Tablets (Infrequent) 3360
▲ Trisenox Injection (8%) 983
Vantin Tablets and Oral Suspension (Less than 1%) 2650
Varivax 2070
VFEND I.V. (Less than 2%) 2543
VFEND Oral Suspension (Less than 2%) 2543
VFEND Tablets (Less than 2%) 2543

Infection, bacterial, ocular, secondary
Poly-Pred Liquifilm Ophthalmic Suspension ⊙ 231
Zylet Ophthalmic Suspension 3508

Infection, bladder
Advate Injection (0.6%) 742
Clindesse Vaginal Cream (Less than 1%) 3296
Vivelle Transdermal System 2288
Vivelle-Dot Transdermal System 2293

Infection, candida albicans
Aerobid/Aerobid-M 1172
Cubicin for Injection (1% to 2%) 1038
Myfortic Tablets (0.6% to 2.3%) 2244
Nasacort HFA Inhalation Aerosol 2939
Zosyn (1% or less) 3492

Infection, corneal, fungal
Blephamide Ophthalmic Ointment 563
HMS Sterile Ophthalmic Suspension .... ⊙228
Pred Forte Ophthalmic Suspension .... ⊙233
Pred Mild Sterile Ophthalmic Suspension .... ⊙236
Pred-G Ophthalmic Suspension .... ⊙234
TobraDex Ophthalmic Ointment 558
TobraDex Ophthalmic Suspension 558

Infection, cryptococcus
Myfortic Tablets (Rare) 2244
Orthoclone OKT3 Sterile Solution (1.6%) 2370

Infection, cytomegalovirus
▲ CellCept Capsules (Less than 4% to 14.1%) 2751
▲ CellCept Intravenous (Less than 4% to 14.1%) 2751
▲ CellCept Oral Suspension (Less than 4% to 14.1%) 2751
▲ CellCept Tablets (Less than 4% to 14.1%) 2751
▲ Doxil Injection (20.1%) 3302
Fuzeon Injection 2772
▲ Gengraf Capsules (4.8%) 458
▲ Myfortic Tablets (1.9% to 21.6%) 2244
▲ Neoral Soft Gelatin Capsules (4.8%) 2247
▲ Neoral Oral Solution (4.8%) 2247
▲ Orthoclone OKT3 Sterile Solution (3% to 19%) 2370
Remicade for IV Injection 987
▲ Sandimmune (4.8% to 12.3%) 2259
▲ Simulect for Injection (14%) 2268
▲ Thymoglobulin for Injection (12.2%) 2848

Infection, decreased resistance
Decadron Tablets 1929
HMS Sterile Ophthalmic Suspension .... ⊙228
Orthoclone OKT3 Sterile Solution 2370
Prograf Capsules and Injection 624
Sandimmune 2259

Infection, ears
Aceon Tablets (2 mg, 4 mg, 8 mg) (Up to 1.3%) 3191
▲ Advair Diskus 100/50 (1% to 4%) 1291
▲ Advair Diskus 250/50 (1% to 4%) 1291
▲ Advair Diskus 500/50 (1% to 4%) 1291
▲ Aerobid/Aerobid-M (3% to 9%) 1172
Amerge Tablets (Frequent) 1312
Avalide Tablets 922
Avalide Tablets 2889
Avapro Tablets (Less than 1%) 925
Avapro Tablets (Less than 1%) 2886
Ciprodex Otic Suspension (0.6%) 555
Colazal Capsules 2845
Cutivate Lotion 0.05% (1%) 1383
Elidel Cream 1% (0.6% to 5.7%) 2198
▲ Entocort EC Capsules (Less than 5%) 2694
▲ Epivir-HBV (25%) 1398
Imitrex Nasal Spray (Infrequent) 1435
Invanz for Injection (Greater than 0.5%) 1974
Lotronex Tablets (Rare) 1479
Neurontin Capsules (Infrequent) 2498
Neurontin Oral Solution (Infrequent) 2498
Neurontin Tablets (Infrequent) 2498
▲ Liquid PedvaxHIB (Among most frequent) 2012
▲ Pulmicort Respules (2% to 5%) 654
Somavert Injection 2648
▲ Strattera Capsules (3%) 1784
Vivelle Transdermal System 2288
Vivelle-Dot Transdermal System 2293
▲ Ziagen (5%) 1600

Infection, Epstein-Barr virus
Rapamune Oral Solution and Tablets (Less frequent) 3472

Infection, eyes
▲ Acular Ophthalmic Solution (Approximately 1% to 10%) 561
▲ Acular LS Ophthalmic Solution (1% to 10%) 562
▲ Advair Diskus 250/50 (1% to 3%) 1291
Aerobid/Aerobid-M (1% to 3%) 1172
Elidel Cream 1% (Up to 1.1%) 2198
▲ Evoxac Capsules (1% to 3%) 1042
Lexapro Oral Solution (Infrequent) 1193
Lexapro Tablets (Infrequent) 1193
Pulmicort Respules (1% to 3%) 654

Infection, fungal
Actiq (1% or greater) 993
Blephamide Ophthalmic Suspension 564
Bravelle for Intramuscular or Subcutaneous Injection (2%) 1140
Campath Ampules 826
Celebrex Capsules (0.1% to 1.9%) 3130
Cleocin Vaginal Ovules (1%) 2613
Clindesse Vaginal Cream (Less than 1%) 3296
Cubicin for Injection (2.6%) 1038
Detrol Tablets (1.1%) 2626
Enbrel for Injection 580
▲ Equetro Extended-Release Capsules (Less than 5%) 3178
▲ Evoxac Capsules (1% to 3%) 1042
Factive Tablets (0.1% to 1%) 2464
Floxin Otic Singles (Reported in a single subject) 1045
Floxin Otic Solution (Single report) 1043
FML Ophthalmic Ointment .... ⊙225
FML Ophthalmic Suspension .... ⊙224
FML Forte Ophthalmic Suspension .... ⊙223
FML-S Liquifilm Sterile Ophthalmic Suspension .... ⊙226
Gengraf Capsules (1% to less than 3%) 458
Humira Injection 464
▲ Intron A for Injection (Less than 5%) 3038
Invirase (Less than 2%) 2776
Keppra Oral Solution (1% or more) 3307
Keppra Tablets (1% or more) 3307
Klonopin (Infrequent) 2782
▲ Leustatin Injection (20%) 2368
Levaquin in 5% Dextrose Injection (0.1% to 0.9%) 2453
Levaquin (0.1% to 0.9%) 2453
Lotronex Tablets (Rare) 1479
Micardis Tablets (More than 0.3%) 884
Micardis HCT Tablets 886
▲ Myfortic Tablets (2.5% to 10.8%) 2244
Neoral Soft Gelatin Capsules (1% to less than 3%) 2247
Neoral Oral Solution (1% to less than 3%) 2247
Omacor Capsules 2735
▲ Orthoclone OKT3 Sterile Solution (4% to 34%) 2370
PEG-Intron Powder for Injection (Less than 1%) 3062
▲ Rebetol (1% to 6%) 3073
Remicade for IV Injection 987
Requip Tablets (Infrequent) 1528
Reyataz Capsules (Less than 3%) 948
▲ Ribavirin, USP Capsules (1% to 6%) 3083
Rituxan I.V. (1%) 1251
Soriatane Capsules (Less than 1%) 1028
Spectracef Tablets (0.1% to 1%) 2706
Tasmar Tablets (Infrequent) 3360
VFEND I.V. (Less than 2%) 2543
VFEND Oral Suspension (Less than 2%) 2543
VFEND Tablets (Less than 2%) 2543
Vivelle Transdermal System 2288
Vivelle-Dot Transdermal System 2293
▲ Xeloda Tablets (Less than 5%) 2825
Zelnorm Tablets (Up to 1%) 2303
Zenapax for Injection 2838
Zithromax for Oral Suspension, 300 mg, 600 mg, 900 mg, 1200 mg (1% or less) 2561
Zithromax Tablets, 250 mg, 500 mg (1% or less) 2561
Zithromax Tri-Pak (1% or less) 2561
Zyvox (0.1% to 1.5%) 2661

Infection, fungal, corneal, secondary
Poly-Pred Liquifilm Ophthalmic Suspension .... ⊙231

Infection, fungal, local
Aceon Tablets (2 mg, 4 mg, 8 mg) (0.3% to 1%) 3191
▲ Aldara Cream, 5% (2% to 11%) 1814
Doxil Injection (Less than 1%) 3302
▲ Gengraf Capsules (7.5%) 458
▲ Neoral Soft Gelatin Capsules (7.5%) 2247
▲ Neoral Oral Solution (7.5%) 2247
▲ Sandimmune (7.5% to 9.6%) 2259
Vantin Tablets and Oral Suspension (Less than 1% to 3.1%) 2650

Infection, fungal, ocular, secondary
Zylet Ophthalmic Suspension 3508

Infection, fungal, systemic
Gengraf Capsules (2.2%) 458
Neoral Soft Gelatin Capsules (2.2%) 2247
Neoral Oral Solution (2.2%) 2247
▲ Sandimmune (2.2% to 3.9%) 2259

Infection, gastrointestinal
Adriamycin for Injection, USP 786
Adriamycin Injection, USP 786
▲ Advair Diskus 100/50 (1% to 3%) 1291
Advair Diskus 250/50 1291
Advair Diskus 500/50 (Up to 3%) 1291
Ceftin for Oral Suspension (0.1% to 1%) 1369
▲ Flovent Diskus 50 mcg (1% to 3%) 1415
Serevent Diskus (1% to 3%) 1540

Infection, genitourinary
depo-subQ provera 104 Injectable Suspension 2622

Infection, gram-negative bacteria
▲ Orthoclone OKT3 (1.6% to 7.5%) 2370

Infection, Legionella
Raptiva for Injection 1247

Infection, localized
▲ Flolan for Injection (21%) 1408
▲ Proleukin for Injection (23%) 1007
▲ Valcyte Tablets (Less than 5%) 2816
Vantas (2 patients) 3367

Infection, lower respiratory tract
▲ Advair Diskus 100/50 (1% to 3%) 1291
▲ Advair Diskus 250/50 (1% to 3%) 1291
▲ Advair Diskus 500/50 (1% to 3%) 1291
▲ Aralast (96.3%) 745
Emend Capsules (Greater than 0.5%) 1944
▲ Flovent Diskus 50 mcg (1% to 3%) 1415
Foradil Aerolizer (2.1%) 3024
Imitrex Injection 1431
Imitrex Tablets 1440
Remicade for IV Injection (Greater than or equal to 0.2%) 987
▲ Velcade for Injection (15%) 2102
▲ Xenical Capsules (7.8%) 2834

Infection, masking signs of
Blephamide Ophthalmic Ointment 563
Blephamide Ophthalmic Suspension 564
FML Ophthalmic Ointment .... ⊙225
FML Ophthalmic Suspension .... ⊙224
FML Forte Ophthalmic Suspension .... ⊙223
FML-S Liquifilm Sterile Ophthalmic Suspension .... ⊙226
HMS Sterile Ophthalmic Suspension .... ⊙228
Pred Forte Ophthalmic Suspension .... ⊙233
Pred Mild Sterile Ophthalmic Suspension .... ⊙236
TobraDex Ophthalmic Ointment 558
TobraDex Ophthalmic Suspension 558

Infection, mononucleosis-like syndrome
Klonopin (Infrequent) 2782
Neurontin Capsules 2498
Neurontin Oral Solution 2498
Neurontin Tablets 2498
Paser Granules 1657

Infection, mycobacterial
CellCept Capsules 2751
CellCept Intravenous 2751
CellCept Oral Suspension 2751
CellCept Tablets 2751
Fuzeon Injection 2772
Myfortic Tablets 2244
Rapamune Oral Solution and Tablets (Less frequent) 3472
Remicade for IV Injection 987

Infection, mycobacterium tuberculosis
Rescriptor Tablets 2535

Infection, nasal
▲ Advair Diskus 100/50 (1% to 4%) 1291
▲ Advair Diskus 250/50 (1% to 4%) 1291
▲ Advair Diskus 500/50 (1% to 4%) 1291
Amerge Tablets (Frequent) 1312
Cutivate Lotion 0.05% (Less than 1%) 1383
▲ Epivir-HBV (25%) 1398
▲ Fortical Nasal Spray (10.6%) 3336
Lotronex Tablets (Rare) 1479
▲ Miacalcin Nasal Spray (1% to 10.6%) 2242
▲ Ziagen (5%) 1600

Infection, neutropenic
Camptosar Injection (1% to 2.2%) 2602

Infection, ocular, secondary
Poly-Pred Liquifilm Ophthalmic Suspension .... ⊙231

Infection, ophthalmic, bacterial
HMS Sterile Ophthalmic Suspension .... ⊙228
Retisert Implant .... ⊙256

Infection, ophthalmic, fungal
Blephamide Ophthalmic Suspension 564
HMS Sterile Ophthalmic Suspension (Rare) .... ⊙228
Pred-G Sterile Ophthalmic Ointment .... ⊙235
Retisert Implant .... ⊙256

Infection, ophthalmic, viral
HMS Sterile Ophthalmic Suspension .... ⊙228
Pred-G Sterile Ophthalmic Ointment .... ⊙235
Retisert Implant .... ⊙256

Infection, opportunistic
Arava Tablets (Rare) 2881
Campath Ampules 826
CellCept Capsules 2751
CellCept Intravenous 2751
CellCept Oral Suspension 2751
CellCept Tablets 2751
▲ Doxil Injection (50.4%) 3302
Fuzeon Injection 2772
Kineret Injection (Rare) 594
Leustatin Injection 2368

Infection, parasitic
▲ Clarinex Syrup (3.1%) 3009
▲ Intron A for Injection (Less than 5%) 3038
Vantin Tablets and Oral Suspension (Less than 1%) 2650

Infection, pelvis
Wellbutrin Tablets (Rare) 1579

Infection, pharyngeal
▲ Epivir-HBV (25%) 1398
Lotronex Tablets (Rare) 1479

Infection, Pneumocystis carinii
(*see under* Pneumocystis carinii, susceptibility)

Infection, post-surgical
Amevive 836
Humira 464

Infection, prosthetic
▲ Myfortic Tablets (3% to less than 20%) 2244

Infection, protozoan
Campath Ampules 826
Enbrel for Injection 580
Orthoclone OKT3 Sterile Solution 2370
Remicade for IV Injection 987

Infection, respiratory
Accutane Capsules 2740
Amnesteem Capsules 2126
▲ Arava Tablets (15%) 2881
▲ Aromasin Tablets (2% to 5%) 2600
Betimol Ophthalmic Solution (1% to 5%) .... ⊙283
Betimol Ophthalmic Solution (1% to 5%) 3371
▲ CellCept Capsules (22% to 37%) 2751
▲ CellCept Intravenous (22% to 37%) 2751

▲ CellCept Oral Suspension (22% to 37%) 2751
▲ CellCept Tablets (22% to 37%) 2751
DDAVP Nasal Spray 2894
▲ Depacon Injection (12% to 20%) 412
▲ Depakene (12% to 20%) 417
▲ Depakote Sprinkle Capsules (12% to 20%) 422
▲ Depakote Tablets (12% to 20%) 427
▲ Depakote ER Tablets (12% to 20%) 433
Desmopressin Acetate Rhinal Tube 1144
▲ Entocort EC Capsules (11%) 2694
Epivir 1394
▲ Epivir-HBV (Among most common) 1398
▲ Flovent Diskus 50 mcg (5%) 1415
▲ Geodon Capsules (8%) 2514
Imitrex Nasal Spray (Infrequent) 1435
Infanrix Vaccine 1444
Lotronex Tablets (Rare) 1479
Neurontin Oral Solution (2.5%) 2498
Pediarix Vaccine 1518
Plendil Extended-Release Tablets (0.5% to 1.5%) 651
▲ Pulmicort Respules (34% to 38%) 654
Relpax Tablets (Infrequent) 2531
Remicade for IV Injection 987
▲ TOBI Solution for Inhalation (5.8%) 1015
▲ Ventolin HFA Inhalation Aerosol (7%) 1576
VFEND I.V. (Less than 2%) 2543
VFEND Oral Suspension (Less than 2%) 2543
VFEND Tablets (Less than 2%) 2543
Viagra Tablets (Greater than 2%) 2552
Xifaxan Tablets (Less than 2%) 2847

Infection, secondary

Aclovate (Infrequent) 1290
Alrex Ophthalmic Suspension 0.2% ⊙243
Analpram-HC 1136
Bactroban Cream (Less than 1%) 1356
Blephamide Ophthalmic Ointment 563
Blephamide Ophthalmic Suspension 564
Clobevate Gel 3213
Clobex Shampoo (Infrequent) 1209
Clobex Lotion 1208
Cutivate Cream (Infrequent) 1381
Cutivate Lotion 0.05% (Rare) 1383
Cutivate Ointment (Infrequent to more frequent) 1384
Diprolene Gel 0.05% 3015
Diprolene Lotion 0.05% (Infrequent) 3016
Diprolene Ointment 0.05% (Infrequent) 3017
Diprolene AF Cream 0.05% (Infrequent) 3014
Diprosone Cream, USP 0.05% 3018
Elocon Cream 0.1% (Infrequent) 3019
Elocon Lotion 0.1% (Infrequent) 3020
Elocon Ointment 0.1% (Infrequent) 3021
EryPed 200 & EryPed 400 445
Ery-Tab Tablets 447
Erythrocin Stearate Filmtab Tablets 452
FML Ophthalmic Ointment ⊙225
FML Ophthalmic Suspension ⊙224
FML Forte Ophthalmic Suspension ⊙223
FML-S Liquifilm Sterile Ophthalmic Suspension ⊙226
HMS Sterile Ophthalmic Suspension ⊙228
Locoid Cream (Infrequent) 1138
Locoid Lipocream Cream (Infrequent) 1138
Locoid (Infrequent) 1138
Lotemax Ophthalmic Suspension 0.5% ⊙249
Lotrisone (Less than 1%) 3054
Luxíq Foam 1026
Olux Foam 1027
Pandel Cream, 0.1% 1017
Pramosone 1139
Pred Forte Ophthalmic Suspension ⊙233
Pred Mild Sterile Ophthalmic Suspension ⊙236
Pred-G Ophthalmic Suspension ⊙234
Pred-G Sterile Ophthalmic Ointment ⊙235
ProctoFoam-HC 3113
Temovate Cream 1549
Temovate Gel (Infrequent) 1550
Temovate Ointment 1549
Temovate Scalp Application (Infrequent) 1551
Temovate E Emollient (Infrequent) 1552
TobraDex Ophthalmic Ointment 558
TobraDex Ophthalmic Suspension 558
Topicort .05% Gel 3288
Topicort .25% Cream 3288
Topicort .25% Ointment 3288
Topicort LP .05% Cream 3288
Tri-Luma Cream 1213
U-cort 1% Cream 3289
Vanos Cream 1864
Varivax 2070

Infection, serious

Raptiva for Injection (0.4%) 1247

Infection, Serratia

Alkeran Tablets 977
Orthoclone OKT3 Sterile Solution (1.6%) 2370

Infection, sinus

Alphagan P Ophthalmic Solution (1% to 4%) 563
▲ Flovent Diskus 50 mcg (10% to 33%) 1415
▲ Flovent HFA (1% to 6%) 1418

Infection, skin

Accutane Capsules 2740
Aceon Tablets (2 mg, 4 mg, 8 mg) (0.3% to 1%) 3191
Bexxar 1360
Cutivate Cream (0.8%) 1381
Cutivate Lotion 0.05% (Less than 1%) 1383
▲ Flovent HFA (1% to 3%) 1418
▲ Gengraf Capsules (7%) 458
▲ Neoral Soft Gelatin Capsules (7.0%) 2247
▲ Neoral Oral Solution (7%) 2247
Prinivil Tablets (0.3% to 1.0%) 2029
Prinzide Tablets 2033
▲ Sandimmune (7.0% to 10.1%) 2259
Zestoretic Tablets 701
Zestril Tablets (0.3% to 1.0%) 704

Infection, skin and soft tissue

AccuNeb Inhalation Solution (Up to 1.7%) 1055
Celebrex Capsules (0.1% to 1.9%) 3130
▲ Elidel Cream 1% (2.2% to 6.4%) 2198
Enbrel for Injection 580
▲ Flovent Diskus 50 mcg (1% to 3%) 1415
▲ Gengraf Capsules (7%) 458
Lotronex Tablets (Rare) 1479
▲ Protopic Ointment (5% to 12%) 629
Varivax 2070

Infection, Staphylococcus epidermidis

▲ Clolar for Intravenous Infusion (13%) 1264
Elidel Cream 1% (0.4% to 2.1%) 2198
▲ Orthoclone OKT3 Sterile Solution (4.8%) 2370

Infection, unspecified

▲ Abelcet Injection (5%) 1119
▲ Accolate Tablets (3.5%) 663
Actiq (1% or greater) 993
▲ Actonel Tablets (19% to 29.9%) 2679
▲ Actonel with Calcium Tablets (19% to 29.9%) 2684
▲ Adderall XR Capsules (2% to 4%) 3169
▲ Advicor Tablets (20%) 1694
▲ Alimta for Injection (Less than 1% to 23%) 1722
Alinia for Oral Suspension (Less than 1%) 2840
Alinia Tablets (Less than 1%) 2840
Alkeran for Injection 976
Aloprim for Injection (Less than 1%) 2156
▲ Altoprev Extended-Release Tablets (11%) 1151
Ambien Tablets (1%) 2867
▲ AmBisome for Injection (11.1%) 615
Amevive (0.7% to 1.5%) 836
▲ Ammonul Injection (12%) 3323
Amnesteem Capsules 2126
Anaprox Tablets (Less than 1%) 2769
Anaprox DS Tablets (Less than 1%) 2769
Angiomax for Injection (Rare) 1856
Antara Capsules 2723
▲ Aranesp for Injection (27%) 576
▲ Arava Tablets (4%) 2881
▲ Argatroban Injection (3.7%) 1321
▲ Arimidex Tablets (2% to 7%) 665
Arthrotec Tablets (Rare) 3126
Asacol Delayed-Release Tablets (2% or greater) 2688
Asmanex Twisthaler (1% to less than 3%) 2981
Atacand HCT (0.5% or greater) 637
▲ Avinza Capsules (5% to 10%) 1714
▲ Avonex (7%) 839
Axid Oral Solution (1.7%) 913
▲ Azasan Tablets (Less than 1% to 20%) 2844
▲ Bexxar (Less than 1% to 21%) 1360
▲ Boniva Tablets (4.3%) 2747
▲ Botox Purified Neurotoxin Complex (3% to 10%) 565
▲ Caduet Tablets (2.8% to 10.3%) 2507
▲ Campath Ampules (1% to 7%) 826
Campral Tablets (Frequent) 1175
▲ Camptosar Injection (0% to 14%) 2602
▲ Carnitor Injection (10% to 24%) 3185
▲ Casodex Tablets (10%) 670
Cataflam Tablets (Occasionally) 2173
▲ CellCept Capsules (18.2% to 27.1%) 2751
▲ CellCept Intravenous (18.2% to 27.1%) 2751
▲ CellCept Oral Suspension (18.2% to 27.1%) 2751
▲ CellCept Tablets (18.2% to 27.1%) 2751
▲ Cenestin Tablets, 0.45mg, 0.625mg, 0.9mg, 1.25mg (1.9% to 14%) 1063
▲ Climara Pro Transdermal System (3.3%) 800
▲ Clolar for Intravenous Infusion (85%) 1264
Clozapine Tablets 2141
Clozaril Tablets 2174
Colazal Capsules 2845
▲ CombiPatch Transdermal System (3% to 5%) 2180
Combunox Tablets (Less than 2%) 1183
▲ Copaxone for Injection (50%) 3292
Cosmegen for Injection 1907
Coumadin for Injection 932
Coumadin Tablets 932
▲ Cozaar Tablets (5%) 1913
Crestor Tablets (Greater than or equal to 2%) 672
▲ Cytovene (9%) 2763
▲ Depakote ER Tablets (12% to 15%) 433
Detrol Tablets (2.1%) 2626
Diastat Rectal Delivery System (Less than 1%) 3344
▲ Doxil Injection (1% to 11.7%) 3302
EC-Naprosyn Delayed-Release Tablets (Less than 1%) 2769
Edex Injection (2%) 3103
▲ Effexor Tablets (2.2% to 6%) 3405
▲ Effexor XR Capsules (10%) 3411
▲ Elestat Ophthalmic Solution (Approximately 10%) 1643
Elitek (Less than or equal to 1%) 2906
▲ Ellence Injection (0% to 21.5%) 2632
▲ Eloxatin for Injection (4% to 25%) 2908
▲ Enbrel for Injection (35% to 64%) 580
▲ Equetro Extended-Release Capsules (12%) 3178
▲ Erbitux (11%) 937
▲ Estrogel 0.06% (17.3%) 3200
▲ Evista Tablets (15.1%) 1735
▲ Evoxac Capsules (1% to 3%) 1042
Exelon Capsules (2% or more) 2204
Ferrlecit Injection (8%) 3379
▲ Flolan for Injection (21%) 1408
▲ Flomax Capsules (9.0% to 10.8%) 881
▲ Fortamet Extended-Release Tablets (20.5%) 1156
▲ Fortical Nasal Spray (1% to 3%) 3336
▲ Gabitril Tablets (1% to 19%) 998
▲ Gemzar for Injection (3% to 16%) 1743
▲ Gengraf Capsules (1% to 24.7%) 458
▲ Hectorol Capsules (Greater than or equal to 5%) 909
▲ Herceptin I.V. (20%) 1234
▲ Hycamtin for Injection (26%) 1427
▲ Idamycin PFS Injection (95%) 2645
▲ Indapamide Tablets (Greater than or equal to 5%) 2119
Infergen (2% to 3%) 1647
▲ Intron A for Injection (Less than 5%) 3038
▲ I.V. Busulfex (51%) 1125
▲ Keppra Oral Solution (2% to 13%) 3307
▲ Keppra Tablets (2% to 13%) 3307
▲ Kineret Injection (39%) 594
▲ Lamictal (5% to 20%) 1449
▲ Leukine (65%) 829
▲ Leustatin Injection (28%) 2368
▲ Lipitor Tablets (2.8% to 10.3%) 2495
Lofibra Capsules 1217
Lotensin Tablets (Less than 1%) 2232
Lotensin HCT Tablets (0.3% or more) 2235
▲ Lunesta Tablets (5% to 10%) 3139
▲ Lupron Depot 7.5 mg (5.4%) 3261
Lupron Depot-PED 7.5 mg, 11.25 mg and 15 mg (Less than 2%) 3266
Lupron Injection Pediatric (Less than 2%) 3256
▲ Lyrica Capsules (3% to 14%) 2524
▲ Megace ES Oral Suspension (1% to 3%) 2492
▲ Menostar Transdermal System (5%) 805
▲ Mepron Suspension (18% to 22%) 1487
Miacalcin Nasal Spray (1% to 3%) 2242
Micardis Tablets (More than 0.3%) 884
Micardis HCT Tablets 886
Mirapex Tablets (Greater than or equal to 1%) 889
Mycamine for Injection 620
Myleran Tablets 1492
▲ Mylotarg for Injection (3% to 10%) 3429
Naprosyn Suspension (Less than 1%) 2769
Naprosyn Tablets (Less than 1%) 2769
Nasacort AQ Nasal Spray 2937
▲ Neoral Soft Gelatin Capsules (1% to 24.7%) 2247
▲ Neoral Oral Solution (1% to 24.7%) 2247
▲ Neumega for Injection (Greater than or equal to 10%) 3433
▲ Neurontin Capsules (5.1%) 2498
▲ Neurontin Oral Solution (5.1%) 2498
▲ Neurontin Tablets (5.1%) 2498
▲ Nipent for Injection (7% to 36%) 3216
Niravam Orally Disintegrating Tablets (1.3%) 3106
▲ Norditropin Cartridges (13%) 2318
▲ Ontak Vials (48%) 1717
▲ Paxil CR Controlled-Release Tablets (5% to 6%) 1509
▲ Paxil (5% to 6%) 1501
PEG-Intron Powder for Injection (Less than or equal to 1%) 3062
Permax Tablets (1.1%) 3357
▲ Pletal Tablets (10% to 14%) 2478
▲ Premarin Tablets (18% to 23%) 3443
▲ Premphase Tablets (16% to 18%) 3452
▲ Prempro Tablets (16% to 18%) 3452
Prevacid Delayed-Release Capsules (Less than 1%) 3268
Prevacid for Delayed-Release Oral Suspension (Less than 1%) 3268
Prevacid NapraPAC (Less than 1%) 3277
Prevacid SoluTab Delayed-Release Orally Disintegrating Tablets (Less than 1%) 3268
PREVPAC (Less than 1%) 3281
Prochieve 4% Gel 1018
Prochieve 8% Gel 1018
▲ Prograf Capsules and Injection (45%) 624
▲ Proleukin for Injection (13%) 1007
Protonix I.V. (Greater than or equal to 1%) 3468
Protonix Tablets (Greater than or equal to 1%) 3465
▲ Protopic Ointment (1% to 14%) 629
Provigil Tablets (At least 1%) 1002
Prozac Pulvules and Liquid 1771
Pulmicort Respules (1% to 3%) 654
▲ Rapamune Oral Solution and Tablets (3% to 20%) 3472
▲ Raptiva for Injection (29%) 1247
Refludan for Injection (1.8%) 815
▲ Renagel Tablets (15%) 1268
Repronex for Intramuscular and Subcutaneous Injection (1%) 1148
Rescriptor Tablets 2535
Reyataz Capsules (Less than 3%) 948
▲ Simulect for Injection (3% to 10%) 2268
▲ Somavert Injection (23%) 2648
▲ Soriatane Capsules (1% to 10%) 1028
▲ Spiriva HandiHaler (1% to 4%) 899
Striant Mucoadhesive 1022
▲ Suboxone Tablets (5.6% to 20%) 2719
▲ Subutex Tablets (11.7% to 20%) 2719
Symbyax Capsules (Frequent) 1788
Synercid I.V. (Less than 1%) 1690
▲ Tarceva Tablets (0% to 24%) 1254
▲ Tarceva Tablets (0% to 24%) 2470
▲ Targretin Capsules (13.1% to 22.6%) 1719
Tasmar Tablets (Frequent) 3360
▲ Taxotere Injection Concentrate (6.1% to 42%) 2947
▲ Thalomid Capsules (6.3% to 8.3%) 979
▲ Thymoglobulin for Injection (17.1%) 2848
Tiazac Capsules (2%) 1204
▲ Topamax Sprinkle Capsules (1% to 7%) 2438
▲ Topamax Tablets (1% to 7%) 2438
▲ Trasylol Injection (6%) 779
Travatan Ophthalmic Solution (1% to 5%) 559

Tricor Tablets 523
Trileptal Oral Suspension (Up to 2%) 2281
Trileptal Tablets (Up to 2%) 2281
▲ Tygacil for Injection (8.3%) 3489
Uniretic Tablets (More than 1%) 3114
▲ Valcyte Tablets (Less than 5%) 2816
▲ Verelan PM Capsules (12.1%) 3120
▲ Vesanoid Capsules (58%) 2823
VFEND I.V. (Less than 2%) 2543
VFEND Oral Suspension (Less than 2%) 2543
VFEND Tablets (Less than 2%) 2543
▲ Vicoprofen Tablets (3% to 9%) 533
▲ Vigamox Ophthalmic Solution (1% to 4%) 560
Voltaren Tablets (Occasionally) 2298
Voltaren-XR Tablets (Occasionally) 2301
▲ WelChol Tablets (10%) 2855
Wellbutrin Tablets (Rare) 1579
▲ Wellbutrin SR Sustained-Release Tablets (8% to 9%) 1583
▲ Wellbutrin XL Extended-Release Tablets (8% to 9%) 1588
Yasmin 28 Tablets (Greater than 1%) 818
Zemaira (0.4%) 3506
▲ Zevalin Injection (29%) 848
▲ Zinecard for Injection (19% to 23%) 2659
▲ Zoladex (13%) 709
Zoladex 3-month 712
▲ Zometa for Intravenous Infusion (5% to 10%) 2306
Zomig Nasal Spray (Infrequent) 718

Infection, upper respiratory tract

Abilify Tablets 916
Abilify Tablets 2472
▲ Aceon Tablets (2 mg, 4 mg, 8 mg) (8.6%) 3191
▲ Activella Tablets (10% to 18%) 2311
▲ ActoPlus Met Tablets (12.4% to 15.5%) 3219
▲ Actos Tablets (13.2%) 3224
▲ Advair Diskus 100/50 (10% to 27%) 1291
▲ Advair Diskus 250/50 (10% To 27%) 1291
▲ Advair Diskus 500/50 (10% to 27%) 1291
▲ Aerobid/Aerobid-M (25%) 1172
Aggrenox Capsules (1%) 855
▲ Aldara Cream, 5% (15.3%) 1814
▲ Aldurazyme for Intravenous Infusion (7%) 1261
▲ Allegra (3.2% to 4.3%) 2857
Allegra-D 12 Hour Extended-Release Tablets (1.4%) 2860
Allegra-D 24 Hour Extended-Release Tablets (1.4%) 2862
Altace Capsules 1673
▲ Ambien Tablets (5%) 2867
▲ Aralast (96.3%) 745
▲ Aranesp for Injection (14%) 576
▲ Aredia for Injection (24.1%) 2168
▲ Asmanex Twisthaler (8% to 15%) 2981
▲ Atacand Tablets (6%) 634
▲ Atacand HCT (3.6%) 637
▲ Atrovent HFA Inhalation Aerosol (9% to 34%) 872
▲ Atrovent Inhalation Solution (13.2%) 868
▲ Atrovent Nasal Spray 0.03% (9.8%) 869
Avalide Tablets (1% or greater) 922
Avalide Tablets (1% or greater) 2889
▲ Avandamet Tablets (16%) 1343
▲ Avandia Tablets (7.3%) 1348
▲ Avapro Tablets (9%) 925
▲ Avapro Tablets (9%) 2886
▲ Avastin IV (40% to 47%) 1229
▲ Avonex (14%) 839
▲ Benicar HCT Tablets (7%) 2852
Bexxar 1360
▲ Boniva Tablets (2% to 33.7%) 2747
▲ Botox Purified Neurotoxin Complex (12%) 565
▲ Caverject Impulse Injection (4%) 2610
Ceftin for Oral Suspension (0.1% to 1%) 1369
▲ Celebrex Capsules (8.1%) 3130
▲ Celexa (5%) 1177
▲ Cenestin Tablets, 0.45mg, 0.625mg, 0.9mg, 1.25mg (13.2%) 1063
▲ Clarinex Syrup (10.8% to 21.2%) 3009
▲ Climara Transdermal System (6% to 17%) 795
▲ Climara Pro Transdermal System (13.2%) 800
Clindesse Vaginal Cream (Less than 1%) 3296
▲ Combivent Inhalation Aerosol (10.9%) 878
Comvax (0.5% to 1.3%) 1904
▲ Concerta Extended-Release Tablets (8%) 1828
Cosopt Sterile Ophthalmic Solution (1% to 5%) 1910
▲ Covera-HS Tablets (5.4%) 3135
▲ Cozaar Tablets (8%) 1913
Crixivan Capsules 1918
▲ Cutivate Lotion 0.05% (3%) 1383
DDAVP Nasal Spray 2894
▲ depo-subQ provera 104 Injectable Suspension (1% to less than 5%) 2622
▲ Detrol Tablets (5.9%) 2626
Diovan HCT Tablets (More than 2%) 2195
Diovan Tablets (More than 1%) 2191
▲ Ditropan XL Extended Release Tablets (2% to less than 5%) 2391
DuoNeb Inhalation Solution 1058
▲ Duragesic Transdermal System (3% to 10%) 2448
▲ Edex Injection (5%) 3103
▲ Elestat Ophthalmic Solution (Approximately 10%) 1643
▲ Elidel Cream 1% (4.3% to 19.4%) 2198
▲ Eloxatin for Injection (7% to 10%) 2908
Emend Capsules (Greater than 0.5%) 1944
▲ Enbrel for Injection (29% to 31%) 580
▲ Epogen for Injection (11%) 586
▲ Evoxac Capsules (11.4%) 1042
Exelon Capsules (2% or more) 2204
▲ Famvir Tablets (0.7% to 3.3%) 2207
▲ Ferrlecit Injection (6%) 3379
▲ Flovent Diskus 50 mcg (18% to 31%) 1415
▲ Flovent HFA (18%) 1418
▲ Follistim AQ Cartridge (5%) 2354
▲ Foradil Aerolizer (7.4%) 3024
▲ Fortical Nasal Spray (1% to 3%) 3336
▲ Gengraf Capsules (7.7%) 458
▲ Gleevec Tablets (3% to 19%) 2221
Havrix Vaccine (Less than 1%) 1425
Herceptin I.V. 1234
▲ Humira Injection (17%) 464
▲ Hyzaar (6.1%) 1964
▲ Infergen (16% to 31%) 1647
Invanz for Injection (2.3%) 1974
Invirase (Less than 2%) 2776
▲ Kineret Injection (14%) 594
▲ Klonopin (8%) 2782
▲ Lescol Capsules (16.2%) 2227
▲ Lescol XL Tablets (12.5%) 2227
Levaquin in 5% Dextrose Injection (0.1% to 0.9%) 2453
Levaquin (0.1% to 0.9%) 2453
Lexapro Oral Solution (At least 2%) 1193
Lexapro Tablets (At least 2%) 1193
Lotensin HCT Tablets (More than 1%) 2235
Lotrel Capsules 2238
Lotronex Tablets (1%) 1479
▲ Lumigan Ophthalmic Solution (Approximately 10%) 569
Mavik Tablets (0.3% to 1.0%) 482
Maxalt Tablets (Infrequent) 1983
Maxalt-MLT Orally Disintegrating Tablets (Infrequent) 1983
▲ Menostar Transdermal System (16%) 805
Metrogel 1% (2.5%) 1212
Miacalcin Nasal Spray (1% to 3%) 2242
▲ Micardis Tablets (7%) 884
▲ Micardis HCT Tablets (8%) 886
Migranal Nasal Spray (Infrequent) 3350
▲ Mirena Intrauterine System (5% or more) 810
▲ Mobic Oral Suspension (0% to 8.3%) 893
▲ Mobic Tablets (0% to 8.3%) 893
▲ Myfortic Tablets (3% to less than 20%) 2244
Nalfon Capsules (1.5%) 2504
Namenda (Greater than or equal to 2%) 1199
▲ Nasonex Nasal Spray (5% to 7%) 3058
▲ Neoral Soft Gelatin Capsules (7.7% to 13%) 2247
▲ Neoral Oral Solution (7.7% to 13%) 2247
Neurontin Oral Solution (More than 2%) 2498
▲ Nipent for Injection (13% to 16%) 3216
▲ Niravam Orally Disintegrating Tablets (4.3%) 3106
▲ Novantrone for Injection Concentrate (51% to 53%) 3158
Oncaspar (Less than 1%) 1123
▲ Ortho Evra Transdermal System (9% to 22%) 2402
Parcopa Orally Disintegrating Tablets 3111
▲ Liquid PedvaxHIB (Among most frequent) 2012
▲ Plavix Tablets (8.7%) 940
▲ Plavix Tablets (8.7%) 2942
▲ Plendil Extended-Release Tablets (0.7% to 3.9%) 651
▲ Prandin Tablets (0.5, 1, and 2 mg) (10% to 16%) 2337
▲ Prefest Tablets (21%) 1069
▲ Premarin Tablets (9% to 12%) 3443
▲ Premphase Tablets (9% to 11%) 3452
▲ Prempro Tablets (9% to 11%) 3452
Prevacid Delayed-Release Capsules (Less than 1%) 3268
Prevacid for Delayed-Release Oral Suspension (Less than 1%) 3268
Prevacid NapraPAC (Less than 1%) 3277
Prevacid SoluTab Delayed-Release Orally Disintegrating Tablets (Less than 1%) 3268
PREVPAC (Less than 1%) 3281
Prilosec OTC Tablets (1.9%) 2674
Prinivil Tablets (1.2% to 1.5%) 2029
Prinzide Tablets (2.2%) 2033
Prochieve 4% Gel 1018
Prochieve 8% Gel 1018
▲ Procrit for Injection (11%) 2374
▲ Prometrium Capsules (100 mg, 200 mg) (5%) 3205
Protonix I.V. (Greater than or equal to 1%) 3468
Protonix Tablets (Greater than or equal to 1%) 3465
▲ Proventil HFA Inhalation Aerosol (21%) 3071
▲ Qvar Inhalation Aerosol (5% to 11%) 1654
▲ Rapamune Oral Solution and Tablets (Greater than 20%) 3472
Razadyne ER Extended-Release Capsules (Greater than or equal to 2%) 2434
Razadyne (Greater than or equal to 2%) 2434
Recombivax HB (Equal to or greater than 1%) 2045
ReFacto Vials 3479
▲ Relenza Rotadisk (1% to 5%) 1525
▲ Remicade for IV Injection (32%) 987
▲ Renagel Tablets (5.1%) 1268
Requip Tablets (1% or more) 1528
▲ Rescriptor Tablets (4.7% to 7.6%) 2535
▲ Retisert Implant (5% to 15%) ⊙ 256
Risperdal Consta Long-Acting Injection (Up to 2%) 1664
▲ Risperdal M-Tab Orally Disintegrating Tablets (3%) 1658
▲ Risperdal (3%) 1658
▲ Rozerem Tablets (3%) 3228
▲ Rythmol SR Capsules (8% to 12%) 2736
▲ Serevent Diskus (Greater than 3%) 1540
▲ Simulect for Injection (Greater than or equal to 10%) 2268
Singulair (1% to 1.9%) 2047
Somavert Injection 2648
▲ Spiriva HandiHaler (41% to 43%) 899
Stalevo Tablets 2270
▲ Starlix Tablets (10.5%) 2276
Strattera Capsules (2% or greater) 1784
▲ Synagis (50.6%) 1868
Tarka Tablets (0.3% to 5.4%) 519
▲ Tasmar Tablets (5% to 7%) 3360
▲ Temodar Capsules (8%) 3088
▲ Teveten Tablets (8%) 1707
Teveten HCT Tablets (0.4%) 1710
Thalomid Capsules 979
Timoptic in Ocudose (Less frequent) 2061
Timoptic Sterile Ophthalmic Solution (Less frequent) 2058
Timoptic-XE Sterile Ophthalmic Gel Forming Solution (1% to 5%) 2062
▲ Topamax Sprinkle Capsules (12% to 18%) 2438
▲ Topamax Tablets (12% to 18%) 2438
▲ Trileptal Oral Suspension (5% to 10%) 2281
▲ Trileptal Tablets (5% to 10%) 2281
▲ Trisenox Injection (13%) 983
▲ Twinrix Vaccine (1% to 10%) 1571
Uniretic Tablets (More than 1%) 3114
Univasc Tablets (Greater than 1%) 3118
▲ Uroxatral Tablets (3%) 2957
▲ Vagifem Tablets (5% to 11%) 2340
▲ Valcyte Tablets (Less than 5%) 2816
Valtrex Caplets 1573
▲ Vaqta (1.1% to 10.1%) 2067
Vaseretic Tablets 2073
Vasotec I.V. Injection (0.5% to 1.0%) 2076
▲ Verelan PM Capsules (12.1%) 3120
▲ Vivelle Transdermal System (2.9% to 3.1%) 2288
▲ Vivelle-Dot Transdermal System (2.9% to 3.1%) 2293
▲ Vytorin 10/10 Tablets (3.9%) 2084
▲ Vytorin 10/10 Tablets (3.9%) 3092
▲ Vytorin 10/20 Tablets (3.9%) 2084
▲ Vytorin 10/20 Tablets (3.9%) 3092
▲ Vytorin 10/40 Tablets (3.9%) 2084
▲ Vytorin 10/40 Tablets (3.9%) 3092
▲ Vytorin 10/80 Tablets (3.9%) 2084
▲ Vytorin 10/80 Tablets (3.9%) 3092
▲ Xalatan Sterile Ophthalmic Solution (Approximately 4%) 2654
Xanax XR Tablets (1.9%) 2655
▲ Xeloda Tablets (4%) 2825
▲ Xenical Capsules (26.1% to 38.1%) 2834
Xifaxan Tablets (Less than 2%) 2847
▲ Xolair (20%) 1259
Yasmin 28 Tablets 818
Zegerid Powder for Oral Solution (1.9%) 2972
▲ Zelnorm Tablets (3% to 4%) 2303
Zemaira (1.6%) 3506
Zenapax for Injection 2838
Zestoretic Tablets (2.2%) 701
Zestril Tablets (1.5% to 2.0%) 704
▲ Zetia Tablets (13%) 2090
▲ Zetia Tablets (13%) 3098
Zevalin Injection 848
Zocor Tablets (2.1%) 2078
▲ Zoladex (7%) 709
Zoladex 3-month 712
Zoloft (Infrequent) 2581
▲ Zometa for Intravenous Infusion (10%) 2306
Zyrtec Chewable Tablets (Less than 2%) 2589
Zyrtec (Less than 2%) 2589
Zyrtec-D 12 Hour Extended Release Tablets (Less than 2%) 2591
▲ Zyvox (3.7% to 4.2%) 2661

Infection, urinary tract

Aceon Tablets (2 mg, 4 mg, 8 mg) (2.8%) 3191
Actiq (Less than 1%) 993
▲ Actonel Tablets (2.9% to 10.9%) 2679
▲ Actonel with Calcium Tablets (2.9% to 10.9%) 2684
▲ ActoPlus Met Tablets (5.3% to 5.8%) 3219
▲ Adderall XR Capsules (5%) 3169
Aldara Cream, 5% (1.4%) 1814
Aloprim for Injection (Less than 1%) 2156
Altoprev Extended-Release Tablets (2%) 1151
Ambien Tablets (2%) 2867
▲ Ammonul Injection (3%) 3323
▲ Apokyn Injection (At least 5%) 2132
▲ Arava Tablets (5%) 2881
▲ Aredia for Injection (18.5%) 2168
▲ Argatroban Injection (4.6%) 1321
▲ Arimidex Tablets (2% to 7%) 665
▲ Arixtra Injection (2.3% to 4%) 1325
Aromasin Tablets (Less frequent) 2600
Arthrotec Tablets (Rare) 3126
Asmanex Twisthaler (1% to less than 3%) 2981
Atacand HCT (0.5% or greater) 637
▲ Atrovent HFA Inhalation Aerosol (2% to 10%) 872
Atrovent Inhalation Solution (Less than 3%) 868
Avalide Tablets (1% or greater) 922
Avalide Tablets (1% or greater) 2889
Avapro Tablets (1% or greater) 925
Avapro Tablets (1% or greater) 2886
▲ Avinza Capsules (5% to 10%) 1714
▲ Avonex (17%) 839
▲ Azmacort Inhalation Aerosol (1% to 3%) 1701
Benicar Tablets (Greater than 0.5%) 2850
Benicar HCT Tablets (Greater than 2%) 2852
Betaseron for SC Injection 791
▲ Boniva Tablets (1.8% to 5.5%) 2747
▲ Bravelle for Intramuscular or Subcutaneous Injection (2.7% to 3.3%) 1140
Caduet Tablets (Greater than or equal to 2%) 2507
Campath Ampules 826
Campral Tablets (Infrequent) 1175
Carnitor Injection (2% to 3%) 3185
▲ Casodex Tablets (6%) 670
Ceftin for Oral Suspension (0.1% to 1%) 1369
Celebrex Capsules (0.1% to 1.9%) 3130
▲ CellCept Capsules (37% to 37.2%) 2751
▲ CellCept Intravenous (37% to 37.2%) 2751
▲ CellCept Oral Suspension (37% to 37.2%) 2751
▲ CellCept Tablets (37% to 37.2%) 2751
▲ Clarinex Syrup (3.6%) 3009

▲ Climara Pro Transdermal System (3.3%) 800
Clindesse Vaginal Cream (1.1%) 3296
Combivent Inhalation Aerosol (Less than 2%) 878
Cosopt Sterile Ophthalmic Solution (1% to 5%) 1910
▲ Cozaar Tablets (Less than 1% to 16%) 1913
Crestor Tablets (2.3%) 672
Cubicin for Injection (2.4%) 1038
Depacon Injection 412
Depakene 417
Depakote Sprinkle Capsules 422
Depakote Tablets 427
Depakote ER Tablets 433
▲ depo-subQ provera 104 Injectable Suspension (1% to less than 5%) 2622
▲ Detrol Tablets (5.5%) 2626
Diastat Rectal Delivery System (Less than 1%) 3344
Diovan HCT Tablets (Greater than 0.2%) 2195
▲ Ditropan XL Extended Release Tablets (5%) 2391
▲ Doxil Injection (1% to 10%) 3302
DuoNeb Inhalation Solution (1.6%) 1058
Effexor Tablets 3405
▲ Enablex Extended-Release Tablets (3.7% to 4.7%) 2201
Enbrel for Injection 580
Epivir 1394
▲ Epogen for Injection (3% to 12%) 586
▲ Equetro Extended-Release Capsules (Less than 5%) 3178
▲ Evista Tablets (4%) 1735
▲ Evoxac Capsules (6.1%) 1042
▲ Exelon Capsules (7%) 2204
▲ Faslodex Injection (6.1%) 682
▲ Femara Tablets (6%) 2210
Ferrlecit Injection 3379
▲ Flolan for Injection (7%) 1408
▲ Flovent Diskus 50 mcg (1% to 3%) 1415
▲ Flovent HFA (1% to 3%) 1418
Gabitril Tablets (1% or more) 998
▲ Gengraf Capsules (3% to 21.1%) 458
Hectorol Capsules 909
Hectorol Injection 911
▲ Herceptin I.V. (5%) 1234
▲ Humira Injection (8%) 464
Hytrin Capsules (0.5% to 1.3%) 469
Hyzaar 1964
▲ Imdur Tablets (Less than or equal to 5%) 3032
Imitrex Injection 1431
Imitrex Nasal Spray 1435
▲ Intron A for Injection (Less than 5% to 15%) 3038
Invirase (Less than 2%) 2776
Keppra Oral Solution (1% or more) 3307
Keppra Tablets (1% or more) 3307
Klonopin (1%) 2782
▲ Lamictal (3%) 1449
Lescol Capsules (1.6%) 2227
Lescol Capsules (1.6%) 2730
Lescol XL Tablets (2.7%) 2227
Lescol XL Tablets (2.7%) 2730
Levaquin in 5% Dextrose Injection (0.1% to 0.9%) 2453
Levaquin (0.1% to 0.9%) 2453
Lexapro Oral Solution (Frequent) 1193
Lexapro Tablets (Frequent) 1193
Lipitor Tablets (Greater than or equal to 2%) 2495
Lotensin Tablets (Less than 1%) 2232
Lotensin HCT Tablets (0.3% or more) 2235
Lotronex Tablets (Rare) 1479
▲ Lunesta Tablets (0% to 3%) 3139
Lupron Depot 7.5 mg (Less than 5%) 3261
▲ Megace ES Oral Suspension (1% to 3%) 2492
Meridia Capsules (2.3%) 485
Metrogel 1% (1.1%) 1212
Micardis Tablets (1%) 884
Micardis HCT Tablets (2% or greater) 886
▲ Mirapex Tablets (Greater than or equal to 1% to 4%) 889
▲ Mobic Oral Suspension (0.3% to 4.7%) 893
▲ Mobic Tablets (0.3% to 4.7%) 893
▲ Myfortic Tablets (29.1%) 2244
Namenda (Greater than or equal to 2%) 1199
Naropin Injection (Less than 1%) 640
▲ Neoral Soft Gelatin Capsules (3% to 21.1%) 2247
▲ Neoral Oral Solution (3% to 21.1%) 2247
Neurontin Capsules (Infrequent) 2498
Neurontin Oral Solution (Infrequent) 2498
Neurontin Tablets (Infrequent) 2498
▲ Nipent for Injection (3%) 3216
▲ Novantrone for Injection Concentrate (29% to 32%) 3158
Parcopa Orally Disintegrating Tablets 3111
Paxil CR Controlled-Release Tablets (2%) 1509
Paxil (2%) 1501
Permax Tablets (2.7%) 3357
▲ Photofrin for Injection (7%) 729
▲ Plavix Tablets (3.1%) 940
▲ Plavix Tablets (3.1%) 2942
Pletal Tablets (2% or greater) 2478
▲ Prandin Tablets (0.5, 1, and 2 mg) (2% to 3%) 2337
Prevacid Delayed-Release Capsules (Less than 1%) 3268
Prevacid for Delayed-Release Oral Suspension (Less than 1%) 3268
Prevacid NapraPAC (Less than 1%) 3277
Prevacid SoluTab Delayed-Release Orally Disintegrating Tablets (Less than 1%) 3268
Prevnar for Injection 3460
PREVPAC (Less than 1%) 3281
Prilosec OTC Tablets (Less than 1%) 2674
Prinivil Tablets (0.3% to 1.0%) 2029
Prinzide Tablets (0.3% to 1%) 2033
Prochieve 4% Gel 1018
Prochieve 8% Gel 1018
▲ Procrit for Injection (3% to 12%) 2374
▲ Prograf Capsules and Injection (16% to 34%) 624
▲ Proleukin for Injection (23%) 1007
Prometrium Capsules (100 mg, 200 mg) (Less than 5%) 3205
Protonix I.V. (Greater than or equal to 1%) 3468
Protonix Tablets (Greater than or equal to 1%) 3465
▲ Proventil HFA Inhalation Aerosol (3%) 3071
Provigil Tablets (At least 1%) 1002
▲ Rapamune Oral Solution and Tablets (23% to 33%) 3472
▲ Razadyne ER Extended-Release Capsules (8%) 2434
▲ Razadyne (8%) 2434
▲ Remicade for IV Injection (8%) 987
ReoPro Vials (1.9%) 1779
▲ Requip Tablets (5%) 1528
Rescriptor Tablets 2535
Reyataz Capsules (Less than 3%) 948
▲ Rilutek Tablets (2.5% to 4.5%) 2945
Roferon-A Injection (Infrequent) 2805
▲ Sandimmune (20.2% to 21.1%) 2259
▲ Sandostatin Injection (1% to 4%) 2263
▲ Sandostatin LAR Depot (5% to 15%) 2264
▲ Simulect for Injection (Greater than or equal to 10%) 2268
▲ Spiriva HandiHaler (4% to 7%) 899
Stalevo Tablets 2270
Symbyax Capsules (Frequent) 1788
Targretin Capsules 1719
▲ Tasmar Tablets (5%) 3360
▲ Temodar Capsules (8%) 3088
Testim 1% Gel 722
Teveten Tablets (1%) 1707
Teveten HCT Tablets (Less than 1%) 1710
▲ Thymoglobulin for Injection (18.3%) 2848
▲ Topamax Sprinkle Capsules (1% to 4%) 2438
▲ Topamax Tablets (1% to 4%) 2438
Trasylol Injection (2%) 779
Travatan Ophthalmic Solution (1% to 5%) 559
Trelstar Depot (1.4%) 3385
▲ Trileptal Oral Suspension (1% to 5%) 2281
▲ Trileptal Tablets (1% to 5%) 2281
Uniretic Tablets (More than 1%) 3114
▲ Valcyte Tablets (Less than 5%) 2816
Vaseretic Tablets (0.5% to 2.0%) 2073
Vasotec I.V. Injection (1.3%) 2076
▲ VESIcare Tablets (2.8% to 4.8%) 631
VFEND I.V. (Less than 2%) 2543
VFEND Oral Suspension (Less than 2%) 2543
VFEND Tablets (Less than 2%) 2543
Viadur Implant (Less than 2%) 782
▲ Viagra Tablets (3%) 2552
Vivelle Transdermal System 2288
Vivelle-Dot Transdermal System 2293
Wellbutrin Tablets (Infrequent) 1579
Wellbutrin SR Sustained-Release Tablets (Up to 1%) 1583
Wellbutrin XL Extended-Release Tablets (Up to 1%) 1588
▲ Xeloda Tablets (Less than 1% to 6%) 2825
▲ Xenical Capsules (5.9% to 7.5%) 2834
Yasmin 28 Tablets 818
Zegerid Powder for Oral Solution (2.2%) 2972
Zelnorm Tablets (1% to 2%) 2303
Zenapax for Injection 2838
Zestoretic Tablets (0.3% to 1%) 701
Zestril Tablets (0.3% to 1.0%) 704
Zevalin Injection 848
Zoladex (1% to 5%) 709
Zoladex 3-month (1% to 5%) 712
▲ Zometa for Intravenous Infusion (12% to 14%) 2306
Zomig Nasal Spray (Rare) 718
Zyprexa Tablets (Frequent) 1798
Zyprexa ZYDIS Orally Disintegrating Tablets (Frequent) 1798
Zyrtec Chewable Tablets (Less than 2%) 2589
Zyrtec (Less than 2%) 2589
Zyrtec-D 12 Hour Extended Release Tablets (Less than 2%) 2591

Infection, urinary tract, fungal
Nexium Delayed-Release Capsules (Less than 1%) 645
Nexium I.V. (Less than 1%) 649

Infection, vagina
Cleocin Vaginal Ovules (Less than 1%) 2613
Clindesse Vaginal Cream (Less than 1%) 3296
Clozapine Tablets (Less than 1%) 2141
Clozaril Tablets (Less than 1%) 2174
FazaClo Orally Disintegrating Tablets (Less than 1%) 547
Ortho-Cyclen/Ortho Tri-Cyclen 2414
Ortho Tri-Cyclen Lo Tablets 2421

Infection, viral
▲ Aceon Tablets (2 mg, 4 mg, 8 mg) (0.3% to 3.4%) 3191
Actiq (1% or greater) 993
Activella Tablets (0% to 6%) 2311
Adderall XR Capsules (2%) 3169
▲ Advair Diskus 100/50 (4%) 1291
▲ Advair Diskus 250/50 (1% to 6%) 1291
▲ Advair Diskus 500/50 (4%) 1291
Aldara Cream, 5% (1.4%) 1814
Allegra (2.5%) 2857
Aralast (Greater than or equal to 0.2%) 745
Astelin Nasal Spray (Infrequent) 1876
Atacand HCT (0.5% or greater) 637
▲ Avandamet Tablets (5%) 1343
Bexxar 1360
Blephamide Ophthalmic Ointment 563
Blephamide Ophthalmic Suspension 564
Campath Ampules 826
Celebrex Capsules (0.1% to 1.9%) 3130
Clindesse Vaginal Cream (Less than 1%) 3296
Colazal Capsules 2845
▲ Depakote ER Tablets (1% to 5%) 433
▲ Diovan HCT Tablets (3%) 2195
▲ Diovan Tablets (3%) 2191
Elidel Cream 1% (0.7% to 6.6%) 2198
Enbrel for Injection 580
▲ Epivir-HBV (Among most common) 1398
▲ Equetro Extended-Release Capsules (Less than 5%) 3178
Evoxac Capsules (Less than 1%) 1042
▲ Femara Tablets (5% to 6%) 2210
▲ Flovent Diskus 50 mcg (2% to 9%) 1415
▲ Flovent HFA (1% to 3%) 1418
FML Ophthalmic Ointment ⊙ 225
FML Ophthalmic Suspension ⊙ 224
FML Forte Ophthalmic Suspension ⊙ 223
▲ Foradil Aerolizer (17.2%) 3024
▲ Gengraf Capsules (1% to 15.9%) 458
Gonal-f RFF Pen for Injection (2.4%) 3155
▲ Imdur Tablets (Less than or equal to 5%) 3032
▲ Intron A for Injection (Less than 5% to 7%) 3038
Kaletra (Less than 2%) 474
Keppra Oral Solution (2%) 3307
Keppra Tablets (2%) 3307
Klonopin (Infrequent) 2782
▲ Leustatin Injection (20%) 2368
Lotronex Tablets (Rare) 1479
▲ Lunesta Tablets (3%) 3139
▲ Nasonex Nasal Spray (8% to 14%) 3058
▲ Neoral Soft Gelatin Capsules (1% to 15.9%) 2247
▲ Neoral Oral Solution (1% to 15.9%) 2247
Neurontin Capsules (Rare) 2498
Neurontin Oral Solution (Rare) 2498
Neurontin Tablets (Rare) 2498
▲ Nipent for Injection (Up to 8%) 3216
Omacor Capsules 2735
Orthoclone OKT3 Sterile Solution (1.5%) 2370
▲ PEG-Intron Powder for Injection (11%) 3062
▲ Prefest Tablets (6%) 1069
Prinivil Tablets (0.3% to 1.0%) 2029
Prinzide Tablets (0.3% to 1%) 2033
Prolastin 3252
▲ Prometrium Capsules (100 mg, 200 mg) (7% to 12%) 3205
Provigil Tablets (Greater than or equal to 1%) 1002
▲ Pulmicort Respules (3% to 5%) 654
▲ Rebetol (12%) 3073
Remicade for IV Injection 987
▲ Requip Tablets (11%) 1528
Rescriptor Tablets 2535
▲ Ribavirin, USP Capsules (12%) 3083
Rituxan for Infusion 845
▲ Rituxan I.V. (10%) 1251
▲ Sandimmune (15.9% to 18.4%) 2259
▲ Sandostatin LAR Depot (5% to 15%) 2264
▲ Simulect for Injection (Greater than or equal to 10%) 2268
Singulair (Greater than or equal to 2%) 2047
Synagis (More than 1%) 1868
Tasmar Tablets (Infrequent) 3360
▲ Temodar Capsules (11%) 3088
Teveten Tablets (2%) 1707
Teveten HCT Tablets (Less than 1%) 1710
Thalomid Capsules 979
▲ Topamax Sprinkle Capsules (Less than 1% to 9%) 2438
▲ Topamax Tablets (Less than 1% to 9%) 2438
▲ Trileptal Oral Suspension (5% to 7%) 2281
▲ Trileptal Tablets (5% to 7%) 2281
▲ Ventolin HFA Inhalation Aerosol (7%) 1576
▲ Voltaren Ophthalmic Solution (Less than or equal to 3%) 2300
Vytorin 10/10 Tablets 2084
Vytorin 10/10 Tablets 3092
Vytorin 10/20 Tablets 2084
Vytorin 10/20 Tablets 3092
Vytorin 10/40 Tablets 2084
Vytorin 10/40 Tablets 3092
Vytorin 10/80 Tablets 2084
Vytorin 10/80 Tablets 3092
▲ Xolair (23%) 1259
▲ Xopenex HFA Inhalation Aerosol (6.9% to 12.3%) 3151
▲ Xopenex Inhalation Solution (6.9% to 12.3%) 3143
▲ Xopenex Inhalation Solution Concentrate (6.9% to 12.3%) 3147
Zenapax for Injection 2838
Zestoretic Tablets (0.3% to 1%) 701
Zestril Tablets (0.3% to 1.0%) 704
Zetia Tablets (2.2%) 2090
Zetia Tablets (2.2%) 3098
▲ Ziagen (5%) 1600

Infection, yersinia
Desferal Vials (Rare) 2190

Infection at injection site
▲ Aranesp for Injection (6%) 576
▲ Cytovene-IV (9%) 2763
Depo-Medrol Single-Dose Vial 2617
I.V. Busulfex 1125
▲ Valcyte Tablets (3%) 2816
VFEND I.V. (Less than 2%) 2543
VFEND Oral Suspension (Less than 2%) 2543
VFEND Tablets (Less than 2%) 2543
Xolair 1259

Infection with grade 3/4 neutropenia
▲ Alimta (Up to 6%) 1722

Infectious disorders, life-threatening, aggravation of
Roferon-A Injection 2805

Infectious-mononucleosis-like syndrome
Dapsone Tablets USP 1656

Infertility
Cytovene 2763
Leukeran Tablets 1472

Levoxyl Tablets 1680
Lo/Ovral-28 Tablets 3423
Unithroid Tablets 3521

Infertility, male
Dapsone Tablets USP 1656

Infertility, temporary
Alesse-28 Tablets 3392
Ortho-Cept Tablets 2395
Ortho-Cyclen Tablets 2414
Ortho Evra Transdermal System 2402
Ortho Tri-Cyclen Tablets 2414
Seasonale Tablets 1073
Triphasil-28 Tablets 3483
Yasmin 28 Tablets 818

Inflammation, ear
Reyataz Capsules (Less than 3%) 948

Inflammation, mucosal
▲ Clolar for Intravenous Infusion (18%) 1264

Inflammation, mycosal
Mycamine for Injection (0.2%) 620

Inflammation, nasal
Imitrex Nasal Spray 1435

Inflammation, ocular
▲ Acular Ophthalmic Solution (1% to 10%) 561
▲ Acular LS Ophthalmic Solution (1% to 10%) 562
Betoptic S Ophthalmic Suspension (Small number of patients) 554
Depo-Medrol Single-Dose Vial 2617
Enbrel for Injection 580
▲ Retisert Implant (10% to 35%) ⊙256
Rilutek Tablets (Infrequent) 2945
Rythmol SR Capsules 2736
Tasmar Tablets (1%) 3360
Zyprexa Tablets (Infrequent) 1798
Zyprexa ZYDIS Orally Disintegrating Tablets (Infrequent) 1798

Inflammation, oral
(*see under* Stomatitis)

Inflammation, periocular
Depo-Medrol Single-Dose Vial 2617

Inflammation, unspecified
Amvisc Plus (Rare) ⊙289
Floxin Otic Singles 1045
Floxin Otic Solution (Single report) 1043
Klonopin (Infrequent) 2782
Permax Tablets 3357
Prilosec OTC Tablets (Less than 1%) 2674
ReoPro Vials (0.1%) 1779
Zegerid Powder for Oral Solution (Less than 1%) 2972
Zestoretic Tablets (0.3% to 1%) 701

Inflammation, upper respiratory tract
▲ Advair Diskus 100/50 (7%) 1291
▲ Advair Diskus 250/50 (6%) 1291
▲ Advair Diskus 500/50 (6% to 7%) 1291
Amerge Tablets (Infrequent) 1312
▲ Flovent Diskus 50 mcg (5%) 1415
Flovent HFA (2%) 1418
Imitrex Nasal Spray 1435
Prevacid Delayed-Release Capsules (Less than 1%) 3268
Prevacid for Delayed-Release Oral Suspension (Less than 1%) 3268
Prevacid NapraPAC (Less than 1%) 3277
Prevacid SoluTab Delayed-Release Orally Disintegrating Tablets (Less than 1%) 3268
PREVPAC (Less than 1%) 3281
▲ Ventolin HFA Inhalation Aerosol (5%) 1576

Inflammation at application site
Aldara Cream, 5% 1814
▲ Tri-Luma Cream (5.45%) 1213
Vivelle Transdermal System 2288
Vivelle-Dot Transdermal System 2293
Zovirax Cream 853

Inflammation at injection site
Abelcet Injection 1119
Ambien Tablets (Rare) 2867
AmBisome for Injection (Less common) 615
▲ Amevive (4% to common) 836
▲ Aredia for Injection (Up to 41%) 2168
▲ Avonex (6% to 52%) 839
▲ Betaseron for SC Injection (53%) 791
Boostrix 1366
▲ Brevibloc Concentrate (About 8%) 766
▲ Brevibloc Injection (About 8%) 766
▲ Brevibloc Double Strength Injection (About 8%) 766
▲ Brevibloc Premixed Injection (About 8%) 766
▲ Brevibloc Double Strength Premixed Injection (About 8%) 766
▲ Copaxone for Injection (49%) 3292
Cytovene-IV (At least 3 subjects) 2763
Delatestryl Injection (Rare) 2976
Depacon Injection (0.6%) 412
Diprivan Injectable Emulsion (Less than 1%) 676
Doxil Injection (Less than 1%) 3302
Estratest Tablets 3196
Estratest H.S. Tablets 3196
Fortaz (1 in 69 patients) 1422
Genotropin Lyophilized Powder (Infrequent) 2642
▲ Gonal-f RFF Pen for Injection (2.4% to 4.2%) 3155
▲ Havrix Vaccine (1% to 10%) 1425
HibTITER 3419
Humalog-Pen 1751
Humulin 50/50, 100 Units 1760
Humulin 70/30 Pen 1761
Humulin L, 100 Units 1763
Humulin R (U-500) 1768
Humulin N Pen 1765
Imitrex Injection 1431
▲ Infanrix Vaccine (1.0% to 39.5%) 1444
Infed Injection 3381
▲ Intron A for Injection (Up to 5%) 3038
▲ I.V. Busulfex (25%) 1125
Levaquin in 5% Dextrose Injection (0.1%) 2453
Levaquin (0.1%) 2453
Maxipime for Injection (0.6%) 1093
Merrem I.V. (2.4%) 687
▲ Miacalcin Injection (About 10%) 2241
Mycamine for Injection (1.5%) 620
Nubain Injection 1111
▲ PEG-Intron Powder for Injection (47%) 3062
▲ Rebetron Combination Therapy (5%) 3078
▲ Ribavirin, USP Capsules (6% to 18%) 3083
Roferon-A Injection (Rare) 2805
Sandostatin LAR Depot (1% to 4%) 2264
▲ Synercid I.V. (42%) 1690
Taxotere Injection Concentrate 2947
Tygacil for Injection (0% to less than 2%) 3489
Varivax (Less than 0.05%) 2070
VFEND I.V. (Less than 2%) 2543
VFEND Oral Suspension (Less than 2%) 2543
VFEND Tablets (Less than 2%) 2543
Xolair 1259
▲ Zithromax for IV Infusion (3.1%) 2573
▲ Zofran Injection (4%) 1607
Zosyn (0.2% to 1.3%) 3492
▲ Zovirax for Injection (Approximately 9%) 1618

Inflammation at insertion site
Vantas (2 patients) 3367

Influenza
Advair Diskus 100/50 1291
Advair Diskus 250/50 1291
Advair Diskus 500/50 1291
▲ Boniva Tablets (3.8% to 4%) 2747
Clindesse Vaginal Cream (Less than 1%) 3296
Cutivate Lotion 0.05% (2%) 1383
▲ depo-subQ provera 104 Injectable Suspension (1% to less than 5%) 2622
Fuzeon Injection (2.4%) 2772
Invirase (2.7%) 2776
Metrogel 1% (1.4%) 1212
▲ Myfortic Tablets (3% to less than 20%) 2244
▲ Requip Tablets (3%) 1528
▲ Retisert Implant (5% to 15%) ⊙256
Rozerem Tablets (1%) 3228
▲ Singulair (4.2%) 2047
▲ Strattera Capsules (2% to 3%) 1784
VESIcare Tablets (0.9% to 2.2%) 631
Vytorin 10/10 Tablets (2.6%) 2084
Vytorin 10/10 Tablets (2.6%) 3092
Vytorin 10/20 Tablets (2.6%) 2084
Vytorin 10/20 Tablets (2.6%) 3092
Vytorin 10/40 Tablets (2.6%) 2084
Vytorin 10/40 Tablets (2.6%) 3092
Vytorin 10/80 Tablets (2.6%) 2084
Vytorin 10/80 Tablets (2.6%) 3092
Xanax XR Tablets (2.4%) 2655

Infused vein complications
▲ Cancidas for Injection (1.5% to 12%) 1894

Infusion reaction
▲ Erbitux (2% to 3%) 937

Inhalation site sensation
▲ Proventil HFA Inhalation Aerosol (6%) 3071

Injury, accidental
▲ Abilify Tablets (5%) 916
▲ Abilify Tablets (5%) 2472
▲ Advate Injection (17.3%) 742
▲ Arimidex Tablets (2% to 7%) 665
Bravelle for Intramuscular or Subcutaneous Injection (2.7%) 1140
▲ Climara Pro Transdermal System (3.3%) 800
▲ Concerta Extended-Release Tablets (6%) 1828
▲ Effexor XR Capsules (5%) 3411
▲ Equetro Extended-Release Capsules (7%) 3178
▲ Flumist Vaccine (2.3%) 1872
▲ Humira Injection (10%) 464
▲ Levitra Tablets (3%) 3048
▲ Lunesta Tablets (0% to 3%) 3139
▲ Lyrica Capsules (2% to 11%) 2524
▲ Menostar Transdermal System (8%) 805
▲ Premarin Tablets (6% to 12%) 3443
▲ Premphase Tablets (4% to 5%) 3452
▲ Prempro Tablets (4% to 5%) 3452
▲ Prilosec OTC Tablets (3.8%) 2674
Prozac Pulvules and Liquid 1771
Relpax Tablets (Rare) 2531
▲ Suboxone Tablets (3%) 2719
▲ Subutex Tablets (3%) 2719
▲ Symbyax Capsules (3% to 5%) 1788
▲ Zegerid Powder for Oral Solution (3.8%) 2972
Zemaira (0.2% to 0.4%) 3506

Injury, intentional
▲ Aldara Cream, 5% (8.8%) 1814
Campral Tablets (Infrequent) 1175
Lyrica Capsules (Rare) 2524
Symbyax Capsules (Infrequent) 1788

Injury, limb
▲ Advate Injection (34.7%) 742

INR, increase
Avelox (0.1% to less than 2%) 2984
Cubicin for Injection (Less than 1%) 1038
Tygacil for Injection (0% to less than 2%) 3489

Insomnia
▲ Abilify Tablets (20%) 916
▲ Abilify Tablets (20%) 2472
Accolate Tablets 663
Accutane Capsules 2740
Aciphex Tablets 1081
Actiq (1% to 2%) 993
Activella Tablets (0% to 6%) 2311
▲ Actonel Tablets (4.7%) 2679
▲ Actonel with Calcium Tablets (4.3%) 2684
Adalat CC Tablets (Less than 1%) 2978
Adderall Tablets 3168
▲ Adderall XR Capsules (1.5% to 27%) 3169
Adipex-P 1216
Advicor Tablets 1694
Advil Allergy Sinus Caplets ▣737
Advil Multi-Symptom Cold Caplets ▣738
Aerobid/Aerobid-M (1% to 3%) 1172
Agrylin Capsules (1% to 5%) 3172
Alacol DM Syrup 739
Alavert Allergy & Sinus D-12 Hour Tablets ▣743
Aldara Cream, 5% 1814
Alferon N Injection (2%) 1640
Alinia for Oral Suspension (Less than 1%) 2840
Alinia Tablets (Less than 1%) 2840
Allegra (Less than 1%) 2857
▲ Allegra-D 12 Hour Extended-Release Tablets (12.6%) 2860
▲ Allegra-D 24 Hour Extended-Release Tablets (12.6%) 2862
Aloxi Injection (Less than 1%) 2099
Alphagan P Ophthalmic Solution (Less than 1%) 563
Altace Capsules (Less than 1%) 1673
Altoprev Extended-Release Tablets 1151
Ambien Tablets (Frequent) 2867
Amnesteem Capsules 2126
Amoxil Capsules (Rare) 1315
Amoxil Chewable Tablets (Rare) 1315
Amoxil Pediatric Drops for Oral Suspension (Rare) 1315
Amoxil Powder for Oral Suspension (Rare) 1315
Amoxil Tablets (Rare) 1315
Anadrol-50 Tablets 3329
Anaprox Tablets (Less than 1%) 2769
Anaprox DS Tablets (Less than 1%) 2769
▲ Angiomax for Injection (7%) 1856
Antara Capsules 2723
▲ Apokyn Injection (At least 5%) 2132
Aptivus Capsules (1.2% to less than 2%) 859
▲ Arava Tablets (1% to 3%) 2881
▲ Aredia for Injection (22.2%) 2168
▲ Aricept Tablets (6% to 14%) 1086
▲ Aricept ODT Tablets (6% to 14%) 1086
▲ Arimidex Tablets (2% to 6%) 665
▲ Arixtra Injection (0.9% to 5%) 1325
▲ Aromasin Tablets (11%) 2600
Arthrotec Tablets (Rare) 3126
Asacol Delayed-Release Tablets (2%) 2688
Asmanex Twisthaler (1% to less than 3%) 2981
Atacand HCT (0.5% or greater) 637
Atrovent Inhalation Solution (0.9%) 868
Augmentin (Rare) 1331
Augmentin Tablets (Rare) 1334
Augmentin XR Extended-Release Tablets (Rare) 1340
Augmentin ES-600 Powder for Oral Suspension (Rare) 1337
Avelox (0.1% to less than 2%) 2984
▲ Avinza Capsules (5% to 10%) 1714
Axert Tablets (Infrequent) 2430
Axid Oral Solution (2.7%) 913
Aygestin Tablets 1062
Balamine DM 739
Baraclude (Less than 1%) 928
Benicar Tablets (Greater than 0.5%) 2850
Bentyl Capsules 724
Bentyl Injection 724
Bentyl Syrup 724
Bentyl Tablets 724
▲ Betaseron for SC Injection (24%) 791
Betoptic S Ophthalmic Suspension (Rare) 554
Biaxin/Biaxin XL 402
Blocadren Tablets (Less than 1%) 1891
Boniva Tablets (0.8% to 2%) 2747
Brimonidine Tartrate Ophthalmic Solution 0.2% (Less than 3%) ⊙245
Caduet Tablets (Greater than 0.1%) 2507
▲ Campath Ampules (10%) 826
▲ Campral Tablets (6% to 9%) 1175
▲ Camptosar Injection (0% to 19%) 2602
Cancidas for Injection (0% to 1.2%) 1894
Captopril Tablets (About 0.5 to 2%) 2114
Carafate Suspension (Less than 0.5%) 727
Carafate Tablets (Less than 0.5%) 728
Cardizem LA Extended Release Tablets (Less than 2%) 1699
Carnitor Injection (1% to 3%) 3185
Carteolol Hydrochloride Ophthalmic Solution USP, 1% (Occasional) ⊙246
▲ Casodex Tablets (5%) 670
Cataflam Tablets (Occasionally) 2173
Catapres Tablets (About 5 in 1,000 patients) 874
Catapres-TTS (2 of 101 patients) 875
Celebrex Capsules (2.3%) 3130
▲ Celexa (15%) 1177
▲ CellCept Capsules (40.8%) 2751
▲ CellCept Intravenous (40.8%) 2751
▲ CellCept Oral Suspension (40.8%) 2751
▲ CellCept Tablets (40.8%) 2751
▲ Cenestin Tablets, 0.45mg, 0.625mg, 0.9mg, 1.25mg (5.7% to 42%) 1063
Cialis Tablets (Less than 2%) 1806
Cipro I.V. (1% or less) 2998
Cipro I.V. Pharmacy Bulk Package (1% or less) 3509
Cipro (Less than 1%) 2991
Cipro XR Tablets (Less than 1%) 3004
▲ Clarinex Syrup (4.5%) 3009
▲ Clarinex-D 24-Hour Extended-Release Tablets (5%) 3012
Clinoril Tablets (Less than 1%) 1899
Clorpres Tablets (About 5 in 1,000) 2139
Clozapine Tablets (2%) 2141
▲ Clozaril Tablets (2% to 20%) 2174
Colazal Capsules (2%) 2845
▲ CombiPatch Transdermal System (8% to 6%) 2180

Combivent Inhalation Aerosol (Less than 2%) 878
▲ Combivir Tablets (11%) 1373
Combunox Tablets (Less than 1%) 1183
▲ Concerta Extended-Release Tablets (1.5% to 5%) 1828
Contac Non-Drowsy 12 Hour Cold Caplets ▣ 614
Contac Non-Drowsy Timed Release 12 Hour Cold Caplets ▣ 615
Contac Severe Cold and Flu Caplets Maximum Strength ▣ 615
Copaxone for Injection (At least 2%) 3292
▲ Copegus Tablets (30%) 2759
Coreg Tablets (2%) 1376
Cosopt Sterile Ophthalmic Solution 1910
Covera-HS Tablets (Less than 2%) 3135
Cozaar Tablets (1% or greater) 1913
Crestor Tablets (Greater than or equal to 2%) 672
▲ Cubicin for Injection (4.5%) 1038
▲ Cymbalta Delayed-Release Capsules (8% to 13%) 1729
Cytovene (At least 3 subjects) 2763
Dantrium Capsules (Less frequent) 2690
Dapsone Tablets USP 1656
Decadron Phosphate Injection 1931
Decadron Tablets 1929
Demser Capsules 1933
▲ Depacon Injection (9% to 15%) 412
▲ Depakene (15%) 417
▲ Depakote Sprinkle Capsules (9% to 15%) 422
▲ Depakote Tablets (1% to 15%) 427
▲ Depakote ER Tablets (1% to 15%) 433
▲ DepoDur Extended-Release Injection (5% to 10%) 1098
▲ Depo-Provera Contraceptive Injection (1% to 5%) 2619
▲ depo-subQ provera 104 Injectable Suspension (1% to less than 5%) 2622
Desoxyn Tablets, USP 2482
Dexedrine 1386
DextroStat Tablets 3177
Dilaudid 439
Dilaudid Oral Liquid (Less frequent) 443
Dilaudid Non-Sterile Powder 439
Dilaudid Rectal Suppositories 439
Dilaudid Tablets 439
Dilaudid Tablets - 8 mg (Less frequent) 443
Dilaudid-HP (Less frequent) 441
Children's Dimetapp Long Acting Cough Plus Cold Syrup ▣ 746
Diovan HCT Tablets (Greater than 0.2%) 2195
Diovan Tablets 2191
Diprivan Injectable Emulsion (Less than 1%) 676
▲ Ditropan XL Extended Release Tablets (2% to less than 5%) 2391
Dolobid Tablets (Greater than 1 in 100) 1937
▲ Dostinex Tablets (1% to less than 10%) 2631
▲ Doxil Injection (Less than 1% to 10%) 3302
▲ Duragesic Transdermal System (3% to 10%) 2448
DynaCirc CR Tablets (0.5% to 1%) 2726
EC-Naprosyn Delayed-Release Tablets (Less than 1%) 2769
▲ Effexor Tablets (3% to 22.5%) 3405
▲ Effexor XR Capsules (3% to 23%) 3411
Efudex 3348
Eldepryl Capsules (1 of 49 patients) 3209
Eligard 7.5 mg (Less than 2%) 2896
Eligard 30 mg (1.1%) 2901
Elmiron Capsules 2393
▲ Eloxatin for Injection (9% to 11%) 2908
▲ Emcyt Capsules (3%) 3137
Emend Capsules (2.9%) 1944
▲ Emtriva Capsules (7% to 16%) 1272
Engerix-B Vaccine (Less than 1%) 1391
▲ Entocort EC Capsules (Less than 5%) 2694
▲ Epivir (11%) 1394
▲ Epogen for Injection (13% to 16%) 586
▲ Epzicom Tablets (7% to 9%) 1402
▲ Equetro Extended-Release Capsules (Less than 5%) 3178
▲ Erbitux (10%) 937
▲ Evista Tablets (5.5%) 1735
Evoxac Capsules (2.4%) 1042
▲ Exelon Capsules (9%) 2204
Factive Tablets (0.1% to 1%) 2464
Famvir Tablets (1.5% to 2.5%) 2207
▲ Faslodex Injection (6.9%) 682
FazaClo Orally Disintegrating Tablets (2%) 547
▲ Femara Tablets (Less than 0.1% to 7%) 2210
Flexeril Tablets (Less than 1%) 1832
▲ Flolan for Injection (4% to 9%) 1408
Flomax Capsules (1.4% to 2.4%) 881
Floxin Otic Singles (Reported in a single subject) 1045
Floxin Otic Solution (Single report) 1043
Flumadine (2.1% to 3.4%) 1186
▲ Focalin Tablets (Among most common) 2214
Focalin XR Capsules 2217
Foradil Aerolizer (1.5%) 3024
▲ Forteo for Injection (4.3%) 1739
Fortical Nasal Spray (Less than 1%) 3336
Frova Tablets (Frequent) 1101
Fuzeon Injection 2772
▲ Gabitril Tablets (6%) 998
Gemzar for Injection (Infrequent) 1743
Gengraf Capsules (1% to less than 3%) 458
Geodon 2514
▲ Gleevec Tablets (10% to 14%) 2221
Grifulvin V Tablets Microsize and Oral Suspension Microsize (Occasional) 2384
Gris-PEG Tablets (Occasional) 2504
Havrix Vaccine (Less than 1%) 1425
▲ Hectorol Capsules (Greater than or equal to 5%) 909
▲ Herceptin I.V. (14%) 1234
Hydrocortone Tablets 1963
Hytrin Capsules (At least 1%) 469
Hyzaar 1964
▲ Imdur Tablets (Less than or equal to 5%) 3032
Indapamide Tablets (Less than 5%) 2119
Inderal LA Long-Acting Capsules 3421
Indocin (Less than 1%) 1968
▲ Infergen (24% to 39%) 1647
InnoPran XL Capsules 2728
▲ Intron A for Injection (Up to 12%) 3038
▲ Invanz for Injection (3% to 3.2%) 1974
Invirase (Greater than or equal to 2%) 2776
▲ I.V. Busulfex (84%) 1125
Kadian Capsules (Less than 3%) 572
Kaletra (Up to 2%) 474
Keppra Oral Solution (1% to 2%) 3307
Keppra Tablets (1% to 2%) 3307
Ketek Tablets (Greater than or equal to 0.2% to less than 2%) 2920
Klonopin (Infrequent) 2782
Kytril Injection (Less than 2%) 2785
▲ Kytril Tablets (3% to 5%) 2788
▲ Lamictal (5.6%) 1449
▲ Lariam Tablets (Among most frequent) 2790
Lescol Capsules (2.7%) 2227
Lescol Capsules (2.7%) 2730
Lescol XL Tablets (1.8%) 2227
Lescol XL Tablets (1.8%) 2730
▲ Leukine (11%) 829
▲ Leustatin Injection (7%) 2368
▲ Levaquin in 5% Dextrose Injection (0.4% to 4.6%) 2453
▲ Levaquin (0.4% to 4.6%) 2453
Levitra Tablets (Less than 2%) 3048
Levothroid Tablets 1189
Levoxyl Tablets 1680
▲ Lexapro Oral Solution (5% to 14%) 1193
▲ Lexapro Tablets (5% to 14%) 1193
Lipitor Tablets (Greater than or equal to 2%) 2495
Lofibra Capsules 1217
Lotensin Tablets (Less than 1%) 2232
Lotensin HCT Tablets (0.3% to 1%) 2235
Lotrel Capsules 2238
Lunesta Tablets (Infrequent) 3139
▲ Lupron Depot 3.75 mg (16%) 3257
Lupron Depot 7.5 mg (Less than 5%) 3261
▲ Lupron Depot–3 Month 11.25 mg (16%) 3262
▲ Malarone Tablets (2% to 3%) 1484
▲ Malarone Pediatric Tablets (2% to 3%) 1484
Matulane Capsules 3188
Mavik Tablets (0.3% to 1.0%) 482
Maxair Autohaler 1820
Maxalt Tablets (Infrequent) 1983
Maxalt-MLT Orally Disintegrating Tablets (Infrequent) 1983
Maxzide 2150
Mebaral Tablets, USP (Less than 1 in 100 patients) 2483
▲ Megace ES Oral Suspension (0% to 6%) 2492
▲ Mepron Suspension (10% to 19%) 1487
▲ Meridia Capsules (10.7%) 485
Merrem I.V. (Greater than 0.1% to 1%) 687
▲ Metadate CD Capsules (5%) 3316
Mevacor Tablets (0.5% to 1.0%) 1996
Miacalcin Nasal Spray (Less than 1%) 2242
Micardis Tablets (More than 0.3%) 884
Micardis HCT Tablets 886
Midamor Tablets (Less than or equal to 1%) 2000
Migranal Nasal Spray (Infrequent) 3350
▲ Mirapex Tablets (17% to 27%) 889
▲ Mobic Oral Suspension (0% to 3.6%) 893
▲ Mobic Tablets (0% to 3.6%) 893
Moduretic Tablets (Less than or equal to 1%) 2003
Motrin Cold & Sinus Caplets 1836
MS Contin Tablets (Less frequent) 2703
▲ Myfortic Tablets (23.5%) 2244
▲ Mylotarg for Injection (11% to 13%) 3429
Nalfon Capsules (Less than 1%) 2504
Namenda (Greater than or equal to 2%) 1199
Naprosyn Suspension (Less than 1%) 2769
Naprosyn Tablets (Less than 1%) 2769
Naropin Injection (Less than 1%) 640
▲ Natrecor for Injection (2% to 6%) 3123
Nembutal Sodium Solution, USP (Less than 1%) 2484
▲ Neoral Soft Gelatin Capsules (1% to 3%) 2247
Neoral Oral Solution (1% to 3%) 2247
▲ Neulasta Injection (15% to 72%) 596
▲ Neumega for Injection (33%) 3433
Neurontin Capsules 2498
Neurontin Oral Solution 2498
Neurontin Tablets 2498
Nexium Delayed-Release Capsules (Less than 1%) 645
Nexium I.V. (Less than 1%) 649
Niaspan Extended-Release Tablets 1703
▲ Nicotrol NS (Greater than 5%) 2596
▲ Nipent for Injection (3% to 10%) 3216
▲ Niravam Orally Disintegrating Tablets (8.9% to 29.5%) 3106
Noroxin Tablets (Less frequent) 2009
Norvasc Tablets (More than 0.1% to 1%) 2529
Norvir (2% to 2.6%) 499
Omacor Capsules 2735
Omnicef Capsules (0.2%) 506
Omnicef for Oral Suspension (0.2%) 506
▲ Ontak Vials (9%) 1717
▲ Orap Tablets (2 of 20 patients) 1220
Ortho-Cyclen/Ortho Tri-Cyclen 2414
Ortho Tri-Cyclen Lo Tablets 2421
Oxandrin Tablets 2977
Oxsoralen-Ultra Capsules 3354
▲ OxyContin Tablets (Between 1% and 5%) 2699
▲ Pacerone Tablets (1% to 3%) 3337
Parcopa Orally Disintegrating Tablets 3111
Parnate Tablets 1499
▲ Paxil CR Controlled-Release Tablets (1.3% to 24%) 1509
▲ Paxil (1.3% to 24%) 1501
Peganone Tablets, USP 2487
▲ Pegasys (19%) 2793
▲ PEG-Intron Powder for Injection (23%) 3062
Pentasa Capsules (Less than 1%) 3182
Pepcid Injection (Infrequent) 2017
Pepcid (Infrequent) 2014
▲ Permax Tablets (7.9%) 3357
Phenergan 3438
Phenytek Capsules 2153
▲ Photofrin for Injection (4% to 14%) 729
Plavix Tablets (1% to 2.5%) 940
Plavix Tablets (1% to 2.5%) 2942
Plendil Extended-Release Tablets (0.5% to 1.5%) 651
Pletal Tablets (Less than 2%) 2478
Pravachol Tablets 943
▲ Premarin Tablets (6% to 7%) 3443
▲ Premphase Tablets (6% to 7%) 3452
▲ Prempro Tablets (6% to 7%) 3452
Prevacid NapraPAC (Less than 1%) 3277
PREVPAC 3281
Prilosec OTC Tablets (Less than 1%) 2674
Primatene Tablets ▣ 749
Prinivil Tablets (0.3% to 1.0%) 2029
Prinzide Tablets 2033
ProAmatine Tablets (Rare) 3183
Prochieve 4% Gel 1018
Prochieve 8% Gel 1018
▲ Procrit for Injection (13% to 21%) 2374
▲ Prograf Capsules and Injection (32% to 64%) 624
Proleukin for Injection 1007
Prometrium Capsules (100 mg, 200 mg) (Less than 5%) 3205
Protonix I.V. (Greater than or equal to 1%) 3468
Protonix Tablets (Less than or equal to 1%) 3465
Protopic Ointment (Up to 4%) 629
Proventil Inhalation Aerosol 3067
Proventil Inhalation Solution 0.083% (1% to 3.1%) 3069
Proventil HFA Inhalation Aerosol 3071
▲ Provigil Tablets (5%) 1002
▲ Prozac Pulvules and Liquid (10% to 33%) 1771
▲ Rapamune Oral Solution and Tablets (13% to 22%) 3472
▲ Razadyne ER Extended-Release Capsules (5%) 2434
▲ Razadyne (5%) 2434
▲ Rebetol (14% to 41%) 3073
▲ Rebetron Combination Therapy (26% to 39%) 3078
Recombivax HB (Less to greater than 1%) 2045
ReFacto Vials 3479
Relafen Tablets (1% to 3%) 1523
Relpax Tablets (Infrequent) 2531
ReoPro Vials (0.3%) 1779
Requip Tablets (1% or more) 1528
▲ Rescriptor Tablets (1.2% to 5%) 2535
▲ Retrovir Capsules (2.4% to 5%) 1533
▲ Retrovir IV Infusion (3% to 5%) 1537
▲ Retrovir (2.4% to 5%) 1533
▲ Revatio Tablets (7%) 2541
▲ Reyataz Capsules (Less than 1% to 5%) 948
▲ Ribavirin, USP Capsules (14% to 41%) 3083
Rilutek Tablets (2.1% to 2.9%) 2945
▲ Risperdal Consta Long-Acting Injection (13% to 16%) 1664
▲ Risperdal M-Tab Orally Disintegrating Tablets (23% to 26%) 1658
▲ Risperdal (23% to 26%) 1658
▲ Ritalin Hydrochloride Tablets (One of the two most common) 2254
▲ Ritalin LA Capsules (3.1%) 2255
▲ Ritalin-SR Tablets (One of the two most common) 2254
▲ Rituxan for Infusion (1% to 5%) 845
▲ Rituxan I.V. (1% to 5%) 1251
Robitussin CF Liquid ▣ 755
Robitussin Maximum Strength Cough & Cold Liquid ▣ 754
Robitussin PE Syrup ▣ 753
Robitussin Pediatric Cough & Cold Liquid ▣ 754
▲ Roferon-A Injection (11% to 14%) 2805
▲ Rozerem Tablets (3%) 3228
Rythmol SR Capsules 2736
▲ Sandostatin LAR Depot (5% to 15%) 2264
▲ Simulect for Injection (Greater than or equal to 10%) 2268
Singulair 2047
Sonata Capsules (Infrequent) 1686
▲ Soriatane Capsules (1% to 10%) 1028
Spectracef Tablets (0.1% to 1%) 2706
Stalevo Tablets 2270
▲ Strattera Capsules (5% to 16%) 1784
▲ Suboxone Tablets (14% to 25%) 2719
▲ Subutex Tablets (21.4% to 25%) 2719
Sudafed 12 Hour Caplets ▣ 708
Sudafed 24 Hour Tablets ▣ 709
Sudafed Nasal Decongestant Tablets ▣ 709
Sular Tablets (Less than or equal to 1%) 1163
Surmontil Capsules 2347
▲ Sustiva Capsules (1% to 7%) 957
Symbyax Capsules 1788
▲ Symmetrel (5% to 10%) 1115
Synercid I.V. (Less than 1%) 1690
Tambocor Tablets (1% to 3%) 1824
Tamiflu Capsules (1.1% to 1.2%) 2810
Tamiflu Oral Suspension (1.1% to 1.2%) 2810
▲ Targretin Capsules (4.8% to 11.3%) 1719
Tarka Tablets (Less frequent) 519
▲ Temodar Capsules (4% to 10%) 3088
▲ Tequin Injection (0.1% to 3%) 964
▲ Tequin Tablets (0.1% to 3%) 964
Testim 1% Gel (1% or less) 722
Teveten Tablets (Less than 1%) 1707
Teveten HCT Tablets (Less than 1%) 1710
Thalomid Capsules 979
TheraFlu Cold & Cough Hot Liquid ▣ 680
TheraFlu Cold & Sore Throat Hot Liquid ▣ 680

TheraFlu Flu & Chest Congestion Non-Drowsy Hot Liquid ▣ 681
TheraFlu Flu & Sore Throat Hot Liquid ▣ 681
TheraFlu Severe Cold Non-Drowsy Hot Liquid ▣ 683
TheraFlu Severe Cold & Cough Hot Liquid ▣ 683
TheraFlu Severe Cold Caplets ▣ 679
TheraFlu Severe Cold Hot Liquid ▣ 682
TheraFlu Severe Cold Non-Drowsy Caplets ▣ 679
Thiothixene Capsules 2124
Thyrolar 1203
Tiazac Capsules (Less than 2%) 1204
Timolide Tablets (Less than 1%) 2056
Timoptic in Ocudose (Less frequent) 2061
Timoptic Sterile Ophthalmic Solution 2058
Timoptic-XE Sterile Ophthalmic Gel Forming Solution 2062
Tindamax 2670
▲ Topamax Sprinkle Capsules (6% to 9%) 2438
▲ Topamax Tablets (6% to 9%) 2438
Toprol-XL Tablets 660
Tranxene 2488
▲ Trasylol Injection (3%) 779
Trelstar Depot (2.1%) 3385
Trelstar LA Suspension (1.7%) 3387
Triaminic Chest & Nasal Congestion Liquid ▣ 685
Triaminic Cold & Allergy Liquid ▣ 685
Triaminic Cold & Cough Liquid ▣ 685
Triaminic Cough Liquid ▣ 687
Triaminic Cough & Nasal Congestion Liquid ▣ 687
Triaminic Cough & Sore Throat Liquid ▣ 687
Triaminic Flu, Cough & Fever Liquid ▣ 685
Triaminic Night Time Cough & Cold Liquid ▣ 685
Triaminic Cough & Sore Throat Softchews ▣ 689
Tricor Tablets 523
▲ Trileptal Oral Suspension (2% to 4%) 2281
▲ Trileptal Tablets (2% to 4%) 2281
▲ Trisenox Injection (43%) 983
▲ Trizivir Tablets (7% to 13%) 1565
Truvada Tablets 1279
Twinrix Vaccine (Less than 1%) 1571
Tygacil for Injection (2.3%) 3489
Children's Tylenol Plus Cold NightTime Suspension Liquid 1851
Children's Tylenol Plus Cold Chewable Tablets 1851
Tylenol Cold & Flu Severe Daytime Liquid with Cool Bust 1846
Tylenol Cold & Flu Severe NightTime Liquid with Cool Burst 1846
Tylenol Flu NightTime Gelcaps 1846
Tylenol Flu Day Non-Drowsy Gelcaps 1846
Concentrated Tylenol Infants' Drops Plus Cold Nasal Congestant, Fever Reducer & Pain Reliever ▣ 668
Concentrated Tylenol Infants' Drops Plus Cold & Cough Nasal Decongestant, Fever Reducer & Pain Reliever ▣ 668
Multi-Symptom Tylenol Cold Night Time Caplets 1845
Multi-Symptom Tylenol Cold Day Non-Drowsy Caplets and Gelcaps 1845
Ultane Liquid for Inhalation (Less than 1%) 526
Ultracet Tablets (2%) 2462
Uniphyl Tablets 2708
Uniretic Tablets (Less than 1%) 3114
Unithroid Tablets 3521
▲ Vagifem Tablets (3% to 5%) 2340
▲ Valcyte Tablets (16%) 2816
Valium Tablets 2822
Vantas (2.9%) 3367
Vantin Tablets and Oral Suspension (Less than 1%) 2650
Vaseretic Tablets (0.5% to 2.0%) 2073
Vasotec I.V. Injection (0.5% to 1.0%) 2076
▲ Velcade for Injection (18%) 2102
▲ Ventavis Inhalation Solution (8%) 1036
Ventolin HFA Inhalation Aerosol 1576
Verelan PM Capsules (2% or less) 3120
▲ Vesanoid Capsules (14%) 2823
VFEND I.V. (Less than 2%) 2543
VFEND Oral Suspension (Less than 2%) 2543
VFEND Tablets (Less than 2%) 2543
Viagra Tablets (Less than 2%) 2552
Vicks 44D Cough & Head Congestion Relief 2676
Pediatric Vicks 44m Cough & Cold Relief 2673
Vicks DayQuil Multi-Symptom Cold/Flu Relief LiquiCaps 2675
Vicks DayQuil Multi-Symptom Cold/Flu Relief Liquid 2675
Children's Vicks NyQuil Cold/Cough Relief 2671
▲ Vicoprofen Tablets (3% to 9%) 533
Viracept (Less than 2%) 2556
▲ Viread Tablets (3% to 4%) 1284
Vivactil Tablets 2350
▲ Vivelle Transdermal System (1.5% to 6.4%) 2288
▲ Vivelle-Dot Transdermal System (1.5% to 6.4%) 2293
▲ Voltaren Ophthalmic Solution (Less than or equal to 3%) 2300
Voltaren Tablets (Occasionally) 2298
Voltaren-XR Tablets (Occasionally) 2301
VoSpire Extended-Release Tablets (2.4%) 2352
Vytorin 10/10 Tablets 2084
Vytorin 10/10 Tablets 3092
Vytorin 10/20 Tablets 2084
Vytorin 10/20 Tablets 3092
Vytorin 10/40 Tablets 2084
Vytorin 10/40 Tablets 3092
Vytorin 10/80 Tablets 2084
Vytorin 10/80 Tablets 3092
▲ Wellbutrin Tablets (18.6%) 1579
▲ Wellbutrin SR Sustained-Release Tablets (5% to 16%) 1583
▲ Wellbutrin XL Extended-Release Tablets (5% to 16%) 1588
▲ Xanax XR Tablets (24.2%) 2655
▲ Xeloda Tablets (Less than 5%) 2825
Xifaxan Tablets (Less than 2%) 2847
Xopenex HFA Inhalation Aerosol 3151
Xopenex Inhalation Solution 3143
Xopenex Inhalation Solution Concentrate 3147
Zantac (Rare) 1597
Zantac Injection 1593
Zantac Injection Pharmacy Bulk Package (Rare) 1595
Zantac Syrup (Rare) 1597
Zegerid Powder for Oral Solution (Less than 1%) 2972
Zelnorm Tablets (1% to 2%) 2303
▲ Zenapax for Injection (Greater than 5%) 2838
▲ Zerit (29%) 971
Zestoretic Tablets 701
Zestril Tablets (0.3% to 1.0%) 704
▲ Zevalin Injection (5%) 848
Zithromax Capsules, 250 mg (1% or less) 2568
Zithromax for IV Infusion (1% or less) 2573
Zithromax for Oral Suspension, 300 mg, 600 mg, 900 mg, 1200 mg (1% or less) 2561
Zithromax Tablets, 250 mg, 500 mg (1% or less) 2561
Zithromax Tri-Pak (1% or less) 2561
Zocor Tablets 2078
▲ Zoladex (5% to 11%) 709
Zoladex 3-month 712
▲ Zoloft (12% to 28%) 2581
▲ Zometa for Intravenous Infusion (15.1% to 16%) 2306
Zomig Nasal Spray (Infrequent to less than 2%) 718
Zomig Tablets (Infrequent) 714
Zomig-ZMT Tablets (Infrequent) 714
▲ Zonegran Capsules (6%) 1089
▲ Zosyn (4.5% to 6.6%) 3492
▲ Zyban Sustained-Release Tablets (31% to 40%) 1620
▲ Zyprexa Tablets (20%) 1798
▲ Zyprexa ZYDIS Orally Disintegrating Tablets (20%) 1798
▲ Zyrtec Chewable Tablets (Less than 2% to 9%) 2589
▲ Zyrtec (Less than 2% to 9%) 2589
▲ Zyrtec-D 12 Hour Extended Release Tablets (4%) 2591
Zyvox (2.5%) 2661

Insomnia, early morning
Strattera Capsules (1% to 3%) 1784

Insomnia, paradoxical
Diastat Rectal Delivery System 3344

Instability, postural
Risperdal Consta Long-Acting Injection 1664

Insulin allergy
Novolin 70/30 PenFill 3 ml Cartridges (Rare) 2325
Novolin N PenFill 3 ml Cartridges (Rare) 2325
Novolin R PenFill (Rare) 2325

Insulin reaction
Novolin 70/30 InnoLet 2322
Novolin N InnoLet 2322
Novolin R InnoLet 2322

Insulin requirement, changes
Decadron Phosphate Injection 1931
Decadron Tablets 1929
Depo-Medrol Single-Dose Vial 2617
Hydrocortone Tablets 1963
Maxzide 2150
Pediapred Oral Solution 3319
Prinzide Tablets 2033
Vaseretic Tablets 2073

Insulin resistance

Interstitial lung disease
Arava Tablets (Rare) 2881
Erbitux (0.5%) 937
Myfortic Tablets (Rare) 2244
Rapamune Oral Solution and Tablets 3472
Tarceva Tablets (Infrequent) 1254
Tarceva Tablets (Infrequent) 2470
Zemaira (1 Patient) 3506

Intervertebral disk disorder, unspecified
Imitrex Nasal Spray (Rare) 1435

Intervertebral disk herniation
Remicade for IV Injection (Greater than or equal to 0.2%) 987

Intestinal obstruction
Abilify Tablets (Rare) 916
Abilify Tablets (Rare) 2472
Aloprim for Injection (Less than 1%) 2156
Ambien Tablets (Rare) 2867
Avastin IV (Rare) 1229
Campath Ampules 826
Celebrex Capsules (Less than 0.1%) 3130
Clozapine Tablets 2141
Clozaril Tablets 2174
Dantrium Capsules (Rare) 2690
▲ Doxil Injection (11.3%) 3302
Effexor Tablets (Rare) 3405
Effexor XR Capsules (Rare) 3411
Elitek (Less than or equal to 1%) 2906
▲ Eloxatin for Injection (2% to 5%) 2908
▲ Entocort EC Capsules (Less than 5%) 2694
Evoxac Capsules 1042
Exelon Capsules (Infrequent) 2204
FazaClo Orally Disintegrating Tablets 547
Gleevec Tablets (Rare) 2221
Herceptin I.V. (At least one of the 958 patients) 1234
▲ Hycamtin for Injection (1.1% to 4.5%) 1427
Imitrex Injection 1431
Imitrex Nasal Spray (Rare) 1435
Imitrex Tablets 1440
Invirase (Rare) 2776
Levaquin in 5% Dextrose Injection (0.1% to 0.9%) 2453
Levaquin (0.1% to 0.9%) 2453
Meridia Capsules 485
Merrem I.V. (Greater than 0.1% to 1%) 687
MS Contin Tablets (Less frequent) 2703
Navelbine Injection 1494
Neurontin Capsules (Rare) 2498
Neurontin Oral Solution (Rare) 2498
Neurontin Tablets (Rare) 2498
Omacor Capsules 2735
▲ Pancrease MT Capsules (Among most frequent) 1839
Paxil CR Controlled-Release Tablets (Rare) 1509
Paxil (Rare) 1501
Permax Tablets (Infrequent) 3357
Proleukin for Injection 1007
Prozac Pulvules and Liquid (Rare) 1771
Pulmozyme Inhalation Solution 1245
Remicade for IV Injection (Greater than or equal to 0.2%) 987
Rilutek Tablets (Infrequent) 2945
Risperdal M-Tab Orally Disintegrating Tablets 1658
Risperdal 1658
Rythmol SR Capsules 2736
Sandostatin LAR Depot (Rare) 2264
Seroquel Tablets (Rare) 691
Sonata Capsules (Rare) 1686
Symbyax Capsules (Rare) 1788
Taxotere Injection Concentrate 2947
Thalomid Capsules 979
VESIcare Tablets 631
Xeloda Tablets 2825
Zomig Nasal Spray (Rare) 718
Zyprexa Tablets (Rare) 1798
Zyprexa ZYDIS Orally Disintegrating Tablets (Rare) 1798

Intestinal obstruction, pseudo
Catapres Tablets (Rare) 874
Nimotop Capsules (Rare) 774

Intestinal perforation
Arthrotec Tablets (Rare) 3126
Campath Ampules 826
Celebrex Capsules (Less than 0.1%) 3130
Cipro I.V. (Less than 1%) 2998
Cipro I.V. Pharmacy Bulk Package (Less than 1%) 3509
Cipro (Less than 1%) 2991
Cipro XR Tablets 3004
Enbrel for Injection 580
Hydrocortone Tablets 1963
Mobic Oral Suspension (Less than 2%) 893
Mobic Tablets (Less than 2%) 893
Myfortic Tablets 2244
Navelbine Injection 1494
Proleukin for Injection (Less than 1%) 1007
Remicade for IV Injection (Greater than or equal to 0.2%) 987
Tabloid Tablets 1545
VFEND I.V. (Less than 2%) 2543
VFEND Oral Suspension (Less than 2%) 2543
VFEND Tablets (Less than 2%) 2543
Wellbutrin Tablets (Rare) 1579
Wellbutrin SR Sustained-Release Tablets 1583
Wellbutrin XL Extended-Release Tablets 1588
Zyban Sustained-Release Tablets 1620

Intestinal strictures
Clinoril Tablets (Rare) 1899
Indocin Capsules (Less than 1%) 1968
Indocin I.V. (Less than 1%) 1973
▲ Pancrease MT Capsules (Among most frequent) 1839

Intestinal villous atrophy
CellCept Capsules (Isolated cases) 2751
CellCept Intravenous (Isolated cases) 2751
CellCept Oral Suspension (Isolated cases) 2751
CellCept Tablets (Isolated cases) 2751

Intestines, hemorrhagic necrosis of
Digitek Tablets 2146
Lanoxicaps Capsules 1458
Lanoxin Injection 1462
Lanoxin Tablets 1468
Lanoxin Injection Pediatric 1465

Intracranial hypertension with papilledema
Norditropin Cartridges (Small number of patients) 2318
Nutropin for Injection (A small number of patients) 1238
Nutropin AQ Injection (A small number of patients) 1241
Nutropin AQ Pen (A small number of patients) 1241
Nutropin AQ Pen Cartridge (A small number of patients) 1241
Tev-Tropin for Injection (Small number of patients) 1224

Intracranial pressure, increase
Albenza Tablets (Up to 1.5%) 1310
Ammonul Injection 3323
Cipro I.V. 2998
Cipro I.V. Pharmacy Bulk Package 3509
Cipro 2991
Cipro XR Tablets 3004
Decadron Phosphate Injection 1931
Decadron Tablets 1929
Depo-Medrol Injectable Suspension 2615
Depo-Medrol Single-Dose Vial 2617
Dilaudid 439
Dilaudid Oral Liquid (Less frequent) 443

Dilaudid Non-Sterile Powder............ 439
Dilaudid Rectal Suppositories........... 439
Dilaudid Tablets............................... 439
Dilaudid Tablets - 8 mg (Less frequent)............................... 443
Dilaudid-HP (Less frequent)............ 441
Eskalith.. 1406
Gleevec Tablets (Rare).................... 2221
Hydrocortone Tablets...................... 1963
Levaquin in 5% Dextrose Injection (0.1% to 0.9%)............................ 2453
Levaquin (0.1% to 0.9%)................. 2453
MS Contin Tablets (Less frequent).... 2703
Noroxin Tablets.............................. 2009
Tequin Injection.............................. 964
Tequin Tablets................................ 964

Intraocular disorders
Amerge Tablets (Rare).................... 1312
Imitrex Tablets............................... 1440

Intraocular pressure, increase
(*see under* Glaucoma)
Advair Diskus 100/50...................... 1291

Intraocular pressure, paradoxical increase
Pulmicort Respules (Rare)................ 654

Intravascular coagulation, disseminated
Aggrenox Capsules.......................... 855
Aloprim for Injection (Less than 1%).. 2156
▲ Ammonul Injection (3%) 3323
Bayer Aspirin Tablets...................... 3515
Cafcit (2.2%).................................. 1854
Campath Ampules........................... 826
Clinoril Tablets (Less than 1 in 100).. 1899
Dolobid Tablets (Less than 1 in 100).. 1937
Ecotrin Enteric Coated Aspirin Low, Regular and Maximum Strength Tablets........................... 1627
Indocin Capsules (Less than 1%)...... 1968
Indocin I.V..................................... 1973
Indocin (Less than 1%).................... 1968
Lamictal... 1449
Mylotarg for Injection (1%).............. 3429
NovoSeven..................................... 2335
Omnicef Capsules........................... 506
Omnicef for Oral Suspension........... 506
Oncaspar (Greater than 1% but less than 5%)................................ 1123
St. Joseph 81 mg Aspirin Chewable and Enteric Coated Tablets.. 1841
Sulfamylon Cream.......................... 2154
Sulfamylon for 5% Topical Solution.... 2155
Trasylol Injection (1% to 2%)........... 779
▲ Trisenox Injection (8%) 983
Vantin Tablets and Oral Suspension................................... 2650
▲ Vesanoid Capsules (26%) 2823
VFEND I.V. (Less than 2%)............... 2543
VFEND Oral Suspension (Less than 2%).. 2543
VFEND Tablets (Less than 2%).......... 2543
Zovirax for Injection....................... 1618

Intussusception, gastrointestinal
Infanrix Vaccine............................. 1444
Lotronex Tablets (Rare).................. 1479
Pediarix Vaccine............................. 1518

Involuntary movements, abnormal
Carbatrol Capsules......................... 3174
Clozapine Tablets (Less than 1%)..... 2141
Clozaril Tablets (Less than 1%)......... 2174
Effexor Tablets............................... 3405
Eldepryl Capsules........................... 3209
▲ Equetro Extended-Release Capsules (Less than 5%)............... 3178
FazaClo Orally Disintegrating Tablets (Less than 1%)................ 547
Moban Tablets................................ 1108
▲ Niravam Orally Disintegrating Tablets (14.8% to 17.3%).............. 3106
Omnicef Capsules........................... 506
Omnicef for Oral Suspension........... 506
Orap Tablets.................................. 1220
Pacerone Tablets............................ 3337
▲ Roferon-A Injection (7%) 2805
Seroquel Tablets (Infrequent)........... 691
Symmetrel (Uncommon).................. 1115
Tegretol/Tegretol-XR....................... 2278

Involuntary movements, extremities
Moban Tablets................................ 1108

Orap Tablets.................................. 1220

IOP, elevation of
Albalon Ophthalmic Solution .... ⊙216
Alrex Ophthalmic Suspension 0.2% (2%).................................. ⊙243
Amvisc Plus.................................. ⊙289
Beconase AQ Nasal Spray (Rare)..... 1359
Blephamide Ophthalmic Ointment.... 563
Blephamide Ophthalmic Suspension.................................. 564
Caduet Tablets (Less than 2%)........ 2507
Depo-Medrol Injectable Suspension.................................. 2615
Effexor Tablets (Rare)..................... 3405
Flonase Nasal Spray....................... 1412
FML Ophthalmic Ointment............... ⊙225
FML Ophthalmic Suspension........... ⊙224
FML Forte Ophthalmic Suspension.................................. ⊙223
FML-S Liquifilm Sterile Ophthalmic Suspension.................................. ⊙226
Gleevec Tablets (Rare).................... 2221
HMS Sterile Ophthalmic Suspension.................................. ⊙228
Lotemax Ophthalmic Suspension 0.5%.. ⊙249
Meridia Capsules............................ 485
Ocucoat (Some cases).................... ⊙290
Paxil CR Controlled-Release Tablets (Rare).............................. 1509
Paxil (Rare)..................................... 1501
Permax Tablets (Infrequent)............ 3357
Poly-Pred Liquifilm Ophthalmic Suspension.................................. ⊙231
Pred Forte Ophthalmic Suspension.................................. ⊙233
Pred Mild Sterile Ophthalmic Suspension.................................. ⊙236
Pred-G Ophthalmic Suspension....... ⊙234
Sandostatin Injection (Less than 1%).. 2263
TobraDex Ophthalmic Ointment....... 558
TobraDex Ophthalmic Suspension.... 558
Viagra Tablets................................ 2552
▲ Voltaren Ophthalmic Solution (Less than or equal to 5% to 15%).. 2300
▲ Zylet Ophthalmic Suspension (2% to 10%).. 3508

Iridocyclitis
(*see also under* Iritis)
Betagan Ophthalmic Solution, USP (Rare).................................... ⊙217
Cosopt Sterile Ophthalmic Solution (Less than 1%)............. 1910
Trusopt Sterile Ophthalmic Solution (Rare)............................ 2065

Iris pigmentation, increase in
▲ Lumigan Ophthalmic Solution (1% to 3%).. 569
Travatan Ophthalmic Solution (1% to 4%).. 559
▲ Xalatan Sterile Ophthalmic Solution (5% to 15%)................... 2654

Iritis
(*see also under* Uveitis)
▲ Acular Ophthalmic Solution (1% to 10%).. 561
▲ Acular LS Ophthalmic Solution (1% to 10%)................................ 562
Alphagan P Ophthalmic Solution....... 563
Aredia for Injection (Rare)................ 2168
Arthrotec Tablets (Rare)................... 3126
Brimonidine Tartrate Ophthalmic Solution 0.2%............................ ⊙245
Colazal Capsules............................ 2845
Lumigan Ophthalmic Solution (Less than 1%)............................. 569
Lunesta Tablets (Rare)..................... 3139
Lyrica Capsules (Rare)..................... 2524
Neurontin Capsules (Rare)................ 2498
Neurontin Oral Solution (Rare).......... 2498
Neurontin Tablets (Rare).................. 2498
Norvir (Less than 2%)...................... 499
Ocucoat (Rare)............................... ⊙290
Ophthetic Ophthalmic Solution (Sometimes)............................... ⊙230
Prozac Pulvules and Liquid (Rare)..... 1771
Topamax Sprinkle Capsules (Rare)... 2438
Topamax Tablets (Rare)................... 2438
Uniretic Tablets (Less than 1%)........ 3114
Viracept (Less than 2%).................. 2556
Xalatan Sterile Ophthalmic Solution...................................... 2654
Zonegran Capsules (Rare)................ 1089

Iron deficiency
Cuprimine Capsules........................ 1925
Epogen for Injection........................ 586
Prozac Pulvules and Liquid (Rare)..... 1771
Risperdal M-Tab Orally Disintegrating Tablets (Rare).......... 1658
Risperdal (Rare).............................. 1658
Sandostatin Injection (Less than 1%).. 2263
Syprine Capsules............................ 2055

Irritability
▲ Aerobid/Aerobid-M (3% to 9%) 1172
Alacol DM Syrup............................. 739
Aricept Tablets (Frequent)................ 1086
Aricept ODT Tablets (Frequent)........ 1086
Arthrotec Tablets (Rare)................... 3126
Attenuvax...................................... 1889
Cafcit... 1854
Catapres-TTS (0.5% or less)............ 875
Ceftin for Oral Suspension (0.1% to 1%)... 1369
Cenestin Tablets, 0.45mg, 0.625mg, 0.9mg, 1.25mg........... 1063
Cenestin Tablets, 0.3mg.................. 1063
Cipro I.V. (1% or less)..................... 2998
Cipro I.V. Pharmacy Bulk Package (1% or less)................................. 3509
Cipro (Less than 1%)....................... 2991
Cipro XR Tablets............................ 3004
Ciprodex Otic Suspension (0.5%)...... 555
▲ Clarinex Syrup (12.1%) 3009
Climara Transdermal System........... 795
Climara Pro Transdermal System..... 800
▲ Clolar for Intravenous Infusion (11%).. 1264
Clozapine Tablets (Less than 1%)..... 2141
Clozaril Tablets (Less than 1%)......... 2174
▲ Comvax (32.2% to 57.0%) 1904
▲ Copegus Tablets (33%) 2759
Cymbalta Delayed-Release Capsules (Frequent)...................... 1729
Cytovene.. 2763
Dalmane Capsules.......................... 3343
▲ DAPTACEL (36.9% to 41.4%) 2964
▲ depo-subQ provera 104 Injectable Suspension (1% to less than 5%)............................... 2622
Effexor Tablets............................... 3405
Effexor XR Capsules....................... 3411
Efudex... 3348
Eldepryl Capsules........................... 3209
Elspar for Injection.......................... 1943
Engerix-B Vaccine (Less than 1%)..... 1391
Estratest Tablets............................. 3196
Estratest H.S. Tablets...................... 3196
Estrogel 0.06%............................... 3200
FazaClo Orally Disintegrating Tablets (Less than 1%)................ 547
▲ Flumist Vaccine (9.9% to 17.8%) 1872
▲ Gabitril Tablets (10%) 998
Guanidine Hydrochloride Tablets...... 3030
HibTITER (133 of 1,118 vaccinations)................................ 3419
▲ Indapamide Tablets (Greater than or equal to 5%).............................. 2119
▲ Infanrix Vaccine (28.8% to 61.5%) ... 1444
▲ Intron A for Injection (Up to 16%) 3038
Invirase (Less than 2%)................... 2776
▲ Lamictal (3.0%)............................... 1449
Levothroid Tablets.......................... 1189
Levoxyl Tablets.............................. 1680
Lexapro Oral Solution (Frequent)...... 1193
Lexapro Tablets (Frequent).............. 1193
Maxalt Tablets (Infrequent).............. 1983
Maxalt-MLT Orally Disintegrating Tablets (Infrequent)..................... 1983
Menostar Transdermal System........ 805
Meruvax II..................................... 1994
M-M-R II.. 1980
Mumpsvax..................................... 2005
Narcan Injection............................. 1109
▲ Nicotrol NS (Greater than 5%) 2596
▲ Niravam Orally Disintegrating Tablets (10.5% to 33.1%)............. 3106
Novarel for Injection........................ 1147
Paxil CR Controlled-Release Tablets.. 1509
Paxil Tablets.................................. 1501
▲ Pediarix Vaccine (1.7% to 63.8%) 1518
Liquid PedvaxHIB........................... 2012
▲ Pegasys (19%) 2793
▲ PEG-Intron Powder for Injection (28%).. 3062
Plendil Extended-Release Tablets (0.5% to 1.5%).............................. 651
Prefest Tablets............................... 1069
Premarin Tablets............................ 3443
Premarin Vaginal Cream................. 3449
Premphase Tablets......................... 3452
Prempro Tablets............................. 3452

▲ Prevnar for Injection (44.2% to 58.7%).. 3460
Prinivil Tablets (0.3% to 1.0%)......... 2029
Prinzide Tablets............................. 2033
Proleukin for Injection..................... 1007
▲ Prometrium Capsules (100 mg, 200 mg) (5% to 8%).................... 3205
Prozac Pulvules and Liquid.............. 1771
Pulmicort Respules (Less than 1%).. 654
▲ Rebetol (10% to 47%) 3073
▲ Rebetron Combination Therapy (23% to 32%)............................... 3078
Recombivax HB (Greater than 1%).... 2045
Retrovir Capsules (1.6%)................. 1533
Retrovir IV Infusion (2%)................. 1537
Retrovir (1.6%)............................... 1533
▲ Ribavirin, USP Capsules (10% to 47%)... 3083
▲ Roferon-A Injection (Less than 5% to 15%).. 2805
Singulair (Very rare)....................... 2047
▲ Skelaxin Tablets (Most frequent) 1685
▲ Strattera Capsules (0.5% to 8%) 1784
Surmontil Capsules 2347
Symbyax Capsules 1788
Symmetrel (1% to 5%) 1115
Tasmar Tablets (1%) 3360
Tranxene 2488
Twinrix Vaccine (Less than 1%) 1571
Uniphyl Tablets 2708
Unithroid Tablets 3521
Vantas (Less than 2%) 3367
▲ Vaqta (10.8%)................................ 2067
Varivax (Greater than or equal to 1%) 2070
Vivactil Tablets 2350
Vivelle Transdermal System 2288
Vivelle-Dot Transdermal System 2293
VoSpire Extended-Release Tablets (Less frequent)........................... 2352
▲ Wellbutrin SR Sustained-Release Tablets (2% to 3%).................... 1583
▲ Wellbutrin XL Extended-Release Tablets (2% to 3%).................... 1588
Xanax XR Tablets (Rare to frequent)..................................... 2655
▲ Xeloda Tablets (Less than 5%) 2825
Zestoretic Tablets 701
Zestril Tablets (0.3% to 1.0%) 704
Zoloft 2581
Zomig Nasal Spray (Rare) 718
Zomig Tablets (Rare) 714
Zomig-ZMT Tablets (Rare) 714
▲ Zonegran Capsules (9%) 1089
Zyban Sustained-Release Tablets (Frequent) 1620
Zyrtec Chewable Tablets 2589
Zyrtec 2589

Irritation
Aclovate Cream (Approximately 2%) 1290
Analpram-HC 1136
Bleph-10 Ophthalmic Solution 10% .... ⊙219
Climara Pro Transdermal System 800
Cutivate Cream (Infrequent) 1381
Cutivate Lotion 0.05% (Rare) 1383
Cutivate Ointment (Less than 1%) 1384
Diprolene Gel 0.05% 3015
Diprolene Lotion 0.05% (Less than 1%) 3016
▲ Dovonex Scalp Solution 0.005% (1% to 5%) 3375
▲ Efudex (Among most frequent) 3348
Locoid (Infrequent) 1138
Lotrisone 3054
Nizoral 2% Shampoo (Less than 1%) 1838
Olux Foam (Less than 2%) 1027
Pandel Cream, 0.1% 1017
Pramosone 1139
Pred-G Ophthalmic Suspension .... ⊙234
Temovate Cream 1549
▲ Temovate Gel (Among most frequent) 1550
Temovate Ointment (0.5%) 1549
Temovate Scalp Application (Infrequent) 1551
Temovate E Emollient (Less than 2%) 1552
U-Kera Cream 3290
Vanos Cream 1864

Irritation, anal
Colyte with Flavor Packs for Oral Solution (Less frequent) 3102
Fleet Glycerin Laxatives 1168
TriLyte with Flavor Packs for Oral Solution 3114
Zosyn (1.0% or less) 3492

Irritation, gastric
Aldoclor Tablets 1881
Aldoril Tablets 1884

Atacand HCT ... 637
Avalide Tablets ... 922
Avalide Tablets ... 2889
Captopril Tablets (About 0.5% to 2%) ... 2114
Clorpres Tablets ... 2139
Cymbalta Delayed-Release Capsules (Infrequent) ... 1729
Dantrium Capsules (Rare) ... 2690
Diovan HCT Tablets ... 2195
Diuril Oral ... 1936
Diuril Sodium Intravenous ... 1934
Furosemide Tablets ... 2117
Guanidine Hydrochloride Tablets ... 3030
Hyzaar ... 1964
Indapamide Tablets (Less than 5%) .. 2119
Lotensin HCT Tablets ... 2235
Maxzide ... 2150
Micardis HCT Tablets ... 886
Moduretic Tablets ... 2003
Norflex Injection ... 1824
Prinzide Tablets ... 2033
Teveten HCT Tablets ... 1710
Timolide Tablets ... 2056
Uniretic Tablets ... 3114
Vaseretic Tablets ... 2073
Zestoretic Tablets ... 701

Irritation, gastrointestinal
Dibenzyline Capsules ... 3390
▲ K-Lor Powder Packets (Among most common) ... 472
Urocit-K Tablets (Some patients) ... 2109

Irritation, glossal
(*see under* Irritation, oral)

Irritation, local
Aldara Cream, 5% (More than 1%) ... 1814
Arixtra Injection ... 1325
Avar Cleanser (Rare) ... 3189
Avar Gel (Rare) ... 3189
Avar Green ... 3189
Avar-e Emollient Cream (Rare) ... 3189
Avar-e Green Cream (Rare) ... 3189
Bentyl Injection ... 724
Betasept Surgical Scrub ... 2715
Bleph-10 Ophthalmic Solution 10% ... ⊙ 219
Blephamide Ophthalmic Ointment ... 563
Blephamide Ophthalmic Suspension ... 564
▲ Carac Cream, 0.5% (94.6%) ... 1048
Climara Transdermal System ... 795
Desenex ... ▣ 674
Desenex Jock Itch Spray Powder ... ▣ 674
Desferal Vials ... 2190
Edecrin Sodium Intravenous (Occasionally) ... 1941
Elidel Cream 1% (0.4% to 6.4%) ... 2198
Garamycin Injectable (Rare) ... 3028
HibTITER ... 3419
Klaron Lotion 10% ... 1050
Lidoderm Patch ... 1107
Locoid Lipocream Cream (Infrequent) ... 1138
Lovenox Injection ... 2931
Mentax Cream (Less than 2%) ... 2152
Metrogel 1% ... 1212
Naftin Cream (2%) ... 2097
▲ Nicotrol Inhaler (40% to 66%) ... 2594
Nitro-Dur Transdermal Infusion System ... 3060
Plexion (Rare) ... 1863
▲ Polytrim Ophthalmic Solution (Most frequent) ... 570
Rosac Cream with Sunscreens (Rare) ... 3216
▲ Solage Topical Solution (5% to 7.3%) ... 740
▲ Striant Mucoadhesive (9.2%) ... 1022
Thera-Gesic Plus Creme ... ▣ 673
Topicort .05% Gel ... 3288
Topicort .25% Cream ... 3288
Topicort .25% Ointment ... 3288
Topicort LP .05% Cream ... 3288
U-cort 1% Cream ... 3289
Ultralytic 2 Cream 20% ... 1651
Ultralytic 2 Foam 20% ... 1652
Vivelle Transdermal System (1.9%) ... 2288
Vivelle-Dot Transdermal System (1.9%) ... 2293

Irritation, nasal
▲ Advair Diskus 100/50 (1% to 3%) ... 1291
▲ Advair Diskus 250/50 (1% to 3%) ... 1291
▲ Advair Diskus 500/50 (1% to 3%) ... 1291
Aerobid/Aerobid-M (1% to 3%) ... 1172
Asmanex Twisthaler (1% to less than 3%) ... 2981
Atrovent Nasal Spray 0.03% (2.0%) ... 869
Beconase AQ Nasal Spray ... 1359
Efudex (Infrequent) ... 3348
▲ Flonase Nasal Spray (1% to 3%) ... 1412
▲ Fortical Nasal Spray (10.6%) ... 3336
Maxalt Tablets (Infrequent) ... 1983
Maxalt-MLT Orally Disintegrating Tablets (Infrequent) ... 1983
▲ Miacalcin Nasal Spray (10.6%) ... 2242
▲ Nasacort HFA Inhalation Aerosol (6.2% to 7.5%) ... 2939
Nasonex Nasal Spray (Greater than or equal to 2%) ... 3058
▲ Nicotrol NS (81% to 94%) ... 2596
Xifaxan Tablets (Less than 2%) ... 2847

Irritation, nasopharyngeal
▲ Beconase AQ Nasal Spray (24% of patients) ... 1359
Rhinocort Aqua Nasal Spray (2%) ... 658

Irritation, oral
Aerobid/Aerobid-M (1% to 3%) ... 1172
Amerge Tablets (Rare) ... 1312
Axert Tablets (Rare) ... 2430
Furosemide Tablets ... 2117
Imitrex Nasal Spray ... 1435
Sandimmune (Rare) ... 2259
▲ Striant Mucoadhesive (9.2%) ... 1022

Irritation, oropharynx
Proventil Inhalation Aerosol ... 3067
Proventil HFA Inhalation Aerosol ... 3071
Serevent Diskus ... 1540
Ventolin HFA Inhalation Aerosol ... 1576
VoSpire Extended-Release Tablets ... 2352

Irritation, perianal
(*see under* Irritation, anal)

Irritation, scalp
Men's Rogaine Extra Strength Topical Solution, Ocean Rush Scent and Original Unscented ... ▣ 706
Women's Rogaine Topical Solution, Spring Bloom Scent and Original Unscented ... ▣ 707

Irritation, sinus
Nicotrol NS ... 2596

Irritation, skin
(*see under* Irritation, local)

Irritation, vaginal
Ceftin for Oral Suspension (0.1% to 1%) ... 1369
Clindesse Vaginal Cream (Less than 1%) ... 3296
▲ MetroGel-Vaginal Gel (9%) ... 1822
Nystatin Vaginal Tablets, USP (Rare) ... 2347

Irritation, vulvovaginal
(*see under* Irritation, vaginal)

Irritation at injection site
▲ Eligard 22.5 mg (21.7%) ... 2899
▲ Eligard 30 mg (20%) ... 2901
▲ Eulexin Capsules (3%) ... 3023
▲ Gammagard S/D (16%) ... 754
Nembutal Sodium Solution, USP ... 2484
▲ Pegasys (22%) ... 2793
Pepcid Injection Premixed (Infrequent) ... 2017
Repronex for Intramuscular and Subcutaneous Injection ... 1148
Retrovir IV Infusion (Infrequent) ... 1537
Xolair ... 1259

Ischemia
Aldara Cream, 5% ... 1814
Camptosar Injection ... 2602
Gammagard S/D ... 754
▲ Prandin Tablets (0.5, 1, and 2 mg) (4%) ... 2337
Sandostatin Injection (Less than 1%) ... 2263
▲ Vesanoid Capsules (3%) ... 2823

Ischemia, arteria basilaris
Fluorescite Injection ... ⊙ 207

Ischemia, cerebral
Abilify Tablets (Infrequent) ... 916
Abilify Tablets (Infrequent) ... 2472
Actiq (Less than 1%) ... 993
Angiomax for Injection (Rare) ... 1856
Apokyn Injection ... 2132
Arimidex Tablets (1%) ... 665
Betagan Ophthalmic Solution, USP ... ⊙ 217
Betimol Ophthalmic Solution ... ⊙ 283
Betimol Ophthalmic Solution ... 3371
Carteolol Hydrochloride Ophthalmic Solution USP, 1% ... ⊙ 246
Cosopt Sterile Ophthalmic Solution ... 1910
Effexor Tablets (Rare) ... 3405
Effexor XR Capsules (Rare) ... 3411
Enbrel for Injection (Infrequent) ... 580
Gabitril Tablets (Infrequent) ... 998
Hyperstat I.V. Injection ... 3031
Imitrex Injection ... 1431
Imitrex Nasal Spray ... 1435
Imitrex Tablets (Rare) ... 1440
Nitrolingual Pumpspray (Occasional) ... 1161
Paxil CR Controlled-Release Tablets (Rare) ... 1509
Paxil (Rare) ... 1501
Permax Tablets (Infrequent) ... 3357
Pletal Tablets (Less than 2%) ... 2478
Prozac Pulvules and Liquid (Rare) ... 1771
ReoPro Vials (0.3%) ... 1779
Rilutek Tablets (Rare) ... 2945
Seroquel Tablets (Infrequent) ... 691
Sonata Capsules (Rare) ... 1686
Sular Tablets (Less than or equal to 1%) ... 1163
Symbyax Capsules (Infrequent) ... 1788
Tasmar Tablets (Infrequent) ... 3360
Thalomid Capsules ... 979
Timolide Tablets ... 2056
Timoptic in Ocudose ... 2061
Timoptic Sterile Ophthalmic Solution (Less frequent) ... 2058
Timoptic-XE Sterile Ophthalmic Gel Forming Solution ... 2062
VFEND I.V. (Less than 2%) ... 2543
VFEND Oral Suspension (Less than 2%) ... 2543
VFEND Tablets (Less than 2%) ... 2543
Zoladex 3-month (1% to 5%) ... 712
Zomig Tablets (Rare) ... 714
Zomig-ZMT Tablets (Rare) ... 714

Ischemia, colonic
Imitrex Tablets ... 1440

Ischemia, gastrointestinal
Zomig Nasal Spray (Very rare) ... 718
Zomig Tablets ... 714

Ischemia, intestinal
Amerge Tablets ... 1312
Digitek Tablets (Rare) ... 2146
Imitrex Nasal Spray ... 1435
Lanoxicaps Capsules ... 1458
Lanoxin Injection ... 1462
Lanoxin Tablets ... 1468
Lanoxin Injection Pediatric ... 1465
Zelnorm Tablets ... 2303

Ischemia, mesenteric
Lotronex Tablets ... 1479
Zelnorm Tablets ... 2303

Ischemia, myocardial
Abilify Tablets (Infrequent) ... 916
Abilify Tablets (Infrequent) ... 2472
▲ Alimta for Injection (1% to 3%) ... 1722
Aloxi Injection (Less than 1%) ... 2099
Anzemet Injection (Rare) ... 2871
Anzemet Tablets (Rare) ... 2874
Apokyn Injection ... 2132
Argatroban Injection (1.8%) ... 1321
▲ Arimidex Tablets (3%) ... 665
BiDil Tablets ... 2161
Camptosar Injection ... 2602
Coreg Tablets (Less than or equal to 0.1%) ... 1376
Diprivan Injectable Emulsion (Less than 1%) ... 676
Enbrel for Injection (Infrequent) ... 580
Ethyol for Injection ... 1869
Femara Tablets (Less than or equal to 2%) ... 2210
Flolan for Injection (2%) ... 1408
Frova Tablets ... 1101
Hyperstat I.V. Injection ... 3031
Imitrex Injection (Extremely rare) ... 1431
Imitrex Nasal Spray ... 1435
Imitrex Tablets (Rare) ... 1440
Levitra Tablets (Less than 2%) ... 3048
Maxalt Tablets (Very rare) ... 1983
Maxalt-MLT Orally Disintegrating Tablets (Very rare) ... 1983
Omacor Capsules ... 2735
Paxil CR Controlled-Release Tablets (Rare) ... 1509
Paxil (Rare) ... 1501
PEG-Intron Powder for Injection ... 3062
Pletal Tablets (Less than 2%) ... 2478
▲ Proleukin for Injection (3%) ... 1007
Protonix I.V. (Less than 1%) ... 3468
Protonix Tablets (Less than 1%) ... 3465
Razadyne (Infrequent) ... 2434
Relpax Tablets (Rare) ... 2531
Rilutek Tablets (Infrequent) ... 2945
Risperdal Consta Long-Acting Injection (Infrequent) ... 1664
Suprane Liquid for Inhalation (Less than 1%) ... 770
Tasmar Tablets (Infrequent) ... 3360
TNKase I.V. ... 1256
Trasylol Injection (1% to 2%) ... 779
Ultracet Tablets ... 2462
Uniretic Tablets (Less than 1%) ... 3114
Viagra Tablets (Less than 2%) ... 2552
Zomig Nasal Spray ... 718
Zomig Tablets ... 714
Zomig-ZMT Tablets ... 714

Ischemia, peripheral
Anzemet Injection (Rare) ... 2871
Anzemet Tablets (Rare) ... 2874
Brevibloc Concentrate (About 1%) ... 766
Brevibloc Injection (About 1%) ... 766
Brevibloc Double Strength Injection (About 1%) ... 766
Brevibloc Premixed Injection (About 1%) ... 766
Brevibloc Double Strength Premixed Injection (About 1%) ... 766
Caduet Tablets (Greater than 0.1% to less than or equal to 1%) ... 2507
Coreg Tablets (Greater than 0.1% to 1%) ... 1376
Cytovene ... 2763
Evoxac Capsules (Less than 1%) ... 1042
Exelon Capsules (Infrequent) ... 2204
Gengraf Capsules (1% to less than 3%) ... 458
Imitrex Tablets ... 1440
▲ Intron A for Injection (Less than 5%) ... 3038
Migranal Nasal Spray (Rare) ... 3350
Neoral Soft Gelatin Capsules (1% to less than 3%) ... 2247
Neoral Oral Solution (1% to less than 3%) ... 2247
Norvasc Tablets (More than 0.1% to 1%) ... 2529
▲ Requip Tablets (3%) ... 1528
Soriatane Capsules (Less than 1%) .. 1028
Teveten Tablets (Less than 1%) ... 1707
Teveten HCT Tablets (Less than 1%) ... 1710
Zoloft (Infrequent) ... 2581
Zomig Tablets ... 714

Ischemia, recurrent
Activase I.V. ... 1225
Retavase ... 1131

Ischemia, small bowel
Lotronex Tablets ... 1479

Ischemia, transient
Imitrex Tablets ... 1440

Ischemia of digits
Zovirax for Injection (Less than 1%) ... 1618

Ischemic attacks, transient
Abilify Tablets ... 916
Abilify Tablets ... 2472
Actimmune (Rare) ... 1646
Amerge Tablets ... 1312
Aranesp for Injection (1%) ... 576
Aricept Tablets (Infrequent) ... 1086
Aricept ODT Tablets (Infrequent) ... 1086
Avalide Tablets ... 922
Avalide Tablets ... 2889
Avapro Tablets (Less than 1%) ... 925
Avapro Tablets (Less than 1%) ... 2886
Celexa (Rare) ... 1177
Clozapine Tablets (Several patients) ... 2141
Clozaril Tablets (Several patients) ... 2174
DynaCirc CR Tablets (0.5% to 1%) ... 2726
Epogen for Injection (0.4%) ... 586
▲ Femara Tablets (6.8%) ... 2210
Gammagard S/D ... 754
Imitrex Injection ... 1431
Meridia Capsules ... 485
Namenda (Frequent) ... 1199
Orthoclone OKT3 Sterile Solution (Less than 1%) ... 2370
PEG-Intron Powder for Injection (Less than or equal to 1%) ... 3062
Prinivil Tablets (0.3% to 1.0%) ... 2029
Prinzide Tablets ... 2033
Procrit for Injection (0.4%) ... 2374
Proleukin for Injection (Less than 1%) ... 1007
Razadyne (Infrequent) ... 2434
Revatio Tablets ... 2541
Risperdal Consta Long-Acting Injection ... 1664
Risperdal M-Tab Orally Disintegrating Tablets ... 1658

Risperdal ... 1658
Roferon-A Injection (Infrequent) ... 2805
Viagra Tablets ... 2552
Zestoretic Tablets ... 701
Zestril Tablets (0.3% to 1.0%) ... 704

Ischemic colitis
Imitrex Injection ... 1431
Imitrex Nasal Spray ... 1435
Imitrex Tablets ... 1440
Inderal LA Long-Acting Capsules ... 3421
Timolide Tablets ... 2056
Timoptic in Ocudose ... 2061
Timoptic Sterile Ophthalmic Solution ... 2058

Ischemic disorders, life-threatening, aggravation of
Roferon-A Injection ... 2805

Itching
(*see under* Pruritus)

Itching, eyes
(*see under* Pruritus, ocular)

Itching, vulvovaginal
Ceftin Tablets (0.1% to 1%) ... 1369
Clozapine Tablets (Less than 1%) ... 2141
Clozaril Tablets (Less than 1%) ... 2174

Itching at application site
Ultralytic 2 Cream 20% ... 1651
Ultralytic 2 Foam 20% ... 1652

Itching at injection site
▲ Humira Injection (20%) ... 464
Symlin Injection ... 608
Xolair ... 1259

J

Jarisch-Herxheimer's reaction
(*see under* Herxheimer's reaction)

Jaundice
Abelcet Injection ... 1119
Aceon Tablets (2 mg, 4 mg, 8 mg) ... 3191
Aciphex Tablets ... 1081
Actiq (1% or greater) ... 993
Adalat CC Tablets (Rare) ... 2978
Advicor Tablets ... 1694
Aggrenox Capsules (Less than 1%) .. 855
Aldoclor Tablets ... 1881
Aldoril Tablets ... 1884
Alkeran for Injection ... 976
Alkeran Tablets ... 977
Aloprim for Injection (Less than 1%) ... 2156
Altace Capsules ... 1673
Amaryl Tablets (Isolated cases) ... 2864
Ammonul Injection ... 3323
Anadrol-50 Tablets ... 3329
Anaprox Tablets (Rare; less than 1%) ... 2769
Anaprox DS Tablets (Rare; less than 1%) ... 2769
Antabuse Tablets ... 2343
AquaMEPHYTON Injection ... 1887
Arava Tablets (Rare) ... 2881
Aricept Tablets (Infrequent) ... 1086
Aricept ODT Tablets (Infrequent) ... 1086
Arthrotec Tablets (Rare) ... 3126
Asacol Delayed-Release Tablets (Rare) ... 2688
Atacand HCT ... 637
Avalide Tablets ... 922
Avalide Tablets ... 2889
Avandia Tablets (Very rare) ... 1348
Avapro Tablets ... 925
Avapro Tablets (Very rare) ... 2886
Avelox (Less than 0.1%) ... 2984
Axid Oral Solution ... 913
Biaxin/Biaxin XL (Infrequent) ... 402
Caduet Tablets ... 2507
▲ Camptosar Injection (9%) ... 2602
Cancidas for Injection (0.9%) ... 1894
Captopril Tablets ... 2114
Casodex Tablets (Rare) ... 670
Cataflam Tablets (Occasionally) ... 2173
Ceftin ... 1369
Celebrex Capsules ... 3130
Celexa (Rare) ... 1177
▲ CellCept Capsules (3% to less than 20%) ... 2751
▲ CellCept Intravenous (3% to less than 20%) ... 2751
▲ CellCept Oral Suspension (3% to less than 20%) ... 2751
▲ CellCept Tablets (3% to less than 20%) ... 2751
Cipro I.V. (1% or less) ... 2998
Cipro I.V. Pharmacy Bulk Package (1% or less) ... 3509
Cipro (Rare) ... 2991
Cipro XR Tablets (Rare) ... 3004
Cleocin Vaginal Ovules ... 2613
Clindesse Vaginal Cream (Rare) ... 3296
Clinoril Tablets (Less than 1%) ... 1899
▲ Clolar for Intravenous Infusion (15%) ... 1264
Clorpres Tablets ... 2139
Clozapine Tablets ... 2141
Clozaril Tablets ... 2174
Colazal Capsules ... 2845
Coumadin for Injection (Infrequent) ... 932
Coumadin Tablets (Infrequent) ... 932
Crestor Tablets (Very rare) ... 672
Crixivan Capsules (1.5%) ... 1918
Cubicin for Injection (Less than 1%) ... 1038
Dantrium Capsules ... 2690
Dapsone Tablets USP ... 1656
Darvocet A 500 Tablets (Rare) ... 3497
Depo-Provera Contraceptive Injection (Less than 1%) ... 2619
depo-subQ provera 104 Injectable Suspension ... 2622
Diastat Rectal Delivery System (Infrequent) ... 3344
Diovan HCT Tablets ... 2195
Dolobid Tablets (Less than 1 in 100) ... 1937
Doxil Injection (Less than 1%) ... 3302
Dyazide Capsules ... 1389
Dyrenium Capsules (Rare) ... 3390
EC-Naprosyn Delayed-Release Tablets (Rare; less than 1%) ... 2769
Edecrin (Rare) ... 1941
Effexor Tablets (Rare) ... 3405
Effexor XR Capsules (Rare) ... 3411
Epivir ... 1394
EryPed ... 445
Ery-Tab Tablets ... 447
Erythrocin Stearate Filmtab Tablets ... 452
Eulexin Capsules (Less than 1%) ... 3023
FazaClo Orally Disintegrating Tablets ... 547
Flexeril Tablets (Rare) ... 1832
Fortaz ... 1422
Furosemide Tablets ... 2117
Geodon Capsules (Rare) ... 2514
Havrix Vaccine (Rare) ... 1425
Hyzaar ... 1964
Indapamide Tablets ... 2119
Indocin Capsules (Less than 1%) ... 1968
Indocin I.V. (Less than 1%) ... 1973
Indocin (Less than 1%) ... 1968
▲ Intron A for Injection (Less than 5%) ... 3038
Invanz for Injection (Greater than 0.1%) ... 1974
Invirase (Rare) ... 2776
▲ I.V. Busulfex (12%) ... 1125
Kaletra (Less than 2%) ... 474
Lamisil Tablets ... 2226
Leukeran Tablets ... 1472
Levaquin in 5% Dextrose Injection (0.1% to 0.9%) ... 2453
Levaquin (0.1% to 0.9%) ... 2453
Librium Capsules ... 3349
Lotensin HCT Tablets ... 2235
Matulane Capsules ... 3188
Mavik Tablets (Rare) ... 482
Maxzide ... 2150
Mefoxin for Injection ... 1987
Mefoxin Premixed Intravenous Solution ... 1990
Merrem I.V. (Greater than 0.1% to 1%) ... 687
Micardis HCT Tablets ... 886
Midamor Tablets (Less than or equal to 1%) ... 2000
Mintezol ... 2002
Miradon Tablets ... 3056
Mobic Oral Suspension (Less than 0.1%) ... 893
Mobic Tablets (Less than 0.1%) ... 893
Moduretic Tablets ... 2003
Mustargen for Injection (Infrequent) .. 2007
Mycamine for Injection ... 620
Mylotarg for Injection ... 3429
Nalfon Capsules (Less than 1%) ... 2504
Naprosyn Suspension (Rare; less than 1%) ... 2769
Naprosyn Tablets (Rare; less than 1%) ... 2769
Naropin Injection (Less than 1%) ... 640
Neurontin Capsules ... 2498
Neurontin Oral Solution ... 2498
Neurontin Tablets ... 2498
Nexium Delayed-Release Capsules (Very rare) ... 645
Nexium I.V. (Very rare) ... 649
Niaspan Extended-Release Tablets ... 1703
Nimotop Capsules (Less than 1%) ... 774
Niravam Orally Disintegrating Tablets ... 3106
Noroxin Tablets ... 2009
Norvasc Tablets (Infrequent) ... 2529
Norvir ... 499
Omnicef Capsules ... 506
Omnicef for Oral Suspension ... 506
Oncaspar (Greater than 1% but less than 5%) ... 1123
Ortho-Cyclen/Ortho Tri-Cyclen ... 2414
Ortho Tri-Cyclen Lo Tablets ... 2421
Oxandrin Tablets ... 2977
Paser Granules ... 1657
Paxil CR Controlled-Release Tablets (Rare) ... 1509
Paxil (Rare) ... 1501
Pediarix Vaccine ... 1518
Pentasa Capsules ... 3182
Permax Tablets (Rare) ... 3357
Phenergan ... 3438
▲ Photofrin for Injection (Less than 5%) ... 729
Pletal Tablets (Very rare) ... 2478
Precose Tablets ... 776
Prevacid NapraPAC (Less than 1%) .. 3277
PREVPAC (Infrequent) ... 3281
Prilosec OTC Tablets (Rare) ... 2674
Primaxin I.M. ... 2022
Primaxin I.V. (Less than 0.2%) ... 2024
Prinivil Tablets ... 2029
Prinzide Tablets ... 2033
▲ Prograf Capsules and Injection (3% to 15%) ... 624
▲ Proleukin for Injection (11%) ... 1007
Protonix I.V. ... 3468
Protonix Tablets ... 3465
Raptiva for Injection ... 1247
Rebif Prefilled Syringe for Injection (Rare) ... 3163
Relafen Tablets (Less than 1%) ... 1523
Remicade for IV Injection (Rare) ... 987
Rescriptor Tablets ... 2535
Retrovir IV Infusion ... 1537
▲ Reyataz Capsules (Less than 1% to 7%) ... 948
Rilutek Tablets (Infrequent) ... 2945
Risperdal Consta Long-Acting Injection (Rare) ... 1664
Risperdal M-Tab Orally Disintegrating Tablets ... 1658
Risperdal ... 1658
Rocephin Injectable Vials, ADD-Vantage, Galaxy, Bulk (Rare) ... 2801
Sandostatin Injection (Less than 1%) ... 2263
Sandostatin LAR Depot (1% to 4%) .. 2264
Skelaxin Tablets ... 1685
Soriatane Capsules (2 of 525 patients) ... 1028
Suprax ... 1811
Surmontil Capsules ... 2347
Tabloid Tablets (A few cases) ... 1545
Tambocor Tablets ... 1824
Tasmar Tablets ... 3360
Teveten HCT Tablets ... 1710
Thioridazine Hydrochloride Tablets .. 2122
Tracleer Tablets ... 539
Trasylol Injection (1% to 2%) ... 779
Twinrix Vaccine ... 1571
Tygacil for Injection (0% to less than 2%) ... 3489
Ultane Liquid for Inhalation (Less than 1%) ... 526
Uniretic Tablets (Less than 1%) ... 3114
Valium Tablets (Isolated reports) ... 2822
Vaseretic Tablets ... 2073
Vasotec I.V. Injection ... 2076
VFEND I.V. (Less than 2%) ... 2543
VFEND Oral Suspension (Less than 2%) ... 2543
VFEND Tablets (Less than 2%) ... 2543
Viracept ... 2556
Viramune Oral Suspension ... 903
Viramune Tablets ... 903
Vivactil Tablets ... 2350
Voltaren Tablets (Occasionally) ... 2298
Voltaren-XR Tablets (Occasionally) ... 2301
Wellbutrin Tablets (Infrequent) ... 1579
Wellbutrin SR Sustained-Release Tablets (Infrequent) ... 1583
Wellbutrin XL Extended-Release Tablets (Infrequent) ... 1588
▲ Xeloda Tablets (Less than 5%) ... 2825
Zantac (Occasional) ... 1597
Zantac Injection ... 1593
Zantac Injection Pharmacy Bulk Package (Infrequent) ... 1595
Zantac Syrup (Occasional) ... 1597
Zegerid Powder for Oral Solution (Rare) ... 2972
Zestoretic Tablets ... 701
Zithromax for Oral Suspension, 300 mg, 600 mg, 900 mg, 1200 mg (1% or less) ... 2561
Zithromax Tablets, 250 mg, 500 mg (1% or less) ... 2561
Zithromax Tri-Pak (1% or less) ... 2561
Zoloft (One or more patients) ... 2581
Zomig Nasal Spray (Rare) ... 718
Zovirax ... 1616
Zyban Sustained-Release Tablets (Infrequent) ... 1620

Jaundice, cholestatic
Aceon Tablets (2 mg, 4 mg, 8 mg) (Rare) ... 3191
Activella Tablets ... 2311
Alesse-28 Tablets ... 3392
Altace Capsules (Rare) ... 1673
Altoprev Extended-Release Tablets ... 1151
Amoxil Capsules ... 1315
Amoxil Chewable Tablets ... 1315
Amoxil Pediatric Drops for Oral Suspension ... 1315
Amoxil Powder for Oral Suspension ... 1315
Amoxil Tablets ... 1315
Asacol Delayed-Release Tablets (Rare) ... 2688
Augmentin ... 1331
Augmentin Tablets ... 1334
Augmentin XR Extended-Release Tablets ... 1340
Augmentin ES-600 Powder for Oral Suspension ... 1337
Avelox (Less than 0.1%) ... 2984
Axid Oral Solution (Rare) ... 913
Aygestin Tablets ... 1062
Caduet Tablets (Less than 2%) ... 2507
Captopril Tablets (Rare) ... 2114
Carbatrol Capsules ... 3174
Ceftin ... 1369
▲ CellCept Capsules (3% to less than 20%) ... 2751
▲ CellCept Intravenous (3% to less than 20%) ... 2751
▲ CellCept Oral Suspension (3% to less than 20%) ... 2751
▲ CellCept Tablets (3% to less than 20%) ... 2751
Cenestin Tablets, 0.45mg, 0.625mg, 0.9mg, 1.25mg ... 1063
Cenestin Tablets, 0.3mg ... 1063
Cipro ... 2991
Cipro XR Tablets ... 3004
Climara Transdermal System ... 795
Climara Pro Transdermal System ... 800
Colazal Capsules ... 2845
Dapsone Tablets USP ... 1656
Darvocet A 500 Tablets (Rare) ... 3497
Delatestryl Injection ... 2976
Doxil Injection (Less than 1%) ... 3302
Equetro Extended-Release Capsules ... 3178
Estratest Tablets ... 3196
Estratest H.S. Tablets ... 3196
Estrogel 0.06% ... 3200
Eulexin Capsules (Less than 1%) ... 3023
Geodon Capsules (Rare) ... 2514
Lescol Capsules ... 2227
Lescol Capsules ... 2730
Lescol XL Tablets ... 2227
Lescol XL Tablets ... 2730
Lipitor Tablets (Less than 2%) ... 2495
Lo/Ovral-28 Tablets ... 3423
Lotrel Capsules (Rare) ... 2238
Mavik Tablets (Rare) ... 482
Menostar Transdermal System ... 805
Merrem I.V. (Greater than 0.1% to 1%) ... 687
Mevacor Tablets ... 1996
Myleran Tablets (Rare) ... 1492
Noroxin Tablets ... 2009
Ortho-Cept Tablets ... 2395
Ortho-Cyclen Tablets ... 2414
Ortho Evra Transdermal System ... 2402
Ortho Tri-Cyclen Tablets ... 2414
Ortho Tri-Cyclen Lo Tablets ... 2421
Oxandrin Tablets ... 2977
Pentasa Capsules ... 3182
Pepcid Injection (Infrequent) ... 2017
Pepcid (Infrequent) ... 2014
Phenergan ... 3438
Pravachol Tablets ... 943
Prefest Tablets ... 1069
Premarin Intravenous ... 3440
Premarin Tablets ... 3443
Premarin Vaginal Cream ... 3449
Premphase Tablets ... 3452
Prempro Tablets ... 3452

PREVPAC 3281
Prilosec OTC Tablets (Rare) 2674
Prinivil Tablets (0.3% to 1.0%) 2029
Prinzide Tablets (Rare) 2033
▲ Prograf Capsules and Injection (3% to 15%) 624
Prometrium Capsules (100 mg, 200 mg) 3205
Protonix I.V. (Less than 1%) 3468
Protonix Tablets (Less than 1%) 3465
Prozac Pulvules and Liquid 1771
Relafen Tablets (1%) 1523
Seasonale Tablets 1073
Tarka Tablets (Rare) 519
Tegretol/Tegretol-XR 2278
Thalomid Capsules 979
Ticlid Tablets (Rare) 2813
Timentin ADD-Vantage (Rare) 1556
Timentin Injection Galaxy Container (Rare) 1559
Timentin IV Infusion (Rare) 1553
Timentin Pharmacy Bulk Package (Rare) 1562
Triphasil-28 Tablets 3483
Uniretic Tablets (Rare) 3114
Vaseretic Tablets (Rare) 2073
Vasotec I.V. Injection (0.5% to 1.0%) 2076
VFEND I.V. (1% to 1.7%) 2543
VFEND Oral Suspension (1% to 1.7%) 2543
VFEND Tablets (1% to 1.7%) 2543
Vivelle Transdermal System 2288
Vivelle-Dot Transdermal System 2293
Vytorin 10/10 Tablets 2084
Vytorin 10/10 Tablets 3092
Vytorin 10/20 Tablets 2084
Vytorin 10/20 Tablets 3092
Vytorin 10/40 Tablets 2084
Vytorin 10/40 Tablets 3092
Vytorin 10/80 Tablets 2084
Vytorin 10/80 Tablets 3092
Yasmin 28 Tablets 818
Zegerid Powder for Oral Solution (Rare) 2972
Zestoretic Tablets (Rare) 701
Zestril Tablets (0.3% to 1.0%) 704
Zithromax Capsules, 250 mg (1% or less; rare) 2568
Zithromax for IV Infusion 2573
Zithromax for Oral Suspension, 1 g (1% or less; rare) 2568
Zithromax for Oral Suspension, 300 mg, 600 mg, 900 mg, 1200 mg (1% or less; rare) 2561
Zithromax Tablets, 250 mg, 500 mg (1% or less; rare) 2561
Zithromax Tablets, 600 mg (1% or less; rare) 2568
Zithromax Tri-Pak (1% or less; rare) 2561
Zithromax Z-Pak (1% or less; rare) 2568
Zmax for Oral Suspension 2577
Zocor Tablets 2078
Zonegran Capsules (Rare) 1089
Zosyn 3492

Jaundice, fetal

Diuril Oral 1936
Diuril Sodium Intravenous 1934

Jaundice, hepatocellular

Aceon Tablets (2 mg, 4 mg, 8 mg) 3191
Augmentin 1331
Augmentin Tablets 1334
Augmentin XR Extended-Release Tablets 1340
Augmentin ES-600 Powder for Oral Suspension 1337
Axid Oral Solution (Rare) 913
Biaxin/Biaxin XL (Infrequent) 402
Carbatrol Capsules 3174
Equetro Extended-Release Capsules 3178
PREVPAC (Infrequent) 3281
Prilosec OTC Tablets (Rare) 2674
Prinivil Tablets (0.3% to 1.0%) 2029
Prinzide Tablets 2033
Tegretol/Tegretol-XR 2278
Ticlid Tablets (Rare) 2813
Vaseretic Tablets 2073
Vasotec I.V. Injection (0.5% to 1.0%) 2076
Zantac (Occasional) 1597
Zegerid Powder for Oral Solution (Rare) 2972
Zestoretic Tablets 701
Zestril Tablets (0.3% to 1.0%) 704

Jaundice, intrahepatic cholestatic

Aldoclor Tablets 1881
Atacand HCT 637
Augmentin 1331
Augmentin Tablets 1334
Augmentin XR Extended-Release Tablets 1340
Augmentin ES-600 Powder for Oral Suspension 1337
Avalide Tablets 922
Avalide Tablets 2889
Clorpres Tablets 2139
Diovan HCT Tablets 2195
Diuril Oral 1936
Diuril Sodium Intravenous 1934
Furosemide Tablets 2117
Hyzaar 1964
Indapamide Tablets 2119
Lotensin HCT Tablets 2235
Maxzide 2150
Micardis HCT Tablets 886
Moduretic Tablets 2003
Prinzide Tablets 2033
Teveten HCT Tablets 1710
Timolide Tablets 2056
Uniretic Tablets 3114
Vaseretic Tablets 2073
Zestoretic Tablets 701

Jaundice, neonatal

Aldoclor Tablets 1881
Aldoril Tablets 1884
AquaMEPHYTON Injection 1887
Diuril Oral 1936
Diuril Sodium Intravenous 1934
Dyazide Capsules 1389
Maxzide 2150
Mephyton Tablets 1993
Moduretic Tablets 2003
▲ Naropin Injection (3.6%) 640
Prinzide Tablets 2033
Timolide Tablets 2056
Vaseretic Tablets 2073
Zestoretic Tablets 701

Jaw tightness

Abilify Tablets (Infrequent) 916
Abilify Tablets (Infrequent) 2472
Imitrex Injection (Relatively common) 1431
Imitrex Tablets 1440
Lexapro Oral Solution (Infrequent) 1193
Lexapro Tablets (Infrequent) 1193
Zomig Nasal Spray (Infrequent) 718
▲ Zomig Tablets (4% to 10%) 714
▲ Zomig-ZMT Tablets (4% to 10%) 714

Jerks

(*see under* Twitching)

Jitteriness

▲ Byetta Injection (9%) 605
Cafcit 1854
Cubicin for Injection (Less than 1%) 1038
Cymbalta Delayed-Release Capsules (Infrequent) 1729
▲ Focalin XR Capsules (12%) 2217
Guanidine Hydrochloride Tablets 3030
Lexapro Oral Solution (Infrequent) 1193
Lexapro Tablets (Infrequent) 1193

Joint dislocation

Evoxac Capsules (Less than 1%) 1042

Joint disorder, unspecified

Actiq (1% or greater) 993
▲ Actonel Tablets (6.8%) 2679
▲ Actonel with Calcium Tablets (6.8%) 2684
Adalat CC Tablets (Less than 1%) 2978
Antara Capsules 2723
▲ Arava Tablets (4%) 2881
Asacol Delayed-Release Tablets (2% or greater) 2688
▲ Boniva Tablets (3.6%) 2747
▲ CellCept Capsules (3% to less than 20%) 2751
▲ CellCept Intravenous (3% to less than 20%) 2751
▲ CellCept Oral Suspension (3% to less than 20%) 2751
▲ CellCept Tablets (3% to less than 20%) 2751
▲ Humatrope Vials and Cartridges (2.3% to 5.8%) 1756
▲ Humira Injection (Less than 5%) 464
Hytrin Capsules (At least 1%) 469
Imitrex Nasal Spray (Infrequent) 1435
Lamictal (1.3%) 1449
Lofibra Capsules 1217
Lunesta Tablets (Infrequent) 3139
▲ Lupron Depot 3.75 mg (7.8%) 3257
▲ Lupron Depot–3 Month 11.25 mg (7.8% to 8%) 3262
Meridia Capsules (1.1%) 485
Mirapex Tablets (Less than 1%) 889
Mobic Oral Suspension (1.5% to 2.3%) 893
Mobic Tablets (1.5% to 2.3%) 893
Neurontin Capsules (Rare) 2498
Neurontin Oral Solution (Rare) 2498
Neurontin Tablets (Rare) 2498
Norvir (Less than 2%) 499
Oncaspar (Less than 1%) 1123
Orthovisc Injection (0.4%) 3518
Prevacid Delayed-Release Capsules (Less than 1%) 3268
Prevacid for Delayed-Release Oral Suspension (Less than 1%) 3268
Prevacid NapraPAC (Less than 1%) 3277
Prevacid SoluTab Delayed-Release Orally Disintegrating Tablets (Less than 1%) 3268
PREVPAC (Less than 1%) 3281
▲ Prograf Capsules and Injection (3% to 15%) 624
Protonix I.V. (Less than 1%) 3468
Protonix Tablets (Less than 1%) 3465
Provigil Tablets (1%) 1002
Relpax Tablets (Rare) 2531
Rythmol SR Capsules 2736
Sonata Capsules (Infrequent) 1686
Symbyax Capsules (1% to 2%) 1788
Tasmar Tablets (Infrequent) 3360
Thalomid Capsules 979
Tricor Tablets 523
Xenical Capsules (2.3%) 2834
Zoladex (1% or greater) 709
Zoladex 3-month 712
Zomig Nasal Spray (Infrequent) 718
Zyprexa IntraMuscular (Infrequent) 1798

Joint effusion

Orthovisc Injection (0.4%) 3518
Sandostatin Injection (Less than 1%) 2263
Sandostatin LAR Depot (Rare) 2264

Joint pain

(*see under* Arthralgia)

Joint stiffness

Amerge Tablets (Infrequent) 1312
Arimidex Tablets 665
Avalide Tablets 922
Avalide Tablets 2889
Avapro Tablets (Less than 1%) 925
Avapro Tablets (Less than 1%) 2886
Cipro I.V. (1% or less) 2998
Cipro I.V. Pharmacy Bulk Package (1% or less) 3509
Cipro (Less than 1%) 2991
Cipro XR Tablets 3004
Gleevec Tablets (Infrequent) 2221
Imitrex Injection (Infrequent) 1431
Lexapro Oral Solution (Infrequent) 1193
Lexapro Tablets (Infrequent) 1193
Lunesta Tablets (Infrequent) 3139
Nabi-HB (2%) 2159
Neurontin Capsules (Infrequent) 2498
Neurontin Oral Solution (Infrequent) 2498
Neurontin Tablets (Infrequent) 2498
Oncaspar 1123
Orthovisc Injection (0.5%) 3518
Xeloda Tablets 2825
Zyprexa Tablets 1798
Zyprexa ZYDIS Orally Disintegrating Tablets 1798

Joints, swollen

▲ Adacel Vaccine (0.3% to 14%) 2959
Lithobid Tablets 1670

K

Kawasaki-like syndrome

Asacol Delayed-Release Tablets (One case) 2688
Pentasa Capsules (Less than 1%) 3182

Keratitis

Acular Ophthalmic Solution (Less than 5%) 561
▲ Advair Diskus 100/50 (1% to 3%) 1291
▲ Advair Diskus 250/50 (1% to 3%) 1291
▲ Advair Diskus 500/50 (1% to 3%) 1291
Amnesteem Capsules 2126
Azopt Ophthalmic Suspension (1% to 5%) 553
Betagan Ophthalmic Solution, USP ⊙ 217
Betimol Ophthalmic Solution (1% to 5%) ⊙ 283
Betimol Ophthalmic Solution (1% to 5%) 3371
Betoptic S Ophthalmic Suspension (Rare) 554
Botox Purified Neurotoxin Complex (Less than 1%) 565
Carteolol Hydrochloride Ophthalmic Solution USP, 1% ⊙ 246
Celexa (Rare) 1177
Ciloxan Ophthalmic Ointment (Less than 1%) 554
Effexor Tablets (Rare) 3405
Effexor XR Capsules (Rare) 3411
▲ Ellence Injection (0% to 14.8%) 2632
Engerix-B Vaccine 1391
Evoxac Capsules (Less than 1%) 1042
▲ Flovent Diskus 50 mcg (1% to 3%) 1415
FML Ophthalmic Ointment (Occasional) ⊙ 225
FML Ophthalmic Suspension (Occasional) ⊙ 224
FML Forte Ophthalmic Suspension (Occasional) ⊙ 223
FML-S Liquifilm Sterile Ophthalmic Suspension ⊙ 226
Geodon Capsules (Rare) 2514
HMS Sterile Ophthalmic Suspension ⊙ 228
Imitrex Injection 1431
Imitrex Nasal Spray 1435
Lyrica Capsules (Rare) 2524
Patanol Ophthalmic Solution (Less than 5%) 557
Poly-Pred Liquifilm Ophthalmic Suspension ⊙ 231
Pred Forte Ophthalmic Suspension (Occasional) ⊙ 233
Pred Mild Sterile Ophthalmic Suspension (Occasional) ⊙ 236
Serevent Diskus (1% to 3%) 1540
Stromectol Tablets 2053
Symmetrel 1115
Tarceva Tablets (Infrequent) 1254
Tarceva Tablets (Infrequent) 2470
Targretin Capsules 1719
Timoptic Sterile Ophthalmic Solution (Less frequent) 2058
Timoptic-XE Sterile Ophthalmic Gel Forming Solution 2062
Travatan Ophthalmic Solution (1% to 4%) 559
Twinrix Vaccine 1571
VFEND I.V. (Less than 2%) 2543
VFEND Oral Suspension (Less than 2%) 2543
VFEND Tablets (Less than 2%) 2543
▲ Vigamox Ophthalmic Solution (1% to 6%) 560
▲ Voltaren Ophthalmic Solution (28%) 2300
Zaditor Ophthalmic Solution (Less than 5%) 2302
▲ Zymar Ophthalmic Solution (5% to 10%) 571

Keratitis, bacterial

Trusopt Sterile Ophthalmic Solution 2065
Xalatan Sterile Ophthalmic Solution 2654

Keratitis, epithelial

Ophthetic Ophthalmic Solution ⊙ 230

Keratitis, punctate

Albalon Ophthalmic Solution ⊙ 216
▲ Cosopt Sterile Ophthalmic Solution (5% to 30%) 1910
▲ Lumigan Ophthalmic Solution (3% to 10%) 569
Pred-G Ophthalmic Suspension (Occasional) ⊙ 234
Pred-G Sterile Ophthalmic Ointment ⊙ 235
▲ Rēv-Eyes Ophthalmic Eyedrops 0.5% (10% to 40%) ⊙ 256

Keratitis, superficial punctate

Acular Ophthalmic Solution 561
▲ Acular LS Ophthalmic Solution (1% to 10%) 562
▲ Trusopt Sterile Ophthalmic Solution (10% to 15%) 2065
▲ Zylet Ophthalmic Suspension (15%) 3508

Keratitis nigricans

Timoptic in Ocudose (Less frequent) 2061

Keratoconjunctivitis

Alrex Ophthalmic Suspension 0.2% (Less than 5%) ⊙ 243

Azopt Ophthalmic Suspension (Less than 1%)............... 553
Evoxac Capsules (Less than 1%)...... 1042
Gabitril Tablets (Infrequent)............ 998
Geodon Capsules (Rare).................. 2514
Lotemax Ophthalmic Suspension 0.5% (Less than 5%).................... ⊙249
Lyrica Capsules (Rare)..................... 2524
Paxil CR Controlled-Release Tablets (Rare)............................. 1509
Paxil (Rare).. 1501
Sular Tablets (Less than or equal to 1%).. 1163
VFEND I.V. (Less than 2%)................ 2543
VFEND Oral Suspension (Less than 2%).. 2543
VFEND Tablets (Less than 2%).......... 2543
▲ Xeloda Tablets (Less than 5%) 2825
Zyprexa Tablets (Rare)..................... 1798
Zyprexa ZYDIS Orally Disintegrating Tablets (Rare)......... 1798

Keratoconjunctivitis sicca
▲ Tarceva Tablets (0% to 12%) 1254
▲ Tarceva Tablets (0% to 12%) 2470

Keratopathy
Alphagan P Ophthalmic Solution (1% to 4%).. 563
Ciloxan Ophthalmic Ointment (Less than 1%)................................ 554

Keratopathy, epithelial
▲ Xalatan Sterile Ophthalmic Solution (5% to 15%)..................... 2654

Keratopathy, vortex
Mepron Suspension......................... 1487

Keratosis
Gengraf Capsules (1% to less than 3%).. 458
Neoral Soft Gelatin Capsules (1% to less than 3%).......................... 2247
Neoral Oral Solution (1% to less than 3%)...................................... 2247

Keratosis pilaris
Finacea Gel (Rare)........................... 1644

Kernicterus, neonatal
Blephamide Ophthalmic Ointment.... 563

Ketoacidosis
FazaClo Orally Disintegrating Tablets 547

Ketoniuria
Amerge Tablets (Rare)...................... 1312

Ketosis
Clozapine Tablets (Sometimes)........ 2141
Clozaril Tablets (Sometimes)............ 2174
Doxil Injection (Less than 1%)........... 3302
Geodon Capsules (Rare).................. 2514
▲ Humira Injection (Less than 5%) 464
Paxil CR Controlled-Release Tablets (Rare)............................. 1509
Paxil (Rare).. 1501
Sonata Capsules (Rare).................. 1686
Zyprexa Tablets (Infrequent)............ 1798
Zyprexa ZYDIS Orally Disintegrating Tablets (Infrequent)................................ 1798

Kidney calculus
Lyrica Capsules (0.1% to 1%).......... 2524

Kidney damage
Furosemide Tablets 2117
▲ Zenapax for Injection (2% to 5%) 2838

Kidney failure, acute
Lyrica Capsules (Rare)..................... 2524

Kidney function, abnormal
Antara Capsules 2723
Avelox (0.1% to less than 2%).......... 2984
Cipro XR Tablets (Less than 1%)....... 3004
Tricor Tablets.................................. 523
VFEND I.V. (0.5% to 1.3%)................ 2543
VFEND Oral Suspension (0.5% to 1.3%)... 2543
VFEND Tablets (0.5% to 1.3%)......... 2543

Kidney pain
(*see under* Pain, renal)

Kidney stones
(*see under* Nephrolithiasis)

Kussmaul respiration
Ammonul Injection 3323

L

Lab test, abnormal, unspecified
▲ Ventavis Inhalation Solution (7%) 1036

Labor, premature
Bravelle for Intramuscular or Subcutaneous Injection................ 1140
Gonal-f RFF Pen for Injection 3155

Labor, prolonged
Bayer Aspirin Tablets 3515

Labor, slowing
Aggrenox Capsules......................... 855
Kadian Capsules (Less than 3%)....... 572
Naropin Injection (Less than 1%)...... 640
Proventil Inhalation Solution 0.083% (Some reports)............... 3069

Laboratory abnormalities, unspecified
Adalat CC Tablets (Less than 1%)..... 2978
Zomig Nasal Spray (Infrequent)........ 718

Labyrinth disorder
▲ Intron A for Injection (Less than 5%).. 3038
Zoloft (Rare) 2581

Labyrinthitis
Amerge Tablets (Rare)..................... 1312
Effexor Tablets (Rare)..................... 3405
Effexor XR Capsules (Rare)............. 3411
Neurontin Capsules (Rare)............... 2498
Neurontin Oral Solution (Rare)......... 2498
Neurontin Tablets (Rare).................. 2498
Nipent for Injection (Less than 3%)... 3216
Sonata Capsules (Rare) 1686

Laceration
▲ Advair Diskus 100/50 (1% to 3%) ... 1291
▲ Advair Diskus 250/50 (1% to 3%) ... 1291
▲ Advair Diskus 500/50 (1% to 3%) ... 1291
Asmanex Twisthaler (1% to less than 3%)...................................... 2981
Elidel Cream 1% (0.7% to 1.5%)....... 2198
▲ Flovent Diskus 50 mcg (1% to 3%).. 1415

Laceration, vulvar
Clindesse Vaginal Cream (Less than 1%).. 3296

Lacrimal duct, stenosis
Taxotere Injection Concentrate (Rare).. 2947
Xeloda Tablets 2825

Lacrimal gland, disorders
DDAVP Nasal Spray (Up to 2%)........ 2894
▲ Intron A for Injection (Less than 5%).. 3038
Neurontin Capsules (Rare)............... 2498
Neurontin Oral Solution (Rare)......... 2498
Neurontin Tablets (Rare).................. 2498

Lacrimation
Adriamycin for Injection, USP (Rare).. 786
Adriamycin Injection, USP (Rare)...... 786
Albalon Ophthalmic Solution .... ⊙216
▲ Avastin IV (6% to 18%) 1229
Azopt Ophthalmic Suspension (Less than 1%)................................ 553
BiDil Tablets................................... 2161
▲ Botox Purified Neurotoxin Complex (10.0%).......................... 565
Camptosar Injection........................ 2602
Ciloxan Ophthalmic Ointment (Less than 1%).............................. 554
Crolom Cromolyn Sodium Sterile Ophthalmic Solution USP 4% (Infrequent).................................. ⊙248
Efudex.. 3348
▲ Eloxatin for Injection (1% to 7%) 2908
Hyperstat I.V. Injection 3031
Imitrex Injection (Infrequent)............ 1431
Imitrex Nasal Spray (Infrequent)....... 1435
Imitrex Tablets (Infrequent).............. 1440
Maxalt Tablets (Infrequent)............... 1983
Maxalt-MLT Orally Disintegrating Tablets (Infrequent)...................... 1983
Neurontin Capsules (Rare)............... 2498
Neurontin Oral Solution (Rare)......... 2498
Neurontin Tablets (Rare).................. 2498
Nipent for Injection (Less than 3%)... 3216
OptiPranolol Metipranolol Ophthalmic Solution 0.3% (A small number of patients)............ ⊙254
Tasmar Tablets (Infrequent).............. 3360
Taxotere Injection Concentrate 2947
Testim 1% Gel (1% or less)............... 722
Trusopt Sterile Ophthalmic Solution (Approximately 1% to 5%)... 2065
Urecholine Tablets 2349
Vaseretic Tablets 2073
Vasotec I.V. Injection (0.5% to 1.0%).. 2076
▲ Vigamox Ophthalmic Solution (1% to 6%).. 560
▲ Voltaren Ophthalmic Solution (Less than or equal to 5% to 30%).. 2300
Zomig Tablets (Rare)........................ 714
Zomig-ZMT Tablets (Rare)................ 714

Lacrimation, abnormal
Ambien Tablets (Rare)...................... 2867
Arthrotec Tablets (Rare)................... 3126
Celexa (Infrequent).......................... 1177
▲ CellCept Capsules (3% to less than 20%) 2751
▲ CellCept Intravenous (3% to less than 20%) 2751
▲ CellCept Oral Suspension (3% to less than 20%) 2751
▲ CellCept Tablets (3% to less than 20%) 2751
Desmopressin Acetate Rhinal Tube (Up to 2%) 1144
Flumadine 1186
▲ Fortical Nasal Spray (1% to 3%) 3336
Frova Tablets (Infrequent) 1101
▲ Gleevec Tablets (6% to 11%) 2221
Lamictal (Rare) 1449
Miacalcin Nasal Spray (1% to 3%) 2242
Migranal Nasal Spray (Infrequent) 3350
Mirapex Tablets (Greater than or equal to 1%) 889
Namenda (Infrequent) 1199
Relpax Tablets (Infrequent) 2531
Requip Tablets (Infrequent) 1528
Risperdal M-Tab Orally Disintegrating Tablets (Rare) 1658
Risperdal (Rare) 1658
▲ Rituxan for Infusion (1% to 5%) 845
▲ Rituxan I.V. (1% to 5%) 1251
Soriatane Capsules (Less than 1%) .. 1028
Topamax Sprinkle Capsules (1%) 2438
Topamax Tablets (1%) 2438
▲ Visudyne for Injection (1% to 10%) .. 2286
Zaditor Ophthalmic Solution (Less than 5%) 2302
Zoloft (Rare) 2581
Zomig Nasal Spray (Infrequent) 718

Lacrimation, increased
Cialis Tablets (Less than 2%) 1806
▲ Zymar Ophthalmic Solution (5% to 10%) 571

Lacrimation disorder, unspecified
▲ Zylet Ophthalmic Suspension (Less than 4%) 3508

Lactation
Abilify Tablets (Rare) 916
Abilify Tablets (Rare) 2472
Aldoclor Tablets 1881
Aldoril Tablets 1884
Effexor Tablets (Rare) 3405
Effexor XR Capsules (Rare) 3411
Geodon Capsules (Infrequent) 2514
Lamictal (Rare) 1449
▲ Lupron Depot 3.75 mg (Among most frequent) 3257
Lupron Depot–3 Month 11.25 mg (Less than 5%) 3262
Paxil CR Controlled-Release Tablets (Rare) 1509
Paxil (Rare) 1501
Permax Tablets (Infrequent) 3357
Prozac Pulvules and Liquid (Infrequent) 1771
Symbyax Capsules (Infrequent) 1788
Thioridazine Hydrochloride Tablets .. 2122
Thiothixene Capsules 2124
Zyprexa Tablets (Infrequent) 1798
Zyprexa ZYDIS Orally Disintegrating Tablets (Infrequent) 1798

Lactation, female
Lunesta Tablets (Infrequent) 3139
Lyrica Capsules (Rare) 2524

Lactation, non-puerperal
Flumadine (Less than 0.3%) 1186
Risperdal Consta Long-Acting Injection (Infrequent) 1664
Risperdal M-Tab Orally Disintegrating Tablets (Infrequent) 1658
Risperdal (Infrequent) 1658
Sandostatin LAR Depot (Rare).......... 2264

Lactation, possible diminution
Alesse-28 Tablets............................ 3392
Lo/Ovral-28 Tablets.......................... 3423
Ortho-Cept Tablets........................... 2395
Ortho-Cyclen Tablets........................ 2414
Ortho Evra Transdermal System 2402
Ortho Tri-Cyclen Tablets................... 2414
Ortho Tri-Cyclen Lo Tablets 2421
Seasonale Tablets 1073
Triphasil-28 Tablets.......................... 3483

Lactation, prevention of
depo-subQ provera 104 Injectable Suspension 2622

Lactation, suppression
Bentyl Capsules............................... 724
Bentyl Injection................................ 724
Bentyl Syrup.................................... 724
Bentyl Tablets.................................. 724
Depo-Provera Contraceptive Injection (Less than 1%) 2619
Ditropan XL Extended Release Tablets 2391

Lactation abnormalities
Seroquel Tablets (Infrequent) 691

Lactic acidosis
ActoPlus Met Tablets 3219
Aloprim for Injection (Less than 1%) 2156
Combivir Tablets 1373
Epivir 1394
Epivir-HBV 1398
Epzicom Tablets 1402
Kaletra (Less than 2%) 474
Retrovir Capsules (Rare) 1533
Retrovir IV Infusion (Rare) 1537
Retrovir (Rare) 1533
Reyataz Capsules (Less than 3%) 948
Trizivir Tablets 1565
Truvada Tablets 1279
Viread Tablets 1284
Zerit 971
Ziagen 1600
Zyvox 2661

Lactic dehydrogenase increased
Abilify Tablets (Rare) 916
Abilify Tablets (Rare) 2472
Campral Tablets (Rare) 1175
Mycamine for Injection (0.5% to 0.8%) 620
▲ Tygacil for Injection (4%) 3489
Viracept (Less than 2%) 2556

Lactose, intolerance to
Sonata Capsules (Rare) 1686

Lagophthalmos
Botox Purified Neurotoxin Complex 565

Language problems, unspecified
▲ Topamax Sprinkle Capsules (2% to 10%) 2438
▲ Topamax Tablets (2% to 10%) 2438

Laryngeal stridor
Lotrel Capsules (About 0.5%) 2238

Laryngismus
Axert Tablets (Infrequent) 2430
Bexxar 1360
Campral Tablets (Rare) 1175
▲ Copaxone for Injection (5%) 3292
Effexor Tablets (Infrequent) 3405
Effexor XR Capsules (Infrequent) 3411
Lyrica Capsules (Rare) 2524
Paxil CR Controlled-Release Tablets 1509
Paxil 1501
Rescriptor Tablets 2535
Symbyax Capsules (Rare) 1788
Trileptal Oral Suspension 2281
Trileptal Tablets 2281
Zoloft (Rare) 2581

Laryngitis
Abilify Tablets (Infrequent) 916
Abilify Tablets (Infrequent) 2472
Aciphex Tablets 1081
▲ Advair Diskus 250/50 (1% to 3%) ... 1291
Aerobid/Aerobid-M (1% to 3%) 1172
Ambien Tablets (Rare) 2867
Antara Capsules 2723
Astelin Nasal Spray (Infrequent) 1876
Axert Tablets (Rare) 2430
Celebrex Capsules (0.1% to 1.9%) ... 3130
Celexa (Rare) 1177

Clozapine Tablets (Less than 1%) 2141
Clozaril Tablets (Less than 1%) 2174
Copaxone for Injection (At least 2%) 3292
Doxil Injection (Less than 1%) 3302
Effexor Tablets (Infrequent) 3405
Effexor XR Capsules (Infrequent) 3411
Evista Tablets (2.2%) 1735
Evoxac Capsules (Less than 1%) 1042
Exelon Capsules (Infrequent) 2204
Fabrazyme for Intravenous Infusion (2%) 1267
FazaClo Orally Disintegrating Tablets (Less than 1%) 547
▲ Flovent Diskus 50 mcg (1% to 3%) 1415
▲ Flovent HFA (1% to 3%) 1418
Frova Tablets (Infrequent) 1101
Gabitril Tablets (Infrequent) 998
Herceptin I.V. (At least one of the 958 patients) 1234
Invirase (Less than 2%) 2776
Lexapro Oral Solution (Infrequent) 1193
Lexapro Tablets (Infrequent) 1193
Lofibra Capsules 1217
Lotronex Tablets (Rare) 1479
Lunesta Tablets (Infrequent) 3139
Lupron Depot–3 Month 11.25 mg 3262
Meridia Capsules (1.3%) 485
Neurontin Capsules (Rare) 2498
Neurontin Oral Solution (Rare) 2498
Neurontin Tablets (Rare) 2498
▲ Norditropin Cartridges (6%) 2318
Omacor Capsules 2735
Permax Tablets (Infrequent) 3357
Prinivil Tablets (0.3% to 1.0%) 2029
Prinzide Tablets 2033
ProSom Tablets (Rare) 512
Protonix I.V. (Less than 1%) 3468
Protonix Tablets (Less than 1%) 3465
Protopic Ointment (Greater than or equal to 1%) 629
▲ Pulmozyme Inhalation Solution (3% to 4%) 1245
Relpax Tablets (Rare) 2531
Requip Tablets (Infrequent) 1528
Rilutek Tablets (Infrequent) 2945
Singulair (Greater than or equal to 2%) 2047
Sonata Capsules (Infrequent) 1686
Soriatane Capsules (Less than 1%) 1028
▲ Spiriva HandiHaler (1% to 3%) 899
Sular Tablets (Less than or equal to 1%) 1163
Symbyax Capsules (Infrequent) 1788
Tasmar Tablets (Infrequent) 3360
Tricor Tablets 523
Uniretic Tablets (Less than 1%) 3114
Ventolin HFA Inhalation Aerosol (Less than 3%) 1576
Viagra Tablets (Less than 2%) 2552
▲ Xeloda Tablets (Less than 5%) 2825
Zestoretic Tablets 701
Zestril Tablets (0.3% to 1.0%) 704
Zoloft (Rare) 2581
Zomig Nasal Spray (Rare) 718
Zomig Tablets (Infrequent) 714
Zomig-ZMT Tablets (Infrequent) 714
Zyprexa Tablets (Rare) 1798
Zyprexa ZYDIS Orally Disintegrating Tablets (Rare) 1798

Laryngospasm
Abilify Tablets (Rare) 916
Abilify Tablets (Rare) 2472
Advair Diskus 100/50 1291
Advair Diskus 250/50 1291
Advair Diskus 500/50 1291
Atrovent HFA Inhalation Aerosol 872
Atrovent Nasal Spray 0.06% 870
Blocadren Tablets 1891
Carafate Suspension 727
Carafate Tablets 728
Combivent Inhalation Aerosol (Less than 2%) 878
Cosopt Sterile Ophthalmic Solution 1910
Dilaudid 439
Dilaudid Oral Liquid 443
Dilaudid Non-Sterile Powder 439
Dilaudid Rectal Suppositories 439
Dilaudid Tablets 439
Dilaudid Tablets - 8 mg 443
Dilaudid-HP (Less frequent) 441
Diprivan Injectable Emulsion (Less than 1%) 676
Inderal LA Long-Acting Capsules 3421
InnoPran XL Capsules 2728
Lidoderm Patch 1107
MS Contin Tablets (Less frequent) 2703
Nadolol Tablets 2121
Numorphan 1112
Orthoclone OKT3 Sterile Solution (Less than 1%) 2370
Raptiva for Injection 1247
Serevent Diskus (Rare) 1540
▲ Suprane Liquid for Inhalation (3% to 50%) 770
Tenormin I.V. Injection 698
Tenormin Tablets 695
Tessalon Capsules 1202
Tessalon Perles 1202
Timolide Tablets 2056
Timoptic in Ocudose 2061
Timoptic Sterile Ophthalmic Solution 2058
Timoptic-XE Sterile Ophthalmic Gel Forming Solution 2062
Toprol-XL Tablets 660
▲ Ultane Liquid for Inhalation (2% to 8%) 526
Zofran Injection 1607
Zofran 1613
Zofran ODT Orally Disintegrating Tablets 1613

Laryngotracheobronchitis
Flumist Vaccine 1872
Prevnar for Injection 3460
Synagis (More than 1%) 1868
Vaqta (1.2%) 2067

Lassitude
Azmacort Inhalation Aerosol 1701
Beconase AQ Nasal Spray 1359
Daranide Tablets 1928
Dexedrine 1386
▲ Hytrin Capsules (7.4% to 11.3%) 469
Inderal LA Long-Acting Capsules 3421
InnoPran XL Capsules 2728
Neurontin Capsules (Rare) 2498
Neurontin Oral Solution (Rare) 2498
Neurontin Tablets (Rare) 2498
Phenergan 3438
Risperdal M-Tab Orally Disintegrating Tablets 1658
Risperdal 1658

Laughing, easy
▲ Marinol Capsules (8% to 24%) 3334

Laxative effect
Beelith Tablets 784

LDH abnormalities
Ceftin Tablets (1.0%) 1369
▲ Emcyt Capsules (2% to 31%) 3137
Nimotop Capsules (0.4%; rare) 774
Parcopa Orally Disintegrating Tablets 3111
Zithromax Capsules, 250 mg (Less than 1%) 2568
▲ Zithromax for IV Infusion (1% to 3%) 2573
Zithromax for Oral Suspension, 1 g (Less than 1%) 2568
Zithromax for Oral Suspension, 300 mg, 600 mg, 900 mg, 1200 mg (Less than 1%) 2561
Zithromax Tablets, 250 mg, 500 mg (Less than 1%) 2561
Zithromax Tablets, 600 mg (Less than 1%) 2568
Zithromax Tri-Pak (Less than 1%) 2561
Zithromax Z-Pak (Less than 1%) 2568
Zyvox (0.2% to 1.8%) 2661

LDH increase
Abelcet Injection 1119
Accutane Capsules 2740
Adalat CC Tablets (Rare) 2978
Advicor Tablets 1694
AmBisome for Injection (Less common) 615
Amnesteem Capsules 2126
Aricept Tablets (Infrequent) 1086
Aricept ODT Tablets (Infrequent) 1086
Arthrotec Tablets (Rare) 3126
Asacol Delayed-Release Tablets 2688
Avelox (0.1% to less than 2%) 2984
Biaxin/Biaxin XL (Less than 1%) 402
Cardizem LA Extended Release Tablets (Less than 2%) 1699
▲ CellCept Capsules (3% to 23.2%) 2751
▲ CellCept Intravenous (3% to 23.2%) 2751
▲ CellCept Oral Suspension (3% to 23.2%) 2751
▲ CellCept Tablets (3% to 23.2%) 2751
▲ Cipro I.V. (Among most frequent) 2998
▲ Cipro I.V. Pharmacy Bulk Package (Among most frequent) 3509
Cipro (0.4%) 2991
Colazal Capsules 2845
Cubicin for Injection (Less than 1%) 1038
Cuprimine Capsules (Few cases) 1925
Depacon Injection (Frequent) 412
Depakene (Frequent) 417
Depakote Sprinkle Capsules 422
▲ Depakote Tablets (Frequent) 427
Depakote ER Tablets (Frequent) 433
Doxil Injection (Less than 1%) 3302
Effexor Tablets 3405
Effexor XR Capsules 3411
Evoxac Capsules 1042
▲ Fortaz (1 in 18) 1422
Garamycin Injectable 3028
Geodon Capsules (Infrequent) 2514
Gleevec Tablets (Infrequent) 2221
Increlex Injection 3290
▲ Intron A for Injection (Less than 5%) 3038
Levaquin in 5% Dextrose Injection (0.1% to 0.9%) 2453
Levaquin (0.1% to 0.9%) 2453
▲ Lupron Depot 3.75 mg (Approximately 5% to 8%) 3257
Lupron Depot 7.5 mg (Greater than or equal to 5%) 3261
Mefoxin for Injection 1987
Mefoxin Premixed Intravenous Solution 1990
▲ Megace ES Oral Suspension (1% to 3%) 2492
Meridia Capsules (1.6%) 485
Merrem I.V. (Greater than 0.2%) 687
▲ Mylotarg for Injection (14% to 18%) 3429
Nalfon Capsules (Less than 1%) 2504
▲ Neulasta Injection (19%) 596
▲ Neupogen for Injection (27% to 58%) 598
Neurontin Capsules (Rare) 2498
Neurontin Oral Solution (Rare) 2498
Neurontin Tablets (Rare) 2498
Niaspan Extended-Release Tablets 1703
Noroxin Tablets (Less frequent) 2009
Omnicef Capsules (0.2%) 506
Omnicef for Oral Suspension (1%) 506
Paxil CR Controlled-Release Tablets (Rare) 1509
Paxil (Rare) 1501
Pentasa Capsules (Less than 1%) 3182
Prevacid Delayed-Release Capsules 3268
Prevacid for Delayed-Release Oral Suspension 3268
Prevacid NapraPAC 3277
Prevacid SoluTab Delayed-Release Orally Disintegrating Tablets 3268
PREVPAC (Less than 1%) 3281
Primaxin I.M. 2022
Primaxin I.V. 2024
▲ Prograf Capsules and Injection (3% to 15%) 624
▲ Rapamune Oral Solution and Tablets (3% to 20%) 3472
Requip Tablets (Infrequent) 1528
Retrovir IV Infusion 1537
Rilutek Tablets (Rare) 2945
▲ Rituxan for Infusion (1% to 5%) 845
▲ Rituxan I.V. (7%) 1251
Roferon-A Injection (Less than 1%) 2805
Rythmol SR Capsules 2736
▲ Soriatane Capsules (Approximately 1 in 3 patients) 1028
Suprax 1811
Symmetrel 1115
▲ Targretin Capsules (7.1% to 13.2%) 1719
Tarka Tablets 519
Thalomid Capsules 979
Tiazac Capsules (Less than 2%) 1204
Timentin ADD-Vantage 1556
Timentin Injection Galaxy Container 1559
Timentin IV Infusion 1553
Timentin Pharmacy Bulk Package 1562
Toprol-XL Tablets 660
Ultane Liquid for Inhalation (Less than 1%) 526
Vantin Tablets and Oral Suspension 2650
VFEND I.V. (Less than 2%) 2543
VFEND Oral Suspension (Less than 2%) 2543
VFEND Tablets (Less than 2%) 2543
Viracept 2556
WinRho SDF 763
Zinacef Injection (1 in 75 patients) 1604
Zinacef for Injection (1 in 75 patients) 1604
Zonegran Capsules (Rare) 1089

LDL, increase
Anadrol-50 Tablets (Sometimes) 3329
Premphase Tablets 3452
Prempro Tablets 3452

LDL, decrease
CombiPatch Transdermal System 2180
Premarin Tablets 3443
Premphase Tablets 3452
Prempro Tablets 3452

LE cells test positive
(*see under* Lupus erythematosus)

Left ventricular dysfunction
▲ Clolar for Intravenous Infusion (27%) 1264
Orthoclone OKT3 Sterile Solution (Less than 1%) 2370

Left ventricular ejection fraction, asymptomatic declines in
Idamycin PFS Injection 2645

Left ventricular ejection fraction, decrease
Novantrone for Injection Concentrate 3158

Leg cramps, nocturnal
▲ Actonel with Calcium Tablets (3.5%) 2684
Niaspan Extended-Release Tablets 1703
▲ Roferon-A Injection (5%) 2805
Trelstar LA Suspension (1.7%) 3387

Legs, heaviness
Uroqid-Acid No. 2 Tablets 785
▲ Zavesca Capsules (8%) 543

Legs, restless
Abilify Tablets (Infrequent) 916
Abilify Tablets (Infrequent) 2472
Ambien Tablets (Rare) 2867
Lexapro Oral Solution (Infrequent) 1193
Lexapro Tablets (Infrequent) 1193

Legs, stiffness
Colazal Capsules 2845

Leiomyoma
(*see also under* Uterine fibroids)
Prefest Tablets 1069

LE-like reactions
(*see under* Lupus erythematosus)

Lens, pigmentation
Zyprexa Tablets (Rare) 1798
Zyprexa ZYDIS Orally Disintegrating Tablets (Rare) 1798

Lens changes, unspecified
Myleran Tablets 1492

Lens opacities, changes
Altoprev Extended-Release Tablets 1151
Cosopt Sterile Ophthalmic Solution (1% to 5%) 1910
Lamisil Tablets 2226
Lescol Capsules 2227
Lescol Capsules 2730
Lescol XL Tablets 2227
Lescol XL Tablets 2730
Levaquin in 5% Dextrose Injection 2453
Levaquin 2453
Mevacor Tablets 1996
Pacerone Tablets 3337
Pravachol Tablets 943
Vytorin 10/10 Tablets 2084
Vytorin 10/10 Tablets 3092
Vytorin 10/20 Tablets 2084
Vytorin 10/20 Tablets 3092
Vytorin 10/40 Tablets 2084
Vytorin 10/40 Tablets 3092
Vytorin 10/80 Tablets 2084
Vytorin 10/80 Tablets 3092
Zocor Tablets 2078

Lens opacities, irregular
Thioridazine Hydrochloride Tablets 2122

Lenticular deposits
Thioridazine Hydrochloride Tablets 2122

Lesions, anogenital
Dynacin Tablets 1859

Lesions, bullous
Parcopa Orally Disintegrating Tablets ... 3111
Stalevo Tablets ... 2270

Lesions, cerebrovascular
Imitrex Nasal Spray ... 1435

Lesions, corneal
Effexor Tablets (Infrequent) ... 3405
Effexor XR Capsules (Infrequent) ... 3411
▲ Soriatane Capsules (1% to 5%) ... 1028
Targretin Capsules ... 1719
▲ Voltaren Ophthalmic Solution (Less than or equal to 5%) ... 2300
Zyprexa Tablets (Rare) ... 1798
Zyprexa ZYDIS Orally Disintegrating Tablets (1%) ... 1798

Lesions, cutaneous
Zestril Tablets (0.3% to 1.0%) ... 704

Lesions, erythema perstans-like
AquaMEPHYTON Injection ... 1887

Lesions, gastrointestinal
K-Dur Extended-Relase Tablets ... 3047
K-Tab Filmtab Tablets ... 473
Lotronex Tablets (Infrequent) ... 1479

Lesions, nerve root
Boniva Tablets (2.2%) ... 2747

Lesions, neuro-ocular
Activella Tablets ... 2311
Prefest Tablets ... 1069
Premphase Tablets ... 3452
Prempro Tablets ... 3452

Lesions, oral
Advair Diskus 250/50 (1% to 3%) ... 1291
Avapro Tablets (Less than 1%) ... 925
Avapro Tablets (Less than 1%) ... 2886
Striant Mucoadhesive ... 1022
Vantin Tablets and Oral Suspension (Less than 1%) ... 2650
Viramune Oral Suspension ... 903
Viramune Tablets ... 903

Lesions, retinal vascular
Activella Tablets ... 2311
Ortho-Cyclen/Ortho Tri-Cyclen ... 2414
Ortho Tri-Cyclen Lo Tablets ... 2421
Premphase Tablets ... 3452
Prempro Tablets ... 3452

Lesions, sceloderma-like
AquaMEPHYTON Injection ... 1887

Lesions, upper motor neuron
Topamax Sprinkle Capsules (Rare) ... 2438
Topamax Tablets (Rare) ... 2438

Lethargy
Accutane Capsules ... 2740
▲ Ambien Tablets (3%) ... 2867
Amnesteem Capsules ... 2126
Arimidex Tablets (1%) ... 665
Asacol Delayed-Release Tablets ... 2688
Avinza Capsules (Less than 5%) ... 1714
Bayer Aspirin Tablets ... 3515
BeneFix for Injection ... 3402
Bentyl Capsules ... 724
Bentyl Injection ... 724
Bentyl Syrup ... 724
Bentyl Tablets ... 724
Betagan Ophthalmic Solution, USP (Rare) ... ⊙ 217
Betoptic S Ophthalmic Suspension (Rare) ... 554
Catapres-TTS (3 of 101 patients) ... 875
Cathflo Activase ... 1232
Celebrex Capsules ... 3130
Cipro I.V. (1% or less) ... 2998
Cipro I.V. Pharmacy Bulk Package (1% or less) ... 3509
Cipro (Less than 1%) ... 2991
Cipro XR Tablets ... 3004
▲ Clolar for Intravenous Infusion (11%) ... 1264
Clozapine Tablets (1%) ... 2141
Clozaril Tablets (1%) ... 2174
Copegus Tablets ... 2759
Cosmegen for Injection ... 1907
Coumadin for Injection (Infrequent) ... 932
Coumadin Tablets (Infrequent) ... 932
Cymbalta Delayed-Release Capsules (Frequent) ... 1729
Dalmane Capsules ... 3343
Depacon Injection ... 412
Depakote Sprinkle Capsules ... 422
Depakote Tablets ... 427
Depakote ER Tablets ... 433
Diastat Rectal Delivery System ... 3344
Dilaudid ... 439
Dilaudid Non-Sterile Powder ... 439
Dilaudid Rectal Suppositories ... 439
Dilaudid Tablets ... 439
Diovan HCT Tablets ... 2195
Diuril Sodium Intravenous ... 1934
Dyazide Capsules ... 1389
DynaCirc CR Tablets (0.5% to 1%) ... 2726
Ecotrin Enteric Coated Aspirin Low, Regular and Maximum Strength Tablets ... 1627
Eldepryl Capsules (1 of 49 patients) ... 3209
Eligard 22.5 mg (Less than 2%) ... 2899
Eligard 30 mg (1.1%) ... 2901
Eligard 45 mg (1%) ... 2904
▲ Ellence Injection (0% to 45.8%) ... 2632
▲ Emcyt Capsules (4%) ... 3137
Eskalith ... 1406
FazaClo Orally Disintegrating Tablets (1%) ... 547
Furosemide Tablets ... 2117
Garamycin Injectable ... 3028
Gengraf Capsules (Rare) ... 458
HibTITER ... 3419
Hycodan ... 1104
Hycomine Compound Tablets ... 1105
Hycotuss Expectorant Syrup ... 1106
Hyperstat I.V. Injection ... 3031
Inderal LA Long-Acting Capsules ... 3421
Invirase (Less than 2%) ... 2776
▲ I.V. Busulfex (7%) ... 1125
Kadian Capsules (Less than 3%) ... 572
▲ Lexapro Oral Solution (3%) ... 1193
▲ Lexapro Tablets (3%) ... 1193
Lithobid Tablets ... 1670
Lortab ... 3315
Lortab Elixir ... 3312
Matulane Capsules ... 3188
Maxzide ... 2150
▲ Navelbine Injection (Up to 67%) ... 1494
Neoral Soft Gelatin Capsules (Rare) ... 2247
Neoral Oral Solution (Rare) ... 2247
Orthoclone OKT3 Sterile Solution (Less than 1%) ... 2370
Pediarix Vaccine ... 1518
Prinzide Tablets ... 2033
Proleukin for Injection ... 1007
ReFacto Vials ... 3479
RhoGAM Ultra-Filtered ... 2429
▲ Roferon-A Injection (1% to 6%) ... 2805
Sandimmune (Rare) ... 2259
St. Joseph 81 mg Aspirin Chewable and Enteric Coated Tablets ... 1841
Stromectol Tablets ... 2053
Tasmar Tablets (1% or more) ... 3360
▲ Tenormin I.V. Injection (1% to 3%) ... 698
Tenormin Tablets (1% to 3%) ... 695
Thioridazine Hydrochloride Tablets (Extremely rare) ... 2122
Tracleer Tablets ... 539
Trizivir Tablets ... 1565
Tussionex Pennkinetic Extended-Release Suspension ... 3322
Vantas (Less than 2%) ... 3367
Vaseretic Tablets ... 2073
Vicodin Tablets ... 530
Vicodin ES Tablets ... 531
Vicodin HP Tablets ... 532
Xanax XR Tablets (1.7%) ... 2655
▲ Xeloda Tablets (Up to 7%) ... 2825
Zestoretic Tablets ... 701
Ziagen ... 1600
▲ Zoladex (5% to 8%) ... 709
Zoladex 3-month ... 712
Zovirax for Injection (Approximately 1%) ... 1618
Zydone Tablets ... 1118

Leucocytosis
Lithobid Tablets ... 1670
Ultane Liquid for Inhalation (Less than 1%) ... 526

Leukemia, acute
Herceptin I.V. (At least one of the 958 patients) ... 1234
I.V. Busulfex (Four cases) ... 1125
Leukeran Tablets ... 1472
Nipent for Injection (Less than 3%) ... 3216
Novantrone for Injection Concentrate ... 3158

Leukemia, lymphoblastic
Permax Tablets (Rare) ... 3357

Leukemia, lymphocytic
Mustargen for Injection ... 2007

Leukemia, myeloblastic, acute
Azasan Tablets ... 2844
Invirase (Rare) ... 2776

Leukemia, myelogenous
Ellence Injection ... 2632
Novantrone for Injection Concentrate ... 3158
Temodar Capsules ... 3088
Thalomid Capsules ... 979
Zevalin Injection ... 848

Leukemia, unspecified
Genotropin Lyophilized Powder (A small number of children) ... 2642
Humatrope Vials and Cartridges ... 1756
Indocin (Rare) ... 1968
Norditropin Cartridges (A small number of children) ... 2318
Nutropin for Injection (A small number of patients) ... 1238
Nutropin AQ Injection (A small number of patients) ... 1241
Nutropin AQ Pen (A small number of patients) ... 1241
Nutropin AQ Pen Cartridge (A small number of patients) ... 1241
Plavix Tablets (Less than 1%) ... 940
Plavix Tablets (Less than 1%) ... 2942
Tasmar Tablets (Rare) ... 3360
Tev-Tropin for Injection ... 1224
Thalomid Capsules ... 979
Ticlid Tablets (Rare) ... 2813

Leukemia, myelocytic, acute
Matulane Capsules ... 3188

Leukemia, polymorphocytic
Campath Ampules ... 826

Leukemia, secondary
Bexxar ... 1360
Campath Ampules ... 826
Novantrone for Injection Concentrate ... 3158

Leukocyte agglutinins
Miradon Tablets ... 3056

Leukocyte count, abnormal
▲ Zyvox (0.2% to 12.4%) ... 2661

Leukocyte count, elevated
Agrylin Capsules ... 3172

Leukocytosis
Abelcet Injection ... 1119
Abilify Tablets (Infrequent) ... 916
Abilify Tablets (Infrequent) ... 2472
Aceon Tablets (2 mg, 4 mg, 8 mg) ... 3191
Aciphex Tablets ... 1081
▲ Adriamycin for Injection, USP (High incidence) ... 786
▲ Adriamycin Injection, USP (High incidence) ... 786
Alinia for Oral Suspension (Less than 1%) ... 2840
Alinia Tablets (Less than 1%) ... 2840
Amerge Tablets (Infrequent) ... 1312
Arthrotec Tablets (Rare) ... 3126
Attenuvax ... 1889
▲ Buphenyl Powder (4%) ... 3327
▲ Buphenyl Tablets (4%) ... 3327
Capastat Sulfate for Injection ... 1728
Carbatrol Capsules ... 3174
Celexa (Infrequent) ... 1177
▲ CellCept Capsules (22.4% to 40.5%) ... 2751
▲ CellCept Intravenous (22.4% to 40.5%) ... 2751
▲ CellCept Oral Suspension (22.4% to 40.5%) ... 2751
▲ CellCept Tablets (22.4% to 40.5%) ... 2751
Cipro I.V. (Rare) ... 2998
Cipro I.V. Pharmacy Bulk Package (Rare) ... 3509
Cipro (Less than 0.1%) ... 2991
Clinoril Tablets (Less than 1 in 100) ... 1899
Clozapine Tablets (Less than 1%) ... 2141
Clozaril Tablets (Less than 1%) ... 2174
Colazal Capsules ... 2845
Cubicin for Injection (Less than 1%) ... 1038
Cuprimine Capsules ... 1925
Diprivan Injectable Emulsion (Less than 1%) ... 676
Effexor Tablets (Infrequent) ... 3405
Effexor XR Capsules (Infrequent) ... 3411
▲ Efudex (Among most frequent) ... 3348
Emend Capsules (Greater than 0.5%) ... 1944
▲ Entocort EC Capsules (Less than 5%) ... 2694
Equetro Extended-Release Capsules ... 3178
Eskalith ... 1406
Evoxac Capsules (Less than 1%) ... 1042
Exelon Capsules (Infrequent) ... 2204
FazaClo Orally Disintegrating Tablets (Less than 1%) ... 547
Ferrlecit Injection ... 3379
Geodon Capsules (Infrequent) ... 2514
Infed Injection ... 3381
Lamictal (Infrequent) ... 1449
Lariam Tablets (Occasional) ... 2790
Levaquin in 5% Dextrose Injection (0.1% to 0.9%) ... 2453
Levaquin (0.1% to 0.9%) ... 2453
Lyrica Capsules (0.1% to 1%) ... 2524
Meruvax II ... 1994
MetroGel-Vaginal Gel (1.7%) ... 1822
Miradon Tablets ... 3056
M-M-R II ... 1980
Moban Tablets ... 1108
Mumpsvax ... 2005
Neulasta Injection (Less than 1%) ... 596
Neupogen for Injection (Approximately 2%) ... 598
Nexium Delayed-Release Capsules (Less than 1%) ... 645
Nexium I.V. (Less than 1%) ... 649
Omnicef Capsules (0.7%) ... 506
Omnicef for Oral Suspension (0.3%) ... 506
Orthoclone OKT3 Sterile Solution (Less than 1%) ... 2370
Panhematin for Injection ... 2487
▲ Paser Granules (79% of 38 patients with drug-induced hepatitis) ... 1657
Paxil CR Controlled-Release Tablets (Rare) ... 1509
Paxil (Rare) ... 1501
Permax Tablets (Infrequent) ... 3357
Prilosec OTC Tablets (Rare) ... 2674
Primaxin I.V. ... 2024
Prinivil Tablets (0.3% to 1.0%) ... 2029
Prinzide Tablets ... 2033
▲ Prograf Capsules and Injection (3% to 32%) ... 624
Prolastin ... 3252
▲ Proleukin for Injection (9%) ... 1007
Protonix I.V. (Less than 1%) ... 3468
Protonix Tablets (Less than 1%) ... 3465
Protopic Ointment (Greater than or equal to 1%) ... 629
Provigil Tablets (At least 1%) ... 1002
Prozac Pulvules and Liquid ... 1771
▲ Rapamune Oral Solution and Tablets (3% to 20%) ... 3472
▲ Raptiva for Injection (26%) ... 1247
ReoPro Vials (1.0%) ... 1779
Requip Tablets (Infrequent) ... 1528
Rilutek Tablets (Infrequent) ... 2945
Risperdal Consta Long-Acting Injection (Rare) ... 1664
Risperdal M-Tab Orally Disintegrating Tablets (Rare) ... 1658
Risperdal (Rare) ... 1658
Rocephin Injectable Vials, ADD-Vantage, Galaxy, Bulk (Less than 0.1%) ... 2801
Seroquel Tablets (Infrequent) ... 691
Sonata Capsules (Rare) ... 1686
Suprane Liquid for Inhalation ... 770
Symbyax Capsules (Infrequent) ... 1788
Symmetrel ... 1115
Tegretol/Tegretol-XR ... 2278
Thiothixene Capsules (Occasional) ... 2124
Trasylol Injection (1% to 2%) ... 779
▲ Trisenox Injection (50%) ... 983
▲ Tygacil for Injection (3.7%) ... 3489
Vantin Tablets and Oral Suspension ... 2650
Vaseretic Tablets ... 2073
Vasotec I.V. Injection (0.5% to 1.0%) ... 2076
▲ Vesanoid Capsules (About 40%) ... 2823
Wellbutrin Tablets ... 1579
Wellbutrin SR Sustained-Release Tablets ... 1583
Wellbutrin XL Extended-Release Tablets ... 1588
Zegerid Powder for Oral Solution (Rare) ... 2972
Zestoretic Tablets ... 701
Zestril Tablets (0.3% to 1.0%) ... 704
Zovirax for Injection (Less than 1%) ... 1618
Zyban Sustained-Release Tablets ... 1620
Zyprexa Tablets (Infrequent) ... 1798
Zyprexa ZYDIS Orally Disintegrating Tablets (Infrequent) ... 1798

Leukocyturia
Amnesteem Capsules ... 2126
Crixivan Capsules ... 1918
Emend Capsules (Greater than 0.5%) ... 1944
Omnicef Capsules (2%) ... 506
Primaxin I.M. ... 2022
Primaxin I.V. ... 2024

Leukoderma
Effexor Tablets (Rare) ... 3405
Effexor XR Capsules (Rare) ... 3411
Lamictal (Rare) ... 1449

Leukoencephalopathy, multifocal progressive
Invirase (Less than 2%) ... 2776

Leukoencephalopathy, unspecified
Prograf Capsules and Injection ... 624

Leukopenia
▲ Abelcet Injection (4%) ... 1119
Abilify Tablets (Infrequent) ... 916
Abilify Tablets (Infrequent) ... 2472
Accutane Capsules ... 2740
Aceon Tablets (2 mg, 4 mg, 8 mg) (0.1%) ... 3191
Aciphex Tablets ... 1081
Actiq (Less than 1%) ... 993
Adalat CC Tablets (Rare) ... 2978
Adriamycin for Injection, USP ... 786
Adriamycin Injection, USP ... 786
Advicor Tablets ... 1694
Aldara Cream, 5% ... 1814
Aldoclor Tablets ... 1881
Aldoril Tablets ... 1884
▲ Alferon N Injection (11%) ... 1640
▲ Alimta for Injection (Less than 1% to 55%) ... 1722
Alkeran Tablets ... 977
Aloprim for Injection (Less than 1%) ... 2156
Altace Capsules ... 1673
Altoprev Extended-Release Tablets ... 1151
Amaryl Tablets ... 2864
Ambien Tablets (Rare) ... 2867
Amnesteem Capsules ... 2126
Amoxil Capsules ... 1315
Amoxil Chewable Tablets ... 1315
Amoxil Pediatric Drops for Oral Suspension ... 1315
Amoxil Powder for Oral Suspension ... 1315
Amoxil Tablets ... 1315
Anaprox Tablets (Less than 1%) ... 2769
Anaprox DS Tablets (Less than 1%) ... 2769
Ancef for Injection ... 1318
Antara Capsules ... 2723
▲ Aptivus Capsules (3.6%) ... 859
Arava Tablets (Rare) ... 2881
Aredia for Injection (Up to 4%) ... 2168
▲ Arimidex Tablets (2% to 5%) ... 665
Arthrotec Tablets (Rare) ... 3126
Asacol Delayed-Release Tablets ... 2688
Atacand Tablets (Very rare) ... 634
Atacand HCT ... 637
Augmentin ... 1331
Augmentin Tablets ... 1334
Augmentin XR Extended-Release Tablets ... 1340
Augmentin ES-600 Powder for Oral Suspension ... 1337
Avalide Tablets ... 922
Avalide Tablets ... 2889
▲ Avastin IV (37%) ... 1229
Avelox (0.1% to less than 2%) ... 2984
▲ Azasan Tablets (28% to greater than 50%) ... 2844
▲ Betaseron for SC Injection (14%) ... 791
▲ Buphenyl Powder (4%) ... 3327
▲ Buphenyl Tablets (4%) ... 3327
Caduet Tablets (Greater than 0.1% to less than or equal to 1%) ... 2507
Campral Tablets (Rare) ... 1175
▲ Camptosar Injection (14% to 96.4%) ... 2602
Canasa Rectal Suppositories (One patient) ... 726
▲ Cancidas for Injection (4.6% to 6.2%) ... 1894
Capastat Sulfate for Injection ... 1728
Carbatrol Capsules ... 3174
Cardizem LA Extended Release Tablets (Infrequent) ... 1699
Carimune NF ... 3501
▲ Casodex Tablets (2% to 5%) ... 670
Cataflam Tablets (Occasionally) ... 2173
Ceftin ... 1369
Celexa (Infrequent) ... 1177
▲ CellCept Capsules (23.2% to 45.8%) ... 2751
▲ CellCept Intravenous (23.2% to 45.8%) ... 2751
▲ CellCept Oral Suspension (23.2% to 45.8%) ... 2751
▲ CellCept Tablets (23.2% to 45.8%) ... 2751
Cipro I.V. (Infrequent) ... 2998
Cipro I.V. Pharmacy Bulk Package (Infrequent) ... 3509
Cipro (0.4%) ... 2991
Cleocin Vaginal Ovules ... 2613
Clindesse Vaginal Cream (Rare) ... 3296
Clinoril Tablets (Less than 1%) ... 1899
Clolar for Intravenous Infusion ... 1264
Clorpres Tablets ... 2139
▲ Clozapine Tablets (3%) ... 2141
▲ Clozaril Tablets (3%) ... 2174
Colazal Capsules ... 2845
Concerta Extended-Release Tablets ... 1828
Copaxone for Injection (Infrequent) ... 3292
Coreg Tablets (Greater than 0.1% to 1%) ... 1376
Cosmegen for Injection ... 1907
Crestor Tablets (Less than 1%) ... 672
Cuprimine Capsules (2%) ... 1925
Cutivate Lotion 0.05% (Rare) ... 1383
▲ Cytovene (29%) ... 2763
Dalmane Capsules (Rare) ... 3343
Dantrium Capsules (Less frequent) ... 2690
Dantrium Intravenous ... 2691
Daranide Tablets ... 1928
Daraprim Tablets ... 1385
Depacon Injection ... 412
Depakene ... 417
Depakote Sprinkle Capsules ... 422
Depakote Tablets ... 427
Depakote ER Tablets (Greater than 1%) ... 433
Didronel Tablets (One report) ... 2693
Diovan HCT Tablets ... 2195
Diuril Oral ... 1936
Diuril Sodium Intravenous ... 1934
Dolobid Tablets (Less than 1 in 100) ... 1937
▲ Doxil Injection (About 42.2% to 60%) ... 3302
Dyazide Capsules ... 1389
DynaCirc CR Tablets (0.5% to 1%) ... 2726
EC-Naprosyn Delayed-Release Tablets (Less than 1%) ... 2769
Effexor Tablets (Infrequent) ... 3405
Effexor XR Capsules (Infrequent) ... 3411
▲ Ellence Injection (1.5% to 80.3%) ... 2632
Elmiron Capsules (Less than or equal to 1%) ... 2393
▲ Eloxatin for Injection (0% to 85%) ... 2908
Elspar for Injection ... 1943
▲ Emcyt Capsules (4%) ... 3137
Enbrel for Injection ... 580
▲ Equetro Extended-Release Capsules (Up to 5%) ... 3178
Erbitux (1%) ... 937
▲ Eulexin Capsules (3%) ... 3023
Evoxac Capsules (Less than 1%) ... 1042
Factive Tablets (0.1% to 1%) ... 2464
Famvir Tablets (1.3%) ... 2207
Faslodex Injection (Less than 1%) ... 682
▲ FazaClo Orally Disintegrating Tablets (3%) ... 547
Flexeril Tablets (Rare) ... 1832
Focalin Tablets ... 2214
Focalin XR Capsules ... 2217
Fortaz (Very rare) ... 1422
Furosemide Tablets ... 2117
Gabitril Tablets (Infrequent) ... 998
Gammagard Liquid ... 751
Gammagard S/D (Rare) ... 754
Gamunex Immune Globulin I.V., 10% (Rare) ... 3232
Garamycin Injectable ... 3028
▲ Gemzar for Injection (15% to 71%) ... 1743
▲ Gengraf Capsules (1% to 6%) ... 458
Geodon Capsules (Infrequent) ... 2514
Grifulvin V Tablets Microsize and Oral Suspension Microsize (Rare) ... 2384
Gris-PEG Tablets (Rare) ... 2504
Guanidine Hydrochloride Tablets ... 3030
▲ Herceptin I.V. (3%) ... 1234
▲ Hexalen Capsules (1% to 15%) ... 2101
▲ Humira Injection (Less than 5%) ... 464
▲ Hycamtin for Injection (32% to 98%) ... 1427
Hyperstat I.V. Injection ... 3031
Hyzaar ... 1964
Indapamide Tablets ... 2119
Indocin Capsules (Less than 1%) ... 1968
Indocin I.V. (Less than 1%) ... 1973
Indocin (Less than 1%) ... 1968
▲ Infergen (15% to 19%) ... 1647
▲ Intron A for Injection (Less than 5% to 68%) ... 3038
▲ Invirase (1% to 8%) ... 2776
Iveegam EN (Rare) ... 759
Kadian Capsules (Less than 3%) ... 572
Kaletra (Less than 2%) ... 474
Keppra Oral Solution ... 3307
Keppra Tablets ... 3307
Klonopin ... 2782
▲ Kytril Tablets (11%) ... 2788
Lamictal (Infrequent) ... 1449
▲ Lariam Tablets (Among most frequent) ... 2790
Lescol Capsules (Rare) ... 2227
Lescol Capsules (Rare) ... 2730
Lescol XL Tablets ... 2227
Lescol XL Tablets ... 2730
▲ Leukine (17%) ... 829
Levaquin in 5% Dextrose Injection (0.1% to 0.9%) ... 2453
Levaquin (0.1% to 0.9%) ... 2453
Lofibra Capsules ... 1217
Lotensin HCT Tablets ... 2235
Lupron Depot 7.5 mg (Greater than or equal to 5%) ... 3261
Lyrica Capsules (0.1% to 1%) ... 2524
Matulane Capsules (Frequent) ... 3188
Mavik Tablets (Rare) ... 482
Maxipime for Injection (Greater than 0.1% to less than 1%) ... 1093
Maxzide ... 2150
Mefoxin for Injection ... 1987
Mefoxin Premixed Intravenous Solution ... 1990
▲ Megace ES Oral Suspension (1% to 3%) ... 2492
▲ Mepron Suspension (4%) ... 1487
Meridia Capsules ... 485
Metadate CD Capsules ... 3316
MetroGel-Vaginal Gel (1.7%) ... 1822
Mevacor Tablets (Rare) ... 1996
Micardis HCT Tablets ... 886
Mintezol ... 2002
Miradon Tablets ... 3056
Moban Tablets ... 1108
Mobic Oral Suspension (Less than 2%) ... 893
Mobic Tablets (Less than 2%) ... 893
Moduretic Tablets ... 2003
Mycamine for Injection (0.9% to 2.7%) ... 620
▲ Myfortic Tablets (3% to less than 20%) ... 2244
Myleran Tablets ... 1492
▲ Mylotarg for Injection (43% to 52%) ... 3429
Namenda (Infrequent) ... 1199
Naprosyn Suspension (Less than 1%) ... 2769
Naprosyn Tablets (Less than 1%) ... 2769
▲ Navelbine Injection (19% to 88%) ... 1494
▲ Neoral Soft Gelatin Capsules (1% to 6%) ... 2247
▲ Neoral Oral Solution (1% to 6%) ... 2247
Neurontin Capsules (1.1%) ... 2498
Neurontin Oral Solution (1.1%) ... 2498
Neurontin Tablets (1.1%) ... 2498
Nexium Delayed-Release Capsules (Less than 1%) ... 645
Nexium I.V. (Less than 1%) ... 649
▲ Nipent for Injection (22% to 60%) ... 3216
Noroxin Tablets ... 2009
Norvasc Tablets (More than 0.1% to 1%) ... 2529
▲ Norvir (0.9% to 36.9%) ... 499
▲ Novantrone for Injection Concentrate (9% to 19%) ... 3158
Omnicef Capsules (0.9%) ... 506
Omnicef for Oral Suspension (0.3%) ... 506
Oncaspar (Greater than 1% but less than 5%) ... 1123
▲ Ontak Vials (6%) ... 1717
Orthoclone OKT3 Sterile Solution (Less than 1%) ... 2370
Parcopa Orally Disintegrating Tablets ... 3111
Parnate Tablets ... 1499
Paser Granules ... 1657
Paxil CR Controlled-Release Tablets (Infrequent) ... 1509
Paxil (Infrequent) ... 1501
▲ PEG-Intron Powder for Injection (4%) ... 3062
Pentasa Capsules ... 3182
Pepcid Injection (Rare) ... 2017
Pepcid (Rare) ... 2014
Permax Tablets (Infrequent) ... 3357
Phenergan ... 3438
Phenytek Capsules (Occasional) ... 2153
Plavix Tablets (Less than 1%) ... 940
Plavix Tablets (Less than 1%) ... 2942
Pletal Tablets (Very rare) ... 2478
Prandin Tablets (0.5, 1, and 2 mg) (Less than 1%) ... 2337
Pravachol Tablets (Rare) ... 943
Prevacid Delayed-Release Capsules (Less than 1%) ... 3268
Prevacid for Delayed-Release Oral Suspension (Less than 1%) ... 3268
Prevacid NapraPAC (Less than 1%) ... 3277
Prevacid SoluTab Delayed-Release Orally Disintegrating Tablets (Less than 1%) ... 3268
PREVPAC ... 3281
Primaxin I.M. ... 2022
Primaxin I.V. (Less than 0.2%) ... 2024
Prinivil Tablets (Rare) ... 2029
Prinzide Tablets ... 2033
▲ Prograf Capsules and Injection (3% to 15%) ... 624
▲ Proleukin for Injection (16%) ... 1007
ProSom Tablets (Rare) ... 512
Protonix I.V. (Less than 1%) ... 3468
Protonix Tablets (Less than 1%) ... 3465
Protopic Ointment (Greater than or equal to 1%) ... 629
Prozac Pulvules and Liquid (Rare) ... 1771
Purinethol Tablets (Frequent) ... 1222
▲ Rapamune Oral Solution and Tablets (9% to 13%) ... 3472
▲ Rebetol (5% to 6%) ... 3073
▲ Rebif Prefilled Syringe for Injection (6% to 36%) ... 3163
Relafen Tablets (Less than 1%) ... 1523
Relpax Tablets (Rare) ... 2531
Remicade for IV Injection (Greater than or equal to 0.2%) ... 987
Requip Tablets (Infrequent) ... 1528
Rescriptor Tablets ... 2535
Retrovir Capsules ... 1533
Retrovir IV Infusion ... 1537
Retrovir ... 1533
▲ Ribavirin, USP Capsules (5% to 6%) ... 3083
Rilutek Tablets (Infrequent) ... 2945
Risperdal Consta Long-Acting Injection (Infrequent) ... 1664
Risperdal M-Tab Orally Disintegrating Tablets (Rare) ... 1658
Risperdal (Rare) ... 1658
Ritalin Hydrochloride Tablets ... 2254
Ritalin LA Capsules ... 2255
Ritalin-SR Tablets ... 2254
▲ Rituxan for Infusion (13%) ... 845
▲ Rituxan I.V. (14%; Among most frequent) ... 1251
Rocephin Injectable Vials, ADD-Vantage, Galaxy, Bulk (2.1%) ... 2801
▲ Roferon-A Injection (1.5% to 45%) ... 2805
▲ Sandimmune (Up to 6%) ... 2259
Seroquel Tablets ... 691
▲ Simulect for Injection (3% to 10%) ... 2268
Skelaxin Tablets ... 1685
Spectracef Tablets (0.1% to 1%) ... 2706
Stalevo Tablets ... 2270
Stromectol Tablets (One patient) ... 2053
Sular Tablets (Less than or equal to 1%) ... 1163
Suprax (Less than 2%) ... 1811
Symbyax Capsules (Rare) ... 1788
Symmetrel (Less than 0.1%) ... 1115
Tabloid Tablets ... 1545
Tagamet Tablets (Approximately 1 per 100,000) ... 1547
Tambocor Tablets (Less than 1%) ... 1824
▲ Targretin Capsules (16.7% to 47.2%) ... 1719
Tarka Tablets (0.3% or more) ... 519
▲ Taxotere Injection Concentrate (6.1% to 98.6%) ... 2947
Tegretol/Tegretol-XR ... 2278
▲ Temodar Capsules (58%) ... 3088
Teveten Tablets (0.3%) ... 1707
Teveten HCT Tablets ... 1710
▲ Thalomid Capsules (16.7% to 25.5%) ... 979
Thioridazine Hydrochloride Tablets (Infrequent) ... 2122
Thiothixene Capsules (Occasional) ... 2124
▲ Thymoglobulin for Injection (57.3%) ... 2848
Tiazac Capsules (Infrequent) ... 1204
Timentin ADD-Vantage ... 1556
Timentin Injection Galaxy Container ... 1559
Timentin IV Infusion ... 1553
Timentin Pharmacy Bulk Package ... 1562
Timolide Tablets ... 2056
Topamax Sprinkle Capsules (1% to 2%) ... 2438
Topamax Tablets (1% to 2%) ... 2438
Tricor Tablets ... 523
Triglide Tablets ... 1165
Trileptal Oral Suspension ... 2281

Trileptal Tablets 2281
Uniretic Tablets (Less than 1%) 3114
Urso 250 Tablets (2%) 737
Urso Forte Tablets (2%) 737
Valtrex Caplets (0.7% to 1.3%) 1573
Vantin Tablets and Oral Suspension 2650
Vaseretic Tablets 2073
VFEND I.V. (Less than 2%) 2543
VFEND Oral Suspension (Less than 2%) 2543
VFEND Tablets (Less than 2%) 2543
Viagra Tablets (Less than 2%) 2552
Viracept (Less than 2%) 2556
Vivactil Tablets 2350
Voltaren Tablets (Occasionally) 2298
Voltaren-XR Tablets (Occasionally) 2301
Vytorin 10/10 Tablets 2084
Vytorin 10/10 Tablets 3092
Vytorin 10/20 Tablets 2084
Vytorin 10/20 Tablets 3092
Vytorin 10/40 Tablets 2084
Vytorin 10/40 Tablets 3092
Vytorin 10/80 Tablets 2084
Vytorin 10/80 Tablets 3092
Wellbutrin Tablets 1579
Wellbutrin SR Sustained-Release Tablets 1583
Wellbutrin XL Extended-Release Tablets 1588
▲ Xeloda Tablets (24% to 91%) 2825
Zantac (A few patients) 1597
Zantac Injection (Few patients) 1593
Zantac Injection Pharmacy Bulk Package (Infrequent) 1595
Zantac Syrup (A few patients) 1597
Zestoretic Tablets (Rare) 701
Zestril Tablets (Rare) 704
Ziagen (<1%) 1600
Zinacef Injection (1 in 750 patients) 1604
Zinacef for Injection (1 in 750 patients) 1604
Zinecard for Injection 2659
Zithromax Capsules, 250 mg (Less than 1%) 2568
Zithromax for IV Infusion (Less than 1%) 2573
Zithromax for Oral Suspension, 1 g (Less than 1%) 2568
Zithromax for Oral Suspension, 300 mg, 600 mg, 900 mg, 1200 mg (Less than 1%) 2561
Zithromax Tablets, 250 mg, 500 mg (Less than 1%) 2561
Zithromax Tablets, 600 mg (Less than 1%) 2568
Zithromax Tri-Pak (Less than 1%) 2561
Zithromax Z-Pak (Less than 1%) 2568
Zmax for Oral Suspension (Less then 1%) 2577
Zocor Tablets (Rare) 2078
Zoloft 2581
Zomig Nasal Spray (Rare) 718
Zomig Tablets (Rare) 714
Zomig-ZMT Tablets (Rare) 714
Zonegran Capsules (Infrequent) 1089
Zosyn 3492
Zovirax Capsules 1616
Zovirax for Injection 1618
Zovirax 1616
Zyban Sustained-Release Tablets 1620
Zyprexa Tablets (Infrequent) 1798
Zyprexa ZYDIS Orally Disintegrating Tablets (Frequent) 1798

Leukopenia, transient

Maxipime for Injection 1093
Tindamax 2670

Leukoplakia, oral

Doxil Injection (Less than 1%) 3302
Geodon Capsules (Rare) 2514
▲ Intron A for Injection (Less than 5%) 3038

Leukorrhea

Abilify Tablets (Infrequent) 916
Abilify Tablets (Infrequent) 2472
Aciphex Tablets (Rare) 1081
▲ Arimidex Tablets (2% to 9%) 665
Arthrotec Tablets (Rare) 3126
▲ Climara Transdermal System (1% to 7%) 795
▲ CombiPatch Transdermal System (8% to 10%) 2180
▲ Depo-Provera Contraceptive Injection (1% to 5%) 2619
▲ Doxil Injection (1% to 10%) 3302
Effexor Tablets (Infrequent) 3405
Effexor XR Capsules (Infrequent) 3411
▲ Evista Tablets (3.3%) 1735
Evoxac Capsules (Less than 1%) 1042
Gengraf Capsules (1%) 458
▲ Intron A for Injection (Less than 5%) 3038
Levaquin in 5% Dextrose Injection (0.1% to 0.9%) 2453
Levaquin (0.1% to 0.9%) 2453
Lyrica Capsules (0.1% to 1%) 2524
▲ Menostar Transdermal System (11%) 805
▲ Mirena Intrauterine System (5% or more) 810
Neoral Soft Gelatin Capsules (1%) 2247
Neoral Oral Solution (1%) 2247
Neurontin Capsules (Rare) 2498
Neurontin Oral Solution (Rare) 2498
Neurontin Tablets (Rare) 2498
Omnicef Capsules (0.2%) 506
Omnicef for Oral Suspension (0.2%) 506
Paxil CR Controlled-Release Tablets (Rare) 1509
Paxil (Rare) 1501
Permax Tablets (Rare) 3357
▲ Premarin Tablets (4% to 7%) 3443
▲ Premphase Tablets (3% to 9%) 3452
▲ Prempro Tablets (3% to 9%) 3452
Prevacid Delayed-Release Capsules (Less than 1%) 3268
Prevacid for Delayed-Release Oral Suspension (Less than 1%) 3268
Prevacid NapraPAC (Less than 1%) 3277
Prevacid SoluTab Delayed-Release Orally Disintegrating Tablets (Less than 1%) 3268
PREVPAC (Less than 1%) 3281
Prometrium Capsules (100 mg, 200 mg) (Less than 5%) 3205
Prozac Pulvules and Liquid (Infrequent) 1771
Relpax Tablets (Rare) 2531
Risperdal Consta Long-Acting Injection (Infrequent) 1664
Risperdal M-Tab Orally Disintegrating Tablets (Infrequent) 1658
Risperdal (Infrequent) 1658
Seroquel Tablets (Infrequent) 691
Sonata Capsules (Rare) 1686
Soriatane Capsules (Less than 1%) 1028
Spectracef Tablets (0.1% to 1%) 2706
Symbyax Capsules (Infrequent) 1788
Topamax Sprinkle Capsules (2% to frequent) 2438
Topamax Tablets (2% to frequent) 2438
Trileptal Oral Suspension 2281
Trileptal Tablets 2281
Tygacil for Injection (0% to less than 2%) 3489
Uniretic Tablets (Less than 1%) 3114
Yasmin 28 Tablets (Greater than 1%) 818
Zoloft (Infrequent) 2581
Zosyn (1.0% or less) 3492
Zyrtec Chewable Tablets (Less than 2%) 2589
Zyrtec (Less than 2%) 2589
Zyrtec-D 12 Hour Extended Release Tablets (Less than 2%) 2591

Lhermitte's sign

Copaxone for Injection (At least 2%) 3292
Eloxatin for Injection 2908

Libido, changes

Activella Tablets 2311
Adderall Tablets 3168
Adderall XR Capsules 3169
Adipex-P 1216
Alesse-28 Tablets 3392
Avalide Tablets 922
Avalide Tablets 2889
Avapro Tablets (Less than 1%) 925
Avapro Tablets (Less than 1%) 2886
Cenestin Tablets, 0.45mg, 0.625mg, 0.9mg, 1.25mg 1063
Cenestin Tablets, 0.3mg 1063
Climara Transdermal System 795
Climara Pro Transdermal System 800
CombiPatch Transdermal System 2180
Desoxyn Tablets, USP 2482
Dexedrine 1386
DextroStat Tablets 3177
Diastat Rectal Delivery System (Infrequent) 3344
Estratest Tablets 3196
Estratest H.S. Tablets 3196
Estrogel 0.06% 3200
Flexeril Tablets (Rare) 1832
Invirase (Greater than or equal to 2%) 2776
Lo/Ovral-28 Tablets 3423
▲ Lupron Depot 3.75 mg (16%) 3257
▲ Lupron Depot–3 Month 11.25 mg (16%) 3262
Menostar Transdermal System 805
Neurontin Capsules (Infrequent) 2498
Neurontin Oral Solution (Infrequent) 2498
Neurontin Tablets (Infrequent) 2498
Nipent for Injection (Less than 3%) 3216
▲ Niravam Orally Disintegrating Tablets (7.1%) 3106
Ortho-Cept Tablets 2395
Ortho-Cyclen Tablets 2414
Ortho Evra Transdermal System 2402
Ortho Tri-Cyclen Tablets 2414
Ortho Tri-Cyclen Lo Tablets 2421
Oxandrin Tablets 2977
Prefest Tablets 1069
Premarin Intravenous 3440
Premarin Tablets 3443
Premarin Vaginal Cream 3449
Premphase Tablets 3452
Prempro Tablets 3452
▲ Roferon-A Injection (Less than 4%) 2805
Seasonale Tablets 1073
Thioridazine Hydrochloride Tablets 2122
Triphasil-28 Tablets 3483
Valium Tablets (Infrequent) 2822
Vivactil Tablets 2350
Vivelle Transdermal System 2288
Vivelle-Dot Transdermal System 2293
Yasmin 28 Tablets 818

Libido, decreased

Abilify Tablets (Infrequent) 916
Abilify Tablets (Infrequent) 2472
Aciphex Tablets 1081
Actiq (Less than 1%) 993
Adalat CC Tablets (Less than 1%) 2978
▲ Adderall XR Capsules (2% to 4%) 3169
Aldoclor Tablets 1881
Aldoril Tablets 1884
Ambien Tablets (Rare) 2867
Amerge Tablets (Rare) 1312
Anadrol-50 Tablets 3329
AndroGel (Up to 3%) 3330
Antara Capsules 2723
Aricept Tablets (Infrequent) 1086
Aricept ODT Tablets (Infrequent) 1086
Asacol Delayed-Release Tablets 2688
Avinza Capsules (Less than 5%) 1714
Avodart Soft Gelatin Capsules (0.3% to 3%) 1353
Axid Oral Solution 913
Blocadren Tablets (0.6%) 1891
Caduet Tablets (Less than 2%) 2507
Calcijex Injection 411
Campral Tablets (Frequent) 1175
▲ Casodex Tablets (2% to 5%) 670
Celexa (2%) 1177
Clozapine Tablets (Less than 1%) 2141
Clozaril Tablets (Less than 1%) 2174
Copaxone for Injection (Infrequent) 3292
Coreg Tablets (Greater than 0.1% to 1%) 1376
Cosopt Sterile Ophthalmic Solution 1910
Cozaar Tablets (Less than 1%) 1913
▲ Cymbalta Delayed-Release Capsules (1% to 6%) 1729
Delatestryl Injection 2976
▲ Depo-Provera Contraceptive Injection (1% to 5%) 2619
▲ depo-subQ provera 104 Injectable Suspension (1% to less than 5%) 2622
Diovan HCT Tablets (Greater than 0.2%) 2195
Duragesic Transdermal System (Less than 1%) 2448
DynaCirc CR Tablets (0.5% to 1%) 2726
▲ Effexor Tablets (2% to 5.7%) 3405
▲ Effexor XR Capsules (3% to 9%) 3411
Eligard 7.5 mg (Less than 2%) 2896
▲ Eligard 30 mg (3.3%) 2901
Eligard 45 mg (1%) 2904
Exelon Capsules (Infrequent) 2204
FazaClo Orally Disintegrating Tablets (Less than 1%) 547
Flomax Capsules (1.0% to 2.0%) 881
Gabitril Tablets (Infrequent) 998
Gengraf Capsules (1% to less than 3%) 458
Hectorol Capsules 909
Hectorol Injection 911
Hyperstat I.V. Injection 3031
Hytrin Capsules (0.6%) 469
Hyzaar 1964
▲ Imdur Tablets (Less than or equal to 5%) 3032
Indapamide Tablets (Less than 5%) 2119
▲ Infergen (5%) 1647
▲ Intron A for Injection (Up to 5%) 3038
Inversine Tablets 3286
Kadian Capsules (Less than 3%) 572
Kaletra (Up to 2%) 474
Klonopin (1%) 2782
Lamictal (Rare) 1449
▲ Lexapro Oral Solution (3% to 7%) 1193
▲ Lexapro Tablets (3% to 7%) 1193
Librium Capsules 3349
Lipitor Tablets (Less than 2%) 2495
Lofibra Capsules 1217
Lotensin HCT Tablets (0.3% to 1%) 2235
Lotrel Capsules 2238
▲ Lunesta Tablets (0% to 3%) 3139
Lupron Depot 3.75 mg (Less than 5%) 3257
▲ Lupron Depot 7.5 mg (5.4%) 3261
▲ Lupron Depot–3 Month 11.25 mg (1.8% to 11%) 3262
Lyrica Capsules (Greater than or equal to 1%) 2524
Mavik Tablets (0.3% to 1.0%) 482
▲ Megace ES Oral Suspension (0% to 5%) 2492
Meridia Capsules 485
Midamor Tablets (Less than or equal to 1%) 2000
Mirapex Tablets (1%) 889
▲ Mirena Intrauterine System (5% or more) 810
Moduretic Tablets 2003
MS Contin Tablets (Less frequent) 2703
Nadolol Tablets (1 to 5 of 1000 patients) 2121
Neoral Soft Gelatin Capsules (1% to less than 3%) 2247
Neoral Oral Solution (1% to less than 3%) 2247
Neurontin Capsules (Infrequent) 2498
Neurontin Oral Solution (Infrequent) 2498
Neurontin Tablets (Infrequent) 2498
▲ Niravam Orally Disintegrating Tablets (14.4%) 3106
Norvir (Less than 2%) 499
OxyContin Tablets 2699
▲ Pacerone Tablets (1% to 3%) 3337
▲ Paxil CR Controlled-Release Tablets (3% to 9%) 1509
▲ Paxil (3% to 9%) 1501
Pepcid Injection (Infrequent) 2017
Pepcid (Infrequent) 2014
Permax Tablets (Infrequent) 3357
Plendil Extended-Release Tablets (0.5% to 1.5%) 651
Prevacid Delayed-Release Capsules (Less than 1%) 3268
Prevacid for Delayed-Release Oral Suspension (Less than 1%) 3268
Prevacid NapraPAC (Less than 1%) 3277
Prevacid SoluTab Delayed-Release Orally Disintegrating Tablets (Less than 1%) 3268
PREVPAC (Less than 1%) 3281
Prinivil Tablets (0.4%) 2029
Prinzide Tablets (0.3% to 1%) 2033
▲ Prochieve 4% Gel (10%) 1018
▲ Prochieve 8% Gel (10%) 1018
▲ Propecia Tablets (1.8% - 6.4%) 2036
▲ Proscar Tablets (2.6% to 6.4%) 2040
ProSom Tablets (Rare) 512
Protonix I.V. (Less than 1%) 3468
Protonix Tablets (Less than 1%) 3465
Provigil Tablets (At least 1%) 1002
▲ Prozac Pulvules and Liquid (1% to 11%) 1771
Requip Tablets (Infrequent) 1528
Rescriptor Tablets 2535
Reyataz Capsules (Less than 3%) 948
Rilutek Tablets (Infrequent) 2945
Risperdal Consta Long-Acting Injection (Infrequent) 1664
Rythmol SR Capsules 2736
Sandostatin Injection (Less than 1%) 2263
Sandostatin LAR Depot (Rare) 2264
Seroquel Tablets (Rare) 691
Sonata Capsules (Infrequent) 1686
Soriatane Capsules (Less than 1%) 1028
▲ Strattera Capsules (5% or greater) 1784
Sular Tablets (Less than or equal to 1%) 1163
Surmontil Capsules 2347
▲ Symbyax Capsules (2% to 4%) 1788
Symmetrel (0.1% to 1%) 1115
Tambocor Tablets (Less than 1%) 1824
Tarka Tablets 519
Tasmar Tablets (Infrequent) 3360
Thalomid Capsules 979
Timolide Tablets (Less than 1%) 2056
Timoptic in Ocudose 2061
Timoptic Sterile Ophthalmic Solution 2058

Timoptic-XE Sterile Ophthalmic Gel Forming Solution 2062
▲ Topamax Sprinkle Capsules (0% to 3%) 2438
▲ Topamax Tablets (0% to 3%) 2438
Toprol-XL Tablets 660
Trelstar LA Suspension (2.3%) 3387
Tricor Tablets 523
Trileptal Oral Suspension 2281
Trileptal Tablets 2281
Uniretic Tablets (Less than 1%) 3114
Vantas (2.3%) 3367
Vaseretic Tablets (0.5% to 2.0%) 2073
VFEND I.V. (Less than 2%) 2543
VFEND Oral Suspension (Less than 2%) 2543
VFEND Tablets (Less than 2%) 2543
Vicoprofen Tablets (Less than 1%) 533
▲ Wellbutrin Tablets (3.1%) 1579
Wellbutrin SR Sustained-Release Tablets (Infrequent) 1583
Wellbutrin XL Extended-Release Tablets (Infrequent) 1588
▲ Xanax XR Tablets (6%) 2655
Zantac Injection 1593
Zantac Injection Pharmacy Bulk Package (Infrequent) 1595
Zestoretic Tablets (0.3% to 1%) 701
Zestril Tablets (0.4%) 704
▲ Zoladex (61%) 709
▲ Zoloft (1% to 11%) 2581
Zonegran Capsules (Infrequent) 1089
Zyban Sustained-Release Tablets (Infrequent) 1620
Zyprexa Tablets (Infrequent) 1798
Zyprexa ZYDIS Orally Disintegrating Tablets (Infrequent) 1798
Zyrtec Chewable Tablets (Less than 2%) 2589
Zyrtec (Less than 2%) 2589
Zyrtec-D 12 Hour Extended Release Tablets (Less than 2%) 2591

Libido, increased

Abilify Tablets (Infrequent) 916
Abilify Tablets (Infrequent) 2472
Anadrol-50 Tablets 3329
AndroGel (One patient) 3330
Apokyn Injection 2132
Aricept Tablets (Frequent) 1086
Aricept ODT Tablets (Frequent) 1086
Campral Tablets (Infrequent) 1175
Celexa (Infrequent) 1177
Clozapine Tablets (Less than 1%) 2141
Clozaril Tablets (Less than 1%) 2174
Delatestryl Injection 2976
Depo-Provera Contraceptive Injection (Less than 1%) 2619
depo-subQ provera 104 Injectable Suspension 2622
▲ Dostinex Tablets (Less than 10%) 2631
Effexor Tablets (Infrequent) 3405
Effexor XR Capsules (Infrequent) 3411
Exelon Capsules (Infrequent) 2204
FazaClo Orally Disintegrating Tablets (Less than 1%) 547
Gabitril Tablets (Infrequent) 998
Gengraf Capsules (1% to less than 3%) 458
Klonopin (Infrequent) 2782
Lamictal (Rare) 1449
Librium Capsules 3349
Lotensin Tablets (Less than 1%) 2232
Lyrica Capsules (0.1% to 1%) 2524
Meridia Capsules 485
Moban Tablets 1108
Namenda (Infrequent) 1199
Neoral Soft Gelatin Capsules (1% to less than 3%) 2247
Neoral Oral Solution (1% to less than 3%) 2247
Neurontin Capsules (Rare) 2498
Neurontin Oral Solution (Rare) 2498
Neurontin Tablets (Rare) 2498
▲ Niravam Orally Disintegrating Tablets (7.7%) 3106
Parcopa Orally Disintegrating Tablets 3111
Paxil CR Controlled-Release Tablets (Rare) 1509
Paxil (Rare) 1501
Permax Tablets (Infrequent) 3357
Prevacid Delayed-Release Capsules (Less than 1%) 3268
Prevacid for Delayed-Release Oral Suspension (Less than 1%) 3268
Prevacid NapraPAC (Less than 1%) 3277
Prevacid SoluTab Delayed-Release Orally Disintegrating Tablets (Less than 1%) 3268
PREVPAC (Less than 1%) 3281
Prozac Pulvules and Liquid (Infrequent) 1771
Razadyne ER Extended-Release Capsules (Infrequent) 2434
Razadyne (Infrequent) 2434
Requip Tablets (Infrequent) 1528
Rilutek Tablets (Infrequent) 2945
Risperdal M-Tab Orally Disintegrating Tablets (Infrequent) 1658
Risperdal (Infrequent) 1658
Seroquel Tablets (Infrequent) 691
Stalevo Tablets 2270
Surmontil Capsules 2347
Symbyax Capsules (Rare) 1788
Tasmar Tablets (Infrequent) 3360
Topamax Sprinkle Capsules (Rare) 2438
Topamax Tablets (Rare) 2438
Trileptal Oral Suspension 2281
Trileptal Tablets 2281
Wellbutrin Tablets (Frequent) 1579
Wellbutrin SR Sustained-Release Tablets 1583
Wellbutrin XL Extended-Release Tablets 1588
Xanax XR Tablets (Frequent) 2655
▲ Zoladex (12%) 709
Zoloft (Rare) 2581
Zyban Sustained-Release Tablets 1620
Zyprexa Tablets 1798
Zyprexa ZYDIS Orally Disintegrating Tablets 1798

Libido, loss of

Advicor Tablets 1694
Altoprev Extended-Release Tablets 1151
Catapres Tablets (About 3 in 100 patients) 874
Catapres-TTS (0.5% or less) 875
Clorpres Tablets (About 3%) 2139
▲ Eulexin Capsules (36%) 3023
Klonopin (Infrequent) 2782
Lescol Capsules 2227
Lescol Capsules 2730
Lescol XL Tablets 2227
Lescol XL Tablets 2730
Mevacor Tablets (0.5% to 1.0%) 1996
Orap Tablets 1220
Pravachol Tablets 943
Roferon-A Injection (Infrequent) 2805
Vytorin 10/10 Tablets 2084
Vytorin 10/10 Tablets 3092
Vytorin 10/20 Tablets 2084
Vytorin 10/20 Tablets 3092
Vytorin 10/40 Tablets 2084
Vytorin 10/40 Tablets 3092
Vytorin 10/80 Tablets 2084
Vytorin 10/80 Tablets 3092
Zantac (Occasional) 1597
Zocor Tablets 2078

Lichen planus

Cuprimine Capsules 1925
Evoxac Capsules (Less than 1%) 1042
Pentasa Capsules (Less than 1%) 3182
Plavix Tablets 940
Plavix Tablets 2942

Ligaments, calcification of

Accutane Capsules 2740
Amnesteem Capsules 2126

Light-headedness

▲ Abilify Tablets (11%) 916
▲ Abilify Tablets (11%) 2472
Adenocard Injection (2%) 612
▲ Adenoscan (12%) 613
Aldoclor Tablets 1881
Alferon N Injection (One patient to 3%) 1640
Altace Capsules 1673
Ambien Tablets (2%) 2867
Anaprox Tablets (Less than 3%) 2769
Anaprox DS Tablets (Less than 3%) 2769
Beconase AQ Nasal Spray (Fewer than 5 per 100 patients) 1359
Benicar HCT Tablets 2852
▲ Bentyl Capsules (11%) 724
▲ Bentyl Injection (11%) 724
▲ Bentyl Syrup (11%) 724
▲ Bentyl Tablets (11%) 724
Brevibloc Concentrate (Less than 1%) 766
Brevibloc Injection (Less than 1%) 766
Brevibloc Double Strength Injection (Less than 1%) 766
Brevibloc Premixed Injection (Less than 1%) 766
Brevibloc Double Strength Premixed Injection (Less than 1%) 766
Buphenyl Powder 3327
Buphenyl Tablets 3327
Captopril Tablets 2114
Cipro I.V. (1% or less) 2998
Cipro I.V. Pharmacy Bulk Package (1% or less) 3509
Cipro (Less than 1%) 2991
Cipro XR Tablets 3004
Cutivate Ointment (Less than 1%) 1384
Dalmane Capsules 3343
Dantrium Capsules (Less frequent) 2690
Dantrium Intravenous 2691
Darvocet A 500 Tablets 3497
Dilaudid 439
Dilaudid Oral Liquid 443
Dilaudid Non-Sterile Powder 439
Dilaudid Rectal Suppositories 439
Dilaudid Tablets 439
Dilaudid Tablets - 8 mg 443
▲ Dilaudid-HP (Among most frequent) 441
Diovan HCT Tablets 2195
Dolobid Tablets (Less than 1 in 100) 1937
Dynacin Tablets 1859
EC-Naprosyn Delayed-Release Tablets (Less than 3%) 2769
▲ Eldepryl Capsules (7 of 49 patients) 3209
▲ Gabitril Tablets (27%) 998
Gammagard S/D (Occasional) 754
Guanidine Hydrochloride Tablets 3030
Hyperstat I.V. Injection 3031
▲ Hytrin Capsules (28%) 469
Hyzaar 1964
Indapamide Tablets (Less than 5%) 2119
Inderal LA Long-Acting Capsules 3421
Indocin (Less than 1%) 1968
InnoPran XL Capsules 2728
Inversine Tablets 3286
Invirase (Less than 2%) 2776
Levaquin in 5% Dextrose Injection 2453
Levaquin 2453
Lexapro Oral Solution (Frequent) 1193
Lexapro Tablets (Frequent) 1193
Lidoderm Patch 1107
▲ Lortab (Among most frequent) 3315
▲ Lortab Elixir (Among most frequent) 3312
Lotensin HCT Tablets 2235
Mavik Tablets 482
Micardis HCT Tablets 886
▲ MS Contin Tablets (Among most frequent) 2703
Naprosyn Suspension (Less than 3%) 2769
Naprosyn Tablets (Less than 3%) 2769
Neumega for Injection 3433
Nimotop Capsules (Less than 1%) 774
▲ Niravam Orally Disintegrating Tablets (19.3% to 29.8%) 3106
▲ Nitro-Dur Transdermal Infusion System (6%) 3060
Norflex Injection 1824
Noroxin Tablets 2009
Numorphan 1112
▲ OxyFast Oral Concentrate Solution (Among most frequent) 2704
▲ OxyIR Capsules (Among most frequent) 2704
▲ Percocet Tablets (Among most frequent) 1114
▲ Percodan Tablets (Among most frequent) 1115
Prevacid NapraPAC (Less than 3%) 3277
Prinivil Tablets 2029
Prinzide Tablets 2033
Prolastin (0.19%) 3252
Raptiva for Injection 1247
Recombivax HB (Less than 1%) 2045
▲ Sedapap Tablets 50 mg/650 mg (Among the most frequent) 2098
▲ Symmetrel (5% to 10%) 1115
Tambocor Tablets 1824
▲ Tenormin I.V. Injection (1% to 3%) 698
Tenormin Tablets (1% to 3%) 695
Tequin Injection 964
Tequin Tablets 964
Thiothixene Capsules 2124
▲ Thrombate III (1 of 17) 3254
▲ Tylenol with Codeine (Among most frequent) 2461
Uniretic Tablets (Less than 1%) 3114
Vaseretic Tablets 2073
Vasotec I.V. Injection 2076
▲ Vicodin Tablets (Among most frequent) 530
▲ Vicodin ES Tablets (Among most frequent) 531
▲ Vicodin HP Tablets (Among most frequent) 532
▲ Zemplar Capsules (5%) 535
▲ Zemplar Injection (5%) 538
Zestoretic Tablets 701
Zestril Tablets 704
Zovirax for Injection (Less than 1%) 1618
▲ Zydone Tablets (Among most frequent) 1118

Limb ischemia

Lovenox Injection 2931

Limb reduction defects

Altace Capsules 1673
Captopril Tablets 2114
Cozaar Tablets 1913
Hyzaar 1964
Lo/Ovral-28 Tablets 3423
Lotrel Capsules 2238
Prinivil Tablets 2029
Prinzide Tablets 2033
Proventil Inhalation Aerosol 3067
Proventil Inhalation Solution 0.083% 3069
Vaseretic Tablets 2073
Vasotec I.V. Injection 2076
Zestoretic Tablets 701
Zestril Tablets 704

Limbitis

▲ Stromectol Tablets (3.5% to 5.5%) 2053

Lipoatrophy

Aptivus Capsules (Less than 2%) 859
Imitrex Injection (Rare) 1431

Lipodystrophy

Apidra Injection 2876
Aptivus Capsules (Less than 2%) 859
Genotropin Lyophilized Powder (Infrequent) 2642
Humalog-Pen 1751
Humalog Mix 75/25-Pen 1754
Humulin 50/50, 100 Units (Rare) 1760
Humulin 70/30 Pen (Rare) 1761
Humulin L, 100 Units (Rare) 1763
Humulin R (U-500) (Rare) 1768
Humulin N Pen (Rare) 1765
▲ Invirase (5.4%) 2776
Lantus Injection 2925
NovoLog Injection 2326
NovoLog Mix 70/30 2331
▲ Reyataz Capsules (1% to 8%) 948

Lipohypertrophy

Aptivus Capsules (Less than 2%) 859
Imitrex Injection (Rare) 1431
▲ Increlex Injection (Greater than or equal to 5%) 3290
Reyataz Capsules (Less than 3%) 948

Lipoma

Copaxone for Injection (Infrequent) 3292
▲ Intron A for Injection (Less than 5%) 3038
Lexapro Oral Solution (Infrequent) 1193
Lexapro Tablets (Infrequent) 1193
Requip Tablets (Infrequent) 1528

Lipoprotein levels, changes

Accutane Capsules 2740
Carbatrol Capsules (Occasional) 3174
Prefest Tablets 1069
▲ Soriatane Capsules (25% to 50%) 1028
Tegretol/Tegretol-XR (Occasional) 2278
Timolide Tablets 2056
Triphasil-28 Tablets 3483
Vivelle Transdermal System 2288
Vivelle-Dot Transdermal System 2293
Zoladex 709
Zoladex 3-month 712

Lipoproteins, electrophoretic abnormalities

Sandimmune 2259

Lipotrophy

Humulin 50/50, 100 Units (Rare) 1760
Humulin 70/30 Pen (Rare) 1761
Humulin L, 100 Units (Rare) 1763
Humulin R (U-500) (Rare) 1768
Humulin N Pen (Rare) 1765
Somavert Injection 2648

Lips, cracked

Zovirax Cream (Less than 1%) 853

Lips, dry

(*see under* Xerochilia)

Lips, enlargement

Eskalith 1406
Phenytek Capsules 2153

Lips, swelling

Altace Capsules 1673
Levaquin in 5% Dextrose Injection 2453
Levaquin 2453

Lithobid Tablets 1670
Propecia Tablets 2036
Proscar Tablets 2040
Tambocor Tablets (Less than 1%) 1824

Listeriosis
Remicade for IV Injection 987

Listlessness
Aricept Tablets (Infrequent) 1086
Aricept ODT Tablets (Infrequent) 1086
Indocin (Greater than 1%) 1968

Livedo reticularis
Activase I.V. 1225
Symmetrel (1% to 5%) 1115

Liver, enlarged
VFEND I.V. (Less than 2%) 2543
VFEND Oral Suspension (Less than 2%) 2543
VFEND Tablets (Less than 2%) 2543

Liver, fatty
Aciphex Tablets (Rare) 1081
Advicor Tablets 1694
Copegus Tablets (Less than 1%) 2759
Effexor Tablets 3405
Effexor XR Capsules 3411
Geodon Capsules (Rare) 2514
Lescol Capsules 2227
Lescol Capsules 2730
Lescol XL Tablets 2227
Lescol XL Tablets 2730
Lofibra Capsules 1217
Pegasys (Less than 1%) 2793
Plavix Tablets (Less than 1%) 940
Plavix Tablets (Less than 1%) 2942
Prozac Pulvules and Liquid (Rare) 1771
Reyataz Capsules (Less than 3%) 948
Risperdal Consta Long-Acting Injection (Rare) 1664
Sandostatin LAR Depot (Rare) 2264
Symbyax Capsules (Rare) 1788
Tricor Tablets 523
Triglide Tablets 1165
Vytorin 10/10 Tablets 2084
Vytorin 10/10 Tablets 3092
Vytorin 10/20 Tablets 2084
Vytorin 10/20 Tablets 3092
Vytorin 10/40 Tablets 2084
Vytorin 10/40 Tablets 3092
Vytorin 10/80 Tablets 2084
Vytorin 10/80 Tablets 3092
Zyprexa Tablets (Rare) 1798
Zyprexa ZYDIS Orally Disintegrating Tablets (Rare) 1798

Liver abnormalities
Catapres Tablets (About 1 in 100 patients) 874
Clorpres Tablets 2139
Clozapine Tablets (1%) 2141
Clozaril Tablets (1%) 2174
Effexor Tablets 3405
Oncaspar (Less than 1%) 1123
Pepcid Injection (Infrequent) 2017
Pepcid (Infrequent) 2014
Pravachol Tablets 943
Relafen Tablets (1%) 1523
▲ Tarka Tablets (3.2%) 519
Ziagen 1600
Zocor Tablets 2078

Liver damage
(*see under* Hepatotoxicity)

Liver disorders
Aldoclor Tablets 1881
Aldoril Tablets 1884
Cosmegen for Injection 1907
Invirase (Rare) 2776
▲ Leukine (77%) 829
Lo/Ovral-28 Tablets 3423
Mycamine for Injection 620
Pulmozyme Inhalation Solution 1245
Triphasil-28 Tablets 3483
▲ Vesanoid Capsules (3%) 2823

Liver dysfunction
(*see under* Hepatic dysfunction)

Liver enzymes, elevated
Bayer Aspirin Tablets 3515
Clarinex-D 24-Hour Extended-Release Tablets 3012
Strattera Capsules 1784
Ultane Liquid for Inhalation (Less than 1%) 526
Zetia Tablets 3098

Liver fatty deposit
Antara Capsules 2723

Liver function, changes
(*see under* Hepatic dysfunction)

Liver function, impaired
(*see under* Hepatic dysfunction)

Liver function tests, abnormal
▲ Advair Diskus 100/50 (1% to 3%) 1291
Advair Diskus 250/50 (1% to 3%) 1291
▲ Advair Diskus 500/50 (1% to 3%) 1291
Anaprox Tablets (Less than 1%) 2769
Anaprox DS Tablets (Less than 1%) 2769
▲ Antara Capsules (7.5%) 2723
Aptivus Capsules (Less than 2%) 859
Avelox (0.1% to less than 2%) 2984
Caduet Tablets (Less than 2%) 2507
Campral Tablets (Infrequent) 1175
Cialis Tablets (Less than 2%) 1806
Cipro I.V. (Greater than 1% to 1.3%) 2998
Cipro I.V. Pharmacy Bulk Package (Greater than 1% to 1.3%) 3509
Cipro (1.3%) 2991
Cipro XR Tablets (Less than 1%) 3004
Concerta Extended-Release Tablets 1828
Cosmegen for Injection 1907
▲ Cubicin for Injection (3%) 1038
EC-Naprosyn Delayed-Release Tablets (Less than 1%) 2769
Epzicom Tablets 1402
▲ Equetro Extended-Release Capsules (Less than 5%) 3178
Erythromycin Delayed-Release Capsules, USP (Rare) 456
FazaClo Orally Disintegrating Tablets (1%) 547
Ketek Tablets (Greater than or equal to 0.2% to less than 2%) 2920
Levitra Tablets (Less than 2%) 3048
Mycamine for Injection (0.7% to 1.5%) 620
▲ Myfortic Tablets (3% to less than 20%) 2244
▲ Mylotarg for Injection (20% to 29%) 3429
Naprosyn Suspension (Less than 1%) 2769
Naprosyn Tablets (Less than 1%) 2769
Oxandrin Tablets 2977
Plavix Tablets 2942
Pletal Tablets (Very rare) 2478
Prevacid NapraPAC (Less than 1%) 3277
Rythmol SR Capsules 2736
Tamiflu Capsules 2810
Tamiflu Oral Suspension 2810
Tarceva Tablets 1254
Tarceva Tablets 2470
▲ Tricor Tablets (7.5%) 523
▲ Triglide Tablets (7.5%) 1165
▲ VFEND I.V. (2.7% to 3.2%) 2543
▲ VFEND Oral Suspension (2.7% to 3.2%) 2543
▲ VFEND Tablets (2.7% to 3.2%) 2543
Viracept (Less than 2%) 2556
Zyvox (0.4% to 1.3%) 2661

Liver function tests, elevated
▲ Anaprox Tablets (1% to 10%) 2769
▲ Anaprox DS Tablets (1% to 10%) 2769
Decadron Tablets 1929
Dolobid Tablets 1937
▲ EC-Naprosyn Delayed-Release Tablets (1% to 10%) 2769
▲ Elmiron Capsules (11.8%) 2393
Levothroid Tablets 1189
▲ Naprosyn Suspension (1% to 10%) 2769
▲ Naprosyn Tablets (1% to 10%) 2769
Neurontin Capsules 2498
Neurontin Oral Solution 2498
Neurontin Tablets 2498
▲ Raptiva for Injection (3.1%) 1247
Trizivir Tablets 1565

Liver injury
Arava Tablets (Rare) 2881
Eulexin Capsules 3023
Pacerone Tablets (Common) 3337
Singulair (Rare) 2047
Strattera Capsules (Rare) 1784
Tasmar Tablets 3360
Vantin Tablets and Oral Suspension 2650

Liver pain
▲ Roferon-A Injection (3%) 2805

Liver tenderness
Actiq (Less than 1%) 993

Liver transplant, need for
Lamisil Tablets 2226

Liver tumors
(*see under* Hepatomas)

Loffler's syndrome
Paser Granules 1657

Loss of balance
(*see under* Balance, loss of)

Lumbago
Klonopin (Infrequent) 2782
Prinivil Tablets (0.3% to 1.0%) 2029
Prinzide Tablets 2033
Zestoretic Tablets 701
Zestril Tablets (0.3% to 1.0%) 704

Lung development, hypoplastic
Altace Capsules 1673
Captopril Tablets 2114
Cozaar Tablets 1913
Hyzaar 1964
Lotrel Capsules 2238
Prinivil Tablets 2029
Prinzide Tablets 2033
Vaseretic Tablets 2073
Vasotec I.V. Injection 2076
Zestoretic Tablets 701
Zestril Tablets 704

Lung disorders, unspecified
Actiq (Less than 1%) 993
Alinia for Oral Suspension (Less than 1%) 2840
Alinia Tablets (Less than 1%) 2840
▲ AmBisome for Injection (13.6% to 17.8%) 615
▲ Arava Tablets (1% to 3%) 2881
BeneFix for Injection (1.5%) 3402
Bravelle for Intramuscular or Subcutaneous Injection 1140
▲ Casodex Tablets (2% to 5%) 670
▲ CellCept Capsules (3% to less than 20%) 2751
▲ CellCept Intravenous (3% to less than 20%) 2751
▲ CellCept Oral Suspension (3% to less than 20%) 2751
▲ CellCept Tablets (3% to less than 20%) 2751
Combunox Tablets (Less than 1%) 1183
▲ DuoNeb Inhalation Solution (6.4%) 1058
▲ Humira Injection (Less than 5%) 464
▲ I.V. Busulfex (34%) 1125
▲ Leukine (20%) 829
▲ Megace ES Oral Suspension (1% to 3%) 2492
Neurontin Capsules (Infrequent) 2498
Neurontin Oral Solution (Infrequent) 2498
Neurontin Tablets (Infrequent) 2498
▲ Nipent for Injection (Up to 12%) 3216
Norvir (Less than 2%) 499
▲ Ontak Vials (8%) 1717
▲ Prograf Capsules and Injection (3% to 15%) 624
▲ Proleukin for Injection (24%) 1007
Protonix I.V. (Less than 1%) 3468
Protonix Tablets (Less than 1%) 3465
Protopic Ointment (Greater than or equal to 1%) 629
Provigil Tablets (2%) 1002
Pulmozyme Inhalation Solution 1245
Rythmol SR Capsules 2736
Symbyax Capsules (Frequent) 1788
Thalomid Capsules 979
▲ Trasylol Injection (7%) 779
Ventolin HFA Inhalation Aerosol (Less than 3%) 1576
Zemaira (0.2% to 0.4%) 3506

Lung function, decreased
▲ Humira Injection (Less than 5%) 464

Lung injury, acute, infusion related
Gammagard Liquid 751

Lung injury, transfusion-associated
Carimune NF 3501
Gammagard S/D (Rare) 754
Gamunex Immune Globulin I.V., 10% (Rare) 3232
Iveegam EN (Rare) 759

Lung neoplasms, malignant
Prinzide Tablets 2033
Zestoretic Tablets 701
Zestril Tablets (0.3% to 1.0%) 704

Lupus erythematosus
Advicor Tablets 1694
Aldoclor Tablets 1881
Aldoril Tablets 1884
Carbatrol Capsules (Isolated cases) 3174
Cosopt Sterile Ophthalmic Solution 1910
Cuprimine Capsules 1925
Dapsone Tablets USP 1656
Depacon Injection 412
Depakene 417
Depakote Sprinkle Capsules 422
▲ Depakote Tablets (1% to 5%) 427
Depakote ER Tablets (Greater than 1%) 433
Evoxac Capsules (Less than 1%) 1042
Gris-PEG Tablets 2504
▲ Humira Injection (Less than 5%) 464
Inderal LA Long-Acting Capsules (Rare) 3421
Lo/Ovral-28 Tablets 3423
Permax Tablets (Rare) 3357
Phenytek Capsules 2153
Recombivax HB 2045
Roferon-A Injection (Rare) 2805
Syprine Capsules 2055
Tegretol/Tegretol-XR (Isolated cases) 2278
Timoptic in Ocudose (Less frequent) 2061
Timoptic Sterile Ophthalmic Solution (Less frequent) 2058
Timoptic-XE Sterile Ophthalmic Gel Forming Solution 2062
Trileptal Oral Suspension 2281
Trileptal Tablets 2281
Triphasil-28 Tablets 3483
Zonegran Capsules (Rare) 1089

Lupus erythematosus, discoid
Enbrel for Injection 580
VFEND I.V. (Less than 2%) 2543
VFEND Oral Suspension (Less than 2%) 2543
VFEND Tablets (Less than 2%) 2543

Lupus erythematosus, disseminated, aggravation of
Equetro Extended-Release Capsules 3178

Lupus erythematosus, systemic
Benicar HCT Tablets 2852
CombiPatch Transdermal System 2180
Copegus Tablets (Less than 1%) 2759
Cosopt Sterile Ophthalmic Solution 1910
Inderal LA Long-Acting Capsules (Extremely rare) 3421
InnoPran XL Capsules (Rare) 2728
Lamisil Tablets (Infrequently) 2226
Peganone Tablets, USP 2487
Pegasys (Less than 1%) 2793
Phenytek Capsules 2153
Recombivax HB 2045
Syprine Capsules 2055
Timoptic in Ocudose (Less frequent) 2061
Timoptic Sterile Ophthalmic Solution (Less frequent) 2058
Timoptic-XE Sterile Ophthalmic Gel Forming Solution 2062

Lupus erythematosus, systemic, exacerbation or activation of
Alesse-28 Tablets 3392
Carbatrol Capsules 3174
Dyazide Capsules 1389
Dynacin Tablets 1859
Furosemide Tablets 2117
Lo/Ovral-28 Tablets 3423
Maxzide 2150
Prefest Tablets 1069
Premphase Tablets 3452
Prempro Tablets 3452
Prinzide Tablets 2033
Seasonale Tablets 1073
Tegretol/Tegretol-XR 2278
Triphasil-28 Tablets 3483
Vaseretic Tablets 2073
Zestoretic Tablets 701

Lupus-like syndrome
Aldoclor Tablets 1881
Aldoril Tablets 1884
Altoprev Extended-Release Tablets (Rare) 1151
Asacol Delayed-Release Tablets 2688
Cuprimine Capsules 1925
Dynacin Tablets 1859
Enbrel for Injection 580
Equetro Extended-Release Capsules 3178

Gris-PEG Tablets ... 2504
Humira Injection ... 464
InnoPran XL Capsules (Rare) ... 2728
Lamictal ... 1449
Lescol Capsules (Rare) ... 2227
Lescol Capsules (Rare) ... 2730
Lescol XL Tablets ... 2227
Lescol XL Tablets ... 2730
Mevacor Tablets (Rare) ... 1996
PEG-Intron Powder for Injection (Less than or equal to 1%) ... 3062
Pravachol Tablets (Rare) ... 943
Recombivax HB ... 2045
Rituxan for Infusion (Less than 0.1%) ... 845
Rituxan I.V. (Less than 0.1%) ... 1251
Tegretol-XR Tablets (Isolated cases) ... 2278
Tenormin I.V. Injection ... 698
Tenormin Tablets ... 695
Tricor Tablets ... 523
Vytorin 10/10 Tablets ... 2084
Vytorin 10/10 Tablets ... 3092
Vytorin 10/20 Tablets ... 2084
Vytorin 10/20 Tablets ... 3092
Vytorin 10/40 Tablets ... 2084
Vytorin 10/40 Tablets ... 3092
Vytorin 10/80 Tablets ... 2084
Vytorin 10/80 Tablets ... 3092
Zocor Tablets (Rare) ... 2078
Zoloft ... 2581

Lyell's syndrome

(*see under* Necrolysis, epidermal, toxic)

Lymph nodes, swelling

▲ Adacel Vaccine (0.1% to 6.6%) ... 2959

Lymph nodes, tender

Clindesse Vaginal Cream (Less than 1%) ... 3296
ProSom Tablets (Rare) ... 512
Stromectol Tablets (1.9%) ... 2053

Lymphadenitis

Boostrix ... 1366
▲ Intron A for Injection (Less than or equal to 5%) ... 3038

Lymphadenopathy

Abilify Tablets (Infrequent) ... 916
Abilify Tablets (Infrequent) ... 2472
AccuNeb Inhalation Solution (0.9% to 2.6%) ... 1055
Accutane Capsules ... 2740
Aciphex Tablets ... 1081
Actiq (1% or greater) ... 993
Adalat CC Tablets (Less than 1%) ... 2978
Aerobid/Aerobid-M (1% to 3%) ... 1172
Alferon N Injection (1%) ... 1640
Ambien Tablets (Rare) ... 2867
Anaprox Tablets (Less than 1%) ... 2769
Anaprox DS Tablets (Less than 1%) ... 2769
Antara Capsules ... 2723
Arthrotec Tablets (Rare) ... 3126
Asacol Delayed-Release Tablets ... 2688
Attenuvax (Less common) ... 1889
▲ Betaseron for SC Injection (8%) ... 791
Boostrix ... 1366
Caduet Tablets (Less than 2%) ... 2507
Campath Ampules ... 826
Campral Tablets (Rare) ... 1175
Carbatrol Capsules ... 3174
Cataflam Tablets (Rarely) ... 2173
Celexa (Infrequent) ... 1177
Cipro I.V. (1% or less) ... 2998
Cipro I.V. Pharmacy Bulk Package (1% or less) ... 3509
Cipro (0.3% to 1%) ... 2991
Cipro XR Tablets ... 3004
Colazal Capsules ... 2845
Combivir Tablets ... 1373
Comvax ... 1904
▲ Copaxone for Injection (12%) ... 3292
Cuprimine Capsules ... 1925
Diastat Rectal Delivery System (Less than 1%) ... 3344
Doxil Injection (Less than 1%) ... 3302
EC-Naprosyn Delayed-Release Tablets (Less than 1%) ... 2769
Effexor Tablets (Infrequent) ... 3405
Effexor XR Capsules (Infrequent) ... 3411
Enbrel for Injection ... 580
Engerix-B Vaccine (Less than 1%) ... 1391
Epivir ... 1394
Epivir-HBV ... 1398
Epzicom Tablets ... 1402
▲ Equetro Extended-Release Capsules (Less than 5%) ... 3178
Evoxac Capsules (Less than 1%) ... 1042
Exelon Capsules (Infrequent) ... 2204
Ferrlecit Injection ... 3379
▲ Fortical Nasal Spray (1% to 3%) ... 3336
Fuzeon Injection ... 2772
Gabitril Tablets (Frequent) ... 998
Gengraf Capsules (1% to less than 3%) ... 458
Geodon Capsules (Infrequent) ... 2514
Havrix Vaccine (Rare) ... 1425
Imitrex Nasal Spray (Rare) ... 1435
Imitrex Tablets (Rare) ... 1440
Infanrix Vaccine ... 1444
Infed Injection ... 3381
▲ Infergen (4% to 6%) ... 1647
▲ Intron A for Injection (Less than or equal to 5%) ... 3038
Invirase (Less than 2%) ... 2776
Kaletra (Less than 2%) ... 474
Klonopin ... 2782
Lamictal (2%) ... 1449
Levaquin in 5% Dextrose Injection (0.1% to 0.9%) ... 2453
Levaquin (0.1% to 0.9%) ... 2453
Lipitor Tablets (Less than 2%) ... 2495
Lofibra Capsules ... 1217
Lunesta Tablets (Infrequent) ... 3139
▲ Lupron Depot 3.75 mg (Among most frequent) ... 3257
Lupron Depot–3 Month 11.25 mg (Less than 5%) ... 3262
Lyrica Capsules (0.1% to 1%) ... 2524
Meridia Capsules ... 485
Meruvax II ... 1994
Miacalcin Nasal Spray (1% to 3%) ... 2242
Mintezol ... 2002
M-M-R II ... 1980
Mumpsvax ... 2005
Nalfon Capsules (Less than 1%) ... 2504
Naprosyn Suspension (Less than 1%) ... 2769
Naprosyn Tablets (Less than 1%) ... 2769
Neoral Soft Gelatin Capsules (1% to less than 3%) ... 2247
Neoral Oral Solution (1% to less than 3%) ... 2247
Neurontin Capsules (Infrequent) ... 2498
Neurontin Oral Solution (Infrequent) ... 2498
Neurontin Tablets (Infrequent) ... 2498
Norvir (Less than 2%) ... 499
Omacor Capsules ... 2735
Orthoclone OKT3 Sterile Solution (Less than 1%) ... 2370
OxyContin Tablets (Less than 1%) ... 2699
▲ Paser Granules (46% of 38 patients with drug-induced hepatitis) ... 1657
Paxil CR Controlled-Release Tablets (Infrequent) ... 1509
Paxil (Infrequent) ... 1501
Pediarix Vaccine ... 1518
Liquid PedvaxHIB ... 2012
Peganone Tablets, USP ... 2487
Permax Tablets (Infrequent) ... 3357
Phenytek Capsules ... 2153
Prevacid Delayed-Release Capsules (Less than 1%) ... 3268
Prevacid for Delayed-Release Oral Suspension (Less than 1%) ... 3268
Prevacid NapraPAC (Less than 1%) ... 3277
Prevacid SoluTab Delayed-Release Orally Disintegrating Tablets (Less than 1%) ... 3268
PREVPAC (Less than 1%) ... 3281
Prometrium Capsules (100 mg, 200 mg) (Less than 5%) ... 3205
Protopic Ointment (1% to 3%) ... 629
Prozac Pulvules and Liquid ... 1771
▲ Rabies Vaccine RabAvert (15%) ... 1011
▲ Rapamune Oral Solution and Tablets (3% to 20%) ... 3472
▲ Rebif Prefilled Syringe for Injection (11% to 12%) ... 3163
Recombivax HB (Less than 1%) ... 2045
Relpax Tablets (Rare) ... 2531
Remicade for IV Injection (Greater than or equal to 0.2%) ... 987
Retrovir Capsules ... 1533
Retrovir IV Infusion ... 1537
Retrovir ... 1533
Rilutek Tablets (Rare) ... 2945
Risperdal Consta Long-Acting Injection (Infrequent) ... 1664
Risperdal M-Tab Orally Disintegrating Tablets (Rare) ... 1658
Risperdal (Rare) ... 1658
Rythmol SR Capsules ... 2736
Seroquel Tablets (Infrequent) ... 691
Sonata Capsules (Infrequent) ... 1686
Symbyax Capsules (Infrequent) ... 1788
Tamiflu Capsules (1%) ... 2810
Tamiflu Oral Suspension (1%) ... 2810
Tegretol/Tegretol-XR ... 2278
Tequin Injection (Less than 0.1%) ... 964
Tequin Tablets (Less than 0.1%) ... 964
▲ Thalomid Capsules (5.6% to 12.5%) ... 979
Topamax Sprinkle Capsules (Infrequent) ... 2438
Topamax Tablets (Infrequent) ... 2438
Tricor Tablets ... 523
Triglide Tablets ... 1165
Trileptal Oral Suspension (Up to 2%) ... 2281
Trileptal Tablets (Up to 2%) ... 2281
▲ Trisenox Injection (8%) ... 983
Trizivir Tablets ... 1565
Twinrix Vaccine (Less than 1%) ... 1571
Uniretic Tablets (Less than 1%) ... 3114
Varivax (Greater than or equal to 1%) ... 2070
VFEND I.V. (Less than 2%) ... 2543
VFEND Oral Suspension (Less than 2%) ... 2543
VFEND Tablets (Less than 2%) ... 2543
Viramune Oral Suspension ... 903
Viramune Tablets ... 903
Voltaren Tablets (Rarely) ... 2298
Voltaren-XR Tablets (Rarely) ... 2301
Wellbutrin Tablets (Rare) ... 1579
Wellbutrin SR Sustained-Release Tablets ... 1583
Wellbutrin XL Extended-Release Tablets ... 1588
Xopenex HFA Inhalation Aerosol ... 3151
Xopenex Inhalation Solution ... 3143
Xopenex Inhalation Solution Concentrate ... 3147
Ziagen ... 1600
Zomig Nasal Spray (Rare) ... 718
Zonegran Capsules (Infrequent) ... 1089
Zovirax Capsules ... 1616
Zovirax for Injection ... 1618
Zovirax ... 1616
Zyban Sustained-Release Tablets ... 1620
Zyprexa Tablets (Infrequent) ... 1798
Zyprexa ZYDIS Orally Disintegrating Tablets (Infrequent) ... 1798
Zyrtec Chewable Tablets (Less than 2%) ... 2589
Zyrtec (Less than 2%) ... 2589
Zyrtec-D 12 Hour Extended Release Tablets (Less than 2%) ... 2591

Lymphadenopathy, cervical

Lexapro Oral Solution (Infrequent) ... 1193
Lexapro Tablets (Infrequent) ... 1193
Nexium Delayed-Release Capsules (Less than 1%) ... 645
Nexium I.V. (Less than 1%) ... 649
Pulmicort Respules (1% to 3%) ... 654
Risperdal Consta Long-Acting Injection (Infrequent) ... 1664

Lymphadenopathy, localized

Prevnar for Injection ... 3460

Lymphadenopathy, post-cervical

Evoxac Capsules (Less than 1%) ... 1042

Lymphangitis, regional

Doxil Injection (Less than 1%) ... 3302
Herceptin I.V. (At least one of the 958 patients) ... 1234

Lymphangitis, unspecified

VFEND I.V. (Less than 2%) ... 2543
VFEND Oral Suspension (Less than 2%) ... 2543
VFEND Tablets (Less than 2%) ... 2543

Lymphatic disorders, unspecified

▲ Ammonul Injection (11%) ... 3323

Lymphedema

Actiq (1% or greater) ... 993
▲ Arimidex Tablets (9% to 10%) ... 665
Aromasin Tablets (Less frequent) ... 2600
Copaxone for Injection (Infrequent) ... 3292
Doxil Injection (Less than 1%) ... 3302
Humatrope Vials and Cartridges ... 1756
Paxil CR Controlled-Release Tablets (Rare) ... 1509
Paxil (Rare) ... 1501
Prozac Pulvules and Liquid (Rare) ... 1771
Rabies Vaccine RabAvert (Uncommon) ... 1011
Requip Tablets (Infrequent) ... 1528
Thalomid Capsules ... 979
▲ Xeloda Tablets (Less than 1% to 3%) ... 2825

Lymphedema, post-mastectomy

▲ Femara Tablets (7%) ... 2210

Lymphocele

▲ Myfortic Tablets (3% to less than 20%) ... 2244
▲ Rapamune Oral Solution and Tablets (3% to 20%) ... 3472
▲ Zenapax for Injection (Greater than 5%) ... 2838

Lymphocytes, decrease

(*see under* Lymphocytopenia)

Lymphocytes, increase

(*see under* Lymphocytosis)

Lymphocytes, atypical

Coreg Tablets (Less than or equal to 0.1%) ... 1376

Lymphocytopenia

▲ Amevive (2% to 59%) ... 836
▲ Betaseron for SC Injection (88%) ... 791
Camptosar Injection ... 2602
Colazal Capsules ... 2845
▲ Copegus Tablets (14%) ... 2759
I.V. Busulfex ... 1125
Leukeran Tablets ... 1472
Levaquin in 5% Dextrose Injection (2.3%) ... 2453
Levaquin (2.3%) ... 2453
Mavik Tablets (0.3% to 1.0%) ... 482
Mustargen for Injection ... 2007
Mycamine for Injection (0.8%) ... 620
Nabi-HB (2%) ... 2159
Omnicef Capsules (1%) ... 506
Omnicef for Oral Suspension (0.8%) ... 506
Orthoclone OKT3 Sterile Solution (Less than 1%) ... 2370
Paxil CR Controlled-Release Tablets (Rare) ... 1509
Paxil (Rare) ... 1501
▲ Pegasys (3% to 86%) ... 2793
Requip Tablets (Infrequent) ... 1528
Risperdal Consta Long-Acting Injection (Rare) ... 1664
▲ Rituxan I.V. (48%) ... 1251
Rocephin Injectable Vials, ADD-Vantage, Galaxy, Bulk (Less than 1%) ... 2801
Tarka Tablets ... 519
▲ Temodar Capsules (55% to 60%) ... 3088
Topamax Sprinkle Capsules (Infrequent) ... 2438
Topamax Tablets (Infrequent) ... 2438
Trizivir Tablets ... 1565
Vantin Tablets and Oral Suspension ... 2650
▲ Xeloda Tablets (13% to 99%) ... 2825
Ziagen ... 1600
Zithromax for Oral Suspension, 300 mg, 600 mg, 900 mg, 1200 mg (Greater than 1%) ... 2561
Zithromax Tablets, 250 mg, 500 mg (Greater than 1%) ... 2561
Zithromax Tri-Pak (Greater than 1%) ... 2561
Zmax for Oral Suspension (Greater then or equal to 1%) ... 2577

Lymphocytosis

Campral Tablets (Infrequent) ... 1175
Celexa (Rare) ... 1177
Cipro I.V. (Infrequent) ... 2998
Cipro I.V. Pharmacy Bulk Package (Infrequent) ... 3509
Depacon Injection ... 412
Depakene ... 417
Depakote Sprinkle Capsules ... 422
Depakote Tablets ... 427
Depakote ER Tablets ... 433
Effexor Tablets (Rare) ... 3405
Evoxac Capsules ... 1042
Fortaz (Very rare) ... 1422
Geodon Capsules (Rare) ... 2514
▲ Infergen (5% to 11%) ... 1647
▲ Intron A for Injection (Less than 5%) ... 3038
Neurontin Capsules (Rare) ... 2498
Neurontin Oral Solution (Rare) ... 2498
Neurontin Tablets (Rare) ... 2498
Norvir (Less than 2%) ... 499
Omnicef Capsules (0.2%) ... 506
Omnicef for Oral Suspension (2%) ... 506
Paxil CR Controlled-Release Tablets (Rare) ... 1509
Paxil (Rare) ... 1501
Permax Tablets (Rare) ... 3357
Primaxin I.M. ... 2022
Primaxin I.V. ... 2024
Prozac Pulvules and Liquid (Rare) ... 1771
▲ Raptiva for Injection (40%) ... 1247
Requip Tablets (Infrequent) ... 1528

Rocephin Injectable Vials, ADD-Vantage, Galaxy, Bulk (Less than 0.1%) 2801
Sonata Capsules (Rare) 1686
Targretin Capsules 1719
Thalomid Capsules 979
Topamax Sprinkle Capsules (Rare) 2438
Topamax Tablets (Rare) 2438
Uniretic Tablets (Less than 1%) 3114
Vantin Tablets and Oral Suspension 2650
Xifaxan Tablets (Less than 2%) 2847
Zithromax for Oral Suspension, 300 mg, 600 mg, 900 mg, 1200 mg (Greater than 1%) 2561
Zithromax Tablets, 250 mg, 500 mg (Greater than 1%) 2561
Zithromax Tri-Pak (Greater than 1%) 2561

Lymphoma
Amevive (Less than 0.1%) 836
Azasan Tablets (0.5%) 2844
Campath Ampules 826
CellCept Capsules (0.4% to 1%) 2751
CellCept Intravenous (0.4% to 1%) 2751
CellCept Oral Suspension (0.4% to 1%) 2751
CellCept Tablets (0.4% to 1%) 2751
▲ Gengraf Capsules (Less than 1% to 6%) 458
Humira Injection 464
Myfortic Tablets (0.9% to 1.3%) 2244
▲ Neoral Soft Gelatin Capsules (Less than 1% to 6%) 2247
▲ Neoral Oral Solution (Less than 1% to 6%) 2247
Orthoclone OKT3 Sterile Solution (Less than 1%) 2370
Phenytek Capsules 2153
Prograf Capsules and Injection 624
▲ Rapamune Oral Solution and Tablets (0.6% to 3.2%) 3472
Remicade for IV Injection (Greater than or equal to 0.2%) 987
▲ Sandimmune (Less than 1% to 6%) 2259
Simulect for Injection (0.3%) 2268
Zenapax for Injection (1.5% or less) 2838

Lymphoma, Hodgkin's
Raptiva for Injection 1247

Lymphoma, lymphocytic
Dantrium Capsules (Less frequent) 2690
Dantrium Intravenous 2691

Lymphoma, non-Hodgkin's
Neurontin Capsules (Rare) 2498
Neurontin Oral Solution (Rare) 2498
Neurontin Tablets (Rare) 2498
Raptiva for Injection 1247

Lymphoma-like disorder
Colazal Capsules 2845
▲ Humira Injection (Less than 5%) 464
Paser Granules 1657
Peganone Tablets, USP 2487
Tegretol/Tegretol-XR 2278

Lymphopenia
(*see under* Lymphocytopenia)

Lymphoproliferative disorder
CellCept Capsules (0.4% to 1%) 2751
CellCept Intravenous (0.4% to 1%) 2751
CellCept Oral Suspension (0.4% to 1%) 2751
CellCept Tablets (0.4% to 1%) 2751
Orthoclone OKT3 Sterile Solution 2370
▲ Rapamune Oral Solution and Tablets (0.6% to 3.2%) 3472
Simulect for Injection 2268

M

Maceration
Aquacel AG with Hydrofiber 1035
Oxistat Cream (0.1%) 1498

Maceration, skin
Analpram-HC 1136
Diprolene Lotion 0.05% (Infrequent) 3016
Diprolene Ointment 0.05% (Infrequent) 3017
Diprolene AF Cream 0.05% (Infrequent) 3014
Locoid Cream (Infrequent) 1138
Locoid Lipocream Cream (Infrequent) 1138
Locoid (Infrequent) 1138
Neurontin Capsules (Rare) 2498
Neurontin Oral Solution (Rare) 2498
Neurontin Tablets (Rare) 2498
Olux Foam 1027
Pramosone 1139
ProctoFoam-HC 3113
Sulfamylon for 5% Topical Solution 2155
Temovate Scalp Application (Infrequent) 1551
Topicort .05% Gel 3288
Topicort .25% Cream 3288
Topicort .25% Ointment 3288
Topicort LP .05% Cream 3288
U-cort 1% Cream 3289
Vanos Cream 1864

Macrocytosis
Depacon Injection 412
Depakene 417
Depakote Sprinkle Capsules 422
▲ Depakote Tablets (1% to 5%) 427
Depakote ER Tablets 433
Phenytek Capsules 2153
Retrovir Capsules 1533
Retrovir IV Infusion 1537
Retrovir 1533

Macula lutea degeneration
Namenda (Infrequent) 1199

Maculae
Covera-HS Tablets (Less than 2%) 3135
Tarka Tablets 519
Verelan PM Capsules (2% or less) 3120

Macular degeneration
Cymbalta Delayed-Release Capsules (Infrequent) 1729
Pacerone Tablets 3337

Macular hypopigmentation
Zyprexa Tablets (Rare) 1798
Zyprexa ZYDIS Orally Disintegrating Tablets (Rare) 1798

Maculopathy
▲ Retisert Implant (10% to 35%) ⊙256

Malabsorption syndrome
Elspar for Injection 1943
Purinethol Tablets (Occasional) 1222
Sustiva Capsules 957

Malaise
Abelcet Injection 1119
Abilify Tablets (Frequent) 916
Abilify Tablets (Frequent) 2472
Accolate Tablets 663
Accutane Capsules 2740
Aceon Tablets (2 mg, 4 mg, 8 mg) (0.3% to 1%) 3191
Aciphex Tablets 1081
Actiq (1% or greater) 993
Adalat CC Tablets (Less than 1%) 2978
▲ Advair Diskus 250/50 (3%) 1291
Advicor Tablets 1694
Aerobid/Aerobid-M (1% to 3%) 1172
Aggrenox Capsules (1.6%) 855
▲ Agrylin Capsules (6.4%) 3172
Aldara Cream, 5% 1814
▲ Alferon N Injection (9% to 65%) 1640
Alinia for Oral Suspension (Less than 1%) 2840
Alinia Tablets (Less than 1%) 2840
Altace Capsules (Less than 1%) 1673
Altoprev Extended-Release Tablets (Rare) 1151
Ambien Tablets (Infrequent) 2867
AmBisome for Injection (Less common) 615
Amerge Tablets (2%) 1312
Amnesteem Capsules 2126
Anaprox Tablets (Less than 1%) 2769
Anaprox DS Tablets (Less than 1%) 2769
Antara Capsules 2723
Aptivus Capsules (Less than 2%) 859
▲ Arava Tablets (1% to 3%) 2881
▲ Arimidex Tablets (2% to 5%) 665
Arthrotec Tablets (Rare) 3126
Asacol Delayed-Release Tablets (1% to 2%) 2688
Astelin Nasal Spray (Infrequent) 1876
Attenuvax 1889
Avelox (0.1% to less than 2%) 2984
Avinza Capsules (Less than 5%) 1714
Azasan Tablets 2844
▲ Betaseron for SC Injection (8%) 791
BiDil Tablets (1% to less than 2%) 2161
Biltricide Tablets 2990
Buprenex Injectable (Infrequent) 2718
Caduet Tablets (Greater than 0.1% to less than 2%) 2507
Calcium Disodium Versenate Injection 1819
▲ Campath Ampules (1% to 9%) 826
Campral Tablets (Infrequent) 1175
Cancidas for Injection (0%) 1894
Captopril Tablets (0.5% to 2%) 2114
Cataflam Tablets (Occasionally) 2173
Catapres Tablets (About 1 in 100 patients) 874
Catapres-TTS (0.5% or less) 875
▲ CellCept Capsules (3% to less than 20%) 2751
▲ CellCept Intravenous (3% to less than 20%) 2751
▲ CellCept Oral Suspension (3% to less than 20%) 2751
▲ CellCept Tablets (3% to less than 20%) 2751
Cipro I.V. (1% or less) 2998
Cipro I.V. Pharmacy Bulk Package (1% or less) 3509
Cipro (Less than 1%) 2991
Cipro XR Tablets (Less than 1%) 3004
Clinoril Tablets (Less than 1 in 100) 1899
Clorpres Tablets (About 1%) 2139
Clozapine Tablets (Less than 1%) 2141
Clozaril Tablets (Less than 1%) 2174
Colazal Capsules 2845
▲ Combivir Tablets (27%) 1373
Copaxone for Injection (At least 2%) 3292
▲ Coreg Tablets (Greater than 1% to 3%) 1376
Cosmegen for Injection 1907
Coumadin for Injection (Infrequent) 932
Coumadin Tablets (Infrequent) 932
Crixivan Capsules (2.1%) 1918
Cytovene (At least 3 subjects) 2763
▲ Dantrium Capsules (Among most frequent) 2690
Decadron Phosphate Injection 1931
Decadron Tablets 1929
▲ Depacon Injection (1% to 5%) 412
▲ Depakene (1% to 5%) 417
▲ Depakote Sprinkle Capsules (1% to 5%) 422
▲ Depakote Tablets (1% to 5%) 427
Depakote ER Tablets (Greater than 1%) 433
Dolobid Tablets (Less than 1 in 100) 1937
▲ Dostinex Tablets (1% to less than 10%) 2631
▲ Doxil Injection (1% to 5%) 3302
EC-Naprosyn Delayed-Release Tablets (Less than 1%) 2769
Edecrin 1941
Effexor Tablets (Infrequent) 3405
Effexor XR Capsules (Infrequent) 3411
Eldepryl Capsules 3209
▲ Eligard 7.5 mg (17.5%) 2896
Emend Capsules (Greater than 0.5%) 1944
Engerix-B Vaccine (Less than 1%) 1391
▲ Entocort EC Capsules (Less than 5%) 2694
▲ Epivir (27%) 1394
▲ Epivir-HBV (24%) 1398
▲ Erbitux (49%) 937
Evoxac Capsules (Less than 1%) 1042
▲ Exelon Capsules (5%) 2204
FazaClo Orally Disintegrating Tablets (Less than 1%) 547
Ferrlecit Injection 3379
Flexeril Tablets (Less than 1%) 1832
▲ Flovent Diskus 50 mcg (1% to 16%) 1415
Follistim AQ Cartridge 2354
Foradil Aerolizer 3024
Fosamax 1949
Fosamax Plus D Tablets 1956
Frova Tablets (Infrequent) 1101
Gabitril Tablets (Frequent) 998
Gemzar for Injection (Infrequent) 1743
Gengraf Capsules (1% to less than 3%) 458
Gonal-f RFF Pen for Injection (2.4%) 3155
▲ Havrix Vaccine (1% to 10%) 1425
▲ Hectorol Capsules (27.9%) 909
▲ Hectorol Injection (27.9%) 911
HibTITER 3419
Hycamtin for Injection (0.5% to 1.8%) 1427
Hydrocortone Tablets 1963
Hyperstat I.V. Injection 3031
▲ Imdur Tablets (Less than or equal to 5%) 3032
Imitrex Injection (1.1%) 1431
Imitrex Tablets 1440
▲ Indapamide Tablets (Greater than or equal to 5%) 2119
Indocin (Greater than 1%) 1968
Infed Injection 3381
▲ Infergen (2% to 11%) 1647
▲ Intron A for Injection (Up to 14%) 3038
Invanz for Injection (Greater than 0.1%) 1974
Iveegam EN (0.3% to 0.8%) 759
Kadian Capsules (Less than 3%) 572
Kaletra (Less than 2%) 474
Klonopin (Infrequent) 2782
Lamictal (2.3%) 1449
Lamisil Tablets 2226
Lariam Tablets 2790
Lescol Capsules (Rare) 2227
Lescol Capsules (Rare) 2730
▲ Lescol XL Tablets (3.8%) 2227
▲ Lescol XL Tablets (3.8%) 2730
▲ Leukine (57%) 829
▲ Leustatin Injection (5% to 7%) 2368
Levaquin in 5% Dextrose Injection (0.1% to 0.9%) 2453
Levaquin (0.1% to 0.9%) 2453
Lexapro Oral Solution (Infrequent) 1193
Lexapro Tablets (Infrequent) 1193
Lipitor Tablets (Less than 2%) 2495
Lofibra Capsules 1217
Lotronex Tablets (Rare) 1479
Lunesta Tablets (Infrequent) 3139
Lyrica Capsules (0.1% to 1%) 2524
Marinol Capsules (Less than 1%) 3334
▲ Menactra Vaccine (1.1% to 23.6%) 2968
Menopur for Subcutaneous Injection (2.6%) 1145
Meruvax II 1994
Mevacor Tablets (Rare) 1996
Micardis Tablets (More than 0.3%) 884
Micardis HCT Tablets 886
▲ Mirapex Tablets (2% to 3%) 889
M-M-R II 1980
Mobic Oral Suspension (Less than 2%) 893
Mobic Tablets (Less than 2%) 893
Moduretic Tablets (Less than or equal to 1%) 2003
▲ Nabi-HB (6%) 2159
Nalfon Capsules (Less than 1%) 2504
Namenda 1199
Naprosyn Suspension (Less than 1%) 2769
Naprosyn Tablets (Less than 1%) 2769
Naropin Injection (Less than 1%) 640
▲ Navelbine Injection (Up to 67%) 1494
Neoral Soft Gelatin Capsules (1% to less than 3%) 2247
Neoral Oral Solution (1% to less than 3%) 2247
Neurontin Capsules (Frequent) 2498
Neurontin Oral Solution (Frequent) 2498
Neurontin Tablets (Frequent) 2498
Nexium Delayed-Release Capsules (Less than 1%) 645
Nexium I.V. (Less than 1%) 649
Norvasc Tablets (More than 0.1% to 1%) 2529
Norvir (0.7% to 1.7%) 499
Omacor Capsules 2735
▲ Oncaspar (Greater than 5%) 1123
Orthoclone OKT3 Sterile Solution (Less than 1%) 2370
Oxsoralen-Ultra Capsules 3354
OxyContin Tablets (Less than 1%) 2699
▲ Pacerone Tablets (4% to 9%) 3337
Parcopa Orally Disintegrating Tablets 3111
Paxil CR Controlled-Release Tablets (Frequent) 1509
Paxil (Frequent) 1501
Pediarix Vaccine 1518
▲ PEG-Intron Powder for Injection (7%) 3062
Pentasa Capsules (Less than 1%) 3182
Permax Tablets (Infrequent) 3357
Persantine Tablets (Rare) 898
Pletal Tablets (Less than 2%) 2478
Pneumovax 23 2020
Pravachol Tablets (Rare) 943
Prevacid Delayed-Release Capsules (Less than 1%) 3268
Prevacid for Delayed-Release Oral Suspension (Less than 1%) 3268
Prevacid NapraPAC (Less than 1%) 3277
Prevacid SoluTab Delayed-Release Orally Disintegrating Tablets (Less than 1%) 3268
PREVPAC (Less than 1%) 3281
Prilosec OTC Tablets (Less than 1%) 2674
Prinivil Tablets (0.3% to 1.0%) 2029
Prinzide Tablets 2033
▲ Proleukin for Injection (27%) 1007

▲ ProSom Tablets (5%) 512
Protonix I.V. (Less than 1%) 3468
Protonix Tablets (Less than 1%) 3465
Protopic Ointment (Greater than or equal to 1%) 629
Proventil Inhalation Solution 0.083% (1.5%) 3069
Prozac Pulvules and Liquid (Infrequent) 1771
Pulmozyme Inhalation Solution 1245
▲ Rabies Vaccine RabAvert (15% to 20%) 1011
▲ Rapamune Oral Solution and Tablets (3% to 20%) 3472
Razadyne (Frequent) 2434
▲ Rebetol (4% to 6%) 3073
▲ Rebif Prefilled Syringe for Injection (4% to 5%) 3163
Recombivax HB (Equal to or greater than 1%) 2045
Relafen Tablets (1%) 1523
Relenza Rotadisk (Less than 1.5%) 1525
Relpax Tablets (Infrequent) 2531
Repronex for Intramuscular and Subcutaneous Injection 1148
▲ Requip Tablets (3%) 1528
Rescriptor Tablets 2535
▲ Retrovir Capsules (8% to 53.2%) 1533
▲ Retrovir IV Infusion (8% to 53.2%) 1537
▲ Retrovir (8% to 53.2%) 1533
Reyataz Capsules (Less than 3%) 948
Rhophylac (Occasionally) 3504
▲ Ribavirin, USP Capsules (4% to 6%) 3083
Rilutek Tablets (0.4% to 1.2%) 2945
Risperdal Consta Long-Acting Injection (Infrequent) 1664
Risperdal M-Tab Orally Disintegrating Tablets (Infrequent) 1658
Risperdal (Infrequent) 1658
▲ Rituxan for Infusion (1% to 5%) 845
▲ Rituxan I.V. (1% to 5%) 1251
Roferon-A Injection (1%) 2805
Rythmol SR Capsules 2736
Seroquel Tablets (Infrequent) 691
▲ Simulect for Injection (3% to 10%) 2268
Sonata Capsules (Less than 1% to 2%) 1686
Soriatane Capsules (Less than 1%) 1028
Stalevo Tablets 2270
Sular Tablets (Less than or equal to 1%) 1163
Surmontil Capsules 2347
Sustiva Capsules (Less than 2%) 957
Symbyax Capsules (Infrequent) 1788
Tambocor Tablets (1% to 3%) 1824
Tarka Tablets (0.3% or more) 519
Tasmar Tablets (1%) 3360
Teveten Tablets (Less than 1%) 1707
Teveten HCT Tablets (Less than 1%) 1710
▲ Thalomid Capsules (8.3%) 979
▲ Thymoglobulin for Injection (13.4%) 2848
Tindamax (1.1% to 2.1%) 2670
▲ TOBI Solution for Inhalation (6.2%) 1015
Tricor Tablets 523
Triglide Tablets 1165
Trileptal Oral Suspension 2281
Trileptal Tablets 2281
▲ Trizivir Tablets (44%) 1565
Univasc Tablets (Less than 1%) 3118
Urecholine Tablets 2349
Vantas (Less than 2%) 3367
Vantin Tablets and Oral Suspension (Less than 1%) 2650
Varivax (Greater than or equal to 1%) 2070
▲ Velcade for Injection (65%) 2102
Verelan PM Capsules 3120
▲ Vesanoid Capsules (66%) 2823
Viadur Implant (Less than 2%) 782
Viracept (Less than 2%) 2556
Viramune Oral Suspension 903
Viramune Tablets 903
Voltaren Tablets (Occasionally) 2298
Voltaren-XR Tablets (Occasionally) 2301
Vytorin 10/10 Tablets 2084
Vytorin 10/10 Tablets 3092
Vytorin 10/20 Tablets 2084
Vytorin 10/20 Tablets 3092
Vytorin 10/40 Tablets 2084
Vytorin 10/40 Tablets 3092
Vytorin 10/80 Tablets 2084
Vytorin 10/80 Tablets 3092
Wellbutrin SR Sustained-Release Tablets (Rare) 1583
Wellbutrin XL Extended-Release Tablets (Rare) 1588
Xanax XR Tablets (Frequent) 2655
Xifaxan Tablets (Less than 2%) 2847
Zantac (Rare) 1597
Zantac Injection (Rare) 1593
Zantac Injection Pharmacy Bulk Package (Rare) 1595
Zantac Syrup (Rare) 1597
Zegerid Powder for Oral Solution (Less than 1%) 2972
Zestoretic Tablets 701
Zestril Tablets (0.3% to 1.0%) 704
▲ Ziagen (12%) 1600
▲ Zinecard for Injection (48% to 61%) 2659
Zithromax Capsules, 250 mg (1% or less) 2568
Zithromax for Oral Suspension, 300 mg, 600 mg, 900 mg, 1200 mg (1% or less) 2561
Zithromax Tablets, 250 mg, 500 mg (1% or less) 2561
Zithromax Tri-Pak (1% or less) 2561
Zmax for Oral Suspension 2577
Zocor Tablets (Rare) 2078
▲ Zofran Injection (5%) 1607
▲ Zofran (9% to 13%) 1613
▲ Zofran ODT Orally Disintegrating Tablets (9% to 13%) 1613
Zoladex (1% to 5%) 709
Zoladex 3-month 712
▲ Zoloft (1% to 10%) 2581
Zomig Tablets (Infrequent) 714
Zomig-ZMT Tablets (Infrequent) 714
Zonegran Capsules (Infrequent) 1089
Zosyn (1.0% or less) 3492
▲ Zovirax (11.5%) 1616
Zyban Sustained-Release Tablets (Rare) 1620
Zyprexa Tablets (Infrequent) 1798
Zyprexa ZYDIS Orally Disintegrating Tablets (Infrequent) 1798
▲ Zyrtec Chewable Tablets (Less than 2% to 3.6%) 2589
▲ Zyrtec (Less than 2% to 3.6%) 2589
Zyrtec-D 12 Hour Extended Release Tablets (Less than 2%) 2591

Malaria relapse

Aramine Injection 1889

Male pattern baldness

(*see under* Alopecia hereditaria)

Malignancies, secondary

I.V. Busulfex 1125
Leukeran Tablets 1472
Temodar Capsules 3088
Xolair 1259
Zevalin Injection (2%) 848

Malignancies, various types

Enbrel for Injection 580
Kineret Injection (45 patients) 594
Rapamune Oral Solution and Tablets (1.1% to 2.2%) 3472
Remicade for IV Injection (18 of 1678 patients) 987
Xolair 1259

Malignancy

Amevive (1.3% to 1.8%) 836
Myfortic Tablets (0.5%) 2244
Raptiva for Injection 1247
▲ Zenapax for Injection (2.7% to 7.8%) 2838

Malignant hyperthermia

Proleukin for Injection (Less than 1%) 1007
Sandostatin LAR Depot (Rare) 2264
Ultane Liquid for Inhalation (Less than 1%) 526

Malignant melanoma

Parcopa Orally Disintegrating Tablets 3111
Raptiva for Injection 1247
Xolair 1259

Malignant neoplasms

CellCept Capsules (0.7% to 2.1%) 2751
CellCept Intravenous (0.7% to 2.1%) 2751
CellCept Oral Suspension (0.7% to 2.1%) 2751
CellCept Tablets (0.7% to 2.1%) 2751
Emend Capsules (Greater than 0.5%) 1944
Orthoclone OKT3 Sterile Solution (Less than 1%) 2370
Xolair 1259

Malignant neoplasms, aggravated

Zometa for Intravenous Infusion 2306

Mania

Cymbalta Delayed-Release Capsules (Infrequent) 1729
Paxil CR Controlled-Release Tablets 1509
Paxil 1501
Prozac Pulvules and Liquid 1771
Surmontil Capsules 2347
Symbyax Capsules 1788
Vivactil Tablets 2350
Zoloft 2581

Manic behavior

Abilify Tablets (Frequent) 916
Abilify Tablets (Frequent) 2472
Ambien Tablets (Rare) 2867
Campral Tablets (Rare) 1175
Celexa 1177
Cipro I.V. (1% or less) 2998
Cipro I.V. Pharmacy Bulk Package (1% or less) 3509
Cipro (Less than 1%) 2991
Cipro XR Tablets 3004
Copaxone for Injection (Infrequent) 3292
Effexor Tablets (0.5%) 3405
Effexor XR Capsules (0.5%) 3411
Evoxac Capsules (Less than 1%) 1042
Herceptin I.V. (At least one of the 958 patients) 1234
▲ Intron A for Injection (Less than 5%) 3038
Lamictal (Rare) 1449
Levaquin in 5% Dextrose Injection (0.1% to 0.9%) 2453
Levaquin (0.1% to 0.9%) 2453
Neurontin Capsules (Rare) 2498
Neurontin Oral Solution (Rare) 2498
Neurontin Tablets (Rare) 2498
Orthoclone OKT3 Sterile Solution (Less than 1%) 2370
Parnate Tablets 1499
Paxil CR Controlled-Release Tablets (Infrequent) 1509
Paxil (Infrequent) 1501
Permax Tablets (Infrequent) 3357
Provigil Tablets 1002
Relpax Tablets (Rare) 2531
Requip Tablets (Infrequent) 1528
Rescriptor Tablets 2535
Retrovir IV Infusion 1537
Rilutek Tablets (Infrequent) 2945
Risperdal Consta Long-Acting Injection (Infrequent) 1664
▲ Risperdal M-Tab Orally Disintegrating Tablets (8%) 1658
▲ Risperdal (8%) 1658
Roferon-A Injection 2805
Seroquel Tablets (Infrequent) 691
Sustiva Capsules (0.2%) 957
Symmetrel 1115
Tasmar Tablets (Infrequent) 3360
Topamax Sprinkle Capsules (Rare) 2438
Topamax Tablets (Rare) 2438
Trileptal Oral Suspension 2281
Trileptal Tablets 2281
Valtrex Caplets 1573
Wellbutrin Tablets (Frequent) 1579
Wellbutrin SR Sustained-Release Tablets 1583
Wellbutrin XL Extended-Release Tablets 1588
Xanax XR Tablets (Infrequent) 2655
Zomig Nasal Spray (Rare) 718
Zyban Sustained-Release Tablets 1620
Zyprexa Tablets (Frequent) 1798

Manic reaction

▲ Equetro Extended-Release Capsules (Less than 5%) 3178
Lyrica Capsules (Rare) 2524

Manic-depressive reaction

Abilify Tablets (Infrequent) 916
Abilify Tablets (Infrequent) 2472
▲ Equetro Extended-Release Capsules (7%) 3178

Marrow aplasia

Aloprim for Injection (Less than 1%) 2156

Masculinization, female fetus

Oxandrin Tablets 2977

Mass, abdominal

(*see under* Abdominal mass)

Mass at injection site

Amevive (1%) 836
Betaseron for SC Injection (2%) 791
Boostrix 1366
HibTITER 3419
Xolair 1259

Mastalgia

(*see under* Mastodynia)

Mastitis

Amerge Tablets (Rare) 1312
Aricept Tablets (Infrequent) 1086
Aricept ODT Tablets (Infrequent) 1086
Doxil Injection (Less than 1%) 3302
Effexor Tablets (Rare) 3405
Effexor XR Capsules (Rare) 3411
▲ Intron A for Injection (Less than or equal to 5%) 3038
Lunesta Tablets (Infrequent) 3139
Paxil CR Controlled-Release Tablets (Rare) 1509
Paxil (Rare) 1501
Requip Tablets (Rare) 1528
Risperdal M-Tab Orally Disintegrating Tablets (Infrequent) 1658
Risperdal (Infrequent) 1658
Zoloft (Rare) 2581
Zonegran Capsules (Rare) 1089

Mastodynia

Climara Transdermal System 795
Estratest Tablets 3196
Estratest H.S. Tablets 3196
Inspra Tablets (0.1%) 2520
Nalfon Capsules (Less than 1%) 2504
Premarin Intravenous 3440
Premarin Vaginal Cream 3449

Mazzotti reactions, worsening of

Stromectol Tablets 2053

Mediastinal disorders, unspecified

▲ Ammonul Injection (15%) 3323
▲ Focalin XR Capsules (9% to 16%) 2217

Megacolon, toxic

Camptosar Injection (Rare) 2602
Numorphan 1112

Megaloblastic anemia

(*see under* Anemia, megaloblastic)

Megaloblastosis

Maxzide 2150

Melancholia

Celexa (Rare) 1177

Melanoma, malignant, activation of

Stalevo Tablets 2270

Melanoma, skin

Paxil CR Controlled-Release Tablets 1509
Paxil 1501
Rapamune Oral Solution and Tablets (0.4% to 1.4%) 3472

Melanoma, unspecified

Bexxar 1360
Humira Injection 464

Melanosis

Celexa (Rare) 1177
Copaxone for Injection (Infrequent) 3292
▲ Intron A for Injection (Less than 5%) 3038
Lyrica Capsules (Rare) 2524
Neurontin Capsules (Rare) 2498
Neurontin Oral Solution (Rare) 2498
Neurontin Tablets (Rare) 2498
Sonata Capsules (Rare) 1686
VFEND I.V. (Less than 2%) 2543
VFEND Oral Suspension (Less than 2%) 2543
VFEND Tablets (Less than 2%) 2543

Melasma

(*see under* Chloasma)

Melasma, possibly persistent

Estratest Tablets 3196
Estratest H.S. Tablets 3196
Estrogel 0.06% 3200
Premarin Tablets 3443
Premphase Tablets 3452
Prempro Tablets 3452
Yasmin 28 Tablets 818

Melena

Abelcet Injection 1119
Abilify Tablets (Rare) 916
Abilify Tablets (Rare) 2472

Aciphex Tablets 1081
Aggrenox Capsules (1.9%) 855
Agrylin Capsules (1% to 5%) 3172
Anaprox Tablets (Less than 1%) 2769
Anaprox DS Tablets (Less than 1%) 2769
▲ Arava Tablets (1% to 3%) 2881
Aricept Tablets (Infrequent) 1086
Aricept ODT Tablets (Infrequent) 1086
Arthrotec Tablets (Rare) 3126
Caduet Tablets (Less than 2%) 2507
Campath Ampules 826
Campral Tablets (Rare) 1175
▲ Carnitor Injection (2% to 6%) 3185
▲ Casodex Tablets (2% to 5%) 670
Cataflam Tablets (Occasionally) 2173
Celebrex Capsules (0.1% to 1.9%) 3130
▲ CellCept Capsules (3% to less than 20%) 2751
▲ CellCept Intravenous (3% to less than 20%) 2751
▲ CellCept Oral Suspension (3% to less than 20%) 2751
▲ CellCept Tablets (3% to less than 20%) 2751
Colazal Capsules 2845
Copaxone for Injection (Infrequent) 3292
▲ Coreg Tablets (Greater than 1% to 3%) 1376
Cymbalta Delayed-Release Capsules (Infrequent) 1729
Doxil Injection (Less than 1%) 3302
EC-Naprosyn Delayed-Release Tablets (Less than 1%) 2769
Effexor Tablets (Infrequent) 3405
Effexor XR Capsules (Infrequent) 3411
▲ Eloxatin for Injection (2% to 5%) 2908
Evoxac Capsules (Less than 1%) 1042
Exelon Capsules (Infrequent) 2204
Ferrlecit Injection 3379
Fosamax (Up to 1.3%) 1949
Fosamax Plus D Tablets (0% to 1.3%) 1956
Gabitril Tablets (Infrequent) 998
Geodon Capsules (Rare) 2514
▲ Imdur Tablets (Less than or equal to 5%) 3032
Imitrex Injection 1431
Imitrex Nasal Spray (Rare) 1435
Imitrex Tablets (Rare) 1440
▲ Intron A for Injection (Less than 5%) 3038
Invirase (Less than 2%) 2776
Lamictal (Rare) 1449
Levaquin in 5% Dextrose Injection (0.1% to 0.9%) 2453
Levaquin (0.1% to 0.9%) 2453
Lipitor Tablets (Less than 2%) 2495
Lotensin Tablets (Less than 1%) 2232
Lotensin HCT Tablets 2235
Lunesta Tablets (Infrequent) 3139
Lyrica Capsules (0.1% to 1%) 2524
Matulane Capsules 3188
Merrem I.V. (0.3%) 687
Mobic Oral Suspension (Less than 2%) 893
Mobic Tablets (Less than 2%) 893
Mylotarg for Injection (1%) 3429
Namenda (Infrequent) 1199
Naprosyn Suspension (Less than 1%) 2769
Naprosyn Tablets (Less than 1%) 2769
Neurontin Capsules (Rare) 2498
Neurontin Oral Solution (Rare) 2498
Neurontin Tablets (Rare) 2498
Nexium Delayed-Release Capsules (Less than 1%) 645
Nexium I.V. (Less than 1%) 649
Omacor Capsules 2735
Omnicef Capsules 506
Omnicef for Oral Suspension 506
Paxil CR Controlled-Release Tablets (Rare) 1509
Paxil (Rare) 1501
Permax Tablets (Infrequent) 3357
▲ Photofrin for Injection (5%) 729
Pletal Tablets (Less than 2%) 2478
Prevacid Delayed-Release Capsules (Less than 1%) 3268
Prevacid for Delayed-Release Oral Suspension (Less than 1%) 3268
Prevacid NapraPAC (Less than 1%) 3277
Prevacid SoluTab Delayed-Release Orally Disintegrating Tablets (Less than 1%) 3268
PREVPAC (Less than 1%) 3281
ProSom Tablets (Rare) 512
Protonix I.V. (Less than 1%) 3468
Protonix Tablets (Less than 1%) 3465
Prozac Pulvules and Liquid (Infrequent) 1771
Razadyne ER Extended-Release Capsules (Infrequent) 2434
Razadyne (Infrequent) 2434
Relafen Tablets (Less than 1%) 1523
Requip Tablets (Infrequent) 1528
Rilutek Tablets (Rare) 2945
Risperdal Consta Long-Acting Injection (Infrequent) 1664
Risperdal M-Tab Orally Disintegrating Tablets (Infrequent) 1658
Risperdal (Infrequent) 1658
Rythmol SR Capsules 2736
Sandostatin LAR Depot (1% to 4%) 2264
Seroquel Tablets (Rare) 691
▲ Simulect for Injection (3% to 10%) 2268
Sonata Capsules (Infrequent) 1686
Soriatane Capsules (Less than 1%) 1028
Sular Tablets (Less than or equal to 1%) 1163
Targretin Capsules 1719
Topamax Sprinkle Capsules (Infrequent) 2438
Topamax Tablets (Infrequent) 2438
Ultracet Tablets (Less than 1%) 2462
Uniretic Tablets (Less than 1%) 3114
Vaseretic Tablets 2073
Vasotec I.V. Injection (0.5% to 1.0%) 2076
VFEND I.V. (Less than 2%) 2543
VFEND Oral Suspension (Less than 2%) 2543
VFEND Tablets (Less than 2%) 2543
Vicoprofen Tablets (Less than 3%) 533
Voltaren Tablets (Occasionally) 2298
Voltaren-XR Tablets (Occasionally) 2301
Zevalin Injection (2%) 848
Zithromax (1% or less) 2568
Zithromax for Oral Suspension, 300 mg, 600 mg, 900 mg, 1200 mg (1% or less) 2561
Zithromax Tablets, 250 mg, 500 mg (1% or less) 2561
Zithromax Tablets, 600 mg (1% or less) 2568
Zithromax Tri-Pak (1% or less) 2561
Zithromax Z-Pak (1% or less) 2568
Zoloft (Rare) 2581
Zomig Tablets (Rare) 714
Zomig-ZMT Tablets (Rare) 714
Zonegran Capsules (Infrequent) 1089
Zosyn (1.0% or less) 3492
Zyprexa Tablets (Infrequent) 1798
Zyprexa ZYDIS Orally Disintegrating Tablets (Infrequent) 1798
Zyrtec Chewable Tablets (Less than 2%) 2589
Zyrtec (Less than 2%) 2589
Zyrtec-D 12 Hour Extended Release Tablets (Less than 2%) 2591

Memory impairment

Abilify Tablets (Infrequent) 916
Abilify Tablets (Infrequent) 2472
Buphenyl Powder 3327
Buphenyl Tablets 3327
Cogentin Injection 1903
Copaxone for Injection (Infrequent) 3292
▲ Copegus Tablets (6%) 2759
Cozaar Tablets (Less than 1%) 1913
Eldepryl Capsules 3209
Eskalith 1406
Gleevec Tablets (Infrequent) 2221
Hyzaar 1964
Imitrex Nasal Spray (Rare) 1435
Imitrex Tablets (Rare) 1440
▲ Klonopin (4%) 2782
Lamictal (2.4%) 1449
Lithobid Tablets 1670
Lunesta Tablets (Infrequent) 3139
▲ Lupron Depot 3.75 mg (Among most frequent) 3257
Lupron Depot–3 Month 11.25 mg (Less than 5%) 3262
Maxalt Tablets (Infrequent) 1983
Maxalt-MLT Orally Disintegrating Tablets (Infrequent) 1983
▲ Niravam Orally Disintegrating Tablets (5.5% to 33.1%) 3106
Parcopa Orally Disintegrating Tablets 3111
▲ Pegasys (5%) 2793
Prinivil Tablets (0.3% to 1.0%) 2029
Prinzide Tablets 2033
Roferon-A Injection (Less than 4%) 2805
Seromycin Capsules 1783
Stalevo Tablets 2270
▲ Temodar Capsules (7%) 3088
Timolide Tablets 2056
▲ Topamax Sprinkle Capsules (2% to 14%) 2438
▲ Topamax Tablets (2% to 14%) 2438
Transderm Scōp Transdermal Therapeutic System (Infrequent) 2166
▲ Vesanoid Capsules (3%) 2823
Wellbutrin Tablets (Infrequent) 1579
Wellbutrin SR Sustained-Release Tablets (Up to 3%) 1583
Wellbutrin XL Extended-Release Tablets (Up to 3%) 1588
▲ Xanax XR Tablets (15.4%) 2655
Zestoretic Tablets 701
▲ Zonegran Capsules (6%) 1089
Zyban Sustained-Release Tablets (Infrequent) 1620

Memory loss, short-term

Altoprev Extended-Release Tablets 1151
Blocadren Tablets 1891
Clozapine Tablets (Less than 1%) 2141
Clozaril Tablets (Less than 1%) 2174
Cosopt Sterile Ophthalmic Solution 1910
Cytovene 2763
Inderal LA Long-Acting Capsules 3421
InnoPran XL Capsules 2728
Lescol Capsules 2227
Lescol Capsules 2730
Lescol XL Tablets 2227
Lescol XL Tablets 2730
Meridia Capsules 485
Mevacor Tablets (0.5% to 1.0%) 1996
Nadolol Tablets 2121
Parnate Tablets 1499
Pravachol Tablets 943
Tenormin I.V. Injection 698
Tenormin Tablets 695
Timoptic in Ocudose 2061
Timoptic Sterile Ophthalmic Solution 2058
Timoptic-XE Sterile Ophthalmic Gel Forming Solution 2062
Toprol-XL Tablets 660
▲ Zavesca Capsules (8%) 543
Zocor Tablets 2078

Mendelson's syndrome

Abilify Tablets (Rare) 916
Abilify Tablets (Rare) 2472

Meniere's syndrome

Imitrex Nasal Spray (Rare) 1435
Imitrex Tablets 1440

Meningioma

Zevalin Injection 848

Meningism

Albenza Tablets (Up to 1.0%) 1310
Neurontin Capsules (Rare) 2498
Neurontin Oral Solution (Rare) 2498
Neurontin Tablets (Rare) 2498
Nipent for Injection (Less than 3%) 3216

Meningismus

Naropin Injection 640

Meningitis

Arthrotec Tablets (Rare) 3126
Campath Ampules 826
Cataflam Tablets (Rarely) 2173
CellCept Capsules (Occasional) 2751
CellCept Intravenous (Occasional) 2751
CellCept Oral Suspension (Occasional) 2751
CellCept Tablets (Occasional) 2751
Depo-Medrol Single-Dose Vial 2617
Myfortic Tablets (Occasionally) 2244
Orthoclone OKT3 Sterile Solution (Less than 1%) 2370
Paxil CR Controlled-Release Tablets (Rare) 1509
Paxil (Rare) 1501
Permax Tablets (Infrequent) 3357
Proleukin for Injection (Less than 1%) 1007
Rabies Vaccine RabAvert 1011
Remicade for IV Injection (Greater than or equal to 0.2%) 987
Tasmar Tablets (Rare) 3360
Voltaren Tablets (Rarely) 2298
Voltaren-XR Tablets (Rarely) 2301

Meningitis, aseptic

Anaprox Tablets (Less than 1%) 2769
Anaprox DS Tablets (Less than 1%) 2769
Arthrotec Tablets (Rare) 3126
Carbatrol Capsules (One case) 3174
Celebrex Capsules (Less than 0.1%) 3130
EC-Naprosyn Delayed-Release Tablets (Less than 1%) 2769
Gammagard Liquid 751
Gamunex Immune Globulin I.V., 10% (Very rare) 3232
Mumpsvax 2005
Naprosyn Suspension (Less than 1%) 2769
Naprosyn Tablets (Less than 1%) 2769
Prevacid NapraPAC (Less than 1%) 3277
Raptiva for Injection (1 case) 1247
Tegretol/Tegretol-XR (One case) 2278
Vicoprofen Tablets (Rare) 533

Meningitis, septic

Naropin Injection 640

Meningitis, infectious

DepoCyt Injection 1121

Menometrorrhagia

▲ depo-subQ provera 104 Injectable Suspension (1% to less than 5%) 2622

Menopause

Effexor Tablets (Rare) 3405
Effexor XR Capsules (Rare) 3411
Permax Tablets (Infrequent) 3357
Sonata Capsules (Rare) 1686
Symbyax Capsules (Infrequent) 1788
Wellbutrin Tablets (Rare) 1579
Wellbutrin SR Sustained-Release Tablets 1583
Wellbutrin XL Extended-Release Tablets 1588
Zyban Sustained-Release Tablets 1620

Menorrhagia

Abilify Tablets (Rare) 916
Abilify Tablets (Rare) 2472
Aciphex Tablets (Rare) 1081
Arthrotec Tablets (Rare) 3126
Asacol Delayed-Release Tablets 2688
Avonex 839
▲ Betaseron for SC Injection (8%) 791
Campral Tablets (Rare) 1175
▲ CombiPatch Transdermal System (2% to 5%) 2180
▲ depo-subQ provera 104 Injectable Suspension (1% to less than 5%) 2622
Effexor Tablets (Infrequent) 3405
Effexor XR Capsules (Infrequent) 3411
Evoxac Capsules (Less than 1%) 1042
Gabitril Tablets (Infrequent) 998
Geodon Capsules (Infrequent) 2514
Gleevec Tablets (Infrequent) 2221
▲ Intron A for Injection (Less than 5%) 3038
Lamictal (Rare) 1449
Lunesta Tablets (Infrequent) 3139
Lyrica Capsules (0.1% to 1%) 2524
Neurontin Capsules (Infrequent) 2498
Neurontin Oral Solution (Infrequent) 2498
Neurontin Tablets (Infrequent) 2498
Paxil CR Controlled-Release Tablets (Infrequent) 1509
Paxil (Infrequent) 1501
Pentasa Capsules (Less than 1%) 3182
Permax Tablets (Infrequent) 3357
Plavix Tablets (Less than 1%) 940
Plavix Tablets (Less than 1%) 2942
Prevacid Delayed-Release Capsules (Less than 1%) 3268
Prevacid for Delayed-Release Oral Suspension (Less than 1%) 3268
Prevacid NapraPAC (Less than 1%) 3277
Prevacid SoluTab Delayed-Release Orally Disintegrating Tablets (Less than 1%) 3268
PREVPAC (Less than 1%) 3281
Prozac Pulvules and Liquid (At least 2%) 1771
▲ Rapamune Oral Solution and Tablets (3% to 20%) 3472
Relpax Tablets (Rare) 2531
Risperdal M-Tab Orally Disintegrating Tablets (Frequent) 1658
Risperdal (Frequent) 1658
Seroquel Tablets (Infrequent) 691
Sonata Capsules (Infrequent) 1686
Symbyax Capsules (Frequent) 1788
Topamax Sprinkle Capsules (1% to 2%) 2438
Topamax Tablets (1% to 2%) 2438
Trileptal Oral Suspension 2281
Trileptal Tablets 2281
Zelnorm Tablets 2303
▲ Zoladex (4%) 709
Zoloft (Rare) 2581
Zomig Nasal Spray (Infrequent) 718
Zonegran Capsules (Rare) 1089
Zyprexa Tablets (Infrequent) 1798
Zyprexa ZYDIS Orally Disintegrating Tablets (Infrequent) 1798
Zyrtec Chewable Tablets (Less than 2%) 2589
Zyrtec (Less than 2%) 2589
Zyrtec-D 12 Hour Extended Release Tablets (Less than 2%) 2591

Menstrual cramps
Lexapro Oral Solution (Frequent) 1193
Lexapro Tablets (Frequent) 1193
▲ Ortho Evra Transdermal System (9% to 22%) 2402

Menstrual disorders
Aceon Tablets (2 mg, 4 mg, 8 mg) (1.1%) 3191
▲ Aerobid/Aerobid-M (3% to 9%) 1172
Ambien Tablets (Infrequent) 2867
Anaprox Tablets (Less than 1%) 2769
Anaprox DS Tablets (Less than 1%) 2769
▲ Arava Tablets (1% to 3%) 2881
Asmanex Twisthaler (1% to less than 3%) 2981
▲ Avonex (6%) 839
Celebrex Capsules (0.1% to 1.9%) 3130
Cleocin Vaginal Ovules (Less than 1%) 2613
Colazal Capsules 2845
▲ CombiPatch Transdermal System (17% to 19%) 2180
Depakote ER Tablets (Greater than 1%) 433
EC-Naprosyn Delayed-Release Tablets (Less than 1%) 2769
Effexor Tablets (1%) 3405
▲ Entocort EC Capsules (Less than 5%) 2694
Evoxac Capsules (Less than 1%) 1042
Gengraf Capsules (1%) 458
▲ Humira Injection (Less than 5%) 464
Lamictal (More than 1%) 1449
Lexapro Oral Solution (2% to frequent) 1193
Lexapro Tablets (2% to frequent) 1193
Lotronex Tablets (Infrequent) 1479
Lupron Depot 3.75 mg (1%) 3257
Lupron Depot–3 Month 11.25 mg (1%) 3262
Maxalt Tablets (Infrequent) 1983
Maxalt-MLT Orally Disintegrating Tablets (Infrequent) 1983
▲ Menopur for Subcutaneous Injection (3.2%) 1145
Meridia Capsules (Greater than or equal to 1%) 485
Mustargen for Injection 2007
Naprosyn Suspension (Less than 1%) 2769
Naprosyn Tablets (Less than 1%) 2769
Neoral Soft Gelatin Capsules (1%) 2247
Neoral Oral Solution (1%) 2247
Neurontin Capsules (Infrequent) 2498
Neurontin Oral Solution (Infrequent) 2498
Neurontin Tablets (Infrequent) 2498
Nexium Delayed-Release Capsules (Less than 1%) 645
Nexium I.V. (Less than 1%) 649
▲ Nicotrol NS (4%) 2596
▲ Niravam Orally Disintegrating Tablets (10.4%) 3106
▲ Novantrone for Injection Concentrate (51% to 61%) 3158
▲ PEG-Intron Powder for Injection (4%) 3062
Prevacid Delayed-Release Capsules (Less than 1%) 3268
Prevacid for Delayed-Release Oral Suspension (Less than 1%) 3268
Prevacid NapraPAC (Less than 1%) 3277
Prevacid SoluTab Delayed-Release Orally Disintegrating Tablets (Less than 1%) 3268
PREVPAC (Less than 1%) 3281
Provigil Tablets (At least 1%) 1002
▲ Rebetol (6% to 7%) 3073
Relpax Tablets (Rare) 2531
Reyataz Capsules (Less than 3%) 948
▲ Ribavirin, USP Capsules (6% to 7%) 3083
Sonata Capsules (Rare) 1686
▲ Strattera Capsules (3%) 1784
▲ Topamax Sprinkle Capsules (1% to 3%) 2438
▲ Topamax Tablets (1% to 3%) 2438
Vaqta (1.1%) 2067
▲ Wellbutrin Tablets (4.7%) 1579
Yasmin 28 Tablets (Greater than 1%) 818
Zoladex 709
Zoloft (Infrequent) 2581

Menstrual dysfunction
▲ Buphenyl Powder (23%) 3327
▲ Buphenyl Tablets (23%) 3327
▲ Zavesca Capsules (6%) 543

Menstrual flow, changes
Alesse-28 Tablets 3392
Aygestin Tablets 1062
Cenestin Tablets, 0.45mg, 0.625mg, 0.9mg, 1.25mg 1063
Cenestin Tablets, 0.3mg 1063
Coumadin for Injection 932
Coumadin Tablets 932
Estratest Tablets 3196
Estratest H.S. Tablets 3196
Estrogel 0.06% 3200
Lo/Ovral-28 Tablets 3423
Moban Tablets 1108
Ortho-Cept Tablets 2395
Ortho-Cyclen Tablets 2414
Ortho Evra Transdermal System 2402
Ortho Tri-Cyclen Tablets 2414
Ortho Tri-Cyclen Lo Tablets 2421
▲ Plan B Tablets (12.5% to 13.8%) 1068
Premarin Intravenous 3440
Premarin Tablets 3443
Premarin Vaginal Cream 3449
Seasonale Tablets 1073
Strattera Capsules (2%) 1784
Tarka Tablets 519
Triphasil-28 Tablets 3483
Vivelle Transdermal System 2288
Vivelle-Dot Transdermal System 2293

Menstrual irregularities
Accutane Capsules 2740
Advair Diskus 100/50 1291
Advair Diskus 250/50 1291
Advair Diskus 500/50 1291
Amnesteem Capsules 2126
Anadrol-50 Tablets 3329
Arthrotec Tablets (Rare) 3126
Covera-HS Tablets (Less than 2%) 3135
Decadron Phosphate Injection 1931
Decadron Tablets 1929
▲ Delatestryl Injection (Among most frequent) 2976
Depacon Injection 412
Depakene 417
Depakote Sprinkle Capsules 422
Depakote Tablets 427
Depakote ER Tablets 433
Depo-Medrol Injectable Suspension 2615
Depo-Medrol Single-Dose Vial 2617
▲ Depo-Provera Contraceptive Injection (Greater than 5%) 2619
▲ depo-subQ provera 104 Injectable Suspension (1% to less than 5%) 2622
▲ Estratest Tablets (Among most common) 3196
▲ Estratest H.S. Tablets (Among most common) 3196
Hydrocortone Tablets 1963
Imitrex Nasal Spray 1435
▲ Infergen (2% to 6%) 1647
▲ Intron A for Injection (Less than 5%) 3038
Klonopin (Infrequent) 2782
Levothroid Tablets 1189
Levoxyl Tablets 1680
Librium Capsules 3349
Niravam Orally Disintegrating Tablets 3106
▲ Ortho Micronor Tablets (Among most frequent) 2411
Oxandrin Tablets 2977
Pediapred Oral Solution 3319
Premphase Tablets 3452
Prempro Tablets 3452
Prevacid Delayed-Release Capsules (Less than 1%) 3268
Prevacid for Delayed-Release Oral Suspension (Less than 1%) 3268
Prevacid NapraPAC (Less than 1%) 3277
Prevacid SoluTab Delayed-Release Orally Disintegrating Tablets (Less than 1%) 3268
PREVPAC (Less than 1%) 3281
Prometrium Capsules (100 mg, 200 mg) 3205
Remicade for IV Injection (Greater than or equal to 0.2%) 987
Roferon-A Injection (2%) 2805
Sandostatin LAR Depot (1% to 4%) 2264
Strattera Capsules (2%) 1784
Thioridazine Hydrochloride Tablets 2122
Unithroid Tablets 3521
Vantin Tablets and Oral Suspension (Less than 1%) 2650
▲ Xenical Capsules (9.8%) 2834
Zyprexa Tablets (Infrequent) 1798
Zyprexa ZYDIS Orally Disintegrating Tablets (Infrequent) 1798

Menstruation, painful
ProSom Tablets (Infrequent) 512

Mental acuity, loss of
Parcopa Orally Disintegrating Tablets 3111
Retrovir Capsules 1533
Retrovir IV Infusion 1537
Retrovir 1533
Stalevo Tablets 2270
Tasmar Tablets (1%) 3360

Mental clouding
Dilaudid Ampules 439
Dilaudid Non-Sterile Powder 439
Dilaudid Rectal Suppositories 439
Dilaudid Tablets 439
Hycodan 1104
Hycomine Compound Tablets 1105
Hycotuss Expectorant Syrup 1106
Lortab 3315
Lortab Elixir 3312
Numorphan 1112
Tussionex Pennkinetic Extended-Release Suspension 3322
Vicodin Tablets 530
Vicodin ES Tablets 531
Vicodin HP Tablets 532
Zydone Tablets 1118

Mental confusion
(*see under* Confusion)

Mental depression
(*see under* Depression)

Mental performance, impairment
Aldoclor Tablets 1881
Aldoril Tablets 1884
Alferon N Injection (1%) 1640
Ambien Tablets (Infrequent) 2867
Amerge Tablets (Infrequent) 1312
▲ Ammonul Injection (6%) 3323
Anaprox Tablets (Less than 1%) 2769
Anaprox DS Tablets (Less than 1%) 2769
Arthrotec Tablets (Rare) 3126
Celexa (Frequent) 1177
Clozapine Tablets 2141
Clozaril Tablets 2174
Copaxone for Injection (Infrequent) 3292
Cosopt Sterile Ophthalmic Solution 1910
Dilaudid 439
Dilaudid Non-Sterile Powder 439
Dilaudid Rectal Suppositories 439
Dilaudid Tablets 439
Dostinex Tablets (1%) 2631
EC-Naprosyn Delayed-Release Tablets (Less than 1%) 2769
Eskalith 1406
Exelon Capsules (Infrequent) 2204
Flumadine (0.3% to 2.1%) 1186
Frova Tablets (Infrequent) 1101
▲ Gabitril Tablets (6%) 998
Gengraf Capsules (1% to less than 3%) 458
Grifulvin V Tablets Microsize and Oral Suspension Microsize 2384
Hycodan 1104
Hycomine Compound Tablets 1105
Hycotuss Expectorant Syrup 1106
Imitrex Injection (Rare) 1431
Imitrex Nasal Spray (Rare) 1435
Imitrex Tablets (Infrequent) 1440
▲ Intron A for Injection (Up to 14%) 3038
Inversine Tablets 3286
Invirase (Less than 2%) 2776
Kadian Capsules (Less than 3%) 572
Klonopin (1% to 2%) 2782
Lamictal (1.7%) 1449
Levaquin in 5% Dextrose Injection (0.1% to 0.9%) 2453
Levaquin (0.1% to 0.9%) 2453
Lexapro Oral Solution (Frequent) 1193
Lexapro Tablets (Frequent) 1193
Lortab 3315
Lortab Elixir 3312
Maxalt Tablets (Frequent) 1983
Maxalt-MLT Orally Disintegrating Tablets (Infrequent) 1983
Meridia Capsules 485
Migranal Nasal Spray (Infrequent) 3350
MS Contin Tablets 2703
Naprosyn Suspension (Less than 1%) 2769
Naprosyn Tablets (Less than 1%) 2769
Neoral Soft Gelatin Capsules (1% to less than 3%) 2247
Neoral Oral Solution (1% to less than 3%) 2247
Orap Tablets 1220
Paxil CR Controlled-Release Tablets (Frequent) 1509
Paxil (Frequent) 1501
Percocet Tablets 1114
Percodan Tablets 1115
Phenergan 3438
Prometrium Capsules (100 mg, 200 mg) (Less than 5%) 3205
ProSom Tablets 512
Rebetron Combination Therapy 3078
Requip Tablets (Infrequent) 1528
Risperdal M-Tab Orally Disintegrating Tablets (Infrequent) 1658
Risperdal (Infrequent) 1658
▲ Roferon-A Injection (4%) 2805
Seroquel Tablets 691
Surmontil Capsules 2347
▲ Sustiva Capsules (1% to 9%) 957
Tarka Tablets (Less frequent) 519
Timolide Tablets 2056
Timoptic in Ocudose 2061
Timoptic Sterile Ophthalmic Solution 2058
Timoptic-XE Sterile Ophthalmic Gel Forming Solution 2062
▲ Topamax Sprinkle Capsules (5% to 14%) 2438
▲ Topamax Tablets (5% to 14%) 2438
Tussionex Pennkinetic Extended-Release Suspension 3322
Tylenol with Codeine 2461
Ultracet Tablets 2462
Vicodin Tablets 530
Vicodin ES Tablets 531
Vicodin HP Tablets 532
Vivactil Tablets 2350
▲ Xanax XR Tablets (7.2%) 2655
Zelnorm Tablets 2303
Zestril Tablets (0.3% to 1.0%) 704
Zoloft (1.3% to 2%) 2581
▲ Zonegran Capsules (6%) 1089
▲ Zyban Sustained-Release Tablets (9%) 1620
Zydone Tablets 1118
Zyrtec Chewable Tablets (Less than 2%) 2589
Zyrtec (Less than 2%) 2589
Zyrtec-D 12 Hour Extended Release Tablets (Less than 2%) 2591

Mental slowness
▲ Topamax Sprinkle Capsules (8% to 15.4%) 2438
▲ Topamax Tablets (8% to 15.4%) 2438
▲ Zonegran Capsules (4%) 1089

Mental status, altered
Clozapine Tablets 2141
Clozaril Tablets 2174
Cubicin for Injection (Less than 1%) 1038
Cuprimine Capsules 1925
▲ Digitek Tablets (5%) 2146
Eldepryl Capsules 3209
▲ Idamycin PFS Injection (41%) 2645
▲ Invanz for Injection (3.3% to 5.1%) 1974
Lanoxicaps Capsules 1458
Lanoxin Injection 1462
Lanoxin Tablets 1468
Lanoxin Injection Pediatric 1465
Moban Tablets 1108
Neumega for Injection 3433
Oncaspar 1123
Orap Tablets 1220
Orthoclone OKT3 Sterile Solution (Less than 1%) 2370
▲ Prograf Capsules and Injection (Approximately 55%) 624
▲ Proleukin for Injection (73%) 1007
Risperdal M-Tab Orally Disintegrating Tablets 1658
Risperdal 1658
▲ Roferon-A Injection (10% to 16%) 2805
Seroquel Tablets 691
Stalevo Tablets 2270
Stromectol Tablets 2053

Mesenteric arterial thrombosis
Blocadren Tablets 1891
Inderal LA Long-Acting Capsules 3421
InnoPran XL Capsules 2728
Lo/Ovral-28 Tablets 3423
Rilutek Tablets (Rare) 2945
Tenormin I.V. Injection 698
Tenormin Tablets 695
Timolide Tablets 2056
Timoptic in Ocudose 2061
Timoptic Sterile Ophthalmic Solution 2058
Triphasil-28 Tablets 3483

Metabolic acidosis
(*see under* Acidosis, metabolic)

Metabolic changes
Clinoril Tablets (Rare) 1899
▲ Leukine (58%) 829
▲ Menostar Transdermal System (12%) 805

▲ Neoral Soft Gelatin Capsules (9.3%) 2247
▲ Neoral Oral Solution (9.3%) 2247
Pravachol Tablets 943

Metabolism disorders, unspecified

▲ Ammonul Injection (21%) 3323
▲ Focalin XR Capsules (34%) 2217

Methemoglobinemia

Cipro I.V. 2998
Cipro I.V. Pharmacy Bulk Package ... 3509
Cipro 2991
Elitek (Less than 1%) 2906
Eulexin Capsules 3023
Hurricaine Topical Anesthetic Aerosol Spray, 2 oz. Wild Cherry (Extremely rare) 835
Hurricaine Topical Anesthetic Aerosol Spray Kit, 2 oz. Wild Cherry with 200 Disposable Extension Tubes (Extremely rare) 835
Hurricaine Topical Anesthetic Gel: 1 oz. Wild Cherry, Pina Colada, Watermelon, Fresh Mint, 0.18 oz. Wild Cherry (Extremely rare) 835
Hurricaine Topical Anesthetic Gel, 1 oz. Fresh Mint, Wild Cherry, Pina Colada, Watermelon, 1/6 oz. Wild Cherry (Extremely rare) .... ▣ 607
Hurricaine Topical Anesthetic Liquid: 1 oz. Wild Cherry and Pina Colada, Swab Applicator Wild Cherry (Extremely rare) 835
Hurricaine Topical Anesthetic Liquid, 1 oz. Wild Cherry, Pina Colada, .25 ml Swab Applicator Wild Cherry (Extremely rare) .... ▣ 607
Hurricaine Topical Anesthetic Spray Extension Tubes (200) (Extremely rare) .... ▣ 607
Hurricaine Topical Anesthetic Spray Kit, 2 oz. Wild Cherry (Extremely rare) .... ▣ 607
Hurricaine Topical Anesthetic Spray, 2 oz. Wild Cherry (Extremely rare) .... ▣ 607
Mepron Suspension 1487
Nitro-Dur Transdermal Infusion System (Very rare) 3060

Metrorrhagia

Aciphex Tablets 1081
Alinia for Oral Suspension (Less than 1%) 2840
Alinia Tablets (Less than 1%) 2840
Aricept Tablets (Infrequent) 1086
Aricept ODT Tablets (Infrequent) 1086
Avonex 839
▲ Betaseron for SC Injection (11%) 791
Caduet Tablets (Less than 2%) 2507
Campral Tablets (Infrequent) 1175
▲ Cenestin Tablets, 0.45mg, 0.625mg, 0.9mg, 1.25mg (14%) 1063
Copaxone for Injection (At least 2%) 3292
Depacon Injection (1% or more) 412
Depakene (1% or more) 417
Depakote Sprinkle Capsules 422
▲ Depakote Tablets (1% to 5%) 427
▲ Depakote ER Tablets (1% to 5%) 433
▲ Estrogel 0.06% (3%) 3200
Gabitril Tablets (Frequent) 998
Geodon Capsules (Infrequent) 2514
Lipitor Tablets (Less than 2%) 2495
Lunesta Tablets (Infrequent) 3139
Lyrica Capsules (0.1% to 1%) 2524
Meridia Capsules (1%) 485
▲ Mylotarg for Injection (2% to 10%) ... 3429
Paxil CR Controlled-Release Tablets (Rare) 1509
Paxil (Rare) 1501
Pentasa Capsules (Less than 1%) 3182
Permax Tablets (Infrequent) 3357
Prozac Pulvules and Liquid (Infrequent) 1771
▲ Rapamune Oral Solution and Tablets (3% to 20%) 3472
Rescriptor Tablets 2535
Rilutek Tablets (Infrequent) 2945
Sonata Capsules (Infrequent) 1686
Symbyax Capsules (Infrequent) 1788
Tequin Injection (Less than 0.1%) 964
Tequin Tablets (Less than 0.1%) 964
Thalomid Capsules 979
Vantin Tablets and Oral Suspension (Less than 1%) 2650
VFEND I.V. (Less than 2%) 2543
VFEND Oral Suspension (Less than 2%) 2543
VFEND Tablets (Less than 2%) 2543
Zomig Nasal Spray (Rare) 718
Zyprexa Tablets (Infrequent) 1798
Zyprexa ZYDIS Orally Disintegrating Tablets (Frequent) ... 1798

Metyrapone test, altered results

Aygestin Tablets 1062
Estratest Tablets 3196
Estratest H.S. Tablets 3196
Premarin Tablets 3443
Premphase Tablets 3452
Prempro Tablets 3452

Microcephaly, fetal

Accutane Capsules 2740
Phenytek Capsules 2153

Microphthalmia, fetal

Accutane Capsules 2740

Microphthalmos

Thalomid Capsules 979

Micropinna, fetal

Accutane Capsules 2740

Micturition, difficulty

Alacol DM Syrup 739
BiDil Tablets 2161
Blocadren Tablets 1891
▲ Casodex Tablets (2% to 5%) 670
Catapres Tablets (About 2 in 1,000 patients) 874
Catapres-TTS (0.5% or less) 875
▲ Chemet Capsules (Up to 3.7%) 2480
Clorpres Tablets (About 2 in 1,000) 2139
Combivent Inhalation Aerosol 878
Cosopt Sterile Ophthalmic Solution 1910
Dantrium Capsules (Less frequent) .. 2690
Effexor Tablets (2%) 3405
Effexor XR Capsules (Frequent) 3411
Eligard 22.5 mg (Less than 2%) 2899
Flexeril Tablets (Rare) 1832
▲ Niravam Orally Disintegrating Tablets (12.2%) 3106
OxyContin Tablets (Less than 1%) 2699
▲ Paxil CR Controlled-Release Tablets (3%) 1509
▲ Paxil (3%) 1501
ProAmatine Tablets (Rare) 3183
▲ Prometrium Capsules (100 mg, 200 mg) (11%) 3205
Timolide Tablets 2056
Timoptic in Ocudose 2061
Timoptic Sterile Ophthalmic Solution 2058
Timoptic-XE Sterile Ophthalmic Gel Forming Solution 2062
Transderm Scōp Transdermal Therapeutic System (Infrequent) ... 2166
Uroqid-Acid No. 2 Tablets (Occasional) 785
Vivactil Tablets 2350
VoSpire Extended-Release Tablets (Less frequent) 2352
Xanax XR Tablets (Frequent) 2655
Zonegran Capsules (Infrequent) 1089
Zovirax for Injection (Less than 1%) 1618
Zyprexa Tablets (Infrequent) 1798
Zyprexa ZYDIS Orally Disintegrating Tablets (Infrequent) 1798

Micturition, frequent

Caduet Tablets (Greater than 0.1% to less than or equal to 1%) 2507
Campral Tablets (Infrequent) 1175
▲ Doxil Injection (1% to 10%) 3302
Gonal-f RFF Pen for Injection (2.4%) 3155
Namenda (Frequent) 1199

Micturition, painful

Eligard 22.5 mg (Less than 2%) 2899
Uroqid-Acid No. 2 Tablets (Occasional) 785
Zoloft (Rare) 2581
Zovirax for Injection (Less than 1%) 1618

Micturition, urgency

Cymbalta Delayed-Release Capsules (Infrequent) 1729
▲ Doxil Injection (1% to 10%) 3302

Micturition disturbances

Abilify Tablets (Infrequent) 916
Abilify Tablets (Infrequent) 2472
Aceon Tablets (2 mg, 4 mg, 8 mg) (0.3% to 1%) 3191
Aciphex Tablets 1081
▲ Adalat CC Tablets (3% or less) 2978
Alacol DM Syrup 739
Ambien Tablets (Rare) 2867
Antara Capsules 2723
▲ Arava Tablets (1% to 3%) 2881
Aricept Tablets (2%) 1086
Aricept ODT Tablets (2%) 1086
Arthrotec Tablets (Rare) 3126
Astelin Nasal Spray (Infrequent) 1876
Avalide Tablets (2%) 922
Avalide Tablets (2%) 2889
Caduet Tablets (Greater than 0.1% to less than 2%) 2507
Captopril Tablets (Approximately 1 to 2 of 1000 patients) 2114
Carbatrol Capsules 3174
Cardene I.V. (Rare) 1129
▲ Casodex Tablets (6%) 670
Caverject Impulse Injection (Less than 1%) 2610
Celebrex Capsules (0.1% to 1.9%) ... 3130
Celexa (At least 2%) 1177
▲ CellCept Capsules (3% to less than 20%) 2751
▲ CellCept Intravenous (3% to less than 20%) 2751
▲ CellCept Oral Suspension (3% to less than 20%) 2751
▲ CellCept Tablets (3% to less than 20%) 2751
Cipro I.V. (1% or less) 2998
Cipro I.V. Pharmacy Bulk Package (1% or less) 3509
Clozapine Tablets (1%) 2141
Clozaril Tablets (1%) 2174
Colazal Capsules 2845
Combunox Tablets (Less than 2%) ... 1183
Copaxone for Injection (At least 2%) 3292
Covera-HS Tablets (Less than 2%) 3135
Cozaar Tablets (Less than 1%) 1913
Cytovene (At least 3 subjects) 2763
Dantrium Capsules (Less frequent) .. 2690
Daranide Tablets 1928
▲ Depacon Injection (1% to 5%) 412
▲ Depakene (1% to 5%) 417
▲ Depakote Sprinkle Capsules (1% to 5%) 422
▲ Depakote Tablets (1% to 5%) 427
▲ Depakote ER Tablets (1% to 5%) 433
Detrol Tablets (1.7%) 2626
Diovan HCT Tablets (Greater than 0.2%) 2195
Duragesic Transdermal System (Greater than 1%) 2448
▲ Effexor Tablets (3%) 3405
Effexor XR Capsules (Frequent) 3411
Eldepryl Capsules 3209
▲ Eloxatin for Injection (2% to 5%) 2908
▲ Entocort EC Capsules (Less than 5%) 2694
Equetro Extended-Release Capsules 3178
Eskalith 1406
Evoxac Capsules (0.9%; less than 1%) 1042
Exelon Capsules (Infrequent) 2204
FazaClo Orally Disintegrating Tablets (1%) 547
Flexeril Tablets (Less than 1%) 1832
Flumadine 1186
Frova Tablets (Infrequent) 1101
Gabitril Tablets (1% or more) 998
Gengraf Capsules (1% to less than 3%) 458
Hytrin Capsules (At least 1%) 469
Hyzaar 1964
Imitrex Injection (Rare) 1431
Imitrex Nasal Spray (Infrequent) 1435
Imitrex Tablets (Infrequent) 1440
Indapamide Tablets (Less than 5%) .. 2119
Indocin (Rare) 1968
▲ Intron A for Injection (Less than 5%) 3038
Invirase (Less than 2%) 2776
Klonopin (1%) 2782
▲ Lamictal (1% to 5%) 1449
Lexapro Oral Solution (Frequent) 1193
Lexapro Tablets (Frequent) 1193
Lipitor Tablets (Less than 2%) 2495
Lofibra Capsules 1217
Lotensin HCT Tablets (0.3% to 1%) .. 2235
Lotronex Tablets (Rare) 1479
Lunesta Tablets (Infrequent) 3139
Lupron Depot 7.5 mg (Less than 5%) 3261
Lyrica Capsules (Greater than or equal to 1%) 2524
Matulane Capsules 3188
Maxalt Tablets (Infrequent) 1983
Maxalt-MLT Orally Disintegrating Tablets (Infrequent) 1983
Megace ES Oral Suspension (0% to 2%) 2492
Meridia Capsules 485
Micardis Tablets (More than 0.3%) 884
Micardis HCT Tablets 886
Midamor Tablets (Less than or equal to 1%) 2000
Migranal Nasal Spray (Infrequent) 3350
▲ Mirapex Tablets (Greater than or equal to 1% to 6%) 889
Mobic Oral Suspension (0.1% to 2.4%) 893
Mobic Tablets (0.1% to 2.4%) 893
Moduretic Tablets 2003
Naropin Injection (Less than 1%) 640
Neoral Soft Gelatin Capsules (1% to less than 3%) 2247
Neoral Oral Solution (1% to less than 3%) 2247
Neurontin Capsules (Infrequent) 2498
Neurontin Oral Solution (Infrequent) 2498
Neurontin Tablets (Infrequent) 2498
Nexium Delayed-Release Capsules (Less than 1%) 645
Nexium I.V. (Less than 1%) 649
Norvasc Tablets (More than 0.1% to 1%) 2529
Norvir (Less than 2%) 499
Oncaspar (Less than 1%) 1123
Orap Tablets 1220
Parcopa Orally Disintegrating Tablets 3111
Parnate Tablets 1499
▲ Paxil CR Controlled-Release Tablets (3%) 1509
▲ Paxil (3%) 1501
Pentasa Capsules (Less than 1%) 3182
Permax Tablets (2.7%) 3357
Plendil Extended-Release Tablets (0.5% to 1.5%) 651
Pletal Tablets (Less than 2%) 2478
Prevacid Delayed-Release Capsules (Less than 1%) 3268
Prevacid for Delayed-Release Oral Suspension (Less than 1%) 3268
Prevacid NapraPAC (Less than 1%) .. 3277
Prevacid SoluTab Delayed-Release Orally Disintegrating Tablets (Less than 1%) 3268
PREVPAC (Less than 1%) 3281
Prilosec OTC Tablets (Less than 1%) 2674
▲ ProAmatine Tablets (Among most frequent) 3183
Prochieve 4% Gel 1018
Prochieve 8% Gel 1018
▲ Prograf Capsules and Injection (3% to 15%) 624
Proleukin for Injection (1%) 1007
ProSom Tablets (Infrequent) 512
Protonix I.V. (Less than 1%) 3468
Protonix Tablets (Less than 1%) 3465
▲ Rapamune Oral Solution and Tablets (3% to 20%) 3472
Razadyne ER Extended-Release Capsules (Infrequent) 2434
Razadyne (Infrequent) 2434
▲ Rebif Prefilled Syringe for Injection (2% to 7%) 3163
Reishimax Capsules 2669
Relpax Tablets (Infrequent) 2531
ReoPro Vials (0.1%) 1779
Requip Tablets (Infrequent) 1528
Retrovir Capsules 1533
Retrovir IV Infusion 1537
Retrovir 1533
Risperdal Consta Long-Acting Injection (Infrequent) 1664
Risperdal M-Tab Orally Disintegrating Tablets 1658
Risperdal 1658
Rythmol SR Capsules 2736
Seroquel Tablets (Infrequent) 691
▲ Simulect for Injection (3% to 10%) ... 2268
Sonata Capsules (Infrequent) 1686
▲ Strattera Capsules (5% or greater) 1784
Surmontil Capsules 2347
Symbyax Capsules (Frequent) 1788
Tarka Tablets 519
Tasmar Tablets (1% to 2%) 3360
Tegretol/Tegretol-XR 2278
▲ Temodar Capsules (6%) 3088
Teveten Tablets (Less than 1%) 1707
Teveten HCT Tablets (Less than 1%) 1710
Topamax Sprinkle Capsules (0% to 2%) 2438
Topamax Tablets (0% to 2%) 2438

Tricor Tablets.................................... 523
Trileptal Oral Suspension (1% to 2%)... 2281
Trileptal Tablets (1% to 2%)............. 2281
Ultracet Tablets (Less than 1%)........ 2462
Uniretic Tablets (Less than 1%)........ 3114
Univasc Tablets (Greater than 1%).... 3118
Urecholine Tablets............................. 2349
Vantas (Less than 2%)...................... 3367
Verelan PM Capsules (2% or less).... 3120
▲ Vesanoid Capsules (3%) 2823
▲ Viadur Implant (3.8%) 782
Viagra Tablets (Less than 2%).......... 2552
Vicoprofen Tablets (Less than 3%).... 533
Vivactil Tablets................................... 2350
Wellbutrin Tablets (2.5%).................. 1579
▲ Wellbutrin SR Sustained-Release Tablets (2% to 5%)......................... 1583
▲ Wellbutrin XL Extended-Release Tablets (2% to 5%)......................... 1588
Xanax XR Tablets (Infrequent)........... 2655
Xifaxan Tablets (Less than 2%)......... 2847
Zegerid Powder for Oral Solution (Less than 1%)............................. 2972
Zoladex (1% or greater)..................... 709
Zoladex 3-month (1% to 5%)............. 712
Zoloft (Infrequent)............................. 2581
Zomig Nasal Spray (Rare)................... 718
Zomig Tablets (Infrequent)................. 714
Zomig-ZMT Tablets (Infrequent)........ 714
Zyban Sustained-Release Tablets (Frequent)...................................... 1620
Zyprexa Tablets (Infrequent)............. 1798
Zyprexa ZYDIS Orally Disintegrating Tablets (Infrequent)...................................... 1798
Zyrtec Chewable Tablets (Less than 2%)... 2589
Zyrtec (Less than 2%)........................ 2589
Zyrtec-D 12 Hour Extended Release Tablets (Less than 2%)..... 2591

Middle ear, fluid in

▲ Increlex Injection (Greater than or equal to 5%)................................. 3290

Migraine

Abilify Tablets (Infrequent)............... 916
Abilify Tablets (Infrequent)............... 2472
AccuNeb Inhalation Solution (0.9% to 1.7%).. 1055
Aciphex Tablets................................. 1081
Actiq (1% or greater)......................... 993
Activella Tablets................................. 2311
Adacel Vaccine (1.5%)...................... 2959
Adalat CC Tablets (Less than 1%)..... 2978
Advicor Tablets.................................. 1694
Agrylin Capsules (1% to 5%)............ 3172
Alesse-28 Tablets.............................. 3392
Ambien Tablets (Infrequent).............. 2867
Antara Capsules................................. 2723
▲ Arava Tablets (1% to 3%) 2881
Arthrotec Tablets (Rare).................... 3126
Asacol Delayed-Release Tablets (2% or greater)............................... 2688
▲ Avonex (5%) 839
Aygestin Tablets................................ 1062
Caduet Tablets (Less than 2%)......... 2507
Campral Tablets (Infrequent)............ 1175
Celexa (Frequent).............................. 1177
Cenestin Tablets, 0.45mg, 0.625mg, 0.9mg, 1.25mg............ 1063
Cenestin Tablets, 0.3mg.................... 1063
Cipro I.V. (1% or less)...................... 2998
Cipro I.V. Pharmacy Bulk Package (1% or less)...................................... 3509
Cipro (Less than 1%).......................... 2991
Cipro XR Tablets (Less than 1%)....... 3004
Climara Transdermal System........... 795
Climara Pro Transdermal System..... 800
▲ Copaxone for Injection (5%) 3292
Coreg Tablets (Less than or equal to 0.1%).. 1376
Cozaar Tablets (Less than 1%)......... 1913
Doxil Injection (Less than 1%).......... 3302
Effexor Tablets (Frequent)................ 3405
Effexor XR Capsules (Frequent)........ 3411
Eldepryl Capsules............................. 3209
Engerix-B Vaccine............................. 1391
▲ Epzicom Tablets (6% to 7%) 1402
Estratest Tablets............................... 3196
Estratest H.S. Tablets....................... 3196
Estrogel 0.06%.................................. 3200
Evista Tablets (2.4%)........................ 1735
▲ Evoxac Capsules (1% to 3%) 1042
Exelon Capsules (Infrequent)............ 2204
▲ Famvir Tablets (0.7% to 3.1%) 2207
▲ Flovent Diskus 50 mcg (1% to 3%)... 1415
▲ Flovent HFA (1% to 3%) 1418
Fortical Nasal Spray (Less than 1%).. 3336
Gabitril Tablets (Frequent)................ 998
▲ Gengraf Capsules (3%) 458
Gleevec Tablets (Infrequent)............ 2221
▲ Gonal-f RFF Pen for Injection (3.6%).. 3155
Hyzaar... 1964
▲ Imdur Tablets (Less than or equal to 5%)... 3032
Imitrex Tablets................................... 1440
▲ Intron A for Injection (Less than 5%).. 3038
Kaletra (Less than 2%)...................... 474
Klonopin (Infrequent)........................ 2782
▲ Lamictal (1% to 5%) 1449
Levaquin in 5% Dextrose Injection (0.1% to 0.9%)............................. 2453
Levaquin (0.1% to 0.9%).................. 2453
Lexapro Oral Solution (Frequent)...... 1193
Lexapro Tablets (Frequent)............... 1193
Lipitor Tablets (Less than 2%).......... 2495
Lofibra Capsules 1217
Lo/Ovral-28 Tablets 3423
Lunesta Tablets (Frequent) 3139
▲ Lupron Depot 3.75 mg (33%) 3257
▲ Lupron Depot–3 Month 11.25 mg (33%) 3262
Maxair Autohaler 1820
Menopur for Subcutaneous Injection (2.4%) 1145
Menostar Transdermal System 805
Meridia Capsules (2.4%) 485
Miacalcin Nasal Spray (Less than 1%) 2242
Micardis Tablets (More than 0.3%) ... 884
Micardis HCT Tablets 886
▲ Neoral Soft Gelatin Capsules (3%) ... 2247
▲ Neoral Oral Solution (3%) 2247
Neurontin Capsules (Infrequent) 2498
Neurontin Oral Solution (Infrequent) 2498
Neurontin Tablets (Infrequent) 2498
Nexium Delayed-Release Capsules (Less than 1%) 645
Nexium I.V. (Less than 1%) 649
Niaspan Extended-Release Tablets ... 1703
Nicotrol NS (Less than 1%) 2596
Norvasc Tablets (Less than or equal to 0.1%) 2529
Norvir (Less than 2%) 499
Omacor Capsules 2735
Ortho-Cept Tablets 2395
Ortho-Cyclen Tablets 2414
Ortho Evra Transdermal System 2402
Ortho Tri-Cyclen Tablets 2414
Ortho Tri-Cyclen Lo Tablets 2421
OxyContin Tablets (Less than 1%) 2699
Paxil CR Controlled-Release Tablets (Infrequent) 1509
Paxil (Infrequent) 1501
Permax Tablets (Rare) 3357
Prefest Tablets 1069
Premarin Intravenous 3440
Premarin Tablets 3443
Premarin Vaginal Cream 3449
Premphase Tablets 3452
Prempro Tablets 3452
Prevacid Delayed-Release Capsules (Less than 1%) 3268
Prevacid for Delayed-Release Oral Suspension (Less than 1%) 3268
Prevacid NapraPAC (Less than 1%) .. 3277
Prevacid SoluTab Delayed-Release Orally Disintegrating Tablets (Less than 1%) 3268
PREVPAC (Less than 1%) 3281
Prochieve 4% Gel 1018
Prochieve 8% Gel 1018
Protonix I.V. (Greater than or equal to 1%) 3468
Protonix Tablets (Greater than or equal to 1%) 3465
Protopic Ointment (Greater than or equal to 1%) 629
Provigil Tablets (At least 1%) 1002
Prozac Pulvules and Liquid (Infrequent) 1771
Recombivax HB 2045
Relpax Tablets (Infrequent) 2531
Requip Tablets (Infrequent) 1528
Rescriptor Tablets 2535
Rilutek Tablets (Infrequent) 2945
Risperdal Consta Long-Acting Injection (Infrequent) 1664
Risperdal M-Tab Orally Disintegrating Tablets (Rare) 1658
Risperdal (Rare) 1658
Sandostatin LAR Depot (Rare) 2264
Seasonale Tablets 1073
Serevent Diskus (1% to 3%) 1540
Seroquel Tablets (Infrequent) 691
Soriatane Capsules (Less than 1%).. 1028
Sular Tablets (Less than or equal to 1%)... 1163
Sustiva Capsules (Less than 2%)...... 957
Symbyax Capsules (Frequent).......... 1788
Tasmar Tablets (Infrequent)............. 3360
Tequin Injection (Less than 0.1%)..... 964
Tequin Tablets (Less than 0.1%)...... 964
Teveten Tablets (Less than 1%)........ 1707
Teveten HCT Tablets (Less than 1%).. 1710
Thalomid Capsules........................... 979
Tricor Tablets.................................... 523
Triglide Tablets................................. 1165
Trileptal Oral Suspension.................. 2281
Trileptal Tablets................................ 2281
Triphasil-28 Tablets.......................... 3483
Ultracet Tablets (Less than 1%)........ 2462
Uniretic Tablets (Less than 1%)........ 3114
Vantin Tablets and Oral Suspension (Less than 1%)........... 2650
Viagra Tablets (Less than 2%) 2552
Viracept (Less than 2%) 2556
Vivelle Transdermal System 2288
Vivelle-Dot Transdermal System 2293
▲ Wellbutrin Tablets (25.7%) 1579
▲ Wellbutrin SR Sustained-Release Tablets (1% to 4%) 1583
▲ Wellbutrin XL Extended-Release Tablets (1% to 4%) 1588
▲ Xeloda Tablets (Less than 5%) 2825
Xifaxan Tablets (Less than 2%) 2847
Xopenex HFA Inhalation Aerosol (2.7%) 3151
Xopenex Inhalation Solution (2.7%) .. 3143
Xopenex Inhalation Solution Concentrate (2.7%) 3147
Yasmin 28 Tablets (Greater than 1%) 818
▲ Zavesca Capsules (6%) 543
Zelnorm Tablets (2%) 2303
Zemaira (0.2% to 0.4%) 3506
▲ Ziagen (7%) 1600
▲ Zoladex (1% to 7%) 709
Zoladex 3-month 712
Zoloft (Infrequent) 2581
Zyban Sustained-Release Tablets (Infrequent) 1620
Zyprexa Tablets (Infrequent) 1798
Zyprexa ZYDIS Orally Disintegrating Tablets (Infrequent) 1798
Zyrtec Chewable Tablets (Less than 2%) 2589
Zyrtec (Less than 2%) 2589
Zyrtec-D 12 Hour Extended Release Tablets (Less than 2%) 2591

Migraine, aggravated

CombiPatch Transdermal System 2180
Frova Tablets (Infrequent) 1101
Migranal Nasal Spray (Rare) 3350
Nexium Delayed-Release Capsules (Less than 1%) 645
Nexium I.V. (Less than 1%) 649
Premphase Tablets 3452
Prempro Tablets 3452
Topamax Sprinkle Capsules (Greater than 1%) 2438
Topamax Tablets (Greater than 1%) 2438

Migration of implant

Viadur Implant (Rare) 782

Miliaria

Aclovate (Infrequent) 1290
Analpram-HC 1136
Clobevate Gel 3213
Clobex Shampoo (Infrequent) 1209
Clobex Lotion 1208
Cutivate Cream (Infrequent) 1381
Cutivate Lotion 0.05% (Rare) 1383
Cutivate Ointment (Infrequent to more frequent) 1384
Diprolene Gel 0.05% 3015
Diprolene Lotion 0.05% (Infrequent) 3016
Diprolene Ointment 0.05% (Infrequent) 3017
Diprolene AF Cream 0.05% (Infrequent) 3014
Diprosone Cream, USP 0.05% 3018
Elocon Cream 0.1% (Infrequent) 3019
Elocon Lotion 0.1% (Infrequent) 3020
Elocon Ointment 0.1% (Infrequent) 3021
Locoid Cream (Infrequent) 1138
Locoid Lipocream Cream (Infrequent) 1138
Locoid (Infrequent) 1138
Lotrisone 3054
Luxíq Foam 1026
Olux Foam 1027
Oxsoralen-Ultra Capsules................. 3354
Pandel Cream, 0.1%........................ 1017
Pramosone....................................... 1139
ProctoFoam-HC................................. 3113
Temovate Cream 1549
Temovate Gel (Infrequent)................ 1550
Temovate Ointment........................... 1549
Temovate Scalp Application (Infrequent)..................................... 1551
Temovate E Emollient (Infrequent)..... 1552
Topicort .05% Gel............................. 3288
Topicort .25% Cream........................ 3288
Topicort .25% Ointment.................... 3288
Topicort LP .05% Cream.................... 3288
Tri-Luma Cream................................ 1213
U-cort 1% Cream 3289
Vanos Cream.................................... 1864

Miosis

Actiq (Less than 1%)......................... 993
Alphagan P Ophthalmic Solution....... 563
Brimonidine Tartrate Ophthalmic Solution 0.2%.............................. ⊙245
▲ Buprenex Injectable (1% to 5%) 2718
Camptosar Injection.......................... 2602
Dibenzyline Capsules........................ 3390
Dilaudid... 439
Dilaudid Oral Liquid (Less frequent).. 443
Dilaudid Non-Sterile Powder............. 439
Dilaudid Rectal Suppositories........... 439
Dilaudid Tablets 439
Dilaudid Tablets - 8 mg (Less frequent)... 443
Dilaudid-HP (Less frequent).............. 441
Effexor Tablets (Rare)....................... 3405
Effexor XR Capsules (Rare)............... 3411
Kadian Capsules (Less than 3%)....... 572
Lyrica Capsules (Rare)...................... 2524
MS Contin Tablets (Less frequent).... 2703
Neurontin Capsules (Rare)................ 2498
Neurontin Oral Solution (Rare).......... 2498
Neurontin Tablets (Rare)................... 2498
Numorphan.. 1112
Ocufen Ophthalmic Solution............. ⊙230
Rythmol SR Capsules........................ 2736
Symbyax Capsules (Infrequent)........ 1788
Thioridazine Hydrochloride Tablets... 2122
Thiothixene Capsules....................... 2124
Urecholine Tablets............................ 2349
Zyprexa Tablets (Rare)...................... 1798
Zyprexa ZYDIS Orally Disintegrating Tablets (Rare)......... 1798

Miscarriage

Efudex... 3348
Vantin Tablets and Oral Suspension....................................... 2650
Zelnorm Tablets................................ 2303

Mitral insufficiency

Requip Tablets (Infrequent)............... 1528

Mitral regurgitation

Activase I.V....................................... 1225
Retavase... 1131
TNKase I.V.. 1256

Mitral valve disease

Effexor XR (Rare).............................. 3411

Moaning

Diprivan Injectable Emulsion (Less than 1%)... 676

Mobility disorders, non-site specific

Amerge Tablets (Rare)....................... 1312

Molluscum contagiosum

Elidel Cream 1% (Up to 1.8%).......... 2198
Norvir (Less than 2%)........................ 499

Moniliasis

(*see under* Candidiasis)

Moniliasis, enteric

Rescriptor Tablets 2535

Moniliasis, genital

(*see under* Candidiasis, genital)

Moniliasis, oral

(*see under* Candidiasis, oral)

Moniliasis, vaginal

Abilify Tablets (Infrequent)............... 916
Abilify Tablets (Infrequent)............... 2472
Antara Capsules................................ 2723
Cipro... 2991
Cipro XR Tablets (1% to 2%)............ 3004
Cleocin Vaginal Ovules (1.5%).......... 2613
Lamictal (Rare).................................. 1449

Merrem I.V. (Greater than 0.1% to 1%) 687
▲ Omnicef Capsules (4%) 506
Omnicef for Oral Suspension (0.3%) 506
▲ Premarin Tablets (5% to 6%) 3443
▲ Premphase Tablets (4% to 8%) 3452
▲ Prempro Tablets (4% to 8%) 3452
Rescriptor Tablets 2535
▲ Spectracef Tablets (3% to 6%) 2706
Symbyax Capsules (Infrequent) 1788
Tricor Tablets 523
Tygacil for Injection (0% to less than 2%) 3489
Zyvox (1% to 1.6%) 2661

Monocytosis
Campral Tablets (Rare) 1175
Cipro (Less than 0.1%) 2991
Cuprimine Capsules 1925
Geodon Capsules (Rare) 2514
Paxil CR Controlled-Release Tablets (Rare) 1509
Paxil (Rare) 1501
Primaxin I.M. 2022
Primaxin I.V. 2024
Relpax Tablets (Rare) 2531
Rocephin Injectable Vials, ADD-Vantage, Galaxy, Bulk (Rare) 2801
Rythmol SR Capsules 2736
Vantin Tablets and Oral Suspension 2650
Xifaxan Tablets (Less than 2%) 2847
Zithromax for Oral Suspension, 300 mg, 600 mg, 900 mg, 1200 mg (Less than 1%) 2561
Zithromax Tablets, 250 mg, 500 mg (Less than 1%) 2561
Zithromax Tri-Pak (Less than 1%) 2561

Mononeuropathy
Adacel Vaccine 2959
Infanrix Vaccine 1444

Mononuclear cells, atypical
Miradon Tablets 3056

Monoplegia
Imitrex Injection (Rare) 1431
Imitrex Nasal Spray (Rare) 1435
Imitrex Tablets (Infrequent) 1440

Mood changes
Adalat CC Tablets (Rare) 2978
Aerobid/Aerobid-M (1% to 3%) 1172
▲ Agenerase Oral Solution (4% to 16%) 1304
Alesse-28 Tablets 3392
▲ Alimta for Injection (Up to 14%) 1722
Aloxi Injection (Less than 1%) 2099
▲ Arimidex Tablets (17%) 665
Aygestin Tablets 1062
Cenestin Tablets, 0.45mg, 0.625mg, 0.9mg, 1.25mg 1063
Cenestin Tablets, 0.3mg 1063
Climara Transdermal System 795
Climara Pro Transdermal System 800
▲ Copegus Tablets (5% to 9%) 2759
Cymbalta Delayed-Release Capsules (Infrequent) 1729
Decadron Phosphate Injection 1931
Decadron Tablets 1929
Dilaudid 439
Dilaudid Oral Liquid (Less frequent) 443
Dilaudid Non-Sterile Powder 439
Dilaudid Rectal Suppositories 439
Dilaudid Tablets 439
Dilaudid Tablets - 8 mg (Less frequent) 443
Dilaudid-HP (Less frequent) 441
Eldepryl Capsules 3209
Enbrel for Injection 580
Estratest Tablets 3196
Estratest H.S. Tablets 3196
Estrogel 0.06% 3200
Guanidine Hydrochloride Tablets 3030
Hexalen Capsules 2101
Hycodan 1104
Hycomine Compound Tablets 1105
Hycotuss Expectorant Syrup 1106
Hydrocortone Tablets 1963
Lariam Tablets (Occasional) 2790
▲ Lexiva Tablets (Less than 1% to 11%) 1473
Lo/Ovral-28 Tablets 3423
Lortab 3315
Lortab Elixir 3312
Lupron Depot 3.75 mg 3257
Marinol Capsules 3334
Meridia Capsules 485
MS Contin Tablets (Less frequent) 2703
Oncaspar 1123
Ortho-Cyclen/Ortho Tri-Cyclen 2414
Ortho Tri-Cyclen Lo Tablets 2421
Orthoclone OKT3 Sterile Solution 2370
Paxil CR Controlled-Release Tablets 1509
Paxil 1501
▲ Pegasys (3%) 2793
Prefest Tablets 1069
Premarin Tablets 3443
Premarin Vaginal Cream 3449
Premphase Tablets 3452
Prempro Tablets 3452
Seasonale Tablets 1073
▲ Strattera Capsules (2% to 5%) 1784
Testim 1% Gel (1% or less) 722
▲ Topamax Sprinkle Capsules (2% to 11%) 2438
▲ Topamax Tablets (2% to 11%) 2438
Triphasil-28 Tablets 3483
Tussionex Pennkinetic Extended-Release Suspension 3322
Univasc Tablets (Less than 1%) 3118
Vicodin Tablets 530
Vicodin ES Tablets 531
Vicodin HP Tablets 532
Vicoprofen Tablets (Less than 1%) 533
Vivelle Transdermal System 2288
Vivelle-Dot Transdermal System 2293
Wellbutrin Tablets (Infrequent) 1579
Xanax XR Tablets (Infrequent) 2655
▲ Xeloda Tablets (5%) 2825
Zydone Tablets 1118

Moon face
Copaxone for Injection (Infrequent) 3292
Decadron Tablets 1929

Motion sickness
Aloxi Injection (Less than 1%) 2099
Aricept Tablets 1086
Aricept ODT Tablets 1086
Evoxac Capsules (Less than 1%) 1042
Klonopin (Infrequent) 2782
Xifaxan Tablets (Less than 2%) 2847

Motor and phonic tics, exacerbations
Adderall Tablets 3168
Adderall XR Capsules 3169
Dexedrine 1386
DextroStat Tablets 3177

Motor disturbances, reversible involuntary
Zantac (Rare) 1597
Zantac Injection (Rare) 1593
Zantac Injection Pharmacy Bulk Package (Rare) 1595
Zantac Syrup (Rare) 1597

Motor function, loss of
Neoral Soft Gelatin Capsules 2247
Neoral Oral Solution 2247
Sandimmune 2259

Motor restlessness
Moban Tablets 1108
Orap Tablets (Less frequent) 1220
Paxil CR Controlled-Release Tablets 1509
Paxil Tablets 1501
▲ Pediarix Vaccine (0.6% to 41.4%) 1518
Thioridazine Hydrochloride Tablets 2122

Motor skills, impairment
Ambien Tablets 2867
Amerge Tablets (Rare) 1312
Cogentin Injection 1903
Dapsone Tablets USP 1656
Effexor Tablets 3405
Moban Tablets 1108
Neurontin Capsules (Rare) 2498
Neurontin Oral Solution (Rare) 2498
Neurontin Tablets (Rare) 2498
Orap Tablets 1220
▲ Prograf Capsules and Injection (Approximately 55%) 624
Proleukin for Injection (2%) 1007
Risperdal M-Tab Orally Disintegrating Tablets 1658
Risperdal 1658

Mouth, burning
Eldepryl Capsules 3209

Mouth, discoloration
▲ Kepivance (17%) 592

Mouth, dry
(*see under* Xerostomia)

Mouth, fissuring in corner of
Parnate Tablets 1499

Mouth, puckering
Moban Tablets 1108
Orap Tablets 1220

Mouth, sore
Alferon N Injection (One patient) 1640
▲ Flovent Diskus 50 mcg (1% to 3%) 1415
Gengraf Capsules (Rare) 458
▲ Imitrex Injection (4.9%) 1431
Miradon Tablets 3056
Neoral Soft Gelatin Capsules (Rare) 2247
Neoral Oral Solution (Rare) 2247
Oncaspar 1123

Mouth, thickening of
▲ Kepivance (17%) 592

Mouth ulceration
▲ Doxil Injection (1% to 10%) 3302
Lyrica Capsules (0.1% to 1%) 2524

Movement, abnormal
▲ Diprivan Injectable Emulsion (3% to 17%) 676
Gabitril Tablets (Infrequent) 998
Lamictal (Rare) 1449
Neoral Soft Gelatin Capsules 2247
Neoral Oral Solution 2247
Orthoclone OKT3 Sterile Solution 2370
Phenergan 3438
Prozac Pulvules and Liquid 1771
Sandimmune 2259
Zonegran Capsules (Infrequent) 1089
▲ Zyprexa Tablets (1% to 5%) 1798
Zyprexa ZYDIS Orally Disintegrating Tablets (1% to 5%) 1798

Movement, unspecified
Ultane Liquid for Inhalation (1%) 526

Movement disorder
Symbyax Capsules (Infrequent) 1788

Mucocutaneous lymph node syndrome
(*see under* Kawasaki-like syndrome)

Mucormycosis
Desferal Vials (Rare) 2190

Mucosa damage
Invirase (Greater than or equal to 2%) 2776

Mucosal pigmentation, changes
Dynacin Tablets 1859
▲ Intron A for Injection (Less than 5%) 3038

Mucositis
Adriamycin for Injection, USP 786
Adriamycin Injection, USP 786
Alferon N Injection (One patient) 1640
Aloprim for Injection (Less than 1%) 2156
AmBisome for Injection (Less common) 615
▲ Campath Ampules (1% to 14%) 826
▲ Camptosar Injection (2% to 29.6%) 2602
Cerubidine for Injection 788
▲ Elitek (2% to 15%) 2906
▲ Ellence Injection (0% to 58.5%) 2632
▲ Eloxatin for Injection (2% to 7%) 2908
Evoxac Capsules (Less than 1%) 1042
▲ Idamycin PFS Injection (50%) 2645
▲ Intron A for Injection (Less than 5%) 3038
▲ I.V. Busulfex (97%) 1125
Myleran Tablets 1492
▲ Mylotarg for Injection (25%) 3429
Navelbine Injection 1494
▲ Neulasta Injection (15% to 72%) 596
▲ Neumega for Injection (43%) 3433
▲ Neupogen for Injection (12%) 598
Neurontin Capsules (Rare) 2498
Neurontin Oral Solution (Rare) 2498
Neurontin Tablets (Rare) 2498
Oncaspar 1123
▲ Vesanoid Capsules (26%) 2823
Zithromax for IV Infusion (1% or less) 2573
▲ Zometa for Intravenous Infusion (5% to 10%) 2306

Mucous membrane, abnormalities
Aceon Tablets (2 mg, 4 mg, 8 mg) (0.3% to 1%) 3191
Actiq (Less than 1%) 993
Altoprev Extended-Release Tablets 1151
Captopril Tablets (Approximately 1 in 1000 patients) 2114
Clinoril Tablets 1899
Emend Capsules (2.6%) 1944
Lescol Capsules 2227
Lescol Capsules 2730
Lescol XL Tablets 2227
Lescol XL Tablets 2730
▲ Leukine (75%) 829
Mevacor Tablets 1996
Mintezol 2002
Neurontin Capsules (Infrequent) 2498
Neurontin Oral Solution (Infrequent) 2498
Neurontin Tablets (Infrequent) 2498
Zocor Tablets 2078

Mucus, blood-tinted
Atrovent Nasal Spray 0.03% (2.0%) 869
▲ Flonase Nasal Spray (1% to 3%) 1412

Multiorgan failure
Ammonul Injection 3323

Multiorgan system failure
Clolar for Intravenous Infusion 1264
Cosmegen for Injection 1907
Lamictal 1449
Levaquin in 5% Dextrose Injection (0.1% to 0.9%) 2453
Levaquin (0.1% to 0.9%) 2453
Tasmar Tablets (One case) 3360
VFEND I.V. (Less than 2%) 2543
VFEND Oral Suspension (Less than 2%) 2543
VFEND Tablets (Less than 2%) 2543

Muscle atrophy
Actiq (Less than 1%) 993
Campath Ampules 826
Copaxone for Injection (Infrequent) 3292
Eligard 30 mg (1.1%) 2901
Permax Tablets (Rare) 3357
Reyataz Capsules (Less than 3%) 948
Virazole for Inhalation Solution 3365

Muscle contractions, involuntary
Dilaudid 439
Dilaudid Non-Sterile Powder 439
Dilaudid Rectal Suppositories 439
Dilaudid Tablets 439
Levaquin in 5% Dextrose Injection (0.1% to 0.9%) 2453
Levaquin (0.1% to 0.9%) 2453
Lexapro Oral Solution (Infrequent) 1193
Lexapro Tablets (Infrequent) 1193
Namenda (Infrequent) 1199
Risperdal Consta Long-Acting Injection (Infrequent) 1664
▲ Topamax Sprinkle Capsules (2% to 4%) 2438
▲ Topamax Tablets (2% to 4%) 2438

Muscle cramp
(*see under* Cramping, muscular)

Muscle hypertonia
Lexapro Oral Solution (Infrequent) 1193
Lexapro Tablets (Infrequent) 1193
Trileptal Oral Suspension 2281
Trileptal Tablets 2281

Muscle mass, loss
Decadron Phosphate Injection 1931
Decadron Tablets 1929
Depo-Medrol Injectable Suspension 2615
Depo-Medrol Single-Dose Vial 2617
Hydrocortone Tablets 1963
Pediapred Oral Solution 3319

Muscle movement, intraoperative
Dilaudid Oral Liquid (Less frequent) 443
Dilaudid Tablets - 8 mg (Less frequent) 443

Muscle rigidity
▲ Advair Diskus 100/50 (1% to 3%) 1291
▲ Advair Diskus 250/50 (1% to 3%) 1291
▲ Advair Diskus 500/50 (1% to 3%) 1291
Amerge Tablets (Infrequent) 1312
Ceftin Tablets (0.1% to 1%) 1369
Clozapine Tablets 2141

Clozaril Tablets 2174
Comtan Tablets 2186
Cozaar Tablets (Less than 1%) 1913
Dilaudid 439
Dilaudid Oral Liquid (Less frequent) 443
Dilaudid Non-Sterile Powder 439
Dilaudid Rectal Suppositories 439
Dilaudid Tablets 439
Dilaudid Tablets - 8 mg (Less frequent) 443
Dilaudid-HP (Less frequent) 441
▲ Flovent HFA (1% to 3%) 1418
Imitrex Injection (Rare) 1431
Invirase (Less than 2%) 2776
Lexapro Oral Solution (Infrequent) 1193
Lexapro Tablets (Infrequent) 1193
Lotronex Tablets (Rare) 1479
Miacalcin Nasal Spray (Less than 1%) 2242
Migranal Nasal Spray (1%; Rare) 3350
MS Contin Tablets (Less frequent) 2703
▲ Orap Tablets (3 of 20 patients) 1220
Orthoclone OKT3 Sterile Solution 2370
Permax Tablets 3357
Phenergan 3438
ProSom Tablets (1%) 512
Risperdal M-Tab Orally Disintegrating Tablets 1658
Risperdal 1658
Serevent Diskus (1% to 3%) 1540
Seroquel Tablets 691
Symmetrel (Uncommon) 1115
Tasmar Tablets (2%) 3360
Thioridazine Hydrochloride Tablets 2122
Thiothixene Capsules 2124
Wellbutrin Tablets 1579
Wellbutrin SR Sustained-Release Tablets 1583
Wellbutrin XL Extended-Release Tablets 1588
Zyban Sustained-Release Tablets 1620

Muscle spasms

Abilify Tablets (Infrequent) 916
Abilify Tablets (Infrequent) 2472
Advair Diskus 100/50 1291
▲ Advair Diskus 250/50 (3%) 1291
Advair Diskus 500/50 1291
Aldoclor Tablets 1881
Aldoril Tablets 1884
Amerge Tablets (Infrequent) 1312
Aricept Tablets (Infrequent) 1086
Aricept ODT Tablets (Infrequent) 1086
Atacand HCT 637
Avalide Tablets 922
Avalide Tablets 2889
Celexa 1177
Clorpres Tablets 2139
Clozapine Tablets (1%) 2141
Clozaril Tablets (1%) 2174
Diovan HCT Tablets 2195
Diuril Oral 1936
Diuril Sodium Intravenous 1934
FazaClo Orally Disintegrating Tablets (1%) 547
Furosemide Tablets 2117
Hyzaar 1964
▲ Indapamide Tablets (Greater than or equal to 5%) 2119
Indocin I.V. (Less than 1%) 1973
Lamictal (1.0%) 1449
Lotensin HCT Tablets 2235
Maxalt Tablets (Infrequent) 1983
Maxalt-MLT Orally Disintegrating Tablets (Infrequent) 1983
Micardis HCT Tablets 886
Migranal Nasal Spray (Rare) 3350
Mivacron Injection (Less than 1%) 489
Moduretic Tablets (Less than or equal to 1%) 2003
Parnate Tablets 1499
Prinzide Tablets 2033
Proleukin for Injection (1%) 1007
ProSom Tablets (Infrequent) 512
Requip Tablets (1% or more) 1528
Retrovir Capsules 1533
Retrovir IV Infusion 1537
Retrovir 1533
Rythmol SR Capsules 2736
Syprine Capsules 2055
Teveten HCT Tablets 1710
Timolide Tablets 2056
Uniretic Tablets 3114
Valium Tablets 2822
Vancocin HCl Capsules, USP 3370
Vaseretic Tablets 2073
Vivelle Transdermal System (1.9% to 2.3%) 2288
Vivelle-Dot Transdermal System (1.9% to 2.3%) 2293
Wellbutrin Tablets (1.9%) 1579
Xanax XR Tablets (Rare) 2655
Xifaxan Tablets (Less than 2%) 2847
Zestoretic Tablets 701

Muscle spasms, paradoxical

Diastat Rectal Delivery System 3344
Niravam Orally Disintegrating Tablets (Rare) 3106

Muscle stiffness

▲ Advair Diskus 100/50 (1% to 3%) 1291
▲ Advair Diskus 250/50 (1% to 3%) 1291
▲ Advair Diskus 500/50 (1% to 3%) 1291
▲ Flovent HFA (1% to 3%) 1418
Gleevec Tablets (Infrequent) 2221
Niravam (2.2%) 3106

Muscle twitching

(*see under* Fasciculations)

Muscle weakness

(*see under* Myasthenia)

Muscular disturbances

Copaxone for Injection (Infrequent) 3292
▲ Gengraf Capsules (12%) 458
Lescol Capsules 2227
Lescol Capsules 2730
Lescol XL Tablets 2227
Lescol XL Tablets 2730
▲ Neoral Soft Gelatin Capsules (12%) 2247
▲ Neoral Oral Solution (12%) 2247
Prometrium Capsules (100 mg, 200 mg) (Less than 5%) 3205
▲ Risperdal M-Tab Orally Disintegrating Tablets (17% to 34%) 1658
▲ Risperdal (17% to 34%) 1658
Zosyn (1.0% or less) 3492

Musculoskeletal aches

Follistim AQ Cartridge 2354

Musculoskeletal contracture

Neurontin Capsules (Rare) 2498
Neurontin Oral Solution (Rare) 2498
Neurontin Tablets (Rare) 2498

Musculoskeletal symptoms, unspecified

Accutane Capsules 2740
Amnesteem Capsules 2126
▲ Arimidex Tablets (30%) 665
▲ Epivir (12%) 1394
Flovent Diskus 50 mcg 1415
▲ Gengraf Capsules (13.2%) 458
▲ Imdur Tablets (Less than or equal to 5%) 3032
▲ Infergen (4% to 7%) 1647
Invirase (0.6% to 2.0%) 2776
Mobic Oral Suspension (1.7% to 2.9%) 893
Mobic Tablets (1.7% to 2.9%) 893
▲ Neoral Soft Gelatin Capsules (13.2%) 2247
▲ Neoral Oral Solution (13.2%) 2247
Trasylol Injection (2%) 779

Musculoskeletal trauma

Avalide Tablets 922
Avalide Tablets 2889
Avapro Tablets (2%) 925
Avapro Tablets (2%) 2886

Myalgia

Abelcet Injection 1119
▲ Abilify Tablets (4%) 916
▲ Abilify Tablets (4%) 2472
Accolate Tablets (1.6%) 663
Aceon Tablets (2 mg, 4 mg, 8 mg) (0.3% to 1.1%) 3191
Aciphex Tablets 1081
▲ Actimmune (6%) 1646
Actiq (Less than 1%) 993
Activella Tablets 2311
▲ Actonel Tablets (4.6% to 6.6%) 2679
▲ Actonel with Calcium Tablets (4.6% to 6.6%) 2684
▲ ActoPlus Met Tablets (5.4%) 3219
▲ Actos Tablets (5.4%) 3224
Adalat CC Tablets (Less than 1%) 2978
▲ Advicor Tablets (3%) 1694
Aggrenox Capsules (1.2%) 855
Agrylin Capsules (1% to 5%) 3172
Aldara Cream, 5% (1% to 1.4%) 1814
Aldoclor Tablets 1881
Aldoril Tablets 1884
▲ Alferon N Injection (One patient to 45%) 1640
▲ Alimta for Injection (Up to 13%) 1722
Alinia for Oral Suspension (Less than 1%) 2840
Alinia Tablets (Less than 1%) 2840
Altace Capsules (Less than 1%) 1673
▲ Altoprev Extended-Release Tablets (3%) 1151
▲ Ambien Tablets (1% to 7%) 2867
AmBisome for Injection (Less common) 615
Amerge Tablets (Infrequent) 1312
Amevive (Common) 836
Anaprox Tablets (Less than 1%) 2769
Anaprox DS Tablets (Less than 1%) 2769
Antara Capsules 2723
Anzemet Injection (Rare) 2871
Anzemet Tablets (Rare) 2874
Aptivus Capsules (Less than 2%) 859
▲ Aranesp for Injection (8% to 21%) 576
▲ Arava Tablets (1% to 3%) 2881
▲ Aredia for Injection (26%) 2168
▲ Arimidex Tablets (2% to 5%) 665
Arthrotec Tablets (Rare) 3126
▲ Asacol Delayed-Release Tablets (3%) 2688
▲ Asmanex Twisthaler (2% to 3%) 2981
Astelin Nasal Spray (1.5%) 1876
Atacand Tablets (0.5% or greater) 634
Atacand HCT (0.5% or greater) 637
Augmentin 1331
Augmentin Tablets 1334
Augmentin XR Extended-Release Tablets 1340
Augmentin ES-600 Powder for Oral Suspension 1337
Avalide Tablets 922
Avalide Tablets 2889
Avapro Tablets (1% or greater) 925
Avapro Tablets (1% or greater) 2886
▲ Avastin IV (8% to 15%) 1229
Avelox (0.1% to less than 2%) 2984
▲ Avonex (29%) 839
Axert Tablets (Infrequent) 2430
Axid Oral Solution (1.7%) 913
Azasan Tablets 2844
▲ Azmacort Inhalation Aerosol (1% to 3%) 1701
Beconase AQ Nasal Spray 1359
Benicar Tablets (Greater than 0.5%) 2850
Benicar HCT Tablets 2852
▲ Betaseron for SC Injection (27%) 791
▲ Bexxar (Less than 1% to 13%) 1360
BiDil Tablets (1% to less than 2%) 2161
Biltricide Tablets 2990
▲ Boniva Tablets (0.8% to 5.7%) 2747
Boostrix 1366
▲ Brimonidine Tartrate Ophthalmic Solution 0.2% (3% to 9%) ⊙ 245
▲ Caduet Tablets (Greater than 0.1% to 5.6%) 2507
Calcijex Injection 411
Calcium Disodium Versenate Injection 1819
▲ Campath Ampules (11%) 826
Campral Tablets (Frequent) 1175
▲ Cancidas for Injection (0% to 3.1%) 1894
Captopril Tablets 2114
Carbatrol Capsules 3174
▲ Casodex Tablets (5%) 670
Catapres Tablets (About 6 in 1,000 patients) 874
Catapres-TTS (0.5% or less) 875
Celebrex Capsules (0.1% to 1.9%) 3130
Celexa (2%) 1177
▲ CellCept Capsules (3% to less than 20%) 2751
▲ CellCept Intravenous (3% to less than 20%) 2751
▲ CellCept Oral Suspension (3% to less than 20%) 2751
▲ CellCept Tablets (3% to less than 20%) 2751
▲ Cenestin Tablets, 0.45mg, 0.625mg, 0.9mg, 1.25mg (3.8% to 28%) 1063
▲ Cialis Tablets (1% to 4%) 1806
Cipro I.V. 2998
Cipro I.V. Pharmacy Bulk Package 3509
Cipro 2991
Cipro XR Tablets 3004
▲ Clarinex Tablets (2.1% to 3%) 3009
▲ Clarinex Reditabs Tablets (2.1% to 3%) 3009
Clindesse Vaginal Cream (Less than 1%) 3296
Clinoril Tablets (Less than 1 in 100) 1899
▲ Clolar for Intravenous Infusion (14%) 1264
Clorpres Tablets (About 6 in 1,000) 2139
Clozapine Tablets (1%) 2141
Clozaril Tablets (1%) 2174
Colazal Capsules (1%) 2845
▲ Combivir Tablets (8%) 1373
Copaxone for Injection (At least 2%) 3292
▲ Copegus Tablets (40%) 2759
Cosmegen for Injection 1907
Coumadin for Injection 932
Coumadin Tablets 932
Cozaar Tablets (1% or greater) 1913
Crestor Tablets (2.8%) 672
Cubicin for Injection (Less than 1%) 1038
▲ Cymbalta Delayed-Release Capsules (1% to 4%) 1729
Cytovene (At least 3 subjects) 2763
Dantrium Capsules (Less frequent) 2690
▲ Depacon Injection (1% to 5%) 412
▲ Depakene (1% to 5%) 417
▲ Depakote Sprinkle Capsules (1% to 5%) 422
▲ Depakote Tablets (1% to 5%) 427
▲ Depakote ER Tablets (1% to 5%) 433
Desferal Vials 2190
Didronel Tablets (Infrequent) 2693
Diovan Tablets 2191
Diprivan Injectable Emulsion (Less than 1%) 676
Dolobid Tablets (Less than 1 in 100) 1937
Dostinex Tablets (2%) 2631
▲ Doxil Injection (Less than 1% to 10%) 3302
Dyazide Capsules 1389
EC-Naprosyn Delayed-Release Tablets (Less than 1%) 2769
Effexor Tablets 3405
▲ Effexor XR Capsules (4%) 3411
Eligard 30 mg (2.2%) 2901
▲ Eligard 45 mg (4.5%) 2904
▲ Eloxatin for Injection (2% to 5%) 2908
Emend Capsules (Greater than 0.5%) 1944
▲ Emtriva Capsules (4% to 6%) 1272
Engerix-B Vaccine (Less than 1%) 1391
▲ Entocort EC Capsules (Less than 5%) 2694
▲ Epivir (8%) 1394
▲ Epivir-HBV (14%) 1398
Epogen for Injection (Rare) 586
Equetro Extended-Release Capsules 3178
▲ Evista Tablets (7.7%) 1735
▲ Evoxac Capsules (1% to 3%) 1042
Exelon Capsules (Frequent) 2204
Factive Tablets (Less than or equal to 0.1%) 2464
Faslodex Injection (Less than 1%) 682
FazaClo Orally Disintegrating Tablets (1%) 547
▲ Femara Tablets (0.3% to 6.7%) 2210
Ferrlecit Injection 3379
Flexeril Tablets (Rare) 1832
▲ Flolan for Injection (3% to 44%) 1408
▲ Flovent Diskus 50 mcg (1% to 12%) 1415
▲ Flovent HFA (1% to 3%) 1418
▲ Flumist Vaccine (5% to 16.7%) 1872
▲ Fortical Nasal Spray (1% to 3%) 3336
▲ Fosamax (0.4% to approximately 6%) 1949
▲ Fosamax Plus D Tablets (0.4% to 4.1%) 1956
Frova Tablets (Infrequent) 1101
Furosemide Tablets 2117
Fuzeon Injection (2.7%) 2772
▲ Gabitril Tablets (1% to 5%) 998
Gemzar for Injection (Common) 1743
Gengraf Capsules (1% to less than 3%) 458
Genotropin Lyophilized Powder 2642
Geodon Capsules (2% to frequent) 2514
▲ Gleevec Tablets (0.2% to 38.6%) 2221
Havrix Vaccine (Less than 1%) 1425
Hectorol Capsules 909
Hectorol Injection 911
▲ Humatrope Vials and Cartridges (9.1% to 24.3%) 1756
Hytrin Capsules (At least 1%) 469
Hyzaar 1964
▲ Imdur Tablets (Less than or equal to 5%) 3032
Imitrex Injection (1.8%) 1431
Imitrex Nasal Spray (Infrequent) 1435
Imitrex Tablets (Frequent) 1440
Infed Injection 3381
▲ Infergen (51% to 58%) 1647
▲ Intron A for Injection (3% to 75%) 3038
Invirase (0.3% to greater than or equal to 2%) 2776
▲ I.V. Busulfex (16%) 1125
Kaletra (Up to 2%) 474
Klonopin (1%) 2782
Lamictal (More than 1%) 1449
Lamisil Tablets 2226

▲ Lariam Tablets (Among most frequent) 2790
▲ Lescol Capsules (5.0%) 2227
▲ Lescol Capsules (5.0%) 2730
▲ Lescol XL Tablets (3.8%) 2227
▲ Lescol XL Tablets (3.8%) 2730
▲ Leukine (18%) 829
▲ Leustatin Injection (7%) 2368
Levaquin in 5% Dextrose Injection (0.1% to 0.9%) 2453
Levaquin (0.1% to 0.9%) 2453
Levitra Tablets (Less than 2%) 3048
Lexapro Oral Solution (Frequent) 1193
Lexapro Tablets (Frequent) 1193
▲ Lipitor Tablets (Up to 5.6%) 2495
Lithobid Tablets 1670
Lofibra Capsules 1217
Lotensin Tablets (Less than 1%) 2232
Lotensin HCT Tablets (0.3% to 1%) 2235
Lotrel Capsules 2238
Lotronex Tablets (Rare) 1479
Lunesta Tablets 3139
Lupron Depot 3.75 mg (Less than 5%) 3257
Lupron Depot 7.5 mg (Less than 5%) 3261
Lupron Depot–3 Month 11.25 mg (0.6% to 1%) 3262
Lupron Injection Pediatric 3256
Lyrica Capsules (Greater than or equal to 1%) 2524
Marinol Capsules (Less than 1%) 3334
Matulane Capsules 3188
▲ Mavik Tablets (4.7%) 482
Maxalt Tablets (Infrequent) 1983
Maxalt-MLT Orally Disintegrating Tablets (Infrequent) 1983
Maxzide 2150
Meridia Capsules (1.9%) 485
Meruvax II 1994
Mevacor Tablets (1.8% to 2.4%) 1996
Miacalcin Nasal Spray (1% to 3%) 2242
Micardis Tablets (1%) 884
Micardis HCT Tablets 886
Migranal Nasal Spray (Infrequent) 3350
Mirapex Tablets (Greater than or equal to 1%) 889
M-M-R II 1980
▲ Myfortic Tablets (3% to less than 20%) 2244
▲ Mylotarg for Injection (3% to 11%) 3429
▲ Nabi-HB (10%) 2159
Naprosyn Suspension (Less than 1%) 2769
Naprosyn Tablets (Less than 1%) 2769
Naropin Injection (Less than 1%) 640
Nasonex Nasal Spray (Greater than or equal to 2%) 3058
▲ Navelbine Injection (Up to 12%) 1494
Neoral Soft Gelatin Capsules (1% to less than 3%) 2247
Neoral Oral Solution (1% to less than 3%) 2247
▲ Neulasta Injection (15% to 72%) 596
▲ Neumega for Injection (Greater than or equal to 10%) 3433
Neupogen for Injection 598
Neurontin Capsules (2.0%) 2498
Neurontin Oral Solution (2.0%) 2498
Neurontin Tablets (2.0%) 2498
Nexium Delayed-Release Capsules (Rare) 645
Nexium I.V. (Rare) 649
Niaspan Extended-Release Tablets 1703
▲ Nicotrol Inhaler (Greater than 3%) 2594
Nicotrol NS (3%) 2596
Nimotop Capsules (Up to 1.4%) 774
▲ Nipent for Injection (11% to 19%) 3216
▲ Norditropin Cartridges (15%) 2318
Noroxin Tablets 2009
Norvasc Tablets (More than 0.1% to 1%) 2529
Norvir (1.7% to 2.4.%) 499
Omacor Capsules 2735
Oncaspar (Greater than 1% but less than 5%) 1123
▲ Ontak Vials (17%) 1717
OptiPranolol Metipranolol Ophthalmic Solution 0.3% (A small number of patients) ⊙ 254
Orap Tablets (2.7%) 1220
Orthoclone OKT3 Sterile Solution (Less than 1%) 2370
Paxil CR Controlled-Release Tablets (2%) 1509
Paxil (2%) 1501
▲ Pegasys (37%) 2793
▲ PEG-Intron Powder for Injection (54%) 3062
Pentasa Capsules (Less than 1%) 3182
Pepcid Injection (Infrequent) 2017
Pepcid (Infrequent) 2014
Permax Tablets (1.1%) 3357
Persantine Tablets (Rare) 898
Plavix Tablets 940
Plavix Tablets 2942
Plendil Extended-Release Tablets (0.5% to 1.5%) 651
▲ Pletal Tablets (2% to 3%) 2478
Pneumovax 23 2020
Pravachol Tablets (0.6% to 2.7%) 943
▲ Prefest Tablets (5%) 1069
▲ Premarin Tablets (5% to 9%) 3443
▲ Premphase Tablets (4% to 5%) 3452
▲ Prempro Tablets (4% to 5%) 3452
Prevacid Delayed-Release Capsules (Less than 1%) 3268
Prevacid for Delayed-Release Oral Suspension (Less than 1%) 3268
Prevacid NapraPAC (Less than 1%) 3277
Prevacid SoluTab Delayed-Release Orally Disintegrating Tablets (Less than 1%) 3268
▲ PREVPAC (Less than 1% to 3%) 3281
Prilosec OTC Tablets (Less than 1%) 2674
Prinivil Tablets (0.3% to greater than 1%) 2029
Prinzide Tablets (0.3% to 1%) 2033
Prochieve 4% Gel 1018
Prochieve 8% Gel 1018
Procrit for Injection (Rare) 2374
▲ Prograf Capsules and Injection (3% to 15%) 624
▲ Proleukin for Injection (6%) 1007
Prometrium Capsules (100 mg, 200 mg) (Less than 5%) 3205
ProSom Tablets (Infrequent) 512
Protonix I.V. (Less than 1%) 3468
Protonix Tablets (Less than 1%) 3465
Protopic Ointment (Up to 3%) 629
Provigil Tablets (At least 1%) 1002
Prozac Pulvules and Liquid 1771
Pulmicort Respules (1% to 3%) 654
▲ Rabies Vaccine RabAvert (53%) 1011
▲ Rapamune Oral Solution and Tablets (3% to 20%) 3472
▲ Raptiva for Injection (8%) 1247
▲ Rebetol (32% to 64%) 3073
▲ Rebetron Combination Therapy (61% to 64%) 3078
▲ Rebif Prefilled Syringe for Injection (25%) 3163
Recombivax HB (Less than 1%) 2045
ReFacto Vials 3479
Relenza Rotadisk (Less than 1.5%) 1525
Relpax Tablets (Infrequent) 2531
Remicade for IV Injection 987
ReoPro Vials (0.3%) 1779
Requip Tablets (1% or more) 1528
Rescriptor Tablets 2535
▲ Retrovir Capsules (8%) 1533
▲ Retrovir IV Infusion (8%) 1537
▲ Retrovir (8%) 1533
▲ Revatio Tablets (7%) 2541
Reyataz Capsules (Less than 3%) 948
RhoGAM Ultra-Filtered 2429
▲ Ribavirin, USP Capsules (32% to 64%) 3083
▲ Risperdal Consta Long-Acting Injection (2% to 4%) 1664
▲ Risperdal M-Tab Orally Disintegrating Tablets (Infrequent to 5%) 1658
▲ Risperdal (Infrequent to 5%) 1658
▲ Rituxan for Infusion (7%) 845
▲ Rituxan I.V. (10%) 1251
▲ Roferon-A Injection (51% to 73%) 2805
Rozerem Tablets (2%) 3228
Rythmol SR Capsules 2736
Sandimmune (2% or less) 2259
Sandostatin Injection (Less than 1%) 2263
▲ Sandostatin LAR Depot (5% to 15%) 2264
▲ Sensipar Tablets (15%) 603
Serevent Diskus (1% to 3%) 1540
▲ Simulect for Injection (3% to 10%) 2268
Singulair 2047
Sonata Capsules (Frequent) 1686
▲ Soriatane Capsules (1% to 10%) 1028
Spectracef Tablets (0.1% to 1%) 2706
▲ Spiriva HandiHaler (4%) 899
▲ Strattera Capsules (3%) 1784
Stromectol Tablets (0.4%) 2053
Sular Tablets (Less than or equal to 1%) 1163
Suprane Liquid for Inhalation (Less than 1%) 770
Sustiva Capsules (Less than 2%) 957
Synercid I.V. (Less than 1%) 1690
Tagamet Tablets (Rare) 1547
Tambocor Tablets (Less than 1%) 1824
Targretin Capsules 1719
Tarka Tablets (0.3% or more) 519
Tasmar Tablets (Frequent) 3360
▲ Taxotere Injection Concentrate (Less than 1% to 21.1%) 2947
Tegretol/Tegretol-XR 2278
▲ Temodar Capsules (5%) 3088
Tequin Injection (Less than 0.1%) 964
Tequin Tablets (Less than 0.1%) 964
Teveten Tablets (1% or greater) 1707
Teveten HCT Tablets (0.4%) 1710
Thalomid Capsules 979
Thyrolar 1203
Tiazac Capsules (2%) 1204
Timentin ADD-Vantage 1556
Timentin Injection Galaxy Container 1559
Timentin IV Infusion 1553
Timentin Pharmacy Bulk Package 1562
Timolide Tablets (Less than 1%) 2056
Tindamax 2670
Topamax Sprinkle Capsules (Greater than 1% to 2%) 2438
Topamax Tablets (Greater than 1% to 2%) 2438
Toprol-XL Tablets 660
Trelstar LA Suspension (1.1%) 3387
Tricor Tablets 523
▲ Trisenox Injection (25%) 983
▲ Trizivir Tablets (8%) 1565
Truvada Tablets 1279
Twinrix Vaccine (Less than 1%) 1571
Uniretic Tablets (Less than 1%) 3114
Univasc Tablets (1.3%) 3118
Vantas (Less than 2%) 3367
Vantin Tablets and Oral Suspension (Less than 1%) 2650
Vaqta (1.9%) 2067
Varivax (Greater than or equal to 1%) 2070
Vaseretic Tablets 2073
Vasotec I.V. Injection (0.5% to 1.0%) 2076
▲ Velcade for Injection (14%) 2102
▲ Vesanoid Capsules (14%) 2823
VFEND I.V. (Less than 2%) 2543
VFEND Oral Suspension (Less than 2%) 2543
VFEND Tablets (Less than 2%) 2543
Viagra Tablets (Less than 2%) 2552
Vicoprofen Tablets (Less than 1%) 533
Viracept (Less than 2%) 2556
Viramune Oral Suspension 903
Viramune Tablets 903
▲ Viread Tablets (3% to 4%) 1284
Vivelle Transdermal System 2288
Vivelle-Dot Transdermal System 2293
▲ Vytorin 10/10 Tablets (3.5%) 2084
▲ Vytorin 10/10 Tablets (3.5%) 3092
▲ Vytorin 10/20 Tablets (3.5%) 2084
▲ Vytorin 10/20 Tablets (3.5%) 3092
▲ Vytorin 10/40 Tablets (3.5%) 2084
▲ Vytorin 10/40 Tablets (3.5%) 3092
▲ Vytorin 10/80 Tablets (3.5%) 2084
▲ Vytorin 10/80 Tablets (3.5%) 3092
WelChol Tablets (2%) 2855
Wellbutrin Tablets 1579
▲ Wellbutrin SR Sustained-Release Tablets (2% to 6%) 1583
▲ Wellbutrin XL Extended-Release Tablets (2% to 6%) 1588
WinRho SDF 763
Xalatan Sterile Ophthalmic Solution (1% to 2%) 2654
Xanax XR Tablets (1.5%) 2655
▲ Xeloda Tablets (Less than 5% to 9%) 2825
▲ Xenical Capsules (4.2%) 2834
Xifaxan Tablets (Less than 2%) 2847
Xopenex HFA Inhalation Aerosol (1.5%) 3151
Xopenex Inhalation Solution (1.5%) 3143
Xopenex Inhalation Solution Concentrate (1.5%) 3147
Zantac (Rare) 1597
Zantac Injection (Rare) 1593
Zantac Injection Pharmacy Bulk Package (Rare) 1595
Zantac Syrup (Rare) 1597
Zegerid Powder for Oral Solution (Less than 1%) 2972
Zelnorm Tablets (1%) 2303
Zemaira (0.2% to 0.4%) 3506
▲ Zenapax for Injection (2% to 5%) 2838
▲ Zerit (32%) 971
Zestoretic Tablets (0.3% to 1%) 701
Zestril Tablets (0.3% to 1.0%) 704
▲ Zetia Tablets (5%) 2090
▲ Zetia Tablets (5%) 3098
▲ Zevalin Injection (7%) 848
Ziagen 1600
Zocor Tablets 2078
▲ Zofran Injection (10%) 1607
▲ Zoladex (3%) 709
Zoladex 3-month 712
Zoloft (Frequent) 2581
▲ Zometa for Intravenous Infusion (23%) 2306
Zomig Nasal Spray (Infrequent) 718
Zomig Tablets (1% to 2%) 714
Zomig-ZMT Tablets (1% to 2%) 714
Zonegran Capsules (Infrequent) 1089
Zosyn (1.0% or less) 3492
Zovirax Capsules 1616
Zovirax for Injection 1618
Zovirax 1616
▲ Zyban Sustained-Release Tablets (2% to 4%) 1620
Zyprexa Tablets 1798
Zyprexa ZYDIS Orally Disintegrating Tablets 1798
Zyrtec Chewable Tablets (Less than 2%) 2589
Zyrtec (Less than 2%) 2589
Zyrtec-D 12 Hour Extended Release Tablets (Less than 2%) 2591

Myasthenia

Abilify Tablets (Infrequent) 916
Abilify Tablets (Infrequent) 2472
Actiq (Less than 1%) 993
▲ Actonel Tablets (3.3%) 2679
Adalat CC Tablets (Less than 1%) 2978
Altoprev Extended-Release Tablets 1151
Ambien Tablets (Rare) 2867
Anaprox Tablets (Less than 1%) 2769
Anaprox DS Tablets (Less than 1%) 2769
Antara Capsules 2723
Aricept Tablets (Infrequent) 1086
Aricept ODT Tablets (Infrequent) 1086
Avalide Tablets 922
Avalide Tablets 2889
Avonex 839
Axert Tablets (Infrequent) 2430
Betagan Ophthalmic Solution, USP ⊙ 217
▲ Betaseron for SC Injection (46%) 791
Caduet Tablets (Less than 2%) 2507
Campath Ampules 826
Carnitor Tablets and Oral Solution 3187
Carteolol Hydrochloride Ophthalmic Solution USP, 1% ⊙ 246
Celexa (Infrequent) 1177
▲ CellCept Capsules (3% to less than 20%) 2751
▲ CellCept Intravenous (3% to less than 20%) 2751
▲ CellCept Oral Suspension (3% to less than 20%) 2751
▲ CellCept Tablets (3% to less than 20%) 2751
Cipro I.V. 2998
Cipro I.V. Pharmacy Bulk Package 3509
Cipro 2991
Cipro XR Tablets 3004
Clozapine Tablets (1%) 2141
Clozaril Tablets (1%) 2174
Combivir Tablets 1373
Copaxone for Injection (At least 2%) 3292
Cozaar Tablets (Less than 1%) 1913
Crestor Tablets (Less than 1%) 672
Decadron Phosphate Injection 1931
Decadron Tablets 1929
▲ Depakene (1% to 5%) 417
Depakote Tablets 427
▲ Depakote ER Tablets (1% to 5%) 433
Depo-Medrol Injectable Suspension 2615
Depo-Medrol Single-Dose Vial 2617
Doxil Injection (Less than 1%) 3302
EC-Naprosyn Delayed-Release Tablets (Less than 1%) 2769
Effexor XR Capsules (Infrequent) 3411
Emend Capsules (Greater than 0.5%) 1944
Epivir 1394
Epzicom Tablets 1402
Eskalith 1406
Evoxac Capsules (Less than 1%) 1042
Exelon Capsules (Infrequent) 2204
FazaClo Orally Disintegrating Tablets (1%) 547
▲ Flumist Vaccine (25.7%) 1872
Frova Tablets (Infrequent) 1101
Gabitril Tablets (1%) 998
Garamycin Injectable 3028
▲ Humira Injection (Less than 5%) 464
Hydrocortone Tablets 1963
Hyzaar 1964
▲ Imdur Tablets (Less than or equal to 5%) 3032
▲ Intron A for Injection (Less than 5%) 3038
Klonopin 2782
Lariam Tablets (Infrequent) 2790
Lescol Capsules 2227
Lescol Capsules 2730
Lescol XL Tablets 2227

Lescol XL Tablets 2730
Levoxyl Tablets 1680
Lexapro Oral Solution (Infrequent) 1193
Lexapro Tablets (Infrequent) 1193
Lofibra Capsules 1217
Lotensin HCT Tablets 2235
Lunesta Tablets (Infrequent) 3139
Lyrica Capsules (Greather than or equal to 1%) 2524
Maxzide 2150
Mevacor Tablets 1996
Migranal Nasal Spray (Infrequent) 3350
Mirapex Tablets (Less than or equal to 1%) 889
Naprosyn Suspension (Less than 1%) 2769
Naprosyn Tablets (Less than 1%) 2769
▲ Navelbine Injection (Up to 15% to 20%) 1494
Neurontin Capsules (Infrequent) 2498
Neurontin Oral Solution (Infrequent) 2498
Neurontin Tablets (Infrequent) 2498
Niaspan Extended-Release Tablets 1703
Nimbex Injection 494
Norvasc Tablets (Less than or equal to 0.1%) 2529
Norvir (Less than 2%) 499
Pediapred Oral Solution 3319
Pravachol Tablets 943
Prevacid Delayed-Release Capsules (Less than 1%) 3268
Prevacid for Delayed-Release Oral Suspension (Less than 1%) 3268
Prevacid NapraPAC (Less than 1%) 3277
Prevacid SoluTab Delayed-Release Orally Disintegrating Tablets (Less than 1%) 3268
PREVPAC (Less than 1%) 3281
Prilosec OTC Tablets (Less than 1%) 2674
Prozac Pulvules and Liquid (Rare) 1771
Recombivax HB 2045
ReFacto Vials 3479
Relpax Tablets (Infrequent) 2531
Requip Tablets (Infrequent) 1528
Retrovir Capsules 1533
Retrovir IV Infusion 1537
Retrovir 1533
Reyataz Capsules (Less than 3%) 948
Risperdal Consta Long-Acting Injection (Infrequent) 1664
▲ Rythmol SR Capsules (1% to 4%) 2736
Sonata Capsules (Infrequent) 1686
Soriatane Capsules (Less than 1%) 1028
Symbyax Capsules (Rare) 1788
Synercid I.V. (Less than 1%) 1690
Targretin Capsules 1719
Tequin Injection (Less than 0.1%) 964
Tequin Tablets (Less than 0.1%) 964
Thalomid Capsules 979
Timolide Tablets 2056
Topamax Sprinkle Capsules (More than 1%) 2438
Topamax Tablets (More than 1%) 2438
Tricor Tablets 523
Trileptal Oral Suspension (1% to 2%) 2281
Trileptal Tablets (1% to 2%) 2281
Trizivir Tablets 1565
Unithroid Tablets 3521
VFEND I.V. (Less than 2%) 2543
VFEND Oral Suspension (Less than 2%) 2543
VFEND Tablets (Less than 2%) 2543
Viagra Tablets (Less than 2%) 2552
Viracept (Less than 2%) 2556
▲ Visudyne for Injection (1% to 10%) 2286
Wellbutrin Tablets 1579
▲ Xeloda Tablets (Less than 5%) 2825
Zegerid Powder for Oral Solution (Less than 1%) 2972
Zocor Tablets 2078
Zoloft (Infrequent) 2581
Zomig Tablets (1% to 2%) 714
Zomig-ZMT Tablets (1% to 2%) 714
Zonegran Capsules (Infrequent) 1089
Zyrtec Chewable Tablets (Less than 2%) 2589
Zyrtec (Less than 2%) 2589
Zyrtec-D 12 Hour Extended Release Tablets (Less than 2%) 2591

Myasthenia gravis

Abelcet Injection 1119
Blocadren Tablets (Less than 1%) 1891
Captopril Tablets 2114
▲ Casodex Tablets (7%) 670
Cuprimine Capsules 1925
Cytovene (At least 3 subjects) 2763
▲ Depacon Injection (1% to 5%) 412
▲ Depakote Sprinkle Capsules (1% to 5%) 422
▲ Depakote Tablets (1% to 5%) 427
Effexor Tablets (Infrequent) 3405
Eskalith (Rare) 1406
Lamictal (1.3%) 1449
Lipitor Tablets (Less than 2%) 2495
Myleran Tablets (Rare) 1492
Paxil CR Controlled-Release Tablets (1%) 1509
Paxil (1%) 1501
▲ Prograf Capsules and Injection (3% to 15%) 624
Rilutek Tablets (Infrequent) 2945
Sular Tablets (Less than or equal to 1%) 1163
Syprine Capsules 2055

Myasthenia gravis, exacerbation of

Betoptic S Ophthalmic Suspension 554
Cipro I.V. 2998
Cipro I.V. Pharmacy Bulk Package 3509
Cipro 2991
Cipro XR Tablets 3004
Cosopt Sterile Ophthalmic Solution 1910
Ketek Tablets 2920
Mefoxin for Injection (A possibility) 1987
Mefoxin Premixed Intravenous Solution 1990
Noroxin Tablets 2009
Timolide Tablets 2056
Timoptic Sterile Ophthalmic Solution (Less frequent) 2058
Timoptic-XE Sterile Ophthalmic Gel Forming Solution 2062

Myasthenia gravis, increase

Betagan Ophthalmic Solution, USP ⊙217
Betimol Ophthalmic Solution ⊙283
Betimol Ophthalmic Solution 3371
Timoptic in Ocudose (Less frequent) 2061

Myasthenia gravis-like syndrome

Clozapine Tablets 2141
Clozaril Tablets 2174
Garamycin Injectable 3028
Seroquel Tablets (Infrequent) 691

Myasthenic syndrome

FazaClo Orally Disintegrating Tablets 547

Mydriasis

Albalon Ophthalmic Solution ⊙216
Atrovent HFA Inhalation Aerosol 872
Bentyl Capsules 724
Bentyl Injection 724
Bentyl Syrup 724
Bentyl Tablets 724
Blephamide Ophthalmic Ointment (Occasional) 563
Blephamide Ophthalmic Suspension 564
Caverject Impulse Injection (Less than 1%) 2610
Celexa (Rare) 1177
Clozapine Tablets (Less than 1%) 2141
Clozaril Tablets (Less than 1%) 2174
Cogentin Injection 1903
Copaxone for Injection (Infrequent) 3292
Diastat Rectal Delivery System (Less than 1%) 3344
Ditropan XL Extended Release Tablets 2391
Effexor Tablets (2%) 3405
Effexor XR Capsules (Frequent) 3411
Evoxac Capsules (Less than 1%) 1042
FazaClo Orally Disintegrating Tablets (Less than 1%) 547
FML Ophthalmic Ointment (Occasional) ⊙225
FML Ophthalmic Suspension (Occasional) ⊙224
FML Forte Ophthalmic Suspension (Occasional) ⊙223
HMS Sterile Ophthalmic Suspension ⊙228
Imitrex Nasal Spray 1435
Imitrex Tablets (Rare) 1440
Inversine Tablets 3286
Lexapro Oral Solution (Infrequent) 1193
Lexapro Tablets (Infrequent) 1193
Lunesta Tablets (Rare) 3139
Lyrica Capsules (Rare) 2524
Meridia Capsules 485
Norflex Injection 1824
Ocufen Ophthalmic Solution ⊙230
Parcopa Orally Disintegrating Tablets 3111
Paxil CR Controlled-Release Tablets (Infrequent) 1509
Paxil (Infrequent) 1501
Pred Forte Ophthalmic Suspension (Occasional) ⊙233
Pred Mild Sterile Ophthalmic Suspension (Occasional) ⊙236
Propine Ophthalmic Solution ⊙237
Prozac Pulvules and Liquid (Infrequent) 1771
Stalevo Tablets 2270
Strattera Capsules (1% to 2%) 1784
Surmontil Capsules 2347
Symmetrel 1115
Thioridazine Hydrochloride Tablets 2122
Thiothixene Capsules 2124
Topamax Sprinkle Capsules (Rare) 2438
Topamax Tablets (Rare) 2438
Transderm Scōp Transdermal Therapeutic System 2166
Trileptal Oral Suspension 2281
Trileptal Tablets 2281
VFEND I.V. (Less than 2%) 2543
VFEND Oral Suspension (Less than 2%) 2543
VFEND Tablets (Less than 2%) 2543
Viagra Tablets (Less than 2%) 2552
Vivactil Tablets 2350
Wellbutrin Tablets (Infrequent) 1579
Wellbutrin SR Sustained-Release Tablets 1583
Wellbutrin XL Extended-Release Tablets 1588
Xanax XR Tablets (Infrequent) 2655
Zaditor Ophthalmic Solution (Less than 5%) 2302
Zoloft (Infrequent) 2581
Zyban Sustained-Release Tablets 1620
Zyprexa Tablets (Rare) 1798
Zyprexa ZYDIS Orally Disintegrating Tablets (Rare) 1798

Myelitis

Havrix Vaccine (Rare) 1425
Paxil CR Controlled-Release Tablets (Rare) 1509
Paxil (Rare) 1501
Permax Tablets (Rare) 3357
Rabies Vaccine RabAvert 1011
Recombivax HB 2045
Twinrix Vaccine 1571
Zyrtec Chewable Tablets (Less than 2%) 2589
Zyrtec (Less than 2%) 2589
Zyrtec-D 12 Hour Extended Release Tablets (Less than 2%) 2591

Myelitis, transverse

Asacol Delayed-Release Tablets (Rare) 2688
Enbrel for Injection (Rare) 580
Engerix-B Vaccine 1391
Raptiva for Injection (1 case) 1247
Recombivax HB 2045
Remicade for IV Injection 987
Twinrix Vaccine 1571
Varivax 2070

Myelodysplastic syndrome

Bexxar 1360
Neupogen for Injection (Approximately 3%) 598
Temodar Capsules 3088
Zevalin Injection 848

Myelofibrosis

Lyrica Capsules (Rare) 2524

Myeloid immaturity

Miradon Tablets 3056

Myeloma, multiple

Effexor XR Capsules (Rare) 3411

Myelopathy

Cytovene 2763

Myelopolyradiculoneuritis

Invirase (Less than 2%) 2776

Myelosclerosis, malignant

Matulane Capsules 3188

Myelosuppression

Adriamycin for Injection, USP 786
Adriamycin Injection, USP 786
Alkeran for Injection 976
Camptosar Injection 2602
▲ Cerubidine for Injection (All patients) 788
Doxil Injection 3302
Gemzar for Injection 1743
Hexalen Capsules 2101
Idamycin PFS Injection 2645
▲ I.V. Busulfex (100%, most frequent, occurring in all patients) 1125
Leukeran Tablets 1472
Leustatin Injection (Frequent) 2368
▲ Myleran Tablets (Most frequent) 1492
Mylotarg for Injection 3429
▲ Navelbine Injection (53%) 1494
Purinethol Tablets 1222
Roferon-A Injection 2805
▲ Tabloid Tablets (Most frequent) 1545
Temodar Capsules 3088
Zinecard for Injection 2659

Myelosuppression, persistent severe

Adriamycin for Injection, USP 786
Adriamycin Injection, USP 786

Myesthenia

▲ Eloxatin for Injection (2% to 5%) 2908

Myocardial hypertrophy

Prograf Capsules and Injection (Rare) 624

Myocardial infarction

▲ Abelcet Injection (3%) 1119
Abilify Tablets (Infrequent) 916
Abilify Tablets (Infrequent) 2472
Aceon Tablets (2 mg, 4 mg, 8 mg) (0.3% to 1%) 3191
Aciphex Tablets 1081
Actimmune (Rare) 1646
Activella Tablets 2311
Adderall Tablets 3168
Adderall XR Capsules 3169
Adenoscan (Less than 1%) 613
Agrylin Capsules 3172
Aldara Cream, 5% 1814
Alesse-28 Tablets 3392
Altace Capsules (1.7%) 1673
Ambien Tablets (Rare) 2867
Amerge Tablets 1312
Amevive (Less than 1%) 836
Anaprox Tablets (Less than 1%) 2769
Anaprox DS Tablets (Less than 1%) 2769
Antara Capsules 2723
▲ Apokyn Injection (4%) 2132
Aranesp for Injection (2%) 576
▲ Argatroban Injection (3.6%) 1321
Aricept Tablets (Infrequent) 1086
Aricept ODT Tablets (Infrequent) 1086
Arimidex Tablets (0.8%) 665
Arthrotec Tablets (Rare) 3126
Atacand Tablets (Less frequently) 634
Atacand HCT (Less than 0.5%) 637
Avalide Tablets 922
Avalide Tablets 2889
Avapro Tablets (Less than 1%) 925
Avapro Tablets (Less than 1%) 2886
Caduet Tablets 2507
Campath Ampules 826
Campral Tablets (Infrequent) 1175
Camptosar Injection (0.4% to 1.3%) 2602
Captopril Tablets (2 to 3 of 1000 patients) 2114
Carbatrol Capsules 3174
Cardene I.V. 1129
Cardizem LA Extended Release Tablets 1699
Cataflam Tablets (Rarely) 2173
Celebrex Capsules (0.1% to 1.9%) 3130
Celexa (Infrequent) 1177
Cenestin Tablets, 0.45mg, 0.625mg, 0.9mg, 1.25mg 1063
Cenestin Tablets, 0.3mg 1063
Cialis Tablets (Less than 2%) 1806
Cipro I.V. (1% or less) 2998
Cipro I.V. Pharmacy Bulk Package (1% or less) 3509
Cipro (Less than 1%) 2991
Cipro XR Tablets 3004
Climara Transdermal System 795
Climara Pro Transdermal System 800
Clozapine Tablets (Several patients) 2141
Clozaril Tablets (Several patients) 2174
CombiPatch Transdermal System 2180
Coreg Tablets (0.1% to 1%) 1376
Cosopt Sterile Ophthalmic Solution (Less than 1%) 1910
Covera-HS Tablets (Less than 2%) 3135
Cozaar Tablets (Less than 1%) 1913
Crixivan Capsules 1918
Cymbalta Delayed-Release Capsules (Infrequent) 1729
DDAVP Injection 4 mcg/mL (Rare) 2893
Desmopressin Acetate Injection (Rare) 1143

Diprivan Injectable Emulsion (Less than 1%) 676
Dolobid Tablets 1937
DynaCirc CR Tablets (0.5% to 1%) 2726
EC-Naprosyn Delayed-Release Tablets (Less than 1%) 2769
Edex Injection (1%) 3103
Effexor Tablets (Rare) 3405
Effexor XR Capsules (Infrequent) 3411
Elitek (Less than or equal to 1%) 2906
▲ Emcyt Capsules (3%) 3137
Emend Capsules (Greater than 0.5%) 1944
Enbrel for Injection (Infrequent) 580
Epogen for Injection (0.4%) 586
Estratest Tablets 3196
Estratest H.S. Tablets 3196
Estrogel 0.06% 3200
Ethyol for Injection (Rare) 1869
Evoxac Capsules (Less than 1%) 1042
Exelon Capsules (Frequent) 2204
Feiba VH 749
Femara Tablets (Less than or equal to 2%) 2210
Ferrlecit Injection 3379
Flexeril Tablets (Rare) 1832
▲ Flolan for Injection (4%) 1408
Fortical Nasal Spray (Less than 1%) 3336
Frova Tablets 1101
Gabitril Tablets (Infrequent) 998
Gammagard S/D 754
Gemzar for Injection (Very rare) 1743
Gengraf Capsules (1% to less than 3%) 458
▲ Humira Injection (Less than 5%) 464
Hyperstat I.V. Injection 3031
Hyzaar 1964
Idamycin PFS Injection 2645
▲ Imdur Tablets (Less than or equal to 5%) 3032
Imitrex Injection (Extremely rare) 1431
Imitrex Nasal Spray 1435
Imitrex Tablets (Rare) 1440
Inspra Tablets 2520
Lamictal (Rare) 1449
Levaquin in 5% Dextrose Injection (0.1% to 0.9%) 2453
Levaquin (0.1% to 0.9%) 2453
Levitra Tablets (Less than 2%) 3048
Levothroid Tablets 1189
Levoxyl Tablets 1680
Lexapro Oral Solution 1193
Lexapro Tablets 1193
Lofibra Capsules 1217
Lo/Ovral-28 Tablets 3423
Lotrel Capsules (Rare) 2238
Maxalt Tablets (Very rare) 1983
Maxalt-MLT Orally Disintegrating Tablets (Very rare) 1983
Menostar Transdermal System 805
Meridia Capsules 485
Merrem I.V. (Greater than 0.1% to 1%) 687
Miacalcin Nasal Spray (Less than 1%) 2242
Micardis Tablets 884
Micardis HCT Tablets 886
Mirapex Tablets (Less than 1%) 889
Mobic Oral Suspension (Less than 2%) 893
Mobic Tablets (Less than 2%) 893
Mycamine for Injection 620
Namenda (Infrequent) 1199
Naprosyn Suspension (Less than 1%) 2769
Naprosyn Tablets (Less than 1%) 2769
Naropin Injection (Less than 1%) 640
Navelbine Injection (Rare) 1494
Neoral Soft Gelatin Capsules (1% to less than 3%) 2247
Neoral Oral Solution (1% to less than 3%) 2247
▲ Neupogen for Injection (11 of 375 cancer patients) 598
Neurontin Capsules (Rare) 2498
Neurontin Oral Solution (Rare) 2498
Neurontin Tablets (Rare) 2498
Noroxin Tablets (Less frequent) 2009
Norvasc Tablets (Rare) 2529
Omacor Capsules 2735
Omnicef Capsules 506
Omnicef for Oral Suspension 506
Ontak Vials (Two patients) 1717
OptiPranolol Metipranolol Ophthalmic Solution 0.3% (A small number of patients) ⊙ 254
Ortho-Cept Tablets 2395
Ortho-Cyclen Tablets 2414
Ortho Evra Transdermal System 2402
Ortho Tri-Cyclen Tablets 2414
Ortho Tri-Cyclen Lo Tablets 2421
Orthoclone OKT3 Sterile Solution (Less than 1%) 2370
Parcopa Orally Disintegrating Tablets 3111
Paxil CR Controlled-Release Tablets (Rare) 1509
Paxil (Rare) 1501
Pegasys 2793
PEG-Intron Powder for Injection (Less than or equal to 1%) 3062
Permax Tablets (1.1%) 3357
Photofrin for Injection 729
Plendil Extended-Release Tablets (0.5% to 1.5%) 651
Pletal Tablets (Less than 2%) 2478
Prandin Tablets (0.5, 1, and 2 mg) (Less than or equal to 1%) 2337
Prefest Tablets 1069
Premarin Intravenous 3440
Premarin Tablets 3443
Premarin Vaginal Cream 3449
Premphase Tablets 3452
Prempro Tablets 3452
Prevacid Delayed-Release Capsules (Less than 1%) 3268
Prevacid for Delayed-Release Oral Suspension (Less than 1%) 3268
Prevacid NapraPAC (Less than 1%) 3277
Prevacid SoluTab Delayed-Release Orally Disintegrating Tablets (Less than 1%) 3268
PREVPAC (Less than 1%) 3281
Prinivil Tablets (0.3% to 1.0%) 2029
Prinzide Tablets 2033
Procrit for Injection (0.4%) 2374
Proleukin for Injection (2%) 1007
Protonix I.V. 3468
Protonix Tablets (Less than 1%) 3465
Prozac Pulvules and Liquid (Infrequent) 1771
Razadyne (Infrequent) 2434
Rebetol 3073
Relafen Tablets (Less than 1%) 1523
Relpax Tablets (Rare) 2531
Remicade for IV Injection (Greater than or equal to 0.2%) 987
Revatio Tablets 2541
Rilutek Tablets (Infrequent) 2945
Risperdal Consta Long-Acting Injection (Infrequent) 1664
Risperdal M-Tab Orally Disintegrating Tablets (Infrequent) 1658
Risperdal (Infrequent) 1658
Rituxan for Infusion 845
Rituxan I.V. 1251
Roferon-A Injection (Rare to infrequent) 2805
Rythmol SR Capsules 2736
Sandimmune (Rare) 2259
Sandostatin LAR Depot (Rare) 2264
Seasonale Tablets 1073
Soriatane Capsules 1028
Stalevo Tablets 2270
Sular Tablets (Less than or equal to 1%) 1163
Suprane Liquid for Inhalation (Less than 1%) 770
Surmontil Capsules 2347
Symbyax Capsules (Rare) 1788
Tarka Tablets (Less frequent) 519
Tasmar Tablets (Infrequent) 3360
Taxotere Injection Concentrate 2947
Tegretol/Tegretol-XR 2278
Thalomid Capsules 979
Thyrogen for Injection (One patient) 1270
Tiazac Capsules 1204
Toprol-XL Tablets (Greater than 1%) 660
▲ Trasylol Injection (6%) 779
Tricor Tablets 523
Triglide Tablets 1165
Triphasil-28 Tablets 3483
Uniretic Tablets (Less than 1%) 3114
Unithroid Tablets 3521
Univasc Tablets (Less than 1%) 3118
Vaseretic Tablets 2073
Vasotec I.V. Injection (0.5% to 1.2%) 2076
Verelan PM Capsules (2% or less) 3120
▲ Vesanoid Capsules (3%) 2823
VFEND I.V. (Less than 2%) 2543
VFEND Oral Suspension (Less than 2%) 2543
VFEND Tablets (Less than 2%) 2543
Viagra Tablets 2552
Vivactil Tablets 2350
Vivelle Transdermal System 2288
Vivelle-Dot Transdermal System 2293
Voltaren Tablets (Rarely) 2298
Voltaren-XR Tablets (Rarely) 2301
Wellbutrin Tablets (Rare) 1579
Wellbutrin SR Sustained-Release Tablets 1583
Wellbutrin XL Extended-Release Tablets 1588
Yasmin 28 Tablets 818
Zestoretic Tablets 701
Zestril Tablets (0.3% to 1.0%) 704
Zoladex (1% to 5%) 709
Zoladex 3-month 712
Zoloft (Rare) 2581
Zomig Nasal Spray (Rare) 718
Zomig Tablets 714
Zomig-ZMT Tablets 714
Zosyn (1.0% or less) 3492
Zyban Sustained-Release Tablets 1620

Myocardial infarction, post-abrupt discontinuation
Inderal LA Long-Acting Capsules (Some cases) 3421
Tenormin I.V. Injection 698
Tenormin Tablets 695

Myocardial insufficiency
Idamycin PFS Injection 2645
Orthoclone OKT3 Sterile Solution 2370

Myocardial reinfarction
Activase I.V. 1225
Retavase 1131
TNKase I.V. 1256

Myocardial rupture
Activase I.V. 1225
Decadron Phosphate Injection 1931
Decadron Tablets 1929
Hydrocortone Tablets 1963
Retavase 1131
TNKase I.V. 1256

Myocarditis
Aldoclor Tablets 1881
Aldoril Tablets 1884
Asacol Delayed-Release Tablets (Rare) 2688
Boostrix 1366
Cerubidine for Injection (Rare) 788
Clozapine Tablets 2141
Clozaril Tablets 2174
Cytovene-IV (One report) 2763
Geodon Capsules (Rare) 2514
Pentasa Capsules (Infrequent) 3182
Proleukin for Injection (Less than 1% to 1%) 1007
Reyataz Capsules (Less than 3%) 948
Risperdal M-Tab Orally Disintegrating Tablets (Rare) 1658
Risperdal (Rare) 1658
▲ Vesanoid Capsules (3%) 2823
▲ Xeloda Tablets (Less than 5%) 2825

Myocardium, depression
Naropin Injection 640

Myoclonia
Abilify Tablets (Infrequent) 916
Abilify Tablets (Infrequent) 2472
Aloprim for Injection (Less than 1%) 2156
Celexa 1177
Cipro I.V. 2998
Cipro I.V. Pharmacy Bulk Package 3509
Cipro 2991
Cipro XR Tablets 3004
Clozapine Tablets (1%) 2141
Clozaril Tablets (1%) 2174
Copaxone for Injection (Infrequent) 3292
Dilaudid 439
Dilaudid Oral Liquid 443
Dilaudid Non-Sterile Powder 439
Dilaudid Tablets - 8 mg 443
Dilaudid-HP Injection 441
Diprivan Injectable Emulsion (Less than 1%) 676
Effexor Tablets (Infrequent) 3405
Effexor XR Capsules (Infrequent) 3411
Eldepryl Capsules 3209
Fortaz 1422
Gabitril Tablets (Frequent) 998
Geodon Capsules (Rare) 2514
Imitrex Injection (Rare) 1431
Kadian Capsules (Less than 3%) 572
Lamictal (Infrequent) 1449
Leukeran Tablets (Rare) 1472
Lexapro Oral Solution 1193
Lexapro Tablets 1193
Mirapex Tablets (1%) 889
Neurontin Capsules (Rare) 2498
Neurontin Oral Solution (Rare) 2498
Neurontin Tablets (Rare) 2498
Noroxin Tablets 2009
Orthoclone OKT3 Sterile Solution 2370
▲ Paxil CR Controlled-Release Tablets (3%) 1509
▲ Paxil (3%) 1501
Permax Tablets (Infrequent) 3357
Primaxin I.M. 2022
Primaxin I.V. (Less than 0.2%) 2024
▲ Prograf Capsules and Injection (3% to 15%) 624
Rilutek Tablets (Infrequent) 2945
Seroquel Tablets (Infrequent) 691
Sonata Capsules (Rare) 1686
Symbyax Capsules (Infrequent) 1788
Tasmar Tablets (Infrequent) 3360
Wellbutrin Tablets (Frequent) 1579
Zonegran Capsules (Rare) 1089
▲ Zyprexa Tablets (1% to 5%) 1798
Zyprexa ZYDIS Orally Disintegrating Tablets (1% to 5%) 1798

Myoclonus
FazaClo Orally Disintegrating Tablets 547
▲ Lyrica Capsules (0.1% to 4%) 2524
Maxipime for Injection 1093

Myoglobinemia
Symmetrel (Uncommon) 1115

Myoglobinuria
Orap Tablets 1220
Risperdal M-Tab Orally Disintegrating Tablets 1658
Risperdal 1658
Seroquel Tablets 691
Zocor Tablets (Rare) 2078

Myolysis
Trizivir Tablets 1565
Ziagen 1600

Myopathy
Abilify Tablets (Infrequent) 916
Abilify Tablets (Infrequent) 2472
Actiq (Less than 1%) 993
Advicor Tablets 1694
Altoprev Extended-Release Tablets 1151
Antara Capsules 2723
Axert Tablets (Rare) 2430
Campral Tablets (Frequent) 1175
Copaxone for Injection (Infrequent) 3292
Crestor Tablets (Less than 1%) 672
Darvocet A 500 Tablets 3497
Effexor Tablets (Rare) 3405
Effexor XR Capsules (Rare) 3411
Geodon Capsules (Rare) 2514
Herceptin I.V. (At least one of the 958 patients) 1234
Lescol Capsules (Occasional) 2227
Lescol Capsules (Occasional) 2730
Lescol XL Tablets 2227
Lescol XL Tablets 2730
Lofibra Capsules 1217
Lunesta Tablets (Rare) 3139
Mevacor Tablets 1996
Nimbex Injection 494
Paxil CR Controlled-Release Tablets (2%) 1509
Paxil (2%) 1501
Pediapred Oral Solution 3319
Pravachol Tablets (Rare) 943
Proleukin for Injection 1007
Prozac Pulvules and Liquid (Rare) 1771
Relpax Tablets (Rare) 2531
ReoPro Vials (0.4%) 1779
Retrovir Capsules 1533
Retrovir IV Infusion 1537
Retrovir 1533
Reyataz Capsules (Less than 3%) 948
Soriatane Capsules 1028
Sustiva Capsules 957
Symbyax Capsules (Rare) 1788
Trizivir Tablets 1565
VFEND I.V. (Less than 2%) 2543
VFEND Oral Suspension (Less than 2%) 2543
VFEND Tablets (Less than 2%) 2543
Viracept (Less than 2%) 2556
Vytorin 10/10 Tablets 2084
Vytorin 10/10 Tablets 3092
Vytorin 10/20 Tablets 2084
Vytorin 10/20 Tablets 3092
Vytorin 10/40 Tablets 2084
Vytorin 10/40 Tablets 3092
Vytorin 10/80 Tablets 2084
Vytorin 10/80 Tablets 3092
Zetia Tablets 2090
Zocor Tablets 2078
Zyprexa Tablets (Rare) 1798
Zyprexa ZYDIS Orally Disintegrating Tablets (Rare) 1798

Myopathy, steroid
Decadron Phosphate Injection 1931

Decadron Tablets 1929
Depo-Medrol Injectable Suspension 2615
Depo-Medrol Single-Dose Vial 2617
Hydrocortone Tablets 1963

Myopia
Evoxac Capsules (Less than 1%) 1042
Namenda (Infrequent) 1199
Topamax Sprinkle Capsules (1%) 2438
Topamax Tablets (1%) 2438

Myopia, transient
Clorpres Tablets (Occasional) 2139
Cosopt Sterile Ophthalmic Solution 1910
Trusopt Sterile Ophthalmic Solution 2065

Myosis
Doxil Injection (Less than 1%) 3302

Myositis
Advair Diskus 100/50 1291
Advair Diskus 250/50 1291
Advair Diskus 500/50 1291
Antara Capsules 2723
Caduet Tablets (Less than 2%) 2507
Campath Ampules 826
Copegus Tablets (Less than 1%) 2759
Crestor Tablets (Less than 1%) 672
▲ Imdur Tablets (Less than or equal to 5%) 3032
Lipitor Tablets (Less than 2%) 2495
Lofibra Capsules 1217
Norvir (Less than 2%) 499
Paxil CR Controlled-Release Tablets (Rare) 1509
Paxil (Rare) 1501
Pegasys (Less than 1%) 2793
Permax Tablets (Infrequent) 3357
Proleukin for Injection 1007
Prozac Pulvules and Liquid (Rare) 1771
Retrovir Capsules 1533
Retrovir IV Infusion 1537
Retrovir 1533
Sonata Capsules (Rare) 1686
Sular Tablets (Less than or equal to 1%) 1163
Ticlid Tablets (Rare) 2813
Tricor Tablets 523
Vaseretic Tablets 2073
Vasotec I.V. Injection (0.5% to 1.0%) 2076
Vesanoid Capsules (Isolated cases) 2823

Myxedema
Eskalith 1406
Thalomid Capsules 979

N

Nail discoloration
Evoxac Capsules (Less than 1%) 1042
Lithobid Tablets 1670
Retrovir Capsules 1533
Retrovir IV Infusion 1537
Retrovir 1533

Nail disorders, unspecified
Amnesteem Capsules 2126
Antara Capsules 2723
▲ Avastin IV (2% to 8%) 1229
Celebrex Capsules (0.1% to 1.9%) 3130
▲ Erbitux (16%) 937
Evoxac Capsules (Less than 1%) 1042
Gleevec Tablets (Infrequent) 2221
Kaletra (Less than 2%) 474
Lofibra Capsules 1217
Lotronex Tablets (Rare) 1479
Neurontin Capsules (Rare) 2498
Neurontin Oral Solution (Rare) 2498
Neurontin Tablets (Rare) 2498
Penlac Nail Lacquer, Topical Solution, 8% (2%) 1051
Prevacid Delayed-Release Capsules (Less than 1%) 3268
Prevacid for Delayed-Release Oral Suspension (Less than 1%) 3268
Prevacid NapraPAC (Less than 1%) 3277
Prevacid SoluTab Delayed-Release Orally Disintegrating Tablets (Less than 1%) 3268
PREVPAC (Less than 1%) 3281
Reyataz Capsules (Less than 3%) 948
Rythmol SR Capsules 2736
Soriatane Capsules 1028
Sustiva Capsules 957
Tricor Tablets 523

Nails, changes of
Accutane Capsules 2740
Advicor Tablets 1694
Altoprev Extended-Release Tablets 1151
▲ Arava Tablets (1% to 3%) 2881
Copaxone for Injection (At least 2%) 3292
Effexor Tablets (Infrequent) 3405
Effexor XR Capsules (Infrequent) 3411
Gengraf Capsules (1% to less than 3%) 458
▲ Intron A for Injection (Less than 5%) 3038
Invirase (Less than 2%) 2776
Lescol Capsules 2227
Lescol Capsules 2730
Lescol XL Tablets 2227
Lescol XL Tablets 2730
Lupron Depot 3.75 mg (Less than 5%) 3257
Lupron Depot–3 Month 11.25 mg (Less than 5%) 3262
Mevacor Tablets 1996
Neoral Soft Gelatin Capsules (1% to less than 3%) 2247
Neoral Oral Solution (1% to less than 3%) 2247
Oncaspar 1123
Pentasa Capsules (Less than 1%) 3182
Pravachol Tablets 943
Rescriptor Tablets 2535
▲ Soriatane Capsules (25% to 50%) 1028
▲ Taxotere Injection Concentrate (Less than 1% to 40.5%) 2947
▲ Thalomid Capsules (4.2%) 979
Vytorin 10/10 Tablets 2084
Vytorin 10/10 Tablets 3092
Vytorin 10/20 Tablets 2084
Vytorin 10/20 Tablets 3092
Vytorin 10/40 Tablets 2084
Vytorin 10/40 Tablets 3092
Vytorin 10/80 Tablets 2084
Vytorin 10/80 Tablets 3092
▲ Xeloda Tablets (Less than 5%) 2825
Zocor Tablets 2078

Nasal burning
▲ Astelin Nasal Spray (4.1%) 1876
Atrovent Nasal Spray 0.03% (2.0%) 869
Atrovent Nasal Spray 0.06% (Less than 1%) 870
▲ Flonase Nasal Spray (2.4% to 3.2%) 1412
▲ Nasacort HFA Inhalation Aerosol (Greater than or equal to 3%) 2939
▲ Nasarel Nasal Spray (13% to 44%) 1652
Nasonex Nasal Spray 3058
Nicotrol NS 2596
Vicks Sinex Nasal Spray and Ultra Fine Mist for Sinus Relief 2677
Zicam Cold Remedy Nasal Pump ▣
Zicam Cold Remedy Swabs ▣
Zicam Cold Remedy Swabs Kids Size ▣
Zicam Extreme Congestion Relief Nasal Pump ▣
Zicam Sinus Relief Nasal Pump ▣

Nasal congestion
Adenoscan (Less than 1%) 613
▲ Advair Diskus 250/50 (1% to 3%) 1291
▲ Aerobid/Aerobid-M (15%) 1172
Alamast Ophthalmic Solution (Less than 5%) 3371
Aldoclor Tablets 1881
Aldoril Tablets 1884
Asacol Delayed-Release Tablets 2688
Astelin Nasal Spray 1876
▲ Atrovent Nasal Spray 0.03% (3.1%) 869
Atrovent Nasal Spray 0.06% (1.1%) 870
Bentyl Capsules 724
Bentyl Injection 724
Bentyl Syrup 724
Bentyl Tablets 724
Betagan Ophthalmic Solution, USP ⊙ 217
Betimol Ophthalmic Solution ⊙ 283
Betimol Ophthalmic Solution 3371
BiDil Tablets 2161
Brevibloc Concentrate (Less than 1%) 766
Brevibloc Injection (Less than 1%) 766
Brevibloc Double Strength Injection (Less than 1%) 766
Brevibloc Premixed Injection (Less than 1%) 766
Brevibloc Double Strength Premixed Injection (Less than 1%) 766
Calcium Disodium Versenate Injection 1819
Cardizem LA Extended Release Tablets (Less than 2%) 1699
Caverject Impulse Injection (1%) 2610
▲ Chemet Capsules (0.7% to 3.7%) 2480
▲ Cialis Tablets (2% to 3%) 1806
Clozapine Tablets (1%) 2141
Clozaril Tablets (1%) 2174
Combivent Inhalation Aerosol 878
Cosopt Sterile Ophthalmic Solution (1% to 5%) 1910
Cozaar Tablets (2%) 1913
DDAVP Nasal Spray (Occasional) 2894
Demser Capsules (Infrequent) 1933
Desmopressin Acetate Rhinal Tube (Occasional) 1144
Dibenzyline Capsules 3390
DynaCirc CR Tablets (0.5% to 1%) 2726
Elidel Cream 1% (0.6% to 2.6%) 2198
FazaClo Orally Disintegrating Tablets (1%) 547
▲ Flovent Diskus 50 mcg (16%) 1415
▲ Flumist Vaccine (9.2% to 48.1%) 1872
▲ Fortical Nasal Spray (10.6%) 3336
▲ Hytrin Capsules (0.6% to 5.9%) 469
Hyzaar 1964
▲ Imdur Tablets (Less than or equal to 5%) 3032
▲ Intron A for Injection (Up to 10%) 3038
Iveegam EN 759
Lexapro Oral Solution (Frequent) 1193
Lexapro Tablets (Frequent) 1193
Maxalt Tablets (Infrequent) 1983
Maxalt-MLT Orally Disintegrating Tablets (Infrequent) 1983
Meridia Capsules 485
Metrogel 1% (1.1%) 1212
▲ Miacalcin Nasal Spray (10.6%) 2242
Midamor Tablets (Less than or equal to 1%) 2000
Moduretic Tablets (Less than or equal to 1%) 2003
Nicotrol NS 2596
▲ Niravam Orally Disintegrating Tablets (7.3% to 17.4%) 3106
Orthoclone OKT3 Sterile Solution 2370
Prinivil Tablets (0.4%) 2029
Prinzide Tablets (0.3% to 1%) 2033
Prometrium Capsules (100 mg, 200 mg) (Less than 5%) 3205
Proventil Inhalation Solution 0.083% (1%) 3069
Requip Tablets (2%) 1528
Sedapap Tablets 50 mg/650 mg (Infrequent) 2098
▲ Serevent Diskus (9%) 1540
Singulair (1.6%) 2047
▲ Strattera Capsules (2% or greater) 1784
Tessalon Capsules 1202
Tessalon Perles 1202
Thiothixene Capsules 2124
Tiazac Capsules (Less than 2%) 1204
Timoptic in Ocudose (Less frequent) 2061
Timoptic Sterile Ophthalmic Solution (Less frequent) 2058
Timoptic-XE Sterile Ophthalmic Gel Forming Solution 2062
Vanos Cream (0% to 1.4%) 1864
Vaqta (1.2%) 2067
▲ Viagra Tablets (4%) 2552
Xanax XR Tablets (Frequent) 2655
Zestoretic Tablets (0.3% to 1%) 701
Zestril Tablets (0.4%) 704

Nasal crusts
▲ Fortical Nasal Spray (10.6%) 3336

Nasal discharge, increase
Aredia for Injection (One patient) 2168
Emend Capsules (Greater than 0.5%) 1944
▲ Flovent Diskus 50 mcg (1% to 3%) 1415
▲ Flumist Vaccine (9.2% to 48.1%) 1872
▲ Miacalcin Nasal Spray (10.6%) 2242
Vicks Sinex Nasal Spray and Ultra Fine Mist for Sinus Relief 2677
Zicam Cold Remedy Nasal Pump ▣
Zicam Cold Remedy Swabs ▣
Zicam Cold Remedy Swabs Kids Size ▣
Zicam Extreme Congestion Relief Nasal Pump ▣
Zicam Sinus Relief Nasal Pump ▣

Nasal drainage
Alferon N Injection (2%) 1640

Nasal drip, posterior
Aceon Tablets (2 mg, 4 mg, 8 mg) (0.3% to 1%) 3191
▲ Advair Diskus 100/50 (1% to 3%) 1291
▲ Advair Diskus 250/50 (1% to 3%) 1291
▲ Advair Diskus 500/50 (1% to 3%) 1291
Aricept Tablets (Infrequent) 1086
Aricept ODT Tablets (Infrequent) 1086
▲ Atrovent Nasal Spray 0.03% (3.1%) 869
▲ Flovent HFA (1% to 3%) 1418
▲ Trisenox Injection (13%) 983

Nasal itching
(*see under* Pruritus, rhinal)

Nasal mucosa, dryness
(*see under* Xeromycteria)

Nasal obstruction
▲ Advair Diskus 250/50 (1% to 3%) 1291
Neurontin Oral Solution (Rare) 2498

Nasal passages, dry
Abilify Tablets (Rare) 916
Abilify Tablets (Rare) 2472

Nasal septum, perforation
Beconase AQ Nasal Spray (Rare) 1359
Flonase Nasal Spray (Rare) 1412
Nasacort HFA Inhalation Aerosol 2939
Nasacort AQ Nasal Spray (One patient) 2937
Nasarel Nasal Spray (Rare) 1652
Nasonex Nasal Spray (Rare) 3058
Rhinocort Aqua Nasal Spray (Rare) 658

Nasal sores
▲ Fortical Nasal Spray (10.6%) 3336

Nasal stinging
▲ Nasarel Nasal Spray (13% to 44%) 1652
Vicks Sinex Nasal Spray and Ultra Fine Mist for Sinus Relief 2677
Zicam Cold Remedy Nasal Pump ▣
Zicam Cold Remedy Swabs ▣
Zicam Cold Remedy Swabs Kids Size ▣
Zicam Extreme Congestion Relief Nasal Pump ▣
Zicam Sinus Relief Nasal Pump ▣

Nasal stuffiness
Beconase AQ Nasal Spray (Fewer than 3 per 100 patients) 1359
▲ Dostinex Tablets (Less than 10%) 2631
Nadolol Tablets (1 to 5 of 1000 patients) 2121
Phenergan 3438
Thioridazine Hydrochloride Tablets 2122

Nasal symptoms
▲ Fortical Nasal Spray (10.6%) 3336

Nasal ulceration
Beconase AQ Nasal Spray (Rare) 1359
Fortical Nasal Spray (2.8%) 3336
Nasarel Nasal Spray (1% or less) 1652
Nasonex Nasal Spray (Rare) 3058
Nicotrol NS 2596

Nasopharyngitis
▲ Advate Injection (14.7%) 742
▲ Boniva Tablets (3.5% to 4.3%) 2747
Clindesse Vaginal Cream (1.1%) 3296
▲ Cymbalta Delayed-Release Capsules (7% to 9%) 1729
▲ depo-subQ provera 104 Injectable Suspension (1% to less than 5%) 2622
▲ Elidel Cream 1% (7.6% to 26.5%) 2198
▲ Gleevec Tablets (10% to 22%) 2221
Invanz for Injection (1.6%) 1974
▲ Metrogel 1% (3.1%) 1212
▲ Myfortic Tablets (3% to less than 20%) 2244
Nalfon Capsules (1.2%) 2504
▲ Requip Tablets (9%) 1528
▲ Retisert Implant (5% to 15%) ⊙ 256
Strattera Capsules (2% or greater) 1784
▲ Tracleer Tablets (11%) 539
▲ Trisenox Injection (5%) 983
Valtrex Caplets 1573
Vanos Cream (0.9% to 1.4%) 1864
▲ Velcade for Injection (14%) 2102
Vivelle Transdermal System 2288
Vivelle-Dot Transdermal System 2293
Xifaxan Tablets (Less than 2%) 2847

Nausea
▲ Abelcet Injection (9%) 1119
▲ Abilify Tablets (Frequent to 16%) 916
▲ Abilify Tablets (Frequent to 16%) 2472
▲ Accolate Tablets (3.1%) 663
AccuNeb Inhalation Solution (0.9% to 1.7%) 1055
Accutane Capsules 2740
Aceon Tablets (2 mg, 4 mg, 8 mg) (2.3%) 3191
Aciphex Tablets 1081

(▣ Described in PDR For Nonprescription Drugs) Incidence data in parenthesis; ▲ 3% or more (⊙ Described in PDR For Ophthalmic Medicines™)

▲ Actimmune (10%) ... **1646**
▲ Actiq (11% to 23%) ... **993**
Activase I.V. ... **1225**
▲ Activella Tablets (3% to 10%) ... **2311**
▲ Actonel Tablets (6.2% to 10.9%) ... **2679**
▲ Actonel with Calcium Tablets (6.2% to 10.9%) ... **2684**
▲ ActoPlus Met Tablets (3.6% to 5.8%) ... **3219**
▲ Adacel Vaccine (0.8% to 13.3%) ... **2959**
Adalat CC Tablets (2%) ... **2978**
▲ Adderall XR Capsules (5%) ... **3169**
▲ Adenocard Injection (3%) ... **612**
Adriamycin for Injection, USP (Frequent) ... **786**
Adriamycin Injection, USP (Frequent) ... **786**
▲ Advair Diskus 100/50 (4% to 5%) ... **1291**
▲ Advair Diskus 250/50 (4% to 5%) ... **1291**
▲ Advair Diskus 500/50 (4% to 5%) ... **1291**
Advate Injection (0.6%) ... **742**
▲ Advicor Tablets (7%) ... **1694**
▲ Aerobid/Aerobid-M (25%) ... **1172**
▲ Agenerase Capsules (23% to 74%) ... **1299**
▲ Agenerase Oral Solution (23% to 74%) ... **1304**
Aggrastat (Less than 1%) ... **1878**
▲ Aggrenox Capsules (16%) ... **855**
▲ Agrylin Capsules (17.1%) ... **3172**
Alacol DM Syrup ... **739**
Albalon Ophthalmic Solution ... ⊙ **216**
▲ Albenza Tablets (3.7% to 6.2%) ... **1310**
Aldara Cream, 5% (1.4%) ... **1814**
Aldoclor Tablets ... **1881**
Aldoril Tablets ... **1884**
Alesse-28 Tablets ... **3392**
▲ Alferon N Injection (4% to 48%) ... **1640**
▲ Alimta for Injection (Up to 84%) ... **1722**
Alinia for Oral Suspension (Less than 1%) ... **2840**
Alinia Tablets (Less than 1%) ... **2840**
Alkeran for Injection (Infrequent) ... **976**
Alkeran Tablets (Infrequent) ... **977**
Allegra (1.6%) ... **2857**
▲ Allegra-D 12 Hour Extended-Release Tablets (7.4%) ... **2860**
▲ Allegra-D 24 Hour Extended-Release Tablets (7.4%) ... **2862**
Aloprim for Injection (1.3%) ... **2156**
Altace Capsules (Less than 1% to 2.2%) ... **1673**
Altoprev Extended-Release Tablets (1.9% to 2.2%) ... **1151**
▲ Alupent Inhalation Aerosol (Up to 14%) ... **858**
Amaryl Tablets (1.1%) ... **2864**
▲ Ambien Tablets (2% to 6%) ... **2867**
▲ AmBisome for Injection (25.9% to 39.7%) ... **615**
▲ Amerge Tablets (4% to 5%) ... **1312**
▲ Amevive (0.2% to common) ... **836**
Aminohippurate Sodium "PAH" Injection ... **1886**
▲ Ammonul Injection (3%) ... **3323**
Amnesteem Capsules ... **2126**
Amoxil Capsules ... **1315**
Amoxil Chewable Tablets ... **1315**
Amoxil Pediatric Drops for Oral Suspension ... **1315**
Amoxil Powder for Oral Suspension ... **1315**
Amoxil Tablets ... **1315**
Anadrol-50 Tablets ... **3329**
▲ Anaprox Tablets (3% to 9%) ... **2769**
▲ Anaprox DS Tablets (3% to 9%) ... **2769**
Ancef for Injection (Rare) ... **1318**
▲ Angiomax for Injection (3% to 15%) ... **1856**
Antara Capsules (2.3%) ... **2723**
▲ Apokyn Injection (30%) ... **2132**
▲ Aptivus Capsules (6.7%) ... **859**
▲ Aranesp for Injection (14%) ... **576**
▲ Arava Tablets (9%) ... **2881**
▲ Aredia for Injection (53.5%) ... **2168**
▲ Argatroban Injection (4.8% to 7.1%) ... **1321**
▲ Aricept Tablets (5% to 19%) ... **1086**
▲ Aricept ODT Tablets (5% to 19%) ... **1086**
▲ Arimidex Tablets (10% to 20%) ... **665**
▲ Arixtra Injection (0.3% to 11.3%) ... **1325**
▲ Aromasin Tablets (18%) ... **2600**
▲ Arthrotec Tablets (11%) ... **3126**
▲ Asacol Delayed-Release Tablets (13%) ... **2688**
▲ Asmanex Twisthaler (1% to 3%) ... **2981**
Astelin Nasal Spray (2.8%) ... **1876**
Atacand Tablets (More than 1%) ... **634**
Atacand HCT (0.5% or greater) ... **637**
▲ Atrovent HFA Inhalation Aerosol (4%) ... **872**
▲ Atrovent Inhalation Solution (4.1%) ... **868**
Atrovent Nasal Spray 0.03% (2.2%) ... **869**
▲ Augmentin (3%) ... **1331**
▲ Augmentin Tablets (3%) ... **1334**
▲ Augmentin XR Extended-Release Tablets (2.2%) ... **1340**
Augmentin ES-600 Powder for Oral Suspension ... **1337**
▲ Avalide Tablets (3%) ... **922**
▲ Avalide Tablets (3%) ... **2889**
Avapro Tablets (1% or greater) ... **925**
Avapro Tablets (1% or greater) ... **2886**
Avastin IV ... **1229**
▲ Avelox (6%) ... **2984**
▲ Avinza Capsules (Greater than 10%) ... **1714**
▲ Avonex (23%) ... **839**
Axert Tablets (1% to 2%) ... **2430**
▲ Axid Oral Solution (1.2% to 5.4%) ... **913**
Aygestin Tablets ... **1062**
▲ Azasan Tablets (12%) ... **2844**
Azopt Ophthalmic Suspension (Less than 1%) ... **553**
Bactroban Cream (1.1% to 4.9%) ... **1356**
Bactroban Nasal (Less than 1%) ... **1357**
Bactroban Ointment (Less than 1%) ... **1358**
Balamine DM ... **739**
Baraclude (Less than 1%) ... **928**
▲ Bayer Aspirin (7.6%) ... **3515**
Beconase AQ Nasal Spray (Fewer than 5 in 100 patients) ... **1359**
▲ BeneFix for Injection (6.2%) ... **3402**
Benicar Tablets (Greater than 0.5%) ... **2850**
▲ Benicar HCT Tablets (3%) ... **2852**
▲ Bentyl Capsules (14%) ... **724**
▲ Bentyl Injection (14%) ... **724**
▲ Bentyl Syrup (14%) ... **724**
▲ Bentyl Tablets (14%) ... **724**
Betagan Ophthalmic Solution, USP ... ⊙ **217**
▲ Betaseron for SC Injection (27%) ... **791**
Betimol Ophthalmic Solution (1% to 5%) ... ⊙ **283**
Betimol Ophthalmic Solution (1% to 5%) ... **3371**
▲ Bexxar (3% to 36%) ... **1360**
▲ Biaxin/Biaxin XL (3%) ... **402**
▲ BiDil Tablets (10%) ... **2161**
Biltricide Tablets ... **2990**
Blocadren Tablets (0.6%) ... **1891**
▲ Boniva Tablets (4.8% to 5.1%) ... **2747**
▲ Boostrix (3% to 26%) ... **1366**
▲ Bravelle for Intramuscular or Subcutaneous Injection (5.7% to 8.7%) ... **1140**
▲ Brevibloc Concentrate (7%) ... **766**
▲ Brevibloc Injection (7%) ... **766**
▲ Brevibloc Double Strength Injection (7%) ... **766**
▲ Brevibloc Premixed Injection (7%) ... **766**
▲ Brevibloc Double Strength Premixed Injection (7%) ... **766**
Buminate 5% Solution, USP (Occasional) ... **747**
Buminate 25% Solution, USP (Occasional) ... **748**
Buphenyl Powder (Less than or equal to 2%) ... **3327**
Buphenyl Tablets (Less than or equal to 2%) ... **3327**
▲ Buprenex Injectable (5% to 10%) ... **2718**
▲ Byetta Injection (44%) ... **605**
Caduet Tablets (Greater than or equal to 2%) ... **2507**
Calcijex Injection ... **411**
Calcium Disodium Versenate Injection ... **1819**
▲ Campath Ampules (2% to 54%) ... **826**
▲ Campral Tablets (3% to 4%) ... **1175**
▲ Camptosar Injection (11% to 86%) ... **2602**
▲ Canasa Rectal Suppositories (3.1%) ... **726**
▲ Cancidas for Injection (1.8% to 6%) ... **1894**
Captopril Tablets (About 0.5% to 2%) ... **2114**
Carafate Suspension (Less than 0.5%) ... **727**
Carafate Tablets (Less than 0.5%) ... **728**
▲ Carbatrol Capsules (Among most frequent) ... **3174**
▲ Cardene I.V. (4.9%) ... **1129**
Cardizem LA Extended Release Tablets (1.4%) ... **1699**
Carimune NF ... **3501**
▲ Carnitor Injection (5% to 12%) ... **3185**
Carnitor Tablets and Oral Solution ... **3187**
Carteolol Hydrochloride Ophthalmic Solution USP, 1% ... ⊙ **246**
▲ Casodex Tablets (11%) ... **670**
▲ Cataflam Tablets (1% to 10%) ... **2173**
▲ Catapres Tablets (About 5 in 100 patients) ... **874**
Catapres-TTS (1 of 101 patients) ... **875**
Caverject Impulse Injection (Less than 1%) ... **2610**
Ceftin (2.6%) ... **1369**
▲ Celebrex Capsules (3.5%) ... **3130**
▲ Celexa (21%) ... **1177**
▲ CellCept Capsules (19.9% to 54.5%) ... **2751**
▲ CellCept Intravenous (19.9% to 54.5%) ... **2751**
▲ CellCept Oral Suspension (19.9% to 54.5%) ... **2751**
▲ CellCept Tablets (19.9% to 54.5%) ... **2751**
▲ Cenestin Tablets, 0.45mg, 0.625mg, 0.9mg, 1.25mg (9.4% to 18%) ... **1063**
Cenestin Tablets, 0.3mg ... **1063**
▲ Cerezyme for Injection (Approximately 6.5%) ... **1263**
Cerubidine for Injection ... **788**
Cervidil Vaginal Insert (Less than 1%) ... **1182**
▲ Chemet Capsules (12.0% to 20.9%) ... **2480**
Chromagen Soft Gelatin Capsules ... **3296**
Chromagen Forte Soft Gelatin Capsules ... **3296**
Cialis Tablets (Less than 2%) ... **1806**
Ciloxan Ophthalmic Ointment (Less than 1%) ... **554**
Cipro I.V. (Greater than 1% to 2.7%) ... **2998**
Cipro I.V. Pharmacy Bulk Package (Greater than 1% to 2.7%) ... **3509**
Cipro (2.5% to 2.7%) ... **2991**
▲ Cipro XR Tablets (3% to 4%) ... **3004**
▲ Clarinex Syrup (3%) ... **3009**
▲ Clarinex Tablets (5%) ... **3009**
▲ Clarinex Reditabs Tablets (5%) ... **3009**
Clarinex-D 24-Hour Extended-Release Tablets (2%) ... **3012**
Cleocin Vaginal Ovules (Less than 1%) ... **2613**
Climara Transdermal System (1% to 6%) ... **795**
Climara Pro Transdermal System ... **800**
Clindesse Vaginal Cream (1.4%) ... **3296**
▲ Clinoril Tablets (3% to 9%) ... **1899**
▲ Clolar for Intravenous Infusion (75%) ... **1264**
▲ Clorpres Tablets (About 5%) ... **2139**
▲ Clozapine Tablets (3% to 5% or more) ... **2141**
▲ Clozaril Tablets (3% to 17%) ... **2174**
Cogentin Injection ... **1903**
Colace Capsules 50 mg ... **2715**
Colace Capsules 100 mg ... **2715**
Colace Glycerin Suppositories, USP 1.2 grams - Infants and Children ... **2715**
Colace Glycerin Suppositories, USP 2.1 grams - Adults and Children ... **2716**
Colace Liquid 1% Solution ... **2716**
Colace Syrup ... 🅾 **729**
▲ Colazal Capsules (5%) ... **2845**
▲ Colyte with Flavor Packs for Oral Solution (Up to 50%) ... **3102**
▲ CombiPatch Transdermal System (8% to 12%) ... **2180**
Combivent Inhalation Aerosol (2.0%) ... **878**
▲ Combivir Tablets (13% to 33%) ... **1373**
▲ Combunox Tablets (8.8% to 25.4%) ... **1183**
▲ Comtan Tablets (14%) ... **2186**
Concerta Extended-Release Tablets ... **1828**
▲ Copaxone for Injection (22%) ... **3292**
▲ Copegus Tablets (25%) ... **2759**
▲ Coreg Tablets (4% to 9%) ... **1376**
Cosmegen for Injection (Common) ... **1907**
Cosopt Sterile Ophthalmic Solution (1% to 5%) ... **1910**
Coumadin for Injection (Infrequent) ... **932**
Coumadin Tablets (Infrequent) ... **932**
Covera-HS Tablets (2.1% to 2.7%) ... **3135**
Cozaar Tablets (1% or greater) ... **1913**
▲ Creon 5 Capsules (Among most frequent) ... **3195**
▲ Creon 10 Capsules (Among most frequent) ... **3195**
▲ Creon 20 Capsules (Among most frequent) ... **3196**
▲ Crestor Tablets (3.4%) ... **672**
▲ Crixivan Capsules (11.7%) ... **1918**
▲ Cubicin for Injection (5.8%) ... **1038**
Cuprimine Capsules (Greater than 1%) ... **1925**
▲ Cymbalta Delayed-Release Capsules (5% to 30%) ... **1729**
CytoGam Intravenous (Less than 5.0%) ... **1866**
Cytovene ... **2763**
Dalmane Capsules ... **3343**
Dantrium Capsules (Rare) ... **2690**
Dapsone Tablets USP ... **1656**
▲ Daranide Tablets (Among the most common effects) ... **1928**
▲ Darvocet A 500 Tablets (Among most frequent) ... **3497**
DDAVP Injection 4 mcg/mL (Infrequent) ... **2893**
DDAVP Nasal Spray (Up to 2%) ... **2894**
DDAVP Tablets ... **2895**
Decadron Phosphate Injection ... **1931**
Decadron Tablets ... **1929**
Delatestryl Injection ... **2976**
Demser Capsules (Infrequent) ... **1933**
▲ Depacon Injection (3.2% to 48%) ... **412**
▲ Depakene (34% to 48%) ... **417**
▲ Depakote Sprinkle Capsules (26% to 48%) ... **422**
▲ Depakote Tablets (22% to 48%) ... **427**
▲ Depakote ER Tablets (15% to 48%) ... **433**
▲ DepoCyt Injection (11%) ... **1121**
▲ DepoDur Extended-Release Injection (Greater than 10%) ... **1098**
▲ Depo-Provera Contraceptive Injection (1% to 5%) ... **2619**
▲ depo-subQ provera 104 Injectable Suspension (1% to less than 5%) ... **2622**
Desferal Vials ... **2190**
Desmopressin Acetate Injection (Infrequent) ... **1143**
Desmopressin Acetate Rhinal Tube (Up to 2%) ... **1144**
▲ Detrol Tablets (4.2%) ... **2626**
▲ Didronel Tablets (About 1 patient in 15; possibly 2 or 3 in 10) ... **2693**
▲ Digitek Tablets (4%) ... **2146**
Dilaudid (Infrequent) ... **439**
Dilaudid Oral Liquid ... **443**
Dilaudid Non-Sterile Powder (Infrequent) ... **439**
Dilaudid Rectal Suppositories (Infrequent) ... **439**
Dilaudid Tablets (Infrequent) ... **439**
Dilaudid Tablets - 8 mg ... **443**
▲ Dilaudid-HP (Among most frequent) ... **441**
Diovan HCT Tablets (Greater than 0.2%) ... **2195**
Diovan Tablets (More than 1%) ... **2191**
Diprivan Injectable Emulsion (Less than 1%) ... **676**
▲ Ditropan XL Extended Release Tablets (2% to 9%) ... **2391**
Diuril Oral ... **1936**
Diuril Sodium Intravenous ... **1934**
▲ Dolobid Tablets (3% to 9%) ... **1937**
▲ Dostinex Tablets (27% to 29%) ... **2631**
▲ Doxil Injection (16.9% to 46%) ... **3302**
DuoNeb Inhalation Solution (1.4%) ... **1058**
▲ Duragesic Transdermal System (Greater than 10% to 24%) ... **2448**
Dyazide Capsules ... **1389**
Dynacin Tablets ... **1859**
DynaCirc CR Tablets ... **2726**
Dyrenium Capsules (Rare) ... **3390**
▲ EC-Naprosyn Delayed-Release Tablets (3% to 9%) ... **2769**
Ecotrin Enteric Coated Aspirin Low, Regular and Maximum Strength Tablets ... **1627**
Edecrin ... **1941**
▲ E.E.S. (Among most frequent) ... **449**
▲ Effexor Tablets (6% to 58.0%) ... **3405**
▲ Effexor XR Capsules (4% to 35%) ... **3411**
▲ Eldepryl Capsules (10 of 49 patients) ... **3209**
Elidel Cream 1% (0.4% to 6.7%) ... **2198**
▲ Eligard 22.5 mg (3.4%) ... **2899**
Eligard 30 mg (2.2%) ... **2901**
▲ Elitek (27%) ... **2906**
▲ Ellence Injection (22.1% to 92.4%) ... **2632**
▲ Elmiron Capsules (4%) ... **2393**
▲ Eloxatin for Injection (5% to 74%) ... **2908**
Elspar for Injection ... **1943**
▲ Emcyt Capsules (15%) ... **3137**
▲ Emend Capsules (12.7%) ... **1944**
▲ Emtriva Capsules (13% to 18%) ... **1272**
▲ Enablex Extended-Release Tablets (1.5% to 4.1%) ... **2201**
▲ Enbrel for Injection (9% to 15%) ... **580**
Engerix-B Vaccine (Less than 1%) ... **1391**
▲ Entocort EC Capsules (11%) ... **2694**
EpiPen ... **1061**
▲ Epivir (13% to 33%) ... **1394**
▲ Epivir-HBV (15%) ... **1398**
▲ Epogen for Injection (0.26% to 48%) ... **586**
▲ Epzicom Tablets (5% to 6%) ... **1402**

▲ Equetro Extended-Release Capsules (10% to 29%) 3178
▲ Erbitux (29%) 937
▲ EryPed (Among most frequent) 445
▲ Ery-Tab Tablets (Among most frequent) 447
▲ Erythrocin Stearate Filmtab Tablets (Among most frequent) 452
▲ Erythromycin Base Filmtab Tablets (Among most frequent) 454
▲ Erythromycin Delayed-Release Capsules, USP (Among most frequent) 456
Eskalith 1406
Estratest Tablets 3196
Estratest H.S. Tablets 3196
▲ Estrogel 0.06% (6.0%) 3200
▲ Ethyol for Injection (8% to 96%) 1869
▲ Eulexin Capsules (9% to 11%) 3023
▲ Evista Tablets (8.3% to 8.8%) 1735
▲ Evoxac Capsules (13.8%) 1042
▲ Exelon Capsules (47%) 2204
▲ Fabrazyme for Intravenous Infusion (8%) 1267
Factive Tablets (2.7%) 2464
▲ Famvir Tablets (7.2% to 12.5%) 2207
▲ Faslodex Injection (26%) 682
▲ FazaClo Orally Disintegrating Tablets (Greater than or equal to 5%) 547
▲ Femara Tablets (0.1% to 17%) 2210
Feosol Caplets 1629
Feosol Tablets (Occasional) 1629
▲ Ferrlecit Injection (2% to 35%) 3379
▲ Flexeril Tablets (1% to 3%) 1832
▲ Flolan for Injection (32% to 67%) 1408
Flomax Capsules (2.0% to 3.9%) 881
▲ Flonase Nasal Spray (2.6% to 4.8%) 1412
▲ Flovent Diskus 50 mcg (4% to 9%) 1415
Floxin Otic Singles (Reported in a single subject) 1045
Floxin Otic Solution (Single report to 0.3%) 1043
Flumadine (2.8%) 1186
Flumist Vaccine 1872
Fluorescite Injection ⊙ 207
▲ Focalin Tablets (9%) 2214
Focalin XR Capsules 2217
▲ Follistim AQ Cartridge (17%) 2354
Foradil Aerolizer 3024
▲ Fortamet Extended-Release Tablets (8.5%) 1156
Fortaz (1 in 156 patients) 1422
▲ Forteo for Injection (8.5%) 1739
▲ Fortical Nasal Spray (1% to 3%) 3336
▲ Fosamax (Up to 3.6%) 1949
▲ Fosamax Plus D Tablets (0% to 3.6%) 1956
▲ Fosrenol Chewable Tablets (11% to 36%) 3180
Frova Tablets (Greater than or equal to 2%) 1101
Furosemide Tablets 2117
▲ Fuzeon Injection (22.8%) 2772
▲ Gabitril Tablets (11%) 998
▲ Gammagard Liquid (1.09% to 9.8%) 751
Gammagard S/D (Occasional) 754
▲ Gamunex Immune Globulin I.V., 10% (0.5% to 21%) 3232
Garamycin Injectable 3028
▲ Gemzar for Injection (58% to 71%) 1743
▲ Gengraf Capsules (2% to 18%) 458
Genotropin Lyophilized Powder (A small number of patients) 2642
▲ Geodon (10%) 2514
▲ Gleevec Tablets (42.5% to 73%) 2221
GlucaGen for Injection (Occassional) 790
Glucagon for Injection Vials and Emergency Kit (Occasional) 1749
▲ Gonal-f RFF Pen for Injection (3.6% to 8%) 3155
Grifulvin V Tablets Microsize and Oral Suspension Microsize (Occasional) 2384
Gris-PEG Tablets (Occasional) 2504
Guanidine Hydrochloride Tablets 3030
▲ HalfLytely and Bisacodyl Tablets Bowel Prep Kit with Flavors Packs (17.1% to 50%) 915
▲ Havrix Vaccine (1% to 10%) 1425
▲ Hectorol Capsules (21.3%) 909
▲ Hectorol Injection (21.3%) 911
Hemofil M (Extremely rare) 757
▲ Hepsera Tablets (2% to 5%) 1275
▲ Herceptin I.V. (8% to 33%) 1234
▲ Hexalen Capsules (1% to 33%) 2101
Humatrope Vials and Cartridges 1756
▲ Humira Injection (9%) 464
▲ Hycamtin for Injection (Less than 1% to 77%) 1427
Hycodan 1104
Hycomine Compound Tablets 1105
Hycotuss Expectorant Syrup 1106
Hydrocortone Tablets 1963
▲ Hyperstat I.V. Injection (4%) 3031
▲ Hytrin Capsules (0.5% to 4.4%) 469
Hyzaar (1% or greater) 1964
▲ Idamycin PFS Injection (82%) 2645
▲ Imdur Tablets (Less than or equal to 5%) 3032
▲ Imitrex Injection (4%) 1431
▲ Imitrex Nasal Spray (11% to 13.5%) 1435
Imitrex Tablets 1440
Imodium Capsules 1834
Increlex Injection 3290
Indapamide Tablets (Less than 5%) 2119
Inderal LA Long-Acting Capsules 3421
▲ Indocin (3% to 9%) 1968
Infed Injection 3381
▲ Infergen (30% to 40%) 1647
InnoPran XL Capsules 2728
▲ Intron A for Injection (1% to 66%) 3038
▲ Invanz for Injection (1.6% to 8.5%) 1974
Inversine Tablets 3286
▲ Invirase (Greater than or equal to 2% to 10.8%) 2776
▲ Iressa Tablets (13% to 20%) 684
▲ I.V. Busulfex (7% to 98%) 1125
Iveegam EN (0.3% to 0.8%) 759
▲ Kadian Capsules (Among most frequent) 572
▲ Kaletra (7% to 16%) 474
K-Dur Extended-Relase Tablets 3047
Keppra Oral Solution (1% to 2%) 3307
Keppra Tablets (1% to 2%) 3307
▲ Ketek Tablets (7% to 7.9%) 2920
▲ Kineret Injection (8%) 594
Klonopin 2782
▲ K-Lor Powder Packets (Among most common) 472
Koāte-DVI (0.7%) 3247
Kogenate FS 3517
K-Phos Neutral Tablets 785
K-Phos Original (Sodium Free) Tablets 785
Kristalose for Oral Solution 2149
▲ K-Tab Filmtab Tablets (Most common) 473
▲ Kytril Tablets (15% to 20%) 2788
▲ Lamictal (5% to 25%) 1449
Lamisil Tablets (2.6%) 2226
Lanoxicaps Capsules (Common) 1458
Lanoxin Injection 1462
Lanoxin Tablets (Common) 1468
Lanoxin Injection Pediatric 1465
▲ Lariam Tablets (Among most frequent) 2790
▲ Lescol Capsules (3.2%) 2227
▲ Lescol Capsules (3.2%) 2730
Lescol XL Tablets (2.5%) 2227
Lescol XL Tablets (2.5%) 2730
Leukeran Tablets (Infrequent) 1472
▲ Leukine (58% to 90%) 829
▲ Leustatin Injection (28%) 2368
▲ Levaquin in 5% Dextrose Injection (1.5% to 6.8%) 2453
▲ Levaquin (1.5% to 6.8%) 2453
Levothroid Tablets 1189
▲ Lexapro Oral Solution (Greater than 5% to 18%) 1193
▲ Lexapro Tablets (Greater than 5% to 18%) 1193
▲ Lexiva Tablets (3% to 39%) 1473
Librium Capsules 3349
Lidoderm Patch 1107
Lipitor Tablets (Greater than or equal to 2%) 2495
Lithobid Tablets 1670
Lofibra Capsules (2.3%) 1217
Lo/Ovral-28 Tablets 3423
▲ Lortab (Among most frequent) 3315
▲ Lortab Elixir (Among most frequent) 3312
Lotensin Tablets (1.5%) 2232
Lotensin HCT Tablets (1.4%) 2235
Lotrel Capsules 2238
▲ Lotronex Tablets (6%) 1479
▲ Lovenox Injection (2.5% to 3%) 2931
▲ Lunesta Tablets (4% to 5%) 3139
▲ Lupron Depot 3.75 mg (13%) 3257
▲ Lupron Depot 7.5 mg (5.4%) 3261
▲ Lupron Depot–3 Month 11.25 mg (4.8% to 13.8%) 3262
Lupron Depot-PED 7.5 mg, 11.25 mg and 15 mg (Less than 2%) 3266
Lupron Injection Pediatric (Less than 2%) 3256
▲ Malarone Tablets (Less than 1% to 12%) 1484
▲ Malarone Pediatric Tablets (Less than 1% to 12%) 1484
▲ Marinol Capsules (3% to 10%) 3334
▲ Matulane Capsules (Among most frequent) 3188
Maxair Autohaler (1.3% to 1.7%) 1820
▲ Maxalt Tablets (4% to 6%) 1983
▲ Maxalt-MLT Orally Disintegrating Tablets (4% to 6%) 1983
Maxipime for Injection (Greater than 0.1% to 2%) 1093
Maxzide 2150
Mebaral Tablets, USP (Less than 1 in 100 patients) 2483
Mefoxin for Injection (Rare) 1987
Mefoxin Premixed Intravenous Solution (Rare) 1990
▲ Megace ES Oral Suspension (0% to 5%) 2492
▲ Menopur for Subcutaneous Injection (7.9% to 12%) 1145
Menostar Transdermal System 805
▲ Mepron Suspension (2.5% to 32%) 1487
▲ Meridia Capsules (5.9%) 485
▲ Merrem I.V. (0.8% to 7.8%) 687
Meruvax II 1994
Metadate CD Capsules 3316
Metrogel 1% 1212
▲ MetroGel-Vaginal Gel (4%) 1822
▲ Mevacor Tablets (1.9% to 4.7%) 1996
▲ Miacalcin Injection (About 10%) 2241
Miacalcin Nasal Spray (1% to 3%) 2242
Micardis Tablets (1%) 884
Micardis HCT Tablets (2%) 886
▲ Midamor Tablets (3% to 8%) 2000
▲ Migranal Nasal Spray (10%) 3350
Mineral Oil 2716
Mintezol 2002
Miradon Tablets 3056
▲ Mirapex Tablets (28%) 889
▲ Mirena Intrauterine System (5% or more) 810
M-M-R II 1980
Moban Tablets (Occasional) 1108
▲ Mobic Oral Suspension (2.4% to 4.7%) 893
▲ Mobic Tablets (2.4% to 4.7%) 893
▲ Moduretic Tablets (3% to 8%) 2003
▲ MS Contin Tablets (Among most frequent) 2703
Mustargen for Injection 2007
Mycamine for Injection (2.3% to 2.8%) 620
▲ Myfortic Tablets (24.5% to 29.1%) 2244
Myleran Tablets 1492
▲ Mylotarg for Injection (63% to 74%) 3429
▲ Nabi-HB (4%) 2159
Nadolol Tablets (1 to 5 of 1000 patients) 2121
▲ Nalfon Capsules (7.7%) 2504
Namenda (Greater than or equal to 2%) 1199
▲ Naprosyn Suspension (3% to 9%) 2769
▲ Naprosyn Tablets (3% to 9%) 2769
Narcan Injection 1109
▲ Naropin Injection (More than 5% to 29.4%) 640
Nasacort HFA Inhalation Aerosol 2939
Nasarel Nasal Spray (Greater than 1%) 1652
Nasonex Nasal Spray (Greater than or equal to 2%) 3058
▲ Natrecor for Injection (4% to 13%) 3123
▲ Navelbine Injection (6% to 58%) 1494
Nembutal Sodium Solution, USP (Less than 1%) 2484
▲ Neoral Soft Gelatin Capsules (2% to 18%) 2247
▲ Neoral Oral Solution (2% to 18%) 2247
▲ Neulasta Injection (15% to 72%) 596
▲ Neumega for Injection (77%) 3433
▲ Neupogen for Injection (10% to 57%) 598
▲ Neurontin Capsules (3.9%) 2498
▲ Neurontin Oral Solution (3.9%) 2498
▲ Neurontin Tablets (3.9%) 2498
Nexium Delayed-Release Capsules (Greater than or equal to 1%) 645
Nexium I.V. (Greater than or equal to 1%) 649
▲ Niaspan Extended-Release Tablets (2% to 8%) 1703
Nicomide Tablets 3190
▲ Nicotrol Inhaler (Greater than 3%) 2594
▲ Nicotrol NS (5%) 2596
Niferex-150 Forte Capsules 3299
Nimotop Capsules (Up to 1.4%) 774
▲ Nipent for Injection (53% to 63%) 3216
▲ Niravam Orally Disintegrating Tablets (9.6% to 22%) 3106
Nitrolingual Pumpspray (Uncommon) 1161
Norditropin Cartridges (Small number of patients) 2318
Norflex Injection 1824
Noritate Cream, 1% (Uncommon) 1051
▲ Noroxin Tablets (2.6% to 4.2%) 2009
Norvasc Tablets (2.9%) 2529
▲ Norvir (25.6% to 29.8%) 499
▲ Novantrone for Injection Concentrate (55% to 76%) 3158
▲ Nubain Injection (6%) 1111
Numorphan 1112
Nutropin for Injection (A small number of patients) 1238
Nutropin AQ Injection (A small number of patients) 1241
Nutropin AQ Pen (A small number of patients) 1241
Nutropin AQ Pen Cartridge (A small number of patients) 1241
▲ Omnicef Capsules (3%) 506
Omnicef for Oral Suspension (0.2%) 506
▲ Oncaspar (Greater than 5%) 1123
▲ Ontak Vials (64%) 1717
OptiPranolol Metipranolol Ophthalmic Solution 0.3% (A small number of patients) ⊙ 254
Orap Tablets 1220
Ortho-Cept Tablets 2395
Ortho-Cyclen Tablets 2414
▲ Ortho Evra Transdermal System (9% to 22%) 2402
Ortho Micronor Tablets 2411
Ortho Tri-Cyclen Tablets 2414
Ortho Tri-Cyclen Lo Tablets 2421
▲ Orthoclone OKT3 Sterile Solution (19%) 2370
Oxandrin Tablets 2977
▲ Oxsoralen-Ultra Capsules (10%) 3354
▲ OxyContin Tablets (Less than 1% to 23%) 2699
▲ OxyFast Oral Concentrate Solution (Among most frequent) 2704
▲ OxyIR Capsules (Among most frequent) 2704
▲ Oxytrol Transdermal System (Greater than 1%) 3383
▲ Pacerone Tablets (10% to 33%) 3337
Parcopa Orally Disintegrating Tablets (Common) 3111
Parnate Tablets 1499
▲ Paser Granules (Among most common) 1657
Patanol Ophthalmic Solution (Less than 5%) 557
▲ Paxil CR Controlled-Release Tablets (1.9% to 36.3%) 1509
▲ Paxil (1.9% to 36.3%) 1501
▲ PCE Dispertab Tablets (Among most frequent) 510
Pediarix Vaccine 1518
Peganone Tablets, USP 2487
▲ Pegasys (24%) 2793
▲ PEG-Intron Powder for Injection (26%) 3062
Pentasa Capsules (1.8% to 3.1%) 3182
Pepcid Injection (Infrequent) 2017
Pepcid (Infrequent) 2014
▲ Percocet Tablets (Among most frequent) 1114
▲ Percodan Tablets (Among most frequent) 1115
Peri-Colace Tablets 2716
▲ Permax Tablets (24.3%) 3357
Persantine Tablets (Rare) 898
Phenergan 3438
Phenytek Capsules 2153
PhosLo GelCaps (Occasional) 2158
▲ Photofrin for Injection (24% to 39%) 729
▲ Plan B Tablets (23.1%) 1068
Plasmanate (Occasional) 3252
▲ Plavix Tablets (3.4%) 940
▲ Plavix Tablets (3.4%) 2942
Plendil Extended-Release Tablets (1.0% to 1.7%) 651
▲ Pletal Tablets (6% to 7%) 2478
Pneumovax 23 2020
Potaba (Infrequent) 1634
▲ Prandin Tablets (0.5, 1, and 2 mg) (3% to 5%) 2337
▲ Pravachol Tablets (2.9% to 7.3%) 943
▲ Prefest Tablets (6%) 1069
Premarin Intravenous 3440
▲ Premarin Tablets (6% to 9%) 3443
Premarin Vaginal Cream 3449
▲ Premphase Tablets (7% to 11%) 3452
▲ Prempro Tablets (7% to 11%) 3452
▲ Prevacid Delayed-Release Capsules (1.3% to 3%) 3268
▲ Prevacid for Delayed-Release Oral Suspension (1.3% to 3%) 3268
Prevacid I.V. for Injection (1.3%) 3274
▲ Prevacid NapraPAC (Less than 1% to 9%) 3277

▲ Prevacid SoluTab Delayed-Release Orally Disintegrating Tablets (1.3% to 3%) 3268
▲ PREVPAC (1.4% to 3%) 3281
▲ Prilosec OTC Tablets (2.2% to 4.0%) 2674
Primaxin I.M. (0.6%) 2022
Primaxin I.V. (2.0%) 2024
Prinivil Tablets (Greater than 1% to 2.0%) 2029
Prinzide Tablets (2.2%) 2033
ProAmatine Tablets (Rare) 3183
▲ Prochieve 4% Gel (7% to 22%) 1018
▲ Prochieve 8% Gel (7% to 22%) 1018
▲ Procrit for Injection (0.26% to 58%) 2374
▲ Prograf Capsules and Injection (32% to 46%) 624
▲ Proleukin for Injection (35%) 1007
▲ Prometrium Capsules (100 mg, 200 mg) (8%) 3205
▲ ProSom Tablets (4%) 512
Protonix I.V. (Greater than 1%) 3468
Protonix Tablets (2%) 3465
Protopic Ointment (1% to 3%) 629
▲ Proventil Inhalation Aerosol (Less than 15%) 3067
▲ Proventil Inhalation Solution 0.083% (3.1% to 4%) 3069
▲ Proventil HFA Inhalation Aerosol (10%) 3071
▲ Provigil Tablets (11%) 1002
▲ Prozac Pulvules and Liquid (12% to 22%) 1771
Purinethol Tablets (Uncommon) 1222
Qvar Inhalation Aerosol (Less than 1% to 2%) 1654
Rabies Vaccine RabAvert (Common) 1011
▲ Rapamune Oral Solution and Tablets (25% to 36%) 3472
▲ Raptiva for Injection (11%) 1247
▲ Razadyne ER Extended-Release Capsules (13% to 24%) 2434
▲ Razadyne (13% to 24%) 2434
▲ Rebetol (33% to 47%) 3073
▲ Rebetron Combination Therapy (38% to 47%) 3078
Recombinate (Extremely rare) 762
Recombivax HB (Equal to or greater than 1%) 2045
ReFacto Vials 3479
▲ Relafen Tablets (3% to 9%) 1523
Relenza Rotadisk (Less than 3%) 1525
▲ Relpax Tablets (4% to 8%) 2531
▲ Remicade for IV Injection (21%) 987
▲ Renagel Tablets (7% to 20.2%) 1268
▲ ReoPro Vials (18.4%) 1779
Repliva 21/7 Tablets 3301
▲ Repronex for Intramuscular and Subcutaneous Injection (4% to 7.3%) 1148
▲ Requip Tablets (30% to 60%) 1528
▲ Rescriptor Tablets (14% to 20.3%) 2535
Retavase 1131
▲ Retisert Implant (5% to 15%) ⊙ 256
▲ Retrovir Capsules (0.8% to 61%) 1533
▲ Retrovir IV Infusion (1% to 61%) 1537
▲ Retrovir (0.8% to 61%) 1533
▲ Reyataz Capsules (6% to 16%) 948
▲ R-Gene 10 for Intravenous Use (3%) 2647
▲ Ribavirin, USP Capsules (33% to 47%) 3083
▲ Rilutek Tablets (12.2% to 20.5%) 2945
Risperdal Consta Long-Acting Injection (Frequent) 1664
▲ Risperdal M-Tab Orally Disintegrating Tablets (4% to 11%) 1658
▲ Risperdal (4% to 11%) 1658
Ritalin Hydrochloride Tablets 2254
Ritalin LA Capsules 2255
Ritalin-SR Tablets 2254
▲ Rituxan for Infusion (18%) 845
▲ Rituxan I.V. (23%) 1251
Rocephin Injectable Vials, ADD-Vantage, Galaxy, Bulk (Less than 1%) 2801
▲ Roferon-A Injection (33% to 39%) 2805
▲ Rozerem Tablets (3%) 3228
▲ Rythmol SR Capsules (9% to 17%) 2736
▲ Sandimmune (2% to 10%) 2259
▲ Sandostatin Injection (34% to 61%) 2263
▲ Sandostatin LAR Depot (10.3%) 2264
Seasonale Tablets 1073
▲ Sedapap Tablets 50 mg/650 mg (Among the most frequent) 2098
▲ Sensipar Tablets (31%) 603
Serevent Diskus (1% to 3%) 1540
▲ Simulect for Injection (Greater than or equal to 10%) 2268
Singulair (Greater than or equal to 2%) 2047
▲ Skelaxin Tablets (Most frequent) 1685
▲ Somavert Injection (8% to 14%) 2648
▲ Sonata Capsules (6% to 8%) 1686
▲ Soriatane Capsules (1% to 10%) 1028
▲ Spectracef Tablets (4% to 6%) 2706
St. Joseph 81 mg Aspirin Chewable and Enteric Coated Tablets 1841
▲ Stalevo Tablets (5% to 14%) 2270
Starlix Tablets 2276
▲ Strattera Capsules (7% to 12%) 1784
Striant Mucoadhesive 1022
Stromectol Tablets (1.8%) 2053
▲ Suboxone Tablets (10% to 15%) 2719
▲ Subutex Tablets (10% to 13.6%) 2719
Sular Tablets (2%) 1163
▲ Suprane Liquid for Inhalation (27%) 770
▲ Suprax (7%) 1811
Surmontil Capsules 2347
▲ Sustiva Capsules (2% to 16%) 957
Symbyax Capsules (Infrequent) 1788
▲ Symlin Injection (37% to 48%) 608
▲ Symmetrel (5% to 10%) 1115
▲ Synercid I.V. (4.6%) 1690
Tabloid Tablets (Less frequent) 1545
▲ Tambocor Tablets (8.9%) 1824
▲ Tamiflu Capsules (3.3% to 9.9%) 2810
▲ Tamiflu Oral Suspension (3.3% to 9.9%) 2810
▲ Tarceva Tablets (0% to 33%) 1254
▲ Tarceva Tablets (0% to 33%) 2470
▲ Targretin Capsules (7.5% to 15.5%) 1719
Tarka Tablets (0.3% to 1.5%) 519
▲ Tasmar Tablets (30% to 35%) 3360
▲ Taxotere Injection Concentrate (5.1% to 42.1%) 2947
▲ Tegretol/Tegretol-XR (Among most frequent) 2278
▲ Temodar Capsules (46% to 53%) 3088
▲ Tenormin I.V. Injection (3% to 4%) 698
▲ Tenormin Tablets (3% to 4%) 695
▲ Tequin Injection (8%) 964
▲ Tequin Tablets (8%) 964
Tessalon Capsules 1202
Tessalon Perles 1202
Teveten Tablets (Less than 1%) 1707
Teveten HCT Tablets (Less than 1%) 1710
Tev-Tropin for Injection (Small number of patients) 1224
▲ Thalomid Capsules (4.2%) 979
Thioridazine Hydrochloride Tablets 2122
Thiothixene Capsules 2124
▲ Thrombate III (3 of 17) 3254
▲ Thymoglobulin for Injection (36.6%) 2848
▲ Thyrogen for Injection (10.5%) 1270
Thyrolar 1203
Tiazac Capsules (2%) 1204
▲ Ticlid Tablets (7.0%) 2813
Timentin ADD-Vantage 1556
Timentin Injection Galaxy Container 1559
Timentin IV Infusion 1553
Timentin Pharmacy Bulk Package 1562
Timolide Tablets (Less than 1%) 2056
Timoptic in Ocudose (Less frequent) 2061
Timoptic Sterile Ophthalmic Solution (Less frequent) 2058
Timoptic-XE Sterile Ophthalmic Gel Forming Solution 2062
▲ Tindamax (3.2% to 4.5%) 2670
TNKase I.V. 1256
▲ TOBI Solution for Inhalation (11.2%) 1015
▲ Topamax Sprinkle Capsules (6% to 14%) 2438
▲ Topamax Tablets (6% to 14%) 2438
Toprol-XL Tablets (About 1 of 100 patients) 660
Tracleer Tablets 539
Transderm Scōp Transdermal Therapeutic System (Few patients) 2166
▲ Trasylol Injection (11%) 779
Trecator Tablets 3482
Trelstar LA Suspension (2.9%) 3387
Tricor Tablets (2.3%) 523
Triglide Tablets (2.3%) 1165
▲ Trileptal Oral Suspension (10% to 29%) 2281
▲ Trileptal Tablets (10% to 29%) 2281
▲ TriLyte with Flavor Packs for Oral Solution (Up to 50%) 3114
Triphasil-28 Tablets 3483
▲ Trisenox Injection (75%) 983
▲ Trizivir Tablets (12% to 60%) 1565
Trusopt Sterile Ophthalmic Solution (Infrequent) 2065
▲ Truvada Tablets (Greater than 5%) 1279
Tussionex Pennkinetic Extended-Release Suspension 3322
Twinrix Vaccine (2% to 4%) 1571
▲ Tygacil for Injection (25.3% to 35%) 3489
▲ Tylenol with Codeine (Among most frequent) 2461
▲ Ultane Liquid for Inhalation (25%) 526
▲ Ultracet Tablets (3%) 2462
Uniphyl Tablets 2708
Uniretic Tablets (More than 1%) 3114
Univasc Tablets (Greater than 1%) 3118
Urecholine Tablets 2349
Urocit-K Tablets (Some patients) 2109
Uroqid-Acid No. 2 Tablets 785
Uroxatral Tablets (1% to 2%) 2957
▲ Urso 250 Tablets (8.3%) 737
▲ Urso Forte Tablets (8.3%) 737
▲ Valcyte Tablets (8% to 30%) 2816
Valium Tablets (Infrequent) 2822
▲ Valtrex Caplets (5% to 15%) 1573
Vancocin HCl Capsules, USP (Infrequent) 3370
Vantas (Less than 2%) 3367
Vantin Tablets and Oral Suspension (1.4% to 3.8%) 2650
Vaqta (2.3%) 2067
Varivax (Greater than or equal to 1%) 2070
Vaseretic Tablets (2.5%) 2073
Vasotec I.V. Injection (1.3% to 1.4%) 2076
▲ Velcade for Injection (57%) 2102
▲ Ventavis Inhalation Solution (13%) 1036
Verelan PM Capsules (1.7% to 2.7%) 3120
▲ Vesanoid Capsules (57%) 2823
▲ VESIcare Tablets (1.7% to 3.3%) 631
▲ VFEND I.V. (1% to 5.4%) 2543
▲ VFEND Oral Suspension (1% to 5.4%) 2543
▲ VFEND Tablets (1% to 5.4%) 2543
Viadur Implant (Less than 2%) 782
▲ Vicodin Tablets (Among most frequent) 530
▲ Vicodin ES Tablets (Among most frequent) 531
▲ Vicodin HP Tablets (Among most frequent) 532
▲ Vicoprofen Tablets (21%) 533
▲ Viracept (3% to 7%) 2556
▲ Viramune Oral Suspension (5%) 903
▲ Viramune Tablets (5%) 903
▲ Viread Tablets (8% to 11%) 1284
▲ Visudyne for Injection (1% to 10%) 2286
Vivactil Tablets 2350
▲ Vivelle Transdermal System (3.9% to 6.2%) 2288
▲ Vivelle-Dot Transdermal System (3.9% to 6.2%) 2293
Vivotif (Infrequent) 834
▲ Voltaren Ophthalmic Solution (Less than or equal to 3%) 2300
▲ Voltaren Tablets (1% to 10%) 2298
▲ Voltaren-XR Tablets (1% to 10%) 2301
▲ VoSpire Extended-Release Tablets (4.2%) 2352
Vytorin 10/10 Tablets 2084
Vytorin 10/10 Tablets 3092
Vytorin 10/20 Tablets 2084
Vytorin 10/20 Tablets 3092
Vytorin 10/40 Tablets 2084
Vytorin 10/40 Tablets 3092
Vytorin 10/80 Tablets 2084
Vytorin 10/80 Tablets 3092
▲ WelChol Tablets (4%) 2855
▲ Wellbutrin Tablets (22.9%) 1579
▲ Wellbutrin SR Sustained-Release Tablets (5% to 18%) 1583
▲ Wellbutrin XL Extended-Release Tablets (5% to 18%) 1588
▲ Xanax XR Tablets (6%) 2655
▲ Xeloda Tablets (4% to 43%) 2825
▲ Xenical Capsules (3.6% to 8.1%) 2834
▲ Xifaxan Tablets (5.3%) 2847
Xopenex HFA Inhalation Aerosol 3151
Xopenex Inhalation Solution 3143
Xopenex Inhalation Solution Concentrate 3147
Yasmin 28 Tablets (Greater than 1%) 818
Zantac 1597
Zantac Injection 1593
Zantac Injection Pharmacy Bulk Package (Frequent) 1595
Zantac Syrup 1597
▲ Zavesca Capsules (8% to 22%) 543
▲ Zegerid Powder for Oral Solution (2.2% to 4.0%) 2972
▲ Zelnorm Tablets (5% to 8%) 2303
Zemaira (0.2% to 0.4%) 3506
▲ Zemplar Capsules (13%) 535
▲ Zemplar Injection (13%) 538
Zemuron Injection (Less than 1%) 2363
▲ Zenapax for Injection (Greater than 5%) 2838
▲ Zerit (39% to 53%) 971
Zestoretic Tablets (2.2%) 701
Zestril Tablets (Greater than 1% to 2.0%) 704
Zetia Tablets 2090
Zetia Tablets 3098
▲ Zevalin Injection (31%) 848
▲ Ziagen (9% to 19%) 1600
Zinacef Injection (1 in 440 patients) 1604
Zinacef for Injection (1 in 440 patients) 1604
▲ Zinecard for Injection (51% to 77%) 2659
▲ Zithromax Capsules, 250 mg (1% to 18%) 2568
▲ Zithromax for IV Infusion (3.9% to 10.3%) 2573
▲ Zithromax for Oral Suspension, 1 g (3% to 5%) 2568
▲ Zithromax for Oral Suspension, 300 mg, 600 mg, 900 mg, 1200 mg (1% to 18%) 2561
▲ Zithromax Tablets, 250 mg, 500 mg (1% to 18%) 2561
▲ Zithromax Tablets, 600 mg (3% to 5%) 2568
▲ Zithromax Tri-Pak (1% to 18%) 2561
▲ Zithromax Z-Pak (3% to 5%) 2568
▲ Zmax for Oral Suspension (3.9%) 2577
Zocor Tablets (1.3%) 2078
▲ Zoladex (5% to 11%) 709
▲ Zoladex 3-month (9%) 712
▲ Zoloft (13% to 30%) 2581
▲ Zometa for Intravenous Infusion (29.1% to 46%) 2306
▲ Zomig Nasal Spray (0% to 4%) 718
▲ Zomig Tablets (4% to 9%) 714
▲ Zomig-ZMT Tablets (4% to 9%) 714
▲ Zonegran Capsules (9%) 1089
▲ Zosyn (5.8% to 6.9%) 3492
Zovirax Capsules (2.4% to 4.8%) 1616
▲ Zovirax for Injection (Approximately 7%) 1618
Zovirax (2.4% to 4.8%) 1616
▲ Zyban Sustained-Release Tablets (9%) 1620
▲ Zydone Tablets (Among most frequent) 1118
▲ Zyprexa Tablets (Up to 9%) 1798
Zyprexa IntraMuscular (Infrequent) 1798
▲ Zyprexa ZYDIS Orally Disintegrating Tablets (Up to 9%) 1798
Zyrtec Chewable Tablets (1.9% to 2.8%) 2589
Zyrtec (1.9% to 2.8%) 2589
Zyrtec-D 12 Hour Extended Release Tablets (1.9% to 2.8%) 2591
▲ Zyvox (1.4% to 6.2%) 2661

Neck, rigidity of

Abilify Tablets (Frequent) 916
Abilify Tablets (Frequent) 2472
Aciphex Tablets 1081
Amerge Tablets 1312
Axert Tablets (Infrequent) 2430
Caduet Tablets (Less than 2%) 2507
Cardizem LA Extended Release Tablets (Less than 2%) 1699
Depacon Injection (1% or more) 412
Depakene (1% or more) 417
Depakote Sprinkle Capsules 422
▲ Depakote Tablets (1% to 5%) 427
Depakote ER Tablets (Greater than 1%) 433
Diprivan Injectable Emulsion (Less than 1%) 676
Effexor Tablets (Infrequent) 3405
Effexor XR Capsules (Infrequent) 3411
Eldepryl Capsules 3209
▲ Imitrex Injection (4.8%) 1431
Imitrex Nasal Spray 1435
Imitrex Tablets 1440
Lipitor Tablets (Less than 2%) 2495
Lunesta Tablets (Infrequent) 3139
Lyrica Capsules (0.1% to 1%) 2524
Maxalt Tablets (Less than 2%) 1983
Maxalt-MLT Orally Disintegrating Tablets (Less than 2%) 1983
Norvir (Less than 2%) 499
Paxil CR Controlled-Release Tablets (Rare) 1509
Paxil (Rare) 1501
Pletal Tablets (Less than 2%) 2478
Prevacid Delayed-Release Capsules (Less than 1%) 3268
Prevacid for Delayed-Release Oral Suspension (Less than 1%) 3268
Prevacid NapraPAC (Less than 1%) 3277
Prevacid SoluTab Delayed-Release Orally Disintegrating Tablets (Less than 1%) 3268
PREVPAC (Less than 1%) 3281
Protonix I.V. (Less than 1%) 3468
Protonix Tablets (Less than 1%) 3465

Provigil Tablets (1%) ... 1002
Rescriptor Tablets ... 2535
Symbyax Capsules (Frequent) ... 1788
▲ Thalomid Capsules (4.2%) ... 979
Uniretic Tablets (Less than 1%) ... 3114
Varivax (Greater than or equal to 1%) ... 2070
Zonegran Capsules (Infrequent) ... 1089
▲ Zyprexa Tablets (2% to 3%) ... 1798
Zyprexa ZYDIS Orally Disintegrating Tablets (2% to 3%) ... 1798

Neck, redistribution/accumulation of body fat

Kaletra ... 474
Retrovir ... 1533

Neck tightness

Abilify Tablets (Infrequent) ... 916
Abilify Tablets (Infrequent) ... 2472
Imitrex Injection (Relatively common) ... 1431
Zomig Nasal Spray (Infrequent) ... 718

Necrolysis, digitus

Sustiva Capsules (Up to 3.5%) ... 957

Necrolysis, epidermal

Amnesteem Capsules ... 2126
Celexa ... 1177
▲ Dovonex Ointment 0.005% (1% to 10%) ... 3375
Prevacid NapraPAC (Less than 1%) .. 3277
Prozac Pulvules and Liquid ... 1771
Zevalin Injection ... 848

Necrolysis, epidermal, toxic

Aciphex Tablets ... 1081
Advicor Tablets ... 1694
Aldoclor Tablets ... 1881
Aldoril Tablets ... 1884
Altoprev Extended-Release Tablets (Rare) ... 1151
Amoxil Capsules ... 1315
Amoxil Chewable Tablets ... 1315
Amoxil Pediatric Drops for Oral Suspension ... 1315
Amoxil Powder for Oral Suspension ... 1315
Amoxil Tablets ... 1315
Anaprox Tablets (Less than 1%) ... 2769
Anaprox DS Tablets (Less than 1%) .. 2769
Antara Capsules (Rare) ... 2723
Arava Tablets (Rare) ... 2881
Arthrotec Tablets (Rare) ... 3126
Atacand HCT ... 637
Augmentin (Occasional) ... 1331
Augmentin Tablets (Occasional) ... 1334
Augmentin ES-600 Powder for Oral Suspension ... 1337
Avalide Tablets ... 922
Avalide Tablets ... 2889
Betoptic S Ophthalmic Suspension (Rare) ... 554
Biaxin/Biaxin XL ... 402
▲ Blephamide Ophthalmic Ointment (Among most often) ... 563
Blephamide Ophthalmic Suspension ... 564
Caduet Tablets ... 2507
Carbatrol Capsules (Extremely rare) ... 3174
Cataflam Tablets (Rarely) ... 2173
Ceftin ... 1369
Celebrex Capsules (Less than 0.1%) ... 3130
Celexa (3 cases) ... 1177
Cipro I.V. (1% or less) ... 2998
Cipro I.V. Pharmacy Bulk Package (1% or less) ... 3509
Cipro ... 2991
Cipro XR Tablets ... 3004
▲ Clindets Pledgets (Up to 11%) ... 3212
Clinoril Tablets (Less than 1%) ... 1899
Clorpres Tablets ... 2139
Cuprimine Capsules ... 1925
Daraprim Tablets ... 1385
Depacon Injection (Rare) ... 412
Depakene (Rare) ... 417
Depakote Sprinkle Capsules (Rare) .. 422
Depakote Tablets (Rare) ... 427
Depakote ER Tablets (Rare) ... 433
Diovan HCT Tablets ... 2195
Diuril Oral ... 1936
Diuril Sodium Intravenous ... 1934
Dolobid Tablets (Less than 1 in 100) ... 1937
▲ Duac Topical Gel (0% to 17%) ... 3214
EC-Naprosyn Delayed-Release Tablets (Less than 1%) ... 2769
E.E.S. (Rare) ... 449
Effexor Tablets ... 3405
Effexor XR Capsules ... 3411
Emcyt Capsules (1%) ... 3137
Epzicom Tablets ... 1402
Equetro Extended-Release Capsules ... 3178
EryPed (Rare) ... 445
Erythromycin Delayed-Release Capsules, USP (Rare) ... 456
Ethyol for Injection ... 1869
Eulexin Capsules ... 3023
FML-S Liquifilm Sterile Ophthalmic Suspension ... ⊙ 226
Fortaz ... 1422
Fosamax (Rare) ... 1949
Fosamax Plus D Tablets ... 1956
Imodium Capsules (Extremely rare) ... 1834
Inderal LA Long-Acting Capsules ... 3421
Indocin Capsules (Less than 1%) ... 1968
Indocin I.V. (Less than 1%) ... 1973
Indocin (Less than 1%) ... 1968
▲ Intron A for Injection (Less than 5%) ... 3038
Iressa Tablets (Very rare) ... 684
Lamictal (Rare) ... 1449
Lamisil Tablets (Isolated reports) ... 2226
Lescol Capsules (Rare) ... 2227
Lescol Capsules (Rare) ... 2730
Lescol XL Tablets ... 2227
Lescol XL Tablets ... 2730
Leukeran Tablets (Rare) ... 1472
Leustatin Injection (Isolated cases) .. 2368
Levaquin in 5% Dextrose Injection (Rare) ... 2453
Levaquin (Rare) ... 2453
Lexapro Oral Solution ... 1193
Lexapro Tablets ... 1193
Lipitor Tablets ... 2495
Lofibra Capsules (Rare) ... 1217
Maxalt Tablets ... 1983
Maxalt-MLT Orally Disintegrating Tablets ... 1983
Maxipime for Injection ... 1093
Mefoxin for Injection ... 1987
Mefoxin Premixed Intravenous Solution ... 1990
Merrem I.V. ... 687
Mevacor Tablets (Rare) ... 1996
Micardis HCT Tablets ... 886
Mobic Oral Suspension (Less than 0.1%) ... 893
Mobic Tablets (Less than 0.1%) ... 893
Moduretic Tablets ... 2003
Nalfon Capsules (Less than 1%) ... 2504
Naprosyn Suspension (Less than 1%) ... 2769
Naprosyn Tablets (Less than 1%) ... 2769
Nexium Delayed-Release Capsules (Rare) ... 645
Nexium I.V. (Rare) ... 649
Noroxin Tablets ... 2009
Omnicef Capsules ... 506
Omnicef for Oral Suspension ... 506
Pacerone Tablets ... 3337
Paxil CR Controlled-Release Tablets ... 1509
Paxil ... 1501
PCE Dispertab Tablets (Rare) ... 510
PEG-Intron Powder for Injection ... 3062
Pepcid Injection (Very rare) ... 2017
Pepcid (very rare) ... 2014
Phenytek Capsules ... 2153
Plavix Tablets ... 940
Pravachol Tablets (Rare) ... 943
Prevacid NapraPAC ... 3277
PREVPAC ... 3281
Prilosec OTC Tablets (Very rare) ... 2674
Primaxin I.M. ... 2022
Primaxin I.V. (Less than 0.2%) ... 2024
Prinivil Tablets (Rare) ... 2029
Prinzide Tablets (Rare) ... 2033
Protonix I.V. ... 3468
Protonix Tablets ... 3465
Raptiva for Injection ... 1247
Relafen Tablets (Less than 1%) ... 1523
Retrovir IV Infusion ... 1537
Rituxan for Infusion (Less than 0.1%) ... 845
Rituxan I.V. (Less than 0.1%) ... 1251
Sedapap Tablets 50 mg/650 mg (Several cases) ... 2098
Stromectol Tablets ... 2053
Suprax ... 1811
Sustiva Capsules (Up to 3.5%) ... 957
Tagamet Tablets (Very rare) ... 1547
Tamiflu Capsules ... 2810
Tamiflu Oral Suspension ... 2810
Tegretol/Tegretol-XR (Extremely rare) ... 2278
Teveten HCT Tablets ... 1710
Tiazac Capsules (Less than 2%) ... 1204
Timentin ADD-Vantage ... 1556
Timentin Injection Galaxy Container ... 1559
Timentin IV Infusion ... 1553
Timentin Pharmacy Bulk Package ... 1562
Timolide Tablets ... 2056
Topamax Sprinkle Capsules ... 2438
Topamax Tablets ... 2438
Tricor Tablets (Rare) ... 523
Trileptal Oral Suspension ... 2281
Trileptal Tablets ... 2281
Trizivir Tablets ... 1565
Trusopt Sterile Ophthalmic Solution (Rare) ... 2065
Ultracet Tablets ... 2462
Vancocin HCl Capsules, USP (Infrequent) ... 3370
Vantin Tablets and Oral Suspension (Less than 1%) ... 2650
Vaseretic Tablets ... 2073
Vasotec I.V. Injection (0.5% to 1.0%) ... 2076
VFEND I.V. (Rare) ... 2543
VFEND Oral Suspension (Rare) ... 2543
VFEND Tablets (Rare) ... 2543
Viramune Oral Suspension ... 903
Viramune Tablets ... 903
Voltaren Tablets (Rarely) ... 2298
Voltaren-XR Tablets (Rarely) ... 2301
Vytorin 10/10 Tablets ... 2084
Vytorin 10/10 Tablets ... 3092
Vytorin 10/20 Tablets ... 2084
Vytorin 10/20 Tablets ... 3092
Vytorin 10/40 Tablets ... 2084
Vytorin 10/40 Tablets ... 3092
Vytorin 10/80 Tablets ... 2084
Vytorin 10/80 Tablets ... 3092
Xalatan Sterile Ophthalmic Solution ... 2654
Zegerid Powder for Oral Solution (Very rare) ... 2972
Zestoretic Tablets ... 701
Zestril Tablets (Rare) ... 704
Ziagen ... 1600
Zinacef Injection (Rare) ... 1604
Zinacef for Injection (Rare) ... 1604
Zithromax Capsules, 250 mg (Rare) ... 2568
Zithromax for IV Infusion (Rare) ... 2573
Zithromax for Oral Suspension, 300 mg, 600 mg, 900 mg, 1200 mg (Rare) ... 2561
Zithromax Tablets, 250 mg, 500 mg (Rare) ... 2561
Zithromax Tri-Pak (Rare) ... 2561
Zmax for Oral Suspension (Rare) ... 2577
Zocor Tablets (Rare) ... 2078
Zonegran Capsules (Rare) ... 1089
Zosyn ... 3492
Zovirax Capsules ... 1616
Zovirax for Injection ... 1618
Zovirax ... 1616

Necrosis

Captopril Tablets (Rare) ... 2114
Fortaz ... 1422
Invanz for Injection (Greater than 0.1%) ... 1974
Miradon Tablets ... 3056
Sustiva Capsules (Up to 3.5%) ... 957

Necrosis, bone

▲ Arava Tablets (1% to 3%) ... 2881
Herceptin I.V. (At least one of the 958 patients) ... 1234
▲ Humira Injection (Less than 5%) ... 464
▲ Rapamune Oral Solution and Tablets (3% to 20%) ... 3472
Rilutek Tablets (Rare) ... 2945
VFEND I.V. (Less than 2%) ... 2543
VFEND Oral Suspension (Less than 2%) ... 2543
VFEND Tablets (Less than 2%) ... 2543

Necrosis, bowel

Proleukin for Injection (Less than 1%) ... 1007

Necrosis, cecal

Adriamycin for Injection, USP ... 786
Adriamycin Injection, USP ... 786

Necrosis, colon

Adriamycin for Injection, USP ... 786
Adriamycin Injection, USP ... 786

Necrosis, cutaneous

Aramine Injection ... 1889
Brevibloc Concentrate (Less than 1%) ... 766
Brevibloc Injection (Less than 1%) ... 766
Brevibloc Double Strength Injection (Less than 1%) ... 766
Brevibloc Premixed Injection (Less than 1%) ... 766
Brevibloc Double Strength Premixed Injection (Less than 1%) ... 766
Coumadin for Injection (Less frequent) ... 932
Coumadin Tablets (Less frequent) ... 932
Doxil Injection (Less than 1%) ... 3302
Effexor Tablets ... 3405
Ellence Injection ... 2632
Lovenox Injection ... 2931
Neurontin Capsules (Rare) ... 2498
Neurontin Oral Solution (Rare) ... 2498
Neurontin Tablets (Rare) ... 2498
Thalomid Capsules ... 979

Necrosis, fat

Garamycin Injectable (Rare) ... 3028

Necrosis, femoral head avascular

Evoxac Capsules (Less than 1%) ... 1042
Pulmicort Respules (Less than 1%) .. 654

Necrosis, gastrointestinal

Zomig Nasal Spray (Very rare) ... 718
Zomig Tablets (Very rare) ... 714

Necrosis, injection sites

Avonex ... 839
▲ Betaseron for SC Injection (5%) ... 791
Eloxatin for Injection ... 2908
PEG-Intron Powder for Injection (Less than or equal to 1%) ... 3062
▲ Rebif Prefilled Syringe for Injection (1% to 3%) ... 3163

Necrosis, intestinal

Avastin IV (Rare) ... 1229
Lanoxicaps Capsules (Very rare) ... 1458
Navelbine Injection ... 1494
Tabloid Tablets ... 1545

Necrosis, ischemic

Plavix Tablets (Less than 1%) ... 940
Plavix Tablets (Less than 1%) ... 2942

Necrosis, papillary

Aggrenox Capsules ... 855
Arthrotec Tablets (Rare) ... 3126
Bayer Aspirin Tablets ... 3515
Ecotrin Enteric Coated Aspirin Low, Regular and Maximum Strength Tablets ... 1627
Nalfon Capsules (Less than 1%) ... 2504
St. Joseph 81 mg Aspirin Chewable and Enteric Coated Tablets ... 1841

Necrosis, renal papillary

Anaprox Tablets (Less than 1%) ... 2769
Anaprox DS Tablets (Less than 1%) .. 2769
Dapsone Tablets USP ... 1656
Darvocet A 500 Tablets ... 3497
Dolobid Tablets ... 1937
EC-Naprosyn Delayed-Release Tablets (Less than 1%) ... 2769
Mobic Oral Suspension ... 893
Mobic Tablets ... 893
Naprosyn Suspension (Less than 1%) ... 2769
Naprosyn Tablets (Less than 1%) ... 2769
Prevacid NapraPAC (Less than 1%) .. 3277
Relafen Tablets ... 1523
Vicoprofen Tablets ... 533

Necrosis, renal tubular

Calcium Disodium Versenate Injection ... 1819
Capastat Sulfate for Injection ... 1728
Carimune NF ... 3501
▲ CellCept Capsules (3% to less than 20%) ... 2751
▲ CellCept Intravenous (3% to less than 20%) ... 2751
▲ CellCept Oral Suspension (3% to less than 20%) ... 2751
▲ CellCept Tablets (3% to less than 20%) ... 2751
Fuzeon Injection ... 2772
Gammagard S/D ... 754
Guanidine Hydrochloride Tablets ... 3030
Iveegam EN (0.3% to 0.8%) ... 759
Miradon Tablets ... 3056
Mycamine for Injection ... 620
▲ Myfortic Tablets (3% to less than 20%) ... 2244
▲ Prograf Capsules and Injection (3% to 15%) ... 624
▲ Rapamune Oral Solution and Tablets (3% to 20%) ... 3472
▲ Simulect for Injection (3% to 10%) ... 2268
Trasylol Injection (1% to 2%) ... 779
Truvada Tablets ... 1279

▲ Vesanoid Capsules (3%) 2823
VFEND I.V. (Less than 2%) 2543
VFEND Oral Suspension (Less than 2%) 2543
VFEND Tablets (Less than 2%) 2543
▲ Zenapax for Injection (Greater than 5%) 2838

Necrosis, skin

Augmentin XR Extended-Release Tablets 1340
Depakote ER Tablets (One patient) 433
Lyrica Capsules (Rare) 2524
Miradon Tablets 3056
Mycamine for Injection 620

Necrosis, tissue

Adriamycin for Injection, USP 786
Adriamycin Injection, USP 786
Cerubidine for Injection 788
Coumadin for Injection (Less frequent) 932
Coumadin Tablets (Less frequent) 932
Ellence Injection 2632
Fragmin Injection (Rare) 2638
Idamycin PFS Injection 2645
Miradon Tablets 3056
Phenergan Tablets 3438
Zovirax for Injection 1618

Necrosis, tumor

Gleevec Tablets (Rare) 2221

Necrotizing angiitis

Aldoclor Tablets 1881
Aldoril Tablets 1884
Atacand HCT 637
Avalide Tablets 922
Avalide Tablets 2889
Clorpres Tablets 2139
Diovan HCT Tablets 2195
Diuril Sodium Intravenous 1934
Dyazide Capsules 1389
Furosemide Tablets 2117
Hyzaar 1964
Indapamide Tablets 2119
Lotensin HCT Tablets 2235
Maxzide 2150
Micardis HCT Tablets 886
Moduretic Tablets 2003
Prinzide Tablets 2033
Teveten HCT Tablets 1710
Uniretic Tablets 3114
Vaseretic Tablets 2073
Zestoretic Tablets 701

Necrotizing cellulitis

Amevive 836

Neonatal morbidity

Aceon Tablets (2 mg, 4 mg, 8 mg) 3191
Altace Capsules 1673
Avalide Tablets 922
Avalide Tablets 2889
Avapro Tablets 925
Avapro Tablets 2886
Captopril Tablets 2114
Cozaar Tablets 1913
Hyzaar 1964
Lotrel Capsules 2238
Mavik Tablets 482
Prinivil Tablets 2029
Prinzide Tablets 2033
Uniretic Tablets (Several dozen cases) 3114
Vaseretic Tablets 2073
Vasotec I.V. Injection 2076
Zestoretic Tablets 701
Zestril Tablets 704

Neonatal prematurity

Adderall Tablets 3168
Altace Capsules 1673
Captopril Tablets 2114
Cozaar Tablets 1913
Hyzaar 1964
Prinivil Tablets 2029
Prinzide Tablets 2033
Vaseretic Tablets 2073
Vasotec I.V. Injection 2076
Zestoretic Tablets 701
Zestril Tablets 704

Neoplasic, hepatic

Lo/Ovral-28 Tablets 3423

Neoplasm
(*see under* Carcinoma, unspecified)

Neoplasm, bladder

Lyrica Capsules (Rare) 2524

Neoplasm, bone

Relpax Tablets (Rare) 2531

Neoplasm, brain, benign

Requip Tablets (Infrequent) 1528

Neoplasm, breast

Lunesta Tablets (Infrequent) 3139

Neoplasm, breast, male

Eulexin Capsules 3023

Neoplasm, breast malignant

Evoxac Capsules (Less than 1%) 1042
Symbyax Capsules (Infrequent) 1788
Xolair 1259

Neoplasm, laryngeal, malignant

Requip Tablets (Infrequent) 1528

Neoplasm, malignant

Estratest Tablets 3196
Estratest H.S. Tablets 3196
Orthoclone OKT3 Sterile Solution 2370
Repronex for Intramuscular and Subcutaneous Injection (Infrequent) 1148
Xolair 1259

Neoplasm, ovarian

Follistim AQ Cartridge 2354
Gonal-f RFF Pen for Injection (Infrequent) 3155

Neoplasm, prostatic malignant

Xolair 1259

Neoplasm, unspecified

Topamax Sprinkle Capsules (Less than 1% to 2%) 2438
Topamax Tablets (Less than 1% to 2%) 2438

Neoplasm, urogenital

Zomig Nasal Spray (Rare) 718

Neoplasms, hepatic

Estratest Tablets (Rare) 3196
Estratest H.S. Tablets (Rare) 3196
Ortho-Cyclen/Ortho Tri-Cyclen 2414
Ortho Tri-Cyclen Lo Tablets 2421
Oxandrin Tablets 2977
Zomig Nasal Spray (Rare) 718

Nephritis

Aceon Tablets (2 mg, 4 mg, 8 mg) 3191
Caduet Tablets (Less than 2%) 2507
Capastat Sulfate for Injection (1 patient) 1728
Cipro I.V. (1% or less) 2998
Cipro I.V. Pharmacy Bulk Package (1% or less) 3509
Cipro (Less than 1%) 2991
Cipro XR Tablets 3004
Lipitor Tablets (Less than 2%) 2495
Lyrica Capsules (0.1% to 1%) 2524
Paxil CR Controlled-Release Tablets (Rare) 1509
Paxil (Rare) 1501
Rilutek Tablets (Rare) 2945
Timolide Tablets 2056
VFEND I.V. (Less than 2%) 2543
VFEND Oral Suspension (Less than 2%) 2543
VFEND Tablets (Less than 2%) 2543
Zithromax (1% or less) 2568
Zithromax for Oral Suspension, 300 mg, 600 mg, 900 mg, 1200 mg (1% or less) 2561
Zithromax Tablets, 250 mg, 500 mg (1% or less) 2561
Zithromax Tablets, 600 mg (1% or less) 2568
Zithromax Tri-Pak (1% or less) 2561
Zithromax Z-Pak (1% or less) 2568

Nephritis, interstitial

Aciphex Tablets 1081
Aggrenox Capsules 855
Aldoclor Tablets 1881
Aldoril Tablets 1884
Anaprox Tablets (Less than 1%) 2769
Anaprox DS Tablets (Less than 1%) 2769
Arthrotec Tablets (Rare) 3126
Asacol Delayed-Release Tablets 2688
Atacand HCT 637
Augmentin (Rare) 1331
Augmentin Tablets (Rare) 1334
Augmentin XR Extended-Release Tablets (Rare) 1340
Augmentin ES-600 Powder for Oral Suspension (Rare) 1337
Avalide Tablets 922
Avalide Tablets 2889
Bayer Aspirin Tablets 3515
Biaxin/Biaxin XL 402
Captopril Tablets 2114
Cataflam Tablets (Occasionally) 2173
Celebrex Capsules (Less than 0.1%) 3130
Cipro I.V. (1% or less) 2998
Cipro I.V. Pharmacy Bulk Package (1% or less) 3509
Cipro (Less than 1%) 2991
Cipro XR Tablets 3004
Clinoril Tablets (Less than 1 in 100) 1899
Clozapine Tablets 2141
Clozaril Tablets 2174
Colazal Capsules 2845
Crixivan Capsules 1918
Diovan HCT Tablets 2195
Diuril Oral 1936
Diuril Sodium Intravenous 1934
Dolobid Tablets (Less than 1 in 100) 1937
Dyazide Capsules 1389
Dyrenium Capsules (Rare) 3390
EC-Naprosyn Delayed-Release Tablets (Less than 1%) 2769
Ecotrin Enteric Coated Aspirin Low, Regular and Maximum Strength Tablets 1627
FazaClo Orally Disintegrating Tablets 547
Furosemide Tablets 2117
Guanidine Hydrochloride Tablets 3030
Hyzaar 1964
Indocin (Less than 1%) 1968
Levaquin in 5% Dextrose Injection (Rare) 2453
Levaquin (Rare) 2453
Maxzide 2150
Mefoxin for Injection 1987
Mefoxin Premixed Intravenous Solution 1990
Meridia Capsules (One patient) 485
Micardis HCT Tablets 886
Mobic Oral Suspension (Less than 0.1%) 893
Mobic Tablets (Less than 0.1%) 893
Moduretic Tablets 2003
Nalfon Capsules (Less than 1%) 2504
Naprosyn Suspension (Less than 1%) 2769
Naprosyn Tablets (Less than 1%) 2769
Noroxin Tablets 2009
Orthoclone OKT3 Sterile Solution 2370
Pegasys 2793
PEG-Intron Powder for Injection (Less than or equal to 1%) 3062
Pentasa Capsules (Infrequent) 3182
Prevacid NapraPAC (Less than 1%) 3277
Prilosec OTC Tablets (Less than 1%) 2674
Prinzide Tablets 2033
Proleukin for Injection (Less than 1%) 1007
Protonix I.V. 3468
Protonix Tablets 3465
Relafen Tablets (Less than 1%) 1523
St. Joseph 81 mg Aspirin Chewable and Enteric Coated Tablets 1841
Tagamet Tablets (Rare) 1547
Teveten HCT Tablets 1710
Vancocin HCl Capsules, USP (Rare) 3370
Vaseretic Tablets 2073
Voltaren Tablets (Occasionally) 2298
Voltaren-XR Tablets (Occasionally) 2301
Zegerid Powder for Oral Solution (Less than 1%) 2972
Zestoretic Tablets 701
Zinacef Injection (Rare) 1604
Zinacef for Injection (Rare) 1604
Zithromax Capsules, 250 mg 2568
Zithromax for IV Infusion 2573
Zithromax for Oral Suspension, 300 mg, 600 mg, 900 mg, 1200 mg 2561
Zithromax Tablets, 250 mg, 500 mg 2561
Zithromax Tri-Pak 2561
Zmax for Oral Suspension 2577
Zosyn (Rare) 3492

Nephritis, purpuric

Vantin Tablets and Oral Suspension 2650

Nephrocalcinosis

Fleet Phospho-soda 1170
Fleet Prep Kits 1172

Nephrolithiasis

Aceon Tablets (2 mg, 4 mg, 8 mg) (0.3% to 1%) 3191
Aciphex Tablets 1081
Axid Oral Solution 913
Caduet Tablets (Less than 2%) 2507
Celebrex Capsules (0.1% to 1.9%) 3130
Celexa (Rare) 1177
Cipro I.V. (1% or less) 2998
Cipro I.V. Pharmacy Bulk Package (1% or less) 3509
Cipro 2991
Cipro XR Tablets 3004
Clinoril Tablets 1899
Copaxone for Injection (Infrequent) 3292
▲ Crixivan Capsules (8.7% to 12.4%) 1918
Daranide Tablets 1928
Dyazide Capsules 1389
Dyrenium Capsules (Rare) 3390
Effexor Tablets (Infrequent) 3405
Effexor XR Capsules (Infrequent) 3411
Evoxac Capsules (Less than 1%) 1042
Exelon Capsules (Infrequent) 2204
▲ Humira Injection (Less than 5%) 464
▲ Imdur Tablets (Less than or equal to 5%) 3032
Imitrex Injection (Rare) 1431
Imitrex Nasal Spray 1435
Imitrex Tablets 1440
Invirase (Rare) 2776
Kaletra (Less than 2%) 474
Lexapro Oral Solution (Infrequent) 1193
Lexapro Tablets (Infrequent) 1193
Lipitor Tablets (Less than 2%) 2495
Lunesta Tablets (Infrequent) 3139
Maxzide 2150
Miacalcin Nasal Spray (Less than 1%) 2242
Neurontin Capsules (Rare) 2498
Neurontin Oral Solution (Rare) 2498
Neurontin Tablets (Rare) 2498
Nipent for Injection (Less than 3%) 3216
Norvir (Less than 2%) 499
Paxil CR Controlled-Release Tablets (Rare) 1509
Paxil (Rare) 1501
Permax Tablets (Infrequent) 3357
Prevacid Delayed-Release Capsules (Less than 1%) 3268
Prevacid for Delayed-Release Oral Suspension (Less than 1%) 3268
Prevacid NapraPAC (Less than 1%) 3277
Prevacid SoluTab Delayed-Release Orally Disintegrating Tablets (Less than 1%) 3268
PREVPAC (Less than 1%) 3281
Protonix I.V. (Less than 1%) 3468
Protonix Tablets (Less than 1%) 3465
Razadyne ER Extended-Release Capsules (Infrequent) 2434
Razadyne (Infrequent) 2434
Relafen Tablets (Less than 1%) 1523
Remicade for IV Injection (Greater than or equal to 0.2%) 987
Requip Tablets (Infrequent) 1528
Rescriptor Tablets 2535
Reyataz Capsules (Less than 3%) 948
Rilutek Tablets (Infrequent) 2945
Rocephin Injectable Vials, ADD-Vantage, Galaxy, Bulk 2801
Sandostatin Injection (Less than 1%) 2263
▲ Sandostatin LAR Depot (5% to 15%) 2264
Sonata Capsules (Infrequent) 1686
Sustiva Capsules (Up to 1%) 957
Symbyax Capsules (Rare) 1788
Tasmar Tablets (Infrequent) 3360
Teveten Tablets (Less than 1%) 1707
Teveten HCT Tablets (Less than 1%) 1710
Topamax Sprinkle Capsules (Frequent) 2438
Topamax Tablets (Frequent) 2438
Tricor Tablets 523
Trileptal Oral Suspension 2281
Trileptal Tablets 2281
Uniretic Tablets (Less than 1%) 3114
Viracept (Less than 2%) 2556
Zonegran Capsules (Rare) 1089

Nephropathy

AmBisome for Injection (Less common) 615
Asacol Delayed-Release Tablets 2688
Campath Ampules 826
Ceftin 1369
Cymbalta Delayed-Release Capsules (Infrequent) 1729
Fortaz 1422
Maxipime for Injection 1093

Mefoxin for Injection 1987
Mefoxin Premixed Intravenous Solution 1990
Nipent for Injection (Less than 3%)... 3216
Omnicef Capsules 506
Omnicef for Oral Suspension 506
▲ Rapamune Oral Solution and Tablets (3% to 20%) 3472
Suprax 1811
Vantin Tablets and Oral Suspension 2650
Zinacef Injection 1604
Zinacef for Injection 1604

Nephropathy, acute uric acid
Oncaspar 1123

Nephropathy, proximal tubular
Carimune NF 3501
CytoGam Intravenous 1866
Gammagard S/D 754
Iveegam EN (0.3% to 0.8%) 759

Nephrosis, osmotic
Carimune NF 3501
CytoGam Intravenous 1866
Gammagard S/D 754
Iveegam EN (0.3% to 0.8%) 759

Nephrosis, toxic
Calcium Disodium Versenate Injection 1819
Evoxac Capsules (Less than 1%) 1042
Neurontin Capsules (Rare) 2498
Neurontin Oral Solution (Rare) 2498
Neurontin Tablets (Rare) 2498
Permax Tablets (Rare) 3357
VFEND I.V. (Less than 2%) 2543
VFEND Oral Suspension (Less than 2%) 2543
VFEND Tablets (Less than 2%) 2543

Nephrosis, unspecified
Nalfon Capsules (Less than 1%) 2504

Nephrotic syndrome
Anaprox Tablets (Occasional; less than 1%) 2769
Anaprox DS Tablets (Occasional; less than 1%) 2769
Arthrotec Tablets (Rare) 3126
Avastin IV 1229
Captopril Tablets (Approximately 1 to 2 of 1000 patients) 2114
Clinoril Tablets (Less than 1 in 100) 1899
Cuprimine Capsules 1925
Dapsone Tablets USP 1656
Dolobid Tablets (Rare) 1937
EC-Naprosyn Delayed-Release Tablets (Occasional; less than 1%) 2769
Fabrazyme for Intravenous Infusion 1267
HyperRAB (Rare) 3239
HyperTET (Few isolated cases) 3245
Indocin (Less than 1%) 1968
Naprosyn Suspension (Occasional; less than 1%) 2769
Naprosyn Tablets (Occasional; less than 1%) 2769
Pentasa Capsules (Infrequent) 3182
Prevacid NapraPAC (Less than 1%) .. 3277
Relafen Tablets (Less than 1%) 1523
Ticlid Tablets (Rare) 2813

Nephrotoxicity
Anaprox Tablets 2769
Anaprox DS Tablets 2769
Aredia for Injection 2168
Canasa Rectal Suppositories 726
Capastat Sulfate for Injection 1728
Dolobid Tablets 1937
EC-Naprosyn Delayed-Release Tablets 2769
Garamycin Injectable 3028
▲ Gengraf Capsules (25% to 38%) 458
Leustatin Injection 2368
Naprosyn Suspension 2769
Naprosyn Tablets 2769
▲ Neoral Soft Gelatin Capsules (25% to 38%) 2247
▲ Neoral Oral Solution (25% to 38%) 2247
▲ Prograf Capsules and Injection (36% to 52%) 624
Relafen Tablets 1523
Roferon-A Injection (Unusual) 2805
▲ Sandimmune (25% to 38%) 2259
TOBI Solution for Inhalation 1015
Vancocin HCl Capsules, USP 3370
Vicoprofen Tablets 533
Zinacef Injection 1604
Zinacef for Injection 1604

Nerve compression, arm
Adacel (1.5%) 2959

Nerve deafness
M-M-R II 1980
Mumpsvax 2005

Nerve paralysis
Ammonul Injection 3323

Nerve syndromes, compressed
▲ Advair Diskus 100/50 (1% to 3%) 1291
▲ Advair Diskus 250/50 (1% to 3%) 1291
▲ Advair Diskus 500/50 (1% to 3%) 1291
Amerge Tablets (Rare) 1312

Nervous system disorders, unspecified
▲ Ammonul Injection (22%) 3323
▲ Focalin XR Capsules (30% to 50%) 2217

Nervousness
Abilify Tablets (Frequent) 916
Abilify Tablets (Frequent) 2472
Accutane Capsules 2740
Aceon Tablets (2 mg, 4 mg, 8 mg) (1.1%) 3191
Aciphex Tablets 1081
Actiq (1% to 2%) 993
Activella Tablets 2311
Adalat CC Tablets (Rare) 2978
▲ Adderall XR Capsules (6%) 3169
Adenoscan (2%) 613
Advil Allergy Sinus Caplets .... ▣ 737
Advil Multi-Symptom Cold Caplets .. ▣ 738
▲ Aerobid/Aerobid-M (3% to 9%) 1172
Agrylin Capsules (1% to 5%) 3172
Alacol DM Syrup 739
Alavert Allergy & Sinus D-12 Hour Tablets .... ▣ 743
Albalon Ophthalmic Solution .... ⊙ 216
Alesse-28 Tablets 3392
Alferon N Injection (1%) 1640
Allegra (Less than 1%) 2857
Allegra-D 12 Hour Extended-Release Tablets (1.4%).. 2860
Allegra-D 24 Hour Extended-Release Tablets (1.4%).. 2862
Altace Capsules (Less than 1%) 1673
▲ Alupent Inhalation Aerosol (14.1%) 858
Ambien Tablets (1%) 2867
AmBisome for Injection (Less common) 615
Amnesteem Capsules 2126
Anaprox Tablets (Less than 1%) 2769
Anaprox DS Tablets (Less than 1%).. 2769
AndroGel (Up to 3%) 3330
▲ Angiomax for Injection (5%) 1856
Antara Capsules 2723
Aricept Tablets (Frequent) 1086
Aricept ODT Tablets (Frequent) 1086
▲ Arimidex Tablets (2% to 5%) 665
Arthrotec Tablets (Rare) 3126
Asacol Delayed-Release Tablets (2% or greater) 2688
Astelin Nasal Spray (Infrequent) 1876
Atrovent Inhalation Solution (0.5%) 868
Avalide Tablets (1% or greater) 922
Avalide Tablets (1% or greater) 2889
Avapro Tablets (1% or greater) 925
Avapro Tablets (1% or greater) 2886
Avelox (0.1% to less than 2%) 2984
Avinza Capsules (Less than 5%) 1714
Axert Tablets (Rare) 2430
Axid Oral Solution (1.1%) 913
Balamine DM 739
▲ Bentyl Capsules (6%) 724
▲ Bentyl Injection (6%) 724
▲ Bentyl Syrup (6%) 724
▲ Bentyl Tablets (6%) 724
▲ Betaseron for SC Injection (7%) 791
Blocadren Tablets (Less than 1%) 1891
Caduet Tablets (Greater than 0.1% to less than or equal to 1%) 2507
Campath Ampules 826
Captopril Tablets 2114
Cardizem LA Extended Release Tablets (Less than 2%) 1699
▲ Casodex Tablets (2% to 5%) 670
Cataflam Tablets (Occasionally) 2173
▲ Catapres Tablets (About 3 in 100 patients) 874
Catapres-TTS (1 of 101 patients) 875
Celebrex Capsules (0.1% to 1.9%) ... 3130
▲ CellCept Capsules (3% to less than 20%) 2751
▲ CellCept Intravenous (3% to less than 20%) 2751
▲ CellCept Oral Suspension (3% to less than 20%) 2751
▲ CellCept Tablets (3% to less than 20%) 2751
▲ Cenestin Tablets, 0.45mg, 0.625mg, 0.9mg, 1.25mg (3.8% to 28%) 1063
Cenestin Tablets, 0.3mg 1063
Cipro I.V. 2998
Cipro I.V. Pharmacy Bulk Package 3509
Cipro 2991
Cipro XR Tablets 3004
Clarinex-D 24-Hour Extended-Release Tablets (2%) 3012
Climara Transdermal System 795
Climara Pro Transdermal System 800
Clinoril Tablets (Greater than 1%) 1899
▲ Clorpres Tablets (About 3%) 2139
Cogentin Injection 1903
Colazal Capsules 2845
▲ CombiPatch Transdermal System (5% to 6%) 2180
Combivent Inhalation Aerosol (Less than 2%) 878
Combunox Tablets (Less than 1%) ... 1183
▲ Concerta Extended-Release Tablets (Greater than 0.7%) 1828
Contac Non-Drowsy 12 Hour Cold Caplets .... ▣ 614
Contac Non-Drowsy Timed Release 12 Hour Cold Caplets .... ▣ 615
Contac Severe Cold and Flu Caplets Maximum Strength .... ▣ 615
Contac Severe Cold and Flu Caplets Non-Drowsy .... ▣ 615
Copaxone for Injection (2%) 3292
▲ Copegus Tablets (33%) 2759
Coreg Tablets (Greater than 0.1% to 1%) 1376
Cosopt Sterile Ophthalmic Solution 1910
▲ Cozaar Tablets (Less than 1% to 4%) 1913
Cymbalta Delayed-Release Capsules (Frequent) 1729
Dalmane Capsules 3343
Dantrium Capsules (Less frequent) .. 2690
Daranide Tablets 1928
▲ Depacon Injection (0.9% to 11%) 412
▲ Depakene (11%) 417
▲ Depakote Sprinkle Capsules (7% to 11%) 422
▲ Depakote Tablets (1% to 11%) 427
▲ Depakote ER Tablets (1% to 11%) ... 433
▲ Depo-Provera Contraceptive Injection (Greater than 5%) 2619
depo-subQ provera 104 Injectable Suspension 2622
Detrol Tablets (1.1%) 2626
Diastat Rectal Delivery System (Greater than or equal to 1%) 3344
Dilaudid Oral Liquid (Less frequent) 443
Dilaudid Tablets - 8 mg (Less frequent) 443
Dilaudid-HP 441
Children's Dimetapp Long Acting Cough Plus Cold Syrup .... ▣ 746
▲ Ditropan XL Extended Release Tablets (2% to less than 5%) 2391
Dolobid Tablets (Less than 1 in 100) 1937
▲ Dostinex Tablets (1% to less than 10%) 2631
Doxil Injection (Less than 1%) 3302
▲ Duragesic Transdermal System (3% to 10%) 2448
DynaCirc CR Tablets (0.5% to 1%) 2726
EC-Naprosyn Delayed-Release Tablets (Less than 1%) 2769
▲ Effexor Tablets (2% to 21.3%) 3405
▲ Effexor XR Capsules (5% to 11%) 3411
Eldepryl Capsules 3209
▲ Eloxatin for Injection (2% to 5%) 2908
▲ Entocort EC Capsules (Less than 5%) 2694
EpiPen Jr. Auto-Injector 1061
▲ Equetro Extended-Release Capsules (Less than 5%) 3178
Estratest Tablets 3196
Estratest H.S. Tablets 3196
Estrogel 0.06% (2.4%) 3200
Eulexin Capsules (1%) 3023
Exelon Capsules (2% or more) 2204
Factive Tablets (Less than or equal to 0.1%) 2464
Ferrlecit Injection (Two or more patients) 3379
▲ Flexeril Tablets (1% to 3%) 1832
▲ Flolan for Injection (7% to 21%) 1408
Flumadine (1.3% to 2.1%) 1186
▲ Focalin Tablets (Among most common) 2214
Focalin XR Capsules 2217
Foradil Aerolizer 3024
Frova Tablets (Infrequent) 1101
▲ Gabitril Tablets (10%) 998
Gengraf Capsules (1% to less than 3%) 458
Hytrin Capsules (2.3%) 469
Hyzaar 1964
▲ Imdur Tablets (Less than or equal to 5%) 3032
Indapamide Tablets (Less than 5%).. 2119
Indocin (Less than 1%) 1968
▲ Infergen (16% to 31%) 1647
▲ Intron A for Injection (Up to 3%) 3038
Invanz for Injection (Greater than 0.1%) 1974
Kaletra (Less than 2%) 474
▲ Keppra Oral Solution (4% to 9.9%) .. 3307
▲ Keppra Tablets (4% to 9.9%) 3307
Klonopin (1% to 3%) 2782
Lamictal (2%) 1449
Levaquin in 5% Dextrose Injection (0.1% to 0.9%) 2453
Levaquin (0.1% to 0.9%) 2453
Levothroid Tablets 1189
Levoxyl Tablets 1680
Lexapro Oral Solution (Infrequent) 1193
Lexapro Tablets (Infrequent) 1193
Lidoderm Patch 1107
Lofibra Capsules 1217
Lo/Ovral-28 Tablets 3423
Lotensin Tablets (Less than 1%) 2232
Lotensin HCT Tablets (0.3% to 1%) .. 2235
Lotrel Capsules 2238
▲ Lunesta Tablets (0% to 5%) 3139
▲ Lupron Depot 3.75 mg (4%) 3257
▲ Lupron Depot–3 Month 11.25 mg (4%) 3262
Lupron Depot-PED 7.5 mg, 11.25 mg and 15 mg (Less than 2%) 3266
Lupron Injection Pediatric (Less than 2%) 3256
Lyrica Capsules (1% to greater than or equal to 2%) 2524
Marinol Capsules (Greater than 1%) 3334
Matulane Capsules 3188
▲ Maxair Autohaler (4.5% to 6.9%) 1820
Maxalt Tablets (Infrequent) 1983
Maxalt-MLT Orally Disintegrating Tablets (Infrequent) 1983
Mebaral Tablets, USP (Less than 1 in 100 patients) 2483
Menostar Transdermal System 805
▲ Meridia Capsules (5.2%) 485
Merrem I.V. (Greater than 0.1% to 1%) 687
▲ Metadate CD Capsules (Among most common) 3316
Micardis HCT Tablets 886
Midamor Tablets (Less than or equal to 1%) 2000
Migranal Nasal Spray (Infrequent) 3350
Mirapex Tablets (1% or more) 889
▲ Mirena Intrauterine System (5% or more) 810
Mobic Oral Suspension (Less than 2%) 893
Mobic Tablets (Less than 2%) 893
Moduretic Tablets (Less than or equal to 1%) 2003
Motrin Cold & Sinus Caplets 1836
MS Contin Tablets (Less frequent) 2703
▲ Nalfon Capsules (5.7%) 2504
Namenda (Infrequent) 1199
Naprosyn Suspension (Less than 1%) 2769
Naprosyn Tablets (Less than 1%) 2769
Narcan Injection 1109
Naropin Injection (Less than 1%) 640
Nembutal Sodium Solution, USP (Less than 1%) 2484
Neoral Soft Gelatin Capsules (1% to less than 3%) 2247
Neoral Oral Solution (1% to less than 3%) 2247
▲ Neumega for Injection (Greater than or equal to 10%) 3433
Neurontin Capsules (2.4%) 2498
Neurontin Oral Solution (2.4%) 2498
Neurontin Tablets (2.4%) 2498
Nexium Delayed-Release Capsules (Less than 1%) 645
Nexium I.V. (Less than 1%) 649
Niaspan Extended-Release Tablets... 1703
▲ Nipent for Injection (3% to 10%) 3216
▲ Niravam Orally Disintegrating Tablets (4.1%) 3106
Norvasc Tablets (More than 0.1% to 1%) 2529
Norvir (Less than 2%) 499
Nubain Injection (1% or less) 1111
Numorphan 1112
▲ Ontak Vials (11%) 1717

OptiPranolol Metipranolol Ophthalmic Solution 0.3% (A small number of patients) ⊙ 254
▲ Orap Tablets (8.3%) 1220
Ortho-Cept Tablets 2395
Ortho-Cyclen Tablets 2414
Ortho Evra Transdermal System 2402
Ortho Tri-Cyclen Tablets 2414
Ortho Tri-Cyclen Lo Tablets 2421
Oxsoralen-Ultra Capsules 3354
▲ OxyContin Tablets (Between 1% and 5%) 2699
Parcopa Orally Disintegrating Tablets 3111
▲ Paxil CR Controlled-Release Tablets (4% to 9%) 1509
▲ Paxil (4% to 9%) 1501
▲ Pegasys (19%) 2793
▲ PEG-Intron Powder for Injection (4%) 3062
Permax Tablets (Frequent) 3357
Phenergan 3438
Phenytek Capsules 2153
Plendil Extended-Release Tablets (0.5% to 1.5%) 651
Prefest Tablets 1069
Premarin Intravenous 3440
▲ Premarin Tablets (2% to 5%) 3443
Premarin Vaginal Cream 3449
▲ Premphase Tablets (2% to 3%) 3452
▲ Prempro Tablets (2% to 3%) 3452
Prevacid Delayed-Release Capsules (Less than 1%) 3268
Prevacid for Delayed-Release Oral Suspension (Less than 1%) 3268
Prevacid NapraPAC (Less than 1%) 3277
Prevacid SoluTab Delayed-Release Orally Disintegrating Tablets (Less than 1%) 3268
PREVPAC (Less than 1%) 3281
Prilosec OTC Tablets (Less than 1%) 2674
Primatene Tablets ▣ 749
Prinivil Tablets (0.3% to 1.0%) 2029
Prinzide Tablets 2033
ProAmatine Tablets (Less frequent) 3183
▲ Prochieve 4% Gel (16%) 1018
▲ Prochieve 8% Gel (16%) 1018
▲ Prograf Capsules and Injection (3%) 624
Prometrium Capsules (100 mg, 200 mg) 3205
▲ ProSom Tablets (8%) 512
Protonix I.V. (Less than 1%) 3468
Protonix Tablets (Less than 1%) 3465
▲ Proventil Inhalation Aerosol (Less than 10%) 3067
▲ Proventil Inhalation Solution 0.083% (4%) 3069
▲ Proventil HFA Inhalation Aerosol (7%) 3071
▲ Provigil Tablets (7%) 1002
▲ Prozac Pulvules and Liquid (8% to 16%) 1771
▲ Rebetol (3% to 6%) 3073
▲ Rebetron Combination Therapy (4% to 5%) 3078
Relafen Tablets (1% to 3%) 1523
Relpax Tablets (Infrequent) 2531
Requip Tablets (1% or more) 1528
Rescriptor Tablets 2535
Retrovir Capsules (1.6%) 1533
Retrovir IV Infusion (2%) 1537
Retrovir (1.6%) 1533
Reyataz Capsules (Less than 3%) 948
▲ Ribavirin, USP Capsules (3% to 6%) 3083
Risperdal Consta Long-Acting Injection (Frequent) 1664
Risperdal M-Tab Orally Disintegrating Tablets (Frequent) 1658
Risperdal (Frequent) 1658
▲ Ritalin Hydrochloride Tablets (One of the two most common) 2254
▲ Ritalin LA Capsules (Among most common) 2255
▲ Ritalin-SR Tablets (One of the two most common) 2254
▲ Rituxan for Infusion (1% to 5%) 845
▲ Rituxan I.V. (1% to 5%) 1251
Robitussin CF Liquid ▣ 755
Robitussin Maximum Strength Cough & Cold Liquid ▣ 754
Robitussin PE Syrup ▣ 753
Robitussin Pediatric Cough & Cold Liquid ▣ 754
▲ Roferon-A Injection (Less than 5%) 2805
Sandostatin LAR Depot (1% to 4%) 2264
Seasonale Tablets 1073
▲ Skelaxin Tablets (Most frequent) 1685
Sonata Capsules (Frequent) 1686
Spectracef Tablets (0.1% to 1%) 2706
Stalevo Tablets 2270
▲ Suboxone Tablets (6%) 2719
▲ Subutex Tablets (6%) 2719
Sudafed 12 Hour Caplets ▣ 708
Sudafed 24 Hour Tablets ▣ 709
Sudafed Nasal Decongestant Tablets ▣ 709
Sular Tablets (Less than or equal to 1%) 1163
▲ Sustiva Capsules (1% to 7%) 957
Symmetrel (1% to 5%) 1115
Synagis (More than 1%) 1868
Tasmar Tablets (Infrequent) 3360
Tequin Injection (Less than 0.1%) 964
Tequin Tablets (Less than 0.1%) 964
Teveten Tablets (Less than 1%) 1707
Teveten HCT Tablets (Less than 1%) 1710
▲ Thalomid Capsules (2.8% to 9.4%) 979
TheraFlu Cold & Cough Hot Liquid ▣ 680
TheraFlu Cold & Sore Throat Hot Liquid ▣ 680
TheraFlu Flu & Chest Congestion Non-Drowsy Hot Liquid ▣ 681
TheraFlu Flu & Sore Throat Hot Liquid ▣ 681
TheraFlu Severe Cold Non-Drowsy Hot Liquid ▣ 683
TheraFlu Severe Cold & Cough Hot Liquid ▣ 683
TheraFlu Severe Cold Caplets ▣ 679
TheraFlu Severe Cold Hot Liquid ▣ 682
TheraFlu Severe Cold Non-Drowsy Caplets ▣ 679
Tiazac Capsules (Less than 2%) 1204
Timolide Tablets (Less than 1%) 2056
Timoptic in Ocudose (Less frequent) 2061
Timoptic Sterile Ophthalmic Solution (Less frequent) 2058
Timoptic-XE Sterile Ophthalmic Gel Forming Solution 2062
▲ Topamax Sprinkle Capsules (4% to 19%) 2438
▲ Topamax Tablets (4% to 19%) 2438
Toprol-XL Tablets 660
Tranxene (Less common) 2488
Triaminic Chest & Nasal Congestion Liquid ▣ 685
Triaminic Cold & Allergy Liquid ▣ 685
Triaminic Cold & Cough Liquid ▣ 685
Triaminic Cough Liquid ▣ 687
Triaminic Cough & Nasal Congestion Liquid ▣ 687
Triaminic Cough & Sore Throat Liquid ▣ 687
Triaminic Flu, Cough & Fever Liquid ▣ 685
Triaminic Night Time Cough & Cold Liquid ▣ 685
Triaminic Cough & Sore Throat Softchews ▣ 689
Tricor Tablets 523
▲ Trileptal Oral Suspension (2% to 4%) 2281
▲ Trileptal Tablets (2% to 4%) 2281
Triphasil-28 Tablets 3483
Children's Tylenol Plus Cold NightTime Suspension Liquid 1851
Children's Tylenol Plus Cold Chewable Tablets 1851
Tylenol Cold & Flu Severe Daytime Liquid with Cool Bust 1846
Tylenol Cold & Flu Severe NightTime Liquid with Cool Burst 1846
Tylenol Flu NightTime Gelcaps 1846
Tylenol Flu Day Non-Drowsy Gelcaps 1846
Concentrated Tylenol Infants' Drops Plus Cold Nasal Congestant, Fever Reducer & Pain Reliever ▣ 668
Concentrated Tylenol Infants' Drops Plus Cold & Cough Nasal Decongestant, Fever Reducer & Pain Reliever ▣ 668
Multi-Symptom Tylenol Cold Night Time Caplets 1845
Multi-Symptom Tylenol Cold Day Non-Drowsy Caplets and Gelcaps 1845
Ultane Liquid for Inhalation (Less than 1%) 526
Ultracet Tablets (At least 1%) 2462
Uniretic Tablets (Less than 1%) 3114
Unithroid Tablets 3521
Univasc Tablets (Less than 1%) 3118
Vantin Tablets and Oral Suspension (Less than 1%) 2650
Varivax (Greater than or equal to 1%) 2070
Vaseretic Tablets (0.5% to 2.0%) 2073
Vasotec I.V. Injection (0.5% to 1.0%) 2076
Vicks 44D Cough & Head Congestion Relief 2676
Pediatric Vicks 44m Cough & Cold Relief 2673
Vicks DayQuil Multi-Symptom Cold/Flu Relief LiquiCaps 2675
Vicks DayQuil Multi-Symptom Cold/Flu Relief Liquid 2675
Children's Vicks NyQuil Cold/Cough Relief 2671
▲ Vicoprofen Tablets (3% to 9%) 533
Vivelle Transdermal System 2288
Vivelle-Dot Transdermal System 2293
Voltaren Tablets (Occasionally) 2298
Voltaren-XR Tablets (Occasionally) 2301
▲ VoSpire Extended-Release Tablets (8.5%) 2352
▲ Wellbutrin SR Sustained-Release Tablets (3% to 5%) 1583
▲ Wellbutrin XL Extended-Release Tablets (3% to 5%) 1588
▲ Xanax XR Tablets (22%) 2655
▲ Xopenex HFA Inhalation Aerosol (2.8% to 9.6%) 3151
▲ Xopenex Inhalation Solution (2.8% to 9.6%) 3143
▲ Xopenex Inhalation Solution Concentrate (2.8% to 9.6%) 3147
Yasmin 28 Tablets (Greater than 1%) 818
Zegerid Powder for Oral Solution (Less than 1%) 2972
Zestoretic Tablets 701
Zestril Tablets (0.3% to 1.0%) 704
Zithromax Capsules, 250 mg (1% or less) 2568
Zithromax for IV Infusion (1% or less) 2573
Zithromax for Oral Suspension, 300 mg, 600 mg, 900 mg, 1200 mg (1% or less) 2561
Zithromax Tablets, 250 mg, 500 mg (1% or less) 2561
Zithromax Tri-Pak (1% or less) 2561
Zmax for Oral Suspension 2577
▲ Zoladex (3% to 5%) 709
Zoladex 3-month 712
▲ Zoloft (6%) 2581
Zomig Nasal Spray (Infrequent) 718
Zonegran Capsules (2%) 1089
▲ Zyban Sustained-Release Tablets (4%) 1620
▲ Zyprexa Tablets (16%) 1798
▲ Zyprexa ZYDIS Orally Disintegrating Tablets (16%) 1798
Zyrtec Chewable Tablets (Less than 2%) 2589
Zyrtec (Less than 2%) 2589
Zyrtec-D 12 Hour Extended Release Tablets (Less than 2%) 2591

Neuralgia

Aciphex Tablets 1081
▲ Actonel Tablets (3.8%) 2679
▲ Actonel with Calcium Tablets (3.8%) 2684
Altace Capsules (Less than 1%) 1673
Ambien Tablets (Rare) 2867
Amerge Tablets (Rare) 1312
Antara Capsules 2723
▲ Arava Tablets (1% to 3%) 2881
Aricept Tablets (Infrequent) 1086
Aricept ODT Tablets (Infrequent) 1086
Arthrotec Tablets (Rare) 3126
Campral Tablets (Infrequent) 1175
Celebrex Capsules (0.1% to 1.9%) 3130
Celexa (Infrequent) 1177
Coreg Tablets (Less than or equal to 0.1%) 1376
Crestor Tablets (Greater than or equal to 1%) 672
▲ Doxil Injection (1% to 10%) 3302
Effexor Tablets (Infrequent) 3405
Effexor XR Capsules (Infrequent) 3411
Evoxac Capsules (Less than 1%) 1042
Exelon Capsules (Infrequent) 2204
Fortical Nasal Spray (Less than 1%) 3336
Imitrex Injection 1431
Imitrex Nasal Spray (Infrequent) 1435
Imitrex Tablets (Rare) 1440
▲ Intron A for Injection (Less than 5%) 3038
Lamictal (Rare) 1449
Lofibra Capsules 1217
▲ Lunesta Tablets (0% to 3%) 3139
Lyrica Capsules (0.1% to 1%) 2524
Miacalcin Nasal Spray (Less than 1%) 2242
Namenda (Infrequent) 1199
Nipent for Injection (Less than 3%) 3216
Norvir (Less than 2%) 499
Paxil CR Controlled-Release Tablets (Rare) 1509
Paxil (Rare) 1501
Permax Tablets (1.1%) 3357
Plavix Tablets (1% to 2.5%) 940
Plavix Tablets (1% to 2.5%) 2942
Pletal Tablets (Less than 2%) 2478
Proleukin for Injection 1007
Protonix I.V. (Less than 1%) 3468
Protonix Tablets (Less than 1%) 3465
Prozac Pulvules and Liquid (Infrequent) 1771
Requip Tablets (Frequent) 1528
Sandostatin LAR Depot (1% to 4%) 2264
Seroquel Tablets (Rare) 691
Sonata Capsules (Infrequent) 1686
Sustiva Capsules (Less than 2%) 957
Symbyax Capsules (Infrequent) 1788
Tasmar Tablets (Infrequent) 3360
Thalomid Capsules 979
Tricor Tablets 523
Trileptal Oral Suspension 2281
Trileptal Tablets 2281
Uniretic Tablets (Less than 1%) 3114
VFEND I.V. (Less than 2%) 2543
VFEND Oral Suspension (Less than 2%) 2543
VFEND Tablets (Less than 2%) 2543
Viagra Tablets (Less than 2%) 2552
Vicoprofen Tablets (Less than 1%) 533
Wellbutrin SR Sustained-Release Tablets 1583
Wellbutrin XL Extended-Release Tablets 1588
Zyban Sustained-Release Tablets 1620
Zyprexa Tablets (Rare) 1798
Zyprexa ZYDIS Orally Disintegrating Tablets (Rare) 1798

Neuralgia, occipital

Neurontin Capsules 2498
Neurontin Oral Solution 2498
Neurontin Tablets 2498

Neuralgia, trigeminal

Nalfon Capsules (Less than 1%) 2504

Neuritis

Ambien Tablets (Rare) 2867
Amerge Tablets (Rare) 1312
▲ Arava Tablets (1% to 3%) 2881
Clinoril Tablets (Rare) 1899
Decadron Tablets 1929
Effexor Tablets (Rare) 3405
Effexor XR Capsules (Rare) 3411
Fluorescite Injection ⊙ 207
Gabitril Tablets (Infrequent) 998
▲ Imdur Tablets (Less than or equal to 5%) 3032
Infanrix Vaccine 1444
▲ Intron A for Injection (Less than 5%) 3038
Lotrel Capsules (Infrequent) 2238
Lunesta Tablets (Rare) 3139
Nipent for Injection (Less than 3%) 3216
Permax Tablets (Rare) 3357
Proleukin for Injection 1007
ProSom Tablets (Rare) 512
Protonix I.V. (Less than 1%) 3468
Protonix Tablets (Less than 1%) 3465
Protopic Ointment (Greater than or equal to 1%) 629
Prozac Pulvules and Liquid (Rare) 1771
Remicade for IV Injection (Greater than or equal to 0.2%) 987
Sandostatin Injection (Less than 1%) 2263
Soriatane Capsules (Less than 1%) 1028
Teveten Tablets (Less than 1%) 1707
Teveten HCT Tablets (Less than 1%) 1710
Thalomid Capsules 979
Uniretic Tablets (Less than 1%) 3114

Neuritis, brachial

Adacel Vaccine 2959
Boostrix 1366
DAPTACEL 2964
Pediarix Vaccine 1518

Neuritis, optic

Accutane Capsules 2740
Activella Tablets 2311
Alesse-28 Tablets 3392
Amnesteem Capsules 2126
Antabuse Tablets 2343
Attenuvax 1889
Aygestin Tablets 1062
Copaxone for Injection (Infrequent) 3292
Cuprimine Capsules 1925
Desferal Vials 2190
▲ Doxil Injection (1% to 5%) 3302
Elmiron Capsules (Less than or equal to 1%) 2393

Eloxatin for Injection 2908
Enbrel for Injection 580
Engerix-B Vaccine 1391
Estratest Tablets 3196
Estratest H.S. Tablets 3196
Intron A for Injection 3038
Lo/Ovral-28 Tablets 3423
Meruvax II 1994
M-M-R II (Infrequent) 1980
Mumpsvax 2005
Nalfon Capsules (Less than 1%) 2504
Ortho Evra Transdermal System 2402
Pacerone Tablets 3337
Paser Granules 1657
Paxil CR Controlled-Release Tablets 1509
Paxil 1501
Pegasys 2793
PEG-Intron Powder for Injection (Less than or equal to 1%) 3062
Premarin Intravenous 3440
Premarin Vaginal Cream 3449
Premphase Tablets 3452
Prempro Tablets 3452
Prilosec OTC Tablets (Less than 1%) 2674
Proleukin for Injection (Less than 1%) 1007
Prozac Pulvules and Liquid 1771
Recombivax HB 2045
Remicade for IV Injection (Rare) 987
Rituxan for Infusion (Less than 0.1%) 845
▲ Rituxan I.V. (1% to 5%) 1251
Seasonale Tablets 1073
Trecator Tablets 3482
Twinrix Vaccine 1571
VFEND I.V. (Less than 2%) 2543
VFEND Oral Suspension (Less than 2%) 2543
VFEND Tablets (Less than 2%) 2543
Yasmin 28 Tablets 818
Zegerid Powder for Oral Solution (Less than 1%) 2972
Zoloft 2581

Neuritis, peripheral
Antabuse Tablets 2343
BiDil Tablets 2161
Carbatrol Capsules 3174
▲ Doxil Injection (1% to 10%) 3302
▲ Emtriva Capsules (4%) 1272
Equetro Extended-Release Capsules 3178
Gabitril Tablets (Infrequent) 998
Herceptin I.V. (2%) 1234
Kaletra (Less than 2%) 474
Lamictal (Rare) 1449
Lyrica Capsules (Rare) 2524
Paxil CR Controlled-Release Tablets (Rare) 1509
Paxil (Rare) 1501
Rilutek Tablets (Rare) 2945
Tegretol/Tegretol-XR 2278
Thalomid Capsules 979
Trecator Tablets 3482
Truvada Tablets 1279
Zonegran Capsules (Infrequent) 1089

Neuritis, retrobulbar
Attenuvax 1889
Meruvax II 1994
M-M-R II 1980
Mumpsvax (Infrequent) 2005
Rabies Vaccine RabAvert 1011

Neurodermatitis
Aricept Tablets (Infrequent) 1086
Aricept ODT Tablets (Infrequent) 1086

Neuroleptic malignant syndrome
Celexa 1177
Clozapine Tablets (Several cases) 2141
Clozaril Tablets (Several cases) 2174
Comtan Tablets 2186
Concerta Extended-Release Tablets (Very rare) 1828
Effexor Tablets 3405
Effexor XR Capsules 3411
Focalin Tablets (Very rare) 2214
Focalin XR Capsules 2217
Geodon 2514
Lexapro Oral Solution 1193
Lexapro Tablets 1193
Metadate CD Capsules (Very rare) 3316
Moban Tablets 1108
Namenda 1199
Orap Tablets 1220
Parcopa Orally Disintegrating Tablets 3111
Paxil CR Controlled-Release Tablets 1509
Paxil 1501
Permax Tablets 3357
Phenergan 3438
Prozac Pulvules and Liquid (Rare) 1771
Risperdal Consta Long-Acting Injection (Rare) 1664
Risperdal M-Tab Orally Disintegrating Tablets 1658
Risperdal 1658
Ritalin Hydrochloride Tablets 2254
Ritalin LA Capsules (Very rare) 2255
Ritalin-SR Tablets 2254
Seroquel Tablets (Rare) 691
Stalevo Tablets 2270
Symmetrel 1115
Tegretol-XR Tablets (Isolated cases) 2278
Thioridazine Hydrochloride Tablets 2122
Thiothixene Capsules 2124
Zoloft 2581

Neurological disability, unspecified
Abelcet Injection 1119
▲ Nipent for Injection (1% to 11%) 3216

Neuromuscular block, inadequate
Nimbex 494

Neuromuscular blockade
Capastat Sulfate for Injection 1728
Mivacron Injection (3 of 2,074 patients) 489
Zemuron Injection 2363

Neuromuscular disorders, unspecified
Eulexin Capsules (2%) 3023
Lupron Depot 3.75 mg (1%) 3257
Lupron Depot 7.5 mg (Less than 5%) 3261
Lupron Depot–3 Month 11.25 mg (1%) 3262

Neuromuscular excitability
Fortaz 1422
Zosyn 3492

Neuro-ocular lesions
Triphasil-28 Tablets 3483

Neuropathy
Abilify Tablets (Infrequent) 916
Abilify Tablets (Infrequent) 2472
Accolate Tablets (Rare) 663
Aciphex Tablets 1081
Actiq (Less than 1%) 993
▲ Alimta for Injection (Up to 29%) 1722
Altace Capsules (Less than 1%) 1673
Ambien Tablets (Rare) 2867
Axert Tablets (Rare) 2430
▲ Casodex Tablets (2% to 5%) 670
Celebrex Capsules (0.1% to 1.9%) 3130
▲ CellCept Capsules (3% to less than 20%) 2751
▲ CellCept Intravenous (3% to less than 20%) 2751
▲ CellCept Oral Suspension (3% to less than 20%) 2751
▲ CellCept Tablets (3% to less than 20%) 2751
▲ Chemet Capsules (1.0% to 12.7%) 2480
▲ Combivir Tablets (12%) 1373
Cuprimine Capsules 1925
▲ Cytovene (8%) 2763
Decadron Tablets 1929
Diprivan Injectable Emulsion (Less than 1%) 676
▲ Doxil Injection (1% to 10%) 3302
Effexor Tablets (Infrequent) 3405
Effexor XR Capsules (Infrequent) 3411
▲ Eloxatin for Injection (12% to 92%) 2908
▲ Emtriva Capsules (4%) 1272
Engerix-B Vaccine 1391
▲ Epivir (12%) 1394
Evoxac Capsules (Less than 1%) 1042
Flovent Diskus 50 mcg 1415
Gengraf Capsules (1% to less than 3%) 458
Geodon Capsules (Frequent) 2514
Havrix Vaccine (Rare) 1425
Herceptin I.V. (1%) 1234
▲ Intron A for Injection (Less than 5%) 3038
Kaletra (Less than 2%) 474
Lariam Tablets (Occasional) 2790
Lunesta Tablets (Rare) 3139
▲ Lyrica Capsules (2% to 9%) 2524
Matulane Capsules 3188
▲ Megace ES Oral Suspension (1% to 3%) 2492
Namenda (Infrequent) 1199
Naropin Injection (Less than 1%) 640
Neoral Soft Gelatin Capsules (1% to less than 3%) 2247
Neoral Oral Solution (1% to less than 3%) 2247
Nimotop Capsules (Less than 1%) 774
Nipent for Injection (Less than 3%) 3216
Norvir (Less than 2%) 499
Paxil CR Controlled-Release Tablets (Rare) 1509
Paxil (Rare) 1501
Permax Tablets (Infrequent) 3357
▲ Prograf Capsules and Injection (3%) 624
Proleukin for Injection 1007
Protonix I.V. 3468
Protonix Tablets 3465
Prozac Pulvules and Liquid (Infrequent) 1771
▲ Rapamune Oral Solution and Tablets (3% to 20%) 3472
ReFacto Vials 3479
Relpax Tablets (Rare) 2531
Rescriptor Tablets 2535
▲ Rituxan I.V. (1% to 5%) 1251
Sandostatin LAR Depot (1% to 4%) 2264
▲ Simulect for Injection (3% to 10%) 2268
Singulair 2047
Sonata Capsules (Rare) 1686
Sustiva Capsules 957
Tambocor Tablets (Less than 1%) 1824
Targretin Capsules 1719
Tasmar Tablets (Infrequent) 3360
▲ Thalomid Capsules (8.3%) 979
Topamax Sprinkle Capsules (Infrequent) 2438
Topamax Tablets (Infrequent) 2438
▲ Trizivir Tablets (12%) 1565
Truvada Tablets 1279
Twinrix Vaccine 1571
VFEND I.V. (Less than 2%) 2543
VFEND Oral Suspension (Less than 2%) 2543
VFEND Tablets (Less than 2%) 2543
Viagra Tablets (Less than 2%) 2552
Wellbutrin SR Sustained-Release Tablets 1583
Wellbutrin XL Extended-Release Tablets 1588
Zerit 971
Zomig Nasal Spray (Rare) 718
Zonegran Capsules (Infrequent) 1089
Zyban Sustained-Release Tablets 1620
Zyprexa Tablets (Rare) 1798
Zyprexa ZYDIS Orally Disintegrating Tablets (Rare) 1798

Neuropathy, optic
Campath Ampules 826
Decadron Phosphate Injection 1931
Imitrex Injection 1431
Imitrex Nasal Spray 1435
Imitrex Tablets 1440
Pacerone Tablets 3337
Prilosec OTC Tablets (Less than 1%) 2674
Protonix I.V. 3468
Protonix Tablets 3465
Zegerid Powder for Oral Solution (Less than 1%) 2972
Zyvox 2661

Neuropathy, optic, anterior ischemic, non-arteritic
Cialis Tablets 1806
Levitra Tablets 3048
Viagra Tablets 2552

Neuropathy, peripheral
Abelcet Injection 1119
Advicor Tablets 1694
Altoprev Extended-Release Tablets 1151
Antabuse Tablets 2343
Aptivus Capsules (Less than 2%) 859
Arava Tablets (Rare) 2881
Asacol Delayed-Release Tablets (Rare) 2688
Caduet Tablets (Greater than 0.1% to less than 2%) 2507
Cipro I.V. 2998
Cipro I.V. Pharmacy Bulk Package 3509
Cipro 2991
Cipro XR Tablets 3004
Combivir Tablets 1373
Copegus Tablets (Less than 1%) 2759
Cozaar Tablets (Less than 1%) 1913
Cuprimine Capsules 1925
Dapsone Tablets USP 1656
DepoCyt Injection 1121
Emend Capsules (Greater than 0.5%) 1944
▲ Epivir (13%) 1394
Epivir-HBV 1398
Epzicom Tablets 1402
Exelon Capsules (Infrequent) 2204
Flexeril Tablets (Rare) 1832
Fuzeon Injection 2772
Garamycin Injectable 3028
Gleevec Tablets (Infrequent) 2221
▲ Hexalen Capsules (9% to 31%) 2101
Hyzaar 1964
▲ Idamycin PFS Injection (7%) 2645
Indocin Capsules (Less than 1%) 1968
Indocin I.V. (Less than 1%) 1973
Indocin (Less than 1%) 1968
Infanrix Vaccine 1444
Invirase (1% to greater than or equal to 2%) 2776
Lescol Capsules 2227
Lescol Capsules 2730
Lescol XL Tablets 2227
Lescol XL Tablets 2730
Leukeran Tablets 1472
Levaquin in 5% Dextrose Injection 2453
Levaquin 2453
Lipitor Tablets (Less than 2%) 2495
Lupron Depot 3.75 mg 3257
Lupron Depot 7.5 mg 3261
Lupron Depot–3 Month 11.25 mg 3262
Lupron Depot-PED 7.5 mg, 11.25 mg and 15 mg 3266
Lupron Injection Pediatric 3256
Mevacor Tablets (0.5% to 1.0%) 1996
▲ Navelbine Injection (Up to 20%) 1494
Noroxin Tablets 2009
Norvasc Tablets (More than 0.1% to 1%) 2529
Norvir (Less than 2%) 499
Pacerone Tablets (Common) 3337
Parcopa Orally Disintegrating Tablets 3111
Pegasys (Less than 1%) 2793
PEG-Intron Powder for Injection 3062
Pravachol Tablets 943
Prinivil Tablets (0.3% to 1.0%) 2029
Prinzide Tablets 2033
Recombivax HB 2045
Remicade for IV Injection (Greater than or equal to 0.2%) 987
Requip Tablets (Infrequent) 1528
Rythmol SR Capsules 2736
Soriatane Capsules 1028
Stalevo Tablets 2270
Surmontil Capsules 2347
Sustiva Capsules (Less than 2%) 957
Tequin Injection 964
Tequin Tablets 964
Thalomid Capsules 979
Ticlid Tablets (Rare) 2813
Trizivir Tablets 1565
Truvada Tablets 1279
▲ Valcyte Tablets (9%) 2816
Vaseretic Tablets 2073
Vasotec I.V. Injection (0.5% to 1.0%) 2076
▲ Velcade for Injection (36%) 2102
▲ Viread Tablets (3% to 5%) 1284
Vivactil Tablets 2350
Vytorin 10/10 Tablets 2084
Vytorin 10/10 Tablets 3092
Vytorin 10/20 Tablets 2084
Vytorin 10/20 Tablets 3092
Vytorin 10/40 Tablets 2084
Vytorin 10/40 Tablets 3092
Vytorin 10/80 Tablets 2084
Vytorin 10/80 Tablets 3092
▲ Xeloda Tablets (Less than 5%) 2825
Zavesca Capsules 543
▲ Zerit (4% to 52%) 971
Zestoretic Tablets 701
Zestril Tablets (0.3% to 1.0%) 704
Zocor Tablets 2078
Zyvox 2661

Neuropathy, peripheral sensory
Desferal Vials 2190
Emend Capsules (Greater than 0.5%) 1944
Lariam Tablets (Occasional) 2790
Norvir (Less than 2%) 499
▲ Velcade for Injection (36%) 2102
▲ Xeloda Tablets (10%) 2825

Neuropsychiatric disorders
Pegasys 2793

Neuropsychiatric disorders, life-threatening, aggravation of
Roferon-A Injection 2805

Neuropsychiatric disorders, transient
Floxin Otic Solution (Uncommon) 1043

Neuropsychometrics performance, decrease
Blocadren Tablets ... 1891
Cosopt Sterile Ophthalmic Solution ... 1910
Inderal LA Long-Acting Capsules ... 3421
InnoPran XL Capsules ... 2728
Nadolol Tablets ... 2121
Tenormin I.V. Injection ... 698
Tenormin Tablets ... 695
Timoptic in Ocudose ... 2061
Timoptic Sterile Ophthalmic Solution ... 2058
Timoptic-XE Sterile Ophthalmic Gel Forming Solution ... 2062
Toprol-XL Tablets ... 660

Neurosensory, unspecified
▲ Alimta for Injection (Up to 29%) ... 1722
▲ Taxotere Injection Concentrate (Up to 58.3%) ... 2947

Neurosis, unspecified
Ambien Tablets (Rare) ... 2867
Campral Tablets (Infrequent) ... 1175
Evoxac Capsules ... 1042
Exelon Capsules (Infrequent) ... 2204
Gabitril Tablets (Infrequent) ... 998
▲ Intron A for Injection (Less than 5%) ... 3038
Keppra Oral Solution ... 3307
Keppra Tablets ... 3307
Lamictal (Rare) ... 1449
Lunesta Tablets (Infrequent) ... 3139
Namenda (Infrequent) ... 1199
Neurontin Capsules (Rare) ... 2498
Neurontin Oral Solution (Rare) ... 2498
Neurontin Tablets (Rare) ... 2498
Nipent for Injection (Less than 3%) ... 3216
Paxil CR Controlled-Release Tablets (Infrequent) ... 1509
Paxil (Infrequent) ... 1501
Permax Tablets (Infrequent) ... 3357
Prevacid Delayed-Release Capsules (Less than 1%) ... 3268
Prevacid for Delayed-Release Oral Suspension (Less than 1%) ... 3268
Prevacid NapraPAC (Less than 1%) ... 3277
Prevacid SoluTab Delayed-Release Orally Disintegrating Tablets (Less than 1%) ... 3268
PREVPAC (Less than 1%) ... 3281
Prozac Pulvules and Liquid (Infrequent) ... 1771
Relpax Tablets (Rare) ... 2531
Requip Tablets (Infrequent) ... 1528
Rythmol SR Capsules ... 2736
Sustiva Capsules ... 957
Symbyax Capsules (Infrequent) ... 1788
Topamax Sprinkle Capsules (1%) ... 2438
Topamax Tablets (1%) ... 2438
Uniretic Tablets (Less than 1%) ... 3114

Neurotoxicity
Buphenyl Powder ... 3327
Buphenyl Tablets ... 3327
Garamycin Injectable ... 3028
Hexalen Capsules ... 2101
Leustatin Injection (Rare) ... 2368
▲ Prograf Capsules and Injection (Approximately 55%) ... 624
▲ Zinecard for Injection (10% to 17%) ... 2659

Neurotoxicity, peripheral
Navelbine Injection ... 1494

Neutropenia
Abilify Tablets (Infrequent) ... 916
Abilify Tablets (Infrequent) ... 2472
Accutane Capsules ... 2740
Aceon Tablets (2 mg, 4 mg, 8 mg) (0.1%) ... 3191
▲ Alimta for Injection (2% to 58%) ... 1722
Aloprim for Injection (Less than 1%) ... 2156
Altace Capsules ... 1673
Amnesteem Capsules ... 2126
Ancef for Injection ... 1318
Aptivus Capsules (Less than 2%) ... 859
Arava Tablets (Rare) ... 2881
Aredia for Injection (Up to 1%) ... 2168
Asacol Delayed-Release Tablets ... 2688
Atacand Tablets (Very rare) ... 634
Atacand HCT ... 637
▲ Avastin IV (21%) ... 1229
▲ Betaseron for SC Injection (14%) ... 791
Bexxar ... 1360
▲ Campath Ampules (64% to 85%) ... 826
▲ Camptosar Injection (12% to 96.4%) ... 2602
▲ Cancidas for Injection (1.9% to 3.1%) ... 1894
Captopril Tablets ... 2114
Ceftin ... 1369
▲ CellCept Capsules (2% to 3.6%) ... 2751
▲ CellCept Intravenous (2% to 3.6%) ... 2751
▲ CellCept Oral Suspension (2% to 3.6%) ... 2751
▲ CellCept Tablets (2% to 3.6%) ... 2751
Chemet Capsules (0.5% to 1.5%) ... 2480
Cleocin Vaginal Ovules ... 2613
Clindesse Vaginal Cream (Rare) ... 3296
Clinoril Tablets (Less than 1 in 100) ... 1899
▲ Clolar for Intravenous Infusion (10%) ... 1264
▲ Clozapine Tablets (3%) ... 2141
▲ Clozaril Tablets (3%) ... 2174
▲ Combivir Tablets (7.2%) ... 1373
▲ Copegus Tablets (27% to 40%) ... 2759
Crixivan Capsules (1.1%) ... 1918
▲ Cytovene (6% to 22%) ... 2763
▲ DepoCyt Injection (8% to 9%) ... 1121
Diastat Rectal Delivery System (Infrequent) ... 3344
Diovan HCT Tablets ... 2195
Diovan Tablets (1.9%) ... 2191
▲ Doxil Injection (12.1% to 45.9%) ... 3302
Dynacin Tablets ... 1859
Edecrin ... 1941
Effexor Tablets ... 3405
Effexor XR Capsules (Rare) ... 3411
Elitek (2%) ... 2906
▲ Ellence Injection (10.5% to 80.3%) ... 2632
▲ Eloxatin for Injection (0% to 81%) ... 2908
▲ Emend Capsules (3.1%) ... 1944
Enbrel for Injection ... 580
▲ Epivir (7.2% to 22%) ... 1394
Epivir-HBV ... 1398
Epzicom Tablets ... 1402
Factive Tablets (0.5%) ... 2464
▲ Famvir Tablets (3.2%) ... 2207
▲ FazaClo Orally Disintegrating Tablets (3%) ... 547
Fortaz (Very rare) ... 1422
Fuzeon Injection ... 2772
▲ Gemzar for Injection (18% to 63%) ... 1743
▲ Gleevec Tablets (2.2% to 48%) ... 2221
▲ Hycamtin for Injection (26% to 98%) ... 1427
▲ Intron A for Injection (Less than 5% to 92%) ... 3038
Invanz for Injection (1% to 1.5%) ... 1974
Invirase (1% to 2%) ... 2776
▲ I.V. Busulfex (100%) ... 1125
Iveegam EN ... 759
▲ Kaletra (1% to 5%) ... 474
Keppra Oral Solution ... 3307
Keppra Tablets ... 3307
Kineret Injection (0.4%) ... 594
Lamictal ... 1449
Lamisil Tablets (Isolated case) ... 2226
Leukeran Tablets ... 1472
▲ Leustatin Injection (70%) ... 2368
▲ Lexiva Tablets (3%) ... 1473
Lotrel Capsules ... 2238
Mavik Tablets (Rare) ... 482
Maxipime for Injection (Greater than 0.1% to less than 1%) ... 1093
Mefoxin for Injection ... 1987
Mefoxin Premixed Intravenous Solution ... 1990
▲ Mepron Suspension (5%) ... 1487
Midamor Tablets (Rare) ... 2000
Moduretic Tablets ... 2003
Mycamine for Injection (1.2%) ... 620
Mylotarg for Injection ... 3429
Neumega for Injection ... 3433
Noroxin Tablets (1.4%) ... 2009
▲ Norvir (6%) ... 499
Omnicef Capsules ... 506
Omnicef for Oral Suspension ... 506
Orthoclone OKT3 Sterile Solution (Less than 1%) ... 2370
Pacerone Tablets ... 3337
Parcopa Orally Disintegrating Tablets ... 3111
▲ Pegasys (21% to 95%) ... 2793
▲ PEG-Intron Powder for Injection (6%) ... 3062
Plavix Tablets (Less than 1%) ... 940
Plavix Tablets (Less than 1%) ... 2942
Prevacid Delayed-Release Capsules (Less than 1%) ... 3268
Prevacid for Delayed-Release Oral Suspension (Less than 1%) ... 3268
Prevacid NapraPAC ... 3277
Prevacid SoluTab Delayed-Release Orally Disintegrating Tablets (Less than 1%) ... 3268
PREVPAC ... 3281
Prilosec OTC Tablets (Rare) ... 2674
Primaxin I.M. ... 2022
Primaxin I.V. (Less than 0.2%) ... 2024
Prinivil Tablets (Rare) ... 2029
Prinzide Tablets (Rare) ... 2033
Proleukin for Injection ... 1007
Rapamune Oral Solution and Tablets ... 3472
Raptiva for Injection ... 1247
▲ Rebetol (14% to 26%) ... 3073
Rebif Prefilled Syringe for Injection ... 3163
Remicade for IV Injection ... 987
▲ Rescriptor Tablets (Less than 2% to 5.7%) ... 2535
Retrovir Capsules ... 1533
Retrovir IV Infusion ... 1537
Retrovir ... 1533
▲ Ribavirin, USP Capsules (14% to 26%) ... 3083
Rilutek Tablets (Three cases) ... 2945
▲ Rituxan for Infusion (1.9% to 7%) ... 845
▲ Rituxan I.V. (14%) ... 1251
Rocephin Injectable Vials, ADD-Vantage, Galaxy, Bulk (Less than 1%) ... 2801
▲ Roferon-A Injection (0% to 68%) ... 2805
Seroquel Tablets ... 691
Suprax ... 1811
Symmetrel (Less than 0.1%) ... 1115
Tarka Tablets (Less frequent) ... 519
▲ Taxotere Injection Concentrate (6.3% to 98.5%) ... 2947
▲ Temodar Capsules (51%) ... 3088
Tequin Injection (Less than 0.1%) ... 964
Tequin Tablets (Less than 0.1%) ... 964
Teveten Tablets (1.3%) ... 1707
Teveten HCT Tablets ... 1710
Thalomid Capsules ... 979
Ticlid Tablets (0.8% to 2.4%) ... 2813
Timentin ADD-Vantage ... 1556
Timentin Injection Galaxy Container ... 1559
Timentin IV Infusion ... 1553
Timentin Pharmacy Bulk Package ... 1562
▲ Trisenox Injection (10%) ... 983
▲ Trizivir Tablets (7.2%) ... 1565
▲ Truvada Tablets (1% to 12%) ... 1279
Uniretic Tablets (More than 1%) ... 3114
▲ Valcyte Tablets (11% to 27%) ... 2816
Valium Tablets (Isolated reports) ... 2822
▲ Valtrex Caplets (18%) ... 1573
Vancocin HCl Capsules, USP (Several dozen cases) ... 3370
Vantin Tablets and Oral Suspension ... 2650
Vaseretic Tablets (Rare) ... 2073
Vasotec I.V. Injection (Rare) ... 2076
▲ Velcade for Injection (19%) ... 2102
Vermox Chewable Tablets (Rare) ... 1853
▲ Viramune Oral Suspension (11.1%) ... 903
▲ Viramune Tablets (11.1%) ... 903
Viread Tablets (1%) ... 1284
▲ Xeloda Tablets (2.2% to 86%) ... 2825
Xifaxan Tablets (Less than 2%) ... 2847
Zegerid Powder for Oral Solution (Rare) ... 2972
▲ Zerit (5%) ... 971
Zestoretic Tablets (Rare) ... 701
Zestril Tablets (Rare) ... 704
▲ Zevalin Injection (77%) ... 848
Ziagen (2%) ... 1600
Zinacef Injection (Fewer than 1 in 100) ... 1604
Zinacef for Injection (Fewer than 1 in 100) ... 1604
Zithromax Capsules, 250 mg (Less than 1%) ... 2568
Zithromax for IV Infusion (Less than 1%) ... 2573
Zithromax for Oral Suspension, 1 g (Less than 1%) ... 2568
Zithromax for Oral Suspension, 300 mg, 600 mg, 900 mg, 1200 mg (Less than 1%) ... 2561
Zithromax Tablets, 250 mg, 500 mg (Less than 1%) ... 2561
Zithromax Tablets, 600 mg (Less than 1%) ... 2568
Zithromax Tri-Pak (Less than 1%) ... 2561
Zithromax Z-Pak (Less than 1%) ... 2568
Zmax for Oral Suspension (Less then 1%) ... 2577
▲ Zometa for Intravenous Infusion (12%) ... 2306
Zosyn ... 3492
Zovirax for Injection (Less than 1%) ... 1618

Neutropenia, febrile
▲ Alimta for Injection (Up to 9%) ... 1722
▲ Clolar for Intravenous Infusion (57%) ... 1264
▲ Elitek (4%) ... 2906
▲ Ellence Injection (0% to 6.1%) ... 2632
Eloxatin for Injection ... 2908
Emend Capsules (Greater than 0.5%) ... 1944
Mycamine for Injection (0.9%) ... 620
▲ Trisenox Injection (8%) ... 983
Zevalin Injection (2%) ... 848

Neutropenia, transient
Tindamax ... 2670

Neutrophil count, abnormal
▲ Zyvox (0% to 5.9%) ... 2661

Neutrophil count, low
Rythmol SR Capsules ... 2736
Zelnorm Tablets ... 2303

Neutrophilia
▲ Emtriva Capsules (5%) ... 1272
Factive Tablets (0.5%) ... 2464
Zovirax for Injection (Less than 1%) ... 1618

Neutrophils, decrease
(*see under* Neutropenia)

Nevi, pre-existing, increased growth of
Humatrope Vials and Cartridges (Rare) ... 1756
Nutropin for Injection (Rare) ... 1238
Nutropin AQ Injection (Rare) ... 1241
Nutropin AQ Pen (Rare) ... 1241
Nutropin AQ Pen Cartridge (Rare) ... 1241

Night blindness
(*see under* Nyctalopia)

Night sweat
Aricept Tablets (Infrequent) ... 1086
Aricept ODT Tablets (Infrequent) ... 1086
Cymbalta Delayed-Release Capsules (Frequent) ... 1729
Effexor Tablets (Rare) ... 3405
Effexor XR Capsules (Rare) ... 3411
Eligard 22.5 mg (Less than 2%) ... 2899
▲ Eligard 30 mg (3.3%) ... 2901
Eligard 45 mg (2.7%) ... 2904
Gengraf Capsules (Rare) ... 458
▲ Gleevec Tablets (13% to 17%) ... 2221
Invirase (Less than 2%) ... 2776
Neoral Soft Gelatin Capsules (Rare) ... 2247
Neoral Oral Solution (Rare) ... 2247
Oncaspar (Greater than 1% but less than 5%) ... 1123
▲ Prometrium Capsules (100 mg, 200 mg) (7%) ... 3205
▲ Rituxan for Infusion (Among most frequent) ... 845
▲ Rituxan I.V. (15%) ... 1251
Sandimmune (Rare) ... 2259
▲ Trisenox Injection (8%) ... 983
Vantas (Less than 2%) ... 3367
▲ Zenapax for Injection (2% to 5%) ... 2838

Nightmares
Aldoclor Tablets ... 1881
Aldoril Tablets ... 1884
Axert Tablets (Rare) ... 2430
Biaxin/Biaxin XL ... 402
Blocadren Tablets ... 1891
Catapres Tablets ... 874
Catapres-TTS (0.5% or less) ... 875
Cipro I.V. (1% or less) ... 2998
Cipro I.V. Pharmacy Bulk Package (1% or less) ... 3509
Cipro (Less than 1%) ... 2991
Cipro XR Tablets ... 3004
Clorpres Tablets ... 2139
▲ Clozapine Tablets (4%) ... 2141
▲ Clozaril Tablets (4%) ... 2174
Cosopt Sterile Ophthalmic Solution ... 1910
Cymbalta Delayed-Release Capsules (Frequent) ... 1729
▲ Effexor XR Capsules (4% to 7%) ... 3411
Eldepryl Capsules ... 3209
▲ FazaClo Orally Disintegrating Tablets (4%) ... 547
Klonopin (Infrequent) ... 2782
Levaquin in 5% Dextrose Injection ... 2453
Levaquin ... 2453
Marinol Capsules (Less than 1%) ... 3334
Matulane Capsules ... 3188
Mebaral Tablets, USP (Less than 1 in 100 patients) ... 2483
Meridia Capsules ... 485
Naropin Injection (Less than 1%) ... 640
Nembutal Sodium Solution, USP (Less than 1%) ... 2484
Parcopa Orally Disintegrating Tablets ... 3111
Phenergan ... 3438
PREVPAC ... 3281
Relafen Tablets (Less than 1%) ... 1523
Risperdal M-Tab Orally Disintegrating Tablets (Rare) ... 1658

Risperdal (Rare) 1658
Rythmol SR Capsules 2736
Stalevo Tablets 2270
Surmontil Capsules 2347
Tequin Injection 964
Tequin Tablets 964
Timolide Tablets 2056
Timoptic in Ocudose 2061
Timoptic Sterile Ophthalmic Solution 2058
Timoptic-XE Sterile Ophthalmic Gel Forming Solution 2062
Toprol-XL Tablets 660
Vantin Tablets and Oral Suspension (Less than 1%) 2650
Vivactil Tablets 2350
Xanax XR Tablets (Frequent) 2655

Nipples, sensitive
Testim 1% Gel (Less than 1%) 722

Nitrogen balance, changes
(*see under* BUN levels, changes)

NMS
(*see under* Neuroleptic malignant syndrome)

Nocardiosis
Remicade for IV Injection 987

Nocturia
Abilify Tablets (Rare) 916
Abilify Tablets (Rare) 2472
Actiq (Less than 1%) 993
Adalat CC Tablets (Less than 1%) 2978
Ambien Tablets (Rare) 2867
Aricept Tablets (Frequent) 1086
Aricept ODT Tablets (Frequent) 1086
Arthrotec Tablets (Rare) 3126
Caduet Tablets (Greater than 0.1% to less than 2%) 2507
Calcijex Injection 411
Campral Tablets (Rare) 1175
Cardizem LA Extended Release Tablets (Less than 2%) 1699
▲ Casodex Tablets (9%) 670
Catapres Tablets (About 1 in 100 patients) 874
Clorpres Tablets (About 1%) 2139
Copaxone for Injection (Infrequent) 3292
Cozaar Tablets (Less than 1%) 1913
Dantrium Capsules (Less frequent) 2690
Doxil Injection (Less than 1%) 3302
DynaCirc CR Tablets (0.5% to 1%) 2726
Effexor Tablets (Infrequent) 3405
Effexor XR Capsules (Infrequent) 3411
Eldepryl Capsules 3209
Eligard 30 mg (2.2%) 2901
Eligard 45 mg (1%) 2904
▲ Entocort EC Capsules (Less than 5%) 2694
Evoxac Capsules (Less than 1%) 1042
Exelon Capsules (Infrequent) 2204
Frova Tablets (Rare) 1101
Gabitril Tablets (Infrequent) 998
Gengraf Capsules (1% to less than 3%) 458
Geodon Capsules (Rare) 2514
Hectorol Capsules 909
Hectorol Injection 911
Hyperstat I.V. Injection 3031
Hyzaar 1964
Indapamide Tablets (Less than 5%) 2119
▲ Intron A for Injection (Less than 5%) 3038
Klonopin 2782
Lamictal (Rare) 1449
Lipitor Tablets (Less than 2%) 2495
Matulane Capsules 3188
Miacalcin Injection 2241
Moduretic Tablets (Less than or equal to 1%) 2003
Neoral Soft Gelatin Capsules (1% to less than 3%) 2247
Neoral Oral Solution (1% to less than 3%) 2247
Neurontin Capsules (Rare) 2498
Neurontin Oral Solution (Rare) 2498
Neurontin Tablets (Rare) 2498
Norvasc Tablets (More than 0.1% to 1%) 2529
Norvir (0% to 0.2%) 499
Orap Tablets 1220
Paxil CR Controlled-Release Tablets (Infrequent) 1509
Paxil (Infrequent) 1501
▲ Prochieve 4% Gel (13%) 1018
▲ Prochieve 8% Gel (13%) 1018
▲ Prograf Capsules and Injection (3% to 15%) 624
ProSom Tablets (Rare) 512
Protonix I.V. (Less than 1%) 3468
Protonix Tablets (Less than 1%) 3465
Prozac Pulvules and Liquid (Infrequent) 1771
▲ Rapamune Oral Solution and Tablets (3% to 20%) 3472
Razadyne ER Extended-Release Capsules (Infrequent) 2434
Razadyne (Infrequent) 2434
Requip Tablets (Infrequent) 1528
Rescriptor Tablets 2535
Rilutek Tablets (Rare) 2945
Rythmol SR Capsules 2736
Seroquel Tablets (Rare) 691
Sular Tablets (Less than or equal to 1%) 1163
Tarka Tablets (Less frequent) 519
Tasmar Tablets (Infrequent) 3360
Tiazac Capsules (Less than 2%) 1204
Topamax Sprinkle Capsules (1%) 2438
Topamax Tablets (1%) 2438
Uniretic Tablets (Less than 1%) 3114
Vantin Tablets and Oral Suspension (Less than 1%) 2650
▲ Viadur Implant (3.8%) 782
Viagra Tablets (Less than 2%) 2552
Vivactil Tablets 2350
Wellbutrin Tablets (Frequent) 1579
Xeloda Tablets 2825
Zoloft (Infrequent) 2581
Zonegran Capsules (Infrequent) 1089

Nodal rhythm
Covera-HS Tablets 3135
Digitek Tablets 2146
Lanoxicaps Capsules (Common) 1458
Lanoxin Injection (Common) 1462
Lanoxin Tablets (Common) 1468
Lanoxin Injection Pediatric (Common) 1465
Suprane Liquid for Inhalation (Greater than 1%) 770

Nodule, subcutaneous
▲ Arava Tablets (1% to 3%) 2881
Enbrel for Injection 580
Gabitril Tablets (Infrequent) 998
Lyrica Capsules (Rare) 2524
Neurontin Capsules (Rare) 2498
Neurontin Oral Solution (Rare) 2498
Neurontin Tablets (Rare) 2498
Permax Tablets (Rare) 3357
Uniretic Tablets (Less than 1%) 3114

Nodule at injection site
Adacel Vaccine 2959
Boostrix 1366
▲ Fuzeon Injection (80%) 2772
Genotropin Lyophilized Powder (Infrequent) 2642
Lovenox Injection 2931

Nodulosis
Advicor Tablets 1694

Noise intolerance
Neurontin Capsules (Rare) 2498
Neurontin Oral Solution (Rare) 2498
Neurontin Tablets (Rare) 2498

Nose, runny
▲ Fortical Nasal Spray (10.6%) 3336

NPN elevation
Celebrex Capsules (0.1% to 1.9%) 3130
▲ Coreg Tablets (6%) 1376
Garamycin Injectable 3028
▲ Gengraf Capsules (18%) 458
▲ Neoral Soft Gelatin Capsules (18%) 2247
▲ Neoral Oral Solution (18%) 2247

Nuchal rigidity
CytoGam Intravenous (Infrequent) 1866

Numbness
Acticin Cream 2125
Adenocard Injection (1%) 612
Aerobid/Aerobid-M (1% to 3%) 1172
Alferon N Injection (One patient to 3%) 1640
Aricept Tablets (Infrequent) 1086
Aricept ODT Tablets (Infrequent) 1086
Avalide Tablets 922
Avalide Tablets 2889
Avapro Tablets (Less than 1%) 925
Avapro Tablets (Less than 1%) 2886
Bentyl Capsules 724
Bentyl Injection 724
Bentyl Syrup 724
Bentyl Tablets 724
BiDil Tablets 2161
Botox Purified Neurotoxin Complex (Rare) 565
Calcium Disodium Versenate Injection 1819
Catapres-TTS (0.5% or less) 875
Clozapine Tablets (Less than 1%) 2141
Clozaril Tablets (Less than 1%) 2174
DepoCyt Injection 1121
DynaCirc CR Tablets (0.5% to 1%) 2726
FazaClo Orally Disintegrating Tablets (Less than 1%) 547
Garamycin Injectable 3028
▲ Imitrex Injection (4.6%) 1431
Imitrex Nasal Spray (Infrequent) 1435
Imitrex Tablets (Frequent) 1440
Infed Injection 3381
K-Phos Neutral Tablets 785
K-Phos Original (Sodium Free) Tablets (Less frequent) 785
Lidoderm Patch 1107
Metrogel 1% 1212
Mintezol 2002
Moduretic Tablets (Less than or equal to 1%) 2003
Nicotrol NS (Less than 1%) 2596
Nubain Injection (1% or less) 1111
Parcopa Orally Disintegrating Tablets 3111
Parnate Tablets 1499
Peganone Tablets, USP 2487
▲ R-Gene 10 for Intravenous Use (3%) 2647
▲ Roferon-A Injection (12%) 2805
Sedapap Tablets 50 mg/650 mg (Infrequent) 2098
Stalevo Tablets 2270
Surmontil Capsules 2347
Tindamax 2670
Vivactil Tablets 2350
Xeloda Tablets 2825

Numbness, buccal mucosa
Clozapine Tablets (1%) 2141
Clozaril Tablets (1%) 2174
FazaClo Orally Disintegrating Tablets (1%) 547
Imitrex Injection 1431
Imitrex Nasal Spray (Infrequent) 1435
Nicotrol NS 2596
Rythmol SR Capsules 2736

Numbness, extremities
Cogentin Injection 1903
▲ Indapamide Tablets (Greater than or equal to 5%) 2119
Invirase (0.6% to greater than or equal to 2%) 2776
Maxair Autohaler 1820
▲ Navelbine Injection (Up to 11%) 1494
Noritate Cream, 1% (Uncommon) 1051
Ortho-Cyclen/Ortho Tri-Cyclen 2414
Ortho Tri-Cyclen Lo Tablets 2421
Zerit 971

Numbness, face
Invirase (Less than 2%) 2776

Numbness, feet
Uroqid-Acid No. 2 Tablets 785

Numbness, fingers
Alferon N Injection (One patient) 1640
Cutivate Cream (1.0%) 1381
Olux Foam (Less than 2%) 1027
▲ Temovate Gel (Among most frequent) 1550
Temovate Ointment (Less frequent) 1549
Temovate E Emollient (Less than 2%) 1552

Numbness, hands
Alferon N Injection (One patient) 1640
Hyperstat I.V. Injection 3031
Uroqid-Acid No. 2 Tablets 785

Numbness, lips
K-Phos Neutral Tablets 785
K-Phos Original (Sodium Free) Tablets (Less frequent) 785
Oncaspar 1123
Uroqid-Acid No. 2 Tablets 785

Numbness, mouth
(*see under* Numbness, buccal mucosa)

Numbness, nose
Nicotrol NS 2596

Numbness, skin
Eskalith 1406

Numbness/tingling, fingers and toes
Eldepryl Capsules 3209

Nutrition disorders, unspecified
▲ Ammonul Injection (21%) 3323
▲ Focalin XR Capsules (34%) 2217

Nyctalopia
Accutane Capsules 2740
Amnesteem Capsules 2126
Arthrotec Tablets (Rare) 3126
Desferal Vials 2190
Lyrica Capsules (Rare) 2524
Paxil CR Controlled-Release Tablets (Rare) 1509
Paxil (Rare) 1501
▲ Soriatane Capsules (1% to 10%) 1028
VFEND I.V. (Less than 2%) 2543
VFEND Oral Suspension (Less than 2%) 2543
VFEND Tablets (Less than 2%) 2543

Nystagmus
Aricept Tablets (Infrequent) 1086
Aricept ODT Tablets (Infrequent) 1086
Axert Tablets (Rare) 2430
Carbatrol Capsules 3174
Celexa 1177
Cipro I.V. (1% or less) 2998
Cipro I.V. Pharmacy Bulk Package (1% or less) 3509
Cipro 2991
Cipro XR Tablets 3004
Clozapine Tablets (Less than 1%) 2141
Clozaril Tablets (Less than 1%) 2174
▲ Depacon Injection (1% to 8%) 412
▲ Depakene (7% to 8%) 417
▲ Depakote Sprinkle Capsules (1% to 8%) 422
▲ Depakote Tablets (7% to 8%) 427
▲ Depakote ER Tablets (1% to 8%) 433
Diastat Rectal Delivery System (Infrequent) 3344
Dilaudid 439
Dilaudid Oral Liquid (Less frequent) 443
Dilaudid Non-Sterile Powder 439
Dilaudid Rectal Suppositories 439
Dilaudid Tablets 439
Dilaudid Tablets - 8 mg (Less frequent) 443
Dilaudid-HP (Less frequent) 441
Diprivan Injectable Emulsion (Less than 1%) 676
Effexor Tablets (Rare) 3405
Effexor XR Capsules (Rare) 3411
Equetro Extended-Release Capsules 3178
Eskalith 1406
Exelon Capsules (Infrequent) 2204
FazaClo Orally Disintegrating Tablets (Less than 1%) 547
Gabitril Tablets (2%) 998
Geodon Capsules (Rare) 2514
Kadian Capsules (Less than 3%) 572
Klonopin 2782
Lamictal (1.0%) 1449
Lexapro Oral Solution 1193
Lexapro Tablets 1193
Lithobid Tablets 1670
Lunesta Tablets (Infrequent) 3139
Lyrica Capsules (Greater than or equal to 2%) 2524
Matulane Capsules 3188
MS Contin Tablets (Less frequent) 2703
▲ Neurontin Capsules (8.3%) 2498
▲ Neurontin Oral Solution (8.3%) 2498
▲ Neurontin Tablets (8.3%) 2498
Noroxin Tablets 2009
Paxil CR Controlled-Release Tablets (Rare) 1509
Paxil (Rare) 1501
Peganone Tablets, USP 2487
▲ Phenytek Capsules (Among most common) 2153
ProSom Tablets (Rare) 512
Rescriptor Tablets 2535
Sonata Capsules (Infrequent) 1686
Tambocor Tablets (Less than 1%) 1824
Tegretol/Tegretol-XR 2278
Thalomid Capsules 979
▲ Topamax Sprinkle Capsules (10% to 11%) 2438
▲ Topamax Tablets (10% to 11%) 2438
▲ Trileptal Oral Suspension (5% to 26%) 2281
▲ Trileptal Tablets (5% to 26%) 2281
VFEND I.V. (Less than 2%) 2543
VFEND Oral Suspension (Less than 2%) 2543
VFEND Tablets (Less than 2%) 2543
Zoloft (Infrequent) 2581
▲ Zonegran Capsules (4%) 1089
Zyprexa Tablets (Rare) 1798
Zyprexa ZYDIS Orally Disintegrating Tablets (Rare) 1798

Nystagmus, horizontal
(*see also under* Nystagmus)

O

Obesity
Abilify Tablets (Infrequent) 916
Abilify Tablets (Infrequent) 2472
Aptivus Capsules 859
Celexa (Rare) 1177
Crixivan Capsules 1918
Invirase 2776
Kaletra (Less than 2%) 474
Reyataz Capsules (Less than 3%) 948
Risperdal Consta Long-Acting Injection (Infrequent) 1664
Symbyax Capsules (Infrequent) 1788
Truvada Tablets 1279

Obsessive compulsive symptoms
Zyprexa Tablets (Infrequent) 1798
Zyprexa ZYDIS Orally Disintegrating Tablets (Infrequent) 1798

Obsessive thoughts
Abilify Tablets (Rare) 916
Abilify Tablets (Rare) 2472

Obstipation
Emend Capsules (Greater than 0.5%) 1944
Thioridazine Hydrochloride Tablets 2122

Obtundation
Orthoclone OKT3 Sterile Solution (Less than 1%) 2370
Risperdal Consta Long-Acting Injection 1664
Roferon-A Injection (Rare) 2805
Zovirax for Injection (Approximately 1%) 1618

Ocular, foreign body sensation
Azopt Ophthalmic Suspension (1% to 5%) 553
▲ Betimol Ophthalmic Solution (More than 5%) ⊙ 283
▲ Betimol Ophthalmic Solution (More than 5%) 3371
Betoptic S Ophthalmic Suspension (Small number of patients) 554
▲ Brimonidine Tartrate Ophthalmic Solution 0.2% (10% to 30%) ⊙ 245
Cosopt Sterile Ophthalmic Solution (1% to 5%) 1910
Patanol Ophthalmic Solution (Less than 5%) 557
Quixin Ophthalmic Solution (1% to 3%) 3373
▲ Restasis Ophthalmic Emulsion (1% to 5%) 570
Timoptic in Ocudose (Less frequent) 2061
Timoptic Sterile Ophthalmic Solution (Less frequent) 2058
Timoptic-XE Sterile Ophthalmic Gel Forming Solution (1% to 5%) 2062

Ocular allergy
▲ Trusopt Sterile Ophthalmic Solution (Approximately 10%) 2065
▲ Voltaren Ophthalmic Solution (Less than or equal to 5%) 2300

Ocular discomfort
Alamast Ophthalmic Solution (Less than 5%) 3371
Amerge Tablets (Rare) 1312
Azopt Ophthalmic Suspension (1% to 5%) 553
▲ Betoptic S Ophthalmic Suspension (Most frequent) 554
▲ Brimonidine Tartrate Ophthalmic Solution 0.2% (3% to 9%) ⊙ 245
▲ Evoxac Capsules (1% to 3%) 1042
HMS Sterile Ophthalmic Suspension ⊙ 228
Photofrin for Injection 729
Quixin Ophthalmic Solution (1% to 3%) 3373
▲ Travatan Ophthalmic Solution (5% to 10%) 559
▲ Trusopt Sterile Ophthalmic Solution (Approximately one-third of patients) 2065
▲ Vigamox Ophthalmic Solution (1% to 6%) 560
▲ Zylet Ophthalmic Suspension (Less than 4%) 3508

Ocular exudate
Betoptic S Ophthalmic Suspension (Small number of patients) 554
Cosopt Sterile Ophthalmic Solution (1% to 5%) 1910
▲ Restasis Ophthalmic Emulsion (1% to 5%) 570
Timoptic in Ocudose (Less frequent) 2061
Timoptic Sterile Ophthalmic Solution (Less frequent) 2058
Timoptic-XE Sterile Ophthalmic Gel Forming Solution (1% to 5%) 2062
Xalatan Sterile Ophthalmic Solution (Less than 1%) 2654

Ocular hypotony
▲ Retisert Implant (10% to 35%) ⊙ 256

Ocular irritation
Pred-G Sterile Ophthalmic Ointment ⊙ 235

Ocular palsies
Attenuvax (Rare) 1889
M-M-R II (Rare) 1980
Mumpsvax 2005

Ocular perforation
HMS Sterile Ophthalmic Suspension ⊙ 228

Ocular tension, increase
Bentyl Capsules 724
Bentyl Injection 724
Bentyl Syrup 724
Bentyl Tablets 724
Norflex Injection 1824

Ocular toxicity
TobraDex Ophthalmic Ointment (Less than 4%) 558
TobraDex Ophthalmic Suspension (Less than 4%) 558
▲ Zylet Ophthalmic Suspension (Less than 4%) 3508

Oculogyric crisis
Abilify Tablets (Rare) 916
Abilify Tablets (Rare) 2472
Geodon Capsules (Frequent) 2514
Orap Tablets (Less frequent) 1220
Parcopa Orally Disintegrating Tablets 3111
Paxil CR Controlled-Release Tablets 1509
Paxil 1501
Phenergan 3438
Relpax Tablets (Rare) 2531
Risperdal Consta Long-Acting Injection (Infrequent) 1664
▲ Risperdal M-Tab Orally Disintegrating Tablets (17% to 34%) 1658
▲ Risperdal (17% to 34%) 1658
Stalevo Tablets 2270
Symmetrel (Less than 0.1%) 1115
Thioridazine Hydrochloride Tablets 2122
Thiothixene Capsules 2124
Timolide Tablets 2056
Trileptal Oral Suspension 2281
Trileptal Tablets 2281
VFEND I.V. (Less than 2%) 2543
VFEND Oral Suspension (Less than 2%) 2543
VFEND Tablets (Less than 2%) 2543
Zofran Injection 1607
Zofran 1613
Zofran ODT Orally Disintegrating Tablets 1613
Zoloft 2581
Zonegran Capsules (Rare) 1089
▲ Zyprexa Tablets (2% to 3%) 1798
Zyprexa ZYDIS Orally Disintegrating Tablets (2% to 3%) 1798

Oculomotor disturbances
Carbatrol Capsules 3174
Equetro Extended-Release Capsules 3178
Pravachol Tablets 943
Tegretol/Tegretol-XR 2278

Odynophagia
▲ Alimta for Injection (Up to 6%) 1722
▲ Photofrin for Injection (5%) 729

Oily evacuation
▲ Xenical Capsules (2.3% to 11.9%) 2834

Oligohydramnios
Aceon Tablets (2 mg, 4 mg, 8 mg) 3191
Altace Capsules 1673
Avalide Tablets 922
Avalide Tablets 2889
Avapro Tablets 925
Avapro Tablets 2886
Captopril Tablets 2114
Clinoril Tablets 1899
Cozaar Tablets 1913
Dolobid Tablets 1937
Hyzaar 1964
Lotensin Tablets 2232
Lotrel Capsules 2238
Prinivil Tablets 2029
Prinzide Tablets 2033
Uniretic Tablets 3114
Vaseretic Tablets 2073
Vasotec I.V. Injection 2076
Zestoretic Tablets 701
Zestril Tablets 704

Oligomenorrhea
depo-subQ provera 104 Injectable Suspension 2622
Mustargen for Injection 2007
Ortho-Cyclen/Ortho Tri-Cyclen 2414
Ortho Tri-Cyclen Lo Tablets 2421
Sandostatin Injection (Less than 1%) 2263

Oligospermia
Anadrol-50 Tablets 3329
Avodart Soft Gelatin Capsules 1353
Oxandrin Tablets 2977
Purinethol Tablets 1222

Oliguria
Abelcet Injection 1119
Actiq (Less than 1%) 993
Aloprim for Injection (Less than 1%) 2156
Altace Capsules 1673
Anaprox Tablets (Less than 1%) 2769
Anaprox DS Tablets (Less than 1%) 2769
Angiomax for Injection (Rare) 1856
Anzemet Injection (2.6%) 2871
Anzemet Tablets (2.6%) 2874
Arthrotec Tablets (Rare) 3126
Avinza Capsules (Less than 5%) 1714
Bravelle for Intramuscular or Subcutaneous Injection 1140
Capastat Sulfate for Injection (1 patient) 1728
Captopril Tablets (Approximately 1 to 2 of 1000 patients) 2114
Carbatrol Capsules 3174
Carimune NF 3501
Cataflam Tablets (Occasionally) 2173
Celexa (Rare) 1177
▲ CellCept Capsules (3% to less than 20%) 2751
▲ CellCept Intravenous (3% to less than 20%) 2751
▲ CellCept Oral Suspension (3% to less than 20%) 2751
▲ CellCept Tablets (3% to less than 20%) 2751
Cleocin Vaginal Ovules (Rare) 2613
Clindesse Vaginal Cream (Rare) 3296
CytoGam Intravenous 1866
▲ DepoDur Extended-Release Injection (2% to 5%) 1098
Diovan HCT Tablets 2195
Diprivan Injectable Emulsion (Less than 1%) 676
Doxil Injection (Less than 1%) 3302
Duragesic Transdermal System (Less than 1%) 2448
Dyazide Capsules 1389
EC-Naprosyn Delayed-Release Tablets (Less than 1%) 2769
Effexor Tablets (Rare) 3405
Equetro Extended-Release Capsules 3178
Eskalith 1406
Evoxac Capsules 1042
Exelon Capsules (Infrequent) 2204
Follistim AQ Cartridge 2354
Furosemide Tablets 2117
Gammagard S/D (Some patients) 754
Garamycin Injectable 3028
Geodon Capsules (Rare) 2514
Hyzaar 1964
Invanz for Injection (Greater than 0.1%) 1974
▲ I.V. Busulfex (15%) 1125
Iveegam EN (0.3% to 0.8%) 759
Levaquin in 5% Dextrose Injection (0.1% to 0.9%) 2453
Levaquin (0.1% to 0.9%) 2453
Lithobid Tablets 1670
Lotrel Capsules 2238
Lunesta Tablets (Rare) 3139
Lyrica Capsules (0.1% to 1%) 2524
Maxzide 2150
Mycamine for Injection 620
Nalfon Capsules (Less than 1%) 2504
Naprosyn Suspension (Less than 1%) 2769
Naprosyn Tablets (Less than 1%) 2769
▲ Naropin Injection (1% to 5%) 640
Orthoclone OKT3 Sterile Solution (Less than 1%) 2370
Paxil CR Controlled-Release Tablets (Rare) 1509
Paxil (Rare) 1501
Primaxin I.M. 2022
Primaxin I.V. (2.2%) 2024
Prinivil Tablets (0.3% to 1.0%) 2029
Prinzide Tablets 2033
▲ Prograf Capsules and Injection (3% to 19%) 624
▲ Proleukin for Injection (63%) 1007
ProSom Tablets (Rare) 512
Prozac Pulvules and Liquid (Rare) 1771
▲ Rapamune Oral Solution and Tablets (3% to 20%) 3472
Reyataz Capsules (Less than 3%) 948
Rythmol SR Capsules 2736
▲ Simulect for Injection (3% to 10%) 2268
Symbyax Capsules (Infrequent) 1788
Tasmar Tablets (Infrequent) 3360
Tegretol/Tegretol-XR 2278
Thalomid Capsules 979
Topamax Sprinkle Capsules (Infrequent) 2438
Topamax Tablets (Infrequent) 2438
Trasylol Injection (1% to 2%) 779
▲ Trisenox Injection (5%) 983
Ultane Liquid for Inhalation (Less than 1%) 526
Univasc Tablets (Less than 1%) 3118
Vaseretic Tablets 2073
Vasotec I.V. Injection (0.5% to 1.0%) 2076
VFEND I.V. (Less than 2%) 2543
VFEND Oral Suspension (Less than 2%) 2543
VFEND Tablets (Less than 2%) 2543
Voltaren Tablets (Occasionally) 2298
Voltaren-XR Tablets (Occasionally) 2301
▲ Zenapax for Injection (Greater than 5%) 2838
Zestoretic Tablets 701
Zestril Tablets (0.3% to 1.0%) 704
Zoloft (Rare) 2581
Zosyn (1.0% or less) 3492

Oliguria, neonatal
Altace Capsules 1673
Captopril Tablets 2114
Zestril Tablets 704

"On-off" phenomenon
Stalevo Tablets 2270

Onychia
Evoxac Capsules (Less than 1%) 1042

Onycholysis
Adriamycin for Injection, USP (A few cases) 786
Adriamycin Injection, USP (A few cases) 786
Taxotere Injection Concentrate (0.8%) 2947
▲ Xeloda Tablets (1% to 5%) 2825

Onychomycosis
Evoxac Capsules (Less than 1%) 1042

Opacity, punctate
Stromectol Tablets (1.4% to 1.8%) 2053

Ophthalmitis
Campral Tablets (Rare) 1175

Ophthalmoplegia
Advicor Tablets 1694
Altoprev Extended-Release Tablets 1151
Lescol Capsules 2227
Lescol Capsules 2730
Lescol XL Tablets 2227
Lescol XL Tablets 2730
Lyrica Capsules (Rare) 2524
Mevacor Tablets 1996
Pravachol Tablets 943
Vytorin 10/10 Tablets 2084
Vytorin 10/10 Tablets 3092
Vytorin 10/20 Tablets 2084
Vytorin 10/20 Tablets 3092
Vytorin 10/40 Tablets 2084
Vytorin 10/40 Tablets 3092
Vytorin 10/80 Tablets 2084
Vytorin 10/80 Tablets 3092
Zocor Tablets 2078

Opisthotonos
Diprivan Injectable Emulsion (Rare) 676
Geodon Capsules (Rare) 2514

Orap Tablets (Less frequent)............ 1220
Thioridazine Hydrochloride Tablets... 2122
▲ Zyprexa Tablets (2% to 3%) 1798
Zyprexa ZYDIS Orally Disintegrating Tablets (2% to 3%)............ 1798

Optic atrophy
Eskalith 1406
Lyrica Capsules (Rare)............ 2524
Prilosec OTC Tablets (Less than 1%)............ 2674
VFEND I.V. (Less than 2%)............ 2543
VFEND Oral Suspension (Less than 2%)............ 2543
VFEND Tablets (Less than 2%)............ 2543
Zegerid Powder for Oral Solution (Less than 1%)............ 2972

Optic disorders
Effexor Tablets (Rare)............ 3405

Optic nerve, damage
Alrex Ophthalmic Suspension 0.2% .... ⊙ 243
Blephamide Ophthalmic Ointment (Infrequent) 563
Blephamide Ophthalmic Suspension (Infrequent) 564
Dapsone Tablets USP 1656
FML Ophthalmic Ointment (Infrequent) .... ⊙ 225
FML Ophthalmic Suspension (Infrequent) .... ⊙ 224
FML Forte Ophthalmic Suspension (Infrequent) .... ⊙ 223
FML-S Liquifilm Sterile Ophthalmic Suspension (Infrequent) .... ⊙ 226
HMS Sterile Ophthalmic Suspension (Rare) .... ⊙ 228
Lotemax Ophthalmic Suspension 0.5% .... ⊙ 249
Poly-Pred Liquifilm Ophthalmic Suspension (Infrequent) .... ⊙ 231
Pred Forte Ophthalmic Suspension (Infrequent) .... ⊙ 233
Pred Mild Sterile Ophthalmic Suspension (Infrequent) .... ⊙ 236
Pred-G Ophthalmic Suspension (Infrequent) .... ⊙ 234
Pred-G Sterile Ophthalmic Ointment .... ⊙ 235
Retisert Implant .... ⊙ 256
TobraDex Ophthalmic Ointment (Infrequent) 558
TobraDex Ophthalmic Suspension (Infrequent) 558
Zylet Ophthalmic Suspension 3508

Optic nerve, infarction
Hyperstat I.V. Injection 3031

Orchitis
Aciphex Tablets (Rare) 1081
Effexor Tablets (Rare) 3405
Effexor XR Capsules (Rare) 3411
M-M-R II 1980
Mumpsvax (Rare) 2005
Seroquel Tablets (Infrequent) 691

Organic brain syndrome
Eskalith 1406

Organomegaly
▲ Vesanoid Capsules (3%) 2823

Orgasm, abnormal
▲ Cymbalta Delayed-Release Capsules (2% to 4%) 1729
Strattera Capsules (2%) 1784

Orgasmic dysfunction, female
▲ Effexor XR Capsules (2% to 8%) 3411

Oropharyngitis
▲ Roferon-A Injection (6%) 2805

Oropharynx, dry
Proventil Inhalation Aerosol 3067
Proventil HFA Inhalation Aerosol 3071
▲ Roferon-A Injection (6%) 2805
Tussionex Pennkinetic Extended-Release Suspension 3322
Ventolin HFA Inhalation Aerosol 1576
VoSpire Extended-Release Tablets 2352

Orthopnea
Clozaril Tablets 2174
▲ Intron A for Injection (Less than or equal to 5%) 3038
Prinivil Tablets (0.3% to 1.0%) 2029
Prinzide Tablets 2033
Zestoretic Tablets 701
Zestril Tablets (0.3% to 1.0%) 704

Oscillopsia
Lamictal (Rare) 1449

Osteoarthritis
Vivelle Transdermal System............ 2288
Vivelle-Dot Transdermal System............ 2293

Osteoarthritis, aggravated
Orthovisc Injection (0.4%)............ 3518

Osteoarthritis, localized
▲ Boniva Tablets (1.3% to 3%) 2747
Orthovisc Injection (0.9%)............ 3518

Osteoarticular pain
Cardizem LA Extended Release Tablets (Less than 2%)............ 1699
Tiazac Capsules (Less than 2%)............ 1204

Osteomalacia
Didronel Tablets............ 2693
Phenytek Capsules............ 2153
VFEND I.V. (Less than 2%)............ 2543
VFEND Oral Suspension (Less than 2%)............ 2543
VFEND Tablets (Less than 2%)............ 2543

Osteomalacia, phosphate-induced
K-Phos Neutral Tablets............ 785
K-Phos Original (Sodium Free) Tablets 785
Uroqid-Acid No. 2 Tablets............ 785

Osteomalacia syndromes
Maalox Regular Strength Antacid/Anti-Gas Liquid............ ⊡ 677
Maalox Max Maximum Strength Antacid/Anti-Gas Liquid............ 2165
Maalox Regular Strength Antacid/Antigas Liquid............ 2164

Osteomyelitis
Campath Ampules 826
Copaxone for Injection (Infrequent)... 3292
▲ Copegus Tablets (3% to 5%) 2759
Cubicin for Injection (Less than 1%)............ 1038
Enbrel for Injection............ 580
Evoxac Capsules (Less than 1%)...... 1042
Levaquin in 5% Dextrose Injection (0.1% to 0.9%)............ 2453
Levaquin (0.1% to 0.9%)............ 2453
Nipent for Injection (1%)............ 3216
▲ Pegasys (3% to 5%) 2793
Permax Tablets (Rare)............ 3357
Prozac Pulvules and Liquid (Rare)...... 1771
Zevalin Injection............ 848

Osteomyelitis, vertebral
Raptiva for Injection............ 1247

Osteonecrosis
Boniva Tablets............ 2747
Zometa for Intravenous Infusion............ 2306

Osteonecrosis, jaw
Actonel Tablets............ 2679
Actonel with Calcium Tablets............ 2684
Didronel Tablets............ 2693
Fosamax Tablets 1949
Fosamax Plus D Tablets (Rarely)............ 1956
Zometa for Intravenous Infusion............ 2306

Osteoporosis
Advair Diskus 100/50............ 1291
Advair Diskus 250/50............ 1291
Advair Diskus 500/50............ 1291
▲ Arimidex Tablets (6% to 7%) 665
Celexa (Rare)............ 1177
▲ CellCept Capsules (3% to less than 20%)............ 2751
▲ CellCept Intravenous (3% to less than 20%)............ 2751
▲ CellCept Oral Suspension (3% to less than 20%)............ 2751
▲ CellCept Tablets (3% to less than 20%) 2751
Decadron Phosphate Injection 1931
Decadron Tablets 1929
Depo-Medrol Injectable Suspension 2615
Depo-Medrol Single-Dose Vial............ 2617
Depo-Provera Contraceptive Injection (Less than 1%)............ 2619
depo-subQ provera 104 Injectable Suspension (Rare)............ 2622
Effexor Tablets (Rare)............ 3405
Effexor XR Capsules (Rare)............ 3411
Evoxac Capsules (Less than 1%)...... 1042
▲ Femara Tablets (6.9%) 2210
Flovent Diskus 50 mcg............ 1415
Flovent HFA............ 1418
Hydrocortone Tablets............ 1963
Neupogen for Injection (Infrequent).. 598
Neurontin Capsules (Rare)............ 2498
Neurontin Oral Solution (Rare)............ 2498
Neurontin Tablets (Rare)............ 2498
Paxil CR Controlled-Release Tablets (Rare)............ 1509
Paxil (Rare)............ 1501
Pediapred Oral Solution............ 3319
Permax Tablets (Rare)............ 3357
▲ Prograf Capsules and Injection (3% to 15%)............ 624
Prozac Pulvules and Liquid (Rare)..... 1771
Pulmicort Respules (Less than 1%).. 654
▲ Rapamune Oral Solution and Tablets (3% to 20%)............ 3472
Requip Tablets (Infrequent)............ 1528
Rilutek Tablets (Rare)............ 2945
Sonata Capsules (Rare) 1686
Symbyax Capsules (Rare) 1788
VFEND I.V. (Less than 2%) 2543
VFEND Oral Suspension (Less than 2%) 2543
VFEND Tablets (Less than 2%) 2543
Zoladex 3-month (1% to 5%) 712
Zomig Nasal Spray (Rare) 718
Zyprexa Tablets (Rare) 1798
Zyprexa ZYDIS Orally Disintegrating Tablets (Rare) 1798

Osteosclerosis
Effexor XR Capsules (Rare) 3411

Otitis
Vaqta (1.8%) 2067

Otitis externa
Abilify Tablets (Rare) 916
Abilify Tablets (Rare) 2472
Ambien Tablets (Rare) 2867
Aricept Tablets (Infrequent) 1086
Aricept ODT Tablets (Infrequent) 1086
Copaxone for Injection (Infrequent) .. 3292
Effexor Tablets (Rare)............ 3405
Effexor XR Capsules (Rare) 3411
Floxin Otic Singles (Reported in a single subject) 1045
Floxin Otic Solution (Single report) ... 1043
Gabitril Tablets (Infrequent) 998
Imitrex Nasal Spray 1435
Infergen (1% to 2%) 1647
Lunesta Tablets (Infrequent) 3139
Meridia Capsules 485
Neurontin Capsules (Rare) 2498
Neurontin Oral Solution (Rare) 2498
Neurontin Tablets (Rare) 2498
Paxil CR Controlled-Release Tablets (Rare) 1509
Paxil (Rare) 1501
Protonix I.V. (Less than 1%) 3468
Protonix Tablets (Less than 1%) 3465
Singulair (Greater than or equal to 2%) 2047
Soriatane Capsules (Less than 1%) .. 1028
Targretin Capsules 1719
Teveten Tablets (Less than 1%) 1707
Teveten HCT Tablets (Less than 1%) 1710
Trileptal Oral Suspension 2281
Trileptal Tablets 2281
VFEND I.V. (Less than 2%)............ 2543
VFEND Oral Suspension (Less than 2%) 2543
VFEND Tablets (Less than 2%) 2543

Otitis media
Abilify Tablets (Infrequent) 916
Abilify Tablets (Infrequent) 2472
AccuNeb Inhalation Solution (0.9% to 4.3%)............ 1055
Aciphex Tablets 1081
Actonel Tablets (2.5%)............ 2679
Actonel with Calcium Tablets (2.5%)............ 2684
Allegra (2.4%)............ 2857
Ambien Tablets (Rare)............ 2867
Antara Capsules 2723
Aricept Tablets (Infrequent) 1086
Aricept ODT Tablets (Infrequent) 1086
Attenuvax 1889
Axert Tablets (Rare) 2430
Campath Ampules 826
Celebrex Capsules (0.1% to 1.9%) ... 3130
▲ Chemet Capsules (1.0% to 3.7%) 2480
▲ Clarinex Syrup (6.1%) 3009
Comvax (0.5% to 2.7%)............ 1904
▲ Depacon Injection (1% to 5%) 412
▲ Depakene (1% to 5%) 417
▲ Depakote Sprinkle Capsules (1% to 5%) 422
▲ Depakote Tablets (1% to 5%) 427
Depakote ER Tablets 433
Doxil Injection (Less than 1%)............ 3302
Effexor Tablets (Infrequent)............ 3405
Effexor XR Capsules (Infrequent)...... 3411
Elidel Cream 1% (0.6% to 3%)............ 2198
▲ Evoxac Capsules (1% to 3%) 1042
Exelon Capsules (Infrequent)............ 2204
▲ Flovent Diskus 50 mcg (1% to 3%)............ 1415
Floxin Otic Singles (Reported in a single subject)............ 1045
Floxin Otic Solution (Single report)... 1043
Flumist Vaccine 1872
Gabitril Tablets (Frequent)............ 998
▲ Humatrope Vials and Cartridges (16.2% to 35.3%)............ 1756
▲ Increlex Injection (Greater than or equal to 5%)............ 3290
Infergen (1% to 2%)............ 1647
Invirase (Less than 2%)............ 2776
Kaletra (Less than 2%)............ 474
Keppra Oral Solution (1% to 2%)...... 3307
Keppra Tablets (1% to 2%)............ 3307
Klonopin (Infrequent)............ 2782
Levaquin in 5% Dextrose Injection (0.1% to 0.9%)............ 2453
Levaquin (0.1% to 0.9%)............ 2453
Lofibra Capsules 1217
Lunesta Tablets (Infrequent)............ 3139
Lyrica Capsules (Greater than or equal to 1%)............ 2524
Meridia Capsules............ 485
Meruvax II............ 1994
Micardis Tablets (More than 0.3%).... 884
Micardis HCT Tablets............ 886
M-M-R II............ 1980
Mumpsvax............ 2005
Namenda (More than one patient).... 1199
Nasacort AQ Nasal Spray............ 2937
Nasonex Nasal Spray (Greater than or equal to 2%)............ 3058
Neurontin Capsules (1.2%)............ 2498
Neurontin Oral Solution (1.2%)............ 2498
Neurontin Tablets (1.2%)............ 2498
Nexium Delayed-Release Capsules (Less than 1%)............ 645
Nexium I.V. (Less than 1%)............ 649
Orthoclone OKT3 Sterile Solution (Less than 1%)............ 2370
Paxil CR Controlled-Release Tablets (Infrequent)............ 1509
Paxil (Infrequent)............ 1501
▲ Liquid PedvaxHIB (Among most frequent)............ 2012
Permax Tablets (Infrequent)............ 3357
Prevacid Delayed-Release Capsules (Less than 1%)............ 3268
Prevacid for Delayed-Release Oral Suspension (Less than 1%)............ 3268
Prevacid NapraPAC (Less than 1%).. 3277
Prevacid SoluTab Delayed-Release Orally Disintegrating Tablets (Less than 1%)............ 3268
Prevnar for Injection............ 3460
PREVPAC (Less than 1%)............ 3281
▲ Prilosec OTC Tablets (22.6%) 2674
▲ Prograf Capsules and Injection (3% to 15%)............ 624
▲ Protopic Ointment (Up to 7%) 629
▲ Pulmicort Respules (9% to 12%) 654
▲ Rapamune Oral Solution and Tablets (3% to 20%)............ 3472
Relpax Tablets (Rare)............ 2531
Requip Tablets (Infrequent)............ 1528
Rescriptor Tablets 2535
Sandostatin Injection (Less than 1%)............ 2263
▲ Sandostatin LAR Depot (5% to 15%)............ 2264
Singulair (Greater than or equal to 2%)............ 2047
Soriatane Capsules (Less than 1%).. 1028
Sular Tablets (Less than or equal to 1%)............ 1163
Symbyax Capsules (Up to 2%)............ 1788
▲ Synagis (36.4%)............ 1868
▲ Tamiflu Capsules (8.9%)............ 2810
▲ Tamiflu Oral Suspension (8.9%) 2810
Tasmar Tablets (Infrequent)............ 3360
Teveten Tablets (Less than 1%)............ 1707
Teveten HCT Tablets (Less than 1%)............ 1710
Topamax Sprinkle Capsules (1% to 2%)............ 2438
Topamax Tablets (1% to 2%)............ 2438
Tricor Tablets............ 523
Uniretic Tablets (Less than 1%)............ 3114
▲ Vaqta (7.6%)............ 2067
Varivax (Greater than or equal to 1%)............ 2070
▲ Vigamox Ophthalmic Solution (1% to 4%)............ 560

▲ Xenical Capsules (2.9% to 4.3%) **2834**
▲ Zegerid Powder for Oral Solution (22.6%) **2972**

Otitis media, serous
Kogenate FS **3517**

Otorrhea
Floxin Otic Singles (0.6%) **1045**
Floxin Otic Solution (0.6%) **1043**

Ototoxicity
Furosemide Tablets **2117**
Garamycin Injectable **3028**
TOBI Solution for Inhalation **1015**
Vancocin HCl Capsules, USP **3370**
Zyrtec Chewable Tablets (Less than 2%) **2589**
Zyrtec (Less than 2%) **2589**
Zyrtec-D 12 Hour Extended Release Tablets (Less than 2%) **2591**

Ovarian cyst
Activella Tablets (0% to 7%) **2311**
Copaxone for Injection (Infrequent) ... **3292**
Effexor Tablets (Rare) **3405**
Effexor XR Capsules (Rare) **3411**
Evoxac Capsules (Less than 1%) **1042**
▲ Gonal-f RFF Pen for Injection (3.6%) **3155**
Repronex for Intramuscular and Subcutaneous Injection **1148**

Ovarian disorder, unspecified
▲ Bravelle for Intramuscular or Subcutaneous Injection (2% to 8.1%) **1140**
Evoxac Capsules (Less than 1%) **1042**
▲ Repronex for Intramuscular and Subcutaneous Injection (3% to 8.3%) **1148**
Symbyax Capsules (Infrequent) **1788**
Wellbutrin Tablets (Rare) **1579**

Ovarian enlargement
Bravelle for Intramuscular or Subcutaneous Injection **1140**
Follistim AQ Cartridge **2354**
Gonal-f RFF Pen for Injection **3155**
▲ Repronex for Intramuscular and Subcutaneous Injection (Approximately 20%) **1148**

Ovarian failure
Neurontin Capsules (Rare) **2498**
Neurontin Oral Solution (Rare) **2498**
Neurontin Tablets (Rare) **2498**

Ovarian hyperstimulation syndrome
▲ Bravelle for Intramuscular or Subcutaneous Injection (5.4% to 11.4%) **1140**
▲ Follistim AQ Cartridge (9%) **2354**
▲ Gonal-f RFF Pen for Injection (4.6% to 7.2%) **3155**
▲ Menopur for Subcutaneous Injection (3.8% to 13.2%) **1145**
▲ Repronex for Intramuscular and Subcutaneous Injection (2% to 5.2%) **1148**

Overstimulation
Adderall Tablets **3168**
Adderall XR Capsules **3169**
Adipex-P **1216**
Desoxyn Tablets, USP **2482**
Dexedrine **1386**
DextroStat Tablets **3177**
Eldepryl Capsules **3209**
Parnate Tablets **1499**

Ovulation
ActoPlus Met Tablets **3219**

Oxygen saturation, decreased
▲ DepoDur Extended-Release Injection (Greater than 10%) **1098**

Oxyhemoglobin desaturation
▲ Suprane Liquid for Inhalation (3% to 26%) **770**

P

Pain
▲ Abelcet Injection (5%) **1119**
Accolate Tablets (1.9%) **663**
Aceon Tablets (2 mg, 4 mg, 8 mg) (0.3% to 1%) **3191**
Actiq (1% or greater) **993**
▲ Actonel Tablets (7.7% to 13.6%) **2679**
▲ Actonel with Calcium Tablets (7.7% to 13.6%) **2684**
Adalat CC Tablets (Less than 1%) **2978**
▲ Advair Diskus 100/50 (1% to 3%) ... **1291**
▲ Advair Diskus 250/50 (1% to 3%) ... **1291**
▲ Advair Diskus 500/50 (1% to 3%) ... **1291**
▲ Advicor Tablets (8%) **1694**
▲ Aggrenox Capsules (6.4%) **855**
▲ Agrylin Capsules (15%) **3172**
Aldara Cream, 5% (1.4%) **1814**
Alinia for Oral Suspension (Less than 1%) **2840**
Alinia Tablets (Less than 1%) **2840**
Aloprim for Injection (Less than 1%) **2156**
▲ Altoprev Extended-Release Tablets (3%) **1151**
Ambien Tablets (Rare) **2867**
▲ AmBisome for Injection (14%) **615**
▲ Angiomax for Injection (3.4% to 15%) **1856**
Anzemet Injection (2.4%) **2871**
Aralast (Greater than or equal to 0.2%) **745**
Arava Tablets (2%) **2881**
▲ Aredia for Injection (14.3%) **2168**
▲ Argatroban Injection (4.6%) **1321**
▲ Aricept Tablets (9%) **1086**
▲ Aricept ODT Tablets (9%) **1086**
▲ Arimidex Tablets (11% to 15%) **665**
Arixtra Injection (0% to 1.7%) **1325**
▲ Aromasin Tablets (13%) **2600**
▲ Asacol Delayed-Release Tablets (14%) **2688**
Asmanex Twisthaler **2981**
Atacand HCT (0.5% or greater) **637**
▲ Atrovent Inhalation Solution (4.1%) **868**
▲ Avastin IV (8% to 62%) **1229**
Avelox (0.1% to less than 2%) **2984**
▲ Avonex (23%) **839**
▲ Axid Oral Solution (4.2%) **913**
▲ Azmacort Inhalation Aerosol (1% to 3%) **1701**
Bactroban Ointment (1.5%) **1358**
Benicar Tablets (Greater than 0.5%) **2850**
▲ Betaseron for SC Injection (51%) **791**
▲ Bexxar (1% to 19%) **1360**
▲ Bravelle for Intramuscular or Subcutaneous Injection (5.3% to 5.7%) **1140**
Caduet Tablets (Greater than 0.1% to less than or equal to 1%) **2507**
▲ Campath Ampules (2% to 24%) **826**
▲ Campral Tablets (2% to 4%) **1175**
▲ Camptosar Injection (2% to 24%) **2602**
▲ Cancidas for Injection (1.3% to 4.6%) **1894**
Cardizem LA Extended Release Tablets (Less than 2%) **1699**
▲ Carnitor Injection (21% to 35%) **3185**
▲ Casodex Tablets (27%) **670**
Celebrex Capsules (0.1% to 1.9%) ... **3130**
▲ CellCept Capsules (3% to 75.8%) **2751**
▲ CellCept Intravenous (3% to 75.8%) **2751**
▲ CellCept Oral Suspension (3% to 75.8%) **2751**
▲ CellCept Tablets (3% to 75.8%) **2751**
▲ Cenestin Tablets, 0.45mg, 0.625mg, 0.9mg, 1.25mg (11% to 11.3%) **1063**
Cialis Tablets (Less than 2%) **1806**
Cipro I.V. (1% or less) **2998**
Cipro I.V. Pharmacy Bulk Package (1% or less) **3509**
Cipro (Less than 1%) **2991**
Cleocin Vaginal Ovules (Less than 1%) **2613**
▲ Climara Transdermal System (1% to 11%) **795**
▲ Climara Pro Transdermal System (5.2%) **800**
Clindesse Vaginal Cream (Less than 1%) **3296**
▲ Clolar for Intravenous Infusion (19%) **1264**
Colazal Capsules (2%) **2845**
▲ CombiPatch Transdermal System (15% to 19%) **2180**
Combivent Inhalation Aerosol (2.5%) **878**
▲ Combivir Tablets (12%) **1373**
▲ Copaxone for Injection (28%) **3292**
▲ Copegus Tablets (10%) **2759**
Coumadin for Injection (Infrequent) ... **932**
Coumadin Tablets (Infrequent) **932**
Crestor Tablets (Greater than or equal to 2%) **672**
Crixivan Capsules **1918**
Cytovene (At least 3 subjects) **2763**
Denavir Cream **2163**
Depacon Injection (1.3%) **412**
▲ DepoCyt Injection (3% to 11%) **1121**
Desferal Vials **2190**
Diastat Rectal Delivery System (1% or more) **3344**
▲ Ditropan XL Extended Release Tablets (4% to 7%) **2391**
▲ Doxil Injection (3.4% to 7.2%) **3302**
DuoNeb Inhalation Solution (1.3%) ... **1058**
DynaCirc CR Tablets (0.5% to 1%) **2726**
Edex Injection (2%) **3103**
Effexor Tablets **3405**
▲ Efudex (Among most frequent) **3348**
▲ Eloxatin for Injection (5% to 15%) **2908**
Enablex Extended-Release Tablets (Greater than or equal to 1%) **2201**
Enbrel for Injection **580**
▲ Entocort EC Capsules (5%) **2694**
▲ Equetro Extended-Release Capsules (12%) **3178**
▲ Erbitux (19%) **937**
▲ Estrogel 0.06% (7.1%) **3200**
▲ Evoxac Capsules (3.3%) **1042**
Exelon Capsules (2% or more) **2204**
▲ Fabrazyme for Intravenous Infusion (6%) **1267**
Factive Tablets (Less than or equal to 0.1%) **2464**
Famvir Tablets (2.0% to 2.6%) **2207**
▲ Faslodex Injection (18.9%) **682**
▲ Femara Tablets (5%) **2210**
▲ Ferrlecit Injection (0.7% to 10%) **3379**
▲ Flonase Nasal Spray (1% to 3%) **1412**
▲ Flovent Diskus 50 mcg (1% to 10%) **1415**
▲ Flovent HFA (1% to 3%) **1418**
Floxin Otic Singles (Reported in a single subject) **1045**
Floxin Otic Solution (Single report) ... **1043**
Fluorescite Injection ..... ⊙ **207**
▲ Forteo for Injection (21.3%) **1739**
Frova Tablets (Frequent) **1101**
▲ Gabitril Tablets (2% to 7%) **998**
▲ Gemzar for Injection (7% to 48%) **1743**
▲ Gengraf Capsules (6% to 13%) **458**
▲ Gonal-f RFF Pen for Injection (2.4% to 3%) **3155**
Hectorol Injection **911**
▲ Herceptin I.V. (47%) **1234**
▲ Humatrope Vials and Cartridges (6.25% to 13.6%) **1756**
Hyalgan Solution **2917**
▲ Hycamtin for Injection (1.1% to 5.4%) **1427**
▲ Indapamide Tablets (Greater than or equal to 5%) **2119**
▲ Infergen (39% to 54%) **1647**
▲ Intron A for Injection (Up to 18%) **3038**
Invanz for Injection (Greater than 0.1%) **1974**
▲ I.V. Busulfex (2% to 44%) **1125**
Kadian Capsules (Less than 3%) **572**
Kaletra (0.6%) **474**
▲ Kepivance (16%) **592**
▲ Keppra Oral Solution (6% to 7%) **3307**
▲ Keppra Tablets (6% to 7%) **3307**
Klonopin (Infrequent) **2782**
K-Phos Neutral Tablets **785**
K-Phos Original (Sodium Free) Tablets (Less frequent) **785**
▲ Lamictal (More than 5%) **1449**
▲ Leukine (17%) **829**
Levaquin in 5% Dextrose Injection (1.3%) **2453**
Levaquin (1.3%) **2453**
Levitra Tablets (Less than 2%) **3048**
Lofibra Capsules **1217**
Lotronex Tablets (Rare) **1479**
Lovenox Injection **2931**
▲ Lunesta Tablets (4% to 5%) **3139**
▲ Lupron Depot 3.75 mg (12%) **3257**
▲ Lupron Depot 7.5 mg (23.2%) **3261**
▲ Lupron Depot–3 Month 11.25 mg (12%) **3262**
Lupron Depot-PED 7.5 mg, 11.25 mg and 15 mg (2%) **3266**
Lupron Injection Pediatric **3256**
▲ Lyrica Capsules (2% to 5%) **2524**
Matulane Capsules **3188**
▲ Megace ES Oral Suspension (0% to 6%) **2492**
▲ Menopur for Subcutaneous Injection (2.6% to 3.2%) **1145**
▲ Menostar Transdermal System (13%) **805**
▲ Mepron Suspension (10%) **1487**
▲ Merrem I.V. (Greater than 1% to 5.1%) **687**
Micardis Tablets (1%) **884**
Micardis HCT Tablets (2% or greater) **886**
Mirapex Tablets (1% or more) **889**
▲ Mobic Oral Suspension (0.9% to 3.6%) **893**
▲ Mobic Tablets (0.9% to 3.6%) **893**
▲ Myfortic Tablets (3% to less than 20%) **2244**
▲ Mylotarg for Injection (18%) **3429**
▲ Namenda (3%) **1199**
▲ Naropin Injection (1% to 5%) **640**
▲ Neoral Soft Gelatin Capsules (4.4% to 13%) **2247**
▲ Neoral Oral Solution (4.4% to 13%) **2247**
▲ Neumega for Injection (Greater than or equal to 10%) **3433**
Neupogen for Injection (2%) **598**
Neurontin Capsules (More than 1%) **2498**
Neurontin Oral Solution (More than 1%) **2498**
Neurontin Tablets (More than 1%) **2498**
Nexium Delayed-Release Capsules (Less than 1%) **645**
Nexium I.V. (Less than 1%) **649**
▲ Niaspan Extended-Release Tablets (1% to 5%) **1703**
▲ Nicotrol Inhaler (Greater than 3%) **2594**
Nicotrol NS (Less than 1%) **2596**
▲ Nipent for Injection (8% to 20%) **3216**
Norvasc Tablets (More than 0.1% to 1%) **2529**
Norvir (1.7% to 2.2%) **499**
NovoSeven (1%) **2335**
Omacor Capsules (1.8%) **2735**
▲ Oncaspar (Greater than 5%) **1123**
▲ Ontak Vials (48%) **1717**
Orthoclone OKT3 Sterile Solution (Less than 1%) **2370**
Orthovisc Injection (2.5%) **3518**
Oxistat Lotion (0.4%) **1498**
OxyContin Tablets (Less than 1%) **2699**
▲ Pediarix Vaccine (0.3% to 30.5%) **1518**
▲ Pegasys (11%) **2793**
▲ Permax Tablets (7.0%) **3357**
▲ Photofrin for Injection (8% to 22%) **729**
▲ Plavix Tablets (6.4%) **940**
▲ Plavix Tablets (6.4%) **2942**
Pletal Tablets (Very rare) **2478**
▲ Pravachol Tablets (1.4% to 10.0%) **943**
▲ Prefest Tablets (6%) **1069**
▲ Premarin Tablets (17% to 20%) **3443**
Premarin Vaginal Cream **3449**
▲ Premphase Tablets (11% to 20%) **3452**
▲ Prempro Tablets (11% to 20%) **3452**
Prevacid Delayed-Release Capsules (Less than 1%) **3268**
Prevacid for Delayed-Release Oral Suspension **3268**
Prevacid NapraPAC (Less than 1%) .. **3277**
Prevacid SoluTab Delayed-Release Orally Disintegrating Tablets (Less than 1%) **3268**
PREVPAC (Less than 1%) **3281**
Prilosec OTC Tablets (Less than 1%) **2674**
Prinivil Tablets (0.3% to 1.0%) **2029**
Prinzide Tablets **2033**
▲ ProAmatine Tablets (4.9%) **3183**
▲ Prochieve 4% Gel (8%) **1018**
▲ Prochieve 8% Gel (8%) **1018**
▲ Prograf Capsules and Injection (24% to 63%) **624**
▲ Proleukin for Injection (12%) **1007**
ProSom Tablets (2%) **512**
Protonix Tablets (Greater than or equal to 1%) **3465**
Protopic Ointment (1% to 4%) **629**
Prozac Pulvules and Liquid **1771**
Qvar Inhalation Aerosol (1% to 5%) ... **1654**
▲ Rapamune Oral Solution and Tablets (24% to 33%) **3472**
▲ Raptiva for Injection (10%) **1247**
ReFacto Vials **3479**
Relpax Tablets (Frequent) **2531**
▲ Remicade for IV Injection (8%) **987**
Renagel Tablets **1268**
▲ ReoPro Vials (3.4% to 5.4%) **1779**
▲ Requip Tablets (3% to 8%) **1528**
Rescriptor Tablets **2535**
▲ Retisert Implant (5% to 15%) ..... ⊙ **256**
▲ Reyataz Capsules (1% to 3%) **948**
▲ Risperdal Consta Long-Acting Injection (3% to 10%) **1664**
▲ Risperdal M-Tab Orally Disintegrating Tablets (5%) **1658**
▲ Risperdal (5%) **1658**
Rituxan for Infusion (0.3%) **845**
▲ Rituxan I.V. (12%) **1251**
▲ Roferon-A Injection (24%) **2805**
Rythmol SR Capsules **2736**
Serevent Diskus (1% to 3%) **1540**
▲ Seroquel Tablets (7%) **691**
▲ Simulect for Injection (Greater than or equal to 10%) **2268**
▲ Somavert Injection (4% to 14%) **2648**
▲ Soriatane Capsules (1% to 10%) **1028**
Spectracef Tablets (0.1% to 1%) **2706**
▲ Suboxone Tablets (22.4% to 24%) .. **2719**
▲ Subutex Tablets (18.4% to 24%) **2719**
Sulfamylon for 5% Topical Solution .. **2155**
▲ Sustiva Capsules (2% to 14%) **957**
▲ Synagis (8.5%) **1868**
Synercid I.V. (1.5%) **1690**
Tasmar Tablets (Infrequent) **3360**

▲ Taxotere Injection Concentrate (7 of 134 patients).......... 2947
Teveten Tablets (Less than 1%).......... 1707
Teveten HCT Tablets (Less than 1%).......... 1710
▲ Thalomid Capsules (8.3%).......... 979
▲ Thymoglobulin for Injection (46.3%).......... 2848
Thyrogen for Injection (4 patients out of 55).......... 1270
▲ Tiazac Capsules (3% to 6%).......... 1204
Ticlid Tablets (0.5% to 1.0%).......... 2813
▲ TOBI Solution for Inhalation (8.1%).......... 1015
Topamax Sprinkle Capsules (More than 1%).......... 2438
Topamax Tablets (More than 1%).......... 2438
Travatan Ophthalmic Solution (1% to 5%).......... 559
Trelstar Depot (2.1%).......... 3385
▲ Trelstar LA Suspension (3.4%).......... 3387
Tricor Tablets.......... 523
Triglide Tablets.......... 1165
▲ Trisenox Injection (15%).......... 983
Truvada Tablets.......... 1279
▲ Tygacil for Injection (3.7%).......... 3489
Ultane Liquid for Inhalation (Less than 1%).......... 526
Uniretic Tablets (More than 1%).......... 3114
Univasc Tablets (Greater than 1%).......... 3118
Uroxatral Tablets (1% to 2%).......... 2957
▲ Vagifem Tablets (3% to 5%).......... 2340
▲ Valcyte Tablets (Less than 5%).......... 2816
Vantas (Less than 2%).......... 3367
Vantin Tablets and Oral Suspension (Less than 1%).......... 2650
Verelan PM Capsules (2.4%).......... 3120
▲ Vesanoid Capsules (37%).......... 2823
VFEND I.V. (Less than 2%).......... 2543
VFEND Oral Suspension (Less than 2%).......... 2543
VFEND Tablets (Less than 2%).......... 2543
Viadur Implant (Less than 2%).......... 782
Viagra Tablets (Less than 2%).......... 2552
Vicoprofen Tablets (Less than 3%).......... 533
Viracept (Less than 2%).......... 2556
▲ Viread Tablets (7% to 12%).......... 1284
Vivelle Transdermal System.......... 2288
Vivelle-Dot Transdermal System.......... 2293
▲ Voltaren Ophthalmic Solution (Less than or equal to 3%).......... 2300
▲ WelChol Tablets (5%).......... 2855
Wellbutrin Tablets (Infrequent).......... 1579
▲ Wellbutrin SR Sustained-Release Tablets (2% to 3%).......... 1583
▲ Wellbutrin XL Extended-Release Tablets (2% to 3%).......... 1588
▲ Xeloda Tablets (Less than 5%).......... 2825
Xifaxan Tablets (Less than 2%).......... 2847
▲ Xolair (7%).......... 1259
Xopenex HFA Inhalation Aerosol (1.4% to 2.8%).......... 3151
Xopenex Inhalation Solution (1.4% to 2.8%).......... 3143
▲ Xopenex Inhalation Solution Concentrate (1.4% to 3%).......... 3147
Zegerid Powder for Oral Solution (Less than 1%).......... 2972
Zemaira (0.5%).......... 3506
▲ Zenapax for Injection (Greater than 5%).......... 2838
Zestoretic Tablets.......... 701
Zestril Tablets (0.3% to 1.0%).......... 704
▲ Zevalin Injection (13%).......... 848
Ziagen (<1%).......... 1600
Zithromax for Oral Suspension, 300 mg, 600 mg, 900 mg, 1200 mg (1% or less).......... 2561
Zithromax Tablets, 250 mg, 500 mg (1% or less).......... 2561
Zithromax Tri-Pak (1% or less).......... 2561
▲ Zoladex (8% to 17%).......... 709
▲ Zoladex 3-month (14%).......... 712
▲ Zoloft (1% to 6%).......... 2581
Zomig Tablets (2% to 3%).......... 714
▲ Zomig-ZMT Tablets (2% to 3%).......... 714
▲ Zosyn (1.7% to 3.2%).......... 3492
Zovirax Capsules.......... 1616
Zovirax for Injection.......... 1618
Zovirax Ointment.......... 854
Zovirax.......... 1616
Zyban Sustained-Release Tablets (Infrequent).......... 1620
Zyrtec Chewable Tablets (Less than 2%).......... 2589
Zyrtec (Less than 2%).......... 2589
Zyrtec-D 12 Hour Extended Release Tablets (Less than 2%).......... 2591

Pain, abdominal
(*see under* Abdominal pain/cramps)

Pain, arm
Cipro XR Tablets.......... 3004
Cozaar Tablets (Less than 1%).......... 1913
Diovan HCT Tablets (Greater than 0.2%).......... 2195
▲ Femara Tablets (21% to 22%).......... 2210
Ferrlecit Injection.......... 3379
Hyzaar.......... 1964
Plendil Extended-Release Tablets (0.5% to 1.5%).......... 651
Prinzide Tablets.......... 2033
Vaqta (1.3%).......... 2067
Xolair (2%).......... 1259
Zestoretic Tablets.......... 701
Zestril Tablets (0.3% to 1.0%).......... 704

Pain, back
(*see under* Backache)

Pain, biliary
Avinza Capsules (Less than 5%).......... 1714
Caduet Tablets (Less than 2%).......... 2507
Campath Ampules.......... 826
Lipitor Tablets (Less than 2%).......... 2495
Protonix I.V. (Less than 1%).......... 3468
Protonix Tablets (Less than 1%).......... 3465
Prozac Pulvules and Liquid (Rare).......... 1771
Remicade for IV Injection (Greater than or equal to 0.2%).......... 987
Requip Tablets (Rare).......... 1528
Rilutek Tablets (Rare).......... 2945
Sonata Capsules (Rare).......... 1686
Trileptal Oral Suspension.......... 2281
Trileptal Tablets.......... 2281

Pain, bone
Abelcet Injection.......... 1119
Abilify Tablets (Infrequent).......... 916
Abilify Tablets (Infrequent).......... 2472
Aciphex Tablets.......... 1081
Actiq (Less than 1%).......... 993
Actonel Tablets (1.4% to 2.9%).......... 2679
▲ Actonel with Calcium Tablets (1.4% to 4.6%).......... 2684
AmBisome for Injection (Less common).......... 615
Amerge Tablets (Rare).......... 1312
▲ Aranesp for Injection (10%).......... 576
▲ Arava Tablets (1% to 3%).......... 2881
▲ Aredia for Injection (At least 5% to 59.4%).......... 2168
▲ Arimidex Tablets (5% to 12%).......... 665
Benicar Tablets (Greater than 0.5%).......... 2850
Boniva Tablets.......... 2747
Calcijex Injection.......... 411
▲ Casodex Tablets (4%).......... 670
Celexa (Infrequent).......... 1177
Copaxone for Injection (Infrequent).......... 3292
Depacon Injection.......... 412
Depakene.......... 417
Depakote Sprinkle Capsules.......... 422
Depakote Tablets.......... 427
Depakote ER Tablets.......... 433
▲ Didronel Tablets (About 1 patient in 10 to about 2 in 10).......... 2693
Doxil Injection (Less than 1%).......... 3302
Effexor Tablets (Infrequent).......... 3405
Effexor XR Capsules (Infrequent).......... 3411
▲ Fabrazyme for Intravenous Infusion (6%).......... 1267
▲ Faslodex Injection (15.8%).......... 682
▲ Femara Tablets (22%).......... 2210
▲ Fosamax (0.4% to approximately 6%).......... 1949
▲ Fosamax Plus D Tablets (0.4% to 4.1%).......... 1956
▲ Frova Tablets (3%).......... 1101
Hectorol Capsules.......... 909
Hectorol Injection.......... 911
▲ Herceptin I.V. (7%).......... 1234
▲ Infergen (13% to 26%).......... 1647
▲ Intron A for Injection (Less than 5%).......... 3038
Kadian Capsules (Less than 3%).......... 572
K-Phos Neutral Tablets.......... 785
K-Phos Original (Sodium Free) Tablets (Less frequent).......... 785
▲ Leukine (21%).......... 829
Levaquin in 5% Dextrose Injection (0.1% to 0.9%).......... 2453
Levaquin (0.1% to 0.9%).......... 2453
Lexapro Oral Solution (Frequent).......... 1193
Lexapro Tablets (Frequent).......... 1193
Lotronex Tablets (Rare).......... 1479
Lupron Depot 7.5 mg (Less than 5%).......... 3261
▲ Neulasta Injection (15% to 72%).......... 596
▲ Neumega for Injection (Greater than or equal to 10%).......... 3433
▲ Neupogen for Injection (22% to 33%).......... 598
Neurontin Capsules (Rare).......... 2498
Neurontin Oral Solution (Rare).......... 2498
Neurontin Tablets (Rare).......... 2498
Oncaspar (Less than 1%).......... 1123
Permax Tablets (Infrequent).......... 3357
Pletal Tablets (Less than 2%).......... 2478
Protonix I.V. (Less than 1%).......... 3468
Protonix Tablets (Less than 1%).......... 3465
Prozac Pulvules and Liquid (Infrequent).......... 1771
Relpax Tablets (Infrequent).......... 2531
Rescriptor Tablets.......... 2535
Reyataz Capsules (Less than 3%).......... 948
Risperdal M-Tab Orally Disintegrating Tablets (Rare).......... 1658
Risperdal (Rare).......... 1658
▲ Roferon-A Injection (25% to 47%).......... 2805
Serevent Diskus (1% to 3%).......... 1540
Seroquel Tablets (Infrequent).......... 691
▲ Soriatane Capsules (1% to 10%).......... 1028
Targretin Capsules.......... 1719
Tasmar Tablets (1% or more).......... 3360
Tequin Injection (Less than 0.1%).......... 964
Tequin Tablets (Less than 0.1%).......... 964
Teveten HCT Tablets (Less than 1%).......... 1710
▲ Trelstar Depot (12.1%).......... 3385
▲ Trisenox Injection (23%).......... 983
Uroqid-Acid No. 2 Tablets.......... 785
Vantas (Less than 2%).......... 3367
▲ Velcade for Injection (16%).......... 2102
▲ Vesanoid Capsules (77%).......... 2823
VFEND I.V. (Less than 2%).......... 2543
VFEND Oral Suspension (Less than 2%).......... 2543
VFEND Tablets (Less than 2%).......... 2543
Viadur Implant (Less than 2%).......... 782
Viagra Tablets (Less than 2%).......... 2552
▲ Vivelle Transdermal System (4.3% to 7.7%).......... 2288
▲ Vivelle-Dot Transdermal System (4.3% to 7.7%).......... 2293
▲ Xeloda Tablets (Less than 5%).......... 2825
Zoladex (Small number of patients).......... 709
▲ Zoladex 3-month (6%).......... 712
▲ Zometa for Intravenous Infusion (11.6% to 55%).......... 2306
Zomig Nasal Spray (Rare).......... 718
Zyprexa Tablets (Rare).......... 1798
Zyprexa ZYDIS Orally Disintegrating Tablets (Rare).......... 1798

Pain, cancer related
Zoladex (Occasional).......... 709
Zoladex 3-month.......... 712

Pain, catheter
Natrecor for Injection (Greater than or equal to 1%).......... 3123

Pain, dental
Abilify Tablets.......... 916
Abilify Tablets.......... 2472
▲ Advair Diskus 100/50 (1% to 3%).......... 1291
▲ Advair Diskus 250/50 (1% to 3%).......... 1291
▲ Advair Diskus 500/50 (1% to 3%).......... 1291
▲ Azmacort Inhalation Aerosol (1% to 3%).......... 1701
Cozaar Tablets (Less than 1%).......... 1913
Elidel Cream 1% (0.4% to 2.6%).......... 2198
▲ Evoxac Capsules (1% to 3%).......... 1042
▲ Flovent Diskus 50 mcg (1% to 3%).......... 1415
Frova Tablets (Rare).......... 1101
Hyzaar.......... 1964
Imitrex Nasal Spray.......... 1435
▲ Infergen (3% to 7%).......... 1647
Klonopin (Infrequent).......... 2782
Lexapro Oral Solution (Frequent).......... 1193
Lexapro Tablets (Frequent).......... 1193
Micardis Tablets (More than 0.3%).......... 884
Micardis HCT Tablets.......... 886
Requip Tablets (Infrequent).......... 1528
Reyataz Capsules (Less than 3%).......... 948
Risperdal M-Tab Orally Disintegrating Tablets (Up to 2%).......... 1658
Risperdal (Up to 2%).......... 1658
Serevent Diskus (1% to 3%).......... 1540
Singulair (1.7%).......... 2047
Teveten Tablets (Less than 1%).......... 1707
Teveten HCT Tablets (Less than 1%).......... 1710
▲ Thalomid Capsules (4.2%).......... 979
Trileptal Oral Suspension (1% to 2%).......... 2281
Trileptal Tablets (1% to 2%).......... 2281
Vantin Tablets and Oral Suspension (Less than 1%).......... 2650
▲ Vivelle Transdermal System (1.5% to 3.9%).......... 2288
▲ Vivelle-Dot Transdermal System (1.5% to 3.9%).......... 2293
Wellbutrin Tablets (Infrequent).......... 1579
Zyprexa Tablets (Frequent).......... 1798
Zyprexa ZYDIS Orally Disintegrating Tablets (Frequent).......... 1798

Pain, ear
Abilify Tablets (Infrequent).......... 916
Abilify Tablets (Infrequent).......... 2472
Aceon Tablets (2 mg, 4 mg, 8 mg) (0.3% to 1%).......... 3191
Actiq (Less than 1%).......... 993
Adenoscan (Less than 1%).......... 613
Advair Diskus 100/50.......... 1291
Advair Diskus 250/50.......... 1291
Advair Diskus 500/50.......... 1291
Alinia for Oral Suspension (Less than 1%).......... 2840
Alinia Tablets (Less than 1%).......... 2840
Antara Capsules.......... 2723
Aricept Tablets (Infrequent).......... 1086
Aricept ODT Tablets (Infrequent).......... 1086
Asacol Delayed-Release Tablets (2% or greater).......... 2688
Asmanex Twisthaler (1% to less than 3%).......... 2981
Avalide Tablets.......... 922
Avalide Tablets.......... 2889
Avapro Tablets (Less than 1%).......... 925
Avapro Tablets (Less than 1%).......... 2886
Axert Tablets (Infrequent).......... 2430
Bactroban Nasal (Less than 1%).......... 1357
Celebrex Capsules (0.1% to 1.9%).......... 3130
▲ CellCept Capsules (3% to less than 20%).......... 2751
▲ CellCept Intravenous (3% to less than 20%).......... 2751
▲ CellCept Oral Suspension (3% to less than 20%).......... 2751
▲ CellCept Tablets (3% to less than 20%).......... 2751
Ciprodex Otic Suspension (0.4% to 2.3%).......... 555
Colazal Capsules.......... 2845
Depacon Injection.......... 412
Depakene.......... 417
Depakote Sprinkle Capsules.......... 422
▲ Depakote Tablets (1% to 5%).......... 427
Depakote ER Tablets.......... 433
Diprivan Injectable Emulsion (Less than 1%).......... 676
▲ Doxil Injection (1% to 10%).......... 3302
Effexor Tablets (Frequent).......... 3405
Elidel Cream 1% (Up to 2.9%).......... 2198
Engerix-B Vaccine.......... 1391
▲ Equetro Extended-Release Capsules (Less than 5%).......... 3178
▲ Evoxac Capsules (1% to 3%).......... 1042
▲ Flovent Diskus 50 mcg (1% to 3%).......... 1415
Floxin Otic Singles (0.6% to 1%).......... 1045
Floxin Otic Solution (0.6% to 1%).......... 1043
Frova Tablets (Infrequent).......... 1101
Gabitril Tablets (Frequent).......... 998
▲ Gamunex Immune Globulin I.V., 10% (18%).......... 3232
▲ Imdur Tablets (Less than or equal to 5%).......... 3032
Imitrex Nasal Spray (Rare).......... 1435
Imitrex Tablets (Infrequent).......... 1440
▲ Increlex Injection (Greater than or equal to 5%).......... 3290
Infanrix Vaccine.......... 1444
▲ Infergen (5%).......... 1647
▲ Intron A for Injection (Less than or equal to 5%).......... 3038
Invirase (Less than 2%).......... 2776
Keppra Oral Solution (2%).......... 3307
Keppra Tablets (2%).......... 3307
Klonopin (Infrequent).......... 2782
Lamictal (1.8%).......... 1449
Lexapro Oral Solution (Frequent).......... 1193
Lexapro Tablets (Frequent).......... 1193
Lofibra Capsules.......... 1217
Lunesta Tablets (Infrequent).......... 3139
Lupron Depot–3 Month 11.25 mg.......... 3262
Maxalt Tablets (Infrequent).......... 1983
Maxalt-MLT Orally Disintegrating Tablets (Infrequent).......... 1983
Meridia Capsules (1.1%).......... 485
Miacalcin Nasal Spray (Less than 1%).......... 2242
Micardis Tablets (More than 0.3%).......... 884
Micardis HCT Tablets.......... 886
Migranal Nasal Spray (Infrequent).......... 3350
Nasonex Nasal Spray (Greater than or equal to 2%).......... 3058
Neurontin Capsules (Infrequent).......... 2498
Neurontin Oral Solution (Infrequent).......... 2498
Neurontin Tablets (Infrequent).......... 2498
Nexium Delayed-Release Capsules (Less than 1%).......... 645
Nexium I.V. (Less than 1%).......... 649
Nipent for Injection (Less than 3%).......... 3216
Norvir (Less than 2%).......... 499

Paxil CR Controlled-Release Tablets (Infrequent) 1509
Paxil (Infrequent) 1501
Pediarix Vaccine 1518
Permax Tablets (Infrequent) 3357
Pletal Tablets (Less than 2%) 2478
Prinzide Tablets (0.3% to 1%) 2033
▲ Prograf Capsules and Injection (3% to 15%) 624
Prometrium Capsules (100 mg, 200 mg) (Less than 5%) 3205
ProSom Tablets (Infrequent) 512
Protonix I.V. (Less than 1%) 3468
Protonix Tablets (Less than 1%) 3465
Protopic Ointment (Greater than or equal to 1%) 629
Provigil Tablets (At least 1%) 1002
Prozac Pulvules and Liquid (Frequent) 1771
Pulmicort Respules (1% to 3%) 654
Recombivax HB (Less than 1%) 2045
Relpax Tablets (Infrequent) 2531
Requip Tablets (Infrequent) 1528
Rescriptor Tablets 2535
Rilutek Tablets (Rare) 2945
Risperdal Consta Long-Acting Injection (Infrequent) 1664
Roferon-A Injection (Less than 1%) 2805
▲ Sandostatin LAR Depot (5% to 15%) 2264
Sedapap Tablets 50 mg/650 mg (Infrequent) 2098
Singulair (Greater than or equal to 2%) 2047
Sonata Capsules (Less than 1%) 1686
▲ Soriatane Capsules (1% to 10%) 1028
Sular Tablets (Less than or equal to 1%) 1163
Symbyax Capsules (1% to 2%) 1788
Targretin Capsules 1719
Tasmar Tablets (Infrequent) 3360
Tequin Injection (Less than 0.1%) 964
Tequin Tablets (Less than 0.1%) 964
Timolide Tablets 2056
▲ TOBI Solution for Inhalation (7.4%) 1015
Tricor Tablets 523
Trileptal Oral Suspension (1% to 2%) 2281
Trileptal Tablets (1% to 2%) 2281
▲ Trisenox Injection (8%) 983
Twinrix Vaccine 1571
Uniretic Tablets (Less than 1%) 3114
▲ Vesanoid Capsules (23%) 2823
VFEND I.V. (Less than 2%) 2543
VFEND Oral Suspension (Less than 2%) 2543
VFEND Tablets (Less than 2%) 2543
Viagra Tablets (Less than 2%) 2552
Xanax XR Tablets (Infrequent) 2655
Xifaxan Tablets (Less than 2%) 2847
Xolair (2%) 1259
Zestoretic Tablets (0.3% to 1%) 701
Zoloft (Infrequent) 2581
Zomig Nasal Spray (Infrequent) 718
Zomig Tablets (Infrequent) 714
Zomig-ZMT Tablets (Infrequent) 714
Zyprexa Tablets (Infrequent) 1798
Zyprexa ZYDIS Orally Disintegrating Tablets (Infrequent) 1798
Zyrtec Chewable Tablets (Less than 2%) 2589
Zyrtec (Less than 2%) 2589
Zyrtec-D 12 Hour Extended Release Tablets (Less than 2%) 2591

Pain, epigastric
(*see under* Distress, epigastric)

Pain, esophageal
▲ Photofrin for Injection (8%) 729

Pain, exacerbation of
Vantas (Less than 2%) 3367

Pain, extremities
Astelin Nasal Spray (Infrequent) 1876
Betimol Ophthalmic Solution (1% to 5%) ⊙ 283
Betimol Ophthalmic Solution (1% to 5%) 3371
Blocadren Tablets 1891
▲ Boniva Tablets (1.3% to 7.8%) 2747
Cipro I.V. (1% or less) 2998
Cipro I.V. Pharmacy Bulk Package (1% or less) 3509
Cipro (Less than 1%) 2991
Cipro XR Tablets 3004
Cosopt Sterile Ophthalmic Solution 1910
Diprivan Injectable Emulsion (Less than 1%) 676
▲ Gammagard Liquid (0.85% to 8.2%) 751
▲ Humira Injection (Less than 5%) 464
▲ Hytrin Capsules (3.5%) 469
▲ Increlex Injection (Greater than or equal to 5%) 3290
Mavik Tablets (0.3% to 1.0%) 482
Oncaspar (Greater than 1% but less than 5%) 1123
Reyataz Capsules (Less than 3%) 948
Tarka Tablets (1.1%) 519
Timoptic-XE Sterile Ophthalmic Gel Forming Solution 2062
Uroqid-Acid No. 2 Tablets 785
▲ Valcyte Tablets (Less than 5%) 2816
▲ Viadur Implant (3.1%) 782
Vytorin 10/10 Tablets (2.3%) 2084
Vytorin 10/10 Tablets (2.3%) 3092
Vytorin 10/20 Tablets (2.3%) 2084
Vytorin 10/20 Tablets (2.3%) 3092
Vytorin 10/40 Tablets (2.3%) 2084
Vytorin 10/40 Tablets (2.3%) 3092
Vytorin 10/80 Tablets (2.3%) 2084
Vytorin 10/80 Tablets (2.3%) 3092
Zerit 971
▲ Zyprexa Tablets (4%) 1798
▲ Zyprexa ZYDIS Orally Disintegrating Tablets (4%) 1798

Pain, eye
Abilify Tablets (Infrequent) 916
Abilify Tablets (Infrequent) 2472
Aciphex Tablets 1081
▲ Acular LS Ophthalmic Solution (1% to 5%) 562
Alphagan P Ophthalmic Solution (1% to 4%) 563
Alrex Ophthalmic Suspension 0.2% (Less than 5%) ⊙ 243
Ambien Tablets (Infrequent) 2867
Amerge Tablets (Rare) 1312
Asacol Delayed-Release Tablets 2688
Astelin Nasal Spray (Infrequent) 1876
Atrovent HFA Inhalation Aerosol 872
Atrovent Inhalation Solution (Less than 3%) 868
Atrovent Nasal Spray 0.06% 870
Avinza Capsules (Less than 5%) 1714
Axert Tablets (Rare) 2430
Azopt Ophthalmic Suspension (1% to 5%) 553
Betimol Ophthalmic Solution (1% to 5%) ⊙ 283
Betimol Ophthalmic Solution (1% to 5%) 3371
Betoptic S Ophthalmic Suspension (Small number of patients) 554
▲ Brimonidine Tartrate Ophthalmic Solution 0.2% (3% to 9%) ⊙ 245
Caduet Tablets (Greater than 0.1% to less than or equal to 1%) 2507
Celebrex Capsules (0.1% to 1.9%) 3130
Celexa (Infrequent) 1177
Cialis Tablets (Less than 2%) 1806
Ciloxan Ophthalmic Ointment (Less than 1%) 554
Cipro I.V. (1% or less) 2998
Cipro I.V. Pharmacy Bulk Package (1% or less) 3509
Cipro (Less than 1%) 2991
Cipro XR Tablets 3004
Combivent Inhalation Aerosol 878
▲ Copaxone for Injection (7%) 3292
Cosopt Sterile Ophthalmic Solution (1% to 5%) 1910
Depacon Injection (1% or more) 412
Depakene (1% or more) 417
Depakote Sprinkle Capsules 422
▲ Depakote Tablets (1% to 5%) 427
Depakote ER Tablets (Greater than 1%) 433
Diprivan Injectable Emulsion (Less than 1%) 676
Doxil Injection (Less than 1%) 3302
DuoNeb Inhalation Solution 1058
Effexor Tablets (Infrequent) 3405
Effexor XR Capsules (Infrequent) 3411
Eldepryl Capsules 3209
▲ Evoxac Capsules (1% to 3%) 1042
Exelon Capsules 2204
Flumadine 1186
Frova Tablets (Infrequent) 1101
Gabitril Tablets (Infrequent) 998
Gengraf Capsules (1% to less than 3%) 458
Imitrex Nasal Spray 1435
▲ Infergen (4% to 5%) 1647
▲ Intron A for Injection (Less than 5%) 3038
Iressa Tablets 684
Levaquin in 5% Dextrose Injection (0.1% to 0.9%) 2453
Levaquin (0.1% to 0.9%) 2453
Levitra Tablets (Less than 2%) 3048
Loprox Gel 1861
Lotemax Ophthalmic Suspension 0.5% (Less than 5%) ⊙ 249
▲ Lumigan Ophthalmic Solution (3% to 10%) 569
Maxalt Tablets (Infrequent) 1983
Maxalt-MLT Orally Disintegrating Tablets (Infrequent) 1983
Meridia Capsules 485
Miacalcin Injection 2241
Migranal Nasal Spray (Rare) 3350
Namenda (Infrequent) 1199
Neoral Soft Gelatin Capsules (1% to less than 3%) 2247
Neoral Oral Solution (1% to less than 3%) 2247
Neurontin Capsules (Infrequent) 2498
Neurontin Oral Solution (Infrequent) 2498
Neurontin Tablets (Infrequent) 2498
Norvasc Tablets (More than 0.1% to 1%) 2529
Norvir (Less than 2%) 499
▲ Optivar Ophthalmic Solution (1% to 10%) 1877
Paxil CR Controlled-Release Tablets (Infrequent) 1509
Paxil (Infrequent) 1501
Permax Tablets (Infrequent) 3357
Photofrin for Injection 729
Prevacid Delayed-Release Capsules (Less than 1%) 3268
Prevacid for Delayed-Release Oral Suspension (Less than 1%) 3268
Prevacid NapraPAC (Less than 1%) 3277
Prevacid SoluTab Delayed-Release Orally Disintegrating Tablets (Less than 1%) 3268
PREVPAC (Less than 1%) 3281
ProSom Tablets (Infrequent) 512
Protopic Ointment (Greater than or equal to 1%) 629
Provigil Tablets (1%) 1002
Quixin Ophthalmic Solution (1% to 3%) 3373
Relpax Tablets (Infrequent) 2531
Requip Tablets (Infrequent) 1528
▲ Restasis Ophthalmic Emulsion (1% to 5%) 570
▲ Retisert Implant (50% to 90%) ⊙ 256
Risperdal Consta Long-Acting Injection (Infrequent) 1664
Risperdal M-Tab Orally Disintegrating Tablets (Rare) 1658
Risperdal (Rare) 1658
Roferon-A Injection (Infrequent) 2805
▲ Sonata Capsules (3% to 4%) 1686
▲ Soriatane Capsules (1% to 10%) 1028
Symbyax Capsules (Infrequent) 1788
Tambocor Tablets (Less than 1%) 1824
Tasmar Tablets (Infrequent) 3360
Tequin Injection (Less than 0.1%) 964
Tequin Tablets (Less than 0.1%) 964
Thalomid Capsules 979
Timoptic in Ocudose (Less frequent) 2061
Timoptic Sterile Ophthalmic Solution (Less frequent) 2058
Timoptic-XE Sterile Ophthalmic Gel Forming Solution (1% to 5%) 2062
Topamax Sprinkle Capsules (More than 1%) 2438
Topamax Tablets (More than 1%) 2438
▲ Travatan Ophthalmic Solution (5% to 10%) 559
Trelstar LA Suspension (1.1%) 3387
Trusopt Sterile Ophthalmic Solution 2065
VFEND I.V. (Less than 2%) 2543
VFEND Oral Suspension (Less than 2%) 2543
VFEND Tablets (Less than 2%) 2543
Viagra Tablets (Less than 2%) 2552
▲ Vigamox Ophthalmic Solution (1% to 6%) 560
Xalatan Sterile Ophthalmic Solution (1% to 4%) 2654
Zaditor Ophthalmic Solution (Less than 5%) 2302
Zoloft (Infrequent) 2581
Zomig Tablets (Infrequent) 714
Zomig-ZMT Tablets (Infrequent) 714
▲ Zymar Ophthalmic Solution (1% to 4%) 571
Zyprexa Tablets (Infrequent) 1798
Zyprexa ZYDIS Orally Disintegrating Tablets (Infrequent) 1798
Zyrtec Chewable Tablets (Less than 2%) 2589
Zyrtec (Less than 2%) 2589
Zyrtec-D 12 Hour Extended Release Tablets (Less than 2%) 2591

Pain, facial
▲ Carac Cream, 0.5% (43.6%) 1048
Imitrex Injection (Infrequent) 1431
Imitrex Nasal Spray (Rare) 1435
Imitrex Tablets (Infrequent) 1440
Invirase (Less than 2%) 2776
Norvir (Less than 2%) 499

Pain, feet
Cipro (Less than 1%) 2991

Pain, flank
Aceon Tablets (2 mg, 4 mg, 8 mg) (0.3% to 1%) 3191
Actiq (Less than 1%) 993
▲ Chemet Capsules (5.2% to 15.7%) 2480
Cleocin Vaginal Ovules (Less than 1%) 2613
Copaxone for Injection (Infrequent) 3292
Crixivan Capsules (Less than 2%) 1918
Ferrlecit Injection 3379
Geodon Capsules (Frequent) 2514
Invanz for Injection (Greater than 0.1%) 1974
Neupogen for Injection (Infrequent) 598
Prinivil Tablets (0.3% to 1.0%) 2029
Prinzide Tablets 2033
Tasmar Tablets (Frequent) 3360
Vaseretic Tablets 2073
Vasotec I.V. Injection (0.5% to 1.0%) 2076
▲ Vesanoid Capsules (9%) 2823
VFEND I.V. (Less than 2%) 2543
VFEND Oral Suspension (Less than 2%) 2543
VFEND Tablets (Less than 2%) 2543
Zestoretic Tablets 701
Zestril Tablets (0.3% to 1.0%) 704
Zonegran Capsules (Infrequent) 1089

Pain, gastrointestinal
▲ Advair Diskus 100/50 (7%) 1291
▲ Advair Diskus 250/50 (7%) 1291
▲ Advair Diskus 500/50 (7%) 1291
▲ Coreg Tablets (Greater than 1% to 3%) 1376
Parcopa Orally Disintegrating Tablets 3111
Stalevo Tablets 2270

Pain, gynecological
Gonal-f RFF Pen for Injection (2.4%) 3155

Pain, hip
Cozaar Tablets (Less than 1%) 1913
Humatrope Vials and Cartridges (2.7%) 1756
Hyzaar 1964
Plendil Extended-Release Tablets (0.5% to 1.5%) 651
Prinivil Tablets (0.3% to 1.0%) 2029
Prinzide Tablets 2033
Zestoretic Tablets 701
Zestril Tablets (0.3% to 1.0%) 704
Zyprexa Tablets (Infrequent) 1798
Zyprexa ZYDIS Orally Disintegrating Tablets (Infrequent) 1798

Pain, jaw
Abilify Tablets (Infrequent) 916
Abilify Tablets (Infrequent) 2472
Cipro I.V. (1% or less) 2998
Cipro I.V. Pharmacy Bulk Package (1% or less) 3509
Cipro XR Tablets 3004
▲ Flolan for Injection (54% to 75%) 1408
Klonopin (Infrequent) 2782
Navelbine Injection (Less than 5%) 1494
▲ Nicotrol Inhaler (Greater than 3%) 2594
Permax Tablets (Infrequent) 3357
ProSom Tablets (Rare) 512
Rythmol SR Capsules 2736
Zomig Nasal Spray (Infrequent) 718

Pain, knee
▲ Cozaar Tablets (Less than 1% to 5%) 1913
Hyzaar 1964
Klonopin (Infrequent) 2782
Plendil Extended-Release Tablets (0.5% to 1.5%) 651
Prinivil Tablets (0.3% to 1.0%) 2029
Zestril Tablets (0.3% to 1.0%) 704

Pain, leg
Arixtra Injection (1.4%) 1325
Edex Injection (1%) 3103
FazaClo Orally Disintegrating Tablets (1%) 547
Levaquin in 5% Dextrose Injection (0.1% to 0.9%) 2453

Levaquin (0.1% to 0.9%) ... 2453
Parcopa Orally Disintegrating Tablets ... 3111
Prochieve 4% Gel ... 1018
Prochieve 8% Gel ... 1018
▲ Risperdal Consta Long-Acting Injection (1% to 4%) ... 1664
Trelstar Depot (2.1%) ... 3385
▲ Trelstar LA Suspension (5.2%) ... 3387
▲ Xolair (4%) ... 1259

Pain, limb
▲ Apokyn Injection (At least 5%) ... 2132
▲ Cialis Tablets (1% to 3%) ... 1806
▲ Clolar for Intravenous Infusion (29%) ... 1264
Cubicin for Injection (1.5%) ... 1038
▲ depo-subQ provera 104 Injectable Suspension (1% to less than 5%) ... 2622
Eligard 30 mg (1.1%) ... 2901
Eligard 45 mg (2.7%) ... 2904
▲ Femara Tablets (10%) ... 2210
Fuzeon Injection (2.9%) ... 2772
Meridia Capsules ... 485
Rabies Vaccine RabAvert (Uncommon) ... 1011
▲ Renagel Tablets (13.1%) ... 1268
▲ Retisert Implant (5% to 15%) ... ⊙256
Stalevo Tablets ... 2270
▲ Trisenox Injection (13%) ... 983
Vantas (Less than 2%) ... 3367
▲ Velcade for Injection (15%) ... 2102
Xanax XR Tablets (1.1%) ... 2655
▲ Zometa for Intravenous Infusion (14%) ... 2306

Pain, localized
▲ Rescriptor Tablets (1.8% to 5.7%) ... 2535
▲ Zomig Nasal Spray (0% to 4%) ... 718
Zyvox (0.9% to 2%) ... 2661

Pain, lower extremities
▲ Aceon Tablets (2 mg, 4 mg, 8 mg) (4.7%) ... 3191
▲ Adalat CC Tablets (3% or less) ... 2978
▲ Aggrastat (3%) ... 1878
Altoprev Extended-Release Tablets (0.5% to 1%) ... 1151
Avelox (Less than 0.1%) ... 2984
▲ Chemet Capsules (Up to 3.0%) ... 2480
Cipro (0.3% to 1%) ... 2991
Cipro XR Tablets ... 3004
Clozapine Tablets (1%) ... 2141
Clozaril Tablets (1%) ... 2174
▲ Cozaar Tablets (1% to 5%) ... 1913
Diovan HCT Tablets (Greater than 0.2%) ... 2195
DynaCirc CR Tablets (0.5% to 1%) ... 2726
Eldepryl Capsules (1 of 49 patients) ... 3209
▲ Femara Tablets (21% to 22%) ... 2210
Frova Tablets (Rare) ... 1101
Hyzaar ... 1964
Invanz for Injection (0.4% to 1.1%) ... 1974
Klonopin (Infrequent) ... 2782
Lexapro Oral Solution (Infrequent) ... 1193
Lexapro Tablets (Infrequent) ... 1193
Mevacor Tablets (0.5% to 1.0%) ... 1996
Micardis Tablets (More than 0.3%) ... 884
Micardis HCT Tablets ... 886
Midamor Tablets (Less than or equal to 1%) ... 2000
Moduretic Tablets ... 2003
▲ Myfortic Tablets (3% to less than 20%) ... 2244
Plendil Extended-Release Tablets (0.5% to 1.5%) ... 651
Prilosec OTC Tablets (Less than 1%) ... 2674
Prinivil Tablets (0.3% to 1.0%) ... 2029
Prinzide Tablets (0.3% to 1%) ... 2033
▲ ProSom Tablets (3%) ... 512
Sedapap Tablets 50 mg/650 mg (Infrequent) ... 2098
Seroquel Tablets (Infrequent) ... 691
▲ Simulect for Injection (3% to 10%) ... 2268
▲ Spiriva HandiHaler (1% to 3%) ... 899
Tenormin I.V. Injection (Up to 3%) ... 698
Tenormin Tablets (Up to 3%) ... 695
Timolide Tablets ... 2056
Timoptic in Ocudose ... 2061
Timoptic Sterile Ophthalmic Solution ... 2058
▲ Topamax Sprinkle Capsules (2% to 4%) ... 2438
▲ Topamax Tablets (2% to 4%) ... 2438
Vivelle Transdermal System ... 2288
Vivelle-Dot Transdermal System ... 2293
▲ Xenical Capsules (10.8%) ... 2834
Zegerid Powder for Oral Solution (Less than 1%) ... 2972
Zelnorm Tablets (1%) ... 2303
Zestoretic Tablets (0.3% to 1%) ... 701
Zestril Tablets (0.3% to 1.0%) ... 704

Pain, medullary bone
▲ Neulasta Injection (26%) ... 596
▲ Neupogen for Injection (33%) ... 598

Pain, muscle
(*see under* Myalgia)

Pain, musculoskeletal
▲ Advair Diskus 100/50 (4%) ... 1291
▲ Advair Diskus 250/50 (2% to 9%) ... 1291
▲ Advair Diskus 500/50 (2% to 4%) ... 1291
▲ Asmanex Twisthaler (4% to 22%) ... 2981
▲ Avalide Tablets (7%) ... 922
▲ Avalide Tablets (7%) ... 2889
Cancidas for Injection (0% to 1.3%) ... 1894
Emend Capsules (Greater than 0.5%) ... 1944
Evoxac Capsules (2.8%) ... 1042
▲ Femara Tablets (21% to 22%) ... 2210
▲ Flovent Diskus 50 mcg (3%) ... 1415
▲ Flovent HFA (1% to 3%) ... 1418
▲ Fosamax (0.4% to approximately 6%) ... 1949
▲ Fosamax Plus D Tablets (0.4% to 4.1%) ... 1956
▲ Gleevec Tablets (11% to 49%) ... 2221
Invirase (Greater than or equal to 2%) ... 2776
Maxalt Tablets (Infrequent) ... 1983
Maxalt-MLT Orally Disintegrating Tablets (Infrequent) ... 1983
▲ Nasonex Nasal Spray (1% to 5%) ... 3058
▲ PEG-Intron Powder for Injection (28%) ... 3062
Prevacid NapraPAC (Less than 1%) ... 3277
Prochieve 4% Gel ... 1018
Prochieve 8% Gel ... 1018
▲ Prometrium Capsules (100 mg, 200 mg) (12%) ... 3205
▲ Rebetol (19% to 28%) ... 3073
▲ Rebetron Combination Therapy (20% to 28%) ... 3078
▲ Rebif Prefilled Syringe for Injection (10% to 15%) ... 3163
▲ Ribavirin, USP Capsules (19% to 28%) ... 3083
Risperdal Consta Long-Acting Injection (Frequent) ... 1664
Risperdal M-Tab Orally Disintegrating Tablets (2%) ... 1658
Risperdal (2%) ... 1658
▲ Spiriva HandiHaler (1% to 3%) ... 899
▲ Trizivir Tablets (12%) ... 1565
▲ Ventolin HFA Inhalation Aerosol (5%) ... 1576
Visudyne for Injection (Less than 1%) ... 2286
▲ Zenapax for Injection (Greater than 5%) ... 2838
▲ Ziagen (5% to 6%) ... 1600

Pain, neck
(*see under* Torticollis)

Pain, nostril
DDAVP Nasal Spray (Up to 2%) ... 2894
Desmopressin Acetate Rhinal Tube (Up to 2%) ... 1144

Pain, oral mucosa
▲ Advair Diskus 100/50 (1% to 3%) ... 1291
▲ Advair Diskus 250/50 (1% to 3%) ... 1291
▲ Advair Diskus 500/50 (1% to 3%) ... 1291
Cipro I.V. (1% or less) ... 2998
Cipro I.V. Pharmacy Bulk Package (1% or less) ... 3509
Cipro (Less than 1%) ... 2991
Cipro XR Tablets ... 3004
▲ Flovent Diskus 50 mcg (1% to 3%) ... 1415

Pain, ovarian
▲ Follistim AQ Cartridge (5%) ... 2354

Pain, paranasal sinus
Advair Diskus 100/50 ... 1291
Advair Diskus 250/50 ... 1291
Advair Diskus 500/50 ... 1291

Pain, pelvic
Abilify Tablets (Frequent) ... 916
Abilify Tablets (Frequent) ... 2472
Actiq (1% or greater) ... 993
Adalat CC Tablets (Less than 1%) ... 2978
▲ Aggrastat (6%) ... 1878
Alinia for Oral Suspension (Less than 1%) ... 2840
Alinia Tablets (Less than 1%) ... 2840
▲ Angiomax for Injection (6%) ... 1856
▲ Arava Tablets (1% to 3%) ... 2881
▲ Arimidex Tablets (5% to 7%) ... 665
Avelox (Less than 1%) ... 2984
▲ Bravelle for Intramuscular or Subcutaneous Injection (6.7%) ... 1140
▲ Casodex Tablets (13%) ... 670
Caverject Impulse Injection (Less than 1%) ... 2610
▲ CellCept Capsules (3% to less than 20%) ... 2751
▲ CellCept Intravenous (3% to less than 20%) ... 2751
▲ CellCept Oral Suspension (3% to less than 20%) ... 2751
▲ CellCept Tablets (3% to less than 20%) ... 2751
Clindesse Vaginal Cream (Less than 1%) ... 3296
Crestor Tablets (Greater than or equal to 1%) ... 672
▲ Depo-Provera Contraceptive Injection (1% to 5%) ... 2619
▲ Doxil Injection (1% to 10%) ... 3302
Effexor Tablets (Infrequent) ... 3405
Effexor XR Capsules (Infrequent) ... 3411
Emend Capsules (Greater than 0.5%) ... 1944
▲ Faslodex Injection (9.9%) ... 682
Follistim AQ Cartridge ... 2354
Gabitril Tablets (Infrequent) ... 998
▲ Gynazole-1 Vaginal Cream (5.7%) ... 3298
▲ Humira Injection (Less than 5%) ... 464
▲ Intron A for Injection (Less than 5%) ... 3038
Invirase (Less than 2%) ... 2776
Klonopin (Infrequent) ... 2782
Lyrica Capsules (0.1% to 1%) ... 2524
Merrem I.V. (Greater than 0.1% to 1%) ... 687
Neurontin Capsules (Rare) ... 2498
Neurontin Oral Solution (Rare) ... 2498
Neurontin Tablets (Rare) ... 2498
Paxil CR Controlled-Release Tablets (Rare) ... 1509
Paxil (Rare) ... 1501
Permax Tablets (Infrequent) ... 3357
Pletal Tablets (Less than 2%) ... 2478
▲ Premphase Tablets (4% to 5%) ... 3452
▲ Prempro Tablets (4% to 5%) ... 3452
Prevacid Delayed-Release Capsules (Less than 1%) ... 3268
Prevacid for Delayed-Release Oral Suspension (Less than 1%) ... 3268
Prevacid NapraPAC (Less than 1%) ... 3277
Prevacid SoluTab Delayed-Release Orally Disintegrating Tablets (Less than 1%) ... 3268
PREVPAC (Less than 1%) ... 3281
Prinivil Tablets (0.3% to 1.0%) ... 2029
Prinzide Tablets ... 2033
Prozac Pulvules and Liquid (Infrequent) ... 1771
▲ Rapamune Oral Solution and Tablets (3% to 20%) ... 3472
▲ Repronex for Intramuscular and Subcutaneous Injection (1% to 3%) ... 1148
Reyataz Capsules (Less than 3%) ... 948
Seroquel Tablets (Infrequent) ... 691
Symbyax Capsules (Infrequent) ... 1788
VFEND I.V. (Less than 2%) ... 2543
VFEND Oral Suspension (Less than 2%) ... 2543
VFEND Tablets (Less than 2%) ... 2543
Zestoretic Tablets ... 701
Zestril Tablets (0.3% to 1.0%) ... 704
▲ Zoladex (9%) ... 709
▲ Zoladex 3-month (6%) ... 712
Zyprexa Tablets (Infrequent) ... 1798
Zyprexa ZYDIS Orally Disintegrating Tablets (Infrequent) ... 1798

Pain, penile
▲ Caverject Impulse Injection (2% to 37%) ... 2610
▲ Edex Injection (11% to 35%) ... 3103

Pain, perineal
Arthrotec Tablets (Rare) ... 3126
▲ Prochieve 4% Gel (17%) ... 1018
▲ Prochieve 8% Gel (17%) ... 1018
Requip Tablets (Infrequent) ... 1528
Risperdal M-Tab Orally Disintegrating Tablets (Infrequent) ... 1658
Risperdal (Infrequent) ... 1658

Pain, peripheral
Celebrex Capsules (0.1% to 1.9%) ... 3130

Pain, pharyngeal
▲ Gammagard Liquid (0.61% to 6.5%) ... 751
Parcopa Orally Disintegrating Tablets ... 3111

Pain, pharynx
▲ Advate Injection (11.3%) ... 742
Prilosec OTC Tablets (Less than 1%) ... 2674
Primaxin I.M. ... 2022
Primaxin I.V. (Less than 0.2%) ... 2024
Prinivil Tablets (0.3% to 1.0%) ... 2029
Prinzide Tablets (0.3% to 1%) ... 2033
Stalevo Tablets ... 2270
Vivelle Transdermal System ... 2288
Vivelle-Dot Transdermal System ... 2293
Zegerid Powder for Oral Solution (Less than 1%) ... 2972
Zestoretic Tablets (0.3% to 1%) ... 701
Zestril Tablets (0.3% to 1.0%) ... 704

Pain, pleural
Invanz for Injection (Greater than 0.1%) ... 1974
Migranal Nasal Spray (Rare) ... 3350

Pain, post retrieval
▲ Bravelle for Intramuscular or Subcutaneous Injection (8%) ... 1140

Pain, postoperative
Aldara Cream, 5% (1.4%) ... 1814
▲ Evoxac Capsules (1% to 3%) ... 1042
▲ Myfortic Tablets (3% to 23.9%) ... 2244
Zenapax for Injection ... 2838

Pain, post-procedure
Asmanex Twisthaler (1% to less than 3%) ... 2981
Zofran Injection (1%) ... 1607

Pain, precordium
Imitrex Tablets ... 1440
Trileptal Oral Suspension ... 2281
Trileptal Tablets ... 2281
Zoloft (Rare) ... 2581

Pain, prostate
Caverject Impulse Injection (2%) ... 2610
Lupron Depot 3.75 mg ... 3257
Lupron Depot 7.5 mg ... 3261
Lupron Depot–3 Month 11.25 mg ... 3262
Lupron Depot-PED 7.5 mg, 11.25 mg and 15 mg ... 3266
Lupron Injection Pediatric ... 3256

Pain, rectum
Canasa Rectal Suppositories (1.8%) ... 726
Noroxin Tablets (0.3% to 1.0%) ... 2009
▲ Xeloda Tablets (Less than 5%) ... 2825
▲ Xenical Capsules (3.3% to 5.2%) ... 2834

Pain, renal
Actiq (Less than 1%) ... 993
Alinia for Oral Suspension (Less than 1%) ... 2840
Alinia Tablets (Less than 1%) ... 2840
Ambien Tablets (Rare) ... 2867
Azopt Ophthalmic Suspension (Less than 1%) ... 553
Ceftin Tablets (0.1% to 1%) ... 1369
Celexa (Rare) ... 1177
Copaxone for Injection (Infrequent) ... 3292
Effexor Tablets (Infrequent) ... 3405
Effexor XR Capsules (Rare) ... 3411
Evoxac Capsules (Less than 1%) ... 1042
Frova Tablets (Rare) ... 1101
Lamictal (Rare) ... 1449
Lunesta Tablets (Infrequent) ... 3139
Neurontin Capsules (Rare) ... 2498
Neurontin Oral Solution (Rare) ... 2498
Neurontin Tablets (Rare) ... 2498
Norvir (Less than 2%) ... 499
Paxil CR Controlled-Release Tablets (Rare) ... 1509
Paxil (Rare) ... 1501
Prevacid Delayed-Release Capsules (Less than 1%) ... 3268
Prevacid for Delayed-Release Oral Suspension (Less than 1%) ... 3268
Prevacid NapraPAC (Less than 1%) ... 3277
Prevacid SoluTab Delayed-Release Orally Disintegrating Tablets (Less than 1%) ... 3268
PREVPAC (Less than 1%) ... 3281
Protonix I.V. (Less than 1%) ... 3468
Protonix Tablets (Less than 1%) ... 3465
Prozac Pulvules and Liquid (Rare) ... 1771
▲ Rapamune Oral Solution and Tablets (3% to 20%) ... 3472
Relpax Tablets (Rare) ... 2531
Rescriptor Tablets ... 2535
Reyataz Capsules (Less than 3%) ... 948
Rilutek Tablets (Infrequent) ... 2945
Risperdal Consta Long-Acting Injection (Infrequent) ... 1664
Topamax Sprinkle Capsules (Infrequent) ... 2438
Topamax Tablets (Infrequent) ... 2438
Trileptal Oral Suspension ... 2281

Trileptal Tablets ... 2281
VFEND I.V. (Less than 2%) ... 2543
VFEND Oral Suspension (Less than 2%) ... 2543
VFEND Tablets (Less than 2%) ... 2543
Zoloft (Rare) ... 2581
Zomig Nasal Spray (Rare) ... 718

Pain, retrosternal
Invirase (Less than 2%) ... 2776
Zofran Injection (2%) ... 1607

Pain, right hypochondrium
Trileptal Oral Suspension ... 2281
Trileptal Tablets ... 2281

Pain, right upper quadrant
Casodex Tablets ... 670
▲ Intron A for Injection (Less than 5% to 15%) ... 3038
Invirase (Rare) ... 2776
Lamisil Tablets ... 2226
▲ PEG-Intron Powder for Injection (8%) ... 3062
▲ Rebetol (6% to 12%) ... 3073
▲ Ribavirin, USP Capsules (6% to 12%) ... 3083
Tarka Tablets (Several cases) ... 519

Pain, salivary gland
▲ Evoxac Capsules (1% to 3%) ... 1042
Frova Tablets (Rare) ... 1101

Pain, shoulder
Altoprev Extended-Release Tablets (0.5% to 1%) ... 1151
Brevibloc Concentrate (Less than 1%) ... 766
Brevibloc Injection (Less than 1%) ... 766
Brevibloc Double Strength Injection (Less than 1%) ... 766
Brevibloc Premixed Injection (Less than 1%) ... 766
Brevibloc Double Strength Premixed Injection (Less than 1%) ... 766
Cozaar Tablets (Less than 1%) ... 1913
Engerix-B Vaccine (Less than 1%) ... 1391
Hytrin Capsules (At least 1%) ... 469
Hyzaar ... 1964
Klonopin (Infrequent) ... 2782
▲ Lexapro Oral Solution (3%) ... 1193
▲ Lexapro Tablets (3%) ... 1193
Mevacor Tablets (0.5% to 1.0%) ... 1996
Moduretic Tablets ... 2003
Parcopa Orally Disintegrating Tablets ... 3111
Prinivil Tablets (0.3% to 1.0%) ... 2029
Prinzide Tablets (0.3% to 1%) ... 2033
Recombivax HB (Less than 1%) ... 2045
Stalevo Tablets ... 2270
Zestoretic Tablets (0.3% to 1%) ... 701
Zestril Tablets (0.3% to 1.0%) ... 704
Zofran Injection (2%) ... 1607

Pain, skeletal
▲ Norditropin Cartridges (11%) ... 2318

Pain, stomach
(*see under* Stomachache)

Pain, substernal
Evoxac Capsules (Less than 1%) ... 1042
Levaquin in 5% Dextrose Injection (Less than 0.5%) ... 2453
Levaquin (Less than 0.5%) ... 2453
Sonata Capsules (Infrequent) ... 1686
Teveten Tablets (Less than 1%) ... 1707
Teveten HCT Tablets (Less than 1%) ... 1710

Pain, testicular
Caverject Impulse Injection (Less than 1%) ... 2610
Edex Injection (1%) ... 3103
Eligard 7.5 mg (Less than 2%) ... 2896
Eligard 22.5 mg (Less than 2%) ... 2899
Eligard 30 mg (2.2%) ... 2901
Fabrazyme for Intravenous Infusion (2%) ... 1267
Lupron Depot 7.5 mg (Less than 5%) ... 3261
Neurontin Capsules (Rare) ... 2498
Neurontin Oral Solution (Rare) ... 2498
Neurontin Tablets (Rare) ... 2498
Prilosec OTC Tablets (Less than 1%) ... 2674
Propecia Tablets ... 2036
Proscar Tablets ... 2040
Rescriptor Tablets ... 2535
▲ Viadur Implant (3.8%) ... 782
Zegerid Powder for Oral Solution (Less than 1%) ... 2972

Pain, thoracic spine
▲ Chemet Capsules (5.2% to 15.7%) ... 2480
Primaxin I.M. ... 2022
Primaxin I.V. (Less than 0.2%) ... 2024

Pain, throat
Abilify Tablets (Infrequent) ... 916
Abilify Tablets (Infrequent) ... 2472
DDAVP Nasal Spray ... 2894
Desmopressin Acetate Rhinal Tube ... 1144
Lotronex Tablets (1%) ... 1479
▲ Zomig Nasal Spray (1% to 4%) ... 718

Pain, tongue
▲ Ventavis Inhalation Solution (4%) ... 1036

Pain, trunk
Diprivan Injectable Emulsion (Less than 1%) ... 676
▲ Epogen for Injection (3%) ... 586
▲ Leustatin Injection (6%) ... 2368
▲ Procrit for Injection (3%) ... 2374
Requip Tablets (Infrequent) ... 1528

Pain, tumor site
▲ Aromasin Tablets (8%) ... 2600
Herceptin I.V. ... 1234
Navelbine Injection ... 1494
Zevalin Injection (1%) ... 848

Pain, unspecified
Antara Capsules ... 2723

Pain, upper extremities
Aceon Tablets (2 mg, 4 mg, 8 mg) (0.2% to 2.8%) ... 3191
Cipro I.V. (1% or less) ... 2998
Cipro I.V. Pharmacy Bulk Package (1% or less) ... 3509
Engerix-B Vaccine (Less than 1%) ... 1391
Midamor Tablets (Less than or equal to 1%) ... 2000
Moduretic Tablets ... 2003
Prinivil Tablets (0.3% to 1.0%) ... 2029
ProSom Tablets (Infrequent) ... 512
Thalomid Capsules ... 979
Timolide Tablets ... 2056
Timoptic in Ocudose ... 2061
Timoptic Sterile Ophthalmic Solution ... 2058

Pain, urethral
Ceftin Tablets (0.1% to 1%) ... 1369
Permax Tablets (Rare) ... 3357
Prevacid Delayed-Release Capsules (Less than 1%) ... 3268
Prevacid for Delayed-Release Oral Suspension (Less than 1%) ... 3268
Prevacid NapraPAC (Less than 1%) ... 3277
Prevacid SoluTab Delayed-Release Orally Disintegrating Tablets (Less than 1%) ... 3268
PREVPAC (Less than 1%) ... 3281
Protonix I.V. (Less than 1%) ... 3468
Protonix Tablets (Less than 1%) ... 3465

Pain, urinary bladder
Duragesic Transdermal System (Less than 1%) ... 2448
Effexor Tablets (Infrequent) ... 3405
Effexor XR Capsules (Infrequent) ... 3411
▲ Rapamune Oral Solution and Tablets (3% to 20%) ... 3472
ReoPro Vials (0.1%) ... 1779
Sonata Capsules (Infrequent) ... 1686
Zonegran Capsules (Rare) ... 1089

Pain, urinary tract
Trileptal Oral Suspension ... 2281
Trileptal Tablets ... 2281

Pain, vaginal
Cleocin Vaginal Ovules (1.9%) ... 2613
Neurontin Capsules (Rare) ... 2498
Neurontin Oral Solution (Rare) ... 2498
Neurontin Tablets (Rare) ... 2498
Vantin Tablets and Oral Suspension (Less than 1%) ... 2650

Pain, vulva
DDAVP Injection 4 mcg/mL (Infrequent) ... 2893
Desmopressin Acetate Injection (Infrequent) ... 1143

Pain at application site
▲ Aldara Cream, 5% (Up to 12%) ... 1814
Aquacel AG with Hydrofiber ... 1035
Cleocin Vaginal Ovules (Less than 1%) ... 2613
Loprox Gel ... 1861
▲ Sulfamylon Cream (One of two most frequent) ... 2154
Zovirax Ointment ... 854

Pain at injection site
Actimmune ... 1646
Actiq (Less than 1%) ... 993
▲ Adacel Vaccine (1.1% to 80%) ... 2959
Aldurazyme for Intravenous Infusion (2%) ... 1261
▲ Alferon N Injection (12%) ... 1640
▲ Amevive (7% to common) ... 836
Ancef for Injection (Infrequent) ... 1318
▲ Angiomax for Injection (2.7% to 8%) ... 1856
Anzemet Injection ... 2871
AquaMEPHYTON Injection ... 1887
▲ Aranesp for Injection (7%) ... 576
▲ Aredia for Injection (Up to 41%) ... 2168
Attenuvax ... 1889
▲ Avonex (8%) ... 839
▲ Betaseron for SC Injection (18%) ... 791
▲ Boostrix (4.6% to 75.3%) ... 1366
▲ Botox Purified Neurotoxin Complex (2% to 10%) ... 565
Calcijex Injection (Occasional) ... 411
Calcium Disodium Versenate Injection ... 1819
Capastat Sulfate for Injection ... 1728
Cardene I.V. (0.7%) ... 1129
Cipro I.V. (1% or less) ... 2998
Cipro I.V. Pharmacy Bulk Package (1% or less) ... 3509
▲ Clolar for Intravenous Infusion (14%) ... 1264
▲ Comvax (23.9% to 34.5%) ... 1904
▲ Copaxone for Injection (73%) ... 3292
Delatestryl Injection (Rare) ... 2976
Depacon Injection (2.6%) ... 412
Depo-Provera Contraceptive Injection (Less than 1%) ... 2619
▲ depo-subQ provera 104 Injectable Suspension (1% to less than 5%) ... 2622
Desferal Vials ... 2190
Dilaudid-HP (Rare) ... 441
▲ Diprivan Injectable Emulsion (10% to 17.6%) ... 676
Doxil Injection (Less than 1%) ... 3302
Edecrin Sodium Intravenous (Occasional) ... 1941
▲ Eligard 22.5 mg (6%) ... 2899
▲ Eligard 30 mg (3.3%) ... 2901
Eligard 45 mg (2.7%) ... 2904
▲ Eloxatin for Injection (9% to 10%) ... 2908
▲ Enbrel for Injection (34% to 37%) ... 580
Engerix-B Vaccine (Less than 1%) ... 1391
▲ Faslodex Injection (10.9%) ... 682
▲ Flolan for Injection (13%) ... 1408
Fluorescite Injection ... ⊙207
Fortaz ... 1422
▲ Fragmin Injection (Up to 4.5%) ... 2638
▲ Fuzeon Injection (95%) ... 2772
GamaSTAN ... 3231
▲ Gammagard S/D (16%) ... 754
Garamycin Injectable (Occasional) ... 3028
Genotropin Lyophilized Powder (Infrequent) ... 2642
▲ Geodon for Injection (7% to 9%) ... 2514
▲ Gonal-f RFF Pen for Injection (4.8% to 5.5%) ... 3155
Humatrope Vials and Cartridges (Infrequent) ... 1756
▲ Humira Injection (12 to 20%) ... 464
▲ Hyalgan Solution (23%) ... 2917
HyperHep B S/D ... 3237
Hyperstat I.V. Injection ... 3031
Imitrex Injection ... 1431
▲ Infanrix Vaccine (0.9% to 10.5%) ... 1444
Infed Injection ... 3381
▲ Infergen (8% to 9%) ... 1647
▲ Intron A for Injection (Less than 5%) ... 3038
▲ Invanz for Injection (7%) ... 1974
▲ I.V. Busulfex (15%) ... 1125
Lantus Injection (2.7%) ... 2925
▲ Leustatin Injection (9% to 19%) ... 2368
Levaquin in 5% Dextrose Injection (0.2%) ... 2453
Levaquin (0.2%) ... 2453
Lovenox Injection (2%) ... 2931
Maxipime for Injection (0.6%) ... 1093
▲ Menactra Vaccine (0.2% to 59.2%) ... 2968
▲ Menopur for Subcutaneous Injection (5.4%) ... 1145
Merrem I.V. (0.4%) ... 687
Meruvax II ... 1994
Mycamine for Injection (0.9%) ... 620
▲ Nabi-HB (4%) ... 2159
Naropin Injection (Less than 1%) ... 640
▲ Navelbine Injection (Up to 13%) ... 1494
Neumega for Injection ... 3433
Novarel for Injection ... 1147
Nubain Injection ... 1111
Nutropin for Injection (Infrequent) ... 1238
Nutropin AQ Pen (Infrequent) ... 1241
Nutropin AQ Pen Cartridge (Infrequent) ... 1241
Oncaspar (Greater than 1% but less than 5%) ... 1123
Orthovisc Injection (2.5%) ... 3518
Pediarix Vaccine ... 1518
Liquid PedvaxHIB ... 2012
Pneumovax 23 (Common) ... 2020
Premarin Intravenous ... 3440
Prevacid I.V. for Injection (1%) ... 3274
Primaxin I.M. (1.2%) ... 2022
Primaxin I.V. (0.7%) ... 2024
Protonix I.V. (Greater than 1%) ... 3468
▲ Rabies Vaccine RabAvert (34%) ... 1011
Recombivax HB (Equal to or greater than 1%) ... 2045
ReoPro Vials (0.1%) ... 1779
Repronex for Intramuscular and Subcutaneous Injection ... 1148
Retrovir IV Infusion (Infrequent) ... 1537
Rhophylac ... 3504
Risperdal Consta Long-Acting Injection (Frequent) ... 1664
▲ Rituxan for Infusion (1% to 5%) ... 845
▲ Rituxan I.V. (1% to 5%) ... 1251
Rocephin Injectable Vials, ADD-Vantage, Galaxy, Bulk (1%) ... 2801
▲ Sandostatin Injection (7.7%) ... 2263
▲ Sandostatin LAR Depot (2% to 11%) ... 2264
▲ Synercid I.V. (40%) ... 1690
Timentin ADD-Vantage ... 1556
Timentin Injection Galaxy Container ... 1559
Timentin IV Infusion ... 1553
Timentin Pharmacy Bulk Package ... 1562
▲ Trelstar Depot (3.6%) ... 3385
▲ Trelstar LA Suspension (4%) ... 3387
▲ Trisenox Injection (20%) ... 983
Tygacil for Injection (0% to less than 2%) ... 3489
▲ Vaqta (1.2% to 51.1%) ... 2067
▲ Varivax (19.3% to 32.5%; less than 0.05%) ... 2070
VFEND I.V. (Less than 2%) ... 2543
VFEND Oral Suspension (Less than 2%) ... 2543
VFEND Tablets (Less than 2%) ... 2543
Xolair ... 1259
Zantac Injection ... 1593
Zantac Injection Pharmacy Bulk Package (Frequent) ... 1595
▲ Zinecard for Injection (12% to 13%) ... 2659
▲ Zithromax for IV Infusion (6.5%) ... 2573
▲ Zofran Injection (4%) ... 1607
Zosyn (0.2%) ... 3492
Zyprexa IntraMuscular (Frequent) ... 1798

Pain at insertion site
▲ Vantas (3.6%) ... 3367

Pain secondary to eczema
Bactroban Cream (One report) ... 1356

Pain, pharyngolaryngeal
▲ Focalin XR Capsules (4% to 7%) ... 2217
▲ Myfortic Tablets (3% to less than 20%) ... 2244
▲ Xanax XR Tablets (3.2%) ... 2655
Xifaxan Tablets (Less than 2%) ... 2847
Zelnorm Tablets ... 2303

Pain, thorax
▲ Humira Injection (Less than 5%) ... 464

Pallor
Abilify Tablets (Infrequent) ... 916
Abilify Tablets (Infrequent) ... 2472
Advair Diskus 100/50 ... 1291
Advair Diskus 250/50 ... 1291
Advair Diskus 500/50 ... 1291
Allegra-D 12 Hour Extended-Release Tablets ... 2860
Allegra-D 24 Hour Extended-Release Tablets ... 2862
Ambien Tablets (Infrequent) ... 2867
Apokyn Injection (Common) ... 2132
Balamine DM ... 739
Brevibloc Concentrate (Less than 1%) ... 766
Brevibloc Injection (Less than 1%) ... 766
Brevibloc Double Strength Injection (Less than 1%) ... 766
Brevibloc Premixed Injection (Less than 1%) ... 766
Brevibloc Double Strength Premixed Injection (Less than 1%) ... 766
Buprenex Injectable (Infrequent) ... 2718
Captopril Tablets (2 to 5 of 1000 patients) ... 2114
Catapres Tablets ... 874

Catapres-TTS (0.5% or less) 875
▲ CellCept Capsules (3% to less than 20%) 2751
▲ CellCept Intravenous (3% to less than 20%) 2751
▲ CellCept Oral Suspension (3% to less than 20%) 2751
▲ CellCept Tablets (3% to less than 20%) 2751
Clorpres Tablets 2139
Clozapine Tablets (Less than 1%) 2141
Clozaril Tablets (Less than 1%) 2174
Dapsone Tablets USP 1656
▲ Doxil Injection (1% to 10%) 3302
Effexor Tablets (Rare) 3405
Effexor XR Capsules (Rare) 3411
Enbrel for Injection 580
EpiPen 1061
Evoxac Capsules (Less than 1%) 1042
▲ Fabrazyme for Intravenous Infusion (4%) 1267
FazaClo Orally Disintegrating Tablets (Less than 1%) 547
Ferrlecit Injection 3379
▲ Flolan for Injection (21% to 32%) 1408
Flumadine (Less than 0.3%) 1186
Gabitril Tablets (Infrequent) 998
Imitrex Injection (Rare) 1431
Imitrex Nasal Spray (Rare) 1435
Imitrex Tablets (Infrequent) 1440
Kadian Capsules (Less than 3%) 572
Kogenate FS 3517
▲ Miacalcin Nasal Spray (10.6%) 2242
Nitrolingual Pumpspray 1161
Paxil CR Controlled-Release Tablets (Rare) 1509
Paxil (Rare) 1501
Pediarix Vaccine 1518
Prozac Pulvules and Liquid (Rare) 1771
ReoPro Vials (0.1%) 1779
Rescriptor Tablets 2535
Reyataz Capsules (Less than 3%) 948
Risperdal M-Tab Orally Disintegrating Tablets (Rare) 1658
Risperdal (Rare) 1658
Rythmol SR Capsules 2736
▲ Serevent Diskus (9%) 1540
Thioridazine Hydrochloride Tablets 2122
Topamax Sprinkle Capsules (1%) 2438
Topamax Tablets (1%) 2438
▲ Trisenox Injection (10%) 983
▲ Vesanoid Capsules (6%) 2823
Wellbutrin Tablets (Rare) 1579
WinRho SDF 763
Zoloft (Rare) 2581
Zyprexa Tablets 1798
Zyprexa ZYDIS Orally Disintegrating Tablets 1798
Zyrtec Chewable Tablets (Less than 2%) 2589
Zyrtec (Less than 2%) 2589
Zyrtec-D 12 Hour Extended Release Tablets (Less than 2%) 2591

Pallor, nasal

▲ Fortical Nasal Spray (10.6%) 3336

Palmar-plantar erythrodysesthesia syndrome

▲ Clolar for Intravenous Infusion (13%) 1264
▲ Doxil Injection (3.4% to 50.6%) 3302
▲ Eloxatin for Injection (1% to 11%) 2908
▲ Xeloda Tablets (17% to 54%) 2825

Palpitations

Abilify Tablets (Infrequent) 916
Abilify Tablets (Infrequent) 2472
Accutane Capsules 2740
Aceon Tablets (2 mg, 4 mg, 8 mg) (0.9% to 1.1%) 3191
Aciphex Tablets 1081
Actiq (1% or greater) 993
Adalat CC Tablets (Less than 1%) 2978
Adderall Tablets 3168
▲ Adderall XR Capsules (2% to 4%) 3169
Adenocard Injection (Less than 1%) 612
Adenoscan (Less than 1%) 613
Adipex-P 1216
▲ Advair Diskus 100/50 (1% to 3%) 1291
▲ Advair Diskus 250/50 (1% to 3%) 1291
▲ Advair Diskus 500/50 (1% to 3%) 1291
Advicor Tablets 1694
▲ Aerobid/Aerobid-M (3% to 9%) 1172
Aggrenox Capsules (Less than 1%) 855
▲ Agrylin Capsules (26.1%) 3172
Aldara Cream, 5% 1814
Allegra-D 12 Hour Extended-Release Tablets (1.9%) 2860
Allegra-D 24 Hour Extended-Release Tablets (1.9%) 2862
Altace Capsules (Less than 1%) 1673
Alupent Inhalation Aerosol (Less frequent) 858
Ambien Tablets (2%) 2867
Amerge Tablets (Infrequent) 1312
Amnesteem Capsules 2126
Anaprox Tablets (Less than 3%) 2769
Anaprox DS Tablets (Less than 3%) 2769
Antara Capsules 2723
Anzemet Injection (Rare) 2871
Anzemet Tablets (Rare) 2874
Apokyn Injection 2132
▲ Arava Tablets (1% to 3%) 2881
Arthrotec Tablets (Rare) 3126
Atacand Tablets (0.5% or greater) 634
Atacand HCT (0.5% or greater) 637
Atrovent Inhalation Solution (Less than 3%) 868
Atrovent Nasal Spray 0.06% (Less than 1%) 870
Avelox (0.1% to less than 2%) 2984
Avinza Capsules (Less than 5%) 1714
Axert Tablets (Infrequent) 2430
Bentyl Capsules 724
Bentyl Injection 724
Bentyl Syrup 724
Bentyl Tablets 724
Betagan Ophthalmic Solution, USP ⊙217
▲ Betaseron for SC Injection (4%) 791
Betimol Ophthalmic Solution ⊙283
Betimol Ophthalmic Solution 3371
▲ BiDil Tablets (4%) 2161
Blocadren Tablets 1891
Brimonidine Tartrate Ophthalmic Solution 0.2% (Less than 3%) ⊙245
▲ Caduet Tablets (Less than 2% to 4.5%) 2507
Campral Tablets (Frequent) 1175
Captopril Tablets (Approximately 1 of 100 patients) 2114
Cardizem LA Extended Release Tablets (Less than 2%) 1699
▲ Carnitor Injection (3% to 8%) 3185
Carteolol Hydrochloride Ophthalmic Solution USP, 1% (Occasional) ⊙246
Cataflam Tablets (Rarely) 2173
Catapres Tablets (About 5 in 1,000 patients) 874
Catapres-TTS (0.5% or less) 875
Celebrex Capsules (0.1% to 1.9%) 3130
Celexa (At least 2%) 1177
▲ CellCept Capsules (3% to less than 20%) 2751
▲ CellCept Intravenous (3% to less than 20%) 2751
▲ CellCept Oral Suspension (3% to less than 20%) 2751
▲ CellCept Tablets (3% to less than 20%) 2751
▲ Cenestin Tablets, 0.45mg, 0.625mg, 0.9mg, 1.25mg (5.7% to 21%) 1063
Cialis Tablets (Less than 2%) 1806
Cipro I.V. (1% or less) 2998
Cipro I.V. Pharmacy Bulk Package (1% or less) 3509
Cipro (Less than 1%) 2991
Cipro XR Tablets 3004
Clarinex Syrup 3009
Clarinex Tablets 3009
Clarinex Reditabs Tablets 3009
Clarinex-D 24-Hour Extended-Release Tablets 3012
Clinoril Tablets (Less than 1 in 100) 1899
Clorpres Tablets (About 5 in 1,000) 2139
Clozapine Tablets (Less than 1%) 2141
Clozaril Tablets (Less than 1%) 2174
Colazal Capsules 2845
Combivent Inhalation Aerosol (Less than 2%) 878
Concerta Extended-Release Tablets 1828
▲ Copaxone for Injection (17%) 3292
▲ Coreg Tablets (Greater than 1% to 3%) 1376
Cosopt Sterile Ophthalmic Solution 1910
Covera-HS Tablets (Less than 2%) 3135
Cozaar Tablets (Less than 1%) 1913
Crestor Tablets (Greater than or equal to 1%) 672
Dalmane Capsules 3343
▲ Depacon Injection (1% to 5%) 412
▲ Depakene (1% to 5%) 417
▲ Depakote Sprinkle Capsules (1% to 5%) 422
▲ Depakote Tablets (1% to 5%) 427
Depakote ER Tablets (Greater than 1%) 433
Desoxyn Tablets, USP 2482
Detrol LA Capsules 2629
Dexedrine 1386
DextroStat Tablets 3177
Digitek Tablets (1%) 2146
Dilaudid Oral Liquid 443
Dilaudid Tablets - 8 mg 443
Dilaudid-HP (Less frequent) 441
Diovan HCT Tablets (Greater than 0.2%) 2195
Diovan Tablets 2191
▲ Ditropan XL Extended Release Tablets (2% to less than 5%) 2391
Dolobid Tablets (Rare) 1937
▲ Dostinex Tablets (1% to less than 10%) 2631
Doxil Injection (Less than 1%) 3302
DuoNeb Inhalation Solution 1058
DynaCirc CR Tablets (1.2%) 2726
EC-Naprosyn Delayed-Release Tablets (Less than 3%) 2769
Effexor Tablets 3405
Effexor XR Capsules (3%) 3411
Eldepryl Capsules (1 of 49 patients) 3209
Engerix-B Vaccine 1391
▲ Entocort EC Capsules (Less than 5%) 2694
EpiPen 1061
Ery-Tab Tablets (Isolated reports) 447
Erythrocin Stearate Filmtab Tablets (Isolated reports) 452
Erythromycin Base Filmtab Tablets (Isolated reports) 454
Erythromycin Delayed-Release Capsules, USP (Isolated reports) 456
Estrogel 0.06% (0.6%) 3200
▲ Evoxac Capsules (1% to 3%) 1042
Exelon Capsules (Frequent) 2204
FazaClo Orally Disintegrating Tablets (Less than 1%) 547
Flexeril Tablets (Less than 1%) 1832
▲ Flolan for Injection (63%) 1408
Flomax Capsules (Infrequent) 881
▲ Flovent Diskus 50 mcg (1% to 3%) 1415
Flumadine (Less than 0.3%) 1186
Focalin Tablets 2214
Focalin XR Capsules 2217
Foradil Aerolizer 3024
Fortical Nasal Spray (Less than 1%) 3336
Frova Tablets (Frequent) 1101
Gabitril Tablets (Frequent) 998
Guanidine Hydrochloride Tablets 3030
▲ Humira Injection (Less than 5%) 464
Hycomine Compound Tablets 1105
Hycotuss Expectorant Syrup 1106
Hyperstat I.V. Injection 3031
▲ Hytrin Capsules (0.9% to 28%) 469
Hyzaar (1.4%) 1964
▲ Imdur Tablets (Less than or equal to 5%) 3032
Imitrex Injection (Infrequent) 1431
Imitrex Nasal Spray (Infrequent) 1435
Imitrex Tablets (Up to 2%) 1440
Indapamide Tablets (Less than 5%) 2119
Indocin (Less than 1%) 1968
▲ Infergen (3% to 5%) 1647
▲ Intron A for Injection (Less than 5%) 3038
Kadian Capsules (Less than 3%) 572
Kaletra (Less than 2%) 474
Klonopin (Infrequent) 2782
Lamictal (1.0%) 1449
Lanoxicaps Capsules 1458
Lanoxin Injection 1462
Lanoxin Tablets 1468
Lanoxin Injection Pediatric 1465
Lariam Tablets (Infrequent) 2790
Levaquin in 5% Dextrose Injection (0.1% to 0.9%) 2453
Levaquin (0.1% to 0.9%) 2453
Levitra Tablets (Less than 2%) 3048
Levothroid Tablets 1189
Levoxyl Tablets 1680
Lexapro Oral Solution (Frequent) 1193
Lexapro Tablets (Frequent) 1193
Lipitor Tablets (Less than 2%) 2495
Lofibra Capsules 1217
Lotensin HCT Tablets (0.3% to 1%) 2235
Lotrel Capsules (0.5% to 0.3%) 2238
▲ Lupron Depot 3.75 mg (Among most frequent) 3257
Lupron Depot–3 Month 11.25 mg (Less than 5%) 3262
Marinol Capsules (Greater than 1%) 3334
Mavik Tablets (0.3% to 1.0%) 482
Maxair Autohaler (1.3% to 1.7%) 1820
Maxalt Tablets (Frequent) 1983
Maxalt-MLT Orally Disintegrating Tablets (Frequent) 1983
▲ Megace ES Oral Suspension (1% to 3%) 2492
Meridia Capsules (2%) 485
Metadate CD Capsules 3316
Miacalcin Nasal Spray (Less than 1%) 2242
Micardis Tablets (More than 0.3%) 884
Micardis HCT Tablets 886
Midamor Tablets (Less than or equal to 1%) 2000
Migranal Nasal Spray (Infrequent) 3350
Mirapex Tablets (Greater than or equal to 1%) 889
Mobic Oral Suspension (Less than 2%) 893
Mobic Tablets (Less than 2%) 893
Moduretic Tablets 2003
MS Contin Tablets (Less frequent) 2703
Nalfon Capsules (2.5%) 2504
Naprosyn Suspension (Less than 3%) 2769
Naprosyn Tablets (Less than 3%) 2769
▲ Neumega for Injection (14%) 3433
Neurontin Capsules (Infrequent) 2498
Neurontin Oral Solution (Infrequent) 2498
Neurontin Tablets (Infrequent) 2498
Niaspan Extended-Release Tablets 1703
Nicotrol Inhaler 2594
▲ Nicotrol NS (4%) 2596
Nimotop Capsules (Less than 1%) 774
Niravam Orally Disintegrating Tablets (7.7%) 3106
Norflex Injection 1824
Noroxin Tablets (Less frequent) 2009
Norvasc Tablets (0.7% to 4.5%) 2529
Norvir (Less than 2%) 499
Numorphan 1112
OptiPranolol Metipranolol Ophthalmic Solution 0.3% (A small number of patients) ⊙254
Orap Tablets 1220
Parcopa Orally Disintegrating Tablets 3111
Parnate Tablets 1499
▲ Paxil CR Controlled-Release Tablets (2% to 3%) 1509
▲ Paxil (2% to 3%) 1501
Pentasa Capsules (Less than 1%) 3182
Pepcid Injection (Infrequent) 2017
Pepcid (Infrequent) 2014
Permax Tablets (2.1%) 3357
Persantine Tablets (Rare) 898
Plavix Tablets (1% to 2.5%) 940
Plavix Tablets (1% to 2.5%) 2942
Plendil Extended-Release Tablets (0.4% to 2.5%) 651
▲ Pletal Tablets (5% to 10%) 2478
Prandin Tablets (0.5, 1, and 2 mg) (Less than or equal to 1%) 2337
Prevacid Delayed-Release Capsules (Less than 1%) 3268
Prevacid for Delayed-Release Oral Suspension (Less than 1%) 3268
Prevacid NapraPAC (Less than 3%) 3277
Prevacid SoluTab Delayed-Release Orally Disintegrating Tablets (Less than 1%) 3268
PREVPAC (Less than 1%) 3281
Prilosec OTC Tablets (Less than 1%) 2674
Primaxin I.M. 2022
Primaxin I.V. (Less than 0.2%) 2024
Prinivil Tablets (0.3% to 1.0%) 2029
Prinzide Tablets (0.3% to 1%) 2033
Prometrium Capsules (100 mg, 200 mg) (Less than 5%) 3205
ProSom Tablets (Infrequent) 512
Protonix I.V. (Less than 1%) 3468
Protonix Tablets (Less than 1%) 3465
Protopic Ointment (Greater than or equal to 1%) 629
▲ Proventil Inhalation Aerosol (Less than 10%) 3067
Proventil HFA Inhalation Aerosol (Less than 3%) 3071
Provigil Tablets (2%) 1002
Prozac Pulvules and Liquid (Frequent) 1771
Rabies Vaccine RabAvert 1011
▲ Rapamune Oral Solution and Tablets (3% to 20%) 3472
Razadyne ER Extended-Release Capsules (Infrequent) 2434
Razadyne (Infrequent) 2434
Recombivax HB (Less than 1%) 2045
ReFacto Vials 3479
Relafen Tablets (Less than 1%) 1523
Relpax Tablets (Frequent) 2531
ReoPro Vials (0.7%) 1779
▲ Requip Tablets (3%) 1528
Reyataz Capsules (Less than 3%) 948

Rhinocort Aqua Nasal Spray (Rare) 658
Rilutek Tablets (0.4% to 1.2%) 2945
Risperdal Consta Long-Acting Injection (Infrequent) 1664
Risperdal M-Tab Orally Disintegrating Tablets (Infrequent) 1658
Risperdal (Infrequent) 1658
Ritalin Hydrochloride Tablets 2254
Ritalin LA Capsules 2255
Ritalin-SR Tablets 2254
Rocephin Injectable Vials, ADD-Vantage, Galaxy, Bulk (Rare) 2801
Rythmol SR Capsules 2736
Sanctura Tablets 1133
Sandostatin Injection (Less than 1%) 2263
▲ Sandostatin LAR Depot (5% to 15%) 2264
Seroquel Tablets (Frequent) 691
Singulair 2047
Sonata Capsules (Infrequent) 1686
Spiriva HandiHaler 899
Stalevo Tablets 2270
▲ Strattera Capsules (0.7% to 4%) 1784
▲ Sular Tablets (3%) 1163
Surmontil Capsules 2347
Sustiva Capsules (Less than 2%) 957
Synercid I.V. (Less than 1%) 1690
▲ Tambocor Tablets (6.1%) 1824
Tarka Tablets (0.3% or more) 519
Tasmar Tablets (Frequent) 3360
▲ Tequin Injection (0.1% to 3%) 964
▲ Tequin Tablets (0.1% to 3%) 964
Teveten Tablets (Less than 1%) 1707
Teveten HCT Tablets (Less than 1%) 1710
Thalomid Capsules 979
Thyrolar 1203
Tiazac Capsules (Less than 2%) 1204
Timolide Tablets 2056
Timoptic in Ocudose (Less frequent) 2061
Timoptic Sterile Ophthalmic Solution (Less frequent) 2058
Timoptic-XE Sterile Ophthalmic Gel Forming Solution 2062
Tindamax 2670
Toprol-XL Tablets (About 1 of 100 patients) 660
▲ Tracleer Tablets (5%) 539
Tricor Tablets 523
Triglide Tablets 1165
Trileptal Oral Suspension 2281
Trileptal Tablets 2281
▲ Trisenox Injection (10%) 983
Twinrix Vaccine 1571
Ultracet Tablets (Less than 1%) 2462
Uniretic Tablets (Less than 1%) 3114
Unithroid Tablets 3521
Univasc Tablets (Less than 1%) 3118
Vantas (Less than 2%) 3367
Vantin Tablets and Oral Suspension (Less than 1%) 2650
Vaseretic Tablets (0.5% to 2.0%) 2073
Vasotec I.V. Injection (0.5% to 1.0%) 2076
▲ Ventavis Inhalation Solution (7%) 1036
Ventolin HFA Inhalation Aerosol (Less than 3%) 1576
Verelan PM Capsules (2% or less) 3120
VFEND I.V. (Less than 2%) 2543
VFEND Oral Suspension (Less than 2%) 2543
VFEND Tablets (Less than 2%) 2543
Viagra Tablets (Less than 2%) 2552
Vicoprofen Tablets (Less than 3%) 533
Vivactil Tablets 2350
Voltaren Tablets (Rarely) 2298
Voltaren-XR Tablets (Rarely) 2301
VoSpire Extended-Release Tablets (2.4%) 2352
▲ Wellbutrin Tablets (3.7%) 1579
▲ Wellbutrin SR Sustained-Release Tablets (2% to 6%) 1583
▲ Wellbutrin XL Extended-Release Tablets (2% to 6%) 1588
Xanax XR Tablets (Frequent) 2655
Zegerid Powder for Oral Solution (Less than 1%) 2972
▲ Zemplar Capsules (3%) 535
▲ Zemplar Injection (3%) 538
Zestoretic Tablets (0.3% to 1%) 701
Zestril Tablets (0.3% to 1.0%) 704
Zithromax (1% or less) 2568
Zithromax for Oral Suspension, 300 mg, 600 mg, 900 mg, 1200 mg (1% or less) 2561
Zithromax Tablets, 250 mg, 500 mg (1% or less) 2561
Zithromax Tablets, 600 mg (1% or less) 2568
Zithromax Tri-Pak (1% or less) 2561
Zithromax Z-Pak (1% or less) 2568
Zmax for Oral Suspension (Less then 1%) 2577
Zofran Injection 1607
Zoladex (1% or greater) 709
Zoladex 3-month 712
Zoloft (Frequent) 2581
Zomig Nasal Spray (1% to 2%) 718
Zomig Tablets (Less than 1% to 2%) 714
Zomig-ZMT Tablets (Less than 1% to 2%) 714
Zonegran Capsules (Infrequent) 1089
Zyban Sustained-Release Tablets (2%) 1620
Zyprexa Tablets (Infrequent) 1798
Zyprexa ZYDIS Orally Disintegrating Tablets (Infrequent) 1798
Zyrtec Chewable Tablets (Less than 2%) 2589
Zyrtec (Less than 2%) 2589
Zyrtec-D 12 Hour Extended Release Tablets (Less than 2%) 2591

Palsy, cranial nerve
DepoCyt Injection 1121
Naropin Injection 640
Orthoclone OKT3 Sterile Solution (Less than 1%) 2370

Palsy, extraocular
Lyrica Capsules (Rare) 2524
Protonix I.V. (Less than 1%) 3468
Protonix Tablets (Less than 1%) 3465

Palsy, facial
Boostrix 1366
depo-subQ provera 104 Injectable Suspension 2622

Palsy, nerve
Fuzeon Injection 2772
Neurontin Capsules (Rare) 2498
Neurontin Oral Solution (Rare) 2498
Neurontin Tablets (Rare) 2498

Palsy, optic nerve
Symmetrel (0.1% to 1%) 1115

Palsy, peripheral nerve
Altoprev Extended-Release Tablets 1151
Lescol Capsules 2227
Lescol Capsules 2730
Lescol XL Tablets 2227
Lescol XL Tablets 2730
Mevacor Tablets 1996
Pravachol Tablets 943
Vytorin 10/10 Tablets 2084
Vytorin 10/10 Tablets 3092
Vytorin 10/20 Tablets 2084
Vytorin 10/20 Tablets 3092
Vytorin 10/40 Tablets 2084
Vytorin 10/40 Tablets 3092
Vytorin 10/80 Tablets 2084
Vytorin 10/80 Tablets 3092
Zocor Tablets 2078

Pancolitis
Canasa Rectal Suppositories 726

Pancreatic disease, unspecified
Pulmozyme Inhalation Solution 1245

Pancreatic enzymes, increased
Camptosar Injection (Rare) 2602
Emtriva Capsules (Less than 1%) 1272

Pancreatitis
Abilify Tablets (Rare) 916
Abilify Tablets (Rare) 2472
Accutane Capsules 2740
Aciphex Tablets 1081
Actimmune (Rare) 1646
Activase I.V. 1225
Advicor Tablets 1694
Aggrenox Capsules 855
Agrylin Capsules 3172
Aldoclor Tablets 1881
Aldoril Tablets 1884
Altace Capsules (Less than 1%) 1673
Altoprev Extended-Release Tablets 1151
Amnesteem Capsules 2126
Anaprox Tablets (Less than 1%) 2769
Anaprox DS Tablets (Less than 1%) 2769
Antara Capsules 2723
Anzemet Injection (Rare) 2871
Anzemet Tablets (Rare) 2874
Aptivus Capsules (Less than 2%) 859
Arava Tablets (Rare) 2881
Aricept Tablets 1086
Aricept ODT Tablets 1086
Arthrotec Tablets (Rare) 3126
Asacol Delayed-Release Tablets 2688
Atacand HCT 637
Avalide Tablets 922
Avalide Tablets 2889
Azasan Tablets 2844
Bayer Aspirin Tablets 3515
Betaseron for SC Injection 791
Biaxin/Biaxin XL 402
Buphenyl Powder (One patient) 3327
Buphenyl Tablets (One patient) 3327
Caduet Tablets (Greater than 0.1% to less than 2%) 2507
Calcijex Injection 411
Campath Ampules 826
Campral Tablets (Infrequent) 1175
Camptosar Injection (Rare) 2602
Canasa Rectal Suppositories 726
Captopril Tablets 2114
Carbatrol Capsules 3174
Cataflam Tablets (Rarely) 2173
Celebrex Capsules (Less than 0.1%) 3130
Celexa 1177
CellCept Capsules 2751
CellCept Intravenous 2751
CellCept Oral Suspension 2751
CellCept Tablets 2751
Cenestin Tablets, 0.45mg, 0.625mg, 0.9mg, 1.25mg 1063
Cenestin Tablets, 0.3mg 1063
Cipro I.V. (1% or less) 2998
Cipro I.V. Pharmacy Bulk Package (1% or less) 3509
Cipro 2991
Cipro XR Tablets 3004
Climara Transdermal System 795
Climara Pro Transdermal System 800
Clinoril Tablets (Less than 1 in 100) 1899
Clorpres Tablets 2139
Clozapine Tablets 2141
Clozaril Tablets 2174
Colazal Capsules 2845
Combivir Tablets (Less than 0.5%) 1373
Copaxone for Injection (Infrequent) 3292
Copegus Tablets (Less than 1%) 2759
Crestor Tablets (Less than 1%) 672
Crixivan Capsules 1918
Cuprimine Capsules 1925
Cytovene 2763
Dapsone Tablets USP 1656
Decadron Phosphate Injection 1931
Decadron Tablets 1929
▲ Depacon Injection (1% to 5%) 412
Depakene 417
▲ Depakote Sprinkle Capsules (1% to 5%) 422
▲ Depakote Tablets (1% to 5%) 427
▲ Depakote ER Tablets (1% to 5%) 433
Depo-Medrol Injectable Suspension 2615
Depo-Medrol Single-Dose Vial 2617
Diovan HCT Tablets 2195
Diprivan Injectable Emulsion (Very rare) 676
Diuril Oral 1936
Diuril Sodium Intravenous 1934
Doxil Injection (Less than 1%) 3302
Dyazide Capsules 1389
Dynacin Tablets 1859
EC-Naprosyn Delayed-Release Tablets (Less than 1%) 2769
Ecotrin Enteric Coated Aspirin Low, Regular and Maximum Strength Tablets 1627
Edecrin (Rare) 1941
E.E.S. 449
Effexor Tablets 3405
Effexor XR Capsules 3411
Eloxatin for Injection 2908
Elspar for Injection 1943
Enbrel for Injection (Infrequent) 580
Epivir (Less than 0.5%) 1394
▲ Epivir-HBV (14% to 15%) 1398
Epzicom Tablets 1402
Erythrocin Stearate Filmtab Tablets (Rare) 452
Erythromycin Delayed-Release Capsules, USP (Rare) 456
Estratest Tablets 3196
Estratest H.S. Tablets 3196
Estrogel 0.06% 3200
Exelon Capsules (Infrequent) 2204
FazaClo Orally Disintegrating Tablets 547
Furosemide Tablets 2117
▲ Fuzeon Injection (3%) 2772
Gengraf Capsules (Rare) 458
Gleevec Tablets (Rare) 2221
Hectorol Capsules 909
Hectorol Injection 911
Herceptin I.V. (At least one of the 958 patients) 1234
Humatrope Vials and Cartridges (Rare) 1756
Hydrocortone Tablets 1963
Hyperstat I.V. Injection 3031
Hyzaar 1964
Imitrex Injection 1431
Imitrex Nasal Spray (Rare) 1435
Imitrex Tablets 1440
Invanz for Injection (Greater than 0.1%) 1974
Invirase (Rare) 2776
Iressa Tablets (Rare) 684
I.V. Busulfex (2%) 1125
Kaletra (Less than 2%) 474
Keppra Oral Solution 3307
Keppra Tablets 3307
Lamictal 1449
Lescol Capsules 2227
Lescol Capsules 2730
Lescol XL Tablets 2227
Lescol XL Tablets 2730
Levaquin in 5% Dextrose Injection (0.1% to 0.9%) 2453
Levaquin (0.1% to 0.9%) 2453
Lexapro Oral Solution 1193
Lexapro Tablets 1193
Lipitor Tablets (Less than 2%) 2495
Lofibra Capsules (Less than 1%) 1217
Lo/Ovral-28 Tablets 3423
Lotensin Tablets (Less than 1%) 2232
Lotensin HCT Tablets (Rare) 2235
Lotrel Capsules (Rare) 2238
Lyrica Capsules (0.1% to 1%) 2524
Mavik Tablets (Rare) 482
Maxzide 2150
Menostar Transdermal System 805
Mepron Suspension 1487
Mevacor Tablets 1996
Micardis HCT Tablets 886
M-M-R II 1980
Mobic Oral Suspension (Less than 2%) 893
Mobic Tablets (Less than 2%) 893
Moduretic Tablets 2003
Mumpsvax 2005
Myfortic Tablets 2244
Nalfon Capsules (Less than 1%) 2504
Namenda 1199
Naprosyn Suspension (Less than 1%) 2769
Naprosyn Tablets (Less than 1%) 2769
Navelbine Injection 1494
Neoral Soft Gelatin Capsules (Rare) 2247
Neoral Oral Solution (Rare) 2247
Neurontin Capsules (Rare) 2498
Neurontin Oral Solution (Rare) 2498
Neurontin Tablets (Rare) 2498
Nexium Delayed-Release Capsules (Rare) 645
Nexium I.V. (Rare) 649
Noroxin Tablets (Rare) 2009
Norvasc Tablets (More than 0.1% to 1%) 2529
Norvir (Less than 2%) 499
Nutropin for Injection (Rare) 1238
Nutropin AQ Injection (Rare) 1241
Nutropin AQ Pen (Rare) 1241
Nutropin AQ Pen Cartridge (Rare) 1241
Omacor Capsules 2735
Oncaspar (1%) 1123
▲ Ontak Vials (Less than 5%) 1717
Pacerone Tablets 3337
Paxil CR Controlled-Release Tablets 1509
Paxil 1501
PCE Dispertab Tablets (Rare) 510
Pediapred Oral Solution 3319
Pegasys (Less than 1%) 2793
PEG-Intron Powder for Injection (Less than or equal to 1%) 3062
Pentasa Capsules (Infrequent to less than 1%) 3182
Permax Tablets (Rare) 3357
Plavix Tablets 940
Plavix Tablets 2942
Prandin Tablets (0.5, 1, and 2 mg) (Rare) 2337
Pravachol Tablets 943
Prefest Tablets 1069
Premarin Intravenous 3440
Premarin Tablets 3443
Premarin Vaginal Cream 3449
Premphase Tablets 3452
Prempro Tablets 3452
Prevacid NapraPAC (Less than 1%) 3277

PREVPAC ... 3281
Prilosec OTC Tablets (Less than 1%) ... 2674
Prinivil Tablets (0.3% to 1.0%) ... 2029
Prinzide Tablets ... 2033
Prograf Capsules and Injection ... 624
Proleukin for Injection (Less than 1%) ... 1007
Protonix I.V. ... 3468
Protonix Tablets ... 3465
Prozac Pulvules and Liquid (Rare) ... 1771
Purinethol Tablets ... 1222
Rapamune Oral Solution and Tablets (Less frequent) ... 3472
Rebetron Combination Therapy ... 3078
Relafen Tablets (Less than 1%) ... 1523
Remicade for IV Injection (Greater than or equal to 0.2%) ... 987
Requip Tablets (Infrequent) ... 1528
Rescriptor Tablets ... 2535
Retrovir Capsules (Rare) ... 1533
Retrovir IV Infusion (Rare) ... 1537
Retrovir (Rare) ... 1533
Reyataz Capsules (Less than 3%) ... 948
Rilutek Tablets (Infrequent) ... 2945
Risperdal M-Tab Orally Disintegrating Tablets ... 1658
Risperdal ... 1658
Roferon-A Injection (Infrequent) ... 2805
Rythmol SR Capsules ... 2736
Sandimmune (Rare) ... 2259
Sandostatin Injection (Less than 1%) ... 2263
Sandostatin LAR Depot (Rare) ... 2264
Seasonale Tablets ... 1073
Seroquel Tablets (Rare) ... 691
Singulair (Very rare) ... 2047
Soriatane Capsules ... 1028
St. Joseph 81 mg Aspirin Chewable and Enteric Coated Tablets ... 1841
Sustiva Capsules (Less than 2%) ... 957
Symbyax Capsules (Rare) ... 1788
Synercid I.V. (Less than 1%) ... 1690
Tagamet Tablets (Rare) ... 1547
Targretin Capsules ... 1719
Tarka Tablets ... 519
Tegretol/Tegretol-XR ... 2278
Tequin Injection ... 964
Tequin Tablets ... 964
Teveten HCT Tablets ... 1710
Thalomid Capsules ... 979
Timolide Tablets ... 2056
Topamax Sprinkle Capsules ... 2438
Topamax Tablets ... 2438
Tricor Tablets ... 523
Triphasil-28 Tablets ... 3483
Trizivir Tablets (3 of 656 patients) ... 1565
Truvada Tablets ... 1279
Tygacil for Injection ... 3489
Uniretic Tablets ... 3114
Univasc Tablets (Less than 1%) ... 3118
Vaseretic Tablets ... 2073
Vasotec I.V. Injection (0.5% to 1.0%) ... 2076
Vesanoid Capsules (Isolated cases) ... 2823
VFEND I.V. (Less than 2%) ... 2543
VFEND Oral Suspension (Less than 2%) ... 2543
VFEND Tablets (Less than 2%) ... 2543
Viracept (Less than 2%) ... 2556
Viread Tablets ... 1284
Vivelle Transdermal System ... 2288
Vivelle-Dot Transdermal System ... 2293
Voltaren Tablets (Rarely) ... 2298
Voltaren-XR Tablets (Rarely) ... 2301
Vytorin 10/10 Tablets ... 2084
Vytorin 10/10 Tablets ... 3092
Vytorin 10/20 Tablets ... 2084
Vytorin 10/20 Tablets ... 3092
Vytorin 10/40 Tablets ... 2084
Vytorin 10/40 Tablets ... 3092
Vytorin 10/80 Tablets ... 2084
Vytorin 10/80 Tablets ... 3092
Wellbutrin SR Sustained-Release Tablets ... 1583
Wellbutrin XL Extended-Release Tablets ... 1588
Zantac (Rare) ... 1597
Zantac Injection (Rare) ... 1593
Zantac Injection Pharmacy Bulk Package (Rare) ... 1595
Zantac Syrup (Rare) ... 1597
Zegerid Powder for Oral Solution (Less than 1%) ... 2972
Zerit (Fewer than 1%) ... 971
Zestoretic Tablets ... 701
Zestril Tablets (0.3% to 1.0%) ... 704
Zetia Tablets ... 2090
Zetia Tablets ... 3098
Ziagen ... 1600
Zithromax ... 2568
Zithromax for Oral Suspension, 300 mg, 600 mg, 900 mg, 1200 mg ... 2561
Zithromax Tablets, 250 mg, 500 mg ... 2561
Zithromax Tablets, 600 mg ... 2568
Zithromax Tri-Pak ... 2561
Zithromax Z-Pak ... 2568
Zmax for Oral Suspension ... 2577
Zocor Tablets ... 2078
Zoloft (Rare) ... 2581
Zomig Tablets (Rare) ... 714
Zomig-ZMT Tablets (Rare) ... 714
Zyban Sustained-Release Tablets ... 1620
Zyprexa Tablets ... 1798
Zyprexa ZYDIS Orally Disintegrating Tablets ... 1798

Pancreatitis, hemorrhagic

Amnesteem Capsules ... 2126

Pancytopenia

Aceon Tablets (2 mg, 4 mg, 8 mg) ... 3191
Actiq (1% or greater) ... 993
Aggrenox Capsules ... 855
Albenza Tablets (Rare) ... 1310
Aloprim for Injection (Less than 1%) ... 2156
Altace Capsules (Less than 1%) ... 1673
Amaryl Tablets ... 2864
Ammonul Injection ... 3323
Anaprox Tablets (Less than 1%) ... 2769
Anaprox DS Tablets (Less than 1%) ... 2769
Arava Tablets (Rare) ... 2881
Arthrotec Tablets (Rare) ... 3126
Asacol Delayed-Release Tablets ... 2688
Avastin IV (Rare) ... 1229
Avonex (Rare) ... 839
Azasan Tablets ... 2844
▲ Campath Ampules (3% to 5%) ... 826
Captopril Tablets ... 2114
Carbatrol Capsules ... 3174
Carimune NF ... 3501
Cataflam Tablets (Rarely) ... 2173
Ceftin ... 1369
▲ CellCept Capsules (3% to less than 20%) ... 2751
▲ CellCept Intravenous (3% to less than 20%) ... 2751
▲ CellCept Oral Suspension (3% to less than 20%) ... 2751
▲ CellCept Tablets (3% to less than 20%) ... 2751
Cipro I.V. (Rare) ... 2998
Cipro I.V. Pharmacy Bulk Package (Rare) ... 3509
Cipro (0.1%) ... 2991
Cipro XR Tablets ... 3004
Copaxone for Injection (Infrequent) ... 3292
Coreg Tablets (Less than or equal to 0.1%) ... 1376
Cosmegen for Injection ... 1907
Cytovene (At least 3 subjects) ... 2763
Daraprim Tablets ... 1385
Depacon Injection ... 412
Depakene ... 417
Depakote Sprinkle Capsules ... 422
Depakote Tablets ... 427
Depakote ER Tablets ... 433
Didronel Tablets (Rare) ... 2693
EC-Naprosyn Delayed-Release Tablets (Less than 1%) ... 2769
Effexor Tablets ... 3405
Effexor XR Capsules (Rare) ... 3411
Elitek (Less than or equal to 1%) ... 2906
Enbrel for Injection (Rare) ... 580
Equetro Extended-Release Capsules ... 3178
Flolan for Injection ... 1408
Fortaz ... 1422
Gammagard Liquid ... 751
Gammagard S/D (Rare) ... 754
Gamunex Immune Globulin I.V., 10% (Rare) ... 3232
Gleevec Tablets (Infrequent) ... 2221
Herceptin I.V. (At least one of the 958 patients) ... 1234
▲ Humira Injection (Less than 5%) ... 464
Imitrex Injection ... 1431
Imitrex Nasal Spray ... 1435
Imitrex Tablets ... 1440
Invirase (Less than 2%) ... 2776
Iveegam EN (Rare) ... 759
Keppra Oral Solution ... 3307
Keppra Tablets ... 3307
Lamictal ... 1449
Leustatin Injection ... 2368
Levaquin in 5% Dextrose Injection (Rare) ... 2453
Levaquin (Rare) ... 2453
Matulane Capsules ... 3188
Maxipime for Injection ... 1093
Mefoxin for Injection ... 1987
Mefoxin Premixed Intravenous Solution ... 1990
Mustargen for Injection ... 2007
Mycamine for Injection ... 620
Myleran Tablets ... 1492
Nalfon Capsules (Less than 1%) ... 2504
Naprosyn Suspension (Less than 1%) ... 2769
Naprosyn Tablets (Less than 1%) ... 2769
Omnicef Capsules ... 506
Omnicef for Oral Suspension ... 506
Oncaspar (Greater than 1% but less than 5%) ... 1123
Orthoclone OKT3 Sterile Solution (Less than 1%) ... 2370
Pacerone Tablets ... 3337
Paxil CR Controlled-Release Tablets ... 1509
Paxil ... 1501
Pentasa Capsules ... 3182
Pepcid Injection (Rare) ... 2017
Pepcid (Rare) ... 2014
Phenytek Capsules (Occasional) ... 2153
Plavix Tablets ... 940
Plavix Tablets ... 2942
Prevacid Delayed-Release Capsules (Less than 1%) ... 3268
Prevacid for Delayed-Release Oral Suspension (Less than 1%) ... 3268
Prevacid NapraPAC ... 3277
Prevacid SoluTab Delayed-Release Orally Disintegrating Tablets (Less than 1%) ... 3268
PREVPAC ... 3281
Prilosec OTC Tablets (Rare) ... 2674
Primaxin I.M. ... 2022
Primaxin I.V. ... 2024
Protonix I.V. ... 3468
Protonix Tablets ... 3465
Prozac Pulvules and Liquid ... 1771
Rapamune Oral Solution and Tablets (Rare) ... 3472
Remicade for IV Injection (Greater than or equal to 0.2%) ... 987
Rescriptor Tablets ... 2535
Retrovir Capsules ... 1533
Retrovir IV Infusion ... 1537
Retrovir ... 1533
Rituxan for Infusion ... 845
Rituxan I.V. ... 1251
Sandostatin LAR Depot (Rare) ... 2264
Suprax ... 1811
▲ Tabloid Tablets (Nearly all patients) ... 1545
Tagamet Tablets (Very rare) ... 1547
Tegretol/Tegretol-XR ... 2278
Temodar Capsules ... 3088
Thalomid Capsules ... 979
Thioridazine Hydrochloride Tablets ... 2122
Thiothixene Capsules ... 2124
Ticlid Tablets (Rare) ... 2813
Topamax Sprinkle Capsules (Rare) ... 2438
Topamax Tablets (Rare) ... 2438
▲ Valcyte Tablets (Less than 5%) ... 2816
Vantin Tablets and Oral Suspension ... 2650
VFEND I.V. (Less than 2%) ... 2543
VFEND Oral Suspension (Less than 2%) ... 2543
VFEND Tablets (Less than 2%) ... 2543
Voltaren Tablets (Rarely) ... 2298
Voltaren-XR Tablets (Rarely) ... 2301
Wellbutrin Tablets (Rare) ... 1579
Wellbutrin SR Sustained-Release Tablets ... 1583
Wellbutrin XL Extended-Release Tablets ... 1588
▲ Xeloda Tablets (Less than 5%) ... 2825
Zantac (Rare) ... 1597
Zantac Injection (Rare) ... 1593
Zantac Injection Pharmacy Bulk Package (Rare) ... 1595
Zantac Syrup (Rare) ... 1597
Zegerid Powder for Oral Solution (Rare) ... 2972
Zevalin Injection (2%) ... 848
Zinacef Injection ... 1604
Zinacef for Injection ... 1604
Zoloft ... 2581
▲ Zometa for Intravenous Infusion (5% to 10%) ... 2306
Zosyn (1% or less) ... 3492
Zyban Sustained-Release Tablets ... 1620

Panencephalitis, sclerosing, subacute

Attenuvax ... 1889
M-M-R II ... 1980

Panic attack

Abilify Tablets (Infrequent) ... 916
Abilify Tablets (Infrequent) ... 2472
Ambien Tablets (Rare) ... 2867
Amerge Tablets (Rare) ... 1312
Celexa (Infrequent) ... 1177
Cozaar Tablets (Less than 1%) ... 1913
Effexor Tablets ... 3405
Effexor XR Capsules ... 3411
Hyzaar ... 1964
Imitrex Injection ... 1431
Imitrex Nasal Spray ... 1435
Imitrex Tablets ... 1440
Lamictal (Infrequent) ... 1449
Lariam Tablets (Occasional) ... 2790
Lexapro Oral Solution (Infrequent) ... 1193
Lexapro Tablets (Infrequent) ... 1193
Paxil CR Controlled-Release Tablets ... 1509
Paxil Tablets ... 1501
Prozac Pulvules and Liquid ... 1771
Surmontil Capsules ... 2347
Symbyax Capsules ... 1788
Tasmar Tablets (1%) ... 3360
Trileptal Oral Suspension ... 2281
Trileptal Tablets ... 2281
Vivactil Tablets ... 2350
Zoloft ... 2581

Panniculitis

Attenuvax ... 1889
M-M-R II ... 1980

Papilledema

Accutane Capsules ... 2740
Decadron Phosphate Injection ... 1931
Depo-Medrol Injectable Suspension ... 2615
Effexor Tablets (Rare) ... 3405
Effexor XR Capsules (Rare) ... 3411
Eskalith ... 1406
Genotropin Lyophilized Powder (A small number of patients) ... 2642
Gleevec Tablets (Rare) ... 2221
Humatrope Vials and Cartridges ... 1756
Hydrocortone Tablets ... 1963
Hyperstat I.V. Injection (1 patient) ... 3031
Increlex Injection ... 3290
Intron A for Injection ... 3038
Lithobid Tablets ... 1670
Lyrica Capsules (Rare) ... 2524
Matulane Capsules ... 3188
▲ Neumega for Injection (1% to 16%) ... 3433
Ortho-Cyclen/Ortho Tri-Cyclen ... 2414
Ortho Tri-Cyclen Lo Tablets ... 2421
Pacerone Tablets ... 3337
Pegasys ... 2793
PEG-Intron Powder for Injection ... 3062
Premphase Tablets ... 3452
Prempro Tablets ... 3452
Roferon-A Injection ... 2805
Soriatane Capsules (Less than 1%) ... 1028
VFEND I.V. (Less than 2%) ... 2543
VFEND Oral Suspension (Less than 2%) ... 2543
VFEND Tablets (Less than 2%) ... 2543

Papilledema, exacerbation of

Intron A for Injection ... 3038

Papillitis

Attenuvax ... 1889
Meruvax II ... 1994
M-M-R II (Infrequent) ... 1980
Mumpsvax (Infrequent) ... 2005

Papillomatosis

Invirase (Less than 2%) ... 2776

Papules

Catapres-TTS (1 of 101 patients) ... 875
Duragesic Transdermal System (1% or greater) ... 2448
Oxistat Cream (0.1%) ... 1498
Tri-Luma Cream (1%) ... 1213

Papules, erythematous

(*see under* Erythema multiforme)

Papules at application site

Lidoderm Patch ... 1107

Paralysis

Aloprim for Injection (Less than 1%) ... 2156
Campath Ampules ... 826
Carbatrol Capsules ... 3174
Coumadin for Injection ... 932
Coumadin Tablets ... 932
Depo-Provera Contraceptive Injection (Less than 1%) ... 2619
depo-subQ provera 104 Injectable Suspension ... 2622

Equetro Extended-Release Capsules ... 3178
Evoxac Capsules ... 1042
Gabitril Tablets (Infrequent) ... 998
▲ Geodon Capsules (14%) ... 2514
Hyperstat I.V. Injection ... 3031
Imitrex Injection ... 1431
Imitrex Tablets (Rare) ... 1440
Lamictal (Rare) ... 1449
Levaquin in 5% Dextrose Injection (0.1% to 0.9%) ... 2453
Levaquin (0.1% to 0.9%) ... 2453
Lovenox Injection (Rare) ... 2931
Lupron Depot 7.5 mg ... 3261
Lupron Depot-PED 7.5 mg, 11.25 mg and 15 mg ... 3266
Lupron Injection Pediatric ... 3256
Mirapex Tablets (1% or more) ... 889
Nipent for Injection (Less than 3%) ... 3216
Norvir (Less than 2%) ... 499
Paxil CR Controlled-Release Tablets (Infrequent) ... 1509
Paxil (Infrequent) ... 1501
Permax Tablets (Infrequent) ... 3357
Prozac Pulvules and Liquid (Rare) ... 1771
Rabies Vaccine RabAvert ... 1011
Relpax Tablets (Rare) ... 2531
Requip Tablets (Infrequent) ... 1528
Rescriptor Tablets ... 2535
Rythmol SR Capsules ... 2736
Tegretol/Tegretol-XR ... 2278
Trileptal Oral Suspension ... 2281
Trileptal Tablets ... 2281
Zyprexa Tablets (Rare) ... 1798
Zyprexa ZYDIS Orally Disintegrating Tablets (Rare) ... 1798
Zyrtec Chewable Tablets (Less than 2%) ... 2589
Zyrtec (Less than 2%) ... 2589
Zyrtec-D 12 Hour Extended Release Tablets (Less than 2%) ... 2591

Paralysis, extraocular muscles
Pravachol Tablets ... 943

Paralysis, facial
Actiq (Less than 1%) ... 993
Altoprev Extended-Release Tablets ... 1151
Angiomax for Injection (Rare) ... 1856
Caduet Tablets (Less than 2%) ... 2507
Copaxone for Injection (Infrequent) ... 3292
Effexor Tablets (Rare) ... 3405
Effexor XR Capsules (Rare) ... 3411
Imitrex Tablets (Rare) ... 1440
Kaletra (Less than 2%) ... 474
Lescol Capsules ... 2227
Lescol Capsules ... 2730
Lescol XL Tablets ... 2227
Lescol XL Tablets ... 2730
Lipitor Tablets (Less than 2%) ... 2495
Neurontin Capsules (Infrequent) ... 2498
Neurontin Oral Solution (Infrequent) ... 2498
Neurontin Tablets (Infrequent) ... 2498
Omacor Capsules ... 2735
Rilutek Tablets (Infrequent) ... 2945
Sonata Capsules (Rare) ... 1686
Uniretic Tablets (Less than 1%) ... 3114
▲ Vesanoid Capsules (3%) ... 2823
Zonegran Capsules (Rare) ... 1089
Zyprexa Tablets (Rare) ... 1798
Zyprexa ZYDIS Orally Disintegrating Tablets (Rare) ... 1798

Paralysis, legs
(*see under* Paralysis, lower extremities)

Paralysis, lower extremities
Naropin Injection ... 640

Paralysis, oculomotor nerve
Cytovene ... 2763

Paralysis, radial nerve
DAPTACEL ... 2964

Paralysis, spinal cord
Lupron Depot 3.75 mg ... 3257
Lupron Depot–3 Month 11.25 mg ... 3262

Paralysis, tongue
Frova Tablets (Rare) ... 1101
Maxalt Tablets (Rare) ... 1983
Maxalt-MLT Orally Disintegrating Tablets (Rare) ... 1983
Topamax Sprinkle Capsules (Rare) ... 2438
Topamax Tablets (Rare) ... 2438

Paralysis, vocal cord
Uniretic Tablets (Less than 1%) ... 3114

Paralysis agitans
(*see under* Parkinsonism)

Paranoia
Adalat CC Tablets (Rare) ... 2978
Allegra-D 12 Hour Extended-Release Tablets (Less than 1%) ... 2860
Allegra-D 24 Hour Extended-Release Tablets (Less than 1%) ... 2862
Aricept Tablets (Infrequent) ... 1086
Aricept ODT Tablets (Infrequent) ... 1086
Arthrotec Tablets (Rare) ... 3126
Avelox ... 2984
Celexa (Infrequent) ... 1177
Cipro I.V. (1% or less) ... 2998
Cipro I.V. Pharmacy Bulk Package (1% or less) ... 3509
Cipro ... 2991
Cipro XR Tablets ... 3004
Clozapine Tablets (Less than 1%) ... 2141
Clozaril Tablets (Less than 1%) ... 2174
Copaxone for Injection (Infrequent) ... 3292
Duragesic Transdermal System (1% or greater) ... 2448
Effexor Tablets (Infrequent) ... 3405
Effexor XR Capsules (Infrequent) ... 3411
Evoxac Capsules ... 1042
Exelon Capsules (2% or more) ... 2204
FazaClo Orally Disintegrating Tablets (Less than 1%) ... 547
Flexeril Tablets ... 1832
Gabitril Tablets (Frequent) ... 998
Lamictal (Infrequent) ... 1449
Lariam Tablets (Occasional) ... 2790
Levaquin in 5% Dextrose Injection (0.1% to 0.9%) ... 2453
Levaquin (0.1% to 0.9%) ... 2453
▲ Marinol Capsules (3% to 10%) ... 3334
Neurontin Capsules (Infrequent) ... 2498
Neurontin Oral Solution (Infrequent) ... 2498
Neurontin Tablets (Infrequent) ... 2498
Orthoclone OKT3 Sterile Solution (Less than 1%) ... 2370
Paxil CR Controlled-Release Tablets (Infrequent) ... 1509
Paxil (Infrequent) ... 1501
Permax Tablets (Frequent) ... 3357
Prozac Pulvules and Liquid (Infrequent) ... 1771
Razadyne ER Extended-Release Capsules (Infrequent) ... 2434
Razadyne (Infrequent) ... 2434
Requip Tablets (Infrequent) ... 1528
Rescriptor Tablets ... 2535
Rilutek Tablets (Infrequent) ... 2945
Sandostatin Injection (Less than 1%) ... 2263
Sandostatin LAR Depot (Rare) ... 2264
Seroquel Tablets (Infrequent) ... 691
Stalevo Tablets ... 2270
Sustiva Capsules (0.4%) ... 957
Symmetrel ... 1115
Tasmar Tablets (Infrequent) ... 3360
Tequin Injection (Less than 0.1%) ... 964
Tequin Tablets (Less than 0.1%) ... 964
Topamax Sprinkle Capsules (Infrequent) ... 2438
Topamax Tablets (Infrequent) ... 2438
Trileptal Oral Suspension ... 2281
Trileptal Tablets ... 2281
Ultracet Tablets (Less than 1%) ... 2462
Wellbutrin Tablets (Infrequent) ... 1579
Wellbutrin SR Sustained-Release Tablets ... 1583
Wellbutrin XL Extended-Release Tablets ... 1588
Zoloft (Infrequent) ... 2581
Zyban Sustained-Release Tablets ... 1620
Zyprexa Tablets ... 1798
Zyprexa ZYDIS Orally Disintegrating Tablets ... 1798

Paranoid ideation
Parcopa Orally Disintegrating Tablets ... 3111

Paraparesis
Depo-Medrol Single-Dose Vial ... 2617
Leustatin Injection ... 2368
Orthoclone OKT3 Sterile Solution (Less than 1%) ... 2370

Paraplegia
Copaxone for Injection (Infrequent) ... 3292
Orthoclone OKT3 Sterile Solution ... 2370

Paraproteinemia
▲ Humira Injection (Less than 5%) ... 464

Parathyroid disorder, unspecified
▲ Carnitor Injection (2% to 6%) ... 3185
▲ CellCept Capsules (3% to less than 20%) ... 2751
▲ CellCept Intravenous (3% to less than 20%) ... 2751
▲ CellCept Oral Suspension (3% to less than 20%) ... 2751
▲ CellCept Tablets (3% to less than 20%) ... 2751
▲ Humira Injection (Less than 5%) ... 464

Parathyroid hormone deficiency, fetal
Accutane Capsules ... 2740

Parathyroid neoplasm
Amerge Tablets (Rare) ... 1312

Parenchymatous organs, toxic damage
Gemzar for Injection (Rare) ... 1743
Tagamet Tablets (Highly unlikely) ... 1547

Paresis
Aldara Cream, 5% ... 1814
Ambien Tablets (Rare) ... 2867
Colazal Capsules ... 2845
Coreg Tablets (Less than or equal to 0.1%) ... 1376
Engerix-B Vaccine ... 1391
Exelon Capsules (Infrequent) ... 2204
▲ Imdur Tablets (Less than or equal to 5%) ... 3032
▲ Intron A for Injection (Less than 5%) ... 3038
Invirase (Less than 2%) ... 2776
Klonopin (Infrequent) ... 2782
Leukeran Tablets (Rare) ... 1472
Naropin Injection (Less than 1%) ... 640
Neurontin Capsules (Infrequent) ... 2498
Neurontin Oral Solution (Infrequent) ... 2498
Neurontin Tablets (Infrequent) ... 2498
▲ Requip Tablets (3%) ... 1528
Sandostatin LAR Depot (Rare) ... 2264
Seromycin Capsules ... 1783
Tambocor Tablets (1% to 3%) ... 1824
Tasmar Tablets (1% or more) ... 3360
▲ Temodar Capsules (8%) ... 3088
Twinrix Vaccine ... 1571

Paresthesia
Abilify Tablets (Infrequent) ... 916
Abilify Tablets (Infrequent) ... 2472
Accutane Capsules ... 2740
Aceon Tablets (2 mg, 4 mg, 8 mg) (2.3%) ... 3191
Aciphex Tablets ... 1081
Actiq (Less than 1%) ... 993
Actonel Tablets (2.1%) ... 2679
Actonel with Calcium Tablets (2.1%) ... 2684
▲ Adalat CC Tablets (3% or less) ... 2978
Adenoscan (2%) ... 613
Advair Diskus 100/50 ... 1291
Advair Diskus 250/50 ... 1291
Advair Diskus 500/50 ... 1291
Advicor Tablets ... 1694
▲ Agenerase Capsules (9% to 11%) ... 1299
▲ Agenerase Oral Solution (9% to 11%) ... 1304
Aggrenox Capsules (Less than 1%) ... 855
▲ Agrylin Capsules (5.9%) ... 3172
Aldoclor Tablets ... 1881
Aldoril Tablets ... 1884
▲ Aldurazyme for Intravenous Infusion (3%) ... 1261
Aloxi Injection (Less than 1%) ... 2099
Altace Capsules (Less than 1%) ... 1673
Altoprev Extended-Release Tablets ... 1151
Ambien Tablets (Infrequent) ... 2867
AmBisome for Injection (Less common) ... 615
Amerge Tablets (1% to 2%) ... 1312
Amnesteem Capsules ... 2126
Anaprox Tablets (Less than 1%) ... 2769
Anaprox DS Tablets (Less than 1%) ... 2769
AndroGel (Fewer than 1%) ... 3330
Antara Capsules ... 2723
Anzemet Injection (Infrequently) ... 2871
Anzemet Tablets (Infrequently) ... 2874
Arava Tablets (2%) ... 2881
Aredia for Injection ... 2168
Aricept Tablets (Frequent) ... 1086
Aricept ODT Tablets (Frequent) ... 1086
▲ Arimidex Tablets (4% to 6%) ... 665
Aromasin Tablets (Less frequent) ... 2600
Arthrotec Tablets (Rare) ... 3126
Asacol Delayed-Release Tablets (2% or greater) ... 2688
Astelin Nasal Spray ... 1876
Atacand Tablets (0.5% or greater) ... 634
Atacand HCT (0.5% or greater) ... 637
Avalide Tablets ... 922
Avalide Tablets ... 2889
Avapro Tablets (Less than 1%) ... 925
Avapro Tablets (Less than 1%) ... 2886
Avelox (Less than 0.1%) ... 2984
▲ Avinza Capsules (5% to 10%) ... 1714
Avonex ... 839
Axert Tablets (1%) ... 2430
Betagan Ophthalmic Solution, USP ... ⊙ 217
Betaseron for SC Injection ... 791
Betimol Ophthalmic Solution ... ⊙ 283
Betimol Ophthalmic Solution ... 3371
▲ BiDil Tablets (4%) ... 2161
Blocadren Tablets (0.6%) ... 1891
Boostrix ... 1366
Brevibloc Concentrate (Less than 1%) ... 766
Brevibloc Injection (Less than 1%) ... 766
Brevibloc Double Strength Injection (Less than 1%) ... 766
Brevibloc Premixed Injection (Less than 1%) ... 766
Brevibloc Double Strength Premixed Injection (Less than 1%) ... 766
Caduet Tablets (Greater than 0.1%) ... 2507
▲ Campral Tablets (2% to 3%) ... 1175
▲ Cancidas for Injection (0% to 3.1%) ... 1894
Captopril Tablets (About 0.5% to 2%) ... 2114
Carbatrol Capsules ... 3174
Cardene I.V. (0.7%) ... 1129
Cardizem LA Extended Release Tablets (Less than 2%) ... 1699
▲ Carnitor Injection (3% to 12%) ... 3185
▲ Casodex Tablets (6%) ... 670
Cataflam Tablets (Occasionally) ... 2173
Celebrex Capsules (0.1% to 1.9%) ... 3130
Celexa (Frequent) ... 1177
▲ CellCept Capsules (3% to 20.8%) ... 2751
▲ CellCept Intravenous (3% to 20.8%) ... 2751
▲ CellCept Oral Suspension (3% to 20.8%) ... 2751
▲ CellCept Tablets (3% to 20.8%) ... 2751
▲ Cenestin Tablets, 0.45mg, 0.625mg, 0.9mg, 1.25mg (7.5% to 33%) ... 1063
▲ Chemet Capsules (1.0% to 12.7%) ... 2480
Cialis Tablets (Less than 2%) ... 1806
Cipro I.V. (1% or less) ... 2998
Cipro I.V. Pharmacy Bulk Package (1% or less) ... 3509
Cipro (Less than 1%) ... 2991
Cipro XR Tablets ... 3004
Clinoril Tablets (Less than 1%) ... 1899
Clorpres Tablets ... 2139
Clozapine Tablets ... 2141
Clozaril Tablets ... 2174
Combivent Inhalation Aerosol (Less than 2%) ... 878
Combivir Tablets ... 1373
Copaxone for Injection (At least 2%) ... 3292
▲ Coreg Tablets (Greater than 1% to 3%) ... 1376
Cosopt Sterile Ophthalmic Solution (1% to 5%) ... 1910
Coumadin for Injection (Infrequent) ... 932
Coumadin Tablets (Infrequent) ... 932
Covera-HS Tablets (1%) ... 3135
Cozaar Tablets (Less than 1%) ... 1913
Crestor Tablets (Greater than or equal to 2%) ... 672
Cubicin for Injection (Less than 1%) ... 1038
Cytovene ... 2763
▲ Daranide Tablets (Among the most common effects) ... 1928
Decadron Tablets ... 1929
Delatestryl Injection ... 2976
Denavir Cream ... 2163
▲ Depacon Injection (0.9% to 5%) ... 412
▲ Depakene (1% to 5%) ... 417
▲ Depakote Sprinkle Capsules (1% to 5%) ... 422
▲ Depakote Tablets (1% to 5%) ... 427
▲ Depakote ER Tablets (1% to 5%) ... 433
DepoCyt Injection ... 1121
▲ DepoDur Extended-Release Injection (2% to 5%) ... 1098
Depo-Provera Contraceptive Injection (Less than 1%) ... 2619
depo-subQ provera 104 Injectable Suspension ... 2622
Detrol Tablets (1.1%) ... 2626
Didronel Tablets ... 2693
Dilaudid ... 439

Dilaudid Oral Liquid (Less frequent)........ 443
Dilaudid Non-Sterile Powder........ 439
Dilaudid Rectal Suppositories........ 439
Dilaudid Tablets........ 439
Dilaudid Tablets - 8 mg (Less frequent)........ 443
Dilaudid-HP (Less frequent)........ 441
Diovan HCT Tablets (Greater than 0.2%)........ 2195
Diovan Tablets........ 2191
Diprivan Injectable Emulsion (Less than 1%)........ 676
Diuril Oral........ 1936
Diuril Sodium Intravenous........ 1934
Dolobid Tablets (Less than 1 in 100)........ 1937
▲ Dostinex Tablets (1% to less than 10%)........ 2631
▲ Doxil Injection (Less than 1% to 10%)........ 3302
Duragesic Transdermal System (1% or greater)........ 2448
Dyazide Capsules........ 1389
DynaCirc CR Tablets (0.5% to 1%)........ 2726
EC-Naprosyn Delayed-Release Tablets (Less than 1%)........ 2769
▲ Effexor Tablets (3%)........ 3405
▲ Effexor XR Capsules (2% to 3%)........ 3411
Elitek (Less than or equal to 1%)........ 2906
Elocon Cream 0.1% (2 in 182 patients)........ 3019
Elocon Lotion 0.1% (2 in 65 patients)........ 3020
▲ Emtriva Capsules (5% to 6%)........ 1272
Enbrel for Injection........ 580
Engerix-B Vaccine........ 1391
▲ Entocort EC Capsules (Less than 5%)........ 2694
▲ Epivir (13%)........ 1394
Epivir-HBV........ 1398
▲ Epogen for Injection (11%)........ 586
Epzicom Tablets........ 1402
Equetro Extended-Release Capsules........ 3178
Estratest Tablets........ 3196
Estratest H.S. Tablets........ 3196
Evoxac Capsules (Less than 1%)........ 1042
Exelon Capsules (Frequent)........ 2204
▲ Fabrazyme for Intravenous Infusion (4%)........ 1267
Factive Tablets (Rare)........ 2464
Famvir Tablets (0.9% to 2.6%)........ 2207
▲ Faslodex Injection (6.4%)........ 682
FazaClo Orally Disintegrating Tablets........ 547
▲ Ferrlecit Injection (6%)........ 3379
Flexeril Tablets (Less than 1%)........ 1832
▲ Flolan for Injection (1% to 12%)........ 1408
Floxin Otic Singles (1%)........ 1045
Floxin Otic Solution (1%)........ 1043
Fortaz (Less than 1%)........ 1422
▲ Fortical Nasal Spray (1% to 3%)........ 3336
▲ Frova Tablets (4%)........ 1101
Furosemide Tablets........ 2117
▲ Gabitril Tablets (3%)........ 998
Gemzar for Injection (Less than 1%)........ 1743
▲ Gengraf Capsules (1% to 11%)........ 458
Geodon (Frequent)........ 2514
Gleevec Tablets (Less common)........ 2221
Havrix Vaccine (Rare)........ 1425
▲ Hectorol Capsules (Greater than or equal to 5%)........ 909
▲ Herceptin I.V. (9%)........ 1234
▲ Humatrope Vials and Cartridges (13.6% to 17.3%)........ 1756
▲ Humira Injection (Less than 5%)........ 464
▲ Hycamtin for Injection (9%)........ 1427
Hytrin Capsules (0.8% to 1.9%)........ 469
Hyzaar........ 1964
▲ Imdur Tablets (Less than or equal to 5%)........ 3032
▲ Imitrex Injection (5%)........ 1431
Imitrex Nasal Spray (Infrequent)........ 1435
Imitrex Tablets (Frequent)........ 1440
Indapamide Tablets........ 2119
Indocin (Less than 1%)........ 1968
Infed Injection........ 3381
▲ Infergen (9% to 13%)........ 1647
▲ Intron A for Injection (1% to 21%)........ 3038
Invanz for Injection (Greater than 0.1%)........ 1974
Inversine Tablets........ 3286
Invirase (0.3% to greater than or equal to 2%)........ 2776
Kadian Capsules (Less than 3%)........ 572
Kaletra (Up to 2%)........ 474
▲ Kepivance (12%)........ 592
Keppra Oral Solution (2%)........ 3307
Keppra Tablets (2%)........ 3307
Ketek Tablets (Less than 0.2%)........ 2920
Klonopin (Infrequent)........ 2782
Lamictal (More than 1%)........ 1449
Lariam Tablets (Occasional)........ 2790
Lescol Capsules........ 2227
Lescol Capsules........ 2730
Lescol XL Tablets........ 2227
Lescol XL Tablets........ 2730
▲ Leukine (11%)........ 829
Levaquin in 5% Dextrose Injection (0.1% to 0.9%)........ 2453
Levaquin (0.1% to 0.9%)........ 2453
Levitra Tablets (Less than 2%)........ 3048
Lexapro Oral Solution (2%)........ 1193
Lexapro Tablets (2%)........ 1193
Lidoderm Patch........ 1107
Lipitor Tablets (Less than 2%)........ 2495
Lofibra Capsules........ 1217
Lotensin Tablets (Less than 1%)........ 2232
Lotensin HCT Tablets (0.3% to 1%)........ 2235
Lotrisone (1.9%)........ 3054
Lunesta Tablets (Infrequent)........ 3139
Lupron Depot 3.75 mg (Less than 5%)........ 3257
Lupron Depot 7.5 mg (Less than 5%)........ 3261
▲ Lupron Depot–3 Month 11.25 mg (1.2% to 7%)........ 3262
Luxíq Foam (One patient)........ 1026
Lyrica Capsules (Greater than or equal to 2%)........ 2524
Matulane Capsules........ 3188
Mavik Tablets (0.3% to 1.0%)........ 482
▲ Maxalt Tablets (3% to 4%)........ 1983
▲ Maxalt-MLT Orally Disintegrating Tablets (3% to 4%)........ 1983
Maxzide........ 2150
▲ Megace ES Oral Suspension (1% to 3%)........ 2492
Meridia Capsules (2%)........ 485
Merrem I.V. (Greater than 0.1% to 1%)........ 687
Meruvax II........ 1994
Mevacor Tablets (0.5% to 1.0%)........ 1996
Miacalcin Nasal Spray (1% to 3%)........ 2242
Micardis Tablets (More than 0.3%)........ 884
Micardis HCT Tablets........ 886
Midamor Tablets (Less than or equal to 1%)........ 2000
Migranal Nasal Spray (2%)........ 3350
Mirapex Tablets (1% or more)........ 889
M-M-R II........ 1980
Mobic Oral Suspension (Less than 2%)........ 893
Mobic Tablets (Less than 2%)........ 893
Moduretic Tablets (Less than or equal to 1%)........ 2003
MS Contin Tablets (Less frequent)........ 2703
Nadolol Tablets (6 of 1000 patients)........ 2121
Namenda (Infrequent)........ 1199
Naprosyn Suspension (Less than 1%)........ 2769
Naprosyn Tablets (Less than 1%)........ 2769
Narcan Injection........ 1109
▲ Naropin Injection (More than 5% to 6.9%)........ 640
Nasacort HFA Inhalation Aerosol........ 2939
Natrecor for Injection (Greater than or equal to 1%)........ 3123
▲ Navelbine Injection (Up to 17%)........ 1494
▲ Neoral Soft Gelatin Capsules (1% to 11%)........ 2247
▲ Neoral Oral Solution (1% to 11%)........ 2247
Neumega for Injection........ 3433
Neurontin Capsules (Frequent)........ 2498
Neurontin Oral Solution (Infrequent)........ 2498
Neurontin Tablets (Frequent)........ 2498
Nexium Delayed-Release Capsules (Less than 1%)........ 645
Nexium I.V. (Less than 1%)........ 649
Niaspan Extended-Release Tablets........ 1703
▲ Nicotrol Inhaler (Greater than 3%)........ 2594
Nicotrol NS........ 2596
▲ Nipent for Injection (3% to 10%)........ 3216
Niravam Orally Disintegrating Tablets (2.4%)........ 3106
▲ Norditropin Cartridges (11%)........ 2318
Noroxin Tablets........ 2009
Norvasc Tablets (More than 0.1% to 1%)........ 2529
▲ Norvir (2.6% to 3%)........ 499
Oncaspar (Greater than 1% but less than 5%)........ 1123
▲ Ontak Vials (13%)........ 1717
OxyContin Tablets (Less than 1%)........ 2699
▲ Pacerone Tablets (4% to 9%)........ 3337
Pandel Cream, 0.1% (0.4%)........ 1017
Parcopa Orally Disintegrating Tablets........ 3111
Parnate Tablets........ 1499
▲ Paxil CR Controlled-Release Tablets (1.0% to 5.9%)........ 1509
▲ Paxil (1.0% to 5.9%)........ 1501
Pentasa Capsules (Less than 1%)........ 3182
Pepcid Injection (Infrequent)........ 2017
Pepcid (Infrequent)........ 2014
Permax Tablets (1.6%)........ 3357
Persantine Tablets (Rare)........ 898
Plavix Tablets (1% to 2.5%)........ 940
Plavix Tablets (1% to 2.5%)........ 2942
Plendil Extended-Release Tablets (1.2% to 1.6%)........ 651
Pletal Tablets (2% or greater)........ 2478
Pneumovax 23 (Rare)........ 2020
▲ Prandin Tablets (0.5, 1, and 2 mg) (2% to 3%)........ 2337
Pravachol Tablets........ 943
Prevacid Delayed-Release Capsules (Less than 1%)........ 3268
Prevacid for Delayed-Release Oral Suspension (Less than 1%)........ 3268
Prevacid I.V. for Injection (Less than 1%)........ 3274
Prevacid NapraPAC (Less than 1%)........ 3277
Prevacid SoluTab Delayed-Release Orally Disintegrating Tablets (Less than 1%)........ 3268
PREVPAC (Less than 1%)........ 3281
Prilosec OTC Tablets (Less than 1%)........ 2674
Primaxin I.M.........2022
Primaxin I.V. (Less than 0.2%)........ 2024
Prinivil Tablets (0.3% to 1.0%)........ 2029
Prinzide Tablets (1.5%)........ 2033
▲ ProAmatine Tablets (18.3%)........ 3183
▲ Procrit for Injection (11%)........ 2374
▲ Prograf Capsules and Injection (17% to 40%)........ 624
ProSom Tablets (Infrequent)........ 512
Protonix I.V. (Less than 1%)........ 3468
Protonix Tablets (Less than 1%)........ 3465
Protopic Ointment (Greater than or equal to 1%)........ 629
Provigil Tablets (2%)........ 1002
Prozac Pulvules and Liquid........ 1771
Rabies Vaccine RabAvert (Rare)........ 1011
▲ Rapamune Oral Solution and Tablets (3% to 20%)........ 3472
Razadyne ER Extended-Release Capsules (Infrequent)........ 2434
Razadyne (Infrequent)........ 2434
Relafen Tablets (Less than 1%)........ 1523
▲ Relpax Tablets (3% to 4%)........ 2531
▲ Requip Tablets (3% to 5%)........ 1528
▲ Retrovir Capsules (6%)........ 1533
▲ Retrovir IV Infusion (6%)........ 1537
▲ Retrovir (6%)........ 1533
▲ Revatio Tablets (3%)........ 2541
Risperdal Consta Long-Acting Injection (Infrequent)........ 1664
Risperdal M-Tab Orally Disintegrating Tablets (Infrequent)........ 1658
Risperdal (Infrequent)........ 1658
▲ Rituxan for Infusion (1% to 5%)........ 845
▲ Rituxan I.V. (1% to 5%)........ 1251
▲ Roferon-A Injection (7% to 12%)........ 2805
Rythmol SR Capsules........ 2736
▲ Sandimmune (1% to 3%)........ 2259
▲ Sandostatin LAR Depot (5% to 15%)........ 2264
Serevent Diskus (1% to 3%)........ 1540
Seromycin Capsules........ 1783
▲ Simulect for Injection (3% to 10%)........ 2268
Singulair........ 2047
▲ Somavert Injection (7%)........ 2648
▲ Sonata Capsules (3%)........ 1686
▲ Soriatane Capsules (10% to 25%)........ 1028
▲ Spiriva HandiHaler (1% to 3%)........ 899
Stalevo Tablets........ 2270
▲ Strattera Capsules (4%)........ 1784
Sular Tablets (Less than or equal to 1%)........ 1163
Sustiva Capsules (Less than 2%)........ 957
Symmetrel........ 1115
Synercid I.V. (Less than 1%)........ 1690
Tambocor Tablets (1% to 3%)........ 1824
Tarka Tablets (Less frequent)........ 519
Tasmar Tablets (1% to 3%)........ 3360
▲ Taxotere Injection Concentrate (7 of 134 patients)........ 2947
Tegretol/Tegretol-XR........ 2278
▲ Temodar Capsules (9%)........ 3088
▲ Tequin Injection (0.1% to 3%)........ 964
▲ Tequin Tablets (0.1% to 3%)........ 964
Teveten Tablets (Less than 1%)........ 1707
Teveten HCT Tablets (Less than 1%)........ 1710
▲ Thalomid Capsules (5.6% to 15.6%)........ 979
Thyrogen for Injection (1.6%)........ 1270
Tiazac Capsules (Less than 2%)........ 1204
Timolide Tablets........ 2056
Timoptic in Ocudose (Less frequent)........ 2061
Timoptic Sterile Ophthalmic Solution (Less frequent)........ 2058
Timoptic-XE Sterile Ophthalmic Gel Forming Solution........ 2062
Tindamax........ 2670
▲ Topamax Sprinkle Capsules (1% to 51%)........ 2438
▲ Topamax Tablets (1% to 51%)........ 2438
Toprol-XL Tablets........ 660
Tricor Tablets........ 523
▲ Tri-Luma Cream (3%)........ 1213
▲ Trisenox Injection (33%)........ 983
Trizivir Tablets........ 1565
Trusopt Sterile Ophthalmic Solution........ 2065
Truvada Tablets........ 1279
Twinrix Vaccine (Less than 1%)........ 1571
Ultracet Tablets (Less than 1%)........ 2462
Uniretic Tablets (Less than 1%)........ 3114
▲ Valcyte Tablets (8%)........ 2816
Vantin Tablets and Oral Suspension (Less than 1%)........ 2650
Varivax........ 2070
Vaseretic Tablets (0.5% to 2.0%)........ 2073
Vasotec I.V. Injection (0.5% to 1.0%)........ 2076
▲ Velcade for Injection (27%)........ 2102
Verelan PM Capsules (2% or less)........ 3120
▲ Vesanoid Capsules (17%)........ 2823
VFEND I.V. (Less than 2%)........ 2543
VFEND Oral Suspension (Less than 2%)........ 2543
VFEND Tablets (Less than 2%)........ 2543
Viadur Implant (Less than 2%)........ 782
Viagra Tablets (Less than 2%)........ 2552
Vicoprofen Tablets (Less than 3%)........ 533
Viracept (Less than 2%)........ 2556
Viramune Oral Suspension........ 903
Viramune Tablets........ 903
Voltaren Tablets (Occasionally)........ 2298
Voltaren-XR Tablets (Occasionally)........ 2301
Vytorin 10/10 Tablets........ 2084
Vytorin 10/10 Tablets........ 3092
Vytorin 10/20 Tablets........ 2084
Vytorin 10/20 Tablets........ 3092
Vytorin 10/40 Tablets........ 2084
Vytorin 10/40 Tablets........ 3092
Vytorin 10/80 Tablets........ 2084
Vytorin 10/80 Tablets........ 3092
Wellbutrin Tablets........ 1579
Wellbutrin SR Sustained-Release Tablets (1% to 2%)........ 1583
Wellbutrin XL Extended-Release Tablets (1% to 2%)........ 1588
▲ Xanax XR Tablets (2.4% to 7.1%)........ 2655
▲ Xeloda Tablets (1% to 21%)........ 2825
Xopenex HFA Inhalation Aerosol........ 3151
Xopenex Inhalation Solution........ 3143
Xopenex Inhalation Solution Concentrate........ 3147
▲ Zavesca Capsules (7%)........ 543
Zegerid Powder for Oral Solution (Less than 1%)........ 2972
Zemaira (0.2% to 0.4%)........ 3506
▲ Zenapax for Injection (2% to 5%)........ 2838
Zestoretic Tablets (1.5%)........ 701
Zestril Tablets (0.3% to 1.0%)........ 704
Ziagen........ 1600
Zithromax Capsules, 250 mg........ 2568
Zithromax for IV Infusion........ 2573
Zithromax for Oral Suspension, 1 g........ 2568
Zithromax for Oral Suspension, 300 mg, 600 mg, 900 mg, 1200 mg........ 2561
Zithromax Tablets, 250 mg, 500 mg........ 2561
Zithromax Tablets, 600 mg........ 2568
Zithromax Tri-Pak........ 2561
Zithromax Z-Pak........ 2568
Zmax for Oral Suspension........ 2577
Zocor Tablets........ 2078
Zofran Injection (2%)........ 1607
Zoladex (1% or greater)........ 709
Zoladex 3-month (1% to 5%)........ 712
▲ Zoloft (3%)........ 2581
▲ Zometa for Intravenous Infusion (15%)........ 2306
▲ Zomig Nasal Spray (5% to 10%)........ 718
▲ Zomig Tablets (5% to 9%)........ 714
▲ Zomig-ZMT Tablets (5% to 9%)........ 714
▲ Zonegran Capsules (4%)........ 1089
Zovirax Capsules........ 1616
Zovirax for Injection........ 1618
Zovirax........ 1616
Zyban Sustained-Release Tablets (Infrequent)........ 1620
Zyprexa Tablets........ 1798
Zyprexa ZYDIS Orally Disintegrating Tablets........ 1798
Zyrtec Chewable Tablets (Less than 2%)........ 2589
Zyrtec (Less than 2%)........ 2589
Zyrtec-D 12 Hour Extended Release Tablets (Less than 2%)........ 2591

Paresthesia, circumoral
▲ Agenerase Oral Solution (26% to 31%) 1304
Copaxone for Injection (Infrequent) 3292
Effexor Tablets (Infrequent) 3405
Effexor XR Capsules (Infrequent) 3411
Gabitril Tablets (Infrequent) 998
Geodon Capsules (Rare) 2514
Lyrica Capsules (0.1% to 1%) 2524
Neurontin Capsules (Infrequent) 2498
Neurontin Oral Solution (Infrequent) 2498
Neurontin Tablets (Infrequent) 2498
▲ Norvir (3.4% to 6.7%) 499
Paxil CR Controlled-Release Tablets (Rare) 1509
Paxil (Rare) 1501
ProSom Tablets (Rare) 512
Prozac Pulvules and Liquid (Rare) 1771
▲ Rilutek Tablets (1.3% to 3.3%) 2945
Sonata Capsules (Infrequent) 1686
Thalomid Capsules 979
Zomig Nasal Spray (Infrequent) 718
Zonegran Capsules (Rare) 1089
Zyprexa Tablets (Rare) 1798
Zyprexa ZYDIS Orally Disintegrating Tablets (Rare) 1798

Paresthesia, extremities
Surmontil Capsules 2347
Vivactil Tablets 2350

Paresthesia, facial
Guanidine Hydrochloride Tablets 3030

Paresthesia, feet
Grifulvin V Tablets Microsize and Oral Suspension Microsize (Rare) 2384
Gris-PEG Tablets (Rare) 2504
Guanidine Hydrochloride Tablets 3030
Lupron Depot 7.5 mg 3261

Paresthesia, hands
Grifulvin V Tablets Microsize and Oral Suspension Microsize (Rare) 2384
Gris-PEG Tablets (Rare) 2504
Guanidine Hydrochloride Tablets 3030
Inderal LA Long-Acting Capsules 3421
InnoPran XL Capsules 2728
Oncaspar 1123

Paresthesia, head
Nicotrol NS 2596

Paresthesia, lip
Guanidine Hydrochloride Tablets 3030

Paresthesia, nose
Nicotrol NS 2596

Paresthesia, oral
▲ Agenerase Capsules (26% to 31%) 1299
▲ Agenerase Oral Solution (26% to 31%) 1304
Crixivan Capsules 1918
▲ Lexiva Tablets (Less than 1% to 10%) 1473
Nicotrol NS 2596

Paresthesia, peripheral
▲ Agenerase Capsules (10% to 14%) 1299
▲ Agenerase Oral Solution (10% to 14%) 1304
▲ Norvir (5% to 6%) 499

Parkinsonism
Aldoclor Tablets 1881
Aldoril Tablets 1884
Clozapine Tablets (Less than 1%) 2141
Clozaril Tablets (Less than 1%) 2174
Demser Capsules 1933
Depakene 417
Depakote Tablets 427
Depakote ER Tablets 433
FazaClo Orally Disintegrating Tablets (Less than 1%) 547
Indocin (Less than 1%) 1968
Orap Tablets 1220
▲ Risperdal Consta Long-Acting Injection (4% to 10%) 1664
▲ Risperdal M-Tab Orally Disintegrating Tablets (0.6% to 6%) 1658
▲ Risperdal (0.6% to 6%) 1658
Seroquel Tablets 691
▲ Zyprexa Tablets (8% to 20%) 1798
▲ Zyprexa IntraMuscular (2% to 4%) 1798
▲ Zyprexa ZYDIS Orally Disintegrating Tablets (8% to 20%) 1798

Parkinsonism, aggravation of
▲ Apokyn Injection (At least 5%) 2132
Lamictal 1449
Requip Tablets (1% or more) 1528
Risperdal M-Tab Orally Disintegrating Tablets 1658
Risperdal 1658

Parkinson-like symptoms
Actimmune (Rare) 1646
Elspar for Injection (Rare) 1943
Moban Tablets 1108
Oncaspar 1123
Orap Tablets (Frequent) 1220

Paroniria
Allegra (Less than 1%) 2857
Celexa (Infrequent) 1177
Coreg Tablets (Greater than 0.1% to 1%) 1376
Evoxac Capsules (Less than 1%) 1042
Gengraf Capsules (1% to less than 3%) 458
▲ Imdur Tablets (Less than or equal to 5%) 3032
▲ Intron A for Injection (Less than 5%) 3038
Namenda (Infrequent) 1199
Neoral Soft Gelatin Capsules (1% to less than 3%) 2247
Neoral Oral Solution (1% to less than 3%) 2247
Razadyne ER Extended-Release Capsules (Infrequent) 2434
Razadyne (Infrequent) 2434
Risperdal Consta Long-Acting Injection (Infrequent) 1664
Zoloft (Infrequent) 2581
Zyrtec Chewable Tablets (Less than 2%) 2589
Zyrtec (Less than 2%) 2589
Zyrtec-D 12 Hour Extended Release Tablets (Less than 2%) 2591

Paronychia
Accutane Capsules 2740
Amnesteem Capsules 2126
Crixivan Capsules 1918
Evoxac Capsules (Less than 1%) 1042
▲ Soriatane Capsules (10% to 25%) 1028

Parosmia
Ambien Tablets (Rare) 2867
Astelin Nasal Spray 1876
Avelox (Less than 0.1%) 2984
Axert Tablets (Rare) 2430
Caduet Tablets (Less than 2%) 2507
Colazal Capsules 2845
Denavir Cream 2163
Doxil Injection (Less than 1%) 3302
Effexor Tablets (Infrequent) 3405
Effexor XR Capsules (Infrequent) 3411
Evoxac Capsules (Less than 1%) 1042
Flumadine (Less than 0.3%) 1186
Fortical Nasal Spray (Less than 1%) 3336
Gabitril Tablets (Infrequent) 998
▲ Intron A for Injection (Less than 5%) 3038
Lamictal (Rare) 1449
Levaquin in 5% Dextrose Injection (0.1% to 0.9%) 2453
Levaquin (0.1% to 0.9%) 2453
Lipitor Tablets (Less than 2%) 2495
Lyrica Capsules (Rare) 2524
Miacalcin Nasal Spray (Less than 1%) 2242
Nexium Delayed-Release Capsules (Less than 1%) 645
Nexium I.V. (Less than 1%) 649
Norvasc Tablets (Less than or equal to 0.1%) 2529
Norvir (Less than 2%) 499
Paxil CR Controlled-Release Tablets (Rare) 1509
Paxil (Rare) 1501
Prevacid Delayed-Release Capsules (Less than 1%) 3268
Prevacid for Delayed-Release Oral Suspension (Less than 1%) 3268
Prevacid NapraPAC (Less than 1%) 3277
Prevacid SoluTab Delayed-Release Orally Disintegrating Tablets (Less than 1%) 3268
PREVPAC (Less than 1%) 3281
Prozac Pulvules and Liquid (Rare) 1771
Relpax Tablets (Rare) 2531
Rescriptor Tablets 2535
Sonata Capsules (Less than 1% to 2%) 1686
Sustiva Capsules (Less than 2%) 957
Tasmar Tablets (Infrequent) 3360
Tequin Injection (Less than 0.1%) 964
Tequin Tablets (Less than 0.1%) 964
Topamax Sprinkle Capsules (Infrequent) 2438
Topamax Tablets (Infrequent) 2438
Zomig Nasal Spray (Infrequent) 718
Zomig Tablets (Infrequent) 714
Zomig-ZMT Tablets (Infrequent) 714
Zonegran Capsules (Infrequent) 1089
Zyrtec Chewable Tablets (Less than 2%) 2589
Zyrtec (Less than 2%) 2589
Zyrtec-D 12 Hour Extended Release Tablets (Less than 2%) 2591

Parotid gland enlargement
Depacon Injection 412
Depakene 417
Depakote Sprinkle Capsules 422
Depakote Tablets 427
Depakote ER Tablets 433
Diprivan Injectable Emulsion (Less than 1%) 676
Hyperstat I.V. Injection 3031
Surmontil Capsules 2347
Thalomid Capsules 979
Thioridazine Hydrochloride Tablets (Rare) 2122
VFEND I.V. (Less than 2%) 2543
VFEND Oral Suspension (Less than 2%) 2543
VFEND Tablets (Less than 2%) 2543

Parotitis
Catapres Tablets (Rare) 874
Clorpres Tablets (Rare) 2139
Effexor Tablets (Rare) 3405
Effexor XR Capsules (Rare) 3411
M-M-R II 1980
Mumpsvax (Very low) 2005
Vivactil Tablets 2350

Partial thromboplastin time, prolonged
Tygacil for Injection (0% to less than 2%) 3489

Partial thromboplastin time, accelerated
Premphase Tablets 3452

Partial thromboplastin time, decrease
Prempro Tablets 3452

Patent ductus arteriosus
Altace Capsules 1673
Captopril Tablets 2114
Cozaar Tablets 1913
Hyzaar 1964
▲ Infasurf Intratracheal Suspension (45% to 47%) 1188
Lotrel Capsules 2238
Prinivil Tablets 2029
Prinzide Tablets 2033
Vaseretic Tablets 2073
Vasotec I.V. Injection 2076
Zestoretic Tablets 701
Zestril Tablets 704

PBI decrease
Dyazide Capsules 1389
Estratest Tablets 3196
Estratest H.S. Tablets 3196
Maxzide 2150

PBI increase
Aygestin Tablets 1062

Peeling, epidermal
Accutane Capsules 2740
Avita Cream 2136
Avita Gel 2138
Benzaclin Topical Gel (2%) 1046
▲ Brevoxyl-4 Creamy Wash (5 of 100 patients) 3212
▲ Brevoxyl-4 Gel (5 of 100 patients) 3211
▲ Brevoxyl-8 Creamy Wash (5 of 100 patients) 3212
▲ Brevoxyl-8 Gel (5 of 100 patients) 3211
Clindagel (0.6%) 1207
▲ Clindets Pledgets (11%) 3212
Cozaar Tablets (One subject) 1913
Erygel Topical Gel (Occasional) 2096
Hyzaar (One subject) 1964
Imitrex Injection (Rare) 1431
Imitrex Nasal Spray (Rare) 1435
Lotrimin 3053
Lotrisone 3054
▲ Renova 0.02% Cream (Almost all subjects) 2384
▲ Renova 0.05% Cream (Almost all subjects) 2387
Retin-A Micro 0.1%/0.04% 2388
Solage Topical Solution 740
▲ Soriatane Capsules (50% to 75%) 1028

Pelger-Huet anomaly
Risperdal M-Tab Orally Disintegrating Tablets (Rare) 1658
Risperdal (Rare) 1658

Peliosis hepatis
Anadrol-50 Tablets 3329
Delatestryl Injection 2976
Estratest Tablets 3196
Estratest H.S. Tablets 3196
Oxandrin Tablets 2977

Pellagra-like syndrome
Trecator Tablets 3482

Pelvic discomfort
Menopur for Subcutaneous Injection (0.4% to 2.6%) 1145

Pelvic inflammation
Lexapro Oral Solution (Infrequent) 1193
Lexapro Tablets (Infrequent) 1193

Pelvic inflammatory disease
Advair Diskus 100/50 1291
Advair Diskus 250/50 1291
Advair Diskus 500/50 1291
Migranal Nasal Spray (Rare) 3350
Mirena Intrauterine System 810

Pelvic pressure
▲ MetroGel-Vaginal Gel (3%) 1822
▲ Zoladex (18%) 709

Pemphigoid-like lesion
Captopril Tablets 2114
Parcopa Orally Disintegrating Tablets 3111
Timoptic in Ocudose 2061
Timoptic Sterile Ophthalmic Solution 2058
Timoptic-XE Sterile Ophthalmic Gel Forming Solution 2062

Pemphigus
Arthrotec Tablets (Rare) 3126
Cuprimine Capsules 1925
Lotensin Tablets (Less than 1%) 2232
Lotensin HCT Tablets (Rare) 2235
Lotrel Capsules (Rare) 2238
Mavik Tablets (0.3% to 1.0%) 482
Prinivil Tablets (0.3% to 1.0%) 2029
Prinzide Tablets 2033
Rituxan for Infusion (Less than 0.1%) 845
Topamax Sprinkle Capsules 2438
Topamax Tablets 2438
Uniretic Tablets (Less than 1%) 3114
Univasc Tablets (Less than 1%) 3118
Vaseretic Tablets 2073
Vasotec I.V. Injection (0.5% to 1.0%) 2076
Zestril Tablets (0.3% to 1.0%) 704

Pemphigus, bullous
Aceon Tablets (2 mg, 4 mg, 8 mg) 3191
Captopril Tablets 2114
Efudex (Infrequent) 3348

Penile angulation
▲ Edex Injection (7%) 3103

Penile discharge, unspecified
Alferon N Injection (1%) 1640
▲ Edex Injection (3%) 3103
ProSom Tablets (Rare) 512

Penile disorder, unspecified
AndroGel (Fewer than 1%) 3330
▲ Caverject Impulse Injection (3%) 2610
▲ Edex Injection (3%) 3103
Eligard 30 mg (1.1%) 2901
Lamictal (2%) 1449
Norvir (Less than 2%) 499
Prevacid Delayed-Release Capsules (Less than 1%) 3268
Prevacid for Delayed-Release Oral Suspension (Less than 1%) 3268
Prevacid NapraPAC (Less than 1%) 3277
Prevacid SoluTab Delayed-Release Orally Disintegrating Tablets (Less than 1%) 3268
PREVPAC (Less than 1%) 3281
Requip Tablets (Infrequent) 1528
Soriatane Capsules (Less than 1%) 1028
Testim 1% Gel (1% or less) 722

Penile erection, decrease
▲ Zoladex (18%) 709
▲ Zoladex 3-month (One of the two most common) 712

Penile erection, increase
(*see under* Priapism)

Penile erection, prolonged or inappropriate
Oxandrin Tablets 2977

Striant Mucoadhesive 1022
Viagra Tablets 2552

Penile erection, spontaneous
Cialis Tablets (Less than 2%) 1806

Penile head, discoloration of
▲ Caverject Impulse (3%) 2610

Penile shrinkage
Eligard 45 mg (1%) 2904

Penile skin tear
▲ Caverject Impulse Injection (3%) 2610

Penis, decreased sensation
Eldepryl Capsules 3209

Penis, enlargement
▲ Intron A for Injection (Less than or equal to 5%) 3038
Oxandrin Tablets 2977

Penis, fibrotic plaques
(*see under* Peyronie's disease)

Penis, strange feeling of
▲ Caverject Impulse Injection (3%) 2610

Penis, swollen
Neurontin Capsules (Rare) 2498
Neurontin Oral Solution (Rare) 2498
Neurontin Tablets (Rare) 2498

Perforation, cervix (total)
Omacor Capsules 2735

Perforation, gastrointestinal
Nalfon Capsules 2504

Periarteritis nodosum
Phenytek Capsules 2153

Pericardial effusion
Activase I.V. 1225
Agrylin Capsules 3172
Ammonul Injection 3323
▲ CellCept Capsules (3% to less than 20%) 2751
▲ CellCept Intravenous (3% to less than 20%) 2751
▲ CellCept Oral Suspension (3% to less than 20%) 2751
▲ CellCept Tablets (3% to less than 20%) 2751
▲ Clolar for Intravenous Infusion (35%) 1264
Clozapine Tablets 2141
Clozaril Tablets 2174
▲ Doxil Injection (1% to 5%) 3302
▲ Gleevec Tablets (2% to 16%) 2221
Herceptin I.V. (At least one of the 958 patients) 1234
▲ Humira Injection (Less than 5%) 464
I.V. Busulfex (2%) 1125
▲ Leukine (25%) 829
Neurontin Capsules (Rare) 2498
Neurontin Oral Solution (Rare) 2498
Neurontin Tablets (Rare) 2498
Nipent for Injection (Less than 3%) 3216
PEG-Intron Powder for Injection (Less than or equal to 1%) 3062
Permax Tablets (Rare) 3357
Proleukin for Injection (1%) 1007
Refludan for Injection 815
Remicade for IV Injection 987
ReoPro Vials (0.4%) 1779
Retavase 1131
Sonata Capsules (Rare) 1686
Tasmar Tablets 3360
Taxotere Injection Concentrate (Less frequent) 2947
TNKase I.V. 1256
Trasylol Injection (1% to 2%) 779
Vesanoid Capsules 2823
▲ Xeloda Tablets (Less than 5%) 2825

Pericardial rub
Neurontin Capsules (Rare) 2498
Neurontin Oral Solution (Rare) 2498
Neurontin Tablets (Rare) 2498

Pericarditis
Activase I.V. 1225
Agrylin Capsules 3172
Aldoclor Tablets 1881
Aldoril Tablets 1884
Asacol Delayed-Release Tablets (Rare) 2688
Campath Ampules 826
Canasa Rectal Suppositories (Rare) 726
Cerubidine for Injection (Rare) 788
Clozapine Tablets 2141
Clozaril Tablets 2174
Colazal Capsules 2845
Cytovene-IV (Two or more reports) 2763
Dynacin Tablets 1859
Evoxac Capsules (Less than 1%) 1042
▲ Humira Injection (Less than 5%) 464
Neurontin Capsules (Rare) 2498
Neurontin Oral Solution (Rare) 2498
Neurontin Tablets (Rare) 2498
Paser Granules 1657
Pentasa Capsules (Infrequent to less than 1%) 3182
Permax Tablets (Rare) 3357
Proleukin for Injection (Less than 1%) 1007
Retavase 1131
Rilutek Tablets (Infrequent) 2945
Rythmol SR Capsules 2736
Thalomid Capsules 979
TNKase I.V. 1256
▲ Trasylol Injection (5%) 779
▲ Vesanoid Capsules (3%) 2823
Zevalin Injection 848

Pericarditis, constrictive
Dostinex Tablets (One case) 2631

Perifollicular thickening
Thalomid Capsules 979

Perihilar infiltrate
Zevalin Injection (2%) 848

Perinatal disorder, unspecified
Diprivan Injectable Emulsion (Less than 1%) 676

Periodontal destruction
Evoxac Capsules (Less than 1%) 1042

Periodontitis
▲ Coreg Tablets (Greater than 1% to 3%) 1376
Effexor Tablets (Rare) 3405
Effexor XR Capsules (Rare) 3411
Kaletra (Less than 2%) 474
Protonix I.V. (Less than 1%) 3468
Protonix Tablets (Less than 1%) 3465
Requip Tablets (Infrequent) 1528
Teveten Tablets (Less than 1%) 1707
Teveten HCT Tablets (Less than 1%) 1710
Thalomid Capsules 979
VFEND I.V. (Less than 2%) 2543
VFEND Oral Suspension (Less than 2%) 2543
VFEND Tablets (Less than 2%) 2543

Periosteal disorder, unspecified
▲ Neumega for Injection (11%) 3433
Thalomid Capsules 979

Peripheral nerve symptoms
▲ Reyataz Capsules (1% to 8%) 948

Peripheral vascular disease
Antara Capsules 2723
Mirapex Tablets (Less than 1%) 889

Peripheral vascular disorder, unspecified
Actiq (Less than 1%) 993
Aricept Tablets (Infrequent) 1086
Aricept ODT Tablets (Infrequent) 1086
▲ Betaseron for SC Injection (6%) 791
Camptosar Injection 2602
Caverject Impulse Injection (Less than 1%) 2610
▲ CellCept Capsules (3% to less than 20%) 2751
▲ CellCept Intravenous (3% to less than 20%) 2751
▲ CellCept Oral Suspension (3% to less than 20%) 2751
▲ CellCept Tablets (3% to less than 20%) 2751
▲ Coreg Tablets (Greater than 1% to 3%) 1376
Effexor Tablets (Infrequent) 3405
Effexor XR Capsules (Infrequent) 3411
▲ Flolan for Injection (96%) 1408
Gabitril Tablets (Infrequent) 998
Lofibra Capsules 1217
Lotensin HCT Tablets (0.3% or more) 2235
Merrem I.V. (Greater than 1%) 687
Neurontin Capsules (Infrequent) 2498
Neurontin Oral Solution (Infrequent) 2498
Neurontin Tablets (Infrequent) 2498
Norvir (Less than 2%) 499
Omacor Capsules 2735
Paxil CR Controlled-Release Tablets (Infrequent) 1509
Paxil (Infrequent) 1501
▲ Prograf Capsules and Injection (3% to 15%) 624
Protopic Ointment (Greater than or equal to 1%) 629
Prozac Pulvules and Liquid (Rare) 1771
▲ Rapamune Oral Solution and Tablets (3% to 20%) 3472
Relpax Tablets (Infrequent) 2531
Rescriptor Tablets 2535
Rilutek Tablets (Infrequent) 2945
Rythmol SR Capsules 2736
Symbyax Capsules (Rare) 1788
Thalomid Capsules 979
Tricor Tablets 523
Triglide Tablets 1165
Uniretic Tablets (Less than 1%) 3114
▲ Visudyne for Injection (1% to 10%) 2286
Zoladex (1% to 5%) 709
Zoladex 3-month 712

Peripheral wasting
Aptivus Capsules 859
Combivir Tablets 1373
Crixivan Capsules 1918
Invirase 2776
Norvir 499
Retrovir 1533
Trizivir Tablets 1565
Truvada Tablets 1279
Viracept 2556
Viramune Oral Suspension 903
Viramune Tablets 903
Viread Tablets 1284
Zerit 971
Ziagen 1600

Peritonitis
▲ Aranesp for Injection (27%) 576
Campath Ampules 826
▲ CellCept Capsules (3% to less than 20%) 2751
▲ CellCept Intravenous (3% to less than 20%) 2751
▲ CellCept Oral Suspension (3% to less than 20%) 2751
▲ CellCept Tablets (3% to less than 20%) 2751
Epogen for Injection 586
Neupogen for Injection (2%) 598
Paxil CR Controlled-Release Tablets (Rare) 1509
Paxil (Rare) 1501
▲ Photofrin for Injection (Less than 5%) 729
▲ Prograf Capsules and Injection (3% to 15%) 624
▲ Rapamune Oral Solution and Tablets (3% to 20%) 3472
Remicade for IV Injection (Greater than or equal to 0.2%) 987
Rilutek Tablets (Infrequent) 2945

Perleche
Neurontin Capsules (Rare) 2498
Neurontin Oral Solution (Rare) 2498
Neurontin Tablets (Rare) 2498

Personality changes
Ambien Tablets (Rare) 2867
Cardizem LA Extended Release Tablets (Less than 2%) 1699
Decadron Tablets 1929
▲ Depacon Injection (1% to 5%) 412
▲ Depakene (1% to 5%) 417
▲ Depakote Sprinkle Capsules (1% to 5%) 422
▲ Depakote Tablets (1% to 5%) 427
▲ Depakote ER Tablets (1% to 5%) 433
Eldepryl Capsules 3209
Enbrel for Injection 580
Evoxac Capsules 1042
Exelon Capsules (Infrequent) 2204
Frova Tablets (Rare) 1101
Gabitril Tablets (Frequent) 998
Geodon for Injection (Up to 2%) 2514
Hydrocortone Tablets 1963
Imitrex Tablets (Rare) 1440
▲ Intron A for Injection (Less than 5%) 3038
▲ Keppra Oral Solution (8%) 3307
▲ Keppra Tablets (8%) 3307
Lamictal (Infrequent) 1449
▲ Lupron Depot 3.75 mg (Among most frequent) 3257
Lupron Depot–3 Month 11.25 mg (Less than 5%) 3262
Lupron Depot-PED 7.5 mg, 11.25 mg and 15 mg (Less than 2%) 3266
Lupron Injection Pediatric (Less than 2%) 3256
Nalfon Capsules (Less than 1%) 2504
Namenda (Infrequent) 1199
Neurontin Capsules (Rare) 2498
Neurontin Oral Solution (2.8%) 2498
Neurontin Tablets (Rare) 2498
Norvir (Less than 2%) 499
Permax Tablets (2.1%) 3357
Prometrium Capsules (100 mg, 200 mg) (Less than 5%) 3205
Prozac Pulvules and Liquid (At least 2%) 1771
Requip Tablets (Infrequent) 1528
Rilutek Tablets (Infrequent) 2945
Tiazac Capsules (Less than 2%) 1204
Topamax Sprinkle Capsules (Frequent) 2438
Topamax Tablets (Frequent) 2438
Trileptal Oral Suspension 2281
Trileptal Tablets 2281
▲ Zyprexa Tablets (8%) 1798
▲ Zyprexa ZYDIS Orally Disintegrating Tablets (8%) 1798

Personality disorder
Symbyax Capsules (1% to 2%) 1788
▲ Topamax Sprinkle Capsules (11%) 2438
▲ Topamax Tablets (11%) 2438

Perspiration
(*see under* Diaphoresis)

Petechia at application site
Lidoderm Patch 1107

Petechiae
Abilify Tablets (Rare) 916
Abilify Tablets (Rare) 2472
AmBisome for Injection (Less common) 615
Caduet Tablets (Less than 2%) 2507
Cardizem LA Extended Release Tablets (Less than 2%) 1699
▲ CellCept Capsules (3% to less than 20%) 2751
▲ CellCept Intravenous (3% to less than 20%) 2751
▲ CellCept Oral Suspension (3% to less than 20%) 2751
▲ CellCept Tablets (3% to less than 20%) 2751
Cipro I.V. (1% or less) 2998
Cipro I.V. Pharmacy Bulk Package (1% or less) 3509
Cipro (Less than 1%) 2991
Cipro XR Tablets 3004
▲ Clolar for Intravenous Infusion (29%) 1264
Clozapine Tablets (Less than 1%) 2141
Clozaril Tablets (Less than 1%) 2174
Decadron Phosphate Injection 1931
▲ Depacon Injection (1% to 5%) 412
▲ Depakene (1% to 5%) 417
▲ Depakote Sprinkle Capsules (1% to 5%) 422
▲ Depakote Tablets (1% to 5%) 427
Depakote ER Tablets (Greater than 1%) 433
Depo-Medrol Injectable Suspension 2615
Depo-Medrol Single-Dose Vial 2617
Doxil Injection (Less than 1%) 3302
Engerix-B Vaccine (Less than 1%) 1391
FazaClo Orally Disintegrating Tablets (Less than 1%) 547
Gabitril Tablets (Infrequent) 998
▲ Gamunex Immune Globulin I.V., 10% (21%) 3232
▲ Gemzar for Injection (16%) 1743
▲ Gleevec Tablets (0.9% to 10%) 2221
Guanidine Hydrochloride Tablets 3030
Hydrocortone Tablets 1963
Indocin Capsules (Less than 1%) 1968
Indocin I.V. (Less than 1%) 1973
Indocin (Less than 1%) 1968
Lamictal (Rare to infrequent) 1449
▲ Leukine (6%) 829
▲ Leustatin Injection (8%) 2368
Lipitor Tablets (Less than 2%) 2495
Matulane Capsules 3188
Meridia Capsules 485
Migranal Nasal Spray (Infrequent) 3350
Mustargen for Injection 2007
▲ Mylotarg for Injection (1% to 20%) 3429
▲ Neupogen for Injection (17%) 598
Nipent for Injection (Less than 3%) 3216
Oncaspar (Less than 1%) 1123
Pediarix Vaccine 1518
Permax Tablets (Infrequent) 3357
Prilosec OTC Tablets 2674
▲ Proleukin for Injection (4%) 1007
Prozac Pulvules and Liquid (Rare) 1771
Raptiva for Injection 1247
Recombivax HB 2045
ReoPro Vials (0.3%) 1779
Rescriptor Tablets 2535
Rilutek Tablets (Rare) 2945

▲ Roferon-A Injection (Less than 5%) 2805
Rythmol SR Capsules 2736
Sandostatin Injection (Less than 1%) 2263
Sandostatin LAR Depot (Rare) 2264
Sular Tablets (Less than or equal to 1%) 1163
Surmontil Capsules 2347
Thalomid Capsules 979
Tiazac Capsules (Less than 2%) 1204
▲ Trisenox Injection (8%) 983
Twinrix Vaccine (Less than 1%) 1571
Uniretic Tablets (Less than 1%) 3114
VFEND I.V. (Less than 2%) 2543
VFEND Oral Suspension (Less than 2%) 2543
VFEND Tablets (Less than 2%) 2543
Vivactil Tablets 2350
Zegerid Powder for Oral Solution 2972
▲ Zevalin Injection (3%) 848
Zonegran Capsules (Rare) 1089

Petechiae and ecchymosis

Decadron Tablets 1929
Pediapred Oral Solution 3319

Petechial hemorrhage

Carbatrol Capsules 3174
Tegretol/Tegretol-XR 2278

Peyronie's disease

Blocadren Tablets 1891
Cosopt Sterile Ophthalmic Solution 1910
Edex Injection (1%) 3103
Inderal LA Long-Acting Capsules (Rare) 3421
InnoPran XL Capsules (Rare) 2728
Nadolol Tablets 2121
Phenytek Capsules 2153
Requip Tablets (Rare) 1528
Tenormin I.V. Injection 698
Tenormin Tablets 695
Timolide Tablets 2056
Timoptic in Ocudose 2061
Timoptic Sterile Ophthalmic Solution 2058
Timoptic-XE Sterile Ophthalmic Gel Forming Solution 2062
Toprol-XL Tablets (Fewer than 1 of 100,000 patients) 660

Pharyngeal discomfort

Cozaar Tablets (Less than 1%) 1913
FazaClo Orally Disintegrating Tablets (1%) 547
Hyzaar 1964
Invanz for Injection (Greater than 0.1%) 1974
Nexium Delayed-Release Capsules (Less than 1%) 645
Nexium I.V. (Less than 1%) 649
Prinzide Tablets (0.3% to 1.0%) 2033
Zestoretic Tablets (0.3% to 1.0%) 701

Pharyngitis

▲ Abilify Tablets (4%) 916
▲ Abilify Tablets (4%) 2472
▲ Aceon Tablets (2 mg, 4 mg, 8 mg) (3.3%) 3191
Actiq (1% or greater) 993
▲ Actonel Tablets (2.9% to 5.8%) 2679
▲ Actonel with Calcium Tablets (2.9% to 5.8%) 2684
▲ ActoPlus Met Tablets (5.1%) 3219
▲ Actos Tablets (5.1%) 3224
Adalat CC Tablets (Less than 1%) 2978
▲ Advair Diskus 100/50 (3% to 13%) 1291
▲ Advair Diskus 250/50 (3% to 13%) 1291
▲ Advair Diskus 500/50 (3% to 13%) 1291
Aerobid/Aerobid-M (1% to 3%) 1172
▲ Agrylin Capsules (6.8%) 3172
Aldara Cream, 5% (1.9%) 1814
Alferon N Injection (1%) 1640
▲ Alimta for Injection (Up to 28%) 1722
Alinia for Oral Suspension (Less than 1%) 2840
Alinia Tablets (Less than 1%) 2840
Aloprim for Injection (Less than 1%) 2156
Alphagan P Ophthalmic Solution (1% to 4%) 563
▲ Ambien Tablets (3%) 2867
AmBisome for Injection (Less common) 615
Amevive (Common) 836
Antara Capsules 2723
Aralast (1.6%) 745
▲ Arava Tablets (3%) 2881
Aricept Tablets (Infrequent) 1086
Aricept ODT Tablets (Infrequent) 1086
▲ Arimidex Tablets (10% to 23%) 665
▲ Aromasin Tablets (2% to 5%) 2600
▲ Asacol Delayed-Release Tablets (11%) 2688
▲ Asmanex Twisthaler (8% to 13%) 2981
▲ Astelin Nasal Spray (3.8%) 1876
Atacand Tablets (2%) 634
Atacand HCT (0.5% or greater) 637
▲ Atrovent Inhalation Solution (3.7%) 868
▲ Atrovent Nasal Spray 0.03% (8.1%) 869
Atrovent Nasal Spray 0.06% (Less than 1%) 870
Avalide Tablets (1% or greater) 922
Avalide Tablets (1% or greater) 2889
Avapro Tablets (1% or greater) 925
Avapro Tablets (1% or greater) 2886
Axert Tablets (Infrequent) 2430
▲ Axid Oral Solution (3.3%) 913
▲ Azmacort Inhalation Aerosol (7% to 25%) 1701
Azopt Ophthalmic Suspension (Less than 1%) 553
Bactroban Nasal (0.5% to 4%) 1357
▲ Bexxar (0% to 12%) 1360
Boniva Tablets (2.5%) 2747
▲ Botox Purified Neurotoxin Complex (3% to 10%) 565
Caduet Tablets (1.3% to 2.5%) 2507
▲ Campath Ampules (12%) 826
Campral Tablets (Frequent) 1175
▲ Carnitor Injection (15% to 27%) 3185
▲ Casodex Tablets (8%) 670
Celebrex Capsules (2.3%) 3130
Celexa (At least 2%) 1177
▲ CellCept Capsules (3% to less than 20%) 2751
▲ CellCept Intravenous (3% to less than 20%) 2751
▲ CellCept Oral Suspension (3% to less than 20%) 2751
▲ CellCept Tablets (3% to less than 20%) 2751
▲ Cenestin Tablets, 0.45mg, 0.625mg, 0.9mg, 1.25mg (1.9% to 8%) 1063
Cialis Tablets (Less than 2%) 1806
▲ Clarinex Syrup (3.1% to 4.5%) 3009
▲ Clarinex Tablets (3% to 4.1%) 3009
▲ Clarinex Reditabs Tablets (3% to 4.1%) 3009
▲ Clarinex-D 24-Hour Extended-Release Tablets (3%) 3012
Climara Transdermal System (0.5% to 7%) 795
Clindesse Vaginal Cream (Less than 1%) 3296
Colazal Capsules (2%) 2845
▲ CombiPatch Transdermal System (9%) 2180
Combivent Inhalation Aerosol (2.2%) 878
Combunox Tablets (Less than 1%) 1183
▲ Concerta Extended-Release Tablets (2% to 4%) 1828
Copaxone for Injection (At least 2%) 3292
Cosmegen for Injection 1907
Cosopt Sterile Ophthalmic Solution (1% to 5%) 1910
Cozaar Tablets (1% or greater) 1913
▲ Crestor Tablets (9%) 672
Crixivan Capsules (Less than 2%) 1918
▲ Depacon Injection (0.6% to 8%) 412
▲ Depakene (8%) 417
▲ Depakote Sprinkle Capsules (2% to 8%) 422
▲ Depakote Tablets (At least 5% to 8%) 427
▲ Depakote ER Tablets (2% to 8%) 433
▲ depo-subQ provera 104 Injectable Suspension (1% to less than 5%) 2622
Detrol Tablets (1.5%) 2626
▲ Diovan HCT Tablets (3%) 2195
Diovan Tablets (More than 1%) 2191
Diprivan Injectable Emulsion (Less than 1%) 676
▲ Ditropan XL Extended Release Tablets (2% to less than 5%) 2391
▲ Doxil Injection (Less than 1% to 15.9%) 3302
▲ DuoNeb Inhalation Solution (4.4%) 1058
Duragesic Transdermal System (1% or greater) 2448
Effexor Tablets 3405
▲ Effexor XR Capsules (7%) 3411
▲ Elestat Ophthalmic Solution (1% to 3%) 1643
▲ Elidel Cream 1% (0.9% to 8.1%) 2198
Elmiron Capsules (Less than or equal to 1%) 2393
▲ Eloxatin for Injection (2% to 9%) 2908
Emend Capsules (Greater than 0.5%) 1944
Enablex Extended-Release Tablets (Greater than or equal to 1%) 2201
▲ Enbrel for Injection (6% to 7%) 580
Epogen for Injection 586
▲ Equetro Extended-Release Capsules (Less than 5%) 3178
▲ Evista Tablets (5.3% to 7.6%) 1735
▲ Evoxac Capsules (5.2%) 1042
Exelon Capsules (2% or more) 2204
▲ Fabrazyme for Intravenous Infusion (8%) 1267
Factive Tablets (Less than or equal to 0.1%) 2464
Famvir Tablets (2.6% to 2.7%) 2207
▲ Faslodex Injection (16.1%) 682
▲ Ferrlecit Injection (6% to 12%) 3379
▲ Flolan for Injection (5%) 1408
▲ Flomax Capsules (5.1% to 5.8%) 881
▲ Flonase Nasal Spray (6% to 7.8%) 1412
▲ Flovent HFA (1% to 3%) 1418
Floxin Otic Singles (Reported in a single subject) 1045
Floxin Otic Solution (Single report) 1043
▲ Foradil Aerolizer (3.5%) 3024
▲ Forteo for Injection (5.5%) 1739
Fortical Nasal Spray (Less than 1%) 3336
Frova Tablets (Infrequent) 1101
▲ Gabitril Tablets (7%) 998
▲ Gamunex Immune Globulin I.V., 10% (0.8% to 41%) 3232
▲ Gengraf Capsules (4%) 458
▲ Geodon Capsules (3%) 2514
▲ Gleevec Tablets (10% to 15%) 2221
▲ Gonal-f RFF Pen for Injection (7.2%) 3155
Havrix Vaccine (Less than 1%) 1425
Hepsera Tablets (2% or greater) 1275
▲ Herceptin I.V. (12%) 1234
▲ Humatrope Vials and Cartridges (3.13% to 6.67%) 1756
Hytrin Capsules (At least 1%) 469
Hyzaar (1% or greater) 1964
▲ Imdur Tablets (Less than or equal to 5%) 3032
Indapamide Tablets (Less than 5%) 2119
Inderal LA Long-Acting Capsules 3421
▲ Infergen (17% to 34%) 1647
InnoPran XL Capsules 2728
▲ Intron A for Injection (1% to 31%) 3038
Invanz for Injection (0.7% to 1.1%) 1974
Invirase (Less than 2%) 2776
▲ I.V. Busulfex (18%) 1125
Kaletra (Less than 2%) 474
▲ Keppra Oral Solution (6% to 10%) 3307
▲ Keppra Tablets (6% to 10%) 3307
Klonopin (2%) 2782
▲ Lamictal (10% to 14%) 1449
▲ Lescol Capsules (3.8%) 2227
Lescol XL Tablets (2.4%) 2227
▲ Leukine (23%) 829
Levaquin in 5% Dextrose Injection (1.1%) 2453
Levaquin (1.1%) 2453
Levitra Tablets (Less than 2%) 3048
Lexapro Oral Solution (At least 2%) 1193
Lexapro Tablets (At least 2%) 1193
Lipitor Tablets (Up to 2.5%) 2495
Lofibra Capsules 1217
▲ Lotemax Ophthalmic Suspension 0.5% (Less than 15%) ⊙249
Lotrel Capsules 2238
Lunesta Tablets 3139
Maxalt Tablets (Infrequent) 1983
Maxalt-MLT Orally Disintegrating Tablets (Infrequent) 1983
▲ Megace ES Oral Suspension (1% to 3%) 2492
▲ Meridia Capsules (10%) 485
Merrem I.V. (Greater than 1%) 687
Miacalcin Nasal Spray (Less than 1%) 2242
Micardis Tablets (1%) 884
Micardis HCT Tablets (Less than 2%) 886
▲ Migranal Nasal Spray (3%) 3350
Mirapex Tablets (Greater than or equal to 1%) 889
▲ Mobic Oral Suspension (0.6% to 3.2%) 893
▲ Mobic Tablets (0.6% to 3.2%) 893
▲ Mylotarg for Injection (10% to 14%) 3429
▲ Nasacort AQ Nasal Spray (5.1%) 2937
▲ Nasarel Nasal Spray (3% to 9%) 1652
▲ Nasonex Nasal Spray (10 % to 12%) 3058
▲ Neoral Soft Gelatin Capsules (4%) 2247
▲ Neoral Oral Solution (4%) 2247
▲ Neumega for Injection (25%) 3433
Neurontin Capsules (1.2% to 2.8%) 2498
Neurontin Oral Solution (1.2% to 2.8%) 2498
Neurontin Tablets (1.2% To 2.8%) 2498
Nexium Delayed-Release Capsules (Less than 1%) 645
Nexium I.V. (Less than 1%) 649
Nicotrol NS 2596
▲ Nipent for Injection (8% to 10%) 3216
Norvir (0.4% to 2.6%) 499
Omacor Capsules 2735
▲ Ontak Vials (17%) 1717
▲ Optivar Ophthalmic Solution (1% to 10%) 1877
OxyContin Tablets (Less than 1%) 2699
Patanol Ophthalmic Solution (Less than 5%) 557
Paxil CR Controlled-Release Tablets (2.1%) 1509
Paxil (2.1%) 1501
▲ PEG-Intron Powder for Injection (10%) 3062
Permax Tablets (Frequent) 3357
▲ Photofrin for Injection (11%) 729
Plendil Extended-Release Tablets (0.5% to 1.5%) 651
▲ Pletal Tablets (7% to 10%) 2478
▲ Prefest Tablets (7%) 1069
▲ Premarin Tablets (10% to 12%) 3443
▲ Premphase Tablets (8% to 13%) 3452
▲ Prempro Tablets (8% to 13%) 3452
Prevacid Delayed-Release Capsules (Less than 1%) 3268
Prevacid for Delayed-Release Oral Suspension (Less than 1%) 3268
Prevacid NapraPAC (Less than 1%) 3277
Prevacid SoluTab Delayed-Release Orally Disintegrating Tablets (Less than 1%) 3268
Prevnar for Injection 3460
PREVPAC (Less than 1%) 3281
Prilosec OTC Tablets (1%) 2674
Prinivil Tablets (0.3% to 1.0%) 2029
Prinzide Tablets 2033
Prochieve 4% Gel 1018
Prochieve 8% Gel 1018
▲ Prograf Capsules and Injection (3% to 15%) 624
Prometrium Capsules (100 mg, 200 mg) (Less than 5%) 3205
ProSom Tablets (1%) 512
Protonix I.V. (Greater than or equal to 1%) 3468
Protonix Tablets (Greater than or equal to 1%) 3465
▲ Protopic Ointment (3% to 12%) 629
Proventil Inhalation Solution 0.083% (Less than 1%) 3069
▲ Provigil Tablets (4%) 1002
▲ Prozac Pulvules and Liquid (3% to 11%) 1771
▲ Pulmozyme Inhalation Solution (32% to 40%) 1245
Quixin Ophthalmic Solution (1% to 3%) 3373
▲ Qvar Inhalation Aerosol (8% to 27%) 1654
▲ Rapamune Oral Solution and Tablets (16% to 21%) 3472
▲ Rebetol (12% to 13%) 3073
Recombivax HB (Equal to or greater than 1%) 2045
ReFacto Vials 3479
Relpax Tablets (Frequent) 2531
▲ Remicade for IV Injection (12%) 987
▲ Requip Tablets (6%) 1528
▲ Rescriptor Tablets (1.6% to 5%) 2535
Retrovir Capsules 1533
Retrovir IV Infusion 1537
Retrovir 1533
▲ Rhinocort Aqua Nasal Spray (4%) 658
▲ Ribavirin, USP Capsules (12% to 13%) 3083
▲ Risperdal M-Tab Orally Disintegrating Tablets (2% to 3%) 1658
▲ Risperdal (2% to 3%) 1658
▲ Sandostatin LAR Depot (5% to 15%) 2264
▲ Serevent Diskus (3% to 6%) 1540
▲ Seroquel Tablets (Frequent to 4%) 691
▲ Simulect for Injection (3% to 10%) 2268
Singulair (Greater than or equal to 2%) 2047
Soriatane Capsules (Less than 1%) 1028
Spectracef Tablets (0.1% to 1%) 2706
▲ Spiriva HandiHaler (7% to 9%) 899
▲ Suboxone Tablets (4%) 2719
▲ Subutex Tablets (4%) 2719
Sular Tablets (Less than 1% to 5%) 1163
▲ Suprane Liquid for Inhalation (3% to 10%) 770
▲ Symbyax Capsules (4% to 6%) 1788
Synagis (2.6%) 1868
Targretin Capsules 1719
Tasmar Tablets (Frequent) 3360
▲ Temodar Capsules (8%) 3088
▲ Tequin Injection (0.1% to 3%) 964
▲ Tequin Tablets (0.1% to 3%) 964

▲ Teveten Tablets (4%) 1707
Teveten HCT Tablets (Less than 1%) 1710
▲ Thalomid Capsules (4.2%) 979
▲ Tiazac Capsules (3%) 1204
Tindamax (Rare) 2670
▲ TOBI Solution for Inhalation (38.1%) 1015
▲ Topamax Sprinkle Capsules (2% to 6%) 2438
▲ Topamax Tablets (2% to 6%) 2438
Trelstar LA Suspension (1.1%) 3387
Tricor Tablets 523
▲ Trileptal Oral Suspension (Up to 3%) 2281
▲ Trileptal Tablets (Up to 3%) 2281
Trizivir Tablets 1565
Ultane Liquid for Inhalation (Less than 1%) 526
Uniretic Tablets (More than 1%) 3114
Univasc Tablets (1.8%) 3118
Uroxatral Tablets (1% to 2%) 2957
▲ Valcyte Tablets (Less than 5%) 2816
Vaqta (Up to 2.7%) 2067
Varivax 2070
▲ Verelan PM Capsules (3%) 3120
VESIcare Tablets (0.3% to 1.1%) 631
VFEND I.V. (Less than 2%) 2543
VFEND Oral Suspension (Less than 2%) 2543
VFEND Tablets (Less than 2%) 2543
Viagra Tablets (Less than 2%) 2552
Vicoprofen Tablets (Less than 3%) 533
▲ Vigamox Ophthalmic Solution (1% to 4%) 560
Viracept (Less than 2%) 2556
▲ Visudyne for Injection (1% to 10%) 2286
Vivelle Transdermal System 2288
Vivelle-Dot Transdermal System 2293
Vytorin 10/10 Tablets 2084
Vytorin 10/10 Tablets 3092
Vytorin 10/20 Tablets 2084
Vytorin 10/20 Tablets 3092
Vytorin 10/40 Tablets 2084
Vytorin 10/40 Tablets 3092
Vytorin 10/80 Tablets 2084
Vytorin 10/80 Tablets 3092
▲ WelChol Tablets (3%) 2855
▲ Wellbutrin SR Sustained-Release Tablets (3% to 11%) 1583
▲ Wellbutrin XL Extended-Release Tablets (3% to 11%) 1588
Xifaxan Tablets (Less than 2%) 2847
▲ Xolair (11%) 1259
▲ Xopenex HFA Inhalation Aerosol (10.4%) 3151
▲ Xopenex Inhalation Solution (10.4%) 3143
▲ Xopenex Inhalation Solution Concentrate (3% to 10.4%) 3147
Yasmin 28 Tablets (Greater than 1%) 818
Zaditor Ophthalmic Solution (Less than 5%) 2302
Zegerid Powder for Oral Solution (1%) 2972
Zelnorm Tablets (1%) 2303
▲ Zenapax for Injection (2% to 5%) 2838
Zestoretic Tablets 701
Zestril Tablets (0.3% to 1.0%) 704
▲ Zetia Tablets (2.3% to 3.1%) 2090
▲ Zetia Tablets (2.3% to 3.1%) 3098
Ziagen 1600
Zithromax for Oral Suspension, 300 mg, 600 mg, 900 mg, 1200 mg (1% or less) 2561
Zithromax Tablets, 250 mg, 500 mg (1% or less) 2561
Zithromax Tri-Pak (1% or less) 2561
▲ Zoladex (5% to 6%) 709
▲ Zoloft (4%) 2581
Zomig Nasal Spray (Infrequent) 718
Zonegran Capsules (Frequent) 1089
Zosyn (1.0% or less) 3492
▲ Zyban Sustained-Release Tablets (3%) 1620
▲ Zyprexa Tablets (5%) 1798
▲ Zyprexa ZYDIS Orally Disintegrating Tablets (5%) 1798
▲ Zyrtec Chewable Tablets (2% to 6.2%) 2589
▲ Zyrtec (2% to 6.2%) 2589
▲ Zyrtec-D 12 Hour Extended Release Tablets (2% to 6.2%) 2591
Zyvox (0.5% to 2.9%) 2661

Pharyngitis, streptococcal

Elidel Cream 1% (Up to 3%) 2198

Pharyngolaryngeal pain

▲ Cymbalta Delayed-Release Capsules (1% to 6%) 1729
▲ Gleevec Tablets (0.2% to 14.2%) 2221

Pharyngoxerosis

Carbatrol Capsules 3174
Tegretol/Tegretol-XR 2278

Pharynix, dryness of

Equetro Extended-Release Capsules 3178

Phimosis

▲ Caverject Impulse Injection (3%) 2610

Phlebitis

Abilify Tablets (Infrequent) 916
Abilify Tablets (Infrequent) 2472
Adalat CC Tablets (Less than 1%) 2978
Ambien Tablets (Rare) 2867
Ancef for Injection (Rare) 1318
Antara Capsules 2723
Anzemet Injection (Rare) 2871
Anzemet Tablets (Rare) 2874
Arthrotec Tablets (Rare) 3126
BeneFix for Injection (1.5%) 3402
Caduet Tablets (Less than 2%) 2507
Campath Ampules 826
Campral Tablets (Infrequent) 1175
▲ Cancidas for Injection (3.5% to 15.7%) 1894
Celexa (Rare) 1177
▲ CellCept Intravenous (4%) 2751
Cipro (Less than 1%) 2991
Cipro XR Tablets 3004
Clozapine Tablets (Less than 1%) 2141
Clozaril Tablets (Less than 1%) 2174
Cymbalta Delayed-Release Capsules (Infrequent) 1729
Cytovene (At least 3 subjects) 2763
Dantrium Capsules (Less frequent) 2690
Diprivan Injectable Emulsion (Rare) 676
Doxil Injection (Less than 1%) 3302
Evoxac Capsules (Less than 1%) 1042
FazaClo Orally Disintegrating Tablets (Less than 1%) 547
Ferrlecit Injection 3379
Fluorescite Injection ⊙ 207
Fortaz (1 in 69 patients) 1422
Gabitril Tablets (Infrequent) 998
Geodon Capsules (Rare) 2514
Imitrex Injection 1431
Imitrex Nasal Spray (Rare) 1435
Imitrex Tablets 1440
Infed Injection 3381
▲ Intron A for Injection (Less than or equal to 5%) 3038
Invanz for Injection (Greater than 0.5% to 1.9%) 1974
Leustatin Injection (2%) 2368
Levaquin in 5% Dextrose Injection (0.1% to 0.9%) 2453
Levaquin (0.1% to 0.9%) 2453
Lipitor Tablets (Less than 2%) 2495
Lofibra Capsules 1217
Maxipime for Injection (1.3%) 1093
Merrem I.V. (0.8%) 687
Mivacron Injection (Less than 1%) 489
▲ Mycamine for Injection (1.6% to 4.2%) 620
Naropin Injection (Less than 1%) 640
▲ Navelbine Injection (Up to 10%) 1494
Neurontin Capsules (Rare) 2498
Neurontin Oral Solution (Rare) 2498
Neurontin Tablets (Rare) 2498
Nipent for Injection (Less than 3%) 3216
Novantrone for Injection Concentrate 3158
Panhematin for Injection 2487
Parcopa Orally Disintegrating Tablets 3111
Paxil CR Controlled-Release Tablets (Rare) 1509
Paxil (Rare) 1501
Premarin Intravenous 3440
▲ Primaxin I.V. (3.1%) 2024
▲ Prograf Capsules and Injection (3% to 15%) 624
▲ Proleukin for Injection (23%) 1007
Prozac Pulvules and Liquid (Rare) 1771
Requip Tablets (Infrequent) 1528
Retrovir Capsules (1.6%) 1533
Retrovir IV Infusion (2%) 1537
Retrovir (1.6%) 1533
Rilutek Tablets (0.4% to 0.8%) 2945
Risperdal Consta Long-Acting Injection (Infrequent) 1664
Risperdal M-Tab Orally Disintegrating Tablets (Rare) 1658
Risperdal (Rare) 1658
Rocephin Injectable Vials, ADD-Vantage, Galaxy, Bulk (Less than 1%) 2801
Sandostatin LAR Depot (1% to 4%) 2264
Stalevo Tablets 2270
Synercid I.V. (Less than 1%) 1690
Taxotere Injection Concentrate 2947
Topamax Sprinkle Capsules (Infrequent) 2438
Topamax Tablets (Infrequent) 2438
Trasylol Injection (1.0%) 779
Tricor Tablets 523
Triglide Tablets 1165
Tygacil for Injection (1.8%) 3489
▲ Vesanoid Capsules (11%) 2823
VFEND I.V. (Less than 2%) 2543
VFEND Oral Suspension (Less than 2%) 2543
VFEND Tablets (Less than 2%) 2543
Wellbutrin Tablets (Rare) 1579
Wellbutrin SR Sustained-Release Tablets 1583
Wellbutrin XL Extended-Release Tablets 1588
▲ Xeloda Tablets (Less than 5%) 2825
▲ Zinecard for Injection (3% to 6%) 2659
Zosyn (1.3%) 3492
▲ Zovirax for Injection (Approximately 9%) 1618
Zyban Sustained-Release Tablets 1620

Phlebitis, injection site

Avelox (0.1% to less than 2%) 2984
Tygacil for Injection (0% to less than 2%) 3489

Phlebosclerosis

Adriamycin for Injection, USP 786
Adriamycin Injection, USP 786

Phlebothrombosis

Ammonul Injection 3323

Phobia, unspecified

Cipro XR Tablets 3004
Imitrex Injection 1431

Phobic disorder

Cipro I.V. (1% or less) 2998
Cipro I.V. Pharmacy Bulk Package (1% or less) 3509
Cipro (Less than 1%) 2991
Imitrex Tablets (Rare) 1440
Zyprexa Tablets (Infrequent) 1798
Zyprexa ZYDIS Orally Disintegrating Tablets (Infrequent) 1798

Phocomelia

Thalomid Capsules 979

Phonophobia

Imitrex Tablets (Frequent) 1440

Phosphate metabolism, disorders of

Lotronex Tablets (Rare) 1479

Phosphaturia

Daranide Tablets 1928

Phospholipid concentration, increase

Estratest Tablets 3196
Estratest H.S. Tablets 3196
Triphasil-28 Tablets 3483

Phosphorus, decrease

Actonel with Calcium Tablets (2.7%) 2684
Maxipime for Injection (2.8%) 1093
Omnicef Capsules (0.3%) 506
Omnicef for Oral Suspension (0.4%) 506
Thalomid Capsules 979

Photodermatosis

Advair Diskus 100/50 1291
Advair Diskus 250/50 1291
Advair Diskus 500/50 1291

Photophobia

Abilify Tablets (Rare) 916
Abilify Tablets (Rare) 2472
Accutane Capsules 2740
Alphagan P Ophthalmic Solution (1% to 4%) 563
▲ Alrex Ophthalmic Suspension 0.2% (5% to 15%) ⊙ 243
Amerge Tablets (Frequent) 1312
Amnesteem Capsules 2126
▲ Betimol Ophthalmic Solution (More than 5%) ⊙ 283
▲ Betimol Ophthalmic Solution (More than 5%) 3371
Betoptic S Ophthalmic Suspension (Small number of patients) 554
Botox Purified Neurotoxin Complex 565
▲ Brimonidine Tartrate Ophthalmic Solution 0.2% (3% to 9%) ⊙ 245
Calcijex Injection 411
Campral Tablets (Rare) 1175
Carteolol Hydrochloride Ophthalmic Solution USP, 1% (Occasional) ⊙ 246
Celexa (Infrequent) 1177
Ciloxan Ophthalmic Ointment (Less than 1%) 554
Copaxone for Injection (Infrequent) 3292
Cosopt Sterile Ophthalmic Solution (Less than 1%) 1910
CytoGam Intravenous (Infrequent) 1866
Depakote ER Tablets (Greater than 1%) 433
Effexor Tablets (Infrequent) 3405
Effexor XR Capsules (Infrequent) 3411
Gabitril Tablets (Infrequent) 998
Geodon Capsules (Infrequent) 2514
Havrix Vaccine (Less than 1%) 1425
Hectorol Capsules 909
Hectorol Injection 911
▲ Imdur Tablets (Less than or equal to 5%) 3032
Imitrex Injection (Infrequent) 1431
Imitrex Tablets (Frequent) 1440
▲ Intron A for Injection (Less than 5%) 3038
Lacrisert Sterile Ophthalmic Insert 1979
Lamictal (Infrequent) 1449
Levitra Tablets (Less than 2%) 3048
▲ Lotemax Ophthalmic Suspension 0.5% (5% to 15%) ⊙ 249
Lotronex Tablets (Rare) 1479
▲ Lumigan Ophthalmic Solution (1% to 3%) 569
Lunesta Tablets (Rare) 3139
Lyrica Capsules (0.1% to 1%) 2524
Matulane Capsules 3188
Maxalt Tablets (Rare) 1983
Maxalt-MLT Orally Disintegrating Tablets (Rare) 1983
Migranal Nasal Spray (Infrequent) 3350
Neurontin Capsules (Infrequent) 2498
Neurontin Oral Solution (Infrequent) 2498
Neurontin Tablets (Infrequent) 2498
Nipent for Injection (Less than 3%) 3216
Norvir (Less than 2%) 499
OptiPranolol Metipranolol Ophthalmic Solution 0.3% (A small number of patients) ⊙ 254
▲ Orthoclone OKT3 Sterile Solution (10%) 2370
▲ Pacerone Tablets (4% to 9%) 3337
Paxil CR Controlled-Release Tablets (Rare) 1509
Paxil (Rare) 1501
Permax Tablets (Infrequent) 3357
Photofrin for Injection 729
Prevacid Delayed-Release Capsules (Less than 1%) 3268
Prevacid for Delayed-Release Oral Suspension (Less than 1%) 3268
Prevacid NapraPAC (Less than 1%) 3277
Prevacid SoluTab Delayed-Release Orally Disintegrating Tablets (Less than 1%) 3268
PREVPAC (Less than 1%) 3281
Prinivil Tablets (0.3% to 1.0%) 2029
Prinzide Tablets 2033
ProSom Tablets (Infrequent) 512
Prozac Pulvules and Liquid (Infrequent) 1771
Quixin Ophthalmic Solution (1% to 3%) 3373
Relpax Tablets (Infrequent) 2531
Requip Tablets (Infrequent) 1528
Rescriptor Tablets 2535
▲ Retisert Implant (5% to 9%) ⊙ 256
Retrovir Capsules 1533
Retrovir IV Infusion 1537
Retrovir 1533
▲ Rēv-Eyes Ophthalmic Eyedrops 0.5% (10% to 40%) ⊙ 256
Rilutek Tablets (Rare) 2945
Risperdal M-Tab Orally Disintegrating Tablets (Rare) 1658
Risperdal (Rare) 1658
Sonata Capsules (Infrequent) 1686
▲ Soriatane Capsules (1% to 10%) 1028
Tambocor Tablets (Less than 1%) 1824
Tequin Injection (Less than 0.1%) 964
Tequin Tablets (Less than 0.1%) 964
Topamax Sprinkle Capsules (Infrequent) 2438
Topamax Tablets (Infrequent) 2438
Travatan Ophthalmic Solution (1% to 4%) 559
Trileptal Oral Suspension 2281
Trileptal Tablets 2281
Trusopt Sterile Ophthalmic Solution (Approximately 1% to 5%) 2065

Twinrix Vaccine (Less than 1%) 1571
▲ VFEND I.V. (1.7% to 21%) 2543
▲ VFEND Oral Suspension (1.7% to 21%) 2543
▲ VFEND Tablets (1.7% to 21%) 2543
Viagra Tablets (Less than 2%) 2552
Visine For Contacts Rewetting Drops ⊙ 278
Xalatan Sterile Ophthalmic Solution (1% to 4%) 2654
Xanax XR Tablets (Infrequent) 2655
Zaditor Ophthalmic Solution (Less than 5%) 2302
Zestoretic Tablets 701
Zestril Tablets (0.3% to 1.0%) 704
Zoloft (Rare) 2581
Zomig Nasal Spray (Rare) 718
Zonegran Capsules (Rare) 1089
Zosyn (1.0% or less) 3492
▲ Zylet Ophthalmic Suspension (Less than 4%) 3508

Photopsia

Ambien Tablets (Rare) 2867
Cymbalta Delayed-Release Capsules (Infrequent) 1729
Evoxac Capsules (Less than 1%) 1042
Maxalt Tablets (Rare) 1983
Maxalt-MLT Orally Disintegrating Tablets (Rare) 1983
▲ Retisert Implant (5% to 9%) ⊙ 256
Risperdal M-Tab Orally Disintegrating Tablets (Rare) 1658
Risperdal (Rare) 1658

Photosensitivity

Abilify Tablets (Infrequent) 916
Abilify Tablets (Infrequent) 2472
Accutane Capsules 2740
Aciphex Tablets 1081
Agrylin Capsules (1% to 5%) 3172
Alacol DM Syrup 739
Aldoclor Tablets 1881
Aldoril Tablets 1884
Alferon N Injection (1%) 1640
Altace Capsules (Less than 1%) 1673
Altoprev Extended-Release Tablets (Rare) 1151
Amaryl Tablets (Less than 1%) 2864
Ambien Tablets (Rare) 2867
Amerge Tablets (Rare) 1312
Amnesteem Capsules 2126
Anaprox Tablets (Less than 1%) 2769
Anaprox DS Tablets (Less than 1%) 2769
Arthrotec Tablets (Rare) 3126
Atacand HCT 637
Avalide Tablets 922
Avalide Tablets 2889
Axert Tablets (Rare) 2430
▲ Azmacort Inhalation Aerosol (1% to 3%) 1701
Caduet Tablets (Less than 2%) 2507
Captopril Tablets 2114
Carbatrol Capsules 3174
Cardizem LA Extended Release Tablets (Less than 2%) 1699
Cataflam Tablets (Occasionally) 2173
Celebrex Capsules (0.1% to 1.9%) 3130
Celexa (Infrequent) 1177
Cipro I.V. (1% or less) 2998
Cipro I.V. Pharmacy Bulk Package (1% or less) 3509
Cipro (Less than 1%) 2991
Cipro XR Tablets (Less than 1%) 3004
Clindagel 1207
Clinoril Tablets (Less than 1 in 100) 1899
Clorpres Tablets 2139
Clozapine Tablets 2141
Clozaril Tablets 2174
Copaxone for Injection (Infrequent) 3292
Coreg Tablets (Greater than 0.1% to 1%) 1376
Cozaar Tablets (Less than 1%) 1913
Dantrium Capsules 2690
Depacon Injection 412
Depakene 417
Depakote Sprinkle Capsules 422
Depakote Tablets 427
Depakote ER Tablets 433
Diovan HCT Tablets 2195
Diuril Oral 1936
Diuril Sodium Intravenous 1934
Dolobid Tablets (Less than 1 in 100) 1937
Dyazide Capsules 1389
Dynacin Tablets 1859
Dyrenium Capsules (Rare) 3390
EC-Naprosyn Delayed-Release Tablets (Less than 1%) 2769
Effexor Tablets (Infrequent) 3405
Effexor XR Capsules (Infrequent) 3411
▲ Efudex (Among most frequent) 3348
Eldepryl Capsules 3209
Elmiron Capsules (Less than or equal to 1%) 2393
Eulexin Capsules 3023
Evoxac Capsules (Less than 1%) 1042
Factive Tablets (0.039%) 2464
FazaClo Orally Disintegrating Tablets 547
Flexeril Tablets (Rare) 1832
Fosamax (Occasional) 1949
Furosemide Tablets 2117
Gabitril Tablets (Infrequent) 998
Geodon Capsules (Frequent) 2514
Gleevec Tablets (Infrequent) 2221
Grifulvin V Tablets Microsize and Oral Suspension Microsize 2384
Gris-PEG Tablets (Occasional) 2504
Hyzaar 1964
Imitrex Injection 1431
Imitrex Nasal Spray 1435
Imitrex Tablets 1440
Indapamide Tablets 2119
▲ Intron A for Injection (Less than 5%) 3038
Invirase (Less than 2%) 2776
Lamictal (2%) 1449
Lescol Capsules (Rare) 2227
Lescol Capsules (Rare) 2730
Lescol XL Tablets 2227
Lescol XL Tablets 2730
Lipitor Tablets (Less than 2%) 2495
Lofibra Capsules 1217
Lotensin Tablets (Less than 1%) 2232
Lotensin HCT Tablets (0.3% or more) 2235
Lunesta Tablets (Infrequent) 3139
Lupron Depot 3.75 mg 3257
Lupron Depot 7.5 mg 3261
Lupron Depot–3 Month 11.25 mg 3262
Lupron Depot-PED 7.5 mg, 11.25 mg and 15 mg 3266
Lupron Injection Pediatric 3256
Malarone Tablets 1484
Malarone Pediatric Tablets 1484
Maxalt Tablets (Infrequent) 1983
Maxalt-MLT Orally Disintegrating Tablets (Infrequent) 1983
Maxzide 2150
Meridia Capsules 485
Mevacor Tablets (Rare) 1996
Micardis HCT Tablets 886
Mobic Oral Suspension (Less than 2%) 893
Mobic Tablets (Less than 2%) 893
Moduretic Tablets 2003
Naprosyn Suspension (Less than 1%) 2769
Naprosyn Tablets (Less than 1%) 2769
Neurontin Capsules (Rare) 2498
Neurontin Oral Solution (Rare) 2498
Neurontin Tablets (Rare) 2498
Nipent for Injection (Less than 3%) 3216
Noroxin Tablets 2009
Norvir (Less than 2%) 499
▲ Pacerone Tablets (4% to 9%) 3337
Paxil CR Controlled-Release Tablets (Rare) 1509
Paxil (Rare) 1501
Pentasa Capsules (Less than 1%) 3182
Phenergan 3438
▲ Photofrin for Injection (19% to 68%) 729
Polytrim Ophthalmic Solution 570
Pravachol Tablets (Rare) 943
Prinivil Tablets (0.3% to 1.0%) 2029
Prinzide Tablets 2033
▲ Prograf Capsules and Injection (3% to 15%) 624
ProSom Tablets (Rare) 512
Protopic Ointment (Greater than or equal to 1%) 629
Prozac Pulvules and Liquid (Rare) 1771
Rapamune Oral Solution and Tablets 3472
Relafen Tablets (Less than 1%) 1523
Requip Tablets (Infrequent) 1528
Reyataz Capsules (Less than 3%) 948
Rilutek Tablets (Infrequent) 2945
Risperdal M-Tab Orally Disintegrating Tablets (Frequent) 1658
Risperdal (Frequent) 1658
Seroquel Tablets (Infrequent) 691
Sonata Capsules (Less than 1%) 1686
Soriatane Capsules (Less than 1%) 1028
Sular Tablets (One case) 1163
Surmontil Capsules 2347
Targretin Capsules 1719
Tegretol/Tegretol-XR 2278
Tequin Injection (Less than 0.1%) 964
Tequin Tablets (Less than 0.1%) 964
Teveten HCT Tablets 1710
Thalomid Capsules 979
Thioridazine Hydrochloride Tablets (Extremely rare) 2122
Thiothixene Capsules 2124
Tiazac Capsules (Less than 2%) 1204
Timolide Tablets 2056
Topamax Sprinkle Capsules (Infrequent) 2438
Topamax Tablets (Infrequent) 2438
Toprol-XL Tablets 660
Trecator Tablets (Rare) 3482
Tricor Tablets 523
Triglide Tablets 1165
Trileptal Oral Suspension 2281
Trileptal Tablets 2281
Tygacil for Injection 3489
Uniretic Tablets (Less than 1%) 3114
Univasc Tablets (Less than 1%) 3118
Valtrex Caplets 1573
Vaseretic Tablets 2073
Vasotec I.V. Injection (0.5% to 1.0%) 2076
VFEND I.V. (Less than 2%) 2543
VFEND Oral Suspension (Less than 2%) 2543
VFEND Tablets (Less than 2%) 2543
Viagra Tablets (Less than 2%) 2552
▲ Visudyne for Injection (1% to 10%) 2286
Vivactil Tablets 2350
Voltaren Tablets (Occasionally) 2298
Voltaren-XR Tablets (Occasionally) 2301
Vytorin 10/10 Tablets 2084
Vytorin 10/10 Tablets 3092
Vytorin 10/20 Tablets 2084
Vytorin 10/20 Tablets 3092
Vytorin 10/40 Tablets 2084
Vytorin 10/40 Tablets 3092
Vytorin 10/80 Tablets 2084
Vytorin 10/80 Tablets 3092
Wellbutrin SR Sustained-Release Tablets (Infrequent) 1583
Wellbutrin XL Extended-Release Tablets (Infrequent) 1588
▲ Xeloda Tablets (Less than 5%) 2825
Zestoretic Tablets 701
Zestril Tablets (0.3% to 1.0%) 704
Zithromax (1% or less) 2568
Zithromax for Oral Suspension, 300 mg, 600 mg, 900 mg, 1200 mg (1% or less) 2561
Zithromax Tablets, 250 mg, 500 mg (1% or less) 2561
Zithromax Tablets, 600 mg (1% or less) 2568
Zithromax Tri-Pak (1% or less) 2561
Zithromax Z-Pak (1% or less) 2568
Zmax for Oral Suspension 2577
Zocor Tablets (Rare) 2078
Zoloft (Infrequent) 2581
Zomig Tablets (Infrequent) 714
Zomig-ZMT Tablets (Infrequent) 714
Zovirax Capsules 1616
Zovirax for Injection 1618
Zovirax 1616
Zyban Sustained-Release Tablets (Infrequent) 1620
Zyprexa Tablets (Infrequent) 1798
Zyprexa ZYDIS Orally Disintegrating Tablets (Infrequent) 1798
Zyrtec Chewable Tablets (Less than 2%) 2589
Zyrtec (Less than 2%) 2589
Zyrtec-D 12 Hour Extended Release Tablets (Less than 2%) 2591

Photosensitivity, cutaneous

Agrylin Capsules 3172
Fosamax Plus D Tablets 1956

Photosensitivity reaction

Adalat CC Tablets (Less than 1%) 2978
▲ Adderall XR Capsules (2% to 4%) 3169
Aldara Cream, 5% (0.9%) 1814
Antara Capsules 2723
BeneFix for Injection (1.6%) 3402
Campral Tablets (Rare) 1175
Crestor Tablets (Less than 1%) 672
Cymbalta Delayed-Release Capsules (Infrequent) 1729
▲ Equetro Extended-Release Capsules (Less than 5%) 3178
Levitra Tablets (Less than 2%) 3048
Lyrica Capsules (0.1% to 1%) 2524
Protonix I.V. 3468
Raptiva for Injection 1247
Risperdal Consta Long-Acting Injection (Infrequent) 1664
Symbyax Capsules (Frequent) 1788

Phototoxicity

Cipro 2991
Cipro XR Tablets 3004
Dapsone Tablets USP 1656
Levaquin in 5% Dextrose Injection (Less than 0.1%) 2453
Levaquin (Less than 0.1%) 2453
Noroxin Tablets 2009
PEG-Intron Powder for Injection (Less than or equal to 1%) 3062
Protonix Tablets (Less than 1%) 3465
Zyrtec Chewable Tablets (Less than 2%) 2589
Zyrtec (Less than 2%) 2589
Zyrtec-D 12 Hour Extended Release Tablets (Less than 2%) 2591

Physical performance, impairment

Adipex-P 1216
Clozapine Tablets 2141
Clozaril Tablets 2174
Dilaudid Ampules 439
Dilaudid Non-Sterile Powder 439
Dilaudid Rectal Suppositories 439
Dilaudid Tablets 439
Gris-PEG Tablets (Occasional) 2504
Hycodan 1104
Hycomine Compound Tablets 1105
Hycotuss Expectorant Syrup 1106
Kadian Capsules 572
Lortab 3315
Lortab Elixir 3312
MS Contin Tablets 2703
Percocet Tablets 1114
Percodan Tablets 1115
Phenergan 3438
Surmontil Capsules 2347
Tussionex Pennkinetic Extended-Release Suspension 3322
Tylenol with Codeine 2461
Vicodin Tablets 530
Vicodin ES Tablets 531
Vicodin HP Tablets 532
Vivactil Tablets 2350
Zydone Tablets 1118

Pigmentation

Copaxone for Injection (Infrequent) 3292
Cosmegen for Injection 1907
Cosopt Sterile Ophthalmic Solution 1910
Dynacin Tablets 1859
Genotropin Lyophilized Powder (Infrequent) 2642
Risperdal M-Tab Orally Disintegrating Tablets (Frequent) 1658
Risperdal (Frequent) 1658
Timolide Tablets (Less than 1%) 2056
Timoptic in Ocudose 2061
Timoptic Sterile Ophthalmic Solution 2058
Timoptic-XE Sterile Ophthalmic Gel Forming Solution 2062

Pigmentation disorders

Accutane Capsules 2740
Carbatrol Capsules 3174
Equetro Extended-Release Capsules 3178
Gengraf Capsules (1% to less than 3%) 458
Gleevec Tablets (Infrequent) 2221
Neoral Soft Gelatin Capsules (1% to less than 3%) 2247
Neoral Oral Solution (1% to less than 3%) 2247
Pacerone Tablets (Occasional) 3337
Retrovir Capsules 1533
Retrovir IV Infusion 1537
Retrovir 1533
Tegretol/Tegretol-XR 2278
▲ Tri-Luma Cream (2% to 4.04%) 1213
▲ Xalatan Sterile Ophthalmic Solution (5% to 15%) 2654

Pill rolling motion

Thioridazine Hydrochloride Tablets 2122
Thiothixene Capsules 2124

Piloerection

Narcan Injection 1109
▲ ProAmatine Tablets (13.4%) 3183

Pituitary apoplexy

Sandostatin Injection (Less than 1%) 2263

Pituitary tumors

Imitrex Nasal Spray (Rare) 1435

Pituitary unresponsiveness, secondary

Decadron Phosphate Injection 1931
Decadron Tablets 1929
Depo-Medrol Injectable Suspension 2615
Depo-Medrol Single-Dose Vial 2617

Hydrocortone Tablets 1963
Pediapred Oral Solution 3319

Plantar fasciitis
Effexor Tablets (Rare) 3405
Effexor XR Capsules (Rare) 3411
Evoxac Capsules (Less than 1%) 1042

Plaques, erythematous
AquaMEPHYTON 1887

Plasminogen, increase
Premarin Tablets 3443
Premphase Tablets 3452
Prempro Tablets 3452

Platelet, decrease
(*see under* Thrombocytopenia)

Platelet, increase
(*see under* Thrombocytosis)

Platelet aggregation time, decrease
Premarin Tablets 3443
Premphase Tablets 3452
Prempro Tablets 3452

Platelet disorder, unspecified
Levaquin in 5% Dextrose Injection (0.1% to 0.9%) 2453
Levaquin (0.1% to 0.9%) 2453
Prevacid NapraPAC 3277
Zoloft (Rare) 2581

Pleural disorder, unspecified
Prevacid Delayed-Release Capsules (Less than 1%) 3268
Prevacid for Delayed-Release Oral Suspension (Less than 1%) 3268
Prevacid NapraPAC (Less than 1%) 3277
Prevacid SoluTab Delayed-Release Orally Disintegrating Tablets (Less than 1%) 3268
PREVPAC (Less than 1%) 3281

Pleural effusion
Abelcet Injection 1119
Actiq (Less than 1%) 993
Activase I.V. 1225
Agrylin Capsules 3172
▲ AmBisome for Injection (12.5%) 615
Apokyn Injection 2132
▲ Aredia for Injection (10.7%) 2168
Bexxar 1360
Campath Ampules 826
▲ CellCept Capsules (3% to 34.3%) 2751
▲ CellCept Intravenous (3% to 34.3%) 2751
▲ CellCept Oral Suspension (3% to 34.3%) 2751
▲ CellCept Tablets (3% to 34.3%) 2751
Cipro I.V. (1% or less) 2998
Cipro I.V. Pharmacy Bulk Package (1% or less) 3509
Cipro XR Tablets 3004
Clinoril Tablets (Less than 1 in 100) 1899
▲ Clolar for Intravenous Infusion (10%) 1264
Clozapine Tablets 2141
Clozaril Tablets 2174
Dostinex Tablets (Rare) 2631
▲ Doxil Injection (1% to 10%) 3302
Ellence Injection 2632
Evoxac Capsules (Less than 1%) 1042
FazaClo Orally Disintegrating Tablets 547
Femara Tablets (Less frequent) 2210
▲ Flolan for Injection (4% to 7%) 1408
Follistim AQ Cartridge 2354
▲ Gleevec Tablets (2% to 16%) 2221
Herceptin I.V. 1234
▲ Humira Injection (Less than 5%) 464
Invanz for Injection (Greater than 0.1%) 1974
▲ I.V. Busulfex (3%) 1125
Leukine 829
Levaquin in 5% Dextrose Injection (0.1% to 0.9%) 2453
Levaquin (0.1% to 0.9%) 2453
Matulane Capsules 3188
Merrem I.V. (Greater than 0.1% to 1%) 687
▲ Neumega for Injection (10%) 3433
Permax Tablets (Rare to infrequent) 3357
▲ Photofrin for Injection (13% to 32%) 729
Prinivil Tablets (0.3% to 1.0%) 2029
Prinzide Tablets 2033
▲ Prograf Capsules and Injection (30% to 36%) 624
▲ Proleukin for Injection (7%) 1007
▲ Rapamune Oral Solution and Tablets (3% to 20%) 3472
Remicade for IV Injection (Greater than or equal to 0.2%) 987
ReoPro Vials (1.3%) 1779
Rilutek Tablets (Infrequent) 2945
Rythmol SR Capsules 2736
Sandostatin LAR Depot (1% to 4%) 2264
Sonata Capsules (Rare) 1686
Stalevo Tablets (Rare) 2270
Sular Tablets (Less than or equal to 1%) 1163
Synercid I.V. (Less than 1%) 1690
Targretin Capsules 1719
Tasmar Tablets (Rare) 3360
▲ Taxotere Injection Concentrate (6%) 2947
▲ Trasylol Injection (7%) 779
▲ Trisenox Injection (20%) 983
▲ Valcyte Tablets (Less than 5%) 2816
Vantin Tablets and Oral Suspension (Less than 1%) 2650
▲ Vesanoid Capsules (20%) 2823
VFEND I.V. (Less than 2%) 2543
VFEND Oral Suspension (Less than 2%) 2543
VFEND Tablets (Less than 2%) 2543
Xeloda Tablets (1% to 2%) 2825
▲ Zenapax for Injection (2% to 5%) 2838
Zestoretic Tablets 701
Zestril Tablets (0.3% to 1.0%) 704
Zithromax for Oral Suspension, 300 mg, 600 mg, 900 mg, 1200 mg (1% or less) 2561
Zithromax Tablets, 250 mg, 500 mg (1% or less) 2561
Zithromax Tri-Pak (1% or less) 2561
▲ Zometa for Intravenous Infusion (5% to 10%) 2306
Zosyn (1.3%) 3492

Pleural effusion, exacerbation of
Neumega for Injection 3433

Pleural effusion with pericarditis
Dantrium Capsules (Less frequent) 2690

Pleural thickening
Apokyn Injection 2132
Stalevo Tablets (Rare) 2270

Pleuralgia
▲ Intron A for Injection (Less than 5%) 3038

Pleurisy
Aerobid/Aerobid-M (1% to 3%) 1172
Aricept Tablets (Infrequent) 1086
Aricept ODT Tablets (Infrequent) 1086
Campath Ampules 826
Effexor Tablets (Rare) 3405
Effexor XR Capsules (Rare) 3411
Evoxac Capsules (Less than 1%) 1042
Klonopin (Infrequent) 2782
Remicade for IV Injection (Greater than or equal to 0.2%) 987
ReoPro Vials (1.3%) 1779
Requip Tablets (Infrequent) 1528
Trileptal Oral Suspension 2281
Trileptal Tablets 2281

Pleuritis
Amerge Tablets (Rare) 1312
Asacol Delayed-Release Tablets 2688
Pacerone Tablets 3337
Permax Tablets (Rare) 3357
Rituxan for Infusion (Less than 0.1%) 845

Pneumocystis carinii
Campath Ampules 826
CellCept Capsules (Less than 4%) 2751
CellCept Intravenous (Less than 4%) 2751
CellCept Oral Suspension (Less than 4%) 2751
CellCept Tablets (Less than 4%) 2751
Cutivate Lotion 0.05% (Rare) 1383

Pneumocystis carinii, susceptibility
▲ Doxil Injection (9.2%) 3302
▲ Orthoclone OKT3 Sterile Solution (3.1%) 2370

Pneumocytosis
Remicade for IV Injection 987

Pneumonia
Abilify Tablets (Frequent) 916
Abilify Tablets (Frequent) 2472
Actiq (Less than 1%) 993
▲ Actonel Tablets (0.8% to 3.1%) 2679
▲ Actonel with Calcium Tablets (0.8% to 3.1%) 2684
▲ Advair Diskus 100/50 (1% to 3%) 1291
▲ Advair Diskus 250/50 (1% to 3%) 1291
▲ Advair Diskus 500/50 (1% to 3%) 1291
Aerobid/Aerobid-M (1% to 3%) 1172
Agrylin Capsules (1% to 5%) 3172
Ambien Tablets (Rare) 2867
AmBisome for Injection (Less common) 615
Amerge Tablets (Infrequent) 1312
Amevive 836
Anaprox Tablets (Less than 1%) 2769
Anaprox DS Tablets (Less than 1%) 2769
Antara Capsules 2723
▲ Apokyn Injection (At least 5%) 2132
▲ Aranesp for Injection (27%) 576
Arava Tablets (2%) 2881
▲ Argatroban Injection (3.3%) 1321
Aricept Tablets (Infrequent) 1086
Aricept ODT Tablets (Infrequent) 1086
Arixtra Injection (2.3%) 1325
Arthrotec Tablets (Rare) 3126
Betaseron for SC Injection 791
▲ Bexxar (0% to 6%) 1360
▲ Boniva Tablets (5.9%) 2747
Caduet Tablets (Less than 2%) 2507
▲ Campath Ampules (10% to 16%) 826
Campral Tablets (Infrequent) 1175
▲ Camptosar Injection (1.3% to 3.6%) 2602
Carbatrol Capsules 3174
▲ Casodex Tablets (4%) 670
Cataflam Tablets (Rarely) 2173
Celebrex Capsules (0.1% to 1.9%) 3130
Celexa (Infrequent) 1177
▲ CellCept Capsules (3% to less than 20%) 2751
▲ CellCept Intravenous (3% to less than 20%) 2751
▲ CellCept Oral Suspension (3% to less than 20%) 2751
▲ CellCept Tablets (3% to less than 20%) 2751
▲ Clolar for Intravenous Infusion (10%) 1264
Clozapine Tablets (Less than 1%) 2141
Clozaril Tablets (Less than 1%) 2174
Combivent Inhalation Aerosol (1.4%) 878
Comvax 1904
Copaxone for Injection (Infrequent) 3292
▲ Copegus Tablets (3% to 5%) 2759
Crestor Tablets (Greater than or equal to 1%) 672
▲ Cytovene (13%) 2763
▲ Depacon Injection (1% to 5%) 412
▲ Depakene (1% to 5%) 417
▲ Depakote Sprinkle Capsules (1% to 5%) 422
▲ Depakote Tablets (1% to 5%) 427
Depakote ER Tablets (1%) 433
▲ Doxil Injection (1% to 10%) 3302
DuoNeb Inhalation Solution 1058
EC-Naprosyn Delayed-Release Tablets (Less than 1%) 2769
Effexor Tablets (Infrequent) 3405
Effexor XR Capsules (Infrequent) 3411
Elidel Cream 1% (0.3% to 1.5%) 2198
Elitek (Less than or equal to 1%) 2906
▲ Eloxatin for Injection (2% to 5%) 2908
Enbrel for Injection 580
Equetro Extended-Release Capsules 3178
Evista Tablets (2.6%) 1735
▲ Evoxac Capsules (1% to 3%) 1042
Factive Tablets (Less than or equal to 0.1%) 2464
FazaClo Orally Disintegrating Tablets 547
Ferrlecit Injection 3379
▲ Flolan for Injection (5%) 1408
Flovent Diskus 50 mcg 1415
Flovent HFA 1418
Flumist Vaccine 1872
▲ Forteo for Injection (3.9%) 1739
Fortical Nasal Spray (Less than 1%) 3336
Fuzeon Injection (2.7%) 2772
Gabitril Tablets (Frequent) 998
▲ Gengraf Capsules (1% to 6.2%) 458
Geodon Capsules (Infrequent) 2514
▲ Gleevec Tablets (4% to 13%) 2221
▲ Humira Injection (Less than 5%) 464
Hycamtin for Injection (2%) 1427
▲ Imdur Tablets (Less than or equal to 5%) 3032
Intron A for Injection (Rare) 3038
▲ Invirase (Less than 2% to 5.4%) 2776
I.V. Busulfex 1125
Kineret Injection 594
Klonopin (Infrequent) 2782
Lamictal (Rare) 1449
▲ Leustatin Injection (6%) 2368
Levaquin in 5% Dextrose Injection (0.1% to 0.9%) 2453
Levaquin (0.1% to 0.9%) 2453
Lexapro Oral Solution (Infrequent) 1193
Lexapro Tablets (Infrequent) 1193
Lipitor Tablets (Less than 2%) 2495
Lofibra Capsules 1217
Lovenox Injection (0.82%) 2931
Megace ES Oral Suspension (0% to 2%) 2492
Merrem I.V. (Greater than 1%) 687
Miacalcin Nasal Spray (Less than 1%) 2242
Mirapex Tablets (Less than 1% to 2%) 889
Mycamine for Injection 620
▲ Myfortic Tablets (3% to less than 20%) 2244
Myleran Tablets 1492
▲ Mylotarg for Injection (8% to 13%) 3429
Namenda (Frequent) 1199
Naprosyn Suspension (Less than 1%) 2769
Naprosyn Tablets (Less than 1%) 2769
Navelbine Injection 1494
▲ Neoral Soft Gelatin Capsules (1% to 6.2%) 2247
▲ Neoral Oral Solution (1% to 6.2%) 2247
Neumega for Injection (Frequent) 3433
Neurontin Capsules (Frequent) 2498
Neurontin Oral Solution (Frequent) 2498
Neurontin Tablets (Frequent) 2498
▲ Nipent for Injection (5%) 3216
NovoSeven (1%) 2335
Omacor Capsules 2735
Omnicef Capsules 506
Omnicef for Oral Suspension 506
Orthoclone OKT3 Sterile Solution 2370
Paxil CR Controlled-Release Tablets (Infrequent) 1509
Paxil (Infrequent) 1501
▲ Pegasys (3% to 5%) 2793
PEG-Intron Powder for Injection 3062
Permax Tablets (Frequent) 3357
▲ Photofrin for Injection (18%) 729
Plavix Tablets (1% to 2.5%) 940
Plavix Tablets (1% to 2.5%) 2942
Pletal Tablets (Less than 2%) 2478
Prevacid Delayed-Release Capsules (Less than 1%) 3268
Prevacid for Delayed-Release Oral Suspension (Less than 1%) 3268
Prevacid NapraPAC (Less than 1%) 3277
Prevacid SoluTab Delayed-Release Orally Disintegrating Tablets (Less than 1%) 3268
Prevnar for Injection 3460
PREVPAC (Less than 1%) 3281
Prinivil Tablets (0.3% to 1.0%) 2029
Prinzide Tablets 2033
▲ Prograf Capsules and Injection (3% to 15%) 624
Proleukin for Injection 1007
Protonix I.V. (Less than 1%) 3468
Protonix Tablets (Less than 1%) 3465
Protopic Ointment (1% to 2%) 629
Provigil Tablets (At least 1%) 1002
Pulmicort Respules 654
Pulmozyme Inhalation Solution 1245
▲ Rapamune Oral Solution and Tablets (3% to 20%) 3472
Raptiva for Injection 1247
Rebetol 3073
Rebetron Combination Therapy 3078
▲ Refludan for Injection (4.4%) 815
Remicade for IV Injection 987
ReoPro Vials (1.0%) 1779
Rescriptor Tablets 2535
Rilutek Tablets (More than 2%) 2945
Risperdal Consta Long-Acting Injection (Infrequent) 1664
Risperdal M-Tab Orally Disintegrating Tablets (Infrequent) 1658
Risperdal (Infrequent) 1658
▲ Roferon-A Injection (11%) 2805
▲ Sandimmune (6.2% to 9.2%) 2259
Sandostatin Injection (Less than 1%) 2263
Sandostatin LAR Depot (1% to 4%) 2264
Seroquel Tablets (Infrequent) 691
▲ Simulect for Injection (3% to 10%) 2268
Singulair (Greater than or equal to 2%) 2047
Sonata Capsules (Infrequent) 1686
Symbyax Capsules (Infrequent) 1788
Synagis (More than 1%) 1868
Tamiflu Capsules (Less than 1.9%) 2810

Tamiflu Oral Suspension (Less than 1.9%) 2810
Tasmar Tablets (1% or more) 3360
Tegretol/Tegretol-XR 2278
Testim 1% Gel 722
Thalomid Capsules 979
▲ Topamax Sprinkle Capsules (Greater than 1% to 5%) 2438
▲ Topamax Tablets (Greater than 1% to 5%) 2438
Toprol-XL Tablets (Greater than 1%) 660
▲ Trasylol Injection (4%) 779
Tricor Tablets 523
Trileptal Oral Suspension (1% to 2%) 2281
Trileptal Tablets (1% to 2%) 2281
Truvada Tablets 1279
Uniretic Tablets (Less than 1%) 3114
Vantin Tablets and Oral Suspension (Less than 1%) 2650
Vaqta 2067
Varivax 2070
Vaseretic Tablets 2073
Vasotec I.V. Injection (1.0%) 2076
▲ Velcade for Injection (10%) 2102
▲ Ventavis Inhalation Solution (4%) 1036
▲ Vesanoid Capsules (14%) 2823
VFEND I.V. (Less than 2%) 2543
VFEND Oral Suspension (Less than 2%) 2543
VFEND Tablets (Less than 2%) 2543
Vicoprofen Tablets (Less than 1%) 533
Virazole for Inhalation Solution 3365
▲ Viread Tablets (2% to 3%) 1284
▲ Visudyne for Injection (1% to 10%) 2286
Voltaren Tablets (Rarely) 2298
Voltaren-XR Tablets (Rarely) 2301
Wellbutrin Tablets (Rare) 1579
Wellbutrin SR Sustained-Release Tablets 1583
Wellbutrin XL Extended-Release Tablets 1588
▲ Xeloda Tablets (Less than 5%) 2825
▲ Zemplar Capsules (5%) 535
▲ Zemplar Injection (5%) 538
▲ Zerit (3% to 4%) 971
Zestoretic Tablets 701
Zestril Tablets (0.3% to 1.0%) 704
Zevalin Injection (2%) 848
▲ Ziagen (4%) 1600
Zoladex 3-month (1% to 5%) 712
Zomig Nasal Spray (Rare) 718
Zyban Sustained-Release Tablets 1620
Zyprexa ZYDIS Orally Disintegrating Tablets (Infrequent) 1798
Zyrtec Chewable Tablets (Less than 2%) 2589
Zyrtec (Less than 2%) 2589
Zyrtec-D 12 Hour Extended Release Tablets (Less than 2%) 2591
Zyvox (0% to 2.8%) 2661

Pneumonia, aspiration
Abilify Tablets (Infrequent) 916
Abilify Tablets (Infrequent) 2472
Ammonul Injection 3323
Namenda 1199
Neurontin Capsules (Rare) 2498
Neurontin Oral Solution (Rare) 2498
Neurontin Tablets (Rare) 2498
Zyprexa ZYDIS Orally Disintegrating Tablets (Infrequent) 1798

Pneumonia, eosinophilic
▲ Asacol Delayed-Release Tablets (5% or greater) 2688
Eloxatin for Injection 2908
Omnicef Capsules 506
Omnicef for Oral Suspension 506
Prozac Pulvules and Liquid 1771
Relafen Tablets (Less than 1%) 1523

Pneumonia, interstitial
Aciphex Tablets 1081
Leukeran Tablets 1472
Norvir (Less than 2%) 499
Omnicef Capsules 506
Omnicef for Oral Suspension 506
Pletal Tablets (Very rare) 2478
Tarceva Tablets 1254
Tarceva Tablets 2470
Taxotere Injection Concentrate 2947

Pneumonia, nosocomial
Zegerid Powder for Oral Solution (1.2%) 2972

Pneumonia, pneumocystis carinii
Temodar Capsules (Rare) 3088
Thalomid Capsules 979

Pneumonia, tuberculous
Raptiva for Injection 1247

Pneumonia, viral
Zevalin Injection (2%) 848

Pneumonia-like symptoms
FazaClo Orally Disintegrating Tablets (Less than 1%) 547

Pneumonitis
Aldoclor Tablets 1881
Aldoril Tablets 1884
Atacand HCT 637
Attenuvax 1889
Avalide Tablets 922
Avalide Tablets 2889
▲ Campath Ampules (13% to 21%) 826
Carbatrol Capsules 3174
Celexa (Rare) 1177
Clinoril Tablets (Less than 1 in 100) 1899
Cosmegen for Injection 1907
Diovan HCT Tablets 2195
Diuril Oral 1936
Diuril Sodium Intravenous 1934
Emend Capsules (Greater than 0.5%) 1944
Herceptin I.V. (Rare) 1234
Hyzaar 1964
Indapamide Tablets 2119
Intron A for Injection (Rare) 3038
Lotensin HCT Tablets 2235
Matulane Capsules 3188
Maxzide 2150
Micardis HCT Tablets 886
M-M-R II 1980
Moduretic Tablets 2003
Orthoclone OKT3 Sterile Solution 2370
PEG-Intron Powder for Injection (Less than or equal to 1%) 3062
Photofrin for Injection 729
Prinzide Tablets 2033
Prometrium Capsules (100 mg, 200 mg) (Less than 5%) 3205
Rapamune Oral Solution and Tablets (Infrequent) 3472
Rebetol 3073
Rebetron Combination Therapy 3078
Rituxan for Infusion 845
Rituxan I.V. 1251
Rocephin Injectable Vials, ADD-Vantage, Galaxy, Bulk (Rare) 2801
Roferon-A Injection (Infrequent) 2805
Tarceva Tablets 1254
Tarceva Tablets 2470
Tegretol/Tegretol-XR 2278
Teveten HCT Tablets 1710
Timolide Tablets 2056
Uniretic Tablets 3114
Varivax (Less than 1%) 2070
Vaseretic Tablets 2073
Zestoretic Tablets 701

Pneumonitis, allergic
Dyazide Capsules 1389
Equetro Extended-Release Capsules 3178
Levaquin in 5% Dextrose Injection 2453
Levaquin 2453
Relafen Tablets (Less than 1%) 1523
Rocephin Injectable Vials, ADD-Vantage, Galaxy, Bulk (Rare) 2801
Ticlid Tablets (Rare) 2813

Pneumonitis, eosinophilic
Aceon Tablets (2 mg, 4 mg, 8 mg) 3191
Anaprox Tablets (Less than 1%) 2769
Anaprox DS Tablets (Less than 1%) 2769
Captopril Tablets 2114
EC-Naprosyn Delayed-Release Tablets (Less than 1%) 2769
Lotensin HCT Tablets 2235
Lotrel Capsules 2238
Naprosyn Suspension (Less than 1%) 2769
Naprosyn Tablets (Less than 1%) 2769
Prevacid NapraPAC (Less than 1%) 3277
Prinivil Tablets 2029
Prinzide Tablets 2033
Raptiva for Injection 1247
Uniretic Tablets 3114
Univasc Tablets (Less than 1%) 3118
Vaseretic Tablets 2073
Vasotec I.V. Injection 2076
Zestoretic Tablets 701
Zestril Tablets (0.3% to 1.0%) 704

Pneumonitis, interstitial
Actimmune (Rare) 1646
Alkeran for Injection 976
Alkeran Tablets 977
Arava Tablets (Rare) 2881
Aredia for Injection (One case) 2168
Asacol Delayed-Release Tablets 2688
Casodex Tablets (Rare) 670
Cuprimine Capsules (Rare) 1925
Gleevec Tablets (Rare) 2221
Pacerone Tablets 3337
Pegasys 2793
PEG-Intron Powder for Injection 3062
Plavix Tablets 940
Plavix Tablets 2942
Raptiva for Injection 1247
Relafen Tablets (Less than 1%) 1523
Remicade for IV Injection 987
Rituxan for Infusion 845
Rituxan I.V. 1251

Pneumonitis, hypersensitivity
Pentasa Capsules (Infrequent) 3182
Relafen Tablets (Rarer) 1523

Pneumothorax
Actiq (Less than 1%) 993
Ammonul Injection 3323
Campath Ampules 826
▲ CellCept Capsules (3% to less than 20%) 2751
▲ CellCept Intravenous (3% to less than 20%) 2751
▲ CellCept Oral Suspension (3% to less than 20%) 2751
▲ CellCept Tablets (3% to less than 20%) 2751
Doxil Injection (Less than 1%) 3302
▲ Flolan for Injection (4%) 1408
Herceptin I.V. (At least one of the 958 patients) 1234
▲ Intron A for Injection (Less than or equal to 5%) 3038
Levaquin in 5% Dextrose Injection (0.1% to 0.9%) 2453
Levaquin (0.1% to 0.9%) 2453
Permax Tablets (Rare) 3357
▲ Prograf Capsules and Injection (3% to 15%) 624
Proleukin for Injection (1%) 1007
Prozac Pulvules and Liquid (Rare) 1771
Pulmozyme Inhalation Solution 1245
Rilutek Tablets (Infrequent) 2945
Sandostatin LAR Depot (Rare) 2264
▲ Trasylol Injection (4%) 779
Virazole for Inhalation Solution 3365
Zegerid Powder for Oral Solution (0.6%) 2972
Zosyn (1.3%) 3492

Poliomyelitis
Invirase (Less than 2%) 2776

Pollakiuria
▲ Cymbalta Delayed-Release Capsules (1% to 5%) 1729
DynaCirc CR Tablets (0.5% to 1%) 2726

Polyarteritis nodosa
▲ Intron A for Injection (Less than 5%) 3038

Polyarthralgia
Dynacin Tablets 1859
Eskalith 1406
Lithobid Tablets 1670
Primaxin I.M. 2022
Primaxin I.V. (Less than 0.2%) 2024

Polyarthralgia, migratory
Cuprimine Capsules (Some patients) 1925

Polyarthritis
Cleocin Vaginal Ovules (Rare) 2613
Clindesse Vaginal Cream (Rare) 3296
Invirase (Rare) 2776
▲ Roferon-A Injection (5%) 2805

Polycythemia
▲ CellCept Capsules (3% to less than 20%) 2751
▲ CellCept Intravenous (3% to less than 20%) 2751
▲ CellCept Oral Suspension (3% to less than 20%) 2751
▲ CellCept Tablets (3% to less than 20%) 2751
Delatestryl Injection 2976
Estratest Tablets 3196
Estratest H.S. Tablets 3196
Factive Tablets (0.1%) 2464
Geodon Capsules (Rare) 2514
▲ Humira Injection (Less than 5%) 464
Lyrica Capsules (Rare) 2524
Oxandrin Tablets 2977
Permax Tablets (Rare) 3357
Pletal Tablets (Less than 2%) 2478
▲ Prograf Capsules and Injection (3% to 15%) 624
▲ Rapamune Oral Solution and Tablets (3% to 20%) 3472
▲ Simulect for Injection (3% to 10%) 2268
Striant Mucoadhesive 1022
Topamax Sprinkle Capsules (Rare) 2438
Topamax Tablets (Rare) 2438

Polydipsia
Amerge Tablets (Infrequent) 1312
Aricept Tablets (Infrequent) 1086
Aricept ODT Tablets (Infrequent) 1086
Calcijex Injection 411
Clozapine Tablets (Less than 1%) 2141
Clozaril Tablets (Less than 1%) 2174
Eskalith 1406
FazaClo Orally Disintegrating Tablets (Less than 1%) 547
Hectorol Capsules 909
Hectorol Injection 911
Imitrex Injection (Rare) 1431
Imitrex Nasal Spray 1435
Imitrex Tablets (Rare) 1440
Lithobid Tablets 1670
Risperdal M-Tab Orally Disintegrating Tablets (Frequent) 1658
Risperdal (Frequent) 1658
Thiothixene Capsules 2124

Polymenorrhea
Sandostatin Injection (Less than 1%) 2263

Polymyalgia rheumatica
Advicor Tablets 1694
Altoprev Extended-Release Tablets (Rare) 1151
Fortical Nasal Spray (Less than 1%) 3336
Lescol Capsules (Rare) 2227
Lescol Capsules (Rare) 2730
Lescol XL Tablets 2227
Lescol XL Tablets 2730
Mevacor Tablets (Rare) 1996
Miacalcin Nasal Spray (Less than 1%) 2242
Nexium Delayed-Release Capsules (Less than 1%) 645
Nexium I.V. (Less than 1%) 649
Pravachol Tablets (Rare) 943
Requip Tablets (Infrequent) 1528
Vytorin 10/10 Tablets 2084
Vytorin 10/10 Tablets 3092
Vytorin 10/20 Tablets 2084
Vytorin 10/20 Tablets 3092
Vytorin 10/40 Tablets 2084
Vytorin 10/40 Tablets 3092
Vytorin 10/80 Tablets 2084
Vytorin 10/80 Tablets 3092
Zocor Tablets (Rare) 2078

Polymyositis
Campath Ampules 826
Cuprimine Capsules (Rare) 1925
Enbrel for Injection (Infrequent) 580
Tagamet Tablets (Rare) 1547

Polyneuritis
Antabuse Tablets 2343
Meruvax II 1994
M-M-R II 1980

Polyneuropathy
▲ Intron A for Injection (Less than 5%) 3038
Meruvax II (Isolated reports) 1994
M-M-R II 1980
Phenytek Capsules 2153
▲ Xeloda Tablets (Less than 5%) 2825

Polyneuropathy, axonal
Avelox 2984
Factive Tablets (Rare) 2464
Tequin Injection 964
Tequin Tablets 964

Polyneuropathy, peripheral
Leustatin Injection 2368

Polyphagia
Clozapine Tablets 2141

Polyposis, gastric
Lexapro Oral Solution (Infrequent) 1193
Lexapro Tablets (Infrequent) 1193

Polyps, cervical
▲ Menostar Transdermal System (6%) 805

Polyps, fundic gland
Prevacid NapraPAC (Less than 1%) 3277

Polyps, gallbladder
- Sandostatin Injection (Less than 1%) 2263
- Sandostatin LAR Depot (Rare) 2264

Polyps, nasal
- ▲ Atrovent Nasal Spray 0.03% (3.1%) 869
- Pulmozyme Inhalation Solution 1245
- Zyrtec Chewable Tablets (Less than 2%) 2589
- Zyrtec (Less than 2%) 2589
- Zyrtec-D 12 Hour Extended Release Tablets (Less than 2%) 2591

Polyserositis
- Avastin IV (Rare) 1229
- Biltricide Tablets 2990

Polyuria
- Abilify Tablets (Rare) 916
- Abilify Tablets (Rare) 2472
- Aciphex Tablets 1081
- Adalat CC Tablets (Less than 1%) 2978
- Ambien Tablets (Rare) 2867
- Amerge Tablets (Infrequent) 1312
- Anaprox Tablets (Less than 1%) 2769
- Anaprox DS Tablets (Less than 1%) 2769
- Anzemet Injection (Rare) 2871
- Anzemet Tablets (Rare) 2874
- Arthrotec Tablets (Rare) 3126
- ▲ Avastin IV (3% to 6%) 1229
- Balamine DM 739
- ▲ Betaseron for SC Injection (7%) 791
- Caduet Tablets (Less than or equal to 0.1%) 2507
- Calcijex Injection 411
- Campral Tablets (Rare) 1175
- Captopril Tablets (Approximately 1 to 2 of 1000 patients) 2114
- Cardene I.V. (1.4%) 1129
- Cardizem LA Extended Release Tablets (Less than 2%) 1699
- Cataflam Tablets (Occasionally) 2173
- Celexa (Frequent) 1177
- Cipro I.V. (1% or less) 2998
- Cipro I.V. Pharmacy Bulk Package (1% or less) 3509
- Cipro (Less than 1%) 2991
- Cipro XR Tablets 3004
- Clozapine Tablets 2141
- Colazal Capsules 2845
- Coreg Tablets (Greater than 0.1% to 1%) 1376
- EC-Naprosyn Delayed-Release Tablets (Less than 1%) 2769
- Effexor Tablets (Infrequent) 3405
- Effexor XR Capsules (Infrequent) 3411
- Elspar for Injection (Low) 1943
- Eskalith 1406
- Evoxac Capsules (0.1%) 1042
- Exelon Capsules (Infrequent) 2204
- Frova Tablets (Infrequent) 1101
- Gabitril Tablets (Infrequent) 998
- Gengraf Capsules (1% to less than 3%) 458
- Geodon Capsules (Infrequent) 2514
- Gleevec Tablets (Infrequent) 2221
- Hectorol Capsules 909
- Hectorol Injection 911
- ▲ Imdur Tablets (Less than or equal to 5%) 3032
- Indapamide Tablets (Less than 5%) 2119
- ▲ Intron A for Injection (Less than 5%) 3038
- Klonopin (Infrequent) 2782
- Lamictal (Infrequent) 1449
- Lithobid Tablets 1670
- Lofibra Capsules (1%) 1217
- Lotrel Capsules 2238
- Lotronex Tablets (Rare) 1479
- Maxalt Tablets (Infrequent) 1983
- Maxalt-MLT Orally Disintegrating Tablets (Infrequent) 1983
- Midamor Tablets (Less than or equal to 1%) 2000
- Moduretic Tablets 2003
- Naprosyn Suspension (Less than 1%) 2769
- Naprosyn Tablets (Less than 1%) 2769
- Neoral Soft Gelatin Capsules (1% to less than 3%) 2247
- Neoral Oral Solution (1% to less than 3%) 2247
- Neurontin Capsules (Infrequent) 2498
- Neurontin Oral Solution (Infrequent) 2498
- Neurontin Tablets (Infrequent) 2498
- Nexium Delayed-Release Capsules (Less than 1%) 645
- Nexium I.V. (Less than 1%) 649
- Norvasc Tablets (Less than or equal to 0.1%) 2529
- Norvir (Less than 2%) 499
- OxyContin Tablets (Less than 1%) 2699
- Paxil CR Controlled-Release Tablets (Infrequent) 1509
- Paxil (Infrequent) 1501
- Plendil Extended-Release Tablets (0.5% to 1.5%) 651
- Prevacid Delayed-Release Capsules (Less than 1%) 3268
- Prevacid for Delayed-Release Oral Suspension (Less than 1%) 3268
- Prevacid NapraPAC (Less than 1%) 3277
- Prevacid SoluTab Delayed-Release Orally Disintegrating Tablets (Less than 1%) 3268
- PREVPAC (Less than 1%) 3281
- Primaxin I.M. 2022
- Primaxin I.V. (Less than 0.2%) 2024
- Prozac Pulvules and Liquid (At least 2%) 1771
- ▲ Rapamune Oral Solution and Tablets (3% to 20%) 3472
- ▲ Rebif Prefilled Syringe for Injection (2% to 7%) 3163
- Relpax Tablets (Infrequent) 2531
- Requip Tablets (Infrequent) 1528
- Rescriptor Tablets 2535
- Retrovir Capsules 1533
- Retrovir IV Infusion 1537
- Retrovir 1533
- Reyataz Capsules (Less than 3%) 948
- Risperdal M-Tab Orally Disintegrating Tablets (Frequent) 1658
- Risperdal (Frequent) 1658
- Seroquel Tablets (Rare) 691
- Stalevo Tablets 2270
- Symbyax Capsules (Infrequent) 1788
- Tambocor Tablets (Less than 1%) 1824
- Tarka Tablets (Less frequent) 519
- Tasmar Tablets (Infrequent) 3360
- Teveten Tablets (Less than 1%) 1707
- Teveten HCT Tablets (Less than 1%) 1710
- Tiazac Capsules (Less than 2%) 1204
- Topamax Sprinkle Capsules (Infrequent) 2438
- Topamax Tablets (Infrequent) 2438
- Tricor Tablets 523
- Trileptal Oral Suspension 2281
- Trileptal Tablets 2281
- Uniretic Tablets (Less than 1%) 3114
- Voltaren Tablets (Occasionally) 2298
- Voltaren-XR Tablets (Occasionally) 2301
- Wellbutrin SR Sustained-Release Tablets (Infrequent) 1583
- Wellbutrin XL Extended-Release Tablets (Infrequent) 1588
- Xifaxan Tablets (Less than 2%) 2847
- Zoloft (Infrequent) 2581
- Zomig Nasal Spray (Infrequent) 718
- Zomig Tablets (Infrequent) 714
- Zomig-ZMT Tablets (Infrequent) 714
- Zonegran Capsules (Infrequent) 1089
- Zyban Sustained-Release Tablets (Infrequent) 1620
- Zyprexa Tablets (Infrequent) 1798
- Zyprexa ZYDIS Orally Disintegrating Tablets (Infrequent) 1798
- Zyrtec Chewable Tablets (Less than 2%) 2589
- Zyrtec (Less than 2%) 2589
- Zyrtec-D 12 Hour Extended Release Tablets (Less than 2%) 2591

Porphyria
- Alesse-28 Tablets 3392
- Arthrotec Tablets (Rare) 3126
- Lo/Ovral-28 Tablets 3423
- Ortho-Cept Tablets 2395
- Ortho-Cyclen Tablets 2414
- Ortho Evra Transdermal System 2402
- Ortho Tri-Cyclen Tablets 2414
- Ortho Tri-Cyclen Lo Tablets 2421
- Paxil CR Controlled-Release Tablets 1509
- Paxil 1501
- Sulfamylon Cream (A single case) 2154
- Sulfamylon for 5% Topical Solution 2155
- Triphasil-28 Tablets 3483
- Yasmin 28 Tablets 818

Porphyria, aggravation of
- Activella Tablets 2311
- Alesse-28 Tablets 3392
- Cenestin Tablets, 0.45mg, 0.625mg, 0.9mg, 1.25mg 1063
- Cenestin Tablets, 0.3mg 1063
- Climara Transdermal System 795
- Climara Pro Transdermal System 800
- CombiPatch Transdermal System 2180
- Epogen for Injection (Rare) 586
- Estratest Tablets 3196
- Estratest H.S. Tablets 3196
- Estrogel 0.06% 3200
- Lo/Ovral-28 Tablets 3423
- Menostar Transdermal System 805
- Phenytek Capsules (Isolated reports) 2153
- Prefest Tablets 1069
- Premarin Intravenous 3440
- Premarin Tablets 3443
- Premarin Vaginal Cream 3449
- Premphase Tablets 3452
- Prempro Tablets 3452
- Procrit for Injection (Rare) 2374
- Seasonale Tablets 1073
- Triphasil-28 Tablets 3483
- Vivelle Transdermal System 2288
- Vivelle-Dot Transdermal System 2293
- Zantac (Rare) 1597
- Zantac Injection (Rare) 1593
- Zantac Syrup (Rare) 1597

Porphyria, cutaneous, drug-induced
- Photofrin for Injection 729

Porphyria, intermittent, acute
- Carbatrol Capsules 3174
- Depacon Injection 412
- Depakene 417
- Depakote Sprinkle Capsules 422
- Depakote Tablets 427
- Depakote ER Tablets 433
- Equetro Extended-Release Capsules 3178
- Tegretol/Tegretol-XR 2278

Porphyria cutanea tarda
- Amaryl Tablets (Less than 1%) 2864
- Anaprox Tablets (Less than 1%) 2769
- Anaprox DS Tablets (Less than 1%) 2769
- EC-Naprosyn Delayed-Release Tablets (Less than 1%) 2769
- Myleran Tablets (Rare) 1492
- Naprosyn Suspension (Less than 1%) 2769
- Naprosyn Tablets (Less than 1%) 2769

Porphyria cutanea tarda, pseudo
- Prevacid NapraPAC (Less than 1%) 3277
- Relafen Tablets (Less than 1%) 1523

Potassium loss
(*see under* Hypokalemia)

Potassium retention
(*see under* Hyperkalemia)

Potentia, decrease
- Kadian Capsules (Less than 3%) 572

Precocious puberty
- Novarel for Injection 1147
- Premarin Vaginal Cream 3449

Pregnancy, accidental
- Antara Capsules 2723
- Depo-Provera Contraceptive Injection (Less than 1%) 2619
- depo-subQ provera 104 Injectable Suspension 2622
- Lofibra Capsules 1217
- Tricor Tablets 523
- Zomig Nasal Spray (Rare) 718

Pregnancy, ectopic
- Bravelle for Intramuscular or Subcutaneous Injection 1140
- Gonal-f RFF Pen for Injection 3155
- Mirena Intrauterine System 810
- Repronex for Intramuscular and Subcutaneous Injection (1%) 1148

Pregnancy, multiple
- Bravelle for Intramuscular or Subcutaneous Injection 1140

Pregnancy, sensation of
- Depo-Provera Contraceptive Injection (Less than 1%) 2619

Pregnancy tests, false positive
- Thioridazine Hydrochloride Tablets 2122
- Thiothixene Capsules 2124

Pregnancy, prolonged
- Aggrenox Capsules 855
- Bayer Aspirin Tablets 3515

Premature depolarizations, ventricular
- Retavase 1131

Premature ventricular contractions
- Diprivan Injectable Emulsion (Less than 1%) 676
- Imitrex Injection (Infrequent) 1431
- Prinivil Tablets (0.3% to 1.0%) 2029
- Prinzide Tablets 2033
- Tarka Tablets (0.3% or more) 519
- Zestril Tablets (0.3% to 1.0%) 704

Premenstrual-like syndrome
- Activella Tablets 2311
- Alesse-28 Tablets 3392
- Estratest Tablets 3196
- Estratest H.S. Tablets 3196
- Lexapro Oral Solution (Infrequent) 1193
- Lexapro Tablets (Infrequent) 1193
- Lo/Ovral-28 Tablets 3423
- Ortho-Cept Tablets 2395
- Ortho-Cyclen Tablets 2414
- Ortho Evra Transdermal System 2402
- Ortho Tri-Cyclen Tablets 2414
- Ortho Tri-Cyclen Lo Tablets 2421
- Premarin Intravenous 3440
- Premarin Vaginal Cream 3449
- Premphase Tablets 3452
- Prempro Tablets 3452
- Seasonale Tablets 1073
- Triphasil-28 Tablets 3483
- Xanax XR Tablets (1.7%) 2655
- Yasmin 28 Tablets 818
- Zyprexa Tablets (2%) 1798
- Zyprexa ZYDIS Orally Disintegrating Tablets (2%) 1798

Pressor response, paradoxical
- BiDil Tablets 2161

Priapism
- Abilify Tablets (Rare) 916
- Abilify Tablets (Rare) 2472
- Anadrol-50 Tablets 3329
- Apokyn Injection (Less than 1%) 2132
- ▲ Caverject Impulse Injection (4%) 2610
- Celexa 1177
- Cialis Tablets (Less than 2%) 1806
- Clozapine Tablets 2141
- Clozaril Tablets 2174
- Copaxone for Injection (Infrequent) 3292
- Coumadin for Injection 932
- Coumadin Tablets 932
- Delatestryl Injection 2976
- ▲ Edex Injection (Less than 1% to 4%) 3103
- Effexor XR Capsules (Rare) 3411
- FazaClo Orally Disintegrating Tablets 547
- Flomax Capsules (Rare) 881
- Geodon for Injection (Up to 1%) 2514
- Hytrin Capsules (Rare) 469
- Levitra Tablets (Less than 2%) 3048
- Lexapro Oral Solution 1193
- Lexapro Tablets 1193
- Miradon Tablets 3056
- Moban Tablets 1108
- Oxandrin Tablets 2977
- Parcopa Orally Disintegrating Tablets 3111
- Paxil CR Controlled-Release Tablets 1509
- Paxil 1501
- Permax Tablets (Infrequent) 3357
- Prozac Pulvules and Liquid (Rare) 1771
- Rilutek Tablets (Infrequent) 2945
- Risperdal M-Tab Orally Disintegrating Tablets (Rare) 1658
- Risperdal (Rare) 1658
- Seroquel Tablets (One case) 691
- Stalevo Tablets 2270
- Testim 1% Gel (1% or less) 722
- Thioridazine Hydrochloride Tablets 2122
- Trileptal Oral Suspension 2281
- Trileptal Tablets 2281
- Uroxatral Tablets 2957
- Viagra Tablets 2552
- Zoloft (Rare) 2581
- Zyprexa Tablets 1798
- Zyprexa ZYDIS Orally Disintegrating Tablets 1798

Proarrhythmia
- Apokyn Injection 2132

Proctalgia
- Remicade for IV Injection (Greater than or equal to 0.2%) 987
- Zelnorm Tablets 2303

Proctitis
- Aciphex Tablets 1081
- Aloprim for Injection (Less than 1%) 2156
- Cosmegen for Injection 1907

Doxil Injection (Less than 1%) 3302
Effexor Tablets (Rare) 3405
Effexor XR Capsules (Rare) 3411
▲ Eloxatin for Injection (2% to 5%) 2908
▲ Eulexin Capsules (8%) 3023
Indocin Capsules (Less than 1%) 1968
Indocin I.V. (Less than 1%) 1973
Indocin (Less than 1%) 1968
Lotronex Tablets (Rare) 1479
Neurontin Capsules (Rare) 2498
Neurontin Oral Solution (Rare) 2498
Neurontin Tablets (Rare) 2498
Rilutek Tablets (Rare) 2945
VFEND I.V. (Less than 2%) 2543
VFEND Oral Suspension (Less than 2%) 2543
VFEND Tablets (Less than 2%) 2543
▲ Zoladex (8%) 709
▲ Zoladex 3-month (8%) 712
Zoloft (Rare) 2581

Proctitis, ulceration
Doxil Injection (Less than 1%) 3302

Prolactin levels, elevated
(*see under* Hyperprolactinemia)

Prolactinemia
Celexa 1177

Proptosis
Ortho-Cyclen/Ortho Tri-Cyclen 2414
Ortho Tri-Cyclen Lo Tablets 2421
Premphase Tablets 3452
Prempro Tablets 3452

Prostate disorders, unspecified
▲ AndroGel (3% to 5%) 3330
Antara Capsules 2723
▲ Arava Tablets (1% to 3%) 2881
Atrovent Nasal Spray 0.03% 869
Atrovent Nasal Spray 0.06% 870
Avalide Tablets 922
Avalide Tablets 2889
Avapro Tablets (Less than 1%) 925
Avapro Tablets (Less than 1%) 2886
Avonex 839
▲ Betaseron for SC Injection (3%) 791
Caverject Impulse Injection (2%) 2610
Celebrex Capsules (0.1% to 1.9%) 3130
Edex Injection (1%) 3103
Evoxac Capsules (Less than 1%) 1042
Lofibra Capsules 1217
Mirapex Tablets (Less than 1%) 889
Protonix I.V. (Less than 1%) 3468
Protonix Tablets (Less than 1%) 3465
Requip Tablets (Infrequent) 1528
Tasmar Tablets (Infrequent) 3360
Testim 1% Gel (1%) 722
Travatan Ophthalmic Solution (1% to 5%) 559
Tricor Tablets 523
Ultracet Tablets (2%) 2462
Viadur Implant (Less than 2%) 782
▲ Visudyne for Injection (1% to 10%) 2286
Wellbutrin SR Sustained-Release Tablets (Infrequent) 1583
Wellbutrin XL Extended-Release Tablets (Infrequent) 1588
Zyban Sustained-Release Tablets 1620

Prostate enlargement
AndroGel (Five patients) 3330
Caverject Impulse Injection (2%) 2610
Effexor Tablets (Frequent) 3405

Prostate specific antigen decrease
▲ Avodart Soft Gelatin Capsules (Approximately 40% to 50%) 1353

Prostate specific antigen increase
Aciphex Tablets 1081
Rythmol SR Capsules 2736
Striant Mucoadhesive 1022

Prostatic acid phosphatase, decreased
Lupron Depot (Greater than or equal to 5%) 3261

Prostatic acid phosphatase, increased
Vantas (Less than 2%) 3367

Prostatic cancer, transient worsening symptoms
Zoladex (A small percentage) 709
Zoladex 3-month (A small percentage) 712

Prostatic hypertrophy
Aricept Tablets (Infrequent) 1086
Aricept ODT Tablets (Infrequent) 1086
Caverject Impulse Injection (2%) 2610
Eldepryl Capsules 3209
Invirase (Less than 2%) 2776
Striant Mucoadhesive 1022
Testim 1% Gel (1% or less) 722
▲ Vesanoid Capsules (3%) 2823

Prostatism
Rythmol SR Capsules 2736

Prostatitis
Caverject Impulse Injection (2%) 2610
Effexor Tablets (Frequent) 3405
Effexor XR Capsules (Infrequent) 3411
ReoPro Vials (0.1%) 1779
▲ Strattera Capsules (3%) 1784

Protein bound iodine, lowered
(*see under* PBI decrease)

Protein catabolism
Depo-Medrol Injectable Suspension 2615
Depo-Medrol Single-Dose Vial 2617
Hydrocortone Tablets 1963

Proteinuria
Accutane Capsules 2740
Aceon Tablets (2 mg, 4 mg, 8 mg) (1.0% to 1.5%) 3191
Aggrenox Capsules 855
Aldara Cream, 5% 1814
Altace Capsules 1673
Amnesteem Capsules 2126
Anaprox Tablets (Less than 1%) 2769
Anaprox DS Tablets (Less than 1%) 2769
Arthrotec Tablets (Rare) 3126
▲ Avastin IV (36%) 1229
Bayer Aspirin Tablets 3515
Calcium Disodium Versenate Injection 1819
Captopril Tablets (Approximately 1 of 100 patients) 2114
Cataflam Tablets (Occasionally) 2173
Cleocin Vaginal Ovules (Rare) 2613
Clindesse Vaginal Cream (Rare) 3296
Clinoril Tablets (Less than 1 in 100) 1899
▲ Cuprimine Capsules (6%) 1925
Dolobid Tablets (Less than 1 in 100) 1937
EC-Naprosyn Delayed-Release Tablets (Less than 1%) 2769
Ecotrin Enteric Coated Aspirin Low, Regular and Maximum Strength Tablets 1627
Elspar for Injection (Infrequent) 1943
▲ Emend Capsules (6.8%) 1944
Garamycin Injectable 3028
▲ Gemzar for Injection (2% to 45%) 1743
Grifulvin V Tablets Microsize and Oral Suspension Microsize (Rare) 2384
Gris-PEG Tablets (Rare) 2504
Indocin (Less than 1%) 1968
▲ Intron A for Injection (Less than 5%) 3038
Kepivance (9 patients) 592
Lotensin HCT Tablets 2235
Naprosyn Suspension (Less than 1%) 2769
Naprosyn Tablets (Less than 1%) 2769
Neupogen for Injection (Infrequent) 598
Parcopa Orally Disintegrating Tablets 3111
Prilosec OTC Tablets (Less than 1%) 2674
Primaxin I.M. 2022
Primaxin I.V. 2024
▲ Proleukin for Injection (12%) 1007
Prozac Pulvules and Liquid 1771
Rescriptor Tablets 2535
Reyataz Capsules (Less than 3%) 948
▲ Roferon-A Injection (0% to 10%) 2805
Rythmol SR Capsules 2736
St. Joseph 81 mg Aspirin Chewable and Enteric Coated Tablets 1841
Tarka Tablets (Less frequent) 519
Truvada Tablets 1279
Vantin Tablets and Oral Suspension (Less than 1%) 2650
Vaqta (Isolated reports) 2067
Voltaren Tablets (Occasionally) 2298
Voltaren-XR Tablets (Occasionally) 2301
Xifaxan Tablets (Less than 2%) 2847
Zegerid Powder for Oral Solution (Less than 1%) 2972
Zosyn 3492

Proteinuria, increased
Cancidas for Injection (0% to 1.2%) 1894
▲ Chemet Capsules (Up to 3.7%) 2480
Noroxin Tablets (1.0%) 2009
Omnicef Capsules (2%) 506
Omnicef for Oral Suspension (1%) 506

Prothrombin, abnormal
Maxipime for Injection (1.4%) 1093

Prothrombin, decrease
(*see under* Hypoprothrombinemia)

Prothrombin, increase
(*see under* Hyperprothrombinemia)

Prothrombin time, deviation
Avelox (Less than 0.1%) 2984
Maxipime for Injection (1.6%) 1093
Thrombin-JMI 1693

Prothrombin time, elevation
Advicor Tablets 1694
Cancidas for Injection (1.3% to 1.5%) 1894
Ecotrin Enteric Coated Aspirin Low, Regular and Maximum Strength Tablets 1627
St. Joseph 81 mg Aspirin Chewable and Enteric Coated Tablets 1841

Prothrombin time, increase
(*see under* Prothrombin time prolongation)

Prothrombin time prolongation
Aggrenox Capsules 855
Anadrol-50 Tablets 3329
Avelox (0.1% to less than 2%) 2984
Bayer Aspirin Tablets 3515
Biaxin/Biaxin XL (1%) 402
Ceftin 1369
▲ CellCept Capsules (3% to less than 20%) 2751
▲ CellCept Intravenous (3% to less than 20%) 2751
▲ CellCept Oral Suspension (3% to less than 20%) 2751
▲ CellCept Tablets (3% to less than 20%) 2751
Cipro I.V. 2998
Cipro I.V. Pharmacy Bulk Package 3509
Cipro 2991
Cipro XR Tablets 3004
Clinoril Tablets 1899
Colazal Capsules 2845
Elmiron Capsules (Less than or equal to 1%) 2393
Fortaz 1422
Infergen (1% to 3%) 1647
Invanz for Injection (0.3% to 1.2%) 1974
I.V. Busulfex (2%) 1125
Levaquin in 5% Dextrose Injection 2453
Levaquin 2453
Mefoxin for Injection 1987
Mefoxin Premixed Intravenous Solution 1990
Merrem I.V. (Greater than 0.2%) 687
Niaspan Extended-Release Tablets 1703
Noroxin Tablets 2009
Oncaspar 1123
Ortho-Cyclen/Ortho Tri-Cyclen 2414
Ortho Tri-Cyclen Lo Tablets 2421
Oxandrin Tablets 2977
Panhematin for Injection 2487
PREVPAC (1%) 3281
Primaxin I.M. 2022
Primaxin I.V. 2024
Rescriptor Tablets 2535
Rocephin Injectable Vials, ADD-Vantage, Galaxy, Bulk (Less than 1%) 2801
Suprax (Rare) 1811
Testim 1% Gel (1% or less) 722
Timentin ADD-Vantage 1556
Timentin Injection Galaxy Container 1559
Timentin IV Infusion 1553
Timentin Pharmacy Bulk Package 1562
Tygacil for Injection (0% to less than 2%) 3489
Vantin Tablets and Oral Suspension 2650
Zinacef Injection 1604
Zinacef for Injection 1604
Zoloft 2581
Zosyn 3492

Prothrombin time, decrease
Cipro I.V. 2998
Cipro I.V. Pharmacy Bulk Package 3509
Cipro 2991
Premarin Tablets 3443
Premphase Tablets 3452
Prempro Tablets 3452

Pruritis, ear
Ciprodex Otic Suspension (1.5%) 555

Pruritus
Abelcet Injection 1119
Abilify Tablets (Infrequent) 916
Abilify Tablets (Infrequent) 2472
Accolate Tablets 663
Accutane Capsules 2740
Aceon Tablets (2 mg, 4 mg, 8 mg) (0.3% to 1%) 3191
Aciphex Tablets 1081
Aclovate (Approximately 2%) 1290
▲ Acticin Cream (7%) 2125
Actiq (Up to 5%) 993
Activella Tablets 2311
▲ Actonel Tablets (1.9% to 3%) 2679
▲ Actonel with Calcium Tablets (1.9% to 3%) 2684
Adacel Vaccine (Very rare) 2959
Adalat CC Tablets (Less than 1%) 2978
Advate Injection (0.6%) 742
▲ Advicor Tablets (7%) 1694
▲ Aerobid/Aerobid-M (3% to 9%) 1172
Agenerase Capsules 1299
Agenerase Oral Solution (1%) 1304
Aggrenox Capsules (Less than 1%) 855
▲ Agrylin Capsules (5.5%) 3172
Alacol DM Syrup 739
Aldara Cream, 5% (0.9%) 1814
Aldurazyme for Intravenous Infusion 1261
Alferon N Injection (2%) 1640
Alinia for Oral Suspension (Less than 1%) 2840
Alinia Tablets (Less than 1%) 2840
Alkeran for Injection 976
Allegra (Rare) 2857
Allegra-D 12 Hour Extended-Release Tablets (Rare) 2860
Allegra-D 24 Hour Extended-Release Tablets (Rare) 2862
Aloprim for Injection (Less than 1%) 2156
Altace Capsules (Less than 1%) 1673
Altoprev Extended-Release Tablets (0.5% to 1%) 1151
Amaryl Tablets (Less than 1%) 2864
Ambien Tablets (Infrequent) 2867
▲ AmBisome for Injection (10.8%) 615
Amerge Tablets (Infrequent) 1312
Amevive (Common) 836
Ammonul Injection 3323
Amnesteem Capsules 2126
Analpram-HC 1136
▲ Anaprox Tablets (3% to 9%) 2769
▲ Anaprox DS Tablets (3% to 9%) 2769
Ancef for Injection 1318
Antara Capsules 2723
▲ Anzemet Injection (3.1%) 2871
▲ Anzemet Tablets (3.1%) 2874
Apidra Injection 2876
Apokyn Injection (2%) 2132
Aptivus Capsules (Less than 2%) 859
Aralast (0.1%) 745
▲ Aranesp for Injection (8%) 576
▲ Arava Tablets (4%) 2881
Aricept Tablets (Frequent) 1086
Aricept ODT Tablets (Frequent) 1086
▲ Arimidex Tablets (2% to 5%) 665
Aromasin Tablets (Less frequent) 2600
Arthrotec Tablets (Rare) 3126
▲ Asacol Delayed-Release Tablets (3%) 2688
Astelin Nasal Spray 1876
Atacand Tablets 634
Atacand HCT (0.5% or greater) 637
Augmentin 1331
Augmentin Tablets 1334
Augmentin XR Extended-Release Tablets 1340
Augmentin ES-600 Powder for Oral Suspension 1337
Avalide Tablets 922
Avalide Tablets 2889
Avapro Tablets (Less than 1%) 925
Avapro Tablets (Less than 1%) 2886
Avelox (0.1% to less than 2%) 2984
Avodart Soft Gelatin Capsules 1353
Avonex 839
Axert Tablets (Rare) 2430
Axid Oral Solution (1.7%) 913
Aygestin Tablets 1062
Bactroban Cream (Less than 1%) 1356
Bactroban Nasal (1%) 1357
Bactroban Ointment (1%) 1358
Beano ▣ 764
Benicar Tablets 2850
Benicar HCT Tablets (Rare) 2852

Bentyl Capsules 724
Bentyl Injection 724
Bentyl Syrup 724
Bentyl Tablets 724
▲ Benzaclin Topical Gel (12%) 1046
Betagan Ophthalmic Solution, USP (Rare) ⊙ 217
Betaseron for SC Injection 791
▲ Bexxar (0% to 10%) 1360
Blocadren Tablets (1.1%) 1891
▲ Botox Purified Neurotoxin Complex (3% to 10%) 565
Buprenex Injectable (Less than 1%) 2718
Caduet Tablets (Less than 1% to 2%) 2507
Calcijex Injection 411
▲ Campath Ampules (1% to 24%) 826
▲ Campral Tablets (3% to 4%) 1175
Cancidas for Injection (1.2% to 2.5%) 1894
Captopril Tablets (About 2 of 100 patients) 2114
Carafate Suspension (Less than 0.5%) 727
Carafate Tablets (Less than 0.5%) 728
Cardizem LA Extended Release Tablets (Less than 2%) 1699
▲ Carnitor Injection (3% to 8%) 3185
Casodex Tablets (2% to 5%) 670
▲ Cataflam Tablets (1% to 10%) 2173
Catapres Tablets (About 7 in 1,000 patients) 874
▲ Catapres-TTS (51 of 101 patients) 875
Caverject Impulse Injection (Less than 1%) 2610
Ceftin (0.1% to 1%) 1369
Celebrex Capsules (0.1% to 1.9%) 3130
Celexa (Frequent) 1177
▲ CellCept Capsules (3% to less than 20%) 2751
▲ CellCept Intravenous (3% to less than 20%) 2751
▲ CellCept Oral Suspension (3% to less than 20%) 2751
▲ CellCept Tablets (3% to less than 20%) 2751
Cenestin Tablets, 0.3mg 1063
Centany Ointment, 2% (1%) 2382
▲ Cerezyme for Injection (Approximately 6.6%) 1263
▲ Chemet Capsules (2.6% to 11.2%) 2480
Cialis Tablets (Less than 2%) 1806
Cipro I.V. (1% or less) 2998
Cipro I.V. Pharmacy Bulk Package (1% or less) 3509
Cipro (Less than 1%) 2991
Cipro XR Tablets (Less than 1%) 3004
Clarinex Syrup (Rare) 3009
Clarinex Tablets (Rare) 3009
Clarinex Reditabs Tablets (Rare) 3009
Clarinex-D 24-Hour Extended-Release Tablets 3012
Cleocin Vaginal Ovules (Less than 1%) 2613
Climara Transdermal System (0.5% to 6%) 795
Climara Pro Transdermal System 800
Clindagel (0.6%) 1207
▲ Clindets Pledgets (7% to 11%) 3212
Clinoril Tablets (Greater than 1%) 1899
Clobevate Gel (Less than 2%) 3213
Clobex Shampoo (0.5%) 1209
Clobex Lotion 1208
Clorpres Tablets (About 7 in 1,000) 2139
Clozapine Tablets (Less than 1%) 2141
Clozaril Tablets (Less than 1%) 2174
Colazal Capsules 2845
CombiPatch Transdermal System 2180
Combivent Inhalation Aerosol 878
Combunox Tablets (Greater than or equal to 1%) 1183
Comvax 1904
▲ Copaxone for Injection (18%) 3292
▲ Copegus Tablets (19%) 2759
Coreg Tablets (Greater than 0.1% to 1%) 1376
Cosopt Sterile Ophthalmic Solution 1910
Coumadin for Injection (Infrequent) 932
Coumadin Tablets (Infrequent) 932
Cozaar Tablets (Less than 1%) 1913
Crestor Tablets (Greater than or equal to 1%) 672
▲ Crixivan Capsules (4.2%) 1918
Cubicin for Injection (2.8%) 1038
▲ Cuprimine Capsules (5%) 1925
Cutivate Cream (1.5% to 2.9%) 1381
Cutivate Lotion 0.05% (Less than 1%) 1383
Cutivate Ointment (Less than 1%) 1384
Cymbalta Delayed-Release Capsules (Frequent) 1729
▲ Cytovene (6%) 2763
Dalmane Capsules (Rare) 3343
Dantrium Capsules (Less frequent) 2690
Daranide Tablets 1928
Denavir Cream 2163
▲ Depacon Injection (1% to 5%) 412
▲ Depakene (1% to 5%) 417
▲ Depakote Sprinkle Capsules (1% to 5%) 422
▲ Depakote Tablets (1% to 5%) 427
▲ Depakote ER Tablets (1% to 5%) 433
▲ DepoDur Extended-Release Injection (Greater than 10%) 1098
depo-subQ provera 104 Injectable Suspension 2622
Desferal Vials 2190
Detrol Tablets (1.3%) 2626
Diastat Rectal Delivery System (Less than 1%) 3344
Didronel Tablets 2693
▲ Differin Cream (Less than 1% to 21%) 1210
▲ Differin Gel (10% to 40%) 1211
Dilaudid 439
Dilaudid Oral Liquid 443
Dilaudid Non-Sterile Powder 439
Dilaudid Rectal Suppositories 439
Dilaudid Tablets 439
Dilaudid Tablets - 8 mg 443
Dilaudid-HP (Less frequent) 441
Diovan Tablets 2191
Diprivan Injectable Emulsion (2%) 676
Diprolene Gel 0.05% (2%) 3015
Diprolene Lotion 0.05% (Infrequent) 3016
Diprolene Ointment 0.05% (2 per 767 patients) 3017
Diprolene AF Cream 0.05% (Infrequent) 3014
Diprosone Cream, USP 0.05% 3018
Dolobid Tablets (Less than 1 in 100) 1937
▲ Dostinex Tablets (1% to less than 10%) 2631
▲ Dovonex Cream 0.005% (1% to 10%) 3374
▲ Dovonex Ointment 0.005% (Approximately 10% to 15%) 3375
▲ Doxil Injection (1% to 10%) 3302
Drysol Solution 2506
DuoNeb Inhalation Solution (0.3%) 1058
▲ Duragesic Transdermal System (1% to 10%) 2448
DynaCirc CR Tablets (0.5% to 1%) 2726
▲ EC-Naprosyn Delayed-Release Tablets (3% to 9%) 2769
Effexor Tablets (1%) 3405
Effexor XR Capsules (Frequent) 3411
▲ Efudex (Among most frequent) 3348
Elidel Cream 1% (0.6% to 5.5%) 2198
Eligard 22.5 mg (2.6%) 2899
▲ Ellence Injection (0% to 8.9%) 2632
Elmiron Capsules (Less than or equal to 1%) 2393
▲ Elocon Cream 0.1% (1.6% to approximately 7%) 3019
Elocon Lotion 0.1% (1 in 209 patients) 3020
▲ Elocon Ointment 0.1% (4.8% to approximately 7%) 3021
▲ Eloxatin for Injection (2% to 5%) 2908
Emcyt Capsules (2%) 3137
Enablex Extended-Release Tablets (Greater than or equal to 1%) 2201
Enbrel for Injection 580
Engerix-B Vaccine (Less than 1%) 1391
Epivir 1394
Epivir-HBV 1398
▲ Epogen for Injection (16%) 586
▲ Equetro Extended-Release Capsules (5% to 8%) 3178
▲ Erbitux (10%) 937
Ertaczo Cream, 2% 2383
Erygel Topical Gel (Occasional) 2096
Estratest Tablets 3196
Estratest H.S. Tablets 3196
▲ Estrogel 0.06% (4.8%) 3200
Eulexin Capsules 3023
▲ Evoxac Capsules (1% to 3%) 1042
Fabrazyme for Intravenous Infusion 1267
Factive Tablets (0.1% to 1%) 2464
▲ Famvir Tablets (0.9% to 3.7%) 2207
FazaClo Orally Disintegrating Tablets (Less than 1%) 547
Femara Tablets (1% to 2%) 2210
▲ Ferrlecit Injection (0.5% to 6%) 3379
▲ Finacea Gel (1% to 7%) 1644
Flexeril Tablets (Rare) 1832
▲ Flolan for Injection (4%) 1408
Flomax Capsules 881
Flonase Nasal Spray 1412
▲ Flovent Diskus 50 mcg (1% to 6%) 1415
Flovent HFA 1418
Floxin Otic Singles (1% to 4%) 1045
▲ Floxin Otic Solution (1% to 4%) 1043
Fluorescite Injection ⊙ 207
Fortaz (2%) 1422
Fortical Nasal Spray (Less than 1%) 3336
Fosamax 1949
Fosamax Plus D Tablets 1956
Fragmin Injection (Rare) 2638
Frova Tablets (Infrequent) 1101
Furosemide Tablets 2117
Fuzeon Injection 2772
Gabitril Tablets (2%) 998
▲ Gammagard Liquid (0.61% to 6.5%) 751
▲ Gamunex Immune Globulin I.V., 10% (4%) 3232
Garamycin Injectable 3028
▲ Gemzar for Injection (13%) 1743
Gengraf Capsules (1% to less than 3%) 458
▲ Gleevec Tablets (8% to 14%) 2221
Havrix Vaccine (Less than 1%) 1425
▲ Hectorol Capsules (8.2%) 909
▲ Hectorol Injection (8.2%) 911
Hepsera Tablets (2% or greater) 1275
Hexalen Capsules (Less than 1%) 2101
Humalog-Pen (Less common) 1751
Humalog Mix 75/25-Pen 1754
▲ Hyalgan Solution (7%) 2917
Hycamtin for Injection (Rare) 1427
Hycodan 1104
Hytrin Capsules (At least 1%) 469
Hyzaar 1964
▲ Imdur Tablets (Less than or equal to 5%) 3032
Imitrex Injection (Infrequent) 1431
Imitrex Nasal Spray (Infrequent) 1435
Imitrex Tablets (Infrequent) 1440
Indocin (Less than 1%) 1968
Infanrix Vaccine 1444
Infed Injection 3381
▲ Infergen (11% to 14%) 1647
▲ Intron A for Injection (Up to 11%) 3038
Invanz for Injection (1% to 2%) 1974
▲ Invirase (Greater than or equal to 2% to 3.4%) 2776
▲ Iressa Tablets (8% to 10%) 684
▲ I.V. Busulfex (28%) 1125
Iveegam EN (0.36%) 759
Kadian Capsules (Less than 3%) 572
Kaletra (Less than 2%) 474
▲ Kepivance (35%) 592
Keppra Oral Solution (2%) 3307
Keppra Tablets (2%) 3307
Ketek Tablets (Less than 0.2%) 2920
Klaron Lotion 10% (One of 105 patients) 1050
Klonopin (Infrequent) 2782
Kogenate FS 3517
▲ Lamictal (2% to 3%) 1449
Lamisil Tablets (2.8%) 2226
Lantus Injection 2925
Lariam Tablets (Occasional) 2790
Lescol Capsules 2227
Lescol Capsules 2730
Lescol XL Tablets 2227
Lescol XL Tablets 2730
▲ Leukine (23%) 829
▲ Leustatin Injection (6%) 2368
Levaquin in 5% Dextrose Injection (0.2% to 1.2%) 2453
Levaquin (0.2% to 1.2%) 2453
Levitra Tablets (Less than 2%) 3048
Levothroid Tablets 1189
Levoxyl Tablets 1680
Lexapro Oral Solution (Infrequent) 1193
Lexapro Tablets (Infrequent) 1193
▲ Lexiva Tablets (Up to 8%) 1473
Lidoderm Patch 1107
Lipitor Tablets (Less than 2%) 2495
Lithobid Tablets 1670
Locoid Cream (Infrequent) 1138
Locoid Lipocream Cream (Infrequent) 1138
Locoid (Infrequent) 1138
Lofibra Capsules 1217
Loprox Gel (1% to 5%) 1861
Loprox Shampoo (1%) 1862
Lortab 3315
Lortab Elixir 3312
Lotensin Tablets (Less than 1%) 2232
Lotensin HCT Tablets (0.3% or more) 2235
Lotrimin 3053
Lotrisone 3054
Lovenox Injection 2931
▲ Lunesta Tablets (1% to 4%) 3139
▲ Luxíq Foam (2% to 44%) 1026
Lyrica Capsules (Greater than or equal to 1%) 2524
▲ Malarone Tablets (1% to 6%) 1484
▲ Malarone Pediatric Tablets (1% to 6%) 1484
Mavik Tablets (0.3% to 1.0%) 482
Maxair Autohaler 1820
Maxalt Tablets (Infrequent) 1983
Maxalt-MLT Orally Disintegrating Tablets (Infrequent) 1983
Maxipime for Injection (Greater than 0.1% to 1%) 1093
Mefoxin for Injection 1987
Mefoxin Premixed Intravenous Solution 1990
▲ Megace ES Oral Suspension (1% to 3%) 2492
Menostar Transdermal System 805
▲ Mepron Suspension (5%) 1487
Meridia Capsules (Greater than or equal to 1%) 485
Merrem I.V. (1.2%) 687
▲ Metrogel 1% (1.1 to 9.7%) 1212
MetroGel-Vaginal Gel (Less than 1%) 1822
▲ Mevacor Tablets (0.5% to 5.2%) 1996
Miacalcin Nasal Spray (Less than 1%) 2242
Micardis Tablets (More than 0.3%) 884
Micardis HCT Tablets (Less than 2%) 886
Midamor Tablets (Less than or equal to 1%) 2000
Migranal Nasal Spray (Infrequent) 3350
Mintezol 2002
Mirapex Tablets (1% or more) 889
Mobic Oral Suspension (0.4% to 2.4%) 893
Mobic Tablets (0.4% to 2.4%) 893
Moduretic Tablets (Greater than 1%, less than 3%) 2003
MS Contin Tablets (Less frequent) 2703
Mycamine for Injection (0.7% to 1.2%) 620
▲ Myfortic Tablets (3% to less than 20%) 2244
▲ Mylotarg for Injection (4% to 10%) 3429
Nadolol Tablets (1 to 5 of 1000 patients) 2121
Naftin Cream (2%) 2097
Naftin Gel (1.0%) 2097
▲ Nalfon Capsules (4.2%) 2504
Namenda (Infrequent) 1199
▲ Naprosyn Suspension (3% to 9%) 2769
▲ Naprosyn Tablets (3% to 9%) 2769
▲ Naropin Injection (1% to 5%) 640
Nasacort HFA Inhalation Aerosol 2939
Natrecor for Injection (Greater than or equal to 1%) 3123
Navelbine Injection 1494
Neoral Soft Gelatin Capsules (1% to less than 3%) 2247
Neoral Oral Solution (1% to less than 3%) 2247
Neurontin Capsules (1.3%) 2498
Neurontin Oral Solution (1.3%) 2498
Neurontin Tablets (1.3%) 2498
▲ Niaspan Extended-Release Tablets (1% to 6%) 1703
Nicotrol NS (2%) 2596
Nimotop Capsules (Less than 1%) 774
▲ Nipent for Injection (10% to 21%) 3216
Niravam Orally Disintegrating Tablets 3106
Nizoral 2% Shampoo (One occurrence in 41 patients) 1838
Norflex Injection 1824
Noroxin Tablets (0.3% to 1.0%) 2009
Norvasc Tablets (Less than 1% to 2%) 2529
Norvir (Less than 2%) 499
NovoLog Injection 2326
NovoSeven (1%) 2335
Nubain Injection (1% or less) 1111
Numorphan 1112
Olux Foam (Less than 2%) 1027
Omacor Capsules 2735
Omnicef Capsules (0.2%) 506
Omnicef for Oral Suspension (0.2%) 506
Oncaspar (Less than 1%) 1123
▲ Ontak Vials (20%) 1717
▲ Optivar Ophthalmic Solution (1% to 10%) 1877
Orthoclone OKT3 Sterile Solution 2370
Oxistat (1.6%) 1498
▲ Oxsoralen-Ultra Capsules (10%) 3354
▲ OxyContin Tablets (13%) 2699
OxyFast Oral Concentrate Solution 2704
OxyIR Capsules 2704
Pandel Cream, 0.1% 1017

(▭ Described in PDR For Nonprescription Drugs) Incidence data in parenthesis; ▲ 3% or more (⊙ Described in PDR For Ophthalmic Medicines™)

Parcopa Orally Disintegrating Tablets 3111
Patanol Ophthalmic Solution (Less than 5%) 557
Paxil CR Controlled-Release Tablets (Frequent) 1509
Paxil (Frequent) 1501
Pediarix Vaccine 1518
▲ Pegasys (12%) 2793
▲ PEG-Intron Powder for Injection (12%) 3062
Pentasa Capsules (Less than 1%) 3182
Pepcid Injection (Infrequent) 2017
Pepcid (Infrequent) 2014
Percocet Tablets 1114
Percodan Tablets 1115
Permax Tablets (Infrequent) 3357
Persantine Tablets 898
PhosLo GelCaps (Isolated cases) 2158
▲ Photofrin for Injection (4%) 729
▲ Plavix Tablets (3.3%) 940
▲ Plavix Tablets (3.3%) 2942
Pletal Tablets (Very rare) 2478
Poly-Pred Liquifilm Ophthalmic Suspension .... ⊙ 231
Pramosone 1139
Pravachol Tablets 943
Prefest Tablets 1069
Premarin Intravenous 3440
▲ Premarin Tablets (4% to 5%) 3443
Premarin Vaginal Cream 3449
▲ Premphase Tablets (5% to 10%) 3452
▲ Prempro Tablets (5% to 10%) 3452
Prevacid Delayed-Release Capsules (Less than 1%) 3268
Prevacid for Delayed-Release Oral Suspension (Less than 1%) 3268
▲ Prevacid NapraPAC (Less than 1% to 9%) 3277
Prevacid SoluTab Delayed-Release Orally Disintegrating Tablets (Less than 1%) 3268
Prevnar for Injection 3460
PREVPAC (Less than 1%) 3281
Prilosec OTC Tablets (Less than 1%) 2674
Primaxin I.M. 2022
Primaxin I.V. (0.3%) 2024
Prinivil Tablets (Greater than 1%) 2029
Prinzide Tablets (0.3% to 1%) 2033
▲ ProAmatine Tablets (12.2%) 3183
Prochieve 4% Gel 1018
Prochieve 8% Gel 1018
▲ Procrit for Injection (14% to 22%) 2374
▲ Prograf Capsules and Injection (15% to 36%) 624
▲ Proleukin for Injection (24%) 1007
Prometrium Capsules (100 mg, 200 mg) 3205
Proscar Tablets 2040
ProSom Tablets (1%) 512
▲ Protonix I.V. (4%) 3468
Protonix Tablets (Less than 1%) 3465
▲ Protopic Ointment (25% to 46%) 629
Provigil Tablets (At least 1%) 1002
▲ Prozac Pulvules and Liquid (3%) 1771
Pulmicort Respules (1% to 3%) 654
Rabies Vaccine RabAvert 1011
▲ Rapamune Oral Solution and Tablets (3% to 20%) 3472
▲ Rebetol (12% to 29%) 3073
▲ Rebetron Combination Therapy (13% to 21%) 3078
Recombivax HB (Less than 1%) 2045
ReFacto Vials 3479
Refludan for Injection (Uncommon) 815
▲ Relafen Tablets (3% to 9%) 1523
Relpax Tablets (Infrequent) 2531
▲ Remicade for IV Injection (7%) 987
▲ Renagel Tablets (13.1%) 1268
▲ Renova 0.02% Cream (Almost all subjects) 2384
▲ Renova 0.05% Cream (Almost all subjects) 2387
ReoPro Vials (0.3%) 1779
Requip Tablets (Infrequent) 1528
▲ Rescriptor Tablets (2.2% to 3.1%) 2535
▲ Retisert Implant (10% to 35%) .... ⊙ 256
Retrovir Capsules 1533
Retrovir IV Infusion 1537
Retrovir 1533
▲ Rēv-Eyes Ophthalmic Eyedrops 0.5% (10% to 40%) .... ⊙ 256
Reyataz Capsules (Less than 3%) 948
▲ Ribavirin, USP Capsules (12% to 29%) 3083
▲ Rilutek Tablets (2.5% to 3.8%) 2945
Risperdal Consta Long-Acting Injection (Infrequent) 1664
Risperdal M-Tab Orally Disintegrating Tablets (Infrequent to 2%) 1658
Risperdal (Infrequent) 1658
▲ Rituxan for Infusion (10%) 845
▲ Rituxan I.V. (14%) 1251
Rocephin Injectable Vials, ADD-Vantage, Galaxy, Bulk (Less than 1%) 2801
▲ Roferon-A Injection (5% to 13%) 2805
Rythmol SR Capsules 2736
Sandimmune (Rare) 2259
▲ Sandostatin Injection (1% to 4%) 2263
▲ Sandostatin LAR Depot (5% to 15%) 2264
Sedapap Tablets 50 mg/650 mg (Infrequent) 2098
Seroquel Tablets (Infrequent) 691
▲ Simulect for Injection (3% to 10%) 2268
Singulair 2047
Skelaxin Tablets 1685
▲ Solage Topical Solution (11% to 12%) 740
Sonata Capsules (Frequent) 1686
▲ Soriatane Capsules (25% to 50%) 1028
▲ Spectazole Cream (3%) 2390
Spectracef Tablets (0.1% to 1%) 2706
Spiriva HandiHaler 899
Stalevo Tablets 2270
▲ Strattera Capsules (1% or greater) 1784
Striant Mucoadhesive 1022
▲ Stromectol Tablets (2.8% to 27.5%) 2053
Sular Tablets (Less than or equal to 1%) 1163
Sulfamylon Cream (2.8%) 2154
Sulfamylon for 5% Topical Solution (2.3%) 2155
Suprane Liquid for Inhalation (Less than 1%) 770
Suprax (Less than 2%) 1811
Surmontil Capsules 2347
Sustiva Capsules (Less than 1% to 2%) 957
Symbyax Capsules (Infrequent) 1788
Symmetrel 1115
Synercid I.V. (1.5%) 1690
Tambocor Tablets (Less than 1%) 1824
▲ Tarceva Tablets (0% to 13%) 1254
▲ Tarceva Tablets (0% to 13%) 2470
Tarka Tablets (Less frequent) 519
Tasmar Tablets (Infrequent) 3360
Taxotere Injection Concentrate 2947
▲ Temodar Capsules (5% to 8%) 3088
Temovate Cream (Less frequent) 1549
▲ Temovate Gel (Among most frequent) 1550
Temovate Ointment (0.5%) 1549
Temovate Scalp Application (1 of 294 patients; infrequent) 1551
Temovate E Emollient (Less than 2%) 1552
Tequin Injection (Less than 0.1%) 964
Tequin Tablets (Less than 0.1%) 964
Tessalon Capsules 1202
Tessalon Perles 1202
Teveten Tablets (Less than 1%) 1707
Teveten HCT Tablets (Less than 1%) 1710
▲ Thalomid Capsules (8.3%) 979
Thiothixene Capsules 2124
Thyrogen for Injection 1270
Thyrolar 1203
Tiazac Capsules (Less than 2%) 1204
Ticlid Tablets (1.3%) 2813
Timentin ADD-Vantage 1556
Timentin Injection Galaxy Container 1559
Timentin IV Infusion 1553
Timentin Pharmacy Bulk Package 1562
Timolide Tablets 2056
Timoptic-XE Sterile Ophthalmic Gel Forming Solution 2062
Tindamax 2670
▲ Topamax Sprinkle Capsules (1% to 4%) 2438
▲ Topamax Tablets (1% to 4%) 2438
▲ Toprol-XL Tablets (About 5 of 100 patients) 660
▲ Tracleer Tablets (4%) 539
Trasylol Injection 779
Trelstar Depot (1.4%) 3385
Tricor Tablets 523
▲ Tri-Luma Cream (4.22% to 11%) 1213
▲ Trisenox Injection (33%) 983
Trusopt Sterile Ophthalmic Solution 2065
▲ Truvada Tablets (Greater than 5%) 1279
Tussionex Pennkinetic Extended-Release Suspension 3322
Twinrix Vaccine (Less than 1%) 1571
Tygacil for Injection (2.6%) 3489
Tylenol with Codeine 2461
U-Kera Cream 3290
Ultane Liquid for Inhalation (Less than 1%) 526
Ultracet Tablets (2%) 2462
Uniretic Tablets (Less than 1%) 3114
Unithroid Tablets 3521
Univasc Tablets (Less than 1%) 3118
▲ Urso 250 Tablets (5%) 737
▲ Urso Forte Tablets (5%) 737
▲ Valcyte Tablets (Less than 5%) 2816
Valtrex Caplets 1573
Vancocin HCl Capsules, USP 3370
Vanos Cream 1864
Vantas (Less than 2%) 3367
Vaqta (Less than 1%) 2067
Varivax (Greater than or equal to 1%) 2070
Vaseretic Tablets (0.5% to 2.0%) 2073
Vasotec I.V. Injection (0.5% to 1.0%) 2076
▲ Velcade for Injection (11%) 2102
▲ Vesanoid Capsules (20%) 2823
VFEND I.V. (1% to 1.1%) 2543
VFEND Oral Suspension (1% to 1.1%) 2543
VFEND Tablets (1% to 1.1%) 2543
Viadur Implant (Less than 2%) 782
Viagra Tablets (Less than 2%) 2552
Vicodin Tablets 530
Vicodin ES Tablets 531
Vicodin HP Tablets 532
▲ Vicoprofen Tablets (3% to 9%) 533
Viracept (Less than 2%) 2556
Viramune Oral Suspension 903
Viramune Tablets 903
Vivactil Tablets 2350
Vivelle Transdermal System (One of the two most common) 2288
Vivelle-Dot Transdermal System (One of the two most common) 2293
▲ Voltaren Tablets (1% to 10%) 2298
▲ Voltaren-XR Tablets (1% to 10%) 2301
Vytorin 10/10 Tablets 2084
Vytorin 10/10 Tablets 3092
Vytorin 10/20 Tablets 2084
Vytorin 10/20 Tablets 3092
Vytorin 10/40 Tablets 2084
Vytorin 10/40 Tablets 3092
Vytorin 10/80 Tablets 2084
Vytorin 10/80 Tablets 3092
Wellbutrin Tablets (2.2%) 1579
▲ Wellbutrin SR Sustained-Release Tablets (2% to 4%) 1583
▲ Wellbutrin XL Extended-Release Tablets (2% to 4%) 1588
WinRho SDF 763
Xanax XR Tablets (1.1%) 2655
▲ Xeloda Tablets (Less than 5%) 2825
Xenical Capsules 2834
Xerac AC Solution 2507
Xifaxan Tablets 2847
Xolair (2%) 1259
Yasmin 28 Tablets 818
Zantac Injection 1593
Zegerid Powder for Oral Solution (Less than 1%) 2972
Zelnorm Tablets (Up to 1%) 2303
Zemaira (0.2% to 0.4%) 3506
Zemuron Injection (Less than 1%) 2363
▲ Zenapax for Injection (2% to 5%) 2838
Zestoretic Tablets (0.3% to 1%) 701
Zestril Tablets (Greater than 1%) 704
▲ Zevalin Injection (9%) 848
Zinacef Injection (Fewer than 1 in 250 patients) 1604
Zinacef for Injection (Fewer than 1 in 250 patients) 1604
Zithromax Capsules, 250 mg (1% or less) 2568
Zithromax for IV Infusion (1.9%) 2573
Zithromax for Oral Suspension, 300 mg, 600 mg, 900 mg, 1200 mg (1% or less) 2561
Zithromax Tablets, 250 mg, 500 mg (1% or less) 2561
Zithromax Tri-Pak (1% or less) 2561
Zmax for Oral Suspension (Less then 1%) 2577
Zocor Tablets 2078
Zofran Injection (2%) 1607
▲ Zofran (5%) 1613
▲ Zofran ODT Orally Disintegrating Tablets (5%) 1613
Zoladex (2%) 709
Zoladex 3-month (1% to 5%) 712
Zoloft (Infrequent) 2581
Zometa for Intravenous Infusion 2306
Zomig Nasal Spray (Infrequent) 718
Zomig Tablets (Infrequent) 714
Zomig-ZMT Tablets (Infrequent) 714
Zonegran Capsules (Frequent) 1089
▲ Zosyn (3.1% to 3.2%) 3492
Zovirax Capsules 1616
Zovirax Cream 853
Zovirax for Injection (Approximately 2%) 1618
Zovirax Ointment 854
Zovirax 1616
▲ Zyban Sustained-Release Tablets (3%) 1620
Zyprexa Tablets 1798
Zyprexa ZYDIS Orally Disintegrating Tablets 1798
Zyrtec Chewable Tablets (Less than 2%) 2589
Zyrtec (Less than 2%) 2589
Zyrtec-D 12 Hour Extended Release Tablets (Less than 2%) 2591
Zyvox (0% to 0.4%) 2661

Pruritus, ear lobes

Miacalcin Injection 2241

Pruritus, exacerbation of

Cutivate Cream (0.8% to 3.0%) 1381

Pruritus, genital

Ancef for Injection 1318
Ceftin Tablets (0.1% to 1%) 1369
Cipro I.V. (1%) 2998
Cipro I.V. Pharmacy Bulk Package (1%) 3509
Cipro (1%) 2991
Evoxac Capsules (Less than 1%) 1042
▲ Gynazole-1 Vaginal Cream (5.7%) 3298
Levaquin in 5% Dextrose Injection (0.1% to 0.9%) 2453
Levaquin (0.1% to 0.9%) 2453
Neurontin Capsules (Rare) 2498
Neurontin Oral Solution (Rare) 2498
Neurontin Tablets (Rare) 2498
Primaxin I.M. 2022
Primaxin I.V. (Less than 0.2%) 2024
▲ Prochieve 4% Gel (5%) 1018
▲ Prochieve 8% Gel (5%) 1018
ProSom Tablets (Infrequent) 512
Risperdal M-Tab Orally Disintegrating Tablets (Rare) 1658
Risperdal (Rare) 1658
Suprax (Les than 2%) 1811
Trileptal Oral Suspension 2281
Trileptal Tablets 2281
▲ Vagifem Tablets (6%) 2340
Vantin Tablets and Oral Suspension (Less than 1%) 2650
Zosyn (1.0% or less) 3492

Pruritus, genital, male

Vantas (Less than 2%) 3367

Pruritus, injection site

▲ Alferon N Injection (12%) 1640
Cerezyme for Injection (Less than 1%) 1263
Cipro I.V. (1% or less) 2998
Cipro I.V. Pharmacy Bulk Package (1% or less) 3509
▲ Copaxone for Injection (40%) 3292
Desferal Vials 2190
Diprivan Injectable Emulsion (Less than 1%) 676
▲ Enbrel for Injection (37%) 580
Engerix-B Vaccine (Less than 1%) 1391
▲ Fuzeon Injection (65%) 2772
Humalog-Pen 1751
Humulin 50/50, 100 Units 1760
Humulin 70/30 Pen 1761
Humulin L, 100 Units 1763
Humulin R (U-500) 1768
Humulin N Pen 1765
▲ Intron A for Injection (Less than 5%) 3038
Invanz for Injection (Greater than 0.5%) 1974
Vaqta (Less than 1%) 2067
▲ Varivax (19.3% to 32.5%) 2070

Pruritus, localized

▲ Aldara Cream, 5% (22% to 32%) 1814
Cleocin Vaginal Ovules (Less than 1%) 2613
Eskalith 1406
Mentax Cream (Less than 2%) 2152
▲ Oxytrol Transdermal System (14% to 16.8%) 3383
▲ Polytrim Ophthalmic Solution (Among most frequent) 570
ProctoFoam-HC 3113
Topicort .05% Gel 3288
Topicort .25% Cream 3288
Topicort .25% Ointment 3288
Topicort LP .05% Cream 3288
U-cort 1% Cream 3289
▲ Zylet Ophthalmic Suspension (Less than 4%) 3508

Pruritus, ocular

▲ Alphagan P Ophthalmic Solution (Approximately 10% to 20%) 563
▲ Alrex Ophthalmic Suspension 0.2% (5% to 15%) .... ⊙ 243
Aredia for Injection (One patient) 2168

Azopt Ophthalmic Suspension (1% to 5%) ... 553
▲ Betimol Ophthalmic Solution (More than 5%) ... ⊙ 283
▲ Betimol Ophthalmic Solution (More than 5%) ... 3371
Betoptic S Ophthalmic Suspension (Small number of patients) ... 554
▲ Brimonidine Tartrate Ophthalmic Solution 0.2% (10% to 30%) ... ⊙ 245
▲ Carac Cream, 0.5% (5.4%) ... 1048
▲ Ciloxan Ophthalmic Ointment (Less than 10%) ... 554
Clorpres Tablets ... 2139
▲ Cosopt Sterile Ophthalmic Solution (5% to 15%) ... 1910
Crolom Cromolyn Sodium Sterile Ophthalmic Solution USP 4% (Infrequent) ... ⊙ 248
▲ Elestat Ophthalmic Solution (1% to 10%) ... 1643
Imitrex Nasal Spray ... 1435
▲ Lotemax Ophthalmic Suspension 0.5% (5% to 15%) ... ⊙ 249
▲ Lumigan Ophthalmic Solution (15% to 45%) ... 569
Maxalt Tablets (Infrequent) ... 1983
Maxalt-MLT Orally Disintegrating Tablets (Infrequent) ... 1983
Neurontin Capsules (Rare) ... 2498
Neurontin Oral Solution (Rare) ... 2498
Neurontin Tablets (Rare) ... 2498
Quixin Ophthalmic Solution (Less than 1%) ... 3373
▲ Restasis Ophthalmic Emulsion (1% to 5%) ... 570
▲ Soriatane Capsules (1% to 5%) ... 1028
Sular Tablets (Less than or equal to 1%) ... 1163
Timoptic in Ocudose ... 2061
Timoptic Sterile Ophthalmic Solution ... 2058
Timoptic-XE Sterile Ophthalmic Gel Forming Solution ... 2062
TobraDex Ophthalmic Ointment (Less than 4%) ... 558
TobraDex Ophthalmic Suspension (Less than 4%) ... 558
Transderm Scōp Transdermal Therapeutic System (Infrequent) ... 2166
▲ Travatan Ophthalmic Solution (5% to 10%) ... 559
Vantin Tablets and Oral Suspension (Less than 1%) ... 2650
Vaqta (Less than 1%) ... 2067
▲ Vigamox Ophthalmic Solution (1% to 6%) ... 560
Visine For Contacts Rewetting Drops ... ⊙ 278
▲ Visudyne for Injection (1% to 10%) .. 2286
▲ Voltaren Ophthalmic Solution (Less than or equal to 5%) ... 2300
▲ Xalatan Sterile Ophthalmic Solution (5% to 15%) ... 2654
Xopenex Inhalation Solution Concentrate (Less than 2%) ... 3147
Zaditor Ophthalmic Solution (Less than 5%) ... 2302

Pruritus, oral
Imitrex Nasal Spray ... 1435

Pruritus, penile
▲ Caverject Impulse Injection (3%) ... 2610

Pruritus, rhinal
Atrovent Nasal Spray 0.03% (2.0%) ... 869
▲ Miacalcin Nasal Spray (10.6%) ... 2242

Pruritus, vaginal
Ancef for Injection ... 1318
Cipro XR Tablets ... 3004
▲ Clindesse Vaginal Cream (3.3%) ... 3296
FazaClo Orally Disintegrating Tablets (Less than 1%) ... 547
Invanz for Injection (Greater than 0.1%) ... 1974

Pruritus ani
Ancef for Injection ... 1318
Arthrotec Tablets (Rare) ... 3126
Celexa (Rare) ... 1177
Colazal Capsules ... 2845
Nexium Delayed-Release Capsules (Less than 1%) ... 645
Nexium I.V. (Less than 1%) ... 649
Noroxin Tablets (Less frequent) ... 2009
PREVPAC (Less than 3%) ... 3281

Pruritus at application site
Evoclin Foam, 1% (1%) ... 1025
Lidoderm Patch ... 1107

Pseudoaneurysm
ReoPro Vials (0.8%) ... 1779

Pseudolymphoma
Phenytek Capsules ... 2153

Pseudomembranous colitis
Amoxil Capsules ... 1315
Amoxil Chewable Tablets ... 1315
Amoxil Pediatric Drops for Oral Suspension ... 1315
Amoxil Powder for Oral Suspension ... 1315
Amoxil Tablets ... 1315
Ancef for Injection ... 1318
Augmentin ... 1331
Augmentin Tablets ... 1334
Augmentin XR Extended-Release Tablets ... 1340
Augmentin ES-600 Powder for Oral Suspension ... 1337
Avelox (Less than 0.1%) ... 2984
Benzaclin Topical Gel ... 1046
Biaxin/Biaxin XL ... 402
Campath Ampules ... 826
Ceftin ... 1369
Cipro I.V. (1% or less) ... 2998
Cipro I.V. Pharmacy Bulk Package (1% or less) ... 3509
Cipro ... 2991
Cipro XR Tablets ... 3004
Cleocin Vaginal Ovules ... 2613
Clindagel ... 1207
Clindesse Vaginal Cream (Rare) ... 3296
Duac Topical Gel ... 3214
E.E.S. ... 449
EryPed ... 445
Ery-Tab Tablets (Rare) ... 447
Erythrocin Stearate Filmtab Tablets (Rare) ... 452
Erythromycin Base Filmtab Tablets (Rare) ... 454
Erythromycin Delayed-Release Capsules, USP (Rare) ... 456
Evoclin Foam, 1% (Rarely) ... 1025
Fortaz (Less frequent) ... 1422
Invanz for Injection ... 1974
Levaquin in 5% Dextrose Injection (0.1% to 0.9%) ... 2453
Levaquin (0.1% to 0.9%) ... 2453
Maxipime for Injection (Greater than 0.1% to less than 1%) ... 1093
Mefoxin for Injection ... 1987
Mefoxin Premixed Intravenous Solution ... 1990
Merrem I.V. ... 687
Noroxin Tablets ... 2009
Omnicef Capsules ... 506
Omnicef for Oral Suspension ... 506
PCE Dispertab Tablets ... 510
PREVPAC ... 3281
Primaxin I.M. ... 2022
Primaxin I.V. (Less than 0.2%) ... 2024
Rocephin Injectable Vials, ADD-Vantage, Galaxy, Bulk ... 2801
Spectracef Tablets (0.1% to 1%) ... 2706
Suprax (Several patients) ... 1811
Tamiflu Capsules (Less than 1%) ... 2810
Tamiflu Oral Suspension (Less than 1%) ... 2810
Tequin Injection (Less than 0.1%) ... 964
Tequin Tablets (Less than 0.1%) ... 964
Timentin ADD-Vantage ... 1556
Timentin Injection Galaxy Container ... 1559
Timentin IV Infusion ... 1553
Timentin Pharmacy Bulk Package ... 1562
Tygacil for Injection ... 3489
Vantin Tablets and Oral Suspension (Less than 1%) ... 2650
VFEND I.V. (Less than 2%) ... 2543
VFEND Oral Suspension (Less than 2%) ... 2543
VFEND Tablets (Less than 2%) ... 2543
Zinacef Injection ... 1604
Zinacef for Injection ... 1604
Zithromax Capsules, 250 mg ... 2568
Zithromax for IV Infusion ... 2573
Zithromax for Oral Suspension, 1 g ... 2568
Zithromax for Oral Suspension, 300 mg, 600 mg, 900 mg, 1200 mg ... 2561
Zithromax Tablets, 250 mg, 500 mg ... 2561
Zithromax Tablets, 600 mg ... 2568
Zithromax Tri-Pak ... 2561
Zithromax Z-Pak ... 2568
Zmax for Oral Suspension ... 2577
Zosyn (One patient) ... 3492
Zyvox ... 2661

Pseudomembranous enterocolitis
Rilutek Tablets (Rare) ... 2945
Synercid I.V. (Less than 1%) ... 1690

Pseudoparkinsonism
Thioridazine Hydrochloride Tablets (Infrequent) ... 2122
Thiothixene Capsules ... 2124
Wellbutrin Tablets (1.5%) ... 1579

Pseudotumor cerebri
Accutane Capsules ... 2740
Amnesteem Capsules ... 2126
Decadron Phosphate Injection ... 1931
Depo-Medrol Injectable Suspension ... 2615
Dynacin Tablets ... 1859
Eskalith ... 1406
Garamycin Injectable ... 3028
Hydrocortone Tablets ... 1963
Levothroid Tablets ... 1189
Levoxyl Tablets ... 1680
Pacerone Tablets (Rare) ... 3337
Pediapred Oral Solution ... 3319
Soriatane Capsules (Less than 1%) .. 1028
Synthroid Tablets ... 515
Tygacil for Injection ... 3489
Unithroid Tablets ... 3521
Vesanoid Capsules ... 2823

Psoriasis
Abilify Tablets (Infrequent) ... 916
Abilify Tablets (Infrequent) ... 2472
Aciphex Tablets (Rare) ... 1081
Asacol Delayed-Release Tablets (Rare) ... 2688
Campral Tablets (Rare) ... 1175
Celexa (Infrequent) ... 1177
Colazal Capsules ... 2845
Copaxone for Injection (Infrequent) .. 3292
Doxil Injection (Less than 1%) ... 3302
Effexor Tablets (Infrequent) ... 3405
Effexor XR Capsules (Infrequent) ... 3411
Eskalith ... 1406
Gabitril Tablets (Infrequent) ... 998
▲ Intron A for Injection (Less than 5%) ... 3038
Neurontin Capsules (Rare) ... 2498
Neurontin Oral Solution (Rare) ... 2498
Neurontin Tablets (Rare) ... 2498
Norvir (Less than 2%) ... 499
Pegasys ... 2793
Provigil Tablets (At least 1%) ... 1002
Prozac Pulvules and Liquid (Rare) ... 1771
Raptiva for Injection (0.7%) ... 1247
Relpax Tablets (Rare) ... 2531
Requip Tablets (Infrequent) ... 1528
Rilutek Tablets (Infrequent) ... 2945
Roferon-A Injection (Less than 1%) ... 2805
Seroquel Tablets (Rare) ... 691
Sonata Capsules (Rare) ... 1686
Symbyax Capsules (Infrequent) ... 1788
Thalomid Capsules ... 979
Trileptal Oral Suspension ... 2281
Trileptal Tablets ... 2281
Uniretic Tablets (Less than 1%) ... 3114
VFEND I.V. (Less than 2%) ... 2543
VFEND Oral Suspension (Less than 2%) ... 2543
VFEND Tablets (Less than 2%) ... 2543

Psoriasis, exacerbation of
Cosopt Sterile Ophthalmic Solution ... 1910
▲ Dovonex Cream 0.005% (1% to 10%) ... 3374
▲ Dovonex Ointment 0.005% (1% to 10%) ... 3375
▲ Dovonex Scalp Solution 0.005% (1% to 5%) ... 3375
Eskalith ... 1406
▲ Intron A for Injection (Less than 5%) ... 3038
Lamisil Tablets ... 2226
Lithobid Tablets ... 1670
Neupogen for Injection (Infrequent) .. 598
Oxsoralen-Ultra Capsules ... 3354
PEG-Intron Powder for Injection (Less than or equal to 1%) ... 3062
Risperdal M-Tab Orally Disintegrating Tablets (Rare) ... 1658
Risperdal (Rare) ... 1658
Soriatane Capsules (Less than 1%) .. 1028
Temovate Cream ... 1549
Temovate Scalp Application (Rare) ... 1551
Tenormin I.V. Injection ... 698
Tenormin Tablets ... 695
Timoptic in Ocudose ... 2061
Timoptic Sterile Ophthalmic Solution ... 2058
Timoptic-XE Sterile Ophthalmic Gel Forming Solution ... 2062
Toprol-XL Tablets ... 660

Psoriasis, pustular
Cutivate Cream ... 1381
Cutivate Lotion 0.05% (Rare) ... 1383
Cutivate Ointment ... 1384

Psoriasis, worsening of
Enbrel for Injection ... 580

Psychiatric disorders, worsening of
Avonex ... 839

Psychiatric disturbances
Accutane Capsules ... 2740
Advicor Tablets ... 1694
Aldoclor Tablets ... 1881
Aldoril Tablets ... 1884
Altoprev Extended-Release Tablets ... 1151
▲ Ammonul Injection (5%) ... 3323
Arthrotec Tablets (Rare) ... 3126
Avonex ... 839
Clinoril Tablets (Less than 1 in 100) ... 1899
Cogentin Injection ... 1903
Cosopt Sterile Ophthalmic Solution ... 1910
Cuprimine Capsules ... 1925
Decadron Phosphate Injection ... 1931
Decadron Tablets ... 1929
Didronel Tablets ... 2693
Floxin Otic Singles ... 1045
▲ Focalin XR Capsules (26% to 46%) ... 2217
▲ Gengraf Capsules (5.0%) ... 458
Hydrocortone Tablets ... 1963
Indocin (Less than 1%) ... 1968
Infergen ... 1647
Invirase (Less than 2%) ... 2776
Lariam Tablets (Occasional) ... 2790
Lescol Capsules ... 2227
Lescol Capsules ... 2730
Lescol XL Tablets ... 2227
Lescol XL Tablets ... 2730
▲ Leukine (15%) ... 829
Mebaral Tablets, USP (Less than 1 in 100 patients) ... 2483
Mintezol ... 2002
Nembutal Sodium Solution, USP (Less than 1%) ... 2484
Neoral Soft Gelatin Capsules ... 2247
Neoral Oral Solution ... 2247
Noroxin Tablets ... 2009
Pepcid Injection (Infrequent) ... 2017
Pepcid (Infrequent) ... 2014
Prilosec OTC Tablets (Less than 1%) ... 2674
Primaxin I.M. ... 2022
Primaxin I.V. (Less than 0.2%) ... 2024
Pulmicort Respules (Less than 1%) .. 654
Sandimmune ... 2259
Thioridazine Hydrochloride Tablets (Extremely rare) ... 2122
Timoptic in Ocudose (Less frequent) ... 2061
Timoptic Sterile Ophthalmic Solution (Less frequent) ... 2058
Timoptic-XE Sterile Ophthalmic Gel Forming Solution ... 2062
Vytorin 10/10 Tablets ... 2084
Vytorin 10/10 Tablets ... 3092
Vytorin 10/20 Tablets ... 2084
Vytorin 10/20 Tablets ... 3092
Vytorin 10/40 Tablets ... 2084
Vytorin 10/40 Tablets ... 3092
Vytorin 10/80 Tablets ... 2084
Vytorin 10/80 Tablets ... 3092
Zegerid Powder for Oral Solution (Less than 1%) ... 2972

Psychic dependence

(*see under* Dependence, psychological)

Psychomotor retardation
Lithobid Tablets ... 1670
Sonata Capsules (Rare) ... 1686
▲ Topamax Sprinkle Capsules (2% to 21%) ... 2438
▲ Topamax Tablets (2% to 21%) ... 2438
Xanax XR Tablets (Infrequent) ... 2655

Psychoses
Abilify Tablets ... 916
Abilify Tablets ... 2472
Accutane Capsules ... 2740
Adderall Tablets (Rare) ... 3168
Adderall XR Capsules ... 3169
Adipex-P ... 1216
Aldoclor Tablets ... 1881
Aldoril Tablets ... 1884
Ammonul Injection ... 3323

Antabuse Tablets 2343
Aredia for Injection (Up to 4%) 2168
Avelox 2984
Avonex 839
Biaxin/Biaxin XL 402
BiDil Tablets 2161
Buprenex Injectable (Less than 1%) 2718
Campral Tablets (Rare) 1175
Celexa (Infrequent) 1177
▲ CellCept Capsules (3% to less than 20%) 2751
▲ CellCept Intravenous (3% to less than 20%) 2751
▲ CellCept Oral Suspension (3% to less than 20%) 2751
▲ CellCept Tablets (3% to less than 20%) 2751
Clinoril Tablets (Less than 1 in 100) 1899
Copegus Tablets (Less than 1%) 2759
Covera-HS Tablets (Less than 2%) 3135
Dapsone Tablets USP 1656
Decadron Phosphate Injection 1931
Decadron Tablets 1929
Depacon Injection 412
Depakene 417
Depakote Sprinkle Capsules 422
Depakote Tablets 427
Depakote ER Tablets (Greater than 1%) 433
Desoxyn Tablets, USP (Rare) 2482
Dexedrine (Rare at recommended doses) 1386
DextroStat Tablets (Rare) 3177
Effexor Tablets (Rare) 3405
Effexor XR Capsules (Infrequent) 3411
Exelon Capsules (Infrequent) 2204
Flexeril Tablets (Less than 1%) 1832
Gabitril Tablets (Infrequent) 998
Geodon for Injection (Up to 1%) 2514
Guanidine Hydrochloride Tablets 3030
Hydrocortone Tablets 1963
Indocin (Less than 1%) 1968
Invirase (Less than 2%) 2776
Klonopin 2782
Lamictal (Infrequent) 1449
Lanoxicaps Capsules 1458
Lanoxin Injection 1462
Lanoxin Injection Pediatric 1465
Lariam Tablets (Occasional) 2790
Mirapex Tablets (Less than 1%) 889
Namenda (Infrequent) 1199
Neurontin Capsules (Infrequent) 2498
Neurontin Oral Solution (Infrequent) 2498
Neurontin Tablets (Infrequent) 2498
Noroxin Tablets 2009
Orthoclone OKT3 Sterile Solution 2370
Paxil CR Controlled-Release Tablets (Rare) 1509
Paxil (Rare) 1501
Pediapred Oral Solution 3319
PEG-Intron Powder for Injection (Less than or equal to 1%) 3062
Permax Tablets (2.1%; frequent) 3357
PREVPAC 3281
▲ Prograf Capsules and Injection (3% to 15%) 624
Provigil Tablets 1002
Prozac Pulvules and Liquid (Infrequent) 1771
Pulmicort Respules (Less than 1%) 654
Reyataz Capsules (Less than 3%) 948
Rilutek Tablets (Rare) 2945
Ritalin Hydrochloride Tablets 2254
Ritalin LA Capsules 2255
Ritalin-SR Tablets 2254
Roferon-A Injection 2805
Seromycin Capsules 1783
Stalevo Tablets 2270
Sustiva Capsules (Less than 2%) 957
Symmetrel (0.1% to 1%) 1115
Tagamet Tablets 1547
Tarka Tablets 519
Tasmar Tablets (Infrequent) 3360
Tenormin I.V. Injection 698
Tenormin Tablets 695
Tequin Injection (Less than 0.1%) 964
Tequin Tablets (Less than 0.1%) 964
Thalomid Capsules 979
Topamax Sprinkle Capsules (Frequent) 2438
Topamax Tablets (Frequent) 2438
Trecator Tablets 3482
▲ Valcyte Tablets (Less than 5%) 2816
Valtrex Caplets 1573
▲ Velcade for Injection (35%) 2102
Verelan PM Capsules (2% or less) 3120
VFEND I.V. (Less than 2%) 2543
VFEND Oral Suspension (Less than 2%) 2543
VFEND Tablets (Less than 2%) 2543
Wellbutrin Tablets (Infrequent) 1579
Wellbutrin SR Sustained-Release Tablets 1583
Wellbutrin XL Extended-Release Tablets 1588
Zoloft 2581
Zomig Nasal Spray (Rare) 718
Zovirax Capsules 1616
Zovirax for Injection 1618
Zovirax 1616
Zyban Sustained-Release Tablets 1620

Psychoses, aggravation

Clozapine Tablets 2141
Clozaril Tablets 2174
Decadron Phosphate Injection 1931
Decadron Tablets 1929
FazaClo Orally Disintegrating Tablets 547
Hydrocortone Tablets 1963
Pediapred Oral Solution 3319
Seroquel Tablets (Infrequent) 691
Surmontil Capsules 2347
Thioridazine Hydrochloride Tablets 2122
Vivactil Tablets 2350

Psychoses, toxic

Cipro I.V. (1% or less) 2998
Cipro I.V. Pharmacy Bulk Package (1% or less) 3509
Cipro 2991
Cipro XR Tablets 3004
Concerta Extended-Release Tablets 1828
Focalin Tablets (Rare) 2214
Focalin XR Capsules 2217
Levaquin in 5% Dextrose Injection 2453
Levaquin 2453
Metadate CD Capsules 3316
Ritalin Hydrochloride Tablets 2254
Ritalin LA Capsules 2255
Ritalin-SR Tablets 2254

Psychosis, activation

Amnesteem Capsules 2126
Carbatrol Capsules 3174
FazaClo Orally Disintegrating Tablets 547
Pegasys (Less than 1%) 2793
Risperdal Consta Long-Acting Injection (Frequent) 1664
Tegretol/Tegretol-XR 2278
Wellbutrin SR Sustained-Release Tablets 1583
Wellbutrin XL Extended-Release Tablets 1588
Zyban Sustained-Release Tablets 1620

Psychosis, overt

Calcijex Injection (Rare) 411
Hectorol Capsules 909
Hectorol Injection (Rare) 911
Pediapred Oral Solution 3319

Psychotic episodes
(*see under* Psychoses)

Psychotic symptoms, paradoxical exacerbation

Thiothixene Capsules 2124

Ptosis

Abilify Tablets (Rare) 916
Abilify Tablets (Rare) 2472
HMS Sterile Ophthalmic Suspension ⊙228
Lunesta Tablets (Rare) 3139
Lyrica Capsules (Rare) 2524
Namenda (Infrequent) 1199
Relpax Tablets (Rare) 2531
▲ Retisert Implant (10% to 35%) ⊙256
Topamax Sprinkle Capsules (Infrequent) 2438
Topamax Tablets (Infrequent) 2438

Ptosis, eyelids

Betagan Ophthalmic Solution, USP ⊙217
Betimol Ophthalmic Solution ⊙283
Betimol Ophthalmic Solution 3371
Blephamide Ophthalmic Ointment (Occasional) 563
Blephamide Ophthalmic Suspension 564
Blocadren Tablets 1891
▲ Botox Purified Neurotoxin Complex (0.3% to 15.7%) 565
Carteolol Hydrochloride Ophthalmic Solution USP, 1% (Occasional) ⊙246
Celexa (Rare) 1177
Clozapine Tablets (Less than 1%) 2141
Clozaril Tablets (Less than 1%) 2174
Copaxone for Injection (Infrequent) 3292
Cosopt Sterile Ophthalmic Solution 1910
FML Ophthalmic Ointment (Occasional) ⊙225
FML Ophthalmic Suspension (Occasional) ⊙224
FML Forte Ophthalmic Suspension (Occasional) ⊙223
▲ Imdur Tablets (Less than or equal to 5%) 3032
Lamictal (Rare) 1449
Lexapro Oral Solution (Frequent) 1193
Lexapro Tablets (Frequent) 1193
Naropin Injection (Less than 1%) 640
Neurontin Capsules (Infrequent) 2498
Neurontin Oral Solution (Infrequent) 2498
Neurontin Tablets (Infrequent) 2498
Paxil CR Controlled-Release Tablets (Rare) 1509
Paxil (Rare) 1501
Pred Forte Ophthalmic Suspension (Occasional) ⊙233
Pred Mild Sterile Ophthalmic Suspension (Occasional) ⊙236
▲ Rēv-Eyes Ophthalmic Eyedrops 0.5% (10% to 40%) ⊙256
Rythmol SR Capsules 2736
Sonata Capsules (Rare) 1686
Tequin Injection (Less than 0.1%) 964
Tequin Tablets (Less than 0.1%) 964
Timolide Tablets 2056
Timoptic in Ocudose (Less frequent) 2061
Timoptic Sterile Ophthalmic Solution (Less frequent) 2058
Timoptic-XE Sterile Ophthalmic Gel Forming Solution 2062
Trileptal Oral Suspension 2281
Trileptal Tablets 2281
Zoloft (Rare) 2581
Zyrtec Chewable Tablets (Less than 2%) 2589
Zyrtec (Less than 2%) 2589
Zyrtec-D 12 Hour Extended Release Tablets (Less than 2%) 2591

Pulmonary allergy, unspecified

Idamycin PFS Injection (2%) 2645

Pulmonary apoplexy

Sandostatin LAR Depot (Rare) 2264

Pulmonary collapse

Levaquin in 5% Dextrose Injection (0.1% to 0.9%) 2453
Levaquin (0.1% to 0.9%) 2453

Pulmonary complications, unspecified

Follistim AQ Cartridge 2354
Gonal-f RFF Pen for Injection 3155

Pulmonary congestion

Aldara Cream, 5% (0.5%) 1814
Aricept Tablets (Infrequent) 1086
Aricept ODT Tablets (Infrequent) 1086
Avalide Tablets 922
Avalide Tablets 2889
Avapro Tablets (Less than 1%) 925
Avapro Tablets (Less than 1%) 2886
Evoxac Capsules (Less than 1%) 1042
Prinzide Tablets 2033
▲ Proleukin for Injection (54%) 1007
Rythmol SR Capsules 2736
Vicoprofen Tablets (Less than 1%) 533
Zestoretic Tablets (0.3% to 1%) 701

Pulmonary disease, chronic obstructive

Campath Ampules 826
Rythmol SR Capsules 2736
▲ Zoladex (5%) 709
Zoladex 3-month 712

Pulmonary disease, chronic obstructive, exacerbation of

▲ Atrovent HFA Inhalation Aerosol (8% to 23%) 872
▲ Zemaira (7 of 30 Patients) 3506

Pulmonary disorder, unspecified

▲ Taxotere Injection Concentrate (21% to 40.9%) 2947

Pulmonary distress

Betoptic S Ophthalmic Suspension (Rare) 554
Follistim AQ Cartridge 2354

Pulmonary edema
(*see under* Edema, pulmonary)

Pulmonary embolism
(*see under* Embolism, pulmonary)

Pulmonary emphysema, interstitial

▲ Infasurf Intratracheal Suspension (7% to 10%) 1188

Pulmonary events, unspecified

▲ Mylotarg for Injection (8% to 10%) 3429

Pulmonary fibrosis

Aceon Tablets (2 mg, 4 mg, 8 mg) (Less than 0.1%) 3191
Agrylin Capsules 3172
Alkeran for Injection 976
Alkeran Tablets 977
Arava Tablets (Rare) 2881
Campath Ampules 826
Casodex Tablets (Rare) 670
CellCept Capsules (Rare) 2751
CellCept Intravenous (Rare) 2751
CellCept Oral Suspension (Rare) 2751
CellCept Tablets (Rare) 2751
Cuprimine Capsules (Rare) 1925
Cytovene 2763
Dostinex Tablets (Rare) 2631
Eloxatin for Injection 2908
Evoxac Capsules (Less than 1%) 1042
Garamycin Injectable 3028
Gleevec Tablets (Rare) 2221
Herceptin I.V. (Rare) 1234
Inversine Tablets 3286
I.V. Busulfex (Rare) 1125
Leukeran Tablets 1472
Lyrica Capsules (Rare) 2524
Myfortic Tablets (Rare) 2244
Myleran Tablets (Rare) 1492
▲ Pacerone Tablets (4% to 9%) 3337
Paxil CR Controlled-Release Tablets (Rare) 1509
Paxil (Rare) 1501
Pentasa Capsules (One case) 3182
Permax Tablets (Rare) 3357
Rapamune Oral Solution and Tablets 3472
Tarceva Tablets 1254
Tarceva Tablets 2470
Tasmar Tablets (One case) 3360
Taxotere Injection Concentrate (Rare) 2947

Pulmonary function, changes

Diprivan Injectable Emulsion (Less than 1%) 676
Eulexin Capsules (Less than 1%) 3023
Intron A for Injection 3038
▲ Leukine (48%) 829
Navelbine Injection (A few patients) 1494
Repronex for Intramuscular and Subcutaneous Injection 1148
Virazole for Inhalation Solution 3365

Pulmonary function, decreased

Relenza Rotadisk 1525
▲ Rilutek Tablets (13.1% to 16%) 2945

Pulmonary hemorrhage
(*see under* Hemorrhage, pulmonary)

Pulmonary hypersensitivity

Carbatrol Capsules 3174
Equetro Extended-Release Capsules 3178
Tegretol/Tegretol-XR 2278

Pulmonary hypersensitivity, chronic

Timolide Tablets 2056

Pulmonary hypertension

Adipex-P (Rare) 1216
Agrylin Capsules 3172
▲ CellCept Capsules (3% to less than 20%) 2751
▲ CellCept Intravenous (3% to less than 20%) 2751
▲ CellCept Oral Suspension (3% to less than 20%) 2751
▲ CellCept Tablets (3% to less than 20%) 2751
Elitek (Less than or equal to 1%) 2906
Indocin I.V. (1% to 3%) 1973
Paxil CR Controlled-Release Tablets 1509
Paxil 1501
Permax Tablets (Rare) 3357

Prozac Pulvules and Liquid.............. 1771
Sandostatin LAR Depot (Rare).......... 2264
Trasylol Injection (1% to 2%)............ 779
▲ Vesanoid Capsules (3%) 2823
Zoloft....................................... 2581

Pulmonary infarction
Prinivil Tablets (0.3% to 1.0%).......... 2029
Prinzide Tablets 2033
Vaseretic Tablets 2073
Vasotec I.V. Injection (0.5% to 1.0%)...................................... 2076
Zestoretic Tablets.......................... 701
Zestril Tablets (0.3% to 1.0%).......... 704

Pulmonary infiltrates
Agrylin Capsules........................... 3172
Apokyn Injection 2132
Campath Ampules 826
Dynacin Tablets 1859
Herceptin I.V................................ 1234
▲ Imdur Tablets (Less than or equal to 5%)..................................... 3032
Intron A for Injection (Rare).............. 3038
Leustatin Injection.......................... 2368
Pegasys 2793
PEG-Intron Powder for Injection........ 3062
Pentasa Capsules (Less than 1%).... 3182
Prinivil Tablets (0.3% to 1.0%).......... 2029
Prinzide Tablets............................ 2033
Rebetol....................................... 3073
Rebetron Combination Therapy........ 3078
Rituxan for Infusion 845
Rituxan I.V. 1251
Stalevo Tablets (Rare).................... 2270
Tarceva Tablets 1254
Tarceva Tablets 2470
Vantin Tablets and Oral Suspension 2650
Vaseretic Tablets 2073
Vasotec I.V. Injection (0.5% to 1.0%)...................................... 2076
▲ Vesanoid Capsules (6%) 2823
Zestoretic Tablets.......................... 701
Zestril Tablets (0.3% to 1.0%).......... 704

Pulmonary inflammation
Pacerone Tablets.......................... 3337

Pulmonary insufficiency
Herceptin I.V............................... 1234

Pulmonary nodule
Sandostatin Injection (Less than 1%)...................................... 2263
Sandostatin LAR Depot (Rare).......... 2264

Pulmonary physical finding
Tygacil for Injection (1.9%).............. 3489

Pulmonary reembolism
Activase I.V................................. 1225

Pulmonary symptoms, worsening
Accolate Tablets (Rare).................. 663
Flovent Diskus 50 mcg.................. 1415
Singulair.................................... 2047

Pulmonary toxicity, unspecified
Alkeran for Injection 976
Alkeran Tablets 977
▲ Idamycin PFS Injection (39%) 2645
Myleran Tablets 1492
▲ Pacerone Tablets (10% to 17%) 3337

Pulse, fast
Caverject Impulse Injection (Less than 1%).................................. 2610
Humalog-Pen (Less common).......... 1751
Humulin 50/50, 100 Units.............. 1760
Humulin 70/30 Pen (Less common)................................... 1761
Humulin L, 100 Units (Less common)................................... 1763
Humulin R (U-500)........................ 1768
Humulin N Pen (Less common)........ 1765
Levoxyl Tablets............................ 1680
Children's Motrin Oral Suspension and Chewable Tablets .... ▣647
Children's Motrin Non-Staining Dye-Free Oral Suspension .... ▣647
Children's Motrin Oral Suspension and Chewable Tablets................ 1837
Children's Motrin Non-Staining Dye-Free Oral Suspension............. 1837
Infants' Motrin Concentrated Drops.. 1837
Infants' Motrin Non-Staining Dye-Free Drops........................... 1837
Junior Strength Motrin Caplets and Chewable Tablets 1837

Novolin 70/30 PenFill 3 ml Cartridges (Rare)......................... 2325
Novolin N PenFill 3 ml Cartridges (Rare).................................... 2325
Novolin R PenFill (Rare)................. 2325
Unithroid Tablets.......................... 3521

Pulse changes
AquaMEPHYTON Injection............... 1887
Clozapine Tablets 2141
Clozaril Tablets 2174
Concerta Extended-Release Tablets 1828
Effexor Tablets 3405
Focalin Tablets............................. 2214
Focalin XR Capsules 2217
Imitrex Injection (Rare).................. 1431
Imitrex Nasal Spray 1435
Mephyton Tablets (Rare)................ 1993
Metadate CD Capsules 3316
Moban Tablets 1108
Norvasc Tablets (Less than or equal to 0.1%)......................... 2529
Orap Tablets 1220
Plasbumin-5 (Rare)....................... 3249
Plasbumin-20 (Rare)..................... 3249
Plasbumin-25 (Rare)..................... 3251
Risperdal M-Tab Orally Disintegrating Tablets................. 1658
Risperdal.................................... 1658
Ritalin Hydrochloride Tablets.......... 2254
Ritalin LA Capsules 2255
Ritalin-SR Tablets 2254
Rituxan for Infusion (Two cases)....... 845
Seroquel Tablets (Infrequent)........... 691

Pulse rate, decreased
Focalin XR Capsules 2217

Pulse rate, depression
Acthrel for Injection (One patient)..... 3528
Lanoxicaps Capsules..................... 1458
Lanoxin Injection.......................... 1462
ReoPro Vials (1.0%)...................... 1779

Pulse rate, increased
Agrylin Capsules.......................... 3172
Focalin XR Capsules 2217

Pulse, irregular
Caduet Tablets (Less than or equal to 0.1%)................................. 2507
Lariam Tablets (Infrequent)............. 2790
Phenergan.................................. 3438
Rythmol SR Capsules.................... 2736

Purple toes syndrome
Activase I.V................................. 1225
Coumadin for Injection (Infrequent)... 932
Coumadin Tablets (Infrequent)......... 932
Miradon Tablets 3056

Purpura
Aceon Tablets (2 mg, 4 mg, 8 mg) (0.1%).................................... 3191
Adalat CC Tablets (Rare)................ 2978
Advicor Tablets............................ 1694
Aggrenox Capsules (1.4%).............. 855
Aldoclor Tablets........................... 1881
Aldoril Tablets.............................. 1884
Altace Capsules (Less than 1%)....... 1673
Altoprev Extended-Release Tablets (Rare).................................... 1151
Ambien Tablets (Rare).................... 2867
AmBisome for Injection (Less common)................................... 615
Amerge Tablets (Rare).................... 1312
Anaprox Tablets (Less than 3%)....... 2769
Anaprox DS Tablets (Less than 3%).. 2769
Anzemet Injection (Infrequently)....... 2871
Anzemet Tablets (Infrequently)......... 2874
▲ Arixtra Injection (0% to 3.5%) 1325
Arthrotec Tablets (Rare)................. 3126
Attenuvax (Rare).......................... 1889
Avalide Tablets............................. 922
Avalide Tablets............................. 2889
BiDil Tablets................................ 2161
Caduet Tablets (Greater than 0.1% to less than or equal to 1%).......... 2507
▲ Campath Ampules (8%) 826
Carbatrol Capsules....................... 3174
Cardizem LA Extended Release Tablets (Infrequent)................... 1699
Cataflam Tablets (Occasionally)....... 2173
Celexa (Infrequent)....................... 1177
Cipro I.V. (1% or less)................... 2998
Cipro I.V. Pharmacy Bulk Package (1% or less).............................. 3509
Cipro XR Tablets 3004
Clinoril Tablets (Less than 1 in 100)....................................... 1899
Clorpres Tablets (Few)................... 2139

Comtan Tablets (2%)...................... 2186
▲ Coreg Tablets (Greater than 1% to 3%).. 1376
Covera-HS Tablets (Less than 2%).... 3135
Dapsone Tablets USP 1656
Diovan HCT Tablets....................... 2195
Diuril Oral 1936
Diuril Sodium Intravenous 1934
Dyazide Capsules......................... 1389
EC-Naprosyn Delayed-Release Tablets (Less than 3%).............. 2769
Effexor XR Capsules (Rare)............. 3411
▲ Eloxatin for Injection (2% to 5%) 2908
Engerix-B Vaccine 1391
Equetro Extended-Release Capsules.................................. 3178
Evoxac Capsules (Less than 1%)...... 1042
Exelon Capsules (Infrequent)........... 2204
Flexeril Tablets (Rare).................... 1832
Frova Tablets (Rare)...................... 1101
Furosemide Tablets 2117
▲ Gamunex Immune Globulin I.V., 10% (40%) 3232
Garamycin Injectable 3028
Gengraf Capsules (2%) 458
Gleevec Tablets (Infrequent)............ 2221
Guanidine Hydrochloride Tablets 3030
Hyzaar 1964
▲ Imdur Tablets (Less than or equal to 5%) 3032
Indapamide Tablets 2119
Indocin Capsules (Less than 1%) 1968
Indocin I.V. (Less than 1%) 1973
Indocin (Less than 1%) 1968
Infed Injection 3381
▲ Intron A for Injection (Less than or equal to 5%) 3038
Lescol Capsules (Rare) 2227
Lescol Capsules (Rare) 2730
Lescol XL Tablets 2227
Lescol XL Tablets 2730
▲ Leustatin Injection (10%) 2368
Levaquin in 5% Dextrose Injection (0.1% to 0.9%) 2453
Levaquin (0.1% to 0.9%) 2453
Lotensin HCT Tablets 2235
Lovenox Injection 2931
Lyrica Capsules (Rare) 2524
Matulane Capsules 3188
Maxzide 2150
Meruvax II 1994
Mevacor Tablets (Rare) 1996
Micardis HCT Tablets 886
M-M-R II 1980
Mobic Oral Suspension (Less than 2%) 893
Mobic Tablets (Less than 2%) 893
Moduretic Tablets 2003
Mumpsvax (Extremely rare) 2005
Nalfon Capsules (Less than 1%) 2504
Naprosyn Suspension (Less than 3%) 2769
Naprosyn Tablets (Less than 3%) 2769
Neoral Soft Gelatin Capsules (2%) 2247
Neoral Oral Solution (2%) 2247
Neurontin Capsules (Frequent) 2498
Neurontin Oral Solution (Frequent) ... 2498
Neurontin Tablets (Frequent) 2498
Nicotrol NS (Less than 1%) 2596
Norvasc Tablets (More than 0.1% to 1%) 2529
NovoSeven (1%) 2335
Oncaspar (Less than 1%) 1123
Paxil CR Controlled-Release Tablets (Infrequent) 1509
Paxil (Infrequent) 1501
Permax Tablets (Rare) 3357
▲ Plavix Tablets (5.3%) 940
▲ Plavix Tablets (5.3%) 2942
Pletal Tablets (Less than 2%) 2478
Pravachol Tablets (Rare) 943
Prevacid NapraPAC (Less than 3%) .. 3277
Prilosec OTC Tablets 2674
Prinzide Tablets 2033
Prochieve 4% Gel 1018
Prochieve 8% Gel 1018
▲ Proleukin for Injection (4%) 1007
ProSom Tablets (Rare) 512
Prozac Pulvules and Liquid (Rare) 1771
Pulmicort Respules (1% to 3%) 654
Razadyne ER Extended-Release Capsules (Infrequent) 2434
Razadyne (Infrequent) 2434
Relpax Tablets (Rare) 2531
Requip Tablets (Infrequent) 1528
Rescriptor Tablets 2535
Reyataz Capsules (Less than 3%) 948
Rilutek Tablets (Rare) 2945
Risperdal Consta Long-Acting Injection (Infrequent) 1664

Risperdal M-Tab Orally Disintegrating Tablets (Infrequent)............................ 1658
Risperdal (Infrequent).................... 1658
▲ Simulect for Injection (3% to 10%) ... 2268
Sonata Capsules (Rare).................. 1686
▲ Soriatane Capsules (1% to 10%) 1028
Stalevo Tablets (2%)...................... 2270
Surmontil Capsules....................... 2347
Symbyax Capsules (Rare)............... 1788
Tarka Tablets 519
Tegretol/Tegretol-XR..................... 2278
Tenormin I.V. Injection................... 698
Tenormin Tablets.......................... 695
Teveten Tablets (Less than 1%)........ 1707
Teveten HCT Tablets (Less than 1%)....................................... 1710
Thalomid Capsules....................... 979
Tiazac Capsules (Infrequent)........... 1204
Ticlid Tablets (2.2%)...................... 2813
Timolide Tablets 2056
▲ Topamax Sprinkle Capsules (8%) 2438
▲ Topamax Tablets (8%) 2438
Trecator Tablets (Rare) 3482
Trileptal Oral Suspension (Up to 2%) 2281
Trileptal Tablets (Up to 2%) 2281
Uniretic Tablets 3114
Vaseretic Tablets 2073
Verelan PM Capsules (2% or less) 3120
VFEND I.V. (Less than 2%) 2543
VFEND Oral Suspension (Less than 2%) 2543
VFEND Tablets (Less than 2%) 2543
Vivactil Tablets 2350
Voltaren Tablets (Occasionally) 2298
Voltaren-XR Tablets (Occasionally) 2301
Vytorin 10/10 Tablets 2084
Vytorin 10/10 Tablets 3092
Vytorin 10/20 Tablets 2084
Vytorin 10/20 Tablets 3092
Vytorin 10/40 Tablets 2084
Vytorin 10/40 Tablets 3092
Vytorin 10/80 Tablets 2084
Vytorin 10/80 Tablets 3092
Zegerid Powder for Oral Solution 2972
Zestoretic Tablets 701
Zocor Tablets (Rare) 2078
Zoloft (2%) 2581
Zosyn (1.0% or less) 3492
Zyrtec Chewable Tablets (Less than 2%) 2589
Zyrtec (Less than 2%) 2589
Zyrtec-D 12 Hour Extended Release Tablets (Less than 2%) 2591

Purpura, allergic
Plavix Tablets (Less than 1%) 940
Plavix Tablets (Less than 1%) 2942

Purpura, anaphylactoid
Dynacin Tablets 1859

Purpura, fulminous
Zovirax for Injection (Less than 1%) 1618

Purpura, nonthrombocytopenic
Blocadren Tablets 1891
Cosopt Sterile Ophthalmic Solution 1910
Edecrin (Rare) 1941
Inderal LA Long-Acting Capsules 3421
InnoPran XL Capsules 2728
Nadolol Tablets 2121
Timolide Tablets 2056
Timoptic in Ocudose 2061
Timoptic Sterile Ophthalmic Solution 2058
Timoptic-XE Sterile Ophthalmic Gel Forming Solution 2062
Toprol-XL Tablets 660

Purpura, thrombocytopenic
Amoxil Capsules 1315
Amoxil Chewable Tablets 1315
Amoxil Pediatric Drops for Oral Suspension 1315
Amoxil Powder for Oral Suspension 1315
Amoxil Tablets 1315
Augmentin 1331
Augmentin Tablets 1334
Augmentin XR Extended-Release Tablets 1340
Augmentin ES-600 Powder for Oral Suspension 1337
Axid Oral Solution (Rare) 913
Blocadren Tablets 1891
Concerta Extended-Release Tablets 1828
Cosopt Sterile Ophthalmic Solution 1910

Cuprimine Capsules ... 1925
Evoxac Capsules (Less than 1%) ... 1042
Focalin Tablets ... 2214
Focalin XR Capsules ... 2217
Genoptic Sterile Ophthalmic Solution (Rare) ... ⊙ 227
Inderal LA Long-Acting Capsules ... 3421
Indocin Capsules (Less than 1%) ... 1968
Indocin I.V. (Less than 1%) ... 1973
Indocin (Less than 1%) ... 1968
Infanrix Vaccine ... 1444
InnoPran XL Capsules ... 2728
▲ Intron A for Injection (Less than 5%) ... 3038
Metadate CD Capsules ... 3316
Nadolol Tablets ... 2121
Omnicef Capsules ... 506
Omnicef for Oral Suspension ... 506
Pediarix Vaccine ... 1518
PEG-Intron Powder for Injection (Less than or equal to 1%) ... 3062
Phenergan Tablets ... 3438
PREVPAC ... 3281
Prograf Capsules and Injection ... 624
Prozac Pulvules and Liquid ... 1771
Remicade for IV Injection ... 987
Ritalin Hydrochloride Tablets ... 2254
Ritalin LA Capsules ... 2255
Ritalin-SR Tablets ... 2254
Timolide Tablets ... 2056
Timoptic in Ocudose ... 2061
Timoptic Sterile Ophthalmic Solution ... 2058
Timoptic-XE Sterile Ophthalmic Gel Forming Solution ... 2062
Toprol-XL Tablets ... 660
▲ Xeloda Tablets (Less than 5%) ... 2825

Purpura, thrombocytopenic, idiopathic
Pegasys (Less than 1%) ... 2793

Purpura, thrombocytopenic thrombotic
Cuprimine Capsules ... 1925
Levaquin in 5% Dextrose Injection (Rare) ... 2453
Levaquin (Rare) ... 2453
Mycamine for Injection ... 620
Plavix Tablets (Rare) ... 940
Plavix Tablets (Rare) ... 2942
Prevacid Delayed-Release Capsules (Less than 1%) ... 3268
Prevacid for Delayed-Release Oral Suspension (Less than 1%) ... 3268
Prevacid NapraPAC ... 3277
Prevacid SoluTab Delayed-Release Orally Disintegrating Tablets (Less than 1%) ... 3268
▲ Rapamune Oral Solution and Tablets (3% to 20%) ... 3472
Remicade for IV Injection ... 987
Risperdal M-Tab Orally Disintegrating Tablets (A single case) ... 1658
Risperdal (A single case) ... 1658
Ticlid Tablets (Rare) ... 2813
Valtrex Caplets ... 1573
VFEND I.V. (Less than 2%) ... 2543
VFEND Oral Suspension (Less than 2%) ... 2543
VFEND Tablets (Less than 2%) ... 2543

Pustules
Cutivate Lotion 0.05% (Less than 1%) ... 1383

Pustules, scalp
Nizoral 2% Shampoo (One occurrence in 41 patients) ... 1838
Temovate Scalp Application (3 of 294 patients) ... 1551

Pustules, unspecified
Duragesic Transdermal System (Less than 1%) ... 2448
Klonopin (Infrequent) ... 2782

Pustulosis, exanthematous
Augmentin ... 1331
Augmentin Tablets ... 1334
Augmentin XR Extended-Release Tablets ... 1340
Augmentin ES-600 Powder for Oral Suspension ... 1337
Gleevec Tablets (Rare) ... 2221
Lamisil Tablets ... 2226
PREVPAC ... 3281

Pustulosis, provocation
Temovate Scalp Application (Rare) ... 1551

Pyelitis
Amerge Tablets (Rare) ... 1312

Pyelonephritis
Actiq (Less than 1%) ... 993
Ambien Tablets (Rare) ... 2867
Aricept Tablets (Infrequent) ... 1086
Aricept ODT Tablets (Infrequent) ... 1086
Avonex ... 839
Celexa (Rare) ... 1177
▲ CellCept Capsules (3% to less than 20%) ... 2751
▲ CellCept Intravenous (3% to less than 20%) ... 2751
▲ CellCept Oral Suspension (3% to less than 20%) ... 2751
▲ CellCept Tablets (3% to less than 20%) ... 2751
Cleocin Vaginal Ovules (Less than 1%) ... 2613
Copaxone for Injection (Infrequent) ... 3292
▲ Copegus Tablets (3% to 5%) ... 2759
Crixivan Capsules ... 1918
Effexor Tablets (Rare) ... 3405
Effexor XR Capsules (Infrequent) ... 3411
Enbrel for Injection ... 580
Evoxac Capsules (Less than 1%) ... 1042
Fortical Nasal Spray (Less than 1%) ... 3336
Gabitril Tablets (Infrequent) ... 998
Gengraf Capsules (1% to less than 3%) ... 458
Herceptin I.V. (At least one of the 958 patients) ... 1234
Humira Injection (Less than 5%) ... 464
Lunesta Tablets (Rare) ... 3139
Lupron Depot 3.75 mg ... 3257
Lupron Depot–3 Month 11.25 mg ... 3262
Miacalcin Nasal Spray (Less than 1%) ... 2242
Neoral Soft Gelatin Capsules (1% to less than 3%) ... 2247
Neoral Oral Solution (1% to less than 3%) ... 2247
Neurontin Capsules (Rare) ... 2498
Neurontin Oral Solution (Rare) ... 2498
Neurontin Tablets (Rare) ... 2498
Norvir (Less than 2%) ... 499
▲ Pegasys (3% to 5%) ... 2793
Permax Tablets (Rare) ... 3357
Prinivil Tablets (0.3% to 1.0%) ... 2029
Prinzide Tablets ... 2033
Protonix I.V. (Less than 1%) ... 3468
Protonix Tablets (Less than 1%) ... 3465
▲ Rapamune Oral Solution and Tablets (Less than 20%) ... 3472
Requip Tablets (Rare) ... 1528
Rilutek Tablets (Rare) ... 2945
Uniretic Tablets (Less than 1%) ... 3114
Zestril Tablets (0.3% to 1.0%) ... 704
Zoloft (Rare) ... 2581
Zomig Nasal Spray (Rare) ... 718

Pyloric stenosis
EryPed ... 445
Invanz for Injection (Greater than 0.1%) ... 1974
PCE Dispertab Tablets ... 510

Pyoderma gangrenosum
Asacol Delayed-Release Tablets (Rare) ... 2688

Pyogenic granuloma
Accutane Capsules ... 2740
Amnesteem Capsules ... 2126
▲ Soriatane Capsules (1% to 10%) ... 1028

Pyrexia
(*see under* Fever)

Pyrosis
(*see under* Heartburn)

Pyuria
Aricept Tablets (Infrequent) ... 1086
Aricept ODT Tablets (Infrequent) ... 1086
Colazal Capsules ... 2845
Effexor Tablets (Infrequent) ... 3405
Effexor XR Capsules (Infrequent) ... 3411
Evoxac Capsules (Less than 1%) ... 1042
Neurontin Capsules (Rare) ... 2498
Neurontin Oral Solution (Rare) ... 2498
Neurontin Tablets (Rare) ... 2498
▲ Ontak Vials (10%) ... 1717
Paxil CR Controlled-Release Tablets (Rare) ... 1509
Paxil (Rare) ... 1501
Permax Tablets (Infrequent) ... 3357
Prilosec OTC Tablets (Less than 1%) ... 2674
▲ Prograf Capsules and Injection (3% to 15%) ... 624
Provigil Tablets (1%) ... 1002
▲ Rapamune Oral Solution and Tablets (3% to 20%) ... 3472
Requip Tablets (2%) ... 1528
Rythmol SR Capsules ... 2736
Singulair (1%) ... 2047
Uniretic Tablets (More than 1%) ... 3114
Zegerid Powder for Oral Solution (Less than 1%) ... 2972
Zosyn ... 3492
Zyprexa Tablets (Infrequent) ... 1798
Zyprexa ZYDIS Orally Disintegrating Tablets (Infrequent) ... 1798

Q

Quadriplegia
Orthoclone OKT3 Sterile Solution ... 2370

Quncke's edema
(*see also under* Angioedema)
Protonix I.V. ... 3468
Protonix Tablets ... 3465

R

Radiation recall syndrome
Taxotere Injection Concentrate ... 2947
▲ Xeloda Tablets (Less than 5%) ... 2825

Radiculoneuropathy
Imitrex Injection ... 1431
Imitrex Tablets (Rare) ... 1440
Pneumovax 23 (Rare) ... 2020
Recombivax HB ... 2045

Rage
Niravam Orally Disintegrating Tablets (Rare) ... 3106
Valium Tablets ... 2822
Xanax XR Tablets (Rare) ... 2655

Rage, paradoxical
Diastat Rectal Delivery System ... 3344

Rales
Adalat CC Tablets (Less than 1%) ... 2978
▲ Aredia for Injection (Up to 6%) ... 2168
Blocadren Tablets (0.6%) ... 1891
Brevibloc Concentrate (Less than 1%) ... 766
Brevibloc Injection (Less than 1%) ... 766
Brevibloc Double Strength Injection (Less than 1%) ... 766
Brevibloc Premixed Injection (Less than 1%) ... 766
Brevibloc Double Strength Premixed Injection (Less than 1%) ... 766
▲ Coreg Tablets (4%) ... 1376
Cosopt Sterile Ophthalmic Solution ... 1910
▲ Imdur Tablets (Less than or equal to 5%) ... 3032
Invanz for Injection (0.5% to 1.1%) ... 1974
ReoPro Vials (0.4%) ... 1779
Rythmol SR Capsules (1% to 2%) ... 2736
Sular Tablets (Less than or equal to 1%) ... 1163
Thalomid Capsules ... 979
Timolide Tablets (Less than 1%) ... 2056
Timoptic in Ocudose ... 2061
Timoptic Sterile Ophthalmic Solution ... 2058
Timoptic-XE Sterile Ophthalmic Gel Forming Solution ... 2062
▲ Trisenox Injection (10%) ... 983
▲ Vesanoid Capsules (14%) ... 2823
▲ Zenapax for Injection (2% to 5%) ... 2838

Rash
▲ Abelcet Injection (4%) ... 1119
▲ Abilify Tablets (6%) ... 916
▲ Abilify Tablets (6%) ... 2472
Accolate Tablets ... 663
Accutane Capsules ... 2740
Aceon Tablets (2 mg, 4 mg, 8 mg) (2.3%) ... 3191
Aciphex Tablets ... 1081
Acticin Cream ... 2125
▲ Actimmune (17%) ... 1646
Actiq (1% to 2%) ... 993
Activase I.V. (Very rare) ... 1225
Activella Tablets ... 2311
▲ Actonel Tablets (3.1% to 11.5%) ... 2679
▲ Actonel with Calcium Tablets (3.1% to 7.7%) ... 2684
Adacel Vaccine (2% to 2.7%) ... 2959
▲ Adalat CC Tablets (3% or less) ... 2978
▲ Advicor Tablets (5%) ... 1694
▲ Aerobid/Aerobid-M (3% to 9%) ... 1172
▲ Agenerase Capsules (20% to 27%) ... 1299
▲ Agenerase Oral Solution (9% to 27%) ... 1304
Aggrastat ... 1878
Aggrenox Capsules ... 855
▲ Agrylin Capsules (8.3%) ... 3172
Alacol DM Syrup ... 739
Albenza Tablets (Rare) ... 1310
Aldara Cream, 5% (More than 1%) ... 1814
Aldoclor Tablets ... 1881
Aldoril Tablets ... 1884
▲ Aldurazyme for Intravenous Infusion (8%) ... 1261
▲ Alimta for Injection (Up to 22%) ... 1722
Alinia for Oral Suspension (Less than 1%) ... 2840
Alinia Tablets (Less than 1%) ... 2840
Alkeran for Injection ... 976
Alkeran Tablets ... 977
Allegra (Rare) ... 2857
Allegra-D 12 Hour Extended-Release Tablets (Rare) ... 2860
Allegra-D 24 Hour Extended-Release Tablets (Rare) ... 2862
Aloprim for Injection (1.5%) ... 2156
Aloxi Injection (Less than 1%) ... 2099
Alphagan P Ophthalmic Solution (1% to 4%) ... 563
Altace Capsules (Less than 1%) ... 1673
Altoprev Extended-Release Tablets (0.8% to 1.3%) ... 1151
Ambien Tablets (2%) ... 2867
▲ AmBisome for Injection (22.2% to 24.8%) ... 615
Amerge Tablets (Infrequent) ... 1312
Ammonul Injection ... 3323
Amoxil Capsules ... 1315
Amoxil Chewable Tablets ... 1315
Amoxil Pediatric Drops for Oral Suspension ... 1315
Amoxil Powder for Oral Suspension ... 1315
Amoxil Tablets ... 1315
▲ Anaprox Tablets (1% to 10%) ... 2769
▲ Anaprox DS Tablets (1% to 10%) ... 2769
Ancef for Injection ... 1318
Antara Capsules ... 2723
Anzemet Injection (Rare) ... 2871
Anzemet Tablets (Rare) ... 2874
Apidra Injection ... 2876
Aptivus Capsules (2%) ... 859
Aralast (0.1% to greater than or equal to 0.2%) ... 745
▲ Aranesp for Injection (7%) ... 576
▲ Arava Tablets (10%) ... 2881
▲ Argatroban Injection (1% to 10%) ... 1321
Aricept Tablets ... 1086
Aricept ODT Tablets ... 1086
▲ Arimidex Tablets (6% to 10%) ... 665
▲ Arixtra Injection (0.6% to 7.5%) ... 1325
Aromasin Tablets (Less frequent) ... 2600
Arthrotec Tablets (Rare) ... 3126
▲ Asacol Delayed-Release Tablets (6%) ... 2688
Astelin Nasal Spray ... 1876
Atacand Tablets (0.5% or greater) ... 634
Atacand HCT (0.5% or greater) ... 637
Atrovent HFA Inhalation Aerosol ... 872
Atrovent Nasal Spray 0.03% (Infrequent) ... 869
Atrovent Nasal Spray 0.06% (Rare) ... 870
Attenuvax (Occasional) ... 1889
▲ Augmentin (3%) ... 1331
▲ Augmentin Tablets (3%) ... 1334
Augmentin XR Extended-Release Tablets ... 1340
Augmentin ES-600 Powder for Oral Suspension (1.1%) ... 1337
Avalide Tablets (1% or greater) ... 922
Avalide Tablets (1% or greater) ... 2889
Avapro Tablets (1% or greater) ... 925
Avapro Tablets (1% or greater) ... 2886
Avelox (0.1% to less than 2%) ... 2984
▲ Avinza Capsules (5% to 10%) ... 1714
Avodart Soft Gelatin Capsules ... 1353
Avonex ... 839
Axert Tablets (Rare) ... 2430
Axid Oral Solution (1.9%) ... 913
Azasan Tablets (2%) ... 2844
▲ Azmacort Inhalation Aerosol (1% to 3%) ... 1701
Bactroban Cream (1.1%) ... 1356
Bactroban Nasal (Less than 1%) ... 1357
Bactroban Ointment (Less than 1%) ... 1358
Beano ... ▣ 764
Beconase AQ Nasal Spray (Rare) ... 1359
▲ BeneFix for Injection (1.6% to 7.7%) ... 3402
Benicar Tablets (Greater than 0.5%) ... 2850
Benicar HCT Tablets (Greater than 1%) ... 2852
Bentyl Capsules ... 724
Bentyl Injection ... 724
Bentyl Syrup ... 724
Bentyl Tablets ... 724

Betagan Ophthalmic Solution, USP ⊙ 217
▲ Betaseron for SC Injection (24%) 791
▲ Betimol Ophthalmic Solution (More than 5%) ⊙ 283
▲ Betimol Ophthalmic Solution (More than 5%) 3371
▲ Bexxar (Less than 1% to 17%) 1360
▲ Biaxin/Biaxin XL (3%) 402
Blocadren Tablets (Less than 1%) 1891
Boniva Tablets (1.3% to 2.3%) 2747
Boostrix 1366
Botox Purified Neurotoxin Complex (7 cases) 565
Brimonidine Tartrate Ophthalmic Solution 0.2% ⊙ 245
Buphenyl Powder (Less than or equal to 2%) 3327
Buphenyl Tablets (Less than or equal to 2%) 3327
Buprenex Injectable (Infrequent) 2718
▲ Caduet Tablets (Less than 1% to 3.9%) 2507
▲ Cafcit (8.7%) 1854
Calcium Disodium Versenate Injection 1819
▲ Campath Ampules (3% to 40%) 826
Campral Tablets (Frequent) 1175
▲ Camptosar Injection (0.4% to 14.3%) 2602
Canasa Rectal Suppositories (1.2%) 726
▲ Cancidas for Injection (0% to 6.2%) 1894
▲ Captopril Tablets (About 4 to 7 of 100 patients) 2114
Carafate Suspension (Less than 0.5%) 727
Carafate Tablets (Less than 0.5%) 728
Carbatrol Capsules 3174
▲ Cardizem LA Extended Release Tablets (1% to 4%) 1699
▲ Carnitor Injection (3% to 5%) 3185
Carteolol Hydrochloride Ophthalmic Solution USP, 1% ⊙ 246
▲ Casodex Tablets (6%) 670
Catapres Tablets (About 1 in 100 patients) 874
Catapres-TTS (0.5% or less) 875
Caverject Impulse Injection (Less than 1%) 2610
Ceftin (0.1% to 1%) 1369
Celebrex Capsules 3130
Celexa (Frequent) 1177
▲ CellCept Capsules (3% to 22.1%) 2751
▲ CellCept Intravenous (3% to 22.1%) 2751
▲ CellCept Oral Suspension (3% to 22.1%) 2751
▲ CellCept Tablets (3% to 22.1%) 2751
▲ Cenestin Tablets, 0.45mg, 0.625mg, 0.9mg, 1.25mg (4%) 1063
Cenestin Tablets, 0.3mg 1063
Centany Ointment, 2% (0.3%) 2382
▲ Cerezyme for Injection (Approximately 6.5%) 1263
Cerubidine for Injection (Rare) 788
▲ Chemet Capsules (2.6% to 11.2%) 2480
Cialis Tablets (Less than 2%) 1806
Cipro I.V. (Greater than or equal to 1%) 2998
Cipro I.V. Pharmacy Bulk Package (Greater than or equal to 1%) 3509
Cipro (1% to 1.8%) 2991
Cipro XR Tablets (Less than 1%) 3004
Clarinex Syrup (Rare) 3009
Clarinex Tablets (Rare) 3009
Clarinex Reditabs Tablets (Rare) 3009
Clarinex-D 24-Hour Extended-Release Tablets 3012
Cleocin Vaginal Ovules (Less than 1%) 2613
Climara Transdermal System 795
Climara Pro Transdermal System (2.4%) 800
▲ Clinoril Tablets (3% to 9%) 1899
Clorpres Tablets (1%) 2139
Clozapine Tablets (2%) 2141
Clozaril Tablets (2%) 2174
Cogentin Injection 1903
▲ CombiPatch Transdermal System (5% to 6%) 2180
Combivent Inhalation Aerosol (Less than 2%; rare) 878
▲ Combivir Tablets (9%) 1373
Combunox Tablets (Less than 2%) 1183
Comvax (0.8% to 0.9%) 1904
Concerta Extended-Release Tablets 1828
▲ Copaxone for Injection (18%) 3292
▲ Copegus Tablets (8%) 2759
Cosopt Sterile Ophthalmic Solution (1% to 5%) 1910
Coumadin for Injection (Infrequent) 932
Coumadin Tablets (Infrequent) 932
Covera-HS Tablets (1.2% to 2%) 3135
Cozaar Tablets (Less than 1%) 1913
Crestor Tablets (Greater than or equal to 2%) 672
Crixivan Capsules (1.2%) 1918
Crolom Cromolyn Sodium Sterile Ophthalmic Solution USP 4% ⊙ 248
▲ Cubicin for Injection (4.3%) 1038
▲ Cuprimine Capsules (5%) 1925
Cutivate Lotion 0.05% (Less than 1%) 1383
Cymbalta Delayed-Release Capsules (Frequent) 1729
Cytovene 2763
Dalmane Capsules (Rare) 3343
Darvocet A 500 Tablets 3497
DDAVP Nasal Spray 2894
Decadron Tablets 1929
▲ Depacon Injection (1% to 5%) 412
▲ Depakene (1% to 5%) 417
▲ Depakote Sprinkle Capsules (1% to 5%) 422
▲ Depakote Tablets (1% to 6%) 427
▲ Depakote ER Tablets (1% to 5%) 433
▲ Depo-Provera Contraceptive Injection (1% to 5%) 2619
Desferal Vials (Very rare) 2190
Desmopressin Acetate Rhinal Tube 1144
Detrol Tablets (1.9%) 2626
▲ Diastat Rectal Delivery System (3%) 3344
Differin Cream (Less than 1%) 1210
Digitek Tablets 2146
Dilaudid Oral Liquid 443
Dilaudid Tablets - 8 mg 443
Dilaudid-HP (Less frequent) 441
Diovan HCT Tablets (Greater than 0.2%) 2195
Diovan Tablets (0.2%) 2191
Diprivan Injectable Emulsion (Less than 1% to 5%) 676
▲ Ditropan XL Extended Release Tablets (2% to less than 5%) 2391
Diuril Oral 1936
Diuril Sodium Intravenous 1934
▲ Dolobid Tablets (3% to 9%) 1937
▲ Dovonex Cream 0.005% (1% to 10%) 3374
▲ Dovonex Ointment 0.005% (1% to 10%) 3375
▲ Dovonex Scalp Solution 0.005% (About 11%) 3375
▲ Doxil Injection (1% to 28.5%) 3302
DuoNeb Inhalation Solution (0.3%) 1058
Duragesic Transdermal System (1% or greater) 2448
Dyazide Capsules 1389
DynaCirc CR Tablets (1.3% to 2.6%) 2726
Dyrenium Capsules (Rare) 3390
▲ EC-Naprosyn Delayed-Release Tablets (1% to 10%) 2769
Edecrin 1941
▲ Effexor Tablets (3%) 3405
Effexor XR Capsules (Frequent) 3411
▲ Efudex (Among most frequent) 3348
Eldepryl Capsules 3209
▲ Elitek (1% to 13%) 2906
▲ Ellence Injection (0% to 8.9%) 2632
▲ Elmiron Capsules (3%) 2393
▲ Eloxatin for Injection (5% to 9%) 2908
Elspar for Injection 1943
Emcyt Capsules (1%) 3137
Emend Capsules (Greater than 0.5%) 1944
Emtriva Capsules 1272
Enablex Extended-Release Tablets (Greater than or equal to 1%) 2201
▲ Enbrel for Injection (5% to 14%) 580
Engerix-B Vaccine (Less than 1%) 1391
▲ Epivir (9%) 1394
▲ Epivir-HBV (5%) 1398
▲ Epogen for Injection (16%) 586
▲ Epzicom Tablets (5%) 1402
▲ Equetro Extended-Release Capsules (13%) 3178
Ery-Tab Tablets 447
Eskalith 1406
Estratest Tablets 3196
Estratest H.S. Tablets 3196
▲ Estrogel 0.06% (7.1%) 3200
▲ Eulexin Capsules (3% to 8%) 3023
▲ Evista Tablets (5.5%) 1735
▲ Evoxac Capsules (4.3%) 1042
Exelon Capsules (2% or more) 2204
Fabrazyme for Intravenous Infusion 1267
▲ Factive Tablets (0.9% to 5.0%) 2464
▲ Famvir Tablets (0.4% to 3.3%) 2207
▲ Faslodex Injection (7.3%) 682
FazaClo Orally Disintegrating Tablets (2%) 547
Feiba VH 749
▲ Femara Tablets (4% to 5%) 2210
Ferrlecit Injection 3379
Flexeril Tablets (Less than 1%) 1832
▲ Flolan for Injection (10% to 25%) 1408
Flomax Capsules 881
Flonase Nasal Spray 1412
▲ Flovent Diskus 50 mcg (8%) 1415
Floxin Otic Singles (1%) 1045
Floxin Otic Solution (1%) 1043
Flumadine (0.3% to 1%) 1186
Flumist Vaccine 1872
Focalin Tablets 2214
Focalin XR Capsules 2217
Follistim AQ Cartridge 2354
Foradil Aerolizer (1.1%) 3024
Fortaz (2%) 1422
▲ Forteo for Injection (4.9%) 1739
Fosamax (Rare) 1949
Fosamax Plus D Tablets 1956
Fragmin Injection (Rare) 2638
Furosemide Tablets 2117
▲ Gabitril Tablets (5%) 998
▲ Gamunex Immune Globulin I.V., 10% (6%) 3232
Garamycin Injectable 3028
▲ Gemzar for Injection (28% to 30%) 1743
▲ Gengraf Capsules (1% to 8%) 458
Genotropin Lyophilized Powder (Infrequent) 2642
▲ Geodon (4%) 2514
▲ Gleevec Tablets (2% to 44%) 2221
GlucaGen for Injection 790
Grifulvin V Tablets Microsize and Oral Suspension Microsize 2384
Gris-PEG Tablets (Rare) 2504
Guanidine Hydrochloride Tablets 3030
Havrix Vaccine (Less than 1%) 1425
Hepsera Tablets (2% or greater) 1275
▲ Herceptin I.V. (18%) 1234
Hexalen Capsules (Less than 1%) 2101
HibTITER (1 of 1,118 vaccinations) 3419
Humalog-Pen (Less common) 1751
Humalog Mix 75/25-Pen 1754
▲ Humira Injection (Less than 1% to 12%) 464
Humulin 50/50, 100 Units 1760
Humulin 70/30 Pen (Less common) 1761
Humulin L, 100 Units (Less common) 1763
Humulin R (U-500) 1768
Humulin N Pen (Less common) 1765
▲ Hyalgan Solution (14%) 2917
Hycamtin for Injection (Less than 1%) 1427
Hycodan 1104
HyperRAB (Rare) 3239
Hyperstat I.V. Injection 3031
Hytrin Capsules (At least 1%) 469
Hyzaar (1.4%) 1964
Idamycin PFS Injection 2645
▲ Imdur Tablets (Less than or equal to 5%) 3032
Imitrex Injection (Infrequent) 1431
Imitrex Nasal Spray (Infrequent) 1435
Imitrex Tablets (Rare to infrequent) 1440
Imodium Capsules 1834
Indocin Capsules (Less than 1%) 1968
Indocin I.V. (Less than 1%) 1973
Indocin (Less than 1%) 1968
Infanrix Vaccine 1444
Infed Injection 3381
▲ Infergen (13%) 1647
▲ Intron A for Injection (Up to 25%) 3038
Invanz for Injection (2.3% to 2.9%) 1974
▲ Invirase (Greater than or equal to 2% to 3.4%) 2776
▲ Iressa Tablets (44% to 61%) 684
▲ I.V. Busulfex (57%) 1125
Iveegam EN (0.3% to 0.8%) 759
Kadian Capsules (Less than 3%) 572
▲ Kaletra (1% to 4%) 474
▲ Kepivance (Less than 1% to 62%) 592
Keppra Oral Solution (1% to 2%) 3307
Keppra Tablets (1% to 2%) 3307
Ketek Tablets (Greater than or equal to 0.2% to less than 2%) 2920
Klonopin 2782
K-Lor Powder Packets (Rare) 472
Kogenate FS 3517
K-Tab Filmtab Tablets (Rare) 473
Kytril Injection (Rare) 2785
▲ Lamictal (5% to 14%) 1449
▲ Lamisil Tablets (5.6%) 2226
Lantus Injection 2925
▲ Lariam Tablets (Among most frequent) 2790
Lescol Capsules (2.3%) 2227
Lescol XL Tablets (1.6%) 2227
Leukeran Tablets (Rare) 1472
▲ Leukine (44% to 70%) 829
▲ Leustatin Injection (10% to 27%) 2368
Levaquin in 5% Dextrose Injection (0.3% to 1.4%) 2453
Levaquin (0.3% to 1.4%) 2453
Levitra Tablets (Less than 2%) 3048
Levothroid Tablets 1189
Levoxyl Tablets 1680
Lexapro Oral Solution (Frequent) 1193
Lexapro Tablets (Frequent) 1193
▲ Lexiva Tablets (8% to 35%) 1473
▲ Lipitor Tablets (1.1% to 3.9%) 2495
Lithobid Tablets 1670
Lofibra Capsules 1217
Lo/Ovral-28 Tablets 3423
Loprox Gel (Less than 1%) 1861
Loprox Shampoo 1862
Lortab 3315
Lortab Elixir 3312
Lotensin Tablets (Less than 1%) 2232
Lotensin HCT Tablets (0.3% to 1%) 2235
Lotrel Capsules 2238
Lotrisone Cream (Less than 1%) 3054
Lotronex Tablets 1479
▲ Lunesta Tablets (3% to 4%) 3139
Lupron Depot 3.75 mg 3257
Lupron Depot 7.5 mg 3261
Lupron Depot–3 Month 11.25 mg 3262
Lupron Depot-PED 7.5 mg, 11.25 mg and 15 mg (2%) 3266
Lupron Injection Pediatric 3256
Malarone Tablets 1484
Malarone Pediatric Tablets 1484
Matulane Capsules 3188
Mavik Tablets (0.3% to 1.0%) 482
Maxair Autohaler 1820
Maxalt Tablets (Infrequent) 1983
Maxalt-MLT Orally Disintegrating Tablets (Infrequent) 1983
▲ Maxipime for Injection (1.1% to 4%) 1093
Maxzide 2150
Mefoxin for Injection 1987
Mefoxin Premixed Intravenous Solution 1990
▲ Megace ES Oral Suspension (2% to 12%) 2492
Menactra Vaccine (1.4% to 1.6%) 2968
Menostar Transdermal System 805
▲ Mepron Suspension (6.3% to 46%) 1487
▲ Meridia Capsules (3.8%) 485
▲ Merrem I.V. (1.6% to 3.1%) 687
Meruvax II 1994
Metadate CD Capsules 3316
MetroGel-Vaginal Gel (Less than 1%) 1822
▲ Mevacor Tablets (0.8% to 5.2%) 1996
Miacalcin Injection 2241
Micardis Tablets (More than 0.3%) 884
Micardis HCT Tablets (2% or greater) 886
Midamor Tablets (Less than or equal to 1%) 2000
Migranal Nasal Spray (Infrequent) 3350
Mintezol 2002
Miradon Tablets 3056
Mirapex Tablets (Greater than or equal to 1%) 889
Mivacron Injection (Less than 1%) 489
M-M-R II (Infrequent) 1980
Moban Tablets 1108
▲ Mobic Oral Suspension (0.3% to 3%) 893
▲ Mobic Tablets (0.3% to 3%) 893
▲ Moduretic Tablets (3% to 8%) 2003
Children's Motrin Oral Suspension and Chewable Tablets 1837
Children's Motrin Cold Non-Staining Dye-Free Oral Suspension 1838
Children's Motrin Cold Oral Suspension 1838
Children's Motrin Non-Staining Dye-Free Oral Suspension 1837
Motrin Cold & Sinus Caplets 1836
Motrin IB Tablets and Caplets 1836
Infants' Motrin Concentrated Drops 1837
Infants' Motrin Non-Staining Dye-Free Drops 1837
Junior Strength Motrin Caplets and Chewable Tablets 1837
MS Contin Tablets (Less frequent) 2703
▲ Mycamine for Injection (1.4% to 3.1%) 620
▲ Myfortic Tablets (3% to less than 20%) 2244
▲ Mylotarg for Injection (18%) 3429
Nadolol Tablets (1 to 5 of 1000 patients) 2121
Naftin Gel (0.5%) 2097

▲ Nalfon Capsules (3.7%) 2504
Namenda (Frequent) 1199
▲ Naprosyn Suspension (1% to 10%) 2769
▲ Naprosyn Tablets (1% to 10%) 2769
Naropin Injection (Less than 1%) 640
Nasacort HFA Inhalation Aerosol 2939
Natrecor for Injection (Greater than or equal to 1%) 3123
Navelbine Injection (Less than 5%) 1494
Nembutal Sodium Solution, USP 2484
▲ Neoral Soft Gelatin Capsules (1% to 8%) 2247
▲ Neoral Oral Solution (1% to 8%) 2247
Neosporin Scar Solution .... ▣702
Neulasta Injection 596
▲ Neumega for Injection (25%) 3433
▲ Neupogen for Injection (6% to 12%) 598
Neurontin Capsules (1.2%) 2498
Neurontin Oral Solution (1.2%) 2498
Neurontin Tablets (1.2%) 2498
Nexium Delayed-Release Capsules (Less than 1%) 645
Nexium I.V. (Less than 1%) 649
▲ Niaspan Extended-Release Tablets (1% to 5%) 1703
Nicomide Tablets 3190
Nicotrol NS (Less than 1%) 2596
Nimbex Injection (0.1%) 494
Nimotop Capsules (Up to 2.4%) 774
▲ Nipent for Injection (26% to 43%) 3216
▲ Niravam Orally Disintegrating Tablets (10.8%) 3106
Norditropin Cartridges 2318
Noritate Cream, 1% (Uncommon) 1051
Noroxin Tablets (0.3% to 1.0%) 2009
Norvasc Tablets (Less than 1% to 2%) 2529
▲ Norvir (0% to 3.5%) 499
Novantrone for Injection Concentrate 3158
Novarel for Injection 1147
Novolin 70/30 PenFill 3 ml Cartridges (Rare) 2325
Novolin N PenFill 3 ml Cartridges (Rare) 2325
Novolin R PenFill (Rare) 2325
NovoLog Injection 2326
NovoSeven (1%) 2335
Numorphan 1112
Omacor Capsules (1.8%) 2735
Omnicef Capsules (0.9%) 506
▲ Omnicef for Oral Suspension (3%) 506
▲ Oncaspar (Greater than 5%) 1123
▲ Ontak Vials (34%) 1717
OptiPranolol Metipranolol Ophthalmic Solution 0.3% (A small number of patients) .... ⊙254
▲ Orap Tablets (8.3%) 1220
Ortho-Cyclen/Ortho Tri-Cyclen 2414
Ortho Tri-Cyclen Lo Tablets 2421
Orthoclone OKT3 Sterile Solution 2370
Oxistat Cream (0.1%) 1498
Oxsoralen-Ultra Capsules 3354
▲ OxyContin Tablets (Between 1% and 5%) 2699
OxyFast Oral Concentrate Solution 2704
OxyIR Capsules 2704
Pacerone Tablets (Less than 1%) 3337
Parcopa Orally Disintegrating Tablets 3111
Parnate Tablets (Rare) 1499
▲ Paser Granules (Among most common) 1657
▲ Paxil CR Controlled-Release Tablets (2% to 3%) 1509
▲ Paxil (2% to 3%) 1501
Peganone Tablets, USP 2487
▲ Pegasys (5%) 2793
▲ PEG-Intron Powder for Injection (6%) 3062
Penlac Nail Lacquer, Topical Solution, 8% 1051
Pentasa Capsules (1.0% to 1.3%) 3182
Pepcid Injection (Infrequent) 2017
Pepcid (Infrequent) 2014
Percocet Tablets 1114
▲ Permax Tablets (3.2%) 3357
Persantine Tablets (2.3%) 898
Phenergan Suppositories 3438
Phenytek Capsules 2153
▲ Photofrin for Injection (7%) 729
▲ Plavix Tablets (4.2%) 940
▲ Plavix Tablets (4.2%) 2942
Plendil Extended-Release Tablets (0.2% to 2.0%) 651
Pletal Tablets (2% or greater) 2478
Pneumovax 23 (Rare) 2020
Potaba (Infrequent) 1634
▲ Pravachol Tablets (1.3% to 4.0%) 943
Precose Tablets (Rare) 776
Prefest Tablets 1069
Premarin Intravenous 3440
Premarin Tablets 3443
Premarin Vaginal Cream 3449
▲ Premphase Tablets (4% to 6%) 3452
▲ Prempro Tablets (4% to 6%) 3452
Prevacid Delayed-Release Capsules (Less than 1%) 3268
Prevacid for Delayed-Release Oral Suspension (Less than 1%) 3268
Prevacid I.V. for Injection (Less than 1%) 3274
Prevacid NapraPAC (Less than 1%) 3277
Prevacid SoluTab Delayed-Release Orally Disintegrating Tablets (Less than 1%) 3268
PREVPAC (Less than 1%) 3281
Prilosec OTC Tablets (Less than 1% to 1.5%) 2674
Primaxin I.M. (0.4%) 2022
Primaxin I.V. (1.5%) 2024
Prinivil Tablets (0.3% to 1.7%) 2029
Prinzide Tablets (1.2%) 2033
ProAmatine Tablets (2.4%; less frequent) 3183
Prochieve 4% Gel 1018
Prochieve 8% Gel 1018
▲ Procrit for Injection (Rare to 16%) 2374
▲ Prograf Capsules and Injection (10% to 24%) 624
Prolastin (Occasional) 3252
Proleukin for Injection (1%) 1007
Propecia Tablets (0.5%) 2036
Proscar Tablets (0.5%) 2040
ProSom Tablets (Infrequent) 512
▲ Protonix I.V. (6%) 3468
Protonix Tablets (Less than 1% to 2%) 3465
▲ Protopic Ointment (2% to 5%) 629
Proventil Inhalation Aerosol 3067
Proventil Inhalation Solution 0.083% (Rare) 3069
Proventil HFA Inhalation Aerosol (Less than 3%) 3071
Provigil Tablets (At least 1%) 1002
▲ Prozac Pulvules and Liquid (2% to 6%) 1771
Pulmicort Respules (Less than 1% to 4%) 654
▲ Pulmozyme Inhalation Solution (3% to 12%) 1245
Purinethol Tablets 1222
Qvar Inhalation Aerosol (Rare) 1654
Rabies Vaccine RabAvert (Common) 1011
▲ Rapamune Oral Solution and Tablets (10% to 20%) 3472
▲ Rebetol (17% to 28%) 3073
▲ Rebetron Combination Therapy (20% to 28%) 3078
Recombivax HB (Less than 1%) 2045
ReFacto Vials 3479
Refludan for Injection (Uncommon) 815
Reishimax Capsules 2669
▲ Relafen Tablets (3% to 9%) 1523
Relpax Tablets (Infrequent) 2531
▲ Remicade for IV Injection (10%) 987
Renagel Tablets 1268
Repronex for Intramuscular and Subcutaneous Injection 1148
Requip Tablets (Infrequent) 1528
▲ Rescriptor Tablets (13.4% to 19.5%) 2535
▲ Retisert Implant (5% to 15%) .... ⊙256
▲ Retrovir Capsules (17%) 1533
▲ Retrovir IV Infusion (17%) 1537
▲ Retrovir (17%) 1533
▲ Reyataz Capsules (3% to 21%) 948
▲ Ribavirin, USP Capsules (17% to 28%) 3083
Risperdal Consta Long-Acting Injection (Frequent) 1664
▲ Risperdal M-Tab Orally Disintegrating Tablets (2% to 5%) 1658
▲ Risperdal (2% to 5%) 1658
Ritalin Hydrochloride Tablets 2254
Ritalin LA Capsules 2255
Ritalin-SR Tablets 2254
▲ Rituxan for Infusion (10%) 845
▲ Rituxan I.V. (15%) 1251
Rocephin Injectable Vials, ADD-Vantage, Galaxy, Bulk (1.7%) 2801
▲ Roferon-A Injection (8% to 44%) 2805
Sandostatin Injection (Less than 1%) 2263
▲ Sandostatin LAR Depot (5% to 15%) 2264
Sedapap Tablets 50 mg/650 mg 2098
▲ Serevent Diskus (4%) 1540
Seromycin Capsules 1783
▲ Seroquel Tablets (4%) 691
▲ Simulect for Injection (3% to 10%) 2268
Singulair (1.6% to 2% or greater) 2047
Skelaxin Tablets 1685
Solage Topical Solution (2.5%) 740
Sonata Capsules (Frequent) 1686
▲ Soriatane Capsules (1% to 10%) 1028
Spectracef Tablets (0.1% to 1%) 2706
▲ Spiriva HandiHaler (2% to 4%) 899
Stromectol Tablets (0.9%) 2053
Sular Tablets (Very rare) 1163
▲ Sulfamylon Cream (4.6%) 2154
▲ Sulfamylon for 5% Topical Solution (4.6%) 2155
Suprax (Less than 2%) 1811
Surmontil Capsules 2347
▲ Sustiva Capsules (5% to 46%) 957
Symmetrel (0.1% to 1%) 1115
▲ Synagis (25.6%) 1868
Synercid I.V. (2.5%) 1690
Synthroid Tablets 515
Tagamet Tablets 1547
Tambocor Tablets (1% to 3%) 1824
Tamiflu Capsules 2810
Tamiflu Oral Suspension 2810
▲ Tarceva Tablets (Less than 1% to 75%) 1254
▲ Tarceva Tablets (Less than 1% to 75%) 2470
▲ Targretin Capsules (16.7% to 22.6%) 1719
Tarka Tablets (0.3% or more) 519
Tasmar Tablets (Frequent) 3360
Taxotere Injection Concentrate (0.9%) 2947
Tegretol/Tegretol-XR 2278
▲ Temodar Capsules (8% to 13%) 3088
Tenormin I.V. Injection 698
Tenormin Tablets 695
▲ Tequin Injection (0.1% to 3%) 964
▲ Tequin Tablets (0.1% to 3%) 964
Teveten Tablets (Less than 1%) 1707
Teveten HCT Tablets (Less than 1%) 1710
▲ Thalomid Capsules (20.8%) 979
Thiothixene Capsules 2124
Thyrogen for Injection 1270
Tiazac Capsules (2%) 1204
▲ Ticlid Tablets (5.1%) 2813
Timentin ADD-Vantage 1556
Timentin Injection Galaxy Container 1559
Timentin IV Infusion 1553
Timentin Pharmacy Bulk Package 1562
Timolide Tablets (Less than 1%) 2056
Timoptic in Ocudose (Less frequent) 2061
Timoptic Sterile Ophthalmic Solution (Less frequent) 2058
Timoptic-XE Sterile Ophthalmic Gel Forming Solution 2062
Tindamax 2670
TNKase I.V. (Rare) 1256
▲ TOBI Solution for Inhalation (5.4%) 1015
Topamax Sprinkle Capsules (More than 1%) 2438
Topamax Tablets (More than 1%) 2438
▲ Toprol-XL Tablets (About 5 of 100 patients) 660
Transderm Scōp Transdermal Therapeutic System (Infrequent) 2166
Tranxene 2488
Trasylol Injection (2%) 779
Trecator Tablets (Rare) 3482
Trelstar LA Suspension (1.7%) 3387
▲ Tricor Tablets (1.4% to 6%) 523
▲ Trileptal Oral Suspension (2% to 5.3%) 2281
▲ Trileptal Tablets (2% to 5.3%) 2281
▲ Tri-Luma Cream (1% to 5.27%) 1213
Triphasil-28 Tablets 3483
▲ Trizivir Tablets (9%) 1565
Trusopt Sterile Ophthalmic Solution (Rare) 2065
▲ Truvada Tablets (Greater than 5%) 1279
Tussionex Pennkinetic Extended-Release Suspension 3322
Twinrix Vaccine (Less than 1%) 1571
Tygacil for Injection (2.4%) 3489
Ultane Liquid for Inhalation (Less than 1%) 526
Ultracet Tablets (At least 1%) 2462
Uniretic Tablets (More than 1%) 3114
Unithroid Tablets 3521
Univasc Tablets (Less than 1% to 1.6%) 3118
Uroqid-Acid No. 2 Tablets (Occasional) 785
Urso 250 Tablets (1%) 737
Urso Forte Tablets (1%) 737
Valium Tablets (Infrequent) 2822
▲ Valtrex Caplets (0.4% to 8%) 1573
Vancocin HCl Capsules, USP (Infrequent) 3370
Vantin Tablets and Oral Suspension (Less than 1% to 1.4%) 2650
Vaqta (1% to 4.5%) 2067
Varivax (Greater than or equal to 1%) 2070
Vaseretic Tablets (0.5% to 2.0%) 2073
Vasotec I.V. Injection (0.5% to 1.4%) 2076
▲ Velcade for Injection (18%) 2102
Ventolin HFA Inhalation Aerosol 1576
Verelan PM Capsules (1.2% to 2%) 3120
Vermox Chewable Tablets (Rare) 1853
▲ Vesanoid Capsules (54%) 2823
▲ VFEND I.V. (1.5% to 5.3%) 2543
▲ VFEND Oral Suspension (1.5% to 5.3%) 2543
▲ VFEND Tablets (1.5% to 5.3%) 2543
Viadur Implant (Less than 2%) 782
Viagra Tablets (2%) 2552
Vicodin Tablets 530
Vicodin ES Tablets 531
Vicodin HP Tablets 532
Vicoprofen Tablets (Less than 1%) 533
▲ Vigamox Ophthalmic Solution (1% to 4%) 560
▲ Viracept (1% to 3%) 2556
▲ Viramune Oral Suspension (8% to 37%) 903
▲ Viramune Tablets (8% to 37%) 903
Virazole for Inhalation Solution 3365
▲ Viread Tablets (5% to 7%) 1284
▲ Visudyne for Injection (10% to 30%) 2286
Vivactil Tablets 2350
▲ Vivelle Transdermal System (3% to 4.9%) 2288
▲ Vivelle-Dot Transdermal System (3% to 4.9%) 2293
Vivotif 834
VoSpire Extended-Release Tablets (Rare) 2352
Vytorin 10/10 Tablets 2084
Vytorin 10/10 Tablets 3092
Vytorin 10/20 Tablets 2084
Vytorin 10/20 Tablets 3092
Vytorin 10/40 Tablets 2084
Vytorin 10/40 Tablets 3092
Vytorin 10/80 Tablets 2084
Vytorin 10/80 Tablets 3092
▲ Wellbutrin Tablets (8.0%) 1579
▲ Wellbutrin SR Sustained-Release Tablets (4% to greater than or equal to 5%) 1583
▲ Wellbutrin XL Extended-Release Tablets (4% to greater than or equal to 5%) 1588
WinRho SDF 763
Xalatan Sterile Ophthalmic Solution (1% to 2%) 2654
Xanax XR Tablets (Infrequent) 2655
▲ Xenical Capsules (4.3%) 2834
Xifaxan Tablets (Less than 2%) 2847
▲ Xopenex HFA Inhalation Aerosol (7.5%) 3151
▲ Xopenex Inhalation Solution (7.5%) 3143
▲ Xopenex Inhalation Solution Concentrate (7.5%) 3147
Yasmin 28 Tablets 818
Zaditor Ophthalmic Solution (Less than 5%) 2302
Zantac (Rare) 1597
Zantac Injection 1593
Zantac Injection Pharmacy Bulk Package (Rare) 1595
Zantac Syrup (Rare) 1597
Zegerid Powder for Oral Solution (Less than 1% to 1.5%) 2972
Zelnorm Tablets (1%) 2303
Zemaira (0.4%) 3506
Zemuron Injection (Less than 1%) 2363
Zenapax for Injection (Greater than 2%) 2838
▲ Zerit (18% to 40%) 971
Zestoretic Tablets (1.2%) 701
Zestril Tablets (0.01% to 1.7%) 704
Zetia Tablets 2090
Zetia Tablets 3098
▲ Zevalin Injection (8%) 848
▲ Ziagen (5% to 7%) 1600
Zinacef Injection (1 in 125 patients) 1604
Zinacef for Injection (1 in 125 patients) 1604
Zithromax Capsules, 250 mg (1% or less to 1.6%) 2568
Zithromax for IV Infusion (1.9%) 2573
Zithromax for Oral Suspension, 1 g (1% or less) 2568
Zithromax for Oral Suspension, 300 mg, 600 mg, 900 mg, 1200 mg (1% or less to 1.6%) 2561
Zithromax Tablets, 250 mg, 500 mg (1% or less to 1.6%) 2561
Zithromax Tablets, 600 mg (1% or less) 2568

Zithromax Tri-Pak (1% or less to 1.6%) ... 2561
Zithromax Z-Pak (1% or less) ... 2568
Zmax for Oral Suspension (Less then 1%) ... 2577
Zofran Injection (Approximately 1%) ... 1607
Zofran (Approximately 1%) ... 1613
Zofran ODT Orally Disintegrating Tablets (Approximately 1%) ... 1613
▲ Zoladex (1% to 6%) ... 709
▲ Zoladex 3-month (8%) ... 712
▲ Zoloft (3%) ... 2581
Zometa for Intravenous Infusion ... 2306
Zomig Nasal Spray (Infrequent) ... 718
Zomig Tablets (Infrequent) ... 714
Zomig-ZMT Tablets (Infrequent) ... 714
▲ Zonegran Capsules (3%) ... 1089
▲ Zosyn (1.3% to 4.2%) ... 3492
Zovirax Capsules ... 1616
Zovirax for Injection (Approximately 2%) ... 1618
Zovirax Ointment ... 854
Zovirax ... 1616
▲ Zyban Sustained-Release Tablets (3% to 4%) ... 1620
Zyprexa Tablets ... 1798
Zyprexa ZYDIS Orally Disintegrating Tablets ... 1798
Zyrtec Chewable Tablets (Less than 2%) ... 2589
Zyrtec (Less than 2%) ... 2589
Zyrtec-D 12 Hour Extended Release Tablets (Less than 2%) ... 2591
▲ Zyvox (0.4% to 7%) ... 2661

Rash, allergic
Alesse-28 Tablets ... 3392
Aygestin Tablets ... 1062
Lo/Ovral-28 Tablets ... 3423
Ortho-Cept Tablets ... 2395
Ortho-Cyclen Tablets ... 2414
Ortho Evra Transdermal System ... 2402
Ortho Tri-Cyclen Tablets ... 2414
Ortho Tri-Cyclen Lo Tablets ... 2421
Premphase Tablets ... 3452
Prempro Tablets ... 3452
Prometrium Capsules (100 mg, 200 mg) ... 3205
Seasonale Tablets ... 1073
Triphasil-28 Tablets ... 3483
Varivax (Greater than or equal to 1%) ... 2070

Rash, bullous
Actonel with Calcium Tablets ... 2684
Caduet Tablets ... 2507
Exelon Capsules (Frequent) ... 2204
Lipitor Tablets ... 2495
Topamax Sprinkle Capsules ... 2438
Topamax Tablets ... 2438
▲ Zosyn (4.2%) ... 3492

Rash, bullous erythrodermatous
Idamycin PFS Injection ... 2645

Rash, circumocular
Polytrim Ophthalmic Solution (Multiple reports) ... 570

Rash, diaper
▲ Augmentin ES-600 Powder for Oral Suspension (3.5%) ... 1337
▲ Ceftin for Oral Suspension (3.4%) ... 1369
Comvax (0.2% to 0.5%) ... 1904
▲ Invanz for Injection (4.7%) ... 1974

Rash, drug
Nitrolingual Pumpspray ... 1161

Rash, eczematous
Exelon Capsules (Frequent) ... 2204
▲ Ontak Vials (34%) ... 1717
Thalomid Capsules ... 979

Rash, erythematous
Blocadren Tablets ... 1891
Caduet Tablets (Greater than 0.1% to less than or equal to 1%) ... 2507
▲ Campath Ampules (3% to 40%) ... 826
Carbatrol Capsules ... 3174
Celebrex Capsules (0.1% to 1.9%) ... 3130
Clindagel ... 1207
Colazal Capsules ... 2845
Coreg Tablets (Greater than 0.1% to 1%) ... 1376
Cosopt Sterile Ophthalmic Solution ... 1910
Cymbalta Delayed-Release Capsules (Infrequent) ... 1729
Denavir Cream (0.1%) ... 2163
Duragesic Transdermal System (1% or greater) ... 2448
Dynacin Tablets ... 1859
▲ Eloxatin for Injection (2% to 5%) ... 2908
Equetro Extended-Release Capsules ... 3178
▲ Evoxac Capsules (1% to 3%) ... 1042
Exelon Capsules (Frequent) ... 2204
▲ Femara Tablets (4% to 5%) ... 2210
Floxin Otic Singles ... 1045
Floxin Otic Solution (Single report) ... 1043
▲ Fortical Nasal Spray (1% to 3%) ... 3336
Hycamtin for Injection (Less than 1%) ... 1427
Inderal LA Long-Acting Capsules ... 3421
InnoPran XL Capsules ... 2728
▲ Intron A for Injection (Less than 5%) ... 3038
Invanz for Injection (Greater than 0.5%) ... 1974
Levaquin in 5% Dextrose Injection (0.1% to 0.9%) ... 2453
Levaquin (0.1% to 0.9%) ... 2453
Miacalcin Nasal Spray (1% to 3%) ... 2242
▲ Mobic Oral Suspension (0.3% to 3%) ... 893
▲ Mobic Tablets (0.3% to 3%) ... 893
Namenda (Infrequent) ... 1199
Nexium Delayed-Release Capsules (Less than 1%) ... 645
Nexium I.V. (Less than 1%) ... 649
Norvasc Tablets (More than 0.1% to 1%) ... 2529
Plavix Tablets (Less than 1%) ... 940
Plavix Tablets (Less than 1%) ... 2942
▲ Rebif Prefilled Syringe for Injection (5% to 7%) ... 3163
Remicade for IV Injection (Less than 1%) ... 987
Risperdal Consta Long-Acting Injection (Infrequent) ... 1664
▲ Soriatane Capsules (10% to 25%) ... 1028
Tegretol/Tegretol-XR ... 2278
Tenormin I.V. Injection ... 698
Tenormin Tablets ... 695
Thalomid Capsules ... 979
Timolide Tablets ... 2056
Timoptic in Ocudose ... 2061
Timoptic Sterile Ophthalmic Solution ... 2058
Timoptic-XE Sterile Ophthalmic Gel Forming Solution ... 2062
Topamax Sprinkle Capsules (Less than 1% to 2%) ... 2438
Topamax Tablets (Less than 1% to 2%) ... 2438
Trileptal Oral Suspension ... 2281
Trileptal Tablets ... 2281
▲ Xeloda Tablets (Less than 1% to 9%) ... 2825
Zoloft (Infrequent) ... 2581
▲ Zosyn (3.9%) ... 3492
Zyrtec Chewable Tablets (Less than 2%) ... 2589
Zyrtec (Less than 2%) ... 2589
Zyrtec-D 12 Hour Extended Release Tablets (Less than 2%) ... 2591

Rash, erythematous maculopapular
Amoxil Capsules ... 1315
Amoxil Chewable Tablets ... 1315
Amoxil Pediatric Drops for Oral Suspension ... 1315
Amoxil Powder for Oral Suspension ... 1315
Amoxil Tablets ... 1315
PREVPAC ... 3281
Viramune Oral Suspension ... 903
Viramune Tablets ... 903

Rash, exfoliative
Exelon Capsules (Frequent) ... 2204

Rash, follicular
Diprolene Gel 0.05% ... 3015
Floxin Otic Singles ... 1045
Floxin Otic Solution (Single report) ... 1043
Zoloft (Rare) ... 2581

Rash, heat
Trileptal Oral Suspension ... 2281
Trileptal Tablets ... 2281

Rash, herpetic
(*see under* Eruptions, herpetic)

Rash, leg
DDAVP Nasal Spray ... 2894
Desmopressin Acetate Rhinal Tube ... 1144

Rash, lichenoid
Permax Tablets (Rare) ... 3357

Rash, lupus erythematosus
Evoxac Capsules (Less than 1%) ... 1042

Rash, maculopapular
Abelcet Injection ... 1119
Abilify Tablets (Infrequent) ... 916
Abilify Tablets (Infrequent) ... 2472
Actiq (Less than 1%) ... 993
Agenerase Capsules ... 1299
Agenerase Oral Solution (1%) ... 1304
Ammonul Injection ... 3323
Antara Capsules ... 2723
▲ Arava Tablets (1% to 3%) ... 2881
Avelox (0.1% to less than 2%) ... 2984
Caduet Tablets (Greater than 0.1% to less than or equal to 1%) ... 2507
▲ Campath Ampules (3% to 40%) ... 826
Campral Tablets (Infrequent) ... 1175
Capastat Sulfate for Injection ... 1728
Captopril Tablets ... 2114
Catapres-TTS ... 875
Celebrex Capsules (0.1% to 1.9%) ... 3130
Cipro XR Tablets (Less than 1%) ... 3004
▲ Clarinex Syrup (3.1%) ... 3009
Cleocin Vaginal Ovules ... 2613
Clindesse Vaginal Cream (Rare) ... 3296
Copaxone for Injection (Infrequent) ... 3292
Coreg Tablets (Greater than 0.1% to 1%) ... 1376
Depacon Injection (1% or more) ... 412
Depakene (1% or more) ... 417
Depakote Sprinkle Capsules ... 422
▲ Depakote Tablets (1% to 5%) ... 427
Depakote ER Tablets (Greater than 1%) ... 433
Didronel Tablets ... 2693
Digitek Tablets ... 2146
▲ Doxil Injection (Less than 1% to 10%) ... 3302
Dynacin Tablets ... 1859
Effexor Tablets (Infrequent) ... 3405
Effexor XR Capsules (Infrequent) ... 3411
Epivir ... 1394
Exelon Capsules (Frequent) ... 2204
▲ Femara Tablets (4% to 5%) ... 2210
Gabitril Tablets (Infrequent) ... 998
Geodon Capsules (Infrequent) ... 2514
Hycamtin for Injection (Less than 1%) ... 1427
▲ Intron A for Injection (Less than 5%) ... 3038
Invirase (Less than 2%) ... 2776
▲ I.V. Busulfex (8%) ... 1125
Kaletra (Less than 2%) ... 474
Lamictal (Infrequent) ... 1449
Lanoxicaps Capsules (Rare) ... 1458
Lanoxin Injection (Rare) ... 1462
Lanoxin Tablets (Rare) ... 1468
Lanoxin Injection Pediatric (Rare) ... 1465
Levaquin in 5% Dextrose Injection (Less than 0.1%) ... 2453
Levaquin (Less than 0.1%) ... 2453
Lofibra Capsules ... 1217
Lunesta Tablets (Rare) ... 3139
▲ Mobic Oral Suspension (0.3% to 3%) ... 893
▲ Mobic Tablets (0.3% to 3%) ... 893
Neurontin Capsules (Rare) ... 2498
Neurontin Oral Solution (Rare) ... 2498
Neurontin Tablets (Rare) ... 2498
Nexium Delayed-Release Capsules (Less than 1%) ... 645
Nexium I.V. (Less than 1%) ... 649
Norvasc Tablets (More than 0.1% to 1%) ... 2529
Norvir (Less than 2%) ... 499
Omnicef for Oral Suspension (0.2%) ... 506
▲ Ontak Vials (34%) ... 1717
Paxil CR Controlled-Release Tablets (Rare) ... 1509
Paxil (Rare) ... 1501
Plavix Tablets (Less than 1%) ... 940
Plavix Tablets (Less than 1%) ... 2942
Prevacid Delayed-Release Capsules (Less than 1%) ... 3268
Prevacid for Delayed-Release Oral Suspension (Less than 1%) ... 3268
Prevacid NapraPAC (Less than 1%) ... 3277
Prevacid SoluTab Delayed-Release Orally Disintegrating Tablets (Less than 1%) ... 3268
PREVPAC (Less than 1%) ... 3281
Protonix I.V. (Less than 1%) ... 3468
Protonix Tablets (Less than 1%) ... 3465
Protopic Ointment (2% to 4%) ... 629
Prozac Pulvules and Liquid (Infrequent) ... 1771
Raptiva for Injection ... 1247
▲ Rebif Prefilled Syringe for Injection (4% to 5%) ... 3163
Relpax Tablets (Rare) ... 2531
Requip Tablets (Infrequent) ... 1528
▲ Rescriptor Tablets (4.5% to 6.6%) ... 2535
Seroquel Tablets (Infrequent) ... 691
Sonata Capsules (Infrequent) ... 1686
Sular Tablets (Less than or equal to 1%) ... 1163
▲ Sustiva Capsules (16.7% to 24.5%) ... 957
Symbyax Capsules (Rare) ... 1788
Synercid I.V. (Less than 1%) ... 1690
Targretin Capsules ... 1719
Tequin Injection (Less than 0.1%) ... 964
Tequin Tablets (Less than 0.1%) ... 964
Teveten Tablets (Less than 1%) ... 1707
Teveten HCT Tablets (Less than 1%) ... 1710
▲ Thalomid Capsules (4.2%) ... 979
Ticlid Tablets ... 2813
Tricor Tablets ... 523
Trileptal Oral Suspension (1.3%) ... 2281
Trileptal Tablets (1.3%) ... 2281
Trizivir Tablets ... 1565
▲ Truvada Tablets (Greater than 5%) ... 1279
Uniretic Tablets (Less than 1%) ... 3114
Vantin Tablets and Oral Suspension (Less than 1%) ... 2650
VFEND I.V. (0.5% to 1.5%) ... 2543
VFEND Oral Suspension (0.5% to 1.5%) ... 2543
VFEND Tablets (0.5% to 1.5%) ... 2543
Viracept (Less than 2%) ... 2556
Wellbutrin SR Sustained-Release Tablets (Rare) ... 1583
Wellbutrin XL Extended-Release Tablets (Rare) ... 1588
Ziagen ... 1600
Zoloft (Infrequent) ... 2581
Zonegran Capsules (Infrequent) ... 1089
▲ Zosyn (4.2%) ... 3492
Zyban Sustained-Release Tablets (Rare) ... 1620
Zyprexa Tablets (Rare) ... 1798
Zyprexa ZYDIS Orally Disintegrating Tablets (Rare) ... 1798
Zyrtec Chewable Tablets (Less than 2%) ... 2589
Zyrtec (Less than 2%) ... 2589
Zyrtec-D 12 Hour Extended Release Tablets (Less than 2%) ... 2591

Rash, morbilliform
▲ Cleocin Vaginal Ovules (Among most frequent) ... 2613
▲ Phenytek Capsules (Among most common) ... 2153

Rash, oral
▲ Advair Diskus 100/50 (1% to 3%) ... 1291
▲ Advair Diskus 250/50 (1% to 3%) ... 1291
▲ Advair Diskus 500/50 (1% to 3%) ... 1291

Rash, papular
Aclovate Cream (Approximately 2%) ... 1290
▲ Chemet Capsules (2.6% to 11.2%) ... 2480
Migranal Nasal Spray (Rare) ... 3350
▲ Stromectol Tablets (22.7%) ... 2053

Rash, papular, neck
Alferon N Injection (1%) ... 1640

Rash, pemphigoid
Nadolol Tablets ... 2121
Stalevo Tablets ... 2270

Rash, penile
Caverject Impulse Injection (1%) ... 2610

Rash, perianal
Mintezol ... 2002

Rash, petechial
Adalat CC Tablets (Less than 1%) ... 2978
Effexor XR Capsules (Rare) ... 3411
Lyrica Capsules (Rare) ... 2524
▲ Ontak Vials (34%) ... 1717
Prozac Pulvules and Liquid (Rare) ... 1771

Rash, pruritic
Amerge Tablets (Rare) ... 1312
▲ Captopril Tablets (About 4 to 7 of 100 patients) ... 2114
Carbatrol Capsules ... 3174
Clindesse Vaginal Cream (Less than 1%) ... 3296
Cymbalta Delayed-Release Capsules (Infrequent) ... 1729
Equetro Extended-Release Capsules ... 3178
Premphase Tablets ... 3452
Prempro Tablets ... 3452
Skelaxin Tablets ... 1685
Spectazole Cream (One case) ... 2390
Tegretol/Tegretol-XR ... 2278

Rash, psoriaform
Coreg Tablets (Less than or equal to 0.1% to 1%) ... 1376

Cosopt Sterile Ophthalmic Solution 1910
Exelon Capsules (Frequent) 2204
▲ Femara Tablets (4% to 5%) 2210
Inderal LA Long-Acting Capsules (Rare) 3421
InnoPran XL Capsules (Rare) 2728
Lamisil Tablets 2226
Requip Tablets (Infrequent) 1528
▲ Soriatane Capsules (1% to 10%) 1028
Tenormin I.V. Injection 698
Tenormin Tablets 695
Timoptic in Ocudose 2061
Timoptic Sterile Ophthalmic Solution 2058
Timoptic-XE Sterile Ophthalmic Gel Forming Solution 2062

Rash, purpuric
Avelox (0.1% to less than 2%) 2984
Campath Ampules 826
Lyrica Capsules (Rare) 2524
Phenytek Capsules 2153
Prozac Pulvules and Liquid (Rare) 1771
Uniretic Tablets (Less than 1%) 3114

Rash, pustular
Avelox (0.1% to less than 2%) 2984
Copaxone for Injection (Frequent) 3292
Doxil Injection (Less than 1%) 3302
Effexor Tablets (Rare) 3405
Effexor XR Capsules (Rare) 3411
Lamictal (Rare) 1449
Lyrica Capsules (Rare) 2524
▲ Protopic Ointment (3% to 8%) 629
Prozac Pulvules and Liquid (Rare) 1771
Pulmicort Respules (1% to 3%) 654
Sonata Capsules (Rare) 1686
▲ Stromectol Tablets (22.7%) 2053
Sular Tablets (Less than or equal to 1%) 1163
Targretin Capsules 1719
▲ Truvada Tablets (Greater than 5%) 1279
Zoloft (Rare) 2581
Zonegran Capsules (Infrequent) 1089
Zyprexa Tablets (Rare) 1798
Zyprexa ZYDIS Orally Disintegrating Tablets (Rare) 1798

Rash, scarlatiniform
Phenytek Capsules 2153

Rash, unspecified
▲ Cataflam Tablets (1% to 10%) 2173
Chromagen Forte Soft Gelatin Capsules 3296
Dilaudid 439
Dilaudid Non-Sterile Powder 439
Dilaudid Rectal Suppositories 439
Dilaudid Tablets 439
▲ Emtriva Capsules (17% to 30%) 1272
▲ Oxytrol Transdermal System (Greater than 1%) 3383
Uroxatral Tablets 2957
Viramune Oral Suspension (2%) 903
Viramune Tablets (2%) 903
▲ Voltaren Tablets (1% to 10%) 2298
▲ Voltaren-XR Tablets (1% to 10%) 2301

Rash, urticarial
Captopril Tablets (Rare) 2114
▲ Ontak Vials (34%) 1717
Prevnar for Injection (0.4% to 1.4%) 3460
ProNutra Protein Supplement 1643
▲ Stromectol Tablets (22.7%) 2053
Ticlid Tablets 2813
Trizivir Tablets 1565
Ziagen 1600
▲ Zosyn (4.2%) 3492

Rash, varicella-like
▲ Varivax (0.9% to 5.5%) 2070

Rash, vasculitic
Accolate Tablets (Rare) 663
Flovent Diskus 50 mcg 1415
Gleevec Tablets (Rare) 2221
Paxil CR Controlled-Release Tablets 1509
Paxil 1501
Singulair 2047

Rash, vesiculobullous
Abilify Tablets (Infrequent) 916
Abilify Tablets (Infrequent) 2472
Actiq (Less than 1%) 993
AmBisome for Injection (Less common) 615
Avonex 839
Campral Tablets (Infrequent) 1175
▲ CellCept Capsules (3% to less than 20%) 2751
▲ CellCept Intravenous (3% to less than 20%) 2751
▲ CellCept Oral Suspension (3% to less than 20%) 2751
▲ CellCept Tablets (3% to less than 20%) 2751
Cipro XR Tablets (Less than 1%) 3004
Cleocin Vaginal Ovules 2613
Clindesse Vaginal Cream (Rare) 3296
Copaxone for Injection (Infrequent) 3292
Crestor Tablets (Less than 1%) 672
Depakote ER Tablets (Greater than 1%) 433
▲ Doxil Injection (Less than 1% to 10%) 3302
Effexor Tablets (Rare) 3405
Effexor XR Capsules (Rare) 3411
Gabitril Tablets (Infrequent) 998
Geodon Capsules (Infrequent) 2514
Iressa Tablets (1%) 684
▲ I.V. Busulfex (10%) 1125
Lamictal (Infrequent) 1449
Lovenox Injection 2931
Lunesta Tablets (Rare) 3139
Lyrica Capsules (0.1% to 1%) 2524
▲ Megace ES Oral Suspension (1% to 3%) 2492
Neurontin Capsules (Infrequent) 2498
Neurontin Oral Solution (Infrequent) 2498
Neurontin Tablets (Infrequent) 2498
Norvir (Less than 2%) 499
▲ Ontak Vials (34%) 1717
Paxil CR Controlled-Release Tablets (Rare) 1509
Paxil (Rare) 1501
Permax Tablets (Rare) 3357
Protopic Ointment (2% to 3%) 629
Prozac Pulvules and Liquid (Infrequent) 1771
Rescriptor Tablets 2535
Reyataz Capsules (Less than 3%) 948
Sonata Capsules (Infrequent) 1686
Symbyax Capsules (Infrequent) 1788
Targretin Capsules 1719
Tequin Injection (Less than 0.1%) 964
Tequin Tablets (Less than 0.1%) 964
Thalomid Capsules 979
▲ Truvada Tablets (Greater than 5%) 1279
Vantin Tablets and Oral Suspension (Less than 1%) 2650
Zithromax for Oral Suspension, 300 mg, 600 mg, 900 mg, 1200 mg (1% or less) 2561
Zithromax Tablets, 250 mg, 500 mg (1% or less) 2561
Zithromax Tri-Pak (1% or less) 2561
Zonegran Capsules (Infrequent) 1089
Zyprexa Tablets (2%) 1798
Zyprexa ZYDIS Orally Disintegrating Tablets (2%) 1798

Rash vesicular bullae
Solage Topical Solution (2.1%) 740

Rash, macular
Amerge Tablets (Rare) 1312
R-Gene 10 for Intravenous Use (One patient) 2647

Raynaud's phenomenon
Blocadren Tablets 1891
Captopril Tablets (2 to 3 of 1000 patients) 2114
Catapres Tablets (Rare) 874
Catapres-TTS (0.5% or less) 875
Clorpres Tablets (Rare) 2139
Cosopt Sterile Ophthalmic Solution 1910
Imitrex Injection (Rare) 1431
Imitrex Nasal Spray 1435
Imitrex Tablets 1440
Inderal LA Long-Acting Capsules 3421
Nadolol Tablets (2 of 100 patients) 2121
Roferon-A Injection (Infrequent) 2805
Sandostatin Injection (Less than 1%) 2263
Sandostatin LAR Depot (Rare) 2264
Tenormin I.V. Injection 698
Tenormin Tablets 695
Thalomid Capsules 979
Timolide Tablets 2056
Timoptic in Ocudose 2061
Timoptic Sterile Ophthalmic Solution 2058
Timoptic-XE Sterile Ophthalmic Gel Forming Solution 2062
Toprol-XL Tablets (About 1 of 100 patients) 660
Vaseretic Tablets 2073
Vasotec I.V. Injection (0.5% to 1.0%) 2076

Reaction, aggravated
Zomig Nasal Spray (0% to 2%) 718

Reaction, local
▲ Tygacil for Injection (9%) 3489

Reaction, paranoid
Abilify Tablets (Frequent) 916
Abilify Tablets (Frequent) 2472
Campral Tablets (Rare) 1175
Lyrica Capsules (Rare) 2524
Mirapex Tablets (2%) 889
Namenda (Infrequent) 1199
Risperdal Consta Long-Acting Injection (Frequent) 1664
Wellbutrin SR Sustained-Release Tablets 1583
Wellbutrin XL Extended-Release Tablets 1588

Reaction, schizophrenic
Abilify Tablets (Frequent) 916
Abilify Tablets (Frequent) 2472
Lyrica Capsules (Rare) 2524

Reaction at injection site
▲ Aldurazyme for Intravenous Infusion (4%) 1261
▲ Amevive (2% to 16%) 836
▲ Ammonul Injection (3%) 3323
▲ Apidra Injection (10.3%) 2876
▲ Apokyn Injection (5% to 26%) 2132
Avelox (0.1% to less than 2%) 2984
▲ BeneFix for Injection (1.6% to 7.7%) 3402
▲ Betaseron for SC Injection (86%) 791
▲ Bravelle for Intramuscular or Subcutaneous Injection (4%) 1140
Cipro I.V. (Greater than 1%) 2998
Cipro I.V. Pharmacy Bulk Package (Greater than 1%) 3509
▲ Copegus Tablets (23%) 2759
▲ Cubicin for Injection (5.8%) 1038
▲ depo-subQ provera 104 Injectable Suspension (5%) 2622
▲ Eloxatin for Injection (3% to 11%) 2908
▲ Enbrel for Injection (7% to 37%) 580
▲ Ferrlecit Injection (33.3%) 3379
▲ Follistim AQ Cartridge (5% to 10%) 2354
▲ Fuzeon Injection (98%) 2772
▲ Gamunex Immune Globulin I.V., 10% (5%) 3232
Gemzar for Injection (Rare) 1743
▲ Gonal-f RFF Pen for Injection (4.2%) 3155
HibTITER 3419
Humira Injection (8% to 20%) 464
Infanrix Vaccine 1444
▲ Kineret Injection (71%) 594
Levaquin in 5% Dextrose Injection (0.2%) 2453
Levaquin (0.2%) 2453
▲ Maxipime for Injection (3%) 1093
▲ Menopur for Subcutaneous Injection (9.6% to 11.8%) 1145
Merrem I.V. (0.9%) 687
Mivacron Injection (Less than 1%) 489
Narcan Injection 1109
Natrecor for Injection (Greater than or equal to 1%) 3123
Norditropin Cartridges 2318
Novolin 70/30 InnoLet 2322
Novolin N InnoLet 2322
Novolin R InnoLet 2322
▲ NovoLog Mix 70/30 (7%) 2331
Orthovisc Injection (0.2%) 3518
Pediarix Vaccine 1518
▲ Pegasys (22%) 2793
▲ PEG-Intron Powder for Injection (47%) 3062
Prevacid I.V. for Injection (1%) 3274
Rabies Vaccine RabAvert (Common) 1011
▲ Rebif Prefilled Syringe for Injection (89% to 92%) 3163
▲ Ribavirin, USP Capsules (5% to 58%) 3083
Risperdal Consta Long-Acting Injection (Infrequent) 1664
▲ Somavert Injection (4% to 11%) 2648
▲ Synercid I.V. (13.4%) 1690
▲ Taxotere Injection Concentrate (3% to 4.4%) 2947
▲ Tev-Tropin for Injection (8 out of 164 patients) 1224
Tygacil for Injection (0% to less than 2%) 3489
Vaqta 2067
▲ Xolair (12% to 45%) 1259
Zemaira (0.2% to 0.4%) 3506
▲ Zyvox (0% to 3.3%) 2661

Reactions, allergic contact
Penlac Nail Lacquer, Topical Solution, 8% (Four subjects) 1051

Reactions, infusion site
▲ Gammagard Liquid (0.97% to 13.1%) 751

Reactions, local, unspecified
Boostrix 1366

Reactive airway disease
▲ Flumist Vaccine (1.4% to 3.1%) 1872

Rectal bleeding
Abilify Tablets (Infrequent) 916
Abilify Tablets (Infrequent) 2472
Accutane Capsules 2740
Aciphex Tablets 1081
Actiq (1% or greater) 993
Aggrenox Capsules (1.6%) 855
Ambien Tablets (Rare) 2867
Anaprox Tablets (Less than 1%) 2769
Anaprox DS Tablets (Less than 1%) 2769
Arthrotec Tablets (Rare) 3126
Asacol Delayed-Release Tablets (2% or greater) 2688
Buphenyl Powder (One patient) 3327
Buphenyl Tablets (One patient) 3327
▲ Casodex Tablets (2% to 5%) 670
Cataflam Tablets (Occasionally) 2173
Celexa (Rare) 1177
Clozapine Tablets (Less than 1%) 2141
Clozaril Tablets (Less than 1%) 2174
Colace Capsules 50 mg 2715
Colace Capsules 100 mg 2715
Colace Glycerin Suppositories, USP 1.2 grams - Infants and Children 2715
Colace Glycerin Suppositories, USP 2.1 grams - Adults and Children 2716
Colace Liquid 1% Solution 2716
Colace Syrup 729
Colazal Capsules (2%) 2845
Copaxone for Injection (Infrequent) 3292
Depo-Provera Contraceptive Injection (Less than 1%) 2619
▲ Doxil Injection (1% to 10%) 3302
EC-Naprosyn Delayed-Release Tablets (Less than 1%) 2769
Effexor Tablets (Infrequent) 3405
Effexor XR Capsules (Infrequent) 3411
Eldepryl Capsules 3209
▲ Elmiron Capsules (6.3% to 15%) 2393
▲ Eloxatin for Injection (2% to 5%) 2908
▲ Eulexin Capsules (14%) 3023
Evoxac Capsules (Less than 1%) 1042
Exelon Capsules (Infrequent) 2204
FazaClo Orally Disintegrating Tablets (Less than 1%) 547
▲ Flolan for Injection (11%) 1408
Gabitril Tablets (Infrequent) 998
Gengraf Capsules (1%) 458
Geodon (Infrequent) 2514
Imitrex Nasal Spray 1435
Indocin Capsules (Less than 1%) 1968
Indocin I.V. (Less than 1%) 1973
Indocin (Less than 1%) 1968
▲ Intron A for Injection (Less than 5%) 3038
Invirase (Less than 2%) 2776
Lipitor Tablets (Less than 2%) 2495
Lofibra Capsules 1217
Lunesta Tablets (Rare) 3139
Mineral Oil 2716
Naprosyn Suspension (Less than 1%) 2769
Naprosyn Tablets (Less than 1%) 2769
Neoral Soft Gelatin Capsules (1%) 2247
Neoral Oral Solution (1%) 2247
Neurontin Capsules (Rare) 2498
Neurontin Oral Solution (Rare) 2498
Neurontin Tablets (Rare) 2498
Paxil CR Controlled-Release Tablets (Infrequent) 1509
Paxil (Infrequent) 1501
Pentasa Capsules (Less than 1%) 3182
Peri-Colace Tablets 2716
Pletal Tablets (Less than 2%) 2478
Prevacid Delayed-Release Capsules (Less than 1%) 3268
Prevacid for Delayed-Release Oral Suspension (Less than 1%) 3268
Prevacid SoluTab Delayed-Release Orally Disintegrating Tablets (Less than 1%) 3268
PREVPAC (Less than 1%) 3281
Prometrium Capsules (100 mg, 200 mg) (Less than 5%) 3205
Protonix I.V. (Greater than or equal to 1%) 3468
Protonix Tablets (Less than 1%) 3465
Razadyne ER Extended-Release Capsules (Infrequent) 2434
Razadyne (Infrequent) 2434
▲ Refludan for Injection (5.3%) 815

Relafen Tablets (Less than 1%) 1523
Requip Tablets (Infrequent) 1528
Retrovir Capsules 1533
Retrovir IV Infusion 1537
Retrovir 1533
Rythmol SR Capsules 2736
Sandostatin LAR Depot (1% to 4%) 2264
Seroquel Tablets (Infrequent) 691
Sonata Capsules (Infrequent) 1686
Tequin Injection (Less than 0.1%) 964
Tequin Tablets (Less than 0.1%) 964
Tricor Tablets 523
Triglide Tablets 1165
Trileptal Oral Suspension (Up to 2%) 2281
Trileptal Tablets (Up to 2%) 2281
Uniretic Tablets (Less than 1%) 3114
Vantin Tablets and Oral Suspension 2650
VFEND I.V. (Less than 2%) 2543
VFEND Oral Suspension (Less than 2%) 2543
VFEND Tablets (Less than 2%) 2543
Viagra Tablets (Less than 2%) 2552
Voltaren Tablets (Occasionally) 2298
Voltaren-XR Tablets (Occasionally) 2301
Xeloda Tablets 2825
Zelnorm Tablets 2303
▲ Zoladex (14%) 709
▲ Zoladex 3-month (14%) 712
Zoloft (Rare) 2581
Zonegran Capsules (Infrequent) 1089
Zyprexa Tablets (Infrequent) 1798
Zyprexa ZYDIS Orally Disintegrating Tablets (Infrequent) 1798
Zyrtec Chewable Tablets (Less than 2%) 2589
Zyrtec (Less than 2%) 2589
Zyrtec-D 12 Hour Extended Release Tablets (Less than 2%) 2591

Rectal burning
Colace Glycerin Suppositories, USP 1.2 grams - Infants and Children 2715
Colace Glycerin Suppositories, USP 2.1 grams - Adults and Children 2716

Rectal discomfort
Colace Glycerin Suppositories, USP 1.2 grams - Infants and Children 2715
Colace Glycerin Suppositories, USP 2.1 grams - Adults and Children 2716
Fleet Glycerin Laxatives 1168
▲ I.V. Busulfex (24%) 1125
▲ Xenical Capsules (3.3% to 5.2%) 2834

Rectal disorders, unspecified
Actiq (1% or greater) 993
Actonel Tablets (2.2%) 2679
Actonel with Calcium Tablets (2.2%) 2684
Antara Capsules 2723
Asacol Delayed-Release Tablets (2% or greater) 2688
Avinza Capsules (Less than 5%) 1714
▲ CellCept Capsules (3% to less than 20%) 2751
▲ CellCept Intravenous (3% to less than 20%) 2751
▲ CellCept Oral Suspension (3% to less than 20%) 2751
▲ CellCept Tablets (3% to less than 20%) 2751
▲ Entocort EC Capsules (Less than 5%) 2694
Evoxac Capsules (Less than 1%) 1042
Ferrlecit Injection 3379
▲ I.V. Busulfex (25%) 1125
Lofibra Capsules 1217
Meridia Capsules (1.2%) 485
Neurontin Capsules (Rare) 2498
Neurontin Oral Solution (Rare) 2498
Neurontin Tablets (Rare) 2498
Nexium Delayed-Release Capsules (Less than 1%) 645
Nexium I.V. (Less than 1%) 649
Norvir (Less than 2%) 499
Prevacid Delayed-Release Capsules (Less than 1%) 3268
Prevacid for Delayed-Release Oral Suspension (Less than 1%) 3268
Prevacid NapraPAC (Less than 1%) 3277
Prevacid SoluTab Delayed-Release Orally Disintegrating Tablets (Less than 1%) 3268
PREVPAC (Less than 1%) 3281
▲ Prograf Capsules and Injection (3% to 15%) 624
Protonix I.V. (Greater than or equal to 1%) 3468
Protonix Tablets (Greater than or equal to 1%) 3465
Rapamune Oral Solution and Tablets 3472
Relpax Tablets (Rare) 2531
Rescriptor Tablets 2535
Tasmar Tablets (Infrequent) 3360
Tricor Tablets 523
Triglide Tablets 1165
Vantin Tablets and Oral Suspension (Less than 1%) 2650
VFEND I.V. (Less than 2%) 2543
VFEND Oral Suspension (Less than 2%) 2543
VFEND Tablets (Less than 2%) 2543
Wellbutrin Tablets (Rare) 1579

Rectal urgency
(*see under* Defecate, desire to)

Red blood cell, aplasia
Rituxan for Infusion (One case) 845

Red blood cell count, decrease
Aldara Cream, 5% 1814
Neumega for Injection 3433
▲ Norvir (18.6%) 499
Rythmol SR Capsules 2736

Red blood cells excretion, increase
Invanz for Injection (1.1% to 2.5%) 1974

"Red man" syndrome
Vancocin HCl Capsules, USP 3370

Redness, local
▲ Menactra Vaccine (0.6% to 14.4%) 2968
Striant Mucoadhesive 1022

Redness, nasal
▲ Fortical Nasal Spray (10.6%) 3336

Redness at injection site
▲ Boostrix (1.7% to 22.5%) 1366
Symlin Injection 608

Reflexes, abnormal
Frova Tablets (Rare) 1101
Neurontin Capsules (Frequent) 2498
Neurontin Oral Solution (Frequent) 2498
Neurontin Tablets (Frequent) 2498

Reflexes, increased
(*see under* Hyperreflexia)

Refraction disorder, unspecified
Antara Capsules 2723
Caduet Tablets (Less than 2%) 2507
Lofibra Capsules 1217
Tricor Tablets 523

Regurgitation
Altoprev Extended-Release Tablets (0.5% to 1%) 1151
Amerge Tablets (Rare) 1312
Invanz for Injection (1.1% to 1.6%) 1974
Lotronex Tablets (2%) 1479
Maxalt Tablets (Infrequent) 1983
Maxalt-MLT Orally Disintegrating Tablets (Infrequent) 1983
Mevacor Tablets (0.5% to 1.0%) 1996
Plendil Extended-Release Tablets (0.5% to 1.5%) 651
Zyban Sustained-Release Tablets (Infrequent) 1620

Renal agenesis, unilateral, neonatal
Leukeran Tablets 1472

Renal calculi
(*see under* Nephrolithiasis)

Renal colic
Crixivan Capsules (Less than 2%) 1918
Daranide Tablets 1928
Noroxin Tablets (Less frequent) 2009
Timolide Tablets (Less than 1%) 2056

Renal disease
Anaprox Tablets (Less than 1%) 2769
Anaprox DS Tablets (Less than 1%) 2769
EC-Naprosyn Delayed-Release Tablets (Less than 1%) 2769
Naprosyn Suspension (Less than 1%) 2769
Naprosyn Tablets (Less than 1%) 2769
Prevacid NapraPAC (Less than 1%) 3277

Renal disorders, unspecified
▲ Ammonul Injection (4%) 3323

Renal dysfunction
(*see under* Renal impairment)

Renal failure
▲ Abelcet Injection (5%) 1119
Abilify Tablets (Infrequent) 916
Abilify Tablets (Infrequent) 2472
Actiq (1% or greater) 993
Aggrenox Capsules (Less than 1%) 855
Agrylin Capsules (6 of 551 patients) 3172
Aldoclor Tablets 1881
Aldoril Tablets 1884
Alimta for Injection (Up to 2%) 1722
Aloprim for Injection (1.2%) 2156
AmBisome for Injection (Less common) 615
Ammonul Injection 3323
Anaprox Tablets (Less than 1%) 2769
Anaprox DS Tablets (Less than 1%) 2769
Ancef for Injection 1318
Angiomax for Injection (Rare) 1856
Aricept Tablets (Infrequent) 1086
Aricept ODT Tablets (Infrequent) 1086
Arthrotec Tablets (Rare) 3126
Atacand Tablets 634
Atacand HCT (Very rare) 637
Avalide Tablets 922
Avalide Tablets 2889
Bayer Aspirin Tablets 3515
Benicar Tablets 2850
Benicar HCT Tablets (Rare) 2852
Cafcit (2.2%) 1854
Captopril Tablets (Approximately 1 to 2 of 1000 patients) 2114
Carbatrol Capsules 3174
▲ Carnitor Injection (6%) 3185
Cataflam Tablets (Occasionally) 2173
▲ CellCept Capsules (3% to less than 20%) 2751
▲ CellCept Intravenous (3% to less than 20%) 2751
▲ CellCept Oral Suspension (3% to less than 20%) 2751
▲ CellCept Tablets (3% to less than 20%) 2751
Cipro I.V. (1% or less) 2998
Cipro I.V. Pharmacy Bulk Package (1% or less) 3509
Cipro (Less than 1%) 2991
Cipro XR Tablets 3004
Clinoril Tablets (Less than 1 in 100) 1899
Crestor Tablets (Less than 1%) 672
Cubicin for Injection (2.2%) 1038
Cytovene (At least 3 subjects) 2763
Diovan HCT Tablets 2195
Diprivan Injectable Emulsion (Less than 1%) 676
Diuril Oral 1936
Diuril Sodium Intravenous 1934
Dolobid Tablets (Less than 1 in 100) 1937
Dyrenium Capsules (One case) 3390
EC-Naprosyn Delayed-Release Tablets (Less than 1%) 2769
Ecotrin Enteric Coated Aspirin Low, Regular and Maximum Strength Tablets 1627
Effexor Tablets 3405
Effexor XR Capsules 3411
Elitek (Less than or equal to 1%) 2906
Equetro Extended-Release Capsules 3178
Erbitux (2%) 937
Ethyol for Injection 1869
Fleet Prep Kits 1172
Fuzeon Injection 2772
Gabitril Tablets (Infrequent) 998
Gemzar for Injection (Rare) 1743
Gleevec Tablets (Infrequent) 2221
Hepsera Tablets (2% or greater) 1275
Herceptin I.V. (At least one of the 958 patients) 1234
Hyzaar 1964
Indocin (Less than 1%) 1968
Iveegam EN (0.3% to 0.8%) 759
Lamictal (Rare) 1449
Merrem I.V. (Greater than 0.1% to 1%) 687
Micardis HCT Tablets 886
Mobic Oral Suspension (Less than 2%) 893
Mobic Tablets (Less than 2%) 893
Moduretic Tablets (Less than or equal to 1%) 2003
Mylotarg for Injection 3429
Nalfon Capsules (Less than 1%) 2504
Namenda 1199
Naprosyn Suspension (Less than 1%) 2769
Naprosyn Tablets (Less than 1%) 2769
Nipent for Injection (Less than 3%) 3216
Noroxin Tablets 2009
Norvir (Less than 2%) 499
Oncaspar 1123
Orthoclone OKT3 Sterile Solution 2370
PEG-Intron Powder for Injection 3062
Permax Tablets (Infrequent) 3357
Prevacid NapraPAC (Less than 1%) 3277
Prinzide Tablets 2033
▲ Prograf Capsules and Injection (3% to 15%) 624
Prozac Pulvules and Liquid 1771
Relafen Tablets (Less than 1%) 1523
Remicade for IV Injection (Greater than or equal to 0.2%) 987
Reyataz Capsules (Less than 3%) 948
Rythmol SR Capsules 2736
Sandostatin LAR Depot (Rare) 2264
St. Joseph 81 mg Aspirin Chewable and Enteric Coated Tablets 1841
Tegretol/Tegretol-XR 2278
Tenormin I.V. Injection (0.4%) 698
Tenormin Tablets (0.4%) 695
Teveten HCT Tablets 1710
Ticlid Tablets (Rare) 2813
Timolide Tablets 2056
Trasylol Injection (1% to 2%) 779
▲ Trisenox Injection (8%) 983
Trizivir Tablets 1565
Truvada Tablets 1279
Valtrex Caplets 1573
Vancocin HCl Capsules, USP (Rare) 3370
Vaseretic Tablets 2073
Vasotec I.V. Injection (0.5% to 1.0%) 2076
Ventavis Inhalation Solution 1036
Viread Tablets 1284
Voltaren Tablets (Occasionally) 2298
Voltaren-XR Tablets (Occasionally) 2301
▲ Xeloda Tablets (Less than 5%) 2825
Zestoretic Tablets 701
Ziagen 1600
Zosyn 3492
Zovirax Capsules 1616
Zovirax for Injection 1618
Zovirax 1616

Renal failure, acute
Abelcet Injection 1119
Aceon Tablets (2 mg, 4 mg, 8 mg) 3191
Activase I.V. 1225
Albenza Tablets 1310
Altace Capsules (Less than 1%) 1673
Ambien Tablets (Rare) 2867
AmBisome for Injection (Less common) 615
Anzemet Injection (Rare) 2871
Anzemet Tablets (Rare) 2874
Campath Ampules 826
Camptosar Injection (Rare) 2602
Carimune NF 3501
Celebrex Capsules (Less than 0.1%) 3130
Celexa 1177
▲ CellCept Capsules (3% to less than 20%) 2751
▲ CellCept Intravenous (3% to less than 20%) 2751
▲ CellCept Oral Suspension (3% to less than 20%) 2751
▲ CellCept Tablets (3% to less than 20%) 2751
Crixivan Capsules 1918
CytoGam Intravenous 1866
Dyazide Capsules 1389
Dynacin Tablets (Rarely reported) 1859
Dyrenium Capsules 3390
Elspar for Injection 1943
Exelon Capsules (Infrequent) 2204
Gammagard S/D 754
Imitrex Injection 1431
Imitrex Nasal Spray 1435
Imitrex Tablets 1440
Indocin I.V. (Less than 1%) 1973
Lamictal (Rare) 1449
Levaquin in 5% Dextrose Injection (0.1% to 0.9%) 2453
Levaquin (0.1% to 0.9%) 2453
Lexapro Oral Solution 1193
Lexapro Tablets 1193
Lipitor Tablets (Rare) 2495
Lotrel Capsules (Rare) 2238
Maxzide 2150
Mefoxin for Injection (Rare) 1987
Mefoxin Premixed Intravenous Solution (Rare) 1990
Mevacor Tablets 1996
Mycamine for Injection 620
Neurontin Capsules (Rare) 2498
Neurontin Oral Solution (Rare) 2498
Neurontin Tablets (Rare) 2498

Omnicef Capsules 506
Omnicef for Oral Suspension 506
Orap Tablets 1220
Paxil CR Controlled-Release Tablets 1509
Paxil 1501
Plavix Tablets (1% to 2.5%) 940
Plavix Tablets (1% to 2.5%) 2942
Pravachol Tablets (Rare) 943
Primaxin I.M. 2022
Primaxin I.V. (Less than 0.2%) 2024
Prinivil Tablets (0.3% to 1.3%) 2029
Prinzide Tablets 2033
Prograf Capsules and Injection 624
Proleukin for Injection (Less than 1%) 1007
Requip Tablets (Rare) 1528
Rescriptor Tablets 2535
Risperdal M-Tab Orally Disintegrating Tablets 1658
Risperdal 1658
Rituxan for Infusion 845
Rituxan I.V. 1251
Roferon-A Injection 2805
Seroquel Tablets (Rare) 691
Suprax 1811
Thalomid Capsules 979
Trasylol Injection (1% to 2%) 779
Vaseretic Tablets (Rare) 2073
Vasotec I.V. Injection (Rare) 2076
▲ Vesanoid Capsules (3%) 2823
VFEND I.V. (0% to 0.4%) 2543
VFEND Oral Suspension (0% to 0.4%) 2543
VFEND Tablets (0% to 0.4%) 2543
Zestoretic Tablets (Rare) 701
Zestril Tablets (0.3% to 1.0%) 704
Zithromax Capsules, 250 mg 2568
Zithromax for IV Infusion 2573
Zithromax for Oral Suspension, 300 mg, 600 mg, 900 mg, 1200 mg 2561
Zithromax Tablets, 250 mg, 500 mg 2561
Zithromax Tri-Pak 2561
Zmax for Oral Suspension 2577
Zocor Tablets (Rare) 2078
Zoloft 2581

Renal failure, aggravated
Vantas (Less than 2%) 3367

Renal failure, neonatal
Aceon Tablets (2 mg, 4 mg, 8 mg) 3191
Altace Capsules 1673
Captopril Tablets 2114
Cozaar Tablets 1913
Hyzaar 1964
Lotrel Capsules 2238
Prinivil Tablets 2029
Prinzide Tablets 2033
Vaseretic Tablets 2073
Vasotec I.V. Injection 2076
Zestoretic Tablets 701
Zestril Tablets 704

Renal function impairment
(*see under* Renal impairment)

Renal impairment
Abelcet Injection 1119
Agrylin Capsules (10 of 551 patients) 3172
Aldoclor Tablets 1881
Aldoril Tablets 1884
Alesse-28 Tablets 3392
Aloprim for Injection (Less than 1%) 2156
Altace Capsules (Rare) 1673
▲ Anaprox Tablets (1% to 10%) 2769
▲ Anaprox DS Tablets (1% to 10%) 2769
Aredia for Injection 2168
Argatroban Injection (2.8%) 1321
Asacol Delayed-Release Tablets 2688
Atacand Tablets 634
Atacand HCT (Very rare) 637
Avalide Tablets 922
Avalide Tablets 2889
Benicar HCT Tablets 2852
Campath Ampules 826
Camptosar Injection (Rare) 2602
Ceftin 1369
▲ CellCept Capsules (21.8% to 25.6%) 2751
▲ CellCept Intravenous (21.8% to 25.6%) 2751
▲ CellCept Oral Suspension (21.8% to 25.6%) 2751
▲ CellCept Tablets (21.8% to 25.6%) 2751
Cleocin Vaginal Ovules (Rare) 2613
Clinoril Tablets (Less than 1 in 100) 1899
Cytovene (At least 3 subjects) 2763
Desferal Vials 2190
Diovan HCT Tablets 2195
Diovan Tablets 2191
Diuril Oral 1936
Diuril Sodium Intravenous 1934
Dolobid Tablets (Less than 1 in 100) 1937
Doxil Injection (Less than 1%) 3302
▲ EC-Naprosyn Delayed-Release Tablets (1% to 10%) 2769
Effexor XR Capsules (Rare) 3411
Evoxac Capsules (Less than 1%) 1042
Fortaz 1422
Garamycin Injectable 3028
▲ Gengraf Capsules (25% to 38%) 458
Hyzaar 1964
Idamycin PFS Injection (No more than 1%) 2645
▲ Indocin I.V. (41% of infants) 1973
Lescol Capsules 2227
Lescol Capsules 2730
Lescol XL Tablets 2227
Lescol XL Tablets 2730
▲ Leukine (8%) 829
Levaquin in 5% Dextrose Injection (0.1% to 0.9%) 2453
Levaquin (0.1% to 0.9%) 2453
Lofibra Capsules 1217
Lo/Ovral-28 Tablets 3423
Maxipime for Injection 1093
Mefoxin for Injection 1987
Mefoxin Premixed Intravenous Solution 1990
Mepron Suspension 1487
Micardis HCT Tablets 886
Moduretic Tablets (Less than or equal to 1%) 2003
Mycamine for Injection 620
▲ Myfortic Tablets (3% to less than 20%) 2244
▲ Naprosyn Suspension (1% to 10%) 2769
▲ Naprosyn Tablets (1% to 10%) 2769
▲ Neoral Soft Gelatin Capsules (25% to 38%) 2247
▲ Neoral Oral Solution (25% to 38%) 2247
Nipent for Injection (Less than 3%) 3216
Omnicef Capsules 506
Omnicef for Oral Suspension 506
Oncaspar 1123
Ortho-Cept Tablets 2395
Ortho-Cyclen Tablets 2414
Ortho Evra Transdermal System 2402
Ortho Tri-Cyclen Tablets 2414
Ortho Tri-Cyclen Lo Tablets 2421
Panhematin for Injection 2487
Paxil CR Controlled-Release Tablets (Rare) 1509
Paxil (Rare) 1501
Plavix Tablets 940
Plavix Tablets 2942
Prinivil Tablets (0.3% to 1.0%) 2029
Prinzide Tablets 2033
▲ Prograf Capsules and Injection (36% to 40%) 624
Proleukin for Injection (2%) 1007
Refludan for Injection (1.8%) 815
ReoPro Vials (0.3%) 1779
Roferon-A Injection 2805
▲ Sandimmune (25% to 38%) 2259
Seasonale Tablets 1073
▲ Simulect for Injection (3% to 10%) 2268
Striant Mucoadhesive 1022
Suprax 1811
Tequin Injection 964
Tequin Tablets 964
Teveten HCT Tablets 1710
Timolide Tablets 2056
Tranxene 2488
▲ Trasylol Injection (5% to 30%) 779
Tricor Tablets 523
Triphasil-28 Tablets 3483
▲ Trisenox Injection (8%) 983
▲ Valcyte Tablets (Less than 5%) 2816
▲ Vantas (4.7%) 3367
Vantin Tablets and Oral Suspension 2650
Vaseretic Tablets 2073
Vasotec I.V. Injection (0.5% to 1.0%) 2076
VFEND I.V. (0.5%) 2543
VFEND Oral Suspension (0.5%) 2543
VFEND Tablets (0.5%) 2543
Viramune Oral Suspension 903
Viramune Tablets 903
Yasmin 28 Tablets 818
Zestoretic Tablets 701
Zestril Tablets (0.3% to 1.0%) 704

Renal infarct
BeneFix for Injection (1.5%) 3402
Vesanoid Capsules 2823

Renal injury
Capastat Sulfate for Injection 1728

Renal insufficiency
Aggrenox Capsules (Less than 1%) 855
Aloprim for Injection (1.2%) 2156
Aptivus Capsules (Less than 2%) 859
Bayer Aspirin Tablets 3515
Cancidas for Injection (0% to 0.9%) 1894
Capastat Sulfate for Injection (1 patient) 1728
Captopril Tablets (Approximately 1 to 2 of 1000 patients) 2114
▲ Cataflam Tablets (1% to 10%) 2173
▲ Coreg Tablets (Greater than 1% to 3%) 1376
Crixivan Capsules (Some cases) 1918
Ecotrin Enteric Coated Aspirin Low, Regular and Maximum Strength Tablets 1627
Elspar for Injection 1943
Emend Capsules (Greater than 0.5%) 1944
Erythrocin Stearate Filmtab Tablets (Isolated reports) 452
Fleet Prep Kits 1172
Fuzeon Injection 2772
Hepsera Tablets (2% or greater) 1275
Indocin Capsules (Less than 1%) 1968
Indocin I.V. (Less than 1%) 1973
Indocin (Less than 1%) 1968
Invanz for Injection (Greater than 0.1%) 1974
Neupogen for Injection (Two events) 598
Nipent for Injection (Less than 3%) 3216
Norvir 499
▲ Ontak Vials (Less than 5%) 1717
Orthoclone OKT3 Sterile Solution 2370
PEG-Intron Powder for Injection 3062
Proleukin for Injection 1007
Risperdal M-Tab Orally Disintegrating Tablets (Rare) 1658
Risperdal (Rare) 1658
Sandostatin LAR Depot (Rare) 2264
St. Joseph 81 mg Aspirin Chewable and Enteric Coated Tablets 1841
Taxotere Injection Concentrate 2947
Truvada Tablets 1279
Univasc Tablets (Less than 1%) 3118
▲ Vesanoid Capsules (11%) 2823
Viread Tablets 1284
▲ Voltaren Tablets (1% to 10%) 2298
▲ Voltaren-XR Tablets (1% to 10%) 2301
▲ Zenapax for Injection (2% to 5%) 2838
Zoladex (1% to 5%) 709
Zoladex 3-month 712

Renal insufficiency, reversible
Actimmune (Rare) 1646

Renal precipitation
Rocephin Injectable Vials, ADD-Vantage, Galaxy, Bulk 2801

Renal stones
Abilify Tablets (Infrequent) 916
Abilify Tablets (Infrequent) 2472
Campral Tablets (Rare) 1175
Enbrel for Injection 580
Fortical Nasal Spray (Less than 1%) 3336
▲ Topamax Sprinkle Capsules (0% to 3%) 2438
▲ Topamax Tablets (0% to 3%) 2438
Vantas (Less than 2%) 3367
▲ Zonegran Capsules (4%) 1089

Renal toxicity
(*see under* Nephrotoxicity)

Renal tubular damage
Cytovene 2763

Reproductive disorders, female
Amerge Tablets (Rare) 1312

Resistance mechanism
▲ Aldara Cream, 5% (4.2%) 1814

Resistance mechanism disorders
▲ Copegus Tablets (12%) 2759

Respiration, painful
Prinivil Tablets (0.3% to 1.0%) 2029
Prinzide Tablets 2033
Zestoretic Tablets 701
Zestril Tablets (0.3% to 1.0%) 704

Respiratory alkalosis
Aggrenox Capsules 855
AmBisome for Injection (Less common) 615
Campath Ampules 826
Coreg Tablets (Less than or equal to 0.1%) 1376
Ecotrin Enteric Coated Aspirin Low, Regular and Maximum Strength Tablets 1627
Geodon Capsules (Rare) 2514
St. Joseph 81 mg Aspirin Chewable and Enteric Coated Tablets 1841

Respiratory arrest
Actiq 993
Ammonul Injection 3323
AquaMEPHYTON Injection 1887
Campath Ampules 826
Cipro I.V. (1% or less) 2998
Cipro I.V. Pharmacy Bulk Package (1% or less) 3509
Cipro XR Tablets 3004
Clozapine Tablets (Rare) 2141
Clozaril Tablets (Rare) 2174
Dilaudid Oral Liquid 443
Dilaudid Tablets - 8 mg 443
Dilaudid-HP 441
Infed Injection 3381
Kadian Capsules 572
Lidoderm Patch 1107
MS Contin Tablets 2703
Naropin Injection 640
Nubain Injection (1% or less) 1111
Orthoclone OKT3 Sterile Solution 2370
OxyContin Tablets 2699
Proleukin for Injection (Less than 1%) 1007

Respiratory congestion, unspecified
Comvax (0.3% to 1.2%) 1904
Cozaar Tablets (Less than 1%) 1913
▲ Epogen for Injection (15%) 586
Hyzaar 1964
Maxalt Tablets (Infrequent) 1983
Maxalt-MLT Orally Disintegrating Tablets (Infrequent) 1983
▲ Procrit for Injection (15%) 2374
Vaqta (1.6%) 2067

Respiratory depression
Actiq 993
Anaprox Tablets (Less than 1%) 2769
Anaprox DS Tablets (Less than 1%) 2769
Arthrotec Tablets (Rare) 3126
Campath Ampules 826
Cataflam Tablets (Rarely) 2173
Dantrium Capsules (Less frequent) 2690
▲ DepoDur Extended-Release Injection (2% to 5%) 1098
Dilaudid 439
Dilaudid Oral Liquid 443
Dilaudid Non-Sterile Powder 439
Dilaudid Rectal Suppositories 439
Dilaudid Tablets 439
Dilaudid Tablets - 8 mg 443
Dilaudid-HP 441
EC-Naprosyn Delayed-Release Tablets (Less than 1%) 2769
Garamycin Injectable 3028
Hycodan 1104
Hycomine Compound Tablets 1105
Hycotuss Expectorant Syrup 1106
Kadian Capsules 572
Klonopin 2782
Levaquin in 5% Dextrose Injection (0.1% to 0.9%) 2453
Levaquin (0.1% to 0.9%) 2453
Lidoderm Patch 1107
Lortab 3315
Lortab Elixir 3312
MS Contin Tablets 2703
Naprosyn Suspension (Less than 1%) 2769
Naprosyn Tablets (Less than 1%) 2769
Narcan Injection 1109
Numorphan 1112
OxyContin Tablets 2699
OxyFast Oral Concentrate Solution 2704
OxyIR Capsules 2704
Percocet Tablets 1114
Phenergan 3438
ProSom Tablets 512
Tussionex Pennkinetic Extended-Release Suspension 3322
Tylenol with Codeine 2461
Vicodin Tablets 530
Vicodin ES Tablets 531
Vicodin HP Tablets 532
Vicoprofen Tablets 533
Voltaren Tablets (Rarely) 2298
Voltaren-XR Tablets (Rarely) 2301
Zydone Tablets 1118

Respiratory desaturation
Curosurf Intratracheal Suspension ... 1057

Respiratory difficulty
▲ Abelcet Injection (4%) ... 1119
▲ Acthrel for Injection (6%) ... 3528
Allegra-D 12 Hour Extended-Release Tablets ... 2860
Allegra-D 24 Hour Extended-Release Tablets ... 2862
Ambien Tablets ... 2867
Balamine DM ... 739
Carafate Suspension ... 727
Carafate Tablets ... 728
Cardene I.V. (Rare) ... 1129
EpiPen ... 1061
Infed Injection ... 3381
Invirase (Less than 2%) ... 2776
Kadian Capsules (Less than 3%) ... 572
▲ Photofrin for Injection (10%) ... 729
Rilutek Tablets (More than 2%) ... 2945
Thyrogen for Injection ... 1270
▲ Trasylol Injection (3%) ... 779
▲ Vesanoid Capsules (26%) ... 2823
Zyrtec-D 12 Hour Extended Release Tablets ... 2591

Respiratory discharge, upper, unspecified
Emcyt Capsules (1%) ... 3137

Respiratory disorders, unspecified
▲ Ammonul Injection (15%) ... 3323
▲ Antara Capsules (6.2%) ... 2723
Asmanex Twisthaler (1% to less than 3%) ... 2981
▲ Bravelle for Intramuscular or Subcutaneous Injection (4% to 5.7%) ... 1140
▲ CellCept Capsules (3% to less than 20%) ... 2751
▲ CellCept Intravenous (3% to less than 20%) ... 2751
▲ CellCept Oral Suspension (3% to less than 20%) ... 2751
▲ CellCept Tablets (3% to less than 20%) ... 2751
▲ Colazal Capsules (4%) ... 2845
▲ CombiPatch Transdermal System (9% to 13%) ... 2180
▲ Enbrel for Injection (5%) ... 580
Evoxac Capsules (Less than 1%) ... 1042
▲ Flolan for Injection (7%) ... 1408
▲ Focalin XR Capsules (9% to 16%) ... 2217
Gabitril Tablets (Infrequent) ... 998
▲ Geodon Capsules (8%) ... 2514
▲ Intron A for Injection (Less than or equal to 5%) ... 3038
Levaquin in 5% Dextrose Injection (0.1% to 0.9%) ... 2453
Levaquin (0.1% to 0.9%) ... 2453
▲ Lofibra Capsules (6.2%) ... 1217
▲ Lupron Depot 7.5 mg (10.7%) ... 3261
Lupron Injection Pediatric ... 3256
▲ Menopur for Subcutaneous Injection (3.9% to 5.8%) ... 1145
Meridia Capsules ... 485
Merrem I.V. (Greater than 0.1% to 1%) ... 687
▲ Paxil CR Controlled-Release Tablets (7%) ... 1509
▲ Paxil (7%) ... 1501
Plasbumin-5 (Rare) ... 3249
Plasbumin-20 (Rare) ... 3249
Plasbumin-25 (Rare) ... 3251
Prevacid Delayed-Release Capsules (Less than 1%) ... 3268
Prevacid for Delayed-Release Oral Suspension (Less than 1%) ... 3268
Prevacid NapraPAC (Less than 1%) ... 3277
Prevacid SoluTab Delayed-Release Orally Disintegrating Tablets (Less than 1%) ... 3268
PREVPAC (Less than 1%) ... 3281
▲ Prilosec OTC Tablets (18.5% to 46.2%) ... 2674
▲ Proleukin for Injection (11%) ... 1007
▲ Proventil HFA Inhalation Aerosol (6%) ... 3071
Relpax Tablets (Infrequent) ... 2531
▲ Rituxan for Infusion (Among most frequent) ... 845
▲ Rituxan I.V. (Among most frequent) ... 1251
▲ Simulect for Injection (3% to 10%) ... 2268
▲ TOBI Solution for Inhalation (31.4%) ... 1015
Topamax Sprinkle Capsules (1%) ... 2438
Topamax Tablets (1%) ... 2438
▲ Tricor Tablets (6.2%) ... 523
▲ Triglide Tablets (6.2%) ... 1165
VFEND I.V. (Less than 2%) ... 2543
VFEND Oral Suspension (Less than 2%) ... 2543
VFEND Tablets (Less than 2%) ... 2543
Wellbutrin SR Sustained-Release Tablets (At least 1%) ... 1583
Wellbutrin XL Extended-Release Tablets (At least 1%) ... 1588
▲ Zegerid Powder for Oral Solution (18.5% to 46.2%) ... 2972
Zyrtec-D 12 Hour Extended Release Tablets (Less than 2%) ... 2591

Respiratory distress
Agrylin Capsules (1% to 5%) ... 3172
Aldoclor Tablets ... 1881
Aldoril Tablets ... 1884
Aloprim for Injection (Less than 1%) ... 2156
▲ Ammonul Injection (3%) ... 3323
Aredia for Injection (One case) ... 2168
Atacand HCT ... 637
Atrovent Inhalation Solution (1.4%) ... 868
Blocadren Tablets ... 1891
Cipro I.V. (1% or less) ... 2998
Cipro I.V. Pharmacy Bulk Package (1% or less) ... 3509
Cipro XR Tablets ... 3004
▲ Clolar for Intravenous Infusion (14%) ... 1264
Combivent Inhalation Aerosol (2.5%) ... 878
Comvax ... 1904
Cosopt Sterile Ophthalmic Solution ... 1910
Desferal Vials ... 2190
Diovan HCT Tablets ... 2195
Diuril Oral ... 1936
Diuril Sodium Intravenous ... 1934
Duragesic Transdermal System (Less than 1%) ... 2448
Dyazide Capsules ... 1389
▲ Elitek (3%) ... 2906
Elspar for Injection ... 1943
Ethyol for Injection (Rare) ... 1869
Fuzeon Injection ... 2772
Glucagon for Injection Vials and Emergency Kit ... 1749
Herceptin I.V. ... 1234
▲ Humatrope Vials and Cartridges (3.13% to 6.67%) ... 1756
Hyzaar ... 1964
Indapamide Tablets ... 2119
Inderal LA Long-Acting Capsules ... 3421
Indocin Capsules (Less than 1%) ... 1968
Indocin I.V. (Less than 1%) ... 1973
Indocin (Less than 1%) ... 1968
InnoPran XL Capsules ... 2728
Lamictal (More than 1%) ... 1449
Leukine ... 829
Levaquin in 5% Dextrose Injection ... 2453
Levaquin ... 2453
Lotensin HCT Tablets ... 2235
Maxzide ... 2150
Micardis HCT Tablets ... 886
Moduretic Tablets ... 2003
Nadolol Tablets ... 2121
Nubain Injection (1% or less) ... 1111
Paxil CR Controlled-Release Tablets ... 1509
Paxil ... 1501
Prinzide Tablets ... 2033
▲ Prograf Capsules and Injection (3% to 15%) ... 624
Prozac Pulvules and Liquid ... 1771
Repronex for Intramuscular and Subcutaneous Injection ... 1148
Rituxan for Infusion ... 845
Sandimmune ... 2259
Tenormin I.V. Injection ... 698
Tenormin Tablets ... 695
Teveten HCT Tablets ... 1710
Timolide Tablets ... 2056
Timoptic in Ocudose ... 2061
Timoptic Sterile Ophthalmic Solution (Less frequent) ... 2058
Timoptic-XE Sterile Ophthalmic Gel Forming Solution ... 2062
Topamax Sprinkle Capsules (1%) ... 2438
Topamax Tablets (1%) ... 2438
Toprol-XL Tablets ... 660
Uniretic Tablets ... 3114
Vaseretic Tablets ... 2073
Virazole for Inhalation Solution ... 3365
▲ Xeloda Tablets (Less than 5%) ... 2825
Zestoretic Tablets ... 701

Respiratory distress, neonatal
Hycodan ... 1104
Hycotuss Expectorant Syrup ... 1106
Naropin Injection (1.5%) ... 640

Respiratory distress syndrome
Ammonul Injection ... 3323
Bravelle for Intramuscular or Subcutaneous Injection ... 1140
Campath Ampules ... 826
Carimune NF ... 3501
Gammagard Liquid ... 751
Gammagard S/D (Rare) ... 754
Gamunex Immune Globulin I.V., 10% (Rare) ... 3232
Iveegam EN (Rare) ... 759
Levaquin in 5% Dextrose Injection (0.1% to 0.9%) ... 2453
Levaquin (0.1% to 0.9%) ... 2453
Neulasta Injection ... 596
Neupogen for Injection ... 598
Remicade for IV Injection (Greater than or equal to 0.2%) ... 987
Tarceva Tablets ... 1254
Tarceva Tablets ... 2470
Taxotere Injection Concentrate ... 2947
Trizivir Tablets ... 1565
VFEND I.V. (Less than 2%) ... 2543
VFEND Oral Suspension (Less than 2%) ... 2543
VFEND Tablets (Less than 2%) ... 2543
▲ Zegerid Powder for Oral Solution (3.4%) ... 2972
Ziagen ... 1600

Respiratory failure
▲ Abelcet Injection (8%) ... 1119
Abilify Tablets (Rare) ... 916
Abilify Tablets (Rare) ... 2472
Actiq (Less than 1%) ... 993
Aloprim for Injection (Less than 1%) ... 2156
AmBisome for Injection (Less common) ... 615
Ammonul Injection ... 3323
Betagan Ophthalmic Solution, USP ... ⊙217
Betimol Ophthalmic Solution ... ⊙283
Betimol Ophthalmic Solution ... 3371
Betoptic S Ophthalmic Suspension (Rare) ... 554
Carteolol Hydrochloride Ophthalmic Solution USP, 1% ... ⊙246
CellCept Capsules ... 2751
CellCept Intravenous ... 2751
CellCept Oral Suspension ... 2751
CellCept Tablets ... 2751
Cosopt Sterile Ophthalmic Solution ... 1910
Gemzar for Injection (Very rare) ... 1743
Omnicef Capsules ... 506
Omnicef for Oral Suspension ... 506
Orthoclone OKT3 Sterile Solution ... 2370
PEG-Intron Powder for Injection ... 3062
Photofrin for Injection ... 729
▲ Proleukin for Injection (Less than 1% to 9%) ... 1007
Pulmozyme Inhalation Solution ... 1245
Rythmol SR Capsules ... 2736
Simulect for Injection ... 2268
Symmetrel ... 1115
Timoptic in Ocudose (Less frequent) ... 2061
Timoptic Sterile Ophthalmic Solution (Less frequent) ... 2058
Timoptic-XE Sterile Ophthalmic Gel Forming Solution ... 2062
Trizivir Tablets ... 1565
Ziagen ... 1600

Respiratory insufficiency
Aloprim for Injection (Less than 1%) ... 2156
Campath Ampules ... 826
Emend Capsules (Greater than 0.5%) ... 1944
Levaquin in 5% Dextrose Injection (0.1% to 0.9%) ... 2453
Levaquin (0.1% to 0.9%) ... 2453
Remicade for IV Injection (Greater than or equal to 0.2%) ... 987

Respiratory moniliasis
▲ CellCept Capsules (3% to less than 20%) ... 2751
▲ CellCept Intravenous (3% to less than 20%) ... 2751
▲ CellCept Oral Suspension (3% to less than 20%) ... 2751
▲ CellCept Tablets (3% to less than 20%) ... 2751
Rilutek Tablets (Infrequent) ... 2945
Tricor Tablets ... 523

Respiratory rate, increased
Ammonul Injection ... 3323

Respiratory secretions, increased
▲ Suprane Liquid for Inhalation (3% to 21%) ... 770

Restless Legs Syndrome
Requip Tablets ... 1528

Restlessness
(*see under* Dysphoria)

Retardation, psychomotor
Eskalith ... 1406
Roferon-A Injection (Infrequent) ... 2805

Retching
Imitrex Injection (Rare) ... 1431
Imitrex Nasal Spray ... 1435
Imitrex Tablets ... 1440
Trileptal Oral Suspension ... 2281
Trileptal Tablets ... 2281

Reticulocytopenia
Cosmegen for Injection ... 1907
Garamycin Injectable ... 3028

Reticulocytosis
▲ Dapsone Tablets USP (Almost all patients) ... 1656
Garamycin Injectable ... 3028
Ticlid Tablets (Rare) ... 2813
Virazole for Inhalation Solution ... 3365

Retinal artery occlusion
Activase I.V. ... 1225
Imitrex Nasal Spray ... 1435
Imitrex Tablets ... 1440

Retinal atrophy
Clinoril Tablets ... 1899

Retinal damage
Dapsone Tablets USP ... 1656
Neurontin Capsules (Rare) ... 2498
Neurontin Oral Solution (Rare) ... 2498
Neurontin Tablets (Rare) ... 2498

Retinal degeneration
Aciphex Tablets ... 1081
Prevacid Delayed-Release Capsules (Less than 1%) ... 3268
Prevacid for Delayed-Release Oral Suspension (Less than 1%) ... 3268
Prevacid NapraPAC (Less than 1%) ... 3277
Prevacid SoluTab Delayed-Release Orally Disintegrating Tablets (Less than 1%) ... 3268
PREVPAC (Less than 1%) ... 3281
Uniretic Tablets (Less than 1%) ... 3114

Retinal detachment
Cymbalta Delayed-Release Capsules (Infrequent) ... 1729
▲ Cytovene (8%) ... 2763
Namenda (Infrequent) ... 1199
Permax Tablets (Rare) ... 3357
Sonata Capsules (Rare) ... 1686
Sular Tablets (Less than or equal to 1%) ... 1163
▲ Valcyte Tablets (15%) ... 2816
Visudyne for Injection (Less than 1%) ... 2286
Xalatan Sterile Ophthalmic Solution (Extremely rare) ... 2654

Retinal disorder, unspecified
Evoxac Capsules (Less than 1%) ... 1042
Lamisil Tablets ... 2226
Lotensin HCT Tablets (0.3% or more) ... 2235
Rythmol SR Capsules ... 2736

Retinal ischemia
PEG-Intron Powder for Injection (Less than or equal to 1%) ... 3062

Retinal pigmentation disorders
Desferal Vials ... 2190

Retinal vascular disorder
Betimol Ophthalmic Solution ... ⊙283
Betimol Ophthalmic Solution ... 3371
Climara Transdermal System ... 795
Climara Pro Transdermal System ... 800
CombiPatch Transdermal System ... 2180
Intron A for Injection (Rare) ... 3038
Lyrica Capsules (0.1% to 1%) ... 2524
Menostar Transdermal System ... 805
Permax Tablets ... 3357
Protonix I.V. (Less than 1%) ... 3468
Protonix Tablets (Less than 1%) ... 3465
Viagra Tablets ... 2552
Virazole for Inhalation Solution ... 3365
Visudyne for Injection (Less than 1%) ... 2286

Retinal vein occlusion
Cialis Tablets ... 1806
Evista Tablets (Very rare) ... 1735
Levitra Tablets (Rare) ... 3048

Retinitis
Attenuvax (Infrequent) ... 1889

Cytovene 2763
▲ Doxil Injection (1% to 5%) 3302
Indocin (Less than 1%) 1968
M-M-R II (Infrequent) 1980
VFEND I.V. (Less than 2%) 2543
VFEND Oral Suspension (Less than 2%) 2543
VFEND Tablets (Less than 2%) 2543

Retinoic-acid-APL syndrome
▲ Vesanoid Capsules (Up to 25%) 2823

Retinopathy
Cardizem LA Extended Release Tablets (Infrequent) 1699
Clinoril Tablets 1899
Desferal Vials 2190
Intron A for Injection 3038
Neurontin Capsules (Rare) 2498
Neurontin Oral Solution (Rare) 2498
Neurontin Tablets (Rare) 2498
Nipent for Injection (Less than 3%) 3216
Pegasys 2793
PEG-Intron Powder for Injection 3062
Roferon-A Injection (Rare) 2805
Tiazac Capsules (Infrequent) 1204

Retinopathy, pigmentary
Thioridazine Hydrochloride Tablets 2122

Retinopathy of prematurity
Cafcit (2.2%) 1854
Decadron Phosphate Injection 1931

Retrolental fibroplasia
▲ Indocin I.V. (3% to 9%) 1973

Retroperitoneal fibrosis
Apokyn Injection 2132
Blocadren Tablets 1891
Cosopt Sterile Ophthalmic Solution 1910
Stalevo Tablets (Rare) 2270
Timolide Tablets 2056
Timoptic in Ocudose (Less frequent) 2061
Timoptic Sterile Ophthalmic Solution (Less frequent) 2058
Timoptic-XE Sterile Ophthalmic Gel Forming Solution 2062

Retroperitoneum, redistribution/accumulation of body fat
Retrovir 1533

Reye's Syndrome, potential for development of
Aggrenox Capsules 855
Bayer, Aspirin Regimen ■□ 606
Bayer Aspirin 3515
BC Powder ■□ 612
BC Allergy Sinus Cold Powder ■□ 612
Arthritis Strength BC Powder ■□ 612
BC Sinus Cold Powder ■□ 612
Dolobid Tablets 1937
Ecotrin Enteric Coated Aspirin Low, Regular and Maximum Strength Tablets 1627
Goody's Body Pain Formula Powder ■□ 621
Goody's Extra Strength Headache Powder ■□ 621
Goody's Extra Strength Pain Relief Tablets ■□ 621
Kaopectate Anti-Diarrheal/Upset Stomach Reliever Liquid ■□ 701
Extra Strength Kaopectate Anti-Diarrheal Liquid ■□ 701
Maalox Maximum Strength Total Stomach Relief Peppermint Liquid (Rare) ■□ 677
Maalox Maximum Strength Total Stomach Relief Strawberry Liquid (Rare) ■□ 678
Pepto-Bismol Maximum Strength Liquid (Rare) ■□ 718
Pepto-Bismol Original Liquid, Maximum Strength Liquid, Original and Cherry Tablets and Easy-To-Swallow Caplets (Rare) 2673
Percodan Tablets 1115
St. Joseph 81 mg Aspirin Chewable and Enteric Coated Tablets 1841

Rhabdomyolysis
Abilify Tablets (Rare) 916
Abilify Tablets (Rare) 2472
Accutane Capsules (Rare) 2740
Aciphex Tablets 1081
Activase I.V. 1225
Advicor Tablets 1694
Aggrenox Capsules 855
Altoprev Extended-Release Tablets 1151
Amnesteem Capsules (Rare) 2126
Antara Capsules 2723
Atacand Tablets 634
Atacand HCT (Rare) 637
Avalide Tablets 922
Avalide Tablets 2889
Avapro Tablets (Rare) 925
Avapro Tablets (Rare) 2886
Bayer Aspirin Tablets 3515
Benicar Tablets 2850
Benicar HCT Tablets (Rare) 2852
Caduet Tablets 2507
Celexa 1177
Clozapine Tablets 2141
Clozaril Tablets 2174
Combivir Tablets 1373
Comtan Tablets 2186
Cozaar Tablets (Rare) 1913
Crestor Tablets (Less than 1%) 672
Cytovene 2763
Diovan Tablets 2191
Diprivan Injectable Emulsion (Very rare) 676
Ecotrin Enteric Coated Aspirin Low, Regular and Maximum Strength Tablets 1627
Effexor Tablets 3405
Epivir 1394
Epivir-HBV 1398
Epzicom Tablets 1402
FazaClo Orally Disintegrating Tablets 547
Hyzaar 50-12.5 Tablets (Rare) 1964
Lamictal 1449
Lescol Capsules 2227
Lescol Capsules 2730
Lescol XL Tablets 2227
Lescol XL Tablets 2730
Levaquin in 5% Dextrose Injection (0.1% to 0.9%) 2453
Levaquin (0.1% to 0.9%) 2453
Lexapro Oral Solution 1193
Lexapro Tablets 1193
Lipitor Tablets (Rare) 2495
Lofibra Capsules (Rare) 1217
Mevacor Tablets 1996
Micardis Tablets (Rare) 884
Mirapex Tablets (One case) 889
Omnicef Capsules 506
Omnicef for Oral Suspension 506
Orap Tablets 1220
PEG-Intron Powder for Injection 3062
Pravachol Tablets (Rare) 943
Proleukin for Injection 1007
Protonix I.V. 3468
Protonix Tablets 3465
Rescriptor Tablets 2535
Retrovir IV Infusion 1537
Risperdal M-Tab Orally Disintegrating Tablets 1658
Risperdal 1658
Sanctura Tablets 1133
Seroquel Tablets 691
St. Joseph 81 mg Aspirin Chewable and Enteric Coated Tablets 1841
Stalevo Tablets (Rare) 2270
Tasmar Tablets 3360
Teveten Tablets (Rare) 1707
Tricor Tablets 523
Trizivir Tablets 1565
Vytorin 10/10 Tablets 2084
Vytorin 10/10 Tablets 3092
Vytorin 10/20 Tablets 2084
Vytorin 10/20 Tablets 3092
Vytorin 10/40 Tablets 2084
Vytorin 10/40 Tablets 3092
Vytorin 10/80 Tablets 2084
Vytorin 10/80 Tablets 3092
Wellbutrin Tablets 1579
Wellbutrin SR Sustained-Release Tablets 1583
Wellbutrin XL Extended-Release Tablets 1588
Zetia Tablets 2090
Zetia Tablets (Very rare) 3098
Zocor Tablets (Rare) 2078
Zyban Sustained-Release Tablets 1620

Rheumatism, articular
▲ Advair Diskus 100/50 (1% to 3%) 1291
▲ Advair Diskus 250/50 (1% to 3%) 1291
▲ Advair Diskus 500/50 (1% to 3%) 1291
▲ Flovent Diskus 50 mcg (1% to 17%) 1415
Serevent Diskus (1% to 3%) 1540

Rheumatoid arthritis
Abilify Tablets (Rare) 916
Abilify Tablets (Rare) 2472
Asacol Delayed-Release Tablets 2688
Campral Tablets (Frequent) 1175
Copegus Tablets (Less than 1%) 2759
Effexor Tablets (Rare) 3405
Effexor XR Capsules (Rare) 3411
Evoxac Capsules (Less than 1%) 1042
Pegasys (Less than 1%) 2793
PEG-Intron Powder for Injection (Less than or equal to 1%) 3062
Prozac Pulvules and Liquid (Rare) 1771
Relpax Tablets (Rare) 2531
Rilutek Tablets (Rare) 2945
Symbyax Capsules (Rare) 1788
Zyprexa Tablets (Infrequent) 1798
Zyprexa ZYDIS Orally Disintegrating Tablets (Infrequent) 1798

Rheumatoid arthritis, worsening of
▲ Kineret Injection (19%) 594

Rheumatoid factor, positive
Aldoclor Tablets 1881
Aldoril Tablets 1884

Rhinitis
▲ Abilify Tablets (4%) 916
▲ Abilify Tablets (4%) 2472
▲ Aceon Tablets (2 mg, 4 mg, 8 mg) (4.8%) 3191
Actiq (Less than 1%) 993
▲ Actonel Tablets (2.1% to 5.7%) 2679
▲ Actonel with Calcium Tablets (2.1% to 5.7%) 2684
▲ Adalat CC Tablets (3% or less) 2978
▲ Advair Diskus 100/50 (1% to 3%) 1291
▲ Advair Diskus 250/50 (1% to 3%) 1291
▲ Advair Diskus 500/50 (1% to 3%) 1291
Advicor Tablets 1694
▲ Aerobid/Aerobid-M (3% to 9%) 1172
Agrylin Capsules (1% to 5%) 3172
▲ Alamast Ophthalmic Solution (10% to 25%) 3371
▲ Aldara Cream, 5% (3.3%) 1814
Alinia for Oral Suspension (Less than 1%) 2840
Alinia Tablets (Less than 1%) 2840
Alphagan P Ophthalmic Solution (1% to 4%) 563
Ambien Tablets (1%) 2867
▲ AmBisome for Injection (11.1%) 615
Amerge Tablets (Rare) 1312
Antara Capsules (2.3%) 2723
Aralast (Greater than or equal to 0.2%) 745
Arava Tablets (2%) 2881
▲ Aredia for Injection (Up to 6%) 2168
▲ Arimidex Tablets (2% to 5%) 665
▲ Aromasin Tablets (2% to 5%) 2600
▲ Asacol Delayed-Release Tablets (5% or greater) 2688
▲ Astelin Nasal Spray (5.6%) 1876
Atacand Tablets (2%) 634
Atacand HCT (0.5% or greater) 637
▲ Atrovent HFA Inhalation Aerosol (4% to 6%) 872
Atrovent Inhalation Solution (2.3%) 868
Atrovent Nasal Spray 0.03% (2.0% to 5.1%) 869
Attenuvax 1889
Avalide Tablets (1% or greater) 922
Avalide Tablets (1% or greater) 2889
Avapro Tablets (1% or greater) 925
Avapro Tablets (1% or greater) 2886
Axert Tablets (Infrequent) 2430
▲ Axid Oral Solution (9.8%) 913
Azopt Ophthalmic Suspension (1% to 5%) 553
▲ Bactroban Nasal (1.0% to 6%) 1357
▲ Bexxar (0% to 10%) 1360
▲ BiDil Tablets (4%) 2161
Caduet Tablets (Greater than or equal to 2%) 2507
▲ Campath Ampules (7%) 826
Campral Tablets (Frequent) 1175
▲ Camptosar Injection (0% to 16%) 2602
Captopril Tablets 2114
Carafate Suspension 727
Carafate Tablets 728
Cardizem LA Extended Release Tablets (Less than 2%) 1699
▲ Carnitor Injection (6% to 11%) 3185
▲ Casodex Tablets (4%) 670
Celebrex Capsules (2%) 3130
▲ Celexa (5%) 1177
▲ CellCept Capsules (3% to less than 20%) 2751
▲ CellCept Intravenous (3% to less than 20%) 2751
▲ CellCept Oral Suspension (3% to less than 20%) 2751
▲ CellCept Tablets (3% to less than 20%) 2751
▲ Cenestin Tablets, 0.45mg, 0.625mg, 0.9mg, 1.25mg (5.7% to 8%) 1063
▲ Cipro I.V. (3%) 2998
▲ Cipro I.V. Pharmacy Bulk Package (3%) 3509
▲ Cipro (3%) 2991
▲ Climara Transdermal System (2% to 6%) 795
Colazal Capsules (2%) 2845
▲ CombiPatch Transdermal System (19% to 22%) 2180
Combivent Inhalation Aerosol (1.1%) 878
▲ Concerta Extended-Release Tablets (3%) 1828
▲ Copaxone for Injection (14%) 3292
Cozaar Tablets (Less than 1%) 1913
Crestor Tablets (2.2%) 672
Cutivate Lotion 0.05% (Less than 1%) 1383
▲ DDAVP Nasal Spray (3% to 8%) 2894
▲ Depacon Injection (5%) 412
▲ Depakene (5%) 417
▲ Depakote Sprinkle Capsules (5%) 422
▲ Depakote Tablets (1% to 5%) 427
▲ Depakote ER Tablets (5%) 433
Depo-Medrol Single-Dose Vial 2617
▲ Desmopressin Acetate Rhinal Tube (3% to 8%) 1144
Detrol Tablets (1.1%) 2626
Diastat Rectal Delivery System (Greater than or equal to 1%) 3344
Diovan Tablets (More than 1%) 2191
▲ Ditropan XL Extended Release Tablets (2% to 6%) 2391
Dostinex Tablets (1%) 2631
▲ Doxil Injection (Less than 1% to 10%) 3302
Duragesic Transdermal System (1% or greater) 2448
Effexor Tablets 3405
▲ Effexor XR Capsules (8%) 3411
▲ Elestat Ophthalmic Solution (1% to 3%) 1643
Elidel Cream 1% (0.4% to 4.4%) 2198
Elmiron Capsules (Less than or equal to 1%) 2393
▲ Eloxatin for Injection (5% to 15%) 2908
▲ Emtriva Capsules (12% to 18%) 1272
Enablex Extended-Release Tablets (Greater than or equal to 1%) 2201
▲ Enbrel for Injection (12% to 16%) 580
▲ Equetro Extended-Release Capsules (Less than 5%) 3178
Estrogel 0.06% (2.4%) 3200
▲ Evoxac Capsules (11.2%) 1042
▲ Exelon Capsules (4%) 2204
▲ Fabrazyme for Intravenous Infusion (11%) 1267
▲ Ferrlecit Injection (3% to 9%) 3379
▲ Flolan for Injection (21%) 1408
▲ Flomax Capsules (13.1% to 17.9%) 881
▲ Flovent Diskus 50 mcg (3% to 13%) 1415
▲ Flovent HFA (1% to 3%) 1418
Floxin Otic Singles (Reported in a single subject) 1045
Floxin Otic Solution (Single report) 1043
▲ Flumist Vaccine (6.3%) 1872
▲ Fortamet Extended-Release Tablets (4.2%) 1156
▲ Forteo for Injection (9.6%) 1739
▲ Fortical Nasal Spray (12%) 3336
▲ Fosrenol Chewable Tablets (5% to 7%) 3180
Frova Tablets (Frequent) 1101
Gabitril Tablets (1% or more) 998
▲ Gamunex Immune Globulin I.V., 10% (51%) 3232
Gemzar for Injection (Infrequent) 1743
▲ Gengraf Capsules (1% to 5%) 458
▲ Geodon (4%) 2514
▲ Gonal-f RFF Pen for Injection (7.2%) 3155
▲ Hectorol Capsules (Greater than or equal to 5%) 909
▲ Herceptin I.V. (14%) 1234
▲ Humatrope Vials and Cartridges (6.25% to 13.5%) 1756
Hytrin Capsules (At least 1% to 1.9%) 469
Hyzaar 1964
▲ Imdur Tablets (Less than or equal to 5%) 3032
▲ Indapamide Tablets (Greater than or equal to 5%) 2119
▲ Infergen (7% to 13%) 1647
▲ Intron A for Injection (Less than 5%) 3038
Invanz for Injection (Greater than 0.5%) 1974
Invirase (Less than 2%) 2776

▲ I.V. Busulfex (44%) ... 1125
Kadian Capsules (Less than 3%) ... 572
Kaletra (Less than 2%) ... 474
▲ Keppra Oral Solution (4% to 13%) ... 3307
▲ Keppra Tablets (4% to 13%) ... 3307
Klonopin (2%) ... 2782
Kogenate FS ... 3517
▲ Lamictal (13.6%) ... 1449
▲ Lescol Capsules (4.7%) ... 2227
▲ Lescol Capsules (4.7%) ... 2730
Lescol XL Tablets (1.5%) ... 2227
Lescol XL Tablets (1.5%) ... 2730
▲ Leukine (11%) ... 829
Levaquin in 5% Dextrose Injection (1.2%) ... 2453
Levaquin (1.2%) ... 2453
▲ Levitra Tablets (9%) ... 3048
▲ Lexapro Oral Solution (5%) ... 1193
▲ Lexapro Tablets (5%) ... 1193
Lipitor Tablets (Greater than or equal to 2%) ... 2495
Lofibra Capsules (2.3%) ... 1217
▲ Lotemax Ophthalmic Suspension 0.5% (Less than 15%) ... ⊙ 249
Lotensin HCT Tablets (More than 1%) ... 2235
Lunesta Tablets ... 3139
Lupron Depot 3.75 mg (Less than 5%) ... 3257
Lupron Depot–3 Month 11.25 mg (Less than 5%) ... 3262
Marinol Capsules (Less than 1%) ... 3334
▲ Mepron Suspension (5% to 24%) ... 1487
▲ Meridia Capsules (10.2%) ... 485
Meruvax II ... 1994
▲ Miacalcin Nasal Spray (12%) ... 2242
Micardis Tablets (More than 0.3%) ... 884
Micardis HCT Tablets ... 886
▲ Migranal Nasal Spray (26%) ... 3350
▲ Mirapex Tablets (Greater than or equal to 1% to 3%) ... 889
M-M-R II ... 1980
Mumpsvax ... 2005
▲ Mylotarg for Injection (7% to 10%) ... 3429
▲ Nasacort HFA Inhalation Aerosol (Greater than or equal to 3% to 4.7%) ... 2939
Nasacort AQ Nasal Spray (2% or greater) ... 2937
Nasonex Nasal Spray (Greater than or equal to 2%) ... 3058
▲ Neoral Soft Gelatin Capsules (1% to 5%) ... 2247
Neoral Oral Solution (1% to 5%) ... 2247
▲ Neumega for Injection (42%) ... 3433
▲ Neurontin Capsules (4.1%) ... 2498
▲ Neurontin Oral Solution (4.1%) ... 2498
▲ Neurontin Tablets (4.1%) ... 2498
Nexium Delayed-Release Capsules (Less than 1%) ... 645
Nexium I.V. (Less than 1%) ... 649
▲ Niaspan Extended-Release Tablets (2% to 5%) ... 1703
▲ Nicotrol Inhaler (23%) ... 2594
Nicotrol NS ... 2596
▲ Nipent for Injection (10% to 11%) ... 3216
Norvasc Tablets (Less than or equal to 0.1%) ... 2529
Norvir (Less than 2%) ... 499
Omacor Capsules ... 2735
▲ Ontak Vials (13%) ... 1717
OptiPranolol Metipranolol Ophthalmic Solution 0.3% (A small number of patients) ... ⊙ 254
▲ Optivar Ophthalmic Solution (1% to 10%) ... 1877
Patanol Ophthalmic Solution (Less than 5%) ... 557
Paxil CR Controlled-Release Tablets (Frequent) ... 1509
Paxil (Frequent) ... 1501
PEG-Intron Powder for Injection (2%) ... 3062
▲ Permax Tablets (12.2%) ... 3357
▲ Plavix Tablets (4.2%) ... 940
▲ Plavix Tablets (4.2%) ... 2942
▲ Pletal Tablets (7% to 12%) ... 2478
▲ Prandin Tablets (0.5, 1, and 2 mg) (3% to 7%) ... 2337
▲ Pravachol Tablets (0.1% to 4.0%) ... 943
▲ Premarin Tablets (6% to 10%) ... 3443
▲ Premphase Tablets (6% to 10%) ... 3452
▲ Prempro Tablets (6% to 10%) ... 3452
Prevacid Delayed-Release Capsules (Less than 1%) ... 3268
Prevacid for Delayed-Release Oral Suspension (Less than 1%) ... 3268
Prevacid NapraPAC (Less than 1%) ... 3277
Prevacid SoluTab Delayed-Release Orally Disintegrating Tablets (Less than 1%) ... 3268
PREVPAC (Less than 1%) ... 3281
Prilosec OTC Tablets (2%) ... 2674
Prinivil Tablets (0.3% to 1.0%) ... 2029
Prinzide Tablets (0.3% to 1%) ... 2033
Prochieve 4% Gel ... 1018
Prochieve 8% Gel ... 1018
▲ Prograf Capsules and Injection (3% to 15%) ... 624
▲ Proleukin for Injection (10%) ... 1007
ProSom Tablets (Infrequent) ... 512
Protonix I.V. (Greater than 1%) ... 3468
Protonix Tablets (Greater than or equal to 1%) ... 3465
▲ Protopic Ointment (3% to 5%) ... 629
▲ Proventil HFA Inhalation Aerosol (16%) ... 3071
▲ Provigil Tablets (7%) ... 1002
Prozac Pulvules and Liquid ... 1771
▲ Pulmicort Respules (7% to 12%) ... 654
▲ Pulmozyme Inhalation Solution (30%) ... 1245
▲ Qvar Inhalation Aerosol (3% to 8%) ... 1654
▲ Rapamune Oral Solution and Tablets (3% to 20%) ... 3472
▲ Razadyne ER Extended-Release Capsules (4%) ... 2434
▲ Razadyne (4%) ... 2434
▲ Rebetol (6% to 8%) ... 3073
Recombivax HB (Greater than 1%) ... 2045
ReFacto Vials ... 3479
Relpax Tablets (Infrequent) ... 2531
▲ Remicade for IV Injection (8%) ... 987
▲ Requip Tablets (4%) ... 1528
Rescriptor Tablets ... 2535
Retrovir Capsules ... 1533
Retrovir IV Infusion ... 1537
Retrovir ... 1533
▲ Revatio Tablets (4%) ... 2541
▲ Ribavirin, USP Capsules (6% to 8%) ... 3083
▲ Rilutek Tablets (7.8% to 8.9%) ... 2945
▲ Risperdal Consta Long-Acting Injection (4% to 14%) ... 1664
▲ Risperdal M-Tab Orally Disintegrating Tablets (3% to 10%) ... 1658
▲ Risperdal (3% to 10%) ... 1658
▲ Rituxan for Infusion (0.3% to 8%) ... 845
▲ Rituxan I.V. (12%) ... 1251
▲ Roferon-A Injection (3%) ... 2805
Rythmol SR Capsules ... 2736
▲ Sandostatin LAR Depot (5% to 15%) ... 2264
▲ Serevent Diskus (5%) ... 1540
▲ Seroquel Tablets (3%) ... 691
▲ Simulect for Injection (3% to 10%) ... 2268
Singulair (Greater than or equal to 2%) ... 2047
▲ Soriatane Capsules (25% to 50%) ... 1028
Spectracef Tablets (0.1% to 1%) ... 2706
▲ Spiriva HandiHaler (3% to 6%) ... 899
▲ Suboxone Tablets (4.7% to 11%) ... 2719
▲ Subutex Tablets (9.7% to 11%) ... 2719
Sular Tablets (Less than or equal to 1%) ... 1163
▲ Synagis (26.8%) ... 1868
Targretin Capsules ... 1719
Tasmar Tablets (Infrequent) ... 3360
▲ Teveten Tablets (4%) ... 1707
Teveten HCT Tablets (Less than 1%) ... 1710
▲ Thalomid Capsules (4.2%) ... 979
Tiazac Capsules (2%) ... 1204
▲ TOBI Solution for Inhalation (34.5%) ... 1015
▲ Topamax Sprinkle Capsules (1% to 7%) ... 2438
▲ Topamax Tablets (1% to 7%) ... 2438
Tricor Tablets (2.3%) ... 523
Triglide Tablets (2.3%) ... 1165
▲ Trileptal Oral Suspension (2% to 10%) ... 2281
▲ Trileptal Tablets (2% to 10%) ... 2281
Truvada Tablets ... 1279
Uniretic Tablets (More than 1%) ... 3114
Univasc Tablets (Greater than 1%) ... 3118
Vantin Tablets and Oral Suspension (Less than 1%) ... 2650
Verelan PM Capsules (2.7%) ... 3120
VFEND I.V. (Less than 2%) ... 2543
VFEND Oral Suspension (Less than 2%) ... 2543
VFEND Tablets (Less than 2%) ... 2543
Vicoprofen Tablets (Less than 3%) ... 533
▲ Vigamox Ophthalmic Solution (1% to 4%) ... 560
Viracept (Less than 2%) ... 2556
Vivelle Transdermal System ... 2288
Vivelle-Dot Transdermal System ... 2293
▲ Voltaren Ophthalmic Solution (Less than or equal to 3%) ... 2300
▲ WelChol Tablets (3%) ... 2855
Wellbutrin SR Sustained-Release Tablets (At least 1%) ... 1583
Wellbutrin XL Extended-Release Tablets (At least 1%) ... 1588
Xifaxan Tablets (Less than 2%) ... 2847
▲ Xopenex HFA Inhalation Aerosol (2.7% to 11.1%) ... 3151
▲ Xopenex Inhalation Solution (2.7% to 11.1%) ... 3143
▲ Xopenex Inhalation Solution Concentrate (2.7% to 11.1%) ... 3147
▲ Zaditor Ophthalmic Solution (10% to 25%) ... 2302
Zegerid Powder for Oral Solution (2%) ... 2972
Zemaira (0.5%) ... 3506
▲ Zenapax for Injection (2% to 5%) ... 2838
Zestoretic Tablets (0.3% to 1%) ... 701
Zestril Tablets (0.3% to 1.0%) ... 704
▲ Zevalin Injection (6%) ... 848
Zithromax for Oral Suspension, 300 mg, 600 mg, 900 mg, 1200 mg (1% or less) ... 2561
Zithromax Tablets, 250 mg, 500 mg (1% or less) ... 2561
Zithromax Tri-Pak (1% or less) ... 2561
Zoladex (1% or greater) ... 709
Zoladex 3-month ... 712
Zoloft (Frequent) ... 2581
Zomig Nasal Spray (Infrequent) ... 718
Zonegran Capsules (2%) ... 1089
Zosyn (1.2%) ... 3492
▲ Zyban Sustained-Release Tablets (12%) ... 1620
▲ Zyprexa Tablets (10%) ... 1798
▲ Zyprexa ZYDIS Orally Disintegrating Tablets (10%) ... 1798
Zyrtec Chewable Tablets (Less than 2%) ... 2589
Zyrtec (Less than 2%) ... 2589
Zyrtec-D 12 Hour Extended Release Tablets (Less than 2%) ... 2591

Rhinitis, allergic

▲ Asmanex Twisthaler (11% to 20%) ... 2981
▲ BeneFix for Injection (4.6%) ... 3402
Imitrex Injection ... 1431
Imitrex Nasal Spray ... 1435
Lotronex Tablets (2%) ... 1479
Xanax XR Tablets (1.1%) ... 2655

Rhinitis, ulcerative

Atrovent Nasal Spray 0.03% (2.0%) ... 869

Rhinorrhea

Aceon Tablets (2 mg, 4 mg, 8 mg) (0.3% to 1%) ... 3191
▲ Advair Diskus 100/50 (1% to 3%) ... 1291
▲ Advair Diskus 250/50 (1% to 3%) ... 1291
▲ Advair Diskus 500/50 (1% to 3%) ... 1291
▲ Aerobid/Aerobid-M (3% to 9%) ... 1172
▲ Apokyn Injection (20%) ... 2132
▲ Atrovent Nasal Spray 0.03% (3.1%) ... 869
Beconase AQ Nasal Spray (Fewer than 3 per 100 patients) ... 1359
Calcijex Injection ... 411
▲ Chemet Capsules (0.7% to 3.7%) ... 2480
▲ Clarinex Syrup (4.5%) ... 3009
Clindesse Vaginal Cream (Less than 1%) ... 3296
Clozapine Tablets (Less than 1%) ... 2141
Clozaril Tablets (Less than 1%) ... 2174
Colyte with Flavor Packs for Oral Solution (Isolated cases) ... 3102
Comvax (0.2% to 1.3%) ... 1904
Elidel Cream 1% (Up to 1.9%) ... 2198
FazaClo Orally Disintegrating Tablets (Less than 1%) ... 547
▲ Flonase Nasal Spray (1% to 3%) ... 1412
▲ Flovent Diskus 50 mcg (1% to 3%) ... 1415
▲ Flovent HFA (1% to 3%) ... 1418
HalfLytely and Bisacodyl Tablets Bowel Prep Kit with Flavors Packs ... 915
Hectorol Capsules ... 909
Hectorol Injection ... 911
Indapamide Tablets (Less than 5%) ... 2119
▲ Intron A for Injection (Less than 5%) ... 3038
Invanz for Injection (Greater than 0.5%) ... 1974
Klonopin ... 2782
Maxalt Tablets (Rare) ... 1983
Maxalt-MLT Orally Disintegrating Tablets (Rare) ... 1983
Plendil Extended-Release Tablets (0.2% to 1.6%) ... 651
Prinivil Tablets (0.3% to 1.0%) ... 2029
Prinzide Tablets ... 2033
▲ Roferon-A Injection (12%) ... 2805
Singulair (Greater than or equal to 2%) ... 2047
▲ Strattera Capsules (4%) ... 1784
TriLyte with Flavor Packs for Oral Solution ... 3114
▲ Valcyte Tablets (Less than 5%) ... 2816
▲ Vaqta (5.7%) ... 2067
Vaseretic Tablets ... 2073
Vasotec I.V. Injection (0.5% to 1.0%) ... 2076
Xanax XR Tablets (Infrequent) ... 2655
▲ Xeloda Tablets (5%) ... 2825
Xifaxan Tablets (Less than 2%) ... 2847
Zestoretic Tablets ... 701
Zestril Tablets (0.3% to 1.0%) ... 704

Rhonchi

Brevibloc Concentrate (Less than 1%) ... 766
Brevibloc Injection (Less than 1%) ... 766
Brevibloc Double Strength Injection (Less than 1%) ... 766
Brevibloc Premixed Injection (Less than 1%) ... 766
Brevibloc Double Strength Premixed Injection (Less than 1%) ... 766
Invanz for Injection (0.5% to 1.1%) ... 1974
ReoPro Vials (0.1%) ... 1779
▲ Trisenox Injection (8%) ... 983
Zemuron Injection (Less than 1%) ... 2363

Rigidity

Ambien Tablets (Rare) ... 2867
Brevibloc Concentrate (Less than 1%) ... 766
Brevibloc Injection (Less than 1%) ... 766
Brevibloc Double Strength Injection (Less than 1%) ... 766
Brevibloc Premixed Injection (Less than 1%) ... 766
Brevibloc Double Strength Premixed Injection (Less than 1%) ... 766
▲ Clozapine Tablets (3%) ... 2141
▲ Clozaril Tablets (3%) ... 2174
Diprivan Injectable Emulsion (Less than 1%) ... 676
Ethyol for Injection (Rare) ... 1869
Famvir Tablets (0.5% to 1.5%) ... 2207
▲ FazaClo Orally Disintegrating Tablets (3%) ... 547
Flumadine ... 1186
Gengraf Capsules (1% to less than 3%) ... 458
Hyzaar ... 1964
Imitrex Tablets (Rare) ... 1440
▲ Infergen (57% to 62%) ... 1647
▲ Intron A for Injection (Up to 42%) ... 3038
Moban Tablets ... 1108
▲ Naropin Injection (1% to 5%) ... 640
Neoral Soft Gelatin Capsules (1% to less than 3%) ... 2247
Neoral Oral Solution (1% to less than 3%) ... 2247
▲ Niravam Orally Disintegrating Tablets (4.2%) ... 3106
Norvasc Tablets (More than 0.1% to 1%) ... 2529
▲ Orap Tablets (2 of 20 patients) ... 1220
▲ Orthoclone OKT3 Sterile Solution (8%) ... 2370
Proleukin for Injection ... 1007
Risperdal M-Tab Orally Disintegrating Tablets (Infrequent) ... 1658
Risperdal (Infrequent) ... 1658
▲ Soriatane Capsules (10% to 25%) ... 1028
Zoloft (Infrequent) ... 2581
Zosyn (1.0% or less) ... 3492
Zovirax for Injection (Less than 1%) ... 1618
Zyrtec Chewable Tablets (Less than 2%) ... 2589
Zyrtec (Less than 2%) ... 2589
Zyrtec-D 12 Hour Extended Release Tablets (Less than 2%) ... 2591

Rigors

Advate Injection (0.6%) ... 742
Aldara Cream, 5% (1.4%) ... 1814
AmBisome for Injection (Less common) ... 615
BeneFix for Injection (1.6%) ... 3402
Bexxar ... 1360
Caduet Tablets (Greater than 0.1% to less than or equal to 1%) ... 2507
▲ Campath Ampules (16% to 86%) ... 826
Carimune NF ... 3501
Celexa (Infrequent) ... 1177
▲ Clolar for Intravenous Infusion (38%) ... 1264
▲ Copegus Tablets (25%) ... 2759
Cubicin for Injection (Less than 1%) ... 1038
Cymbalta Delayed-Release Capsules (Frequent) ... 1729

▲ DepoDur Extended-Release Injection (2% to 5%) 1098
Duragesic Transdermal System (Greater than or less than 1%) 2448
Eligard 22.5 mg (Less than 2%) 2899
Elitek (Less than or equal to 1%) 2906
▲ Eloxatin for Injection (7% to 9%) 2908
Evoxac Capsules (1.3%) 1042
Exelon Capsules (Frequent) 2204
▲ Fabrazyme for Intravenous Infusion (15%) 1267
Ferrlecit Injection 3379
Frova Tablets (Infrequent) 1101
Gammagard Liquid 751
Gammagard S/D 754
Gamunex Immune Globulin I.V., 10% 3232
▲ Gengraf Capsules (3%) 458
▲ Gleevec Tablets (10% to 12%) 2221
Herceptin I.V. 1234
▲ Imdur Tablets (Less than or equal to 5%) 3032
▲ Intron A for Injection (2% to 42%) 3038
Iveegam EN 759
Levaquin in 5% Dextrose Injection (0.1% to 0.9%) 2453
Levaquin (0.1% to 0.9%) 2453
Migranal Nasal Spray (Infrequent) 3350
Mycamine for Injection (0.2% to 2.3%) 620
▲ Neoral Soft Gelatin Capsules (3%) 2247
▲ Neoral Oral Solution (3%) 2247
Nexium Delayed-Release Capsules (Less than 1%) 645
Nexium I.V. (Less than 1%) 649
▲ Pegasys (35%) 2793
▲ PEG-Intron Powder for Injection (23%) 3062
Proventil HFA Inhalation Aerosol (Less than 3%) 3071
▲ Rebetol (25% to 48%) 3073
▲ Rebetron Combination Therapy (32% to 42%) 3078
▲ Rebif Prefilled Syringe for Injection (6% to 13%) 3163
Requip Tablets (1% or more) 1528
▲ Ribavirin, USP Capsules (25% to 48%) 3083
▲ Sandostatin LAR Depot (5% to 15%) 2264
▲ Simulect for Injection (3% to 10%) 2268
▲ Strattera Capsules (3%) 1784
Teveten Tablets (Less than 1%) 1707
Teveten HCT Tablets (Less than 1%) 1710
Topamax Sprinkle Capsules (Less than or equal to 1%) 2438
Topamax Tablets (Less than or equal to 1%) 2438
Trileptal Oral Suspension 2281
Trileptal Tablets 2281
▲ Trisenox Injection (38%) 983
Ultracet Tablets (Less than 1%) 2462
▲ Velcade for Injection (11%) 2102
Xanax XR Tablets (Infrequent) 2655
▲ Zometa for Intravenous Infusion (11% to less than 15%) 2306

Romberg test, positive
Neurontin Capsules (Infrequent) 2498
Neurontin Oral Solution (Infrequent) 2498
Neurontin Tablets (Infrequent) 2498

Rosacea
Elocon Cream 0.1% 3019
Elocon Ointment 0.1% 3021
Evoxac Capsules (Less than 1%) 1042
Tri-Luma Cream (1%) 1213

Rosacea, worsening of
Noritate Cream, 1% (One patient) 1051

Roseola
Prevnar for Injection 3460

Rupture, Achilles tendon
Cipro XR Tablets 3004
Factive Tablets 2464

S

S_3 gallop
(*see under* Ventricular gallop)

Saliva, discoloration
Parcopa Orally Disintegrating Tablets 3111
Stalevo Tablets 2270

Salivary gland enlargement
Aciphex Tablets (Rare) 1081
Alinia for Oral Suspension (Less than 1%) 2840
Alinia Tablets (Less than 1%) 2840
▲ Arava Tablets (1% to 3%) 2881
Clozapine Tablets 2141
Clozaril Tablets 2174
Copaxone for Injection (Frequent) 3292
▲ Evoxac Capsules (1% to 3%) 1042
FazaClo Orally Disintegrating Tablets 547
Gengraf Capsules (1% to less than 3%) 458
Imitrex Nasal Spray 1435
Lithobid Tablets 1670
Neoral Soft Gelatin Capsules (1% to less than 3%) 2247
Neoral Oral Solution (1% to less than 3%) 2247
Neurontin Capsules (Rare) 2498
Neurontin Oral Solution (Rare) 2498
Neurontin Tablets (Rare) 2498
Permax Tablets (Infrequent) 3357
Prozac Pulvules and Liquid (Rare) 1771
Rilutek Tablets (Rare) 2945

Salivation
(*see under* Sialism)

Salivation, increase
(*see under* Sialism)

Salpingitis
Amerge Tablets (Rare) 1312
Effexor Tablets (Rare) 3405
Effexor XR Capsules (Rare) 3411
Gabitril Tablets (Infrequent) 998
Permax Tablets (Infrequent) 3357
Wellbutrin SR Sustained-Release Tablets 1583
Wellbutrin XL Extended-Release Tablets 1588
Zyban Sustained-Release Tablets 1620

Sarcoidosis
Copegus Tablets (Less than 1%) 2759
Enbrel for Injection 580
Intron A for Injection (Very rare) 3038
Pegasys (Less than 1%) 2793
PEG-Intron Powder for Injection 3062
Rebetol 3073
Rebetron Combination Therapy 3078
Risperdal M-Tab Orally Disintegrating Tablets (Rare) 1658
Risperdal (Rare) 1658
Roferon-A Injection 2805

Sarcoidosis, exacerbation of
Intron A for Injection (Very rare) 3038
Rebetol 3073
Rebetron Combination Therapy 3078

Sarcoma, bone
Permax Tablets (Infrequent) 3357

Sarcoma, unspecified
▲ Megace ES Oral Suspension (1% to 3%) 2492
Thalomid Capsules 979

Scabbing
▲ Aldara Cream, 5% (Up to 13%) 1814
Avita Cream 2136

Scalp, dry
Nizoral Shampoo 1838

Scalp, tightness
Temovate Scalp Application (1 of 294 patients) 1551

Scalp hair, thinning
Decadron Tablets 1929

Scarring
▲ Efudex (Among most frequent) 3348

Schizophrenia, precipitation
Zyprexa Tablets 1798
Zyprexa ZYDIS Orally Disintegrating Tablets 1798

Sciatica
Ambien Tablets (Rare) 2867
Atacand HCT (0.5% or greater) 637
Clindesse Vaginal Cream (Less than 1%) 3296
Gleevec Tablets (Infrequent) 2221
Rythmol SR Capsules 2736
Wellbutrin Tablets (Rare) 1579

Sclera, discoloration
Ticlid Tablets 2813

Scleral perforation
HMS ⊙ 228

Scleral thinning
Pred-G Sterile Ophthalmic Ointment ⊙ 235

Scleritis
Ambien Tablets (Infrequent) 2867
Aredia for Injection (Rare) 2168
Effexor Tablets (Rare) 3405
Effexor XR Capsules (Rare) 3411
Evoxac Capsules (Less than 1%) 1042
Fosamax 1949
Fosamax Plus D Tablets (Rarely) 1956
Prozac Pulvules and Liquid (Rare) 1771
VFEND I.V. (Less than 2%) 2543
VFEND Oral Suspension (Less than 2%) 2543
VFEND Tablets (Less than 2%) 2543

Scleroderma
Depo-Provera Contraceptive Injection (Less than 1%) 2619
depo-subQ provera 104 Injectable Suspension 2622
Evoxac Capsules (Less than 1%) 1042
Soriatane Capsules (Less than 1%) 1028

Sclerosis, multiple
Enbrel for Injection 580
Engerix-B Vaccine (Less than 1%) 1391
Evoxac Capsules (Less than 1%) 1042
Havrix Vaccine (Rare) 1425
▲ Humira Injection (Less than 5%) 464
Rabies Vaccine RabAvert 1011
Recombivax HB 2045
Remicade for IV Injection 987
Twinrix Vaccine 1571

Sclerosis, multiple, aggravation
Aldara Cream, 5% 1814

Sclerosis, skin
Parnate Tablets 1499

Scoliosis
▲ Humatrope Vials and Cartridges (18.9%) 1756

Scotomata
Adenoscan (Less than 1%) 613
Amerge Tablets (Rare) 1312
Axert Tablets (Rare) 2430
Desferal Vials 2190
Eskalith 1406
Lithobid Tablets 1670
Pacerone Tablets 3337
ProSom Tablets (Rare) 512
Requip Tablets (Rare) 1528
Sandostatin LAR Depot (Rare) 2264
Topamax Sprinkle Capsules (Infrequent) 2438
Topamax Tablets (Infrequent) 2438
Trileptal Oral Suspension 2281
Trileptal Tablets 2281

Scrotal disorder, unspecified
Caverject Impulse Injection (Less than 1%) 2610

Scrotum, swollen
Neurontin Capsules (Rare) 2498
Neurontin Oral Solution (Rare) 2498
Neurontin Tablets (Rare) 2498

Seborrhea
Abilify Tablets (Infrequent) 916
Abilify Tablets (Infrequent) 2472
Accutane Capsules 2740
Caduet Tablets (Less than 2%) 2507
Depacon Injection (1% or more) 412
Depakene (1% or more) 417
Depakote Sprinkle Capsules 422
▲ Depakote Tablets (1% to 5%) 427
Depakote ER Tablets (Greater than 1%) 433
Effexor Tablets (Rare) 3405
Effexor XR Capsules (Rare) 3411
Evoxac Capsules (Less than 1%) 1042
Finacea Gel (1% or less) 1644
Floxin Otic Singles (Reported in a single subject) 1045
Floxin Otic Solution (Single report) 1043
Invirase (Less than 2%) 2776
Kaletra (Less than 2%) 474
Lamictal (Rare) 1449
Lipitor Tablets (Less than 2%) 2495
Lupron Depot-PED 7.5 mg, 11.25 mg and 15 mg (2%) 3266
Lupron Injection Pediatric 3256
Neurontin Capsules (Infrequent) 2498
Neurontin Oral Solution (Infrequent) 2498
Neurontin Tablets (Infrequent) 2498
Norvir (Less than 2%) 499
Paxil CR Controlled-Release Tablets (Rare) 1509
Paxil (Rare) 1501
Permax Tablets (Infrequent) 3357
Prochieve 4% Gel 1018
Prochieve 8% Gel 1018
Prozac Pulvules and Liquid (Rare) 1771
Requip Tablets (Infrequent) 1528
Rescriptor Tablets 2535
Reyataz Capsules (Less than 3%) 948
Rilutek Tablets (Infrequent) 2945
Risperdal Consta Long-Acting Injection (Infrequent) 1664
Risperdal M-Tab Orally Disintegrating Tablets (Up to 1%) 1658
Risperdal (Up to 1%) 1658
Roferon-A Injection (Less than 1%) 2805
Seroquel Tablets (Infrequent) 691
▲ Soriatane Capsules (1% to 10%) 1028
Symbyax Capsules (Rare) 1788
Synagis (More than 1%) 1868
Tasmar Tablets (Infrequent) 3360
Thalomid Capsules 979
Topamax Sprinkle Capsules (1%) 2438
Topamax Tablets (1%) 2438
▲ Zoladex (26%) 709
Zoladex 3-month 712
Zyprexa Tablets (Infrequent) 1798
Zyprexa ZYDIS Orally Disintegrating Tablets (Infrequent) 1798
Zyrtec Chewable Tablets (Less than 2%) 2589
Zyrtec (Less than 2%) 2589
Zyrtec-D 12 Hour Extended Release Tablets (Less than 2%) 2591

Sedation
▲ Alacol DM Syrup (Among most frequent) 739
Aldoclor Tablets 1881
Aldoril Tablets 1884
Amerge Tablets (Rare) 1312
Balamine DM 739
▲ Buprenex Injectable (Most frequent) 2718
▲ Catapres Tablets (About 10 in 100 patients) 874
Catapres-TTS (3 of 101 patients) 875
▲ Clorpres Tablets (About 10%) 2139
▲ Clozapine Tablets (More than 5% to 39%) 2141
▲ Clozaril Tablets (More than 5% to 39%) 2174
Dalmane Capsules 3343
▲ Darvocet A 500 Tablets (Among most frequent) 3497
▲ Demser Capsules (Almost all patients) 1933
Depacon Injection 412
Depakene 417
Depakote Tablets 427
Depakote ER Tablets 433
Dilaudid 439
Dilaudid Oral Liquid 443
Dilaudid Non-Sterile Powder 439
Dilaudid Rectal Suppositories 439
Dilaudid Tablets 439
Dilaudid Tablets - 8 mg 443
▲ Dilaudid-HP (Among most frequent) 441
▲ FazaClo Orally Disintegrating Tablets (Greater than 5% to 39%) 547
Hycodan 1104
Hycomine Compound Tablets 1105
Hycotuss Expectorant Syrup 1106
Imitrex Injection (2.7%) 1431
Imitrex Nasal Spray (Infrequent) 1435
Imitrex Tablets 1440
Inversine Tablets 3286
Kadian Capsules (Less than 3%) 572
▲ Lortab (Among most frequent) 3315
▲ Lortab Elixir (Among most frequent) 3312
Lotronex Tablets (Rare) 1479
▲ MS Contin Tablets (Among most frequent) 2703
Nadolol Tablets (6 of 1000 patients) 2121
Niravam Orally Disintegrating Tablets 3106
▲ Nubain Injection (36%) 1111
▲ Orap Tablets (14 of 20 patients) 1220
▲ OxyFast Oral Concentrate Solution (Among most frequent) 2704
▲ OxyIR Capsules (Among most frequent) 2704
▲ Percocet Tablets (Among most frequent) 1114
▲ Percodan Tablets (Among most frequent) 1115
Phenergan Suppositories 3438
Roferon-A Injection (Infrequent) 2805
▲ Sedapap Tablets 50 mg/650 mg (Among the most frequent) 2098
Sonata Capsules 1686
▲ Strattera Capsules (2% to 4%) 1784
Tessalon Capsules 1202

Tessalon Perles 1202
Thiothixene Capsules 2124
Tussionex Pennkinetic Extended-Release Suspension 3322
▲ Tylenol with Codeine (Among most frequent) 2461
Valcyte Tablets 2816
▲ Vicodin Tablets (Among most frequent) 530
▲ Vicodin ES Tablets (Among most frequent) 531
▲ Vicodin HP Tablets (Among most frequent) 532
▲ Wellbutrin Tablets (19.8%) 1579
▲ Xanax XR Tablets (45.2%) 2655
▲ Xeloda Tablets (Less than 5%) 2825
▲ Zofran Injection (8%) 1607
▲ Zofran (20%) 1613
▲ Zofran ODT Orally Disintegrating Tablets (20%) 1613
▲ Zydone Tablets (Among most frequent) 1118

Seizure control, loss of

Depakote Sprinkle Capsules 422

Seizures

(*see also under* Convulsions)

Abilify Tablets (0.1% to 0.3%) 916
Abilify Tablets (0.1% to 0.3%) 2472
Accutane Capsules 2740
Actimmune (Rare) 1646
Activase I.V. 1225
Adderall Tablets 3168
Adderall XR Capsules 3169
Agrylin Capsules 3172
Allegra-D 12 Hour Extended-Release Tablets 2860
Allegra-D 24 Hour Extended-Release Tablets 2862
Aloprim for Injection (Less than 1%) 2156
Amnesteem Capsules 2126
Aranesp for Injection (0.6% to 1%) 576
▲ Aredia for Injection (3% to 4%) 2168
Attenuvax (Rare) 1889
Avonex (4 in 351 patients) 839
Bayer Aspirin Tablets 3515
Carbatrol Capsules 3174
Carimune NF 3501
Carnitor Injection 3185
Carnitor Tablets and Oral Solution 3187
Ceftin Tablets 1369
Celexa (0.3%) 1177
Cipro XR Tablets 3004
▲ Clozapine Tablets (3% to 5%) 2141
▲ Clozaril Tablets (3% to approximately 5%) 2174
Combivir Tablets 1373
Comvax 1904
Dantrium Capsules (Less frequent) 2690
DDAVP Injection 4 mcg/mL (Rare) 2893
DDAVP Nasal Spray (Rare) 2894
▲ DepoCyt Injection (6.3%) 1121
Depo-Medrol Single-Dose Vial 2617
Desmopressin Acetate Injection (Rare) 1143
Dilaudid 439
Dilaudid Oral Liquid 443
Dilaudid Non-Sterile Powder 439
Dilaudid Tablets - 8 mg 443
Dilaudid-HP Injection 441
Diprivan Injectable Emulsion (Less than 1%) 676
Ecotrin Enteric Coated Aspirin Low, Regular and Maximum Strength Tablets 1627
Effexor XR Capsules (Infrequent) 3411
Eldepryl Capsules 3209
Enbrel for Injection 580
Engerix-B Vaccine (Less than 1%) 1391
Epogen for Injection (1.1% to approximately 2.5%) 586
Ery-Tab Tablets (Isolated reports) 447
Erythrocin Stearate Filmtab Tablets (Isolated reports) 452
Erythromycin Base Filmtab Tablets (Isolated reports) 454
Erythromycin Delayed-Release Capsules, USP (Isolated reports) 456
Ethyol for Injection (Rare) 1869
Flexeril Tablets (Less than 1%) 1832
Flumist Vaccine 1872
Focalin XR Capsules 2217
Fortaz 1422
Gammagard Liquid 751
Gammagard S/D 754
Gamunex Immune Globulin I.V., 10% 3232
Geodon Capsules (0.4%) 2514
Hexalen Capsules (1%) 2101
HibTITER (One case) 3419
▲ Idamycin PFS Injection (4%) 2645
Imitrex Nasal Spray (Rare) 1435
Imitrex Tablets (Rare) 1440
Infanrix Vaccine 1444
Infed Injection 3381
Invanz for Injection (Greater than 0.1%) 1974
I.V. Busulfex (2%, one patient) 1125
Iveegam EN 759
K-Phos Neutral Tablets 785
Lariam Tablets 2790
Leukeran Tablets (Rare) 1472
Levothroid Tablets 1189
Levoxyl Tablets (Rare) 1680
Maxipime for Injection 1093
Mefoxin for Injection 1987
Mefoxin Premixed Intravenous Solution 1990
Meridia Capsules (0.1%) 485
Merrem I.V. (Greater than 0.1% to 1%) 687
MS Contin Tablets (Less frequent) 2703
Myleran Tablets 1492
Nalfon Capsules (Less than 1%) 2504
Narcan Injection 1109
Niravam Orally Disintegrating Tablets 3106
Noroxin Tablets 2009
Norvir 499
Nubain Injection 1111
Omnicef Capsules 506
Omnicef for Oral Suspension 506
Orap Tablets 1220
Orthoclone OKT3 Sterile Solution 2370
OxyContin Tablets (Less than 1%) 2699
Pediarix Vaccine 1518
Liquid PedvaxHIB (Infrequent) 2012
PEG-Intron Powder for Injection 3062
Primaxin I.M. 2022
Primaxin I.V. (0.4%) 2024
Prinzide Tablets 2033
▲ Procrit for Injection (1.1% to 10%) 2374
ProSom Tablets (Infrequent) 512
Recombivax HB 2045
Remicade for IV Injection (Rare) 987
Retrovir Capsules (Rare; 0.8%) 1533
Retrovir IV Infusion (Rare; 1%) 1537
Retrovir (Rare; 0.8%) 1533
Risperdal M-Tab Orally Disintegrating Tablets (0.3%) 1658
Risperdal (0.3%) 1658
Rocephin Injectable Vials, ADD-Vantage, Galaxy, Bulk (Rare) 2801
▲ Roferon-A Injection (Less than 4%) 2805
Sandostatin Injection (Less than 1%) 2263
Seromycin Capsules 1783
Seroquel Tablets (0.6%) 691
Singulair (Very rare) 2047
St. Joseph 81 mg Aspirin Chewable and Enteric Coated Tablets 1841
Suprax 1811
Surmontil Capsules 2347
Tamiflu Capsules 2810
Tamiflu Oral Suspension 2810
Taxotere Injection Concentrate (Rare) 2947
Tegretol/Tegretol-XR 2278
Thiothixene Capsules 2124
Trizivir Tablets 1565
Ultane Liquid for Inhalation (Less than 1%) 526
Ultracet Tablets 2462
Unithroid Tablets (Rare) 3521
Urecholine Tablets 2349
Uroqid-Acid No. 2 Tablets 785
Valtrex Caplets 1573
Vaseretic Tablets 2073
Viagra Tablets 2552
Viracept (Less than 2%) 2556
Vivactil Tablets 2350
Wellbutrin Tablets (Frequent) 1579
Wellbutrin SR Sustained-Release Tablets (Approximately 0.1% to 0.4%) 1583
Wellbutrin XL Extended-Release Tablets (Approximately 0.1% to 0.4%) 1588
Xanax XR Tablets (Infrequent) 2655
Zinacef Injection 1604
Zinacef for Injection 1604
Zovirax Capsules 1616
Zovirax for Injection (Approximately 1%) 1618
Zovirax 1616
Zyban Sustained-Release Tablets 1620
Zyprexa Tablets (0.9%) 1798
Zyprexa ZYDIS Orally Disintegrating Tablets (0.9%) 1798
Zyrtec-D 12 Hour Extended Release Tablets 2591

Seizures, afebrile

Attenuvax 1889
M-M-R II 1980

Seizures, convulsive

Cipro I.V. (1% or less) 2998
Cipro I.V. Pharmacy Bulk Package (1% or less) 3509
Cipro (Less than 1%) 2991
Phenergan 3438
Thioridazine Hydrochloride Tablets (Infrequent) 2122
Timentin ADD-Vantage 1556
Timentin Injection Galaxy Container 1559
Timentin IV Infusion 1553
Timentin Pharmacy Bulk Package 1562

Seizures, epileptiform

Eskalith 1406
Lithobid Tablets 1670

Seizures, exacerbation of

Enbrel for Injection (Rare) 580
Lamictal (2.3%) 1449
Topamax Sprinkle Capsules (More than 1%) 2438
Topamax Tablets (More than 1%) 2438

Seizures, febrile

Attenuvax 1889
Comvax 1904
Flumist Vaccine 1872
HibTITER 3419
M-M-R II 1980
Mumpsvax 2005
Prevnar for Injection 3460
Recombivax HB 2045

Seizures, generalized

Leukeran Tablets (Rare) 1472
Noroxin Tablets 2009

Seizures, grand mal

Cipro I.V. (1% or less) 2998
Cipro I.V. Pharmacy Bulk Package (1% or less) 3509
Cipro XR Tablets 3004
Orap Tablets 1220
Pepcid Injection (Infrequent) 2017
Pepcid (Infrequent) 2014
Proleukin for Injection (1%) 1007
Topamax Sprinkle Capsules (1%) 2438
Topamax Tablets (1%) 2438
Zofran Injection (Rare) 1607
Zofran (Rare) 1613
Zofran ODT Orally Disintegrating Tablets (Rare) 1613

Seizures, neonatal

Captopril Tablets 2114

Seizures, non-febrile

Varivax 2070

Seminal volume, decrease in

Anadrol-50 Tablets 3329

Sensation, abnormal

(*see under* Paresthesia)

Sensation, abnormal, ocular

▲ Retisert Implant (10% to 35%) .... ⊙256

Sensation, disturbance of temperature

Amerge Tablets (Frequent) 1312
▲ Fabrazyme for Intravenous Infusion (5%) 1267
▲ Frova Tablets (3%) 1101
▲ Imitrex Injection (10.8%) 1431
Imitrex Nasal Spray (Infrequent) 1435
Imitrex Tablets (2% to 3%) 1440
Lidoderm Patch 1107
Maxalt Tablets (Infrequent) 1983
Maxalt-MLT Orally Disintegrating Tablets (Infrequent) 1983
Xanax XR Tablets (Infrequent) 2655
▲ Zomig Tablets (5% to 7%) 714
▲ Zomig-ZMT Tablets (5% to 7%) 714

Sensation, heavy

Amerge Tablets (Frequent) 1312
▲ Imitrex Injection (7.3%) 1431
Imitrex Nasal Spray (Infrequent) 1435
Imitrex Tablets (Less than 1% to 2%) 1440
Nubain Injection (1% or less) 1111

Sensation, lightness

Imitrex Nasal Spray (Infrequent) 1435

Sensation of pressure/tightness

Amerge Tablets (Frequent) 1312
▲ Imitrex Injection (5.1 to 7.1%) 1431
Imitrex Nasal Spray (Infrequent) 1435
Imitrex Tablets (Less than 1% to 2%) 1440
Maxalt Tablets (Less than 2%) 1983
Maxalt-MLT Orally Disintegrating Tablets (Less than 2%) 1983
Zomig Nasal Spray (Infrequent) 718
▲ Zomig Tablets (2% to 4%) 714
▲ Zomig-ZMT Tablets (2% to 4%) 714

Sensations, numbness

Lidoderm Patch 1107

Sensations, pulsating

Imitrex Injection (Infrequent) 1431
Imitrex Nasal Spray 1435
Imitrex Tablets (Infrequent) 1440

Sensitivity, light

Cipro 2991
Cipro XR Tablets 3004
▲ Orap Tablets (1 of 20 patients) 1220
Revatio Tablets 2541
Symmetrel (0.1% to 1%) 1115

Sensitivity, sun

Avita Cream (Some individuals) 2136
Avita Gel (Some individuals) 2138
Cipro 2991
Cipro XR Tablets 3004
Dantrium Capsules 2690
Renova 0.02% Cream 2384
Renova 0.05% Cream 2387
Retin-A Micro 0.1%/0.04% 2388
Tegrin Dandruff Shampoo - Extra Conditioning .... ▣637
Tegrin Dandruff Shampoo - Fresh Herbal .... ▣638
Tegrin Skin Cream .... ▣638

Sensitivity reactions

Aldara Cream, 5% (More than 1%) 1814
Bactroban Ointment 1358
Betadine 5% Ophthalmic Solution .... ⊙202
Betadine Skin Cleanser (Rare) 2714
Betasept Surgical Scrub 2715
Bleph-10 Ophthalmic Solution 10% (Rare) .... ⊙219
Brevoxyl-4 Creamy Wash 3212
Brevoxyl-4 Gel 3211
Brevoxyl-8 Creamy Wash 3212
Brevoxyl-8 Gel 3211
Combivir Tablets 1373
Creon 10 Capsules 3195
Creon 20 Capsules 3196
FML-S Liquifilm Sterile Ophthalmic Suspension .... ⊙226
HyperRAB (Occasional) 3239
HyperRho S/D Full Dose (Extremely rare) 3243
HyperRho S/D Mini-Dose (Extremely rare) 3241
HyperTET (Extremely rare) 3245
Polytrim Ophthalmic Solution (Rare) 570
Prinzide Tablets 2033
Repronex for Intramuscular and Subcutaneous Injection 1148
Retrovir Capsules (Rare) 1533
Retrovir IV Infusion (Rare) 1537
Retrovir 1533
Trusopt Sterile Ophthalmic Solution 2065
Children's Tylenol Suspension Liquid and Meltaways (Rare) 1850
Concentrated Tylenol Infants' Drops (Rare) 1850
Junior Tylenol Meltaways (Rare) 1850
Tylenol Allergy Complete Multi-Symptom Caplets and Gelcaps with Cool Burst (Rare) 1844
Tylenol Severe Allergy Caplets (Rare) 1844
Vaseretic Tablets 2073
Zestoretic Tablets 701

Sensorium, clouded

Blocadren Tablets 1891
Cosopt Sterile Ophthalmic Solution 1910
Inderal LA Long-Acting Capsules 3421
InnoPran XL Capsules 2728
Nadolol Tablets 2121
Tenormin I.V. Injection 698
Tenormin Tablets 695
Timolide Tablets 2056
Timoptic in Ocudose 2061
Timoptic Sterile Ophthalmic Solution 2058
Timoptic-XE Sterile Ophthalmic Gel Forming Solution 2062
Toprol-XL Tablets 660

Sensory disturbances

- Depo-Medrol Single-Dose Vial 2617
- ▲ Eloxatin for Injection (8%) 2908
- Hectorol Capsules 909
- Hectorol Injection 911
- ▲ Leukine (6%) 829
- Paxil CR Controlled-Release Tablets 1509
- Paxil 1501
- ▲ Prograf Capsules and Injection (Approximately 55%) 624
- ▲ Proleukin for Injection (10%) 1007
- Topamax Sprinkle Capsules (Greater than 1%) 2438
- Topamax Tablets (Greater than 1%) 2438
- ▲ Wellbutrin Tablets (4.0%) 1579

Sepsis

- ▲ Abelcet Injection (7%) 1119
- Actiq (1% or greater) 993
- Aloprim for Injection (Less than 1%) 2156
- ▲ AmBisome for Injection (7.4% to 14%) 615
- Ammonul Injection 3323
- Anaprox Tablets (Less than 1%) 2769
- Anaprox DS Tablets (Less than 1%) 2769
- Angiomax for Injection (Rare) 1856
- ▲ Aranesp for Injection (27%) 576
- Arava Tablets (Rare) 2881
- ▲ Argatroban Injection (6%) 1321
- Arthrotec Tablets (Rare) 3126
- Bexxar 1360
- ▲ Cafcit (4.3%) 1854
- ▲ Campath Ampules (10% to 15%) 826
- Camptosar Injection 2602
- ▲ Casodex Tablets (2% to 5%) 670
- Cataflam Tablets (Occasionally) 2173
- Cathflo Activase 1232
- ▲ CellCept Capsules (2% to 27.4%) 2751
- ▲ CellCept Intravenous (2% to 27.4%) 2751
- ▲ CellCept Oral Suspension (2% to 27.4%) 2751
- ▲ CellCept Tablets (2% to 27.4%) 2751
- ▲ Clolar for Intravenous Infusion (15%) 1264
- Clozapine Tablets 2141
- Clozaril Tablets 2174
- ▲ Copegus Tablets (3% to 5%) 2759
- ▲ Cytovene (4%) 2763
- Diprivan Injectable Emulsion (Less than 1%) 676
- ▲ Doxil Injection (Less than 1% to 5%) 3302
- EC-Naprosyn Delayed-Release Tablets (Less than 1%) 2769
- ▲ Elitek (3%) 2906
- Enbrel for Injection 580
- Epivir 1394
- ▲ Erbitux (3%) 937
- Evoxac Capsules (Less than 1%) 1042
- FazaClo Orally Disintegrating Tablets 547
- Ferrlecit Injection 3379
- ▲ Flolan for Injection (13% to 25%) 1408
- Gabitril Tablets (Infrequent) 998
- Gemzar for Injection (Less than 1%) 1743
- Gleevec Tablets (Infrequent) 2221
- ▲ Humira Injection (Less than 5%) 464
- ▲ Hycamtin for Injection (26%) 1427
- ▲ Infasurf Intratracheal Suspension (20% to 28%) 1188
- ▲ Intron A for Injection (Less than 5%) 3038
- ▲ Leukine (11%) 829
- Levaquin in 5% Dextrose Injection (0.1% to 0.9%) 2453
- Levaquin (0.1% to 0.9%) 2453
- Merrem I.V. (1.6%) 687
- Mycamine for Injection 620
- Myleran Tablets 1492
- ▲ Mylotarg for Injection (17% to 28%) 3429
- Naprosyn Suspension (Less than 1%) 2769
- Naprosyn Tablets (Less than 1%) 2769
- ▲ Navelbine Injection (8%) 1494
- Neurontin Capsules (Rare) 2498
- Neurontin Oral Solution (Rare) 2498
- Neurontin Tablets (Rare) 2498
- ▲ Nipent for Injection (3%) 3216
- Oncaspar (Less than 1%) 1123
- Orthoclone OKT3 Sterile Solution 2370
- Paxil CR Controlled-Release Tablets (Rare) 1509
- Paxil (Rare) 1501
- ▲ Pegasys (3% to 5%) 2793
- PEG-Intron Powder for Injection (Less than or equal to 1%) 3062
- Permax Tablets (Infrequent) 3357
- Photofrin for Injection (Occasional) 729
- Pravachol Tablets 943
- Prevnar for Injection 3460
- ▲ Prograf Capsules and Injection (3% to 15%) 624
- ▲ Proleukin for Injection (23%) 1007
- Pulmozyme Inhalation Solution 1245
- ▲ Rapamune Oral Solution and Tablets (3% to 20%) 3472
- Raptiva for Injection 1247
- ▲ Refludan for Injection (3.5%) 815
- Remicade for IV Injection (Greater than or equal to 0.2%) 987
- Requip Tablets (Infrequent) 1528
- Rilutek Tablets (Infrequent) 2945
- Rituxan for Infusion 845
- Rituxan I.V. (2%) 1251
- ▲ Simulect for Injection (3% to 10%) 2268
- Targretin Capsules 1719
- Thalomid Capsules 979
- ▲ Thymoglobulin for Injection (12.2%) 2848
- Ticlid Tablets (Rare) 2813
- Trasylol Injection (1% to 2%) 779
- ▲ Trisenox Injection (5%) 983
- ▲ Valcyte Tablets (Less than 5%) 2816
- VFEND I.V. (Less than 2%) 2543
- VFEND Oral Suspension (Less than 2%) 2543
- VFEND Tablets (Less than 2%) 2543
- Voltaren Tablets (Occasionally) 2298
- Voltaren-XR Tablets (Occasionally) 2301
- ▲ Xeloda Tablets (Less than 5%) 2825
- ▲ Zegerid Powder for Oral Solution (5.1%) 2972
- ▲ Zemplar Capsules (5%) 535
- ▲ Zemplar Injection (5%) 538
- Zevalin Injection (2%) 848
- ▲ Zinecard for Injection (12% to 17%) 2659
- Zoladex 3-month (1% to 5%) 712
- ▲ Zyvox (0% to 8%) 2661

Sepsis, neutropenic

- ▲ Alimta for Injection (6%) 1722
- Camptosar Injection 2602
- ▲ Xeloda Tablets (Less than 5%) 2825

Septic shock

- Aloprim for Injection (Less than 1%) 2156
- Ammonul Injection 3323
- Emend Capsules (Greater than 0.5%) 1944
- Enbrel for Injection 580
- Invanz for Injection (Greater than 0.1%) 1974
- Oncaspar (Less than 1%) 1123
- Tygacil for Injection (0% to less than 2%) 3489

Septicemia

- Bexxar 1360
- ▲ Gengraf Capsules (5.3%) 458
- Invanz for Injection (Greater than 0.1%) 1974
- ▲ Leustatin Injection (6%) 2368
- ▲ Neoral Soft Gelatin Capsules (5.3%) 2247
- ▲ Neoral Oral Solution (5.3%) 2247
- ▲ Sandimmune (4.8% to 5.3%) 2259
- Vesanoid Capsules 2823
- Zenapax for Injection 2838

Serositis

- Aceon Tablets (2 mg, 4 mg, 8 mg) 3191
- Vaseretic Tablets 2073
- Vasotec I.V. Injection (0.5% to 1.0%) 2076

Serotonin syndrome

- Celexa 1177
- Effexor Tablets 3405
- Effexor XR Capsules 3411
- Imitrex Injection 1431
- Imitrex Tablets 1440
- Lexapro Oral Solution 1193
- Lexapro Tablets 1193
- Meridia Capsules 485
- Paxil CR Controlled-Release Tablets 1509
- Paxil 1501
- Prozac Pulvules and Liquid 1771
- Zoloft 2581

Serous drainage

- Targretin Capsules 1719

Serum alkaline phosphatase, abnormal

- Invirase 2776
- Parcopa Orally Disintegrating Tablets 3111
- Vytorin 10/10 Tablets 2084
- Vytorin 10/10 Tablets 3092
- Vytorin 10/20 Tablets 2084
- Vytorin 10/20 Tablets 3092
- Vytorin 10/40 Tablets 2084
- Vytorin 10/40 Tablets 3092
- Vytorin 10/80 Tablets 2084
- Vytorin 10/80 Tablets 3092
- ▲ Zyvox (0.2% to 3.5%) 2661

Serum alkaline phosphatase, elevation

- Abelcet Injection 1119
- Abilify Tablets (Infrequent) 916
- Abilify Tablets (Infrequent) 2472
- Accutane Capsules 2740
- Aceon Tablets (2 mg, 4 mg, 8 mg) (0.3% to 1%) 3191
- Adalat CC Tablets (Rare) 2978
- Advicor Tablets 1694
- Altoprev Extended-Release Tablets 1151
- Ambien Tablets (Rare) 2867
- ▲ AmBisome for Injection (7.1% to 22.2%) 615
- Anadrol-50 Tablets 3329
- Ancef for Injection 1318
- ▲ Arimidex Tablets (2% to 5%) 665
- Arthrotec Tablets (Rare) 3126
- Asacol Delayed-Release Tablets 2688
- Augmentin (Infrequent) 1331
- Augmentin Tablets (Infrequent) 1334
- Augmentin XR Extended-Release Tablets (Infrequent) 1340
- Augmentin ES-600 Powder for Oral Suspension (Infrequently) 1337
- Axid Oral Solution (Less common) 913
- Azasan Tablets 2844
- BeneFix for Injection (1.6%) 3402
- Biaxin/Biaxin XL (Less than 1%) 402
- ▲ Buphenyl Powder (6%) 3327
- ▲ Buphenyl Tablets (6%) 3327
- Campath Ampules 826
- Campral Tablets (Rare) 1175
- ▲ Camptosar Injection (4% to 13%) 2602
- ▲ Cancidas for Injection (2.9% to 10.5%) 1894
- Captopril Tablets 2114
- Cardizem LA Extended Release Tablets (Less than 2%) 1699
- ▲ Casodex Tablets (2% to 5%) 670
- Ceftin 1369
- Celebrex Capsules (0.1% to 1.9%) 3130
- Celexa (Infrequent) 1177
- ▲ CellCept Capsules (3% to less than 20%) 2751
- ▲ CellCept Intravenous (3% to less than 20%) 2751
- ▲ CellCept Oral Suspension (3% to less than 20%) 2751
- ▲ CellCept Tablets (3% to less than 20%) 2751
- ▲ Chemet Capsules (4.2% to 10.4%) 2480
- ▲ Cipro I.V. (Among most frequent) 2998
- ▲ Cipro I.V. Pharmacy Bulk Package (Among most frequent) 3509
- Cipro (0.8%) 2991
- Colazal Capsules 2845
- ▲ Coreg Tablets (Greater than 1% to 3%) 1376
- Covera-HS Tablets 3135
- Cubicin for Injection (1% to 2%) 1038
- Cymbalta Delayed-Release Capsules 1729
- Depo-Medrol Single-Dose Vial 2617
- ▲ Doxil Injection (1.3% to 7.8%) 3302
- Effexor Tablets (Infrequent) 3405
- Effexor XR Capsules (Infrequent) 3411
- ▲ Eloxatin for Injection (0% to 4%) 2908
- Elspar for Injection 1943
- Emend Capsules (Greater than 0.5%) 1944
- Evoxac Capsules 1042
- Factive Tablets (0.3%) 2464
- ▲ Fortaz (1 in 23) 1422
- ▲ Gemzar for Injection (55% to 77%) 1743
- Geodon Capsules (Infrequent) 2514
- ▲ Gleevec Tablets (Up to 5.1%) 2221
- ▲ Hexalen Capsules (9%) 2101
- ▲ Humira Injection (5%) 464
- ▲ Intron A for Injection (Up to 13%) 3038
- ▲ Invanz for Injection (4.3% to 6.6%) 1974
- ▲ I.V. Busulfex (15%) 1125
- Ketek Tablets (Less than 0.2%) 2920
- Klonopin 2782
- Lamictal (Infrequent) 1449
- Lescol Capsules 2227
- Lescol Capsules 2730
- Lescol XL Tablets 2227
- Lescol XL Tablets 2730
- ▲ Leukine (8%) 829
- Lotronex Tablets 1479
- Maxipime for Injection (Greater than 0.1% to less than 1%) 1093
- Mefoxin for Injection 1987
- Mefoxin Premixed Intravenous Solution 1990
- ▲ Mepron Suspension (5% to 8%) 1487
- Meridia Capsules (1.6%) 485
- Merrem I.V. (Greater than 0.2%) 687
- Mevacor Tablets 1996
- Mycamine for Injection (1.5% to 2%) 620
- ▲ Mylotarg for Injection (5% to 10%) 3429
- ▲ Nabi-HB (4%) 2159
- Nalfon Capsules (Less than 1%) 2504
- Namenda (Frequent) 1199
- ▲ Neulasta Injection (9%) 596
- ▲ Neupogen for Injection (21% to 58%) 598
- Neurontin Capsules (Rare) 2498
- Neurontin Oral Solution (Rare) 2498
- Neurontin Tablets (Rare) 2498
- Nexium Delayed-Release Capsules (Less than 1%) 645
- Nexium I.V. (Less than 1%) 649
- Nimotop Capsules (0.2%; rare) 774
- Noroxin Tablets (1.1%) 2009
- NovoLog Mix 70/30 2331
- Nutropin for Injection 1238
- Nutropin AQ Injection 1241
- Nutropin AQ Pen 1241
- Nutropin AQ Pen Cartridge 1241
- Omnicef Capsules (0.3%) 506
- Omnicef for Oral Suspension (1%) 506
- Oxandrin Tablets 2977
- Paxil CR Controlled-Release Tablets (Rare) 1509
- Paxil (Rare) 1501
- Pentasa Capsules (Less than 1%) 3182
- Pravachol Tablets 943
- Prevacid Delayed-Release Capsules 3268
- Prevacid for Delayed-Release Oral Suspension 3268
- Prevacid NapraPAC 3277
- Prevacid SoluTab Delayed-Release Orally Disintegrating Tablets 3268
- PREVPAC (Less than 1%) 3281
- Prilosec OTC Tablets (Rare) 2674
- Primaxin I.M. 2022
- Primaxin I.V. 2024
- ▲ Prograf Capsules and Injection (3% to 15%) 624
- ▲ Proleukin for Injection (10%) 1007
- Protonix I.V. (Less than 1%) 3468
- Protonix Tablets (Less than 1%) 3465
- Prozac Pulvules and Liquid (Rare) 1771
- ▲ Rapamune Oral Solution and Tablets (3% to 20%) 3472
- ▲ Raptiva for Injection (4%) 1247
- Razadyne ER Extended-Release Capsules (Infrequent) 2434
- Razadyne (Infrequent) 2434
- Relpax Tablets (Rare) 2531
- Requip Tablets (Infrequent) 1528
- Rescriptor Tablets 2535
- Rilutek Tablets (Infrequent) 2945
- Rocephin Injectable Vials, ADD-Vantage, Galaxy, Bulk (Less than 1%) 2801
- ▲ Roferon-A Injection (0% to 3%) 2805
- ▲ Rythmol SR Capsules (3%) 2736
- Seroquel Tablets (Infrequent) 691
- Somavert Injection (Minimal) 2648
- Suprax (Less than 2%) 1811
- Symmetrel 1115
- Tabloid Tablets 1545
- Tambocor Tablets (Rare) 1824
- Tarka Tablets (2.8%) 519
- ▲ Taxotere Injection Concentrate (4.3%) 2947
- Tequin Injection (Less than 0.1%) 964
- Tequin Tablets (Less than 0.1%) 964
- Teveten Tablets 1707
- Teveten HCT Tablets 1710
- Thalomid Capsules 979
- Thiothixene Capsules 2124
- Tiazac Capsules (Less than 2%) 1204
- Timentin ADD-Vantage 1556
- Timentin Injection Galaxy Container 1559
- Timentin IV Infusion 1553
- Timentin Pharmacy Bulk Package 1562
- Topamax Sprinkle Capsules (Infrequent) 2438
- Topamax Tablets (Infrequent) 2438
- Toprol-XL Tablets 660
- Trelstar LA Suspension (1.7%) 3387
- ▲ Tygacil for Injection (3.5%) 3489
- Ultane Liquid for Inhalation (Less than 1%) 526
- Uniretic Tablets (Less than 1%) 3114
- ▲ Valtrex Caplets (4%) 1573
- Vantin Tablets and Oral Suspension 2650
- ▲ Ventavis Inhalation Solution (6%) 1036
- Verelan PM Capsules 3120

▲ VFEND I.V. (3.6% to 22.6%) 2543
▲ VFEND Oral Suspension (3.6% to 22.6%) 2543
▲ VFEND Tablets (3.6% to 22.6%) 2543
Viracept (Less than 2%) 2556
Zegerid Powder for Oral Solution (Rare) 2972
Zinacef Injection (1 in 50 patients).... 1604
Zinacef for Injection (1 in 50 patients) 1604
Zithromax Capsules, 250 mg (Less than 1%) 2568
Zithromax for IV Infusion (Less than 1%) 2573
Zithromax for Oral Suspension, 1 g (Less than 1%) 2568
Zithromax for Oral Suspension, 300 mg, 600 mg, 900 mg, 1200 mg (Less than 1%) 2561
Zithromax Tablets, 250 mg, 500 mg (Less than 1%) 2561
Zithromax Tablets, 600 mg (Less than 1%) 2568
Zithromax Tri-Pak (Less than 1%) 2561
Zithromax Z-Pak (Less than 1%) 2568
Zocor Tablets 2078
Zomig Tablets (Rare) 714
Zomig-ZMT Tablets (Rare) 714
Zonegran Capsules 1089
Zosyn 3492
Zyprexa Tablets (Infrequent) 1798
Zyprexa ZYDIS Orally Disintegrating Tablets (Infrequent) 1798

Serum alkaline phosphatase, changes
Oxandrin Tablets 2977

Serum aminotransferase, elevation
Arixtra Injection (1.7% to 2.6%) 1325

Serum amylase, abnormal
Zyvox (0.2% to 2.4%) 2661

Serum amylase, elevation
Abelcet Injection 1119
AmBisome for Injection (Less common) 615
Aptivus Capsules (2.9%) 859
Avelox (0.1% to less than 2%) 2984
▲ Baraclude (2% to 3%) 928
Cipro I.V. (1% or less) 2998
Cipro I.V. Pharmacy Bulk Package (1% or less) 3509
Cipro (Less than 1%) 2991
Cipro XR Tablets 3004
Colazal Capsules 2845
Combunox Tablets 1183
Crixivan Capsules (2.1%) 1918
Cuprimine Capsules (Few cases) 1925
▲ Emtriva Capsules (2% to 5%) 1272
▲ Epivir (3% to 4.2%) 1394
Epivir-HBV (Less than 1%) 1398
Epzicom Tablets 1402
▲ Evoxac Capsules (1% to 3%) 1042
Famvir Tablets (1.5%) 2207
Fuzeon Injection 2772
▲ Hepsera Tablets (4%) 1275
Invirase (1% to 2%) 2776
Kadian Capsules 572
▲ Kaletra (3% to 8%) 474
▲ Kepivance (38% to 62%) 592
▲ Mepron Suspension (1% to 8%) 1487
Niaspan Extended-Release Tablets ... 1703
Omnicef Capsules 506
Omnicef for Oral Suspension 506
Oncaspar (Less than 1%) 1123
Pentasa Capsules (Less than 1%) 3182
Rescriptor Tablets (2.5% to 2.9%) 2535
▲ Sustiva Capsules (10%) 957
Targretin Capsules 1719
Tequin Injection (Less than 0.1%) 964
Tequin Tablets (Less than 0.1%) 964
▲ Truvada Tablets (1% to 12%) 1279
▲ Tygacil for Injection (3.1%) 3489
Uniretic Tablets (Less than 1%) 3114
Viracept (Less than 2%) 2556
▲ Viread Tablets (6% to 7%) 1284
▲ Zerit (14%) 971
▲ Ziagen (4%) 1600

Serum bicarbonate, decrease
Cancidas for Injection (0% to 0.9%) 1894
Omnicef Capsules (0.6%) 506
Omnicef for Oral Suspension (1%) 506
Zmax for Oral Suspension (Greater than or equal to 1%) 2577

Serum bicarbonate, increase
Cubicin for Injection (Less than 1%) 1038
Zithromax for Oral Suspension, 300 mg, 600 mg, 900 mg, 1200 mg (Less than 1%) 2561
Zithromax Tablets, 250 mg, 500 mg (Less than 1%) 2561
Zithromax Tri-Pak (Less than 1%) 2561

Serum bicarbonate content, variations
▲ Prograf Capsules and Injection (3% to 15%) 624

Serum bilirubin, elevation
(*see under* Hyperbilirubinemia)

Serum bilirubin levels, abnormalities
Amerge Tablets (Rare) 1312
Emcyt Capsules (1% to 2%) 3137
Parcopa Orally Disintegrating Tablets 3111
Vytorin 10/10 Tablets 2084
Vytorin 10/10 Tablets 3092
Vytorin 10/20 Tablets 2084
Vytorin 10/20 Tablets 3092
Vytorin 10/40 Tablets 2084
Vytorin 10/40 Tablets 3092
Vytorin 10/80 Tablets 2084
Vytorin 10/80 Tablets 3092
▲ Zyvox (0.2% to 6.3%) 2661

Serum calcium, depression
(*see under* Hypocalcemia)

Serum calcium decrease
(*see under* Hypocalcemia)

Serum cholesterol, increase
(*see under* Hypercholesterolemia)

Serum creatine phosphokinase, elevation
Abilify Tablets (Frequent) 916
Abilify Tablets (Frequent) 2472
Accutane Capsules 2740
ActoPlus Met Tablets 3219
▲ Antara Capsules (3%) 2723
Aricept Tablets (Infrequent) 1086
Aricept ODT Tablets (Infrequent) 1086
Arthrotec Tablets (Rare) 3126
Benicar HCT Tablets (Greater than 1%) 2852
Caduet Tablets (Less than 2%) 2507
Catapres Tablets (Rare) 874
▲ Cipro I.V. (Among most frequent) 2998
▲ Cipro I.V. Pharmacy Bulk Package (Among most frequent) 3509
Clorpres Tablets (Rare) 2139
Cymbalta Delayed-Release Capsules 1729
Epzicom Tablets 1402
Factive Tablets (0.6%) 2464
FazaClo Orally Disintegrating Tablets 547
▲ Fuzeon Injection (2.3% to 5.9%) 2772
Geodon Capsules (Infrequent) 2514
Gleevec Tablets (Infrequent) 2221
Havrix Vaccine (Less than 1%) 1425
▲ Invirase (7% to 12%) 2776
Lipitor Tablets (Less than 2%) 2495
Mirapex Tablets (1% or more) 889
▲ Norvir (0.9% to 3.4%) 499
Protonix I.V. 3468
Protonix Tablets 3465
Prozac Pulvules and Liquid (Rare) 1771
Relpax Tablets (Infrequent) 2531
Requip Tablets (Infrequent) 1528
Risperdal M-Tab Orally Disintegrating Tablets (Infrequent) 1658
Risperdal (Infrequent) 1658
Sular Tablets (Less than or equal to 1%) 1163
Suprane Liquid for Inhalation (Less than 1%) 770
Symmetrel (Uncommon) 1115
Trasylol Injection (2%) 779
▲ Triglide Tablets (3%) 1165
Trizivir Tablets 1565
Viracept (Less than 2%) 2556
Zelnorm Tablets 2303
▲ Ziagen (8%) 1600
Zithromax (1% to 2%) 2568
Zithromax for Oral Suspension, 300 mg, 600 mg, 900 mg, 1200 mg (1% to 2%) 2561
Zithromax Tablets, 250 mg, 500 mg (1% to 2%) 2561
Zithromax Tablets, 600 mg (1% to 2%) 2568
Zithromax Tri-Pak (1% to 2%) 2561
Zithromax Z-Pak (1% to 2%) 2568
▲ Zocor Tablets (About 5% of patients) 2078
Zyprexa IntraMuscular (Infrequent)... 1798

Serum creatinine, abnormal
Zyvox (0.4% to 2.4%) 2661

Serum creatinine, elevation
▲ Abelcet Injection (11%) 1119
Abilify Tablets (Infrequent) 916
Abilify Tablets (Infrequent) 2472
Aceon Tablets (2 mg, 4 mg, 8 mg) (0.3% to 1%) 3191
▲ Alimta for Injection (Up to 16%) 1722
Alinia for Oral Suspension (Less than 1%) 2840
Alinia Tablets (Less than 1%) 2840
Aloprim for Injection (Less than 1%) 2156
Altace Capsules (1.2% to 1.5%) 1673
▲ AmBisome for Injection (18.5% to 22.4%) 615
Amnesteem Capsules 2126
Anadrol-50 Tablets 3329
Ancef for Injection (Very rare) 1318
▲ AndroGel (3% to 6%) 3330
Antara Capsules 2723
▲ Aredia for Injection (9.1%) 2168
Asacol Delayed-Release Tablets 2688
Atacand Tablets (Infrequent) 634
Avalide Tablets (Less than 0.7%) 922
Avalide Tablets (Less than 0.7%) 2889
Avapro Tablets (Less than 0.7%) 925
Avapro Tablets (Less than 0.7%) 2886
Baraclude (0% to 2%) 928
Benicar Tablets 2850
Benicar HCT Tablets (Rare) 2852
Biaxin/Biaxin XL (Less than 1%) 402
Campral Tablets (Rare) 1175
▲ Cancidas for Injection (0% to 3.7%) 1894
Capastat Sulfate for Injection (A significant number of patients) 1728
Captopril Tablets 2114
Carimune NF 3501
▲ Casodex Tablets (2% to 5%) 670
Caverject Impulse Injection (Less than 1%) 2610
Ceftin 1369
Celebrex Capsules (0.1% to 1.9%) ... 3130
▲ CellCept Capsules (3% to 39.4%) 2751
▲ CellCept Intravenous (3% to 39.4%) 2751
▲ CellCept Oral Suspension (3% to 39.4%) 2751
▲ CellCept Tablets (3% to 39.4%) 2751
▲ Cipro I.V. (Among most frequent) 2998
▲ Cipro I.V. Pharmacy Bulk Package (Among most frequent) 3509
Cipro (1.1%) 2991
▲ Clolar for Intravenous Infusion (6%) 1264
▲ Coreg Tablets (Greater than 1% to 3%) 1376
Cozaar Tablets (Less than 0.1%) 1913
Crixivan Capsules 1918
Cymbalta Delayed-Release Capsules (Infrequent) 1729
CytoGam Intravenous 1866
▲ Cytovene (Up to 43%) 2763
Didronel Tablets 2693
Diovan HCT Tablets 2195
▲ Diovan Tablets (0.6% to 4.2%) 2191
Diprivan Injectable Emulsion (Less than 1%) 676
Doxil Injection (Less than 1%) 3302
Dyazide Capsules 1389
Dyrenium Capsules (Rare) 3390
Effexor Tablets (Infrequent) 3405
Effexor XR Capsules (Infrequent) 3411
▲ Eloxatin for Injection (5% to 10%) ... 2908
▲ Emend Capsules (3.7%) 1944
Eulexin Capsules 3023
Factive Tablets (0.2%) 2464
Famvir Tablets (0.2%) 2207
Fortaz (Occasional) 1422
Gammagard S/D 754
Garamycin Injectable 3028
▲ Gemzar for Injection (Up to 8%) 1743
▲ Gengraf Capsules (18% to 48%) 458
Geodon Capsules (Rare) 2514
▲ Gleevec Tablets (Up to 3%) 2221
Guanidine Hydrochloride Tablets 3030
▲ Hepsera Tablets (2% to 4%) 1275
▲ Hexalen Capsules (7%) 2101
Hyzaar (0.8%) 1964
Indapamide Tablets (Less than 5%) .. 2119
Indocin I.V. 1973
▲ Inspra Tablets (0.2% to 6.5%) 2520
▲ Intron A for Injection (Up to 3%) 3038
Invanz for Injection (0.9% to 1.1%) ... 1974
▲ I.V. Busulfex (21%) 1125
Iveegam EN (0.3% to 0.8%) 759
Lamictal (Rare) 1449
▲ Leukine (15%) 829
Lofibra Capsules 1217
Lotensin Tablets (2%) 2232
Lotensin HCT Tablets 2235
Lotrel Capsules 2238
Lupron Depot 7.5 mg (Greater than or equal to 5%) 3261
▲ Mavik Tablets (1.1% to 4.7%) 482
Maxipime for Injection (Greater than 0.1% to less than 1%) 1093
Maxzide 2150
Mefoxin for Injection 1987
Mefoxin Premixed Intravenous Solution 1990
Mepron Suspension (1%) 1487
Merrem I.V. (Greater than 0.2%) 687
Mobic Oral Suspension (Less than 2%) 893
Mobic Tablets (Less than 2%) 893
Mycamine for Injection (0.2% to 0.6%) 620
▲ Myfortic Tablets (3% to less than 20%) 2244
Nabi-HB (2%) 2159
Natrecor for Injection (Greater than or equal to 1%) 3123
▲ Navelbine Injection (2% to 37%) 1494
▲ Neoral Soft Gelatin Capsules (18% to 48%) 2247
▲ Neoral Oral Solution (18% to 48%) 2247
▲ Nipent for Injection (3% to 10%) 3216
Noroxin Tablets (Less frequent) 2009
Oncaspar 1123
▲ Ontak Vials (7%) 1717
Oxandrin Tablets 2977
Parcopa Orally Disintegrating Tablets 3111
Plavix Tablets 940
Plavix Tablets 2942
Pletal Tablets (Less than 2%) 2478
Prevacid Delayed-Release Capsules 3268
Prevacid for Delayed-Release Oral Suspension 3268
Prevacid NapraPAC 3277
Prevacid SoluTab Delayed-Release Orally Disintegrating Tablets 3268
PREVPAC (Less than 1%) 3281
Prilosec OTC Tablets (Less than 1%) 2674
Primaxin I.M. 2022
Primaxin I.V. 2024
▲ Prinivil Tablets (About 2.0% to approximately 11.6%) 2029
Prinzide Tablets 2033
▲ Prograf Capsules and Injection (24% to 39%) 624
▲ Proleukin for Injection (33%) 1007
Protopic Ointment (Greater than or equal to 1%) 629
▲ Rapamune Oral Solution and Tablets (35% to 40%) 3472
Rescriptor Tablets 2535
Rocephin Injectable Vials, ADD-Vantage, Galaxy, Bulk (Less than 1%) 2801
Roferon-A Injection 2805
Rythmol SR Capsules 2736
Sandimmune 2259
Sandostatin LAR Depot (Rare) 2264
Sular Tablets (Less than or equal to 1%) 1163
Suprax (Less than 2%) 1811
Symbyax Capsules (Rare) 1788
Symmetrel 1115
Tagamet Tablets 1547
Targretin Capsules 1719
Testim 1% Gel (Less than 1%) 722
Teveten Tablets (1.3%) 1707
Teveten HCT Tablets (0.6%) 1710
Thalomid Capsules 979
Timentin ADD-Vantage 1556
Timentin Injection Galaxy Container 1559
Timentin IV Infusion 1553
Timentin Pharmacy Bulk Package 1562
Topamax Sprinkle Capsules (Rare) 2438
Topamax Tablets (Rare) 2438
▲ Trasylol Injection (18% to 21%) 779
Tricor Tablets 523
Trizivir Tablets 1565
Truvada Tablets 1279
Tygacil for Injection (0% to less than 2%) 3489
Ultane Liquid for Inhalation (Less than 1%) 526
Ultracet Tablets 2462
Uniretic Tablets (Less than 1%) 3114
Univasc Tablets (1%) 3118
Urso 250 Tablets (1%) 737
Urso Forte Tablets (1%) 737
Valtrex Caplets (Up to 0.7%) 1573

Vancocin HCl Capsules, USP (Rare) ... 3370
Vantin Tablets and Oral Suspension ... 2650
▲ Vaseretic Tablets (About 0.6% to 20%) ... 2073
▲ Vasotec I.V. Injection (About 0.2% to 20%) ... 2076
▲ VFEND I.V. (0% to 21.4%) ... 2543
▲ VFEND Oral Suspension (0% to 21.4%) ... 2543
▲ VFEND Tablets (0% to 21.4%) ... 2543
Viread Tablets ... 1284
▲ Visudyne for Injection (1% to 10%) .. 2286
Zantac (Rare) ... 1597
Zantac Injection ... 1593
Zantac Injection Pharmacy Bulk Package (Rare) ... 1595
Zantac Syrup (Rare) ... 1597
Zegerid Powder for Oral Solution (Less than 1%) ... 2972
Zestoretic Tablets ... 701
Zestril Tablets (About 2.0%) ... 704
Ziagen ... 1600
Zinacef Injection ... 1604
Zinacef for Injection ... 1604
Zithromax Capsules, 250 mg (Less than 1%) ... 2568
▲ Zithromax for IV Infusion (4% to 6%) ... 2573
Zithromax for Oral Suspension, 1 g (Less than 1%) ... 2568
Zithromax for Oral Suspension, 300 mg, 600 mg, 900 mg, 1200 mg (Less than 1%) ... 2561
Zithromax Tablets, 250 mg, 500 mg (Less than 1%) ... 2561
Zithromax Tablets, 600 mg (Less than 1%) ... 2568
Zithromax Tri-Pak (Less than 1%) ... 2561
Zithromax Z-Pak (Less than 1%) ... 2568
Zometa for Intravenous Infusion (0.4% to 1.3%) ... 2306
Zonegran Capsules ... 1089
Zosyn ... 3492
Zovirax Capsules ... 1616
▲ Zovirax for Injection (5% to 10%) ... 1618
Zovirax ... 1616

Serum electrolyte changes
(*see under* Electrolyte imbalance)

Serum folate levels, decreased
Lo/Ovral-28 Tablets ... 3423
Seasonale Tablets ... 1073

Serum gastrin levels, increased
Nexium Delayed-Release Capsules (Less than 1%) ... 645
Nexium I.V. (Less than 1%) ... 649
Prevacid NapraPAC ... 3277

Serum lipase, abnormal
Zyvox (0.4% to 2.3%) ... 2661

Serum lipase, elevation
Aptivus Capsules (Less than 2%) ... 859
▲ Baraclude (7% to 8%) ... 928
Cipro I.V. (1% or less) ... 2998
Cipro I.V. Pharmacy Bulk Package (1% or less) ... 3509
Cipro (Less than 1%) ... 2991
Cipro XR Tablets ... 3004
Emtriva Capsules (Less than 1%) ... 1272
▲ Epivir-HBV (10%) ... 1398
Epzicom Tablets ... 1402
▲ Famvir Tablets (4.9%) ... 2207
▲ Fuzeon Injection (2.3% to 5.9%) ... 2772
▲ Kepivance (11% to 28%) ... 592
▲ Lexiva Tablets (8%) ... 1473
Oncaspar ... 1123
Pentasa Capsules (Less than 1%) ... 3182
Rescriptor Tablets ... 2535
▲ Truvada Tablets (1% to 12%) ... 1279

Serum Lipids, changes in
Avandamet Tablets ... 1343
Aygestin Tablets ... 1062
Reyataz Capsules (Less than 3%) ... 948
Striant Mucoadhesive ... 1022

Serum PBI levels, decrease
(*see under* PBI decrease)

Serum phosphorus, elevation
▲ Lupron Depot 3.75 mg (Approximately 5% to 8%) ... 3257
Maxipime for Injection (Greater than 0.1% to less than 1%) ... 1093
Nutropin for Injection ... 1238
Nutropin AQ Injection ... 1241
Nutropin AQ Pen ... 1241
Nutropin AQ Pen Cartridge ... 1241
Omnicef Capsules (0.6%) ... 506
Omnicef for Oral Suspension (0.9%) ... 506

Serum potassium, reduction
(*see under* Hypokalemia)

Serum proteins, changes
▲ Cancidas for Injection (Up to 3.1%) ... 1894
Premarin Tablets ... 3443
Premphase Tablets ... 3452
Prempro Tablets ... 3452

Serum sickness
Amoxil Capsules ... 1315
Amoxil Chewable Tablets ... 1315
Amoxil Pediatric Drops for Oral Suspension ... 1315
Amoxil Powder for Oral Suspension ... 1315
Amoxil Tablets ... 1315
Antivenin (Black Widow Spider Antivenin) ... 1887
Augmentin ... 1331
Augmentin Tablets ... 1334
Augmentin XR Extended-Release Tablets ... 1340
Augmentin ES-600 Powder for Oral Suspension ... 1337
Axid Oral Solution (Rare) ... 913
Bexxar ... 1360
Campath Ampules ... 826
Ceftin ... 1369
Copaxone for Injection (Infrequent) .. 3292
Dynacin Tablets ... 1859
Engerix-B Vaccine (Less than 1%) ... 1391
Levaquin in 5% Dextrose Injection (Rare) ... 2453
Levaquin (Rare) ... 2453
Levothroid Tablets ... 1189
Levoxyl Tablets ... 1680
Mefoxin for Injection ... 1987
Mefoxin Premixed Intravenous Solution ... 1990
Orthoclone OKT3 Sterile Solution ... 2370
Plavix Tablets ... 940
Pneumovax 23 (Rare) ... 2020
PREVPAC ... 3281
Recombivax HB (Less than 1%) ... 2045
Remicade for IV Injection (Greater than or equal to 0.2%) ... 987
Rituxan for Infusion (Less than 0.1%) ... 845
Rituxan I.V. (Less than 0.1%) ... 1251
Rocephin Injectable Vials, ADD-Vantage, Galaxy, Bulk (Rare) ... 2801
Suprax (Less than 2%) ... 1811
Ticlid Tablets (Rare) ... 2813
Twinrix Vaccine ... 1571
Unithroid Tablets ... 3521
Vantin Tablets and Oral Suspension ... 2650
Wellbutrin Tablets ... 1579
Wellbutrin SR Sustained-Release Tablets ... 1583
Wellbutrin XL Extended-Release Tablets ... 1588
Zoloft ... 2581

Serum sickness-like reaction
Cipro I.V. ... 2998
Cipro I.V. Pharmacy Bulk Package ... 3509
Cipro ... 2991
Cipro XR Tablets ... 3004
Raptiva for Injection (1 patient) ... 1247

Serum transaminase, elevation
Advicor Tablets ... 1694
Altoprev Extended-Release Tablets .. 1151
Aricept Tablets (Infrequent) ... 1086
Aricept ODT Tablets (Infrequent) ... 1086
Augmentin (Infrequent) ... 1331
Augmentin Tablets (Infrequent) ... 1334
Augmentin XR Extended-Release Tablets (Infrequent) ... 1340
Augmentin ES-600 Powder for Oral Suspension (Infrequently) ... 1337
Azasan Tablets ... 2844
Benicar Tablets ... 2850
▲ Buphenyl Powder (4%) ... 3327
▲ Buphenyl Tablets (4%) ... 3327
Captopril Tablets ... 2114
▲ Chemet Capsules (6% to 10%) ... 2480
Concerta Extended-Release Tablets ... 1828
Covera-HS Tablets ... 3135
Depacon Injection (Frequent) ... 412
Depakene (Frequent) ... 417
Depakote Tablets (Frequent) ... 427
Depakote ER Tablets (Frequent) ... 433
Dynacin Tablets ... 1859
Enbrel for Injection ... 580
Eulexin Capsules ... 3023
Focalin Tablets ... 2214
Focalin XR Capsules ... 2217
Garamycin Injectable ... 3028
▲ Gemzar for Injection (Approximately two-thirds) ... 1743
Geodon Capsules (Infrequent) ... 2514
▲ Gleevec Tablets (3% to 6%) ... 2221
▲ Intron A for Injection (Less than 5%) ... 3038
Invirase (Isolated cases) ... 2776
Ketek Tablets (Greater than or equal to 0.2% to less than 2%) ... 2920
Klonopin ... 2782
▲ Lariam Tablets (Among most frequent) ... 2790
Lescol Capsules ... 2227
Lescol Capsules ... 2730
Lescol XL Tablets ... 2227
Lescol XL Tablets ... 2730
Leustatin Injection ... 2368
Lofibra Capsules ... 1217
▲ Lupron Depot–3 Month 11.25 mg (3%) ... 3262
Marinol Capsules (Less than 1%) ... 3334
Mavik Tablets (0.8% of patients) ... 482
Metadate CD Capsules ... 3316
Mevacor Tablets (1.9%) ... 1996
Mycamine for Injection (0.2% to 0.8%) ... 620
Mylotarg for Injection (13 Patients) .. 3429
Navelbine Injection ... 1494
Niaspan Extended-Release Tablets ... 1703
Norvir ... 499
▲ Ontak Vials (61%) ... 1717
Pacerone Tablets ... 3337
Paxil CR Controlled-Release Tablets ... 1509
Paxil ... 1501
Plendil Extended-Release Tablets (Two episodes) ... 651
Pravachol Tablets ... 943
Precose Tablets ... 776
▲ Proleukin for Injection (56%) ... 1007
Prometrium Capsules (100 mg, 200 mg) ... 3205
Prozac Pulvules and Liquid ... 1771
Remicade for IV Injection ... 987
Ritalin Hydrochloride Tablets (Some instances) ... 2254
Ritalin LA Capsules ... 2255
Ritalin-SR Tablets (Some instances) ... 2254
▲ Roferon-A Injection (Up to 50%) ... 2805
Seromycin Capsules ... 1783
Somavert Injection ... 2648
Tagamet Tablets ... 1547
Tambocor Tablets (Rare) ... 1824
Thiothixene Capsules ... 2124
Ticlid Tablets (Rare) ... 2813
Tindamax ... 2670
Toprol-XL Tablets ... 660
▲ Trasylol Injection (5%) ... 779
Tricor Tablets ... 523
Trileptal Oral Suspension ... 2281
Trileptal Tablets ... 2281
Verelan PM Capsules ... 3120
▲ Viramune Oral Suspension (8.8%) ... 903
▲ Viramune Tablets (8.8%) ... 903
Vytorin 10/10 Tablets ... 2084
Vytorin 10/10 Tablets ... 3092
Vytorin 10/20 Tablets ... 2084
Vytorin 10/20 Tablets ... 3092
Vytorin 10/40 Tablets ... 2084
Vytorin 10/40 Tablets ... 3092
Vytorin 10/80 Tablets ... 2084
Vytorin 10/80 Tablets ... 3092
Zelnorm Tablets ... 2303
Zetia Tablets (0.5%) ... 2090
Zetia Tablets (0.5%) ... 3098
Zocor Tablets (1%) ... 2078
Zofran ... 1613
Zofran ODT Orally Disintegrating Tablets ... 1613
Zovirax for Injection (1% to 2%) ... 1618
Zyrtec Chewable Tablets (Occasional) ... 2589
Zyrtec (Occasional) ... 2589
Zyrtec-D 12 Hour Extended Release Tablets (Occasional) ... 2591

Serum triglyceride, elevation
(*see under* Hypertriglyceridemia)

Serum vitamin B_{12} levels, subnormal
▲ Avandamet Tablets (7%) ... 1343

Sex hormone binding globulin, elevated
Prempro Tablets ... 3452

Sexual activity, decrease
▲ Catapres Tablets (About 3 in 100 patients) ... 874
Catapres-TTS (0.5% or less) ... 875
Clorpres Tablets (About 3%) ... 2139
Risperdal M-Tab Orally Disintegrating Tablets (Frequent) ... 1658
Risperdal (Frequent) ... 1658

Sexual dysfunction
Aceon Tablets (2 mg, 4 mg, 8 mg) (0.3% to 1.4%) ... 3191
Avalide Tablets ... 922
Avalide Tablets ... 2889
Avapro Tablets (Less than 1%) ... 925
Avapro Tablets (Less than 1%) ... 2886
Bentyl Capsules ... 724
Bentyl Injection ... 724
Bentyl Syrup ... 724
Bentyl Tablets ... 724
Caduet Tablets (Greater that 0.1% to 2%) ... 2507
Campral Tablets (Infrequent) ... 1175
Cardizem LA Extended Release Tablets (Less than 2%) ... 1699
Catapres-TTS (2 of 101 patients) ... 875
Celexa ... 1177
Copaxone for Injection (Infrequent) .. 3292
Effexor Tablets (2%) ... 3405
Effexor XR Capsules ... 3411
Eldepryl Capsules ... 3209
Eskalith ... 1406
Evoxac Capsules (Less than 1%) ... 1042
Geodon Capsules (Infrequent) ... 2514
Gleevec Tablets (Infrequent) ... 2221
Lexapro Oral Solution ... 1193
Lexapro Tablets ... 1193
Lithobid Tablets ... 1670
Lotronex Tablets (Rare) ... 1479
Maxzide ... 2150
Micardis HCT Tablets ... 886
Naropin Injection ... 640
Neurontin Capsules (Infrequent) ... 2498
Neurontin Oral Solution (Infrequent) ... 2498
Neurontin Tablets (Infrequent) ... 2498
▲ Niravam Orally Disintegrating Tablets (7.4%) ... 3106
Norvasc Tablets (Less than 1% to 2%) ... 2529
▲ Paxil CR Controlled-Release Tablets (3.7% to 10.0%) ... 1509
▲ Paxil (3.7% to 10.0%) ... 1501
Risperdal M-Tab Orally Disintegrating Tablets (Frequent) ... 1658
Risperdal (Frequent) ... 1658
Roferon-A Injection (Infrequent) ... 2805
▲ Strattera Capsules (3% or greater) ... 1784
Tiazac Capsules (Less than 2%) ... 1204
Vantas (Less than 2%) ... 3367
Viracept (Less than 2%) ... 2556
Wellbutrin Tablets (Frequent) ... 1579
Xanax XR Tablets (2.4%) ... 2655
▲ Zoladex (21%) ... 709
▲ Zoladex 3-month (One of the two most common) ... 712
Zoloft (Frequent) ... 2581

Sexual maturity, accelerated
Lupron Depot-PED 7.5 mg, 11.25 mg and 15 mg (Less than 2%) ... 3266
Lupron Injection Pediatric (Less than 2%) ... 3256

SGOT changes
(*see under* Aspartate aminotransferase levels, changes in)

SGOT elevation
(*see under* Aspartate aminotransferase levels, elevation of)

SGPT changes
(*see under* Alanine aminotransferase levels, changes in)

SGPT elevation
(*see under* Alanine aminotransferase levels, elevation of)

Shaking
(*see under* Tremors)

Shivering
(*see under* Tremors)

Shock
Abelcet Injection (Rare) ... 1119

Actiq 993
Adacel Vaccine 2959
AquaMEPHYTON Injection 1887
Boostrix (Rarely) 1366
Campral Tablets (Rare) 1175
Coumadin for Injection 932
Coumadin Tablets 932
Desferal Vials 2190
Dilaudid 439
Dilaudid Oral Liquid 443
Dilaudid Non-Sterile Powder 439
Dilaudid Rectal Suppositories 439
Dilaudid Tablets 439
Dilaudid Tablets - 8 mg 443
Dilaudid-HP 441
Doxil Injection (Less than 1%) 3302
Effexor Tablets 3405
Effexor XR Capsules 3411
Elitek 2906
Ellence Injection 2632
Ferrlecit Injection 3379
▲ Flolan for Injection (5%) 1408
Fluorescite Injection ⊙ 207
Herceptin I.V. (At least one of the 958 patients) 1234
Hyalgan Solution (One case) 2917
Hyperstat I.V. Injection 3031
Imitrex Injection 1431
Imitrex Nasal Spray 1435
Imitrex Tablets 1440
Indocin Capsules (Less than 1%) 1968
Indocin I.V. (Less than 1%) 1973
Indocin (Less than 1%) 1968
Infanrix Vaccine 1444
Infed Injection 3381
Kadian Capsules 572
Lidoderm Patch (Rare) 1107
Lyrica Capsules (Rare) 2524
Merrem I.V. (1.2%) 687
Midamor Tablets 2000
Migranal Nasal Spray (Rare) 3350
Mobic Oral Suspension (Less than 0.1%) 893
Mobic Tablets (Less than 0.1%) 893
Children's Motrin Oral Suspension and Chewable Tablets ▣ 647
Children's Motrin Non-Staining Dye-Free Oral Suspension ▣ 647
Children's Motrin Oral Suspension and Chewable Tablets 1837
Children's Motrin Cold Non-Staining Dye-Free Oral Suspension 1838
Children's Motrin Cold Oral Suspension 1838
Children's Motrin Non-Staining Dye-Free Oral Suspension 1837
Motrin Cold & Sinus Caplets 1836
Motrin IB Tablets and Caplets 1836
Infants' Motrin Concentrated Drops 1837
Infants' Motrin Non-Staining Dye-Free Drops 1837
Junior Strength Motrin Caplets and Chewable Tablets 1837
MS Contin Tablets 2703
Mycamine for Injection 620
▲ Mylotarg for Injection (4%) 3429
Nubain Injection (1% or less) 1111
Omnicef Capsules 506
Omnicef for Oral Suspension 506
Orthoclone OKT3 Sterile Solution (Less than 1%) 2370
OxyContin Tablets 2699
Pediarix Vaccine (Rare) 1518
Permax Tablets (Infrequent) 3357
Prevacid NapraPAC (Less than 1%) 3277
Prevnar for Injection 3460
Proleukin for Injection (Less than 1%) 1007
Prozac Pulvules and Liquid (Rare) 1771
Relpax Tablets (Rare) 2531
Rhophylac (Rare) 3504
Rilutek Tablets (Infrequent) 2945
Trasylol Injection (1% to 2%) 779
Viagra Tablets (Less than 2%) 2552
Zofran Injection (Rare) 1607
Zofran 1613
Zofran ODT Orally Disintegrating Tablets 1613

Shock, anaphylactic

(*see under* Anaphylactic shock)

Shock, hypovolemic

Prevacid Delayed-Release Capsules (Less than 1%) 3268
Prevacid for Delayed-Release Oral Suspension (Less than 1%) 3268
Prevacid SoluTab Delayed-Release Orally Disintegrating Tablets (Less than 1%) 3268
PREVPAC (Less than 1%) 3281

Shortness of breath

▲ Adenocard Injection (12%) 612
Aerobid/Aerobid-M (Less than 1%) 1172
Alacol DM Syrup 739
Ceftin Tablets (0.1% to 1%) 1369
Clozapine Tablets (1%) 2141
Clozaril Tablets (1%) 2174
Coumadin for Injection 932
Coumadin Tablets 932
Dalmane Capsules (Rare) 3343
▲ Doxil Injection (Approximately 6.8%) 3302
DynaCirc CR Tablets (0.5% to 1%) 2726
Eldepryl Capsules 3209
▲ Epogen for Injection (0.14% to 14%) 586
Flumist Vaccine 1872
Humalog-Pen (Less common) 1751
Humalog Mix 75/25-Pen (Less common) 1754
Humulin 50/50, 100 Units 1760
Humulin 70/30 Pen (Less common) 1761
Humulin L, 100 Units (Less common) 1763
Humulin R (U-500) (Less common) 1768
Humulin N Pen (Less common) 1765
Imitrex Injection 1431
Imitrex Nasal Spray 1435
Imitrex Tablets 1440
Klonopin 2782
K-Phos Neutral Tablets 785
K-Phos Original (Sodium Free) Tablets (Less frequent) 785
Kytril Injection (Rare) 2785
Kytril Tablets (Rare) 2788
▲ Leustatin Injection (7%) 2368
Lexapro Oral Solution (Infrequent) 1193
Lexapro Tablets (Infrequent) 1193
Lupron Depot–3 Month 11.25 mg 3262
Lupron Injection Pediatric 3256
Maxzide 2150
Midamor Tablets (Less than or equal to 1%) 2000
Moduretic Tablets 2003
Children's Motrin Oral Suspension and Chewable Tablets ▣ 647
Children's Motrin Non-Staining Dye-Free Oral Suspension ▣ 647
Children's Motrin Oral Suspension and Chewable Tablets 1837
Children's Motrin Non-Staining Dye-Free Oral Suspension 1837
Infants' Motrin Concentrated Drops 1837
Infants' Motrin Non-Staining Dye-Free Drops 1837
Junior Strength Motrin Caplets and Chewable Tablets 1837
▲ Navelbine Injection (3%; infrequent) 1494
Neumega for Injection 3433
Niaspan Extended-Release Tablets 1703
Novarel for Injection 1147
Novolin 70/30 PenFill 3 ml Cartridges (Rare) 2325
Novolin N PenFill 3 ml Cartridges (Rare) 2325
Novolin R PenFill (Rare) 2325
NovoLog Injection 2326
Ortho-Cyclen/Ortho Tri-Cyclen 2414
Ortho Tri-Cyclen Lo Tablets 2421
Orthoclone OKT3 Sterile Solution (Less than 1%) 2370
▲ Procrit for Injection (0.14% to 14%) 2374
Retrovir Capsules 1533
Retrovir IV Infusion 1537
Retrovir 1533
Sandostatin Injection (Less than 1%) 2263
▲ Sedapap Tablets 50 mg/650 mg (Among the most frequent) 2098
Sular Tablets (Very rare) 1163
▲ Thrombate III (1 of 17) 3254
▲ Toprol-XL Tablets (Approximately 3 of 100 patients) 660
▲ Tylenol with Codeine (Among most frequent) 2461
Uroqid-Acid No. 2 Tablets 785
Vivelle Transdermal System 2288
Vivelle-Dot Transdermal System 2293
Wellbutrin Tablets (Infrequent) 1579
Ziagen 1600
Zofran Injection (Rare) 1607
Zofran 1613
Zofran ODT Orally Disintegrating Tablets 1613

SIADH secretion syndrome

(*see under* ADH syndrome, inappropriate)

Sialadenitis

Aldoclor Tablets 1881
Aldoril Tablets 1884
Amerge Tablets (Rare) 1312
Atacand HCT 637
Avalide Tablets 922
Avalide Tablets 2889
Diovan HCT Tablets 2195
Diuril Oral 1936
Diuril Sodium Intravenous 1934
Dyazide Capsules 1389
▲ Evoxac Capsules (1% to 3%) 1042
Hyzaar 1964
Indapamide Tablets 2119
Kaletra (Less than 2%) 474
Lotensin HCT Tablets 2235
Maxzide 2150
Micardis HCT Tablets 886
Moduretic Tablets 2003
Paxil CR Controlled-Release Tablets (Rare) 1509
Paxil (Rare) 1501
Permax Tablets (Rare) 3357
Prinzide Tablets 2033
Raptiva for Injection (1 case) 1247
Rescriptor Tablets 2535
Teveten HCT Tablets 1710
Timolide Tablets 2056
Trileptal Oral Suspension 2281
Trileptal Tablets 2281
Uniretic Tablets 3114
Vaseretic Tablets 2073
Zestoretic Tablets 701
Zomig Nasal Spray (Rare) 718

Sialism

▲ Abilify Tablets (3%) 916
▲ Abilify Tablets (3%) 2472
Alferon N Injection (1%) 1640
Altace Capsules (Less than 1%) 1673
Ambien Tablets (Rare) 2867
Aricept Tablets (Infrequent) 1086
Aricept ODT Tablets (Infrequent) 1086
Axert Tablets (Rare) 2430
Campral Tablets (Rare) 1175
Camptosar Injection 2602
Ceftin for Oral Suspension (0.1% to 1%) 1369
Celexa (Frequent) 1177
▲ Clozapine Tablets (More than 5% to 31%) 2141
▲ Clozaril Tablets (More than 5% to 48%) 2174
Dalmane Capsules (Rare) 3343
Diprivan Injectable Emulsion (Less than 1%) 676
Doxil Injection (Less than 1%) 3302
Effexor Tablets (Rare) 3405
Effexor XR Capsules (Rare) 3411
Emend Capsules (Greater than 0.5%) 1944
Eskalith 1406
Evoxac Capsules (2.2%) 1042
Exelon Capsules (Infrequent) 2204
▲ FazaClo Orally Disintegrating Tablets (Greater than 5% to 31%) 547
Frova Tablets (Infrequent) 1101
Gabitril Tablets (Infrequent) 998
Garamycin Injectable 3028
▲ Geodon Capsules (4%) 2514
Hyperstat I.V. Injection 3031
Imitrex Injection 1431
Imitrex Nasal Spray 1435
▲ Intron A for Injection (Less than 5%) 3038
Klonopin 2782
Lamictal (Infrequent) 1449
Lithobid Tablets 1670
▲ Megace ES Oral Suspension (1% to 3%) 2492
Meridia Capsules 485
Mirapex Tablets (1% or more) 889
Moban Tablets (Occasional) 1108
Neurontin Capsules (Infrequent) 2498
Neurontin Oral Solution (Infrequent) 2498
Neurontin Tablets (Infrequent) 2498
▲ Niravam Orally Disintegrating Tablets (4.2% to 5.6%) 3106
▲ Orap Tablets (13.8%) 1220
▲ Pacerone Tablets (1% to 3%) 3337
Parcopa Orally Disintegrating Tablets 3111
Paxil CR Controlled-Release Tablets (Infrequent) 1509
Paxil (Infrequent) 1501
Prevacid Delayed-Release Capsules (Less than 1%) 3268
Prevacid for Delayed-Release Oral Suspension (Less than 1%) 3268
Prevacid NapraPAC (Less than 1%) 3277
Prevacid SoluTab Delayed-Release Orally Disintegrating Tablets (Less than 1%) 3268
PREVPAC (Less than 1%) 3281
Primaxin I.M. 2022
Primaxin I.V. (Less than 0.2%) 2024
Prinivil Tablets (Greater than 1%) 2029
Prinzide Tablets 2033
Protonix I.V. 3468
Protonix Tablets 3465
Prozac Pulvules and Liquid (Infrequent) 1771
Razadyne ER Extended-Release Capsules (Infrequent) 2434
Razadyne (Infrequent) 2434
Relpax Tablets (Infrequent) 2531
Requip Tablets (1% or more) 1528
Rescriptor Tablets 2535
▲ Risperdal Consta Long-Acting Injection (2% to 6%) 1664
▲ Risperdal M-Tab Orally Disintegrating Tablets (Up to 2% to 5%) 1658
▲ Risperdal (Up to 2% to 5%) 1658
Roferon-A Injection (Rare to infrequent) 2805
Seroquel Tablets (Infrequent) 691
Sonata Capsules (Rare) 1686
▲ Soriatane Capsules (1% to 10%) 1028
Stalevo Tablets 2270
Suprane Liquid for Inhalation (Greater than 1%) 770
Symbyax Capsules (Frequent) 1788
Tasmar Tablets (Infrequent) 3360
Thiothixene Capsules (Infrequently) 2124
Tindamax 2670
▲ Topamax Sprinkle Capsules (6%) 2438
▲ Topamax Tablets (6%) 2438
Trecator Tablets 3482
▲ Ultane Liquid for Inhalation (2% to 4%) 526
Urecholine Tablets 2349
Valium Tablets (Infrequent) 2822
▲ Wellbutrin Tablets (3.4%) 1579
Wellbutrin SR Sustained-Release Tablets (Infrequent) 1583
Wellbutrin XL Extended-Release Tablets (Infrequent) 1588
Xanax XR Tablets (Infrequent) 2655
Zestril Tablets (Greater than 1%) 704
Zoloft (Infrequent) 2581
Zomig Nasal Spray (Infrequent) 718
Zyban Sustained-Release Tablets 1620
Zyprexa Tablets (Frequent) 1798
Zyprexa ZYDIS Orally Disintegrating Tablets (Frequent) 1798
Zyrtec Chewable Tablets (Less than 2%) 2589
Zyrtec (Less than 2%) 2589
Zyrtec-D 12 Hour Extended Release Tablets (Less than 2%) 2591

Sialorrhea

(*see under* Sialism)

Sialosis

(*see under* Sialism)

SICCA syndrome

(*see under* Sjögren's syndrome)

Sickle cell crises

Neupogen for Injection 598

Sickle cell disease

Lo/Ovral-28 Tablets 3423
Neulasta Injection 596
Triphasil-28 Tablets 3483

Sinoatrial block

Blocadren Tablets (Less than 1%) 1891
Flumadine (Less than 0.3%) 1186
Neurontin Capsules (Rare) 2498
Neurontin Oral Solution (Rare) 2498
Neurontin Tablets (Rare) 2498
Rythmol SR Capsules 2736
Timoptic in Ocudose (Less frequent) 2061
Timoptic-XE Sterile Ophthalmic Gel Forming Solution 2062

Sinoatrial node dysfunction

Cardene I.V. 1129
Eskalith 1406
Pacerone Tablets 3337

Sinus arrest

Catapres Tablets (Rare) 874
Nipent for Injection (Less than 3%) 3216
Pacerone Tablets 3337
Rythmol SR Capsules 2736

Tambocor Tablets (1% to 3%)............ 1824

Sinus bradycardia

Aciphex Tablets 1081
Activase I.V. 1225
Adenocard Injection 612
Adenoscan 613
Catapres Tablets (Rare) 874
Catapres-TTS (0.5% or less) 875
Clorpres Tablets (Rare) 2139
Cozaar Tablets (Less than 1%) 1913
Digitek Tablets 2146
Eldepryl Capsules 3209
Hyzaar 1964
Kytril Injection (Rare) 2785
Lanoxicaps Capsules 1458
Lanoxin Injection 1462
Lanoxin Tablets 1468
Lanoxin Injection Pediatric 1465
▲ Pacerone Tablets (2% to 5%) 3337
Retavase 1131
Rythmol SR Capsules (Greater than 2%) 2736
▲ Sandostatin Injection (25%) 2263
Sonata Capsules (Rare) 1686
Uniretic Tablets (Less than 1%) 3114

Sinus congestion

▲ Aerobid/Aerobid-M (3% to 9%) 1172
▲ Asmanex Twisthaler (9%) 2981
Cardizem LA Extended Release Tablets (1% to 2%) 1699
Elidel Cream 1% (0.6% to 1.1%) 2198
Lexapro Oral Solution (Frequent) 1193
Lexapro Tablets (Frequent) 1193
▲ Myfortic Tablets (3% to less than 20%) 2244
▲ Serevent Diskus (9%) 1540
▲ Strattera Capsules (2% or greater) 1784
Tasmar Tablets (1% to 2%) 3360
Vivelle Transdermal System 2288
Vivelle-Dot Transdermal System 2293
Zelnorm Tablets (Up to 1%) 2303

Sinus discomfort

Aerobid/Aerobid-M (1% to 3%) 1172
Avalide Tablets 922
Avalide Tablets 2889
Avapro Tablets (1% or greater) 925
Avapro Tablets (1% or greater) 2886
Cozaar Tablets (1% or greater) 1913
Imitrex Injection (2.2%) 1431
Imitrex Nasal Spray (0.8% to 2.4%) 1435
Maxalt Tablets (Infrequent) 1983
Maxalt-MLT Orally Disintegrating Tablets (Infrequent) 1983

Sinus drainage

▲ Aerobid/Aerobid-M (3% to 9%) 1172
Alferon N Injection (2%) 1640

Sinus exit block

Adenoscan (Less than 1%) 613

Sinus node dysfunction

Cardene I.V. 1129
Eskalith 1406
Lithobid Tablets 1670

Sinus pause

Adenoscan (Less than 1%) 613

Sinus syndrome, sick

Exelon Capsules (Infrequent) 2204
Photofrin for Injection 729

Sinus tachycardia

Adenocard Injection 612
Aloxi Injection (Less than 1%) 2099
Aramine Injection 1889
Ellence Injection 2632
▲ Proleukin for Injection (70%) 1007
Strattera Capsules 1784
Taxotere Injection Concentrate (Rare) 2947
Xanax XR Tablets (Infrequent) 2655

Sinusitis

Abilify Tablets (Frequent) 916
Abilify Tablets (Frequent) 2472
▲ Aceon Tablets (2 mg, 4 mg, 8 mg) (0.6% to 5.2%) 3191
Actiq (1% or greater) 993
▲ Activella Tablets (7% to 11%) 2311
▲ Actonel Tablets (4.5% to 4.9%) 2679
▲ Actonel with Calcium Tablets (4.5% to 4.6%) 2684
▲ ActoPlus Met Tablets (4.4% to 5%) 3219
▲ Actos Tablets (6.3%) 3224
▲ Advair Diskus 100/50 (3% to 4%) 1291
▲ Advair Diskus 250/50 (3% to 4%) 1291
▲ Advair Diskus 500/50 (3% To 4%) 1291
▲ Aerobid/Aerobid-M (3% to 9%) 1172
Agrylin Capsules (1% to 5%) 3172
Alamast Ophthalmic Solution (Less than 5%) 3371
▲ Aldara Cream, 5% (7.4%) 1814
Allegra (2.2%) 2857
Alphagan P Ophthalmic Solution (1% to 4%) 563
▲ Altoprev Extended-Release Tablets (4%) 1151
▲ Ambien Tablets (4%) 2867
AmBisome for Injection (Less common) 615
Amerge Tablets (Infrequent) 1312
Antara Capsules 2723
Aralast (Greater than or equal to 0.2%) 745
Arava Tablets (2%) 2881
▲ Aredia for Injection (15.6%) 2168
▲ Arimidex Tablets (2% to 5%) 665
Aromasin Tablets (Less frequent) 2600
Asacol Delayed-Release Tablets (2% or greater) 2688
▲ Asmanex Twisthaler (5% to 22%) 2981
▲ Astelin Nasal Spray (3.2%) 1876
Atacand Tablets (More than 1%) 634
Atacand HCT (0.5% or greater) 637
▲ Atrovent HFA Inhalation Aerosol (1% to 11%) 872
Atrovent Inhalation Solution (2.3%) 868
▲ Avandia Tablets (3.2%) 1348
▲ Avonex (14%) 839
Axert Tablets (Infrequent) 2430
Axid Oral Solution (2.4%) 913
▲ Azmacort Inhalation Aerosol (2% to 9%) 1701
Betimol Ophthalmic Solution (1% to 5%) .... ⊙283
Betimol Ophthalmic Solution (1% to 5%) 3371
▲ BiDil Tablets (4%) 2161
Bravelle for Intramuscular or Subcutaneous Injection (2%) 1140
▲ Caduet Tablets (2.5% to 6.4%) 2507
Campath Ampules 826
Carac Cream, 0.5% (1.6%) 1048
Carnitor Injection (2% to 3%) 3185
Carteolol Hydrochloride Ophthalmic Solution USP, 1% (Occasional) .... ⊙246
▲ Casodex Tablets (2% to 5%) 670
Caverject Impulse Injection (2%) 2610
Ceftin for Oral Suspension (0.1% to 1%) 1369
▲ Celebrex Capsules (5%) 3130
▲ Celexa (3%) 1177
▲ CellCept Capsules (3% to 26%) 2751
▲ CellCept Intravenous (3% to 26%) 2751
▲ CellCept Oral Suspension (3% to 26%) 2751
▲ CellCept Tablets (3% to 26%) 2751
▲ Climara Transdermal System (4% to 5%) 795
▲ Climara Pro Transdermal System (3.8%) 800
Clindesse Vaginal Cream (Less than 1%) 3296
Colazal Capsules (1%) 2845
▲ CombiPatch Transdermal System (10% to 12%) 2180
Combivent Inhalation Aerosol (2.3%) 878
▲ Concerta Extended-Release Tablets (3%) 1828
Copaxone for Injection (At least 2%) 3292
Cosopt Sterile Ophthalmic Solution (1% to 5%) 1910
▲ Cozaar Tablets (1% to 6%) 1913
Crestor Tablets (2%) 672
▲ Depacon Injection (1% to 5%) 412
▲ Depakene (1% to 5%) 417
▲ Depakote Sprinkle Capsules (1% to 5%) 422
▲ Depakote Tablets (1% to 5%) 427
▲ Depakote ER Tablets (1% to 5%) 433
▲ depo-subQ provera 104 Injectable Suspension (1% to less than 5%) 2622
Detrol Tablets (1.1%) 2626
Detrol LA Capsules (2%) 2629
Diovan HCT Tablets (More than 2%) 2195
Diovan Tablets (More than 1%) 2191
▲ Ditropan XL Extended Release Tablets (2% to less than 5%) 2391
▲ Doxil Injection (1% to 10%) 3302
DuoNeb Inhalation Solution 1058
Duragesic Transdermal System (Greater than or less than 1%) 2448
Edex Injection (1%) 3103
Effexor XR Capsules (2%) 3411
▲ Elestat Ophthalmic Solution (1% to 3%) 1643
Elidel Cream 1% (0.6% to 3.3%) 2198
Enablex Extended-Release Tablets (Greater than or equal to 1%) 2201
▲ Enbrel for Injection (3% to 5%) 580
▲ Equetro Extended-Release Capsules (Less than 5%) 3178
▲ Estrogel 0.06% (3.6%) 3200
▲ Evista Tablets (7.9% to 10.3%) 1735
▲ Evoxac Capsules (12.3%) 1042
Fabrazyme for Intravenous Infusion (2%) 1267
Famvir Tablets (1.3% to 2.6%) 2207
▲ Flolan for Injection (4%) 1408
Flomax Capsules (2.2% to 3.7%) 881
▲ Flovent Diskus 50 mcg (10% to 33%) 1415
▲ Flovent HFA (1% to 6%) 1418
Floxin Otic Singles (Reported in a single subject) 1045
Floxin Otic Solution (Single report) 1043
▲ Flumist Vaccine (4.1%) 1872
▲ Follistim AQ Cartridge (5%) 2354
Foradil Aerolizer (2.7%) 3024
▲ Fortical Nasal Spray (1% to 3%) 3336
Frova Tablets (Frequent) 1101
▲ Fuzeon Injection (6%) 2772
Gabitril Tablets (1% or more) 998
Gengraf Capsules (Less than 1%) 458
▲ Gleevec Tablets (4% to 11%) 2221
▲ Gonal-f RFF Pen for Injection (6%) 3155
Hepsera Tablets (2% or greater) 1275
▲ Herceptin I.V. (9%) 1234
▲ Humira Injection (11%) 464
Hytrin Capsules (2.6%) 469
Hyzaar (1.2%) 1964
▲ Imdur Tablets (Less than or equal to 5%) 3032
Imitrex Nasal Spray 1435
Indapamide Tablets (Less than 5%) 2119
▲ Infergen (12% to 17%) 1647
▲ Intron A for Injection (Up to 21%) 3038
Invirase (Less than 2% to 2.7%) 2776
▲ I.V. Busulfex (3%) 1125
Kaletra (Less than 2%) 474
Keppra Oral Solution (2%) 3307
Keppra Tablets (2%) 3307
▲ Kineret Injection (7%) 594
▲ Klonopin (4%) 2782
Lamictal (2%) 1449
Lescol Capsules (2.6%) 2227
Lescol Capsules (2.6%) 2730
▲ Lescol XL Tablets (3.5%) 2227
▲ Lescol XL Tablets (3.5%) 2730
Levaquin in 5% Dextrose Injection (1.1%) 2453
Levaquin (1.1%) 2453
▲ Levitra Tablets (3%) 3048
▲ Lexapro Oral Solution (3%) 1193
▲ Lexapro Tablets (3%) 1193
▲ Lipitor Tablets (Up to 6.4%) 2495
Lofibra Capsules 1217
Lotensin Tablets (Less than 1%) 2232
Lotensin HCT Tablets (More than 1%) 2235
Marinol Capsules (Less than 1%) 3334
▲ Mepron Suspension (7%) 1487
▲ Meridia Capsules (5%) 485
Metrogel 1% (1.4%) 1212
Miacalcin Nasal Spray (1% to 3%) 2242
▲ Micardis Tablets (3%) 884
▲ Micardis HCT Tablets (4%) 886
Migranal Nasal Spray (1%) 3350
Mirapex Tablets (1% or more) 889
▲ Mirena Intrauterine System (5% or more) 810
▲ Myfortic Tablets (3% to less than 20%) 2244
Nasacort AQ Nasal Spray 2937
Nasarel Nasal Spray (1% or less) 1652
▲ Nasonex Nasal Spray (4% to 5%) 3058
▲ Neoral Soft Gelatin Capsules (1% to 7%) 2247
▲ Neoral Oral Solution (1% to 7%) 2247
Neurontin Capsules (Infrequent) 2498
Neurontin Oral Solution (Infrequent) 2498
Neurontin Tablets (Infrequent) 2498
Nexium Delayed-Release Capsules (Less than 1%) 645
Nexium I.V. (Less than 1%) 649
▲ Nicotrol Inhaler (Greater than 3%) 2594
▲ Nipent for Injection (6%) 3216
▲ Novantrone for Injection Concentrate (3% to 6%) 3158
Omacor Capsules 2735
Patanol Ophthalmic Solution (Less than 5%) 557
▲ Paxil CR Controlled-Release Tablets (Infrequent to 4%) 1509
▲ Paxil (Infrequent to 4%) 1501
▲ PEG-Intron Powder for Injection (7%) 3062
Permax Tablets (Infrequent) 3357
▲ Photofrin for Injection (4%) 729
Plavix Tablets (1% to 2.5%) 940
Plavix Tablets (1% to 2.5%) 2942
Plendil Extended-Release Tablets (0.5% to 1.5%) 651
Pletal Tablets (Less than 2%) 2478
▲ Prandin Tablets (0.5, 1, and 2 mg) (3% to 6%) 2337
▲ Prefest Tablets (8%) 1069
▲ Premarin Tablets (6% to 11%) 3443
▲ Premphase Tablets (7% to 10%) 3452
▲ Prempro Tablets (7% to 10%) 3452
Prevacid Delayed-Release Capsules (Less than 1%) 3268
Prevacid for Delayed-Release Oral Suspension (Less than 1%) 3268
Prevacid NapraPAC (Less than 1%) 3277
Prevacid SoluTab Delayed-Release Orally Disintegrating Tablets (Less than 1%) 3268
PREVPAC (Less than 1%) 3281
Prinivil Tablets (0.3% to 1.0%) 2029
Prinzide Tablets (0.3% to 1%) 2033
Prochieve 4% Gel 1018
Prochieve 8% Gel 1018
▲ Prograf Capsules and Injection (3% to 15%) 624
Prometrium Capsules (100 mg, 200 mg) (Less than 5%) 3205
ProSom Tablets (Infrequent) 512
Protonix I.V. (Greater than or equal to 1%) 3468
Protonix Tablets (Greater than or equal to 1%) 3465
▲ Protopic Ointment (2% to 7%) 629
Provigil Tablets (At least 1%) 1002
▲ Prozac Pulvules and Liquid (1% to 6%) 1771
Pulmozyme Inhalation Solution 1245
Qvar Inhalation Aerosol (Up to 3%) 1654
▲ Rapamune Oral Solution and Tablets (3% to 20%) 3472
Raptiva for Injection 1247
▲ Rebetol (Less than 1% to 12%) 3073
▲ Rebetron Combination Therapy (9% to 12%) 3078
ReFacto Vials 3479
Relenza Rotadisk (2% to 3%) 1525
Relpax Tablets (Rare) 2531
▲ Remicade for IV Injection (14%) 987
▲ Requip Tablets (4%) 1528
▲ Rescriptor Tablets (1.2% to 7.3%) 2535
Retisert Implant (5% to 15%) .... ⊙256
Retrovir Capsules 1533
Retrovir IV Infusion 1537
Retrovir 1533
▲ Revatio Tablets (3%) 2541
▲ Ribavirin, USP Capsules (Less than 1% to 12%) 3083
Rilutek Tablets (0.4% to 1.6%) 2945
▲ Risperdal Consta Long-Acting Injection (1% to 3%) 1664
▲ Risperdal M-Tab Orally Disintegrating Tablets (1% to 4%) 1658
▲ Risperdal (1% to 4%) 1658
▲ Rituxan for Infusion (1% to 5%) 845
▲ Rituxan I.V. (6%) 1251
▲ Roferon-A Injection (Less than 1% to 11%) 2805
▲ Sandimmune (Less than 1% to 7%) 2259
▲ Sandostatin LAR Depot (5% to 15%) 2264
▲ Serevent Diskus (Greater than 3%) 1540
▲ Simulect for Injection (3% to 10%) 2268
Singulair (Greater than or equal to 1%) 2047
▲ Somavert Injection (4% to 8%) 2648
▲ Soriatane Capsules (1% to 10%) 1028
Spectracef Tablets (0.1% to 1%) 2706
▲ Spiriva HandiHaler (3% to 11%) 899
▲ Strattera Capsules (6%) 1784
▲ Sular Tablets (3%) 1163
Synagis (More than 1%) 1868
Tamiflu Capsules (1.7%) 2810
Tamiflu Oral Suspension (1.7%) 2810
Tasmar Tablets (1% or more) 3360
▲ Temodar Capsules (6%) 3088
Teveten Tablets (1% or greater) 1707
Teveten HCT Tablets 1710
▲ Thalomid Capsules (4.2%) 979
▲ TOBI Solution for Inhalation (8.1%) 1015
▲ Topamax Sprinkle Capsules (2% to 10%) 2438
▲ Topamax Tablets (2% to 10%) 2438
Travatan Ophthalmic Solution (1% to 5%) 559
Tricor Tablets 523
▲ Trileptal Oral Suspension (2% to 4%) 2281
▲ Trileptal Tablets (2% to 4%) 2281
▲ Trisenox Injection (20%) 983
Twinrix Vaccine 1571
Uniretic Tablets (More than 1%) 3114

Univasc Tablets (Greater than 1%).... 3118
Uroxatral Tablets (1% to 2%)............ 2957
▲ Vagifem Tablets (3% to 5%) 2340
Vantin Tablets and Oral Suspension (Less than 1%)........... 2650
▲ Verelan PM Capsules (3%) 3120
VFEND I.V. (Less than 2%)................ 2543
VFEND Oral Suspension (Less than 2%).. 2543
VFEND Tablets (Less than 2%)........... 2543
Viagra Tablets (Less than 2%)........... 2552
Vicoprofen Tablets (Less than 1%).... 533
Viracept (Less than 2%).................... 2556
▲ Vivelle Transdermal System (2.6% to 8.5%).. 2288
▲ Vivelle-Dot Transdermal System (2.6% to 8.5%).............................. 2293
Vytorin 10/10 Tablets........................ 2084
Vytorin 10/10 Tablets........................ 3092
Vytorin 10/20 Tablets........................ 2084
Vytorin 10/20 Tablets........................ 3092
Vytorin 10/40 Tablets........................ 2084
Vytorin 10/40 Tablets........................ 3092
Vytorin 10/80 Tablets........................ 2084
Vytorin 10/80 Tablets........................ 3092
WelChol Tablets (2%)......................... 2855
▲ Wellbutrin SR Sustained-Release Tablets (1% to 3%)........................ 1583
▲ Wellbutrin XL Extended-Release Tablets (1% to 3%)........................ 1588
▲ Xolair (16%) 1259
▲ Xopenex HFA Inhalation Aerosol (1.4% to 4.2%)............................. 3151
▲ Xopenex Inhalation Solution (1.4% to 4.2%)...................................... 3143
▲ Xopenex Inhalation Solution Concentrate (1.4% to 4.2%).............. 3147
Yasmin 28 Tablets (Greater than 1%).. 818
▲ Zelnorm Tablets (3%) 2303
Zemaira (1.5%).................................. 3506
Zestoretic Tablets (0.3% to 1%)....... 701
Zestril Tablets (0.3% to 1.0%).......... 704
▲ Zetia Tablets (3.6% to 4.6%) 2090
▲ Zetia Tablets (3.6% to 4.6%) 3098
Zoladex (1% to 3%)............................ 709
Zoladex 3-month................................ 712
Zoloft (Infrequent to 2%)................... 2581
Zomig Nasal Spray (Infrequent)........ 718
Zyban Sustained-Release Tablets (2%)... 1620
Zyrtec Chewable Tablets (Less than 2%).. 2589
Zyrtec (Less than 2%)......................... 2589
Zyrtec-D 12 Hour Extended Release Tablets (Less than 2%)..... 2591

Sjögren's syndrome

Mintezol 2002

Skin, anesthesia

(*see under* Numbness, skin)

Skin, burning of

▲ Clindets Pledgets (10% to 11%) 3212
Clobex Lotion 1208
▲ Differin Cream (Less than 1% to 24%).. 1210
▲ Differin Gel (10% to 40%) 1211
▲ Diprolene Gel 0.05% (6%) 3015
Diprolene Lotion 0.05% (1%)............ 3016
Diprolene Ointment 0.05% (Infrequent) 3017
Diprolene AF Cream 0.05% (Infrequent) 3014
Diprosone Cream, USP 0.05%.......... 3018
▲ Dovonex Ointment 0.005% (Approximately 10% to 15%).......... 3375
Drysol Solution.................................. 2506
▲ Duac Topical Gel (0% to 5%) 3214
Ertaczo Cream, 2%............................ 2383
▲ Erygel Topical Gel (Approximately 25%)... 2096
Klonopin (Infrequent)........................ 2782
▲ Loprox Gel (34%) 1861
Lotrisone (1.6%)................................ 3054
▲ Luxíq Foam (2% to 44%) 1026
Nubain Injection (1% or less)............ 1111
Oxistat (1.7%).................................... 1498
Oxsoralen Lotion 1%......................... 3354
Oxsoralen-Ultra Capsules................. 3354
ProctoFoam-HC.................................. 3113
▲ Protopic Ointment (25% to 58%) 629
▲ Tri-Luma Cream (6.68% to 18%) 1213
Zovirax Cream (Less than 1%)......... 853

Skin, cracking

Clobevate Gel (Less than 2%)........... 3213
Diprolene Gel 0.05%......................... 3015
Olux Foam (Less than 2%)................ 1027
Soriatane Capsules 1028
Temovate Cream (Less frequent)..... 1549
▲ Temovate Gel (Among most frequent).. 1550
Temovate Ointment (Less frequent).. 1549
Temovate E Emollient (Less than 2%).. 1552

Skin, darkening

Claripel Cream (Rare)........................ 3212

Skin, dryness of

(*see under* Xerosis cutis)

Skin, eruptions of

▲ Anaprox Tablets (3% to 9%) 2769
▲ Anaprox DS Tablets (3% to 9%) 2769
Antabuse Tablets............................... 2343
Biaxin/Biaxin XL................................ 402
Cosmegen for Injection..................... 1907
Daranide Tablets................................ 1928
▲ EC-Naprosyn Delayed-Release Tablets (3% to 9%)........................ 2769
E.E.S.. 449
Ery-Tab Tablets 447
Erythrocin Stearate Filmtab Tablets 452
Erythromycin Delayed-Release Capsules, USP (Rare) 456
Imitrex Injection (Infrequent) 1431
Imitrex Nasal Spray (Infrequent) 1435
▲ Naprosyn Suspension (3% to 9%) 2769
▲ Naprosyn Tablets (3% to 9%) 2769
Norvir 499
Paser Granules 1657
PCE Dispertab Tablets (Rare) 510
PREVPAC 3281
Tessalon Capsules 1202
Tessalon Perles 1202
Thioridazine Hydrochloride Tablets (Infrequent) 2122
Trasylol Injection 779

Skin, exfoliation

Levaquin in 5% Dextrose Injection (0.1% to 0.9%) 2453
Levaquin (0.1% to 0.9%) 2453

Skin, exfoliation, application site

Lidoderm Patch 1107

Skin, flakiness

▲ Advair Diskus 100/50 (1% to 3%) ... 1291
▲ Advair Diskus 250/50 (1% to 3%) ... 1291
▲ Advair Diskus 500/50 (1% to 3%) ... 1291
Zovirax Cream (Less than 1%) 853

Skin, fragile

Accutane Capsules 2740
Amnesteem Capsules 2126
Depo-Medrol Injectable Suspension 2615
Depo-Medrol Single-Dose Vial 2617
Photofrin for Injection 729
Soriatane Capsules 1028

Skin, fragility

Cuprimine Capsules 1925
Decadron Phosphate Injection 1931
Decadron Tablets 1929
Hydrocortone Tablets 1963
Pediapred Oral Solution 3319

Skin, irritation of

Accuzyme Debriding Ointment (Occasional) 1636
Accuzyme Spray (Occasional) 1637
BenGay Pain Relieving Patch .... ▣698
Betadine Solution 2715
Betadine Surgical Scrub (Rare) 2715
Blocadren Tablets 1891
Carac Cream, 0.5% (1.2%) 1048
Clobevate Gel (Less than 2%) 3213
▲ Clobex Shampoo (4.7%) 1209
Clobex Lotion 1208
Cosopt Sterile Ophthalmic Solution 1910
Cutivate Cream (0.8% to 4.5%) 1381
Differin Cream (1%) 1210
Differin Gel (Approximately 1% or less) 1211
Diprolene Gel 0.05% 3015
Diprolene Lotion 0.05% (Less than 1%) 3016
Diprolene Ointment 0.05% (Infrequent) 3017
Diprolene AF Cream 0.05% (Infrequent) 3014
Diprosone Cream, USP 0.05% 3018
▲ Dovonex Cream 0.005% (Approximately 10% to 15%) 3374
▲ Dovonex Ointment 0.005% (Approximately 10% to 15%) 3375
Elocon Cream 0.1% (Infrequent) 3019
Elocon Lotion 0.1% (Infrequent) 3020
Elocon Ointment 0.1% (Infrequent)... 3021
Lotrimin.. 3053
Lotrisone.. 3054
Luxíq Foam... 1026
Noritate Cream, 1% (Uncommon)..... 1051
Orap Tablets....................................... 1220
Ovide .5% Lotion 3287
Oxistat Cream (0.4%)......................... 1498
Panafil Ointment (Occasional)........... 1637
Panafil Spray (Occasional) 1637
ProctoFoam-HC.................................. 3113
Soriatane Capsules (Less than 1%).. 1028
ThermaCare Heat Wraps 2674
Timolide Tablets 2056
Timoptic in Ocudose.......................... 2061
Timoptic Sterile Ophthalmic Solution... 2058
Timoptic-XE Sterile Ophthalmic Gel Forming Solution 2062
Tri-Luma Cream (2%)......................... 1213
Xerac AC Solution.............................. 2507

Skin, lesions non-specific

Invanz for Injection (Greater than 0.5%)... 1974
Prinivil Tablets (0.3% to 1.0%).......... 2029
Prinzide Tablets................................. 2033
Roferon-A Injection (Infrequent)........ 2805
▲ Trisenox Injection (8%) 983
Zestoretic Tablets 701

Skin, oiliness

▲ Clindets Pledgets (1% to 18%) 3212
Erygel Topical Gel (Occasional)........ 2096

Skin, reddening

Children's Motrin Oral Suspension and Chewable Tablets.................... 1837
Children's Motrin Cold Non-Staining Dye-Free Oral Suspension 1838
Children's Motrin Cold Oral Suspension 1838
Children's Motrin Non-Staining Dye-Free Oral Suspension............. 1837
Motrin Cold & Sinus Caplets............. 1836
Motrin IB Tablets and Caplets........... 1836
Infants' Motrin Concentrated Drops 1837
Infants' Motrin Non-Staining Dye-Free Drops................................ 1837
Junior Strength Motrin Caplets and Chewable Tablets 1837
Rosac Cream with Sunscreens......... 3216
ThermaCare Heat Wraps 2674
Xolair.. 1259

Skin, tenderness

Efudex.. 3348
Ertaczo Cream, 2% 2383
Erygel Topical Gel.............................. 2096
Imitrex Injection (Rare)...................... 1431
Imitrex Nasal Spray 1435
Imitrex Tablets (Infrequent)............... 1440
Naftin Gel (0.5%)................................ 2097

Skin, tightness of

Diprolene Gel 0.05%........................... 3015

Skin, wrinkling

Amerge Tablets (Rare)........................ 1312
Imitrex Nasal Spray 1435
Imitrex Tablets (Rare)......................... 1440
Photofrin for Injection........................ 729

Skin atrophy

Aclovate (Infrequent).......................... 1290
Analpram-HC 1136
Clobevate Gel (Less than 2%)............ 3213
Clobex Shampoo (Infrequent)............ 1209
▲ Clobex Lotion (4.2%) 1208
Copaxone for Injection (Frequent)..... 3292
Cutivate Cream (Infrequent)............... 1381
Cutivate Lotion 0.05% (Rare)............. 1383
Cutivate Ointment (Infrequent to more frequent)................................ 1384
Diprolene Gel 0.05%........................... 3015
Diprolene Lotion 0.05% (Infrequent)....................................... 3016
Diprolene Ointment 0.05% (Infrequent)....................................... 3017
Diprolene AF Cream 0.05% (Infrequent)....................................... 3014
Diprosone Cream, USP 0.05%........... 3018
Dovonex Ointment 0.005% (Less than 1%)... 3375
Dovonex Scalp Solution 0.005%....... 3375
Effexor Tablets (Rare)........................ 3405
Effexor XR Capsules (Rare)............... 3411
Elocon Cream 0.1% (1.6%)................ 3019
Elocon Lotion 0.1% (Infrequent)........ 3020
▲ Elocon Ointment 0.1% (4.8%) 3021
Locoid Cream (Infrequent).................. 1138
Locoid Lipocream Cream (Infrequent) 1138
Locoid (Infrequent).............................. 1138
Lotrisone... 3054
Luxíq Foam.. 1026
Lyrica Capsules (Rare)........................ 2524
Olux Foam (Less than 2%)................. 1027
Pandel Cream, 0.1%............................ 1017
Pramosone.. 1139
ProctoFoam-HC................................... 3113
Soriatane Capsules 1028
Temovate Cream (Less frequent)...... 1549
▲ Temovate Gel (Among most frequent).. 1550
Temovate Ointment (Less frequent).. 1549
Temovate Scalp Application (Infrequent) 1551
Temovate E Emollient (Less than 2%)... 1552
Topicort .05% Gel 3288
Topicort .25% Cream 3288
Topicort .25% Ointment 3288
Topicort LP .05% Cream 3288
Tri-Luma Cream 1213
U-cort 1% Cream 3289
Vanos Cream 1864

Skin discoloration

Abilify Tablets (Infrequent) 916
Abilify Tablets (Infrequent) 2472
Aciphex Tablets (Rare) 1081
Actiq (Less than 1%) 993
Altoprev Extended-Release Tablets .. 1151
AmBisome for Injection (Less common) 615
Aricept Tablets (Infrequent) 1086
Aricept ODT Tablets (Infrequent) 1086
▲ Avastin IV (2% to 16%) 1229
Betaseron for SC Injection 791
Brevibloc Concentrate (Less than 1%) 766
Brevibloc Injection (Less than 1%) 766
Brevibloc Double Strength Injection (Less than 1%) 766
Brevibloc Premixed Injection (Less than 1%) 766
Brevibloc Double Strength Premixed Injection (Less than 1%) 766
Caduet Tablets (Less than 0.1%) 2507
Carbatrol Capsules 3174
Celexa (Infrequent) 1177
Denavir Cream 2163
Differin Cream (Less than 1%) 1210
▲ Doxil Injection (Less than 1% to 10%) 3302
Effexor Tablets (Rare) 3405
Effexor XR Capsules (Rare) 3411
Emtriva Capsules 1272
Estratest Tablets 3196
Estratest H.S. Tablets 3196
Evoxac Capsules (Less than 1%) 1042
Ferrlecit Injection 3379
Fluorescite Injection .... ⊙207
Gabitril Tablets (Infrequent) 998
Infed Injection 3381
▲ Intron A for Injection (Less than 5%) 3038
Invirase (Less than 2%) 2776
▲ I.V. Busulfex (8%) 1125
Kaletra (Less than 2%) 474
Keppra Oral Solution (2%) 3307
Keppra Tablets (2%) 3307
Lamictal (Rare) 1449
Lescol Capsules 2227
Lescol Capsules 2730
Lescol XL Tablets 2227
Lescol XL Tablets 2730
Lunesta Tablets (Infrequent) 3139
Mevacor Tablets 1996
Neumega for Injection 3433
Neurontin Capsules (Rare) 2498
Neurontin Oral Solution (Rare) 2498
Neurontin Tablets (Rare) 2498
Norvasc Tablets (Less than or equal to 0.1%) 2529
Oxandrin Tablets 2977
Pacerone Tablets (Less than 1%) 3337
Paxil CR Controlled-Release Tablets (Rare) 1509
Paxil (Rare) 1501
Permax Tablets (Infrequent) 3357
Photofrin for Injection 729
Pravachol Tablets 943
Prochieve 4% Gel 1018
Prochieve 8% Gel 1018
▲ Prograf Capsules and Injection (3% to 15%) 624
Protopic Ointment (Greater than or equal to 1%) 629

Prozac Pulvules and Liquid (Infrequent) 1771
Psoriatec Cream 3191
Relpax Tablets (Rare) 2531
Rescriptor Tablets 2535
Retrovir IV Infusion 1537
Seroquel Tablets (Rare) 691
Sonata Capsules (Rare) 1686
Striant Mucoadhesive 1022
Sular Tablets (Less than or equal to 1%) 1163
Sustiva Capsules 957
Symbyax Capsules (Infrequent) 1788
Tasmar Tablets (Infrequent) 3360
Tegretol/Tegretol-XR 2278
Thalomid Capsules 979
Ticlid Tablets 2813
Topamax Sprinkle Capsules (1%) 2438
Topamax Tablets (1%) 2438
Trasylol Injection (1% to 2%) 779
Truvada Tablets 1279
VFEND I.V. (Less than 2%) 2543
VFEND Oral Suspension (Less than 2%) 2543
VFEND Tablets (Less than 2%) 2543
Vytorin 10/10 Tablets 2084
Vytorin 10/10 Tablets 3092
Vytorin 10/20 Tablets 2084
Vytorin 10/20 Tablets 3092
Vytorin 10/40 Tablets 2084
Vytorin 10/40 Tablets 3092
Vytorin 10/80 Tablets 2084
Vytorin 10/80 Tablets 3092
Zocor Tablets 2078
Zoladex (1% or greater) 709
Zoladex 3-month 712
Zoloft (Very rare) 2581
Zyprexa Tablets (Infrequent) 1798
Zyprexa ZYDIS Orally Disintegrating Tablets (Rare) 1798

Skin disorder, unspecified

Advicor Tablets 1694
Agrylin Capsules (1% to 5%) 3172
AmBisome for Injection (Less common) 615
▲ Ammonul Injection (6%) 3323
Antara Capsules 2723
▲ Betaseron for SC Injection (12%) 791
▲ Catapres-TTS (51 of 101 patients) 875
▲ CellCept Capsules (3% to less than 20%) 2751
▲ CellCept Intravenous (3% to less than 20%) 2751
▲ CellCept Oral Suspension (3% to less than 20%) 2751
▲ CellCept Tablets (3% to less than 20%) 2751
Cipro XR Tablets (Less than 1%) 3004
depo-subQ provera 104 Injectable Suspension (1%) 2622
▲ Doxil Injection (1% to 5%) 3302
Edex Injection (1%) 3103
▲ Ellence Injection (0% to 4.7%) 2632
Elocon Lotion 0.1% (1 in 65 patients) 3020
Elocon Ointment 0.1% (1 in 63 patients) 3021
▲ Eloxatin for Injection (2% to 32%) 2908
▲ Epogen for Injection (7% to 10%) 586
▲ Erbitux (5%) 937
EryPed 445
▲ Evoxac Capsules (1% to 3%) 1042
Invirase (Rare) 2776
Klonopin (Infrequent) 2782
Lamisil Tablets (Isolated reports) 2226
Lanoxicaps Capsules (Rare) 1458
Lanoxin Injection (Rare) 1462
Lanoxin Injection Pediatric (Rare) 1465
▲ Leukine (77%) 829
Levaquin in 5% Dextrose Injection (0.1% to 0.9%) 2453
Levaquin (0.1% to 0.9%) 2453
Lofibra Capsules 1217
Loprox Shampoo 1862
Lupron Depot 3.75 mg (2%) 3257
Lupron Depot 7.5 mg (Less than 5%) 3261
Lupron Depot–3 Month 11.25 mg (2%) 3262
▲ Megace ES Oral Suspension (1% to 3%) 2492
Mirapex Tablets (2%) 889
▲ Mirena Intrauterine System (5% or more) 810
▲ Neoral Soft Gelatin Capsules (1% to 17.6%) 2247
▲ Neoral Oral Solution (1% to 17.6%) 2247
▲ Nipent for Injection (4% to 17%) 3216
Prevacid Delayed-Release Capsules (Less than 1%) 3268
Prevacid for Delayed-Release Oral Suspension (Less than 1%) 3268
Prevacid NapraPAC (Less than 1%) 3277
Prevacid SoluTab Delayed-Release Orally Disintegrating Tablets (Less than 1%) 3268
PREVPAC (Less than 1%) 3281
Prilosec OTC Tablets (Very rare) 2674
Primaxin I.M. 2022
Primaxin I.V. (Less than 0.2%) 2024
Prinivil Tablets (Rare) 2029
Prinzide Tablets (Rare) 2033
Prochieve 4% Gel 1018
Prochieve 8% Gel 1018
▲ Prograf Capsules and Injection (3% to 15%) 624
Protonix I.V. (Less than 1%) 3468
Protonix Tablets (Less than 1%) 3465
Relpax Tablets (Infrequent) 2531
Rescriptor Tablets 2535
Rilutek Tablets (Infrequent) 2945
Soriatane Capsules (Less than 1%) 1028
▲ Taxotere Injection Concentrate (0.6% to 54.1%) 2947
Thyrolar 1203
▲ Topamax Sprinkle Capsules (1% to 3%) 2438
▲ Topamax Tablets (1% to 3%) 2438
Tricor Tablets 523
▲ Vesanoid Capsules (14%) 2823
VFEND I.V. (Less than 2%) 2543
VFEND Oral Suspension (Less than 2%) 2543
VFEND Tablets (Less than 2%) 2543
Xalatan Sterile Ophthalmic Solution (1% to 2%) 2654
Zegerid Powder for Oral Solution (Very rare) 2972
Zestoretic Tablets (Rare) 701
Zestril Tablets (Rare) 704
Zinecard for Injection (1%) 2659
Zithromax Capsules, 250 mg (Rare) 2568
Zithromax for IV Infusion (Rare) 2573
Zithromax for Oral Suspension, 300 mg, 600 mg, 900 mg, 1200 mg (Rare) 2561
Zithromax Tablets, 250 mg, 500 mg (Rare) 2561
Zithromax Tri-Pak (Rare) 2561
Zoloft 2581
Zomig Nasal Spray (Infrequent) 718
Zyrtec Chewable Tablets (Less than 2%) 2589
Zyrtec (Less than 2%) 2589
Zyrtec-D 12 Hour Extended Release Tablets (Less than 2%) 2591
Zyvox (0.9% to 2%) 2661

Skin eruptions

Guanidine Hydrochloride Tablets 3030
Librium Capsules 3349
▲ Prevacid NapraPAC (3% to 9%) 3277

Skin hypertrophy

▲ CellCept Capsules (3% to less than 20%) 2751
▲ CellCept Intravenous (3% to less than 20%) 2751
▲ CellCept Oral Suspension (3% to less than 20%) 2751
▲ CellCept Tablets (3% to less than 20%) 2751
Copaxone for Injection (Infrequent) 3292
Effexor Tablets (Infrequent) 3405
Effexor XR Capsules (Infrequent) 3411
Evoxac Capsules (Less than 1%) 1042
Neurontin Capsules (Rare) 2498
Neurontin Oral Solution (Rare) 2498
Neurontin Tablets (Rare) 2498
Olux Foam (One case) 1027
Paxil CR Controlled-Release Tablets (Rare) 1509
Paxil (Rare) 1501
Pletal Tablets (Less than 2%) 2478
▲ Rapamune Oral Solution and Tablets (3% to 20%) 3472
Relpax Tablets (Rare) 2531
Rescriptor Tablets 2535
Sonata Capsules (Infrequent) 1686
Soriatane Capsules (Less than 1%) 1028

Skin nodule

Altoprev Extended-Release Tablets 1151
▲ Arava Tablets (1% to 3%) 2881
Celebrex Capsules (0.1% to 1.9%) 3130
Copaxone for Injection (2%) 3292
Doxil Injection (Less than 1%) 3302
Gabitril Tablets (Infrequent) 998
▲ Imdur Tablets (Less than or equal to 5%) 3032
Imitrex Nasal Spray 1435
Imitrex Tablets (Rare) 1440
Invirase (Less than 2%) 2776
Lescol Capsules 2227
Lescol Capsules 2730
Lescol XL Tablets 2227
Lescol XL Tablets 2730
Lexapro Oral Solution (Infrequent) 1193
Lexapro Tablets (Infrequent) 1193
Lotrel Capsules 2238
Lyrica Capsules (Rare) 2524
Mevacor Tablets 1996
Neurontin Capsules (Rare) 2498
Neurontin Oral Solution (Rare) 2498
Neurontin Tablets (Rare) 2498
Permax Tablets (Rare) 3357
Photofrin for Injection 729
Pravachol Tablets 943
Rescriptor Tablets 2535
Rilutek Tablets (Rare) 2945
Soriatane Capsules (Less than 1%) 1028
Targretin Capsules 1719
Vytorin 10/10 Tablets 2084
Vytorin 10/10 Tablets 3092
Vytorin 10/20 Tablets 2084
Vytorin 10/20 Tablets 3092
Vytorin 10/40 Tablets 2084
Vytorin 10/40 Tablets 3092
Vytorin 10/80 Tablets 2084
Vytorin 10/80 Tablets 3092
Zocor Tablets 2078
Zyrtec Chewable Tablets (Less than 2%) 2589
Zyrtec (Less than 2%) 2589
Zyrtec-D 12 Hour Extended Release Tablets (Less than 2%) 2591

Skin odor, abnormal

▲ Soriatane Capsules (1% to 10%) 1028

Skin papilloma

Elidel Cream 1% (Up to 3.3%) 2198
▲ Fuzeon Injection (4.2%) 2772

Skin reactions, unspecified

Aldara Cream, 5% 1814
Alphagan P Ophthalmic Solution 563
Brimonidine Tartrate Ophthalmic Solution 0.2% ⊙ 245
Duragesic Transdermal System (1% or greater) 2448
Ethyol for Injection (Rare) 1869
Fosamax Plus D Tablets (Rarely) 1956
▲ Gengraf Capsules (1% to 17.6%) 458
Inderal LA Long-Acting Capsules 3421
Protopic Ointment (1% to 4%) 629
▲ Tri-Luma Cream (5.45%) 1213
▲ Ultrase MT Capsules (0.2%) 736
Xalatan Sterile Ophthalmic Solution (1% to 2%) 2654

Skin redness

Thera-Gesic Plus Creme ▣ 673

Skin test reactions, suppression

Decadron Phosphate Injection 1931
Decadron Tablets 1929
Depo-Medrol Single-Dose Vial 2617
Hydrocortone Tablets 1963
Pediapred Oral Solution 3319

Skin trauma

Nasonex Nasal Spray (Greater than or equal to 2%) 3058

Skull abnormalities, fetal

Accutane Capsules 2740
Aceon Tablets (2 mg, 4 mg, 8 mg) 3191
Altace Capsules 1673
Captopril Tablets 2114
Cozaar Tablets 1913
Hyzaar 1964
Lotrel Capsules 2238
Prinivil Tablets 2029
Prinzide Tablets 2033
Vaseretic Tablets 2073
Vasotec I.V. Injection 2076
Zestoretic Tablets 701
Zestril Tablets 704

Sleep disturbances

Aceon Tablets (2 mg, 4 mg, 8 mg) (2.5%) 3191
Adalat CC Tablets (Rare) 2978
▲ Advair Diskus 100/50 (1% to 3%) 1291
▲ Advair Diskus 250/50 (1% to 3%) 1291
▲ Advair Diskus 500/50 (1% to 3%) 1291
Allegra-D 12 Hour Extended-Release Tablets (Less than 1%) 2860
Allegra-D 24 Hour Extended-Release Tablets (Less than 1%) 2862
Ambien Tablets (Infrequent) 2867
Amerge Tablets (Infrequent) 1312
Anzemet Injection (Infrequently) 2871
Anzemet Tablets (Infrequently) 2874
Aptivus Capsules (Less than 2%) 859
▲ Arava Tablets (1% to 3%) 2881
Astelin Nasal Spray (Infrequent) 1876
Avalide Tablets 922
Avalide Tablets 2889
Avapro Tablets (Less than 1%) 925
Avapro Tablets (Less than 1%) 2886
Avelox (Less than 0.1%) 2984
Celexa (At least 2%) 1177
▲ Clozapine Tablets (4%) 2141
▲ Clozaril Tablets (4%) 2174
▲ Combivir Tablets (11%) 1373
Copaxone for Injection (At least 2%) 3292
Coreg Tablets (Greater than 0.1% to 1%) 1376
Cozaar Tablets (Less than 1%) 1913
Cymbalta Delayed-Release Capsules (Frequent) 1729
Depakote ER Tablets (Greater than 1%) 433
Effexor Tablets (Infrequent) 3405
Eldepryl Capsules 3209
▲ Entocort EC Capsules (Less than 5%) 2694
▲ Epivir (11%) 1394
▲ FazaClo Orally Disintegrating Tablets (4%) 547
▲ Flovent Diskus 50 mcg (1% to 3%) 1415
▲ Hectorol Capsules (3.3%) 909
▲ Hectorol Injection (3.3%) 911
HibTITER 3419
Hyzaar 1964
Imitrex Injection (Rare) 1431
Imitrex Nasal Spray (Infrequent) 1435
Imitrex Tablets (Rare to infrequent) 1440
Klonopin (Infrequent) 2782
Lamictal (1.4%) 1449
▲ Lariam Tablets (Among most frequent) 2790
Levaquin in 5% Dextrose Injection (0.1% to 0.9%) 2453
Levaquin (0.1% to 0.9%) 2453
▲ Lotronex Tablets (3%) 1479
▲ Lupron Depot 3.75 mg (16%) 3257
Lupron Depot 7.5 mg (Less than 5%) 3261
▲ Lupron Depot–3 Month 11.25 mg (16%) 3262
Lupron Injection Pediatric 3256
Mirapex Tablets (Less than or equal to 1%) 889
Nadolol Tablets 2121
Namenda (Infrequent) 1199
Nexium Delayed-Release Capsules (Less than 1%) 645
Nexium I.V. (Less than 1%) 649
▲ Nicotrol Inhaler (Greater than 3%) 2594
Noroxin Tablets (Less frequent) 2009
Numorphan 1112
▲ Pacerone Tablets (1% to 3%) 3337
▲ Pediarix Vaccine (0.4% to 46.7%) 1518
Prevacid Delayed-Release Capsules (Less than 1%) 3268
Prevacid for Delayed-Release Oral Suspension (Less than 1%) 3268
Prevacid NapraPAC (Less than 1%) 3277
Prevacid SoluTab Delayed-Release Orally Disintegrating Tablets (Less than 1%) 3268
▲ Prevnar for Injection (15.3% to 25.2%) 3460
PREVPAC (Less than 1%) 3281
Prochieve 4% Gel 1018
Prochieve 8% Gel 1018
ProSom Tablets (Infrequent) 512
Protonix I.V. (Less than 1%) 3468
Protonix Tablets (Less than 1%) 3465
Provigil Tablets (At least 1%) 1002
Prozac Pulvules and Liquid (Frequent) 1771
Recombivax HB (Less than 1%) 2045
Relpax Tablets (Rare) 2531
Rescriptor Tablets 2535
Reyataz Capsules (Less than 3%) 948
Risperdal M-Tab Orally Disintegrating Tablets (Frequent) 1658
Risperdal (Frequent) 1658
▲ Roferon-A Injection (10% to 11%) 2805
Rythmol SR Capsules 2736
Serevent Diskus (1% to 3%) 1540
Sonata Capsules (Rare) 1686
▲ Strattera Capsules (4%) 1784
Symbyax Capsules (1% to 2%) 1788
▲ Tasmar Tablets (24% to 25%) 3360
Tricor Tablets 523
▲ Trizivir Tablets (7% to 11%) 1565
Univasc Tablets (Less than 1%) 3118

Valium Tablets ... 2822
Varivax (Greater than or equal to 1%) ... 2070
Viracept (Less than 2%) ... 2556
▲ Visudyne for Injection (1% to 10%) .. 2286
▲ Wellbutrin Tablets (4.0%) ... 1579
Xanax XR Tablets (Rare) ... 2655
▲ Xenical Capsules (3.9%) ... 2834
Zelnorm Tablets ... 2303
▲ Ziagen (10%) ... 1600
Zyrtec Chewable Tablets (Less than 2%) ... 2589
Zyrtec (Less than 2%) ... 2589
Zyrtec-D 12 Hour Extended Release Tablets (Less than 2%) ... 2591

Sleep disturbances, paradoxical
Diastat Rectal Delivery System (Infrequent) ... 3344
Niravam Orally Disintegrating Tablets (Rare) ... 3106

Sleep talking
Sonata Capsules (Rare) ... 1686
Xanax XR Tablets (Infrequent) ... 2655

Sleep walking
Neurontin Capsules ... 2498
Neurontin Oral Solution ... 2498
Neurontin Tablets ... 2498
Sonata Capsules (Rare) ... 1686

Sleepiness
(*see under* Drowsiness)

Sleeplessness
(*see under* Insomnia)

SLE-like syndrome
(*see under* Lupus erythematosus, systemic)

Slipped capital femoral epiphysis
Levothroid Tablets ... 1189

Sloughing
Aramine Injection ... 1889
Brevibloc Concentrate ... 766
Brevibloc Injection ... 766
Brevibloc Double Strength Injection ... 766
Brevibloc Premixed Injection ... 766
Brevibloc Double Strength Premixed Injection ... 766
Efudex ... 3348
Fluorescite Injection ... ⊙ 207
Navelbine Injection ... 1494
Ophthetic Ophthalmic Solution ... ⊙ 230

Sloughing at injection site
Depo-Medrol Single-Dose Vial ... 2617
Iveegam EN ... 759

Sluggishness
Cymbalta Delayed-Release Capsules (Infrequent) ... 1729
Lexapro Oral Solution (Infrequent) ... 1193
Lexapro Tablets (Infrequent) ... 1193
Sedapap Tablets 50 mg/650 mg (Infrequent) ... 2098
Thyrolar ... 1203
Xanax XR Tablets (Infrequent) ... 2655

Smell, loss of the sense
(*see under* Anosmia)

Smell disturbances
Amerge Tablets (Infrequent) ... 1312
Beconase AQ Nasal Spray (Rare) ... 1359
Biaxin/Biaxin XL ... 402
Eligard 7.5 mg (Less than 2%) ... 2896
Flonase Nasal Spray ... 1412
Imitrex Injection (Rare) ... 1431
Imitrex Nasal Spray (Infrequent) ... 1435
Imitrex Tablets (Infrequent) ... 1440
Lotronex Tablets (Rare) ... 1479
Maxair Autohaler (0.6%) ... 1820
Maxalt Tablets (Rare) ... 1983
Maxalt-MLT Orally Disintegrating Tablets (Rare) ... 1983
Migranal Nasal Spray (Infrequent) ... 3350
Nasonex Nasal Spray (Very rare) ... 3058
Nicotrol NS ... 2596
▲ Pacerone Tablets (1% to 3%) ... 3337
PREVPAC ... 3281
▲ Roferon-A Injection (3%) ... 2805
Testim 1% Gel (1% or less) ... 722
Timentin ADD-Vantage ... 1556
Timentin Injection Galaxy Container ... 1559
Timentin IV Infusion ... 1553
Timentin Pharmacy Bulk Package ... 1562

Smoker's tongue
(*see under* Leukoplakia, oral)

Sneezing
Aceon Tablets (2 mg, 4 mg, 8 mg) (0.3% to 1%) ... 3191
▲ Advair Diskus 100/50 (1% to 3%) ... 1291
▲ Advair Diskus 250/50 (1% to 3%) ... 1291
▲ Advair Diskus 500/50 (1% to 3%) ... 1291
▲ Aerobid/Aerobid-M (3% to 9%) ... 1172
Alamast Ophthalmic Solution (Less than 5%) ... 3371
▲ Astelin Nasal Spray (3.1%) ... 1876
▲ Atrovent Nasal Spray 0.03% (3.1%) ... 869
Axert Tablets (Rare) ... 2430
▲ Beconase AQ Nasal Spray (4%) ... 1359
Bentyl Capsules ... 724
Bentyl Injection ... 724
Bentyl Syrup ... 724
Bentyl Tablets ... 724
Calcium Disodium Versenate Injection ... 1819
Clozapine Tablets (Less than 1%) ... 2141
Clozaril Tablets (Less than 1%) ... 2174
Diprivan Injectable Emulsion (Less than 1%) ... 676
Ethyol for Injection ... 1869
FazaClo Orally Disintegrating Tablets (Less than 1%) ... 547
▲ Intron A for Injection (Less than or equal to 5%) ... 3038
Klonopin (Infrequent) ... 2782
Maxalt Tablets (Rare) ... 1983
Maxalt-MLT Orally Disintegrating Tablets (Rare) ... 1983
Naropin Injection ... 640
▲ Nasacort HFA Inhalation Aerosol (Greater than or equal to 3% to 15.9%) ... 2939
Nicotrol NS ... 2596
Plendil Extended-Release Tablets (Up to 1.6%) ... 651
Simulect for Injection ... 2268
Vicks NyQuil LiquiCaps/Liquid Multi-Symptom Cold/Flu Relief ... ▣ 725
Vicks Sinex Nasal Spray and Ultra Fine Mist for Sinus Relief ... 2677
Zicam Cold Remedy Nasal Pump ... ▣
Zicam Cold Remedy Swabs ... ▣
Zicam Cold Remedy Swabs Kids Size ... ▣
Zicam Extreme Congestion Relief Nasal Pump ... ▣
Zicam Sinus Relief Nasal Pump ... ▣

Snoring
Aricept Tablets (Infrequent) ... 1086
Aricept ODT Tablets (Infrequent) ... 1086
▲ Increlex Injection (Greater than or equal to 5%) ... 3290
Neurontin Capsules (Rare) ... 2498
Neurontin Oral Solution (Rare) ... 2498
Neurontin Tablets (Rare) ... 2498
Sonata Capsules (Infrequent) ... 1686

Social reaction, anti
(*see under* Sociopathy)

Sociopathy
DextroStat Tablets ... 3177
Neurontin Capsules (Rare) ... 2498
Neurontin Oral Solution (Rare) ... 2498
Neurontin Tablets (Rare) ... 2498
Paxil CR Controlled-Release Tablets (Rare) ... 1509
Paxil (Rare) ... 1501
Zyprexa Tablets (Infrequent) ... 1798
Zyprexa ZYDIS Orally Disintegrating Tablets (Infrequent) ... 1798

Sodium depletion
(*see under* Hyponatremia)

Sodium loss
(*see under* Hyponatremia)

Sodium retention
Decadron Phosphate Injection ... 1931
Decadron Tablets ... 1929
Delatestryl Injection ... 2976
Depo-Medrol Injectable Suspension ... 2615
Depo-Medrol Single-Dose Vial ... 2617
▲ Estratest Tablets (Among most common) ... 3196
▲ Estratest H.S. Tablets (Among most common) ... 3196
Hydrocortone Tablets ... 1963
Hyperstat I.V. Injection ... 3031
Oxandrin Tablets ... 2977
Pediapred Oral Solution ... 3319

Somatization
Zyprexa Tablets (Infrequent) ... 1798
Zyprexa ZYDIS Orally Disintegrating Tablets (Infrequent) ... 1798

Somnambulism
Ambien Tablets (Rare) ... 2867
Requip Tablets (Infrequent) ... 1528
Zoloft (Rare) ... 2581

Somnolence
(*see under* Drowsiness)

Sore throat
(*see under* Throat soreness)

Soreness, injection site
▲ Alferon N Injection (10%) ... 1640
▲ Comvax (23.9% to 34.5%) ... 1904
▲ Engerix-B Vaccine (22%) ... 1391
▲ Havrix Vaccine (21% to 56%) ... 1425
HyperRAB ... 3239
HyperRho S/D Full Dose ... 3243
HyperRho S/D Mini-Dose ... 3241
HyperTET ... 3245
Infed Injection ... 3381
Pneumovax 23 (Common) ... 2020
▲ Vaqta (1.2% to 3.5%) ... 2067
▲ Varivax (19.3% to 32.5%) ... 2070

Soreness, nasal
▲ Fortical Nasal Spray (10.6%) ... 3336

Soreness, vaginal
▲ Gynazole-1 Vaginal Cream (5.7%) ... 3298

Soreness at insertion site
▲ Vantas (3.6%) ... 3367

Spasm, biliary tract
Dilaudid ... 439
Dilaudid Oral Liquid ... 443
Dilaudid Non-Sterile Powder ... 439
Dilaudid Rectal Suppositories ... 439
Dilaudid Tablets ... 439
Dilaudid Tablets - 8 mg ... 443
Dilaudid-HP (Less frequent) ... 441
MS Contin Tablets (Less frequent) ... 2703
Numorphan ... 1112

Spasm, gastrointestinal
Lotronex Tablets (Infrequent) ... 1479

Spasm, generalized
Colazal Capsules ... 2845
Gabitril Tablets (Infrequent) ... 998
Invirase (Less than 2%) ... 2776
Lyrica Capsules (Rare) ... 2524
Paxil CR Controlled-Release Tablets (Rare) ... 1509
Paxil (Rare) ... 1501
Prinivil Tablets (0.3% to 1.0%) ... 2029
Prinzide Tablets ... 2033
▲ Prograf Capsules and Injection (3% to 15%) ... 624
Symbyax Capsules (Infrequent) ... 1788
Zestoretic Tablets ... 701
Zestril Tablets (0.3% to 1.0%) ... 704
▲ Zyprexa Tablets (2% to 3%) ... 1798
Zyprexa ZYDIS Orally Disintegrating Tablets (2% to 3%) ... 1798

Spasm, non-site specific
Amerge Tablets (Rare) ... 1312
Invanz for Injection (Greater than 0.1%) ... 1974

Spasm, sphincter of Oddi
Combunox Tablets ... 1183
Zelnorm Tablets ... 2303

Spasm, urinary bladder
Eligard 22.5 mg (Less than 2%) ... 2899

Spasm, vesical sphincters
Hycomine Compound Tablets ... 1105
Hycotuss Expectorant Syrup ... 1106
Lortab ... 3315
Lortab Elixir ... 3312
Tussionex Pennkinetic Extended-Release Suspension ... 3322
Vicodin Tablets ... 530
Vicodin ES Tablets ... 531
Vicodin HP Tablets ... 532
Zydone Tablets ... 1118

Speech, incoherent
Clozapine Tablets (Less than 1%) ... 2141
Clozaril Tablets (Less than 1%) ... 2174

Speech, pressure of
Cymbalta Delayed-Release Capsules (Infrequent) ... 1729

Speech, slurring
Clozapine Tablets (1%) ... 2141
Clozaril Tablets (1%) ... 2174
Dalmane Capsules (Rare) ... 3343
Diastat Rectal Delivery System (Infrequent) ... 3344
Eskalith ... 1406
FazaClo Orally Disintegrating Tablets (1%) ... 547
Kadian Capsules (Less than 3%) ... 572
Klonopin ... 2782
Lithobid Tablets ... 1670
Matulane Capsules ... 3188
Nadolol Tablets (1 to 5 of 1000 patients) ... 2121
Niravam Orally Disintegrating Tablets ... 3106
▲ Phenytek Capsules (Among most common) ... 2153
Sonata Capsules (Rare) ... 1686
Symmetrel (0.1% to 1%) ... 1115
Tranxene ... 2488
Valium Tablets (Infrequent) ... 2822
Vicoprofen Tablets (Less than 1%) ... 533

Speech difficulties
Clozapine Tablets (Less than 1%) ... 2141
Clozaril Tablets (Less than 1%) ... 2174
▲ Demser Capsules (10%) ... 1933
FazaClo Orally Disintegrating Tablets (Less than 1%) ... 547
Geodon for Injection (Up to 2%) ... 2514
Marinol Capsules (Less than 1%) ... 3334
Nubain Injection (1% or less) ... 1111
Zyprexa Tablets (2%) ... 1798
Zyprexa ZYDIS Orally Disintegrating Tablets (2%) ... 1798

Speech disorder
▲ Lyrica Capsules (1% to 7%) ... 2524

Speech disturbances
Actiq (Less than 1%) ... 993
▲ Adderall XR Capsules (2% to 4%) ... 3169
Ambien Tablets (Infrequent) ... 2867
Avelox (Less than 0.1%) ... 2984
Bentyl Capsules ... 724
Bentyl Injection ... 724
Bentyl Syrup ... 724
Bentyl Tablets ... 724
Brevibloc Concentrate (Less than 1%) ... 766
Brevibloc Injection (Less than 1%) ... 766
Brevibloc Double Strength Injection (Less than 1%) ... 766
Brevibloc Premixed Injection (Less than 1%) ... 766
Brevibloc Double Strength Premixed Injection (Less than 1%) ... 766
Carbatrol Capsules ... 3174
Copaxone for Injection (2%) ... 3292
Dantrium Capsules (Less frequent) .. 2690
▲ Depakote Tablets (1% to 5%) ... 427
▲ Depakote ER Tablets (1% to 5%) ... 433
Diastat Rectal Delivery System (Greater than or equal to 1%) ... 3344
Duragesic Transdermal System (1% or greater) ... 2448
Effexor Tablets (Infrequent) ... 3405
Effexor XR Capsules (Infrequent) ... 3411
Eldepryl Capsules ... 3209
▲ Equetro Extended-Release Capsules (6%) ... 3178
Evoxac Capsules (Less than 1%) ... 1042
Frova Tablets (Infrequent) ... 1101
▲ Gabitril Tablets (4%) ... 998
Geodon Capsules (2%) ... 2514
Imitrex Injection ... 1431
▲ Intron A for Injection (Less than 5%) ... 3038
Invirase (Less than 2%) ... 2776
Lamictal (2.5%) ... 1449
Levaquin in 5% Dextrose Injection (0.1% to 0.9%) ... 2453
Levaquin (0.1% to 0.9%) ... 2453
Meridia Capsules ... 485
Migranal Nasal Spray (Rare) ... 3350
Neurontin Capsules (Infrequent) ... 2498
Neurontin Oral Solution (Infrequent) ... 2498
Neurontin Tablets (Infrequent) ... 2498
▲ Orap Tablets (2 of 20 patients) ... 1220
Ortho-Cyclen/Ortho Tri-Cyclen ... 2414
Ortho Tri-Cyclen Lo Tablets ... 2421
OxyContin Tablets (Less than 1%) ... 2699
Permax Tablets (1.1%) ... 3357
Prevacid Delayed-Release Capsules (Less than 1%) ... 3268

Prevacid for Delayed-Release Oral Suspension (Less than 1%) ... 3268
Prevacid NapraPAC ... 3277
Prevacid SoluTab Delayed-Release Orally Disintegrating Tablets (Less than 1%) ... 3268
PREVPAC ... 3281
▲ Proleukin for Injection (7%) ... 1007
Prometrium Capsules (100 mg, 200 mg) (Less than 5%) ... 3205
Protonix I.V. ... 3468
Protonix Tablets ... 3465
Relpax Tablets (Infrequent) ... 2531
Rythmol SR Capsules ... 2736
Symbyax Capsules (Up to 2%) ... 1788
Tambocor Tablets (Less than 1%) ... 1824
Tasmar Tablets (Frequent) ... 3360
Tegretol/Tegretol-XR ... 2278
▲ Topamax Sprinkle Capsules (Less than 1% to 13%) ... 2438
▲ Topamax Tablets (Less than 1% to 13%) ... 2438
▲ Trileptal Oral Suspension (1% to 3%) ... 2281
▲ Trileptal Tablets (1% to 3%) ... 2281
▲ Vesanoid Capsules (3%) ... 2823
Zomig Nasal Spray (Infrequent) ... 718
▲ Zonegran Capsules (5%) ... 1089
Zyprexa Tablets (2%) ... 1798
Zyprexa ZYDIS Orally Disintegrating Tablets (2%) ... 1798

Spermatogenesis, changes
Cytovene-IV ... 2763

Spermatogenesis, defective
Mustargen for Injection ... 2007

Spermatogenesis, inhibition
Cytovene-IV ... 2763

Spermatozoa, changes
Decadron Tablets ... 1929

Spinal block
Naropin Injection ... 640

Spinal cord, compression
Zoladex ... 709
Zoladex 3-month (Isolated cases) ... 712

Spinal cord infarction
Activase I.V. ... 1225

Spinal fracture
Lupron Depot 3.75 mg ... 3257
Lupron Depot 7.5 mg ... 3261
Lupron Depot–3 Month 11.25 mg ... 3262
Lupron Depot-PED 7.5 mg, 11.25 mg and 15 mg ... 3266

Spleen disorder
Rescriptor Tablets ... 2535
Rythmol SR Capsules ... 2736

Spleen palpable
Thalomid Capsules ... 979

Spleenomegaly
BiDil Tablets ... 2161
Flolan for Injection ... 1408
VFEND I.V. (Less than 2%) ... 2543
VFEND Oral Suspension (Less than 2%) ... 2543
VFEND Tablets (Less than 2%) ... 2543

Splenic infarction
Campath Ampules ... 826
Zomig Nasal Spray (Very rare) ... 718
Zomig Tablets ... 714
Zomig-ZMT Tablets ... 714

Splenic rupture
Neulasta Injection (Rare) ... 596
Neupogen for Injection (Rare) ... 598

Splenomegaly
Aloprim for Injection (Less than 1%) ... 2156
Campath Ampules ... 826
Combivir Tablets ... 1373
Copaxone for Injection (Infrequent) ... 3292
Epivir ... 1394
Epivir-HBV ... 1398
Epzicom Tablets ... 1402
Garamycin Injectable ... 3028
Invirase (Less than 2%) ... 2776
Iveegam EN ... 759
▲ Neupogen for Injection (Approximately 30%) ... 598
Orthoclone OKT3 Sterile Solution ... 2370
Permax Tablets (Rare) ... 3357
Retrovir IV Infusion ... 1537
RhoGAM Ultra-Filtered (One patient) ... 2429
Tabloid Tablets ... 1545
Trizivir Tablets ... 1565

Spotting
Activella Tablets ... 2311
Alesse-28 Tablets ... 3392
Aygestin Tablets ... 1062
Bravelle for Intramuscular or Subcutaneous Injection (2.7%) ... 1140
Cenestin Tablets, 0.45mg, 0.625mg, 0.9mg, 1.25mg ... 1063
Cenestin Tablets, 0.3mg ... 1063
Climara Transdermal System ... 795
Climara Pro Transdermal System ... 800
Estratest Tablets ... 3196
Estratest H.S. Tablets ... 3196
Estrogel 0.06% ... 3200
Lexapro Oral Solution (Infrequent) ... 1193
Lexapro Tablets (Infrequent) ... 1193
Lo/Ovral-28 Tablets ... 3423
Menostar Transdermal System ... 805
Ortho-Cept Tablets ... 2395
Ortho-Cyclen Tablets ... 2414
Ortho Evra Transdermal System ... 2402
Ortho Tri-Cyclen Tablets ... 2414
Ortho Tri-Cyclen Lo Tablets ... 2421
Prefest Tablets ... 1069
Premarin Intravenous ... 3440
Premarin Tablets ... 3443
Premarin Vaginal Cream ... 3449
Premphase Tablets ... 3452
Prempro Tablets ... 3452
Prometrium Capsules (100 mg, 200 mg) ... 3205
Seasonale Tablets ... 1073
Triphasil-28 Tablets ... 3483
Verelan PM Capsules (2% or less) ... 3120
Vivelle Transdermal System ... 2288
Vivelle-Dot Transdermal System ... 2293

Spotting, irregular
depo-subQ provera 104 Injectable Suspension ... 2622

Spotting, oily
▲ Xenical Capsules (4.4% to 26.6%) ... 2834

Spotting, prolonged
depo-subQ provera 104 Injectable Suspension ... 2622

Sputum, discoloration
▲ TOBI Solution for Inhalation (21.3%) ... 1015

Sputum increased
Abilify Tablets (Rare) ... 916
Abilify Tablets (Rare) ... 2472
Actiq (Less than 1%) ... 993
▲ Aerobid/Aerobid-M (3% to 9%) ... 1172
Atrovent Inhalation Solution (1.4%) ... 868
Celexa (Rare) ... 1177
▲ CellCept Capsules (3% to less than 20%) ... 2751
▲ CellCept Intravenous (3% to less than 20%) ... 2751
▲ CellCept Oral Suspension (3% to less than 20%) ... 2751
▲ CellCept Tablets (3% to less than 20%) ... 2751
Combivent Inhalation Aerosol (Less than 2%) ... 878
Foradil Aerolizer (1.5%) ... 3024
▲ Imdur Tablets (Less than or equal to 5%) ... 3032
Lupron Depot 7.5 mg (Less than 5%) ... 3261
Nicotrol NS (Less than 1%) ... 2596
Paxil CR Controlled-Release Tablets (Rare) ... 1509
Paxil (Rare) ... 1501
Proventil Inhalation Solution 0.083% (1.5%) ... 3069
Pulmozyme Inhalation Solution ... 1245
Relpax Tablets (Rare) ... 2531
Rilutek Tablets (More than 2%) ... 2945
Risperdal M-Tab Orally Disintegrating Tablets (Rare) ... 1658
Risperdal (Rare) ... 1658
Sonata Capsules (Rare) ... 1686
Soriatane Capsules (Less than 1%) ... 1028
▲ TOBI Solution for Inhalation (37.6%) ... 1015
Ultane Liquid for Inhalation (Less than 1%) ... 526
Viagra Tablets (Less than 2%) ... 2552
Zomig Nasal Spray (Rare) ... 718
Zyrtec Chewable Tablets (Less than 2%) ... 2589
Zyrtec (Less than 2%) ... 2589
Zyrtec-D 12 Hour Extended Release Tablets (Less than 2%) ... 2591

S-T depressed
Lyrica Capsules (Rare) ... 2524
Ultane Liquid for Inhalation (Less than 1%) ... 526

ST section changes
(*see under* EKG changes, ST section)

Standing, difficulty in
Stromectol Tablets ... 2053

Status asthmaticus
Sandostatin Injection (Less than 1%) ... 2263
Sandostatin LAR Depot (Rare) ... 2264

Status epilepticus
Aloprim for Injection (Less than 1%) ... 2156
Carbatrol Capsules ... 3174
Clozapine Tablets ... 2141
Clozaril Tablets ... 2174
FazaClo Orally Disintegrating Tablets ... 547
Gabitril Tablets ... 998
Keppra Oral Solution (2%) ... 3307
Keppra Tablets (2%) ... 3307
Oncaspar ... 1123
Paxil CR Controlled-Release Tablets ... 1509
Paxil ... 1501
Tegretol/Tegretol-XR ... 2278

Steatorrhea
Azasan Tablets (Less than 1%) ... 2844
Miradon Tablets ... 3056
▲ Sandostatin Injection (22% to 35%) ... 2263
▲ Sandostatin LAR Depot (4% to 6%) ... 2264

Steatosis, hepatic
Combivir Tablets ... 1373
Cymbalta Delayed-Release Capsules (Infrequent) ... 1729
Epivir ... 1394
Epivir-HBV ... 1398
Epzicom Tablets ... 1402
Retrovir Capsules ... 1533
Retrovir IV Infusion (Rare) ... 1537
Retrovir ... 1533
Trizivir Tablets ... 1565
Viread Tablets ... 1284
Zerit ... 971
Ziagen ... 1600

Stenosis, aortic
Argatroban Injection (0.9%) ... 1321
Tasmar Tablets (Infrequent) ... 3360

Stenosis, intestinal
Remicade for IV Injection (Greater than or equal to 0.2%) ... 987

Stenosis, hepatic artery
Ammonul Injection ... 3323

Stenosis, nasal
▲ Fortical Nasal Spray (10.6%) ... 3336

Stevens-Johnson syndrome
Aciphex Tablets ... 1081
Advicor Tablets ... 1694
Agenerase Capsules (1%) ... 1299
Agenerase Oral Solution (1%) ... 1304
Aggrenox Capsules ... 855
Aldoclor Tablets ... 1881
Aldoril Tablets ... 1884
Altoprev Extended-Release Tablets ... 1151
Amoxil Capsules ... 1315
Amoxil Chewable Tablets ... 1315
Amoxil Pediatric Drops for Oral Suspension ... 1315
Amoxil Powder for Oral Suspension ... 1315
Amoxil Tablets ... 1315
Anaprox Tablets (Less than 1%) ... 2769
Anaprox DS Tablets (Less than 1%) ... 2769
Ancef for Injection ... 1318
Antara Capsules (Rare) ... 2723
Arava Tablets (Rare) ... 2881
Arimidex Tablets (Very rare) ... 665
Arthrotec Tablets (Rare) ... 3126
Atacand HCT ... 637
Attenuvax ... 1889
Augmentin (Rare) ... 1331
Augmentin Tablets (Rare) ... 1334
Augmentin XR Extended-Release Tablets (Rare) ... 1340
Augmentin ES-600 Powder for Oral Suspension ... 1337
Avalide Tablets ... 922
Avalide Tablets ... 2889
Avelox ... 2984
Betagan Ophthalmic Solution, USP ... ⊙217
Biaxin/Biaxin XL (Rare) ... 402
Bleph-10 Ophthalmic Solution 10% (Isolated incident) ... ⊙219
▲ Blephamide Ophthalmic Ointment (Among most often) ... 563
Blephamide Ophthalmic Suspension ... 564
Caduet Tablets ... 2507
Captopril Tablets ... 2114
Carbatrol Capsules (Extremely rare) ... 3174
Carimune NF ... 3501
Cataflam Tablets (Rarely) ... 2173
Ceftin ... 1369
Celebrex Capsules (Less than 0.1%) ... 3130
Cialis Tablets ... 1806
Cipro I.V. (1% or less) ... 2998
Cipro I.V. Pharmacy Bulk Package (1% or less) ... 3509
Cipro ... 2991
Cipro XR Tablets ... 3004
Cleocin Vaginal Ovules ... 2613
Clindesse Vaginal Cream (Rare) ... 3296
Clinoril Tablets (Less than 1 in 100) ... 1899
Clozapine Tablets ... 2141
Clozaril Tablets ... 2174
Combivir Tablets ... 1373
Comvax ... 1904
Covera-HS Tablets (Less than 2%) ... 3135
Crixivan Capsules ... 1918
Cytovene ... 2763
Daraprim Tablets ... 1385
Depacon Injection ... 412
Depakene ... 417
Depakote Sprinkle Capsules ... 422
Depakote Tablets ... 427
Depakote ER Tablets ... 433
Didronel Tablets (A single case) ... 2693
Diovan HCT Tablets ... 2195
Diuril Oral ... 1936
Diuril Sodium Intravenous ... 1934
Dolobid Tablets (Less than 1 in 100) ... 1937
Dynacin Tablets (Rarely reported) ... 1859
EC-Naprosyn Delayed-Release Tablets (Less than 1%) ... 2769
E.E.S. (Rare) ... 449
Effexor Tablets ... 3405
Effexor XR Capsules ... 3411
Emend Capsules (One patient) ... 1944
Engerix-B Vaccine ... 1391
Epzicom Tablets ... 1402
Equetro Extended-Release Capsules ... 3178
EryPed (Rare) ... 445
Erythromycin Delayed-Release Capsules, USP (Rare) ... 456
Ethyol for Injection (Rare) ... 1869
Exelon Capsules ... 2204
FazaClo Orally Disintegrating Tablets ... 547
FML-S Liquifilm Sterile Ophthalmic Suspension (Rare) ... ⊙226
Fortaz ... 1422
Fosamax (Rare) ... 1949
Fosamax Plus D Tablets (Rarely) ... 1956
Gammagard Liquid ... 751
Gammagard S/D (Rare) ... 754
Gamunex Immune Globulin I.V., 10% (Rare) ... 3232
Gleevec Tablets (Rare) ... 2221
Hyzaar ... 1964
Indapamide Tablets ... 2119
Inderal LA Long-Acting Capsules ... 3421
Indocin Capsules (Less than 1%) ... 1968
Indocin I.V. (Less than 1%) ... 1973
Indocin (Less than 1%) ... 1968
Invirase (Rare) ... 2776
Iveegam EN (Rare) ... 759
Lamictal (Rare) ... 1449
Lamisil Tablets (Isolated reports) ... 2226
Lariam Tablets ... 2790
Lescol Capsules (Rare) ... 2227
Lescol Capsules (Rare) ... 2730
Lescol XL Tablets ... 2227
Lescol XL Tablets ... 2730
Leukeran Tablets (Rare) ... 1472
Leustatin Injection (Isolated cases) ... 2368
Levaquin in 5% Dextrose Injection (Rare) ... 2453
Levaquin (Rare) ... 2453
Lexiva Tablets (One case) ... 1473
Lipitor Tablets ... 2495
Lofibra Capsules (Rare) ... 1217
Lotensin Tablets (Less than 1%) ... 2232
Lotensin HCT Tablets (Rare) ... 2235
Lotrel Capsules (Rare) ... 2238

Lyrica Capsules (Rare) 2524
Malarone Tablets (One case) 1484
Malarone Pediatric Tablets (One case) 1484
Maxipime for Injection 1093
Mefoxin for Injection 1987
Mefoxin Premixed Intravenous Solution 1990
Merrem I.V. 687
Meruvax II 1994
Mevacor Tablets (Rare) 1996
Micardis HCT Tablets 886
Mintezol 2002
M-M-R II 1980
Mobic Oral Suspension (Less than 0.1%) 893
Mobic Tablets (Less than 0.1%) 893
Moduretic Tablets 2003
Mumpsvax 2005
Nalfon Capsules (Less than 1%) 2504
Namenda 1199
Naprosyn Suspension (Less than 1%) 2769
Naprosyn Tablets (Less than 1%) 2769
Neurontin Capsules 2498
Neurontin Oral Solution 2498
Neurontin Tablets 2498
Nexium Delayed-Release Capsules (Rare) 645
Nexium I.V. (Rare) 649
Niravam Orally Disintegrating Tablets 3106
Noroxin Tablets 2009
Norvir (Rare) 499
Omnicef Capsules 506
Omnicef for Oral Suspension 506
Orthoclone OKT3 Sterile Solution 2370
PCE Dispertab Tablets (Rare) 510
PEG-Intron Powder for Injection 3062
Phenytek Capsules 2153
Plavix Tablets 940
Plavix Tablets 2942
Pletal Tablets (Very rare) 2478
Prandin Tablets (0.5, 1, and 2 mg) (Rare) 2337
Pravachol Tablets (Rare) 943
Prevacid NapraPAC (Less than 1%) 3277
PREVPAC (Rare) 3281
Prilosec OTC Tablets (Very rare) 2674
Primaxin I.M. 2022
Primaxin I.V. 2024
Prinivil Tablets (Rare) 2029
Prinzide Tablets (Rare) 2033
Prograf Capsules and Injection 624
ProSom Tablets (Rare) 512
Protonix I.V. 3468
Protonix Tablets 3465
Provigil Tablets (Rare) 1002
Prozac Pulvules and Liquid 1771
Recombivax HB 2045
Relafen Tablets (Less than 1%) 1523
Rescriptor Tablets 2535
Retrovir IV Infusion 1537
Reyataz Capsules 948
Sanctura Tablets 1133
Seroquel Tablets 691
Stromectol Tablets 2053
Suprax (Less than 2%) 1811
Sustiva Capsules (Up to 3.5%) 957
Tagamet Tablets (Very Rare) 1547
Tarka Tablets 519
Taxotere Injection Concentrate 2947
Tegretol/Tegretol-XR (Extremely rare) 2278
Tequin Injection 964
Tequin Tablets 964
Teveten HCT Tablets 1710
Thalomid Capsules 979
Tiazac Capsules (Less than 2%) 1204
Ticlid Tablets (Rare) 2813
Timentin ADD-Vantage 1556
Timentin Injection Galaxy Container 1559
Timentin IV Infusion 1553
Timentin Pharmacy Bulk Package 1562
Timolide Tablets 2056
Topamax Sprinkle Capsules 2438
Topamax Tablets 2438
Tricor Tablets (Rare) 523
Trileptal Oral Suspension 2281
Trileptal Tablets 2281
Trizivir Tablets 1565
Trusopt Sterile Ophthalmic Solution (Rare) 2065
Twinrix Vaccine 1571
Ultracet Tablets 2462
Uniretic Tablets 3114
Vancocin HCl Capsules, USP (Infrequent) 3370
Vantin Tablets and Oral Suspension 2650
Varivax 2070
Vaseretic Tablets 2073
Vasotec I.V. Injection (0.5% to 1.0%) 2076
Verelan PM Capsules (2% or less) 3120
VFEND I.V. (Rare) 2543
VFEND Oral Suspension (Rare) 2543
VFEND Tablets (Rare) 2543
Viramune Oral Suspension 903
Viramune Tablets 903
Voltaren Tablets (Rarely) 2298
Voltaren-XR Tablets (Rarely) 2301
Vytorin 10/10 Tablets 2084
Vytorin 10/10 Tablets 3092
Vytorin 10/20 Tablets 2084
Vytorin 10/20 Tablets 3092
Vytorin 10/40 Tablets 2084
Vytorin 10/40 Tablets 3092
Vytorin 10/80 Tablets 2084
Vytorin 10/80 Tablets 3092
Wellbutrin Tablets (Rare) 1579
Wellbutrin SR Sustained-Release Tablets (Rare) 1583
Wellbutrin XL Extended-Release Tablets (Rare) 1588
Xanax XR Tablets 2655
Zegerid Powder for Oral Solution (Very rare) 2972
Zestoretic Tablets 701
Zevalin Injection 848
Ziagen 1600
Zinacef Injection (Rare) 1604
Zinacef for Injection (Rare) 1604
Zithromax Capsules, 250 mg (Rare) 2568
Zithromax for IV Infusion (Rare) 2573
Zithromax for Oral Suspension, 300 mg, 600 mg, 900 mg, 1200 mg (Rare) 2561
Zithromax Tablets, 250 mg, 500 mg (Rare) 2561
Zithromax Tri-Pak (Rare) 2561
Zmax for Oral Suspension (Rare) 2577
Zocor Tablets (Rare) 2078
Zoloft 2581
Zonegran Capsules (Rare) 1089
Zosyn (Rare) 3492
Zovirax Capsules 1616
Zovirax for Injection 1618
Zovirax 1616
Zyban Sustained-Release Tablets 1620

Stiffness, unspecified

Fortical Nasal Spray (Less than 1%) 3336

Stillbirths

Aggrenox Capsules 855
Bayer Aspirin Tablets 3515
Ecotrin Enteric Coated Aspirin Low, Regular and Maximum Strength Tablets 1627
St. Joseph 81 mg Aspirin Chewable and Enteric Coated Tablets 1841
Zyrtec-D 12 Hour Extended Release Tablets (Rare) 2591

Stimulation

Dalmane Capsules (Rare) 3343
Parcopa Orally Disintegrating Tablets 3111
Sonata Capsules (Rare) 1686
Stalevo Tablets 2270
Valium Tablets 2822
Xanax XR Tablets (Rare) 2655

Stinging

Acticin Cream 2125
▲ Acular Ophthalmic Solution (Up to 40%) 561
▲ Acular LS Ophthalmic Solution (20% to 40%) 562
Adriamycin for Injection, USP 786
Adriamycin Injection, USP 786
Aldara Cream, 5% (More than 1%) 1814
Attenuvax 1889
Bactroban Nasal (2%) 1357
Bactroban Ointment (1.5%) 1358
▲ Betagan Ophthalmic Solution, USP (About 1 in 3 patients) ⊙ 217
▲ Betimol Ophthalmic Solution (1 in 8 patients) ⊙ 283
▲ Betimol Ophthalmic Solution (1 in 8 patients) 3371
Bleph-10 Ophthalmic Solution 10% ⊙ 219
▲ Brimonidine Tartrate Ophthalmic Solution 0.2% (10% to 30%) ⊙ 245
Clobevate Gel (Less than 2%) 3213
Clobex Shampoo 1209
▲ Cosopt Sterile Ophthalmic Solution (Up to 30%) 1910
Cozaar Tablets (Less than 1%) 1913
Cutivate Cream (0.8%) 1381
Cutivate Lotion 0.05% (2%) 1383
▲ Differin Cream (Less than 1% to 24%) 1210
Differin Gel (Approximately 1% or less) 1211
▲ Diprivan Injectable Emulsion (10% to 17.6%) 676
Diprolene AF Cream 0.05% (0.4%) 3014
▲ Dovonex Scalp Solution 0.005% (Approximately 23%) 3375
Doxil Injection 3302
Drysol Solution 2506
▲ Elocon Cream 0.1% (1.6% to approximately 7%) 3019
▲ Elocon Ointment 0.1% (4.8% to approximately 7%) 3021
▲ Finacea Gel (4% to 20%) 1644
FML Ophthalmic Suspension ⊙ 224
FML Forte Ophthalmic Suspension ⊙ 223
HMS Sterile Ophthalmic Suspension (Occasional) ⊙ 228
Hyzaar 1964
Idamycin PFS Injection 2645
Imitrex Injection (Infrequent) 1431
Klaron Lotion 10% 1050
Lotrimin 3053
Lotrisone (Less than 1%) 3054
▲ Luxíq Foam (2% to 44%) 1026
Mentax Cream (Approximately 1%) 2152
Meruvax II 1994
▲ Metrogel 1% (1.3% to 7.2%) 1212
M-M-R II 1980
Mumpsvax 2005
▲ Naftin Cream (6%) 2097
▲ Naftin Gel (5.0%) 2097
Ocufen Ophthalmic Solution ⊙ 230
Olux Foam (Less than 2%) 1027
Ophthetic Ophthalmic Solution (Occasional) ⊙ 230
▲ Optivar Ophthalmic Solution (Approximately 30%) 1877
Oxistat (0.1%) 1498
Pandel Cream, 0.1% (0.9%) 1017
Patanol Ophthalmic Solution (Less than 5%) 557
Polytrim Ophthalmic Solution 570
Pred Forte Ophthalmic Suspension ⊙ 233
Pred Mild Sterile Ophthalmic Suspension ⊙ 236
Pred-G Ophthalmic Suspension ⊙ 234
▲ Propine Ophthalmic Solution (6%) ⊙ 237
▲ Renova 0.02% Cream (Almost all subjects) 2384
▲ Renova 0.05% Cream (Almost all subjects) 2387
▲ Solage Topical Solution (21.9% to 26%) 740
▲ Spectazole Cream (3%) 2390
Temovate Cream (1%) 1549
▲ Temovate Gel (Among most frequent) 1550
Temovate Ointment (Less frequent) 1549
▲ Temovate Scalp Application (29 of 294 patients) 1551
▲ Temovate E Emollient (5%) 1552
▲ Timoptic in Ocudose (Approximately 1 in 8 patients) 2061
▲ Timoptic Sterile Ophthalmic Solution (Approximately 1 in 8 patients) 2058
▲ Timoptic-XE Sterile Ophthalmic Gel Forming Solution (1 in 8 patients) 2062
▲ Trusopt Sterile Ophthalmic Solution (Approximately one-third of patients) 2065
▲ Xalatan Sterile Ophthalmic Solution (5% to 15%) 2654
Xerac AC Solution 2507
▲ Zovirax Ointment (28.3%) 854

Stinging at application site

▲ Diprolene Gel 0.05% (6%) 3015
Ultralytic 2 Cream 20% 1651
Ultralytic 2 Foam 20% 1652

Stinging at injection site

▲ Eligard 45 mg (16%) 2904

Stomach, nervous

Clozapine Tablets (Less than 1%) 2141
Clozaril Tablets (Less than 1%) 2174
FazaClo Orally Disintegrating Tablets (Less than 1%) 547

Stomach atony

Tasmar Tablets (Rare) 3360

Stomachache

▲ Aerobid/Aerobid-M (10%) 1172
▲ Bayer Aspirin Tablets (14.5%) 3515
▲ Chemet Capsules (5.2% to 15.7%) 2480
Ecotrin Enteric Coated Aspirin Low, Regular and Maximum Strength Tablets 1627
Invirase (Less than 2%) 2776
Klonopin (Infrequent) 2782
Koāte-DVI (0.7%) 3247
K-Phos Neutral Tablets 785
K-Phos Original (Sodium Free) Tablets 785
Ortho-Cyclen/Ortho Tri-Cyclen 2414
Ortho Tri-Cyclen Lo Tablets 2421
St. Joseph 81 mg Aspirin Chewable and Enteric Coated Tablets 1841
Uroqid-Acid No. 2 Tablets 785
Zofran Injection (2%) 1607

Stomatitis

Abilify Tablets (Infrequent) 916
Abilify Tablets (Infrequent) 2472
Aciphex Tablets 1081
Actiq (1% or greater) 993
Adriamycin for Injection, USP 786
Adriamycin Injection, USP 786
▲ Alferon N Injection (6%) 1640
▲ Alimta for Injection (Up to 28%) 1722
AmBisome for Injection (Less common) 615
Anaprox Tablets (Less than 3%) 2769
Anaprox DS Tablets (Less than 3%) 2769
▲ Arava Tablets (1% to 3%) 2881
Aredia for Injection (Up to 1%) 2168
Arthrotec Tablets (Rare) 3126
Asacol Delayed-Release Tablets 2688
Augmentin 1331
Augmentin Tablets 1334
Augmentin XR Extended-Release Tablets 1340
Augmentin ES-600 Powder for Oral Suspension 1337
▲ Avastin IV (30% to 32%) 1229
Avelox (0.1% to less than 2%) 2984
Biaxin/Biaxin XL 402
Caduet Tablets (Less than 2%) 2507
▲ Campath Ampules (1% to 14%) 826
▲ Camptosar Injection (1% to 12%) 2602
Carbatrol Capsules 3174
Cataflam Tablets (Occasionally) 2173
Celebrex Capsules (0.1% to 1.9%) 3130
Celexa (Infrequent) 1177
▲ CellCept Capsules (3% to less than 20%) 2751
▲ CellCept Intravenous (3% to less than 20%) 2751
▲ CellCept Oral Suspension (3% to less than 20%) 2751
▲ CellCept Tablets (3% to less than 20%) 2751
Clinoril Tablets (Less than 1 in 100) 1899
Combivir Tablets 1373
Copaxone for Injection (Infrequent) 3292
Cubicin for Injection (Less than 1%) 1038
Depacon Injection (1% or more) 412
Depakene (1% or more) 417
Depakote Sprinkle Capsules 422
▲ Depakote Tablets (1% to 5%) 427
▲ Depakote ER Tablets (1% to 5%) 433
Dolobid Tablets (Less than 1 in 100) 1937
▲ Doxil Injection (5.2% to 41.4%) 3302
EC-Naprosyn Delayed-Release Tablets (Less than 3%) 2769
Effexor Tablets (Infrequent) 3405
Effexor XR Capsules (Infrequent) 3411
Efudex 3348
Ellence Injection 2632
▲ Eloxatin for Injection (3% to 42%) 2908
Epivir 1394
Epivir-HBV 1398
Epzicom Tablets 1402
Equetro Extended-Release Capsules 3178
▲ Erbitux (11%) 937
Estratest Tablets 3196
Estratest H.S. Tablets 3196
Evoxac Capsules (Less than 1%) 1042
Flexeril Tablets (Rare) 1832
Flumadine 1186
Frova Tablets (Rare) 1101
Gabitril Tablets (Frequent) 998
Garamycin Injectable 3028
▲ Gemzar for Injection (10% to 15%) 1743
▲ Gengraf Capsules (6%) 458
Herceptin I.V. (At least one of the 958 patients) 1234
▲ Hycamtin for Injection (Less than 1% to 24%) 1427
▲ Intron A for Injection (Less than 5%) 3038

Invanz for Injection (Greater than 0.1%)....... 1974
Invirase (Less than 2%)....... 2776
▲ I.V. Busulfex (26% to 97%)....... 1125
Kaletra (Less than 2%)....... 474
Ketek Tablets (Greater than or equal to 0.2% to less than 2%)....... 2920
Lamictal (Infrequent)....... 1449
▲ Leukine (24% to 62%)....... 829
Levaquin in 5% Dextrose Injection (0.1% to 0.9%)....... 2453
Levaquin (0.1% to 0.9%)....... 2453
Lipitor Tablets (Less than 2%)....... 2495
Lunesta Tablets (Rare)....... 3139
Matulane Capsules....... 3188
Maxair Autohaler....... 1820
▲ Mylotarg for Injection (2% to 29%)....... 3429
Naprosyn Suspension (Less than 3%)....... 2769
Naprosyn Tablets (Less than 3%)....... 2769
▲ Navelbine Injection (Less than 20%)....... 1494
▲ Neoral Soft Gelatin Capsules (6%)....... 2247
▲ Neoral Oral Solution (6%)....... 2247
▲ Neulasta Injection (15% to 72%)....... 596
▲ Neupogen for Injection (5%)....... 598
Neurontin Capsules (Infrequent)....... 2498
Neurontin Oral Solution (Infrequent)....... 2498
Neurontin Tablets (Infrequent)....... 2498
Nicotrol NS....... 2596
▲ Nipent for Injection (5% to 12%)....... 3216
Noroxin Tablets....... 2009
▲ Novantrone for Injection Concentrate (15% to 19%)....... 3158
Omnicef Capsules....... 506
Omnicef for Oral Suspension....... 506
OxyContin Tablets (Less than 1%)....... 2699
Paxil CR Controlled-Release Tablets (Rare)....... 1509
Paxil (Rare)....... 1501
PEG-Intron Powder for Injection....... 3062
Plavix Tablets....... 940
Prevacid Delayed-Release Capsules (Less than 1%)....... 3268
Prevacid for Delayed-Release Oral Suspension (Less than 1%)....... 3268
Prevacid NapraPAC (Less than 3%)....... 3277
Prevacid SoluTab Delayed-Release Orally Disintegrating Tablets (Less than 1%)....... 3268
▲ PREVPAC (Less than 1% to 3%)....... 3281
▲ Prograf Capsules and Injection (3% to 15%)....... 624
▲ Proleukin for Injection (22%)....... 1007
Protonix I.V. (Less than 1%)....... 3468
Protonix Tablets (Less than 1%)....... 3465
Prozac Pulvules and Liquid (Infrequent)....... 1771
▲ Rapamune Oral Solution and Tablets (3% to 20%)....... 3472
Relafen Tablets (1% to 3%)....... 1523
Relpax Tablets (Rare)....... 2531
Requip Tablets (Infrequent)....... 1528
Rescriptor Tablets....... 2535
Retrovir IV Infusion....... 1537
Rilutek Tablets (0.8% to 1.2%)....... 2945
Risperdal Consta Long-Acting Injection (Infrequent)....... 1664
Risperdal M-Tab Orally Disintegrating Tablets (Infrequent)....... 1658
Risperdal (Infrequent)....... 1658
Roferon-A Injection (Infrequent)....... 2805
Sandostatin LAR Depot (1% to 4%)....... 2264
Seroquel Tablets (Infrequent)....... 691
Sonata Capsules (Infrequent)....... 1686
▲ Soriatane Capsules (1% to 10%)....... 1028
Spectracef Tablets (0.1% to 1%)....... 2706
▲ Spiriva HandiHaler (1% to 3%)....... 899
Striant Mucoadhesive....... 1022
Surmontil Capsules....... 2347
Symbyax Capsules (Infrequent)....... 1788
Synercid I.V. (Less than 1%)....... 1690
Tabloid Tablets (Less frequent)....... 1545
▲ Tarceva Tablets (0% to 17%)....... 1254
▲ Tarceva Tablets (0% to 17%)....... 2470
▲ Taxotere Injection Concentrate (1.1% to 51.7%)....... 2947
Tegretol/Tegretol-XR....... 2278
▲ Temodar Capsules (1% to 9%)....... 3088
▲ Tequin Injection (0.1% to 3%)....... 964
▲ Tequin Tablets (0.1% to 3%)....... 964
Thalomid Capsules....... 979
Timentin ADD-Vantage....... 1556
Timentin Injection Galaxy Container....... 1559
Timentin IV Infusion....... 1553
Timentin Pharmacy Bulk Package....... 1562
Tindamax....... 2670
Topamax Sprinkle Capsules (Infrequent)....... 2438
Topamax Tablets (Infrequent)....... 2438
Trecator Tablets....... 3482
Trileptal Oral Suspension....... 2281
Trileptal Tablets....... 2281
Trizivir Tablets....... 1565
Uniretic Tablets (Less than 1%)....... 3114
Vantin Tablets and Oral Suspension (Less than 1%)....... 2650
Vaseretic Tablets....... 2073
Vasotec I.V. Injection (0.5% to 1.0%)....... 2076
VFEND I.V. (Less than 2%)....... 2543
VFEND Oral Suspension (Less than 2%)....... 2543
VFEND Tablets (Less than 2%)....... 2543
Viagra Tablets (Less than 2%)....... 2552
Vivactil Tablets....... 2350
Voltaren Tablets (Occasionally)....... 2298
Voltaren-XR Tablets (Occasionally)....... 2301
Wellbutrin Tablets (Frequent)....... 1579
Wellbutrin SR Sustained-Release Tablets (Infrequent)....... 1583
Wellbutrin XL Extended-Release Tablets (Infrequent)....... 1588
▲ Xeloda Tablets (2% to 25%)....... 2825
▲ Zinecard for Injection (26% to 34%)....... 2659
Zithromax for IV Infusion (1.9%)....... 2573
Zoloft (Rare)....... 2581
▲ Zometa for Intravenous Infusion (8%)....... 2306
Zomig Nasal Spray (Rare)....... 718
Zonegran Capsules (Infrequent)....... 1089
Zyban Sustained-Release Tablets (Infrequent)....... 1620
Zyprexa Tablets (Infrequent)....... 1798
Zyprexa ZYDIS Orally Disintegrating Tablets (Infrequent)....... 1798
Zyrtec Chewable Tablets (Less than 2%)....... 2589
Zyrtec (Less than 2%)....... 2589
Zyrtec-D 12 Hour Extended Release Tablets (Less than 2%)....... 2591

Stomatitis, ulcerative

Agrylin Capsules (1% to 5%)....... 3172
AmBisome for Injection (Less common)....... 615
Anaprox Tablets (Less than 1%)....... 2769
Anaprox DS Tablets (Less than 1%)....... 2769
Arthrotec Tablets (Rare)....... 3126
Astelin Nasal Spray (Infrequent)....... 1876
Bactroban Cream (Less than 1%)....... 1356
Caduet Tablets (Less than 2%)....... 2507
▲ Campath Ampules (1% to 14%)....... 826
Colazal Capsules....... 2845
Copaxone for Injection (Frequent)....... 3292
Cosmegen for Injection....... 1907
Cymbalta Delayed-Release Capsules (Infrequent)....... 1729
Cytovene (At least 3 subjects)....... 2763
▲ Doxil Injection (1% to 5%)....... 3302
EC-Naprosyn Delayed-Release Tablets (Less than 1%)....... 2769
▲ Evoxac Capsules (1% to 3%)....... 1042
Exelon Capsules (Infrequent)....... 2204
Gabitril Tablets (Infrequent)....... 998
Gonal-f RFF Pen for Injection (2.4%)....... 3155
Indocin Capsules (Less than 1%)....... 1968
Indocin I.V. (Less than 1%)....... 1973
Indocin (Less than 1%)....... 1968
▲ Intron A for Injection (Less than 5%)....... 3038
Kaletra (Less than 2%)....... 474
Lipitor Tablets (Less than 2%)....... 2495
Lunesta Tablets (Infrequent)....... 3139
Lyrica Capsules (Rare)....... 2524
Mobic Oral Suspension (Less than 2%)....... 893
Mobic Tablets (Less than 2%)....... 893
Naprosyn Suspension (Less than 1%)....... 2769
Naprosyn Tablets (Less than 1%)....... 2769
Neurontin Capsules (Rare)....... 2498
Neurontin Oral Solution (Rare)....... 2498
Neurontin Tablets (Rare)....... 2498
Nexium Delayed-Release Capsules (Less than 1%)....... 645
Nexium I.V. (Less than 1%)....... 649
Paxil CR Controlled-Release Tablets (Rare to infrequent)....... 1509
Paxil (Rare to infrequent)....... 1501
Permax Tablets (Rare)....... 3357
Prevacid Delayed-Release Capsules (Less than 1%)....... 3268
Prevacid for Delayed-Release Oral Suspension (Less than 1%)....... 3268
Prevacid NapraPAC (Less than 1%)....... 3277
Prevacid SoluTab Delayed-Release Orally Disintegrating Tablets (Less than 1%)....... 3268
PREVPAC (Less than 1%)....... 3281
Protonix I.V. (Less than 1%)....... 3468
Protonix Tablets (Less than 1%)....... 3465
Prozac Pulvules and Liquid (Infrequent)....... 1771
Requip Tablets (Infrequent)....... 1528
Reyataz Capsules (Less than 3%)....... 948
Risperdal Consta Long-Acting Injection (Infrequent)....... 1664
▲ Simulect for Injection (3% to 10%)....... 2268
Sonata Capsules (Rare)....... 1686
▲ Soriatane Capsules (1% to 10%)....... 1028
▲ Spiriva HandiHaler (1% to 3%)....... 899
Symbyax Capsules (Rare)....... 1788
Trileptal Oral Suspension....... 2281
Trileptal Tablets....... 2281
Viramune Oral Suspension....... 903
Viramune Tablets....... 903
Zoloft (Rare)....... 2581
Zonegran Capsules (Infrequent)....... 1089
Zosyn (1.0% or less)....... 3492
Zyprexa Tablets (Infrequent)....... 1798
Zyprexa ZYDIS Orally Disintegrating Tablets (Infrequent)....... 1798
Zyrtec Chewable Tablets (Less than 2%)....... 2589
Zyrtec (Less than 2%)....... 2589
Zyrtec-D 12 Hour Extended Release Tablets (Less than 2%)....... 2591

Stool, bloody

(*see under* Hematochezia)

Stool, color changes

Coumadin for Injection....... 932
Coumadin Tablets....... 932
Invirase (Less than 2%)....... 2776
Kaopectate Anti-Diarrheal/Upset Stomach Reliever Liquid....... ▣701
Extra Strength Kaopectate Anti-Diarrheal Liquid....... ▣701
Lamisil Tablets....... 2226
Niferex-150 Forte Capsules....... 3299
Ortho-Cyclen/Ortho Tri-Cyclen....... 2414
Ortho Tri-Cyclen Lo Tablets....... 2421
Pepto-Bismol Maximum Strength Liquid....... ▣718
Pepto-Bismol Original Liquid, Maximum Strength Liquid, Original and Cherry Tablets and Easy-To-Swallow Caplets....... 2673
Prevacid NapraPAC (Less than 1%)....... 3277
PREVPAC (Less than 3%)....... 3281
▲ Sandostatin LAR Depot (4% to 6%)....... 2264
Tasmar Tablets....... 3360
Ticlid Tablets....... 2813

Stool, oily

▲ Xenical Capsules (5.5% to 20%)....... 2834

Stool frequency, increased

Lexapro Oral Solution (Infrequent)....... 1193
Lexapro Tablets (Infrequent)....... 1193

Stools, abnormal

Aciphex Tablets....... 1081
Asacol Delayed-Release Tablets (2% or greater)....... 2688
Clozapine Tablets (Less than 1%)....... 2141
Clozaril Tablets (Less than 1%)....... 2174
Colazal Capsules (1%)....... 2845
Effexor Tablets (Rare)....... 3405
Effexor XR Capsules (Rare)....... 3411
FazaClo Orally Disintegrating Tablets (Less than 1%)....... 547
Gabitril Tablets (Infrequent)....... 998
▲ Kaletra (Up to 6%)....... 474
Neurontin Capsules (Infrequent)....... 2498
Neurontin Oral Solution (Infrequent)....... 2498
Neurontin Tablets (Infrequent)....... 2498
Nexium Delayed-Release Capsules (Less than 1%)....... 645
Nexium I.V. (Less than 1%)....... 649
Norvir (Less than 2%)....... 499
Omnicef Capsules (0.3%)....... 506
Omnicef for Oral Suspension (0.2%)....... 506
Pentasa Capsules (Less than 1%)....... 3182
▲ Pletal Tablets (12% to 15%)....... 2478
Prevacid Delayed-Release Capsules (Less than 1%)....... 3268
Prevacid for Delayed-Release Oral Suspension (Less than 1%)....... 3268
Prevacid NapraPAC (Less than 1%)....... 3277
Prevacid SoluTab Delayed-Release Orally Disintegrating Tablets (Less than 1%)....... 3268
PREVPAC (Less than 1%)....... 3281
Protonix I.V. (Less than 1%)....... 3468
Protonix Tablets (Less than 1%)....... 3465
▲ Relafen Tablets (3% to 9%)....... 1523
▲ Sandostatin Injection (Less than 10%)....... 2263
Tasmar Tablets (Infrequent)....... 3360
Tygacil for Injection (0% to less than 2%)....... 3489
Ultrase MT Capsules (1.5%)....... 736
Vicoprofen Tablets (Less than 1%)....... 533
Zosyn (1.9% to 2.4%)....... 3492
Zyban Sustained-Release Tablets....... 1620

Stools, dark

Repliva 21/7 Tablets....... 3301

Stools, loose

▲ Agenerase Capsules (28% to 60%)....... 1299
▲ Agenerase Oral Solution (28% to 56%)....... 1304
▲ Augmentin (9%)....... 1331
▲ Augmentin Tablets (9%)....... 1334
Caduet Tablets (Less than or equal to 0.1%)....... 2507
▲ Ceftin (8.6%)....... 1369
▲ Chemet Capsules (12.0% to 20.9%)....... 2480
Cialis Tablets (Less than 2%)....... 1806
▲ Cymbalta Delayed-Release Capsules (2% to 3%)....... 1729
Elidel Cream 1% (Up to 1.2%)....... 2198
▲ Imdur Tablets (Less than or equal to 5%)....... 3032
▲ Intron A for Injection (Up to 10%)....... 3038
Invanz for Injection (2.1%)....... 1974
Ketek Tablets (Greater than or equal to 0.2% to less than 2%)....... 2920
▲ Lariam Tablets (Among most frequent)....... 2790
MetroGel-Vaginal Gel (1%)....... 1822
▲ Myfortic Tablets (3% to less than 20%)....... 2244
Noroxin Tablets (0.3% to 1.0%)....... 2009
Norvasc Tablets (Less than or equal to 0.1%)....... 2529
Reishimax Capsules....... 2669
▲ Sandostatin Injection (34% to 61%)....... 2263
▲ Suprax (6%)....... 1811
▲ Sustiva Capsules (39%)....... 957
▲ Trisenox Injection (10%)....... 983
Urocit-K Tablets (Some patients)....... 2109
▲ Vantin Tablets and Oral Suspension (5.9% to 10.6%)....... 2650
▲ Zithromax Capsules, 250 mg (2% to 14%)....... 2568
▲ Zithromax for IV Infusion (4.3%)....... 2573
▲ Zithromax for Oral Suspension, 1 g (5% to 7%)....... 2568
▲ Zithromax for Oral Suspension, 300 mg, 600 mg, 900 mg, 1200 mg (2% to 14%)....... 2561
▲ Zithromax Tablets, 250 mg, 500 mg (2% to 14%)....... 2561
▲ Zithromax Tablets, 600 mg (5% to 7%)....... 2568
▲ Zithromax Tri-Pak (2% to 14%)....... 2561
▲ Zithromax Z-Pak (5% to 7%)....... 2568
Zmax for Oral Suspension (Less then 1%)....... 2577
▲ Zoloft (20% to 24%)....... 2581
Zyvox (1.2% to 2.3%)....... 2661

Strabismus

Aciphex Tablets....... 1081
Lamictal (Rare)....... 1449
Neurontin Capsules (Rare)....... 2498
Neurontin Oral Solution (Rare)....... 2498
Neurontin Tablets (Rare)....... 2498
Prozac Pulvules and Liquid (Rare)....... 1771
Topamax Sprinkle Capsules (Infrequent)....... 2438
Topamax Tablets (Infrequent)....... 2438

Strangury

Evoxac Capsules (Less than 1%)....... 1042

Striae

Aclovate (Infrequent)....... 1290
Analpram-HC....... 1136
Aricept Tablets (Infrequent)....... 1086
Aricept ODT Tablets (Infrequent)....... 1086
Clobevate Gel....... 3213
Clobex Shampoo (Infrequent)....... 1209
Clobex Lotion....... 1208
Copaxone for Injection (Infrequent)....... 3292
Cutivate Cream (Infrequent)....... 1381
Cutivate Lotion 0.05% (Rare)....... 1383
Cutivate Ointment (Infrequent to more frequent)....... 1384
Decadron Tablets....... 1929
Diprolene Gel 0.05%....... 3015
Diprolene Lotion 0.05% (Infrequent)....... 3016
Diprolene Ointment 0.05% (Infrequent)....... 3017

Diprolene AF Cream 0.05% (Infrequent) 3014
Diprosone Cream, USP 0.05% 3018
Effexor Tablets (Rare) 3405
Elocon Cream 0.1% (Infrequent) 3019
Elocon Lotion 0.1% (Infrequent) 3020
Elocon Ointment 0.1% (Infrequent) 3021
Entocort EC Capsules (1%) 2694
Locoid Cream (Infrequent) 1138
Locoid Lipocream Cream (Infrequent) 1138
Locoid (Infrequent) 1138
Lotrisone 3054
Lupron Depot-PED 7.5 mg, 11.25 mg and 15 mg (Less than 2%) 3266
Lupron Injection Pediatric (Less than 2%) 3256
Luxíq Foam 1026
Olux Foam 1027
Pandel Cream, 0.1% 1017
Pramosone 1139
ProctoFoam-HC 3113
Temovate Cream 1549
Temovate Gel (Infrequent) 1550
Temovate Ointment 1549
Temovate Scalp Application (Infrequent) 1551
Temovate E Emollient (Infrequent) 1552
Topicort .05% Gel 3288
Topicort .25% Cream 3288
Topicort .25% Ointment 3288
Topicort LP .05% Cream 3288
Tri-Luma Cream 1213
U-cort 1% Cream 3289
Vanos Cream 1864

Stridor
Adalat CC Tablets (Less than 1%) 2978
Advair Diskus 100/50 1291
Advair Diskus 250/50 1291
Advair Diskus 500/50 1291
Campath Ampules 826
Fortaz 1422
Nubain Injection (1% or less) 1111
Paxil CR Controlled-Release Tablets (Rare) 1509
Paxil (Rare) 1501
Photofrin for Injection 729
Prevacid Delayed-Release Capsules (Less than 1%) 3268
Prevacid for Delayed-Release Oral Suspension (Less than 1%) 3268
Prevacid NapraPAC (Less than 1%) 3277
Prevacid SoluTab Delayed-Release Orally Disintegrating Tablets (Less than 1%) 3268
PREVPAC (Less than 1%) 3281
Prozac Pulvules and Liquid (Rare) 1771
Pulmicort Respules (1% to 3%) 654
Refludan for Injection (Common) 815
Rilutek Tablets (Infrequent) 2945
Risperdal Consta Long-Acting Injection (Infrequent) 1664
Risperdal M-Tab Orally Disintegrating Tablets (Infrequent) 1658
Risperdal (Infrequent) 1658
Serevent Diskus (Rare) 1540
Ultane Liquid for Inhalation (Less than 1%) 526
Zofran Injection 1607
Zofran 1613
Zofran ODT Orally Disintegrating Tablets 1613
Zoloft (Rare) 2581
Zyprexa Tablets (Rare) 1798
Zyprexa ZYDIS Orally Disintegrating Tablets (Rare) 1798

Stroke
Abilify Tablets 916
Abilify Tablets 2472
Accutane Capsules 2740
Activase I.V. (0.9%) 1225
Adderall Tablets 3168
Adderall XR Capsules 3169
Aloprim for Injection (Less than 1%) 2156
Amerge Tablets 1312
Amnesteem Capsules 2126
Aranesp for Injection (1%) 576
Cenestin Tablets, 0.45mg, 0.625mg, 0.9mg, 1.25mg 1063
Cenestin Tablets, 0.3mg 1063
Cialis Tablets 1806
Climara Transdermal System 795
Climara Pro Transdermal System 800
CombiPatch Transdermal System 2180
Cytovene 2763
Dolobid Tablets 1937
DynaCirc CR Tablets (0.5% to 1%) 2726
Enbrel for Injection 580
Estratest Tablets 3196
Estratest H.S. Tablets 3196
Estrogel 0.06% 3200
Fabrazyme for Intravenous Infusion 1267
Flexeril Tablets (Rare) 1832
Imitrex Injection 1431
Imitrex Tablets 1440
Integrilin Injection (0.5%) 3034
▲ Intron A for Injection (Less than 5%) 3038
▲ Mavik Tablets (3.3%) 482
Maxalt Tablets 1983
Maxalt-MLT Orally Disintegrating Tablets 1983
Menostar Transdermal System 805
Mobic Oral Suspension 893
Mobic Tablets 893
Neumega for Injection 3433
Ortho-Cyclen/Ortho Tri-Cyclen 2414
Prefest Tablets 1069
Premarin Intravenous 3440
Premarin Tablets 3443
Premarin Vaginal Cream 3449
Premphase Tablets (1.4%) 3452
Prempro Tablets (1.4%) 3452
Prinivil Tablets (0.3% to 1.0%) 2029
Prinzide Tablets 2033
Proleukin for Injection (Less than 1%) 1007
Risperdal Consta Long-Acting Injection 1664
Risperdal M-Tab Orally Disintegrating Tablets 1658
Risperdal 1658
Roferon-A Injection (Infrequent) 2805
Soriatane Capsules 1028
Surmontil Capsules 2347
▲ Vesanoid Capsules (3%) 2823
Vivactil Tablets 2350
Vivelle Transdermal System 2288
Vivelle-Dot Transdermal System 2293
Wellbutrin SR Sustained-Release Tablets (Infrequent) 1583
Wellbutrin XL Extended-Release Tablets (Infrequent) 1588
Zestoretic Tablets 701
Zestril Tablets (0.3% to 1.0%) 704
Zomig Tablets 714
Zomig-ZMT Tablets 714
Zyban Sustained-Release Tablets (Infrequent) 1620

Stroke, hemorrhagic
Activase I.V. (0.7%) 1225
Femara Tablets (Less than or equal to 2%) 2210
Ortho-Cyclen/Ortho Tri-Cyclen 2414
Triphasil-28 Tablets 3483

Stroke, new ischemic
Activase I.V. 1225

Stroke, thrombotic
Ortho-Cyclen/Ortho Tri-Cyclen 2414
Triphasil-28 Tablets 3483

Strongyloidiasis hyperinfection
Tagamet Tablets (Extremely rare) 1547

Stuffiness, nasal
(*see under* Nasal congestion)

Stupor
Abilify Tablets (Infrequent) 916
Abilify Tablets (Infrequent) 2472
Ambien Tablets (Infrequent) 2867
Celexa (Rare) 1177
Copaxone for Injection (Frequent) 3292
Duragesic Transdermal System (Less than 1%) 2448
Effexor Tablets (Infrequent) 3405
Effexor XR Capsules (Infrequent) 3411
Eskalith 1406
Gabitril Tablets (Frequent) 998
▲ Invanz for Injection (3.3% to 5.1%) 1974
Lamictal (Infrequent) 1449
Levaquin in 5% Dextrose Injection (0.1% to 0.9%) 2453
Levaquin (0.1% to 0.9%) 2453
Lithobid Tablets 1670
Lunesta Tablets (Rare) 3139
Lyrica Capsules (Greater than or equal to 1%) 2524
Maxipime for Injection 1093
Migranal Nasal Spray (Rare) 3350
Moduretic Tablets (Less than or equal to 1%) 2003
Namenda (Infrequent) 1199
Naropin Injection (Less than 1%) 640
Neurontin Capsules (Infrequent) 2498
Neurontin Oral Solution (Infrequent) 2498
Neurontin Tablets (Infrequent) 2498
Orthoclone OKT3 Sterile Solution 2370
OxyContin Tablets (Less than 1%) 2699
Paxil CR Controlled-Release Tablets (Rare) 1509
Paxil (Rare) 1501
Permax Tablets (Rare) 3357
PhosLo GelCaps 2158
ProSom Tablets (Infrequent) 512
Prozac Pulvules and Liquid (Rare) 1771
Relpax Tablets (Infrequent) 2531
Requip Tablets (Infrequent) 1528
Rilutek Tablets (Infrequent) 2945
Risperdal M-Tab Orally Disintegrating Tablets (Infrequent) 1658
Risperdal (Infrequent) 1658
Seroquel Tablets (Infrequent) 691
Sonata Capsules (Rare) 1686
Stromectol Tablets 2053
Symmetrel 1115
Tambocor Tablets (Less than 1%) 1824
Topamax Sprinkle Capsules (1% to 2%) 2438
Topamax Tablets (1% to 2%) 2438
Trileptal Oral Suspension 2281
Trileptal Tablets 2281
Ultracet Tablets (Less than 1%) 2462
Xanax XR Tablets (Infrequent) 2655
Zyprexa Tablets (Infrequent) 1798
Zyprexa ZYDIS Orally Disintegrating Tablets (Infrequent) 1798

Stuttering
FazaClo Orally Disintegrating Tablets (Less than 1%) 547
Seroquel Tablets (Rare) 691
Zyprexa Tablets (Infrequent) 1798
Zyprexa ZYDIS Orally Disintegrating Tablets (Infrequent) 1798

Stye
Crolom Cromolyn Sodium Sterile Ophthalmic Solution USP 4% (Infrequent) ⊙ 248
▲ Intron A for Injection (Less than 5%) 3038
Klonopin (Infrequent) 2782
Neurontin Capsules (Infrequent) 2498
Neurontin Oral Solution (Infrequent) 2498
Neurontin Tablets (Infrequent) 2498

Subcutaneous tissue disorders, unspecified
▲ Ammonul Injection (6%) 3323

Sudden Infant Death Syndrome
Infanrix Vaccine 1444
Pediarix Vaccine 1518

Suicidal ideation
Abilify Tablets (Frequent) 916
Abilify Tablets (Frequent) 2472
Accutane Capsules 2740
Ambien Tablets 2867
Amnesteem Capsules 2126
Avelox 2984
▲ Avonex (4%) 839
Betaseron for SC Injection 791
Campral Tablets (Infrequent) 1175
Cipro XR Tablets (Rare) 3004
Copegus Tablets (Less than 1%) 2759
Depakote Tablets 427
Effexor Tablets (Rare) 3405
Effexor XR Capsules (Rare) 3411
Exelon Capsules (Infrequent) 2204
Infergen 1647
Intron A for Injection (Rare) 3038
Keppra Oral Solution (Rare) 3307
Keppra Tablets (Rare) 3307
Klonopin (Infrequent) 2782
Lamictal (Rare) 1449
Lariam Tablets (Rare) 2790
Levaquin in 5% Dextrose Injection (Rare) 2453
Levaquin (Rare) 2453
Lexapro Oral Solution (Infrequent) 1193
Lexapro Tablets (Infrequent) 1193
Lupron Depot 3.75 mg (Very rare) 3257
Lupron Depot–3 Month 11.25 mg (Very rare) 3262
Meridia Capsules 485
Neurontin Capsules (Infrequent) 2498
Neurontin Oral Solution (Infrequent) 2498
Neurontin Tablets (Infrequent) 2498
Parcopa Orally Disintegrating Tablets 3111
▲ Parnate Tablets (4%) 1499
Paxil CR Controlled-Release Tablets 1509
Paxil 1501
Pegasys (Less than 1%) 2793
PEG-Intron Powder for Injection (Less than or equal to 1%) 3062
Prozac Pulvules and Liquid 1771
Razadyne (Rare) 2434
Rebetron Combination Therapy (Less than 1%) 3078
Rebif Prefilled Syringe for Injection 3163
Roferon-A Injection 2805
Seromycin Capsules 1783
Soriatane Capsules 1028
Stalevo Tablets 2270
Surmontil Capsules 2347
Sustiva Capsules (0.7%) 957
Symbyax Capsules 1788
Symmetrel (Less than 0.1%) 1115
VFEND I.V. (Less than 2%) 2543
VFEND Oral Suspension (Less than 2%) 2543
VFEND Tablets (Less than 2%) 2543
Viracept (Less than 2%) 2556
Vivactil Tablets 2350
Wellbutrin Tablets (Rare) 1579
Wellbutrin SR Sustained-Release Tablets (Infrequent) 1583
Wellbutrin XL Extended-Release Tablets (Infrequent) 1588
Xanax XR Tablets (Infrequent) 2655
Zoloft (Rare) 2581
Zyban Sustained-Release Tablets (Infrequent) 1620
Zyrtec Chewable Tablets (Rare) 2589
Zyrtec (Rare) 2589
Zyrtec-D 12 Hour Extended Release Tablets (Rare) 2591

Suicidality
Paxil CR Controlled-Release Tablets 1509
Paxil 1501
Prozac Pulvules and Liquid 1771
Surmontil Capsules 2347
Symbyax Capsules 1788
Vivactil Tablets 2350
Zoloft 2581

Suicide
Aldara Cream, 5% 1814
Amnesteem Capsules (Rare) 2126
Cipro XR Tablets (Less than 1%) 3004
Copegus Tablets (Less than 1%) 2759
Cymbalta Delayed-Release Capsules (Infrequent) 1729
Lyrica Capsules (Rare) 2524
Meridia Capsules 485
Omacor Capsules 2735
Pegasys (Less than 1%) 2793
Razadyne (Very rare) 2434
Zyrtec Chewable Tablets (Rare) 2589
Zyrtec (Rare) 2589
Zyrtec-D 12 Hour Extended Release Tablets (Rare) 2591

Suicide, attempt of
Abilify Tablets (Infrequent) 916
Abilify Tablets (Infrequent) 2472
Accutane Capsules 2740
Ambien Tablets (Rare) 2867
Amnesteem Capsules (Rare) 2126
Campral Tablets (Frequent) 1175
Celexa (Frequent) 1177
Copaxone for Injection (Infrequent) 3292
Cymbalta Delayed-Release Capsules (Infrequent) 1729
Effexor Tablets (Infrequent) 3405
Effexor XR Capsules (Infrequent) 3411
▲ Equetro Extended-Release Capsules (Less than 5%) 3178
Exelon Capsules (Infrequent) 2204
Fuzeon Injection 2772
Gabitril Tablets (Infrequent) 998
Imitrex Tablets (Rare) 1440
Infergen 1647
▲ Intron A for Injection (Rare; less than 5%) 3038
Invirase (Rare) 2776
Klonopin (Infrequent) 2782
Lamictal (Rare) 1449
Lariam Tablets (Rare) 2790
Levaquin in 5% Dextrose Injection (Rare) 2453
Levaquin (Rare) 2453
Lexapro Oral Solution (Infrequent) 1193
Lexapro Tablets (Infrequent) 1193
Lupron Depot 3.75 mg (Very rare) 3257
Lupron Depot–3 Month 11.25 mg (Very rare) 3262
Lyrica Capsules (0.1% to 1%) 2524
Mirapex Tablets (Less than 1%) 889

Namenda (Infrequent) 1199
Neurontin Capsules (Rare) 2498
Neurontin Oral Solution (Rare) 2498
Neurontin Tablets (Rare) 2498
▲ Parnate Tablets (4%) 1499
Paxil CR Controlled-Release Tablets 1509
Paxil 1501
PEG-Intron Powder for Injection (Less than or equal to 1%) 3062
Proleukin for Injection 1007
Prozac Pulvules and Liquid (Infrequent) 1771
Rebetron Combination Therapy (Less than 1%) 3078
Rebif Prefilled Syringe for Injection 3163
Remicade for IV Injection (Greater than or equal to 0.2%) 987
Requip Tablets (Rare) 1528
Reyataz Capsules (Less than 3%) 948
Rilutek Tablets (Infrequent) 2945
▲ Risperdal Consta Long-Acting Injection (1% to 4%) 1664
Risperdal M-Tab Orally Disintegrating Tablets (1.2%) 1658
Risperdal (1.2%) 1658
Roferon-A Injection 2805
Sandostatin LAR Depot (Rare) 2264
Seroquel Tablets (Infrequent) 691
Sustiva Capsules (0.5%) 957
Symbyax Capsules (Infrequent) 1788
Symmetrel (Less than 0.1%) 1115
Thalomid Capsules 979
Topamax Sprinkle Capsules (Frequent) 2438
Topamax Tablets (Frequent) 2438
Vivactil Tablets 2350
Zoloft 2581
Zyprexa Tablets (Infrequent) 1798
Zyprexa ZYDIS Orally Disintegrating Tablets (Frequent) 1798

Sulfhemoglobinemia
Eulexin Capsules 3023

Sulfite, sensitivity to
Aramine Injection 1889
Decadron Phosphate Injection 1931
Dilaudid Oral Liquid 443
Dilaudid Tablets - 8 mg 443
EpiPen 1061
Garamycin Injectable 3028
Moban Tablets 1108
Norflex Injection 1824
Pred Forte Ophthalmic Suspension ⊙233
Pred Mild Sterile Ophthalmic Suspension ⊙236
Tylenol with Codeine (Probably low) 2461

Sunburn
Accutane Capsules 2740
Benzaclin Topical Gel (1%) 1046
Differin Cream (2%) 1210
Differin Gel (Approximately 1% or less) 1211
Diovan HCT Tablets (Greater than 0.2%) 2195
Dynacin Tablets 1859
▲ Photofrin for Injection (4%) 729
Protopic Ointment (1% to 4%) 629
▲ Soriatane Capsules (1% to 10%) 1028
Xifaxan Tablets (Less than 2%) 2847

Sunburn, exacerbation of
Amnesteem Capsules 2126
Imitrex Injection 1431
Imitrex Nasal Spray 1435
Imitrex Tablets 1440

Superinfection
Adriamycin for Injection, USP 786
Adriamycin Injection, USP 786
Ancef for Injection 1318
Augmentin 1331
Augmentin Tablets 1334
Augmentin XR Extended-Release Tablets 1340
Ceftin 1369
Fortaz 1422
Mefoxin for Injection 1987
Mefoxin Premixed Intravenous Solution 1990
PREVPAC 3281
Primaxin I.M. 2022
Suprax 1811
Zinacef Injection 1604
Zinacef for Injection 1604

Suppuration
Efudex 3348

Supraventricular contractions, premature
Paxil CR Controlled-Release Tablets (Rare) 1509
Paxil (Rare) 1501

Surgery
▲ Humira Injection (Less than 5%) 464

Surgical site reaction, unspecified
▲ Arixtra Injection (0.8% to 3.2%) 1325

Swallowing
Diprivan Injectable Emulsion (Less than 1%) 676

Swallowing, impairment
Captopril Tablets 2114
Coumadin for Injection 932
Coumadin Tablets 932
Dantrium Capsules (Rare) 2690
Dantrium Intravenous 2691
Emend Capsules (Greater than 0.5%) 1944
Gengraf Capsules (Rare) 458
Imitrex Injection 1431
Imitrex Nasal Spray 1435
Levaquin in 5% Dextrose Injection 2453
Levaquin 2453
Lexapro Oral Solution (Infrequent) 1193
Lexapro Tablets (Infrequent) 1193
Mavik Tablets 482
Neoral Soft Gelatin Capsules (Rare) 2247
Neoral Oral Solution (Rare) 2247
Orthoclone OKT3 Sterile Solution 2370
Prinivil Tablets 2029
Prinzide Tablets 2033
Sandimmune (Rare) 2259
Sedapap Tablets 50 mg/650 mg (Infrequent) 2098
Thioridazine Hydrochloride Tablets 2122
Vaseretic Tablets 2073
Vasotec I.V. Injection 2076
Zestoretic Tablets 701
Zestril Tablets 704

Sweat, cold
Cymbalta Delayed-Release Capsules (Infrequent) 1729

Sweat discoloration
Parcopa Orally Disintegrating Tablets 3111
Stalevo Tablets 2270

Sweat gland disorder
▲ Advair Diskus 100/50 (1% to 3%) 1291
▲ Advair Diskus 250/50 (1% to 3%) 1291
▲ Advair Diskus 500/50 (1% to 3%) 1291
Soriatane Capsules (Less than 1%) 1028

Sweating
(*see under* Diaphoresis)

Sweating, axillary
depo-subQ provera 104 Injectable Suspension 2622

Sweating, decreased
(*see under* Hypohidrosis)

Sweating, increased
Advate Injection (0.6%) 742
▲ Apokyn Injection (At least 5%) 2132
Caduet Tablets (Greater than 0.1% to less than or equal to 1%) 2507
Cataflam Tablets (Occasionally) 2173
▲ Copegus Tablets (6%) 2759
▲ Cymbalta Delayed-Release Capsules (6%) 1729
Decadron Tablets 1929
▲ DepoDur Extended-Release Injection (2% to 5%) 1098
Depo-Provera Contraceptive Injection (Less than 1%) 2619
Eligard 22.5 mg (Less than 2%) 2899
Ketek Tablets (Greater than or equal to 0.2% to less than 2%) 2920
Levothroid Tablets 1189
▲ Lexapro Oral Solution (3% to 8%) 1193
▲ Lexapro Tablets (3% to 8%) 1193
▲ Nalfon Capsules (4.6%) 2504
▲ Nicotrol NS (Greater than 5%) 2596
▲ Norditropin Cartridges (8%) 2318
Parcopa Orally Disintegrating Tablets 3111
Prochieve 4% Gel 1018
Prochieve 8% Gel 1018
▲ Ribavirin, USP Capsules (7% to 11%) 3083
Risperdal Consta Long-Acting Injection (Infrequent) 1664
Rythmol SR Capsules 2736
Stalevo Tablets (2%) 2270
▲ Strattera Capsules (4%) 1784
Topamax Sprinkle Capsules (Less than or equal to 1%) 2438
Topamax Tablets (Less than or equal to 1%) 2438
Toprol-XL Tablets 660
Vantas (Less than 2%) 3367
Voltaren Tablets (Occasionally) 2298
Voltaren-XR Tablets (Occasionally) 2301
Xanax XR Tablets (Frequent) 2655
Xifaxan Tablets (Less than 2%) 2847
▲ Zoloft (3% to 11%) 2581

Sweating, non-axillary
▲ Botox Purified Neurotoxin Complex (3% to 10%) 565

Sweet's syndrome
▲ Vesanoid Capsules (3%) 2823

Swelling, axillary
Depo-Provera Contraceptive Injection (Less than 1%) 2619

Swelling, edematous, ankles
Eskalith 1406
Estratest Tablets 3196
Estratest H.S. Tablets 3196
Klonopin (Infrequent) 2782
Lo/Ovral-28 Tablets 3423
Ortho-Cyclen/Ortho Tri-Cyclen 2414
Striant Mucoadhesive 1022
Triphasil-28 Tablets 3483

Swelling, edematous, wrists
Eskalith 1406

Swelling, extremities
▲ Apokyn Injection (10%) 2132
Avalide Tablets 922
Avalide Tablets 2889
Avapro Tablets (Less than 1%) 925
Avapro Tablets (Less than 1%) 2886
Imitrex Injection (Rare) 1431
Imitrex Nasal Spray (Rare) 1435
Infanrix Vaccine 1444
Noroxin Tablets (Less frequent) 2009
Pediarix Vaccine 1518
Rabies Vaccine RabAvert 1011
Men's Rogaine Extra Strength Topical Solution, Ocean Rush Scent and Original Unscented ▣706
Women's Rogaine Topical Solution, Spring Bloom Scent and Original Unscented ▣707

Swelling, feet
K-Phos Neutral Tablets 785
▲ Prometrium Capsules (100 mg, 200 mg) (6%) 3205
Men's Rogaine Extra Strength Topical Solution, Ocean Rush Scent and Original Unscented ▣706
Women's Rogaine Topical Solution, Spring Bloom Scent and Original Unscented ▣707
Uroqid-Acid No. 2 Tablets 785

Swelling, hands
▲ Prometrium Capsules (100 mg, 200 mg) (6%) 3205

Swelling, joint
Advate Injection (0.6%) 742
Ceftin for Oral Suspension (0.1% to 1%) 1369
Cozaar Tablets (Less than 1%) 1913
Gleevec Tablets (Less common) 2221
Hyzaar 1964
Imitrex Injection (Infrequent) 1431
Lunesta Tablets (Infrequent) 3139
Neurontin Capsules (Infrequent) 2498
Neurontin Oral Solution (Infrequent) 2498
Neurontin Tablets (Infrequent) 2498
Orthovisc Injection (0.7%) 3518

Swelling, legs
K-Phos Neutral Tablets 785
Uroqid-Acid No. 2 Tablets 785

Swelling, lower legs
(*see under* Swelling, legs)

Swelling, mouth
Adacel Vaccine 2959
Boostrix (Rarely) 1366
Infanrix Vaccine 1444
Pediarix Vaccine (Rare) 1518
Tambocor Tablets (Less than 1%) 1824

Swelling, non-site specific
▲ Advair Diskus 250/50 (1% to 3%) 1291
Amerge Tablets (Infrequent) 1312
Bactroban Ointment (Less than 1%) 1358
Coumadin for Injection 932
Coumadin Tablets 932
▲ Doxil Injection (3.4%) 3302
Efudex 3348
Hyzaar (1.3%) 1964
Oncaspar 1123
Oxandrin Tablets 2977
Recombivax HB (Equal to or greater than 1%) 2045
Serevent Diskus (1% to 3%) 1540
Sulfamylon Cream 2154
Sulfamylon for 5% Topical Solution 2155
TobraDex Ophthalmic Ointment (Less than 4%) 558
TobraDex Ophthalmic Suspension (Less than 4%) 558
Vaqta (Less than 1%) 2067
Viramune Oral Suspension 903
Viramune Tablets 903

Swelling, oropharyngeal
Cymbalta Delayed-Release Capsules (Infrequent) 1729

Swelling, parotid
Surmontil Capsules 2347

Swelling, salivary gland
Eskalith 1406
Flexeril Tablets (Rare) 1832

Swelling, unspecified
▲ Pediarix Vaccine (1% to 22.3%) 1518
ThermaCare Heat Wraps 2674

Swelling at injection site
▲ Adacel Vaccine (2.8% to 21%) 2959
▲ Aredia for Injection (Up to 41%) 2168
Attenuvax 1889
Avonex 839
▲ Boostrix (0.5% to 28.3%) 1366
Cerezyme for Injection (Less than 1%) 1263
Cipro I.V. (1% or less) 2998
Cipro I.V. Pharmacy Bulk Package (1% or less) 3509
▲ Comvax (27.2% to 27.6%) 1904
DAPTACEL 2964
DDAVP Injection 4 mcg/mL (Occasional) 2893
Desferal Vials 2190
Desmopressin Acetate Injection (Occasional) 1143
▲ Enbrel for Injection (37%) 580
▲ Engerix-B Vaccine (1% to 10%) 1391
▲ Havrix Vaccine (1% to 10%) 1425
HibTITER (Less than 1% to 1.7%) 3419
Humalog-Pen 1751
▲ Humira Injection (20%) 464
Humulin 50/50, 100 Units 1760
Humulin 70/30 Pen (Occasional) 1761
Humulin L, 100 Units (Occasional) 1763
Humulin R (U-500) 1768
Humulin N Pen (Occasional) 1765
Hyalgan Solution (Common) 2917
Imitrex Injection 1431
▲ Infanrix Vaccine (0.7% to 32.9%) 1444
Infed Injection 3381
Invanz for Injection (1.8%) 1974
▲ Leustatin Injection (9% to 19%) 2368
▲ Menactra Vaccine (0.5% to12.6%) 2968
Merrem I.V. (0.2%) 687
M-M-R II 1980
Nubain Injection 1111
Pediarix Vaccine 1518
Liquid PedvaxHIB (0.9% to 2.5%) 2012
Pneumovax 23 (Common) 2020
Repronex for Intramuscular and Subcutaneous Injection 1148
Risperdal Consta Long-Acting Injection (1%) 1664
Symlin Injection 608
Timentin ADD-Vantage 1556
Timentin Injection Galaxy Container 1559
Timentin IV Infusion 1553
Timentin Pharmacy Bulk Package 1562
▲ Trisenox Injection (10%) 983
▲ Vaqta (1.3% to 13.8%) 2067
▲ Varivax (19.3% to 32.5%) 2070
Zemuron Injection (Less than 1%) 2363

Swelling at insertion site
Vantas (0.7%) 3367

Syncope
Accutane Capsules 2740
Aceon Tablets (2 mg, 4 mg, 8 mg) (0.3% to 1%) 3191
Aciphex Tablets 1081

Actimmune (Rare) 1646
Actonel Tablets (0.6% to 2.1%) 2679
Actonel with Calcium Tablets (0.6% to 2.1%) 2684
Adalat CC Tablets (Rare) 2978
▲ Advair Diskus 250/50 (1% to 3%) 1291
Advicor Tablets 1694
Aerobid/Aerobid-M (1% to 3%) 1172
Aggrenox Capsules (1%) 855
Agrylin Capsules (1% to 5%) 3172
Aldara Cream, 5% 1814
Alinia for Oral Suspension (Less than 1%) 2840
Alinia Tablets (Less than 1%) 2840
Altace Capsules (Less than 1% to 2.1%) 1673
Ambien Tablets (Infrequent) 2867
Amerge Tablets (Infrequent) 1312
Amnesteem Capsules 2126
Anaprox Tablets (Less than 1%) 2769
Anaprox DS Tablets (Less than 1%) 2769
Angiomax for Injection (Rare) 1856
Anzemet Injection (Rare) 2871
Anzemet Tablets (Rare) 2874
Apokyn Injection (2%) 2132
▲ Aredia for Injection (Up to 6%) 2168
Aricept Tablets (2%) 1086
Aricept ODT Tablets (2%) 1086
Arthrotec Tablets (Rare) 3126
Attenuvax 1889
Avalide Tablets 922
Avalide Tablets 2889
Avapro Tablets 925
Avapro Tablets 2886
▲ Avastin IV (3%) 1229
Avelox (Less than 0.1%) 2984
Avinza Capsules (Less than 5%) 1714
Axert Tablets (Rare) 2430
Bentyl Capsules 724
Bentyl Injection 724
Bentyl Syrup 724
Bentyl Tablets 724
Betagan Ophthalmic Solution, USP ⊙ 217
Betimol Ophthalmic Solution ⊙ 283
Betimol Ophthalmic Solution 3371
Blocadren Tablets (0.6%) 1891
Brevibloc Concentrate (Less than 1%) 766
Brevibloc Injection (Less than 1%) 766
Brevibloc Double Strength Injection (Less than 1%) 766
Brevibloc Premixed Injection (Less than 1%) 766
Brevibloc Double Strength Premixed Injection (Less than 1%) 766
Brimonidine Tartrate Ophthalmic Solution 0.2% (Less than 3%) ⊙ 245
Buphenyl Powder (Less than or equal to 2%) 3327
Buphenyl Tablets (Less than or equal to 2%) 3327
Caduet Tablets (Greater than 0.1% to less than 2%) 2507
Campath Ampules 826
Campral Tablets (Frequent) 1175
Camptosar Injection 2602
Captopril Tablets 2114
Carbatrol Capsules 3174
Cardene I.V. (0.7%) 1129
Cardizem LA Extended Release Tablets (Less than 2%) 1699
Carteolol Hydrochloride Ophthalmic Solution USP, 1% ⊙ 246
▲ Casodex Tablets (2% to 5%) 670
Cataflam Tablets (Occasionally) 2173
Catapres Tablets (Rare) 874
Catapres-TTS (0.5% or less) 875
Celebrex Capsules (Less than 0.1%) 3130
Celexa (Infrequent) 1177
▲ CellCept Capsules (3% to less than 20%) 2751
▲ CellCept Intravenous (3% to less than 20%) 2751
▲ CellCept Oral Suspension (3% to less than 20%) 2751
▲ CellCept Tablets (3% to less than 20%) 2751
Cialis Tablets (Less than 2%) 1806
Cipro I.V. (1% or less) 2998
Cipro I.V. Pharmacy Bulk Package (1% or less) 3509
Cipro (Less than 1%) 2991
Cipro XR Tablets (Less than 1%) 3004
Clinoril Tablets (Less than 1%) 1899
▲ Clozapine Tablets (More than 5% to 6%) 2141
▲ Clozaril Tablets (More than 5% to 6%) 2174
Combunox Tablets (Less than 1%) 1183
Comtan Tablets 2186
Comvax 1904
▲ Copaxone for Injection (5 %) 3292
▲ Coreg Tablets (3% to 8%) 1376
Cosopt Sterile Ophthalmic Solution 1910
Covera-HS Tablets (Less than 2%) 3135
Cozaar Tablets (Less than 1%) 1913
Crestor Tablets (Less than 1%) 672
Dalmane Capsules (Rare) 3343
Decadron Tablets 1929
Depo-Provera Contraceptive Injection (Less than 1%) 2619
depo-subQ provera 104 Injectable Suspension 2622
Diastat Rectal Delivery System (Infrequent) 3344
Dilaudid Multiple Dose Vials 439
Dilaudid Oral Liquid 443
Dilaudid Tablets - 8 mg 443
Dilaudid-HP (Less frequent) 441
Diovan HCT Tablets (Greater than 0.2%) 2195
Diovan Tablets (Less frequent) 2191
Diprivan Injectable Emulsion (Less than 1%) 676
Dolobid Tablets (Rare) 1937
▲ Dostinex Tablets (1% to less than 10%) 2631
Doxil Injection (Less than 1%) 3302
Duragesic Transdermal System (1% or greater) 2448
DynaCirc CR Tablets (0.5% to 1%) 2726
EC-Naprosyn Delayed-Release Tablets (Less than 1%) 2769
Edex Injection (Less than 1%) 3103
Effexor Tablets (Infrequent) 3405
Effexor XR Capsules (Infrequent) 3411
▲ Eldepryl Capsules (7 of 49 patients) 3209
Eligard 7.5 mg (Less than 2%) 2896
Engerix-B Vaccine 1391
Equetro Extended-Release Capsules 3178
Eskalith 1406
Evoxac Capsules (Less than 1%) 1042
▲ Exelon Capsules (3%) 2204
▲ FazaClo Orally Disintegrating Tablets (Greater than 5% to 6%) 547
▲ Ferrlecit Injection (6%) 3379
Fleet Bisacodyl Laxatives 1169
Flexeril Tablets (Less than 1%) 1832
▲ Flolan for Injection (7%) 1408
Flomax Capsules (0.2% to 0.4%) 881
Flumadine (Less than 0.3%) 1186
Fluorescite Injection ⊙ 207
Forteo for Injection (2.6%) 1739
Frova Tablets (Rare) 1101
Gabitril Tablets (Frequent) 998
Geodon Capsules (0.6%) 2514
Gleevec Tablets (Infrequent) 2221
Havrix Vaccine (Rare) 1425
Herceptin I.V. (At least one of the 958 patients) 1234
▲ Humira Injection (Less than 5%) 464
▲ Hytrin Capsules (0.5% to 21%) 469
Hyzaar 1964
Imdur Tablets 3032
Imitrex Injection (Infrequent) 1431
Imitrex Nasal Spray (Infrequent) 1435
Imitrex Tablets (Rare to infrequent) 1440
Indocin (Less than 1%) 1968
Infed Injection 3381
▲ Intron A for Injection (Less than 5%) 3038
Invanz for Injection (Greater than 0.1%) 1974
Inversine Tablets 3286
Invirase (Less than 2%) 2776
Kadian Capsules (Less than 3%) 572
Kytril Tablets (Rare) 2788
Lamictal (Infrequent) 1449
Lariam Tablets (Occasional) 2790
Leukine 829
Levaquin in 5% Dextrose Injection (0.1% to 0.9%) 2453
Levaquin (0.1% to 0.9%) 2453
Levitra Tablets (Less than 2%) 3048
Lexapro Oral Solution (Infrequent) 1193
Lexapro Tablets (Infrequent) 1193
Lipitor Tablets (Less than 2%) 2495
Lithobid Tablets 1670
Lotensin Tablets (0.1%) 2232
Lotensin HCT Tablets (0.3% or more) 2235
▲ Lupron Depot 3.75 mg (Among most frequent) 3257
Lupron Depot–3 Month 11.25 mg (Less than 5%) 3262
Lupron Depot-PED 7.5 mg, 11.25 mg and 15 mg (Less than 2%) 3266
Lupron Injection Pediatric (Less than 2%) 3256
Lyrica Capsules (0.1% to 1%) 2524
Matulane Capsules 3188
▲ Mavik Tablets (0.2% to 5.9%) 482
Maxair Autohaler 1820
Maxalt Tablets (Rare) 1983
Maxalt-MLT Orally Disintegrating Tablets (Rare) 1983
Mebaral Tablets, USP (Less than 1 in 100 patients) 2483
Meridia Capsules 485
Merrem I.V. (Greater than 0.1% to 1%) 687
Meruvax II 1994
Micardis Tablets 884
Micardis HCT Tablets 886
Mirapex Tablets (1% or more) 889
Mirena Intrauterine System 810
M-M-R II 1980
Mobic Oral Suspension (Less than 2%) 893
Mobic Tablets (Less than 2%) 893
Moduretic Tablets (Less than or equal to 1%) 2003
MS Contin Tablets (Less frequent) 2703
Mumpsvax 2005
Namenda (Frequent) 1199
Naprosyn Suspension (Less than 1%) 2769
Naprosyn Tablets (Less than 1%) 2769
Naropin Injection (Less than 1%) 640
Nembutal Sodium Solution, USP (Less than 1%) 2484
▲ Neumega for Injection (13%) 3433
Neurontin Capsules (Infrequent) 2498
Neurontin Oral Solution (Infrequent) 2498
Neurontin Tablets (Infrequent) 2498
Niaspan Extended-Release Tablets 1703
Nipent for Injection (Less than 3%) 3216
▲ Niravam Orally Disintegrating Tablets (3% to 3.8%) 3106
▲ Nitro-Dur Transdermal Infusion System (4%) 3060
Norflex Injection 1824
Norvasc Tablets (More than 0.1% to 1%) 2529
Norvir (0.6% to 1.7%) 499
Nubain Injection (1% or less) 1111
Omacor Capsules 2735
Orap Tablets 1220
Ortho-Cyclen/Ortho Tri-Cyclen 2414
OxyContin Tablets (Less than 1%) 2699
Parcopa Orally Disintegrating Tablets 3111
Paxil CR Controlled-Release Tablets (Frequent) 1509
Paxil (Frequent) 1501
Permax Tablets (2.1%) 3357
Phenergan 3438
Plavix Tablets (1% to 2.5%) 940
Plavix Tablets (1% to 2.5%) 2942
Plendil Extended-Release Tablets (0.5% to 1.5%) 651
Pletal Tablets (Less than 2%) 2478
Prevacid Delayed-Release Capsules (Less than 1%) 3268
Prevacid for Delayed-Release Oral Suspension (Less than 1%) 3268
Prevacid NapraPAC (Less than 1%) 3277
Prevacid SoluTab Delayed-Release Orally Disintegrating Tablets (Less than 1%) 3268
PREVPAC (Less than 1%) 3281
Prinivil Tablets (0.3% to 1.0%) 2029
Prinzide Tablets (0.8% to 0.1%) 2033
Prochieve 4% Gel 1018
Prochieve 8% Gel 1018
Proleukin for Injection (Less than 1%) 1007
Prometrium Capsules (100 mg, 200 mg) (Rare) 3205
ProSom Tablets (Rare) 512
Protonix I.V. (Less than 1%) 3468
Protonix Tablets (Less than 1%) 3465
Provigil Tablets (1%) 1002
Prozac Pulvules and Liquid (Infrequent) 1771
▲ Rapamune Oral Solution and Tablets (3% to 20%) 3472
Razadyne ER Extended-Release Capsules (0.4% to 2.2%) 2434
Razadyne (0.4% to 2.2%) 2434
Recombivax HB 2045
Relafen Tablets (Less than 1%) 1523
Relpax Tablets (Rare) 2531
Remicade for IV Injection (Greater than or equal to 0.2%) 987
▲ Requip Tablets (3% to 12%) 1528
Retrovir Capsules 1533
Retrovir IV Infusion 1537
Retrovir 1533
Reyataz Capsules (Less than 3%) 948
Rilutek Tablets (Infrequent) 2945
Risperdal Consta Long-Acting Injection (Up to 2%) 1664
Risperdal M-Tab Orally Disintegrating Tablets (0.2%) 1658
Risperdal (0.2%) 1658
▲ Roferon-A Injection (Less than 5%) 2805
Rythmol SR Capsules 2736
Sanctura Tablets 1133
Sandostatin Injection (Less than 1%) 2263
Sandostatin LAR Depot (1% to 4%) 2264
Sedapap Tablets 50 mg/650 mg (Infrequent) 2098
Seroquel Tablets (1%) 691
Sonata Capsules (Infrequent) 1686
Stalevo Tablets (1.2%) 2270
Sular Tablets (Less than or equal to 1%) 1163
Sustiva Capsules (Less than 2%) 957
Tambocor Tablets (1% to 3%) 1824
Targretin Capsules 1719
Tarka Tablets (0.1% to 0.3% or more) 519
▲ Tasmar Tablets (4% to 5%) 3360
Taxotere Injection Concentrate 2947
Tegretol/Tegretol-XR 2278
Tenormin I.V. Injection 698
Tenormin Tablets 695
Tequin Injection 964
Tequin Tablets 964
Thalomid Capsules 979
Thiothixene Capsules 2124
Tiazac Capsules (Less than 2%) 1204
Timolide Tablets (Less than 1%) 2056
Timoptic in Ocudose (Less frequent) 2061
Timoptic Sterile Ophthalmic Solution (Less frequent) 2058
Timoptic-XE Sterile Ophthalmic Gel Forming Solution 2062
Topamax Sprinkle Capsules (Frequent) 2438
Topamax Tablets (Frequent) 2438
Toprol-XL Tablets (Greater than 1%) 660
Trileptal Oral Suspension 2281
Trileptal Tablets 2281
Twinrix Vaccine (Less than 1%) 1571
Ultane Liquid for Inhalation (Less than 1%) 526
Uniretic Tablets (Less than 1%) 3114
Univasc Tablets (0.51%) 3118
Uroxatral Tablets (0.2%) 2957
Vantin Tablets and Oral Suspension (Less than 1%) 2650
Vaseretic Tablets (0.5% to 2.0%) 2073
Vasotec I.V. Injection (0.5% to 2.2%) 2076
▲ Ventavis Inhalation Solution (8%) 1036
Verelan PM Capsules (2% or less) 3120
Viadur Implant (Rare) 782
Viagra Tablets (Less than 2%) 2552
Visudyne for Injection (Less than 1%) 2286
Vivelle Transdermal System 2288
Vivelle-Dot Transdermal System 2293
Voltaren Tablets (Occasionally) 2298
Voltaren-XR Tablets (Occasionally) 2301
Wellbutrin Tablets (1.2%) 1579
Wellbutrin SR Sustained-Release Tablets (Rare) 1583
Wellbutrin XL Extended-Release Tablets (Rare) 1588
Xanax XR Tablets (Infrequent) 2655
▲ Xeloda Tablets (Less than 5%) 2825
Xifaxan Tablets (Less than 2%) 2847
Xopenex HFA Inhalation Aerosol 3151
Xopenex Inhalation Solution 3143
Xopenex Inhalation Solution Concentrate 3147
Zelnorm Tablets 2303
Zestoretic Tablets (0.1% to 0.8%) 701
Zestril Tablets (0.1% to 1.8%) 704
Zithromax 2568
Zithromax for Oral Suspension, 300 mg, 600 mg, 900 mg, 1200 mg 2561
Zithromax Tablets, 250 mg, 500 mg 2561
Zithromax Tablets, 600 mg 2568
Zithromax Tri-Pak 2561
Zithromax Z-Pak 2568
Zmax for Oral Suspension 2577
Zofran Injection (Rare) 1607
Zoloft (Infrequent) 2581
Zomig Nasal Spray (Infrequent) 718
Zomig Tablets (Infrequent) 714
Zomig-ZMT Tablets (Infrequent) 714
Zonegran Capsules (Infrequent) 1089

Zosyn (1.0% or less) ... 3492
Zyban Sustained-Release Tablets (Rare) ... 1620
Zyprexa Tablets (0.6%) ... 1798
Zyprexa IntraMuscular (Infrequent) ... 1798
Zyprexa ZYDIS Orally Disintegrating Tablets (0.6%) ... 1798
Zyrtec Chewable Tablets (Less than 2%) ... 2589
Zyrtec (Less than 2%) ... 2589
Zyrtec-D 12 Hour Extended Release Tablets (Less than 2%) ... 2591

Synovitis
Actiq (Less than 1%) ... 993
Arava Tablets (2%) ... 2881
Celebrex Capsules (0.1% to 1.9%) ... 3130
Cuprimine Capsules (Some patients) ... 1925
Evoxac Capsules (Less than 1%) ... 1042
▲ Humira Injection (Less than 5%) ... 464
Levaquin in 5% Dextrose Injection (0.1% to 0.9%) ... 2453
Levaquin (0.1% to 0.9%) ... 2453
Prevacid Delayed-Release Capsules (Less than 1%) ... 3268
Prevacid for Delayed-Release Oral Suspension (Less than 1%) ... 3268
Prevacid NapraPAC (Less than 1%) ... 3277
Prevacid SoluTab Delayed-Release Orally Disintegrating Tablets (Less than 1%) ... 3268
PREVPAC (Less than 1%) ... 3281
▲ Stromectol Tablets (9.3%) ... 2053
Viagra Tablets (Less than 2%) ... 2552

Systemic inflammatory response syndrome
Clolar for Intravenous Infusion ... 1264

Systolic blood pressure, decreased
Agrylin Capsules ... 3172

T

T3, decrease
Aygestin Tablets ... 1062
Eskalith ... 1406
Estratest Tablets ... 3196
Estratest H.S. Tablets ... 3196
Premarin Tablets ... 3443

T3, increase
Premphase Tablets ... 3452
Prempro Tablets ... 3452
Striant Mucoadhesive ... 1022

T4, decrease
Eskalith ... 1406
Striant Mucoadhesive ... 1022

T4, increase
CombiPatch Transdermal System ... 2180
Estratest Tablets ... 3196
Estratest H.S. Tablets ... 3196
Ortho-Cyclen/Ortho Tri-Cyclen ... 2414
Premarin Tablets ... 3443
Premphase Tablets ... 3452
Prempro Tablets ... 3452
Striant Mucoadhesive ... 1022

Tachyarrhythmia
Actimmune (Rare) ... 1646
Amerge Tablets (Infrequent) ... 1312
Ellence Injection ... 2632
Lotronex Tablets (Infrequent) ... 1479

Tachyarrhythmia, ventricular
Avelox ... 2984
Frova Tablets ... 1101
Zmax for Oral Suspension ... 2577

Tachyarrhythmias, supraventricular
Digitek Tablets ... 2146
Lanoxicaps Capsules ... 1458
Lanoxin Injection ... 1462
Lanoxin Tablets ... 1468
Lanoxin Injection Pediatric ... 1465

Tachycardia
Abilify Tablets (Frequent) ... 916
Abilify Tablets (Frequent) ... 2472
AccuNeb Inhalation Solution ... 1055
Accutane Capsules ... 2740
Aciphex Tablets ... 1081
Acthrel for Injection ... 3528
Actiq (Less than 1%) ... 993
Adalat CC Tablets (Less than 1%) ... 2978
Adderall Tablets ... 3168
▲ Adderall XR Capsules (6%) ... 3169
Adipex-P ... 1216
Advicor Tablets ... 1694
Aerobid/Aerobid-M (1% to 3%) ... 1172
Aggrenox Capsules (Less than 1%) ... 855
▲ Agrylin Capsules (7.5%) ... 3172
Aldara Cream, 5% ... 1814
Alinia for Oral Suspension (Less than 1%) ... 2840
Alinia Tablets (Less than 1%) ... 2840
Alkeran for Injection (In some patients) ... 976
Allegra-D 12 Hour Extended-Release Tablets ... 2860
Allegra-D 24 Hour Extended-Release Tablets ... 2862
Aloxi Injection (1%) ... 2099
Alphagan P Ophthalmic Solution ... 563
▲ Alupent Inhalation Aerosol (2.5% to 16.6%) ... 858
Ambien Tablets (Infrequent) ... 2867
▲ AmBisome for Injection (9.4% to 18.5%) ... 615
Amnesteem Capsules ... 2126
Anaprox Tablets (Less than 1%) ... 2769
Anaprox DS Tablets (Less than 1%) ... 2769
Antara Capsules ... 2723
Anzemet Injection (2.2% to 3.3%) ... 2871
Anzemet Tablets (2.2% to 3.3%) ... 2874
▲ Arava Tablets (1% to 3%) ... 2881
▲ Aredia for Injection (Up to 6%) ... 2168
Arthrotec Tablets (Rare) ... 3126
Astelin Nasal Spray (Infrequent) ... 1876
Atacand Tablets (0.5% or greater) ... 634
Atacand HCT (0.5% or greater) ... 637
Atrovent HFA Inhalation Aerosol ... 872
Atrovent Inhalation Solution (Less than 3%) ... 868
Atrovent Nasal Spray 0.03% ... 869
Atrovent Nasal Spray 0.06% (Less than 1%) ... 870
Avalide Tablets (1%) ... 922
Avalide Tablets (1%) ... 2889
Avapro Tablets (1% or greater) ... 925
Avapro Tablets (1% or greater) ... 2886
Avelox (0.1% to less than 2%) ... 2984
Avinza Capsules (Less than 5%) ... 1714
Axert Tablets (Infrequent) ... 2430
Bayer Aspirin Tablets ... 3515
Benicar Tablets (Greater than 0.5%) ... 2850
Bentyl Capsules ... 724
Bentyl Injection ... 724
Bentyl Syrup ... 724
Bentyl Tablets ... 724
▲ Betaseron for SC Injection (4%) ... 791
BiDil Tablets (2%) ... 2161
Brimonidine Tartrate Ophthalmic Solution 0.2% ... ⊙ 245
Buprenex Injectable (Less than 1%) ... 2718
Caduet Tablets (Greater than 0.1% to less than or equal to 1%) ... 2507
Cafcit ... 1854
Campral Tablets (Infrequent) ... 1175
Cancidas for Injection (0% to 1.8%) ... 1894
Captopril Tablets (Approximately 1 of 100 patients) ... 2114
▲ Cardene I.V. (3.5%) ... 1129
Cardizem LA Extended Release Tablets (Less than 2%) ... 1699
▲ Carnitor Injection (5% to 9%) ... 3185
Cataflam Tablets (Occasionally) ... 2173
Catapres Tablets (About 5 in 1,000 patients) ... 874
Catapres-TTS (0.5% or less) ... 875
Ceftin Tablets (0.1% to 1%) ... 1369
Celebrex Capsules (0.1% to 1.9%) ... 3130
Celexa (Frequent) ... 1177
▲ CellCept Capsules (3% to 22%) ... 2751
▲ CellCept Intravenous (3% to 22%) ... 2751
▲ CellCept Oral Suspension (3% to 22%) ... 2751
▲ CellCept Tablets (3% to 22%) ... 2751
▲ Cerezyme for Injection (Approximately 6.5%) ... 1263
Cialis Tablets (Less than 2%) ... 1806
Cipro I.V. (1% or less) ... 2998
Cipro I.V. Pharmacy Bulk Package (1% or less) ... 3509
Cipro (Less than 1%) ... 2991
Cipro XR Tablets ... 3004
Clarinex Syrup ... 3009
Clarinex Tablets ... 3009
Clarinex Reditabs Tablets ... 3009
Clarinex-D 24-Hour Extended-Release Tablets ... 3012
Clinoril Tablets (Less than 1 in 100) ... 1899
▲ Clolar for Intravenous Infusion (34%) ... 1264
Clorpres Tablets (About 5 in 1,000) ... 2139
▲ Clozapine Tablets (More than 5% to 25%) ... 2141
▲ Clozaril Tablets (More than 5% to 25%) ... 2174
Cogentin Injection ... 1903
Combivent Inhalation Aerosol (Less than 2%) ... 878
Combunox Tablets (Less than 1%) ... 1183
Comvax ... 1904
Concerta Extended-Release Tablets ... 1828
▲ Copaxone for Injection (5%) ... 3292
Coreg Tablets (Greater than 0.1% to 1%) ... 1376
Cozaar Tablets (Less than 1%) ... 1913
Dantrium Capsules (Less frequent) ... 2690
Dapsone Tablets USP ... 1656
Decadron Tablets ... 1929
▲ Depacon Injection (1% to 5%) ... 412
▲ Depakene (1% to 5%) ... 417
▲ Depakote Sprinkle Capsules (1% to 5%) ... 422
▲ Depakote Tablets (1% to 5%) ... 427
▲ Depakote ER Tablets (1% to 5%) ... 433
▲ DepoDur Extended-Release Injection (5% to 10%) ... 1098
Depo-Provera Contraceptive Injection (Less than 1%) ... 2619
depo-subQ provera 104 Injectable Suspension ... 2622
Desferal Vials ... 2190
Desoxyn Tablets, USP ... 2482
Detrol Tablets ... 2626
Detrol LA Capsules ... 2629
Dexedrine ... 1386
DextroStat Tablets ... 3177
Dibenzyline Capsules ... 3390
Digitek Tablets (2%) ... 2146
Dilaudid ... 439
Dilaudid Oral Liquid ... 443
Dilaudid Non-Sterile Powder ... 439
Dilaudid Rectal Suppositories ... 439
Dilaudid Tablets ... 439
Dilaudid Tablets - 8 mg ... 443
Dilaudid-HP (Less frequent) ... 441
Diovan HCT Tablets (Greater than 0.2%) ... 2195
Diprivan Injectable Emulsion (Less than 1%) ... 676
Ditropan XL Extended Release Tablets (Rare) ... 2391
▲ Doxil Injection (1% to 10%) ... 3302
Duragesic Transdermal System ... 2448
Dyazide Capsules ... 1389
DynaCirc CR Tablets (0.5% to 1%) ... 2726
EC-Naprosyn Delayed-Release Tablets (Less than 1%) ... 2769
Ecotrin Enteric Coated Aspirin Low, Regular and Maximum Strength Tablets ... 1627
Effexor Tablets (2%) ... 3405
Effexor XR Capsules (Frequent) ... 3411
Eldepryl Capsules ... 3209
Ellence Injection ... 2632
▲ Eloxatin for Injection (2% to 5%) ... 2908
Emend Capsules (Greater than 0.5%) ... 1944
Engerix-B Vaccine ... 1391
▲ Entocort EC Capsules (Less than 5%) ... 2694
EpiPen ... 1061
Epogen for Injection (0.31%) ... 586
Ethyol for Injection ... 1869
Evoxac Capsules (Less than 1%) ... 1042
Exelon Capsules (Infrequent) ... 2204
▲ FazaClo Orally Disintegrating Tablets (Greater than 5% to 25%) ... 547
▲ Ferrlecit Injection (5% to 21%) ... 3379
Flexeril Tablets (Less than 1%) ... 1832
▲ Flolan for Injection (1% to 43%) ... 1408
Floxin Otic Singles (Reported in a single subject) ... 1045
Floxin Otic Solution (Single report) ... 1043
Flumadine (Less than 0.3%) ... 1186
▲ Focalin Tablets (Among more frequent) ... 2214
Focalin XR Capsules ... 2217
Follistim AQ Cartridge ... 2354
Foradil Aerolizer ... 3024
Fortical Nasal Spray (Less than 1%) ... 3336
Frova Tablets (Infrequent) ... 1101
Furosemide Tablets ... 2117
Gabitril Tablets (Frequent) ... 998
Geodon (Frequent) ... 2514
Gleevec Tablets (Infrequent) ... 2221
GlucaGen for Injection ... 790
Guanidine Hydrochloride Tablets ... 3030
▲ Herceptin I.V. (5%) ... 1234
▲ Humira Injection (Less than 5%) ... 464
Hycomine Compound Tablets ... 1105
Hytrin Capsules (0.6% to 1.9%) ... 469
Hyzaar ... 1964
▲ Imdur Tablets (Less than or equal to 5%) ... 3032
Imitrex Injection (Infrequent) ... 1431
Imitrex Nasal Spray (Infrequent) ... 1435
Imitrex Tablets (Infrequent) ... 1440
Indocin Capsules (Less than 1%) ... 1968
Indocin I.V. (Less than 1%) ... 1973
Indocin (Less than 1%) ... 1968
Infed Injection ... 3381
▲ Infergen (4%) ... 1647
▲ Intron A for Injection (Less than 5%) ... 3038
Invanz for Injection (1.3% to 1.6%) ... 1974
▲ I.V. Busulfex (44%) ... 1125
Kadian Capsules (Less than 3%) ... 572
K-Phos Neutral Tablets ... 785
Kytril Injection (Rare) ... 2785
Lamictal (Infrequent) ... 1449
Lanoxicaps Capsules ... 1458
Lanoxin Injection ... 1462
Lanoxin Tablets ... 1468
Lanoxin Injection Pediatric ... 1465
Lariam Tablets (Infrequent) ... 2790
▲ Leukine (11%) ... 829
▲ Leustatin Injection (6%) ... 2368
Levaquin in 5% Dextrose Injection (0.1% to 0.9%) ... 2453
Levaquin (0.1% to 0.9%) ... 2453
Levitra Tablets (Less than 2%) ... 3048
Levothroid Tablets ... 1189
Levoxyl Tablets ... 1680
Lexapro Oral Solution (Infrequent) ... 1193
Lexapro Tablets (Infrequent) ... 1193
Lofibra Capsules ... 1217
Lotensin HCT Tablets (0.3% or more) ... 2235
Lupron Depot 3.75 mg (Less than 5%) ... 3257
Lupron Depot–3 Month 11.25 mg (Less than 5%) ... 3262
Marinol Capsules (Greater than 1%) ... 3334
Matulane Capsules ... 3188
Maxair Autohaler (1.2% to 1.3%) ... 1820
Maxalt Tablets (Infrequent) ... 1983
Maxalt-MLT Orally Disintegrating Tablets (Infrequent) ... 1983
Maxzide ... 2150
Meridia Capsules (2.6%) ... 485
Merrem I.V. (Greater than 0.1% to 1%) ... 687
Metadate CD Capsules ... 3316
Miacalcin Nasal Spray (Less than 1%) ... 2242
Micardis Tablets (More than 0.3%) ... 884
Micardis HCT Tablets (Less than 2%) ... 886
Migranal Nasal Spray (Infrequent) ... 3350
▲ Mirapex Tablets (Greater than or equal to 1%) ... 889
Mivacron Injection (Less than 1%) ... 489
Moban Tablets ... 1108
Mobic Oral Suspension (Less than 2%) ... 893
Mobic Tablets (Less than 2%) ... 893
Moduretic Tablets (Less than or equal to 1%) ... 2003
MS Contin Tablets (Less frequent) ... 2703
Mycamine for Injection ... 620
▲ Myfortic Tablets (3% to less than 20%) ... 2244
▲ Mylotarg for Injection (9% to 11%) ... 3429
Nalfon Capsules (Less than 1%) ... 2504
Namenda ... 1199
Naprosyn Suspension (Less than 1%) ... 2769
Naprosyn Tablets (Less than 1%) ... 2769
Narcan Injection ... 1109
▲ Naropin Injection (1% to 5%) ... 640
Natrecor for Injection (Greater than or equal to 1%) ... 3123
Navelbine Injection ... 1494
▲ Neumega for Injection (20% to 84%) ... 3433
Neupogen for Injection ... 598
Neurontin Capsules (Infrequent) ... 2498
Neurontin Oral Solution (Infrequent) ... 2498
Neurontin Tablets (Infrequent) ... 2498
Nexium Delayed-Release Capsules (Less than 1%) ... 645
Nexium I.V. (Less than 1%) ... 649
Niaspan Extended-Release Tablets ... 1703
Nicotrol Inhaler ... 2594
Nicotrol NS ... 2596
Nimotop Capsules (Up to 1.4%) ... 774
Nipent for Injection (Less than 3%) ... 3216
▲ Niravam Orally Disintegrating Tablets (7.7% to 15.4%) ... 3106
Norflex Injection ... 1824
Norvasc Tablets (More than 0.1% to 1%) ... 2529

- Norvir (Less than 2%) 499
- Nubain Injection (1% or less) 1111
- Numorphan 1112
- Omacor Capsules 2735
- Oncaspar (Greater than 1% but less than 5%) 1123
- ▲ Ontak Vials (12%) 1717
- Orap Tablets 1220
- ▲ Orthoclone OKT3 Sterile Solution (10%) 2370
- Parnate Tablets 1499
- Paxil CR Controlled-Release Tablets (Frequent) 1509
- Paxil (Frequent) 1501
- Permax Tablets (Infrequent) 3357
- Persantine Tablets (Rare) 898
- Phenergan 3438
- ▲ Photofrin for Injection (6%) 729
- Plendil Extended-Release Tablets (0.5% to 1.5%) 651
- ▲ Pletal Tablets (4%) 2478
- Prevacid Delayed-Release Capsules (Less than 1%) 3268
- Prevacid for Delayed-Release Oral Suspension (Less than 1%) 3268
- Prevacid NapraPAC (Less than 1%) 3277
- Prevacid SoluTab Delayed-Release Orally Disintegrating Tablets (Less than 1%) 3268
- PREVPAC (Less than 1%) 3281
- Prilosec OTC Tablets (Less than 1%) 2674
- Primaxin I.M. 2022
- Primaxin I.V. (1.5%) 2024
- Prinzide Tablets 2033
- Procrit for Injection (0.31%) 2374
- ▲ Prograf Capsules and Injection (3% to 15%) 624
- Prolastin (Occasional) 3252
- ▲ Proleukin for Injection (23%) 1007
- Propine Ophthalmic Solution ⊙ 237
- Protonix I.V. (Less than 1%) 3468
- Protonix Tablets (Less than 1%) 3465
- ▲ Proventil Inhalation Aerosol (10%) 3067
- Proventil Inhalation Solution 0.083% (1%) 3069
- ▲ Proventil HFA Inhalation Aerosol (7%) 3071
- Provigil Tablets (2%) 1002
- Prozac Pulvules and Liquid (Infrequent) 1771
- ▲ Rapamune Oral Solution and Tablets (3% to 20%) 3472
- Recombivax HB 2045
- ReFacto Vials 3479
- Relpax Tablets (Infrequent) 2531
- Remicade for IV Injection (Greater than or equal to 0.2%) 987
- Repronex for Intramuscular and Subcutaneous Injection 1148
- Requip Tablets (2%) 1528
- Rhophylac (Rare) 3504
- Rilutek Tablets (1.3% to 2.0%) 2945
- Risperdal Consta Long-Acting Injection (Frequent to 2%) 1664
- ▲ Risperdal M-Tab Orally Disintegrating Tablets (3% to 5%) 1658
- ▲ Risperdal (3% to 5%) 1658
- Ritalin Hydrochloride Tablets 2254
- Ritalin LA Capsules 2255
- Ritalin-SR Tablets 2254
- ▲ Rituxan for Infusion (Among most frequent) 845
- Rituxan I.V. 1251
- Sanctura Tablets (Greater than or equal to 0.5%) 1133
- Sandimmune 2259
- Sandostatin Injection (Less than 1%) 2263
- Sandostatin LAR Depot (1% to 4%) 2264
- Sedapap Tablets 50 mg/650 mg (Infrequent) 2098
- ▲ Seroquel Tablets (6%) 691
- ▲ Simulect for Injection (3% to 10%) 2268
- Sonata Capsules (Infrequent) 1686
- St. Joseph 81 mg Aspirin Chewable and Enteric Coated Tablets 1841
- ▲ Stromectol Tablets (3.5%) 2053
- Sular Tablets (Very rare) 1163
- Suprane Liquid for Inhalation (Greater than 1%) 770
- Surmontil Capsules 2347
- Sustiva Capsules (Less than 2%) 957
- Symbyax Capsules (2%) 1788
- Symmetrel 1115
- Tagamet Tablets (Rare) 1547
- Tambocor Tablets (1% to 3%) 1824
- Targretin Capsules 1719
- Tarka Tablets (0.3% or more) 519
- Tasmar Tablets (Infrequent) 3360
- Taxotere Injection Concentrate 2947
- Tenormin I.V. Injection 698
- Tenormin Tablets 695
- Tequin Injection (Less than 0.1%) 964
- Tequin Tablets (Less than 0.1%) 964
- Teveten Tablets (Less than 1%) 1707
- Teveten HCT Tablets (Less than 1%) 1710
- Thalomid Capsules 979
- Thiothixene Capsules 2124
- ▲ Thymoglobulin for Injection (26.8%) 2848
- Tiazac Capsules (Less than 2%) 1204
- Trasylol Injection (2%) 779
- Tricor Tablets 523
- Triglide Tablets 1165
- Trileptal Oral Suspension 2281
- Trileptal Tablets 2281
- ▲ Trisenox Injection (55%) 983
- Twinrix Vaccine 1571
- Tygacil for Injection (0% to less than 2%) 3489
- ▲ Ultane Liquid for Inhalation (2% to 6%) 526
- Ultracet Tablets (Less than 1%) 2462
- Uniretic Tablets (Less than 1%) 3114
- Unithroid Tablets 3521
- Uroqid-Acid No. 2 Tablets 785
- Uroxatral Tablets 2957
- Valtrex Caplets 1573
- Vaseretic Tablets (0.5% to 2.0%) 2073
- Ventolin HFA Inhalation Aerosol (Less than 3%) 1576
- VFEND I.V. (0% to 2.4%) 2543
- VFEND Oral Suspension (0% to 2.4%) 2543
- VFEND Tablets (0% to 2.4%) 2543
- Viagra Tablets (Less than 2%) 2552
- Vicoprofen Tablets (Less than 1%) 533
- Virazole for Inhalation Solution (Infrequent) 3365
- Vivactil Tablets 2350
- Voltaren Tablets (Occasionally) 2298
- Voltaren-XR Tablets (Occasionally) 2301
- VoSpire Extended-Release Tablets (2.7%) 2352
- ▲ Wellbutrin Tablets (10.8%) 1579
- Wellbutrin SR Sustained-Release Tablets (Infrequent) 1583
- Wellbutrin XL Extended-Release Tablets (Infrequent) 1588
- ▲ Xeloda Tablets (Less than 5%) 2825
- Xopenex HFA Inhalation Aerosol (2.7%) 3151
- Xopenex Inhalation Solution (2.7%) 3143
- Xopenex Inhalation Solution Concentrate (2.7%) 3147
- Zantac (Rare) 1597
- Zantac Injection (Rare) 1593
- Zantac Injection Pharmacy Bulk Package (Rare) 1595
- Zantac Syrup (Rare) 1597
- ▲ Zegerid Powder for Oral Solution (3.4%) 2972
- Zemuron Injection (Less than 1%) 2363
- ▲ Zenapax for Injection (Greater than 5%) 2838
- Zestoretic Tablets 701
- Zevalin Injection (Less than 1%) 848
- Zofran Injection (Rare) 1607
- Zofran (Rare) 1613
- Zofran ODT Orally Disintegrating Tablets (Rare) 1613
- Zoladex (1% or greater) 709
- Zoladex 3-month 712
- Zoloft (Infrequent) 2581
- Zomig Nasal Spray (Infrequent) 718
- Zomig Tablets (Rare) 714
- Zomig-ZMT Tablets (Rare) 714
- Zonegran Capsules (Infrequent) 1089
- Zosyn (1.0% or less) 3492
- Zyban Sustained-Release Tablets (Infrequent) 1620
- ▲ Zyprexa Tablets (4%) 1798
- Zyprexa IntraMuscular 1798
- ▲ Zyprexa ZYDIS Orally Disintegrating Tablets (4%) 1798
- Zyrtec Chewable Tablets (Less than 2%) 2589
- Zyrtec (Less than 2%) 2589
- Zyrtec-D 12 Hour Extended Release Tablets (Less than 2%) 2591

Tachycardia, junctional
- Digitek Tablets 2146
- ▲ Lanoxicaps Capsules (Among most common) 1458
- Lanoxin Injection 1462
- Lanoxin Tablets 1468
- ▲ Lanoxin Injection Pediatric (Among most common) 1465

Tachycardia, nodal
- Diprivan Injectable Emulsion (1.6%) 676

Tachycardia, reflex
- Plendil Extended-Release Tablets 651
- Urecholine Tablets 2349

Tachycardia, supraventricular
- Abilify Tablets (Frequent) 916
- Abilify Tablets (Frequent) 2472
- Aciphex Tablets (Rare) 1081
- Advair Diskus 100/50 1291
- Advair Diskus 250/50 1291
- Advair Diskus 500/50 1291
- Aggrenox Capsules (Less than 1%) 855
- Aricept Tablets (Infrequent) 1086
- Aricept ODT Tablets (Infrequent) 1086
- Atrovent HFA Inhalation Aerosol 872
- Avelox (Less than 0.1%) 2984
- ▲ Campath Ampules (3% to 11%) 826
- Cardene I.V. (0.7%) 1129
- ▲ CellCept Capsules (3% to less than 20%) 2751
- ▲ CellCept Intravenous (3% to less than 20%) 2751
- ▲ CellCept Oral Suspension (3% to less than 20%) 2751
- ▲ CellCept Tablets (3% to less than 20%) 2751
- Diprivan Injectable Emulsion (Less than 1%) 676
- Effexor Tablets 3405
- Effexor XR Capsules 3411
- Ethyol for Injection (Rare) 1869
- Evoxac Capsules (Less than 1%) 1042
- Exelon Capsules (Infrequent) 2204
- ▲ Flolan for Injection (8%) 1408
- Hytrin Capsules (Occasional) 469
- Levaquin in 5% Dextrose Injection (0.1% to 0.9%) 2453
- Levaquin (0.1% to 0.9%) 2453
- Meridia Capsules 485
- Nalfon Capsules (Less than 1%) 2504
- Namenda 1199
- Photofrin for Injection 729
- Pletal Tablets (Less than 2%) 2478
- ▲ Proleukin for Injection (12%) 1007
- Proventil Inhalation Aerosol 3067
- Razadyne ER Extended-Release Capsules (Infrequent) 2434
- Razadyne (Infrequent) 2434
- ReoPro Vials (1.0%) 1779
- Requip Tablets (Infrequent) 1528
- Retavase 1131
- Rilutek Tablets (Rare) 2945
- Rituxan for Infusion 845
- Rituxan I.V. 1251
- Rythmol SR Capsules 2736
- Serevent Diskus 1540
- Spiriva HandiHaler (Less than 1%) 899
- Sular Tablets (Less than or equal to 1%) 1163
- ▲ Tenormin I.V. Injection (11.5%) 698
- ▲ Tenormin Tablets (11.5%) 695
- ▲ Trasylol Injection (4%) 779
- Ventavis Inhalation Solution 1036
- Ventolin HFA Inhalation Aerosol 1576
- VFEND I.V. (Less than 2%) 2543
- VFEND Oral Suspension (Less than 2%) 2543
- VFEND Tablets (Less than 2%) 2543
- ▲ Xeloda Tablets (Less than 5%) 2825
- Xopenex HFA Inhalation Aerosol 3151
- Xopenex Inhalation Solution 3143
- Xopenex Inhalation Solution Concentrate 3147
- Zelnorm Tablets 2303
- Zofran Injection 1607
- Zosyn (1.0% or less to 1.3%) 3492

Tachycardia, ventricular
- Abilify Tablets (Frequent) 916
- Abilify Tablets (Frequent) 2472
- Aciphex Tablets (Rare) 1081
- Activase I.V. 1225
- Adenocard Injection 612
- Adenoscan 613
- Advair Diskus 100/50 1291
- Advair Diskus 250/50 1291
- Advair Diskus 500/50 1291
- Ambien Tablets (Rare) 2867
- Aramine Injection 1889
- ▲ Argatroban Injection (4.8%) 1321
- Avelox (Less than 0.1%) 2984
- Axid Oral Solution (2 individuals) 913
- Biaxin/Biaxin XL (Rare) 402
- ▲ BiDil Tablets (4%) 2161
- Caduet Tablets (Greater than 0.1% to less than or equal to 1%) 2507
- Campath Ampules 826
- Cardene I.V. (0.7%) 1129
- ▲ CellCept Capsules (3% to less than 20%) 2751
- ▲ CellCept Intravenous (3% to less than 20%) 2751
- ▲ CellCept Oral Suspension (3% to less than 20%) 2751
- ▲ CellCept Tablets (3% to less than 20%) 2751
- Cozaar Tablets (Less than 1%) 1913
- Cytovene 2763
- Digitek Tablets 2146
- Diprivan Injectable Emulsion (Less than 1%) 676
- E.E.S. (Rare) 449
- Effexor Tablets 3405
- Effexor XR Capsules 3411
- Ellence Injection 2632
- EryPed (Rare) 445
- Ery-Tab Tablets (Occasional reports) 447
- Erythrocin Stearate Filmtab Tablets (Occasional reports) 452
- Erythromycin Base Filmtab Tablets (Occasional reports) 454
- Erythromycin Delayed-Release Capsules, USP (Occasional reports) 456
- Hyperstat I.V. Injection 3031
- Hyzaar 1964
- ▲ Imdur Tablets (Less than or equal to 5%) 3032
- Imitrex Injection (Extremely rare) 1431
- Imitrex Tablets (Rare) 1440
- Invanz for Injection (Greater than 0.1%) 1974
- Lanoxicaps Capsules 1458
- Lanoxin Injection 1462
- Lanoxin Tablets 1468
- Lanoxin Injection Pediatric 1465
- Levaquin in 5% Dextrose Injection (0.1% to 0.9%) 2453
- Levaquin (0.1% to 0.9%) 2453
- Lexapro Oral Solution 1193
- Lexapro Tablets 1193
- Loprox Shampoo 1862
- Meridia Capsules 485
- Narcan Injection 1109
- Naropin Injection 640
- ▲ Natrecor for Injection (2% to 10%) 3123
- Norvasc Tablets (More than 0.1% to 1%) 2529
- Paxil CR Controlled-Release Tablets 1509
- Paxil 1501
- PCE Dispertab Tablets 510
- Permax Tablets (Infrequent) 3357
- Pletal Tablets (Less than 2%) 2478
- PREVPAC (Rare) 3281
- Prinivil Tablets (0.3% to 1.0%) 2029
- Prinzide Tablets 2033
- Prozac Pulvules and Liquid 1771
- Razadyne ER Extended-Release Capsules (Infrequent) 2434
- Razadyne (Infrequent) 2434
- Relpax Tablets (Infrequent) 2531
- ReoPro Vials (1.4%) 1779
- Requip Tablets (Rare) 1528
- Retavase 1131
- Rilutek Tablets (Rare) 2945
- Risperdal M-Tab Orally Disintegrating Tablets (Rare) 1658
- Risperdal (Rare) 1658
- Rituxan for Infusion 845
- Rituxan I.V. 1251
- Sonata Capsules (Rare) 1686
- Tambocor Tablets (0.4%) 1824
- ▲ Tenormin I.V. Injection (16%) 698
- ▲ Tenormin Tablets (16%) 695
- Thioridazine Hydrochloride Tablets 2122
- Toprol-XL Tablets (Greater than 1%) 660
- Trasylol Injection (1% to 2%) 779
- VFEND I.V. (Less than 2%) 2543
- VFEND Oral Suspension (Less than 2%) 2543
- VFEND Tablets (Less than 2%) 2543
- Zestril Tablets (0.3% to 1.0%) 704
- Zithromax Capsules, 250 mg 2568
- Zithromax for IV Infusion 2573
- Zithromax for Oral Suspension, 300 mg, 600 mg, 900 mg, 1200 mg 2561
- Zithromax Tablets, 250 mg, 500 mg 2561
- Zithromax Tri-Pak 2561
- Zofran Injection 1607
- Zoloft 2581
- Zomig Nasal Spray 718
- Zomig Tablets 714
- Zomig-ZMT Tablets 714
- Zosyn (1.0% or less) 3492

Tachyphylaxis
- ▲ Sandostatin Injection (35%) 2263

Tachypnea
- Abelcet Injection 1119
- Actimmune (Rare) 1646
- Aggrenox Capsules 855

Bayer Aspirin Tablets ... 3515
Cancidas for Injection (0% to 1.3%) ... 1894
Clolar for Intravenous Infusion ... 1264
Diprivan Injectable Emulsion (Less than 1%) ... 676
Follistim AQ Cartridge ... 2354
Maxalt Tablets (Rare) ... 1983
Maxalt-MLT Orally Disintegrating Tablets (Rare) ... 1983
Orthoclone OKT3 Sterile Solution ... 2370
▲ Proleukin for Injection (8%) ... 1007
Repronex for Intramuscular and Subcutaneous Injection ... 1148
Retrovir Capsules ... 1533
Retrovir IV Infusion ... 1537
Retrovir ... 1533
Roferon-A Injection (Rare to infrequent) ... 2805
Sulfamylon Cream ... 2154
Sulfamylon for 5% Topical Solution ... 2155
Symmetrel ... 1115
▲ Trisenox Injection (8%) ... 983

Talkativeness

Carbatrol Capsules ... 3174
Dalmane Capsules ... 3343
Equetro Extended-Release Capsules ... 3178
▲ Niravam Orally Disintegrating Tablets (2.2%) ... 3106
Tegretol/Tegretol-XR ... 2278
Xanax XR Tablets (Infrequent) ... 2655

Tardive dyskinesia

Abilify Tablets (Infrequent) ... 916
Abilify Tablets (Infrequent) ... 2472
Clozapine Tablets ... 2141
Clozaril Tablets ... 2174
Depacon Injection (1% or more) ... 412
Depakene (1% or more) ... 417
Depakote Sprinkle Capsules ... 422
▲ Depakote Tablets (1% to 5%) ... 427
Depakote ER Tablets (Greater than 1%) ... 433
Effexor Tablets ... 3405
Effexor XR Capsules ... 3411
Eldepryl Capsules ... 3209
FazaClo Orally Disintegrating Tablets ... 547
Geodon Capsules ... 2514
Moban Tablets ... 1108
Namenda ... 1199
Orap Tablets ... 1220
Risperdal Consta Long-Acting Injection (Infrequent) ... 1664
Risperdal M-Tab Orally Disintegrating Tablets ... 1658
Risperdal ... 1658
Seroquel Tablets ... 691
Thioridazine Hydrochloride Tablets ... 2122
Thiothixene Capsules ... 2124
Wellbutrin Tablets ... 1579
Wellbutrin SR Sustained-Release Tablets ... 1583
Wellbutrin XL Extended-Release Tablets ... 1588
Zomig Nasal Spray (Rare) ... 718
Zyban Sustained-Release Tablets ... 1620
Zyprexa Tablets (Up to 2%) ... 1798
Zyprexa ZYDIS Orally Disintegrating Tablets (Up to 2%) ... 1798

Tardive dyskinesia, unmasking of

Wellbutrin Tablets ... 1579

Tardive dystonia

(*see under* Dystonia, tardive)

Taste, altered

Abilify Tablets (Infrequent) ... 916
Abilify Tablets (Infrequent) ... 2472
Actiq (Less than 1%) ... 993
Adalat CC Tablets (Rare) ... 2978
▲ Advair Diskus 100/50 (1% to 3%) ... 1291
▲ Advair Diskus 250/50 (1% to 3%) ... 1291
▲ Advair Diskus 500/50 (1% to 3%) ... 1291
▲ Agenerase Capsules (2% to 10%) ... 1299
▲ Agenerase Oral Solution (2% to 10%) ... 1304
Alferon N Injection (1%) ... 1640
Alphagan P Ophthalmic Solution (Less than 1%) ... 563
Altace Capsules (Less than 1%) ... 1673
Altoprev Extended-Release Tablets ... 1151
Ambien Tablets (Infrequent) ... 2867
Amerge Tablets (Rare) ... 1312
Antabuse Tablets ... 2343
Anzemet Injection (Infrequently) ... 2871
Anzemet Tablets (Infrequently) ... 2874
AquaMEPHYTON Injection ... 1887
▲ Arava Tablets (1% to 3%) ... 2881
Arthrotec Tablets (Rare) ... 3126
Asacol Delayed-Release Tablets ... 2688
Atrovent HFA Inhalation Aerosol (0.9%) ... 872
Atrovent Nasal Spray 0.03% (Less than 2%) ... 869
Atrovent Nasal Spray 0.06% (Less than 1%) ... 870
▲ Avastin IV (14% to 21%) ... 1229
Avelox (0.1% to less than 2%) ... 2984
Avinza Capsules (Less than 5%) ... 1714
Axert Tablets (Infrequent) ... 2430
Bactroban Nasal (0.8% to 3%) ... 1357
▲ BeneFix for Injection (4.6%) ... 3402
▲ Biaxin/Biaxin XL (3%) ... 402
Brevibloc Concentrate ... 766
Brevibloc Injection ... 766
Brevibloc Double Strength Injection ... 766
Brevibloc Premixed Injection ... 766
Brevibloc Double Strength Premixed Injection ... 766
Brimonidine Tartrate Ophthalmic Solution 0.2% (Less than 3%) ... ⊙ 245
▲ Buphenyl Powder (3%) ... 3327
▲ Buphenyl Tablets (3%) ... 3327
Caduet Tablets (Less than 2%) ... 2507
Campral Tablets (Frequent) ... 1175
Captopril Tablets (Approximately 2 to 4 of 100 patients) ... 2114
▲ Carnitor Injection (2% to 9%) ... 3185
Carteolol Hydrochloride Ophthalmic Solution USP, 1% (Occasional) ... ⊙ 246
Catapres-TTS (1 of 101 patients) ... 875
Celebrex Capsules (0.1% to 1.9%) ... 3130
Celexa (Frequent) ... 1177
Cipro XR Tablets (Less than 1%) ... 3004
Ciprodex Otic Suspension (0.5%) ... 555
Colazal Capsules ... 2845
Combivent Inhalation Aerosol (Less than 2%) ... 878
Combunox Tablets (Less than 2%) ... 1183
Comtan Tablets (1%) ... 2186
Copaxone for Injection (At least 2%) ... 3292
▲ Cosopt Sterile Ophthalmic Solution (Up to 30%) ... 1910
Coumadin for Injection (Infrequent) ... 932
Coumadin Tablets (Infrequent) ... 932
Cozaar Tablets (Less than 1%) ... 1913
Crixivan Capsules (2.7%) ... 1918
Cubicin for Injection (Less than 1%) ... 1038
▲ Cuprimine Capsules (12%) ... 1925
Cytovene (At least 3 subjects) ... 2763
Dantrium Capsules (Less frequent) ... 2690
Denavir Cream (0.2%) ... 2163
▲ Depacon Injection (1% to 5%) ... 412
▲ Depakene (1% to 5%) ... 417
▲ Depakote Sprinkle Capsules (1% to 5%) ... 422
▲ Depakote Tablets (1% to 5%) ... 427
Depakote ER Tablets (Greater than 1%) ... 433
Dilaudid ... 439
Dilaudid Oral Liquid ... 443
Dilaudid Non-Sterile Powder ... 439
Dilaudid Rectal Suppositories ... 439
Dilaudid Tablets ... 439
Dilaudid Tablets - 8 mg ... 443
Dilaudid-HP (Less frequent) ... 441
Diprivan Injectable Emulsion (Less than 1%) ... 676
▲ Doxil Injection (Less than 1% to 10%) ... 3302
DuoNeb Inhalation Solution ... 1058
Effexor Tablets (2%) ... 3405
Effexor XR Capsules (Frequent) ... 3411
Eldepryl Capsules ... 3209
Eligard 7.5 mg (Less than 2%) ... 2896
▲ Eloxatin for Injection (5% to 12%) ... 2908
Emend Capsules (Greater than 0.5%) ... 1944
Enbrel for Injection ... 580
Eskalith ... 1406
Evoxac Capsules (Less than 1%) ... 1042
Exelon Capsules (Infrequent) ... 2204
Factive Tablets (0.3%) ... 2464
Flonase Nasal Spray ... 1412
Floxin Otic Singles ... 1045
▲ Floxin Otic Solution (7%) ... 1043
Flumadine (Less than 0.3%) ... 1186
FML Ophthalmic Suspension ... ⊙ 224
FML Forte Ophthalmic Suspension ... ⊙ 223
Fortical Nasal Spray (Less than 1%) ... 3336
Fosamax (0.1% to 0.5%) ... 1949
Fosamax Plus D Tablets (0.1% to 0.5%) ... 1956
Frova Tablets (Infrequent) ... 1101
Fuzeon Injection ... 2772
Gabitril Tablets (Infrequent) ... 998
Gengraf Capsules (1% to less than 3%) ... 458
▲ Gleevec Tablets (1% to 14%) ... 2221
Hyperstat I.V. Injection ... 3031
Hyzaar ... 1964
Imitrex Injection (Infrequent) ... 1431
▲ Imitrex Nasal Spray (13.5% to 24.5%) ... 1435
Imitrex Tablets ... 1440
Infed Injection ... 3381
▲ Infergen (3%) ... 1647
▲ Intron A for Injection (Up to 24%) ... 3038
Invanz for Injection (Greater than 0.1%) ... 1974
Invirase (Greater than or equal to 2%) ... 2776
Kaletra (Less than 2%) ... 474
▲ Kepivance (16%) ... 592
Kogenate FS ... 3517
Kytril Injection (2%) ... 2785
Lamictal (Infrequent) ... 1449
Lamisil Tablets (2.8%) ... 2226
Lescol Capsules ... 2227
Lescol Capsules ... 2730
Lescol XL Tablets ... 2227
Lescol XL Tablets ... 2730
Levaquin in 5% Dextrose Injection (0.1% to 0.9%) ... 2453
Levaquin (0.1% to 0.9%) ... 2453
Lexapro Oral Solution (Infrequent) ... 1193
Lexapro Tablets (Infrequent) ... 1193
Lidoderm Patch ... 1107
Lipitor Tablets (Less than 2%) ... 2495
Lithobid Tablets ... 1670
Lotensin HCT Tablets (0.3% to 1%) ... 2235
Lotronex Tablets (Rare) ... 1479
Lupron Depot 3.75 mg (Less than 5%) ... 3257
Lupron Depot–3 Month 11.25 mg (Less than 5%) ... 3262
Lyrica Capsules (0.1% to 1%) ... 2524
Maxair Autohaler (0.6%) ... 1820
Maxzide ... 2150
▲ Mepron Suspension (3%) ... 1487
Meridia Capsules (2.2%) ... 485
MetroGel-Vaginal Gel (2%) ... 1822
Mevacor Tablets ... 1996
Miacalcin Nasal Spray (Less than 1%) ... 2242
▲ Migranal Nasal Spray (8%) ... 3350
Mirapex Tablets (Greater than or equal to 1%) ... 889
Mobic Oral Suspension (Less than 2%) ... 893
Mobic Tablets (Less than 2%) ... 893
MS Contin Tablets (Less frequent) ... 2703
Nasonex Nasal Spray (Very rare) ... 3058
▲ Navelbine Injection (Up to 17%) ... 1494
Neoral Soft Gelatin Capsules (1% to less than 3%) ... 2247
Neoral Oral Solution (1% to less than 3%) ... 2247
▲ Neulasta Injection (15% to 72%) ... 596
Neurontin Capsules (Infrequent) ... 2498
Neurontin Oral Solution (Infrequent) ... 2498
Neurontin Tablets (Infrequent) ... 2498
Nexium Delayed-Release Capsules (Less than 1% to 6.6%) ... 645
Nexium I.V. (Less than 1% to 6.6%) ... 649
▲ Nicotrol Inhaler (Greater than 3%) ... 2594
Nicotrol NS ... 2596
Nipent for Injection (Less than 3%) ... 3216
Niravam Orally Disintegrating Tablets ... 3106
Norvasc Tablets (Less than or equal to 0.1%) ... 2529
▲ Norvir (7% to 11.1%) ... 499
Omacor Capsules (2.7%) ... 2735
▲ Orap Tablets (1 of 20 patients) ... 1220
OxyContin Tablets (Less than 1%) ... 2699
▲ Pacerone Tablets (1% to 3%) ... 3337
Parcopa Orally Disintegrating Tablets ... 3111
Patanol Ophthalmic Solution (Less than 5%) ... 557
Paxil CR Controlled-Release Tablets (2%) ... 1509
Paxil (2%) ... 1501
PEG-Intron Powder for Injection (Less than 1%) ... 3062
Pepcid Injection (Infrequent) ... 2017
Pepcid (Infrequent) ... 2014
Permax Tablets (1.6%) ... 3357
Plavix Tablets ... 940
Plavix Tablets ... 2942
Pravachol Tablets ... 943
Prevacid Delayed-Release Capsules (Less than 1%) ... 3268
Prevacid for Delayed-Release Oral Suspension (Less than 1%) ... 3268
Prevacid I.V. for Injection (Less than 1%) ... 3274
Prevacid NapraPAC (Less than 1%) ... 3277
Prevacid SoluTab Delayed-Release Orally Disintegrating Tablets (Less than 1%) ... 3268
▲ PREVPAC (3% to 5%) ... 3281
▲ Prilosec OTC Tablets (Less than 1% to 15%) ... 2674
Primaxin I.M. ... 2022
Primaxin I.V. (Less than 0.2%) ... 2024
Prinivil Tablets ... 2029
Prinzide Tablets ... 2033
▲ Proleukin for Injection (7%) ... 1007
ProSom Tablets (Infrequent) ... 512
Protonix I.V. (Less than 1%) ... 3468
Protonix Tablets (Less than 1%) ... 3465
Protopic Ointment (Greater than or equal to 1%) ... 629
Proventil Inhalation Aerosol ... 3067
▲ Proventil HFA Inhalation Aerosol (4%) ... 3071
Provigil Tablets (1%) ... 1002
Prozac Pulvules and Liquid (Frequent) ... 1771
▲ Rebetol (Less than 1% to 9%) ... 3073
▲ Rebetron Combination Therapy (6% to 8%) ... 3078
ReFacto Vials ... 3479
Relafen Tablets (Less than 1%) ... 1523
Relpax Tablets (Infrequent) ... 2531
Rescriptor Tablets ... 2535
▲ Retrovir Capsules (5%) ... 1533
▲ Retrovir IV Infusion (5%) ... 1537
▲ Retrovir (5%) ... 1533
Reyataz Capsules (Less than 3%) ... 948
▲ Ribavirin, USP Capsules (Less than 1% to 9%) ... 3083
▲ Rituxan for Infusion (1% to 5%) ... 845
▲ Roferon-A Injection (3% to less than 4%) ... 2805
▲ Rythmol SR Capsules (6% to 22%) ... 2736
Sandostatin LAR Depot (1% to 4%) ... 2264
Seroquel Tablets (Infrequent) ... 691
Sonata Capsules (Frequent) ... 1686
▲ Soriatane Capsules (1% to 10%) ... 1028
Spectracef Tablets (0.1% to 1%) ... 2706
Stalevo Tablets (1%) ... 2270
Striant Mucoadhesive (2.0%) ... 1022
Sular Tablets (Less than or equal to 1%) ... 1163
Surmontil Capsules ... 2347
Sustiva Capsules (Less than 2%) ... 957
Symbyax Capsules (Frequent) ... 1788
Tambocor Tablets (Less than 1%) ... 1824
Tasmar Tablets (1% or more) ... 3360
▲ Taxotere Injection Concentrate (0.6% to 5.7%) ... 2947
▲ Temodar Capsules (5%) ... 3088
▲ Tequin Injection (0.1% to 3%) ... 964
▲ Tequin Tablets (0.1% to 3%) ... 964
Testim 1% Gel (1%) ... 722
Timentin ADD-Vantage ... 1556
Timentin Injection Galaxy Container ... 1559
Timentin IV Infusion ... 1553
Timentin Pharmacy Bulk Package ... 1562
Tindamax ... 2670
▲ TOBI Solution for Inhalation (6.6%) ... 1015
▲ Topamax Sprinkle Capsules (2% to 15%) ... 2438
▲ Topamax Tablets (2% to 15%) ... 2438
Toprol-XL Tablets ... 660
Trileptal Oral Suspension ... 2281
Trileptal Tablets ... 2281
Tygacil for Injection (0% to less than 2%) ... 3489
Ultane Liquid for Inhalation (Less than 1%) ... 526
Univasc Tablets (Less than 1%) ... 3118
Vantin Tablets and Oral Suspension (Less than 1%) ... 2650
Vaseretic Tablets ... 2073
Vasotec I.V. Injection (0.5% to 1.0%) ... 2076
VFEND I.V. (Less than 2%) ... 2543
VFEND Oral Suspension (Less than 2%) ... 2543
VFEND Tablets (Less than 2%) ... 2543
VoSpire Extended-Release Tablets ... 2352
Vytorin 10/10 Tablets ... 2084
Vytorin 10/10 Tablets ... 3092
Vytorin 10/20 Tablets ... 2084
Vytorin 10/20 Tablets ... 3092
Vytorin 10/40 Tablets ... 2084
Vytorin 10/40 Tablets ... 3092
Vytorin 10/80 Tablets ... 2084
Vytorin 10/80 Tablets ... 3092
▲ Wellbutrin SR Sustained-Release Tablets (2% to 4%) ... 1583
▲ Wellbutrin XL Extended-Release Tablets (2% to 4%) ... 1588
▲ Zegerid Powder for Oral Solution (Less than 1% to 15%) ... 2972

Zemplar Capsules (Rare) 535
Zemplar Injection (Rare) 538
Zestoretic Tablets 701
Zestril Tablets (0.3% to 1.0%) 704
Zithromax Capsules, 250 mg (Rare) 2568
Zithromax for IV Infusion (Rare) 2573
Zithromax for Oral Suspension, 300 mg, 600 mg, 900 mg, 1200 mg (Rare) 2561
Zithromax Tablets, 250 mg, 500 mg (Rare) 2561
Zithromax Tri-Pak (Rare) 2561
Zmax for Oral Suspension (Less then 1%) 2577
Zocor Tablets 2078
▲ Zomig Nasal Spray (5% to 21%) 718
Zonegran Capsules (2%) 1089
Zosyn (1.0% or less) 3492
▲ Zyban Sustained-Release Tablets (2% to 3%) 1620
▲ Zymar Ophthalmic Solution (1% to 4%) 571
Zyprexa Tablets (Infrequent) 1798
Zyprexa ZYDIS Orally Disintegrating Tablets (Infrequent) 1798
Zyrtec Chewable Tablets (Less than 2%) 2589
Zyrtec (Less than 2%) 2589
Zyrtec-D 12 Hour Extended Release Tablets (Less than 2%) 2591
Zyvox (0.9% to 1.8%) 2661

Taste, bad
Alupent Inhalation Aerosol (Less frequent) 858
Aricept Tablets (Infrequent) 1086
Aricept ODT Tablets (Infrequent) 1086
▲ Buphenyl Powder (3%) 3327
▲ Buphenyl Tablets (3%) 3327
▲ Ciloxan Ophthalmic Ointment (Less than 10%) 554
Cipro I.V. (1% or less) 2998
Cipro I.V. Pharmacy Bulk Package (1% or less) 3509
Cipro (Less than 1%) 2991
Fluorescite Injection ⊙ 207
Imitrex Injection 1431
▲ Imitrex Nasal Spray (13.5% to 24.5%) 1435
Imitrex Tablets 1440
Moduretic Tablets (Less than or equal to 1%) 2003
▲ Thrombate III (3 of 17) 3254
Vicoprofen Tablets (Less than 1%) 533

Taste, bitter
▲ Astelin Nasal Spray (19.4%) 1876
▲ Azopt Ophthalmic Suspension (5% to 10%) 553
Ceftin Tablets 1369
Clinoril Tablets (Less than 1 in 100) 1899
Clozapine Tablets (Less than 1%) 2141
Clozaril Tablets (Less than 1%) 2174
▲ Cosopt Sterile Ophthalmic Solution (Up to 30%) 1910
Dalmane Capsules (Rare) 3343
FazaClo Orally Disintegrating Tablets (Less than 1%) 547
Noroxin Tablets (Less frequent) 2009
Nubain Injection (1% or less) 1111
▲ Optivar Ophthalmic Solution (Approximately 10%) 1877
Risperdal M-Tab Orally Disintegrating Tablets (Rare) 1658
Risperdal (Rare) 1658
▲ Striant Mucoadhesive (4.1%) 1022
▲ Tindamax (3.7% to 6.3%) 2670
▲ Trusopt Sterile Ophthalmic Solution (Approximately one-quarter of patients) 2065

Taste, changes
(*see under* Taste, altered)

Taste, loss
(*see under* Ageusia)

Taste, metallic
Adenocard Injection (Less than 1%) 612
Adenoscan (Less than 1%) 613
Antabuse Tablets 2343
Calcijex Injection 411
▲ Chemet Capsules (12.0% to 20.9%) 2480
Clinoril Tablets (Less than 1 in 100) 1899
Eskalith 1406
Hectorol Capsules 909
Hectorol Injection 911
Lexapro Oral Solution (Infrequent) 1193
Lexapro Tablets (Infrequent) 1193
Lidoderm Patch 1107
Lithobid Tablets 1670
Metrogel 1% 1212
Nalfon Capsules (Less than 1%) 2504
▲ Tindamax (3.7% to 6.3%) 2670
Trecator Tablets 3482

Taste, salty
Miacalcin Injection 2241

Taste, unpleasant
Adderall Tablets 3168
Adderall XR Capsules 3169
Adipex-P 1216
▲ Aerobid/Aerobid-M (10%) 1172
▲ Azopt Ophthalmic Suspension (5% to 10%) 553
Beconase AQ Nasal Spray 1359
▲ Ceftin for Oral Suspension (5.0%) 1369
Cipro XR Tablets 3004
Desoxyn Tablets, USP 2482
Dexedrine 1386
DextroStat Tablets 3177
Efudex 3348
▲ Flexeril Tablets (1% to 3%) 1832
Flonase Nasal Spray (Less than 1%) 1412
▲ Lunesta Tablets (8% to 34%) 3139
Mephyton Tablets 1993
Vivactil Tablets 2350

Teeth, discoloration
Neurontin Capsules (Rare) 2498
Neurontin Oral Solution (Rare) 2498
Neurontin Tablets (Rare) 2498
Primaxin I.M. 2022
Primaxin I.V. (Less than 0.2%) 2024

Teeth, mottling of enamel
(*see under* Teeth, discoloration)

Teeth grinding
Celexa (Infrequent) 1177
Zoloft (Infrequent) 2581

Telangiectasia
Clobevate Gel (Less than 2%) 3213
Clobex Shampoo 1209
▲ Clobex Lotion (3.2%) 1208
Cutivate Ointment 1384
Diprolene Gel 0.05% 3015
Diprolene AF Cream 0.05% 3014
Efudex 3348
Lofibra Capsules (Less than 1%) 1217
Olux Foam (Less than 2%) 1027
▲ Temovate Gel (Among most frequent) 1550
Temovate Ointment (Less frequent) 1549
Temovate E Emollient (Less than 2%) 1552
Tricor Tablets 523
▲ Tri-Luma Cream (3%) 1213

Telogen effluvium
Lariam Tablets 2790

Temperature disturbances, cutaneous
Wellbutrin Tablets (1.9%) 1579

Temperature elevation
(*see under* Hyperthermia)

Tenderness
Aldara Cream, 5% (More than 1%) 1814
Altoprev Extended-Release Tablets 1151
Bactroban Ointment (Less than 1%) 1358
Efudex (Infrequent) 3348
▲ HibTITER (0.3% to 3.7%) 3419
Mevacor Tablets 1996
▲ Miacalcin Nasal Spray (10.6%) 2242
M-M-R II 1980
Oncaspar 1123
Recombivax HB (Equal to or greater than 1%) 2045
Tabloid Tablets 1545
Temovate Scalp Application (1 of 294 patients) 1551
Vivelle Transdermal System 2288
Vivelle-Dot Transdermal System 2293
Zocor Tablets 2078

Tenderness, elbow
Temovate E Emollient (Less than 2%) 1552

Tenderness, nasal
▲ Fortical Nasal Spray (10.6%) 3336

Tenderness, right upper quadrant
Celebrex Capsules 3130
Tasmar Tablets 3360

Tenderness at injection site
▲ Actimmune (14%) 1646
▲ DAPTACEL (8% to 10.8%) 2964
GamaSTAN 3231
HyperHep B S/D 3237
▲ Infanrix Vaccine (4.0% to 5.2%) 1444
▲ Prevnar for Injection (0.8% to 82.8%) 3460
Rhophylac 3504
Rocephin Injectable Vials, ADD-Vantage, Galaxy, Bulk (1%) 2801
▲ Vaqta (1.7% to 52.7%) 2067

Tenderness at insertion site
▲ Vantas (3.6%) 3367

Tendinitis
Ambien Tablets (Rare) 2867
Celebrex Capsules (0.1% to 1.9%) 3130
Cipro I.V. 2998
Cipro I.V. Pharmacy Bulk Package 3509
Cipro 2991
Cipro XR Tablets 3004
Evoxac Capsules (Less than 1%) 1042
▲ Intron A for Injection (Less than 5%) 3038
Klonopin (Infrequent) 2782
Levaquin in 5% Dextrose Injection (0.1% to 0.9%) 2453
Levaquin (0.1% to 0.9%) 2453
Neurontin Capsules 2498
Neurontin Oral Solution (Infrequent) 2498
Neurontin Tablets 2498
Noroxin Tablets 2009
Requip Tablets (Infrequent) 1528
Risperdal Consta Long-Acting Injection (Infrequent) 1664
Teveten Tablets (Less than 1%) 1707
Teveten HCT Tablets (Less than 1%) 1710

Tendinous contracture
Caduet Tablets (Less than 2%) 2507
Gabitril Tablets (Infrequent) 998
Lamictal (Rare) 1449
Lipitor Tablets (Less than 2%) 2495
Symbyax Capsules (Infrequent) 1788

Tendon disorder, unspecified
Actiq (Less than 1%) 993
▲ Actonel Tablets (3%) 2679
▲ Actonel with Calcium Tablets (3%) 2684
Avelox (Less than 0.1%) 2984
BiDil Tablets (1% to less than 2%) 2161
Cipro I.V. 2998
Cipro I.V. Pharmacy Bulk Package 3509
Gengraf Capsules (1% to less than 3%) 458
Humira Injection (Less than 5%) 464
▲ Imdur Tablets (Less than or equal to 5%) 3032
Neoral Soft Gelatin Capsules (1% to less than 3%) 2247
Neoral Oral Solution (1% to less than 3%) 2247
Neurontin Capsules (Rare) 2498
Neurontin Oral Solution (Rare) 2498
Neurontin Tablets (Rare) 2498
Omacor Capsules 2735
Remicade for IV Injection (Greater than or equal to 0.2%) 987
Rescriptor Tablets 2535

Tendon rupture
▲ Arava Tablets (1% to 3%) 2881
Avelox 2984
Cipro I.V. 2998
Cipro I.V. Pharmacy Bulk Package 3509
Cipro 2991
Cipro XR Tablets 3004
Decadron Phosphate Injection 1931
Decadron Tablets 1929
Depo-Medrol Single-Dose Vial 2617
Effexor Tablets (Rare) 3405
Effexor XR Capsules (Rare) 3411
Factive Tablets 2464
Hydrocortone Tablets 1963
Levaquin in 5% Dextrose Injection 2453
Levaquin 2453
Noroxin Tablets 2009
Tequin Injection 964
Tequin Tablets 964
Viagra Tablets (Less than 2%) 2552

Tendonitis
Abilify Tablets (Rare) 916
Abilify Tablets (Rare) 2472
Accutane Capsules 2740
Amnesteem Capsules 2126
Rythmol SR Capsules 2736
Soriatane Capsules (Less than 1%) 1028
Xenical Capsules (2%) 2834

Tendons, calcification of
Accutane Capsules 2740
Amnesteem Capsules 2126

Tenesmus
Ambien Tablets (Rare) 2867
Arthrotec Tablets (Rare) 3126
Asacol Delayed-Release Tablets (2% or greater) 2688
Caduet Tablets (Less than 2%) 2507
Celebrex Capsules (0.1% to 1.9%) 3130
Colazal Capsules 2845
Copaxone for Injection (Infrequent) 3292
Doxil Injection (Less than 1%) 3302
▲ Eloxatin for Injection (2% to 5%) 2908
Evoxac Capsules (Less than 1%) 1042
Exelon Capsules (Infrequent) 2204
Lipitor Tablets (Less than 2%) 2495
Naropin Injection (Less than 1%) 640
Norvir (Less than 2%) 499
Omacor Capsules 2735
Prevacid Delayed-Release Capsules (Less than 1%) 3268
Prevacid for Delayed-Release Oral Suspension (Less than 1%) 3268
Prevacid NapraPAC (Less than 1%) 3277
Prevacid SoluTab Delayed-Release Orally Disintegrating Tablets (Less than 1%) 3268
PREVPAC (Less than 1%) 3281
Rilutek Tablets (Infrequent) 2945
▲ Sandostatin LAR Depot (4% to 6%) 2264
Soriatane Capsules (Less than 1%) 1028
▲ Xifaxan Tablets (7.2%) 2847
Zoloft (Rare) 2581

Tenosynovitis
Abilify Tablets (Rare) 916
Abilify Tablets (Rare) 2472
Antara Capsules 2723
▲ Arava Tablets (3%) 2881
▲ Azmacort Inhalation Aerosol (1% to 3%) 1701
Caduet Tablets (Less than 2%) 2507
Copaxone for Injection (Infrequent) 3292
Effexor Tablets (Infrequent) 3405
Effexor XR Capsules (Infrequent) 3411
Evoxac Capsules (Less than 1%) 1042
Geodon Capsules (Infrequent) 2514
Lipitor Tablets (Less than 2%) 2495
Lofibra Capsules 1217
Lupron Depot 3.75 mg 3257
Lupron Depot 7.5 mg 3261
Lupron Depot–3 Month 11.25 mg 3262
Lupron Depot-PED 7.5 mg, 11.25 mg and 15 mg 3266
Lupron Injection Pediatric 3256
Meridia Capsules (1.2%) 485
Paxil CR Controlled-Release Tablets (Rare) 1509
Paxil (Rare) 1501
Permax Tablets (Infrequent) 3357
Protonix I.V. (Less than 1%) 3468
Protonix Tablets (Less than 1%) 3465
Prozac Pulvules and Liquid (Infrequent) 1771
Rescriptor Tablets 2535
Sonata Capsules (Infrequent) 1686
Sular Tablets (Less than or equal to 1%) 1163
Symbyax Capsules (Infrequent) 1788
Tasmar Tablets (Infrequent) 3360
Tricor Tablets 523
Uniretic Tablets (Less than 1%) 3114
Viagra Tablets (Less than 2%) 2552
Zomig Nasal Spray (Rare) 718
Zomig Tablets (Infrequent) 714
Zomig-ZMT Tablets (Infrequent) 714

Tenseness
Allegra-D 12 Hour Extended-Release Tablets 2860
Allegra-D 24 Hour Extended-Release Tablets 2862
▲ Indapamide Tablets (Greater than or equal to 5%) 2119
Zelnorm Tablets 2303
Zyrtec-D 12 Hour Extended Release Tablets 2591

Tensosynovitis
Relpax Tablets (Rare) 2531

Testes, size decrease
▲ Lupron Depot 7.5 mg (5.4%) 3261

Testicular atrophy
Anadrol-50 Tablets 3329
▲ Eligard 7.5 mg (5%) 2896
Eligard 22.5 mg (Less than 2%) 2899
▲ Eligard 30 mg (4.4%) 2901

▲ Lupron Depot 7.5 mg (5.4%) 3261
Oxandrin Tablets 2977
▲ Viadur Implant (3.8%) 782

Testicular disorder, unspecified
AndroGel (Up to 3%) 3330
Caverject Impulse Injection (Less than 1%) 2610
Prevacid Delayed-Release Capsules (Less than 1%) 3268
Prevacid for Delayed-Release Oral Suspension (Less than 1%) 3268
Prevacid NapraPAC (Less than 1%) .. 3277
Prevacid SoluTab Delayed-Release Orally Disintegrating Tablets (Less than 1%) 3268
PREVPAC (Less than 1%) 3281
▲ Rapamune Oral Solution and Tablets (3% to 20%) 3472
Vivelle Transdermal System 2288
Vivelle-Dot Transdermal System 2293

Testicular function, inhibited
Alkeran for Injection 976
Anadrol-50 Tablets 3329
Oxandrin Tablets 2977

Testicular hypotrophy
Cytovene 2763

Testicular swelling
Flexeril Tablets (Rare) 1832
Neurontin Capsules (Rare) 2498
Neurontin Oral Solution (Rare) 2498
Neurontin Tablets (Rare) 2498
Surmontil Capsules 2347
Vivactil Tablets 2350
Wellbutrin Tablets (Infrequent) 1579

Testosterone, decreased physiologic effects
Zoladex 709

Testosterone serum levels, transient increase
Avodart Soft Gelatin Capsules 1353
Vantas (Less than 2%) 3367
Zoladex 709
Zoladex 3-month 712

Tetany
Ambien Tablets (Rare) 2867
Ammonul Injection 3323
Aredia for Injection (Rare) 2168
Furosemide Tablets 2117
Garamycin Injectable 3028
Imitrex Injection 1431
Imitrex Nasal Spray (Rare) 1435
Imitrex Tablets (Rare) 1440
Paxil CR Controlled-Release Tablets (Rare) 1509
Paxil (Rare) 1501
▲ Rapamune Oral Solution and Tablets (3% to 20%) 3472
Rescriptor Tablets 2535
Rilutek Tablets (Rare) 2945
Risperdal Consta Long-Acting Injection (Infrequent) 1664
Trileptal Oral Suspension 2281
Trileptal Tablets 2281
Zomig Tablets (Rare) 714
Zomig-ZMT Tablets (Rare) 714

Thick feeling, nasal
▲ Fortical Nasal Spray (10.6%) 3336

Thickening, facial tissue
Increlex Injection (Several patients) .. 3290

Thinking, slowed
Abilify Tablets (Infrequent) 916
Abilify Tablets (Infrequent) 2472
Lithobid Tablets 1670
Xanax XR Tablets (Infrequent) 2655

Thinking abnormality
Actiq (1% to 2%) 993
Ambien Tablets (Rare) 2867
AmBisome for Injection (Less common) 615
Astelin Nasal Spray (Infrequent) 1876
Avelox (Less than 0.1%) 2984
Avinza Capsules (Less than 5%) 1714
Brevibloc Concentrate (Less than 1%) 766
Brevibloc Injection (Less than 1%) 766
Brevibloc Double Strength Injection (Less than 1%) 766
Brevibloc Premixed Injection (Less than 1%) 766
Brevibloc Double Strength Premixed Injection (Less than 1%) 766
Campath Ampules 826
Campral Tablets (Frequent) 1175
▲ CellCept Capsules (3% to less than 20%) 2751
▲ CellCept Intravenous (3% to less than 20%) 2751
▲ CellCept Oral Suspension (3% to less than 20%) 2751
▲ CellCept Tablets (3% to less than 20%) 2751
Combunox Tablets (Less than 2%) 1183
Coreg Tablets (Greater than 0.1% to 1%) 1376
Cytovene (At least 3 subjects) 2763
DDAVP Tablets 2895
▲ Depacon Injection (6%) 412
▲ Depakene (6%) 417
▲ Depakote Sprinkle Capsules (6%) 422
▲ Depakote Tablets (1% to 6%) 427
▲ Depakote ER Tablets (6%) 433
Diastat Rectal Delivery System (Greater than or equal to 1%) 3344
Diprivan Injectable Emulsion (Less than 1%) 676
Doxil Injection (Less than 1%) 3302
Duragesic Transdermal System (1% or greater) 2448
Effexor Tablets (2%) 3405
Effexor XR Capsules (Frequent) 3411
Evoxac Capsules (Less than 1%) 1042
Flexeril Tablets (Less than 1%) 1832
Frova Tablets (Infrequent) 1101
▲ Gabitril Tablets (6%) 998
▲ Infergen (8% to 10%) 1647
▲ Intron A for Injection (Less than 5%) 3038
Kadian Capsules (Less than 3%) 572
Kaletra (Less than 2%) 474
Keppra Oral Solution (1% to 2%) 3307
Keppra Tablets (1% to 2%) 3307
▲ Lamictal (3%) 1449
Lunesta Tablets 3139
▲ Lyrica Capsules (1% to 9%) 2524
▲ Marinol Capsules (3% to 10%) 3334
Mebaral Tablets, USP (Less than 1 in 100 patients) 2483
▲ Megace ES Oral Suspension (1% to 3%) 2492
Meridia Capsules (Greater than or equal to 1%) 485
▲ Mirapex Tablets (2% to 3%) 889
Namenda (Infrequent) 1199
Nembutal Sodium Solution, USP (Less than 1%) 2484
Neurontin Capsules (1.7% to 2.7%) 2498
Neurontin Oral Solution (1.7% to 2.7%) 2498
Neurontin Tablets (1.7% to 2.7%) 2498
Nipent for Injection (Less than 3%) ... 3216
Norvir (0% to 0.9%) 499
▲ OxyContin Tablets (Between 1% and 5%) 2699
Paxil CR Controlled-Release Tablets (Infrequent) 1509
Paxil (Infrequent) 1501
Permax Tablets (Frequent) 3357
Prevacid Delayed-Release Capsules (Less than 1%) 3268
Prevacid for Delayed-Release Oral Suspension (Less than 1%) 3268
Prevacid NapraPAC (Less than 1%) .. 3277
Prevacid SoluTab Delayed-Release Orally Disintegrating Tablets (Less than 1%) 3268
PREVPAC (Less than 1%) 3281
ProAmatine Tablets (Less frequent) 3183
▲ Prograf Capsules and Injection (3% to 15%) 624
ProSom Tablets (2%) 512
Protonix I.V. (Less than 1%) 3468
Protonix Tablets (Less than 1%) 3465
Provigil Tablets (At least 1%) 1002
Prozac Pulvules and Liquid (2%) 1771
Relpax Tablets (Infrequent) 2531
ReoPro Vials (2.1%) 1779
Rilutek Tablets (Infrequent) 2945
▲ Risperdal Consta Long-Acting Injection (Up to 3%) 1664
Seroquel Tablets (Infrequent) 691
Sonata Capsules (Frequent) 1686
Sular Tablets (Less than or equal to 1%) 1163
▲ Symbyax Capsules (Greater than or equal to 5% to 6%) 1788
Symmetrel (0.1% to 1%) 1115
Tasmar Tablets (Infrequent) 3360
Tequin Injection (Less than 0.1%) 964
Tequin Tablets (Less than 0.1%) 964
Thalomid Capsules 979
Trileptal Oral Suspension (2%) 2281
Trileptal Tablets (2%) 2281
Ultracet Tablets (Less than 1%) 2462
Vicoprofen Tablets (Less than 3%) 533
Wellbutrin Tablets (Infrequent) 1579
Zoladex (1% or greater) 709
Zoladex 3-month 712
Zomig Nasal Spray (Infrequent) 718
Zyban Sustained-Release Tablets (1%) 1620
Zyprexa Tablets 1798
Zyprexa ZYDIS Orally Disintegrating Tablets 1798
Zyrtec Chewable Tablets (Less than 2%) 2589
Zyrtec (Less than 2%) 2589
Zyrtec-D 12 Hour Extended Release Tablets (Less than 2%) 2591

Thirst
(*see under* Dipsesis)

Thoracic disorders, unspecified
▲ Focalin XR (9% to 16%) 2217

Thrashing
Diprivan Injectable Emulsion (Less than 1%) 676

Throacic disorders, unspecified
▲ Ammonul Injection (15%) 3323

Throat, aching
InnoPran XL Capsules 2728
Zomig Nasal Spray (Infrequent) 718

Throat, burning
Astelin Nasal Spray (Infrequent) 1876
Diprivan Injectable Emulsion (Less than 1%) 676
Eldepryl Capsules 3209
Emcyt Capsules (1%) 3137
Rhinocort Aqua Nasal Spray (Rare) .. 658

Throat, congestion
Bentyl Capsules 724
Bentyl Injection 724
Bentyl Syrup 724
Bentyl Tablets 724

Throat, dryness of
Aerobid/Aerobid-M (1% to 3%) 1172
▲ Alacol DM Syrup (Among most frequent) 739
Asmanex Twisthaler (1% to less than 3%) 2981
Atrovent Nasal Spray 0.03% (Less than 2%) 869
Atrovent Nasal Spray 0.06% (1.4%) 870
Azmacort Inhalation Aerosol 1701
Beconase AQ Nasal Spray 1359
Catapres-TTS (2 of 101 patients) 875
Clozapine Tablets (Less than 1%) 2141
Clozaril Tablets (Less than 1%) 2174
FazaClo Orally Disintegrating Tablets (Less than 1%) 547
Flonase Nasal Spray 1412
Maxalt Tablets (Infrequent) 1983
Maxalt-MLT Orally Disintegrating Tablets (Infrequent) 1983
Neurontin Capsules (1.7%) 2498
Neurontin Oral Solution (1.7%) 2498
Neurontin Tablets (1.7%) 2498
Rythmol SR Capsules 2736
Sanctura Tablets (Greater than or equal to 0.5%) 1133
Vantin Tablets and Oral Suspension (Less than 1%) 2650
Xifaxan Tablets (Less than 2%) 2847
Xopenex HFA Inhalation Aerosol 3151
Xopenex Inhalation Solution 3143
Xopenex Inhalation Solution Concentrate 3147

Throat, presence of hard nodule
Lupron Depot 7.5 mg (Less than 5%) 3261
Lupron Injection Pediatric 3256

Throat, swelling of
Cutivate Lotion 0.05% (Rare) 1383
Fortical Nasal Spray 3336
Miacalcin Injection (A few cases) 2241
Miacalcin Nasal Spray (Few reports) 2242
Rhinocort Aqua Nasal Spray (Rare) .. 658

Throat, tightness
Abilify Tablets (Rare) 916
Abilify Tablets (Rare) 2472
Adenocard Injection (Less than 1%) 612
Alferon N Injection (1%) 1640
Campath Ampules 826
▲ Doxil Injection (Approximately 6.8%) 3302
Levaquin in 5% Dextrose Injection 2453
Levaquin 2453
Maxalt Tablets (Less than 2%) 1983
Maxalt-MLT Orally Disintegrating Tablets (Less than 2%) 1983
Neumega for Injection 3433
Paxil CR Controlled-Release Tablets (2%) 1509
Paxil (2%) 1501
Rythmol SR Capsules 2736
Zomig Nasal Spray (0% to 2%) 718

Throat irritation
▲ Advair Diskus 100/50 (4% to 8%) ... 1291
▲ Advair Diskus 250/50 (4% To 8%) ... 1291
▲ Advair Diskus 500/50 (4% to 8%) ... 1291
Aerobid/Aerobid-M (1% to 3%) 1172
Allegra (Greater than 1%) 2857
Allegra-D 12 Hour Extended-Release Tablets (2.3%) .. 2860
Allegra-D 24 Hour Extended-Release Tablets (2.3%) .. 2862
Alupent Inhalation Aerosol (1 to 4%) 858
Aredia for Injection (One patient) 2168
Azmacort Inhalation Aerosol 1701
Clozapine Tablets (1%) 2141
Clozaril Tablets (1%) 2174
Cosopt Sterile Ophthalmic Solution 1910
Dostinex Tablets (1%) 2631
▲ Epivir-HBV (13%) 1398
Flonase Nasal Spray 1412
▲ Flovent Diskus 50 mcg (10% to 13%) 1415
▲ Flovent HFA (8%) 1418
Nicotrol NS 2596
Norvir (1.7% to 2.8%) 499
Paxil CR Controlled-Release Tablets (2%) 1509
Paxil (2%) 1501
Rhinocort Aqua Nasal Spray (Rare) ... 658
▲ Rituxan for Infusion (6%) 845
▲ Rituxan I.V. (9%) 1251
▲ Roferon-A Injection (21%) 2805
Trusopt Sterile Ophthalmic Solution 2065
▲ Ventolin HFA Inhalation Aerosol (10%) 1576
▲ Zevalin Injection (10%) 848

Throat soreness
Aceon Tablets (2 mg, 4 mg, 8 mg) ... 3191
▲ Adenoscan (15%) 613
Advair Diskus 100/50 1291
Advair Diskus 250/50 1291
Advair Diskus 500/50 1291
▲ Aerobid/Aerobid-M (20%) 1172
Altace Capsules 1673
Aricept Tablets (Frequent) 1086
Aricept ODT Tablets (Frequent) 1086
Blocadren Tablets 1891
Captopril Tablets 2114
Carbatrol Capsules 3174
▲ Chemet Capsules (0.7% to 3.7%) 2480
▲ Clolar for Intravenous Infusion (14%) 1264
Clozapine Tablets 2141
Clozaril Tablets 2174
Cosopt Sterile Ophthalmic Solution 1910
Cubicin for Injection (1% to 2%) 1038
Dapsone Tablets USP 1656
DDAVP Nasal Spray 2894
DuoNeb Inhalation Solution 1058
▲ Elidel Cream 1% (3.4% to 8.1%) 2198
Flovent Diskus 50 mcg 1415
Flovent HFA 1418
▲ Flumist Vaccine (9.3% to 27.8%) 1872
▲ Gleevec Tablets (Up to 11%) 2221
Guanidine Hydrochloride Tablets 3030
▲ Imitrex Injection (3.3%) 1431
Inderal LA Long-Acting Capsules 3421
InnoPran XL Capsules 2728
Mavik Tablets (0.3% to 1.0%) 482
Maxair Autohaler 1820
Meruvax II 1994
Miradon Tablets 3056
M-M-R II 1980
▲ Myfortic Tablets (3% to less than 20%) 2244
Nadolol Tablets 2121
▲ Neupogen for Injection (4%) 598
Prinivil Tablets 2029

Prinzide Tablets 2033
Remicade for IV Injection 987
Rythmol SR Capsules 2736
▲ Strattera Capsules (2% or greater) 1784
Tegretol/Tegretol-XR 2278
Tenormin I.V. Injection 698
Tenormin Tablets 695
Ticlid Tablets 2813
Timoptic in Ocudose 2061
Timoptic Sterile Ophthalmic Solution 2058
Timoptic-XE Sterile Ophthalmic Gel Forming Solution 2062
Toprol-XL Tablets 660
▲ Trisenox Injection (40%) 983
Vaseretic Tablets 2073
Vasotec I.V. Injection (0.5% to 1.0%) 2076
▲ Xeloda Tablets (2% to 12%) 2825
Zemaira (0.9%) 3506
Zestoretic Tablets 701
Zestril Tablets 704
▲ Zometa for Intravenous Infusion (8%) 2306

Throbbing, localized

Catapres-TTS (1 of 101 patients) 875

Thrombocythemia

(*see under* Thrombocytosis)

Thrombocytopenia

▲ Abelcet Injection (5%) 1119
Abilify Tablets (Infrequent) 916
Abilify Tablets (Infrequent) 2472
Accutane Capsules 2740
Aceon Tablets (2 mg, 4 mg, 8 mg) 3191
Aciphex Tablets 1081
Actiq (1% or greater) 993
Adalat CC Tablets (Rare) 2978
Advicor Tablets 1694
Aggrastat 1878
Aggrenox Capsules 855
Agrylin Capsules (1% to 5%) 3172
Alacol DM Syrup 739
Albenza Tablets (Rare) 1310
Aldara Cream, 5% 1814
Aldoclor Tablets 1881
Aldoril Tablets 1884
Aldurazyme for Intravenous Infusion (2%) 1261
▲ Alimta for Injection (Up to 27%) 1722
Alkeran Tablets 977
Aloprim for Injection (Less than 1%) 2156
Altace Capsules (Less than 1%) 1673
Altoprev Extended-Release Tablets (Rare) 1151
Amaryl Tablets 2864
AmBisome for Injection (Less common) 615
Amerge Tablets (Rare) 1312
Ammonul Injection 3323
Amnesteem Capsules 2126
Amoxil Capsules 1315
Amoxil Chewable Tablets 1315
Amoxil Pediatric Drops for Oral Suspension 1315
Amoxil Powder for Oral Suspension 1315
Amoxil Tablets 1315
Anaprox Tablets (Less than 1%) 2769
Anaprox DS Tablets (Less than 1%) 2769
Ancef for Injection 1318
Angiomax for Injection (0.3% to 0.7%) 1856
Antara Capsules 2723
Anzemet Injection (Infrequently) 2871
Anzemet Tablets (Infrequently) 2874
Aptivus Capsules (Less than 2%) 859
Arava Tablets (Rare) 2881
▲ Aredia for Injection (14%) 2168
Aricept Tablets (Infrequent) 1086
Aricept ODT Tablets (Infrequent) 1086
Arixtra Injection (2.9%) 1325
Arthrotec Tablets (Rare) 3126
Asacol Delayed-Release Tablets 2688
Atacand Tablets 634
Atacand HCT 637
Attenuvax (Rare) 1889
Augmentin 1331
Augmentin Tablets 1334
Augmentin XR Extended-Release Tablets 1340
Augmentin ES-600 Powder for Oral Suspension 1337
Avalide Tablets 922
Avalide Tablets 2889
▲ Avastin IV (5%) 1229
Avelox (Less than 0.1%) 2984
Avinza Capsules (Less than 5%) 1714
Avonex (Rare) 839
Axid Oral Solution (One patient) 913
Azasan Tablets 2844
Baraclude (Less than 1%) 928
Bayer Aspirin Tablets 3515
Betaseron for SC Injection 791
Bexxar 1360
▲ Buphenyl Powder (3%) 3327
▲ Buphenyl Tablets (3%) 3327
Caduet Tablets (Greater than 0.1% to less than 2%) 2507
▲ Campath Ampules (50% to 72%) 826
Campral Tablets (Infrequent) 1175
▲ Camptosar Injection (1% to 96%) 2602
Canasa Rectal Suppositories (One patient) 726
▲ Cancidas for Injection (1.5% to 3.1%) 1894
Capastat Sulfate for Injection (Rare) 1728
Captopril Tablets 2114
Carbatrol Capsules 3174
Cardene I.V. (Rare) 1129
Cardizem LA Extended Release Tablets (Infrequent) 1699
Cataflam Tablets (Occasionally) 2173
Catapres Tablets (Rare) 874
Cathflo Activase 1232
Ceftin 1369
Celebrex Capsules (0.1% to 1.9%) 3130
Celexa 1177
▲ CellCept Capsules (23.5% to 38.3%) 2751
▲ CellCept Intravenous (23.5% to 38.3%) 2751
▲ CellCept Oral Suspension (23.5% to 38.3%) 2751
▲ CellCept Tablets (23.5% to 38.3%) 2751
▲ Cipro I.V. (Among most frequent) 2998
▲ Cipro I.V. Pharmacy Bulk Package (Among most frequent) 3509
Cipro (0.1%) 2991
Cleocin Vaginal Ovules 2613
Clindesse Vaginal Cream (Rare) 3296
Clinoril Tablets (Less than 1 in 100) 1899
Clolar for Intravenous Infusion 1264
Clorpres Tablets 2139
Clozapine Tablets 2141
Clozaril Tablets 2174
Combivir Tablets (0.4%) 1373
Comvax 1904
Concerta Extended-Release Tablets 1828
▲ Copegus Tablets (5% to 8%) 2759
▲ Coreg Tablets (1% to 3%) 1376
Cosmegen for Injection 1907
Cozaar Tablets 1913
Crestor Tablets (Less than 1%) 672
Crixivan Capsules (0.9%) 1918
Cubicin for Injection (Less than 1%) 1038
▲ Cuprimine Capsules (4%) 1925
Cutivate Lotion 0.05% (Rare) 1383
▲ Cytovene (5%) 2763
Dantrium Capsules (Less frequent) 2690
Daranide Tablets 1928
Daraprim Tablets 1385
Demser Capsules (Rare) 1933
▲ Depacon Injection (1% to 24%) 412
▲ Depakene (24%) 417
▲ Depakote Sprinkle Capsules (1% to 24%) 422
▲ Depakote Tablets (24%) 427
▲ Depakote ER Tablets (24%) 433
▲ DepoCyt Injection (5% to 8%) 1121
Digitek Tablets 2146
Diovan HCT Tablets 2195
Diuril Oral 1936
Diuril Sodium Intravenous 1934
Dolobid Tablets (Less than 1 in 100) 1937
▲ Doxil Injection (1.3% to 24.2%) 3302
Dyazide Capsules 1389
Dynacin Tablets 1859
Dyrenium Capsules (Rare) 3390
EC-Naprosyn Delayed-Release Tablets (Less than 1%) 2769
Ecotrin Enteric Coated Aspirin Low, Regular and Maximum Strength Tablets 1627
Edecrin (Rare) 1941
Effexor Tablets (Infrequent) 3405
Efudex 3348
▲ Ellence Injection (0% to 48.8%) 2632
Elmiron Capsules (Less than or equal to 1%) 2393
▲ Eloxatin for Injection (2% to 77%) 2908
Emcyt Capsules (1%) 3137
Emend Capsules (Greater than 0.5%) 1944
Enbrel for Injection 580
Engerix-B Vaccine 1391
Epivir (Up to 0.4%) 1394
▲ Epivir-HBV (4%) 1398
Epzicom Tablets 1402
Equetro Extended-Release Capsules 3178
Eulexin Capsules (1%) 3023
Evoxac Capsules (Less than 1%) 1042
Exelon Capsules (Infrequent) 2204
Factive Tablets (Less than or equal to 0.1% to 0.2%) 2464
FazaClo Orally Disintegrating Tablets 547
Flexeril Tablets (Rare) 1832
▲ Flolan for Injection (4%) 1408
Fortaz (Very rare) 1422
Fragmin Injection (Less than 1%) 2638
Furosemide Tablets 2117
Fuzeon Injection 2772
Gabitril Tablets (Infrequent) 998
▲ Gamunex Immune Globulin I.V., 10% (15%) 3232
Garamycin Injectable 3028
▲ Gemzar for Injection (15% to 47%) 1743
Gengraf Capsules (2% or less) 458
Geodon Capsules (Rare) 2514
▲ Gleevec Tablets (Up to 33%) 2221
Guanidine Hydrochloride Tablets 3030
▲ Hexalen Capsules (3% to 10%) 2101
Humira Injection (Infrequent) 464
▲ Hycamtin for Injection (26% to 63%) 1427
Hyperstat I.V. Injection 3031
Hytrin Capsules 469
Hyzaar 1964
▲ Imdur Tablets (Less than or equal to 5%) 3032
Imitrex Injection 1431
Imitrex Nasal Spray 1435
Imitrex Tablets 1440
Indapamide Tablets 2119
Indocin I.V. (1% to 3%) 1973
Infanrix Vaccine 1444
▲ Infergen (18% to 19%) 1647
Integrilin Injection 3034
▲ Intron A for Injection (Less than 5% to 15%) 3038
Invanz for Injection (1.1%) 1974
Invirase (Less than or equal to 2%) 2776
▲ I.V. Busulfex (100%) 1125
Kadian Capsules (Less than 3%) 572
Keppra Oral Solution 3307
Keppra Tablets 3307
Klonopin 2782
▲ Kytril Tablets (3%) 2788
Lamictal (Rare) 1449
Lamisil Tablets (Rare) 2226
Lariam Tablets (Occasional) 2790
Lescol Capsules (Rare) 2227
Lescol Capsules (Rare) 2730
Lescol XL Tablets 2227
Lescol XL Tablets 2730
▲ Leukine (19%) 829
▲ Leustatin Injection (12%) 2368
Levaquin in 5% Dextrose Injection (0.1% to 0.9%) 2453
Levaquin (0.1% to 0.9%) 2453
Lexapro Oral Solution 1193
Lexapro Tablets 1193
Lipitor Tablets (Less than 2%) 2495
Lofibra Capsules (Rare) 1217
Lortab 3315
Lortab Elixir 3312
Lotensin Tablets (Less than 1%) 2232
Lotensin HCT Tablets (Rare) 2235
Lotrel Capsules (Rare) 2238
Lovenox Injection (1.8% to 2.8%) 2931
Lyrica Capsules (0.1% to 1%) 2524
Matulane Capsules (Frequent) 3188
Mavik Tablets (0.3% to 1.0%) 482
Maxipime for Injection (Greater than 0.1% to less than 1%) 1093
Maxzide 2150
Mefoxin for Injection 1987
Mefoxin Premixed Intravenous Solution 1990
Mepron Suspension 1487
Meridia Capsules 485
Merrem I.V. (Greater than 0.2%) 687
Meruvax II 1994
Mevacor Tablets (Rare) 1996
Micardis HCT Tablets 886
Miradon Tablets 3056
M-M-R II 1980
Mobic Oral Suspension (Less than 2%) 893
Mobic Tablets (Less than 2%) 893
Moduretic Tablets 2003
Mumpsvax 2005
Mustargen for Injection 2007
Mycamine for Injection (0.8% to 1.2%) 620
▲ Myfortic Tablets (3% to less than 20%) 2244
Myleran Tablets 1492
▲ Mylotarg for Injection (49% to 52%) 3429
Nalfon Capsules (Less than 1%) 2504
Namenda (More than one patient) 1199
Naprosyn Suspension (Less than 1%) 2769
Naprosyn Tablets (Less than 1%) 2769
▲ Navelbine Injection (1% to 29%) 1494
Neoral Soft Gelatin Capsules (2% or less) 2247
Neoral Oral Solution (2% or less) 2247
▲ Neupogen for Injection (Fewer than 6% to 12%) 598
Neurontin Capsules (Infrequent) 2498
Neurontin Oral Solution (Infrequent) 2498
Neurontin Tablets (Infrequent) 2498
Nexium Delayed-Release Capsules (Less than 1%) 645
Nexium I.V. (Less than 1%) 649
Niaspan Extended-Release Tablets 1703
Nimotop Capsules (0.3%; rare) 774
▲ Nipent for Injection (6% to 32%) 3216
Noroxin Tablets (1.0%) 2009
Norvasc Tablets (More than 0.1% to 1%) 2529
Norvir (Less than 2%) 499
Omnicef Capsules 506
Omnicef for Oral Suspension 506
▲ Oncaspar (Greater than 1% but less than 5%) 1123
▲ Ontak Vials (8%) 1717
Orthoclone OKT3 Sterile Solution 2370
Pacerone Tablets 3337
Panhematin for Injection 2487
Parcopa Orally Disintegrating Tablets 3111
Parnate Tablets 1499
Paser Granules 1657
Paxil CR Controlled-Release Tablets 1509
Paxil 1501
Pediarix Vaccine 1518
Liquid PedvaxHIB (One child) 2012
▲ Pegasys (5% to 52%) 2793
▲ PEG-Intron Powder for Injection (7%) 3062
Pentasa Capsules (Less than 1%) 3182
Pepcid Injection (Rare) 2017
Pepcid (Rare) 2014
Permax Tablets (Infrequent) 3357
Persantine Tablets (Rare) 898
Phenergan 3438
Phenytek Capsules (Occasional) 2153
Plavix Tablets (1% to 2.5%) 940
Plavix Tablets (1% to 2.5%) 2942
Pletal Tablets (Very rare) 2478
Pneumovax 23 2020
Prandin Tablets (0.5, 1, and 2 mg) (Less than 1%) 2337
Pravachol Tablets (Rare) 943
Prevacid Delayed-Release Capsules (Less than 1%) 3268
Prevacid for Delayed-Release Oral Suspension (Less than 1%) 3268
Prevacid NapraPAC (Less than 1%) 3277
Prevacid SoluTab Delayed-Release Orally Disintegrating Tablets (Less than 1%) 3268
PREVPAC 3281
Prilosec OTC Tablets (Rare) 2674
Primaxin I.M. 2022
Primaxin I.V. (Less than 0.2%) 2024
Prinivil Tablets (Rare) 2029
Prinzide Tablets (Rare) 2033
▲ Prograf Capsules and Injection (3% to 24%) 624
▲ Proleukin for Injection (37%) 1007
Protonix I.V. (Less than 1%) 3468
Protonix Tablets (Less than 1%) 3465
Prozac Pulvules and Liquid (Rare) 1771
Purinethol Tablets (Frequent) 1222
▲ Rapamune Oral Solution and Tablets (13% to 30%) 3472
Raptiva for Injection (0.3%) 1247
Razadyne ER Extended-Release Capsules (Infrequent) 2434
Razadyne (Infrequent) 2434
Rebetol (2%) 3073
▲ Rebif Prefilled Syringe for Injection (2% to 8%) 3163
Recombivax HB 2045
Relafen Tablets (Less than 1%) 1523
Remicade for IV Injection (Greater than or equal to 0.2%) 987
ReoPro Vials (0.7% to 5.2%) 1779
Requip Tablets (Infrequent) 1528
Rescriptor Tablets 2535
▲ Retrovir Capsules (12%) 1533
▲ Retrovir IV Infusion (12%) 1537

▲ Retrovir (12%) 1533
R-Gene 10 for Intravenous Use (One patient) 2647
▲ Ribavirin, USP Capsules (2% to 5%) 3083
Risperdal Consta Long-Acting Injection (Rare) 1664
Risperdal M-Tab Orally Disintegrating Tablets (Rare) 1658
Risperdal (Rare) 1658
▲ Rituxan for Infusion (1.3% to 8%) 845
▲ Rituxan I.V. (12%) 1251
Rocephin Injectable Vials, ADD-Vantage, Galaxy, Bulk (Less than 1%) 2801
▲ Roferon-A Injection (4.5% to 62%) 2805
Rythmol SR Capsules 2736
Sandimmune (2% or less; occasional) 2259
Sandostatin LAR Depot (Rare) 2264
Sedapap Tablets 50 mg/650 mg 2098
Seroquel Tablets (Rare) 691
▲ Simulect for Injection (3% to 10%) 2268
St. Joseph 81 mg Aspirin Chewable and Enteric Coated Tablets 1841
Stalevo Tablets 2270
Suprax (Less than 2%) 1811
Surmontil Capsules 2347
Tabloid Tablets 1545
Tagamet Tablets (Approximately 3 per 1,000,000) 1547
Tambocor Tablets (Less than 1%) 1824
Targretin Capsules 1719
Tarka Tablets 519
Tasmar Tablets (Rare) 3360
▲ Taxotere Injection Concentrate (2.8% to 24.6%) 2947
Tegretol/Tegretol-XR 2278
▲ Temodar Capsules (5% to 58%) 3088
Tenormin I.V. Injection 698
Tenormin Tablets 695
Tequin Injection 964
Tequin Tablets 964
Teveten Tablets (0.3%) 1707
Teveten HCT Tablets 1710
Thalomid Capsules 979
Thioridazine Hydrochloride Tablets 2122
Thiothixene Capsules 2124
▲ Thymoglobulin for Injection (36.6%) 2848
Tiazac Capsules (Infrequent) 1204
Ticlid Tablets (Rare) 2813
Timentin ADD-Vantage 1556
Timentin Injection Galaxy Container 1559
Timentin IV Infusion 1553
Timentin Pharmacy Bulk Package 1562
Timolide Tablets 2056
Tindamax (Rare) 2670
Topamax Sprinkle Capsules (Infrequent to 1%) 2438
Topamax Tablets (Infrequent to 1%) 2438
Toprol-XL Tablets 660
Trasylol Injection (2%) 779
Trecator Tablets (Rare) 3482
Tricor Tablets (Rare) 523
Triglide Tablets 1165
Trileptal Oral Suspension 2281
Trileptal Tablets 2281
▲ Trisenox Injection (13%) 983
Trizivir Tablets (0.4%) 1565
Twinrix Vaccine 1571
Tygacil for Injection (0% to less than 2%) 3489
Ultane Liquid for Inhalation (Less than 1%) 526
Uniretic Tablets 3114
Urso 250 Tablets 737
Urso Forte Tablets 737
▲ Valcyte Tablets (6%) 2816
▲ Valtrex Caplets (0.1% to 3%) 1573
Vancocin HCl Capsules, USP (Rare) 3370
Vantin Tablets and Oral Suspension 2650
Vaqta (Very rare) 2067
Varivax 2070
Vaseretic Tablets (Rare) 2073
Vasotec I.V. Injection (Rare) 2076
▲ Velcade for Injection (35%-43%) 2102
VFEND I.V. (Less than 2%) 2543
VFEND Oral Suspension (Less than 2%) 2543
VFEND Tablets (Less than 2%) 2543
Vicodin Tablets 530
Vicodin ES Tablets 531
Vicodin HP Tablets 532
Viracept (Less than 2%) 2556
Viramune Oral Suspension (0.8%) 903
Viramune Tablets (0.8%) 903
Vivactil Tablets 2350
Voltaren Tablets (Occasionally) 2298
Voltaren-XR Tablets (Occasionally) 2301
Vytorin 10/10 Tablets 2084
Vytorin 10/10 Tablets 3092
Vytorin 10/20 Tablets 2084
Vytorin 10/20 Tablets 3092
Vytorin 10/40 Tablets 2084
Vytorin 10/40 Tablets 3092
Vytorin 10/80 Tablets 2084
Vytorin 10/80 Tablets 3092
Wellbutrin Tablets 1579
Wellbutrin SR Sustained-Release Tablets 1583
Wellbutrin XL Extended-Release Tablets 1588
▲ Xeloda Tablets (1% to 41%) 2825
Zantac (A few patients) 1597
Zantac Injection (Few patients) 1593
Zantac Injection Pharmacy Bulk Package (Infrequent) 1595
Zantac Syrup (A few patients) 1597
▲ Zavesca Capsules (7%) 543
Zegerid Powder for Oral Solution (0.1%) 2972
▲ Zerit (3%) 971
Zestoretic Tablets (Rare) 701
Zestril Tablets (Rare) 704
Zetia Tablets 2090
Zetia Tablets 3098
▲ Zevalin Injection (95%) 848
Ziagen (1%) 1600
Zinacef Injection (Rare) 1604
Zinacef for Injection (Rare) 1604
Zinecard for Injection 2659
Zithromax Capsules, 250 mg (Less than 1%) 2568
Zithromax for IV Infusion (Less than 1%) 2573
Zithromax for Oral Suspension, 1 g (Less than 1%) 2568
Zithromax for Oral Suspension, 300 mg, 600 mg, 900 mg, 1200 mg (Less than 1%) 2561
Zithromax Tablets, 250 mg, 500 mg (Less than 1%) 2561
Zithromax Tablets, 600 mg (Less than 1%) 2568
Zithromax Tri-Pak (Less than 1%) 2561
Zithromax Z-Pak (Less than 1%) 2568
Zocor Tablets (Rare) 2078
Zoloft 2581
▲ Zometa for Intravenous Infusion (5% to 10%) 2306
Zomig Tablets (Rare) 714
Zomig-ZMT Tablets (Rare) 714
Zonegran Capsules (Rare) 1089
Zosyn 3492
Zovirax Capsules 1616
Zovirax for Injection (Less than 1%) 1618
Zovirax 1616
Zyban Sustained-Release Tablets 1620
Zyrtec Chewable Tablets (Rare) 2589
Zyrtec (Rare) 2589
Zyrtec-D 12 Hour Extended Release Tablets (Rare) 2591
▲ Zyvox (0% to 4.7%) 2661

Thrombocytopenia, immune

PEG-Intron Powder for Injection (Less than or equal to 1%) 3062
Ticlid Tablets (Rare) 2813

Thrombocytopenia, immuno-allergic

Eloxatin for Injection 2908

Thrombocytopenia, neonatal

Dyazide Capsules (Rare) 1389
Prinzide Tablets 2033
Zestoretic Tablets 701

Thrombocytopenia, autoimmune idiopathic

Avonex 839
Campath Ampules 826

Thrombocytopenic purpura

(*see under* Purpura, thrombocytopenic)

Thrombocytosis

Abilify Tablets (Rare) 916
Abilify Tablets (Rare) 2472
Accutane Capsules 2740
Aggrenox Capsules 855
Ancef for Injection 1318
Aricept Tablets (Infrequent) 1086
Aricept ODT Tablets (Infrequent) 1086
Arthrotec Tablets (Rare) 3126
Augmentin (Less than 1%) 1331
Augmentin Tablets (Less than 1%) 1334
▲ Augmentin XR Extended-Release Tablets (3.6%) 1340
Avelox (0.1% to less than 2%) 2984
Buphenyl Powder (1%) 3327
Buphenyl Tablets (1%) 3327
Campath Ampules 826
Celebrex Capsules (0.1% to 1.9%) 3130
Chemet Capsules (0.5% to 1.5%) 2480
▲ Cipro I.V. (Among most frequent) 2998
▲ Cipro I.V. Pharmacy Bulk Package (Among most frequent) 3509
Cipro (0.1%) 2991
Clozapine Tablets 2141
Clozaril Tablets 2174
Colazal Capsules 2845
Cubicin for Injection (Less than 1%) 1038
Cuprimine Capsules 1925
Demser Capsules (Rare) 1933
Effexor Tablets (Infrequent) 3405
Estratest Tablets 3196
Estratest H.S. Tablets 3196
Evoxac Capsules (Less than 1%) 1042
Factive Tablets (0.1% to 1%) 2464
FazaClo Orally Disintegrating Tablets 547
Fortaz (1 in 45) 1422
Geodon Capsules (Rare) 2514
▲ Invanz for Injection (4.3% to 6.5%) 1974
Ketek Tablets (Greater than or equal to 0.2% to less than 2%) 2920
Lovenox Injection 2931
Lyrica Capsules (Rare) 2524
Merrem I.V. (Greater than 0.2%) 687
Neumega for Injection 3433
Omnicef Capsules (0.2%) 506
Omnicef for Oral Suspension (1%) 506
Paxil CR Controlled-Release Tablets (Rare) 1509
Paxil (Rare) 1501
Pentasa Capsules (Less than 1%) 3182
Permax Tablets (Rare) 3357
Premarin Tablets 3443
Prevacid Delayed-Release Capsules 3268
Prevacid for Delayed-Release Oral Suspension 3268
Prevacid NapraPAC 3277
Prevacid SoluTab Delayed-Release Orally Disintegrating Tablets 3268
PREVPAC 3281
Primaxin I.M. 2022
Primaxin I.V. 2024
Prozac Pulvules and Liquid (Rare) 1771
▲ Rocephin Injectable Vials, ADD-Vantage, Galaxy, Bulk (5.1%) 2801
Spectracef Tablets (0.1% to 1%) 2706
Symbyax Capsules (Rare) 1788
Targretin Capsules 1719
Ticlid Tablets 2813
Topamax Sprinkle Capsules (Infrequent) 2438
Topamax Tablets (Infrequent) 2438
▲ Tygacil for Injection (6.1%) 3489
Vantin Tablets and Oral Suspension 2650
Vesanoid Capsules 2823
Zosyn (1% or less) 3492
Zovirax for Injection (Less than 1%) 1618
Zyprexa Tablets (Rare) 1798
Zyprexa ZYDIS Orally Disintegrating Tablets (Infrequent) 1798
Zyvox (0% to 2.8%) 2661

Thromboembolic complications

Activella Tablets 2311
▲ Arimidex Tablets (2% to 4%) 665
▲ Camptosar Injection (5.4%) 2602
Cenestin Tablets, 0.45mg, 0.625mg, 0.9mg, 1.25mg 1063
Cenestin Tablets, 0.3mg 1063
Estratest Tablets 3196
Estratest H.S. Tablets 3196
Faslodex Injection (Less than 1%) 682
Femara Tablets (Less than or equal to 2%) 2210
Follistim AQ Cartridge 2354
Ortho-Cyclen/Ortho Tri-Cyclen 2414
Ortho Tri-Cyclen Lo Tablets 2421
Premarin Intravenous 3440
Premarin Vaginal Cream 3449
Premphase Tablets 3452
Prempro Tablets 3452
Ticlid Tablets 2813
Triphasil-28 Tablets 3483

Thromboembolic disease

(*see under* Thromboembolic complications)

Thromboembolism

Activase I.V. 1225
▲ Aranesp for Injection (5.6%) 576
Camptosar Injection 2602
Carimune NF 3501
CombiPatch Transdermal System 2180
Decadron Phosphate Injection 1931
Decadron Tablets 1929
▲ Eloxatin for Injection (2% to 9%) 2908
Equetro Extended-Release Capsules 3178
Estratest Tablets 3196
Estratest H.S. Tablets 3196
Gammagard Liquid 751
Gammagard S/D 754
Gamunex Immune Globulin I.V., 10% 3232
Hydrocortone Tablets 1963
Iveegam EN 759
Lo/Ovral-28 Tablets 3423
Ortho-Cyclen/Ortho Tri-Cyclen 2414
Ortho Tri-Cyclen Lo Tablets 2421
Premarin Vaginal Cream 3449
Soriatane Capsules 1028
Tegretol-XR Tablets 2278
Triphasil-28 Tablets 3483

Thromboembolism, arterial

Alesse-28 Tablets 3392
Ortho-Cept Tablets 2395
Ortho-Cyclen Tablets 2414
Ortho Evra Transdermal System 2402
Ortho Tri-Cyclen Tablets 2414
Ortho Tri-Cyclen Lo Tablets 2421
Repronex for Intramuscular and Subcutaneous Injection 1148
Seasonale Tablets 1073
Yasmin 28 Tablets 818

Thromboembolism, venous

Cenestin Tablets, 0.45mg, 0.625mg, 0.9mg, 1.25mg 1063
Cenestin Tablets, 0.3mg 1063
Premarin Intravenous 3440
Premphase Tablets 3452
▲ Rapamune Oral Solution and Tablets (3% to less than 20%) 3472
Vivelle-Dot Transdermal System 2293

Thrombopenia

(*see under* Thrombocytopenia)

Thrombophlebitis

Abelcet Injection 1119
Abilify Tablets (Rare) 916
Abilify Tablets (Rare) 2472
Aciphex Tablets (Rare) 1081
Actiq (Less than 1%) 993
Activella Tablets 2311
Alesse-28 Tablets 3392
Aloprim for Injection (Less than 1%) 2156
Anzemet Injection (Rare) 2871
Anzemet Tablets (Rare) 2874
▲ Aranesp for Injection (5.6%) 576
▲ Arimidex Tablets (2% to 5%) 665
Brevibloc Concentrate (Less than 1%) 766
Brevibloc Injection (Less than 1%) 766
Brevibloc Double Strength Injection (Less than 1%) 766
Brevibloc Premixed Injection (Less than 1%) 766
Brevibloc Double Strength Premixed Injection (Less than 1%) 766
Campath Ampules 826
Campral Tablets (Rare) 1175
Camptosar Injection (1.3% to 5.3%) 2602
▲ Cancidas for Injection (3.5% to 15.7%) 1894
Carbatrol Capsules 3174
Celebrex Capsules (Less than 0.1%) 3130
Cenestin Tablets, 0.45mg, 0.625mg, 0.9mg, 1.25mg 1063
Cenestin Tablets, 0.3mg 1063
Cipro I.V. (1% or less) 2998
Cipro I.V. Pharmacy Bulk Package (1% or less) 3509
Climara Transdermal System 795
Climara Pro Transdermal System 800
Clozapine Tablets (Less than 1%) 2141
Clozaril Tablets (Less than 1%) 2174
CombiPatch Transdermal System 2180
Combunox Tablets (Less than 2%) 1183
Cuprimine Capsules (Rare) 1925
Dantrium Intravenous 2691

Decadron Tablets 1929
Depo-Provera Contraceptive Injection (Less than 1%) 2619
depo-subQ provera 104 Injectable Suspension 2622
▲ Doxil Injection (1% to 10%) 3302
Effexor Tablets (Infrequent) 3405
Effexor XR Capsules (Infrequent) 3411
Elitek (Less than or equal to 1%) 2906
▲ Emcyt Capsules (3%) 3137
Enbrel for Injection (Infrequent) 580
Epogen for Injection (Rare) 586
Equetro Extended-Release Capsules 3178
Estratest Tablets 3196
Estratest H.S. Tablets 3196
Estrogel 0.06% 3200
FazaClo Orally Disintegrating Tablets (Less than 1%) 547
Femara Tablets (Less than or equal to 2%) 2210
Fluorescite Injection .... ⊙ 207
Fortical Nasal Spray (Less than 1%) 3336
Furosemide Tablets 2117
Gabitril Tablets (Infrequent) 998
Geodon Capsules (Rare) 2514
Imitrex Nasal Spray 1435
Imitrex Tablets 1440
Indocin Capsules (Rare) 1968
Indocin I.V. (Less than 1%) 1973
Indocin (Rare) 1968
Invanz for Injection (1.6% to 1.9%) 1974
Invirase (Rare; up to 1%) 2776
Kaletra (Less than 2%) 474
Klonopin (Infrequent) 2782
Lo/Ovral-28 Tablets 3423
Lunesta Tablets (Rare) 3139
Mefoxin for Injection 1987
Mefoxin Premixed Intravenous Solution 1990
Megace ES Oral Suspension 2492
Menostar Transdermal System 805
Merrem I.V. (0.8%) 687
Miacalcin Nasal Spray (Less than 1%) 2242
Mustargen for Injection 2007
Namenda (Infrequent) 1199
Neurontin Capsules (Rare) 2498
Neurontin Oral Solution (Rare) 2498
Neurontin Tablets (Rare) 2498
Ortho-Cept Tablets 2395
Ortho-Cyclen Tablets 2414
Ortho Evra Transdermal System 2402
Ortho Tri-Cyclen Tablets 2414
Ortho Tri-Cyclen Lo Tablets 2421
Paxil CR Controlled-Release Tablets (Rare) 1509
Paxil (Rare) 1501
Permax Tablets (Infrequent) 3357
Prefest Tablets 1069
Premarin Intravenous 3440
Premarin Tablets 3443
Premarin Vaginal Cream 3449
Premphase Tablets 3452
Prempro Tablets 3452
▲ Primaxin I.V. (3.1%) 2024
Procrit for Injection (Rare) 2374
Protonix I.V. (Less than 1%) 3468
Protonix Tablets (Less than 1%) 3465
Prozac Pulvules and Liquid (Rare) 1771
▲ Rapamune Oral Solution and Tablets (3% to 20%) 3472
ReFacto Vials 3479
Relafen Tablets (Less than 1%) 1523
Relpax Tablets (Rare) 2531
Remicade for IV Injection (Greater than or equal to 0.2%) 987
ReoPro Vials (0.1%) 1779
Risperdal Consta Long-Acting Injection (Rare) 1664
Risperdal M-Tab Orally Disintegrating Tablets (Rare) 1658
Risperdal (Rare) 1658
▲ Roferon-A Injection (Less than 5%) 2805
Sandostatin Injection (Less than 1%) 2263
Seasonale Tablets 1073
Seroquel Tablets (Infrequent) 691
Sonata Capsules (Rare) 1686
Sustiva Capsules (Less than 2%) 957
Synercid I.V. (2.4%) 1690
Taxotere Injection Concentrate 2947
Tegretol/Tegretol-XR 2278
Thalomid Capsules 979
Timentin ADD-Vantage 1556
Timentin Injection Galaxy Container 1559
Timentin IV Infusion 1553
Timentin Pharmacy Bulk Package 1562
Trasylol Injection (1% to 2%) 779
Triphasil-28 Tablets 3483
Tygacil for Injection (0% to less than 2%) 3489
VFEND I.V. (Less than 2%) 2543
VFEND Oral Suspension (Less than 2%) 2543
VFEND Tablets (Less than 2%) 2543
Vivelle Transdermal System 2288
Vivelle-Dot Transdermal System 2293
Yasmin 28 Tablets 818
Zinacef Injection (1 in 60 patients) 1604
Zinacef for Injection (1 in 60 patients) 1604
Zomig Nasal Spray (Infrequent) 718
Zomig Tablets (Rare) 714
Zomig-ZMT Tablets (Rare) 714
Zonegran Capsules (Infrequent) 1089
Zosyn (0.2% to 1.3%) 3492

Thrombophlebitis, deep-vein

▲ Avastin IV (6% to 34%) 1229
Cardene I.V. (Rare) 1129
Effexor Tablets 3405
Effexor XR Capsules 3411
Estratest Tablets 3196
Estratest H.S. Tablets 3196
Evoxac Capsules (Less than 1%) 1042
Exelon Capsules (Infrequent) 2204
Lamictal (Rare) 1449
Lyrica Capsules (0.1% to 1%) 2524
Nipent for Injection (Less than 3%) 3216
▲ Prograf Capsules and Injection (3% to 15%) 624
Requip Tablets (Rare) 1528
VFEND I.V. (Less than 2%) 2543
VFEND Oral Suspension (Less than 2%) 2543
VFEND Tablets (Less than 2%) 2543

Thrombophlebitis, leg

Requip Tablets (Rare) 1528

Thromboplastin decrease

Avelox (Less than 0.1%) 2984

Thromboplastin time, increase

▲ CellCept Capsules (3% to less than 20%) 2751
▲ CellCept Intravenous (3% to less than 20%) 2751
▲ CellCept Oral Suspension (3% to less than 20%) 2751
▲ CellCept Tablets (3% to less than 20%) 2751
Elmiron Capsules (Less than or equal to 1%) 2393
Merrem I.V. (Greater than 0.2%) 687
Oncaspar (Greater than 1% but less than 5%) 1123
Panhematin for Injection 2487
Testim 1% Gel (Less than 1%) 722
Viramune Oral Suspension 903
Viramune Tablets 903
Zosyn 3492

Thrombosis

▲ Alimta for Injection (1% to 7%) 1722
Ambien Tablets (Rare) 2867
Ammonul Injection 3323
▲ Aranesp for Injection (5.6%) 576
▲ Avastin IV (15.1%) 1229
BeneFix for Injection 3402
Camptosar Injection 2602
Celexa 1177
▲ CellCept Capsules (3% to less than 20%) 2751
▲ CellCept Intravenous (4%) 2751
▲ CellCept Oral Suspension (3% to less than 20%) 2751
▲ CellCept Tablets (3% to less than 20%) 2751
Colazal Capsules 2845
Diprivan Injectable Emulsion (Rare) 676
Doxil Injection (Less than 1%) 3302
Elitek (Less than or equal to 1%) 2906
Emcyt Capsules 3137
Estratest Tablets 3196
Estratest H.S. Tablets 3196
Exelon Capsules (Infrequent) 2204
▲ Ferrlecit Injection (6%) 3379
Gamunex Immune Globulin I.V., 10% 3232
Herceptin I.V. (At least one of the 958 patients) 1234
Imitrex Nasal Spray 1435
Imitrex Tablets (Rare) 1440
▲ I.V. Busulfex (33%) 1125
Leukine 829
Leustatin Injection (2%) 2368
Lexapro Oral Solution 1193
Lexapro Tablets 1193
Lovenox Injection (Rare) 2931
Mustargen for Injection 2007
▲ Navelbine Injection (Up to 10%) 1494
NovoSeven (Two patients) 2335
Oncaspar (Greater than 1% but less than 5%) 1123
Paxil CR Controlled-Release Tablets (Rare) 1509
Paxil (Rare) 1501
Premarin Intravenous 3440
Premarin Vaginal Cream 3449
Proleukin for Injection (1%) 1007
Protonix I.V. (Less than 1%) 3468
Protonix Tablets (Less than 1%) 3465
Prozac Pulvules and Liquid (Rare) 1771
▲ Rapamune Oral Solution and Tablets (3% to 20%) 3472
Renagel Tablets 1268
Requip Tablets (Rare) 1528
Rilutek Tablets (Rare) 2945
Rythmol SR Capsules 2736
▲ Simulect for Injection (3% to 10%) 2268
Tasmar Tablets (Rare) 3360
Thalomid Capsules 979
Thrombin-JMI 1693
TNKase I.V. 1256
Trasylol Injection (1% to 2%) 779
▲ Zenapax for Injection (Greater than 5%) 2838

Thrombosis, arterial

Argatroban Injection (1.8%) 1321
Orthoclone OKT3 Sterile Solution 2370
Sandostatin LAR Depot (Rare) 2264
Trasylol Injection (1% to 2%) 779

Thrombosis, cerebral

(*see under* Cerebral thrombosis)

Thrombosis, coronary

(*see under* Coronary thrombosis)

Thrombosis, deep-vein

Aygestin Tablets 1062
Cenestin Tablets, 0.45mg, 0.625mg, 0.9mg, 1.25mg 1063
Cenestin Tablets, 0.3mg 1063
Climara Transdermal System 795
Climara Pro Transdermal System 800
Depo-Provera Contraceptive Injection (Less than 1%) 2619
depo-subQ provera 104 Injectable Suspension 2622
Emend Capsules (Greater than 0.5%) 1944
Estrogel 0.06% 3200
FazaClo Orally Disintegrating Tablets 547
Menostar Transdermal System 805
Mycamine for Injection 620
Prefest Tablets 1069
Premarin Intravenous 3440
Premarin Tablets 3443
Premarin Vaginal Cream 3449
Premphase Tablets 3452
Prempro Tablets 3452
Rythmol SR Capsules 2736
Topamax Sprinkle Capsules (Infrequent) 2438
Topamax Tablets (Infrequent) 2438
Vivelle Transdermal System 2288
Vivelle-Dot Transdermal System 2293

Thrombosis, glomerular capillary

Gengraf Capsules 458
Neoral Soft Gelatin Capsules 2247
Neoral Oral Solution 2247
Sandimmune 2259

Thrombosis, intraabdominal

▲ Avastin IV (3% to 10%) 1229

Thrombosis, leg

▲ Humira Injection (Less than 5%) 464

Thrombosis, mesenteric

Alesse-28 Tablets 3392
Estratest Tablets 3196
Estratest H.S. Tablets 3196
Lo/Ovral-28 Tablets 3423
Ortho-Cept Tablets 2395
Ortho Evra Transdermal System 2402
Premarin Intravenous 3440
Premarin Vaginal Cream 3449
Seasonale Tablets 1073
Triphasil-28 Tablets 3483
Yasmin 28 Tablets 818

Thrombosis, mesenteric venous

Avastin IV (Rare) 1229

Thrombosis, mesenteric arterial

Campral Tablets (Rare) 1175
Cosopt Sterile Ophthalmic Solution 1910
Nadolol Tablets 2121
Timoptic-XE Sterile Ophthalmic Gel Forming Solution 2062

Thrombosis, portal vein

Femara Tablets (Less than or equal to 2%) 2210

Thrombosis, pulmonary

Estratest Tablets 3196
Estratest H.S. Tablets 3196
Neurontin Capsules (Rare) 2498
Neurontin Oral Solution (Rare) 2498
Neurontin Tablets (Rare) 2498
Trasylol Injection (1% to 2%) 779

Thrombosis, renal artery

Epogen for Injection (Rare) 586
Procrit for Injection (Rare) 2374

Thrombosis, retinal artery

Roferon-A Injection 2805

Thrombosis, retinal vascular

Activella Tablets 2311
Alesse-28 Tablets 3392
Aygestin Tablets 1062
Cenestin Tablets, 0.45mg, 0.625mg, 0.9mg, 1.25mg 1063
Cenestin Tablets, 0.3mg 1063
CombiPatch Transdermal System 2180
Epogen for Injection (Rare) 586
Estratest Tablets 3196
Estratest H.S. Tablets 3196
Estrogel 0.06% 3200
Imitrex Tablets 1440
Intron A for Injection 3038
Lo/Ovral-28 Tablets 3423
Neurontin Capsules (Rare) 2498
Neurontin Oral Solution (Rare) 2498
Neurontin Tablets (Rare) 2498
Ortho-Cept Tablets 2395
Ortho-Cyclen Tablets 2414
Ortho Evra Transdermal System 2402
Ortho Tri-Cyclen Tablets 2414
Ortho Tri-Cyclen Lo Tablets 2421
Pegasys 2793
PEG-Intron Powder for Injection (Less than or equal to 1%) 3062
Prefest Tablets 1069
Premarin Intravenous 3440
Premarin Tablets 3443
Premarin Vaginal Cream 3449
Premphase Tablets 3452
Prempro Tablets 3452
Procrit for Injection (Rare) 2374
Sandostatin LAR Depot (Rare) 2264
Seasonale Tablets 1073
Triphasil-28 Tablets 3483
Vivelle Transdermal System 2288
Vivelle-Dot Transdermal System 2293
Yasmin 28 Tablets 818

Thrombosis, sagittal sinus

Oncaspar 1123

Thrombosis, venous

Abilify Tablets (Infrequent) 916
Abilify Tablets (Infrequent) 2472
Actimmune (Rare) 1646
Activase I.V. 1225
▲ Aranesp for Injection (5.6%) 576
Aricept Tablets (Infrequent) 1086
Aricept ODT Tablets (Infrequent) 1086
Aygestin Tablets 1062
Betaseron for SC Injection 791
Campath Ampules 826
Cathflo Activase 1232
Climara Transdermal System 795
Climara Pro Transdermal System 800
Clozapine Tablets 2141
Clozaril Tablets 2174
CombiPatch Transdermal System 2180
Enbrel for Injection (Infrequent) 580
Epogen for Injection (Rare) 586
Estrogel 0.06% 3200
Femara Tablets (Less than or equal to 2%) 2210
Kaletra (Less than 2%) 474
Lo/Ovral-28 Tablets 3423
Menostar Transdermal System 805
Naropin Injection (Less than 1%) 640
Navelbine Injection 1494
Nimotop Capsules (Less than 1%) 774
Oncaspar 1123
Ortho-Cept Tablets 2395
Ortho-Cyclen Tablets 2414
Ortho Evra Transdermal System 2402
Ortho Tri-Cyclen Tablets 2414
Ortho Tri-Cyclen Lo Tablets 2421
Orthoclone OKT3 Sterile Solution 2370
Prefest Tablets 1069
Premarin Tablets 3443
Premarin Vaginal Cream 3449

Premphase Tablets 3452
Prempro Tablets 3452
▲ Procrit for Injection (Up to 10%) 2374
Retavase 1131
Taxotere Injection Concentrate 2947
▲ Xeloda Tablets (Less than 1% to 8%) 2825
Yasmin 28 Tablets 818

Thrombosis at injection site
Mycamine for Injection 620

Thrombosis of vascular access
▲ Aranesp for Injection (5.6% to 8%) 576
Epogen for Injection (0.25%) 586
Furosemide Tablets 2117
Procrit for Injection 2374

Thrombotic events, unspecified
Apokyn Injection 2132
Aygestin Tablets 1062
DDAVP Injection 4 mcg/mL (Rare) 2893
Desmopressin Acetate Injection (Rare) 1143
Dolobid Tablets 1937
Gammagard S/D 754
Lo/Ovral-28 Tablets 3423
Mobic Oral Suspension 893
Mobic Tablets 893
Neumega for Injection 3433
▲ Ontak Vials (7%) 1717
Procrit for Injection 2374

Thrombotic vascular disease
Accutane Capsules 2740
Amnesteem Capsules 2126
Ortho-Cyclen/Ortho Tri-Cyclen 2414
Ortho Tri-Cyclen Lo Tablets 2421

Thrush, oral
(*see under* Candidiasis, oral)

Thymol turbidity test, positive
Cuprimine Capsules 1925

Thymus gland abnormalities, fetal
Accutane Capsules 2740

Thyroid adenoma
Permax Tablets (Rare) 3357
Relpax Tablets (Rare) 2531

Thyroid binding globulin, increase
(*see under* T4, increase)

Thyroid disease, exacerbation
Proleukin for Injection 1007

Thyroid disorder, unspecified
Betaseron for SC Injection 791
Dynacin Tablets 1859
▲ Rebif Prefilled Syringe for Injection (4% to 6%) 3163
Vytorin 10/10 Tablets 2084
Vytorin 10/10 Tablets 3092
Vytorin 10/20 Tablets 2084
Vytorin 10/20 Tablets 3092
Vytorin 10/40 Tablets 2084
Vytorin 10/40 Tablets 3092
Vytorin 10/80 Tablets 2084
Vytorin 10/80 Tablets 3092

Thyroid disorders
(*see under* T3, decrease; T4, decrease; T4, increase)

Thyroid function test, abnormal
Altoprev Extended-Release Tablets 1151
Depacon Injection 412
Depakene 417
Depakote Sprinkle Capsules 422
Depakote Tablets 427
Depakote ER Tablets 433
▲ Infergen (4% to 9%) 1647
Lescol Capsules 2227
Lescol Capsules 2730
Lescol XL Tablets 2227
Lescol XL Tablets 2730
Mevacor Tablets 1996
Pegasys 2793
Pravachol Tablets 943
Proleukin for Injection 1007
Roferon-A Injection (Infrequent) 2805
Zocor Tablets 2078

Thyroid gland discoloration
Dynacin Tablets 1859

Thyroid hormone, changes
(*see under* T3, decrease; T4, decrease; T4, increase)

Thyroid nodule
Effexor Tablets (Rare) 3405
Effexor XR Capsules (Rare) 3411
ProSom Tablets (Rare) 512

Thyroid stimulating hormone elevation
Aciphex Tablets 1081
Avodart Soft Gelatin Capsules 1353

Thyroiditis
Aldara Cream, 5% 1814
Cuprimine Capsules 1925
Effexor Tablets (Rare) 3405
Effexor XR Capsules (Rare) 3411
▲ Ontak Vials (Less than 5%) 1717
Paxil CR Controlled-Release Tablets (Rare) 1509
Paxil (Rare) 1501
Pegasys 2793
Relpax Tablets (Rare) 2531
Sular Tablets (Less than or equal to 1%) 1163

Thyrotoxicosis
▲ Ontak Vials (Less than 5%) 1717
Synthroid Tablets 515

Thyroxin-binding globulin, decrease
Striant Mucoadhesive 1022
Testim 1% Gel 722

Tics
FazaClo Orally Disintegrating Tablets (Less than 1%) 547
Lamictal 1449
Lexapro Oral Solution (Infrequent) 1193
Lexapro Tablets (Infrequent) 1193
Lithobid Tablets 1670

Tightness, abdominal
Abilify Tablets (Infrequent) 916
Abilify Tablets (Infrequent) 2472

Tightness, back
Abilify Tablets (Infrequent) 916
Abilify Tablets (Infrequent) 2472

Tightness, extremities
Abilify Tablets (Infrequent) 916
Abilify Tablets (Infrequent) 2472

Tightness, head
Abilify Tablets (Infrequent) 916
Abilify Tablets (Infrequent) 2472

Tightness, tongue
Abilify Tablets (Infrequent) 916
Abilify Tablets (Infrequent) 2472

Tingling
Acticin Cream 2125
Bentyl Capsules 724
Bentyl Injection 724
Bentyl Syrup 724
Bentyl Tablets 724
BiDil Tablets 2161
Calcium Disodium Versenate Injection 1819
Cipro I.V. 2998
Cipro I.V. Pharmacy Bulk Package 3509
Cipro 2991
Decadron Phosphate Injection 1931
DynaCirc CR Tablets (0.5% to 1%) 2726
▲ Elocon Ointment 0.1% (4.8%) 3021
Engerix-B Vaccine (Less than 1%) 1391
▲ Finacea Gel (4% to 20%) 1644
Gengraf Capsules (Rare) 458
▲ Imitrex Injection (13.5%) 1431
Imitrex Nasal Spray (Infrequent) 1435
▲ Imitrex Tablets (4% to 8%) 1440
K-Phos Neutral Tablets 785
K-Phos Original (Sodium Free) Tablets (Less frequent) 785
Levaquin in 5% Dextrose Injection 2453
Levaquin 2453
Metrogel 1% 1212
Neoral Soft Gelatin Capsules (Rare) 2247
Neoral Oral Solution (Rare) 2247
▲ Niaspan Extended-Release Tablets (Among most common) 1703
Noroxin Tablets 2009
Nubain Injection (1% or less) 1111
Oxistat Lotion (0.4%) 1498
▲ Protopic Ointment (1% to 8%) 629
Rescriptor Tablets 2535
Sandimmune (Rare) 2259
Sedapap Tablets 50 mg/650 mg (Infrequent) 2098
▲ Solage Topical Solution (21.9% to 26%) 740
Twinrix Vaccine (Less than 1%) 1571
U-Kera Cream 3290

Tingling, ears
Ciprodex Otic Suspension (1 patient) 555
Koāte-DVI (0.7%) 3247

Tingling, extremities
Indapamide Tablets (Less than 5%) 2119
Surmontil Capsules 2347
Vivactil Tablets 2350
Zerit 971

Tingling, feet
Alferon N Injection (1%) 1640
Uroqid-Acid No. 2 Tablets 785

Tingling, fingers
Noroxin Tablets (0.3% to 1.0%) 2009

Tingling, hands
Adenocard Injection (1%) 612
Koāte-DVI (0.7%) 3247
Uroqid-Acid No. 2 Tablets 785

Tingling, legs
Alferon N Injection (1%) 1640

Tingling, limbs

Tingling, lips
K-Phos Neutral Tablets 785
K-Phos Original (Sodium Free) Tablets (Less frequent) 785
Striant Mucoadhesive 1022
Uroqid-Acid No. 2 Tablets 785

Tingling, scalp
▲ Dovonex Scalp Solution 0.005% (Approximately 23%) 3375
Temovate Scalp Application (2 of 294 patients) 1551

Tingling, skin
Garamycin Injectable 3028

Tinnitus
Abelcet Injection 1119
Abilify Tablets (Infrequent) 916
Abilify Tablets (Infrequent) 2472
Accutane Capsules 2740
Aceon Tablets (2 mg, 4 mg, 8 mg) (1.5%) 3191
Aciphex Tablets 1081
Actiq (1% or greater) 993
▲ Actonel Tablets (3.3%) 2679
Adalat CC Tablets (Less than 1%) 2978
Aggrenox Capsules (Less than 1%) 855
Agrylin Capsules (1% to 5%) 3172
Alferon N Injection (One patient) 1640
Aloxi Injection (Less than 1%) 2099
Altace Capsules (Less than 1%) 1673
Ambien Tablets (Infrequent) 2867
Amerge Tablets (Infrequent) 1312
Amnesteem Capsules 2126
▲ Anaprox Tablets (3% to 9%) 2769
▲ Anaprox DS Tablets (3% to 9%) 2769
Anzemet Injection (Infrequently) 2871
Anzemet Tablets (Infrequently) 2874
Aricept Tablets (Infrequent) 1086
Aricept ODT Tablets (Infrequent) 1086
Arthrotec Tablets (Rare) 3126
Asacol Delayed-Release Tablets 2688
Atacand HCT (0.5% or greater) 637
Atrovent Nasal Spray 0.06% (Less than 1%) 870
Avelox (Less than 0.1%) 2984
Axert Tablets (Rare) 2430
Bayer, Aspirin Regimen ▣ 606
Bayer Aspirin 3515
BC Powder ▣ 612
BC Allergy Sinus Cold Powder ▣ 612
Arthritis Strength BC Powder ▣ 612
BC Sinus Cold Powder ▣ 612
Biaxin/Biaxin XL 402
Blocadren Tablets (Less than 1%) 1891
Buprenex Injectable (Less than 1%) 2718
Caduet Tablets (Greater than 0.1% to less than 2%) 2507
Campral Tablets (Infrequent) 1175
Capastat Sulfate for Injection 1728
Carbatrol Capsules 3174
Cardene I.V. (Rare) 1129
Cardizem LA Extended Release Tablets (Less than 2%) 1699
▲ Cataflam Tablets (1% to 10%) 2173
Celebrex Capsules (0.1% to 1.9%) 3130
Celexa (Infrequent) 1177
▲ CellCept Capsules (3% to less than 20%) 2751
▲ CellCept Intravenous (3% to less than 20%) 2751
▲ CellCept Oral Suspension (3% to less than 20%) 2751
▲ CellCept Tablets (3% to less than 20%) 2751
Cipro I.V. (1% or less) 2998
Cipro I.V. Pharmacy Bulk Package (1% or less) 3509
Cipro (Less than 1%) 2991
Cipro XR Tablets 3004
Clinoril Tablets (Greater than 1%) 1899
Colazal Capsules 2845
Copaxone for Injection (At least 2%) 3292
Coreg Tablets (Greater than 0.1% to 1%) 1376
Cosopt Sterile Ophthalmic Solution 1910
Covera-HS Tablets (Less than 2%) 3135
Cozaar Tablets (Less than 1%) 1913
Cuprimine Capsules (Greater than 1%) 1925
Cytovene (At least 3 subjects) 2763
Dapsone Tablets USP 1656
Daranide Tablets 1928
▲ Depacon Injection (1% to 7%) 412
▲ Depakene (7%) 417
▲ Depakote Sprinkle Capsules (1% to 7%) 422
▲ Depakote Tablets (1% to 7%) 427
▲ Depakote ER Tablets (1% to 7%) 433
Desferal Vials 2190
Diovan HCT Tablets (Greater than 0.2%) 2195
Diprivan Injectable Emulsion (Less than 1%) 676
Dolobid Tablets (Greater than 1 in 100) 1937
Doxil Injection (Less than 1%) 3302
Dynacin Tablets (Rarely reported) 1859
▲ EC-Naprosyn Delayed-Release Tablets (3% to 9%) 2769
Ecotrin Enteric Coated Aspirin Low, Regular and Maximum Strength Tablets 1627
Edecrin 1941
Effexor Tablets (2%) 3405
Effexor XR Capsules (Frequent) 3411
Eldepryl Capsules 3209
Elmiron Capsules (Less than or equal to 1%) 2393
▲ Emend Capsules (3.7%) 1944
Engerix-B Vaccine 1391
Equetro Extended-Release Capsules 3178
Eskalith 1406
Evoxac Capsules (Less than 1%) 1042
Exelon Capsules (Frequent) 2204
Flexeril Tablets (Less than 1%) 1832
Floxin Otic Singles (0.3%) 1045
Floxin Otic Solution (Single report to 0.3%) 1043
Flumadine (0.3% to 1%) 1186
Fortical Nasal Spray (Less than 1%) 3336
Frova Tablets (Frequent) 1101
Furosemide Tablets 2117
Gabitril Tablets (Frequent) 998
Garamycin Injectable 3028
Gengraf Capsules (1% to less than 3%) 458
Geodon Capsules (Infrequent) 2514
Gleevec Tablets (Infrequent) 2221
Hyperstat I.V. Injection 3031
Hytrin Capsules (At least 1%) 469
Hyzaar 1964
▲ Imdur Tablets (Less than or equal to 5%) 3032
Imitrex Nasal Spray 1435
Indocin (Greater than 1%) 1968
▲ Infergen (4% to 6%) 1647
▲ Intron A for Injection (Less than 5%) 3038
Invirase (Less than 2%) 2776
Kaletra (Less than 2%) 474
Kaopectate Anti-Diarrheal/Upset Stomach Reliever Liquid ▣ 701
Extra Strength Kaopectate Anti-Diarrheal Liquid ▣ 701
Lamictal (1.1%) 1449
▲ Lariam Tablets (Among most frequent) 2790
Levaquin in 5% Dextrose Injection (0.1% to 0.9%) 2453
Levaquin (0.1% to 0.9%) 2453

Levitra Tablets (Less than 2%) 3048
Lexapro Oral Solution (Frequent) 1193
Lexapro Tablets (Frequent) 1193
Lidoderm Patch 1107
Lipitor Tablets (Less than 2%) 2495
Lithobid Tablets 1670
Lotensin HCT Tablets (0.3% to 1%) 2235
Lotrel Capsules (Infrequent) 2238
Lunesta Tablets (Infrequent) 3139
Lyrica Capsules (Greater than or equal to 1%) 2524
Maalox Maximum Strength Total Stomach Relief Peppermint Liquid ■ 677
Maalox Maximum Strength Total Stomach Relief Strawberry Liquid ■ 678
Marinol Capsules (Less than 1%) 3334
Maxalt Tablets (Infrequent) 1983
Maxalt-MLT Orally Disintegrating Tablets (Infrequent) 1983
Meridia Capsules 485
Miacalcin Nasal Spray (Less than 1%) 2242
Micardis Tablets (More than 0.3%) 884
Micardis HCT Tablets 886
Midamor Tablets (Less than or equal to 1%) 2000
Migranal Nasal Spray (Infrequent) 3350
Mintezol 2002
Mirapex Tablets (Greater than or equal to 1%) 889
Mobic Oral Suspension (Less than 2%) 893
Mobic Tablets (Less than 2%) 893
Moduretic Tablets 2003
Mustargen for Injection (Infrequent) 2007
Nadolol Tablets (1 to 5 of 1000 patients) 2121
▲ Nalfon Capsules (4.5%) 2504
Namenda (Infrequent) 1199
▲ Naprosyn Suspension (3% to 9%) 2769
▲ Naprosyn Tablets (3% to 9%) 2769
Naropin Injection (Less than 1%) 640
Neoral Soft Gelatin Capsules (1% to less than 3%) 2247
Neoral Oral Solution (1% to less than 3%) 2247
Neurontin Capsules (Infrequent) 2498
Neurontin Oral Solution (Infrequent) 2498
Neurontin Tablets (Infrequent) 2498
Nexium Delayed-Release Capsules (Less than 1%) 645
Nexium I.V. (Less than 1%) 649
Nipent for Injection (Less than 3%) 3216
▲ Niravam Orally Disintegrating Tablets (6.6%) 3106
Noroxin Tablets 2009
Norvasc Tablets (More than 0.1% to 1%) 2529
Norvir (Less than 2%) 499
Orthoclone OKT3 Sterile Solution 2370
OxyContin Tablets (Less than 1%) 2699
Parnate Tablets 1499
Paxil CR Controlled-Release Tablets (Frequent) 1509
Paxil (Frequent) 1501
Pepcid Injection (Infrequent) 2017
Pepcid (Infrequent) 2014
Pepto-Bismol Maximum Strength Liquid ■ 718
Pepto-Bismol Original Liquid, Maximum Strength Liquid, Original and Cherry Tablets and Easy-To-Swallow Caplets 2673
Permax Tablets (Infrequent) 3357
Phenergan 3438
Pletal Tablets (Less than 2%) 2478
Prevacid Delayed-Release Capsules (Less than 1%) 3268
Prevacid for Delayed-Release Oral Suspension (Less than 1%) 3268
▲ Prevacid NapraPAC (Less than 1% to 9%) 3277
Prevacid SoluTab Delayed-Release Orally Disintegrating Tablets (Less than 1%) 3268
PREVPAC (Less than 1%) 3281
Prilosec OTC Tablets (Less than 1%) 2674
Primaxin I.M. 2022
Primaxin I.V. (Less than 0.2%) 2024
Prinivil Tablets (0.3% to 1.0%) 2029
Prinzide Tablets (0.3% to 1%) 2033
▲ Prograf Capsules and Injection (3% to 15%) 624
ProSom Tablets (Infrequent) 512
Protonix I.V. (Less than 1%) 3468
Protonix Tablets (Less than 1%) 3465
Proventil HFA Inhalation Aerosol (Less than 3%) 3071
Prozac Pulvules and Liquid (Frequent) 1771
▲ Rapamune Oral Solution and Tablets (3% to 20%) 3472
Razadyne (Infrequent) 2434
Recombivax HB (Less than 1%) 2045
▲ Relafen Tablets (3% to 9%) 1523
Relpax Tablets (Infrequent) 2531
Requip Tablets (Infrequent) 1528
Rescriptor Tablets 2535
Reyataz Capsules (Less than 3%) 948
Risperdal M-Tab Orally Disintegrating Tablets (Rare) 1658
Risperdal (Rare) 1658
Rythmol SR Capsules 2736
Sandimmune (2% or less) 2259
Sandostatin LAR Depot (1% to 4%) 2264
Sedapap Tablets 50 mg/650 mg (Infrequent) 2098
Seroquel Tablets (Infrequent) 691
Sonata Capsules (Infrequent) 1686
▲ Soriatane Capsules (Less than 1% to 10%) 1028
St. Joseph 81 mg Aspirin Chewable and Enteric Coated Tablets 1841
Sular Tablets (Less than or equal to 1%) 1163
Surmontil Capsules 2347
Sustiva Capsules (Less than 2%) 957
Symbyax Capsules (Frequent) 1788
Tambocor Tablets (1% to 3%) 1824
Tarka Tablets (Less frequent) 519
Tasmar Tablets (Frequent) 3360
Tegretol/Tegretol-XR 2278
▲ Tequin Injection (0.1% to 3%) 964
▲ Tequin Tablets (0.1% to 3%) 964
Teveten Tablets (Less than 1%) 1707
Teveten HCT Tablets (Less than 1%) 1710
Thalomid Capsules 979
Tiazac Capsules (Less than 2%) 1204
Ticlid Tablets (0.5% to 1.0%) 2813
Timolide Tablets 2056
Timoptic in Ocudose 2061
Timoptic Sterile Ophthalmic Solution 2058
Timoptic-XE Sterile Ophthalmic Gel Forming Solution 2062
▲ TOBI Solution for Inhalation (3%) 1015
Topamax Sprinkle Capsules (Less than 1% to 2%) 2438
Topamax Tablets (Less than 1% to 2%) 2438
Toprol-XL Tablets 660
Tricor Tablets 523
Trileptal Oral Suspension 2281
Trileptal Tablets 2281
▲ Trisenox Injection (5%) 983
Twinrix Vaccine 1571
Ultracet Tablets (Less than 1%) 2462
Uniretic Tablets (Less than 1%) 3114
Univasc Tablets (Less than 1%) 3118
Vancocin HCl Capsules, USP (Rare) 3370
Vantin Tablets and Oral Suspension (Less than 1%) 2650
Vaseretic Tablets (0.5% to 2.0%) 2073
Vasotec I.V. Injection (0.5% to 1.0%) 2076
Verelan PM Capsules (2% or less) 3120
VFEND I.V. (Less than 2%) 2543
VFEND Oral Suspension (Less than 2%) 2543
VFEND Tablets (Less than 2%) 2543
Viagra Tablets (Less than 2%) 2552
Vicoprofen Tablets (Less than 3%) 533
Vivactil Tablets 2350
▲ Voltaren Tablets (1% to 10%) 2298
▲ Voltaren-XR Tablets (1% to 10%) 2301
Wellbutrin Tablets 1579
▲ Wellbutrin SR Sustained-Release Tablets (5% to 6%) 1583
▲ Wellbutrin XL Extended-Release Tablets (5% to 6%) 1588
Xanax XR Tablets (Infrequent) 2655
Xifaxan Tablets (Less than 2%) 2847
Zegerid Powder for Oral Solution (Less than 1%) 2972
Zestoretic Tablets (0.3% to 1%) 701
Zestril Tablets (0.3% to 1.0%) 704
Zithromax Capsules, 250 mg 2568
Zithromax for IV Infusion (Rare) 2573
Zithromax for Oral Suspension, 300 mg, 600 mg, 900 mg, 1200 mg 2561
Zithromax Tablets, 250 mg, 500 mg 2561
Zithromax Tri-Pak 2561
Zmax for Oral Suspension 2577
Zoloft (Frequent) 2581
Zomig Nasal Spray (Infrequent) 718
Zomig Tablets (Infrequent) 714
Zomig-ZMT Tablets (Infrequent) 714
Zonegran Capsules (Frequent) 1089
Zosyn (1.0% or less) 3492
Zyban Sustained-Release Tablets (1%) 1620
Zyprexa Tablets (Infrequent) 1798
Zyprexa ZYDIS Orally Disintegrating Tablets (Infrequent) 1798
Zyrtec Chewable Tablets (Less than 2%) 2589
Zyrtec (Less than 2%) 2589
Zyrtec-D 12 Hour Extended Release Tablets (Less than 2%) 2591

Tiredness
(*see under* Fatigue)

Tobacco misuse

Zyprexa Tablets (Rare) 1798
Zyprexa ZYDIS Orally Disintegrating Tablets (Infrequent) 1798

Toenails, ingrown

Crixivan Capsules 1918
Prevnar for Injection 3460

Toes, discoloration

Eskalith (A few reports) 1406

Tolerance

Adipex-P 1216
Astelin Nasal Spray 1876
Carnitor Tablets and Oral Solution 3187
DextroStat Tablets 3177
Dilaudid Oral Liquid 443
Dilaudid Tablets - 8 mg 443
Duragesic Transdermal System 2448
Hycodan 1104
Hycomine Compound Tablets 1105
Hycotuss Expectorant Syrup 1106
Kadian Capsules (Less than 3%) 572
Lortab 3315
Lortab Elixir 3312
MS Contin Tablets 2703
Nembutal Sodium Solution, USP 2484
Percocet Tablets 1114
Percodan Tablets 1115
Ritalin Hydrochloride Tablets 2254
Ritalin LA Capsules 2255
Ritalin-SR Tablets 2254
Sedapap Tablets 50 mg/650 mg (Infrequent) 2098
Tylenol with Codeine 2461
Vicodin Tablets 530
Vicodin HP Tablets 532
Vicoprofen Tablets 533
Zemuron Injection (Rare) 2363

Tolerance, diminished

Symbyax Capsules (Rare) 1788
Timolide Tablets 2056

Tongue, black "hairy"
(*see under* Glossotrichia)

Tongue, burning

Imitrex Injection 1431
Imitrex Nasal Spray (Infrequent) 1435
Imitrex Tablets 1440
Nalfon Capsules (Less than 1%) 2504
Parcopa Orally Disintegrating Tablets 3111
Stalevo Tablets 2270

Tongue, fine vermicular movements

Eskalith 1406
Lithobid Tablets 1670
Moban Tablets 1108
Orap Tablets 1220
Thioridazine Hydrochloride Tablets 2122
Thiothixene Capsules 2124

Tongue, furry

Tindamax (Rare) 2670

Tongue, geographic

Evoxac Capsules (Less than 1%) 1042

Tongue, mucosal atrophy

Prilosec OTC Tablets (Less than 1%) 2674
Zegerid Powder for Oral Solution (Less than 1%) 2972

Tongue, protrusion

Moban Tablets 1108
Orap Tablets 1220
Phenergan Suppositories 3438
Thioridazine Hydrochloride Tablets 2122
Thiothixene Capsules 2124

Tongue, sore
(*see under* Glossodynia)

Tongue, swelling
(*see under* Glossoncus)

Tongue, thickening of

▲ Kepivance (17%) 592

Tongue discoloration

Avelox (Less than 0.1%) 2984
Biaxin/Biaxin XL 402
Colazal Capsules 2845
Copaxone for Injection (Infrequent) 3292
Effexor Tablets (Rare) 3405
Effexor XR Capsules (Rare) 3411
Evoxac Capsules (Less than 1%) 1042
Kaopectate Anti-Diarrheal/Upset Stomach Reliever Liquid ■ 701
Extra Strength Kaopectate Anti-Diarrheal Liquid ■ 701
▲ Kepivance (17%) 592
Paxil CR Controlled-Release Tablets (Rare) 1509
Paxil (Rare) 1501
Pepto-Bismol Maximum Strength Liquid ■ 718
Pepto-Bismol Original Liquid, Maximum Strength Liquid, Original and Cherry Tablets and Easy-To-Swallow Caplets 2673
PREVPAC (Less than 3%) 3281
Prilosec OTC Tablets (2%) 2674
Primaxin I.M. 2022
Primaxin I.V. (Less than 0.2%) 2024
Protonix I.V. (Less than 1%) 3468
Protonix Tablets (Less than 1%) 3465
Rilutek Tablets (Rare) 2945
Risperdal M-Tab Orally Disintegrating Tablets (Rare) 1658
Risperdal (Rare) 1658
Sonata Capsules (Rare) 1686
Thalomid Capsules 979
Tindamax 2670
Uniretic Tablets (Less than 1%) 3114
Zegerid Powder for Oral Solution (2%) 2972
Zyprexa Tablets (Rare) 1798
Zyprexa ZYDIS Orally Disintegrating Tablets (Rare) 1798
Zyrtec Chewable Tablets (Less than 2%) 2589
Zyrtec (Less than 2%) 2589
Zyrtec-D 12 Hour Extended Release Tablets (Less than 2%) 2591
Zyvox (0.2% to 1.1%) 2661

Tongue disorder, unspecified

Evoxac Capsules (Less than 1%) 1042
▲ Flovent Diskus 50 mcg (1% to 3%) 1415
Gengraf Capsules (1% to less than 3%) 458
Neoral Soft Gelatin Capsules (1% to less than 3%) 2247
Neoral Oral Solution (1% to less than 3%) 2247
Neurontin Capsules (Infrequent) 2498
Neurontin Oral Solution (Infrequent) 2498
Neurontin Tablets (Infrequent) 2498
Nexium Delayed-Release Capsules (Less than 1%) 645
Nexium I.V. (Less than 1%) 649
Prevacid NapraPAC (Less than 1%) 3277
PREVPAC (Less than 3%) 3281
Relpax Tablets (Rare) 2531
▲ Soriatane Capsules (1% to 10%) 1028
Tasmar Tablets (Infrequent) 3360

Tongue numbness
(*see under* Numbness, buccal mucosa)

Tonsillitis

Elidel Cream 1% (0.4% to 6.3%) 2198
▲ Flovent Diskus 50 mcg (1% to 3%) 1415
Foradil Aerolizer (1.2%) 3024
Gengraf Capsules (1% to less than 3%) 458
Neoral Soft Gelatin Capsules (1% to less than 3%) 2247
Neoral Oral Solution (1% to less than 3%) 2247

Singulair (Greater than or equal to 2%) 2047

Tooth discoloration

Amoxil Capsules (Rare) 1315
Amoxil Chewable Tablets (Rare) 1315
Amoxil Pediatric Drops for Oral Suspension (Rare) 1315
Amoxil Powder for Oral Suspension (Rare) 1315
Amoxil Tablets (Rare) 1315
Augmentin (Rare) 1331
Augmentin Tablets (Rare) 1334
Augmentin XR Extended-Release Tablets (Rare) 1340
Augmentin ES-600 Powder for Oral Suspension (Rare) 1337
Biaxin/Biaxin XL 402
Dynacin Tablets 1859
PREVPAC 3281

Tooth disorder

Actiq (Less than 1%) 993
Actonel Tablets (2.1%) 2679
Actonel with Calcium Tablets (2.1%) 2684
▲ ActoPlus Met Tablets (5.3%) 3219
▲ Actos Tablets (5.3%) 3224
▲ Adderall XR Capsules (2% to 4%) 3169
Antara Capsules 2723
▲ Arava Tablets (1% to 3%) 2881
Axid Oral Solution (1.0%) 913
Boniva Tablets (3.5%) 2747
Celebrex Capsules (0.1% to 1.9%) 3130
▲ CombiPatch Transdermal System (4% to 6%) 2180
▲ Depakote ER Tablets (1% to 5%) 433
▲ Entocort EC Capsules (Less than 5%) 2694
▲ Evoxac Capsules (1% to 3%) 1042
Flomax Capsules (1.2% to 2.0%) 881
▲ Flovent Diskus 50 mcg (1% to 3%) 1415
Forteo for Injection (2%) 1739
Gengraf Capsules (1% to less than 3%) 458
Geodon for Injection (Up to 1%) 2514
Invirase (Less than 2%) 2776
▲ Lamictal (2% to 3%) 1449
Lescol Capsules (2.1%) 2227
Lescol XL Tablets (1.4%) 2227
Lofibra Capsules 1217
Lotensin HCT Tablets (0.3% or more) 2235
Meridia Capsules (Greater than or equal to 1%) 485
Mirapex Tablets (1% or more) 889
Neoral Soft Gelatin Capsules (1% to less than 3%) 2247
Neoral Oral Solution (1% to less than 3%) 2247
Neurontin Capsules (Infrequent) 2498
Neurontin Oral Solution (Infrequent) 2498
Neurontin Tablets (Infrequent) 2498
▲ Nicotrol Inhaler (Greater than 3%) 2594
▲ Nicotrol NS (4%) 2596
▲ Nipent for Injection (3% to 10%) 3216
Paxil CR Controlled-Release Tablets (Rare) 1509
Paxil (Rare) 1501
Prandin Tablets (0.5, 1, and 2 mg) (Less than 1% to 2%) 2337
▲ Prefest Tablets (5%) 1069
Prometrium Capsules (100 mg, 200 mg) 3205
Protopic Ointment (Greater than or equal to 1%) 629
Provigil Tablets (At least 1%) 1002
Relpax Tablets (Rare) 2531
Rescriptor Tablets 2535
Rilutek Tablets (Up to 1.2%) 2945
▲ Risperdal Consta Long-Acting Injection (2% to 4%) 1664
Roferon-A Injection (Infrequent) 2805
Symbyax Capsules (1% to 2%) 1788
Tasmar Tablets (Frequent) 3360
Thalomid Capsules 979
Topamax Sprinkle Capsules (Greater than 1%) 2438
Topamax Tablets (Greater than 1%) 2438
Tricor Tablets 523
Triglide Tablets 1165
Vantin Tablets and Oral Suspension (Less than 1%) 2650
Vivelle Transdermal System (2.3%) 2288
Vivelle-Dot Transdermal System (2.3%) 2293
Wellbutrin SR Sustained-Release Tablets (At least 1%) 1583
Wellbutrin XL Extended-Release Tablets (At least 1%) 1588
▲ Xenical Capsules (2.9% to 4.3%) 2834
Zyprexa Tablets 1798
Zyprexa ZYDIS Orally Disintegrating Tablets 1798
Zyrtec Chewable Tablets (Less than 2%) 2589
Zyrtec (Less than 2%) 2589
Zyrtec-D 12 Hour Extended Release Tablets (Less than 2%) 2591

Toothache

Aricept Tablets (Infrequent) 1086
Aricept ODT Tablets (Infrequent) 1086
▲ Avonex (3%) 839
▲ Azmacort Inhalation Aerosol (1% to 3%) 1701
Dostinex Tablets (2%) 2631
Elidel Cream 1% (0.4% to 2.6%) 2198
▲ Evoxac Capsules (1% to 3%) 1042
Frova Tablets (Rare) 1101
▲ Gonal-f RFF Pen for Injection (3.6%) 3155
Klonopin (Infrequent) 2782
Lexapro Oral Solution (2%) 1193
Lexapro Tablets (2%) 1193
Micardis Tablets (More than 0.3%) 884
Micardis HCT Tablets 886
▲ Prochieve 4% Gel (Less than 5%) 1018
▲ Prochieve 8% Gel (Less than 5%) 1018
Requip Tablets (Infrequent) 1528
Rescriptor Tablets 2535
▲ Risperdal Consta Long-Acting Injection (1% to 3%) 1664
Risperdal M-Tab Orally Disintegrating Tablets (2%) 1658
Risperdal (2%) 1658
Striant Mucoadhesive 1022
Teveten Tablets (Less than 1%) 1707
Teveten HCT Tablets (Less than 1%) 1710
Trileptal Oral Suspension (1% to 2%) 2281
Trileptal Tablets (1% to 2%) 2281
Vantin Tablets and Oral Suspension (Infrequent) 2650
Vivelle Transdermal System (2.3%) 2288
Vivelle-Dot Transdermal System (2.3%) 2293
Wellbutrin Tablets (Infrequent) 1579

Torsade de pointes

Avelox (Very rare) 2984
Biaxin/Biaxin XL (Rare) 402
Celexa 1177
Cipro I.V. 2998
Cipro I.V. Pharmacy Bulk Package 3509
Cipro 2991
Cipro XR Tablets 3004
Cytovene 2763
E.E.S. (Rare) 449
Effexor Tablets (Rare) 3405
Effexor XR Capsules (Rare) 3411
EryPed (Rare) 445
Erythrocin Stearate Filmtab Tablets (Rare) 452
Erythromycin Base Filmtab Tablets (Rare) 454
Erythromycin Delayed-Release Capsules, USP 456
Geodon 2514
Levaquin in 5% Dextrose Injection 2453
Levaquin 2453
Lexapro Oral Solution 1193
Lexapro Tablets 1193
Meridia Capsules 485
Noroxin Tablets (Rare) 2009
Paxil CR Controlled-Release Tablets 1509
Paxil 1501
PCE Dispertab Tablets 510
Pletal Tablets (Very rare) 2478
PREVPAC (Rare) 3281
Prograf Capsules and Injection 624
Razadyne ER Extended-Release Capsules 2434
Razadyne 2434
Tambocor Tablets (Rare) 1824
Tequin Injection 964
Tequin Tablets 964
Thioridazine Hydrochloride Tablets 2122
VFEND I.V. (Less than 2%) 2543
VFEND Oral Suspension (Less than 2%) 2543
VFEND Tablets (Less than 2%) 2543
Viracept 2556
Zithromax Capsules, 250 mg (Rare) 2568
Zithromax for IV Infusion 2573
Zithromax for Oral Suspension, 1 g 2568
Zithromax for Oral Suspension, 300 mg, 600 mg, 900 mg, 1200 mg (Rare) 2561
Zithromax Tablets, 250 mg, 500 mg (Rare) 2561
Zithromax Tablets, 600 mg 2568
Zithromax Tri-Pak (Rare) 2561
Zithromax Z-Pak 2568
Zmax for Oral Suspension 2577
Zoloft 2581

Torticollis

Abilify Tablets (Frequent) 916
Abilify Tablets (Frequent) 2472
Aceon Tablets (2 mg, 4 mg, 8 mg) (1.4%) 3191
Actiq (1% or greater) 993
Actonel Tablets (1.2% to 2.7%) 2679
▲ Actonel with Calcium Tablets (1.2% to 5.3%) 2684
Adalat CC Tablets (Less than 1%) 2978
Adenocard Injection (Less than 1%) 612
▲ Adenoscan (15%) 613
Agrylin Capsules (1% to 5%) 3172
AmBisome for Injection (Less common) 615
▲ Arava Tablets (1% to 3%) 2881
▲ Arimidex Tablets (2% to 5%) 665
Asacol Delayed-Release Tablets 2688
Axert Tablets (Infrequent) 2430
▲ Bexxar (1% to 6%) 1360
▲ Botox Purified Neurotoxin Complex (3 % to 11%) 565
Bravelle for Intramuscular or Subcutaneous Injection (2.7%) 1140
Caduet Tablets (Less than 2%) 2507
Campral Tablets (Rare) 1175
Cardene I.V. (Rare) 1129
▲ Casodex Tablets (2% to 5%) 670
▲ CellCept Capsules (3% to less than 20%) 2751
▲ CellCept Intravenous (3% to less than 20%) 2751
▲ CellCept Oral Suspension (3% to less than 20%) 2751
▲ CellCept Tablets (3% to less than 20%) 2751
▲ Cenestin Tablets, 0.45mg, 0.625mg, 0.9mg, 1.25mg (3%) 1063
Cialis Tablets (Less than 2%) 1806
Cipro I.V. (1% or less) 2998
Cipro I.V. Pharmacy Bulk Package (1% or less) 3509
Cipro (Less than 1%) 2991
Cipro XR Tablets 3004
Clindesse Vaginal Cream (Less than 1%) 3296
Clozapine Tablets (1%) 2141
Clozaril Tablets (1%) 2174
▲ Copaxone for Injection (8%) 3292
Crestor Tablets (Greater than or equal to 1%) 672
Depacon Injection (1% or more) 412
Depakene (1% or more) 417
Depakote Sprinkle Capsules 422
▲ Depakote Tablets (1% to 5%) 427
Depakote ER Tablets (1% or more) 433
Diprivan Injectable Emulsion (Less than 1%) 676
Doxil Injection (Less than 1%) 3302
DynaCirc CR Tablets (0.5% to 1%) 2726
Effexor Tablets (Frequent) 3405
▲ Effexor XR Capsules (3%) 3411
Engerix-B Vaccine (Less than 1%) 1391
FazaClo Orally Disintegrating Tablets (1%) 547
▲ Flolan for Injection (84%) 1408
Forteo for Injection (3%) 1739
Gabitril Tablets (Frequent) 998
Geodon Capsules (Rare) 2514
Hytrin Capsules (At least 1%) 469
▲ Imdur Tablets (Less than or equal to 5%) 3032
▲ Imitrex Injection (4.8%) 1431
▲ Infergen (8% to 14%) 1647
Keppra Oral Solution (2%) 3307
Keppra Tablets (2%) 3307
Klonopin (Infrequent) 2782
▲ Lamictal (1% to 5%) 1449
Levitra Tablets (Less than 2%) 3048
▲ Lexapro Oral Solution (3%) 1193
▲ Lexapro Tablets (3%) 1193
Lipitor Tablets (Less than 2%) 2495
Lotensin HCT Tablets (0.3% or more) 2235
Lyrica Capsules (Rare) 2524
Meridia Capsules (1.6%) 485
Mirapex Tablets (Greater than or equal to 1%) 889
Moduretic Tablets 2003
Neurontin Capsules (Infrequent) 2498
Neurontin Oral Solution (Infrequent) 2498
Neurontin Tablets (Infrequent) 2498
▲ Nicotrol Inhaler (Greater than 3%) 2594
Norvir (Less than 2%) 499
Omacor Capsules 2735
Orap Tablets (2.7%) 1220
▲ Orthoclone OKT3 Sterile Solution (14%) 2370
OxyContin Tablets (Less than 1%) 2699
Paxil CR Controlled-Release Tablets (Infrequent) 1509
Paxil (Infrequent) 1501
Permax Tablets (2.7%) 3357
Phenergan Suppositories 3438
Prevacid Delayed-Release Capsules (Less than 1%) 3268
Prevacid for Delayed-Release Oral Suspension (Less than 1%) 3268
Prevacid NapraPAC (Less than 1%) 3277
Prevacid SoluTab Delayed-Release Orally Disintegrating Tablets (Less than 1%) 3268
PREVPAC (Less than 1%) 3281
Prinivil Tablets (0.3% to 1.0%) 2029
Prinzide Tablets 2033
ProSom Tablets (Infrequent) 512
Protonix I.V. (Greater than or equal to 1%) 3468
Protonix Tablets (Greater than or equal to 1%) 3465
Protopic Ointment (Greater than or equal to 1%) 629
Provigil Tablets (Greater than or equal to 1%) 1002
Recombivax HB (Less than 1%) 2045
Requip Tablets (Infrequent) 1528
Risperdal Consta Long-Acting Injection (Infrequent) 1664
Risperdal M-Tab Orally Disintegrating Tablets (Rare) 1658
Risperdal (Rare) 1658
Rythmol SR Capsules 2736
Seroquel Tablets (Infrequent) 691
Sonata Capsules (Infrequent) 1686
Symbyax Capsules (Frequent) 1788
Tasmar Tablets (2%) 3360
Tequin Injection (Less than 0.1%) 964
Tequin Tablets (Less than 0.1%) 964
▲ Thalomid Capsules (4.2%) 979
Thioridazine Hydrochloride Tablets 2122
Tiazac Capsules (1%) 1204
▲ Trisenox Injection (13%) 983
Uniretic Tablets (Less than 1%) 3114
Vantas (Less than 2%) 3367
Vivelle Transdermal System 2288
Vivelle-Dot Transdermal System 2293
Wellbutrin SR Sustained-Release Tablets (At least 1%) 1583
Wellbutrin XL Extended-Release Tablets (At least 1%) 1588
Xifaxan Tablets (Less than 2%) 2847
Zestoretic Tablets 701
Zestril Tablets (0.3% to 1.0%) 704
Zomig Nasal Spray (Infrequent) 718
Zyban Sustained-Release Tablets (2%) 1620
▲ Zyprexa Tablets (2% to 3%) 1798
Zyprexa ZYDIS Orally Disintegrating Tablets (2% to 3%) 1798

Total proteins, decrease

(*see under* Hypoproteinemia)

Tourette's syndrome

Adderall Tablets 3168
Adderall XR Capsules 3169
Concerta Extended-Release Tablets (Rare) 1828
Desoxyn Tablets, USP 2482
Dexedrine 1386
DextroStat Tablets 3177
Focalin Tablets (Rare) 2214
Focalin XR Capsules 2217
Meridia Capsules 485
Metadate CD Capsules (Rare) 3316
Ritalin Hydrochloride Tablets (Rare) 2254
Ritalin LA Capsules (Rare) 2255
Ritalin-SR Tablets (Rare) 2254

Toxic granulation

Efudex 3348

Toxic shock syndrome

Amevive 836

Toxicity, bone marrow

Pegasys 2793

Toxicity, hepatic

Hexalen Capsules (Less than 1%) 2101
Pacerone Tablets 3337

Toxicity, local

▲ Ellence Injection (0.3% to 19.5%) 2632

Toxicity, vascular
Gemzar for Injection (Very rare)........ 1743

Toxoplasmosis
Doxil Injection.................................. 3302

Tracheitis
Advair Diskus 100/50 1291
Advair Diskus 250/50 1291
Advair Diskus 500/50 1291
Amerge Tablets (Rare)...................... 1312
Lexapro Oral Solution (Infrequent).... 1193
Lexapro Tablets (Infrequent)............. 1193
Liquid PedvaxHIB (One case)............ 2012
▲ Serevent Diskus (7%) 1540

Tracheobronchitis
Avalide Tablets................................ 922
Avalide Tablets................................ 2889
Avapro Tablets (Less than 1%).......... 925
Avapro Tablets (Less than 1%).......... 2886

Transaminase, elevation
(*see under* Serum transaminase, elevation)

Transfusion reactions
▲ Clolar for Intravenous Infusion (10%)... 1264

Trauma
Caverject Impulse Injection (2%)....... 2610
▲ Cozaar Tablets (4%) 1913
Exelon Capsules (Frequent).............. 2204
Foradil Aerolizer (1.2%).................... 3024
▲ Gengraf Capsules (4%) 458
▲ Neoral Soft Gelatin Capsules (4%) ... 2247
▲ Neoral Oral Solution (4%) 2247
▲ Simulect for Injection (3% to 10%) ... 2268
Singulair (1%).................................. 2047
Starlix Tablets (2.9%)....................... 2276
▲ Zelnorm Tablets (3%) 2303

Trauma, unspecified
Ambien Tablets (Infrequent).............. 2867
Effexor Tablets (2%)......................... 3405
Invirase (Less than 2%).................... 2776
▲ Lescol Capsules (5.1%) 2227
▲ Lescol Capsules (5.1%) 2730
▲ Lescol XL Tablets (4.2%) 2227
▲ Lescol XL Tablets (4.2%) 2730
Neurontin Capsules (Frequent).......... 2498
Neurontin Oral Solution (Frequent).... 2498
Neurontin Tablets (Frequent)............ 2498
Paxil CR Controlled-Release Tablets (1.4%).................................. 1509
▲ Paxil (1.4% to 6%) 1501
Pravachol Tablets............................. 943
Prinzide Tablets (0.3% to 1%)............ 2033
Zestoretic Tablets (0.3% to 1%)......... 701
▲ Zyvox (2.8% to 3.3%) 2661

Trembling
(*see under* Tremors)

Tremor, fine hand
Eskalith 1406
Lithobid Tablets............................... 1670

Tremors
▲ Abilify Tablets (3% to 9%) 916
▲ Abilify Tablets (3% to 9%) 2472
Aciphex Tablets 1081
Adalat CC Tablets (Rare)................... 2978
Adderall Tablets............................... 3168
Adderall XR Capsules....................... 3169
Adenoscan (Less than 1%)................ 613
Adipex-P.. 1216
▲ Advair Diskus 100/50 (1% to 3%) ... 1291
▲ Advair Diskus 250/50 (1% to 3%) ... 1291
▲ Advair Diskus 500/50 (1% to 3%) ... 1291
Advicor Tablets 1694
▲ Aerobid/Aerobid-M (3% to 9%) 1172
Alacol DM Syrup 739
Alferon N Injection (One patient)....... 1640
Alimta for Injection (Less than 1%).... 1722
Alinia for Oral Suspension (Less than 1%).. 2840
Alinia Tablets (Less than 1%)............ 2840
Aloprim for Injection (Less than 1%)... 2156
Altace Capsules (Less than 1%)........ 1673
Altoprev Extended-Release Tablets.... 1151
▲ Alupent Inhalation Aerosol (About 1 in 20 patients)........................... 858
Ambien Tablets (Infrequent).............. 2867
AmBisome for Injection (Less common)... 615
Amerge Tablets (Infrequent).............. 1312
Ammonul Injection 3323
Anaprox Tablets (Less than 1%)....... 2769
Anaprox DS Tablets (Less than 1%).. 2769
Anzemet Injection (Infrequently)........ 2871
Anzemet Tablets (Infrequently)......... 2874
Aricept Tablets (Frequent)................ 1086
Aricept ODT Tablets (Frequent)........ 1086
Arthrotec Tablets (Rare)................... 3126
Asacol Delayed-Release Tablets........ 2688
Atrovent Inhalation Solution (0.9%)... 868
Avalide Tablets................................ 922
Avalide Tablets................................ 2889
Avapro Tablets (Less than 1%)......... 925
Avapro Tablets (Less than 1%)......... 2886
Avelox (0.1% to less than 2%).......... 2984
Avinza Capsules (Less than 5%)....... 1714
Axert Tablets (Infrequent)................ 2430
Balamine DM 739
▲ BeneFix for Injection (3.1%) 3402
Biaxin/Biaxin XL.............................. 402
Buprenex Injectable (Infrequent)....... 2718
Caduet Tablets (Greater than 0.1% to less than or equal to 1%).......... 2507
Calcium Disodium Versenate Injection 1819
▲ Campath Ampules (7%) 826
Campral Tablets (Frequent) 1175
Cancidas for Injection (0% to 1.8%)... 1894
Cardizem LA Extended Release Tablets (Less than 2%) 1699
Carimune NF 3501
Cataflam Tablets (Occasionally) 2173
▲ Celexa (8%) 1177
▲ CellCept Capsules (24.2% to 33.9%) 2751
▲ CellCept Intravenous (24.2% to 33.9%) 2751
▲ CellCept Oral Suspension (24.2% to 33.9%) 2751
▲ CellCept Tablets (24.2% to 33.9%) 2751
Cipro I.V. (1% or less) 2998
Cipro I.V. Pharmacy Bulk Package (1% or less) 3509
Cipro (Less than 1%) 2991
Cipro XR Tablets (Less than 1%) 3004
▲ Clolar for Intravenous Infusion (10%) 1264
▲ Clozapine Tablets (More than 5% to 6%) 2141
▲ Clozaril Tablets (More than 5% to 6%) 2174
Colazal Capsules 2845
Combivent Inhalation Aerosol (Less than 2%) 878
▲ Copaxone for Injection (7%) 3292
Covera-HS Tablets (Less than 2%) 3135
Cozaar Tablets (Less than 1%) 1913
▲ Cymbalta Delayed-Release Capsules (Up to 5%) 1729
Cytovene (At least 3 subjects) 2763
Daranide Tablets 1928
▲ Demser Capsules (10%) 1933
▲ Depacon Injection (0.6% to 57%) 412
▲ Depakene (25% to 57%) 417
▲ Depakote Sprinkle Capsules (19% to 57%) 422
▲ Depakote Tablets (9% to 57%) 427
▲ Depakote ER Tablets (9% to 57%) ... 433
Desoxyn Tablets, USP 2482
Dexedrine 1386
DextroStat Tablets 3177
Dilaudid 439
Dilaudid Oral Liquid (Less frequent) 443
Dilaudid Non-Sterile Powder 439
Dilaudid Rectal Suppositories 439
Dilaudid Tablets 439
Dilaudid Tablets - 8 mg (Less frequent) 443
Dilaudid-HP (Less frequent) 441
Diprivan Injectable Emulsion (Less than 1%) 676
Duragesic Transdermal System (1% or greater) 2448
Dyazide Capsules 1389
EC-Naprosyn Delayed-Release Tablets (Less than 1%) 2769
▲ Effexor Tablets (5% to 10.2%) 3405
▲ Effexor XR Capsules (4% to 5%) 3411
Eldepryl Capsules 3209
Eligard 7.5 mg (Less than 2%) 2896
Elspar for Injection 1943
▲ Entocort EC Capsules (Less than 5%) 2694
EpiPen 1061
Eskalith 1406
▲ Evoxac Capsules (1% to 3%) 1042
▲ Exelon Capsules (4%) 2204
Factive Tablets (Less than or equal to 0.1%) 2464
▲ FazaClo Orally Disintegrating Tablets (Less than 1% to 6%) 547
Flexeril Tablets (Less than 1%) 1832
▲ Flolan for Injection (7% to 21%) 1408
Floxin Otic Singles (Reported in a single subject) 1045
Floxin Otic Solution (Single report)... 1043
Flumadine (Less than 0.3%)............. 1186
Foradil Aerolizer (1.9%)................... 3024
Frova Tablets (Infrequent)................ 1101
▲ Gabitril Tablets (9%) 998
Gammagard Liquid 751
Gammagard S/D 754
Gamunex Immune Globulin I.V., 10%... 3232
▲ Gengraf Capsules (13%) 458
▲ Geodon Capsules (14%) 2514
Guanidine Hydrochloride Tablets 3030
▲ Humira Injection (Less than 5%) 464
Hyzaar.. 1964
▲ Imdur Tablets (Less than or equal to 5%).. 3032
Imitrex Injection (Infrequent)............ 1431
Imitrex Nasal Spray (Infrequent)....... 1435
Imitrex Tablets (Rare to infrequent)... 1440
Infed Injection................................. 3381
▲ Intron A for Injection (Less than 5%)... 3038
Invanz for Injection (Greater than 0.1%).. 1974
Inversine Tablets............................. 3286
Invirase (Less than 2%).................... 2776
Iveegam EN.................................... 759
Kadian Capsules (Less than 3%)....... 572
Kaletra (Less than 2%)..................... 474
Keppra Oral Solution (1% to 2%)...... 3307
Keppra Tablets (1% to 2%).............. 3307
Klonopin (Infrequent)....................... 2782
▲ Lamictal (4% to 10%) 1449
Lariam Tablets (Occasional)............. 2790
Lescol Capsules.............................. 2227
Lescol Capsules.............................. 2730
Lescol XL Tablets 2227
Lescol XL Tablets 2730
Leukeran Tablets (Rare)................... 1472
Levaquin in 5% Dextrose Injection (0.1% to 0.9%)............................... 2453
Levaquin (0.1% to 0.9%).................. 2453
Levothroid Tablets........................... 1189
Levoxyl Tablets 1680
Lexapro Oral Solution (Infrequent).... 1193
Lexapro Tablets (Infrequent)............ 1193
Lidoderm Patch 1107
Lithobid Tablets 1670
Lotrel Capsules 2238
Lotronex Tablets (Rare).................... 1479
Lunesta Tablets (Rare)..................... 3139
▲ Lyrica Capsules (1% to 11%) 2524
Matulane Capsules 3188
▲ Maxair Autohaler (1.3% to 6.0%) 1820
Maxalt Tablets (Frequent)................. 1983
Maxalt-MLT Orally Disintegrating Tablets (Frequent)......................... 1983
Meridia Capsules............................. 485
Mevacor Tablets (0.5% to 1.0%)....... 1996
Midamor Tablets (Less than or equal to 1%)................................... 2000
Migranal Nasal Spray (Infrequent)..... 3350
Mirapex Tablets (1% or more)........... 889
Moban Tablets 1108
Mobic Oral Suspension (Less than 2%)... 893
Mobic Tablets (Less than 2%)........... 893
Moduretic Tablets 2003
MS Contin Tablets (Less frequent).... 2703
▲ Myfortic Tablets (3% to less than 20%)... 2244
Nalfon Capsules (2.2%).................... 2504
Namenda (Infrequent)...................... 1199
Naprosyn Suspension (Less than 1%)... 2769
Naprosyn Tablets (Less than 1%)..... 2769
Narcan Injection.............................. 1109
Naropin Injection (Less than 1%)...... 640
Natrecor for Injection (Greater than or equal to 1%)......................... 3123
▲ Neoral Soft Gelatin Capsules (12% to 55%)...................................... 2247
▲ Neoral Oral Solution (12% to 55%)... 2247
▲ Neurontin Capsules (1% to 6.8%) 2498
▲ Neurontin Oral Solution (1% to 6.8%)... 2498
▲ Neurontin Tablets (1% to 6.8%) 2498
Nexium Delayed-Release Capsules (Less than 1%)............................ 645
Nexium I.V. (Less than 1%)............... 649
▲ Nicotrol NS (Greater than 5%) 2596
▲ Niravam Orally Disintegrating Tablets (4%)................................. 3106
Norflex Injection.............................. 1824
Noroxin Tablets............................... 2009
Norvasc Tablets (More than 0.1% to 1%).. 2529
Norvir (Less than 2%)...................... 499
Nubain Injection (1% or less)............ 1111
Orap Tablets (2.7%)........................ 1220
▲ Orthoclone OKT3 Sterile Solution (13%).. 2370
OxyContin Tablets (Less than 1%).... 2699
▲ Pacerone Tablets (4% to 9%) 3337
Parnate Tablets 1499
▲ Paxil CR Controlled-Release Tablets (5% to 14.7%).................... 1509
▲ Paxil (1% to 14.7%) 1501
▲ Permax Tablets (4.2%) 3357
Phenergan....................................... 3438
Phenytek Capsules (Rare)................ 2153
Pravachol Tablets 943
Prevacid Delayed-Release Capsules (Less than 1%)................ 3268
Prevacid for Delayed-Release Oral Suspension (Less than 1%)........... 3268
Prevacid NapraPAC (Less than 1%).. 3277
Prevacid SoluTab Delayed-Release Orally Disintegrating Tablets (Less than 1%).............................. 3268
PREVPAC (Less than 1%)................. 3281
Prilosec OTC Tablets (Less than 1%)... 2674
Primaxin I.M. 2022
Primaxin I.V. (Less than 0.2%).......... 2024
Prinivil Tablets (0.3% to 1.0%).......... 2029
Prinzide Tablets 2033
Prochieve 4% Gel 1018
Prochieve 8% Gel 1018
▲ Prograf Capsules and Injection (48% to 56%)................................. 624
ProSom Tablets (Rare)..................... 512
Protonix I.V. (Less than 1%)............. 3468
Protonix Tablets (Less than 1%) 3465
▲ Proventil Inhalation Aerosol (Less than 15%)...................................... 3067
▲ Proventil Inhalation Solution 0.083% (10.7% to 20%) 3069
▲ Proventil HFA Inhalation Aerosol (7%)... 3071
Provigil Tablets (1%) 1002
▲ Prozac Pulvules and Liquid (3% to 13%)... 1771
▲ Rapamune Oral Solution and Tablets (21% to 31%)..................... 3472
▲ Razadyne ER Extended-Release Capsules (3%)............................... 2434
▲ Razadyne (3%) 2434
Relafen Tablets (Less than 1%) 1523
Relpax Tablets (Infrequent) 2531
Requip Tablets (1% or more) 1528
Rescriptor Tablets 2535
Retrovir Capsules 1533
Retrovir IV Infusion 1537
Retrovir 1533
Rilutek Tablets (Frequent) 2945
▲ Risperdal Consta Long-Acting Injection (Up to 3%) 1664
▲ Risperdal M-Tab Orally Disintegrating Tablets (17% to 34%)... 1658
▲ Risperdal (17% to 34%) 1658
▲ Roferon-A Injection (Less than 3%) .. 2805
Rythmol SR Capsules (2%) 2736
▲ Sandimmune (12% to 55%) 2259
Sandostatin Injection (Less than 1%) 2263
Sandostatin LAR Depot (1% to 4%) .. 2264
Sedapap Tablets 50 mg/650 mg (Infrequent) 2098
Seromycin Capsules 1783
▲ Simulect for Injection (Greater than or equal to 10%) 2268
Sonata Capsules (2%) 1686
Stalevo Tablets 2270
▲ Strattera Capsules (1% to 4%) 1784
Stromectol Tablets (0.9%) 2053
Sular Tablets (Less than or equal to 1%) 1163
Surmontil Capsules 2347
Sustiva Capsules (Less than 2%) 957
▲ Symbyax Capsules (Greater than or equal to 5% to 9%) 1788
Symmetrel 1115
▲ Tambocor Tablets (4.7%) 1824
Tarka Tablets 519
Tasmar Tablets (Frequent) 3360
▲ Tequin Injection (0.1% to 3%) 964
▲ Tequin Tablets (0.1% to 3%) 964
Teveten Tablets (Less than 1%) 1707
Teveten HCT Tablets (Less than 1%) 1710
▲ Thalomid Capsules (4.2%) 979
Thioridazine Hydrochloride Tablets .. 2122
Thyrolar 1203
Tiazac Capsules (Less than 2%) 1204
▲ Topamax Sprinkle Capsules (Greater than 1% to 9%) 2438
▲ Topamax Tablets (Greater than 1% to 9%) 2438
Tranxene 2488
▲ Trileptal Oral Suspension (3% to 16%) 2281
▲ Trileptal Tablets (3% to 16%) 2281
▲ Trisenox Injection (13%) 983
▲ Ultane Liquid for Inhalation (6%) 526
Ultracet Tablets (At least 1%) 2462

Unithroid Tablets 3521
Valium Tablets (Infrequent) 2822
Vantas (Less than 2%) 3367
Vantin Tablets and Oral Suspension (Less than 1%) 2650
Verelan PM Capsules (2% or less) 3120
▲ Vesanoid Capsules (3%) 2823
VFEND I.V. (Less than 2%) 2543
VFEND Oral Suspension (Less than 2%) 2543
VFEND Tablets (Less than 2%) 2543
Viadur Implant (Rare) 782
Viagra Tablets (Less than 2%) 2552
Vicoprofen Tablets (Less than 1%) 533
Vivactil Tablets 2350
Voltaren Tablets (Occasionally) 2298
Voltaren-XR Tablets (Occasionally) 2301
▲ VoSpire Extended-Release Tablets (24.2% to 37.9%) 2352
Vytorin 10/10 Tablets 2084
Vytorin 10/10 Tablets 3092
Vytorin 10/20 Tablets 2084
Vytorin 10/20 Tablets 3092
Vytorin 10/40 Tablets 2084
Vytorin 10/40 Tablets 3092
Vytorin 10/80 Tablets 2084
Vytorin 10/80 Tablets 3092
▲ Wellbutrin Tablets (21.1%) 1579
▲ Wellbutrin SR Sustained-Release Tablets (3% to 6%) 1583
▲ Wellbutrin XL Extended-Release Tablets (3% to 6%) 1588
▲ Xanax XR Tablets (28.2%) 2655
▲ Xeloda Tablets (Less than 5%) 2825
▲ Xopenex HFA Inhalation Aerosol (6.8%) 3151
▲ Xopenex Inhalation Solution (6.8%) 3143
▲ Xopenex Inhalation Solution Concentrate (6.8%) 3147
▲ Zavesca Capsules (11% to 30%) 543
Zegerid Powder for Oral Solution (Less than 1%) 2972
▲ Zenapax for Injection (Greater than 5%) 2838
Zestoretic Tablets 701
Zestril Tablets (0.3% to 1.0%) 704
Zocor Tablets 2078
▲ Zofran Injection (7%) 1607
▲ Zofran (5%) 1613
▲ Zofran ODT Orally Disintegrating Tablets (5%) 1613
▲ Zoloft (Less than 1% to 11%) 2581
Zomig Nasal Spray (Infrequent) 718
Zonegran Capsules (Frequent) 1089
Zosyn (1.0% or less) 3492
Zovirax Capsules 1616
Zovirax for Injection (Approximately 1%) 1618
Zovirax 1616
Zyban Sustained-Release Tablets (1% to 2%) 1620
▲ Zyprexa Tablets (Up to 20%) 1798
Zyprexa IntraMuscular (1%) 1798
▲ Zyprexa ZYDIS Orally Disintegrating Tablets (Up to 20%) 1798
Zyrtec Chewable Tablets (Less than 2%) 2589
Zyrtec (Less than 2%) 2589
Zyrtec-D 12 Hour Extended Release Tablets (Less than 2%) 2591

Tremors, extremities
Abilify Tablets (Infrequent) 916
Abilify Tablets (Infrequent) 2472

Tremulousness
(*see under* Tremors)

Trichomoniasis, vulvovaginal
Clindesse Vaginal Cream (Less than 1%) 3296

Trigeminal neuralgia
(*see under* Neuralgia, trigeminal)

Trigeminy
Digitek Tablets 2146
Lanoxicaps Capsules 1458
Lanoxin Injection 1462
Lanoxin Tablets 1468
Lanoxin Injection Pediatric 1465
Rituxan for Infusion (One case) 845

Triglycerides, increase
(*see under* Hypertriglyceridemia)

Trismus
Ceftin Tablets (0.1% to 1%) 1369
Demser Capsules 1933
Effexor Tablets (Frequent) 3405
Effexor XR Capsules (2%) 3411
Geodon Capsules (Rare) 2514
Lyrica Capsules (Rare) 2524
Parcopa Orally Disintegrating Tablets 3111
Paxil CR Controlled-Release Tablets (Rare) 1509
Paxil (Rare) 1501
Rilutek Tablets (Rare) 2945
Sonata Capsules (Rare) 1686
Stalevo Tablets 2270
Thioridazine Hydrochloride Tablets 2122
▲ Ventavis Inhalation Solution (12%) 1036

TSH, decrease
Thyrolar 1203

Tuberculosis
Campath Ampules 826
CellCept Capsules 2751
CellCept Intravenous 2751
CellCept Oral Suspension 2751
CellCept Tablets 2751
Enbrel for Injection 580
Fuzeon Injection 2772
Humira Injection 464
Myfortic Tablets 2244
Remicade for IV Injection 987

Tubulopathy
Truvada Tablets 1279

Tumor flare
▲ Arimidex Tablets (3%) 665
Gengraf Capsules (1% to less than 3%) 458
Invirase (Less than 2%) 2776
Neoral Soft Gelatin Capsules (1% to less than 3%) 2247
Neoral Oral Solution (1% to less than 3%) 2247
▲ Zoladex (23%) 709

Tumor lysis syndrome
Aloprim for Injection (Less than 1%) 2156
Campath Ampules 826
Ellence Injection 2632
Leustatin Injection (Rare) 2368
Mylotarg for Injection 3429
Rituxan for Infusion 845
Rituxan I.V. 1251
Velcade for Injection 2102

Tumors, solid, non-cutaneous
Raptiva 1247

T-wave, inverted
Ultane Liquid for Inhalation (Less than 1%) 526

T-wave flattening
(*see under* EKG changes, T-wave)

Twitching
Abilify Tablets (Infrequent) 916
Abilify Tablets (Infrequent) 2472
Aciphex Tablets (Rare) 1081
▲ Adderall XR Capsules (2% to 4%) 3169
Aloprim for Injection (Less than 1%) 2156
Anzemet Injection (Rare) 2871
Anzemet Tablets (Rare) 2874
Caduet Tablets (Less than or equal to 0.1%) 2507
Campral Tablets (Rare) 1175
Cipro I.V. 2998
Cipro I.V. Pharmacy Bulk Package 3509
Cipro 2991
Cipro XR Tablets 3004
Clozapine Tablets (Less than 1%) 2141
Clozaril Tablets (Less than 1%) 2174
Concerta Extended-Release Tablets (1%) 1828
▲ Depacon Injection (1% to 5%) 412
▲ Depakene (1% to 5%) 417
▲ Depakote Tablets (1% to 5%) 427
Depakote ER Tablets (Greater than 1%) 433
Desoxyn Tablets, USP 2482
Diprivan Injectable Emulsion (Less than 1%) 676
Effexor Tablets (1%) 3405
Effexor XR Capsules (2%) 3411
Eskalith 1406
FazaClo Orally Disintegrating Tablets (Less than 1%) 547
Focalin XR Capsules 2217
Gabitril Tablets (1% or more) 998
▲ Geodon Capsules (14%) 2514
Imitrex Tablets (Rare) 1440
Klonopin (Infrequent) 2782
Lamictal (Infrequent) 1449
Lexapro Oral Solution (Infrequent) 1193
Lexapro Tablets (Infrequent) 1193
Lidoderm Patch 1107
Lunesta Tablets (Infrequent) 3139
▲ Lyrica Capsules (4% to 5%) 2524
Meridia Capsules 485
Mirapex Tablets (Greater than or equal to 1% to 2%) 889
Neurontin Capsules (1.3%) 2498
Neurontin Oral Solution (1.3%) 2498
Neurontin Tablets (1.3%) 2498
Nipent for Injection (Less than 3%) 3216
Norvasc Tablets (Less than or equal to 0.1%) 2529
Norvir (Less than 2%) 499
▲ OxyContin Tablets (Between 1% and 5%) 2699
Permax Tablets (1.1%) 3357
Phenytek Capsules 2153
ProSom Tablets (Infrequent) 512
Relpax Tablets (Rare) 2531
Retrovir Capsules 1533
Retrovir IV Infusion 1537
Retrovir 1533
Reyataz Capsules (Less than 3%) 948
Seroquel Tablets (Infrequent) 691
▲ Symbyax Capsules (2% to 6%) 1788
Tambocor Tablets (Less than 1%) 1824
Tasmar Tablets (Infrequent) 3360
Wellbutrin SR Sustained-Release Tablets (1% to 2%) 1583
Wellbutrin XL Extended-Release Tablets (1% to 2%) 1588
Zoloft (Infrequent) 2581
Zomig Nasal Spray (Rare) 718
Zomig Tablets (Rare) 714
Zomig-ZMT Tablets (Rare) 714
Zonegran Capsules (Infrequent) 1089
Zyban Sustained-Release Tablets (Infrequent) 1620
▲ Zyprexa Tablets (1% to 5%) 1798
Zyprexa IntraMuscular (Infrequent) 1798
Zyprexa ZYDIS Orally Disintegrating Tablets (1% to 5%) 1798
Zyrtec Chewable Tablets (Less than 2%) 2589
Zyrtec (Less than 2%) 2589
Zyrtec-D 12 Hour Extended Release Tablets (Less than 2%) 2591

Twitching, lid muscle
Neurontin Capsules (Infrequent) 2498
Neurontin Oral Solution (Infrequent) 2498
Neurontin Tablets (Infrequent) 2498

Tympanic membrane perforation
▲ Imdur Tablets (Less than or equal to 5%) 3032

Tympanometry, abnormal
▲ Increlex Injection (Greater than or equal to 5%) 3290

Typhlitis
Adriamycin for Injection, USP 786
Adriamycin Injection, USP 786

U

Ulceration
Adriamycin for Injection, USP 786
Adriamycin Injection, USP 786
▲ Aldara Cream, 5% (Up to 8%) 1814
▲ Efudex (Among most frequent) 3348
Eulexin Capsules 3023
K-Tab Filmtab Tablets 473

Ulceration, bucial mucosa
Invirase (Greater than or equal to 2%) 2776
Nalfon Capsules (Less than 1%) 2504

Ulceration, tongue
Evoxac Capsules (Less than 1%) 1042
▲ Invirase (Up to 3.8%) 2776
Rescriptor Tablets 2535
Soriatane Capsules (Less than 1%) 1028
Zoloft (Rare) 2581

Ulcers
Paxil CR Controlled-Release Tablets (Rare) 1509
Paxil (Rare) 1501
▲ Vesanoid Capsules (3%) 2823
Zoladex (1% to 5%) 709
Zoladex 3-month 712

Ulcers, aphthous
Captopril Tablets (About 0.5% to 2%) 2114

Ulcers, corneal
Copaxone for Injection (Infrequent) 3292
FML Ophthalmic Ointment (Occasional) ⊙ 225
FML Ophthalmic Suspension (Occasional) ⊙ 224
FML Forte Ophthalmic Suspension (Occasional) ⊙ 223
FML-S Liquifilm Sterile Ophthalmic Suspension ⊙ 226
Genoptic Sterile Ophthalmic Solution ⊙ 227
HMS Sterile Ophthalmic Suspension ⊙ 228
Lyrica Capsules (Rare) 2524
Poly-Pred Liquifilm Ophthalmic Suspension ⊙ 231

Ulcers, cutaneous
Actiq (1% or greater) 993
AmBisome for Injection (Less common) 615
▲ Arava Tablets (1% to 3%) 2881
Aricept Tablets (Infrequent) 1086
Aricept ODT Tablets (Infrequent) 1086
Arthrotec Tablets (Rare) 3126
▲ CellCept Capsules (3% to less than 20%) 2751
▲ CellCept Intravenous (3% to less than 20%) 2751
▲ CellCept Oral Suspension (3% to less than 20%) 2751
▲ CellCept Tablets (3% to less than 20%) 2751
Colazal Capsules 2845
Doxil Injection (Less than 1%) 3302
Enbrel for Injection 580
Eskalith 1406
Evoxac Capsules (Less than 1%) 1042
Exelon Capsules (Infrequent) 2204
▲ Flolan for Injection (39%) 1408
Gabitril Tablets (Infrequent) 998
Gengraf Capsules 458
Herceptin I.V. (At least one of the 958 patients) 1234
Invirase (Less than 2%) 2776
Kaletra (Less than 2%) 474
Levaquin in 5% Dextrose Injection (0.1% to 0.9%) 2453
Levaquin (0.1% to 0.9%) 2453
Lipitor Tablets (Less than 2%) 2495
Lithobid Tablets 1670
Lofibra Capsules 1217
Miacalcin Nasal Spray (Less than 1%) 2242
Neoral Soft Gelatin Capsules 2247
Neoral Oral Solution 2247
Neurontin Capsules (Infrequent) 2498
Neurontin Oral Solution (Infrequent) 2498
Neurontin Tablets (Infrequent) 2498
Paxil CR Controlled-Release Tablets (Rare) 1509
Paxil (Rare) 1501
Permax Tablets (Infrequent) 3357
Plavix Tablets (1% to 2.5%) 940
Plavix Tablets (1% to 2.5%) 2942
▲ Prograf Capsules and Injection (3% to 15%) 624
Protonix I.V. (Less than 1%) 3468
Protonix Tablets (Less than 1%) 3465
Prozac Pulvules and Liquid (Infrequent) 1771
▲ Rapamune Oral Solution and Tablets (3% to 20%) 3472
Remicade for IV Injection (Greater than or equal to 0.2%) 987
Requip Tablets (Infrequent) 1528
Rilutek Tablets (Infrequent) 2945
Risperdal M-Tab Orally Disintegrating Tablets (Rare) 1658
Risperdal (Rare) 1658
▲ Simulect for Injection (3% to 10%) 2268
▲ Soriatane Capsules (1% to 10%) 1028
Sular Tablets (Less than or equal to 1%) 1163
Tricor Tablets 523
Viagra Tablets (Less than 2%) 2552
▲ Xeloda Tablets (Less than 5%) 2825
Zyprexa Tablets (Infrequent) 1798
Zyprexa ZYDIS Orally Disintegrating Tablets (Infrequent) 1798

Ulcers, duodenal
Abilify Tablets (Rare) 916
Abilify Tablets (Rare) 2472
Agrylin Capsules 3172
▲ Anaprox Tablets (1% to 10%) 2769
▲ Anaprox DS Tablets (1% to 10%) 2769
Antara Capsules 2723
Aricept Tablets (Infrequent) 1086
Aricept ODT Tablets (Infrequent) 1086
Caduet Tablets (Less than 2%) 2507
Campath Ampules 826
Campral Tablets (Rare) 1175

▲ Cataflam Tablets (1% to 10%) 2173
Celexa (Rare) 1177
Copaxone for Injection (Infrequent) 3292
Dostinex Tablets (Rare) 2631
▲ EC-Naprosyn Delayed-Release Tablets (1% to 10%) 2769
Exelon Capsules (Infrequent) 2204
Fosamax 1949
Fosamax Plus D Tablets 1956
Indocin Capsules (Less than 1%) 1968
Indocin I.V. (Less than 1%) 1973
Indocin (Less than 1%) 1968
Lipitor Tablets (Less than 2%) 2495
Lofibra Capsules 1217
Meridia Capsules 485
Mobic Oral Suspension (Less than 2%) 893
Mobic Tablets (Less than 2%) 893
Myfortic Tablets 2244
▲ Naprosyn Suspension (1% to 10%) 2769
▲ Naprosyn Tablets (1% to 10%) 2769
Neurontin Capsules (Rare) 2498
Neurontin Oral Solution (Rare) 2498
Neurontin Tablets (Rare) 2498
Parcopa Orally Disintegrating Tablets 3111
Pentasa Capsules (Less than 1%) 3182
Pletal Tablets (Less than 2%) 2478
Proleukin for Injection (Less than 1%) 1007
Prozac Pulvules and Liquid (Rare) 1771
Relafen Tablets (Less than 1%) 1523
Sonata Capsules (Rare) 1686
Stalevo Tablets 2270
Tasmar Tablets (Rare) 3360
Taxotere Injection Concentrate 2947
Tricor Tablets 523
Triglide Tablets 1165
Trileptal Oral Suspension 2281
Trileptal Tablets 2281
VFEND I.V. (Less than 2%) 2543
VFEND Oral Suspension (Less than 2%) 2543
VFEND Tablets (Less than 2%) 2543
▲ Voltaren Tablets (1% to 10%) 2298
▲ Voltaren-XR Tablets (1% to 10%) 2301
Zonegran Capsules (Infrequent) 1089
Zosyn (1.3%) 3492

Ulcers, duodenal, hemorrhagic

Mobic Oral Suspension (Less than 2%) 893
Mobic Tablets (Less than 2%) 893

Ulcers, esophageal

Accutane Capsules 2740
Actonel Tablets 2679
Amnesteem Capsules 2126
Copaxone for Injection (Infrequent) 3292
Doxil Injection (Less than 1%) 3302
Effexor Tablets (Rare) 3405
Fosamax (0.1% to 1.5%) 1949
Herceptin I.V. (At least one of the 958 patients) 1234
Lyrica Capsules (Rare) 2524
Namenda (Infrequent) 1199
Nexium Delayed-Release Capsules (Less than 1%) 645
Nexium I.V. (Less than 1%) 649
Pentasa Capsules (Less than 1%) 3182
Permax Tablets (Rare) 3357
Prevacid NapraPAC (Less than 1%) 3277
Prozac Pulvules and Liquid (Rare) 1771
Reyataz Capsules (Less than 3%) 948
VFEND I.V. (Less than 2%) 2543
VFEND Oral Suspension (Less than 2%) 2543
VFEND Tablets (Less than 2%) 2543
Zyprexa Tablets (Rare) 1798
Zyprexa ZYDIS Orally Disintegrating Tablets (Rare) 1798

Ulcers, gastric

Actonel Tablets 2679
Actonel with Calcium Tablets 2684
Agrylin Capsules 3172
Amerge Tablets (Rare) 1312
▲ Anaprox Tablets (1% to 10%) 2769
▲ Anaprox DS Tablets (1% to 10%) 2769
Campral Tablets (Rare) 1175
▲ Cataflam Tablets (1% to 10%) 2173
Celexa (Rare) 1177
Cymbalta Delayed-Release Capsules (Infrequent) 1729
▲ EC-Naprosyn Delayed-Release Tablets (1% to 10%) 2769
Evoxac Capsules (Less than 1%) 1042
Exelon Capsules (Infrequent) 2204
FazaClo Orally Disintegrating Tablets (Less than 1%) 547
Fosamax (Up to 1.1%) 1949
Fosamax Plus D Tablets (0% to 1.1%) 1956
Gengraf Capsules (1% to less than 3%) 458
Lunesta Tablets (Rare) 3139
Meridia Capsules 485
Mobic Oral Suspension (Less than 2%) 893
Mobic Tablets (Less than 2%) 893
Myfortic Tablets 2244
▲ Naprosyn Suspension (1% to 10%) 2769
▲ Naprosyn Tablets (1% to 10%) 2769
Neoral Soft Gelatin Capsules (1% to less than 3%) 2247
Neoral Oral Solution (1% to less than 3%) 2247
Nexium Delayed-Release Capsules (Less than 1%) 645
Nexium I.V. (Less than 1%) 649
Plavix Tablets (Less than 1%) 940
Plavix Tablets (Less than 1%) 2942
Pletal Tablets (Less than 2%) 2478
Prozac Pulvules and Liquid (Infrequent) 1771
Requip Tablets (Infrequent) 1528
Risperdal Consta Long-Acting Injection (Infrequent) 1664
Sandostatin Injection (Less than 1%) 2263
Sandostatin LAR Depot (Rare) 2264
Thalomid Capsules 979
Trileptal Oral Suspension 2281
Trileptal Tablets 2281
▲ Voltaren Tablets (1% to 10%) 2298
▲ Voltaren-XR Tablets (1% to 10%) 2301
Wellbutrin SR Sustained-Release Tablets 1583
Wellbutrin XL Extended-Release Tablets 1588
Zonegran Capsules (Infrequent) 1089

Ulcers, gastrointestinal

Adriamycin for Injection, USP 786
Adriamycin Injection, USP 786
Aggrenox Capsules (Less than 1%) 855
▲ Anaprox Tablets (1% to 10%) 2769
▲ Anaprox DS Tablets (1% to 10%) 2769
Arthrotec Tablets 3126
Bayer Aspirin Tablets 3515
▲ Cataflam Tablets (1% to 10%) 2173
CellCept Capsules (Infrequent) 2751
CellCept Intravenous (Infrequent) 2751
CellCept Oral Suspension (Infrequent) 2751
CellCept Tablets (Infrequent) 2751
Clinoril Tablets 1899
Clozapine Tablets (Less than 1%) 2141
Clozaril Tablets (Less than 1%) 2174
Combunox Tablets 1183
Cosmegen for Injection 1907
Dolobid Tablets 1937
Dostinex Tablets (Rare) 2631
▲ EC-Naprosyn Delayed-Release Tablets (1% to 10%) 2769
Ecotrin Enteric Coated Aspirin Low, Regular and Maximum Strength Tablets 1627
Effexor Tablets (Infrequent) 3405
Effexor XR Capsules (Infrequent) 3411
Gleevec Tablets (Infrequent) 2221
Indocin Capsules (Less than 1%) 1968
Indocin I.V. (Less than 1%) 1973
Indocin (Less than 1%) 1968
▲ Intron A for Injection (Less than 5%) 3038
K-Dur Extended-Relase Tablets 3047
K-Tab Filmtab Tablets 473
Lotronex Tablets 1479
Mobic Oral Suspension 893
Mobic Tablets 893
Nalfon Capsules 2504
▲ Naprosyn Suspension (1% to 10%) 2769
▲ Naprosyn Tablets (1% to 10%) 2769
Paxil CR Controlled-Release Tablets (Rare) 1509
Paxil (Rare) 1501
▲ Photofrin for Injection (Less than 5%) 729
Plavix Tablets (Less than 1%) 940
Plavix Tablets (Less than 1%) 2942
Prevacid NapraPAC (Less than 1%) 3277
Purinethol Tablets 1222
Relafen Tablets (1%) 1523
Rilutek Tablets (Infrequent) 2945
Sandostatin Injection (Less than 1%) 2263
Sandostatin LAR Depot (Rare) 2264
St. Joseph 81 mg Aspirin Chewable and Enteric Coated Tablets 1841
▲ Voltaren Tablets (1% to 10%) 2298
▲ Voltaren-XR Tablets (1% to 10%) 2301
Wellbutrin Tablets (Rare) 1579
Zomig Tablets (Rare) 714
Zomig-ZMT Tablets (Rare) 714

Ulcers, intestinal

Cytovene 2763
Neurontin Capsules (Rare) 2498
Neurontin Oral Solution (Rare) 2498
Neurontin Tablets (Rare) 2498
VFEND I.V. (Less than 2%) 2543
VFEND Oral Suspension (Less than 2%) 2543
VFEND Tablets (Less than 2%) 2543

Ulcers, leg

Colazal Capsules 2845
Enbrel for Injection 580
▲ Imdur Tablets (Less than or equal to 5%) 3032
Neurontin Capsules (Rare) 2498
Neurontin Oral Solution (Rare) 2498
Neurontin Tablets (Rare) 2498

Ulcers, oral mucosal

Abilify Tablets (Infrequent) 916
Abilify Tablets (Infrequent) 2472
Aciphex Tablets 1081
Actiq (Less than 1%) 993
▲ Advair Diskus 100/50 (1% to 3%) 1291
▲ Advair Diskus 250/50 (1% to 3%) 1291
▲ Advair Diskus 500/50 (1% to 3%) 1291
Alkeran for Injection (Infrequent) 976
Alkeran Tablets (Infrequent) 977
▲ Arava Tablets (3%) 2881
Asacol Delayed-Release Tablets 2688
Caduet Tablets (Less than 2%) 2507
Campral Tablets (Rare) 1175
Carbatrol Capsules 3174
Ceftin Tablets (0.1% to 1%) 1369
▲ CellCept Capsules (3% to less than 20%) 2751
▲ CellCept Intravenous (3% to less than 20%) 2751
▲ CellCept Oral Suspension (3% to less than 20%) 2751
▲ CellCept Tablets (3% to less than 20%) 2751
Cipro I.V. (1% or less) 2998
Cipro I.V. Pharmacy Bulk Package (1% or less) 3509
Cipro XR Tablets 3004
Clozapine Tablets 2141
Clozaril Tablets 2174
Combivent Inhalation Aerosol 878
Copaxone for Injection (Infrequent) 3292
Cuprimine Capsules (Some patients) 1925
Depakote ER Tablets (Greater than 1%) 433
▲ Doxil Injection (1% to 5%) 3302
Effexor Tablets (Infrequent) 3405
Effexor XR Capsules (Infrequent) 3411
Elmiron Capsules (Less than or equal to 1%) 2393
▲ Enbrel for Injection (2% to 6%) 580
▲ Flovent Diskus 50 mcg (1% to 3%) 1415
Gabitril Tablets (1%) 998
Gleevec Tablets (Less common) 2221
▲ Intron A for Injection (Less than 5%) 3038
Invanz for Injection (Greater than 0.1%) 1974
Iressa Tablets (1%) 684
Kaletra (Less than 2%) 474
Lamictal (Infrequent) 1449
Leukeran Tablets (Infrequent) 1472
Lipitor Tablets (Less than 2%) 2495
Lunesta Tablets (Infrequent) 3139
▲ Malarone Tablets (2% to 6%) 1484
▲ Malarone Pediatric Tablets (2% to 6%) 1484
Meridia Capsules 485
Miradon Tablets 3056
Neurontin Capsules (Rare) 2498
Neurontin Oral Solution (Rare) 2498
Neurontin Tablets (Rare) 2498
Noroxin Tablets (Less frequent) 2009
Norvir (Less than 2%) 499
▲ Ontak Vials (Less than 5%) 1717
Paxil CR Controlled-Release Tablets (Infrequent) 1509
Paxil (Infrequent) 1501
Pentasa Capsules (Less than 1%) 3182
Prevacid Delayed-Release Capsules (Less than 1%) 3268
Prevacid for Delayed-Release Oral Suspension (Less than 1%) 3268
Prevacid NapraPAC (Less than 1%) 3277
Prevacid SoluTab Delayed-Release Orally Disintegrating Tablets (Less than 1%) 3268
PREVPAC (Less than 1%) 3281
ProAmatine Tablets (Rare) 3183
ProSom Tablets (Rare) 512
Protonix I.V. (Less than 1%) 3468
Protonix Tablets (Less than 1%) 3465
Provigil Tablets (1%) 1002
Prozac Pulvules and Liquid (Infrequent) 1771
▲ Rapamune Oral Solution and Tablets (3% to 20%) 3472
Rescriptor Tablets 2535
Retrovir Capsules 1533
Retrovir IV Infusion 1537
Retrovir 1533
Reyataz Capsules (Less than 3%) 948
Rythmol SR Capsules 2736
Seroquel Tablets (Infrequent) 691
Sonata Capsules (Infrequent) 1686
Sular Tablets (Less than or equal to 1%) 1163
Tasmar Tablets (Infrequent) 3360
Tegretol/Tegretol-XR 2278
▲ Tequin Injection (0.1% to 3%) 964
▲ Tequin Tablets (0.1% to 3%) 964
Trizivir Tablets 1565
Vantin Tablets and Oral Suspension (Less than 1%) 2650
VFEND I.V. (Less than 2%) 2543
VFEND Oral Suspension (Less than 2%) 2543
VFEND Tablets (Less than 2%) 2543
Vicoprofen Tablets (Less than 3%) 533
Viracept (Less than 2%) 2556
Wellbutrin SR Sustained-Release Tablets (Infrequent) 1583
Wellbutrin XL Extended-Release Tablets (Infrequent) 1588
Ziagen 1600
Zonegran Capsules (Rare) 1089
Zyban Sustained-Release Tablets (2%) 1620
Zyprexa Tablets (Infrequent) 1798
Zyprexa ZYDIS Orally Disintegrating Tablets (Infrequent) 1798

Ulcers, oropharyngeal

Fosamax 1949
Fosamax Plus D Tablets (Rarely) 1956

Ulcers, peptic

Abilify Tablets (Rare) 916
Abilify Tablets (Rare) 2472
Advicor Tablets 1694
Antara Capsules 2723
Aricept Tablets (Infrequent) 1086
Aricept ODT Tablets (Infrequent) 1086
Arthrotec Tablets (Rare) 3126
Buphenyl Powder (One patient) 3327
Buphenyl Tablets (One patient) 3327
Caduet Tablets (Less than 2%) 2507
Campath Ampules 826
Captopril Tablets (About 0.5% to 2%) 2114
▲ CellCept Capsules (3% to less than 20%) 2751
▲ CellCept Intravenous (3% to less than 20%) 2751
▲ CellCept Oral Suspension (3% to less than 20%) 2751
▲ CellCept Tablets (3% to less than 20%) 2751
Clinoril Tablets (Less than 1 in 100) 1899
Copegus Tablets (Less than 1%) 2759
Cuprimine Capsules (Less than 1%) 1925
Depo-Medrol Single-Dose Vial 2617
Dolobid Tablets (Less than 1 in 100) 1937
Effexor Tablets (Infrequent) 3405
Effexor XR Capsules 3411
Evoxac Capsules (Less than 1%) 1042
Frova Tablets (Rare) 1101
Gengraf Capsules (1% to less than 3%) 458
Hydrocortone Tablets 1963
▲ Imdur Tablets (Less than or equal to 5%) 3032
Imitrex Injection (Rare) 1431
Imitrex Nasal Spray 1435
Imitrex Tablets (Rare) 1440
Indocin Capsules (Less than 1%) 1968
Indocin I.V. (Less than 1%) 1973
Indocin (Less than 1%) 1968
Lamictal (Rare) 1449
Lipitor Tablets (Less than 2%) 2495
Lofibra Capsules 1217
Lupron Depot 7.5 mg (Less than 5%) 3261
Midamor Tablets (Rare) 2000
Moduretic Tablets 2003
Nalfon Capsules (Less than 1%) 2504

Neoral Soft Gelatin Capsules (1% to less than 3%) 2247
Neoral Oral Solution (1% to less than 3%) 2247
Neurontin Capsules (Rare) 2498
Neurontin Oral Solution (Rare) 2498
Neurontin Tablets (Rare) 2498
Niaspan Extended-Release Tablets 1703
Omnicef Capsules 506
Omnicef for Oral Suspension 506
Paxil CR Controlled-Release Tablets (Rare) 1509
Paxil (Rare) 1501
Pegasys (Less than 1%) 2793
Permax Tablets (Rare to infrequent) 3357
Pletal Tablets (Less than 2%) 2478
Prograf Capsules and Injection 624
Protonix I.V. (Less than 1%) 3468
Protonix Tablets (Less than 1%) 3465
Prozac Pulvules and Liquid (Rare) 1771
Relafen Tablets (0.3%) 1523
Requip Tablets (Infrequent) 1528
Reyataz Capsules (Less than 3%) 948
Rythmol SR Capsules 2736
Sandimmune (2% or less) 2259
Sandostatin Injection (Less than 1%) 2263
Sandostatin LAR Depot (Rare) 2264
Sonata Capsules (Rare) 1686
Symbyax Capsules (Infrequent) 1788
Ticlid Tablets (Rare) 2813
Tricor Tablets 523
Triglide Tablets 1165
Urso 250 Tablets (1%) 737
Urso Forte Tablets (1%) 737
VFEND I.V. (Less than 2%) 2543
VFEND Oral Suspension (Less than 2%) 2543
VFEND Tablets (Less than 2%) 2543
Zosyn (1.0% or less) 3492
Zyban Sustained-Release Tablets 1620

Ulcers, peptic, aggravation of
Eldepryl Capsules 3209
Niaspan Extended-Release Tablets 1703

Ulcers, peptic, hemorrhagic
▲ Imdur Tablets (Less than or equal to 5%) 3032
Mobic Oral Suspension (Less than 2%) 893
Mobic Tablets (Less than 2%) 893
Prozac Pulvules and Liquid (Rare) 1771
Zoloft (Rare) 2581

Ulcers, peptic, reactivation of
Didronel Tablets (A few patients) 2693

Ulcers, peptic with or without perforation
Asacol Delayed-Release Tablets (Rare) 2688
Didronel Tablets (One report) 2693

Ulcers, peptic with perforation and hemorrhage
▲ Anaprox Tablets (Approximately 1% to 4%) 2769
▲ Anaprox DS Tablets (Approximately 1% to 4%) 2769
Decadron Phosphate Injection 1931
Decadron Tablets 1929
Depo-Medrol Injectable Suspension 2615
▲ EC-Naprosyn Delayed-Release Tablets (Approximately 1% to 4%) 2769
Hydrocortone Tablets 1963
Mobic Oral Suspension (Less than 2%) 893
Mobic Tablets (Less than 2%) 893
▲ Naprosyn Suspension (Approximately 1% to 4%) 2769
▲ Naprosyn Tablets (Approximately 1% to 4%) 2769
Pediapred Oral Solution 3319

Ulcers, skin
Abilify Tablets (Frequent) 916
Abilify Tablets (Frequent) 2472
Antara Capsules 2723
▲ Avastin IV (6%) 1229
Caduet Tablets (Less than 2%) 2507
Cymbalta Delayed-Release Capsules (Frequent) 1729
Fortical Nasal Spray (Less than 1%) 3336
Levaquin in 5% Dextrose Injection (0.1% to 0.9%) 2453
Levaquin (0.1% to 0.9%) 2453
Lyrica Capsules (0.1% to 1%) 2524
Merrem I.V. (Greater than 0.1% to 1%) 687
Namenda (Infrequent) 1199
Symbyax Capsules (Rare) 1788

Unconsciousness
(*see under* Consciousness, loss of)

Underventilation
(*see under* Hypoventilation)

Unsteadiness
▲ Carbatrol Capsules (Among most frequent) 3174
Equetro Extended-Release Capsules 3178
Kadian Capsules 572
Matulane Capsules 3188
Tambocor Tablets 1824
▲ Tegretol/Tegretol-XR (Among most frequent) 2278

Upper respiratory symptoms
▲ Bactroban Nasal (5%) 1357
▲ Brimonidine Tartrate Ophthalmic Solution 0.2% (3% to 9%) ⊙ 245
Engerix-B Vaccine (Less than 1%) 1391
▲ Neoral Soft Gelatin Capsules (13%) 2247
▲ Neoral Oral Solution (13%) 2247
Tarka Tablets (2.4%) 519
Varivax (Greater than or equal to 1%) 2070
▲ Vesanoid Capsules (63%) 2823
▲ Wellbutrin Tablets (5.0%) 1579

Uremia
(*see under* Azotemia)

Ureteral obstruction
Zoladex 709
Zoladex 3-month (Isolated cases) 712

Ureteral spasm
Dilaudid 439
Dilaudid Non-Sterile Powder 439
Dilaudid Rectal Suppositories 439
Dilaudid Tablets 439
Hycodan 1104
Hycomine Compound Tablets 1105
Hycotuss Expectorant Syrup 1106
Lortab 3315
Lortab Elixir 3312
Tussionex Pennkinetic Extended-Release Suspension 3322
Vicodin Tablets 530
Vicodin ES Tablets 531
Vicodin HP Tablets 532
Zydone Tablets 1118

Urethral disorder
Evoxac Capsules (Less than 1%) 1042

Urethritis
Copaxone for Injection (Infrequent) 3292
Gabitril Tablets (Infrequent) 998
Imitrex Injection 1431
Imitrex Nasal Spray 1435
Lunesta Tablets (Rare) 3139
Norvir (Less than 2%) 499
Paxil CR Controlled-Release Tablets (Rare to infrequent) 1509
Paxil (Rare to infrequent) 1501
Protonix I.V. (Less than 1%) 3468
Protonix Tablets (Less than 1%) 3465
Sonata Capsules (Rare) 1686

Uric acid, reduction of
Timentin ADD-Vantage 1556
Timentin IV Infusion 1553

Uric acid level, increase
(*see under* Hyperuricemia)

Uricaciduria
Permax Tablets (Rare) 3357

Urinary bladder, inflammation of
Amerge Tablets (Infrequent) 1312

Urinary bladder malignancies
Permax Tablets (Rare) 3357

Urinary calculi
Adalat CC Tablets (Less than 1%) 2978

Urinary casts
Garamycin Injectable 3028
Primaxin I.M. 2022
Primaxin I.V. 2024
Rocephin Injectable Vials, ADD-Vantage, Galaxy, Bulk (Less than 1%) 2801
Rythmol SR Capsules 2736
Uniretic Tablets (Less than 1%) 3114

Urinary cytology, abnormal
Orthoclone OKT3 Sterile Solution 2370

Urinary difficulty
(*see under* Micturition, difficulty)

Urinary disorders, unspecified
▲ Ammonul Injection (4%) 3323
Enablex Extended-Release Tablets (Greater than or equal to 1%) 2201

Urinary disturbances
Avapro Tablets (Less than 1%) 925
Avapro Tablets (Less than 1%) 2886
Eldepryl Capsules 3209
FazaClo Orally Disintegrating Tablets (2%) 547
▲ Lupron Depot 7.5 mg (12.5%) 3261
Lupron Depot–3 Month 11.25 mg 3262
▲ Neoral Soft Gelatin Capsules (24.2%) 2247
▲ Neoral Oral Solution (24.2%) 2247

Urinary findings, abnormal
Capastat Sulfate for Injection 1728
Clozapine Tablets (2%) 2141
Clozaril Tablets (2%) 2174

Urinary frequency
(*see under* Polyuria)

Urinary glucose, false-positive
Augmentin 1331
Augmentin Tablets 1334
Augmentin XR Extended-Release Tablets 1340
Ceftin 1369
Fortaz 1422
Mefoxin for Injection 1987
Mefoxin Premixed Intravenous Solution 1990

Urinary hesitancy
Cymbalta Delayed-Release Capsules (Infrequent) 1729
Dilaudid Oral Liquid 443
Dilaudid Tablets - 8 mg 443
Dilaudid-HP (Less frequent) 441
▲ Ditropan XL Extended Release Tablets (2% to less than 5%) 2391
Eldepryl Capsules 3209
Kadian Capsules (Less than 3%) 572
MS Contin Tablets (Less frequent) 2703
Norflex Injection 1824
Numorphan 1112
▲ Paxil CR Controlled-Release Tablets (3%) 1509
▲ Paxil (3%) 1501
ProSom Tablets (Infrequent) 512
Retrovir Capsules 1533
Retrovir IV Infusion 1537
Retrovir 1533
▲ Strattera Capsules (5% or greater) 1784
Valium Tablets (Infrequent) 2822

Urinary incontinence
Abilify Tablets (Frequent) 916
Abilify Tablets (Frequent) 2472
Aciphex Tablets (Rare) 1081
Actiq (Less than 1%) 993
Ambien Tablets (Infrequent) 2867
AmBisome for Injection (Less common) 615
Amerge Tablets (Rare) 1312
Aricept Tablets (Frequent) 1086
Aricept ODT Tablets (Frequent) 1086
Caduet Tablets (Less than 2%) 2507
Campral Tablets (Infrequent) 1175
Casodex Tablets (2%) 670
Celebrex Capsules (0.1% to 1.9%) 3130
Celexa (Infrequent) 1177
▲ CellCept Capsules (3% to less than 20%) 2751
▲ CellCept Intravenous (3% to less than 20%) 2751
▲ CellCept Oral Suspension (3% to less than 20%) 2751
▲ CellCept Tablets (3% to less than 20%) 2751
Clozapine Tablets (1%) 2141
Clozaril Tablets (1%) 2174
Copaxone for Injection (At least 2%) 3292
Cymbalta Delayed-Release Capsules (Infrequent) 1729
Dantrium Capsules (Less frequent) 2690
▲ Depacon Injection (1% to 5%) 412
▲ Depakene (1% to 5%) 417
▲ Depakote Sprinkle Capsules (1% to 5%) 422
▲ Depakote Tablets (1% to 5%) 427
Depakote ER Tablets (Greater than 1%) 433
DepoCyt Injection (Less than 3%) 1121
▲ Doxil Injection (1% to 10%) 3302
Effexor Tablets (Infrequent) 3405
Effexor XR Capsules (Infrequent) 3411
Eligard 30 mg (1.1%) 2901
▲ Eloxatin for Injection (2% to 5%) 2908
Eskalith 1406
Evoxac Capsules (Less than 1%) 1042
Exelon Capsules (2% or more) 2204
FazaClo Orally Disintegrating Tablets (1%) 547
Gabitril Tablets (Frequent) 998
Gengraf Capsules (1% to less than 3%) 458
Hytrin Capsules (At least 1%) 469
▲ Intron A for Injection (Less than 5%) 3038
Klonopin (Infrequent) 2782
Lamictal (Infrequent) 1449
Levaquin in 5% Dextrose Injection (0.1% to 0.9%) 2453
Levaquin (0.1% to 0.9%) 2453
Lipitor Tablets (Less than 2%) 2495
Lithobid Tablets 1670
Lunesta Tablets (Infrequent) 3139
Lupron Depot-PED 7.5 mg, 11.25 mg and 15 mg (Less than 2%) 3266
Lupron Injection Pediatric (Less than 2%) 3256
Lyrica Capsules (1% to 2%) 2524
▲ Megace ES Oral Suspension (1% to 3%) 2492
Merrem I.V. (Greater than 0.1% to 1%) 687
Mirapex Tablets (2%) 889
Naropin Injection (Less than 1%) 640
Neoral Soft Gelatin Capsules (1% to less than 3%) 2247
Neoral Oral Solution (1% to less than 3%) 2247
Neurontin Capsules (Infrequent) 2498
Neurontin Oral Solution (Infrequent) 2498
Neurontin Tablets (Infrequent) 2498
Parcopa Orally Disintegrating Tablets 3111
Parnate Tablets 1499
Paxil CR Controlled-Release Tablets (Infrequent) 1509
Paxil (Infrequent) 1501
Permax Tablets (Frequent) 3357
▲ Prograf Capsules and Injection (3% to 15%) 624
ProSom Tablets (Rare) 512
Prozac Pulvules and Liquid (Infrequent) 1771
▲ Rapamune Oral Solution and Tablets (3% to 20%) 3472
Razadyne ER Extended-Release Capsules (Greater than or equal to 2%) 2434
Razadyne (Greater than or equal to 2%) 2434
▲ Rebif Prefilled Syringe for Injection (2% to 4%) 3163
ReoPro Vials (0.1%) 1779
Requip Tablets (2%) 1528
Rilutek Tablets (Infrequent) 2945
Risperdal Consta Long-Acting Injection (Frequent) 1664
Risperdal M-Tab Orally Disintegrating Tablets (Infrequent) 1658
Risperdal (Infrequent) 1658
Rythmol SR Capsules 2736
Seroquel Tablets (Infrequent) 691
Sonata Capsules (Infrequent) 1686
Stalevo Tablets 2270
Stromectol Tablets 2053
Symbyax Capsules (Frequent) 1788
Targretin Capsules 1719
Tasmar Tablets (Frequent) 3360
▲ Temodar Capsules (8%) 3088
Teveten Tablets (Less than 1%) 1707
Teveten HCT Tablets (Less than 1%) 1710
Thioridazine Hydrochloride Tablets 2122
▲ Topamax Sprinkle Capsules (1% to 4%) 2438
▲ Topamax Tablets (1% to 4%) 2438
Travatan Ophthalmic Solution (1% to 5%) 559
▲ Trisenox Injection (5%) 983
VFEND I.V. (Less than 2%) 2543
VFEND Oral Suspension (Less than 2%) 2543
VFEND Tablets (Less than 2%) 2543
Viagra Tablets (Less than 2%) 2552
Vicoprofen Tablets (Less than 1%) 533
Wellbutrin Tablets (Rare) 1579
Wellbutrin SR Sustained-Release Tablets 1583

Wellbutrin XL Extended-Release Tablets ... 1588
Xanax XR Tablets (Infrequent) ... 2655
Zoladex 3-month (1% to 5%) ... 712
Zoloft (Infrequent to 2%) ... 2581
Zomig Nasal Spray (Rare) ... 718
Zonegran Capsules (Infrequent) ... 1089
Zosyn (1.0% or less) ... 3492
Zyban Sustained-Release Tablets ... 1620
Zyprexa Tablets (Frequent) ... 1798
Zyprexa ZYDIS Orally Disintegrating Tablets (Frequent) ... 1798
Zyrtec Chewable Tablets (Less than 2%) ... 2589
Zyrtec (Less than 2%) ... 2589
Zyrtec-D 12 Hour Extended Release Tablets (Less than 2%) ... 2591

Urinary obstruction

Campath Ampules ... 826

Urinary retention

Abilify Tablets (Infrequent) ... 916
Abilify Tablets (Infrequent) ... 2472
Aceon Tablets (2 mg, 4 mg, 8 mg) (0.3% to 1%) ... 3191
Actiq (Less than 1%) ... 993
Aloxi Injection (Less than 1%) ... 2099
Ambien Tablets (Rare) ... 2867
Ammonul Injection ... 3323
▲ Angiomax for Injection (4%) ... 1856
Anzemet Injection (2%) ... 2871
Arixtra Injection (Up to 2.9%) ... 1325
Astelin Nasal Spray ... 1876
Atrovent HFA Inhalation Aerosol ... 872
Atrovent Inhalation Solution (Less than 3%) ... 868
Atrovent Nasal Spray 0.03% ... 869
Atrovent Nasal Spray 0.06% ... 870
Avinza Capsules (Less than 5%) ... 1714
Balamine DM ... 739
Bentyl Capsules ... 724
Bentyl Injection ... 724
Bentyl Syrup ... 724
Bentyl Tablets ... 724
Brevibloc Concentrate (Less than 1%) ... 766
Brevibloc Injection (Less than 1%) ... 766
Brevibloc Double Strength Injection (Less than 1%) ... 766
Brevibloc Premixed Injection (Less than 1%) ... 766
Brevibloc Double Strength Premixed Injection (Less than 1%) ... 766
Buprenex Injectable (Less than 1%) ... 2718
Caduet Tablets (Less than 2%) ... 2507
Campath Ampules ... 826
Carbatrol Capsules ... 3174
▲ Casodex Tablets (2% to 5%) ... 670
Catapres Tablets (About 1 in 1,000 patients) ... 874
Celexa (Infrequent) ... 1177
▲ CellCept Capsules (3% to less than 20%) ... 2751
▲ CellCept Intravenous (3% to less than 20%) ... 2751
▲ CellCept Oral Suspension (3% to less than 20%) ... 2751
▲ CellCept Tablets (3% to less than 20%) ... 2751
Cipro I.V. (1% or less) ... 2998
Cipro I.V. Pharmacy Bulk Package (1% or less) ... 3509
Cipro (Less than 1%) ... 2991
Cipro XR Tablets ... 3004
Clorpres Tablets (About 1 in 1,000) ... 2139
Clozapine Tablets (1%) ... 2141
Clozaril Tablets (1%) ... 2174
Cogentin Injection ... 1903
Combunox Tablets (Less than 1%) ... 1183
Copaxone for Injection (At least 2%) ... 3292
Cymbalta Delayed-Release Capsules (Infrequent) ... 1729
Dantrium Capsules (Less frequent) ... 2690
▲ DepoDur Extended-Release Injection (Greater than 10%) ... 1098
Detrol Tablets (1.7%) ... 2626
Detrol LA Capsules ... 2629
Diastat Rectal Delivery System (Infrequent) ... 3344
Dilaudid ... 439
Dilaudid Oral Liquid ... 443
Dilaudid Non-Sterile Powder ... 439
Dilaudid Rectal Suppositories ... 439
Dilaudid Tablets ... 439
Dilaudid Tablets - 8 mg ... 443
Dilaudid-HP (Less frequent) ... 441
Diprivan Injectable Emulsion (Less than 1%) ... 676
▲ Ditropan XL Extended Release Tablets (2% to less than 5%) ... 2391
▲ Duragesic Transdermal System (3% to 10%) ... 2448
Effexor Tablets (1%) ... 3405
Effexor XR Capsules (Frequent) ... 3411
Eldepryl Capsules (1 of 49 patients) ... 3209
Eligard 22.5 mg (Less than 2%) ... 2899
Enablex Extended-Release Tablets (16 patients) ... 2201
Equetro Extended-Release Capsules ... 3178
Evoxac Capsules ... 1042
Exelon Capsules (Infrequent) ... 2204
FazaClo Orally Disintegrating Tablets (1%) ... 547
Flexeril Tablets (Less than 1%) ... 1832
Gabitril Tablets (Infrequent) ... 998
Geodon Capsules (Infrequent) ... 2514
Hycodan ... 1104
Hycomine Compound Tablets ... 1105
Hycotuss Expectorant Syrup ... 1106
Invanz for Injection (Greater than 0.1%) ... 1974
Inversine Tablets ... 3286
Kadian Capsules (Less than 3%) ... 572
Klonopin (Infrequent) ... 2782
Lamictal (Infrequent) ... 1449
Levaquin in 5% Dextrose Injection (0.1% to 0.9%) ... 2453
Levaquin (0.1% to 0.9%) ... 2453
Lortab ... 3315
Lortab Elixir ... 3312
Lyrica Capsules (0.1% to 1%) ... 2524
Moban Tablets ... 1108
MS Contin Tablets (Less frequent) ... 2703
▲ Myfortic Tablets (3% to less than 20%) ... 2244
Namenda (Infrequent) ... 1199
▲ Naropin Injection (1% to 5%) ... 640
Neurontin Capsules (Infrequent) ... 2498
Neurontin Oral Solution (Infrequent) ... 2498
Neurontin Tablets (Infrequent) ... 2498
Niravam Orally Disintegrating Tablets ... 3106
Norflex Injection ... 1824
Norvir (Less than 2%) ... 499
Numorphan ... 1112
OxyContin Tablets (Less than 1%) ... 2699
Parcopa Orally Disintegrating Tablets ... 3111
Parnate Tablets ... 1499
Paxil CR Controlled-Release Tablets (Infrequent) ... 1509
Paxil (Infrequent) ... 1501
Permax Tablets (Infrequent) ... 3357
Prevacid Delayed-Release Capsules (Less than 1%) ... 3268
Prevacid for Delayed-Release Oral Suspension (Less than 1%) ... 3268
Prevacid NapraPAC ... 3277
Prevacid SoluTab Delayed-Release Orally Disintegrating Tablets (Less than 1%) ... 3268
PREVPAC ... 3281
▲ ProAmatine Tablets (Among most frequent) ... 3183
Proleukin for Injection (1%) ... 1007
Provigil Tablets (1%) ... 1002
Prozac Pulvules and Liquid (Infrequent) ... 1771
▲ Rapamune Oral Solution and Tablets (3% to 20%) ... 3472
Razadyne ER Extended-Release Capsules (Infrequent) ... 2434
Razadyne (Infrequent) ... 2434
ReoPro Vials (0.4%) ... 1779
Rilutek Tablets (Infrequent) ... 2945
Risperdal Consta Long-Acting Injection (Infrequent) ... 1664
Risperdal M-Tab Orally Disintegrating Tablets (Rare) ... 1658
Risperdal (Rare) ... 1658
Rythmol SR Capsules ... 2736
Sanctura Tablets (1.2%) ... 1133
Seroquel Tablets (Infrequent) ... 691
▲ Simulect for Injection (3% to 10%) ... 2268
Sonata Capsules (Rare) ... 1686
Spiriva HandiHaler (Less than 1%) ... 899
Stalevo Tablets ... 2270
▲ Strattera Capsules (0.7% or greater) ... 1784
Surmontil Capsules ... 2347
Symbyax Capsules (Infrequent) ... 1788
Symmetrel (0.1% to 1%) ... 1115
Tagamet Tablets (Rare) ... 1547
Tambocor Tablets (Less than 1%) ... 1824
Tasmar Tablets (Infrequent) ... 3360
Tegretol/Tegretol-XR ... 2278
Thioridazine Hydrochloride Tablets ... 2122
Topamax Sprinkle Capsules (Infrequent) ... 2438
Topamax Tablets (Infrequent) ... 2438
▲ Trasylol Injection (3%) ... 779
Trelstar Depot (1.4%) ... 3385
Trelstar LA Suspension (1.1%) ... 3387
Tussionex Pennkinetic Extended-Release Suspension ... 3322
Ultane Liquid for Inhalation (Less than 1%) ... 526
Ultracet Tablets (Less than 1%) ... 2462
Uniretic Tablets (Less than 1%) ... 3114
Vantas (Less than 2%) ... 3367
VESIcare Tablets (0% to 1.4%) ... 631
VFEND I.V. (Less than 2%) ... 2543
VFEND Oral Suspension (Less than 2%) ... 2543
VFEND Tablets (Less than 2%) ... 2543
Viadur Implant (Less than 2%) ... 782
Vicodin Tablets ... 530
Vicodin ES Tablets ... 531
Vicodin HP Tablets ... 532
Vicoprofen Tablets (Less than 1%) ... 533
Vivactil Tablets ... 2350
Wellbutrin Tablets (1.9%) ... 1579
Wellbutrin SR Sustained-Release Tablets ... 1583
Wellbutrin XL Extended-Release Tablets ... 1588
▲ Zenapax for Injection (2% to 5%) ... 2838
▲ Zofran Injection (3%) ... 1607
▲ Zofran (5%) ... 1613
▲ Zofran ODT Orally Disintegrating Tablets (5%) ... 1613
Zoladex 3-month (1% to 5%) ... 712
Zoloft (Infrequent) ... 2581
Zonegran Capsules (Infrequent) ... 1089
Zosyn (1.0% or less) ... 3492
Zyban Sustained-Release Tablets ... 1620
Zydone Tablets ... 1118
Zyprexa Tablets (Infrequent) ... 1798
Zyprexa ZYDIS Orally Disintegrating Tablets (Infrequent) ... 1798
Zyrtec Chewable Tablets (Less than 2%) ... 2589
Zyrtec (Less than 2%) ... 2589
Zyrtec-D 12 Hour Extended Release Tablets (Less than 2%) ... 2591

Urinary sediment, abnormalities

Capastat Sulfate for Injection ... 1728
Dyazide Capsules ... 1389
Roferon-A Injection (Infrequent) ... 2805

Urinary tract, burning of

Abilify Tablets (Infrequent) ... 916
Abilify Tablets (Infrequent) ... 2472

Urinary tract, obstruction

Zoladex (1% to 5%) ... 709
Zoladex 3-month (1% to 5%) ... 712

Urinary tract dilatation

Surmontil Capsules ... 2347

Urinary tract disorder, unspecified

Amnesteem Capsules ... 2126
▲ Casodex Tablets (2% to 5%) ... 670
▲ CellCept Capsules (3% to less than 20%) ... 2751
▲ CellCept Intravenous (3% to less than 20%) ... 2751
▲ CellCept Oral Suspension (3% to less than 20%) ... 2751
▲ CellCept Tablets (3% to less than 20%) ... 2751
▲ Leukine (14%) ... 829
Lupron Depot 3.75 mg ... 3257
Pravachol Tablets (0.7% to 2.4%) ... 943
Protonix I.V. (Less than 1%) ... 3468
Protonix Tablets (Less than 1%) ... 3465
Relpax Tablets (Infrequent) ... 2531
Tasmar Tablets (Infrequent) ... 3360
▲ Zenapax for Injection (2% to 5%) ... 2838
▲ Zoladex (13%) ... 709
Zoladex 3-month (1% to 5%) ... 712
Zomig Nasal Spray (Rare) ... 718
Zyban Sustained-Release Tablets ... 1620

Urinary urgency

Abilify Tablets (Infrequent) ... 916
Abilify Tablets (Infrequent) ... 2472
Actiq (1% or greater) ... 993
Adenoscan (Less than 1%) ... 613
Amerge Tablets (Rare) ... 1312
Aricept Tablets (Infrequent) ... 1086
Aricept ODT Tablets (Infrequent) ... 1086
Asacol Delayed-Release Tablets ... 2688
▲ Avastin IV (3% to 6%) ... 1229
▲ Betaseron for SC Injection (13%) ... 791
Caduet Tablets (Less than 2%) ... 2507
Campral Tablets (Rare) ... 1175
▲ Casodex Tablets (2% to 5%) ... 670
Caverject Impulse Injection (Less than 1%) ... 2610
Clozapine Tablets (1%) ... 2141
Clozaril Tablets (1%) ... 2174
▲ Copaxone for Injection (10%) ... 3292
Effexor Tablets (Infrequent) ... 3405
Effexor XR Capsules (Infrequent) ... 3411
Eligard 22.5 mg (2.6%) ... 2899
Eligard 30 mg (1.1%) ... 2901
FazaClo Orally Disintegrating Tablets (1%) ... 547
Gabitril Tablets (Infrequent) ... 998
Keppra Oral Solution (2%) ... 3307
Keppra Tablets (2%) ... 3307
Lexapro Oral Solution (Infrequent) ... 1193
Lexapro Tablets (Infrequent) ... 1193
Lipitor Tablets (Less than 2%) ... 2495
Lupron Depot 7.5 mg (Less than 5%) ... 3261
Neurontin Capsules (Rare) ... 2498
Neurontin Oral Solution (Infrequent) ... 2498
Neurontin Tablets (Rare) ... 2498
Nubain Injection (1% or less) ... 1111
Paxil CR Controlled-Release Tablets (Infrequent) ... 1509
Paxil (Infrequent) ... 1501
Plendil Extended-Release Tablets (0.5% to 1.5%) ... 651
Prevacid Delayed-Release Capsules (Less than 1%) ... 3268
Prevacid for Delayed-Release Oral Suspension (Less than 1%) ... 3268
Prevacid NapraPAC (Less than 1%) ... 3277
Prevacid SoluTab Delayed-Release Orally Disintegrating Tablets (Less than 1%) ... 3268
PREVPAC (Less than 1%) ... 3281
▲ ProAmatine Tablets (Among most frequent) ... 3183
ProSom Tablets (Infrequent) ... 512
Prozac Pulvules and Liquid (Infrequent) ... 1771
Rilutek Tablets (Infrequent) ... 2945
Sonata Capsules (Infrequent) ... 1686
Symbyax Capsules (Infrequent) ... 1788
Targretin Capsules ... 1719
Viadur Implant (Less than 2%) ... 782
Wellbutrin SR Sustained-Release Tablets (Up to 2%) ... 1583
Wellbutrin XL Extended-Release Tablets (Up to 2%) ... 1588
Zomig Tablets (Infrequent) ... 714
Zomig-ZMT Tablets (Infrequent) ... 714
Zyban Sustained-Release Tablets (Infrequent) ... 1620
Zyprexa Tablets (Infrequent) ... 1798

Urination, difficult

(*see under* Micturition, difficulty)

Urination, impaired

Actiq (1% or greater) ... 993
AndroGel (Fewer than 1%) ... 3330
Eligard 22.5 mg (Less than 2%) ... 2899
Prevacid Delayed-Release Capsules (Less than 1%) ... 3268
Prevacid for Delayed-Release Oral Suspension (Less than 1%) ... 3268
Prevacid NapraPAC (Less than 1%) ... 3277
Prevacid SoluTab Delayed-Release Orally Disintegrating Tablets (Less than 1%) ... 3268
PREVPAC (Less than 1%) ... 3281
Rescriptor Tablets ... 2535
Symbyax Capsules (Infrequent) ... 1788
Ultane Liquid for Inhalation (Less than 1%) ... 526

Urination, painful

(*see under* Micturition, painful)

Urine, abnormal

Aciphex Tablets ... 1081
▲ Avonex (3%) ... 839
Diprivan Injectable Emulsion (Less than 1%) ... 676
Evoxac Capsules (Less than 1%) ... 1042
Factive Tablets (Less than or equal to 0.1%) ... 2464
Frova Tablets (Rare) ... 1101
Gengraf Capsules (1% to less than 3%) ... 458
Kaletra (Less than 2%) ... 474
Keppra Oral Solution (2%) ... 3307
Keppra Tablets (2%) ... 3307
Lamictal (Rare) ... 1449
Neoral Soft Gelatin Capsules (1% to less than 3%) ... 2247

Neoral Oral Solution (1% to less than 3%) ... 2247
Neurontin Capsules (Rare) ... 2498
Neurontin Oral Solution (Rare) ... 2498
Neurontin Tablets (Rare) ... 2498
▲ Novantrone for Injection Concentrate (5% to 11%) ... 3158
Provigil Tablets (1%) ... 1002
Reyataz Capsules (Less than 3%) ... 948
Rilutek Tablets (Infrequent) ... 2945
Rythmol SR Capsules ... 2736
Soriatane Capsules (Less than 1%) .. 1028
Ultane Liquid for Inhalation (Less than 1%) ... 526
Viracept (Less than 2%) ... 2556

Urine, cells in
Accutane Capsules ... 2740
Garamycin Injectable ... 3028
Merrem I.V. (Greater than 0.2%) ... 687
Parcopa Orally Disintegrating Tablets ... 3111
Zovirax for Injection (Less than 1%) ... 1618

Urine, color change
Adriamycin for Injection, USP ... 786
Adriamycin Injection, USP ... 786
Alinia for Oral Suspension (Less than 1%) ... 2840
Alinia Tablets (Less than 1%) ... 2840
Casodex Tablets ... 670
Cerubidine for Injection ... 788
Clinoril Tablets (Less than 1%) ... 1899
▲ Comtan Tablets (10%) ... 2186
Coumadin for Injection ... 932
Coumadin Tablets ... 932
Desferal Vials ... 2190
Diprivan Injectable Emulsion (Less than 1%) ... 676
Eulexin Capsules ... 3023
Fluorescite Injection ... ⊙ 207
Klonopin (Infrequent) ... 2782
Lamisil Tablets ... 2226
Maxzide ... 2150
MetroGel-Vaginal Gel (Less than 1%) ... 1822
Ortho-Cyclen/Ortho Tri-Cyclen ... 2414
Ortho Tri-Cyclen Lo Tablets ... 2421
Parcopa Orally Disintegrating Tablets ... 3111
Primaxin I.M. ... 2022
Primaxin I.V. (Less than 0.2%) ... 2024
▲ Stalevo Tablets (5% to 10%) ... 2270
▲ Tasmar Tablets (2% to 7%) ... 3360
Ticlid Tablets ... 2813
Tindamax ... 2670

Urine, microscopic deposits
Carbatrol Capsules ... 3174
Equetro Extended-Release Capsules ... 3178
Tegretol/Tegretol-XR ... 2278

Urine, output low
(*see under* Hypouresis)

Urine, presence of RBC's
(*see under* Hematuria)

Urine, presence of urobilinogen
Primaxin I.M. ... 2022
Primaxin I.V. ... 2024

Urine flow decreased
Cymbalta Delayed-Release Capsules (infrequent) ... 1729
Evoxac Capsules (Less than 1%) ... 1042

Urolithiasis
Abilify Tablets (Rare) ... 916
Abilify Tablets (Rare) ... 2472
Antara Capsules ... 2723
Cosopt Sterile Ophthalmic Solution (Less than 1%) ... 1910
▲ Crixivan Capsules (Approximately 12.4%) ... 1918
Effexor Tablets (Rare) ... 3405
Effexor XR Capsules (Rare) ... 3411
Kytril Injection (Rare) ... 2785
Lofibra Capsules ... 1217
Paxil CR Controlled-Release Tablets (Rare) ... 1509
Paxil (Rare) ... 1501
Permax Tablets (Infrequent) ... 3357
Tricor Tablets ... 523
Trusopt Sterile Ophthalmic Solution (Rare) ... 2065

Urticaria
Abilify Tablets (Infrequent) ... 916
Abilify Tablets (Infrequent) ... 2472
Accolate Tablets ... 663
AccuNeb Inhalation Solution (0.9% to 1.7%) ... 1055
Accutane Capsules ... 2740
Aciphex Tablets ... 1081
Actiq (Less than 1%) ... 993
Activase I.V. (Very rare) ... 1225
Adacel Vaccine (Very rare) ... 2959
Adalat CC Tablets (Rare) ... 2978
Adderall Tablets ... 3168
Adderall XR Capsules ... 3169
Adipex-P ... 1216
Adriamycin for Injection, USP (Occasional) ... 786
Adriamycin Injection, USP (Occasional) ... 786
▲ Advair Diskus 100/50 (1% to 3%) ... 1291
▲ Advair Diskus 250/50 (1% to 3%) ... 1291
▲ Advair Diskus 500/50 (1% to 3%) ... 1291
Advicor Tablets ... 1694
Aerobid/Aerobid-M (1% to 3%) ... 1172
Aggrastat ... 1878
Aggrenox Capsules (Less than 1%) .. 855
▲ Agrylin Capsules (8.3%) ... 3172
Alacol DM Syrup ... 739
Albenza Tablets (Rare) ... 1310
Aldoclor Tablets ... 1881
Aldoril Tablets ... 1884
Aldurazyme for Intravenous Infusion ... 1261
Alesse-28 Tablets ... 3392
Alferon N Injection ... 1640
Alkeran for Injection ... 976
Allegra (Rare) ... 2857
Allegra-D 12 Hour Extended-Release Tablets (Rare) ... 2860
Allegra-D 24 Hour Extended-Release Tablets (Rare) ... 2862
Aloprim for Injection (Less than 1%) ... 2156
Altace Capsules (Less than 1%) ... 1673
Altoprev Extended-Release Tablets (Rare) ... 1151
Amaryl Tablets (Less than 1%) ... 2864
Ambien Tablets (Rare) ... 2867
AmBisome for Injection (Less common) ... 615
Amerge Tablets (Infrequent) ... 1312
Amevive (Less than 1%) ... 836
Aminohippurate Sodium "PAH" Injection ... 1886
Ammonul Injection ... 3323
Amnesteem Capsules ... 2126
Amoxil Capsules ... 1315
Amoxil Chewable Tablets ... 1315
Amoxil Pediatric Drops for Oral Suspension ... 1315
Amoxil Powder for Oral Suspension ... 1315
Amoxil Tablets ... 1315
Anaprox Tablets (Less than 1%) ... 2769
Anaprox DS Tablets (Less than 1%) .. 2769
Antara Capsules ... 2723
Anzemet Injection (Rare) ... 2871
Anzemet Tablets (Rare) ... 2874
Appearex Tablets ... 2095
Arava Tablets (Rare) ... 2881
Aricept Tablets (Frequent) ... 1086
Aricept ODT Tablets (Frequent) ... 1086
Arimidex Tablets (Very rare) ... 665
Arthrotec Tablets (Rare) ... 3126
Asacol Delayed-Release Tablets ... 2688
Atacand Tablets ... 634
Atacand HCT ... 637
Atrovent HFA Inhalation Aerosol ... 872
Atrovent Inhalation Solution (Less than 3%) ... 868
Atrovent Nasal Spray 0.06% (Rare) .. 870
Attenuvax (Rare) ... 1889
▲ Augmentin (3%) ... 1331
▲ Augmentin Tablets (3%) ... 1334
Augmentin XR Extended-Release Tablets ... 1340
Augmentin ES-600 Powder for Oral Suspension ... 1337
Avalide Tablets (Rare) ... 922
Avalide Tablets (Rare) ... 2889
Avapro Tablets (Rare) ... 925
Avapro Tablets (Less than 1%) ... 2886
Avelox (0.1% to less than 2%) ... 2984
Avinza Capsules (Less than 5%) ... 1714
Avodart Soft Gelatin Capsules ... 1353
Avonex ... 839
Axid Oral Solution (More frequent) ... 913
Aygestin Tablets ... 1062
Azmacort Inhalation Aerosol (Rare) .. 1701
Azopt Ophthalmic Suspension (Less than 1%) ... 553
Bactroban Cream (One report) ... 1356
Bayer Aspirin Tablets ... 3515
Beconase AQ Nasal Spray (Rare) ... 1359
▲ BeneFix for Injection (3.1% to 4.8%) ... 3402
Benicar Tablets ... 2850
Benicar HCT Tablets (Rare) ... 2852
Bentyl Capsules ... 724
Bentyl Injection ... 724
Bentyl Syrup ... 724
Bentyl Tablets ... 724
Betagan Ophthalmic Solution, USP (Rare) ... ⊙ 217
Betaseron for SC Injection ... 791
Betimol Ophthalmic Solution ... ⊙ 283
Betimol Ophthalmic Solution ... 3371
Betoptic S Ophthalmic Suspension (Rare) ... 554
Biaxin/Biaxin XL ... 402
Biltricide Tablets (Rare) ... 2990
Boostrix (Rarely) ... 1366
Bravelle for Intramuscular or Subcutaneous Injection ... 1140
Buminate 5% Solution, USP (Occasional) ... 747
Buminate 25% Solution, USP (Occasional) ... 748
Buprenex Injectable (Rare) ... 2718
Caduet Tablets (Less than 2%) ... 2507
▲ Campath Ampules (5% to 30%) ... 826
Campral Tablets (Infrequent) ... 1175
Capastat Sulfate for Injection ... 1728
Carafate Suspension ... 727
Carafate Tablets ... 728
Carbatrol Capsules ... 3174
Cataflam Tablets (Rarely) ... 2173
Catapres Tablets (About 5 in 1,000 patients) ... 874
Catapres-TTS (2 cases of 3,539 patients) ... 875
Ceftin (0.1% to 1%) ... 1369
Celebrex Capsules (0.1% to 1.9%) ... 3130
Celexa (Infrequent) ... 1177
Cenestin Tablets, 0.45mg, 0.625mg, 0.9mg, 1.25mg ... 1063
Cenestin Tablets, 0.3mg ... 1063
▲ Cerezyme for Injection (Approximately 6.6%) ... 1263
Cialis Tablets ... 1806
Cipro I.V. (1% or less) ... 2998
Cipro I.V. Pharmacy Bulk Package (1% or less) ... 3509
Cipro (Less than 1%) ... 2991
Cipro XR Tablets (Less than 1%) ... 3004
Clarinex Syrup (Rare) ... 3009
Clarinex Tablets (Rare) ... 3009
Clarinex Reditabs Tablets (Rare) ... 3009
Clarinex-D 24-Hour Extended-Release Tablets ... 3012
Cleocin Vaginal Ovules ... 2613
Climara Transdermal System ... 795
Climara Pro Transdermal System ... 800
Clindesse Vaginal Cream (Rare) ... 3296
Clobex Shampoo ... 1209
Clorpres Tablets (About 5 in 1,000) ... 2139
Clozapine Tablets (Less than 1%) ... 2141
Clozaril Tablets (Less than 1%) ... 2174
Colyte with Flavor Packs for Oral Solution (Isolated cases) ... 3102
CombiPatch Transdermal System ... 2180
Combivent Inhalation Aerosol (Less than 2%; rare) ... 878
Combivir Tablets ... 1373
Comvax ... 1904
Concerta Extended-Release Tablets ... 1828
▲ Copaxone for Injection (5%) ... 3292
Cosopt Sterile Ophthalmic Solution ... 1910
Coumadin for Injection (Infrequent) ... 932
Coumadin Tablets (Infrequent) ... 932
Covera-HS Tablets (Less than 2%) ... 3135
Cozaar Tablets (Less than 1%) ... 1913
Crestor Tablets (Less than 1%) ... 672
Crixivan Capsules (Less than 2%) ... 1918
Cuprimine Capsules ... 1925
Cutivate Lotion 0.05% (Rare) ... 1383
Cutivate Ointment (Less than 1%) ... 1384
Dantrium Capsules (Less frequent) ... 2690
Dantrium Intravenous (Rare) ... 2691
Decadron Phosphate Injection ... 1931
Decadron Tablets ... 1929
Demser Capsules (Rare) ... 1933
Denavir Cream ... 2163
Depo-Medrol Single-Dose Vial ... 2617
depo-subQ provera 104 Injectable Suspension ... 2622
Desferal Vials ... 2190
Desoxyn Tablets, USP ... 2482
Dexedrine ... 1386
DextroStat Tablets ... 3177
Diastat Rectal Delivery System (Infrequent) ... 3344
Didronel Tablets ... 2693
Dilaudid ... 439
Dilaudid Oral Liquid ... 443
Dilaudid Non-Sterile Powder ... 439
Dilaudid Rectal Suppositories ... 439
Dilaudid Tablets ... 439
Dilaudid Tablets - 8 mg ... 443
Dilaudid-HP (Less frequent) ... 441
Diovan HCT Tablets ... 2195
Diprivan Injectable Emulsion (Less than 1%) ... 676
Diuril Oral ... 1936
Diuril Sodium Intravenous ... 1934
Dolobid Tablets (Less than 1 in 100) ... 1937
▲ Doxil Injection (1% to 5%) ... 3302
DuoNeb Inhalation Solution (0.3%) ... 1058
Dyazide Capsules ... 1389
Dynacin Tablets ... 1859
DynaCirc CR Tablets (0.5% to 1%) ... 2726
EC-Naprosyn Delayed-Release Tablets (Less than 1%) ... 2769
Ecotrin Enteric Coated Aspirin Low, Regular and Maximum Strength Tablets ... 1627
E.E.S. ... 449
Effexor Tablets (Infrequent) ... 3405
Effexor XR Capsules ... 3411
Efudex ... 3348
Elidel Cream 1% (0.3% to 1.1%) ... 2198
Elitek ... 2906
Ellence Injection ... 2632
Elmiron Capsules (Less than or equal to 1%) ... 2393
Eloxatin for Injection (Less than 1%) ... 2908
Elspar for Injection ... 1943
Emend Capsules (One patient) ... 1944
Enbrel for Injection ... 580
Engerix-B Vaccine (Less than 1%) ... 1391
Epivir ... 1394
Epivir-HBV ... 1398
Epogen for Injection (Rare) ... 586
Epzicom Tablets ... 1402
Equetro Extended-Release Capsules ... 3178
Erygel Topical Gel ... 2096
EryPed ... 445
Ery-Tab Tablets ... 447
Erythrocin Stearate Filmtab Tablets ... 452
Erythromycin Base Filmtab Tablets ... 454
Erythromycin Delayed-Release Capsules, USP ... 456
Estratest Tablets ... 3196
Estratest H.S. Tablets ... 3196
Ethyol for Injection ... 1869
Evoxac Capsules (Less than 1%) ... 1042
Exelon Capsules (Infrequent) ... 2204
Fabrazyme for Intravenous Infusion ... 1267
Factive Tablets (0.1% to 1%) ... 2464
Famvir Tablets (Infrequent) ... 2207
Faslodex Injection (Less than 1%) ... 682
FazaClo Orally Disintegrating Tablets (Less than 1%) ... 547
Feiba VH ... 749
Flexeril Tablets (Less than 1%) ... 1832
▲ Flolan for Injection (25%) ... 1408
Flomax Capsules ... 881
Flonase Nasal Spray (Less than 1%) ... 1412
Flovent Diskus 50 mcg ... 1415
Flovent HFA (Rare) ... 1418
Floxin Otic Singles (Reported in a single subject) ... 1045
Floxin Otic Solution (Single report) ... 1043
Flumist Vaccine ... 1872
Fluorescite Injection (Very rare) ... ⊙ 207
Focalin Tablets ... 2214
Focalin XR Capsules ... 2217
Follistim AQ Cartridge ... 2354
Fortaz ... 1422
Fosamax ... 1949
Fosamax Plus D Tablets ... 1956
Furosemide Tablets ... 2117
Gabitril Tablets (Infrequent) ... 998
GamaSTAN ... 3231
Gammagard Liquid ... 751
Gammagard S/D (Occasional) ... 754
▲ Gamunex Immune Globulin I.V., 10% (0.5% to 5%) ... 3232
Garamycin Injectable ... 3028
Gengraf Capsules (1% to less than 3%) ... 458
Geodon Capsules (Infrequent) ... 2514
Glucagon for Injection Vials and Emergency Kit ... 1749
Grifulvin V Tablets Microsize and Oral Suspension Microsize (Occasional) ... 2384
Gris-PEG Tablets ... 2504

HalfLytely and Bisacodyl Tablets Bowel Prep Kit with Flavors Packs 915
Havrix Vaccine (Less than 1%) 1425
Hemofil M (Extremely rare) 757
HibTITER 3419
Hycamtin for Injection (Less than 1%) 1427
Hydrocortone Tablets 1963
HyperHep B S/D 3237
Hyzaar 1964
Idamycin PFS Injection 2645
Imitrex Injection 1431
Imitrex Nasal Spray 1435
Imitrex Tablets 1440
Imodium Capsules 1834
Inderal LA Long-Acting Capsules 3421
Indocin Capsules (Less than 1%) 1968
Indocin I.V. (Less than 1%) 1973
Indocin (Less than 1%) 1968
Infanrix Vaccine 1444
Infed Injection 3381
▲ Intron A for Injection (Rare; Less than 5%) 3038
Invanz for Injection (Greater than 0.1%) 1974
Invirase (Less than 2%) 2776
Ketek Tablets (Less than 0.2%) 2920
Kogenate FS (Rare) 3517
Kytril Injection (Rare) 2785
Kytril Tablets (Rare) 2788
Lamictal (Infrequent) 1449
Lamisil Tablets (1.1%) 2226
Lescol Capsules (Rare) 2227
Lescol Capsules (Rare) 2730
Lescol XL Tablets 2227
Lescol XL Tablets 2730
Leukeran Tablets 1472
Leustatin Injection 2368
Levaquin in 5% Dextrose Injection (0.1% to 0.9%) 2453
Levaquin (0.1% to 0.9%) 2453
Levothroid Tablets 1189
Levoxyl Tablets 1680
Lidoderm Patch (Rare) 1107
Lipitor Tablets (Less than 2%) 2495
Lofibra Capsules 1217
Lotensin HCT Tablets 2235
Lotrimin 3053
Lotrisone 3054
Lotronex Tablets (Infrequent) 1479
Lovenox Injection 2931
Lunesta Tablets (Infrequent) 3139
Lupron Depot 3.75 mg 3257
Lupron Depot 7.5 mg 3261
Lupron Depot–3 Month 11.25 mg 3262
Lupron Depot-PED 7.5 mg, 11.25 mg and 15 mg 3266
Lupron Injection Pediatric 3256
Lyrica Capsules (0.1% to 1%) 2524
Malarone Tablets 1484
Malarone Pediatric Tablets 1484
Matulane Capsules 3188
Maxalt Tablets (Infrequent) 1983
Maxalt-MLT Orally Disintegrating Tablets (Infrequent) 1983
Maxipime for Injection (Greater than 0.1% to less than 1%) 1093
Maxzide 2150
Mefoxin for Injection 1987
Mefoxin Premixed Intravenous Solution 1990
Menostar Transdermal System 805
Meridia Capsules 485
Merrem I.V. (Greater than 0.1% to 1%) 687
Meruvax II 1994
Metadate CD Capsules 3316
Mevacor Tablets (Rare) 1996
Micardis Tablets 884
Micardis HCT Tablets 886
Migranal Nasal Spray (Rare) 3350
Miradon Tablets 3056
Mivacron Injection (Less than 1%) 489
M-M-R II 1980
Mobic Oral Suspension (Less than 2%) 893
Mobic Tablets (Less than 2%) 893
Moduretic Tablets 2003
Children's Motrin Oral Suspension and Chewable Tablets ▣ 647
Children's Motrin Non-Staining Dye-Free Oral Suspension ▣ 647
Children's Motrin Oral Suspension and Chewable Tablets 1837
Children's Motrin Cold Non-Staining Dye-Free Oral Suspension 1838
Children's Motrin Cold Oral Suspension 1838
Children's Motrin Non-Staining Dye-Free Oral Suspension 1837
Motrin Cold & Sinus Caplets 1836
Motrin IB Tablets and Caplets 1836
Infants' Motrin Concentrated Drops 1837
Infants' Motrin Non-Staining Dye-Free Drops 1837
Junior Strength Motrin Caplets and Chewable Tablets 1837
MS Contin Tablets (Less frequent) 2703
Mumpsvax (Extremely rare) 2005
Mycamine for Injection 620
Myleran Tablets 1492
Nalfon Capsules (Less than 1%) 2504
Namenda (Infrequent) 1199
Naprosyn Suspension (Less than 1%) 2769
Naprosyn Tablets (Less than 1%) 2769
Naropin Injection (Less than 1%) 640
Nasacort HFA Inhalation Aerosol 2939
Navelbine Injection 1494
Neoral Soft Gelatin Capsules (1% to less than 3%) 2247
Neoral Oral Solution (1% to less than 3%) 2247
Neulasta Injection 596
Neumega for Injection 3433
Neupogen for Injection 598
Neurontin Capsules (Infrequent) 2498
Neurontin Oral Solution (Infrequent) 2498
Neurontin Tablets (Infrequent) 2498
Nexium Delayed-Release Capsules (Less than 1%) 645
Nexium I.V. (Less than 1%) 649
Niaspan Extended-Release Tablets 1703
▲ Nipent for Injection (3% to 10%) 3216
Norflex Injection (Rare) 1824
Noroxin Tablets (Less frequent) 2009
Norvasc Tablets (Less than or equal to 0.1%) 2529
Norvir (Less than 2%) 499
Novantrone for Injection Concentrate 3158
Novarel for Injection 1147
Nubain Injection (1% or less) 1111
Numorphan 1112
▲ Oncaspar (Greater than 5%) 1123
Orthoclone OKT3 Sterile Solution 2370
Oxsoralen-Ultra Capsules 3354
Parcopa Orally Disintegrating Tablets 3111
Parnate Tablets 1499
Paxil CR Controlled-Release Tablets (Infrequent) 1509
Paxil (Infrequent) 1501
PCE Dispertab Tablets 510
Pediarix Vaccine (Rare) 1518
Liquid PedvaxHIB (Two children) 2012
Pegasys 2793
PEG-Intron Powder for Injection (Less than or equal to 1%) 3062
Pentasa Capsules (Less than 1%) 3182
Pepcid Injection (Infrequent) 2017
Pepcid (Infrequent) 2014
Persantine Tablets (Rare) 898
Phenergan 3438
Plasbumin-5 (Rare) 3249
Plasbumin-20 (Rare) 3249
Plasbumin-25 (Rare) 3251
Plasmanate (Occasional) 3252
Plavix Tablets (Less than 1%) 940
Plavix Tablets (Less than 1%) 2942
Plendil Extended-Release Tablets (0.5% to 1.5%) 651
Pletal Tablets (Less than 2%) 2478
Pneumovax 23 (Rare) 2020
Pravachol Tablets (Rare) 943
Prefest Tablets 1069
Premarin Intravenous 3440
Premarin Tablets 3443
Premarin Vaginal Cream 3449
Premphase Tablets 3452
Prempro Tablets 3452
Prevacid Delayed-Release Capsules (Less than 1%) 3268
Prevacid for Delayed-Release Oral Suspension (Less than 1%) 3268
Prevacid NapraPAC (Less than 1%) 3277
Prevacid SoluTab Delayed-Release Orally Disintegrating Tablets (Less than 1%) 3268
PREVPAC (Less than 1%) 3281
Prilosec OTC Tablets (Less than 1%) 2674
Primaxin I.M. 2022
Primaxin I.V. (0.2%) 2024
Prinivil Tablets (0.3% to 1.0%) 2029
Prinzide Tablets 2033
Prochieve 4% Gel 1018
Prochieve 8% Gel 1018
Procrit for Injection (Rare) 2374
Proleukin for Injection (2%) 1007
Propecia Tablets 2036
Proscar Tablets 2040
ProSom Tablets (Infrequent) 512
Protonix I.V. (Less than 1%) 3468
Protonix Tablets (Less than 1%) 3465
▲ Protopic Ointment (3% to 5%) 629
Proventil Inhalation Aerosol 3067
Proventil Inhalation Solution 0.083% (Rare) 3069
Proventil HFA Inhalation Aerosol (Rare) 3071
Prozac Pulvules and Liquid 1771
Pulmozyme Inhalation Solution 1245
Qvar Inhalation Aerosol (Rare) 1654
Rabies Vaccine RabAvert 1011
Raptiva for Injection (1%) 1247
Rebetron Combination Therapy 3078
Recombinate (Extremely rare) 762
Recombivax HB (Less than 1%) 2045
ReFacto Vials 3479
Refludan for Injection (Uncommon) 815
Relafen Tablets (1%) 1523
Relenza Rotadisk (Less than 1.5%) 1525
Relpax Tablets (Rare) 2531
Remicade for IV Injection (Less than 1%) 987
Repronex for Intramuscular and Subcutaneous Injection 1148
Requip Tablets (Infrequent) 1528
Rescriptor Tablets 2535
Retin-A Micro 0.1%/0.04% 2388
Retrovir Capsules 1533
Retrovir IV Infusion 1537
Retrovir 1533
Reyataz Capsules (Less than 3%) 948
Rilutek Tablets (Infrequent) 2945
Risperdal M-Tab Orally Disintegrating Tablets (Rare) 1658
Risperdal (Rare) 1658
Ritalin Hydrochloride Tablets 2254
Ritalin LA Capsules 2255
Ritalin-SR Tablets 2254
▲ Rituxan for Infusion (1% to 8%) 845
▲ Rituxan I.V. (1% to 8%) 1251
Roferon-A Injection (Rare) 2805
Rythmol SR Capsules 2736
Sandostatin Injection (Less than 1%) 2263
Sandostatin LAR Depot (1% to 4%) 2264
Seasonale Tablets 1073
▲ Serevent Diskus (3%) 1540
Singulair (Greater than or equal to 2%) 2047
Sonata Capsules (Infrequent) 1686
Soriatane Capsules (Less than 1%) 1028
Spectracef Tablets (0.1% to 1%) 2706
Spiriva HandiHaler 899
St. Joseph 81 mg Aspirin Chewable and Enteric Coated Tablets 1841
Stalevo Tablets 2270
Stromectol Tablets (0.9%) 2053
Sular Tablets (Less than or equal to 1%) 1163
Sulfamylon Cream 2154
Sulfamylon for 5% Topical Solution 2155
Suprax (Less than 2%) 1811
Surmontil Capsules 2347
Sustiva Capsules (Less than 2%) 957
Synercid I.V. (Less than 1%) 1690
Synthroid Tablets 515
Tambocor Tablets (Less than 1%) 1824
Tarka Tablets 519
Tasmar Tablets (Infrequent) 3360
Tegretol/Tegretol-XR 2278
Teveten HCT Tablets 1710
Thalomid Capsules 979
Thioridazine Hydrochloride Tablets (Infrequent) 2122
Thiothixene Capsules 2124
▲ Thrombate III (1 of 17) 3254
Thyrogen for Injection 1270
Thyrolar 1203
Ticlid Tablets (0.5% to 1.0%) 2813
Timentin ADD-Vantage 1556
Timentin Injection Galaxy Container 1559
Timentin IV Infusion 1553
Timentin Pharmacy Bulk Package 1562
Timolide Tablets 2056
Timoptic in Ocudose (Less frequent) 2061
Timoptic Sterile Ophthalmic Solution (Less frequent) 2058
Timoptic-XE Sterile Ophthalmic Gel Forming Solution 2062
Tindamax 2670
TNKase I.V. (Rare) 1256
Topamax Sprinkle Capsules (Infrequent) 2438
Topamax Tablets (Infrequent) 2438
Toprol-XL Tablets 660
Tricor Tablets (1.1%) 523
TriLyte with Flavor Packs for Oral Solution 3114
▲ Trisenox Injection (8%) 983
Trizivir Tablets 1565
Trusopt Sterile Ophthalmic Solution 2065
▲ Truvada Tablets (Greater than 5%) 1279
Twinrix Vaccine (Less than 1%) 1571
Ultane Liquid for Inhalation (Less than 1%) 526
Ultracet Tablets 2462
Uniretic Tablets (Less than 1%) 3114
Unithroid Tablets 3521
Univasc Tablets (Less than 1%) 3118
Valtrex Caplets 1573
Vancocin HCl Capsules, USP 3370
Vantin Tablets and Oral Suspension (Less than 1%) 2650
Vaqta (Less than 1%) 2067
Varivax (Greater than or equal to 1%) 2070
Vaseretic Tablets 2073
Vasotec I.V. Injection (0.5% to 1.0%) 2076
Ventolin HFA Inhalation Aerosol 1576
Verelan PM Capsules (2% or less) 3120
Vermox Chewable Tablets (Rare) 1853
VFEND I.V. (Less than 2%) 2543
VFEND Oral Suspension (Less than 2%) 2543
VFEND Tablets (Less than 2%) 2543
Viagra Tablets (Less than 2%) 2552
Vicoprofen Tablets (Less than 1%) 533
Viracept (Less than 2%) 2556
Viramune Oral Suspension 903
Viramune Tablets 903
Vivactil Tablets 2350
Vivelle Transdermal System 2288
Vivelle-Dot Transdermal System 2293
Vivotif (Infrequent) 834
Voltaren Tablets (Rarely) 2298
Voltaren-XR Tablets (Rarely) 2301
VoSpire Extended-Release Tablets (Rare) 2352
Vytorin 10/10 Tablets 2084
Vytorin 10/10 Tablets 3092
Vytorin 10/20 Tablets 2084
Vytorin 10/20 Tablets 3092
Vytorin 10/40 Tablets 2084
Vytorin 10/40 Tablets 3092
Vytorin 10/80 Tablets 2084
Vytorin 10/80 Tablets 3092
Wellbutrin Tablets 1579
Wellbutrin SR Sustained-Release Tablets (1% to 2%) 1583
Wellbutrin XL Extended-Release Tablets (1% to 2%) 1588
Xanax XR Tablets (Infrequent) 2655
Xenical Capsules 2834
Xifaxan Tablets 2847
Xolair 1259
▲ Xopenex HFA Inhalation Aerosol (3%) 3151
▲ Xopenex Inhalation Solution (3%) 3143
▲ Xopenex Inhalation Solution Concentrate (3%) 3147
Zegerid Powder for Oral Solution (Less than 1%) 2972
Zelnorm Tablets 2303
Zestoretic Tablets 701
Zestril Tablets (0.3% to 1.0%) 704
Zetia Tablets 2090
▲ Zevalin Injection (4%) 848
Zinacef Injection (Fewer than 1 in 250 patients) 1604
Zinacef for Injection (Fewer than 1 in 250 patients) 1604
Zinecard for Injection (2%) 2659
Zithromax Capsules, 250 mg (1% or less) 2568
Zithromax for IV Infusion 2573
Zithromax for Oral Suspension, 300 mg, 600 mg, 900 mg, 1200 mg (1% or less) 2561
Zithromax Tablets, 250 mg, 500 mg (1% or less) 2561
Zithromax Tri-Pak (1% or less) 2561
Zmax for Oral Suspension (Less then 1%) 2577
Zocor Tablets (Rare) 2078
Zofran Injection (Rare) 1607
Zofran 1613
Zofran ODT Orally Disintegrating Tablets 1613
Zoladex (Rare) 709
Zoladex 3-month (Rare) 712
Zoloft (Infrequent) 2581

Zomig Tablets (Infrequent)............... 714
Zomig-ZMT Tablets (Infrequent)........ 714
Zonegran Capsules (Infrequent)....... 1089
Zovirax Capsules.......................... 1616
Zovirax for Injection...................... 1618
Zovirax.. 1616
Zyban Sustained-Release Tablets (1% to 2%)................................ 1620
Zyprexa Tablets (Infrequent)........... 1798
Zyprexa ZYDIS Orally Disintegrating Tablets (Infrequent)........................... 1798
Zyrtec Chewable Tablets (Less than 2%)................................... 2589
Zyrtec (Less than 2%).................... 2589
Zyrtec-D 12 Hour Extended Release Tablets (Less than 2%)..... 2591

Urticaria pigmentosa

Rabies Vaccine RabAvert (One case).. 1011

Uterine contractions, abnormal

Cervidil Vaginal Insert (2.0% to 4.7%).. 1182

Uterine contractions, altered

Proventil Inhalation Solution 0.083%.. 3069

Uterine disorder, unspecified

Evista Tablets.............................. 1735
Zomig Nasal Spray (Rare)............... 718

Uterine fibroids

Activella Tablets (0% to 5%)............ 2311
Zomig Nasal Spray (Rare)............... 718

Uterine fibroids, enlarged

Symbyax Capsules (Rare)............... 1788

Uterine fibromyomata, increase in size

Activella Tablets............................ 2311
Climara Transdermal System........... 795
Estratest Tablets........................... 3196
Estratest H.S. Tablets.................... 3196
Premarin Intravenous..................... 3440
Premarin Tablets........................... 3443
Premarin Vaginal Cream.................. 3449
Premphase Tablets......................... 3452
Prempro Tablets............................ 3452
Prozac Pulvules and Liquid (Rare)..... 1771
Vivelle Transdermal System............ 2288
Vivelle-Dot Transdermal System....... 2293
Zyprexa Tablets (Infrequent)........... 1798
Zyprexa ZYDIS Orally Disintegrating Tablets (Infrequent)........................... 1798

Uterine inertia

Tasmar Tablets (Infrequent)............ 3360

Uterine leiomyomata, enlargement

Cenestin Tablets, 0.45mg, 0.625mg, 0.9mg, 1.25mg.......... 1063
Cenestin Tablets, 0.3mg................. 1063
Climara Transdermal System........... 795
Climara Pro Transdermal System..... 800
Estrogel 0.06%.............................. 3200
Menostar Transdermal System........ 805
Vivelle Transdermal System............ 2288
Vivelle-Dot Transdermal System....... 2293

Uterine rupture

Cervidil Vaginal Insert................... 1182

Uterine spasm

Bravelle for Intramuscular or Subcutaneous Injection (2.7%)...... 1140
Clindesse Vaginal Cream (Less than 1%)................................... 3296
Effexor Tablets (Rare)................... 3405
Effexor XR Capsules (Rare)............ 3411
▲ Menopur for Subcutaneous Injection (1.6% to 3.9%).............. 1145
Paxil CR Controlled-Release Tablets (Rare)............................ 1509
Paxil (Rare).................................. 1501

Uveitis

Alrex Ophthalmic Suspension 0.2% (Less than 5%)................... ⊙243
Aredia for Injection (Rare)............. 2168
Blephamide Ophthalmic Ointment.... 563
Blephamide Ophthalmic Suspension.................................. 564
Effexor Tablets (Rare)................... 3405
Effexor XR Capsules (Rare)............ 3411
FML Ophthalmic Ointment.............. ⊙225
FML Ophthalmic Suspension........... ⊙224
FML Forte Ophthalmic Suspension.................................. ⊙223
Fosamax (Rare)............................. 1949
Fosamax Plus D Tablets (Rarely)....... 1956
HMS Sterile Ophthalmic Suspension.................................. ⊙228
Lamictal (Rare)............................. 1449
Lotemax Ophthalmic Suspension 0.5% (Less than 5%).................... ⊙249
Lyrica Capsules (Rare).................... 2524
Nipent for Injection (Less than 3%)... 3216
Norvir (Less than 2%)...................... 499
OptiPranolol Metipranolol Ophthalmic Solution 0.3%........... ⊙254
Pred Forte Ophthalmic Suspension.................................. ⊙233
Pred Mild Sterile Ophthalmic Suspension.................................. ⊙236
Rituxan for Infusion (Less than 0.1%).. 845
Rituxan I.V................................... 1251
Stromectol Tablets 2053
VFEND I.V. (Less than 2%) 2543
VFEND Oral Suspension (Less than 2%).. 2543
VFEND Tablets (Less than 2%) 2543
▲ Voltaren Ophthalmic Solution (Less than or equal to 5%) 2300
Xalatan Sterile Ophthalmic Solution 2654

V

Vagina, dryness

Arimidex Tablets (1% to 2%) 665
▲ Intron A for Injection (Less than 5%).. 3038
Prochieve 4% Gel 1018
Prochieve 8% Gel 1018
Prometrium Capsules (100 mg, 200 mg) (Less than 6%) 3205
Risperdal M-Tab Orally Disintegrating Tablets (Frequent) ... 1658
Risperdal (Frequent) 1658

Vaginal adenosis

Vivelle Transdermal System 2288
Vivelle-Dot Transdermal System 2293

Vaginal burning

Clindesse Vaginal Cream (Less than 1%) 3296
▲ Gynazole-1 Vaginal Cream (5.7%) 3298

Vaginal candidiasis

Abilify Tablets (Infrequent) 916
Abilify Tablets (Infrequent) 2472
Activella Tablets 2311
Advair Diskus 100/50 1291
Advair Diskus 250/50 1291
Advair Diskus 500/50 1291
Alesse-28 Tablets 3392
▲ Arava Tablets (1% to 3%) 2881
Ceftin (Less frequent) 1369
Cenestin Tablets, 0.45mg, 0.625mg, 0.9mg, 1.25mg 1063
Cenestin Tablets, 0.3mg 1063
Cipro I.V. 2998
Cipro I.V. Pharmacy Bulk Package 3509
Cipro 2991
Cipro XR Tablets 3004
Climara Transdermal System 795
Climara Pro Transdermal System 800
Clozapine Tablets (Less than 1%) 2141
Clozaril Tablets (Less than 1%) 2174
▲ Copaxone for Injection (8%) 3292
▲ depo-subQ provera 104 Injectable Suspension (1% to less than 5%) 2622
Doxil Injection (Less than 1%) 3302
Estratest Tablets 3196
Estratest H.S. Tablets 3196
Estrogel 0.06% 3200
Invanz for Injection (Greater than 0.1%) 1974
Ketek Tablets (Greater than or equal to 0.2% to less than 2%) 2920
Lamictal (Infrequent) 1449
Lofibra Capsules 1217
Lo/Ovral-28 Tablets 3423
Menostar Transdermal System 805
Meridia Capsules (1.2%) 485
Metrogel 1% (0.2%) 1212
▲ MetroGel-Vaginal Gel (10%) 1822
Neurontin Capsules (Infrequent) 2498
Neurontin Oral Solution (Infrequent) 2498
Neurontin Tablets (Infrequent) 2498
Noroxin Tablets 2009
▲ Omnicef Capsules (5%) 506
Omnicef for Oral Suspension (0.3%) 506
Ortho-Cept Tablets 2395
Ortho-Cyclen Tablets...................... 2414
Ortho Evra Transdermal System...... 2402
Ortho Tri-Cyclen Tablets.................. 2414
Ortho Tri-Cyclen Lo Tablets............. 2421
Prefest Tablets.............................. 1069
Premarin Tablets........................... 3443
Premarin Vaginal Cream.................. 3449
Premphase Tablets......................... 3452
Prempro Tablets............................ 3452
Prometrium Capsules (100 mg, 200 mg) (Less than 5%)............... 3205
Protopic Ointment (Greater than or equal to 1%)............................... 629
Seroquel Tablets (Infrequent)........... 691
Soriatane Capsules 1028
Tricor Tablets................................ 523
Triphasil-28 Tablets........................ 3483
▲ Vantin Tablets and Oral Suspension (3.1%)....................... 2650
Vivelle Transdermal System............ 2288
Vivelle-Dot Transdermal System 2293
Yasmin 28 Tablets (Greater than 1%) 818
Zinacef Injection 1604
Zinacef for Injection 1604
Zyvox (1% to 1.6%) 2661

Vaginal discharge

▲ Arimidex Tablets (3%) 665
Bravelle for Intramuscular or Subcutaneous Injection (2.7%) 1140
Ceftin Tablets (0.1% to 1%) 1369
Cleocin Vaginal Ovules (Less than 1%) 2613
Clindesse Vaginal Cream (1.1%) 3296
Invirase (Less than 2%) 2776
Lupron Depot-PED 7.5 mg, 11.25 mg and 15 mg (2%) 3266
Lupron Injection Pediatric 3256
▲ MetroGel-Vaginal Gel (12%) 1822
▲ Prochieve 4% Gel (7%) 1018
▲ Prochieve 8% Gel (7%) 1018
▲ Prometrium Capsules (100 mg, 200 mg) (10%) 3205
ProSom Tablets (Infrequent) 512
Tindamax 2670
▲ Vivelle Transdermal System (1.5% to 4.3%) 2288
▲ Vivelle-Dot Transdermal System (1.5% to 4.3%) 2293

Vaginal hemorrhage

▲ Femara Tablets (Less than 0.1% to 4.8%) 2210

Vaginal pressure

Adenoscan (Less than 1%) 613

Vaginitis

Abilify Tablets 916
Abilify Tablets 2472
Aceon Tablets (2 mg, 4 mg, 8 mg) (0.3% to 1%) 3191
Actiq (1% or greater) 993
Advair Diskus 100/50 1291
Advair Diskus 250/50 1291
Advair Diskus 500/50 1291
Alesse-28 Tablets 3392
Ambien Tablets (Infrequent) 2867
Amerge Tablets (Rare) 1312
Ancef for Injection 1318
Aricept Tablets (Infrequent) 1086
Aricept ODT Tablets (Infrequent) 1086
Augmentin (1%) 1331
Augmentin Tablets (1%) 1334
Augmentin XR Extended-Release Tablets (1%) 1340
Avelox (0.1% to less than 2%) 2984
Campral Tablets (Infrequent) 1175
▲ Ceftin Tablets (0.1% to 5.4%) 1369
Celebrex Capsules (0.1% to 1.9%) ... 3130
▲ Cenestin Tablets, 0.45mg, 0.625mg, 0.9mg, 1.25mg (7.5%) 1063
Cenestin Tablets, 0.3mg 1063
Cipro I.V. (1% or less) 2998
Cipro I.V. Pharmacy Bulk Package (1% or less) 3509
Cipro (Less than 1% to 2%) 2991
Cipro XR Tablets (Less than 1%) 3004
Cleocin Vaginal Ovules (Less than 1%) 2613
Climara Transdermal System 795
Climara Pro Transdermal System (1.9%) 800
▲ CombiPatch Transdermal System (9% to 13%) 2180
Copaxone for Injection (At least 2%) 3292
▲ Depacon Injection (1% to 5%) 412
▲ Depakene (1% to 5%) 417
▲ Depakote Sprinkle Capsules (1% to 5%) 422
▲ Depakote Tablets (1% to 5%) 427
Depakote ER Tablets (Greater than 1%) 433
▲ Depo-Provera Contraceptive Injection (1% to 5%) 2619
▲ depo-subQ provera 104 Injectable Suspension (1% to less than 5%) 2622
Doxil Injection (Less than 1%) 3302
Effexor Tablets (Frequent) 3405
Effexor XR Capsules (Frequent) 3411
Enablex Extended-Release Tablets (Greater than or equal to 1%) 2201
▲ Estrogel 0.06% (8.9%) 3200
▲ Evista Tablets (4.3%) 1735
▲ Evoxac Capsules (1% to 3%) 1042
Factive Tablets (0.1% to 1%) 2464
Fortaz (Less than 1%) 1422
Gabitril Tablets (Frequent) 998
▲ Infergen (5% to 8%) 1647
▲ Invanz for Injection (1.4% to 3.3%) 1974
Ketek Tablets (Greater than or equal to 0.2% to less than 2%) 2920
Klonopin (1%) 2782
▲ Lamictal (4.1%) 1449
Levaquin in 5% Dextrose Injection (0.5% to 1.3%) 2453
Levaquin (0.5% to 1.3%) 2453
Lo/Ovral-28 Tablets 3423
Lunesta Tablets (Infrequent) 3139
▲ Lupron Depot 3.75 mg (10%) 3257
▲ Lupron Depot–3 Month 11.25 mg (10%) 3262
Lupron Depot-PED 7.5 mg, 11.25 mg and 15 mg (2%) 3266
Lupron Injection Pediatric 3256
Maxipime for Injection (Greater than 0.1% to less than 1%) 1093
Mefoxin for Injection 1987
Mefoxin Premixed Intravenous Solution 1990
Menostar Transdermal System 805
Migranal Nasal Spray (Rare) 3350
▲ Mirena Intrauterine System (5% or more) 810
Nexium Delayed-Release Capsules (Less than 1%) 645
Nexium I.V. (Less than 1%) 649
Omnicef Capsules (1%) 506
Omnicef for Oral Suspension (0.3%) 506
Ortho-Cept Tablets 2395
Ortho-Cyclen Tablets 2414
Ortho Evra Transdermal System 2402
Ortho Tri-Cyclen Tablets 2414
Ortho Tri-Cyclen Lo Tablets 2421
Paxil CR Controlled-Release Tablets (Infrequent) 1509
Paxil (Infrequent) 1501
Permax Tablets (Infrequent) 3357
Pletal Tablets (Less than 2%) 2478
▲ Prefest Tablets (7%) 1069
▲ Premarin Tablets (5% to 7%) 3443
Premarin Vaginal Cream 3449
▲ Premphase Tablets (4% to 7%) 3452
▲ Prempro Tablets (4% to 7%) 3452
Prevacid Delayed-Release Capsules (Less than 1%) 3268
Prevacid for Delayed-Release Oral Suspension (Less than 1%) 3268
Prevacid NapraPAC (Less than 1%) .. 3277
Prevacid SoluTab Delayed-Release Orally Disintegrating Tablets (Less than 1%) 3268
PREVPAC (Less than 3%) 3281
▲ Prograf Capsules and Injection (3% to 15%) 624
Prometrium Capsules (100 mg, 200 mg) (Less than 5%) 3205
Protonix I.V. (Less than 1%) 3468
Protonix Tablets (Less than 1%) 3465
Relpax Tablets (Rare) 2531
Risperdal Consta Long-Acting Injection (Infrequent) 1664
Rocephin Injectable Vials, ADD-Vantage, Galaxy, Bulk (Occasional) 2801
Sandostatin Injection (Less than 1%) 2263
Seasonale Tablets 1073
Seroquel Tablets (Infrequent) 691
Sonata Capsules (Infrequent) 1686
Spectracef Tablets (0.1% to 1%) 2706
Sular Tablets (Less than or equal to 1%) 1163
Suprax (Less than 2%) 1811
Symbyax Capsules (Infrequent) 1788
Synercid I.V. (Less than 1%) 1690
Tasmar Tablets (Infrequent) 3360
▲ Tequin Injection (6%) 964
▲ Tequin Tablets (6%) 964
Trileptal Oral Suspension (Up to 2%) 2281

Trileptal Tablets (Up to 2%)............... 2281
Triphasil-28 Tablets........................ 3483
Tygacil for Injection (0% to less than 2%).................................... 3489
Uniretic Tablets (Less than 1%)......... 3114
▲ Vagifem Tablets (3% to 5%) 2340
Vantin Tablets and Oral Suspension (Less than 1%)........... 2650
Vivelle Transdermal System............. 2288
Vivelle-Dot Transdermal System....... 2293
Wellbutrin Tablets (Infrequent).......... 1579
Wellbutrin SR Sustained-Release Tablets 1583
Wellbutrin XL Extended-Release Tablets 1588
Xenical Capsules (2.6% to 3.8%)...... 2834
Yasmin 28 Tablets (Greater than 1%).. 818
Zinacef Injection............................ 1604
Zinacef for Injection........................ 1604
Zithromax Capsules, 250 mg (1% or less to 2%)............................. 2568
Zithromax for IV Infusion (2.8%) 2573
Zithromax for Oral Suspension, 1 g (1% or less to 1%) 2568
Zithromax for Oral Suspension, 300 mg, 600 mg, 900 mg, 1200 mg (1% or less to 2%) 2561
Zithromax Tablets, 250 mg, 500 mg (1% or less to 2%) 2561
Zithromax Tablets, 600 mg (1% or less to 1%) 2568
Zithromax Tri-Pak (1% or less to 2%) 2561
Zithromax Z-Pak (1% or less to 1%) .. 2568
Zmax for Oral Suspension (Less then 1%) 2577
▲ Zoladex (1% to 75%) 709
Zomig Nasal Spray (Rare) 718
Zosyn (1.0% or less) 3492
Zyban Sustained-Release Tablets 1620
Zyprexa Tablets 1798
Zyprexa ZYDIS Orally Disintegrating Tablets 1798
Zyrtec Chewable Tablets (Less than 2%) 2589
Zyrtec (Less than 2%) 2589
Zyrtec-D 12 Hour Extended Release Tablets (Less than 2%) 2591

Vaginitis, atrophic

Clindesse Vaginal Cream (Less than 1%) 3296
Evoxac Capsules (Less than 1%) 1042
Exelon Capsules (Infrequent) 2204
▲ Imdur Tablets (Less than or equal to 5%) 3032
Soriatane Capsules (Less than 1%) .. 1028
Zoloft (Rare) 2581

Vaginitis, bacterial

▲ depo-subQ provera 104 Injectable Suspension (1% to less than 5%) 2622

Vaginosis, fungal

▲ Clindesse Vaginal Cream (14.1%) ... 3296
Ketek Tablets (Greater than or equal to 0.2% to less than 2%) 2920

Varicella

▲ Clarinex Syrup (3.6%) 3009
Elidel Cream 1% (0.7% to 2.9%)....... 2198
Singulair (Greater than or equal to 2%) 2047

Varices, esophageal

Myleran Tablets 1492
Nexium Delayed-Release Capsules (Less than 1%) 645
Nexium I.V. (Less than 1%) 649
Tabloid Tablets 1545

Vascular access, clotting

▲ Epogen for Injection (0.25% to 7%) 586
▲ Procrit for Injection (0.25 to 7%) 2374

Vascular collapse

Carimune NF 3501
Gammagard Liquid 751
Gammagard S/D (Rare) 754
Gamunex Immune Globulin I.V., 10% (Rare) 3232
Iveegam EN (Rare) 759

Vascular complications, unspecified

Angiomax for Injection (Rare) 1856
Bravelle for Intramuscular or Subcutaneous Injection 1140
Camptosar Injection 2602
▲ Carnitor Injection (2% to 6%) 3185
▲ Cozaar Tablets (4%) 1913
▲ Flolan for Injection (95%) 1408
Follistim AQ Cartridge...................... 2354
Gonal-f RFF Pen for Injection 3155
▲ Humira Injection (Less than 5%) 464
Lofibra Capsules 1217
Ortho-Cyclen/Ortho Tri-Cyclen 2414
Ortho Tri-Cyclen Lo Tablets............. 2421
ReoPro Vials (1.8%)......................... 1779
Repronex for Intramuscular and Subcutaneous Injection............. 1148
Sandostatin LAR Depot (1% to 4%)... 2264
Tricor Tablets.................................. 523
Zofran (Rare)................................... 1613
Zofran ODT Orally Disintegrating Tablets (Rare)............................ 1613
Zomig Nasal Spray (Rare)................. 718

Vascular disorder

Antara Capsules.............................. 2723

Vascular disorders, unspecified

▲ Ammonul Injection (6%) 3323

Vascular insufficiency

Zonegran Capsules (Infrequent) 1089

Vascular leak syndrome

▲ Ontak Vials (27%) 1717

Vasculitis

Accutane Capsules 2740
Aceon Tablets (2 mg, 4 mg, 8 mg) ... 3191
Advair Diskus 100/50 1291
Advair Diskus 250/50 1291
Advair Diskus 500/50 1291
Advicor Tablets 1694
Aldoclor Tablets 1881
Aldoril Tablets 1884
Alkeran for Injection 976
Alkeran Tablets 977
Altace Capsules (Less than 1%) 1673
Altoprev Extended-Release Tablets (Rare) 1151
Amnesteem Capsules 2126
Anaprox Tablets (Less than 1%) 2769
Anaprox DS Tablets (Less than 1%) .. 2769
▲ Arava Tablets (1% to 3%) 2881
Arthrotec Tablets (Rare) 3126
Atacand HCT 637
Attenuvax 1889
Avalide Tablets 922
Avalide Tablets 2889
Axid Oral Solution (Rare) 913
Caduet Tablets (Greater than 0.1% to less than or equal to 1%) 2507
Cancidas for Injection (0%) 1894
Captopril Tablets 2114
Cataflam Tablets (Rarely) 2173
Celebrex Capsules (Less than 0.1%) 3130
Cipro I.V. (1% or less) 2998
Cipro I.V. Pharmacy Bulk Package (1% or less) 3509
Cipro 2991
Cipro XR Tablets 3004
Clorpres Tablets 2139
Clozapine Tablets 2141
Clozaril Tablets 2174
Combivir Tablets 1373
Coumadin for Injection (Infrequent) ... 932
Coumadin Tablets (Infrequent) 932
Covera-HS Tablets (Less than 2%) 3135
Cozaar Tablets 1913
Crixivan Capsules 1918
Cytovene Capsules 2763
Decadron Tablets 1929
Diovan HCT Tablets 2195
Diuril Oral 1936
Diuril Sodium Intravenous 1934
Dyazide Capsules 1389
EC-Naprosyn Delayed-Release Tablets (Less than 1%) 2769
Evoxac Capsules (Less than 1%) 1042
FazaClo Orally Disintegrating Tablets 547
Furosemide Tablets 2117
Hyzaar 1964
Kaletra (Less than 2%) 474
Lamictal 1449
Lescol Capsules (Rare) 2227
Lescol Capsules (Rare) 2730
Lescol XL Tablets 2227
Lescol XL Tablets 2730
Levaquin in 5% Dextrose Injection (Rare) 2453
Levaquin (Rare) 2453
Maxzide 2150
Meruvax II 1994
Mevacor Tablets (Rare) 1996
Micardis HCT Tablets 886
M-M-R II 1980
Mobic Oral Suspension (Less than 2%) 893
Mobic Tablets (Less than 2%)............ 893
Moduretic Tablets............................ 2003
Mumpsvax (Rare)............................. 2005
Naprosyn Suspension (Less than 1%).. 2769
Naprosyn Tablets (Less than 1%)..... 2769
Nipent for Injection (Less than 3%)... 3216
Noroxin Tablets............................... 2009
Norvasc Tablets (More than 0.1% to 1%)... 2529
Orthoclone OKT3 Sterile Solution..... 2370
Pacerone Tablets (Rare)................... 3337
Paser Granules................................ 1657
PEG-Intron Powder for Injection (Less than or equal to 1%)........... 3062
Permax Tablets (Rare)...................... 3357
Plavix Tablets.................................. 940
Plavix Tablets.................................. 2942
Pravachol Tablets (Rare).................. 943
Prevacid NapraPAC (Less than 1%).. 3277
Prinivil Tablets (0.3% to 1.0%) 2029
Prinzide Tablets 2033
Recombivax HB 2045
Relafen Tablets (Less than 1%) 1523
Remicade for IV Injection 987
Retrovir Capsules (Rare) 1533
Retrovir IV Infusion (Rare) 1537
Retrovir (Rare) 1533
Ritalin Hydrochloride Tablets 2254
Ritalin LA Capsules 2255
Ritalin-SR Tablets 2254
Rituxan for Infusion (Less than 0.1%) 845
Rituxan I.V. (Less than 0.1%) 1251
Roferon-A Injection (Rare) 2805
Tarka Tablets 519
Tegretol/Tegretol-XR 2278
Teveten HCT Tablets 1710
Ticlid Tablets (Rare) 2813
Timolide Tablets 2056
Trizivir Tablets 1565
Vancocin HCl Capsules, USP (Rare) 3370
Vaseretic Tablets 2073
Vasotec I.V. Injection (0.5% to 1.0%) 2076
Verelan PM Capsules (2% or less) 3120
Vesanoid Capsules 2823
Voltaren Tablets (Rarely) 2298
Voltaren-XR Tablets (Rarely) 2301
Vytorin 10/10 Tablets 2084
Vytorin 10/10 Tablets 3092
Vytorin 10/20 Tablets 2084
Vytorin 10/20 Tablets 3092
Vytorin 10/40 Tablets 2084
Vytorin 10/40 Tablets 3092
Vytorin 10/80 Tablets 2084
Vytorin 10/80 Tablets 3092
Zantac (Rare) 1597
Zantac Injection (Rare) 1593
Zantac Injection Pharmacy Bulk Package (Rare) 1595
Zantac Syrup (Rare) 1597
Zestoretic Tablets 701
Zestril Tablets (0.3% to 1.0%) 704
Zocor Tablets (Rare) 2078
Zoloft 2581

Vasculitis, allergic

Aggrenox Capsules 855
Amaryl Tablets (Rare) 2864
Amoxil Capsules 1315
Amoxil Chewable Tablets 1315
Amoxil Pediatric Drops for Oral Suspension 1315
Amoxil Powder for Oral Suspension 1315
Amoxil Tablets 1315
Imitrex Nasal Spray 1435
Imitrex Tablets 1440
Omnicef Capsules 506
Omnicef for Oral Suspension 506

Vasculitis, central nervous system

Imitrex Nasal Spray 1435
Imitrex Tablets 1440

Vasculitis, cutaneous

Atacand HCT 637
Avalide Tablets 922
Avalide Tablets 2889
Clorpres Tablets 2139
Depacon Injection 412
Depakene 417
Depakote Sprinkle Capsules 422
Depakote Tablets 427
Depakote ER Tablets 433
Diovan HCT Tablets 2195
Diuril Oral 1936
Diuril Sodium Intravenous 1934
Enbrel for Injection 580
Hyzaar 1964
Maxzide... 2150
Micardis HCT Tablets....................... 886
Moduretic Tablets............................ 2003
Neupogen for Injection (Infrequent).. 598
Prinzide Tablets.............................. 2033
Remicade for IV Injection................. 987
Teveten HCT Tablets........................ 1710
Timolide Tablets.............................. 2056
Vaseretic Tablets............................. 2073
Zestoretic Tablets............................ 701

Vasculitis, eosinophilic

Accolate Tablets (Rare)..................... 663

Vasculitis, leukocytoclastic

Plendil Extended-Release Tablets..... 651
Rescriptor Tablets........................... 2535
Tiazac Capsules.............................. 1204
Valtrex Caplets................................ 1573
Zovirax Capsules............................. 1616
Zovirax for Injection........................ 1618
Zovirax.. 1616

Vasculitis, necrotizing

Arava Tablets.................................. 2881
Concerta Extended-Release Tablets 1828
Focalin Tablets................................ 2214
Focalin XR Capsules........................ 2217
Metadate CD Capsules..................... 3316

Vasculitis, renal

Cuprimine Capsules (Rare)............... 1925

Vasoconstriction

Invirase (Rare)................................ 2776

Vasodilation

Abilify Tablets (Infrequent)............... 916
Abilify Tablets (Infrequent)............... 2472
Aceon Tablets (2 mg, 4 mg, 8 mg) (0.3% to 1%)................................ 3191
Aciphex Tablets (Rare)..................... 1081
Actiq (Up to 2%).............................. 993
Actonel Tablets (1.4% to 2.3%)......... 2679
Actonel with Calcium Tablets (1.4% to 2.3%).......................... 2684
Agrylin Capsules (1% to 5%)............. 3172
Alphagan P Ophthalmic Solution....... 563
AmBisome for Injection (Less common).. 615
AndroGel (Fewer than 1%)................ 3330
Antara Capsules.............................. 2723
Aralast (0.1%)................................. 745
Arava Tablets (1% to less than 3%)... 2881
▲ Argatroban Injection (1% to 10%) 1321
Aricept Tablets (Frequent)................ 1086
Aricept ODT Tablets (Frequent)........ 1086
▲ Arimidex Tablets (25% to 41%) 665
Asacol Delayed-Release Tablets (2% or greater).............................. 2688
Avelox (0.1% to less than 2%).......... 2984
Avinza Capsules (Less than 5%)....... 1714
Avonex (2%)................................... 839
Axert Tablets (Infrequent)................. 2430
▲ Betaseron for SC Injection (8%) 791
▲ Bexxar (0% to 5%) 1360
Brimonidine Tartrate Ophthalmic Solution 0.2%............................ ⊙ 245
Caduet Tablets (Less than 2%)......... 2507
Campral Tablets (Frequent).............. 1175
▲ Camptosar Injection (0% to 11%) 2602
Cardene I.V. (0.7%)......................... 1129
Caverject Impulse Injection (Less than 1%)...................................... 2610
▲ CellCept Capsules (3% to less than 20%)...................................... 2751
▲ CellCept Intravenous (3% to less than 20%).................................. 2751
▲ CellCept Oral Suspension (3% to less than 20%).......................... 2751
▲ CellCept Tablets (3% to less than 20%).. 2751
▲ Cenestin Tablets, 0.45mg, 0.625mg, 0.9mg, 1.25mg (1% to 3.8%)................................... 1063
Cipro I.V. (1% or less)..................... 2998
Cipro I.V. Pharmacy Bulk Package (1% or less).............................. 3509
▲ Combunox Tablets (Less than 1% to 3%)....................................... 1183
▲ Copaxone for Injection (27%) 3292
Cosopt Sterile Ophthalmic Solution....................................... 1910
Crestor Tablets (Greater than or equal to 1%)................................ 672
Cytovene (At least 3 subjects).......... 2763
DDAVP Nasal Spray......................... 2894
Depacon Injection (0.9%)................. 412
Depakene (1% or more)................... 417
Depakote Sprinkle Capsules............ 422
▲ Depakote Tablets (1% to 5%) 427
▲ Depakote ER Tablets (1% to 5%) 433

Desmopressin Acetate Rhinal Tube 1144
Diastat Rectal Delivery System (1% to 2%) 3344
▲ Ditropan XL Extended Release Tablets (2% to less than 5%) 2391
▲ Doxil Injection (1% to 10%) 3302
▲ Effexor Tablets (2.3% to 5.6%) 3405
▲ Effexor XR Capsules (3% to 5%) 3411
Enbrel for Injection 580
▲ Faslodex Injection (17.7%) 682
Ferrlecit Injection 3379
Flexeril Tablets (Less than 1%) 1832
▲ Flolan for Injection (Most common) 1408
Gabitril Tablets (2%) 998
Geodon for Injection (Up to 1%) 2514
Hyperstat I.V. Injection 3031
Hytrin Capsules (At least 1%) 469
Imitrex Injection (Rare) 1431
Imitrex Nasal Spray 1435
Imitrex Tablets (Rare) 1440
▲ I.V. Busulfex (25%) 1125
Kadian Capsules (Less than 3%) 572
Lamictal (Infrequent) 1449
Levaquin in 5% Dextrose Injection 2453
Levaquin 2453
Lipitor Tablets (Less than 2%) 2495
Lofibra Capsules 1217
Lotrel Capsules 2238
Lupron Depot-PED 7.5 mg, 11.25 mg and 15 mg (Less than 2%) 3266
Lupron Injection Pediatric (Less than 2%) 3256
Marinol Capsules (Greater than 1%) 3334
Meridia Capsules (2.4%) 485
Mirapex Tablets (1% or more) 889
Navelbine Injection 1494
▲ Neumega for Injection (19%) 3433
Neurontin Capsules (1.1%) 2498
Neurontin Oral Solution (1.1%) 2498
Neurontin Tablets (1.1%) 2498
Norvir (1.7%) 499
Omacor Capsules 2735
▲ Ontak Vials (22%) 1717
OxyContin Tablets (Less than 1%) 2699
▲ Paxil CR Controlled-Release Tablets (3% to 4%) 1509
▲ Paxil (3% to 4%) 1501
Pentasa Capsules (Less than 1%) 3182
▲ Permax Tablets (3.2%) 3357
Pletal Tablets (Less than 2%) 2478
Prevacid Delayed-Release Capsules (Less than 1%) 3268
Prevacid for Delayed-Release Oral Suspension (Less than 1%) 3268
Prevacid I.V. for Injection (Less than 1%) 3274
Prevacid NapraPAC (Less than 1%) 3277
Prevacid SoluTab Delayed-Release Orally Disintegrating Tablets (Less than 1%) 3268
PREVPAC (Less than 1%) 3281
ProAmatine Tablets (Less frequent) 3183
▲ Proleukin for Injection (13%) 1007
Protonix I.V. (Less than 1%) 3468
Protonix Tablets (Less than 1%) 3465
Protopic Ointment (Greater than or equal to 1%) 629
Provigil Tablets (2%) 1002
▲ Prozac Pulvules and Liquid (1% to 5%) 1771
▲ Rapamune Oral Solution and Tablets (3% to 20%) 3472
ReFacto Vials 3479
Retrovir Capsules 1533
Retrovir IV Infusion 1537
Retrovir 1533
Reyataz Capsules (Less than 3%) 948
Seroquel Tablets (Infrequent) 691
Sonata Capsules (Infrequent) 1686
▲ Suboxone Tablets (9.30%) 2719
▲ Subutex Tablets (3.9%) 2719
▲ Sular Tablets (4%) 1163
Suprane Liquid for Inhalation (Less than 1%) 770
Symbyax Capsules (Frequent) 1788
Synercid I.V. (Less than 1%) 1690
Tasmar Tablets (Infrequent) 3360
▲ Tequin Injection (0.1% to 3%) 964
▲ Tequin Tablets (0.1% to 3%) 964
Thalomid Capsules 979
▲ Tiazac Capsules (4%) 1204
Timolide Tablets 2056
Timoptic in Ocudose 2061
Timoptic Sterile Ophthalmic Solution 2058
Timoptic-XE Sterile Ophthalmic Gel Forming Solution 2062
Topamax Sprinkle Capsules (Infrequent) 2438
Topamax Tablets (Infrequent) 2438
Tricor Tablets 523
Triglide Tablets 1165
Tygacil for Injection (0% to less than 2%) 3489
Ultracet Tablets 2462
Vantin Tablets and Oral Suspension (Less than 1%) 2650
▲ Ventavis Inhalation Solution (27%) 1036
VFEND I.V. (1% to 1.5%) 2543
VFEND Oral Suspension (1% to 1.5%) 2543
VFEND Tablets (1% to 1.5%) 2543
▲ Viadur Implant (67.9%) 782
Vicoprofen Tablets (Less than 3%) 533
Wellbutrin SR Sustained-Release Tablets (Infrequent) 1583
Wellbutrin XL Extended-Release Tablets (Infrequent) 1588
WinRho SDF 763
Zemaira (0.2% to 0.4%) 3506
▲ Zoladex (57%) 709
Zoloft (Rare) 2581
Zomig Nasal Spray (Rare) 718
Zyban Sustained-Release Tablets (Infrequent) 1620
Zyprexa Tablets (Infrequent) 1798
Zyprexa ZYDIS Orally Disintegrating Tablets (Infrequent) 1798

Vasodilation, peripheral
Aggrenox Capsules 855
Persantine Tablets 898

Vasomotor disturbances
Aminohippurate Sodium "PAH" Injection 1886
Niravam Orally Disintegrating Tablets (2%) 3106
Urecholine Tablets 2349

Vasospasm, coronary artery
Amerge Tablets 1312
Frova Tablets 1101
Imitrex Tablets 1440
Migranal Nasal Spray 3350
Relpax Tablets (Rare) 2531
Zomig Nasal Spray 718
Zomig Tablets 714
Zomig-ZMT Tablets 714

Vasospasm, rebound
Nimotop Capsules (Less than 1%) 774

Vasospasm, unspecified
▲ CellCept Capsules (3% to less than 20%) 2751
▲ CellCept Intravenous (3% to less than 20%) 2751
▲ CellCept Oral Suspension (3% to less than 20%) 2751
▲ CellCept Tablets (3% to less than 20%) 2751
Prozac Pulvules and Liquid (Rare) 1771
Relpax Tablets (Rare) 2531
Topamax Sprinkle Capsules (Rare) 2438
Topamax Tablets (Rare) 2438

Vasospastic reactions
Imitrex Tablets 1440
Zomig Tablets 714
Zomig-ZMT Tablets 714

Vasovagal episode
Abilify Tablets (Rare) 916
Abilify Tablets (Rare) 2472
Aggrastat (2%) 1878
Alferon N Injection (2%) 1640
Caverject Impulse Injection (Less than 1%) 2610
Naropin Injection (Less than 1%) 640
Visudyne for Injection (Less than 1%) 2286

Vein, pigmentation of
Aloxi Injection (Less than 1%) 2099

Vein disorder, unspecified
▲ Aldurazyme for Intravenous Infusion (3%) 1261

Vein distention
Aloxi Injection (Less than 1%) 2099

Veins, varicosis
Alesse-28 Tablets 3392
Ambien Tablets (Rare) 2867
Amerge Tablets (Rare) 1312
Antara Capsules 2723
▲ Arava Tablets (1% to 3%) 2881
Campral Tablets (Infrequent) 1175
Copaxone for Injection (Infrequent) 3292
Depo-Provera Contraceptive Injection (Less than 1%) 2619
▲ Imdur Tablets (Less than or equal to 5%) 3032
Kaletra (Less than 2%) 474
Lexapro Oral Solution (Infrequent) 1193
Lexapro Tablets (Infrequent) 1193
Lofibra Capsules 1217
Lo/Ovral-28 Tablets 3423
Neurontin Capsules (Rare) 2498
Neurontin Oral Solution (Rare) 2498
Neurontin Tablets (Rare) 2498
Paxil CR Controlled-Release Tablets (Rare) 1509
Paxil (Rare) 1501
Permax Tablets (Infrequent) 3357
Pletal Tablets (Less than 2%) 2478
Requip Tablets (Infrequent) 1528
Seasonale Tablets 1073
Tricor Tablets 523
Triglide Tablets 1165
Triphasil-28 Tablets 3483
▲ Visudyne for Injection (1% to 10%) 2286
Zoladex 3-month (1% to 5%) 712

Veno-occlusive disease, unspecified
Eloxatin for Injection 2908
▲ Mylotarg for Injection (1% to 20%) 3429

Venous infection at injection site
Primaxin I.V. (0.1%) 2024

Venous irritation
▲ R-Gene 10 for Intravenous Use (3%) 2647

Venous leak
▲ Caverject Impulse Injection (3%) 2610

Venous thromboembolism
Arimidex Tablets (1% to 2%) 665
Prempro Tablets 3452

Venous thrombophlebitis
▲ Xeloda Tablets (Less than 5%) 2825

Ventilator dependence
Virazole for Inhalation Solution 3365

Ventricular arrhythmias
Adenoscan (Less than 1%) 613
Biaxin/Biaxin XL 402
Campath Ampules 826
Celexa 1177
Digitek Tablets 2146
Doxil Injection (Less than 1%) 3302
E.E.S. (Rare) 449
EryPed (Rare) 445
Erythrocin Stearate Filmtab Tablets (Rare) 452
Erythromycin Base Filmtab Tablets (Rare) 454
Erythromycin Delayed-Release Capsules, USP 456
Hyperstat I.V. Injection 3031
Lanoxicaps Capsules (Less common) 1458
Lanoxin Injection 1462
Lanoxin Tablets (Less common) 1468
Lanoxin Injection Pediatric (Less common) 1465
Lexapro Oral Solution 1193
Lexapro Tablets 1193
Naropin Injection 640
Noroxin Tablets (Rare) 2009
PCE Dispertab Tablets 510
PREVPAC (Rare) 3281
▲ Proleukin for Injection (3%) 1007
Prozac Pulvules and Liquid (Rare) 1771
Relpax Tablets (Rare) 2531
ReoPro Vials (0.3%) 1779
Revatio Tablets 2541
Rituxan for Infusion (Four patients) 845
Rituxan I.V. (Four patients) 1251
Rythmol SR Capsules 2736
▲ Tambocor Tablets (7% to 13%) 1824
Tequin Injection 964
Tequin Tablets 964
Trasylol Injection (1% to 2%) 779
VFEND I.V. (Less than 2%) 2543
VFEND Oral Suspension (Less than 2%) 2543
VFEND Tablets (Less than 2%) 2543
Viagra Tablets 2552

Ventricular arrhythmias, post-abrupt discontinuation
Tenormin I.V. Injection 698
Tenormin Tablets 695

Ventricular contractions, premature
Adenocard Injection 612
Amerge Tablets (Infrequent) 1312
Arthrotec Tablets (Rare) 3126
Clozapine Tablets (Less than 1%) 2141
Clozaril Tablets (Less than 1%) 2174
Diprivan Injectable Emulsion (Less than 1%) 676
Ellence Injection 2632
FazaClo Orally Disintegrating Tablets (Less than 1%) 547
Indapamide Tablets (Less than 5%) 2119
Lanoxin Injection (Less common) 1462
Lanoxin Injection Pediatric (Less common) 1465
▲ Proleukin for Injection (5%) 1007
Zantac (Rare) 1597
Zantac Injection (Rare) 1593
Zantac Injection Pharmacy Bulk Package (Rare) 1595
Zantac Syrup (Rare) 1597
Zofran Injection 1607

Ventricular contractions, premature, multifocal
Digitek Tablets 2146
Lanoxicaps Capsules (Common) 1458
Lanoxin Injection 1462
▲ Lanoxin Tablets (Among most common) 1468
Lanoxin Injection Pediatric (Less common) 1465

Ventricular contractions, premature, unifocal
Digitek Tablets 2146
Lanoxicaps Capsules (Common) 1458
Lanoxin Injection 1462
▲ Lanoxin Tablets (Among most common) 1468
Lanoxin Injection Pediatric (Less common) 1465

Ventricular dilation, left-side
Retrovir Capsules (0.8%) 1533
Retrovir IV Infusion (1%) 1537
Retrovir (0.8%) 1533

Ventricular dysfunction
Herceptin I.V. 1234
Prograf Capsules and Injection (Rare) 624
Taxotere Injection Concentrate 2947

Ventricular ectopic beats
Cipro I.V. (1% or less) 2998
Cipro I.V. Pharmacy Bulk Package (1% or less) 3509
Cipro (Less than 1%) 2991
Cipro XR Tablets 3004
Digibind for Injection 1388
Imitrex Tablets 1440
Kytril Injection (Rare) 2785

Ventricular extrasystoles
Aceon Tablets (2 mg, 4 mg, 8 mg) (0.3% to 1%) 3191
Antara Capsules 2723
Cardene I.V. (1.4%) 1129
Cardizem LA Extended Release Tablets (Less than 2%) 1699
▲ CellCept Capsules (3% to less than 20%) 2751
▲ CellCept Intravenous (3% to less than 20%) 2751
▲ CellCept Oral Suspension (3% to less than 20%) 2751
▲ CellCept Tablets (3% to less than 20%) 2751
Digitek Tablets (1%) 2146
Effexor Tablets 3405
Effexor XR Capsules 3411
I.V. Busulfex (2%) 1125
Lanoxicaps Capsules 1458
Lanoxin Injection 1462
Lanoxin Tablets 1468
Lanoxin Injection Pediatric 1465
Lofibra Capsules 1217
Lotrel Capsules (Infrequent) 2238
▲ Natrecor for Injection (3% to 4%) 3123
Neurontin Capsules (Rare) 2498
Neurontin Oral Solution (Rare) 2498
Neurontin Tablets (Rare) 2498
Nipent for Injection (Less than 3%) 3216
Paxil CR Controlled-Release Tablets (Rare) 1509
Paxil (Rare) 1501
Permax Tablets (Infrequent) 3357
Pletal Tablets (Less than 2%) 2478
Proleukin for Injection (Less than 1%) 1007
Provigil Tablets (At least 1%) 1002
Prozac Pulvules and Liquid (Rare) 1771
Rilutek Tablets (Infrequent) 2945
Risperdal M-Tab Orally Disintegrating Tablets (Rare) 1658

Risperdal (Rare) 1658
Rythmol SR Capsules 2736
Sonata Capsules (Infrequent) 1686
Sular Tablets (Less than or equal to 1%) 1163
Tiazac Capsules (Less than 2%) 1204
▲ Trasylol Injection (6%) 779
Tricor Tablets 523
Ultane Liquid for Inhalation (Less than 1%) 526
Uniretic Tablets (Less than 1%) 3114
Vantas (Less than 2%) 3367
▲ Xeloda Tablets (Less than 5%) 2825
Zonegran Capsules (Rare) 1089
Zyprexa Tablets (Infrequent) 1798
Zyprexa ZYDIS Orally Disintegrating Tablets (Infrequent) 1798

Ventricular failure
Flolan for Injection 1408

Ventricular fibrillations
Abelcet Injection 1119
Adenocard Injection (Rare) 612
Aloprim for Injection (Less than 1%) 2156
Angiomax for Injection (Rare) 1856
Biltricide Tablets 2990
Celebrex Capsules (Less than 0.1%) 3130
Clozapine Tablets 2141
Clozaril Tablets 2174
Covera-HS Tablets 3135
Digitek Tablets 2146
Diprivan Injectable Emulsion (Less than 1%) 676
DynaCirc CR Tablets (0.5% to 1%) 2726
Effexor Tablets (Rare) 3405
Effexor XR Capsules (Rare) 3411
FazaClo Orally Disintegrating Tablets 547
Frova Tablets 1101
Hyzaar 1964
Imitrex Injection (Rare) 1431
Imitrex Tablets (Rare) 1440
Lanoxicaps Capsules 1458
Lanoxin Injection 1462
Lanoxin Tablets 1468
Lanoxin Injection Pediatric 1465
Levaquin in 5% Dextrose Injection (0.1% to 0.9%) 2453
Levaquin (0.1% to 0.9%) 2453
Lyrica Capsules (Rare) 2524
Meridia Capsules 485
Narcan Injection 1109
Naropin Injection 640
Paxil CR Controlled-Release Tablets 1509
Paxil 1501
Prozac Pulvules and Liquid (Rare) 1771
Refludan for Injection 815
Relpax Tablets (Rare) 2531
Retavase 1131
Rilutek Tablets (Rare) 2945
Rituxan for Infusion 845
Rituxan I.V. 1251
Trasylol Injection (2%) 779
Uniretic Tablets (Less than 1%) 3114
VFEND I.V. (Less than 2%) 2543
VFEND Oral Suspension (Less than 2%) 2543
VFEND Tablets (Less than 2%) 2543
Zomig Nasal Spray 718
Zomig Tablets 714
Zomig-ZMT Tablets 714
Zosyn (1.0% or less) 3492

Ventricular gallop
Herceptin I.V. 1234
Retrovir Capsules (0.8%) 1533
Retrovir IV Infusion (1%) 1537
Retrovir (0.8%) 1533

Ventricular hypertrophy
Rythmol SR Capsules 2736

Ventricular irregularities
Cerubidine for Injection 788

Ventricular irritation
Timolide Tablets 2056
Vaseretic Tablets 2073
Zestoretic Tablets 701

Ventricular response, rapid
Verelan PM Capsules 3120

Venus sequelae
Diprivan Injectable Emulsion (Rare) 676

Verruca
Aldara Cream, 5% (0.5%) 1814
Copaxone for Injection (Frequent) 3292
Evoxac Capsules (Less than 1%) 1042
Invirase (Greater than or equal to 2%) 2776
Prometrium Capsules (100 mg, 200 mg) (Less than 5%) 3205
Rescriptor Tablets 2535
Risperdal M-Tab Orally Disintegrating Tablets (Rare) 1658
Risperdal (Rare) 1658
Soriatane Capsules (Less than 1%) 1028

Vertebral compression fractures
Decadron Phosphate Injection 1931
Depo-Medrol Injectable Suspension 2615
Pediapred Oral Solution 3319

Vertical deviation
▲ Botox Purified Neurotoxin Complex (2.1% to 16.9%) 565

Vertigo
Abelcet Injection 1119
Abilify Tablets (Infrequent) 916
Abilify Tablets (Infrequent) 2472
Aceon Tablets (2 mg, 4 mg, 8 mg) (0.3% to 1%) 3191
Aciphex Tablets 1081
Actiq (Up to 1%) 993
▲ Actonel Tablets (1.6% to 3.3%) 2679
▲ Actonel with Calcium Tablets (1.6% to 3.3%) 2684
▲ Adalat CC Tablets (3% or less) 2978
Advicor Tablets 1694
Aerobid/Aerobid-M (1% to 3%) 1172
Albenza Tablets (Less than 1.0% to 1.2%) 1310
Aldoclor Tablets 1881
Aldoril Tablets 1884
Altace Capsules (Less than 1% to 1.5%) 1673
Altoprev Extended-Release Tablets 1151
Ambien Tablets (Frequent) 2867
Amerge Tablets (Frequent) 1312
Anaprox Tablets (Less than 3%) 2769
Anaprox DS Tablets (Less than 3%) 2769
Antara Capsules 2723
Anzemet Injection (Infrequently) 2871
Anzemet Tablets (Infrequently) 2874
▲ Arava Tablets (1% to 3%) 2881
Aricept Tablets (Frequent) 1086
Aricept ODT Tablets (Frequent) 1086
Arthrotec Tablets (Rare) 3126
Asacol Delayed-Release Tablets 2688
Astelin Nasal Spray (Infrequent) 1876
Atacand Tablets (0.5% or greater) 634
Atacand HCT (0.5% or greater) 637
Avalide Tablets 922
Avalide Tablets 2889
Avapro Tablets 925
Avapro Tablets 2886
Avelox (0.1% to less than 2%) 2984
Avinza Capsules (Less than 5%) 1714
Axert Tablets (Infrequent) 2430
Benicar Tablets (Greater than 0.5%) 2850
Benicar HCT Tablets (Greater than 1%) 2852
Betoptic S Ophthalmic Suspension (Rare) 554
Biaxin/Biaxin XL 402
Biltricide Tablets 2990
Blocadren Tablets (0.6%) 1891
▲ Boniva Tablets (3%) 2747
▲ Buprenex Injectable (5% to 10%) 2718
Caduet Tablets (Greater than 0.1% to less than or equal to 1%) 2507
Campral Tablets (Infrequent) 1175
Camptosar Injection 2602
Capastat Sulfate for Injection 1728
Carafate Suspension (Less than 0.5%) 727
Carafate Tablets (Less than 0.5%) 728
▲ Carnitor Injection (2% to 6%) 3185
Cataflam Tablets (Occasionally) 2173
Celebrex Capsules (0.1% to 1.9%) 3130
Celexa (Infrequent) 1177
▲ CellCept Capsules (3% to less than 20%) 2751
▲ CellCept Intravenous (3% to less than 20%) 2751
▲ CellCept Oral Suspension (3% to less than 20%) 2751
▲ CellCept Tablets (3% to less than 20%) 2751
▲ Cenestin Tablets, 0.45mg, 0.625mg, 0.9mg, 1.25mg (5.7% to 17%) 1063
Cialis Tablets (Less than 2%) 1806
Cipro XR Tablets (Less than 1%) 3004
Clinoril Tablets (Less than 1 in 100) 1899
Clorpres Tablets 2139
▲ Clozapine Tablets (More than 5% to 19%) 2141
▲ Clozaril Tablets (More than 5% to 27%) 2174
▲ Copaxone for Injection (6%) 3292
▲ Coreg Tablets (Greater than 1% to 3%) 1376
Cosopt Sterile Ophthalmic Solution 1910
Cozaar Tablets (Less than 1%) 1913
Crestor Tablets (Greater than or equal to 1%) 672
Cubicin for Injection (Less than 1%) 1038
Dapsone Tablets USP 1656
Decadron Phosphate Injection 1931
Decadron Tablets 1929
Depacon Injection (1% or more) 412
Depakene (1% or more) 417
Depakote Sprinkle Capsules 422
▲ Depakote Tablets (1% to 5%) 427
▲ Depakote ER Tablets (1% to 5%) 433
Depo-Medrol Injectable Suspension 2615
Depo-Medrol Single-Dose Vial 2617
▲ Detrol Tablets (8.6%) 2626
Diastat Rectal Delivery System (Greater than or equal to 1%) 3344
Diovan HCT Tablets (Greater than 0.2%) 2195
Diovan Tablets 2191
Diuril Oral 1936
Diuril Sodium Intravenous 1934
Dolobid Tablets (Less than 1 in 100) 1937
Dostinex Tablets (1% to 4%) 2631
▲ Doxil Injection (1% to 10%) 3302
Duragesic Transdermal System (Less than 1%) 2448
Dyazide Capsules 1389
Dynacin Tablets 1859
EC-Naprosyn Delayed-Release Tablets (Less than 3%) 2769
Edecrin 1941
Effexor Tablets (Frequent) 3405
Effexor XR Capsules (Frequent) 3411
Eldepryl Capsules 3209
Eligard 7.5 mg (Less than 2%) 2896
Engerix-B Vaccine 1391
▲ Entocort EC Capsules (Less than 5%) 2694
▲ Epzicom Tablets (6%) 1402
Ery-Tab Tablets (Isolated reports) 447
Erythrocin Stearate Filmtab Tablets (Isolated reports) 452
Erythromycin Base Filmtab Tablets (Isolated reports) 454
Erythromycin Delayed-Release Capsules, USP (Isolated reports) 456
Eskalith 1406
▲ Evoxac Capsules (1% to 3%) 1042
Exelon Capsules (2% or more) 2204
Fabrazyme for Intravenous Infusion 1267
Factive Tablets (Less than or equal to 0.1%) 2464
Faslodex Injection (Less than 1%) 682
▲ FazaClo Orally Disintegrating Tablets (Greater than 5% to 19%) 547
Femara Tablets (Less frequent) 2210
Flexeril Tablets (Less than 1%) 1832
Flomax Capsules (0.6% to 1.0%) 881
Floxin Otic Singles (0.3% to 1%) 1045
Floxin Otic Solution (0.5% to 1%) 1043
▲ Forteo for Injection (3.8%) 1739
Fortical Nasal Spray (Less than 1%) 3336
Frova Tablets (Infrequent) 1101
Furosemide Tablets 2117
Gabitril Tablets (Frequent) 998
Garamycin Injectable 3028
Gengraf Capsules (1% to less than 3%) 458
Geodon Capsules (Frequent) 2514
Gleevec Tablets (Infrequent) 2221
Havrix Vaccine (Less than 1%) 1425
Hexalen Capsules 2101
Hydrocortone Tablets 1963
▲ Hytrin Capsules (0.5% to 21%) 469
Hyzaar 1964
▲ Imdur Tablets (Less than or equal to 5%) 3032
▲ Imitrex Injection (11.9%) 1431
Imitrex Nasal Spray (1% to 1.7%) 1435
Imitrex Tablets 1440
Indapamide Tablets (Less than 5%) 2119
Indocin (Greater than 1%) 1968
▲ Intron A for Injection (Less than 5% to 23%) 3038
Invanz for Injection (Greater than 0.1%) 1974
Kadian Capsules (Less than 3%) 572
Kaletra (Less than 2%) 474
▲ Keppra Oral Solution (3%) 3307
▲ Keppra Tablets (3%) 3307
Ketek Tablets (Greater than or equal to 0.2% to less than 2%) 2920
Klonopin (Infrequent) 2782
Lamictal (2%) 1449
▲ Lariam Tablets (Among most frequent) 2790
Lescol Capsules 2227
Lescol Capsules 2730
Lescol XL Tablets 2227
Lescol XL Tablets 2730
Levaquin in 5% Dextrose Injection (0.1% to 0.9%) 2453
Levaquin (0.1% to 0.9%) 2453
Levitra Tablets (Less than 2%) 3048
Lexapro Oral Solution (Infrequent) 1193
Lexapro Tablets (Infrequent) 1193
Lithobid Tablets 1670
Lofibra Capsules 1217
Lotensin HCT Tablets (1.5%) 2235
Lunesta Tablets (Infrequent) 3139
▲ Lupron Depot 3.75 mg (8%) 3257
▲ Lupron Depot–3 Month 11.25 mg (8%) 3262
▲ Lyrica Capsules (1% to 4%) 2524
Mavik Tablets (0.3% to 1.0%) 482
Maxalt Tablets (Infrequent) 1983
Maxalt-MLT Orally Disintegrating Tablets (Infrequent) 1983
Maxzide 2150
Meridia Capsules 485
Mevacor Tablets (0.5% to 1.0%) 1996
Miacalcin Nasal Spray (Less than 1%) 2242
Micardis Tablets (More than 0.3%) 884
Micardis HCT Tablets 886
Midamor Tablets (Less than or equal to 1%) 2000
Migranal Nasal Spray (Infrequent) 3350
Mirapex Tablets (1% or more) 889
Mobic Oral Suspension (Less than 2%) 893
Mobic Tablets (Less than 2%) 893
Moduretic Tablets (Less than or equal to 1%) 2003
Mustargen for Injection (Infrequent) 2007
Namenda (Frequent) 1199
Naprosyn Suspension (Less than 3%) 2769
Naprosyn Tablets (Less than 3%) 2769
Naropin Injection (Less than 1%) 640
Neoral Soft Gelatin Capsules (1% to less than 3%) 2247
Neoral Oral Solution (1% to less than 3%) 2247
Neurontin Capsules (Frequent) 2498
Neurontin Oral Solution (Frequent) 2498
Neurontin Tablets (Frequent) 2498
Nexium Delayed-Release Capsules (Less than 1%) 645
Nexium I.V. (Less than 1%) 649
Nipent for Injection (Less than 3%) 3216
Norvasc Tablets (More than 0.1% to 1%) 2529
Norvir (Less than 2%) 499
▲ Nubain Injection (5%) 1111
Omacor Capsules 2735
Orthoclone OKT3 Sterile Solution 2370
OxyContin Tablets (Less than 1%) 2699
Paxil CR Controlled-Release Tablets (Frequent) 1509
Paxil (Frequent) 1501
Pediapred Oral Solution 3319
PEG-Intron Powder for Injection 3062
Permax Tablets (Infrequent) 3357
Plavix Tablets (1% to 2.5%) 940
Plavix Tablets (1% to 2.5%) 2942
▲ Pletal Tablets (1% to 3%) 2478
Pravachol Tablets 943
Prevacid NapraPAC (Less than 3%) 3277
PREVPAC 3281
Prilosec OTC Tablets (Less than 1%) 2674
Primaxin I.M. 2022
Primaxin I.V. (Less than 0.2%) 2024
Prinivil Tablets (0.2%) 2029
Prinzide Tablets (0.3% to 1%) 2033
Protonix I.V. (Less than 1%) 3468
Protonix Tablets (Less than 1%) 3465
Protopic Ointment (Greater than or equal to 1%) 629
Proventil Inhalation Aerosol 3067
Proventil HFA Inhalation Aerosol 3071
Provigil Tablets (1%) 1002
Prozac Pulvules and Liquid (Infrequent) 1771
Rabies Vaccine RabAvert 1011
Razadyne ER Extended-Release Capsules (Infrequent) 2434

Razadyne (Infrequent) 2434
Rebetol 3073
Relafen Tablets (Less than 1%) 1523
Relpax Tablets (Frequent) 2531
Requip Tablets (2%) 1528
Rescriptor Tablets 2535
Retrovir Capsules 1533
Retrovir IV Infusion 1537
Retrovir 1533
Ribavirin, USP Capsules 3083
▲ Rilutek Tablets (2.5% to 4.5%) 2945
Risperdal Consta Long-Acting Injection (Infrequent) 1664
Risperdal M-Tab Orally Disintegrating Tablets (Infrequent) 1658
Risperdal (Infrequent) 1658
▲ Rituxan I.V. (1% to 5%) 1251
▲ Roferon-A Injection (Less than 5%) 2805
Rythmol SR Capsules 2736
Sandostatin LAR Depot (1% to 4%) 2264
Seromycin Capsules 1783
Seroquel Tablets (Infrequent) 691
Sonata Capsules (Less than 1%) 1686
Stromectol Tablets (0.9%) 2053
Sular Tablets (Less than or equal to 1%) 1163
Sustiva Capsules (Less than 2%) 957
Symbyax Capsules (Infrequent) 1788
Tambocor Tablets (1% to 3%) 1824
Tamiflu Capsules (0.3% to 1%) 2810
Tamiflu Oral Suspension (0.3% to 1%) 2810
Tarka Tablets (Less frequent) 519
Tasmar Tablets (Frequent) 3360
Tenormin I.V. Injection (2%) 698
Tenormin Tablets (2%) 695
▲ Tequin Injection (0.1% to 3%) 964
▲ Tequin Tablets (0.1% to 3%) 964
Testim 1% Gel 722
Teveten Tablets (Less than 1%) 1707
Teveten HCT Tablets (Less than 1%) 1710
▲ Thalomid Capsules (8.3%) 979
Timolide Tablets 2056
Timoptic in Ocudose 2061
Timoptic Sterile Ophthalmic Solution 2058
Timoptic-XE Sterile Ophthalmic Gel Forming Solution 2062
Tindamax 2670
Topamax Sprinkle Capsules (1% to 2%) 2438
Topamax Tablets (1% to 2%) 2438
Toprol-XL Tablets (1.8%) 660
Tricor Tablets 523
▲ Trileptal Oral Suspension (2% to 15%) 2281
▲ Trileptal Tablets (2% to 15%) 2281
Twinrix Vaccine (Less than 1%) 1571
Ultracet Tablets (Less than 1%) 2462
Uniretic Tablets (More than 1%) 3114
Valium Tablets (Infrequent) 2822
Vancocin HCl Capsules, USP (Rare) 3370
Vantin Tablets and Oral Suspension (Less than 1%) 2650
Vaseretic Tablets (0.5% to 2.0%) 2073
Vasotec I.V. Injection (1.6%) 2076
▲ Velcade for Injection (21%) 2102
VFEND I.V. (Less than 2%) 2543
VFEND Oral Suspension (Less than 2%) 2543
VFEND Tablets (Less than 2%) 2543
Viagra Tablets (Less than 2%) 2552
Vicoprofen Tablets (Less than 1%) 533
▲ Visudyne for Injection (1% to 10%) 2286
Voltaren Tablets (Occasionally) 2298
Voltaren-XR Tablets (Occasionally) 2301
VoSpire Extended-Release Tablets 2352
Vytorin 10/10 Tablets 2084
Vytorin 10/10 Tablets 3092
Vytorin 10/20 Tablets 2084
Vytorin 10/20 Tablets 3092
Vytorin 10/40 Tablets 2084
Vytorin 10/40 Tablets 3092
Vytorin 10/80 Tablets 2084
Vytorin 10/80 Tablets 3092
Wellbutrin Tablets (Infrequent) 1579
Wellbutrin SR Sustained-Release Tablets (Infrequent) 1583
Wellbutrin XL Extended-Release Tablets (Infrequent) 1588
Xanax XR Tablets (Frequent) 2655
▲ Xeloda Tablets (Less than 5%) 2825
Zantac (Rare) 1597
Zantac Injection 1593
Zantac Injection Pharmacy Bulk Package (Rare) 1595
Zantac Syrup (Rare) 1597
Zegerid Powder for Oral Solution (Less than 1%) 2972
Zelnorm Tablets 2303
Zestoretic Tablets (0.3% to 1%) 701
Zestril Tablets (0.2%) 704
Zithromax (1% or less) 2568
Zithromax for Oral Suspension, 300 mg, 600 mg, 900 mg, 1200 mg (1% or less) 2561
Zithromax Tablets, 250 mg, 500 mg (1% or less) 2561
Zithromax Tablets, 600 mg (1% or less) 2568
Zithromax Tri-Pak (1% or less) 2561
Zithromax Z-Pak (1% or less) 2568
Zmax for Oral Suspension (Less then 1%) 2577
Zocor Tablets 2078
Zoloft (Infrequent) 2581
▲ Zometa for Intravenous Infusion (14%) 2306
Zomig Nasal Spray (Infrequent) 718
Zomig Tablets (2%) 714
Zomig-ZMT Tablets (2%) 714
Zonegran Capsules (Infrequent) 1089
Zosyn (1.0% or less) 3492
Zyban Sustained-Release Tablets (Infrequent) 1620
Zyprexa Tablets (Infrequent) 1798
Zyprexa ZYDIS Orally Disintegrating Tablets (Infrequent) 1798
Zyrtec Chewable Tablets (Less than 2%) 2589
Zyrtec (Less than 2%) 2589
Zyrtec-D 12 Hour Extended Release Tablets (Less than 2%) 2591
Zyvox (0% to 1.2%) 2661

Vesical spasm
Dilaudid 439
Dilaudid Non-Sterile Powder 439
Dilaudid Rectal Suppositories 439
Dilaudid Tablets 439
Hycodan 1104

Vesicles at application site
Lidoderm Patch 1107
▲ Oxytrol Transdermal System (3.2%) 3383

Vesiculation
Adriamycin for Injection, USP 786
Adriamycin Injection, USP 786
▲ Aldara Cream, 5% (Up to 3%) 1814
Attenuvax 1889
▲ Catapres-TTS (7 of 101 patients) 875
Cipro I.V. (1% or less) 2998
Cipro I.V. Pharmacy Bulk Package (1% or less) 3509
Cipro XR Tablets 3004
Diprolene Ointment 0.05% (1 per 767 patients) 3017
Ertaczo Cream, 2% 2383
M-M-R II 1980
Oxsoralen-Ultra Capsules 3354
Tri-Luma Cream (1%) 1213

Vesiculobullous reaction
▲ I.V. Busulfex (10%) 1125

Vestibular disturbances
Lunesta Tablets (Infrequent) 3139
Navelbine Injection 1494
Neurontin Capsules (Rare) 2498
Neurontin Oral Solution (Rare) 2498
Neurontin Tablets (Rare) 2498
Rebetron Combination Therapy 3078

Vestibular dysfunction
Gengraf Capsules (1% to less than 3%) 458
Neoral Soft Gelatin Capsules (1% to less than 3%) 2247
Neoral Oral Solution (1% to less than 3%) 2247
Rilutek Tablets (Rare) 2945

Viral syndrome
Flumist Vaccine 1872

Virilization
Anadrol-50 Tablets 3329
▲ Delatestryl Injection (Among most frequent) 2976
▲ Estratest Tablets (Among most common) 3196
▲ Estratest H.S. Tablets (Among most common) 3196
▲ Intron A for Injection (Less than 5%) 3038
Oxandrin Tablets 2977

Virilization, female fetus
Delatestryl Injection 2976

Vision, blurred
▲ Abilify Tablets (3%) 916
▲ Abilify Tablets (3%) 2472
Aciphex Tablets 1081
Acular Ophthalmic Solution (Rare) 561
Adenocard Injection (Less than 1%) 612
Adenoscan (Less than 1%) 613
Aerobid/Aerobid-M (1% to 3%) 1172
Albalon Ophthalmic Solution ⊙ 216
Aldoclor Tablets 1881
Aldoril Tablets 1884
▲ Alferon N Injection (3% to 6%) 1640
▲ Alrex Ophthalmic Suspension 0.2% (5% to 15%) ⊙ 243
Altoprev Extended-Release Tablets (0.9% to 1.2%) 1151
Amaryl Tablets (0.4%) 2864
Amerge Tablets (Infrequent) 1312
Anaprox Tablets (Less than 1%) 2769
Anaprox DS Tablets (Less than 1%) 2769
▲ Arava Tablets (1% to 3%) 2881
Aricept Tablets (Frequent) 1086
Aricept ODT Tablets (Frequent) 1086
Arthrotec Tablets (Rare) 3126
Asacol Delayed-Release Tablets 2688
Atacand HCT 637
Atrovent Nasal Spray 0.03% (Less than 2%) 869
Atrovent Nasal Spray 0.06% (Less than 1%) 870
Avalide Tablets 922
Avalide Tablets 2889
▲ Azopt Ophthalmic Suspension (5% to 10%) 553
▲ Bentyl Capsules (27%) 724
▲ Bentyl Injection (27%) 724
▲ Bentyl Syrup (27%) 724
▲ Bentyl Tablets (27%) 724
Betimol Ophthalmic Solution (1% to 5%) ⊙ 283
Betimol Ophthalmic Solution (1% to 5%) 3371
Betoptic S Ophthalmic Suspension (Small number of patients) 554
▲ Brimonidine Tartrate Ophthalmic Solution 0.2% (10% to 30%) ⊙ 245
Captopril Tablets 2114
Carbatrol Capsules 3174
Carteolol Hydrochloride Ophthalmic Solution USP, 1% (Occasional) ⊙ 246
Cataflam Tablets (Occasionally) 2173
Catapres Tablets 874
Catapres-TTS (0.5% or less) 875
Celebrex Capsules (0.1% to 1.9%) 3130
Cialis Tablets (Less than 2%) 1806
Ciloxan Ophthalmic Ointment (Less than 1%) 554
Cipro I.V. (1% or less) 2998
Cipro I.V. Pharmacy Bulk Package (1% or less) 3509
Cipro (Less than 1%) 2991
Cipro XR Tablets 3004
Clinoril Tablets (Less than 1 in 100) 1899
Clorpres Tablets 2139
Cogentin Injection 1903
Combivent Inhalation Aerosol 878
Concerta Extended-Release Tablets 1828
▲ Copegus Tablets (5%) 2759
▲ Coreg Tablets (Greater than 1% to 3%) 1376
▲ Cosopt Sterile Ophthalmic Solution (5% to 15%) 1910
Covera-HS Tablets (Less than 2%) 3135
Cozaar Tablets (Less than 1%) 1913
Cutivate Lotion 0.05% (Rare) 1383
▲ Cymbalta Delayed-Release Capsules (4%) 1729
Dalmane Capsules (Rare) 3343
Dapsone Tablets USP 1656
▲ Depacon Injection (8% to 12%) 412
▲ Depakene (8% to 12%) 417
▲ Depakote Sprinkle Capsules (4% to 12%) 422
▲ Depakote Tablets (8% to 12%) 427
▲ Depakote ER Tablets (12%) 433
Desferal Vials 2190
Detrol Tablets 2626
Detrol LA Capsules 2629
Digitek Tablets 2146
Dilaudid 439
Dilaudid Oral Liquid (Less frequent) 443
Dilaudid Non-Sterile Powder 439
Dilaudid Rectal Suppositories 439
Dilaudid Tablets 439
Dilaudid Tablets - 8 mg (Less frequent) 443
Dilaudid-HP (Less frequent) 441
Diovan HCT Tablets 2195
▲ Ditropan XL Extended Release Tablets (1% to 8%) 2391
Diuril Oral 1936
Diuril Sodium Intravenous 1934
Dolobid Tablets (Less than 1 in 100) 1937
DuoNeb Inhalation Solution 1058
Duragesic Transdermal System 2448
Dyazide Capsules 1389
Dynacin Tablets 1859
EC-Naprosyn Delayed-Release Tablets (Less than 1%) 2769
Edecrin 1941
▲ Effexor Tablets (6%) 3405
▲ Effexor XR Capsules (4% to 8%) 3411
Eldepryl Capsules 3209
Equetro Extended-Release Capsules 3178
Eskalith 1406
Femara Tablets (Less than 1%) 2210
▲ Flexeril Tablets (1% to 3%) 1832
Flonase Nasal Spray 1412
FML Ophthalmic Suspension ⊙ 224
FML Forte Ophthalmic Suspension ⊙ 223
Focalin Tablets 2214
Focalin XR Capsules 2217
Fortical Nasal Spray (Less than 1%) 3336
Furosemide Tablets 2117
Gleevec Tablets (Less common) 2221
HMS Sterile Ophthalmic Suspension ⊙ 228
Hycomine Compound Tablets 1105
Hycotuss Expectorant Syrup 1106
Hyperstat I.V. Injection 3031
Hytrin Capsules (0.6% to 1.6%) 469
Hyzaar 1964
Indocin (Less than 1%) 1968
▲ Intron A for Injection (Less than 5%) 3038
Inversine Tablets 3286
Kadian Capsules (Less than 3%) 572
Ketek Tablets (Greater than or equal to 0.2% to less than 2%) 2920
Klonopin (1%) 2782
Koāte-DVI (0.7%) 3247
Lacrisert Sterile Ophthalmic Insert 1979
▲ Lamictal (4% to 25%) 1449
Lanoxicaps Capsules 1458
Lanoxin Injection 1462
Lanoxin Tablets 1468
Lanoxin Injection Pediatric 1465
Levitra Tablets (Less than 2%) 3048
Lexapro Oral Solution (Frequent) 1193
Lexapro Tablets (Frequent) 1193
Lidoderm Patch 1107
Lithobid Tablets 1670
Lofibra Capsules 1217
▲ Lotemax Ophthalmic Suspension 0.5% (5% to 15%) ⊙ 249
Lotensin HCT Tablets 2235
▲ Lyrica Capsules (1% to 12%) 2524
Maxalt Tablets (Infrequent) 1983
Maxalt-MLT Orally Disintegrating Tablets (Infrequent) 1983
Maxzide 2150
Meridia Capsules 485
Metadate CD Capsules 3316
Mevacor Tablets (0.9% to 1.5%) 1996
Miacalcin Nasal Spray (Less than 1%) 2242
Micardis HCT Tablets 886
Mintezol 2002
Miradon Tablets 3056
Moban Tablets (Occasional) 1108
Moduretic Tablets 2003
MS Contin Tablets (Less frequent) 2703
▲ Myfortic Tablets (3% to less than 20%) 2244
Nadolol Tablets (1 to 5 of 1000 patients) 2121
Nalfon Capsules (2.2%) 2504
Namenda (Infrequent) 1199
Naprosyn Suspension (Less than 1%) 2769
Naprosyn Tablets (Less than 1%) 2769
Naropin Injection 640
Neumega for Injection 3433
Neurontin Capsules (2.7%) 2498
Neurontin Oral Solution (2.7%) 2498
Neurontin Tablets (2.7%) 2498
Nicomide Tablets 3190
▲ Niravam Orally Disintegrating Tablets (6.2% to 21%) 3106
Norflex Injection 1824
Noroxin Tablets (Less frequent) 2009
Norvir (Less than 2%) 499
Nubain Injection (1% or less) 1111
OptiPranolol Metipranolol Ophthalmic Solution 0.3% (A small number of patients) ⊙ 254
▲ Optivar Ophthalmic Solution (1% to 10%) 1877

Orap Tablets ... 1220
Orthoclone OKT3 Sterile Solution ... 2370
Parcopa Orally Disintegrating Tablets ... 3111
Parnate Tablets ... 1499
Patanol Ophthalmic Solution (Less than 5%) ... 557
▲ Paxil CR Controlled-Release Tablets (2.0% to 7.8%) ... 1509
▲ Paxil (2.0% to 7.8%) ... 1501
▲ Pegasys (4%) ... 2793
PEG-Intron Powder for Injection (2%) ... 3062
Phenergan ... 3438
Pred Forte Ophthalmic Suspension ... ⊙ 233
Prevacid NapraPAC (Less than 1%) .. 3277
Prilosec OTC Tablets (Less than 1%) ... 2674
Prinivil Tablets (0.3% to 1.0%) ... 2029
Prinzide Tablets (0.3% to 1%) ... 2033
Propine Ophthalmic Solution ... ⊙ 237
Protonix I.V. ... 3468
Protonix Tablets ... 3465
▲ Rebetol (5% to 6%) ... 3073
Rescriptor Tablets ... 2535
▲ Restasis Ophthalmic Emulsion (1% to 5%) ... 570
▲ Retisert Implant (10% to 35%) ... ⊙ 256
Revatio Tablets ... 2541
Rēv-Eyes Ophthalmic Eyedrops 0.5% (Less frequently) ... ⊙ 256
▲ Ribavirin, USP Capsules (5% to 6%) ... 3083
Ritalin Hydrochloride Tablets ... 2254
Ritalin LA Capsules ... 2255
Ritalin-SR Tablets ... 2254
▲ Rythmol SR Capsules (1% to 6%) ... 2736
Sanctura Tablets (Greater than or equal to 0.5%) ... 1133
▲ Sandostatin Injection (1% to 4%) ... 2263
▲ Soriatane Capsules (1% to 10%) ... 1028
Stalevo Tablets ... 2270
Surmontil Capsules ... 2347
Tambocor Tablets ... 1824
Tarka Tablets (Less frequent) ... 519
Tasmar Tablets (1% or more) ... 3360
Tegretol/Tegretol-XR ... 2278
▲ Temodar Capsules (8%) ... 3088
Teveten HCT Tablets ... 1710
Thioridazine Hydrochloride Tablets .. 2122
Thiothixene Capsules (Infrequently) .. 2124
Timolide Tablets ... 2056
Timoptic-XE Sterile Ophthalmic Gel Forming Solution ... 2062
▲ Topamax Sprinkle Capsules (2% to 4%) ... 2438
▲ Topamax Tablets (2% to 4%) ... 2438
Toprol-XL Tablets ... 660
Transderm Scōp Transdermal Therapeutic System ... 2166
Tranxene (Less common) ... 2488
Travatan Ophthalmic Solution (1% to 4%) ... 559
Trecator Tablets ... 3482
▲ Trisenox Injection (10%) ... 983
Trusopt Sterile Ophthalmic Solution (Approximately 1% to 5%) ... 2065
Uniretic Tablets ... 3114
Valium Tablets (Infrequent) ... 2822
Vaseretic Tablets ... 2073
Vasotec I.V. Injection (0.5% to 1.0%) ... 2076
▲ Velcade for Injection (11%) ... 2102
Verelan PM Capsules (2% or less) ... 3120
▲ VESIcare Tablets (3.8% to 4.8%) ... 631
▲ VFEND I.V. (Approximately 30%) ... 2543
▲ VFEND Oral Suspension (Approximately 30%) ... 2543
▲ VFEND Tablets (Approximately 30%) ... 2543
▲ Viagra Tablets (3%) ... 2552
Visine For Contacts Rewetting Drops ... ⊙ 278
▲ Visudyne for Injection (10% to 30%) ... 2286
Vivactil Tablets ... 2350
▲ Voltaren Ophthalmic Solution (Less than or equal to 5%) ... 2300
Voltaren Tablets (Occasionally) ... 2298
Voltaren-XR Tablets (Occasionally) ... 2301
▲ Wellbutrin Tablets (14.6%) ... 1579
▲ Xalatan Sterile Ophthalmic Solution (5% to 15%) ... 2654
Xanax XR Tablets (Frequent) ... 2655
Zantac (Rare) ... 1597
Zantac Injection (Rare) ... 1593
Zantac Injection Pharmacy Bulk Package (Rare) ... 1595
Zantac Syrup (Rare) ... 1597
Zegerid Powder for Oral Solution (Less than 1%) ... 2972
▲ Zenapax for Injection (2% to 5%) ... 2838
Zestoretic Tablets (0.3% to 1%) ... 701
Zestril Tablets (0.3% to 1.0%) ... 704
Zofran Injection ... 1607

Vision, changes
(*see under* Visual disturbances)

Vision, color tinge to
▲ Viagra Tablets (3%) ... 2552

Vision, complete loss
Alesse-28 Tablets ... 3392
Ortho-Cyclen/Ortho Tri-Cyclen ... 2414
Ortho Tri-Cyclen Lo Tablets ... 2421
Premphase Tablets ... 3452
Prempro Tablets ... 3452

Vision, double
(*see under* Diplopia)

Vision, loss of
Desferal Vials ... 2190
Imitrex Injection ... 1431
Imitrex Nasal Spray ... 1435
Imitrex Tablets ... 1440
Intron A for Injection ... 3038
Levitra Tablets (Rare) ... 3048
Lo/Ovral-28 Tablets ... 3423
Nipent for Injection (Less than 3%) ... 3216
Pacerone Tablets ... 3337
Pegasys ... 2793
PEG-Intron Powder for Injection ... 3062
Prinivil Tablets (0.3% to 1.0%) ... 2029
Prinzide Tablets ... 2033
Triphasil-28 Tablets ... 3483
Viagra Tablets ... 2552
▲ Visudyne for Injection (1% to 10%) .. 2286
Zestoretic Tablets ... 701
Zestril Tablets (0.3% to 1.0%) ... 704
Zyvox ... 2661

Vision, loss of color
Cipro I.V. (1% or less) ... 2998
Cipro I.V. Pharmacy Bulk Package (1% or less) ... 3509
Cipro (Less than 1%) ... 2991
Cipro XR Tablets ... 3004

Vision, partial loss
Imitrex Tablets ... 1440
Lo/Ovral-28 Tablets ... 3423
Mintezol ... 2002
Ortho-Cyclen/Ortho Tri-Cyclen ... 2414
Ortho Tri-Cyclen Lo Tablets ... 2421
Premphase Tablets ... 3452
Prempro Tablets ... 3452
Triphasil-28 Tablets ... 3483

Vision, temporary loss of
Sular Tablets (Less than or equal to 1%) ... 1163
Viagra Tablets ... 2552

Vision abnormalities
(*see under* Visual disturbances)

Visual acuity, decreased
Ketek Tablets (Greater than or equal to 0.2% to less than 2%) ... 2920
Levitra Tablets (Rare) ... 3048
Namenda (Infrequent) ... 1199
▲ Retisert Implant (10% to 35%) ... ⊙ 256
Rythmol SR Capsules ... 2736
▲ Vigamox Ophthalmic Solution (1% to 6%) ... 560

Visual acuity, defects
Alphagan P Ophthalmic Solution (1% to 4%) ... 563
Alrex Ophthalmic Suspension 0.2% ... ⊙ 243
Betoptic S Ophthalmic Suspension (Small number of patients) ... 554
Blephamide Ophthalmic Ointment ... 563
Blephamide Ophthalmic Suspension ... 564
Cipro I.V. (1% or less) ... 2998
Cipro I.V. Pharmacy Bulk Package (1% or less) ... 3509
Cipro (Less than 1%) ... 2991
Cozaar Tablets (Less than 1%) ... 1913
Desferal Vials ... 2190
Eloxatin for Injection ... 2908
FML Ophthalmic Ointment ... ⊙ 225
FML Ophthalmic Suspension ... ⊙ 224
FML Forte Ophthalmic Suspension ... ⊙ 223
FML-S Liquifilm Sterile Ophthalmic Suspension ... ⊙ 226
HMS Sterile Ophthalmic Suspension ... ⊙ 228
Hyzaar ... 1964
Intron A for Injection ... 3038
Lotemax Ophthalmic Suspension 0.5% ... ⊙ 249
PEG-Intron Powder for Injection (Less than or equal to 1%) ... 3062
Pred Forte Ophthalmic Suspension ... ⊙ 233
Pred Mild Sterile Ophthalmic Suspension ... ⊙ 236
Pred-G Ophthalmic Suspension ... ⊙ 234
Pred-G Sterile Ophthalmic Ointment ... ⊙ 235
Retisert Implant ... ⊙ 256
Roferon-A Injection (Less than 1%) ... 2805
Symmetrel (0.1% to 1%) ... 1115
TobraDex Ophthalmic Ointment ... 558
TobraDex Ophthalmic Suspension ... 558
▲ Travatan Ophthalmic Solution (5% to 10%) ... 559
▲ Vesanoid Capsules (6%) ... 2823
▲ Vigamox Ophthalmic Solution (1% to 6%) ... ⊙ 212
Visine For Contacts Rewetting Drops ... ⊙ 278
▲ Visudyne for Injection (10% to 30%) ... 2286
Zylet Ophthalmic Suspension ... 3508
▲ Zymar Ophthalmic Solution (1% to 4%) ... 571

Visual disturbances
Accutane Capsules ... 2740
Aciphex Tablets ... 1081
Actiq (1% to 2%) ... 993
Activella Tablets ... 2311
Acular Ophthalmic Solution (Rare) ... 561
Adalat CC Tablets (Less than 1%) ... 2978
Agrylin Capsules (1% to 5%) ... 3172
Alacol DM Syrup ... 739
Alferon N Injection (1%) ... 1640
▲ Alphagan P Ophthalmic Solution (Approximately 5% to 9%) ... 563
▲ Alrex Ophthalmic Suspension 0.2% (5% to 15%) ... ⊙ 243
Altace Capsules (Less than 1%) ... 1673
Ambien Tablets (Frequent) ... 2867
Amnesteem Capsules ... 2126
Anaprox Tablets (Less than 3%) ... 2769
Anaprox DS Tablets (Less than 3%) .. 2769
Antara Capsules ... 2723
Anzemet Injection (Infrequently) ... 2871
Anzemet Tablets (Infrequently) ... 2874
Aralast (0.1%) ... 745
Arthrotec Tablets (Rare) ... 3126
Asacol Delayed-Release Tablets (2% or greater) ... 2688
Astelin Nasal Spray ... 1876
Avalide Tablets ... 922
Avalide Tablets ... 2889
Avapro Tablets (Less than 1%) ... 925
Avapro Tablets (Less than 1%) ... 2886
Avelox (Less than 0.1%) ... 2984
BeneFix for Injection (1.5%) ... 3402
Betagan Ophthalmic Solution, USP ... ⊙ 217
▲ Betimol Ophthalmic Solution (More than 5%) ... ⊙ 283
▲ Betimol Ophthalmic Solution (More than 5%) ... 3371
Blephamide Ophthalmic Suspension ... 564
Blocadren Tablets ... 1891
Brevibloc Concentrate (Less than 1%) ... 766
Brevibloc Injection (Less than 1%) ... 766
Brevibloc Double Strength Injection (Less than 1%) ... 766
Brevibloc Premixed Injection (Less than 1%) ... 766
Brevibloc Double Strength Premixed Injection (Less than 1%) ... 766
▲ Brimonidine Tartrate Ophthalmic Solution 0.2% (3% to 9%) ... ⊙ 245
Buprenex Injectable (Less than 1%) ... 2718
Caduet Tablets (Greater than 0.1% to less than or equal to 1%) ... 2507
Campral Tablets (Frequent) ... 1175
Carteolol Hydrochloride Ophthalmic Solution USP, 1% (Occasional) ... ⊙ 246
Celexa (At least 2%) ... 1177
▲ CellCept Capsules (3% to less than 20%) ... 2751
▲ CellCept Intravenous (3% to less than 20%) ... 2751
▲ CellCept Oral Suspension (3% to less than 20%) ... 2751
▲ CellCept Tablets (3% to less than 20%) ... 2751
Cenestin Tablets, 0.45mg, 0.625mg, 0.9mg, 1.25mg ... 1063
Cenestin Tablets, 0.3mg ... 1063
Cipro I.V. (1% or less) ... 2998
Cipro I.V. Pharmacy Bulk Package (1% or less) ... 3509
Cipro (Less than 1%) ... 2991
Cipro XR Tablets ... 3004
Clinoril Tablets (Less than 1 in 100) ... 1899
▲ Clozapine Tablets (5% or more) ... 2141
▲ Clozaril Tablets (5% or more) ... 2174
Colazal Capsules ... 2845
Comvax ... 1904
Concerta Extended-Release Tablets ... 1828
Copaxone for Injection (At least 2%) ... 3292
▲ Coreg Tablets (5%) ... 1376
Cosopt Sterile Ophthalmic Solution ... 1910
Cuprimine Capsules ... 1925
Cytovene (At least 3 subjects) ... 2763
Dantrium Capsules (Less frequent) .. 2690
Darvocet A 500 Tablets ... 3497
▲ Depacon Injection (1% to 5%) ... 412
▲ Depakene (1% to 5%) ... 417
▲ Depakote Sprinkle Capsules (1% to 5%) ... 422
▲ Depakote Tablets (1% to 5%) ... 427
▲ Depakote ER Tablets (1% to 5%) ... 433
DepoCyt Injection ... 1121
Desferal Vials ... 2190
▲ Detrol Tablets (4.7%) ... 2626
Detrol LA Capsules (1%) ... 2629
Digitek Tablets ... 2146
Dilaudid ... 439
Dilaudid Oral Liquid (Less frequent) ... 443
Dilaudid Non-Sterile Powder ... 439
Dilaudid Rectal Suppositories ... 439
Dilaudid Tablets ... 439
Dilaudid Tablets - 8 mg (Less frequent) ... 443
Dilaudid-HP (Less frequent) ... 441
Diovan HCT Tablets (Greater than 0.2%) ... 2195
Diprivan Injectable Emulsion (Less than 1%) ... 676
Dolobid Tablets (Less than 1 in 100) ... 1937
▲ Dostinex Tablets (1% to less than 10%) ... 2631
Doxil Injection (Less than 1%) ... 3302
DynaCirc CR Tablets (0.5% to 1%) ... 2726
EC-Naprosyn Delayed-Release Tablets (Less than 3%) ... 2769
Edex Injection (1%) ... 3103
Effexor Tablets (Frequent) ... 3405
▲ Effexor XR Capsules (4% to 5%) ... 3411
Eloxatin for Injection ... 2908
Enablex Extended-Release Tablets (Greater than or equal to 1%) ... 2201
Engerix-B Vaccine ... 1391
▲ Entocort EC Capsules (Less than 5%) ... 2694
Estratest Tablets ... 3196
Estratest H.S. Tablets ... 3196
▲ Evoxac Capsules (1% to 3%) ... 1042
Factive Tablets (Less than or equal to 0.1%) ... 2464
▲ FazaClo Orally Disintegrating Tablets (Greater than 5%) ... 547
Ferrlecit Injection ... 3379
▲ Flolan for Injection (4%) ... 1408
FML Ophthalmic Suspension ... ⊙ 224
FML Forte Ophthalmic Suspension ... ⊙ 223
FML-S Liquifilm Sterile Ophthalmic Suspension ... ⊙ 226
Focalin Tablets (Rare) ... 2214
Focalin XR Capsules ... 2217
Frova Tablets (Frequent) ... 1101
Gabitril Tablets (Frequent) ... 998
Garamycin Injectable ... 3028
Gengraf Capsules (1% to less than 3%) ... 458
Genotropin Lyophilized Powder (A small number of patients) ... 2642
▲ Geodon Capsules (3% to 6%) ... 2514
Humatrope Vials and Cartridges ... 1756
Hytrin Capsules (At least 1%) ... 469
▲ Imdur Tablets (Less than or equal to 5%) ... 3032
Imitrex Injection (1.1%) ... 1431
Imitrex Nasal Spray (Infrequent) ... 1435
Imitrex Tablets (Up to 3%) ... 1440
Increlex Injection ... 3290
Inderal LA Long-Acting Capsules ... 3421
▲ Infergen (3% to 5%) ... 1647
InnoPran XL Capsules ... 2728
▲ Intron A for Injection (Less than 5%) ... 3038
Invirase (Less than 2%) ... 2776
Kaletra (Less than 2%) ... 474
Klonopin (Infrequent) ... 2782
▲ Lamictal (2% to 3%) ... 1449

Lamisil Tablets (1.1%) 2226
Lanoxicaps Capsules 1458
Lanoxin Injection 1462
Lanoxin Tablets 1468
Lanoxin Injection Pediatric 1465
Lariam Tablets 2790
Levaquin in 5% Dextrose Injection (0.1% to 0.9%) 2453
Levaquin (0.1% to 0.9%) 2453
Levitra Tablets (Less than 2%) 3048
Lexapro Oral Solution (Infrequent) 1193
Lexapro Tablets (Infrequent) 1193
Lidoderm Patch 1107
Lofibra Capsules 1217
▲ Lotemax Ophthalmic Suspension 0.5% (5% to 15%) ⊙ 249
Lotensin HCT Tablets (0.3% or more) 2235
▲ Lumigan Ophthalmic Solution (3% to 10%) 569
▲ Lyrica Capsules (1% to 5%) 2524
Malarone Tablets (2%) 1484
Malarone Pediatric Tablets (2%) 1484
Marinol Capsules (Less than 1%) 3334
Meridia Capsules 485
Metadate CD Capsules 3316
Micardis Tablets (More than 0.3%) 884
Micardis HCT Tablets 886
Midamor Tablets (Less than or equal to 1%) 2000
Migranal Nasal Spray (Infrequent) 3350
▲ Mirapex Tablets (3%) 889
Mobic Oral Suspension (Less than 2%) 893
Mobic Tablets (Less than 2%) 893
Moduretic Tablets (Less than or equal to 1%) 2003
MS Contin Tablets (Less frequent) 2703
Nadolol Tablets 2121
Naprosyn Suspension (Less than 3%) 2769
Naprosyn Tablets (Less than 3%) 2769
Naropin Injection (Less than 1%) 640
Neoral Soft Gelatin Capsules (1% to less than 3%) 2247
Neoral Oral Solution (1% to less than 3%) 2247
Neurontin Capsules (Frequent) 2498
Neurontin Oral Solution (Frequent) 2498
Neurontin Tablets (Frequent) 2498
Nexium Delayed-Release Capsules (Less than 1%) 645
Nexium I.V. (Less than 1%) 649
Nicotrol NS (Less than 1%) 2596
Nipent for Injection (Less than 3%) 3216
Norditropin Cartridges (Small number of patients) 2318
Noroxin Tablets 2009
Norvasc Tablets (More than 0.1% to 1%) 2529
Norvir (Less than 2%) 499
Nutropin for Injection (A small number of patients) 1238
Nutropin AQ Injection (A small number of patients) 1241
Nutropin AQ Pen (A small number of patients) 1241
Nutropin AQ Pen Cartridge (A small number of patients) 1241
OptiPranolol Metipranolol Ophthalmic Solution 0.3% (A small number of patients) ⊙ 254
▲ Orap Tablets (5.5%) 1220
Ortho-Cyclen/Ortho Tri-Cyclen 2414
Ortho Tri-Cyclen Lo Tablets 2421
OxyContin Tablets (Less than 1%) 2699
Oxytrol Transdermal System (2.5%) 3383
▲ Pacerone Tablets (4% to 9%) 3337
▲ Paxil CR Controlled-Release Tablets (2% to 4%) 1509
▲ Paxil (2% to 4%) 1501
Pegasys 2793
PEG-Intron Powder for Injection 3062
▲ Permax Tablets (5.8%) 3357
Photofrin for Injection 729
Plendil Extended-Release Tablets (0.5% to 1.5%) 651
Pred Forte Ophthalmic Suspension ⊙ 233
Premarin Tablets 3443
Premphase Tablets 3452
Prempro Tablets 3452
Prevacid Delayed-Release Capsules (Less than 1%) 3268
Prevacid for Delayed-Release Oral Suspension (Less than 1%) 3268
Prevacid NapraPAC (Less than 3%) 3277
Prevacid SoluTab Delayed-Release Orally Disintegrating Tablets (Less than 1%) 3268
PREVPAC (Less than 1%) 3281
▲ Prograf Capsules and Injection (3% to 15%) 624
▲ Proleukin for Injection (7%) 1007
Prometrium Capsules (100 mg, 200 mg) (Less than 5%) 3205
ProSom Tablets (Infrequent) 512
Protonix I.V. (Less than 1%) 3468
Protonix Tablets (Less than 1%) 3465
Provigil Tablets (1%) 1002
Prozac Pulvules and Liquid (2%) 1771
Quixin Ophthalmic Solution (1% to 3%) 3373
Rabies Vaccine RabAvert 1011
▲ Rapamune Oral Solution and Tablets (3% to 20%) 3472
▲ Rebif Prefilled Syringe for Injection (7% to 13%) 3163
Recombivax HB (Less than 1%) 2045
ReFacto Vials 3479
Relafen Tablets (Less than 1%) 1523
Relpax Tablets (Infrequent) 2531
ReoPro Vials (0.7%) 1779
▲ Requip Tablets (6%) 1528
▲ Restasis Ophthalmic Emulsion (1% to 5%) 570
▲ Retisert Implant (5% to 9%) ⊙ 256
▲ Risperdal Consta Long-Acting Injection (2% to 3%) 1664
▲ Risperdal M-Tab Orally Disintegrating Tablets (1% to 6%) 1658
▲ Risperdal (1% to 6%) 1658
Ritalin Hydrochloride Tablets (Rare) 2254
Ritalin LA Capsules 2255
Ritalin-SR Tablets 2254
▲ Roferon-A Injection (6%) 2805
Sanctura Tablets 1133
Sandimmune (Rare) 2259
▲ Sandostatin Injection (1% to 4%) 2263
Sandostatin LAR Depot (1% to 4%) 2264
Seroquel Tablets (Infrequent) 691
▲ Simulect for Injection (3% to 10%) 2268
Sonata Capsules (Less than 1% to 2%) 1686
▲ Soriatane Capsules (1% to 10%) 1028
Sular Tablets (Less than or equal to 1%) 1163
Sustiva Capsules 957
Symbyax Capsules (Frequent) 1788
Symmetrel (0.1% to 1%) 1115
▲ Tambocor Tablets (15.9%) 1824
Taxotere Injection Concentrate (Rare) 2947
▲ Temodar Capsules (5%) 3088
Tenormin I.V. Injection 698
Tenormin Tablets 695
▲ Tequin Injection (0.1% to 3%) 964
▲ Tequin Tablets (0.1% to 3%) 964
Teveten Tablets (Less than 1%) 1707
Teveten HCT Tablets (Less than 1%) 1710
Tev-Tropin for Injection (Small number of patients) 1224
Timolide Tablets 2056
Timoptic in Ocudose (Less frequent) 2061
Timoptic Sterile Ophthalmic Solution (Less frequent) 2058
Timoptic-XE Sterile Ophthalmic Gel Forming Solution 2062
▲ Topamax Sprinkle Capsules (1% to 13%) 2438
▲ Topamax Tablets (1% to 13%) 2438
Travatan Ophthalmic Solution (1% to 4%) 559
Tricor Tablets 523
▲ Trileptal Oral Suspension (2% to 14%) 2281
▲ Trileptal Tablets (2% to 14%) 2281
Twinrix Vaccine 1571
Ultracet Tablets (Less than 1%) 2462
Uniretic Tablets (Less than 1%) 3114
Valtrex Caplets 1573
▲ Vesanoid Capsules (17%) 2823
▲ VFEND I.V. (13.5% to 21%) 2543
▲ VFEND Oral Suspension (13.5% to 21%) 2543
▲ VFEND Tablets (13.5% to 21%) 2543
▲ Viagra Tablets (3%) 2552
Vicoprofen Tablets (Less than 1%) 533
Visine For Contacts Rewetting Drops ⊙ 278
▲ Visudyne for Injection (10% to 30%) 2286
Vivelle Transdermal System 2288
Vivelle-Dot Transdermal System 2293
▲ Voltaren Ophthalmic Solution (Less than or equal to 5%) 2300
Wellbutrin Tablets (Infrequent) 1579
▲ Xeloda Tablets (5%) 2825
▲ Zavesca Capsules (17%) 543
Zelnorm Tablets 2303
▲ Zoloft (4%) 2581
Zovirax Capsules 1616
Zovirax for Injection 1618
Zovirax 1616
▲ Zylet Ophthalmic Suspension (Less than 4%) 3508

Visual disturbances, flashing lights

Cipro XR Tablets 3004

Visual field defect

Agrylin Capsules (1% to 5%) 3172
Alphagan P Ophthalmic Solution (1% to 4%) 563
Alrex Ophthalmic Suspension 0.2% ⊙ 243
Blephamide Ophthalmic Ointment 563
Blephamide Ophthalmic Suspension 564
Cialis Tablets 1806
Cosopt Sterile Ophthalmic Solution (1% to 5%) 1910
Doxil Injection (Less than 1%) 3302
Effexor Tablets (Infrequent) 3405
Effexor XR Capsules (Infrequent) 3411
Eskalith 1406
FML Ophthalmic Ointment ⊙ 225
FML Ophthalmic Suspension ⊙ 224
FML Forte Ophthalmic Suspension ⊙ 223
FML-S Liquifilm Sterile Ophthalmic Suspension ⊙ 226
Gabitril Tablets (Infrequent) 998
Geodon Capsules (Rare) 2514
HMS Sterile Ophthalmic Suspension ⊙ 228
Intron A for Injection 3038
Klonopin (Infrequent) 2782
Levitra Tablets (Rare) 3048
Lotemax Ophthalmic Suspension 0.5% ⊙ 249
Lyrica Capsules (Greater than or equal to 2%) 2524
Neurontin Capsules (Infrequent) 2498
Neurontin Oral Solution (Infrequent) 2498
Neurontin Tablets (Infrequent) 2498
Nexium Delayed-Release Capsules (Less than 1%) 645
Nexium I.V. (Less than 1%) 649
Norvir (Less than 2%) 499
Paxil CR Controlled-Release Tablets (Infrequent) 1509
Paxil (Infrequent) 1501
Permax Tablets (Infrequent) 3357
Pred Forte Ophthalmic Suspension ⊙ 233
Pred Mild Sterile Ophthalmic Suspension ⊙ 236
Pred-G Ophthalmic Suspension ⊙ 234
Prevacid Delayed-Release Capsules (Less than 1%) 3268
Prevacid for Delayed-Release Oral Suspension (Less than 1%) 3268
Prevacid NapraPAC (Less than 1%) 3277
Prevacid SoluTab Delayed-Release Orally Disintegrating Tablets (Less than 1%) 3268
PREVPAC (Less than 1%) 3281
ProAmatine Tablets (Rare) 3183
Prozac Pulvules and Liquid (Rare) 1771
Retisert Implant ⊙ 256
Sandostatin LAR Depot (Rare) 2264
Sonata Capsules (Rare) 1686
Targretin Capsules 1719
TobraDex Ophthalmic Ointment 558
TobraDex Ophthalmic Suspension 558
Topamax Sprinkle Capsules (Infrequent) 2438
Topamax Tablets (Infrequent) 2438
▲ Vesanoid Capsules (3%) 2823
VFEND I.V. (Less than 2%) 2543
VFEND Oral Suspension (Less than 2%) 2543
VFEND Tablets (Less than 2%) 2543
▲ Visudyne for Injection (10% to 30%) 2286
Zoloft (Rare) 2581
Zomig Nasal Spray (Rare) 718
Zonegran Capsules (Infrequent) 1089
Zylet Ophthalmic Suspension 3508
Zyrtec Chewable Tablets (Less than 2%) 2589
Zyrtec (Less than 2%) 2589
Zyrtec-D 12 Hour Extended Release Tablets (Less than 2%) 2591

Visual impairment

Abelcet Injection 1119
Ciloxan Ophthalmic Ointment (Less than 1%) 554
Cipro XR Tablets 3004
Depo-Medrol Single-Dose Vial 2617
Ortho-Cyclen/Ortho Tri-Cyclen (Rare) 2414
Ortho Tri-Cyclen Lo Tablets 2421
Pacerone Tablets 3337

Vitamin B12 deficiency

Nexium Delayed-Release Capsules (Less than 1%) 645
Nexium I.V. (Less than 1%) 649

Vitiligo

▲ Intron A for Injection (Less than 5%) 3038
Proleukin for Injection 1007
Trileptal Oral Suspension 2281
Trileptal Tablets 2281

Vitreous detachment

Cosopt Sterile Ophthalmic Solution (1% to 5%) 1910
Evoxac Capsules (Less than 1%) 1042
Viagra Tablets 2552

Vitreous disorder, unspecified

Cytovene (At least 3 subjects) 2763

Vitreous floaters

Alphagan P Ophthalmic Solution (1% to 4%) 563
Fortical Nasal Spray (Less than 1%) 3336
Miacalcin Nasal Spray (Less than 1%) 2242
▲ Retisert Implant (10% to 35%) ⊙ 256
Sular Tablets (Less than or equal to 1%) 1163

Vitreous opacity

▲ Retisert Implant (5% to 9%) ⊙ 256

Voice, deepening of

Anadrol-50 Tablets 3329
▲ Delatestryl Injection (Among most frequent) 2976
Estratest Tablets 3196
Estratest H.S. Tablets 3196
Oxandrin Tablets 2977

Voice, hoarseness

Estratest Tablets 3196
Estratest H.S. Tablets 3196

Voice, loss of

(*see under* Aphonia)

Voice alteration

Accutane Capsules 2740
Actiq (Less than 1%) 993
Amnesteem Capsules 2126
▲ Avastin IV (6% to 9%) 1229
Avinza Capsules (Less than 5%) 1714
▲ Azmacort Inhalation Aerosol (1% to 3%) 1701
▲ CellCept Capsules (3% to less than 20%) 2751
▲ CellCept Intravenous (3% to less than 20%) 2751
▲ CellCept Oral Suspension (3% to less than 20%) 2751
▲ CellCept Tablets (3% to less than 20%) 2751
Copaxone for Injection (Infrequent) 3292
Doxil Injection (Less than 1%) 3302
DuoNeb Inhalation Solution (More than 1%) 1058
Effexor Tablets (Infrequent) 3405
Effexor XR Capsules (Infrequent) 3411
Emend Capsules (Greater than 0.5%) 1944
Flonase Nasal Spray 1412
Gabitril Tablets (Infrequent) 998
Imitrex Injection 1431
Imitrex Nasal Spray (Rare) 1435
Imitrex Tablets (Rare) 1440
Invanz for Injection (Greater than 0.1%) 1974
Kadian Capsules (Less than 3%) 572
Lotensin HCT Tablets 2235
▲ Mirapex Tablets (Greater than or equal to 1%) 889
Neurontin Capsules (Rare) 2498
Neurontin Oral Solution (Rare) 2498
Neurontin Tablets (Rare) 2498
OxyContin Tablets (Less than 1%) 2699
Paxil CR Controlled-Release Tablets (Infrequent) 1509
Paxil (Infrequent) 1501
Permax Tablets (Infrequent) 3357
▲ Prograf Capsules and Injection (3% to 15%) 624
Protonix I.V. (Less than 1%) 3468
Protonix Tablets (Less than 1%) 3465

▲ Pulmozyme Inhalation Solution (12% to 18%) 1245
Relpax Tablets (Infrequent) 2531
Sonata Capsules (Infrequent) 1686
Symbyax Capsules (Infrequent) 1788
Thalomid Capsules 979
▲ TOBI Solution for Inhalation (13%) 1015
Uniretic Tablets (Less than 1%) 3114
VFEND I.V. (Less than 2%) 2543
VFEND Oral Suspension (Less than 2%) 2543
VFEND Tablets (Less than 2%) 2543
▲ Zoladex (3%) 709
Zoladex 3-month 712
Zomig Nasal Spray (Infrequent) 718
Zomig Tablets (Rare) 714
Zomig-ZMT Tablets (Rare) 714
Zyprexa Tablets (Infrequent) 1798
Zyprexa ZYDIS Orally Disintegrating Tablets (Infrequent) 1798

Vomiting

▲ Abelcet Injection (3% to 8%) 1119
▲ Abilify Tablets (Frequent to 11%) 916
▲ Abilify Tablets (Frequent to 11%) 2472
Accolate Tablets (1.5%) 663
Accutane Capsules 2740
Aceon Tablets (2 mg, 4 mg, 8 mg) (1.5%) 3191
Aciphex Tablets 1081
▲ Actimmune (13%) 1646
▲ Actiq (6% to 15%) 993
Activase I.V. 1225
Activella Tablets 2311
Actonel Tablets (1.9% to 2.5%) 2679
Actonel with Calcium Tablets (1.9% to 2.5%) 2684
▲ Adacel Vaccine (0.5% to 4.6%) 2959
Adalat CC Tablets (Less than 1%) 2978
▲ Adderall XR Capsules (7%) 3169
Adriamycin for Injection, USP (Frequent) 786
Adriamycin Injection, USP (Frequent) 786
▲ Advair Diskus 100/50 (4% to 5%) 1291
▲ Advair Diskus 250/50 (4% To 5%) 1291
▲ Advair Diskus 500/50 (4% to 5%) 1291
▲ Advicor Tablets (3%) 1694
▲ Aerobid/Aerobid-M (25%) 1172
▲ Agenerase Capsules (9% to 34%) 1299
▲ Agenerase Oral Solution (9% to 34%) 1304
▲ Aggrenox Capsules (8.4%) 855
▲ Agrylin Capsules (9.7%) 3172
Alacol DM Syrup 739
▲ Albenza Tablets (3.7% to 6.2%) 1310
Aldara Cream, 5% (1.4%) 1814
Aldoclor Tablets 1881
Aldoril Tablets 1884
Alesse-28 Tablets 3392
▲ Alferon N Injection (3% to 29%) 1640
▲ Alimta for Injection (Up to 58%) 1722
Alinia for Oral Suspension (1.1%) 2840
Alinia Tablets (1.1%) 2840
Alkeran for Injection (Infrequent) 976
Alkeran Tablets (Infrequent) 977
Aloprim for Injection (1.2%) 2156
Altace Capsules (Less than 1% to 2%) 1673
Altoprev Extended-Release Tablets (0.5% to 1%) 1151
Alupent Inhalation Aerosol (Approximately 1 in 300 patients) 858
Amaryl Tablets (Less than 1%) 2864
Ambien Tablets (1%) 2867
▲ AmBisome for Injection (22.4% to 31.8%) 615
Amerge Tablets (Frequent) 1312
Aminohippurate Sodium "PAH" Injection 1886
▲ Ammonul Injection (9%) 3323
Amoxil Capsules 1315
Amoxil Chewable Tablets 1315
Amoxil Pediatric Drops for Oral Suspension 1315
Amoxil Powder for Oral Suspension 1315
Amoxil Tablets 1315
Anadrol-50 Tablets 3329
▲ Anaprox Tablets (1% to 10%) 2769
▲ Anaprox DS Tablets (1% to 10%) 2769
Ancef for Injection (Rare) 1318
▲ Angiomax for Injection (6%) 1856
Antara Capsules 2723
▲ Apokyn Injection (11% to 30%) 2132
▲ Aptivus Capsules (3.4%) 859
▲ Arava Tablets (3%) 2881
▲ Aredia for Injection (35.7%) 2168
▲ Argatroban Injection (4.2% to 6.3%) 1321
▲ Aricept Tablets (3% to 8%) 1086
▲ Aricept ODT Tablets (3% to 8%) 1086
▲ Arimidex Tablets (8% to 11%) 665
▲ Arixtra Injection (0.6% to 5.9%) 1325
▲ Aromasin Tablets (7%) 2600
Arthrotec Tablets (Rare) 3126
▲ Asacol Delayed-Release Tablets (5%) 2688
Asmanex Twisthaler (1% to less than 3%) 2981
Astelin Nasal Spray (Infrequent) 1876
Atacand Tablets (More than 1%) 634
Atacand HCT (0.5% or greater) 637
Augmentin (1%) 1331
Augmentin Tablets (1%) 1334
Augmentin XR Extended-Release Tablets 1340
Augmentin ES-600 Powder for Oral Suspension (2.2%) 1337
▲ Avalide Tablets (3%) 922
▲ Avalide Tablets (3%) 2889
Avapro Tablets (1% or greater) 925
Avapro Tablets (1% or greater) 2886
▲ Avastin IV (47% to 52%) 1229
Avelox (0.1% to less than 2%) 2984
▲ Avinza Capsules (Greater than 10%) 1714
Avonex 839
Axert Tablets (Infrequent) 2430
▲ Axid Oral Solution (1.2% to 3.6%) 913
▲ Azasan Tablets (12%) 2844
▲ Azmacort Inhalation Aerosol (1% to 3%) 1701
Balamine DM 739
Baraclude (Less than 1%) 928
Bayer Aspirin 3515
BeneFix for Injection (1.5%) 3402
Benicar Tablets 2850
Benicar HCT Tablets (Rare) 2852
Bentyl Capsules 724
Bentyl Injection 724
Bentyl Syrup 724
Bentyl Tablets 724
Betaseron for SC Injection 791
▲ Bexxar (1% to 15%) 1360
▲ Biaxin/Biaxin XL (6%) 402
▲ BiDil Tablets (4%) 2161
Biltricide Tablets 2990
Blocadren Tablets (Less than 1%) 1891
Boniva Tablets (2.7%) 2747
▲ Boostrix (3% to 26%) 1366
Bravelle for Intramuscular or Subcutaneous Injection (2.7%) 1140
Brevibloc Concentrate (About 1%) 766
Brevibloc Injection (About 1%) 766
Brevibloc Double Strength Injection (About 1%) 766
Brevibloc Premixed Injection (About 1%) 766
Brevibloc Double Strength Premixed Injection (About 1%) 766
Buphenyl Powder (Less than or equal to 2%) 3327
Buphenyl Tablets (Less than or equal to 2%) 3327
▲ Buprenex Injectable (1% to 5%) 2718
▲ Byetta Injection (13%) 605
Caduet Tablets (Greater than 0.1% to less than 2%) 2507
Calcijex Injection 411
Calcium Disodium Versenate Injection 1819
▲ Campath Ampules (4% to 41%) 826
Campral Tablets 1175
▲ Camptosar Injection (12% to 67%) 2602
▲ Cancidas for Injection (1.2% to 3.5%) 1894
Captopril Tablets (About 0.5% to 2%) 2114
Carafate Suspension (Less than 0.5%) 727
Carafate Tablets (Less than 0.5%) 728
▲ Carbatrol Capsules (Among most frequent) 3174
▲ Cardene I.V. (4.9%) 1129
▲ Carnitor Injection (9% to 12%) 3185
Carnitor Tablets and Oral Solution 3187
▲ Casodex Tablets (5%) 670
▲ Cataflam Tablets (1% to 10%) 2173
▲ Catapres Tablets (About 5 in 100 patients) 874
Catapres-TTS (0.5% or less) 875
Ceftin (2.6%) 1369
Celebrex Capsules (0.1% to 1.9%) 3130
▲ Celexa (4%) 1177
▲ CellCept Capsules (32.9% to 33.9%) 2751
▲ CellCept Intravenous (32.9% to 33.9%) 2751
▲ CellCept Oral Suspension (32.9% to 33.9%) 2751
▲ CellCept Tablets (32.9% to 33.9%) 2751
▲ Cenestin Tablets, 0.45mg, 0.625mg, 0.9mg, 1.25mg (7%) 1063
Cenestin Tablets, 0.3mg 1063
▲ Cerezyme for Injection (Approximately 6.5%) 1263
Cerubidine for Injection 788
Cervidil Vaginal Insert (Less than 1%) 1182
▲ Chemet Capsules (12.0% to 20.9%) 2480
Chromagen Soft Gelatin Capsules 3296
Chromagen Forte Soft Gelatin Capsules 3296
Cialis Tablets (Less than 2%) 1806
▲ Cipro I.V. (1% to 4.8%) 2998
▲ Cipro I.V. Pharmacy Bulk Package (1% to 4.8%) 3509
▲ Cipro (1% to 4.8%) 2991
Cipro XR Tablets (1% to 2%) 3004
▲ Clarinex Syrup (6.1%) 3009
Cleocin Vaginal Ovules (Less than 1%) 2613
Climara Transdermal System 795
Climara Pro Transdermal System 800
Clindesse Vaginal Cream (Less than 1%) 3296
Clinoril Tablets (Greater than 1%) 1899
▲ Clolar for Intravenous Infusion (83%) 1264
▲ Clorpres Tablets (About 5%) 2139
▲ Clozapine Tablets (3%) 2141
▲ Clozaril Tablets (3% to 17%) 2174
Cogentin Injection 1903
Colace Capsules 50 mg 2715
Colace Capsules 100 mg 2715
Colace Glycerin Suppositories, USP 1.2 grams - Infants and Children 2715
Colace Glycerin Suppositories, USP 2.1 grams - Adults and Children 2716
Colace Liquid 1% Solution 2716
Colace Syrup ▣ 729
▲ Colazal Capsules (4%) 2845
Colyte with Flavor Packs for Oral Solution (Less frequent) 3102
Combivent Inhalation Aerosol (Less than 2%) 878
▲ Combivir Tablets (13%) 1373
▲ Combunox Tablets (4.5% to 5.3%) 1183
▲ Comtan Tablets (4%) 2186
Comvax (1.0% to 2.5%) 1904
▲ Concerta Extended-Release Tablets (3% to 4%) 1828
▲ Copaxone for Injection (6%) 3292
▲ Copegus Tablets (25%) 2759
▲ Coreg Tablets (1% to 6%) 1376
Cosmegen for Injection (Common) 1907
Cosopt Sterile Ophthalmic Solution (1% to 5%) 1910
Coumadin for Injection (Infrequent) 932
Coumadin Tablets (Infrequent) 932
Cozaar Tablets (Less than 1%) 1913
▲ Creon 5 Capsules (Among most frequent) 3195
▲ Creon 10 Capsules (Among most frequent) 3195
▲ Creon 20 Capsules (Among most frequent) 3196
Crestor Tablets (Greater than or equal to 1%) 672
▲ Crixivan Capsules (8.4%) 1918
▲ Cubicin for Injection (3.2%) 1038
Cuprimine Capsules (Greater than 1%) 1925
Cutivate Lotion 0.05% (1%) 1383
▲ Cymbalta Delayed-Release Capsules (5% to 6%) 1729
CytoGam Intravenous (Less than 5.0%) 1866
▲ Cytovene (13%) 2763
Dalmane Capsules 3343
Dantrium Capsules (Rare) 2690
Dapsone Tablets USP 1656
▲ DAPTACEL (4.3% to 6.9%) 2964
▲ Daranide Tablets (Among the most common effects) 1928
Daraprim Tablets 1385
▲ Darvocet A 500 Tablets (Among most frequent) 3497
Demser Capsules (Infrequent) 1933
▲ Depacon Injection (1.3% to 27%) 412
▲ Depakene (23% to 27%) 417
▲ Depakote Sprinkle Capsules (15% to 27%) 422
▲ Depakote Tablets (11% to 27%) 427
▲ Depakote ER Tablets (7% to 27%) 433
▲ DepoCyt Injection (3% to 12%) 1121
▲ DepoDur Extended-Release Injection (Greater than 10%) 1098
Desferal Vials 2190
▲ Detrol Tablets (4.2%) 2626
Diastat Rectal Delivery System (Less than 1%) 3344
Digitek Tablets (2%) 2146
Dilaudid (Infrequent) 439
Dilaudid Oral Liquid 443
Dilaudid Non-Sterile Powder (Infrequent) 439
Dilaudid Rectal Suppositories (Infrequent) 439
Dilaudid Tablets (Infrequent) 439
Dilaudid Tablets - 8 mg 443
▲ Dilaudid-HP (Among most frequent) 441
Diovan HCT Tablets (Greater than 0.2%) 2195
Diovan Tablets (Less frequent) 2191
Diprivan Injectable Emulsion (Less than 1%) 676
Diuril Oral 1936
Diuril Sodium Intravenous 1934
Dolobid Tablets (Greater than 1 in 100) 1937
Dostinex Tablets (2% to 4%) 2631
▲ Doxil Injection (7.8% to 32.6%) 3302
▲ Duragesic Transdermal System (Greater than 10% to 33%) 2448
Dyazide Capsules 1389
Dynacin Tablets 1859
DynaCirc CR Tablets (0.5% to 1%) 2726
Dyrenium Capsules (Rare) 3390
▲ EC-Naprosyn Delayed-Release Tablets (1% to 10%) 2769
Ecotrin Enteric Coated Aspirin Low, Regular and Maximum Strength Tablets 1627
Edecrin 1941
▲ E.E.S. (Among most frequent) 449
▲ Effexor Tablets (6% to 7.9%) 3405
▲ Effexor XR Capsules (3% to 5%) 3411
Eldepryl Capsules 3209
▲ Elidel Cream 1% (0.6% to 8%) 2198
▲ Elitek (50%) 2906
▲ Ellence Injection (22.1% to 92.4%) 2632
Elmiron Capsules (Less than or equal to 1%) 2393
▲ Eloxatin for Injection (6% to 47%) 2908
Elspar for Injection 1943
Emcyt Capsules (1%) 3137
▲ Emend Capsules (7.5%) 1944
▲ Emtriva Capsules (9%) 1272
Enablex Extended-Release Tablets (Greater than or equal to 1%) 2201
▲ Enbrel for Injection (3% to 5%) 580
Engerix-B Vaccine (Less than 1%) 1391
▲ Entocort EC Capsules (6%) 2694
EpiPen 1061
▲ Epivir (13%) 1394
▲ Epivir-HBV (15%) 1398
▲ Epogen for Injection (0.26% to 22%) 586
▲ Equetro Extended-Release Capsules (18%) 3178
▲ Erbitux (25%) 937
▲ EryPed (Among most frequent) 445
▲ Ery-Tab Tablets (Among most frequent) 447
▲ Erythrocin Stearate Filmtab Tablets (Among most frequent) 452
▲ Erythromycin Base Filmtab Tablets (Among most frequent) 454
▲ Erythromycin Delayed-Release Capsules, USP (Among most frequent) 456
Eskalith 1406
Estratest Tablets 3196
Estratest H.S. Tablets 3196
Estrogel 0.06% 3200
▲ Ethyol for Injection (8% to 96%) 1869
▲ Eulexin Capsules (11%) 3023
▲ Evista Tablets (3.4% to 4.8%) 1735
▲ Evoxac Capsules (4.6%) 1042
▲ Exelon Capsules (31%) 2204
Fabrazyme for Intravenous Infusion 1267
Factive Tablets (0.9%) 2464
▲ Famvir Tablets (1.3% to 4.8%) 2207
▲ Faslodex Injection (13%) 682
▲ FazaClo Orally Disintegrating Tablets (3%) 547
▲ Femara Tablets (7%) 2210
▲ Ferrlecit Injection (2% to 35%) 3379
Flexeril Tablets (Less than 1%) 1832
▲ Flolan for Injection (32% to 67%) 1408
Flomax Capsules (Infrequent) 881
▲ Flonase Nasal Spray (2.6% to 4.8%) 1412
▲ Flovent Diskus 50 mcg (4% to 9%) 1415
Floxin Otic Singles (0.3%) 1045
Floxin Otic Solution (0.3%) 1043
Flumadine (1.7%) 1186
▲ Flumist Vaccine (4.7% to 5.6%) 1872
Fluorescite Injection ⊙ 207
Focalin Tablets 2214
Follistim AQ Cartridge 2354
Fortaz (1 in 500 patients) 1422
▲ Forteo for Injection (3%) 1739

Fortical Nasal Spray (Less than 1%) 3336
Fosamax (0.2% to 1%) 1949
Fosamax Plus D Tablets (0.2% to 1%) 1956
▲ Fosrenol Chewable Tablets (9% to 26%) 3180
Frova Tablets (Frequent) 1101
Furosemide Tablets 2117
▲ Gabitril Tablets (7%) 998
▲ Gammagard Liquid (1.21% to 14.8%) 751
Gammagard S/D (Occasional) 754
▲ Gamunex Immune Globulin I.V., 10% (13% to 21%) 3232
Garamycin Injectable 3028
▲ Gemzar for Injection (58% to 71%) 1743
▲ Gengraf Capsules (2% to 10%) 458
Genotropin Lyophilized Powder (A small number of patients) 2642
▲ Geodon (5%) 2514
▲ Gleevec Tablets (14.7% to 58%) 2221
GlucaGen for Injection (Occassional) 790
Glucagon for Injection Vials and Emergency Kit (Occasional) 1749
Grifulvin V Tablets Microsize and Oral Suspension Microsize (Occasional) 2384
Gris-PEG Tablets (Occasional) 2504
▲ HalfLytely and Bisacodyl Tablets Bowel Prep Kit with Flavors Packs (5.9%) 915
Havrix Vaccine (Less than 1%) 1425
▲ Hectorol Capsules (21.3%) 909
▲ Hectorol Injection (21.3%) 911
Hepsera Tablets (2% or greater) 1275
▲ Herceptin I.V. (8% to 23%) 1234
▲ Hexalen Capsules (1% to 33%) 2101
HibTITER (9 of 1,118 vaccinations) 3419
Humatrope Vials and Cartridges 1756
▲ Humira Injection (Less than 5%) 464
▲ Hycamtin for Injection (Less than 1% to 58%) 1427
Hycodan 1104
Hycomine Compound Tablets 1105
Hycotuss Expectorant Syrup 1106
▲ Hyperstat I.V. Injection (4%) 3031
Hytrin Capsules (At least 1%) 469
Hyzaar 1964
▲ Idamycin PFS Injection (82%) 2645
▲ Imdur Tablets (Less than or equal to 5%) 3032
▲ Imitrex Injection (4%) 1431
▲ Imitrex Nasal Spray (11% to 13.5%) 1435
Imitrex Tablets 1440
Imodium Capsules 1834
▲ Increlex Injection (Greater than or equal to 5%) 3290
Indapamide Tablets (Less than 5%) 2119
Inderal LA Long-Acting Capsules 3421
Indocin I.V. (1% to 3%) 1973
▲ Infanrix Vaccine (3.3% to 6.6.%) 1444
Infed Injection 3381
▲ Infergen (12% to 13%) 1647
InnoPran XL Capsules 2728
▲ Intron A for Injection (1% to 66%) 3038
▲ Invanz for Injection (3.7% to 10.2%) 1974
Inversine Tablets 3286
▲ Invirase (Less than 2% to 7.4%) 2776
▲ Iressa Tablets (10% to 12%) 684
▲ I.V. Busulfex (43% to 95%) 1125
Iveegam EN (0.3% to 0.8%) 759
Kadian Capsules (Less than 3%) 572
▲ Kaletra (2% to 6%) 474
K-Dur Extended-Relase Tablets 3047
▲ Keppra Oral Solution (1% to 15%) 3307
▲ Keppra Tablets (1% to 15%) 3307
Ketek Tablets (2.4% to 2.9%) 2920
▲ K-Lor Powder Packets (Among most common) 472
K-Phos Neutral Tablets 785
K-Phos Original (Sodium Free) Tablets 785
Kristalose for Oral Solution 2149
▲ K-Tab Filmtab Tablets (Most common) 473
▲ Kytril Tablets (9% to 12%) 2788
▲ Lamictal (5% to 20%) 1449
Lamisil Tablets 2226
Lanoxicaps Capsules (Common) 1458
Lanoxin Injection (Common) 1462
Lanoxin Tablets (Common) 1468
Lanoxin Injection Pediatric 1465
▲ Lariam Tablets (Among most frequent) 2790
Lescol Capsules 2227
Lescol Capsules 2730
Lescol XL Tablets 2227
Lescol XL Tablets 2730
Leukeran Tablets (Infrequent) 1472
▲ Leukine (46% to 85%) 829
▲ Leustatin Injection (13%) 2368
Levaquin in 5% Dextrose Injection (0.3% to 2.4%) 2453
Levaquin (0.3% to 2.4%) 2453
Levitra Tablets (Less than 2%) 3048
Levothroid Tablets 1189
Levoxyl Tablets 1680
▲ Lexapro Oral Solution (3%) 1193
▲ Lexapro Tablets (3%) 1193
▲ Lexiva Tablets (2% to 20%) 1473
Lidoderm Patch 1107
Lipitor Tablets (Less than 2%) 2495
Lithobid Tablets 1670
Lofibra Capsules 1217
Lo/Ovral-28 Tablets 3423
▲ Lortab (Among most frequent) 3315
▲ Lortab Elixir (Among most frequent) 3312
Lotensin Tablets (Less than 1%) 2232
Lotensin HCT Tablets (0.3% to 1%) 2235
▲ Lunesta Tablets (0% to 3%) 3139
▲ Lupron Depot 3.75 mg (13%) 3257
▲ Lupron Depot 7.5 mg (5.4%) 3261
▲ Lupron Depot–3 Month 11.25 mg (13%) 3262
Lupron Depot-PED 7.5 mg, 11.25 mg and 15 mg (Less than 2%) 3266
Lupron Injection Pediatric (Less than 2%) 3256
▲ Lyrica Capsules (1% to 3%) 2524
▲ Malarone Tablets (Less than 1% to 13%) 1484
▲ Malarone Pediatric Tablets (Less than 1% to 13%) 1484
▲ Marinol Capsules (3% to 10%) 3334
▲ Matulane Capsules (Among most frequent) 3188
Mavik Tablets (0.3% to 1.0%) 482
Maxair Autohaler 1820
Maxalt Tablets (Frequent) 1983
Maxalt-MLT Orally Disintegrating Tablets (Frequent) 1983
Maxipime for Injection (Greater than 0.1% to 1%) 1093
Maxzide 2150
Mebaral Tablets, USP (Less than 1 in 100 patients) 2483
Mefoxin for Injection (Rare) 1987
Mefoxin Premixed Intravenous Solution (Rarely) 1990
▲ Megace ES Oral Suspension (0% to 6%) 2492
Menactra Vaccine (0.2% to 2.3%) 2968
▲ Menopur for Subcutaneous Injection (2.6% to 4.2%) 1145
Menostar Transdermal System 805
▲ Mepron Suspension (1.3% to 22%) 1487
Meridia Capsules (1.5%) 485
▲ Merrem I.V. (0.8% to 3.6%) 687
Meruvax II 1994
▲ MetroGel-Vaginal Gel (4%) 1822
Mevacor Tablets (0.5% to 1.0%) 1996
▲ Miacalcin Injection (About 10%) 2241
Miacalcin Nasal Spray (Less than 1% to 1.8%) 2242
Micardis Tablets (More than 0.3%) 884
Micardis HCT Tablets (Less than 2%) 886
▲ Midamor Tablets (3% to 8%) 2000
▲ Migranal Nasal Spray (4%) 3350
Mineral Oil 2716
Mintezol 2002
Miradon Tablets 3056
Mirapex Tablets (1% or more) 889
M-M-R II 1980
Mobic Oral Suspension (0.6% to 1.8%) 893
Mobic Tablets (0.6% to 1.8%) 893
Moduretic Tablets (Less than or equal to 1%) 2003
▲ MS Contin Tablets (Among most frequent) 2703
Mustargen for Injection 2007
Mycamine for Injection (1.2% to 2.4%) 620
▲ Myfortic Tablets (3% to 23%) 2244
Myleran Tablets 1492
▲ Mylotarg for Injection (53% to 66%) 3429
Nadolol Tablets (1 to 5 of 1000 patients) 2121
Nalfon Capsules (2.6%) 2504
▲ Namenda (3%) 1199
▲ Naprosyn Suspension (1% to 10%) 2769
▲ Naprosyn Tablets (1% to 10%) 2769
Narcan Injection 1109
▲ Naropin Injection (More than 5% to 14.6%) 640
Nasacort AQ Nasal Spray 2937
▲ Nasonex Nasal Spray (1% to 5%) 3058
▲ Natrecor for Injection (1% to 4%) 3123
▲ Navelbine Injection (6% to 60%) 1494
Nembutal Sodium Solution, USP (Less than 1%) 2484
▲ Neoral Soft Gelatin Capsules (2% to 10%) 2247
▲ Neoral Oral Solution (2% to 10%) 2247
▲ Neulasta Injection (15% to 72%) 596
▲ Neumega for Injection (77%) 3433
▲ Neupogen for Injection (7% to 57%) 598
Neurontin Capsules (1% to 3.3%) 2498
Neurontin Oral Solution (1% to 3.3%) 2498
Neurontin Tablets (1% to 3.3%) 2498
Nexium Delayed-Release Capsules (Less than 1%) 645
Nexium I.V. (Less than 1%) 649
Nicomide Tablets 3190
Niferex-150 Forte Capsules 3299
Nimotop Capsules (Less than 1%) 774
▲ Nipent for Injection (53% to 63%) 3216
▲ Niravam Orally Disintegrating Tablets (9.6% to 22%) 3106
Nitrolingual Pumpspray (Uncommon) 1161
Norditropin Cartridges (Small number of patients) 2318
Norflex Injection 1824
Noroxin Tablets (0.3 to 1.0%) 2009
Norvasc Tablets (More than 0.1% to 1%) 2529
▲ Norvir (13.7% to 17.4%) 499
Novantrone for Injection Concentrate (Mild to moderate) 3158
NovoSeven (1%) 2335
▲ Nubain Injection (6%) 1111
Numorphan 1112
Nutropin for Injection (A small number of patients) 1238
Nutropin AQ Injection (A small number of patients) 1241
Nutropin AQ Pen (A small number of patients) 1241
Nutropin AQ Pen Cartridge (A small number of patients) 1241
Omacor Capsules 2735
Omnicef Capsules (0.7%) 506
Omnicef for Oral Suspension (1%) 506
▲ Oncaspar (Greater than 5%) 1123
▲ Ontak Vials (64%) 1717
Orap Tablets 1220
Ortho-Cept Tablets 2395
Ortho-Cyclen Tablets 2414
Ortho Evra Transdermal System 2402
Ortho Tri-Cyclen Tablets 2414
Ortho Tri-Cyclen Lo Tablets 2421
▲ Orthoclone OKT3 Sterile Solution (19%) 2370
Oxandrin Tablets 2977
▲ OxyContin Tablets (Less than 1% to 12%) 2699
▲ OxyFast Oral Concentrate Solution (Among most frequent) 2704
▲ OxyIR Capsules (Among most frequent) 2704
▲ Pacerone Tablets (10% to 33%) 3337
▲ Pancrease MT Capsules (Among most frequent) 1839
Parcopa Orally Disintegrating Tablets 3111
▲ Paser Granules (Among most common) 1657
▲ Paxil CR Controlled-Release Tablets (1% to 3%) 1509
▲ Paxil (1% to 3%) 1501
▲ PCE Dispertab Tablets (Among most frequent) 510
Pediarix Vaccine 1518
Peganone Tablets, USP 2487
▲ Pegasys (24%) 2793
▲ PEG-Intron Powder for Injection (7%) 3062
Pentasa Capsules (1.5%) 3182
Pepcid Injection (Infrequent) 2017
Pepcid (Infrequent) 2014
▲ Percocet Tablets (Among most frequent) 1114
▲ Percodan Tablets (Among most frequent) 1115
Peri-Colace Tablets 2716
Permax Tablets (2.7%; frequent) 3357
Persantine Tablets 898
Phenergan 3438
Phenytek Capsules 2153
PhosLo GelCaps 2158
▲ Photofrin for Injection (17% to 34%) 729
▲ Plan B Tablets (5.6%) 1068
Plavix Tablets (1% to 2.5%) 940
Plavix Tablets (1% to 2.5%) 2942
Plendil Extended-Release Tablets (0.5% to 1.5%) 651
Pletal Tablets (2% or greater) 2478
Pneumovax 23 2020
▲ Prandin Tablets (0.5, 1, and 2 mg) (2% to 3%) 2337
▲ Pravachol Tablets (2.9% to 7.3%) 943
Prefest Tablets 1069
Premarin Intravenous 3440
Premarin Tablets 3443
Premarin Vaginal Cream 3449
Premphase Tablets 3452
Prempro Tablets 3452
Prevacid Delayed-Release Capsules (Less than 1%) 3268
Prevacid for Delayed-Release Oral Suspension (Less than 1%) 3268
Prevacid I.V. for Injection (Less than 1%) 3274
Prevacid NapraPAC (Less than 1%) 3277
Prevacid SoluTab Delayed-Release Orally Disintegrating Tablets (Less than 1%) 3268
▲ Prevnar for Injection (4.9% to 16.8%) 3460
▲ PREVPAC (3% to 6%) 3281
▲ Prilosec OTC Tablets (1.5% to 3.2%) 2674
Primaxin I.M. (0.3%) 2022
Primaxin I.V. (Up to 1.5%) 2024
Prinivil Tablets (0.3% to 1.0%) 2029
Prinzide Tablets (1.4%) 2033
▲ Prochieve 4% Gel (5%) 1018
▲ Prochieve 8% Gel (5%) 1018
▲ Procrit for Injection (0.26% to 29%) 2374
▲ Prograf Capsules and Injection (14% to 29%) 624
▲ Proleukin for Injection (50%) 1007
▲ Prometrium Capsules (100 mg, 200 mg) (5% to 8%) 3205
ProSom Tablets (Infrequent) 512
Protonix I.V. (Greater than 1%) 3468
Protonix Tablets (2%) 3465
Protopic Ointment (1% to 5%) 629
Proventil Inhalation Aerosol 3067
▲ Proventil HFA Inhalation Aerosol (7%) 3071
Provigil Tablets (Greater than or equal to 1%) 1002
▲ Prozac Pulvules and Liquid (3%) 1771
Pulmicort Respules (2% to 4%) 654
Purinethol Tablets (Uncommon) 1222
▲ Rapamune Oral Solution and Tablets (19% to 25%) 3472
▲ Razadyne ER Extended-Release Capsules (6% to 13%) 2434
▲ Razadyne (6% to 13%) 2434
▲ Rebetol (9% to 42%) 3073
▲ Rebetron Combination Therapy (9% to 12%) 3078
Recombivax HB (Less to greater than 1%) 2045
ReFacto Vials 3479
Relafen Tablets (1% to 3%) 1523
Relenza Rotadisk (1% to 2%) 1525
▲ Renagel Tablets (22.2%) 1268
▲ ReoPro Vials (11.4%) 1779
Repliva 21/7 Tablets 3301
Repronex for Intramuscular and Subcutaneous Injection 1148
▲ Requip Tablets (7% to 12%) 1528
▲ Rescriptor Tablets (2.5% to 6.5%) 2535
Retavase 1131
▲ Retisert Implant (5% to 15%) ⊙256
▲ Retrovir Capsules (4.8% to 25%) 1533
▲ Retrovir IV Infusion (6% to 25%) 1537
▲ Retrovir (4.8% to 25%) 1533
▲ Reyataz Capsules (6% to 8%) 948
▲ R-Gene 10 for Intravenous Use (3%) 2647
Rhophylac (Rare) 3504
▲ Ribavirin, USP Capsules (9% to 42%) 3083
▲ Rilutek Tablets (4.2% to 4.5%) 2945
Risperdal Consta Long-Acting Injection (Frequent) 1664
▲ Risperdal M-Tab Orally Disintegrating Tablets (5% to 7%) 1658
▲ Risperdal (5% to 7%) 1658
▲ Rituxan for Infusion (7%) 845
▲ Rituxan I.V. (10%) 1251
Rocephin Injectable Vials, ADD-Vantage, Galaxy, Bulk (Less than 1%) 2801
▲ Roferon-A Injection (33% to 39%) 2805
▲ Rythmol SR Capsules (1% to 6%) 2736
Sanctura Tablets (Greater than or equal to 0.5%) 1133
▲ Sandimmune (2% to 10%) 2259
▲ Sandostatin Injection (Less than 10% to 35%) 2263
▲ Sandostatin LAR Depot (6.5%) 2264
Seasonale Tablets 1073
▲ Sedapap Tablets 50 mg/650 mg (Among the most frequent) 2098
▲ Sensipar Tablets (27%) 603

▲ Seroquel Tablets (6%) ... 691
▲ Simulect for Injection (Greater than or equal to 10%) ... 2268
Singulair ... 2047
▲ Skelaxin Tablets (Most frequent) ... 1685
Soriatane Capsules ... 1028
Spectracef Tablets (1%) ... 2706
▲ Spiriva HandiHaler (1% to 4%) ... 899
St. Joseph 81 mg Aspirin Chewable and Enteric Coated Tablets ... 1841
▲ Stalevo Tablets (4%) ... 2270
▲ Strattera Capsules (0.5% to 15%) ... 1784
Striant Mucoadhesive ... 1022
Stromectol Tablets (0.9%) ... 2053
▲ Suboxone Tablets (5% to 7.5%) ... 2719
▲ Subutex Tablets (5% to 7.8%) ... 2719
▲ Suprane Liquid for Inhalation (16%) ... 770
Suprax (Less than 2%) ... 1811
Surmontil Capsules ... 2347
▲ Sustiva Capsules (3% to 16%) ... 957
Symbyax Capsules (Infrequent) ... 1788
▲ Symlin Injection (7% to 11%) ... 608
Symmetrel (0.1% to 1%) ... 1115
Synagis (More than 1%) ... 1868
Synercid I.V. (2.7%) ... 1690
Tabloid Tablets (Less frequent) ... 1545
Tambocor Tablets (1% to 3%) ... 1824
▲ Tamiflu Capsules (2.1% to 15%) ... 2810
▲ Tamiflu Oral Suspension (2.1% to 15%) ... 2810
▲ Tarceva Tablets (Less than 1% to 23%) ... 1254
▲ Tarceva Tablets (Less than 1% to 23%) ... 2470
▲ Targretin Capsules (3.6% to 13.2%) ... 1719
▲ Tasmar Tablets (8% to 10%) ... 3360
▲ Taxotere Injection Concentrate (2.8% to 23.4%) ... 2947
▲ Tegretol/Tegretol-XR (Among most frequent) ... 2278
▲ Temodar Capsules (29% to 51%) ... 3088
▲ Tequin Injection (0.1% to 3%) ... 964
▲ Tequin Tablets (0.1% to 3%) ... 964
Teveten Tablets (Less than 1%) ... 1707
Teveten HCT Tablets (Less than 1%) ... 1710
Tev-Tropin for Injection (Small number of patients) ... 1224
Thalomid Capsules ... 979
Thioridazine Hydrochloride Tablets ... 2122
Thiothixene Capsules ... 2124
Thyrogen for Injection (2.1%) ... 1270
Tiazac Capsules (Less than 2%) ... 1204
Ticlid Tablets (1.9%) ... 2813
Timentin ADD-Vantage ... 1556
Timentin Injection Galaxy Container ... 1559
Timentin IV Infusion ... 1553
Timentin Pharmacy Bulk Package ... 1562
Timolide Tablets ... 2056
Timoptic in Ocudose ... 2061
Timoptic Sterile Ophthalmic Solution ... 2058
Timoptic-XE Sterile Ophthalmic Gel Forming Solution ... 2062
Tindamax (0.9% to 1.5%) ... 2670
TNKase I.V. ... 1256
▲ TOBI Solution for Inhalation (14%) ... 1015
▲ Topamax Sprinkle Capsules (1% to 3%) ... 2438
▲ Topamax Tablets (1% to 3%) ... 2438
Toprol-XL Tablets ... 660
Tracleer Tablets ... 539
Transderm Scōp Transdermal Therapeutic System (Few patients) ... 2166
▲ Trasylol Injection (3%) ... 779
Trecator Tablets ... 3482
Trelstar Depot (2.1%) ... 3385
Tricor Tablets ... 523
Triglide Tablets ... 1165
▲ Trileptal Oral Suspension (5% to 36%) ... 2281
▲ Trileptal Tablets (5% to 36%) ... 2281
TriLyte with Flavor Packs for Oral Solution ... 3114
Triphasil-28 Tablets ... 3483
▲ Trisenox Injection (58%) ... 983
▲ Trizivir Tablets (12% to 30%) ... 1565
▲ Truvada Tablets (Greater than 5%) ... 1279
Tussionex Pennkinetic Extended-Release Suspension ... 3322
Twinrix Vaccine (Up to 1%) ... 1571
▲ Tygacil for Injection (19.5% to 20%) ... 3489
▲ Tylenol with Codeine (Among most frequent) ... 2461
▲ Ultane Liquid for Inhalation (18%) ... 526
Ultracet Tablets (At least 1%) ... 2462
Uniphyl Tablets ... 2708
Uniretic Tablets (Less than 1%) ... 3114
Unithroid Tablets ... 3521
Univasc Tablets (Less than 1%) ... 3118
Urocit-K Tablets (Some patients) ... 2109
Uroqid-Acid No. 2 Tablets ... 785
Urso 250 Tablets ... 737
Urso Forte Tablets ... 737
▲ Valcyte Tablets (21%) ... 2816
▲ Valtrex Caplets (Less than 1% to 6%) ... 1573
Vantin Tablets and Oral Suspension (1%) ... 2650
▲ Vaqta (1% to 4%) ... 2067
Varivax (Greater than or equal to 1%) ... 2070
Vaseretic Tablets (0.5% to 2.0%) ... 2073
Vasotec I.V. Injection (1.3%) ... 2076
▲ Velcade for Injection (35%) ... 2102
▲ Ventavis Inhalation Solution (7%) ... 1036
▲ Vesanoid Capsules (57%) ... 2823
VESIcare Tablets (0.2% to 1.1%) ... 631
▲ VFEND I.V. (1% to 4.4%) ... 2543
▲ VFEND Oral Suspension (1% to 4.4%) ... 2543
▲ VFEND Tablets (1% to 4.4%) ... 2543
Viadur Implant (Rare) ... 782
Viagra Tablets (Less than 2%) ... 2552
▲ Vicodin Tablets (Among most frequent) ... 530
▲ Vicodin ES Tablets (Among most frequent) ... 531
▲ Vicodin HP Tablets (Among most frequent) ... 532
▲ Vicoprofen Tablets (3% to 9%) ... 533
Viracept (Less than 2%) ... 2556
▲ Viramune Oral Suspension (2% to 15%) ... 903
▲ Viramune Tablets (2% to 15%) ... 903
▲ Viread Tablets (4% to 7%) ... 1284
Vivactil Tablets ... 2350
Vivelle Transdermal System (1.5% to 2.3%) ... 2288
Vivelle-Dot Transdermal System (1.5% to 2.3%) ... 2293
Vivotif (Infrequent) ... 834
▲ Voltaren Ophthalmic Solution (Less than or equal to 3%) ... 2300
▲ Voltaren Tablets (1% to 10%) ... 2298
▲ Voltaren-XR Tablets (1% to 10%) ... 2301
▲ VoSpire Extended-Release Tablets (4.2%) ... 2352
Vytorin 10/10 Tablets ... 2084
Vytorin 10/10 Tablets ... 3092
Vytorin 10/20 Tablets ... 2084
Vytorin 10/20 Tablets ... 3092
Vytorin 10/40 Tablets ... 2084
Vytorin 10/40 Tablets ... 3092
Vytorin 10/80 Tablets ... 2084
Vytorin 10/80 Tablets ... 3092
▲ Wellbutrin Tablets (22.9%) ... 1579
▲ Wellbutrin SR Sustained-Release Tablets (2% to 4%) ... 1583
▲ Wellbutrin XL Extended-Release Tablets (2% to 4%) ... 1588
Xanax XR Tablets (Frequent) ... 2655
▲ Xeloda Tablets (4% to 27%) ... 2825
▲ Xenical Capsules (3.8%) ... 2834
Xifaxan Tablets (2.2%) ... 2847
Xopenex HFA Inhalation Aerosol ... 3151
Xopenex Inhalation Solution ... 3143
Xopenex Inhalation Solution Concentrate ... 3147
Yasmin 28 Tablets (Greater than 1%) ... 818
Zantac ... 1597
Zantac Injection ... 1593
Zantac Injection Pharmacy Bulk Package (Frequent) ... 1595
Zantac Syrup ... 1597
▲ Zavesca Capsules (4% to 11%) ... 543
▲ Zegerid Powder for Oral Solution (1.5% to 3.2%) ... 2972
Zelnorm Tablets (1% to 2%) ... 2303
▲ Zemplar Capsules (8%) ... 535
▲ Zemplar Injection (8%) ... 538
Zemuron Injection (Less than 1%) ... 2363
▲ Zenapax for Injection (Greater than 5%) ... 2838
▲ Zerit (18% to 39%) ... 971
Zestoretic Tablets (1.4%) ... 701
Zestril Tablets (0.3% to 1.0%) ... 704
▲ Zevalin Injection (12%) ... 848
▲ Ziagen (2% to 10%) ... 1600
Zinacef Injection ... 1604
Zinacef for Injection ... 1604
▲ Zinecard for Injection (42% to 59%) ... 2659
▲ Zithromax Capsules, 250 mg (1% or less to 7%) ... 2568
Zithromax for IV Infusion (1.4% to 2.8%) ... 2573
Zithromax for Oral Suspension, 1 g (1% or less to 2%) ... 2568
▲ Zithromax for Oral Suspension, 300 mg, 600 mg, 900 mg, 1200 mg (1% or less to 7%) ... 2561
▲ Zithromax Tablets, 250 mg, 500 mg (1% or less to 7%) ... 2561
Zithromax Tablets, 600 mg (1% or less to 2%) ... 2568
▲ Zithromax Tri-Pak (1% or less to 7%) ... 2561
Zithromax Z-Pak (1% or less to 2%) ... 2568
Zmax for Oral Suspension (1.1%) ... 2577
Zocor Tablets ... 2078
Zoladex (1% to 5%) ... 709
Zoladex 3-month ... 712
▲ Zoloft (4%) ... 2581
▲ Zometa for Intravenous Infusion (14% to 32%) ... 2306
Zomig Nasal Spray (1% to less than 2%) ... 718
Zonegran Capsules (Frequent) ... 1089
▲ Zosyn (2.6% to 3.3%) ... 3492
Zovirax Capsules (2.7%) ... 1616
▲ Zovirax for Injection (Approximately 7%) ... 1618
Zovirax (2.7%) ... 1616
Zyban Sustained-Release Tablets (Frequent) ... 1620
▲ Zydone Tablets (Among most frequent) ... 1118
Zyprexa Tablets (Frequent) ... 1798
Zyprexa ZYDIS Orally Disintegrating Tablets (Frequent) ... 1798
Zyrtec Chewable Tablets (2.3% to 2.5%) ... 2589
Zyrtec (2.3% to 2.5%) ... 2589
Zyrtec-D 12 Hour Extended Release Tablets (2.3% to 2.5%) ... 2591
▲ Zyvox (0.9% to 9.4%) ... 2661

Vulva, dryness
(*see under* Vagina, dryness)

Vulvitis
Clindesse Vaginal Cream (Less than 1%) ... 3296
Zovirax Ointment (0.3%) ... 854

Vulvovaginal disorder, unspecified
▲ Cleocin Vaginal Ovules (3.4%) ... 2613

Vulvovaginitis
Advair Diskus 100/50 ... 1291
Advair Diskus 250/50 ... 1291
Advair Diskus 500/50 ... 1291
▲ Arimidex Tablets (4% to 6%) ... 665
Clindesse Vaginal Cream (Less than 1%) ... 3296
Invanz for Injection (Greater than 0.1%) ... 1974
Seroquel Tablets (Infrequent) ... 691
▲ Zoladex (5%) ... 709

W

Walking disorders
Imitrex Nasal Spray (Rare) ... 1435

Warmth
Aceon Tablets (2 mg, 4 mg, 8 mg) (0.3% to 1%) ... 3191
▲ Adalat CC Tablets (4%) ... 2978
Buprenex Injectable (Less than 1%) ... 2718
Cancidas for Injection (0% to 1.5%) ... 1894
Ethyol for Injection ... 1869
Hyperstat I.V. Injection ... 3031
▲ Imitrex Injection (10.8%) ... 1431
Imitrex Nasal Spray (Infrequent) ... 1435
Miacalcin Injection ... 2241
▲ Niaspan Extended-Release Tablets (Among most common) ... 1703
Niravam Orally Disintegrating Tablets (1.3%) ... 3106
Nubain Injection (1% or less) ... 1111
Plendil Extended-Release Tablets (Up to 1.5%) ... 651
Recombivax HB (Less than 1%) ... 2045
Urecholine Tablets ... 2349
▲ Zomig Nasal Spray (0% to 4%) ... 718

Warmth at injection site
Boostrix ... 1366
HibTITER (Less than 1% to 1.8%) ... 3419
Hyalgan Solution ... 2917
Nubain Injection ... 1111
Pneumovax 23 (Common) ... 2020
Rocephin Injectable Vials, ADD-Vantage, Galaxy, Bulk ... 2801
▲ Vaqta (0.6% to 17.4%) ... 2067
Xolair ... 1259

Warts
(*see under* Verruca)

Wasting syndrome
Invirase (Less than 2%) ... 2776

Water intoxication
Aloprim for Injection (Less than 1%) ... 2156
Carbatrol Capsules ... 3174
DDAVP Injection 4 mcg/mL ... 2893
DDAVP Nasal Spray ... 2894
DDAVP Tablets ... 2895
Desmopressin Acetate Injection ... 1143
Equetro Extended-Release Capsules ... 3178
Seroquel Tablets (Infrequent) ... 691
Tegretol/Tegretol-XR ... 2278
Zyprexa Tablets (Rare) ... 1798
Zyprexa ZYDIS Orally Disintegrating Tablets (Infrequent) ... 1798

Water retention
(*see also under* Edema)
Hyperstat I.V. Injection ... 3031
Prochieve 4% Gel ... 1018
Prochieve 8% Gel ... 1018

WBC, immature
Cipro I.V. (Infrequent) ... 2998
Cipro I.V. Pharmacy Bulk Package (Infrequent) ... 3509
▲ Clozapine Tablets (3%) ... 2141
▲ Clozaril Tablets (3%) ... 2174
Lupron Depot 3.75 mg ... 3257
Lupron Depot 7.5 mg ... 3261
Lupron Depot–3 Month 11.25 mg ... 3262
Lupron Depot-PED 7.5 mg, 11.25 mg and 15 mg ... 3266
Merrem I.V. (Greater than 0.2%) ... 687
Neurontin Capsules (1.1%) ... 2498
Neurontin Oral Solution (Rare) ... 2498
Neurontin Tablets (1.1%) ... 2498

WBC counts, fluctuation
Aciphex Tablets ... 1081
Effexor Tablets (Infrequent) ... 3405
Invanz for Injection (0.8% to 1.5%) ... 1974
Levaquin in 5% Dextrose Injection (0.1% to 0.9%) ... 2453
Levaquin (0.1% to 0.9%) ... 2453
▲ Lupron Depot 3.75 mg (Approximately 5% to 8%) ... 3257
Neurontin Capsules (Rare) ... 2498
Neurontin Oral Solution (1.1%) ... 2498
Neurontin Tablets (Rare) ... 2498
Noroxin Tablets (1.3% to 1.4%) ... 2009
Prevacid Delayed-Release Capsules ... 3268
Prevacid for Delayed-Release Oral Suspension ... 3268
Prevacid NapraPAC ... 3277
Prevacid SoluTab Delayed-Release Orally Disintegrating Tablets ... 3268
PREVPAC ... 3281
Primaxin I.M. ... 2022
Uniretic Tablets (Less than 1%) ... 3114
▲ Visudyne for Injection (1% to 10%) ... 2286

Weakness
(*see under* Asthenia)

Weakness, feet
K-Phos Neutral Tablets ... 785
K-Phos Original (Sodium Free) Tablets (Less frequent) ... 785
Roferon-A Injection (Infrequent) ... 2805
Uroqid-Acid No. 2 Tablets ... 785

Weakness, hands
K-Phos Neutral Tablets ... 785
K-Phos Original (Sodium Free) Tablets (Less frequent) ... 785
Roferon-A Injection (Infrequent) ... 2805
Uroqid-Acid No. 2 Tablets ... 785

Weakness, legs
Dantrium Intravenous ... 2691
K-Phos Neutral Tablets ... 785
K-Phos Original (Sodium Free) Tablets (Less frequent) ... 785
Uroqid-Acid No. 2 Tablets ... 785
▲ Vesanoid Capsules (3%) ... 2823

Weakness, local
Cosopt Sterile Ophthalmic Solution ... 1910
Timoptic in Ocudose (Less frequent) ... 2061
Timoptic Sterile Ophthalmic Solution ... 2058
Timoptic-XE Sterile Ophthalmic Gel Forming Solution ... 2062

Weakness, musculoskeletal
Niravam Orally Disintegrating Tablets ... 3106

weeping, skin
Aldara Cream, 5% ... 1814

Weight change, unspecified

Anaprox Tablets (Less than 1%) 2769
Anaprox DS Tablets (Less than 1%) 2769
Arthrotec Tablets (Rare) 3126
Aygestin Tablets 1062
Cataflam Tablets (Occasionally) 2173
▲ Depo-Provera Contraceptive Injection (Greater than 5%) 2619
EC-Naprosyn Delayed-Release Tablets (Less than 1%) 2769
Flexeril Tablets (Rare) 1832
Focalin XR Capsules 2217
Lo/Ovral-28 Tablets 3423
▲ Lupron Depot 3.75 mg (6%) 3257
▲ Lupron Depot–3 Month 11.25 mg (6%) 3262
Naprosyn Suspension (Less than 1%) 2769
Naprosyn Tablets (Less than 1%) 2769
Triphasil-28 Tablets 3483
Univasc Tablets (Less than 1%) 3118
Vivactil Tablets 2350
Voltaren Tablets (Occasionally) 2298
Voltaren-XR Tablets (Occasionally) 2301

Weight changes, increase or decrease

Activella Tablets 2311
Alesse-28 Tablets 3392
▲ Avastin IV (15% to 16%) 1229
Cenestin Tablets, 0.45mg, 0.625mg, 0.9mg, 1.25mg 1063
Cenestin Tablets, 0.3mg 1063
Climara Transdermal System 795
▲ Clolar for Intravenous Infusion (15%) 1264
Estratest Tablets 3196
Estratest H.S. Tablets 3196
Estrogel 0.06% 3200
Klonopin (Infrequent) 2782
Moban Tablets 1108
Ortho-Cept Tablets 2395
Ortho-Cyclen Tablets 2414
Ortho Evra Transdermal System 2402
Ortho Tri-Cyclen Tablets 2414
Ortho Tri-Cyclen Lo Tablets 2421
Prefest Tablets 1069
Premphase Tablets 3452
Prempro Tablets 3452
Prometrium Capsules (100 mg, 200 mg) 3205
Rescriptor Tablets 2535
Seasonale Tablets 1073
Yasmin 28 Tablets 818

Weight decrease

(*see under* Weight loss)

Weight gain

▲ Abilify Tablets (5.1% to 30%) 916
▲ Abilify Tablets (5.1% to 30%) 2472
Aciphex Tablets 1081
Activella Tablets (0% to 9%) 2311
▲ ActoPlus Met Tablets (2.9% to 6.7%) 3219
▲ Actos Tablets (0.9% to 3.6%) 3224
Advair Diskus 100/50 1291
Advair Diskus 250/50 1291
Advair Diskus 500/50 1291
Aerobid/Aerobid-M (1% to 3%) 1172
Aldoclor Tablets 1881
Aldoril Tablets 1884
Altace Capsules (Less than 1%) 1673
Antara Capsules 2723
Aricept Tablets (Infrequent) 1086
Aricept ODT Tablets (Infrequent) 1086
▲ Arimidex Tablets (2% to 13%) 665
Astelin Nasal Spray (2.0%) 1876
Avandia Tablets 1348
▲ Azmacort Inhalation Aerosol (1% to 3%) 1701
Betaseron for SC Injection 791
Bravelle for Intramuscular or Subcutaneous Injection (2.9%) 1140
Buphenyl Powder (Less than or equal to 2%) 3327
Buphenyl Tablets (Less than or equal to 2%) 3327
Caduet Tablets (Greater than 0.1% to less than 2%) 2507
Campral Tablets (Frequent) 1175
Cardizem LA Extended Release Tablets (Less than 2%) 1699
▲ Carnitor Injection (2% to 6%) 3185
▲ Casodex Tablets (2% to 5%) 670
Catapres Tablets (About 1 in 100 patients) 874
Catapres-TTS (0.5% or less) 875
Celebrex Capsules (0.1% to 1.9%) 3130
Celexa (Frequent) 1177
▲ CellCept Capsules (3% to less than 20%) 2751
▲ CellCept Intravenous (3% to less than 20%) 2751
▲ CellCept Oral Suspension (3% to less than 20%) 2751
▲ CellCept Tablets (3% to less than 20%) 2751
▲ Cenestin Tablets, 0.45mg, 0.625mg, 0.9mg, 1.25mg (5.7%) 1063
Climara Pro Transdermal System (2.8%) 800
Clorpres Tablets (About 1%) 2139
▲ Clozapine Tablets (4%) 2141
▲ Clozaril Tablets (4% to 31%) 2174
Colazal Capsules 2845
▲ Copaxone for Injection (3%) 3292
▲ Coreg Tablets (10% to 12%) 1376
▲ Cozaar Tablets (4%) 1913
Cymbalta Delayed-Release Capsules (Frequent) 1729
DDAVP Tablets 2895
Decadron Phosphate Injection 1931
Decadron Tablets 1929
▲ Depacon Injection (4% to 9%) 412
▲ Depakene (9%) 417
▲ Depakote Sprinkle Capsules (4% to 9%) 422
▲ Depakote Tablets (8% to 9%) 427
▲ Depakote ER Tablets (8% to 9%) 433
▲ depo-subQ provera 104 Injectable Suspension (6%) 2622
Detrol Tablets (1.5%) 2626
▲ Dostinex Tablets (Less than 10%) 2631
Doxil Injection (Less than 1%) 3302
DynaCirc CR Tablets (0.5% to 1%) 2726
Effexor Tablets (Frequent) 3405
Effexor XR Capsules (Frequent) 3411
Eligard 7.5 mg (Less than 2%) 2896
▲ Eloxatin for Injection (10%) 2908
Enablex Extended-Release Tablets (Greater than or equal to 1%) 2201
Enbrel for Injection 580
▲ Entocort EC Capsules (Less than 5%) 2694
Eskalith 1406
Estrogel 0.06% (2.4%) 3200
▲ Evista Tablets (8.8%) 1735
Evoxac Capsules (Less than 1%) 1042
Femara Tablets (2%) 2210
▲ Flolan for Injection (6%) 1408
▲ Flovent Diskus 50 mcg (1% to 3%) 1415
Flovent HFA 1418
Follistim AQ Cartridge 2354
Fortical Nasal Spray (Less than 1%) 3336
Gabitril Tablets (Frequent) 998
Gengraf Capsules (1% to less than 3%) 458
▲ Geodon Capsules (10%) 2514
▲ Gleevec Tablets (5% to 32%) 2221
▲ Hectorol Capsules (4.9%) 909
▲ Hectorol Injection (4.9%) 911
Hydrocortone Tablets 1963
Hytrin Capsules (0.5%) 469
Imitrex Injection 1431
Imitrex Nasal Spray 1435
Imitrex Tablets (Rare) 1440
Indocin Capsules (Less than 1%) 1968
Indocin I.V. (Less than 1%) 1973
Indocin (Less than 1%) 1968
▲ Intron A for Injection (Less than or equal to 5%) 3038
Invirase (Less than 2%) 2776
▲ I.V. Busulfex (8%) 1125
Kaletra (Less than 2%) 474
Keppra Oral Solution (1% or more) 3307
Keppra Tablets (1% or more) 3307
K-Phos Neutral Tablets 785
Lamictal (Frequent) 1449
▲ Leukine (8%) 829
Lexapro Oral Solution (Frequent) 1193
Lexapro Tablets (Frequent) 1193
Lipitor Tablets (Less than 2%) 2495
Lithobid Tablets 1670
Lofibra Capsules 1217
Lunesta Tablets (Infrequent) 3139
Lupron Depot 7.5 mg (Less than 5%) 3261
Lupron Depot-PED 7.5 mg, 11.25 mg and 15 mg (Less than 2%) 3266
Lupron Injection Pediatric (Less than 2%) 3256
▲ Lyrica Capsules (4% to 16%) 2524
Maxair Autohaler 1820
Menostar Transdermal System 805
Miacalcin Nasal Spray (Less than 1%) 2242
▲ Mirena Intrauterine System (5% or more) 810
Mobic Oral Suspension (Less than 2%) 893
Mobic Tablets (Less than 2%) 893
▲ Myfortic Tablets (3% to less than 20%) 2244
Nadolol Tablets (1 to 5 of 1000 patients) 2121
Neoral Soft Gelatin Capsules (1% to less than 3%) 2247
Neoral Oral Solution (1% to less than 3%) 2247
Neurontin Capsules (1.8% to 2.9%) 2498
Neurontin Oral Solution (1.8% to 2.9%) 2498
Neurontin Tablets (1.8% to 2.9%) 2498
Nexium Delayed-Release Capsules (Less than 1%) 645
Nexium I.V. (Less than 1%) 649
▲ Nicotrol NS (Greater than 5%) 2596
▲ Niravam Orally Disintegrating Tablets (2.7% to 27.2%) 3106
Norvasc Tablets (More than 0.1% to 1%) 2529
Orap Tablets 1220
Ortho Micronor Tablets (Rare) 2411
Parcopa Orally Disintegrating Tablets 3111
Paxil CR Controlled-Release Tablets (Frequent) 1509
Paxil (Frequent) 1501
Permax Tablets (1.6%; frequent) 3357
Premarin Intravenous 3440
Premarin Tablets 3443
Premarin Vaginal Cream 3449
Prevacid Delayed-Release Capsules (Less than 1%) 3268
Prevacid for Delayed-Release Oral Suspension (Less than 1%) 3268
Prevacid NapraPAC (Less than 1%) 3277
Prevacid SoluTab Delayed-Release Orally Disintegrating Tablets (Less than 1%) 3268
PREVPAC (Less than 1%) 3281
Prilosec OTC Tablets (Less than 1%) 2674
Prinivil Tablets (0.3% to 1.0%) 2029
Prinzide Tablets 2033
▲ Prograf Capsules and Injection (3% to 15%) 624
▲ Proleukin for Injection (16%) 1007
ProSom Tablets (Rare) 512
Protonix I.V. (Less than 1%) 3468
Protonix Tablets (Less than 1%) 3465
Provigil Tablets (At least 1%) 1002
Prozac Pulvules and Liquid (Frequent) 1771
▲ Rapamune Oral Solution and Tablets (8% to 21%) 3472
Relafen Tablets (Less than 1%) 1523
Relpax Tablets (Rare) 2531
Requip Tablets (Infrequent) 1528
Rescriptor Tablets 2535
Reyataz Capsules (Less than 3%) 948
Rilutek Tablets (Infrequent) 2945
▲ Risperdal Consta Long-Acting Injection (4% to 9%) 1664
▲ Risperdal M-Tab Orally Disintegrating Tablets (2% to 18%) 1658
▲ Risperdal (2% to 18%) 1658
Men's Rogaine Extra Strength Topical Solution, Ocean Rush Scent and Original Unscented ▣ 706
Women's Rogaine Topical Solution, Spring Bloom Scent and Original Unscented ▣ 707
Rythmol SR Capsules 2736
▲ Seroquel Tablets (5% to 23%) 691
▲ Simulect for Injection (3% to 10%) 2268
Somavert Injection 2648
Sonata Capsules (Infrequent) 1686
Soriatane Capsules (Less than 1%) 1028
Stalevo Tablets 2270
Sular Tablets (Less than or equal to 1%) 1163
Surmontil Capsules 2347
▲ Symbyax Capsules (Up to 21%) 1788
Targretin Capsules 1719
Taxotere Injection Concentrate 2947
▲ Temodar Capsules (5%) 3088
Thalomid Capsules 979
Thioridazine Hydrochloride Tablets 2122
Thiothixene Capsules 2124
Thyrolar 1203
Tiazac Capsules (Less than 2%) 1204
Topamax Sprinkle Capsules (1%) 2438
Topamax Tablets (1%) 2438
Tricor Tablets 523
Triglide Tablets 1165
Trileptal Oral Suspension (1% to 2%) 2281
Trileptal Tablets (1% to 2%) 2281
▲ Trisenox Injection (13%) 983
Uniretic Tablets (Less than 1%) 3114
Uroqid-Acid No. 2 Tablets 785
Vantas (2.3%) 3367
Vantin Tablets and Oral Suspension (Less than 1%) 2650
▲ Vesanoid Capsules (23%) 2823
Viadur Implant (2.3%) 782
▲ Vivelle Transdermal System (1.9% to 8.5%) 2288
▲ Vivelle-Dot Transdermal System (1.9% to 8.5%) 2293
▲ Wellbutrin Tablets (9.4% to 13.6%) 1579
▲ Wellbutrin SR Sustained-Release Tablets (2% to 3%) 1583
▲ Wellbutrin XL Extended-Release Tablets (2% to 3%) 1588
▲ Xanax XR Tablets (5.1%) 2655
Zegerid Powder for Oral Solution (Less than 1%) 2972
Zestoretic Tablets 701
Zestril Tablets (0.3% to 1.0%) 704
Zoladex (1% to 5%) 709
Zoladex 3-month 712
Zoloft (Frequent) 2581
Zomig Nasal Spray (Rare) 718
Zonegran Capsules (Infrequent) 1089
Zyban Sustained-Release Tablets (Infrequent) 1620
▲ Zyprexa Tablets (5.6% to 6%) 1798
▲ Zyprexa ZYDIS Orally Disintegrating Tablets (5.6% to 6%) 1798
Zyrtec Chewable Tablets (Less than 2%) 2589
Zyrtec (Less than 2%) 2589
Zyrtec-D 12 Hour Extended Release Tablets (Less than 2%) 2591

Weight gain, delayed

Elocon Cream 0.1% 3019
Elocon Lotion 0.1% 3020
Elocon Ointment 0.1% 3021
▲ Sandostatin Injection (32%) 2263

Weight loss

Abelcet Injection 1119
Abilify Tablets (Frequent) 916
Abilify Tablets (Frequent) 2472
Accutane Capsules 2740
Aciphex Tablets 1081
▲ Actimmune (6%) 1646
Actiq (Less than 1%) 993
Adalat CC Tablets (Less than 1%) 2978
Adderall Tablets 3168
▲ Adderall XR Capsules (1.2% to 11%) 3169
Alferon N Injection (1%) 1640
Alkeran for Injection 976
Alkeran Tablets 977
Ambien Tablets (Rare) 2867
Antara Capsules 2723
Aptivus Capsules (Less than 2%) 859
▲ Arava Tablets (4%) 2881
▲ Aricept Tablets (3%) 1086
▲ Aricept ODT Tablets (3%) 1086
Avinza Capsules (Less than 5%) 1714
▲ Bexxar (Less than 1% to 6%) 1360
Blocadren Tablets 1891
Caduet Tablets (Greater than 0.1% to less than or equal to 1%) 2507
Calcijex Injection 411
Campral Tablets (Infrequent) 1175
▲ Camptosar Injection (1% to 30%) 2602
Captopril Tablets 2114
▲ Carnitor Injection (3% to 8%) 3185
▲ Casodex Tablets (4%) 670
Celexa (Frequent) 1177
▲ CellCept Capsules (3% to less than 20%) 2751
▲ CellCept Intravenous (3% to less than 20%) 2751
▲ CellCept Oral Suspension (3% to less than 20%) 2751
▲ CellCept Tablets (3% to less than 20%) 2751
Climara Pro Transdermal System 800
Clozapine Tablets 2141
Clozaril Tablets 2174
Cogentin Injection 1903
Colazal Capsules 2845
Concerta Extended-Release Tablets 1828
Copaxone for Injection (Infrequent) 3292
▲ Copegus Tablets (10% to 16%) 2759
▲ Coreg Tablets (Greater than 1% to 3%) 1376
Cosopt Sterile Ophthalmic Solution 1910
Cymbalta Delayed-Release Capsules (2%) 1729
Cytovene (At least 3 subjects) 2763
Daranide Tablets 1928
▲ Depacon Injection (6%) 412
▲ Depakene (6%) 417
▲ Depakote Sprinkle Capsules (6%) 422
▲ Depakote Tablets (6%) 427

▲ Depakote ER Tablets (6%) 433
Dexedrine 1386
DextroStat Tablets 3177
▲ Dostinex Tablets (Less than 10%) 2631
▲ Doxil Injection (1% to 10%) 3302
Duragesic Transdermal System 2448
Effexor Tablets (1%) 3405
▲ Effexor XR Capsules (3% to 4%) 3411
Eldepryl Capsules (1 of 49 patients) 3209
▲ Eloxatin for Injection (2% to 5%) 2908
Elspar for Injection 1943
Emend Capsules (Greater than 0.5%) 1944
▲ Erbitux (9%) 937
Eskalith 1406
Evoxac Capsules (Less than 1%) 1042
▲ Exelon Capsules (3%) 2204
FazaClo Orally Disintegrating Tablets 547
▲ Femara Tablets (7%) 2210
▲ Flolan for Injection (27% to 45%) 1408
▲ Focalin Tablets (Among more frequent) 2214
Focalin XR Capsules 2217
▲ Fuzeon Injection (6.6%) 2772
Gabitril Tablets (Frequent) 998
Garamycin Injectable 3028
Gengraf Capsules (1% to less than 3%) 458
Gleevec Tablets (Infrequent) 2221
Hectorol Capsules 909
Hectorol Injection 911
Herceptin I.V. (At least one of the 958 patients) 1234
Imitrex Injection 1431
Imitrex Nasal Spray (Rare) 1435
Imitrex Tablets (Rare) 1440
Indapamide Tablets (Less than 5%) 2119
▲ Infergen (5%) 1647
▲ Intron A for Injection (Less than 1% to 10%) 3038
Invanz for Injection (Greater than 0.1%) 1974
Invirase (Less than 2%) 2776
▲ Iressa Tablets (3% to 6%) 684
▲ Kaletra (Up to 3%) 474
Lamictal (Infrequent) 1449
Lamisil Tablets 2226
▲ Leukine (37%) 829
Levaquin in 5% Dextrose Injection (0.1% to 0.9%) 2453
Levaquin (0.1% to 0.9%) 2453
Levothroid Tablets 1189
Levoxyl Tablets 1680
Lexapro Oral Solution (Infrequent) 1193
Lexapro Tablets (Infrequent) 1193
Lithobid Tablets 1670
Lofibra Capsules 1217
Lunesta Tablets (Infrequent) 3139
Menostar Transdermal System 805
Metadate CD Capsules 3316
Mirapex Tablets (2%) 889
Mobic Oral Suspension (Less than 2%) 893
Mobic Tablets (Less than 2%) 893
Myleran Tablets 1492
Namenda (Frequent) 1199
▲ Navelbine Injection (Up to 34%) 1494
Neoral Soft Gelatin Capsules (1% to less than 3%) 2247
Neoral Oral Solution (1% to less than 3%) 2247
Neurontin Capsules (Infrequent) 2498
Neurontin Oral Solution (Infrequent) 2498
Neurontin Tablets (Infrequent) 2498
Nexium Delayed-Release Capsules (Less than 1%) 645
Nexium I.V. (Less than 1%) 649
▲ Niravam Orally Disintegrating Tablets (2.3% to 22.6%) 3106
Norvir (0 to 2.4%) 499
Oncaspar (Less than 1%) 1123
▲ Ontak Vials (14%) 1717
Orap Tablets 1220
Parcopa Orally Disintegrating Tablets 3111
Paxil CR Controlled-Release Tablets (Frequent) 1509
Paxil (Frequent) 1501
▲ Pegasys (4%) 2793
▲ PEG-Intron Powder for Injection (11%) 3062
Permax Tablets (Frequent) 3357
▲ Photofrin for Injection (6% to 9%) 729
Premarin Intravenous 3440
Premarin Tablets 3443
Premarin Vaginal Cream 3449
Prevacid Delayed-Release Capsules (Less than 1%) 3268
Prevacid for Delayed-Release Oral Suspension (Less than 1%) 3268
Prevacid NapraPAC (Less than 1%) 3277
Prevacid SoluTab Delayed-Release Orally Disintegrating Tablets (Less than 1%) 3268
PREVPAC (Less than 1%) 3281
Prinivil Tablets (0.3% to 1.0%) 2029
Prinzide Tablets 2033
▲ Proleukin for Injection (5%) 1007
ProSom Tablets (Rare) 512
Protonix I.V. (Less than 1%) 3468
Protonix Tablets (Less than 1%) 3465
Provigil Tablets (Greater than or equal to 1%) 1002
Prozac Pulvules and Liquid (1.4% to 2%) 1771
Pulmozyme Inhalation Solution 1245
▲ Rapamune Oral Solution and Tablets (3% to 20%) 3472
▲ Razadyne ER Extended-Release Capsules (5% to 7%) 2434
▲ Razadyne (5% to 7%) 2434
▲ Rebetol (20% to 29%) 3073
Relafen Tablets (Less than 1%) 1523
Relpax Tablets (Rare) 2531
Requip Tablets (1% or more) 1528
Rescriptor Tablets 2535
Retrovir Capsules (0.8%) 1533
Retrovir IV Infusion (1%) 1537
Retrovir (0.8%) 1533
Reyataz Capsules (Less than 3%) 948
▲ Ribavirin, USP Capsules (20% to 29%) 3083
▲ Rilutek Tablets (3.7% to 4.6%) 2945
▲ Risperdal Consta Long-Acting Injection (1% to 4%) 1664
Risperdal M-Tab Orally Disintegrating Tablets (Infrequent) 1658
Risperdal (Infrequent) 1658
Ritalin Hydrochloride Tablets 2254
Ritalin LA Capsules 2255
Ritalin-SR Tablets 2254
▲ Rituxan I.V. (1% to 5%) 1251
▲ Roferon-A Injection (25% to 33%) 2805
Rythmol SR Capsules 2736
Sandimmune (Rare) 2259
Sandostatin Injection (Less than 1%) 2263
▲ Sandostatin LAR Depot (5% to 15%) 2264
Seroquel Tablets (Infrequent) 691
Sonata Capsules (Rare) 1686
Stalevo Tablets 2270
Strattera Capsules (2%) 1784
Sular Tablets (Less than or equal to 1%) 1163
Surmontil Capsules 2347
Symbyax Capsules (Frequent) 1788
Targretin Capsules 1719
Timolide Tablets 2056
Timoptic in Ocudose 2061
Timoptic Sterile Ophthalmic Solution 2058
Timoptic-XE Sterile Ophthalmic Gel Forming Solution 2062
▲ TOBI Solution for Inhalation (10.1%) 1015
▲ Topamax Sprinkle Capsules (4% to 21%) 2438
▲ Topamax Tablets (4% to 21%) 2438
Trecator Tablets 3482
Tricor Tablets 523
Triglide Tablets 1165
Trileptal Oral Suspension 2281
Trileptal Tablets 2281
▲ Trisenox Injection (8%) 983
Truvada Tablets 1279
Ultracet Tablets (Less than 1%) 2462
Unithroid Tablets 3521
Vantas (Less than 2%) 3367
▲ Vesanoid Capsules (17%) 2823
Vicoprofen Tablets (Less than 1%) 533
▲ Viread Tablets (2% to 4%) 1284
Vivelle Transdermal System 2288
Vivelle-Dot Transdermal System 2293
▲ Wellbutrin Tablets (23.2% to 28%) 1579
▲ Wellbutrin SR Sustained-Release Tablets (14% to 19%) 1583
▲ Wellbutrin XL Extended-Release Tablets (14% to 19%) 1588
▲ Xanax XR Tablets (4.3%) 2655
▲ Xeloda Tablets (Up to 7%) 2825
Xifaxan Tablets (Less than 2%) 2847
▲ Zavesca Capsules (39% to 85%) 543
Zestoretic Tablets 701
Zestril Tablets (0.3% to 1.0%) 704
Zoloft 2581
▲ Zometa for Intravenous Infusion (16%) 2306
▲ Zonegran Capsules (3%) 1089
Zyprexa Tablets (Frequent) 1798
Zyprexa ZYDIS Orally Disintegrating Tablets (Frequent) 1798

Wenckebach block

Buprenex Injectable (Less than 1%) 2718
Digitek Tablets 2146
Lanoxin Injection 1462
Lanoxin Tablets 1468
Lanoxin Injection Pediatric 1465

Wenckebach's period

(*see under* A-V conduction, prolongation)

Wheals

Attenuvax (Rare) 1889
Desferal Vials 2190
Dilaudid-HP (Less frequent) 441
Meruvax II 1994
M-M-R II 1980
Mumpsvax (Extremely rare) 2005

Wheezing

Abelcet Injection 1119
▲ Advair Diskus 100/50 (1% to 3%) 1291
▲ Advair Diskus 250/50 (1% to 3%) 1291
▲ Advair Diskus 500/50 (1% to 3%) 1291
▲ Aerobid/Aerobid-M (3% to 9%) 1172
Alacol DM Syrup 739
Alferon N Injection 1640
Aricept Tablets (Infrequent) 1086
Aricept ODT Tablets (Infrequent) 1086
Avalide Tablets 922
Avalide Tablets 2889
Avapro Tablets (Less than 1%) 925
Avapro Tablets (Less than 1%) 2886
Azmacort Inhalation Aerosol 1701
Beconase AQ Nasal Spray (Rare) 1359
Brevibloc Concentrate (Less than 1%) 766
Brevibloc Injection (Less than 1%) 766
Brevibloc Double Strength Injection (Less than 1%) 766
Brevibloc Premixed Injection (Less than 1%) 766
Brevibloc Double Strength Premixed Injection (Less than 1%) 766
Clindesse Vaginal Cream (Less than 1%) 3296
Clozapine Tablets (Less than 1%) 2141
Clozaril Tablets (Less than 1%) 2174
Combivent Inhalation Aerosol 878
Combivir Tablets 1373
CytoGam Intravenous (Less than 5.0%) 1866
Diprivan Injectable Emulsion (Less than 1%) 676
DuoNeb Inhalation Solution 1058
Elidel Cream 1% (Up to 1.2%) 2198
Epivir 1394
Epivir-HBV 1398
Epzicom Tablets 1402
FazaClo Orally Disintegrating Tablets (Less than 1%) 547
Flonase Nasal Spray 1412
Flovent Diskus 50 mcg 1415
Flovent HFA 1418
Flumist Vaccine 1872
Gammagard Liquid 751
Humalog-Pen (Less common) 1751
Humalog Mix 75/25-Pen (Less common) 1754
Humulin 50/50, 100 Units 1760
Humulin 70/30 Pen (Less common) 1761
Humulin L, 100 Units (Less common) 1763
Humulin R (U-500) 1768
Humulin N Pen (Less common) 1765
Imitrex Tablets 1440
Infed Injection 3381
▲ Intron A for Injection (Less than or equal to 5%) 3038
Invanz for Injection (1%) 1974
Levothroid Tablets 1189
Levoxyl Tablets 1680
Maxair Autohaler 1820
Maxalt Tablets 1983
Maxalt-MLT Orally Disintegrating Tablets 1983
Mivacron Injection (Less than 1%) 489
Children's Motrin Oral Suspension and Chewable Tablets 1837
Children's Motrin Cold Non-Staining Dye-Free Oral Suspension 1838
Children's Motrin Cold Oral Suspension 1838
Children's Motrin Non-Staining Dye-Free Oral Suspension 1837
Motrin Cold & Sinus Caplets 1836
Motrin IB Tablets and Caplets 1836
Infants' Motrin Concentrated Drops 1837
Infants' Motrin Non-Staining Dye-Free Drops 1837
Junior Strength Motrin Caplets and Chewable Tablets 1837
Nasacort HFA Inhalation Aerosol 2939
Nasonex Nasal Spray (Greater than or equal to 2%) 3058
Neumega for Injection 3433
Neupogen for Injection 598
Nimotop Capsules (Less than 1%) 774
NovoLog Injection 2326
Nubain Injection (1% or less) 1111
▲ Orthoclone OKT3 Sterile Solution (13%) 2370
Prevnar for Injection 3460
Prinivil Tablets (0.3% to 1.0%) 2029
Prinzide Tablets 2033
▲ Proleukin for Injection (6%) 1007
Proventil Inhalation Solution 0.083% (1% to 1.5%) 3069
Pulmozyme Inhalation Solution 1245
Rhinocort Aqua Nasal Spray (Rare) 658
Rythmol SR Capsules (2%) 2736
Sandimmune 2259
Simulect for Injection 2268
Singulair (Greater than or equal to 2%) 2047
Sular Tablets (Less than or equal to 1%) 1163
Synagis (More than 1%) 1868
Tenormin I.V. Injection (Up to 3%) 698
Tenormin Tablets (Up to 3%) 695
Toprol-XL Tablets (About 1 of 100 patients) 660
▲ Trisenox Injection (13%) 983
Trizivir Tablets 1565
Ultane Liquid for Inhalation (Less than 1%) 526
Unithroid Tablets 3521
Vancocin HCl Capsules, USP 3370
Vantin Tablets and Oral Suspension (Less than 1%) 2650
Vaqta (Less than 1%) 2067
▲ Vesanoid Capsules (14%) 2823
Xopenex HFA Inhalation Aerosol 3151
Xopenex Inhalation Solution 3143
Xopenex Inhalation Solution Concentrate 3147
Zemuron Injection (Less than 1%) 2363
Zestoretic Tablets 701
Zestril Tablets (0.3% to 1.0%) 704

White blood cell count, decreased

Mycamine for Injection 620

Withdrawal reactions

Ambien Tablets (Rare) 2867
Aricept Tablets (Infrequent) 1086
Aricept ODT Tablets (Infrequent) 1086
Avinza Capsules (Less than 5%) 1714
Catapres Tablets 874
Catapres-TTS (0.5% or less) 875
Celexa 1177
Darvocet A 500 Tablets 3497
Dexedrine 1386
Dilaudid 439
Dilaudid Non-Sterile Powder 439
Dilaudid Rectal Suppositories 439
Dilaudid Tablets 439
Effexor Tablets (Rare) 3405
Effexor XR Capsules (Infrequent) 3411
Kadian Capsules (Less than 3%) 572
Klonopin 2782
Levaquin in 5% Dextrose Injection (0.1% to 0.9%) 2453
Levaquin (0.1% to 0.9%) 2453
Lortab 3315
Lortab Elixir 3312
MS Contin Tablets 2703
Nembutal Sodium Solution, USP 2484
▲ Nicotrol Inhaler (Greater than 3%) 2594
▲ Nicotrol NS (Greater than 5%) 2596
OxyContin Tablets (Less than 1%) 2699
Paxil CR Controlled-Release Tablets (Rare) 1509
Paxil (Rare) 1501
ProSom Tablets 512
Risperdal M-Tab Orally Disintegrating Tablets (Rare) 1658
Risperdal (Rare) 1658
▲ Suboxone Tablets (22% to 25.2%) 2719
▲ Subutex Tablets (18.4% to 22%) 2719
Tranxene 2488
Ultracet Tablets (Less than 1%) 2462
Valium Tablets 2822
Xanax XR Tablets 2655
Zoloft (Rare) 2581
Zyprexa Tablets (Infrequent) 1798

Zyprexa ZYDIS Orally Disintegrating Tablets (Infrequent) 1798

Withdrawal syndrome

Campral Tablets (Infrequent) 1175
▲ Nicotrol Inhaler (Greater than 3%) 2594
Symbyax Capsules (Rare) 1788

Worsening of underlying illness

Synercid I.V. (Less than 1%) 1690

Wound, nasal

▲ Fortical Nasal Spray (10.6%) 3336

Wound dehiscence

▲ Valcyte Tablets (Less than 5%) 2816

Wound drainage, increased

▲ Arixtra Injection (0.6% to 4.5%) 1325
▲ Valcyte Tablets (Less than 5%) 2816

Wound healing, impaired

Blephamide Ophthalmic Ointment (Infrequent) 563
Blephamide Ophthalmic Suspension 564
Decadron Phosphate Injection 1931
Decadron Tablets 1929
Depo-Medrol Injectable Suspension 2615
Depo-Medrol Single-Dose Vial 2617
FML Ophthalmic Ointment (Infrequent) ⊙ 225
FML Ophthalmic Suspension ⊙ 224
FML Forte Ophthalmic Suspension (Infrequent) ⊙ 223
FML-S Liquifilm Sterile Ophthalmic Suspension ⊙ 226
HMS Sterile Ophthalmic Suspension ⊙ 228
Hydrocortone Tablets 1963
Ocufen Ophthalmic Solution ⊙ 230
Pediapred Oral Solution 3319
Poly-Pred Liquifilm Ophthalmic Suspension ⊙ 231
Pred Forte Ophthalmic Suspension ⊙ 233
Pred Mild Sterile Ophthalmic Suspension (Infrequent) ⊙ 236
Pred-G Ophthalmic Suspension ⊙ 234
Pred-G Sterile Ophthalmic Ointment ⊙ 235
▲ Rapamune Oral Solution and Tablets (3% to less than 20%) 3472
Retisert Implant ⊙ 256
TobraDex Ophthalmic Ointment 558
TobraDex Ophthalmic Suspension 558
▲ Zenapax for Injection (Greater than 5%) 2838
▲ Zofran (28%) 1613
▲ Zofran ODT Orally Disintegrating Tablets (28%) 1613
Zylet Ophthalmic Suspension 3508

Wound infection

▲ Arixtra Injection (4.9%) 1325
Enbrel for Injection 580
▲ Gengraf Capsules (7%) 458
▲ Infergen (3% to 4%) 1647
▲ Myfortic Tablets (3% to less than 20%) 2244
▲ Neoral Soft Gelatin Capsules (7.0%) 2247
▲ Neoral Oral Solution (7.0%) 2247
▲ Sandimmune (7.0% to 10.1%) 2259
▲ Valcyte Tablets (Less than 5%) 2816

Wrist-drop

Rilutek Tablets (Rare) 2945

X

Xanthomas, eruptive

Accutane Capsules 2740
Amnesteem Capsules 2126

Xanthopsia

Aldoclor Tablets 1881
Aldoril Tablets 1884
Atacand HCT 637
Avalide Tablets 922
Avalide Tablets 2889
Clorpres Tablets 2139
Digitek Tablets 2146
Diovan HCT Tablets 2195
Diuril Oral 1936
Diuril Sodium Intravenous 1934
Dyazide Capsules 1389
Furosemide Tablets 2117
Hyzaar (One subject) 1964
Indapamide Tablets 2119
Lanoxicaps Capsules 1458
Lanoxin Injection 1462
Lanoxin Tablets 1468
Lanoxin Injection Pediatric 1465
Lotensin HCT Tablets 2235
Maxzide 2150
Micardis HCT Tablets 886
Mintezol 2002
Moduretic Tablets 2003
Prinzide Tablets 2033
Teveten HCT Tablets 1710
Timolide Tablets 2056
Uniretic Tablets 3114
Vaseretic Tablets 2073
Zestoretic Tablets 701

Xerochilia

Invirase (2%) 2776
Lexapro Oral Solution (Infrequent) 1193
Lexapro Tablets (Infrequent) 1193
Xifaxan Tablets (Less than 2%) 2847
Zovirax Cream (Less than 1%) 853

Xeroderma
(*see under* Xerosis cutis)

Xeromycteria

Accutane Capsules 2740
▲ Alacol DM Syrup (Among most frequent) 739
Alphagan P Ophthalmic Solution (Less than 1%) 563
AmBisome for Injection (Less common) 615
Amnesteem Capsules 2126
▲ Atrovent Nasal Spray 0.03% (5.1%) 869
▲ Atrovent Nasal Spray 0.06% (4.8%) 870
Beconase AQ Nasal Spray 1359
Brimonidine Tartrate Ophthalmic Solution 0.2% (Less than 3%) ⊙ 245
Catapres Tablets 874
Clorpres Tablets 2139
▲ Ditropan XL Extended Release Tablets (2% to less than 5%) 2391
Flonase Nasal Spray (Less than 1%) 1412
▲ Fortical Nasal Spray (10.6%) 3336
Maxalt Tablets (Infrequent) 1983
Maxalt-MLT Orally Disintegrating Tablets (Infrequent) 1983
▲ Miacalcin Nasal Spray (10.6%) 2242
▲ Nasarel Nasal Spray (3% to 9%) 1652
Symmetrel (1% to 5%) 1115

Xerophthalmia

Abilify Tablets (Infrequent) 916
Abilify Tablets (Infrequent) 2472
Accutane Capsules 2740
Aciphex Tablets 1081
▲ Actonel Tablets (3.3%) 2679
Acular Ophthalmic Solution (Rare) 561
▲ Advair Diskus 250/50 (1% to 3%) 1291
Alamast Ophthalmic Solution (Less than 5%) 3371
Alphagan P Ophthalmic Solution (1% to 4%) 563
▲ Alrex Ophthalmic Suspension 0.2% (5% to 15%) ⊙ 243
AmBisome for Injection (Less common) 615
Amerge Tablets (Rare) 1312
Amnesteem Capsules 2126
Aricept Tablets (Infrequent) 1086
Aricept ODT Tablets (Infrequent) 1086
Astelin Nasal Spray 1876
Axert Tablets (Rare) 2430
Azopt Ophthalmic Suspension (1% to 5%) 553
▲ Betimol Ophthalmic Solution (More than 5%) ⊙ 283
▲ Betimol Ophthalmic Solution (More than 5%) 3371
Betoptic S Ophthalmic Suspension (Small number of patients) 554
Blocadren Tablets 1891
Botox Purified Neurotoxin Complex 565
▲ Brimonidine Tartrate Ophthalmic Solution 0.2% (3% to 9%) ⊙ 245
Caduet Tablets (Less than 2%) 2507
Catapres Tablets 874
Catapres-TTS (0.5% or less) 875
Celexa (Infrequent) 1177
Ciloxan Ophthalmic Ointment (Less than 1%) 554
Clorpres Tablets 2139
Copaxone for Injection (Infrequent) 3292
Cosopt Sterile Ophthalmic Solution (1% to 5%) 1910
Cytovene 2763
Depacon Injection (1% or more) 412
Depakene (1% or more) 417
Depakote Sprinkle Capsules 422
▲ Depakote Tablets (1% to 5%) 427
Depakote ER Tablets (Greater than 1%) 433
▲ Detrol Tablets (3.8%) 2626
▲ Detrol LA Capsules (3%) 2629
▲ Ditropan XL Extended Release Tablets (3% to 6%) 2391
▲ Doxil Injection (1% to 10%) 3302
Effexor Tablets (Infrequent) 3405
Effexor XR Capsules (Infrequent) 3411
Enablex Extended-Release Tablets (1.5% to 2.1%) 2201
Enbrel for Injection 580
▲ Evoxac Capsules (1% to 3%) 1042
Flonase Nasal Spray 1412
Geodon Capsules (Infrequent) 2514
Gleevec Tablets (Infrequent) 2221
Inderal LA Long-Acting Capsules (Rare) 3421
InnoPran XL Capsules (Rare) 2728
▲ Intron A for Injection (Less than 5%) 3038
Invirase (Less than 2%) 2776
Klonopin (Infrequent) 2782
Lamictal (Infrequent) 1449
Lexapro Oral Solution (Infrequent) 1193
Lexapro Tablets (Infrequent) 1193
Lipitor Tablets (Less than 2%) 2495
▲ Lotemax Ophthalmic Suspension 0.5% (5% to 15%) ⊙ 249
▲ Lumigan Ophthalmic Solution (3% to 10%) 569
Lunesta Tablets (Infrequent) 3139
Lyrica Capsules (0.1% to 1%) 2524
Maxalt Tablets (Infrequent) 1983
Maxalt-MLT Orally Disintegrating Tablets (Infrequent) 1983
Meridia Capsules 485
Mintezol 2002
Nadolol Tablets (1 to 5 of 1000 patients) 2121
Namenda (Infrequent) 1199
Neurontin Capsules (Infrequent) 2498
Neurontin Oral Solution (Infrequent) 2498
Neurontin Tablets (Infrequent) 2498
Nipent for Injection (Less than 3%) 3216
Norvasc Tablets (Less than or equal to 0.1%) 2529
Pacerone Tablets 3337
Patanol Ophthalmic Solution (Less than 5%) 557
Prevacid Delayed-Release Capsules (Less than 1%) 3268
Prevacid for Delayed-Release Oral Suspension (Less than 1%) 3268
Prevacid NapraPAC (Less than 1%) 3277
Prevacid SoluTab Delayed-Release Orally Disintegrating Tablets (Less than 1%) 3268
PREVPAC (Less than 1%) 3281
Prilosec OTC Tablets (Less than 1%) 2674
Prochieve 4% Gel 1018
Prochieve 8% Gel 1018
Prozac Pulvules and Liquid (Infrequent) 1771
Quixin Ophthalmic Solution (Less than 1%) 3373
▲ Rebif Prefilled Syringe for Injection (1% to 3%) 3163
Relpax Tablets (Rare) 2531
Requip Tablets (2%) 1528
Rescriptor Tablets 2535
▲ Retisert Implant (10 % to 35%) ⊙ 256
Rēv-Eyes Ophthalmic Eyedrops 0.5% (Less frequently) ⊙ 256
Risperdal M-Tab Orally Disintegrating Tablets (Infrequent) 1658
Risperdal (Infrequent) 1658
Sanctura Tablets (1.2%) 1133
Seroquel Tablets (Infrequent) 691
Sonata Capsules (Infrequent) 1686
▲ Soriatane Capsules (10% to 25%) 1028
Symbyax Capsules (Infrequent) 1788
Targretin Capsules 1719
Tenormin I.V. Injection 698
Tenormin Tablets 695
Teveten Tablets (Less than 1%) 1707
Teveten HCT Tablets (Less than 1%) 1710
Timolide Tablets 2056
Timoptic in Ocudose 2061
Timoptic Sterile Ophthalmic Solution 2058
Timoptic-XE Sterile Ophthalmic Gel Forming Solution 2062
Topamax Sprinkle Capsules (Infrequent) 2438
Topamax Tablets (Infrequent) 2438
Toprol-XL Tablets (Rare) 660
Transderm Scōp Transdermal Therapeutic System (Infrequent) 2166
Travatan Ophthalmic Solution (1% to 4%) 559
Trileptal Oral Suspension 2281
Trileptal Tablets 2281
▲ Trisenox Injection (8%) 983
Trusopt Sterile Ophthalmic Solution (Approximately 1% to 5%) 2065
Vaseretic Tablets 2073
Vasotec I.V. Injection (0.5% to 1.0%) 2076
VESIcare Tablets (0.3% to 1.6%) 631
VFEND I.V. (Less than 2%) 2543
VFEND Oral Suspension (Less than 2%) 2543
VFEND Tablets (Less than 2%) 2543
Viagra Tablets (Less than 2%) 2552
Vicoprofen Tablets (Less than 1%) 533
▲ Vigamox Ophthalmic Solution (1% to 6%) 560
Visine For Contacts Rewetting Drops ⊙ 278
▲ Visudyne for Injection (1% to 10%) 2286
Wellbutrin SR Sustained-Release Tablets (Infrequent) 1583
Wellbutrin XL Extended-Release Tablets (Infrequent) 1588
Xalatan Sterile Ophthalmic Solution (1% to 4%) 2654
Zegerid Powder for Oral Solution (Less than 1%) 2972
Zoladex (1% or greater) 709
Zoladex 3-month 712
Zoloft (Rare) 2581
Zomig Nasal Spray (Rare) 718
Zomig Tablets (Infrequent) 714
Zomig-ZMT Tablets (Infrequent) 714
Zyban Sustained-Release Tablets (Infrequent) 1620
▲ Zymar Ophthalmic Solution (1% to 4%) 571
Zyprexa Tablets (Infrequent) 1798
Zyprexa ZYDIS Orally Disintegrating Tablets (Infrequent) 1798
Zyrtec Chewable Tablets (Less than 2%) 2589
Zyrtec (Less than 2%) 2589
Zyrtec-D 12 Hour Extended Release Tablets (Less than 2%) 2591

Xerosis cutis

Abilify Tablets (Frequent) 916
Abilify Tablets (Frequent) 2472
Accutane Capsules 2740
Aceon Tablets (2 mg, 4 mg, 8 mg) (0.3% to 1%) 3191
Aciphex Tablets (Rare) 1081
Advicor Tablets 1694
Aldara Cream, 5% 1814
Altoprev Extended-Release Tablets 1151
AmBisome for Injection (Less common) 615
Amerge Tablets (Rare) 1312
Amnesteem Capsules 2126
AndroGel (Fewer than 1%) 3330
Arava Tablets (2%) 2881
Asacol Delayed-Release Tablets 2688
▲ Avastin IV (7% to 20%) 1229
Avinza Capsules (Less than 5%) 1714
Bactroban Cream (One report) 1356
Bactroban Ointment (Less than 1%) 1358
▲ Benzaclin Topical Gel (3%) 1046
Caduet Tablets (Less than 2%) 2507
Cafcit (2.2%) 1854
Campral Tablets (Infrequent) 1175
▲ Carac Cream, 0.5% (83.4%) 1048
▲ Casodex Tablets (2% to 5%) 670
Celebrex Capsules (0.1% to 1.9%) 3130
Celexa (Infrequent) 1177
Cipro XR Tablets (Less than 1%) 3004
Clinac BPO 7 Gel USP 1137
Clindagel 1207
Clindesse Vaginal Cream (Less than 1%) 3296
▲ Clindets Pledgets (18% to 23%) 3212
Clobevate Gel 3213
Clobex Shampoo 1209
Clobex Lotion (1%) 1208
▲ Clolar for Intravenous Infusion (10%) 1264
Copaxone for Injection (Infrequent) 3292
▲ Copegus Tablets (10%) 2759
Cozaar Tablets (Less than 1%) 1913
Crixivan Capsules 1918
Cutivate Cream (0.8%) 1381
▲ Cutivate Lotion 0.05% (7%) 1383
Cytovene (At least 3 subjects) 2763
Decadron Tablets 1929
▲ Depacon Injection (1% to 5%) 412

▲ Depakene (1% to 5%) 417
▲ Depakote Sprinkle Capsules (1% to 5%) 422
▲ Depakote Tablets (1% to 5%) 427
Depakote ER Tablets (Greater than 1%) 433
Depo-Provera Contraceptive Injection (Less than 1%) 2619
depo-subQ provera 104 Injectable Suspension 2622
Detrol Tablets (1.7%) 2626
▲ Differin Cream (Less than 1% to 38%) 1210
▲ Differin Gel (10% to 40%) 1211
▲ Diprolene Gel 0.05% (4%) 3015
Diprolene Lotion 0.05% (Infrequent) 3016
Diprolene Ointment 0.05% (Infrequent) 3017
Diprolene AF Cream 0.05% (Infrequent) 3014
Diprosone Cream, USP 0.05% 3018
▲ Ditropan XL Extended Release Tablets (2% to less than 5%) 2391
▲ Dovonex Ointment 0.005% (1% to 10%) 3375
▲ Dovonex Scalp Solution 0.005% (1% to 5%) 3375
▲ Doxil Injection (1% to 10%) 3302
▲ Duac Topical Gel (3%) 3214
Effexor Tablets (Infrequent) 3405
Effexor XR Capsules (Infrequent) 3411
Elocon Cream 0.1% (Infrequent) 3019
Elocon Ointment 0.1% (Infrequent) 3021
▲ Eloxatin for Injection (2% to 5%) 2908
Emcyt Capsules (2%) 3137
Enablex Extended-Release Tablets (Greater than or equal to 1%) 2201
Ertaczo Cream, 2% 2383
Erygel Topical Gel (Occasional) 2096
Eskalith 1406
Evoxac Capsules (Less than 1%) 1042
▲ Finacea Gel (1% to 6%) 1644
Follistim AQ Cartridge 2354
Gabitril Tablets (Frequent) 998
Gengraf Capsules (1% to less than 3%) 458
Gleevec Tablets (Less common) 2221
Guanidine Hydrochloride Tablets 3030
Hyzaar 1964
Imitrex Injection 1431
Imitrex Nasal Spray 1435
Imitrex Tablets (Rare) 1440
▲ Infergen (2% to 6%) 1647
▲ Intron A for Injection (Up to 10%) 3038
Invirase (Less than or equal to 2%) 2776
▲ Iressa Tablets (13% to 30%) 684
Kaletra (Less than 2%) 474
Klonopin (Infrequent) 2782
▲ Lamictal (2% to 5%) 1449
Lescol Capsules 2227
Lescol Capsules 2730
Lescol XL Tablets 2227
Lescol XL Tablets 2730
Levaquin in 5% Dextrose Injection (0.1% to 0.9%) 2453
Levaquin (0.1% to 0.9%) 2453
Lexapro Oral Solution (Infrequent) 1193
Lexapro Tablets (Infrequent) 1193
Lipitor Tablets (Less than 2%) 2495
Lithobid Tablets 1670
Loprox Gel 1861
Lotrisone (1.6%) 3054
Lunesta Tablets (Infrequent) 3139
Luxíq Foam 1026
Lyrica Capsules (0.1% to 1%) 2524
▲ Metrogel 1% (0.6% to 17.1%) 1212
Mevacor Tablets 1996
Myleran Tablets (Rare) 1492
Neoral Soft Gelatin Capsules (1% to less than 3%) 2247
Neoral Oral Solution (1% to less than 3%) 2247
Neurontin Capsules (Infrequent) 2498
Neurontin Oral Solution (Infrequent) 2498
Neurontin Tablets (Infrequent) 2498
Niaspan Extended-Release Tablets 1703
▲ Nipent for Injection (3% to 10%) 3216
Nizoral 2% Shampoo (One occurrence in 41 patients) 1838
Norvasc Tablets (Less than or equal to 0.1%) 2529
Norvir (Less than 2%) 499
Olux Foam (One case) 1027
OxyContin Tablets (Less than 1%) 2699
Paxil CR Controlled-Release Tablets (Infrequent) 1509
Paxil (Infrequent) 1501
▲ Pegasys (4%) 2793
▲ PEG-Intron Powder for Injection (11%) 3062
Pentasa Capsules (Less than 1%) 3182
Pepcid Injection (Infrequent) 2017
Pepcid (Infrequent) 2014
Permax Tablets (Infrequent) 3357
Pletal Tablets (Less than 2%) 2478
Pravachol Tablets 943
Prevacid Delayed-Release Capsules (Less than 1%) 3268
Prevacid for Delayed-Release Oral Suspension (Less than 1%) 3268
Prevacid NapraPAC (Less than 1%) 3277
Prevacid SoluTab Delayed-Release Orally Disintegrating Tablets (Less than 1%) 3268
PREVPAC (Less than 1%) 3281
Prilosec OTC Tablets (Less than 1%) 2674
ProAmatine Tablets (Rare) 3183
ProctoFoam-HC 3113
▲ Proleukin for Injection (15%) 1007
ProSom Tablets (Rare) 512
Protonix Tablets (Less than 1%) 3465
Protopic Ointment (Up to 3%) 629
Provigil Tablets (1%) 1002
▲ Rebetol (23% to 24%) 3073
Relpax Tablets 2531
▲ Renova 0.02% Cream (Almost all subjects) 2384
▲ Renova 0.05% Cream (Almost all subjects) 2387
Rescriptor Tablets 2535
Reyataz Capsules (Less than 3%) 948
▲ Ribavirin, USP Capsules (23% to 24%) 3083
Risperdal Consta Long-Acting Injection (Up to 2%) 1664
▲ Risperdal M-Tab Orally Disintegrating Tablets (2% to 4%) 1658
▲ Risperdal (2% to 4%) 1658
▲ Roferon-A Injection (7% to 17%) 2805
Rythmol SR Capsules 2736
Sanctura Tablets (Greater than or equal to 0.5%) 1133
▲ Solage Topical Solution (3.1%) 740
Sonata Capsules (Infrequent) 1686
▲ Soriatane Capsules (25% to 50%) 1028
Sular Tablets (Less than or equal to 1%) 1163
Symbyax Capsules (Infrequent) 1788
▲ Tarceva Tablets (0% to 12%) 1254
▲ Tarceva Tablets (0% to 12%) 2470
▲ Targretin Capsules (9.4% to 10.7%) 1719
Taxotere Injection Concentrate 2947
▲ Temodar Capsules (5%) 3088
Tequin Injection (Less than 0.1%) 964
Tequin Tablets (Less than 0.1%) 964
Thalomid Capsules 979
Topamax Sprinkle Capsules (Infrequent) 2438
Topamax Tablets (Infrequent) 2438
Triaz 1864
Triaz Pads 1864
▲ Tri-Luma Cream (8.08% to 14%) 1213
▲ Trisenox Injection (15%) 983
Uniretic Tablets (Less than 1%) 3114
Varivax (Greater than or equal to 1%) 2070
▲ Vesanoid Capsules (77%) 2823
VFEND I.V. (Less than 2%) 2543
VFEND Oral Suspension (Less than 2%) 2543
VFEND Tablets (Less than 2%) 2543
Vytorin 10/10 Tablets 2084
Vytorin 10/10 Tablets 3092
Vytorin 10/20 Tablets 2084
Vytorin 10/20 Tablets 3092
Vytorin 10/40 Tablets 2084
Vytorin 10/40 Tablets 3092
Vytorin 10/80 Tablets 2084
Vytorin 10/80 Tablets 3092
Wellbutrin Tablets (Infrequent) 1579
Xenical Capsules (2.1%) 2834
▲ Zavesca Capsules (8%) 543
Zegerid Powder for Oral Solution (Less than 1%) 2972
Zocor Tablets 2078
Zoladex (1% or greater) 709
Zoladex 3-month 712
Zoloft (Infrequent) 2581
Zonegran Capsules (Infrequent) 1089
Zovirax Cream (Less than 1%) 853
Zyban Sustained-Release Tablets (2%) 1620
Zyprexa Tablets (Infrequent) 1798
Zyprexa ZYDIS Orally Disintegrating Tablets (Infrequent) 1798
Zyrtec Chewable Tablets (Less than 2%) 2589
Zyrtec (Less than 2%) 2589
Zyrtec-D 12 Hour Extended Release Tablets (Less than 2%) 2591

Xerostomia

Abilify Tablets 916
Abilify Tablets 2472
Accutane Capsules 2740
Aceon Tablets (2 mg, 4 mg, 8 mg) (0.3% to 1%) 3191
Aciphex Tablets 1081
Actiq (1% to 2%) 993
Actonel Tablets (1.4% to 2.5%) 2679
Actonel with Calcium Tablets (1.4% to 2.5%) 2684
Adalat CC Tablets (Less than 1%) 2978
Adderall Tablets 3168
▲ Adderall XR Capsules (35%) 3169
Adenoscan (Less than 1%) 613
Adipex-P 1216
Advair Diskus 100/50 1291
Advair Diskus 250/50 1291
Advair Diskus 500/50 1291
Advicor Tablets 1694
▲ Alacol DM Syrup (Among most frequent) 739
Aldoclor Tablets 1881
Aldoril Tablets 1884
Alferon N Injection (One patient) 1640
Alimta for Injection (Less than 1%) 1722
Allegra-D 12 Hour Extended-Release Tablets (2.8%) 2860
Allegra-D 24 Hour Extended-Release Tablets (2.8%) 2862
Aloxi Injection (Less than 1%) 2099
▲ Alphagan P Ophthalmic Solution (Approximately 5% to 9%) 563
Altace Capsules (Less than 1%) 1673
Altoprev Extended-Release Tablets (0.5% to 1%) 1151
▲ Ambien Tablets (3%) 2867
AmBisome for Injection (Less common) 615
Amnesteem Capsules 2126
Anaprox Tablets (Less than 1%) 2769
Anaprox DS Tablets (Less than 1%) 2769
Antara Capsules 2723
▲ Arava Tablets (1% to 3%) 2881
Aricept Tablets (Infrequent) 1086
Aricept ODT Tablets (Infrequent) 1086
▲ Arimidex Tablets (4% to 6%) 665
Arthrotec Tablets (Rare) 3126
Asacol Delayed-Release Tablets 2688
Astelin Nasal Spray (2.8%) 1876
▲ Atrovent HFA Inhalation Aerosol (1.6% to 4%) 872
▲ Atrovent Inhalation Solution (3.2%) 868
Atrovent Nasal Spray 0.03% (Less than 2%) 869
Atrovent Nasal Spray 0.06% (1.4%) 870
Avalide Tablets 922
Avalide Tablets 2889
▲ Avastin IV (4% to 7%) 1229
Avelox (0.1% to less than 2%) 2984
▲ Avinza Capsules (5% to 10%) 1714
Axert Tablets (1%) 2430
Axid Oral Solution (1.4%) 913
▲ Azmacort Inhalation Aerosol (1% to 3%) 1701
Azopt Ophthalmic Suspension (Less than 1%) 553
Bactroban Nasal (Less than 1%) 1357
Balamine DM 739
▲ Bentyl Capsules (33%) 724
▲ Bentyl Injection (33%) 724
▲ Bentyl Syrup (33%) 724
▲ Bentyl Tablets (33%) 724
▲ Betimol Ophthalmic Solution (More than 5%) ⊙283
▲ Betimol Ophthalmic Solution (More than 5%) 3371
Brevibloc Concentrate (Less than 1%) 766
Brevibloc Injection (Less than 1%) 766
Brevibloc Double Strength Injection (Less than 1%) 766
Brevibloc Premixed Injection (Less than 1%) 766
Brevibloc Double Strength Premixed Injection (Less than 1%) 766
▲ Brimonidine Tartrate Ophthalmic Solution 0.2% (10% to 30%) ⊙245
Caduet Tablets (Greater than 0.1% to less than 2%) 2507
Calcijex Injection 411
▲ Campral Tablets (1% to 3%) 1175
Captopril Tablets (About 0.5% to 2%) 2114
Carafate Suspension (Less than 0.5%) 727
Carafate Tablets (Less than 0.5%) 728
Carbatrol Capsules 3174
Cardizem LA Extended Release Tablets (Less than 2%) 1699
▲ Casodex Tablets (2% to 5%) 670
Cataflam Tablets (Occasionally) 2173
▲ Catapres Tablets (40 of 100 patients) 874
▲ Catapres-TTS (25 of 101 patients) 875
Caverject Impulse Injection (Less than 1%) 2610
Celebrex Capsules (0.1% to 1.9%) 3130
▲ Celexa (20%) 1177
▲ CellCept Capsules (3% to less than 20%) 2751
▲ CellCept Intravenous (3% to less than 20%) 2751
▲ CellCept Oral Suspension (3% to less than 20%) 2751
▲ CellCept Tablets (3% to less than 20%) 2751
Cialis Tablets (Less than 2%) 1806
Cipro I.V. (1% or less) 2998
Cipro I.V. Pharmacy Bulk Package (1% or less) 3509
Cipro XR Tablets (Less than 1%) 3004
▲ Clarinex Tablets (3%) 3009
▲ Clarinex Reditabs Tablets (3%) 3009
▲ Clarinex-D 24-Hour Extended-Release Tablets (8%) 3012
Clinoril Tablets (Less than 1%) 1899
▲ Clorpres Tablets (40%) 2139
▲ Clozapine Tablets (More than 5% to 6%) 2141
▲ Clozaril Tablets (More than 5% to 6%) 2174
Cogentin Injection 1903
Colazal Capsules (1%) 2845
Combivent Inhalation Aerosol (Less than 2%) 878
Combunox Tablets (Less than 1%) 1183
▲ Comtan Tablets (3%) 2186
Copaxone for Injection (At least 2%) 3292
▲ Copegus Tablets (4%) 2759
Coreg Tablets (Greater than 0.1% to 1%) 1376
Cosopt Sterile Ophthalmic Solution (Less than 1%) 1910
Covera-HS Tablets (Less than 2%) 3135
Cozaar Tablets (Less than 1%) 1913
▲ Cymbalta Delayed-Release Capsules (5% to 20%) 1729
Cytovene (At least 3 subjects) 2763
Dalmane Capsules (Rare) 3343
Demser Capsules (Infrequent) 1933
Depacon Injection (1% or more) 412
Depakene (1% or more) 417
Depakote Sprinkle Capsules 422
▲ Depakote Tablets (1% to 5%) 427
▲ Depakote ER Tablets (1% to 5%) 433
Desoxyn Tablets, USP 2482
▲ Detrol Tablets (39.5%) 2626
▲ Detrol LA Capsules (23.4%) 2629
Dexedrine 1386
DextroStat Tablets 3177
Dilaudid 439
Dilaudid Oral Liquid 443
Dilaudid Non-Sterile Powder 439
Dilaudid Rectal Suppositories 439
Dilaudid Tablets 439
Dilaudid Tablets - 8 mg 443
Dilaudid-HP (Less frequent) 441
Diovan HCT Tablets (Greater than 0.2%) 2195
Diovan Tablets 2191
Diprivan Injectable Emulsion (Less than 1%) 676
▲ Ditropan XL Extended Release Tablets (29% to 61%) 2391
Diuril Sodium Intravenous 1934
▲ Dostinex Tablets (2% to less than 10%) 2631
▲ Doxil Injection (1% to 10%) 3302
▲ Duragesic Transdermal System (10% or more) 2448
Dyazide Capsules 1389
DynaCirc CR Tablets (0.5% to 1%) 2726
Dyrenium Capsules (Rare) 3390
EC-Naprosyn Delayed-Release Tablets (Less than 1%) 2769
▲ Effexor Tablets (2% to 22%) 3405
▲ Effexor XR Capsules (5% to 17%) 3411
▲ Eldepryl Capsules (3 of 49 patients) 3209
Elocon Lotion 0.1% (1 in 65 patients) 3020
▲ Eloxatin for Injection (2% to 5%) 2908
▲ Enablex Extended-Release Tablets (18.7% to 35.3%) 2201
Enbrel for Injection 580
▲ Equetro Extended-Release Capsules (8%) 3178
Eskalith 1406
▲ Evoxac Capsules (1% to 3%) 1042
Exelon Capsules (Infrequent) 2204
Factive Tablets (0.1% to 1%) 2464

▲ FazaClo Orally Disintegrating Tablets (Greater than 5% to 6%).... 547
Ferrlecit Injection (Two or more patients)........ 3379
▲ Flexeril Tablets (7% to 32%) 1832
Floxin Otic Singles (0.5%)........ 1045
Floxin Otic Solution (0.5%)........ 1043
Flumadine (1.5%)........ 1186
▲ Focalin XR Capsules (7% to 20%) 2217
Foradil Aerolizer (1.2%)........ 3024
Fortical Nasal Spray (Less than 1%)........ 3336
▲ Frova Tablets (3%) 1101
Furosemide Tablets 2117
Fuzeon Injection (2.1%)........ 2772
Gabitril Tablets (1% or more)........ 998
Gengraf Capsules (1% to less than 3%)........ 458
▲ Geodon (4% to 5%) 2514
Guanidine Hydrochloride Tablets...... 3030
Hectorol Capsules 909
Hectorol Injection........ 911
Hyperstat I.V. Injection........ 3031
Hytrin Capsules (At least 1%)........ 469
Hyzaar........ 1964
▲ Imdur Tablets (Less than or equal to 5%)........ 3032
Imitrex Injection 1431
Imitrex Nasal Spray (Infrequent)....... 1435
Imitrex Tablets........ 1440
Imodium Capsules........ 1834
▲ Infergen (4% to 6%) 1647
▲ Intron A for Injection (Up to 28%) 3038
Inversine Tablets........ 3286
Invirase (Less than 2%)........ 2776
▲ I.V. Busulfex (26%) 1125
Kadian Capsules (Less than 3%)....... 572
Kaletra (Less than 2%)........ 474
Ketek Tablets (Greater than or equal to 0.2% to less than 2%)...... 2920
Klonopin........ 2782
▲ Lamictal (2% to 6%) 1449
Levaquin in 5% Dextrose Injection (0.2%)........ 2453
Levaquin (0.2%)........ 2453
Levitra Tablets (Less than 2%)........ 3048
▲ Lexapro Oral Solution (4% to 9%) 1193
▲ Lexapro Tablets (4% to 9%) 1193
Lipitor Tablets (Less than 2%)........ 2495
Lithobid Tablets........ 1670
Lofibra Capsules 1217
Lotensin HCT Tablets (0.3% to 1%).. 2235
Lotrel Capsules 2238
▲ Lunesta Tablets (3% to 7%) 3139
Lupron Depot 3.75 mg (Less than 5%)........ 3257
Lupron Depot–3 Month 11.25 mg (Less than 5%)........ 3262
▲ Lyrica Capsules (3% to 15%) 2524
Matulane Capsules 3188
Maxair Autohaler (1.3%)........ 1820
▲ Maxalt Tablets (3%) 1983
▲ Maxalt-MLT Orally Disintegrating Tablets (3%)........ 1983
Maxzide........ 2150
▲ Megace ES Oral Suspension (1% to 3%)........ 2492
▲ Meridia Capsules (17.2%) 485
MetroGel-Vaginal Gel (Less than 1%)........ 1822
Mevacor Tablets (0.5% to 1.0%)....... 1996
Miacalcin Nasal Spray (Less than 1%)........ 2242
Micardis Tablets (More than 0.3%).... 884
Micardis HCT Tablets........ 886
Midamor Tablets (Less than or equal to 1%)........ 2000
Migranal Nasal Spray (1%)........ 3350
Mintezol........ 2002
▲ Mirapex Tablets (Greater than or equal to 1% to 7%)........ 889
Moban Tablets (Occasional)........ 1108
Mobic Oral Suspension (Less than 2%)........ 893
Mobic Tablets (Less than 2%)........ 893
Moduretic Tablets........ 2003
MS Contin Tablets (Less frequent).... 2703
Nadolol Tablets (1 to 5 of 1000 patients)........ 2121
Nalfon Capsules (Less than 1%)....... 2504
Naprosyn Suspension (Less than 1%)........ 2769
Naprosyn Tablets (Less than 1%)..... 2769
Nasacort HFA Inhalation Aerosol...... 2939
Neoral Soft Gelatin Capsules (1% to less than 3%)........ 2247
Neoral Oral Solution (1% to less than 3%)........ 2247
Neurontin Capsules (1.7% to 4.8%)........ 2498
Neurontin Oral Solution (1.7% to 4.8%)........ 2498
Neurontin Tablets (1.7% to 4.8%)..... 2498
Nexium Delayed-Release Capsules (Greater than or equal to 1%)........ 645
Nexium I.V. (Greater than or equal to 1%)........ 649
Niaspan Extended-Release Tablets... 1703
Nicotrol NS (Less than 1%)........ 2596
▲ Niravam Orally Disintegrating Tablets (14.7%)........ 3106
Norflex Injection........ 1824
Noritate Cream, 1% (Uncommon)..... 1051
Noroxin Tablets (0.3 to 1.0%)........ 2009
Norvasc Tablets (More than 0.1% to 1%)........ 2529
Norvir (Less than 2%)........ 499
▲ Nubain Injection (4%) 1111
Numorphan........ 1112
Omacor Capsules........ 2735
Omnicef Capsules (0.3%)........ 506
▲ Orap Tablets (5 of 20 patients) 1220
▲ OxyContin Tablets (6%) 2699
▲ Oxytrol Transdermal System (4.1% to 9.6%)........ 3383
Parcopa Orally Disintegrating Tablets 3111
Parnate Tablets 1499
▲ Paxil CR Controlled-Release Tablets (1.0% to 20.6%)........ 1509
▲ Paxil (1.0% to 20.6%) 1501
▲ Pegasys (6%) 2793
▲ PEG-Intron Powder for Injection (6%)........ 3062
Pepcid Injection (Infrequent)........ 2017
Pepcid (Infrequent)........ 2014
▲ Permax Tablets (3.7%; frequent) 3357
Phenergan........ 3438
Plendil Extended-Release Tablets (0.5% to 1.5%)........ 651
Prevacid Delayed-Release Capsules (Less than 1%)........ 3268
Prevacid for Delayed-Release Oral Suspension (Less than 1%)........ 3268
Prevacid NapraPAC (Less than 1%).. 3277
Prevacid SoluTab Delayed-Release Orally Disintegrating Tablets (Less than 1%)........ 3268
PREVPAC (Less than 1% to 3%)........ 3281
Prilosec OTC Tablets (Less than 1%)........ 2674
Prinivil Tablets (0.3% to 1.0%)........ 2029
Prinzide Tablets (0.3% to 1%)........ 2033
ProAmatine Tablets (Less frequent)........ 3183
Prochieve 4% Gel........ 1018
Prochieve 8% Gel........ 1018
Prometrium Capsules (100 mg, 200 mg) (Less than 5%)........ 3205
ProSom Tablets (Frequent)........ 512
Protonix I.V. (Less than 1%)........ 3468
Protonix Tablets (Less than 1%)........ 3465
Proventil HFA Inhalation Aerosol (Less than 3%)........ 3071
▲ Provigil Tablets (4%) 1002
▲ Prozac Pulvules and Liquid (4% to 12%)........ 1771
Razadyne ER Extended-Release Capsules (Infrequent)........ 2434
Razadyne (Infrequent)........ 2434
▲ Rebetol (8% to 12%) 3073
▲ Rebif Prefilled Syringe for Injection (1% to 5%)........ 3163
Relafen Tablets (1% to 3%)........ 1523
▲ Relpax Tablets (2% to 4%) 2531
ReoPro Vials (0.1%)........ 1779
▲ Requip Tablets (3% to 5%) 1528
Rescriptor Tablets 2535
▲ Ribavirin, USP Capsules (8% to 12%)........ 3083
▲ Rilutek Tablets (2.0% to 3.0%) 2945
▲ Risperdal Consta Long-Acting Injection (Up to 7%)........ 1664
▲ Risperdal M-Tab Orally Disintegrating Tablets (3%)........ 1658
▲ Risperdal (3%) 1658
▲ Rythmol SR Capsules (1% to 4%) 2736
▲ Sanctura Tablets (20.1%) 1133
Sandostatin LAR Depot (1% to 4%)... 2264
Sedapap Tablets 50 mg/650 mg (Infrequent)........ 2098
▲ Seroquel Tablets (9%) 691
Sonata Capsules (Frequent)........ 1686
Spectracef Tablets (0.1% to 1%)...... 2706
▲ Spiriva HandiHaler (12% to 16%) 899
▲ Stalevo Tablets (3%) 2270
▲ Strattera Capsules (21%) 1784
Striant Mucoadhesive........ 1022
Sular Tablets (Less than or equal to 1%)........ 1163
Surmontil Capsules (Rare)........ 2347
▲ Symbyax Capsules (11% to 16%) 1788
Symmetrel (1% to 5%)........ 1115
Tambocor Tablets (Less than 1%)...... 1824
Targretin Capsules........ 1719
Tarka Tablets (0.3% or more)........ 519
▲ Tasmar Tablets (5% to 6%) 3360
Tegretol/Tegretol-XR........ 2278
Tenormin I.V. Injection........ 698
Tenormin Tablets 695
Teveten Tablets (Less than 1%)........ 1707
Teveten HCT Tablets (Less than 1%)........ 1710
▲ Thalomid Capsules (8.3% to 9.4%)........ 979
Thioridazine Hydrochloride Tablets... 2122
Thiothixene Capsules........ 2124
Tiazac Capsules (Less than 2%)........ 1204
Timoptic in Ocudose (Less frequent)........ 2061
Timoptic Sterile Ophthalmic Solution (Less frequent)........ 2058
Timoptic-XE Sterile Ophthalmic Gel Forming Solution 2062
Tindamax 2670
▲ Topamax Sprinkle Capsules (2% to 5%)........ 2438
▲ Topamax Tablets (2% to 5%) 2438
Toprol-XL Tablets (About 1 of 100 patients)........ 660
▲ Transderm Scōp Transdermal Therapeutic System (About two-thirds)........ 2166
Tranxene (Less common)........ 2488
Tricor Tablets........ 523
▲ Trileptal Oral Suspension (Up to 3%)........ 2281
▲ Trileptal Tablets (Up to 3%) 2281
Tri-Luma Cream (1%)........ 1213
▲ Trisenox Injection (8%) 983
Trusopt Sterile Ophthalmic Solution........ 2065
Tygacil for Injection (0% to less than 2%)........ 3489
Ultane Liquid for Inhalation (Less than 1%)........ 526
Ultracet Tablets (2%)........ 2462
Uniretic Tablets (Less than 1%)........ 3114
Univasc Tablets (Less than 1%)........ 3118
Vantin Tablets and Oral Suspension (Less than 1%)........ 2650
Vaseretic Tablets (0.5% to 2.0%)...... 2073
Vasotec I.V. Injection (0.5% to 1.0%)........ 2076
Verelan PM Capsules (2% or less).... 3120
▲ VESIcare Tablets (10.9% to 27.6%)........ 631
VFEND I.V. (Less than 2%)........ 2543
VFEND Oral Suspension (Less than 2%)........ 2543
VFEND Tablets (Less than 2%)........ 2543
Viadur Implant (Less than 2%)........ 782
Viagra Tablets (Less than 2%)........ 2552
▲ Vicoprofen Tablets (3% to 9%) 533
Vivactil Tablets........ 2350
Voltaren Tablets (Occasionally)........ 2298
Voltaren-XR Tablets (Occasionally).... 2301
▲ Wellbutrin Tablets (27.6%) 1579
▲ Wellbutrin SR Sustained-Release Tablets (5% to 24%)........ 1583
▲ Wellbutrin XL Extended-Release Tablets (5% to 24%)........ 1588
▲ Xanax XR Tablets (10.2%) 2655
▲ Xeloda Tablets (Less than 1% to 6%)........ 2825
Xopenex HFA Inhalation Aerosol....... 3151
Xopenex Inhalation Solution........ 3143
Xopenex Inhalation Solution Concentrate........ 3147
Zaditor Ophthalmic Solution (Less than 5%)........ 2302
Zegerid Powder for Oral Solution (Less than 1%)........ 2972
▲ Zemplar Capsules (3%) 535
▲ Zemplar Injection (3%) 538
Zestoretic Tablets (0.3% to 1%)........ 701
Zestril Tablets (0.3% to 1.0%)........ 704
Zofran (1% to 2%)........ 1613
Zofran ODT Orally Disintegrating Tablets (1% to 2%)........ 1613
Zoladex (1% or greater)........ 709
Zoladex 3-month........ 712
▲ Zoloft (6% to 16%) 2581
▲ Zomig Nasal Spray (1% to 3%) 718
▲ Zomig Tablets (3% to 5%) 714
▲ Zomig-ZMT Tablets (3% to 5%) 714
Zonegran Capsules (2%)........ 1089
▲ Zyban Sustained-Release Tablets (10% to 11%)........ 1620
▲ Zyprexa Tablets (3% to 22%) 1798
▲ Zyprexa ZYDIS Orally Disintegrating Tablets (3% to 22%)........ 1798
▲ Zyrtec Chewable Tablets (Less than 2% to 5%)........ 2589
▲ Zyrtec (Less than 2% to 5%) 2589
▲ Zyrtec-D 12 Hour Extended Release Tablets (3.6% to 5%)........ 2591

Y

Yawning

Ambien Tablets (Rare)........ 2867
▲ Apokyn Injection (40%) 2132
Celexa (2%)........ 1177
▲ Effexor Tablets (3% to 8%) 3405
▲ Effexor XR Capsules (3% to 5%) 3411
Evoxac Capsules........ 1042
Imitrex Injection (Rare)........ 1431
Imitrex Nasal Spray........ 1435
Imitrex Tablets........ 1440
Klonopin (Infrequent)........ 2782
Lamictal (Infrequent)........ 1449
Lexapro Oral Solution (2%)........ 1193
Lexapro Tablets (2%)........ 1193
Lyrica Capsules (Rare)........ 2524
Maxalt Tablets (Infrequent)........ 1983
Maxalt-MLT Orally Disintegrating Tablets (Infrequent)........ 1983
Meridia Capsules........ 485
Migranal Nasal Spray (Rare)........ 3350
Narcan Injection........ 1109
▲ Paxil CR Controlled-Release Tablets (4%)........ 1509
▲ Paxil (4%) 1501
▲ Prozac Pulvules and Liquid (3%) 1771
Relpax Tablets (Infrequent)........ 2531
▲ Requip Tablets (3%) 1528
Rilutek Tablets (Infrequent)........ 2945
Risperdal M-Tab Orally Disintegrating Tablets (Rare)........ 1658
Risperdal (Rare)........ 1658
Symbyax Capsules (Infrequent)........ 1788
Zoloft (Frequent)........ 2581
Zomig Nasal Spray (Rare)........ 718
Zomig Tablets (Infrequent)........ 714
Zomig-ZMT Tablets (Infrequent)........ 714

Z

Zinc deficiency

Calcium Disodium Versenate Injection 1819

Zollinger-Ellison syndrome

Zegerid Powder for Oral Solution (Less than 1%)........ 2972

SECTION 4

INDICATIONS INDEX

This section lists in alphabetical order every indication cited in *PDR*® and its companion volumes, with cross-references to each product entry in which the indication is found. For easy comparison, each listing includes the product's brand name, generic ingredients, and manufacturer. Page numbers refer to the 2006 editions of *PDR*® and *PDR for Ophthalmic Medicines*™ and the 2005 edition of *PDR for Nonprescription Drugs and Dietary Supplements*™, which is published later each year. A key to the symbols denoting the companion volumes appears in the bottom margin.

Because *PDR*® publishes only official product labeling, only approved indications are cited here. No unapproved uses are listed.

This index is intended to assist you in identifying the extent and nature of your prescribing alternatives as quickly and easily as possible. However, it is by its nature only an extract of the official labeling as it appears in *PDR*®. For more definitive information, always consult the underlying *PDR*® text.

A

A. baumanii infections
Zosyn (Piperacillin Sodium, Tazobactam Sodium) Wyeth 3492

Abrasions, pain associated with
(*see under* Pain, topical relief of)

Abrasions, skin
(*see also under* Infections, skin, bacterial, minor)
Biafine Topical Emulsion (Propylparaben, Methylparaben, Propylene Glycol, Stearic Acid, Triethanolamine) OrthoNeutrogena 2382

Abscess, cutaneous
(*see also under* Infections, skin and skin structure)
Levaquin in 5% Dextrose Injection (Levofloxacin) Ortho-McNeil 2453
Levaquin (Levofloxacin) Ortho-McNeil 2453
Zosyn (Piperacillin Sodium, Tazobactam Sodium) Wyeth 3492

Abscess, hepatic
(*see under* Infections, intra-abdominal)

Abscess, intra-abdominal
(*see also under* Infections, intra-abdominal)
Cancidas for Injection (Caspofungin acetate) Merck 1894
Cleocin Vaginal Ovules (Clindamycin Hydrochloride) Pharmacia & Upjohn 2613
Mefoxin for Injection (Cefoxitin Sodium) Merck 1987
Mefoxin Premixed Intravenous Solution (Cefoxitin Sodium) Merck 1990

Abscess, lung
(*see also under* Infections, lower respiratory tract)
Cleocin Vaginal Ovules (Clindamycin Hydrochloride) Pharmacia & Upjohn 2613
Mefoxin for Injection (Cefoxitin Sodium) Merck 1987
Mefoxin Premixed Intravenous Solution (Cefoxitin Sodium) Merck 1990

Abscess, tubo-ovarian
(*see under* Infections, gynecologic)

Aches
(*see under* Pain, general)

Aches, muscular
(*see under* Pain, muscular, temporary relief of)

Aches due to common cold
(*see under* Pain associated with upper respiratory infection)

Acid indigestion
(*see under* Hyperacidity, gastric, symptomatic relief of)

Acinetobacter calcoaceticus infections
Primaxin I.M. (Cilastatin Sodium, Imipenem) Merck 2022
Rocephin Injectable Vials, ADD-Vantage, Galaxy, Bulk (Ceftriaxone Sodium) Roche Laboratories 2801

Acinetobacter calcoaceticus infections, ocular
Quixin Ophthalmic Solution (Levofloxacin) Vistakon 3373
TobraDex Ophthalmic Ointment (Dexamethasone, Tobramycin) Alcon 558
TobraDex Ophthalmic Suspension (Dexamethasone, Tobramycin) Alcon 558
Zylet Ophthalmic Suspension (Loteprednol Etabonate, Tobramycin) Bausch & Lomb 3508

Acinetobacter calcoaceticus skin and skin structure infections
Primaxin I.M. (Cilastatin Sodium, Imipenem) Merck 2022

Acinetobacter iwoffi
Vigamox Ophthalmic Solution (Moxifloxacin Hydrochloride) Alcon 560

Acinetobacter species infections
Dynacin Tablets (Minocycline Hydrochloride) Medicis 1859
Primaxin I.M. (Cilastatin Sodium, Imipenem) Merck 2022
Primaxin I.V. (Cilastatin Sodium, Imipenem) Merck 2024

Acinetobacter species skin and skin structure infections
Primaxin I.M. (Cilastatin Sodium, Imipenem) Merck 2022
Primaxin I.V. (Cilastatin Sodium, Imipenem) Merck 2024
Rocephin Injectable Vials, ADD-Vantage, Galaxy, Bulk (Ceftriaxone Sodium) Roche Laboratories 2801

Acne, cystic, severe recalcitrant
Accutane Capsules (Isotretinoin) Roche Laboratories 2740
Amnesteem Capsules (Isotretinoin) Mylan Bertek 2126

Acne rosacea
Avar Cleanser (Sodium Sulfacetamide, Sulfur) Sirius 3189
Avar Gel (Sodium Sulfacetamide, Sulfur) Sirius 3189
Avar Green (Sodium Sulfacetamide, Sulfur) Sirius 3189
Avar-e Emollient Cream (Sodium Sulfacetamide, Sulfur) Sirius 3189
Avar-e Green Cream (Sodium Sulfacetamide, Sulfur) Sirius 3189
Nicomide Tablets (Folic Acid, Nicotinamide, Zinc Oxide) Sirius 3190
Plexion (Sodium Sulfacetamide, Sulfur) Medicis 1863
Rosac Cream with Sunscreens (Sodium Sulfacetamide, Sulfur) Stiefel 3216

Acne rosacea, ocular
Zylet Ophthalmic Suspension (Loteprednol Etabonate, Tobramycin) Bausch & Lomb 3508

Acne vulgaris
Avar Cleanser (Sodium Sulfacetamide, Sulfur) Sirius 3189
Avar Gel (Sodium Sulfacetamide, Sulfur) Sirius 3189
Avar Green (Sodium Sulfacetamide, Sulfur) Sirius 3189
Avar-e Emollient Cream (Sodium Sulfacetamide, Sulfur) Sirius 3189
Avar-e Green Cream (Sodium Sulfacetamide, Sulfur) Sirius 3189
Avita Cream (Tretinoin) Mylan Bertek 2136
Avita Gel (Tretinoin) Mylan Bertek 2138
Benzaclin Topical Gel (Benzoyl Peroxide, Clindamycin Phosphate) Dermik 1046
Brevoxyl-4 Creamy Wash (Benzoyl Peroxide) Stiefel 3212

Brevoxyl-4 Gel (Benzoyl Peroxide) Stiefel 3211
Brevoxyl-8 Creamy Wash (Benzoyl Peroxide) Stiefel 3212
Brevoxyl-8 Gel (Benzoyl Peroxide) Stiefel 3211
Clinac BPO 7 Gel USP (Benzoyl Peroxide) Ferndale 1137
Clindagel (Clindamycin Phosphate) Galderma 1207
Clindets Pledgets (Clindamycin Phosphate) Stiefel 3212
Differin Cream (Adapalene) Galderma 1210
Differin Gel (Adapalene) Galderma 1211
Duac Topical Gel (Benzoyl Peroxide, Clindamycin) Stiefel 3214
Erygel Topical Gel (Erythromycin) Merz 2096
Evoclin Foam, 1% (Clindamycin Phosphate) Connetics 1025
Klaron Lotion 10% (Sulfacetamide Sodium) Dermik 1050
Nicomide Tablets (Folic Acid, Nicotinamide, Zinc Oxide) Sirius 3190
Ortho Tri-Cyclen Tablets (Ethinyl Estradiol, Norgestimate) Ortho Women's Health & Urology 2414
Plexion (Sodium Sulfacetamide, Sulfur) Medicis 1863
Retin-A Micro 0.1%/0.04% (Tretinoin) OrthoNeutrogena 2388
Rosac Cream with Sunscreens (Sodium Sulfacetamide, Sulfur) Stiefel 3216
Triaz (Benzoyl Peroxide) Medicis 1864
Triaz Pads (Benzoyl Peroxide) Medicis 1864

Acneiform eruptions, severe, adjunct in
Dynacin Tablets (Minocycline Hydrochloride) Medicis 1859

Acquired immunodeficiency syndrome
(*see under* Infections, human immunodeficiency virus)

Acromegaly
Sandostatin Injection (Octreotide Acetate) Novartis 2263
Sandostatin LAR Depot (Octreotide Acetate) Novartis 2264
Somavert Injection (Pegvisomant) Pharmacia & Upjohn 2648

Actinomyces species infection
(*see under* Actinomycosis)

Actinomycosis
Dynacin Tablets (Minocycline Hydrochloride) Medicis 1859

Addison's disease
(*see under* Adrenocortical insufficiency)

Adenomatous polyposis, familial
Celebrex Capsules (Celecoxib) Searle 3130

Adenosine deaminase, enzyme replacement therapy for
Gamunex Immune Globulin I.V., 10% (Immune Globulin Intravenous (Human)) Talecris 3232

ADHD
(*see under* Attention Deficit Hyperactivity Disorder)

Adrenal hyperplasia, congenital
Decadron Phosphate Injection (Dexamethasone Sodium Phosphate) Merck 1931
Decadron Tablets (Dexamethasone) Merck 1929
Depo-Medrol Injectable Suspension (Methylprednisolone Acetate) Pharmacia & Upjohn 2615
Depo-Medrol Single-Dose Vial (Methylprednisolone Acetate) Pharmacia & Upjohn 2617
Hydrocortone Tablets (Hydrocortisone) Merck 1963
Pediapred Oral Solution (Prednisolone Sodium Phosphate) UCB 3319

Adrenocortical hyperfunction, diagnostic testing of
Decadron Phosphate Injection (Dexamethasone Sodium Phosphate) Merck 1931
Decadron Tablets (Dexamethasone) Merck 1929

Adrenocortical insufficiency
Decadron Phosphate Injection (Dexamethasone Sodium Phosphate) Merck 1931
Decadron Tablets (Dexamethasone) Merck 1929
Depo-Medrol Injectable Suspension (Methylprednisolone Acetate) Pharmacia & Upjohn 2615
Depo-Medrol Single-Dose Vial (Methylprednisolone Acetate) Pharmacia & Upjohn 2617
Hydrocortone Tablets (Hydrocortisone) Merck 1963
Pediapred Oral Solution (Prednisolone Sodium Phosphate) UCB 3319

Aerobacter aerogenes infections
(*see under* Enterobacter aerogenes infections)

Agammaglobulinemias, congenital
Gammagard Liquid (Immune Globulin Intravenous (Human)) Baxter Healthcare 751
Gammagard S/D (Immune Globulin Intravenous (Human)) Baxter Healthcare 754
Gamunex Immune Globulin I.V., 10% (Immune Globulin Intravenous (Human)) Talecris 3232
Iveegam EN (Immune Globulin Intravenous (Human)) Baxter Healthcare 759

AIDS
(*see under* Infections, human immunodeficiency virus)

AIDS related complex
(*see under* Infections, acquired immunodeficiency syndrome-related complex)

Airway obstruction disorders
(*see under* Bronchial asthma; Emphysema)

Albinism
(*see under* Hypopigmentation, skin)

Alcohol withdrawal, acute, symptomatic relief of
Librium Capsules (Chlordiazepoxide Hydrochloride) Valeant 3349
Tranxene (Clorazepate Dipotassium) Ovation 2488
Valium Tablets (Diazepam) Roche Laboratories 2822

Alcoholism, chronic, an aid in the management of
Antabuse Tablets (Disulfiram) Odyssey 2343
Campral Tablets (Acamprosate Calcium) Forest 1175

Allergic reactions, drug-induced
(*see under* Hypersensitivity reactions, drug-induced)

Allergic reactions, general
Decadron Phosphate Injection (Dexamethasone Sodium Phosphate) Merck 1931
Decadron Tablets (Dexamethasone) Merck 1929
Depo-Medrol Injectable Suspension (Methylprednisolone Acetate) Pharmacia & Upjohn 2615
EpiPen (Epinephrine) Dey 1061
Hydrocortone Tablets (Hydrocortisone) Merck 1963
Pediapred Oral Solution (Prednisolone Sodium Phosphate) UCB 3319

Allergic reactions associated with blood or plasma
Phenergan (Promethazine Hydrochloride) Wyeth 3438

Allergic rhinitis
(*see under* Rhinitis, allergic)

Allergies, respiratory
Advil Allergy Sinus Caplets (Chlorpheniramine Maleate, Ibuprofen, Pseudoephedrine Hydrochloride) Wyeth .... ■737
Advil Multi-Symptom Cold Caplets (Chlorpheniramine Maleate, Ibuprofen, Pseudoephedrine Hydrochloride) Wyeth .... ■738
Alavert Allergy & Sinus D-12 Hour Tablets (Loratadine, Pseudoephedrine Sulfate) Wyeth .... ■743
Children's Benadryl Allergy Fastmelt Tablets (Diphenhydramine Citrate) Pfizer Consumer Healthcare .... ■696
PediaCare Decongestant Infants' Drops (Pseudoephedrine Hydrochloride) Pfizer Consumer Healthcare .... ■705
PediaCare Long-Acting Cough Plus Cold Liquid (Dextromethorphan Hydrobromide, Pseudoephedrine Hydrochloride) Pfizer Consumer Healthcare .... ■704
PediaCare NightRest Cough & Cold Liquid (Chlorpheniramine Maleate, Dextromethorphan Hydrobromide, Pseudoephedrine Hydrochloride) Pfizer Consumer Healthcare .... ■704
Triaminic Allerchews (Loratadine) Novartis Consumer .... ■684
Zicam Allergy Relief Nasal Pump (Histanium Hydrochloricum, Luffa operculata, Galphimia Glauca, Sulfur) Matrixx .... ■665
Zicam Extreme Congestion Relief Nasal Pump (Oxymetazoline Hydrochloride) Matrixx .... ■666
Zicam Sinus Relief Nasal Pump (Oxymetazoline Hydrochloride) Matrixx .... ■666

Alopecia, androgenetic
Propecia Tablets (Finasteride) Merck 2036

Alopecia areata
Decadron Phosphate Injection (Dexamethasone Sodium Phosphate) Merck 1931
Depo-Medrol Single-Dose Vial (Methylprednisolone Acetate) Pharmacia & Upjohn 2617

Alpha1-Proteinase inhibitor deficiency
Zemaira (Alpha$_1$-Proteinase Inhibitor (Human)) ZLB Behring 3506

Alzheimer's disease
(*see under* Dementia, Alzheimer's type)

Amebiasis, acute intestinal
E.E.S. (Erythromycin Ethylsuccinate) Abbott 449
EryPed (Erythromycin Ethylsuccinate) Abbott 445
Ery-Tab Tablets (Erythromycin) Abbott 447
Erythrocin Stearate Filmtab Tablets (Erythromycin Stearate) Abbott 452
Erythromycin Base Filmtab Tablets (Erythromycin) Abbott 454
Erythromycin Delayed-Release Capsules, USP (Erythromycin) Abbott 456
PCE Dispertab Tablets (Erythromycin) Abbott 510

Amebiasis, acute intestinal, adjunct in
Dynacin Tablets (Minocycline Hydrochloride) Medicis 1859

Amebiasis, intestinal
Tindamax (Tinidazole) Presutti 2670

Amenorrhea, secondary
Aygestin Tablets (Norethindrone Acetate) Duramed 1062
Prochieve 4% Gel (Progesterone) Columbia 1018
Prochieve 8% Gel (Progesterone) Columbia 1018
Prometrium Capsules (100 mg, 200 mg) (Progesterone) Solvay 3205

Amyotrophic lateral sclerosis
Rilutek Tablets (Riluzole) Sanofi-Aventis 2945

Analgesia
(*see under* Pain, general)

Anaphylactic reactions, adjunctive therapy in
Phenergan (Promethazine Hydrochloride) Wyeth 3438

Anaphylactoid reactions
EpiPen (Epinephrine) Dey 1061

Ancylostoma duodenale infections
Mintezol (Thiabendazole) Merck 2002
Vermox Chewable Tablets (Mebendazole) McNeil Consumer 1853

Androgen, absence or deficiency of
AndroGel (Testosterone) Unimed 3330
Striant Mucoadhesive (Testosterone) Columbia 1022
Testim 1% Gel (Testosterone) Auxilium 722

Anemia, aplastic, acquired
Anadrol-50 (Oxymetholone) Unimed 3329

Anemia, AZT-treated HIV-infected patients, treatment of
Epogen for Injection (Epoetin Alfa) Amgen 586
Procrit for Injection (Epoetin Alfa) Ortho Biotech 2374

Anemia, chemotherapy-induced in cancer patients
Aranesp for Injection (Darbepoetin alfa) Amgen 576
Epogen for Injection (Epoetin Alfa) Amgen 586
Procrit for Injection (Epoetin Alfa) Ortho Biotech 2374

Anemia, hemolytic, acquired
Decadron Phosphate Injection (Dexamethasone Sodium Phosphate) Merck 1931
Decadron Tablets (Dexamethasone) Merck 1929
Depo-Medrol Injectable Suspension (Methylprednisolone Acetate) Pharmacia & Upjohn 2615
Depo-Medrol Single-Dose Vial (Methylprednisolone Acetate) Pharmacia & Upjohn 2617
Hydrocortone Tablets (Hydrocortisone) Merck 1963
Pediapred Oral Solution (Prednisolone Sodium Phosphate) UCB 3319

Anemia, hypoplastic
Anadrol-50 Tablets (Oxymetholone) Unimed 3329

Anemia, hypoplastic, congenital
Decadron Phosphate Injection (Dexamethasone Sodium Phosphate) Merck 1931
Decadron Tablets (Dexamethasone) Merck 1929
Depo-Medrol Injectable Suspension (Methylprednisolone Acetate) Pharmacia & Upjohn 2615
Depo-Medrol Single-Dose Vial (Methylprednisolone Acetate) Pharmacia & Upjohn 2617
Hydrocortone Tablets (Hydrocortisone) Merck 1963
Pediapred Oral Solution (Prednisolone Sodium Phosphate) UCB 3319

Anemia, iron deficiency
Chromagen Soft Gelatin Capsules Ther-Rx 3296
Chromagen Forte Soft Gelatin Capsules (Ferrous Fumarate, Folic Acid, Iron, Vitamin B_{12}, Vitamin C) Ther-Rx 3296
Feosol Caplets (Iron Carbonyl) GlaxoSmithKline Consumer 1629
Feosol Tablets (Ferrous Sulfate) GlaxoSmithKline Consumer 1629
Ferrlecit Injection (Sodium Ferric Gluconate) Watson 3379

Niferex-150 Forte Capsules (Folic Acid, Polysaccharide Iron Complex, Vitamin B_{12}, Vitamin C) Ther-Rx 3299
Nu-Iron 150 Capsules (Polysaccharide Iron Complex) Merz 2098
Slow Fe Iron Tablets (Ferrous Sulfate) Novartis Consumer .... ▣ 772
Slow Fe with Folic Acid Tablets (Ferrous Sulfate, Folic Acid) Novartis Consumer .... ▣ 773

Anemia, iron deficiency, prevention of
Niferex-150 Forte (Folic Acid, Polysaccharide Iron Complex, Vitamin B_{12}, Vitamin C) Ther-Rx 3299

Anemia, myelofibrosis
Anadrol-50 Tablets (Oxymetholone) Unimed 3329

Anemia, oral iron responsive
Repliva 21/7 Tablets (Ferrous Fumarate, Folic Acid, Iron, Vitamin B_{12}, Vitamin C) Ther-Rx 3301

Anemia, RBC
(*see under* Erythroblastopenia)

Anemia, surgical procedure-induced, to reduce the need for allogeneic blood transfusions
Epogen for Injection (Epoetin Alfa) Amgen 586
Procrit for Injection (Epoetin Alfa) Ortho Biotech 2374

Anemia associated with chronic renal failure
Aranesp for Injection (Darbepoetin alfa) Amgen 576
Epogen for Injection (Epoetin Alfa) Amgen 586
Procrit for Injection (Epoetin Alfa) Ortho Biotech 2374

Anemias, deficient red cell production
Anadrol-50 Tablets (Oxymetholone) Unimed 3329

Anesthesia, general
Diprivan Injectable Emulsion (Propofol) AstraZeneca 676
Suprane Liquid for Inhalation (Desflurane) Baxter Anesthesia 770
Ultane Liquid for Inhalation (Sevoflurane) Abbott 526

Anesthesia, general, adjunct in
Mivacron Injection (Mivacurium Chloride) Abbott 489
Nembutal Sodium Solution, USP (Pentobarbital Sodium) Ovation 2484
Nimbex Injection (Cisatracurium Besylate) Abbott 494
Nubain Injection (Nalbuphine Hydrochloride) Endo Labs 1111
Numorphan Injection (Oxymorphone Hydrochloride) Endo Labs 1112
Phenergan (Promethazine Hydrochloride) Wyeth 3438
Zemuron Injection (Rocuronium Bromide) Organon USA 2363

Anesthesia, general, supplement to
(*see under* Anesthesia, general, adjunct in)

Anesthesia, local
Hurricaine Topical Anesthetic Gel, 1 oz. Fresh Mint, Wild Cherry, Pina Colada, Watermelon, 1/6 oz. Wild Cherry (Benzocaine) Beutlich .... ▣ 607
Hurricaine Topical Anesthetic Liquid, 1 oz. Wild Cherry, Pina Colada, .25 ml Swab Applicator Wild Cherry (Benzocaine) Beutlich .... ▣ 607
Hurricaine Topical Anesthetic Spray Extension Tubes (200) (Benzocaine) Beutlich .... ▣ 607
Hurricaine Topical Anesthetic Spray Kit, 2 oz. Wild Cherry (Benzocaine) Beutlich .... ▣ 607
Hurricaine Topical Anesthetic Spray, 2 oz. Wild Cherry (Benzocaine) Beutlich .... ▣ 607
Naropin Injection (Ropivacaine Hydrochloride) AstraZeneca LP 640

Anesthesia, local, adjunct in
Diprivan Injectable Emulsion (Propofol) AstraZeneca 676

Anesthesia, local, obstetrical procedures
Naropin Injection (Ropivacaine Hydrochloride) AstraZeneca LP 640

Anesthesia, local, ocular
Ophthetic Ophthalmic Solution (Proparacaine Hydrochloride) Allergan .... ⊙ 230

Anesthesia, local, oral cavity
Hurricaine Topical Anesthetic Gel, 1 oz. Fresh Mint, Wild Cherry, Pina Colada, Watermelon, 1/6 oz. Wild Cherry (Benzocaine) Beutlich .... ▣ 607
Hurricaine Topical Anesthetic Liquid, 1 oz. Wild Cherry, Pina Colada, .25 ml Swab Applicator Wild Cherry (Benzocaine) Beutlich .... ▣ 607
Hurricaine Topical Anesthetic Spray Extension Tubes (200) (Benzocaine) Beutlich .... ▣ 607
Hurricaine Topical Anesthetic Spray Kit, 2 oz. Wild Cherry (Benzocaine) Beutlich .... ▣ 607
Hurricaine Topical Anesthetic Spray, 2 oz. Wild Cherry (Benzocaine) Beutlich .... ▣ 607
Triaminic Sore Throat Spray (Phenol) Novartis Consumer .... ▣ 689

Anesthesia, local, pharyngeal
Hurricaine Topical Anesthetic Gel, 1 oz. Fresh Mint, Wild Cherry, Pina Colada, Watermelon, 1/6 oz. Wild Cherry (Benzocaine) Beutlich .... ▣ 607
Hurricaine Topical Anesthetic Liquid, 1 oz. Wild Cherry, Pina Colada, .25 ml Swab Applicator Wild Cherry (Benzocaine) Beutlich .... ▣ 607
Hurricaine Topical Anesthetic Spray Extension Tubes (200) (Benzocaine) Beutlich .... ▣ 607
Hurricaine Topical Anesthetic Spray Kit, 2 oz. Wild Cherry (Benzocaine) Beutlich .... ▣ 607
Hurricaine Topical Anesthetic Spray, 2 oz. Wild Cherry (Benzocaine) Beutlich .... ▣ 607

Anesthesia, local, surgical procedures
Naropin Injection (Ropivacaine Hydrochloride) AstraZeneca LP 640

Anesthesia, regional
Naropin Injection (Ropivacaine Hydrochloride) AstraZeneca LP 640

Anesthesia, regional, adjunct in
Diprivan Injectable Emulsion (Propofol) AstraZeneca 676

Anesthesia care sedation, monitored
Diprivan Injectable Emulsion (Propofol) AstraZeneca 676

Angina
(*see under* Angina pectoris)

Angina, chronic stable
Caduet Tablets (Amlodipine Besylate, Atorvastatin Calcium) Pfizer 2507
Ecotrin Enteric Coated Aspirin Low, Regular and Maximum Strength Tablets (Aspirin) GlaxoSmithKline Consumer 1627
Norvasc Tablets (Amlodipine Besylate) Pfizer 2529
St. Joseph 81 mg Aspirin Chewable and Enteric Coated Tablets (Aspirin) McNeil Consumer 1841
Tiazac Capsules (Diltiazem Hydrochloride) Forest 1204

Angina, classic effort-associated
(*see under* Angina, chronic stable)

Angina, crescendo
(*see under* Angina, unstable)

Angina, pre-infarction
(*see under* Angina, unstable)

Angina, Prinzmetal's
Caduet Tablets (Amlodipine Besylate, Atorvastatin Calcium) Pfizer 2507
Norvasc Tablets (Amlodipine Besylate) Pfizer 2529

Angina, unstable
Angiomax for Injection (Bivalirudin) The Medicines Company 1856
Bayer Aspirin Tablets (Aspirin) Bayer Healthcare LLC 3515
Ecotrin Enteric Coated Aspirin Low, Regular and Maximum Strength Tablets (Aspirin) GlaxoSmithKline Consumer 1627
Fragmin Injection (Dalteparin Sodium) Pharmacia & Upjohn 2638
St. Joseph 81 mg Aspirin Chewable and Enteric Coated Tablets (Aspirin) McNeil Consumer 1841

Angina, variant
(*see under* Angina, Prinzmetal's)

Angina, vasospastic
(*see under* Angina, Prinzmetal's)

Angina pectoris
Covera-HS Tablets (Verapamil Hydrochloride) Searle 3135
Imdur Tablets (Isosorbide Mononitrate) Schering 3032
Inderal LA Long-Acting Capsules (Propranolol Hydrochloride) Wyeth 3421
Nitro-Dur Transdermal Infusion System (Nitroglycerin) Schering 3060
Nitrolingual Pumpspray (Nitroglycerin) First Horizon 1161
Tenormin Tablets (Atenolol) AstraZeneca 695
Toprol-XL Tablets (Metoprolol Succinate) AstraZeneca LP 660

Angina pectoris, acute, prophylaxis
Nitrolingual Pumpspray (Nitroglycerin) First Horizon 1161

Angina pectoris, reduce complications from
Bayer Aspirin Tablets (Aspirin) Bayer Healthcare LLC 3515

Angioedema, adjunctive therapy in
Phenergan (Promethazine Hydrochloride) Wyeth 3438

Angiography, fluorescein, fundus
Fluorescite (Fluorescein Sodium) Alcon .... ⊙ 207

Ankylosing spondylitis
Anaprox Tablets (Naproxen Sodium) Roche Laboratories 2769
Anaprox DS Tablets (Naproxen Sodium) Roche Laboratories 2769
Bayer Aspirin Tablets (Aspirin) Bayer Healthcare LLC 3515
Cataflam Tablets (Diclofenac Potassium) Novartis 2173
Celebrex Capsules (Celecoxib) Searle 3130
Clinoril Tablets (Sulindac) Merck 1899
Decadron Phosphate Injection (Dexamethasone Sodium Phosphate) Merck 1931
Decadron Tablets (Dexamethasone) Merck 1929
Depo-Medrol Injectable Suspension (Methylprednisolone Acetate) Pharmacia & Upjohn 2615
Depo-Medrol Single-Dose Vial (Methylprednisolone Acetate) Pharmacia & Upjohn 2617
EC-Naprosyn Delayed-Release Tablets (Naproxen) Roche Laboratories 2769
Ecotrin Enteric Coated Aspirin Low, Regular and Maximum Strength Tablets (Aspirin) GlaxoSmithKline Consumer 1627
Enbrel for Injection (Etanercept) Amgen 580
Hydrocortone Tablets (Hydrocortisone) Merck 1963
Indocin (Indomethacin) Merck 1968
Naprosyn Suspension (Naproxen) Roche Laboratories 2769
Naprosyn Tablets (Naproxen) Roche Laboratories 2769
Pediapred Oral Solution (Prednisolone Sodium Phosphate) UCB 3319
Remicade for IV Injection (Infliximab) Centocor 987
St. Joseph 81 mg Aspirin Chewable and Enteric Coated Tablets (Aspirin) McNeil Consumer 1841
Traumeel Injection Solution (Homeopathic Formulations) Heel 1638
Voltaren Tablets (Diclofenac Sodium) Novartis 2298

Anorectal conditions
Tucks Anti-Itch (Hydrocortisone Acetate) Pfizer Consumer Healthcare .... ▣ 712
Tucks Hemorrhoidal Ointment (Mineral Oil, Pramoxine Hydrochloride, Zinc Oxide, Mineral Oil, Pramoxine Hydrochloride, Zinc Oxide) Pfizer Consumer Healthcare .... ▣ 711
Tucks Hemorrhoidal Suppositories (Starch, topical) Pfizer Consumer Healthcare .... ▣ 712
Tucks Witch Hazel Hemorrhoidal Pad (Witch Hazel) Pfizer Consumer Healthcare .... ▣ 712

Anorexia associated with weight loss, AIDS-induced
Marinol Capsules (Dronabinol) Unimed 3334
Megace ES Oral Suspension (Megestrol Acetate) Par 2492

Anterior segment inflammation
(*see under* Inflammation, anterior segment)

Anthrax
(*see under* B. anthracis infections)

Antithrombin III deficiency, hereditary
Thrombate III (Antithrombin III) Talecris 3254

Anxiety, preoperative
Librium Capsules (Chlordiazepoxide Hydrochloride) Valeant 3349

Anxiety, short-term symptomatic relief of
Effexor XR Capsules (Venlafaxine Hydrochloride) Wyeth 3411
Hyland's Nerve Tonic Tablets and Caplets (Homeopathic Formulations) Standard Homeopathic .... ▣ 735
Librium Capsules (Chlordiazepoxide Hydrochloride) Valeant 3349
Tranxene (Clorazepate Dipotassium) Ovation 2488
Valium Tablets (Diazepam) Roche Laboratories 2822

Anxiety disorder, generalized
Lexapro Oral Solution (Escitalopram Oxalate) Forest 1193
Lexapro Tablets (Escitalopram Oxalate) Forest 1193
Paxil (Paroxetine Hydrochloride) GlaxoSmithKline 1501

Anxiety disorder, social
Effexor XR Capsules (Venlafaxine Hydrochloride) Wyeth 3411
Paxil CR Controlled-Release Tablets (Paroxetine Hydrochloride) GlaxoSmithKline 1509
Paxil (Paroxetine Hydrochloride) GlaxoSmithKline 1501
Zoloft (Sertraline Hydrochloride) Pfizer 2581

Anxiety disorders, management of
Librium Capsules (Chlordiazepoxide Hydrochloride) Valeant 3349
Niravam Orally Disintegrating Tablets (Alprazolam) Schwarz 3106

Phenergan (Promethazine Hydrochloride) Wyeth ... 3438
Tranxene (Clorazepate Dipotassium) Ovation ... 2488
Valium Tablets (Diazepam) Roche Laboratories ... 2822

Aplasia, pure red cell
Decadron Tablets (Dexamethasone) Merck ... 1929

Apnea of prematurity
Cafcit (Caffeine Citrate) Mead Johnson ... 1854

Appendicitis, gangrenous
Primaxin I.M. (Cilastatin Sodium, Imipenem) Merck ... 2022

Appendicitis with peritonitis
Merrem I.V. (Meropenem) AstraZeneca ... 687
Primaxin I.M. (Cilastatin Sodium, Imipenem) Merck ... 2022
Zosyn (Piperacillin Sodium, Tazobactam Sodium) Wyeth ... 3492

Appetite, suppression of
(*see under* Obesity, exogenous)

Apprehension
(*see under* Anxiety disorders, management of)

ARC
(*see under* Infections, acquired immunodeficiency syndrome-related complex)

Arrhythmias, ventricular
Tambocor Tablets (Flecainide Acetate) 3M ... 1824

Arrhythmias, ventricular, life-threatening
Pacerone Tablets (Amiodarone Hydrochloride) Upsher-Smith ... 3337
Tambocor Tablets (Flecainide Acetate) 3M ... 1824

Arteritis, temporal
Decadron Tablets (Dexamethasone) Merck ... 1929

Arthralgia, topical relief of
(*see under* Pain, topical relief of)

Arthritis
(*see also under* Osteoarthritis; Rheumatoid arthritis)
Goody's Body Pain Formula Powder (Acetaminophen, Aspirin, Acetaminophen, Aspirin) GlaxoSmithKline ... ▣ 621

Arthritis, acute, gouty
Clinoril Tablets (Sulindac) Merck ... 1899
Decadron Phosphate Injection (Dexamethasone Sodium Phosphate) Merck ... 1931
Decadron Tablets (Dexamethasone) Merck ... 1929
Depo-Medrol Injectable Suspension (Methylprednisolone Acetate) Pharmacia & Upjohn ... 2615
Depo-Medrol Single-Dose Vial (Methylprednisolone Acetate) Pharmacia & Upjohn ... 2617
Hydrocortone Tablets (Hydrocortisone) Merck ... 1963
Indocin (Indomethacin) Merck ... 1968
Pediapred Oral Solution (Prednisolone Sodium Phosphate) UCB ... 3319

Arthritis, juvenile
Anaprox Tablets (Naproxen Sodium) Roche Laboratories ... 2769
Anaprox DS Tablets (Naproxen Sodium) Roche Laboratories ... 2769
EC-Naprosyn Delayed-Release Tablets (Naproxen) Roche Laboratories ... 2769
Naprosyn Suspension (Naproxen) Roche Laboratories ... 2769
Naprosyn Tablets (Naproxen) Roche Laboratories ... 2769

Arthritis, osteo-
(*see under* Osteoarthritis)

Arthritis, psoriatic
Bayer Aspirin Tablets (Aspirin) Bayer Healthcare LLC ... 3515
Decadron Phosphate Injection (Dexamethasone Sodium Phosphate) Merck ... 1931
Decadron Tablets (Dexamethasone) Merck ... 1929
Depo-Medrol Injectable Suspension (Methylprednisolone Acetate) Pharmacia & Upjohn ... 2615
Depo-Medrol Single-Dose Vial (Methylprednisolone Acetate) Pharmacia & Upjohn ... 2617
Ecotrin Enteric Coated Aspirin Low, Regular and Maximum Strength Tablets (Aspirin) GlaxoSmithKline Consumer ... 1627
Enbrel for Injection (Etanercept) Amgen ... 580
Hydrocortone Tablets (Hydrocortisone) Merck ... 1963
Pediapred Oral Solution (Prednisolone Sodium Phosphate) UCB ... 3319
Remicade for IV Injection (Infliximab) Centocor ... 987
St. Joseph 81 mg Aspirin Chewable and Enteric Coated Tablets (Aspirin) McNeil Consumer ... 1841

Arthritis, rheumatoid
(*see under* Rheumatoid arthritis)

Arthritis, topical adjunct to
BenGay External Analgesic Products (Menthol, Methyl Salicylate) Pfizer Consumer Healthcare ... ▣ 698
BenGay Pain Relieving Patch (Menthol) Pfizer Consumer Healthcare ... ▣ 698
BenGay Ultra Strength Pain Relieving Patch (Menthol) Pfizer Consumer Healthcare ... ▣ 698
Thera-Gesic Creme (Menthol, Methyl Salicylate) Mission ... 2108
Thera-Gesic Plus Creme (Menthol, Methyl Salicylate) Mission ... ▣ 673

Ascariasis, as secondary therapy in
Mintezol (Thiabendazole) Merck ... 2002

Ascaris lumbricoides infections
Vermox Chewable Tablets (Mebendazole) McNeil Consumer ... 1853

Aspergillosis
Abelcet Injection (Amphotericin B Lipid Complex) Enzon ... 1119
AmBisome for Injection (Amphotericin B, liposomal) Astellas ... 615
Cancidas for Injection (Caspofungin acetate) Merck ... 1894
VFEND I.V. (Voriconazole) Pfizer ... 2543
VFEND Oral Suspension (Voriconazole) Pfizer ... 2543
VFEND Tablets (Voriconazole) Pfizer ... 2543

Aspergillus fumigatus infections
(*see under* Aspergillosis)

Asthma, allergen induced
Xolair (Omalizumab) Genentech ... 1259

Asthma, bronchial
(*see under* Bronchial asthma)

Astrocytoma, anaplastic
Temodar Capsules (Temozolomide) Schering ... 3088

Athetosis, adjunctive therapy in
Valium Tablets (Diazepam) Roche Laboratories ... 2822

Athlete's foot
(*see under* Tinea pedis infections)

Atrial fibrillation
Brevibloc Concentrate (Esmolol Hydrochloride) Baxter Anesthesia ... 766
Brevibloc Injection (Esmolol Hydrochloride) Baxter Anesthesia ... 766
Brevibloc Double Strength Injection (Esmolol Hydrochloride) Baxter Anesthesia ... 766
Brevibloc Premixed Injection (Esmolol Hydrochloride) Baxter Anesthesia ... 766
Brevibloc Double Strength Premixed Injection (Esmolol Hydrochloride) Baxter Anesthesia ... 766
Digitek Tablets (Digoxin) Mylan Bertek ... 2146
Lanoxicaps Capsules (Digoxin) GlaxoSmithKline ... 1458
Lanoxin Injection (Digoxin) GlaxoSmithKline ... 1462
Lanoxin Tablets (Digoxin) GlaxoSmithKline ... 1468
Lanoxin Injection Pediatric (Digoxin) GlaxoSmithKline ... 1465
Rythmol SR Capsules (Propafenone Hydrochloride) Reliant ... 2736

Atrial fibrillation, paroxysmal
Tambocor Tablets (Flecainide Acetate) 3M ... 1824

Atrial fibrillation with embolism
Coumadin for Injection (Warfarin Sodium) Bristol-Myers Squibb ... 932
Coumadin Tablets (Warfarin Sodium) Bristol-Myers Squibb ... 932
Miradon Tablets (Anisindione) Schering ... 3056

Atrial flutter
Brevibloc Concentrate (Esmolol Hydrochloride) Baxter Anesthesia ... 766
Brevibloc Injection (Esmolol Hydrochloride) Baxter Anesthesia ... 766
Brevibloc Double Strength Injection (Esmolol Hydrochloride) Baxter Anesthesia ... 766
Brevibloc Premixed Injection (Esmolol Hydrochloride) Baxter Anesthesia ... 766
Brevibloc Double Strength Premixed Injection (Esmolol Hydrochloride) Baxter Anesthesia ... 766

Attention Deficit Hyperactivity Disorder
Adderall Tablets (Amphetamine Aspartate, Amphetamine Sulfate, Dextroamphetamine Saccharate, Dextroamphetamine Sulfate) Shire US ... 3168
Adderall XR Capsules (Amphetamine Aspartate, Amphetamine Sulfate, Dextroamphetamine Saccharate, Dextroamphetamine Sulfate) Shire US ... 3169
Concerta Extended-Release Tablets (Methylphenidate Hydrochloride) McNeil Consumer ... 1828
Desoxyn Tablets, USP (Methamphetamine Hydrochloride) Ovation ... 2482
Dexedrine (Dextroamphetamine Sulfate) GlaxoSmithKline ... 1386
DextroStat Tablets (Dextroamphetamine Sulfate) Shire US ... 3177
Focalin Tablets (Dexmethylphenidate Hydrochloride) Novartis ... 2214
Focalin XR Capsules (Dexmethylphenidate Hydrochloride) Novartis ... 2217
Metadate CD Capsules (Methylphenidate Hydrochloride) UCB ... 3316
Ritalin Hydrochloride Tablets (Methylphenidate Hydrochloride) Novartis ... 2254
Ritalin LA Capsules (Methylphenidate Hydrochloride) Novartis ... 2255
Ritalin-SR Tablets (Methylphenidate Hydrochloride) Novartis ... 2254
Strattera Capsules (Atomoxetine Hydrochloride) Lilly ... 1784

B

B. anthracis infections
Cipro (Ciprofloxacin) Schering ... 2991
Dynacin Tablets (Minocycline Hydrochloride) Medicis ... 1859
Levaquin in 5% Dextrose Injection (Levofloxacin) Ortho-McNeil ... 2453
Levaquin (Levofloxacin) Ortho-McNeil ... 2453

B. distasonis infections
Invanz for Injection (Ertapenem) Merck ... 1974
Primaxin I.M. (Cilastatin Sodium, Imipenem) Merck ... 2022

B. distasonis intra-abdominal infections
Invanz for Injection (Ertapenem) Merck ... 1974
Primaxin I.M. (Cilastatin Sodium, Imipenem) Merck ... 2022

B. fragilis endomyometritis
Invanz for Injection (Ertapenem) Merck ... 1974

B. fragilis gynecologic infections
Mefoxin for Injection (Cefoxitin Sodium) Merck ... 1987
Mefoxin Premixed Intravenous Solution (Cefoxitin Sodium) Merck ... 1990
Primaxin I.V. (Cilastatin Sodium, Imipenem) Merck ... 2024

B. fragilis infections
Cipro I.V. (Ciprofloxacin) Schering ... 2998
Cipro I.V. Pharmacy Bulk Package (Ciprofloxacin) Bayer ... 3509
Cipro (Ciprofloxacin) Schering ... 2991
Invanz for Injection (Ertapenem) Merck ... 1974
Mefoxin for Injection (Cefoxitin Sodium) Merck ... 1987
Mefoxin Premixed Intravenous Solution (Cefoxitin Sodium) Merck ... 1990
Merrem I.V. (Meropenem) AstraZeneca ... 687
Primaxin I.M. (Cilastatin Sodium, Imipenem) Merck ... 2022
Primaxin I.V. (Cilastatin Sodium, Imipenem) Merck ... 2024
Rocephin Injectable Vials, ADD-Vantage, Galaxy, Bulk (Ceftriaxone Sodium) Roche Laboratories ... 2801
Timentin ADD-Vantage (Clavulanate Potassium, Ticarcillin Disodium) GlaxoSmithKline ... 1556
Timentin Injection Galaxy Container (Clavulanate Potassium, Ticarcillin Disodium) GlaxoSmithKline ... 1559
Timentin IV Infusion (Clavulanate Potassium, Ticarcillin Disodium) GlaxoSmithKline ... 1553
Timentin Pharmacy Bulk Package (Clavulanate Potassium, Ticarcillin Disodium) GlaxoSmithKline ... 1562
Tygacil for Injection (Tigecycline) Wyeth ... 3489
Zosyn (Piperacillin Sodium, Tazobactam Sodium) Wyeth ... 3492

B. fragilis intra-abdominal infections
Cipro I.V. (Ciprofloxacin) Schering ... 2998
Cipro I.V. Pharmacy Bulk Package (Ciprofloxacin) Bayer ... 3509
Cipro (Ciprofloxacin) Schering ... 2991
Fortaz (Ceftazidime Sodium) GlaxoSmithKline ... 1422
Invanz for Injection (Ertapenem) Merck ... 1974
Maxipime for Injection (Cefepime Hydrochloride) Elan ... 1093
Mefoxin for Injection (Cefoxitin Sodium) Merck ... 1987
Mefoxin Premixed Intravenous Solution (Cefoxitin Sodium) Merck ... 1990
Merrem I.V. (Meropenem) AstraZeneca ... 687
Primaxin I.M. (Cilastatin Sodium, Imipenem) Merck ... 2022
Primaxin I.V. (Cilastatin Sodium, Imipenem) Merck ... 2024
Rocephin Injectable Vials, ADD-Vantage, Galaxy, Bulk (Ceftriaxone Sodium) Roche Laboratories ... 2801
Timentin ADD-Vantage (Clavulanate Potassium, Ticarcillin Disodium) GlaxoSmithKline ... 1556
Timentin Injection Galaxy Container (Clavulanate Potassium, Ticarcillin Disodium) GlaxoSmithKline ... 1559
Timentin IV Infusion (Clavulanate Potassium, Ticarcillin Disodium) GlaxoSmithKline ... 1553
Timentin Pharmacy Bulk Package (Clavulanate Potassium, Ticarcillin Disodium) GlaxoSmithKline ... 1562
Tygacil for Injection (Tigecycline) Wyeth ... 3489

B. fragilis peritonitis
Mefoxin for Injection (Cefoxitin Sodium) Merck ... 1987
Mefoxin Premixed Intravenous Solution (Cefoxitin Sodium) Merck ... 1990
Merrem I.V. (Meropenem) AstraZeneca ... 687
Timentin ADD-Vantage (Clavulanate Potassium, Ticarcillin Disodium) GlaxoSmithKline ... 1556
Timentin Injection Galaxy Container (Clavulanate Potassium, Ticarcillin Disodium) GlaxoSmithKline ... 1559
Timentin IV Infusion (Clavulanate Potassium, Ticarcillin Disodium) GlaxoSmithKline ... 1553
Timentin Pharmacy Bulk Package (Clavulanate Potassium, Ticarcillin Disodium) GlaxoSmithKline ... 1562
Zosyn (Piperacillin Sodium, Tazobactam Sodium) Wyeth ... 3492

B. fragilis septicemia
Mefoxin for Injection (Cefoxitin Sodium) Merck ... 1987
Mefoxin Premixed Intravenous Solution (Cefoxitin Sodium) Merck ... 1990
Primaxin I.V. (Cilastatin Sodium, Imipenem) Merck ... 2024

B. fragilis skin and skin structure infections
Mefoxin for Injection (Cefoxitin Sodium) Merck ... 1987
Mefoxin Premixed Intravenous Solution (Cefoxitin Sodium) Merck ... 1990
Merrem I.V. (Meropenem) AstraZeneca ... 687
Primaxin I.M. (Cilastatin Sodium, Imipenem) Merck ... 2022
Primaxin I.V. (Cilastatin Sodium, Imipenem) Merck ... 2024
Rocephin Injectable Vials, ADD-Vantage, Galaxy, Bulk (Ceftriaxone Sodium) Roche Laboratories ... 2801
Tygacil for Injection (Tigecycline) Wyeth ... 3489

B. intermedius infections
Primaxin I.M. (Cilastatin Sodium, Imipenem) Merck ... 2022

B. melaninogenicus endometritis
Timentin ADD-Vantage (Clavulanate Potassium, Ticarcillin Disodium) GlaxoSmithKline ... 1556
Timentin Injection Galaxy Container (Clavulanate Potassium, Ticarcillin Disodium) GlaxoSmithKline ... 1559
Timentin IV Infusion (Clavulanate Potassium, Ticarcillin Disodium) GlaxoSmithKline ... 1553
Timentin Pharmacy Bulk Package (Clavulanate Potassium, Ticarcillin Disodium) GlaxoSmithKline ... 1562

B. melaninogenicus infections
Timentin ADD-Vantage (Clavulanate Potassium, Ticarcillin Disodium) GlaxoSmithKline ... 1556
Timentin Injection Galaxy Container (Clavulanate Potassium, Ticarcillin Disodium) GlaxoSmithKline ... 1559
Timentin IV Infusion (Clavulanate Potassium, Ticarcillin Disodium) GlaxoSmithKline ... 1553
Timentin Pharmacy Bulk Package (Clavulanate Potassium, Ticarcillin Disodium) GlaxoSmithKline ... 1562

B. ovatus infections
Zosyn (Piperacillin Sodium, Tazobactam Sodium) Wyeth ... 3492

B. pertussis infections
E.E.S. (Erythromycin Ethylsuccinate) Abbott ... 449
EryPed (Erythromycin Ethylsuccinate) Abbott ... 445
Ery-Tab Tablets (Erythromycin) Abbott ... 447
Erythrocin Stearate Filmtab Tablets (Erythromycin Stearate) Abbott ... 452
Erythromycin Base Filmtab Tablets (Erythromycin) Abbott ... 454
Erythromycin Delayed-Release Capsules, USP (Erythromycin) Abbott ... 456
PCE Dispertab Tablets (Erythromycin) Abbott ... 510

B. pertussis respiratory tract infections
E.E.S. (Erythromycin Ethylsuccinate) Abbott ... 449
EryPed (Erythromycin Ethylsuccinate) Abbott ... 445
Ery-Tab Tablets (Erythromycin) Abbott ... 447
Erythrocin Stearate Filmtab Tablets (Erythromycin Stearate) Abbott ... 452
Erythromycin Base Filmtab Tablets (Erythromycin) Abbott ... 454
Erythromycin Delayed-Release Capsules, USP (Erythromycin) Abbott ... 456
PCE Dispertab Tablets (Erythromycin) Abbott ... 510

B. thetaiotaomicron infections
Merrem I.V. (Meropenem) AstraZeneca ... 687
Primaxin I.M. (Cilastatin Sodium, Imipenem) Merck ... 2022
Tygacil for Injection (Tigecycline) Wyeth ... 3489
Zosyn (Piperacillin Sodium, Tazobactam Sodium) Wyeth ... 3492

B. thetaiotaomicron intra-abdominal infections
Merrem I.V. (Meropenem) AstraZeneca ... 687
Primaxin I.M. (Cilastatin Sodium, Imipenem) Merck ... 2022
Tygacil for Injection (Tigecycline) Wyeth ... 3489

B. thetaiotaomicron peritonitis
Merrem I.V. (Meropenem) AstraZeneca ... 687
Zosyn (Piperacillin Sodium, Tazobactam Sodium) Wyeth ... 3492

B. uniformis infections
Tygacil (Tigecycline) Wyeth ... 3489

B. vulgatus infections
Zosyn (Piperacillin Sodium, Tazobactam Sodium) Wyeth ... 3492

B. vulgatus intra-abdominal infections
Tygacil for Injection (Tigecycline) Wyeth ... 3489

B. vulgatus peritonitis
Zosyn (Piperacillin Sodium, Tazobactam Sodium) Wyeth ... 3492

Backache
Hyland's BackAche with Arnica Caplets (Homeopathic Formulations) Standard Homeopathic ... ■733
Thera-Gesic Plus Creme (Menthol, Methyl Salicylate) Mission ... ■673
Extra Strength Tylenol Rapid Release Gels (Acetaminophen) McNeil Consumer ... 1843
Women's Tylenol Menstrual Relief Caplets (Acetaminophen, Pamabrom) McNeil Consumer ... 1849

Backache, systemic, symptomatic relief of
Advil (Ibuprofen) Wyeth ... ■737
Aleve Tablets, Caplets and Gelcaps (Naproxen Sodium) Bayer Healthcare ... ■605
Goody's Extra Strength Headache Powder (Acetaminophen, Aspirin, Caffeine) GlaxoSmithKline ... ■621
Goody's Extra Strength Pain Relief Tablets (Acetaminophen, Aspirin, Caffeine) GlaxoSmithKline ... ■621
Motrin IB Tablets and Caplets (Ibuprofen) McNeil Consumer ... 1836
Traumeel Injection Solution (Homeopathic Formulations) Heel ... 1638
Tylenol 8 Hour Extended Release Geltabs and Caplets (Acetaminophen) McNeil Consumer ... 1843
Tylenol 8-Hour Extended Release Geltabs/Caplets (Acetaminophen) McNeil Consumer ... ■655
Tylenol (Acetaminophen) McNeil Consumer ... 1843

Backache, temporary relief of
(*see under* Pain, topical relief of)

Bacteremia
(*see under* Septicemia, bacterial)

Bacteriuria associated with cystitis, elimination or suppression of
(*see also under* Infections, urinary tract)
Uroqid-Acid No. 2 Tablets (Methenamine Mandelate, Sodium Acid Phosphate) Beach ... 785

Bacteriuria associated with polynephritis, elimination or suppression of
(*see under* Infections, urinary tract)

Bacteroides distasonis infections
(*see under* B. distasonis infections)

Bacteroides fragilis infections
(*see under* B. fragilis infections)

Bacteroides ovatus infections
(*see under* B. ovatus infections)

Bacteroides species gynecologic infections
Mefoxin for Injection (Cefoxitin Sodium) Merck ... 1987
Mefoxin Premixed Intravenous Solution (Cefoxitin Sodium) Merck ... 1990
Primaxin I.M. (Cilastatin Sodium, Imipenem) Merck ... 2022
Primaxin I.V. (Cilastatin Sodium, Imipenem) Merck ... 2024

Bacteroides species infections
(*see also under* B. distasonis infections; B. fragilis infections; B. ovatus infections; B. thetaiotaomicron infections; B. vulgatus infections)
Fortaz (Ceftazidime Sodium) GlaxoSmithKline ... 1422
Invanz for Injection (Ertapenem) Merck ... 1974
Mefoxin for Injection (Cefoxitin Sodium) Merck ... 1987
Mefoxin Premixed Intravenous Solution (Cefoxitin Sodium) Merck ... 1990
Primaxin I.M. (Cilastatin Sodium, Imipenem) Merck ... 2022
Primaxin I.V. (Cilastatin Sodium, Imipenem) Merck ... 2024
Tygacil for Injection (Tigecycline) Wyeth ... 3489

Bacteroides species intra-abdominal infections
Fortaz (Ceftazidime Sodium) GlaxoSmithKline ... 1422
Invanz for Injection (Ertapenem) Merck ... 1974
Mefoxin for Injection (Cefoxitin Sodium) Merck ... 1987
Mefoxin Premixed Intravenous Solution (Cefoxitin Sodium) Merck ... 1990
Primaxin I.M. (Cilastatin Sodium, Imipenem) Merck ... 2022
Primaxin I.V. (Cilastatin Sodium, Imipenem) Merck ... 2024

Bacteroides species lower respiratory tract infections
Mefoxin for Injection (Cefoxitin Sodium) Merck ... 1987
Mefoxin Premixed Intravenous Solution (Cefoxitin Sodium) Merck ... 1990

Bacteroides species lung abscess
Mefoxin for Injection (Cefoxitin Sodium) Merck ... 1987
Mefoxin Premixed Intravenous Solution (Cefoxitin Sodium) Merck ... 1990

Bacteroides species peritonitis
Mefoxin for Injection (Cefoxitin Sodium) Merck ... 1987
Mefoxin Premixed Intravenous Solution (Cefoxitin Sodium) Merck ... 1990
Primaxin I.M. (Cilastatin Sodium, Imipenem) Merck ... 2022

Bacteroides species pneumonia
Mefoxin for Injection (Cefoxitin Sodium) Merck ... 1987
Mefoxin Premixed Intravenous Solution (Cefoxitin Sodium) Merck ... 1990

Bacteroides species septicemia
Mefoxin for Injection (Cefoxitin Sodium) Merck ... 1987
Mefoxin Premixed Intravenous Solution (Cefoxitin Sodium) Merck ... 1990
Primaxin I.V. (Cilastatin Sodium, Imipenem) Merck ... 2024

Bacteroides species skin and skin structure infections
Mefoxin for Injection (Cefoxitin Sodium) Merck ... 1987
Mefoxin Premixed Intravenous Solution (Cefoxitin Sodium) Merck ... 1990
Primaxin I.M. (Cilastatin Sodium, Imipenem) Merck ... 2022
Primaxin I.V. (Cilastatin Sodium, Imipenem) Merck ... 2024

Bacteroides thetaiotaomicron infections
(*see under* B. thetaiotaomicron infections)

Bacteroides vulgatus infections
(*see under* B. vulgatus infections)

Baldness, male pattern of vertex of scalp
Propecia Tablets (Finasteride) Merck ... 2036
Men's Rogaine Extra Strength Topical Solution, Ocean Rush Scent and Original Unscented (Minoxidil) Pfizer Consumer Healthcare ... ■706

Barber's itch
(*see under* Folliculitis barbae)

Barrett's esophagus
Photofrin for Injection (Porfimer Sodium) Axcan Scandipharm ... 729

Bartonella bacilliformis infections
Dynacin (Minocycline Hydrochloride) Medicis ... 1859

Bedsores
(*see under* Ulcers, decubitus, adjunctive therapy in)

Berylliosis
Decadron Phosphate Injection (Dexamethasone Sodium Phosphate) Merck ... 1931
Decadron Tablets (Dexamethasone) Merck ... 1929
Depo-Medrol Injectable Suspension (Methylprednisolone Acetate) Pharmacia & Upjohn ... 2615
Depo-Medrol Single-Dose Vial (Methylprednisolone Acetate) Pharmacia & Upjohn ... 2617
Hydrocortone Tablets (Hydrocortisone) Merck ... 1963
Pediapred Oral Solution (Prednisolone Sodium Phosphate) UCB ... 3319

Bifidobacterium species gynecologic infections
Primaxin I.V. (Cilastatin Sodium, Imipenem) Merck ... 2024

Biotin, deficiency of
Appearex Tablets (Biotin) Merz ... 2095

Bipolar disorder
Lamictal (Lamotrigine) GlaxoSmithKline ... 1449

Bipolar disorder, acute mixed
Abilify Tablets (Aripiprazole) Bristol-Myers Squibb ... 916

Abilify Tablets (Aripiprazole) Otsuka America ... 2472
Equetro Extended-Release Capsules (Carbamazepine) Shire US ... 3178
Risperdal M-Tab Orally Disintegrating Tablets (Risperidone) Janssen ... 1658
Risperdal (Risperidone) Janssen ... 1658
Zyprexa Tablets (Olanzapine) Lilly ... 1798
Zyprexa ZYDIS Orally Disintegrating Tablets (Olanzapine) Lilly ... 1798

Bipolar disorder, manic episodes
(*see also under* Manic episodes associated with bipolar disorder)
Depakote Tablets (Divalproex Sodium) Abbott ... 427
Equetro Extended-Release Capsules (Carbamazepine) Shire US ... 3178
Eskalith Capsules (Lithium Carbonate) GlaxoSmithKline ... 1406
Lithobid Tablets (Lithium Carbonate) JDS ... 1670
Risperdal M-Tab Orally Disintegrating Tablets (Risperidone) Janssen ... 1658
Risperdal (Risperidone) Janssen ... 1658
Zyprexa Tablets (Olanzapine) Lilly ... 1798
Zyprexa ZYDIS Orally Disintegrating Tablets (Olanzapine) Lilly ... 1798

Bites, black widow spider
Antivenin (Black Widow Spider Antivenin) (Black Widow Spider Antivenin (Equine)) Merck ... 1887

Bites, crotalidae
(*see under* Envenomation, pit viper)

Bites, insect
Benadryl Itch Relief Stick Extra Strength (Diphenhydramine Hydrochloride, Zinc Acetate) Pfizer Consumer Healthcare ... ▣696
Benadryl Itch Stopping Cream Extra Strength (Diphenhydramine Hydrochloride, Zinc Acetate) Pfizer Consumer Healthcare ... ▣697
Benadryl Itch Stopping Gel Extra Strength (Diphenhydramine Hydrochloride) Pfizer Consumer Healthcare ... ▣697
Benadryl Itch Stopping Spray Extra Strength (Diphenhydramine Hydrochloride, Zinc Acetate) Pfizer Consumer Healthcare ... ▣697
Cortizone•5 Ointment (Hydrocortisone) Pfizer Consumer Healthcare ... ▣699
Cortizone•10 Creme (Hydrocortisone) Pfizer Consumer Healthcare ... ▣699
Cortizone•10 Ointment (Hydrocortisone) Pfizer Consumer Healthcare ... ▣699
Cortizone•10 Plus Creme (Hydrocortisone) Pfizer Consumer Healthcare ... ▣700
Cortizone•10 Maximum Strength Quick Shot Spray (Hydrocortisone) Pfizer Consumer Healthcare ... ▣700
EpiPen (Epinephrine) Dey ... 1061

Bites, pit vipers
(*see under* Envenomation, pit viper)

Bladder carcinoma, transitional cell
(*see under* Carcinoma, bladder, transitional cell)

Bleeding, upper gastrointestinal, in critically ill
Tagamet Tablets (Cimetidine) GlaxoSmithKline ... 1547
Zegerid Powder for Oral Solution (Omeprazole) Santarus ... 2972

Bleeding associated with hemophilia A
Advate Injection (Antihemophilic Factor (Recombinant)) Baxter Healthcare ... 742
Feiba VH (Anti-Inhibitor Coagulant Complex) Baxter Healthcare ... 749
NovoSeven (Antihemophilic Factor (Recombinant)) Novo Nordisk ... 2335

Blepharitis
Genoptic Sterile Ophthalmic Solution (Gentamicin Sulfate) Allergan ... ⊙227
Pred Mild Sterile Ophthalmic Suspension (Prednisolone Acetate) Allergan ... ⊙236

Blepharitis, fungal
Natacyn Antifungal Ophthalmic Suspension (Natamycin) Alcon ... ⊙207

Blepharoconjunctivitis
Genoptic Sterile Ophthalmic Solution (Gentamicin Sulfate) Allergan ... ⊙227
Polytrim Ophthalmic Solution (Polymyxin B Sulfate, Trimethoprim Sulfate) Allergan ... 570

Blepharospasm
Botox Purified Neurotoxin Complex (Botulinum Toxin Type A) Allergan ... 565

Blood loss, perioperative, reduction of
Trasylol Injection (Aprotinin) Bayer ... 779

Body aches
(*see under* Pain, general)

Boils, symptomatic relief of
(*see under* Furunculosis, symptomatic relief of)

Bone disease, metabolic, with chronic renal failure
(*see under* Osteodystrophy, renal)

Bone marrow transplantation, allogeneic or autologous, delayed or failed
Leukine (Sargramostim) Berlex ... 829

Bone mass, loss of
(*see under* Osteoporosis)

Bone metastases of solid tumors
Zometa for Intravenous Infusion (Zoledronic acid) Novartis ... 2306

Bordetella pertussis
(*see under* B. pertussis infections)

Borrelia burgdorferi infection
Ceftin Tablets (Cefuroxime Axetil) GlaxoSmithKline ... 1369

Borrelia recurrentis infection
Dynacin Tablets (Minocycline Hydrochloride) Medicis ... 1859

Bowel, evacuation of
Colyte with Flavor Packs for Oral Solution (Polyethylene Glycol, Potassium Chloride, Sodium Bicarbonate, Sodium Chloride, Sodium Sulfate) Schwarz ... 3102
Fleet Bisacodyl Laxatives (Bisacodyl) Fleet ... 1169
Fleet Enema (Sodium Phosphate) Fleet ... 1169
Fleet Mineral Oil Enema (Mineral Oil) Fleet ... 1170
Fleet Phospho-soda (Sodium Phosphate) Fleet ... 1170
Fleet Phospho-soda ACCU-PREP (Glycerin, Pramoxine Hydrochloride, Sodium Phosphate) Fleet ... 1171
Fleet Prep Kits (Bisacodyl, Sodium Phosphate) Fleet ... 1172
HalfLytely and Bisacodyl Tablets Bowel Prep Kit with Flavors Packs (Bisacodyl, Polyethylene Glycol, Potassium Chloride, Sodium Bicarbonate, Sodium Chloride) Braintree ... 915
TriLyte with Flavor Packs for Oral Solution (PEG-3350, Potassium Chloride, Sodium Bicarbonate, Sodium Chloride) Schwarz ... 3114

Bowel, irritable, syndrome
Bentyl Capsules (Dicyclomine Hydrochloride) Axcan Scandipharm ... 724
Bentyl Injection (Dicyclomine Hydrochloride) Axcan Scandipharm ... 724
Bentyl Syrup (Dicyclomine Hydrochloride) Axcan Scandipharm ... 724
Bentyl Tablets (Dicyclomine Hydrochloride) Axcan Scandipharm ... 724
Citrucel Caplets (Methylcellulose) GlaxoSmithKline ... ▣614
Citrucel Orange Flavor Powder (Methylcellulose) GlaxoSmithKline ... ▣613
Citrucel Sugar Free Orange Flavor Powder (Methylcellulose) GlaxoSmithKline ... ▣613
Lotronex Tablets (Alosetron Hydrochloride) GlaxoSmithKline ... 1479
Metamucil Capsules (Psyllium Preparations) Procter & Gamble ... 2672
Metamucil (Psyllium Preparations) Procter & Gamble ... 2672
Zelnorm Tablets (Tegaserod maleate) Novartis ... 2303

Branhamella catarrhalis
(*see under* M. catarrhalis infections)

Breast cancer
(*see under* Carcinoma, breast)

Breast carcinoma
(*see under* Carcinoma, breast)

Bromhidrosis, topical relief of
(*see under* Hyperhidrosis, topical relief of)

Bronchial asthma
Accolate Tablets (Zafirlukast) AstraZeneca ... 663
AccuNeb Inhalation Solution (Albuterol Sulfate) Dey ... 1055
Advair Diskus 100/50 (Fluticasone Propionate, Salmeterol Xinafoate) GlaxoSmithKline ... 1291
Advair Diskus 250/50 (Fluticasone Propionate, Salmeterol Xinafoate) GlaxoSmithKline ... 1291
Advair Diskus 500/50 (Fluticasone Propionate, Salmeterol Xinafoate) GlaxoSmithKline ... 1291
Aerobid/Aerobid-M (Flunisolide) Forest ... 1172
Alupent Inhalation Aerosol (Metaproterenol Sulfate) Boehringer Ingelheim ... 858
Asmanex Twisthaler (Mometasone Furoate) Schering ... 2981
Atrovent HFA Inhalation Aerosol (Ipratropium Bromide) Boehringer Ingelheim ... 872
Azmacort Inhalation Aerosol (Triamcinolone Acetonide) Kos ... 1701
Combivent Inhalation Aerosol (Albuterol Sulfate, Ipratropium Bromide) Boehringer Ingelheim ... 878
Decadron Phosphate Injection (Dexamethasone Sodium Phosphate) Merck ... 1931
Decadron Tablets (Dexamethasone) Merck ... 1929
Depo-Medrol Injectable Suspension (Methylprednisolone Acetate) Pharmacia & Upjohn ... 2615
Depo-Medrol Single-Dose Vial (Methylprednisolone Acetate) Pharmacia & Upjohn ... 2617
DuoNeb Inhalation Solution (Albuterol Sulfate, Ipratropium Bromide) Dey ... 1058
Flovent Diskus 50 mcg (Fluticasone Propionate) GlaxoSmithKline ... 1415
Flovent HFA (Fluticasone Propionate HFA) GlaxoSmithKline ... 1418
Foradil Aerolizer (Formoterol Fumarate) Schering ... 3024
Hydrocortone Tablets (Hydrocortisone) Merck ... 1963
Maxair Autohaler (Pirbuterol Acetate) 3M ... 1820
Pediapred Oral Solution (Prednisolone Sodium Phosphate) UCB ... 3319
Primatene Mist (Epinephrine) Wyeth ... ▣749
Primatene Tablets (Ephedrine Hydrochloride, Guaifenesin) Wyeth ... ▣749
Proventil Inhalation Aerosol (Albuterol) Schering ... 3067
Proventil Inhalation Solution 0.083% (Albuterol Sulfate) Schering ... 3069
Pulmicort Respules (Budesonide) AstraZeneca LP ... 654
Qvar Inhalation Aerosol (Beclomethasone Dipropionate) IVAX ... 1654
Serevent Diskus (Salmeterol Xinafoate) GlaxoSmithKline ... 1540
Singulair (Montelukast Sodium) Merck ... 2047
Uniphyl Tablets (Theophylline Anhydrous) Purdue Pharmaceutical ... 2708
Ventolin HFA Inhalation Aerosol (Albuterol Sulfate) GlaxoSmithKline ... 1576
Xopenex HFA Inhalation Aerosol (Levalbuterol Tartrate) Sepracor ... 3151
Xopenex Inhalation Solution (Levalbuterol Hydrochloride) Sepracor ... 3143
Xopenex Inhalation Solution Concentrate (Levalbuterol Hydrochloride) Sepracor ... 3147

Bronchial congestion
Mucinex 600mg Extended-Release Tablets (Guaifenesin) Adams ... ▣602
Mucinex DM Tablets (Dextromethorphan Hydrobromide, Guaifenesin) Adams ... ▣602
Robitussin Expectorant (Guaifenesin) Wyeth ... ▣749
Robitussin DM Infant Drops (Dextromethorphan Hydrobromide, Guaifenesin) Wyeth ... ▣753
Robitussin DM Liquid (Dextromethorphan Hydrobromide, Guaifenesin) Wyeth ... ▣753
Robitussin PE Syrup (Guaifenesin, Pseudoephedrine Hydrochloride) Wyeth ... ▣753
Robitussin Severe Congestion Liquid-filled Capsules (Guaifenesin, Pseudoephedrine Hydrochloride) Wyeth ... ▣751
Robitussin Sugar Free Cough Liquid (Dextromethorphan Hydrobromide, Guaifenesin) Wyeth ... ▣753
Sudafed Non-Drying Sinus Liquid Caps (Guaifenesin, Pseudoephedrine Hydrochloride) Pfizer Consumer Healthcare ... ▣709
TheraFlu Flu & Chest Congestion Non-Drowsy Hot Liquid (Acetaminophen, Dextromethorphan Hydrobromide, Guaifenesin, Pseudoephedrine Hydrochloride) Novartis Consumer ... ▣681
Triaminic Chest & Nasal Congestion Liquid (Guaifenesin, Pseudoephedrine Hydrochloride) Novartis Consumer ... ▣685
Vicks 44E Cough & Chest Congestion Relief (Dextromethorphan Hydrobromide, Guaifenesin) Procter & Gamble ... 2676
Pediatric Vicks 44e Cough & Chest Congestion Relief Liquid (Dextromethorphan Hydrobromide, Guaifenesin) Procter & Gamble ... 2673

Bronchial secretions, thinning of
Tylenol Cold Severe Congestion Non-Drowsy Caplets with Cool Burst (Acetaminophen, Dextromethorphan Hydrobromide, Guaifenesin, Pseudoephedrine Hydrochloride) McNeil Consumer ... 1846
Tylenol Sinus Severe Congestion Caplets with Cool Burst (Acetaminophen, Doxylamine Succinate, Pseudoephedrine Hydrochloride) McNeil Consumer ... 1848

Bronchitis, acute
Omnicef Capsules (Cefdinir) Abbott ... 506
Omnicef for Oral Suspension (Cefdinir) Abbott ... 506
Suprax (Cefixime) Lupin ... 1811

Bronchitis, chronic
Advair Diskus 250/50 (Fluticasone Propionate, Salmeterol Xinafoate) GlaxoSmithKline ... 1291
Atrovent HFA Inhalation Aerosol (Ipratropium Bromide) Boehringer Ingelheim ... 872
Serevent Diskus (Salmeterol Xinafoate) GlaxoSmithKline ... 1540
Spiriva HandiHaler (Tiotropium bromide) Boehringer Ingelheim ... 899
Uniphyl Tablets (Theophylline Anhydrous) Purdue Pharmaceutical ... 2708

Bronchitis, chronic, acute exacerbation of
Avelox (Moxifloxacin Hydrochloride) Schering ... 2984
Biaxin/Biaxin XL (Clarithromycin) Abbott ... 402
Ceftin Tablets (Cefuroxime Axetil) GlaxoSmithKline ... 1369
Cipro (Ciprofloxacin) Schering ... 2991
Factive Tablets (Gemifloxacin Mesylate) Oscient ... 2464
Ketek Tablets (Telithromycin) Sanofi-Aventis ... 2920
Levaquin in 5% Dextrose Injection (Levofloxacin) Ortho-McNeil ... 2453
Levaquin (Levofloxacin) Ortho-McNeil ... 2453
Omnicef Capsules (Cefdinir) Abbott ... 506
Omnicef for Oral Suspension (Cefdinir) Abbott ... 506
Primaxin I.M. (Cilastatin Sodium, Imipenem) Merck ... 2022
Spectracef Tablets (Cefditoren Pivoxil) Purdue Pharmaceutical ... 2706
Suprax (Cefixime) Lupin ... 1811
Tequin Injection (Gatifloxacin) Bristol-Myers Squibb ... 964
Tequin Tablets (Gatifloxacin) Bristol-Myers Squibb ... 964
Vantin Tablets and Oral Suspension (Cefpodoxime Proxetil) Pharmacia & Upjohn ... 2650

Bronchospasm, exercise-induced
Foradil Aerolizer (Formoterol Fumarate) Schering ... 3024
Proventil Inhalation Aerosol (Albuterol) Schering ... 3067
Proventil HFA Inhalation Aerosol (Albuterol Sulfate) Schering ... 3071
Serevent Diskus (Salmeterol Xinafoate) GlaxoSmithKline ... 1540

Bronchospasm, prevention and relief of
Xopenex HFA Inhalation Aerosol (Levalbuterol Tartrate) Sepracor ... 3151
Xopenex Inhalation Solution (Levalbuterol Hydrochloride) Sepracor ... 3143
Xopenex Inhalation Solution Concentrate (Levalbuterol Hydrochloride) Sepracor ... 3147

Bronchospasm, reversible
(*see also under* Bronchial asthma)
AccuNeb Inhalation Solution (Albuterol Sulfate) Dey ... 1055
Alupent Inhalation Aerosol (Metaproterenol Sulfate) Boehringer Ingelheim ... 858
Atrovent HFA Inhalation Aerosol (Ipratropium Bromide) Boehringer Ingelheim ... 872
Atrovent Inhalation Solution (Ipratropium Bromide) Boehringer Ingelheim ... 868
Proventil Inhalation Aerosol (Albuterol) Schering ... 3067
Proventil Inhalation Solution 0.083% (Albuterol Sulfate) Schering ... 3069
Proventil HFA Inhalation Aerosol (Albuterol Sulfate) Schering ... 3071
Uniphyl Tablets (Theophylline Anhydrous) Purdue Pharmaceutical ... 2708
Ventolin HFA Inhalation Aerosol (Albuterol Sulfate) GlaxoSmithKline ... 1576
VoSpire Extended-Release Tablets (Albuterol Sulfate) Odyssey ... 2352
Xopenex HFA Inhalation Aerosol (Levalbuterol Tartrate) Sepracor ... 3151
Xopenex Inhalation Solution (Levalbuterol Hydrochloride) Sepracor ... 3143
Xopenex Inhalation Solution Concentrate (Levalbuterol Hydrochloride) Sepracor ... 3147

Bronchospasm associated with chronic obstructive pulmonary disease
Alupent Inhalation Aerosol (Metaproterenol Sulfate) Boehringer Ingelheim ... 858
Atrovent HFA Inhalation Aerosol (Ipratropium Bromide) Boehringer Ingelheim ... 872
Atrovent Inhalation Solution (Ipratropium Bromide) Boehringer Ingelheim ... 868
Foradil Aerolizer (Formoterol Fumarate) Schering ... 3024
Maxair Autohaler (Pirbuterol Acetate) 3M ... 1820
Serevent Diskus (Salmeterol Xinafoate) GlaxoSmithKline ... 1540
Spiriva HandiHaler (Tiotropium bromide) Boehringer Ingelheim ... 899
Uniphyl Tablets (Theophylline Anhydrous) Purdue Pharmaceutical ... 2708

Bronchospasm associated with reversible obstructive airways disease
Foradil Aerolizer (Formoterol Fumarate) Schering ... 3024

Brucella species infections, adjunct in
Dynacin Tablets (Minocycline Hydrochloride) Medicis ... 1859

Bruises
Thera-Gesic Plus Creme (Menthol, Methyl Salicylate) Mission ... ▣673

Bruises, topical relief of
(*see under* Pain, topical relief of)

Bruising
Hyland's Bumps 'n Bruises Tablets (Homeopathic Formulations) Standard Homeopathic ... ▣734

"Bubble boy" disease
(*see under* Adenosine deaminase, enzyme replacement therapy for)

Bulbar conjunctiva inflammation
Blephamide Ophthalmic Suspension (Prednisolone Acetate, Sulfacetamide Sodium) Allergan ... 564
FML Ophthalmic Ointment (Fluorometholone) Allergan ... ⊙225
FML Ophthalmic Suspension (Fluorometholone) Allergan ... ⊙224
FML Forte Ophthalmic Suspension (Fluorometholone) Allergan ... ⊙223
FML-S Liquifilm Sterile Ophthalmic Suspension (Fluorometholone, Sulfacetamide Sodium) Allergan ... ⊙226
Lotemax Ophthalmic Suspension 0.5% (Loteprednol Etabonate) Bausch & Lomb ... ⊙249
Poly-Pred Liquifilm Ophthalmic Suspension (Neomycin Sulfate, Polymyxin B Sulfate, Prednisolone Acetate) Allergan ... ⊙231
Pred Forte Ophthalmic Suspension (Prednisolone Acetate) Allergan ... ⊙233
Pred-G Ophthalmic Suspension (Gentamicin Sulfate, Prednisolone Acetate) Allergan ... ⊙234
Pred-G Sterile Ophthalmic Ointment (Gentamicin Sulfate, Prednisolone Acetate) Allergan ... ⊙235
TobraDex Ophthalmic Ointment (Dexamethasone, Tobramycin) Alcon ... 558
TobraDex Ophthalmic Suspension (Dexamethasone, Tobramycin) Alcon ... 558
Zylet Ophthalmic Suspension (Loteprednol Etabonate, Tobramycin) Bausch & Lomb ... 3508

Bulimia nervosa
Prozac Pulvules and Liquid (Fluoxetine Hydrochloride) Lilly ... 1771

Burn wound infections
(*see under* Infections, burn wound)

Burns, adjunctive therapy in
Accuzyme Spray (Papain, Urea) Healthpoint ... 1637
Panafil Ointment (Chlorophyllin Copper Complex Sodium, Papain, Urea) Healthpoint ... 1637
Panafil Spray (Chlorophyllin Copper Complex Sodium, Papain, Urea) Healthpoint ... 1637

Burns, maintenance of electrolyte balance
Buminate 5% Solution, USP (Albumin (human)) Baxter Healthcare ... 747
Buminate 25% Solution, USP (Albumin (human)) Baxter Healthcare ... 748
Plasbumin-5 (Albumin (human)) Talecris ... 3249
Plasbumin-20 (Albumin (human)) Talecris ... 3249
Plasbumin-25 (Albumin (human)) Talecris ... 3251

Burns, minor
Aquacel AG with Hydrofiber (Silver impregnated antimicrobial dressing) ConvaTec ... 1035
Betadine Solution (Povidone Iodine) Purdue Products ... 2715
Desitin Ointment (Zinc Oxide) Pfizer Consumer Healthcare ... ▣700
Neosporin Ointment (Bacitracin, Neomycin, Polymyxin B Sulfate) Pfizer Consumer Healthcare ... ▣702
Neosporin + Pain Relief Maximum Strength Cream (Neomycin, Polymyxin B Sulfate, Pramoxine Hydrochloride) Pfizer Consumer Healthcare ... ▣703
Neosporin + Pain Relief Maximum Strength Ointment (Bacitracin, Neomycin, Polymyxin B Sulfate, Pramoxine Hydrochloride) Pfizer Consumer Healthcare ... ▣703
Polysporin Ointment (Bacitracin, Polymyxin B Sulfate) Pfizer Consumer Healthcare ... ▣706

Burns, pain associated with
(*see under* Pain, topical relief of)

Burns, second- and third-degree, adjunctive therapy in
Sulfamylon for 5% Topical Solution (Mafenide Acetate) Mylan Bertek ... 2155

Burns, superficial
Biafine Topical Emulsion (Propylparaben, Methylparaben, Propylene Glycol, Stearic Acid, Triethanolamine) OrthoNeutrogena ... 2382

Burns, to prevent hemoconcentration
Plasbumin-5 (Albumin (human)) Talecris ... 3249
Plasbumin-20 (Albumin (human)) Talecris ... 3249
Plasbumin-25 (Albumin (human)) Talecris ... 3251

Burns, wound healing of
Biafine Topical Emulsion (Propylparaben, Methylparaben, Propylene Glycol, Stearic Acid, Triethanolamine) OrthoNeutrogena ... 2382

Bursitis
Anaprox Tablets (Naproxen Sodium) Roche Laboratories ... 2769
Anaprox DS Tablets (Naproxen Sodium) Roche Laboratories ... 2769
Decadron Phosphate Injection (Dexamethasone Sodium Phosphate) Merck ... 1931
Depo-Medrol Injectable Suspension (Methylprednisolone Acetate) Pharmacia & Upjohn ... 2615
Depo-Medrol Single-Dose Vial (Methylprednisolone Acetate) Pharmacia & Upjohn ... 2617
Hydrocortone Tablets (Hydrocortisone) Merck ... 1963
Indocin (Indomethacin) Merck ... 1968
Naprosyn Suspension (Naproxen) Roche Laboratories ... 2769
Naprosyn Tablets (Naproxen) Roche Laboratories ... 2769
Pediapred Oral Solution (Prednisolone Sodium Phosphate) UCB ... 3319
Traumeel Injection Solution (Homeopathic Formulations) Heel ... 1638

Bursitis, subacromial, acute, symptomatic relief of
Clinoril Tablets (Sulindac) Merck ... 1899
Indocin (Indomethacin) Merck ... 1968

C

C. difficile infection
(*see under* Colitis, pseudomembranous, antibiotic-associated)

C. diphtheriae infections
E.E.S. (Erythromycin Ethylsuccinate) Abbott ... 449
EryPed (Erythromycin Ethylsuccinate) Abbott ... 445
Ery-Tab Tablets (Erythromycin) Abbott ... 447
Erythrocin Stearate Filmtab Tablets (Erythromycin Stearate) Abbott ... 452
Erythromycin Base Filmtab Tablets (Erythromycin) Abbott ... 454
Erythromycin Delayed-Release Capsules, USP (Erythromycin) Abbott ... 456
PCE Dispertab Tablets (Erythromycin) Abbott ... 510

C. minutissimum infections
E.E.S. (Erythromycin Ethylsuccinate) Abbott ... 449
EryPed (Erythromycin Ethylsuccinate) Abbott ... 445
Ery-Tab Tablets (Erythromycin) Abbott ... 447
Erythrocin Stearate Filmtab Tablets (Erythromycin Stearate) Abbott ... 452
Erythromycin Base Filmtab Tablets (Erythromycin) Abbott ... 454
Erythromycin Delayed-Release Capsules, USP (Erythromycin) Abbott ... 456
PCE Dispertab Tablets (Erythromycin) Abbott ... 510

C. perfringens infections
Tygacil (Tigecycline) Wyeth ... 3489

Cachexia associated with weight loss, AIDS-induced
Megace ES Oral Suspension (Megestrol Acetate) Par ... 2492

Calcium deficiency
(*see under* Hypocalcemia)

Calluses
(*see under* Hyperkeratosis skin disorders)

Calymmatobacterium granulomatis infections
Dynacin Tablets (Minocycline Hydrochloride) Medicis ... 1859

Campylobacter fetus infections
Dynacin Tablets (Minocycline Hydrochloride) Medicis ... 1859

Campylobacter jejuni infectious diarrhea
Cipro (Ciprofloxacin) Schering ... 2991

Cancer, prostatic
(*see under* Carcinoma, prostate, palliative treatment of)

Candida albicans infections
Gynazole-1 Vaginal Cream (Butoconazole Nitrate) Ther-Rx ... 3298
Loprox Gel (Ciclopirox) Medicis ... 1861
Lotrimin (Clotrimazole) Schering ... 3053
Nystop Topical Powder USP (Nystatin) Paddock ... 2490

Candida infections, abdomen
VFEND I.V. (Voriconazole) Pfizer ... 2543
VFEND Oral Suspension (Voriconazole) Pfizer ... 2543
VFEND Tablets (Voriconazole) Pfizer ... 2543

Candida infections, bladder wall
VFEND I.V. (Voriconazole) Pfizer ... 2543
VFEND Oral Suspension (Voriconazole) Pfizer ... 2543
VFEND Tablets (Voriconazole) Pfizer ... 2543

Candida infections, disseminated, skin
VFEND I.V. (Voriconazole) Pfizer ... 2543
VFEND Oral Suspension (Voriconazole) Pfizer ... 2543
VFEND Tablets (Voriconazole) Pfizer ... 2543

Candida infections, kidney
VFEND I.V. (Voriconazole) Pfizer ... 2543
VFEND Oral Suspension (Voriconazole) Pfizer ... 2543

VFEND Tablets (Voriconazole) Pfizer 2543

Candida infections, prophylaxis in hematopoietic stem cell transplantation
Mycamine for Injection (Micafungin Sodium) Astellas 620

Candida infections, wounds
VFEND I.V. (Voriconazole) Pfizer 2543
VFEND Oral Suspension (Voriconazole) Pfizer 2543
VFEND Tablets (Voriconazole) Pfizer 2543

Candidemia
Cancidas for Injection (Caspofungin acetate) Merck 1894

Candidemia, non-neutropenic patients
VFEND I.V. (Voriconazole) Pfizer 2543
VFEND Oral Suspension (Voriconazole) Pfizer 2543
VFEND Tablets (Voriconazole) Pfizer 2543

Candidiasis, cutaneous
Loprox Gel (Ciclopirox) Medicis 1861
Lotrimin (Clotrimazole) Schering 3053
Nystop Topical Powder USP (Nystatin) Paddock 2490
Spectazole Cream (Econazole Nitrate) OrthoNeutrogena 2390

Candidiasis, esophageal
Cancidas for Injection (Caspofungin acetate) Merck 1894
Mycamine for Injection (Micafungin Sodium) Astellas 620
VFEND I.V. (Voriconazole) Pfizer 2543
VFEND Oral Suspension (Voriconazole) Pfizer 2543
VFEND Tablets (Voriconazole) Pfizer 2543

Candidiasis, systemic
Abelcet Injection (Amphotericin B Lipid Complex) Enzon 1119
AmBisome for Injection (Amphotericin B, liposomal) Astellas 615

Candidiasis, vaginal
Gynazole-1 Vaginal Cream (Butoconazole Nitrate) Ther-Rx 3298
Nystatin Vaginal Tablets, USP (Nystatin) Odyssey 2347

Carbuncles
(*see under* Furunculosis, symptomatic relief of)

Carbuncles, adjunctive therapy in
Accuzyme Spray (Papain, Urea) Healthpoint 1637
Panafil Ointment (Chlorophyllin Copper Complex Sodium, Papain, Urea) Healthpoint 1637

Carcinoma, bladder, transitional cell
Adriamycin for Injection, USP (Doxorubicin Hydrochloride) Bedford 786
Adriamycin Injection, USP (Doxorubicin Hydrochloride) Bedford 786

Carcinoma, breast
Adriamycin for Injection, USP (Doxorubicin Hydrochloride) Bedford 786
Adriamycin Injection, USP (Doxorubicin Hydrochloride) Bedford 786
Arimidex Tablets (Anastrozole) AstraZeneca 665
Aromasin Tablets (Exemestane) Pharmacia & Upjohn 2600
Ellence Injection (Epirubicin Hydrochloride) Pharmacia & Upjohn 2632
Faslodex Injection (Fulvestrant) AstraZeneca 682
Femara Tablets (Letrozole) Novartis 2210
Taxotere Injection Concentrate (Docetaxel) Sanofi-Aventis 2947
Xeloda Tablets (Capecitabine) Roche Laboratories 2825

Carcinoma, breast, adjunctive therapy in
Femara Tablets (Letrozole) Novartis 2210

Carcinoma, breast, metastatic, resistant, treatment of (Monotherapy)
Xeloda Tablets (Capecitabine) Roche Laboratories 2825

Carcinoma, breast, metastatic, treatment of
Delatestryl Injection (Testosterone Enanthate) Savient 2976
Faslodex Injection (Fulvestrant) AstraZeneca 682
Gemzar for Injection (Gemcitabine Hydrochloride) Lilly 1743
Herceptin I.V. (Trastuzumab) Genentech 1234
Taxotere Injection Concentrate (Docetaxel) Sanofi-Aventis 2947
Xeloda Tablets (Capecitabine) Roche Laboratories 2825

Carcinoma, breast, osteolytic bone metastases of
Aredia for Injection (Pamidronate Disodium) Novartis 2168

Carcinoma, breast, palliative therapy in
Premarin Tablets (Estrogens, Conjugated) Wyeth 3443
Zoladex (Goserelin Acetate) AstraZeneca 709

Carcinoma, bronchogenic
Adriamycin for Injection, USP (Doxorubicin Hydrochloride) Bedford 786
Adriamycin Injection, USP (Doxorubicin Hydrochloride) Bedford 786
Mustargen for Injection (Mechlorethamine Hydrochloride) Merck 2007

Carcinoma, colon, Dukes' stage C, adjunctive treatment in
Xeloda Tablets (Capecitabine) Roche Laboratories 2825

Carcinoma, colon, metastatic
Camptosar Injection (Irinotecan Hydrochloride) Pharmacia & Upjohn 2602
Xeloda Tablets (Capecitabine) Roche Laboratories 2825

Carcinoma, colorectal
Eloxatin for Injection (Oxaliplatin) Sanofi-Aventis 2908
Erbitux (Cetuximab) Bristol-Myers Squibb 937
Xeloda Tablets (Capecitabine) Roche Laboratories 2825

Carcinoma, colorectal, adjunctive therapy in
Avastin IV (Bevacizumab) Genentech 1229
Erbitux (Cetuximab) Bristol-Myers Squibb 937

Carcinoma, esophageal, obstructing, palliative treatment of
Photofrin for Injection (Porfimer Sodium) Axcan Scandipharm 729

Carcinoma, gastric
Adriamycin for Injection, USP (Doxorubicin Hydrochloride) Bedford 786
Adriamycin Injection, USP (Doxorubicin Hydrochloride) Bedford 786

Carcinoma, lung, non-small cell
Alimta for Injection (Pemetrexed) Lilly 1722
Gemzar for Injection (Gemcitabine Hydrochloride) Lilly 1743
Iressa Tablets (Gefitinib) AstraZeneca 684
Navelbine Injection (Vinorelbine Tartrate) GlaxoSmithKline 1494
Photofrin for Injection (Porfimer Sodium) Axcan Scandipharm 729
Tarceva Tablets (Erlotinib) Genentech 1254
Tarceva Tablets (Erlotinib) OSI 2470
Taxotere Injection Concentrate (Docetaxel) Sanofi-Aventis 2947

Carcinoma, lung, small cell
Hycamtin for Injection (Topotecan Hydrochloride) GlaxoSmithKline 1427

Carcinoma, metastatic, palliative treatment of
Mustargen for Injection (Mechlorethamine Hydrochloride) Merck 2007

Carcinoma, ovary
Adriamycin for Injection, USP (Doxorubicin Hydrochloride) Bedford 786
Adriamycin Injection, USP (Doxorubicin Hydrochloride) Bedford 786
Alkeran Tablets (Melphalan) Celgene 977
Doxil Injection (Doxorubicin Hydrochloride Liposome) Tibotec 3302
Hexalen Capsules (Altretamine) MGI 2101
Hycamtin for Injection (Topotecan Hydrochloride) GlaxoSmithKline 1427

Carcinoma, pancreas
Gemzar for Injection (Gemcitabine Hydrochloride) Lilly 1743

Carcinoma, prostate
Eulexin Capsules (Flutamide) Schering 3023
Taxotere Injection Concentrate (Docetaxel) Sanofi-Aventis 2947

Carcinoma, prostate, adjunctive therapy in
Casodex Tablets (Bicalutamide) AstraZeneca 670
Eulexin Capsules (Flutamide) Schering 3023
Novantrone for Injection Concentrate (Mitoxantrone Hydrochloride) Serono 3158
Zoladex (Goserelin Acetate) AstraZeneca 709
Zoladex 3-month (Goserelin Acetate) AstraZeneca 712

Carcinoma, prostate, palliative treatment of
Eligard 7.5 mg (Leuprolide Acetate) Sanofi-Aventis 2896
Eligard 22.5 mg (Leuprolide Acetate) Sanofi-Aventis 2899
Eligard 30 mg (Leuprolide Acetate) Sanofi-Aventis 2901
Eligard 45 mg (Leuprolide Acetate) Sanofi-Aventis 2904
Emcyt Capsules (Estramustine Phosphate Sodium) Searle 3137
Lupron Depot 7.5 mg (Leuprolide Acetate) TAP 3261
Premarin Tablets (Estrogens, Conjugated) Wyeth 3443
Trelstar Depot (Triptorelin Pamoate) Watson 3385
Trelstar LA Suspension (Triptorelin Pamoate) Watson 3387
Vantas (Histrelin Acetate) Valera 3367
Viadur Implant (Leuprolide Acetate) Bayer 782
Zoladex (Goserelin Acetate) AstraZeneca 709
Zoladex 3-month (Goserelin Acetate) AstraZeneca 712

Carcinoma, rectal, metastatic
Camptosar Injection (Irinotecan Hydrochloride) Pharmacia & Upjohn 2602

Carcinoma, renal cell, metastatic, in adults
Proleukin for Injection (Aldesleukin) Chiron 1007

Carcinoma, superficial basal cell
Efudex (Fluorouracil) Valeant 3348

Carcinoma, testis, advanced
Cosmegen for Injection (Dactinomycin) Merck 1907

Carcinoma, thyroid
Adriamycin for Injection, USP (Doxorubicin Hydrochloride) Bedford 786
Adriamycin Injection, USP (Doxorubicin Hydrochloride) Bedford 786
Cytomel Tablets (Liothyronine Sodium) King 1678
Levothroid Tablets (Levothyroxine Sodium) Forest 1189
Levoxyl Tablets (Levothyroxine Sodium) King 1680
Synthroid Tablets (Levothyroxine Sodium) Abbott 515
Thyrolar (Liotrix) Forest 1203
Unithroid Tablets (Levothyroxine Sodium) Lannett 3521

Carcinoma, thyroid, adjunctive diagnostic tool for serum thyroglobulin testing
Thyrogen for Injection (Thyrotropin alfa) Genzyme 1270

Cardiac failure
(*see under* Congestive heart failure, adjunct in)

Cardiac ischemic complications, acute, prevention of, adjunct to PTCA
ReoPro Vials (Abciximab) Lilly 1779

Cardiomyopathy, doxorubicin-induced, to reduce the incidence and severity of
Zinecard for Injection (Dexrazoxane) Pharmacia & Upjohn 2659

Cardiopulmonary bypass surgery, adjunct in
Buminate 5% Solution, USP (Albumin (human)) Baxter Healthcare 747
Buminate 25% Solution, USP (Albumin (human)) Baxter Healthcare 748
Plasbumin-5 (Albumin (human)) Talecris 3249
Plasbumin-20 (Albumin (human)) Talecris 3249
Plasbumin-25 (Albumin (human)) Talecris 3251

Cardiovascular disease, prevention of
Caduet Tablets (Amlodipine Besylate, Atorvastatin Calcium) Pfizer 2507
Lipitor Tablets (Atorvastatin Calcium) Parke-Davis 2495

Cardiovascular mortality, reduction of, post-MI
Diovan Tablets (Valsartan) Novartis 2191

Carnitine, deficiency of
Carnitor Injection (Levocarnitine) Sigma-Tau 3185
Carnitor Tablets and Oral Solution (Levocarnitine) Sigma-Tau 3187

Catabolic or tissue depleting processes, adjunctive therapy
Oxandrin Tablets (Oxandrolone) Savient 2977

Cataract extraction, surgical aid in
Amvisc Plus (Sodium Hyaluronate) Bausch & Lomb .... ⊙ 289
Ocucoat (Hydroxypropyl Methylcellulose) Bausch & Lomb .... ⊙ 290

Cellulitis, adjunctive therapy
Plasbumin-20 (Albumin (human)) Talecris 3249

Cellulitis, pelvic
(*see under* Pelvic cellulitis)

Central cranial diabetes insipidus
(*see under* Diabetes insipidus)

Cephalalgia, histaminic
Imitrex Injection (Sumatriptan Succinate) GlaxoSmithKline 1431

Cerebral edema
(*see under* Edema, cerebral)

Cerebral palsy
Decadron Phosphate Injection (Dexamethasone Sodium Phosphate) Merck 1931

Cerumen, removal of
Debrox Drops (Carbamide Peroxide) GlaxoSmithKline 616

Cervicitis
Zithromax (Azithromycin Dihydrate) Pfizer 2568
Zithromax for Oral Suspension, 300 mg, 600 mg, 900 mg, 1200 mg (Azithromycin Dihydrate) Pfizer 2561
Zithromax Tablets, 250 mg, 500 mg (Azithromycin Dihydrate) Pfizer 2561
Zithromax Tablets, 600 mg (Azithromycin Dihydrate) Pfizer 2568
Zithromax Tri-Pak (Azithromycin Dihydrate) Pfizer 2561
Zithromax Z-Pak (Azithromycin Dihydrate) Pfizer 2568

Cervix, ripening of, in pregnant women at or near term
Cervidil Vaginal Insert (Dinoprostone) Forest 1182

Chancroid
Dynacin Tablets (Minocycline Hydrochloride) Medicis 1859
Zithromax Capsules, 250 mg (Azithromycin Dihydrate) Pfizer 2568
Zithromax for Oral Suspension, 300 mg, 600 mg, 900 mg, 1200 mg (Azithromycin Dihydrate) Pfizer 2561
Zithromax Tablets, 250 mg, 500 mg (Azithromycin Dihydrate) Pfizer 2561
Zithromax Tri-Pak (Azithromycin Dihydrate) Pfizer 2561

Chickenpox
(*see under* Varicella, acute, treatment of)

Chlamydia pneumoniae infections
Avelox (Moxifloxacin Hydrochloride) Schering 2984
Biaxin/Biaxin XL (Clarithromycin) Abbott 402
Factive Tablets (Gemifloxacin Mesylate) Oscient 2464
Levaquin in 5% Dextrose Injection (Levofloxacin) Ortho-McNeil 2453
Levaquin (Levofloxacin) Ortho-McNeil 2453
Tequin Injection (Gatifloxacin) Bristol-Myers Squibb 964
Tequin Tablets (Gatifloxacin) Bristol-Myers Squibb 964
Zithromax Capsules, 250 mg (Azithromycin Dihydrate) Pfizer 2568
Zithromax for IV Infusion (Azithromycin Dihydrate) Pfizer 2573
Zithromax for Oral Suspension, 300 mg, 600 mg, 900 mg, 1200 mg (Azithromycin Dihydrate) Pfizer 2561
Zithromax Tablets, 250 mg, 500 mg (Azithromycin Dihydrate) Pfizer 2561
Zithromax Tri-Pak (Azithromycin Dihydrate) Pfizer 2561
Zmax for Oral Suspension (Azithromycin) Pfizer 2577

Chlamydia pneumoniae lower respiratory tract infections
Avelox (Moxifloxacin Hydrochloride) Schering 2984
Biaxin/Biaxin XL (Clarithromycin) Abbott 402
Ketek Tablets (Telithromycin) Sanofi-Aventis 2920
Levaquin in 5% Dextrose Injection (Levofloxacin) Ortho-McNeil 2453
Levaquin (Levofloxacin) Ortho-McNeil 2453
Tequin Injection (Gatifloxacin) Bristol-Myers Squibb 964
Tequin Tablets (Gatifloxacin) Bristol-Myers Squibb 964
Zithromax Capsules, 250 mg (Azithromycin Dihydrate) Pfizer 2568
Zithromax for IV Infusion (Azithromycin Dihydrate) Pfizer 2573
Zithromax for Oral Suspension, 300 mg, 600 mg, 900 mg, 1200 mg (Azithromycin Dihydrate) Pfizer 2561
Zithromax Tablets, 250 mg, 500 mg (Azithromycin Dihydrate) Pfizer 2561
Zithromax Tri-Pak (Azithromycin Dihydrate) Pfizer 2561
Zmax for Oral Suspension (Azithromycin) Pfizer 2577

Chlamydia psittaci infection
Dynacin Tablets (Minocycline Hydrochloride) Medicis 1859

Chlamydia trachomatis conjunctivitis of the newborn
E.E.S. (Erythromycin Ethylsuccinate) Abbott 449
EryPed (Erythromycin Ethylsuccinate) Abbott 445
Ery-Tab Tablets (Erythromycin) Abbott 447
Erythrocin Stearate Filmtab Tablets (Erythromycin Stearate) Abbott 452
Erythromycin Base Filmtab Tablets (Erythromycin) Abbott 454
Erythromycin Delayed-Release Capsules, USP (Erythromycin) Abbott 456
PCE Dispertab Tablets (Erythromycin) Abbott 510

Chlamydia trachomatis endocervical infections
Dynacin Tablets (Minocycline Hydrochloride) Medicis 1859
E.E.S. (Erythromycin Ethylsuccinate) Abbott 449
EryPed (Erythromycin Ethylsuccinate) Abbott 445
Ery-Tab Tablets (Erythromycin) Abbott 447
Erythrocin Stearate Filmtab Tablets (Erythromycin Stearate) Abbott 452
Erythromycin Base Filmtab Tablets (Erythromycin) Abbott 454
Erythromycin Delayed-Release Capsules, USP (Erythromycin) Abbott 456
PCE Dispertab Tablets (Erythromycin) Abbott 510

Chlamydia trachomatis infections
Dynacin Tablets (Minocycline Hydrochloride) Medicis 1859
E.E.S. (Erythromycin Ethylsuccinate) Abbott 449
EryPed (Erythromycin Ethylsuccinate) Abbott 445
Ery-Tab Tablets (Erythromycin) Abbott 447
Erythrocin Stearate Filmtab Tablets (Erythromycin Stearate) Abbott 452
Erythromycin Base Filmtab Tablets (Erythromycin) Abbott 454
Erythromycin Delayed-Release Capsules, USP (Erythromycin) Abbott 456
PCE Dispertab Tablets (Erythromycin) Abbott 510
Vigamox Ophthalmic Solution (Moxifloxacin Hydrochloride) Alcon 560
Zithromax Capsules, 250 mg (Azithromycin Dihydrate) Pfizer 2568
Zithromax for IV Infusion (Azithromycin Dihydrate) Pfizer 2573
Zithromax for Oral Suspension, 1 g (Azithromycin Dihydrate) Pfizer 2568
Zithromax for Oral Suspension, 300 mg, 600 mg, 900 mg, 1200 mg (Azithromycin Dihydrate) Pfizer 2561
Zithromax Tablets, 250 mg, 500 mg (Azithromycin Dihydrate) Pfizer 2561
Zithromax Tablets, 600 mg (Azithromycin Dihydrate) Pfizer 2568
Zithromax Tri-Pak (Azithromycin Dihydrate) Pfizer 2561
Zithromax Z-Pak (Azithromycin Dihydrate) Pfizer 2568

Chlamydia trachomatis infections, ocular
(*see under* Trachoma)

Chlamydia trachomatis nongonococcal cervicitis
Zithromax (Azithromycin Dihydrate) Pfizer 2568
Zithromax for Oral Suspension, 300 mg, 600 mg, 900 mg, 1200 mg (Azithromycin Dihydrate) Pfizer 2561
Zithromax Tablets, 250 mg, 500 mg (Azithromycin Dihydrate) Pfizer 2561
Zithromax Tablets, 600 mg (Azithromycin Dihydrate) Pfizer 2568
Zithromax Tri-Pak (Azithromycin Dihydrate) Pfizer 2561
Zithromax Z-Pak (Azithromycin Dihydrate) Pfizer 2568

Chlamydia trachomatis nongonococcal urethritis
Zithromax (Azithromycin Dihydrate) Pfizer 2568
Zithromax for Oral Suspension, 300 mg, 600 mg, 900 mg, 1200 mg (Azithromycin Dihydrate) Pfizer 2561
Zithromax Tablets, 250 mg, 500 mg (Azithromycin Dihydrate) Pfizer 2561
Zithromax Tablets, 600 mg (Azithromycin Dihydrate) Pfizer 2568
Zithromax Tri-Pak (Azithromycin Dihydrate) Pfizer 2561
Zithromax Z-Pak (Azithromycin Dihydrate) Pfizer 2568

Chlamydia trachomatis pneumonia of infancy
E.E.S. (Erythromycin Ethylsuccinate) Abbott 449
EryPed (Erythromycin Ethylsuccinate) Abbott 445
Ery-Tab Tablets (Erythromycin) Abbott 447
Erythrocin Stearate Filmtab Tablets (Erythromycin Stearate) Abbott 452
Erythromycin Base Filmtab Tablets (Erythromycin) Abbott 454
Erythromycin Delayed-Release Capsules, USP (Erythromycin) Abbott 456
PCE Dispertab Tablets (Erythromycin) Abbott 510

Chlamydia trachomatis rectal infections
Dynacin Tablets (Minocycline Hydrochloride) Medicis 1859
E.E.S. (Erythromycin Ethylsuccinate) Abbott 449
EryPed (Erythromycin Ethylsuccinate) Abbott 445
Ery-Tab Tablets (Erythromycin) Abbott 447
Erythrocin Stearate Filmtab Tablets (Erythromycin Stearate) Abbott 452
Erythromycin Base Filmtab Tablets (Erythromycin) Abbott 454
Erythromycin Delayed-Release Capsules, USP (Erythromycin) Abbott 456
PCE Dispertab Tablets (Erythromycin) Abbott 510

Chlamydia trachomatis urethral infections
E.E.S. (Erythromycin Ethylsuccinate) Abbott 449
EryPed (Erythromycin Ethylsuccinate) Abbott 445
Ery-Tab Tablets (Erythromycin) Abbott 447
Erythrocin Stearate Filmtab Tablets (Erythromycin Stearate) Abbott 452
Erythromycin Base Filmtab Tablets (Erythromycin) Abbott 454
Erythromycin Delayed-Release Capsules, USP (Erythromycin) Abbott 456
PCE Dispertab Tablets (Erythromycin) Abbott 510

Chlamydia trachomatis urogenital infections during pregnancy
E.E.S. (Erythromycin Ethylsuccinate) Abbott 449
EryPed (Erythromycin Ethylsuccinate) Abbott 445
Ery-Tab Tablets (Erythromycin) Abbott 447
Erythrocin Stearate Filmtab Tablets (Erythromycin Stearate) Abbott 452
Erythromycin Base Filmtab Tablets (Erythromycin) Abbott 454
Erythromycin Delayed-Release Capsules, USP (Erythromycin) Abbott 456
PCE Dispertab Tablets (Erythromycin) Abbott 510

Chloasma
(*see under* Hyperpigmentation, skin, bleaching of)

Cholangitis
(*see under* Infections, intra-abdominal)

Cholecystitis, acute
(*see under* Infections, intra-abdominal)

Cholesterol levels, elevated
(*see under* Hypercholesterolemia, primary, adjunct to diet)

Chorioretinitis
Decadron Phosphate Injection (Dexamethasone Sodium Phosphate) Merck 1931
Depo-Medrol Injectable Suspension (Methylprednisolone Acetate) Pharmacia & Upjohn 2615
Hydrocortone Tablets (Hydrocortisone) Merck 1963
Pediapred Oral Solution (Prednisolone Sodium Phosphate) UCB 3319

Choroidal neovascularization, secondary to macular degeneration
Visudyne for Injection (Verteporfin) Novartis 2286

Choroiditis
Decadron Phosphate Injection (Dexamethasone Sodium Phosphate) Merck 1931
Depo-Medrol Injectable Suspension (Methylprednisolone Acetate) Pharmacia & Upjohn 2615
Hydrocortone Tablets (Hydrocortisone) Merck 1963
Pediapred Oral Solution (Prednisolone Sodium Phosphate) UCB 3319

Christmas disease
(*see under* Hemophilia B)

Cirrhosis, biliary
Urso 250 Tablets (Ursodiol) Axcan Scandipharm 737
Urso Forte Tablets (Ursodiol) Axcan Scandipharm 737

Citrobacter diversus infections
Cipro I.V. (Ciprofloxacin) Schering 2998
Cipro I.V. Pharmacy Bulk Package (Ciprofloxacin) Bayer 3509
Cipro (Ciprofloxacin) Schering 2991

Citrobacter diversus urinary tract infections
Cipro I.V. (Ciprofloxacin) Schering 2998
Cipro I.V. Pharmacy Bulk Package (Ciprofloxacin) Bayer 3509
Cipro (Ciprofloxacin) Schering 2991

Citrobacter freundii infections
Cipro I.V. (Ciprofloxacin) Schering 2998
Cipro I.V. Pharmacy Bulk Package (Ciprofloxacin) Bayer 3509
Cipro (Ciprofloxacin) Schering 2991
Noroxin Tablets (Norfloxacin) Merck 2009
Tygacil (Tigecycline) Wyeth 3489

Citrobacter freundii skin and skin structure infections
Cipro I.V. (Ciprofloxacin) Schering 2998
Cipro I.V. Pharmacy Bulk Package (Ciprofloxacin) Bayer 3509
Cipro (Ciprofloxacin) Schering 2991

Citrobacter freundii urinary tract infections
Cipro I.V. (Ciprofloxacin) Schering 2998
Cipro I.V. Pharmacy Bulk Package (Ciprofloxacin) Bayer 3509
Cipro (Ciprofloxacin) Schering 2991
Noroxin Tablets (Norfloxacin) Merck 2009

Citrobacter species infections
- Fortaz (Ceftazidime Sodium) GlaxoSmithKline ... 1422
- Garamycin Injectable (Gentamicin Sulfate) Schering ... 3028
- Primaxin I.M. (Cilastatin Sodium, Imipenem) Merck ... 2022
- Primaxin I.V. (Cilastatin Sodium, Imipenem) Merck ... 2024
- Timentin ADD-Vantage (Clavulanate Potassium, Ticarcillin Disodium) GlaxoSmithKline ... 1556
- Timentin Injection Galaxy Container (Clavulanate Potassium, Ticarcillin Disodium) GlaxoSmithKline ... 1559
- Timentin IV Infusion (Clavulanate Potassium, Ticarcillin Disodium) GlaxoSmithKline ... 1553
- Timentin Pharmacy Bulk Package (Clavulanate Potassium, Ticarcillin Disodium) GlaxoSmithKline ... 1562

Citrobacter species intra-abdominal infections
- Primaxin I.V. (Cilastatin Sodium, Imipenem) Merck ... 2024

Citrobacter species lower respiratory tract infections
- Fortaz (Ceftazidime Sodium) GlaxoSmithKline ... 1422

Citrobacter species skin and skin structure infections
- Primaxin I.M. (Cilastatin Sodium, Imipenem) Merck ... 2022
- Primaxin I.V. (Cilastatin Sodium, Imipenem) Merck ... 2024

Citrobacter species urinary tract infections
- Timentin ADD-Vantage (Clavulanate Potassium, Ticarcillin Disodium) GlaxoSmithKline ... 1556
- Timentin Injection Galaxy Container (Clavulanate Potassium, Ticarcillin Disodium) GlaxoSmithKline ... 1559
- Timentin IV Infusion (Clavulanate Potassium, Ticarcillin Disodium) GlaxoSmithKline ... 1553
- Timentin Pharmacy Bulk Package (Clavulanate Potassium, Ticarcillin Disodium) GlaxoSmithKline ... 1562

Claudication, intermittent
- Pletal Tablets (Cilostazol) Otsuka America ... 2478

Clonorchiasis
- Biltricide (Praziquantel) Schering ... 2990

Clostridium species gynecologic infections
- Mefoxin for Injection (Cefoxitin Sodium) Merck ... 1987
- Mefoxin Premixed Intravenous Solution (Cefoxitin Sodium) Merck ... 1990

Clostridium species infections
- Dynacin Tablets (Minocycline Hydrochloride) Medicis ... 1859
- Mefoxin for Injection (Cefoxitin Sodium) Merck ... 1987
- Mefoxin Premixed Intravenous Solution (Cefoxitin Sodium) Merck ... 1990
- Primaxin I.V. (Cilastatin Sodium, Imipenem) Merck ... 2024
- Rocephin Injectable Vials, ADD-Vantage, Galaxy, Bulk (Ceftriaxone Sodium) Roche Laboratories ... 2801

Clostridium species intra-abdominal infections
- Invanz for Injection (Ertapenem) Merck ... 1974
- Mefoxin for Injection (Cefoxitin Sodium) Merck ... 1987
- Mefoxin Premixed Intravenous Solution (Cefoxitin Sodium) Merck ... 1990
- Primaxin I.V. (Cilastatin Sodium, Imipenem) Merck ... 2024
- Rocephin Injectable Vials, ADD-Vantage, Galaxy, Bulk (Ceftriaxone Sodium) Roche Laboratories ... 2801

Clostridium species peritonitis
- Mefoxin for Injection (Cefoxitin Sodium) Merck ... 1987
- Mefoxin Premixed Intravenous Solution (Cefoxitin Sodium) Merck ... 1990

Clostridium species skin and skin structure infections
- Mefoxin for Injection (Cefoxitin Sodium) Merck ... 1987
- Mefoxin Premixed Intravenous Solution (Cefoxitin Sodium) Merck ... 1990

Cold, common, symptomatic relief of
(*see also under* Influenza syndrome, symptomatic relief of)
- Advil Allergy Sinus Caplets (Chlorpheniramine Maleate, Ibuprofen, Pseudoephedrine Hydrochloride) Wyeth ... ▣737
- Advil (Ibuprofen) Wyeth ... ▣737
- Children's Advil Suspension (Ibuprofen) Wyeth ... ▣742
- Children's Advil Chewable Tablets (Ibuprofen) Wyeth ... ▣741
- Advil Cold & Sinus (Ibuprofen, Pseudoephedrine Hydrochloride) Wyeth ... ▣739
- Advil Flu & Body Ache Caplets (Ibuprofen, Pseudoephedrine Hydrochloride) Wyeth ... ▣739
- Children's Advil Cold Suspension (Ibuprofen, Pseudoephedrine Hydrochloride) Wyeth ... ▣741
- Infants' Advil Concentrated Drops (Ibuprofen) Wyeth ... ▣743
- Advil Multi-Symptom Cold Caplets (Chlorpheniramine Maleate, Ibuprofen, Pseudoephedrine Hydrochloride) Wyeth ... ▣738
- BC Cold Powder (Aspirin, Chlorpheniramine Maleate, Pseudoephedrine Hydrochloride) GlaxoSmithKline ... ▣612
- Benadryl Allergy & Cold Tablets (Acetaminophen, Diphenhydramine Hydrochloride, Pseudoephedrine Hydrochloride) Pfizer Consumer Healthcare ... ▣692
- Benadryl Allergy & Sinus Headache Caplets & Gelcaps (Acetaminophen, Diphenhydramine Hydrochloride, Pseudoephedrine Hydrochloride) Pfizer Consumer Healthcare ... ▣693
- Children's Benadryl Allergy Liquid (Diphenhydramine Hydrochloride) Pfizer Consumer Healthcare ... ▣695
- Children's Benadryl Allergy & Cold Fastmelt Tablets (Diphenhydramine Citrate, Pseudoephedrine Hydrochloride) Pfizer Consumer Healthcare ... ▣695
- Benadryl Dye-Free Allergy Liqui-Gels Softgels (Diphenhydramine Hydrochloride) Pfizer Consumer Healthcare ... ▣692
- Children's Benadryl D Allergy & Sinus Fastmelt Tablets (Diphenhydramine Citrate, Pseudoephedrine Hydrochloride) Pfizer, Consumer Healthcare ... ▣694
- Children's Benadryl D Liquid Medication (Diphenhydramine Hydrochloride, Pseudoephedrine Hydrochloride) Pfizer Consumer Healthcare ... ▣693
- Benadryl D Tablets (Diphenhydramine Hydrochloride, Pseudoephedrine Hydrochloride) Pfizer Consumer Healthcare ... ▣694
- Children's Benadryl Allergy Fastmelt Tablets (Diphenhydramine Citrate) Pfizer Consumer Healthcare ... ▣696
- Claritin-D Non-Drowsy 12 Hour Tablets (Loratadine, Pseudoephedrine Sulfate) Schering-Plough ... ▣731
- Claritin-D Non-Drowsy 24 Hour Tablets (Loratadine, Pseudoephedrine Sulfate) Schering-Plough ... ▣731
- Contac Non-Drowsy 12 Hour Cold Caplets (Pseudoephedrine Hydrochloride) GlaxoSmithKline ... ▣614
- Contac Non-Drowsy Timed Release 12 Hour Cold Caplets (Pseudoephedrine Hydrochloride) GlaxoSmithKline ... ▣615
- Children's Dimetapp Cold & Allergy Elixir (Brompheniramine Maleate, Pseudoephedrine Hydrochloride) Wyeth ... ▣745
- Dimetapp Infant Drops Decongestant Plus Cough (Dextromethorphan Hydrobromide, Pseudoephedrine Hydrochloride) Wyeth ... ▣746
- Mucinex DM Tablets (Dextromethorphan Hydrobromide, Guaifenesin) Adams ... ▣602
- PediaCare Freezer Pops Long-Acting Cough-Glacier Grape and Polar Berry Blue (Dextromethorphan Hydrobromide) Pfizer Consumer Healthcare ... ▣706
- PediaCare Decongestant Infants' Drops (Pseudoephedrine Hydrochloride) Pfizer Consumer Healthcare ... ▣705
- PediaCare Long-Acting Cough Infant Drops (Dextromethorphan Hydrobromide) Pfizer Consumer Healthcare ... ▣705
- PediaCare Long-Acting Cough Plus Cold Liquid (Dextromethorphan Hydrobromide, Pseudoephedrine Hydrochloride) Pfizer Consumer Healthcare ... ▣704
- PediaCare Multi-Symptom Cold Liquid (Chlorpheniramine Maleate, Dextromethorphan Hydrobromide, Pseudoephedrine Hydrochloride) Pfizer Consumer Healthcare ... ▣704
- PediaCare NightRest Cough & Cold Liquid (Chlorpheniramine Maleate, Dextromethorphan Hydrobromide, Pseudoephedrine Hydrochloride) Pfizer Consumer Healthcare ... ▣704
- Robitussin PE Syrup (Guaifenesin, Pseudoephedrine Hydrochloride) Wyeth ... ▣753
- Simply Stuffy Liquid (Pseudoephedrine Hydrochloride) McNeil Consumer ... 1841
- Sudafed Nasal Decongestant Tablets (Pseudoephedrine Hydrochloride) Pfizer Consumer Healthcare ... ▣709
- Sudafed Non-Drowsy Severe Cold Tablets (Acetaminophen, Dextromethorphan Hydrobromide, Pseudoephedrine Hydrochloride) Pfizer Consumer Healthcare ... ▣710
- Sudafed PE Tablets (Phenylephrine Hydrochloride) Pfizer Consumer Healthcare ... ▣711
- Sudafed Sinus & Allergy Tablets (Chlorpheniramine Maleate, Pseudoephedrine Hydrochloride) Pfizer Consumer Healthcare ... ▣710
- TheraFlu Cold & Cough Hot Liquid (Acetaminophen, Chlorpheniramine Maleate, Dextromethorphan Hydrobromide, Pseudoephedrine Hydrochloride) Novartis Consumer ... ▣680
- TheraFlu Cold & Sore Throat Hot Liquid (Acetaminophen, Chlorpheniramine Maleate, Pseudoephedrine Hydrochloride) Novartis Consumer ... ▣680
- TheraFlu Flu & Chest Congestion Non-Drowsy Hot Liquid (Acetaminophen, Dextromethorphan Hydrobromide, Guaifenesin, Pseudoephedrine Hydrochloride) Novartis Consumer ... ▣681
- TheraFlu Flu & Sore Throat Hot Liquid (Acetaminophen, Chlorpheniramine Maleate, Pseudoephedrine Hydrochloride) Novartis Consumer ... ▣681
- TheraFlu Severe Cold Non-Drowsy Hot Liquid (Acetaminophen, Dextromethorphan Hydrobromide, Pseudoephedrine Hydrochloride) Novartis Consumer ... ▣683
- TheraFlu Severe Cold & Cough Hot Liquid (Acetaminophen, Chlorpheniramine Maleate, Dextromethorphan Hydrobromide, Pseudoephedrine Hydrochloride) Novartis Consumer ... ▣683
- TheraFlu Severe Cold Caplets (Acetaminophen, Chlorpheniramine Maleate, Dextromethorphan Hydrobromide, Pseudoephedrine Hydrochloride) Novartis Consumer ... ▣679
- TheraFlu Severe Cold Hot Liquid (Acetaminophen, Chlorpheniramine Maleate, Dextromethorphan Hydrobromide, Pseudoephedrine Hydrochloride) Novartis Consumer ... ▣682
- TheraFlu Severe Cold Non-Drowsy Caplets (Acetaminophen, Dextromethorphan Hydrobromide, Pseudoephedrine Hydrochloride) Novartis Consumer ... ▣679
- TheraFlu Thin Strips Multi Symptom (Diphenhydramine Hydrochloride) Novartis Consumer ... ▣684
- Triaminic Cold & Allergy Liquid (Chlorpheniramine Maleate, Pseudoephedrine Hydrochloride) Novartis Consumer ... ▣685
- Triaminic Allergy Runny Nose & Congestion Softchews (Chlorpheniramine Maleate, Pseudoephedrine Hydrochloride) Novartis Consumer ... ▣688
- Triaminic Thin Strips Cough & Runny Nose (Diphenhydramine Hydrochloride) Novartis Consumer ... ▣690
- Children's Tylenol Plus Cold & Allergy Suspension Liquid (Acetaminophen, Diphenhydramine Hydrochloride, Pseudoephedrine Hydrochloride) McNeil Consumer ... 1850
- Children's Tylenol Plus Cold NightTime Suspension Liquid (Acetaminophen, Chlorpheniramine Maleate, Pseudoephedrine Hydrochloride) McNeil Consumer ... 1851
- Children's Tylenol Plus Cold & Cough Suspension Liquid and Chewable Tablets (Acetaminophen, Chlorpheniramine Maleate, Dextromethorphan Hydrobromide, Pseudoephedrine Hydrochloride) McNeil Consumer ... 1851
- Children's Tylenol Plus Cold Chewable Tablets (Acetaminophen, Chlorpheniramine Maleate, Pseudoephedrine Hydrochloride) McNeil Consumer ... 1851
- Concentrated Tylenol Infants' Drops Plus Cold (Acetaminophen, Pseudoephedrine Hydrochloride) McNeil Consumer ... 1851
- Concentrated Tylenol Infants' Drops Plus Cold and Cough (Acetaminophen, Dextromethorphan Hydrobromide, Pseudoephedrine Hydrochloride) McNeil Consumer ... 1851
- Tylenol Cold Severe Congestion Non-Drowsy Caplets with Cool Burst (Acetaminophen, Dextromethorphan Hydrobromide, Guaifenesin, Pseudoephedrine Hydrochloride) McNeil Consumer ... 1846
- Vicks NyQuil Cough Liquid (Dextromethorphan Hydrobromide, Doxylamine Succinate) Procter & Gamble ... 2677
- Vicks NyQuil LiquiCaps/Liquid Multi-Symptom Cold/Flu Relief (Acetaminophen, Dextromethorphan Hydrobromide, Doxylamine Succinate, Pseudoephedrine Hydrochloride) Procter & Gamble ... ▣725
- Vicks Sinex 12-Hour Nasal Spray and Ultra Fine Mist for Sinus Relief (Oxymetazoline Hydrochloride) Procter & Gamble ... 2678
- Vicks Sinex Nasal Spray and Ultra Fine Mist for Sinus Relief (Phenylephrine Hydrochloride) Procter & Gamble ... 2677
- Vicks Vapor Inhaler (Levmetamfetamine) Procter & Gamble ... 2678

Zicam Cold Remedy Chewables (Zincum Aceticum, Zincum Gluconicum) Matrixx ▣ 665
Zicam Cold Remedy Nasal Pump (Zincum Gluconicum) Matrixx ▣ 665
Zicam Cold Remedy Oral Mist (Zincum Aceticum, Zincum Gluconicum) Matrixx ▣ 665
Zicam Cold Remedy RapidMelts (Zincum Aceticum, Zincum Gluconicum) Matrixx ▣ 665
Zicam Cold Remedy Swabs (Zincum Gluconicum) Matrixx ▣ 665
Zicam Cold Remedy Swabs Kids Size (Zincum Gluconicum) Matrixx ▣ 665
Zicam Concentrated Cough Mist for Kids Plus D Cool Cherry (Dextromethorphan Hydrobromide, Phenylephrine Hydrochloride) Matrixx ▣ 643
Zicam Concentrated Cough Mist Plus D Cool Cherry (Dextromethorphan Hydrobromide, Phenylephrine Hydrochloride) Matrixx ▣ 642
Zicam Extreme Congestion Relief Nasal Pump (Oxymetazoline Hydrochloride) Matrixx ▣ 666
Zicam Sinus Relief Nasal Pump (Oxymetazoline Hydrochloride) Matrixx ▣ 666

Cold sores
(*see under* Herpetic manifestations, oral, symptomatic relief of)

Colitis, mucous
(*see under* Bowel, irritable, syndrome)

Colitis, pseudomembranous, antibiotic-associated
Vancocin HCl Capsules, USP (Vancomycin Hydrochloride) ViroPharma 3370

Colitis, ulcerative
Asacol Delayed-Release Tablets (Mesalamine) Procter & Gamble Pharmaceuticals 2688
Colazal Capsules (Balsalazide Disodium) Salix 2845
Decadron Phosphate Injection (Dexamethasone Sodium Phosphate) Merck 1931
Decadron Tablets (Dexamethasone) Merck 1929
Depo-Medrol Injectable Suspension (Methylprednisolone Acetate) Pharmacia & Upjohn 2615
Depo-Medrol Single-Dose Vial (Methylprednisolone Acetate) Pharmacia & Upjohn 2617
Hydrocortone Tablets (Hydrocortisone) Merck 1963
Pediapred Oral Solution (Prednisolone Sodium Phosphate) UCB 3319
Pentasa Capsules (Mesalamine) Shire US 3182

Collagen disease
Decadron Phosphate Injection (Dexamethasone Sodium Phosphate) Merck 1931
Depo-Medrol Injectable Suspension (Methylprednisolone Acetate) Pharmacia & Upjohn 2615
Hydrocortone Tablets (Hydrocortisone) Merck 1963
Pediapred Oral Solution (Prednisolone Sodium Phosphate) UCB 3319

Colon, irritable
(*see under* Bowel, irritable, syndrome)

Colon, spastic
(*see under* Bowel, irritable, syndrome)

Colorectal polyps, adenomatous
Celebrex Capsules (Celecoxib) Searle 3130

Condylomata acuminata
Aldara Cream, 5% (Imiquimod) 3M 1814
Alferon N Injection (Interferon alfa-N3 (Human Leukocyte Derived)) Hemispherx 1640
Intron A for Injection (Interferon alfa-2b, Recombinant) Schering 3038

Congestive heart failure, adjunct in
(*see also under* Edema, adjunctive therapy in)
BiDil Tablets (Hydralazine Hydrochloride, Isosorbide Dinitrate) Nitromed 2161
Captopril Tablets (Captopril) Mylan 2114
Coreg Tablets (Carvedilol) GlaxoSmithKline 1376
Diuril Oral (Chlorothiazide) Merck 1936
Diuril Sodium Intravenous (Chlorothiazide Sodium) Merck 1934
Dyrenium Capsules (Triamterene) WellSpring 3390
Edecrin (Ethacrynic Acid) Merck 1941
Furosemide Tablets (Furosemide) Mylan 2117
Indapamide Tablets (Indapamide) Mylan 2119
Lanoxicaps Capsules (Digoxin) GlaxoSmithKline 1458
Lanoxin Injection (Digoxin) GlaxoSmithKline 1462
Lanoxin Tablets (Digoxin) GlaxoSmithKline 1468
Lanoxin Injection Pediatric (Digoxin) GlaxoSmithKline 1465
Midamor Tablets (Amiloride Hydrochloride) Merck 2000
Moduretic Tablets (Amiloride Hydrochloride, Hydrochlorothiazide) Merck 2003
Natrecor for Injection (Nesiritide) Scios Inc. 3123
Prinivil Tablets (Lisinopril) Merck 2029
Zestril Tablets (Lisinopril) AstraZeneca 704

Congestive heart failure, post-myocardial infarction
Altace Capsules (Ramipril) King 1673
Inspra Tablets (Eplerenone) Pfizer 2520
Mavik Tablets (Trandolapril) Abbott 482

Conjunctival inflammation, bulbar, steroid-responsive
Blephamide (Prednisolone Acetate, Sulfacetamide Sodium) Allergan 563

Conjunctivitis, allergic
Alamast Ophthalmic Solution (Pemirolast Potassium) Vistakon 3371
Alrex Ophthalmic Suspension 0.2% (Loteprednol Etabonate) Bausch & Lomb ⊙ 243
Decadron Phosphate Injection (Dexamethasone Sodium Phosphate) Merck 1931
Depo-Medrol Injectable Suspension (Methylprednisolone Acetate) Pharmacia & Upjohn 2615
Elestat Ophthalmic Solution (Epinastine Hydrochloride) Ispire 1643
Emadine Ophthalmic Solution Alcon
HMS Sterile Ophthalmic Suspension (Medrysone) Allergan ⊙ 228
Hydrocortone Tablets (Hydrocortisone) Merck 1963
Optivar Ophthalmic Solution (Azelastine Hydrochloride) MedPointe 1877
Patanol Ophthalmic Solution (Olopatadine Hydrochloride) Alcon 557
Pediapred Oral Solution (Prednisolone Sodium Phosphate) UCB 3319
Phenergan (Promethazine Hydrochloride) Wyeth 3438
Zaditor Ophthalmic Solution (Ketotifen Fumarate) Novartis 2302
Zylet Ophthalmic Suspension (Loteprednol Etabonate, Tobramycin) Bausch & Lomb 3508

Conjunctivitis, bacterial
Ciloxan Ophthalmic Ointment (Ciprofloxacin Hydrochloride) Alcon 554
Polytrim Ophthalmic Solution (Polymyxin B Sulfate, Trimethoprim Sulfate) Allergan 570
Quixin Ophthalmic Solution (Levofloxacin) Vistakon 3373
Vigamox Ophthalmic Solution (Moxifloxacin Hydrochloride) Alcon 560

Conjunctivitis, fungal
Natacyn Antifungal Ophthalmic Suspension (Natamycin) Alcon ⊙ 207

Conjunctivitis, granular
(*see under* Trachoma)

Conjunctivitis, inclusion
Dynacin Tablets (Minocycline Hydrochloride) Medicis 1859

Conjunctivitis, infective
Blephamide Ophthalmic Ointment (Prednisolone Acetate, Sulfacetamide Sodium) Allergan 563
Blephamide Ophthalmic Suspension (Prednisolone Acetate, Sulfacetamide Sodium) Allergan 564
FML-S Liquifilm Sterile Ophthalmic Suspension (Fluorometholone, Sulfacetamide Sodium) Allergan ⊙ 226
Poly-Pred Liquifilm Ophthalmic Suspension (Neomycin Sulfate, Polymyxin B Sulfate, Prednisolone Acetate) Allergan ⊙ 231
Pred-G Ophthalmic Suspension (Gentamicin Sulfate, Prednisolone Acetate) Allergan ⊙ 234
Pred-G Sterile Ophthalmic Ointment (Gentamicin Sulfate, Prednisolone Acetate) Allergan ⊙ 235
TobraDex Ophthalmic Ointment (Dexamethasone, Tobramycin) Alcon 558
TobraDex Ophthalmic Suspension (Dexamethasone, Tobramycin) Alcon 558
Zylet Ophthalmic Suspension (Loteprednol Etabonate, Tobramycin) Bausch & Lomb 3508

Conjunctivitis, neonatal
Ery-Tab Tablets (Erythromycin) Abbott 447
Erythrocin Stearate Filmtab Tablets (Erythromycin Stearate) Abbott 452
Erythromycin Base Filmtab Tablets (Erythromycin) Abbott 454
Erythromycin Delayed-Release Capsules, USP (Erythromycin) Abbott 456
PCE Dispertab Tablets (Erythromycin) Abbott 510

Conjunctivitis, unspecified
Bleph-10 Ophthalmic Solution 10% (Sulfacetamide Sodium) Allergan ⊙ 219
Genoptic Sterile Ophthalmic Solution (Gentamicin Sulfate) Allergan ⊙ 227
Pred Mild Sterile Ophthalmic Suspension (Prednisolone Acetate) Allergan ⊙ 236

Conjunctivitis, vernal
Crolom Cromolyn Sodium Sterile Ophthalmic Solution USP 4% (Cromolyn Sodium) Bausch & Lomb ⊙ 248
HMS Sterile Ophthalmic Suspension (Medrysone) Allergan ⊙ 228

Constipation
Colace Capsules 50 mg (Docusate Sodium) Purdue Products 2715
Colace Capsules 100 mg (Docusate Sodium) Purdue Products 2715
Colace Glycerin Suppositories, USP 1.2 grams - Infants and Children (Glycerin) Purdue Products 2715
Colace Glycerin Suppositories, USP 2.1 grams - Adults and Children (Glycerin) Purdue Products 2716
Colace Liquid 1% Solution (Docusate Sodium) Purdue Products 2716
Colace Syrup (Docusate Sodium) Purdue Products 2716
Dulcolax Stool Softener (Docusate Sodium) Boehringer Ingelheim ▣ 608
Kaopectate Stool Softener (Docusate Calcium) Pfizer Consumer Healthcare ▣ 702
Metamucil Capsules (Psyllium Preparations) Procter & Gamble ▣ 717
Mineral Oil (Mineral Oil) Purdue Products 2716
Peri-Colace Tablets (Docusate Sodium, Senna) Purdue Products ▣ 730

Constipation, chronic
Kristalose for Oral Solution (Lactulose) Mylan Bertek 2149
Metamucil Capsules (Psyllium Preparations) Procter & Gamble 2672
Metamucil (Psyllium Preparations) Procter & Gamble 2672
Senokot Tablets (Senna) Purdue Products 2717
Senokot-S Tablets (Docusate Sodium, Senna) Purdue Products 2717

Constipation, chronic idiopathic
Zelnorm Tablets (Tegaserod maleate) Novartis 2303

Constipation, temporary
Ceo-Two Evacuant Suppository (Potassium Bitartrate, Sodium Bicarbonate) Beutlich ▣ 607
Citrucel Caplets (Methylcellulose) GlaxoSmithKline ▣ 614
Citrucel Orange Flavor Powder (Methylcellulose) GlaxoSmithKline ▣ 613
Citrucel Sugar Free Orange Flavor Powder (Methylcellulose) GlaxoSmithKline ▣ 613
Dulcolax Suppositories (Bisacodyl) Boehringer Ingelheim ▣ 608
Dulcolax Tablets (Bisacodyl) Boehringer Ingelheim ▣ 607
Ex•Lax Chocolated Laxative Pieces (Sennosides) Novartis Consumer ▣ 674
Ex•Lax Regular Strength Pills (Sennosides) Novartis Consumer ▣ 674
Ex•Lax Maximum Strength Pills (Sennosides) Novartis Consumer ▣ 674
FiberCon Caplets (Calcium Polycarbophil) Wyeth ▣ 747
Fleet Bisacodyl Laxatives (Bisacodyl) Fleet 1169
Fleet Enema (Sodium Phosphate) Fleet 1169
Fleet Glycerin Laxatives (Glycerin) Fleet 1168
Fleet Mineral Oil Enema (Mineral Oil) Fleet 1170
Fleet Phospho-soda (Sodium Phosphate) Fleet 1170
Perdiem Overnight Relief Pills (Calcium, Sennosides) Novartis Consumer 2166
Peri-Colace Tablets (Sennosides, Docusate Sodium) Purdue Products 2716
Senokot Tablets (Senna) Purdue Products 2717
Senokot-S Tablets (Docusate Sodium, Senna) Purdue Products 2717

Contact lenses, fitting of, adjunct in
Fluor-I-Strip A.T. Ophthalmic Strips 1 mg (Fluorescein Sodium) Bausch & Lomb ⊙ 249
Fluor-I-Strip Ophthalmic Strips 9 mg (Fluorescein Sodium) Bausch & Lomb ⊙ 249

Contraception
(*see under* Pregnancy, prevention of)

Convulsive disorders, adjunctive therapy in
Valium Tablets (Diazepam) Roche Laboratories 2822

Convulsive episodes, control of
Nembutal Sodium Solution, USP (Pentobarbital Sodium) Ovation 2484

Corneal erosions, recurrent
Lacrisert Sterile Ophthalmic Insert (Hydroxypropyl Cellulose) Merck 1979

Corneal inflammation, steroid-responsive
Blephamide Ophthalmic Ointment (Prednisolone Acetate, Sulfacetamide Sodium) Allergan 563
Blephamide Ophthalmic Suspension (Prednisolone Acetate, Sulfacetamide Sodium) Allergan 564
FML Ophthalmic Ointment (Fluorometholone) Allergan ⊙ 225
FML Ophthalmic Suspension (Fluorometholone) Allergan ⊙ 224

FML Forte Ophthalmic Suspension (Fluorometholone) Allergan .... ⊙ 223
FML-S Liquifilm Sterile Ophthalmic Suspension (Fluorometholone, Sulfacetamide Sodium) Allergan ... ⊙ 226
Lotemax Ophthalmic Suspension 0.5% (Loteprednol Etabonate) Bausch & Lomb .... ⊙ 249
Poly-Pred Liquifilm Ophthalmic Suspension (Neomycin Sulfate, Polymyxin B Sulfate, Prednisolone Acetate) Allergan .... ⊙ 231
Pred Forte Ophthalmic Suspension (Prednisolone Acetate) Allergan .... ⊙ 233
Pred-G Ophthalmic Suspension (Gentamicin Sulfate, Prednisolone Acetate) Allergan .... ⊙ 234
Pred-G Sterile Ophthalmic Ointment (Gentamicin Sulfate, Prednisolone Acetate) Allergan .... ⊙ 235
TobraDex Ophthalmic Ointment (Dexamethasone, Tobramycin) Alcon 558
TobraDex Ophthalmic Suspension (Dexamethasone, Tobramycin) Alcon 558
Zylet Ophthalmic Suspension (Loteprednol Etabonate, Tobramycin) Bausch & Lomb 3508

Corneal injury, chemical
Blephamide Ophthalmic Ointment (Prednisolone Acetate, Sulfacetamide Sodium) Allergan 563
Blephamide Ophthalmic Suspension (Prednisolone Acetate, Sulfacetamide Sodium) Allergan 564
FML-S Liquifilm Sterile Ophthalmic Suspension (Fluorometholone, Sulfacetamide Sodium) Allergan ... ⊙ 226
Poly-Pred Liquifilm Ophthalmic Suspension (Neomycin Sulfate, Polymyxin B Sulfate, Prednisolone Acetate) Allergan .... ⊙ 231
Pred Mild Sterile Ophthalmic Suspension (Prednisolone Acetate) Allergan .... ⊙ 236
Pred-G Ophthalmic Suspension (Gentamicin Sulfate, Prednisolone Acetate) Allergan .... ⊙ 234
Pred-G Sterile Ophthalmic Ointment (Gentamicin Sulfate, Prednisolone Acetate) Allergan .... ⊙ 235
TobraDex Ophthalmic Ointment (Dexamethasone, Tobramycin) Alcon 558
TobraDex Ophthalmic Suspension (Dexamethasone, Tobramycin) Alcon 558
Zylet Ophthalmic Suspension (Loteprednol Etabonate, Tobramycin) Bausch & Lomb 3508

Corneal injury, foreign bodies
Blephamide Ophthalmic Ointment (Prednisolone Acetate, Sulfacetamide Sodium) Allergan 563
Blephamide Ophthalmic Suspension (Prednisolone Acetate, Sulfacetamide Sodium) Allergan 564
FML-S Liquifilm Sterile Ophthalmic Suspension (Fluorometholone, Sulfacetamide Sodium) Allergan ... ⊙ 226
Poly-Pred Liquifilm Ophthalmic Suspension (Neomycin Sulfate, Polymyxin B Sulfate, Prednisolone Acetate) Allergan .... ⊙ 231
Pred-G Ophthalmic Suspension (Gentamicin Sulfate, Prednisolone Acetate) Allergan .... ⊙ 234
Pred-G Sterile Ophthalmic Ointment (Gentamicin Sulfate, Prednisolone Acetate) Allergan .... ⊙ 235
TobraDex Ophthalmic Ointment (Dexamethasone, Tobramycin) Alcon 558
TobraDex Ophthalmic Suspension (Dexamethasone, Tobramycin) Alcon 558
Zylet Ophthalmic Suspension (Loteprednol Etabonate, Tobramycin) Bausch & Lomb 3508

Corneal injury, radiation
Blephamide Ophthalmic Ointment (Prednisolone Acetate, Sulfacetamide Sodium) Allergan 563
Blephamide Ophthalmic Suspension (Prednisolone Acetate, Sulfacetamide Sodium) Allergan 564
FML-S Liquifilm Sterile Ophthalmic Suspension (Fluorometholone, Sulfacetamide Sodium) Allergan ... ⊙ 226
Poly-Pred Liquifilm Ophthalmic Suspension (Neomycin Sulfate, Polymyxin B Sulfate, Prednisolone Acetate) Allergan .... ⊙ 231
Pred-G Ophthalmic Suspension (Gentamicin Sulfate, Prednisolone Acetate) Allergan .... ⊙ 234
Pred-G Sterile Ophthalmic Ointment (Gentamicin Sulfate, Prednisolone Acetate) Allergan .... ⊙ 235
TobraDex Ophthalmic Ointment (Dexamethasone, Tobramycin) Alcon 558
TobraDex Ophthalmic Suspension (Dexamethasone, Tobramycin) Alcon 558
Zylet Ophthalmic Suspension (Loteprednol Etabonate, Tobramycin) Bausch & Lomb 3508

Corneal injury, thermal burns
Blephamide Ophthalmic Ointment (Prednisolone Acetate, Sulfacetamide Sodium) Allergan 563
Blephamide Ophthalmic Suspension (Prednisolone Acetate, Sulfacetamide Sodium) Allergan 564
FML-S Liquifilm Sterile Ophthalmic Suspension (Fluorometholone, Sulfacetamide Sodium) Allergan ... ⊙ 226
Poly-Pred Liquifilm Ophthalmic Suspension (Neomycin Sulfate, Polymyxin B Sulfate, Prednisolone Acetate) Allergan .... ⊙ 231
Pred Mild Sterile Ophthalmic Suspension (Prednisolone Acetate) Allergan .... ⊙ 236
Pred-G Ophthalmic Suspension (Gentamicin Sulfate, Prednisolone Acetate) Allergan .... ⊙ 234
Pred-G Sterile Ophthalmic Ointment (Gentamicin Sulfate, Prednisolone Acetate) Allergan .... ⊙ 235
TobraDex Ophthalmic Ointment (Dexamethasone, Tobramycin) Alcon 558
TobraDex Ophthalmic Suspension (Dexamethasone, Tobramycin) Alcon 558
Zylet Ophthalmic Suspension (Loteprednol Etabonate, Tobramycin) Bausch & Lomb 3508

Corneal marginal ulcers, allergic
Decadron Phosphate Injection (Dexamethasone Sodium Phosphate) Merck 1931
Depo-Medrol Injectable Suspension (Methylprednisolone Acetate) Pharmacia & Upjohn 2615
Hydrocortone Tablets (Hydrocortisone) Merck 1963
Pediapred Oral Solution (Prednisolone Sodium Phosphate) UCB 3319

Corneal sensitivity, decreased
Lacrisert Sterile Ophthalmic Insert (Hydroxypropyl Cellulose) Merck ... 1979

Corneal ulcers
Bleph-10 Ophthalmic Solution 10% (Sulfacetamide Sodium) Allergan .. ⊙ 219
Ciloxan Ophthalmic Ointment (Ciprofloxacin Hydrochloride) Alcon 554
Genoptic Sterile Ophthalmic Solution (Gentamicin Sulfate) Allergan .... ⊙ 227

Corns
(*see under* Hyperkeratosis skin disorders)

Coronary angioplasty or atherectomy, percutaneous transluminal, adjunct in
Angiomax for Injection (Bivalirudin) The Medicines Company 1856
ReoPro Vials (Abciximab) Lilly 1779

Coronary artery disease, reducing the risk of
Aceon Tablets (2 mg, 4 mg, 8 mg) (Perindopril Erbumine) Solvay 3191
Altoprev Extended-Release Tablets (Lovastatin) First Horizon 1151
Metamucil Dietary Fiber Supplement (Psyllium Preparations) Procter & Gamble .... ▣ 774
Mevacor Tablets (Lovastatin) Merck .. 1996
Zocor Tablets (Simvastatin) Merck 2078

Coronary atherosclerosis, to slow the progression of
(*see also under* Coronary artery disease, reducing the risk of)
Altoprev Extended-Release Tablets (Lovastatin) First Horizon 1151
Lescol Capsules (Fluvastatin Sodium) Novartis 2227
Lescol Capsules (Fluvastatin Sodium) Reliant 2730
Lescol XL Tablets (Fluvastatin Sodium) Novartis 2227
Lescol XL Tablets (Fluvastatin Sodium) Reliant 2730
Mevacor Tablets (Lovastatin) Merck . 1996
Niaspan Extended-Release Tablets (Niacin) Kos 1703
Pravachol (Pravastatin Sodium) Bristol-Myers Squibb 943

Coronary syndrome, acute
(*see also under* Cardiac ischemic complications, acute, prevention of, adjunct to PTCA; Coronary angioplasty or atherectomy, percutaneous transluminal, adjunct in)
Aggrastat (Tirofiban Hydrochloride) Merck 1878
Ecotrin Enteric Coated Aspirin Low, Regular and Maximum Strength Tablets (Aspirin) GlaxoSmithKline Consumer 1627
Fragmin Injection (Dalteparin Sodium) Pharmacia & Upjohn 2638
Integrilin Injection (Eptifibatide) Schering 3034
Lovenox Injection (Enoxaparin Sodium) Sanofi-Aventis 2931
Plavix Tablets (Clopidogrel Bisulfate) Bristol-Myers Squibb 940
Plavix Tablets (Clopidogrel Bisulfate) Sanofi-Aventis 2942
St. Joseph 81 mg Aspirin Chewable and Enteric Coated Tablets (Aspirin) McNeil Consumer 1841

Corynebacterium diphtheriae
(*see under* C. diphtheriae infections)

Corynebacterium infections, ocular
Vigamox Ophthalmic Solution (Moxifloxacin Hydrochloride) Alcon 560

Corynebacterium infections, unspecified
Vigamox Ophthalmic Solution (Moxifloxacin Hydrochloride) Alcon .... ⊙ 212

Corynebacterium minutissimum
(*see under* C. minutissimum infections)

Corynebacterium vaginitis
Metrogel 1% (Metronidazole) Galderma 1212
MetroGel-Vaginal Gel (Metronidazole) 3M 1822

Coryza, acute
(*see under* Cold, common, symptomatic relief of)

Cough, symptomatic relief of
Children's Benadryl Allergy Liquid (Diphenhydramine Hydrochloride) Pfizer Consumer Healthcare .... ▣ 695
Delsym Extended-Release Suspension (Dextromethorphan Polistirex) Celltech .... ▣ 611
Delsym 12 Hour Cough Suppressant for Children (Dextromethorphan Polistirex) Celltech .... ▣ 611
Children's Dimetapp Long Acting Cough Plus Cold Syrup (Dextromethorphan Hydrobromide, Pseudoephedrine Hydrochloride) Wyeth .... ▣ 746
Halls Mentho-Lyptus Drops (Menthol) Cadbury Adams .... ▣ 609
Halls Sugar Free (Menthol) Cadbury Adams .... ▣ 610
Halls Plus Cough Drops (Menthol, Pectin) Cadbury Adams .... ▣ 609
Hycodan (Homatropine Methylbromide, Hydrocodone Bitartrate) Endo Labs 1104
Hycotuss Expectorant Syrup (Guaifenesin, Hydrocodone Bitartrate) Endo Labs 1106
Mucinex DM Tablets (Dextromethorphan Hydrobromide, Guaifenesin) Adams .... ▣ 602
PediaCare Freezer Pops Long-Acting Cough-Glacier Grape and Polar Berry Blue (Dextromethorphan Hydrobromide) Pfizer Consumer Healthcare .... ▣ 706
PediaCare Long-Acting Cough Infant Drops (Dextromethorphan Hydrobromide) Pfizer Consumer Healthcare .... ▣ 705
PediaCare Long-Acting Cough Plus Cold Liquid (Dextromethorphan Hydrobromide, Pseudoephedrine Hydrochloride) Pfizer Consumer Healthcare .... ▣ 704
PediaCare Multi-Symptom Cold Liquid (Chlorpheniramine Maleate, Dextromethorphan Hydrobromide, Pseudoephedrine Hydrochloride) Pfizer Consumer Healthcare .... ▣ 704
PediaCare NightRest Cough & Cold Liquid (Chlorpheniramine Maleate, Dextromethorphan Hydrobromide, Pseudoephedrine Hydrochloride) Pfizer Consumer Healthcare .... ▣ 704
Robitussin Cough Drops (Menthol) Wyeth .... ▣ 751
Robitussin DM Infant Drops (Dextromethorphan Hydrobromide, Guaifenesin) Wyeth .... ▣ 753
Robitussin DM Liquid (Dextromethorphan Hydrobromide, Guaifenesin) Wyeth .... ▣ 753
Robitussin Honey Cough Drops (Menthol) Wyeth .... ▣ 752
Robitussin Maximum Strength Cough Liquid (Dextromethorphan Hydrobromide) Wyeth .... ▣ 754
Robitussin Pediatric Cough Liquid (Dextromethorphan Hydrobromide) Wyeth .... ▣ 754
Robitussin Pediatric Cough & Cold Liquid (Dextromethorphan Hydrobromide, Pseudoephedrine Hydrochloride) Wyeth .... ▣ 754
Robitussin Sugar Free Cough Liquid (Dextromethorphan Hydrobromide, Guaifenesin) Wyeth .... ▣ 753
Robitussin Sugar Free Throat Drops (Menthol) Wyeth .... ▣ 754
Simply Cough Liquid (Dextromethorphan Hydrobromide) McNeil Consumer 1840
Tessalon Capsules (Benzonatate) Forest 1202
Tessalon Perles (Benzonatate) Forest 1202
TheraFlu Cold & Cough Hot Liquid (Acetaminophen, Chlorpheniramine Maleate, Dextromethorphan Hydrobromide, Pseudoephedrine Hydrochloride) Novartis Consumer .... ▣ 680
TheraFlu Severe Cold Non-Drowsy Hot Liquid (Acetaminophen, Dextromethorphan Hydrobromide, Pseudoephedrine Hydrochloride) Novartis Consumer .... ▣ 683
TheraFlu Severe Cold & Cough Hot Liquid (Acetaminophen, Chlorpheniramine Maleate, Dextromethorphan Hydrobromide, Pseudoephedrine Hydrochloride) Novartis Consumer .... ▣ 683

TheraFlu Severe Cold Caplets (Acetaminophen, Chlorpheniramine Maleate, Dextromethorphan Hydrobromide, Pseudoephedrine Hydrochloride) Novartis Consumer ▣ 679
TheraFlu Severe Cold Hot Liquid (Acetaminophen, Chlorpheniramine Maleate, Dextromethorphan Hydrobromide, Pseudoephedrine Hydrochloride) Novartis Consumer ▣ 682
TheraFlu Severe Cold Non-Drowsy Caplets (Acetaminophen, Dextromethorphan Hydrobromide, Pseudoephedrine Hydrochloride) Novartis Consumer ▣ 679
TheraFlu Thin Strips Long Acting Cough (Dextromethorphan Hydrobromide) Novartis Consumer ▣ 684
TheraFlu Thin Strips Multi Symptom (Diphenhydramine Hydrochloride) Novartis Consumer ▣ 684
Triaminic Cough Liquid (Dextromethorphan Hydrobromide, Pseudoephedrine Hydrochloride) Novartis Consumer ▣ 687
Triaminic Cough & Nasal Congestion Liquid (Dextromethorphan Hydrobromide, Pseudoephedrine Hydrochloride) Novartis Consumer ▣ 687
Triaminic Cough & Sore Throat Liquid (Acetaminophen, Dextromethorphan Hydrobromide, Pseudoephedrine Hydrochloride) Novartis Consumer ▣ 687
Triaminic Cough & Sore Throat Softchews (Acetaminophen, Dextromethorphan Hydrobromide, Pseudoephedrine Hydrochloride) Novartis Consumer ▣ 689
Triaminic Thin Strips Cough & Runny Nose (Diphenhydramine Hydrochloride) Novartis Consumer ▣ 690
Triaminic Thin Strips Long Acting Cough (Dextromethorphan Hydrobromide) Novartis Consumer ▣ 689
Tussionex Pennkinetic Extended-Release Suspension (Chlorpheniramine Polistirex, Hydrocodone Polistirex) UCB 3322
Tylenol Cough & Sore Throat Daytime Liquid with Cool Burst (Acetaminophen, Dextromethorphan Hydrobromide) McNeil Consumer ▣ 664
Tylenol Cough & Sore Throat NightTime Liquid with Cool Burst (Acetaminophen, Dextromethorphan Hydrobromide, Doxylamine Succinate) McNeil Consumer ▣ 664
Tylenol Cold & Flu Severe Daytime Liquid with Cool Bust (Acetaminophen, Dextromethorphan Hydrobromide, Pseudoephedrine Hydrochloride) McNeil Consumer 1846
Tylenol Cold & Flu Severe NightTime Liquid with Cool Burst (Acetaminophen, Dextromethorphan Hydrobromide, Doxylamine Succinate, Pseudoephedrine Hydrochloride) McNeil Consumer 1846
Tylenol Cough & Sore Throat Daytime Liquid with Cool Burst (Acetaminophen, Dextromethorphan Hydrobromide) McNeil Consumer 1849
Tylenol Cough & Sore Throat NightTime Liquid with Cool Burst (Acetaminophen, Dextromethorphan Hydrobromide, Doxylamine Succinate) McNeil Consumer 1849
Tylenol Flu Day Non-Drowsy Gelcaps (Acetaminophen, Dextromethorphan Hydrobromide, Pseudoephedrine Hydrochloride) McNeil Consumer 1846
Vicks 44 Cough Relief (Dextromethorphan Hydrobromide) Procter & Gamble 2675
Vicks 44E Cough & Chest Congestion Relief (Dextromethorphan Hydrobromide, Guaifenesin) Procter & Gamble 2676
Pediatric Vicks 44e Cough & Chest Congestion Relief Liquid (Dextromethorphan Hydrobromide, Guaifenesin) Procter & Gamble 2673
Vicks Cough Drops, Menthol & Cherry Flavors (Menthol) Procter & Gamble 2675
Vicks NyQuil Cough Liquid (Dextromethorphan Hydrobromide, Doxylamine Succinate) Procter & Gamble 2677
Zicam Concentrated Cough Mist for Kids Cool Cherry (Dextromethorphan Hydrobromide) Matrixx ▣ 643
Zicam Concentrated Cough Mist for Kids Plus D Cool Cherry (Dextromethorphan Hydrobromide, Phenylephrine Hydrochloride) Matrixx ▣ 643
Zicam Concentrated Cough Mist Nite-Cool Cherry (Dextromethorphan Hydrobromide) Matrixx ▣ 642
Zicam Concentrated Cough Mist Plus D Cool Cherry (Dextromethorphan Hydrobromide, Phenylephrine Hydrochloride) Matrixx ▣ 642
Zicam Concentrated Cough Mist-Honey Lemon & Cool Cherry (Dextromethorphan Hydrobromide) Matrixx ▣ 642

Cough, whooping

(*see under* Pertussis)

Cough and nasal congestion, symptomatic relief of

Alacol DM Syrup (Brompheniramine Maleate, Dextromethorphan Hydrobromide, Phenylephrine Hydrochloride) Ballay 739
Balamine DM (Carbinoxamine Maleate, Dextromethorphan Hydrobromide, Pseudoephedrine Hydrochloride) Ballay 739
Children's Benadryl Allergy & Cold Fastmelt Tablets (Diphenhydramine Citrate, Pseudoephedrine Hydrochloride) Pfizer Consumer Healthcare ▣ 695
Contac Severe Cold and Flu Caplets Maximum Strength (Acetaminophen, Chlorpheniramine Maleate, Dextromethorphan Hydrobromide, Pseudoephedrine Hydrochloride) GlaxoSmithKline ▣ 615
Contac Severe Cold and Flu Caplets Non-Drowsy (Acetaminophen, Dextromethorphan Hydrobromide, Pseudoephedrine Hydrochloride) GlaxoSmithKline ▣ 615
Children's Dimetapp DM Cold & Cough Elixir (Brompheniramine Maleate, Dextromethorphan Hydrobromide, Pseudoephedrine Hydrochloride) Wyeth ▣ 745
Dimetapp Infant Drops Decongestant Plus Cough (Dextromethorphan Hydrobromide, Pseudoephedrine Hydrochloride) Wyeth ▣ 746
Hycomine Compound Tablets (Acetaminophen, Caffeine, Chlorpheniramine Maleate, Hydrocodone Bitartrate, Phenylephrine Hydrochloride) Endo Labs 1105
PediaCare Decongestant & Cough Infant Drops (Dextromethorphan Hydrobromide, Pseudoephedrine Hydrochloride) Pfizer Consumer Healthcare ▣ 705
PediaCare Long-Acting Cough Plus Cold Liquid (Dextromethorphan Hydrobromide, Pseudoephedrine Hydrochloride) Pfizer Consumer Healthcare ▣ 704
PediaCare Multi-Symptom Cold Liquid (Chlorpheniramine Maleate, Dextromethorphan Hydrobromide, Pseudoephedrine Hydrochloride) Pfizer Consumer Healthcare ▣ 704
PediaCare NightRest Cough & Cold Liquid (Chlorpheniramine Maleate, Dextromethorphan Hydrobromide, Pseudoephedrine Hydrochloride) Pfizer Consumer Healthcare ▣ 704
Robitussin Allergy & Cough Syrup (Brompheniramine Maleate, Dextromethorphan Hydrobromide, Pseudoephedrine Hydrochloride) Wyeth ▣ 750
Robitussin CF Liquid (Dextromethorphan Hydrobromide, Guaifenesin, Pseudoephedrine Hydrochloride) Wyeth ▣ 755
Robitussin Cough & Cold Liquid-filled Capsules (Dextromethorphan Hydrobromide, Guaifenesin, Pseudoephedrine Hydrochloride) Wyeth ▣ 750
Robitussin Cough, Cold & Flu Liquid-filled Capsules (Acetaminophen, Dextromethorphan Hydrobromide, Guaifenesin, Pseudoephedrine Hydrochloride) Wyeth ▣ 750
Robitussin Cough & Cold Infant Drops (Dextromethorphan Hydrobromide, Guaifenesin, Pseudoephedrine Hydrochloride) Wyeth ▣ 755
Robitussin Flu Liquid (Acetaminophen, Chlorpheniramine Maleate, Dextromethorphan Hydrobromide, Pseudoephedrine Hydrochloride) Wyeth ▣ 752
Robitussin Maximum Strength Cough & Cold Liquid (Dextromethorphan Hydrobromide, Pseudoephedrine Hydrochloride) Wyeth ▣ 754
Robitussin PM Cough & Cold Liquid (Chlorpheniramine Maleate, Dextromethorphan Hydrobromide, Pseudoephedrine Hydrochloride) Wyeth ▣ 752
Sudafed Non-Drowsy Severe Cold Tablets (Acetaminophen, Dextromethorphan Hydrobromide, Pseudoephedrine Hydrochloride) Pfizer Consumer Healthcare ▣ 710
TheraFlu Cold & Cough Hot Liquid (Acetaminophen, Chlorpheniramine Maleate, Dextromethorphan Hydrobromide, Pseudoephedrine Hydrochloride) Novartis Consumer ▣ 680
TheraFlu Severe Cold & Cough Hot Liquid (Acetaminophen, Chlorpheniramine Maleate, Dextromethorphan Hydrobromide, Pseudoephedrine Hydrochloride) Novartis Consumer ▣ 683
TheraFlu Severe Cold Caplets (Acetaminophen, Chlorpheniramine Maleate, Dextromethorphan Hydrobromide, Pseudoephedrine Hydrochloride) Novartis Consumer ▣ 679
TheraFlu Severe Cold Hot Liquid (Acetaminophen, Chlorpheniramine Maleate, Dextromethorphan Hydrobromide, Pseudoephedrine Hydrochloride) Novartis Consumer ▣ 682
Triaminic Cold & Cough Liquid (Chlorpheniramine Maleate, Dextromethorphan Hydrobromide, Pseudoephedrine Hydrochloride) Novartis Consumer ▣ 685
Triaminic Cough Liquid (Dextromethorphan Hydrobromide, Pseudoephedrine Hydrochloride) Novartis Consumer ▣ 687
Triaminic Cough & Nasal Congestion Liquid (Dextromethorphan Hydrobromide, Pseudoephedrine Hydrochloride) Novartis Consumer ▣ 687
Triaminic Cough & Sore Throat Liquid (Acetaminophen, Dextromethorphan Hydrobromide, Pseudoephedrine Hydrochloride) Novartis Consumer ▣ 687
Triaminic Flu, Cough & Fever Liquid (Acetaminophen, Chlorpheniramine Maleate, Dextromethorphan Hydrobromide, Pseudoephedrine Hydrochloride) Novartis Consumer ▣ 685
Triaminic Night Time Cough & Cold Liquid (Chlorpheniramine Maleate, Dextromethorphan Hydrobromide, Pseudoephedrine Hydrochloride) Novartis Consumer ▣ 685
Triaminic Cold & Cough Softchews (Chlorpheniramine Maleate, Dextromethorphan Hydrobromide, Pseudoephedrine Hydrochloride) Novartis Consumer ▣ 688
Triaminic Cough & Sore Throat Softchews (Acetaminophen, Dextromethorphan Hydrobromide, Pseudoephedrine Hydrochloride) Novartis Consumer ▣ 689
Triaminic Vapor Patch-Cherry Scent (Camphor, Menthol) Novartis Consumer ▣ 690
Triaminic Vapor Patch-Menthol Scent (Camphor, Menthol) Novartis Consumer ▣ 690
Children's Tylenol Plus Cold & Cough Suspension Liquid and Chewable Tablets (Acetaminophen, Chlorpheniramine Maleate, Dextromethorphan Hydrobromide, Pseudoephedrine Hydrochloride) McNeil Consumer 1851
Children's Tylenol Plus Flu Suspension Liquid (Acetaminophen, Chlorpheniramine Maleate, Dextromethorphan Hydrobromide, Pseudoephedrine Hydrochloride) McNeil Consumer 1853
Concentrated Tylenol Infants' Drops Plus Cold and Cough (Acetaminophen, Dextromethorphan Hydrobromide, Pseudoephedrine Hydrochloride) McNeil Consumer 1851
Tylenol Cold & Flu Severe Daytime Liquid with Cool Bust (Acetaminophen, Dextromethorphan Hydrobromide, Pseudoephedrine Hydrochloride) McNeil Consumer 1846
Tylenol Cold & Flu Severe NightTime Liquid with Cool Burst (Acetaminophen, Dextromethorphan Hydrobromide, Doxylamine Succinate, Pseudoephedrine Hydrochloride) McNeil Consumer 1846
Tylenol Cold Severe Congestion Non-Drowsy Caplets with Cool Burst (Acetaminophen, Dextromethorphan Hydrobromide, Guaifenesin, Pseudoephedrine Hydrochloride) McNeil Consumer 1846
Tylenol Flu Day Non-Drowsy Gelcaps (Acetaminophen, Dextromethorphan Hydrobromide, Pseudoephedrine Hydrochloride) McNeil Consumer 1846
Multi-Symptom Tylenol Cold Night Time Caplets (Acetaminophen, Chlorpheniramine Maleate, Dextromethorphan Hydrobromide, Pseudoephedrine Hydrochloride) McNeil Consumer 1845
Multi-Symptom Tylenol Cold Day Non-Drowsy Caplets and Gelcaps (Acetaminophen, Dextromethorphan Hydrobromide, Pseudoephedrine Hydrochloride) McNeil Consumer 1845
Vicks 44D Cough & Head Congestion Relief (Dextromethorphan Hydrobromide, Pseudoephedrine Hydrochloride) Procter & Gamble 2676
Vicks 44M Cough, Cold & Flu Relief (Acetaminophen, Chlorpheniramine Maleate, Dextromethorphan Hydrobromide, Pseudoephedrine Hydrochloride) Procter & Gamble 2676
Vicks DayQuil Multi-Symptom Cold/Flu Relief LiquiCaps (Acetaminophen, Dextromethorphan Hydrobromide, Pseudoephedrine Hydrochloride) Procter & Gamble 2675
Vicks DayQuil Multi-Symptom Cold/Flu Relief Liquid (Acetaminophen, Dextromethorphan Hydrobromide, Pseudoephedrine Hydrochloride) Procter & Gamble 2675
Children's Vicks NyQuil Cold/Cough Relief (Chlorpheniramine Maleate, Dextromethorphan Hydrobromide, Pseudoephedrine Hydrochloride) Procter & Gamble 2671
Vicks NyQuil LiquiCaps (Acetaminophen, Dextromethorphan Hydrobromide, Doxylamine Succinate, Pseudoephedrine Hydrochloride) Procter & Gamble 2677

Vicks NyQuil LiquiCaps/Liquid Multi-Symptom Cold/Flu Relief (Acetaminophen, Dextromethorphan Hydrobromide, Doxylamine Succinate, Pseudoephedrine Hydrochloride) Procter & Gamble ▣ 725
Vicks NyQuil Liquid (Acetaminophen, Dextromethorphan Hydrobromide, Doxylamine Succinate, Pseudoephedrine Hydrochloride) Procter & Gamble 2677
Vicks VapoRub Cream (Camphor, Menthol) Procter & Gamble 2678
Vicks VapoRub Ointment (Camphor, Eucalyptus, Oil of, Menthol) Procter & Gamble 2678
Vicks VapoSteam (Camphor) Procter & Gamble 2679
Zicam Cold Remedy Chewables (Zincum Aceticum, Zincum Gluconicum) Matrixx ▣ 665
Zicam Cold Remedy Nasal Pump (Zincum Gluconicum) Matrixx ▣ 665
Zicam Cold Remedy Oral Mist (Zincum Aceticum, Zincum Gluconicum) Matrixx ▣ 665
Zicam Cold Remedy RapidMelts (Zincum Aceticum, Zincum Gluconicum) Matrixx ▣ 665
Zicam Cold Remedy Swabs (Zincum Gluconicum) Matrixx ▣ 665
Zicam Cold Remedy Swabs Kids Size (Zincum Gluconicum) Matrixx ▣ 665
Zicam Concentrated Cough Mist for Kids Plus D Cool Cherry (Dextromethorphan Hydrobromide, Phenylephrine Hydrochloride) Matrixx ▣ 643
Zicam Concentrated Cough Mist Plus D Cool Cherry (Dextromethorphan Hydrobromide, Phenylephrine Hydrochloride) Matrixx ▣ 642

Cradle cap
(*see under* Dermatitis, seborrheic)

Creeping eruptions
(*see under* Larva migrans, cutaneous)

Cretinism
(*see under* Hypothyroidism, replacement or supplemental therapy in)

Crohn's disease
Entocort EC Capsules (Budesonide) Prometheus 2694
Remicade for IV Injection (Infliximab) Centocor 987

Cryptococcosis
Abelcet Injection (Amphotericin B Lipid Complex) Enzon 1119
AmBisome for Injection (Amphotericin B, liposomal) Astellas 615

Cryptorchidism, prepubertal
Novarel for Injection (Chorionic Gonadotropin) Ferring 1147

Cushing's syndrome, ACTH-dependent, differential diagnosis of
Acthrel for Injection (Corticorelin Ovine Triflutate) Ferring 3528

Cushing's syndrome, diagnosis of
(*see under* Adrenocortical hyperfunction, diagnostic testing of)

Cuts, minor
Aquacel AG with Hydrofiber (Silver impregnated antimicrobial dressing) ConvaTec 1035

Cuts, minor, infection from
(*see under* Infections, skin, bacterial, minor)

Cuts, minor, pain associated with
(*see under* Pain, topical relief of)

Cyclitis
Zylet Ophthalmic Suspension (Loteprednol Etabonate, Tobramycin) Bausch & Lomb 3508

Cystic fibrosis, adjunctive therapy in
Pulmozyme Inhalation Solution (Dornase Alfa) Genentech 1245
TOBI Solution for Inhalation (Tobramycin) Chiron 1015

Cystic tumors
Depo-Medrol Single-Dose Vial (Methylprednisolone Acetate) Pharmacia & Upjohn 2617

Cystinuria
Cuprimine Capsules (Penicillamine) Merck 1925

Cystitis
Cipro (Ciprofloxacin) Schering 2991
Cipro XR Tablets (Ciprofloxacin) Schering 3004
Noroxin Tablets (Norfloxacin) Merck 2009
Tequin Injection (Gatifloxacin) Bristol-Myers Squibb 964
Tequin Tablets (Gatifloxacin) Bristol-Myers Squibb 964
Uroqid-Acid No. 2 Tablets (Methenamine Mandelate, Sodium Acid Phosphate) Beach 785
Vantin Tablets and Oral Suspension (Cefpodoxime Proxetil) Pharmacia & Upjohn 2650

Cystitis, interstitial, symptomatic relief of
Elmiron Capsules (Pentosan Polysulfate Sodium) Ortho Women's Health & Urology 2393

Cytomegalovirus disease associated with renal transplantation, prophylaxis of
CytoGam Intravenous (Cytomegalovirus Immune Globulin) MedImmune 1866

Cytomegalovirus disease associated with transplant patients
Cytovene (Ganciclovir) Roche Laboratories 2763

D

Dacryocystitis
Genoptic Sterile Ophthalmic Solution (Gentamicin Sulfate) Allergan ⊙ 227

Dandruff
(*see also under* Dermatitis, seborrheic)
Nizoral A-D Shampoo, 1% (Ketoconazole) McNeil Consumer 1839
Tegrin Dandruff Shampoo - Extra Conditioning (Coal Tar) GlaxoSmithKline ▣ 637
Tegrin Dandruff Shampoo - Fresh Herbal (Coal Tar) GlaxoSmithKline ▣ 638

Dehydration, prevention of
Pedialyte Oral Electrolyte Maintenance Solution (Electrolyte Solution) Ross 2842

Dementia, Alzheimer's type
Aricept Tablets (Donepezil Hydrochloride) Eisai 1086
Aricept ODT Tablets (Donepezil Hydrochloride) Eisai 1086
Exelon Capsules (Rivastigmine Tartrate) Novartis 2204
Namenda (Memantine Hydrochloride) Forest 1199
Razadyne ER Extended-Release Capsules (Galantamine Hydrobromide) Ortho-McNeil Neurologics 2434
Razadyne (Galantamine Hydrobromide) Ortho-McNeil Neurologics 2434

Dental hygiene, adjunct to
Trident White Sugarless Gum (Mannitol, Sorbitol) Cadbury Adams ▣ 611

Depression, bipolar
(*see under* Depression, manic-depressive)

Depression, major, without melancholia
Parnate Tablets (Tranylcypromine Sulfate) GlaxoSmithKline 1499

Depression, manic-depressive
(*see also under* Mania, bipolar)
Eskalith CR Controlled-Release Tablets (Lithium Carbonate) GlaxoSmithKline 1406
Symbyax Capsules (Fluoxetine Hydrochloride, Olanzapine) Lilly 1788

Depression, relief of symptoms
Vivactil Tablets (Protriptyline Hydrochloride) Odyssey 2350

Depression, treatment of
Celexa (Citalopram Hydrobromide) Forest 1177
Cymbalta Delayed-Release Capsules (Duloxetine Hydrochloride) Lilly 1729
Effexor Tablets (Venlafaxine Hydrochloride) Wyeth 3405
Effexor XR Capsules (Venlafaxine Hydrochloride) Wyeth 3411
Lexapro Oral Solution (Escitalopram Oxalate) Forest 1193
Lexapro Tablets (Escitalopram Oxalate) Forest 1193
Paxil CR Controlled-Release Tablets (Paroxetine Hydrochloride) GlaxoSmithKline 1509
Paxil (Paroxetine Hydrochloride) GlaxoSmithKline 1501
Prozac Pulvules and Liquid (Fluoxetine Hydrochloride) Lilly 1771
Surmontil Capsules (Trimipramine Maleate) Odyssey 2347
Wellbutrin Tablets (Bupropion Hydrochloride) GlaxoSmithKline 1579
Wellbutrin SR Sustained-Release Tablets (Bupropion Hydrochloride) GlaxoSmithKline 1583
Wellbutrin XL Extended-Release Tablets (Bupropion Hydrochloride) GlaxoSmithKline 1588
Zoloft (Sertraline Hydrochloride) Pfizer 2581

Dermatitis, atopic
Cortizone•5 Ointment (Hydrocortisone) Pfizer Consumer Healthcare ▣ 699
Cortizone•10 Creme (Hydrocortisone) Pfizer Consumer Healthcare ▣ 699
Cortizone•10 Ointment (Hydrocortisone) Pfizer Consumer Healthcare ▣ 699
Cortizone•10 Plus Creme (Hydrocortisone) Pfizer Consumer Healthcare ▣ 700
Cortizone•10 Maximum Strength Quick Shot Spray (Hydrocortisone) Pfizer Consumer Healthcare ▣ 700
Cutivate Lotion 0.05% (Fluticasone Propionate) GlaxoSmithKline 1383
Decadron Phosphate Injection (Dexamethasone Sodium Phosphate) Merck 1931
Decadron Tablets (Dexamethasone) Merck 1929
Depo-Medrol Injectable Suspension (Methylprednisolone Acetate) Pharmacia & Upjohn 2615
Depo-Medrol Single-Dose Vial (Methylprednisolone Acetate) Pharmacia & Upjohn 2617
Elidel Cream 1% (Pimecrolimus) Novartis 2198
Hydrocortone Tablets (Hydrocortisone) Merck 1963
Pediapred Oral Solution (Prednisolone Sodium Phosphate) UCB 3319
Protopic Ointment (Tacrolimus) Astellas 629

Dermatitis, contact
(*see also under* Dermatoses, corticosteroid-responsive)
Benadryl Itch Relief Stick Extra Strength (Diphenhydramine Hydrochloride, Zinc Acetate) Pfizer Consumer Healthcare ▣ 696
Benadryl Itch Stopping Cream Extra Strength (Diphenhydramine Hydrochloride, Zinc Acetate) Pfizer Consumer Healthcare ▣ 697
Benadryl Itch Stopping Gel Extra Strength (Diphenhydramine Hydrochloride) Pfizer Consumer Healthcare ▣ 697
Benadryl Itch Stopping Spray Extra Strength (Diphenhydramine Hydrochloride, Zinc Acetate) Pfizer Consumer Healthcare ▣ 697
Cortizone•5 Ointment (Hydrocortisone) Pfizer Consumer Healthcare ▣ 699
Cortizone•10 Creme (Hydrocortisone) Pfizer Consumer Healthcare ▣ 699
Cortizone•10 Ointment (Hydrocortisone) Pfizer Consumer Healthcare ▣ 699
Cortizone•10 Plus Creme (Hydrocortisone) Pfizer Consumer Healthcare ▣ 700
Cortizone•10 Maximum Strength Quick Shot Spray (Hydrocortisone) Pfizer Consumer Healthcare ▣ 700
Decadron Phosphate Injection (Dexamethasone Sodium Phosphate) Merck 1931
Decadron Tablets (Dexamethasone) Merck 1929
Depo-Medrol Injectable Suspension (Methylprednisolone Acetate) Pharmacia & Upjohn 2615
Depo-Medrol Single-Dose Vial (Methylprednisolone Acetate) Pharmacia & Upjohn 2617
Hydrocortone Tablets (Hydrocortisone) Merck 1963
Pediapred Oral Solution (Prednisolone Sodium Phosphate) UCB 3319

Dermatitis, corticosteroid-responsive, anal region
Analpram-HC (Hydrocortisone Acetate, Pramoxine Hydrochloride) Ferndale 1136

Dermatitis, exfoliative
Decadron Phosphate Injection (Dexamethasone Sodium Phosphate) Merck 1931
Depo-Medrol Injectable Suspension (Methylprednisolone Acetate) Pharmacia & Upjohn 2615
Depo-Medrol Single-Dose Vial (Methylprednisolone Acetate) Pharmacia & Upjohn 2617
Hydrocortone Tablets (Hydrocortisone) Merck 1963
Pediapred Oral Solution (Prednisolone Sodium Phosphate) UCB 3319

Dermatitis, herpetiformis
Dapsone Tablets USP (Dapsone) Jacobus 1656

Dermatitis, herpetiformis bullous
Decadron Phosphate Injection (Dexamethasone Sodium Phosphate) Merck 1931
Decadron Tablets (Dexamethasone) Merck 1929
Depo-Medrol Injectable Suspension (Methylprednisolone Acetate) Pharmacia & Upjohn 2615
Depo-Medrol Single-Dose Vial (Methylprednisolone Acetate) Pharmacia & Upjohn 2617
Hydrocortone Tablets (Hydrocortisone) Merck 1963
Pediapred Oral Solution (Prednisolone Sodium Phosphate) UCB 3319

Dermatitis, seborrheic
Avar Cleanser (Sodium Sulfacetamide, Sulfur) Sirius 3189
Avar Gel (Sodium Sulfacetamide, Sulfur) Sirius 3189
Avar Green (Sodium Sulfacetamide, Sulfur) Sirius 3189
Avar-e Emollient Cream (Sodium Sulfacetamide, Sulfur) Sirius 3189
Avar-e Green Cream (Sodium Sulfacetamide, Sulfur) Sirius 3189

Cortizone•10 Creme (Hydrocortisone) Pfizer Consumer Healthcare ▣ 699
Cortizone•10 Ointment (Hydrocortisone) Pfizer Consumer Healthcare ▣ 699
Cortizone•10 Plus Creme (Hydrocortisone) Pfizer Consumer Healthcare ▣ 700
Cortizone•10 Maximum Strength Quick Shot Spray (Hydrocortisone) Pfizer Consumer Healthcare ▣ 700
Loprox Shampoo (Ciclopirox) Medicis 1862
Plexion (Sodium Sulfacetamide, Sulfur) Medicis 1863
Rosac Cream with Sunscreens (Sodium Sulfacetamide, Sulfur) Stiefel 3216
Tegrin Dandruff Shampoo - Extra Conditioning (Coal Tar) GlaxoSmithKline ▣ 637
Tegrin Dandruff Shampoo - Fresh Herbal (Coal Tar) GlaxoSmithKline ▣ 638
Tegrin Skin Cream (Coal Tar) GlaxoSmithKline ▣ 638

Dermatitis, seborrheic, severe
Decadron Phosphate Injection (Dexamethasone Sodium Phosphate) Merck 1931
Depo-Medrol Injectable Suspension (Methylprednisolone Acetate) Pharmacia & Upjohn 2615
Depo-Medrol Single-Dose Vial (Methylprednisolone Acetate) Pharmacia & Upjohn 2617
Hydrocortone Tablets (Hydrocortisone) Merck 1963
Pediapred Oral Solution (Prednisolone Sodium Phosphate) UCB 3319

Dermatitis, unspecified
Ultralytic 2 Cream 20% (Urea) Ivax Dermatologicals 1651
Ultralytic 2 Foam 20% (Urea) Ivax Dermatologicals 1652

Dermatomycosis, systemic
Decadron Tablets (Dexamethasone) Merck 1929

Dermatomyositis, possibly effective in
Potaba (Aminobenzoate Potassium) Glenwood 1634

Dermatomyositis, systemic
Depo-Medrol Injectable Suspension (Methylprednisolone Acetate) Pharmacia & Upjohn 2615
Depo-Medrol Single-Dose Vial (Methylprednisolone Acetate) Pharmacia & Upjohn 2617
Hydrocortone Tablets (Hydrocortisone) Merck 1963
Pediapred Oral Solution (Prednisolone Sodium Phosphate) UCB 3319

Dermatoses, corticosteroid-responsive
(*see also under* Skin, inflammatory conditions)
Aclovate (Alclometasone Dipropionate) GlaxoSmithKline 1290
Clobevate Gel (Clobetasol Propionate) Stiefel 3213
Clobex Lotion (Clobetasol Propionate) Galderma 1208
Cutivate Cream (Fluticasone Propionate) GlaxoSmithKline 1381
Cutivate Ointment (Fluticasone Propionate) GlaxoSmithKline 1384
Diprolene Ointment 0.05% (Betamethasone Dipropionate) Schering 3017
Diprolene AF Cream 0.05% (Betamethasone Dipropionate) Schering 3014
Diprosone Cream, USP 0.05% (Betamethasone Dipropionate) Schering 3018
Elocon Cream 0.1% (Mometasone Furoate) Schering 3019
Elocon Lotion 0.1% (Mometasone Furoate) Schering 3020
Elocon Ointment 0.1% (Mometasone Furoate) Schering 3021
Locoid Cream (Hydrocortisone Butyrate) Ferndale 1138
Locoid Lipocream Cream (Hydrocortisone Butyrate) Ferndale 1138
Locoid (Hydrocortisone Butyrate) Ferndale 1138
Luxíq Foam (Betamethasone Valerate) Connetics 1026
Olux Foam (Clobetasol Propionate) Connetics 1027
Pramosone (Hydrocortisone Acetate, Pramoxine Hydrochloride) Ferndale 1139
ProctoFoam-HC (Hydrocortisone Acetate, Pramoxine Hydrochloride) Schwarz 3113
Temovate Cream (Clobetasol Propionate) GlaxoSmithKline 1549
Temovate Gel (Clobetasol Propionate) GlaxoSmithKline 1550
Temovate Ointment (Clobetasol Propionate) GlaxoSmithKline 1549
Temovate Scalp Application (Clobetasol Propionate) GlaxoSmithKline 1551
Temovate E Emollient (Clobetasol Propionate) GlaxoSmithKline 1552
Topicort .05% Gel (Desoximetasone) TaroPharma 3288
Topicort .25% Cream (Desoximetasone) TaroPharma 3288
Topicort .25% Ointment (Desoximetasone) TaroPharma 3288
Topicort LP .05% Cream (Desoximetasone) TaroPharma 3288
U-cort 1% Cream (Hydrocortisone Acetate) TaroPharma 3289

Dermographism
Phenergan (Promethazine Hydrochloride) Wyeth 3438

Detrusor overactivity
Ditropan XL Extended Release Tablets (Oxybutynin Chloride) Ortho Women's Health & Urology 2391

Diabetes insipidus
DDAVP Injection 4 mcg/mL (Desmopressin Acetate) Sanofi-Aventis 2893
DDAVP Nasal Spray (Desmopressin Acetate) Sanofi-Aventis 2894
DDAVP Tablets (Desmopressin Acetate) Sanofi-Aventis 2895
Desmopressin Acetate Injection (Desmopressin Acetate) Ferring 1143
Desmopressin Acetate Rhinal Tube (Desmopressin Acetate) Ferring 1144

Diabetes mellitus
(*see under* Hyperglycemia, control of, adjunct to diet)

Diabetes mellitus, insulin-dependent
Humalog-Pen (Insulin Lispro, Human) Lilly 1751
Humalog Mix 75/25-Pen (Insulin Lispro, Human, Insulin Lispro Protamine, Human) Lilly 1754
Humulin 50/50, 100 Units (Insulin, Human Regular and Human NPH Mixture) Lilly 1760
Humulin 70/30 Pen (Insulin, Human Regular and Human NPH Mixture) Lilly 1761
Humulin L, 100 Units (Insulin, Human, Zinc Suspension) Lilly 1763
Humulin N, 100 Units (Insulin, Human NPH) Lilly 1764
Humulin R (U-500) (Insulin, Human Regular) Lilly 1768
Humulin R, 100 Units (Insulin, Human Regular) Lilly 1767
Humulin U, 100 Units (Insulin, Human, Zinc Suspension) Lilly 1770
Humulin N Pen (Insulin, Human NPH) Lilly 1765
Innovo (Device) Novo Nordisk 2314
Lantus Injection (Insulin glargine) Sanofi-Aventis 2925
Novolin 70/30 Human Insulin 10 ml Vials (Insulin, Human Regular and Human NPH Mixture) Novo Nordisk 2321
Novolin 70/30 PenFill 3 ml Cartridges (Insulin, Human Regular and Human NPH Mixture) Novo Nordisk 2325
Novolin N Human Insulin 10 ml Vials (Insulin, Human NPH) Novo Nordisk 2322
Novolin N PenFill 3 ml Cartridges (Insulin, Human NPH) Novo Nordisk 2325
Novolin R Human Insulin 10 ml Vials (Insulin, Human Regular) Novo Nordisk 2322
Novolin R PenFill (Insulin, Human Regular) Novo Nordisk 2325
NovoLog Injection (Insulin Aspart, Human Regular) Novo Nordisk 2326
NovoLog Mix 70/30 (Insulin Aspart, Human, Insulin Aspart Protamine, Human) Novo Nordisk 2331
Symlin Injection (Pramlintide Acetate) Amylin 608

Diabetes mellitus, non-insulin-dependent
ActoPlus Met Tablets (Metformin Hydrochloride, Pioglitazone Hydrochloride) Takeda 3219
Actos Tablets (Pioglitazone Hydrochloride) Takeda 3224
Amaryl Tablets (Glimepiride) Sanofi-Aventis 2864
Avandamet Tablets (Rosiglitazone Maleate, Metformin Hydrochloride) GlaxoSmithKline 1343
Avandia Tablets (Rosiglitazone Maleate) GlaxoSmithKline 1348
Byetta Injection (Exenatide) Amylin 605
Lantus Injection (Insulin glargine) Sanofi-Aventis 2925
Prandin Tablets (0.5, 1, and 2 mg) (Repaglinide) Novo Nordisk 2337
Precose Tablets (Acarbose) Bayer 776
Starlix Tablets (Nateglinide) Novartis 2276

Diabetes mellitus, type 1
Lantus Injection (Insulin glargine) Sanofi-Aventis 2925
Novolin 70/30 InnoLet (Insulin, Human Regular and Human NPH Mixture) Novo Nordisk 2322
Novolin N InnoLet (Insulin, Human NPH) Novo Nordisk 2322
Novolin R InnoLet (Insulin, Human NPH) Novo Nordisk 2322

Diabetes mellitus, type 2
Fortamet Extended-Release Tablets (Metformin Hydrochloride) First Horizon 1156
Lantus Injection (Insulin glargine) Sanofi-Aventis 2925
Prandin Tablets (0.5, 1, and 2 mg) (Repaglinide) Novo Nordisk 2337

Diabetic nephropathy
(*see under* Nephropathy, diabetic)

Diarrhea
Kaopectate Anti-Diarrheal/Upset Stomach Reliever Liquid (Bismuth Subsalicylate) Pfizer Consumer Healthcare ▣ 701
Extra Strength Kaopectate Anti-Diarrheal Liquid (Bismuth Subsalicylate) Pfizer Consumer Healthcare ▣ 701

Diarrhea, adjunctive therapy in
Imodium Advanced Caplets and Chewable Tablets (Loperamide Hydrochloride, Simethicone) McNeil Consumer 1835
Pedialyte Oral Electrolyte Maintenance Solution (Electrolyte Solution) Ross 2842

Diarrhea, bacterial
(*see under* Diarrhea, infectious)

Diarrhea, cryptosporidium parvum-induced
Alinia for Oral Suspension (Nitazoxanide) Romark 2840
Alinia Tablets (Nitazoxanide) Romark 2840

Diarrhea, E. coli-induced
Cipro (Ciprofloxacin) Schering 2991

Diarrhea, giardia lamblia-induced
Alinia for Oral Suspension (Nitazoxanide) Romark 2840
Alinia Tablets (Nitazoxanide) Romark 2840

Diarrhea, infectious
Alinia for Oral Suspension (Nitazoxanide) Romark 2840
Alinia Tablets (Nitazoxanide) Romark 2840
Cipro (Ciprofloxacin) Schering 2991

Diarrhea, protozoal
(*see under* Diarrhea, infectious)

Diarrhea, symptomatic relief of
Imodium Capsules (Loperamide Hydrochloride) McNeil Consumer 1834
Imodium A-D Liquid and Caplets (Loperamide Hydrochloride) McNeil Consumer 1835
Imodium Advanced Caplets and Chewable Tablets (Loperamide Hydrochloride, Simethicone) McNeil Consumer 1835
Kaopectate Anti-Diarrheal/Upset Stomach Reliever Liquid (Bismuth Subsalicylate) Pfizer Consumer Healthcare ▣ 701
Extra Strength Kaopectate Anti-Diarrheal Liquid (Bismuth Subsalicylate) Pfizer Consumer Healthcare ▣ 701
Pepto-Bismol Maximum Strength Liquid (Bismuth Subsalicylate) Procter & Gamble ▣ 718
Pepto-Bismol Original Liquid, Maximum Strength Liquid, Original and Cherry Tablets and Easy-To-Swallow Caplets (Bismuth Subsalicylate) Procter & Gamble 2673

Diarrhea, traveler's
Xifaxan Tablets (Rifaximin) Salix 2847

Diarrhea associated with vasoactive intestinal peptide tumors
Sandostatin Injection (Octreotide Acetate) Novartis 2263
Sandostatin LAR Depot (Octreotide Acetate) Novartis 2264

Diet, supplementation of
Active Calcium Tablets (Calcium Citrate, Vitamin D) Usana 3342
All-Basic Capsules (Amino Acid Preparations) Montiff 2110
Alluna Sleep Tablets (Valeriana officinalis) GlaxoSmithKline ▣ 763
Ambrotose AO Capsules (Herbals with Vitamins) Mannatech ▣ 769
Ambrotose Capsules (Herbals, Multiple) Mannatech ▣ 768
Ambrotose Powder (Glucosamine Hydrochloride, Herbals, Multiple) Mannatech ▣ 768
Ambrotose with Lecithin Capsules (Lecithin, Herbals, Multiple) Mannatech ▣ 768
Athena Hair System Supplement (Herbals with Vitamins) Greek Island Labs ▣ 767
Athena Hair System Shampoo (Azelaic Acid, Biotin, Caffeine, Tocopherol Acetate, Lecithin, Serenoa repens, Panthenol, Zinc Sulfate, Phytosterols) Greek Island Labs ▣ 767
Awareness Clear Capsules (Herbals, Multiple) Awareness Corporation/AwarenessLife ▣ 759
Bausch & Lomb PreserVision AREDS Tablets (Vitamins with Minerals) Bausch & Lomb ⊙ 252
Beano (Alpha Galactosidase Enzyme) GlaxoSmithKline ▣ 764
Benefiber Fiber Supplement Caplets (Fiber, dietary) Novartis Consumer ▣ 772
Benefiber Dietary Fiber Supplement Powder (Fiber, dietary) Novartis Consumer ▣ 771
Benefiber Dietary Fiber Supplement Chewable Tablets (Fiber, dietary) Novartis Consumer ▣ 772
Bevitamel Tablets (Folic Acid, Melatonin, Vitamin B_{12}) Westlake 3392
Bios Life 2 Drink Mix (Fiber, Vitamins with Minerals) Unicity 3328
Caltrate 600 PLUS Chewables (Calcium Carbonate, Minerals, Multiple, Vitamin D) Wyeth ▣ 779

Caltrate 600 PLUS Tablets (Calcium Carbonate, Minerals, Multiple, Vitamin D) Wyeth ▣ 779
Caltrate 600 + D Tablets (Calcium Carbonate, Vitamin D) Wyeth ▣ 779
Cardio Essentials Capsules (Coenzyme Q-10) Unicity 3328
Centrum Tablets (Vitamins with Minerals) Wyeth ▣ 780
Centrum Kids Rugrats Complete Children's Chewables (Vitamins with Minerals) Wyeth ▣ 780
Centrum Performance Complete Multivitamin Tablets (Vitamins with Minerals) Wyeth ▣ 781
Centrum Silver Tablets (Vitamins with Minerals) Wyeth ▣ 781
Chelated Mineral Tablets (Minerals, Multiple) Usana 3342
CoQuinone Capsules (Coenzyme Q-10, Lipoic Acid) Usana 3343
CordyMax Cs-4 Capsules (Herbals, Multiple) Pharmanex 2669
Daily Complete Liquid (Aloe vera, Amino Acid Preparations, Herbals with Vitamins & Minerals, Antioxidants) Awareness Corporation/AwarenessLife ▣ 760
Encora Capsules (Calcium Carbonate, Fatty Acids, Folic Acid, Vitamins, Multiple) Ther-Rx 3298
Encora AM Tablets (Calcium Carbonate, Fatty Acids, Folic Acid, Vitamins, Multiple) Ther-Rx 3298
Encora PM Tablets (Calcium Carbonate, Fatty Acids, Folic Acid, Vitamins, Multiple) Ther-Rx 3298
Experience Capsules (Psyllium Preparations, Herbals, Multiple) Awareness Corporation/AwarenessLife ▣ 760
Ferretts IPS Liquid (Iron) Pharmics, Inc. ▣ 773
Ferretts Tablets (Ferrous Fumarate) Pharmics, Inc. ▣ 773
Gluca-Balance Capsules (Amino Acid Preparations) Montiff 2110
Halls Defense Multiblend Supplement Drops (Herbals with Vitamins, Echinacea) Cadbury Adams ▣ 610
Hyland's Complete Flu Care Tablets (Herbals, Multiple) Standard Homeopathic ▣ 734
Hyland's Earache Drops (Herbals, Multiple) Standard Homeopathic ▣ 734
immune^{26} Balance Powder Shake Mix (Egg product, hyperimmune) Legacy for Life ▣ 768
immune^{26} Complete Support Powder Shake Mix (Egg product, hyperimmune) Legacy for Life ▣ 768
immune^{26} Powder, Capsules and Chewable Tablets (Egg product, hyperimmune) Legacy for Life ▣ 768
Immunocal Powder Sachets (Whey Protein Isolate) Immunotec 1642
Intelectol Tablets (Vinpocetine) Memory Secret ▣ 770
Lifepak Capsules (Vitamins with Minerals) Pharmanex 2669
MarineOmega Softgel Capsules (Fatty Acids, Vitamin E) Pharmanex 2669
MDR Vital Factors (Vitamins with Minerals) MDR 1854
Mega Antioxidant Tablets (Vitamins, Multiple) Usana 3343
Metamucil Dietary Fiber Supplement (Psyllium Preparations) Procter & Gamble ▣ 774
Microdiet Dietary Supplement (Multivitamins with Minerals) Sunny Health ▣ 775
Noni Plus Plus Liquid (Multivitamins with Minerals) American Longevity ▣ 759
NutriSure OTC Tablets (Folic Acid, Herbals, Multiple, Vitamins with Minerals) Westlake 3392
Peridin-C Tablets (Bioflavonoids, Hesperidin Complex, Hesperidin Methyl Chalcone, Vitamin C) Beutlich ▣ 761
PLUS with Ambrotose Complex Caplets (Amino Acid Preparations) Mannatech ▣ 769
Prelief Tablets and Powder (Calcium Glycerophosphate) AK Pharma ▣ 758
PremCal Light, Regular, and Extra Strength Tablets (Calcium Carbonate, Magnesium Oxide, Vitamin D_3) Dannmarie ▣ 762
Procosa II Tablets (Glucosamine Sulfate) Usana 3343
Proflavanol 90 Tablets (Dietary Supplement) Usana 3343
PureTrim Whole Food Wellness Shake (Fatty Acids, Rice Protein, Antioxidants) Awareness Corporation/AwarenessLife ▣ 760
Reishimax Capsules (Ganoderma lucinum mushroom extract) Pharmanex 2669
Remifemin Menopause Tablets (Black Cohosh) GlaxoSmithKline ▣ 766
Senokot Wheat Bran (Bran, wheat) Purdue Products 2717
Sen-Sei-Ro Liquid (Dietary Supplement) Kyowa 1713
Sen-Sei-Ro Powder Gold (Dietary Supplement) Kyowa 1713
SinEcch Capsules (Arnica montana) Alpine ▣ 758
SON Formula Tablets (Amino Acid Preparations) International Nutrition Research 1651
Spartan Hair System Supplement (Herbals with Vitamins) Greek Island Labs ▣ 767
Spartan Hair System Shampoo (Azelaic Acid, Biotin, Caffeine, Tocopherol Acetate, Lecithin, Serenoa repens, Panthenol, Zinc Sulfate, Phytosterols) Greek Island Labs ▣ 767
SynergyDefense Capsules (Herbals, Multiple) Awareness Corporation/AwarenessLife ▣ 760
Tahitian Noni Liquid (Dietary Supplement) Tahitian Noni International ▣ 777
Tēgreen 97 Capsules (Camellia sinensis) Pharmanex 2669
4Life Transfer Factor Plus Advanced Formula Capsules (Amino Acid Preparations) 4Life ▣ 763
Unique E Vitamin E Concentrate Capsules (Vitamin E) A. C. Grace ▣ 602
Vemma Nutrition Program - Essential Minerals (Minerals, Multiple) Vemma ▣ 778
Vemma Nutrition Program - Mangosteen Plus (Aloe vera, Phytonutrients, Herbals with Vitamins) Vemma ▣ 778
Wobenzym Tablets (Dietary Supplement) Marlyn 3525
Zinc-220 Capsules (Zinc Sulfate) Alto 576

Digestive disorders, symptomatic relief of
DDS-Acidophilus Capsules, Tablets, and Powder (Lactobacillus Acidophilus) UAS Labs ▣ 736
Maalox Maximum Strength Total Stomach Relief Peppermint Liquid (Bismuth Subsalicylate) Novartis Consumer ▣ 677
Maalox Maximum Strength Total Stomach Relief Strawberry Liquid (Bismuth Subsalicylate) Novartis Consumer ▣ 678
Extra Strength Rolaids Softchews (Calcium Carbonate) Pfizer Consumer Healthcare ▣ 708

Digoxin intoxication, life-threatening
Digibind for Injection (Digoxin Immune Fab (Ovine)) GlaxoSmithKline 1388

Diphtheria
(*see under* C. diphtheriae infections)

Diplococcus pneumoniae infections
(*see under* S. pneumoniae infections)

Diuresis, induction of in edema due to lupus erythematosus
Decadron Phosphate Injection (Dexamethasone Sodium Phosphate) Merck 1931
Decadron Tablets (Dexamethasone) Merck 1929
Depo-Medrol Injectable Suspension (Methylprednisolone Acetate) Pharmacia & Upjohn 2615
Hydrocortone Tablets (Hydrocortisone) Merck 1963
Pediapred Oral Solution (Prednisolone Sodium Phosphate) UCB 3319

Diuresis, induction of in nephrotic syndrome
Decadron Phosphate Injection (Dexamethasone Sodium Phosphate) Merck 1931
Decadron Tablets (Dexamethasone) Merck 1929
Depo-Medrol Injectable Suspension (Methylprednisolone Acetate) Pharmacia & Upjohn 2615
Depo-Medrol Single-Dose Vial (Methylprednisolone Acetate) Pharmacia & Upjohn 2617
Hydrocortone Tablets (Hydrocortisone) Merck 1963
Pediapred Oral Solution (Prednisolone Sodium Phosphate) UCB 3319

Donovania granulomatis infection
(*see under* Granuloma inguinale)

Drowsiness, symptomatic relief of
Vivarin (Caffeine) GlaxoSmithKline ▣ 639

Ductus arteriosus, patent, palliative maintenance
Indocin I.V. (Indomethacin Sodium Trihydrate) Merck 1973

Dukes' stage C colon cancer
(*see under* Carcinoma, colon, Dukes' stage C, adjunctive treatment in)

Duodenal ulcer and H. pylori infection, adjunct in
Aciphex Tablets (Rabeprazole Sodium) Eisai 1081
Amoxil Capsules (Amoxicillin) GlaxoSmithKline 1315
Amoxil Chewable Tablets (Amoxicillin) GlaxoSmithKline 1315
Amoxil Pediatric Drops for Oral Suspension (Amoxicillin) GlaxoSmithKline 1315
Amoxil Powder for Oral Suspension (Amoxicillin) GlaxoSmithKline 1315
Amoxil Tablets (Amoxicillin) GlaxoSmithKline 1315
Biaxin/Biaxin XL (Clarithromycin) Abbott 402
Prevacid Delayed-Release Capsules (Lansoprazole) TAP 3268
Prevacid for Delayed-Release Oral Suspension (Lansoprazole) TAP 3268
Prevacid SoluTab Delayed-Release Orally Disintegrating Tablets (Lansoprazole) TAP 3268
PREVPAC (Amoxicillin, Clarithromycin, Lansoprazole) TAP 3281
Prilosec OTC Tablets (Omeprazole magnesium) Procter & Gamble 2674

Duodenal ulcers, active, short-term treatment of
Aciphex Tablets (Rabeprazole Sodium) Eisai 1081
Axid Oral Solution (Nizatidine) Braintree 913
Carafate Suspension (Sucralfate) Axcan Scandipharm 727
Carafate Tablets (Sucralfate) Axcan Scandipharm 728
Pepcid Injection (Famotidine) Merck 2017
Pepcid (Famotidine) Merck 2014
Prevacid Delayed-Release Capsules (Lansoprazole) TAP 3268
Prevacid for Delayed-Release Oral Suspension (Lansoprazole) TAP 3268
Prevacid SoluTab Delayed-Release Orally Disintegrating Tablets (Lansoprazole) TAP 3268
Prilosec OTC Tablets (Omeprazole magnesium) Procter & Gamble 2674
Tagamet Tablets (Cimetidine) GlaxoSmithKline 1547
Zantac (Ranitidine Hydrochloride) GlaxoSmithKline 1597
Zantac Injection (Ranitidine Hydrochloride) GlaxoSmithKline 1593
Zantac Injection Pharmacy Bulk Package (Ranitidine Hydrochloride) GlaxoSmithKline 1595
Zantac Syrup (Ranitidine Hydrochloride) GlaxoSmithKline 1597
Zegerid Powder for Oral Solution (Omeprazole) Santarus 2972

Duodenal ulcers, maintenance therapy for
Axid Oral Solution (Nizatidine) Braintree 913
Carafate Tablets (Sucralfate) Axcan Scandipharm 728
Pepcid Injection (Famotidine) Merck 2017
Pepcid (Famotidine) Merck 2014
Prevacid Delayed-Release Capsules (Lansoprazole) TAP 3268
Prevacid for Delayed-Release Oral Suspension (Lansoprazole) TAP 3268
Prevacid SoluTab Delayed-Release Orally Disintegrating Tablets (Lansoprazole) TAP 3268
Tagamet Tablets (Cimetidine) GlaxoSmithKline 1547
Zantac (Ranitidine Hydrochloride) GlaxoSmithKline 1597

Duodenal ulcers, to reduce the risk of recurrence
Prilosec OTC Tablets (Omeprazole magnesium) Procter & Gamble 2674

Dysbetalipoproteinemia
Caduet Tablets (Amlodipine Besylate, Atorvastatin Calcium) Pfizer 2507
Lipitor Tablets (Atorvastatin Calcium) Parke-Davis 2495
Zocor Tablets (Simvastatin) Merck 2078

Dysentery, amoebic
(*see under* Amebiasis, acute intestinal)

Dysmenorrhea, primary
Anaprox Tablets (Naproxen Sodium) Roche Laboratories 2769
Anaprox DS Tablets (Naproxen Sodium) Roche Laboratories 2769
Celebrex Capsules (Celecoxib) Searle 3130
EC-Naprosyn Delayed-Release Tablets (Naproxen) Roche Laboratories 2769
Naprosyn Suspension (Naproxen) Roche Laboratories 2769
Naprosyn Tablets (Naproxen) Roche Laboratories 2769

Dysphoric disorder, premenstrual
Paxil CR Controlled-Release Tablets (Paroxetine Hydrochloride) GlaxoSmithKline 1509
Zoloft (Sertraline Hydrochloride) Pfizer 2581

Dyspnea associated with congestive heart failure
Natrecor for Injection (Nesiritide) Scios Inc. 3123

Dystonia, cervical
Botox Purified Neurotoxin Complex (Botulinum Toxin Type A) Allergan 565

E

E. faecalis urinary tract infections
Cipro XR Tablets (Ciprofloxacin) Schering 3004

E. cloacae gynecologic infections
Timentin ADD-Vantage (Clavulanate Potassium, Ticarcillin Disodium) GlaxoSmithKline 1556
Timentin Injection Galaxy Container (Clavulanate Potassium, Ticarcillin Disodium) GlaxoSmithKline 1559
Timentin IV Infusion (Clavulanate Potassium, Ticarcillin Disodium) GlaxoSmithKline 1553
Timentin Pharmacy Bulk Package (Clavulanate Potassium, Ticarcillin Disodium) GlaxoSmithKline 1562

E. coli biliary tract infections
Ancef for Injection (Cefazolin Sodium) GlaxoSmithKline 1318

E. coli bone and joint infections
Rocephin Injectable Vials, ADD-Vantage, Galaxy, Bulk (Ceftriaxone Sodium) Roche Laboratories ... 2801

E. coli genital infections
Ancef for Injection (Cefazolin Sodium) GlaxoSmithKline ... 1318

E. coli gynecological infections
Fortaz (Ceftazidime Sodium) GlaxoSmithKline ... 1422
Invanz for Injection (Ertapenem) Merck ... 1974
Mefoxin for Injection (Cefoxitin Sodium) Merck ... 1987
Mefoxin Premixed Intravenous Solution (Cefoxitin Sodium) Merck ... 1990
Primaxin I.M. (Cilastatin Sodium, Imipenem) Merck ... 2022
Primaxin I.V. (Cilastatin Sodium, Imipenem) Merck ... 2024
Timentin ADD-Vantage (Clavulanate Potassium, Ticarcillin Disodium) GlaxoSmithKline ... 1556
Timentin Injection Galaxy Container (Clavulanate Potassium, Ticarcillin Disodium) GlaxoSmithKline ... 1559
Timentin IV Infusion (Clavulanate Potassium, Ticarcillin Disodium) GlaxoSmithKline ... 1553
Timentin Pharmacy Bulk Package (Clavulanate Potassium, Ticarcillin Disodium) GlaxoSmithKline ... 1562
Zosyn (Piperacillin Sodium, Tazobactam Sodium) Wyeth ... 3492

E. coli infections
Amoxil Capsules (Amoxicillin) GlaxoSmithKline ... 1315
Amoxil Chewable Tablets (Amoxicillin) GlaxoSmithKline ... 1315
Amoxil Pediatric Drops for Oral Suspension (Amoxicillin) GlaxoSmithKline ... 1315
Amoxil Powder for Oral Suspension (Amoxicillin) GlaxoSmithKline ... 1315
Amoxil Tablets (Amoxicillin) GlaxoSmithKline ... 1315
Ancef for Injection (Cefazolin Sodium) GlaxoSmithKline ... 1318
Augmentin (Amoxicillin, Clavulanate Potassium) GlaxoSmithKline ... 1331
Augmentin Tablets (Amoxicillin, Clavulanate Potassium) GlaxoSmithKline ... 1334
Ceftin Tablets (Cefuroxime Axetil) GlaxoSmithKline ... 1369
Cipro I.V. (Ciprofloxacin) Schering ... 2998
Cipro I.V. Pharmacy Bulk Package (Ciprofloxacin) Bayer ... 3509
Cipro (Ciprofloxacin) Schering ... 2991
Dynacin Tablets (Minocycline Hydrochloride) Medicis ... 1859
Fortaz (Ceftazidime Sodium) GlaxoSmithKline ... 1422
Garamycin Injectable (Gentamicin Sulfate) Schering ... 3028
Invanz for Injection (Ertapenem) Merck ... 1974
Levaquin in 5% Dextrose Injection (Levofloxacin) Ortho-McNeil ... 2453
Levaquin (Levofloxacin) Ortho-McNeil ... 2453
Mefoxin for Injection (Cefoxitin Sodium) Merck ... 1987
Mefoxin Premixed Intravenous Solution (Cefoxitin Sodium) Merck ... 1990
Merrem I.V. (Meropenem) AstraZeneca ... 687
Noroxin Tablets (Norfloxacin) Merck ... 2009
Primaxin I.M. (Cilastatin Sodium, Imipenem) Merck ... 2022
Primaxin I.V. (Cilastatin Sodium, Imipenem) Merck ... 2024
Rocephin Injectable Vials, ADD-Vantage, Galaxy, Bulk (Ceftriaxone Sodium) Roche Laboratories ... 2801
Seromycin Capsules (Cycloserine) Lilly ... 1783
Suprax (Cefixime) Lupin ... 1811
Timentin ADD-Vantage (Clavulanate Potassium, Ticarcillin Disodium) GlaxoSmithKline ... 1556
Timentin Injection Galaxy Container (Clavulanate Potassium, Ticarcillin Disodium) GlaxoSmithKline ... 1559
Timentin IV Infusion (Clavulanate Potassium, Ticarcillin Disodium) GlaxoSmithKline ... 1553
Timentin Pharmacy Bulk Package (Clavulanate Potassium, Ticarcillin Disodium) GlaxoSmithKline ... 1562
Tygacil for Injection (Tigecycline) Wyeth ... 3489
Vantin Tablets and Oral Suspension (Cefpodoxime Proxetil) Pharmacia & Upjohn ... 2650
Zinacef Injection (Cefuroxime) GlaxoSmithKline ... 1604
Zinacef for Injection (Cefuroxime) GlaxoSmithKline ... 1604
Zosyn (Piperacillin Sodium, Tazobactam Sodium) Wyeth ... 3492

E. coli infections, ocular
Blephamide Ophthalmic Ointment (Prednisolone Acetate, Sulfacetamide Sodium) Allergan ... 563
Blephamide Ophthalmic Suspension (Prednisolone Acetate, Sulfacetamide Sodium) Allergan ... 564
FML-S Liquifilm Sterile Ophthalmic Suspension (Fluorometholone, Sulfacetamide Sodium) Allergan ... ⊙226
Genoptic Sterile Ophthalmic Solution (Gentamicin Sulfate) Allergan ... ⊙227
Poly-Pred Liquifilm Ophthalmic Suspension (Neomycin Sulfate, Polymyxin B Sulfate, Prednisolone Acetate) Allergan ... ⊙231
Pred-G Ophthalmic Suspension (Gentamicin Sulfate, Prednisolone Acetate) Allergan ... ⊙234
Pred-G Sterile Ophthalmic Ointment (Gentamicin Sulfate, Prednisolone Acetate) Allergan ... ⊙235
TobraDex Ophthalmic Ointment (Dexamethasone, Tobramycin) Alcon ... 558
TobraDex Ophthalmic Suspension (Dexamethasone, Tobramycin) Alcon ... 558
Zylet Ophthalmic Suspension (Loteprednol Etabonate, Tobramycin) Bausch & Lomb ... 3508

E. coli intra-abdominal infections
Cipro I.V. (Ciprofloxacin) Schering ... 2998
Cipro I.V. Pharmacy Bulk Package (Ciprofloxacin) Bayer ... 3509
Cipro (Ciprofloxacin) Schering ... 2991
Fortaz (Ceftazidime Sodium) GlaxoSmithKline ... 1422
Invanz for Injection (Ertapenem) Merck ... 1974
Maxipime for Injection (Cefepime Hydrochloride) Elan ... 1093
Mefoxin for Injection (Cefoxitin Sodium) Merck ... 1987
Mefoxin Premixed Intravenous Solution (Cefoxitin Sodium) Merck ... 1990
Merrem I.V. (Meropenem) AstraZeneca ... 687
Primaxin I.M. (Cilastatin Sodium, Imipenem) Merck ... 2022
Primaxin I.V. (Cilastatin Sodium, Imipenem) Merck ... 2024
Rocephin Injectable Vials, ADD-Vantage, Galaxy, Bulk (Ceftriaxone Sodium) Roche Laboratories ... 2801
Timentin ADD-Vantage (Clavulanate Potassium, Ticarcillin Disodium) GlaxoSmithKline ... 1556
Timentin Injection Galaxy Container (Clavulanate Potassium, Ticarcillin Disodium) GlaxoSmithKline ... 1559
Timentin IV Infusion (Clavulanate Potassium, Ticarcillin Disodium) GlaxoSmithKline ... 1553
Timentin Pharmacy Bulk Package (Clavulanate Potassium, Ticarcillin Disodium) GlaxoSmithKline ... 1562
Tygacil for Injection (Tigecycline) Wyeth ... 3489

E. coli lower respiratory tract infections
Cipro I.V. (Ciprofloxacin) Schering ... 2998
Cipro I.V. Pharmacy Bulk Package (Ciprofloxacin) Bayer ... 3509
Cipro (Ciprofloxacin) Schering ... 2991
Fortaz (Ceftazidime Sodium) GlaxoSmithKline ... 1422
Levaquin in 5% Dextrose Injection (Levofloxacin) Ortho-McNeil ... 2453
Levaquin (Levofloxacin) Ortho-McNeil ... 2453
Mefoxin for Injection (Cefoxitin Sodium) Merck ... 1987
Mefoxin Premixed Intravenous Solution (Cefoxitin Sodium) Merck ... 1990
Primaxin I.V. (Cilastatin Sodium, Imipenem) Merck ... 2024
Rocephin Injectable Vials, ADD-Vantage, Galaxy, Bulk (Ceftriaxone Sodium) Roche Laboratories ... 2801
Zinacef Injection (Cefuroxime) GlaxoSmithKline ... 1604
Zinacef for Injection (Cefuroxime) GlaxoSmithKline ... 1604

E. coli meningitis
Rocephin Injectable Vials, ADD-Vantage, Galaxy, Bulk (Ceftriaxone Sodium) Roche Laboratories ... 2801

E. coli otitis externa
Floxin Otic Singles (Ofloxacin) Daiichi ... 1045
Floxin Otic Solution (Ofloxacin) Daiichi ... 1043

E. coli peritonitis
Fortaz (Ceftazidime Sodium) GlaxoSmithKline ... 1422
Mefoxin for Injection (Cefoxitin Sodium) Merck ... 1987
Mefoxin Premixed Intravenous Solution (Cefoxitin Sodium) Merck ... 1990
Merrem I.V. (Meropenem) AstraZeneca ... 687
Timentin ADD-Vantage (Clavulanate Potassium, Ticarcillin Disodium) GlaxoSmithKline ... 1556
Timentin Injection Galaxy Container (Clavulanate Potassium, Ticarcillin Disodium) GlaxoSmithKline ... 1559
Timentin IV Infusion (Clavulanate Potassium, Ticarcillin Disodium) GlaxoSmithKline ... 1553
Timentin Pharmacy Bulk Package (Clavulanate Potassium, Ticarcillin Disodium) GlaxoSmithKline ... 1562
Zosyn (Piperacillin Sodium, Tazobactam Sodium) Wyeth ... 3492

E. coli prostatitis
Ancef for Injection (Cefazolin Sodium) GlaxoSmithKline ... 1318
Cipro I.V. (Ciprofloxacin) Schering ... 2998
Cipro I.V. Pharmacy Bulk Package (Ciprofloxacin) Bayer ... 3509
Cipro (Ciprofloxacin) Schering ... 2991
Noroxin Tablets (Norfloxacin) Merck ... 2009

E. coli septicemia
Ancef for Injection (Cefazolin Sodium) GlaxoSmithKline ... 1318
Cipro I.V. (Ciprofloxacin) Schering ... 2998
Cipro I.V. Pharmacy Bulk Package (Ciprofloxacin) Bayer ... 3509
Fortaz (Ceftazidime Sodium) GlaxoSmithKline ... 1422
Mefoxin for Injection (Cefoxitin Sodium) Merck ... 1987
Mefoxin Premixed Intravenous Solution (Cefoxitin Sodium) Merck ... 1990
Primaxin I.V. (Cilastatin Sodium, Imipenem) Merck ... 2024
Rocephin Injectable Vials, ADD-Vantage, Galaxy, Bulk (Ceftriaxone Sodium) Roche Laboratories ... 2801
Timentin ADD-Vantage (Clavulanate Potassium, Ticarcillin Disodium) GlaxoSmithKline ... 1556
Timentin Injection Galaxy Container (Clavulanate Potassium, Ticarcillin Disodium) GlaxoSmithKline ... 1559
Timentin IV Infusion (Clavulanate Potassium, Ticarcillin Disodium) GlaxoSmithKline ... 1553
Timentin Pharmacy Bulk Package (Clavulanate Potassium, Ticarcillin Disodium) GlaxoSmithKline ... 1562
Zinacef Injection (Cefuroxime) GlaxoSmithKline ... 1604
Zinacef for Injection (Cefuroxime) GlaxoSmithKline ... 1604

E. coli skin and skin structure infections
Amoxil Capsules (Amoxicillin) GlaxoSmithKline ... 1315
Amoxil Chewable Tablets (Amoxicillin) GlaxoSmithKline ... 1315
Amoxil Pediatric Drops for Oral Suspension (Amoxicillin) GlaxoSmithKline ... 1315
Amoxil Powder for Oral Suspension (Amoxicillin) GlaxoSmithKline ... 1315
Amoxil Tablets (Amoxicillin) GlaxoSmithKline ... 1315
Augmentin (Amoxicillin, Clavulanate Potassium) GlaxoSmithKline ... 1331
Augmentin Tablets (Amoxicillin, Clavulanate Potassium) GlaxoSmithKline ... 1334
Cipro I.V. (Ciprofloxacin) Schering ... 2998
Cipro I.V. Pharmacy Bulk Package (Ciprofloxacin) Bayer ... 3509
Cipro (Ciprofloxacin) Schering ... 2991
Fortaz (Ceftazidime Sodium) GlaxoSmithKline ... 1422
Invanz for Injection (Ertapenem) Merck ... 1974
Mefoxin for Injection (Cefoxitin Sodium) Merck ... 1987
Mefoxin Premixed Intravenous Solution (Cefoxitin Sodium) Merck ... 1990
Merrem I.V. (Meropenem) AstraZeneca ... 687
Primaxin I.M. (Cilastatin Sodium, Imipenem) Merck ... 2022
Primaxin I.V. (Cilastatin Sodium, Imipenem) Merck ... 2024
Rocephin Injectable Vials, ADD-Vantage, Galaxy, Bulk (Ceftriaxone Sodium) Roche Laboratories ... 2801
Timentin ADD-Vantage (Clavulanate Potassium, Ticarcillin Disodium) GlaxoSmithKline ... 1556
Timentin Injection Galaxy Container (Clavulanate Potassium, Ticarcillin Disodium) GlaxoSmithKline ... 1559
Timentin IV Infusion (Clavulanate Potassium, Ticarcillin Disodium) GlaxoSmithKline ... 1553
Timentin Pharmacy Bulk Package (Clavulanate Potassium, Ticarcillin Disodium) GlaxoSmithKline ... 1562
Tygacil for Injection (Tigecycline) Wyeth ... 3489
Zinacef Injection (Cefuroxime) GlaxoSmithKline ... 1604
Zinacef for Injection (Cefuroxime) GlaxoSmithKline ... 1604

E. coli urinary tract infections
Ancef for Injection (Cefazolin Sodium) GlaxoSmithKline ... 1318
Augmentin (Amoxicillin, Clavulanate Potassium) GlaxoSmithKline ... 1331
Augmentin Tablets (Amoxicillin, Clavulanate Potassium) GlaxoSmithKline ... 1334
Ceftin Tablets (Cefuroxime Axetil) GlaxoSmithKline ... 1369
Cipro I.V. (Ciprofloxacin) Schering ... 2998
Cipro I.V. Pharmacy Bulk Package (Ciprofloxacin) Bayer ... 3509
Cipro (Ciprofloxacin) Schering ... 2991
Cipro XR Tablets (Ciprofloxacin) Schering ... 3004
Fortaz (Ceftazidime Sodium) GlaxoSmithKline ... 1422
Invanz for Injection (Ertapenem) Merck ... 1974
Levaquin in 5% Dextrose Injection (Levofloxacin) Ortho-McNeil ... 2453
Levaquin (Levofloxacin) Ortho-McNeil ... 2453
Maxipime for Injection (Cefepime Hydrochloride) Elan ... 1093
Mefoxin for Injection (Cefoxitin Sodium) Merck ... 1987
Mefoxin Premixed Intravenous Solution (Cefoxitin Sodium) Merck ... 1990
Noroxin Tablets (Norfloxacin) Merck ... 2009
Primaxin I.V. (Cilastatin Sodium, Imipenem) Merck ... 2024

Rocephin Injectable Vials, ADD-Vantage, Galaxy, Bulk (Ceftriaxone Sodium) Roche Laboratories 2801
Seromycin Capsules (Cycloserine) Lilly 1783
Suprax (Cefixime) Lupin 1811
Tequin Injection (Gatifloxacin) Bristol-Myers Squibb 964
Tequin Tablets (Gatifloxacin) Bristol-Myers Squibb 964
Timentin ADD-Vantage (Clavulanate Potassium, Ticarcillin Disodium) GlaxoSmithKline 1556
Timentin Injection Galaxy Container (Clavulanate Potassium, Ticarcillin Disodium) GlaxoSmithKline 1559
Timentin IV Infusion (Clavulanate Potassium, Ticarcillin Disodium) GlaxoSmithKline 1553
Timentin Pharmacy Bulk Package (Clavulanate Potassium, Ticarcillin Disodium) GlaxoSmithKline 1562
Vantin Tablets and Oral Suspension (Cefpodoxime Proxetil) Pharmacia & Upjohn 2650
Zinacef Injection (Cefuroxime) GlaxoSmithKline 1604
Zinacef for Injection (Cefuroxime) GlaxoSmithKline 1604

E. coli-induced diarrhea
(*see under* Diarrhea, E. coli-induced)

E. faecalis (vancomycin susceptible strains) skin and skin structure infections
Cubicin for Injection (Daptomycin) Cubist 1038
Tygacil (Tigecycline) Wyeth 3489

E. faecalis infections
Merrem I.V. (Meropenem) AstraZeneca 687
Tygacil for Injection (Tigecycline) Wyeth 3489

E. faecalis skin and skin structure infections
Merrem I.V. (Meropenem) AstraZeneca 687

Ear, infection
(*see under* Otitis externa; Otitis media, acute)

Eaton-Lambert syndrome, symptomatic relief of
Guanidine Hydrochloride Tablets (Guanidine Hydrochloride) Schering 3030

Echinococcus granulosus infections
Albenza Tablets (Albendazole) GlaxoSmithKline 1310

Eczema, unspecified
(*see under* Skin, inflammatory conditions)

Edema, adjunctive therapy in
Diuril Oral (Chlorothiazide) Merck 1936
Diuril Sodium Intravenous (Chlorothiazide Sodium) Merck 1934
Dyazide Capsules (Hydrochlorothiazide, Triamterene) GlaxoSmithKline 1389
Dyrenium Capsules (Triamterene) WellSpring 3390
Edecrin (Ethacrynic Acid) Merck 1941
Furosemide Tablets (Furosemide) Mylan 2117
Indapamide Tablets (Indapamide) Mylan 2119
Maxzide (Hydrochlorothiazide, Triamterene) Mylan Bertek 2150

Edema, cerebral
Decadron Phosphate Injection (Dexamethasone Sodium Phosphate) Merck 1931
Decadron Tablets (Dexamethasone) Merck 1929

Edema, corneal, temporary relief of
Muro 128 Ophthalmic Ointment (Sodium Chloride) Bausch & Lomb .... ⊙251
Muro 128 Ophthalmic Solution 2% and 5% (Sodium Chloride) Bausch & Lomb .... ⊙251

Electrolytes, depletion of
Pedialyte Oral Electrolyte Maintenance Solution (Electrolyte Solution) Ross 2842

Embolism, atrial fibrillation with
(*see under* Atrial fibrillation with embolism)

Embolism, pulmonary
Activase I.V. (Alteplase) Genentech 1225
Arixtra Injection (Fondaparinux Sodium) GlaxoSmithKline 1325
Coumadin for Injection (Warfarin Sodium) Bristol-Myers Squibb 932
Coumadin Tablets (Warfarin Sodium) Bristol-Myers Squibb 932
Lovenox Injection (Enoxaparin Sodium) Sanofi-Aventis 2931
Miradon Tablets (Anisindione) Schering 3056

Embolism, pulmonary, acute, lysis of
Activase I.V. (Alteplase) Genentech 1225

Embolism, pulmonary, prophylaxis of
Coumadin for Injection (Warfarin Sodium) Bristol-Myers Squibb 932
Coumadin Tablets (Warfarin Sodium) Bristol-Myers Squibb 932
Miradon Tablets (Anisindione) Schering 3056

Embolism, systemic, post-myocardial infarction, prophylaxis
Coumadin for Injection (Warfarin Sodium) Bristol-Myers Squibb 932
Coumadin Tablets (Warfarin Sodium) Bristol-Myers Squibb 932

Emphysema
Atrovent HFA Inhalation Aerosol (Ipratropium Bromide) Boehringer Ingelheim 872
Serevent Diskus (Salmeterol Xinafoate) GlaxoSmithKline 1540
Spiriva HandiHaler (Tiotropium bromide) Boehringer Ingelheim 899
Uniphyl Tablets (Theophylline Anhydrous) Purdue Pharmaceutical 2708
Zemaira (Alpha$_1$-Proteinase Inhibitor (Human)) ZLB Behring 3506

Emphysema, panacinar, due to congenital Alpha1-antitrypsin deficiency
Aralast (Alpha$_1$-Proteinase Inhibitor (Human)) Baxter Healthcare 745
Prolastin (Alpha$_1$-Proteinase Inhibitor (Human)) Talecris 3252

Empyema
Cleocin Vaginal Ovules (Clindamycin Hydrochloride) Pharmacia & Upjohn 2613

Encephalopathy, hyperammonemia-associated
Ammonul Injection (Sodium Benzoate, Sodium Phenylacelate) Ucyclyd 3323

Endocarditis, bacterial
Ancef for Injection (Cefazolin Sodium) GlaxoSmithKline 1318
Garamycin Injectable (Gentamicin Sulfate) Schering 3028
Primaxin I.V. (Cilastatin Sodium, Imipenem) Merck 2024

Endocarditis, bacterial, prophylaxis
Erythrocin Stearate Filmtab Tablets (Erythromycin Stearate) Abbott 452
Erythromycin Base Filmtab Tablets (Erythromycin) Abbott 454
Erythromycin Delayed-Release Capsules, USP (Erythromycin) Abbott 456

Endocrine adenomas, multiple
(*see also under* Hypersecretory conditions, pathological)
Pepcid Injection (Famotidine) Merck 2017
Pepcid (Famotidine) Merck 2014
Prilosec OTC Tablets (Omeprazole magnesium) Procter & Gamble 2674
Tagamet Tablets (Cimetidine) GlaxoSmithKline 1547

Endocrine disorders
Decadron Phosphate Injection (Dexamethasone Sodium Phosphate) Merck 1931
Decadron Tablets (Dexamethasone) Merck 1929
Depo-Medrol Injectable Suspension (Methylprednisolone Acetate) Pharmacia & Upjohn 2615
Hydrocortone Tablets (Hydrocortisone) Merck 1963
Pediapred Oral Solution (Prednisolone Sodium Phosphate) UCB 3319

Endometrial hyperplasia, prevention of
Prometrium Capsules (100 mg, 200 mg) (Progesterone) Solvay 3205

Endometrial thinning, prior to endometrial ablation
Zoladex (Goserelin Acetate) AstraZeneca 709

Endometriosis
Aygestin Tablets (Norethindrone Acetate) Duramed 1062
Lupron Depot 3.75 mg (Leuprolide Acetate) TAP 3257
Lupron Depot–3 Month 11.25 mg (Leuprolide Acetate) TAP 3262
Zoladex (Goserelin Acetate) AstraZeneca 709

Endometritis
(*see also under* Infections, gynecologic)
Cleocin Vaginal Ovules (Clindamycin Hydrochloride) Pharmacia & Upjohn 2613
Fortaz (Ceftazidime Sodium) GlaxoSmithKline 1422
Mefoxin for Injection (Cefoxitin Sodium) Merck 1987
Mefoxin Premixed Intravenous Solution (Cefoxitin Sodium) Merck 1990
Timentin ADD-Vantage (Clavulanate Potassium, Ticarcillin Disodium) GlaxoSmithKline 1556
Timentin Injection Galaxy Container (Clavulanate Potassium, Ticarcillin Disodium) GlaxoSmithKline 1559
Timentin IV Infusion (Clavulanate Potassium, Ticarcillin Disodium) GlaxoSmithKline 1553
Timentin Pharmacy Bulk Package (Clavulanate Potassium, Ticarcillin Disodium) GlaxoSmithKline 1562

Endomyometritis
Invanz for Injection (Ertapenem) Merck 1974
Primaxin I.M. (Cilastatin Sodium, Imipenem) Merck 2022

Entamoeba histolytica
(*see under* Amebiasis, acute intestinal)

Entamoeba species infections
Dynacin Tablets (Minocycline Hydrochloride) Medicis 1859

Enteritis, regional, systemic therapy for
Decadron Phosphate Injection (Dexamethasone Sodium Phosphate) Merck 1931
Decadron Tablets (Dexamethasone) Merck 1929
Depo-Medrol Injectable Suspension (Methylprednisolone Acetate) Pharmacia & Upjohn 2615
Depo-Medrol Single-Dose Vial (Methylprednisolone Acetate) Pharmacia & Upjohn 2617
Hydrocortone Tablets (Hydrocortisone) Merck 1963
Pediapred Oral Solution (Prednisolone Sodium Phosphate) UCB 3319

Enterobacter aerogenes infections
Dynacin Tablets (Minocycline Hydrochloride) Medicis 1859
Noroxin Tablets (Norfloxacin) Merck 2009
Rocephin Injectable Vials, ADD-Vantage, Galaxy, Bulk (Ceftriaxone Sodium) Roche Laboratories 2801

Enterobacter aerogenes infections, ocular
Genoptic Sterile Ophthalmic Solution (Gentamicin Sulfate) Allergan .... ⊙227
Pred-G Ophthalmic Suspension (Gentamicin Sulfate, Prednisolone Acetate) Allergan .... ⊙234
Pred-G Sterile Ophthalmic Ointment (Gentamicin Sulfate, Prednisolone Acetate) Allergan .... ⊙235
TobraDex Ophthalmic Ointment (Dexamethasone, Tobramycin) Alcon 558
TobraDex Ophthalmic Suspension (Dexamethasone, Tobramycin) Alcon 558
Zylet Ophthalmic Suspension (Loteprednol Etabonate, Tobramycin) Bausch & Lomb 3508

Enterobacter aerogenes lower respiratory tract infections
Rocephin Injectable Vials, ADD-Vantage, Galaxy, Bulk (Ceftriaxone Sodium) Roche Laboratories 2801

Enterobacter aerogenes urinary tract infections
Noroxin Tablets (Norfloxacin) Merck 2009

Enterobacter cloacae bone and joint infections
Cipro I.V. (Ciprofloxacin) Schering 2998
Cipro I.V. Pharmacy Bulk Package (Ciprofloxacin) Bayer 3509
Cipro (Ciprofloxacin) Schering 2991

Enterobacter cloacae infections
Cipro I.V. (Ciprofloxacin) Schering 2998
Cipro I.V. Pharmacy Bulk Package (Ciprofloxacin) Bayer 3509
Cipro (Ciprofloxacin) Schering 2991
Levaquin in 5% Dextrose Injection (Levofloxacin) Ortho-McNeil 2453
Levaquin (Levofloxacin) Ortho-McNeil 2453
Noroxin Tablets (Norfloxacin) Merck 2009
Primaxin I.M. (Cilastatin Sodium, Imipenem) Merck 2022
Rocephin Injectable Vials, ADD-Vantage, Galaxy, Bulk (Ceftriaxone Sodium) Roche Laboratories 2801
Timentin ADD-Vantage (Clavulanate Potassium, Ticarcillin Disodium) GlaxoSmithKline 1556
Timentin Injection Galaxy Container (Clavulanate Potassium, Ticarcillin Disodium) GlaxoSmithKline 1559
Timentin IV Infusion (Clavulanate Potassium, Ticarcillin Disodium) GlaxoSmithKline 1553
Timentin Pharmacy Bulk Package (Clavulanate Potassium, Ticarcillin Disodium) GlaxoSmithKline 1562
Tygacil (Tigecycline) Wyeth 3489

Enterobacter cloacae lower respiratory tract infections
Cipro I.V. (Ciprofloxacin) Schering 2998
Cipro I.V. Pharmacy Bulk Package (Ciprofloxacin) Bayer 3509
Cipro (Ciprofloxacin) Schering 2991

Enterobacter cloacae skin and skin structure infections
Cipro I.V. (Ciprofloxacin) Schering 2998
Cipro I.V. Pharmacy Bulk Package (Ciprofloxacin) Bayer 3509
Cipro (Ciprofloxacin) Schering 2991
Primaxin I.M. (Cilastatin Sodium, Imipenem) Merck 2022
Rocephin Injectable Vials, ADD-Vantage, Galaxy, Bulk (Ceftriaxone Sodium) Roche Laboratories 2801

Enterobacter cloacae urinary tract infections
Cipro I.V. (Ciprofloxacin) Schering 2998
Cipro I.V. Pharmacy Bulk Package (Ciprofloxacin) Bayer 3509

Cipro (Ciprofloxacin) Schering 2991
Levaquin in 5% Dextrose Injection (Levofloxacin) Ortho-McNeil 2453
Levaquin (Levofloxacin) Ortho-McNeil 2453
Noroxin Tablets (Norfloxacin) Merck 2009
Timentin ADD-Vantage (Clavulanate Potassium, Ticarcillin Disodium) GlaxoSmithKline 1556
Timentin Injection Galaxy Container (Clavulanate Potassium, Ticarcillin Disodium) GlaxoSmithKline 1559
Timentin IV Infusion (Clavulanate Potassium, Ticarcillin Disodium) GlaxoSmithKline 1553
Timentin Pharmacy Bulk Package (Clavulanate Potassium, Ticarcillin Disodium) GlaxoSmithKline 1562

Enterobacter species bone and joint infections
Fortaz (Ceftazidime Sodium) GlaxoSmithKline 1422
Primaxin I.V. (Cilastatin Sodium, Imipenem) Merck 2024
Rocephin Injectable Vials, ADD-Vantage, Galaxy, Bulk (Ceftriaxone Sodium) Roche Laboratories 2801

Enterobacter species gynecologic infections
Primaxin I.V. (Cilastatin Sodium, Imipenem) Merck 2024
Timentin ADD-Vantage (Clavulanate Potassium, Ticarcillin Disodium) GlaxoSmithKline 1556
Timentin Injection Galaxy Container (Clavulanate Potassium, Ticarcillin Disodium) GlaxoSmithKline 1559
Timentin IV Infusion (Clavulanate Potassium, Ticarcillin Disodium) GlaxoSmithKline 1553
Timentin Pharmacy Bulk Package (Clavulanate Potassium, Ticarcillin Disodium) GlaxoSmithKline 1562

Enterobacter species infections
Augmentin (Amoxicillin, Clavulanate Potassium) GlaxoSmithKline 1331
Augmentin Tablets (Amoxicillin, Clavulanate Potassium) GlaxoSmithKline 1334
Fortaz (Ceftazidime Sodium) GlaxoSmithKline 1422
Garamycin Injectable (Gentamicin Sulfate) Schering 3028
Primaxin I.V. (Cilastatin Sodium, Imipenem) Merck 2024
Rocephin Injectable Vials, ADD-Vantage, Galaxy, Bulk (Ceftriaxone Sodium) Roche Laboratories 2801
Seromycin Capsules (Cycloserine) Lilly 1783
Timentin ADD-Vantage (Clavulanate Potassium, Ticarcillin Disodium) GlaxoSmithKline 1556
Timentin Injection Galaxy Container (Clavulanate Potassium, Ticarcillin Disodium) GlaxoSmithKline 1559
Timentin IV Infusion (Clavulanate Potassium, Ticarcillin Disodium) GlaxoSmithKline 1553
Timentin Pharmacy Bulk Package (Clavulanate Potassium, Ticarcillin Disodium) GlaxoSmithKline 1562
Zinacef Injection (Cefuroxime) GlaxoSmithKline 1604
Zinacef for Injection (Cefuroxime) GlaxoSmithKline 1604

Enterobacter species infections, ocular
Pred-G Sterile Ophthalmic Ointment (Gentamicin Sulfate, Prednisolone Acetate) Allergan ⊙ 235

Enterobacter species intra-abdominal infections
Maxipime for Injection (Cefepime Hydrochloride) Elan 1093
Primaxin I.V. (Cilastatin Sodium, Imipenem) Merck 2024

Enterobacter species lower respiratory tract infections
Fortaz (Ceftazidime Sodium) GlaxoSmithKline 1422
Maxipime for Injection (Cefepime Hydrochloride) Elan 1093
Primaxin I.V. (Cilastatin Sodium, Imipenem) Merck 2024

Enterobacter species septicemia
Primaxin I.V. (Cilastatin Sodium, Imipenem) Merck 2024

Enterobacter species skin and skin structure infections
Fortaz (Ceftazidime Sodium) GlaxoSmithKline 1422
Primaxin I.V. (Cilastatin Sodium, Imipenem) Merck 2024
Zinacef Injection (Cefuroxime) GlaxoSmithKline 1604
Zinacef for Injection (Cefuroxime) GlaxoSmithKline 1604

Enterobacter species urinary tract infections
Augmentin (Amoxicillin, Clavulanate Potassium) GlaxoSmithKline 1331
Augmentin Tablets (Amoxicillin, Clavulanate Potassium) GlaxoSmithKline 1334
Fortaz (Ceftazidime Sodium) GlaxoSmithKline 1422
Primaxin I.V. (Cilastatin Sodium, Imipenem) Merck 2024
Seromycin Capsules (Cycloserine) Lilly 1783

Enterobiasis
Reese's Pinworm Treatments (Pyrantel Pamoate) Reese ■□ 730
Vermox Chewable Tablets (Mebendazole) McNeil Consumer 1853

Enterobius vermicularis infestation
(*see under* Enterobiasis)

Enterococci infections
(*see under* Streptococci group D infections)

Enterococcus faecium, vancomycin-resistant bacteremia
Synercid I.V. (Dalfopristin, Quinupristin) King 1690
Zyvox (Linezolid) Pharmacia & Upjohn 2661

Enterococcus faecium, vancomycin-resistant infections
Zyvox (Linezolid) Pharmacia & Upjohn 2661

Enterocolitis, staphylococcal
Vancocin HCl Capsules, USP (Vancomycin Hydrochloride) ViroPharma 3370

Enuresis, nocturnal, primary
DDAVP Nasal Spray (Desmopressin Acetate) Sanofi-Aventis 2894
DDAVP Tablets (Desmopressin Acetate) Sanofi-Aventis 2895
Desmopressin Acetate Rhinal Tube (Desmopressin Acetate) Ferring 1144

Envenomation, Micrurus fulvius
Antivenin (Micrurus fulvius) (Antivenin (Micrurus Fulvius)) Wyeth 3401

Envenomation, pit viper
Antivenin Polyvalent (Antivenin (Crotalidae) Polyvalent) Wyeth 3399

Epicondylitis
Decadron Phosphate Injection (Dexamethasone Sodium Phosphate) Merck 1931
Depo-Medrol Injectable Suspension (Methylprednisolone Acetate) Pharmacia & Upjohn 2615
Depo-Medrol Single-Dose Vial (Methylprednisolone Acetate) Pharmacia & Upjohn 2617
Hydrocortone Tablets (Hydrocortisone) Merck 1963
Pediapred Oral Solution (Prednisolone Sodium Phosphate) UCB 3319
Traumeel Injection Solution (Homeopathic Formulations) Heel 1638

Epidermophyton floccosum infections
Ertaczo Cream, 2% (Sertaconazole Nitrate) OrthoNeutrogena 2383
Grifulvin V Tablets Microsize and Oral Suspension Microsize (Griseofulvin) OrthoNeutrogena 2384
Gris-PEG Tablets (Griseofulvin) Pedinol 2504
Loprox Gel (Ciclopirox) Medicis 1861
Lotrimin (Clotrimazole) Schering 3053
Lotrisone (Betamethasone Dipropionate, Clotrimazole) Schering 3054
Naftin Cream (Naftifine Hydrochloride) Merz 2097
Naftin Gel (Naftifine Hydrochloride) Merz 2097
Oxistat (Oxiconazole Nitrate) GlaxoSmithKline 1498
Spectazole Cream (Econazole Nitrate) OrthoNeutrogena 2390

Epididymitis
Ancef for Injection (Cefazolin Sodium) GlaxoSmithKline 1318

Epilepsy
Lamictal (Lamotrigine) GlaxoSmithKline 1449

Epilepsy, generalized
(*see under* Seizures, generalized, tonic-clonic)

Epilepsy, grand mal
(*see under* Seizures, generalized, tonic-clonic)

Epilepsy, petit mal
(*see under* Seizures, generalized, absence)

Epilepticus, status
Nembutal Sodium Solution, USP (Pentobarbital Sodium) Ovation 2484

Epinephrine sensitivity, ocular, treatment of
HMS (Medrysone) Allergan ⊙ 228

Episiotomy, topical debriding in
(*see under* Wounds, debridement of)

Erectile dysfunction
Caverject Impulse Injection (Alprostadil) Pharmacia & Upjohn 2610
Cialis Tablets (Tadalafil) Lilly ICOS 1806
Edex Injection (Alprostadil) Schwarz 3103
Levitra Tablets (Vardenafil Hydrochloride) Schering 3048
Viagra Tablets (Sildenafil Citrate) Pfizer 2552

Erectile dysfunction, diagnosis of
Caverject Impulse Injection (Alprostadil) Pharmacia & Upjohn 2610

Erythema multiforme, severe
(*see under* Stevens-Johnson syndrome)

Erythema nodosum leprosum
Thalomid Capsules (Thalidomide) Celgene 979

Erythrasma
E.E.S. (Erythromycin Ethylsuccinate) Abbott 449
EryPed (Erythromycin Ethylsuccinate) Abbott 445
Ery-Tab Tablets (Erythromycin) Abbott 447
Erythrocin Stearate Filmtab Tablets (Erythromycin Stearate) Abbott 452
Erythromycin Base Filmtab Tablets (Erythromycin) Abbott 454
Erythromycin Delayed-Release Capsules, USP (Erythromycin) Abbott 456
PCE Dispertab Tablets (Erythromycin) Abbott 510

Erythroblastopenia
Decadron Phosphate Injection (Dexamethasone Sodium Phosphate) Merck 1931
Depo-Medrol Injectable Suspension (Methylprednisolone Acetate) Pharmacia & Upjohn 2615
Depo-Medrol Single-Dose Vial (Methylprednisolone Acetate) Pharmacia & Upjohn 2617
Hydrocortone Tablets (Hydrocortisone) Merck 1963
Pediapred Oral Solution (Prednisolone Sodium Phosphate) UCB 3319

Erythroblastosis fetalis, prevention of
HyperRho S/D Full Dose (Rh_o (D) Immune Globulin (Human)) Talecris 3243

Erythrocyle, resuspension
Plasbumin-20 (Albumin (human)) Talecris 3249

Erythroderma, exfoliative
Decadron Tablets (Dexamethasone) Merck 1929

Escherichia coli
(*see under* E. coli infections)

Esophagitis, erosive
(*see also under* Gastroesophageal reflux disease)
Axid Oral Solution (Nizatidine) Braintree 913
Nexium Delayed-Release Capsules (Esomeprazole Magnesium) AstraZeneca LP 645
Nexium I.V. (Esomeprazole Sodium) AstraZeneca LP 649
Prevacid Delayed-Release Capsules (Lansoprazole) TAP 3268
Prevacid for Delayed-Release Oral Suspension (Lansoprazole) TAP 3268
Prevacid I.V. for Injection (Lansoprazole) TAP 3274
Prevacid SoluTab Delayed-Release Orally Disintegrating Tablets (Lansoprazole) TAP 3268
Prilosec OTC Tablets (Omeprazole magnesium) Procter & Gamble 2674
Protonix Tablets (Pantoprazole Sodium) Wyeth 3465
Tagamet Tablets (Cimetidine) GlaxoSmithKline 1547
Zantac (Ranitidine Hydrochloride) GlaxoSmithKline 1597
Zegerid Powder for Oral Solution (Omeprazole) Santarus 2972

Esophagitis, ulcerative
Axid Oral Solution (Nizatidine) Braintree 913

Estrogen, deficiency
(*see under* Hypoestrogenism)

Eubacterium species infections
Invanz for Injection (Ertapenem) Merck 1974
Primaxin I.V. (Cilastatin Sodium, Imipenem) Merck 2024

Eubacterium species intra-abdominal infections
Invanz for Injection (Ertapenem) Merck 1974
Primaxin I.V. (Cilastatin Sodium, Imipenem) Merck 2024

Ewing's sarcoma, palliative treatment of
Cosmegen for Injection (Dactinomycin) Merck 1907

Extrapyramidal reactions, drug-induced
Cogentin Injection (Benztropine Mesylate) Merck 1903
Symmetrel (Amantadine Hydrochloride) Endo Labs 1115

Eye, anterior segment inflammation
(*see under* Inflammation, anterior segment)

Eye and its adnexa, external infections of
Genoptic Sterile Ophthalmic Solution (Gentamicin Sulfate) Allergan ⊙ 227

Eyes, anterior segment, staining of
Fluor-I-Strip A.T. Ophthalmic Strips 1 mg (Fluorescein Sodium) Bausch & Lomb ⊙ 249

Fluor-I-Strip Ophthalmic Strips 9 mg (Fluorescein Sodium) Bausch & Lomb ... ⊙ 249

Eyes, burning, reduction of

Acular LS Ophthalmic Solution (Ketorolac Tromethamine) Allergan ... 562
Refresh Endura Lubricant Eye Drops (Glycerin, Polysorbate 80) Allergan ... ⊙ 238
Refresh Liquigel (Carboxymethyl-cellulose Sodium) Allergan ... ⊙ 238
Refresh Tears Lubricant Eye Drops (Carboxymethylcellulose Sodium) Allergan ... ⊙ 239
Systane Lubricant Eye Drops (Polyethylene Glycol, Propylene Glycol) Alcon ... 558
Visine Pure Tears Eye Drops Single Drop Dispenser (Hypromellose, Glycerin, Polyethylene Glycol) Pfizer Consumer ... ⊙ 280

Eyes, diagnostic procedures, adjunct in

Fluor-I-Strip A.T. Ophthalmic Strips 1 mg (Fluorescein Sodium) Bausch & Lomb ... ⊙ 249
Fluor-I-Strip Ophthalmic Strips 9 mg (Fluorescein Sodium) Bausch & Lomb ... ⊙ 249

Eyes, dry
(*see under* Keratoconjunctivitis sicca)

Eyes, external infections of

Genoptic Sterile Ophthalmic Solution (Gentamicin Sulfate) Allergan ... ⊙ 227

Eyes, inflammation
(*see under* Ocular inflammation)

Eyes, irrigation of

Betadine 5% Ophthalmic Solution (Povidone Iodine) Alcon ... ⊙ 202

Eyes, irritation, symptomatic relief of

Refresh Endura Lubricant Eye Drops (Glycerin, Polysorbate 80) Allergan ... ⊙ 238
Refresh Liquigel (Carboxymethyl-cellulose Sodium) Allergan ... ⊙ 238
Refresh Tears Lubricant Eye Drops (Carboxymethylcellulose Sodium) Allergan ... ⊙ 239
Systane Lubricant Eye Drops (Polyethylene Glycol, Propylene Glycol) Alcon ... 558
Visine Original Eye Drops (Tetrahydrozoline Hydrochloride) Pfizer Consumer ... ⊙ 279
Visine A.C. Seasonal Itching and Redness Relief Drops (Tetrahydrozoline Hydrochloride, Zinc Sulfate) Pfizer Consumer ... ⊙ 278
Advanced Relief Visine Eye Drops (Dextran 70, Polyethylene Glycol, Povidone, Tetrahydrozoline Hydrochloride) Pfizer Consumer ... ⊙ 278
Visine For Contacts Rewetting Drops (Glycerin, Hydroxypropyl Methylcellulose) Pfizer Consumer ... ⊙ 278
Visine L.R. Long Lasting Eye Drops (Oxymetazoline Hydrochloride) Pfizer Consumer ... ⊙ 279
Visine Pure Tears Eye Drops Single Drop Dispenser (Hypromellose, Glycerin, Polyethylene Glycol) Pfizer Consumer ... ⊙ 280
Visine Pure Tears Portables (Hypromellose, Glycerin, Polyethylene Glycol) Pfizer Consumer ... ⊙ 280
Visine Tears Eye Drops (Hypromellose, Glycerin, Polyethylene Glycol) Pfizer Consumer ... ⊙ 279
Viva Eye Drops (Polysorbate 80) Vision Pharmaceuticals ... ⊙ 282
Zicam Allergy Relief Nasal Pump (Histanium Hydrochloricum, Luffa operculata, Galphimia Glauca, Sulfur) Matrixx ...

Eyes, lubrication of
(*see also under* Keratoconjunctivitis sicca)

Restasis Ophthalmic Emulsion (Cyclosporine) Allergan ... 570

Eyes, surgery, adjunct to

Acular LS Ophthalmic Solution (Ketorolac Tromethamine) Allergan ... 562
Amvisc Plus (Sodium Hyaluronate) Bausch & Lomb ... ⊙ 289
Ocucoat (Hydroxypropyl Methylcellulose) Bausch & Lomb ... ⊙ 290

Eyes, watery
(*see under* Lacrimation, symptomatic relief of)

F

Fabry disease

Fabrazyme for Intravenous Infusion (Agalsidase beta) Genzyme ... 1267

Fatigue, symptomatic relief of

Vivarin (Caffeine) GlaxoSmithKline ... ▣ 639

Female castration
(*see under* Ovaries, castration of)

Fever, reduction of

Advil (Ibuprofen) Wyeth ... ▣ 737
Children's Advil Suspension (Ibuprofen) Wyeth ... ▣ 742
Children's Advil Chewable Tablets (Ibuprofen) Wyeth ... ▣ 741
Children's Advil Cold Suspension (Ibuprofen, Pseudoephedrine Hydrochloride) Wyeth ... ▣ 741
Infants' Advil Concentrated Drops (Ibuprofen) Wyeth ... ▣ 743
Junior Strength Advil Swallow Tablets (Ibuprofen) Wyeth ... ▣ 740
Aleve Tablets, Caplets and Gelcaps (Naproxen Sodium) Bayer Healthcare ... ▣ 605
BC Powder (Aspirin, Caffeine, Salicylamide) GlaxoSmithKline ... ▣ 612
Goody's Extra Strength Headache Powder (Acetaminophen, Aspirin, Caffeine) GlaxoSmithKline ... ▣ 621
Goody's Extra Strength Pain Relief Tablets (Acetaminophen, Aspirin, Caffeine) GlaxoSmithKline ... ▣ 621
Children's Motrin Oral Suspension and Chewable Tablets (Ibuprofen) McNeil Consumer ... ▣ 647
Children's Motrin Non-Staining Dye-Free Oral Suspension (Ibuprofen) McNeil Consumer ... ▣ 647
Children's Motrin Oral Suspension and Chewable Tablets (Ibuprofen) McNeil Consumer ... 1837
Children's Motrin Non-Staining Dye-Free Oral Suspension (Ibuprofen) McNeil Consumer ... 1837
Motrin IB Tablets and Caplets (Ibuprofen) McNeil Consumer ... 1836
Infants' Motrin Concentrated Drops (Ibuprofen) McNeil Consumer ... 1837
Infants' Motrin Non-Staining Dye-Free Drops (Ibuprofen) McNeil Consumer ... 1837
Junior Strength Motrin Caplets and Chewable Tablets (Ibuprofen) McNeil Consumer ... 1837
TheraFlu Cold & Cough Hot Liquid (Acetaminophen, Chlorpheniramine Maleate, Dextromethorphan Hydrobromide, Pseudoephedrine Hydrochloride) Novartis Consumer ... ▣ 680
TheraFlu Cold & Sore Throat Hot Liquid (Acetaminophen, Chlorpheniramine Maleate, Pseudoephedrine Hydrochloride) Novartis Consumer ... ▣ 680
TheraFlu Flu & Chest Congestion Non-Drowsy Hot Liquid (Acetaminophen, Dextromethorphan Hydrobromide, Guaifenesin, Pseudoephedrine Hydrochloride) Novartis Consumer ... ▣ 681
TheraFlu Flu & Sore Throat Hot Liquid (Acetaminophen, Chlorpheniramine Maleate, Pseudoephedrine Hydrochloride) Novartis Consumer ... ▣ 681
TheraFlu Severe Cold & Cough Hot Liquid (Acetaminophen, Chlorpheniramine Maleate, Dextromethorphan Hydrobromide, Pseudoephedrine Hydrochloride) Novartis Consumer ... ▣ 683
TheraFlu Severe Cold Caplets (Acetaminophen, Chlorpheniramine Maleate, Dextromethorphan Hydrobromide, Pseudoephedrine Hydrochloride) Novartis Consumer ... ▣ 679
TheraFlu Severe Cold Hot Liquid (Acetaminophen, Chlorpheniramine Maleate, Dextromethorphan Hydrobromide, Pseudoephedrine Hydrochloride) Novartis Consumer ... ▣ 682
Tylenol 8 Hour Extended Release Geltabs and Caplets (Acetaminophen) McNeil Consumer ... 1843
Tylenol 8-Hour Extended Release Geltabs/Caplets (Acetaminophen) McNeil Consumer ... ▣ 655
Children's Tylenol Suspension Liquid and Meltaways (Acetaminophen) McNeil Consumer ... 1850
Children's Tylenol Plus Cold & Allergy Suspension Liquid (Acetaminophen, Diphenhydramine Hydrochloride, Pseudoephedrine Hydrochloride) McNeil Consumer ... 1850
Children's Tylenol Plus Flu Suspension Liquid (Acetaminophen, Chlorpheniramine Maleate, Dextromethorphan Hydrobromide, Pseudoephedrine Hydrochloride) McNeil Consumer ... 1853
Concentrated Tylenol Infants' Drops (Acetaminophen) McNeil Consumer ... 1850
Junior Tylenol Meltaways (Acetaminophen) McNeil Consumer ... 1850
Tylenol Cold & Flu Severe Daytime Liquid with Cool Bust (Acetaminophen, Dextromethorphan Hydrobromide, Pseudoephedrine Hydrochloride) McNeil Consumer ... 1846
Tylenol Cold & Flu Severe NightTime Liquid with Cool Burst (Acetaminophen, Dextromethorphan Hydrobromide, Doxylamine Succinate, Pseudoephedrine Hydrochloride) McNeil Consumer ... 1846
Tylenol (Acetaminophen) McNeil Consumer ... 1843
Extra Strength Tylenol Rapid Release Gels (Acetaminophen) McNeil Consumer ... 1843
Tylenol (Acetaminophen) McNeil Consumer ... 1843
Tylenol Flu NightTime Gelcaps (Acetaminophen, Diphenhydramine Hydrochloride, Pseudoephedrine Hydrochloride) McNeil Consumer ... 1846
Tylenol Flu Day Non-Drowsy Gelcaps (Acetaminophen, Dextromethorphan Hydrobromide, Pseudoephedrine Hydrochloride) McNeil Consumer ... 1846
Concentrated Tylenol Infants' Drops Plus Cold Nasal Congestant, Fever Reducer & Pain Reliever (Acetaminophen, Pseudoephedrine Hydrochloride) McNeil Consumer ... ▣ 668
Concentrated Tylenol Infants' Drops Plus Cold & Cough Nasal Decongestant, Fever Reducer & Pain Reliever (Acetaminophen, Dextromethorphan Hydrobromide, Pseudoephedrine Hydrochloride) McNeil Consumer ... ▣ 668
Tylenol Sore Throat Daytime Liquid with Cool Burst (Acetaminophen) McNeil Consumer ... 1849
Tylenol Sore Throat NightTime Liquid with Cool Burst (Acetaminophen, Diphenhydramine) McNeil Consumer ... 1849

Fever associated with common cold

Advil Allergy Sinus Caplets (Chlorpheniramine Maleate, Ibuprofen, Pseudoephedrine Hydrochloride) Wyeth ... ▣ 737
Advil Cold & Sinus (Ibuprofen, Pseudoephedrine Hydrochloride) Wyeth ... ▣ 739
Advil Flu & Body Ache Caplets (Ibuprofen, Pseudoephedrine Hydrochloride) Wyeth ... ▣ 739
Children's Advil Cold Suspension (Ibuprofen, Pseudoephedrine Hydrochloride) Wyeth ... ▣ 741
Advil Multi-Symptom Cold Caplets (Chlorpheniramine Maleate, Ibuprofen, Pseudoephedrine Hydrochloride) Wyeth ... ▣ 738
BC Cold Powder (Aspirin, Chlorpheniramine Maleate, Pseudoephedrine Hydrochloride) GlaxoSmithKline ... ▣ 612
Benadryl Allergy & Cold Tablets (Acetaminophen, Diphenhydramine Hydrochloride, Pseudoephedrine Hydrochloride) Pfizer Consumer Healthcare ... ▣ 692
Benadryl Maximum Strength Severe Allergy & Sinus Headache Caplets (Acetaminophen, Diphenhydramine Hydrochloride, Pseudoephedrine Hydrochloride) Pfizer Consumer Healthcare ... ▣ 694
Contac Severe Cold and Flu Caplets Maximum Strength (Acetaminophen, Chlorpheniramine Maleate, Dextromethorphan Hydrobromide, Pseudoephedrine Hydrochloride) GlaxoSmithKline ... ▣ 615
Contac Severe Cold and Flu Caplets Non-Drowsy (Acetaminophen, Dextromethorphan Hydrobromide, Pseudoephedrine Hydrochloride) GlaxoSmithKline ... ▣ 615
Children's Motrin Cold Non-Staining Dye-Free Oral Suspension (Ibuprofen, Pseudoephedrine Hydrochloride) McNeil Consumer ... 1838
Children's Motrin Cold Oral Suspension (Ibuprofen, Pseudoephedrine Hydrochloride) McNeil Consumer ... ▣ 648
Children's Motrin Cold Non-Staining Dye-Free Oral Suspension (Ibuprofen, Pseudoephedrine Hydrochloride) McNeil Consumer ... ▣ 648
Children's Motrin Cold Oral Suspension (Ibuprofen, Pseudoephedrine Hydrochloride) McNeil Consumer ... 1838
Motrin Cold & Sinus Caplets (Ibuprofen, Pseudoephedrine Hydrochloride) McNeil Consumer ... 1836
Triaminic Cough & Sore Throat Softchews (Acetaminophen, Dextromethorphan Hydrobromide, Pseudoephedrine Hydrochloride) Novartis Consumer ... ▣ 689
Children's Tylenol Plus Cold NightTime Suspension Liquid (Acetaminophen, Chlorpheniramine Maleate, Pseudoephedrine Hydrochloride) McNeil Consumer ... 1851
Children's Tylenol Plus Cold Chewable Tablets (Acetaminophen, Chlorpheniramine Maleate, Pseudoephedrine Hydrochloride) McNeil Consumer ... 1851
Children's Tylenol Plus Cold Daytime Non-Drowsy Suspension Liquid (Acetaminophen, Pseudoephedrine Hydrochloride) McNeil Consumer ... 1851
Concentrated Tylenol Infants' Drops Plus Cold (Acetaminophen, Pseudoephedrine Hydrochloride) McNeil Consumer ... 1851
Concentrated Tylenol Infants' Drops Plus Cold and Cough (Acetaminophen, Dextromethorphan Hydrobromide, Pseudoephedrine Hydrochloride) McNeil Consumer ... 1851
Tylenol Cold Severe Congestion Non-Drowsy Caplets with Cool Burst (Acetaminophen, Dextromethorphan Hydrobromide, Guaifenesin, Pseudoephedrine Hydrochloride) McNeil Consumer ... 1846
Multi-Symptom Tylenol Cold Night Time Caplets (Acetaminophen, Chlorpheniramine Maleate, Dextromethorphan Hydrobromide, Pseudoephedrine Hydrochloride) McNeil Consumer ... 1845

Multi-Symptom Tylenol Cold Day Non-Drowsy Caplets and Gelcaps (Acetaminophen, Dextromethorphan Hydrobromide, Pseudoephedrine Hydrochloride) McNeil Consumer **1845**
Vicks NyQuil LiquiCaps/Liquid Multi-Symptom Cold/Flu Relief (Acetaminophen, Dextromethorphan Hydrobromide, Doxylamine Succinate, Pseudoephedrine Hydrochloride) Procter & Gamble .... ▣ **725**

Fever blisters
(*see under* Herpetic manifestations, oral, symptomatic relief of)

Fiber, deficiency of
Metamucil Dietary Fiber Supplement (Psyllium Preparations) Procter & Gamble .... ▣ **774**
Senokot Wheat Bran (Bran, wheat) Purdue Products **2717**

Fissures, skin
Ultralytic 2 Cream 20% (Urea) Ivax Dermatologicals **1651**
Ultralytic 2 Foam 20% (Urea) Ivax Dermatologicals **1652**

Flatulence, relief of
Beano (Alpha Galactosidase Enzyme) GlaxoSmithKline .... ▣ **764**
Gas-X Regular Strength Chewable Tablets (Simethicone) Novartis Consumer .... ▣ **675**
Gas-X Extra Strength (Simethicone) Novartis Consumer .... ▣ **675**
Gas-X Maximum Strength Softgels (Simethicone) Novartis Consumer .... ▣ **675**
Maalox Max Maximum Strength Antacid/Anti-Gas Liquid (Aluminum Hydroxide, Magnesium Hydroxide, Simethicone) Novartis Consumer **2165**
Maalox Regular Strength Antacid/Antigas Liquid (Aluminum Hydroxide, Magnesium Hydroxide, Simethicone) Novartis Consumer **2164**
Phazyme-125 mg Quick Dissolve Chewable Tablets (Simethicone) GlaxoSmithKline .... ▣ **635**
Phazyme-180 mg Ultra Strength Softgels (Simethicone) GlaxoSmithKline .... ▣ **635**
Rolaids Multi-Symptom Antacid & Antigas Tablets (Calcium Carbonate, Magnesium Hydroxide, Simethicone) Pfizer Consumer Healthcare .... ▣ **708**

Flu symptoms
(*see under* Influenza syndrome, symptomatic relief of)

Folic acid deficiency, prevention of
Slow Fe with Folic Acid Tablets (Ferrous Sulfate, Folic Acid) Novartis Consumer .... ▣ **773**

Folliculitis barbae
Grifulvin V Tablets Microsize and Oral Suspension Microsize (Griseofulvin) OrthoNeutrogena **2384**
Gris-PEG Tablets (Griseofulvin) Pedinol **2504**

Francisella tularensis infections
Dynacin Tablets (Minocycline Hydrochloride) Medicis **1859**

Fungal infections, skin
(*see under* Infections, mycotic, cutaneous)

Furunculosis
Levaquin in 5% Dextrose Injection (Levofloxacin) Ortho-McNeil **2453**
Levaquin (Levofloxacin) Ortho-McNeil **2453**

Furunculosis, symptomatic relief of
Panafil Ointment (Chlorophyllin Copper Complex Sodium, Papain, Urea) Healthpoint **1637**
Panafil Spray (Chlorophyllin Copper Complex Sodium, Papain, Urea) Healthpoint **1637**

Fusarium solani infections
VFEND I.V. (Voriconazole) Pfizer **2543**
VFEND Oral Suspension (Voriconazole) Pfizer **2543**
VFEND Tablets (Voriconazole) Pfizer **2543**

Fusobacterium fusiforme infections
Dynacin Tablets (Minocycline Hydrochloride) Medicis **1859**

Fusobacterium species infections
Primaxin I.M. (Cilastatin Sodium, Imipenem) Merck **2022**
Primaxin I.V. (Cilastatin Sodium, Imipenem) Merck **2024**

Fusobacterium species intra-abdominal infections
Primaxin I.M. (Cilastatin Sodium, Imipenem) Merck **2022**
Primaxin I.V. (Cilastatin Sodium, Imipenem) Merck **2024**

Fusospirochetosis
Dynacin Tablets (Minocycline Hydrochloride) Medicis **1859**

G

Gag reflex, suppression
Cetacaine Topical Anesthetic (Benzocaine, Butyl Aminobenzoate, Tetracaine Hydrochloride) Cetylite **1007**
Hurricaine Topical Anesthetic Gel, 1 oz. Fresh Mint, Wild Cherry, Pina Colada, Watermelon, 1/6 oz. Wild Cherry (Benzocaine) Beutlich .... ▣ **607**
Hurricaine Topical Anesthetic Liquid, 1 oz. Wild Cherry, Pina Colada, .25 ml Swab Applicator Wild Cherry (Benzocaine) Beutlich .... ▣ **607**
Hurricaine Topical Anesthetic Spray Extension Tubes (200) (Benzocaine) Beutlich .... ▣ **607**
Hurricaine Topical Anesthetic Spray Kit, 2 oz. Wild Cherry (Benzocaine) Beutlich .... ▣ **607**
Hurricaine Topical Anesthetic Spray, 2 oz. Wild Cherry (Benzocaine) Beutlich .... ▣ **607**

Gardnerella vaginalis infections
Metrogel 1% (Metronidazole) Galderma **1212**
MetroGel-Vaginal Gel (Metronidazole) 3M **1822**
Primaxin I.V. (Cilastatin Sodium, Imipenem) Merck **2024**

Gardnerella vaginalis vaginitis
(*see under* H. vaginalis vaginitis)

Gas
Imodium Advanced Caplets and Chewable Tablets McNeil Consumer .... ▣ **644**
Rolaids Multi-Symptom Antacid & Antigas Tablets (Calcium Carbonate, Magnesium Hydroxide, Simethicone) Pfizer Consumer Healthcare .... ▣ **708**

Gastric ulcer, nonsteroidal anti-inflammatory drug induced
Prevacid Delayed-Release Capsules (Lansoprazole) TAP **3268**
Prevacid for Delayed-Release Oral Suspension (Lansoprazole) TAP **3268**
Prevacid SoluTab Delayed-Release Orally Disintegrating Tablets (Lansoprazole) TAP **3268**

Gastric ulcer, NSAID-associated, risk reductions
Nexium Delayed-Release Capsules (Esomeprazole Magnesium) AstraZeneca LP **645**

Gastric ulcers, active, benign, short-term treatment of
Axid Oral Solution (Nizatidine) Braintree **913**
Pepcid Injection (Famotidine) Merck . **2017**
Pepcid (Famotidine) Merck **2014**
Prevacid Delayed-Release Capsules (Lansoprazole) TAP **3268**
Prevacid for Delayed-Release Oral Suspension (Lansoprazole) TAP **3268**
Prevacid SoluTab Delayed-Release Orally Disintegrating Tablets (Lansoprazole) TAP **3268**
Prilosec OTC Tablets (Omeprazole magnesium) Procter & Gamble **2674**
Tagamet Tablets (Cimetidine) GlaxoSmithKline **1547**
Zantac (Ranitidine Hydrochloride) GlaxoSmithKline **1597**
Zegerid Powder for Oral Solution (Omeprazole) Santarus **2972**

Gastric ulcers, nonsteroidal anti-inflammatory drug-induced, prevention of
Prevacid NapraPAC (Lansoprazole, Naproxen) TAP **3277**

Gastroesophageal reflux, symptomatic
Zegerid Powder for Oral Solution (Omeprazole) Santarus **2972**

Gastroesophageal reflux disease
Aciphex Tablets (Rabeprazole Sodium) Eisai **1081**
Axid Oral Solution (Nizatidine) Braintree **913**
Nexium Delayed-Release Capsules (Esomeprazole Magnesium) AstraZeneca LP **645**
Nexium I.V. (Esomeprazole Sodium) AstraZeneca LP **649**
Pepcid Injection (Famotidine) Merck . **2017**
Pepcid (Famotidine) Merck **2014**
Prevacid Delayed-Release Capsules (Lansoprazole) TAP **3268**
Prevacid for Delayed-Release Oral Suspension (Lansoprazole) TAP **3268**
Prevacid SoluTab Delayed-Release Orally Disintegrating Tablets (Lansoprazole) TAP **3268**
Prilosec OTC Tablets (Omeprazole magnesium) Procter & Gamble **2674**
Protonix I.V. (Pantoprazole Sodium) Wyeth **3468**
Protonix Tablets (Pantoprazole Sodium) Wyeth **3465**
Tagamet Tablets (Cimetidine) GlaxoSmithKline **1547**
Zantac (Ranitidine Hydrochloride) GlaxoSmithKline **1597**
Zegerid Powder for Oral Solution (Omeprazole) Santarus **2972**

Gastrointestinal stromal tumors
(*see under* Tumors, gastrointestinal stromal)

Gaucher disease, Type 1
Cerezyme for Injection (Imiglucerase) Genzyme **1263**
Zavesca Capsules (Miglustat) Actelion **543**

Gelineau's syndrome
(*see under* Narcolepsy)

Genital warts
(*see under* Condylomata acuminata)

GERD
(*see under* Gastroesophageal reflux disease)

German measles
(*see under* Rubella, prophylaxis)

Gestational trophoblastic neoplasia
Cosmegen for Injection (Dactinomycin) Merck **1907**

Giardiasis
Tindamax (Tinidazole) Presutti **2670**

Gingivitis, necrotizing ulcerative
(*see under* Fusospirochetosis)

GIST
(*see under* Tumors, gastrointestinal stromal)

Glaucoma, angle-closure, acute
Daranide Tablets (Dichlorphenamide) Merck **1928**

Glaucoma, chronic open-angle
Betagan Ophthalmic Solution, USP (Levobunolol Hydrochloride) Allergan .... ⊙ **217**
Betoptic S Ophthalmic Suspension (Betaxolol Hydrochloride) Alcon **554**
Carteolol Hydrochloride Ophthalmic Solution USP, 1% (Carteolol Hydrochloride) Bausch & Lomb .... ⊙ **246**
Daranide Tablets (Dichlorphenamide) Merck **1928**
OptiPranolol Metipranolol Ophthalmic Solution 0.3% (Metipranolol) Bausch & Lomb .... ⊙ **254**
Propine Ophthalmic Solution (Dipivefrin Hydrochloride) Allergan .... ⊙ **237**
Timoptic in Ocudose (Timolol Maleate) Merck **2061**
Timoptic Sterile Ophthalmic Solution (Timolol Maleate) Merck **2058**
Timoptic-XE Sterile Ophthalmic Gel Forming Solution (Timolol Maleate) Merck **2062**

Glaucoma, open-angle
Alphagan P Ophthalmic Solution (Brimonidine Tartrate) Allergan **563**
Azopt Ophthalmic Suspension (Brinzolamide) Alcon **553**
Brimonidine Tartrate Ophthalmic Solution 0.2% (Brimonidine Tartrate) Bausch & Lomb .... ⊙ **245**
Cosopt Sterile Ophthalmic Solution (Dorzolamide Hydrochloride, Timolol Maleate) Merck **1910**
Lumigan Ophthalmic Solution (Bimatoprost) Allergan **569**
Travatan Ophthalmic Solution (Travoprost) Alcon **559**
Trusopt Sterile Ophthalmic Solution (Dorzolamide Hydrochloride) Merck **2065**
Xalatan Sterile Ophthalmic Solution (Latanoprost) Pharmacia & Upjohn **2654**

Glaucoma, secondary
Daranide Tablets (Dichlorphenamide) Merck **1928**

Glioblastoma multiforme
Temodar Capsules (Temozolomide) Schering **3088**

Goiter, euthyroid, treatment or prevention of
Synthroid Tablets (Levothyroxine Sodium) Abbott **515**
Thyrolar (Liotrix) Forest **1203**

Goiter, suppression of pituitary TSH in
Cytomel Tablets (Liothyronine Sodium) King **1678**
Levothroid Tablets (Levothyroxine Sodium) Forest **1189**
Levoxyl Tablets (Levothyroxine Sodium) King **1680**
Synthroid Tablets (Levothyroxine Sodium) Abbott **515**
Thyrolar (Liotrix) Forest **1203**
Unithroid Tablets (Levothyroxine Sodium) Lannett **3521**

Gonococcal infections, uncomplicated
Rocephin Injectable Vials, ADD-Vantage, Galaxy, Bulk (Ceftriaxone Sodium) Roche Laboratories **2801**
Vantin Tablets and Oral Suspension (Cefpodoxime Proxetil) Pharmacia & Upjohn **2650**
Zinacef Injection (Cefuroxime) GlaxoSmithKline **1604**
Zinacef for Injection (Cefuroxime) GlaxoSmithKline **1604**

Gonorrhea
(*see also under* N. gonorrhoeae infections)
Amoxil Capsules (Amoxicillin) GlaxoSmithKline ... 1315
Amoxil Chewable Tablets (Amoxicillin) GlaxoSmithKline ... 1315
Amoxil Pediatric Drops for Oral Suspension (Amoxicillin) GlaxoSmithKline ... 1315
Amoxil Powder for Oral Suspension (Amoxicillin) GlaxoSmithKline ... 1315
Amoxil Tablets (Amoxicillin) GlaxoSmithKline ... 1315
Rocephin Injectable Vials, ADD-Vantage, Galaxy, Bulk (Ceftriaxone Sodium) Roche Laboratories ... 2801
Zinacef Injection (Cefuroxime) GlaxoSmithKline ... 1604
Zinacef for Injection (Cefuroxime) GlaxoSmithKline ... 1604

Gonorrhea, cervical/urethral
Cipro (Ciprofloxacin) Schering ... 2991
Noroxin Tablets (Norfloxacin) Merck . 2009
Rocephin Injectable Vials, ADD-Vantage, Galaxy, Bulk (Ceftriaxone Sodium) Roche Laboratories ... 2801
Vantin Tablets and Oral Suspension (Cefpodoxime Proxetil) Pharmacia & Upjohn ... 2650

Gonorrhea, pharyngeal
Rocephin (Ceftriaxone Sodium) Roche Laboratories ... 2801

Gonorrhea, uncomplicated
Ceftin Tablets (Cefuroxime Axetil) GlaxoSmithKline ... 1369
Cipro (Ciprofloxacin) Schering ... 2991
Noroxin Tablets (Norfloxacin) Merck . 2009
Rocephin Injectable Vials, ADD-Vantage, Galaxy, Bulk (Ceftriaxone Sodium) Roche Laboratories ... 2801

Gout, acute
Anaprox Tablets (Naproxen Sodium) Roche Laboratories ... 2769
Anaprox DS Tablets (Naproxen Sodium) Roche Laboratories ... 2769
Naprosyn Suspension (Naproxen) Roche Laboratories ... 2769
Naprosyn Tablets (Naproxen) Roche Laboratories ... 2769

Grand mal epilepsy
(*see under* Seizures, generalized, tonic-clonic)

Granuloma annulare, infiltrated inflammatory lesions of
Decadron Phosphate Injection (Dexamethasone Sodium Phosphate) Merck ... 1931
Depo-Medrol Single-Dose Vial (Methylprednisolone Acetate) Pharmacia & Upjohn ... 2617

Granuloma inguinale
Dynacin Tablets (Minocycline Hydrochloride) Medicis ... 1859

Granulomatous disease, chronic
Actimmune (Interferon Gamma-1B) InterMune ... 1646

Growth, in children, stimulation of
Increlex Injection (Mecasermin [rDNA origin]) Tercica ... 3290

Growth failure, chronic renal insufficiency-induced in children
Nutropin for Injection (Somatropin) Genentech ... 1238
Nutropin AQ Injection (Somatropin) Genentech ... 1241
Nutropin AQ Pen (Somatropin) Genentech ... 1241
Nutropin AQ Pen Cartridge (Somatropin) Genentech ... 1241

Growth hormone secretion, evaluation of the secreting capability of
R-Gene 10 for Intravenous Use (Arginine Hydrochloride) Pharmacia & Upjohn ... 2647

Growth hormone secretion, inadequate
Genotropin Lyophilized Powder (Somatropin) Pharmacia & Upjohn ... 2642
Humatrope Vials and Cartridges (Somatropin) Lilly ... 1756
Norditropin Cartridges (Somatropin) Novo Nordisk ... 2318
Nutropin for Injection (Somatropin) Genentech ... 1238
Nutropin AQ Injection (Somatropin) Genentech ... 1241
Nutropin AQ Pen (Somatropin) Genentech ... 1241
Nutropin AQ Pen Cartridge (Somatropin) Genentech ... 1241
Tev-Tropin for Injection (Somatropin (rDNA Origin)) Gate ... 1224

Gums, sore
(*see under* Pain, dental)

H

H. parainfluenzae infections, ocular
Vigamox Ophthalmic Solution (Moxifloxacin Hydrochloride) Alcon ... 560

H. aegypticus infections, ocular
TobraDex Ophthalmic Ointment (Dexamethasone, Tobramycin) Alcon ... 558
TobraDex Ophthalmic Suspension (Dexamethasone, Tobramycin) Alcon ... 558
Zylet Ophthalmic Suspension (Loteprednol Etabonate, Tobramycin) Bausch & Lomb ... 3508

H. ducreyi infections
Dynacin Tablets (Minocycline Hydrochloride) Medicis ... 1859
Zithromax Capsules, 250 mg (Azithromycin Dihydrate) Pfizer ... 2568
Zithromax for IV Infusion (Azithromycin Dihydrate) Pfizer ... 2573
Zithromax for Oral Suspension, 300 mg, 600 mg, 900 mg, 1200 mg (Azithromycin Dihydrate) Pfizer ... 2561
Zithromax Tablets, 250 mg, 500 mg (Azithromycin Dihydrate) Pfizer ... 2561
Zithromax Tri-Pak (Azithromycin Dihydrate) Pfizer ... 2561

H. influenzae, central nervous system infections
Fortaz (Ceftazidime Sodium) GlaxoSmithKline ... 1422

H. influenzae bronchitis
Avelox (Moxifloxacin Hydrochloride) Schering ... 2984
Biaxin/Biaxin XL (Clarithromycin) Abbott ... 402
Ceftin Tablets (Cefuroxime Axetil) GlaxoSmithKline ... 1369
Factive Tablets (Gemifloxacin Mesylate) Oscient ... 2464
Ketek Tablets (Telithromycin) Sanofi-Aventis ... 2920
Levaquin in 5% Dextrose Injection (Levofloxacin) Ortho-McNeil ... 2453
Levaquin (Levofloxacin) Ortho-McNeil ... 2453
Omnicef Capsules (Cefdinir) Abbott .. 506
Omnicef for Oral Suspension (Cefdinir) Abbott ... 506
Tequin Injection (Gatifloxacin) Bristol-Myers Squibb ... 964
Tequin Tablets (Gatifloxacin) Bristol-Myers Squibb ... 964
Vantin Tablets and Oral Suspension (Cefpodoxime Proxetil) Pharmacia & Upjohn ... 2650

H. influenzae infections
Amoxil Capsules (Amoxicillin) GlaxoSmithKline ... 1315
Amoxil Chewable Tablets (Amoxicillin) GlaxoSmithKline ... 1315
Amoxil Pediatric Drops for Oral Suspension (Amoxicillin) GlaxoSmithKline ... 1315
Amoxil Powder for Oral Suspension (Amoxicillin) GlaxoSmithKline ... 1315
Amoxil Tablets (Amoxicillin) GlaxoSmithKline ... 1315
Augmentin (Amoxicillin, Clavulanate Potassium) GlaxoSmithKline ... 1331
Augmentin Tablets (Amoxicillin, Clavulanate Potassium) GlaxoSmithKline ... 1334
Augmentin XR Extended-Release Tablets (Amoxicillin, Clavulanate Potassium) GlaxoSmithKline ... 1340
Augmentin ES-600 Powder for Oral Suspension (Amoxicillin, Clavulanate Potassium) GlaxoSmithKline 1337
Avelox (Moxifloxacin Hydrochloride) Schering ... 2984
Biaxin/Biaxin XL (Clarithromycin) Abbott ... 402
Ceftin (Cefuroxime Axetil) GlaxoSmithKline ... 1369
Cipro I.V. (Ciprofloxacin) Schering 2998
Cipro I.V. Pharmacy Bulk Package (Ciprofloxacin) Bayer ... 3509
Cipro (Ciprofloxacin) Schering ... 2991
E.E.S. (Erythromycin Ethylsuccinate) Abbott ... 449
EryPed (Erythromycin Ethylsuccinate) Abbott ... 445
Ery-Tab Tablets (Erythromycin) Abbott ... 447
Erythrocin Stearate Filmtab Tablets (Erythromycin Stearate) Abbott ... 452
Erythromycin Base Filmtab Tablets (Erythromycin) Abbott ... 454
Erythromycin Delayed-Release Capsules, USP (Erythromycin) Abbott ... 456
Factive Tablets (Gemifloxacin Mesylate) Oscient ... 2464
Fortaz (Ceftazidime Sodium) GlaxoSmithKline ... 1422
Invanz for Injection (Ertapenem) Merck ... 1974
Levaquin in 5% Dextrose Injection (Levofloxacin) Ortho-McNeil ... 2453
Levaquin (Levofloxacin) Ortho-McNeil ... 2453
Mefoxin for Injection (Cefoxitin Sodium) Merck ... 1987
Mefoxin Premixed Intravenous Solution (Cefoxitin Sodium) Merck ... 1990
Merrem I.V. (Meropenem) AstraZeneca ... 687
Omnicef Capsules (Cefdinir) Abbott .. 506
Omnicef for Oral Suspension (Cefdinir) Abbott ... 506
PCE Dispertab Tablets (Erythromycin) Abbott ... 510
Primaxin I.M. (Cilastatin Sodium, Imipenem) Merck ... 2022
Primaxin I.V. (Cilastatin Sodium, Imipenem) Merck ... 2024
Rocephin Injectable Vials, ADD-Vantage, Galaxy, Bulk (Ceftriaxone Sodium) Roche Laboratories ... 2801
Suprax (Cefixime) Lupin ... 1811
Tequin Injection (Gatifloxacin) Bristol-Myers Squibb ... 964
Tequin Tablets (Gatifloxacin) Bristol-Myers Squibb ... 964
Timentin ADD-Vantage (Clavulanate Potassium, Ticarcillin Disodium) GlaxoSmithKline ... 1556
Timentin Injection Galaxy Container (Clavulanate Potassium, Ticarcillin Disodium) GlaxoSmithKline ... 1559
Timentin IV Infusion (Clavulanate Potassium, Ticarcillin Disodium) GlaxoSmithKline ... 1553
Timentin Pharmacy Bulk Package (Clavulanate Potassium, Ticarcillin Disodium) GlaxoSmithKline ... 1562
Vantin Tablets and Oral Suspension (Cefpodoxime Proxetil) Pharmacia & Upjohn ... 2650
Vigamox Ophthalmic Solution (Moxifloxacin Hydrochloride) Alcon ... ⊙212
Zinacef Injection (Cefuroxime) GlaxoSmithKline ... 1604
Zinacef for Injection (Cefuroxime) GlaxoSmithKline ... 1604
Zithromax Capsules, 250 mg (Azithromycin Dihydrate) Pfizer ... 2568
Zithromax for IV Infusion (Azithromycin Dihydrate) Pfizer ... 2573
Zithromax for Oral Suspension, 1 g (Azithromycin Dihydrate) Pfizer ... 2568
Zithromax for Oral Suspension, 300 mg, 600 mg, 900 mg, 1200 mg (Azithromycin Dihydrate) Pfizer ... 2561
Zithromax Tablets, 250 mg, 500 mg (Azithromycin Dihydrate) Pfizer ... 2561
Zithromax Tablets, 600 mg (Azithromycin Dihydrate) Pfizer ... 2568
Zithromax Tri-Pak (Azithromycin Dihydrate) Pfizer ... 2561
Zithromax Z-Pak (Azithromycin Dihydrate) Pfizer ... 2568
Zmax for Oral Suspension (Azithromycin) Pfizer ... 2577
Zosyn (Piperacillin Sodium, Tazobactam Sodium) Wyeth ... 3492

H. influenzae infections, ocular
Blephamide Ophthalmic Ointment (Prednisolone Acetate, Sulfacetamide Sodium) Allergan ... 563
Blephamide Ophthalmic Suspension (Prednisolone Acetate, Sulfacetamide Sodium) Allergan ... 564
Ciloxan Ophthalmic Ointment (Ciprofloxacin Hydrochloride) Alcon ... 554
FML-S Liquifilm Sterile Ophthalmic Suspension (Fluorometholone, Sulfacetamide Sodium) Allergan ... ⊙226
Genoptic Sterile Ophthalmic Solution (Gentamicin Sulfate) Allergan ... ⊙227
Poly-Pred Liquifilm Ophthalmic Suspension (Neomycin Sulfate, Polymyxin B Sulfate, Prednisolone Acetate) Allergan ... ⊙231
Polytrim Ophthalmic Solution (Polymyxin B Sulfate, Trimethoprim Sulfate) Allergan ... 570
Pred-G Ophthalmic Suspension (Gentamicin Sulfate, Prednisolone Acetate) Allergan ... ⊙234
Pred-G Sterile Ophthalmic Ointment (Gentamicin Sulfate, Prednisolone Acetate) Allergan ... ⊙235
Quixin Ophthalmic Solution (Levofloxacin) Vistakon ... 3373
TobraDex Ophthalmic Ointment (Dexamethasone, Tobramycin) Alcon ... 558
TobraDex Ophthalmic Suspension (Dexamethasone, Tobramycin) Alcon ... 558
Vigamox Ophthalmic Solution (Moxifloxacin Hydrochloride) Alcon ... 560
Zylet Ophthalmic Suspension (Loteprednol Etabonate, Tobramycin) Bausch & Lomb ... 3508
Zymar Ophthalmic Solution (Gatifloxacin) Allergan ... 571

H. influenzae lower respiratory tract infections
Amoxil Capsules (Amoxicillin) GlaxoSmithKline ... 1315
Amoxil Chewable Tablets (Amoxicillin) GlaxoSmithKline ... 1315
Amoxil Pediatric Drops for Oral Suspension (Amoxicillin) GlaxoSmithKline ... 1315
Amoxil Powder for Oral Suspension (Amoxicillin) GlaxoSmithKline ... 1315
Amoxil Tablets (Amoxicillin) GlaxoSmithKline ... 1315
Augmentin (Amoxicillin, Clavulanate Potassium) GlaxoSmithKline ... 1331
Augmentin Tablets (Amoxicillin, Clavulanate Potassium) GlaxoSmithKline ... 1334
Augmentin XR Extended-Release Tablets (Amoxicillin, Clavulanate Potassium) GlaxoSmithKline ... 1340
Biaxin/Biaxin XL (Clarithromycin) Abbott ... 402
Cipro I.V. (Ciprofloxacin) Schering 2998
Cipro I.V. Pharmacy Bulk Package (Ciprofloxacin) Bayer ... 3509
Cipro (Ciprofloxacin) Schering ... 2991
Fortaz (Ceftazidime Sodium) GlaxoSmithKline ... 1422

Invanz for Injection (Ertapenem) Merck ... 1974
Levaquin in 5% Dextrose Injection (Levofloxacin) Ortho-McNeil ... 2453
Levaquin (Levofloxacin) Ortho-McNeil ... 2453
Mefoxin for Injection (Cefoxitin Sodium) Merck ... 1987
Mefoxin Premixed Intravenous Solution (Cefoxitin Sodium) Merck ... 1990
Primaxin I.M. (Cilastatin Sodium, Imipenem) Merck ... 2022
Primaxin I.V. (Cilastatin Sodium, Imipenem) Merck ... 2024
Rocephin Injectable Vials, ADD-Vantage, Galaxy, Bulk (Ceftriaxone Sodium) Roche Laboratories ... 2801
Spectracef Tablets (Cefditoren Pivoxil) Purdue Pharmaceutical ... 2706
Tequin Injection (Gatifloxacin) Bristol-Myers Squibb ... 964
Tequin Tablets (Gatifloxacin) Bristol-Myers Squibb ... 964
Timentin ADD-Vantage (Clavulanate Potassium, Ticarcillin Disodium) GlaxoSmithKline ... 1556
Timentin Injection Galaxy Container (Clavulanate Potassium, Ticarcillin Disodium) GlaxoSmithKline ... 1559
Timentin IV Infusion (Clavulanate Potassium, Ticarcillin Disodium) GlaxoSmithKline ... 1553
Timentin Pharmacy Bulk Package (Clavulanate Potassium, Ticarcillin Disodium) GlaxoSmithKline ... 1562
Vantin Tablets and Oral Suspension (Cefpodoxime Proxetil) Pharmacia & Upjohn ... 2650
Zinacef Injection (Cefuroxime) GlaxoSmithKline ... 1604
Zinacef for Injection (Cefuroxime) GlaxoSmithKline ... 1604
Zithromax Capsules, 250 mg (Azithromycin Dihydrate) Pfizer ... 2568
Zithromax for IV Infusion (Azithromycin Dihydrate) Pfizer ... 2573
Zithromax for Oral Suspension, 1 g (Azithromycin Dihydrate) Pfizer ... 2568
Zithromax for Oral Suspension, 300 mg, 600 mg, 900 mg, 1200 mg (Azithromycin Dihydrate) Pfizer ... 2561
Zithromax Tablets, 250 mg, 500 mg (Azithromycin Dihydrate) Pfizer ... 2561
Zithromax Tablets, 600 mg (Azithromycin Dihydrate) Pfizer ... 2568
Zithromax Tri-Pak (Azithromycin Dihydrate) Pfizer ... 2561
Zithromax Z-Pak (Azithromycin Dihydrate) Pfizer ... 2568
Zmax for Oral Suspension (Azithromycin) Pfizer ... 2577
Zosyn (Piperacillin Sodium, Tazobactam Sodium) Wyeth ... 3492

H. influenzae meningitis
Fortaz (Ceftazidime Sodium) GlaxoSmithKline ... 1422
Merrem I.V. (Meropenem) AstraZeneca ... 687
Rocephin Injectable Vials, ADD-Vantage, Galaxy, Bulk (Ceftriaxone Sodium) Roche Laboratories ... 2801
Zinacef Injection (Cefuroxime) GlaxoSmithKline ... 1604
Zinacef for Injection (Cefuroxime) GlaxoSmithKline ... 1604

H. influenzae otitis media
Augmentin (Amoxicillin, Clavulanate Potassium) GlaxoSmithKline ... 1331
Augmentin Tablets (Amoxicillin, Clavulanate Potassium) GlaxoSmithKline ... 1334
Augmentin XR Extended-Release Tablets (Amoxicillin, Clavulanate Potassium) GlaxoSmithKline ... 1340
Augmentin ES-600 Powder for Oral Suspension (Amoxicillin, Clavulanate Potassium) GlaxoSmithKline ... 1337
Biaxin/Biaxin XL (Clarithromycin) Abbott ... 402
Ceftin (Cefuroxime Axetil) GlaxoSmithKline ... 1369
Floxin Otic Singles (Ofloxacin) Daiichi ... 1045
Floxin Otic Solution (Ofloxacin) Daiichi ... 1043
Omnicef Capsules (Cefdinir) Abbott ... 506
Omnicef for Oral Suspension (Cefdinir) Abbott ... 506
Rocephin Injectable Vials, ADD-Vantage, Galaxy, Bulk (Ceftriaxone Sodium) Roche Laboratories ... 2801
Suprax (Cefixime) Lupin ... 1811
Vantin Tablets and Oral Suspension (Cefpodoxime Proxetil) Pharmacia & Upjohn ... 2650
Zithromax Capsules, 250 mg (Azithromycin Dihydrate) Pfizer ... 2568
Zithromax for Oral Suspension, 300 mg, 600 mg, 900 mg, 1200 mg (Azithromycin Dihydrate) Pfizer ... 2561
Zithromax Tablets, 250 mg, 500 mg (Azithromycin Dihydrate) Pfizer ... 2561
Zithromax Tri-Pak (Azithromycin Dihydrate) Pfizer ... 2561

H. influenzae pneumonia
Avelox (Moxifloxacin Hydrochloride) Schering ... 2984
Biaxin/Biaxin XL (Clarithromycin) Abbott ... 402
Factive Tablets (Gemifloxacin Mesylate) Oscient ... 2464
Invanz for Injection (Ertapenem) Merck ... 1974
Ketek Tablets (Telithromycin) Sanofi-Aventis ... 2920
Omnicef Capsules (Cefdinir) Abbott ... 506
Omnicef for Oral Suspension (Cefdinir) Abbott ... 506
Spectracef Tablets (Cefditoren Pivoxil) Purdue Pharmaceutical ... 2706
Tequin Injection (Gatifloxacin) Bristol-Myers Squibb ... 964
Tequin Tablets (Gatifloxacin) Bristol-Myers Squibb ... 964
Zmax for Oral Suspension (Azithromycin) Pfizer ... 2577

H. influenzae respiratory tract infections
Dynacin Tablets (Minocycline Hydrochloride) Medicis ... 1859
Spectracef Tablets (Cefditoren Pivoxil) Purdue Pharmaceutical ... 2706

H. influenzae septicemia
Fortaz (Ceftazidime Sodium) GlaxoSmithKline ... 1422
Rocephin Injectable Vials, ADD-Vantage, Galaxy, Bulk (Ceftriaxone Sodium) Roche Laboratories ... 2801
Zinacef Injection (Cefuroxime) GlaxoSmithKline ... 1604
Zinacef for Injection (Cefuroxime) GlaxoSmithKline ... 1604

H. influenzae sinusitis
Augmentin (Amoxicillin, Clavulanate Potassium) GlaxoSmithKline ... 1331
Augmentin Tablets (Amoxicillin, Clavulanate Potassium) GlaxoSmithKline ... 1334
Augmentin XR Extended-Release Tablets (Amoxicillin, Clavulanate Potassium) GlaxoSmithKline ... 1340
Avelox (Moxifloxacin Hydrochloride) Schering ... 2984
Biaxin/Biaxin XL (Clarithromycin) Abbott ... 402
Ceftin Tablets (Cefuroxime Axetil) GlaxoSmithKline ... 1369
Cipro I.V. (Ciprofloxacin) Schering ... 2998
Cipro I.V. Pharmacy Bulk Package (Ciprofloxacin) Bayer ... 3509
Cipro (Ciprofloxacin) Schering ... 2991
Ketek Tablets (Telithromycin) Sanofi-Aventis ... 2920
Levaquin in 5% Dextrose Injection (Levofloxacin) Ortho-McNeil ... 2453
Levaquin (Levofloxacin) Ortho-McNeil ... 2453
Omnicef Capsules (Cefdinir) Abbott ... 506
Omnicef for Oral Suspension (Cefdinir) Abbott ... 506
Tequin Injection (Gatifloxacin) Bristol-Myers Squibb ... 964
Tequin Tablets (Gatifloxacin) Bristol-Myers Squibb ... 964
Vantin Tablets and Oral Suspension (Cefpodoxime Proxetil) Pharmacia & Upjohn ... 2650
Zithromax for Oral Suspension, 300 mg, 600 mg, 900 mg, 1200 mg (Azithromycin Dihydrate) Pfizer ... 2561
Zithromax Tablets, 250 mg, 500 mg (Azithromycin Dihydrate) Pfizer ... 2561
Zithromax Tri-Pak (Azithromycin Dihydrate) Pfizer ... 2561
Zmax for Oral Suspension (Azithromycin) Pfizer ... 2577

H. influenzae upper respiratory tract infections
E.E.S. (Erythromycin Ethylsuccinate) Abbott ... 449
EryPed (Erythromycin Ethylsuccinate) Abbott ... 445
Ery-Tab Tablets (Erythromycin) Abbott ... 447
Erythrocin Stearate Filmtab Tablets (Erythromycin Stearate) Abbott ... 452
Erythromycin Base Filmtab Tablets (Erythromycin) Abbott ... 454
Erythromycin Delayed-Release Capsules, USP (Erythromycin) Abbott ... 456
PCE Dispertab Tablets (Erythromycin) Abbott ... 510

H. parainfluenzae bronchitis
Avelox (Moxifloxacin Hydrochloride) Schering ... 2984
Ceftin Tablets (Cefuroxime Axetil) GlaxoSmithKline ... 1369
Factive Tablets (Gemifloxacin Mesylate) Oscient ... 2464
Levaquin in 5% Dextrose Injection (Levofloxacin) Ortho-McNeil ... 2453
Levaquin (Levofloxacin) Ortho-McNeil ... 2453
Tequin Injection (Gatifloxacin) Bristol-Myers Squibb ... 964
Tequin Tablets (Gatifloxacin) Bristol-Myers Squibb ... 964

H. parainfluenzae infections
Augmentin XR Extended-Release Tablets (Amoxicillin, Clavulanate Potassium) GlaxoSmithKline ... 1340
Avelox (Moxifloxacin Hydrochloride) Schering ... 2984
Biaxin/Biaxin XL (Clarithromycin) Abbott ... 402
Ceftin Tablets (Cefuroxime Axetil) GlaxoSmithKline ... 1369
Cipro (Ciprofloxacin) Schering ... 2991
Factive Tablets (Gemifloxacin Mesylate) Oscient ... 2464
Levaquin in 5% Dextrose Injection (Levofloxacin) Ortho-McNeil ... 2453
Levaquin (Levofloxacin) Ortho-McNeil ... 2453
Primaxin I.V. (Cilastatin Sodium, Imipenem) Merck ... 2024
Rocephin Injectable Vials, ADD-Vantage, Galaxy, Bulk (Ceftriaxone Sodium) Roche Laboratories ... 2801
Spectracef Tablets (Cefditoren Pivoxil) Purdue Pharmaceutical ... 2706
Tequin Injection (Gatifloxacin) Bristol-Myers Squibb ... 964
Tequin Tablets (Gatifloxacin) Bristol-Myers Squibb ... 964
Vigamox Ophthalmic Solution (Moxifloxacin Hydrochloride) Alcon ... ⊙ 212

H. parainfluenzae lower respiratory tract infections
Augmentin XR Extended-Release Tablets (Amoxicillin, Clavulanate Potassium) GlaxoSmithKline ... 1340
Biaxin/Biaxin XL (Clarithromycin) Abbott ... 402
Cipro I.V. (Ciprofloxacin) Schering ... 2998
Cipro I.V. Pharmacy Bulk Package (Ciprofloxacin) Bayer ... 3509
Cipro (Ciprofloxacin) Schering ... 2991
Levaquin in 5% Dextrose Injection (Levofloxacin) Ortho-McNeil ... 2453
Levaquin (Levofloxacin) Ortho-McNeil ... 2453
Primaxin I.V. (Cilastatin Sodium, Imipenem) Merck ... 2024
Rocephin Injectable Vials, ADD-Vantage, Galaxy, Bulk (Ceftriaxone Sodium) Roche Laboratories ... 2801
Spectracef Tablets (Cefditoren Pivoxil) Purdue Pharmaceutical ... 2706
Suprax (Cefixime) Lupin ... 1811
Tequin Injection (Gatifloxacin) Bristol-Myers Squibb ... 964
Tequin Tablets (Gatifloxacin) Bristol-Myers Squibb ... 964

H. parainfluenzae pneumonia
Augmentin XR Extended-Release Tablets (Amoxicillin, Clavulanate Potassium) GlaxoSmithKline ... 1340
Biaxin/Biaxin XL (Clarithromycin) Abbott ... 402
Omnicef Capsules (Cefdinir) Abbott ... 506
Omnicef for Oral Suspension (Cefdinir) Abbott ... 506
Spectracef Tablets (Cefditoren Pivoxil) Purdue Pharmaceutical ... 2706
Tequin Injection (Gatifloxacin) Bristol-Myers Squibb ... 964
Tequin Tablets (Gatifloxacin) Bristol-Myers Squibb ... 964

H. pylori infection and duodenal ulcer, adjunct in
Aciphex Tablets (Rabeprazole Sodium) Eisai ... 1081
Amoxil Capsules (Amoxicillin) GlaxoSmithKline ... 1315
Amoxil Chewable Tablets (Amoxicillin) GlaxoSmithKline ... 1315
Amoxil Pediatric Drops for Oral Suspension (Amoxicillin) GlaxoSmithKline ... 1315
Amoxil Powder for Oral Suspension (Amoxicillin) GlaxoSmithKline ... 1315
Amoxil Tablets (Amoxicillin) GlaxoSmithKline ... 1315
Biaxin/Biaxin XL (Clarithromycin) Abbott ... 402
Nexium Delayed-Release Capsules (Esomeprazole Magnesium) AstraZeneca LP ... 645
Prevacid Delayed-Release Capsules (Lansoprazole) TAP ... 3268
Prevacid for Delayed-Release Oral Suspension (Lansoprazole) TAP ... 3268
Prevacid SoluTab Delayed-Release Orally Disintegrating Tablets (Lansoprazole) TAP ... 3268
PREVPAC (Amoxicillin, Clarithromycin, Lansoprazole) TAP ... 3281
Prilosec OTC Tablets (Omeprazole magnesium) Procter & Gamble ... 2674

H. vaginalis vaginitis
Metrogel 1% (Metronidazole) Galderma ... 1212
MetroGel-Vaginal Gel (Metronidazole) 3M ... 1822

Haemophilus influenzae
(*see under* H. influenzae infections)

Hair loss or thinning of the frontoparietal areas, females
Women's Rogaine Topical Solution, Spring Bloom Scent and Original Unscented (Minoxidil) Pfizer Consumer Healthcare ... ▣ 707

Hairy cell leukemias
(*see under* Leukemia, hairy cell)

Hansen's disease
(*see under* Leprosy)

Hashimoto's thyroiditis
Synthroid Tablets (Levothyroxine Sodium) Abbott ... 515
Thyrolar (Liotrix) Forest ... 1203

Hay fever
(*see under* Pollinosis)

Headache
Children's Advil Suspension (Ibuprofen) Wyeth ... ▣ 742
Children's Advil Chewable Tablets (Ibuprofen) Wyeth ... ▣ 741
Children's Advil Cold Suspension (Ibuprofen, Pseudoephedrine Hydrochloride) Wyeth ... ▣ 741
Infants' Advil Concentrated Drops (Ibuprofen) Wyeth ... ▣ 743
Junior Strength Advil Swallow Tablets (Ibuprofen) Wyeth ... ▣ 740
Aleve Tablets, Caplets and Gelcaps (Naproxen Sodium) Bayer Healthcare ... ▣ 605
BC Powder (Aspirin, Caffeine, Salicylamide) GlaxoSmithKline ... ▣ 612

Benadryl Allergy & Cold Tablets (Acetaminophen, Diphenhydramine Hydrochloride, Pseudoephedrine Hydrochloride) Pfizer Consumer Healthcare ▣692
Ecotrin Enteric Coated Aspirin Low, Regular and Maximum Strength Tablets (Aspirin) GlaxoSmithKline Consumer 1627
Goody's Body Pain Formula Powder (Acetaminophen, Aspirin, Acetaminophen, Aspirin) GlaxoSmithKline ▣621
Goody's Extra Strength Headache Powder (Acetaminophen, Aspirin, Caffeine) GlaxoSmithKline ▣621
Goody's Extra Strength Pain Relief Tablets (Acetaminophen, Aspirin, Caffeine) GlaxoSmithKline ▣621
Goody's PM Powder (Acetaminophen, Diphenhydramine Citrate) GlaxoSmithKline ▣622
Children's Motrin Oral Suspension and Chewable Tablets (Ibuprofen) McNeil Consumer ▣647
Children's Motrin Non-Staining Dye-Free Oral Suspension (Ibuprofen) McNeil Consumer ▣647
Children's Motrin Oral Suspension and Chewable Tablets (Ibuprofen) McNeil Consumer 1837
Children's Motrin Non-Staining Dye-Free Oral Suspension (Ibuprofen) McNeil Consumer 1837
Motrin IB Tablets and Caplets (Ibuprofen) McNeil Consumer 1836
Infants' Motrin Concentrated Drops (Ibuprofen) McNeil Consumer 1837
Infants' Motrin Non-Staining Dye-Free Drops (Ibuprofen) McNeil Consumer 1837
Junior Strength Motrin Caplets and Chewable Tablets (Ibuprofen) McNeil Consumer 1837
St. Joseph 81 mg Aspirin Chewable and Enteric Coated Tablets (Aspirin) McNeil Consumer 1841
TheraFlu Cold & Cough Hot Liquid (Acetaminophen, Chlorpheniramine Maleate, Dextromethorphan Hydrobromide, Pseudoephedrine Hydrochloride) Novartis Consumer ▣680
TheraFlu Cold & Sore Throat Hot Liquid (Acetaminophen, Chlorpheniramine Maleate, Pseudoephedrine Hydrochloride) Novartis Consumer ▣680
TheraFlu Flu & Chest Congestion Non-Drowsy Hot Liquid (Acetaminophen, Dextromethorphan Hydrobromide, Guaifenesin, Pseudoephedrine Hydrochloride) Novartis Consumer ▣681
TheraFlu Flu & Sore Throat Hot Liquid (Acetaminophen, Chlorpheniramine Maleate, Pseudoephedrine Hydrochloride) Novartis Consumer ▣681
TheraFlu Severe Cold & Cough Hot Liquid (Acetaminophen, Chlorpheniramine Maleate, Dextromethorphan Hydrobromide, Pseudoephedrine Hydrochloride) Novartis Consumer ▣683
TheraFlu Severe Cold Caplets (Acetaminophen, Chlorpheniramine Maleate, Dextromethorphan Hydrobromide, Pseudoephedrine Hydrochloride) Novartis Consumer ▣679
TheraFlu Severe Cold Hot Liquid (Acetaminophen, Chlorpheniramine Maleate, Dextromethorphan Hydrobromide, Pseudoephedrine Hydrochloride) Novartis Consumer ▣682
Tylenol 8 Hour Extended Release Geltabs and Caplets (Acetaminophen) McNeil Consumer 1843
Tylenol 8-Hour Extended Release Geltabs/Caplets (Acetaminophen) McNeil Consumer ▣655
Tylenol Cough & Sore Throat Daytime Liquid with Cool Burst (Acetaminophen, Dextromethorphan Hydrobromide) McNeil Consumer ▣664
Tylenol Cough & Sore Throat NightTime Liquid with Cool Burst (Acetaminophen, Dextromethorphan Hydrobromide, Doxylamine Succinate) McNeil Consumer ▣664
Children's Tylenol Plus Cold & Allergy Suspension Liquid (Acetaminophen, Diphenhydramine Hydrochloride, Pseudoephedrine Hydrochloride) McNeil Consumer 1850
Children's Tylenol Plus Flu Suspension Liquid (Acetaminophen, Chlorpheniramine Maleate, Dextromethorphan Hydrobromide, Pseudoephedrine Hydrochloride) McNeil Consumer 1853
Junior Tylenol Meltaways (Acetaminophen) McNeil Consumer 1850
Tylenol Cold & Flu Severe Daytime Liquid with Cool Bust (Acetaminophen, Dextromethorphan Hydrobromide, Pseudoephedrine Hydrochloride) McNeil Consumer 1846
Tylenol Cold & Flu Severe NightTime Liquid with Cool Burst (Acetaminophen, Dextromethorphan Hydrobromide, Doxylamine Succinate, Pseudoephedrine Hydrochloride) McNeil Consumer 1846
Tylenol Cough & Sore Throat Daytime Liquid with Cool Burst (Acetaminophen, Dextromethorphan Hydrobromide) McNeil Consumer 1849
Tylenol Cough & Sore Throat NightTime Liquid with Cool Burst (Acetaminophen, Dextromethorphan Hydrobromide, Doxylamine Succinate) McNeil Consumer 1849
Tylenol (Acetaminophen) McNeil Consumer 1843
Extra Strength Tylenol Rapid Release Gels (Acetaminophen) McNeil Consumer 1843
Regular Strength Tylenol Tablets (Acetaminophen) McNeil Consumer 1843
Tylenol Flu NightTime Gelcaps (Acetaminophen, Diphenhydramine Hydrochloride, Pseudoephedrine Hydrochloride) McNeil Consumer 1846
Tylenol Flu Day Non-Drowsy Gelcaps (Acetaminophen, Dextromethorphan Hydrobromide, Pseudoephedrine Hydrochloride) McNeil Consumer 1846
Concentrated Tylenol Infants' Drops Plus Cold Nasal Congestant, Fever Reducer & Pain Reliever (Acetaminophen, Pseudoephedrine Hydrochloride) McNeil Consumer ▣668
Concentrated Tylenol Infants' Drops Plus Cold & Cough Nasal Decongestant, Fever Reducer & Pain Reliever (Acetaminophen, Dextromethorphan Hydrobromide, Pseudoephedrine Hydrochloride) McNeil Consumer ▣668
Tylenol Sinus Day Non-Drowsy (Acetaminophen, Pseudoephedrine Hydrochloride) McNeil Consumer 1848
Tylenol Sinus Night Time Caplets (Acetaminophen, Doxylamine Succinate, Pseudoephedrine Hydrochloride) McNeil Consumer 1848
Tylenol Sore Throat Daytime Liquid with Cool Burst (Acetaminophen) McNeil Consumer 1849
Tylenol Sore Throat NightTime Liquid with Cool Burst (Acetaminophen, Diphenhydramine) McNeil Consumer 1849
Women's Tylenol Menstrual Relief Caplets (Acetaminophen, Pamabrom) McNeil Consumer 1849

Headache, cluster
(*see under* Cephalalgia, histaminic)

Headache, migraine
Advil Migraine Liquigels (Ibuprofen) Wyeth ▣740
Amerge Tablets (Naratriptan Hydrochloride) GlaxoSmithKline 1312
Axert Tablets (Almotriptan Malate) Ortho-McNeil Neurologics 2430
Frova Tablets (Frovatriptan Succinate) Endo Labs 1101
Imitrex Injection (Sumatriptan Succinate) GlaxoSmithKline 1431
Imitrex Nasal Spray (Sumatriptan) GlaxoSmithKline 1435
Imitrex Tablets (Sumatriptan Succinate) GlaxoSmithKline 1440
Maxalt Tablets (Rizatriptan Benzoate) Merck 1983
Maxalt-MLT Orally Disintegrating Tablets (Rizatriptan Benzoate) Merck 1983
Migranal Nasal Spray (Dihydroergotamine Mesylate) Valeant 3350
Relpax Tablets (Eletriptan Hydrobromide) Pfizer 2531
Zomig Nasal Spray (Zolmitriptan) AstraZeneca 718
Zomig Tablets (Zolmitriptan) AstraZeneca 714
Zomig-ZMT Tablets (Zolmitriptan) AstraZeneca 714

Headache, migraine, prophylaxis of
Blocadren Tablets (Timolol Maleate) Merck 1891
Depakote Tablets (Divalproex Sodium) Abbott 427
Depakote ER Tablets (Divalproex Sodium) Abbott 433
Inderal LA Long-Acting Capsules (Propranolol Hydrochloride) Wyeth 3421
Topamax Sprinkle Capsules (Topiramate) Ortho-McNeil Neurologics 2438
Topamax Tablets (Topiramate) Ortho-McNeil Neurologics 2438

Headache, sinus, symptomatic relief of
(*see under* Sinus headache)

Headache, tension
(*see also under* Pain, unspecified)
Sedapap Tablets 50 mg/650 mg (Acetaminophen, Butalbital) Merz 2098

Headache, vascular
(*see under* Headache, migraine)

Headache accompanied by insomnia
Goody's PM Powder (Acetaminophen, Diphenhydramine Citrate) GlaxoSmithKline ▣622
Extra Strength Tylenol PM Caplets, Geltabs, Gelcaps and Liquid (Acetaminophen, Diphenhydramine Hydrochloride) McNeil Consumer 1847

Headache associated with common cold
(*see also under* Sinus headache)
Advil Allergy Sinus Caplets (Chlorpheniramine Maleate, Ibuprofen, Pseudoephedrine Hydrochloride) Wyeth ▣737
Advil Cold & Sinus (Ibuprofen, Pseudoephedrine Hydrochloride) Wyeth ▣739
Advil Flu & Body Ache Caplets (Ibuprofen, Pseudoephedrine Hydrochloride) Wyeth ▣739
Children's Advil Cold Suspension (Ibuprofen, Pseudoephedrine Hydrochloride) Wyeth ▣741
Advil Multi-Symptom Cold Caplets (Chlorpheniramine Maleate, Ibuprofen, Pseudoephedrine Hydrochloride) Wyeth ▣738
Benadryl Maximum Strength Severe Allergy & Sinus Headache Caplets (Acetaminophen, Diphenhydramine Hydrochloride, Pseudoephedrine Hydrochloride) Pfizer Consumer Healthcare ▣694
Children's Motrin Cold Non-Staining Dye-Free Oral Suspension (Ibuprofen; Pseudoephedrine Hydrochloride) McNeil Consumer 1838
Children's Motrin Cold Oral Suspension (Ibuprofen, Pseudoephedrine Hydrochloride) McNeil Consumer ▣648
Children's Motrin Cold Non-Staining Dye-Free Oral Suspension (Ibuprofen, Pseudoephedrine Hydrochloride) McNeil Consumer ▣648
Children's Motrin Cold Oral Suspension (Ibuprofen, Pseudoephedrine Hydrochloride) McNeil Consumer 1838
Motrin Cold & Sinus Caplets (Ibuprofen, Pseudoephedrine Hydrochloride) McNeil Consumer 1836
Triaminic Cough & Sore Throat Softchews (Acetaminophen, Dextromethorphan Hydrobromide, Pseudoephedrine Hydrochloride) Novartis Consumer ▣689
Children's Tylenol Plus Cold NightTime Suspension Liquid (Acetaminophen, Chlorpheniramine Maleate, Pseudoephedrine Hydrochloride) McNeil Consumer 1851
Children's Tylenol Plus Cold & Cough Suspension Liquid and Chewable Tablets (Acetaminophen, Chlorpheniramine Maleate, Dextromethorphan Hydrobromide, Pseudoephedrine Hydrochloride) McNeil Consumer 1851
Children's Tylenol Plus Cold Chewable Tablets (Acetaminophen, Chlorpheniramine Maleate, Pseudoephedrine Hydrochloride) McNeil Consumer 1851
Concentrated Tylenol Infants' Drops Plus Cold (Acetaminophen, Pseudoephedrine Hydrochloride) McNeil Consumer 1851
Concentrated Tylenol Infants' Drops Plus Cold and Cough (Acetaminophen, Dextromethorphan Hydrobromide, Pseudoephedrine Hydrochloride) McNeil Consumer 1851
Tylenol Cold Severe Congestion Non-Drowsy Caplets with Cool Burst (Acetaminophen, Dextromethorphan Hydrobromide, Guaifenesin, Pseudoephedrine Hydrochloride) McNeil Consumer 1846

Heart, allogeneic transplants, prophylaxis of organ rejection in
CellCept Capsules (Mycophenolate Mofetil) Roche Laboratories 2751
CellCept Intravenous (Mycophenolate Mofetil Hydrochloride) Roche Laboratories 2751
CellCept Oral Suspension (Mycophenolate Mofetil) Roche Laboratories 2751
CellCept Tablets (Mycophenolate Mofetil) Roche Laboratories 2751
Gengraf Capsules (Cyclosporine) Abbott 458
Neoral Soft Gelatin Capsules (Cyclosporine) Novartis 2247
Neoral Oral Solution (Cyclosporine) Novartis 2247
Orthoclone OKT3 Sterile Solution (Muromonab-CD3) Ortho Biotech 2370
Sandimmune (Cyclosporine) Novartis 2259

Heart failure
(*see under* Congestive heart failure, adjunct in)

Heart failure, congestive
(*see under* Congestive heart failure, adjunct in)

Heart failure, NYHA Class II - IV
Atacand Tablets (Candesartan Cilexetil) AstraZeneca LP 634
Diovan Tablets (Valsartan) Novartis 2191
Toprol-XL Tablets (Metoprolol Succinate) AstraZeneca LP 660

Heart transplantation, donor organ perfusion and flushing of
Custodiol HTK Solution (Electrolyte Solution) Odyssey 2344

Heartburn
(*see under* Hyperacidity, gastric, symptomatic relief of)

Heartburn, frequent
Prilosec OTC Tablets (Omeprazole magnesium) Procter & Gamble 2674

Hematopoietic progenitor cells, mobilization of
Neupogen for Injection (Filgrastim) Amgen 598

Hemolytic disease, newborn
Buminate 25% Solution, USP (Albumin (human)) Baxter Healthcare 748
Plasbumin-20 (Albumin (human)) Talecris 3249

Hemolytic disease, Rh, prevention of
(*see under* Erythroblastosis fetalis, prevention of)

Hemolytic disease, unspecified
Plasbumin-20 (Albumin (human)) Talecris 3249
Plasbumin-25 (Albumin (human)) Talecris 3251

Hemophilia A
Advate Injection (Antihemophilic Factor (Recombinant)) Baxter Healthcare 742
DDAVP Injection 4 mcg/mL (Desmopressin Acetate) Sanofi-Aventis 2893
Desmopressin Acetate Injection (Desmopressin Acetate) Ferring 1143
Hemofil M (Antihemophilic Factor (Human)) Baxter Healthcare 757
Koāte-DVI (Antihemophilic Factor (Human)) Talecris 3247
Kogenate FS (Antihemophilic Factor (Recombinant)) Bayer Healthcare Biologicals 3517
Recombinate (Antihemophilic Factor (Recombinant)) Baxter Healthcare 762
ReFacto Vials (Antihemophilic Factor (Recombinant)) Wyeth 3479

Hemophilia A, perioperative management of
Advate Injection (Antihemophilic Factor (Recombinant)) Baxter Healthcare 742

Hemophilia B
BeneFix for Injection (Antihemophilic Factor (Recombinant)) Wyeth 3402
NovoSeven (Antihemophilic Factor (Recombinant)) Novo Nordisk 2335

Hemorrhage, postpartum, control of
AquaMEPHYTON Injection (Vitamin K_1) Merck 1887

Hemorrhage, subarachnoid, resulting in neurological deficits
Nimotop Capsules (Nimodipine) Bayer 774

Hemorrhoids
Preparation H Maximum Strength Cream (Glycerin, Petrolatum, Phenylephrine Hydrochloride, Pramoxine Hydrochloride) Wyeth .... ▣747
Preparation H Cooling Gel (Phenylephrine Hydrochloride) Wyeth .... ▣747
Preparation H (Mineral Oil, Petrolatum, Phenylephrine Hydrochloride, Shark Liver Oil) Wyeth .... ▣747
Preparation H Medicated Wipes (Witch Hazel) Wyeth .... ▣748

Hemorrhoids, symptomatic relief of
Tucks Anti-Itch (Hydrocortisone Acetate) Pfizer Consumer Healthcare .... ▣712
Tucks Hemorrhoidal Ointment (Mineral Oil, Pramoxine Hydrochloride, Zinc Oxide, Mineral Oil, Pramoxine Hydrochloride, Zinc Oxide) Pfizer Consumer Healthcare .... ▣711
Tucks Hemorrhoidal Suppositories (Starch, topical) Pfizer Consumer Healthcare .... ▣712
Tucks Witch Hazel Hemorrhoidal Pad (Witch Hazel) Pfizer Consumer Healthcare .... ▣712

Hemostasis, an aid in
DDAVP Injection 4 mcg/mL (Desmopressin Acetate) Sanofi-Aventis 2893
Desmopressin Acetate Injection (Desmopressin Acetate) Ferring 1143
Thrombin-JMI (Thrombin) King 1693
Trasylol Injection (Aprotinin) Bayer 779

Hepatitis A, prophylaxis
GamaSTAN (Globulin, Immune (Human)) Talecris 3231

Hepatitis B, chronic
Baraclude (Entecavir) Bristol-Myers Squibb 928
Epivir-HBV (Lamivudine) GlaxoSmithKline 1398
Hepsera Tablets (Adefovir dipivoxil) Gilead 1275
Intron A for Injection (Interferon alfa-2b, Recombinant) Schering 3038
Pegasys (Peginterferon alfa-2a) Roche Laboratories 2793

Hepatitis B virus, postexposure prophylaxis
HyperHep B S/D (Hepatitis B Immune Globulin (Human)) Talecris 3237
Nabi-HB (Hepatitis B Immune Globulin (Human)) Nabi 2159

Hepatitis C, chronic
Copegus Tablets (Ribavirin) Roche Laboratories 2759
Infergen (Interferon Alfacon-1) InterMune 1647
Intron A for Injection (Interferon alfa-2b, Recombinant) Schering 3038
Pegasys (Peginterferon alfa-2a) Roche Laboratories 2793
PEG-Intron Powder for Injection (Peginterferon Alfa-2b) Schering 3062
Rebetol (Ribavirin) Schering 3073
Rebetron Combination Therapy (Interferon alfa-2b, Recombinant, Ribavirin) Schering 3078
Ribavirin, USP Capsules (Ribavirin) Schering 3083
Roferon-A Injection (Interferon alfa-2a, Recombinant) Roche Laboratories 2805

Hepatitis C, chronic, HIV co-infection
Copegus Tablets (Ribavirin) Roche Laboratories 2759

Herellea vaginicola
(*see under* Acinetobacter calcoaceticus infections, ocular)

Herpes, genital, initial and recurrent episodes
Famvir Tablets (Famciclovir) Novartis 2207
Zovirax Capsules (Acyclovir) GlaxoSmithKline 1616
Zovirax for Injection (Acyclovir Sodium) GlaxoSmithKline 1618
Zovirax (Acyclovir) GlaxoSmithKline 1616

Herpes genitalis
Valtrex Caplets (Valacyclovir Hydrochloride) GlaxoSmithKline 1573
Zovirax Capsules (Acyclovir) GlaxoSmithKline 1616
Zovirax Cream (Acyclovir) Biovail 853
Zovirax for Injection (Acyclovir Sodium) GlaxoSmithKline 1618
Zovirax Ointment (Acyclovir) Biovail 854
Zovirax (Acyclovir) GlaxoSmithKline 1616

Herpes labialis
Valtrex Caplets (Valacyclovir Hydrochloride) GlaxoSmithKline 1573

Herpes labialis, recurrent
Zovirax Cream (Acyclovir) Biovail 853

Herpes simplex virus encephalitis
Zovirax for Injection (Acyclovir Sodium) GlaxoSmithKline 1618

Herpes simplex virus infections
Denavir Cream (Penciclovir) Novartis Consumer 2163
Famvir Tablets (Famciclovir) Novartis 2207
Zovirax Cream (Acyclovir) Biovail 853
Zovirax for Injection (Acyclovir Sodium) GlaxoSmithKline 1618
Zovirax Ointment (Acyclovir) Biovail 854

Herpes simplex virus mucocutaneous infection
Famvir Tablets (Famciclovir) Novartis 2207
Zovirax Cream (Acyclovir) Biovail 853
Zovirax for Injection (Acyclovir Sodium) GlaxoSmithKline 1618
Zovirax Ointment (Acyclovir) Biovail 854

Herpes zoster infections
Famvir Tablets (Famciclovir) Novartis 2207
Valtrex Caplets (Valacyclovir Hydrochloride) GlaxoSmithKline 1573
Zovirax (Acyclovir) GlaxoSmithKline 1616

Herpes zoster ophthalmicus
Decadron Phosphate Injection (Dexamethasone Sodium Phosphate) Merck 1931
Depo-Medrol Injectable Suspension (Methylprednisolone Acetate) Pharmacia & Upjohn 2615
Hydrocortone Tablets (Hydrocortisone) Merck 1963
Pediapred Oral Solution (Prednisolone Sodium Phosphate) UCB 3319

Herpetic manifestations, oral, symptomatic relief of
(*see also under* Herpes simplex virus infections)
Abreva Cream (Docosanol) GlaxoSmithKline .... ▣612
Anbesol Cold Sore Therapy Ointment (Allantoin, Benzocaine, Camphor, Petrolatum, White) Wyeth .... ▣745
Denavir Cream (Penciclovir) Novartis Consumer 2163
Valtrex Caplets (Valacyclovir Hydrochloride) GlaxoSmithKline 1573

HIV Infection
(*see under* Infections, human immunodeficiency virus)

Hodgkin's disease
Adriamycin for Injection, USP (Doxorubicin Hydrochloride) Bedford 786
Adriamycin Injection, USP (Doxorubicin Hydrochloride) Bedford 786
Leukeran Tablets (Chlorambucil) GlaxoSmithKline 1472

Hodgkin's disease, adjunctive therapy in
Leukine (Sargramostim) Berlex 829

Hodgkin's disease, stages III and IV, palliative treatment of
Matulane Capsules (Procarbazine Hydrochloride) Sigma-Tau 3188
Mustargen for Injection (Mechlorethamine Hydrochloride) Merck 2007

Hookworm, American
(*see under* Necator americanus infections)

Hookworm infections
(*see under* Ancylostoma duodenale infections)

Horton's headache
(*see under* Cephalalgia, histaminic)

Hot flashes
Peridin-C Tablets (Bioflavonoids, Hesperidin Complex, Hesperidin Methyl Chalcone, Vitamin C) Beutlich .... ▣761

Hydatid disease, cystic
Albenza Tablets (Albendazole) GlaxoSmithKline 1310

Hyperacidity, gastric, symptomatic relief of
Gas-X with Maalox (Calcium Carbonate, Simethicone) Novartis Consumer .... ▣675
Gaviscon Regular Strength Liquid (Aluminum Hydroxide, Magnesium Carbonate) GlaxoSmithKline .... ▣620
Gaviscon Regular Strength Tablets (Aluminum Hydroxide, Magnesium Trisilicate) GlaxoSmithKline .... ▣619
Gaviscon Extra Strength Liquid (Aluminum Hydroxide, Magnesium Carbonate) GlaxoSmithKline .... ▣620
Gaviscon Extra Strength Tablets (Aluminum Hydroxide, Magnesium Carbonate) GlaxoSmithKline .... ▣619
Maalox Regular Strength Antacid/Anti-Gas Liquid (Aluminum Hydroxide, Magnesium Hydroxide, Simethicone) Novartis Consumer .... ▣677
Maalox Regular Strength Antacid Tablets (Calcium Carbonate) Novartis Consumer 2166
Maalox Max Maximum Strength Antacid/Anti-Gas Liquid (Aluminum Hydroxide, Magnesium Hydroxide, Simethicone) Novartis Consumer 2165
Maalox Regular Strength Antacid/Antigas Liquid (Aluminum Hydroxide, Magnesium Hydroxide, Simethicone) Novartis Consumer 2164
Quick Dissolve Maalox Max Maximum Strength Antacid/Antigas Tablets (Calcium Carbonate) Novartis Consumer 2165
Maalox Maximum Strength Total Stomach Relief Peppermint Liquid (Bismuth Subsalicylate) Novartis Consumer .... ▣677
Maalox Maximum Strength Total Stomach Relief Strawberry Liquid (Bismuth Subsalicylate) Novartis Consumer .... ▣678
Nexium Delayed-Release Capsules (Esomeprazole Magnesium) AstraZeneca LP 645
Pepcid AC Tablets, Chewable Tablets, and Gelcaps (Famotidine) J&J – Merck .... ▣640
Pepcid AC Chewable Tablets (Famotidine) J&J – Merck 1672
Pepcid AC Gelcaps (Famotidine) J&J – Merck 1672
Maximum Strength Pepcid AC Tablets (Famotidine) J&J – Merck .... ▣640
Pepcid AC Tablets (Famotidine) J&J – Merck 1672
Maximum Strength Pepcid AC Tablets (Famotidine) J&J – Merck 1672
Pepcid Complete Chewable Tablets (Calcium Carbonate, Famotidine, Magnesium Hydroxide) J&J – Merck 1672
Prilosec OTC Tablets (Omeprazole magnesium) Procter & Gamble 2674
Rolaids Tablets (Calcium Carbonate, Magnesium Hydroxide) Pfizer Consumer Healthcare .... ▣707
Extra Strength Rolaids Softchews (Calcium Carbonate) Pfizer Consumer Healthcare .... ▣708
Extra Strength Rolaids Tablets (Calcium Carbonate, Magnesium Hydroxide) Pfizer Consumer Healthcare .... ▣707
Rolaids Multi-Symptom Antacid & Antigas Tablets (Calcium Carbonate, Magnesium Hydroxide, Simethicone) Pfizer Consumer Healthcare .... ▣708
Tagamet HB 200 Tablets (Cimetidine) GlaxoSmithKline .... ▣637
Tums (Calcium Carbonate) GlaxoSmithKline .... ▣639
Zantac 75 Tablets (Ranitidine Hydrochloride) Pfizer Consumer Healthcare .... ▣715
Zantac 150 Maximum Strength Tablets (Ranitidine Hydrochloride) Pfizer Consumer Healthcare .... ▣715

Hyperammonemia, acute
Ammonul Injection (Sodium Benzoate, Sodium Phenylacelate) Ucyclyd 3323

Hyperbetalipoproteinemia
(*see under* Hyperlipoproteinemia, types IIa and IIb, adjunct to diet)

Hypercalcemia associated with cancer
Aredia for Injection (Pamidronate Disodium) Novartis 2168

Decadron Phosphate Injection (Dexamethasone Sodium Phosphate) Merck 1931
Decadron Tablets (Dexamethasone) Merck 1929
Depo-Medrol Injectable Suspension (Methylprednisolone Acetate) Pharmacia & Upjohn 2615
Depo-Medrol Single-Dose Vial (Methylprednisolone Acetate) Pharmacia & Upjohn 2617
Hydrocortone Tablets (Hydrocortisone) Merck 1963
Pediapred Oral Solution (Prednisolone Sodium Phosphate) UCB 3319
Sensipar Tablets (Cinacalcet Hydrochloride) Amgen 603
Zometa for Intravenous Infusion (Zoledronic acid) Novartis 2306

Hypercalcemic emergencies, adjunct in
Miacalcin Injection (Calcitonin-Salmon) Novartis 2241

Hypercholesterolemia
Niaspan Extended-Release Tablets (Niacin) Kos 1703
Zetia Tablets (Ezetimibe) Merck/Schering Plough 2090
Zetia Tablets (Ezetimibe) Schering 3098

Hypercholesterolemia, homozygous, familial, adjunct to other agents
Crestor Tablets (Rosuvastatin Calcium) AstraZeneca 672
Vytorin 10/10 Tablets (Ezetimibe, Simvastatin) Merck/Schering Plough 2084
Vytorin 10/10 Tablets (Ezetimibe, Simvastatin) Schering 3092
Vytorin 10/20 Tablets (Ezetimibe, Simvastatin) Merck/Schering Plough 2084
Vytorin 10/20 Tablets (Ezetimibe, Simvastatin) Schering 3092
Vytorin 10/40 Tablets (Ezetimibe, Simvastatin) Merck/Schering Plough 2084
Vytorin 10/40 Tablets (Ezetimibe, Simvastatin) Schering 3092
Vytorin 10/80 Tablets (Ezetimibe, Simvastatin) Merck/Schering Plough 2084
Vytorin 10/80 Tablets (Ezetimibe, Simvastatin) Schering 3092

Hypercholesterolemia, primary, adjunct to diet
Advicor Tablets (Lovastatin, Niacin) Kos 1694
Altoprev Extended-Release Tablets (Lovastatin) First Horizon 1151
Antara Capsules (Fenofibrate) Reliant 2723
Caduet Tablets (Amlodipine Besylate, Atorvastatin Calcium) Pfizer 2507
Crestor Tablets (Rosuvastatin Calcium) AstraZeneca 672
Lescol Capsules (Fluvastatin Sodium) Novartis 2227
Lescol Capsules (Fluvastatin Sodium) Reliant 2730
Lescol XL Tablets (Fluvastatin Sodium) Novartis 2227
Lescol XL Tablets (Fluvastatin Sodium) Reliant 2730
Lipitor Tablets (Atorvastatin Calcium) Parke-Davis 2495
Lofibra Capsules (Fenofibrate) Gate 1217
Mevacor Tablets (Lovastatin) Merck 1996
Niaspan Extended-Release Tablets (Niacin) Kos 1703
Pravachol Tablets (Pravastatin Sodium) Bristol-Myers Squibb 943
Tricor Tablets (Fenofibrate) Abbott 523
Triglide Tablets (Fenofibrate) First Horizon 1165
Vytorin 10/10 Tablets (Ezetimibe, Simvastatin) Merck/Schering Plough 2084
Vytorin 10/10 Tablets (Ezetimibe, Simvastatin) Schering 3092
Vytorin 10/20 Tablets (Ezetimibe, Simvastatin) Merck/Schering Plough 2084
Vytorin 10/20 Tablets (Ezetimibe, Simvastatin) Schering 3092
Vytorin 10/40 Tablets (Ezetimibe, Simvastatin) Merck/Schering Plough 2084
Vytorin 10/40 Tablets (Ezetimibe, Simvastatin) Schering 3092
Vytorin 10/80 Tablets (Ezetimibe, Simvastatin) Merck/Schering Plough 2084
Vytorin 10/80 Tablets (Ezetimibe, Simvastatin) Schering 3092
WelChol Tablets (Colesevelam Hydrochloride) Sankyo 2855
Zetia Tablets (Ezetimibe) Merck/Schering Plough 2090
Zetia Tablets (Ezetimibe) Schering 3098
Zocor Tablets (Simvastatin) Merck 2078

Hyperglycemia, control of, adjunct to diet
(*see also under* Diabetes mellitus, insulin-dependent; Diabetes mellitus, non-insulin-dependent)
ActoPlus Met Tablets (Metformin Hydrochloride, Pioglitazone Hydrochloride) Takeda 3219
Actos Tablets (Pioglitazone Hydrochloride) Takeda 3224
Amaryl Tablets (Glimepiride) Sanofi-Aventis 2864
Apidra Injection (Insulin Glulisine) Sanofi-Aventis 2876
Avandamet Tablets (Rosiglitazone Maleate, Metformin Hydrochloride) GlaxoSmithKline 1343
Avandia Tablets (Rosiglitazone Maleate) GlaxoSmithKline 1348
Byetta Injection (Exenatide) Amylin 605
Fortamet Extended-Release Tablets (Metformin Hydrochloride) First Horizon 1156
Prandin Tablets (0.5, 1, and 2 mg) (Repaglinide) Novo Nordisk 2337
Precose Tablets (Acarbose) Bayer 776
Starlix Tablets (Nateglinide) Novartis 2276

Hyperhidrosis
Botox Purified Neurotoxin Complex (Botulinum Toxin Type A) Allergan 565

Hyperhidrosis, topical relief of
Drysol Solution (Aluminum Chloride) Person & Covey 2506
Xerac AC Solution (Aluminum Chloride) Person & Covey 2507

Hyperkeratosis skin disorders
U-Kera Cream (Urea) TaroPharma 3290
Ultralytic 2 Cream 20% (Urea) Ivax Dermatologicals 1651
Ultralytic 2 Foam 20% (Urea) Ivax Dermatologicals 1652

Hyperlipoproteinemia, type III, adjunct to diet
Zocor Tablets (Simvastatin) Merck 2078

Hyperlipoproteinemia, types IIa and IIb, adjunct to diet
Advicor Tablets (Lovastatin, Niacin) Kos 1694
Altoprev Extended-Release Tablets (Lovastatin) First Horizon 1151
Caduet Tablets (Amlodipine Besylate, Atorvastatin Calcium) Pfizer 2507
Crestor Tablets (Rosuvastatin Calcium) AstraZeneca 672
Lescol Capsules (Fluvastatin Sodium) Novartis 2227
Lescol Capsules (Fluvastatin Sodium) Reliant 2730
Lescol XL Tablets (Fluvastatin Sodium) Novartis 2227
Lescol XL Tablets (Fluvastatin Sodium) Reliant 2730
Lipitor Tablets (Atorvastatin Calcium) Parke-Davis 2495
Mevacor Tablets (Lovastatin) Merck 1996
Niaspan Extended-Release Tablets (Niacin) Kos 1703
Pravachol Tablets (Pravastatin Sodium) Bristol-Myers Squibb 943
Triglide Tablets (Fenofibrate) First Horizon 1165
Zocor Tablets (Simvastatin) Merck 2078

Hyperlipoproteinemia, types IV and V, adjunct to diet
Antara Capsules (Fenofibrate) Reliant 2723
Lofibra Capsules (Fenofibrate) Gate 1217
Niaspan Extended-Release Tablets (Niacin) Kos 1703
Tricor Tablets (Fenofibrate) Abbott 523
Triglide Tablets (Fenofibrate) First Horizon 1165

Hyperparathyroidism, secondary
Hectorol Capsules (Doxercalciferol) Bone Care 909
Hectorol Injection (Doxercalciferol) Bone Care 911
Sensipar Tablets (Cinacalcet Hydrochloride) Amgen 603
Zemplar Capsules (Paricalcitol) Abbott 535
Zemplar Injection (Paricalcitol) Abbott 538

Hyperphosphatemia
Fosrenol Chewable Tablets (Lanthanum Carbonate) Shire US 3180
PhosLo GelCaps (Calcium Acetate) Nabi 2158
Renagel Tablets (Sevelamer Hydrochloride) Genzyme 1268

Hyperpigmentation, mottled, adjunct in
Renova 0.02% Cream (Tretinoin) OrthoNeutrogena 2384
Renova 0.05% Cream (Tretinoin) OrthoNeutrogena 2387

Hyperpigmentation, skin, bleaching of
Claripel Cream (Hydroquinone) Stiefel 3212
Lustra Cream (Hydroquinone) TaroPharma 3287
Lustra-AF Cream (Hydroquinone) TaroPharma 3287
Lustra-Ultra Cream (Hydroquinone) TaroPharma 3287
Pure Gardens Cream (Herbals with Vitamins) Awareness Corporation/AwarenessLife ▣ 760
Solage Topical Solution (Mequinol, Tretinoin) Barrier 740
Tri-Luma Cream (Fluocinolone Acetonide, Hydroquinone, Tretinoin) Galderma 1213

Hyperprolactinemia-associated dysfunctions
Dostinex Tablets (Cabergoline) Pharmacia & Upjohn 2631

Hypersecretory conditions, pathological
Aciphex Tablets (Rabeprazole Sodium) Eisai 1081
Pepcid Injection (Famotidine) Merck 2017
Pepcid (Famotidine) Merck 2014
Prevacid Delayed-Release Capsules (Lansoprazole) TAP 3268
Prevacid for Delayed-Release Oral Suspension (Lansoprazole) TAP 3268
Prevacid SoluTab Delayed-Release Orally Disintegrating Tablets (Lansoprazole) TAP 3268
Prilosec OTC Tablets (Omeprazole magnesium) Procter & Gamble 2674
Protonix I.V. (Pantoprazole Sodium) Wyeth 3468
Protonix Tablets (Pantoprazole Sodium) Wyeth 3465
Tagamet Tablets (Cimetidine) GlaxoSmithKline 1547
Zantac (Ranitidine Hydrochloride) GlaxoSmithKline 1597
Zantac Injection (Ranitidine Hydrochloride) GlaxoSmithKline 1593
Zantac Injection Pharmacy Bulk Package (Ranitidine Hydrochloride) GlaxoSmithKline 1595
Zantac Syrup (Ranitidine Hydrochloride) GlaxoSmithKline 1597

Hypersensitivity reactions, drug-induced
Decadron Phosphate Injection (Dexamethasone Sodium Phosphate) Merck 1931
Decadron Tablets (Dexamethasone) Merck 1929
Depo-Medrol Injectable Suspension (Methylprednisolone Acetate) Pharmacia & Upjohn 2615
Depo-Medrol Single-Dose Vial (Methylprednisolone Acetate) Pharmacia & Upjohn 2617
EpiPen (Epinephrine) Dey 1061
Hydrocortone Tablets (Hydrocortisone) Merck 1963
Pediapred Oral Solution (Prednisolone Sodium Phosphate) UCB 3319

Hypersensitivity reactions, general
HibTITER (Haemophilus B Conjugate Vaccine) Wyeth 3419

Hypertension
Aceon Tablets (2 mg, 4 mg, 8 mg) (Perindopril Erbumine) Solvay 3191
Adalat CC Tablets (Nifedipine) Schering 2978
Aldoclor Tablets (Chlorothiazide, Methyldopa) Merck 1881
Aldoril Tablets (Hydrochlorothiazide, Methyldopa) Merck 1884
Altace Capsules (Ramipril) King 1673
Atacand Tablets (Candesartan Cilexetil) AstraZeneca LP 634
Atacand HCT (Hydrochlorothiazide, Candesartan Cilexetil) AstraZeneca LP 637
Avalide Tablets (Irbesartan, Hydrochlorothiazide) Bristol-Myers Squibb 922
Avalide Tablets (Irbesartan, Hydrochlorothiazide) Sanofi-Aventis 2889
Avapro Tablets (Irbesartan) Bristol-Myers Squibb 925
Avapro Tablets (Irbesartan) Sanofi-Aventis 2886
Benicar Tablets (Olmesartan Medoxomil) Sankyo 2850
Benicar HCT Tablets (Olmesartan Medoxomil, Hydrochlorothiazide) Sankyo 2852
Blocadren Tablets (Timolol Maleate) Merck 1891
Caduet Tablets (Amlodipine Besylate, Atorvastatin Calcium) Pfizer 2507
Captopril Tablets (Captopril) Mylan 2114
Cardene I.V. (Nicardipine Hydrochloride) ESP Pharma 1129
Cardizem LA Extended Release Tablets (Diltiazem Hydrochloride) Kos 1699
Catapres Tablets (Clonidine Hydrochloride) Boehringer Ingelheim 874
Catapres-TTS (Clonidine) Boehringer Ingelheim 875
Clorpres Tablets (Chlorthalidone, Clonidine Hydrochloride) Mylan Bertek 2139
Coreg Tablets (Carvedilol) GlaxoSmithKline 1376
Covera-HS Tablets (Verapamil Hydrochloride) Searle 3135
Cozaar Tablets (Losartan Potassium) Merck 1913
Diovan HCT Tablets (Hydrochlorothiazide, Valsartan) Novartis 2195
Diovan Tablets (Valsartan) Novartis 2191
Diuril Oral (Chlorothiazide) Merck 1936
Dyazide Capsules (Hydrochlorothiazide, Triamterene) GlaxoSmithKline 1389
DynaCirc CR Tablets (Isradipine) Reliant 2726
Furosemide Tablets (Furosemide) Mylan 2117
Hytrin Capsules (Terazosin Hydrochloride) Abbott 469
Hyzaar (Hydrochlorothiazide, Losartan Potassium) Merck 1964
Indapamide Tablets (Indapamide) Mylan 2119
Inderal LA Long-Acting Capsules (Propranolol Hydrochloride) Wyeth 3421
InnoPran XL Capsules (Propranolol Hydrochloride) Reliant 2728
Inspra Tablets (Eplerenone) Pfizer 2520
Inversine Tablets (Mecamylamine Hydrochloride) Targacept 3286
Lotensin Tablets (Benazepril Hydrochloride) Novartis 2232
Lotensin HCT Tablets (Benazepril Hydrochloride, Hydrochlorothiazide) Novartis 2235
Lotrel Capsules (Amlodipine Besylate, Benazepril Hydrochloride) Novartis 2238
Mavik Tablets (Trandolapril) Abbott 482

(▣ Described in PDR For Nonprescription Drugs) (⊙ Described in PDR For Ophthalmic Medicines™)

Maxzide (Hydrochlorothiazide, Triamterene) Mylan Bertek ... 2150
Micardis Tablets (Telmisartan) Boehringer Ingelheim ... 884
Micardis HCT Tablets (Hydrochlorothiazide, Telmisartan) Boehringer Ingelheim ... 886
Midamor Tablets (Amiloride Hydrochloride) Merck ... 2000
Moduretic Tablets (Amiloride Hydrochloride, Hydrochlorothiazide) Merck ... 2003
Nadolol Tablets (Nadolol) Mylan ... 2121
Norvasc Tablets (Amlodipine Besylate) Pfizer ... 2529
Plendil Extended-Release Tablets (Felodipine) AstraZeneca LP ... 651
Prinivil Tablets (Lisinopril) Merck ... 2029
Prinzide Tablets (Hydrochlorothiazide, Lisinopril) Merck ... 2033
Sular Tablets (Nisoldipine) First Horizon ... 1163
Tarka Tablets (Trandolapril, Verapamil Hydrochloride) Abbott ... 519
Tenormin Tablets (Atenolol) AstraZeneca ... 695
Teveten Tablets (Eprosartan Mesylate) Kos ... 1707
Teveten HCT Tablets (Eprosartan Mesylate, Hydrochlorothiazide) Kos ... 1710
Tiazac Capsules (Diltiazem Hydrochloride) Forest ... 1204
Timolide Tablets (Hydrochlorothiazide, Timolol Maleate) Merck ... 2056
Toprol-XL Tablets (Metoprolol Succinate) AstraZeneca LP ... 660
Uniretic Tablets (Hydrochlorothiazide, Moexipril Hydrochloride) Schwarz ... 3114
Univasc Tablets (Moexipril Hydrochloride) Schwarz ... 3118
Vaseretic Tablets (Enalapril Maleate, Hydrochlorothiazide) Merck ... 2073
Vasotec I.V. Injection (Enalapril Maleate) Merck ... 2076
Verelan PM Capsules (Verapamil Hydrochloride) Schwarz ... 3120
Zestoretic Tablets (Hydrochlorothiazide, Lisinopril) AstraZeneca ... 701
Zestril Tablets (Lisinopril) AstraZeneca ... 704

Hypertension, adjunctive treatment
RESPeRATE Device (Device) InterCure ... 1645

Hypertension, essential
(*see under* Hypertension)

Hypertension, malignant
Hyperstat I.V. Injection (Diazoxide) Schering ... 3031
Inversine Tablets (Mecamylamine Hydrochloride) Targacept ... 3286

Hypertension, non-malignant
Hyperstat I.V. Injection (Diazoxide) Schering ... 3031

Hypertension, ocular
(*see also under* Glaucoma, chronic open-angle; Glaucoma, secondary)
Alphagan P Ophthalmic Solution (Brimonidine Tartrate) Allergan ... 563
Azopt Ophthalmic Suspension (Brinzolamide) Alcon ... 553
Betagan Ophthalmic Solution, USP (Levobunolol Hydrochloride) Allergan ... ⊙ 217
Betimol Ophthalmic Solution (Timolol Hemihydrate) Vistakon ... ⊙ 283
Betimol Ophthalmic Solution (Timolol Hemihydrate) Vistakon ... 3371
Betoptic S Ophthalmic Suspension (Betaxolol Hydrochloride) Alcon ... 554
Brimonidine Tartrate Ophthalmic Solution 0.2% (Brimonidine Tartrate) Bausch & Lomb ... ⊙ 245
Carteolol Hydrochloride Ophthalmic Solution USP, 1% (Carteolol Hydrochloride) Bausch & Lomb ... ⊙ 246
Cosopt Sterile Ophthalmic Solution (Dorzolamide Hydrochloride, Timolol Maleate) Merck ... 1910
Lumigan Ophthalmic Solution (Bimatoprost) Allergan ... 569
OptiPranolol Metipranolol Ophthalmic Solution 0.3% (Metipranolol) Bausch & Lomb ... ⊙ 254
Timoptic in Ocudose (Timolol Maleate) Merck ... 2061
Timoptic Sterile Ophthalmic Solution (Timolol Maleate) Merck ... 2058
Timoptic-XE Sterile Ophthalmic Gel Forming Solution (Timolol Maleate) Merck ... 2062
Travatan Ophthalmic Solution (Travoprost) Alcon ... 559
Trusopt Sterile Ophthalmic Solution (Dorzolamide Hydrochloride) Merck ... 2065
Xalatan Sterile Ophthalmic Solution (Latanoprost) Pharmacia & Upjohn ... 2654

Hypertension, pulmonary
Flolan for Injection (Epoprostenol Sodium) GlaxoSmithKline ... 1408
Tracleer Tablets (Bosentan) Actelion ... 539

Hypertension, pulmonary arterial
Revatio Tablets (Sildenafil Citrate) Pfizer ... 2541
Ventavis Inhalation Solution (Iloprost) Cotherix ... 1036

Hypertension, severe
Hyperstat I.V. Injection (Diazoxide) Schering ... 3031

Hypertension associated with anesthesia
Brevibloc Concentrate (Esmolol Hydrochloride) Baxter Anesthesia ... 766
Brevibloc Injection (Esmolol Hydrochloride) Baxter Anesthesia ... 766
Brevibloc Double Strength Injection (Esmolol Hydrochloride) Baxter Anesthesia ... 766
Brevibloc Premixed Injection (Esmolol Hydrochloride) Baxter Anesthesia ... 766
Brevibloc Double Strength Premixed Injection (Esmolol Hydrochloride) Baxter Anesthesia ... 766

Hypertension associated with intratracheal intubation
Brevibloc Concentrate (Esmolol Hydrochloride) Baxter Anesthesia ... 766
Brevibloc Injection (Esmolol Hydrochloride) Baxter Anesthesia ... 766
Brevibloc Double Strength Injection (Esmolol Hydrochloride) Baxter Anesthesia ... 766
Brevibloc Premixed Injection (Esmolol Hydrochloride) Baxter Anesthesia ... 766
Brevibloc Double Strength Premixed Injection (Esmolol Hydrochloride) Baxter Anesthesia ... 766

Hypertension associated with surgical procedures
Brevibloc Concentrate (Esmolol Hydrochloride) Baxter Anesthesia ... 766
Brevibloc Injection (Esmolol Hydrochloride) Baxter Anesthesia ... 766
Brevibloc Double Strength Injection (Esmolol Hydrochloride) Baxter Anesthesia ... 766
Brevibloc Premixed Injection (Esmolol Hydrochloride) Baxter Anesthesia ... 766
Brevibloc Double Strength Premixed Injection (Esmolol Hydrochloride) Baxter Anesthesia ... 766

Hypertensive crises
(*see under* Hypertension)

Hypertensive episodes, control of, in pheochromocytoma
(*see also under* Pheochromocytoma, adjunctive therapy)
Dibenzyline Capsules (Phenoxybenzamine Hydrochloride) WellSpring ... 3390

Hyperthermia, malignant, prophylaxis
Dantrium Capsules (Dantrolene Sodium) Procter & Gamble Pharmaceuticals ... 2690
Dantrium Intravenous (Dantrolene Sodium) Procter & Gamble Pharmaceuticals ... 2691

Hypertriglyceridemia, adjunct to diet
(*see also under* Dysbetalipoproteinemia)
Antara Capsules (Fenofibrate) Reliant ... 2723
Caduet Tablets (Amlodipine Besylate, Atorvastatin Calcium) Pfizer ... 2507
Crestor Tablets (Rosuvastatin Calcium) AstraZeneca ... 672
Lescol Capsules (Fluvastatin Sodium) Novartis ... 2227
Lescol Capsules (Fluvastatin Sodium) Reliant ... 2730
Lescol XL Tablets (Fluvastatin Sodium) Novartis ... 2227
Lescol XL Tablets (Fluvastatin Sodium) Reliant ... 2730
Lipitor Tablets (Atorvastatin Calcium) Parke-Davis ... 2495
Lofibra Capsules (Fenofibrate) Gate ... 1217
Omacor Capsules (Omega-3-acid ethyl esters) Reliant ... 2735
Pravachol Tablets (Pravastatin Sodium) Bristol-Myers Squibb ... 943
Tricor Tablets (Fenofibrate) Abbott ... 523
Triglide Tablets (Fenofibrate) First Horizon ... 1165
Zocor Tablets (Simvastatin) Merck ... 2078

Hyperuricemia
Elitek (Rasburicase) Sanofi-Aventis ... 2906

Hypnotic
(*see under* Sleep, induction of)

Hypoalbuminemia
Buminate 5% Solution, USP (Albumin (human)) Baxter Healthcare ... 747
Buminate 25% Solution, USP (Albumin (human)) Baxter Healthcare ... 748

Hypocalcemia
Citracal Tablets (Calcium Citrate) Mission ... 2108
Os-Cal Chewable Tablets (Calcium Carbonate) GlaxoSmithKline ... ▣ 765
Os-Cal 500 Tablets (Calcium) GlaxoSmithKline ... ▣ 765

Hypocalcemia associated with chronic renal failure
Calcijex Injection (Calcitriol) Abbott ... 411

Hypocalcemia with vitamin D, deficiency of
Caltrate 600 PLUS Chewables (Calcium Carbonate, Minerals, Multiple, Vitamin D) Wyeth ... ▣ 779
Caltrate 600 PLUS Tablets (Calcium Carbonate, Minerals, Multiple, Vitamin D) Wyeth ... ▣ 779
Caltrate 600 + D Tablets (Calcium Carbonate, Vitamin D) Wyeth ... ▣ 779
Os-Cal 250 + D Tablets (Calcium, Vitamin D) GlaxoSmithKline ... ▣ 765
Os-Cal 500 + D Tablets (Calcium, Vitamin D) GlaxoSmithKline ... ▣ 766

Hypoestrogenism
Climara Transdermal System (Estradiol) Berlex ... 795
CombiPatch Transdermal System (Estradiol, Norethindrone Acetate) Novartis ... 2180
Premarin Intravenous (Estrogens, Conjugated) Wyeth ... 3440
Premarin Tablets (Estrogens, Conjugated) Wyeth ... 3443
Vivelle Transdermal System (Estradiol) Novartis ... 2288
Vivelle-Dot Transdermal System (Estradiol) Novartis ... 2293

Hypoglycemia
GlucaGen for Injection (Glucagon) Bedford ... 790
Glucagon for Injection Vials and Emergency Kit (Glucagon) Lilly ... 1749

Hypogonadism, female
Vivelle-Dot Transdermal System (Estradiol) Novartis ... 2293

Hypogonadism, hypogonadotropic, in males
AndroGel (Testosterone) Unimed ... 3330
Delatestryl Injection (Testosterone Enanthate) Savient ... 2976
Novarel for Injection (Chorionic Gonadotropin) Ferring ... 1147
Repronex for Intramuscular and Subcutaneous Injection (Menotropins) Ferring ... 1148
Striant Mucoadhesive (Testosterone) Columbia ... 1022
Testim 1% Gel (Testosterone) Auxilium ... 722

Hypogonadism, hypogonadotropic, secondary, adjunctive therapy in
Repronex for Intramuscular and Subcutaneous Injection (Menotropins) Ferring ... 1148

Hypogonadism, male, primary
AndroGel (Testosterone) Unimed ... 3330
Delatestryl Injection (Testosterone Enanthate) Savient ... 2976
Striant Mucoadhesive (Testosterone) Columbia ... 1022
Testim 1% Gel (Testosterone) Auxilium ... 722

Hypokalemia
K-Dur Extended-Relase Tablets (Potassium Chloride) Schering ... 3047
K-Lor Powder Packets (Potassium Chloride) Abbott ... 472
K-Tab Filmtab Tablets (Potassium Chloride) Abbott ... 473

Hypomagnesemia
Slow-Mag Tablets (Calcium, Magnesium Chloride) Purdue Products ... 2717

Hypophosphatemia
K-Phos Neutral Tablets (Potassium Phosphate, Sodium Phosphate) Beach ... 785

Hypopigmentation, skin
Oxsoralen Lotion 1% (Methoxsalen) Valeant ... 3354

Hypoproteinemia
Buminate 5% Solution, USP (Albumin (human)) Baxter Healthcare ... 747
Buminate 25% Solution, USP (Albumin (human)) Baxter Healthcare ... 748
Plasbumin-20 (Albumin (human)) Talecris ... 3249
Plasbumin-25 (Albumin (human)) Talecris ... 3251

Hypoprothrombinemia, drug-induced
AquaMEPHYTON Injection (Vitamin K_1) Merck ... 1887
Mephyton Tablets (Vitamin K_1) Merck ... 1993

Hypoprothrombinemia, salicylate-induced
AquaMEPHYTON Injection (Vitamin K_1) Merck ... 1887
Mephyton Tablets (Vitamin K_1) Merck ... 1993

Hypoprothrombinemia, secondary factors-induced
AquaMEPHYTON Injection (Vitamin K_1) Merck ... 1887
Mephyton Tablets (Vitamin K_1) Merck ... 1993

Hypoprothrombinemia due to antibacterial therapy
AquaMEPHYTON Injection (Vitamin K_1) Merck ... 1887

Hypotension, orthostatic
ProAmatine Tablets (Midodrine Hydrochloride) Shire US ... 3183

Hypotension, shock associated with brain damage due to trauma, adjunct to
Aramine (Metaraminol Bitartrate) Merck ... 1889

Hypothyroidism, ordinary
(*see under* Hypothyroidism, replacement or supplemental therapy in)

Hypothyroidism, primary
(*see under* Hypothyroidism, replacement or supplemental therapy in)

Hypothyroidism, replacement or supplemental therapy in
Cytomel Tablets (Liothyronine Sodium) King ... 1678
Levothroid Tablets (Levothyroxine Sodium) Forest ... 1189
Levoxyl Tablets (Levothyroxine Sodium) King ... 1680
Synthroid Tablets (Levothyroxine Sodium) Abbott ... 515
Thyrolar (Liotrix) Forest ... 1203
Unithroid Tablets (Levothyroxine Sodium) Lannett ... 3521

Hypothyroidism, secondary
(*see under* Hypothyroidism, replacement or supplemental therapy in)

Hypothyroidism, tertiary
(*see under* Hypothyroidism, replacement or supplemental therapy in)

Hypovolemia
Buminate 5% Solution, USP (Albumin (human)) Baxter Healthcare ... 747
Buminate 25% Solution, USP (Albumin (human)) Baxter Healthcare ... 748
Plasbumin-5 (Albumin (human)) Talecris ... 3249

I

Ichthyosis, unspecified
Ultralytic 2 Cream 20% (Urea) Ivax Dermatologicals ... 1651
Ultralytic 2 Foam 20% (Urea) Ivax Dermatologicals ... 1652

Idiopathic thrombocytopenic purpura
(*see under* Purpura, idiopathic thrombocytopenic)

Ileostomies, reducing the volume of discharge
Imodium Capsules (Loperamide Hydrochloride) McNeil Consumer .. 1834

Immunization, diphtheria, tetanus and pertussis
Adacel Vaccine (Diphtheria & Tetanus Toxoids and Acellular Pertussis Vaccine Adsorbed) Sanofi Pasteur ... 2959
Boostrix (Diphtheria & Tetanus Toxoids and Acellular Pertussis Vaccine Adsorbed) GlaxoSmithKline ... 1366
DAPTACEL (Diphtheria & Tetanus Toxoids and Acellular Pertussis Vaccine Adsorbed) Sanofi Pasteur ... 2964
Infanrix Vaccine (Diphtheria & Tetanus Toxoids and Acellular Pertussis Vaccine Adsorbed) GlaxoSmithKline ... 1444
Pediarix Vaccine (Diphtheria & Tetanus Toxoids and Pertussis Vaccine Adsorbed, Hepatitis B Vaccine, Recombinant, Poliovirus Vaccine Inactivated, Trivalent Types 1,2,3) GlaxoSmithKline ... 1518

Immunization, haemophilus influenzae type b
HibTITER (Haemophilus B Conjugate Vaccine) Wyeth ... 3419
Liquid PedvaxHIB (Haemophilus B Conjugate Vaccine) Merck ... 2012

Immunization, haemophilus influenzae type B and hepatitis B virus
Comvax (Haemophilus B Conjugate Vaccine, Hepatitis B Vaccine, Recombinant) Merck ... 1904

Immunization, hepatitis A and B virus
Twinrix Vaccine (Hepatitis A Vaccine, Inactivated, Hepatitis B Vaccine, Recombinant) GlaxoSmithKline ... 1571

Immunization, hepatitis A virus
Havrix Vaccine (Hepatitis A Vaccine, Inactivated) GlaxoSmithKline ... 1425
Vaqta (Hepatitis A Vaccine, Inactivated) Merck ... 2067

Immunization, hepatitis B virus
Engerix-B Vaccine (Hepatitis B Vaccine, Recombinant) GlaxoSmithKline ... 1391
Pediarix Vaccine (Diphtheria & Tetanus Toxoids and Pertussis Vaccine Adsorbed, Hepatitis B Vaccine, Recombinant, Poliovirus Vaccine Inactivated, Trivalent Types 1,2,3) GlaxoSmithKline ... 1518
Recombivax HB (Hepatitis B Vaccine, Recombinant) Merck ... 2045

Immunization, influenza virus, types A and B
Flumist Vaccine (Influenza Virus Vaccine) Medimmune ... 1872

Immunization, meningococcal
Menactra Vaccine (Meningoccal Polysaccharide Diphtheria Toxoid Conjugate Vaccine) Sanofi Pasteur ... 2968

Immunization, poliovirus 1, 2, and 3
Pediarix Vaccine (Diphtheria & Tetanus Toxoids and Pertussis Vaccine Adsorbed, Hepatitis B Vaccine, Recombinant, Poliovirus Vaccine Inactivated, Trivalent Types 1,2,3) GlaxoSmithKline ... 1518

Immunization, rabies
Rabies Vaccine RabAvert (Rabies Vaccine) Chiron ... 1011

Immunization, tetanus
HyperTET (Tetanus Immune Globulin (Human)) Talecris ... 3245

Immunization, typhoid fever
Vivotif (Typhoid Vaccine Live Oral TY21a) Berna ... 834

Immunization, varicella
Varivax (Varicella Virus Vaccine Live) Merck ... 2070

Immunodeficiencies
GamaSTAN (Globulin, Immune (Human)) Talecris ... 3231
Gammagard Liquid (Immune Globulin Intravenous (Human)) Baxter Healthcare ... 751
Gammagard S/D (Immune Globulin Intravenous (Human)) Baxter Healthcare ... 754
Gamunex Immune Globulin I.V., 10% (Immune Globulin Intravenous (Human)) Talecris ... 3232
Iveegam EN (Immune Globulin Intravenous (Human)) Baxter Healthcare ... 759

Immunodeficiency, common variable
Gamunex Immune Globulin I.V., 10% (Immune Globulin Intravenous (Human)) Talecris ... 3232
Iveegam EN (Immune Globulin Intravenous (Human)) Baxter Healthcare ... 759

Immunodeficiency, unspecified
(*see under* Infection, tendency to)

Immunodeficiency disease, severe combined
(*see under* Adenosine deaminase, enzyme replacement therapy for)

Impetigo contagiosa
Bactroban Ointment (Mupirocin) GlaxoSmithKline ... 1358
Ceftin for Oral Suspension (Cefuroxime Axetil) GlaxoSmithKline ... 1369
Centany Ointment, 2% (Mupirocin) OrthoNeutrogena ... 2382
Levaquin in 5% Dextrose Injection (Levofloxacin) Ortho-McNeil ... 2453
Levaquin (Levofloxacin) Ortho-McNeil ... 2453

Impotence, male
(*see under* Erectile dysfunction)

Infection, tendency to
Carimune NF (Immune Globulin Intravenous (Human)) ZLB Behring ... 3501

Infections, acquired immunodeficiency syndrome-related complex
AmBisome for Injection (Amphotericin B, liposomal) Astellas ... 615
Biaxin/Biaxin XL (Clarithromycin) Abbott ... 402
Cytovene (Ganciclovir) Roche Laboratories ... 2763
Doxil Injection (Doxorubicin Hydrochloride Liposome) Tibotec ... 3302
Famvir Tablets (Famciclovir) Novartis ... 2207
Intron A for Injection (Interferon alfa-2b, Recombinant) Schering ... 3038
Marinol Capsules (Dronabinol) Unimed ... 3334
Retrovir IV Infusion (Zidovudine) GlaxoSmithKline ... 1537
Roferon-A Injection (Interferon alfa-2a, Recombinant) Roche Laboratories ... 2805
Valcyte Tablets (Valganciclovir Hydrochloride) Roche Laboratories ... 2816
WinRho SDF (Rh_o (D) Immune Globulin (Human)) Baxter Healthcare ... 763

Infections, aerobic organisms
Fortaz (Ceftazidime Sodium) GlaxoSmithKline ... 1422
Mefoxin for Injection (Cefoxitin Sodium) Merck ... 1987
Mefoxin Premixed Intravenous Solution (Cefoxitin Sodium) Merck ... 1990

Infections, anaerobic organisms
Cleocin Vaginal Ovules (Clindamycin Hydrochloride) Pharmacia & Upjohn ... 2613
Fortaz (Ceftazidime Sodium) GlaxoSmithKline ... 1422
Garamycin Injectable (Gentamicin Sulfate) Schering ... 3028
Mefoxin for Injection (Cefoxitin Sodium) Merck ... 1987
Mefoxin Premixed Intravenous Solution (Cefoxitin Sodium) Merck ... 1990
Primaxin I.V. (Cilastatin Sodium, Imipenem) Merck ... 2024

Infections, bacterial, various types
Synercid I.V. (Dalfopristin, Quinupristin) King ... 1690

Infections, beta-lactamase producing organisms
Augmentin (Amoxicillin, Clavulanate Potassium) GlaxoSmithKline ... 1331
Augmentin Tablets (Amoxicillin, Clavulanate Potassium) GlaxoSmithKline ... 1334
Augmentin XR Extended-Release Tablets (Amoxicillin, Clavulanate Potassium) GlaxoSmithKline ... 1340
Ceftin (Cefuroxime Axetil) GlaxoSmithKline ... 1369
Merrem I.V. (Meropenem) AstraZeneca ... 687
Vantin Tablets and Oral Suspension (Cefpodoxime Proxetil) Pharmacia & Upjohn ... 2650
Zosyn (Piperacillin Sodium, Tazobactam Sodium) Wyeth ... 3492

Infections, biliary tract
Ancef (Cefazolin Sodium) GlaxoSmithKline ... 1318

Infections, bone and joint
Cipro I.V. (Ciprofloxacin) Schering ... 2998
Cipro I.V. Pharmacy Bulk Package (Ciprofloxacin) Bayer ... 3509
Cipro (Ciprofloxacin) Schering ... 2991
Fortaz (Ceftazidime Sodium) GlaxoSmithKline ... 1422
Garamycin Injectable (Gentamicin Sulfate) Schering ... 3028
Mefoxin for Injection (Cefoxitin Sodium) Merck ... 1987
Mefoxin Premixed Intravenous Solution (Cefoxitin Sodium) Merck ... 1990
Primaxin I.V. (Cilastatin Sodium, Imipenem) Merck ... 2024
Rocephin Injectable Vials, ADD-Vantage, Galaxy, Bulk (Ceftriaxone Sodium) Roche Laboratories ... 2801
Timentin ADD-Vantage (Clavulanate Potassium, Ticarcillin Disodium) GlaxoSmithKline ... 1556
Timentin Injection Galaxy Container (Clavulanate Potassium, Ticarcillin Disodium) GlaxoSmithKline ... 1559
Timentin IV Infusion (Clavulanate Potassium, Ticarcillin Disodium) GlaxoSmithKline ... 1553
Timentin Pharmacy Bulk Package (Clavulanate Potassium, Ticarcillin Disodium) GlaxoSmithKline ... 1562
Zinacef Injection (Cefuroxime) GlaxoSmithKline ... 1604
Zinacef for Injection (Cefuroxime) GlaxoSmithKline ... 1604

Infections, burn wound
(*see also under* Infections, skin, bacterial, minor)
Garamycin Injectable (Gentamicin Sulfate) Schering ... 3028
Sulfamylon Cream (Mafenide Acetate) Mylan Bertek ... 2154

Infections, central nervous system
Fortaz (Ceftazidime Sodium) GlaxoSmithKline ... 1422
Garamycin Injectable (Gentamicin Sulfate) Schering ... 3028

Infections, ear, nose and throat
Amoxil Capsules (Amoxicillin) GlaxoSmithKline ... 1315
Amoxil Chewable Tablets (Amoxicillin) GlaxoSmithKline ... 1315
Amoxil Pediatric Drops for Oral Suspension (Amoxicillin) GlaxoSmithKline ... 1315
Amoxil Powder for Oral Suspension (Amoxicillin) GlaxoSmithKline ... 1315
Amoxil Tablets (Amoxicillin) GlaxoSmithKline ... 1315

Infections, fungal, systemic
Abelcet Injection (Amphotericin B Lipid Complex) Enzon ... 1119

Infections, genitourinary tract
Amoxil Capsules (Amoxicillin) GlaxoSmithKline ... 1315
Amoxil Chewable Tablets (Amoxicillin) GlaxoSmithKline ... 1315
Amoxil Pediatric Drops for Oral Suspension (Amoxicillin) GlaxoSmithKline ... 1315
Amoxil Powder for Oral Suspension (Amoxicillin) GlaxoSmithKline ... 1315
Amoxil Tablets (Amoxicillin) GlaxoSmithKline ... 1315
Ancef for Injection (Cefazolin Sodium) GlaxoSmithKline ... 1318

Infections, gram-negative bacteria
Amoxil Capsules (Amoxicillin) GlaxoSmithKline ... 1315
Amoxil Chewable Tablets (Amoxicillin) GlaxoSmithKline ... 1315
Amoxil Pediatric Drops for Oral Suspension (Amoxicillin) GlaxoSmithKline ... 1315
Amoxil Powder for Oral Suspension (Amoxicillin) GlaxoSmithKline ... 1315
Amoxil Tablets (Amoxicillin) GlaxoSmithKline ... 1315
Garamycin Injectable (Gentamicin Sulfate) Schering ... 3028
Mefoxin for Injection (Cefoxitin Sodium) Merck ... 1987
Mefoxin Premixed Intravenous Solution (Cefoxitin Sodium) Merck ... 1990
Primaxin I.V. (Cilastatin Sodium, Imipenem) Merck ... 2024
Seromycin Capsules (Cycloserine) Lilly ... 1783

Infections, gram-positive anaerobic cocci
Mefoxin for Injection (Cefoxitin Sodium) Merck ... 1987
Mefoxin Premixed Intravenous Solution (Cefoxitin Sodium) Merck ... 1990

Infections, gram-positive bacteria
Amoxil Capsules (Amoxicillin) GlaxoSmithKline ... 1315
Amoxil Chewable Tablets (Amoxicillin) GlaxoSmithKline ... 1315
Amoxil Pediatric Drops for Oral Suspension (Amoxicillin) GlaxoSmithKline ... 1315
Amoxil Powder for Oral Suspension (Amoxicillin) GlaxoSmithKline ... 1315
Amoxil Tablets (Amoxicillin) GlaxoSmithKline ... 1315
Primaxin I.V. (Cilastatin Sodium, Imipenem) Merck ... 2024
Seromycin Capsules (Cycloserine) Lilly ... 1783

Infections, gynecologic
Cleocin Vaginal Ovules (Clindamycin Hydrochloride) Pharmacia & Upjohn ... 2613
Ery-Tab Tablets (Erythromycin) Abbott ... 447
Erythrocin Stearate Filmtab Tablets (Erythromycin Stearate) Abbott ... 452
Erythromycin Base Filmtab Tablets (Erythromycin) Abbott ... 454
Erythromycin Delayed-Release Capsules, USP (Erythromycin) Abbott ... 456
Fortaz (Ceftazidime Sodium) GlaxoSmithKline ... 1422
Mefoxin for Injection (Cefoxitin Sodium) Merck ... 1987
Mefoxin Premixed Intravenous Solution (Cefoxitin Sodium) Merck ... 1990
PCE Dispertab Tablets (Erythromycin) Abbott ... 510
Primaxin I.M. (Cilastatin Sodium, Imipenem) Merck ... 2022
Primaxin I.V. (Cilastatin Sodium, Imipenem) Merck ... 2024
Timentin ADD-Vantage (Clavulanate Potassium, Ticarcillin Disodium) GlaxoSmithKline ... 1556
Timentin Injection Galaxy Container (Clavulanate Potassium, Ticarcillin Disodium) GlaxoSmithKline ... 1559
Timentin IV Infusion (Clavulanate Potassium, Ticarcillin Disodium) GlaxoSmithKline ... 1553
Timentin Pharmacy Bulk Package (Clavulanate Potassium, Ticarcillin Disodium) GlaxoSmithKline ... 1562
Vantin Tablets and Oral Suspension (Cefpodoxime Proxetil) Pharmacia & Upjohn ... 2650
Zosyn (Piperacillin Sodium, Tazobactam Sodium) Wyeth ... 3492

Infections, human immunodeficiency virus
Agenerase Capsules (Amprenavir) GlaxoSmithKline ... 1299
Agenerase Oral Solution (Amprenavir) GlaxoSmithKline ... 1304
Aptivus Capsules (Tipranavir) Boehringer Ingelheim ... 859
Combivir Tablets (Lamivudine, Zidovudine) GlaxoSmithKline ... 1373
Crixivan Capsules (Indinavir Sulfate) Merck ... 1918
Emtriva Capsules (Emtricitabine) Gilead ... 1272
Epivir (Lamivudine) GlaxoSmithKline ... 1394
Epzicom Tablets (Lamivudine, Abacavir Sulfate) GlaxoSmithKline ... 1402
Fuzeon Injection (Enfuvirtide) Roche Laboratories ... 2772
Invirase (Saquinavir Mesylate) Roche Laboratories ... 2776
Kaletra (Lopinavir, Ritonavir) Abbott ... 474
Lexiva Tablets (Fosamprenavir Calcium) GlaxoSmithKline ... 1473
Norvir (Ritonavir) Abbott ... 499
Rescriptor Tablets (Delavirdine Mesylate) Pfizer ... 2535
Retrovir Capsules (Zidovudine) GlaxoSmithKline ... 1533
Retrovir IV Infusion (Zidovudine) GlaxoSmithKline ... 1537
Retrovir (Zidovudine) GlaxoSmithKline ... 1533
Reyataz Capsules (Atazanavir sulfate) Bristol-Myers Squibb ... 948
Sustiva Capsules (Efavirenz) Bristol-Myers Squibb ... 957
Trizivir Tablets (Lamivudine, Abacavir Sulfate, Zidovudine) GlaxoSmithKline ... 1565
Truvada Tablets (Tenofovir Disoproxil Fumarate, Emtricitabine) Gilead ... 1279
Viracept (Nelfinavir Mesylate) Pfizer ... 2556
Viramune Oral Suspension (Nevirapine) Boehringer Ingelheim ... 903
Viramune Tablets (Nevirapine) Boehringer Ingelheim ... 903
Viread Tablets (Tenofovir Disoproxil Fumarate) Gilead ... 1284
Zerit (Stavudine) Bristol-Myers Squibb ... 971
Ziagen (Abacavir Sulfate) GlaxoSmithKline ... 1600

Infections, intra-abdominal
Cipro I.V. (Ciprofloxacin) Schering ... 2998
Cipro I.V. Pharmacy Bulk Package (Ciprofloxacin) Bayer ... 3509
Cipro (Ciprofloxacin) Schering ... 2991
Cleocin Vaginal Ovules (Clindamycin Hydrochloride) Pharmacia & Upjohn ... 2613
Fortaz (Ceftazidime Sodium) GlaxoSmithKline ... 1422
Garamycin Injectable (Gentamicin Sulfate) Schering ... 3028
Invanz for Injection (Ertapenem) Merck ... 1974
Maxipime for Injection (Cefepime Hydrochloride) Elan ... 1093
Mefoxin for Injection (Cefoxitin Sodium) Merck ... 1987
Mefoxin Premixed Intravenous Solution (Cefoxitin Sodium) Merck ... 1990
Merrem I.V. (Meropenem) AstraZeneca ... 687
Primaxin I.M. (Cilastatin Sodium, Imipenem) Merck ... 2022
Primaxin I.V. (Cilastatin Sodium, Imipenem) Merck ... 2024
Rocephin Injectable Vials, ADD-Vantage, Galaxy, Bulk (Ceftriaxone Sodium) Roche Laboratories ... 2801
Timentin ADD-Vantage (Clavulanate Potassium, Ticarcillin Disodium) GlaxoSmithKline ... 1556
Timentin Injection Galaxy Container (Clavulanate Potassium, Ticarcillin Disodium) GlaxoSmithKline ... 1559
Timentin IV Infusion (Clavulanate Potassium, Ticarcillin Disodium) GlaxoSmithKline ... 1553
Timentin Pharmacy Bulk Package (Clavulanate Potassium, Ticarcillin Disodium) GlaxoSmithKline ... 1562

Infections, liver flukes
(*see under* Clonorchiasis)

Infections, lower respiratory tract
Amoxil Capsules (Amoxicillin) GlaxoSmithKline ... 1315
Amoxil Chewable Tablets (Amoxicillin) GlaxoSmithKline ... 1315
Amoxil Pediatric Drops for Oral Suspension (Amoxicillin) GlaxoSmithKline ... 1315
Amoxil Powder for Oral Suspension (Amoxicillin) GlaxoSmithKline ... 1315
Amoxil Tablets (Amoxicillin) GlaxoSmithKline ... 1315
Augmentin (Amoxicillin, Clavulanate Potassium) GlaxoSmithKline ... 1331
Augmentin Tablets (Amoxicillin, Clavulanate Potassium) GlaxoSmithKline ... 1334
Augmentin XR Extended-Release Tablets (Amoxicillin, Clavulanate Potassium) GlaxoSmithKline ... 1340
Avelox (Moxifloxacin Hydrochloride) Schering ... 2984
Biaxin/Biaxin XL (Clarithromycin) Abbott ... 402
Cipro I.V. (Ciprofloxacin) Schering ... 2998
Cipro I.V. Pharmacy Bulk Package (Ciprofloxacin) Bayer ... 3509
Cipro (Ciprofloxacin) Schering ... 2991
Cleocin Vaginal Ovules (Clindamycin Hydrochloride) Pharmacia & Upjohn ... 2613
E.E.S. (Erythromycin Ethylsuccinate) Abbott ... 449
EryPed (Erythromycin Ethylsuccinate) Abbott ... 445
Ery-Tab Tablets (Erythromycin) Abbott ... 447
Erythrocin Stearate Filmtab Tablets (Erythromycin Stearate) Abbott ... 452
Erythromycin Base Filmtab Tablets (Erythromycin) Abbott ... 454
Erythromycin Delayed-Release Capsules, USP (Erythromycin) Abbott ... 456
Fortaz (Ceftazidime Sodium) GlaxoSmithKline ... 1422
Invanz for Injection (Ertapenem) Merck ... 1974
Mefoxin for Injection (Cefoxitin Sodium) Merck ... 1987
Mefoxin Premixed Intravenous Solution (Cefoxitin Sodium) Merck ... 1990
Omnicef Capsules (Cefdinir) Abbott ... 506
Omnicef for Oral Suspension (Cefdinir) Abbott ... 506
PCE Dispertab Tablets (Erythromycin) Abbott ... 510
Primaxin I.M. (Cilastatin Sodium, Imipenem) Merck ... 2022
Primaxin I.V. (Cilastatin Sodium, Imipenem) Merck ... 2024
Rocephin Injectable Vials, ADD-Vantage, Galaxy, Bulk (Ceftriaxone Sodium) Roche Laboratories ... 2801
Tequin Injection (Gatifloxacin) Bristol-Myers Squibb ... 964
Tequin Tablets (Gatifloxacin) Bristol-Myers Squibb ... 964
Timentin ADD-Vantage (Clavulanate Potassium, Ticarcillin Disodium) GlaxoSmithKline ... 1556
Timentin Injection Galaxy Container (Clavulanate Potassium, Ticarcillin Disodium) GlaxoSmithKline ... 1559
Timentin IV Infusion (Clavulanate Potassium, Ticarcillin Disodium) GlaxoSmithKline ... 1553
Timentin Pharmacy Bulk Package (Clavulanate Potassium, Ticarcillin Disodium) GlaxoSmithKline ... 1562
Vantin Tablets and Oral Suspension (Cefpodoxime Proxetil) Pharmacia & Upjohn ... 2650
Zinacef Injection (Cefuroxime) GlaxoSmithKline ... 1604
Zinacef for Injection (Cefuroxime) GlaxoSmithKline ... 1604
Zithromax Capsules, 250 mg (Azithromycin Dihydrate) Pfizer ... 2568
Zithromax for IV Infusion (Azithromycin Dihydrate) Pfizer ... 2573
Zithromax for Oral Suspension, 1 g (Azithromycin Dihydrate) Pfizer ... 2568
Zithromax for Oral Suspension, 300 mg, 600 mg, 900 mg, 1200 mg (Azithromycin Dihydrate) Pfizer ... 2561
Zithromax Tablets, 250 mg, 500 mg (Azithromycin Dihydrate) Pfizer ... 2561
Zithromax Tablets, 600 mg (Azithromycin Dihydrate) Pfizer ... 2568
Zithromax Tri-Pak (Azithromycin Dihydrate) Pfizer ... 2561
Zithromax Z-Pak (Azithromycin Dihydrate) Pfizer ... 2568
Zosyn (Piperacillin Sodium, Tazobactam Sodium) Wyeth ... 3492

Infections, lower respiratory tract, RSV-induced
Virazole for Inhalation Solution (Ribavirin) Valeant ... 3365

Infections, lower respiratory tract, RSV-induced, prevention of
Synagis (Palivizumab) MedImmune ... 1868

Infections, manifested by febrile neutropenia, to decrease incidence of
Maxipime for Injection (Cefepime Hydrochloride) Elan ... 1093

Infections, mycotic, cutaneous
Nystop (Nystatin) Paddock ... 2490

Infections, ocular, bacterial
Bleph-10 Ophthalmic Solution 10% (Sulfacetamide Sodium) Allergan ... ⊙219
Polytrim Ophthalmic Solution (Polymyxin B Sulfate, Trimethoprim Sulfate) Allergan ... 570
Quixin Ophthalmic Solution (Levofloxacin) Vistakon ... 3373

Infections, perioperative, reduction of the incidence of
Ancef for Injection (Cefazolin Sodium) GlaxoSmithKline ... 1318
Rocephin Injectable Vials, ADD-Vantage, Galaxy, Bulk (Ceftriaxone Sodium) Roche Laboratories ... 2801
Zinacef Injection (Cefuroxime) GlaxoSmithKline ... 1604
Zinacef for Injection (Cefuroxime) GlaxoSmithKline ... 1604

Infections, polymicrobic
Fortaz (Ceftazidime Sodium) GlaxoSmithKline ... 1422
Primaxin I.V. (Cilastatin Sodium, Imipenem) Merck ... 2024

Infections, respiratory tract, unspecified
Ancef for Injection (Cefazolin Sodium) GlaxoSmithKline ... 1318
E.E.S. (Erythromycin Ethylsuccinate) Abbott ... 449
EryPed (Erythromycin Ethylsuccinate) Abbott ... 445
Erythrocin Stearate Filmtab Tablets (Erythromycin Stearate) Abbott ... 452
Erythromycin Base Filmtab Tablets (Erythromycin) Abbott ... 454
Erythromycin Delayed-Release Capsules, USP (Erythromycin) Abbott ... 456
Garamycin Injectable (Gentamicin Sulfate) Schering ... 3028
Omnicef Capsules (Cefdinir) Abbott ... 506
Omnicef for Oral Suspension (Cefdinir) Abbott ... 506
PCE Dispertab Tablets (Erythromycin) Abbott ... 510

Infections, skin, bacterial, minor
Aquacel AG with Hydrofiber (Silver impregnated antimicrobial dressing) ConvaTec ... 1035
Bactroban Ointment (Mupirocin) GlaxoSmithKline ... 1358
Betadine Solution (Povidone Iodine) Purdue Products ... 2715
Clorpactin WCS-90 (Sodium Oxychlorosene) Guardian ... 1636
Garamycin Injectable (Gentamicin Sulfate) Schering ... 3028
Neosporin Ointment (Bacitracin, Neomycin, Polymyxin B Sulfate) Pfizer Consumer Healthcare ... [PDR Nonprescription]702
Neosporin + Pain Relief Maximum Strength Cream (Neomycin, Polymyxin B Sulfate, Pramoxine Hydrochloride) Pfizer Consumer Healthcare ... [PDR Nonprescription]703
Neosporin + Pain Relief Maximum Strength Ointment (Bacitracin, Neomycin, Polymyxin B Sulfate, Pramoxine Hydrochloride) Pfizer Consumer Healthcare ... [PDR Nonprescription]703
Polysporin Ointment (Bacitracin, Polymyxin B Sulfate) Pfizer Consumer Healthcare ... [PDR Nonprescription]706

Infections, skin and skin structure
Amoxil Capsules (Amoxicillin) GlaxoSmithKline ... 1315
Amoxil Chewable Tablets (Amoxicillin) GlaxoSmithKline ... 1315
Amoxil Pediatric Drops for Oral Suspension (Amoxicillin) GlaxoSmithKline ... 1315
Amoxil Powder for Oral Suspension (Amoxicillin) GlaxoSmithKline ... 1315
Amoxil Tablets (Amoxicillin) GlaxoSmithKline ... 1315
Ancef for Injection (Cefazolin Sodium) GlaxoSmithKline ... 1318
Augmentin (Amoxicillin, Clavulanate Potassium) GlaxoSmithKline ... 1331
Augmentin Tablets (Amoxicillin, Clavulanate Potassium) GlaxoSmithKline ... 1334

Avelox (Moxifloxacin Hydrochloride) Schering ... 2984
Bactroban Cream (Mupirocin Calcium) GlaxoSmithKline ... 1356
Biaxin/Biaxin XL (Clarithromycin) Abbott ... 402
Ceftin Tablets (Cefuroxime Axetil) GlaxoSmithKline ... 1369
Cipro I.V. (Ciprofloxacin) Schering ... 2998
Cipro I.V. Pharmacy Bulk Package (Ciprofloxacin) Bayer ... 3509
Cipro (Ciprofloxacin) Schering ... 2991
Cleocin Vaginal Ovules (Clindamycin Hydrochloride) Pharmacia & Upjohn ... 2613
E.E.S. (Erythromycin Ethylsuccinate) Abbott ... 449
EryPed (Erythromycin Ethylsuccinate) Abbott ... 445
Ery-Tab Tablets (Erythromycin) Abbott ... 447
Erythrocin Stearate Filmtab Tablets (Erythromycin Stearate) Abbott ... 452
Erythromycin Base Filmtab Tablets (Erythromycin) Abbott ... 454
Erythromycin Delayed-Release Capsules, USP (Erythromycin) Abbott ... 456
Fortaz (Ceftazidime Sodium) GlaxoSmithKline ... 1422
Garamycin Injectable (Gentamicin Sulfate) Schering ... 3028
Invanz for Injection (Ertapenem) Merck ... 1974
Levaquin in 5% Dextrose Injection (Levofloxacin) Ortho-McNeil ... 2453
Levaquin (Levofloxacin) Ortho-McNeil ... 2453
Maxipime for Injection (Cefepime Hydrochloride) Elan ... 1093
Mefoxin for Injection (Cefoxitin Sodium) Merck ... 1987
Mefoxin Premixed Intravenous Solution (Cefoxitin Sodium) Merck ... 1990
Merrem I.V. (Meropenem) AstraZeneca ... 687
Omnicef Capsules (Cefdinir) Abbott ... 506
Omnicef for Oral Suspension (Cefdinir) Abbott ... 506
PCE Dispertab Tablets (Erythromycin) Abbott ... 510
Primaxin I.M. (Cilastatin Sodium, Imipenem) Merck ... 2022
Primaxin I.V. (Cilastatin Sodium, Imipenem) Merck ... 2024
Rocephin Injectable Vials, ADD-Vantage, Galaxy, Bulk (Ceftriaxone Sodium) Roche Laboratories ... 2801
Spectracef Tablets (Cefditoren Pivoxil) Purdue Pharmaceutical ... 2706
Tequin Injection (Gatifloxacin) Bristol-Myers Squibb ... 964
Tequin Tablets (Gatifloxacin) Bristol-Myers Squibb ... 964
Timentin ADD-Vantage (Clavulanate Potassium, Ticarcillin Disodium) GlaxoSmithKline ... 1556
Timentin Injection Galaxy Container (Clavulanate Potassium, Ticarcillin Disodium) GlaxoSmithKline ... 1559
Timentin IV Infusion (Clavulanate Potassium, Ticarcillin Disodium) GlaxoSmithKline ... 1553
Timentin Pharmacy Bulk Package (Clavulanate Potassium, Ticarcillin Disodium) GlaxoSmithKline ... 1562
Vantin Tablets and Oral Suspension (Cefpodoxime Proxetil) Pharmacia & Upjohn ... 2650
Zinacef Injection (Cefuroxime) GlaxoSmithKline ... 1604
Zinacef for Injection (Cefuroxime) GlaxoSmithKline ... 1604
Zithromax (Azithromycin Dihydrate) Pfizer ... 2568
Zithromax for Oral Suspension, 300 mg, 600 mg, 900 mg, 1200 mg (Azithromycin Dihydrate) Pfizer ... 2561
Zithromax Tablets, 250 mg, 500 mg (Azithromycin Dihydrate) Pfizer ... 2561
Zithromax Tablets, 600 mg (Azithromycin Dihydrate) Pfizer ... 2568
Zithromax Tri-Pak (Azithromycin Dihydrate) Pfizer ... 2561
Zithromax Z-Pak (Azithromycin Dihydrate) Pfizer ... 2568
Zosyn (Piperacillin Sodium, Tazobactam Sodium) Wyeth ... 3492
Zyvox (Linezolid) Pharmacia & Upjohn ... 2661

Infections, soft tissues
(*see under* Infections, skin and skin structure)

Infections, superficial, external auditory canal
(*see under* Otitis externa)

Infections, surgical, ophthalmic, prevention of
Betadine 5% Ophthalmic Solution (Povidone Iodine) Alcon ... ⊙202

Infections, tapeworm
Albenza Tablets (Albendazole) GlaxoSmithKline ... 1310

Infections, upper respiratory tract
Amoxil Capsules (Amoxicillin) GlaxoSmithKline ... 1315
Amoxil Chewable Tablets (Amoxicillin) GlaxoSmithKline ... 1315
Amoxil Pediatric Drops for Oral Suspension (Amoxicillin) GlaxoSmithKline ... 1315
Amoxil Powder for Oral Suspension (Amoxicillin) GlaxoSmithKline ... 1315
Amoxil Tablets (Amoxicillin) GlaxoSmithKline ... 1315
Avelox (Moxifloxacin Hydrochloride) Schering ... 2984
Biaxin/Biaxin XL (Clarithromycin) Abbott ... 402
E.E.S. (Erythromycin Ethylsuccinate) Abbott ... 449
EryPed (Erythromycin Ethylsuccinate) Abbott ... 445
Ery-Tab Tablets (Erythromycin) Abbott ... 447
Erythrocin Stearate Filmtab Tablets (Erythromycin Stearate) Abbott ... 452
Erythromycin Base Filmtab Tablets (Erythromycin) Abbott ... 454
Erythromycin Delayed-Release Capsules, USP (Erythromycin) Abbott ... 456
Omnicef Capsules (Cefdinir) Abbott ... 506
Omnicef for Oral Suspension (Cefdinir) Abbott ... 506
PCE Dispertab Tablets (Erythromycin) Abbott ... 510
Suprax (Cefixime) Lupin ... 1811
Tequin Injection (Gatifloxacin) Bristol-Myers Squibb ... 964
Tequin Tablets (Gatifloxacin) Bristol-Myers Squibb ... 964
Vantin Tablets and Oral Suspension (Cefpodoxime Proxetil) Pharmacia & Upjohn ... 2650
Zithromax (Azithromycin Dihydrate) Pfizer ... 2568
Zithromax for Oral Suspension, 300 mg, 600 mg, 900 mg, 1200 mg (Azithromycin Dihydrate) Pfizer ... 2561
Zithromax Tablets, 250 mg, 500 mg (Azithromycin Dihydrate) Pfizer ... 2561
Zithromax Tablets, 600 mg (Azithromycin Dihydrate) Pfizer ... 2568
Zithromax Tri-Pak (Azithromycin Dihydrate) Pfizer ... 2561
Zithromax Z-Pak (Azithromycin Dihydrate) Pfizer ... 2568

Infections, urinary tract
Amoxil Capsules (Amoxicillin) GlaxoSmithKline ... 1315
Amoxil Chewable Tablets (Amoxicillin) GlaxoSmithKline ... 1315
Amoxil Pediatric Drops for Oral Suspension (Amoxicillin) GlaxoSmithKline ... 1315
Amoxil Powder for Oral Suspension (Amoxicillin) GlaxoSmithKline ... 1315
Amoxil Tablets (Amoxicillin) GlaxoSmithKline ... 1315
Ancef for Injection (Cefazolin Sodium) GlaxoSmithKline ... 1318
Augmentin (Amoxicillin, Clavulanate Potassium) GlaxoSmithKline ... 1331
Augmentin Tablets (Amoxicillin, Clavulanate Potassium) GlaxoSmithKline ... 1334
Ceftin Tablets (Cefuroxime Axetil) GlaxoSmithKline ... 1369
Cipro I.V. (Ciprofloxacin) Schering ... 2998
Cipro I.V. Pharmacy Bulk Package (Ciprofloxacin) Bayer ... 3509
Cipro (Ciprofloxacin) Schering ... 2991
Cipro XR Tablets (Ciprofloxacin) Schering ... 3004
Fortaz (Ceftazidime Sodium) GlaxoSmithKline ... 1422
Garamycin Injectable (Gentamicin Sulfate) Schering ... 3028
Invanz for Injection (Ertapenem) Merck ... 1974
Levaquin in 5% Dextrose Injection (Levofloxacin) Ortho-McNeil ... 2453
Levaquin (Levofloxacin) Ortho-McNeil ... 2453
Maxipime for Injection (Cefepime Hydrochloride) Elan ... 1093
Mefoxin for Injection (Cefoxitin Sodium) Merck ... 1987
Mefoxin Premixed Intravenous Solution (Cefoxitin Sodium) Merck ... 1990
Noroxin Tablets (Norfloxacin) Merck ... 2009
Primaxin I.V. (Cilastatin Sodium, Imipenem) Merck ... 2024
Rocephin Injectable Vials, ADD-Vantage, Galaxy, Bulk (Ceftriaxone Sodium) Roche Laboratories ... 2801
Seromycin Capsules (Cycloserine) Lilly ... 1783
Suprax (Cefixime) Lupin ... 1811
Tequin Injection (Gatifloxacin) Bristol-Myers Squibb ... 964
Tequin Tablets (Gatifloxacin) Bristol-Myers Squibb ... 964
Timentin ADD-Vantage (Clavulanate Potassium, Ticarcillin Disodium) GlaxoSmithKline ... 1556
Timentin Injection Galaxy Container (Clavulanate Potassium, Ticarcillin Disodium) GlaxoSmithKline ... 1559
Timentin IV Infusion (Clavulanate Potassium, Ticarcillin Disodium) GlaxoSmithKline ... 1553
Timentin Pharmacy Bulk Package (Clavulanate Potassium, Ticarcillin Disodium) GlaxoSmithKline ... 1562
Uroqid-Acid No. 2 Tablets (Methenamine Mandelate, Sodium Acid Phosphate) Beach ... 785
Vantin Tablets and Oral Suspension (Cefpodoxime Proxetil) Pharmacia & Upjohn ... 2650
Zinacef Injection (Cefuroxime) GlaxoSmithKline ... 1604
Zinacef for Injection (Cefuroxime) GlaxoSmithKline ... 1604

Infections, vaginal cuff, post-surgical
Cleocin Vaginal Ovules (Clindamycin Hydrochloride) Pharmacia & Upjohn ... 2613

Infections, venereal
(*see under* Gonorrhea; Yaws)

Infectious diarrhea
(*see under* Diarrhea, infectious)

Infertility, progesterone deficiency-induced
Prochieve 8% Gel (Progesterone) Columbia ... 1018

Inflammation, anorectal
Analpram-HC (Hydrocortisone Acetate, Pramoxine Hydrochloride) Ferndale ... 1136
Cortizone•5 Ointment (Hydrocortisone) Pfizer Consumer Healthcare ... ■699
Cortizone•10 Creme (Hydrocortisone) Pfizer Consumer Healthcare ... ■699
Cortizone•10 Ointment (Hydrocortisone) Pfizer Consumer Healthcare ... ■699
Cortizone•10 Plus Creme (Hydrocortisone) Pfizer Consumer Healthcare ... ■700
ProctoFoam-HC (Hydrocortisone Acetate, Pramoxine Hydrochloride) Schwarz ... 3113

Inflammation, anterior segment
Blephamide Ophthalmic Ointment (Prednisolone Acetate, Sulfacetamide Sodium) Allergan ... 563
Blephamide Ophthalmic Suspension (Prednisolone Acetate, Sulfacetamide Sodium) Allergan ... 564
Decadron Phosphate Injection (Dexamethasone Sodium Phosphate) Merck ... 1931
Depo-Medrol Injectable Suspension (Methylprednisolone Acetate) Pharmacia & Upjohn ... 2615
FML Ophthalmic Ointment (Fluorometholone) Allergan ... ⊙225
FML Ophthalmic Suspension (Fluorometholone) Allergan ... ⊙224
FML Forte Ophthalmic Suspension (Fluorometholone) Allergan ... ⊙223
FML-S Liquifilm Sterile Ophthalmic Suspension (Fluorometholone, Sulfacetamide Sodium) Allergan ... ⊙226
Hydrocortone Tablets (Hydrocortisone) Merck ... 1963
Lotemax Ophthalmic Suspension 0.5% (Loteprednol Etabonate) Bausch & Lomb ... ⊙249
Pediapred Oral Solution (Prednisolone Sodium Phosphate) UCB ... 3319
Poly-Pred Liquifilm Ophthalmic Suspension (Neomycin Sulfate, Polymyxin B Sulfate, Prednisolone Acetate) Allergan ... ⊙231
Pred Forte Ophthalmic Suspension (Prednisolone Acetate) Allergan ... ⊙233
Pred-G Ophthalmic Suspension (Gentamicin Sulfate, Prednisolone Acetate) Allergan ... ⊙234
Pred-G Sterile Ophthalmic Ointment (Gentamicin Sulfate, Prednisolone Acetate) Allergan ... ⊙235
TobraDex Ophthalmic Ointment (Dexamethasone, Tobramycin) Alcon ... 558
TobraDex Ophthalmic Suspension (Dexamethasone, Tobramycin) Alcon ... 558
Zylet Ophthalmic Suspension (Loteprednol Etabonate, Tobramycin) Bausch & Lomb ... 3508

Influenza A virus, acute illness, treatment of
Relenza Rotadisk (Zanamivir) GlaxoSmithKline ... 1525
Tamiflu Capsules (Oseltamivir Phosphate) Roche Laboratories ... 2810
Tamiflu Oral Suspension (Oseltamivir Phosphate) Roche Laboratories ... 2810

Influenza A virus, respiratory tract illness, chemoprophylaxis of
Flumadine (Rimantadine Hydrochloride) Forest ... 1186
Symmetrel (Amantadine Hydrochloride) Endo Labs ... 1115
Tamiflu Capsules (Oseltamivir Phosphate) Roche Laboratories ... 2810
Tamiflu Oral Suspension (Oseltamivir Phosphate) Roche Laboratories ... 2810

Influenza A virus, respiratory tract illness, treatment of
Flumadine (Rimantadine Hydrochloride) Forest ... 1186
Symmetrel (Amantadine Hydrochloride) Endo Labs ... 1115

Influenza syndrome, symptomatic relief of
Advil Cold & Sinus (Ibuprofen, Pseudoephedrine Hydrochloride) Wyeth ... ■739
Advil Flu & Body Ache Caplets (Ibuprofen, Pseudoephedrine Hydrochloride) Wyeth ... ■739
Children's Advil Cold Suspension (Ibuprofen, Pseudoephedrine Hydrochloride) Wyeth ... ■741
Benadryl Allergy & Cold Tablets (Acetaminophen, Diphenhydramine Hydrochloride, Pseudoephedrine Hydrochloride) Pfizer Consumer Healthcare ... ■692

(■ Described in PDR For Nonprescription Drugs)   (⊙ Described in PDR For Ophthalmic Medicines™)

Benadryl Allergy (Diphenhydramine Hydrochloride) Pfizer Consumer Healthcare ▣ 691
Children's Benadryl Dye-Free Allergy Liquid (Diphenhydramine Hydrochloride) Pfizer Consumer Healthcare ▣ 695
Benadryl Maximum Strength Severe Allergy & Sinus Headache Caplets (Acetaminophen, Diphenhydramine Hydrochloride, Pseudoephedrine Hydrochloride) Pfizer Consumer Healthcare ▣ 694
Contac Severe Cold and Flu Caplets Maximum Strength (Acetaminophen, Chlorpheniramine Maleate, Dextromethorphan Hydrobromide, Pseudoephedrine Hydrochloride) GlaxoSmithKline ▣ 615
Contac Severe Cold and Flu Caplets Non-Drowsy (Acetaminophen, Dextromethorphan Hydrobromide, Pseudoephedrine Hydrochloride) GlaxoSmithKline ▣ 615
Children's Motrin Cold Non-Staining Dye-Free Oral Suspension (Ibuprofen, Pseudoephedrine Hydrochloride) McNeil Consumer 1838
Children's Motrin Cold Oral Suspension (Ibuprofen, Pseudoephedrine Hydrochloride) McNeil Consumer ▣ 648
Children's Motrin Cold Non-Staining Dye-Free Oral Suspension (Ibuprofen, Pseudoephedrine Hydrochloride) McNeil Consumer ▣ 648
Children's Motrin Cold Oral Suspension (Ibuprofen, Pseudoephedrine Hydrochloride) McNeil Consumer 1838
Motrin Cold & Sinus Caplets (Ibuprofen, Pseudoephedrine Hydrochloride) McNeil Consumer 1836
PediaCare NightRest Cough & Cold Liquid (Chlorpheniramine Maleate, Dextromethorphan Hydrobromide, Pseudoephedrine Hydrochloride) Pfizer Consumer Healthcare ▣ 704
Robitussin Cough, Cold & Flu Liquid-filled Capsules (Acetaminophen, Dextromethorphan Hydrobromide, Guaifenesin, Pseudoephedrine Hydrochloride) Wyeth ▣ 750
Robitussin Flu Liquid (Acetaminophen, Chlorpheniramine Maleate, Dextromethorphan Hydrobromide, Pseudoephedrine Hydrochloride) Wyeth ▣ 752
Robitussin PM Cough & Cold Liquid (Chlorpheniramine Maleate, Dextromethorphan Hydrobromide, Pseudoephedrine Hydrochloride) Wyeth ▣ 752
Sudafed Severe Cold (Acetaminophen, Dextromethorphan Hydrobromide, Pseudoephedrine Hydrochloride) Pfizer Consumer Healthcare ▣ 710
TheraFlu Cold & Cough Hot Liquid (Acetaminophen, Chlorpheniramine Maleate, Dextromethorphan Hydrobromide, Pseudoephedrine Hydrochloride) Novartis Consumer ▣ 680
TheraFlu Flu & Sore Throat Hot Liquid (Acetaminophen, Chlorpheniramine Maleate, Pseudoephedrine Hydrochloride) Novartis Consumer ▣ 681
TheraFlu Severe Cold & Cough Hot Liquid (Acetaminophen, Chlorpheniramine Maleate, Dextromethorphan Hydrobromide, Pseudoephedrine Hydrochloride) Novartis Consumer ▣ 683
TheraFlu Severe Cold Caplets (Acetaminophen, Chlorpheniramine Maleate, Dextromethorphan Hydrobromide, Pseudoephedrine Hydrochloride) Novartis Consumer ▣ 679
TheraFlu Severe Cold Hot Liquid (Acetaminophen, Chlorpheniramine Maleate, Dextromethorphan Hydrobromide, Pseudoephedrine Hydrochloride) Novartis Consumer ▣ 682
Triaminic Cold & Cough Liquid (Chlorpheniramine Maleate, Dextromethorphan Hydrobromide, Pseudoephedrine Hydrochloride) Novartis Consumer ▣ 685
Triaminic Cough & Sore Throat Liquid (Acetaminophen, Dextromethorphan Hydrobromide, Pseudoephedrine Hydrochloride) Novartis Consumer ▣ 687
Triaminic Flu, Cough & Fever Liquid (Acetaminophen, Chlorpheniramine Maleate, Dextromethorphan Hydrobromide, Pseudoephedrine Hydrochloride) Novartis Consumer ▣ 685
Triaminic Night Time Cough & Cold Liquid (Chlorpheniramine Maleate, Dextromethorphan Hydrobromide, Pseudoephedrine Hydrochloride) Novartis Consumer ▣ 685
Triaminic Cough & Sore Throat Softchews (Acetaminophen, Dextromethorphan Hydrobromide, Pseudoephedrine Hydrochloride) Novartis Consumer ▣ 689
Tussionex Pennkinetic Extended-Release Suspension (Chlorpheniramine Polistirex, Hydrocodone Polistirex) UCB 3322
Children's Tylenol Suspension Liquid and Meltaways (Acetaminophen) McNeil Consumer 1850
Children's Tylenol Plus Cold & Allergy Suspension Liquid (Acetaminophen, Diphenhydramine Hydrochloride, Pseudoephedrine Hydrochloride) McNeil Consumer 1850
Tylenol Cold & Flu Severe Daytime Liquid with Cool Bust (Acetaminophen, Dextromethorphan Hydrobromide, Pseudoephedrine Hydrochloride) McNeil Consumer 1846
Tylenol Cold & Flu Severe NightTime Liquid with Cool Burst (Acetaminophen, Dextromethorphan Hydrobromide, Doxylamine Succinate, Pseudoephedrine Hydrochloride) McNeil Consumer 1846
Tylenol Allergy Complete Night Time Caplets (Acetaminophen, Diphenhydramine Hydrochloride, Pseudoephedrine Hydrochloride) McNeil Consumer 1844
Tylenol Flu NightTime Gelcaps (Acetaminophen, Diphenhydramine Hydrochloride, Pseudoephedrine Hydrochloride) McNeil Consumer 1846
Tylenol Flu Day Non-Drowsy Gelcaps (Acetaminophen, Dextromethorphan Hydrobromide, Pseudoephedrine Hydrochloride) McNeil Consumer 1846
Multi-Symptom Tylenol Cold Night Time Caplets (Acetaminophen, Chlorpheniramine Maleate, Dextromethorphan Hydrobromide, Pseudoephedrine Hydrochloride) McNeil Consumer 1845
Multi-Symptom Tylenol Cold Day Non-Drowsy Caplets and Gelcaps (Acetaminophen, Dextromethorphan Hydrobromide, Pseudoephedrine Hydrochloride) McNeil Consumer 1845
Vicks 44M Cough, Cold & Flu Relief (Acetaminophen, Chlorpheniramine Maleate, Dextromethorphan Hydrobromide, Pseudoephedrine Hydrochloride) Procter & Gamble 2676
Pediatric Vicks 44m Cough & Cold Relief (Chlorpheniramine Maleate, Dextromethorphan Hydrobromide, Pseudoephedrine Hydrochloride) Procter & Gamble 2673
Vicks DayQuil Multi-Symptom Cold/Flu Relief LiquiCaps (Acetaminophen, Dextromethorphan Hydrobromide, Pseudoephedrine Hydrochloride) Procter & Gamble 2675
Vicks DayQuil Multi-Symptom Cold/Flu Relief Liquid (Acetaminophen, Dextromethorphan Hydrobromide, Pseudoephedrine Hydrochloride) Procter & Gamble 2675
Children's Vicks NyQuil Cold/Cough Relief (Chlorpheniramine Maleate, Dextromethorphan Hydrobromide, Pseudoephedrine Hydrochloride) Procter & Gamble 2671
Vicks NyQuil Cough Liquid (Dextromethorphan Hydrobromide, Doxylamine Succinate) Procter & Gamble 2677
Vicks NyQuil LiquiCaps (Acetaminophen, Dextromethorphan Hydrobromide, Doxylamine Succinate, Pseudoephedrine Hydrochloride) Procter & Gamble 2677
Vicks NyQuil LiquiCaps/Liquid Multi-Symptom Cold/Flu Relief (Acetaminophen, Dextromethorphan Hydrobromide, Doxylamine Succinate, Pseudoephedrine Hydrochloride) Procter & Gamble ▣ 725
Vicks NyQuil Liquid (Acetaminophen, Dextromethorphan Hydrobromide, Doxylamine Succinate, Pseudoephedrine Hydrochloride) Procter & Gamble 2677

Insect bites, pain due to
(*see under* Pain, topical relief of)

Insomnia
(*see under* Sleep, induction of)

Intermittent claudication
(*see under* Claudication, intermittent)

Intertrigo
(*see under* Skin, inflammatory conditions)

Intraocular pressure, elevation
(*see under* Hypertension, ocular)

Intravascular device, maintenance of patency
Cathflo Activase (Alteplase) Genentech 1232

Intubation, endotracheal
Mivacron Injection (Mivacurium Chloride) Abbott 489
Nimbex Injection (Cisatracurium Besylate) Abbott 494
Zemuron Injection (Rocuronium Bromide) Organon USA 2363

Iridocyclitis
Decadron Phosphate Injection (Dexamethasone Sodium Phosphate) Merck 1931
Depo-Medrol Injectable Suspension (Methylprednisolone Acetate) Pharmacia & Upjohn 2615
Hydrocortone Tablets (Hydrocortisone) Merck 1963
Pediapred Oral Solution (Prednisolone Sodium Phosphate) UCB 3319

Iritis
Decadron Phosphate Injection (Dexamethasone Sodium Phosphate) Merck 1931
Depo-Medrol Injectable Suspension (Methylprednisolone Acetate) Pharmacia & Upjohn 2615
Hydrocortone Tablets (Hydrocortisone) Merck 1963
Pediapred Oral Solution (Prednisolone Sodium Phosphate) UCB 3319
Zylet Ophthalmic Suspension (Loteprednol Etabonate, Tobramycin) Bausch & Lomb 3508

Iron deficiency
Feosol Caplets (Iron Carbonyl) GlaxoSmithKline Consumer 1629
Feosol Tablets (Ferrous Sulfate) GlaxoSmithKline Consumer 1629
Infed Injection (Iron Dextran) Watson 3381
Slow Fe Iron Tablets (Ferrous Sulfate) Novartis Consumer ▣ 772

Iron intoxication, acute
Desferal (Deferoxamine Mesylate) Novartis 2190

Irritable bowel syndrome
(*see under* Bowel, irritable, syndrome)

Ischemic attacks, transient
Bayer Aspirin Tablets (Aspirin) Bayer Healthcare LLC 3515
Ecotrin Enteric Coated Aspirin Low, Regular and Maximum Strength Tablets (Aspirin) GlaxoSmithKline Consumer 1627
Pravachol Tablets (Pravastatin Sodium) Bristol-Myers Squibb 943
St. Joseph 81 mg Aspirin Chewable and Enteric Coated Tablets (Aspirin) McNeil Consumer 1841

Ischemic attacks, transient, reduce risk of
Bayer Aspirin Tablets (Aspirin) Bayer Healthcare LLC 3515

Isoimmunization, prevention of in Rho(D) negative individuals
HyperRho S/D Full Dose (Rh$_0$ (D) Immune Globulin (Human)) Talecris 3243
Rhophylac (Rh$_0$ (D) Immune Globulin (Human)) ZLB Behring 3504

Isoimmunization, prevention of in Rho(D) negative women
HyperRho S/D Mini-Dose (Rh$_0$ (D) Immune Globulin (Human)) Talecris 3241
MICRhoGAM Ultra-Filtered (Rh$_0$ (D) Immune Globulin (Human)) Ortho-Clinical 2429
RhoGAM Ultra-Filtered (Rh$_0$ (D) Immune Globulin (Human)) Ortho-Clinical 2429
Rhophylac (Rh$_0$ (D) Immune Globulin (Human)) ZLB Behring 3504

Itching, eye, reduction of
Advil Allergy Sinus Caplets (Chlorpheniramine Maleate, Ibuprofen, Pseudoephedrine Hydrochloride) Wyeth ▣ 737
Advil Multi-Symptom Cold Caplets (Chlorpheniramine Maleate, Ibuprofen, Pseudoephedrine Hydrochloride) Wyeth ▣ 738
Children's Dimetapp ND Non-Drowsy Allergy Syrup (Loratadine) Wyeth ▣ 746
Optivar Ophthalmic Solution (Azelastine Hydrochloride) MedPointe 1877
TheraFlu Thin Strips Multi Symptom (Diphenhydramine Hydrochloride) Novartis Consumer ▣ 684
Triaminic Thin Strips Cough & Runny Nose (Diphenhydramine Hydrochloride) Novartis Consumer ▣ 690
Tylenol Severe Allergy Caplets (Acetaminophen, Diphenhydramine Hydrochloride) McNeil Consumer 1844

Itching, skin
(*see under* Pruritus, topical relief of)

Itching, sunburn
(*see under* Pruritus, topical relief of)

J

Jock itch
(*see under* Tinea cruris infections)

Joint pain
(*see under* Pain, arthritic, minor)

K

K. pneumoniae bacteremia
Rocephin (Ceftriaxone Sodium) Roche Laboratories 2801

K. pneumoniae gynecologic infections
Primaxin I.M. (Cilastatin Sodium, Imipenem) Merck 2022
Timentin ADD-Vantage (Clavulanate Potassium, Ticarcillin Disodium) GlaxoSmithKline 1556
Timentin Injection Galaxy Container (Clavulanate Potassium, Ticarcillin Disodium) GlaxoSmithKline 1559

Timentin IV Infusion (Clavulanate Potassium, Ticarcillin Disodium) GlaxoSmithKline 1553
Timentin Pharmacy Bulk Package (Clavulanate Potassium, Ticarcillin Disodium) GlaxoSmithKline 1562

K. pneumoniae infections
Augmentin XR Extended-Release Tablets (Amoxicillin, Clavulanate Potassium) GlaxoSmithKline 1340
Avelox (Moxifloxacin Hydrochloride) Schering 2984
Ceftin Tablets (Cefuroxime Axetil) GlaxoSmithKline 1369
Cipro I.V. (Ciprofloxacin) Schering 2998
Cipro I.V. Pharmacy Bulk Package (Ciprofloxacin) Bayer 3509
Cipro (Ciprofloxacin) Schering 2991
Factive Tablets (Gemifloxacin Mesylate) Oscient 2464
Invanz for Injection (Ertapenem) Merck 1974
Levaquin in 5% Dextrose Injection (Levofloxacin) Ortho-McNeil 2453
Levaquin (Levofloxacin) Ortho-McNeil 2453
Merrem I.V. (Meropenem) AstraZeneca 687
Noroxin Tablets (Norfloxacin) Merck 2009
Primaxin I.M. (Cilastatin Sodium, Imipenem) Merck 2022
Rocephin Injectable Vials, ADD-Vantage, Galaxy, Bulk (Ceftriaxone Sodium) Roche Laboratories 2801
Suprax (Cefixime) Lupin 1811
Tequin Injection (Gatifloxacin) Bristol-Myers Squibb 964
Tequin Tablets (Gatifloxacin) Bristol-Myers Squibb 964
Timentin ADD-Vantage (Clavulanate Potassium, Ticarcillin Disodium) GlaxoSmithKline 1556
Timentin Injection Galaxy Container (Clavulanate Potassium, Ticarcillin Disodium) GlaxoSmithKline 1559
Timentin IV Infusion (Clavulanate Potassium, Ticarcillin Disodium) GlaxoSmithKline 1553
Timentin Pharmacy Bulk Package (Clavulanate Potassium, Ticarcillin Disodium) GlaxoSmithKline 1562
Tygacil for Injection (Tigecycline) Wyeth 3489
Vantin Tablets and Oral Suspension (Cefpodoxime Proxetil) Pharmacia & Upjohn 2650
Zosyn (Piperacillin Sodium, Tazobactam Sodium) Wyeth 3492

K. pneumoniae infections, ocular
Genoptic Sterile Ophthalmic Solution (Gentamicin Sulfate) Allergan .... ⊙ 227
Pred-G Sterile Ophthalmic Ointment (Gentamicin Sulfate, Prednisolone Acetate) Allergan .... ⊙ 235

K. pneumoniae intra-abdominal infections
Cipro I.V. (Ciprofloxacin) Schering 2998
Cipro I.V. Pharmacy Bulk Package (Ciprofloxacin) Bayer 3509
Cipro (Ciprofloxacin) Schering 2991
Maxipime for Injection (Cefepime Hydrochloride) Elan 1093
Merrem I.V. (Meropenem) AstraZeneca 687
Primaxin I.M. (Cilastatin Sodium, Imipenem) Merck 2022
Rocephin Injectable Vials, ADD-Vantage, Galaxy, Bulk (Ceftriaxone Sodium) Roche Laboratories 2801
Timentin ADD-Vantage (Clavulanate Potassium, Ticarcillin Disodium) GlaxoSmithKline 1556
Timentin Injection Galaxy Container (Clavulanate Potassium, Ticarcillin Disodium) GlaxoSmithKline 1559
Timentin IV Infusion (Clavulanate Potassium, Ticarcillin Disodium) GlaxoSmithKline 1553
Timentin Pharmacy Bulk Package (Clavulanate Potassium, Ticarcillin Disodium) GlaxoSmithKline 1562

K. pneumoniae lower respiratory tract infections
Augmentin XR Extended-Release Tablets (Amoxicillin, Clavulanate Potassium) GlaxoSmithKline 1340
Cipro I.V. (Ciprofloxacin) Schering 2998
Cipro I.V. Pharmacy Bulk Package (Ciprofloxacin) Bayer 3509
Cipro (Ciprofloxacin) Schering 2991
Invanz for Injection (Ertapenem) Merck 1974
Levaquin in 5% Dextrose Injection (Levofloxacin) Ortho-McNeil 2453
Levaquin (Levofloxacin) Ortho-McNeil 2453
Maxipime for Injection (Cefepime Hydrochloride) Elan 1093
Rocephin Injectable Vials, ADD-Vantage, Galaxy, Bulk (Ceftriaxone Sodium) Roche Laboratories 2801

K. pneumoniae respiratory tract infections
Avelox (Moxifloxacin Hydrochloride) Schering 2984

K. pneumoniae septicemia
Rocephin Injectable Vials, ADD-Vantage, Galaxy, Bulk (Ceftriaxone Sodium) Roche Laboratories 2801

K. pneumoniae skin and skin structure infections
Cipro I.V. (Ciprofloxacin) Schering 2998
Cipro I.V. Pharmacy Bulk Package (Ciprofloxacin) Bayer 3509
Cipro (Ciprofloxacin) Schering 2991
Primaxin I.M. (Cilastatin Sodium, Imipenem) Merck 2022
Rocephin Injectable Vials, ADD-Vantage, Galaxy, Bulk (Ceftriaxone Sodium) Roche Laboratories 2801

K. pneumoniae urinary tract infections
Ceftin Tablets (Cefuroxime Axetil) GlaxoSmithKline 1369
Cipro I.V. (Ciprofloxacin) Schering 2998
Cipro I.V. Pharmacy Bulk Package (Ciprofloxacin) Bayer 3509
Cipro (Ciprofloxacin) Schering 2991
Cipro XR Tablets (Ciprofloxacin) Schering 3004
Levaquin in 5% Dextrose Injection (Levofloxacin) Ortho-McNeil 2453
Levaquin (Levofloxacin) Ortho-McNeil 2453
Maxipime for Injection (Cefepime Hydrochloride) Elan 1093
Noroxin Tablets (Norfloxacin) Merck 2009
Rocephin Injectable Vials, ADD-Vantage, Galaxy, Bulk (Ceftriaxone Sodium) Roche Laboratories 2801
Tequin Injection (Gatifloxacin) Bristol-Myers Squibb 964
Tequin Tablets (Gatifloxacin) Bristol-Myers Squibb 964
Vantin Tablets and Oral Suspension (Cefpodoxime Proxetil) Pharmacia & Upjohn 2650

Kaposi's sarcoma, AIDS-related
Doxil Injection (Doxorubicin Hydrochloride Liposome) Tibotec 3302
Intron A for Injection (Interferon alfa-2b, Recombinant) Schering 3038

Kawasaki syndrome
Gammagard S/D (Immune Globulin Intravenous (Human)) Baxter Healthcare 754
Iveegam EN (Immune Globulin Intravenous (Human)) Baxter Healthcare 759

Keloids
Decadron Phosphate Injection (Dexamethasone Sodium Phosphate) Merck 1931
Depo-Medrol Single-Dose Vial (Methylprednisolone Acetate) Pharmacia & Upjohn 2617

Keratitis
Decadron Phosphate Injection (Dexamethasone Sodium Phosphate) Merck 1931
Depo-Medrol Injectable Suspension (Methylprednisolone Acetate) Pharmacia & Upjohn 2615
Genoptic Sterile Ophthalmic Solution (Gentamicin Sulfate) Allergan .... ⊙ 227
Hydrocortone Tablets (Hydrocortisone) Merck 1963
Pediapred Oral Solution (Prednisolone Sodium Phosphate) UCB 3319

Keratitis, exposure
Lacrisert Sterile Ophthalmic Insert (Hydroxypropyl Cellulose) Merck 1979

Keratitis, fungal
Natacyn (Natamycin) Alcon .... ⊙ 207

Keratitis, herpes zoster
Zylet (Loteprednol Etabonate, Tobramycin) Bausch & Lomb 3508

Keratitis, vernal
Crolom Cromolyn Sodium Sterile Ophthalmic Solution USP 4% (Cromolyn Sodium) Bausch & Lomb .... ⊙ 248

Keratitis sicca
(*see under* Keratoconjunctivitis sicca)

Keratoconjunctivitis, unspecified
Genoptic Sterile Ophthalmic Solution (Gentamicin Sulfate) Allergan .... ⊙ 227
Refresh Endura Lubricant Eye Drops (Glycerin, Polysorbate 80) Allergan .... ⊙ 238
Refresh Liquigel (Carboxymethylcellulose Sodium) Allergan .... ⊙ 238

Keratoconjunctivitis, vernal
Crolom Cromolyn Sodium Sterile Ophthalmic Solution USP 4% (Cromolyn Sodium) Bausch & Lomb .... ⊙ 248

Keratoconjunctivitis sicca
Lacrisert Sterile Ophthalmic Insert (Hydroxypropyl Cellulose) Merck 1979
Refresh Celluvisc Lubricant Eye Drops (Carboxymethylcellulose Sodium) Allergan .... ⊙ 238
Refresh P.M. Lubricant Eye Ointment (Mineral Oil, Petrolatum, White) Allergan .... ⊙ 239
Refresh Plus Lubricant Eye Drops (Carboxymethylcellulose Sodium) Allergan .... ⊙ 238
Refresh Tears Lubricant Eye Drops (Carboxymethylcellulose Sodium) Allergan .... ⊙ 239
Restasis Ophthalmic Emulsion (Cyclosporine) Allergan 570
Systane Lubricant Eye Drops (Polyethylene Glycol, Propylene Glycol) Alcon 558
Visine Pure Tears Eye Drops Single Drop Dispenser (Hypromellose, Glycerin, Polyethylene Glycol) Pfizer Consumer .... ⊙ 280
Viva Eye Drops (Polysorbate 80) Vision Pharmaceuticals .... ⊙ 282

Keratosis, actinic
Aldara Cream, 5% (Imiquimod) 3M 1814
Carac Cream, 0.5% (Fluorouracil) Dermik 1048
Efudex (Fluorouracil) Valeant 3348

Keratosis, solar
Carac Cream, 0.5% (Fluorouracil) Dermik 1048
Efudex (Fluorouracil) Valeant 3348

Keratosis palmaris
(*see under* Hyperkeratosis skin disorders)

Keratosis pilaris
(*see under* Hyperkeratosis skin disorders)

Keratosis plantaris
(*see under* Hyperkeratosis skin disorders)

Klebsiella oxytoca infections
Rocephin Injectable Vials, ADD-Vantage, Galaxy, Bulk (Ceftriaxone Sodium) Roche Laboratories 2801
Tygacil (Tigecycline) Wyeth 3489

Klebsiella oxytoca skin and structure infections
Rocephin Injectable Vials, ADD-Vantage, Galaxy, Bulk (Ceftriaxone Sodium) Roche Laboratories 2801

Klebsiella pneumonia intra-abdominal infections
Tygacil for Injection (Tigecycline) Wyeth 3489

Klebsiella pneumoniae infections
(*see under* K. pneumoniae infections)

Klebsiella species bone and joint infections
Fortaz (Ceftazidime Sodium) GlaxoSmithKline 1422

Klebsiella species gynecologic infections
Primaxin I.V. (Cilastatin Sodium, Imipenem) Merck 2024

Klebsiella species infections
Augmentin (Amoxicillin, Clavulanate Potassium) GlaxoSmithKline 1331
Augmentin Tablets (Amoxicillin, Clavulanate Potassium) GlaxoSmithKline 1334
Dynacin Tablets (Minocycline Hydrochloride) Medicis 1859
Fortaz (Ceftazidime Sodium) GlaxoSmithKline 1422
Garamycin Injectable (Gentamicin Sulfate) Schering 3028
Mefoxin for Injection (Cefoxitin Sodium) Merck 1987
Mefoxin Premixed Intravenous Solution (Cefoxitin Sodium) Merck 1990
Primaxin I.V. (Cilastatin Sodium, Imipenem) Merck 2024
Timentin ADD-Vantage (Clavulanate Potassium, Ticarcillin Disodium) GlaxoSmithKline 1556
Timentin Injection Galaxy Container (Clavulanate Potassium, Ticarcillin Disodium) GlaxoSmithKline 1559
Timentin IV Infusion (Clavulanate Potassium, Ticarcillin Disodium) GlaxoSmithKline 1553
Timentin Pharmacy Bulk Package (Clavulanate Potassium, Ticarcillin Disodium) GlaxoSmithKline 1562
Zinacef Injection (Cefuroxime) GlaxoSmithKline 1604
Zinacef for Injection (Cefuroxime) GlaxoSmithKline 1604

Klebsiella species intra-abdominal infections
Fortaz (Ceftazidime Sodium) GlaxoSmithKline 1422
Mefoxin for Injection (Cefoxitin Sodium) Merck 1987
Mefoxin Premixed Intravenous Solution (Cefoxitin Sodium) Merck 1990
Primaxin I.V. (Cilastatin Sodium, Imipenem) Merck 2024
Tygacil for Injection (Tigecycline) Wyeth 3489

Klebsiella species lower respiratory tract infections
Fortaz (Ceftazidime Sodium) GlaxoSmithKline 1422
Mefoxin for Injection (Cefoxitin Sodium) Merck 1987
Mefoxin Premixed Intravenous Solution (Cefoxitin Sodium) Merck 1990
Primaxin I.V. (Cilastatin Sodium, Imipenem) Merck 2024
Timentin ADD-Vantage (Clavulanate Potassium, Ticarcillin Disodium) GlaxoSmithKline 1556
Timentin Injection Galaxy Container (Clavulanate Potassium, Ticarcillin Disodium) GlaxoSmithKline 1559

Timentin IV Infusion (Clavulanate Potassium, Ticarcillin Disodium) GlaxoSmithKline ... 1553
Timentin Pharmacy Bulk Package (Clavulanate Potassium, Ticarcillin Disodium) GlaxoSmithKline ... 1562
Zinacef Injection (Cefuroxime) GlaxoSmithKline ... 1604
Zinacef for Injection (Cefuroxime) GlaxoSmithKline ... 1604

Klebsiella species respiratory tract infections
Dynacin Tablets (Minocycline Hydrochloride) Medicis ... 1859

Klebsiella species septicemia
Fortaz (Ceftazidime Sodium) GlaxoSmithKline ... 1422
Mefoxin for Injection (Cefoxitin Sodium) Merck ... 1987
Mefoxin Premixed Intravenous Solution (Cefoxitin Sodium) Merck ... 1990
Primaxin I.V. (Cilastatin Sodium, Imipenem) Merck ... 2024
Timentin ADD-Vantage (Clavulanate Potassium, Ticarcillin Disodium) GlaxoSmithKline ... 1556
Timentin Injection Galaxy Container (Clavulanate Potassium, Ticarcillin Disodium) GlaxoSmithKline ... 1559
Timentin IV Infusion (Clavulanate Potassium, Ticarcillin Disodium) GlaxoSmithKline ... 1553
Timentin Pharmacy Bulk Package (Clavulanate Potassium, Ticarcillin Disodium) GlaxoSmithKline ... 1562
Zinacef Injection (Cefuroxime) GlaxoSmithKline ... 1604
Zinacef for Injection (Cefuroxime) GlaxoSmithKline ... 1604

Klebsiella species skin and skin structure infections
Augmentin (Amoxicillin, Clavulanate Potassium) GlaxoSmithKline ... 1331
Augmentin Tablets (Amoxicillin, Clavulanate Potassium) GlaxoSmithKline ... 1334
Fortaz (Ceftazidime Sodium) GlaxoSmithKline ... 1422
Mefoxin for Injection (Cefoxitin Sodium) Merck ... 1987
Mefoxin Premixed Intravenous Solution (Cefoxitin Sodium) Merck ... 1990
Primaxin I.V. (Cilastatin Sodium, Imipenem) Merck ... 2024
Timentin ADD-Vantage (Clavulanate Potassium, Ticarcillin Disodium) GlaxoSmithKline ... 1556
Timentin Injection Galaxy Container (Clavulanate Potassium, Ticarcillin Disodium) GlaxoSmithKline ... 1559
Timentin IV Infusion (Clavulanate Potassium, Ticarcillin Disodium) GlaxoSmithKline ... 1553
Timentin Pharmacy Bulk Package (Clavulanate Potassium, Ticarcillin Disodium) GlaxoSmithKline ... 1562
Zinacef Injection (Cefuroxime) GlaxoSmithKline ... 1604
Zinacef for Injection (Cefuroxime) GlaxoSmithKline ... 1604

Klebsiella species urinary tract infections
Augmentin (Amoxicillin, Clavulanate Potassium) GlaxoSmithKline ... 1331
Augmentin Tablets (Amoxicillin, Clavulanate Potassium) GlaxoSmithKline ... 1334
Dynacin Tablets (Minocycline Hydrochloride) Medicis ... 1859
Fortaz (Ceftazidime Sodium) GlaxoSmithKline ... 1422
Mefoxin for Injection (Cefoxitin Sodium) Merck ... 1987
Mefoxin Premixed Intravenous Solution (Cefoxitin Sodium) Merck ... 1990
Primaxin I.V. (Cilastatin Sodium, Imipenem) Merck ... 2024
Timentin ADD-Vantage (Clavulanate Potassium, Ticarcillin Disodium) GlaxoSmithKline ... 1556
Timentin Injection Galaxy Container (Clavulanate Potassium, Ticarcillin Disodium) GlaxoSmithKline ... 1559
Timentin IV Infusion (Clavulanate Potassium, Ticarcillin Disodium) GlaxoSmithKline ... 1553
Timentin Pharmacy Bulk Package (Clavulanate Potassium, Ticarcillin Disodium) GlaxoSmithKline ... 1562
Zinacef Injection (Cefuroxime) GlaxoSmithKline ... 1604
Zinacef for Injection (Cefuroxime) GlaxoSmithKline ... 1604

Klebsiella-Enterobacter species infections, ocular
Blephamide Ophthalmic Ointment (Prednisolone Acetate, Sulfacetamide Sodium) Allergan ... 563
Blephamide Ophthalmic Suspension (Prednisolone Acetate, Sulfacetamide Sodium) Allergan ... 564
FML-S Liquifilm Sterile Ophthalmic Suspension (Fluorometholone, Sulfacetamide Sodium) Allergan ... ⊙226
Poly-Pred Liquifilm Ophthalmic Suspension (Neomycin Sulfate, Polymyxin B Sulfate, Prednisolone Acetate) Allergan ... ⊙231
Pred-G Ophthalmic Suspension (Gentamicin Sulfate, Prednisolone Acetate) Allergan ... ⊙234
TobraDex Ophthalmic Ointment (Dexamethasone, Tobramycin) Alcon ... 558
TobraDex Ophthalmic Suspension (Dexamethasone, Tobramycin) Alcon ... 558
Zylet Ophthalmic Suspension (Loteprednol Etabonate, Tobramycin) Bausch & Lomb ... 3508

Koch-Weeks bacillus infections, ocular
(*see under* H. aegypticus infections, ocular)

L

Lacerations
Aquacel AG with Hydrofiber (Silver impregnated antimicrobial dressing) ConvaTec ... 1035

Lacrimation, symptomatic relief of
Advil Allergy Sinus Caplets (Chlorpheniramine Maleate, Ibuprofen, Pseudoephedrine Hydrochloride) Wyeth ... ▣737
Advil Multi-Symptom Cold Caplets (Chlorpheniramine Maleate, Ibuprofen, Pseudoephedrine Hydrochloride) Wyeth ... ▣738
Alavert Allergy & Sinus D-12 Hour Tablets (Loratadine, Pseudoephedrine Sulfate) Wyeth ... ▣743
Alavert (Loratadine) Wyeth ... ▣743
Allegra-D 12 Hour Extended-Release Tablets (Fexofenadine Hydrochloride, Pseudoephedrine Hydrochloride) Sanofi-Aventis ... 2860
Benadryl Allergy & Cold Tablets (Acetaminophen, Diphenhydramine Hydrochloride, Pseudoephedrine Hydrochloride) Pfizer Consumer Healthcare ... ▣692
Benadryl Allergy (Diphenhydramine Hydrochloride) Pfizer Consumer Healthcare ... ▣691
Children's Benadryl Allergy Liquid (Diphenhydramine Hydrochloride) Pfizer Consumer Healthcare ... ▣695
Children's Benadryl D Allergy & Sinus Fastmelt Tablets (Diphenhydramine Citrate, Pseudoephedrine Hydrochloride) Pfizer Consumer Healthcare ... ▣694
Children's Benadryl D Liquid Medication (Diphenhydramine Hydrochloride, Pseudoephedrine Hydrochloride) Pfizer Consumer Healthcare ... ▣693
Benadryl D Tablets (Diphenhydramine Hydrochloride, Pseudoephedrine Hydrochloride) Pfizer Consumer Healthcare ... ▣694
Children's Benadryl Allergy Fastmelt Tablets (Diphenhydramine Citrate) Pfizer Consumer Healthcare ... ▣696
Children's Claritin 24 Hour Non-Drowsy Allergy Syrup (Loratadine) Schering-Plough ... ▣732
Claritin Non-Drowsy 24 Hour Tablets (Loratadine) Schering-Plough ... ▣731
Claritin Reditabs 24 Hour Non-Drowsy Tablets (Loratadine) Schering-Plough ... ▣732
Claritin-D Non-Drowsy 12 Hour Tablets (Loratadine, Pseudoephedrine Sulfate) Schering-Plough ... ▣731
Claritin-D Non-Drowsy 24 Hour Tablets (Loratadine, Pseudoephedrine Sulfate) Schering-Plough ... ▣731
Children's Dimetapp Cold & Allergy Elixir (Brompheniramine Maleate, Pseudoephedrine Hydrochloride) Wyeth ... ▣745
Children's Dimetapp ND Non-Drowsy Allergy Syrup (Loratadine) Wyeth ... ▣746
Hyland's Seasonal Allergy Tablets (Homeopathic Formulations) Standard Homeopathic ... ▣735
TheraFlu Cold & Cough Hot Liquid (Acetaminophen, Chlorpheniramine Maleate, Dextromethorphan Hydrobromide, Pseudoephedrine Hydrochloride) Novartis Consumer ... ▣680
TheraFlu Cold & Sore Throat Hot Liquid (Acetaminophen, Chlorpheniramine Maleate, Pseudoephedrine Hydrochloride) Novartis Consumer ... ▣680
TheraFlu Flu & Sore Throat Hot Liquid (Acetaminophen, Chlorpheniramine Maleate, Pseudoephedrine Hydrochloride) Novartis Consumer ... ▣681
TheraFlu Severe Cold & Cough Hot Liquid (Acetaminophen, Chlorpheniramine Maleate, Dextromethorphan Hydrobromide, Pseudoephedrine Hydrochloride) Novartis Consumer ... ▣683
TheraFlu Severe Cold Caplets (Acetaminophen, Chlorpheniramine Maleate, Dextromethorphan Hydrobromide, Pseudoephedrine Hydrochloride) Novartis Consumer ... ▣679
TheraFlu Severe Cold Hot Liquid (Acetaminophen, Chlorpheniramine Maleate, Dextromethorphan Hydrobromide, Pseudoephedrine Hydrochloride) Novartis Consumer ... ▣682
TheraFlu Thin Strips Multi Symptom (Diphenhydramine Hydrochloride) Novartis Consumer ... ▣684
Triaminic Allerchews (Loratadine) Novartis Consumer ... ▣684
Triaminic Thin Strips Cough & Runny Nose (Diphenhydramine Hydrochloride) Novartis Consumer ... ▣690
Children's Tylenol Plus Cold & Allergy Suspension Liquid (Acetaminophen, Diphenhydramine Hydrochloride, Pseudoephedrine Hydrochloride) McNeil Consumer ... 1850
Tylenol Severe Allergy Caplets (Acetaminophen, Diphenhydramine Hydrochloride) McNeil Consumer ... 1844
Tylenol Sinus Night Time Caplets (Acetaminophen, Doxylamine Succinate, Pseudoephedrine Hydrochloride) McNeil Consumer ... 1848
Zicam Allergy Relief Nasal Pump (Histanium Hydrochloricum, Luffa operculata, Galphimia Glauca, Sulfur) Matrixx ...

Lactobacillus acidophilus, deficiency of
DDS-Acidophilus Capsules, Tablets, and Powder (Lactobacillus Acidophilus) UAS Labs ... ▣736

Lactose intolerance
Lactaid Original Strength Caplets (Lactase (beta-d-Galactosidase)) McNeil Consumer ... 1836
Lactaid Fast Act Caplets and Chewable Tablets (Lactase (beta-d-Galactosidase)) McNeil Consumer ... 1836

Larva migrans, cutaneous
Mintezol (Thiabendazole) Merck ... 2002

Laryngeal edema, acute noninfectious, adjunctive therapy in
Decadron Phosphate Injection (Dexamethasone Sodium Phosphate) Merck ... 1931
Depo-Medrol Injectable Suspension (Methylprednisolone Acetate) Pharmacia & Upjohn ... 2615
Depo-Medrol Single-Dose Vial (Methylprednisolone Acetate) Pharmacia & Upjohn ... 2617

LDL cholesterol, elevation
(*see under* Hyperlipoproteinemia, types IIa and IIb, adjunct to diet)

Lead encephalopathy
Calcium Disodium Versenate (Calcium Disodium Edetate) 3M ... 1819

Lead poisoning
Chemet Capsules (Succimer) Ovation ... 2480

Leg muscle cramps
Hyland's Leg Cramps Ointment (Homeopathic Formulations) Standard Homeopathic ... ▣735
Hyland's Leg Cramps with Quinine Tablets and Caplets (Homeopathic Formulations) Standard Homeopathic ... ▣735

Legionella pneumophila infections
(*see under* Legionnaires' disease)

Legionnaires' disease
E.E.S. (Erythromycin Ethylsuccinate) Abbott ... 449
EryPed (Erythromycin Ethylsuccinate) Abbott ... 445
Ery-Tab Tablets (Erythromycin) Abbott ... 447
Erythrocin Stearate Filmtab Tablets (Erythromycin Stearate) Abbott ... 452
Erythromycin Base Filmtab Tablets (Erythromycin) Abbott ... 454
Erythromycin Delayed-Release Capsules, USP (Erythromycin) Abbott ... 456
Levaquin in 5% Dextrose Injection (Levofloxacin) Ortho-McNeil ... 2453
Levaquin (Levofloxacin) Ortho-McNeil ... 2453
PCE Dispertab Tablets (Erythromycin) Abbott ... 510
Tequin Injection (Gatifloxacin) Bristol-Myers Squibb ... 964
Tequin Tablets (Gatifloxacin) Bristol-Myers Squibb ... 964
Zithromax for IV Infusion (Azithromycin Dihydrate) Pfizer ... 2573

Lennox-Gastaut syndrome
Klonopin (Clonazepam) Roche Laboratories ... 2782
Lamictal (Lamotrigine) GlaxoSmithKline ... 1449
Topamax Sprinkle Capsules (Topiramate) Ortho-McNeil Neurologics ... 2438
Topamax Tablets (Topiramate) Ortho-McNeil Neurologics ... 2438

Lens, intraocular, implantation of, surgical aid in
Ocucoat (Hydroxypropyl Methylcellulose) Bausch & Lomb ... ⊙290

Leprosy
Dapsone Tablets USP (Dapsone) Jacobus ... 1656

Leukemia, acute, nonlymphocytic, adjunctive therapy
Novantrone for Injection Concentrate (Mitoxantrone Hydrochloride) Serono ... 3158

Leukemia, acute, palliative management of in childhood
Decadron Phosphate Injection (Dexamethasone Sodium Phosphate) Merck ... 1931
Depo-Medrol Single-Dose Vial (Methylprednisolone Acetate) Pharmacia & Upjohn ... 2617
Hydrocortone Tablets (Hydrocortisone) Merck ... 1963
Pediapred Oral Solution (Prednisolone Sodium Phosphate) UCB ... 3319

Leukemia, acute, promyelocytic
Trisenox Injection (Arsenic Trioxide) Cell Therapeutics ... 983
Vesanoid Capsules (Tretinoin) Roche Laboratories ... 2823

Leukemia, acute erythroid
Cerubidine for Injection (Daunorubicin Hydrochloride) Bedford ... 788

Leukemia, acute lymphoblastic
Adriamycin for Injection, USP (Doxorubicin Hydrochloride) Bedford ... 786
Adriamycin Injection, USP (Doxorubicin Hydrochloride) Bedford ... 786
Clolar for Intravenous Infusion (Clofarabine) Genzyme ... 1264
Oncaspar (Pegaspargase) Enzon ... 1123
Purinethol Tablets (Mercaptopurine) Gate ... 1222

Leukemia, acute lymphocytic
Cerubidine for Injection (Daunorubicin Hydrochloride) Bedford ... 788
Elspar for Injection (Asparaginase) Merck ... 1943
Purinethol Tablets (Mercaptopurine) Gate ... 1222

Leukemia, acute monocytic
Cerubidine for Injection (Daunorubicin Hydrochloride) Bedford ... 788

Leukemia, acute myeloblastic
Adriamycin for Injection, USP (Doxorubicin Hydrochloride) Bedford ... 786
Adriamycin Injection, USP (Doxorubicin Hydrochloride) Bedford ... 786

Leukemia, acute myelogenous
Cerubidine for Injection (Daunorubicin Hydrochloride) Bedford ... 788
Idamycin PFS Injection (Idarubicin Hydrochloride) Pharmacia & Upjohn ... 2645
Leukine (Sargramostim) Berlex ... 829

Leukemia, acute myeloid, adjunctive therapy in
Neupogen for Injection (Filgrastim) Amgen ... 598

Leukemia, acute myeloid, CD33 positive
Mylotarg for Injection (Gemtuzumab Ozogamicin) Wyeth ... 3429

Leukemia, acute nonlymphocytic
Cerubidine for Injection (Daunorubicin Hydrochloride) Bedford ... 788
Tabloid Tablets (Thioguanine) GlaxoSmithKline ... 1545

Leukemia, adjunctive therapy in
Aloprim for Injection (Allopurinol Sodium) Nabi ... 2156
Elitek (Rasburicase) Sanofi-Aventis ... 2906

Leukemia, chronic lymphocytic
Leukeran Tablets (Chlorambucil) GlaxoSmithKline ... 1472
Mustargen for Injection (Mechlorethamine Hydrochloride) Merck ... 2007

Leukemia, chronic lymphocytic, B-cell
Campath Ampules (Alemtuzumab) Berlex ... 826

Leukemia, chronic lymphocytic, B-cell, prevention of bacterial infection in
Gammagard S/D (Immune Globulin Intravenous (Human)) Baxter Healthcare ... 754

Leukemia, chronic myeloid
Gleevec Tablets (Imatinib Mesylate) Novartis ... 2221
I.V. Busulfex (Busulfan) ESP Pharma ... 1125
Mustargen for Injection (Mechlorethamine Hydrochloride) Merck ... 2007
Myleran Tablets (Busulfan) GlaxoSmithKline ... 1492
Roferon-A Injection (Interferon alfa-2a, Recombinant) Roche Laboratories ... 2805

Leukemia, hairy cell
Intron A for Injection (Interferon alfa-2b, Recombinant) Schering ... 3038
Leustatin Injection (Cladribine) Ortho Biotech ... 2368
Roferon-A Injection (Interferon alfa-2a, Recombinant) Roche Laboratories ... 2805

Leukemia, hairy cell, alpha-interferon-refractory
Nipent for Injection (Pentostatin) SuperGen ... 3216

Leukemia, lymphoblastic, adjunctive therapy in
Leukine (Sargramostim) Berlex ... 829

Leukemias, palliative management of
Decadron Phosphate Injection (Dexamethasone Sodium Phosphate) Merck ... 1931
Decadron Tablets (Dexamethasone) Merck ... 1929
Depo-Medrol Injectable Suspension (Methylprednisolone Acetate) Pharmacia & Upjohn ... 2615
Depo-Medrol Single-Dose Vial (Methylprednisolone Acetate) Pharmacia & Upjohn ... 2617
Hydrocortone Tablets (Hydrocortisone) Merck ... 1963
Pediapred Oral Solution (Prednisolone Sodium Phosphate) UCB ... 3319

Lice, body
(*see under* Pediculosis, human)

Lice, head
(*see under* Pediculosis, human)

Lice, pubic
(*see under* Pediculosis, human)

Lichen planus
Decadron Phosphate Injection (Dexamethasone Sodium Phosphate) Merck ... 1931
Depo-Medrol Single-Dose Vial (Methylprednisolone Acetate) Pharmacia & Upjohn ... 2617

Lichen simplex chronicus
Decadron Phosphate Injection (Dexamethasone Sodium Phosphate) Merck ... 1931
Depo-Medrol Single-Dose Vial (Methylprednisolone Acetate) Pharmacia & Upjohn ... 2617

Listeria monocytogenes infections
E.E.S. (Erythromycin Ethylsuccinate) Abbott ... 449
EryPed (Erythromycin Ethylsuccinate) Abbott ... 445
Ery-Tab Tablets (Erythromycin) Abbott ... 447
Erythrocin Stearate Filmtab Tablets (Erythromycin Stearate) Abbott ... 452
Erythromycin Base Filmtab Tablets (Erythromycin) Abbott ... 454
Erythromycin Delayed-Release Capsules, USP (Erythromycin) Abbott ... 456
PCE Dispertab Tablets (Erythromycin) Abbott ... 510

Listeriosis
Dynacin Tablets (Minocycline Hydrochloride) Medicis ... 1859
E.E.S. (Erythromycin Ethylsuccinate) Abbott ... 449
EryPed (Erythromycin Ethylsuccinate) Abbott ... 445
Erythromycin Delayed-Release Capsules, USP (Erythromycin) Abbott ... 456
PCE Dispertab Tablets (Erythromycin) Abbott ... 510

Liver, allogeneic transplants, prophylaxis of organ rejection in
CellCept Capsules (Mycophenolate Mofetil) Roche Laboratories ... 2751
CellCept Intravenous (Mycophenolate Mofetil Hydrochloride) Roche Laboratories ... 2751
CellCept Oral Suspension (Mycophenolate Mofetil) Roche Laboratories ... 2751
CellCept Tablets (Mycophenolate Mofetil) Roche Laboratories ... 2751
Gengraf Capsules (Cyclosporine) Abbott ... 458
Neoral Soft Gelatin Capsules (Cyclosporine) Novartis ... 2247
Neoral Oral Solution (Cyclosporine) Novartis ... 2247
Orthoclone OKT3 Sterile Solution (Muromonab-CD3) Ortho Biotech ... 2370
Prograf Capsules and Injection (Tacrolimus) Astellas ... 624
Sandimmune (Cyclosporine) Novartis ... 2259

Liver abscess, amebic
(*see under* Amebic liver abscess)

Liver failure, acute
Plasbumin-5 (Albumin (human)) Talecris ... 3249
Plasbumin-20 (Albumin (human)) Talecris ... 3249
Plasbumin-25 (Albumin (human)) Talecris ... 3251

Liver transplantation, donor organ perfusion and flushing of
Custodiol HTK Solution (Electrolyte Solution) Odyssey ... 2344

Locoregional solid malignancies
Cosmegen for Injection (Dactinomycin) Merck ... 1907

Loeffler's syndrome
Decadron Phosphate Injection (Dexamethasone Sodium Phosphate) Merck ... 1931
Depo-Medrol Injectable Suspension (Methylprednisolone Acetate) Pharmacia & Upjohn ... 2615
Depo-Medrol Single-Dose Vial (Methylprednisolone Acetate) Pharmacia & Upjohn ... 2617
Hydrocortone Tablets (Hydrocortisone) Merck ... 1963
Pediapred Oral Solution (Prednisolone Sodium Phosphate) UCB ... 3319

Lou Gehrig's disease
(*see under* Amyotrophic lateral sclerosis)

Lung abscess
(*see under* Abscess, lung)

Lupus erythematosus, systemic
Bayer Aspirin Tablets (Aspirin) Bayer Healthcare LLC ... 3515
Decadron Phosphate Injection (Dexamethasone Sodium Phosphate) Merck ... 1931
Decadron Tablets (Dexamethasone) Merck ... 1929
Depo-Medrol Injectable Suspension (Methylprednisolone Acetate) Pharmacia & Upjohn ... 2615
Depo-Medrol Single-Dose Vial (Methylprednisolone Acetate) Pharmacia & Upjohn ... 2617
Ecotrin Enteric Coated Aspirin Low, Regular and Maximum Strength Tablets (Aspirin) GlaxoSmithKline Consumer ... 1627
Hydrocortone Tablets (Hydrocortisone) Merck ... 1963
Pediapred Oral Solution (Prednisolone Sodium Phosphate) UCB ... 3319
St. Joseph 81 mg Aspirin Chewable and Enteric Coated Tablets (Aspirin) McNeil Consumer ... 1841

Lupus erythematosus discoides
Decadron Phosphate Injection (Dexamethasone Sodium Phosphate) Merck ... 1931
Depo-Medrol Single-Dose Vial (Methylprednisolone Acetate) Pharmacia & Upjohn ... 2617

Lyme disease
(*see under* Borrelia burgdorferi infection)

Lymphogranuloma venereum
Dynacin Tablets (Minocycline Hydrochloride) Medicis ... 1859

Lymphoma, cutaneous T-cell
Ontak Vials (Denileukin Diftitox) Ligand ... 1717
Targretin Capsules (Bexarotene) Ligand ... 1719

Lymphoma, non-Hodgkin's, B-cell
Zevalin Injection (Ibritumomab Tiuxetan) Biogen Idec ... 848

Lymphoma, non-Hodgkin's, follicular
Bexxar (Iodine I 131 Tositumomab, Tositumomab) GlaxoSmithKline ... 1360
Intron A for Injection (Interferon alfa-2b, Recombinant) Schering ... 3038
Zevalin Injection (Ibritumomab Tiuxetan) Biogen Idec ... 848

Lymphoma, unspecified, adjunctive therapy in
Aloprim for Injection (Allopurinol Sodium) Nabi ... 2156
Elitek (Rasburicase) Sanofi-Aventis ... 2906

Lymphomas, giant follicular
Leukeran Tablets (Chlorambucil) GlaxoSmithKline ... 1472

Lymphomas, Hodgkin's
(*see under* Hodgkin's disease)

Lymphomas, malignant
Adriamycin for Injection, USP (Doxorubicin Hydrochloride) Bedford ... 786
Adriamycin Injection, USP (Doxorubicin Hydrochloride) Bedford ... 786
Leukeran Tablets (Chlorambucil) GlaxoSmithKline ... 1472

Lymphomas, non-Hodgkin's
Bexxar (Iodine I 131 Tositumomab, Tositumomab) GlaxoSmithKline ... 1360
Leukeran Tablets (Chlorambucil) GlaxoSmithKline ... 1472
Rituxan for Infusion (Rituximab) Biogen Idec ... 845
Rituxan I.V. (Rituximab) Genentech ... 1251

Lymphomas, non-Hodgkin's, adjunctive therapy in
Leukine (Sargramostim) Berlex ... 829

Lymphomas, non-Hodgkin's, refractory
Bexxar (Iodine I 131 Tositumomab, Tositumomab) GlaxoSmithKline ... 1360

Lymphomas, palliative management of
Decadron Tablets (Dexamethasone) Merck ... 1929

Lymphomas, palliative management of in adults
Decadron Phosphate Injection (Dexamethasone Sodium Phosphate) Merck ... 1931
Depo-Medrol Injectable Suspension (Methylprednisolone Acetate) Pharmacia & Upjohn ... 2615
Depo-Medrol Single-Dose Vial (Methylprednisolone Acetate) Pharmacia & Upjohn ... 2617
Hydrocortone Tablets (Hydrocortisone) Merck ... 1963

Pediapred Oral Solution (Prednisolone Sodium Phosphate) UCB........ **3319**

Lymphomatous meningitis
DepoCyt Injection (Cytarabine Liposome) Enzon **1121**

Lymphosarcoma
(*see under* Lymphomas, non-Hodgkin's)

M

M. catarrhalis, otitis media
Augmentin (Amoxicillin, Clavulanate Potassium) GlaxoSmithKline **1331**
Augmentin Tablets (Amoxicillin, Clavulanate Potassium) GlaxoSmithKline **1334**
Augmentin ES-600 Powder for Oral Suspension (Amoxicillin, Clavulanate Potassium) GlaxoSmithKline **1337**
Biaxin/Biaxin XL (Clarithromycin) Abbott **402**
Ceftin (Cefuroxime Axetil) GlaxoSmithKline **1369**
Floxin Otic Singles (Ofloxacin) Daiichi **1045**
Floxin Otic Solution (Ofloxacin) Daiichi **1043**
Omnicef Capsules (Cefdinir) Abbott .. **506**
Omnicef for Oral Suspension (Cefdinir) Abbott **506**
Rocephin Injectable Vials, ADD-Vantage, Galaxy, Bulk (Ceftriaxone Sodium) Roche Laboratories **2801**
Suprax (Cefixime) Lupin **1811**
Vantin Tablets and Oral Suspension (Cefpodoxime Proxetil) Pharmacia & Upjohn **2650**
Zithromax Capsules, 250 mg (Azithromycin Dihydrate) Pfizer **2568**
Zithromax for Oral Suspension, 300 mg, 600 mg, 900 mg, 1200 mg (Azithromycin Dihydrate) Pfizer **2561**
Zithromax Tablets, 250 mg, 500 mg (Azithromycin Dihydrate) Pfizer **2561**
Zithromax Tri-Pak (Azithromycin Dihydrate) Pfizer **2561**

M. catarrhalis bronchitis
Factive Tablets (Gemifloxacin Mesylate) Oscient **2464**
Ketek Tablets (Telithromycin) Sanofi-Aventis **2920**

M. catarrhalis infections
Augmentin (Amoxicillin, Clavulanate Potassium) GlaxoSmithKline **1331**
Augmentin Tablets (Amoxicillin, Clavulanate Potassium) GlaxoSmithKline **1334**
Augmentin XR Extended-Release Tablets (Amoxicillin, Clavulanate Potassium) GlaxoSmithKline **1340**
Avelox (Moxifloxacin Hydrochloride) Schering **2984**
Biaxin/Biaxin XL (Clarithromycin) Abbott **402**
Ceftin (Cefuroxime Axetil) GlaxoSmithKline **1369**
Cipro (Ciprofloxacin) Schering **2991**
Factive Tablets (Gemifloxacin Mesylate) Oscient **2464**
Invanz for Injection (Ertapenem) Merck **1974**
Levaquin in 5% Dextrose Injection (Levofloxacin) Ortho-McNeil **2453**
Levaquin (Levofloxacin) Ortho-McNeil **2453**
Omnicef Capsules (Cefdinir) Abbott .. **506**
Omnicef for Oral Suspension (Cefdinir) Abbott **506**
Spectracef Tablets (Cefditoren Pivoxil) Purdue Pharmaceutical **2706**
Suprax (Cefixime) Lupin **1811**
Tequin Injection (Gatifloxacin) Bristol-Myers Squibb **964**
Tequin Tablets (Gatifloxacin) Bristol-Myers Squibb **964**
Vantin Tablets and Oral Suspension (Cefpodoxime Proxetil) Pharmacia & Upjohn **2650**
Zithromax Capsules, 250 mg (Azithromycin Dihydrate) Pfizer **2568**
Zithromax for IV Infusion (Azithromycin Dihydrate) Pfizer **2573**
Zithromax for Oral Suspension, 1 g (Azithromycin Dihydrate) Pfizer **2568**
Zithromax for Oral Suspension, 300 mg, 600 mg, 900 mg, 1200 mg (Azithromycin Dihydrate) Pfizer **2561**
Zithromax Tablets, 250 mg, 500 mg (Azithromycin Dihydrate) Pfizer....................................... **2561**
Zithromax Tablets, 600 mg (Azithromycin Dihydrate) Pfizer...... **2568**
Zithromax Tri-Pak (Azithromycin Dihydrate) Pfizer **2561**
Zithromax Z-Pak (Azithromycin Dihydrate) Pfizer **2568**
Zmax for Oral Suspension (Azithromycin) Pfizer................................ **2577**

M. catarrhalis lower respiratory tract infections
Augmentin (Amoxicillin, Clavulanate Potassium) GlaxoSmithKline **1331**
Augmentin Tablets (Amoxicillin, Clavulanate Potassium) GlaxoSmithKline **1334**
Augmentin XR Extended-Release Tablets (Amoxicillin, Clavulanate Potassium) GlaxoSmithKline **1340**
Avelox (Moxifloxacin Hydrochloride) Schering **2984**
Biaxin/Biaxin XL (Clarithromycin) Abbott **402**
Cipro (Ciprofloxacin) Schering **2991**
Invanz for Injection (Ertapenem) Merck **1974**
Levaquin in 5% Dextrose Injection (Levofloxacin) Ortho-McNeil **2453**
Levaquin (Levofloxacin) Ortho-McNeil **2453**
Omnicef Capsules (Cefdinir) Abbott .. **506**
Omnicef for Oral Suspension (Cefdinir) Abbott **506**
Spectracef Tablets (Cefditoren Pivoxil) Purdue Pharmaceutical **2706**
Tequin Injection (Gatifloxacin) Bristol-Myers Squibb **964**
Tequin Tablets (Gatifloxacin) Bristol-Myers Squibb **964**
Vantin Tablets and Oral Suspension (Cefpodoxime Proxetil) Pharmacia & Upjohn **2650**
Zithromax Capsules, 250 mg (Azithromycin Dihydrate) Pfizer **2568**
Zithromax for IV Infusion (Azithromycin Dihydrate) Pfizer **2573**
Zithromax for Oral Suspension, 1 g (Azithromycin Dihydrate) Pfizer **2568**
Zithromax for Oral Suspension, 300 mg, 600 mg, 900 mg, 1200 mg (Azithromycin Dihydrate) Pfizer **2561**
Zithromax Tablets, 250 mg, 500 mg (Azithromycin Dihydrate) Pfizer **2561**
Zithromax Tablets, 600 mg (Azithromycin Dihydrate) Pfizer **2568**
Zithromax Tri-Pak (Azithromycin Dihydrate) Pfizer **2561**
Zithromax Z-Pak (Azithromycin Dihydrate) Pfizer **2568**

M. catarrhalis pneumonia
Avelox (Moxifloxacin Hydrochloride) Schering **2984**
Factive Tablets (Gemifloxacin Mesylate) Oscient **2464**
Invanz for Injection (Ertapenem) Merck **1974**
Ketek Tablets (Telithromycin) Sanofi-Aventis **2920**
Omnicef Capsules (Cefdinir) Abbott .. **506**
Omnicef for Oral Suspension (Cefdinir) Abbott **506**
Spectracef Tablets (Cefditoren Pivoxil) Purdue Pharmaceutical **2706**
Tequin Injection (Gatifloxacin) Bristol-Myers Squibb **964**
Tequin Tablets (Gatifloxacin) Bristol-Myers Squibb **964**

M. catarrhalis sinusitis
Augmentin (Amoxicillin, Clavulanate Potassium) GlaxoSmithKline **1331**
Augmentin Tablets (Amoxicillin, Clavulanate Potassium) GlaxoSmithKline **1334**
Augmentin XR Extended-Release Tablets (Amoxicillin, Clavulanate Potassium) GlaxoSmithKline **1340**
Avelox (Moxifloxacin Hydrochloride) Schering **2984**
Biaxin/Biaxin XL (Clarithromycin) Abbott **402**
Cipro I.V. (Ciprofloxacin) Schering **2998**
Cipro I.V. Pharmacy Bulk Package (Ciprofloxacin) Bayer **3509**
Cipro (Ciprofloxacin) Schering **2991**
Ketek Tablets (Telithromycin) Sanofi-Aventis **2920**
Levaquin in 5% Dextrose Injection (Levofloxacin) Ortho-McNeil **2453**
Levaquin (Levofloxacin) Ortho-McNeil **2453**
Vantin Tablets and Oral Suspension (Cefpodoxime Proxetil) Pharmacia & Upjohn **2650**
Zithromax for Oral Suspension, 300 mg, 600 mg, 900 mg, 1200 mg (Azithromycin Dihydrate) Pfizer **2561**
Zithromax Tablets, 250 mg, 500 mg (Azithromycin Dihydrate) Pfizer.. **2561**
Zithromax Tri-Pak (Azithromycin Dihydrate) Pfizer **2561**
Zmax for Oral Suspension (Azithromycin) Pfizer **2577**

Magnesium deficiency
(*see under* Hypomagnesemia)

Malaria
(*see under* P. falciparum infections; P. malariae infections; P. ovale infections; P. vivax infections)

Malaria, prophylaxis of
Daraprim Tablets (Pyrimethamine) GlaxoSmithKline **1385**
Lariam Tablets (Mefloquine Hydrochloride) Roche Laboratories **2790**
Malarone Tablets (Atovaquone, Proguanil Hydrochloride) GlaxoSmithKline **1484**
Malarone Pediatric Tablets (Atovaquone, Proguanil Hydrochloride) GlaxoSmithKline **1484**

Malassezia furfur
(*see under* Pityrosporon orbiculare infections)

Mania, bipolar
Depakote Tablets (Divalproex Sodium) Abbott **427**
Geodon (Ziprasidone Hydrochloride) Pfizer **2514**
Zyprexa Tablets (Olanzapine) Lilly **1798**
Zyprexa IntraMuscular (Olanzapine) Lilly **1798**
Zyprexa ZYDIS Orally Disintegrating Tablets (Olanzapine) Lilly **1798**

Manic episodes associated with bipolar disorder
Depakote Tablets (Divalproex Sodium) Abbott **427**
Eskalith CR Controlled-Release Tablets (Lithium Carbonate) GlaxoSmithKline **1406**
Seroquel Tablets (Quetiapine Fumarate) AstraZeneca **691**

Mastocytosis, systemic
Prilosec OTC Tablets (Omeprazole magnesium) Procter & Gamble **2674**
Tagamet Tablets (Cimetidine) GlaxoSmithKline **1547**
Zantac (Ranitidine Hydrochloride) GlaxoSmithKline **1597**

Measles, prevention or modification of
GamaSTAN (Globulin, Immune (Human)) Talecris **3231**

Measles, prophylaxis
Attenuvax (Measles Virus Vaccine Live) Merck **1889**
M-M-R II (Measles, Mumps & Rubella Virus Vaccine, Live) Merck **1980**

Mediastinitis, adjunctive therapy
Plasbumin-20 (Albumin (human)) Talecris **3249**

Meibomianitis, acute
Genoptic Sterile Ophthalmic Solution (Gentamicin Sulfate) Allergan ....⊙**227**

Melanin hyperpigmentation
(*see under* Hyperpigmentation, skin, bleaching of)

Melanoma
Intron A for Injection (Interferon alfa-2b, Recombinant) Schering..... **3038**
Proleukin for Injection (Aldesleukin) Chiron **1007**

Melasma
(*see under* Hyperpigmentation, skin, bleaching of)

Meningitis
Fortaz (Ceftazidime Sodium) GlaxoSmithKline **1422**
Garamycin Injectable (Gentamicin Sulfate) Schering **3028**
Merrem I.V. (Meropenem) AstraZeneca **687**
Rocephin Injectable Vials, ADD-Vantage, Galaxy, Bulk (Ceftriaxone Sodium) Roche Laboratories **2801**
Zinacef for Injection (Cefuroxime) GlaxoSmithKline **1604**
Zinacef for Injection (Cefuroxime) GlaxoSmithKline **1604**

Meningitis, tuberculous
Decadron Phosphate Injection (Dexamethasone Sodium Phosphate) Merck **1931**
Decadron Tablets (Dexamethasone) Merck **1929**
Depo-Medrol Injectable Suspension (Methylprednisolone Acetate) Pharmacia & Upjohn **2615**
Depo-Medrol Single-Dose Vial (Methylprednisolone Acetate) Pharmacia & Upjohn **2617**
Hydrocortone Tablets (Hydrocortisone) Merck **1963**
Pediapred Oral Solution (Prednisolone Sodium Phosphate) UCB **3319**

Menopause, vasomotor symptoms of
Activella Tablets (Estradiol, Norethindrone Acetate) Novo Nordisk **2311**
Cenestin Tablets, 0.45mg, 0.625mg, 0.9mg, 1.25mg (Estrogens, Conjugated, Synthetic A) Duramed **1063**
Climara Transdermal System (Estradiol) Berlex **795**
Climara Pro Transdermal System (Estradiol, Levonorgestrel) Berlex .. **800**
CombiPatch Transdermal System (Estradiol, Norethindrone Acetate) Novartis **2180**
Estratest Tablets (Estrogens, Esterified, Methyltestosterone) Solvay ...**3196**
Estratest H.S. Tablets (Estrogens, Esterified, Methyltestosterone) Solvay **3196**
Estrogel 0.06% (Estradiol) Solvay **3200**
Prefest Tablets (Estradiol, Norgestimate) Duramed **1069**
Premarin Tablets (Estrogens, Conjugated) Wyeth **3443**
Premphase Tablets (Estrogens, Conjugated, Medroxyprogesterone Acetate) Wyeth **3452**
Prempro Tablets (Estrogens, Conjugated, Medroxyprogesterone Acetate) Wyeth **3452**
Vivelle Transdermal System (Estradiol) Novartis **2288**
Vivelle-Dot Transdermal System (Estradiol) Novartis **2293**

Menstrual cramps
(*see under* Pain, menstrual)

Micrococcus luteus
Vigamox Ophthalmic Solution (Moxifloxacin Hydrochloride) Alcon **560**

Microsporum audouinii infections
Grifulvin V Tablets Microsize and Oral Suspension Microsize (Griseofulvin) OrthoNeutrogena **2384**
Gris-PEG Tablets (Griseofulvin) Pedinol **2504**
Spectazole Cream (Econazole Nitrate) OrthoNeutrogena **2390**

Microsporum canis infections
Grifulvin V Tablets Microsize and Oral Suspension Microsize (Griseofulvin) OrthoNeutrogena 2384
Gris-PEG Tablets (Griseofulvin) Pedinol 2504
Loprox Gel (Ciclopirox) Medicis 1861
Lotrimin (Clotrimazole) Schering 3053
Spectazole Cream (Econazole Nitrate) OrthoNeutrogena 2390

Microsporum gypseum infections
Grifulvin V Tablets Microsize and Oral Suspension Microsize (Griseofulvin) OrthoNeutrogena 2384
Gris-PEG Tablets (Griseofulvin) Pedinol 2504
Spectazole Cream (Econazole Nitrate) OrthoNeutrogena 2390

Migraine headache
(*see under* Headache, migraine)

Mima-Herellea species infections
(*see under* Acinetobacter species infections)

Miosis, intraoperative, inhibition of
Ocufen Ophthalmic Solution (Flurbiprofen Sodium) Allergan .... ⊙230

Miosis, production of
Rēv-Eyes Ophthalmic Eyedrops 0.5% (Dapiprazole Hydrochloride) Bausch & Lomb .... ⊙256

Moraxella catarrhalis
(*see under* M. catarrhalis infections)

Moraxella lacunata infections, ocular
TobraDex Ophthalmic Ointment (Dexamethasone, Tobramycin) Alcon 558
TobraDex Ophthalmic Suspension (Dexamethasone, Tobramycin) Alcon 558
Zylet Ophthalmic Suspension (Loteprednol Etabonate, Tobramycin) Bausch & Lomb 3508

Morganella morganii infections
Cipro I.V. (Ciprofloxacin) Schering 2998
Cipro I.V. Pharmacy Bulk Package (Ciprofloxacin) Bayer 3509
Cipro (Ciprofloxacin) Schering 2991
Fortaz (Ceftazidime Sodium) GlaxoSmithKline 1422
Mefoxin for Injection (Cefoxitin Sodium) Merck 1987
Mefoxin Premixed Intravenous Solution (Cefoxitin Sodium) Merck 1990
Primaxin I.V. (Cilastatin Sodium, Imipenem) Merck 2024
Rocephin Injectable Vials, ADD-Vantage, Galaxy, Bulk (Ceftriaxone Sodium) Roche Laboratories 2801

Morganella morganii infections, ocular
TobraDex Ophthalmic Ointment (Dexamethasone, Tobramycin) Alcon 558
TobraDex Ophthalmic Suspension (Dexamethasone, Tobramycin) Alcon 558
Zylet Ophthalmic Suspension (Loteprednol Etabonate, Tobramycin) Bausch & Lomb 3508

Morganella morganii skin and skin structure infections
Cipro I.V. (Ciprofloxacin) Schering 2998
Cipro I.V. Pharmacy Bulk Package (Ciprofloxacin) Bayer 3509
Cipro (Ciprofloxacin) Schering 2991
Primaxin I.V. (Cilastatin Sodium, Imipenem) Merck 2024
Rocephin Injectable Vials, ADD-Vantage, Galaxy, Bulk (Ceftriaxone Sodium) Roche Laboratories 2801

Morganella morganii urinary tract infections
Cipro I.V. (Ciprofloxacin) Schering 2998
Cipro I.V. Pharmacy Bulk Package (Ciprofloxacin) Bayer 3509
Cipro (Ciprofloxacin) Schering 2991
Mefoxin for Injection (Cefoxitin Sodium) Merck 1987
Mefoxin Premixed Intravenous Solution (Cefoxitin Sodium) Merck 1990
Primaxin I.V. (Cilastatin Sodium, Imipenem) Merck 2024
Rocephin Injectable Vials, ADD-Vantage, Galaxy, Bulk (Ceftriaxone Sodium) Roche Laboratories 2801

Morphea, possibly effective in
Potaba (Aminobenzoate Potassium) Glenwood 1634

Motion sickness
Phenergan (Promethazine Hydrochloride) Wyeth 3438
Transderm Scōp Transdermal Therapeutic System (Scopolamine) Novartis Consumer 2166

Mouth and throat disorders
Hurricaine Topical Anesthetic Aerosol Spray, 2 oz. Wild Cherry (Benzocaine) Beutlich 835
Hurricaine Topical Anesthetic Aerosol Spray Kit, 2 oz. Wild Cherry with 200 Disposable Extension Tubes (Benzocaine) Beutlich 835
Hurricaine Topical Anesthetic Gel: 1 oz. Wild Cherry, Pina Colada, Watermelon, Fresh Mint, 0.18 oz. Wild Cherry (Benzocaine) Beutlich 835
Hurricaine Topical Anesthetic Liquid: 1 oz. Wild Cherry and Pina Colada, Swab Applicator Wild Cherry (Benzocaine) Beutlich 835

Mucopolysaccharidosis
Aldurazyme for Intravenous Infusion (Laronidase) Genzyme 1261

Mucormycosis
(*see under* Zygomycosis)

Mucositis
Kepivance (Palifermin) Amgen 592

Multiple follicles, development of in an ART program
Bravelle for Intramuscular or Subcutaneous Injection (Urofollitropin) Ferring 1140
Menopur for Subcutaneous Injection (Menotropins) Ferring 1145

Multiple sclerosis, acute exacerbations
Copaxone for Injection (Glatiramer Acetate) Teva Neuroscience 3292
Decadron Tablets (Dexamethasone) Merck 1929
Depo-Medrol Injectable Suspension (Methylprednisolone Acetate) Pharmacia & Upjohn 2615
Depo-Medrol Single-Dose Vial (Methylprednisolone Acetate) Pharmacia & Upjohn 2617
Pediapred Oral Solution (Prednisolone Sodium Phosphate) UCB 3319

Multiple sclerosis, alleviation of signs and symptoms
Dantrium Capsules (Dantrolene Sodium) Procter & Gamble Pharmaceuticals 2690

Multiple sclerosis, chronic progressive
Novantrone for Injection Concentrate (Mitoxantrone Hydrochloride) Serono 3158

Multiple sclerosis, relapsing-remitting
Avonex (Interferon Beta-1a) Biogen Idec 839
Betaseron for SC Injection (Interferon Beta-1b) Berlex 791
Copaxone for Injection (Glatiramer Acetate) Teva Neuroscience 3292
Novantrone for Injection Concentrate (Mitoxantrone Hydrochloride) Serono 3158
Rebif Prefilled Syringe for Injection (Interferon Beta-1a) Serono 3163

Mumps, prophylaxis
M-M-R II (Measles, Mumps & Rubella Virus Vaccine, Live) Merck 1980
Mumpsvax (Mumps Virus Vaccine, Live) Merck 2005

Muscle spasm
(*see under* Spasticity, muscle, symptomatic alleviation of)

Muscles, skeletal, relaxation, preoperative
Mivacron Injection (Mivacurium Chloride) Abbott 489
Nimbex Injection (Cisatracurium Besylate) Abbott 494
Zemuron Injection (Rocuronium Bromide) Organon USA 2363

Musculo-skeletal discomfort, adjunct in
Flexeril Tablets (Cyclobenzaprine Hydrochloride) McNeil Consumer 1832
Norflex Injection (Orphenadrine Citrate) 3M 1824
Skelaxin Tablets (Metaxalone) King 1685

Myalgia
(*see under* Pain, muscular, temporary relief of)

Myalgia, topical relief of
(*see under* Pain, topical relief of)

Mycobacterium avium complex (MAC) disease, disseminated
Biaxin/Biaxin XL (Clarithromycin) Abbott 402

Mycobacterium avium complex (MAC) disease, disseminated, prophylaxis of
Zithromax (Azithromycin Dihydrate) Pfizer 2568
Zithromax Z-Pak (Azithromycin Dihydrate) Pfizer 2568

Mycobacterium intracellulare infections
Biaxin/Biaxin XL (Clarithromycin) Abbott 402

Mycobacterium leprae infections
(*see under* Leprosy)

Mycobacterium tuberculosis infection, pulmonary
Capastat Sulfate for Injection (Capreomycin Sulfate) Lilly 1728

Mycoplasma hominis pelvic inflammatory disease
Zithromax for IV Infusion (Azithromycin Dihydrate) Pfizer 2573

Mycoplasma pneumoniae infection
Avelox (Moxifloxacin Hydrochloride) Schering 2984
Biaxin/Biaxin XL (Clarithromycin) Abbott 402
Dynacin Tablets (Minocycline Hydrochloride) Medicis 1859
E.E.S. (Erythromycin Ethylsuccinate) Abbott 449
EryPed (Erythromycin Ethylsuccinate) Abbott 445
Ery-Tab Tablets (Erythromycin) Abbott 447
Erythrocin Stearate Filmtab Tablets (Erythromycin Stearate) Abbott 452
Erythromycin Base Filmtab Tablets (Erythromycin) Abbott 454
Erythromycin Delayed-Release Capsules, USP (Erythromycin) Abbott 456
Factive Tablets (Gemifloxacin Mesylate) Oscient 2464
Levaquin in 5% Dextrose Injection (Levofloxacin) Ortho-McNeil 2453
Levaquin (Levofloxacin) Ortho-McNeil 2453
PCE Dispertab Tablets (Erythromycin) Abbott 510
Tequin Injection (Gatifloxacin) Bristol-Myers Squibb 964
Tequin Tablets (Gatifloxacin) Bristol-Myers Squibb 964
Zithromax Capsules, 250 mg (Azithromycin Dihydrate) Pfizer 2568
Zithromax for IV Infusion (Azithromycin Dihydrate) Pfizer 2573
Zithromax for Oral Suspension, 300 mg, 600 mg, 900 mg, 1200 mg (Azithromycin Dihydrate) Pfizer 2561
Zithromax Tablets, 250 mg, 500 mg (Azithromycin Dihydrate) Pfizer 2561
Zithromax Tri-Pak (Azithromycin Dihydrate) Pfizer 2561

Mycoplasma pneumoniae respiratory tract infections
Biaxin/Biaxin XL (Clarithromycin) Abbott 402
E.E.S. (Erythromycin Ethylsuccinate) Abbott 449
EryPed (Erythromycin Ethylsuccinate) Abbott 445
Ery-Tab Tablets (Erythromycin) Abbott 447
Erythrocin Stearate Filmtab Tablets (Erythromycin Stearate) Abbott 452
Erythromycin Base Filmtab Tablets (Erythromycin) Abbott 454
Erythromycin Delayed-Release Capsules, USP (Erythromycin) Abbott 456
Ketek Tablets (Telithromycin) Sanofi-Aventis 2920
Levaquin in 5% Dextrose Injection (Levofloxacin) Ortho-McNeil 2453
Levaquin (Levofloxacin) Ortho-McNeil 2453
PCE Dispertab Tablets (Erythromycin) Abbott 510
Zithromax Capsules, 250 mg (Azithromycin Dihydrate) Pfizer 2568
Zithromax for IV Infusion (Azithromycin Dihydrate) Pfizer 2573
Zithromax for Oral Suspension, 300 mg, 600 mg, 900 mg, 1200 mg (Azithromycin Dihydrate) Pfizer 2561
Zithromax Tablets, 250 mg, 500 mg (Azithromycin Dihydrate) Pfizer 2561
Zithromax Tri-Pak (Azithromycin Dihydrate) Pfizer 2561

Mycosis fungoides
Decadron Phosphate Injection (Dexamethasone Sodium Phosphate) Merck 1931
Decadron Tablets (Dexamethasone) Merck 1929
Depo-Medrol Injectable Suspension (Methylprednisolone Acetate) Pharmacia & Upjohn 2615
Depo-Medrol Single-Dose Vial (Methylprednisolone Acetate) Pharmacia & Upjohn 2617
Hydrocortone Tablets (Hydrocortisone) Merck 1963
Mustargen for Injection (Mechlorethamine Hydrochloride) Merck 2007
Pediapred Oral Solution (Prednisolone Sodium Phosphate) UCB 3319

Myeloid recovery, acceleration of
Leukine (Sargramostim) Berlex 829

Myeloma, multiple
Alkeran Tablets (Melphalan) Celgene 977
Velcade for Injection (Bortezomib) Millennium 2102
Zometa for Intravenous Infusion (Zoledronic acid) Novartis 2306

Myeloma, multiple, adjunct in
Alkeran for Injection (Melphalan Hydrochloride) Celgene 976
Aredia for Injection (Pamidronate Disodium) Novartis 2168

Myocardial infarction, acute
Activase I.V. (Alteplase) Genentech 1225
Bayer Aspirin Tablets (Aspirin) Bayer Healthcare LLC 3515
Ecotrin Enteric Coated Aspirin Low, Regular and Maximum Strength Tablets (Aspirin) GlaxoSmithKline Consumer 1627
Integrilin Injection (Eptifibatide) Schering 3034

Plavix Tablets (Clopidogrel Bisulfate) Bristol-Myers Squibb 940
Plavix Tablets (Clopidogrel Bisulfate) Sanofi-Aventis 2942
Retavase (Reteplase) ESP Pharma ... 1131
St. Joseph 81 mg Aspirin Chewable and Enteric Coated Tablets (Aspirin) McNeil Consumer.. 1841
TNKase I.V. (Tenecteplase) Genentech 1256

Myocardial infarction, non-Q-wave

Aggrastat (Tirofiban Hydrochloride) Merck 1878
Fragmin Injection (Dalteparin Sodium) Pharmacia & Upjohn 2638
Integrilin Injection (Eptifibatide) Schering.. 3034
Lovenox Injection (Enoxaparin Sodium) Sanofi-Aventis 2931
ReoPro Vials (Abciximab) Lilly 1779

Myocardial infarction, post, left ventricular dysfunction

Captopril Tablets (Captopril) Mylan ...2114
Coreg Tablets (Carvedilol) GlaxoSmithKline 1376
Mavik Tablets (Trandolapril) Abbott ... 482

Myocardial infarction, prophylaxis, adjunct in

Altoprev Extended-Release Tablets (Lovastatin) First Horizon 1151
Mevacor Tablets (Lovastatin) Merck .1996

Myocardial infarction, to reduce the risk of

Altace Capsules (Ramipril) King 1673
Bayer Aspirin Tablets (Aspirin) Bayer Healthcare LLC 3515
Niaspan Extended-Release Tablets (Niacin) Kos 1703
Pravachol Tablets (Pravastatin Sodium) Bristol-Myers Squibb 943
Zocor Tablets (Simvastatin) Merck ...2078

Myocardial infarction, treatment adjunct

Altace Capsules (Ramipril) King 1673
Mavik Tablets (Trandolapril) Abbott ... 482
Prinivil Tablets (Lisinopril) Merck 2029
Zestril Tablets (Lisinopril) AstraZeneca 704

Myocardial perfusion imaging, thallium, adjunct in

Adenoscan (Adenosine) Astellas 613

Myocardial reinfarction, prophylaxis

Bayer Aspirin Tablets (Aspirin) Bayer Healthcare LLC 3515
Blocadren Tablets (Timolol Maleate) Merck 1891
Coumadin for Injection (Warfarin Sodium) Bristol-Myers Squibb 932
Coumadin Tablets (Warfarin Sodium) Bristol-Myers Squibb 932
Ecotrin Enteric Coated Aspirin Low, Regular and Maximum Strength Tablets (Aspirin) GlaxoSmithKline Consumer 1627
Plavix Tablets (Clopidogrel Bisulfate) Bristol-Myers Squibb 940
Plavix Tablets (Clopidogrel Bisulfate) Sanofi-Aventis 2942
St. Joseph 81 mg Aspirin Chewable and Enteric Coated Tablets (Aspirin) McNeil Consumer 1841
Tenormin I.V. Injection (Atenolol) AstraZeneca 698
Tenormin Tablets (Atenolol) AstraZeneca 695

Myocardial revascularization procedures, to reduce the risk of

Bayer Aspirin Tablets (Aspirin) Bayer Healthcare LLC 3515
Lescol Capsules (Fluvastatin Sodium) Novartis 2227
Lescol XL Tablets (Fluvastatin Sodium) Novartis 2227
Pravachol Tablets (Pravastatin Sodium) Bristol-Myers Squibb 943
St. Joseph 81 mg Aspirin Chewable and Enteric Coated Tablets (Aspirin) McNeil Consumer.................................... 1841
Zocor Tablets (Simvastatin) Merck.... 2078

Myxedema
(*see under* Hypothyroidism, replacement or supplemental therapy in)

Myxedema coma/precoma
(*see under* Hypothyroidism, replacement or supplemental therapy in)

N

N. gonorrhoeae endocervical infections

Ceftin Tablets (Cefuroxime Axetil) GlaxoSmithKline.......................... 1369
Cipro (Ciprofloxacin) Schering 2991
Noroxin Tablets (Norfloxacin) Merck . 2009
Rocephin Injectable Vials, ADD-Vantage, Galaxy, Bulk (Ceftriaxone Sodium) Roche Laboratories 2801
Vantin Tablets and Oral Suspension (Cefpodoxime Proxetil) Pharmacia & Upjohn 2650
Zithromax Capsules, 250 mg (Azithromycin Dihydrate) Pfizer 2568
Zithromax for Oral Suspension, 300 mg, 600 mg, 900 mg, 1200 mg (Azithromycin Dihydrate) Pfizer 2561
Zithromax Tablets, 250 mg, 500 mg (Azithromycin Dihydrate) Pfizer 2561
Zithromax Tri-Pak (Azithromycin Dihydrate) Pfizer 2561

N. gonorrhoeae gynecologic infections

Dynacin Tablets (Minocycline Hydrochloride) Medicis 1859
Erythrocin Stearate Filmtab Tablets (Erythromycin Stearate) Abbott 452
Erythromycin Base Filmtab Tablets (Erythromycin) Abbott 454
Erythromycin Delayed-Release Capsules, USP (Erythromycin) Abbott 456
Mefoxin for Injection (Cefoxitin Sodium) Merck 1987
Mefoxin Premixed Intravenous Solution (Cefoxitin Sodium) Merck 1990
Noroxin Tablets (Norfloxacin) Merck .2009
PCE Dispertab Tablets (Erythromycin) Abbott 510

N. gonorrhoeae infections

Amoxil Capsules (Amoxicillin) GlaxoSmithKline 1315
Amoxil Chewable Tablets (Amoxicillin) GlaxoSmithKline 1315
Amoxil Pediatric Drops for Oral Suspension (Amoxicillin) GlaxoSmithKline 1315
Amoxil Powder for Oral Suspension (Amoxicillin) GlaxoSmithKline 1315
Amoxil Tablets (Amoxicillin) GlaxoSmithKline 1315
Ceftin Tablets (Cefuroxime Axetil) GlaxoSmithKline 1369
Cipro (Ciprofloxacin) Schering 2991
E.E.S. (Erythromycin Ethylsuccinate) Abbott 449
EryPed (Erythromycin Ethylsuccinate) Abbott 445
Ery-Tab Tablets (Erythromycin) Abbott 447
Erythrocin Stearate Filmtab Tablets (Erythromycin Stearate) Abbott 452
Erythromycin Base Filmtab Tablets (Erythromycin) Abbott 454
Erythromycin Delayed-Release Capsules, USP (Erythromycin) Abbott 456
Fortaz (Ceftazidime Sodium) GlaxoSmithKline 1422
Mefoxin for Injection (Cefoxitin Sodium) Merck 1987
Mefoxin Premixed Intravenous Solution (Cefoxitin Sodium) Merck 1990
Noroxin Tablets (Norfloxacin) Merck .2009
PCE Dispertab Tablets (Erythromycin) Abbott................................. 510
Rocephin Injectable Vials, ADD-Vantage, Galaxy, Bulk (Ceftriaxone Sodium) Roche Laboratories 2801
Tequin Injection (Gatifloxacin) Bristol-Myers Squibb 964
Tequin Tablets (Gatifloxacin) Bristol-Myers Squibb 964
Vantin Tablets and Oral Suspension (Cefpodoxime Proxetil) Pharmacia & Upjohn 2650
Zinacef Injection (Cefuroxime) GlaxoSmithKline........................... 1604
Zinacef for Injection (Cefuroxime) GlaxoSmithKline........................... 1604
Zithromax Capsules, 250 mg (Azithromycin Dihydrate) Pfizer...... 2568
Zithromax for IV Infusion (Azithromycin Dihydrate) Pfizer 2573
Zithromax for Oral Suspension, 300 mg, 600 mg, 900 mg, 1200 mg (Azithromycin Dihydrate) Pfizer 2561
Zithromax Tablets, 250 mg, 500 mg (Azithromycin Dihydrate) Pfizer 2561
Zithromax Tri-Pak (Azithromycin Dihydrate) Pfizer 2561

N. gonorrhoeae infections, ocular

Genoptic Sterile Ophthalmic Solution (Gentamicin Sulfate) Allergan ....⊙227
Pred-G Ophthalmic Suspension (Gentamicin Sulfate, Prednisolone Acetate) Allergan ....⊙234
Pred-G Sterile Ophthalmic Ointment (Gentamicin Sulfate, Prednisolone Acetate) Allergan .....⊙235

N. gonorrhoeae pelvic inflammatory disease

E.E.S. (Erythromycin Ethylsuccinate) Abbott 449
EryPed (Erythromycin Ethylsuccinate) Abbott 445
Ery-Tab Tablets (Erythromycin) Abbott 447
Erythromycin Delayed-Release Capsules, USP (Erythromycin) Abbott 456
Mefoxin for Injection (Cefoxitin Sodium) Merck 1987
Mefoxin Premixed Intravenous Solution (Cefoxitin Sodium) Merck 1990
Rocephin Injectable Vials, ADD-Vantage, Galaxy, Bulk (Ceftriaxone Sodium) Roche Laboratories 2801
Zithromax for IV Infusion (Azithromycin Dihydrate) Pfizer 2573

N. gonorrhoeae pharyngeal infections

Rocephin Injectable Vials, ADD-Vantage, Galaxy, Bulk (Ceftriaxone Sodium) Roche Laboratories 2801

N. gonorrhoeae rectal infections

Ceftin Tablets (Cefuroxime Axetil) GlaxoSmithKline 1369
Rocephin Injectable Vials, ADD-Vantage, Galaxy, Bulk (Ceftriaxone Sodium) Roche Laboratories 2801
Vantin Tablets and Oral Suspension (Cefpodoxime Proxetil) Pharmacia & Upjohn 2650

N. gonorrhoeae urethral infections

Ceftin Tablets (Cefuroxime Axetil) GlaxoSmithKline 1369
Cipro (Ciprofloxacin) Schering 2991
Dynacin Tablets (Minocycline Hydrochloride) Medicis 1859
Noroxin Tablets (Norfloxacin) Merck .2009
Rocephin Injectable Vials, ADD-Vantage, Galaxy, Bulk (Ceftriaxone Sodium) Roche Laboratories 2801
Tequin Injection (Gatifloxacin) Bristol-Myers Squibb 964
Tequin Tablets (Gatifloxacin) Bristol-Myers Squibb 964
Vantin Tablets and Oral Suspension (Cefpodoxime Proxetil) Pharmacia & Upjohn 2650
Zithromax Capsules, 250 mg (Azithromycin Dihydrate) Pfizer...... 2568
Zithromax for Oral Suspension, 300 mg, 600 mg, 900 mg, 1200 mg (Azithromycin Dihydrate) Pfizer 2561
Zithromax Tablets, 250 mg, 500 mg (Azithromycin Dihydrate) Pfizer... 2561
Zithromax Tri-Pak (Azithromycin Dihydrate) Pfizer 2561

N. meningitidis, asymptomatic carriers of

Dynacin Tablets (Minocycline Hydrochloride) Medicis................. 1859

N. meningitidis infections

Dynacin Tablets (Minocycline Hydrochloride) Medicis................. 1859
Fortaz (Ceftazidime Sodium) GlaxoSmithKline.......................... 1422
Merrem I.V. (Meropenem) AstraZeneca 687
Rocephin Injectable Vials, ADD-Vantage, Galaxy, Bulk (Ceftriaxone Sodium) Roche Laboratories 2801
Zinacef Injection (Cefuroxime) GlaxoSmithKline.......................... 1604
Zinacef for Injection (Cefuroxime) GlaxoSmithKline.......................... 1604

N. meningitidis meningitis

Fortaz (Ceftazidime Sodium) GlaxoSmithKline.......................... 1422
Merrem I.V. (Meropenem) AstraZeneca 687
Rocephin Injectable Vials, ADD-Vantage, Galaxy, Bulk (Ceftriaxone Sodium) Roche Laboratories 2801
Zinacef Injection (Cefuroxime) GlaxoSmithKline.......................... 1604
Zinacef for Injection (Cefuroxime) GlaxoSmithKline.......................... 1604

Nail, dry brittle

Appearex Tablets (Biotin) Merz 2095

Narcolepsy

Adderall Tablets (Amphetamine Aspartate, Amphetamine Sulfate, Dextroamphetamine Saccharate, Dextroamphetamine Sulfate) Shire US.. 3168
Dexedrine (Dextroamphetamine Sulfate) GlaxoSmithKline 1386
DextroStat Tablets (Dextroamphetamine Sulfate) Shire US 3177
Provigil Tablets (Modafinil) Cephalon 1002
Ritalin (Methylphenidate Hydrochloride) Novartis.............................. 2254

Nasal congestion, symptomatic relief of

Advil Allergy Sinus Caplets (Chlorpheniramine Maleate, Ibuprofen, Pseudoephedrine Hydrochloride) Wyeth .... ▣737
Advil Cold & Sinus (Ibuprofen, Pseudoephedrine Hydrochloride) Wyeth .... ▣739
Advil Flu & Body Ache Caplets (Ibuprofen, Pseudoephedrine Hydrochloride) Wyeth .... ▣739
Children's Advil Cold Suspension (Ibuprofen, Pseudoephedrine Hydrochloride) Wyeth .... ▣741
Advil Multi-Symptom Cold Caplets (Chlorpheniramine Maleate, Ibuprofen, Pseudoephedrine Hydrochloride) Wyeth............................ ▣738
Alavert Allergy & Sinus D-12 Hour Tablets (Loratadine, Pseudoephedrine Sulfate) Wyeth .... ▣743
Allegra-D 12 Hour Extended-Release Tablets (Fexofenadine Hydrochloride, Pseudoephedrine Hydrochloride) Sanofi-Aventis 2860
Allegra-D 24 Hour Extended-Release Tablets (Fexofenadine Hydrochloride, Pseudoephedrine Hydrochloride) Sanofi-Aventis 2862

BC Cold Powder (Aspirin, Chlorpheniramine Maleate, Pseudoephedrine Hydrochloride) GlaxoSmithKline ▣ 612
Benadryl Allergy & Sinus Headache Caplets & Gelcaps (Acetaminophen, Diphenhydramine Hydrochloride, Pseudoephedrine Hydrochloride) Pfizer Consumer Healthcare ▣ 693
Benadryl Maximum Strength Severe Allergy & Sinus Headache Caplets (Acetaminophen, Diphenhydramine Hydrochloride, Pseudoephedrine Hydrochloride) Pfizer Consumer Healthcare ▣ 694
Children's Benadryl D Allergy & Sinus Fastmelt Tablets (Diphenhydramine Citrate, Pseudoephedrine Hydrochloride) Pfizer Consumer Healthcare ▣ 694
Children's Benadryl D Liquid Medication (Diphenhydramine Hydrochloride, Pseudoephedrine Hydrochloride) Pfizer Consumer Healthcare ▣ 693
Benadryl D Tablets (Diphenhydramine Hydrochloride, Pseudoephedrine Hydrochloride) Pfizer Consumer Healthcare ▣ 694
Clarinex-D 24-Hour Extended-Release Tablets (Desloratadine, Pseudoephedrine Sulfate) Schering 3012
Claritin-D Non-Drowsy 12 Hour Tablets (Loratadine, Pseudoephedrine Sulfate) Schering-Plough ▣ 731
Claritin-D Non-Drowsy 24 Hour Tablets (Loratadine, Pseudoephedrine Sulfate) Schering-Plough ▣ 731
Contac Non-Drowsy 12 Hour Cold Caplets (Pseudoephedrine Hydrochloride) GlaxoSmithKline ▣ 614
Contac Non-Drowsy Timed Release 12 Hour Cold Caplets (Pseudoephedrine Hydrochloride) GlaxoSmithKline ▣ 615
Children's Dimetapp Cold & Allergy Elixir (Brompheniramine Maleate, Pseudoephedrine Hydrochloride) Wyeth ▣ 745
Children's Dimetapp Long Acting Cough Plus Cold Syrup (Dextromethorphan Hydrobromide, Pseudoephedrine Hydrochloride) Wyeth ▣ 746
Dimetapp Infant Drops Decongestant Plus Cough (Dextromethorphan Hydrobromide, Pseudoephedrine Hydrochloride) Wyeth ▣ 746
Motrin Cold & Sinus Caplets (Ibuprofen, Pseudoephedrine Hydrochloride) McNeil Consumer 1836
PediaCare Decongestant Infants' Drops (Pseudoephedrine Hydrochloride) Pfizer Consumer Healthcare ▣ 705
PediaCare Long-Acting Cough Plus Cold Liquid (Dextromethorphan Hydrobromide, Pseudoephedrine Hydrochloride) Pfizer Consumer Healthcare ▣ 704
PediaCare Multi-Symptom Cold Liquid (Chlorpheniramine Maleate, Dextromethorphan Hydrobromide, Pseudoephedrine Hydrochloride) Pfizer Consumer Healthcare ▣ 704
PediaCare NightRest Cough & Cold Liquid (Chlorpheniramine Maleate, Dextromethorphan Hydrobromide, Pseudoephedrine Hydrochloride) Pfizer Consumer Healthcare ▣ 704
Robitussin PE Syrup (Guaifenesin, Pseudoephedrine Hydrochloride) Wyeth ▣ 753
Robitussin Pediatric Cough & Cold Liquid (Dextromethorphan Hydrobromide, Pseudoephedrine Hydrochloride) Wyeth ▣ 754
Robitussin PM Cough & Cold Liquid (Chlorpheniramine Maleate, Dextromethorphan Hydrobromide, Pseudoephedrine Hydrochloride) Wyeth ▣ 752
Robitussin Severe Congestion Liquid-filled Capsules (Guaifenesin, Pseudoephedrine Hydrochloride) Wyeth ▣ 751
Simply Stuffy Liquid (Pseudoephedrine Hydrochloride) McNeil Consumer 1841
Singlet Caplets (Acetaminophen, Chlorpheniramine Maleate, Pseudoephedrine Hydrochloride) GlaxoSmithKline ▣ 636
Sudafed 12 Hour Caplets (Pseudoephedrine Hydrochloride) Pfizer Consumer Healthcare ▣ 708
Sudafed 24 Hour Tablets (Pseudoephedrine Hydrochloride) Pfizer Consumer Healthcare ▣ 709
Sudafed Nasal Decongestant Tablets (Pseudoephedrine Hydrochloride) Pfizer Consumer Healthcare ▣ 709
Sudafed Non-Drowsy Severe Cold Tablets (Acetaminophen, Dextromethorphan Hydrobromide, Pseudoephedrine Hydrochloride) Pfizer Consumer Healthcare ▣ 710
Sudafed Non-Drying Sinus Liquid Caps (Guaifenesin, Pseudoephedrine Hydrochloride) Pfizer Consumer Healthcare ▣ 709
Sudafed PE Tablets (Phenylephrine Hydrochloride) Pfizer Consumer Healthcare ▣ 711
Sudafed Sinus Headache (Acetaminophen, Pseudoephedrine Hydrochloride) Pfizer Consumer Healthcare ▣ 711
TheraFlu Cold & Cough Hot Liquid (Acetaminophen, Chlorpheniramine Maleate, Dextromethorphan Hydrobromide, Pseudoephedrine Hydrochloride) Novartis Consumer ▣ 680
TheraFlu Cold & Sore Throat Hot Liquid (Acetaminophen, Chlorpheniramine Maleate, Pseudoephedrine Hydrochloride) Novartis Consumer ▣ 680
TheraFlu Flu & Chest Congestion Non-Drowsy Hot Liquid (Acetaminophen, Dextromethorphan Hydrobromide, Guaifenesin, Pseudoephedrine Hydrochloride) Novartis Consumer ▣ 681
TheraFlu Flu & Sore Throat Hot Liquid (Acetaminophen, Chlorpheniramine Maleate, Pseudoephedrine Hydrochloride) Novartis Consumer ▣ 681
TheraFlu Severe Cold Non-Drowsy Hot Liquid (Acetaminophen, Dextromethorphan Hydrobromide, Pseudoephedrine Hydrochloride) Novartis Consumer ▣ 683
TheraFlu Severe Cold & Cough Hot Liquid (Acetaminophen, Chlorpheniramine Maleate, Dextromethorphan Hydrobromide, Pseudoephedrine Hydrochloride) Novartis Consumer ▣ 683
TheraFlu Severe Cold Caplets (Acetaminophen, Chlorpheniramine Maleate, Dextromethorphan Hydrobromide, Pseudoephedrine Hydrochloride) Novartis Consumer ▣ 679
TheraFlu Severe Cold Hot Liquid (Acetaminophen, Chlorpheniramine Maleate, Dextromethorphan Hydrobromide, Pseudoephedrine Hydrochloride) Novartis Consumer ▣ 682
TheraFlu Severe Cold Non-Drowsy Caplets (Acetaminophen, Dextromethorphan Hydrobromide, Pseudoephedrine Hydrochloride) Novartis Consumer ▣ 679
Triaminic Chest & Nasal Congestion Liquid (Guaifenesin, Pseudoephedrine Hydrochloride) Novartis Consumer ▣ 685
Triaminic Allergy Runny Nose & Congestion Softchews (Chlorpheniramine Maleate, Pseudoephedrine Hydrochloride) Novartis Consumer ▣ 688
Triaminic Cough & Sore Throat Softchews (Acetaminophen, Dextromethorphan Hydrobromide, Pseudoephedrine Hydrochloride) Novartis Consumer ▣ 689
Children's Tylenol Plus Cold NightTime Suspension Liquid (Acetaminophen, Chlorpheniramine Maleate, Pseudoephedrine Hydrochloride) McNeil Consumer 1851
Children's Tylenol Plus Cold Chewable Tablets (Acetaminophen, Chlorpheniramine Maleate, Pseudoephedrine Hydrochloride) McNeil Consumer 1851
Children's Tylenol Plus Cold Daytime Non-Drowsy Suspension Liquid (Acetaminophen, Pseudoephedrine Hydrochloride) McNeil Consumer 1851
Children's Tylenol Plus Flu Suspension Liquid (Acetaminophen, Chlorpheniramine Maleate, Dextromethorphan Hydrobromide, Pseudoephedrine Hydrochloride) McNeil Consumer 1853
Concentrated Tylenol Infants' Drops Plus Cold (Acetaminophen, Pseudoephedrine Hydrochloride) McNeil Consumer 1851
Tylenol Cold & Flu Severe Daytime Liquid with Cool Bust (Acetaminophen, Dextromethorphan Hydrobromide, Pseudoephedrine Hydrochloride) McNeil Consumer 1846
Tylenol Cold & Flu Severe NightTime Liquid with Cool Burst (Acetaminophen, Dextromethorphan Hydrobromide, Doxylamine Succinate, Pseudoephedrine Hydrochloride) McNeil Consumer 1846
Tylenol Allergy Complete Multi-Symptom Caplets and Gelcaps with Cool Burst (Acetaminophen, Chlorpheniramine Maleate, Pseudoephedrine Hydrochloride) McNeil Consumer 1844
Tylenol Flu NightTime Gelcaps (Acetaminophen, Diphenhydramine Hydrochloride, Pseudoephedrine Hydrochloride) McNeil Consumer 1846
Tylenol Flu Day Non-Drowsy Gelcaps (Acetaminophen, Dextromethorphan Hydrobromide, Pseudoephedrine Hydrochloride) McNeil Consumer 1846
Concentrated Tylenol Infants' Drops Plus Cold Nasal Congestant, Fever Reducer & Pain Reliever (Acetaminophen, Pseudoephedrine Hydrochloride) McNeil Consumer ▣ 668
Concentrated Tylenol Infants' Drops Plus Cold & Cough Nasal Decongestant, Fever Reducer & Pain Reliever (Acetaminophen, Dextromethorphan Hydrobromide, Pseudoephedrine Hydrochloride) McNeil Consumer ▣ 668
Tylenol Sinus Day Non-Drowsy (Acetaminophen, Pseudoephedrine Hydrochloride) McNeil Consumer 1848
Tylenol Sinus Night Time Caplets (Acetaminophen, Doxylamine Succinate, Pseudoephedrine Hydrochloride) McNeil Consumer 1848
Tylenol Sinus Severe Congestion Caplets with Cool Burst (Acetaminophen, Doxylamine Succinate, Pseudoephedrine Hydrochloride) McNeil Consumer 1848
Vicks Sinex 12-Hour Nasal Spray and Ultra Fine Mist for Sinus Relief (Oxymetazoline Hydrochloride) Procter & Gamble 2678
Vicks Sinex Nasal Spray and Ultra Fine Mist for Sinus Relief (Phenylephrine Hydrochloride) Procter & Gamble 2677
Zicam Allergy Relief Nasal Pump (Histanium Hydrochloricum, Luffa operculata, Galphimia Glauca, Sulfur) Matrixx ▣ 665
Zicam Concentrated Cough Mist for Kids Plus D Cool Cherry (Dextromethorphan Hydrobromide, Phenylephrine Hydrochloride) Matrixx ▣ 643
Zicam Concentrated Cough Mist Plus D Cool Cherry (Dextromethorphan Hydrobromide, Phenylephrine Hydrochloride) Matrixx ▣ 642
Zicam Extreme Congestion Relief Nasal Pump (Oxymetazoline Hydrochloride) Matrixx ▣ 666
Zicam Sinus Relief Nasal Pump (Oxymetazoline Hydrochloride) Matrixx ▣ 666

Nasal dryness
Zicam No-Drip Liquid Nasal Moisturizer (Glycerin) Matrixx ▣ 643

Nausea
(*see also under* Motion sickness)
Maalox Maximum Strength Total Stomach Relief Peppermint Liquid (Bismuth Subsalicylate) Novartis Consumer ▣ 677
Maalox Maximum Strength Total Stomach Relief Strawberry Liquid (Bismuth Subsalicylate) Novartis Consumer ▣ 678

Nausea, emetogenic, cancer chemotherapy-induced
Aloxi Injection (Palonosetron Hydrochloride) MGI 2099
Anzemet Injection (Dolasetron Mesylate) Sanofi-Aventis 2871
Anzemet Tablets (Dolasetron Mesylate) Sanofi-Aventis 2874
Kytril Injection (Granisetron Hydrochloride) Roche Laboratories 2785
Kytril (Granisetron Hydrochloride) Roche Laboratories 2788
Marinol Capsules (Dronabinol) Unimed 3334
Zofran Injection (Ondansetron Hydrochloride) GlaxoSmithKline 1607
Zofran (Ondansetron Hydrochloride) GlaxoSmithKline 1613
Zofran ODT Orally Disintegrating Tablets (Ondansetron) GlaxoSmithKline 1613

Nausea, emetogenic, cancer chemotherapy-induced, adjunct in
Emend Capsules (Aprepitant) Merck 1944

Nausea, emetogenic, radiation therapy-induced
Kytril (Granisetron Hydrochloride) Roche Laboratories 2788
Zofran (Ondansetron Hydrochloride) GlaxoSmithKline 1613
Zofran ODT Orally Disintegrating Tablets (Ondansetron) GlaxoSmithKline 1613

Nausea, postoperative
Anzemet Injection (Dolasetron Mesylate) Sanofi-Aventis 2871
Anzemet Tablets (Dolasetron Mesylate) Sanofi-Aventis 2874
Kytril Injection (Granisetron Hydrochloride) Roche Laboratories 2785
Phenergan (Promethazine Hydrochloride) Wyeth 3438
Zofran Injection (Ondansetron Hydrochloride) GlaxoSmithKline 1607
Zofran (Ondansetron Hydrochloride) GlaxoSmithKline 1613
Zofran ODT Orally Disintegrating Tablets (Ondansetron) GlaxoSmithKline 1613

Necator americanus infections
Mintezol (Thiabendazole) Merck 2002
Vermox Chewable Tablets (Mebendazole) McNeil Consumer 1853

Necrobiosis lipoidica diabeticorum
Decadron Phosphate Injection (Dexamethasone Sodium Phosphate) Merck 1931
Depo-Medrol Single-Dose Vial (Methylprednisolone Acetate) Pharmacia & Upjohn 2617

Necrotic tissue, debridement of
Accuzyme Spray (Papain, Urea) Healthpoint 1637
Panafil Ointment (Chlorophyllin Copper Complex Sodium, Papain, Urea) Healthpoint 1637
Panafil Spray (Chlorophyllin Copper Complex Sodium, Papain, Urea) Healthpoint 1637
U-Kera Cream (Urea) TaroPharma 3290

Neisseria gonorrhoeae
(*see under* N. gonorrhoeae infections)

Neisseria meningitidis
(*see under* N. gonorrhoeae infections)

Neisseria species infections, ocular
Poly-Pred Liquifilm Ophthalmic Suspension (Neomycin Sulfate, Polymyxin B Sulfate, Prednisolone Acetate) Allergan ⊙ 231
Pred-G Ophthalmic Suspension (Gentamicin Sulfate, Prednisolone Acetate) Allergan ⊙ 234
TobraDex Ophthalmic Ointment (Dexamethasone, Tobramycin) Alcon 558
TobraDex Ophthalmic Suspension (Dexamethasone, Tobramycin) Alcon 558
Zylet Ophthalmic Suspension (Loteprednol Etabonate, Tobramycin) Bausch & Lomb 3508

Nephroblastoma
(*see under* Wilms' tumor)

Nephrolithiasis, calcium
Urocit-K Tablets (Potassium Citrate) Mission 2109

Nephropathy, diabetic
Avapro Tablets (Irbesartan) Bristol-Myers Squibb 925
Avapro Tablets (Irbesartan) Sanofi-Aventis 2886
Cozaar Tablets (Losartan Potassium) Merck 1913

Nephrosis, acute, adjunctive therapy
Buminate 25% Solution, USP (Albumin (human)) Baxter Healthcare 748
Plasbumin-20 (Albumin (human)) Talecris 3249
Plasbumin-25 (Albumin (human)) Talecris 3251

Neuralgia
(*see under* Pain, neurogenic)

Neuralgia, glossopharyngeal
Carbatrol Capsules (Carbamazepine) Shire US 3174
Tegretol/Tegretol-XR (Carbamazepine) Novartis 2278

Neuralgia, postherpetic
Lidoderm Patch (Lidocaine) Endo Labs 1107
Lyrica Capsules (Pregabalin) Pfizer 2524
Neurontin Capsules (Gabapentin) Parke-Davis 2498
Neurontin Oral Solution (Gabapentin) Parke-Davis 2498
Neurontin Tablets (Gabapentin) Parke-Davis 2498

Neuralgia, trigeminal
Carbatrol Capsules (Carbamazepine) Shire US 3174
Tegretol/Tegretol-XR (Carbamazepine) Novartis 2278

Neuritis, peripheral, acute
(*see under* Pain, neurogenic)

Neuroblastoma
Adriamycin for Injection, USP (Doxorubicin Hydrochloride) Bedford 786
Adriamycin Injection, USP (Doxorubicin Hydrochloride) Bedford 786

Neurocysticercosis
Albenza Tablets (Albendazole) GlaxoSmithKline 1310

Neurodermatitis
(*see under* Lichen simplex chronicus)

Neurological deficits, post-SAH, improvement of
Nimotop Capsules (Nimodipine) Bayer 774

Neutropenia, chemotherapy-induced
Neulasta Injection (Pegfilgrastim) Amgen 596
Neupogen for Injection (Filgrastim) Amgen 598

Neutropenia, febrile, to decrease the incidence of infection
AmBisome for Injection (Amphotericin B, liposomal) Astellas 615
Cipro I.V. (Ciprofloxacin) Schering 2998
Cipro I.V. Pharmacy Bulk Package (Ciprofloxacin) Bayer 3509
Neulasta Injection (Pegfilgrastim) Amgen 596
Neupogen (Filgrastim) Amgen 598

Neutropenia-related clinical sequelae, post-bone marrow transplant
Neupogen for Injection (Filgrastim) Amgen 598

Nicolas-Favre disease
(*see under* Lymphogranuloma venereum)

Nose, itchy
(*see under* Pruritus, rhinopharyngeal, symptomatic relief of)

Nose, runny
(*see under* Rhinorrhea)

Nutrients, deficiency of
Beelith Tablets (Magnesium Oxide, Vitamin B_6) Beach 784
Marlyn Formula 50 Capsules (Amino Acid Preparations, Vitamin B_6) Marlyn 3525
PediaSure (Entereal Nutrition) Ross 2843
ProNutra Protein Supplement (Vitamins with Minerals, Whey Protein Isolate) Immunotec 1643

Nutrients, deficiency of, stress-induced
(*see under* Nutrients, deficiency of)

Nutrients, deficiency of, surgery-induced
(*see under* Nutrients, deficiency of)

O

Obesity, exogenous
Adipex-P (Phentermine Hydrochloride) Gate 1216
Desoxyn Tablets, USP (Methamphetamine Hydrochloride) Ovation 2482
Meridia Capsules (Sibutramine Hydrochloride Monohydrate) Abbott 485
Xenical Capsules (Orlistat) Roche Laboratories 2834

Obsessive compulsive disorder
Paxil (Paroxetine Hydrochloride) GlaxoSmithKline 1501
Prozac Pulvules and Liquid (Fluoxetine Hydrochloride) Lilly 1771
Zoloft (Sertraline Hydrochloride) Pfizer 2581

Ocular congestion, symptomatic relief of
Albalon Ophthalmic Solution (Naphazoline Hydrochloride) Allergan ⊙ 216

Ocular health, maintenance
Bausch & Lomb PreserVision AREDS Softgels (Vitamins with Minerals) Bausch & Lomb ⊙ 244
Bausch & Lomb PreserVision Lutein Softgels (Lutein, Vitamins with Minerals) Bausch & Lomb ⊙ 245
Bausch & Lomb PreserVision AREDS Eye Vitamin and Mineral Supplement Softgels (Vitamins with Minerals) Bausch & Lomb ▣ 760
Bausch & Lomb PreserVision Lutein Eye Vitamin and Mineral Supplement Softgels (Lutein, Vitamins with Minerals) Bausch & Lomb ▣ 760
Visutein Capsules (Lutein, Acetylcysteine, Carotenoids, Vitamin A, Vitamin B_2, Zinc) Unicity 3328

Ocular inflammation
Decadron Tablets (Dexamethasone) Merck 1929
Poly-Pred Liquifilm Ophthalmic Suspension (Neomycin Sulfate, Polymyxin B Sulfate, Prednisolone Acetate) Allergan ⊙ 231
Pred Mild Sterile Ophthalmic Suspension (Prednisolone Acetate) Allergan ⊙ 236

Ocular inflammation, postoperative
Acular Ophthalmic Solution (Ketorolac Tromethamine) Allergan 561
Voltaren Ophthalmic Solution (Diclofenac Sodium) Novartis 2300

Ocular inflammation, steroid-responsive
FML Ophthalmic Suspension (Fluorometholone) Allergan ⊙ 224
Lotemax Ophthalmic Suspension 0.5% (Loteprednol Etabonate) Bausch & Lomb ⊙ 249
Pred Forte Ophthalmic Suspension (Prednisolone Acetate) Allergan ⊙ 233

Ocular inflammation with bacterial infection, steroid-responsive
Blephamide Ophthalmic Ointment (Prednisolone Acetate, Sulfacetamide Sodium) Allergan 563
Blephamide Ophthalmic Suspension (Prednisolone Acetate, Sulfacetamide Sodium) Allergan 564
FML-S Liquifilm Sterile Ophthalmic Suspension (Fluorometholone, Sulfacetamide Sodium) Allergan ⊙ 226
Poly-Pred Liquifilm Ophthalmic Suspension (Neomycin Sulfate, Polymyxin B Sulfate, Prednisolone Acetate) Allergan ⊙ 231
Pred-G Ophthalmic Suspension (Gentamicin Sulfate, Prednisolone Acetate) Allergan ⊙ 234
Pred-G Sterile Ophthalmic Ointment (Gentamicin Sulfate, Prednisolone Acetate) Allergan ⊙ 235
TobraDex Ophthalmic Ointment (Dexamethasone, Tobramycin) Alcon 558
TobraDex Ophthalmic Suspension (Dexamethasone, Tobramycin) Alcon 558
Zylet Ophthalmic Suspension (Loteprednol Etabonate, Tobramycin) Bausch & Lomb 3508

Ocular redness
Visine Original Eye Drops (Tetrahydrozoline Hydrochloride) Pfizer Consumer ⊙ 279
Visine A.C. Seasonal Itching and Redness Relief Drops (Tetrahydrozoline Hydrochloride, Zinc Sulfate) Pfizer Consumer ⊙ 278
Advanced Relief Visine Eye Drops (Dextran 70, Polyethylene Glycol, Povidone, Tetrahydrozoline Hydrochloride) Pfizer Consumer ⊙ 278
Visine L.R. Long Lasting Eye Drops (Oxymetazoline Hydrochloride) Pfizer Consumer ⊙ 279
Visine-A Eye Allergy Relief Eye Drops (Naphazoline Hydrochloride, Pheniramine Maleate) Pfizer Consumer ⊙ 278
Visine-A Eye Drops (Naphazoline Hydrochloride, Pheniramine Maleate) Pfizer Consumer Healthcare ▣ 713

Onchocerciasis
Stromectol Tablets (Ivermectin) Merck 2053

Onychomycosis
(*see under* Tinea unguium infections)

Ophthalmia, Egyptian
(*see under* Trachoma)

Ophthalmia, sympathetic
Decadron Phosphate Injection (Dexamethasone Sodium Phosphate) Merck 1931
Decadron Tablets (Dexamethasone) Merck 1929
Depo-Medrol Injectable Suspension (Methylprednisolone Acetate) Pharmacia & Upjohn 2615
Hydrocortone Tablets (Hydrocortisone) Merck 1963
Pediapred Oral Solution (Prednisolone Sodium Phosphate) UCB 3319

Ophthalmic disorders
Depo-Medrol Single-Dose Vial (Methylprednisolone Acetate) Pharmacia & Upjohn 2617

Opioid dependence, treatment of
Suboxone Tablets (Buprenorphine Hydrochloride, Naloxone Hydrochloride) Reckitt Benckiser 2719
Subutex Tablets (Buprenorphine Hydrochloride) Reckitt Benckiser 2719

Opioids, acute overdosage, diagnosis of
Narcan Injection (Naloxone Hydrochloride) Endo Labs 1109

Optic neuritis
Decadron Phosphate Injection (Dexamethasone Sodium Phosphate) Merck 1931
Depo-Medrol Injectable Suspension (Methylprednisolone Acetate) Pharmacia & Upjohn 2615
Hydrocortone Tablets (Hydrocortisone) Merck 1963
Pediapred Oral Solution (Prednisolone Sodium Phosphate) UCB 3319

Ornithosis
(*see under* Chlamydia psittaci infection)

Ossification, heterotopic
Didronel Tablets (Etidronate Disodium) Procter & Gamble Pharmaceuticals 2693

Osteitis deformans
(*see under* Paget's disease of bone)

Osteoarthritis
Anaprox Tablets (Naproxen Sodium) Roche Laboratories 2769
Anaprox DS Tablets (Naproxen Sodium) Roche Laboratories 2769
Arthrotec Tablets (Diclofenac Sodium, Misoprostol) Searle 3126
Bayer Aspirin (Aspirin) Bayer Healthcare LLC 3515
Cataflam Tablets (Diclofenac Potassium) Novartis 2173
Celebrex Capsules (Celecoxib) Searle 3130
Clinoril Tablets (Sulindac) Merck 1899
CM Plex (Cetyl Myristate, Cetyl Myristoleate, Fatty Acids) Unicity 3328
Dolobid Tablets (Diflunisal) Merck 1937
EC-Naprosyn Delayed-Release Tablets (Naproxen) Roche Laboratories 2769
Ecotrin Enteric Coated Aspirin Low, Regular and Maximum Strength Tablets (Aspirin) GlaxoSmithKline Consumer 1627
Hyalgan Solution (Sodium Hyaluronate) Sanofi-Aventis 2917
Indocin (Indomethacin) Merck 1968
Mobic Oral Suspension (Meloxicam) Boehringer Ingelheim 893
Mobic Tablets (Meloxicam) Boehringer Ingelheim 893
Nalfon Capsules (Fenoprofen Calcium) Pedinol 2504
Naprosyn Suspension (Naproxen) Roche Laboratories 2769
Naprosyn Tablets (Naproxen) Roche Laboratories 2769
Orthovisc Injection (Hyaluronan) Depuy Mitek 3518
Relafen Tablets (Nabumetone) GlaxoSmithKline 1523
St. Joseph 81 mg Aspirin Chewable and Enteric Coated Tablets (Aspirin) McNeil Consumer 1841

Traumeel Injection Solution (Homeopathic Formulations) Heel 1638
Tylenol 8 Hour Extended Release Geltabs and Caplets (Acetaminophen) McNeil Consumer 1843
Tylenol 8-Hour Extended Release Geltabs/Caplets (Acetaminophen) McNeil Consumer .... ▣655
Tylenol (Acetaminophen) McNeil Consumer 1843
Extra Strength Tylenol Rapid Release Gels (Acetaminophen) McNeil Consumer 1843
Tylenol (Acetaminophen) McNeil Consumer 1843
Voltaren Tablets (Diclofenac Sodium) Novartis 2298
Voltaren-XR Tablets (Diclofenac Sodium) Novartis 2301

Osteoarthritis, post-traumatic
Decadron Phosphate Injection (Dexamethasone Sodium Phosphate) Merck 1931
Depo-Medrol Injectable Suspension (Methylprednisolone Acetate) Pharmacia & Upjohn 2615
Depo-Medrol Single-Dose Vial (Methylprednisolone Acetate) Pharmacia & Upjohn 2617
Hydrocortone Tablets (Hydrocortisone) Merck 1963

Osteoarthritis, synovitis of
Decadron Phosphate Injection (Dexamethasone Sodium Phosphate) Merck 1931
Depo-Medrol Injectable Suspension (Methylprednisolone Acetate) Pharmacia & Upjohn 2615
Depo-Medrol Single-Dose Vial (Methylprednisolone Acetate) Pharmacia & Upjohn 2617
Hydrocortone Tablets (Hydrocortisone) Merck 1963

Osteoarthritis, symptoms of
Zeel Solution (Arnica montana, Sulfur, Herbals, Multiple) Heel 1639

Osteodystrophy, renal
Calcijex Injection (Calcitriol) Abbott ... 411

Osteolytic bone lesions, multiple myeloma-induced
Aredia for Injection (Pamidronate Disodium) Novartis 2168

Osteoporosis
Activella Tablets (Estradiol, Norethindrone Acetate) Novo Nordisk 2311
Actonel Tablets (Risedronate Sodium) Procter & Gamble Pharmaceuticals 2679
Boniva Tablets (Ibandronate Sodium) Roche Laboratories 2747
Evista Tablets (Raloxifene Hydrochloride) Lilly 1735
Forteo for Injection (Teriparatide) Lilly 1739
Fosamax (Alendronate Sodium) Merck 1949
Fosamax Plus D Tablets (Alendronate Sodium, Cholecalciferol) Merck 1956
Premarin Tablets (Estrogens, Conjugated) Wyeth 3443
Premphase Tablets (Estrogens, Conjugated, Medroxyprogesterone Acetate) Wyeth 3452
Prempro Tablets (Estrogens, Conjugated, Medroxyprogesterone Acetate) Wyeth 3452
Vivelle Transdermal System (Estradiol) Novartis 2288
Vivelle-Dot Transdermal System (Estradiol) Novartis 2293

Osteoporosis, corticosteroid-induced
Actonel Tablets (Risedronate Sodium) Procter & Gamble Pharmaceuticals 2679
Fosamax (Alendronate Sodium) Merck 1949

Osteoporosis, postmenopausal, prevention of
Actonel with Calcium Tablets (Risedronate Sodium, Calcium Carbonate) Procter & Gamble Pharmaceuticals 2684
Boniva Tablets (Ibandronate Sodium) Roche Laboratories 2747
Climara Transdermal System (Estradiol) Berlex 795
Menostar Transdermal System (Estradiol) Berlex 805
Prefest Tablets (Estradiol, Norgestimate) Duramed 1069
Vivelle Transdermal System (Estradiol) Novartis 2288
Vivelle-Dot Transdermal System (Estradiol) Novartis 2293

Osteoporosis, postmenopausal, treatment adjunct
Fortical Nasal Spray (Calcitonin-Salmon) Upsher-Smith 3336
Miacalcin Injection (Calcitonin-Salmon) Novartis 2241
Miacalcin Nasal Spray (Calcitonin-Salmon) Novartis 2242
Premarin Tablets (Estrogens, Conjugated) Wyeth 3443

Osteoporosis, postmenopausal, treatment of
Actonel with Calcium Tablets (Risedronate Sodium, Calcium Carbonate) Procter & Gamble Pharmaceuticals 2684

Otitis externa
Floxin Otic Singles (Ofloxacin) Daiichi 1045
Floxin Otic Solution (Ofloxacin) Daiichi 1043

Otitis externa, acute
Ciprodex Otic Suspension (Ciprofloxacin, Dexamethasone) Alcon 555

Otitis media, acute
Amoxil Capsules (Amoxicillin) GlaxoSmithKline 1315
Amoxil Chewable Tablets (Amoxicillin) GlaxoSmithKline 1315
Amoxil Pediatric Drops for Oral Suspension (Amoxicillin) GlaxoSmithKline 1315
Amoxil Powder for Oral Suspension (Amoxicillin) GlaxoSmithKline 1315
Amoxil Tablets (Amoxicillin) GlaxoSmithKline 1315
Augmentin (Amoxicillin, Clavulanate Potassium) GlaxoSmithKline 1331
Augmentin Tablets (Amoxicillin, Clavulanate Potassium) GlaxoSmithKline 1334
Augmentin XR Extended-Release Tablets (Amoxicillin, Clavulanate Potassium) GlaxoSmithKline 1340
Augmentin ES-600 Powder for Oral Suspension (Amoxicillin, Clavulanate Potassium) GlaxoSmithKline 1337
Biaxin/Biaxin XL (Clarithromycin) Abbott 402
Ceftin (Cefuroxime Axetil) GlaxoSmithKline 1369
Ciprodex Otic Suspension (Ciprofloxacin, Dexamethasone) Alcon 555
Floxin Otic Singles (Ofloxacin) Daiichi 1045
Floxin Otic Solution (Ofloxacin) Daiichi 1043
Omnicef Capsules (Cefdinir) Abbott .. 506
Omnicef for Oral Suspension (Cefdinir) Abbott 506
Rocephin Injectable Vials, ADD-Vantage, Galaxy, Bulk (Ceftriaxone Sodium) Roche Laboratories 2801
Suprax (Cefixime) Lupin 1811
Vantin Tablets and Oral Suspension (Cefpodoxime Proxetil) Pharmacia & Upjohn 2650
Zithromax Capsules, 250 mg (Azithromycin Dihydrate) Pfizer 2568
Zithromax for Oral Suspension, 300 mg, 600 mg, 900 mg, 1200 mg (Azithromycin Dihydrate) Pfizer 2561
Zithromax Tablets, 250 mg, 500 mg (Azithromycin Dihydrate) Pfizer 2561
Zithromax Tri-Pak (Azithromycin Dihydrate) Pfizer 2561

Otitis media, adjunctive therapy
Hyland's Earache Tablets (Homeopathic Formulations) Standard Homeopathic .... ▣734

Otitis media, chronic suppurative
Floxin Otic Singles (Ofloxacin) Daiichi 1045
Floxin Otic Solution (Ofloxacin) Daiichi 1043

Otitis media, H. influenzae-induced
(*see under* H. influenzae otitis media)

Otitis media, S. pneumoniae-induced
(*see under* S. pneumoniae otitis media)

Otitis media, S. pyogenes-induced
(*see under* S. pyogenes otitis media)

Otitis media, Staphylococci-induced
(*see under* Staphylococci otitis media)

Ovarian failure, primary
CombiPatch Transdermal System (Estradiol, Norethindrone Acetate) Novartis 2180
Premarin Tablets (Estrogens, Conjugated) Wyeth 3443
Vivelle Transdermal System (Estradiol) Novartis 2288
Vivelle-Dot Transdermal System (Estradiol) Novartis 2293

Ovaries, castration of
CombiPatch Transdermal System (Estradiol, Norethindrone Acetate) Novartis 2180
Premarin Tablets (Estrogens, Conjugated) Wyeth 3443
Vivelle Transdermal System (Estradiol) Novartis 2288
Vivelle-Dot Transdermal System (Estradiol) Novartis 2293

Ovary, adenocarcinoma
(*see under* Carcinoma, ovary)

Ovulation, induction of
Bravelle for Intramuscular or Subcutaneous Injection (Urofollitropin) Ferring 1140
Follistim AQ Cartridge (Follitropin Beta) Organon USA 2354
Gonal-f RFF Pen for Injection (Follitropin Alfa) Serono 3155
Novarel for Injection (Chorionic Gonadotropin) Ferring 1147
Repronex for Intramuscular and Subcutaneous Injection (Menotropins) Ferring 1148

Oxyuriasis
(*see under* Enterobiasis)

P

P. aeruginosa bone and joint infections
Cipro I.V. (Ciprofloxacin) Schering 2998
Cipro I.V. Pharmacy Bulk Package (Ciprofloxacin) Bayer 3509
Cipro (Ciprofloxacin) Schering 2991
Fortaz (Ceftazidime Sodium) GlaxoSmithKline 1422
Primaxin I.V. (Cilastatin Sodium, Imipenem) Merck 2024

P. aeruginosa infection, cystic fibrosis
TOBI Solution for Inhalation (Tobramycin) Chiron 1015

P. aeruginosa infections
Cipro I.V. (Ciprofloxacin) Schering 2998
Cipro I.V. Pharmacy Bulk Package (Ciprofloxacin) Bayer 3509
Cipro (Ciprofloxacin) Schering 2991
Fortaz (Ceftazidime Sodium) GlaxoSmithKline 1422
Garamycin Injectable (Gentamicin Sulfate) Schering 3028
Levaquin in 5% Dextrose Injection (Levofloxacin) Ortho-McNeil 2453
Levaquin (Levofloxacin) Ortho-McNeil 2453
Merrem I.V. (Meropenem) AstraZeneca 687
Noroxin Tablets (Norfloxacin) Merck . 2009
Primaxin I.M. (Cilastatin Sodium, Imipenem) Merck 2022
Primaxin I.V. (Cilastatin Sodium, Imipenem) Merck 2024
Rocephin Injectable Vials, ADD-Vantage, Galaxy, Bulk (Ceftriaxone Sodium) Roche Laboratories 2801
Timentin ADD-Vantage (Clavulanate Potassium, Ticarcillin Disodium) GlaxoSmithKline 1556
Timentin Injection Galaxy Container (Clavulanate Potassium, Ticarcillin Disodium) GlaxoSmithKline 1559
Timentin IV Infusion (Clavulanate Potassium, Ticarcillin Disodium) GlaxoSmithKline 1553
Timentin Pharmacy Bulk Package (Clavulanate Potassium, Ticarcillin Disodium) GlaxoSmithKline 1562
TOBI Solution for Inhalation (Tobramycin) Chiron 1015
Zosyn (Piperacillin Sodium, Tazobactam Sodium) Wyeth 3492

P. aeruginosa infections, ocular
Ciloxan Ophthalmic Ointment (Ciprofloxacin Hydrochloride) Alcon 554
Genoptic Sterile Ophthalmic Solution (Gentamicin Sulfate) Allergan .... ⊙227
Poly-Pred Liquifilm Ophthalmic Suspension (Neomycin Sulfate, Polymyxin B Sulfate, Prednisolone Acetate) Allergan .... ⊙231
Polytrim Ophthalmic Solution (Polymyxin B Sulfate, Trimethoprim Sulfate) Allergan 570
Pred-G Ophthalmic Suspension (Gentamicin Sulfate, Prednisolone Acetate) Allergan .... ⊙234
Pred-G Sterile Ophthalmic Ointment (Gentamicin Sulfate, Prednisolone Acetate) Allergan ..... ⊙235
TobraDex Ophthalmic Ointment (Dexamethasone, Tobramycin) Alcon 558
TobraDex Ophthalmic Suspension (Dexamethasone, Tobramycin) Alcon 558
Zylet Ophthalmic Suspension (Loteprednol Etabonate, Tobramycin) Bausch & Lomb 3508

P. aeruginosa intra-abdominal infections
Cipro I.V. (Ciprofloxacin) Schering 2998
Cipro I.V. Pharmacy Bulk Package (Ciprofloxacin) Bayer 3509
Cipro (Ciprofloxacin) Schering 2991
Maxipime for Injection (Cefepime Hydrochloride) Elan 1093
Merrem I.V. (Meropenem) AstraZeneca 687
Primaxin I.M. (Cilastatin Sodium, Imipenem) Merck 2022
Primaxin I.V. (Cilastatin Sodium, Imipenem) Merck 2024

P. aeruginosa lower respiratory tract infections
Cipro I.V. (Ciprofloxacin) Schering 2998
Cipro I.V. Pharmacy Bulk Package (Ciprofloxacin) Bayer 3509
Cipro (Ciprofloxacin) Schering 2991
Fortaz (Ceftazidime Sodium) GlaxoSmithKline 1422
Levaquin in 5% Dextrose Injection (Levofloxacin) Ortho-McNeil 2453
Levaquin (Levofloxacin) Ortho-McNeil 2453
Maxipime for Injection (Cefepime Hydrochloride) Elan 1093

P. aeruginosa meningitis
Fortaz (Ceftazidime Sodium) GlaxoSmithKline 1422

P. aeruginosa otitis externa
Floxin Otic Singles (Ofloxacin) Daiichi 1045
Floxin Otic Solution (Ofloxacin) Daiichi 1043

P. aeruginosa septicemia
Fortaz (Ceftazidime Sodium) GlaxoSmithKline 1422
Primaxin I.V. (Cilastatin Sodium, Imipenem) Merck 2024
Timentin ADD-Vantage (Clavulanate Potassium, Ticarcillin Disodium) GlaxoSmithKline 1556

Timentin Injection Galaxy Container (Clavulanate Potassium, Ticarcillin Disodium) GlaxoSmithKline 1559
Timentin IV Infusion (Clavulanate Potassium, Ticarcillin Disodium) GlaxoSmithKline 1553
Timentin Pharmacy Bulk Package (Clavulanate Potassium, Ticarcillin Disodium) GlaxoSmithKline 1562

P. aeruginosa skin and skin structure infections
Cipro I.V. (Ciprofloxacin) Schering 2998
Cipro I.V. Pharmacy Bulk Package (Ciprofloxacin) Bayer 3509
Cipro (Ciprofloxacin) Schering 2991
Fortaz (Ceftazidime Sodium) GlaxoSmithKline 1422
Merrem I.V. (Meropenem) AstraZeneca 687
Primaxin I.M. (Cilastatin Sodium, Imipenem) Merck 2022
Primaxin I.V. (Cilastatin Sodium, Imipenem) Merck 2024
Rocephin Injectable Vials, ADD-Vantage, Galaxy, Bulk (Ceftriaxone Sodium) Roche Laboratories 2801

P. aeruginosa urinary tract infections
Cipro I.V. (Ciprofloxacin) Schering 2998
Cipro I.V. Pharmacy Bulk Package (Ciprofloxacin) Bayer 3509
Cipro (Ciprofloxacin) Schering 2991
Cipro XR Tablets (Ciprofloxacin) Schering 3004
Fortaz (Ceftazidime Sodium) GlaxoSmithKline 1422
Levaquin in 5% Dextrose Injection (Levofloxacin) Ortho-McNeil 2453
Levaquin (Levofloxacin) Ortho-McNeil 2453
Noroxin Tablets (Norfloxacin) Merck .2009
Primaxin I.V. (Cilastatin Sodium, Imipenem) Merck 2024
Timentin ADD-Vantage (Clavulanate Potassium, Ticarcillin Disodium) GlaxoSmithKline 1556
Timentin Injection Galaxy Container (Clavulanate Potassium, Ticarcillin Disodium) GlaxoSmithKline 1559
Timentin IV Infusion (Clavulanate Potassium, Ticarcillin Disodium) GlaxoSmithKline 1553
Timentin Pharmacy Bulk Package (Clavulanate Potassium, Ticarcillin Disodium) GlaxoSmithKline 1562

P. falciparum infections
Daraprim Tablets (Pyrimethamine) GlaxoSmithKline 1385
Lariam Tablets (Mefloquine Hydrochloride) Roche Laboratories 2790
Malarone Tablets (Atovaquone, Proguanil Hydrochloride) GlaxoSmithKline 1484
Malarone Pediatric Tablets (Atovaquone, Proguanil Hydrochloride) GlaxoSmithKline 1484

P. malariae infections
Daraprim Tablets (Pyrimethamine) GlaxoSmithKline 1385

P. mirabilis biliary tract infections
Ancef for Injection (Cefazolin Sodium) GlaxoSmithKline 1318

P. mirabilis bone and joint infections
Rocephin Injectable Vials, ADD-Vantage, Galaxy, Bulk (Ceftriaxone Sodium) Roche Laboratories 2801

P. mirabilis genitourinary tract infections
Ancef for Injection (Cefazolin Sodium) GlaxoSmithKline 1318

P. mirabilis infections
Amoxil Capsules (Amoxicillin) GlaxoSmithKline 1315
Amoxil Chewable Tablets (Amoxicillin) GlaxoSmithKline 1315
Amoxil Pediatric Drops for Oral Suspension (Amoxicillin) GlaxoSmithKline 1315
Amoxil Powder for Oral Suspension (Amoxicillin) GlaxoSmithKline 1315
Amoxil Tablets (Amoxicillin) GlaxoSmithKline 1315
Ancef for Injection (Cefazolin Sodium) GlaxoSmithKline 1318
Cipro I.V. (Ciprofloxacin) Schering 2998
Cipro I.V. Pharmacy Bulk Package (Ciprofloxacin) Bayer 3509
Cipro (Ciprofloxacin) Schering 2991
Fortaz (Ceftazidime Sodium) GlaxoSmithKline 1422
Levaquin in 5% Dextrose Injection (Levofloxacin) Ortho-McNeil 2453
Levaquin (Levofloxacin) Ortho-McNeil 2453
Mefoxin for Injection (Cefoxitin Sodium) Merck 1987
Mefoxin Premixed Intravenous Solution (Cefoxitin Sodium) Merck 1990
Merrem I.V. (Meropenem) AstraZeneca 687
Noroxin Tablets (Norfloxacin) Merck .2009
Rocephin Injectable Vials, ADD-Vantage, Galaxy, Bulk (Ceftriaxone Sodium) Roche Laboratories 2801
Suprax (Cefixime) Lupin 1811
Tequin Injection (Gatifloxacin) Bristol-Myers Squibb 964
Tequin Tablets (Gatifloxacin) Bristol-Myers Squibb 964
Vantin Tablets and Oral Suspension (Cefpodoxime Proxetil) Pharmacia & Upjohn 2650

P. mirabilis infections, ocular
TobraDex Ophthalmic Ointment (Dexamethasone, Tobramycin) Alcon 558
TobraDex Ophthalmic Suspension (Dexamethasone, Tobramycin) Alcon 558
Zylet Ophthalmic Suspension (Loteprednol Etabonate, Tobramycin) Bausch & Lomb 3508

P. mirabilis intra-abdominal infections
Cipro I.V. (Ciprofloxacin) Schering 2998
Cipro I.V. Pharmacy Bulk Package (Ciprofloxacin) Bayer 3509
Cipro (Ciprofloxacin) Schering 2991

P. mirabilis lower respiratory tract infections
Cipro I.V. (Ciprofloxacin) Schering 2998
Cipro I.V. Pharmacy Bulk Package (Ciprofloxacin) Bayer 3509
Cipro (Ciprofloxacin) Schering 2991
Fortaz (Ceftazidime Sodium) GlaxoSmithKline 1422
Rocephin Injectable Vials, ADD-Vantage, Galaxy, Bulk (Ceftriaxone Sodium) Roche Laboratories 2801

P. mirabilis otitis media
Floxin Otic Singles (Ofloxacin) Daiichi 1045
Floxin Otic Solution (Ofloxacin) Daiichi 1043

P. mirabilis prostatitis
Ancef for Injection (Cefazolin Sodium) GlaxoSmithKline 1318
Cipro I.V. (Ciprofloxacin) Schering 2998
Cipro I.V. Pharmacy Bulk Package (Ciprofloxacin) Bayer 3509
Cipro (Ciprofloxacin) Schering 2991

P. mirabilis septicemia
Ancef for Injection (Cefazolin Sodium) GlaxoSmithKline 1318

P. mirabilis skin and skin structure infections
Cipro I.V. (Ciprofloxacin) Schering 2998
Cipro I.V. Pharmacy Bulk Package (Ciprofloxacin) Bayer 3509
Cipro (Ciprofloxacin) Schering 2991
Fortaz (Ceftazidime Sodium) GlaxoSmithKline 1422
Mefoxin for Injection (Cefoxitin Sodium) Merck 1987
Mefoxin Premixed Intravenous Solution (Cefoxitin Sodium) Merck 1990
Merrem I.V. (Meropenem) AstraZeneca 687
Rocephin Injectable Vials, ADD-Vantage, Galaxy, Bulk (Ceftriaxone Sodium) Roche Laboratories 2801

P. mirabilis urinary tract infections
Ancef for Injection (Cefazolin Sodium) GlaxoSmithKline 1318
Cipro I.V. (Ciprofloxacin) Schering 2998
Cipro I.V. Pharmacy Bulk Package (Ciprofloxacin) Bayer 3509
Cipro (Ciprofloxacin) Schering 2991
Cipro XR Tablets (Ciprofloxacin) Schering 3004
Fortaz (Ceftazidime Sodium) GlaxoSmithKline 1422
Levaquin in 5% Dextrose Injection (Levofloxacin) Ortho-McNeil 2453
Levaquin (Levofloxacin) Ortho-McNeil 2453
Maxipime for Injection (Cefepime Hydrochloride) Elan 1093
Mefoxin for Injection (Cefoxitin Sodium) Merck 1987
Mefoxin Premixed Intravenous Solution (Cefoxitin Sodium) Merck 1990
Noroxin Tablets (Norfloxacin) Merck .2009
Rocephin Injectable Vials, ADD-Vantage, Galaxy, Bulk (Ceftriaxone Sodium) Roche Laboratories 2801
Suprax (Cefixime) Lupin 1811
Tequin Injection (Gatifloxacin) Bristol-Myers Squibb 964
Tequin Tablets (Gatifloxacin) Bristol-Myers Squibb 964
Vantin Tablets and Oral Suspension (Cefpodoxime Proxetil) Pharmacia & Upjohn 2650

P. ovale infections
Daraprim (Pyrimethamine) GlaxoSmithKline 1385

P. vivax infections
Lariam Tablets (Mefloquine Hydrochloride) Roche Laboratories 2790

P. vulgaris infections
Cipro I.V. (Ciprofloxacin) Schering 2998
Cipro I.V. Pharmacy Bulk Package (Ciprofloxacin) Bayer 3509
Cipro (Ciprofloxacin) Schering 2991
Mefoxin for Injection (Cefoxitin Sodium) Merck 1987
Mefoxin Premixed Intravenous Solution (Cefoxitin Sodium) Merck 1990
Noroxin Tablets (Norfloxacin) Merck .2009
Primaxin I.V. (Cilastatin Sodium, Imipenem) Merck 2024
Rocephin Injectable Vials, ADD-Vantage, Galaxy, Bulk (Ceftriaxone Sodium) Roche Laboratories 2801

P. vulgaris infections, ocular
TobraDex Ophthalmic Ointment (Dexamethasone, Tobramycin) Alcon 558
TobraDex Ophthalmic Suspension (Dexamethasone, Tobramycin) Alcon 558
Zylet Ophthalmic Suspension (Loteprednol Etabonate, Tobramycin) Bausch & Lomb 3508

P. vulgaris skin and skin structure infections
Cipro I.V. (Ciprofloxacin) Schering 2998
Cipro I.V. Pharmacy Bulk Package (Ciprofloxacin) Bayer 3509
Cipro (Ciprofloxacin) Schering 2991
Primaxin I.V. (Cilastatin Sodium, Imipenem) Merck 2024

P. vulgaris urinary tract infections
Mefoxin for Injection (Cefoxitin Sodium) Merck 1987
Mefoxin Premixed Intravenous Solution (Cefoxitin Sodium) Merck 1990
Noroxin Tablets (Norfloxacin) Merck .2009
Primaxin I.V. (Cilastatin Sodium, Imipenem) Merck 2024
Rocephin Injectable Vials, ADD-Vantage, Galaxy, Bulk (Ceftriaxone Sodium) Roche Laboratories 2801

Paget's disease of bone
Actonel Tablets (Risedronate Sodium) Procter & Gamble Pharmaceuticals 2679
Aredia for Injection (Pamidronate Disodium) Novartis 2168
Didronel Tablets (Etidronate Disodium) Procter & Gamble Pharmaceuticals 2693
Fosamax (Alendronate Sodium) Merck 1949
Miacalcin Injection (Calcitonin-Salmon) Novartis 2241

Pain, anogenital
Preparation H Maximum Strength Cream (Glycerin, Petrolatum, Phenylephrine Hydrochloride, Pramoxine Hydrochloride) Wyeth . ■ 747
Preparation H Cooling Gel (Phenylephrine Hydrochloride) Wyeth...... ■ 747
Preparation H (Mineral Oil, Petrolatum, Phenylephrine Hydrochloride, Shark Liver Oil) Wyeth ....■ 747
Tucks Witch Hazel Hemorrhoidal Pad (Witch Hazel) Pfizer Consumer Healthcare ....■ 712

Pain, arthritic, minor
Advil (Ibuprofen) Wyeth ....■ 737
Aleve Tablets, Caplets and Gelcaps (Naproxen Sodium) Bayer Healthcare ....■ 605
Bayer, Aspirin Regimen (Aspirin) Bayer Healthcare ....■ 606
BC Powder (Aspirin, Caffeine, Salicylamide) GlaxoSmithKline ....■ 612
Arthritis Strength BC Powder (Aspirin, Caffeine, Salicylamide) GlaxoSmithKline ....■ 612
Biofreeze Pain Relieving Gel (Camphor, Menthol) Performance Health ....■ 691
Ecotrin Enteric Coated Aspirin Low, Regular and Maximum Strength Tablets (Aspirin) GlaxoSmithKline Consumer 1627
Goody's Extra Strength Headache Powder (Acetaminophen, Aspirin, Caffeine) GlaxoSmithKline ....■ 621
Goody's Extra Strength Pain Relief Tablets (Acetaminophen, Aspirin, Caffeine) GlaxoSmithKline ....■ 621
Motrin IB Tablets and Caplets (Ibuprofen) McNeil Consumer 1836
St. Joseph 81 mg Aspirin Chewable and Enteric Coated Tablets (Aspirin) McNeil Consumer 1841
ThermaCare Heat Wraps (Device) Procter & Gamble 2674
Traumeel Injection Solution (Homeopathic Formulations) Heel 1638
Tylenol 8 Hour Extended Release Geltabs and Caplets (Acetaminophen) McNeil Consumer 1843
Tylenol 8-Hour Extended Release Geltabs/Caplets (Acetaminophen) McNeil Consumer ....■ 655
Tylenol (Acetaminophen) McNeil Consumer 1843
Extra Strength Tylenol Rapid Release Gels (Acetaminophen) McNeil Consumer 1843
Tylenol (Acetaminophen) McNeil Consumer 1843

Pain, dental
Advil (Ibuprofen) Wyeth ....■ 737
Children's Advil Suspension (Ibuprofen) Wyeth ....■ 742
Children's Advil Chewable Tablets (Ibuprofen) Wyeth ....■ 741
Infants' Advil Concentrated Drops (Ibuprofen) Wyeth ....■ 743
Junior Strength Advil Swallow Tablets (Ibuprofen) Wyeth ....■ 740
Aleve Tablets, Caplets and Gelcaps (Naproxen Sodium) Bayer Healthcare ....■ 605
Anbesol Cold Sore Therapy Ointment (Allantoin, Benzocaine, Camphor, Petrolatum, White) Wyeth ....■ 745
Baby Anbesol Gel (Benzocaine) Wyeth ....■ 744
Junior Anbesol Gel (Benzocaine) Wyeth ....■ 744
Anbesol (Benzocaine) Wyeth ....■ 744
BC Powder (Aspirin, Caffeine, Salicylamide) GlaxoSmithKline ....■ 612

Arthritis Strength BC Powder (Aspirin, Caffeine, Salicylamide) GlaxoSmithKline ▣ 612
Celebrex Capsules (Celecoxib) Searle 3130
Goody's Extra Strength Headache Powder (Acetaminophen, Aspirin, Caffeine) GlaxoSmithKline ▣ 621
Goody's Extra Strength Pain Relief Tablets (Acetaminophen, Aspirin, Caffeine) GlaxoSmithKline ▣ 621
Hurricaine Topical Anesthetic Aerosol Spray, 2 oz. Wild Cherry (Benzocaine) Beutlich 835
Hurricaine Topical Anesthetic Aerosol Spray Kit, 2 oz. Wild Cherry with 200 Disposable Extension Tubes (Benzocaine) Beutlich 835
Hurricaine Topical Anesthetic Gel: 1 oz. Wild Cherry, Pina Colada, Watermelon, Fresh Mint, 0.18 oz. Wild Cherry (Benzocaine) Beutlich 835
Hurricaine Topical Anesthetic Liquid: 1 oz. Wild Cherry and Pina Colada, Swab Applicator Wild Cherry (Benzocaine) Beutlich 835
Hyland's Teething Gel (Homeopathic Formulations) Standard Homeopathic ▣ 736
Hyland's Teething Tablets (Belladonna Alkaloids, Homeopathic Formulations) Standard Homeopathic ▣ 736
Children's Motrin Oral Suspension and Chewable Tablets (Ibuprofen) McNeil Consumer ▣ 647
Children's Motrin Non-Staining Dye-Free Oral Suspension (Ibuprofen) McNeil Consumer ▣ 647
Children's Motrin Oral Suspension and Chewable Tablets (Ibuprofen) McNeil Consumer 1837
Children's Motrin Non-Staining Dye-Free Oral Suspension (Ibuprofen) McNeil Consumer 1837
Motrin IB Tablets and Caplets (Ibuprofen) McNeil Consumer 1836
Infants' Motrin Concentrated Drops (Ibuprofen) McNeil Consumer 1837
Infants' Motrin Non-Staining Dye-Free Drops (Ibuprofen) McNeil Consumer 1837
Junior Strength Motrin Caplets and Chewable Tablets (Ibuprofen) McNeil Consumer 1837
Triaminic Sore Throat Spray (Phenol) Novartis Consumer ▣ 689
Tylenol 8 Hour Extended Release Geltabs and Caplets (Acetaminophen) McNeil Consumer 1843
Tylenol 8-Hour Extended Release Geltabs/Caplets (Acetaminophen) McNeil Consumer ▣ 655
Children's Tylenol Suspension Liquid and Meltaways (Acetaminophen) McNeil Consumer 1850
Concentrated Tylenol Infants' Drops (Acetaminophen) McNeil Consumer 1850
Tylenol (Acetaminophen) McNeil Consumer 1843
Extra Strength Tylenol Rapid Release Gels (Acetaminophen) McNeil Consumer 1843
Tylenol (Acetaminophen) McNeil Consumer 1843

Pain, endometriosis-associated

depo-subQ provera 104 Injectable Suspension (Medroxyprogesterone Acetate) Pharmacia & Upjohn 2622

Pain, general

Advil (Ibuprofen) Wyeth ▣ 737
Children's Advil Cold Suspension (Ibuprofen, Pseudoephedrine Hydrochloride) Wyeth ▣ 741
Junior Strength Advil Swallow Tablets (Ibuprofen) Wyeth ▣ 740
Aleve Tablets, Caplets and Gelcaps (Naproxen Sodium) Bayer Healthcare ▣ 605
Bayer, Aspirin Regimen (Aspirin) Bayer Healthcare ▣ 606
Bayer Aspirin Tablets (Aspirin) Bayer Healthcare LLC 3515
Benadryl Allergy & Cold Tablets (Acetaminophen, Diphenhydramine Hydrochloride, Pseudoephedrine Hydrochloride) Pfizer Consumer Healthcare ▣ 692
Goody's Body Pain Formula Powder (Acetaminophen, Aspirin, Acetaminophen, Aspirin) GlaxoSmithKline ▣ 621
Hyland's Leg Cramps Ointment (Homeopathic Formulations) Standard Homeopathic ▣ 735
Children's Motrin Oral Suspension and Chewable Tablets (Ibuprofen) McNeil Consumer ▣ 647
Children's Motrin Non-Staining Dye-Free Oral Suspension (Ibuprofen) McNeil Consumer ▣ 647
Children's Motrin Oral Suspension and Chewable Tablets (Ibuprofen) McNeil Consumer 1837
Children's Motrin Non-Staining Dye-Free Oral Suspension (Ibuprofen) McNeil Consumer 1837
Motrin IB Tablets and Caplets (Ibuprofen) McNeil Consumer 1836
Infants' Motrin Concentrated Drops (Ibuprofen) McNeil Consumer 1837
Infants' Motrin Non-Staining Dye-Free Drops (Ibuprofen) McNeil Consumer 1837
TheraFlu Cold & Cough Hot Liquid (Acetaminophen, Chlorpheniramine Maleate, Dextromethorphan Hydrobromide, Pseudoephedrine Hydrochloride) Novartis Consumer ▣ 680
TheraFlu Cold & Sore Throat Hot Liquid (Acetaminophen, Chlorpheniramine Maleate, Pseudoephedrine Hydrochloride) Novartis Consumer ▣ 680
TheraFlu Flu & Chest Congestion Non-Drowsy Hot Liquid (Acetaminophen, Dextromethorphan Hydrobromide, Guaifenesin, Pseudoephedrine Hydrochloride) Novartis Consumer ▣ 681
TheraFlu Flu & Sore Throat Hot Liquid (Acetaminophen, Chlorpheniramine Maleate, Pseudoephedrine Hydrochloride) Novartis Consumer ▣ 681
TheraFlu Severe Cold Non-Drowsy Hot Liquid (Acetaminophen, Dextromethorphan Hydrobromide, Pseudoephedrine Hydrochloride) Novartis Consumer ▣ 683
TheraFlu Severe Cold & Cough Hot Liquid (Acetaminophen, Chlorpheniramine Maleate, Dextromethorphan Hydrobromide, Pseudoephedrine Hydrochloride) Novartis Consumer ▣ 683
TheraFlu Severe Cold Caplets (Acetaminophen, Chlorpheniramine Maleate, Dextromethorphan Hydrobromide, Pseudoephedrine Hydrochloride) Novartis Consumer ▣ 679
TheraFlu Severe Cold Hot Liquid (Acetaminophen, Chlorpheniramine Maleate, Dextromethorphan Hydrobromide, Pseudoephedrine Hydrochloride) Novartis Consumer ▣ 682
TheraFlu Severe Cold Non-Drowsy Caplets (Acetaminophen, Dextromethorphan Hydrobromide, Pseudoephedrine Hydrochloride) Novartis Consumer ▣ 679
Traumeel Injection Solution (Homeopathic Formulations) Heel 1638
Tylenol 8 Hour Extended Release Geltabs and Caplets (Acetaminophen) McNeil Consumer 1843
Tylenol 8-Hour Extended Release Geltabs/Caplets (Acetaminophen) McNeil Consumer ▣ 655
Tylenol Cough & Sore Throat Daytime Liquid with Cool Burst (Acetaminophen, Dextromethorphan Hydrobromide) McNeil Consumer ▣ 664
Tylenol Cough & Sore Throat NightTime Liquid with Cool Burst (Acetaminophen, Dextromethorphan Hydrobromide, Doxylamine Succinate) McNeil Consumer ▣ 664
Children's Tylenol Suspension Liquid and Meltaways (Acetaminophen) McNeil Consumer 1850
Concentrated Tylenol Infants' Drops (Acetaminophen) McNeil Consumer 1850
Junior Tylenol Meltaways (Acetaminophen) McNeil Consumer 1850
Tylenol Cold & Flu Severe Daytime Liquid with Cool Bust (Acetaminophen, Dextromethorphan Hydrobromide, Pseudoephedrine Hydrochloride) McNeil Consumer 1846
Tylenol Cold & Flu Severe NightTime Liquid with Cool Burst (Acetaminophen, Dextromethorphan Hydrobromide, Doxylamine Succinate, Pseudoephedrine Hydrochloride) McNeil Consumer 1846
Tylenol Cough & Sore Throat Daytime Liquid with Cool Burst (Acetaminophen, Dextromethorphan Hydrobromide) McNeil Consumer 1849
Tylenol Cough & Sore Throat NightTime Liquid with Cool Burst (Acetaminophen, Dextromethorphan Hydrobromide, Doxylamine Succinate) McNeil Consumer 1849
Tylenol (Acetaminophen) McNeil Consumer 1843
Extra Strength Tylenol Rapid Release Gels (Acetaminophen) McNeil Consumer 1843
Regular Strength Tylenol Tablets (Acetaminophen) McNeil Consumer 1843
Tylenol Flu NightTime Gelcaps (Acetaminophen, Diphenhydramine Hydrochloride, Pseudoephedrine Hydrochloride) McNeil Consumer 1846
Tylenol Flu Day Non-Drowsy Gelcaps (Acetaminophen, Dextromethorphan Hydrobromide, Pseudoephedrine Hydrochloride) McNeil Consumer 1846
Extra Strength Tylenol PM Caplets, Geltabs, Gelcaps and Liquid (Acetaminophen, Diphenhydramine Hydrochloride) McNeil Consumer 1847
Tylenol Sinus Severe Congestion Caplets with Cool Burst (Acetaminophen, Doxylamine Succinate, Pseudoephedrine Hydrochloride) McNeil Consumer 1848
Tylenol Sore Throat NightTime Liquid with Cool Burst (Acetaminophen, Diphenhydramine) McNeil Consumer 1849

Pain, intractable chronic

(*see under* Pain, severe)

Pain, joint

Biofreeze Pain Relieving Gel (Camphor, Menthol) Performance Health ▣ 691

Pain, major surgical

DepoDur Extended-Release Injection (Morphine sulfate, liposomal) Endo Labs 1098

Pain, menstrual

Advil (Ibuprofen) Wyeth ▣ 737
Aleve Tablets, Caplets and Gelcaps (Naproxen Sodium) Bayer Healthcare ▣ 605
BC Powder (Aspirin, Caffeine, Salicylamide) GlaxoSmithKline ▣ 612
Goody's Extra Strength Headache Powder (Acetaminophen, Aspirin, Caffeine) GlaxoSmithKline ▣ 621
Goody's Extra Strength Pain Relief Tablets (Acetaminophen, Aspirin, Caffeine) GlaxoSmithKline ▣ 621
Motrin IB Tablets and Caplets (Ibuprofen) McNeil Consumer 1836
ThermaCare Heat Wraps (Device) Procter & Gamble 2674
Tylenol 8 Hour Extended Release Geltabs and Caplets (Acetaminophen) McNeil Consumer 1843
Tylenol 8-Hour Extended Release Geltabs/Caplets (Acetaminophen) McNeil Consumer ▣ 655
Tylenol (Acetaminophen) McNeil Consumer 1843
Extra Strength Tylenol Rapid Release Gels (Acetaminophen) McNeil Consumer 1843
Tylenol (Acetaminophen) McNeil Consumer 1843
Women's Tylenol Menstrual Relief Caplets (Acetaminophen, Pamabrom) McNeil Consumer 1849

Pain, mild

Advil (Ibuprofen) Wyeth ▣ 737
Children's Advil Suspension (Ibuprofen) Wyeth ▣ 742
Children's Advil Chewable Tablets (Ibuprofen) Wyeth ▣ 741
Children's Advil Cold Suspension (Ibuprofen, Pseudoephedrine Hydrochloride) Wyeth ▣ 741
Infants' Advil Concentrated Drops (Ibuprofen) Wyeth ▣ 743
Junior Strength Advil Swallow Tablets (Ibuprofen) Wyeth ▣ 740
Aleve Tablets, Caplets and Gelcaps (Naproxen Sodium) Bayer Healthcare ▣ 605
Ecotrin Enteric Coated Aspirin Low, Regular and Maximum Strength Tablets (Aspirin) GlaxoSmithKline Consumer 1627
Goody's Body Pain Formula Powder (Acetaminophen, Aspirin, Acetaminophen, Aspirin) GlaxoSmithKline ▣ 621
Goody's Extra Strength Headache Powder (Acetaminophen, Aspirin, Caffeine) GlaxoSmithKline ▣ 621
Goody's Extra Strength Pain Relief Tablets (Acetaminophen, Aspirin, Caffeine) GlaxoSmithKline ▣ 621
Goody's PM Powder (Acetaminophen, Diphenhydramine Citrate) GlaxoSmithKline ▣ 622
Motrin IB Tablets and Caplets (Ibuprofen) McNeil Consumer 1836
Junior Strength Motrin Caplets and Chewable Tablets (Ibuprofen) McNeil Consumer 1837
St. Joseph 81 mg Aspirin Chewable and Enteric Coated Tablets (Aspirin) McNeil Consumer 1841
Tylenol 8 Hour Extended Release Geltabs and Caplets (Acetaminophen) McNeil Consumer 1843
Tylenol 8-Hour Extended Release Geltabs/Caplets (Acetaminophen) McNeil Consumer ▣ 655
Children's Tylenol Plus Cold & Allergy Suspension Liquid (Acetaminophen, Diphenhydramine Hydrochloride, Pseudoephedrine Hydrochloride) McNeil Consumer 1850
Children's Tylenol Plus Flu Suspension Liquid (Acetaminophen, Chlorpheniramine Maleate, Dextromethorphan Hydrobromide, Pseudoephedrine Hydrochloride) McNeil Consumer 1853
Junior Tylenol Meltaways (Acetaminophen) McNeil Consumer 1850
Extra Strength Tylenol Geltabs, Caplets, Cool Caplets and EZ Tabs (Acetaminophen) McNeil Consumer 1843
Extra Strength Tylenol Rapid Release Gels (Acetaminophen) McNeil Consumer 1843
Regular Strength Tylenol Tablets (Acetaminophen) McNeil Consumer 1843
Concentrated Tylenol Infants' Drops Plus Cold Nasal Congestant, Fever Reducer & Pain Reliever (Acetaminophen, Pseudoephedrine Hydrochloride) McNeil Consumer ▣ 668
Concentrated Tylenol Infants' Drops Plus Cold & Cough Nasal Decongestant, Fever Reducer & Pain Reliever (Acetaminophen, Dextromethorphan Hydrobromide, Pseudoephedrine Hydrochloride) McNeil Consumer ▣ 668

Pain, mild to moderate

Anaprox Tablets (Naproxen Sodium) Roche Laboratories 2769
Anaprox DS Tablets (Naproxen Sodium) Roche Laboratories 2769
Darvocet A 500 Tablets (Acetaminophen, Propoxyphene Napsylate) Xanodyne 3497

Dolobid Tablets (Diflunisal) Merck 1937
Nalfon Capsules (Fenoprofen Calcium) Pedinol 2504
Naprosyn Suspension (Naproxen) Roche Laboratories 2769
Naprosyn Tablets (Naproxen) Roche Laboratories 2769
Tylenol with Codeine Elixir (Acetaminophen, Codeine Phosphate) Ortho-McNeil 2461

Pain, mild to moderate, acute musculo-skeletal
Biofreeze Pain Relieving Gel (Camphor, Menthol) Performance Health ..... ▣ 691

Pain, moderate to moderately severe
Lortab (Acetaminophen, Hydrocodone Bitartrate) UCB 3315
Lortab Elixir (Acetaminophen, Hydrocodone Bitartrate) UCB 3312
OxyFast Oral Concentrate Solution (Oxycodone Hydrochloride) Purdue Pharma 2704
OxyIR Capsules (Oxycodone Hydrochloride) Purdue Pharma 2704
Percocet Tablets (Acetaminophen, Oxycodone Hydrochloride) Endo Labs 1114
Percodan Tablets (Aspirin, Oxycodone Hydrochloride, Oxycodone Terephthalate) Endo Labs 1115
Tylenol with Codeine Tablets (Acetaminophen, Codeine Phosphate) Ortho-McNeil 2461
Vicodin Tablets (Acetaminophen, Hydrocodone Bitartrate) Abbott 530
Vicodin ES Tablets (Acetaminophen, Hydrocodone Bitartrate) Abbott 531
Vicodin HP Tablets (Acetaminophen, Hydrocodone Bitartrate) Abbott 532
Zydone Tablets (Acetaminophen, Hydrocodone Bitartrate) Endo Labs 1118

Pain, moderate to severe
Avinza Capsules (Morphine Sulfate) Ligand 1714
Buprenex Injectable (Buprenorphine Hydrochloride) Reckitt Benckiser 2718
Celebrex Capsules (Celecoxib) Searle 3130
Combunox Tablets (Ibuprofen, Oxycodone Hydrochloride) Forest 1183
Dilaudid (Hydromorphone Hydrochloride) Abbott 439
Dilaudid Oral Liquid (Hydromorphone Hydrochloride) Abbott 443
Dilaudid Non-Sterile Powder (Hydromorphone Hydrochloride) Abbott 439
Dilaudid Rectal Suppositories (Hydromorphone Hydrochloride) Abbott 439
Dilaudid Tablets (Hydromorphone Hydrochloride) Abbott 439
Dilaudid Tablets - 8 mg (Hydromorphone Hydrochloride) Abbott 443
Dilaudid-HP (Hydromorphone Hydrochloride) Abbott 441
Duragesic Transdermal System (Fentanyl) Ortho-McNeil 2448
Kadian Capsules (Morphine Sulfate) Alpharma Branded Products 572
MS Contin Tablets (Morphine Sulfate) Purdue Pharma 2703
Nubain Injection (Nalbuphine Hydrochloride) Endo Labs 1111
Numorphan (Oxymorphone Hydrochloride) Endo Labs 1112
OxyContin Tablets (Oxycodone Hydrochloride) Purdue Pharma 2699
Vicoprofen Tablets (Hydrocodone Bitartrate, Ibuprofen) Abbott 533

Pain, muscular, temporary relief of
Aleve Tablets, Caplets and Gelcaps (Naproxen Sodium) Bayer Healthcare ..... ▣ 605
Bayer, Aspirin Regimen (Aspirin) Bayer Healthcare ..... ▣ 606
Benadryl Allergy & Cold Tablets (Acetaminophen, Diphenhydramine Hydrochloride, Pseudoephedrine Hydrochloride) Pfizer Consumer Healthcare ..... ▣ 692
Goody's Body Pain Formula Powder (Acetaminophen, Aspirin, Acetaminophen, Aspirin) GlaxoSmithKline ..... ▣ 621
Motrin IB Tablets and Caplets (Ibuprofen) McNeil Consumer 1836
Thera-Gesic Plus Creme (Menthol, Methyl Salicylate) Mission ..... ▣ 673
ThermaCare Heat Wraps (Device) Procter & Gamble 2674
Traumeel Injection Solution (Homeopathic Formulations) Heel 1638
Tylenol 8 Hour Extended Release Geltabs and Caplets (Acetaminophen) McNeil Consumer 1843
Tylenol 8-Hour Extended Release Geltabs/Caplets (Acetaminophen) McNeil Consumer ..... ▣ 655
Junior Tylenol Meltaways (Acetaminophen) McNeil Consumer 1850
Tylenol (Acetaminophen) McNeil Consumer 1843
Extra Strength Tylenol Rapid Release Gels (Acetaminophen) McNeil Consumer 1843
Tylenol (Acetaminophen) McNeil Consumer 1843
Tylenol Sore Throat Daytime Liquid with Cool Burst (Acetaminophen) McNeil Consumer 1849

Pain, neurogenic
BC Powder (Aspirin, Caffeine, Salicylamide) GlaxoSmithKline ..... ▣ 612
Arthritis Strength BC Powder (Aspirin, Caffeine, Salicylamide) GlaxoSmithKline ..... ▣ 612
Tegretol/Tegretol-XR (Carbamazepine) Novartis 2278

Pain, neuropathic
Cymbalta Delayed-Release Capsules (Duloxetine Hydrochloride) Lilly 1729

Pain, neuropathic, associated with diabetic peripheral neuropathy
Lyrica Capsules (Pregabalin) Pfizer 2524

Pain, obstetrical
Nubain Injection (Nalbuphine Hydrochloride) Endo Labs 1111

Pain, ocular
Acular LS Ophthalmic Solution (Ketorolac Tromethamine) Allergan 562

Pain, oral
Hurricaine Topical Anesthetic Aerosol Spray, 2 oz. Wild Cherry (Benzocaine) Beutlich 835
Hurricaine Topical Anesthetic Aerosol Spray Kit, 2 oz. Wild Cherry with 200 Disposable Extension Tubes (Benzocaine) Beutlich 835
Hurricaine Topical Anesthetic Gel: 1 oz. Wild Cherry, Pina Colada, Watermelon, Fresh Mint, 0.18 oz. Wild Cherry (Benzocaine) Beutlich 835
Hurricaine Topical Anesthetic Liquid: 1 oz. Wild Cherry and Pina Colada, Swab Applicator Wild Cherry (Benzocaine) Beutlich 835

Pain, oral mucosal and gingival
Cetacaine Topical Anesthetic (Benzocaine, Butyl Aminobenzoate, Tetracaine Hydrochloride) Cetylite 1007
Hurricaine Topical Anesthetic Aerosol Spray, 2 oz. Wild Cherry (Benzocaine) Beutlich 835
Hurricaine Topical Anesthetic Aerosol Spray Kit, 2 oz. Wild Cherry with 200 Disposable Extension Tubes (Benzocaine) Beutlich 835
Hurricaine Topical Anesthetic Gel: 1 oz. Wild Cherry, Pina Colada, Watermelon, Fresh Mint, 0.18 oz. Wild Cherry (Benzocaine) Beutlich 835
Hurricaine Topical Anesthetic Liquid: 1 oz. Wild Cherry and Pina Colada, Swab Applicator Wild Cherry (Benzocaine) Beutlich 835
Triaminic Sore Throat Spray (Phenol) Novartis Consumer ..... ▣ 689

Pain, postoperative, relief of
Celebrex Capsules (Celecoxib) Searle 3130
Naropin Injection (Ropivacaine Hydrochloride) AstraZeneca LP 640
Voltaren Ophthalmic Solution (Diclofenac Sodium) Novartis 2300

Pain, pre- and postoperative, relief of
Nubain Injection (Nalbuphine Hydrochloride) Endo Labs 1111

Pain, prepartum
(*see under* Pain, obstetrical)

Pain, severe
Actiq (Fentanyl Citrate) Cephalon 993
Kadian Capsules (Morphine Sulfate) Alpharma Branded Products 572

Pain, short-term management of
Ultracet Tablets (Acetaminophen, Tramadol Hydrochloride) Ortho-McNeil 2462

Pain, teething
(*see under* Pain, dental)

Pain, topical relief of
Benadryl Itch Relief Stick Extra Strength (Diphenhydramine Hydrochloride, Zinc Acetate) Pfizer Consumer Healthcare ..... ▣ 696
Benadryl Itch Stopping Cream Extra Strength (Diphenhydramine Hydrochloride, Zinc Acetate) Pfizer Consumer Healthcare ..... ▣ 697
Benadryl Itch Stopping Gel Extra Strength (Diphenhydramine Hydrochloride) Pfizer Consumer Healthcare ..... ▣ 697
Benadryl Itch Stopping Spray Extra Strength (Diphenhydramine Hydrochloride, Zinc Acetate) Pfizer Consumer Healthcare ..... ▣ 697
BenGay External Analgesic Products (Menthol, Methyl Salicylate) Pfizer Consumer Healthcare ..... ▣ 698
BenGay Pain Relieving Patch (Menthol) Pfizer Consumer Healthcare ..... ▣ 698
BenGay Ultra Strength Pain Relieving Patch (Menthol) Pfizer Consumer Healthcare ..... ▣ 698
Biofreeze Pain Relieving Gel (Camphor, Menthol) Performance Health ..... ▣ 691
Lidoderm Patch (Lidocaine) Endo Labs 1107
Smile's Prid Salve (Homeopathic Formulations) Standard Homeopathic ..... ▣ 735
Thera-Gesic Creme (Menthol, Methyl Salicylate) Mission 2108
Thera-Gesic Plus Creme (Menthol, Methyl Salicylate) Mission ..... ▣ 673
ThermaCare Heat Wraps (Device) Procter & Gamble 2674
Vicks VapoRub Cream (Camphor, Menthol) Procter & Gamble 2678
Vicks VapoRub Ointment (Camphor, Eucalyptus, Oil of, Menthol) Procter & Gamble 2678

Pain, unspecified
Cataflam Tablets (Diclofenac Potassium) Novartis 2173
Ecotrin Enteric Coated Aspirin Low, Regular and Maximum Strength Tablets (Aspirin) GlaxoSmithKline Consumer 1627
St. Joseph 81 mg Aspirin Chewable and Enteric Coated Tablets (Aspirin) McNeil Consumer 1841

Pain associated with arthritis, topical
(*see under* Pain, topical relief of)

Pain associated with sports injuries
(*see under* Pain, topical relief of)

Pain associated with upper respiratory infection
Advil Allergy Sinus Caplets (Chlorpheniramine Maleate, Ibuprofen, Pseudoephedrine Hydrochloride) Wyeth ..... ▣ 737
Advil (Ibuprofen) Wyeth ..... ▣ 737
Children's Advil Suspension (Ibuprofen) Wyeth ..... ▣ 742
Children's Advil Chewable Tablets (Ibuprofen) Wyeth ..... ▣ 741
Advil Cold & Sinus (Ibuprofen, Pseudoephedrine Hydrochloride) Wyeth ..... ▣ 739
Advil Flu & Body Ache Caplets (Ibuprofen, Pseudoephedrine Hydrochloride) Wyeth ..... ▣ 739
Infants' Advil Concentrated Drops (Ibuprofen) Wyeth ..... ▣ 743
Junior Strength Advil Swallow Tablets (Ibuprofen) Wyeth ..... ▣ 740
Advil Multi-Symptom Cold Caplets (Chlorpheniramine Maleate, Ibuprofen, Pseudoephedrine Hydrochloride) Wyeth ..... ▣ 738
BC Cold Powder (Aspirin, Chlorpheniramine Maleate, Pseudoephedrine Hydrochloride) GlaxoSmithKline ..... ▣ 612
Benadryl Allergy & Cold Tablets (Acetaminophen, Diphenhydramine Hydrochloride, Pseudoephedrine Hydrochloride) Pfizer Consumer Healthcare ..... ▣ 692
Benadryl Maximum Strength Severe Allergy & Sinus Headache Caplets (Acetaminophen, Diphenhydramine Hydrochloride, Pseudoephedrine Hydrochloride) Pfizer Consumer Healthcare ..... ▣ 694
Contac Severe Cold and Flu Caplets Maximum Strength (Acetaminophen, Chlorpheniramine Maleate, Dextromethorphan Hydrobromide, Pseudoephedrine Hydrochloride) GlaxoSmithKline ..... ▣ 615
Contac Severe Cold and Flu Caplets Non-Drowsy (Acetaminophen, Dextromethorphan Hydrobromide, Pseudoephedrine Hydrochloride) GlaxoSmithKline ..... ▣ 615
Children's Motrin Oral Suspension and Chewable Tablets (Ibuprofen) McNeil Consumer ..... ▣ 647
Children's Motrin Non-Staining Dye-Free Oral Suspension (Ibuprofen) McNeil Consumer ..... ▣ 647
Children's Motrin Oral Suspension and Chewable Tablets (Ibuprofen) McNeil Consumer 1837
Children's Motrin Cold Non-Staining Dye-Free Oral Suspension (Ibuprofen, Pseudoephedrine Hydrochloride) McNeil Consumer 1838
Children's Motrin Cold Oral Suspension (Ibuprofen, Pseudoephedrine Hydrochloride) McNeil Consumer ..... ▣ 648
Children's Motrin Cold Non-Staining Dye-Free Oral Suspension (Ibuprofen, Pseudoephedrine Hydrochloride) McNeil Consumer ..... ▣ 648
Children's Motrin Cold Oral Suspension (Ibuprofen, Pseudoephedrine Hydrochloride) McNeil Consumer 1838
Children's Motrin Non-Staining Dye-Free Oral Suspension (Ibuprofen) McNeil Consumer 1837
Motrin Cold & Sinus Caplets (Ibuprofen, Pseudoephedrine Hydrochloride) McNeil Consumer 1836
Infants' Motrin Concentrated Drops (Ibuprofen) McNeil Consumer 1837
Infants' Motrin Non-Staining Dye-Free Drops (Ibuprofen) McNeil Consumer 1837
Junior Strength Motrin Caplets and Chewable Tablets (Ibuprofen) McNeil Consumer 1837

TheraFlu Cold & Cough Hot Liquid (Acetaminophen, Chlorpheniramine Maleate, Dextromethorphan Hydrobromide, Pseudoephedrine Hydrochloride) Novartis Consumer ..... ▣ 680
TheraFlu Cold & Sore Throat Hot Liquid (Acetaminophen, Chlorpheniramine Maleate, Pseudoephedrine Hydrochloride) Novartis Consumer ..... ▣ 680
TheraFlu Flu & Sore Throat Hot Liquid (Acetaminophen, Chlorpheniramine Maleate, Pseudoephedrine Hydrochloride) Novartis Consumer ..... ▣ 681
TheraFlu Severe Cold & Cough Hot Liquid (Acetaminophen, Chlorpheniramine Maleate, Dextromethorphan Hydrobromide, Pseudoephedrine Hydrochloride) Novartis Consumer ..... ▣ 683
TheraFlu Severe Cold Caplets (Acetaminophen, Chlorpheniramine Maleate, Dextromethorphan Hydrobromide, Pseudoephedrine Hydrochloride) Novartis Consumer ..... ▣ 679
TheraFlu Severe Cold Hot Liquid (Acetaminophen, Chlorpheniramine Maleate, Dextromethorphan Hydrobromide, Pseudoephedrine Hydrochloride) Novartis Consumer ..... ▣ 682
Triaminic Cough & Sore Throat Softchews (Acetaminophen, Dextromethorphan Hydrobromide, Pseudoephedrine Hydrochloride) Novartis Consumer ..... ▣ 689
Tylenol 8 Hour Extended Release Geltabs and Caplets (Acetaminophen) McNeil Consumer 1843
Children's Tylenol Plus Cold NightTime Suspension Liquid (Acetaminophen, Chlorpheniramine Maleate, Pseudoephedrine Hydrochloride) McNeil Consumer 1851
Children's Tylenol Plus Cold & Cough Suspension Liquid and Chewable Tablets (Acetaminophen, Chlorpheniramine Maleate, Dextromethorphan Hydrobromide, Pseudoephedrine Hydrochloride) McNeil Consumer 1851
Children's Tylenol Plus Cold Chewable Tablets (Acetaminophen, Chlorpheniramine Maleate, Pseudoephedrine Hydrochloride) McNeil Consumer 1851
Children's Tylenol Plus Cold Daytime Non-Drowsy Suspension Liquid (Acetaminophen, Pseudoephedrine Hydrochloride) McNeil Consumer 1851
Concentrated Tylenol Infants' Drops Plus Cold (Acetaminophen, Pseudoephedrine Hydrochloride) McNeil Consumer 1851
Concentrated Tylenol Infants' Drops Plus Cold and Cough (Acetaminophen, Dextromethorphan Hydrobromide, Pseudoephedrine Hydrochloride) McNeil Consumer 1851
Tylenol Cold Severe Congestion Non-Drowsy Caplets with Cool Burst (Acetaminophen, Dextromethorphan Hydrobromide, Guaifenesin, Pseudoephedrine Hydrochloride) McNeil Consumer 1846
Tylenol (Acetaminophen) McNeil Consumer 1843
Extra Strength Tylenol Rapid Release Gels (Acetaminophen) McNeil Consumer 1843
Tylenol (Acetaminophen) McNeil Consumer 1843
Tylenol Flu Day Non-Drowsy Gelcaps (Acetaminophen, Dextromethorphan Hydrobromide, Pseudoephedrine Hydrochloride) McNeil Consumer 1846
Concentrated Tylenol Infants' Drops Plus Cold Nasal Congestant, Fever Reducer & Pain Reliever (Acetaminophen, Pseudoephedrine Hydrochloride) McNeil Consumer ..... ▣ 668
Concentrated Tylenol Infants' Drops Plus Cold & Cough Nasal Decongestant, Fever Reducer & Pain Reliever (Acetaminophen, Dextromethorphan Hydrobromide, Pseudoephedrine Hydrochloride) McNeil Consumer ..... ▣ 668
Multi-Symptom Tylenol Cold Night Time Caplets (Acetaminophen, Chlorpheniramine Maleate, Dextromethorphan Hydrobromide, Pseudoephedrine Hydrochloride) McNeil Consumer 1845
Multi-Symptom Tylenol Cold Day Non-Drowsy Caplets and Gelcaps (Acetaminophen, Dextromethorphan Hydrobromide, Pseudoephedrine Hydrochloride) McNeil Consumer 1845
Tylenol Sore Throat Daytime Liquid with Cool Burst (Acetaminophen) McNeil Consumer 1849
Vicks NyQuil LiquiCaps/Liquid Multi-Symptom Cold/Flu Relief (Acetaminophen, Dextromethorphan Hydrobromide, Doxylamine Succinate, Pseudoephedrine Hydrochloride) Procter & Gamble ..... ▣ 725

Pain due to common cold
(*see under* Pain associated with upper respiratory infection)

Palpebral conjunctiva inflammation
Blephamide Ophthalmic Suspension (Prednisolone Acetate, Sulfacetamide Sodium) Allergan 564
FML Ophthalmic Ointment (Fluorometholone) Allergan ..... ⊙ 225
FML Ophthalmic Suspension (Fluorometholone) Allergan ..... ⊙ 224
FML Forte Ophthalmic Suspension (Fluorometholone) Allergan ..... ⊙ 223
FML-S Liquifilm Sterile Ophthalmic Suspension (Fluorometholone, Sulfacetamide Sodium) Allergan ..... ⊙ 226
Lotemax Ophthalmic Suspension 0.5% (Loteprednol Etabonate) Bausch & Lomb ..... ⊙ 249
Poly-Pred Liquifilm Ophthalmic Suspension (Neomycin Sulfate, Polymyxin B Sulfate, Prednisolone Acetate) Allergan ..... ⊙ 231
Pred Forte Ophthalmic Suspension (Prednisolone Acetate) Allergan ..... ⊙ 233
Pred-G Ophthalmic Suspension (Gentamicin Sulfate, Prednisolone Acetate) Allergan ..... ⊙ 234
Pred-G Sterile Ophthalmic Ointment (Gentamicin Sulfate, Prednisolone Acetate) Allergan ..... ⊙ 235
TobraDex Ophthalmic Ointment (Dexamethasone, Tobramycin) Alcon 558
TobraDex Ophthalmic Suspension (Dexamethasone, Tobramycin) Alcon 558
Zylet Ophthalmic Suspension (Loteprednol Etabonate, Tobramycin) Bausch & Lomb 3508

Pancreas, disseminated adenocarcinoma
(*see under* Carcinoma, pancreas)

Pancreatic cystic fibrosis
Pancrease MT Capsules (Pancrelipase) McNeil Consumer 1839
Viokase (Pancrelipase) Axcan Scandipharm 738

Pancreatic insufficiency
Creon 5 Capsules (Pancrelipase) Solvay 3195
Creon 10 Capsules (Pancrelipase) Solvay 3195
Creon 20 Capsules (Pancrelipase) Solvay 3196
Pancrease MT Capsules (Pancrelipase) McNeil Consumer 1839
Ultrase Capsules (Pancrelipase) Axcan Scandipharm 735
Ultrase MT Capsules (Pancrelipase) Axcan Scandipharm 736
Viokase (Pancrelipase) Axcan Scandipharm 738

Pancreatitis, adjunctive therapy
Plasbumin-5 (Albumin (human)) Talecris 3249
Plasbumin-20 (Albumin (human)) Talecris 3249
Plasbumin-25 (Albumin (human)) Talecris 3251

Panic disorder
Klonopin (Clonazepam) Roche Laboratories 2782
Niravam Orally Disintegrating Tablets (Alprazolam) Schwarz 3106
Paxil CR Controlled-Release Tablets (Paroxetine Hydrochloride) GlaxoSmithKline 1509
Paxil (Paroxetine Hydrochloride) GlaxoSmithKline 1501
Prozac Pulvules and Liquid (Fluoxetine Hydrochloride) Lilly 1771
Xanax XR Tablets (Alprazolam) Pharmacia & Upjohn 2655
Zoloft (Sertraline Hydrochloride) Pfizer 2581

Papillitis
(*see under* Optic neuritis)

Paralysis agitans
(*see under* Parkinson's disease)

Parkinsonism
Parcopa Orally Disintegrating Tablets (Carbidopa, Levodopa) Schwarz 3111

Parkinson's disease
Apokyn Injection (Apomorphine Hydrochloride) Mylan Bertek 2132
Cogentin Injection (Benztropine Mesylate) Merck 1903
Comtan Tablets (Entacapone) Novartis 2186
Eldepryl Capsules (Selegiline Hydrochloride) Somerset 3209
Mirapex Tablets (Pramipexole Dihydrochloride) Boehringer Ingelheim 889
Parcopa Orally Disintegrating Tablets (Carbidopa, Levodopa) Schwarz 3111
Permax Tablets (Pergolide Mesylate) Valeant 3357
Requip Tablets (Ropinirole Hydrochloride) GlaxoSmithKline 1528
Stalevo Tablets (Carbidopa, Levodopa, Entacapone) Novartis 2270
Symmetrel (Amantadine Hydrochloride) Endo Labs 1115
Tasmar Tablets (Tolcapone) Valeant 3360

Pasteurella pestis
(*see under* Yersinia pestis infections)

Pasteurella tularensis
(*see under* Francisella tularensis infections)

PCP
(*see under* Pneumocystis carinii pneumonia)

Pediculosis, human
Ovide .5% Lotion (Malathion) TaroPharma 3287

Pediculosis capitis infestation
Permethrin Lotion (Permethrin) Alpharma ..... ▣ 603

Pelvic cellulitis
(*see also under* Infections, gynecologic)
Cleocin Vaginal Ovules (Clindamycin Hydrochloride) Pharmacia & Upjohn 2613
Fortaz (Ceftazidime Sodium) GlaxoSmithKline 1422
Mefoxin for Injection (Cefoxitin Sodium) Merck 1987
Mefoxin Premixed Intravenous Solution (Cefoxitin Sodium) Merck 1990

Pelvic inflammatory disease
(*see also under* Infections, gynecologic)
E.E.S. (Erythromycin Ethylsuccinate) Abbott 449
EryPed (Erythromycin Ethylsuccinate) Abbott 445
Mefoxin for Injection (Cefoxitin Sodium) Merck 1987
Mefoxin Premixed Intravenous Solution (Cefoxitin Sodium) Merck 1990
PCE Dispertab Tablets (Erythromycin) Abbott 510
Rocephin Injectable Vials, ADD-Vantage, Galaxy, Bulk (Ceftriaxone Sodium) Roche Laboratories 2801
Zithromax for IV Infusion (Azithromycin Dihydrate) Pfizer 2573

Pemphigus
Decadron Phosphate Injection (Dexamethasone Sodium Phosphate) Merck 1931
Decadron Tablets (Dexamethasone) Merck 1929
Depo-Medrol Injectable Suspension (Methylprednisolone Acetate) Pharmacia & Upjohn 2615
Depo-Medrol Single-Dose Vial (Methylprednisolone Acetate) Pharmacia & Upjohn 2617
Hydrocortone Tablets (Hydrocortisone) Merck 1963
Pediapred Oral Solution (Prednisolone Sodium Phosphate) UCB 3319

Pemphigus, possibly effective in
Potaba (Aminobenzoate Potassium) Glenwood 1634

Penicillin therapy, an adjuvant to
E.E.S. (Erythromycin Ethylsuccinate) Abbott 449
EryPed (Erythromycin Ethylsuccinate) Abbott 445
PCE Dispertab Tablets (Erythromycin) Abbott 510

Peptococcus niger gynecologic infections
Mefoxin Premixed IV (Cefoxitin Sodium) Merck 1990

Peptococcus species gynecologic infections
Primaxin I.V. (Cilastatin Sodium, Imipenem) Merck 2024

Peptococcus species intra-abdominal infections
Primaxin I.M. (Cilastatin Sodium, Imipenem) Merck 2022
Primaxin I.V. (Cilastatin Sodium, Imipenem) Merck 2024

Peptostreptococcus species endometritis
Mefoxin for Injection (Cefoxitin Sodium) Merck 1987
Mefoxin Premixed Intravenous Solution (Cefoxitin Sodium) Merck 1990

Peptostreptococcus species endomyometritis
Invanz for Injection (Ertapenem) Merck 1974

Peptostreptococcus species gynecologic infections
Mefoxin for Injection (Cefoxitin Sodium) Merck 1987
Mefoxin Premixed Intravenous Solution (Cefoxitin Sodium) Merck 1990
Primaxin I.M. (Cilastatin Sodium, Imipenem) Merck 2022
Primaxin I.V. (Cilastatin Sodium, Imipenem) Merck 2024

Peptostreptococcus species infections
Invanz for Injection (Ertapenem) Merck 1974
Mefoxin for Injection (Cefoxitin Sodium) Merck 1987
Mefoxin Premixed Intravenous Solution (Cefoxitin Sodium) Merck 1990
Merrem I.V. (Meropenem) AstraZeneca 687

Primaxin I.M. (Cilastatin Sodium, Imipenem) Merck ... 2022
Primaxin I.V. (Cilastatin Sodium, Imipenem) Merck ... 2024
Rocephin Injectable Vials, ADD-Vantage, Galaxy, Bulk (Ceftriaxone Sodium) Roche Laboratories ... 2801
Tygacil for Injection (Tigecycline) Wyeth ... 3489

Peptostreptococcus species intra-abdominal infections
Invanz for Injection (Ertapenem) Merck ... 1974
Merrem I.V. (Meropenem) AstraZeneca ... 687
Primaxin I.M. (Cilastatin Sodium, Imipenem) Merck ... 2022
Primaxin I.V. (Cilastatin Sodium, Imipenem) Merck ... 2024
Rocephin Injectable Vials, ADD-Vantage, Galaxy, Bulk (Ceftriaxone Sodium) Roche Laboratories ... 2801
Tygacil for Injection (Tigecycline) Wyeth ... 3489

Peptostreptococcus species peritonitis
Merrem I.V. (Meropenem) AstraZeneca ... 687

Peptostreptococcus species skin and skin structure infections
Invanz for Injection (Ertapenem) Merck ... 1974
Mefoxin for Injection (Cefoxitin Sodium) Merck ... 1987
Mefoxin Premixed Intravenous Solution (Cefoxitin Sodium) Merck ... 1990
Merrem I.V. (Meropenem) AstraZeneca ... 687
Primaxin I.V. (Cilastatin Sodium, Imipenem) Merck ... 2024
Rocephin Injectable Vials, ADD-Vantage, Galaxy, Bulk (Ceftriaxone Sodium) Roche Laboratories ... 2801

Peripheral blood progenitor cell transplantation
(*see under* Hematopoietic progenitor cells, mobilization of)

Peritonitis
(*see also under* Infections, intra-abdominal)
Cleocin Vaginal Ovules (Clindamycin Hydrochloride) Pharmacia & Upjohn ... 2613
Fortaz (Ceftazidime Sodium) GlaxoSmithKline ... 1422
Garamycin Injectable (Gentamicin Sulfate) Schering ... 3028
Mefoxin for Injection (Cefoxitin Sodium) Merck ... 1987
Mefoxin Premixed Intravenous Solution (Cefoxitin Sodium) Merck ... 1990
Timentin ADD-Vantage (Clavulanate Potassium, Ticarcillin Disodium) GlaxoSmithKline ... 1556
Timentin Injection Galaxy Container (Clavulanate Potassium, Ticarcillin Disodium) GlaxoSmithKline ... 1559
Timentin IV Infusion (Clavulanate Potassium, Ticarcillin Disodium) GlaxoSmithKline ... 1553
Timentin Pharmacy Bulk Package (Clavulanate Potassium, Ticarcillin Disodium) GlaxoSmithKline ... 1562

Peritonitis, adjunctive therapy
Plasbumin-5 (Albumin (human)) Talecris ... 3249
Plasbumin-20 (Albumin (human)) Talecris ... 3249
Plasbumin-25 (Albumin (human)) Talecris ... 3251

Peritonitis, candidal
Cancidas for Injection (Caspofungin acetate) Merck ... 1894

Pertussis
E.E.S. (Erythromycin Ethylsuccinate) Abbott ... 449
EryPed (Erythromycin Ethylsuccinate) Abbott ... 445
Ery-Tab Tablets (Erythromycin) Abbott ... 447
Erythrocin Stearate Filmtab Tablets (Erythromycin Stearate) Abbott ... 452
Erythromycin Base Filmtab Tablets (Erythromycin) Abbott ... 454
Erythromycin Delayed-Release Capsules, USP (Erythromycin) Abbott ... 456
PCE Dispertab Tablets (Erythromycin) Abbott ... 510

Petit mal epilepsy
(*see under* Seizures, generalized, absence)

Peyronie's disease, possibly effective in
Potaba (Aminobenzoate Potassium) Glenwood ... 1634

Pharyngitis, symptomatic relief of
Advil (Ibuprofen) Wyeth ... ■ 737
Children's Advil Suspension (Ibuprofen) Wyeth ... ■ 742
Children's Advil Chewable Tablets (Ibuprofen) Wyeth ... ■ 741
Advil Cold & Sinus (Ibuprofen, Pseudoephedrine Hydrochloride) Wyeth ... ■ 739
Advil Flu & Body Ache Caplets (Ibuprofen, Pseudoephedrine Hydrochloride) Wyeth ... ■ 739
Children's Advil Cold Suspension (Ibuprofen, Pseudoephedrine Hydrochloride) Wyeth ... ■ 741
Infants' Advil Concentrated Drops (Ibuprofen) Wyeth ... ■ 743
Junior Strength Advil Swallow Tablets (Ibuprofen) Wyeth ... ■ 740
Halls Fruit Breezers Pectin Throat Drops (Pectin) Cadbury Adams ... ■ 609
Hurricaine Topical Anesthetic Aerosol Spray, 2 oz. Wild Cherry (Benzocaine) Beutlich ... 835
Hurricaine Topical Anesthetic Aerosol Spray Kit, 2 oz. Wild Cherry with 200 Disposable Extension Tubes (Benzocaine) Beutlich ... 835
Hurricaine Topical Anesthetic Gel: 1 oz. Wild Cherry, Pina Colada, Watermelon, Fresh Mint, 0.18 oz. Wild Cherry (Benzocaine) Beutlich ... 835
Hurricaine Topical Anesthetic Liquid: 1 oz. Wild Cherry and Pina Colada, Swab Applicator Wild Cherry (Benzocaine) Beutlich ... 835
Junior Strength Motrin Caplets and Chewable Tablets (Ibuprofen) McNeil Consumer ... 1837
TheraFlu Cold & Cough Hot Liquid (Acetaminophen, Chlorpheniramine Maleate, Dextromethorphan Hydrobromide, Pseudoephedrine Hydrochloride) Novartis Consumer ... ■ 680
TheraFlu Cold & Sore Throat Hot Liquid (Acetaminophen, Chlorpheniramine Maleate, Pseudoephedrine Hydrochloride) Novartis Consumer ... ■ 680
TheraFlu Flu & Chest Congestion Non-Drowsy Hot Liquid (Acetaminophen, Dextromethorphan Hydrobromide, Guaifenesin, Pseudoephedrine Hydrochloride) Novartis Consumer ... ■ 681
TheraFlu Flu & Sore Throat Hot Liquid (Acetaminophen, Chlorpheniramine Maleate, Pseudoephedrine Hydrochloride) Novartis Consumer ... ■ 681
TheraFlu Severe Cold Non-Drowsy Hot Liquid (Acetaminophen, Dextromethorphan Hydrobromide, Pseudoephedrine Hydrochloride) Novartis Consumer ... ■ 683
TheraFlu Severe Cold & Cough Hot Liquid (Acetaminophen, Chlorpheniramine Maleate, Dextromethorphan Hydrobromide, Pseudoephedrine Hydrochloride) Novartis Consumer ... ■ 683
TheraFlu Severe Cold Caplets (Acetaminophen, Chlorpheniramine Maleate, Dextromethorphan Hydrobromide, Pseudoephedrine Hydrochloride) Novartis Consumer ... ■ 679
TheraFlu Severe Cold Hot Liquid (Acetaminophen, Chlorpheniramine Maleate, Dextromethorphan Hydrobromide, Pseudoephedrine Hydrochloride) Novartis Consumer ... ■ 682
TheraFlu Severe Cold Non-Drowsy Caplets (Acetaminophen, Dextromethorphan Hydrobromide, Pseudoephedrine Hydrochloride) Novartis Consumer ... ■ 679
Triaminic Sore Throat Spray (Phenol) Novartis Consumer ... ■ 689
Tylenol Cold Severe Congestion Non-Drowsy Caplets with Cool Burst (Acetaminophen, Dextromethorphan Hydrobromide, Guaifenesin, Pseudoephedrine Hydrochloride) McNeil Consumer ... 1846
Tylenol Severe Allergy Caplets (Acetaminophen, Diphenhydramine Hydrochloride) McNeil Consumer ... 1844
Multi-Symptom Tylenol Cold Night Time Caplets (Acetaminophen, Chlorpheniramine Maleate, Dextromethorphan Hydrobromide, Pseudoephedrine Hydrochloride) McNeil Consumer ... 1845
Multi-Symptom Tylenol Cold Day Non-Drowsy Caplets and Gelcaps (Acetaminophen, Dextromethorphan Hydrobromide, Pseudoephedrine Hydrochloride) McNeil Consumer ... 1845

Pharyngitis, treatment of
Biaxin/Biaxin XL (Clarithromycin) Abbott ... 402
Ceftin (Cefuroxime Axetil) GlaxoSmithKline ... 1369
E.E.S. (Erythromycin Ethylsuccinate) Abbott ... 449
EryPed (Erythromycin Ethylsuccinate) Abbott ... 445
Ery-Tab Tablets (Erythromycin) Abbott ... 447
Erythrocin Stearate Filmtab Tablets (Erythromycin Stearate) Abbott ... 452
Erythromycin Base Filmtab Tablets (Erythromycin) Abbott ... 454
Omnicef Capsules (Cefdinir) Abbott ... 506
Omnicef for Oral Suspension (Cefdinir) Abbott ... 506
PCE Dispertab Tablets (Erythromycin) Abbott ... 510
Spectracef Tablets (Cefditoren Pivoxil) Purdue Pharmaceutical ... 2706
Suprax (Cefixime) Lupin ... 1811
Vantin Tablets and Oral Suspension (Cefpodoxime Proxetil) Pharmacia & Upjohn ... 2650
Zithromax (Azithromycin Dihydrate) Pfizer ... 2568
Zithromax for Oral Suspension, 300 mg, 600 mg, 900 mg, 1200 mg (Azithromycin Dihydrate) Pfizer ... 2561
Zithromax Tablets, 250 mg, 500 mg (Azithromycin Dihydrate) Pfizer ... 2561
Zithromax Tablets, 600 mg (Azithromycin Dihydrate) Pfizer ... 2568
Zithromax Tri-Pak (Azithromycin Dihydrate) Pfizer ... 2561
Zithromax Z-Pak (Azithromycin Dihydrate) Pfizer ... 2568

Pheochromocytoma
Demser Capsules (Metyrosine) Merck ... 1933
Dibenzyline Capsules (Phenoxybenzamine Hydrochloride) WellSpring ... 3390

Pheochromocytoma, adjunctive therapy
Demser Capsules (Metyrosine) Merck ... 1933

Phosphorus deficiency
(*see under* Hypophosphatemia)

Photophobia
Voltaren Ophthalmic Solution (Diclofenac Sodium) Novartis ... 2300

Phycomycosis
(*see under* Zygomycosis)

Pinworm infestation
(*see under* Enterobiasis)

Pityrosporon orbiculare infections
Loprox Gel (Ciclopirox) Medicis ... 1861
Lotrimin (Clotrimazole) Schering ... 3053
Mentax Cream (Butenafine Hydrochloride) Mylan Bertek ... 2152
Nizoral 2% Shampoo (Ketoconazole) McNeil Consumer ... 1838
Oxistat (Oxiconazole Nitrate) GlaxoSmithKline ... 1498
Spectazole Cream (Econazole Nitrate) OrthoNeutrogena ... 2390

Plague
Dynacin Tablets (Minocycline Hydrochloride) Medicis ... 1859

Plasmodium infection
(*see under* P. falciparum infections; P. malariae infections; P. ovale infections; P. vivax infections)

Platelet transfusions, reduction of the need for
Neumega for Injection (Oprelvekin) Wyeth ... 3433

Pleural effusion, malignant
Alimta for Injection (Pemetrexed) Lilly ... 1722

PMDD
(*see under* Dysphoric disorder, premenstrual)

PMS
(*see under* Pre-Menstrual syndrome, management of)

Pneumococcal disease, immunization against
Pneumovax 23 (Pneumococcal Vaccine, Polyvalent) Merck ... 2020
Prevnar for Injection (Pneumococcal vaccine, diphtheria conjugate) Wyeth ... 3460

Pneumocystis carinii pneumonia
Mepron Suspension (Atovaquone) GlaxoSmithKline ... 1487

Pneumonia
(*see also under* Infections, lower respiratory tract)
Avelox (Moxifloxacin Hydrochloride) Schering ... 2984
Biaxin/Biaxin XL (Clarithromycin) Abbott ... 402
Cleocin Vaginal Ovules (Clindamycin Hydrochloride) Pharmacia & Upjohn ... 2613
Ery-Tab Tablets (Erythromycin) Abbott ... 447
Erythrocin Stearate Filmtab Tablets (Erythromycin Stearate) Abbott ... 452
Erythromycin Base Filmtab Tablets (Erythromycin) Abbott ... 454
Factive Tablets (Gemifloxacin Mesylate) Oscient ... 2464
Fortaz (Ceftazidime Sodium) GlaxoSmithKline ... 1422
Invanz for Injection (Ertapenem) Merck ... 1974
Ketek Tablets (Telithromycin) Sanofi-Aventis ... 2920
Levaquin in 5% Dextrose Injection (Levofloxacin) Ortho-McNeil ... 2453
Levaquin (Levofloxacin) Ortho-McNeil ... 2453
Maxipime for Injection (Cefepime Hydrochloride) Elan ... 1093
Mefoxin for Injection (Cefoxitin Sodium) Merck ... 1987
Mefoxin Premixed Intravenous Solution (Cefoxitin Sodium) Merck ... 1990
Omnicef Capsules (Cefdinir) Abbott ... 506
Omnicef for Oral Suspension (Cefdinir) Abbott ... 506
Tequin Injection (Gatifloxacin) Bristol-Myers Squibb ... 964
Tequin Tablets (Gatifloxacin) Bristol-Myers Squibb ... 964

Vantin Tablets and Oral Suspension (Cefpodoxime Proxetil) Pharmacia & Upjohn 2650
Zinacef Injection (Cefuroxime) GlaxoSmithKline 1604
Zinacef for Injection (Cefuroxime) GlaxoSmithKline 1604
Zithromax Capsules, 250 mg (Azithromycin Dihydrate) Pfizer 2568
Zithromax for IV Infusion (Azithromycin Dihydrate) Pfizer 2573
Zithromax for Oral Suspension, 1 g (Azithromycin Dihydrate) Pfizer 2568
Zithromax for Oral Suspension, 300 mg, 600 mg, 900 mg, 1200 mg (Azithromycin Dihydrate) Pfizer 2561
Zithromax Tablets, 250 mg, 500 mg (Azithromycin Dihydrate) Pfizer 2561
Zithromax Tablets, 600 mg (Azithromycin Dihydrate) Pfizer 2568
Zithromax Tri-Pak (Azithromycin Dihydrate) Pfizer 2561
Zithromax Z-Pak (Azithromycin Dihydrate) Pfizer 2568
Zmax for Oral Suspension (Azithromycin) Pfizer 2577
Zyvox (Linezolid) Pharmacia & Upjohn 2661

Pneumonia, community-acquired
Augmentin XR Extended-Release Tablets (Amoxicillin, Clavulanate Potassium) GlaxoSmithKline 1340
Avelox (Moxifloxacin Hydrochloride) Schering 2984
Factive Tablets (Gemifloxacin Mesylate) Oscient 2464
Invanz for Injection (Ertapenem) Merck 1974
Ketek Tablets (Telithromycin) Sanofi-Aventis 2920
Levaquin (Levofloxacin) Ortho-McNeil 2453
Spectracef Tablets (Cefditoren Pivoxil) Purdue Pharmaceutical 2706
Tequin Injection (Gatifloxacin) Bristol-Myers Squibb 964
Tequin Tablets (Gatifloxacin) Bristol-Myers Squibb 964
Vantin Tablets and Oral Suspension (Cefpodoxime Proxetil) Pharmacia & Upjohn 2650
Zithromax Capsules, 250 mg (Azithromycin Dihydrate) Pfizer 2568
Zithromax for IV Infusion (Azithromycin Dihydrate) Pfizer 2573
Zithromax for Oral Suspension, 1 g (Azithromycin Dihydrate) Pfizer 2568
Zithromax for Oral Suspension, 300 mg, 600 mg, 900 mg, 1200 mg (Azithromycin Dihydrate) Pfizer 2561
Zithromax Tablets, 250 mg, 500 mg (Azithromycin Dihydrate) Pfizer 2561
Zithromax Tablets, 600 mg (Azithromycin Dihydrate) Pfizer 2568
Zithromax Tri-Pak (Azithromycin Dihydrate) Pfizer 2561
Zithromax Z-Pak (Azithromycin Dihydrate) Pfizer 2568
Zmax for Oral Suspension (Azithromycin) Pfizer 2577
Zosyn (Piperacillin Sodium, Tazobactam Sodium) Wyeth 3492
Zyvox (Linezolid) Pharmacia & Upjohn 2661

Pneumonia, idiopathic eosinophilic
Decadron Tablets (Dexamethasone) Merck 1929

Pneumonia, nosocomial
(*see also under* Infections, lower respiratory tract)
Cipro I.V. (Ciprofloxacin) Schering 2998
Cipro I.V. Pharmacy Bulk Package (Ciprofloxacin) Bayer 3509
Zosyn (Piperacillin Sodium, Tazobactam Sodium) Wyeth 3492
Zyvox (Linezolid) Pharmacia & Upjohn 2661

Pneumonia, pneumocystis carinii
(*see under* Pneumocystis carinii pneumonia)

Pneumonitis, aspiration
Decadron Phosphate Injection (Dexamethasone Sodium Phosphate) Merck 1931
Depo-Medrol Injectable Suspension (Methylprednisolone Acetate) Pharmacia & Upjohn 2615
Depo-Medrol Single-Dose Vial (Methylprednisolone Acetate) Pharmacia & Upjohn 2617
Hydrocortone Tablets (Hydrocortisone) Merck 1963
Pediapred Oral Solution (Prednisolone Sodium Phosphate) UCB 3319

Poison ivy
(*see under* Dermatitis, contact)

Poison oak
(*see under* Dermatitis, contact)

Poison sumac
(*see under* Dermatitis, contact)

Poliomyelitis, prevention of
(*see under* Immunization, poliovirus 1, 2, and 3)

Pollinosis
(*see also under* Rhinitis, seasonal allergic)
Advil Allergy Sinus Caplets (Chlorpheniramine Maleate, Ibuprofen, Pseudoephedrine Hydrochloride) Wyeth .... ■ 737
Advil Multi-Symptom Cold Caplets (Chlorpheniramine Maleate, Ibuprofen, Pseudoephedrine Hydrochloride) Wyeth .... ■ 738
Alavert Allergy & Sinus D-12 Hour Tablets (Loratadine, Pseudoephedrine Sulfate) Wyeth .... ■ 743
Alavert (Loratadine) Wyeth .... ■ 743
Benadryl Allergy & Cold Tablets (Acetaminophen, Diphenhydramine Hydrochloride, Pseudoephedrine Hydrochloride) Pfizer Consumer Healthcare .... ■ 692
Benadryl Allergy & Sinus Headache Caplets & Gelcaps (Acetaminophen, Diphenhydramine Hydrochloride, Pseudoephedrine Hydrochloride) Pfizer Consumer Healthcare .... ■ 693
Children's Benadryl Allergy Liquid (Diphenhydramine Hydrochloride) Pfizer Consumer Healthcare .... ■ 695
Children's Benadryl Dye-Free Allergy Liquid (Diphenhydramine Hydrochloride) Pfizer Consumer Healthcare .... ■ 695
Benadryl Dye-Free Allergy Liqui-Gels Softgels (Diphenhydramine Hydrochloride) Pfizer Consumer Healthcare .... ■ 692
Children's Benadryl D Allergy & Sinus Fastmelt Tablets (Diphenhydramine Citrate, Pseudoephedrine Hydrochloride) Pfizer Consumer Healthcare .... ■ 694
Children's Benadryl D Liquid Medication (Diphenhydramine Hydrochloride, Pseudoephedrine Hydrochloride) Pfizer Consumer Healthcare .... ■ 693
Benadryl D Tablets (Diphenhydramine Hydrochloride, Pseudoephedrine Hydrochloride) Pfizer Consumer Healthcare .... ■ 694
Children's Benadryl Allergy Fastmelt Tablets (Diphenhydramine Citrate) Pfizer Consumer Healthcare .... ■ 696
Children's Claritin 24 Hour Non-Drowsy Allergy Syrup (Loratadine) Schering-Plough .... ■ 732
Claritin Non-Drowsy 24 Hour Tablets (Loratadine) Schering-Plough .... ■ 731
Claritin Reditabs 24 Hour Non-Drowsy Tablets (Loratadine) Schering-Plough .... ■ 732
Claritin-D Non-Drowsy 12 Hour Tablets (Loratadine, Pseudoephedrine Sulfate) Schering-Plough .... ■ 731
Claritin-D Non-Drowsy 24 Hour Tablets (Loratadine, Pseudoephedrine Sulfate) Schering-Plough .... ■ 731
Children's Dimetapp Cold & Allergy Elixir (Brompheniramine Maleate, Pseudoephedrine Hydrochloride) Wyeth .... ■ 745
Children's Dimetapp ND Non-Drowsy Allergy Syrup (Loratadine) Wyeth .... ■ 746
PediaCare Decongestant Infants' Drops (Pseudoephedrine Hydrochloride) Pfizer Consumer Healthcare .... ■ 705
PediaCare Long-Acting Cough Plus Cold Liquid (Dextromethorphan Hydrobromide, Pseudoephedrine Hydrochloride) Pfizer Consumer Healthcare .... ■ 704
PediaCare NightRest Cough & Cold Liquid (Chlorpheniramine Maleate, Dextromethorphan Hydrobromide, Pseudoephedrine Hydrochloride) Pfizer Consumer Healthcare .... ■ 704
Sudafed Sinus & Allergy Tablets (Chlorpheniramine Maleate, Pseudoephedrine Hydrochloride) Pfizer Consumer Healthcare .... ■ 710
TheraFlu Thin Strips Multi Symptom (Diphenhydramine Hydrochloride) Novartis Consumer .... ■ 684
Triaminic Allerchews (Loratadine) Novartis Consumer .... ■ 684
Triaminic Cold & Allergy Liquid (Chlorpheniramine Maleate, Pseudoephedrine Hydrochloride) Novartis Consumer .... ■ 685
Triaminic Thin Strips Cough & Runny Nose (Diphenhydramine Hydrochloride) Novartis Consumer .... ■ 690
Children's Tylenol Plus Cold & Allergy Suspension Liquid (Acetaminophen, Diphenhydramine Hydrochloride, Pseudoephedrine Hydrochloride) McNeil Consumer .. 1850
Tylenol Severe Allergy Caplets (Acetaminophen, Diphenhydramine Hydrochloride) McNeil Consumer 1844
Vicks Sinex 12-Hour Nasal Spray and Ultra Fine Mist for Sinus Relief (Oxymetazoline Hydrochloride) Procter & Gamble 2678
Vicks Sinex Nasal Spray and Ultra Fine Mist for Sinus Relief (Phenylephrine Hydrochloride) Procter & Gamble 2677
Zicam Allergy Relief Nasal Pump (Histanium Hydrochloricum, Luffa operculata, Galphimia Glauca, Sulfur) Matrixx .... ■ 665
Zicam Extreme Congestion Relief Nasal Pump (Oxymetazoline Hydrochloride) Matrixx .... ■ 666
Zicam Sinus Relief Nasal Pump (Oxymetazoline Hydrochloride) Matrixx .... ■ 666

Polycythemia vera
Mustargen for Injection (Mechlorethamine Hydrochloride) Merck 2007

Polydipsia, temporary, management of
DDAVP Injection 4 mcg/mL (Desmopressin Acetate) Sanofi-Aventis 2893
DDAVP Nasal Spray (Desmopressin Acetate) Sanofi-Aventis 2894
DDAVP Tablets (Desmopressin Acetate) Sanofi-Aventis 2895
Desmopressin Acetate Rhinal Tube (Desmopressin Acetate) Ferring 1144

Polymyositis
(*see under* Dermatomyositis, systemic)

Polyps, nasal, prevention of recurrence
Beconase AQ Nasal Spray (Beclomethasone Dipropionate Monohydrate) GlaxoSmithKline 1359

Polyps, nasal, treatment of
Nasonex Nasal Spray (Mometasone Furoate Monohydrate) Schering 3058

Polyuria, temporary, management of
DDAVP Injection 4 mcg/mL (Desmopressin Acetate) Sanofi-Aventis 2893
DDAVP Nasal Spray (Desmopressin Acetate) Sanofi-Aventis 2894
DDAVP Tablets (Desmopressin Acetate) Sanofi-Aventis 2895
Desmopressin Acetate Rhinal Tube (Desmopressin Acetate) Ferring 1144

Porphyria, acute intermittent, amelioration of recurrent attacks of
Panhematin (Hemin) Ovation 2487

Porphyromonas asaccharolytica endomyometritis
Invanz for Injection (Ertapenem) Merck 1974

Postnasal drip
(*see under* Cold, common, symptomatic relief of)

Post-traumatic stress disorder
(*see under* Stress disorder, post-traumatic)

Prader-Willi syndrome
Genotropin Lyophilized Powder (Somatropin) Pharmacia & Upjohn 2642

Pregnancy, prevention of
Alesse-28 Tablets (Ethinyl Estradiol, Levonorgestrel) Wyeth 3392
Depo-Provera Contraceptive Injection (Medroxyprogesterone Acetate) Pharmacia & Upjohn 2619
depo-subQ provera 104 Injectable Suspension (Medroxyprogesterone Acetate) Pharmacia & Upjohn 2622
Lo/Ovral-28 Tablets (Ethinyl Estradiol, Norgestrel) Wyeth 3423
Mirena Intrauterine System (Levonorgestrel) Berlex 810
NuvaRing (Etonogestrel, Ethinyl Estradiol) Organon USA 2357
Ortho-Cept Tablets (Desogestrel, Ethinyl Estradiol) Ortho Women's Health & Urology 2395
Ortho-Cyclen Tablets (Ethinyl Estradiol, Norgestimate) Ortho Women's Health & Urology 2414
Ortho Evra Transdermal System (Norelgestromin, Ethinyl Estradiol) Ortho Women's Health & Urology 2402
Ortho Micronor Tablets (Norethindrone) Ortho Women's Health & Urology 2411
Ortho Tri-Cyclen Tablets (Ethinyl Estradiol, Norgestimate) Ortho Women's Health & Urology 2414
Ortho Tri-Cyclen Lo Tablets (Ethinyl Estradiol, Norgestimate) Ortho Women's Health & Urology 2421
Plan B Tablets (Levonorgestrel) Duramed 1068
Seasonale Tablets (Ethinyl Estradiol, Levonorgestrel) Duramed 1073
Triphasil-28 Tablets (Ethinyl Estradiol, Levonorgestrel) Wyeth 3483
Yasmin 28 Tablets (Ethinyl Estradiol, Drospirenone) Berlex 818

Pregnancy, vitamin supplement for
(*see under* Vitamin deficiency, postpartum; Vitamin deficiency, prenatal)

Premenstrual dysphoric disorder
(*see under* Dysphoric disorder, premenstrual)

Premenstrual syndrome
(*see under* Pre-Menstrual syndrome, management of)

Premenstrual syndrome, management of
(*see also under* Dysphoric disorder, premenstrual)

Women's Tylenol Menstrual Relief Caplets (Acetaminophen, Pamabrom) McNeil Consumer 1849

Prevotella bivia endomyometritis

Invanz for Injection (Ertapenem) Merck 1974

Prevotella melaninogenica, endometritis

Timentin ADD-Vantage (Clavulanate Potassium, Ticarcillin Disodium) GlaxoSmithKline 1556

Timentin IV Infusion (Clavulanate Potassium, Ticarcillin Disodium) GlaxoSmithKline 1553

Prevotella melaninogenica, infections

Timentin ADD-Vantage (Clavulanate Potassium, Ticarcillin Disodium) GlaxoSmithKline 1556

Timentin IV Infusion (Clavulanate Potassium, Ticarcillin Disodium) GlaxoSmithKline 1553

Prinzmetal's angina
(*see under* Angina, Prinzmetal's)

Proctitis, ulcerative

Canasa Rectal Suppositories (Mesalamine) Axcan Scandipharm 726

Promote the natural immune system of the body

Ambrotose AO Capsules (Herbals with Vitamins) Mannatech .... ▣ 769

immune[26] Balance Powder Shake Mix (Egg product, hyperimmune) Legacy for Life .... ▣ 768

immune[26] Complete Support Powder Shake Mix (Egg product, hyperimmune) Legacy for Life .... ▣ 768

immune[26] Powder, Capsules and Chewable Tablets (Egg product, hyperimmune) Legacy for Life .... ▣ 768

SynergyDefense Capsules (Herbals, Multiple) Awareness Corporation/AwarenessLife .... ▣ 760

Propionibacterium acnes infections

Dynacin Tablets (Minocycline Hydrochloride) Medicis 1859

Propionibacterium species gynecologic infections

Primaxin I.V. (Cilastatin Sodium, Imipenem) Merck 2024

Prostatic cancer
(*see under* Carcinoma, prostate)

Prostatic cancer, palliative treatment of
(*see under* Carcinoma, prostate, palliative treatment of)

Prostatic hyperplasia, benign, symptomatic treatment

Avodart Soft Gelatin Capsules (Dutasteride) GlaxoSmithKline 1353

Flomax Capsules (Tamsulosin Hydrochloride) Boehringer Ingelheim 881

Hytrin Capsules (Terazosin Hydrochloride) Abbott 469

Proscar Tablets (Finasteride) Merck 2040

Uroxatral Tablets (Alfuzosin Hydrochloride) Sanofi-Aventis 2957

Prostatitis

Ancef for Injection (Cefazolin Sodium) GlaxoSmithKline 1318

Cipro I.V. (Ciprofloxacin) Schering 2998

Cipro I.V. Pharmacy Bulk Package (Ciprofloxacin) Bayer 3509

Cipro (Ciprofloxacin) Schering 2991

Noroxin Tablets (Norfloxacin) Merck 2009

Proteinuria, remission of in lupus erythematosus

Decadron Tablets (Dexamethasone) Merck 1929

Proteinuria, remission of in nephrotic syndrome

Decadron Phosphate Injection (Dexamethasone Sodium Phosphate) Merck 1931

Decadron Tablets (Dexamethasone) Merck 1929

Depo-Medrol Injectable Suspension (Methylprednisolone Acetate) Pharmacia & Upjohn 2615

Depo-Medrol Single-Dose Vial (Methylprednisolone Acetate) Pharmacia & Upjohn 2617

Hydrocortone Tablets (Hydrocortisone) Merck 1963

Pediapred Oral Solution (Prednisolone Sodium Phosphate) UCB 3319

Proteus, indole-positive, infections
(*see under* Morganella morganii infections)

Proteus mirabilis
(*see under* P. mirabilis infections)

Proteus species gynecologic infections

Primaxin I.V. (Cilastatin Sodium, Imipenem) Merck 2024

Proteus species infections

Fortaz (Ceftazidime Sodium) GlaxoSmithKline 1422

Garamycin Injectable (Gentamicin Sulfate) Schering 3028

Primaxin I.V. (Cilastatin Sodium, Imipenem) Merck 2024

Proteus species infections, ocular, indole-negative

Pred-G Ophthalmic Suspension (Gentamicin Sulfate, Prednisolone Acetate) Allergan .... ⊙ 234

Proteus species intra-abdominal infections

Primaxin I.V. (Cilastatin Sodium, Imipenem) Merck 2024

Proteus species skin and skin structure infections

Fortaz (Ceftazidime Sodium) GlaxoSmithKline 1422

Proteus vulgaris
(*see under* P. vulgaris infections)

Prothrombin deficiency, anticoagulant-induced

AquaMEPHYTON Injection (Vitamin K_1) Merck 1887

Mephyton Tablets (Vitamin K_1) Merck 1993

Providencia rettgeri infections

Cipro I.V. (Ciprofloxacin) Schering 2998

Cipro I.V. Pharmacy Bulk Package (Ciprofloxacin) Bayer 3509

Cipro (Ciprofloxacin) Schering 2991

Mefoxin for Injection (Cefoxitin Sodium) Merck 1987

Mefoxin Premixed Intravenous Solution (Cefoxitin Sodium) Merck 1990

Primaxin I.V. (Cilastatin Sodium, Imipenem) Merck 2024

Providencia rettgeri urinary tract infections

Cipro I.V. (Ciprofloxacin) Schering 2998

Cipro I.V. Pharmacy Bulk Package (Ciprofloxacin) Bayer 3509

Cipro (Ciprofloxacin) Schering 2991

Mefoxin for Injection (Cefoxitin Sodium) Merck 1987

Mefoxin Premixed Intravenous Solution (Cefoxitin Sodium) Merck 1990

Primaxin I.V. (Cilastatin Sodium, Imipenem) Merck 2024

Providencia species infections

Mefoxin for Injection (Cefoxitin Sodium) Merck 1987

Mefoxin Premixed Intravenous Solution (Cefoxitin Sodium) Merck 1990

Providencia species urinary tract infections

Mefoxin for Injection (Cefoxitin Sodium) Merck 1987

Mefoxin Premixed Intravenous Solution (Cefoxitin Sodium) Merck 1990

Providencia stuartii infections

Cipro I.V. (Ciprofloxacin) Schering 2998

Cipro I.V. Pharmacy Bulk Package (Ciprofloxacin) Bayer 3509

Cipro (Ciprofloxacin) Schering 2991

Providencia stuartii skin and skin structure infections

Cipro I.V. (Ciprofloxacin) Schering 2998

Cipro I.V. Pharmacy Bulk Package (Ciprofloxacin) Bayer 3509

Cipro (Ciprofloxacin) Schering 2991

Pruritus, anogenital

Analpram-HC (Hydrocortisone Acetate, Pramoxine Hydrochloride) Ferndale 1136

Cortizone•5 Ointment (Hydrocortisone) Pfizer Consumer Healthcare .... ▣ 699

Cortizone•10 Creme (Hydrocortisone) Pfizer Consumer Healthcare .... ▣ 699

Cortizone•10 Ointment (Hydrocortisone) Pfizer Consumer Healthcare .... ▣ 699

Cortizone•10 Plus Creme (Hydrocortisone) Pfizer Consumer Healthcare .... ▣ 700

Preparation H Maximum Strength Cream (Glycerin, Petrolatum, Phenylephrine Hydrochloride, Pramoxine Hydrochloride) Wyeth .... ▣ 747

Preparation H Cooling Gel (Phenylephrine Hydrochloride) Wyeth .... ▣ 747

Preparation H Hydrocortisone Cream (Hydrocortisone) Wyeth .... ▣ 748

Preparation H (Mineral Oil, Petrolatum, Phenylephrine Hydrochloride, Shark Liver Oil) Wyeth .... ▣ 747

Preparation H Medicated Wipes (Witch Hazel) Wyeth .... ▣ 748

ProctoFoam-HC (Hydrocortisone Acetate, Pramoxine Hydrochloride) Schwarz 3113

Tucks Anti-Itch (Hydrocortisone Acetate) Pfizer Consumer Healthcare .... ▣ 712

Tucks Hemorrhoidal Ointment (Mineral Oil, Pramoxine Hydrochloride, Zinc Oxide, Mineral Oil, Pramoxine Hydrochloride, Zinc Oxide) Pfizer Consumer Healthcare .... ▣ 711

Tucks Hemorrhoidal Suppositories (Starch, topical) Pfizer Consumer Healthcare .... ▣ 712

Tucks Witch Hazel Hemorrhoidal Pad (Witch Hazel) Pfizer Consumer Healthcare .... ▣ 712

Pruritus, ocular

Acular Ophthalmic Solution (Ketorolac Tromethamine) Allergan 561

Visine-A Eye Allergy Relief Eye Drops (Naphazoline Hydrochloride, Pheniramine Maleate) Pfizer Consumer .... ⊙ 278

Visine-A Eye Drops (Naphazoline Hydrochloride, Pheniramine Maleate) Pfizer Consumer Healthcare .... ▣ 713

Pruritus, rhinopharyngeal, symptomatic relief of

Advil Allergy Sinus Caplets (Chlorpheniramine Maleate, Ibuprofen, Pseudoephedrine Hydrochloride) Wyeth .... ▣ 737

Advil Multi-Symptom Cold Caplets (Chlorpheniramine Maleate, Ibuprofen, Pseudoephedrine Hydrochloride) Wyeth .... ▣ 738

Alavert Allergy & Sinus D-12 Hour Tablets (Loratadine, Pseudoephedrine Sulfate) Wyeth .... ▣ 743

Alavert (Loratadine) Wyeth .... ▣ 743

Allegra-D 12 Hour Extended-Release Tablets (Fexofenadine Hydrochloride, Pseudoephedrine Hydrochloride) Sanofi-Aventis 2860

Benadryl Allergy (Diphenhydramine Hydrochloride) Pfizer Consumer Healthcare .... ▣ 691

Benadryl Allergy & Sinus Headache Caplets & Gelcaps (Acetaminophen, Diphenhydramine Hydrochloride, Pseudoephedrine Hydrochloride) Pfizer Consumer Healthcare .... ▣ 693

Children's Benadryl Allergy Liquid (Diphenhydramine Hydrochloride) Pfizer Consumer Healthcare .... ▣ 695

Children's Benadryl D Allergy & Sinus Fastmelt Tablets (Diphenhydramine Citrate, Pseudoephedrine Hydrochloride) Pfizer Consumer Healthcare .... ▣ 694

Children's Benadryl D Liquid Medication (Diphenhydramine Hydrochloride, Pseudoephedrine Hydrochloride) Pfizer Consumer Healthcare .... ▣ 693

Benadryl D Tablets (Diphenhydramine Hydrochloride, Pseudoephedrine Hydrochloride) Pfizer Consumer Healthcare .... ▣ 694

Children's Benadryl Allergy Fastmelt Tablets (Diphenhydramine Citrate) Pfizer Consumer Healthcare .... ▣ 696

Children's Claritin 24 Hour Non-Drowsy Allergy Syrup (Loratadine) Schering-Plough .... ▣ 732

Claritin Non-Drowsy 24 Hour Tablets (Loratadine) Schering-Plough .... ▣ 731

Claritin Reditabs 24 Hour Non-Drowsy Tablets (Loratadine) Schering-Plough .... ▣ 732

Claritin-D Non-Drowsy 12 Hour Tablets (Loratadine, Pseudoephedrine Sulfate) Schering-Plough .... ▣ 731

Claritin-D Non-Drowsy 24 Hour Tablets (Loratadine, Pseudoephedrine Sulfate) Schering-Plough .... ▣ 731

Children's Dimetapp ND Non-Drowsy Allergy Syrup (Loratadine) Wyeth .... ▣ 746

TheraFlu Cold & Cough Hot Liquid (Acetaminophen, Chlorpheniramine Maleate, Dextromethorphan Hydrobromide, Pseudoephedrine Hydrochloride) Novartis Consumer .... ▣ 680

TheraFlu Cold & Sore Throat Hot Liquid (Acetaminophen, Chlorpheniramine Maleate, Pseudoephedrine Hydrochloride) Novartis Consumer .... ▣ 680

TheraFlu Flu & Sore Throat Hot Liquid (Acetaminophen, Chlorpheniramine Maleate, Pseudoephedrine Hydrochloride) Novartis Consumer .... ▣ 681

TheraFlu Severe Cold & Cough Hot Liquid (Acetaminophen, Chlorpheniramine Maleate, Dextromethorphan Hydrobromide, Pseudoephedrine Hydrochloride) Novartis Consumer .... ▣ 683

TheraFlu Severe Cold Caplets (Acetaminophen, Chlorpheniramine Maleate, Dextromethorphan Hydrobromide, Pseudoephedrine Hydrochloride) Novartis Consumer .... ▣ 679

TheraFlu Severe Cold Hot Liquid (Acetaminophen, Chlorpheniramine Maleate, Dextromethorphan Hydrobromide, Pseudoephedrine Hydrochloride) Novartis Consumer .... ▣ 682

TheraFlu Thin Strips Multi Symptom (Diphenhydramine Hydrochloride) Novartis Consumer .... ▣ 684

Triaminic Allerchews (Loratadine) Novartis Consumer .... ▣ 684

Triaminic Thin Strips Cough & Runny Nose (Diphenhydramine Hydrochloride) Novartis Consumer .... ▣ 690

Tylenol Severe Allergy Caplets (Acetaminophen, Diphenhydramine Hydrochloride) McNeil Consumer 1844

Tylenol Sinus Night Time Caplets (Acetaminophen, Doxylamine Succinate, Pseudoephedrine Hydrochloride) McNeil Consumer .. 1848

Pruritus, systemic relief of
Non-Drowsy Claritin Hives Relief (Loratadine) Schering-Plough .... ◘733

Pruritus, topical relief of
(*see also under* Pruritus, systemic relief of)
Aclovate (Alclometasone Dipropionate) GlaxoSmithKline 1290
Benadryl Itch Relief Stick Extra Strength (Diphenhydramine Hydrochloride, Zinc Acetate) Pfizer Consumer Healthcare .... ◘696
Benadryl Itch Stopping Cream Extra Strength (Diphenhydramine Hydrochloride, Zinc Acetate) Pfizer Consumer Healthcare .... ◘697
Benadryl Itch Stopping Gel Extra Strength (Diphenhydramine Hydrochloride) Pfizer Consumer Healthcare .... ◘697
Benadryl Itch Stopping Spray Extra Strength (Diphenhydramine Hydrochloride, Zinc Acetate) Pfizer Consumer Healthcare .... ◘697
Clobevate Gel (Clobetasol Propionate) Stiefel 3213
Cortizone•5 Ointment (Hydrocortisone) Pfizer Consumer Healthcare .... ◘699
Cortizone•10 Creme (Hydrocortisone) Pfizer Consumer Healthcare .... ◘699
Cortizone•10 Ointment (Hydrocortisone) Pfizer Consumer Healthcare .... ◘699
Cortizone•10 Plus Creme (Hydrocortisone) Pfizer Consumer Healthcare .... ◘700
Cortizone•10 Maximum Strength Quick Shot Spray (Hydrocortisone) Pfizer Consumer Healthcare .... ◘700
Cutivate Cream (Fluticasone Propionate) GlaxoSmithKline 1381
Cutivate Lotion 0.05% (Fluticasone Propionate) GlaxoSmithKline 1383
Cutivate Ointment (Fluticasone Propionate) GlaxoSmithKline 1384
Diprolene Gel 0.05% (Betamethasone Dipropionate) Schering 3015
Diprolene Lotion 0.05% (Betamethasone Dipropionate) Schering 3016
Diprolene Ointment 0.05% (Betamethasone Dipropionate) Schering 3017
Diprolene AF Cream 0.05% (Betamethasone Dipropionate) Schering 3014
Diprosone Cream, USP 0.05% (Betamethasone Dipropionate) Schering 3018
Elocon Cream 0.1% (Mometasone Furoate) Schering 3019
Elocon Lotion 0.1% (Mometasone Furoate) Schering 3020
Elocon Ointment 0.1% (Mometasone Furoate) Schering 3021
Locoid Cream (Hydrocortisone Butyrate) Ferndale 1138
Locoid Lipocream Cream (Hydrocortisone Butyrate) Ferndale 1138
Locoid (Hydrocortisone Butyrate) Ferndale 1138
Luxíq Foam (Betamethasone Valerate) Connetics 1026
Olux Foam (Clobetasol Propionate) Connetics 1027
Pramosone (Hydrocortisone Acetate, Pramoxine Hydrochloride) Ferndale 1139
Preparation H Hydrocortisone Cream (Hydrocortisone) Wyeth .... ◘748
Temovate Gel (Clobetasol Propionate) GlaxoSmithKline 1550
Temovate Scalp Application (Clobetasol Propionate) GlaxoSmithKline 1551
Topicort .05% Gel (Desoximetasone) TaroPharma 3288
Topicort .25% Cream (Desoximetasone) TaroPharma 3288
Topicort .25% Ointment (Desoximetasone) TaroPharma 3288
Topicort LP .05% Cream (Desoximetasone) TaroPharma 3288
Tucks Anti-Itch (Hydrocortisone Acetate) Pfizer Consumer Healthcare .... ◘712
U-cort 1% Cream (Hydrocortisone Acetate) TaroPharma 3289

Pruritus ani
(*see under* Pruritus, anogenital)

Pseudomonas aeruginosa infections
(*see under* P. aeruginosa infections)

Pseudomonas species infections
Fortaz (Ceftazidime Sodium) GlaxoSmithKline 1422

Pseudomonas species infections, ocular
Blephamide Ophthalmic Suspension (Prednisolone Acetate, Sulfacetamide Sodium) Allergan 564

Pseudomonas species septicemia
Timentin ADD-Vantage (Clavulanate Potassium, Ticarcillin Disodium) GlaxoSmithKline 1556
Timentin Injection Galaxy Container (Clavulanate Potassium, Ticarcillin Disodium) GlaxoSmithKline 1559
Timentin IV Infusion (Clavulanate Potassium, Ticarcillin Disodium) GlaxoSmithKline 1553
Timentin Pharmacy Bulk Package (Clavulanate Potassium, Ticarcillin Disodium) GlaxoSmithKline 1562

Pseudomonas species urinary tract infections
Timentin ADD-Vantage (Clavulanate Potassium, Ticarcillin Disodium) GlaxoSmithKline 1556
Timentin Injection Galaxy Container (Clavulanate Potassium, Ticarcillin Disodium) GlaxoSmithKline 1559
Timentin IV Infusion (Clavulanate Potassium, Ticarcillin Disodium) GlaxoSmithKline 1553
Timentin Pharmacy Bulk Package (Clavulanate Potassium, Ticarcillin Disodium) GlaxoSmithKline 1562

Psittacosis
(*see under* Chlamydia psittaci infection)

Psoriasis
Amevive (Alefacept) Biogen Idec 836
Cortizone•5 Ointment (Hydrocortisone) Pfizer Consumer Healthcare .... ◘699
Cortizone•10 Plus Creme (Hydrocortisone) Pfizer Consumer Healthcare .... ◘700
Cortizone•10 Maximum Strength Quick Shot Spray (Hydrocortisone) Pfizer Consumer Healthcare .... ◘700
Dovonex Cream 0.005% (Calcipotriene) Warner Chilcott 3374
Dovonex Ointment 0.005% (Calcipotriene) Warner Chilcott 3375
Olux Foam (Clobetasol Propionate) Connetics 1027
Oxsoralen-Ultra Capsules (Methoxsalen) Valeant 3354
Psoriatec Cream (Anthralin) Sirius 3191
Raptiva for Injection (Efalizumab) Genentech 1247
Tegrin Dandruff Shampoo - Extra Conditioning (Coal Tar) GlaxoSmithKline .... ◘637
Tegrin Dandruff Shampoo - Fresh Herbal (Coal Tar) GlaxoSmithKline .... ◘638
Tegrin Skin Cream (Coal Tar) GlaxoSmithKline .... ◘638
Ultralytic 2 Cream 20% (Urea) Ivax Dermatologicals 1651
Ultralytic 2 Foam 20% (Urea) Ivax Dermatologicals 1652

Psoriasis, scalp
Clobex Shampoo (Clobetasol Propionate) Galderma 1209
Dovonex Scalp Solution 0.005% (Calcipotriene) Warner Chilcott 3375

Psoriasis, erythrodermic
Soriatane (Acitretin) Connetics 1028

Psoriasis, severe
Decadron Phosphate Injection (Dexamethasone Sodium Phosphate) Merck 1931
Depo-Medrol Injectable Suspension (Methylprednisolone Acetate) Pharmacia & Upjohn 2615
Depo-Medrol Single-Dose Vial (Methylprednisolone Acetate) Pharmacia & Upjohn 2617
Hydrocortone Tablets (Hydrocortisone) Merck 1963
Pediapred Oral Solution (Prednisolone Sodium Phosphate) UCB......... 3319

Psoriasis, severe recalcitrant
Gengraf Capsules (Cyclosporine) Abbott 458
Neoral Soft Gelatin Capsules (Cyclosporine) Novartis 2247
Neoral Oral Solution (Cyclosporine) Novartis 2247

Psoriasis, plaque-type
Vanos Cream (Fluocinonide) Medicis 1864

Psoriatic arthritis
(*see under* Arthritis, psoriatic)

Psoriatic plaques
Amevive (Alefacept) Biogen Idec 836
Clobex Lotion (Clobetasol Propionate) Galderma 1208
Decadron Phosphate Injection (Dexamethasone Sodium Phosphate) Merck 1931
Depo-Medrol Single-Dose Vial (Methylprednisolone Acetate) Pharmacia & Upjohn 2617
Dovonex Cream 0.005% (Calcipotriene) Warner Chilcott 3374
Dovonex Ointment 0.005% (Calcipotriene) Warner Chilcott 3375
Enbrel for Injection (Etanercept) Amgen 580
Gengraf Capsules (Cyclosporine) Abbott 458
Neoral Soft Gelatin Capsules (Cyclosporine) Novartis 2247
Neoral Oral Solution (Cyclosporine) Novartis 2247
Raptiva for Injection (Efalizumab) Genentech 1247

Psychotic disorders, management of the manifestations of
(*see under* Schizophrenia)

Puberty, central precocious
Lupron Depot-PED 7.5 mg, 11.25 mg and 15 mg (Leuprolide Acetate) TAP 3266
Lupron Injection Pediatric (Leuprolide Acetate) TAP 3256

Puberty, delayed, in male
Delatestryl Injection (Testosterone Enanthate) Savient 2976

Pulmonary disease, obstruction, exacerbation of
Zithromax (Azithromycin Dihydrate) Pfizer 2568
Zithromax for Oral Suspension, 300 mg, 600 mg, 900 mg, 1200 mg (Azithromycin Dihydrate) Pfizer 2561
Zithromax Tablets, 250 mg, 500 mg (Azithromycin Dihydrate) Pfizer 2561
Zithromax Tablets, 600 mg (Azithromycin Dihydrate) Pfizer 2568
Zithromax Tri-Pak (Azithromycin Dihydrate) Pfizer 2561
Zithromax Z-Pak (Azithromycin Dihydrate) Pfizer 2568

Pulmonary emphysema
(*see under* Emphysema)

Purpura, idiopathic thrombocytopenic
Carimune NF (Immune Globulin Intravenous (Human)) ZLB Behring 3501
Decadron Phosphate Injection (Dexamethasone Sodium Phosphate) Merck 1931
Decadron Tablets (Dexamethasone) Merck 1929
Depo-Medrol Injectable Suspension (Methylprednisolone Acetate) Pharmacia & Upjohn 2615
Gammagard S/D (Immune Globulin Intravenous (Human)) Baxter Healthcare 754
Gamunex Immune Globulin I.V., 10% (Immune Globulin Intravenous (Human)) Talecris 3232
Hydrocortone Tablets (Hydrocortisone) Merck 1963
Pediapred Oral Solution (Prednisolone Sodium Phosphate) UCB......... 3319
WinRho SDF (Rh_0 (D) Immune Globulin (Human)) Baxter Healthcare 763

Pyelitis
Uroqid-Acid No. 2 Tablets (Methenamine Mandelate, Sodium Acid Phosphate) Beach 785

Pyelonephritis
Cipro I.V. (Ciprofloxacin) Schering 2998
Cipro I.V. Pharmacy Bulk Package (Ciprofloxacin) Bayer 3509
Cipro (Ciprofloxacin) Schering 2991
Cipro XR Tablets (Ciprofloxacin) Schering 3004
Levaquin in 5% Dextrose Injection (Levofloxacin) Ortho-McNeil 2453
Levaquin (Levofloxacin) Ortho-McNeil 2453
Maxipime for Injection (Cefepime Hydrochloride) Elan 1093
Tequin Injection (Gatifloxacin) Bristol-Myers Squibb 964
Tequin Tablets (Gatifloxacin) Bristol-Myers Squibb 964
Uroqid-Acid No. 2 Tablets (Methenamine Mandelate, Sodium Acid Phosphate) Beach 785

Pyoderma gangrenosum
Levaquin in 5% Dextrose Injection (Levofloxacin) Ortho-McNeil 2453
Levaquin (Levofloxacin) Ortho-McNeil 2453

Q

Q fever
Dynacin Tablets (Minocycline Hydrochloride) Medicis 1859

R

Rabies, postexposure prophylaxis
HyperRAB (Rabies Immune Globulin (Human)) Talecris 3239
Rabies Vaccine RabAvert (Rabies Vaccine) Chiron 1011

Radiography, gastrointestinal tract, adjunct in
GlucaGen for Injection (Glucagon) Bedford 790
Glucagon for Injection Vials and Emergency Kit (Glucagon) Lilly 1749

Rash, diaper
Desitin Creamy Ointment (Zinc Oxide) Pfizer Consumer Healthcare .... ◘700
Desitin Ointment (Zinc Oxide) Pfizer Consumer Healthcare .... ◘700

Rash, drug
(*see under* Hypersensitivity reactions, drug-induced)

Rash, unspecified
(*see under* Skin, inflammatory conditions)

RDS
(*see under* Respiratory distress syndrome)

Reiter's syndrome
Bayer Aspirin Tablets (Aspirin) Bayer Healthcare LLC 3515
Ecotrin Enteric Coated Aspirin Low, Regular and Maximum Strength Tablets (Aspirin) GlaxoSmithKline Consumer 1627

Relapsing fever
(*see under* Borrelia recurrentis infection)

Renal allogeneic transplants, prophylaxis of organ rejection in
CellCept Capsules (Mycophenolate Mofetil) Roche Laboratories 2751
CellCept Intravenous (Mycophenolate Mofetil Hydrochloride) Roche Laboratories 2751
CellCept Oral Suspension (Mycophenolate Mofetil) Roche Laboratories 2751
CellCept Tablets (Mycophenolate Mofetil) Roche Laboratories 2751
Zenapax for Injection (Daclizumab) Roche Laboratories 2838

Renal allograft transplants, acute rejection in
Orthoclone OKT3 Sterile Solution (Muromonab-CD3) Ortho Biotech 2370

Renal allograft transplants, prophylaxis of organ rejection
Myfortic Tablets (Mycophenolic Acid) Novartis 2244

Renal dialysis, adjunctive therapy
Plasbumin-20 (Albumin (human)) Talecris 3249
Plasbumin-25 (Albumin (human)) Talecris 3251

Renal homotransplantation, adjunct for the prevention of rejection in
Azasan Tablets (Azathioprine) Salix 2844

Renal plasma flow, estimation of
Aminohippurate Sodium "PAH" Injection (Aminohippurate Sodium) Merck 1886

Renal toxicity, cumulative, cisplatin-induced
Ethyol for Injection (Amifostine) MedImmune Oncology 1869

Renal transplantation, prevention of rejection in
CellCept Capsules (Mycophenolate Mofetil) Roche Laboratories 2751
CellCept Intravenous (Mycophenolate Mofetil Hydrochloride) Roche Laboratories 2751
CellCept Oral Suspension (Mycophenolate Mofetil) Roche Laboratories 2751
CellCept Tablets (Mycophenolate Mofetil) Roche Laboratories 2751
Gengraf Capsules (Cyclosporine) Abbott 458
Neoral Soft Gelatin Capsules (Cyclosporine) Novartis 2247
Neoral Oral Solution (Cyclosporine) Novartis 2247
Prograf Capsules and Injection (Tacrolimus) Astellas 624
Rapamune Oral Solution and Tablets (Sirolimus) Wyeth 3472
Sandimmune (Cyclosporine) Novartis 2259
Simulect for Injection (Basiliximab) Novartis 2268
Thymoglobulin for Injection (Anti-thymocyte Globulin) SangStat 2848

Renal transplantation, donor organ perfusion and flushing of
Custodiol HTK Solution (Electrolyte Solution) Odyssey 2344

Renal tubular acidosis, management of
Urocit-K Tablets (Potassium Citrate) Mission 2109

Renal tubular secretory mechanism, measurement of the functional capacity of
Aminohippurate Sodium "PAH" Injection (Aminohippurate Sodium) Merck 1886

Respiratory distress syndrome
Buminate 25% Solution, USP (Albumin (human)) Baxter Healthcare 748
Curosurf Intratracheal Suspension (Poractant alfa) Dey 1057
Infasurf Intratracheal Suspension (Calfactant) Forest 1188
Plasbumin-20 (Albumin (human)) Talecris 3249
Plasbumin-25 (Albumin (human)) Talecris 3251

Respiratory symptoms, upper, relief of
(*see under* Influenza syndrome, symptomatic relief of)

Respiratory syncytial virus (RSV) infections
(*see under* Infections, lower respiratory tract, RSV-induced)

Restless legs syndrome
Requip Tablets (Ropinirole Hydrochloride) GlaxoSmithKline 1528

Retinitis, cytomegalovirus
Cytovene (Ganciclovir) Roche Laboratories 2763
Valcyte Tablets (Valganciclovir Hydrochloride) Roche Laboratories 2816

Rhabdomyosarcoma
Cosmegen for Injection (Dactinomycin) Merck 1907

Rheumatic carditis, acute
Decadron Phosphate Injection (Dexamethasone Sodium Phosphate) Merck 1931
Decadron Tablets (Dexamethasone) Merck 1929
Depo-Medrol Injectable Suspension (Methylprednisolone Acetate) Pharmacia & Upjohn 2615
Depo-Medrol Single-Dose Vial (Methylprednisolone Acetate) Pharmacia & Upjohn 2617
Hydrocortone Tablets (Hydrocortisone) Merck 1963
Pediapred Oral Solution (Prednisolone Sodium Phosphate) UCB 3319

Rheumatic fever, prophylaxis of
E.E.S. (Erythromycin Ethylsuccinate) Abbott 449
EryPed (Erythromycin Ethylsuccinate) Abbott 445
Erythromycin Base Filmtab Tablets (Erythromycin) Abbott 454
Erythromycin Delayed-Release Capsules, USP (Erythromycin) Abbott 456
PCE Dispertab Tablets (Erythromycin) Abbott 510

Rheumatoid arthritis
Anaprox Tablets (Naproxen Sodium) Roche Laboratories 2769
Anaprox DS Tablets (Naproxen Sodium) Roche Laboratories 2769
Arava Tablets (Leflunomide) Sanofi-Aventis 2881
Arthrotec Tablets (Diclofenac Sodium, Misoprostol) Searle 3126
Azasan Tablets (Azathioprine) Salix 2844
Bayer Aspirin (Aspirin) Bayer Healthcare LLC 3515
Cataflam Tablets (Diclofenac Potassium) Novartis 2173
Celebrex Capsules (Celecoxib) Searle 3130
Clinoril Tablets (Sulindac) Merck 1899
Cuprimine Capsules (Penicillamine) Merck 1925
Decadron Phosphate Injection (Dexamethasone Sodium Phosphate) Merck 1931
Decadron Tablets (Dexamethasone) Merck 1929
Depo-Medrol Injectable Suspension (Methylprednisolone Acetate) Pharmacia & Upjohn 2615
Depo-Medrol Single-Dose Vial (Methylprednisolone Acetate) Pharmacia & Upjohn 2617
Dolobid Tablets (Diflunisal) Merck 1937
EC-Naprosyn Delayed-Release Tablets (Naproxen) Roche Laboratories 2769
Ecotrin Enteric Coated Aspirin Low, Regular and Maximum Strength Tablets (Aspirin) GlaxoSmithKline Consumer 1627
Enbrel for Injection (Etanercept) Amgen 580
Gengraf Capsules (Cyclosporine) Abbott 458
Humira Injection (Adalimumab) Abbott 464
Hydrocortone Tablets (Hydrocortisone) Merck 1963
Indocin (Indomethacin) Merck 1968
Kineret Injection (Anakinra) Amgen 594
Nalfon Capsules (Fenoprofen Calcium) Pedinol 2504
Naprosyn Suspension (Naproxen) Roche Laboratories 2769
Naprosyn Tablets (Naproxen) Roche Laboratories 2769
Neoral Soft Gelatin Capsules (Cyclosporine) Novartis 2247
Neoral Oral Solution (Cyclosporine) Novartis 2247
Pediapred Oral Solution (Prednisolone Sodium Phosphate) UCB 3319
Relafen Tablets (Nabumetone) GlaxoSmithKline 1523
Remicade for IV Injection (Infliximab) Centocor 987
St. Joseph 81 mg Aspirin Chewable and Enteric Coated Tablets (Aspirin) McNeil Consumer 1841
Voltaren Tablets (Diclofenac Sodium) Novartis 2298
Voltaren-XR Tablets (Diclofenac Sodium) Novartis 2301

Rheumatoid arthritis, juvenile
Bayer Aspirin (Aspirin) Bayer Healthcare LLC 3515
Decadron Phosphate Injection (Dexamethasone Sodium Phosphate) Merck 1931
Decadron Tablets (Dexamethasone) Merck 1929
Depo-Medrol Injectable Suspension (Methylprednisolone Acetate) Pharmacia & Upjohn 2615
Ecotrin Enteric Coated Aspirin Low, Regular and Maximum Strength Tablets (Aspirin) GlaxoSmithKline Consumer 1627
Enbrel for Injection (Etanercept) Amgen 580
Hydrocortone Tablets (Hydrocortisone) Merck 1963
Pediapred Oral Solution (Prednisolone Sodium Phosphate) UCB 3319
St. Joseph 81 mg Aspirin Chewable and Enteric Coated Tablets (Aspirin) McNeil Consumer 1841

Rhinitis
Advil (Ibuprofen) Wyeth .... ▣ 737
Children's Advil Suspension (Ibuprofen) Wyeth .... ▣ 742
Children's Advil Chewable Tablets (Ibuprofen) Wyeth .... ▣ 741
Advil Cold & Sinus (Ibuprofen, Pseudoephedrine Hydrochloride) Wyeth .... ▣ 739
Advil Flu & Body Ache Caplets (Ibuprofen, Pseudoephedrine Hydrochloride) Wyeth .... ▣ 739
Children's Advil Cold Suspension (Ibuprofen, Pseudoephedrine Hydrochloride) Wyeth .... ▣ 741
Infants' Advil Concentrated Drops (Ibuprofen) Wyeth .... ▣ 743
TheraFlu Cold & Cough Hot Liquid (Acetaminophen, Chlorpheniramine Maleate, Dextromethorphan Hydrobromide, Pseudoephedrine Hydrochloride) Novartis Consumer .... ▣ 680
TheraFlu Cold & Sore Throat Hot Liquid (Acetaminophen, Chlorpheniramine Maleate, Pseudoephedrine Hydrochloride) Novartis Consumer .... ▣ 680
TheraFlu Flu & Chest Congestion Non-Drowsy Hot Liquid (Acetaminophen, Dextromethorphan Hydrobromide, Guaifenesin, Pseudoephedrine Hydrochloride) Novartis Consumer .... ▣ 681
TheraFlu Flu & Sore Throat Hot Liquid (Acetaminophen, Chlorpheniramine Maleate, Pseudoephedrine Hydrochloride) Novartis Consumer .... ▣ 681
TheraFlu Severe Cold Non-Drowsy Hot Liquid (Acetaminophen, Dextromethorphan Hydrobromide, Pseudoephedrine Hydrochloride) Novartis Consumer .... ▣ 683
TheraFlu Severe Cold & Cough Hot Liquid (Acetaminophen, Chlorpheniramine Maleate, Dextromethorphan Hydrobromide, Pseudoephedrine Hydrochloride) Novartis Consumer .... ▣ 683
TheraFlu Severe Cold Caplets (Acetaminophen, Chlorpheniramine Maleate, Dextromethorphan Hydrobromide, Pseudoephedrine Hydrochloride) Novartis Consumer .... ▣ 679
TheraFlu Severe Cold Hot Liquid (Acetaminophen, Chlorpheniramine Maleate, Dextromethorphan Hydrobromide, Pseudoephedrine Hydrochloride) Novartis Consumer .... ▣ 682
TheraFlu Severe Cold Non-Drowsy Caplets (Acetaminophen, Dextromethorphan Hydrobromide, Pseudoephedrine Hydrochloride) Novartis Consumer .... ▣ 679

Rhinitis, allergic
Atrovent Nasal Spray 0.03% (Ipratropium Bromide) Boehringer Ingelheim 869
Children's Dimetapp Cold & Allergy Elixir (Brompheniramine Maleate, Pseudoephedrine Hydrochloride) Wyeth .... ▣ 745
Nasacort HFA Inhalation Aerosol (Triamcinolone Acetonide) Sanofi-Aventis 2939
Phenergan (Promethazine Hydrochloride) Wyeth 3438
Robitussin Allergy & Cough Syrup (Brompheniramine Maleate, Dextromethorphan Hydrobromide, Pseudoephedrine Hydrochloride) Wyeth .... ▣ 750

Rhinitis, perennial allergic
Atrovent Nasal Spray 0.03% (Ipratropium Bromide) Boehringer Ingelheim 869
Beconase AQ Nasal Spray (Beclomethasone Dipropionate Monohydrate) GlaxoSmithKline 1359
Clarinex Syrup (Desloratadine) Schering 3009
Clarinex Tablets (Desloratadine) Schering 3009
Clarinex Reditabs Tablets (Desloratadine) Schering 3009
Decadron Phosphate Injection (Dexamethasone Sodium Phosphate) Merck 1931
Decadron Tablets (Dexamethasone) Merck 1929
Depo-Medrol Injectable Suspension (Methylprednisolone Acetate) Pharmacia & Upjohn 2615
Depo-Medrol Single-Dose Vial (Methylprednisolone Acetate) Pharmacia & Upjohn 2617
Flonase Nasal Spray (Fluticasone Propionate) GlaxoSmithKline 1412
Hydrocortone Tablets (Hydrocortisone) Merck 1963
Nasacort HFA Inhalation Aerosol (Triamcinolone Acetonide) Sanofi-Aventis 2939
Nasacort AQ Nasal Spray (Triamcinolone Acetonide) Sanofi-Aventis 2937
Nasarel Nasal Spray (Flunisolide) IVAX 1652
Nasonex Nasal Spray (Mometasone Furoate Monohydrate) Schering 3058
Pediapred Oral Solution (Prednisolone Sodium Phosphate) UCB 3319
Rhinocort Aqua Nasal Spray (Budesonide) AstraZeneca LP 658
Singulair (Montelukast Sodium) Merck 2047
Zyrtec Chewable Tablets (Cetirizine Hydrochloride) Pfizer 2589
Zyrtec (Cetirizine Hydrochloride) Pfizer 2589

Zyrtec-D 12 Hour Extended Release Tablets (Cetirizine Hydrochloride, Pseudoephedrine Hydrochloride) Pfizer 2591

Rhinitis, seasonal allergic

Allegra (Fexofenadine Hydrochloride) Sanofi-Aventis 2857
Allegra-D 12 Hour Extended-Release Tablets (Fexofenadine Hydrochloride, Pseudoephedrine Hydrochloride) Sanofi-Aventis 2860
Allegra-D 24 Hour Extended-Release Tablets (Fexofenadine Hydrochloride, Pseudoephedrine Hydrochloride) Sanofi-Aventis 2862
Astelin Nasal Spray (Azelastine Hydrochloride) MedPointe 1876
Beconase AQ Nasal Spray (Beclomethasone Dipropionate Monohydrate) GlaxoSmithKline 1359
Benadryl Allergy & Sinus Headache Caplets & Gelcaps (Acetaminophen, Diphenhydramine Hydrochloride, Pseudoephedrine Hydrochloride) Pfizer Consumer Healthcare .... ■ 693
Children's Benadryl Allergy Liquid (Diphenhydramine Hydrochloride) Pfizer Consumer Healthcare .... ■ 695
Benadryl Maximum Strength Severe Allergy & Sinus Headache Caplets (Acetaminophen, Diphenhydramine Hydrochloride, Pseudoephedrine Hydrochloride) Pfizer Consumer Healthcare .... ■ 694
Children's Benadryl D Allergy & Sinus Fastmelt Tablets (Diphenhydramine Citrate, Pseudoephedrine Hydrochloride) Pfizer Consumer Healthcare .... ■ 694
Children's Benadryl D Liquid Medication (Diphenhydramine Hydrochloride, Pseudoephedrine Hydrochloride) Pfizer Consumer Healthcare .... ■ 693
Benadryl D Tablets (Diphenhydramine Hydrochloride, Pseudoephedrine Hydrochloride) Pfizer Consumer Healthcare .... ■ 694
Clarinex Syrup (Desloratadine) Schering 3009
Clarinex Tablets (Desloratadine) Schering 3009
Clarinex Reditabs Tablets (Desloratadine) Schering 3009
Clarinex-D 24-Hour Extended-Release Tablets (Desloratadine, Pseudoephedrine Sulfate) Schering 3012
Claritin-D Non-Drowsy 12 Hour Tablets (Loratadine, Pseudoephedrine Sulfate) Schering-Plough .... ■ 731
Claritin-D Non-Drowsy 24 Hour Tablets (Loratadine, Pseudoephedrine Sulfate) Schering-Plough .... ■ 731
Decadron Phosphate Injection (Dexamethasone Sodium Phosphate) Merck 1931
Decadron Tablets (Dexamethasone) Merck 1929
Depo-Medrol Injectable Suspension (Methylprednisolone Acetate) Pharmacia & Upjohn 2615
Depo-Medrol Single-Dose Vial (Methylprednisolone Acetate) Pharmacia & Upjohn 2617
Flonase Nasal Spray (Fluticasone Propionate) GlaxoSmithKline 1412
Hydrocortone Tablets (Hydrocortisone) Merck 1963
Nasacort HFA Inhalation Aerosol (Triamcinolone Acetonide) Sanofi-Aventis 2939
Nasacort AQ Nasal Spray (Triamcinolone Acetonide) Sanofi-Aventis 2937
Nasarel Nasal Spray (Flunisolide) IVAX 1652
Nasonex Nasal Spray (Mometasone Furoate Monohydrate) Schering 3058
Pediapred Oral Solution (Prednisolone Sodium Phosphate) UCB 3319
Rhinocort Aqua Nasal Spray (Budesonide) AstraZeneca LP 658
Singulair (Montelukast Sodium) Merck 2047
Zyrtec Chewable Tablets (Cetirizine Hydrochloride) Pfizer 2589
Zyrtec (Cetirizine Hydrochloride) Pfizer 2589
Zyrtec-D 12 Hour Extended Release Tablets (Cetirizine Hydrochloride, Pseudoephedrine Hydrochloride) Pfizer 2591

Rhinitis, vasomotor

Astelin Nasal Spray (Azelastine Hydrochloride) MedPointe 1876
Beconase AQ Nasal Spray (Beclomethasone Dipropionate Monohydrate) GlaxoSmithKline 1359
Phenergan (Promethazine Hydrochloride) Wyeth 3438

Rhinorrhea

Advil Allergy Sinus Caplets (Chlorpheniramine Maleate, Ibuprofen, Pseudoephedrine Hydrochloride) Wyeth .... ■ 737
Advil Multi-Symptom Cold Caplets (Chlorpheniramine Maleate, Ibuprofen, Pseudoephedrine Hydrochloride) Wyeth .... ■ 738
Alavert Allergy & Sinus D-12 Hour Tablets (Loratadine, Pseudoephedrine Sulfate) Wyeth .... ■ 743
Alavert (Loratadine) Wyeth .... ■ 743
Allegra-D 12 Hour Extended-Release Tablets (Fexofenadine Hydrochloride, Pseudoephedrine Hydrochloride) Sanofi-Aventis 2860
Allegra-D 24 Hour Extended-Release Tablets (Fexofenadine Hydrochloride, Pseudoephedrine Hydrochloride) Sanofi-Aventis 2862
Atrovent Nasal Spray 0.03% (Ipratropium Bromide) Boehringer Ingelheim 869
Atrovent Nasal Spray 0.06% (Ipratropium Bromide) Boehringer Ingelheim 870
Benadryl Allergy & Cold Tablets (Acetaminophen, Diphenhydramine Hydrochloride, Pseudoephedrine Hydrochloride) Pfizer Consumer Healthcare .... ■ 692
Benadryl Allergy (Diphenhydramine Hydrochloride) Pfizer Consumer Healthcare .... ■ 691
Benadryl Allergy & Sinus Headache Caplets & Gelcaps (Acetaminophen, Diphenhydramine Hydrochloride, Pseudoephedrine Hydrochloride) Pfizer Consumer Healthcare .... ■ 693
Children's Benadryl Allergy Liquid (Diphenhydramine Hydrochloride) Pfizer Consumer Healthcare .... ■ 695
Children's Benadryl Dye-Free Allergy Liquid (Diphenhydramine Hydrochloride) Pfizer Consumer Healthcare .... ■ 695
Benadryl Dye-Free Allergy Liqui-Gels Softgels (Diphenhydramine Hydrochloride) Pfizer Consumer Healthcare .... ■ 692
Children's Benadryl D Allergy & Sinus Fastmelt Tablets (Diphenhydramine Citrate, Pseudoephedrine Hydrochloride) Pfizer Consumer Healthcare .... ■ 694
Children's Benadryl D Liquid Medication (Diphenhydramine Hydrochloride, Pseudoephedrine Hydrochloride) Pfizer Consumer Healthcare .... ■ 693
Benadryl D Tablets (Diphenhydramine Hydrochloride, Pseudoephedrine Hydrochloride) Pfizer Consumer Healthcare .... ■ 694
Children's Benadryl Allergy Fastmelt Tablets (Diphenhydramine Citrate) Pfizer Consumer Healthcare .... ■ 696
Children's Claritin 24 Hour Non-Drowsy Allergy Syrup (Loratadine) Schering-Plough .... ■ 732
Claritin Non-Drowsy 24 Hour Tablets (Loratadine) Schering-Plough .... ■ 731
Claritin Reditabs 24 Hour Non-Drowsy Tablets (Loratadine) Schering-Plough .... ■ 732
Claritin-D Non-Drowsy 12 Hour Tablets (Loratadine, Pseudoephedrine Sulfate) Schering-Plough .... ■ 731
Claritin-D Non-Drowsy 24 Hour Tablets (Loratadine, Pseudoephedrine Sulfate) Schering-Plough .... ■ 731
Children's Dimetapp Cold & Allergy Elixir (Brompheniramine Maleate, Pseudoephedrine Hydrochloride) Wyeth .... ■ 745
Children's Dimetapp ND Non-Drowsy Allergy Syrup (Loratadine) Wyeth .... ■ 746
Hyland's Seasonal Allergy Tablets (Homeopathic Formulations) Standard Homeopathic .... ■ 735
PediaCare Multi-Symptom Cold Liquid (Chlorpheniramine Maleate, Dextromethorphan Hydrobromide, Pseudoephedrine Hydrochloride) Pfizer Consumer Healthcare .... ■ 704
PediaCare NightRest Cough & Cold Liquid (Chlorpheniramine Maleate, Dextromethorphan Hydrobromide, Pseudoephedrine Hydrochloride) Pfizer Consumer Healthcare .... ■ 704
TheraFlu Cold & Cough Hot Liquid (Acetaminophen, Chlorpheniramine Maleate, Dextromethorphan Hydrobromide, Pseudoephedrine Hydrochloride) Novartis Consumer .... ■ 680
TheraFlu Cold & Sore Throat Hot Liquid (Acetaminophen, Chlorpheniramine Maleate, Pseudoephedrine Hydrochloride) Novartis Consumer .... ■ 680
TheraFlu Flu & Sore Throat Hot Liquid (Acetaminophen, Chlorpheniramine Maleate, Pseudoephedrine Hydrochloride) Novartis Consumer .... ■ 681
TheraFlu Severe Cold & Cough Hot Liquid (Acetaminophen, Chlorpheniramine Maleate, Dextromethorphan Hydrobromide, Pseudoephedrine Hydrochloride) Novartis Consumer .... ■ 683
TheraFlu Severe Cold Caplets (Acetaminophen, Chlorpheniramine Maleate, Dextromethorphan Hydrobromide, Pseudoephedrine Hydrochloride) Novartis Consumer .... ■ 679
TheraFlu Severe Cold Hot Liquid (Acetaminophen, Chlorpheniramine Maleate, Dextromethorphan Hydrobromide, Pseudoephedrine Hydrochloride) Novartis Consumer .... ■ 682
TheraFlu Thin Strips Multi Symptom (Diphenhydramine Hydrochloride) Novartis Consumer .... ■ 684
Triaminic Allerchews (Loratadine) Novartis Consumer .... ■ 684
Triaminic Thin Strips Cough & Runny Nose (Diphenhydramine Hydrochloride) Novartis Consumer .... ■ 690
Tylenol Cough & Sore Throat NightTime Liquid with Cool Burst (Acetaminophen, Dextromethorphan Hydrobromide, Doxylamine Succinate) McNeil Consumer .... ■ 664
Children's Tylenol Plus Cold & Allergy Suspension Liquid (Acetaminophen, Diphenhydramine Hydrochloride, Pseudoephedrine Hydrochloride) McNeil Consumer 1850
Children's Tylenol Plus Cold NightTime Suspension Liquid (Acetaminophen, Chlorpheniramine Maleate, Pseudoephedrine Hydrochloride) McNeil Consumer 1851
Children's Tylenol Plus Cold & Cough Suspension Liquid and Chewable Tablets (Acetaminophen, Chlorpheniramine Maleate, Dextromethorphan Hydrobromide, Pseudoephedrine Hydrochloride) McNeil Consumer 1851
Children's Tylenol Plus Cold Chewable Tablets (Acetaminophen, Chlorpheniramine Maleate, Pseudoephedrine Hydrochloride) McNeil Consumer 1851
Children's Tylenol Plus Flu Suspension Liquid (Acetaminophen, Chlorpheniramine Maleate, Dextromethorphan Hydrobromide, Pseudoephedrine Hydrochloride) McNeil Consumer 1853
Tylenol Cold & Flu Severe NightTime Liquid with Cool Burst (Acetaminophen, Dextromethorphan Hydrobromide, Doxylamine Succinate, Pseudoephedrine Hydrochloride) McNeil Consumer 1846
Tylenol Cough & Sore Throat NightTime Liquid with Cool Burst (Acetaminophen, Dextromethorphan Hydrobromide, Doxylamine Succinate) McNeil Consumer 1849
Tylenol Allergy Complete Multi-Symptom Caplets and Gelcaps with Cool Burst (Acetaminophen, Chlorpheniramine Maleate, Pseudoephedrine Hydrochloride) McNeil Consumer 1844
Tylenol Severe Allergy Caplets (Acetaminophen, Diphenhydramine Hydrochloride) McNeil Consumer 1844
Tylenol Flu NightTime Gelcaps (Acetaminophen, Diphenhydramine Hydrochloride, Pseudoephedrine Hydrochloride) McNeil Consumer 1846
Tylenol Sinus Night Time Caplets (Acetaminophen, Doxylamine Succinate, Pseudoephedrine Hydrochloride) McNeil Consumer 1848
Tylenol Sore Throat NightTime Liquid with Cool Burst (Acetaminophen, Diphenhydramine) McNeil Consumer 1849
Vicks NyQuil LiquiCaps/Liquid Multi-Symptom Cold/Flu Relief (Acetaminophen, Dextromethorphan Hydrobromide, Doxylamine Succinate, Pseudoephedrine Hydrochloride) Procter & Gamble .... ■ 725
Zicam Allergy Relief Nasal Pump (Histanium Hydrochloricum, Luffa operculata, Galphimia Glauca, Sulfur) Matrixx .... ■ 665

Rickettsiae

Dynacin Tablets (Minocycline Hydrochloride) Medicis 1859

Rickettsialpox

Dynacin Tablets (Minocycline Hydrochloride) Medicis 1859

Ringworm infections of the body

(*see under* Tinea corporis infections)

Ringworm infections of the feet

(*see under* Tinea pedis infections)

Ringworm infections of the groin

(*see under* Tinea cruris infections)

Ringworm infections of the nails

(*see under* Tinea unguium infections)

Ringworm infections of the scalp

(*see under* Tinea capitis infections)

Rocky Mountain spotted fever

Dynacin Tablets (Minocycline Hydrochloride) Medicis 1859

Rosacea

Finacea Gel (Azelaic Acid) Intendis 1644
Noritate Cream, 1% (Metronidazole) Dermik 1051

Roundworm, common

(*see under* Ascaris lumbricoides infections)

Rubella, prophylaxis

Meruvax II (Rubella Virus Vaccine Live) Merck 1994
M-M-R II (Measles, Mumps & Rubella Virus Vaccine, Live) Merck 1980

S

S. agalactiae gynecologic infections

Mefoxin for Injection (Cefoxitin Sodium) Merck **1987**
Mefoxin Premixed Intravenous Solution (Cefoxitin Sodium) Merck **1990**

S. agalactiae infections

Invanz for Injection (Ertapenem) Merck **1974**
Mefoxin for Injection (Cefoxitin Sodium) Merck **1987**
Mefoxin Premixed Intravenous Solution (Cefoxitin Sodium) Merck **1990**
Merrem I.V. (Meropenem) AstraZeneca **687**
Noroxin Tablets (Norfloxacin) Merck . **2009**
Tygacil for Injection (Tigecycline) Wyeth **3489**
Zithromax (Azithromycin Dihydrate) Pfizer **2568**
Zithromax for Oral Suspension, 300 mg, 600 mg, 900 mg, 1200 mg (Azithromycin Dihydrate) Pfizer **2561**
Zithromax Tablets, 250 mg, 500 mg (Azithromycin Dihydrate) Pfizer **2561**
Zithromax Tablets, 600 mg (Azithromycin Dihydrate) Pfizer **2568**
Zithromax Tri-Pak (Azithromycin Dihydrate) Pfizer **2561**
Zithromax Z-Pak (Azithromycin Dihydrate) Pfizer **2568**
Zyvox (Linezolid) Pharmacia & Upjohn **2661**

S. agalactiae pelvic inflammatory disease

Invanz for Injection (Ertapenem) Merck **1974**

S. agalactiae skin and skin structure infections

Cubicin for Injection (Daptomycin) Cubist **1038**
Merrem I.V. (Meropenem) AstraZeneca **687**
Tygacil for Injection (Tigecycline) Wyeth **3489**
Zithromax (Azithromycin Dihydrate) Pfizer **2568**
Zithromax for Oral Suspension, 300 mg, 600 mg, 900 mg, 1200 mg (Azithromycin Dihydrate) Pfizer **2561**
Zithromax Tablets, 250 mg, 500 mg (Azithromycin Dihydrate) Pfizer **2561**
Zithromax Tablets, 600 mg (Azithromycin Dihydrate) Pfizer **2568**
Zithromax Tri-Pak (Azithromycin Dihydrate) Pfizer **2561**
Zithromax Z-Pak (Azithromycin Dihydrate) Pfizer **2568**
Zyvox (Linezolid) Pharmacia & Upjohn **2661**

S. agalactiae urinary tract infections

Noroxin Tablets (Norfloxacin) Merck . **2009**

S. anginosus infections

Tygacil (Tigecycline) Wyeth **3489**

S. aureus (non-penicillinase producing) infections

Mefoxin for Injection (Cefoxitin Sodium) Merck **1987**
Mefoxin Premixed Intravenous Solution (Cefoxitin Sodium) Merck **1990**
Primaxin I.V. (Cilastatin Sodium, Imipenem) Merck **2024**

S. aureus (penicillinase and non-penicillinase producing strains) skin and skin structure infections

Mefoxin for Injection (Cefoxitin Sodium) Merck **1987**
Mefoxin Premixed Intravenous Solution (Cefoxitin Sodium) Merck **1990**
Tequin Injection (Gatifloxacin) Bristol-Myers Squibb **964**
Tequin Tablets (Gatifloxacin) Bristol-Myers Squibb **964**
Tygacil for Injection (Tigecycline) Wyeth **3489**
Zinacef Injection (Cefuroxime) GlaxoSmithKline **1604**
Zinacef for Injection (Cefuroxime) GlaxoSmithKline **1604**

S. aureus (penicillinase producing) infections

Mefoxin for Injection (Cefoxitin Sodium) Merck **1987**
Mefoxin Premixed Intravenous Solution (Cefoxitin Sodium) Merck **1990**
Primaxin I.M. (Cilastatin Sodium, Imipenem) Merck **2022**
Primaxin I.V. (Cilastatin Sodium, Imipenem) Merck **2024**

S. aureus biliary tract infections

Ancef (Cefazolin Sodium) GlaxoSmithKline **1318**

S. aureus bone and joint infections

Fortaz (Ceftazidime Sodium) GlaxoSmithKline **1422**
Mefoxin for Injection (Cefoxitin Sodium) Merck **1987**
Mefoxin Premixed Intravenous Solution (Cefoxitin Sodium) Merck **1990**
Primaxin I.V. (Cilastatin Sodium, Imipenem) Merck **2024**
Rocephin Injectable Vials, ADD-Vantage, Galaxy, Bulk (Ceftriaxone Sodium) Roche Laboratories **2801**
Timentin ADD-Vantage (Clavulanate Potassium, Ticarcillin Disodium) GlaxoSmithKline **1556**
Timentin Injection Galaxy Container (Clavulanate Potassium, Ticarcillin Disodium) GlaxoSmithKline **1559**
Timentin IV Infusion (Clavulanate Potassium, Ticarcillin Disodium) GlaxoSmithKline **1553**
Timentin Pharmacy Bulk Package (Clavulanate Potassium, Ticarcillin Disodium) GlaxoSmithKline **1562**
Zinacef Injection (Cefuroxime) GlaxoSmithKline **1604**
Zinacef for Injection (Cefuroxime) GlaxoSmithKline **1604**

S. aureus endocarditis

Ancef for Injection (Cefazolin Sodium) GlaxoSmithKline **1318**
Primaxin I.V. (Cilastatin Sodium, Imipenem) Merck **2024**

S. aureus gynecologic infections

Timentin ADD-Vantage (Clavulanate Potassium, Ticarcillin Disodium) GlaxoSmithKline **1556**
Timentin Injection Galaxy Container (Clavulanate Potassium, Ticarcillin Disodium) GlaxoSmithKline **1559**
Timentin IV Infusion (Clavulanate Potassium, Ticarcillin Disodium) GlaxoSmithKline **1553**
Timentin Pharmacy Bulk Package (Clavulanate Potassium, Ticarcillin Disodium) GlaxoSmithKline **1562**

S. aureus infection, eradication of nasal colonization of

Bactroban Nasal (Mupirocin Calcium) GlaxoSmithKline **1357**

S. aureus infections

Ancef for Injection (Cefazolin Sodium) GlaxoSmithKline **1318**
Augmentin (Amoxicillin, Clavulanate Potassium) GlaxoSmithKline **1331**
Augmentin Tablets (Amoxicillin, Clavulanate Potassium) GlaxoSmithKline **1334**
Augmentin XR Extended-Release Tablets (Amoxicillin, Clavulanate Potassium) GlaxoSmithKline **1340**
Avelox (Moxifloxacin Hydrochloride) Schering **2984**
Bactroban Ointment (Mupirocin) GlaxoSmithKline **1358**
Biaxin/Biaxin XL (Clarithromycin) Abbott **402**
Ceftin (Cefuroxime Axetil) GlaxoSmithKline **1369**
Centany Ointment, 2% (Mupirocin) OrthoNeutrogena **2382**
Cipro I.V. (Ciprofloxacin) Schering **2998**
Cipro I.V. Pharmacy Bulk Package (Ciprofloxacin) Bayer **3509**
Cipro (Ciprofloxacin) Schering **2991**
Cleocin Vaginal Ovules (Clindamycin Hydrochloride) Pharmacia & Upjohn **2613**
E.E.S. (Erythromycin Ethylsuccinate) Abbott **449**
EryPed (Erythromycin Ethylsuccinate) Abbott **445**
Ery-Tab Tablets (Erythromycin) Abbott **447**
Erythrocin Stearate Filmtab Tablets (Erythromycin Stearate) Abbott **452**
Erythromycin Base Filmtab Tablets (Erythromycin) Abbott **454**
Erythromycin Delayed-Release Capsules, USP (Erythromycin) Abbott **456**
Fortaz (Ceftazidime Sodium) GlaxoSmithKline **1422**
Invanz for Injection (Ertapenem) Merck **1974**
Levaquin in 5% Dextrose Injection (Levofloxacin) Ortho-McNeil **2453**
Levaquin (Levofloxacin) Ortho-McNeil **2453**
Mefoxin for Injection (Cefoxitin Sodium) Merck **1987**
Mefoxin Premixed Intravenous Solution (Cefoxitin Sodium) Merck **1990**
Noroxin Tablets (Norfloxacin) Merck . **2009**
PCE Dispertab Tablets (Erythromycin) Abbott **510**
Primaxin I.M. (Cilastatin Sodium, Imipenem) Merck **2022**
Primaxin I.V. (Cilastatin Sodium, Imipenem) Merck **2024**
Rocephin Injectable Vials, ADD-Vantage, Galaxy, Bulk (Ceftriaxone Sodium) Roche Laboratories **2801**
Spectracef Tablets (Cefditoren Pivoxil) Purdue Pharmaceutical **2706**
Tequin Injection (Gatifloxacin) Bristol-Myers Squibb **964**
Tequin Tablets (Gatifloxacin) Bristol-Myers Squibb **964**
Timentin ADD-Vantage (Clavulanate Potassium, Ticarcillin Disodium) GlaxoSmithKline **1556**
Timentin Injection Galaxy Container (Clavulanate Potassium, Ticarcillin Disodium) GlaxoSmithKline **1559**
Timentin IV Infusion (Clavulanate Potassium, Ticarcillin Disodium) GlaxoSmithKline **1553**
Timentin Pharmacy Bulk Package (Clavulanate Potassium, Ticarcillin Disodium) GlaxoSmithKline **1562**
Tygacil for Injection (Tigecycline) Wyeth **3489**
Vantin Tablets and Oral Suspension (Cefpodoxime Proxetil) Pharmacia & Upjohn **2650**
Zinacef Injection (Cefuroxime) GlaxoSmithKline **1604**
Zinacef for Injection (Cefuroxime) GlaxoSmithKline **1604**
Zithromax Capsules, 250 mg (Azithromycin Dihydrate) Pfizer **2568**
Zithromax for IV Infusion (Azithromycin Dihydrate) Pfizer **2573**
Zithromax for Oral Suspension, 1 g (Azithromycin Dihydrate) Pfizer **2568**
Zithromax for Oral Suspension, 300 mg, 600 mg, 900 mg, 1200 mg (Azithromycin Dihydrate) Pfizer **2561**
Zithromax Tablets, 250 mg, 500 mg (Azithromycin Dihydrate) Pfizer **2561**
Zithromax Tablets, 600 mg (Azithromycin Dihydrate) Pfizer **2568**
Zithromax Tri-Pak (Azithromycin Dihydrate) Pfizer **2561**
Zithromax Z-Pak (Azithromycin Dihydrate) Pfizer **2568**
Zosyn (Piperacillin Sodium, Tazobactam Sodium) Wyeth **3492**
Zyvox (Linezolid) Pharmacia & Upjohn **2661**

S. aureus infections, ocular

Blephamide Ophthalmic Ointment (Prednisolone Acetate, Sulfacetamide Sodium) Allergan **563**
Blephamide Ophthalmic Suspension (Prednisolone Acetate, Sulfacetamide Sodium) Allergan **564**
Ciloxan Ophthalmic Ointment (Ciprofloxacin Hydrochloride) Alcon **554**
FML-S Liquifilm Sterile Ophthalmic Suspension (Fluorometholone, Sulfacetamide Sodium) Allergan ... ⊙ **226**
Genoptic Sterile Ophthalmic Solution (Gentamicin Sulfate) Allergan .... ⊙ **227**
Poly-Pred Liquifilm Ophthalmic Suspension (Neomycin Sulfate, Polymyxin B Sulfate, Prednisolone Acetate) Allergan .... ⊙ **231**
Polytrim Ophthalmic Solution (Polymyxin B Sulfate, Trimethoprim Sulfate) Allergan **570**
Pred-G Ophthalmic Suspension (Gentamicin Sulfate, Prednisolone Acetate) Allergan .... ⊙ **234**
Pred-G Sterile Ophthalmic Ointment (Gentamicin Sulfate, Prednisolone Acetate) Allergan ..... ⊙ **235**
Quixin Ophthalmic Solution (Levofloxacin) Vistakon **3373**
TobraDex Ophthalmic Ointment (Dexamethasone, Tobramycin) Alcon **558**
TobraDex Ophthalmic Suspension (Dexamethasone, Tobramycin) Alcon **558**
Vigamox Ophthalmic Solution (Moxifloxacin Hydrochloride) Alcon **560**
Zylet Ophthalmic Suspension (Loteprednol Etabonate, Tobramycin) Bausch & Lomb **3508**
Zymar Ophthalmic Solution (Gatifloxacin) Allergan **571**

S. aureus infections (methicillin-susceptible strains)

Merrem I.V. (Meropenem) AstraZeneca **687**

S. aureus intra-abdominal infections

Fortaz (Ceftazidime Sodium) GlaxoSmithKline **1422**
Primaxin I.V. (Cilastatin Sodium, Imipenem) Merck **2024**

S. aureus lower respiratory tract infections

Augmentin XR Extended-Release Tablets (Amoxicillin, Clavulanate Potassium) GlaxoSmithKline **1340**
Cleocin Vaginal Ovules (Clindamycin Hydrochloride) Pharmacia & Upjohn **2613**
Fortaz (Ceftazidime Sodium) GlaxoSmithKline **1422**
Levaquin in 5% Dextrose Injection (Levofloxacin) Ortho-McNeil **2453**
Levaquin (Levofloxacin) Ortho-McNeil **2453**
Mefoxin for Injection (Cefoxitin Sodium) Merck **1987**
Mefoxin Premixed Intravenous Solution (Cefoxitin Sodium) Merck **1990**
Primaxin I.V. (Cilastatin Sodium, Imipenem) Merck **2024**
Rocephin Injectable Vials, ADD-Vantage, Galaxy, Bulk (Ceftriaxone Sodium) Roche Laboratories **2801**
Tequin Injection (Gatifloxacin) Bristol-Myers Squibb **964**
Tequin Tablets (Gatifloxacin) Bristol-Myers Squibb **964**
Timentin ADD-Vantage (Clavulanate Potassium, Ticarcillin Disodium) GlaxoSmithKline **1556**
Timentin Injection Galaxy Container (Clavulanate Potassium, Ticarcillin Disodium) GlaxoSmithKline **1559**
Timentin IV Infusion (Clavulanate Potassium, Ticarcillin Disodium) GlaxoSmithKline **1553**
Timentin Pharmacy Bulk Package (Clavulanate Potassium, Ticarcillin Disodium) GlaxoSmithKline **1562**

Zinacef Injection (Cefuroxime) GlaxoSmithKline ... 1604
Zinacef for Injection (Cefuroxime) GlaxoSmithKline ... 1604
Zithromax for IV Infusion (Azithromycin Dihydrate) Pfizer ... 2573
Zosyn (Piperacillin Sodium, Tazobactam Sodium) Wyeth ... 3492
Zyvox (Linezolid) Pharmacia & Upjohn ... 2661

S. aureus meningitis
Zinacef Injection (Cefuroxime) GlaxoSmithKline ... 1604
Zinacef for Injection (Cefuroxime) GlaxoSmithKline ... 1604

S. aureus otitis externa
Floxin Otic Solution (Ofloxacin) Daiichi ... 1043

S. aureus respiratory tract infections
Ancef for Injection (Cefazolin Sodium) GlaxoSmithKline ... 1318
Avelox (Moxifloxacin Hydrochloride) Schering ... 2984

S. aureus septicemia
Ancef for Injection (Cefazolin Sodium) GlaxoSmithKline ... 1318
Fortaz (Ceftazidime Sodium) GlaxoSmithKline ... 1422
Mefoxin for Injection (Cefoxitin Sodium) Merck ... 1987
Mefoxin Premixed Intravenous Solution (Cefoxitin Sodium) Merck ... 1990
Primaxin I.V. (Cilastatin Sodium, Imipenem) Merck ... 2024
Rocephin Injectable Vials, ADD-Vantage, Galaxy, Bulk (Ceftriaxone Sodium) Roche Laboratories ... 2801
Timentin ADD-Vantage (Clavulanate Potassium, Ticarcillin Disodium) GlaxoSmithKline ... 1556
Timentin Injection Galaxy Container (Clavulanate Potassium, Ticarcillin Disodium) GlaxoSmithKline ... 1559
Timentin IV Infusion (Clavulanate Potassium, Ticarcillin Disodium) GlaxoSmithKline ... 1553
Timentin Pharmacy Bulk Package (Clavulanate Potassium, Ticarcillin Disodium) GlaxoSmithKline ... 1562
Zinacef Injection (Cefuroxime) GlaxoSmithKline ... 1604
Zinacef for Injection (Cefuroxime) GlaxoSmithKline ... 1604

S. aureus sinusitis
Ketek Tablets (Telithromycin) Sanofi-Aventis ... 2920

S. aureus skin and skin structure infections
Ancef for Injection (Cefazolin Sodium) GlaxoSmithKline ... 1318
Augmentin (Amoxicillin, Clavulanate Potassium) GlaxoSmithKline ... 1331
Augmentin Tablets (Amoxicillin, Clavulanate Potassium) GlaxoSmithKline ... 1334
Avelox (Moxifloxacin Hydrochloride) Schering ... 2984
Bactroban Cream (Mupirocin Calcium) GlaxoSmithKline ... 1356
Bactroban Ointment (Mupirocin) GlaxoSmithKline ... 1358
Biaxin/Biaxin XL (Clarithromycin) Abbott ... 402
Ceftin Tablets (Cefuroxime Axetil) GlaxoSmithKline ... 1369
Centany Ointment, 2% (Mupirocin) OrthoNeutrogena ... 2382
Cipro I.V. (Ciprofloxacin) Schering ... 2998
Cipro I.V. Pharmacy Bulk Package (Ciprofloxacin) Bayer ... 3509
Cipro (Ciprofloxacin) Schering ... 2991
Cleocin Vaginal Ovules (Clindamycin Hydrochloride) Pharmacia & Upjohn ... 2613
Cubicin for Injection (Daptomycin) Cubist ... 1038
Dynacin Tablets (Minocycline Hydrochloride) Medicis ... 1859
E.E.S. (Erythromycin Ethylsuccinate) Abbott ... 449
EryPed (Erythromycin Ethylsuccinate) Abbott ... 445
Ery-Tab Tablets (Erythromycin) Abbott ... 447
Erythrocin Stearate Filmtab Tablets (Erythromycin Stearate) Abbott ... 452
Erythromycin Base Filmtab Tablets (Erythromycin) Abbott ... 454
Erythromycin Delayed-Release Capsules, USP (Erythromycin) Abbott ... 456
Fortaz (Ceftazidime Sodium) GlaxoSmithKline ... 1422
Invanz for Injection (Ertapenem) Merck ... 1974
Levaquin in 5% Dextrose Injection (Levofloxacin) Ortho-McNeil ... 2453
Levaquin (Levofloxacin) Ortho-McNeil ... 2453
Maxipime for Injection (Cefepime Hydrochloride) Elan ... 1093
Mefoxin for Injection (Cefoxitin Sodium) Merck ... 1987
Mefoxin Premixed Intravenous Solution (Cefoxitin Sodium) Merck ... 1990
Merrem I.V. (Meropenem) AstraZeneca ... 687
Omnicef Capsules (Cefdinir) Abbott ... 506
Omnicef for Oral Suspension (Cefdinir) Abbott ... 506
PCE Dispertab Tablets (Erythromycin) Abbott ... 510
Primaxin I.M. (Cilastatin Sodium, Imipenem) Merck ... 2022
Primaxin I.V. (Cilastatin Sodium, Imipenem) Merck ... 2024
Rocephin Injectable Vials, ADD-Vantage, Galaxy, Bulk (Ceftriaxone Sodium) Roche Laboratories ... 2801
Synercid I.V. (Dalfopristin, Quinupristin) King ... 1690
Timentin ADD-Vantage (Clavulanate Potassium, Ticarcillin Disodium) GlaxoSmithKline ... 1556
Timentin Injection Galaxy Container (Clavulanate Potassium, Ticarcillin Disodium) GlaxoSmithKline ... 1559
Timentin IV Infusion (Clavulanate Potassium, Ticarcillin Disodium) GlaxoSmithKline ... 1553
Timentin Pharmacy Bulk Package (Clavulanate Potassium, Ticarcillin Disodium) GlaxoSmithKline ... 1562
Vantin Tablets and Oral Suspension (Cefpodoxime Proxetil) Pharmacia & Upjohn ... 2650
Zinacef Injection (Cefuroxime) GlaxoSmithKline ... 1604
Zinacef for Injection (Cefuroxime) GlaxoSmithKline ... 1604
Zithromax (Azithromycin Dihydrate) Pfizer ... 2568
Zithromax for Oral Suspension, 300 mg, 600 mg, 900 mg, 1200 mg (Azithromycin Dihydrate) Pfizer ... 2561
Zithromax Tablets, 250 mg, 500 mg (Azithromycin Dihydrate) Pfizer ... 2561
Zithromax Tablets, 600 mg (Azithromycin Dihydrate) Pfizer ... 2568
Zithromax Tri-Pak (Azithromycin Dihydrate) Pfizer ... 2561
Zithromax Z-Pak (Azithromycin Dihydrate) Pfizer ... 2568
Zosyn (Piperacillin Sodium, Tazobactam Sodium) Wyeth ... 3492
Zyvox (Linezolid) Pharmacia & Upjohn ... 2661

S. aureus urinary tract infections
Noroxin Tablets (Norfloxacin) Merck ... 2009
Primaxin I.V. (Cilastatin Sodium, Imipenem) Merck ... 2024
Timentin ADD-Vantage (Clavulanate Potassium, Ticarcillin Disodium) GlaxoSmithKline ... 1556
Timentin Injection Galaxy Container (Clavulanate Potassium, Ticarcillin Disodium) GlaxoSmithKline ... 1559
Timentin IV Infusion (Clavulanate Potassium, Ticarcillin Disodium) GlaxoSmithKline ... 1553
Timentin Pharmacy Bulk Package (Clavulanate Potassium, Ticarcillin Disodium) GlaxoSmithKline ... 1562

S. dysgalactiae (subspecies equisimilis) skin and skin structure infections
Cubicin for Injection (Daptomycin) Cubist ... 1038

S. epidermis bone and joint infections
Primaxin I.V. (Cilastatin Sodium, Imipenem) Merck ... 2024

S. epidermis gynecologic infections
Timentin ADD-Vantage (Clavulanate Potassium, Ticarcillin Disodium) GlaxoSmithKline ... 1556
Timentin Injection Galaxy Container (Clavulanate Potassium, Ticarcillin Disodium) GlaxoSmithKline ... 1559
Timentin IV Infusion (Clavulanate Potassium, Ticarcillin Disodium) GlaxoSmithKline ... 1553
Timentin Pharmacy Bulk Package (Clavulanate Potassium, Ticarcillin Disodium) GlaxoSmithKline ... 1562

S. epidermis infections
Cipro I.V. (Ciprofloxacin) Schering ... 2998
Cipro I.V. Pharmacy Bulk Package (Ciprofloxacin) Bayer ... 3509
Cipro (Ciprofloxacin) Schering ... 2991
Mefoxin for Injection (Cefoxitin Sodium) Merck ... 1987
Mefoxin Premixed Intravenous Solution (Cefoxitin Sodium) Merck ... 1990
Noroxin Tablets (Norfloxacin) Merck ... 2009
Primaxin I.V. (Cilastatin Sodium, Imipenem) Merck ... 2024
Rocephin Injectable Vials, ADD-Vantage, Galaxy, Bulk (Ceftriaxone Sodium) Roche Laboratories ... 2801
Timentin ADD-Vantage (Clavulanate Potassium, Ticarcillin Disodium) GlaxoSmithKline ... 1556
Timentin Injection Galaxy Container (Clavulanate Potassium, Ticarcillin Disodium) GlaxoSmithKline ... 1559
Timentin IV Infusion (Clavulanate Potassium, Ticarcillin Disodium) GlaxoSmithKline ... 1553
Timentin Pharmacy Bulk Package (Clavulanate Potassium, Ticarcillin Disodium) GlaxoSmithKline ... 1562
Zymar Ophthalmic Solution (Gatifloxacin) Allergan ... 571

S. epidermis infections, ocular
Ciloxan Ophthalmic Ointment (Ciprofloxacin Hydrochloride) Alcon ... 554
Genoptic Sterile Ophthalmic Solution (Gentamicin Sulfate) Allergan ... ⊙ 227
Polytrim Ophthalmic Solution (Polymyxin B Sulfate, Trimethoprim Sulfate) Allergan ... 570
Quixin Ophthalmic Solution (Levofloxacin) Vistakon ... 3373
TobraDex Ophthalmic Ointment (Dexamethasone, Tobramycin) Alcon ... 558
TobraDex Ophthalmic Suspension (Dexamethasone, Tobramycin) Alcon ... 558
Vigamox Ophthalmic Solution (Moxifloxacin Hydrochloride) Alcon ... 560
Zylet Ophthalmic Suspension (Loteprednol Etabonate, Tobramycin) Bausch & Lomb ... 3508

S. epidermis intra-abdominal infections
Primaxin I.V. (Cilastatin Sodium, Imipenem) Merck ... 2024

S. epidermis meningitis
Rocephin Injectable Vials, ADD-Vantage, Galaxy, Bulk (Ceftriaxone Sodium) Roche Laboratories ... 2801

S. epidermis skin and skin structure infections
Cipro I.V. (Ciprofloxacin) Schering ... 2998
Cipro I.V. Pharmacy Bulk Package (Ciprofloxacin) Bayer ... 3509
Cipro (Ciprofloxacin) Schering ... 2991
Mefoxin for Injection (Cefoxitin Sodium) Merck ... 1987
Mefoxin Premixed Intravenous Solution (Cefoxitin Sodium) Merck ... 1990
Primaxin I.V. (Cilastatin Sodium, Imipenem) Merck ... 2024
Rocephin Injectable Vials, ADD-Vantage, Galaxy, Bulk (Ceftriaxone Sodium) Roche Laboratories ... 2801

S. epidermis urinary tract infections
Cipro I.V. (Ciprofloxacin) Schering ... 2998
Cipro I.V. Pharmacy Bulk Package (Ciprofloxacin) Bayer ... 3509
Cipro (Ciprofloxacin) Schering ... 2991
Noroxin Tablets (Norfloxacin) Merck ... 2009

S. faecalis infections
Amoxil Capsules (Amoxicillin) GlaxoSmithKline ... 1315
Amoxil Chewable Tablets (Amoxicillin) GlaxoSmithKline ... 1315
Amoxil Pediatric Drops for Oral Suspension (Amoxicillin) GlaxoSmithKline ... 1315
Amoxil Powder for Oral Suspension (Amoxicillin) GlaxoSmithKline ... 1315
Amoxil Tablets (Amoxicillin) GlaxoSmithKline ... 1315
Cipro I.V. (Ciprofloxacin) Schering ... 2998
Cipro I.V. Pharmacy Bulk Package (Ciprofloxacin) Bayer ... 3509
Cipro (Ciprofloxacin) Schering ... 2991
Levaquin in 5% Dextrose Injection (Levofloxacin) Ortho-McNeil ... 2453
Levaquin (Levofloxacin) Ortho-McNeil ... 2453
Noroxin Tablets (Norfloxacin) Merck ... 2009

S. faecalis urinary tract infections
Cipro I.V. (Ciprofloxacin) Schering ... 2998
Cipro I.V. Pharmacy Bulk Package (Ciprofloxacin) Bayer ... 3509
Cipro (Ciprofloxacin) Schering ... 2991
Levaquin in 5% Dextrose Injection (Levofloxacin) Ortho-McNeil ... 2453
Levaquin (Levofloxacin) Ortho-McNeil ... 2453
Noroxin Tablets (Norfloxacin) Merck ... 2009

S. haemolyticus
Vigamox (Moxifloxacin Hydrochloride) Alcon ... 560

S. pneumoniae bone and joint infections
Rocephin Injectable Vials, ADD-Vantage, Galaxy, Bulk (Ceftriaxone Sodium) Roche Laboratories ... 2801

S. pneumoniae bronchitis
Avelox (Moxifloxacin Hydrochloride) Schering ... 2984
Biaxin/Biaxin XL (Clarithromycin) Abbott ... 402
Ceftin Tablets (Cefuroxime Axetil) GlaxoSmithKline ... 1369
Factive Tablets (Gemifloxacin Mesylate) Oscient ... 2464
Ketek Tablets (Telithromycin) Sanofi-Aventis ... 2920
Levaquin in 5% Dextrose Injection (Levofloxacin) Ortho-McNeil ... 2453
Levaquin (Levofloxacin) Ortho-McNeil ... 2453
Omnicef Capsules (Cefdinir) Abbott ... 506
Omnicef for Oral Suspension (Cefdinir) Abbott ... 506
Suprax (Cefixime) Lupin ... 1811
Tequin Injection (Gatifloxacin) Bristol-Myers Squibb ... 964
Tequin Tablets (Gatifloxacin) Bristol-Myers Squibb ... 964
Vantin Tablets and Oral Suspension (Cefpodoxime Proxetil) Pharmacia & Upjohn ... 2650

S. pneumoniae central nervous system infections
Fortaz (Ceftazidime Sodium) GlaxoSmithKline ... 1422

S. pneumoniae infections
Amoxil Capsules (Amoxicillin) GlaxoSmithKline ... 1315
Amoxil Chewable Tablets (Amoxicillin) GlaxoSmithKline ... 1315

Amoxil Pediatric Drops for Oral Suspension (Amoxicillin) GlaxoSmithKline 1315
Amoxil Powder for Oral Suspension (Amoxicillin) GlaxoSmithKline 1315
Amoxil Tablets (Amoxicillin) GlaxoSmithKline 1315
Ancef for Injection (Cefazolin Sodium) GlaxoSmithKline 1318
Augmentin Tablets (Amoxicillin, Clavulanate Potassium) GlaxoSmithKline 1334
Augmentin XR Extended-Release Tablets (Amoxicillin, Clavulanate Potassium) GlaxoSmithKline 1340
Augmentin ES-600 Powder for Oral Suspension (Amoxicillin, Clavulanate Potassium) GlaxoSmithKline 1337
Avelox (Moxifloxacin Hydrochloride) Schering 2984
Biaxin/Biaxin XL (Clarithromycin) Abbott 402
Ceftin (Cefuroxime Axetil) GlaxoSmithKline 1369
Cipro I.V. (Ciprofloxacin) Schering 2998
Cipro I.V. Pharmacy Bulk Package (Ciprofloxacin) Bayer 3509
Cipro (Ciprofloxacin) Schering 2991
Cleocin Vaginal Ovules (Clindamycin Hydrochloride) Pharmacia & Upjohn 2613
E.E.S. (Erythromycin Ethylsuccinate) Abbott 449
EryPed (Erythromycin Ethylsuccinate) Abbott 445
Ery-Tab Tablets (Erythromycin) Abbott 447
Erythrocin Stearate Filmtab Tablets (Erythromycin Stearate) Abbott 452
Erythromycin Base Filmtab Tablets (Erythromycin) Abbott 454
Erythromycin Delayed-Release Capsules, USP (Erythromycin) Abbott 456
Factive Tablets (Gemifloxacin Mesylate) Oscient 2464
Fortaz (Ceftazidime Sodium) GlaxoSmithKline 1422
Invanz for Injection (Ertapenem) Merck 1974
Levaquin in 5% Dextrose Injection (Levofloxacin) Ortho-McNeil 2453
Levaquin (Levofloxacin) Ortho-McNeil 2453
Mefoxin for Injection (Cefoxitin Sodium) Merck 1987
Mefoxin Premixed Intravenous Solution (Cefoxitin Sodium) Merck 1990
Merrem I.V. (Meropenem) AstraZeneca 687
Omnicef Capsules (Cefdinir) Abbott 506
Omnicef for Oral Suspension (Cefdinir) Abbott 506
PCE Dispertab Tablets (Erythromycin) Abbott 510
Primaxin I.M. (Cilastatin Sodium, Imipenem) Merck 2022
Primaxin I.V. (Cilastatin Sodium, Imipenem) Merck 2024
Rocephin Injectable Vials, ADD-Vantage, Galaxy, Bulk (Ceftriaxone Sodium) Roche Laboratories 2801
Spectracef Tablets (Cefditoren Pivoxil) Purdue Pharmaceutical 2706
Suprax (Cefixime) Lupin 1811
Tequin Injection (Gatifloxacin) Bristol-Myers Squibb 964
Tequin Tablets (Gatifloxacin) Bristol-Myers Squibb 964
Vantin Tablets and Oral Suspension (Cefpodoxime Proxetil) Pharmacia & Upjohn 2650
Zinacef Injection (Cefuroxime) GlaxoSmithKline 1604
Zinacef for Injection (Cefuroxime) GlaxoSmithKline 1604
Zithromax Capsules, 250 mg (Azithromycin Dihydrate) Pfizer 2568
Zithromax for IV Infusion (Azithromycin Dihydrate) Pfizer 2573
Zithromax for Oral Suspension, 1 g (Azithromycin Dihydrate) Pfizer 2568
Zithromax for Oral Suspension, 300 mg, 600 mg, 900 mg, 1200 mg (Azithromycin Dihydrate) Pfizer 2561
Zithromax Tablets, 250 mg, 500 mg (Azithromycin Dihydrate) Pfizer 2561
Zithromax Tablets, 600 mg (Azithromycin Dihydrate) Pfizer 2568
Zithromax Tri-Pak (Azithromycin Dihydrate) Pfizer 2561
Zithromax Z-Pak (Azithromycin Dihydrate) Pfizer 2568
Zmax for Oral Suspension (Azithromycin) Pfizer 2577
Zyvox (Linezolid) Pharmacia & Upjohn 2661

S. pneumoniae infections, ocular

Blephamide Ophthalmic Ointment (Prednisolone Acetate, Sulfacetamide Sodium) Allergan 563
Blephamide Ophthalmic Suspension (Prednisolone Acetate, Sulfacetamide Sodium) Allergan 564
Ciloxan Ophthalmic Ointment (Ciprofloxacin Hydrochloride) Alcon 554
FML-S Liquifilm Sterile Ophthalmic Suspension (Fluorometholone, Sulfacetamide Sodium) Allergan .... ⊙ 226
Genoptic Sterile Ophthalmic Solution (Gentamicin Sulfate) Allergan .... ⊙ 227
Polytrim Ophthalmic Solution (Polymyxin B Sulfate, Trimethoprim Sulfate) Allergan 570
Pred-G Ophthalmic Suspension (Gentamicin Sulfate, Prednisolone Acetate) Allergan .... ⊙ 234
Pred-G Sterile Ophthalmic Ointment (Gentamicin Sulfate, Prednisolone Acetate) Allergan .... ⊙ 235
Quixin Ophthalmic Solution (Levofloxacin) Vistakon 3373
TobraDex Ophthalmic Ointment (Dexamethasone, Tobramycin) Alcon 558
TobraDex Ophthalmic Suspension (Dexamethasone, Tobramycin) Alcon 558
Vigamox Ophthalmic Solution (Moxifloxacin Hydrochloride) Alcon 560
Zylet Ophthalmic Suspension (Loteprednol Etabonate, Tobramycin) Bausch & Lomb 3508
Zymar Ophthalmic Solution (Gatifloxacin) Allergan 571

S. pneumoniae lower respiratory tract infections

Augmentin XR Extended-Release Tablets (Amoxicillin, Clavulanate Potassium) GlaxoSmithKline 1340
Avelox (Moxifloxacin Hydrochloride) Schering 2984
Biaxin/Biaxin XL (Clarithromycin) Abbott 402
Cipro I.V. (Ciprofloxacin) Schering 2998
Cipro I.V. Pharmacy Bulk Package (Ciprofloxacin) Bayer 3509
Cipro (Ciprofloxacin) Schering 2991
Cleocin Vaginal Ovules (Clindamycin Hydrochloride) Pharmacia & Upjohn 2613
E.E.S. (Erythromycin Ethylsuccinate) Abbott 449
EryPed (Erythromycin Ethylsuccinate) Abbott 445
Ery-Tab Tablets (Erythromycin) Abbott 447
Erythrocin Stearate Filmtab Tablets (Erythromycin Stearate) Abbott 452
Erythromycin Base Filmtab Tablets (Erythromycin) Abbott 454
Erythromycin Delayed-Release Capsules, USP (Erythromycin) Abbott 456
Fortaz (Ceftazidime Sodium) GlaxoSmithKline 1422
Invanz for Injection (Ertapenem) Merck 1974
Ketek Tablets (Telithromycin) Sanofi-Aventis 2920
Levaquin in 5% Dextrose Injection (Levofloxacin) Ortho-McNeil 2453
Levaquin (Levofloxacin) Ortho-McNeil 2453
Maxipime for Injection (Cefepime Hydrochloride) Elan 1093
Mefoxin for Injection (Cefoxitin Sodium) Merck 1987
Mefoxin Premixed Intravenous Solution (Cefoxitin Sodium) Merck 1990
Omnicef Capsules (Cefdinir) Abbott 506
Omnicef for Oral Suspension (Cefdinir) Abbott 506
PCE Dispertab Tablets (Erythromycin) Abbott 510
Primaxin I.M. (Cilastatin Sodium, Imipenem) Merck 2022
Rocephin Injectable Vials, ADD-Vantage, Galaxy, Bulk (Ceftriaxone Sodium) Roche Laboratories 2801
Spectracef Tablets (Cefditoren Pivoxil) Purdue Pharmaceutical 2706
Vantin Tablets and Oral Suspension (Cefpodoxime Proxetil) Pharmacia & Upjohn 2650
Zinacef Injection (Cefuroxime) GlaxoSmithKline 1604
Zinacef for Injection (Cefuroxime) GlaxoSmithKline 1604
Zithromax Capsules, 250 mg (Azithromycin Dihydrate) Pfizer 2568
Zithromax for IV Infusion (Azithromycin Dihydrate) Pfizer 2573
Zithromax for Oral Suspension, 1 g (Azithromycin Dihydrate) Pfizer 2568
Zithromax for Oral Suspension, 300 mg, 600 mg, 900 mg, 1200 mg (Azithromycin Dihydrate) Pfizer 2561
Zithromax Tablets, 250 mg, 500 mg (Azithromycin Dihydrate) Pfizer 2561
Zithromax Tablets, 600 mg (Azithromycin Dihydrate) Pfizer 2568
Zithromax Tri-Pak (Azithromycin Dihydrate) Pfizer 2561
Zithromax Z-Pak (Azithromycin Dihydrate) Pfizer 2568
Zmax for Oral Suspension (Azithromycin) Pfizer 2577
Zyvox (Linezolid) Pharmacia & Upjohn 2661

S. pneumoniae meningitis

Fortaz (Ceftazidime Sodium) GlaxoSmithKline 1422
Merrem I.V. (Meropenem) AstraZeneca 687
Rocephin Injectable Vials, ADD-Vantage, Galaxy, Bulk (Ceftriaxone Sodium) Roche Laboratories 2801
Zinacef Injection (Cefuroxime) GlaxoSmithKline 1604
Zinacef for Injection (Cefuroxime) GlaxoSmithKline 1604

S. pneumoniae otitis media

Augmentin Tablets (Amoxicillin, Clavulanate Potassium) GlaxoSmithKline 1334
Augmentin ES-600 Powder for Oral Suspension (Amoxicillin, Clavulanate Potassium) GlaxoSmithKline 1337
Biaxin/Biaxin XL (Clarithromycin) Abbott 402
Ceftin (Cefuroxime Axetil) GlaxoSmithKline 1369
Floxin Otic Singles (Ofloxacin) Daiichi 1045
Floxin Otic Solution (Ofloxacin) Daiichi 1043
Omnicef Capsules (Cefdinir) Abbott 506
Omnicef for Oral Suspension (Cefdinir) Abbott 506
Prevnar for Injection (Pneumococcal vaccine, diphtheria conjugate) Wyeth 3460
Rocephin Injectable Vials, ADD-Vantage, Galaxy, Bulk (Ceftriaxone Sodium) Roche Laboratories 2801
Suprax (Cefixime) Lupin 1811
Vantin Tablets and Oral Suspension (Cefpodoxime Proxetil) Pharmacia & Upjohn 2650
Zithromax Capsules, 250 mg (Azithromycin Dihydrate) Pfizer 2568
Zithromax for Oral Suspension, 300 mg, 600 mg, 900 mg, 1200 mg (Azithromycin Dihydrate) Pfizer 2561
Zithromax Tablets, 250 mg, 500 mg (Azithromycin Dihydrate) Pfizer 2561
Zithromax Tri-Pak (Azithromycin Dihydrate) Pfizer 2561

S. pneumoniae pharyngitis

EryPed (Erythromycin Ethylsuccinate) Abbott 445
Ery-Tab Tablets (Erythromycin) Abbott 447
Erythrocin Stearate Filmtab Tablets (Erythromycin Stearate) Abbott 452
Erythromycin Base Filmtab Tablets (Erythromycin) Abbott 454
Erythromycin Delayed-Release Capsules, USP (Erythromycin) Abbott 456
PCE Dispertab Tablets (Erythromycin) Abbott 510

S. pneumoniae respiratory tract infections

Ancef for Injection (Cefazolin Sodium) GlaxoSmithKline 1318
Spectracef Tablets (Cefditoren Pivoxil) Purdue Pharmaceutical 2706
Zmax for Oral Suspension (Azithromycin) Pfizer 2577

S. pneumoniae septicemia

Ancef for Injection (Cefazolin Sodium) GlaxoSmithKline 1318
Fortaz (Ceftazidime Sodium) GlaxoSmithKline 1422
Mefoxin for Injection (Cefoxitin Sodium) Merck 1987
Mefoxin Premixed Intravenous Solution (Cefoxitin Sodium) Merck 1990
Rocephin Injectable Vials, ADD-Vantage, Galaxy, Bulk (Ceftriaxone Sodium) Roche Laboratories 2801
Zinacef Injection (Cefuroxime) GlaxoSmithKline 1604
Zinacef for Injection (Cefuroxime) GlaxoSmithKline 1604

S. pneumoniae sinusitis

Augmentin XR Extended-Release Tablets (Amoxicillin, Clavulanate Potassium) GlaxoSmithKline 1340
Avelox (Moxifloxacin Hydrochloride) Schering 2984
Biaxin/Biaxin XL (Clarithromycin) Abbott 402
Ceftin Tablets (Cefuroxime Axetil) GlaxoSmithKline 1369
Cipro I.V. (Ciprofloxacin) Schering 2998
Cipro I.V. Pharmacy Bulk Package (Ciprofloxacin) Bayer 3509
Cipro (Ciprofloxacin) Schering 2991
Ketek Tablets (Telithromycin) Sanofi-Aventis 2920
Levaquin in 5% Dextrose Injection (Levofloxacin) Ortho-McNeil 2453
Levaquin (Levofloxacin) Ortho-McNeil 2453
Tequin Injection (Gatifloxacin) Bristol-Myers Squibb 964
Tequin Tablets (Gatifloxacin) Bristol-Myers Squibb 964
Vantin Tablets and Oral Suspension (Cefpodoxime Proxetil) Pharmacia & Upjohn 2650
Zithromax for Oral Suspension, 300 mg, 600 mg, 900 mg, 1200 mg (Azithromycin Dihydrate) Pfizer 2561
Zithromax Tablets, 250 mg, 500 mg (Azithromycin Dihydrate) Pfizer 2561
Zithromax Tri-Pak (Azithromycin Dihydrate) Pfizer 2561
Zmax for Oral Suspension (Azithromycin) Pfizer 2577

S. pneumoniae upper respiratory tract infections

Biaxin/Biaxin XL (Clarithromycin) Abbott 402
Dynacin Tablets (Minocycline Hydrochloride) Medicis 1859
E.E.S. (Erythromycin Ethylsuccinate) Abbott 449
EryPed (Erythromycin Ethylsuccinate) Abbott 445
Ery-Tab Tablets (Erythromycin) Abbott 447
Erythrocin Stearate Filmtab Tablets (Erythromycin Stearate) Abbott 452
Erythromycin Base Filmtab Tablets (Erythromycin) Abbott 454
Erythromycin Delayed-Release Capsules, USP (Erythromycin) Abbott 456
PCE Dispertab Tablets (Erythromycin) Abbott 510

S. pyogenes endocarditis
Ancef (Cefazolin Sodium) GlaxoSmithKline ... 1318

S. pyogenes infections
Bactroban Ointment (Mupirocin) GlaxoSmithKline ... 1358
Biaxin/Biaxin XL (Clarithromycin) Abbott ... 402
Ceftin (Cefuroxime Axetil) GlaxoSmithKline ... 1369
Centany Ointment, 2% (Mupirocin) OrthoNeutrogena ... 2382
Cipro I.V. (Ciprofloxacin) Schering ... 2998
Cipro I.V. Pharmacy Bulk Package (Ciprofloxacin) Bayer ... 3509
Cipro (Ciprofloxacin) Schering ... 2991
Cleocin Vaginal Ovules (Clindamycin Hydrochloride) Pharmacia & Upjohn ... 2613
E.E.S. (Erythromycin Ethylsuccinate) Abbott ... 449
EryPed (Erythromycin Ethylsuccinate) Abbott ... 445
Ery-Tab Tablets (Erythromycin) Abbott ... 447
Erythrocin Stearate Filmtab Tablets (Erythromycin Stearate) Abbott ... 452
Erythromycin Base Filmtab Tablets (Erythromycin) Abbott ... 454
Erythromycin Delayed-Release Capsules, USP (Erythromycin) Abbott ... 456
Fortaz (Ceftazidime Sodium) GlaxoSmithKline ... 1422
Invanz for Injection (Ertapenem) Merck ... 1974
Levaquin in 5% Dextrose Injection (Levofloxacin) Ortho-McNeil ... 2453
Levaquin (Levofloxacin) Ortho-McNeil ... 2453
Mefoxin for Injection (Cefoxitin Sodium) Merck ... 1987
Mefoxin Premixed Intravenous Solution (Cefoxitin Sodium) Merck ... 1990
Merrem I.V. (Meropenem) AstraZeneca ... 687
Omnicef Capsules (Cefdinir) Abbott ... 506
Omnicef for Oral Suspension (Cefdinir) Abbott ... 506
PCE Dispertab Tablets (Erythromycin) Abbott ... 510
Primaxin I.M. (Cilastatin Sodium, Imipenem) Merck ... 2022
Primaxin I.V. (Cilastatin Sodium, Imipenem) Merck ... 2024
Rocephin Injectable Vials, ADD-Vantage, Galaxy, Bulk (Ceftriaxone Sodium) Roche Laboratories ... 2801
Spectracef Tablets (Cefditoren Pivoxil) Purdue Pharmaceutical ... 2706
Suprax (Cefixime) Lupin ... 1811
Tygacil for Injection (Tigecycline) Wyeth ... 3489
Vantin Tablets and Oral Suspension (Cefpodoxime Proxetil) Pharmacia & Upjohn ... 2650
Zinacef Injection (Cefuroxime) GlaxoSmithKline ... 1604
Zinacef for Injection (Cefuroxime) GlaxoSmithKline ... 1604
Zithromax (Azithromycin Dihydrate) Pfizer ... 2568
Zithromax for Oral Suspension, 300 mg, 600 mg, 900 mg, 1200 mg (Azithromycin Dihydrate) Pfizer ... 2561
Zithromax Tablets, 250 mg, 500 mg (Azithromycin Dihydrate) Pfizer ... 2561
Zithromax Tablets, 600 mg (Azithromycin Dihydrate) Pfizer ... 2568
Zithromax Tri-Pak (Azithromycin Dihydrate) Pfizer ... 2561
Zithromax Z-Pak (Azithromycin Dihydrate) Pfizer ... 2568
Zyvox (Linezolid) Pharmacia & Upjohn ... 2661

S. pyogenes infections, ocular
Genoptic Sterile Ophthalmic Solution (Gentamicin Sulfate) Allergan ... ⊙ 227
Pred-G Sterile Ophthalmic Ointment (Gentamicin Sulfate, Prednisolone Acetate) Allergan ... ⊙ 235

S. pyogenes lower respiratory tract infections
E.E.S. (Erythromycin Ethylsuccinate) Abbott ... 449
EryPed (Erythromycin Ethylsuccinate) Abbott ... 445
Ery-Tab Tablets (Erythromycin) Abbott ... 447
Erythrocin Stearate Filmtab Tablets (Erythromycin Stearate) Abbott ... 452
Erythromycin Base Filmtab Tablets (Erythromycin) Abbott ... 454
Erythromycin Delayed-Release Capsules, USP (Erythromycin) Abbott ... 456
PCE Dispertab Tablets (Erythromycin) Abbott ... 510
Zinacef Injection (Cefuroxime) GlaxoSmithKline ... 1604
Zinacef for Injection (Cefuroxime) GlaxoSmithKline ... 1604

S. pyogenes otitis media
Ceftin (Cefuroxime Axetil) GlaxoSmithKline ... 1369
Suprax (Cefixime) Lupin ... 1811

S. pyogenes pharyngitis
Biaxin/Biaxin XL (Clarithromycin) Abbott ... 402
Ceftin (Cefuroxime Axetil) GlaxoSmithKline ... 1369
Omnicef Capsules (Cefdinir) Abbott ... 506
Omnicef for Oral Suspension (Cefdinir) Abbott ... 506
Suprax (Cefixime) Lupin ... 1811
Vantin Tablets and Oral Suspension (Cefpodoxime Proxetil) Pharmacia & Upjohn ... 2650
Zithromax (Azithromycin Dihydrate) Pfizer ... 2568
Zithromax for Oral Suspension, 300 mg, 600 mg, 900 mg, 1200 mg (Azithromycin Dihydrate) Pfizer ... 2561
Zithromax Tablets, 250 mg, 500 mg (Azithromycin Dihydrate) Pfizer ... 2561
Zithromax Tablets, 600 mg (Azithromycin Dihydrate) Pfizer ... 2568
Zithromax Tri-Pak (Azithromycin Dihydrate) Pfizer ... 2561
Zithromax Z-Pak (Azithromycin Dihydrate) Pfizer ... 2568

S. pyogenes respiratory tract infections
Ancef for Injection (Cefazolin Sodium) GlaxoSmithKline ... 1318

S. pyogenes skin and skin structure infections
Ancef for Injection (Cefazolin Sodium) GlaxoSmithKline ... 1318
Avelox (Moxifloxacin Hydrochloride) Schering ... 2984
Bactroban Cream (Mupirocin Calcium) GlaxoSmithKline ... 1356
Biaxin/Biaxin XL (Clarithromycin) Abbott ... 402
Ceftin Tablets (Cefuroxime Axetil) GlaxoSmithKline ... 1369
Centany Ointment, 2% (Mupirocin) OrthoNeutrogena ... 2382
Cipro I.V. (Ciprofloxacin) Schering ... 2998
Cipro I.V. Pharmacy Bulk Package (Ciprofloxacin) Bayer ... 3509
Cipro (Ciprofloxacin) Schering ... 2991
Cleocin Vaginal Ovules (Clindamycin Hydrochloride) Pharmacia & Upjohn ... 2613
Cubicin for Injection (Daptomycin) Cubist ... 1038
E.E.S. (Erythromycin Ethylsuccinate) Abbott ... 449
EryPed (Erythromycin Ethylsuccinate) Abbott ... 445
Ery-Tab Tablets (Erythromycin) Abbott ... 447
Erythrocin Stearate Filmtab Tablets (Erythromycin Stearate) Abbott ... 452
Erythromycin Base Filmtab Tablets (Erythromycin) Abbott ... 454
Erythromycin Delayed-Release Capsules, USP (Erythromycin) Abbott ... 456
Fortaz (Ceftazidime Sodium) GlaxoSmithKline ... 1422
Invanz for Injection (Ertapenem) Merck ... 1974
Levaquin in 5% Dextrose Injection (Levofloxacin) Ortho-McNeil ... 2453
Levaquin (Levofloxacin) Ortho-McNeil ... 2453
Maxipime for Injection (Cefepime Hydrochloride) Elan ... 1093
Mefoxin for Injection (Cefoxitin Sodium) Merck ... 1987
Mefoxin Premixed Intravenous Solution (Cefoxitin Sodium) Merck ... 1990
Merrem I.V. (Meropenem) AstraZeneca ... 687
Omnicef Capsules (Cefdinir) Abbott ... 506
Omnicef for Oral Suspension (Cefdinir) Abbott ... 506
PCE Dispertab Tablets (Erythromycin) Abbott ... 510
Primaxin I.M. (Cilastatin Sodium, Imipenem) Merck ... 2022
Primaxin I.V. (Cilastatin Sodium, Imipenem) Merck ... 2024
Rocephin Injectable Vials, ADD-Vantage, Galaxy, Bulk (Ceftriaxone Sodium) Roche Laboratories ... 2801
Synercid I.V. (Dalfopristin, Quinupristin) King ... 1690
Tequin Injection (Gatifloxacin) Bristol-Myers Squibb ... 964
Tequin Tablets (Gatifloxacin) Bristol-Myers Squibb ... 964
Tygacil for Injection (Tigecycline) Wyeth ... 3489
Vantin Tablets and Oral Suspension (Cefpodoxime Proxetil) Pharmacia & Upjohn ... 2650
Zinacef Injection (Cefuroxime) GlaxoSmithKline ... 1604
Zinacef for Injection (Cefuroxime) GlaxoSmithKline ... 1604
Zithromax (Azithromycin Dihydrate) Pfizer ... 2568
Zithromax for Oral Suspension, 300 mg, 600 mg, 900 mg, 1200 mg (Azithromycin Dihydrate) Pfizer ... 2561
Zithromax Tablets, 250 mg, 500 mg (Azithromycin Dihydrate) Pfizer ... 2561
Zithromax Tablets, 600 mg (Azithromycin Dihydrate) Pfizer ... 2568
Zithromax Tri-Pak (Azithromycin Dihydrate) Pfizer ... 2561
Zithromax Z-Pak (Azithromycin Dihydrate) Pfizer ... 2568
Zyvox (Linezolid) Pharmacia & Upjohn ... 2661

S. pyogenes tonsillitis
Biaxin/Biaxin XL (Clarithromycin) Abbott ... 402
Ceftin (Cefuroxime Axetil) GlaxoSmithKline ... 1369
Omnicef Capsules (Cefdinir) Abbott ... 506
Omnicef for Oral Suspension (Cefdinir) Abbott ... 506
Suprax (Cefixime) Lupin ... 1811
Vantin Tablets and Oral Suspension (Cefpodoxime Proxetil) Pharmacia & Upjohn ... 2650
Zithromax (Azithromycin Dihydrate) Pfizer ... 2568
Zithromax for Oral Suspension, 300 mg, 600 mg, 900 mg, 1200 mg (Azithromycin Dihydrate) Pfizer ... 2561
Zithromax Tablets, 250 mg, 500 mg (Azithromycin Dihydrate) Pfizer ... 2561
Zithromax Tablets, 600 mg (Azithromycin Dihydrate) Pfizer ... 2568
Zithromax Tri-Pak (Azithromycin Dihydrate) Pfizer ... 2561
Zithromax Z-Pak (Azithromycin Dihydrate) Pfizer ... 2568

S. pyogenes upper respiratory tract infections
Biaxin/Biaxin XL (Clarithromycin) Abbott ... 402
E.E.S. (Erythromycin Ethylsuccinate) Abbott ... 449
EryPed (Erythromycin Ethylsuccinate) Abbott ... 445
Ery-Tab Tablets (Erythromycin) Abbott ... 447
Erythrocin Stearate Filmtab Tablets (Erythromycin Stearate) Abbott ... 452
Erythromycin Base Filmtab Tablets (Erythromycin) Abbott ... 454
Erythromycin Delayed-Release Capsules, USP (Erythromycin) Abbott ... 456
Omnicef Capsules (Cefdinir) Abbott ... 506
Omnicef for Oral Suspension (Cefdinir) Abbott ... 506
PCE Dispertab Tablets (Erythromycin) Abbott ... 510
Suprax (Cefixime) Lupin ... 1811
Zithromax (Azithromycin Dihydrate) Pfizer ... 2568
Zithromax for Oral Suspension, 300 mg, 600 mg, 900 mg, 1200 mg (Azithromycin Dihydrate) Pfizer ... 2561
Zithromax Tablets, 250 mg, 500 mg (Azithromycin Dihydrate) Pfizer ... 2561
Zithromax Tablets, 600 mg (Azithromycin Dihydrate) Pfizer ... 2568
Zithromax Tri-Pak (Azithromycin Dihydrate) Pfizer ... 2561
Zithromax Z-Pak (Azithromycin Dihydrate) Pfizer ... 2568

S. saprophyticus urinary tract infections
Cipro (Ciprofloxacin) Schering ... 2991
Cipro XR Tablets (Ciprofloxacin) Schering ... 3004
Noroxin Tablets (Norfloxacin) Merck ... 2009
Vantin Tablets and Oral Suspension (Cefpodoxime Proxetil) Pharmacia & Upjohn ... 2650

S. viridans endocarditis
Erythrocin Stearate Filmtab Tablets (Erythromycin Stearate) Abbott ... 452
Erythromycin Base Filmtab Tablets (Erythromycin) Abbott ... 454

S. viridans skin and skin structure infections
Merrem I.V. (Meropenem) AstraZeneca ... 687

S. warnerii infections, ocular
Vigamox Ophthalmic Solution (Moxifloxacin Hydrochloride) Alcon ... 560

SAH
(*see under* Hemorrhage, subarachnoid, resulting in neurological deficits)

Salmonella typhi infections
Cipro (Ciprofloxacin) Schering ... 2991

Sarcoidosis, symptomatic
Decadron Phosphate Injection (Dexamethasone Sodium Phosphate) Merck ... 1931
Decadron Tablets (Dexamethasone) Merck ... 1929
Depo-Medrol Injectable Suspension (Methylprednisolone Acetate) Pharmacia & Upjohn ... 2615
Depo-Medrol Single-Dose Vial (Methylprednisolone Acetate) Pharmacia & Upjohn ... 2617
Hydrocortone Tablets (Hydrocortisone) Merck ... 1963
Pediapred Oral Solution (Prednisolone Sodium Phosphate) UCB ... 3319

Sarcoma botryoides
Cosmegen for Injection (Dactinomycin) Merck ... 1907

Sarcomas, soft tissue and bone
Adriamycin for Injection, USP (Doxorubicin Hydrochloride) Bedford ... 786
Adriamycin Injection, USP (Doxorubicin Hydrochloride) Bedford ... 786

Sarcoptes scabiei infestations
Acticin Cream (Permethrin) Mylan Bertek ... 2125

Scabies
(*see under* Sarcoptes scabiei infestations)

Scar tissue
Mederma for Kids Topical Gel (Allantoin, Allium cepa) Merz ... 2097
Mederma Topical Gel (Allantoin, Allium cepa) Merz ... 2096

Scar Tissue Removal
Neosporin Scar Solution (Silicone) Pfizer Consumer Healthcare .... ▣ 702

Scedosporium apiospermum infections
VFEND I.V. (Voriconazole) Pfizer 2543
VFEND Oral Suspension (Voriconazole) Pfizer 2543
VFEND Tablets (Voriconazole) Pfizer.................. 2543

Schistosoma haematobium infections
Biltricide (Praziquantel) Schering 2990

Schizophrenia
Abilify Tablets (Aripiprazole) Bristol-Myers Squibb 916
Abilify Tablets (Aripiprazole) Otsuka America.................. 2472
Clozapine Tablets (Clozapine) Mylan Bertek 2141
Clozaril Tablets (Clozapine) Novartis 2174
FazaClo Orally Disintegrating Tablets (Clozapine) Alamo 547
Geodon (Ziprasidone Hydrochloride) Pfizer 2514
Moban Tablets (Molindone Hydrochloride) Endo Labs 1108
Risperdal Consta Long-Acting Injection (Risperidone) Janssen 1664
Risperdal M-Tab Orally Disintegrating Tablets (Risperidone) Janssen 1658
Risperdal (Risperidone) Janssen 1658
Seroquel Tablets (Quetiapine Fumarate) AstraZeneca 691
Thioridazine Hydrochloride Tablets (Thioridazine Hydrochloride) Mylan 2122
Thiothixene Capsules (Thiothixene) Mylan 2124
Zyprexa Tablets (Olanzapine) Lilly 1798
Zyprexa IntraMuscular (Olanzapine) Lilly 1798
Zyprexa ZYDIS Orally Disintegrating Tablets (Olanzapine) Lilly 1798

Sciatica, temporary relief of
BC Powder (Aspirin, Caffeine, Salicylamide) GlaxoSmithKline ....▣ 612
Arthritis Strength BC Powder (Aspirin, Caffeine, Salicylamide) GlaxoSmithKline ....▣ 612

Scleroderma, linear, possibly effective in
Potaba (Aminobenzoate Potassium) Glenwood 1634

Seborrhea
(*see under* Dandruff)

Sedation
(*see also under* Sleep, induction of)
Nembutal Sodium Solution, USP (Pentobarbital Sodium) Ovation 2484
Phenergan (Promethazine Hydrochloride) Wyeth 3438

Sedation, obstetric
Phenergan (Promethazine Hydrochloride) Wyeth 3438

Seizures, absence, adjunctive therapy in
Depacon Injection (Valproate Sodium) Abbott 412
Depakene (Valproic Acid) Abbott 417
Depakote Sprinkle Capsules (Divalproex Sodium) Abbott 422
Depakote Tablets (Divalproex Sodium) Abbott 427
Depakote ER Tablets (Divalproex Sodium) Abbott 433

Seizures, akinetic
Klonopin (Clonazepam) Roche Laboratories 2782

Seizures, centrencephalic
(*see under* Seizures, generalized, absence; Seizures, generalized, tonic-clonic)

Seizures, focal
Carbatrol Capsules (Carbamazepine) Shire US 3174
Depacon Injection (Valproate Sodium) Abbott 412
Depakene (Valproic Acid) Abbott 417
Depakote Sprinkle Capsules (Divalproex Sodium) Abbott 422
Depakote Tablets (Divalproex Sodium) Abbott 427
Depakote ER Tablets (Divalproex Sodium) Abbott.................. 433
Lamictal (Lamotrigine) GlaxoSmithKline 1449
Lyrica Capsules (Pregabalin) Pfizer... 2524
Phenytek Capsules (Phenytoin Sodium) Mylan Bertek 2153
Tegretol/Tegretol-XR (Carbamazepine) Novartis 2278
Tranxene T-TAB Tablets (Clorazepate Dipotassium) Ovation 2488
Trileptal Oral Suspension (Oxcarbazepine) Novartis.................. 2281
Trileptal Tablets (Oxcarbazepine) Novartis 2281

Seizures, focal, adjunctive therapy in
Depakote Sprinkle Capsules (Divalproex Sodium) Abbott 422
Keppra Oral Solution (Levetiracetam) UCB 3307
Keppra Tablets (Levetiracetam) UCB 3307
Neurontin Capsules (Gabapentin) Parke-Davis 2498
Neurontin Oral Solution (Gabapentin) Parke-Davis 2498
Neurontin Tablets (Gabapentin) Parke-Davis 2498
Topamax Sprinkle Capsules (Topiramate) Ortho-McNeil Neurologics 2438
Topamax Tablets (Topiramate) Ortho-McNeil Neurologics 2438
Tranxene (Clorazepate Dipotassium) Ovation 2488
Trileptal Oral Suspension (Oxcarbazepine) Novartis 2281
Trileptal Tablets (Oxcarbazepine) Novartis 2281

Seizures, generalized, absence
Depacon Injection (Valproate Sodium) Abbott 412
Depakene (Valproic Acid) Abbott 417
Depakote Sprinkle Capsules (Divalproex Sodium) Abbott 422
Depakote Tablets (Divalproex Sodium) Abbott 427
Depakote ER Tablets (Divalproex Sodium) Abbott 433
Klonopin (Clonazepam) Roche Laboratories 2782
Mebaral Tablets, USP (Mephobarbital) Ovation 2483

Seizures, generalized, tonic-clonic
Carbatrol Capsules (Carbamazepine) Shire US 3174
Mebaral Tablets, USP (Mephobarbital) Ovation 2483
Peganone Tablets, USP (Ethotoin) Ovation 2487
Phenytek Capsules (Phenytoin Sodium) Mylan Bertek 2153
Tegretol/Tegretol-XR (Carbamazepine) Novartis 2278
Topamax Sprinkle Capsules (Topiramate) Ortho-McNeil Neurologics 2438
Topamax Tablets (Topiramate) Ortho-McNeil Neurologics 2438

Seizures, multiple, adjunctive therapy in
Depacon Injection (Valproate Sodium) Abbott 412
Depakene (Valproic Acid) Abbott 417
Depakote Tablets (Divalproex Sodium) Abbott 427
Depakote ER Tablets (Divalproex Sodium) Abbott 433

Seizures, myoclonic
Klonopin (Clonazepam) Roche Laboratories 2782

Seizures, neurosurgery-induced
Phenytek Capsules (Phenytoin Sodium) Mylan Bertek 2153

Seizures, partial
(*see under* Seizures, focal)

Seizures, partial, adjunctive therapy in
Depacon Injection (Valproate Sodium) Abbott 412
Depakene (Valproic Acid) Abbott 417
Depakote Sprinkle Capsules (Divalproex Sodium) Abbott 422
Depakote Tablets (Divalproex Sodium) Abbott 427
Depakote ER Tablets (Divalproex Sodium) Abbott.................. 433
Gabitril Tablets (Tiagabine Hydrochloride) Cephalon 998
Lamictal (Lamotrigine) GlaxoSmithKline.................. 1449
Zonegran Capsules (Zonisamide) Eisai 1089

Seizures, psychomotor
Carbatrol Capsules (Carbamazepine) Shire US 3174
Peganone Tablets, USP (Ethotoin) Ovation.................. 2487
Phenytek Capsules (Phenytoin Sodium) Mylan Bertek 2153
Tegretol-XR Tablets (Carbamazepine) Novartis 2278

Seizures, unspecified, adjunctive therapy in
Diastat Rectal Delivery System (Diazepam) Valeant 3344

Senile lentigines
(*see under* Hyperpigmentation, skin, bleaching of)

Sepsis
Zinacef Injection (Cefuroxime) GlaxoSmithKline 1604
Zinacef for Injection (Cefuroxime) GlaxoSmithKline 1604

Sepsis, bacterial, neonatal
Garamycin Injectable (Gentamicin Sulfate) Schering 3028

Sepsis, severe
Xigris Powder for Intravenous Infusion (Drotrecogin alfa (activated)) Lilly 1796

Septic shock, treatment adjunct
Narcan Injection (Naloxone Hydrochloride) Endo Labs 1109

Septicemia, bacterial
Ancef for Injection (Cefazolin Sodium) GlaxoSmithKline 1318
Cipro I.V. (Ciprofloxacin) Schering 2998
Cipro I.V. Pharmacy Bulk Package (Ciprofloxacin) Bayer 3509
Cleocin Vaginal Ovules (Clindamycin Hydrochloride) Pharmacia & Upjohn 2613
Fortaz (Ceftazidime Sodium) GlaxoSmithKline 1422
Garamycin Injectable (Gentamicin Sulfate) Schering 3028
Invanz for Injection (Ertapenem) Merck 1974
Mefoxin for Injection (Cefoxitin Sodium) Merck 1987
Mefoxin Premixed Intravenous Solution (Cefoxitin Sodium) Merck 1990
Primaxin I.V. (Cilastatin Sodium, Imipenem) Merck 2024
Rocephin Injectable Vials, ADD-Vantage, Galaxy, Bulk (Ceftriaxone Sodium) Roche Laboratories 2801
Timentin ADD-Vantage (Clavulanate Potassium, Ticarcillin Disodium) GlaxoSmithKline 1556
Timentin Injection Galaxy Container (Clavulanate Potassium, Ticarcillin Disodium) GlaxoSmithKline 1559
Timentin IV Infusion (Clavulanate Potassium, Ticarcillin Disodium) GlaxoSmithKline 1553
Timentin Pharmacy Bulk Package (Clavulanate Potassium, Ticarcillin Disodium) GlaxoSmithKline 1562
Zinacef Injection (Cefuroxime) GlaxoSmithKline 1604
Zinacef for Injection (Cefuroxime) GlaxoSmithKline 1604
Zyvox (Linezolid) Pharmacia & Upjohn 2661

Serratia marcescens bone and joint infections
Cipro I.V. (Ciprofloxacin) Schering 2998
Cipro I.V. Pharmacy Bulk Package (Ciprofloxacin) Bayer.................. 3509
Cipro (Ciprofloxacin) Schering 2991

Serratia marcescens infections
Cipro I.V. (Ciprofloxacin) Schering 2998
Cipro I.V. Pharmacy Bulk Package (Ciprofloxacin) Bayer 3509
Cipro (Ciprofloxacin) Schering 2991
Noroxin Tablets (Norfloxacin) Merck . 2009
Primaxin I.V. (Cilastatin Sodium, Imipenem) Merck 2024
Rocephin Injectable Vials, ADD-Vantage, Galaxy, Bulk (Ceftriaxone Sodium) Roche Laboratories 2801
Timentin ADD-Vantage (Clavulanate Potassium, Ticarcillin Disodium) GlaxoSmithKline.................. 1556
Timentin Injection Galaxy Container (Clavulanate Potassium, Ticarcillin Disodium) GlaxoSmithKline 1559
Timentin IV Infusion (Clavulanate Potassium, Ticarcillin Disodium) GlaxoSmithKline.................. 1553
Timentin Pharmacy Bulk Package (Clavulanate Potassium, Ticarcillin Disodium) GlaxoSmithKline 1562

Serratia marcescens infections, ocular
Ciloxan Ophthalmic Ointment (Ciprofloxacin Hydrochloride) Alcon.................. 554
Genoptic Sterile Ophthalmic Solution (Gentamicin Sulfate) Allergan .... ⊙ 227
Pred-G Ophthalmic Suspension (Gentamicin Sulfate, Prednisolone Acetate) Allergan.................. ⊙ 234
Pred-G Sterile Ophthalmic Ointment (Gentamicin Sulfate, Prednisolone Acetate) Allergan..... ⊙ 235
Quixin Ophthalmic Solution (Levofloxacin) Vistakon.................. 3373

Serratia marcescens lower respiratory tract infections
Levaquin in 5% Dextrose Injection (Levofloxacin) Ortho-McNeil.......... 2453
Levaquin (Levofloxacin) Ortho-McNeil.................. 2453
Primaxin I.V. (Cilastatin Sodium, Imipenem) Merck 2024
Rocephin Injectable Vials, ADD-Vantage, Galaxy, Bulk (Ceftriaxone Sodium) Roche Laboratories.................. 2801

Serratia marcescens skin and skin structure infections
Rocephin Injectable Vials, ADD-Vantage, Galaxy, Bulk (Ceftriaxone Sodium) Roche Laboratories.................. 2801

Serratia marcescens urinary tract infections
Cipro I.V. (Ciprofloxacin) Schering 2998
Cipro I.V. Pharmacy Bulk Package (Ciprofloxacin) Bayer 3509
Cipro (Ciprofloxacin) Schering 2991
Noroxin Tablets (Norfloxacin) Merck . 2009
Timentin ADD-Vantage (Clavulanate Potassium, Ticarcillin Disodium) GlaxoSmithKline.................. 1556
Timentin Injection Galaxy Container (Clavulanate Potassium, Ticarcillin Disodium) GlaxoSmithKline 1559
Timentin IV Infusion (Clavulanate Potassium, Ticarcillin Disodium) GlaxoSmithKline.................. 1553
Timentin Pharmacy Bulk Package (Clavulanate Potassium, Ticarcillin Disodium) GlaxoSmithKline 1562

Serratia species infections
Fortaz (Ceftazidime Sodium) GlaxoSmithKline.................. 1422
Garamycin Injectable (Gentamicin Sulfate) Schering 3028
Primaxin I.V. (Cilastatin Sodium, Imipenem) Merck 2024

Serratia species lower respiratory tract infections
Fortaz (Ceftazidime Sodium) GlaxoSmithKline.................. 1422

Serratia species septicemia
Primaxin I.V. (Cilastatin Sodium, Imipenem) Merck ... 2024

Serratia species skin and skin structure infections
Fortaz (Ceftazidime Sodium) GlaxoSmithKline ... 1422
Primaxin I.V. (Cilastatin Sodium, Imipenem) Merck ... 2024

Serum sickness
Decadron Phosphate Injection (Dexamethasone Sodium Phosphate) Merck ... 1931
Decadron Tablets (Dexamethasone) Merck ... 1929
Depo-Medrol Injectable Suspension (Methylprednisolone Acetate) Pharmacia & Upjohn ... 2615
Depo-Medrol Single-Dose Vial (Methylprednisolone Acetate) Pharmacia & Upjohn ... 2617
Hydrocortone Tablets (Hydrocortisone) Merck ... 1963
Pediapred Oral Solution (Prednisolone Sodium Phosphate) UCB ... 3319

Shigella flexneri infectious diarrhea
Cipro (Ciprofloxacin) Schering ... 2991

Shigella species infections
Dynacin Tablets (Minocycline Hydrochloride) Medicis ... 1859

Shingles
(*see under* Herpes zoster infections)

Shock, emergency treatment of
Plasbumin-5 (Albumin (human)) Talecris ... 3249
Plasbumin-20 (Albumin (human)) Talecris ... 3249
Plasbumin-25 (Albumin (human)) Talecris ... 3251
Plasmanate (Plasma Protein Fraction (Human)) Talecris ... 3252

Shock, suspected adrenocortical insufficiency
Decadron Phosphate Injection (Dexamethasone Sodium Phosphate) Merck ... 1931

Short stature, idiopathic
Humatrope Vials and Cartridges (Somatropin) Lilly ... 1756

Shoulder, acute painful
(*see under* Bursitis, subacromial, acute, symptomatic relief of)

Sinus congestion, symptomatic relief of
Advil Allergy Sinus Caplets (Chlorpheniramine Maleate, Ibuprofen, Pseudoephedrine Hydrochloride) Wyeth ... ▣737
Children's Advil Cold Suspension (Ibuprofen, Pseudoephedrine Hydrochloride) Wyeth ... ▣741
Advil Multi-Symptom Cold Caplets (Chlorpheniramine Maleate, Ibuprofen, Pseudoephedrine Hydrochloride) Wyeth ... ▣738
Alavert Allergy & Sinus D-12 Hour Tablets (Loratadine, Pseudoephedrine Sulfate) Wyeth ... ▣743
Benadryl Allergy & Cold Tablets (Acetaminophen, Diphenhydramine Hydrochloride, Pseudoephedrine Hydrochloride) Pfizer Consumer Healthcare ... ▣692
Claritin-D Non-Drowsy 12 Hour Tablets (Loratadine, Pseudoephedrine Sulfate) Schering-Plough ... ▣731
Claritin-D Non-Drowsy 24 Hour Tablets (Loratadine, Pseudoephedrine Sulfate) Schering-Plough ... ▣731
Children's Dimetapp Cold & Allergy Elixir (Brompheniramine Maleate, Pseudoephedrine Hydrochloride) Wyeth ... ▣745
Sudafed PE Tablets (Phenylephrine Hydrochloride) Pfizer Consumer Healthcare ... ▣711
TheraFlu Cold & Cough Hot Liquid (Acetaminophen, Chlorpheniramine Maleate, Dextromethorphan Hydrobromide, Pseudoephedrine Hydrochloride) Novartis Consumer ... ▣680
TheraFlu Cold & Sore Throat Hot Liquid (Acetaminophen, Chlorpheniramine Maleate, Pseudoephedrine Hydrochloride) Novartis Consumer ... ▣680
TheraFlu Flu & Sore Throat Hot Liquid (Acetaminophen, Chlorpheniramine Maleate, Pseudoephedrine Hydrochloride) Novartis Consumer ... ▣681
TheraFlu Severe Cold Non-Drowsy Hot Liquid (Acetaminophen, Dextromethorphan Hydrobromide, Pseudoephedrine Hydrochloride) Novartis Consumer ... ▣683
TheraFlu Severe Cold & Cough Hot Liquid (Acetaminophen, Chlorpheniramine Maleate, Dextromethorphan Hydrobromide, Pseudoephedrine Hydrochloride) Novartis Consumer ... ▣683
TheraFlu Severe Cold Caplets (Acetaminophen, Chlorpheniramine Maleate, Dextromethorphan Hydrobromide, Pseudoephedrine Hydrochloride) Novartis Consumer ... ▣679
TheraFlu Severe Cold Hot Liquid (Acetaminophen, Chlorpheniramine Maleate, Dextromethorphan Hydrobromide, Pseudoephedrine Hydrochloride) Novartis Consumer ... ▣682
TheraFlu Severe Cold Non-Drowsy Caplets (Acetaminophen, Dextromethorphan Hydrobromide, Pseudoephedrine Hydrochloride) Novartis Consumer ... ▣679
Triaminic Cold & Allergy Liquid (Chlorpheniramine Maleate, Pseudoephedrine Hydrochloride) Novartis Consumer ... ▣685
Triaminic Cold & Cough Liquid (Chlorpheniramine Maleate, Dextromethorphan Hydrobromide, Pseudoephedrine Hydrochloride) Novartis Consumer ... ▣685
Triaminic Flu, Cough & Fever Liquid (Acetaminophen, Chlorpheniramine Maleate, Dextromethorphan Hydrobromide, Pseudoephedrine Hydrochloride) Novartis Consumer ... ▣685
Triaminic Night Time Cough & Cold Liquid (Chlorpheniramine Maleate, Dextromethorphan Hydrobromide, Pseudoephedrine Hydrochloride) Novartis Consumer ... ▣685
Triaminic Allergy Runny Nose & Congestion Softchews (Chlorpheniramine Maleate, Pseudoephedrine Hydrochloride) Novartis Consumer ... ▣688
Triaminic Cough & Sore Throat Softchews (Acetaminophen, Dextromethorphan Hydrobromide, Pseudoephedrine Hydrochloride) Novartis Consumer ... ▣689
Children's Tylenol Plus Cold Daytime Non-Drowsy Suspension Liquid (Acetaminophen, Pseudoephedrine Hydrochloride) McNeil Consumer ... 1851
Tylenol Allergy Complete Night Time Caplets (Acetaminophen, Diphenhydramine Hydrochloride, Pseudoephedrine Hydrochloride) McNeil Consumer ... 1844
Tylenol Allergy Complete Multi-Symptom Caplets and Gelcaps with Cool Burst (Acetaminophen, Chlorpheniramine Maleate, Pseudoephedrine Hydrochloride) McNeil Consumer ... 1844
Tylenol Sinus Day Non-Drowsy (Acetaminophen, Pseudoephedrine Hydrochloride) McNeil Consumer ... 1848
Tylenol Sinus Night Time Caplets (Acetaminophen, Doxylamine Succinate, Pseudoephedrine Hydrochloride) McNeil Consumer ... 1848
Tylenol Sinus Severe Congestion Caplets with Cool Burst (Acetaminophen, Doxylamine Succinate, Pseudoephedrine Hydrochloride) McNeil Consumer ... 1848
Vicks Sinex 12-Hour Nasal Spray and Ultra Fine Mist for Sinus Relief (Oxymetazoline Hydrochloride) Procter & Gamble ... 2678
Vicks Sinex Nasal Spray and Ultra Fine Mist for Sinus Relief (Phenylephrine Hydrochloride) Procter & Gamble ... 2677
Zicam Allergy Relief Nasal Pump (Histanium Hydrochloricum, Luffa operculata, Galphimia Glauca, Sulfur) Matrixx ... ▣665
Zicam Extreme Congestion Relief Nasal Pump (Oxymetazoline Hydrochloride) Matrixx ... ▣666
Zicam Sinus Relief Nasal Pump (Oxymetazoline Hydrochloride) Matrixx ... ▣666

Sinus headache
Benadryl Maximum Strength Severe Allergy & Sinus Headache Caplets (Acetaminophen, Diphenhydramine Hydrochloride, Pseudoephedrine Hydrochloride) Pfizer Consumer Healthcare ... ▣694
Singlet Caplets (Acetaminophen, Chlorpheniramine Maleate, Pseudoephedrine Hydrochloride) GlaxoSmithKline ... ▣636
Sudafed Sinus Headache (Acetaminophen, Pseudoephedrine Hydrochloride) Pfizer Consumer Healthcare ... ▣711
Children's Tylenol Plus Cold Daytime Non-Drowsy Suspension Liquid (Acetaminophen, Pseudoephedrine Hydrochloride) McNeil Consumer ... 1851
Tylenol Allergy Complete Night Time Caplets (Acetaminophen, Diphenhydramine Hydrochloride, Pseudoephedrine Hydrochloride) McNeil Consumer ... 1844
Tylenol Allergy Complete Multi-Symptom Caplets and Gelcaps with Cool Burst (Acetaminophen, Chlorpheniramine Maleate, Pseudoephedrine Hydrochloride) McNeil Consumer ... 1844
Tylenol Sinus Day Non-Drowsy Caplets (Acetaminophen, Pseudoephedrine Hydrochloride) McNeil Consumer ... 1848
Tylenol Sinus Night Time Caplets (Acetaminophen, Doxylamine Succinate, Pseudoephedrine Hydrochloride) McNeil Consumer ... 1848
Tylenol Sinus Severe Congestion Caplets with Cool Burst (Acetaminophen, Doxylamine Succinate, Pseudoephedrine Hydrochloride) McNeil Consumer ... 1848
Vicks NyQuil LiquiCaps/Liquid Multi-Symptom Cold/Flu Relief (Acetaminophen, Dextromethorphan Hydrobromide, Doxylamine Succinate, Pseudoephedrine Hydrochloride) Procter & Gamble ... ▣725

Sinusitis
Claritin-D Non-Drowsy 12 Hour Tablets (Loratadine, Pseudoephedrine Sulfate) Schering-Plough ... ▣731
Claritin-D Non-Drowsy 24 Hour Tablets (Loratadine, Pseudoephedrine Sulfate) Schering-Plough ... ▣731
Zicam Extreme Congestion Relief Nasal Pump (Oxymetazoline Hydrochloride) Matrixx ... ▣666
Zicam Sinus Relief Nasal Pump (Oxymetazoline Hydrochloride) Matrixx ... ▣666
Zithromax for Oral Suspension, 300 mg, 600 mg, 900 mg, 1200 mg (Azithromycin Dihydrate) Pfizer ... 2561
Zithromax Tablets, 250 mg, 500 mg (Azithromycin Dihydrate) Pfizer ... 2561
Zithromax Tri-Pak (Azithromycin Dihydrate) Pfizer ... 2561
Zmax for Oral Suspension (Azithromycin) Pfizer ... 2577

Sinusitis, adjunctive therapy
Advil (Ibuprofen) Wyeth ... ▣737
Children's Advil Suspension (Ibuprofen) Wyeth ... ▣742
Children's Advil Chewable Tablets (Ibuprofen) Wyeth ... ▣741
Advil Cold & Sinus (Ibuprofen, Pseudoephedrine Hydrochloride) Wyeth ... ▣739
Advil Flu & Body Ache Caplets (Ibuprofen, Pseudoephedrine Hydrochloride) Wyeth ... ▣739
Children's Advil Cold Suspension (Ibuprofen, Pseudoephedrine Hydrochloride) Wyeth ... ▣741
Infants' Advil Concentrated Drops (Ibuprofen) Wyeth ... ▣743
Benadryl Maximum Strength Severe Allergy & Sinus Headache Caplets (Acetaminophen, Diphenhydramine Hydrochloride, Pseudoephedrine Hydrochloride) Pfizer Consumer Healthcare ... ▣694
Contac Non-Drowsy 12 Hour Cold Caplets (Pseudoephedrine Hydrochloride) GlaxoSmithKline ... ▣614
Contac Non-Drowsy Timed Release 12 Hour Cold Caplets (Pseudoephedrine Hydrochloride) GlaxoSmithKline ... ▣615
Children's Motrin Cold Non-Staining Dye-Free Oral Suspension (Ibuprofen, Pseudoephedrine Hydrochloride) McNeil Consumer ... 1838
Children's Motrin Cold Oral Suspension (Ibuprofen, Pseudoephedrine Hydrochloride) McNeil Consumer ... ▣648
Children's Motrin Cold Non-Staining Dye-Free Oral Suspension (Ibuprofen, Pseudoephedrine Hydrochloride) McNeil Consumer ... ▣648
Children's Motrin Cold Oral Suspension (Ibuprofen, Pseudoephedrine Hydrochloride) McNeil Consumer ... 1838
Motrin Cold & Sinus Caplets (Ibuprofen, Pseudoephedrine Hydrochloride) McNeil Consumer ... 1836
Simply Stuffy Liquid (Pseudoephedrine Hydrochloride) McNeil Consumer ... 1841
Sudafed Non-Drying Sinus Liquid Caps (Guaifenesin, Pseudoephedrine Hydrochloride) Pfizer Consumer Healthcare ... ▣709
Sudafed Sinus Headache (Acetaminophen, Pseudoephedrine Hydrochloride) Pfizer Consumer Healthcare ... ▣711
TheraFlu Cold & Cough Hot Liquid (Acetaminophen, Chlorpheniramine Maleate, Dextromethorphan Hydrobromide, Pseudoephedrine Hydrochloride) Novartis Consumer ... ▣680
TheraFlu Cold & Sore Throat Hot Liquid (Acetaminophen, Chlorpheniramine Maleate, Pseudoephedrine Hydrochloride) Novartis Consumer ... ▣680
TheraFlu Flu & Chest Congestion Non-Drowsy Hot Liquid (Acetaminophen, Dextromethorphan Hydrobromide, Guaifenesin, Pseudoephedrine Hydrochloride) Novartis Consumer ... ▣681
TheraFlu Flu & Sore Throat Hot Liquid (Acetaminophen, Chlorpheniramine Maleate, Pseudoephedrine Hydrochloride) Novartis Consumer ... ▣681
TheraFlu Severe Cold Non-Drowsy Hot Liquid (Acetaminophen, Dextromethorphan Hydrobromide, Pseudoephedrine Hydrochloride) Novartis Consumer ... ▣683
TheraFlu Severe Cold & Cough Hot Liquid (Acetaminophen, Chlorpheniramine Maleate, Dextromethorphan Hydrobromide, Pseudoephedrine Hydrochloride) Novartis Consumer ... ▣683

TheraFlu Severe Cold Caplets (Acetaminophen, Chlorpheniramine Maleate, Dextromethorphan Hydrobromide, Pseudoephedrine Hydrochloride) Novartis Consumer .... ▣ 679
TheraFlu Severe Cold Hot Liquid (Acetaminophen, Chlorpheniramine Maleate, Dextromethorphan Hydrobromide, Pseudoephedrine Hydrochloride) Novartis Consumer .... ▣ 682
TheraFlu Severe Cold Non-Drowsy Caplets (Acetaminophen, Dextromethorphan Hydrobromide, Pseudoephedrine Hydrochloride) Novartis Consumer .... ▣ 679
Triaminic Chest & Nasal Congestion Liquid (Guaifenesin, Pseudoephedrine Hydrochloride) Novartis Consumer .... ▣ 685
Tylenol Allergy Complete Multi-Symptom Caplets and Gelcaps with Cool Burst (Acetaminophen, Chlorpheniramine Maleate, Pseudoephedrine Hydrochloride) McNeil Consumer 1844

Sinusitis, treatment of
Augmentin (Amoxicillin, Clavulanate Potassium) GlaxoSmithKline 1331
Augmentin Tablets (Amoxicillin, Clavulanate Potassium) GlaxoSmithKline 1334
Augmentin XR Extended-Release Tablets (Amoxicillin, Clavulanate Potassium) GlaxoSmithKline 1340
Avelox (Moxifloxacin Hydrochloride) Schering 2984
Biaxin/Biaxin XL (Clarithromycin) Abbott 402
Ceftin Tablets (Cefuroxime Axetil) GlaxoSmithKline 1369
Cipro I.V. (Ciprofloxacin) Schering 2998
Cipro I.V. Pharmacy Bulk Package (Ciprofloxacin) Bayer 3509
Cipro (Ciprofloxacin) Schering 2991
Ketek Tablets (Telithromycin) Sanofi-Aventis 2920
Levaquin in 5% Dextrose Injection (Levofloxacin) Ortho-McNeil 2453
Levaquin (Levofloxacin) Ortho-McNeil 2453
Omnicef Capsules (Cefdinir) Abbott 506
Omnicef for Oral Suspension (Cefdinir) Abbott 506
Tequin Injection (Gatifloxacin) Bristol-Myers Squibb 964
Tequin Tablets (Gatifloxacin) Bristol-Myers Squibb 964
Vantin Tablets and Oral Suspension (Cefpodoxime Proxetil) Pharmacia & Upjohn 2650

Sitosterolemia
Zetia Tablets (Ezetimibe) Merck/Schering Plough 2090
Zetia Tablets (Ezetimibe) Schering 3098

Sjogren's syndrome
Evoxac Capsules (Cevimeline Hydrochloride) Daiichi 1042

Skin, bactericidal/virucidal cleansing of
Betadine Skin Cleanser (Povidone Iodine) Purdue Products 2714
Betadine Surgical Scrub (Povidone Iodine) Purdue Products 2715

Skin, bacteriostatic cleansing of
Betasept Surgical Scrub (Chlorhexidine Gluconate) Purdue Products 2715

Skin, dry, moisturization of
Lubriderm Advanced Therapy Moisturizing Lotion (Cetyl Alcohol, Glycerin, Mineral Oil) Pfizer Consumer Healthcare .... ▣ 702
Pure Gardens Cream (Herbals with Vitamins) Awareness Corporation/AwarenessLife .... ▣ 760
Ultralytic 2 Cream 20% (Urea) Ivax Dermatologicals 1651
Ultralytic 2 Foam 20% (Urea) Ivax Dermatologicals 1652

Skin, facial, tactile roughness of, adjunct in
Renova 0.02% Cream (Tretinoin) OrthoNeutrogena 2384
Renova 0.05% Cream (Tretinoin) OrthoNeutrogena 2387

Skin, fine wrinkles, mitigation of
Pure Gardens Cream (Herbals with Vitamins) Awareness Corporation/AwarenessLife .... ▣ 760
Renova 0.02% Cream (Tretinoin) OrthoNeutrogena 2384
Renova 0.05% Cream (Tretinoin) OrthoNeutrogena 2387

Skin, hyperpigmentation
(*see under* Hyperpigmentation, skin, bleaching of)

Skin, inflammatory conditions
(*see also under* Dermatitis, contact; Dermatoses, corticosteroid-responsive)
Cortizone•5 Ointment (Hydrocortisone) Pfizer Consumer Healthcare .... ▣ 699
Cortizone•10 Plus Creme (Hydrocortisone) Pfizer Consumer Healthcare .... ▣ 700
Cortizone•10 Maximum Strength Quick Shot Spray (Hydrocortisone) Pfizer Consumer Healthcare .... ▣ 700
Cutivate Cream (Fluticasone Propionate) GlaxoSmithKline 1381
Cutivate Lotion 0.05% (Fluticasone Propionate) GlaxoSmithKline 1383
Cutivate Ointment (Fluticasone Propionate) GlaxoSmithKline 1384
Diprolene Gel 0.05% (Betamethasone Dipropionate) Schering 3015
Diprolene Lotion 0.05% (Betamethasone Dipropionate) Schering 3016
Pandel Cream, 0.1% (Hydrocortisone Probutate) CollaGenex 1017
Ultralytic 2 Cream 20% (Urea) Ivax Dermatologicals 1651
Ultralytic 2 Foam 20% (Urea) Ivax Dermatologicals 1652

Skin, irritation, minor, pain associated with
(*see under* Pain, topical relief of)

Skin, irritation, minor, temporary relief of
Smile's Prid Salve (Homeopathic Formulations) Standard Homeopathic .... ▣ 735

Skin, radiation damage, treatment of
Biafine Topical Emulsion (Propylparaben, Methylparaben, Propylene Glycol, Stearic Acid, Triethanolamine) OrthoNeutrogena 2382

Skin abscesses
(*see under* Infections, skin and skin structure)

Skin grafting, treatment adjunct
Biafine Topical Emulsion (Propylparaben, Methylparaben, Propylene Glycol, Stearic Acid, Triethanolamine) OrthoNeutrogena 2382

Skin infections, bacterial, minor
(*see under* Infections, skin, bacterial, minor)

Skin lacerations, infected
(*see under* Infections, skin and skin structure)

Skin ulcers, venous insufficiency-induced, non-infected
ProNutra Protein Supplement (Vitamins with Minerals, Whey Protein Isolate) Immunotec 1643

Sleep, induction of
(*see also under* Sedation)
Ambien Tablets (Zolpidem Tartrate) Sanofi-Aventis 2867
Dalmane Capsules (Flurazepam Hydrochloride) Valeant 3343
Hyland's Calms Forté Tablets and Caplets (Homeopathic Formulations) Standard Homeopathic .... ▣ 734
Lunesta Tablets (Eszopiclone) Sepracor 3139
Nembutal Sodium Solution, USP (Pentobarbital Sodium) Ovation 2484
Nytol QuickCaps Caplets (Diphenhydramine Hydrochloride) GlaxoSmithKline .... ▣ 635
Maximum Strength Nytol QuickGels Softgels (Diphenhydramine Hydrochloride) GlaxoSmithKline .... ▣ 635
ProSom Tablets (Estazolam) Abbott 512
Rozerem Tablets (Ramelteon) Takeda 3228
Simply Sleep Caplets (Diphenhydramine Hydrochloride) McNeil Consumer 1841
Sominex Original Formula Tablets (Diphenhydramine Hydrochloride) GlaxoSmithKline .... ▣ 637
Sonata Capsules (Zaleplon) King 1686
Unisom SleepTabs (Doxylamine Succinate) Pfizer Consumer Healthcare .... ▣ 713
Unisom Maximum Strength SleepGels (Diphenhydramine Hydrochloride) Pfizer Consumer Healthcare .... ▣ 712

Sleep disorders
Provigil Tablets (Modafinil) Cephalon 1002

Slough, liquefaction of
Accuzyme Spray (Papain, Urea) Healthpoint 1637

Smoking cessation, temporary aid to
Commit Lozenges (Nicotine Polacrilex) GlaxoSmithKline Consumer 1625
Nicoderm CQ Patch (Nicotine) GlaxoSmithKline Consumer 1629
NicoDerm CQ Clear Patch (Nicotine) GlaxoSmithKline .... ▣ 627
Nicorette Gum (Nicotine Polacrilex) GlaxoSmithKline Consumer 1632
Nicotrol Inhaler (Nicotine) Pfizer Consumer 2594
Nicotrol NS (Nicotine) Pfizer Consumer 2596
Zyban Sustained-Release Tablets (Bupropion Hydrochloride) GlaxoSmithKline 1620

Sneezing
Advil Allergy Sinus Caplets (Chlorpheniramine Maleate, Ibuprofen, Pseudoephedrine Hydrochloride) Wyeth .... ▣ 737
Advil Multi-Symptom Cold Caplets (Chlorpheniramine Maleate, Ibuprofen, Pseudoephedrine Hydrochloride) Wyeth .... ▣ 738
Alavert Allergy & Sinus D-12 Hour Tablets (Loratadine, Pseudoephedrine Sulfate) Wyeth .... ▣ 743
Alavert (Loratadine) Wyeth .... ▣ 743
Allegra-D 12 Hour Extended-Release Tablets (Fexofenadine Hydrochloride, Pseudoephedrine Hydrochloride) Sanofi-Aventis 2860
Benadryl Allergy & Cold Tablets (Acetaminophen, Diphenhydramine Hydrochloride, Pseudoephedrine Hydrochloride) Pfizer Consumer Healthcare .... ▣ 692
Benadryl Allergy (Diphenhydramine Hydrochloride) Pfizer Consumer Healthcare .... ▣ 691
Benadryl Allergy & Sinus Headache Caplets & Gelcaps (Acetaminophen, Diphenhydramine Hydrochloride, Pseudoephedrine Hydrochloride) Pfizer Consumer Healthcare .... ▣ 693
Children's Benadryl Allergy Liquid (Diphenhydramine Hydrochloride) Pfizer Consumer Healthcare .... ▣ 695
Children's Benadryl Dye-Free Allergy Liquid (Diphenhydramine Hydrochloride) Pfizer Consumer Healthcare .... ▣ 695
Benadryl Dye-Free Allergy Liqui-Gels Softgels (Diphenhydramine Hydrochloride) Pfizer Consumer Healthcare .... ▣ 692
Children's Benadryl D Allergy & Sinus Fastmelt Tablets (Diphenhydramine Citrate, Pseudoephedrine Hydrochloride) Pfizer Consumer Healthcare .... ▣ 694
Children's Benadryl D Liquid Medication (Diphenhydramine Hydrochloride, Pseudoephedrine Hydrochloride) Pfizer Consumer Healthcare .... ▣ 693
Benadryl D Tablets (Diphenhydramine Hydrochloride, Pseudoephedrine Hydrochloride) Pfizer Consumer Healthcare .... ▣ 694
Children's Benadryl Allergy Fastmelt Tablets (Diphenhydramine Citrate) Pfizer Consumer Healthcare .... ▣ 696
Children's Claritin 24 Hour Non-Drowsy Allergy Syrup (Loratadine) Schering-Plough .... ▣ 732
Claritin Non-Drowsy 24 Hour Tablets (Loratadine) Schering-Plough .... ▣ 731
Claritin Reditabs 24 Hour Non-Drowsy Tablets (Loratadine) Schering-Plough .... ▣ 732
Claritin-D Non-Drowsy 12 Hour Tablets (Loratadine, Pseudoephedrine Sulfate) Schering-Plough .... ▣ 731
Claritin-D Non-Drowsy 24 Hour Tablets (Loratadine, Pseudoephedrine Sulfate) Schering-Plough .... ▣ 731
Children's Dimetapp Cold & Allergy Elixir (Brompheniramine Maleate, Pseudoephedrine Hydrochloride) Wyeth .... ▣ 745
Children's Dimetapp ND Non-Drowsy Allergy Syrup (Loratadine) Wyeth .... ▣ 746
PediaCare Multi-Symptom Cold Liquid (Chlorpheniramine Maleate, Dextromethorphan Hydrobromide, Pseudoephedrine Hydrochloride) Pfizer Consumer Healthcare .... ▣ 704
TheraFlu Cold & Cough Hot Liquid (Acetaminophen, Chlorpheniramine Maleate, Dextromethorphan Hydrobromide, Pseudoephedrine Hydrochloride) Novartis Consumer .... ▣ 680
TheraFlu Cold & Sore Throat Hot Liquid (Acetaminophen, Chlorpheniramine Maleate, Pseudoephedrine Hydrochloride) Novartis Consumer .... ▣ 680
TheraFlu Flu & Sore Throat Hot Liquid (Acetaminophen, Chlorpheniramine Maleate, Pseudoephedrine Hydrochloride) Novartis Consumer .... ▣ 681
TheraFlu Severe Cold & Cough Hot Liquid (Acetaminophen, Chlorpheniramine Maleate, Dextromethorphan Hydrobromide, Pseudoephedrine Hydrochloride) Novartis Consumer .... ▣ 683
TheraFlu Severe Cold Caplets (Acetaminophen, Chlorpheniramine Maleate, Dextromethorphan Hydrobromide, Pseudoephedrine Hydrochloride) Novartis Consumer .... ▣ 679
TheraFlu Severe Cold Hot Liquid (Acetaminophen, Chlorpheniramine Maleate, Dextromethorphan Hydrobromide, Pseudoephedrine Hydrochloride) Novartis Consumer .... ▣ 682
TheraFlu Thin Strips Multi Symptom (Diphenhydramine Hydrochloride) Novartis Consumer .... ▣ 684
Triaminic Allerchews (Loratadine) Novartis Consumer .... ▣ 684
Triaminic Thin Strips Cough & Runny Nose (Diphenhydramine Hydrochloride) Novartis Consumer .... ▣ 690
Tylenol Cough & Sore Throat NightTime Liquid with Cool Burst (Acetaminophen, Dextromethorphan Hydrobromide, Doxylamine Succinate) McNeil Consumer .... ▣ 664

Children's Tylenol Plus Cold & Allergy Suspension Liquid (Acetaminophen, Diphenhydramine Hydrochloride, Pseudoephedrine Hydrochloride) McNeil Consumer .. 1850
Children's Tylenol Plus Cold NightTime Suspension Liquid (Acetaminophen, Chlorpheniramine Maleate, Pseudoephedrine Hydrochloride) McNeil Consumer .. 1851
Children's Tylenol Plus Cold & Cough Suspension Liquid and Chewable Tablets (Acetaminophen, Chlorpheniramine Maleate, Dextromethorphan Hydrobromide, Pseudoephedrine Hydrochloride) McNeil Consumer 1851
Children's Tylenol Plus Cold Chewable Tablets (Acetaminophen, Chlorpheniramine Maleate, Pseudoephedrine Hydrochloride) McNeil Consumer 1851
Children's Tylenol Plus Flu Suspension Liquid (Acetaminophen, Chlorpheniramine Maleate, Dextromethorphan Hydrobromide, Pseudoephedrine Hydrochloride) McNeil Consumer 1853
Tylenol Cold & Flu Severe NightTime Liquid with Cool Burst (Acetaminophen, Dextromethorphan Hydrobromide, Doxylamine Succinate, Pseudoephedrine Hydrochloride) McNeil Consumer .. 1846
Tylenol Cough & Sore Throat NightTime Liquid with Cool Burst (Acetaminophen, Dextromethorphan Hydrobromide, Doxylamine Succinate) McNeil Consumer 1849
Tylenol Severe Allergy Caplets (Acetaminophen, Diphenhydramine Hydrochloride) McNeil Consumer................................ 1844
Tylenol Flu NightTime Gelcaps (Acetaminophen, Diphenhydramine Hydrochloride, Pseudoephedrine Hydrochloride) McNeil Consumer.................................. 1846
Tylenol Sinus Night Time Caplets (Acetaminophen, Doxylamine Succinate, Pseudoephedrine Hydrochloride) McNeil Consumer .. 1848
Tylenol Sore Throat NightTime Liquid with Cool Burst (Acetaminophen, Diphenhydramine) McNeil Consumer 1849
Vicks NyQuil LiquiCaps/Liquid Multi-Symptom Cold/Flu Relief (Acetaminophen, Dextromethorphan Hydrobromide, Doxylamine Succinate, Pseudoephedrine Hydrochloride) Procter & Gamble .... ▣ 725
Zicam Allergy Relief Nasal Pump (Histanium Hydrochloricum, Luffa operculata, Galphimia Glauca, Sulfur) Matrixx .... ▣ 665
Zicam Cold Remedy Chewables (Zincum Aceticum, Zincum Gluconicum) Matrixx.......................... ▣ 665
Zicam Cold Remedy Nasal Pump (Zincum Gluconicum) Matrixx .... ▣ 665
Zicam Cold Remedy Oral Mist (Zincum Aceticum, Zincum Gluconicum) Matrixx .... ▣ 665
Zicam Cold Remedy RapidMelts (Zincum Aceticum, Zincum Gluconicum) Matrixx........................ ▣ 665
Zicam Cold Remedy Swabs (Zincum Gluconicum) Matrixx .... ▣ 665
Zicam Cold Remedy Swabs Kids Size (Zincum Gluconicum) Matrixx.. ▣ 665

Social phobia
(*see under* Anxiety disorder, social)

Solar lentigines
(*see under* Hyperpigmentation, skin, bleaching of)

Somatotropin deficiency syndrome
Humatrope Vials and Cartridges (Somatropin) Lilly 1756

Sore throat
Children's Advil Cold Suspension (Ibuprofen, Pseudoephedrine Hydrochloride) Wyeth .... ▣ 741
Benadryl Allergy & Cold Tablets (Acetaminophen, Diphenhydramine Hydrochloride, Pseudoephedrine Hydrochloride) Pfizer Consumer Healthcare................. ▣ 692
Halls Fruit Breezers Pectin Throat Drops (Pectin) Cadbury Adams.... ▣ 609
Halls Max Drops (Benzocaine, Menthol) Cadbury Adams .... ▣ 609
Hurricaine Topical Anesthetic Aerosol Spray, 2 oz. Wild Cherry (Benzocaine) Beutlich.................. 835
Hurricaine Topical Anesthetic Aerosol Spray Kit, 2 oz. Wild Cherry with 200 Disposable Extension Tubes (Benzocaine) Beutlich 835
Hurricaine Topical Anesthetic Gel: 1 oz. Wild Cherry, Pina Colada, Watermelon, Fresh Mint, 0.18 oz. Wild Cherry (Benzocaine) Beutlich 835
Hurricaine Topical Anesthetic Liquid: 1 oz. Wild Cherry and Pina Colada, Swab Applicator Wild Cherry (Benzocaine) Beutlich 835
Children's Motrin Oral Suspension and Chewable Tablets (Ibuprofen) McNeil Consumer 1837
Children's Motrin Non-Staining Dye-Free Oral Suspension (Ibuprofen) McNeil Consumer 1837
Infants' Motrin Concentrated Drops (Ibuprofen) McNeil Consumer 1837
Infants' Motrin Non-Staining Dye-Free Drops (Ibuprofen) McNeil Consumer 1837
Junior Strength Motrin Caplets and Chewable Tablets (Ibuprofen) McNeil Consumer 1837
TheraFlu Cold & Cough Hot Liquid (Acetaminophen, Chlorpheniramine Maleate, Dextromethorphan Hydrobromide, Pseudoephedrine Hydrochloride) Novartis Consumer .... ▣ 680
TheraFlu Cold & Sore Throat Hot Liquid (Acetaminophen, Chlorpheniramine Maleate, Pseudoephedrine Hydrochloride) Novartis Consumer .... ▣ 680
TheraFlu Flu & Chest Congestion Non-Drowsy Hot Liquid (Acetaminophen, Dextromethorphan Hydrobromide, Guaifenesin, Pseudoephedrine Hydrochloride) Novartis Consumer .... ▣ 681
TheraFlu Flu & Sore Throat Hot Liquid (Acetaminophen, Chlorpheniramine Maleate, Pseudoephedrine Hydrochloride) Novartis Consumer .... ▣ 681
TheraFlu Severe Cold Non-Drowsy Hot Liquid (Acetaminophen, Dextromethorphan Hydrobromide, Pseudoephedrine Hydrochloride) Novartis Consumer .... ▣ 683
TheraFlu Severe Cold & Cough Hot Liquid (Acetaminophen, Chlorpheniramine Maleate, Dextromethorphan Hydrobromide, Pseudoephedrine Hydrochloride) Novartis Consumer .... ▣ 683
TheraFlu Severe Cold Caplets (Acetaminophen, Chlorpheniramine Maleate, Dextromethorphan Hydrobromide, Pseudoephedrine Hydrochloride) Novartis Consumer .... ▣ 679
TheraFlu Severe Cold Hot Liquid (Acetaminophen, Chlorpheniramine Maleate, Dextromethorphan Hydrobromide, Pseudoephedrine Hydrochloride) Novartis Consumer .... ▣ 682
TheraFlu Severe Cold Non-Drowsy Caplets (Acetaminophen, Dextromethorphan Hydrobromide, Pseudoephedrine Hydrochloride) Novartis Consumer .... ▣ 679
Triaminic Cough & Sore Throat Softchews (Acetaminophen, Dextromethorphan Hydrobromide, Pseudoephedrine Hydrochloride) Novartis Consumer ...... ▣ 689
Tylenol Cough & Sore Throat Daytime Liquid with Cool Burst (Acetaminophen, Dextromethorphan Hydrobromide) McNeil Consumer .... ▣ 664
Tylenol Cough & Sore Throat NightTime Liquid with Cool Burst (Acetaminophen, Dextromethorphan Hydrobromide, Doxylamine Succinate) McNeil Consumer .... ▣ 664
Children's Tylenol Plus Cold NightTime Suspension Liquid (Acetaminophen, Chlorpheniramine Maleate, Pseudoephedrine Hydrochloride) McNeil Consumer .. 1851
Children's Tylenol Plus Cold & Cough Suspension Liquid and Chewable Tablets (Acetaminophen, Chlorpheniramine Maleate, Dextromethorphan Hydrobromide, Pseudoephedrine Hydrochloride) McNeil Consumer 1851
Children's Tylenol Plus Cold Chewable Tablets (Acetaminophen, Chlorpheniramine Maleate, Pseudoephedrine Hydrochloride) McNeil Consumer 1851
Children's Tylenol Plus Flu Suspension Liquid (Acetaminophen, Chlorpheniramine Maleate, Dextromethorphan Hydrobromide, Pseudoephedrine Hydrochloride) McNeil Consumer 1853
Concentrated Tylenol Infants' Drops Plus Cold and Cough (Acetaminophen, Dextromethorphan Hydrobromide, Pseudoephedrine Hydrochloride) McNeil Consumer............................. 1851
Tylenol Cold & Flu Severe Daytime Liquid with Cool Bust (Acetaminophen, Dextromethorphan Hydrobromide, Pseudoephedrine Hydrochloride) McNeil Consumer .. 1846
Tylenol Cold & Flu Severe NightTime Liquid with Cool Burst (Acetaminophen, Dextromethorphan Hydrobromide, Doxylamine Succinate, Pseudoephedrine Hydrochloride) McNeil Consumer .. 1846
Tylenol Cold Severe Congestion Non-Drowsy Caplets with Cool Burst (Acetaminophen, Dextromethorphan Hydrobromide, Guaifenesin, Pseudoephedrine Hydrochloride) McNeil Consumer .. 1846
Tylenol Cough & Sore Throat Daytime Liquid with Cool Burst (Acetaminophen, Dextromethorphan Hydrobromide) McNeil Consumer............................. 1849
Tylenol Cough & Sore Throat NightTime Liquid with Cool Burst (Acetaminophen, Dextromethorphan Hydrobromide, Doxylamine Succinate) McNeil Consumer 1849
Tylenol Flu NightTime Gelcaps (Acetaminophen, Diphenhydramine Hydrochloride, Pseudoephedrine Hydrochloride) McNeil Consumer............................. 1846
Tylenol Flu Day Non-Drowsy Gelcaps (Acetaminophen, Dextromethorphan Hydrobromide, Pseudoephedrine Hydrochloride) McNeil Consumer 1846
Tylenol Sore Throat Daytime Liquid with Cool Burst (Acetaminophen) McNeil Consumer 1849
Tylenol Sore Throat NightTime Liquid with Cool Burst (Acetaminophen, Diphenhydramine) McNeil Consumer 1849
Vicks NyQuil LiquiCaps/Liquid Multi-Symptom Cold/Flu Relief (Acetaminophen, Dextromethorphan Hydrobromide, Doxylamine Succinate, Pseudoephedrine Hydrochloride) Procter & Gamble .... ▣ 725
Zicam Cold Remedy Chewables (Zincum Aceticum, Zincum Gluconicum) Matrixx......................... ▣ 665
Zicam Cold Remedy Nasal Pump (Zincum Gluconicum) Matrixx .... ▣ 665
Zicam Cold Remedy Oral Mist (Zincum Aceticum, Zincum Gluconicum) Matrixx .... ▣ 665
Zicam Cold Remedy RapidMelts (Zincum Aceticum, Zincum Gluconicum) Matrixx......................... ▣ 665
Zicam Cold Remedy Swabs (Zincum Gluconicum) Matrixx .... ▣ 665
Zicam Cold Remedy Swabs Kids Size (Zincum Gluconicum) Matrixx.. ▣ 665

Sour stomach
(*see under* Hyperacidity, gastric, symptomatic relief of)

Spasm, skeletal muscle
Flexeril Tablets (Cyclobenzaprine Hydrochloride) McNeil Consumer .. 1832
Valium Tablets (Diazepam) Roche Laboratories 2822

Spasticity, cerebral palsy-induced
(*see under* Spasticity, upper motor neuron disorder-induced)

Spasticity, multiple sclerosis-induced
(*see under* Spasticity, upper motor neuron disorder-induced)

Spasticity, muscle, symptomatic alleviation of
Flexeril Tablets (Cyclobenzaprine Hydrochloride) McNeil Consumer .. 1832

Spasticity, spinal cord injury-induced
(*see under* Spasticity, upper motor neuron disorder-induced)

Spasticity, stroke-induced
(*see under* Spasticity, upper motor neuron disorder-induced)

Spasticity, upper motor neuron disorder-induced
Dantrium Capsules (Dantrolene Sodium) Procter & Gamble Pharmaceuticals 2690
Valium Tablets (Diazepam) Roche Laboratories 2822

Spirochetes species infections
(*see under* Borrelia recurrentis infection)

Spondyloarthropathy
Bayer Aspirin Tablets (Aspirin) Bayer Healthcare LLC 3515

Sprains, topical relief of
(*see under* Pain, topical relief of)

Staphylococcal enterocolitis
(*see under* Enterocolitis, staphylococcal)

Staphylococci, coagulase-negative, infections, ocular
Pred-G Ophthalmic Suspension (Gentamicin Sulfate, Prednisolone Acetate) Allergan .... ⊙ 234
TobraDex Ophthalmic Ointment (Dexamethasone, Tobramycin) Alcon 558
TobraDex Ophthalmic Suspension (Dexamethasone, Tobramycin) Alcon 558
Zylet Ophthalmic Suspension (Loteprednol Etabonate, Tobramycin) Bausch & Lomb 3508

Staphylococci, coagulase-positive, infections, ocular
Pred-G Ophthalmic Suspension (Gentamicin Sulfate, Prednisolone Acetate) Allergan .... ⊙ 234
TobraDex Ophthalmic Ointment (Dexamethasone, Tobramycin) Alcon 558
TobraDex Ophthalmic Suspension (Dexamethasone, Tobramycin) Alcon 558
Zylet Ophthalmic Suspension (Loteprednol Etabonate, Tobramycin) Bausch & Lomb 3508

Staphylococci, nonpenicillinase-producing, infections
Amoxil Capsules (Amoxicillin) GlaxoSmithKline 1315
Amoxil Chewable Tablets (Amoxicillin) GlaxoSmithKline 1315
Amoxil Pediatric Drops for Oral Suspension (Amoxicillin) GlaxoSmithKline 1315
Amoxil Powder for Oral Suspension (Amoxicillin) GlaxoSmithKline 1315

Amoxil Tablets (Amoxicillin) GlaxoSmithKline ... 1315

Staphylococci, penicillinase-producing, infections
Mefoxin for Injection (Cefoxitin Sodium) Merck ... 1987
Mefoxin Premixed Intravenous Solution (Cefoxitin Sodium) Merck ... 1990

Staphylococci otitis media
Floxin Otic Singles (Ofloxacin) Daiichi ... 1045

Staphylococcus aureus
(*see under* S. aureus infections)

Staphylococcus epidermidis
(*see under* S. epidermis infections)

Staphylococcus species, coagulase-negative, infections
Garamycin (Gentamicin Sulfate) Schering ... 3028

Status epilepticus
(*see under* Epilepticus, status)

Steatorrhea, adjunctive therapy in
Ultrase MT Capsules (Pancrelipase) Axcan Scandipharm ... 736

Stenosis, hypertrophic subaortic
Inderal LA Long-Acting Capsules (Propranolol Hydrochloride) Wyeth ... 3421

Stevens-Johnson syndrome
Decadron Phosphate Injection (Dexamethasone Sodium Phosphate) Merck ... 1931
Decadron Tablets (Dexamethasone) Merck ... 1929
Depo-Medrol Injectable Suspension (Methylprednisolone Acetate) Pharmacia & Upjohn ... 2615
Depo-Medrol Single-Dose Vial (Methylprednisolone Acetate) Pharmacia & Upjohn ... 2617
Hydrocortone Tablets (Hydrocortisone) Merck ... 1963
Pediapred Oral Solution (Prednisolone Sodium Phosphate) UCB ... 3319

Stiff-man syndrome, adjunctive therapy in
Valium Tablets (Diazepam) Roche Laboratories ... 2822

Stomach, sour
(*see under* Hyperacidity, gastric, symptomatic relief of)

Stomatitis
Hurricaine Topical Anesthetic Aerosol Spray, 2 oz. Wild Cherry (Benzocaine) Beutlich ... 835
Hurricaine Topical Anesthetic Aerosol Spray Kit, 2 oz. Wild Cherry with 200 Disposable Extension Tubes (Benzocaine) Beutlich ... 835
Hurricaine Topical Anesthetic Gel: 1 oz. Wild Cherry, Pina Colada, Watermelon, Fresh Mint, 0.18 oz. Wild Cherry (Benzocaine) Beutlich ... 835
Hurricaine Topical Anesthetic Liquid: 1 oz. Wild Cherry and Pina Colada, Swab Applicator Wild Cherry (Benzocaine) Beutlich ... 835

Stomatitis, recurrent aphthous, symptomatic relief of
Gly-Oxide Liquid (Carbamide Peroxide) GlaxoSmithKline ... ▣620
Hurricaine Topical Anesthetic Aerosol Spray, 2 oz. Wild Cherry (Benzocaine) Beutlich ... 835
Hurricaine Topical Anesthetic Aerosol Spray Kit, 2 oz. Wild Cherry with 200 Disposable Extension Tubes (Benzocaine) Beutlich ... 835
Hurricaine Topical Anesthetic Gel: 1 oz. Wild Cherry, Pina Colada, Watermelon, Fresh Mint, 0.18 oz. Wild Cherry (Benzocaine) Beutlich ... 835
Hurricaine Topical Anesthetic Liquid: 1 oz. Wild Cherry and Pina Colada, Swab Applicator Wild Cherry (Benzocaine) Beutlich ... 835
Triaminic Sore Throat Spray (Phenol) Novartis Consumer ... ▣689

Strabismus
Botox Purified Neurotoxin Complex (Botulinum Toxin Type A) Allergan ... 565

Strep throat
(*see under* Streptococci species upper respiratory tract infections)

Streptococcal pharyngitis
E.E.S. (Erythromycin Ethylsuccinate) Abbott ... 449
Omnicef Capsules (Cefdinir) Abbott ... 506
Omnicef for Oral Suspension (Cefdinir) Abbott ... 506
Suprax (Cefixime) Lupin ... 1811

Streptococci biliary tract infections
Ancef (Cefazolin Sodium) GlaxoSmithKline ... 1318

Streptococci group A beta-hemolytic infections
Primaxin I.V. (Cilastatin Sodium, Imipenem) Merck ... 2024

Streptococci group A beta-hemolytic skin and skin structure infections
Fortaz (Ceftazidime Sodium) GlaxoSmithKline ... 1422
Primaxin I.V. (Cilastatin Sodium, Imipenem) Merck ... 2024

Streptococci group A beta-hemolytic species infections, ocular
Pred-G Ophthalmic Suspension (Gentamicin Sulfate, Prednisolone Acetate) Allergan ... ⊙234
Pred-G Sterile Ophthalmic Ointment (Gentamicin Sulfate, Prednisolone Acetate) Allergan ... ⊙235
TobraDex Ophthalmic Ointment (Dexamethasone, Tobramycin) Alcon ... 558
TobraDex Ophthalmic Suspension (Dexamethasone, Tobramycin) Alcon ... 558
Zylet Ophthalmic Suspension (Loteprednol Etabonate, Tobramycin) Bausch & Lomb ... 3508

Streptococci group A beta-hemolytic upper respiratory tract infections
PCE Dispertab Tablets (Erythromycin) Abbott ... 510

Streptococci group B infections
Ancef for Injection (Cefazolin Sodium) GlaxoSmithKline ... 1318
Mefoxin for Injection (Cefoxitin Sodium) Merck ... 1987
Mefoxin Premixed Intravenous Solution (Cefoxitin Sodium) Merck ... 1990
Primaxin I.V. (Cilastatin Sodium, Imipenem) Merck ... 2024

Streptococci group D bone and joint infections
Primaxin I.V. (Cilastatin Sodium, Imipenem) Merck ... 2024

Streptococci group D endocarditis, adjunct in
Garamycin Injectable (Gentamicin Sulfate) Schering ... 3028

Streptococci group D genitourinary tract infections
Primaxin I.V. (Cilastatin Sodium, Imipenem) Merck ... 2024

Streptococci group D gynecologic infections
Primaxin I.M. (Cilastatin Sodium, Imipenem) Merck ... 2022

Streptococci group D infections
Ancef for Injection (Cefazolin Sodium) GlaxoSmithKline ... 1318
Garamycin Injectable (Gentamicin Sulfate) Schering ... 3028
Primaxin I.V. (Cilastatin Sodium, Imipenem) Merck ... 2024

Streptococci group D intra-abdominal infections
Primaxin I.M. (Cilastatin Sodium, Imipenem) Merck ... 2022
Primaxin I.V. (Cilastatin Sodium, Imipenem) Merck ... 2024

Streptococci group D skin and skin structure infections
Primaxin I.M. (Cilastatin Sodium, Imipenem) Merck ... 2022
Primaxin I.V. (Cilastatin Sodium, Imipenem) Merck ... 2024

Streptococci infections, ocular
Quixin Ophthalmic Solution (Levofloxacin) Vistakon ... 3373
TobraDex Ophthalmic Ointment (Dexamethasone, Tobramycin) Alcon ... 558
TobraDex Ophthalmic Suspension (Dexamethasone, Tobramycin) Alcon ... 558
Zylet Ophthalmic Suspension (Loteprednol Etabonate, Tobramycin) Bausch & Lomb ... 3508

Streptococci non-hemolytic species infections, ocular
Pred-G Ophthalmic Suspension (Gentamicin Sulfate, Prednisolone Acetate) Allergan ... ⊙234
TobraDex Ophthalmic Ointment (Dexamethasone, Tobramycin) Alcon ... 558
TobraDex Ophthalmic Suspension (Dexamethasone, Tobramycin) Alcon ... 558
Zylet Ophthalmic Suspension (Loteprednol Etabonate, Tobramycin) Bausch & Lomb ... 3508

Streptococci skin and skin structure infections
Ancef for Injection (Cefazolin Sodium) GlaxoSmithKline ... 1318
Mefoxin for Injection (Cefoxitin Sodium) Merck ... 1987
Mefoxin Premixed Intravenous Solution (Cefoxitin Sodium) Merck ... 1990

Streptococci species infections
Ancef for Injection (Cefazolin Sodium) GlaxoSmithKline ... 1318
Centany Ointment, 2% (Mupirocin) OrthoNeutrogena ... 2382

Streptococci species upper respiratory tract infections
Ceftin (Cefuroxime Axetil) GlaxoSmithKline ... 1369
Omnicef Capsules (Cefdinir) Abbott ... 506
Omnicef for Oral Suspension (Cefdinir) Abbott ... 506
Suprax (Cefixime) Lupin ... 1811

Streptococci (viridans group) infections, ocular
Blephamide Ophthalmic Suspension (Prednisolone Acetate, Sulfacetamide Sodium) Allergan ... 564
Ciloxan Ophthalmic Ointment (Ciprofloxacin Hydrochloride) Alcon ... 554
FML-S Liquifilm Sterile Ophthalmic Suspension (Fluorometholone, Sulfacetamide Sodium) Allergan ... ⊙226
Polytrim Ophthalmic Solution (Polymyxin B Sulfate, Trimethoprim Sulfate) Allergan ... 570
Quixin Ophthalmic Solution (Levofloxacin) Vistakon ... 3373

Streptococci (viridans group) intra-abdominal infections
Maxipime for Injection (Cefepime Hydrochloride) Elan ... 1093

Streptococcus agalactiae infections
(*see under* S. agalactiae infections)

Streptococcus faecalis
(*see under* S. faecalis infections)

Streptococcus pneumoniae
(*see under* S. pneumoniae infections)

Streptococcus pyogenes
(*see under* S. pyogenes infections)

Streptococcus species infections
Amoxil Capsules (Amoxicillin) GlaxoSmithKline ... 1315
Amoxil Chewable Tablets (Amoxicillin) GlaxoSmithKline ... 1315
Amoxil Pediatric Drops for Oral Suspension (Amoxicillin) GlaxoSmithKline ... 1315
Amoxil Powder for Oral Suspension (Amoxicillin) GlaxoSmithKline ... 1315
Amoxil Tablets (Amoxicillin) GlaxoSmithKline ... 1315
Bactroban Ointment (Mupirocin) GlaxoSmithKline ... 1358
Cleocin Vaginal Ovules (Clindamycin Hydrochloride) Pharmacia & Upjohn ... 2613
Garamycin Injectable (Gentamicin Sulfate) Schering ... 3028
Omnicef Capsules (Cefdinir) Abbott ... 506
Omnicef for Oral Suspension (Cefdinir) Abbott ... 506
Suprax (Cefixime) Lupin ... 1811

Streptococcus species lower respiratory tract infections
Mefoxin for Injection (Cefoxitin Sodium) Merck ... 1987
Mefoxin Premixed Intravenous Solution (Cefoxitin Sodium) Merck ... 1990

Streptococcus species respiratory tract infections
Cleocin Vaginal Ovules (Clindamycin Hydrochloride) Pharmacia & Upjohn ... 2613

Streptococcus tonsillitis
(*see under* Streptococci species upper respiratory tract infections)

Streptococcus viridans group infections
Blephamide Ophthalmic Ointment (Prednisolone Acetate, Sulfacetamide Sodium) Allergan ... 563
Merrem I.V. (Meropenem) AstraZeneca ... 687
Primaxin I.M. (Cilastatin Sodium, Imipenem) Merck ... 2022
Rocephin Injectable Vials, ADD-Vantage, Galaxy, Bulk (Ceftriaxone Sodium) Roche Laboratories ... 2801
Vigamox Ophthalmic Solution (Moxifloxacin Hydrochloride) Alcon ... 560

Stress disorder, post-traumatic
Paxil (Paroxetine Hydrochloride) GlaxoSmithKline ... 1501
Zoloft (Sertraline Hydrochloride) Pfizer ... 2581

Stroke, ischemic
Activase I.V. (Alteplase) Genentech ... 1225

Stroke, to reduce the risk of
Aggrenox Capsules (Aspirin, Dipyridamole) Boehringer Ingelheim ... 855
Altace Capsules (Ramipril) King ... 1673
Bayer Aspirin Tablets (Aspirin) Bayer Healthcare LLC ... 3515
Coumadin for Injection (Warfarin Sodium) Bristol-Myers Squibb ... 932
Coumadin Tablets (Warfarin Sodium) Bristol-Myers Squibb ... 932
Hyzaar (Hydrochlorothiazide, Losartan Potassium) Merck ... 1964
Plavix Tablets (Clopidogrel Bisulfate) Bristol-Myers Squibb ... 940

Plavix Tablets (Clopidogrel Bisulfate) Sanofi-Aventis 2942
Pravachol Tablets (Pravastatin Sodium) Bristol-Myers Squibb 943
Ticlid Tablets (Ticlopidine Hydrochloride) Roche Laboratories 2813
Zocor Tablets (Simvastatin) Merck 2078

Strongyloidiasis
Mintezol (Thiabendazole) Merck 2002
Stromectol Tablets (Ivermectin) Merck 2053

Suicidal behavior, recurrent, in schizoaffective disorder
Clozaril (Clozapine) Novartis 2174

Sunburn, pain associated with
(*see under* Pain, topical relief of)

Swelling, unspecified
Hyland's Bumps 'n Bruises Tablets (Homeopathic Formulations) Standard Homeopathic .... ▣ 734

Sympathetic ophthalmia
(*see under* Ophthalmia, sympathetic)

Syphilis
Erythromycin Delayed-Release Capsules, USP (Erythromycin) Abbott 456

T

T. pallidum infections
Dynacin Tablets (Minocycline Hydrochloride) Medicis 1859
E.E.S. (Erythromycin Ethylsuccinate) Abbott 449
EryPed (Erythromycin Ethylsuccinate) Abbott 445
Ery-Tab Tablets (Erythromycin) Abbott 447
Erythrocin Stearate Filmtab Tablets (Erythromycin Stearate) Abbott 452
Erythromycin Base Filmtab Tablets (Erythromycin) Abbott 454
Erythromycin Delayed-Release Capsules, USP (Erythromycin) Abbott 456
PCE Dispertab Tablets (Erythromycin) Abbott 510

T. vaginalis infections
Tindamax (Tinidazole) Presutti 2670

Tachycardia, noncompensatory sinus
Brevibloc Concentrate (Esmolol Hydrochloride) Baxter Anesthesia 766
Brevibloc Injection (Esmolol Hydrochloride) Baxter Anesthesia 766
Brevibloc Double Strength Injection (Esmolol Hydrochloride) Baxter Anesthesia 766
Brevibloc Premixed Injection (Esmolol Hydrochloride) Baxter Anesthesia 766
Brevibloc Double Strength Premixed Injection (Esmolol Hydrochloride) Baxter Anesthesia 766

Tachycardia, paroxysmal supraventricular
Adenocard Injection (Adenosine) Astellas 612
Tambocor Tablets (Flecainide Acetate) 3M 1824

Tachycardia, paroxysmal supraventricular associated with Wolff-Parkinson-White syndrome
(*see under* Wolff-Parkinson-White syndrome)

Tachycardia, supraventricular
Brevibloc Concentrate (Esmolol Hydrochloride) Baxter Anesthesia 766
Brevibloc Injection (Esmolol Hydrochloride) Baxter Anesthesia 766
Brevibloc Double Strength Injection (Esmolol Hydrochloride) Baxter Anesthesia 766
Brevibloc Premixed Injection (Esmolol Hydrochloride) Baxter Anesthesia 766
Brevibloc Double Strength Premixed Injection (Esmolol Hydrochloride) Baxter Anesthesia 766
Tambocor Tablets (Flecainide Acetate) 3M 1824

Tachycardia, ventricular
Tambocor Tablets (Flecainide Acetate) 3M 1824

Tachycardia, ventricular, recurrent hemodynamically unstable
Pacerone Tablets (Amiodarone Hydrochloride) Upsher-Smith 3337

Tachycardia, ventricular, sustained
Tambocor Tablets (Flecainide Acetate) 3M 1824

Tachycardias, paroxysmal atrial
(*see under* Tachycardia, paroxysmal supraventricular)

Taenia solium infections
Albenza Tablets (Albendazole) GlaxoSmithKline 1310

Tapeworm infections
(*see under* Infections, tapeworm)

Tendonitis
Anaprox Tablets (Naproxen Sodium) Roche Laboratories 2769
Anaprox DS Tablets (Naproxen Sodium) Roche Laboratories 2769
Clinoril Tablets (Sulindac) Merck 1899
Indocin (Indomethacin) Merck 1968
Naprosyn Suspension (Naproxen) Roche Laboratories 2769
Naprosyn Tablets (Naproxen) Roche Laboratories 2769
Traumeel Injection Solution (Homeopathic Formulations) Heel 1638

Tenosynovitis, acute nonspecific
Decadron Phosphate Injection (Dexamethasone Sodium Phosphate) Merck 1931
Depo-Medrol Injectable Suspension (Methylprednisolone Acetate) Pharmacia & Upjohn 2615
Depo-Medrol Single-Dose Vial (Methylprednisolone Acetate) Pharmacia & Upjohn 2617
Hydrocortone Tablets (Hydrocortisone) Merck 1963
Pediapred Oral Solution (Prednisolone Sodium Phosphate) UCB 3319

Testis, advanced carcinoma of
(*see under* Carcinoma, testis, advanced)

Testosterone, deficiency of
(*see under* Androgen, absence or deficiency of)

Tetanus
HyperTET (Tetanus Immune Globulin (Human)) Talecris 3245

Threadworm infestations
(*see under* Strongyloidiasis)

Throat, itchy
(*see under* Pruritus, rhinopharyngeal, symptomatic relief of)

Throat, sore
(*see under* Pharyngitis, symptomatic relief of)

Thrombocythemia
Agrylin Capsules (Anagrelide Hydrochloride) Shire US 3172

Thrombocytopenia, heparin-induced
Argatroban Injection (Argatroban) GlaxoSmithKline 1321
Refludan for Injection (Lepirudin) Berlex 815

Thrombocytopenia, prevention of
Neumega for Injection (Oprelvekin) Wyeth 3433

Thrombocytopenia, secondary
Decadron Phosphate Injection (Dexamethasone Sodium Phosphate) Merck 1931
Decadron Tablets (Dexamethasone) Merck 1929
Depo-Medrol Injectable Suspension (Methylprednisolone Acetate) Pharmacia & Upjohn 2615
Depo-Medrol Single-Dose Vial (Methylprednisolone Acetate) Pharmacia & Upjohn 2617
Hydrocortone Tablets (Hydrocortisone) Merck 1963
Pediapred Oral Solution (Prednisolone Sodium Phosphate) UCB 3319

Thromboembolic complications
Coumadin for Injection (Warfarin Sodium) Bristol-Myers Squibb 932
Coumadin Tablets (Warfarin Sodium) Bristol-Myers Squibb 932
Refludan for Injection (Lepirudin) Berlex 815

Thromboembolism, postoperative, adjunct in
Persantine Tablets (Dipyridamole) Boehringer Ingelheim 898

Thrombosis, deep venous, prophylaxis of
Arixtra (Fondaparinux Sodium) GlaxoSmithKline 1325

Thrombosis, venous
Coumadin for Injection (Warfarin Sodium) Bristol-Myers Squibb 932
Coumadin Tablets (Warfarin Sodium) Bristol-Myers Squibb 932
Miradon Tablets (Anisindione) Schering 3056

Thrombosis, venous, prophylaxis of
Coumadin for Injection (Warfarin Sodium) Bristol-Myers Squibb 932
Coumadin Tablets (Warfarin Sodium) Bristol-Myers Squibb 932
Fragmin Injection (Dalteparin Sodium) Pharmacia & Upjohn 2638
Lovenox Injection (Enoxaparin Sodium) Sanofi-Aventis 2931
Miradon Tablets (Anisindione) Schering 3056

Thyroid function, aid in the diagnosis of
Cytomel Tablets (Liothyronine Sodium) King 1678
Levothroid Tablets (Levothyroxine Sodium) Forest 1189
Levoxyl Tablets (Levothyroxine Sodium) King 1680
Synthroid Tablets (Levothyroxine Sodium) Abbott 515
Thyrolar (Liotrix) Forest 1203

Thyroiditis, chronic lymphocytic
(*see under* Hashimoto's thyroiditis)

Thyroiditis, nonsuppurative
Decadron Phosphate Injection (Dexamethasone Sodium Phosphate) Merck 1931
Decadron Tablets (Dexamethasone) Merck 1929
Depo-Medrol Injectable Suspension (Methylprednisolone Acetate) Pharmacia & Upjohn 2615
Depo-Medrol Single-Dose Vial (Methylprednisolone Acetate) Pharmacia & Upjohn 2617
Hydrocortone Tablets (Hydrocortisone) Merck 1963
Pediapred Oral Solution (Prednisolone Sodium Phosphate) UCB 3319

Tick fevers
Dynacin Tablets (Minocycline Hydrochloride) Medicis 1859

Tinea barbae
(*see under* Folliculitis barbae)

Tinea capitis infections
Grifulvin V Tablets Microsize and Oral Suspension Microsize (Griseofulvin) OrthoNeutrogena 2384
Gris-PEG Tablets (Griseofulvin) Pedinol 2504

Tinea corporis infections
Desenex Spray Powder (Miconazole Nitrate) Novartis Consumer .... ▣ 674
Desenex Jock Itch Spray Powder (Miconazole Nitrate) Novartis Consumer .... ▣ 674
Grifulvin V Tablets Microsize and Oral Suspension Microsize (Griseofulvin) OrthoNeutrogena 2384
Gris-PEG Tablets (Griseofulvin) Pedinol 2504
Loprox Gel (Ciclopirox) Medicis 1861
Lotrimin (Clotrimazole) Schering 3053
Lotrimin Ultra Cream 1% (Butenafine Hydrochloride) Schering-Plough .... ▣ 733
Lotrisone (Betamethasone Dipropionate, Clotrimazole) Schering 3054
Naftin Cream (Naftifine Hydrochloride) Merz 2097
Naftin Gel (Naftifine Hydrochloride) Merz 2097
Oxistat (Oxiconazole Nitrate) GlaxoSmithKline 1498
Spectazole Cream (Econazole Nitrate) OrthoNeutrogena 2390

Tinea cruris infections
Desenex Liquid Spray (Miconazole Nitrate) Novartis Consumer .... ▣ 674
Grifulvin V Tablets Microsize and Oral Suspension Microsize (Griseofulvin) OrthoNeutrogena 2384
Gris-PEG Tablets (Griseofulvin) Pedinol 2504
Loprox Gel (Ciclopirox) Medicis 1861
Lotrimin (Clotrimazole) Schering 3053
Lotrimin Ultra Cream 1% (Butenafine Hydrochloride) Schering-Plough .... ▣ 733
Lotrisone (Betamethasone Dipropionate, Clotrimazole) Schering 3054
Naftin Cream (Naftifine Hydrochloride) Merz 2097
Naftin Gel (Naftifine Hydrochloride) Merz 2097
Oxistat (Oxiconazole Nitrate) GlaxoSmithKline 1498
Spectazole Cream (Econazole Nitrate) OrthoNeutrogena 2390

Tinea pedis infections
Desenex (Miconazole Nitrate) Novartis Consumer .... ▣ 674
Desenex Jock Itch Spray Powder (Miconazole Nitrate) Novartis Consumer .... ▣ 674
Ertaczo Cream, 2% (Sertaconazole Nitrate) OrthoNeutrogena 2383
Gordochom Solution (Chloroxylenol, Undecylenic Acid) Gordon 1634
Grifulvin V Tablets Microsize and Oral Suspension Microsize (Griseofulvin) OrthoNeutrogena 2384
Gris-PEG Tablets (Griseofulvin) Pedinol 2504
Lamisil AT Creams (Athlete's Foot & Jock Itch) (Terbinafine Hydrochloride) Novartis Consumer .... ▣ 676
Loprox Gel (Ciclopirox) Medicis 1861
Lotrimin (Clotrimazole) Schering 3053
Lotrimin Ultra Cream 1% (Butenafine Hydrochloride) Schering-Plough .... ▣ 733
Lotrisone (Betamethasone Dipropionate, Clotrimazole) Schering 3054
Naftin Cream (Naftifine Hydrochloride) Merz 2097
Naftin Gel (Naftifine Hydrochloride) Merz 2097
Oxistat (Oxiconazole Nitrate) GlaxoSmithKline 1498
Spectazole Cream (Econazole Nitrate) OrthoNeutrogena 2390

Tinea unguium infections
Grifulvin V Tablets Microsize and Oral Suspension Microsize (Griseofulvin) OrthoNeutrogena 2384
Gris-PEG Tablets (Griseofulvin) Pedinol 2504
Lamisil Tablets (Terbinafine Hydrochloride) Novartis 2226
Penlac Nail Lacquer, Topical Solution, 8% (Ciclopirox) Dermik 1051

Tinea versicolor infections
(*see under* Pityrosporon orbiculare infections)

Tonsillitis
Biaxin/Biaxin XL (Clarithromycin) Abbott ... 402
Ceftin (Cefuroxime Axetil) GlaxoSmithKline ... 1369
E.E.S. (Erythromycin Ethylsuccinate) Abbott ... 449
EryPed (Erythromycin Ethylsuccinate) Abbott ... 445
Hurricaine Topical Anesthetic Aerosol Spray, 2 oz. Wild Cherry (Benzocaine) Beutlich ... 835
Hurricaine Topical Anesthetic Aerosol Spray Kit, 2 oz. Wild Cherry with 200 Disposable Extension Tubes (Benzocaine) Beutlich ... 835
Hurricaine Topical Anesthetic Gel: 1 oz. Wild Cherry, Pina Colada, Watermelon, Fresh Mint, 0.18 oz. Wild Cherry (Benzocaine) Beutlich ... 835
Hurricaine Topical Anesthetic Liquid: 1 oz. Wild Cherry and Pina Colada, Swab Applicator Wild Cherry (Benzocaine) Beutlich ... 835
Omnicef Capsules (Cefdinir) Abbott ... 506
Omnicef for Oral Suspension (Cefdinir) Abbott ... 506
PCE Dispertab Tablets (Erythromycin) Abbott ... 510
Spectracef Tablets (Cefditoren Pivoxil) Purdue Pharmaceutical ... 2706
Suprax (Cefixime) Lupin ... 1811
Vantin Tablets and Oral Suspension (Cefpodoxime Proxetil) Pharmacia & Upjohn ... 2650
Zithromax (Azithromycin Dihydrate) Pfizer ... 2568
Zithromax for Oral Suspension, 300 mg, 600 mg, 900 mg, 1200 mg (Azithromycin Dihydrate) Pfizer ... 2561
Zithromax Tablets, 250 mg, 500 mg (Azithromycin Dihydrate) Pfizer ... 2561
Zithromax Tablets, 600 mg (Azithromycin Dihydrate) Pfizer ... 2568
Zithromax Tri-Pak (Azithromycin Dihydrate) Pfizer ... 2561
Zithromax Z-Pak (Azithromycin Dihydrate) Pfizer ... 2568

Tooth, hypersensitivity of
Sensodyne Original Flavor (Potassium Nitrate, Sodium Fluoride) GlaxoSmithKline ... ▣636
Sensodyne Cool Gel (Potassium Nitrate, Sodium Fluoride) GlaxoSmithKline ... ▣636
Sensodyne Extra Whitening (Potassium Nitrate, Sodium Monofluorophosphate) GlaxoSmithKline ... ▣636
Sensodyne Fresh Mint (Potassium Nitrate, Sodium Fluoride) GlaxoSmithKline ... ▣636
Sensodyne Tartar Control (Potassium Nitrate, Sodium Fluoride) GlaxoSmithKline ... ▣636
Sensodyne Tartar Control Plus Whitening (Potassium Nitrate, Sodium Fluoride) GlaxoSmithKline ... ▣636
Sensodyne with Baking Soda (Potassium Nitrate, Sodium Fluoride) GlaxoSmithKline ... ▣636

Torulosis
(*see under* Cryptococcosis)

Tourette, Gilles de la, syndrome
Orap Tablets (Pimozide) Gate ... 1220

Toxoplasmosis, adjunctive therapy in
Daraprim Tablets (Pyrimethamine) GlaxoSmithKline ... 1385

Trachoma
Dynacin Tablets (Minocycline Hydrochloride) Medicis ... 1859

Trachoma, adjunct in
Bleph-10 Ophthalmic Solution 10% (Sulfacetamide Sodium) Allergan ... ⊙219

Treponema pallidum
(*see under* T. pallidum infections)

Treponema pertenue infections
(*see under* Yaws)

Trichinosis
Mintezol (Thiabendazole) Merck ... 2002

Trichinosis with myocardial involvement
Decadron Phosphate Injection (Dexamethasone Sodium Phosphate) Merck ... 1931
Decadron Tablets (Dexamethasone) Merck ... 1929
Depo-Medrol Injectable Suspension (Methylprednisolone Acetate) Pharmacia & Upjohn ... 2615
Depo-Medrol Single-Dose Vial (Methylprednisolone Acetate) Pharmacia & Upjohn ... 2617
Hydrocortone Tablets (Hydrocortisone) Merck ... 1963
Pediapred Oral Solution (Prednisolone Sodium Phosphate) UCB ... 3319

Trichinosis with neurologic involvement
Decadron Phosphate Injection (Dexamethasone Sodium Phosphate) Merck ... 1931
Decadron Tablets (Dexamethasone) Merck ... 1929
Depo-Medrol Injectable Suspension (Methylprednisolone Acetate) Pharmacia & Upjohn ... 2615
Hydrocortone Tablets (Hydrocortisone) Merck ... 1963
Pediapred Oral Solution (Prednisolone Sodium Phosphate) UCB ... 3319

Trichomoniasis, asymptomatic
Tindamax (Tinidazole) Presutti ... 2670

Trichophyton crateriform infections
Grifulvin V Tablets Microsize and Oral Suspension Microsize (Griseofulvin) OrthoNeutrogena ... 2384
Gris-PEG Tablets (Griseofulvin) Pedinol ... 2504

Trichophyton gallinae infections
Grifulvin V Tablets Microsize and Oral Suspension Microsize (Griseofulvin) OrthoNeutrogena ... 2384
Gris-PEG Tablets (Griseofulvin) Pedinol ... 2504

Trichophyton interdigitalis infections
Grifulvin V Tablets Microsize and Oral Suspension Microsize (Griseofulvin) OrthoNeutrogena ... 2384
Gris-PEG Tablets (Griseofulvin) Pedinol ... 2504

Trichophyton megnini infections
Grifulvin V Tablets Microsize and Oral Suspension Microsize (Griseofulvin) OrthoNeutrogena ... 2384
Gris-PEG Tablets (Griseofulvin) Pedinol ... 2504

Trichophyton mentagrophytes infections
Ertaczo Cream, 2% (Sertaconazole Nitrate) OrthoNeutrogena ... 2383
Grifulvin V Tablets Microsize and Oral Suspension Microsize (Griseofulvin) OrthoNeutrogena ... 2384
Gris-PEG Tablets (Griseofulvin) Pedinol ... 2504
Loprox Gel (Ciclopirox) Medicis ... 1861
Lotrimin (Clotrimazole) Schering ... 3053
Lotrisone (Betamethasone Dipropionate, Clotrimazole) Schering ... 3054
Naftin Cream (Naftifine Hydrochloride) Merz ... 2097
Naftin Gel (Naftifine Hydrochloride) Merz ... 2097
Oxistat (Oxiconazole Nitrate) GlaxoSmithKline ... 1498
Spectazole Cream (Econazole Nitrate) OrthoNeutrogena ... 2390

Trichophyton rubrum infections
Ertaczo Cream, 2% (Sertaconazole Nitrate) OrthoNeutrogena ... 2383
Grifulvin V Tablets Microsize and Oral Suspension Microsize (Griseofulvin) OrthoNeutrogena ... 2384
Gris-PEG Tablets (Griseofulvin) Pedinol ... 2504
Loprox Gel (Ciclopirox) Medicis ... 1861
Lotrimin (Clotrimazole) Schering ... 3053
Lotrisone (Betamethasone Dipropionate, Clotrimazole) Schering ... 3054
Naftin Cream (Naftifine Hydrochloride) Merz ... 2097
Naftin Gel (Naftifine Hydrochloride) Merz ... 2097
Oxistat (Oxiconazole Nitrate) GlaxoSmithKline ... 1498
Penlac Nail Lacquer, Topical Solution, 8% (Ciclopirox) Dermik ... 1051
Spectazole Cream (Econazole Nitrate) OrthoNeutrogena ... 2390

Trichophyton schoenleini infections
Grifulvin V Tablets Microsize and Oral Suspension Microsize (Griseofulvin) OrthoNeutrogena ... 2384
Gris-PEG Tablets (Griseofulvin) Pedinol ... 2504

Trichophyton sulfureum infections
Grifulvin V Tablets Microsize and Oral Suspension Microsize (Griseofulvin) OrthoNeutrogena ... 2384
Gris-PEG Tablets (Griseofulvin) Pedinol ... 2504

Trichophyton tonsurans infections
Grifulvin V Tablets Microsize and Oral Suspension Microsize (Griseofulvin) OrthoNeutrogena ... 2384
Gris-PEG Tablets (Griseofulvin) Pedinol ... 2504
Naftin Gel (Naftifine Hydrochloride) Merz ... 2097
Spectazole Cream (Econazole Nitrate) OrthoNeutrogena ... 2390

Trichophyton verrucosum infections
Grifulvin V Tablets Microsize and Oral Suspension Microsize (Griseofulvin) OrthoNeutrogena ... 2384
Gris-PEG Tablets (Griseofulvin) Pedinol ... 2504

Trichuriasis, as secondary therapy
Mintezol (Thiabendazole) Merck ... 2002

Trichuris trichiura infections
Vermox Chewable Tablets (Mebendazole) McNeil Consumer ... 1853

Triglyceride levels, elevated
(*see under* Hypertriglyceridemia, adjunct to diet)

Tuberculosis, pulmonary
Seromycin Capsules (Cycloserine) Lilly ... 1783

Tuberculosis, pulmonary, disseminated
Decadron Phosphate Injection (Dexamethasone Sodium Phosphate) Merck ... 1931
Decadron Tablets (Dexamethasone) Merck ... 1929
Depo-Medrol Injectable Suspension (Methylprednisolone Acetate) Pharmacia & Upjohn ... 2615
Depo-Medrol Single-Dose Vial (Methylprednisolone Acetate) Pharmacia & Upjohn ... 2617
Hydrocortone Tablets (Hydrocortisone) Merck ... 1963
Pediapred Oral Solution (Prednisolone Sodium Phosphate) UCB ... 3319

Tuberculosis, pulmonary, fulminating
Decadron Phosphate Injection (Dexamethasone Sodium Phosphate) Merck ... 1931
Decadron Tablets (Dexamethasone) Merck ... 1929
Depo-Medrol Injectable Suspension (Methylprednisolone Acetate) Pharmacia & Upjohn ... 2615
Depo-Medrol Single-Dose Vial (Methylprednisolone Acetate) Pharmacia & Upjohn ... 2617
Hydrocortone Tablets (Hydrocortisone) Merck ... 1963
Pediapred Oral Solution (Prednisolone Sodium Phosphate) UCB ... 3319

Tuberculosis, resistant, treatment of
Trecator Tablets (Ethionamide) Wyeth ... 3482

Tuberculosis, treatment
Seromycin Capsules (Cycloserine) Lilly ... 1783

Tuberculosis, treatment adjunct
Capastat Sulfate for Injection (Capreomycin Sulfate) Lilly ... 1728
Paser Granules (Aminosalicylic Acid) Jacobus ... 1657

Tuberculosis meningitis, adjunctive therapy in
(*see under* Meningitis, tuberculous)

Tularemia
Dynacin Tablets (Minocycline Hydrochloride) Medicis ... 1859

Tumors, carcinoid, symptomatic relief of
Sandostatin Injection (Octreotide Acetate) Novartis ... 2263
Sandostatin LAR Depot (Octreotide Acetate) Novartis ... 2264

Tumors, gastrointestinal stromal
Gleevec Tablets (Imatinib Mesylate) Novartis ... 2221

Turner's syndrome
Humatrope Vials and Cartridges (Somatropin) Lilly ... 1756
Nutropin for Injection (Somatropin) Genentech ... 1238
Nutropin AQ Injection (Somatropin) Genentech ... 1241
Nutropin AQ Pen (Somatropin) Genentech ... 1241
Nutropin AQ Pen Cartridge (Somatropin) Genentech ... 1241

Typhoid fever
Cipro (Ciprofloxacin) Schering ... 2991

Typhus fever
Dynacin Tablets (Minocycline Hydrochloride) Medicis ... 1859

U

Ulcerative colitis
(*see under* Colitis, ulcerative)

Ulcers, decubitus, adjunctive therapy in
Panafil Ointment (Chlorophyllin Copper Complex Sodium, Papain, Urea) Healthpoint ... 1637
Panafil Spray (Chlorophyllin Copper Complex Sodium, Papain, Urea) Healthpoint ... 1637

Ulcers, decubitus, reduction of possible occurrence of
Betadine Solution (Povidone Iodine) Purdue Products ... 2715

Ulcers, dermal
Accuzyme Spray (Papain, Urea) Healthpoint ... 1637
Primaxin I.M. (Cilastatin Sodium, Imipenem) Merck ... 2022

Ulcers, diabetic, adjunctive therapy in
Accuzyme Debriding Ointment (Papain, Urea) Healthpoint ... 1636
Accuzyme Spray (Papain, Urea) Healthpoint ... 1637
Panafil Ointment (Chlorophyllin Copper Complex Sodium, Papain, Urea) Healthpoint ... 1637
Panafil Spray (Chlorophyllin Copper Complex Sodium, Papain, Urea) Healthpoint ... 1637

Ulcers, varicose, adjunctive therapy in
Accuzyme Debriding Ointment (Papain, Urea) Healthpoint 1636
Accuzyme Spray (Papain, Urea) Healthpoint 1637
Panafil Ointment (Chlorophyllin Copper Complex Sodium, Papain, Urea) Healthpoint 1637
Panafil Spray (Chlorophyllin Copper Complex Sodium, Papain, Urea) Healthpoint 1637

Uncinariasis, as secondary therapy
Mintezol (Thiabendazole) Merck........ 2002

Urea cycle disorders
Buphenyl Powder (Sodium Phenylbutyrate) Ucyclyd 3327
Buphenyl Tablets (Sodium Phenylbutyrate) Ucyclyd 3327

Ureaplasma urealyticum infections
Dynacin Tablets (Minocycline Hydrochloride) Medicis............ 1859
Erythromycin Delayed-Release Capsules, USP (Erythromycin) Abbott 456

Ureaplasma urealyticum urethritis
E.E.S. Granules (Erythromycin Ethylsuccinate) Abbott 449

Ureaplasma urealyticum urethritis, nongonococcal
Dynacin Tablets (Minocycline Hydrochloride) Medicis............ 1859
E.E.S. (Erythromycin Ethylsuccinate) Abbott............ 449
EryPed (Erythromycin Ethylsuccinate) Abbott............ 445
PCE Dispertab Tablets (Erythromycin) Abbott............ 510

Urethritis
E.E.S. Granules (Erythromycin Ethylsuccinate) Abbott 449
Zithromax (Azithromycin Dihydrate) Pfizer............ 2568
Zithromax for Oral Suspension, 300 mg, 600 mg, 900 mg, 1200 mg (Azithromycin Dihydrate) Pfizer 2561
Zithromax Tablets, 250 mg, 500 mg (Azithromycin Dihydrate) Pfizer............ 2561
Zithromax Tablets, 600 mg (Azithromycin Dihydrate) Pfizer...... 2568
Zithromax Tri-Pak (Azithromycin Dihydrate) Pfizer 2561
Zithromax Z-Pak (Azithromycin Dihydrate) Pfizer 2568

Urethritis, Chlamydia trachomatis, nongonococcal
Dynacin Tablets (Minocycline Hydrochloride) Medicis............ 1859
Zithromax (Azithromycin Dihydrate) Pfizer............ 2568
Zithromax Z-Pak (Azithromycin Dihydrate) Pfizer 2568

Urethritis, nongonococcal
E.E.S. (Erythromycin Ethylsuccinate) Abbott............ 449
EryPed (Erythromycin Ethylsuccinate) Abbott............ 445
PCE Dispertab Tablets (Erythromycin) Abbott............ 510

Uric acid lithiasis
(*see under* Urolithiasis, management of)

Urinary bladder, overactive
Detrol Tablets (Tolterodine Tartrate) Pharmacia & Upjohn 2626
Detrol LA Capsules (Tolterodine Tartrate) Pharmacia & Upjohn 2629
Ditropan XL Extended Release Tablets (Oxybutynin Chloride) Ortho Women's Health & Urology .. 2391
Enablex Extended-Release Tablets (Darifenacin) Novartis............ 2201
Oxytrol Transdermal System (Oxybutynin) Watson 3383
Sanctura Tablets (Trospium Chloride) Esprit 1133
VESIcare Tablets (Solifenacin Succinate) Astellas 631

Urinary bladder with retention, neurogenic atony of
Urecholine Tablets (Bethanechol Chloride) Odyssey............ 2349

Urinary retention, acute postoperative
Urecholine (Bethanechol Chloride) Odyssey 2349

Urine, acidification of
K-Phos Original (Sodium Free) Tablets (Potassium Acid Phosphate) Beach 785

Urolithiasis, management of
Urocit-K Tablets (Potassium Citrate) Mission............ 2109

Urticaria, chronic
(*see also under* Urticarial manifestations, relief of)
Allegra (Fexofenadine Hydrochloride) Sanofi-Aventis 2857
Clarinex Syrup (Desloratadine) Schering 3009
Clarinex Tablets (Desloratadine) Schering 3009
Clarinex Reditabs Tablets (Desloratadine) Schering 3009
Zyrtec Chewable Tablets (Cetirizine Hydrochloride) Pfizer 2589
Zyrtec (Cetirizine Hydrochloride) Pfizer 2589

Urticarial manifestations, relief of
(*see also under* Urticaria, chronic)
Phenergan (Promethazine Hydrochloride) Wyeth 3438

Urticarial transfusion reactions
Decadron Phosphate Injection (Dexamethasone Sodium Phosphate) Merck 1931
Depo-Medrol Single-Dose Vial (Methylprednisolone Acetate) Pharmacia & Upjohn 2617

Uterine bleeding, abnormal
Aygestin Tablets (Norethindrone Acetate) Duramed 1062
Climara Transdermal System (Estradiol) Berlex 795
Premarin Intravenous (Estrogens, Conjugated) Wyeth 3440

Uterine leiomymata
Lupron Depot 3.75 mg (Leuprolide Acetate) TAP 3257
Lupron Depot–3 Month 11.25 mg (Leuprolide Acetate) TAP 3262

Uveitis
Decadron Tablets (Dexamethasone) Merck 1929

Uveitis, chronic anterior, steroid-responsive
Blephamide Ophthalmic Ointment (Prednisolone Acetate, Sulfacetamide Sodium) Allergan 563
Blephamide Ophthalmic Suspension (Prednisolone Acetate, Sulfacetamide Sodium) Allergan 564
FML-S Liquifilm Sterile Ophthalmic Suspension (Fluorometholone, Sulfacetamide Sodium) Allergan ...⊙226
Poly-Pred Liquifilm Ophthalmic Suspension (Neomycin Sulfate, Polymyxin B Sulfate, Prednisolone Acetate) Allergan ....⊙231
Pred-G Ophthalmic Suspension (Gentamicin Sulfate, Prednisolone Acetate) Allergan ....⊙234
Pred-G Sterile Ophthalmic Ointment (Gentamicin Sulfate, Prednisolone Acetate) Allergan .....⊙235
TobraDex Ophthalmic Ointment (Dexamethasone, Tobramycin) Alcon 558
TobraDex Ophthalmic Suspension (Dexamethasone, Tobramycin) Alcon 558
Zylet Ophthalmic Suspension (Loteprednol Etabonate, Tobramycin) Bausch & Lomb 3508

Uveitis, diffuse posterior
Decadron Phosphate Injection (Dexamethasone Sodium Phosphate) Merck............ 1931
Depo-Medrol Injectable Suspension (Methylprednisolone Acetate) Pharmacia & Upjohn 2615
Hydrocortone Tablets (Hydrocortisone) Merck 1963
Pediapred Oral Solution (Prednisolone Sodium Phosphate) UCB........ 3319

Uveitis, non-infectious, chronic posterior
Retisert Implant (Fluocinolone Acetonide) Bausch & Lomb.......... ⊙256

V

Vagina, cleansing of
Massengill Feminine Cleansing Wash (Cleanser) GlaxoSmithKline. ▣622

Vaginal and anogenital areas, external, cleansing of
Massengill Baby Powder Scent Soft Cloth Towelette (Lactic Acid, Potassium Sorbate, Sodium Lactate) GlaxoSmithKline ....▣622
Preparation H Medicated Wipes (Witch Hazel) Wyeth ....▣748

Vaginal atrophy
Activella Tablets (Estradiol, Norethindrone Acetate) Novo Nordisk 2311
Cenestin Tablets, 0.3mg (Estrogens, Conjugated, Synthetic A) Duramed 1063
Climara Transdermal System (Estradiol) Berlex 795
Estrogel 0.06% (Estradiol) Solvay 3200
Prefest Tablets (Estradiol, Norgestimate) Duramed 1069
Premarin Tablets (Estrogens, Conjugated) Wyeth 3443
Premphase Tablets (Estrogens, Conjugated, Medroxyprogesterone Acetate) Wyeth 3452
Prempro Tablets (Estrogens, Conjugated, Medroxyprogesterone Acetate) Wyeth 3452
Vivelle Transdermal System (Estradiol) Novartis 2288
Vivelle-Dot Transdermal System (Estradiol) Novartis 2293

Vaginitis
(*see under* Vaginosis, bacterial)

Vaginitis, atrophic
Climara Transdermal System (Estradiol) Berlex 795
CombiPatch Transdermal System (Estradiol, Norethindrone Acetate) Novartis 2180
Premarin Vaginal Cream (Estrogens, Conjugated) Wyeth 3449
Vagifem Tablets (Estradiol) Novo Nordisk 2340

Vaginosis, bacterial
Cleocin Vaginal Ovules (Clindamycin Hydrochloride) Pharmacia & Upjohn 2613
Clindesse Vaginal Cream (Clindamycin Phosphate) Ther-Rx 3296
Metrogel 1% (Metronidazole) Galderma 1212
MetroGel-Vaginal Gel (Metronidazole) 3M 1822

Varicella, acute, treatment of
Zovirax (Acyclovir) GlaxoSmithKline ..1616

Varicella, prevention or modification of
GamaSTAN (Globulin, Immune (Human)) Talecris 3231

Vasopressin-sensitive diabetes insipidus
(*see under* Diabetes insipidus)

Ventilation, mechanical, facilitation of
Mivacron Injection (Mivacurium Chloride) Abbott 489
Nimbex Injection (Cisatracurium Besylate) Abbott 494
Zemuron Injection (Rocuronium Bromide) Organon USA 2363

Ventricular arrhythmias
(*see under* Arrhythmias, ventricular)

Ventricular dysfunction, left, asymptomatic
(*see under* Myocardial infarction, post, left ventricular dysfunction)

Ventricular fibrillation
Pacerone Tablets (Amiodarone Hydrochloride) Upsher-Smith 3337

Ventricular tachycardia, sustained
(*see under* Tachycardia, ventricular, sustained)

Ventriculitis
(*see under* Infections, central nervous system)

Vibrio cholerae infections
Dynacin Tablets (Minocycline Hydrochloride) Medicis............ 1859

Vibrio comma
(*see under* Vibrio cholerae infections)

Vibrio fetus infections
(*see under* Campylobacter fetus infections)

Vincent's gingivitis
(*see under* Fusospirochetosis)

Vincent's infection
(*see under* Fusospirochetosis)

Vincent's pharyngitis
(*see under* Fusospirochetosis)

VIPomas diarrhea
(*see under* Diarrhea associated with vasoactive intestinal peptide tumors)

Vitamin, multiple, deficiency of
Hep-Forte Capsules (Vitamins with Minerals) Marlyn 3525
Mega Antioxidant Tablets (Vitamins, Multiple) Usana 3343

Vitamin and mineral, multiple, deficiency of
Centrum Tablets (Vitamins with Minerals) Wyeth ....▣780
Centrum Kids Rugrats Complete Children's Chewables (Vitamins with Minerals) Wyeth ....▣780
Centrum Performance Complete Multivitamin Tablets (Vitamins with Minerals) Wyeth ....▣781
Centrum Silver Tablets (Vitamins with Minerals) Wyeth ....▣781
MDR Fitness Tabs for Men and Women (Vitamins with Minerals) MDR 1854
Ocuvite Lutein Vitamin and Mineral Supplement (Vitamins with Minerals) Bausch & Lomb ....⊙252
Ocuvite Vitamin and Mineral Supplement (Vitamins with Minerals) Bausch & Lomb ....⊙251
Ocuvite Extra Vitamin and Mineral Supplement (Vitamins with Minerals) Bausch & Lomb ....⊙252

Vitamin B complex, deficiency of
Eldertonic (Vitamins with Minerals) Merz 2096
Mega-B Tablets (Vitamin B Complex) Arco 612

Vitamin C, deficiency of
Halls Defense Sugarfree Vitamin C Drops (Vitamin C) Cadbury Adams ....▣611

Vitamin deficiency, postpartum
Citracal Prenatal Rx Tablets (Vitamins, Prenatal) Mission 2108
OptiNate (Docosahexaenoic Acid (DHA), Folic Acid, Iron, Multivitamins with Minerals) First Horizon ..1162
PreCare Chewables Tablets (Vitamins, Prenatal) Ther-Rx 3300
PreCare Prenatal Caplets (Vitamins, Prenatal) Ther-Rx 3300
Prenate Elite Tablets (Vitamins, Prenatal) First Horizon 1163
PrimaCare AM Capsules (Vitamins, Prenatal) Ther-Rx 3300

PrimaCare One Capsules (Vitamins, Prenatal) Ther-Rx 3301
PrimaCare PM Tablets (Vitamins, Prenatal) Ther-Rx 3300

Vitamin deficiency, prenatal
Citracal Prenatal Rx Tablets (Vitamins, Prenatal) Mission 2108
OptiNate (Docosahexaenoic Acid (DHA), Folic Acid, Iron, Multivitamins with Minerals) First Horizon... 1162
PreCare Chewables Tablets (Vitamins, Prenatal) Ther-Rx 3300
PreCare Prenatal Caplets (Vitamins, Prenatal) Ther-Rx 3300
PremesisRx Tablets (Vitamin B_6, Vitamins, Prenatal) Ther-Rx.......... 3300
Prenate Elite Tablets (Vitamins, Prenatal) First Horizon 1163
PrimaCare AM Capsules (Vitamins, Prenatal) Ther-Rx 3300
PrimaCare One Capsules (Vitamins, Prenatal) Ther-Rx 3301
PrimaCare PM Tablets (Vitamins, Prenatal) Ther-Rx 3300

Vitiligo
(*see under* Hypopigmentation, skin)

Vomiting
(*see under* Motion sickness)

Vomiting, emetogenic, cancer chemotherapy-induced
Aloxi Injection (Palonosetron Hydrochloride) MGI 2099
Anzemet Injection (Dolasetron Mesylate) Sanofi-Aventis 2871
Anzemet Tablets (Dolasetron Mesylate) Sanofi-Aventis 2874
Kytril Injection (Granisetron Hydrochloride) Roche Laboratories 2785
Kytril (Granisetron Hydrochloride) Roche Laboratories 2788
Marinol Capsules (Dronabinol) Unimed 3334
Zofran Injection (Ondansetron Hydrochloride) GlaxoSmithKline 1607
Zofran (Ondansetron Hydrochloride) GlaxoSmithKline 1613
Zofran ODT Orally Disintegrating Tablets (Ondansetron) GlaxoSmithKline 1613

Vomiting, emetogenic, cancer chemotherapy-induced, adjunct in
Emend Capsules (Aprepitant) Merck 1944

Vomiting, emetogenic, radiation therapy-induced
Kytril (Granisetron Hydrochloride) Roche Laboratories 2788
Zofran (Ondansetron Hydrochloride) GlaxoSmithKline 1613
Zofran ODT Orally Disintegrating Tablets (Ondansetron) GlaxoSmithKline 1613

Vomiting, postoperative
Anzemet Injection (Dolasetron Mesylate) Sanofi-Aventis 2871
Anzemet Tablets (Dolasetron Mesylate) Sanofi-Aventis 2874
Kytril Injection (Granisetron Hydrochloride) Roche Laboratories 2785
Phenergan (Promethazine Hydrochloride) Wyeth 3438
Zofran Injection (Ondansetron Hydrochloride) GlaxoSmithKline 1607
Zofran (Ondansetron Hydrochloride) GlaxoSmithKline 1613
Zofran ODT Orally Disintegrating Tablets (Ondansetron) GlaxoSmithKline 1613

von Willebrand's disease, type 1
DDAVP Injection 4 mcg/mL (Desmopressin Acetate) Sanofi-Aventis 2893
Desmopressin Acetate Injection (Desmopressin Acetate) Ferring 1143

Vulvae, kraurosis
Climara Transdermal System (Estradiol) Berlex 795
Premarin Vaginal Cream (Estrogens, Conjugated) Wyeth 3449

Vulvar atrophy
Activella Tablets (Estradiol, Norethindrone Acetate) Novo Nordisk 2311
Cenestin Tablets, 0.3mg (Estrogens, Conjugated, Synthetic A) Duramed 1063
Climara Transdermal System (Estradiol) Berlex 795
CombiPatch Transdermal System (Estradiol, Norethindrone Acetate) Novartis 2180
Estrogel 0.06% (Estradiol) Solvay 3200
Prefest Tablets (Estradiol, Norgestimate) Duramed 1069
Premarin Tablets (Estrogens, Conjugated) Wyeth 3443
Premphase Tablets (Estrogens, Conjugated, Medroxyprogesterone Acetate) Wyeth 3452
Prempro Tablets (Estrogens, Conjugated, Medroxyprogesterone Acetate) Wyeth 3452
Vivelle Transdermal System (Estradiol) Novartis 2288
Vivelle-Dot Transdermal System (Estradiol) Novartis 2293

Vulvovaginal candidiasis
(*see under* Candidiasis, vaginal)

W

Warts, genital
(*see under* Condylomata acuminata)

Water, body, depletion of
(*see under* Dehydration, prevention of)

Weight, body, management of
Oxandrin Tablets (Oxandrolone) Savient 2977

Wheezing, symptomatic relief of
(*see also under* Bronchial asthma)
Primatene Mist (Epinephrine) Wyeth .... ◼ 749

Whipworm infection
(*see under* Trichuris trichiura infections)

Whooping cough
(*see under* Pertussis)

Wilms' tumor
Adriamycin for Injection, USP (Doxorubicin Hydrochloride) Bedford 786
Adriamycin Injection, USP (Doxorubicin Hydrochloride) Bedford 786
Cosmegen for Injection (Dactinomycin) Merck 1907

Wilson's disease
Cuprimine Capsules (Penicillamine) Merck 1925
Syprine Capsules (Trientine Hydrochloride) Merck 2055

Wiskott-Aldrich syndrome
Gammagard Liquid (Immune Globulin Intravenous (Human)) Baxter Healthcare 751
Gammagard S/D (Immune Globulin Intravenous (Human)) Baxter Healthcare 754
Gamunex Immune Globulin I.V., 10% (Immune Globulin Intravenous (Human)) Talecris 3232
Iveegam EN (Immune Globulin Intravenous (Human)) Baxter Healthcare 759

Wolff-Parkinson-White syndrome
Adenocard Injection (Adenosine) Astellas 612

Wound care, adjunctive therapy in
Aquacel AG with Hydrofiber (Silver impregnated antimicrobial dressing) ConvaTec 1035
Betasept Surgical Scrub (Chlorhexidine Gluconate) Purdue Products 2715
Desitin Ointment (Zinc Oxide) Pfizer Consumer Healthcare .... ◼ 700
Panafil Ointment (Chlorophyllin Copper Complex Sodium, Papain, Urea) Healthpoint 1637
Preparation H Medicated Wipes (Witch Hazel) Wyeth .... ◼ 748
Tucks Hemorrhoidal Ointment (Mineral Oil, Pramoxine Hydrochloride, Zinc Oxide, Mineral Oil, Pramoxine Hydrochloride, Zinc Oxide) Pfizer Consumer Healthcare .... ◼ 711
Tucks Hemorrhoidal Suppositories (Starch, topical) Pfizer Consumer Healthcare .... ◼ 712
Xenaderm Ointment (Balsam Peru, Castor Oil, Trypsin) Healthpoint 1638

Wounds, debridement of
Accuzyme Debriding Ointment (Papain, Urea) Healthpoint 1636
Accuzyme Spray (Papain, Urea) Healthpoint 1637
Panafil Ointment (Chlorophyllin Copper Complex Sodium, Papain, Urea) Healthpoint 1637
Panafil Spray (Chlorophyllin Copper Complex Sodium, Papain, Urea) Healthpoint 1637
U-Kera Cream (Urea) TaroPharma 3290

Wounds, infected, adjunctive therapy in
Accuzyme Spray (Papain, Urea) Healthpoint 1637
Panafil Ointment (Chlorophyllin Copper Complex Sodium, Papain, Urea) Healthpoint 1637
Panafil Spray (Chlorophyllin Copper Complex Sodium, Papain, Urea) Healthpoint 1637

Wounds, pilonidal cyst, adjunctive therapy in
Accuzyme Spray (Papain, Urea) Healthpoint 1637
Panafil Ointment (Chlorophyllin Copper Complex Sodium, Papain, Urea) Healthpoint 1637
Panafil Spray (Chlorophyllin Copper Complex Sodium, Papain, Urea) Healthpoint 1637

Wounds, postoperative, adjunctive therapy in
Accuzyme Spray (Papain, Urea) Healthpoint 1637
Panafil Ointment (Chlorophyllin Copper Complex Sodium, Papain, Urea) Healthpoint 1637
Panafil Spray (Chlorophyllin Copper Complex Sodium, Papain, Urea) Healthpoint 1637

Wounds, removal of exudates, aids in
Aquacel AG with Hydrofiber (Silver impregnated antimicrobial dressing) ConvaTec 1035
Panafil Ointment (Chlorophyllin Copper Complex Sodium, Papain, Urea) Healthpoint 1637

Wounds, superficial
Biafine Topical Emulsion (Propylparaben, Methylparaben, Propylene Glycol, Stearic Acid, Triethanolamine) OrthoNeutrogena 2382

Wounds, traumatic, adjunctive therapy in
Accuzyme Spray (Papain, Urea) Healthpoint 1637
Panafil Ointment (Chlorophyllin Copper Complex Sodium, Papain, Urea) Healthpoint 1637
Panafil Spray (Chlorophyllin Copper Complex Sodium, Papain, Urea) Healthpoint 1637

Wrinkles, fine
(*see under* Skin, fine wrinkles, mitigation of)

X

Xerosis
Ultralytic 2 Cream 20% (Urea) Ivax Dermatologicals 1651
Ultralytic 2 Foam 20% (Urea) Ivax Dermatologicals 1652

Xerostomia, radiotherapy-induced
Ethyol for Injection (Amifostine) MedImmune Oncology 1869

X-linked gammaglobulinemia
Iveegam EN (Immune Globulin Intravenous (Human)) Baxter Healthcare 759

X-linked immunodeficiency with hyper IgM
Gamunex Immune Globulin I.V., 10% (Immune Globulin Intravenous (Human)) Talecris 3232

XO syndrome
(*see under* Turner's syndrome)

Y

Yaws
Dynacin Tablets (Minocycline Hydrochloride) Medicis 1859

Yersinia pestis infections
Dynacin Tablets (Minocycline Hydrochloride) Medicis 1859

Z

Zollinger-Ellison syndrome
Aciphex Tablets (Rabeprazole Sodium) Eisai 1081
Pepcid Injection (Famotidine) Merck 2017
Pepcid (Famotidine) Merck 2014
Prilosec OTC Tablets (Omeprazole magnesium) Procter & Gamble 2674
Protonix I.V. (Pantoprazole Sodium) Wyeth 3468
Protonix Tablets (Pantoprazole Sodium) Wyeth 3465
Tagamet Tablets (Cimetidine) GlaxoSmithKline 1547
Zantac (Ranitidine Hydrochloride) GlaxoSmithKline 1597

Zygomycosis
Abelcet Injection (Amphotericin B Lipid Complex) Enzon 1119

SECTION 5

CONTRAINDICATIONS INDEX

This section lists in alphabetical order every medical condition cited as a contraindication in *PDR®* and its companion volumes, with cross-references to all product entries in which the contraindication is found. Page numbers refer to the 2006 editions of *PDR®* and *PDR For Ophthalmic Medicines™* and the 2005 edition of *PDR For Nonprescription Drugs and Dietary Supplements™*, which is published later in the year. A key to the symbols denoting the companion volumes appears in the bottom margin.

These listings will enable you to quickly identify drugs that generally threaten to be inappropriate in the presence of a given complication. However, a drug's suitability is sometimes affected by the severity of the complicating condition, the age or gender of the patient, and the drug's route of administration. In ambiguous situations, a quick review of the underlying *PDR®* text may therefore prove helpful.

Note, too, that the index does not list other drugs and dietary items whose use would present a contraindication. Contraindicated combinations can be found in the Interactions Index and the Food Interactions Cross-Reference. Hypersensitivity to the product's ingredients—an almost universal contraindication—also has not been indexed here. If the clinical picture includes the risk of allergic reaction, be sure to check individual product labeling for additional information.

A

Abdominal adhesions
Zelnorm Tablets 2303

Abortion, infected
Mirena Intrauterine System 810

Abortion, missed
Aygestin Tablets 1062
Prochieve 4% Gel 1018
Prochieve 8% Gel 1018
Prometrium Capsules (100 mg, 200 mg) 3205

Abortion, threatened
Coumadin for Injection 932
Coumadin Tablets 932
Miradon Tablets 3056

Achalasia, esophageal
Fosamax 1949
Fosamax Plus D Tablets 1956

Acid base imbalance, uncorrected
(*see under* Acidosis, hyperchloremic; Acidosis, metabolic, unspecified; Ketoacidosis, diabetic)

Acidosis, hyperchloremic
Daranide Tablets 1928

Acidosis, metabolic, unspecified
(*see also under* Ketoacidosis, diabetic)
ActoPlus Met Tablets 3219
Avandamet Tablets 1343
Fortamet Extended-Release Tablets 1156

Acquired immune deficiency syndrome
(*see also under* Human immunodeficiency virus)
Attenuvax 1889
Flumist Vaccine 1872
Meruvax II 1994
M-M-R II 1980
Mumpsvax 2005
Varivax 2070

Actinomycosis, genital
Mirena Intrauterine System 810

Adenoma, hepatic
Alesse-28 Tablets 3392
Lo/Ovral-28 Tablets 3423
Ortho-Cept Tablets 2395
Ortho-Cyclen Tablets 2414
Ortho Evra Transdermal System 2402
Ortho Tri-Cyclen Tablets 2414
Ortho Tri-Cyclen Lo Tablets 2421
Seasonale Tablets 1073
Triphasil-28 Tablets 3483
Yasmin 28 Tablets 818

Adrenal cortical insufficiency
(*see under* Adrenal insufficiency, uncorrected; Adrenal insufficiency, unspecified)

Adrenal cortical insufficiency, uncorrected
Thyrolar 1203

Adrenal dysfunction, uncontrolled
Bravelle for Intramuscular or Subcutaneous Injection 1140
Follistim AQ Cartridge 2354
Gonal-f RFF Pen for Injection 3155
Menopur for Subcutaneous Injection 1145

Adrenal dysfunction, uncorrected
(*see also under* Adrenal insufficiency, uncorrected)
Repronex for Intramuscular and Subcutaneous Injection 1148

Adrenal gland failure
(*see under* Adrenal insufficiency, unspecified)

Adrenal insufficiency, uncorrected
(*see also under* Adrenal dysfunction, uncorrected)
Cytomel Tablets 1678
Levothroid Tablets 1189
Levoxyl Tablets 1680
Synthroid Tablets 515
Unithroid Tablets 3521

Adrenal insufficiency, unspecified
Daranide Tablets 1928
Urocit-K Tablets 2109
Yasmin 28 Tablets 818

Adrenocortical insufficiency
(*see under* Adrenal insufficiency, uncorrected; Adrenal insufficiency, unspecified)

Agammaglobulinemia
Flumist Vaccine 1872

Agitated states
(*see under* Agitation)

Agitation
Adderall Tablets 3168
Adderall XR Capsules 3169
Adipex-P 1216
Concerta Extended-Release Tablets 1828
Desoxyn Tablets, USP 2482
Dexedrine 1386
DextroStat Tablets 3177
Focalin Tablets 2214
Focalin XR Capsules 2217
Metadate CD Capsules 3316
Ritalin Hydrochloride Tablets 2254
Ritalin LA Capsules 2255
Ritalin-SR Tablets 2254

Agranulocytosis, history of
Clozapine Tablets 2141
Clozaril Tablets 2174
Cuprimine Capsules 1925
FazaClo Orally Disintegrating Tablets 547

AIDS
(*see under* Acquired immune deficiency syndrome)

Albinism
Oxsoralen-Ultra Capsules 3354

Alcohol discontinuation, abrupt
Zyban Sustained-Release Tablets 1620

Alcoholism
Seromycin Capsules 1783

Alcoholism, unsupervised
Coumadin for Injection 932
Coumadin Tablets 932

Allergic reaction to aspirin
Prevacid NapraPAC 3277
Zomig Nasal Spray 718

Allergic reaction to non-steroidal anti-inflammatory drugs
Prevacid NapraPAC 3277
Zomig Nasal Spray 718

Allograft
(*see under* Organ allograft)

Amino acid metabolism disorders
(*see under* Electrolyte imbalance, uncorrected)

Amniocentesis, genetic
MICRhoGAM Ultra-Filtered 2429

Anastomosis, unspecified
(*see also under* Ileocolostomy)
Urecholine Tablets 2349

Anemia, aplastic, history of
Cuprimine Capsules 1925
Ticlid Tablets 2813

Anemia, hemolytic, history of
Skelaxin Tablets 1685

Anemia, megaloblastic, unspecified
Daraprim Tablets 1385

Anemia, non-iron deficiency, unspecified
Ferrlecit Injection 3379
Infed Injection 3381

Anemia, sickle cell
Caverject Impulse Injection 2610

Anemia, unspecified
Buminate 5% Solution, USP 747
Buminate 25% Solution, USP 748
Plasbumin-5 3249
Plasbumin-20 3249
Plasbumin-25 3251
Plasmanate 3252

Anemia, unspecified, history of
Plasbumin-20 3249
Skelaxin Tablets 1685

Anesthesia, general
Parnate Tablets 1499

Anesthesia, local
(*see also under* Anesthesia, major regional lumbar block)
Parnate Tablets 1499

Anesthesia, major regional lumbar block
Coumadin for Injection 932
Coumadin Tablets 932

Aneurysm
(*see also under* Cerebrovascular accident)
Activase I.V. 1225
Aggrastat 1878
Coumadin for Injection 932
Coumadin Tablets 932
Miradon Tablets 3056
ReoPro Vials 1779
Retavase 1131
TNKase I.V. 1256

Angina pectoris
Amerge Tablets 1312
Axert Tablets 2430
Frova Tablets 1101
Imitrex Injection 1431
Imitrex Nasal Spray 1435
Imitrex Tablets 1440
Maxalt Tablets 1983
Maxalt-MLT Orally Disintegrating Tablets 1983
Migranal Nasal Spray 3350
Relpax Tablets 2531
Zomig Nasal Spray 718
Zomig Tablets 714
Zomig-ZMT Tablets 714

Angina, Prinzmetal's
Amerge Tablets 1312
Axert Tablets 2430
Frova Tablets 1101
Imitrex Injection 1431
Imitrex Nasal Spray 1435
Imitrex Tablets 1440
Maxalt Tablets 1983
Maxalt-MLT Orally Disintegrating Tablets 1983
Migranal Nasal Spray 3350
Relpax Tablets 2531
Zomig Nasal Spray 718
Zomig Tablets 714
Zomig-ZMT Tablets 714

Angina, unspecified, history of
Proleukin for Injection 1007

Angioedema, hereditary
Prinivil Tablets 2029
Prinzide Tablets 2033
Vaseretic Tablets 2073
Vasotec I.V. Injection 2076
Zestril Tablets 704

Angioedema, idiopathic
Prinivil Tablets 2029
Prinzide Tablets 2033
Vaseretic Tablets 2073
Vasotec I.V. Injection 2076
Zestril Tablets 704

Angulation, penile
Caverject Impulse Injection 2610
Edex Injection 3103

Anorexia nervosa
Meridia Capsules 485
Wellbutrin Tablets 1579
Wellbutrin SR Sustained-Release Tablets 1583
Wellbutrin XL Extended-Release Tablets 1588
Zyban Sustained-Release Tablets 1620

Antepartum prophylaxis
MICRhoGAM Ultra-Filtered 2429

Anuria
Aldoclor Tablets 1881
Aldoril Tablets 1884
Atacand HCT 637
Avalide Tablets 922
Avalide Tablets 2889
Benicar HCT Tablets 2852
Calcium Disodium Versenate Injection 1819
Clorpres Tablets 2139
Desferal Vials 2190
Diovan HCT Tablets 2195
Diuril Oral 1936
Diuril Sodium Intravenous 1934
Dyazide Capsules 1389
Dyrenium Capsules 3390
Edecrin 1941
Furosemide Tablets 2117
Hyzaar 1964
Indapamide Tablets 2119
Lotensin HCT Tablets 2235
Maxzide 2150
Micardis HCT Tablets 886
Midamor Tablets 2000
Moduretic Tablets 2003
Prinzide Tablets 2033
Teveten HCT Tablets 1710
Timolide Tablets 2056
Uniretic Tablets 3114
Vaseretic Tablets 2073
Zestoretic Tablets 701

Anxiety
Concerta Extended-Release Tablets 1828
Focalin Tablets 2214
Focalin XR Capsules 2217
Metadate CD Capsules 3316
Ritalin Hydrochloride Tablets 2254
Ritalin LA Capsules 2255
Ritalin-SR Tablets 2254
Seromycin Capsules 1783

Aortic coarctation
(*see under* Stenosis, aortic)

Aortic dissection
Aggrastat 1878

Aortic stenosis
(*see under* Stenosis, aortic)

Aphakia
Oxsoralen-Ultra Capsules 3354

Apoplexy, cerebral
(*see under* Cerebrovascular accident)

Appendicitis
Dulcolax Suppositories .... ▣ 608

Arrhythmia, cardiac, severe
Ellence Injection 2632

Arrhythmia, cardiac, history of
Proleukin for Injection 1007
Thioridazine Hydrochloride Tablets 2122

Arrhythmia, cardiac, unspecified
(*see also under* Bradycardia, sinus; Bradycardia, unspecified; Fibrillation, atrial; Fibrillation, ventricular; Flutter, atrial; Heart block, greater than first degree; Heart block, unspecified; Lown-Ganong-Levine syndrome; Q-T interval prolongation; Sick sinus syndrome; Sinus node dysfunction, unspecified; Tachycardia, unspecified; Tachycardia, ventricular, history of; Wolff-Parkinson-White syndrome)
Flexeril Tablets 1832
Rythmol SR Capsules 2736

Arrhythmia, ventricular, unspecified
(*see under* Fibrillation, ventricular; Tachycardia, ventricular, history of; Ventricular dysfunction, left)

Arterial disease, unspecified
(*see under* Angina pectoris; Angina, Prinzmetal's; Arteriosclerosis, unspecified; Arteriovenous malformation; Coronary artery disease; Coronary artery disease, history of; Coronary artery vasospasm; Stenosis, aortic)

Arteriosclerosis, unspecified
(*see also under* Coronary artery disease; Stenosis, aortic)
Adderall Tablets 3168
Adderall XR Capsules 3169
Adipex-P 1216
Desoxyn Tablets, USP 2482
Dexedrine 1386
DextroStat Tablets 3177

Arteriovenous malformation
Activase I.V. 1225
Aggrastat 1878
ReoPro Vials 1779
Retavase 1131
TNKase I.V. 1256

As primary therapy in patients with cardiogenic shock
Natrecor for Injection 3123

Asthma, acute
(*see also under* Status asthmaticus)
Advair Diskus 100/50 1291
Advair Diskus 250/50 1291
Advair Diskus 500/50 1291
Alacol DM Syrup 739
Asmanex Twisthaler 2981
Avinza Capsules 1714
Azmacort Inhalation Aerosol 1701
Balamine DM 739
Combunox Tablets 1183
DepoDur Extended-Release Injection 1098
Duragesic Transdermal System 2448
Flovent Diskus 50 mcg 1415
InnoPran XL Capsules 2728
Kadian Capsules 572
MS Contin Tablets 2703
OxyContin Tablets 2699
OxyFast Oral Concentrate Solution 2704
OxyIR Capsules 2704
Pulmicort Respules 654
Qvar Inhalation Aerosol 1654
Urecholine Tablets 2349

Asthma, history of
Betagan Ophthalmic Solution, USP .... ⊙ 217
Betimol Ophthalmic Solution 3371
Blocadren Tablets 1891
Carteolol Hydrochloride Ophthalmic Solution USP, 1% .... ⊙ 246
Cosopt Sterile Ophthalmic Solution 1910
Duragesic Transdermal System 2448
InnoPran XL Capsules 2728
OptiPranolol Metipranolol Ophthalmic Solution 0.3% .... ⊙ 254
Timolide Tablets 2056
Timoptic in Ocudose 2061
Timoptic Sterile Ophthalmic Solution 2058
Timoptic-XE Sterile Ophthalmic Gel Forming Solution 2062

Asthma, unspecified
Adenoscan 613
Avinza Capsules 1714
Betagan Ophthalmic Solution, USP .... ⊙ 217
Betimol Ophthalmic Solution 3371
Blocadren Tablets 1891
Carteolol Hydrochloride Ophthalmic Solution USP, 1% .... ⊙ 246
Combunox Tablets 1183
Coreg Tablets 1376
Cosopt Sterile Ophthalmic Solution 1910
DepoDur Extended-Release Injection 1098
Inderal LA Long-Acting Capsules 3421
InnoPran XL Capsules 2728
Kadian Capsules 572
MS Contin Tablets 2703
Nadolol Tablets 2121
OptiPranolol Metipranolol Ophthalmic Solution 0.3% .... ⊙ 254
OxyContin Tablets 2699
OxyFast Oral Concentrate Solution 2704
OxyIR Capsules 2704
Phenergan 3438
Timolide Tablets 2056
Timoptic in Ocudose 2061
Timoptic Sterile Ophthalmic Solution 2058
Timoptic-XE Sterile Ophthalmic Gel Forming Solution 2062
Urecholine Tablets 2349

Asthmatic attack
(*see under* Asthma, acute)

Atresia, pulmonary
Indocin I.V. 1973

Atrial fibrillation
(*see under* Fibrillation, atrial)

Atrial flutter
(*see under* Flutter, atrial)

Atrioventricular block
(*see under* Heart block, greater than first degree; Heart block, unspecified)

AV block
(*see under* Heart block, greater than first degree; Heart block, unspecified)

Azotemia
(*see also under* Uremia)
Edecrin 1941

B

Bacterial endocarditis
(*see under* Endocarditis, bacterial)

Bedridden
(*see under* Debilitation)

Bladder neck obstruction
(*see under* Obstruction, bladder neck)

Bleeding, ulcer, peptic
Pletal Tablets 2478

Bleeding, uterine
Menopur for Subcutaneous Injection 1145

Bleeding disorders, unspecified
(*see also under* Bleeding tendencies; Thrombocytopenia, unspecified)
Indocin I.V. 1973
Ticlid Tablets 2813

Bleeding tendencies
Activase I.V. 1225
Aggrastat 1878
Coumadin for Injection 932
Coumadin Tablets 932
Miradon Tablets 3056
ReoPro Vials 1779
Retavase 1131
TNKase I.V. 1256

Bleeding, abnormal, unspecified
Indocin I.V. 1973
Repronex for Intramuscular and Subcutaneous Injection 1148

Bleeding, arterial
Advicor Tablets 1694
Niaspan Extended-Release Tablets 1703

Bleeding, cerebrovascular
(*see under* Bleeding, intracranial; Cerebrovascular accident)

Bleeding, gastrointestinal
Indocin I.V. 1973
Plavix Tablets 940
Plavix Tablets 2942
ReoPro Vials 1779
Ticlid Tablets 2813

Bleeding, gastrointestinal, history of
Proleukin for Injection 1007

Bleeding, genital, abnormal
(*see also under* Bleeding, genitourinary)
Activella Tablets 2311
Alesse-28 Tablets 3392
Aygestin Tablets 1062
Cenestin Tablets, 0.45mg, 0.625mg, 0.9mg, 1.25mg 1063
Cenestin Tablets, 0.3mg 1063
Cervidil Vaginal Insert 1182
Climara Pro Transdermal System 800
CombiPatch Transdermal System 2180
Depo-Provera Contraceptive Injection 2619
depo-subQ provera 104 Injectable Suspension 2622
Estratest Tablets 3196
Estratest H.S. Tablets 3196
Estrogel 0.06% 3200
Follistim AQ Cartridge 2354
Gonal-f RFF Pen for Injection 3155
Lo/Ovral-28 Tablets 3423
Lupron Depot 3.75 mg 3257
Lupron Depot–3 Month 11.25 mg 3262
Menostar Transdermal System 805
Mirena Intrauterine System 810
Ortho-Cept Tablets 2395
Ortho-Cyclen Tablets 2414
Ortho Evra Transdermal System 2402
Ortho Micronor Tablets 2411
Ortho Tri-Cyclen Tablets 2414
Ortho Tri-Cyclen Lo Tablets 2421
Plan B Tablets 1068
Prefest Tablets 1069
Premarin Intravenous 3440
Premarin Tablets 3443
Premarin Vaginal Cream 3449
Premphase Tablets 3452
Prempro Tablets 3452
Prochieve 4% Gel 1018
Prochieve 8% Gel 1018
Prometrium Capsules (100 mg, 200 mg) 3205
Repronex for Intramuscular and Subcutaneous Injection 1148
Seasonale Tablets 1073
Triphasil-28 Tablets 3483
Vagifem Tablets 2340
Vivelle Transdermal System 2288
Vivelle-Dot Transdermal System 2293
Yasmin 28 Tablets 818

Bleeding, genitourinary
(*see also under* Bleeding, genital, abnormal)
ReoPro Vials 1779

Bleeding, history of
Aggrastat 1878
Integrilin Injection 3034
Oncaspar 1123

Bleeding, internal, unspecified
Activase I.V. 1225
ReoPro Vials 1779
Retavase 1131
TNKase I.V. 1256
Xigris Powder for Intravenous Infusion 1796

Bleeding, intracranial
(*see also under* Cerebrovascular accident)
Activase I.V. 1225
Aggrastat 1878
Coumadin for Injection 932
Coumadin Tablets 932
Indocin I.V. 1973
Miradon Tablets 3056
Plavix Tablets 940
Plavix Tablets 2942
Pletal Tablets 2478
Ticlid Tablets 2813

Bleeding, rectal
Dulcolax Suppositories ■ 608
Indocin Suppositories 1968

Bleeding, unspecified
(*see also under* Bleeding, internal, unspecified)
Angiomax for Injection 1856
Argatroban Injection 1321
Arixtra Injection 1325
Coumadin for Injection 932
Coumadin Tablets 932
Fragmin Injection 2638
Lovenox Injection 2931
Miradon Tablets 3056
Ticlid Tablets 2813

Bleeding, uterine
(*see under* Bleeding, genital, abnormal)

Bleeding, vaginal, abnormal
(*see under* Bleeding, genital, abnormal)

Blood dyscrasias, unspecified
(*see also under* Agranulocytosis, history of; Anemia, aplastic, history of; Anemia, hemolytic, history of; Anemia, megaloblastic, unspecified; Anemia, non-iron deficiency, unspecified; Anemia, sickle cell; Anemia, unspecified; Anemia, unspecified, history of; Bleeding disorders, unspecified; Granulocytopenia, history of; Neutropenia; Thrombocytopenia, unspecified)
Attenuvax 1889
Coumadin for Injection 932
Coumadin Tablets 932
Meruvax II 1994
Miradon Tablets 3056
M-M-R II 1980
Mumpsvax 2005
Peganone Tablets, USP 2487
Thiothixene Capsules 2124
Ticlid Tablets 2813
Varivax 2070

Blood vessel, major, tumors eroding into
Photofrin for Injection 729

Body weight less than 50 kg
Arixtra Injection 1325

Bone marrow aplasia
(*see under* Bone marrow depression)

Bone marrow damage
(*see under* Bone marrow depression)

Bone marrow depression
Adriamycin for Injection, USP 786
Adriamycin Injection, USP 786
Hexalen Capsules 2101
Hycamtin for Injection 1427

Bone marrow depression, history of
Carbatrol Capsules 3174
Equetro Extended-Release Capsules 3178
Tegretol/Tegretol-XR 2278

Bone marrow function impairment
(*see under* Bone marrow depression)

Bone marrow hypoplasia
(*see under* Bone marrow depression)

Bone marrow reserve, inadequate
Matulane Capsules 3188

Bowel disease, inflammatory
(*see under* Inflammation, gastrointestinal tract)

Bowel ischemia, history of
Amerge Tablets 1312
Frova Tablets 1101
Imitrex Nasal Spray 1435
Imitrex Tablets 1440
Lotronex Tablets 1479
Proleukin for Injection 1007
Relpax Tablets 2531

Bowel obstruction
(*see under* Bowel ischemia, history of; Obstruction, gastrointestinal tract)

Bowel perforation
(*see under* Perforation, gastrointestinal tract)

Bowel perforation, history of
(*see under* Perforation, gastrointestinal tract, history of)

Bradycardia, sinus
Adenoscan 613
Betagan Ophthalmic Solution, USP ⊙ 217
Betimol Ophthalmic Solution 3371
Betoptic S Ophthalmic Suspension 554
Blocadren Tablets 1891
Brevibloc Concentrate 766
Brevibloc Injection 766
Brevibloc Double Strength Injection 766
Brevibloc Premixed Injection 766
Brevibloc Double Strength Premixed Injection 766
Inderal LA Long-Acting Capsules 3421
InnoPran XL Capsules 2728
Nadolol Tablets 2121
OptiPranolol Metipranolol Ophthalmic Solution 0.3% ⊙ 254
Pacerone Tablets 3337
Tenormin I.V. Injection 698
Tenormin Tablets 695
Timolide Tablets 2056
Timoptic in Ocudose 2061
Timoptic Sterile Ophthalmic Solution 2058
Timoptic-XE Sterile Ophthalmic Gel Forming Solution 2062
Toprol-XL Tablets 660

Bradycardia, unspecified
Coreg Tablets 1376
Pacerone Tablets 3337
Rythmol SR Capsules 2736
Urecholine Tablets 2349

Brain tumor
(*see under* Tumor, pituitary, unspecified)

Breast cancer
(*see under* Carcinoma, breast, history of; Carcinoma, breast, male; Carcinoma, breast, unspecified)
Vivelle Transdermal System 2288

Breastfeeding
Advicor Tablets 1694
Alacol DM Syrup 739
Altoprev Extended-Release Tablets 1151
Bentyl Capsules 724
Bentyl Injection 724
Bentyl Syrup 724
Bentyl Tablets 724
Caduet Tablets 2507
Crestor Tablets 672
Cuprimine Capsules 1925
Doxil Injection 3302
Estratest Tablets 3196
Estratest H.S. Tablets 3196
Evista Tablets 1735
Hycamtin for Injection 1427
Lescol Capsules 2227
Lescol Capsules 2730
Lescol XL Tablets 2227
Lescol XL Tablets 2730
Lipitor Tablets 2495
Lupron Depot 3.75 mg 3257
Lupron Depot–3 Month 11.25 mg 3262
Mevacor Tablets 1996
Migranal Nasal Spray 3350
Orthoclone OKT3 Sterile Solution 2370
Pravachol Tablets 943
Testim 1% Gel 722
Vytorin 10/10 Tablets 2084
Vytorin 10/10 Tablets 3092
Vytorin 10/20 Tablets 2084
Vytorin 10/20 Tablets 3092
Vytorin 10/40 Tablets 2084
Vytorin 10/40 Tablets 3092
Vytorin 10/80 Tablets 2084
Vytorin 10/80 Tablets 3092
Zocor Tablets 2078
Zoladex 709

Breathing problems, unspecified
(*see under* Pulmonary disorders, unspecified; Respiratory illness, febrile; Respiratory illness, unspecified)

Bronchial asthma
(*see under* Asthma, acute; Asthma, history of; Asthma, unspecified)

Bronchoesophageal, fistula, existence of
Photofrin for Injection 729

Bronchospastic disorders, unspecified
(*see also under* Asthma, acute; Asthma, history of; Asthma, unspecified)
Coreg Tablets 1376
Rythmol SR Capsules 2736

Bulimia
Wellbutrin Tablets 1579
Wellbutrin SR Sustained-Release Tablets 1583
Wellbutrin XL Extended-Release Tablets 1588
Zyban Sustained-Release Tablets 1620

Bundle branch block
(*see under* Heart block, unspecified)

C

CAD
(*see under* Coronary artery disease)

Cancer
(*see under* Carcinoma, breast, history of; Carcinoma, breast, male; Carcinoma, breast, unspecified; Carcinoma, cervical; Carcinoma, endometrium; Carcinoma, female reproductive organs; Carcinoma, genital, unspecified; Carcinoma, hepatic; Carcinoma, prostate; Carcinoma, skin, unspecified; Carcinoma, uterine; Malignancy, generalized; Neoplasm, bone marrow system, malignant; Neoplasm, lymphatic system, malignant)

Carcinoma, visceral
Miradon Tablets 3056

Carcinoma, breast, history of
Alesse-28 Tablets ... 3392
Ortho-Cept Tablets ... 2395
Prefest Tablets ... 1069
Premphase Tablets ... 3452
Prempro Tablets ... 3452

Carcinoma, breast, male
(*see also under* Carcinoma, breast, unspecified)
Anadrol-50 Tablets ... 3329
AndroGel ... 3330
Delatestryl Injection ... 2976
Oxandrin Tablets ... 2977
Striant Mucoadhesive ... 1022
Testim 1% Gel ... 722

Carcinoma, breast, unspecified
(*see also under* Carcinoma, breast, history of; Carcinoma, breast, male; Neoplasm, estrogen dependent)
Activella Tablets ... 2311
Alesse-28 Tablets ... 3392
Anadrol-50 Tablets ... 3329
Aygestin Tablets ... 1062
Cenestin Tablets, 0.45mg, 0.625mg, 0.9mg, 1.25mg ... 1063
Cenestin Tablets, 0.3mg ... 1063
Climara Transdermal System ... 795
Climara Pro Transdermal System ... 800
CombiPatch Transdermal System ... 2180
Depo-Provera Contraceptive Injection ... 2619
depo-subQ provera 104 Injectable Suspension ... 2622
Estratest Tablets ... 3196
Estratest H.S. Tablets ... 3196
Estrogel 0.06% ... 3200
Lo/Ovral-28 Tablets ... 3423
Menostar Transdermal System ... 805
Mirena Intrauterine System ... 810
Ortho-Cept Tablets ... 2395
Ortho-Cyclen Tablets ... 2414
Ortho Evra Transdermal System ... 2402
Ortho Micronor Tablets ... 2411
Ortho Tri-Cyclen Tablets ... 2414
Ortho Tri-Cyclen Lo Tablets ... 2421
Oxandrin Tablets ... 2977
Prefest Tablets ... 1069
Premarin Intravenous ... 3440
Premarin Tablets ... 3443
Premarin Vaginal Cream ... 3449
Premphase Tablets ... 3452
Prempro Tablets ... 3452
Prochieve 4% Gel ... 1018
Prochieve 8% Gel ... 1018
Prometrium Capsules (100 mg, 200 mg) ... 3205
Seasonale Tablets ... 1073
Triphasil-28 Tablets ... 3483
Vagifem Tablets ... 2340
Vivelle Transdermal System ... 2288
Vivelle-Dot Transdermal System ... 2293
Yasmin 28 Tablets ... 818

Carcinoma, cervical
(*see also under* Carcinoma, female reproductive organs; Carcinoma, genital, unspecified)
Mirena Intrauterine System ... 810

Carcinoma, endometrium
(*see also under* Carcinoma, female reproductive organs; Carcinoma, uterine)
Alesse-28 Tablets ... 3392
Lo/Ovral-28 Tablets ... 3423
Ortho-Cept Tablets ... 2395
Ortho-Cyclen Tablets ... 2414
Ortho Evra Transdermal System ... 2402
Ortho Tri-Cyclen Tablets ... 2414
Ortho Tri-Cyclen Lo Tablets ... 2421
Seasonale Tablets ... 1073
Triphasil-28 Tablets ... 3483
Yasmin 28 Tablets ... 818

Carcinoma, female reproductive organs
(*see under* Carcinoma, cervical; Carcinoma, endometrium; Carcinoma, genital, unspecified; Carcinoma, uterine)

Carcinoma, genital, unspecified
(*see also under* Carcinoma, cervical; Carcinoma, female reproductive organs; Carcinoma, prostate)
Prochieve 4% Gel ... 1018
Prochieve 8% Gel ... 1018

Carcinoma, hepatic
Alesse-28 Tablets ... 3392
Lo/Ovral-28 Tablets ... 3423
Mirena Intrauterine System ... 810
Ortho-Cept Tablets ... 2395
Ortho-Cyclen Tablets ... 2414
Ortho Evra Transdermal System ... 2402
Ortho Micronor Tablets ... 2411
Ortho Tri-Cyclen Tablets ... 2414
Ortho Tri-Cyclen Lo Tablets ... 2421
Seasonale Tablets ... 1073
Triphasil-28 Tablets ... 3483
Yasmin 28 Tablets ... 818

Carcinoma, ovarian
(*see under* Carcinoma, female reproductive organs)

Carcinoma, prostate
(*see also under* Carcinoma, genital, unspecified; Neoplasm, androgen dependent)
Anadrol-50 Tablets ... 3329
AndroGel ... 3330
Delatestryl Injection ... 2976
Novarel for Injection ... 1147
Oxandrin Tablets ... 2977
Striant Mucoadhesive ... 1022
Testim 1% Gel ... 722

Carcinoma, skin, unspecified
(*see also under* Melanoma, history of)
Oxsoralen Lotion 1% ... 3354

Carcinoma, squamous cell, unspecified
Oxsoralen-Ultra Capsules ... 3354

Carcinoma, uterine
(*see also under* Carcinoma, endometrium; Carcinoma, female reproductive organs)
Mirena Intrauterine System ... 810

Cardiac arrhythmia
(*see under* Arrhythmia, cardiac, unspecified)

Cardiac decompensation
(*see under* Heart failure, unspecified)

Cardiac dilation
Daranide Tablets ... 1928

Cardiac disease
(*see under* Cardiovascular disorders, unspecified)

Cardiac dysfunction
(*see under* Cardiovascular disorders, unspecified)

Cardiac failure
(*see under* Heart failure, unspecified)

Cardiac failure, NYHA class IV decompensated
Coreg Tablets ... 1376
Toprol-XL Tablets ... 660

Cardiac insufficiency
(*see under* Cardiovascular disorders, unspecified)

Cardiac rhythm disturbances, unspecified
(*see under* Arrhythmia, cardiac, unspecified)

Cardiogenic shock
Betagan Ophthalmic Solution, USP ... ⊙217
Betimol Ophthalmic Solution ... 3371
Betoptic S Ophthalmic Suspension ... 554
Blocadren Tablets ... 1891
Brevibloc Concentrate ... 766
Brevibloc Injection ... 766
Brevibloc Double Strength Injection ... 766
Brevibloc Premixed Injection ... 766
Brevibloc Double Strength Premixed Injection ... 766
Carteolol Hydrochloride Ophthalmic Solution USP, 1% ... ⊙246
Coreg Tablets ... 1376
Cosopt Sterile Ophthalmic Solution ... 1910
Covera-HS Tablets ... 3135
Inderal LA Long-Acting Capsules ... 3421
InnoPran XL Capsules ... 2728
Nadolol Tablets ... 2121
OptiPranolol Metipranolol Ophthalmic Solution 0.3% ... ⊙254
Rythmol SR Capsules ... 2736
Tambocor Tablets ... 1824
Tarka Tablets ... 519
Tenormin I.V. Injection ... 698
Tenormin Tablets ... 695
Timolide Tablets ... 2056
Timoptic in Ocudose ... 2061
Timoptic Sterile Ophthalmic Solution ... 2058
Timoptic-XE Sterile Ophthalmic Gel Forming Solution ... 2062
Toprol-XL Tablets ... 660

Cardiopulmonary bypass
Plasmanate ... 3252

Cardiospasm
Norflex Injection ... 1824

Cardiovascular collapse
(*see under* Shock, unspecified)

Cardiovascular disorders, unspecified
(*see also under* Angina pectoris; Angina, Prinzmetal's; Arrhythmia, cardiac, unspecified; Cardiogenic shock; Cardiospasm; Congestive heart failure, uncontrolled; Congestive heart failure, unspecified; Coronary artery disease; Coronary artery disease, history of; Coronary occlusion; ECG changes, history of; Endocarditis, bacterial; Heart disease, ischemic; Heart failure, unspecified; Hypertension, unspecified; Myocardial infarction; Myocardial infarction, history of; Pericardial effusion)
Adderall Tablets ... 3168
Adderall XR Capsules ... 3169
Adipex-P ... 1216
Antabuse Tablets ... 2343
Desoxyn Tablets, USP ... 2482
Dexedrine ... 1386
DextroStat Tablets ... 3177
Hycomine Compound Tablets ... 1105
Imitrex Injection ... 1431
Indocin I.V. ... 1973
Parnate Tablets ... 1499
Relpax Tablets ... 2531

Cardiovascular status, unstable in acute hemorrhage
Bentyl Capsules ... 724
Bentyl Injection ... 724
Bentyl Syrup ... 724
Bentyl Tablets ... 724

Carnitine deficiency
Spectracef Tablets ... 2706

Cavernosal fibrosis
(*see under* Fibrosis, cavernosal)

Cellular immune deficiency
(*see under* Immunodeficiency, unspecified)

Central nervous system depression
Clozapine Tablets ... 2141
Clozaril Tablets ... 2174
FazaClo Orally Disintegrating Tablets ... 547
Moban Tablets ... 1108
Orap Tablets ... 1220
Thioridazine Hydrochloride Tablets ... 2122
Thiothixene Capsules ... 2124

Cephalopelvic disproportion
Cervidil Vaginal Insert ... 1182

Cerebral apoplexy
(*see under* Cerebrovascular accident)

Cerebral herniation
Xigris Powder for Intravenous Infusion ... 1796

Cerebral vascular accident
(*see under* Cerebrovascular accident)

Cerebral vascular disease
(*see also under* Bleeding, intracranial; Cerebrovascular accident)
Alesse-28 Tablets ... 3392
Depo-Provera Contraceptive Injection ... 2619
depo-subQ provera 104 Injectable Suspension ... 2622
Lo/Ovral-28 Tablets ... 3423
Ortho-Cept Tablets ... 2395
Ortho-Cyclen Tablets ... 2414
Ortho Evra Transdermal System ... 2402
Ortho Tri-Cyclen Tablets ... 2414
Ortho Tri-Cyclen Lo Tablets ... 2421
Parnate Tablets ... 1499
Seasonale Tablets ... 1073
Triphasil-28 Tablets ... 3483
Yasmin 28 Tablets ... 818

Cerebral vascular disease, history of
(*see also under* Cerebrovascular accident, history of)
Alesse-28 Tablets ... 3392
Depo-Provera Contraceptive Injection ... 2619
depo-subQ provera 104 Injectable Suspension ... 2622
Ortho-Cept Tablets ... 2395
Seasonale Tablets ... 1073

Cerebrovascular accident
(*see also under* Bleeding, intracranial)
Amerge Tablets ... 1312
Aygestin Tablets ... 1062
CombiPatch Transdermal System ... 2180
Estratest H.S. Tablets ... 3196
Frova Tablets ... 1101
Imitrex Injection ... 1431
Imitrex Nasal Spray ... 1435
Imitrex Tablets ... 1440
Prefest Tablets ... 1069
Premphase Tablets ... 3452
Prempro Tablets ... 3452
Prometrium Capsules (100 mg, 200 mg) ... 3205
Relpax Tablets ... 2531
ReoPro Vials ... 1779

Cerebrovascular accident, history of
Activase I.V. ... 1225
Aggrastat ... 1878
Aygestin Tablets ... 1062
Estratest H.S. Tablets ... 3196
Integrilin Injection ... 3034
Prefest Tablets ... 1069
Prempro Tablets ... 3452
Prometrium Capsules (100 mg, 200 mg) ... 3205
ReoPro Vials ... 1779
Retavase ... 1131
TNKase I.V. ... 1256

Cerebrovascular defects
(*see under* Cerebral vascular disease)

Cerebrovascular disorders, unspecified
(*see under* Cerebral vascular disease; Neurological disorders, unspecified)

Cerebrovascular hemorrhage
(*see under* Bleeding, intracranial; Cerebrovascular accident)

Cerebrovascular syndrome
Amerge Tablets ... 1312
Imitrex Nasal Spray ... 1435
Imitrex Tablets ... 1440

Relpax Tablets 2531
Zomig Nasal Spray 718

Cervicitis, untreated
Mirena Intrauterine System 810

Cesarean section, history of
Cervidil Vaginal Insert 1182

Chest pain, unspecified, history of
(*see also under* Angina, unspecified, history of)
Proleukin for Injection 1007

CHF
(*see under* Congestive heart failure, uncontrolled; Congestive heart failure, unspecified)

Chicken pox
(*see under* Varicella)

Children
Avodart Soft Gelatin Capsules 1353
Edex Injection 3103
Eligard 22.5 mg 2899
Eligard 30 mg 2901
Vantas 3367

Children below the age of 4 years
Agenerase Capsules 1299
Agenerase Oral Solution 1304

Cholestasis
Xenical Capsules 2834

Chronic obstructive pulmonary disease
(*see also under* Asthma, history of; Asthma, unspecified)
Betagan Ophthalmic Solution, USP .... ⊙ 217
Betimol Ophthalmic Solution 3371
Blocadren Tablets 1891
Carteolol Hydrochloride Ophthalmic Solution USP, 1% .... ⊙ 246
Cosopt Sterile Ophthalmic Solution 1910
OptiPranolol Metipranolol Ophthalmic Solution 0.3% .... ⊙ 254
Timolide Tablets 2056
Timoptic in Ocudose 2061
Timoptic Sterile Ophthalmic Solution 2058
Timoptic-XE Sterile Ophthalmic Gel Forming Solution 2062

Chronic obstructive pulmonary disease, acute
Advair Diskus 100/50 1291
Advair Diskus 250/50 1291
Advair Diskus 500/50 1291

Circulatory collapse
(*see under* Shock, unspecified)

Cirrhosis, primary biliary
Lofibra Capsules 1217
Tricor Tablets 523
Triglide Tablets 1165

Cirrhosis, unspecified
Aldoclor Tablets 1881
Aldoril Tablets 1884
Dantrium Capsules 2690
Precose Tablets 776

Coagulation disorders
(*see under* Bleeding disorders, unspecified)

Colitis, antibiotic-associated
Cleocin Vaginal Ovules 2613
Clindesse Vaginal Cream 3296
Duac Topical Gel 3214
Evoclin Foam, 1% 1025

Colitis, pseudomembranous
Duac Topical Gel 3214

Colitis, ischemic, history of
Lotronex Tablets 1479

Colitis, toxic
Colyte with Flavor Packs for Oral Solution 3102
HalfLytely and Bisacodyl Tablets Bowel Prep Kit with Flavors Packs 915
TriLyte with Flavor Packs for Oral Solution 3114

Colitis, ulcerative
Bentyl Capsules 724
Bentyl Injection 724
Bentyl Syrup 724
Bentyl Tablets 724
Cleocin Vaginal Ovules 2613
Clindesse Vaginal Cream 3296
Evoclin Foam, 1% 1025
Lotronex Tablets 1479
Miradon Tablets 3056
Precose Tablets 776

Colitis, ulcerative, history of
Benzaclin Topical Gel 1046
Clindagel 1207
Clindets Pledgets 3212
Duac Topical Gel 3214
Lotronex Tablets 1479

Colitis, unspecified
(*see under* Colitis, ulcerative; Enterocolitis, necrotizing)

Colitis, unspecified, history of
Benzaclin Topical Gel 1046
Clindagel 1207

Collagen diseases, unspecified
(*see under* Lupus erythematosus)

Colonic ulceration
(*see under* Colitis, ulcerative)

Coma, diabetic
Amaryl Tablets 2864
Avandamet Tablets 1343
FazaClo Orally Disintegrating Tablets 547

Coma, hepatic
FazaClo Orally Disintegrating Tablets 547

Coma, unspecified
Clozapine Tablets 2141
Clozaril Tablets 2174
FazaClo Orally Disintegrating Tablets 547
Moban Tablets 1108
Orap Tablets 1220
Phenergan 3438
Thioridazine Hydrochloride Tablets 2122
Thiothixene Capsules 2124

Coma, unspecified, history of
Proleukin for Injection 1007

Comatose states
(*see under* Coma, diabetic; Coma, hepatic; Coma, unspecified)

Conduction disorders, cardiac
(*see under* Arrhythmia, cardiac, unspecified)

Conduction disturbances
(*see under* Arrhythmia, cardiac, unspecified)

Confusion, drug-induced
Tasmar Tablets 3360

Congestive heart failure, uncontrolled
Rythmol SR Capsules 2736

Congestive heart failure, unspecified
Avandamet Tablets 1343
Flexeril Tablets 1832
Flolan for Injection 1408
Fortamet Extended-Release Tablets 1156
Inderal LA Long-Acting Capsules 3421
Plasbumin-5 3249
Plasbumin-20 3249
Plasbumin-25 3251
Plasmanate 3252
Pletal Tablets 2478
Remicade for IV Injection 987

Constipation
Lotronex Tablets 1479

Constipation, severe chronic
Lotronex Tablets 1479

Convulsions, history of
(*see under* Seizure disorders, history of)

Convulsive disorders
(*see under* Seizure disorders, unspecified)

Convulsive disorders, history of
(*see under* Seizure disorders, history of)

COPD
(*see under* Chronic obstructive pulmonary disease)

Corneal foreign body removal
Blephamide Ophthalmic Suspension 564
Poly-Pred Liquifilm Ophthalmic Suspension .... ⊙ 231
TobraDex Ophthalmic Ointment 558
TobraDex Ophthalmic Suspension 558

Coronary artery disease
(*see also under* Coronary artery vasospasm; Stenosis, aortic)
Alesse-28 Tablets 3392
Allegra-D 24 Hour Extended-Release Tablets 2862
Balamine DM 739
Clarinex-D 24-Hour Extended-Release Tablets 3012
Lo/Ovral-28 Tablets 3423
Ortho-Cept Tablets 2395
Ortho-Cyclen Tablets 2414
Ortho Evra Transdermal System 2402
Ortho Tri-Cyclen Tablets 2414
Ortho Tri-Cyclen Lo Tablets 2421
Seasonale Tablets 1073
Triphasil-28 Tablets 3483
Urecholine Tablets 2349
Yasmin 28 Tablets 818
Zyrtec-D 12 Hour Extended Release Tablets 2591

Coronary artery disease, severe
Allegra-D 12 Hour Extended-Release Tablets 2860

Coronary artery disease, history of
Alesse-28 Tablets 3392
Ortho-Cept Tablets 2395
Seasonale Tablets 1073

Coronary artery vasospasm
(*see also under* Angina pectoris; Angina, Prinzmetal's)
Axert Tablets 2430
Frova Tablets 1101
Imitrex Injection 1431
Maxalt Tablets 1983
Maxalt-MLT Orally Disintegrating Tablets 1983
Migranal Nasal Spray 3350
Zomig Nasal Spray 718
Zomig Tablets 714
Zomig-ZMT Tablets 714

Coronary heart disease
(*see under* Cardiovascular disorders, unspecified)

Coronary insufficiency
(*see under* Cardiovascular disorders, unspecified)

Coronary occlusion
(*see also under* Myocardial infarction)
Antabuse Tablets 2343

Creatinine clearance, abnormal
(*see under* Renal dysfunction)

Critical illness, acute
Genotropin Lyophilized Powder 2642
Humatrope Vials and Cartridges 1756
Norditropin Cartridges 2318
Nutropin for Injection 1238
Nutropin AQ Injection 1241
Nutropin AQ Pen 1241
Nutropin AQ Pen Cartridge 1241
Tev-Tropin for Injection 1224

Crohn's disease
Lotronex Tablets 1479

Cysticercosis, ocular
Biltricide Tablets 2990

Cysts, ovarian
Bravelle for Intramuscular or Subcutaneous Injection 1140
Follistim AQ Cartridge 2354
Gonal-f RFF Pen for Injection 3155
Menopur for Subcutaneous Injection 1145
Repronex for Intramuscular and Subcutaneous Injection 1148

D

Debilitation
Mineral Oil 2716

Deep vein thrombophlebitis, history of
(*see under* Thrombophlebitis, history of)

Deep vein thrombosis
Cenestin Tablets, 0.45mg, 0.625mg, 0.9mg, 1.25mg 1063
Cenestin Tablets, 0.3mg 1063
Climara Transdermal System 795
Climara Pro Transdermal System 800
Estratest Tablets 3196
Estratest H.S. Tablets 3196
Estrogel 0.06% 3200
Menostar Transdermal System 805
Premarin Intravenous 3440
Premarin Tablets 3443
Premarin Vaginal Cream 3449
Prempro Tablets 3452
Prometrium Capsules (100 mg, 200 mg) 3205
Vivelle Transdermal System 2288
Vivelle-Dot Transdermal System 2293

Deep vein thrombosis, history of
Climara Transdermal System 795
Climara Pro Transdermal System 800
Estratest Tablets 3196
Estratest H.S. Tablets 3196
Estrogel 0.06% 3200
Menostar Transdermal System 805
Premarin Intravenous 3440
Premarin Tablets 3443
Premarin Vaginal Cream 3449
Premphase Tablets 3452
Prempro Tablets 3452
Prometrium Capsules (100 mg, 200 mg) 3205
Seasonale Tablets 1073
Vivelle Transdermal System 2288
Vivelle-Dot Transdermal System 2293

Dehydration, unspecified
Urocit-K Tablets 2109
Uroqid-Acid No. 2 Tablets 785

Delivery, unspecified
Dilaudid Oral Liquid 443
Dilaudid Tablets - 8 mg 443
Dilaudid-HP 441

Dendritic keratitis
(*see under* Herpes simplex keratitis)

Depression, mental
Seromycin Capsules 1783

Diabetes, type 2, with microalbuminuria
Inspra Tablets 2520

Diabetes mellitus
Urocit-K Tablets 2109

Diabetes mellitus, type 1, sole therapy
Prandin Tablets (0.5, 1, and 2 mg) 2337
Starlix Tablets 2276

Diabetes with vascular involvement
Alesse-28 Tablets 3392
Lo/Ovral-28 Tablets 3423
Ortho-Cept Tablets 2395
Ortho Evra Transdermal System 2402
Ortho Tri-Cyclen Lo Tablets 2421
Seasonale Tablets 1073
Triphasil-28 Tablets 3483

Diabetes, unspecified
Hycomine Compound Tablets 1105

Diabetic gastroparesis
(*see under* Gastroparesis, diabetic)

Diabetic ketoacidosis
(*see under* Ketoacidosis, diabetic)

Diabetic nephropathy
(*see under* Nephropathy, diabetic)

Diarrhea, severe
Edecrin ... 1941

Dihydropyrimidine Dehydrogenase (DPD) Deficiency
Carac Cream, 0.5% ... 1048
Efudex ... 3348
Xeloda Tablets ... 2825

Disease, infectious, unspecified
Mustargen for Injection ... 2007

Dissecting aorta
Coumadin for Injection ... 932
Coumadin Tablets ... 932

Diverticulitis
Lotronex Tablets ... 1479
Miradon Tablets ... 3056

Drug abuse, history of
Adderall Tablets ... 3168
Adderall XR Capsules ... 3169
Adipex-P ... 1216
Desoxyn Tablets, USP ... 2482
Dexedrine ... 1386
DextroStat Tablets ... 3177

Dysgammaglobulinemia
Attenuvax ... 1889
Meruvax II ... 1994
M-M-R II ... 1980
Mumpsvax ... 2005
Varivax ... 2070

E

ECG, QT syndrome, long
Thioridazine Hydrochloride Tablets ... 2122

ECG changes, history of
Proleukin for Injection ... 1007

Eclampsia
Coumadin for Injection ... 932
Coumadin Tablets ... 932
Miradon Tablets ... 3056

Effusion, pericardial
(*see under* Pericardial effusion)

Electrocardiogram changes
(*see under* ECG changes, history of)

Electrolyte depletion
(*see under* Electrolyte imbalance, uncorrected)

Electrolyte disturbances
(*see under* Electrolyte imbalance, uncorrected)

Electrolyte imbalance, uncorrected
(*see also under* Hypercalcemia; Hyperkalemia; Hyperphosphatemia; Hypocalcemia; Hypokalemia; Hyponatremia)
Edecrin ... 1941
Rythmol SR Capsules ... 2736

Emaciation
Miradon Tablets ... 3056

Encephalopathy, history of
Adacel Vaccine ... 2959
Boostrix ... 1366
DAPTACEL ... 2964
Infanrix Vaccine ... 1444
Pediarix Vaccine ... 1518

Endocarditis, bacterial
Arixtra Injection ... 1325
Coumadin for Injection ... 932
Coumadin Tablets ... 932
Miradon Tablets ... 3056

Endometrial cancer
(*see under* Carcinoma, endometrium)

Endometritis, postpartum
Mirena Intrauterine System ... 810

Enteritis, history of
Benzaclin Topical Gel ... 1046
Cleocin Vaginal Ovules ... 2613
Clindagel ... 1207
Clindesse Vaginal Cream ... 3296
Clindets Pledgets ... 3212
Duac Topical Gel ... 3214
Evoclin Foam, 1% ... 1025

Enterobiasis, prophylactic treatment for
Mintezol ... 2002

Enterocolitis, necrotizing
Indocin I.V. ... 1973

Epidural catheter, presence of
Xigris Powder for Intravenous Infusion ... 1796

Epilepsy
Seromycin Capsules ... 1783
Urecholine Tablets ... 2349

Epilepsy, uncontrolled
Adacel Vaccine ... 2959
Boostrix ... 1366
Clozapine Tablets ... 2141
Clozaril Tablets ... 2174
FazaClo Orally Disintegrating Tablets ... 547
Infanrix Vaccine ... 1444
Pediarix Vaccine ... 1518

Epiphyses, closed
Genotropin Lyophilized Powder ... 2642
Humatrope Vials and Cartridges ... 1756
Increlex Injection ... 3290
Norditropin Cartridges ... 2318
Nutropin for Injection ... 1238
Nutropin AQ Injection ... 1241
Nutropin AQ Pen ... 1241
Nutropin AQ Pen Cartridge ... 1241
Tev-Tropin for Injection ... 1224

Epiphyses, fused
(*see under* Epiphyses, closed)

Epithelial herpes simplex keratitis
(*see under* Herpes simplex keratitis)

Esophageal abnormalities, unspecified
(*see also under* Achalasia, esophageal; Esophageal compression; Esophagitis, reflux; Stricture, esophageal)
Fosamax ... 1949
Fosamax Plus D Tablets ... 1956

Esophageal achalasia
(*see under* Achalasia, esophageal)

Esophageal compression
K-Dur Extended-Relase Tablets ... 3047

Esophageal stricture
(*see under* Stricture, esophageal)

Esophageal ulcers less than 1 cm
Photofrin for Injection ... 729

Esophageal varices
Photofrin for Injection ... 729

Esophagitis, reflux
Bentyl Capsules ... 724
Bentyl Injection ... 724
Bentyl Syrup ... 724
Bentyl Tablets ... 724

Exercise, strenuous physical
Urocit-K Tablets ... 2109

Eye infection
(*see under* Cysticercosis, ocular; Infection, ophthalmic, fungal; Infection, ophthalmic, mycobacterial; Infection, ophthalmic, viral; Iritis, acute)

Eye surgery
(*see under* Surgery, ophthalmic)

F

Fallot's tetralogy
(*see under* Tetralogy of Fallot)

Febrile illness
(*see under* Fever; Infection, febrile; Respiratory illness, febrile)

Fecal impaction
Citrucel Orange Flavor Powder ... ▣ 613
Citrucel Sugar Free Orange Flavor Powder ... ▣ 613

Fetal distress, non-imminent delivery
Cervidil Vaginal Insert ... 1182

Fever
(*see also under* Infection, febrile; Respiratory illness, febrile)
DAPTACEL ... 2964
Tasmar Tablets ... 3360

Fibrillation, atrial
Covera-HS Tablets ... 3135
Verelan PM Capsules ... 3120

Fibrillation, ventricular
Digitek Tablets ... 2146
Lanoxicaps Capsules ... 1458
Lanoxin Injection ... 1462
Lanoxin Tablets ... 1468
Lanoxin Injection Pediatric ... 1465

Fibrosis, cavernosal
Caverject Impulse Injection ... 2610
Edex Injection ... 3103

Fibrosis, unspecified
(*see under* Fibrosis, cavernosal)

Fibrotic processes
(*see under* Fibrosis, cavernosal)

Fluid overload
Orthoclone OKT3 Sterile Solution ... 2370

Flutter, atrial
Covera-HS Tablets ... 3135
Verelan PM Capsules ... 3120

Fungal disease, ophthalmic
Retisert Implant ... ⊙ 256

Fungal infections
(*see under* Actinomycosis, genital; Infection, ophthalmic, fungal; Infection, systemic, fungal)

G

Gallbladder disease, unspecified
Antara Capsules ... 2723
Lofibra Capsules ... 1217
Tricor Tablets ... 523
Triglide Tablets ... 1165
Zelnorm Tablets ... 2303

Gastric retention
Colyte with Flavor Packs for Oral Solution ... 3102
Detrol Tablets ... 2626
Detrol LA Capsules ... 2629
Ditropan XL Extended Release Tablets ... 2391
Enablex Extended-Release Tablets ... 2201
HalfLytely and Bisacodyl Tablets Bowel Prep Kit with Flavors Packs ... 915
Oxytrol Transdermal System ... 3383
Sanctura Tablets ... 1133
TriLyte with Flavor Packs for Oral Solution ... 3114
VESIcare Tablets ... 631

Gastric varices
Photofrin for Injection ... 729

Gastroenteritis
Dulcolax Suppositories ... ▣ 608

Gastrointestinal adhesion, history of
Lotronex Tablets ... 1479

Gastrointestinal disorders
(*see under* Bleeding, gastrointestinal; Esophageal abnormalities, unspecified; Gastric retention; Gastroparesis, diabetic; Inflammation, gastrointestinal tract; Intestinal disorders, unspecified; Obstruction, gastrointestinal tract; Perforation, gastrointestinal tract; Spasms, gastrointestinal; Ulcer, gastrointestinal)

Gastrointestinal obstruction
(*see under* Obstruction, gastrointestinal tract)

Gastrointestinal perforation
(*see under* Perforation, gastrointestinal tract)

Gastroparesis
Symlin Injection ... 608

Gastroparesis, diabetic
K-Tab Filmtab Tablets ... 473

General anesthesia
(*see under* Anesthesia, general)

Genital bleeding
(*see under* Bleeding, genital, abnormal)

Glaucoma, narrow-angle, uncontrolled
Detrol Tablets ... 2626
Detrol LA Capsules ... 2629
Enablex Extended-Release Tablets ... 2201
Sanctura Tablets ... 1133
VESIcare Tablets ... 631

Glaucoma, angle closure
Albalon Ophthalmic Solution ... ⊙ 216
Allegra-D 12 Hour Extended-Release Tablets ... 2860
Allegra-D 24 Hour Extended-Release Tablets ... 2862
Clarinex-D 24-Hour Extended-Release Tablets ... 3012
Cymbalta Delayed-Release Capsules ... 1729
Diastat Rectal Delivery System ... 3344
Ditropan XL Extended Release Tablets ... 2391
Evoxac Capsules ... 1042
Klonopin ... 2782
Niravam Orally Disintegrating Tablets ... 3106
Oxytrol Transdermal System ... 3383
Parcopa Orally Disintegrating Tablets ... 3111
Stalevo Tablets ... 2270
Strattera Capsules ... 1784
Transderm Scōp Transdermal Therapeutic System ... 2166
Tranxene ... 2488
Valium Tablets ... 2822
Xanax XR Tablets ... 2655
Zyrtec-D 12 Hour Extended Release Tablets ... 2591

Glaucoma, narrow angle
(*see under* Glaucoma, angle closure)

Glaucoma, open angle, untreated
Klonopin ... 2782
Niravam Orally Disintegrating Tablets ... 3106
Valium Tablets ... 2822
Xanax XR Tablets ... 2655

Glaucoma, unspecified
Adderall Tablets ... 3168
Adderall XR Capsules ... 3169
Adipex-P ... 1216
Bentyl Capsules ... 724
Bentyl Injection ... 724
Bentyl Syrup ... 724
Bentyl Tablets ... 724
Concerta Extended-Release Tablets ... 1828
Desoxyn Tablets, USP ... 2482
Dexedrine ... 1386
DextroStat Tablets ... 3177
Focalin Tablets ... 2214
Focalin XR Capsules ... 2217
Inversine Tablets ... 3286
Metadate CD Capsules ... 3316
Norflex Injection ... 1824
Ritalin Hydrochloride Tablets ... 2254
Ritalin LA Capsules ... 2255
Ritalin-SR Tablets ... 2254

Glucose-6-phosphate dehydrogenase
Elitek ... 2906

Gonadal failure, primary
Gonal-f RFF Pen for Injection ... 3155

Granulocytopenia, history of
Clozapine Tablets ... 2141
Clozaril Tablets ... 2174
FazaClo Orally Disintegrating Tablets ... 547

Guillain-Barre syndrome, history of
Flumist Vaccine ... 1872

H

Head injury
(*see also under* Trauma, intracranial)
DepoDur Extended-Release Injection ... 1098

Headache
(*see under* Headache, history of; Migraine, basilar; Migraine, hemiplegic)

Headache, history of
Parnate Tablets ... 1499

Headaches with focal neurological symptoms
Alesse-28 Tablets ... 3392
Lo/Ovral-28 Tablets ... 3423
Ortho-Cept Tablets ... 2395
Ortho Evra Transdermal System ... 2402
Ortho Tri-Cyclen Lo Tablets ... 2421
Seasonale Tablets ... 1073
Yasmin 28 Tablets ... 818

Heart attack
(*see under* Myocardial infarction)

Heart block, greater than first degree
Adenocard Injection ... 612
Adenoscan ... 613
Betagan Ophthalmic Solution, USP ... ⊙ 217
Betimol Ophthalmic Solution ... 3371
Betoptic S Ophthalmic Suspension ... 554
Blocadren Tablets ... 1891
Brevibloc Concentrate ... 766
Brevibloc Injection ... 766
Brevibloc Double Strength Injection ... 766
Brevibloc Premixed Injection ... 766
Brevibloc Double Strength Premixed Injection ... 766
Cardizem LA Extended Release Tablets ... 1699
Carteolol Hydrochloride Ophthalmic Solution USP, 1% ... ⊙ 246
Coreg Tablets ... 1376
Covera-HS Tablets ... 3135
Inderal LA Long-Acting Capsules ... 3421
InnoPran XL Capsules ... 2728
Nadolol Tablets ... 2121
OptiPranolol Metipranolol Ophthalmic Solution 0.3% ... ⊙ 254
Pacerone Tablets ... 3337
Tambocor Tablets ... 1824
Tarka Tablets ... 519
Tenormin I.V. Injection ... 698
Tenormin Tablets ... 695
Tiazac Capsules ... 1204
Timolide Tablets ... 2056
Timoptic in Ocudose ... 2061
Timoptic Sterile Ophthalmic Solution ... 2058
Timoptic-XE Sterile Ophthalmic Gel Forming Solution ... 2062
Toprol-XL Tablets ... 660
Verelan PM Capsules ... 3120

Heart block, unspecified
Flexeril Tablets ... 1832
Primaxin I.M. ... 2022
Tambocor Tablets ... 1824

Heart damage
(*see under* Cardiovascular disorders, unspecified)

Heart disease, ischemic
(*see also under* Angina pectoris; Ischemia, silent; Myocardial infarction)
Amerge Tablets ... 1312
Axert Tablets ... 2430
Frova Tablets ... 1101
Imitrex Injection ... 1431
Imitrex Nasal Spray ... 1435
Imitrex Tablets ... 1440
Maxalt Tablets ... 1983
Maxalt-MLT Orally Disintegrating Tablets ... 1983
Migranal Nasal Spray ... 3350
Relpax Tablets ... 2531
Zomig Nasal Spray ... 718
Zomig Tablets ... 714
Zomig-ZMT Tablets ... 714

Heart disease, severe organic
ProAmatine Tablets ... 3183

Heart disease, unspecified
(*see under* Cardiovascular disorders, unspecified)

Heart disease, valvular
Ortho-Cept Tablets ... 2395
Seasonale Tablets ... 1073
Yasmin 28 Tablets ... 818

Heart failure, unspecified
(*see also under* Congestive heart failure, unspecified)
Betagan Ophthalmic Solution, USP ... ⊙ 217
Betimol Ophthalmic Solution ... 3371
Betoptic S Ophthalmic Suspension ... 554
Blocadren Tablets ... 1891
Brevibloc Concentrate ... 766
Brevibloc Injection ... 766
Brevibloc Double Strength Injection ... 766
Brevibloc Premixed Injection ... 766
Brevibloc Double Strength Premixed Injection ... 766
Buminate 5% Solution, USP ... 747
Buminate 25% Solution, USP ... 748
Carteolol Hydrochloride Ophthalmic Solution USP, 1% ... ⊙ 246
Cosopt Sterile Ophthalmic Solution ... 1910
Geodon ... 2514
Inversine Tablets ... 3286
Nadolol Tablets ... 2121
OptiPranolol Metipranolol Ophthalmic Solution 0.3% ... ⊙ 254
Orthoclone OKT3 Sterile Solution ... 2370
Tenormin I.V. Injection ... 698
Tenormin Tablets ... 695
Timolide Tablets ... 2056
Timoptic in Ocudose ... 2061
Timoptic Sterile Ophthalmic Solution ... 2058
Timoptic-XE Sterile Ophthalmic Gel Forming Solution ... 2062
Toprol-XL Tablets ... 660

Hematologic disorders
(*see under* Bleeding disorders, unspecified; Blood dyscrasias, unspecified)

Hematopoietic disorders
(*see under* Blood dyscrasias, unspecified; Bone marrow depression)

Hemochromatosis
Chromagen Soft Gelatin Capsules ... 3296
Chromagen Forte Soft Gelatin Capsules ... 3296
Niferex-150 Forte Capsules ... 3299
Repliva 21/7 Tablets ... 3301

Hemoglobinopathies
Copegus Tablets ... 2759
Rebetol ... 3073
Ribavirin, USP Capsules ... 3083

Hemorrhage
(*see under* Bleeding disorders, unspecified; Bleeding tendencies; Bleeding, abnormal, unspecified; Bleeding, gastrointestinal; Bleeding, gastrointestinal, history of; Bleeding, genital, abnormal; Bleeding, genitourinary; Bleeding, history of; Bleeding, internal, unspecified; Bleeding, intracranial; Bleeding, rectal; Bleeding, unspecified; Cardiovascular status, unstable in acute hemorrhage)

Hemorrhagic diathesis
(*see under* Bleeding tendencies)

Hemorrhagic stroke
(*see under* Stroke, hemorrhagic)

Hemosiderosis
Chromagen Soft Gelatin Capsules ... 3296
Chromagen Forte Soft Gelatin Capsules ... 3296
Niferex-150 Forte Capsules ... 3299
Repliva 21/7 Tablets ... 3301

Hemostatic disorders
(*see under* Bleeding disorders, unspecified)

Hepatic adenoma
(*see under* Adenoma, hepatic)

Hepatic cancer
(*see under* Carcinoma, hepatic)

Hepatic coma
(*see under* Coma, hepatic)

Hepatic damage
(*see under* Liver dysfunction)

Hepatic decompensation
Pegasys ... 2793
Roferon-A Injection ... 2805

Hepatic disease
(*see also under* Liver disease, unspecified)
Vivelle Transdermal System ... 2288

Hepatic dysfunction
(*see also under* Liver dysfunction)
Triglide Tablets ... 1165
Vivelle Transdermal System ... 2288

Hepatic failure
(*see under* Liver failure)

Hepatic impairment
(*see under* Liver dysfunction)

Hepatic impairment, moderate
Aptivus Capsules ... 859

Hepatic impairment, severe
Agrylin Capsules ... 3172
Aptivus Capsules ... 859
Miradon Tablets ... 3056
Trecator Tablets ... 3482

Hepatic injury
(*see under* Liver dysfunction)

Hepatic insufficiency
(*see under* Liver dysfunction)

Hepatitis
Aldoclor Tablets ... 1881
Aldoril Tablets ... 1884
Calcium Disodium Versenate Injection ... 1819
Dantrium Capsules ... 2690

Hepatitis, autoimmune
Pegasys ... 2793
PEG-Intron Powder for Injection ... 3062
Rebetron Combination Therapy ... 3078
Ribavirin, USP Capsules ... 3083
Roferon-A Injection ... 2805

Hepatocellular failure
(*see under* Liver failure)

Herpes simplex keratitis
Alrex Ophthalmic Suspension 0.2% ... ⊙ 243
Blephamide Ophthalmic Ointment ... 563
Blephamide Ophthalmic Suspension ... 564
FML Ophthalmic Ointment ... ⊙ 225
FML Ophthalmic Suspension ... ⊙ 224
FML Forte Ophthalmic Suspension ... ⊙ 223
FML-S Liquifilm Sterile Ophthalmic Suspension ... ⊙ 226
HMS Sterile Ophthalmic Suspension ... ⊙ 228
Lotemax Ophthalmic Suspension 0.5% ... ⊙ 249
Poly-Pred Liquifilm Ophthalmic Suspension ... ⊙ 231
Pred Forte Ophthalmic Suspension ... ⊙ 233
Pred Mild Sterile Ophthalmic Suspension ... ⊙ 236
Pred-G Ophthalmic Suspension ... ⊙ 234
Pred-G Sterile Ophthalmic Ointment ... ⊙ 235
TobraDex Ophthalmic Ointment ... 558
TobraDex Ophthalmic Suspension ... 558
Zylet Ophthalmic Suspension ... 3508

Herpes zoster
Cosmegen for Injection ... 1907

HIV
(*see under* Human immunodeficiency virus)

Human immunodeficiency virus
(*see also under* Acquired immune deficiency syndrome)
Attenuvax ... 1889
Flumist Vaccine ... 1872
Infanrix Vaccine ... 1444
Mumpsvax ... 2005
Pediarix Vaccine ... 1518
Varivax ... 2070

Hyperammonemia, acute
Buphenyl Powder ... 3327
Buphenyl Tablets ... 3327

Hypercalcemia
Actonel with Calcium Tablets ... 2684
Calcijex Injection ... 411
Dovonex Cream 0.005% ... 3374
Dovonex Ointment 0.005% ... 3375
Dovonex Scalp Solution 0.005% ... 3375
Hectorol Capsules ... 909
Hectorol Injection ... 911
Oxandrin Tablets ... 2977
PhosLo GelCaps ... 2158
Zemplar Capsules ... 535
Zemplar Injection ... 538

Hypercarbia
Combunox Tablets ... 1183
OxyContin Tablets ... 2699
OxyFast Oral Concentrate Solution ... 2704
OxyIR Capsules ... 2704

Hypercoagulable state, history of
Lotronex Tablets ... 1479

Hyperkalemia
Dyazide Capsules 1389
Dyrenium Capsules 3390
Inspra Tablets 2520
K-Dur Extended-Relase Tablets 3047
K-Lor Powder Packets 472
K-Phos Original (Sodium Free) Tablets 785
K-Tab Filmtab Tablets 473
Maxzide 2150
Midamor Tablets 2000
Moduretic Tablets 2003
Urocit-K Tablets 2109

Hyperphosphatemia
K-Phos Neutral Tablets 785
K-Phos Original (Sodium Free) Tablets 785
Uroqid-Acid No. 2 Tablets 785

Hypersensitivity to benzyl alcohol
Lovenox Injection 2931

Hypersensitivity to pork products
Lovenox Injection 2931

Hypertension, moderate
Adderall XR Capsules 3169

Hypertension, compensatory
Hyperstat I.V. Injection 3031

Hypertension, excessive supine
ProAmatine Tablets 3183

Hypertension, malignant
Coumadin for Injection 932
Coumadin Tablets 932
Miradon Tablets 3056

Hypertension, pulmonary
Zomig-ZMT Tablets 714

Hypertension, severe
Adderall XR Capsules 3169
Allegra-D 12 Hour Extended-Release Tablets 2860
Miradon Tablets 3056

Hypertension, uncontrolled
Activase I.V. 1225
Aggrastat 1878
Alesse-28 Tablets 3392
Amerge Tablets 1312
Aranesp for Injection 576
Axert Tablets 2430
Dostinex Tablets 2631
Epogen for Injection 586
Frova Tablets 1101
Gengraf Capsules 458
Imitrex Nasal Spray 1435
Imitrex Tablets 1440
Integrilin Injection 3034
Lo/Ovral-28 Tablets 3423
Maxalt Tablets 1983
Maxalt-MLT Orally Disintegrating Tablets 1983
Migranal Nasal Spray 3350
Neoral Soft Gelatin Capsules 2247
Neoral Oral Solution 2247
Orthoclone OKT3 Sterile Solution 2370
Procrit for Injection 2374
Relpax Tablets 2531
ReoPro Vials 1779
Retavase 1131
Seasonale Tablets 1073
TNKase I.V. 1256
Triphasil-28 Tablets 3483
Zomig Nasal Spray 718
Zomig Tablets 714
Zomig-ZMT Tablets 714

Hypertension, unspecified
Adderall Tablets 3168
Adipex-P 1216
Alacol DM Syrup 739
Allegra-D 24 Hour Extended-Release Tablets 2862
Balamine DM 739
Clarinex-D 24-Hour Extended-Release Tablets 3012
Desoxyn Tablets, USP 2482
Dexedrine 1386
DextroStat Tablets 3177
Hycomine Compound Tablets 1105
Imitrex Injection 1431
Inversine Tablets 3286
Ortho-Cept Tablets 2395
Ortho Evra Transdermal System 2402
Ortho Tri-Cyclen Lo Tablets 2421
Parnate Tablets 1499
Yasmin 28 Tablets 818
Zyrtec-D 12 Hour Extended Release Tablets 2591

Hyperthermia, malignant, susceptibility to
Ultane Liquid for Inhalation 526

Hyperthermia, malignant, history of
Suprane Liquid for Inhalation 770

Hyperthyroidism
(*see also under* Thyrotoxicosis; Thyrotoxicosis, untreated)
Adderall Tablets 3168
Adderall XR Capsules 3169
Adipex-P 1216
Desoxyn Tablets, USP 2482
Dexedrine 1386
DextroStat Tablets 3177
Flexeril Tablets 1832
Hycomine Compound Tablets 1105
Urecholine Tablets 2349

Hypervitaminosis D
(*see under* Toxicity, vitamin D)

Hypervolemia
Plasmanate 3252

Hypocalcemia
Actonel Tablets 2679
Actonel with Calcium Tablets 2684
Boniva Tablets 2747
Fosamax 1949
Fosamax Plus D Tablets 1956

Hypogammaglobulinemia
(*see also under* Immunodeficiency, unspecified)
Attenuvax 1889
Meruvax II 1994
M-M-R II 1980
Mumpsvax 2005
Varivax 2070

Hypoglycemia, unspecified
Apidra Injection 2876
Humalog-Pen 1751
Humulin R (U-500) 1768
NovoLog Injection 2326
NovoLog Mix 70/30 2331
Symlin Injection 608

Hypokalemia
Daranide Tablets 1928

Hyponatremia
Daranide Tablets 1928

Hypophosphatemia
Renagel Tablets 1268

Hypotension, history of
Mivacron Injection 489

Hypotension, unspecified
Cardizem LA Extended Release Tablets 1699
Covera-HS Tablets 3135
Rythmol SR Capsules 2736
Tarka Tablets 519
Tiazac Capsules 1204
Urecholine Tablets 2349
Verelan PM Capsules 3120

Hypovolemia
(*see under* Shock, unspecified)

I

IgA deficiencies, selective
(*see under* Immunoglobulin A deficiency)

Ileocolostomy
Activase I.V. 1225

Ileus, paralytic
Avinza Capsules 1714
Clozapine Tablets 2141
Combunox Tablets 1183
DepoDur Extended-Release Injection 1098
Duragesic Transdermal System 2448
Kadian Capsules 572
MS Contin Tablets 2703
OxyContin Tablets 2699
OxyFast Oral Concentrate Solution 2704
OxyIR Capsules 2704

Ileus, unspecified
(*see also under* Ileus, paralytic)
Colyte with Flavor Packs for Oral Solution 3102
HalfLytely and Bisacodyl Tablets Bowel Prep Kit with Flavors Packs 915
TriLyte with Flavor Packs for Oral Solution 3114

Immunodeficiency, family history of
Meruvax II 1994
M-M-R II 1980
Mumpsvax 2005

Immunodeficiency, history of
Attenuvax 1889
Varivax 2070

Immunodeficiency, unspecified
(*see also under* Acquired immune deficiency syndrome; Dysgammaglobulinemia; Human immunodeficiency virus; Hypogammaglobulinemia; Immunodeficiency, family history of; Immunodeficiency, history of; Immunoglobulin A deficiency; Immunosuppression)
Attenuvax 1889
Flumist Vaccine 1872
Meruvax II 1994
M-M-R II 1980
Mumpsvax 2005
Varivax 2070
Vivotif 834

Immunodeficient state
(*see under* Immunodeficiency, unspecified)

Immunoglobulin A deficiency
CytoGam Intravenous 1866
GamaSTAN 3231
Gammagard S/D 754

Immunosuppression
Attenuvax 1889
Flumist Vaccine 1872
Meruvax II 1994
M-M-R II 1980
Mumpsvax 2005
Varivax 2070
Vivotif 834

Impulse generation disorders
(*see under* Arrhythmia, cardiac, unspecified)

Inability to stand or sit upright for at least 30 minutes
Actonel with Calcium Tablets 2684
Fosamax 1949
Fosamax Plus D Tablets 1956

Inability to stand or sit upright for at least 60 minutes
Boniva Tablets 2747

Increased intracranial pressure
(*see under* Intracranial pressure, increased)

Infants
Agenerase Capsules 1299
Agenerase Oral Solution 1304
Bentyl Capsules 724
Bentyl Injection 724
Bentyl Syrup 724
Bentyl Tablets 724
Caverject Impulse Injection 2610
Ovide .5% Lotion 3287
Pegasys 2793

Infants, premature
Alacol DM Syrup 739

Infection, ophthalmic, active
Restasis Ophthalmic Emulsion 570

Infection, viral
Bayer Aspirin Tablets 3515

Infection, viral, external canal
Ciprodex Otic Suspension 555

Infection, bacterial, unspecified
(*see under* Endocarditis, bacterial)

Infection, febrile
Attenuvax 1889
DAPTACEL 2964
Meruvax II 1994
M-M-R II 1980
Mumpsvax 2005
Varivax 2070

Infection, fungal
(*see under* Actinomycosis, genital; Infection, ophthalmic, fungal; Infection, systemic, fungal)

Infection, fungal, unspecified
(*see under* Actinomycosis, genital)

Infection, injection site
Botox Purified Neurotoxin Complex 565
Hyalgan Solution 2917
Orthovisc Injection 3518

Infection, mycobacterial
(*see under* Infection, ophthalmic, mycobacterial; Tuberculosis, unspecified)

Infection, nasal, untreated
Nasarel Nasal Spray 1652

Infection, ophthalmic, cysticercosis
(*see under* Cysticercosis, ocular)

Infection, ophthalmic, fungal
Alrex Ophthalmic Suspension 0.2% ⊙ 243
Blephamide Ophthalmic Ointment 563
Blephamide Ophthalmic Suspension 564
FML Ophthalmic Ointment ⊙ 225
FML Ophthalmic Suspension ⊙ 224
FML Forte Ophthalmic Suspension ⊙ 223
FML-S Liquifilm Sterile Ophthalmic Suspension ⊙ 226
HMS Sterile Ophthalmic Suspension ⊙ 228
Lotemax Ophthalmic Suspension 0.5% ⊙ 249
Poly-Pred Liquifilm Ophthalmic Suspension ⊙ 231
Pred Forte Ophthalmic Suspension ⊙ 233
Pred Mild Sterile Ophthalmic Suspension ⊙ 236
Pred-G Ophthalmic Suspension ⊙ 234
Pred-G Sterile Ophthalmic Ointment ⊙ 235
TobraDex Ophthalmic Ointment 558
TobraDex Ophthalmic Suspension 558
Zylet Ophthalmic Suspension 3508

Infection, ophthalmic, mycobacterial
(*see also under* Tuberculosis, unspecified)
Alrex Ophthalmic Suspension 0.2% ⊙ 243
Blephamide Ophthalmic Ointment 563
Blephamide Ophthalmic Suspension 564
FML Ophthalmic Ointment ⊙ 225
FML Ophthalmic Suspension ⊙ 224
FML Forte Ophthalmic Suspension ⊙ 223
FML-S Liquifilm Sterile Ophthalmic Suspension ⊙ 226
HMS Sterile Ophthalmic Suspension ⊙ 228
Lotemax Ophthalmic Suspension 0.5% ⊙ 249
Poly-Pred Liquifilm Ophthalmic Suspension ⊙ 231
Pred Forte Ophthalmic Suspension ⊙ 233
Pred Mild Sterile Ophthalmic Suspension ⊙ 236
Pred-G Ophthalmic Suspension ⊙ 234
Pred-G Sterile Ophthalmic Ointment ⊙ 235
TobraDex Ophthalmic Ointment 558
TobraDex Ophthalmic Suspension 558
Zylet Ophthalmic Suspension 3508

Infection, ophthalmic, unspecified
(*see under* Cysticercosis, ocular; Iritis, acute)

Infection, ophthalmic, untreated
Pred Forte Ophthalmic Suspension ⊙ 233
Pred Mild Sterile Ophthalmic Suspension ⊙ 236

Infection, ophthalmic, viral
(*see also under* Herpes simplex keratitis)
Blephamide Ophthalmic Ointment 563
Blephamide Ophthalmic Suspension 564
FML Ophthalmic Ointment ⊙ 225
FML Ophthalmic Suspension ⊙ 224
FML Forte Ophthalmic Suspension ⊙ 223
HMS Sterile Ophthalmic Suspension ⊙ 228
Lotemax Ophthalmic Suspension 0.5% ⊙ 249
Poly-Pred Liquifilm Ophthalmic Suspension ⊙ 231
Pred Forte Ophthalmic Suspension ⊙ 233
Pred Mild Sterile Ophthalmic Suspension ⊙ 236
Pred-G Ophthalmic Suspension ⊙ 234
Pred-G Sterile Ophthalmic Ointment ⊙ 235
TobraDex Ophthalmic Ointment 558
TobraDex Ophthalmic Suspension 558
Zylet Ophthalmic Suspension 3508

Infection, respiratory
(*see under* Respiratory illness, febrile; Respiratory illness, unspecified; Tuberculosis, unspecified)

Infection, scalp
Temovate Scalp Application 1551

Infection, systemic, fungal
Decadron Phosphate Injection 1931
Decadron Tablets 1929
Depo-Medrol Injectable Suspension 2615
Depo-Medrol Single-Dose Vial 2617
Hydrocortone Tablets 1963
Pediapred Oral Solution 3319

Infection, untreated
(*see also under* Infection, nasal, untreated; Infection, ophthalmic, untreated)
Indocin I.V. 1973

Infection, urinary tract
(*see under* Nephritis)

Infection, vaginal
(*see under* Cervicitis, untreated; Vaginitis, untreated; Vaginosis, bacterial, untreated)

Infection, viral
(*see under* Herpes simplex keratitis; Herpes zoster; Human immunodeficiency virus; Infection, ophthalmic, viral; Varicella)

Infertility, non-anovulatory
Repronex for Intramuscular and Subcutaneous Injection 1148

Infertility, non-hypogonadotropic
Repronex for Intramuscular and Subcutaneous Injection 1148

Infertility, treatment of
Synthroid Tablets 515

Inflammation, gastrointestinal tract
(*see also under* Colitis, toxic; Colitis, ulcerative; Colitis, ulcerative, history of; Colitis, unspecified, history of; Diverticulitis; Enteritis, history of; Enterocolitis, necrotizing; Esophagitis, reflux; Gastroenteritis; Ulcer, gastrointestinal)
Precose Tablets 776

Inflammatory bowel disease
(*see under* Inflammation, gastrointestinal tract)

Intestinal circulation, impaired
Lotronex Tablets 1479

Intestinal disorders, unspecified
(*see also under* Bowel ischemia, history of; Inflammation, gastrointestinal tract; Megacolon, toxic; Obstruction, gastrointestinal tract; Perforation, gastrointestinal tract)
Precose Tablets 776

Intestinal obstruction
(*see under* Obstruction, gastrointestinal tract)

Intoxication, acute
Ultracet Tablets 2462

Intracranial pressure, increased
DepoDur Extended-Release Injection 1098
Hycomine Compound Tablets 1105
Hycotuss Expectorant Syrup 1106

Intracranial trauma
(*see under* Trauma, intracranial)

Intrathecal administration
Depo-Medrol Single-Dose Vial 2617

Intravenous administration
Increlex Injection 3290

Intubation, history of
Proleukin for Injection 1007

Iritis, acute
Evoxac Capsules 1042
Rēv-Eyes Ophthalmic Eyedrops 0.5% ⊙ 256

Iron overload, evidence of
Ferrlecit Injection 3379

Ischemia, silent
Amerge Tablets 1312
Axert Tablets 2430
Frova Tablets 1101
Imitrex Injection 1431
Imitrex Nasal Spray 1435
Imitrex Tablets 1440
Maxalt Tablets 1983
Maxalt-MLT Orally Disintegrating Tablets 1983
Migranal Nasal Spray 3350
Relpax Tablets 2531
Zomig Nasal Spray 718
Zomig Tablets 714
Zomig-ZMT Tablets 714

Ischemia, unspecified
Imitrex Injection 1431

Ischemic attacks, transient
Amerge Tablets 1312
Frova Tablets 1101
Imitrex Injection 1431
Imitrex Nasal Spray 1435
Imitrex Tablets 1440
Relpax Tablets 2531
Zomig Nasal Spray 718

Ischemic heart disease
(*see under* Heart disease, ischemic)

Ischemic myocardial disease
(*see under* Heart disease, ischemic)

J

Jaundice, cholestatic of pregnancy, history of
Alesse-28 Tablets 3392
Lo/Ovral-28 Tablets 3423
Ortho-Cept Tablets 2395
Ortho-Cyclen Tablets 2414
Ortho Evra Transdermal System 2402
Ortho Tri-Cyclen Tablets 2414
Ortho Tri-Cyclen Lo Tablets 2421
Seasonale Tablets 1073
Triphasil-28 Tablets 3483
Yasmin 28 Tablets 818

Jaundice, history of
Alesse-28 Tablets 3392
Augmentin 1331
Augmentin Tablets 1334
Augmentin XR Extended-Release Tablets 1340
Augmentin ES-600 Powder for Oral Suspension 1337
Lo/Ovral-28 Tablets 3423
Ortho-Cept Tablets 2395
Ortho-Cyclen Tablets 2414
Ortho Evra Transdermal System 2402
Ortho Tri-Cyclen Tablets 2414
Ortho Tri-Cyclen Lo Tablets 2421
Seasonale Tablets 1073
Triphasil-28 Tablets 3483
Yasmin 28 Tablets 818

K

Keratitis, dendritic
(*see under* Herpes simplex keratitis)

Ketoacidosis, diabetic
ActoPlus Met Tablets 3219
Amaryl Tablets 2864
Avandamet Tablets 1343
Prandin Tablets (0.5, 1, and 2 mg) 2337
Precose Tablets 776
Starlix Tablets 2276

Kidney damage
(*see under* Renal dysfunction)

Kidney disease
(*see under* Renal disease, unspecified)

Kidney failure
(*see under* Renal failure)

L

Labor
Dilaudid Oral Liquid 443
Dilaudid Tablets - 8 mg 443
Dilaudid-HP 441

Lactation
(*see under* Breastfeeding)

Left ventricular dysfunction
(*see under* Ventricular dysfunction, left)

Lesions, gastrointestinal, unspecified
(*see also under* Colitis, ulcerative; Colitis, ulcerative, history of; Ulcer, gastrointestinal)
Urecholine Tablets 2349

Lesions, intracranial, unspecified
(*see also under* Tumor, intracranial, unspecified; Tumor, pituitary, unspecified)
Genotropin Lyophilized Powder 2642
Gonal-f RFF Pen for Injection 3155
Hycomine Compound Tablets 1105
Hycotuss Expectorant Syrup 1106
Menopur for Subcutaneous Injection 1145
Repronex for Intramuscular and Subcutaneous Injection 1148
Tev-Tropin for Injection 1224

Lesions, malignant, unspecified
(*see under* Carcinoma, breast, history of; Carcinoma, breast, male; Carcinoma, breast, unspecified; Carcinoma, cervical; Carcinoma, endometrium; Carcinoma, female reproductive organs; Carcinoma, genital, unspecified; Carcinoma, hepatic; Carcinoma, prostate; Carcinoma, skin, unspecified; Carcinoma, squamous cell, unspecified; Melanoma, history of; Melanoma, unspecified; Neoplasm, bone marrow system, malignant; Neoplasm, lymphatic system, malignant)

Lesions, skin, unspecified
(*see also under* Melanoma, unspecified)
Parcopa Orally Disintegrating Tablets 3111
Stalevo Tablets 2270

Lesions, skin, viral
(*see under* Herpes zoster; Varicella)

Leukemia, chronic myelogenous, without definitive diagnosis
Myleran Tablets 1492

Leukemia, unspecified
Attenuvax 1889
Caverject Impulse Injection 2610
Flumist Vaccine 1872
Meruvax II 1994
Miradon Tablets 3056
M-M-R II 1980
Mumpsvax 2005
Varivax 2070

Liver adenoma
(*see under* Adenoma, hepatic)

Liver cancer
(*see under* Carcinoma, hepatic)

Liver damage
(*see under* Liver dysfunction)

Liver disease, decompensated
PEG-Intron Powder for Injection 3062

Liver disease, history of
(*see also under* Liver dysfunction, history of)
Vivelle Transdermal System 2288

Liver disease, unspecified
(*see also under* Cirrhosis, primary biliary; Cirrhosis, unspecified; Hepatitis; Liver dysfunction)
Activella Tablets 2311
Advicor Tablets 1694
Aldoclor Tablets 1881
Aldoril Tablets 1884
Altoprev Extended-Release Tablets 1151
Aygestin Tablets 1062
Caduet Tablets 2507
Cenestin Tablets, 0.45mg, 0.625mg, 0.9mg, 1.25mg 1063
Cenestin Tablets, 0.3mg 1063
Climara Transdermal System 795
Climara Pro Transdermal System 800
Crestor Tablets 672
Dantrium Capsules 2690
Depacon Injection 412
Depakene 417
Depakote Sprinkle Capsules 422
Depakote Tablets 427
Depakote ER Tablets 433
Depo-Provera Contraceptive Injection 2619

depo-subQ provera 104 Injectable Suspension 2622
Dyrenium Capsules 3390
Estratest Tablets 3196
Estratest H.S. Tablets 3196
Estrogel 0.06% 3200
Klonopin 2782
Lescol Capsules 2227
Lescol Capsules 2730
Lescol XL Tablets 2227
Lescol XL Tablets 2730
Lipitor Tablets 2495
Menostar Transdermal System 805
Mevacor Tablets 1996
Mirena Intrauterine System 810
Ortho Micronor Tablets 2411
Pravachol Tablets 943
Prefest Tablets 1069
Premarin Intravenous 3440
Premarin Tablets 3443
Premarin Vaginal Cream 3449
Premphase Tablets 3452
Prempro Tablets 3452
Prochieve 4% Gel 1018
Prochieve 8% Gel 1018
Prometrium Capsules (100 mg, 200 mg) 3205
Seasonale Tablets 1073
Tasmar Tablets 3360
Uroqid-Acid No. 2 Tablets 785
Vivelle Transdermal System 2288
Vivelle-Dot Transdermal System 2293
Vytorin 10/10 Tablets 2084
Vytorin 10/10 Tablets 3092
Vytorin 10/20 Tablets 2084
Vytorin 10/20 Tablets 3092
Vytorin 10/40 Tablets 2084
Vytorin 10/40 Tablets 3092
Vytorin 10/80 Tablets 2084
Vytorin 10/80 Tablets 3092
Ziagen Tablets 1600
Zocor Tablets 2078

Liver disorders, history of
Aldoclor Tablets 1881
Aldoril Tablets 1884
Augmentin 1331
Augmentin ES-600 Powder for Oral Suspension 1337

Liver disorders, unspecified
(*see under* Liver dysfunction)

Liver dysfunction
(*see also under* Jaundice, cholestatic of pregnancy, history of; Jaundice, history of; Liver disease, unspecified; Liver failure; Serum transaminase elevation)
Activella Tablets 2311
Advicor Tablets 1694
Anadrol-50 Tablets 3329
Antara Capsules 2723
Aygestin Tablets 1062
Cenestin Tablets, 0.45mg, 0.625mg, 0.9mg, 1.25mg 1063
Cenestin Tablets, 0.3mg 1063
Climara Transdermal System 795
Climara Pro Transdermal System 800
CombiPatch Transdermal System 2180
Coreg Tablets 1376
Daranide Tablets 1928
Depacon Injection 412
Depakene 417
Depakote Sprinkle Capsules 422
Depakote Tablets 427
Depo-Provera Contraceptive Injection 2619
depo-subQ provera 104 Injectable Suspension 2622
Ellence Injection 2632
Epzicom Tablets 1402
Estratest Tablets 3196
Estratest H.S. Tablets 3196
Estrogel 0.06% 3200
Imitrex Injection 1431
Imitrex Tablets 1440
Lofibra Capsules 1217
Menostar Transdermal System 805
Niaspan Extended-Release Tablets 1703
Peganone Tablets, USP 2487
Prefest Tablets 1069
Premarin Intravenous 3440
Premarin Tablets 3443
Premarin Vaginal Cream 3449
Premphase Tablets 3452
Prempro Tablets 3452
Prochieve 4% Gel 1018
Prochieve 8% Gel 1018
Prometrium Capsules (100 mg, 200 mg) 3205
Relpax Tablets 2531
Skelaxin Tablets 1685
Tasmar Tablets 3360
Ticlid Tablets 2813
Tricor Tablets 523
Trizivir Tablets 1565
Uroxatral Tablets 2957
Vivelle Transdermal System 2288
Vivelle-Dot Transdermal System 2293
Yasmin 28 Tablets 818
Zelnorm Tablets 2303
Ziagen 1600

Liver dysfunction, severe
(*see under* Hepatic impairment, severe)

Liver dysfunction, history of
(*see also under* Liver disease, history of)
Augmentin Tablets 1334
Augmentin XR Extended-Release Tablets 1340
CombiPatch Transdermal System 2180

Liver failure
(*see also under* Coma, hepatic; Liver dysfunction)
Agenerase Capsules 1299
Agenerase Oral Solution 1304
Grifulvin V Tablets Microsize and Oral Suspension Microsize 2384
Gris-PEG Tablets 2504
Soriatane Capsules 1028

Liver function tests, abnormal
(*see under* Serum transaminase elevation)

Liver insufficiency
(*see under* Liver dysfunction)

Liver tumor
(*see under* Adenoma, hepatic; Carcinoma, hepatic; Tumor, liver, benign)

Local anesthesia
(*see under* Anesthesia, local)

Lown-Ganong-Levine syndrome
Covera-HS Tablets 3135
Tarka Tablets 519
Verelan PM Capsules 3120

Lung disease, unspecified
(*see under* Pulmonary disorders, unspecified)

Lupus erythematosus
Oxsoralen Lotion 1% 3354
Oxsoralen-Ultra Capsules 3354

Lymphoma
(*see also under* Neoplasm, lymphatic system, malignant)
Attenuvax 1889
Flumist Vaccine 1872
Meruvax II 1994
M-M-R II 1980
Mumpsvax 2005
Varivax 2070

M

Malabsorption syndrome
Xenical Capsules 2834

Malignancies, unspecified
Gengraf Capsules 458
Neoral Soft Gelatin Capsules 2247
Neoral Oral Solution 2247

Malignancy
(*see under* Carcinoma, breast, history of; Carcinoma, breast, male; Carcinoma, breast, unspecified; Carcinoma, endometrium; Carcinoma, hepatic; Carcinoma, prostate; Carcinoma, skin, unspecified; Hypertension, malignant; Hyperthermia, malignant, history of; Leukemia, unspecified; Lymphoma; Malignancy, generalized; Melanoma, history of; Melanoma, unspecified; Neoplasm, bone marrow system, malignant; Neoplasm, lymphatic system, malignant)

Malignancy, generalized
Flumist Vaccine 1872

Malnutrition
Miradon Tablets 3056

Mechanical disorders of ventilation
(*see under* Asthma, acute; Asthma, history of; Asthma, unspecified; Obstruction, respiratory tract)

Megacolon, toxic
Colyte with Flavor Packs for Oral Solution 3102
HalfLytely and Bisacodyl Tablets Bowel Prep Kit with Flavors Packs 915
Lotronex Tablets 1479
TriLyte with Flavor Packs for Oral Solution 3114

Megaloblastic anemia
(*see under* Anemia, megaloblastic, unspecified)

Melanoma, history of
Oxsoralen Lotion 1% 3354
Oxsoralen-Ultra Capsules 3354
Parcopa Orally Disintegrating Tablets 3111
Stalevo Tablets 2270

Melanoma, unspecified
Oxsoralen Lotion 1% 3354
Oxsoralen-Ultra Capsules 3354

Mental depression
(*see under* Depression, mental)

Metabolic acidosis
(*see under* Acidosis, hyperchloremic; Acidosis, metabolic, unspecified; Ketoacidosis, diabetic)

Migraine, basilar
Amerge Tablets 1312
Axert Tablets 2430
Frova Tablets 1101
Imitrex Injection 1431
Imitrex Nasal Spray 1435
Imitrex Tablets 1440
Maxalt Tablets 1983
Maxalt-MLT Orally Disintegrating Tablets 1983
Migranal Nasal Spray 3350
Relpax Tablets 2531
Zomig Nasal Spray 718
Zomig Tablets 714
Zomig-ZMT Tablets 714

Migraine, hemiplegic
Amerge Tablets 1312
Axert Tablets 2430
Frova Tablets 1101
Imitrex Injection 1431
Imitrex Nasal Spray 1435
Imitrex Tablets 1440
Maxalt Tablets 1983
Maxalt-MLT Orally Disintegrating Tablets 1983
Migranal Nasal Spray 3350
Relpax Tablets 2531
Zomig Nasal Spray 718
Zomig Tablets 714
Zomig-ZMT Tablets 714

Multipara, unspecified
Cervidil Vaginal Insert 1182

Myasthenia gravis
Bentyl Capsules 724
Bentyl Injection 724
Bentyl Syrup 724
Bentyl Tablets 724
Norflex Injection 1824

Mycobacterial infection
(*see under* Infection, ophthalmic, mycobacterial; Tuberculosis, unspecified)

Mycobacterial infections, ophthalmic
Retisert Implant ⊙256

Myeloid blasts, leukemic
Leukine 829

Myeloma, multiple
Caverject Impulse Injection 2610

Myeloproliferative disorders
(*see also under* Leukemia, unspecified; Myeloma, multiple)
Clozapine Tablets 2141
Clozaril Tablets 2174
FazaClo Orally Disintegrating Tablets 547

Myelosuppression
(*see under* Bone marrow depression)

Myocardial damage
(*see under* Cardiovascular disorders, unspecified)

Myocardial disease
(*see under* Cardiovascular disorders, unspecified)

Myocardial infarction
Cardizem LA Extended Release Tablets 1699
Cytomel Tablets 1678
Ellence Injection 2632
Estratest Tablets 3196
Estratest H.S. Tablets 3196
Flexeril Tablets 1832
Geodon 2514
Inversine Tablets 3286
Levothroid Tablets 1189
Levoxyl Tablets 1680
Prefest Tablets 1069
Premphase Tablets 3452
Prempro Tablets 3452
Prometrium Capsules (100 mg, 200 mg) 3205
Surmontil Capsules 2347
Tiazac Capsules 1204
Vivactil Tablets 2350

Myocardial infarction, history of
Amerge Tablets 1312
Axert Tablets 2430
Estratest Tablets 3196
Estratest H.S. Tablets 3196
Frova Tablets 1101
Imitrex Injection 1431
Imitrex Nasal Spray 1435
Imitrex Tablets 1440
Maxalt Tablets 1983
Maxalt-MLT Orally Disintegrating Tablets 1983
Migranal Nasal Spray 3350
Prefest Tablets 1069
Proleukin for Injection 1007
Prometrium Capsules (100 mg, 200 mg) 3205
Relpax Tablets 2531
Zomig Nasal Spray 718
Zomig Tablets 714
Zomig-ZMT Tablets 714

Myocardial insufficiency, severe
Ellence Injection 2632

N

Narrow angle glaucoma
(*see under* Glaucoma, angle closure)

Narrow angles
Propine Ophthalmic Solution .... ⊙ 237

Necrosis
(*see also under* Enterocolitis, necrotizing)
Urocit-K Tablets 2109

Neonates
(*see also under* Infants)
Ovide .5% Lotion 3287
Pegasys 2793

Neonates, premature
(*see under* Infants, premature)

Neoplasia, unspecified
Increlex Injection 3290
Norditropin Cartridges 2318

Neoplasia, estrogen dependent
(*see under* Neoplasm, estrogen dependent)

Neoplasia, hepatic
(*see under* Adenoma, hepatic; Carcinoma, hepatic; Tumor, liver, benign)

Neoplasia, unspecified
(*see under* Neoplasm, unspecified)

Neoplasm, androgen dependent
(*see also under* Carcinoma, prostate)
Novarel for Injection 1147

Neoplasm, bone marrow system, malignant
(*see also under* Myeloid blasts, leukemic; Myeloma, multiple)
Attenuvax 1889
Meruvax II 1994
M-M-R II 1980
Mumpsvax 2005
Varivax 2070

Neoplasm, estrogen dependent
(*see also under* Carcinoma, breast, male; Carcinoma, breast, unspecified)
Activella Tablets 2311
Alesse-28 Tablets 3392
Cenestin Tablets, 0.45mg, 0.625mg, 0.9mg, 1.25mg 1063
Cenestin Tablets, 0.3mg 1063
Climara Transdermal System 795
Climara Pro Transdermal System 800
CombiPatch Transdermal System 2180
Estratest Tablets 3196
Estratest H.S. Tablets 3196
Estrogel 0.06% 3200
Lo/Ovral-28 Tablets 3423
Menostar Transdermal System 805
Ortho-Cept Tablets 2395
Ortho-Cyclen Tablets 2414
Ortho Evra Transdermal System 2402
Ortho Tri-Cyclen Tablets 2414
Ortho Tri-Cyclen Lo Tablets 2421
Prefest Tablets 1069
Premarin Intravenous 3440
Premarin Tablets 3443
Premarin Vaginal Cream 3449
Premphase Tablets 3452
Prempro Tablets 3452
Triphasil-28 Tablets 3483
Vagifem Tablets 2340
Vivelle Transdermal System 2288
Vivelle-Dot Transdermal System 2293
Yasmin 28 Tablets 818

Neoplasm, estrogen dependent, history of
(*see under* Carcinoma, breast, history of)

Neoplasm, hepatic, unspecified
(*see under* Adenoma, hepatic; Carcinoma, hepatic; Tumor, liver, benign)

Neoplasm, intracranial
(*see under* Tumor, intracranial, unspecified)

Neoplasm, lymphatic system, malignant
(*see also under* Lymphoma)
Attenuvax 1889
Meruvax II 1994
M-M-R II 1980
Mumpsvax 2005
Varivax 2070

Neoplasm, ovarian
(*see under* Cysts, ovarian)

Neoplasm, unspecified
Nutropin for Injection 1238
Nutropin AQ Injection 1241
Nutropin AQ Pen 1241
Nutropin AQ Pen Cartridge 1241

Neoplastic activity, unspecified
(*see under* Neoplasm, unspecified; Tumor activity, unspecified)

Nephritis
Anadrol-50 Tablets 3329

Nephropathy, diabetic
Midamor Tablets 2000
Moduretic Tablets 2003

Nephrosis
Anadrol-50 Tablets 3329
Oxandrin Tablets 2977

Neurologic toxicity
(*see under* Toxicity, neurologic)

Neurological disorders, unspecified
(*see also under* Central nervous system depression; Cerebral vascular disease; Cerebral vascular disease, history of; Cerebrovascular accident; Cerebrovascular accident, history of; Depression, mental; Encephalopathy, history of; Epilepsy; Epilepsy, uncontrolled; Guillain-Barre syndrome, history of; Intracranial pressure, increased; Myasthenia gravis; Parkinsonism; Psychosis; Psychosis, toxic, history of; Psychosis, unsupervised; Seizure disorders, history of; Seizure disorders, unspecified; Senility, unsupervised; Tourette's syndrome; Toxicity, neurologic; Vagotonia)
Adacel Vaccine 2959
Boostrix 1366
Infanrix Vaccine 1444
Pediarix Vaccine 1518

Neutropenia
Taxotere Injection Concentrate 2947
Ticlid Tablets 2813

Neutrophil count, baseline, less than 1500 cells/mm3
Ellence Injection 2632

Nursing mothers
(*see under* Breastfeeding)

O

Obesity, therapy of
Synthroid Tablets 515

Obstetrics
(*see under* Delivery, unspecified; Labor)

Obstruction, biliary tract
(*see under* Jaundice, cholestatic of pregnancy, history of; Jaundice, history of)

Obstruction, bladder neck
(*see also under* Obstruction, urinary tract)
Norflex Injection 1824
Urecholine Tablets 2349

Obstruction, gastrointestinal tract
(*see also under* Achalasia, esophageal; Bowel ischemia, history of; Fecal impaction; Ileus, paralytic; Ileus, unspecified; Stenosis, pyloric; Stenosis, pyloroduodenal; Stricture, esophageal)
Bentyl Capsules 724
Bentyl Injection 724
Bentyl Syrup 724
Bentyl Tablets 724
Citrucel Orange Flavor Powder .... ▣ 613
Citrucel Sugar Free Orange Flavor Powder .... ▣ 613
Colyte with Flavor Packs for Oral Solution 3102
Ditropan XL Extended Release Tablets 2391
Dulcolax Suppositories .... ▣ 608
HalfLytely and Bisacodyl Tablets Bowel Prep Kit with Flavors Packs 915
Lotronex Tablets 1479
Norflex Injection 1824
Precose Tablets 776
Renagel Tablets 1268
TriLyte with Flavor Packs for Oral Solution 3114
Urecholine Tablets 2349
Zelnorm Tablets 2303

Obstruction, pulmonary
Daranide Tablets 1928

Obstruction, respiratory tract
(*see also under* Obstruction, pulmonary)
Daranide Tablets 1928
DepoDur Extended-Release Injection 1098

Obstruction, urinary tract
(*see also under* Obstruction, bladder neck; Prostatic hypertrophy; Urinary retention)
Bentyl Capsules 724
Bentyl Injection 724
Bentyl Syrup 724
Bentyl Tablets 724
Urecholine Tablets 2349

Obstruction, urogenital tract
(*see under* Obstruction, urinary tract)

Obstructive uropathy
(*see under* Obstruction, urinary tract)

Occlusion, coronary
(*see under* Coronary occlusion)

Ocular herpes simplex
(*see under* Herpes simplex keratitis)

Oliguria
Edecrin 1941

Opioid intolerance
Duragesic Transdermal System 2448

Organ allograft
Proleukin for Injection 1007

Organic heart disease
(*see under* Cardiovascular disorders, unspecified; Heart disease, ischemic)

Ovarian enlargement, unspecified
Repronex for Intramuscular and Subcutaneous Injection 1148

Ovarian failure, primary
Bravelle for Intramuscular or Subcutaneous Injection 1140
Follistim AQ Cartridge 2354
Repronex for Intramuscular and Subcutaneous Injection 1148

Overt cardiac failure
(*see under* Heart failure, unspecified)

P

Pain, peri-operative, associated with coronary artery bypass graft surgery
Celebrex Capsules 3130
Indocin 1968

Pain, peri-operative, coronary artery bypass graft surgery
Clinoril Tablets 1899
Dolobid Tablets 1937
Mobic Oral Suspension 893
Mobic Tablets 893

Pain, acute
Actiq 993
Duragesic Transdermal System 2448

Pain, intermittent
Actiq 993
Duragesic Transdermal System 2448

Pain, mild
Actiq 993
Duragesic Transdermal System 2448

Pain, post operative
Actiq 993
Duragesic Transdermal System 2448

Pancreatic diseases, unspecified
Ultrase Capsules 735
Ultrase MT Capsules 736

Pancreatitis
Creon 5 Capsules 3195
Creon 10 Capsules 3195
Creon 20 Capsules 3196
Elspar for Injection 1943
Oncaspar 1123
Ultrase Capsules 735
Ultrase MT Capsules 736

Pancreatitis, history of
Elspar for Injection 1943
Oncaspar 1123

Paralytic ileus
(*see under* Ileus, paralytic)

Parkinsonism
Urecholine Tablets 2349

Parkinson's disease
(*see under* Parkinsonism)

Pediatric patients less than 2 years of age
Phenergan 3438

Pelvic inflammatory disease
Mirena Intrauterine System 810

Penile deformation
(*see under* Angulation, penile; Fibrosis, cavernosal; Peyronie's disease)

Peptic ulcer
(*see under* Ulcer, peptic)

Perforation, gastrointestinal tract
(*see also under* Ulcer, gastrointestinal)
Colyte with Flavor Packs for Oral Solution 3102
HalfLytely and Bisacodyl Tablets Bowel Prep Kit with Flavors Packs 915
TriLyte with Flavor Packs for Oral Solution 3114

Perforation, gastrointestinal tract, history of
Lotronex Tablets 1479
Proleukin for Injection 1007

Perforation, intestinal
(*see under* Perforation, gastrointestinal tract)

Pericardial effusion
Coumadin for Injection 932
Coumadin Tablets 932

Pericardial tamponade, history of
Proleukin for Injection 1007

Pericarditis, acute
Aggrastat 1878

Pericarditis, unspecified
Coumadin for Injection 932
Coumadin Tablets 932
Miradon Tablets 3056

Peripheral arterial disease
(*see under* Peripheral vascular disease)

Peripheral vascular disease
(*see also under* Arteriosclerosis, unspecified; Thrombophlebitis)
Amerge Tablets 1312
Frova Tablets 1101
Imitrex Injection 1431
Imitrex Nasal Spray 1435
Imitrex Tablets 1440
Relpax Tablets 2531

Peripheral vascular insufficiency
(*see under* Peripheral vascular disease)

Peritonitis
Urecholine Tablets 2349

Peyronie's disease
Caverject Impulse Injection 2610
Edex Injection 3103

Pheochromocytoma
GlucaGen for Injection 790
Glucagon for Injection Vials and Emergency Kit 1749
Parnate Tablets 1499
ProAmatine Tablets 3183

Phlebitis
(*see under* Thrombophlebitis)

Phosphate stones, infected
K-Phos Neutral Tablets 785
K-Phos Original (Sodium Free) Tablets 785

Photosensitivity diseases, unspecified
(*see also under* Albinism; Lupus erythematosus; Porphyria cutanea tarda; Porphyria, erythropoietic; Porphyria, unspecified; Xeroderma pigmentosum)
Oxsoralen Lotion 1% 3354
Oxsoralen-Ultra Capsules 3354

Pituitary function, normal, male
Repronex for Intramuscular and Subcutaneous Injection 1148

Poly-arthritis
Miradon Tablets 3056

Polycythemia
Miradon Tablets 3056

Poor nutritional state
(*see under* Electrolyte imbalance, uncorrected; Malnutrition)

Porphyria cutanea tarda
Oxsoralen-Ultra Capsules 3354

Porphyria, erythropoietic
Oxsoralen-Ultra Capsules 3354

Porphyria, unspecified
Grifulvin V Tablets Microsize and Oral Suspension Microsize 2384
Gris-PEG Tablets 2504
Nembutal Sodium Solution, USP 2484
Oxsoralen Lotion 1% 3354
Photofrin for Injection 729
Vagifem Tablets 2340
Visudyne for Injection 2286

Porphyria, variegate
Oxsoralen-Ultra Capsules 3354

Prader-Willi Syndrome
Norditropin Cartridges 2318
Nutropin for Injection 1238
Nutropin AQ Injection 1241
Nutropin AQ Pen 1241
Nutropin AQ Pen Cartridge 1241
Tev-Tropin for Injection 1224

Precocious puberty
Novarel for Injection 1147

Preeclampsia
Coumadin for Injection 932
Coumadin Tablets 932
Miradon Tablets 3056

Pregnancy
Accutane Capsules 2740
Activella Tablets 2311
Advicor Tablets 1694
Agenerase Capsules 1299
Agenerase Oral Solution 1304
Alesse-28 Tablets 3392
Altoprev Extended-Release Tablets 1151
Amnesteem Capsules 2126
Anadrol-50 Tablets 3329
Arava Tablets 2881
Arthrotec Tablets 3126
Attenuvax 1889
Aygestin Tablets 1062
Bravelle for Intramuscular or Subcutaneous Injection 1140
Caduet Tablets 2507
Carac Cream, 0.5% 1048
Casodex Tablets 670
Cenestin Tablets, 0.45mg, 0.625mg, 0.9mg, 1.25mg 1063
Cenestin Tablets, 0.3mg 1063
Climara Transdermal System 795
Climara Pro Transdermal System 800
CombiPatch Transdermal System 2180
Copegus Tablets 2759
Coumadin for Injection 932
Coumadin Tablets 932
Crestor Tablets 672
Cuprimine Capsules 1925
Dalmane Capsules 3343
Delatestryl Injection 2976
Depo-Provera Contraceptive Injection 2619
depo-subQ provera 104 Injectable Suspension 2622
Efudex 3348
Eligard 7.5 mg 2896
Eligard 22.5 mg 2899
Eligard 30 mg 2901
Eligard 45 mg 2904
Estratest Tablets 3196
Estratest H.S. Tablets 3196
Estrogel 0.06% 3200
Evista Tablets 1735
Faslodex Injection 682
Follistim AQ Cartridge 2354
Gonal-f RFF Pen for Injection 3155
Grifulvin V Tablets Microsize and Oral Suspension Microsize 2384
Gris-PEG Tablets 2504
Hycamtin for Injection 1427
Lescol Capsules 2227
Lescol Capsules 2730
Lescol XL Tablets 2227
Lescol XL Tablets 2730
Lipitor Tablets 2495
Lo/Ovral-28 Tablets 3423
Lupron Depot 3.75 mg 3257
Lupron Depot 7.5 mg 3261
Lupron Depot–3 Month 11.25 mg 3262
Lupron Depot-PED 7.5 mg, 11.25 mg and 15 mg 3266
Lupron Injection Pediatric 3256
Menopur for Subcutaneous Injection 1145
Menostar Transdermal System 805
Meruvax II 1994
Mevacor Tablets 1996
Migranal Nasal Spray 3350
Mineral Oil 2716
Miradon Tablets 3056
Mirena Intrauterine System 810
M-M-R II 1980
Mumpsvax 2005
Ortho-Cept Tablets 2395
Ortho-Cyclen Tablets 2414
Ortho Evra Transdermal System 2402
Ortho Micronor Tablets 2411
Ortho Tri-Cyclen Tablets 2414
Ortho Tri-Cyclen Lo Tablets 2421
Orthoclone OKT3 Sterile Solution 2370
Oxandrin Tablets 2977
Plan B Tablets 1068
Pravachol Tablets 943
Prefest Tablets 1069
Premarin Intravenous 3440
Premarin Tablets 3443
Premarin Vaginal Cream 3449
Premphase Tablets 3452
Prempro Tablets 3452
Prometrium Capsules (100 mg, 200 mg) 3205
Propecia Tablets 2036
Proscar Tablets 2040
ProSom Tablets 512
Rebetol 3073
Rebetron Combination Therapy 3078
Repronex for Intramuscular and Subcutaneous Injection 1148
Ribavirin, USP Capsules 3083
Seasonale Tablets 1073
Soriatane Capsules 1028
Targretin Capsules 1719
Testim 1% Gel 722
Thalomid Capsules 979
Tindamax 2670
Tracleer Tablets 539
Travatan Ophthalmic Solution 559
Triphasil-28 Tablets 3483
Vagifem Tablets 2340
Varivax 2070
Virazole for Inhalation Solution 3365
Vivelle Transdermal System 2288
Vivelle-Dot Transdermal System 2293
Vytorin 10/10 Tablets 2084
Vytorin 10/10 Tablets 3092
Vytorin 10/20 Tablets 2084
Vytorin 10/20 Tablets 3092
Vytorin 10/40 Tablets 2084
Vytorin 10/40 Tablets 3092
Vytorin 10/80 Tablets 2084
Vytorin 10/80 Tablets 3092
Yasmin 28 Tablets 818
Zavesca Capsules 543
Zocor Tablets 2078
Zoladex 709
Zoladex 3-month 712

Pregnancy, diagnostic test for
Aygestin Tablets 1062
Prometrium Capsules (100 mg, 200 mg) 3205

Previous treatment with anthracyclines up to maximum cumulative dose
Ellence Injection 2632

Priapism, predisposition to
Edex Injection 3103

Proctitis, history of
Indocin Suppositories 1968

Prolactinoma, pituitary
(*see under* Tumor, intracranial, unspecified)

Prostate enlargement
(*see under* Prostatic hypertrophy)

Prostatic hypertrophy
Norflex Injection 1824

Protoporphyria
(*see under* Porphyria, erythropoietic)

Psoriasis, acute
Dovonex Scalp Solution 0.005% 3375
Psoriatec Cream 3191

Psoriatic eruptions, acute
(*see under* Psoriasis, acute)

Psychic disturbances
(*see under* Psychosis)

Psychosis
Antabuse Tablets 2343
Seromycin Capsules 1783

Psychosis, toxic, history of
Proleukin for Injection 1007

Psychosis, unsupervised
Coumadin for Injection 932
Coumadin Tablets 932

Pulmonary atresia
(*see under* Atresia, pulmonary)

Pulmonary congestion
Cardizem LA Extended Release Tablets 1699
Tiazac Capsules 1204

Pulmonary disorders, unspecified
(*see also under* Asthma, acute; Asthma, unspecified; Atresia, pulmonary; Chronic obstructive pulmonary disease; Hypertension, pulmonary; Obstruction, pulmonary; Pulmonary congestion; Pulmonary function test, abnormal; Respiratory tract conditions, lower; Tuberculosis, unspecified)
Adenoscan 613

Pulmonary embolism
Cenestin Tablets, 0.45mg, 0.625mg, 0.9mg, 1.25mg 1063
Cenestin Tablets, 0.3mg 1063
Climara Transdermal System 795
Climara Pro Transdermal System 800
Estratest Tablets 3196
Estratest H.S. Tablets 3196
Estrogel 0.06% 3200
Evista Tablets 1735
Menostar Transdermal System 805
Prefest Tablets 1069
Premarin Intravenous 3440
Premarin Tablets 3443
Premarin Vaginal Cream 3449
Premphase Tablets 3452
Prempro Tablets 3452
Prometrium Capsules (100 mg, 200 mg) 3205
Vivelle Transdermal System 2288
Vivelle-Dot Transdermal System 2293

Pulmonary embolism, history of
Climara Transdermal System 795
Climara Pro Transdermal System 800
Estratest Tablets 3196
Estratest H.S. Tablets 3196
Estrogel 0.06% 3200
Menostar Transdermal System 805
Prefest Tablets 1069
Premarin Intravenous 3440
Premarin Tablets 3443
Premarin Vaginal Cream 3449
Premphase Tablets 3452
Prempro Tablets 3452
Prometrium Capsules (100 mg, 200 mg) 3205
Vivelle Transdermal System 2288
Vivelle-Dot Transdermal System 2293

Pulmonary function test, abnormal
Proleukin for Injection 1007

Pulmonary hypertension
(*see under* Hypertension, pulmonary)

Pyloroduodenal stenosis
(*see under* Stenosis, pyloroduodenal)

Q

Q-T interval prolongation
Geodon 2514
Orap Tablets 1220

R

Radiation therapy
Flumist Vaccine 1872
Leukine 829
Neoral Soft Gelatin Capsules 2247
Neoral Oral Solution 2247

Radiotherapy
(*see under* Radiation therapy)

Rectal bleeding
(*see under* Bleeding, rectal)

Renal decompensation
(*see under* Renal failure)

Renal dialysis
Augmentin XR Extended-Release Tablets 1340
Integrilin Injection 3034

Renal disease, unspecified
(*see also under* Nephritis; Nephropathy, diabetic; Nephrosis; Renal dysfunction)
ActoPlus Met Tablets 3219
Avandamet Tablets 1343
Avar Cleanser 3189
Avar Gel 3189
Avar Green 3189
Avar-e Emollient Cream 3189
Avar-e Green Cream 3189
Calcium Disodium Versenate Injection 1819
Desferal Vials 2190
Dyrenium Capsules 3390
Fortamet Extended-Release Tablets 1156
Paser Granules 1657
ProAmatine Tablets 3183
Rosac Cream with Sunscreens 3216

Renal dysfunction
(*see also under* Anuria; Oliguria; Renal disease, unspecified; Renal failure; Uremia)
ActoPlus Met Tablets 3219
Augmentin XR Extended-Release Tablets 1340
Avandamet Tablets 1343
Cuprimine Capsules 1925
Dyazide Capsules 1389
Dyrenium Capsules 3390
Fortamet Extended-Release Tablets 1156
Gengraf Capsules 458
Indocin I.V. 1973
Inspra Tablets 2520
Integrilin Injection 3034
Inversine Tablets 3286
K-Phos Neutral Tablets 785
K-Phos Original (Sodium Free) Tablets 785
Lofibra Capsules 1217
Maxzide 2150
Midamor Tablets 2000
Moduretic Tablets 2003
Nalfon Capsules 2504
Neoral Soft Gelatin Capsules 2247
Neoral Oral Solution 2247
Plasbumin-5 3249
Plasbumin-20 3249
Plasbumin-25 3251
Seromycin Capsules 1783
Skelaxin Tablets 1685
Tricor Tablets 523
Uroqid-Acid No. 2 Tablets 785
Xeloda Tablets 2825
Yasmin 28 Tablets 818
Zelnorm Tablets 2303

Renal dysfunction, severe
Malarone Tablets 1484
Malarone Pediatric Tablets 1484
Miradon Tablets 3056
Triglide Tablets 1165

Renal dysfunction, history of
Cuprimine Capsules 1925
Proleukin for Injection 1007

Renal excretory function impairment
(*see under* Renal dysfunction)

Renal failure
(*see also under* Renal dysfunction)
Agenerase Capsules 1299
Agenerase Oral Solution 1304
Daranide Tablets 1928
Maxzide 2150
Soriatane Capsules 1028
Urocit-K Tablets 2109

Renal impairment
(*see under* Renal dysfunction)

Renal insufficiency
(*see under* Renal dysfunction)

Respiratory depression
Avinza Capsules 1714
Combunox Tablets 1183
DepoDur Extended-Release Injection 1098
Dilaudid 439
Dilaudid Oral Liquid 443
Dilaudid Non-Sterile Powder 439
Dilaudid Rectal Suppositories 439
Dilaudid Tablets 439
Dilaudid Tablets - 8 mg 443
Dilaudid-HP 441
Duragesic Transdermal System 2448
Hycomine Compound Tablets 1105
Hycotuss Expectorant Syrup 1106
Kadian Capsules 572
MS Contin Tablets 2703
OxyContin Tablets 2699
OxyFast Oral Concentrate Solution 2704
OxyIR Capsules 2704

Respiratory depression, history of
Mivacron Injection 489

Respiratory disease, unspecified
(*see under* Respiratory illness, febrile; Respiratory illness, unspecified)

Respiratory disorders
(*see under* Bronchospastic disorders, unspecified; Obstruction, respiratory tract; Pulmonary disorders, unspecified; Respiratory depression; Respiratory illness, unspecified; Respiratory tract conditions, lower)

Respiratory distress
(*see under* Asthma, acute; Respiratory depression)

Respiratory distress, acute, caused by obstructing endobronchial lesion
Photofrin for Injection 729

Respiratory failure
Norditropin Cartridges 2318

Respiratory illness, febrile
Attenuvax 1889
Meruvax II 1994
M-M-R II 1980
Mumpsvax 2005
Varivax 2070

Respiratory illness, unspecified
(*see also under* Pulmonary disorders, unspecified; Respiratory illness, febrile)
Adenoscan 613

Respiratory insufficiency, unspecified
(*see under* Obstruction, respiratory tract; Pulmonary disorders, unspecified; Respiratory illness, febrile; Respiratory illness, unspecified)

Respiratory obstruction
(*see under* Obstruction, respiratory tract)

Respiratory tract conditions, lower
(*see also under* Pulmonary disorders, unspecified)
Phenergan 3438

Retinopathy, diabetic
Norditropin Cartridges 2318

Rhabdomyolsis, non-traumatic, history of
Tasmar Tablets 3360

S

Seizure disorders, history of
Orthoclone OKT3 Sterile Solution 2370
Proleukin for Injection 1007

Seizure disorders, unspecified
(*see also under* Epilepsy; Epilepsy, uncontrolled)
Wellbutrin Tablets 1579
Wellbutrin SR Sustained-Release Tablets 1583
Wellbutrin XL Extended-Release Tablets 1588
Zyban Sustained-Release Tablets 1620

Seizure disorders, untreated
(*see under* Epilepsy, uncontrolled)

Seizures, history of
(*see under* Seizure disorders, history of)

Senility, unsupervised
Coumadin for Injection 932
Coumadin Tablets 932

Serum creatinine, elevated
Inspra Tablets 2520

Serum transaminase elevation
(*see also under* Liver dysfunction)
Advicor Tablets 1694
Altoprev Extended-Release Tablets 1151
Caduet Tablets 2507
Crestor Tablets 672
Lescol Capsules 2227
Lescol Capsules 2730
Lescol XL Tablets 2227
Lescol XL Tablets 2730
Lipitor Tablets 2495
Mevacor Tablets 1996
Pravachol Tablets 943
Vytorin 10/10 Tablets 2084
Vytorin 10/10 Tablets 3092
Vytorin 10/20 Tablets 2084
Vytorin 10/20 Tablets 3092
Vytorin 10/40 Tablets 2084
Vytorin 10/40 Tablets 3092
Vytorin 10/80 Tablets 2084
Vytorin 10/80 Tablets 3092
Zocor Tablets 2078

Severe left ventricular dysfunction
(*see under* Ventricular dysfunction, left)

Shingles
(*see under* Herpes zoster)

Shock, circulatory
DepoDur Extended-Release Injection 1098

Shock, cardiogenic
(*see under* Cardiogenic shock)

Shock, unspecified
(*see also under* Cardiogenic shock)
Primaxin I.M. 2022
Thiothixene Capsules 2124

Sick sinus node syndrome
(*see under* Sick sinus syndrome)

Sick sinus syndrome
Adenocard Injection 612
Adenoscan 613
Cardizem LA Extended Release Tablets 1699
Coreg Tablets 1376
Covera-HS Tablets 3135
Rythmol SR Capsules 2736
Tarka Tablets 519
Tiazac Capsules 1204
Toprol-XL Tablets 660
Verelan PM Capsules 3120

Sickle cell anemia
(*see under* Anemia, sickle cell)

Sino-atrial block
(*see under* Heart block, greater than first degree; Heart block, unspecified)

Sinus node disease
(*see under* Bradycardia, sinus; Sick sinus syndrome; Sinus node dysfunction, unspecified)

Sinus node dysfunction, unspecified
Adenoscan 613
Pacerone Tablets 3337

Skin disorders, unspecified
(*see under* Lesions, skin, unspecified; Melanoma, history of; Melanoma, unspecified; Psoriasis, acute; Skin, denuded; Xeroderma pigmentosum)

Skin lesions
(*see under* Lesions, skin, unspecified)

Skin, denuded
ThermaCare Heat Wraps 2674

Smoking, heavy
Yasmin 28 Tablets 818

Sodium depletion
(*see under* Hyponatremia)

Spasms, gastrointestinal
Urecholine Tablets 2349

Spasms, infantile, history of
Infanrix Vaccine 1444
Pediarix Vaccine 1518

Sphincter of Oddi dysfunction
Zelnorm Tablets 2303

Spinal puncture
Coumadin for Injection 932
Coumadin Tablets 932

Status asthmaticus
Advair Diskus 100/50 1291
Advair Diskus 250/50 1291
Advair Diskus 500/50 1291
Aerobid/Aerobid-M 1172
Asmanex Twisthaler 2981
Azmacort Inhalation Aerosol 1701
Dilaudid 439
Dilaudid Oral Liquid 443
Dilaudid Non-Sterile Powder 439
Dilaudid Rectal Suppositories 439
Dilaudid Tablets 439
Dilaudid Tablets - 8 mg 443
Dilaudid-HP 441
Flovent HFA 1418
Pulmicort Respules 654
Qvar Inhalation Aerosol 1654

Stenosis, aortic
Cardene I.V. 1129
Indocin I.V. 1973
Inversine Tablets 3286

Stenosis, pyloric
(*see also under* Stenosis, pyloroduodenal)
Inversine Tablets 3286

Stenosis, pyloroduodenal
Norflex Injection 1824

Stress test, abnormal
Proleukin for Injection....1007

Stricture, esophageal
Fosamax....1949
Fosamax Plus D Tablets....1956

Stroke
(*see under* Cerebrovascular accident)

Stroke, hemorrhagic
Aggrastat....1878
Xigris Powder for Intravenous Infusion....1796

Stroke, history of
(*see under* Cerebrovascular accident, history of)

Superficial herpes simplex keratitis
(*see under* Herpes simplex keratitis)

Surgery, major, with prolonged immobilization
Alesse-28 Tablets....3392
Lo/Ovral-28 Tablets....3423
Ortho-Cept Tablets....2395
Ortho Evra Transdermal System....2402
Ortho Tri-Cyclen Lo Tablets....2421
Seasonale Tablets....1073

Surgery, abdominal
(*see also under* Surgery, gastrointestinal)
Dulcolax Suppositories....▣608

Surgery, bladder
Urecholine Tablets....2349

Surgery, central nervous system
(*see also under* Surgery, intracranial; Surgery, intraspinal)
Coumadin for Injection....932
Coumadin Tablets....932
Miradon Tablets....3056

Surgery, elective
Parnate Tablets....1499

Surgery, gastrointestinal
Urecholine Tablets....2349

Surgery, intracranial
Activase I.V....1225
Retavase....1131
TNKase I.V....1256
Xigris Powder for Intravenous Infusion....1796

Surgery, intraspinal
Activase I.V....1225
Miradon Tablets....3056
Retavase....1131
Xigris Powder for Intravenous Infusion....1796

Surgery, ophthalmic
Coumadin for Injection....932
Coumadin Tablets....932
Miradon Tablets....3056

Surgery, traumatic
Coumadin for Injection....932
Coumadin Tablets....932
Miradon Tablets....3056

Surgery, unspecified
Integrilin Injection....3034
ReoPro Vials....1779

Surgery, uterine, history of
(*see also under* Cesarean section, history of)
Cervidil Vaginal Insert....1182

Surgical abdomen
(*see under* Surgery, abdominal)

Syncope
Pacerone Tablets....3337

Systemic lupus erythematosus
(*see under* Lupus erythematosus)

Systolic blood pressure less than 90 mm Hg
Natrecor for Injection....3123

T

Tachyarrhythmia
(*see under* Arrhythmia, cardiac, unspecified; Tachycardia, unspecified)

Tachycardia, unspecified
Alupent Inhalation Aerosol....858

Tachycardia, ventricular, history of
Proleukin for Injection....1007

Tendinitis, history of
Noroxin Tablets....2009

Tendon rupture, history of
Noroxin Tablets....2009

Tension
Concerta Extended-Release Tablets....1828
Focalin Tablets....2214
Focalin XR Capsules....2217
Metadate CD Capsules....3316
Ritalin Hydrochloride Tablets....2254
Ritalin LA Capsules....2255
Ritalin-SR Tablets....2254

Testicular failure, primary
Repronex for Intramuscular and Subcutaneous Injection....1148

Tetralogy of Fallot
Indocin I.V....1973

Thallium stress test, abnormal
(*see under* Stress test, abnormal)

Thrombocytopathy, unspecified
(*see under* Thrombocytopenia, unspecified)

Thrombocytopenia, unspecified
Aggrastat....1878
Arixtra Injection....1325
Fragmin Injection....2638
Indocin I.V....1973
Integrilin Injection....3034
Lovenox Injection....2931
ReoPro Vials....1779
Ticlid Tablets....2813

Thromboembolic disorders
(*see also under* Cerebrovascular accident)
Activella Tablets....2311
Alesse-28 Tablets....3392
Aygestin Tablets....1062
Climara Transdermal System....795
Climara Pro Transdermal System....800
CombiPatch Transdermal System....2180
Depo-Provera Contraceptive Injection....2619
depo-subQ provera 104 Injectable Suspension....2622
Emcyt Capsules....3137
Estratest Tablets....3196
Estratest H.S. Tablets....3196
Estrogel 0.06%....3200
Lo/Ovral-28 Tablets....3423
Menostar Transdermal System....805
Ortho-Cept Tablets....2395
Ortho-Cyclen Tablets....2414
Ortho Evra Transdermal System....2402
Ortho Tri-Cyclen Tablets....2414
Ortho Tri-Cyclen Lo Tablets....2421
Prefest Tablets....1069
Premarin Intravenous....3440
Premarin Tablets....3443
Premarin Vaginal Cream....3449
Premphase Tablets....3452
Prempro Tablets....3452
Prochieve 4% Gel....1018
Prochieve 8% Gel....1018
Prometrium Capsules (100 mg, 200 mg)....3205
Seasonale Tablets....1073
Triphasil-28 Tablets....3483
Vivelle Transdermal System....2288
Vivelle-Dot Transdermal System....2293
Yasmin 28 Tablets....818

Thromboembolic disorders, history of
(*see also under* Cerebrovascular accident, history of)
Activella Tablets....2311
Alesse-28 Tablets....3392
Aygestin Tablets....1062
Climara Transdermal System....795
Depo-Provera Contraceptive Injection....2619
depo-subQ provera 104 Injectable Suspension....2622
Estratest Tablets....3196
Estratest H.S. Tablets....3196
Estrogel 0.06%....3200
Evista Tablets....1735
Lo/Ovral-28 Tablets....3423
Menostar Transdermal System....805
Ortho-Cept Tablets....2395
Ortho-Cyclen Tablets....2414
Ortho Evra Transdermal System....2402
Ortho Tri-Cyclen Tablets....2414
Ortho Tri-Cyclen Lo Tablets....2421
Prefest Tablets....1069
Premarin Intravenous....3440
Premarin Vaginal Cream....3449
Premphase Tablets....3452
Prempro Tablets....3452
Prochieve 4% Gel....1018
Prochieve 8% Gel....1018
Prometrium Capsules (100 mg, 200 mg)....3205
Seasonale Tablets....1073
Triphasil-28 Tablets....3483
Vagifem Tablets....2340
Yasmin 28 Tablets....818

Thrombogenic rhythm disorders
Alesse-28 Tablets....3392
Lo/Ovral-28 Tablets....3423
Triphasil-28 Tablets....3483

Thrombogenic valvulopathies
Alesse-28 Tablets....3392
Lo/Ovral-28 Tablets....3423
Triphasil-28 Tablets....3483

Thrombophlebitis
Activella Tablets....2311
Alesse-28 Tablets....3392
Aygestin Tablets....1062
CombiPatch Transdermal System....2180
Depo-Provera Contraceptive Injection....2619
depo-subQ provera 104 Injectable Suspension....2622
Emcyt Capsules....3137
Lo/Ovral-28 Tablets....3423
Ortho-Cept Tablets....2395
Ortho-Cyclen Tablets....2414
Ortho Evra Transdermal System....2402
Ortho Tri-Cyclen Tablets....2414
Ortho Tri-Cyclen Lo Tablets....2421
Premarin Intravenous....3440
Prochieve 4% Gel....1018
Prochieve 8% Gel....1018
Seasonale Tablets....1073
Triphasil-28 Tablets....3483
Vagifem Tablets....2340
Yasmin 28 Tablets....818

Thrombophlebitis, history of
Activella Tablets....2311
Alesse-28 Tablets....3392
Aygestin Tablets....1062
Lo/Ovral-28 Tablets....3423
Lotronex Tablets....1479
Ortho-Cept Tablets....2395
Ortho-Cyclen Tablets....2414
Ortho Evra Transdermal System....2402
Ortho Tri-Cyclen Tablets....2414
Ortho Tri-Cyclen Lo Tablets....2421
Premarin Intravenous....3440
Prochieve 4% Gel....1018
Prochieve 8% Gel....1018
Seasonale Tablets....1073
Triphasil-28 Tablets....3483
Yasmin 28 Tablets....818

Thrombosis, deep vein
Prefest Tablets....1069
Premphase Tablets....3452

Thrombosis, history of
Estratest Tablets....3196
Estratest H.S. Tablets....3196
Evista Tablets....1735
Prefest Tablets....1069
Premarin Intravenous....3440
Premarin Vaginal Cream....3449

Thrombotic thrombocytopenic purpura, history of
Ticlid Tablets....2813

Thymic abnormalities
Flumist Vaccine....1872

Thyroid dysfunction, uncontrolled
Bravelle for Intramuscular or Subcutaneous Injection....1140
Follistim AQ Cartridge....2354
Gonal-f RFF Pen for Injection....3155
Menopur for Subcutaneous Injection....1145
Repronex for Intramuscular and Subcutaneous Injection....1148

Thyrotoxicosis
ProAmatine Tablets....3183

Thyrotoxicosis, untreated
Cytomel Tablets....1678
Levothroid Tablets....1189
Levoxyl Tablets....1680
Synthroid Tablets....515
Thyrolar....1203
Unithroid Tablets....3521

Tics, motor
Concerta Extended-Release Tablets....1828
Focalin Tablets....2214
Focalin XR Capsules....2217
Metadate CD Capsules....3316
Ritalin Hydrochloride Tablets....2254
Ritalin LA Capsules....2255
Ritalin-SR Tablets....2254

Tics, non-Tourette's disorder
Orap Tablets....1220

Tissue breakdown
(*see under* Necrosis)

Tourette's syndrome
Concerta Extended-Release Tablets....1828
Focalin Tablets....2214
Focalin XR Capsules....2217
Metadate CD Capsules....3316
Ritalin Hydrochloride Tablets....2254
Ritalin LA Capsules....2255
Ritalin-SR Tablets....2254

Tourette's syndrome, history of
Concerta Extended-Release Tablets....1828
Focalin Tablets....2214
Focalin XR Capsules....2217
Metadate CD Capsules....3316
Ritalin Hydrochloride Tablets....2254
Ritalin LA Capsules....2255
Ritalin-SR Tablets....2254

Toxic megacolon
(*see under* Megacolon, toxic)

Toxicity, neurologic
Hexalen Capsules....2101

Toxicity, vitamin D
Calcijex Injection....411
Dovonex Cream 0.005%....3374
Dovonex Ointment 0.005%....3375
Dovonex Scalp Solution 0.005%....3375
Hectorol Capsules....909
Hectorol Injection....911
Zemplar Capsules....535
Zemplar Injection....538

Tracheoesophageal fistula, existence of
Photofrin for Injection....729

Transaminases elevation, serum
(*see under* Serum transaminase elevation)

Transplant
(*see under* Organ allograft)

Trauma, intracranial, unspecified
TNKase I.V....1256
Xigris Powder for Intravenous Infusion....1796

Trauma, intracranial
(*see also under* Cerebrovascular accident; Head injury)
Activase I.V....1225
Retavase....1131
TNKase I.V....1256

Trauma, intraspinal
Activase I.V....1225
Retavase....1131

TNKase I.V. 1256

Trauma, unspecified
ReoPro Vials 1779

Tuberculosis, untreated
Attenuvax 1889
Meruvax II 1994
M-M-R II 1980
Mumpsvax 2005
Varivax 2070

Tuberculosis, unspecified
(*see also under* Infection, ophthalmic, mycobacterial)
HMS Sterile Ophthalmic Suspension .... ⊙ 228

Tumor, breast
Follistim AQ Cartridge 2354

Tumor, breast, malignant
Vivelle Transdermal System 2288

Tumor, hypothalamus
Follistim AQ Cartridge 2354

Tumor, intracranial, unspecified
Retavase 1131

Tumor, ovarian
Follistim AQ Cartridge 2354

Tumor activity, unspecified
Genotropin Lyophilized Powder 2642
Humatrope Vials and Cartridges 1756

Tumor, adrenal
(*see under* Pheochromocytoma)

Tumor, breast, malignant
(*see under* Carcinoma, breast, history of; Carcinoma, breast, male; Carcinoma, breast, unspecified)

Tumor, hepatic
(*see under* Adenoma, hepatic; Carcinoma, hepatic; Tumor, liver, benign)

Tumor, hormone dependent
(*see under* Neoplasm, androgen dependent; Neoplasm, estrogen dependent)

Tumor, intracranial, unspecified
(*see also under* Lesions, intracranial, unspecified; Tumor, pituitary, unspecified)
Activase I.V. 1225
Aggrastat 1878
ReoPro Vials 1779
Repronex for Intramuscular and Subcutaneous Injection 1148
TNKase I.V. 1256
Xigris Powder for Intravenous Infusion 1796

Tumor, liver, benign
Mirena Intrauterine System 810

Tumor, liver, malignant
(*see under* Carcinoma, hepatic)

Tumor, pituitary, unspecified
(*see also under* Tumor, intracranial, unspecified)
Bravelle for Intramuscular or Subcutaneous Injection 1140
Follistim AQ Cartridge 2354
Menopur for Subcutaneous Injection 1145
Repronex for Intramuscular and Subcutaneous Injection 1148

Tumor, unspecified
(*see under* Neoplasm, unspecified)

Tumors, reproductive tract, hormone dependent
Gonal-f RFF Pen for Injection 3155
Menopur for Subcutaneous Injection 1145

Tumors, intracranial, in hypopituitary children
Norditropin Cartridges 2318

U

Ulcer, gastrointestinal
(*see also under* Lesions, gastrointestinal, unspecified; Perforation, gastrointestinal tract; Ulcer, peptic)
Miradon Tablets 3056

Ulcer, peptic
Advicor Tablets 1694
Balamine DM 739
Niaspan Extended-Release Tablets 1703
Norflex Injection 1824
Urecholine Tablets 2349

Ulcer, unspecified
(*see under* Ulceration, unspecified)

Ulceration, unspecified
Coumadin for Injection 932
Coumadin Tablets 932
Miradon Tablets 3056

Ulcerative colitis
(*see under* Colitis, ulcerative)

Unstable cardiovascular status in acute hemorrhage
(*see under* Cardiovascular status, unstable in acute hemorrhage)

Urea cycle disorders
Depacon Injection 412
Depakene 417
Depakote Sprinkle Capsules 422
Depakote Tablets 427
Depakote ER Tablets 433

Uremia
(*see also under* Azotemia)
Inversine Tablets 3286

Urinary obstruction
(*see under* Obstruction, urinary tract)

Urinary retention
(*see also under* Obstruction, urinary tract; Prostatic hypertrophy)
Allegra-D 12 Hour Extended-Release Tablets 2860
Allegra-D 24 Hour Extended-Release Tablets 2862
Balamine DM 739
Clarinex-D 24-Hour Extended-Release Tablets 3012
Detrol Tablets 2626
Detrol LA Capsules 2629
Ditropan XL Extended Release Tablets 2391
Enablex Extended-Release Tablets 2201
Oxytrol Transdermal System 3383
ProAmatine Tablets 3183
Sanctura Tablets 1133
VESIcare Tablets 631
Zyrtec-D 12 Hour Extended Release Tablets 2591

Urinary tract disorders
(*see under* Obstruction, urinary tract; Renal disease, unspecified; Renal dysfunction)

Uropathy, obstructive
(*see under* Obstruction, urinary tract)

Uterine abnormalities, unspecified
Mirena Intrauterine System 810

V

Vaccinia
Alrex Ophthalmic Suspension 0.2% .... ⊙ 243
Blephamide Ophthalmic Ointment 563
Blephamide Ophthalmic Suspension 564
FML Ophthalmic Ointment .... ⊙ 225
FML Ophthalmic Suspension .... ⊙ 224
FML Forte Ophthalmic Suspension .... ⊙ 223
FML-S Liquifilm Sterile Ophthalmic Suspension .... ⊙ 226
HMS Sterile Ophthalmic Suspension .... ⊙ 228
Lotemax Ophthalmic Suspension 0.5% .... ⊙ 249
Poly-Pred Liquifilm Ophthalmic Suspension .... ⊙ 231
Pred Forte Ophthalmic Suspension .... ⊙ 233
Pred Mild Sterile Ophthalmic Suspension .... ⊙ 236
Pred-G Ophthalmic Suspension .... ⊙ 234
Pred-G Sterile Ophthalmic Ointment .... ⊙ 235
TobraDex Ophthalmic Ointment 558
TobraDex Ophthalmic Suspension 558
Zylet Ophthalmic Suspension 3508

Vaginal bleeding, abnormal
(*see under* Bleeding, genital, abnormal)

Vaginitis, untreated
Mirena Intrauterine System 810

Vaginosis, bacterial, untreated
Mirena Intrauterine System 810

Vagotonia
Urecholine Tablets 2349

Varicella
Alrex Ophthalmic Suspension 0.2% .... ⊙ 243
Blephamide Ophthalmic Ointment 563
Blephamide Ophthalmic Suspension 564
Cosmegen for Injection 1907
FML Ophthalmic Ointment .... ⊙ 225
FML Ophthalmic Suspension .... ⊙ 224
FML Forte Ophthalmic Suspension .... ⊙ 223
FML-S Liquifilm Sterile Ophthalmic Suspension .... ⊙ 226
HMS Sterile Ophthalmic Suspension .... ⊙ 228
Lotemax Ophthalmic Suspension 0.5% .... ⊙ 249
Poly-Pred Liquifilm Ophthalmic Suspension .... ⊙ 231
Pred Forte Ophthalmic Suspension .... ⊙ 233
Pred Mild Sterile Ophthalmic Suspension .... ⊙ 236
Pred-G Ophthalmic Suspension .... ⊙ 234
Pred-G Sterile Ophthalmic Ointment .... ⊙ 235
TobraDex Ophthalmic Ointment 558
TobraDex Ophthalmic Suspension 558
Zylet Ophthalmic Suspension 3508

Vascular impairment of extremities
(*see also under* Peripheral vascular disease)
Yasmin 28 Tablets 818

Vasculitis, history of
ReoPro Vials 1779

Vasomotor instability
Urecholine Tablets 2349

Vasospasm, coronary artery
(*see under* Coronary artery vasospasm)

Ventilatory function depression
(*see under* Respiratory depression)

Ventricular dysfunction, left
Covera-HS Tablets 3135
Flolan for Injection 1408
Tarka Tablets 519
Verelan PM Capsules 3120

Ventricular fibrillation
(*see under* Fibrillation, ventricular)

Viral disease, conjunctiva
Retisert Implant .... ⊙ 256

Viral disease, cornea
Retisert Implant .... ⊙ 256

Viral infections
(*see under* Herpes simplex keratitis; Herpes zoster; Human immunodeficiency virus; Infection, ophthalmic, viral; Varicella)

Vitamin C, deficiency of
Miradon Tablets 3056

Vitamin D toxicity
(*see under* Toxicity, vitamin D)

Vitamin K, deficiency of
Miradon Tablets 3056

W

Wolff-Parkinson-White syndrome
Covera-HS Tablets 3135
Tarka Tablets 519
Verelan PM Capsules 3120

Women
Avodart Soft Gelatin Capsules 1353
Edex Injection 3103
Eligard 22.5 mg 2899
Eligard 30 mg 2901
Eligard 45 mg 2904
Striant Mucoadhesive 1022
Vantas 3367

Women of childbearing potential
Solage Topical Solution 740

X

Xeroderma pigmentosum
Oxsoralen Lotion 1% 3354
Oxsoralen-Ultra Capsules 3354

SECTION 6

INTERNATIONAL DRUG NAME INDEX

This section names the *PDR*® equivalents of over 33,000 foreign pharmaceutical products. Organized alphabetically by overseas trade name, it shows the country (or countries) in which the name is used, gives the product's closest U.S. generic equivalent, and lists the associated brand-name prescription drugs described by *PDR*®, together with the page on which they are found.

Products from the following nations are included:

Argentina	Finland	Italy	Singapore
Australia	France	Japan	South Africa
Austria	Germany	Malaysia	Spain
Belgium	Greece	Mexico	Sweden
Brazil	Hong Kong	Monaco	Switzerland
Canada	Hungary	New Zealand	Thailand
Chile	India	Norway	The Netherlands
Czech Republic	Irish Republic	Portugal	United Arab Emirates
Denmark	Israel	Russia	United Kingdom

Page numbers refer to the 2005 editions of *PDR*® and *PDR for Ophthalmic Medicines™*. The symbol denoting an entry in *PDR for Ophthalmic Medicines™* appears in the bottom margin.

These entries are intended only as an aid in approximating the contents of a foreign prescription. For proper dosing guidelines, indications, contraindications, warnings, and precautions of its U.S. equivalents, always consult the underlying *PDR*® text. Foreign trade names are courtesy of *PDR*'s affiliate, MICROMEDEX, Inc.

3-A (Mexico)
DICLOFENAC SODIUM
Voltaren Tablets **2298**
Voltaren-XR Tablets **2301**

3A OFTENO (Chile)
DICLOFENAC SODIUM
Voltaren Tablets **2298**
Voltaren-XR Tablets **2301**

3TC (Argentina, Australia, Canada, Hong Kong, Malaysia, Mexico, New Zealand, South Africa, Switzerland)
LAMIVUDINE
Epivir Oral Solution **1394**
Epivir Tablets **1394**
Epivir-HBV Oral Solution **1398**
Epivir-HBV Tablets **1398**

3TC COMPLEX (Argentina)
LAMIVUDINE
Epivir Oral Solution **1394**
Epivir Tablets **1394**
Epivir-HBV Oral Solution **1398**
Epivir-HBV Tablets **1398**

3TC/AZT (Argentina)
LAMIVUDINE
Epivir Oral Solution **1394**
Epivir Tablets **1394**
Epivir-HBV Oral Solution **1398**
Epivir-HBV Tablets **1398**

3TC/EPIVIR (Chile)
LAMIVUDINE
Epivir Oral Solution **1394**
Epivir Tablets **1394**
Epivir-HBV Oral Solution **1398**
Epivir-HBV Tablets **1398**

5-MONO (India)
ISOSORBIDE MONONITRATE
Imdur Tablets **3032**

9PM (India)
LATANOPROST
Xalatan Ophthalmic Solution . . . . ⊙**280**

A ACIDO (Argentina)
TRETINOIN
Avita Cream **2136**
Avita Gel **2138**
Renova 0.05% Cream **2387**
Retin-A Micro 0.1%/0.04% **2388**
Vesanoid Capsules **2823**

AACIDEXAM (Belgium)
DEXAMETHASONE SODIUM PHOSPHATE
Decadron Phosphate Injection **1931**

ABAGLIN (Argentina)
GABAPENTIN
Neurontin Capsules **2498**

ABAMUNE (India)
ABACAVIR SULFATE
Ziagen Oral Solution **1600**
Ziagen Tablets **1600**

ABBA (Greece)
KETOCONAZOLE
Nizoral 2% Shampoo **1838**

ABBOCALCIJEX (Greece)
CALCITRIOL
Calcijex Injection **411**

ABBONIDAZOLE (South Africa)
METRONIDAZOLE
MetroGel-Vaginal Gel **1822**
Noritate Cream, 1% **1051**

ABBOSYNAGIS (Israel)
PALIVIZUMAB
Synagis Intramuscular Powder **1868**

ABENTEL (Thailand)
ALBENDAZOLE
Albenza Tablets **1310**

ABEREL (France)
TRETINOIN
Avita Cream **2136**
Avita Gel **2138**
Renova 0.05% Cream **2387**
Retin-A Micro 0.1%/0.04% **2388**
Vesanoid Capsules **2823**

ABERELA (Norway, Sweden)
TRETINOIN
Avita Cream **2136**
Avita Gel **2138**
Renova 0.05% Cream **2387**
Retin-A Micro 0.1%/0.04% **2388**
Vesanoid Capsules **2823**

ABERTEN (Greece)
THEOPHYLLINE
Uniphyl Tablets **2708**

ABIOLEX (Chile)
AMOXICILLIN
Amoxil Pediatric Drops for Oral Suspension **1315**
Amoxil Tablets **1315**

ABIOTYL (Argentina)
AMOXICILLIN
Amoxil Pediatric Drops for Oral Suspension **1315**
Amoxil Tablets **1315**

ABITREN (Hong Kong, Israel, Thailand)
DICLOFENAC SODIUM
Voltaren Tablets **2298**
Voltaren-XR Tablets **2301**

ABLOCK (Brazil)
ATENOLOL
Tenormin I.V. Injection **698**

ABLOCK PLUS (Brazil)
ATENOLOL
Tenormin I.V. Injection **698**

ABRILAR (Argentina)
SALMETEROL XINAFOATE
Serevent Diskus **1540**

ABSORLENT (Spain)
ESTRADIOL
Climara Transdermal System **795**
Vivelle Transdermal System **2288**
Vivelle-Dot Transdermal System **2293**

ABTRIM (United Kingdom)
CLOTRIMAZOLE
Lotrimin Cream **3053**
Lotrimin Lotion 1% **3053**
Lotrimin Topical Solution 1% **3053**

ABUTIROI (Mexico)
LEVOTHYROXINE SODIUM
Levothroid Tablets **1189**
Levoxyl Tablets **1680**
Synthroid Tablets **515**

AC VASCULAR (Argentina)
NIMODIPINE
Nimotop Capsules **774**

ACALIX (Argentina)
DILTIAZEM HYDROCHLORIDE
Cardizem LA Extended Release Tablets . . . **1699**
Tiazac Capsules **1204**

ACALKA (Brazil, Chile, Portugal, Spain)
POTASSIUM CITRATE
Urocit-K Tablets **2109**

ACANTEX (Chile)
CEFTRIAXONE SODIUM
Rocephin Injectable Vials, ADD-Vantage, Galaxy, Bulk **2801**

ACARBAY (India)
ACARBOSE
Precose Tablets **776**

ACASMUL (Chile)
DILTIAZEM HYDROCHLORIDE
Cardizem LA Extended Release Tablets . . . **1699**
Tiazac Capsules **1204**

ACCOLATE (Argentina, Australia, Belgium, Brazil, Canada, Chile, Czech Republic, Finland, Hong Kong, Hungary, Irish Republic, Israel, Mexico, Portugal, Singapore, South Africa, Spain, Switzerland, Thailand, United Kingdom)
ZAFIRLUKAST
Accolate Tablets 663

ACCOLEIT (Italy)
ZAFIRLUKAST
Accolate Tablets 663

ACCURE (Australia)
ISOTRETINOIN
Accutane Capsules 2740

ACCUSITE (United Kingdom)
FLUOROURACIL
Efudex Topical Cream 3348
Efudex Topical Solutions 3348

ACCUTANE (Canada)
ISOTRETINOIN
Accutane Capsules 2740

ACCUTIN (Denmark)
ISOTRETINOIN
Accutane Capsules 2740

AC-DE (Mexico)
DACTINOMYCIN
Cosmegen for Injection 1907

ACEA (United Kingdom)
METRONIDAZOLE
MetroGel-Vaginal Gel 1822
Noritate Cream, 1% 1051

ACECOMB (Austria)
HYDROCHLOROTHIAZIDE/LISINOPRIL
Prinzide Tablets 2033
Zestoretic Tablets 701

ACEDIUR (Spain)
ENALAPRIL MALEATE/HYDROCHLOROTHIAZIDE
Vaseretic Tablets 2073

ACEF (Italy)
CEFAZOLIN SODIUM
Ancef for Injection 1318

ACE-HEMMER COMP (Germany)
CAPTOPRIL
Captopril Tablets 2114

ACEMEDROX (Brazil)
MEDROXYPROGESTERONE ACETATE
Depo-Medrol Single-Dose Vial 2617

ACEMIN (Austria)
LISINOPRIL
Prinivil Tablets 2029
Zestril Tablets 704

ACENORM (Australia, Germany)
CAPTOPRIL
Captopril Tablets 2114

ACENORM HCT (Germany)
CAPTOPRIL
Captopril Tablets 2114

ACEOMEL (Hungary, Irish Republic)
CAPTOPRIL
Captopril Tablets 2114

ACEOTO PLUS (Spain)
CIPROFLOXACIN
Cipro Oral Suspension 2991

ACEPRAN (Chile)
CLONAZEPAM
Klonopin Tablets 2782

ACEPRESS (Italy)
CAPTOPRIL
Captopril Tablets 2114

ACEPRIL (Denmark, Hong Kong, Hungary, Switzerland, United Kingdom)
LISINOPRIL
Prinivil Tablets 2029
Zestril Tablets 704

ACEPRILEX (Italy)
CAPTOPRIL
Captopril Tablets 2114

ACERBON (Germany)
LISINOPRIL
Prinivil Tablets 2029
Zestril Tablets 704

ACERCOMP (Finland, Germany)
HYDROCHLOROTHIAZIDE/LISINOPRIL
Prinzide Tablets 2033
Zestoretic Tablets 701

ACERDIL (Chile)
LISINOPRIL
Prinivil Tablets 2029
Zestril Tablets 704

ACERDIL-D (Chile)
HYDROCHLOROTHIAZIDE/LISINOPRIL
Prinzide Tablets 2033
Zestoretic Tablets 701

ACEREN (Denmark)
ENALAPRIL MALEATE
Vasotec I.V. Injection 2076

ACERIL (Israel)
CAPTOPRIL
Captopril Tablets 2114

ACESISTEM (Italy)
ENALAPRIL MALEATE/HYDROCHLOROTHIAZIDE
Vaseretic Tablets 2073

ACETAN (Austria)
LISINOPRIL
Prinivil Tablets 2029
Zestril Tablets 704

ACETEC (Malaysia)
ENALAPRIL MALEATE
Vasotec I.V. Injection 2076

ACETEN (India, South Africa)
CAPTOPRIL
Captopril Tablets 2114

ACETENSIL (Czech Republic, Spain)
ENALAPRIL MALEATE
Vasotec I.V. Injection 2076

ACETENSIL PLUS (Spain)
ENALAPRIL MALEATE/HYDROCHLOROTHIAZIDE
Vaseretic Tablets 2073

ACETOFLUX (Brazil)
MEDROXYPROGESTERONE ACETATE
Depo-Medrol Single-Dose Vial 2617

ACETOPT (Australia, New Zealand)
SULFACETAMIDE SODIUM
Klaron Lotion 10% 1050

ACETOXYL (Canada, United Kingdom)
BENZOYL PEROXIDE
Brevoxyl-4 Creamy Wash 3212
Brevoxyl-4 Gel 3211
Brevoxyl-8 Creamy Wash 3212
Brevoxyl-8 Gel 3211
Triaz Cleanser 1864
Triaz Gel 1864

AC-FA (Thailand)
KETOCONAZOLE
Nizoral 2% Shampoo 1838

ACID A VIT (Belgium, The Netherlands)
TRETINOIN
Avita Cream 2136
Avita Gel 2138
Renova 0.05% Cream 2387
Retin-A Micro 0.1%/0.04% 2388
Vesanoid Capsules 2823

ACID HALT (Canada)
FAMOTIDINE
Pepcid Injection 2017
Pepcid Injection Premixed 2017
Pepcid Tablets 2014
Pepcid for Oral Suspension 2014

ACIDERM (Brazil)
KETOCONAZOLE
Nizoral 2% Shampoo 1838

ACIDEX (Austria)
CIMETIDINE
Tagamet Tablets 1547

ACID-EZE (United Kingdom)
CIMETIDINE
Tagamet Tablets 1547

ACIDINE (Malaysia)
FAMOTIDINE
Pepcid Injection 2017
Pepcid Injection Premixed 2017
Pepcid Tablets 2014
Pepcid for Oral Suspension 2014

ACIDOWN (South Africa)
CIMETIDINE
Tagamet Tablets 1547

ACIFLUX (Chile)
RANITIDINE HYDROCHLORIDE
Zantac 25 EFFERdose Tablets 1597
Zantac 150 EFFERdose Tablets 1597
Zantac 150 Tablets 1597
Zantac 300 Tablets 1597
Zantac Injection 1593
Zantac Injection Premixed 1593
Zantac Syrup 1597

ACILAC (Canada)
LACTULOSE
Kristalose for Oral Solution 2149

ACILOC (Denmark, India, Sweden, Thailand)
CIMETIDINE
Tagamet Tablets 1547

ACILOC RD (India)
RANITIDINE HYDROCHLORIDE
Zantac 25 EFFERdose Tablets 1597
Zantac 150 EFFERdose Tablets 1597
Zantac 150 Tablets 1597
Zantac 300 Tablets 1597
Zantac Injection 1593
Zantac Injection Premixed 1593
Zantac Syrup 1597

ACI-MED (South Africa)
CIMETIDINE
Tagamet Tablets 1547

ACINIL (Denmark, Norway, Sweden)
CIMETIDINE
Tagamet Tablets 1547

ACITAK (United Kingdom)
CIMETIDINE
Tagamet Tablets 1547

ACIVAL (Argentina)
NIMODIPINE
Nimotop Capsules 774

ACLAV (Argentina)
AMOXICILLIN
Amoxil Pediatric Drops for Oral Suspension 1315
Amoxil Tablets 1315

ACLENE (India)
ADAPALENE
Differin Gel 1211

ACLIN (Australia, Hong Kong)
SULINDAC
Clinoril Tablets 1899

ACLINDA (Germany)
CLINDAMYCIN HYDROCHLORIDE
Cleocin Vaginal Ovules 2613

ACLONIUM (Italy)
GABAPENTIN
Neurontin Capsules 2498

ACLORAL (Mexico)
RANITIDINE HYDROCHLORIDE
Zantac 25 EFFERdose Tablets 1597
Zantac 150 EFFERdose Tablets 1597
Zantac 150 Tablets 1597
Zantac 300 Tablets 1597
Zantac Injection 1593
Zantac Injection Premixed 1593
Zantac Syrup 1597

ACLOSAN (Argentina)
TAMSULOSIN HYDROCHLORIDE
Flomax Capsules 881

ACLOSONE (France, South Africa, The Netherlands)
ALCLOMETASONE DIPROPIONATE
Aclovate Cream 1290
Aclovate Ointment 1290

ACNACYL (Australia, Hong Kong, Singapore)
BENZOYL PEROXIDE
Brevoxyl-4 Creamy Wash 3212
Brevoxyl-4 Gel 3211
Brevoxyl-8 Creamy Wash 3212
Brevoxyl-8 Gel 3211
Triaz Cleanser 1864
Triaz Gel 1864

ACNE DERM (Israel)
BENZOYL PEROXIDE
Brevoxyl-4 Creamy Wash 3212
Brevoxyl-4 Gel 3211
Brevoxyl-8 Creamy Wash 3212
Brevoxyl-8 Gel 3211
Triaz Cleanser 1864
Triaz Gel 1864

ACNE HERMAL (Greece)
ERYTHROMYCIN
Ery-Tab Tablets 447
Erythromycin Base Filmtab Tablets 454
Erythromycin Delayed-Release Capsules, USP 456
PCE Dispertab Tablets 510

ACNE MASK (Israel)
BENZOYL PEROXIDE
Brevoxyl-4 Creamy Wash 3212
Brevoxyl-4 Gel 3211
Brevoxyl-8 Creamy Wash 3212
Brevoxyl-8 Gel 3211
Triaz Cleanser 1864
Triaz Gel 1864

ACNE-AID (Spain)
BENZOYL PEROXIDE
Brevoxyl-4 Creamy Wash 3212
Brevoxyl-4 Gel 3211
Brevoxyl-8 Creamy Wash 3212
Brevoxyl-8 Gel 3211
Triaz Cleanser 1864
Triaz Gel 1864

ACNECIDE (Irish Republic, United Kingdom)
BENZOYL PEROXIDE
Brevoxyl-4 Creamy Wash 3212
Brevoxyl-4 Gel 3211
Brevoxyl-8 Creamy Wash 3212
Brevoxyl-8 Gel 3211
Triaz Cleanser 1864
Triaz Gel 1864

ACNECLEAR (Hong Kong)
BENZOYL PEROXIDE
Brevoxyl-4 Creamy Wash 3212
Brevoxyl-4 Gel 3211
Brevoxyl-8 Creamy Wash 3212
Brevoxyl-8 Gel 3211
Triaz Cleanser 1864
Triaz Gel 1864

ACNECOLOR (Switzerland)
CLOTRIMAZOLE
Lotrimin Cream 3053
Lotrimin Lotion 1% 3053
Lotrimin Topical Solution 1% 3053

ACNEFUGE (Switzerland)
BENZOYL PEROXIDE
Brevoxyl-4 Creamy Wash 3212
Brevoxyl-4 Gel 3211
Brevoxyl-8 Creamy Wash 3212
Brevoxyl-8 Gel 3211
Triaz Cleanser 1864
Triaz Gel 1864

ACNEGEL (United Kingdom)
BENZOYL PEROXIDE
Brevoxyl-4 Creamy Wash 3212
Brevoxyl-4 Gel 3211
Brevoxyl-8 Creamy Wash 3212
Brevoxyl-8 Gel 3211
Triaz Cleanser 1864
Triaz Gel 1864

ACNE-MED (Hungary)
BENZOYL PEROXIDE
Brevoxyl-4 Creamy Wash 3212
Brevoxyl-4 Gel 3211
Brevoxyl-8 Creamy Wash 3212
Brevoxyl-8 Gel 3211
Triaz Cleanser 1864
Triaz Gel 1864

ACNEPAS (Argentina)
BENZOYL PEROXIDE
Brevoxyl-4 Creamy Wash 3212
Brevoxyl-4 Gel 3211
Brevoxyl-8 Creamy Wash 3212
Brevoxyl-8 Gel 3211
Triaz Cleanser 1864
Triaz Gel 1864

ACNEPAS E (Argentina)
BENZOYL PEROXIDE
Brevoxyl-4 Creamy Wash 3212
Brevoxyl-4 Gel 3211
Brevoxyl-8 Creamy Wash 3212
Brevoxyl-8 Gel 3211
Triaz Cleanser 1864
Triaz Gel 1864

ACNERYNE (Belgium)
ERYTHROMYCIN
Ery-Tab Tablets 447
Erythromycin Base Filmtab Tablets 454
Erythromycin Delayed-Release Capsules, USP 456
PCE Dispertab Tablets 510

ACNESAN (Argentina, Brazil)
BENZOYL PEROXIDE
Brevoxyl-4 Creamy Wash 3212
Brevoxyl-4 Gel 3211
Brevoxyl-8 Creamy Wash 3212
Brevoxyl-8 Gel 3211
Triaz Cleanser 1864
Triaz Gel 1864

ACNESOL (India)
ERYTHROMYCIN
Ery-Tab Tablets 447
Erythromycin Base Filmtab Tablets 454
Erythromycin Delayed-Release Capsules, USP 456
PCE Dispertab Tablets 510

ACNETANE (South Africa)
ISOTRETINOIN
Accutane Capsules 2740

ACNETRIM (Israel)
ERYTHROMYCIN
Ery-Tab Tablets 447
Erythromycin Base Filmtab Tablets 454
Erythromycin Delayed-Release Capsules, USP 456
PCE Dispertab Tablets 510

ACNEXYL (Thailand)
BENZOYL PEROXIDE
Brevoxyl-4 Creamy Wash 3212
Brevoxyl-4 Gel 3211
Brevoxyl-8 Creamy Wash 3212
Brevoxyl-8 Gel 3211
Triaz Cleanser 1864
Triaz Gel 1864

ACNOTIN (Hong Kong)
ISOTRETINOIN
Accutane Capsules 2740

ACOFLAM (United Kingdom)
DICLOFENAC SODIUM
Voltaren Tablets 2298
Voltaren-XR Tablets 2301

ACOLITIUM (Brazil)
LITHIUM CARBONATE
Eskalith CR Controlled-Release Tablets 1406
Eskalith Capsules 1406

ACONEX (Austria)
NAPHAZOLINE HYDROCHLORIDE
Albalon Ophthalmic Solution . . . . ⊙216

ACOVIL (Spain)
RAMIPRIL
Altace Capsules 1673

ACRIDILOLE (Russia)
CARVEDILOL
Coreg Tablets 1376

ACSACEA (Austria)
METRONIDAZOLE
MetroGel-Vaginal Gel 1822
Noritate Cream, 1% 1051

ACTA (Hong Kong, Singapore)
TRETINOIN
Avita Cream 2136
Avita Gel 2138
Renova 0.05% Cream 2387
Retin-A Micro 0.1%/0.04% 2388
Vesanoid Capsules 2823

ACTICIN (United Kingdom)
TRETINOIN
Avita Cream 2136
Avita Gel 2138
Renova 0.05% Cream 2387
Retin-A Micro 0.1%/0.04% 2388
Vesanoid Capsules 2823

ACTIDINE (Hong Kong)
FAMOTIDINE
Pepcid Injection 2017
Pepcid Injection Premixed 2017
Pepcid Tablets 2014
Pepcid for Oral Suspension 2014

ACTILAX (Australia)
LACTULOSE
Kristalose for Oral Solution 2149

ACTIMAX (Argentina)
ALENDRONATE SODIUM
Fosamax Tablets 1949

ACTIMOL (India)
DICLOFENAC SODIUM
Voltaren Tablets 2298
Voltaren-XR Tablets 2301

ACTINERVAL (Argentina)
CARBAMAZEPINE
Carbatrol Capsules 3174
Tegretol Chewable Tablets 2278
Tegretol Suspension 2278
Tegretol Tablets 2278
Tegretol-XR Tablets 2278

ACTINO-HERMAL (Germany)
FLUOROURACIL
Efudex Topical Cream 3348
Efudex Topical Solutions 3348

ACTIPRAM (Chile)
CITALOPRAM HYDROBROMIDE
Celexa Tablets 1177

ACTIQ (Australia, Denmark, Finland, France, Germany, Irish Republic, Norway, Spain, Sweden, United Kingdom)
FENTANYL CITRATE
Actiq 993

ACTIQUIM (Mexico)
NAPROXEN
EC-Naprosyn Delayed-Release Tablets 2769
Naprosyn Suspension 2769
Naprosyn Tablets 2769

ACTISKENAN (France)
MORPHINE SULFATE
Kadian Capsules 572
MS Contin Tablets 2703

ACTISON (Argentina)
AMANTADINE HYDROCHLORIDE
Symmetrel Syrup 1115
Symmetrel Tablets 1115

ACTIVELLE (Argentina, Brazil, Czech Republic, France, Hong Kong, Hungary, Irish Republic, Israel, Malaysia, Portugal, South Africa, Spain, Thailand, The Netherlands)
ESTRADIOL
Climara Transdermal System 795
Vivelle Transdermal System 2288
Vivelle-Dot Transdermal System 2293

ACTONEL (Argentina, Australia, Austria, Belgium, Brazil, Canada, Chile, Czech Republic, France, Greece, Hong Kong, Hungary, Irish Republic, Israel, Italy, Portugal, Singapore, South Africa, Spain, Switzerland, Thailand, The Netherlands)
RISEDRONATE SODIUM
Actonel Tablets 2679

ACTOPRIL (Irish Republic)
CAPTOPRIL
Captopril Tablets 2114

ACTOS (Argentina, Australia, Austria, Belgium, Brazil, Canada, Chile, Czech Republic, Denmark, Finland, France, Germany, Greece, Hong Kong, Italy, Japan, New Zealand, Norway, Portugal, Russia, South Africa, Spain, Sweden, Switzerland, Thailand, United Kingdom)
PIOGLITAZONE HYDROCHLORIDE
Actos Tablets 3224

ACTUALENE (Italy)
CABERGOLINE
Dostinex Tablets 2631

ACUMOD (South Africa)
AMILORIDE HYDROCHLORIDE/HYDROCHLOROTHIAZIDE
Moduretic Tablets 2003

ACURA (Norway, Sweden)
CETIRIZINE HYDROCHLORIDE
Zyrtec Syrup 2589
Zyrtec Tablets 2589

ACUSPRAIN (South Africa)
NAPROXEN
EC-Naprosyn Delayed-Release Tablets 2769
Naprosyn Suspension 2769
Naprosyn Tablets 2769

ACUTRET (India)
ISOTRETINOIN
Accutane Capsules 2740

ACUZOLE (South Africa)
METRONIDAZOLE
MetroGel-Vaginal Gel 1822
Noritate Cream, 1% 1051

ADAFERIN (Greece, India, Israel, Mexico)
ADAPALENE
Differin Gel 1211

ADALAT (Argentina, Australia, Austria, Belgium, Brazil, Canada, Chile, Czech Republic, Denmark, Finland, Germany, Greece, Hong Kong, Hungary, Irish Republic, Italy, Japan, Malaysia, Mexico, New Zealand, Norway, Portugal, Singapore, South Africa, Spain, Sweden, Switzerland, Thailand, The Netherlands, United Kingdom)
NIFEDIPINE
Adalat CC Tablets 2978

ADALATE (France)
NIFEDIPINE
Adalat CC Tablets 2978

ADALKEN (Mexico)
PENICILLAMINE
Cuprimine Capsules 1925

ADANA (Argentina)
IRBESARTAN
Avapro Tablets 925

ADANT (France, Israel)
SODIUM HYALURONATE
Hyalgan Solution 2917

ADAPINE (Australia)
NIFEDIPINE
Adalat CC Tablets 2978

ADAPRESS (Switzerland)
NIFEDIPINE
Adalat CC Tablets 2978

ADCO-AMOCLAV (South Africa)
AMOXICILLIN
Amoxil Pediatric Drops for Oral Suspension 1315
Amoxil Tablets 1315

ADCO-CIPRIN (South Africa)
CIPROFLOXACIN
Cipro Oral Suspension 2991

ADCO-DERMED (South Africa)
KETOCONAZOLE
Nizoral 2% Shampoo 1838

ADCO-LIQUILAX (South Africa)
LACTULOSE
Kristalose for Oral Solution 2149

ADCO-LOTEN (South Africa)
ATENOLOL
Tenormin I.V. Injection 698

ADCOR (Brazil)
NIFEDIPINE
Adalat CC Tablets 2978

ADCO-RETIC (South Africa)
AMILORIDE HYDROCHLORIDE/HYDROCHLOROTHIAZIDE
Moduretic Tablets 2003

ADCORTYL (Irish Republic, Israel, United Kingdom)
TRIAMCINOLONE ACETONIDE
Azmacort Inhalation Aerosol 1701
Nasacort AQ Nasal Spray 2937

ADCORTYL IN ORABASE (Irish Republic, United Kingdom)
TRIAMCINOLONE ACETONIDE
Azmacort Inhalation Aerosol 1701
Nasacort AQ Nasal Spray 2937

ADCO-WORMEX (South Africa)
MEBENDAZOLE
Vermox Chewable Tablets 1853

ADDI-K (Hong Kong, Singapore, Thailand)
POTASSIUM CHLORIDE
K-Dur Extended-Relase Tablets 3047
K-Lor Powder Packets 472
K-Tab Filmtab Tablets 473

ADECUR (Mexico)
TERAZOSIN HYDROCHLORIDE
Hytrin Capsules 469

ADEFIN (Australia)
NIFEDIPINE
Adalat CC Tablets 2978

ADEKIN (Germany)
AMANTADINE HYDROCHLORIDE
Symmetrel Syrup 1115
Symmetrel Tablets 1115

ADEL (Mexico)
CLARITHROMYCIN
Biaxin Filmtab Tablets 402
Biaxin Granules 402

ADENOCARD (Brazil, Canada)
ADENOSINE
Adenocard Injection 612
Adenoscan 613

ADENOCOR (Australia, Belgium, Czech Republic, Denmark, Finland, Greece, Hungary, Irish Republic, Israel, Malaysia, New Zealand, Norway, Portugal, Singapore, South Africa, Spain, Sweden, Thailand, The Netherlands, United Kingdom)
ADENOSINE
Adenocard Injection 612
Adenoscan 613

ADENOJECT (India)
ADENOSINE
Adenocard Injection 612
Adenoscan 613

ADENOSAN (Greece)
KETOCONAZOLE
Nizoral 2% Shampoo 1838

ADENOSCAN (Australia, Austria, Czech Republic, Finland, France, Germany, Hong Kong, Italy, Japan, Spain, The Netherlands, United Kingdom)
ADENOSINE
Adenocard Injection 612
Adenoscan 613

ADEPRIL (Mexico)
CARBAMAZEPINE
Carbatrol Capsules 3174
Tegretol Chewable Tablets 2278
Tegretol Suspension 2278
Tegretol Tablets 2278
Tegretol-XR Tablets 2278

ADERAN (Argentina)
SIBUTRAMINE HYDROCHLORIDE
Meridia Capsules 485

ADESIPRESS-TTS (Italy)
CLONIDINE
Catapres-TTS 875

ADEXONE (Israel)
DEXAMETHASONE
Decadron Tablets 1929

ADEZAN (Greece)
DIPYRIDAMOLE
Persantine Tablets 898

ADEZIO (Hong Kong, Malaysia, Singapore)
CETIRIZINE HYDROCHLORIDE
Zyrtec Syrup 2589
Zyrtec Tablets 2589

ADGYN ESTRO (United Kingdom)
ESTRADIOL
Climara Transdermal System 795
Vivelle Transdermal System 2288
Vivelle-Dot Transdermal System 2293

ADGYN MEDRO (United Kingdom)
MEDROXYPROGESTERONE ACETATE
Depo-Medrol Single-Dose Vial 2617

ADICLAIR (Germany)
NYSTATIN
Nystop Topical Powder USP 2490

ADIFEN (Malaysia)
NIFEDIPINE
Adalat CC Tablets 2978

ADIFF (India)
ADAPALENE
Differin Gel 1211

ADIPINE (United Kingdom)
NIFEDIPINE
Adalat CC Tablets . . . 2978

ADIPUR (Switzerland)
SIMVASTATIN
Zocor Tablets . . . 2078

ADISAR (Chile)
SIBUTRAMINE HYDROCHLORIDE
Meridia Capsules . . . 485

ADIUVAN (Argentina)
GLIMEPIRIDE
Amaryl Tablets . . . 2864

ADIZEM (Irish Republic, Israel, United Kingdom)
DILTIAZEM HYDROCHLORIDE
Cardizem LA Extended Release Tablets . . . 1699
Tiazac Capsules . . . 1204

ADMON (Spain)
NIMODIPINE
Nimotop Capsules . . . 774

ADOCOMP (Germany)
CAPTOPRIL
Captopril Tablets . . . 2114

ADOCOR (Germany)
CAPTOPRIL
Captopril Tablets . . . 2114

ADOLL (Hong Kong)
ATENOLOL
Tenormin I.V. Injection . . . 698

ADOMAL (Italy)
DIFLUNISAL
Dolobid Tablets . . . 1937

ADRECORT (Mexico)
DEXAMETHASONE
Decadron Tablets . . . 1929

ADREKAR (Austria, Germany)
ADENOSINE
Adenocard Injection . . . 612
Adenoscan . . . 613

ADREXAN (France)
PROPRANOLOL HYDROCHLORIDE
Inderal LA Long-Acting Capsules . . . 3421

ADRONAT (Italy, Portugal)
ALENDRONATE SODIUM
Fosamax Tablets . . . 1949

ADROYD (Australia, India)
OXYMETHOLONE
Anadrol-50 Tablets . . . 3329

ADRUCIL (Canada)
FLUOROURACIL
Efudex Topical Cream . . . 3348
Efudex Topical Solutions . . . 3348

ADUAR (Argentina)
MEBENDAZOLE
Vermox Chewable Tablets . . . 1853

ADUCIN (Denmark)
RANITIDINE HYDROCHLORIDE
Zantac 25 EFFERdose Tablets . . . 1597
Zantac 150 EFFERdose Tablets . . . 1597
Zantac 150 Tablets . . . 1597
Zantac 300 Tablets . . . 1597
Zantac Injection . . . 1593
Zantac Injection Premixed . . . 1593
Zantac Syrup . . . 1597

AERFLU (Italy)
FLUNISOLIDE
Aerobid Inhaler System . . . 1172
Aerobid-M Inhaler System . . . 1172
Nasarel Nasal Spray . . . 1652

AEROCEF (Austria)
CEFIXIME
Suprax . . . 1811

AERODIOL (Argentina, Australia, Austria, Belgium, Brazil, Denmark, France, Germany, Greece, Hong Kong, Irish Republic, Italy, Switzerland, The Netherlands, United Kingdom)
ESTRADIOL
Climara Transdermal System . . . 795
Vivelle Transdermal System . . . 2288
Vivelle-Dot Transdermal System . . . 2293

AEROLID (Italy)
FLUNISOLIDE
Aerobid Inhaler System . . . 1172
Aerobid-M Inhaler System . . . 1172
Nasarel Nasal Spray . . . 1652

AEROMAX (Germany)
SALMETEROL XINAFOATE
Serevent Diskus . . . 1540

AERONIX (Spain)
ZAFIRLUKAST
Accolate Tablets . . . 663

AEROTROP (Argentina)
IPRATROPIUM BROMIDE
Atrovent Inhalation Solution . . . 868
Atrovent Nasal Spray 0.03% . . . 869
Atrovent Nasal Spray 0.06% . . . 870

AEROVENT (Israel)
IPRATROPIUM BROMIDE
Atrovent Inhalation Solution . . . 868
Atrovent Nasal Spray 0.03% . . . 869
Atrovent Nasal Spray 0.06% . . . 870

AEROXINA (Argentina)
CLARITHROMYCIN
Biaxin Filmtab Tablets . . . 402
Biaxin Granules . . . 402

AFAZOL (Mexico)
NAPHAZOLINE HYDROCHLORIDE
Albalon Ophthalmic Solution . . . ⊙216

AFENEXIL (Argentina)
PAROXETINE HYDROCHLORIDE
Paxil Oral Suspension . . . 1501
Paxil Tablets . . . 1501

AFENIL (Greece)
TRANDOLAPRIL
Mavik Tablets . . . 482

AFENOXIN (Greece)
CIPROFLOXACIN HYDROCHLORIDE
Ciloxan Ophthalmic Ointment . . . 554
Ciloxan Ophthalmic Solution . . . ⊙205
Cipro Tablets . . . 2991

AFIANCEN (Argentina)
LEFLUNOMIDE
Arava Tablets . . . 2881

AFLEX (Thailand)
NABUMETONE
Relafen Tablets . . . 1523

AFLODAC (Italy)
SULINDAC
Clinoril Tablets . . . 1899

AFLODERM (Czech Republic)
ALCLOMETASONE DIPROPIONATE
Aclovate Cream . . . 1290
Aclovate Ointment . . . 1290

AFLORIX (Argentina)
CLOTRIMAZOLE
Lotrimin Cream . . . 3053
Lotrimin Lotion 1% . . . 3053
Lotrimin Topical Solution 1% . . . 3053

AFLUON (Spain)
AZELASTINE HYDROCHLORIDE
Astelin Nasal Spray . . . 1876

AFLUTA (Austria)
FLUTAMIDE
Eulexin Capsules . . . 3023

AFONILUM (Austria, Czech Republic, Germany)
THEOPHYLLINE
Uniphyl Tablets . . . 2708

AFPRED-THEO (Germany)
THEOPHYLLINE
Uniphyl Tablets . . . 2708

AFTAB (Finland, Germany, Italy)
TRIAMCINOLONE ACETONIDE
Azmacort Inhalation Aerosol . . . 1701
Nasacort AQ Nasal Spray . . . 2937

AFTACH (Hong Kong, Japan, Portugal)
TRIAMCINOLONE ACETONIDE
Azmacort Inhalation Aerosol . . . 1701
Nasacort AQ Nasal Spray . . . 2937

AFTER BURN (Israel)
LIDOCAINE
Lidoderm Patch . . . 1107

AGELAN (Hong Kong, Irish Republic)
INDAPAMIDE
Indapamide Tablets . . . 2119

AGELMIN (Greece, Singapore)
CETIRIZINE HYDROCHLORIDE
Zyrtec Syrup . . . 2589
Zyrtec Tablets . . . 2589

AGENERASE (Argentina, Australia, Austria, Belgium, Brazil, Canada, Chile, Denmark, Finland, France, Germany, Greece, Irish Republic, Israel, Italy, Mexico, New Zealand, Norway, Portugal, Spain, Sweden, Switzerland, United Kingdom)
AMPRENAVIR
Agenerase Capsules . . . 1299
Agenerase Oral Solution . . . 1304

AGGRASTAT (Australia, Austria, Belgium, Canada, Czech Republic, Denmark, Finland, Germany, Greece, Hong Kong, Hungary, Irish Republic, Israel, Italy, Malaysia, New Zealand, Norway, Singapore, Sweden, Switzerland, Thailand, The Netherlands, United Kingdom)
TIROFIBAN HYDROCHLORIDE
Aggrastat Injection . . . 1878
Aggrastat Injection Premixed . . . 1878

AGGRASTET (South Africa)
TIROFIBAN HYDROCHLORIDE
Aggrastat Injection . . . 1878
Aggrastat Injection Premixed . . . 1878

AGGRENOX (Belgium, Canada, Germany, Hong Kong, Portugal, Thailand)
DIPYRIDAMOLE
Persantine Tablets . . . 898

AGILOMED (Austria)
DICLOFENAC SODIUM
Voltaren Tablets . . . 2298
Voltaren-XR Tablets . . . 2301

AGISTEN (Israel)
CLOTRIMAZOLE
Lotrimin Cream . . . 3053
Lotrimin Lotion 1% . . . 3053
Lotrimin Topical Solution 1% . . . 3053

AGOFENAC (Switzerland)
DICLOFENAC SODIUM
Voltaren Tablets . . . 2298
Voltaren-XR Tablets . . . 2301

AGON (Australia, New Zealand)
FELODIPINE
Plendil Extended-Release Tablets . . . 651

AGOPTON (Austria, Germany, Switzerland)
LANSOPRAZOLE
Prevacid Delayed-Release Capsules . . . 3268

AGOREX (Switzerland)
AMILORIDE HYDROCHLORIDE/HYDROCHLOROTHIAZIDE
Moduretic Tablets . . . 2003

AGRASTAT (Argentina, Brazil, Chile, France, Mexico, Spain)
TIROFIBAN HYDROCHLORIDE
Aggrastat Injection . . . 1878
Aggrastat Injection Premixed . . . 1878

AGREDAMOL (Belgium)
DIPYRIDAMOLE
Persantine Tablets . . . 898

AGREGAMINA (Portugal)
TICLOPIDINE HYDROCHLORIDE
Ticlid Tablets . . . 2813

AGREMOL (Thailand)
DIPYRIDAMOLE
Persantine Tablets . . . 898

AGRENOX (Argentina)
DIPYRIDAMOLE
Persantine Tablets . . . 898

AGRYLIN (Australia, Canada, Israel, South Africa)
ANAGRELIDE HYDROCHLORIDE
Agrylin Capsules . . . 3172

AGUFAM (Thailand)
FAMOTIDINE
Pepcid Injection . . . 2017
Pepcid Injection Premixed . . . 2017
Pepcid Tablets . . . 2014
Pepcid for Oral Suspension . . . 2014

AGYR (Austria)
CIPROFLOXACIN HYDROCHLORIDE
Ciloxan Ophthalmic Ointment . . . 554
Ciloxan Ophthalmic Solution . . . ⊙205
Cipro Tablets . . . 2991

AIDAR (Thailand)
CIMETIDINE
Tagamet Tablets . . . 1547

AIRBRONAL (Argentina)
THEOPHYLLINE
Uniphyl Tablets . . . 2708

AIROL (Australia, Austria, Czech Republic, Germany, Greece, Israel, Italy, Mexico, Norway, South Africa, Switzerland)
TRETINOIN
Avita Cream . . . 2136
Avita Gel . . . 2138
Renova 0.05% Cream . . . 2387
Retin-A Micro 0.1%/0.04% . . . 2388
Vesanoid Capsules . . . 2823

AK-CIDE (Canada)
PREDNISOLONE ACETATE/SULFACETAMIDE SODIUM
Blephamide Ophthalmic Ointment . . . 563
Blephamide Ophthalmic Suspension . . . 564

AK-CON (Canada)
NAPHAZOLINE HYDROCHLORIDE
Albalon Ophthalmic Solution . . . ⊙216

AK-DEX (Canada)
DEXAMETHASONE SODIUM PHOSPHATE
Decadron Phosphate Injection . . . 1931

AK-FLUOR (Canada)
FLUORESCEIN SODIUM
Fluorescite Injection . . . ⊙207

AKILEN (Hong Kong, Malaysia)
VERAPAMIL HYDROCHLORIDE
Covera-HS Tablets . . . 3135
Verelan PM Capsules . . . 3120

AKNE CORDES (Austria, Germany)
ERYTHROMYCIN
Ery-Tab Tablets . . . 447
Erythromycin Base Filmtab Tablets . . . 454
Erythromycin Delayed-Release Capsules, USP . . . 456
PCE Dispertab Tablets . . . 510

AKNE-AID-LOTION MILD (Germany)
BENZOYL PEROXIDE
Brevoxyl-4 Creamy Wash . . . 3212
Brevoxyl-4 Gel . . . 3211
Brevoxyl-8 Creamy Wash . . . 3212
Brevoxyl-8 Gel . . . 3211
Triaz Cleanser . . . 1864
Triaz Gel . . . 1864

AKNECIDE (Czech Republic)
BENZOYL PEROXIDE
Brevoxyl-4 Creamy Wash . . . 3212
Brevoxyl-4 Gel . . . 3211
Brevoxyl-8 Creamy Wash . . . 3212
Brevoxyl-8 Gel . . . 3211
Triaz Cleanser . . . 1864
Triaz Gel . . . 1864

AKNECOLOR (Czech Republic)
CLOTRIMAZOLE
Lotrimin Cream . . . 3053
Lotrimin Lotion 1% . . . 3053
Lotrimin Topical Solution 1% . . . 3053

AKNEDERM ERY (Germany)
ERYTHROMYCIN
Ery-Tab Tablets . . . 447
Erythromycin Base Filmtab Tablets . . . 454
Erythromycin Delayed-Release Capsules, USP . . . 456
PCE Dispertab Tablets . . . 510

AKNEDERM OXID (Germany)
BENZOYL PEROXIDE
Brevoxyl-4 Creamy Wash . . . 3212
Brevoxyl-4 Gel . . . 3211
Brevoxyl-8 Creamy Wash . . . 3212
Brevoxyl-8 Gel . . . 3211
Triaz Cleanser . . . 1864
Triaz Gel . . . 1864

AKNEFUG (Czech Republic)
ESTRADIOL
Climara Transdermal System . . . 795
Vivelle Transdermal System . . . 2288
Vivelle-Dot Transdermal System . . . 2293

AKNEFUG ISO (Germany)
ISOTRETINOIN
Accutane Capsules 2740

AKNEFUG-EL (Czech Republic, Germany, Hungary)
ERYTHROMYCIN
Ery-Tab Tablets 447
Erythromycin Base Filmtab Tablets. 454
Erythromycin Delayed-Release Capsules, USP 456
PCE Dispertab Tablets 510

AKNEFUG-OXID (Czech Republic, Germany, Hungary)
BENZOYL PEROXIDE
Brevoxyl-4 Creamy Wash. 3212
Brevoxyl-4 Gel 3211
Brevoxyl-8 Creamy Wash. 3212
Brevoxyl-8 Gel 3211
Triaz Cleanser 1864
Triaz Gel. 1864

AKNEMAGO (Germany)
ERYTHROMYCIN
Ery-Tab Tablets 447
Erythromycin Base Filmtab Tablets. 454
Erythromycin Delayed-Release Capsules, USP 456
PCE Dispertab Tablets 510

AKNEMYCIN (Austria, Belgium, Czech Republic, Germany, Hong Kong, Hungary, Israel, Malaysia, Singapore, Switzerland, The Netherlands)
ERYTHROMYCIN
Ery-Tab Tablets 447
Erythromycin Base Filmtab Tablets. 454
Erythromycin Delayed-Release Capsules, USP 456
PCE Dispertab Tablets 510

AKNE-MYCIN (Portugal)
ERYTHROMYCIN
Ery-Tab Tablets 447
Erythromycin Base Filmtab Tablets. 454
Erythromycin Delayed-Release Capsules, USP 456
PCE Dispertab Tablets 510

AKNEMYCIN PLUS (Germany, Israel, Malaysia, Singapore, United Kingdom)
ERYTHROMYCIN
Ery-Tab Tablets 447
Erythromycin Base Filmtab Tablets. 454
Erythromycin Delayed-Release Capsules, USP 456
PCE Dispertab Tablets 510

AKNENORMIN (Germany)
ISOTRETINOIN
Accutane Capsules 2740

AKNEROXID (Austria, Belgium, Czech Republic, Germany, Hungary, Malaysia, Singapore, Switzerland, The Netherlands)
BENZOYL PEROXIDE
Brevoxyl-4 Creamy Wash. 3212
Brevoxyl-4 Gel 3211
Brevoxyl-8 Creamy Wash. 3212
Brevoxyl-8 Gel 3211
Triaz Cleanser 1864
Triaz Gel. 1864

AKNESIL (Greece)
ISOTRETINOIN
Accutane Capsules 2740

AKNEX (Switzerland)
BENZOYL PEROXIDE
Brevoxyl-4 Creamy Wash. 3212
Brevoxyl-4 Gel 3211
Brevoxyl-8 Creamy Wash. 3212
Brevoxyl-8 Gel 3211
Triaz Cleanser 1864
Triaz Gel. 1864

AKNILOX (Switzerland)
ERYTHROMYCIN
Ery-Tab Tablets 447
Erythromycin Base Filmtab Tablets. 454
Erythromycin Delayed-Release Capsules, USP 456
PCE Dispertab Tablets 510

AKNIN (Germany)
ERYTHROMYCIN
Ery-Tab Tablets 447
Erythromycin Base Filmtab Tablets. 454
Erythromycin Delayed-Release Capsules, USP 456
PCE Dispertab Tablets 510

AKORAZOL (Mexico)
KETOCONAZOLE
Nizoral 2% Shampoo 1838

AKRATOL (Greece)
NABUMETONE
Relafen Tablets. 1523

AK-SULF (Canada)
SULFACETAMIDE SODIUM
Klaron Lotion 10%. 1050

AKTIOSAN (Argentina)
DICLOFENAC SODIUM
Voltaren Tablets 2298
Voltaren-XR Tablets 2301

AKUDOL (Italy)
NAPROXEN SODIUM
Anaprox DS Tablets 2769
Anaprox Tablets 2769

ALACOR (Denmark)
ENALAPRIL MALEATE
Vasotec I.V. Injection 2076

ALAGER (Argentina)
AZELASTINE HYDROCHLORIDE
Astelin Nasal Spray 1876

ALAMIL (Brazil)
TERBINAFINE HYDROCHLORIDE
Lamisil Tablets 2226

ALANDIEM (Portugal)
DILTIAZEM HYDROCHLORIDE
Cardizem LA Extended Release Tablets. . . 1699
Tiazac Capsules 1204

ALAPREN (South Africa)
ENALAPRIL MALEATE
Vasotec I.V. Injection 2076

ALAPRIL (Austria, Italy)
ENALAPRIL MALEATE
Vasotec I.V. Injection 2076

ALBA-3 (Brazil)
ALBENDAZOLE
Albenza Tablets. 1310

ALBALON (Australia, Belgium, Canada, Hong Kong, Irish Republic, Malaysia, New Zealand, South Africa, Switzerland, Thailand)
NAPHAZOLINE HYDROCHLORIDE
Albalon Ophthalmic Solution . . . . ⊙216

ALBALON LIQUIFILM (The Netherlands)
NAPHAZOLINE HYDROCHLORIDE
Albalon Ophthalmic Solution . . . . ⊙216

ALBALON-A (Australia)
NAPHAZOLINE HYDROCHLORIDE
Albalon Ophthalmic Solution . . . . ⊙216

ALBASOL (Chile)
NAPHAZOLINE HYDROCHLORIDE
Albalon Ophthalmic Solution . . . . ⊙216

ALBATEL (Thailand)
ALBENDAZOLE
Albenza Tablets. 1310

ALBEN (Brazil, Thailand)
ALBENDAZOLE
Albenza Tablets. 1310

ALBENDA (Thailand, United Arab Emirates)
ALBENDAZOLE
Albenza Tablets. 1310

ALBENDOL (Malaysia)
ALBENDAZOLE
Albenza Tablets. 1310

ALBENDROX (Brazil)
ALBENDAZOLE
Albenza Tablets. 1310

ALBENDY (Brazil)
ALBENDAZOLE
Albenza Tablets. 1310

ALBENSIL (Mexico)
ALBENDAZOLE
Albenza Tablets. 1310

ALBENTEL (Brazil)
ALBENDAZOLE
Albenza Tablets. 1310

ALBENZONIL (Brazil)
ALBENDAZOLE
Albenza Tablets. 1310

ALBEOLER (Chile)
FLUTICASONE PROPIONATE
Cutivate Cream. 1381
Cutivate Ointment 1384
Flonase Nasal Spray 1412

ALBESINE BIOTIC (Argentina)
AMOXICILLIN
Amoxil Pediatric Drops for Oral Suspension. 1315
Amoxil Tablets 1315

ALBEZOLE (India)
ALBENDAZOLE
Albenza Tablets. 1310

ALBICAR (Argentina)
LEVOCARNITINE
Carnitor Injection. 3185
Carnitor Tablets and Oral Solution 3187

ALBICORT (Belgium, The Netherlands)
TRIAMCINOLONE ACETONIDE
Azmacort Inhalation Aerosol. 1701
Nasacort AQ Nasal Spray 2937

ALBISTIN (Brazil)
NYSTATIN
Nystop Topical Powder USP. 2490

ALBORAL (Mexico)
DIAZEPAM
Diastat Rectal Delivery System 3344
Valium Tablets 2822

ALBUCID (Germany, India, South Africa, United Kingdom)
SULFACETAMIDE SODIUM
Klaron Lotion 10%. 1050

ALCATEX (Mexico)
CIMETIDINE
Tagamet Tablets 1547

ALCIS (Spain)
ESTRADIOL
Climara Transdermal System 795
Vivelle Transdermal System 2288
Vivelle-Dot Transdermal System 2293

ALCOMICIN (Belgium, Canada, Spain)
GENTAMICIN SULFATE
Garamycin Injectable 3028
Genoptic Sterile Ophthalmic Solution . . . . ⊙227

ALCOPHYLLIN (South Africa)
THEOPHYLLINE
Uniphyl Tablets 2708

ALDA (Thailand)
ALBENDAZOLE
Albenza Tablets. 1310

ALDAR (Mexico)
NIFEDIPINE
Adalat CC Tablets 2978

ALDARA (Argentina, Australia, Belgium, Canada, Chile, Czech Republic, Denmark, Finland, France, Germany, Greece, Hong Kong, Irish Republic, Israel, Italy, Malaysia, Mexico, New Zealand, Norway, Singapore, South Africa, Spain, Sweden, Switzerland, Thailand, The Netherlands, United Kingdom)
IMIQUIMOD
Aldara Cream, 5% 1814

ALDARONE (India)
AMIODARONE HYDROCHLORIDE
Pacerone Tablets 3337

ALDAZINE (Australia, New Zealand)
THIORIDAZINE HYDROCHLORIDE
Thioridazine Hydrochloride Tablets 2122

ALDIC (Thailand)
FUROSEMIDE
Furosemide Tablets 2117

ALDIPIN (Switzerland)
NIFEDIPINE
Adalat CC Tablets 2978

ALDIZEM (Czech Republic)
DILTIAZEM HYDROCHLORIDE
Cardizem LA Extended Release Tablets. . . 1699
Tiazac Capsules 1204

ALDOACNE (Spain)
BENZOYL PEROXIDE
Brevoxyl-4 Creamy Wash. 3212
Brevoxyl-4 Gel 3211
Brevoxyl-8 Creamy Wash. 3212
Brevoxyl-8 Gel 3211
Triaz Cleanser 1864
Triaz Gel. 1864

ALDOCUMAR (Spain)
WARFARIN SODIUM
Coumadin Tablets 932
Coumadin for Injection 932

ALDORETIC (Portugal)
AMILORIDE HYDROCHLORIDE/HYDROCHLOROTHIAZIDE
Moduretic Tablets 2003

ALDORIL (Canada)
HYDROCHLOROTHIAZIDE/METHYLDOPA
Aldoril Tablets. 1884

ALDORON NF (Argentina)
DICLOFENAC SODIUM
Voltaren Tablets 2298
Voltaren-XR Tablets 2301

ALDOTRIDE (Italy)
HYDROCHLOROTHIAZIDE/METHYLDOPA
Aldoril Tablets. 1884

ALDROX (Chile)
ALENDRONATE SODIUM
Fosamax Tablets 1949

ALENATO (Argentina)
ALENDRONATE SODIUM
Fosamax Tablets. 1949

ALENBIT (Greece)
NORFLOXACIN
Noroxin Tablets. 2009

ALENDIL (Brazil)
ALENDRONATE SODIUM
Fosamax Tablets. 1949

ALENDROS (Italy)
ALENDRONATE SODIUM
Fosamax Tablets. 1949

ALENSTRAN (Greece)
CETIRIZINE HYDROCHLORIDE
Zyrtec Syrup 2589
Zyrtec Tablets 2589

ALERCORTIL (Argentina)
HYDROCORTISONE
Hydrocortone Tablets 1963

ALERDUAL (France)
AZELASTINE HYDROCHLORIDE
Astelin Nasal Spray 1876

ALERFEDINE (Argentina)
FEXOFENADINE HYDROCHLORIDE
Allegra Capsules 2857

ALERGI (Argentina)
DEXAMETHASONE
Decadron Tablets 1929

ALERGIDERM (Brazil)
PROMETHAZINE HYDROCHLORIDE
Phenergan Suppositories. 3438
Phenergan Tablets 3438

ALERID (Czech Republic, Germany, India, Sweden)
CETIRIZINE HYDROCHLORIDE
Zyrtec Syrup 2589
Zyrtec Tablets 2589

ALERION (Argentina)
CLONAZEPAM
Klonopin Tablets 2782

ALERLISIN (Spain)
CETIRIZINE HYDROCHLORIDE
Zyrtec Syrup 2589
Zyrtec Tablets 2589

ALERNEX (India)
FEXOFENADINE HYDROCHLORIDE
Allegra Capsules 2857

ALERTEC (Canada)
MODAFINIL
Provigil Tablets 1002

ALERTOP (Chile)
CETIRIZINE HYDROCHLORIDE
Zyrtec Syrup 2589
Zyrtec Tablets 2589

ALETIR (Brazil)
CETIRIZINE HYDROCHLORIDE
Zyrtec Syrup 2589
Zyrtec Tablets 2589

ALEVE (Argentina, Australia, Austria, Belgium, Czech Republic, France, Germany, Hungary, Italy, South Africa, Spain, Switzerland, The Netherlands)
NAPROXEN SODIUM
Anaprox DS Tablets 2769
Anaprox Tablets 2769

ALEXIA (Chile)
FEXOFENADINE HYDROCHLORIDE
Allegra Capsules 2857

ALEXIN (Portugal)
LANSOPRAZOLE
Prevacid Delayed-Release Capsules 3268

ALFACORT (Argentina, United Arab Emirates)
HYDROCORTISONE
Hydrocortone Tablets 1963

ALFAKEN (Mexico)
LISINOPRIL
Prinivil Tablets 2029
Zestril Tablets 704

ALFAPROST (Spain)
TERAZOSIN HYDROCHLORIDE
Hytrin Capsules 469

ALFASIN (Brazil)
FINASTERIDE
Propecia Tablets 2036
Proscar Tablets 2040

ALFASON (Germany)
HYDROCORTISONE BUTYRATE
Locoid Cream 1138
Locoid Lipocream Cream 1138
Locoid Ointment 1138
Locoid Topical Solution 1138

ALFAZOL (Mexico)
ALBENDAZOLE
Albenza Tablets 1310

ALFEROS (Spain)
AZELASTINE HYDROCHLORIDE
Astelin Nasal Spray 1876

ALFIN (Chile)
SILDENAFIL CITRATE
Viagra Tablets 2552

ALFUCA (Thailand)
ALBENDAZOLE
Albenza Tablets 1310

ALGEDOL (Argentina)
MORPHINE SULFATE
Kadian Capsules 572
MS Contin Tablets 2703

ALGEFIT (Austria)
DICLOFENAC SODIUM
Voltaren Tablets 2298
Voltaren-XR Tablets 2301

ALGICORTIS (Italy)
HYDROCORTISONE
Hydrocortone Tablets 1963

ALGIDERM (Argentina)
ERYTHROMYCIN
Ery-Tab Tablets 447
Erythromycin Base Filmtab Tablets 454
Erythromycin Delayed-Release Capsules, USP 456
PCE Dispertab Tablets 510

ALGIOPRUX (Argentina)
NAPROXEN
EC-Naprosyn Delayed-Release Tablets 2769
Naprosyn Suspension 2769
Naprosyn Tablets 2769

ALGOCETIL (Italy)
SULINDAC
Clinoril Tablets 1899

ALGONAPRIL (Italy)
NAPROXEN
EC-Naprosyn Delayed-Release Tablets 2769
Naprosyn Suspension 2769
Naprosyn Tablets 2769

ALGOSENAC (Italy)
DICLOFENAC SODIUM
Voltaren Tablets 2298
Voltaren-XR Tablets 2301

ALGYBREX (Argentina)
CELECOXIB
Celebrex Capsules 3130

ALI VEG (Spain)
CIMETIDINE
Tagamet Tablets 1547

ALIB (Brazil)
ALBENDAZOLE
Albenza Tablets 1310

ALIDASE (Argentina)
NAPROXEN
EC-Naprosyn Delayed-Release Tablets 2769
Naprosyn Suspension 2769
Naprosyn Tablets 2769

ALIFLUS (Italy)
SALMETEROL XINAFOATE
Serevent Diskus 1540

ALIN (Brazil)
ALBENDAZOLE
Albenza Tablets 1310

ALINOR (Norway, Sweden)
ATENOLOL
Tenormin I.V. Injection 698

ALIPASE (France)
PANCRELIPASE
Ultrase Capsules 735
Ultrase MT Capsules 736

ALISEUM (Italy)
DIAZEPAM
Diastat Rectal Delivery System 3344
Valium Tablets 2822

ALIVIOMAS (Spain)
NAPROXEN
EC-Naprosyn Delayed-Release Tablets 2769
Naprosyn Suspension 2769
Naprosyn Tablets 2769

ALKADIL (Czech Republic)
CAPTOPRIL
Captopril Tablets 2114

ALKALIT (Czech Republic)
POTASSIUM CITRATE
Urocit-K Tablets 2109

ALKASTOM (Greece)
CIMETIDINE
Tagamet Tablets 1547

ALKERAN (Australia, Austria, Belgium, Brazil, Canada, Chile, Czech Republic, Denmark, Finland, France, Germany, Hong Kong, India, Irish Republic, Israel, Italy, Malaysia, Mexico, New Zealand, Norway, Portugal, Singapore, South Africa, Switzerland, Thailand, The Netherlands)
MELPHALAN
Alkeran Tablets 977
Alkeran for Injection 976

ALKERANA (Argentina)
MELPHALAN
Alkeran Tablets 977
Alkeran for Injection 976

ALL CLEAR (Hong Kong)
NAPHAZOLINE HYDROCHLORIDE
Albalon Ophthalmic Solution ⊙216

ALLECET (South Africa)
CETIRIZINE HYDROCHLORIDE
Zyrtec Syrup 2589
Zyrtec Tablets 2589

ALLEGRA (Argentina, Brazil, Canada, Chile, India, Mexico)
FEXOFENADINE HYDROCHLORIDE
Allegra Capsules 2857

ALLEGRA-D (Canada, Chile)
FEXOFENADINE HYDROCHLORIDE/PSEUDOEPHEDRINE HYDROCHLORIDE
Allegra-D 12 Hour Extended-Release Tablets 2860

ALLEGRO (Israel)
FLUTICASONE PROPIONATE
Cutivate Cream 1381
Cutivate Ointment 1384
Flonase Nasal Spray 1412

ALLER-EZE (United Kingdom)
AZELASTINE HYDROCHLORIDE
Astelin Nasal Spray 1876

ALLERFEN (Italy)
PROMETHAZINE HYDROCHLORIDE
Phenergan Suppositories 3438
Phenergan Tablets 3438

ALLERGODIL (Argentina, Austria, Belgium, Chile, Czech Republic, Denmark, France, Germany, Hungary, Italy, Portugal, Switzerland, The Netherlands)
AZELASTINE HYDROCHLORIDE
Astelin Nasal Spray 1876

ALLERGY DROPS (Canada)
NAPHAZOLINE HYDROCHLORIDE
Albalon Ophthalmic Solution ⊙216

ALLERGY RELIEF (Canada)
CETIRIZINE HYDROCHLORIDE
Zyrtec Syrup 2589
Zyrtec Tablets 2589

ALLERMAX (Australia)
MOMETASONE FUROATE
Elocon Cream 0.1% 3019
Elocon Lotion 0.1% 3020
Elocon Ointment 0.1% 3021
Nasonex Nasal Spray 3058

ALLERTEC (Russia, Singapore)
CETIRIZINE HYDROCHLORIDE
Zyrtec Syrup 2589
Zyrtec Tablets 2589

ALLVORAN (Germany)
DICLOFENAC SODIUM
Voltaren Tablets 2298
Voltaren-XR Tablets 2301

ALMARION (Thailand)
THEOPHYLLINE
Uniphyl Tablets 2708

ALMARYTM (Italy)
FLECAINIDE ACETATE
Tambocor Tablets 1824

ALMIRAL (Hong Kong)
DICLOFENAC SODIUM
Voltaren Tablets 2298
Voltaren-XR Tablets 2301

ALMODAN (United Kingdom)
AMOXICILLIN
Amoxil Pediatric Drops for Oral Suspension 1315
Amoxil Tablets 1315

ALNA (Austria, Germany)
TAMSULOSIN HYDROCHLORIDE
Flomax Capsules 881

ALNOK (Denmark)
CETIRIZINE HYDROCHLORIDE
Zyrtec Syrup 2589
Zyrtec Tablets 2589

ALONET (Singapore)
ATENOLOL
Tenormin I.V. Injection 698

ALOPRESIN (Spain)
CAPTOPRIL
Captopril Tablets 2114

ALPERTAN (Argentina)
VALSARTAN
Diovan Tablets 2191

ALPHADERM (Belgium, United Kingdom)
HYDROCORTISONE
Hydrocortone Tablets 1963

ALPHADINAL (Mexico)
NAPHAZOLINE HYDROCHLORIDE
Albalon Ophthalmic Solution ⊙216

ALPHADINE (Greece)
RANITIDINE HYDROCHLORIDE
Zantac 25 EFFERdose Tablets 1597
Zantac 150 EFFERdose Tablets 1597
Zantac 150 Tablets 1597
Zantac 300 Tablets 1597
Zantac Injection 1593
Zantac Injection Premixed 1593
Zantac Syrup 1597

ALPHA-LAC (Canada)
LACTULOSE
Kristalose for Oral Solution 2149

ALPHAPRIL (Australia)
ENALAPRIL MALEATE
Vasotec I.V. Injection 2076

ALPOXEN (Denmark, Finland, Norway, Sweden)
NAPROXEN
EC-Naprosyn Delayed-Release Tablets 2769
Naprosyn Suspension 2769
Naprosyn Tablets 2769

ALPROFEN (Spain)
NAPROXEN
EC-Naprosyn Delayed-Release Tablets 2769
Naprosyn Suspension 2769
Naprosyn Tablets 2769

ALPROSTAN (Czech Republic)
ALPROSTADIL
Edex Injection 3103

ALPROSTAPINT (Austria, Czech Republic, Hungary, Israel)
ALPROSTADIL
Edex Injection 3103

ALQUEN (Spain)
RANITIDINE HYDROCHLORIDE
Zantac 25 EFFERdose Tablets 1597
Zantac 150 EFFERdose Tablets 1597
Zantac 150 Tablets 1597
Zantac 300 Tablets 1597
Zantac Injection 1593
Zantac Injection Premixed 1593
Zantac Syrup 1597

ALSARTAN (India)
LOSARTAN POTASSIUM
Cozaar Tablets 1913

ALSARTAN-AM (India)
LOSARTAN POTASSIUM
Cozaar Tablets 1913

ALSARTAN-H (India)
LOSARTAN POTASSIUM
Cozaar Tablets 1913

ALSERINE (Thailand)
CIMETIDINE
Tagamet Tablets 1547

ALSIDEXTEN (Mexico)
DICLOFENAC SODIUM
Voltaren Tablets 2298
Voltaren-XR Tablets 2301

ALSUCRAL (Finland, Malaysia, Singapore)
SUCRALFATE
Carafate Suspension 727
Carafate Tablets 728

ALTACE (Canada)
RAMIPRIL
Altace Capsules 1673

ALTACEF (India)
CEFUROXIME AXETIL
Ceftin Tablets 1369
Ceftin for Oral Suspension 1369

ALTEMOL (Mexico)
INTERFERON ALFA-N3
Alferon N Injection 1640

ALTEN (Hong Kong, Malaysia, Singapore)
TRETINOIN
Avita Cream 2136
Avita Gel 2138
Renova 0.05% Cream 2387
Retin-A Micro 0.1%/0.04% 2388
Vesanoid Capsules 2823

ALTERCOR (The Netherlands)
SIMVASTATIN
Zocor Tablets 2078

ALTERGEN (Italy)
SODIUM HYALURONATE
Hyalgan Solution 2917

ALTER-H2 (Mexico)
RANITIDINE HYDROCHLORIDE
Zantac 25 EFFERdose Tablets 1597
Zantac 150 EFFERdose Tablets 1597
Zantac 150 Tablets 1597
Zantac 300 Tablets 1597
Zantac Injection 1593
Zantac Injection Premixed 1593
Zantac Syrup 1597

ALTIAZEM (Hong Kong, Italy, Singapore, Thailand)
DILTIAZEM HYDROCHLORIDE
Cardizem LA Extended Release Tablets 1699
Tiazac Capsules 1204

ALTICORT (Chile)
CLOBETASOL PROPIONATE
Temovate Cream 1549
Temovate E Emollient 1552
Temovate Gel 1550
Temovate Ointment 1549
Temovate Scalp Application 1551

ALTI-MPA (Canada)
MEDROXYPROGESTERONE ACETATE
Depo-Medrol Single-Dose Vial 2617

ALTOCEL (France)
LOPERAMIDE HYDROCHLORIDE
Imodium Capsules 1834

ALTOSONE (Italy)
MOMETASONE FUROATE
Elocon Cream 0.1% 3019
Elocon Lotion 0.1% 3020
Elocon Ointment 0.1% 3021
Nasonex Nasal Spray 3058

ALTRAMET (Hong Kong)
CIMETIDINE
Tagamet Tablets 1547

ALTRAZ (India)
ANASTROZOLE
Arimidex Tablets 665

ALTRULINE (Mexico)
SERTRALINE HYDROCHLORIDE
Zoloft Tablets 2581

ALUDROX AC (Argentina)
RANITIDINE HYDROCHLORIDE
Zantac 25 EFFERdose Tablets 1597
Zantac 150 EFFERdose Tablets 1597
Zantac 150 Tablets 1597
Zantac 300 Tablets 1597
Zantac Injection 1593
Zantac Injection Premixed 1593
Zantac Syrup 1597

ALUPRAM (United Kingdom)
DIAZEPAM
Diastat Rectal Delivery System 3344
Valium Tablets 2822

ALUSULIN (Hungary)
SUCRALFATE
Carafate Suspension 727
Carafate Tablets 728

ALUTAN (Switzerland)
CITALOPRAM HYDROBROMIDE
Celexa Tablets 1177

ALUZINE (United Kingdom)
FUROSEMIDE
Furosemide Tablets 2117

ALVENT (Brazil)
IPRATROPIUM BROMIDE
Atrovent Inhalation Solution 868
Atrovent Nasal Spray 0.03% 869
Atrovent Nasal Spray 0.06% 870

ALVIDINA (Mexico)
RANITIDINE HYDROCHLORIDE
Zantac 25 EFFERdose Tablets 1597
Zantac 150 EFFERdose Tablets 1597
Zantac 150 Tablets 1597
Zantac 300 Tablets 1597
Zantac Injection 1593
Zantac Injection Premixed 1593
Zantac Syrup 1597

ALXEN (Mexico)
NAPROXEN
EC-Naprosyn Delayed-Release Tablets 2769
Naprosyn Suspension 2769
Naprosyn Tablets 2769

ALZAIMAX (Argentina)
DONEPEZIL HYDROCHLORIDE
Aricept Tablets 1086

ALZEN (Portugal)
QUETIAPINE FUMARATE
Seroquel Tablets 691

ALZENTAL (Singapore)
ALBENDAZOLE
Albenza Tablets 1310

ALZOL (Thailand)
ALBENDAZOLE
Albenza Tablets 1310

ALZOMED-F (Mexico)
BENZONATATE
Tessalon Perles 1202

ALZYR (Finland)
CETIRIZINE HYDROCHLORIDE
Zyrtec Syrup 2589
Zyrtec Tablets 2589

ALZYTEC (Singapore)
CETIRIZINE HYDROCHLORIDE
Zyrtec Syrup 2589
Zyrtec Tablets 2589

AMANTA (Germany)
AMANTADINE HYDROCHLORIDE
Symmetrel Syrup 1115
Symmetrel Tablets 1115

AMANTAGAMMA (Germany)
AMANTADINE HYDROCHLORIDE
Symmetrel Syrup 1115
Symmetrel Tablets 1115

AMANTAN (Belgium)
AMANTADINE HYDROCHLORIDE
Symmetrel Syrup 1115
Symmetrel Tablets 1115

AMAREL (France)
GLIMEPIRIDE
Amaryl Tablets 2864

AMARYL (Argentina, Australia, Austria, Brazil, Canada, Chile, Czech Republic, Denmark, Finland, Germany, Hong Kong, Hungary, India, Irish Republic, Israel, Italy, Malaysia, Mexico, Norway, Portugal, Russia, Singapore, South Africa, Spain, Sweden, Switzerland, Thailand, The Netherlands, United Kingdom)
GLIMEPIRIDE
Amaryl Tablets 2864

AMARYLLE (Belgium)
GLIMEPIRIDE
Amaryl Tablets 2864

AMATINE (Canada)
MIDODRINE HYDROCHLORIDE
ProAmatine Tablets 3183

AMBAMIDA (Argentina)
ERYTHROMYCIN
Ery-Tab Tablets 447
Erythromycin Base Filmtab Tablets 454
Erythromycin Delayed-Release Capsules, USP 456
PCE Dispertab Tablets 510

AMBERIN (Sweden)
HYDROCORTISONE
Hydrocortone Tablets 1963

AMBONEURAL (Austria)
SELEGILINE HYDROCHLORIDE
Eldepryl Capsules 3209

AMBRAL (South Africa)
METRONIDAZOLE
MetroGel-Vaginal Gel 1822
Noritate Cream, 1% 1051

AMCOLD (India)
CETIRIZINE HYDROCHLORIDE
Zyrtec Syrup 2589
Zyrtec Tablets 2589

AMERGE (Canada)
NARATRIPTAN HYDROCHLORIDE
Amerge Tablets 1312

AMERIDE (Spain)
AMILORIDE HYDROCHLORIDE/HYDROCHLOROTHIAZIDE
Moduretic Tablets 2003

AMFAMOX (Australia)
FAMOTIDINE
Pepcid Injection 2017
Pepcid Injection Premixed 2017
Pepcid Tablets 2014
Pepcid for Oral Suspension 2014

AMIAS (United Kingdom)
CANDESARTAN CILEXETIL
Atacand Tablets 634

AMICEL (Italy)
ECONAZOLE NITRATE
Spectazole Cream 2390

AMICLARAN (Czech Republic)
AMILORIDE HYDROCHLORIDE
Midamor Tablets 2000

AMICLOTON (Czech Republic)
AMILORIDE HYDROCHLORIDE
Midamor Tablets 2000

AMICROBIN (Spain)
NORFLOXACIN
Noroxin Tablets 2009

AMIDAL (Australia)
AMILORIDE HYDROCHLORIDE
Midamor Tablets 2000

AMIDOX (United Kingdom)
AMIODARONE HYDROCHLORIDE
Pacerone Tablets 3337

AMIDURET (Germany)
AMILORIDE HYDROCHLORIDE/HYDROCHLOROTHIAZIDE
Moduretic Tablets 2003

AMI-HYDROTRIDE (Malaysia)
AMILORIDE HYDROCHLORIDE
Midamor Tablets 2000

AMIKAL (Denmark, Sweden)
AMILORIDE HYDROCHLORIDE
Midamor Tablets 2000

AMILAMONT (United Kingdom)
AMILORIDE HYDROCHLORIDE
Midamor Tablets 2000

AMILCO (Denmark, Hong Kong, Irish Republic)
AMILORIDE HYDROCHLORIDE/HYDROCHLOROTHIAZIDE
Moduretic Tablets 2003

AMIL-CO (United Kingdom)
AMILORIDE HYDROCHLORIDE/HYDROCHLOROTHIAZIDE
Moduretic Tablets 2003

AMILENE (Chile)
ONDANSETRON
Zofran ODT Orally Disintegrating Tablets . . 1613

AMILIDE (Thailand)
AMILORIDE HYDROCHLORIDE/HYDROCHLOROTHIAZIDE
Moduretic Tablets 2003

AMILMAXCO (United Kingdom)
AMILORIDE HYDROCHLORIDE/HYDROCHLOROTHIAZIDE
Moduretic Tablets 2003

AMILO-BASAN (Switzerland)
AMILORIDE HYDROCHLORIDE/HYDROCHLOROTHIAZIDE
Moduretic Tablets 2003

AMILOCOMP BETA (Germany)
AMILORIDE HYDROCHLORIDE/HYDROCHLOROTHIAZIDE
Moduretic Tablets 2003

AMILOFERM (Sweden)
AMILORIDE HYDROCHLORIDE/HYDROCHLOROTHIAZIDE
Moduretic Tablets 2003

AMILO-OPT (Germany)
AMILORIDE HYDROCHLORIDE/HYDROCHLOROTHIAZIDE
Moduretic Tablets 2003

AMILORAL/HCT (Austria)
AMILORIDE HYDROCHLORIDE/HYDROCHLOROTHIAZIDE
Moduretic Tablets 2003

AMILORETIC (South Africa)
AMILORIDE HYDROCHLORIDE/HYDROCHLOROTHIAZIDE
Moduretic Tablets 2003

AMILORETIK (Austria, Germany)
AMILORIDE HYDROCHLORIDE/HYDROCHLOROTHIAZIDE
Moduretic Tablets 2003

AMILORID COMP (Austria, Germany, Switzerland)
AMILORIDE HYDROCHLORIDE/HYDROCHLOROTHIAZIDE
Moduretic Tablets 2003

AMILORID/HCT (Austria, Czech Republic)
AMILORIDE HYDROCHLORIDE/HYDROCHLOROTHIAZIDE
Moduretic Tablets 2003

AMILORIDE COMPOSTO (Portugal)
AMILORIDE HYDROCHLORIDE/HYDROCHLOROTHIAZIDE
Moduretic Tablets 2003

AMILORIDE/HCTZ (Switzerland)
AMILORIDE HYDROCHLORIDE
Midamor Tablets 2000

AMILOSPARE (United Kingdom)
AMILORIDE HYDROCHLORIDE
Midamor Tablets 2000

AMILOSTAD HCT (Austria)
AMILORIDE HYDROCHLORIDE/HYDROCHLOROTHIAZIDE
Moduretic Tablets 2003

AMILOTHIAZID (Germany)
AMILORIDE HYDROCHLORIDE/HYDROCHLOROTHIAZIDE
Moduretic Tablets 2003

AMILOZID (Germany)
AMILORIDE HYDROCHLORIDE/HYDROCHLOROTHIAZIDE
Moduretic Tablets 2003

AMILOZID-B (Hungary)
AMILORIDE HYDROCHLORIDE
Midamor Tablets 2000

AMIMOX (Norway)
AMOXICILLIN
Amoxil Pediatric Drops for Oral Suspension 1315
Amoxil Tablets 1315

AMINDAN (Germany)
SELEGILINE HYDROCHLORIDE
Eldepryl Capsules 3209

AMINOFILIN (Argentina)
THEOPHYLLINE
Uniphyl Tablets 2708

AMINOMAL (Italy)
THEOPHYLLINE
Uniphyl Tablets 2708

AMINOMUX (Argentina)
PAMIDRONATE DISODIUM
Aredia for Injection 2168

AMIOBAL (Brazil)
AMIODARONE HYDROCHLORIDE
Pacerone Tablets 3337

AMIOBETA (Germany)
AMIODARONE HYDROCHLORIDE
Pacerone Tablets 3337

AMIOD (Germany)
AMIODARONE HYDROCHLORIDE
Pacerone Tablets 3337

AMIODACORE (Israel)
AMIODARONE HYDROCHLORIDE
Pacerone Tablets 3337

AMIODAR (Italy)
AMIODARONE HYDROCHLORIDE
Pacerone Tablets 3337

AMIODAREX (Germany)
AMIODARONE HYDROCHLORIDE
Pacerone Tablets 3337

AMIODURA (Germany)
AMIODARONE HYDROCHLORIDE
Pacerone Tablets 3337

AMIOGAMMA (Germany)
AMIODARONE HYDROCHLORIDE
Pacerone Tablets 3337

AMIOHEXAL (Czech Republic, Germany)
AMIODARONE HYDROCHLORIDE
Pacerone Tablets 3337

AMIOKORDIN (Czech Republic, Hungary)
AMIODARONE HYDROCHLORIDE
Pacerone Tablets 3337

AMIPHOS (India)
AMIFOSTINE
Ethyol for Injection 1869

AMIRETIC (Brazil)
AMILORIDE HYDROCHLORIDE/HYDROCHLOROTHIAZIDE
Moduretic Tablets 2003

AMIRONE (United Arab Emirates)
AMIODARONE HYDROCHLORIDE
Pacerone Tablets 3337

AMITHIAZIDE (Hong Kong)
AMILORIDE HYDROCHLORIDE/HYDROCHLOROTHIAZIDE
Moduretic Tablets 2003

AMITRID (Finland)
AMILORIDE HYDROCHLORIDE/HYDROCHLOROTHIAZIDE
Moduretic Tablets 2003

AMIXEN (Argentina)
AMOXICILLIN
Amoxil Pediatric Drops for Oral Suspension 1315
Amoxil Tablets 1315

AMIXX (Germany)
AMANTADINE HYDROCHLORIDE
Symmetrel Syrup 1115
Symmetrel Tablets 1115

AMIYODAZOL (Mexico)
METRONIDAZOLE
MetroGel-Vaginal Gel 1822
Noritate Cream, 1% 1051

AMIZIDE (Australia, Irish Republic, Malaysia, New Zealand, South Africa)
AMILORIDE HYDROCHLORIDE/HYDROCHLOROTHIAZIDE
Moduretic Tablets 2003

AMMINAC (Thailand)
DICLOFENAC SODIUM
Voltaren Tablets 2298
Voltaren-XR Tablets 2301

AMMI-VOTARA (Thailand)
DICLOFENAC SODIUM
Voltaren Tablets 2298
Voltaren-XR Tablets 2301

AMO VITRAX (Australia, New Zealand, Singapore, South Africa, Sweden, Switzerland, Thailand)
SODIUM HYALURONATE
Hyalgan Solution 2917

AMOBIOTIC (Chile)
AMOXICILLIN
Amoxil Pediatric Drops for Oral Suspension 1315
Amoxil Tablets 1315

AMOFAT (Mexico)
FAMOTIDINE
Pepcid Injection 2017
Pepcid Injection Premixed 2017
Pepcid Tablets 2014
Pepcid for Oral Suspension 2014

AMOLIN (Irish Republic)
ATENOLOL
Tenormin I.V. Injection 698

AMOPEN (United Kingdom)
AMOXICILLIN
Amoxil Pediatric Drops for Oral Suspension 1315
Amoxil Tablets 1315

AMOSPES (Greece)
AMOXICILLIN
Amoxil Pediatric Drops for Oral Suspension 1315
Amoxil Tablets 1315

AMOTEIN (Spain)
METRONIDAZOLE
MetroGel-Vaginal Gel 1822
Noritate Cream, 1% 1051

AMOVAL (Chile)
AMOXICILLIN
Amoxil Pediatric Drops for Oral Suspension 1315
Amoxil Tablets 1315

AMOVAL DUO (Chile)
AMOXICILLIN
Amoxil Pediatric Drops for Oral Suspension 1315
Amoxil Tablets 1315

AMOX (Brazil)
AMOXICILLIN
Amoxil Pediatric Drops for Oral Suspension 1315
Amoxil Tablets 1315

AMOXAPEN (Hong Kong, Singapore)
AMOXICILLIN
Amoxil Pediatric Drops for Oral Suspension 1315
Amoxil Tablets 1315

AMOXCILLIN (Thailand)
AMOXICILLIN
Amoxil Pediatric Drops for Oral Suspension 1315
Amoxil Tablets 1315

AMOX-G (Argentina)
AMOXICILLIN
Amoxil Pediatric Drops for Oral Suspension 1315
Amoxil Tablets 1315

AMOX-G BRONQUIAL (Argentina)
AMOXICILLIN
Amoxil Pediatric Drops for Oral Suspension 1315
Amoxil Tablets 1315

AMOXI (Argentina)
AMOXICILLIN
Amoxil Pediatric Drops for Oral Suspension 1315
Amoxil Tablets 1315

AMOXI RESPIRATORIO (Argentina)
AMOXICILLIN
Amoxil Pediatric Drops for Oral Suspension 1315
Amoxil Tablets 1315

AMOXI-BASAN (Switzerland)
AMOXICILLIN
Amoxil Pediatric Drops for Oral Suspension 1315
Amoxil Tablets 1315

AMOXIBIOCIN (Germany)
AMOXICILLIN
Amoxil Pediatric Drops for Oral Suspension 1315
Amoxil Tablets 1315

AMOXIBIOT (Argentina)
AMOXICILLIN
Amoxil Pediatric Drops for Oral Suspension 1315
Amoxil Tablets 1315

AMOXICINA (Argentina)
AMOXICILLIN
Amoxil Pediatric Drops for Oral Suspension 1315
Amoxil Tablets 1315

AMOXIDAL (Argentina)
AMOXICILLIN
Amoxil Pediatric Drops for Oral Suspension 1315
Amoxil Tablets 1315

AMOXIDENT (United Kingdom)
AMOXICILLIN
Amoxil Pediatric Drops for Oral Suspension 1315
Amoxil Tablets 1315

AMOXIDIL (Brazil)
AMOXICILLIN
Amoxil Pediatric Drops for Oral Suspension 1315
Amoxil Tablets 1315

AMOXIFAR BALSAMICO (Brazil)
AMOXICILLIN
Amoxil Pediatric Drops for Oral Suspension 1315
Amoxil Tablets 1315

AMOXIGRAND (Argentina)
AMOXICILLIN
Amoxil Pediatric Drops for Oral Suspension 1315
Amoxil Tablets 1315

AMOXIGRAND BRONQUIAL (Argentina)
AMOXICILLIN
Amoxil Pediatric Drops for Oral Suspension 1315
Amoxil Tablets 1315

AMOXIGRAND COMPUESTO (Argentina)
AMOXICILLIN
Amoxil Pediatric Drops for Oral Suspension 1315
Amoxil Tablets 1315

AMOXIL (Hong Kong, Singapore)
AMOXICILLIN
Amoxil Pediatric Drops for Oral Suspension 1315
Amoxil Tablets 1315

AMOXINA (Brazil)
AMOXICILLIN
Amoxil Pediatric Drops for Oral Suspension 1315
Amoxil Tablets 1315

AMOXI-PED (Brazil)
AMOXICILLIN
Amoxil Pediatric Drops for Oral Suspension 1315
Amoxil Tablets 1315

AMOXIPOTEN (Argentina)
AMOXICILLIN
Amoxil Pediatric Drops for Oral Suspension 1315
Amoxil Tablets 1315

AMOXITAN (Brazil)
AMOXICILLIN
Amoxil Pediatric Drops for Oral Suspension 1315
Amoxil Tablets 1315

AMOXITENK (Argentina)
AMOXICILLIN
Amoxil Pediatric Drops for Oral Suspension 1315
Amoxil Tablets 1315

AMOXITENK PLUS (Argentina)
AMOXICILLIN
Amoxil Pediatric Drops for Oral Suspension 1315
Amoxil Tablets 1315

AMOXITENK RESPIRATORIO (Argentina)
AMOXICILLIN
Amoxil Pediatric Drops for Oral Suspension 1315
Amoxil Tablets 1315

AMOXIVAN (India)
AMOXICILLIN
Amoxil Pediatric Drops for Oral Suspension 1315
Amoxil Tablets 1315

AMOXOL (Argentina)
AMOXICILLIN
Amoxil Pediatric Drops for Oral Suspension 1315
Amoxil Tablets 1315

AMOXY (Thailand)
AMOXICILLIN
Amoxil Pediatric Drops for Oral Suspension 1315
Amoxil Tablets 1315

AMPINA (Argentina)
NIMODIPINE
Nimotop Capsules 774

AMPLAL (Brazil)
AMOXICILLIN
Amoxil Pediatric Drops for Oral Suspension 1315
Amoxil Tablets 1315

AMPLEXOL (Portugal)
ISOSORBIDE MONONITRATE
Imdur Tablets 3032

AMPLIAR (Argentina)
ATORVASTATIN CALCIUM
Lipitor Tablets 2495

AMPLOMICINA (Brazil)
GENTAMICIN SULFATE
Garamycin Injectable 3028
Genoptic Sterile Ophthalmic Solution . . . . ⊙227

AMPLOZOL (Brazil)
ALBENDAZOLE
Albenza Tablets 1310

AMPRACE (Australia)
ENALAPRIL MALEATE
Vasotec I.V. Injection 2076

AMVISC (Austria, Canada, Israel, Norway, South Africa, Sweden)
SODIUM HYALURONATE
Hyalgan Solution 2917

AMX (Mexico)
AMOXICILLIN
Amoxil Pediatric Drops for Oral Suspension 1315
Amoxil Tablets 1315

AMYBEN (United Kingdom)
AMIODARONE HYDROCHLORIDE
Pacerone Tablets 3337

AMYCIL (Mexico)
MEBENDAZOLE
Vermox Chewable Tablets 1853

AMYCLON (Russia)
CLOTRIMAZOLE
Lotrimin Cream 3053
Lotrimin Lotion 1% 3053
Lotrimin Topical Solution 1% 3053

ANABACT (Irish Republic, Singapore, Thailand, United Kingdom)
METRONIDAZOLE
MetroGel-Vaginal Gel 1822
Noritate Cream, 1% 1051

ANABET (Portugal)
NADOLOL
Nadolol Tablets 2121

ANAEROBEX (Austria)
METRONIDAZOLE
MetroGel-Vaginal Gel 1822
Noritate Cream, 1% 1051

ANAEROBYL (South Africa)
METRONIDAZOLE
MetroGel-Vaginal Gel 1822
Noritate Cream, 1% 1051

ANAEROMET (Belgium, The Netherlands)
METRONIDAZOLE
MetroGel-Vaginal Gel 1822
Noritate Cream, 1% 1051

ANA-FLEX (Brazil)
DICLOFENAC SODIUM
Voltaren Tablets 2298
Voltaren-XR Tablets 2301

ANAFLIN (Mexico)
NAPROXEN
EC-Naprosyn Delayed-Release Tablets 2769
Naprosyn Suspension 2769
Naprosyn Tablets 2769

ANAGREGAL (Italy)
TICLOPIDINE HYDROCHLORIDE
Ticlid Tablets 2813

ANALEPT (Greece)
ENALAPRIL MALEATE
Vasotec I.V. Injection 2076

ANALERGIN (Russia)
CETIRIZINE HYDROCHLORIDE
Zyrtec Syrup 2589
Zyrtec Tablets 2589

ANALERIC (Greece)
DIFLUNISAL
Dolobid Tablets 1937

ANALFIN (Mexico)
MORPHINE SULFATE
Kadian Capsules 572
MS Contin Tablets 2703

ANALPAN (Hong Kong)
DICLOFENAC SODIUM
Voltaren Tablets 2298
Voltaren-XR Tablets 2301

ANAMORPH (Australia)
MORPHINE SULFATE
Kadian Capsules 572
MS Contin Tablets 2703

ANAPOLON (Australia, Canada, South Africa, United Kingdom)
OXYMETHOLONE
Anadrol-50 Tablets 3329

ANAPRIL (Hong Kong, Singapore, Thailand)
ENALAPRIL MALEATE
Vasotec I.V. Injection 2076

ANAPROX (Australia, Canada, Greece, Spain)
NAPROXEN SODIUM
Anaprox DS Tablets 2769
Anaprox Tablets 2769

ANAPSYL (Mexico)
NAPROXEN SODIUM
Anaprox DS Tablets 2769
Anaprox Tablets 2769

ANAPTIVAN (Greece)
CEFUROXIME SODIUM
Zinacef Injection 1604

ANAREX (Malaysia)
ORPHENADRINE CITRATE
Norflex Injection 1824

ANASKEBIR (Argentina)
ANASTROZOLE
Arimidex Tablets 665

ANASTRAZE (Argentina)
ANASTROZOLE
Arimidex Tablets 665

ANATINE (Argentina)
FINASTERIDE
Propecia Tablets 2036
Proscar Tablets 2040

ANAUS (Argentina)
SILDENAFIL CITRATE
Viagra Tablets 2552

ANAX (Singapore)
NAPROXEN SODIUM
Anaprox DS Tablets 2769
Anaprox Tablets 2769

ANCARON (Japan)
AMIODARONE HYDROCHLORIDE
Pacerone Tablets 3337

ANCEF (Canada)
CEFAZOLIN SODIUM
Ancef for Injection 1318

ANCOREN (Portugal)
ATENOLOL
Tenormin I.V. Injection 698

ANCORON (Brazil)
AMIODARONE HYDROCHLORIDE
Pacerone Tablets 3337

ANDAPSIN (Sweden)
SUCRALFATE
Carafate Suspension 727
Carafate Tablets 728

ANDRAXAN (Czech Republic)
FLUTAMIDE
Eulexin Capsules 3023

ANDREGEN (India)
GENTAMICIN SULFATE
Garamycin Injectable 3028
Genoptic Sterile Ophthalmic Solution . . . . ⊙227

ANDRIN (Argentina)
TERAZOSIN HYDROCHLORIDE
Hytrin Capsules 469

ANDROBLOC (Austria)
FLUTAMIDE
Eulexin Capsules 3023

ANDRODOR (Chile)
FLUTAMIDE
Eulexin Capsules 3023

ANDROLIC (Thailand)
OXYMETHOLONE
Anadrol-50 Tablets 3329

ANDROLIP (Brazil)
SIMVASTATIN
Zocor Tablets 2078

ANDROPEL (Argentina)
FINASTERIDE
Propecia Tablets 2036
Proscar Tablets 2040

ANDROSTAT (Irish Republic)
FLUTAMIDE
Eulexin Capsules 3023

ANDROXINON (Argentina)
BICALUTAMIDE
Casodex Tablets 670

ANEMUL MONO (Germany)
DEXAMETHASONE
Decadron Tablets 1929

ANEUROL (Spain)
DIAZEPAM
Diastat Rectal Delivery System 3344
Valium Tablets 2822

ANFENAX (New Zealand, South Africa)
DICLOFENAC SODIUM
Voltaren Tablets 2298
Voltaren-XR Tablets 2301

ANFER (Greece)
NABUMETONE
Relafen Tablets 1523

ANFLAM (United Kingdom)
HYDROCORTISONE
Hydrocortone Tablets 1963

ANFOZAN (Greece)
ETIDRONATE DISODIUM
Didronel Tablets 2693

ANGELIQ (Argentina, South Africa, The Netherlands, United Kingdom)
ESTRADIOL
Climara Transdermal System 795
Vivelle Transdermal System 2288
Vivelle-Dot Transdermal System 2293

ANGEZE (United Kingdom)
ISOSORBIDE MONONITRATE
Imdur Tablets 3032

ANGIACT (Denmark)
DILTIAZEM HYDROCHLORIDE
Cardizem LA Extended Release Tablets . . . 1699
Tiazac Capsules 1204

ANGICONTIN (Denmark)
DILTIAZEM HYDROCHLORIDE
Cardizem LA Extended Release Tablets . . . 1699
Tiazac Capsules 1204

ANGIDIL (Italy)
DILTIAZEM HYDROCHLORIDE
Cardizem LA Extended Release Tablets . . . 1699
Tiazac Capsules 1204

ANGILOL (Hong Kong, New Zealand, United Kingdom)
PROPRANOLOL HYDROCHLORIDE
Inderal LA Long-Acting Capsules 3421

ANGIMON (United Kingdom)
VERAPAMIL HYDROCHLORIDE
Covera-HS Tablets 3135
Verelan PM Capsules 3120

ANGINAMIDE (Belgium)
SULFACETAMIDE SODIUM
Klaron Lotion 10% 1050

ANGINOR (South Africa)
NIFEDIPINE
Adalat CC Tablets 2978

ANGIODROX (Spain)
DILTIAZEM HYDROCHLORIDE
Cardizem LA Extended Release Tablets . . . 1699
Tiazac Capsules 1204

ANGIOFLUOR (Argentina)
FLUORESCEIN SODIUM
Fluorescite Injection . . . . . ⊙207

ANGIOLONG (Brazil)
DILTIAZEM HYDROCHLORIDE
Cardizem LA Extended Release Tablets . . . 1699
Tiazac Capsules 1204

ANGIOPINE (United Kingdom)
NIFEDIPINE
Adalat CC Tablets 2978

ANGIOPRIL (Brazil)
ENALAPRIL MALEATE
Vasotec I.V. Injection 2076

ANGIOSAN (Austria)
VALSARTAN
Diovan Tablets 2191

ANGIOTROFIN (Mexico)
DILTIAZEM HYDROCHLORIDE
Cardizem LA Extended Release Tablets . . . 1699
Tiazac Capsules 1204

ANGIOVAL (Greece)
ISOSORBIDE MONONITRATE
Imdur Tablets 3032

ANGIOZEM (United Kingdom)
DILTIAZEM HYDROCHLORIDE
Cardizem LA Extended Release Tablets . . . 1699
Tiazac Capsules 1204

ANGIPRESS (Brazil, Italy)
ATENOLOL
Tenormin I.V. Injection 698

ANGIPRESS CD (Brazil)
ATENOLOL
Tenormin I.V. Injection 698

ANGITIL (United Kingdom)
DILTIAZEM HYDROCHLORIDE
Cardizem LA Extended Release Tablets . . . 1699
Tiazac Capsules 1204

ANGITRATE (South Africa)
ISOSORBIDE MONONITRATE
Imdur Tablets 3032

ANGIZEM (Italy, Singapore, Thailand)
DILTIAZEM HYDROCHLORIDE
Cardizem LA Extended Release Tablets . . . 1699
Tiazac Capsules 1204

ANGORON (Greece)
AMIODARONE HYDROCHLORIDE
Pacerone Tablets 3337

ANGOTEN (Argentina)
AMIODARONE HYDROCHLORIDE
Pacerone Tablets 3337

ANGYTON (Brazil)
AMIODARONE HYDROCHLORIDE
Pacerone Tablets 3337

ANIDUV (Argentina)
NIMODIPINE
Nimotop Capsules 774

ANIFED (Italy)
NIFEDIPINE
Adalat CC Tablets 2978

ANISTAL (Mexico)
RANITIDINE HYDROCHLORIDE
Zantac 25 EFFERdose Tablets 1597
Zantac 150 EFFERdose Tablets 1597
Zantac 150 Tablets 1597
Zantac 300 Tablets 1597
Zantac Injection 1593
Zantac Injection Premixed 1593
Zantac Syrup 1597

ANNOXEN (Thailand)
NAPROXEN SODIUM
Anaprox DS Tablets 2769
Anaprox Tablets 2769

ANORFIN (Denmark)
BUPRENORPHINE HYDROCHLORIDE
Buprenex Injectable 2718

ANPEC (Australia, Malaysia)
VERAPAMIL HYDROCHLORIDE
Covera-HS Tablets 3135
Verelan PM Capsules 3120

ANPINE (Australia)
NIFEDIPINE
Adalat CC Tablets 2978

ANSELOL (Australia, New Zealand)
ATENOLOL
Tenormin I.V. Injection 698

ANSENTRON (Brazil)
ONDANSETRON HYDROCHLORIDE
Zofran Injection 1607
Zofran Injection Premixed 1607
Zofran Oral Solution 1613
Zofran Tablets 1613

ANSILAN (Greece)
FAMOTIDINE
Pepcid Injection 2017
Pepcid Injection Premixed 2017
Pepcid Tablets 2014
Pepcid for Oral Suspension 2014

ANSILIVE (Brazil)
DIAZEPAM
Diastat Rectal Delivery System 3344
Valium Tablets 2822

ANSIOLIN (Italy)
DIAZEPAM
Diastat Rectal Delivery System 3344
Valium Tablets 2822

ANSIUM (Spain)
DIAZEPAM
Diastat Rectal Delivery System 3344
Valium Tablets 2822

ANSIVEN (Switzerland)
PROPOFOL
Diprivan Injectable Emulsion 676

ANTADINE (Australia, South Africa)
AMANTADINE HYDROCHLORIDE
Symmetrel Syrup 1115
Symmetrel Tablets 1115

ANTAFIT (Thailand)
CARBAMAZEPINE
Carbatrol Capsules 3174
Tegretol Chewable Tablets 2278
Tegretol Suspension 2278
Tegretol Tablets 2278
Tegretol-XR Tablets 2278

ANTAGON (Brazil)
RANITIDINE HYDROCHLORIDE
Zantac 25 EFFERdose Tablets 1597
Zantac 150 EFFERdose Tablets 1597
Zantac 150 Tablets 1597
Zantac 300 Tablets 1597
Zantac Injection 1593
Zantac Injection Premixed 1593
Zantac Syrup 1597

ANTAGOSAN (France, Germany, Italy)
APROTININ
Trasylol Injection 779

ANTAK (Brazil)
RANITIDINE HYDROCHLORIDE
Zantac 25 EFFERdose Tablets 1597
Zantac 150 EFFERdose Tablets 1597
Zantac 150 Tablets 1597
Zantac 300 Tablets 1597
Zantac Injection 1593
Zantac Injection Premixed 1593
Zantac Syrup 1597

ANTALGIN (Spain)
NAPROXEN SODIUM
Anaprox DS Tablets 2769
Anaprox Tablets 2769

ANTALON (Germany)
PIMOZIDE
Orap Tablets 1220

ANTAMEX (Switzerland)
NIFEDIPINE
Adalat CC Tablets 2978

ANTANAZOL (Singapore)
KETOCONAZOLE
Nizoral 2% Shampoo 1838

ANTAROL (Hong Kong, Irish Republic)
PROPRANOLOL HYDROCHLORIDE
Inderal LA Long-Acting Capsules 3421

ANTASTEN (Argentina)
CAPTOPRIL
Captopril Tablets 2114

ANTEBOR (Belgium, France, Switzerland)
SULFACETAMIDE SODIUM
Klaron Lotion 10% 1050

ANTELEPSIN (Czech Republic, Germany)
CLONAZEPAM
Klonopin Tablets 2782

ANTENEX (Australia)
DIAZEPAM
Diastat Rectal Delivery System 3344
Valium Tablets 2822

ANTEPSIN (Argentina, Brazil, Denmark, Finland, Irish Republic, Italy, Norway)
SUCRALFATE
Carafate Suspension 727
Carafate Tablets 728

ANTHEL (Thailand)
ALBENDAZOLE
Albenza Tablets 1310

ANTHEX (South Africa)
MEBENDAZOLE
Vermox Chewable Tablets 1853

ANTHRAXITON (Greece)
DICLOFENAC SODIUM
Voltaren Tablets 2298
Voltaren-XR Tablets 2301

ANTI CD3 (Brazil)
MUROMONAB-CD3
Orthoclone OKT3 Sterile Solution 2370

ANTIBACIN (Greece)
CEFTRIAXONE SODIUM
Rocephin Injectable Vials, ADD-Vantage, Galaxy, Bulk 2801

ANTIBIOCILINA (Argentina)
AMOXICILLIN
Amoxil Pediatric Drops for Oral Suspension 1315
Amoxil Tablets 1315

ANTIBIOPTAL (Argentina)
TOBRAMYCIN
TOBI Solution for Inhalation 1015

ANTIBIOTREX (France)
ISOTRETINOIN
Accutane Capsules 2740

ANTIBLUT (Greece)
NIFEDIPINE
Adalat CC Tablets 2978

(⊙ Described in PDR For Ophthalmic Medicines™)

ANTICHOL (Greece)
SIMVASTATIN
Zocor Tablets . . . 2078

ANTIDIAR (France)
LOPERAMIDE HYDROCHLORIDE
Imodium Capsules . . . 1834

ANTI-DIARRHEAL (Canada)
LOPERAMIDE HYDROCHLORIDE
Imodium Capsules . . . 1834

ANTIDIN (Brazil)
RANITIDINE HYDROCHLORIDE
Zantac 25 EFFERdose Tablets . . . 1597
Zantac 150 EFFERdose Tablets . . . 1597
Zantac 150 Tablets . . . 1597
Zantac 300 Tablets . . . 1597
Zantac Injection . . . 1593
Zantac Injection Premixed . . . 1593
Zantac Syrup . . . 1597

ANTIFUNGOL (Germany)
CLOTRIMAZOLE
Lotrimin Cream . . . 3053
Lotrimin Lotion 1% . . . 3053
Lotrimin Topical Solution 1% . . . 3053

ANTIGREG (Italy, Malaysia, Singapore)
TICLOPIDINE HYDROCHLORIDE
Ticlid Tablets . . . 2813

ANTIL (Mexico)
CIMETIDINE
Tagamet Tablets . . . 1547

ANTILYSIN (Czech Republic)
APROTININ
Trasylol Injection . . . 779

ANTIMICOTICO (Italy)
CLOTRIMAZOLE
Lotrimin Cream . . . 3053
Lotrimin Lotion 1% . . . 3053
Lotrimin Topical Solution 1% . . . 3053

ANTIMIGRIN (Austria)
NARATRIPTAN HYDROCHLORIDE
Amerge Tablets . . . 1312

ANTIMYK (Germany)
CLOTRIMAZOLE
Lotrimin Cream . . . 3053
Lotrimin Lotion 1% . . . 3053
Lotrimin Topical Solution 1% . . . 3053

ANTIOBIOCILINA (Argentina)
AMOXICILLIN
Amoxil Pediatric Drops for Oral Suspension . . . 1315
Amoxil Tablets . . . 1315

ANTIPARKIN (Germany)
SELEGILINE HYDROCHLORIDE
Eldepryl Capsules . . . 3209

ANTIPLAQ (Argentina)
CLOPIDOGREL BISULFATE
Plavix Tablets . . . 940, 2942

ANTIPRESSAN (Hong Kong, Irish Republic, United Kingdom)
ATENOLOL
Tenormin I.V. Injection . . . 698

ANTIPREX (Greece)
ENALAPRIL MALEATE
Vasotec I.V. Injection . . . 2076

ANTITENSIN (Brazil)
PROPRANOLOL HYDROCHLORIDE
Inderal LA Long-Acting Capsules . . . 3421

ANTOPAR (Czech Republic, Hong Kong)
BENZOYL PEROXIDE
Brevoxyl-4 Creamy Wash . . . 3212
Brevoxyl-4 Gel . . . 3211
Brevoxyl-8 Creamy Wash . . . 3212
Brevoxyl-8 Gel . . . 3211
Triaz Cleanser . . . 1864
Triaz Gel . . . 1864

ANTRAL (Mexico)
METRONIDAZOLE
MetroGel-Vaginal Gel . . . 1822
Noritate Cream, 1% . . . 1051

ANULBET (Chile)
FAMOTIDINE
Pepcid Injection . . . 2017
Pepcid Injection Premixed . . . 2017
Pepcid Tablets . . . 2014
Pepcid for Oral Suspension . . . 2014

ANXICALM (Irish Republic)
DIAZEPAM
Diastat Rectal Delivery System . . . 3344
Valium Tablets . . . 2822

ANZEM (South Africa)
DILTIAZEM HYDROCHLORIDE
Cardizem LA Extended Release Tablets . . . 1699
Tiazac Capsules . . . 1204

AORTEN (Brazil)
CAPTOPRIL
Captopril Tablets . . . 2114

AOVA (Greece)
RANITIDINE HYDROCHLORIDE
Zantac 25 EFFERdose Tablets . . . 1597
Zantac 150 EFFERdose Tablets . . . 1597
Zantac 150 Tablets . . . 1597
Zantac 300 Tablets . . . 1597
Zantac Injection . . . 1593
Zantac Injection Premixed . . . 1593
Zantac Syrup . . . 1597

AP INYEC CLORURO POTASIC (Spain)
POTASSIUM CHLORIDE
K-Dur Extended-Relase Tablets . . . 3047
K-Lor Powder Packets . . . 472
K-Tab Filmtab Tablets . . . 473

APARO (Austria)
PAROXETINE HYDROCHLORIDE
Paxil Oral Suspension . . . 1501
Paxil Tablets . . . 1501

APAURIN (Czech Republic)
DIAZEPAM
Diastat Rectal Delivery System . . . 3344
Valium Tablets . . . 2822

APECITAB (Argentina)
CAPECITABINE
Xeloda Tablets . . . 2825

APEPLUS (Chile)
FINASTERIDE
Propecia Tablets . . . 2036
Proscar Tablets . . . 2040

APERAMID (Germany)
LOPERAMIDE HYDROCHLORIDE
Imodium Capsules . . . 1834

APILCAV (Brazil)
ALPROSTADIL
Edex Injection . . . 3103

APIMID (Germany)
FLUTAMIDE
Eulexin Capsules . . . 3023

APIROL (Israel)
NORFLOXACIN
Noroxin Tablets . . . 2009

APLACTIN (Italy)
PRAVASTATIN SODIUM
Pravachol Tablets . . . 943

APLAKET (Czech Republic, Hong Kong, Italy, Malaysia, Portugal, Singapore, Thailand)
TICLOPIDINE HYDROCHLORIDE
Ticlid Tablets . . . 2813

APLATIC (Hungary)
TICLOPIDINE HYDROCHLORIDE
Ticlid Tablets . . . 2813

A-PLEX (Mexico)
TRETINOIN
Avita Cream . . . 2136
Avita Gel . . . 2138
Renova 0.05% Cream . . . 2387
Retin-A Micro 0.1%/0.04% . . . 2388
Vesanoid Capsules . . . 2823

APOACOR (Israel)
VERAPAMIL HYDROCHLORIDE
Covera-HS Tablets . . . 3135
Verelan PM Capsules . . . 3120

APO-AMILZIDE (Canada, Czech Republic, Hong Kong, Malaysia, Singapore)
AMILORIDE HYDROCHLORIDE/HYDROCHLOROTHIAZIDE
Moduretic Tablets . . . 2003

APO-AMOXI (Hong Kong)
AMOXICILLIN
Amoxil Pediatric Drops for Oral Suspension . . . 1315
Amoxil Tablets . . . 1315

APO-ATENOL (Canada, Czech Republic, Hong Kong, Malaysia, Singapore)
ATENOLOL
Tenormin I.V. Injection . . . 698

APOCANDA (Germany)
CLOTRIMAZOLE
Lotrimin Cream . . . 3053
Lotrimin Lotion 1% . . . 3053
Lotrimin Topical Solution 1% . . . 3053

APOCAPEN (Israel)
CAPTOPRIL
Captopril Tablets . . . 2114

APO-CAPTO (Canada, Czech Republic, Hong Kong, Malaysia, Singapore)
CAPTOPRIL
Captopril Tablets . . . 2114

APOCARD (Portugal, Spain)
FLECAINIDE ACETATE
Tambocor Tablets . . . 1824

APO-DICLO (Canada, Czech Republic, Malaysia, New Zealand)
DICLOFENAC POTASSIUM
Cataflam Tablets . . . 2173

APO-DILTIAZ (Canada, Hong Kong)
DILTIAZEM HYDROCHLORIDE
Cardizem LA Extended Release Tablets . . . 1699
Tiazac Capsules . . . 1204

APO-ERYTHRO (Hong Kong)
ERYTHROMYCIN
Ery-Tab Tablets . . . 447
Erythromycin Base Filmtab Tablets . . . 454
Erythromycin Delayed-Release Capsules, USP . . . 456
PCE Dispertab Tablets . . . 510

APO-FENO (Canada, Czech Republic)
FENOFIBRATE
Tricor Tablets . . . 523

APO-FENO-MICRO (Hong Kong, Malaysia)
FENOFIBRATE
Tricor Tablets . . . 523

APOGASTINE (Israel)
FAMOTIDINE
Pepcid Injection . . . 2017
Pepcid Injection Premixed . . . 2017
Pepcid Tablets . . . 2014
Pepcid for Oral Suspension . . . 2014

APO-IPRAVENT (Canada)
IPRATROPIUM BROMIDE
Atrovent Inhalation Solution . . . 868
Atrovent Nasal Spray 0.03% . . . 869
Atrovent Nasal Spray 0.06% . . . 870

APO-K (Canada, Hong Kong, Malaysia)
POTASSIUM CHLORIDE
K-Dur Extended-Relase Tablets . . . 3047
K-Lor Powder Packets . . . 472
K-Tab Filmtab Tablets . . . 473

APOLLONSET (Greece)
DIAZEPAM
Diastat Rectal Delivery System . . . 3344
Valium Tablets . . . 2822

APO-MEDROXY (Canada)
MEDROXYPROGESTERONE ACETATE
Depo-Medrol Single-Dose Vial . . . 2617

APO-METHAZIDE (Canada)
HYDROCHLOROTHIAZIDE/METHYLDOPA
Aldoril Tablets . . . 1884

APOMEX (Israel)
SELEGILINE HYDROCHLORIDE
Eldepryl Capsules . . . 3209

APOMOXYN (Israel)
AMOXICILLIN
Amoxil Pediatric Drops for Oral Suspension . . . 1315
Amoxil Tablets . . . 1315

APONACIN (Israel)
NAPROXEN
EC-Naprosyn Delayed-Release Tablets . . . 2769
Naprosyn Suspension . . . 2769
Naprosyn Tablets . . . 2769

APO-NADOL (Canada, Hong Kong)
NADOLOL
Nadolol Tablets . . . 2121

APO-NAPRO-NA (Canada, Hong Kong, Malaysia, Singapore)
NAPROXEN SODIUM
Anaprox DS Tablets . . . 2769
Anaprox Tablets . . . 2769

APO-NIFED (Canada, Singapore)
NIFEDIPINE
Adalat CC Tablets . . . 2978

APO-NORFLOX (Canada)
NORFLOXACIN
Noroxin Tablets . . . 2009

APONORM (Israel)
ATENOLOL
Tenormin I.V. Injection . . . 698

APO-OFLOX (Canada, Malaysia)
OFLOXACIN
Floxin Otic Solution . . . 1043

A-POR (South Africa)
CLOTRIMAZOLE
Lotrimin Cream . . . 3053
Lotrimin Lotion 1% . . . 3053
Lotrimin Topical Solution 1% . . . 3053

APO-SULIN (Canada, Malaysia)
SULINDAC
Clinoril Tablets . . . 1899

APO-THEO (Canada, Hong Kong, Malaysia, Singapore)
THEOPHYLLINE
Uniphyl Tablets . . . 2708

APO-TIC (Czech Republic)
TICLOPIDINE HYDROCHLORIDE
Ticlid Tablets . . . 2813

APOTIL (Israel)
TIMOLOL MALEATE
Blocadren Tablets . . . 1891
Timoptic Sterile Ophthalmic Solution . . . 2058
Timoptic in Ocudose . . . 2061
Timoptic-XE Sterile Ophthalmic Gel Forming Solution . . . 2062

APO-TIMOL (Canada, New Zealand)
TIMOLOL MALEATE
Blocadren Tablets . . . 1891
Timoptic Sterile Ophthalmic Solution . . . 2058
Timoptic in Ocudose . . . 2061
Timoptic-XE Sterile Ophthalmic Gel Forming Solution . . . 2062

APO-TIMOP (Canada, Hong Kong, New Zealand)
TIMOLOL MALEATE
Blocadren Tablets . . . 1891
Timoptic Sterile Ophthalmic Solution . . . 2058
Timoptic in Ocudose . . . 2061
Timoptic-XE Sterile Ophthalmic Gel Forming Solution . . . 2062

APO-TRIAZIDE (Hong Kong, Singapore)
HYDROCHLOROTHIAZIDE/TRIAMTERENE
Dyazide Capsules . . . 1389
Maxzide Tablets . . . 2150
Maxzide-25 mg Tablets . . . 2150

APO-TRIMIP (Canada, Hong Kong)
TRIMIPRAMINE MALEATE
Surmontil Capsules . . . 2347

APOVEN (Australia)
IPRATROPIUM BROMIDE
Atrovent Inhalation Solution . . . 868
Atrovent Nasal Spray 0.03% . . . 869
Atrovent Nasal Spray 0.06% . . . 870

APOVENT (Israel)
IPRATROPIUM BROMIDE
Atrovent Inhalation Solution . . . 868
Atrovent Nasal Spray 0.03% . . . 869
Atrovent Nasal Spray 0.06% . . . 870

APO-VERAP (Canada, Czech Republic)
VERAPAMIL HYDROCHLORIDE
Covera-HS Tablets . . . 3135
Verelan PM Capsules . . . 3120

APOZAN (Israel)
RANITIDINE HYDROCHLORIDE
Zantac 25 EFFERdose Tablets . . . 1597
Zantac 150 EFFERdose Tablets . . . 1597

Zantac 150 Tablets . . . 1597
Zantac 300 Tablets . . . 1597
Zantac Injection . . . 1593
Zantac Injection Premixed . . . 1593
Zantac Syrup . . . 1597

APOZEPAM (Denmark, Sweden)
DIAZEPAM
Diastat Rectal Delivery System . . . 3344
Valium Tablets . . . 2822

APRACUR BIOTIC (Argentina)
AMOXICILLIN
Amoxil Pediatric Drops for Oral Suspension . . . 1315
Amoxil Tablets . . . 1315

APRA-GEL (Belgium)
NAPROXEN
EC-Naprosyn Delayed-Release Tablets . . . 2769
Naprosyn Suspension . . . 2769
Naprosyn Tablets . . . 2769

APRANAX (Belgium, France, Hungary, Switzerland)
NAPROXEN SODIUM
Anaprox DS Tablets . . . 2769
Anaprox Tablets . . . 2769

APRICAL (Czech Republic, Germany, Israel)
NIFEDIPINE
Adalat CC Tablets . . . 2978

APROVEL (Argentina, Belgium, Brazil, Chile, Czech Republic, Denmark, France, Germany, Greece, Hong Kong, Hungary, Irish Republic, Italy, Malaysia, Mexico, Norway, Russia, Singapore, South Africa, Spain, Sweden, Switzerland, Thailand, The Netherlands, United Kingdom)
IRBESARTAN
Avapro Tablets . . . 925

APROVEL HCT (Hong Kong, Thailand)
IRBESARTAN
Avapro Tablets . . . 925

APROZIDE (Brazil)
IRBESARTAN
Avapro Tablets . . . 925

APSOLOL (United Kingdom)
PROPRANOLOL HYDROCHLORIDE
Inderal LA Long-Acting Capsules . . . 3421

APUZIN (Malaysia)
CAPTOPRIL
Captopril Tablets . . . 2114

AQUACORT (Canada)
HYDROCORTISONE
Hydrocortone Tablets . . . 1963

AQUANIL (Denmark, Finland, Norway, Sweden)
TIMOLOL MALEATE
Blocadren Tablets . . . 1891
Timoptic Sterile Ophthalmic Solution . . . 2058
Timoptic in Ocudose . . . 2061
Timoptic-XE Sterile Ophthalmic Gel Forming Solution . . . 2062

AQUANIL HC (Chile, Mexico)
HYDROCORTISONE
Hydrocortone Tablets . . . 1963

AQUARETIC (Germany)
AMILORIDE HYDROCHLORIDE/HYDROCHLOROTHIAZIDE
Moduretic Tablets . . . 2003

AQUARID (South Africa)
FUROSEMIDE
Furosemide Tablets . . . 2117

AQUARIUS (Greece)
KETOCONAZOLE
Nizoral 2% Shampoo . . . 1838

AQUEDUX (Portugal)
FUROSEMIDE
Furosemide Tablets . . . 2117

ARABLOC (Australia)
LEFLUNOMIDE
Arava Tablets . . . 2881

ARADOIS (Brazil)
LOSARTAN POTASSIUM
Cozaar Tablets . . . 1913

ARADOIS H (Brazil)
LOSARTAN POTASSIUM
Cozaar Tablets . . . 1913

ARAGEST (Israel)
MEDROXYPROGESTERONE ACETATE
Depo-Medrol Single-Dose Vial . . . 2617

ARATAC (Australia, Malaysia, New Zealand, Thailand)
AMIODARONE HYDROCHLORIDE
Pacerone Tablets . . . 3337

ARATAN (Chile)
LOSARTAN POTASSIUM
Cozaar Tablets . . . 1913

ARATAN D (Chile)
HYDROCHLOROTHIAZIDE/LOSARTAN POTASSIUM
Hyzaar 50-12.5 Tablets . . . 1964

ARAVA (Argentina, Australia, Austria, Belgium, Brazil, Canada, Chile, Czech Republic, Denmark, Finland, France, Germany, Greece, Hong Kong, Hungary, India, Irish Republic, Israel, Italy, Malaysia, Mexico, New Zealand, Norway, Portugal, Russia, Singapore, South Africa, Spain, Sweden, Switzerland, Thailand, The Netherlands, United Kingdom)
LEFLUNOMIDE
Arava Tablets . . . 2881

ARBIL (United Kingdom)
CARBAMAZEPINE
Carbatrol Capsules . . . 3174
Tegretol Chewable Tablets . . . 2278
Tegretol Suspension . . . 2278
Tegretol Tablets . . . 2278
Tegretol-XR Tablets . . . 2278

ARCABLOCK (Austria)
ATENOLOL
Tenormin I.V. Injection . . . 698

ARCABLOCK COMP (Austria)
ATENOLOL
Tenormin I.V. Injection . . . 698

ARCANAFENAC (South Africa)
DICLOFENAC SODIUM
Voltaren Tablets . . . 2298
Voltaren-XR Tablets . . . 2301

ARCANAMIDE (South Africa)
FUROSEMIDE
Furosemide Tablets . . . 2117

ARCANARETIC (South Africa)
AMILORIDE HYDROCHLORIDE/HYDROCHLOROTHIAZIDE
Moduretic Tablets . . . 2003

ARCID (Spain)
RANITIDINE HYDROCHLORIDE
Zantac 25 EFFERdose Tablets . . . 1597
Zantac 150 EFFERdose Tablets . . . 1597
Zantac 150 Tablets . . . 1597
Zantac 300 Tablets . . . 1597
Zantac Injection . . . 1593
Zantac Injection Premixed . . . 1593
Zantac Syrup . . . 1597

ARCLONAC (Thailand)
DICLOFENAC SODIUM
Voltaren Tablets . . . 2298
Voltaren-XR Tablets . . . 2301

ARCOIRAN (Spain)
SUMATRIPTAN SUCCINATE
Imitrex Injection . . . 1431
Imitrex Tablets . . . 1440

ARCOLAN (Brazil)
KETOCONAZOLE
Nizoral 2% Shampoo . . . 1838

ARCOLANE (Chile, India)
KETOCONAZOLE
Nizoral 2% Shampoo . . . 1838

ARDORAL (Spain)
RANITIDINE HYDROCHLORIDE
Zantac 25 EFFERdose Tablets . . . 1597
Zantac 150 EFFERdose Tablets . . . 1597
Zantac 150 Tablets . . . 1597
Zantac 300 Tablets . . . 1597
Zantac Injection . . . 1593
Zantac Injection Premixed . . . 1593
Zantac Syrup . . . 1597

AREDIA (Australia, Austria, Belgium, Brazil, Canada, Czech Republic, Denmark, Finland, France, Germany, Greece, Hong Kong, Hungary, Irish Republic, Israel, Italy, Malaysia, Mexico, New Zealand, Norway, Singapore, South Africa, Spain, Sweden, Switzerland, Thailand, The Netherlands, United Kingdom)
PAMIDRONATE DISODIUM
Aredia for Injection . . . 2168

AREDRONET (India)
PAMIDRONATE DISODIUM
Aredia for Injection . . . 2168

AREMIS (Spain)
SERTRALINE HYDROCHLORIDE
Zoloft Tablets . . . 2581

ARENDAL (Argentina, Chile)
ALENDRONATE SODIUM
Fosamax Tablets . . . 1949

ARETENSIN (Germany)
RAMIPRIL
Altace Capsules . . . 1673

AREUZOLIN (Spain)
CEFAZOLIN SODIUM
Ancef for Injection . . . 1318

ARFAREL (Greece)
CLINDAMYCIN PHOSPHATE
Clindets Pledgets . . . 3212

ARFLOXINA (Mexico)
CIPROFLOXACIN
Cipro Oral Suspension . . . 2991

ARGEFLOX (Argentina)
CIPROFLOXACIN HYDROCHLORIDE
Ciloxan Ophthalmic Ointment . . . 554
Ciloxan Ophthalmic Solution . . . ⊙205
Cipro Tablets . . . 2991

ARIAL (Italy)
SALMETEROL XINAFOATE
Serevent Diskus . . . 1540

ARICEPT (Australia, Austria, Belgium, Canada, Czech Republic, Denmark, Finland, France, Greece, Hong Kong, Hungary, Irish Republic, Israel, Italy, Japan, Malaysia, New Zealand, Norway, Portugal, Singapore, South Africa, Spain, Sweden, Switzerland, Thailand, United Kingdom)
DONEPEZIL HYDROCHLORIDE
Aricept Tablets . . . 1086

ARIDIL (United Kingdom)
FUROSEMIDE
Furosemide Tablets . . . 2117

ARIFON (Russia)
INDAPAMIDE
Indapamide Tablets . . . 2119

ARILIN (Germany, Switzerland)
METRONIDAZOLE
MetroGel-Vaginal Gel . . . 1822
Noritate Cream, 1% . . . 1051

ARILINE (Austria)
METRONIDAZOLE
MetroGel-Vaginal Gel . . . 1822
Noritate Cream, 1% . . . 1051

ARIMIDEX (Argentina, Australia, Austria, Belgium, Brazil, Canada, Chile, Czech Republic, Denmark, Finland, France, Germany, Greece, Hong Kong, Hungary, Irish Republic, Israel, Italy, Malaysia, Mexico, New Zealand, Norway, Portugal, Russia, Singapore, South Africa, Spain, Sweden, Switzerland, Thailand, The Netherlands, United Kingdom)
ANASTROZOLE
Arimidex Tablets . . . 665

ARISTIN-C (Greece)
CIPROFLOXACIN
Cipro Oral Suspension . . . 2991

ARISTOCOR (Austria)
FLECAINIDE ACETATE
Tambocor Tablets . . . 1824

ARISTOCORT (Australia, Hong Kong, New Zealand, Thailand)
TRIAMCINOLONE ACETONIDE
Azmacort Inhalation Aerosol . . . 1701
Nasacort AQ Nasal Spray . . . 2937

ARISTOGYL (India)
METRONIDAZOLE
MetroGel-Vaginal Gel . . . 1822
Noritate Cream, 1% . . . 1051

ARISTOGYL-F (India)
METRONIDAZOLE
MetroGel-Vaginal Gel . . . 1822
Noritate Cream, 1% . . . 1051

ARISTROL (India)
CALCITRIOL
Calcijex Injection . . . 411

ARISTROL FORTE (India)
CALCITRIOL
Calcijex Injection . . . 411

ARKAMIN (India)
CLONIDINE HYDROCHLORIDE
Catapres Tablets . . . 874

ARKAMIN-H (India)
CLONIDINE HYDROCHLORIDE
Catapres Tablets . . . 874

ARMAMENT (Greece)
BETAXOLOL HYDROCHLORIDE
Betoptic S Ophthalmic Suspension . . . 554

ARMONIL (Italy)
ESTRADIOL
Climara Transdermal System . . . 795
Vivelle Transdermal System . . . 2288
Vivelle-Dot Transdermal System . . . 2293

ARMOPHYLLINE (France)
THEOPHYLLINE
Uniphyl Tablets . . . 2708

ARMOTRAZ (India)
ANASTROZOLE
Arimidex Tablets . . . 665

ARNELA (Chile)
CLOTRIMAZOLE
Lotrimin Cream . . . 3053
Lotrimin Lotion 1% . . . 3053
Lotrimin Topical Solution 1% . . . 3053

ARNETIN (Czech Republic, Malaysia)
RANITIDINE HYDROCHLORIDE
Zantac 25 EFFERdose Tablets . . . 1597
Zantac 150 EFFERdose Tablets . . . 1597
Zantac 150 Tablets . . . 1597
Zantac 300 Tablets . . . 1597
Zantac Injection . . . 1593
Zantac Injection Premixed . . . 1593
Zantac Syrup . . . 1597

AROMENAL (Argentina)
ANASTROZOLE
Arimidex Tablets . . . 665

AROPAX (Argentina, Australia, Belgium, Brazil, Mexico, New Zealand, South Africa, Spain)
PAROXETINE HYDROCHLORIDE
Paxil Oral Suspension . . . 1501
Paxil Tablets . . . 1501

AROXAT (Chile)
PAROXETINE HYDROCHLORIDE
Paxil Oral Suspension . . . 1501
Paxil Tablets . . . 1501

ARPAMYL LP (France)
VERAPAMIL HYDROCHLORIDE
Covera-HS Tablets . . . 3135
Verelan PM Capsules . . . 3120

ARRET (Irish Republic, United Kingdom)
LOPERAMIDE HYDROCHLORIDE
Imodium Capsules . . . 1834

ARRETIN (Mexico)
TRETINOIN
Avita Cream . . . 2136
Avita Gel . . . 2138
Renova 0.05% Cream . . . 2387
Retin-A Micro 0.1%/0.04% . . . 2388
Vesanoid Capsules . . . 2823

ARSORB (Australia)
ISOSORBIDE MONONITRATE
Imdur Tablets . . . 3032

ARTAGEN (India, Thailand)
NAPROXEN
EC-Naprosyn Delayed-Release Tablets . . . 2769
Naprosyn Suspension . . . 2769
Naprosyn Tablets . . . 2769

(⊙ Described in PDR For Ophthalmic Medicines™)

ARTAMIN (Austria, Malaysia, Singapore)
PENICILLAMINE
Cuprimine Capsules . . . 1925

ARTAXAN (Italy)
NABUMETONE
Relafen Tablets . . . 1523

ARTEROSAN (Chile)
SIMVASTATIN
Zocor Tablets . . . 2078

ARTESOL (Chile)
CILOSTAZOL
Pletal Tablets . . . 2478

ARTFLEX (Argentina)
SODIUM HYALURONATE
Hyalgan Solution . . . 2917

ARTHAXAN (Germany)
NABUMETONE
Relafen Tablets . . . 1523

ARTHOTEC (Germany)
DICLOFENAC SODIUM
Voltaren Tablets . . . 2298
Voltaren-XR Tablets . . . 2301

ARTHREASE (Germany, Israel, United Kingdom)
SODIUM HYALURONATE
Hyalgan Solution . . . 2917

ARTHREX (Germany)
DICLOFENAC SODIUM
Voltaren Tablets . . . 2298
Voltaren-XR Tablets . . . 2301

ARTHREX DUO (Germany)
DICLOFENAC SODIUM
Voltaren Tablets . . . 2298
Voltaren-XR Tablets . . . 2301

ARTHROCINE (France)
SULINDAC
Clinoril Tablets . . . 1899

ARTHROSIN (United Kingdom)
NAPROXEN
EC-Naprosyn Delayed-Release Tablets . . . 2769
Naprosyn Suspension . . . 2769
Naprosyn Tablets . . . 2769

ARTHROTEC (Australia, Austria, Belgium, Canada, Czech Republic, Denmark, Finland, Hong Kong, Irish Republic, Israel, Norway, Portugal, Singapore, South Africa, Sweden, Switzerland, Thailand, The Netherlands, United Kingdom)
DICLOFENAC SODIUM
Voltaren Tablets . . . 2298
Voltaren-XR Tablets . . . 2301

ARTHROXEN (United Kingdom)
NAPROXEN
EC-Naprosyn Delayed-Release Tablets . . . 2769
Naprosyn Suspension . . . 2769
Naprosyn Tablets . . . 2769

ARTHRU-DERM (South Africa)
DICLOFENAC SODIUM
Voltaren Tablets . . . 2298
Voltaren-XR Tablets . . . 2301

ARTHRUM H (France)
SODIUM HYALURONATE
Hyalgan Solution . . . 2917

ARTILOG (Italy)
CELECOXIB
Celebrex Capsules . . . 3130

ARTONIL (Sweden)
RANITIDINE HYDROCHLORIDE
Zantac 25 EFFERdose Tablets . . . 1597
Zantac 150 EFFERdose Tablets . . . 1597
Zantac 150 Tablets . . . 1597
Zantac 300 Tablets . . . 1597
Zantac Injection . . . 1593
Zantac Injection Premixed . . . 1593
Zantac Syrup . . . 1597

ARTOTEC (France)
DICLOFENAC SODIUM
Voltaren Tablets . . . 2298
Voltaren-XR Tablets . . . 2301

ARTREN (Brazil)
DICLOFENAC SODIUM
Voltaren Tablets . . . 2298
Voltaren-XR Tablets . . . 2301

ARTRENAC (Mexico)
DICLOFENAC SODIUM
Voltaren Tablets . . . 2298
Voltaren-XR Tablets . . . 2301

ARTRENAC PRO (Mexico)
DICLOFENAC SODIUM
Voltaren Tablets . . . 2298
Voltaren-XR Tablets . . . 2301

ARTRIBID (Portugal)
SULINDAC
Clinoril Tablets . . . 1899

ARTRODOL (Italy)
DIFLUNISAL
Dolobid Tablets . . . 1937

ARTROFENAC (Italy)
DICLOFENAC SODIUM
Voltaren Tablets . . . 2298
Voltaren-XR Tablets . . . 2301

ARTRON (Mexico)
NAPROXEN
EC-Naprosyn Delayed-Release Tablets . . . 2769
Naprosyn Suspension . . . 2769
Naprosyn Tablets . . . 2769

ARTROSONE (Spain)
DEXAMETHASONE
Decadron Tablets . . . 1929

ARTROTEC (Italy, Mexico, Spain)
DICLOFENAC SODIUM
Voltaren Tablets . . . 2298
Voltaren-XR Tablets . . . 2301

ARTROXEN (Italy)
NAPROXEN
EC-Naprosyn Delayed-Release Tablets . . . 2769
Naprosyn Suspension . . . 2769
Naprosyn Tablets . . . 2769

ARTZ (Denmark, Italy)
SODIUM HYALURONATE
Hyalgan Solution . . . 2917

ARTZAL (Austria, Finland, Sweden)
SODIUM HYALURONATE
Hyalgan Solution . . . 2917

ARU C (Germany)
CLOTRIMAZOLE
Lotrimin Cream . . . 3053
Lotrimin Lotion 1% . . . 3053
Lotrimin Topical Solution 1% . . . 3053

ARUCLONIN (Czech Republic, Germany, Hungary)
CLONIDINE HYDROCHLORIDE
Catapres Tablets . . . 874

ARUDEL (Spain)
SIMVASTATIN
Zocor Tablets . . . 2078

ARUTIMOL (Czech Republic, Germany, Hungary)
TIMOLOL MALEATE
Blocadren Tablets . . . 1891
Timoptic Sterile Ophthalmic Solution . . . 2058
Timoptic in Ocudose . . . 2061
Timoptic-XE Sterile Ophthalmic Gel Forming Solution . . . 2062

ARUTRIN (Germany)
TRIAMCINOLONE ACETONIDE
Azmacort Inhalation Aerosol . . . 1701
Nasacort AQ Nasal Spray . . . 2937

ARUTROPID (Germany)
IPRATROPIUM BROMIDE
Atrovent Inhalation Solution . . . 868
Atrovent Nasal Spray 0.03% . . . 869
Atrovent Nasal Spray 0.06% . . . 870

ARYCOR (South Africa)
AMIODARONE HYDROCHLORIDE
Pacerone Tablets . . . 3337

ARYTHMOL (Irish Republic, United Kingdom)
PROPAFENONE HYDROCHLORIDE
Rythmol SR Capsules . . . 2736

ARZEPAM (Mexico)
DIAZEPAM
Diastat Rectal Delivery System . . . 3344
Valium Tablets . . . 2822

ASASANTIN (Australia, Austria, Denmark, Finland, Hungary, Mexico, Sweden, The Netherlands)
DIPYRIDAMOLE
Persantine Tablets . . . 898

ASASANTINE (France)
DIPYRIDAMOLE
Persantine Tablets . . . 898

ASAUREX (Mexico)
CIMETIDINE
Tagamet Tablets . . . 1547

ASAX (Chile)
FUROSEMIDE
Furosemide Tablets . . . 2117

ASCARIOBEL (Brazil)
MEBENDAZOLE
Vermox Chewable Tablets . . . 1853

ASCARITOR (Brazil)
MEBENDAZOLE
Vermox Chewable Tablets . . . 1853

ASCAROBEX (Brazil)
MEBENDAZOLE
Vermox Chewable Tablets . . . 1853

ASENTA (Israel)
DONEPEZIL HYDROCHLORIDE
Aricept Tablets . . . 1086

ASENTRA (Russia, The Netherlands)
SERTRALINE HYDROCHLORIDE
Zoloft Tablets . . . 2581

ASIAZOLE (Thailand)
METRONIDAZOLE
MetroGel-Vaginal Gel . . . 1822
Noritate Cream, 1% . . . 1051

ASIOLEX (Argentina)
ANASTROZOLE
Arimidex Tablets . . . 665

ASMABIOL (Argentina)
THEOPHYLLINE
Uniphyl Tablets . . . 2708

ASMAFLU (Italy)
FLUNISOLIDE
Aerobid Inhaler System . . . 1172
Aerobid-M Inhaler System . . . 1172
Nasarel Nasal Spray . . . 1652

ASMANEX (Austria, Czech Republic, Denmark, Finland, Germany, Irish Republic, Sweden, The Netherlands, United Kingdom)
MOMETASONE FUROATE
Elocon Cream 0.1% . . . 3019
Elocon Lotion 0.1% . . . 3020
Elocon Ointment 0.1% . . . 3021
Nasonex Nasal Spray . . . 3058

ASMASOLON (Thailand)
THEOPHYLLINE
Uniphyl Tablets . . . 2708

ASMATIL (Portugal)
FLUTICASONE PROPIONATE
Cutivate Cream . . . 1381
Cutivate Ointment . . . 1384
Flonase Nasal Spray . . . 1412

ASMO (Spain)
THEOPHYLLINE
Uniphyl Tablets . . . 2708

ASMO-LAVI (Portugal)
FLUTICASONE PROPIONATE
Cutivate Cream . . . 1381
Cutivate Ointment . . . 1384
Flonase Nasal Spray . . . 1412

ASODOCEL (Argentina)
DOCETAXEL
Taxotere Injection Concentrate . . . 2947

ASOFLUT (Argentina)
FLUTAMIDE
Eulexin Capsules . . . 3023

ASONACOR (Austria)
PROPAFENONE HYDROCHLORIDE
Rythmol SR Capsules . . . 2736

ASPASERINE B6 TRANQ (Spain)
DIAZEPAM
Diastat Rectal Delivery System . . . 3344
Valium Tablets . . . 2822

ASPENIL (Italy)
AMOXICILLIN
Amoxil Pediatric Drops for Oral Suspension . . . 1315
Amoxil Tablets . . . 1315

ASPITRATE (India)
ISOSORBIDE MONONITRATE
Imdur Tablets . . . 3032

ASSIVAL (Israel)
DIAZEPAM
Diastat Rectal Delivery System . . . 3344
Valium Tablets . . . 2822

ASSY CREMA DE ENJUAGUE (Argentina)
PERMETHRIN
Acticin Cream . . . 2125

ASSY ESPUMA (Chile)
PERMETHRIN
Acticin Cream . . . 2125

ASTELIN (Mexico)
AZELASTINE HYDROCHLORIDE
Astelin Nasal Spray . . . 1876

ASTERGYL (Brazil)
METRONIDAZOLE
MetroGel-Vaginal Gel . . . 1822
Noritate Cream, 1% . . . 1051

ASTHMA T (Israel)
THEOPHYLLINE
Uniphyl Tablets . . . 2708

ASTIN (Mexico)
PRAVASTATIN SODIUM
Pravachol Tablets . . . 943

ASTRAMORPH (Brazil)
MORPHINE SULFATE
Kadian Capsules . . . 572
MS Contin Tablets . . . 2703

ASUCROSE (India)
ACARBOSE
Precose Tablets . . . 776

ASYTEC (Denmark)
CETIRIZINE HYDROCHLORIDE
Zyrtec Syrup . . . 2589
Zyrtec Tablets . . . 2589

ATACAND (Argentina, Australia, Austria, Belgium, Brazil, Canada, Chile, Czech Republic, Denmark, Finland, France, Germany, Greece, Hungary, Irish Republic, Israel, Malaysia, Mexico, New Zealand, Norway, Portugal, Singapore, South Africa, Spain, Sweden, Switzerland, The Netherlands)
CANDESARTAN CILEXETIL
Atacand Tablets . . . 634

ATACAND PLUS (Australia, Belgium, Canada, Czech Republic, Hungary, Israel, Malaysia, Norway, Singapore, South Africa, Spain, Switzerland, The Netherlands)
CANDESARTAN CILEXETIL
Atacand Tablets . . . 634

ATACAND-D (Argentina)
CANDESARTAN CILEXETIL
Atacand Tablets . . . 634

ATACANDZID (Denmark)
CANDESARTAN CILEXETIL
Atacand Tablets . . . 634

ATAMIR (Denmark)
PENICILLAMINE
Cuprimine Capsules . . . 1925

ATARIN (Finland)
AMANTADINE HYDROCHLORIDE
Symmetrel Syrup . . . 1115
Symmetrel Tablets . . . 1115

ATARVA (Argentina)
ATORVASTATIN CALCIUM
Lipitor Tablets . . . 2495

ATARVITON (Greece)
DIAZEPAM
Diastat Rectal Delivery System . . . 3344
Valium Tablets . . . 2822

ATAZID (Denmark)
CANDESARTAN CILEXETIL
Atacand Tablets . . . 634

ATE (Germany)
ATENOLOL
Tenormin I.V. Injection . . . 698

ATE LICH (Germany)
ATENOLOL
Tenormin I.V. Injection . . . 698

ATE LICH COMP (Germany)
ATENOLOL
Tenormin I.V. Injection . . . 698

ATEBETA (Germany)
ATENOLOL
Tenormin I.V. Injection 698

ATEBLOCOR (Czech Republic)
ATENOLOL
Tenormin I.V. Injection 698

ATECARD (Brazil, India)
ATENOLOL
Tenormin I.V. Injection 698

ATECARD-D (India)
ATENOLOL
Tenormin I.V. Injection 698

ATECOR (Irish Republic)
ATENOLOL
Tenormin I.V. Injection 698

ATECOR CT (Irish Republic)
ATENOLOL
Tenormin I.V. Injection 698

ATEDON (Czech Republic)
ATENOLOL
Tenormin I.V. Injection 698

ATEDUREX (Switzerland)
ATENOLOL
Tenormin I.V. Injection 698

ATEHEXAL (Australia, Austria, Czech Republic, Germany)
ATENOLOL
Tenormin I.V. Injection 698

ATEHEXAL COMP (Germany)
ATENOLOL
Tenormin I.V. Injection 698

ATEL (Argentina, Germany)
ATENOLOL
Tenormin I.V. Injection 698

ATEL C (Argentina)
ATENOLOL
Tenormin I.V. Injection 698

ATEL N (Argentina)
ATENOLOL
Tenormin I.V. Injection 698

ATEM (Italy)
IPRATROPIUM BROMIDE
Atrovent Inhalation Solution 868
Atrovent Nasal Spray 0.03% 869
Atrovent Nasal Spray 0.06% 870

ATEMUR (Germany)
FLUTICASONE PROPIONATE
Cutivate Cream 1381
Cutivate Ointment 1384
Flonase Nasal Spray 1412

ATEN (India)
ATENOLOL
Tenormin I.V. Injection 698

ATENBLOCK (Finland)
ATENOLOL
Tenormin I.V. Injection 698

ATENDOL (Germany)
ATENOLOL
Tenormin I.V. Injection 698

ATENEO (Brazil)
ATENOLOL
Tenormin I.V. Injection 698

ATENET (Denmark)
ATENOLOL
Tenormin I.V. Injection 698

ATENFAR (Chile)
ATORVASTATIN CALCIUM
Lipitor Tablets 2495

ATENI (Irish Republic)
ATENOLOL
Tenormin I.V. Injection 698

ATENIF BETA (Germany)
ATENOLOL
Tenormin I.V. Injection 698

ATE-NIFE (Irish Republic)
ATENOLOL
Tenormin I.V. Injection 698

ATENIL (Switzerland)
ATENOLOL
Tenormin I.V. Injection 698

ATENIX (Chile, United Kingdom)
SIBUTRAMINE HYDROCHLORIDE
Meridia Capsules 485

ATENO (Germany, Hong Kong)
ATENOLOL
Tenormin I.V. Injection 698

ATENO COMP (Germany)
ATENOLOL
Tenormin I.V. Injection 698

ATENO-BASAN (Switzerland)
ATENOLOL
Tenormin I.V. Injection 698

ATENOBENE (Austria, Czech Republic, Hungary)
ATENOLOL
Tenormin I.V. Injection 698

ATENOBENE COMP (Austria)
ATENOLOL
Tenormin I.V. Injection 698

ATENOBLOCK (Argentina)
ATENOLOL
Tenormin I.V. Injection 698

ATENOBLOK (South Africa)
ATENOLOL
Tenormin I.V. Injection 698

ATENOBLOK CO (South Africa)
ATENOLOL
Tenormin I.V. Injection 698

ATENODAN (Denmark)
ATENOLOL
Tenormin I.V. Injection 698

ATENOGAMMA (Germany)
ATENOLOL
Tenormin I.V. Injection 698

ATENOGAMMA COMP (Germany)
ATENOLOL
Tenormin I.V. Injection 698

ATENOGEN (Irish Republic)
ATENOLOL
Tenormin I.V. Injection 698

ATENOL (Brazil, Finland, Italy, Thailand)
ATENOLOL
Tenormin I.V. Injection 698

ATENOLAN (Austria)
ATENOLOL
Tenormin I.V. Injection 698

ATENOLOL AL COMP (Germany)
ATENOLOL
Tenormin I.V. Injection 698

ATENOLOL COMP (Hungary)
ATENOLOL
Tenormin I.V. Injection 698

ATENOLOL COMPOSITUM (Czech Republic)
ATENOLOL
Tenormin I.V. Injection 698

ATENOMEL (Hungary, Irish Republic)
ATENOLOL
Tenormin I.V. Injection 698

ATENOMERCK (Germany)
ATENOLOL
Tenormin I.V. Injection 698

ATENOMERCK COMP (Germany)
ATENOLOL
Tenormin I.V. Injection 698

ATENOPRESS (Brazil)
ATENOLOL
Tenormin I.V. Injection 698

ATENOR (Denmark)
ATENOLOL
Tenormin I.V. Injection 698

ATENORIC (Brazil)
ATENOLOL
Tenormin I.V. Injection 698

ATENOTYROL (Austria)
ATENOLOL
Tenormin I.V. Injection 698

ATENOTYROL COMP (Austria)
ATENOLOL
Tenormin I.V. Injection 698

ATENS (Brazil)
ENALAPRIL MALEATE
Vasotec I.V. Injection 2076

ATENS H (Brazil)
ENALAPRIL MALEATE/HYDROCHLOROTHIAZIDE
Vaseretic Tablets 2073

ATENSES (Mexico)
NIFEDIPINE
Adalat CC Tablets 2978

ATENSIN (Thailand)
PROPRANOLOL HYDROCHLORIDE
Inderal LA Long-Acting Capsules 3421

ATENSINA (Brazil)
CLONIDINE HYDROCHLORIDE
Catapres Tablets 874

ATENSINE (Irish Republic, United Kingdom)
DIAZEPAM
Diastat Rectal Delivery System 3344
Valium Tablets 2822

ATEREAL (Germany)
ATENOLOL
Tenormin I.V. Injection 698

ATEREN (South Africa)
ATENOLOL
Tenormin I.V. Injection 698

ATERKEY (Spain)
LOVASTATIN
Mevacor Tablets 1996

ATERMIN (Italy)
ATENOLOL
Tenormin I.V. Injection 698

ATEROCLAR (Argentina, Chile)
ATORVASTATIN CALCIUM
Lipitor Tablets 2495

ATEROL (South Africa)
ATENOLOL
Tenormin I.V. Injection 698

ATESIFAR (Switzerland)
ATENOLOL
Tenormin I.V. Injection 698

ATHELMIN (Brazil)
MEBENDAZOLE
Vermox Chewable Tablets 1853

ATHENOL (Belgium)
ATENOLOL
Tenormin I.V. Injection 698

ATHLETES FOOT CREAM (United Kingdom)
CLOTRIMAZOLE
Lotrimin Cream 3053
Lotrimin Lotion 1% 3053
Lotrimin Topical Solution 1% 3053

ATHROFEN (Switzerland)
DICLOFENAC SODIUM
Voltaren Tablets 2298
Voltaren-XR Tablets 2301

ATIBAX C (Argentina)
CIPROFLOXACIN
Cipro Oral Suspension 2991

ATIFLAN (Mexico)
NAPROXEN
EC-Naprosyn Delayed-Release Tablets 2769
Naprosyn Suspension 2769
Naprosyn Tablets 2769

A-TINIC (Thailand)
TRETINOIN
Avita Cream 2136
Avita Gel 2138
Renova 0.05% Cream 2387
Retin-A Micro 0.1%/0.04% 2388
Vesanoid Capsules 2823

ATINORM (Italy)
ATENOLOL
Tenormin I.V. Injection 698

ATLACNE (Argentina)
ISOTRETINOIN
Accutane Capsules 2740

ATLAMICIN (Argentina)
ERYTHROMYCIN
Ery-Tab Tablets 447
Erythromycin Base Filmtab Tablets 454
Erythromycin Delayed-Release Capsules, USP 456
PCE Dispertab Tablets 510

ATLANSIL (Argentina, Brazil, Chile)
AMIODARONE HYDROCHLORIDE
Pacerone Tablets 3337

ATORLIP (India)
ATORVASTATIN CALCIUM
Lipitor Tablets 2495

ATORVA (India)
ATORVASTATIN CALCIUM
Lipitor Tablets 2495

ATOSIL (Germany)
PROMETHAZINE HYDROCHLORIDE
Phenergan Suppositories 3438
Phenergan Tablets 3438

ATRISOL (Mexico)
CAPTOPRIL
Captopril Tablets 2114

ATRIVAL (Argentina)
AMOXICILLIN
Amoxil Pediatric Drops for Oral Suspension 1315
Amoxil Tablets 1315

ATROMBIN (Finland)
DIPYRIDAMOLE
Persantine Tablets 898

ATRONASE (Austria, Belgium, South Africa)
IPRATROPIUM BROMIDE
Atrovent Inhalation Solution 868
Atrovent Nasal Spray 0.03% 869
Atrovent Nasal Spray 0.06% 870

ATROVENT (Argentina, Australia, Austria, Belgium, Brazil, Canada, Chile, Czech Republic, Denmark, Finland, France, Germany, Greece, Hong Kong, Hungary, Irish Republic, Israel, Italy, Japan, Malaysia, Mexico, New Zealand, Norway, Portugal, Russia, Singapore, South Africa, Spain, Sweden, Switzerland, Thailand, The Netherlands, United Kingdom)
IPRATROPIUM BROMIDE
Atrovent Inhalation Solution 868
Atrovent Nasal Spray 0.03% 869
Atrovent Nasal Spray 0.06% 870

ATTENTA (Australia)
METHYLPHENIDATE HYDROCHLORIDE
Ritalin Hydrochloride Tablets 2254
Ritalin-SR Tablets 2254

ATTOR (India)
ATORVASTATIN CALCIUM
Lipitor Tablets 2495

AT-V (Mexico)
DIAZEPAM
Diastat Rectal Delivery System 3344
Valium Tablets 2822

AUGELIT (Brazil)
DICLOFENAC SODIUM
Voltaren Tablets 2298
Voltaren-XR Tablets 2301

AUGMEX (Singapore)
AMOXICILLIN
Amoxil Pediatric Drops for Oral Suspension 1315
Amoxil Tablets 1315

AURODIPINE (Greece)
NIMODIPINE
Nimotop Capsules 774

AUROSTATIN (Greece)
LOVASTATIN
Mevacor Tablets 1996

AUSCARD (Australia)
DILTIAZEM HYDROCHLORIDE
Cardizem LA Extended Release Tablets 1699
Tiazac Capsules 1204

AUSFAM (Australia)
FAMOTIDINE
Pepcid Injection 2017
Pepcid Injection Premixed 2017
Pepcid Tablets 2014
Pepcid for Oral Suspension 2014

AUSPRIL (Australia)
ENALAPRIL MALEATE
Vasotec I.V. Injection 2076

AUSRAN (Australia)
RANITIDINE HYDROCHLORIDE
Zantac 25 EFFERdose Tablets 1597
Zantac 150 EFFERdose Tablets 1597

Zantac 150 Tablets **1597**
Zantac 300 Tablets **1597**
Zantac Injection **1593**
Zantac Injection Premixed **1593**
Zantac Syrup **1597**

AUSTYN (Australia, Singapore)
THEOPHYLLINE
Uniphyl Tablets **2708**

AUTDOL (Chile)
DICLOFENAC SODIUM
Voltaren Tablets **2298**
Voltaren-XR Tablets **2301**

AUXXIL (Chile)
LEVOFLOXACIN
Levaquin Injection **2453**
Levaquin Tablets **2453**

AVANDAMET (Argentina, Canada, Denmark, Finland, France, Irish Republic, Malaysia, Singapore, Sweden, United Kingdom)
ROSIGLITAZONE MALEATE
Avandia Tablets **1348**

AVANDIA (Argentina, Australia, Belgium, Brazil, Canada, Chile, Czech Republic, Denmark, Finland, France, Germany, Greece, Hong Kong, Hungary, Irish Republic, Israel, Italy, Malaysia, Mexico, New Zealand, Norway, Portugal, Singapore, South Africa, Spain, Sweden, Switzerland, Thailand, The Netherlands, United Kingdom)
ROSIGLITAZONE MALEATE
Avandia Tablets **1348**

AVAPRO (Argentina, Australia, Brazil, Mexico)
IRBESARTAN
Avapro Tablets **925**

AVAPRO HCT (Argentina, Australia)
IRBESARTAN
Avapro Tablets **925**

AVERPAN (Brazil)
MEBENDAZOLE
Vermox Chewable Tablets **1853**

AVERTEX (Argentina)
FINASTERIDE
Propecia Tablets **2036**
Proscar Tablets **2040**

AVILAC (Israel)
LACTULOSE
Kristalose for Oral Solution **2149**

AVIROSTAT (Argentina)
INTERFERON ALFA-2A
Roferon-A Injection **2805**

AVITCID (Finland)
TRETINOIN
Avita Cream **2136**
Avita Gel **2138**
Renova 0.05% Cream **2387**
Retin-A Micro 0.1%/0.04% **2388**
Vesanoid Capsules **2823**

AVLOCARDYL (France)
PROPRANOLOL HYDROCHLORIDE
Inderal LA Long-Acting Capsules **3421**

AVLOSULFON (Canada, Israel)
DAPSONE
Dapsone Tablets USP **1656**

AVONEX (Argentina, Australia, Austria, Belgium, Brazil, Chile, Czech Republic, Finland, France, Germany, Greece, Hungary, Irish Republic, Israel, Italy, Mexico, Norway, Portugal, Russia, South Africa, Spain, Sweden, Switzerland, The Netherlands, United Kingdom)
INTERFERON BETA-1A
Avonex **839**

AXACEF (Denmark, Sweden)
CEFUROXIME SODIUM
Zinacef Injection **1604**

AXASOL (Chile)
CLOTRIMAZOLE
Lotrimin Cream **3053**
Lotrimin Lotion 1% **3053**
Lotrimin Topical Solution 1% **3053**

AXCIL (Mexico)
AMOXICILLIN
Amoxil Pediatric Drops for Oral Suspension **1315**
Amoxil Tablets **1315**

AXELVIN (Greece)
LISINOPRIL
Prinivil Tablets **2029**
Zestril Tablets **704**

AXEPIM (France)
CEFEPIME HYDROCHLORIDE
Maxipime for Injection **1093**

AXER (Italy)
NAPROXEN SODIUM
Anaprox DS Tablets **2769**
Anaprox Tablets **2769**

AXETINE (Belgium, Czech Republic, Hong Kong, Thailand)
CEFUROXIME AXETIL
Ceftin Tablets **1369**
Ceftin for Oral Suspension **1369**

AXONE (India)
CEFTRIAXONE SODIUM
Rocephin Injectable Vials, ADD-Vantage, Galaxy, Bulk **2801**

AXOTIDE (Switzerland)
FLUTICASONE PROPIONATE
Cutivate Cream **1381**
Cutivate Ointment **1384**
Flonase Nasal Spray **1412**

AXUROCEF (Thailand)
CEFUROXIME AXETIL
Ceftin Tablets **1369**
Ceftin for Oral Suspension **1369**

AZ (Mexico)
AZELASTINE HYDROCHLORIDE
Astelin Nasal Spray **1876**

AZ OFTENO (Chile)
AZELASTINE HYDROCHLORIDE
Astelin Nasal Spray **1876**

AZANTAC (France, Mexico)
RANITIDINE HYDROCHLORIDE
Zantac 25 EFFERdose Tablets **1597**
Zantac 150 EFFERdose Tablets **1597**
Zantac 150 Tablets **1597**
Zantac 300 Tablets **1597**
Zantac Injection **1593**
Zantac Injection Premixed **1593**
Zantac Syrup **1597**

AZATYL (Greece)
CEFTRIAXONE SODIUM
Rocephin Injectable Vials, ADD-Vantage, Galaxy, Bulk **2801**

AZECTOL (Greece)
ATENOLOL
Tenormin I.V. Injection **698**

AZELAST (Brazil)
AZELASTINE HYDROCHLORIDE
Astelin Nasal Spray **1876**

AZELVIN (Sweden)
AZELASTINE HYDROCHLORIDE
Astelin Nasal Spray **1876**

AZEP (Australia, Hong Kong, India, Malaysia, Portugal, Singapore, Thailand)
AZELASTINE HYDROCHLORIDE
Astelin Nasal Spray **1876**

AZEPAL (Hungary)
CARBAMAZEPINE
Carbatrol Capsules **3174**
Tegretol Chewable Tablets **2278**
Tegretol Suspension **2278**
Tegretol Tablets **2278**
Tegretol-XR Tablets **2278**

AZEPAM (Thailand)
DIAZEPAM
Diastat Rectal Delivery System **3344**
Valium Tablets **2822**

AZEPTIN (Japan)
AZELASTINE HYDROCHLORIDE
Astelin Nasal Spray **1876**

AZERTY (France)
NALBUPHINE HYDROCHLORIDE
Nubain Injection **1111**

AZETAVIR (Mexico)
ZIDOVUDINE
Retrovir Capsules **1533**
Retrovir IV Infusion **1537**
Retrovir Syrup **1533**
Retrovir Tablets **1533**

AZIDE (Australia)
CHLOROTHIAZIDE
Diuril Oral Suspension **1936**
Diuril Tablets **1936**

AZILIV (Brazil)
RANITIDINE HYDROCHLORIDE
Zantac 25 EFFERdose Tablets **1597**
Zantac 150 EFFERdose Tablets **1597**
Zantac 150 Tablets **1597**
Zantac 300 Tablets **1597**
Zantac Injection **1593**
Zantac Injection Premixed **1593**
Zantac Syrup **1597**

AZIMAX (Spain)
ZAFIRLUKAST
Accolate Tablets **663**

AZMACORT (Brazil, Canada, Czech Republic)
TRIAMCINOLONE ACETONIDE
Azmacort Inhalation Aerosol **1701**
Nasacort AQ Nasal Spray **2937**

AZOAZOL (Argentina)
ZIDOVUDINE
Retrovir Capsules **1533**
Retrovir IV Infusion **1537**
Retrovir Syrup **1533**
Retrovir Tablets **1533**

AZOLIN (India)
CEFAZOLIN SODIUM
Ancef for Injection **1318**

AZONA (Mexico)
DEXAMETHASONE
Decadron Tablets **1929**

AZOPT (Argentina, Australia, Austria, Belgium, Brazil, Canada, Chile, Czech Republic, Denmark, Finland, France, Germany, Greece, Hong Kong, Hungary, Irish Republic, Israel, Italy, Malaysia, Mexico, Norway, Portugal, Singapore, Spain, Sweden, Switzerland, Thailand, United Kingdom)
BRINZOLAMIDE
Azopt Ophthalmic Suspension **553**

AZOPTIC (South Africa)
BRINZOLAMIDE
Azopt Ophthalmic Suspension **553**

AZOTINE (Argentina)
ZIDOVUDINE
Retrovir Capsules **1533**
Retrovir IV Infusion **1537**
Retrovir Syrup **1533**
Retrovir Tablets **1533**

AZUCIMET (Germany)
CIMETIDINE
Tagamet Tablets **1547**

AZUPAMIL (Germany)
VERAPAMIL HYDROCHLORIDE
Covera-HS Tablets **3135**
Verelan PM Capsules **3120**

AZUPERAMID (Germany)
LOPERAMIDE HYDROCHLORIDE
Imodium Capsules **1834**

AZURANIT (Germany)
RANITIDINE HYDROCHLORIDE
Zantac 25 EFFERdose Tablets **1597**
Zantac 150 EFFERdose Tablets **1597**
Zantac 150 Tablets **1597**
Zantac 300 Tablets **1597**
Zantac Injection **1593**
Zantac Injection Premixed **1593**
Zantac Syrup **1597**

AZUTRIMAZOL (Germany)
CLOTRIMAZOLE
Lotrimin Cream **3053**
Lotrimin Lotion 1% **3053**
Lotrimin Topical Solution 1% **3053**

B DEXOL (Thailand)
DEXAMETHASONE
Decadron Tablets **1929**

BABY AGISTEN (Israel)
CLOTRIMAZOLE
Lotrimin Cream **3053**
Lotrimin Lotion 1% **3053**
Lotrimin Topical Solution 1% **3053**

BACCIDAL (Japan, Spain)
NORFLOXACIN
Noroxin Tablets **2009**

BACDA-B (Thailand)
CLOTRIMAZOLE
Lotrimin Cream **3053**
Lotrimin Lotion 1% **3053**
Lotrimin Topical Solution 1% **3053**

BACIGYL (India)
NORFLOXACIN
Noroxin Tablets **2009**

BACIGYL-N (India)
NORFLOXACIN
Noroxin Tablets **2009**

BACROCIN (Brazil)
MUPIROCIN
Bactroban Ointment **1358**

BACTIFLOX (Malaysia)
CIPROFLOXACIN HYDROCHLORIDE
Ciloxan Ophthalmic Ointment **554**
Ciloxan Ophthalmic Solution . . . . ⊙**205**
Cipro Tablets **2991**

BACTIO RHIN (Argentina)
NAPHAZOLINE HYDROCHLORIDE
Albalon Ophthalmic Solution . . . . ⊙**216**

BACTIO RHIN PREDNISOLONA (Argentina)
NAPHAZOLINE HYDROCHLORIDE
Albalon Ophthalmic Solution . . . . ⊙**216**

BACTOCIN (Mexico)
OFLOXACIN
Floxin Otic Solution **1043**

BACTODERM (Israel)
MUPIROCIN
Bactroban Ointment **1358**

BACTOFLOX (Portugal)
OFLOXACIN
Floxin Otic Solution **1043**

BACTOQUIN (India)
CIPROFLOXACIN HYDROCHLORIDE
Ciloxan Ophthalmic Ointment **554**
Ciloxan Ophthalmic Solution . . . . ⊙**205**
Cipro Tablets **2991**

BACTRACID (Germany)
NORFLOXACIN
Noroxin Tablets **2009**

BACTROBAN (Argentina, Australia, Belgium, Brazil, Chile, Czech Republic, France, Greece, Hong Kong, Hungary, India, Japan, Malaysia, Mexico, New Zealand, Portugal, Singapore, South Africa, Thailand, United Kingdom)
MUPIROCIN
Bactroban Ointment **1358**

BACTRONEO (Brazil)
MUPIROCIN
Bactroban Ointment **1358**

BAC-ZIDIM (Mexico)
CEFTAZIDIME
Fortaz for Injection **1422**

BAJATEN (Argentina, Chile)
INDAPAMIDE
Indapamide Tablets **2119**

BAJATEN D (Chile)
ENALAPRIL MALEATE/HYDROCHLOROTHIAZIDE
Vaseretic Tablets **2073**

BAKTOZIL (Germany)
CEFAZOLIN SODIUM
Ancef for Injection **1318**

B-ALCERIN (Greece)
RANITIDINE HYDROCHLORIDE
Zantac 25 EFFERdose Tablets **1597**
Zantac 150 EFFERdose Tablets **1597**
Zantac 150 Tablets **1597**
Zantac 300 Tablets **1597**
Zantac Injection **1593**
Zantac Injection Premixed **1593**
Zantac Syrup **1597**

BALCOR (Brazil, Portugal)
DILTIAZEM HYDROCHLORIDE
Cardizem LA Extended Release Tablets . . . **1699**
Tiazac Capsules **1204**

(⊙ Described in PDR For Ophthalmic Medicines™)

BALEPTON (Greece)
CIPROFLOXACIN HYDROCHLORIDE
Ciloxan Ophthalmic Ointment 554
Ciloxan Ophthalmic Solution .... ⊙205
Cipro Tablets 2991

BALMOX (Portugal, Switzerland)
NABUMETONE
Relafen Tablets 1523

BALPRIL (Portugal)
ENALAPRIL MALEATE
Vasotec I.V. Injection 2076

BALSULPH (Canada)
SULFACETAMIDE SODIUM
Klaron Lotion 10% 1050

BAMALITE (Spain)
LANSOPRAZOLE
Prevacid Delayed-Release Capsules 3268

BANAN (Hong Kong, Japan, Thailand)
CEFPODOXIME PROXETIL
Vantin Tablets and Oral Suspension 2650

BANATIN (Greece)
FAMOTIDINE
Pepcid Injection 2017
Pepcid Injection Premixed 2017
Pepcid Tablets 2014
Pepcid for Oral Suspension 2014

BANTENOL (Spain)
MEBENDAZOLE
Vermox Chewable Tablets 1853

BARAZAN (Germany)
NORFLOXACIN
Noroxin Tablets 2009

BARCLYD (France)
CLONIDINE HYDROCHLORIDE
Catapres Tablets 874

BARIPRIL (Spain)
ENALAPRIL MALEATE
Vasotec I.V. Injection 2076

BARIPRIL DIU (Spain)
ENALAPRIL MALEATE/HYDROCHLOROTHIAZIDE
Vaseretic Tablets 2073

BARMICIL (Mexico)
GENTAMICIN SULFATE
Garamycin Injectable 3028
Genoptic Sterile Ophthalmic Solution .... ⊙227

BAROXAL (Greece)
RANITIDINE HYDROCHLORIDE
Zantac 25 EFFERdose Tablets 1597
Zantac 150 EFFERdose Tablets 1597
Zantac 150 Tablets 1597
Zantac 300 Tablets 1597
Zantac Injection 1593
Zantac Injection Premixed 1593
Zantac Syrup 1597

BARRIERE-HC (Canada)
HYDROCORTISONE
Hydrocortone Tablets 1963

BASIRON (Denmark, Finland, Norway, Russia, Sweden, Switzerland, The Netherlands)
BENZOYL PEROXIDE
Brevoxyl-4 Creamy Wash 3212
Brevoxyl-4 Gel 3211
Brevoxyl-8 Creamy Wash 3212
Brevoxyl-8 Gel 3211
Triaz Cleanser 1864
Triaz Gel 1864

BASOCEF (Germany)
CEFAZOLIN SODIUM
Ancef for Injection 1318

BASOCIN (Germany)
CLINDAMYCIN PHOSPHATE
Clindets Pledgets 3212

BAYCUTEN (Brazil, Czech Republic, Mexico, Portugal)
CLOTRIMAZOLE
Lotrimin Cream 3053
Lotrimin Lotion 1% 3053
Lotrimin Topical Solution 1% 3053

BAYCUTEN HC (Germany)
CLOTRIMAZOLE
Lotrimin Cream 3053
Lotrimin Lotion 1% 3053
Lotrimin Topical Solution 1% 3053

BAYCUTEN N (Malaysia)
CLOTRIMAZOLE
Lotrimin Cream 3053
Lotrimin Lotion 1% 3053
Lotrimin Topical Solution 1% 3053

BAYCUTEN SD (Germany)
CLOTRIMAZOLE
Lotrimin Cream 3053
Lotrimin Lotion 1% 3053
Lotrimin Topical Solution 1% 3053

BAYMYCARD (Germany, Hungary)
NISOLDIPINE
Sular Tablets 1163

BEACON K (Malaysia)
POTASSIUM CHLORIDE
K-Dur Extended-Relase Tablets 3047
K-Lor Powder Packets 472
K-Tab Filmtab Tablets 473

BEAGENTA (Malaysia)
GENTAMICIN SULFATE
Garamycin Injectable 3028
Genoptic Sterile Ophthalmic Solution .... ⊙227

BEAMAT (Mexico)
CIMETIDINE
Tagamet Tablets 1547

BEAMODIUM (Malaysia)
LOPERAMIDE HYDROCHLORIDE
Imodium Capsules 1834

BEAMOKEN A (Mexico)
DEXAMETHASONE
Decadron Tablets 1929

BEATIZEM (Singapore)
DILTIAZEM HYDROCHLORIDE
Cardizem LA Extended Release Tablets 1699
Tiazac Capsules 1204

BEATOCONAZOLE (Singapore)
KETOCONAZOLE
Nizoral 2% Shampoo 1838

BECABIL (Spain)
AMOXICILLIN
Amoxil Pediatric Drops for Oral Suspension 1315
Amoxil Tablets 1315

BECACORT (Malaysia)
HYDROCORTISONE
Hydrocortone Tablets 1963

BECARDIN (Hong Kong)
PROPRANOLOL HYDROCHLORIDE
Inderal LA Long-Acting Capsules 3421

BECONASE ALLERGY (Australia)
FLUTICASONE PROPIONATE
Cutivate Cream 1381
Cutivate Ointment 1384
Flonase Nasal Spray 1412

BECTAM (Chile)
PAROXETINE HYDROCHLORIDE
Paxil Oral Suspension 1501
Paxil Tablets 1501

BEDRANOL (Switzerland, United Kingdom)
PROPRANOLOL HYDROCHLORIDE
Inderal LA Long-Acting Capsules 3421

BEFAR (Hong Kong)
ALPROSTADIL
Edex Injection 3103

BEFARIN (Thailand)
WARFARIN SODIUM
Coumadin Tablets 932
Coumadin for Injection 932

BEFIMAT (Greece)
NIMODIPINE
Nimotop Capsules 774

BEFOL (Argentina)
DICLOFENAC POTASSIUM
Cataflam Tablets 2173

BEGLAN (Spain)
SALMETEROL XINAFOATE
Serevent Diskus 1540

BEILANDE (Hong Kong)
FAMOTIDINE
Pepcid Injection 2017
Pepcid Injection Premixed 2017
Pepcid Tablets 2014
Pepcid for Oral Suspension 2014

BEKNOL (Mexico)
BENZONATATE
Tessalon Perles 1202

BEL (Germany)
SIMVASTATIN
Zocor Tablets 2078

BELIDRAL (Belgium)
AMILORIDE HYDROCHLORIDE/HYDROCHLOROTHIAZIDE
Moduretic Tablets 2003

BELIVON (Austria, Italy)
RISPERIDONE
Risperdal Oral Solution 1658
Risperdal Tablets 1658

BELMACINA (Spain)
CIPROFLOXACIN HYDROCHLORIDE
Ciloxan Ophthalmic Ointment 554
Ciloxan Ophthalmic Solution .... ⊙205
Cipro Tablets 2991

BELMALAX (Spain)
LACTULOSE
Kristalose for Oral Solution 2149

BELMALIP (Spain)
SIMVASTATIN
Zocor Tablets 2078

BELMIRAX (Brazil)
MEBENDAZOLE
Vermox Chewable Tablets 1853

BELOC-ZOK (Germany, Switzerland)
METOPROLOL SUCCINATE
Toprol-XL Tablets 660

BELOKEN (Spain)
METOPROLOL SUCCINATE
Toprol-XL Tablets 660

BELOZOK (Argentina)
METOPROLOL SUCCINATE
Toprol-XL Tablets 660

BELTOP (Austria)
KETOCONAZOLE
Nizoral 2% Shampoo 1838

BEMAZ (Chile)
BETAXOLOL HYDROCHLORIDE
Betoptic S Ophthalmic Suspension 554

BEMETRAZOLE (South Africa)
METRONIDAZOLE
MetroGel-Vaginal Gel 1822
Noritate Cream, 1% 1051

BEMPLAS (Argentina)
CLONIDINE HYDROCHLORIDE
Catapres Tablets 874

BENACE (India)
BENAZEPRIL HYDROCHLORIDE
Lotensin Tablets 2232

BENACNE (Portugal)
BENZOYL PEROXIDE
Brevoxyl-4 Creamy Wash 3212
Brevoxyl-4 Gel 3211
Brevoxyl-8 Creamy Wash 3212
Brevoxyl-8 Gel 3211
Triaz Cleanser 1864
Triaz Gel 1864

BENADAY (Denmark)
CETIRIZINE HYDROCHLORIDE
Zyrtec Syrup 2589
Zyrtec Tablets 2589

BENADRYL ALLERGY ORAL SOLUTION (United Kingdom)
CETIRIZINE HYDROCHLORIDE
Zyrtec Syrup 2589
Zyrtec Tablets 2589

BENADRYL ONE A DAY (United Kingdom)
CETIRIZINE HYDROCHLORIDE
Zyrtec Syrup 2589
Zyrtec Tablets 2589

BENALAPRIL (Germany)
ENALAPRIL MALEATE
Vasotec I.V. Injection 2076

BENAPROST (Argentina)
TERAZOSIN HYDROCHLORIDE
Hytrin Capsules 469

BENAXONA (Mexico)
CEFTRIAXONE SODIUM
Rocephin Injectable Vials, ADD-Vantage, Galaxy, Bulk 2801

BENCIL SCAB (Argentina)
PERMETHRIN
Acticin Cream 2125

BENDA (Thailand)
MEBENDAZOLE
Vermox Chewable Tablets 1853

BENDAPAR (Mexico)
ALBENDAZOLE
Albenza Tablets 1310

BENDEX (India, South Africa)
ALBENDAZOLE
Albenza Tablets 1310

BENDRAX (Brazil)
MEBENDAZOLE
Vermox Chewable Tablets 1853

BENECUT (Austria)
NAFTIFINE HYDROCHLORIDE
Naftin Cream 2097
Naftin Gel 2097

BENEDAXOL (Mexico)
MEBENDAZOLE
Vermox Chewable Tablets 1853

BENET (Japan)
RISEDRONATE SODIUM
Actonel Tablets 2679

BENEVRAN (Brazil)
DICLOFENAC POTASSIUM
Cataflam Tablets 2173

BENFOFEN (Germany)
DICLOFENAC SODIUM
Voltaren Tablets 2298
Voltaren-XR Tablets 2301

BENOXID (Italy)
BENZOYL PEROXIDE
Brevoxyl-4 Creamy Wash 3212
Brevoxyl-4 Gel 3211
Brevoxyl-8 Creamy Wash 3212
Brevoxyl-8 Gel 3211
Triaz Cleanser 1864
Triaz Gel 1864

BENOXYGEL (Portugal, Spain)
BENZOYL PEROXIDE
Brevoxyl-4 Creamy Wash 3212
Brevoxyl-4 Gel 3211
Brevoxyl-8 Creamy Wash 3212
Brevoxyl-8 Gel 3211
Triaz Cleanser 1864
Triaz Gel 1864

BENOXYL (Australia, Canada, Irish Republic, Mexico, New Zealand, South Africa, United Kingdom)
BENZOYL PEROXIDE
Brevoxyl-4 Creamy Wash 3212
Brevoxyl-4 Gel 3211
Brevoxyl-8 Creamy Wash 3212
Brevoxyl-8 Gel 3211
Triaz Cleanser 1864
Triaz Gel 1864

BENPH (Irish Republic)
TERAZOSIN HYDROCHLORIDE
Hytrin Capsules 469

BENPINE (Malaysia, Singapore, Thailand)
CHLORDIAZEPOXIDE HYDROCHLORIDE
Librium Capsules 3349

BENSOLMIN (Mexico)
MEBENDAZOLE
Vermox Chewable Tablets 1853

BENTIAMIN (Brazil)
ALBENDAZOLE
Albenza Tablets 1310

BENZAC (Australia, Belgium, Brazil, Canada, Italy, Mexico, New Zealand, Portugal, Singapore, Switzerland, Thailand, The Netherlands)
BENZOYL PEROXIDE
Brevoxyl-4 Creamy Wash 3212
Brevoxyl-4 Gel 3211
Brevoxyl-8 Creamy Wash 3212
Brevoxyl-8 Gel 3211
Triaz Cleanser 1864
Triaz Gel 1864

BENZAC AC (India)
BENZOYL PEROXIDE
Brevoxyl-4 Creamy Wash 3212
Brevoxyl-4 Gel 3211
Brevoxyl-8 Creamy Wash 3212
Brevoxyl-8 Gel 3211
Triaz Cleanser 1864
Triaz Gel 1864

BENZAC ERITROMICINA (Brazil)
ERYTHROMYCIN
Ery-Tab Tablets 447
Erythromycin Base Filmtab Tablets 454
Erythromycin Delayed-Release Capsules, USP 456
PCE Dispertab Tablets 510

BENZAC-AC (Brazil, Hong Kong, Israel, Malaysia, South Africa)
BENZOYL PEROXIDE
Brevoxyl-4 Creamy Wash 3212
Brevoxyl-4 Gel 3211
Brevoxyl-8 Creamy Wash 3212
Brevoxyl-8 Gel 3211
Triaz Cleanser 1864
Triaz Gel 1864

BENZAC-W (Greece)
BENZOYL PEROXIDE
Brevoxyl-4 Creamy Wash 3212
Brevoxyl-4 Gel 3211
Brevoxyl-8 Creamy Wash 3212
Brevoxyl-8 Gel 3211
Triaz Cleanser 1864
Triaz Gel 1864

BENZADERM (Mexico)
BENZOYL PEROXIDE
Brevoxyl-4 Creamy Wash 3212
Brevoxyl-4 Gel 3211
Brevoxyl-8 Creamy Wash 3212
Brevoxyl-8 Gel 3211
Triaz Cleanser 1864
Triaz Gel 1864

BENZAGEL (Brazil, Canada, France, United Kingdom)
BENZOYL PEROXIDE
Brevoxyl-4 Creamy Wash 3212
Brevoxyl-4 Gel 3211
Brevoxyl-8 Creamy Wash 3212
Brevoxyl-8 Gel 3211
Triaz Cleanser 1864
Triaz Gel 1864

BENZAKNEN (Austria, Germany)
BENZOYL PEROXIDE
Brevoxyl-4 Creamy Wash 3212
Brevoxyl-4 Gel 3211
Brevoxyl-8 Creamy Wash 3212
Brevoxyl-8 Gel 3211
Triaz Cleanser 1864
Triaz Gel 1864

BENZAMYCIN (Argentina, Belgium, Canada, Chile, Hong Kong, Israel, Mexico, United Kingdom)
BENZOYL PEROXIDE
Brevoxyl-4 Creamy Wash 3212
Brevoxyl-4 Gel 3211
Brevoxyl-8 Creamy Wash 3212
Brevoxyl-8 Gel 3211
Triaz Cleanser 1864
Triaz Gel 1864

BENZAMYCINE (South Africa)
BENZOYL PEROXIDE
Brevoxyl-4 Creamy Wash 3212
Brevoxyl-4 Gel 3211
Brevoxyl-8 Creamy Wash 3212
Brevoxyl-8 Gel 3211
Triaz Cleanser 1864
Triaz Gel 1864

BENZEVIT (Brazil)
NYSTATIN
Nystop Topical Powder USP 2490

BENZIHEX (Argentina)
BENZOYL PEROXIDE
Brevoxyl-4 Creamy Wash 3212
Brevoxyl-4 Gel 3211
Brevoxyl-8 Creamy Wash 3212
Brevoxyl-8 Gel 3211
Triaz Cleanser 1864
Triaz Gel 1864

BENZODERM MYCO (Germany)
CLOTRIMAZOLE
Lotrimin Cream 3053
Lotrimin Lotion 1% 3053
Lotrimin Topical Solution 1% 3053

BENZODIAPIN (Italy)
CHLORDIAZEPOXIDE HYDROCHLORIDE
Librium Capsules 3349

BENZOMIX (Italy)
BENZOYL PEROXIDE
Brevoxyl-4 Creamy Wash 3212
Brevoxyl-4 Gel 3211
Brevoxyl-8 Creamy Wash 3212
Brevoxyl-8 Gel 3211
Triaz Cleanser 1864
Triaz Gel 1864

BENZONAL (Mexico)
BENZONATATE
Tessalon Perles 1202

BENZOPIN (South Africa)
DIAZEPAM
Diastat Rectal Delivery System 3344
Valium Tablets 2822

BENZOYT (Germany)
BENZOYL PEROXIDE
Brevoxyl-4 Creamy Wash 3212
Brevoxyl-4 Gel 3211
Brevoxyl-8 Creamy Wash 3212
Brevoxyl-8 Gel 3211
Triaz Cleanser 1864
Triaz Gel 1864

BENZPEROX (Germany)
BENZOYL PEROXIDE
Brevoxyl-4 Creamy Wash 3212
Brevoxyl-4 Gel 3211
Brevoxyl-8 Creamy Wash 3212
Brevoxyl-8 Gel 3211
Triaz Cleanser 1864
Triaz Gel 1864

BENZYME (Mexico)
DIAZEPAM
Diastat Rectal Delivery System 3344
Valium Tablets 2822

BEOCID PUROPTAL (Austria)
SULFACETAMIDE SODIUM
Klaron Lotion 10% 1050

BEOF (Chile)
BETAXOLOL HYDROCHLORIDE
Betoptic S Ophthalmic Suspension 554

BEPRANE (France)
PROPRANOLOL HYDROCHLORIDE
Inderal LA Long-Acting Capsules 3421

BEPTAZINE (India)
PROPRANOLOL HYDROCHLORIDE
Inderal LA Long-Acting Capsules 3421

BERAMICINA (Mexico)
GENTAMICIN SULFATE
Garamycin Injectable 3028
Genoptic Sterile Ophthalmic Solution ⊙227

BERAZOLE (South Africa)
METRONIDAZOLE
MetroGel-Vaginal Gel 1822
Noritate Cream, 1% 1051

BERKATENS (Irish Republic, United Kingdom)
VERAPAMIL HYDROCHLORIDE
Covera-HS Tablets 3135
Verelan PM Capsules 3120

BERKOLOL (Hong Kong, Irish Republic, United Kingdom)
PROPRANOLOL HYDROCHLORIDE
Inderal LA Long-Acting Capsules 3421

BERLEX (Argentina)
ALENDRONATE SODIUM
Fosamax Tablets 1949

BERLIPRIL (Czech Republic)
ENALAPRIL MALEATE
Vasotec I.V. Injection 2076

BERLTHYROX (Germany)
LEVOTHYROXINE SODIUM
Levothroid Tablets 1189
Levoxyl Tablets 1680
Synthroid Tablets 515

BERMACIA (Brazil)
THEOPHYLLINE
Uniphyl Tablets 2708

BERTOCIL (Portugal)
BETAXOLOL HYDROCHLORIDE
Betoptic S Ophthalmic Suspension 554

BESIDIN (Greece)
CIMETIDINE
Tagamet Tablets 1547

BESITRAN (Spain)
SERTRALINE HYDROCHLORIDE
Zoloft Tablets 2581

BESTATIN (Thailand)
SIMVASTATIN
Zocor Tablets 2078

BESTELAR (Mexico)
MEBENDAZOLE
Vermox Chewable Tablets 1853

BETA (India)
ATENOLOL
Tenormin I.V. Injection 698

BETA NICARDIA (India, Singapore)
ATENOLOL
Tenormin I.V. Injection 698

BETA-ADALAT (Finland, United Kingdom)
ATENOLOL
Tenormin I.V. Injection 698

BETABLOC (India)
PROPRANOLOL HYDROCHLORIDE
Inderal LA Long-Acting Capsules 3421

BETAC (Russia)
BETAXOLOL HYDROCHLORIDE
Betoptic S Ophthalmic Suspension 554

BETACAINE (Canada)
LIDOCAINE
Lidoderm Patch 1107

BETACAR (Chile)
ATENOLOL
Tenormin I.V. Injection 698

BETACEF (Italy)
CEFOXITIN SODIUM
Mefoxin Premixed Intravenous Solution 1990
Mefoxin for Injection 1987

BETADIUR (Switzerland)
AMILORIDE HYDROCHLORIDE/HYDROCHLOROTHIAZIDE
Moduretic Tablets 2003

BETADUR CR (United Kingdom)
PROPRANOLOL HYDROCHLORIDE
Inderal LA Long-Acting Capsules 3421

BETAFERON (Australia, Austria, Belgium, Brazil, Czech Republic, Denmark, Finland, France, Germany, Hong Kong, Hungary, Irish Republic, Israel, Italy, Malaysia, Mexico, New Zealand, Norway, Portugal, Singapore, South Africa, Spain, Sweden, Switzerland, Thailand, The Netherlands, United Kingdom)
INTERFERON BETA-1B
Betaseron for SC Injection 791

BETAGLIM (India)
GLIMEPIRIDE
Amaryl Tablets 2864

BETAGLIM M (India)
GLIMEPIRIDE
Amaryl Tablets 2864

BETALOC (Czech Republic, Hungary, New Zealand)
METOPROLOL SUCCINATE
Toprol-XL Tablets 660

BETALOC ZOK (Russia)
METOPROLOL SUCCINATE
Toprol-XL Tablets 660

BETALOL (Thailand)
PROPRANOLOL HYDROCHLORIDE
Inderal LA Long-Acting Capsules 3421

BETAMICAN (Spain)
SALMETEROL XINAFOATE
Serevent Diskus 1540

BETAPAM (South Africa)
DIAZEPAM
Diastat Rectal Delivery System 3344
Valium Tablets 2822

BETAPERAMIDE (South Africa)
LOPERAMIDE HYDROCHLORIDE
Imodium Capsules 1834

BETAPLEX (Chile)
CARVEDILOL
Coreg Tablets 1376

BETAPRESS (Thailand)
PROPRANOLOL HYDROCHLORIDE
Inderal LA Long-Acting Capsules 3421

BETA-PROGRANE (United Kingdom)
PROPRANOLOL HYDROCHLORIDE
Inderal LA Long-Acting Capsules 3421

BETAPROL (Switzerland)
PROPRANOLOL HYDROCHLORIDE
Inderal LA Long-Acting Capsules 3421

BETAREN (Israel)
DICLOFENAC SODIUM
Voltaren Tablets 2298
Voltaren-XR Tablets 2301

BETARETIC (South Africa)
AMILORIDE HYDROCHLORIDE/HYDROCHLOROTHIAZIDE
Moduretic Tablets 2003

BETASEL (Argentina)
BETAXOLOL HYDROCHLORIDE
Betoptic S Ophthalmic Suspension 554

BETASERON (Canada)
INTERFERON BETA-1B
Betaseron for SC Injection 791

BETASOL (Malaysia, Thailand)
CLOBETASOL PROPIONATE
Temovate Cream 1549
Temovate E Emollient 1552
Temovate Gel 1550
Temovate Ointment 1549
Temovate Scalp Application 1551

BETASPAN (India)
PROPRANOLOL HYDROCHLORIDE
Inderal LA Long-Acting Capsules 3421

BETASYN (Austria)
ATENOLOL
Tenormin I.V. Injection 698

BETA-TABLINEN (Germany)
PROPRANOLOL HYDROCHLORIDE
Inderal LA Long-Acting Capsules 3421

BETA-TIM (Canada)
TIMOLOL MALEATE
Blocadren Tablets 1891
Timoptic Sterile Ophthalmic Solution 2058
Timoptic in Ocudose 2061
Timoptic-XE Sterile Ophthalmic Gel Forming Solution 2062

BETA-TIMELETS (Germany)
PROPRANOLOL HYDROCHLORIDE
Inderal LA Long-Acting Capsules 3421

BETATOP (France)
ATENOLOL
Tenormin I.V. Injection 698

BETAZOK (Irish Republic)
METOPROLOL SUCCINATE
Toprol-XL Tablets 660

BETIM (Irish Republic, Norway, United Kingdom)
TIMOLOL MALEATE
Blocadren Tablets 1891
Timoptic Sterile Ophthalmic Solution 2058
Timoptic in Ocudose 2061
Timoptic-XE Sterile Ophthalmic Gel Forming Solution 2062

BETOPTIC (Australia, Austria, Belgium, Brazil, Canada, Chile, Czech Republic, Denmark, Finland, France, Greece, Hong Kong, Hungary, Irish Republic, Italy, Malaysia, Mexico, New Zealand, Norway, Portugal, Singapore, South Africa, Spain, Sweden, Thailand, The Netherlands, United Kingdom)
BETAXOLOL HYDROCHLORIDE
Betoptic S Ophthalmic Suspension 554

BETOPTIC S (Greece, Israel, Switzerland)
BETAXOLOL HYDROCHLORIDE
Betoptic S Ophthalmic Suspension 554

BETOPTIMA (Germany)
BETAXOLOL HYDROCHLORIDE
Betoptic S Ophthalmic Suspension 554

BETOQUIN (Australia)
BETAXOLOL HYDROCHLORIDE
Betoptic S Ophthalmic Suspension 554

BETULAC (Sweden)
LACTULOSE
Kristalose for Oral Solution 2149

(⊙ Described in PDR For Ophthalmic Medicines™)

BEURISES (South Africa)
FUROSEMIDE
Furosemide Tablets 2117

BEXID (Sweden)
BENZOYL PEROXIDE
Brevoxyl-4 Creamy Wash 3212
Brevoxyl-4 Gel 3211
Brevoxyl-8 Creamy Wash 3212
Brevoxyl-8 Gel 3211
Triaz Cleanser 1864
Triaz Gel 1864

BEXINE (Mexico)
DEXAMETHASONE
Decadron Tablets 1929

BEXINOR (Singapore)
NORFLOXACIN
Noroxin Tablets 2009

BEXON (Argentina)
METRONIDAZOLE
MetroGel-Vaginal Gel 1822
Noritate Cream, 1% 1051

BGB NORFLOX (Thailand)
NORFLOXACIN
Noroxin Tablets 2009

BI PRETERAX (Belgium)
PERINDOPRIL ERBUMINE
Aceon Tablets (2 mg, 4 mg, 8 mg) 3191

BIALZEPAM (Portugal)
DIAZEPAM
Diastat Rectal Delivery System 3344
Valium Tablets 2822

BIAMOTIL (Brazil)
CIPROFLOXACIN HYDROCHLORIDE
Ciloxan Ophthalmic Ointment 554
Ciloxan Ophthalmic Solution . . . . ⊙205
Cipro Tablets 2991

BIARTAC (Belgium)
DIFLUNISAL
Dolobid Tablets 1937

BIAXIN (Canada, Germany)
CLARITHROMYCIN
Biaxin Filmtab Tablets 402
Biaxin Granules 402

BIAZOLINA (Italy)
CEFAZOLIN SODIUM
Ancef for Injection 1318

BICAPROST (Argentina)
BICALUTAMIDE
Casodex Tablets 670

BICLAR (Belgium)
CLARITHROMYCIN
Biaxin Filmtab Tablets 402
Biaxin Granules 402

BICLOPAN (Singapore)
DICLOFENAC SODIUM
Voltaren Tablets 2298
Voltaren-XR Tablets 2301

BIDECAR (Argentina)
CARVEDILOL
Coreg Tablets 1376

BIDOFLOX (India)
OFLOXACIN
Floxin Otic Solution 1043

BIDOFLOX-OZ (India)
OFLOXACIN
Floxin Otic Solution 1043

BIDROSTAT (Argentina)
BICALUTAMIDE
Casodex Tablets 670

BIDURET (India)
AMILORIDE HYDROCHLORIDE
Midamor Tablets 2000

BIFARDOL S (Mexico)
NAPROXEN SODIUM
Anaprox DS Tablets 2769
Anaprox Tablets 2769

BIFINORMA (Germany)
LACTULOSE
Kristalose for Oral Solution 2149

BIFITERAL (Austria, Belgium, Germany)
LACTULOSE
Kristalose for Oral Solution 2149

BIFORT (Argentina)
SILDENAFIL CITRATE
Viagra Tablets 2552

BIFOSA (India)
ALENDRONATE SODIUM
Fosamax Tablets 1949

BIG-BEN (Thailand)
MEBENDAZOLE
Vermox Chewable Tablets 1853

BILDURETIC (Thailand)
AMILORIDE HYDROCHLORIDE
Midamor Tablets 2000

BILORDYL (Germany)
THEOPHYLLINE
Uniphyl Tablets 2708

BILTRICIDE (Australia, Canada, France, Germany, Greece, Hong Kong, Israel, South Africa, Thailand, The Netherlands)
PRAZIQUANTEL
Biltricide Tablets 2990

BINALDAN (Switzerland)
LOPERAMIDE HYDROCHLORIDE
Imodium Capsules 1834

BINDAZAC (Greece)
RANITIDINE HYDROCHLORIDE
Zantac 25 EFFERdose Tablets 1597
Zantac 150 EFFERdose Tablets 1597
Zantac 150 Tablets 1597
Zantac 300 Tablets 1597
Zantac Injection 1593
Zantac Injection Premixed 1593
Zantac Syrup 1597

BIO CABAL (Argentina)
DEXAMETHASONE
Decadron Tablets 1929

BIO TARBUN (Argentina)
NORFLOXACIN
Noroxin Tablets 2009

BIOACT-D (Brazil)
DACTINOMYCIN
Cosmegen for Injection 1907

BIO-AMOKSICLAV (South Africa)
AMOXICILLIN
Amoxil Pediatric Drops for Oral Suspension 1315
Amoxil Tablets 1315

BIOCARD (Irish Republic)
CARVEDILOL
Coreg Tablets 1376

BIOCARN (Germany)
LEVOCARNITINE
Carnitor Injection 3185
Carnitor Tablets and Oral Solution 3187

BIOCEF (Austria)
CEFPODOXIME PROXETIL
Vantin Tablets and Oral Suspension 2650

BIO-CEST (Mexico)
PRAZIQUANTEL
Biltricide Tablets 2990

BIOCICLIN (Italy)
CEFUROXIME SODIUM
Zinacef Injection 1604

BIOCIP (India)
CIPROFLOXACIN
Cipro Oral Suspension 2991

BIOCIPRO (Greece)
CIPROFLOXACIN
Cipro Oral Suspension 2991

BIOCIP-TZ (India)
CIPROFLOXACIN
Cipro Oral Suspension 2991

BIOCLAR (India)
CLARITHROMYCIN
Biaxin Filmtab Tablets 402
Biaxin Granules 402

BIOCORD (Brazil)
NIFEDIPINE
Adalat CC Tablets 2978

BIOCORTIN (Argentina)
HYDROCORTISONE
Hydrocortone Tablets 1963

BIO-DAC (Mexico)
SULINDAC
Clinoril Tablets 1899

BIODERMIN (Italy)
ECONAZOLE NITRATE
Spectazole Cream 2390

BIODEZIL (Mexico)
CAPTOPRIL
Captopril Tablets 2114

BIODROP (Argentina)
DORZOLAMIDE HYDROCHLORIDE
Trusopt Sterile Ophthalmic Solution 2065

BIOFANAL (Germany)
NYSTATIN
Nystop Topical Powder USP 2490

BIOFERON (Thailand)
INTERFERON ALFA-2B
Intron A for Injection 3038

BIOFF (India)
OFLOXACIN
Floxin Otic Solution 1043

BIOFLOX (Mexico)
CIPROFLOXACIN
Cipro Oral Suspension 2991

BIOFLOXIN (India)
NORFLOXACIN
Noroxin Tablets 2009

BIOFLOX-TZ (India)
NORFLOXACIN
Noroxin Tablets 2009

BIOFUREX (Italy)
CEFUROXIME SODIUM
Zinacef Injection 1604

BIOGARACIN (India)
GENTAMICIN SULFATE
Garamycin Injectable 3028
Genoptic Sterile Ophthalmic Solution . . . . ⊙227

BIOGEL (Chile)
KETOCONAZOLE
Nizoral 2% Shampoo 1838

BIOGEN (Spain)
GENTAMICIN SULFATE
Garamycin Injectable 3028
Genoptic Sterile Ophthalmic Solution . . . . ⊙227

BIOGYL (Thailand)
METRONIDAZOLE
MetroGel-Vaginal Gel 1822
Noritate Cream, 1% 1051

BIOLAC (Italy)
LACTULOSE
Kristalose for Oral Solution 2149

BIOLAN (Germany)
SODIUM HYALURONATE
Hyalgan Solution 2917

BIOLON (Brazil, Canada, Germany, Israel, Italy, Mexico, Switzerland)
SODIUM HYALURONATE
Hyalgan Solution 2917

BIOLONE (South Africa)
SODIUM HYALURONATE
Hyalgan Solution 2917

BIOMAG (Italy)
CIMETIDINE
Tagamet Tablets 1547

BIOMARGEN (Spain)
GENTAMICIN SULFATE
Garamycin Injectable 3028
Genoptic Sterile Ophthalmic Solution . . . . ⊙227

BIOMIDA (Brazil)
FLUTAMIDE
Eulexin Capsules 3023

BIOMISEN (Mexico)
FUROSEMIDE
Furosemide Tablets 2117

BIOMONA (Mexico)
METRONIDAZOLE
MetroGel-Vaginal Gel 1822
Noritate Cream, 1% 1051

BIOMOX (Thailand)
AMOXICILLIN
Amoxil Pediatric Drops for Oral Suspension 1315
Amoxil Tablets 1315

BIOMOXIL (India)
AMOXICILLIN
Amoxil Pediatric Drops for Oral Suspension 1315
Amoxil Tablets 1315

BIOMOXIL-LB (India)
AMOXICILLIN
Amoxil Pediatric Drops for Oral Suspension 1315
Amoxil Tablets 1315

BIONEURYL (Mexico)
CARBAMAZEPINE
Carbatrol Capsules 3174
Tegretol Chewable Tablets 2278
Tegretol Suspension 2278
Tegretol Tablets 2278
Tegretol-XR Tablets 2278

BIONIF (Italy)
NIFEDIPINE
Adalat CC Tablets 2978

BIOPHYLLIN (South Africa)
THEOPHYLLINE
Uniphyl Tablets 2708

BIOPIME (India)
CEFEPIME HYDROCHLORIDE
Maxipime for Injection 1093

BIOPLASMA FDP (South Africa)
PLASMA PROTEIN FRACTION
Plasmanate 3252

BIOPRIL (India)
LISINOPRIL
Prinivil Tablets 2029
Zestril Tablets 704

BIOPRIL-AM (India)
LISINOPRIL
Prinivil Tablets 2029
Zestril Tablets 704

BIOPROFOL (Brazil)
PROPOFOL
Diprivan Injectable Emulsion 676

BIOPTIC (Argentina)
TOBRAMYCIN
TOBI Solution for Inhalation 1015

BIOPTIC DX (Argentina)
TOBRAMYCIN
TOBI Solution for Inhalation 1015

BIOQUIL (Portugal)
OFLOXACIN
Floxin Otic Solution 1043

BIOREUNIL (Mexico)
CARBAMAZEPINE
Carbatrol Capsules 3174
Tegretol Chewable Tablets 2278
Tegretol Suspension 2278
Tegretol Tablets 2278
Tegretol-XR Tablets 2278

BIOSIM (India)
SIMVASTATIN
Zocor Tablets 2078

BIOTAX-O (India)
CEFIXIME
Suprax 1811

BIOTAZOL (Mexico)
METRONIDAZOLE
MetroGel-Vaginal Gel 1822
Noritate Cream, 1% 1051

BIOTECAN (Argentina)
IRINOTECAN HYDROCHLORIDE
Camptosar Injection 2602

BIOTIC (Argentina)
CIPROFLOXACIN HYDROCHLORIDE
Ciloxan Ophthalmic Ointment 554
Ciloxan Ophthalmic Solution . . . . ⊙205
Cipro Tablets 2991

BIOTREDINE (Greece)
ETIDRONATE DISODIUM
Didronel Tablets 2693

BIOTRIL (Mexico)
ERYTHROMYCIN
Ery-Tab Tablets 447
Erythromycin Base Filmtab Tablets 454
Erythromycin Delayed-Release Capsules, USP 456
PCE Dispertab Tablets 510

BIO-VAGIN (Brazil)
METRONIDAZOLE
MetroGel-Vaginal Gel 1822
Noritate Cream, 1% 1051

(⊙ Described in PDR For Ophthalmic Medicines™)

BIOVANCOMIN (Brazil)
VANCOMYCIN HYDROCHLORIDE
Vancocin HCl Capsules, USP 3370

BIOVELBIN (Spain)
VINORELBINE TARTRATE
Navelbine Injection. 1494

BIOVIR (Brazil)
LAMIVUDINE
Epivir Oral Solution 1394
Epivir Tablets 1394
Epivir-HBV Oral Solution 1398
Epivir-HBV Tablets 1398

BIOXAN (Mexico)
NAPROXEN
EC-Naprosyn Delayed-Release Tablets. . . . 2769
Naprosyn Suspension. 2769
Naprosyn Tablets 2769

BIOXILINA (Argentina)
AMOXICILLIN
Amoxil Pediatric Drops for Oral Suspension. 1315
Amoxil Tablets 1315

BIOXILINA PLUS (Argentina)
AMOXICILLIN
Amoxil Pediatric Drops for Oral Suspension. 1315
Amoxil Tablets 1315

BIOXIMA (Italy)
CEFUROXIME SODIUM
Zinacef Injection 1604

BIOZOLIN (Greece)
CEFAZOLIN SODIUM
Ancef for Injection 1318

BIOZORAL (Mexico)
KETOCONAZOLE
Nizoral 2% Shampoo 1838

BIPREDONIUM (Spain)
INDAPAMIDE
Indapamide Tablets 2119

BIPRETERAX (Argentina, Spain)
PERINDOPRIL ERBUMINE
Aceon Tablets (2 mg, 4 mg, 8 mg) 3191

BIPRONYL (Singapore)
NAPROXEN
EC-Naprosyn Delayed-Release Tablets. . . . 2769
Naprosyn Suspension. 2769
Naprosyn Tablets 2769

BIRAC (Argentina)
STAVUDINE
Zerit Capsules 971
Zerit for Oral Solution. 971

BIRVAC (Argentina)
LAMIVUDINE
Epivir Oral Solution 1394
Epivir Tablets 1394
Epivir-HBV Oral Solution 1398
Epivir-HBV Tablets 1398

BISEKO (Czech Republic)
PLASMA PROTEIN FRACTION
Plasmanate 3252

BISMULTIN (Greece)
ECONAZOLE NITRATE
Spectazole Cream. 2390

BISTATIN V (Mexico)
NYSTATIN
Nystop Topical Powder USP. 2490

BISTON (Czech Republic)
CARBAMAZEPINE
Carbatrol Capsules 3174
Tegretol Chewable Tablets 2278
Tegretol Suspension. 2278
Tegretol Tablets 2278
Tegretol-XR Tablets 2278

BITAKEBIR (Argentina)
BICALUTAMIDE
Casodex Tablets 670

BITENSIL (Spain)
ENALAPRIL MALEATE
Vasotec I.V. Injection 2076

BITENSIL DIU (Spain)
ENALAPRIL MALEATE/HYDROCHLOROTHIAZIDE
Vaseretic Tablets. 2073

BI-TILDIEM (France)
DILTIAZEM HYDROCHLORIDE
Cardizem LA Extended Release Tablets. . . 1699
Tiazac Capsules 1204

BIVALEM (Brazil)
MEBENDAZOLE
Vermox Chewable Tablets 1853

B-JEN (Argentina)
PERMETHRIN
Acticin Cream. 2125

BK HC (New Zealand)
HYDROCORTISONE
Hydrocortone Tablets 1963

BLADER (Argentina)
CIPROFLOXACIN
Cipro Oral Suspension 2991

BLEF-10 (Mexico)
SULFACETAMIDE SODIUM
Klaron Lotion 10%. 1050

BLEFAMIDE (Chile)
PREDNISOLONE ACETATE/SULFACETAMIDE SODIUM
Blephamide Ophthalmic Ointment. 563
Blephamide Ophthalmic Suspension 564

BLEFAMIDE SOP (Mexico)
PREDNISOLONE ACETATE/SULFACETAMIDE SODIUM
Blephamide Ophthalmic Ointment. 563
Blephamide Ophthalmic Suspension 564

BLENOX (Spain)
AMOXICILLIN
Amoxil Pediatric Drops for Oral Suspension. 1315
Amoxil Tablets 1315

BLEPH-10 (Australia, Canada, Hong Kong, Irish Republic, New Zealand, South Africa, Thailand)
SULFACETAMIDE SODIUM
Klaron Lotion 10%. 1050

BLEPHAMIDE (Switzerland)
PREDNISOLONE ACETATE/SULFACETAMIDE SODIUM
Blephamide Ophthalmic Ointment. 563
Blephamide Ophthalmic Suspension 564

BLEPHASULF (Austria)
SULFACETAMIDE SODIUM
Klaron Lotion 10%. 1050

BLEZAMONT (Greece)
CETIRIZINE HYDROCHLORIDE
Zyrtec Syrup 2589
Zyrtec Tablets 2589

BLOCACID (India, Mexico, Singapore)
FAMOTIDINE
Pepcid Injection 2017
Pepcid Injection Premixed 2017
Pepcid Tablets 2014
Pepcid for Oral Suspension 2014

BLOCADREN (Australia, Austria, Belgium, Canada, Hong Kong, Irish Republic, Italy, Mexico, Norway, Portugal, South Africa, Spain, Sweden, Switzerland, The Netherlands, United Kingdom)
TIMOLOL MALEATE
Blocadren Tablets 1891
Timoptic Sterile Ophthalmic Solution 2058
Timoptic in Ocudose 2061
Timoptic-XE Sterile Ophthalmic Gel Forming Solution 2062

BLOCALCIN (Czech Republic, Hungary)
DILTIAZEM HYDROCHLORIDE
Cardizem LA Extended Release Tablets. . . 1699
Tiazac Capsules 1204

BLOCAN (Mexico)
CIMETIDINE
Tagamet Tablets 1547

BLOCANOL (Finland)
TIMOLOL MALEATE
Blocadren Tablets 1891
Timoptic Sterile Ophthalmic Solution 2058
Timoptic in Ocudose 2061
Timoptic-XE Sterile Ophthalmic Gel Forming Solution 2062

BLOCAR (Chile)
CARVEDILOL
Coreg Tablets. 1376

BLOCOTENOL (Germany, Greece)
ATENOLOL
Tenormin I.V. Injection. 698

BLOCOTENOL COMP (Germany)
ATENOLOL
Tenormin I.V. Injection. 698

BLOKIUM (Belgium, Hungary, Portugal, Spain)
ATENOLOL
Tenormin I.V. Injection. 698

BLOKIUM DIU (Hungary, Portugal, Spain)
ATENOLOL
Tenormin I.V. Injection. 698

BLOKIUM FLEX (Argentina)
DICLOFENAC SODIUM
Voltaren Tablets 2298
Voltaren-XR Tablets 2301

BLOKIUM GESIC (Argentina)
DICLOFENAC POTASSIUM
Cataflam Tablets 2173

BLOKTUS (Mexico)
BENZONATATE
Tessalon Perles 1202

BLOOTEC (Brazil)
ENALAPRIL MALEATE
Vasotec I.V. Injection 2076

BLOPRESID (Italy)
CANDESARTAN CILEXETIL
Atacand Tablets 634

BLOPRESS (Austria, Brazil, Chile, Czech Republic, Germany, Hong Kong, Italy, Japan, Malaysia, Mexico, Portugal, Switzerland, Thailand)
CANDESARTAN CILEXETIL
Atacand Tablets 634

BLOPRESS 16 MG + 12,5 MG (Portugal)
CANDESARTAN CILEXETIL
Atacand Tablets 634

BLOPRESS PLUS (Germany, Switzerland)
CANDESARTAN CILEXETIL
Atacand Tablets 634

BLOTEX (Mexico)
ATENOLOL
Tenormin I.V. Injection. 698

B-LOVATIN (Greece)
LOVASTATIN
Mevacor Tablets 1996

BLOX (Chile, Italy)
CANDESARTAN CILEXETIL
Atacand Tablets 634

BLUM (Argentina)
PERMETHRIN
Acticin Cream. 2125

BOCATRIOL (Austria, Denmark, Germany, Switzerland)
CALCITRIOL
Calcijex Injection 411

BONALEN (Brazil)
ALENDRONATE SODIUM
Fosamax Tablets 1949

BONCEUR (South Africa)
VERAPAMIL HYDROCHLORIDE
Covera-HS Tablets 3135
Verelan PM Capsules 3120

BONCORDIN (Argentina)
BENAZEPRIL HYDROCHLORIDE
Lotensin Tablets 2232

BONDIL (Norway, Sweden)
ALPROSTADIL
Edex Injection. 3103

BONEMASS (Brazil)
ETIDRONATE DISODIUM
Didronel Tablets 2693

BONJELA TEETHING GEL (United Kingdom)
LIDOCAINE
Lidoderm Patch 1107

BONMAX (India)
RALOXIFENE HYDROCHLORIDE
Evista Tablets. 1735

BONOCEF (Portugal)
CEFIXIME
Suprax 1811

BONYL (Denmark)
NAPROXEN
EC-Naprosyn Delayed-Release Tablets. . . . 2769
Naprosyn Suspension. 2769
Naprosyn Tablets 2769

BOOTS THREADWORM TABLETS 2 YEARS PLUS (United Kingdom)
MEBENDAZOLE
Vermox Chewable Tablets 1853

BOR-CEFAZOL (Italy)
CEFAZOLIN SODIUM
Ancef for Injection 1318

BOSCONAR (Argentina)
BICALUTAMIDE
Casodex Tablets 670

BOTADERM (Greece)
KETOCONAZOLE
Nizoral 2% Shampoo 1838

BOTAMYCIN-N (Greece)
CLINDAMYCIN PHOSPHATE
Clindets Pledgets 3212

BOXOL (Spain)
DALTEPARIN SODIUM
Fragmin Injection. 2638

BOXOLIP (Germany)
LOPERAMIDE HYDROCHLORIDE
Imodium Capsules 1834

BQL (India)
ENALAPRIL MALEATE
Vasotec I.V. Injection 2076

BRADELMIN (Mexico)
ALBENDAZOLE
Albenza Tablets. 1310

BRAINAL (Chile, Czech Republic, Spain)
NIMODIPINE
Nimotop Capsules 774

BRAXAN (Mexico)
AMIODARONE HYDROCHLORIDE
Pacerone Tablets 3337

BREK (Argentina, Italy)
ALENDRONATE SODIUM
Fosamax Tablets 1949

BREMON (Spain)
CLARITHROMYCIN
Biaxin Filmtab Tablets 402
Biaxin Granules 402

BRENOXIL (Mexico)
AMOXICILLIN
Amoxil Pediatric Drops for Oral Suspension. 1315
Amoxil Tablets 1315

BRESBEN (Germany)
ATENOLOL
Tenormin I.V. Injection. 698

BRESEC (Greece)
CEFTRIAXONE SODIUM
Rocephin Injectable Vials, ADD-Vantage, Galaxy, Bulk 2801

BREVIBLOC (Argentina, Australia, Austria, Belgium, Brazil, Canada, Czech Republic, Denmark, Finland, France, Germany, Greece, Hungary, Irish Republic, Israel, Italy, Malaysia, Mexico, New Zealand, Portugal, Singapore, South Africa, Spain, Sweden, Switzerland, United Kingdom)
ESMOLOL HYDROCHLORIDE
Brevibloc Injection 766

BREVOXYL (Australia, Austria, Finland, France, Germany, Greece, Hong Kong, Irish Republic, Malaysia, New Zealand, Norway, Singapore, South Africa, Sweden, Thailand, United Kingdom)
BENZOYL PEROXIDE
Brevoxyl-4 Creamy Wash 3212
Brevoxyl-4 Gel 3211
Brevoxyl-8 Creamy Wash 3212

Brevoxyl-8 Gel . . . 3211
Triaz Cleanser . . . 1864
Triaz Gel . . . 1864

BREXONASE (Chile)
FLUTICASONE PROPIONATE
Cutivate Cream . . . 1381
Cutivate Ointment . . . 1384
Flonase Nasal Spray . . . 1412

BREXOVENT (Chile)
FLUTICASONE PROPIONATE
Cutivate Cream . . . 1381
Cutivate Ointment . . . 1384
Flonase Nasal Spray . . . 1412

BRIAZIDE (France)
BENAZEPRIL HYDROCHLORIDE/HYDROCHLOROTHIAZIDE
Lotensin HCT Tablets . . . 2235

BRIEM (France)
BENAZEPRIL HYDROCHLORIDE
Lotensin Tablets . . . 2232

BRINAF (Czech Republic)
TERBINAFINE HYDROCHLORIDE
Lamisil Tablets . . . 2226

BRINTENAL (Argentina)
SELEGILINE HYDROCHLORIDE
Eldepryl Capsules . . . 3209

BRISOVENT (Portugal)
FLUTICASONE PROPIONATE
Cutivate Cream . . . 1381
Cutivate Ointment . . . 1384
Flonase Nasal Spray . . . 1412

BRISTACOL (Spain)
PRAVASTATIN SODIUM
Pravachol Tablets . . . 943

BRISTAMOX (Sweden)
AMOXICILLIN
Amoxil Pediatric Drops for Oral Suspension . . . 1315
Amoxil Tablets . . . 1315

BRITIAZIM (United Kingdom)
DILTIAZEM HYDROCHLORIDE
Cardizem LA Extended Release Tablets . . . 1699
Tiazac Capsules . . . 1204

BRIXIA (Argentina, Chile)
AZELASTINE HYDROCHLORIDE
Astelin Nasal Spray . . . 1876

BRIXORAL (Greece)
RANITIDINE HYDROCHLORIDE
Zantac 25 EFFERdose Tablets . . . 1597
Zantac 150 EFFERdose Tablets . . . 1597
Zantac 150 Tablets . . . 1597
Zantac 300 Tablets . . . 1597
Zantac Injection . . . 1593
Zantac Injection Premixed . . . 1593
Zantac Syrup . . . 1597

BRIZOLINA (Spain)
CEFAZOLIN SODIUM
Ancef for Injection . . . 1318

BROLIN (Spain)
FAMOTIDINE
Pepcid Injection . . . 2017
Pepcid Injection Premixed . . . 2017
Pepcid Tablets . . . 2014
Pepcid for Oral Suspension . . . 2014

BRONALIDE (Canada, Germany, Greece)
FLUNISOLIDE
Aerobid Inhaler System . . . 1172
Aerobid-M Inhaler System . . . 1172
Nasarel Nasal Spray . . . 1652

BRONCHOPHEN (South Africa)
THEOPHYLLINE
Uniphyl Tablets . . . 2708

BRONCHOPHYLLINE (Israel)
THEOPHYLLINE
Uniphyl Tablets . . . 2708

BRONCHORETARD (Germany)
THEOPHYLLINE
Uniphyl Tablets . . . 2708

BRONCOFOL (India)
THEOPHYLLINE
Uniphyl Tablets . . . 2708

BRONCOFOL-P (India)
THEOPHYLLINE
Uniphyl Tablets . . . 2708

BRONCORT (Belgium, Switzerland)
FLUNISOLIDE
Aerobid Inhaler System . . . 1172
Aerobid-M Inhaler System . . . 1172
Nasarel Nasal Spray . . . 1652

BRONILIDE (Czech Republic, France, Switzerland)
FLUNISOLIDE
Aerobid Inhaler System . . . 1172
Aerobid-M Inhaler System . . . 1172
Nasarel Nasal Spray . . . 1652

BRONKASMA (Argentina)
THEOPHYLLINE
Uniphyl Tablets . . . 2708

BRONQUIASMA (Brazil)
THEOPHYLLINE
Uniphyl Tablets . . . 2708

BROVAFLAMP (South Africa)
DICLOFENAC SODIUM
Voltaren Tablets . . . 2298
Voltaren-XR Tablets . . . 2301

BROVICARPINE (Greece)
VERAPAMIL HYDROCHLORIDE
Covera-HS Tablets . . . 3135
Verelan PM Capsules . . . 3120

BRULAMYCIN (Czech Republic)
TOBRAMYCIN
TOBI Solution for Inhalation . . . 1015

BRUMETIDINA (Italy)
CIMETIDINE
Tagamet Tablets . . . 1547

BRUNAZINE (South Africa)
PROMETHAZINE HYDROCHLORIDE
Phenergan Suppositories . . . 3438
Phenergan Tablets . . . 3438

BUCONIF (Austria)
NIFEDIPINE
Adalat CC Tablets . . . 2978

BUCORT (Finland)
HYDROCORTISONE BUTYRATE
Locoid Cream . . . 1138
Locoid Lipocream Cream . . . 1138
Locoid Ointment . . . 1138
Locoid Topical Solution . . . 1138

BUFIGEN (Mexico)
NALBUPHINE HYDROCHLORIDE
Nubain Injection . . . 1111

BUG PROOF (United Kingdom)
PERMETHRIN
Acticin Cream . . . 2125

BUGAZON (Mexico)
CAPTOPRIL
Captopril Tablets . . . 2114

BUMAFLEX N (Argentina)
NAPROXEN
EC-Naprosyn Delayed-Release Tablets . . . 2769
Naprosyn Suspension . . . 2769
Naprosyn Tablets . . . 2769

BUMETONE (Thailand)
NABUMETONE
Relafen Tablets . . . 1523

BUPREN (Hungary)
BUPRENORPHINE HYDROCHLORIDE
Buprenex Injectable . . . 2718

BUPREX (Portugal, Spain)
BUPRENORPHINE HYDROCHLORIDE
Buprenex Injectable . . . 2718

BUPRINE (Thailand)
BUPRENORPHINE HYDROCHLORIDE
Buprenex Injectable . . . 2718

BURAM (Irish Republic)
AMILORIDE HYDROCHLORIDE
Midamor Tablets . . . 2000

BUROFIX (Hungary)
CALCIUM ACETATE
PhosLo GelCaps . . . 2158

BUSILVEX (Denmark, Sweden, United Kingdom)
BUSULFAN
Myleran Tablets . . . 1492

BUSULFEX (Canada, Hong Kong, Israel)
BUSULFAN
Myleran Tablets . . . 1492

BUTAVATE (Greece)
CLOBETASOL PROPIONATE
Temovate Cream . . . 1549
Temovate E Emollient . . . 1552
Temovate Gel . . . 1550
Temovate Ointment . . . 1549
Temovate Scalp Application . . . 1551

BUTOP (India)
BUTENAFINE HYDROCHLORIDE
Mentax Cream . . . 2152

BUTOSALI (Mexico)
FUROSEMIDE
Furosemide Tablets . . . 2117

BUXON (Chile)
BUPROPION HYDROCHLORIDE
Wellbutrin SR Sustained-Release Tablets . . . 1583
Wellbutrin Tablets . . . 1579
Zyban Sustained-Release Tablets . . . 1620

B-VASC (South Africa)
ATENOLOL
Tenormin I.V. Injection . . . 698

BYANODINE (Hungary)
PENICILLAMINE
Cuprimine Capsules . . . 1925

C-86 (Argentina)
KETOCONAZOLE
Nizoral 2% Shampoo . . . 1838

CABAL (Argentina)
CETIRIZINE HYDROCHLORIDE
Zyrtec Syrup . . . 2589
Zyrtec Tablets . . . 2589

CABASER (Argentina, Australia, Denmark, Finland, Irish Republic, Israel, Italy, Norway, Sweden, Switzerland, United Kingdom)
CABERGOLINE
Dostinex Tablets . . . 2631

CABASERIL (Austria, Germany)
CABERGOLINE
Dostinex Tablets . . . 2631

CADPRES (India)
ATENOLOL
Tenormin I.V. Injection . . . 698

CAGINAL (Thailand)
CLOTRIMAZOLE
Lotrimin Cream . . . 3053
Lotrimin Lotion 1% . . . 3053
Lotrimin Topical Solution 1% . . . 3053

CALANIF (United Kingdom)
NIFEDIPINE
Adalat CC Tablets . . . 2978

CAL-ANTAGON (Portugal)
DILTIAZEM HYDROCHLORIDE
Cardizem LA Extended Release Tablets . . . 1699
Tiazac Capsules . . . 1204

CALAPTIN (India)
VERAPAMIL HYDROCHLORIDE
Covera-HS Tablets . . . 3135
Verelan PM Capsules . . . 3120

CALAZEM (United Kingdom)
DILTIAZEM HYDROCHLORIDE
Cardizem LA Extended Release Tablets . . . 1699
Tiazac Capsules . . . 1204

CALCETAT (Italy)
CALCIUM ACETATE
PhosLo GelCaps . . . 2158

CALCHAN (United Kingdom)
NIFEDIPINE
Adalat CC Tablets . . . 2978

CALCICARD (South Africa, United Kingdom)
VERAPAMIL HYDROCHLORIDE
Covera-HS Tablets . . . 3135
Verelan PM Capsules . . . 3120

CALCIGARD (India, Thailand)
NIFEDIPINE
Adalat CC Tablets . . . 2978

CALCIJEX (Australia, Austria, Canada, Czech Republic, Finland, Hong Kong, Hungary, Irish Republic, Israel, Italy, Malaysia, Mexico, Norway, Singapore, Spain, Sweden, Switzerland, United Kingdom)
CALCITRIOL
Calcijex Injection . . . 411

CALCILAT (United Kingdom)
NIFEDIPINE
Adalat CC Tablets . . . 2978

CALFATE (Portugal)
SUCRALFATE
Carafate Suspension . . . 727
Carafate Tablets . . . 728

CALIDIOL (Hungary)
ESTRADIOL
Climara Transdermal System . . . 795
Vivelle Transdermal System . . . 2288
Vivelle-Dot Transdermal System . . . 2293

CALMANTE DE DENTICION (Chile)
LIDOCAINE
Lidoderm Patch . . . 1107

CALMARIL (Thailand)
THIORIDAZINE HYDROCHLORIDE
Thioridazine Hydrochloride Tablets . . . 2122

CALMAVEN (Spain)
DIAZEPAM
Diastat Rectal Delivery System . . . 3344
Valium Tablets . . . 2822

CALMICORT (France)
HYDROCORTISONE
Hydrocortone Tablets . . . 1963

CALMIDAN (Spain)
SUCRALFATE
Carafate Suspension . . . 727
Carafate Tablets . . . 728

CALMIGEN (Irish Republic)
DIAZEPAM
Diastat Rectal Delivery System . . . 3344
Valium Tablets . . . 2822

CALMOCITENO (Brazil)
DIAZEPAM
Diastat Rectal Delivery System . . . 3344
Valium Tablets . . . 2822

CALMOSERPIN (Germany)
HYDROCHLOROTHIAZIDE/TRIAMTERENE
Dyazide Capsules . . . 1389
Maxzide Tablets . . . 2150
Maxzide-25 mg Tablets . . . 2150

CALMPOSE (India, South Africa)
DIAZEPAM
Diastat Rectal Delivery System . . . 3344
Valium Tablets . . . 2822

CALMURID (Chile)
HYDROCORTISONE
Hydrocortone Tablets . . . 1963

CALNIF (India)
NIFEDIPINE
Adalat CC Tablets . . . 2978

CALNIT (Spain)
NIMODIPINE
Nimotop Capsules . . . 774

CALURAN (India)
BICALUTAMIDE
Casodex Tablets . . . 670

CALUTIDE (India)
BICALUTAMIDE
Casodex Tablets . . . 670

CAMCOLIT (Belgium, Hong Kong, Irish Republic, Singapore, South Africa, The Netherlands, United Kingdom)
LITHIUM CARBONATE
Eskalith CR Controlled-Release Tablets . . . 1406
Eskalith Capsules . . . 1406

CAMIL (Spain)
CEFAZOLIN SODIUM
Ancef for Injection . . . 1318

CAMOXIN (Brazil)
AMOXICILLIN
Amoxil Pediatric Drops for Oral Suspension . . . 1315
Amoxil Tablets . . . 1315

CAMPTO (Austria, Belgium, Czech Republic, Denmark, Finland, France, Germany, Greece, Hong Kong, Hungary, Irish Republic, Israel, Italy, Malaysia, Norway, Portugal, Russia, Singapore, South Africa, Spain, Sweden, Switzerland, Thailand, The Netherlands, United Kingdom)
IRINOTECAN HYDROCHLORIDE
Camptosar Injection . . . 2602

CAMPTOSAR (Argentina, Australia, Brazil, Canada, Chile, Mexico, New Zealand)
IRINOTECAN HYDROCHLORIDE
Camptosar Injection 2602

CANADINE (Thailand)
CLOTRIMAZOLE
Lotrimin Cream 3053
Lotrimin Lotion 1% 3053
Lotrimin Topical Solution 1% 3053

CANALBA (South Africa)
CLOTRIMAZOLE
Lotrimin Cream 3053
Lotrimin Lotion 1% 3053
Lotrimin Topical Solution 1% 3053

CANAZOL (Denmark, Thailand)
CLOTRIMAZOLE
Lotrimin Cream 3053
Lotrimin Lotion 1% 3053
Lotrimin Topical Solution 1% 3053

CANDACIDE (South Africa)
NYSTATIN
Nystop Topical Powder USP 2490

CANDACORT (Malaysia, Singapore)
CLOTRIMAZOLE
Lotrimin Cream 3053
Lotrimin Lotion 1% 3053
Lotrimin Topical Solution 1% 3053

CANDASPOR (South Africa)
CLOTRIMAZOLE
Lotrimin Cream 3053
Lotrimin Lotion 1% 3053
Lotrimin Topical Solution 1% 3053

CANDAZOL (Germany)
CLOTRIMAZOLE
Lotrimin Cream 3053
Lotrimin Lotion 1% 3053
Lotrimin Topical Solution 1% 3053

CANDAZOLE (Malaysia, Singapore)
CLOTRIMAZOLE
Lotrimin Cream 3053
Lotrimin Lotion 1% 3053
Lotrimin Topical Solution 1% 3053

CANDERME (Brazil)
METRONIDAZOLE
MetroGel-Vaginal Gel 1822
Noritate Cream, 1% 1051

CANDERMIL (Argentina)
NYSTATIN
Nystop Topical Powder USP 2490

CANDIBENE (Austria, Czech Republic, Hungary)
CLOTRIMAZOLE
Lotrimin Cream 3053
Lotrimin Lotion 1% 3053
Lotrimin Topical Solution 1% 3053

CANDICORT (Brazil)
KETOCONAZOLE
Nizoral 2% Shampoo 1838

CANDID (India, Malaysia, Portugal, Thailand)
CLOTRIMAZOLE
Lotrimin Cream 3053
Lotrimin Lotion 1% 3053
Lotrimin Topical Solution 1% 3053

CANDID B (India)
CLOTRIMAZOLE
Lotrimin Cream 3053
Lotrimin Lotion 1% 3053
Lotrimin Topical Solution 1% 3053

CANDID EAR DROPS (India)
CLOTRIMAZOLE
Lotrimin Cream 3053
Lotrimin Lotion 1% 3053
Lotrimin Topical Solution 1% 3053

CANDIDA-LOKALICID (Germany)
NYSTATIN
Nystop Topical Powder USP 2490

CANDIDEN (United Kingdom)
CLOTRIMAZOLE
Lotrimin Cream 3053
Lotrimin Lotion 1% 3053
Lotrimin Topical Solution 1% 3053

CANDIDERM (Brazil)
KETOCONAZOLE
Nizoral 2% Shampoo 1838

CANDIDIAS (Argentina)
NYSTATIN
Nystop Topical Powder USP 2490

CANDID-TV (India)
CLOTRIMAZOLE
Lotrimin Cream 3053
Lotrimin Lotion 1% 3053
Lotrimin Topical Solution 1% 3053

CANDIMON (Mexico)
CLOTRIMAZOLE
Lotrimin Cream 3053
Lotrimin Lotion 1% 3053
Lotrimin Topical Solution 1% 3053

CANDINOX (Thailand)
CLOTRIMAZOLE
Lotrimin Cream 3053
Lotrimin Lotion 1% 3053
Lotrimin Topical Solution 1% 3053

CANDIO (Austria, Germany, Switzerland)
NYSTATIN
Nystop Topical Powder USP 2490

CANDISTATIN (Canada)
NYSTATIN
Nystop Topical Powder USP 2490

CANDIZOLE (South Africa)
CLOTRIMAZOLE
Lotrimin Cream 3053
Lotrimin Lotion 1% 3053
Lotrimin Topical Solution 1% 3053

CANDORAL (Brazil)
KETOCONAZOLE
Nizoral 2% Shampoo 1838

CANEF (Denmark, Finland, Mexico, Norway, Portugal, Sweden, The Netherlands)
FLUVASTATIN SODIUM
Lescol Capsules 2227

CANESTEN (Australia, Austria, Brazil, Canada, Chile, Denmark, Finland, Germany, Greece, Hong Kong, Hungary, Irish Republic, Italy, Malaysia, Mexico, New Zealand, Norway, Portugal, Singapore, South Africa, Spain, Sweden, Thailand, The Netherlands, United Kingdom)
CLOTRIMAZOLE
Lotrimin Cream 3053
Lotrimin Lotion 1% 3053
Lotrimin Topical Solution 1% 3053

CANESTEN COMBI (United Kingdom)
CLOTRIMAZOLE
Lotrimin Cream 3053
Lotrimin Lotion 1% 3053
Lotrimin Topical Solution 1% 3053

CANESTEN HC (Germany, Hong Kong, United Kingdom)
CLOTRIMAZOLE
Lotrimin Cream 3053
Lotrimin Lotion 1% 3053
Lotrimin Topical Solution 1% 3053

CANESTENE (Belgium, Switzerland)
CLOTRIMAZOLE
Lotrimin Cream 3053
Lotrimin Lotion 1% 3053
Lotrimin Topical Solution 1% 3053

CANEX (South Africa)
CLOTRIMAZOLE
Lotrimin Cream 3053
Lotrimin Lotion 1% 3053
Lotrimin Topical Solution 1% 3053

CANFERON (Japan)
INTERFERON ALFA-2A
Roferon-A Injection 2805

CANIFUG (Czech Republic, Germany, Hungary)
CLOTRIMAZOLE
Lotrimin Cream 3053
Lotrimin Lotion 1% 3053
Lotrimin Topical Solution 1% 3053

CANSTAT (South Africa)
NYSTATIN
Nystop Topical Powder USP 2490

CANTANIDIN (Austria)
CLONIDINE HYDROCHLORIDE
Catapres Tablets 874

CAPACE (Australia, Austria, India, South Africa)
CAPTOPRIL
Captopril Tablets 2114

CAPEL (Brazil)
KETOCONAZOLE
Nizoral 2% Shampoo 1838

CAPIN (Hungary)
CAPTOPRIL
Captopril Tablets 2114

CAPITIS (Argentina)
PERMETHRIN
Acticin Cream 2125

CAPOCARD (Hong Kong)
CAPTOPRIL
Captopril Tablets 2114

CAPOSTAD (Austria)
CAPTOPRIL
Captopril Tablets 2114

CAPOTEN (Australia, Belgium, Brazil, Canada, Chile, Czech Republic, Denmark, Finland, Greece, Hong Kong, Irish Republic, Italy, Malaysia, New Zealand, Norway, Portugal, Singapore, South Africa, Spain, Sweden, Thailand, The Netherlands, United Kingdom)
CAPTOPRIL
Captopril Tablets 2114

CAPOTENA (Mexico)
CAPTOPRIL
Captopril Tablets 2114

CAPOTRIL (Brazil)
CAPTOPRIL
Captopril Tablets 2114

CAPOZID (Denmark)
CAPTOPRIL
Captopril Tablets 2114

CAPOZIDE (Germany, Mexico, New Zealand, South Africa, United Kingdom)
CAPTOPRIL
Captopril Tablets 2114

CAPRIL (Brazil, Hong Kong)
CAPTOPRIL
Captopril Tablets 2114

CAPROS (Germany)
MORPHINE SULFATE
Kadian Capsules 572
MS Contin Tablets 2703

CAPRYSIN (Finland)
CLONIDINE HYDROCHLORIDE
Catapres Tablets 874

CAPSICOF (Mexico)
BENZONATATE
Tessalon Perles 1202

CAPTI (Israel)
CAPTOPRIL
Captopril Tablets 2114

CAPTIL (Brazil)
CAPTOPRIL
Captopril Tablets 2114

CAPTIREX (France)
CAPTOPRIL
Captopril Tablets 2114

CAPTO PLUS (Germany)
CAPTOPRIL
Captopril Tablets 2114

CAPTO-BASAN (Switzerland)
CAPTOPRIL
Captopril Tablets 2114

CAPTOBETA (Germany)
CAPTOPRIL
Captopril Tablets 2114

CAPTOBETA COMP (Germany)
CAPTOPRIL
Captopril Tablets 2114

CAPTO-CO (United Kingdom)
CAPTOPRIL
Captopril Tablets 2114

CAPTODAN (Denmark)
CAPTOPRIL
Captopril Tablets 2114

CAPTODOC (Germany)
CAPTOPRIL
Captopril Tablets 2114

CAPTODOC COMP (Germany)
CAPTOPRIL
Captopril Tablets 2114

CAPTO-DURA COR (Germany)
CAPTOPRIL
Captopril Tablets 2114

CAPTO-DURA M (Germany)
CAPTOPRIL
Captopril Tablets 2114

CAPTOFLUX (Germany)
CAPTOPRIL
Captopril Tablets 2114

CAPTOGAMMA (Germany, Hungary)
CAPTOPRIL
Captopril Tablets 2114

CAPTOGAMMA HCT (Germany)
CAPTOPRIL
Captopril Tablets 2114

CAPTOHEXAL (Australia, Germany, New Zealand, South Africa)
CAPTOPRIL
Captopril Tablets 2114

CAPTOHEXAL COMP (Austria, Czech Republic, Germany)
CAPTOPRIL
Captopril Tablets 2114

CAPTOL (Denmark)
CAPTOPRIL
Captopril Tablets 2114

CAPTOLANE (France)
CAPTOPRIL
Captopril Tablets 2114

CAPTOMAX (South Africa)
CAPTOPRIL
Captopril Tablets 2114

CAPTOMED (Austria, Brazil)
CAPTOPRIL
Captopril Tablets 2114

CAPTOMERCK (Germany)
CAPTOPRIL
Captopril Tablets 2114

CAPTOMIN (Finland)
CAPTOPRIL
Captopril Tablets 2114

CAPTON (Brazil)
CAPTOPRIL
Captopril Tablets 2114

CAPTOPIRIL (Brazil)
CAPTOPRIL
Captopril Tablets 2114

CAPTOPLUS (Austria)
CAPTOPRIL
Captopril Tablets 2114

CAPTOPRESS (Germany)
CAPTOPRIL
Captopril Tablets 2114

CAPTOPRIL HCT (Germany)
CAPTOPRIL
Captopril Tablets 2114

CAPTOPRIL PLUS (Germany)
CAPTOPRIL
Captopril Tablets 2114

CAPTOPRIL-HCT (Austria)
CAPTOPRIL
Captopril Tablets 2114

CAPTOR (Austria, Irish Republic)
CAPTOPRIL
Captopril Tablets 2114

CAPTOREAL (Germany)
CAPTOPRIL
Captopril Tablets 2114

CAPTORETIC (South Africa)
CAPTOPRIL
Captopril Tablets 2114

CAPTOR-HCT (Irish Republic)
CAPTOPRIL
Captopril Tablets 2114

CAPTOSER (Mexico)
CAPTOPRIL
Captopril Tablets 2114

CAPTOSINA (Spain)
CAPTOPRIL
Captopril Tablets 2114

CAPTOSOL (Switzerland)
CAPTOPRIL
Captopril Tablets 2114

CAPTOSOL COMP (Switzerland)
CAPTOPRIL
Captopril Tablets 2114

CAPTOSTAD (Finland)
CAPTOPRIL
Captopril Tablets 2114

CAPTOTEC (Brazil)
CAPTOPRIL
Captopril Tablets 2114

CAPTOTEC + HCT (Brazil)
CAPTOPRIL
Captopril Tablets 2114

CAPTOTYROL (Austria)
CAPTOPRIL
Captopril Tablets 2114

CAPTRAL (Mexico)
CAPTOPRIL
Captopril Tablets 2114

CAPTRIL (Canada)
CAPTOPRIL
Captopril Tablets 2114

CAPTRIZIN (Brazil)
CAPTOPRIL
Captopril Tablets 2114

CARACE (Irish Republic, United Kingdom)
LISINOPRIL
Prinivil Tablets 2029
Zestril Tablets 704

CARACE PLUS (Irish Republic, United Kingdom)
HYDROCHLOROTHIAZIDE/LISINOPRIL
Prinzide Tablets 2033
Zestoretic Tablets 701

CARAFATE (Australia, New Zealand)
SUCRALFATE
Carafate Suspension 727
Carafate Tablets 728

CARALPHA (United Kingdom)
LISINOPRIL
Prinivil Tablets 2029
Zestril Tablets 704

CARASEL (Spain)
RAMIPRIL
Altace Capsules 1673

CARBA (Germany)
CARBAMAZEPINE
Carbatrol Capsules 3174
Tegretol Chewable Tablets 2278
Tegretol Suspension 2278
Tegretol Tablets 2278
Tegretol-XR Tablets 2278

CARBABETA (Germany)
CARBAMAZEPINE
Carbatrol Capsules 3174
Tegretol Chewable Tablets 2278
Tegretol Suspension 2278
Tegretol Tablets 2278
Tegretol-XR Tablets 2278

CARBACTOL RETARD (Chile)
CARBAMAZEPINE
Carbatrol Capsules 3174
Tegretol Chewable Tablets 2278
Tegretol Suspension 2278
Tegretol Tablets 2278
Tegretol-XR Tablets 2278

CARBADURA (Germany)
CARBAMAZEPINE
Carbatrol Capsules 3174
Tegretol Chewable Tablets 2278
Tegretol Suspension 2278
Tegretol Tablets 2278
Tegretol-XR Tablets 2278

CARBAFLUX (Germany)
CARBAMAZEPINE
Carbatrol Capsules 3174
Tegretol Chewable Tablets 2278
Tegretol Suspension 2278
Tegretol Tablets 2278
Tegretol-XR Tablets 2278

CARBAGAMMA (Germany)
CARBAMAZEPINE
Carbatrol Capsules 3174
Tegretol Chewable Tablets 2278
Tegretol Suspension 2278
Tegretol Tablets 2278
Tegretol-XR Tablets 2278

CARBAGEN (United Kingdom)
CARBAMAZEPINE
Carbatrol Capsules 3174
Tegretol Chewable Tablets 2278
Tegretol Suspension 2278
Tegretol Tablets 2278
Tegretol-XR Tablets 2278

CARBAGRAMON (Argentina)
CARBAMAZEPINE
Carbatrol Capsules 3174
Tegretol Chewable Tablets 2278
Tegretol Suspension 2278
Tegretol Tablets 2278
Tegretol-XR Tablets 2278

CARBALAN (Mexico)
CARBAMAZEPINE
Carbatrol Capsules 3174
Tegretol Chewable Tablets 2278
Tegretol Suspension 2278
Tegretol Tablets 2278
Tegretol-XR Tablets 2278

CARBAMAT (Argentina)
CARBAMAZEPINE
Carbatrol Capsules 3174
Tegretol Chewable Tablets 2278
Tegretol Suspension 2278
Tegretol Tablets 2278
Tegretol-XR Tablets 2278

CARBATIL (Mexico)
MEBENDAZOLE
Vermox Chewable Tablets 1853

CARBATOL (Thailand)
CARBAMAZEPINE
Carbatrol Capsules 3174
Tegretol Chewable Tablets 2278
Tegretol Suspension 2278
Tegretol Tablets 2278
Tegretol-XR Tablets 2278

CARBAVAL (Mexico)
CARBAMAZEPINE
Carbatrol Capsules 3174
Tegretol Chewable Tablets 2278
Tegretol Suspension 2278
Tegretol Tablets 2278
Tegretol-XR Tablets 2278

CARBAZENE (Thailand)
CARBAMAZEPINE
Carbatrol Capsules 3174
Tegretol Chewable Tablets 2278
Tegretol Suspension 2278
Tegretol Tablets 2278
Tegretol-XR Tablets 2278

CARBAZEP (Mexico)
CARBAMAZEPINE
Carbatrol Capsules 3174
Tegretol Chewable Tablets 2278
Tegretol Suspension 2278
Tegretol Tablets 2278
Tegretol-XR Tablets 2278

CARBAZINA (Mexico)
CARBAMAZEPINE
Carbatrol Capsules 3174
Tegretol Chewable Tablets 2278
Tegretol Suspension 2278
Tegretol Tablets 2278
Tegretol-XR Tablets 2278

CARBI (Israel)
CARBAMAZEPINE
Carbatrol Capsules 3174
Tegretol Chewable Tablets 2278
Tegretol Suspension 2278
Tegretol Tablets 2278
Tegretol-XR Tablets 2278

CARBIUM (Australia, Germany)
CARBAMAZEPINE
Carbatrol Capsules 3174
Tegretol Chewable Tablets 2278
Tegretol Suspension 2278
Tegretol Tablets 2278
Tegretol-XR Tablets 2278

CARBLOC (Chile)
NIFEDIPINE
Adalat CC Tablets 2978

CARBOLIM (Brazil)
LITHIUM CARBONATE
Eskalith CR Controlled-Release Tablets . . . 1406
Eskalith Capsules 1406

CARBOLIT (Chile, Mexico)
LITHIUM CARBONATE
Eskalith CR Controlled-Release Tablets . . . 1406
Eskalith Capsules 1406

CARBOLITH (Canada)
LITHIUM CARBONATE
Eskalith CR Controlled-Release Tablets . . . 1406
Eskalith Capsules 1406

CARBOLITHIUM (Italy)
LITHIUM CARBONATE
Eskalith CR Controlled-Release Tablets . . . 1406
Eskalith Capsules 1406

CARBOLITIUM (Brazil)
LITHIUM CARBONATE
Eskalith CR Controlled-Release Tablets . . . 1406
Eskalith Capsules 1406

CARBORON (Chile)
LITHIUM CARBONATE
Eskalith CR Controlled-Release Tablets . . . 1406
Eskalith Capsules 1406

CARBRITAL (Australia)
PENTOBARBITAL SODIUM
Nembutal Sodium Solution, USP 2484

CARDACE (Finland, India)
RAMIPRIL
Altace Capsules 1673

CARDACE COMP (Finland)
RAMIPRIL
Altace Capsules 1673

CARDALIN (Brazil)
NIFEDIPINE
Adalat CC Tablets 2978

CARDAXEN (Switzerland)
ATENOLOL
Tenormin I.V. Injection 698

CARDCAL (Australia)
DILTIAZEM HYDROCHLORIDE
Cardizem LA Extended Release Tablets . . . 1699
Tiazac Capsules 1204

CARDCOR (Brazil)
DIGOXIN
Lanoxicaps Capsules 1458
Lanoxin Injection 1462
Lanoxin Injection Pediatric 1465
Lanoxin Tablets 1468

CARDENOL (Thailand)
PROPRANOLOL HYDROCHLORIDE
Inderal LA Long-Acting Capsules 3421

CARDIACE (South Africa)
CAPTOPRIL
Captopril Tablets 2114

CARDIACTON (Austria)
DILTIAZEM HYDROCHLORIDE
Cardizem LA Extended Release Tablets . . . 1699
Tiazac Capsules 1204

CARDIAGEN (Germany)
CAPTOPRIL
Captopril Tablets 2114

CARDIAGEN HCT (Germany)
CAPTOPRIL
Captopril Tablets 2114

CARDIAGUTT (Germany)
VERAPAMIL HYDROCHLORIDE
Covera-HS Tablets 3135
Verelan PM Capsules 3120

CARDIBELTIN (Germany)
VERAPAMIL HYDROCHLORIDE
Covera-HS Tablets 3135
Verelan PM Capsules 3120

CARDIBLOK (South Africa)
PROPRANOLOL HYDROCHLORIDE
Inderal LA Long-Acting Capsules 3421

CARDICON (Chile)
NIFEDIPINE
Adalat CC Tablets 2978

CARDIFEN (South Africa)
NIFEDIPINE
Adalat CC Tablets 2978

CARDIL (Denmark, Malaysia, Singapore, Thailand)
DILTIAZEM HYDROCHLORIDE
Cardizem LA Extended Release Tablets . . . 1699
Tiazac Capsules 1204

CARDILAT (South Africa)
NIFEDIPINE
Adalat CC Tablets 2978

CARDILATE MR (Hong Kong, United Kingdom)
NIFEDIPINE
Adalat CC Tablets 2978

CARDILOL (Brazil, United Arab Emirates)
CARVEDILOL
Coreg Tablets 1376

CARDINOL (Australia, New Zealand, United Kingdom)
PROPRANOLOL HYDROCHLORIDE
Inderal LA Long-Acting Capsules 3421

CARDINORM (Australia, Italy)
AMIODARONE HYDROCHLORIDE
Pacerone Tablets 3337

CARDIOBIL (Italy)
LEVOCARNITINE
Carnitor Injection 3185
Carnitor Tablets and Oral Solution 3187

CARDIOBRON (Argentina)
ALPROSTADIL
Edex Injection 3103

CARDIOFENONE (Italy)
PROPAFENONE HYDROCHLORIDE
Rythmol SR Capsules 2736

CARDIOGEN (Italy)
LEVOCARNITINE
Carnitor Injection 3185
Carnitor Tablets and Oral Solution 3187

CARDIOGOXIN (Argentina)
DIGOXIN
Lanoxicaps Capsules 1458
Lanoxin Injection 1462
Lanoxin Injection Pediatric 1465
Lanoxin Tablets 1468

CARDIOL (Finland, Portugal)
CARVEDILOL
Coreg Tablets 1376

CARDIOLEN (Chile)
VERAPAMIL HYDROCHLORIDE
Covera-HS Tablets 3135
Verelan PM Capsules 3120

CARDIONIL (Brazil, Spain)
ISOSORBIDE MONONITRATE
Imdur Tablets 3032

CARDIOPINA (Brazil)
NIFEDIPINE
Adalat CC Tablets 2978

CARDIOPINE (United Arab Emirates)
NIFEDIPINE
Adalat CC Tablets 2978

CARDIOPLEN (United Kingdom)
FELODIPINE
Plendil Extended-Release Tablets 651

CARDIOPROTECT (Germany)
VERAPAMIL HYDROCHLORIDE
Covera-HS Tablets 3135
Verelan PM Capsules 3120

CARDIOREG (Italy)
DIGOXIN
Lanoxicaps Capsules 1458
Lanoxin Injection 1462
Lanoxin Injection Pediatric 1465
Lanoxin Tablets 1468

CARDIOVAS (Spain)
ISOSORBIDE MONONITRATE
Imdur Tablets 3032

CARDIOXIN (India)
DIGOXIN
Lanoxicaps Capsules 1458
Lanoxin Injection 1462
Lanoxin Injection Pediatric 1465
Lanoxin Tablets 1468

CARDIPIN (Switzerland)
NIFEDIPINE
Adalat CC Tablets 2978

CARDIPRIL (Mexico)
CAPTOPRIL
Captopril Tablets 2114

CARDISER (Spain)
DILTIAZEM HYDROCHLORIDE
Cardizem LA Extended Release Tablets 1699
Tiazac Capsules 1204

CARDISORB (Hungary)
ISOSORBIDE MONONITRATE
Imdur Tablets 3032

CARDISPAN (Mexico)
LEVOCARNITINE
Carnitor Injection 3185
Carnitor Tablets and Oral Solution 3187

CARDISPARE (South Africa)
PROPRANOLOL HYDROCHLORIDE
Inderal LA Long-Acting Capsules 3421

CARDIUM (Hong Kong, Singapore)
DILTIAZEM HYDROCHLORIDE
Cardizem LA Extended Release Tablets 1699
Tiazac Capsules 1204

CARDIVAS (Russia)
CARVEDILOL
Coreg Tablets 1376

CARDIZEM (Australia, Brazil, Canada, Denmark, Finland, New Zealand, Norway, Sweden)
DILTIAZEM HYDROCHLORIDE
Cardizem LA Extended Release Tablets 1699
Tiazac Capsules 1204

CARDOXIN (Israel)
DIPYRIDAMOLE
Persantine Tablets 898

CARDULES (India)
NIFEDIPINE
Adalat CC Tablets 2978

CARDULES PLUS (India)
ATENOLOL
Tenormin I.V. Injection 698

CARDYL (Spain)
ATORVASTATIN CALCIUM
Lipitor Tablets 2495

CAREFLU (Italy)
FLUNISOLIDE
Aerobid Inhaler System 1172
Aerobid-M Inhaler System 1172
Nasarel Nasal Spray 1652

CARENCIL (Portugal)
CAPTOPRIL
Captopril Tablets 2114

CARICEF (Spain)
CEFAZOLIN SODIUM
Ancef for Injection 1318

CARLOC (India, South Africa)
CARVEDILOL
Coreg Tablets 1376

CARMAPINE (Thailand)
CARBAMAZEPINE
Carbatrol Capsules 3174
Tegretol Chewable Tablets 2278
Tegretol Suspension 2278
Tegretol Tablets 2278
Tegretol-XR Tablets 2278

CARMAZIN (Brazil)
CARBAMAZEPINE
Carbatrol Capsules 3174
Tegretol Chewable Tablets 2278
Tegretol Suspension 2278
Tegretol Tablets 2278
Tegretol-XR Tablets 2278

CARMIAN (Italy)
ATENOLOL
Tenormin I.V. Injection 698

CARMICINA (Portugal)
CIPROFLOXACIN HYDROCHLORIDE
Ciloxan Ophthalmic Ointment 554
Ciloxan Ophthalmic Solution ⊙205
Cipro Tablets 2991

CARNICOR (Chile, Italy)
LEVOCARNITINE
Carnitor Injection 3185
Carnitor Tablets and Oral Solution 3187

CARNIDOSE (Greece)
LEVOCARNITINE
Carnitor Injection 3185
Carnitor Tablets and Oral Solution 3187

CARNIL (Greece)
LEVOCARNITINE
Carnitor Injection 3185
Carnitor Tablets and Oral Solution 3187

CARNITENE (Hong Kong, Italy)
LEVOCARNITINE
Carnitor Injection 3185
Carnitor Tablets and Oral Solution 3187

CARNITOP (Italy)
LEVOCARNITINE
Carnitor Injection 3185
Carnitor Tablets and Oral Solution 3187

CARNITOR (Canada, Hong Kong, United Kingdom)
LEVOCARNITINE
Carnitor Injection 3185
Carnitor Tablets and Oral Solution 3187

CARNOVIS (Italy)
LEVOCARNITINE
Carnitor Injection 3185
Carnitor Tablets and Oral Solution 3187

CARNUM (Italy)
LEVOCARNITINE
Carnitor Injection 3185
Carnitor Tablets and Oral Solution 3187

CARPAZ (South Africa)
CARBAMAZEPINE
Carbatrol Capsules 3174
Tegretol Chewable Tablets 2278
Tegretol Suspension 2278
Tegretol Tablets 2278
Tegretol-XR Tablets 2278

CARPIN (Mexico)
CARBAMAZEPINE
Carbatrol Capsules 3174
Tegretol Chewable Tablets 2278
Tegretol Suspension 2278
Tegretol Tablets 2278
Tegretol-XR Tablets 2278

CARPINE (Thailand)
CARBAMAZEPINE
Carbatrol Capsules 3174
Tegretol Chewable Tablets 2278
Tegretol Suspension 2278
Tegretol Tablets 2278
Tegretol-XR Tablets 2278

CARRELDON (Spain)
DILTIAZEM HYDROCHLORIDE
Cardizem LA Extended Release Tablets 1699
Tiazac Capsules 1204

CARRIER (Italy)
LEVOCARNITINE
Carnitor Injection 3185
Carnitor Tablets and Oral Solution 3187

CARVEDEXXON (Israel)
CARVEDILOL
Coreg Tablets 1376

CARVEDIL (Argentina)
CARVEDILOL
Coreg Tablets 1376

CARVEL (Argentina)
CARVEDILOL
Coreg Tablets 1376

CARVETONE (Denmark)
CARVEDILOL
Coreg Tablets 1376

CARVIL (India)
CARVEDILOL
Coreg Tablets 1376

CARVIPRESS (Italy)
CARVEDILOL
Coreg Tablets 1376

CARZEM (Italy)
DILTIAZEM HYDROCHLORIDE
Cardizem LA Extended Release Tablets 1699
Tiazac Capsules 1204

CARZEPINE (Thailand)
CARBAMAZEPINE
Carbatrol Capsules 3174
Tegretol Chewable Tablets 2278
Tegretol Suspension 2278
Tegretol Tablets 2278
Tegretol-XR Tablets 2278

CASBOL (Spain)
PAROXETINE HYDROCHLORIDE
Paxil Oral Suspension 1501
Paxil Tablets 1501

CASCOR (Malaysia, Thailand)
DILTIAZEM HYDROCHLORIDE
Cardizem LA Extended Release Tablets 1699
Tiazac Capsules 1204

CASODEX (Argentina, Austria, Belgium, Brazil, Canada, Chile, Czech Republic, Denmark, Finland, France, Germany, Greece, Hong Kong, Hungary, Irish Republic, Israel, Italy, Malaysia, Mexico, Norway, Portugal, Russia, Singapore, South Africa, Spain, Sweden, Switzerland, Thailand, The Netherlands, United Kingdom)
BICALUTAMIDE
Casodex Tablets 670

CATAFLAM (Argentina, Greece, Hong Kong, Irish Republic, Israel, Italy, Malaysia, New Zealand, Norway, Portugal, Singapore, South Africa, Thailand, The Netherlands)
DICLOFENAC POTASSIUM
Cataflam Tablets 2173

CATALGEM (Brazil)
DICLOFENAC POTASSIUM
Cataflam Tablets 2173

CATALIP (Portugal)
FENOFIBRATE
Tricor Tablets 523

CATANAC (Thailand)
DICLOFENAC POTASSIUM
Cataflam Tablets 2173

CATAPRES (Australia, Canada, Hong Kong, India, Irish Republic, Japan, New Zealand, South Africa, Thailand, United Kingdom)
CLONIDINE HYDROCHLORIDE
Catapres Tablets 874

CATAPRES DIU (India)
CLONIDINE HYDROCHLORIDE
Catapres Tablets 874

CATAPRESAN (Austria, Chile, Czech Republic, Denmark, Finland, Germany, Greece, Mexico, Norway, Portugal, Spain, Sweden, Switzerland, The Netherlands)
CLONIDINE HYDROCHLORIDE
Catapres Tablets 874

CATAPRESSAN (Belgium, France)
CLONIDINE HYDROCHLORIDE
Catapres Tablets 874

CATAREN (Brazil)
DICLOFENAC POTASSIUM
Cataflam Tablets 2173

CATENOL (Czech Republic)
ATENOLOL
Tenormin I.V. Injection 698

CATEX (Spain)
CIPROFLOXACIN HYDROCHLORIDE
Ciloxan Ophthalmic Ointment 554
Ciloxan Ophthalmic Solution ⊙205
Cipro Tablets 2991

CATEXAN (South Africa)
INDAPAMIDE
Indapamide Tablets 2119

CATONA (Mexico)
CAPTOPRIL
Captopril Tablets 2114

CATONET (Denmark)
CAPTOPRIL
Captopril Tablets 2114

CATOPLIN (Singapore)
CAPTOPRIL
Captopril Tablets 2114

CATOPROL (Brazil)
CAPTOPRIL
Captopril Tablets 2114

CAUSALON PRO (Argentina)
NAPROXEN
EC-Naprosyn Delayed-Release Tablets 2769
Naprosyn Suspension 2769
Naprosyn Tablets 2769

CAVERIL (Thailand)
VERAPAMIL HYDROCHLORIDE
Covera-HS Tablets 3135
Verelan PM Capsules 3120

CAVERJECT (Argentina, Australia, Austria, Belgium, Brazil, Canada, Chile, Czech Republic, Denmark, Finland, France, Germany, Greece, Hong Kong, Hungary, Irish Republic, Israel, Italy, Malaysia, Mexico, New Zealand, Norway, Portugal, Singapore, South Africa, Spain, Sweden, Switzerland, Thailand, The Netherlands, United Kingdom)
ALPROSTADIL
Edex Injection 3103

CAVERTA (India)
SILDENAFIL CITRATE
Viagra Tablets 2552

C-BILDZ (Austria)
CIPROFLOXACIN HYDROCHLORIDE
Ciloxan Ophthalmic Ointment 554
Ciloxan Ophthalmic Solution ⊙205
Cipro Tablets 2991

CEBEDEX (France)
DEXAMETHASONE SODIUM PHOSPHATE
Decadron Phosphate Injection 1931

CEBRALAT (Brazil)
CILOSTAZOL
Pletal Tablets 2478

CEBRILIN (Brazil)
PAROXETINE HYDROCHLORIDE
Paxil Oral Suspension 1501
Paxil Tablets 1501

CEBROCAL (Argentina)
DONEPEZIL HYDROCHLORIDE
Aricept Tablets 1086

CEBROFORT (Argentina)
NIMODIPINE
Nimotop Capsules 774

CECURAL (Greece)
LOVASTATIN
Mevacor Tablets 1996

CEDETRIN-T (Czech Republic)
MUROMONAB-CD3
Orthoclone OKT3 Sterile Solution 2370

CEDINE (Irish Republic)
CIMETIDINE
Tagamet Tablets 1547

CEF-3 (Thailand)
CEFTRIAXONE SODIUM
Rocephin Injectable Vials, ADD-Vantage, Galaxy, Bulk 2801

CEF-4 (Thailand)
CEFTAZIDIME
Fortaz for Injection 1422

CEFA RESAN (Spain)
CEFAZOLIN SODIUM
Ancef for Injection 1318

CEFABIOZIM (Italy)
CEFAZOLIN SODIUM
Ancef for Injection 1318

CEFACENE (Spain)
CEFAZOLIN SODIUM
Ancef for Injection 1318

CEFACIDAL (Belgium, France, Mexico, South Africa, Thailand, The Netherlands)
CEFAZOLIN SODIUM
Ancef for Injection 1318

CEFADREX (Spain)
CEFAZOLIN SODIUM
Ancef for Injection 1318

CEFAKES (Spain)
CEFAZOLIN SODIUM
Ancef for Injection 1318

CEFALIN (Thailand)
CEFAZOLIN SODIUM
Ancef for Injection 1318

CEFAMAR (Italy, Thailand)
CEFUROXIME SODIUM
Zinacef Injection 1604

CEFAMEZIN (Argentina, Australia, Brazil, Hong Kong, Israel, Italy, Japan, Portugal, Spain, Thailand)
CEFAZOLIN SODIUM
Ancef for Injection 1318

CEFAMUSEL (Spain)
CEFAZOLIN SODIUM
Ancef for Injection 1318

CEFASYN (India)
CEFUROXIME AXETIL
Ceftin Tablets 1369
Ceftin for Oral Suspension 1369

CEFAXICINA (Spain)
CEFOXITIN SODIUM
Mefoxin Premixed Intravenous Solution . . . 1990
Mefoxin for Injection 1987

CEFAXONA (Mexico)
CEFTRIAXONE SODIUM
Rocephin Injectable Vials, ADD-Vantage, Galaxy, Bulk 2801

CEFAXONE (Czech Republic, Malaysia, Singapore)
CEFTRIAXONE SODIUM
Rocephin Injectable Vials, ADD-Vantage, Galaxy, Bulk 2801

CEFAZID (India)
CEFTAZIDIME
Fortaz for Injection 1422

CEFAZIL (Italy)
CEFAZOLIN SODIUM
Ancef for Injection 1318

CEFAZILLIN (Thailand)
CEFAZOLIN SODIUM
Ancef for Injection 1318

CEFAZIMA (Brazil)
CEFTAZIDIME
Fortaz for Injection 1422

CEFAZIME (Singapore)
CEFTAZIDIME
Fortaz for Injection 1422

CEFAZINA (Italy)
CEFAZOLIN SODIUM
Ancef for Injection 1318

CEFAZOL (Thailand)
CEFAZOLIN SODIUM
Ancef for Injection 1318

CEFICAD (India)
CEFEPIME HYDROCHLORIDE
Maxipime for Injection 1093

CEFIMEN-K (Argentina)
CEFEPIME HYDROCHLORIDE
Maxipime for Injection 1093

CEFIMIX (Portugal)
CEFIXIME
Suprax 1811

CEFIN (Singapore)
CEFTRIAXONE SODIUM
Rocephin Injectable Vials, ADD-Vantage, Galaxy, Bulk 2801

CEFINE (Thailand)
CEFTRIAXONE SODIUM
Rocephin Injectable Vials, ADD-Vantage, Galaxy, Bulk 2801

CEFITON (Portugal)
CEFIXIME
Suprax 1811

CEFIX (India)
CEFIXIME
Suprax 1811

CEFIX LB (India)
CEFIXIME
Suprax 1811

CEFIXDURA (Germany)
CEFIXIME
Suprax 1811

CEFIXORAL (Italy)
CEFIXIME
Suprax 1811

CEFLOUR (Malaysia)
CEFUROXIME SODIUM
Zinacef Injection 1604

CEFNAX (Brazil)
CEFIXIME
Suprax 1811

CEFOCEF (India)
CEFTRIAXONE SODIUM
Rocephin Injectable Vials, ADD-Vantage, Galaxy, Bulk 2801

CEFOCEF-LB (India)
CEFIXIME
Suprax 1811

CEFOCICLIN (Italy)
CEFOXITIN SODIUM
Mefoxin Premixed Intravenous Solution . . . 1990
Mefoxin for Injection 1987

CEFODIME (Thailand)
CEFTAZIDIME
Fortaz for Injection 1422

CEFODOX (France, Irish Republic, Italy)
CEFPODOXIME PROXETIL
Vantin Tablets and Oral Suspension 2650

CEFOFIX (Portugal)
CEFUROXIME SODIUM
Zinacef Injection 1604

CEFOGEN (India, Thailand)
CEFUROXIME SODIUM
Zinacef Injection 1604

CEFOMAX (Argentina)
CEFTRIAXONE SODIUM
Rocephin Injectable Vials, ADD-Vantage, Galaxy, Bulk 2801

CEFOPRIM (Greece, Italy)
CEFUROXIME SODIUM
Zinacef Injection 1604

CEFOPROX (India)
CEFPODOXIME PROXETIL
Vantin Tablets and Oral Suspension 2650

CEFORTAM (Portugal)
CEFTAZIDIME SODIUM
Fortaz for Injection 1422

CEFOTRIX (Denmark, Hungary)
CEFTRIAXONE SODIUM
Rocephin Injectable Vials, ADD-Vantage, Galaxy, Bulk 2801

CEFOXIM (India)
CEFUROXIME AXETIL
Ceftin Tablets 1369
Ceftin for Oral Suspension 1369

CEFOXIN (Brazil, Thailand)
CEFOXITIN SODIUM
Mefoxin Premixed Intravenous Solution . . . 1990
Mefoxin for Injection 1987

CEFRADEN (Mexico)
CEFTRIAXONE SODIUM
Rocephin Injectable Vials, ADD-Vantage, Galaxy, Bulk 2801

CEFSPAN (Chile, Japan, Thailand)
CEFIXIME
Suprax 1811

CEFT (Brazil)
CEFTRIAXONE SODIUM
Rocephin Injectable Vials, ADD-Vantage, Galaxy, Bulk 2801

CEFTAZ (India)
CEFTAZIDIME
Fortaz for Injection 1422

CEFTAZIDON (Brazil)
CEFTAZIDIME
Fortaz for Injection 1422

CEFTEN (Brazil)
CEFTAZIDIME
Fortaz for Injection 1422

CEFTIDIN (India)
CEFTAZIDIME
Fortaz for Injection 1422

CEFTIM (Italy)
CEFTAZIDIME
Fortaz for Injection 1422

CEFTIN (Canada)
CEFUROXIME AXETIL
Ceftin Tablets 1369
Ceftin for Oral Suspension 1369

CEFTORAL (Greece)
CEFIXIME
Suprax 1811

CEFTRAT (Brazil)
CEFAZOLIN SODIUM
Ancef for Injection 1318

CEFTREX (Malaysia, Mexico, Thailand)
CEFTRIAXONE SODIUM
Rocephin Injectable Vials, ADD-Vantage, Galaxy, Bulk 2801

CEFTRILEM (Mexico)
CEFTRIAXONE SODIUM
Rocephin Injectable Vials, ADD-Vantage, Galaxy, Bulk 2801

CEFTRINAL (Greece)
RANITIDINE HYDROCHLORIDE
Zantac 25 EFFERdose Tablets 1597
Zantac 150 EFFERdose Tablets 1597
Zantac 150 Tablets 1597
Zantac 300 Tablets 1597
Zantac Injection 1593
Zantac Injection Premixed 1593
Zantac Syrup 1597

CEFTRIPHIN (Thailand)
CEFTRIAXONE SODIUM
Rocephin Injectable Vials, ADD-Vantage, Galaxy, Bulk 2801

CEFUDURA (Germany)
CEFUROXIME AXETIL
Ceftin Tablets 1369
Ceftin for Oral Suspension 1369

CEFUHEXAL (Germany)
CEFUROXIME AXETIL
Ceftin Tablets 1369
Ceftin for Oral Suspension 1369

CEFUMAX (Italy)
CEFUROXIME SODIUM
Zinacef Injection 1604

CEFUR (Italy)
CEFUROXIME SODIUM
Zinacef Injection 1604

CEFURACET (Mexico)
CEFUROXIME AXETIL
Ceftin Tablets 1369
Ceftin for Oral Suspension 1369

CEFURAX (Germany)
CEFUROXIME AXETIL
Ceftin Tablets 1369
Ceftin for Oral Suspension 1369

CEFUREX (Italy)
CEFUROXIME SODIUM
Zinacef Injection 1604

CEFURIN (Italy)
CEFUROXIME SODIUM
Zinacef Injection 1604

CEFURO-PUREN (Germany)
CEFUROXIME AXETIL
Ceftin Tablets 1369
Ceftin for Oral Suspension 1369

CEFUROX (Argentina)
CEFUROXIME AXETIL
Ceftin Tablets 1369
Ceftin for Oral Suspension 1369

CEFUROX-REU (Germany)
CEFUROXIME SODIUM
Zinacef Injection 1604

CEFUROX-WOLFF (Germany)
CEFUROXIME AXETIL
Ceftin Tablets 1369
Ceftin for Oral Suspension 1369

CEFUZIME (United Arab Emirates)
CEFUROXIME AXETIL
Ceftin Tablets 1369
Ceftin for Oral Suspension 1369

CEFXITIN (Thailand)
CEFOXITIN SODIUM
Mefoxin Premixed Intravenous Solution . . . 1990
Mefoxin for Injection 1987

CEFZON (Japan)
CEFDINIR
Omnicef Capsules 506
Omnicef for Oral Suspension 506

CEGLUTION (Argentina)
LITHIUM CARBONATE
Eskalith CR Controlled-Release Tablets . . . 1406
Eskalith Capsules 1406

CELAPRAM (Australia)
CITALOPRAM HYDROBROMIDE
Celexa Tablets 1177

CELCOX (Israel)
CELECOXIB
Celebrex Capsules 3130

CELEBRA (Brazil, Chile, Denmark, Finland, Israel)
CELECOXIB
Celebrex Capsules 3130

CELEBREX (Argentina, Australia, Austria, Belgium, Canada, Czech Republic, France, Germany, Hungary, Irish Republic, Italy, Malaysia, Mexico, New Zealand, Portugal, Russia, Singapore, South Africa, Spain, Switzerland, Thailand, The Netherlands, United Kingdom)
CELECOXIB
Celebrex Capsules 3130

CELEDOL (India)
CELECOXIB
Celebrex Capsules 3130

CELEFER (Spain)
MUPIROCIN
Bactroban Ointment 1358

CELEMAX (Argentina)
CELECOXIB
Celebrex Capsules 3130

CELEXA (Canada)
CITALOPRAM HYDROBROMIDE
Celexa Tablets 1177

CELIB (India)
CELECOXIB
Celebrex Capsules 3130

CELKALM (France)
LOPERAMIDE HYDROCHLORIDE
Imodium Capsules 1834

CELLCEPT (Argentina, Belgium, Brazil, Chile, Czech Republic, Denmark, Finland, France, Greece, Hong Kong, Israel, Italy, Japan, Mexico, New Zealand, Norway, Singapore, South Africa, Spain, Sweden, Switzerland, Thailand, The Netherlands)
MYCOPHENOLATE MOFETIL
CellCept Capsules 2751
CellCept Oral Suspension 2751
CellCept Tablets 2751

CELLCEPT (Hungary)
MYCOPHENOLATE MOFETIL HYDROCHLORIDE
CellCept Intravenous 2751

CELLMUNE (India)
MYCOPHENOLATE MOFETIL
CellCept Capsules 2751
CellCept Oral Suspension 2751
CellCept Tablets 2751

CELLOIDS PC 73 (Australia)
POTASSIUM CHLORIDE
K-Dur Extended-Release Tablets 3047
K-Lor Powder Packets 472
K-Tab Filmtab Tablets 473

CELVISTA (Thailand)
RALOXIFENE HYDROCHLORIDE
Evista Tablets 1735

CEMENTIN (Hong Kong, Singapore)
CIMETIDINE
Tagamet Tablets 1547

CEMIDIN (Israel)
CIMETIDINE
Tagamet Tablets 1547

CENCAMET (Thailand)
CIMETIDINE
Tagamet Tablets 1547

CENLIDAC (Thailand)
SULINDAC
Clinoril Tablets 1899

CENPIDINE (Thailand)
TICLOPIDINE HYDROCHLORIDE
Ticlid Tablets 2813

CENTOCORT (Thailand)
TRIAMCINOLONE ACETONIDE
Azmacort Inhalation Aerosol 1701
Nasacort AQ Nasal Spray 2937

CENTRAPRYL (United Kingdom)
SELEGILINE HYDROCHLORIDE
Eldepryl Capsules ... 3209

CENTROMICINA (Argentina)
CLARITHROMYCIN
Biaxin Filmtab Tablets ... 402
Biaxin Granules ... 402

CEPAL (Greece)
FAMOTIDINE
Pepcid Injection ... 2017
Pepcid Injection Premixed ... 2017
Pepcid Tablets ... 2014
Pepcid for Oral Suspension ... 2014

CEPAZINE (France)
CEFUROXIME AXETIL
Ceftin Tablets ... 1369
Ceftin for Oral Suspension ... 1369

CEPHORAL (Germany, Switzerland)
CEFIXIME
Suprax ... 1811

CEPHULAC (Canada)
LACTULOSE
Kristalose for Oral Solution ... 2149

CEPIM (Italy)
CEFEPIME HYDROCHLORIDE
Maxipime for Injection ... 1093

CEPIMEX (Italy)
CEFEPIME HYDROCHLORIDE
Maxipime for Injection ... 1093

CEPODEM (India, South Africa)
CEFPODOXIME PROXETIL
Vantin Tablets and Oral Suspension ... 2650

CEPRAZOL (Chile)
ALBENDAZOLE
Albenza Tablets ... 1310

CEPRIMAX (Spain)
CIPROFLOXACIN HYDROCHLORIDE
Ciloxan Ophthalmic Ointment ... 554
Ciloxan Ophthalmic Solution ... ⊙205
Cipro Tablets ... 2991

CEPTAZ (Canada)
CEFTAZIDIME
Fortaz for Injection ... 1422

CERCON (Mexico)
PRAZIQUANTEL
Biltricide Tablets ... 2990

CEREBRAMED (Germany)
AMANTADINE HYDROCHLORIDE
Symmetrel Syrup ... 1115
Symmetrel Tablets ... 1115

CEREBROVASE (United Kingdom)
DIPYRIDAMOLE
Persantine Tablets ... 898

CERELLA (Germany)
ESTRADIOL
Climara Transdermal System ... 795
Vivelle Transdermal System ... 2288
Vivelle-Dot Transdermal System ... 2293

CERELUC (Argentina)
PIOGLITAZONE HYDROCHLORIDE
Actos Tablets ... 3224

CEREX (Czech Republic)
CETIRIZINE HYDROCHLORIDE
Zyrtec Syrup ... 2589
Zyrtec Tablets ... 2589

CEREZYME (Australia, Austria, Canada, Czech Republic, Denmark, France, Germany, Hong Kong, Israel, Italy, Japan, New Zealand, Norway, Portugal, South Africa, Spain, Sweden, Switzerland, United Kingdom)
IMIGLUCERASE
Cerezyme for Injection ... 1263

CERINA (Switzerland)
ESTRADIOL
Climara Transdermal System ... 795
Vivelle Transdermal System ... 2288
Vivelle-Dot Transdermal System ... 2293

CEROFENE (Greece)
CEFUROXIME SODIUM
Zinacef Injection ... 1604

CEROXIM (Hungary, South Africa)
CEFUROXIME AXETIL
Ceftin Tablets ... 1369
Ceftin for Oral Suspension ... 1369

CERTALAC (Belgium)
LACTULOSE
Kristalose for Oral Solution ... 2149

CERTOVERMIL (Brazil)
MEBENDAZOLE
Vermox Chewable Tablets ... 1853

CERUBIDIN (Australia, Denmark, Irish Republic, Norway, South Africa, Sweden, United Kingdom)
DAUNORUBICIN HYDROCHLORIDE
Cerubidine for Injection ... 788

CERUBIDINE (Belgium, Canada, Czech Republic, France, Israel, New Zealand, Switzerland, The Netherlands)
DAUNORUBICIN HYDROCHLORIDE
Cerubidine for Injection ... 788

CERUXIM (Greece)
CEFUROXIME SODIUM
Zinacef Injection ... 1604

CERVIDIL (Australia, Canada)
DINOPROSTONE
Cervidil Vaginal Insert ... 1182

CERVIPRIME (India)
DINOPROSTONE
Cervidil Vaginal Insert ... 1182

CERVIPROST (Austria, Germany, Norway, Sweden, Switzerland, The Netherlands)
DINOPROSTONE
Cervidil Vaginal Insert ... 1182

CESOL (Chile, Germany, Mexico, Portugal)
PRAZIQUANTEL
Biltricide Tablets ... 2990

CESPLON (Spain)
CAPTOPRIL
Captopril Tablets ... 2114

CESSAVERM (Brazil)
MEBENDAZOLE
Vermox Chewable Tablets ... 1853

CESTOP (Chile)
CLOTRIMAZOLE
Lotrimin Cream ... 3053
Lotrimin Lotion 1% ... 3053
Lotrimin Topical Solution 1% ... 3053

CESTOX (Brazil)
PRAZIQUANTEL
Biltricide Tablets ... 2990

CETA SULFA (Mexico)
SULFACETAMIDE SODIUM
Klaron Lotion 10% ... 1050

CETALERG (Germany)
CETIRIZINE HYDROCHLORIDE
Zyrtec Syrup ... 2589
Zyrtec Tablets ... 2589

CETALLERG (Switzerland)
CETIRIZINE HYDROCHLORIDE
Zyrtec Syrup ... 2589
Zyrtec Tablets ... 2589

CETAMIDE (Canada)
SULFACETAMIDE SODIUM
Klaron Lotion 10% ... 1050

CETAMPRIL (Portugal)
ENALAPRIL MALEATE
Vasotec I.V. Injection ... 2076

CETAPRED (Belgium)
PREDNISOLONE ACETATE/SULFACETAMIDE SODIUM
Blephamide Ophthalmic Ointment ... 563
Blephamide Ophthalmic Suspension ... 564

CETASIL (Thailand)
SULFACETAMIDE SODIUM
Klaron Lotion 10% ... 1050

CETAXIM (Argentina)
CEFIXIME
Suprax ... 1811

CETAZ (Brazil)
CEFTAZIDIME
Fortaz for Injection ... 1422

CETAZIME (Hungary)
CEFTAZIDIME
Fortaz for Injection ... 1422

CETAZIN (Austria)
SULFACETAMIDE SODIUM
Klaron Lotion 10% ... 1050

CETCIP (India)
CETIRIZINE HYDROCHLORIDE
Zyrtec Syrup ... 2589
Zyrtec Tablets ... 2589

CETERIFUG (Germany)
CETIRIZINE HYDROCHLORIDE
Zyrtec Syrup ... 2589
Zyrtec Tablets ... 2589

CETI (Germany)
CETIRIZINE HYDROCHLORIDE
Zyrtec Syrup ... 2589
Zyrtec Tablets ... 2589

CETIDERM (Germany)
CETIRIZINE HYDROCHLORIDE
Zyrtec Syrup ... 2589
Zyrtec Tablets ... 2589

CETIDURA (Germany)
CETIRIZINE HYDROCHLORIDE
Zyrtec Syrup ... 2589
Zyrtec Tablets ... 2589

CETIHIS (Thailand)
CETIRIZINE HYDROCHLORIDE
Zyrtec Syrup ... 2589
Zyrtec Tablets ... 2589

CETIL (Germany)
CETIRIZINE HYDROCHLORIDE
Zyrtec Syrup ... 2589
Zyrtec Tablets ... 2589

CETILICH (Germany)
CETIRIZINE HYDROCHLORIDE
Zyrtec Syrup ... 2589
Zyrtec Tablets ... 2589

CETIRAM (Greece)
CETIRIZINE HYDROCHLORIDE
Zyrtec Syrup ... 2589
Zyrtec Tablets ... 2589

CETIRHEXAL (Austria)
CETIRIZINE HYDROCHLORIDE
Zyrtec Syrup ... 2589
Zyrtec Tablets ... 2589

CETIRIGAMMA (Germany)
CETIRIZINE HYDROCHLORIDE
Zyrtec Syrup ... 2589
Zyrtec Tablets ... 2589

CETIRISTAD (Austria)
CETIRIZINE HYDROCHLORIDE
Zyrtec Syrup ... 2589
Zyrtec Tablets ... 2589

CETIRLAN (Germany)
CETIRIZINE HYDROCHLORIDE
Zyrtec Syrup ... 2589
Zyrtec Tablets ... 2589

CETIROCOL (United Kingdom)
CETIRIZINE HYDROCHLORIDE
Zyrtec Syrup ... 2589
Zyrtec Tablets ... 2589

CETIZINE (Argentina)
CETIRIZINE HYDROCHLORIDE
Zyrtec Syrup ... 2589
Zyrtec Tablets ... 2589

CETOHEXAL (Brazil)
KETOCONAZOLE
Nizoral 2% Shampoo ... 1838

CETOMED (Brazil)
KETOCONAZOLE
Nizoral 2% Shampoo ... 1838

CETONAX (Brazil)
KETOCONAZOLE
Nizoral 2% Shampoo ... 1838

CETONEO (Brazil)
KETOCONAZOLE
Nizoral 2% Shampoo ... 1838

CETONIL (Argentina, Brazil)
KETOCONAZOLE
Nizoral 2% Shampoo ... 1838

CETOZAN (Brazil)
KETOCONAZOLE
Nizoral 2% Shampoo ... 1838

CETOZOL (Brazil)
KETOCONAZOLE
Nizoral 2% Shampoo ... 1838

CETRALON (United Arab Emirates)
CETIRIZINE HYDROCHLORIDE
Zyrtec Syrup ... 2589
Zyrtec Tablets ... 2589

CETRAPHYLLINE (France)
THEOPHYLLINE
Uniphyl Tablets ... 2708

CETRAXAL PLUS (Spain)
CIPROFLOXACIN
Cipro Oral Suspension ... 2991

CETRILER (Argentina)
CETIRIZINE HYDROCHLORIDE
Zyrtec Syrup ... 2589
Zyrtec Tablets ... 2589

CETRIMED (Thailand)
CETIRIZINE HYDROCHLORIDE
Zyrtec Syrup ... 2589
Zyrtec Tablets ... 2589

CETRINE (Singapore, Thailand)
CETIRIZINE HYDROCHLORIDE
Zyrtec Syrup ... 2589
Zyrtec Tablets ... 2589

CETRIWAL (India)
CETIRIZINE HYDROCHLORIDE
Zyrtec Syrup ... 2589
Zyrtec Tablets ... 2589

CETRIZET (India, Thailand)
CETIRIZINE HYDROCHLORIDE
Zyrtec Syrup ... 2589
Zyrtec Tablets ... 2589

CETRIZIN (Brazil, Thailand)
CETIRIZINE HYDROCHLORIDE
Zyrtec Syrup ... 2589
Zyrtec Tablets ... 2589

CETRON (Argentina)
ONDANSETRON
Zofran ODT Orally Disintegrating Tablets ... 1613

CETYROL (Austria)
CETIRIZINE HYDROCHLORIDE
Zyrtec Syrup ... 2589
Zyrtec Tablets ... 2589

CEVAS (India)
CARVEDILOL
Coreg Tablets ... 1376

CEXIDAL OTICO (Spain)
CIPROFLOXACIN
Cipro Oral Suspension ... 2991

CEXIM (Hungary)
CEFUROXIME SODIUM
Zinacef Injection ... 1604

CEZA (Thailand)
CETIRIZINE HYDROCHLORIDE
Zyrtec Syrup ... 2589
Zyrtec Tablets ... 2589

CEZOLIN (Greece)
KETOCONAZOLE
Nizoral 2% Shampoo ... 1838

C-FLOX (Australia)
CIPROFLOXACIN HYDROCHLORIDE
Ciloxan Ophthalmic Ointment ... 554
Ciloxan Ophthalmic Solution ... ⊙205
Cipro Tablets ... 2991

C-FLOXACIN (Thailand)
CIPROFLOXACIN HYDROCHLORIDE
Ciloxan Ophthalmic Ointment ... 554
Ciloxan Ophthalmic Solution ... ⊙205
Cipro Tablets ... 2991

C-G (Argentina)
SULFACETAMIDE SODIUM
Klaron Lotion 10% ... 1050

CHAMPS D-WORMS (Malaysia)
ALBENDAZOLE
Albenza Tablets ... 1310

CHANTALINE (Spain)
THEOPHYLLINE
Uniphyl Tablets ... 2708

CHARLIEU ANTI-POUX (Czech Republic)
PERMETHRIN
Acticin Cream ... 2125

CHEMIONAZOLO (Italy)
ECONAZOLE NITRATE
Spectazole Cream ... 2390

(⊙ Described in PDR For Ophthalmic Medicines™)

CHEMISTS OWN CLOZOLE (Australia)
CLOTRIMAZOLE
Lotrimin Cream. . . . 3053
Lotrimin Lotion 1%. . . . 3053
Lotrimin Topical Solution 1% 3053

CHEMISTS OWN DE WORM (Australia)
MEBENDAZOLE
Vermox Chewable Tablets 1853

CHEMISTS OWN DIARRHOEA RELIEF (Australia)
LOPERAMIDE HYDROCHLORIDE
Imodium Capsules 1834

CHEMISTS OWN PERIOD PAIN TABLETS (Australia)
NAPROXEN SODIUM
Anaprox DS Tablets 2769
Anaprox Tablets 2769

CHEMYDUR (United Kingdom)
ISOSORBIDE MONONITRATE
Imdur Tablets 3032

CHEXID (India)
LANSOPRAZOLE
Prevacid Delayed-Release Capsules 3268

CHIBRETICO (Portugal)
AMILORIDE HYDROCHLORIDE/HYDROCHLOROTHIAZIDE
Moduretic Tablets 2003

CHIBRO-PROSCAR (France)
FINASTERIDE
Propecia Tablets 2036
Proscar Tablets. . . . 2040

CHIBRO-TIMOPTOL (Germany)
TIMOLOL MALEATE
Blocadren Tablets 1891
Timoptic Sterile Ophthalmic Solution 2058
Timoptic in Ocudose 2061
Timoptic-XE Sterile Ophthalmic Gel Forming Solution 2062

CHIBROXIN (Argentina, Brazil, Chile, Germany, Hong Kong, Israel, Malaysia, Singapore, Spain)
NORFLOXACIN
Noroxin Tablets. . . . 2009

CHIBROXINE (France)
NORFLOXACIN
Noroxin Tablets. . . . 2009

CHIBROXOL (Belgium, Portugal, Switzerland, The Netherlands)
NORFLOXACIN
Noroxin Tablets. . . . 2009

CHIMAX (United Kingdom)
FLUTAMIDE
Eulexin Capsules 3023

CHINGAZOL (Thailand)
CLOTRIMAZOLE
Lotrimin Cream. . . . 3053
Lotrimin Lotion 1%. . . . 3053
Lotrimin Topical Solution 1% 3053

CHINOPAMIL (Hungary)
VERAPAMIL HYDROCHLORIDE
Covera-HS Tablets 3135
Verelan PM Capsules 3120

CHINTARAL (Thailand)
KETOCONAZOLE
Nizoral 2% Shampoo 1838

CHIRON IL-2 (South Africa)
ALDESLEUKIN
Proleukin for Injection 1007

CHLORAMINOPHENE (Monaco)
CHLORAMBUCIL
Leukeran Tablets. . . . 1472

CHLOROPOTASSURIL (Belgium)
POTASSIUM CHLORIDE
K-Dur Extended-Relase Tablets 3047
K-Lor Powder Packets 472
K-Tab Filmtab Tablets 473

CHLORVESCENT (New Zealand)
POTASSIUM CHLORIDE
K-Dur Extended-Relase Tablets 3047
K-Lor Powder Packets 472
K-Tab Filmtab Tablets 473

CHLORZIDE (Singapore)
CHLOROTHIAZIDE
Diuril Oral Suspension 1936
Diuril Tablets 1936

CHLOTRIDE (Australia, Denmark, The Netherlands)
CHLOROTHIAZIDE
Diuril Oral Suspension 1936
Diuril Tablets 1936

CHRONADALATE (France)
NIFEDIPINE
Adalat CC Tablets 2978

CHRONOPHYLLIN (South Africa)
THEOPHYLLINE
Uniphyl Tablets 2708

CHRONOVERA (Austria, Canada, The Netherlands)
VERAPAMIL HYDROCHLORIDE
Covera-HS Tablets 3135
Verelan PM Capsules 3120

CHRONULAC (Canada)
LACTULOSE
Kristalose for Oral Solution 2149

CIBACE (South Africa)
BENAZEPRIL HYDROCHLORIDE
Lotensin Tablets 2232

CIBACEN (Austria, Belgium, Denmark, Germany, Greece, Irish Republic, Israel, Italy, New Zealand, Spain, Switzerland, The Netherlands)
BENAZEPRIL HYDROCHLORIDE
Lotensin Tablets 2232

CIBACENE (France)
BENAZEPRIL HYDROCHLORIDE
Lotensin Tablets 2232

CIBADREX (Austria, Denmark, France, Germany, Greece, Italy, South Africa, Sweden, Switzerland, The Netherlands)
BENAZEPRIL HYDROCHLORIDE/HYDROCHLOROTHIAZIDE
Lotensin HCT Tablets 2235

CIBRAL (United Kingdom)
ISOSORBIDE MONONITRATE
Imdur Tablets 3032

CIBRAMICINA (Brazil)
AMOXICILLIN
Amoxil Pediatric Drops for Oral Suspension 1315
Amoxil Tablets 1315

CIBROGAN (Argentina)
CILOSTAZOL
Pletal Tablets 2478

CICLOTAL (Mexico)
MEDROXYPROGESTERONE ACETATE
Depo-Medrol Single-Dose Vial 2617

CICLOTRAN (Argentina)
RALOXIFENE HYDROCHLORIDE
Evista Tablets. . . . 1735

CICLOX (Argentina)
CLONAZEPAM
Klonopin Tablets 2782

CIDANAMOX (Spain)
AMOXICILLIN
Amoxil Pediatric Drops for Oral Suspension. . . . 1315
Amoxil Tablets 1315

CIDINE (Thailand)
CIMETIDINE
Tagamet Tablets 1547

CIDOMYCIN (Australia, Canada, Irish Republic, Israel, South Africa, United Kingdom)
GENTAMICIN SULFATE
Garamycin Injectable 3028
Genoptic Sterile Ophthalmic Solution . . . . ⊙227

CIDRON (Denmark, Finland, Sweden)
CETIRIZINE HYDROCHLORIDE
Zyrtec Syrup 2589
Zyrtec Tablets 2589

CIDROPS (Greece)
CIPROFLOXACIN
Cipro Oral Suspension 2991

CIFIN (Denmark)
CIPROFLOXACIN HYDROCHLORIDE
Ciloxan Ophthalmic Ointment 554
Ciloxan Ophthalmic Solution . . . . ⊙205
Cipro Tablets 2991

CIFLAN (Portugal)
CIPROFLOXACIN HYDROCHLORIDE
Ciloxan Ophthalmic Ointment 554
Ciloxan Ophthalmic Solution . . . . ⊙205
Cipro Tablets 2991

CIFLOC (South Africa)
CIPROFLOXACIN
Cipro Oral Suspension 2991

CIFLOLAN (Thailand)
CIPROFLOXACIN
Cipro Oral Suspension 2991

CIFLOX (Austria, Brazil, Italy)
CIPROFLOXACIN HYDROCHLORIDE
Ciloxan Ophthalmic Ointment 554
Ciloxan Ophthalmic Solution . . . . ⊙205
Cipro Tablets 2991

CIFLOXIN (Chile)
CIPROFLOXACIN
Cipro Oral Suspension 2991

CIFLOXINAL (Czech Republic)
CIPROFLOXACIN HYDROCHLORIDE
Ciloxan Ophthalmic Ointment 554
Ciloxan Ophthalmic Solution . . . . ⊙205
Cipro Tablets 2991

CIFLOXTRON (Brazil)
CIPROFLOXACIN
Cipro Oral Suspension 2991

CIFRAN (Czech Republic, Hungary, Malaysia, South Africa)
CIPROFLOXACIN HYDROCHLORIDE
Ciloxan Ophthalmic Ointment 554
Ciloxan Ophthalmic Solution . . . . ⊙205
Cipro Tablets 2991

CIFRANTIL (Brazil)
ERYTHROMYCIN
Ery-Tab Tablets 447
Erythromycin Base Filmtab Tablets. . . . 454
Erythromycin Delayed-Release Capsules, USP 456
PCE Dispertab Tablets 510

CIGAMET (Thailand)
CIMETIDINE
Tagamet Tablets 1547

CIGANCLOR (Argentina)
GANCICLOVIR
Cytovene Capsules 2763

CIL (Germany)
FENOFIBRATE
Tricor Tablets 523

CILAB (Thailand)
CIPROFLOXACIN
Cipro Oral Suspension 2991

CILAMIN (India)
PENICILLAMINE
Cuprimine Capsules 1925

CILATRON (Argentina)
ISOSORBIDE MONONITRATE
Imdur Tablets 3032

CILEX (Germany)
CITALOPRAM HYDROBROMIDE
Celexa Tablets 1177

CILIFT (South Africa)
CITALOPRAM HYDROBROMIDE
Celexa Tablets 1177

CILOQUIN (Australia)
CIPROFLOXACIN HYDROCHLORIDE
Ciloxan Ophthalmic Ointment 554
Ciloxan Ophthalmic Solution . . . . ⊙205
Cipro Tablets 2991

CILOSTAL (Argentina)
CILOSTAZOL
Pletal Tablets 2478

CILOVAS (Argentina)
CILOSTAZOL
Pletal Tablets 2478

CILOX (Norway)
CIPROFLOXACIN HYDROCHLORIDE
Ciloxan Ophthalmic Ointment 554
Ciloxan Ophthalmic Solution . . . . ⊙205
Cipro Tablets 2991

CILOXACIN (Chile)
CIPROFLOXACIN HYDROCHLORIDE
Ciloxan Ophthalmic Ointment 554
Ciloxan Ophthalmic Solution . . . . ⊙205
Cipro Tablets 2991

CILOXADEX (Argentina)
CIPROFLOXACIN HYDROCHLORIDE
Ciloxan Ophthalmic Ointment 554
Ciloxan Ophthalmic Solution . . . . ⊙205
Cipro Tablets 2991

CILOXAN (Argentina, Australia, Austria, Belgium, Brazil, Canada, Czech Republic, Denmark, France, Germany, Greece, Hong Kong, Hungary, Israel, Malaysia, Mexico, New Zealand, Singapore, South Africa, Sweden, Switzerland, Thailand, The Netherlands, United Kingdom)
CIPROFLOXACIN HYDROCHLORIDE
Ciloxan Ophthalmic Ointment 554
Ciloxan Ophthalmic Solution . . . . ⊙205
Cipro Tablets 2991

CIM (Portugal)
CIMETIDINE
Tagamet Tablets 1547

CIMAG (Thailand)
CIMETIDINE
Tagamet Tablets 1547

CIMAGEN (Irish Republic)
CIMETIDINE
Tagamet Tablets 1547

CIMAL (Chile, Norway, Sweden)
CIMETIDINE
Tagamet Tablets 1547

CIME (Germany)
CIMETIDINE
Tagamet Tablets 1547

CIMEBEC (Mexico)
CIMETIDINE
Tagamet Tablets 1547

CIMEBETA (Germany)
CIMETIDINE
Tagamet Tablets 1547

CIMECARD (Brazil)
DIGOXIN
Lanoxicaps Capsules 1458
Lanoxin Injection 1462
Lanoxin Injection Pediatric 1465
Lanoxin Tablets. . . . 1468

CIMECODAN (Denmark)
CIMETIDINE
Tagamet Tablets 1547

CIMEDINE (Hong Kong)
CIMETIDINE
Tagamet Tablets 1547

CIMEDUL (Mexico)
CIMETIDINE
Tagamet Tablets 1547

CIMEHEXAL (Australia)
CIMETIDINE
Tagamet Tablets 1547

CIMELDINE (Irish Republic)
CIMETIDINE
Tagamet Tablets 1547

CIMEMERCK (Germany)
CIMETIDINE
Tagamet Tablets 1547

CIMEPHIL (Germany)
CIMETIDINE
Tagamet Tablets 1547

CIMET (Germany, India)
CIMETIDINE
Tagamet Tablets 1547

CIMETA (Hong Kong)
CIMETIDINE
Tagamet Tablets 1547

CIMETAG (Israel, United Arab Emirates)
CIMETIDINE
Tagamet Tablets 1547

CIMETASE (Mexico)
CIMETIDINE
Tagamet Tablets 1547

CIMETID (Norway)
CIMETIDINE
Tagamet Tablets 1547

(⊙ Described in PDR For Ophthalmic Medicines™)

CIMETIDAN (Brazil)
CIMETIDINE
Tagamet Tablets 1547

CIMETIL (Brazil)
CIMETIDINE
Tagamet Tablets 1547

CIMETIMAX (Australia)
CIMETIDINE
Tagamet Tablets 1547

CIMETIN (Brazil)
CIMETIDINE
Tagamet Tablets 1547

CIMETINA (Brazil)
CIMETIDINE
Tagamet Tablets 1547

CIMETINAX (Brazil)
CIMETIDINE
Tagamet Tablets 1547

CIMETINE (Thailand)
CIMETIDINE
Tagamet Tablets 1547

CIMETIVAL (Brazil)
CIMETIDINE
Tagamet Tablets 1547

CIMETON (Greece)
CIMETIDINE
Tagamet Tablets 1547

CIMET-P (Thailand)
CIMETIDINE
Tagamet Tablets 1547

CIMEX (Brazil, Finland)
CIMETIDINE
Tagamet Tablets 1547

CIMI (Israel)
CIMETIDINE
Tagamet Tablets 1547

CIMIDINE (Thailand)
CIMETIDINE
Tagamet Tablets 1547

CIMLICH (Czech Republic, Germany)
CIMETIDINE
Tagamet Tablets 1547

CIMLOK (South Africa)
CIMETIDINE
Tagamet Tablets 1547

CIMOGAL (Mexico)
CIPROFLOXACIN HYDROCHLORIDE
Ciloxan Ophthalmic Ointment 554
Ciloxan Ophthalmic Solution . . . . ⊙205
Cipro Tablets 2991

CIMULCER (Hong Kong, Malaysia, Singapore, Thailand)
CIMETIDINE
Tagamet Tablets 1547

CINABEL (Mexico)
CLOTRIMAZOLE
Lotrimin Cream. 3053
Lotrimin Lotion 1%. 3053
Lotrimin Topical Solution 1% 3053

CINADINE (South Africa)
CIMETIDINE
Tagamet Tablets 1547

CINAFLAN (Brazil)
DICLOFENAC POTASSIUM
Cataflam Tablets 2173

CINCO-FU (Argentina)
FLUOROURACIL
Efudex Topical Cream. 3348
Efudex Topical Solutions 3348

CINCORDIL (Brazil)
ISOSORBIDE MONONITRATE
Imdur Tablets 3032

CINFLOXINE (Thailand)
CIPROFLOXACIN HYDROCHLORIDE
Ciloxan Ophthalmic Ointment 554
Ciloxan Ophthalmic Solution . . . . ⊙205
Cipro Tablets 2991

CINKEF-U (Portugal)
FLUOROURACIL
Efudex Topical Cream. 3348
Efudex Topical Solutions 3348

CINOFLAX (Brazil)
CIPROFLOXACIN HYDROCHLORIDE
Ciloxan Ophthalmic Ointment 554
Ciloxan Ophthalmic Solution . . . . ⊙205
Cipro Tablets 2991

CINTON (Brazil)
CIMETIDINE
Tagamet Tablets 1547

CINTSU (Malaysia)
VERAPAMIL HYDROCHLORIDE
Covera-HS Tablets 3135
Verelan PM Capsules 3120

CINULCUS (Spain)
CIMETIDINE
Tagamet Tablets 1547

CIP ECO (Switzerland)
CIPROFLOXACIN HYDROCHLORIDE
Ciloxan Ophthalmic Ointment 554
Ciloxan Ophthalmic Solution . . . . ⊙205
Cipro Tablets 2991

CIPALAT (South Africa)
NIFEDIPINE
Adalat CC Tablets 2978

CIPCORLIN (India)
HYDROCORTISONE
Hydrocortone Tablets 1963

CIPEX (South Africa)
MEBENDAZOLE
Vermox Chewable Tablets 1853

CIPFLOCIN (Thailand)
CIPROFLOXACIN
Cipro Oral Suspension 2991

CIPGEN (India)
CIPROFLOXACIN
Cipro Oral Suspension 2991

CIPGEN TZ (India)
CIPROFLOXACIN
Cipro Oral Suspension 2991

CIPHIN (Czech Republic)
CIPROFLOXACIN
Cipro Oral Suspension 2991

CIPIDE (Hong Kong)
CIPROFLOXACIN HYDROCHLORIDE
Ciloxan Ophthalmic Ointment 554
Ciloxan Ophthalmic Solution . . . . ⊙205
Cipro Tablets 2991

CIPLACEF (India)
CEFTRIAXONE SODIUM
Rocephin Injectable Vials, ADD-Vantage, Galaxy, Bulk 2801

CIPLAR (India)
PROPRANOLOL HYDROCHLORIDE
Inderal LA Long-Acting Capsules 3421

CIPLAR-H (India)
PROPRANOLOL HYDROCHLORIDE
Inderal LA Long-Acting Capsules 3421

CIPLATEC (South Africa)
ENALAPRIL MALEATE
Vasotec I.V. Injection 2076

CIPLOX (Israel, Portugal)
CIPROFLOXACIN
Cipro Oral Suspension 2991

CIPLOX D (India)
CIPROFLOXACIN
Cipro Oral Suspension 2991

CIPLOX TZ (India)
CIPROFLOXACIN
Cipro Oral Suspension 2991

CIPLOXX (South Africa)
CIPROFLOXACIN HYDROCHLORIDE
Ciloxan Ophthalmic Ointment 554
Ciloxan Ophthalmic Solution . . . . ⊙205
Cipro Tablets 2991

CIPOBACTER (Spain)
CIPROFLOXACIN HYDROCHLORIDE
Ciloxan Ophthalmic Ointment 554
Ciloxan Ophthalmic Solution . . . . ⊙205
Cipro Tablets 2991

CIPOFIX (South Africa)
CEFUROXIME SODIUM
Zinacef Injection 1604

CIPRAGER (Irish Republic)
CITALOPRAM HYDROBROMIDE
Celexa Tablets 1177

CIPRAIN (Mexico)
CIPROFLOXACIN
Cipro Oral Suspension 2991

CIPRAM (Hong Kong, Malaysia, Singapore, Thailand)
CITALOPRAM HYDROBROMIDE
Celexa Tablets 1177

CIPRAMIL (Australia, Chile, Germany, Israel, Norway, Russia, South Africa)
CITALOPRAM HYDROBROMIDE
Celexa Tablets 1177

CIPRAPINE (Irish Republic, The Netherlands)
CITALOPRAM HYDROBROMIDE
Celexa Tablets 1177

CIPRENIT OTICO (Spain)
CIPROFLOXACIN HYDROCHLORIDE
Ciloxan Ophthalmic Ointment 554
Ciloxan Ophthalmic Solution . . . . ⊙205
Cipro Tablets 2991

CIPREX (Brazil)
CIPROFLOXACIN HYDROCHLORIDE
Ciloxan Ophthalmic Ointment 554
Ciloxan Ophthalmic Solution . . . . ⊙205
Cipro Tablets 2991

CIPRIL (India)
LISINOPRIL
Prinivil Tablets 2029
Zestril Tablets. 704

CIPRIL-H (India)
LISINOPRIL
Prinivil Tablets 2029
Zestril Tablets. 704

CIPRO HC (Argentina, Brazil, Hong Kong)
CIPROFLOXACIN HYDROCHLORIDE
Ciloxan Ophthalmic Ointment 554
Ciloxan Ophthalmic Solution . . . . ⊙205
Cipro Tablets 2991

CIPROBAY (Czech Republic, Hungary)
CIPROFLOXACIN
Cipro Oral Suspension 2991

CIPROBAY HC (Singapore, South Africa)
CIPROFLOXACIN
Cipro Oral Suspension 2991

CIPROBAY HC OTIC (Czech Republic)
CIPROFLOXACIN HYDROCHLORIDE
Ciloxan Ophthalmic Ointment 554
Ciloxan Ophthalmic Solution . . . . ⊙205
Cipro Tablets 2991

CIPROBETA (Germany)
CIPROFLOXACIN HYDROCHLORIDE
Ciloxan Ophthalmic Ointment 554
Ciloxan Ophthalmic Solution . . . . ⊙205
Cipro Tablets 2991

CIPROBID (Czech Republic, Thailand)
CIPROFLOXACIN HYDROCHLORIDE
Ciloxan Ophthalmic Ointment 554
Ciloxan Ophthalmic Solution . . . . ⊙205
Cipro Tablets 2991

CIPROBIOT (Brazil)
CIPROFLOXACIN HYDROCHLORIDE
Ciloxan Ophthalmic Ointment 554
Ciloxan Ophthalmic Solution . . . . ⊙205
Cipro Tablets 2991

CIPROBIOTIC (Mexico)
CIPROFLOXACIN HYDROCHLORIDE
Ciloxan Ophthalmic Ointment 554
Ciloxan Ophthalmic Solution . . . . ⊙205
Cipro Tablets 2991

CIPRO-CENT (India)
CIPROFLOXACIN HYDROCHLORIDE
Ciloxan Ophthalmic Ointment 554
Ciloxan Ophthalmic Solution . . . . ⊙205
Cipro Tablets 2991

CIPROCEP (Thailand)
CIPROFLOXACIN
Cipro Oral Suspension 2991

CIPROCIN (Brazil)
CIPROFLOXACIN
Cipro Oral Suspension 2991

CIPROCINA (Brazil)
CIPROFLOXACIN
Cipro Oral Suspension 2991

CIPRODAC (India)
CIPROFLOXACIN
Cipro Oral Suspension 2991

CIPRODEX (Israel)
CIPROFLOXACIN HYDROCHLORIDE
Ciloxan Ophthalmic Ointment 554
Ciloxan Ophthalmic Solution . . . . ⊙205
Cipro Tablets 2991

CIPRODINE (Brazil)
CIPROFLOXACIN HYDROCHLORIDE
Ciloxan Ophthalmic Ointment 554
Ciloxan Ophthalmic Solution . . . . ⊙205
Cipro Tablets 2991

CIPRODURA (Germany)
CIPROFLOXACIN HYDROCHLORIDE
Ciloxan Ophthalmic Ointment 554
Ciloxan Ophthalmic Solution . . . . ⊙205
Cipro Tablets 2991

CIPROFAR (Brazil)
CIPROFLOXACIN HYDROCHLORIDE
Ciloxan Ophthalmic Ointment 554
Ciloxan Ophthalmic Solution . . . . ⊙205
Cipro Tablets 2991

CIPROFIN (Thailand)
CIPROFLOXACIN
Cipro Oral Suspension 2991

CIPROFLOX (Brazil, Germany, Switzerland)
CIPROFLOXACIN
Cipro Oral Suspension 2991

CIPROFUR (Mexico)
CIPROFLOXACIN HYDROCHLORIDE
Ciloxan Ophthalmic Ointment 554
Ciloxan Ophthalmic Solution . . . . ⊙205
Cipro Tablets 2991

CIPROGAMMA (Germany)
CIPROFLOXACIN HYDROCHLORIDE
Ciloxan Ophthalmic Ointment 554
Ciloxan Ophthalmic Solution . . . . ⊙205
Cipro Tablets 2991

CIPROGEN (South Africa, Thailand)
CIPROFLOXACIN
Cipro Oral Suspension 2991

CIPROGIS (Israel)
CIPROFLOXACIN
Cipro Oral Suspension 2991

CIPROGLEN (Thailand)
CIPROFLOXACIN
Cipro Oral Suspension 2991

CIPRO-HEXAL (South Africa)
CIPROFLOXACIN
Cipro Oral Suspension 2991

CIPROK (Spain)
CIPROFLOXACIN HYDROCHLORIDE
Ciloxan Ophthalmic Ointment 554
Ciloxan Ophthalmic Solution . . . . ⊙205
Cipro Tablets 2991

CIPROL (Australia)
CIPROFLOXACIN HYDROCHLORIDE
Ciloxan Ophthalmic Ointment 554
Ciloxan Ophthalmic Solution . . . . ⊙205
Cipro Tablets 2991

CIPROLET (Singapore)
CIPROFLOXACIN
Cipro Oral Suspension 2991

CIPRO-LICH (Germany)
CIPROFLOXACIN HYDROCHLORIDE
Ciloxan Ophthalmic Ointment 554
Ciloxan Ophthalmic Solution . . . . ⊙205
Cipro Tablets 2991

CIPROMED (Austria, Finland, Russia)
CIPROFLOXACIN HYDROCHLORIDE
Ciloxan Ophthalmic Ointment 554
Ciloxan Ophthalmic Solution . . . . ⊙205
Cipro Tablets 2991

CIPRO-MED (Switzerland)
CIPROFLOXACIN HYDROCHLORIDE
Ciloxan Ophthalmic Ointment 554
Ciloxan Ophthalmic Solution . . . . ⊙205
Cipro Tablets 2991

CIPROMYCIN (Greece)
CIPROFLOXACIN HYDROCHLORIDE
Ciloxan Ophthalmic Ointment 554
Ciloxan Ophthalmic Solution . . . . ⊙205
Cipro Tablets 2991

CIPRONAL (Brazil)
CIPROFLOXACIN HYDROCHLORIDE
Ciloxan Ophthalmic Ointment 554
Ciloxan Ophthalmic Solution . . . . ⊙205
Cipro Tablets 2991

CIPRO-OTICO (Argentina)
CIPROFLOXACIN HYDROCHLORIDE
Ciloxan Ophthalmic Ointment 554
Ciloxan Ophthalmic Solution . . . . ⊙205
Cipro Tablets 2991

CIPROQUINOL (Portugal)
CIPROFLOXACIN
Cipro Oral Suspension 2991

CIPRO-SAAR (Germany)
CIPROFLOXACIN HYDROCHLORIDE
Ciloxan Ophthalmic Ointment 554
Ciloxan Ophthalmic Solution . . . . ⊙205
Cipro Tablets 2991

CIPROSER (Mexico)
CIPROFLOXACIN
Cipro Oral Suspension 2991

CIPROSTAD (Austria)
CIPROFLOXACIN HYDROCHLORIDE
Ciloxan Ophthalmic Ointment 554
Ciloxan Ophthalmic Solution . . . . ⊙205
Cipro Tablets 2991

CIPROSUN (Thailand)
CIPROFLOXACIN
Cipro Oral Suspension 2991

CIPROVAL (Chile)
CIPROFLOXACIN
Cipro Oral Suspension 2991

CIPROWIN (India)
CIPROFLOXACIN
Cipro Oral Suspension 2991

CIPRO-WOLFF (Germany)
CIPROFLOXACIN HYDROCHLORIDE
Ciloxan Ophthalmic Ointment 554
Ciloxan Ophthalmic Solution . . . . ⊙205
Cipro Tablets 2991

CIPROX (Germany)
CIPROFLOXACIN HYDROCHLORIDE
Ciloxan Ophthalmic Ointment 554
Ciloxan Ophthalmic Solution . . . . ⊙205
Cipro Tablets 2991

CIPROXAN (Brazil, Thailand)
CIPROFLOXACIN
Cipro Oral Suspension 2991

CIPROXIL (Brazil)
CIPROFLOXACIN HYDROCHLORIDE
Ciloxan Ophthalmic Ointment 554
Ciloxan Ophthalmic Solution . . . . ⊙205
Cipro Tablets 2991

CIPROXIN (Israel)
CIPROFLOXACIN
Cipro Oral Suspension 2991

CIPROXIN HC (Australia, Israel, New Zealand, Switzerland)
CIPROFLOXACIN HYDROCHLORIDE
Ciloxan Ophthalmic Ointment 554
Ciloxan Ophthalmic Solution . . . . ⊙205
Cipro Tablets 2991

CIPROXINA (Portugal)
CIPROFLOXACIN HYDROCHLORIDE
Ciloxan Ophthalmic Ointment 554
Ciloxan Ophthalmic Solution . . . . ⊙205
Cipro Tablets 2991

CIPROXINA SIMPLE (Spain)
CIPROFLOXACIN HYDROCHLORIDE
Cilo
Ciloxan Ophthalmic Ointment 554
Ciloxan Ophthalmic Solution . . . . ⊙205
Cipro Tablets 2991

CIPROXINE (Belgium)
CIPROFLOXACIN
Cipro Oral Suspension 2991

CIPROXINO (Chile)
CIPROFLOXACIN
Cipro Oral Suspension 2991

CIPROXYL (Hong Kong, Thailand)
CIPROFLOXACIN
Cipro Oral Suspension 2991

CIPTINI (India)
CIPROFLOXACIN
Cipro Oral Suspension 2991

CIQFADIN (Mexico)
CIPROFLOXACIN
Cipro Oral Suspension 2991

CIRCUVIT (Argentina)
WARFARIN SODIUM
Coumadin Tablets 932
Coumadin for Injection 932

CIRFLOX-G (Argentina)
CIPROFLOXACIN
Cipro Oral Suspension 2991

CIRIAX (Argentina)
CIPROFLOXACIN
Cipro Oral Suspension 2991

CIRIAX OTIC (Argentina)
CIPROFLOXACIN HYDROCHLORIDE
Ciloxan Ophthalmic Ointment 554
Ciloxan Ophthalmic Solution . . . . ⊙205
Cipro Tablets 2991

CIROK (Singapore)
CIPROFLOXACIN HYDROCHLORIDE
Ciloxan Ophthalmic Ointment 554
Ciloxan Ophthalmic Solution . . . . ⊙205
Cipro Tablets 2991

CIROXIN (Singapore)
CIPROFLOXACIN HYDROCHLORIDE
Ciloxan Ophthalmic Ointment 554
Ciloxan Ophthalmic Solution . . . . ⊙205
Cipro Tablets 2991

CISCUTAN (Austria)
ISOTRETINOIN
Accutane Capsules 2740

CISDAY (Germany)
NIFEDIPINE
Adalat CC Tablets 2978

CISTAMINE (Thailand)
CETIRIZINE HYDROCHLORIDE
Zyrtec Syrup 2589
Zyrtec Tablets 2589

CISTICID (Brazil, Chile, Mexico)
PRAZIQUANTEL
Biltricide Tablets 2990

CITADEP (India)
CITALOPRAM HYDROBROMIDE
Celexa Tablets 1177

CITADUR (Denmark)
CITALOPRAM HYDROBROMIDE
Celexa Tablets 1177

CITADURA (Germany)
CITALOPRAM HYDROBROMIDE
Celexa Tablets 1177

CITAHAM (Denmark)
CITALOPRAM HYDROBROMIDE
Celexa Tablets 1177

CITALEC (Czech Republic)
CITALOPRAM HYDROBROMIDE
Celexa Tablets 1177

CITALHEXAL (Austria)
CITALOPRAM HYDROBROMIDE
Celexa Tablets 1177

CITALON (Austria)
CITALOPRAM HYDROBROMIDE
Celexa Tablets 1177

CITARCANA (Austria)
CITALOPRAM HYDROBROMIDE
Celexa Tablets 1177

CITAVIE (Sweden)
CITALOPRAM HYDROBROMIDE
Celexa Tablets 1177

CITIDINE (Hong Kong, Singapore, Thailand)
CIMETIDINE
Tagamet Tablets 1547

CITIDOL (Italy)
DIFLUNISAL
Dolobid Tablets 1937

CITIFLUX (Italy)
FLUNISOLIDE
Aerobid Inhaler System 1172
Aerobid-M Inhaler System 1172
Nasarel Nasal Spray 1652

CITILAT (Italy)
NIFEDIPINE
Adalat CC Tablets 2978

CITIMID (Italy)
CIMETIDINE
Tagamet Tablets 1547

CITIREUMA (Italy)
SULINDAC
Clinoril Tablets 1899

CITIZEM (Italy)
DILTIAZEM HYDROCHLORIDE
Cardizem LA Extended Release Tablets . . . 1699
Tiazac Capsules 1204

CITIZOL (India)
CIPROFLOXACIN
Cipro Oral Suspension 2991

CITOGEL (Austria, Italy)
SUCRALFATE
Carafate Suspension 727
Carafate Tablets 728

CITOR (Austria)
CITALOPRAM HYDROBROMIDE
Celexa Tablets 1177

CITOVIRAX (Italy)
GANCICLOVIR
Cytovene Capsules 2763

CITRIHEXAL (Australia)
CALCITRIOL
Calcijex Injection 411

CITROL (Irish Republic)
CITALOPRAM HYDROBROMIDE
Celexa Tablets 1177

CITROVENOT (Greece)
CIPROFLOXACIN HYDROCHLORIDE
Ciloxan Ophthalmic Ointment 554
Ciloxan Ophthalmic Solution . . . . ⊙205
Cipro Tablts 2991

CIUK (Germany)
CIMETIDINE
Tagamet Tablets 1547

CIVICOR (New Zealand, Singapore)
VERAPAMIL HYDROCHLORIDE
Covera-HS Tablets 3135
Verelan PM Capsules 3120

CIZETOL (India)
CARBAMAZEPINE
Carbatrol Capsules 3174
Tegretol Chewable Tablets 2278
Tegretol Suspension. 2278
Tegretol Tablets 2278
Tegretol-XR Tablets 2278

CLACIN (Hong Kong)
CLARITHROMYCIN
Biaxin Filmtab Tablets 402
Biaxin Granules 402

CLACINA (Portugal)
CLARITHROMYCIN
Biaxin Filmtab Tablets 402
Biaxin Granules 402

CLAMENTIN (South Africa)
AMOXICILLIN
Amoxil Pediatric Drops for Oral Suspension. 1315
Amoxil Tablets 1315

CLAMICIN (Brazil)
CLARITHROMYCIN
Biaxin Filmtab Tablets 402
Biaxin Granules 402

CLAMYCIN (United Arab Emirates)
CLARITHROMYCIN
Biaxin Filmtab Tablets 402
Biaxin Granules 402

CLARAC (Australia)
CLARITHROMYCIN
Biaxin Filmtab Tablets 402
Biaxin Granules 402

CLARBACT (India)
CLARITHROMYCIN
Biaxin Filmtab Tablets 402
Biaxin Granules 402

CLARIBEL (Hong Kong)
CLINDAMYCIN PHOSPHATE
Clindets Pledgets 3212

CLARIBID (India)
CLARITHROMYCIN
Biaxin Filmtab Tablets 402
Biaxin Granules 402

CLARIBIOTIC (Argentina)
CLARITHROMYCIN
Biaxin Filmtab Tablets 402
Biaxin Granules 402

CLARICIP (India)
CLARITHROMYCIN
Biaxin Filmtab Tablets 402
Biaxin Granules 402

CLARIMAC (India)
CLARITHROMYCIN
Biaxin Filmtab Tablets 402
Biaxin Granules 402

CLARIMAX (Brazil, Chile)
CLARITHROMYCIN
Biaxin Filmtab Tablets 402
Biaxin Granules 402

CLARIMID (Argentina)
CLARITHROMYCIN
Biaxin Filmtab Tablets 402
Biaxin Granules 402

CLARIMIR (Chile)
NAPHAZOLINE HYDROCHLORIDE
Albalon Ophthalmic Solution . . . . ⊙216

CLARINEO (Brazil)
CLARITHROMYCIN
Biaxin Filmtab Tablets 402
Biaxin Granules 402

CLARIPEN (Singapore)
CLARITHROMYCIN
Biaxin Filmtab Tablets 402
Biaxin Granules 402

CLARITAB (Brazil)
CLARITHROMYCIN
Biaxin Filmtab Tablets 402
Biaxin Granules 402

CLARITH (Japan, Thailand)
CLARITHROMYCIN
Biaxin Filmtab Tablets 402
Biaxin Granules 402

CLARITIN SKIN ITCH RELIEF (Canada)
HYDROCORTISONE
Hydrocortone Tablets 1963

CLARITUR (Spain)
CLARITHROMYCIN
Biaxin Filmtab Tablets 402
Biaxin Granules 402

CLAROFT (Brazil)
NAPHAZOLINE HYDROCHLORIDE
Albalon Ophthalmic Solution . . . . ⊙216

CLARON (Thailand)
CLARITHROMYCIN
Biaxin Filmtab Tablets 402
Biaxin Granules 402

CLAROPRAM (Switzerland)
CITALOPRAM HYDROBROMIDE
Celexa Tablets 1177

CLAROVIL (Argentina)
CLARITHROMYCIN
Biaxin Filmtab Tablets 402
Biaxin Granules 402

CLATROMICIN (Argentina)
CLARITHROMYCIN
Biaxin Filmtab Tablets 402
Biaxin Granules 402

CLEAN & CLEAR CONTINUOUS CONTROL (Canada)
BENZOYL PEROXIDE
Brevoxyl-4 Creamy Wash 3212
Brevoxyl-4 Gel 3211
Brevoxyl-8 Creamy Wash 3212
Brevoxyl-8 Gel 3211
Triaz Cleanser 1864
Triaz Gel 1864

CLEAN & CLEAR PERSA GEL (Canada)
BENZOYL PEROXIDE
Brevoxyl-4 Creamy Wash 3212
Brevoxyl-4 Gel 3211
Brevoxyl-8 Creamy Wash 3212
Brevoxyl-8 Gel 3211
Triaz Cleanser 1864
Triaz Gel 1864

CLEAN HAIR (Brazil)
PERMETHRIN
Acticin Cream. 2125

CLEAR EYES (Australia, Canada, New Zealand)
NAPHAZOLINE HYDROCHLORIDE
Albalon Ophthalmic Solution . . . . ⊙216

CLEAR EYES ACR (New Zealand)
NAPHAZOLINE HYDROCHLORIDE
Albalon Ophthalmic Solution ⊙216

CLEARAMED (Spain, Sweden)
BENZOYL PEROXIDE
Brevoxyl-4 Creamy Wash 3212
Brevoxyl-4 Gel 3211
Brevoxyl-8 Creamy Wash 3212
Brevoxyl-8 Gel 3211
Triaz Cleanser 1864
Triaz Gel 1864

CLEARASIL B.P. PLUS (Canada)
BENZOYL PEROXIDE
Brevoxyl-4 Creamy Wash 3212
Brevoxyl-4 Gel 3211
Brevoxyl-8 Creamy Wash 3212
Brevoxyl-8 Gel 3211
Triaz Cleanser 1864
Triaz Gel 1864

CLEARASIL BENZOYL P (South Africa)
BENZOYL PEROXIDE
Brevoxyl-4 Creamy Wash 3212
Brevoxyl-4 Gel 3211
Brevoxyl-8 Creamy Wash 3212
Brevoxyl-8 Gel 3211
Triaz Cleanser 1864
Triaz Gel 1864

CLEARASIL EXTRA STRENGTH (Australia)
BENZOYL PEROXIDE
Brevoxyl-4 Creamy Wash 3212
Brevoxyl-4 Gel 3211
Brevoxyl-8 Creamy Wash 3212
Brevoxyl-8 Gel 3211
Triaz Cleanser 1864
Triaz Gel 1864

CLEARASIL MAX 10 (United Kingdom)
BENZOYL PEROXIDE
Brevoxyl-4 Creamy Wash 3212
Brevoxyl-4 Gel 3211
Brevoxyl-8 Creamy Wash 3212
Brevoxyl-8 Gel 3211
Triaz Cleanser 1864
Triaz Gel 1864

CLEARASIL PLUS (Mexico)
BENZOYL PEROXIDE
Brevoxyl-4 Creamy Wash 3212
Brevoxyl-4 Gel 3211
Brevoxyl-8 Creamy Wash 3212
Brevoxyl-8 Gel 3211
Triaz Cleanser 1864
Triaz Gel 1864

CLEARASIL ULTRA (Australia, Italy, New Zealand)
BENZOYL PEROXIDE
Brevoxyl-4 Creamy Wash 3212
Brevoxyl-4 Gel 3211
Brevoxyl-8 Creamy Wash 3212
Brevoxyl-8 Gel 3211
Triaz Cleanser 1864
Triaz Gel 1864

CLEAREX COVER UP (Israel)
BENZOYL PEROXIDE
Brevoxyl-4 Creamy Wash 3212
Brevoxyl-4 Gel 3211
Brevoxyl-8 Creamy Wash 3212
Brevoxyl-8 Gel 3211
Triaz Cleanser 1864
Triaz Gel 1864

CLEARINE (India)
NAPHAZOLINE HYDROCHLORIDE
Albalon Ophthalmic Solution ⊙216

CLEOCIN (Australia, Austria, Italy)
CLINDAMYCIN HYDROCHLORIDE
Cleocin Vaginal Ovules 2613

CLERIDIUM (France)
DIPYRIDAMOLE
Persantine Tablets 898

CLERON (Hong Kong)
CLARITHROMYCIN
Biaxin Filmtab Tablets 402
Biaxin Granules 402

CLETONOL (Argentina)
NIMODIPINE
Nimotop Capsules 774

CLEVERON (Brazil)
ALENDRONATE SODIUM
Fosamax Tablets 1949

CLEXANE (Argentina, Australia, Belgium, Brazil, Chile, Czech Republic, Germany, Greece, Hong Kong, Hungary, India, Irish Republic, Israel, Italy, Malaysia, Mexico, New Zealand, Russia, Singapore, South Africa, Spain, Switzerland, Thailand, The Netherlands, United Kingdom)
ENOXAPARIN SODIUM
Lovenox Injection 2931

CLIANE (Brazil, New Zealand)
ESTRADIOL
Climara Transdermal System 795
Vivelle Transdermal System 2288
Vivelle-Dot Transdermal System 2293

CLIARVAS (Argentina)
LOSARTAN POTASSIUM
Cozaar Tablets 1913

CLIDAM (Austria)
CLINDAMYCIN HYDROCHLORIDE
Cleocin Vaginal Ovules 2613

CLIDETS (Chile)
CLINDAMYCIN PHOSPHATE
Clindets Pledgets 3212

CLIMADAN (Singapore)
CLINDAMYCIN HYDROCHLORIDE
Cleocin Vaginal Ovules 2613

CLIMADERM (Argentina, Brazil, Chile, Mexico)
ESTRADIOL
Climara Transdermal System 795
Vivelle Transdermal System 2288
Vivelle-Dot Transdermal System 2293

CLIMARA (Australia, Austria, Belgium, Canada, Czech Republic, Denmark, Finland, France, Irish Republic, Israel, Italy, New Zealand, Norway, Portugal, South Africa, Sweden, Switzerland, Thailand, The Netherlands)
ESTRADIOL
Climara Transdermal System 795
Vivelle Transdermal System 2288
Vivelle-Dot Transdermal System 2293

CLIMASTON (France)
ESTRADIOL
Climara Transdermal System 795
Vivelle Transdermal System 2288
Vivelle-Dot Transdermal System 2293

CLIMATIDINE (Brazil)
CIMETIDINE
Tagamet Tablets 1547

CLINAC (New Zealand, Portugal)
CLINDAMYCIN PHOSPHATE
Clindets Pledgets 3212

CLINAGEL (Brazil)
CLINDAMYCIN PHOSPHATE
Clindets Pledgets 3212

CLINATEN (South Africa)
ATENOLOL
Tenormin I.V. Injection 698

CLINAZOLE (South Africa)
METRONIDAZOLE
MetroGel-Vaginal Gel 1822
Noritate Cream, 1% 1051

CLINDABETA (Germany)
CLINDAMYCIN HYDROCHLORIDE
Cleocin Vaginal Ovules 2613

CLINDAC (Austria, South Africa)
CLINDAMYCIN HYDROCHLORIDE
Cleocin Vaginal Ovules 2613

CLINDAC A (India)
CLINDAMYCIN PHOSPHATE
Clindets Pledgets 3212

CLINDACIN (Argentina, Russia)
CLINDAMYCIN PHOSPHATE
Clindets Pledgets 3212

CLINDACUR (Argentina)
CLINDAMYCIN PHOSPHATE
Clindets Pledgets 3212

CLINDAGEL (Singapore)
CLINDAMYCIN PHOSPHATE
Clindets Pledgets 3212

CLINDAHEXAL (South Africa)
CLINDAMYCIN HYDROCHLORIDE
Cleocin Vaginal Ovules 2613

CLINDAL (Austria)
CLINDAMYCIN HYDROCHLORIDE
Cleocin Vaginal Ovules 2613

CLINDAMIN C (Brazil)
CLINDAMYCIN HYDROCHLORIDE
Cleocin Vaginal Ovules 2613

CLINDASTAD (Germany)
CLINDAMYCIN HYDROCHLORIDE
Cleocin Vaginal Ovules 2613

CLINDATECH (Australia, Hong Kong, Singapore)
CLINDAMYCIN HYDROCHLORIDE
Cleocin Vaginal Ovules 2613

CLINDAZYN (Mexico)
CLINDAMYCIN PHOSPHATE
Clindets Pledgets 3212

CLINDETS (Canada)
CLINDAMYCIN PHOSPHATE
Clindets Pledgets 3212

CLINDOPAX (Argentina)
CLINDAMYCIN PHOSPHATE
Clindets Pledgets 3212

CLINDOXYL (Argentina, Canada)
BENZOYL PEROXIDE
Brevoxyl-4 Creamy Wash 3212
Brevoxyl-4 Gel 3211
Brevoxyl-8 Creamy Wash 3212
Brevoxyl-8 Gel 3211
Triaz Cleanser 1864
Triaz Gel 1864

CLINFAR (Brazil)
SIMVASTATIN
Zocor Tablets 2078

CLINIFLAM (South Africa)
DICLOFENAC SODIUM
Voltaren Tablets 2298
Voltaren-XR Tablets 2301

CLINIMET (Thailand)
CIMETIDINE
Tagamet Tablets 1547

CLINIRETIC (South Africa)
AMILORIDE HYDROCHLORIDE/HYDROCHLOROTHIAZIDE
Moduretic Tablets 2003

CLINODERM (Thailand)
CLOBETASOL PROPIONATE
Temovate Cream 1549
Temovate E Emollient 1552
Temovate Gel 1550
Temovate Ointment 1549
Temovate Scalp Application 1551

CLINOFEM (Germany)
MEDROXYPROGESTERONE ACETATE
Depo-Medrol Single-Dose Vial 2617

CLINOFUG GEL (Germany)
ERYTHROMYCIN
Ery-Tab Tablets 447
Erythromycin Base Filmtab Tablets 454
Erythromycin Delayed-Release Capsules, USP 456
PCE Dispertab Tablets 510

CLINOLAT (South Africa)
NIFEDIPINE
Adalat CC Tablets 2978

CLINORIL (Australia, Austria, Belgium, Canada, Czech Republic, Denmark, Hong Kong, Irish Republic, Italy, Malaysia, Mexico, New Zealand, Norway, South Africa, Sweden, Switzerland, Thailand, The Netherlands, United Kingdom)
SULINDAC
Clinoril Tablets 1899

CLINOSYN (South Africa)
NAPROXEN
EC-Naprosyn Delayed-Release Tablets 2769
Naprosyn Suspension 2769
Naprosyn Tablets 2769

CLINOTT (Thailand)
CLINDAMYCIN HYDROCHLORIDE
Cleocin Vaginal Ovules 2613

CLINOVIR (Germany)
MEDROXYPROGESTERONE ACETATE
Depo-Medrol Single-Dose Vial 2617

CLIN-SANORANIA (Germany)
CLINDAMYCIN HYDROCHLORIDE
Cleocin Vaginal Ovules 2613

CLINTOPIC (Argentina)
CLINDAMYCIN HYDROCHLORIDE
Cleocin Vaginal Ovules 2613

CLINWAS (Spain)
CLINDAMYCIN PHOSPHATE
Clindets Pledgets 3212

CLIOGAN (Spain)
ESTRADIOL
Climara Transdermal System 795
Vivelle Transdermal System 2288
Vivelle-Dot Transdermal System 2293

CLIPTO (Spain)
ENALAPRIL MALEATE
Vasotec I.V. Injection 2076

CLISUNDAC (Italy)
SULINDAC
Clinoril Tablets 1899

CLIVOTEN (Italy)
ISRADIPINE
DynaCirc CR Tablets 2726

CLOBASOL (Hong Kong)
CLOBETASOL PROPIONATE
Temovate Cream 1549
Temovate E Emollient 1552
Temovate Gel 1550
Temovate Ointment 1549
Temovate Scalp Application 1551

CLOBASONE (Thailand)
CLOBETASOL PROPIONATE
Temovate Cream 1549
Temovate E Emollient 1552
Temovate Gel 1550
Temovate Ointment 1549
Temovate Scalp Application 1551

CLOBEGALEN (Germany)
CLOBETASOL PROPIONATE
Temovate Cream 1549
Temovate E Emollient 1552
Temovate Gel 1550
Temovate Ointment 1549
Temovate Scalp Application 1551

CLOBENDIAN (Spain)
DILTIAZEM HYDROCHLORIDE
Cardizem LA Extended Release Tablets 1699
Tiazac Capsules 1204

CLOBEPLUS (Argentina)
CLOBETASOL PROPIONATE
Temovate Cream 1549
Temovate E Emollient 1552
Temovate Gel 1550
Temovate Ointment 1549
Temovate Scalp Application 1551

CLOBESOL (Argentina, Brazil, Italy)
CLOBETASOL PROPIONATE
Temovate Cream 1549
Temovate E Emollient 1552
Temovate Gel 1550
Temovate Ointment 1549
Temovate Scalp Application 1551

CLOBESOL LA (Argentina)
CLOBETASOL PROPIONATE
Temovate Cream 1549
Temovate E Emollient 1552
Temovate Gel 1550
Temovate Ointment 1549
Temovate Scalp Application 1551

CLOBESON (Singapore)
CLOBETASOL PROPIONATE
Temovate Cream 1549
Temovate E Emollient 1552
Temovate Gel 1550
Temovate Ointment 1549
Temovate Scalp Application 1551

CLOBET (Malaysia, Thailand)
CLOBETASOL PROPIONATE
Temovate Cream 1549
Temovate E Emollient 1552
Temovate Gel 1550
Temovate Ointment 1549
Temovate Scalp Application 1551

CLOBETATE (Thailand)
CLOBETASOL PROPIONATE
Temovate Cream 1549
Temovate E Emollient 1552
Temovate Gel 1550

(⊙ Described in PDR For Ophthalmic Medicines™)

Temovate Ointment 1549
Temovate Scalp Application 1551

CLOBEX (Argentina)
CLOBETASOL PROPIONATE
Temovate Cream 1549
Temovate E Emollient 1552
Temovate Gel 1550
Temovate Ointment 1549
Temovate Scalp Application 1551

CLOB-X (Brazil)
CLOBETASOL PROPIONATE
Temovate Cream 1549
Temovate E Emollient 1552
Temovate Gel 1550
Temovate Ointment 1549
Temovate Scalp Application 1551

CLOCIM (Switzerland)
CLOTRIMAZOLE
Lotrimin Cream 3053
Lotrimin Lotion 1% 3053
Lotrimin Topical Solution 1% 3053

CLOCIP (India)
CLOTRIMAZOLE
Lotrimin Cream 3053
Lotrimin Lotion 1% 3053
Lotrimin Topical Solution 1% 3053

CLOCIP B (India)
CLOTRIMAZOLE
Lotrimin Cream 3053
Lotrimin Lotion 1% 3053
Lotrimin Topical Solution 1% 3053

CLOCREME (Hong Kong, New Zealand)
CLOTRIMAZOLE
Lotrimin Cream 3053
Lotrimin Lotion 1% 3053
Lotrimin Topical Solution 1% 3053

CLODAVAN (Chile)
CLOBETASOL PROPIONATE
Temovate Cream 1549
Temovate E Emollient 1552
Temovate Gel 1550
Temovate Ointment 1549
Temovate Scalp Application 1551

CLODERM (Germany, India, Malaysia, Singapore)
CLOBETASOL PROPIONATE
Temovate Cream 1549
Temovate E Emollient 1552
Temovate Gel 1550
Temovate Ointment 1549
Temovate Scalp Application 1551

CLODIAN (Argentina)
CLOPIDOGREL BISULFATE
Plavix Tablets 940, 2942

CLODREL (Argentina)
CLOPIDOGREL BISULFATE
Plavix Tablets 940, 2942

CLOFAMOX (Argentina)
AMOXICILLIN
Amoxil Pediatric Drops for Oral Suspension 1315
Amoxil Tablets 1315

CLO-FAR (Mexico)
DICLOFENAC POTASSIUM
Cataflam Tablets 2173

CLOFEC (Hong Kong, Malaysia, Singapore, Thailand)
DICLOFENAC SODIUM
Voltaren Tablets 2298
Voltaren-XR Tablets 2301

CLOFEME (Australia)
CLOTRIMAZOLE
Lotrimin Cream 3053
Lotrimin Lotion 1% 3053
Lotrimin Topical Solution 1% 3053

CLOFENAC (Hong Kong, Malaysia, Singapore)
DICLOFENAC SODIUM
Voltaren Tablets 2298
Voltaren-XR Tablets 2301

CLOFENAK (Brazil)
DICLOFENAC POTASSIUM
Cataflam Tablets 2173

CLOFLOW (India)
CLOPIDOGREL BISULFATE
Plavix Tablets 940, 2942

CLOFLOW PLUS (India)
CLOPIDOGREL BISULFATE
Plavix Tablets 940, 2942

CLOFON (Thailand)
DICLOFENAC SODIUM
Voltaren Tablets 2298
Voltaren-XR Tablets 2301

CLOGEN (Brazil)
CLOTRIMAZOLE
Lotrimin Cream 3053
Lotrimin Lotion 1% 3053
Lotrimin Topical Solution 1% 3053

CLOMADERM (South Africa)
CLOTRIMAZOLE
Lotrimin Cream 3053
Lotrimin Lotion 1% 3053
Lotrimin Topical Solution 1% 3053

CLOMAZEN (Brazil)
CLOTRIMAZOLE
Lotrimin Cream 3053
Lotrimin Lotion 1% 3053
Lotrimin Topical Solution 1% 3053

CLOMENT (South Africa)
CLOZAPINE
Clozapine Tablets 2141
Clozaril Tablets 2174

CLOMYCIN (India)
CLOTRIMAZOLE
Lotrimin Cream 3053
Lotrimin Lotion 1% 3053
Lotrimin Topical Solution 1% 3053

CLONAC (Australia, Greece)
DICLOFENAC SODIUM
Voltaren Tablets 2298
Voltaren-XR Tablets 2301

CLONAGIN (Argentina)
CLONAZEPAM
Klonopin Tablets 2782

CLONAPAM (Canada, Chile, Hungary)
CLONAZEPAM
Klonopin Tablets 2782

CLONASTEN (Brazil)
CLOTRIMAZOLE
Lotrimin Cream 3053
Lotrimin Lotion 1% 3053
Lotrimin Topical Solution 1% 3053

CLONAX (Argentina)
CLONAZEPAM
Klonopin Tablets 2782

CLONDEPRYL (Irish Republic)
SELEGILINE HYDROCHLORIDE
Eldepryl Capsules 3209

CLONEA (Australia)
CLOTRIMAZOLE
Lotrimin Cream 3053
Lotrimin Lotion 1% 3053
Lotrimin Topical Solution 1% 3053

CLONER (Argentina)
CLONAZEPAM
Klonopin Tablets 2782

CLONESINA (Brazil)
CLONIDINE HYDROCHLORIDE
Catapres Tablets 874

CLONEX (Israel)
CLONAZEPAM
Klonopin Tablets 2782

CLONID-OPHTAL (Germany)
CLONIDINE HYDROCHLORIDE
Catapres Tablets 874

CLONIDURAL (Argentina)
CLONIDINE
Catapres-TTS 875

CLONILIX (Irish Republic)
INDAPAMIDE
Indapamide Tablets 2119

CLONISTADA (Germany)
CLONIDINE HYDROCHLORIDE
Catapres Tablets 874

CLONNIRIT (Israel)
CLONIDINE HYDROCHLORIDE
Catapres Tablets 874

CLONODIFEN (Mexico)
DICLOFENAC SODIUM
Voltaren Tablets 2298
Voltaren-XR Tablets 2301

CLONOGAL (Hungary)
CLONAZEPAM
Klonopin Tablets 2782

CLONOVATE (Thailand)
CLOBETASOL PROPIONATE
Temovate Cream 1549
Temovate E Emollient 1552
Temovate Gel 1550
Temovate Ointment 1549
Temovate Scalp Application 1551

CLONT (Germany)
METRONIDAZOLE
MetroGel-Vaginal Gel 1822
Noritate Cream, 1% 1051

CLONURETIC (Irish Republic)
AMILORIDE HYDROCHLORIDE/HYDROCHLOROTHIAZIDE
Moduretic Tablets 2003

CLOPACT (India)
CLOPIDOGREL BISULFATE
Plavix Tablets 940, 2942

CLOPACT A (India)
CLOPIDOGREL BISULFATE
Plavix Tablets 940, 2942

CLOPINE (Australia, New Zealand)
CLOZAPINE
Clozapine Tablets 2141
Clozaril Tablets 2174

CLOPIVAS (India)
CLOPIDOGREL BISULFATE
Plavix Tablets 940, 2942

CLOPIVAS AP (India)
CLOPIDOGREL BISULFATE
Plavix Tablets 940, 2942

CLOPOD (India)
CLOPIDOGREL BISULFATE
Plavix Tablets 940, 2942

CLOPOD-A (India)
CLOPIDOGREL BISULFATE
Plavix Tablets 940, 2942

CLOPSINE (Mexico)
CLOZAPINE
Clozapine Tablets 2141
Clozaril Tablets 2174

CLORADEX (Italy)
DEXAMETHASONE
Decadron Tablets 1929

CLOR-K-ZAF (Mexico)
POTASSIUM CHLORIDE
K-Dur Extended-Relase Tablets 3047
K-Lor Powder Packets 472
K-Tab Filmtab Tablets 473

CLORTANOL (Italy)
ATENOLOL
Tenormin I.V. Injection 698

CLOSCRIPT (South Africa)
CLOTRIMAZOLE
Lotrimin Cream 3053
Lotrimin Lotion 1% 3053
Lotrimin Topical Solution 1% 3053

CLOSIN (Germany)
PROMETHAZINE HYDROCHLORIDE
Phenergan Suppositories 3438
Phenergan Tablets 3438

CLOSINA (Australia)
CYCLOSERINE
Seromycin Capsules 1783

CLOSTEDAL (Mexico)
CARBAMAZEPINE
Carbatrol Capsules 3174
Tegretol Chewable Tablets 2278
Tegretol Suspension 2278
Tegretol Tablets 2278
Tegretol-XR Tablets 2278

CLOTASSIO (Brazil)
POTASSIUM CHLORIDE
K-Dur Extended-Relase Tablets 3047
K-Lor Powder Packets 472
K-Tab Filmtab Tablets 473

CLOT-BASAN (Switzerland)
CLOTRIMAZOLE
Lotrimin Cream 3053
Lotrimin Lotion 1% 3053
Lotrimin Topical Solution 1% 3053

CLOTREME (Australia)
CLOTRIMAZOLE
Lotrimin Cream 3053
Lotrimin Lotion 1% 3053
Lotrimin Topical Solution 1% 3053

CLOTREN (Brazil)
CLOTRIMAZOLE
Lotrimin Cream 3053
Lotrimin Lotion 1% 3053
Lotrimin Topical Solution 1% 3053

CLOTRI (Thailand)
CLOTRIMAZOLE
Lotrimin Cream 3053
Lotrimin Lotion 1% 3053
Lotrimin Topical Solution 1% 3053

CLOTRI OPT (Germany)
CLOTRIMAZOLE
Lotrimin Cream 3053
Lotrimin Lotion 1% 3053
Lotrimin Topical Solution 1% 3053

CLOTRICIN (Thailand)
CLOTRIMAZOLE
Lotrimin Cream 3053
Lotrimin Lotion 1% 3053
Lotrimin Topical Solution 1% 3053

CLOTRI-DENK (Hong Kong)
CLOTRIMAZOLE
Lotrimin Cream 3053
Lotrimin Lotion 1% 3053
Lotrimin Topical Solution 1% 3053

CLOTRIFERM (Sweden)
CLOTRIMAZOLE
Lotrimin Cream 3053
Lotrimin Lotion 1% 3053
Lotrimin Topical Solution 1% 3053

CLOTRIFUG (Germany)
CLOTRIMAZOLE
Lotrimin Cream 3053
Lotrimin Lotion 1% 3053
Lotrimin Topical Solution 1% 3053

CLOTRIGALEN (Germany)
CLOTRIMAZOLE
Lotrimin Cream 3053
Lotrimin Lotion 1% 3053
Lotrimin Topical Solution 1% 3053

CLOTRIHEXAL (New Zealand)
CLOTRIMAZOLE
Lotrimin Cream 3053
Lotrimin Lotion 1% 3053
Lotrimin Topical Solution 1% 3053

CLOTRIMADERM (Canada, Israel, New Zealand)
CLOTRIMAZOLE
Lotrimin Cream 3053
Lotrimin Lotion 1% 3053
Lotrimin Topical Solution 1% 3053

CLOTRIMIN (Chile)
CLOTRIMAZOLE
Lotrimin Cream 3053
Lotrimin Lotion 1% 3053
Lotrimin Topical Solution 1% 3053

CLOTRIMIX (Brazil)
CLOTRIMAZOLE
Lotrimin Cream 3053
Lotrimin Lotion 1% 3053
Lotrimin Topical Solution 1% 3053

CLOTRINOLON (Hong Kong)
CLOTRIMAZOLE
Lotrimin Cream 3053
Lotrimin Lotion 1% 3053
Lotrimin Topical Solution 1% 3053

CLOTRIZAN (Brazil)
CLOTRIMAZOLE
Lotrimin Cream 3053
Lotrimin Lotion 1% 3053
Lotrimin Topical Solution 1% 3053

CLOVATE (Spain)
CLOBETASOL PROPIONATE
Temovate Cream 1549
Temovate E Emollient 1552
Temovate Gel 1550
Temovate Ointment 1549
Temovate Scalp Application 1551

CLOX (Italy)
TICLOPIDINE HYDROCHLORIDE
Ticlid Tablets 2813

CLOXIB (Argentina)
CELECOXIB
Celebrex Capsules . . . 3130

CLOZANIL (Chile)
CLONAZEPAM
Klonopin Tablets . . . 2782

CLOZARIL (Australia, Canada, Hong Kong, Irish Republic, Malaysia, New Zealand, Singapore, Thailand, United Kingdom)
CLOZAPINE
Clozapine Tablets . . . 2141
Clozaril Tablets . . . 2174

CLOZOL (India)
CLOTRIMAZOLE
Lotrimin Cream . . . 3053
Lotrimin Lotion 1% . . . 3053
Lotrimin Topical Solution 1% . . . 3053

CLOZOLE (Australia, Hong Kong, Singapore)
CLOTRIMAZOLE
Lotrimin Cream . . . 3053
Lotrimin Lotion 1% . . . 3053
Lotrimin Topical Solution 1% . . . 3053

CLUSINOL (Australia)
SULINDAC
Clinoril Tablets . . . 1899

CMD (Thailand)
CIMETIDINE
Tagamet Tablets . . . 1547

CMP (Argentina)
CARBAMAZEPINE
Carbatrol Capsules . . . 3174
Tegretol Chewable Tablets . . . 2278
Tegretol Suspension . . . 2278
Tegretol Tablets . . . 2278
Tegretol-XR Tablets . . . 2278

C-MYCIN (Malaysia, Singapore)
CLINDAMYCIN PHOSPHATE
Clindets Pledgets . . . 3212

CO-ACEPRIL (Switzerland)
ENALAPRIL MALEATE
Vasotec I.V. Injection . . . 2076

CO-ACETAN (Austria)
HYDROCHLOROTHIAZIDE/LISINOPRIL
Prinzide Tablets . . . 2033
Zestoretic Tablets . . . 701

CO-AMILORID (Switzerland)
AMILORIDE HYDROCHLORIDE/HYDROCHLOROTHIAZIDE
Moduretic Tablets . . . 2003

CO-AMOXYCLAV (South Africa)
AMOXICILLIN
Amoxil Pediatric Drops for Oral Suspension . . . 1315
Amoxil Tablets . . . 1315

COAPROVEL (Argentina, Belgium, Chile, Czech Republic, Denmark, France, Germany, Hong Kong, Hungary, Irish Republic, Italy, Malaysia, Norway, Portugal, Singapore, South Africa, Spain, Sweden, Switzerland, Thailand, The Netherlands)
IRBESARTAN
Avapro Tablets . . . 925

CO-ATENOLOL (Switzerland)
ATENOLOL
Tenormin I.V. Injection . . . 698

COBADEX (United Kingdom)
HYDROCORTISONE
Hydrocortone Tablets . . . 1963

COBAY (Thailand)
CIPROFLOXACIN HYDROCHLORIDE
Ciloxan Ophthalmic Ointment . . . 554
Ciloxan Ophthalmic Solution . . . ⊙205
Cipro Tablets . . . 2991

COBIX (India)
CELECOXIB
Celebrex Capsules . . . 3130

CO-CAPTOPRIL (Austria)
CAPTOPRIL
Captopril Tablets . . . 2114

CO-CAPTOTYROL (Austria)
CAPTOPRIL
Captopril Tablets . . . 2114

CO-CAPTRAL (Mexico)
CAPTOPRIL
Captopril Tablets . . . 2114

CO-DIOVAN (Austria, Czech Republic, Germany, Hong Kong, Irish Republic, Israel, Malaysia, Mexico, Portugal, Russia, Singapore, South Africa, Spain, Switzerland, Thailand, The Netherlands, United Kingdom)
HYDROCHLOROTHIAZIDE/VALSARTAN
Diovan HCT Tablets . . . 2195

CO-DIOVANE (Belgium)
HYDROCHLOROTHIAZIDE/VALSARTAN
Diovan HCT Tablets . . . 2195

CODRINAN (Brazil)
THEOPHYLLINE
Uniphyl Tablets . . . 2708

CO-ENAC (Austria)
ENALAPRIL MALEATE
Vasotec I.V. Injection . . . 2076

CO-ENALAPRIL (Austria, Belgium)
ENALAPRIL MALEATE
Vasotec I.V. Injection . . . 2076

CO-ENARAN (Austria)
ENALAPRIL MALEATE
Vasotec I.V. Injection . . . 2076

CO-ENATEC (Switzerland)
ENALAPRIL MALEATE
Vasotec I.V. Injection . . . 2076

CO-ENATYROL (Austria)
ENALAPRIL MALEATE
Vasotec I.V. Injection . . . 2076

CO-EPRIL (Switzerland)
ENALAPRIL MALEATE
Vasotec I.V. Injection . . . 2076

COFENAC (India)
DICLOFENAC SODIUM
Voltaren Tablets . . . 2298
Voltaren-XR Tablets . . . 2301

COGNITIV (Austria, Czech Republic)
SELEGILINE HYDROCHLORIDE
Eldepryl Capsules . . . 3209

COLATAN (Spain)
NARATRIPTAN HYDROCHLORIDE
Amerge Tablets . . . 1312

COLDAN (Austria)
NAPHAZOLINE HYDROCHLORIDE
Albalon Ophthalmic Solution . . . ⊙216

COLEB (Germany)
ISOSORBIDE MONONITRATE
Imdur Tablets . . . 3032

COLEDIS (Argentina)
SIMVASTATIN
Zocor Tablets . . . 2078

COLEMIN (Spain)
SIMVASTATIN
Zocor Tablets . . . 2078

COLESVIR (Spain)
LOVASTATIN
Mevacor Tablets . . . 1996

COLEVIX (Chile)
LOVASTATIN
Mevacor Tablets . . . 1996

COLIFOSSIM (Italy)
CEFUROXIME SODIUM
Zinacef Injection . . . 1604

COLIMET (Mexico)
CIMETIDINE
Tagamet Tablets . . . 1547

COLIRIOCILINA GENTAM (Spain)
GENTAMICIN SULFATE
Garamycin Injectable . . . 3028
Genoptic Sterile Ophthalmic Solution . . . ⊙227

COLITROMIN (Mexico)
ERYTHROMYCIN
Ery-Tab Tablets . . . 447
Erythromycin Base Filmtab Tablets . . . 454
Erythromycin Delayed-Release Capsules, USP . . . 456
PCE Dispertab Tablets . . . 510

COLODIUM (Hong Kong, Singapore)
LOPERAMIDE HYDROCHLORIDE
Imodium Capsules . . . 1834

COLPISTAR (Brazil)
METRONIDAZOLE
MetroGel-Vaginal Gel . . . 1822
Noritate Cream, 1% . . . 1051

COLPOCIN-T (Greece)
METRONIDAZOLE
MetroGel-Vaginal Gel . . . 1822
Noritate Cream, 1% . . . 1051

COLPROSTERONE (Spain)
PROGESTERONE
Prometrium Capsules (100 mg, 200 mg) . 3205

COLSANAC (Portugal)
LACTULOSE
Kristalose for Oral Solution . . . 2149

COLTHER (Greece)
TOBRAMYCIN
TOBI Solution for Inhalation . . . 1015

COLUMINA (Mexico)
CIMETIDINE
Tagamet Tablets . . . 1547

COMALOSE-R (Canada)
LACTULOSE
Kristalose for Oral Solution . . . 2149

COMAT (Thailand)
CLOTRIMAZOLE
Lotrimin Cream . . . 3053
Lotrimin Lotion 1% . . . 3053
Lotrimin Topical Solution 1% . . . 3053

COMBANTRIN-1 (New Zealand)
MEBENDAZOLE
Vermox Chewable Tablets . . . 1853

COMBANTRIN-1 WITH MEBENDAZOLE (Australia)
MEBENDAZOLE
Vermox Chewable Tablets . . . 1853

COMBID (Thailand)
LAMIVUDINE
Epivir Oral Solution . . . 1394
Epivir Tablets . . . 1394
Epivir-HBV Oral Solution . . . 1398
Epivir-HBV Tablets . . . 1398

COMBINED (Argentina)
OLANZAPINE
Zyprexa Tablets . . . 1798

COMBIPROTECT (Germany)
AMILORIDE HYDROCHLORIDE/HYDROCHLOROTHIAZIDE
Moduretic Tablets . . . 2003

COMBIREX (India)
LAMIVUDINE
Epivir Oral Solution . . . 1394
Epivir Tablets . . . 1394
Epivir-HBV Oral Solution . . . 1398
Epivir-HBV Tablets . . . 1398

COMBISARTAN (Italy)
HYDROCHLOROTHIAZIDE/VALSARTAN
Diovan HCT Tablets . . . 2195

COMBIVENT (Argentina, Australia, Brazil, Malaysia)
IPRATROPIUM BROMIDE
Atrovent Inhalation Solution . . . 868
Atrovent Nasal Spray 0.03% . . . 869
Atrovent Nasal Spray 0.06% . . . 870

COMBIVIR (Australia, Austria, Belgium, Brazil, Canada, Chile, Czech Republic, Denmark, Finland, France, Germany, Greece, Hong Kong, Irish Republic, Israel, Italy, Malaysia, Mexico, New Zealand, Norway, Portugal, Singapore, South Africa, Spain, Sweden, Switzerland, The Netherlands, United Kingdom)
LAMIVUDINE
Epivir Oral Solution . . . 1394
Epivir Tablets . . . 1394
Epivir-HBV Oral Solution . . . 1398
Epivir-HBV Tablets . . . 1398

CO-MEPRIL (Austria)
ENALAPRIL MALEATE/HYDROCHLOROTHIAZIDE
Vaseretic Tablets . . . 2073

CO-MICARDIS (South Africa)
TELMISARTAN
Micardis Tablets . . . 884

COMILORID (Switzerland)
AMILORIDE HYDROCHLORIDE/HYDROCHLOROTHIAZIDE
Moduretic Tablets . . . 2003

COMPAZ (Brazil)
DIAZEPAM
Diastat Rectal Delivery System . . . 3344
Valium Tablets . . . 2822

COMPLUTINE (Spain)
DIAZEPAM
Diastat Rectal Delivery System . . . 3344
Valium Tablets . . . 2822

CONAZOL (Mexico)
KETOCONAZOLE
Nizoral 2% Shampoo . . . 1838

CONCERTA (Argentina, Australia, Austria, Belgium, Canada, Finland, France, Germany, Hong Kong, Irish Republic, Israel, Norway, Portugal, Singapore, Sweden, Switzerland, The Netherlands, United Kingdom)
METHYLPHENIDATE HYDROCHLORIDE
Ritalin Hydrochloride Tablets . . . 2254
Ritalin-SR Tablets . . . 2254

CONDIUREN (Italy)
ENALAPRIL MALEATE/HYDROCHLOROTHIAZIDE
Vaseretic Tablets . . . 2073

CONDROTEC (United Kingdom)
NAPROXEN
EC-Naprosyn Delayed-Release Tablets . . . 2769
Naprosyn Suspension . . . 2769
Naprosyn Tablets . . . 2769

CONEF (Argentina)
FINASTERIDE
Propecia Tablets . . . 2036
Proscar Tablets . . . 2040

CONFOBOS (Spain)
FAMOTIDINE
Pepcid Injection . . . 2017
Pepcid Injection Premixed . . . 2017
Pepcid Tablets . . . 2014
Pepcid for Oral Suspension . . . 2014

CONFORMAL (Argentina)
CARBAMAZEPINE
Carbatrol Capsules . . . 3174
Tegretol Chewable Tablets . . . 2278
Tegretol Suspension . . . 2278
Tegretol Tablets . . . 2278
Tegretol-XR Tablets . . . 2278

CONGEX (Argentina)
NAPROXEN
EC-Naprosyn Delayed-Release Tablets . . . 2769
Naprosyn Suspension . . . 2769
Naprosyn Tablets . . . 2769

CONJUNCTIN-S (Austria)
NEOMYCIN SULFATE/POLYMYXIN B SULFATE/PREDNISOLONE ACETATE
Poly-Pred Liquifilm Ophthalmic Suspension . . . ⊙231

CONNETTIVINA (Austria, Hong Kong, Italy, Thailand)
SODIUM HYALURONATE
Hyalgan Solution . . . 2917

CONPIN (Germany)
ISOSORBIDE MONONITRATE
Imdur Tablets . . . 3032

CONPRES (Hungary)
LISINOPRIL
Prinivil Tablets . . . 2029
Zestril Tablets . . . 704

CONSEC (India)
RANITIDINE HYDROCHLORIDE
Zantac 25 EFFERdose Tablets . . . 1597
Zantac 150 EFFERdose Tablets . . . 1597
Zantac 150 Tablets . . . 1597
Zantac 300 Tablets . . . 1597
Zantac Injection . . . 1593
Zantac Injection Premixed . . . 1593
Zantac Syrup . . . 1597

CONSTILAX (Greece)
NORFLOXACIN
Noroxin Tablets . . . 2009

CONTALGIN (Denmark)
MORPHINE SULFATE
Kadian Capsules . . . 572
MS Contin Tablets . . . 2703

CONTEMNOL (Czech Republic)
LITHIUM CARBONATE
Eskalith CR Controlled-Release Tablets . . . 1406
Eskalith Capsules . . . 1406

CONTIPHYLLIN (Germany)
THEOPHYLLINE
Uniphyl Tablets 2708

CONTRACEP (Brazil, Thailand)
MEDROXYPROGESTERONE ACETATE
Depo-Medrol Single-Dose Vial 2617

CONTRACID (Germany)
CIMETIDINE
Tagamet Tablets 1547

CONTRAFUNGIN (Germany)
CLOTRIMAZOLE
Lotrimin Cream 3053
Lotrimin Lotion 1% 3053
Lotrimin Topical Solution 1% 3053

CONTROL K (Argentina)
POTASSIUM CHLORIDE
K-Dur Extended-Relase Tablets 3047
K-Lor Powder Packets 472
K-Tab Filmtab Tablets 473

CONTROLIP (Mexico)
FENOFIBRATE
Tricor Tablets 523

CONTROLPROS (Argentina)
TAMSULOSIN HYDROCHLORIDE
Flomax Capsules 881

CONTROLVAS (Spain)
ENALAPRIL MALEATE
Vasotec I.V. Injection 2076

CONVADEN (Czech Republic)
ESTRADIOL
Climara Transdermal System 795
Vivelle Transdermal System 2288
Vivelle-Dot Transdermal System 2293

CONVECTAL (Spain)
DILTIAZEM HYDROCHLORIDE
Cardizem LA Extended Release Tablets . . . 1699
Tiazac Capsules 1204

CONVERTAL (Portugal)
CAPTOPRIL
Captopril Tablets 2114

CONVERTEN (Italy)
ENALAPRIL MALEATE
Vasotec I.V. Injection 2076

CONVERTIN (Israel)
ENALAPRIL MALEATE
Vasotec I.V. Injection 2076

CONVULEX (Belgium, Czech Republic, Hungary, Russia, Singapore, United Kingdom)
VALPROIC ACID
Depakene Capsules 417
Depakene Syrup 417

CONVULSAN (Brazil)
CARBAMAZEPINE
Carbatrol Capsules 3174
Tegretol Chewable Tablets 2278
Tegretol Suspension 2278
Tegretol Tablets 2278
Tegretol-XR Tablets 2278

COOLIPS (Chile)
CETIRIZINE HYDROCHLORIDE
Zyrtec Syrup 2589
Zyrtec Tablets 2589

COPAL (Mexico)
SULINDAC
Clinoril Tablets 1899

COPAXONE (Argentina, Australia, Austria, Belgium, Brazil, Canada, Czech Republic, Denmark, Finland, France, Hungary, Irish Republic, Israel, Italy, Norway, Portugal, Russia, Spain, Sweden, Switzerland, The Netherlands)
GLATIRAMER ACETATE
Copaxone for Injection 3292

COPEGUS (Argentina, Austria, Belgium, Denmark, Finland, France, Germany, Hong Kong, Irish Republic, Israel, Italy, New Zealand, Norway, Portugal, Spain, Sweden, Switzerland, The Netherlands, United Kingdom)
RIBAVIRIN
Virazole for Inhalation Solution 3365

COPHADYL (Singapore)
PROMETHAZINE HYDROCHLORIDE
Phenergan Suppositories 3438
Phenergan Tablets 3438

COPOVAN (Italy)
VANCOMYCIN HYDROCHLORIDE
Vancocin HCl Capsules, USP 3370

CO-PRESSOTEC (Brazil)
ENALAPRIL MALEATE
Vasotec I.V. Injection 2076

COR MIO (Brazil)
AMIODARONE HYDROCHLORIDE
Pacerone Tablets 3337

COR TENSOBON (Germany)
CAPTOPRIL
Captopril Tablets 2114

CORACTEN (Greece, Hong Kong, Thailand, United Kingdom)
NIFEDIPINE
Adalat CC Tablets 2978

CORAGOXINE (France)
DIGOXIN
Lanoxicaps Capsules 1458
Lanoxin Injection 1462
Lanoxin Injection Pediatric 1465
Lanoxin Tablets 1468

CORAL (Italy)
NIFEDIPINE
Adalat CC Tablets 2978

CORALEN (Spain)
RANITIDINE HYDROCHLORIDE
Zantac 25 EFFERdose Tablets 1597
Zantac 150 EFFERdose Tablets 1597
Zantac 150 Tablets 1597
Zantac 300 Tablets 1597
Zantac Injection 1593
Zantac Injection Premixed 1593
Zantac Syrup 1597

CORAMIL (Sweden)
DILTIAZEM HYDROCHLORIDE
Cardizem LA Extended Release Tablets . . . 1699
Tiazac Capsules 1204

CORANGIN (Austria, Germany, Hong Kong, New Zealand)
ISOSORBIDE MONONITRATE
Imdur Tablets 3032

CORANGINE (Switzerland)
ISOSORBIDE MONONITRATE
Imdur Tablets 3032

CORAS (Australia)
DILTIAZEM HYDROCHLORIDE
Cardizem LA Extended Release Tablets . . . 1699
Tiazac Capsules 1204

CORATOL (Norway, Thailand)
ATENOLOL
Tenormin I.V. Injection 698

CORAZEM (Austria)
DILTIAZEM HYDROCHLORIDE
Cardizem LA Extended Release Tablets . . . 1699
Tiazac Capsules 1204

CORAZET (Germany)
DILTIAZEM HYDROCHLORIDE
Cardizem LA Extended Release Tablets . . . 1699
Tiazac Capsules 1204

CORBETA (India)
PROPRANOLOL HYDROCHLORIDE
Inderal LA Long-Acting Capsules 3421

CORBIONAX (France)
AMIODARONE HYDROCHLORIDE
Pacerone Tablets 3337

CORDAFEN (Czech Republic)
NIFEDIPINE
Adalat CC Tablets 2978

CORDAFLEX (Hungary, Russia)
NIFEDIPINE
Adalat CC Tablets 2978

CORDAN (Denmark)
AMIODARONE HYDROCHLORIDE
Pacerone Tablets 3337

CORDAREX (Germany)
AMIODARONE HYDROCHLORIDE
Pacerone Tablets 3337

CORDARONE (Belgium, Canada, Chile, Czech Republic, Denmark, Finland, France, Hong Kong, Hungary, India, Italy, Malaysia, Mexico, New Zealand, Norway, Portugal, Russia, Singapore, Sweden, Switzerland, Thailand, The Netherlands)
AMIODARONE HYDROCHLORIDE
Pacerone Tablets 3337

CORDARONE X (Australia, Irish Republic, South Africa, United Kingdom)
AMIODARONE HYDROCHLORIDE
Pacerone Tablets 3337

CORDES BPO (Germany)
BENZOYL PEROXIDE
Brevoxyl-4 Creamy Wash 3212
Brevoxyl-4 Gel 3211
Brevoxyl-8 Creamy Wash 3212
Brevoxyl-8 Gel 3211
Triaz Cleanser 1864
Triaz Gel 1864

CORDES NYSTATIN SOFT (Germany)
NYSTATIN
Nystop Topical Powder USP 2490

CORDES VAS (Germany)
TRETINOIN
Avita Cream 2136
Avita Gel 2138
Renova 0.05% Cream 2387
Retin-A Micro 0.1%/0.04% 2388
Vesanoid Capsules 2823

CORDICANT (Germany)
NIFEDIPINE
Adalat CC Tablets 2978

CORDILAN (Spain)
NIFEDIPINE
Adalat CC Tablets 2978

CORDILAT (Brazil, Mexico)
NIFEDIPINE
Adalat CC Tablets 2978

CORDILOX (Australia, United Kingdom)
VERAPAMIL HYDROCHLORIDE
Covera-HS Tablets 3135
Verelan PM Capsules 3120

CORDIPIN (Czech Republic, Hungary, Russia, Singapore)
NIFEDIPINE
Adalat CC Tablets 2978

COREG (Brazil, Canada)
CARVEDILOL
Coreg Tablets 1376

CORENISTAD (Austria)
ENALAPRIL MALEATE
Vasotec I.V. Injection 2076

CO-RENITEC (Argentina, Austria, Belgium, Brazil, Denmark, France, Greece, Hong Kong, Hungary, Mexico, New Zealand, Russia, Singapore, South Africa, Spain, The Netherlands)
ENALAPRIL MALEATE
Vasotec I.V. Injection 2076

CO-RENITEN (Switzerland)
ENALAPRIL MALEATE/HYDROCHLOROTHIAZIDE
Vaseretic Tablets 2073

CORFLENE (Spain)
FLECAINIDE ACETATE
Tambocor Tablets 1824

CORGARD (Argentina, Belgium, Brazil, Canada, Chile, France, Hong Kong, Irish Republic, Italy, Malaysia, New Zealand, South Africa, Spain, Switzerland, United Kingdom)
NADOLOL
Nadolol Tablets 2121

CORGARETIC (United Kingdom)
NADOLOL
Nadolol Tablets 2121

CORIBON (Italy)
DIPYRIDAMOLE
Persantine Tablets 898

CORIC (Germany)
LISINOPRIL
Prinivil Tablets 2029
Zestril Tablets 704

CORIC PLUS (Germany)
HYDROCHLOROTHIAZIDE/LISINOPRIL
Prinzide Tablets 2033
Zestoretic Tablets 701

CORIDIL (Switzerland)
DILTIAZEM HYDROCHLORIDE
Cardizem LA Extended Release Tablets . . . 1699
Tiazac Capsules 1204

CORIFINA (Spain)
AZELASTINE HYDROCHLORIDE
Astelin Nasal Spray 1876

CORILAX (Thailand)
ORPHENADRINE CITRATE
Norflex Injection 1824

CORINFAR (Czech Republic, Germany, Hungary, Russia)
NIFEDIPINE
Adalat CC Tablets 2978

CORIODAL (Chile)
PROPRANOLOL HYDROCHLORIDE
Inderal LA Long-Acting Capsules 3421

CORISOL (Switzerland)
CLOTRIMAZOLE
Lotrimin Cream 3053
Lotrimin Lotion 1% 3053
Lotrimin Topical Solution 1% 3053

CORITENSIL (Argentina)
CARVEDILOL
Coreg Tablets 1376

CORIXA (Argentina)
CLARITHROMYCIN
Biaxin Filmtab Tablets 402
Biaxin Granules 402

CORNARON (Germany)
AMIODARONE HYDROCHLORIDE
Pacerone Tablets 3337

CORNEL (Spain)
NISOLDIPINE
Sular Tablets 1163

CORODAY (United Kingdom)
NIFEDIPINE
Adalat CC Tablets 2978

CORODIL (Denmark)
ENALAPRIL MALEATE
Vasotec I.V. Injection 2076

CORODIL COMP (Denmark)
ENALAPRIL MALEATE/HYDROCHLOROTHIAZIDE
Vaseretic Tablets 2073

CORODIN (Chile)
LOSARTAN POTASSIUM
Cozaar Tablets 1913

CORODIN D (Chile)
HYDROCHLOROTHIAZIDE/LOSARTAN POTASSIUM
Hyzaar 50-12.5 Tablets 1964

COROGAL (Mexico)
NIFEDIPINE
Adalat CC Tablets 2978

COROLATER (Spain)
DILTIAZEM HYDROCHLORIDE
Cardizem LA Extended Release Tablets . . . 1699
Tiazac Capsules 1204

COROLIN (Finland)
SIMVASTATIN
Zocor Tablets 2078

CORONARINE (France)
DIPYRIDAMOLE
Persantine Tablets 898

CORONORM (Germany)
CAPTOPRIL
Captopril Tablets 2114

CORONOVO (Argentina, Chile)
AMIODARONE HYDROCHLORIDE
Pacerone Tablets 3337

CORONUR (Spain)
ISOSORBIDE MONONITRATE
Imdur Tablets 3032

COROPRES (Spain)
CARVEDILOL
Coreg Tablets 1376

COROSAN (Italy)
DIPYRIDAMOLE
Persantine Tablets 898

COROTENOL (Czech Republic, Hong Kong, Malaysia)
ATENOLOL
Tenormin I.V. Injection 698

COROTREND (Germany, Mexico, Switzerland)
NIFEDIPINE
Adalat CC Tablets 2978

COROXIN (Italy)
DIPYRIDAMOLE
Persantine Tablets 898

COROZELL (Austria)
POTASSIUM CHLORIDE
K-Dur Extended-Relase Tablets 3047
K-Lor Powder Packets 472
K-Tab Filmtab Tablets 473

CORPAMIL (Switzerland)
VERAPAMIL HYDROCHLORIDE
Covera-HS Tablets 3135
Verelan PM Capsules 3120

CORPENDOL (Portugal)
PROPRANOLOL HYDROCHLORIDE
Inderal LA Long-Acting Capsules 3421

CORPRIL (Thailand)
RAMIPRIL
Altace Capsules 1673

CORPRILOR (Singapore, Spain)
ENALAPRIL MALEATE
Vasotec I.V. Injection 2076

CORTALEN C (Brazil)
CLOBETASOL PROPIONATE
Temovate Cream 1549
Temovate E Emollient 1552
Temovate Gel 1550
Temovate Ointment 1549
Temovate Scalp Application 1551

CORTALER NOVO (Argentina)
DEXAMETHASONE
Decadron Tablets 1929

CORTAPAISYL (France)
HYDROCORTISONE
Hydrocortone Tablets 1963

CORTEF (Hungary)
HYDROCORTISONE
Hydrocortone Tablets 1963

CORTENEM (Argentina)
HYDROCORTISONE
Hydrocortone Tablets 1963

CORTENEMA (Canada, United Kingdom)
HYDROCORTISONE
Hydrocortone Tablets 1963

CORTICIN (Hong Kong)
HYDROCORTISONE
Hydrocortone Tablets 1963

CORTICOSAN (Argentina)
LOSARTAN POTASSIUM
Cozaar Tablets 1913

CORTICOTHERAPIQUE (Switzerland)
TRIAMCINOLONE ACETONIDE
Azmacort Inhalation Aerosol 1701
Nasacort AQ Nasal Spray 2937

CORTIDEX (Mexico)
DEXAMETHASONE
Decadron Tablets 1929

CORTIDEXASON (Germany)
DEXAMETHASONE
Decadron Tablets 1929

CORTISEDERMYL (France)
HYDROCORTISONE
Hydrocortone Tablets 1963

CORTISTON (Brazil)
HYDROCORTISONE
Hydrocortone Tablets 1963

CORTISUMMAN (Germany)
DEXAMETHASONE
Decadron Tablets 1929

CORTIZONE (Israel)
HYDROCORTISONE
Hydrocortone Tablets 1963

CORTODERM (Canada)
HYDROCORTISONE
Hydrocortone Tablets 1963

CORTOLA-M (India)
SULFACETAMIDE SODIUM
Klaron Lotion 10% 1050

CORTOPIC (Chile)
CLOBETASOL PROPIONATE
Temovate Cream 1549
Temovate E Emollient 1552
Temovate Gel 1550
Temovate Ointment 1549
Temovate Scalp Application 1551

CORTOPIN (Irish Republic, United Kingdom)
HYDROCORTISONE
Hydrocortone Tablets 1963

CORTRIL (Finland)
HYDROCORTISONE
Hydrocortone Tablets 1963

CORTROPIN (United Kingdom)
HYDROCORTISONE
Hydrocortone Tablets 1963

CORUBIN (Argentina, Greece)
CARVEDILOL
Coreg Tablets 1376

CORUS (Brazil)
LOSARTAN POTASSIUM
Cozaar Tablets 1913

CORUS H (Brazil)
LOSARTAN POTASSIUM
Cozaar Tablets 1913

CORVASAL (Germany)
ISOSORBIDE MONONITRATE
Imdur Tablets 3032

CORVO (Germany)
ENALAPRIL MALEATE
Vasotec I.V. Injection 2076

CORZIDE (Canada)
NADOLOL
Nadolol Tablets 2121

COSAAR (Austria, Switzerland)
LOSARTAN POTASSIUM
Cozaar Tablets 1913

COSAAR PLUS (Austria, Switzerland)
HYDROCHLOROTHIAZIDE/LOSARTAN POTASSIUM
Hyzaar 50-12.5 Tablets 1964

CO-SALT (Argentina)
POTASSIUM CHLORIDE
K-Dur Extended-Relase Tablets 3047
K-Lor Powder Packets 472
K-Tab Filmtab Tablets 473

COSMEGEN (Argentina, Australia, Austria, Brazil, Canada, Finland, France, Greece, Hong Kong, Irish Republic, Italy, Malaysia, New Zealand, Norway, South Africa, Sweden, Switzerland, Thailand, United Kingdom)
DACTINOMYCIN
Cosmegen for Injection 1907

COSMOFER (Denmark, Germany, Greece, Irish Republic, Norway, Thailand, United Kingdom)
IRON DEXTRAN
Infed Injection 3381

COSMOPRIL (Greece)
SELEGILINE HYDROCHLORIDE
Eldepryl Capsules 3209

COSOPT (Argentina, Australia, Brazil, Chile, Czech Republic, Greece, Hong Kong, Hungary, Irish Republic, New Zealand, Portugal, Singapore, Thailand, The Netherlands)
DORZOLAMIDE HYDROCHLORIDE
Trusopt Sterile Ophthalmic Solution 2065

COSUDEX (Australia, New Zealand)
BICALUTAMIDE
Casodex Tablets 670

COTAREG (Brazil, France, Italy)
VALSARTAN
Diovan Tablets 2191

CO-TAREG (Portugal)
VALSARTAN
Diovan Tablets 2191

COTAZYM (Canada, New Zealand)
PANCRELIPASE
Ultrase Capsules 735
Ultrase MT Capsules 736

COTAZYM S FORTE (Australia)
PANCRELIPASE
Ultrase Capsules 735
Ultrase MT Capsules 736

COTAZYM-S (The Netherlands)
PANCRELIPASE
Ultrase Capsules 735
Ultrase MT Capsules 736

COTENOLOL-NEO (Switzerland)
ATENOLOL
Tenormin I.V. Injection 698

COTENOMEL (Irish Republic)
ATENOLOL
Tenormin I.V. Injection 698

COTESIFAR (Switzerland)
ATENOLOL
Tenormin I.V. Injection 698

COTREN (Hong Kong, Malaysia, Singapore, Thailand)
CLOTRIMAZOLE
Lotrimin Cream 3053
Lotrimin Lotion 1% 3053
Lotrimin Topical Solution 1% 3053

COTRISAN (Chile)
CLOTRIMAZOLE
Lotrimin Cream 3053
Lotrimin Lotion 1% 3053
Lotrimin Topical Solution 1% 3053

COUMADIN (Argentina, Australia, Canada, Chile, Germany, Israel, Italy, Malaysia, New Zealand, Singapore, South Africa)
WARFARIN SODIUM
Coumadin Tablets 932
Coumadin for Injection 932

COUMADINE (France)
WARFARIN SODIUM
Coumadin Tablets 932
Coumadin for Injection 932

CO-VALS (Spain)
HYDROCHLOROTHIAZIDE/VALSARTAN
Diovan HCT Tablets 2195

COVANCE (India)
LOSARTAN POTASSIUM
Cozaar Tablets 1913

CO-VASOCOR (Switzerland)
ENALAPRIL MALEATE
Vasotec I.V. Injection 2076

COVASTIN (Hong Kong, Malaysia, Singapore)
SIMVASTATIN
Zocor Tablets 2078

COVERENE (Argentina)
PERINDOPRIL ERBUMINE
Aceon Tablets (2 mg, 4 mg, 8 mg) 3191

COVEREX (Hungary, The Netherlands)
PERINDOPRIL ERBUMINE
Aceon Tablets (2 mg, 4 mg, 8 mg) 3191

COVEREX KOMB (Hungary)
PERINDOPRIL ERBUMINE
Aceon Tablets (2 mg, 4 mg, 8 mg) 3191

COVERSUM (Austria, Germany, Switzerland)
PERINDOPRIL ERBUMINE
Aceon Tablets (2 mg, 4 mg, 8 mg) 3191

COVERSUM COMBI (Germany, Switzerland)
PERINDOPRIL ERBUMINE
Aceon Tablets (2 mg, 4 mg, 8 mg) 3191

COVERSYL (Australia, Belgium, Brazil, Canada, Chile, Denmark, Finland, France, Greece, India, Irish Republic, Italy, Japan, Malaysia, Mexico, New Zealand, Portugal, Singapore, South Africa, Spain, Thailand, The Netherlands, United Kingdom)
PERINDOPRIL ERBUMINE
Aceon Tablets (2 mg, 4 mg, 8 mg) 3191

COVERSYL COMP (Denmark, Finland)
PERINDOPRIL ERBUMINE
Aceon Tablets (2 mg, 4 mg, 8 mg) 3191

COVERSYL PLUS (Australia, Belgium, Canada, India, Irish Republic, Malaysia, South Africa, The Netherlands, United Kingdom)
PERINDOPRIL ERBUMINE
Aceon Tablets (2 mg, 4 mg, 8 mg) 3191

COVOCEF-N (Greece)
CEFIXIME
Suprax 1811

COVOCORT (South Africa)
HYDROCORTISONE
Hydrocortone Tablets 1963

COVOSPOR (South Africa)
CLOTRIMAZOLE
Lotrimin Cream 3053
Lotrimin Lotion 1% 3053
Lotrimin Topical Solution 1% 3053

COVOSULF (South Africa)
SULFACETAMIDE SODIUM
Klaron Lotion 10% 1050

COXEL (Argentina)
CELECOXIB
Celebrex Capsules 3130

COXTENK (Argentina)
CELECOXIB
Celebrex Capsules 3130

COZAAR (Australia, Belgium, Brazil, Canada, Chile, Czech Republic, Denmark, Finland, France, Greece, Hong Kong, Hungary, Irish Republic, Malaysia, Mexico, New Zealand, Norway, Portugal, Russia, Singapore, South Africa, Spain, Sweden, Thailand, The Netherlands, United Kingdom)
LOSARTAN POTASSIUM
Cozaar Tablets 1913

COZAAR COMP (Denmark, Finland, Irish Republic, Norway, South Africa, Sweden, United Kingdom)
HYDROCHLOROTHIAZIDE/LOSARTAN POTASSIUM
Hyzaar 50-12.5 Tablets 1964

COZAAR PLUS (Belgium, Portugal, Spain, The Netherlands)
HYDROCHLOROTHIAZIDE/LOSARTAN POTASSIUM
Hyzaar 50-12.5 Tablets 1964

COZAAREX (Argentina)
LOSARTAN POTASSIUM
Cozaar Tablets 1913

COZAAREX D (Argentina)
LOSARTAN POTASSIUM
Cozaar Tablets 1913

COZEP (Thailand)
CHLORDIAZEPOXIDE HYDROCHLORIDE
Librium Capsules 3349

CP-ATENOL (Hong Kong)
ATENOLOL
Tenormin I.V. Injection 698

CP-CARBA (Hong Kong)
CARBAMAZEPINE
Carbatrol Capsules 3174
Tegretol Chewable Tablets 2278
Tegretol Suspension 2278
Tegretol Tablets 2278
Tegretol-XR Tablets 2278

CP-FURO (Hong Kong)
FUROSEMIDE
Furosemide Tablets 2117

CP-THEO (Hong Kong)
THEOPHYLLINE
Uniphyl Tablets 2708

CRAFILM (Italy)
SUCRALFATE
Carafate Suspension 727
Carafate Tablets 728

CRALSANIC (South Africa)
SUCRALFATE
Carafate Suspension 727
Carafate Tablets 728

CRANOC (Germany)
FLUVASTATIN SODIUM
Lescol Capsules 2227

CRASNITIN (Germany, Italy, The Netherlands)
ASPARAGINASE
Elspar for Injection ... 1943

CRASNITINE (Switzerland)
ASPARAGINASE
Elspar for Injection ... 1943

CRAVERIL (Argentina)
FENOFIBRATE
Tricor Tablets ... 523

CRAVIT (Hong Kong, Japan, Malaysia, Singapore, Thailand)
LEVOFLOXACIN
Levaquin Injection ... 2453
Levaquin Tablets ... 2453

CREMICORT-H (Belgium)
HYDROCORTISONE
Hydrocortone Tablets ... 1963

CREMINEM (Chile)
CLOTRIMAZOLE
Lotrimin Cream ... 3053
Lotrimin Lotion 1% ... 3053
Lotrimin Topical Solution 1% ... 3053

CREMOSAN (Mexico)
KETOCONAZOLE
Nizoral 2% Shampoo ... 1838

CRIMA (Argentina)
CEFTAZIDIME
Fortaz for Injection ... 1422

CRINONE (Argentina, Brazil, Canada, Denmark, Finland, Germany, Greece, Hong Kong, Irish Republic, Israel, Italy, Malaysia, Mexico, Norway, Portugal, Singapore, Spain, Sweden, Switzerland, Thailand, United Kingdom)
PROGESTERONE
Prometrium Capsules (100 mg, 200 mg) . 3205

CRINOREN (Spain)
ENALAPRIL MALEATE
Vasotec I.V. Injection ... 2076

CRINORETIC (Spain)
ENALAPRIL MALEATE/HYDROCHLOROTHIAZIDE
Vaseretic Tablets ... 2073

CRISACIDE (Argentina)
CIPROFLOXACIN
Cipro Oral Suspension ... 2991

CRISASMA (Argentina)
THEOPHYLLINE
Uniphyl Tablets ... 2708

CRISAZET (Argentina)
ZIDOVUDINE
Retrovir Capsules ... 1533
Retrovir IV Infusion ... 1537
Retrovir Syrup ... 1533
Retrovir Tablets ... 1533

CRISDAZOL (Brazil)
MEBENDAZOLE
Vermox Chewable Tablets ... 1853

CRISMOL (Chile)
CLONAZEPAM
Klonopin Tablets ... 2782

CRISOMET (Spain)
LAMOTRIGINE
Lamictal Chewable Dispersible Tablets ... 1449
Lamictal Tablets ... 1449

CRISTACLAR (Argentina)
DONEPEZIL HYDROCHLORIDE
Aricept Tablets ... 1086

CRISTAN (Singapore)
CLOTRIMAZOLE
Lotrimin Cream ... 3053
Lotrimin Lotion 1% ... 3053
Lotrimin Topical Solution 1% ... 3053

CRISTERONA (Argentina)
ESTRADIOL
Climara Transdermal System ... 795
Vivelle Transdermal System ... 2288
Vivelle-Dot Transdermal System ... 2293

CRIXAN (Malaysia, Singapore, Thailand)
CLARITHROMYCIN
Biaxin Filmtab Tablets ... 402
Biaxin Granules ... 402

CRIXIVAN (Argentina, Australia, Austria, Belgium, Brazil, Canada, Chile, Czech Republic, Denmark, Finland, France, Germany, Greece, Hong Kong, Irish Republic, Israel, Italy, Malaysia, Mexico, New Zealand, Norway, Portugal, Singapore, South Africa, Spain, Sweden, Switzerland, Thailand, The Netherlands, United Kingdom)
INDINAVIR SULFATE
Crixivan Capsules ... 1918

CROMEZIN (Italy)
CEFAZOLIN SODIUM
Ancef for Injection ... 1318

CROMYCIN (Austria)
TOBRAMYCIN
TOBI Solution for Inhalation ... 1015

CRONASMA (Germany)
THEOPHYLLINE
Uniphyl Tablets ... 2708

CRONOCOL (Portugal)
GENTAMICIN SULFATE
Garamycin Injectable ... 3028
Genoptic Sterile Ophthalmic Solution ... ⊙227

CRONODINE (Spain)
DILTIAZEM HYDROCHLORIDE
Cardizem LA Extended Release Tablets ... 1699
Tiazac Capsules ... 1204

CRONOL (Spain)
FAMOTIDINE
Pepcid Injection ... 2017
Pepcid Injection Premixed ... 2017
Pepcid Tablets ... 2014
Pepcid for Oral Suspension ... 2014

CRONOVERA (Brazil, Mexico)
VERAPAMIL HYDROCHLORIDE
Covera-HS Tablets ... 3135
Verelan PM Capsules ... 3120

CROTAMITON H (Malaysia)
HYDROCORTISONE
Hydrocortone Tablets ... 1963

CRYOMETASONA (Mexico)
DEXAMETHASONE
Decadron Tablets ... 1929

CRYOPERACID (Mexico)
LOPERAMIDE HYDROCHLORIDE
Imodium Capsules ... 1834

CRYOPRIL (Mexico)
CAPTOPRIL
Captopril Tablets ... 2114

CRYOTOL (Mexico)
PROPOFOL
Diprivan Injectable Emulsion ... 676

CRYOVAL (Mexico)
VALPROIC ACID
Depakene Capsules ... 417
Depakene Syrup ... 417

CRYOZOL (Mexico)
METRONIDAZOLE
MetroGel-Vaginal Gel ... 1822
Noritate Cream, 1% ... 1051

CRYSANAL (Australia)
NAPROXEN SODIUM
Anaprox DS Tablets ... 2769
Anaprox Tablets ... 2769

CRYSTACIT (South Africa)
POTASSIUM CITRATE
Urocit-K Tablets ... 2109

CST (Thailand)
CLOTRIMAZOLE
Lotrimin Cream ... 3053
Lotrimin Lotion 1% ... 3053
Lotrimin Topical Solution 1% ... 3053

CUADEL (Argentina)
DIAZEPAM
Diastat Rectal Delivery System ... 3344
Valium Tablets ... 2822

CUANTIN (Spain)
FAMOTIDINE
Pepcid Injection ... 2017
Pepcid Injection Premixed ... 2017
Pepcid Tablets ... 2014
Pepcid for Oral Suspension ... 2014

CUERPO AMARILLO FUERTE (Mexico)
PROGESTERONE
Prometrium Capsules (100 mg, 200 mg) . 3205

CUNESIN (Spain)
CIPROFLOXACIN HYDROCHLORIDE
Ciloxan Ophthalmic Ointment ... 554
Ciloxan Ophthalmic Solution ... ⊙205
Cipro Tablets ... 2991

CUPAX (Greece)
CEFUROXIME AXETIL
Ceftin Tablets ... 1369
Ceftin for Oral Suspension ... 1369

CUPRIMINE (Argentina, Brazil, Canada, Hong Kong, Israel, Norway, Sweden, Thailand, The Netherlands)
PENICILLAMINE
Cuprimine Capsules ... 1925

CUPRIPEN (Argentina, Spain)
PENICILLAMINE
Cuprimine Capsules ... 1925

CURACNE (France)
ISOTRETINOIN
Accutane Capsules ... 2740

CURAM (Hong Kong, Malaysia)
AMOXICILLIN
Amoxil Pediatric Drops for Oral Suspension ... 1315
Amoxil Tablets ... 1315

CURANTYL N (Czech Republic, Germany)
DIPYRIDAMOLE
Persantine Tablets ... 898

CURATANE (Israel)
ISOTRETINOIN
Accutane Capsules ... 2740

CURBAN (Greece)
NIMODIPINE
Nimotop Capsules ... 774

CURIOSIN (Czech Republic)
SODIUM HYALURONATE
Hyalgan Solution ... 2917

CUROCEF (Austria, Chile)
CEFUROXIME SODIUM
Zinacef Injection ... 1604

CUROXIM (Italy)
CEFUROXIME SODIUM
Zinacef Injection ... 1604

CUROXIMA (Spain)
CEFUROXIME SODIUM
Zinacef Injection ... 1604

CUROXIME (Portugal)
CEFUROXIME SODIUM
Zinacef Injection ... 1604

CUSIMICINA (Spain)
ERYTHROMYCIN STEARATE
Erythrocin Stearate Filmtab Tablets ... 452

CUSIMOLOL (Hong Kong, Hungary, Italy, Malaysia, Mexico, Portugal, Spain)
TIMOLOL MALEATE
Blocadren Tablets ... 1891
Timoptic Sterile Ophthalmic Solution ... 2058
Timoptic in Ocudose ... 2061
Timoptic-XE Sterile Ophthalmic Gel Forming Solution ... 2062

CUSTEY (Argentina)
LOPERAMIDE HYDROCHLORIDE
Imodium Capsules ... 1834

CUTACLIN (Mexico)
CLINDAMYCIN PHOSPHATE
Clindets Pledgets ... 3212

CUTACNYL (France)
BENZOYL PEROXIDE
Brevoxyl-4 Creamy Wash ... 3212
Brevoxyl-4 Gel ... 3211
Brevoxyl-8 Creamy Wash ... 3212
Brevoxyl-8 Gel ... 3211
Triaz Cleanser ... 1864
Triaz Gel ... 1864

CUTADERM (South Africa)
HYDROCORTISONE
Hydrocortone Tablets ... 1963

CUTANUM (Germany)
ESTRADIOL
Climara Transdermal System ... 795
Vivelle Transdermal System ... 2288
Vivelle-Dot Transdermal System ... 2293

CUTIFITOL (Spain)
PROGESTERONE
Prometrium Capsules (100 mg, 200 mg) . 3205

CUTISTAD (Germany, Switzerland)
CLOTRIMAZOLE
Lotrimin Cream ... 3053
Lotrimin Lotion 1% ... 3053
Lotrimin Topical Solution 1% ... 3053

CUTIVAT (Denmark)
FLUTICASONE PROPIONATE
Cutivate Cream ... 1381
Cutivate Ointment ... 1384
Flonase Nasal Spray ... 1412

CUTIVATE (Argentina, Austria, Belgium, Czech Republic, Hong Kong, Hungary, Israel, Malaysia, Mexico, Portugal, Singapore, South Africa, Spain, Switzerland, The Netherlands, United Kingdom)
FLUTICASONE PROPIONATE
Cutivate Cream ... 1381
Cutivate Ointment ... 1384
Flonase Nasal Spray ... 1412

CUXAFENON (Germany)
PROPAFENONE HYDROCHLORIDE
Rythmol SR Capsules ... 2736

CUXANORM (Germany)
ATENOLOL
Tenormin I.V. Injection ... 698

CYCIN (Singapore)
CIPROFLOXACIN HYDROCHLORIDE
Ciloxan Ophthalmic Ointment ... 554
Ciloxan Ophthalmic Solution ... ⊙205
Cipro Tablets ... 2991

CYCLODERM (Austria)
ESTRADIOL
Climara Transdermal System ... 795
Vivelle Transdermal System ... 2288
Vivelle-Dot Transdermal System ... 2293

CYCLOGEST (Hong Kong, Malaysia, Singapore, South Africa, Thailand, United Kingdom)
PROGESTERONE
Prometrium Capsules (100 mg, 200 mg) . 3205

CYCLORINE (India)
CYCLOSERINE
Seromycin Capsules ... 1783

CYCLOSERINE (TM) (United Kingdom)
CYCLOSERINE
Seromycin Capsules ... 1783

CYCRIN (Argentina, Brazil, Mexico)
MEDROXYPROGESTERONE ACETATE
Depo-Medrol Single-Dose Vial ... 2617

CYFLOX (Thailand)
CIPROFLOXACIN
Cipro Oral Suspension ... 2991

CYFLOXIN (Hong Kong)
CIPROFLOXACIN HYDROCHLORIDE
Ciloxan Ophthalmic Ointment ... 554
Ciloxan Ophthalmic Solution ... ⊙205
Cipro Tablets ... 2991

CYKRINA (Finland, Sweden)
MEDROXYPROGESTERONE ACETATE
Depo-Medrol Single-Dose Vial ... 2617

CYLLIND (Germany)
CLARITHROMYCIN
Biaxin Filmtab Tablets ... 402
Biaxin Granules ... 402

CYMALON CRANBERRY (United Kingdom)
POTASSIUM CITRATE
Urocit-K Tablets ... 2109

CYMEVEN (Germany)
GANCICLOVIR
Cytovene Capsules ... 2763

CYMEVENE (Argentina, Australia, Belgium, Brazil, Chile, Czech Republic, Finland, Greece, Hong Kong, Hungary, Irish Republic, Israel, Italy, Mexico, Norway, Portugal, Singapore, South Africa, Spain, Thailand, The Netherlands, United Kingdom)
GANCICLOVIR
Cytovene Capsules ... 2763

CYMI (South Africa)
CIMETIDINE
Tagamet Tablets 1547

CYNOMEL (Brazil, France, Mexico)
LIOTHYRONINE SODIUM
Cytomel Tablets 1678

CYSTICIDE (Germany, South Africa)
PRAZIQUANTEL
Biltricide Tablets 2990

CYSTISTAT (Canada, United Kingdom)
SODIUM HYALURONATE
Hyalgan Solution 2917

CYSTOPURIN (Irish Republic, United Kingdom)
POTASSIUM CITRATE
Urocit-K Tablets 2109

CYTAMID (Hungary)
FLUTAMIDE
Eulexin Capsules 3023

CYTINE (New Zealand)
CIMETIDINE
Tagamet Tablets 1547

CYTOMEL (Belgium, Canada, The Netherlands)
LIOTHYRONINE SODIUM
Cytomel Tablets 1678

CYTOMID (India)
FLUTAMIDE
Eulexin Capsules 3023

CYTOSAFE (Germany)
FLUOROURACIL
Efudex Topical Cream 3348
Efudex Topical Solutions 3348

CYTOVENE (Argentina)
GANCICLOVIR
Cytovene Capsules 2763

CYZINE (Thailand)
CETIRIZINE HYDROCHLORIDE
Zyrtec Syrup 2589
Zyrtec Tablets 2589

DABEN (Mexico)
MEBENDAZOLE
Vermox Chewable Tablets 1853

DABENZOL (Mexico)
ALBENDAZOLE
Albenza Tablets 1310

DABONAL (Spain)
ENALAPRIL MALEATE
Vasotec I.V. Injection 2076

DABONAL PLUS (Spain)
ENALAPRIL MALEATE/HYDROCHLOROTHIAZIDE
Vaseretic Tablets 2073

DABROSON (Greece)
GENTAMICIN SULFATE
Garamycin Injectable 3028
Genoptic Sterile Ophthalmic Solution . . . . ⊙227

DACALA (Spain)
AMOXICILLIN
Amoxil Pediatric Drops for Oral Suspension 1315
Amoxil Tablets 1315

DACIN-F (Thailand)
CLINDAMYCIN HYDROCHLORIDE
Cleocin Vaginal Ovules 2613

DACLIN (Chile, New Zealand)
CLINDAMYCIN PHOSPHATE
Clindets Pledgets 3212

DACMOZEN (India)
DACTINOMYCIN
Cosmegen for Injection 1907

DACOVO (Spain)
CEFAZOLIN SODIUM
Ancef for Injection 1318

DACTEN (Argentina)
CANDESARTAN CILEXETIL
Atacand Tablets 634

DACTEN D (Argentina)
CANDESARTAN CILEXETIL
Atacand Tablets 634

DAFEX (Argentina)
LAMOTRIGINE
Lamictal Chewable Dispersible Tablets . . . 1449
Lamictal Tablets 1449

DAFLOXEN (Mexico)
NAPROXEN
EC-Naprosyn Delayed-Release Tablets 2769
Naprosyn Suspension 2769
Naprosyn Tablets 2769

DAFLOXEN F (Mexico)
NAPROXEN SODIUM
Anaprox DS Tablets 2769
Anaprox Tablets 2769

DAGOTIL (Chile)
RISPERIDONE
Risperdal Oral Solution 1658
Risperdal Tablets 1658

DAIV (Argentina)
DIAZEPAM
Diastat Rectal Delivery System 3344
Valium Tablets 2822

DAKAR (Belgium)
LANSOPRAZOLE
Prevacid Delayed-Release Capsules 3268

DAKTAGOLD (Australia, New Zealand)
KETOCONAZOLE
Nizoral 2% Shampoo 1838

DAKTARIN GOLD (United Kingdom)
KETOCONAZOLE
Nizoral 2% Shampoo 1838

DALACIN (Argentina, Chile, Czech Republic, Hungary, India, Irish Republic, New Zealand, Russia, United Kingdom)
CLINDAMYCIN PHOSPHATE
Clindets Pledgets 3212

DALACIN C (Australia, Brazil, Czech Republic, Irish Republic, Malaysia)
CLINDAMYCIN HYDROCHLORIDE
Cleocin Vaginal Ovules 2613

DALACIN ST (Argentina)
CLINDAMYCIN PHOSPHATE
Clindets Pledgets 3212

DALACIN T (Australia, Brazil, Canada, Chile, Czech Republic, Hong Kong, Hungary, Irish Republic, Italy, Malaysia, Mexico, New Zealand, Portugal, Singapore, South Africa, Switzerland, Thailand, The Netherlands, United Kingdom)
CLINDAMYCIN PHOSPHATE
Clindets Pledgets 3212

DALACIN TOPICAL (Belgium)
CLINDAMYCIN PHOSPHATE
Clindets Pledgets 3212

DALACIN V (Australia, Brazil, Chile, Hong Kong, Mexico, New Zealand, Portugal, Switzerland, The Netherlands)
CLINDAMYCIN PHOSPHATE
Clindets Pledgets 3212

DALACIN VAGINAL (Belgium, Canada, Israel)
CLINDAMYCIN PHOSPHATE
Clindets Pledgets 3212

DALACIN VC (South Africa)
CLINDAMYCIN PHOSPHATE
Clindets Pledgets 3212

DALACINE T (France)
CLINDAMYCIN PHOSPHATE
Clindets Pledgets 3212

DALAGIS T (Israel)
CLINDAMYCIN PHOSPHATE
Clindets Pledgets 3212

DALAMON INYECTABLE (Spain)
DEXAMETHASONE SODIUM PHOSPHATE
Decadron Phosphate Injection 1931

DALCAP (India)
CLINDAMYCIN HYDROCHLORIDE
Cleocin Vaginal Ovules 2613

DALGEX (Brazil)
ORPHENADRINE CITRATE
Norflex Injection 1824

DALMADORM (Brazil, Hong Kong, Singapore, Switzerland, The Netherlands)
FLURAZEPAM HYDROCHLORIDE
Dalmane Capsules 3343

DALMANE (Canada, Irish Republic)
FLURAZEPAM HYDROCHLORIDE
Dalmane Capsules 3343

DALTROID (Mexico)
LEVOTHYROXINE SODIUM
Levothroid Tablets 1189
Levoxyl Tablets 1680
Synthroid Tablets 515

DALZAD (Greece)
VALSARTAN
Diovan Tablets 2191

DALZOLSTON (Brazil)
METRONIDAZOLE
MetroGel-Vaginal Gel 1822
Noritate Cream, 1% 1051

DAMIDE (Italy)
INDAPAMIDE
Indapamide Tablets 2119

DAMOSAL (Mexico)
DIPYRIDAMOLE
Persantine Tablets 898

DANDRAZOL (United Kingdom)
KETOCONAZOLE
Nizoral 2% Shampoo 1838

DANDRID (United Kingdom)
KETOCONAZOLE
Nizoral 2% Shampoo 1838

DANFREE (India)
KETOCONAZOLE
Nizoral 2% Shampoo 1838

DANILAX (Denmark, Hong Kong)
LACTULOSE
Kristalose for Oral Solution 2149

DANLENE (Italy)
DANTROLENE SODIUM
Dantrium Capsules 2690
Dantrium Intravenous 2691

DANRUF (India)
KETOCONAZOLE
Nizoral 2% Shampoo 1838

DANSSAN (Hong Kong)
ENALAPRIL MALEATE
Vasotec I.V. Injection 2076

DANTAMACRIN (Austria, Germany, Switzerland)
DANTROLENE SODIUM
Dantrium Capsules 2690
Dantrium Intravenous 2691

DANTENK (Argentina)
ONDANSETRON HYDROCHLORIDE
Zofran Injection 1607
Zofran Injection Premixed 1607
Zofran Oral Solution 1613
Zofran Tablets 1613

DANTRALEN (Spain)
DANTROLENE SODIUM
Dantrium Capsules 2690
Dantrium Intravenous 2691

DANTRIUM (Australia, Belgium, Canada, Denmark, France, Greece, Hong Kong, Irish Republic, Israel, Italy, New Zealand, Portugal, South Africa, The Netherlands, United Kingdom)
DANTROLENE SODIUM
Dantrium Capsules 2690
Dantrium Intravenous 2691

DANTROLEN (Brazil, Greece)
DANTROLENE SODIUM
Dantrium Capsules 2690
Dantrium Intravenous 2691

DANTRON (PREPARATION) (Thailand)
ONDANSETRON
Zofran ODT Orally Disintegrating Tablets . . 1613

DAPA (Malaysia)
INDAPAMIDE
Indapamide Tablets 2119

DAPAMAX (South Africa)
INDAPAMIDE
Indapamide Tablets 2119

DAPA-TABS (Australia, Hong Kong)
INDAPAMIDE
Indapamide Tablets 2119

DAPRIL (Czech Republic, Singapore)
LISINOPRIL
Prinivil Tablets 2029
Zestril Tablets 704

DAPROX (Denmark)
NAPROXEN
EC-Naprosyn Delayed-Release Tablets 2769
Naprosyn Suspension 2769
Naprosyn Tablets 2769

DAPS (Argentina)
DAPSONE
Dapsone Tablets USP 1656

DAPSODERM-X (Mexico)
DAPSONE
Dapsone Tablets USP 1656

DAPTRIL (South Africa)
INDAPAMIDE
Indapamide Tablets 2119

DARALIX (South Africa)
PROMETHAZINE HYDROCHLORIDE
Phenergan Suppositories 3438
Phenergan Tablets 3438

DARAPRIM (Argentina, Australia, Austria, Belgium, Brazil, Canada, Chile, Germany, Irish Republic, Israel, Mexico, South Africa, Spain, Sweden, Switzerland, Thailand, The Netherlands, United Kingdom)
PYRIMETHAMINE
Daraprim Tablets 1385

DARAPRIN (Brazil)
PYRIMETHAMINE
Daraprim Tablets 1385

DARDEX (Spain)
CAPTOPRIL
Captopril Tablets 2114

DAREN (Singapore)
ENALAPRIL MALEATE
Vasotec I.V. Injection 2076

DARI (Spain)
NIFEDIPINE
Adalat CC Tablets 2978

DARIC (Argentina)
FINASTERIDE
Propecia Tablets 2036
Proscar Tablets 2040

DARMOL LACTULOSE (Austria)
LACTULOSE
Kristalose for Oral Solution 2149

DARSTIN (Spain)
PROGESTERONE
Prometrium Capsules (100 mg, 200 mg) . 3205

DARTROX (Mexico)
NAPROXEN
EC-Naprosyn Delayed-Release Tablets 2769
Naprosyn Suspension 2769
Naprosyn Tablets 2769

DARZITIL (Argentina)
AMOXICILLIN
Amoxil Pediatric Drops for Oral Suspension 1315
Amoxil Tablets 1315

DARZITIL SB (Argentina)
AMOXICILLIN
Amoxil Pediatric Drops for Oral Suspension 1315
Amoxil Tablets 1315

DASKIL (Austria, Italy)
TERBINAFINE HYDROCHLORIDE
Lamisil Tablets 2226

DASKYL (Portugal)
TERBINAFINE HYDROCHLORIDE
Lamisil Tablets 2226

DASMETROL (Mexico)
METRONIDAZOLE
MetroGel-Vaginal Gel 1822
Noritate Cream, 1% 1051

DASOLIN (Mexico)
METRONIDAZOLE
MetroGel-Vaginal Gel 1822
Noritate Cream, 1% 1051

DATEVAN (Argentina)
PAROXETINE HYDROCHLORIDE
Paxil Oral Suspension 1501
Paxil Tablets 1501

(⊙ Described in PDR For Ophthalmic Medicines™)

DATRON (Spain)
ONDANSETRON HYDROCHLORIDE
Zofran Injection . . . 1607
Zofran Injection Premixed . . . 1607
Zofran Oral Solution . . . 1613
Zofran Tablets . . . 1613

DAUNOBLASTIN (Austria, Germany, South Africa)
DAUNORUBICIN HYDROCHLORIDE
Cerubidine for Injection . . . 788

DAUNOBLASTINA (Argentina, Brazil, Hong Kong, Hungary, Italy, Portugal, Singapore, Spain)
DAUNORUBICIN HYDROCHLORIDE
Cerubidine for Injection . . . 788

DAUNOCIN (Brazil)
DAUNORUBICIN HYDROCHLORIDE
Cerubidine for Injection . . . 788

DAUNOTEC (India)
DAUNORUBICIN HYDROCHLORIDE
Cerubidine for Injection . . . 788

DAVIXOLOL (Portugal)
BETAXOLOL HYDROCHLORIDE
Betoptic S Ophthalmic Suspension . . . 554

DAXOTEL (India, Thailand)
DOCETAXEL
Taxotere Injection Concentrate . . . 2947

DAZID (Thailand)
TRIAMTERENE
Dyrenium Capsules . . . 3390

DAZINE (Thailand)
THIORIDAZINE HYDROCHLORIDE
Thioridazine Hydrochloride Tablets . . . 2122

DAZOCAN (Mexico)
ALBENDAZOLE
Albenza Tablets . . . 1310

DAZOL (Brazil)
ALBENDAZOLE
Albenza Tablets . . . 1310

DAZOLIN (Argentina, Mexico)
NAPHAZOLINE HYDROCHLORIDE
Albalon Ophthalmic Solution . . . ⊙216

DAZOMET (Argentina)
MEBENDAZOLE
Vermox Chewable Tablets . . . 1853

DAZOTRON (Argentina)
METRONIDAZOLE
MetroGel-Vaginal Gel . . . 1822
Noritate Cream, 1% . . . 1051

D-CYCLOSERIN (Greece)
CYCLOSERINE
Seromycin Capsules . . . 1783

DDAVP (Brazil, Canada, Chile, Germany, Greece, Irish Republic, Portugal, United Kingdom)
DESMOPRESSIN ACETATE
DDAVP Injection 4 mcg/mL . . . 2893
DDAVP Nasal Spray . . . 2894
DDAVP Tablets . . . 2895
Desmopressin Acetate Injection . . . 1143
Desmopressin Acetate Rhinal Tube . . . 1144

DE ICOL (Malaysia)
DEXAMETHASONE SODIUM PHOSPHATE
Decadron Phosphate Injection . . . 1931

DEALGIC (Italy)
DICLOFENAC SODIUM
Voltaren Tablets . . . 2298
Voltaren-XR Tablets . . . 2301

DEBAX (Austria)
CAPTOPRIL
Captopril Tablets . . . 2114

DEBRIL (Argentina)
NAPROXEN
EC-Naprosyn Delayed-Release Tablets . . . 2769
Naprosyn Suspension . . . 2769
Naprosyn Tablets . . . 2769

DECADRON (Australia, Austria, Belgium, Brazil, Canada, Finland, France, Germany, Greece, Hong Kong, Irish Republic, Malaysia, New Zealand, South Africa, Switzerland, Thailand, The Netherlands, United Kingdom)
DEXAMETHASONE SODIUM PHOSPHATE
Decadron Phosphate Injection . . . 1931

DECADRON CON CIPROFLOXINA (Argentina)
DEXAMETHASONE
Decadron Tablets . . . 1929

DECADRON CON NEOMICINA (Argentina)
DEXAMETHASONE SODIUM PHOSPHATE
Decadron Phosphate Injection . . . 1931

DECADRON CON TOBRAMICINA (Argentina)
DEXAMETHASONE
Decadron Tablets . . . 1929

DECAN (Malaysia)
DEXAMETHASONE
Decadron Tablets . . . 1929

DECDAN (India)
DEXAMETHASONE
Decadron Tablets . . . 1929

DECDAN-N (India)
DEXAMETHASONE SODIUM PHOSPHATE
Decadron Phosphate Injection . . . 1931

DECIPAR (Spain)
ENOXAPARIN SODIUM
Lovenox Injection . . . 2931

DECLOBAN (Spain)
CLOBETASOL PROPIONATE
Temovate Cream . . . 1549
Temovate E Emollient . . . 1552
Temovate Gel . . . 1550
Temovate Ointment . . . 1549
Temovate Scalp Application . . . 1551

DECLOFON (Greece)
DICLOFENAC SODIUM
Voltaren Tablets . . . 2298
Voltaren-XR Tablets . . . 2301

DECOFLUOR (Italy)
DEXAMETHASONE
Decadron Tablets . . . 1929

DECOREX (Mexico)
DEXAMETHASONE
Decadron Tablets . . . 1929

DECOSIL (Mexico)
NAPROXEN SODIUM
Anaprox DS Tablets . . . 2769
Anaprox Tablets . . . 2769

DECOSTRIOL (Germany)
CALCITRIOL
Calcijex Injection . . . 411

DEDILE (Argentina)
FLUTAMIDE
Eulexin Capsules . . . 3023

DEDOLOR (Austria)
DICLOFENAC SODIUM
Voltaren Tablets . . . 2298
Voltaren-XR Tablets . . . 2301

DEFANAC (United Kingdom)
DICLOFENAC SODIUM
Voltaren Tablets . . . 2298
Voltaren-XR Tablets . . . 2301

DEFIRIN (Greece)
DESMOPRESSIN ACETATE
DDAVP Injection 4 mcg/mL . . . 2893
DDAVP Nasal Spray . . . 2894
DDAVP Tablets . . . 2895
Desmopressin Acetate Injection . . . 1143
Desmopressin Acetate Rhinal Tube . . . 1144

DEFLAMAT (Austria, Italy, Switzerland)
DICLOFENAC SODIUM
Voltaren Tablets . . . 2298
Voltaren-XR Tablets . . . 2301

DEFLAMM (Austria)
DICLOFENAC SODIUM
Voltaren Tablets . . . 2298
Voltaren-XR Tablets . . . 2301

DEFLAMON (Czech Republic, Italy)
METRONIDAZOLE
MetroGel-Vaginal Gel . . . 1822
Noritate Cream, 1% . . . 1051

DEFLAMOX (Mexico)
NAPROXEN SODIUM
Anaprox DS Tablets . . . 2769
Anaprox Tablets . . . 2769

DEFLAREN (Brazil)
DEXAMETHASONE
Decadron Tablets . . . 1929

DEFLOX (Spain)
TERAZOSIN HYDROCHLORIDE
Hytrin Capsules . . . 469

DEFLUIN (Argentina)
ENALAPRIL MALEATE
Vasotec I.V. Injection . . . 2076

DEFLUIN PLUS (Argentina)
ENALAPRIL MALEATE
Vasotec I.V. Injection . . . 2076

DEFUNGO (Thailand)
CLOTRIMAZOLE
Lotrimin Cream . . . 3053
Lotrimin Lotion 1% . . . 3053
Lotrimin Topical Solution 1% . . . 3053

DEGEST 2 (Canada)
NAPHAZOLINE HYDROCHLORIDE
Albalon Ophthalmic Solution . . . ⊙216

DEGRANOL (South Africa)
CARBAMAZEPINE
Carbatrol Capsules . . . 3174
Tegretol Chewable Tablets . . . 2278
Tegretol Suspension . . . 2278
Tegretol Tablets . . . 2278
Tegretol-XR Tablets . . . 2278

DELEPTIN (Austria)
CARBAMAZEPINE
Carbatrol Capsules . . . 3174
Tegretol Chewable Tablets . . . 2278
Tegretol Suspension . . . 2278
Tegretol Tablets . . . 2278
Tegretol-XR Tablets . . . 2278

DELIDOSE (France)
ESTRADIOL
Climara Transdermal System . . . 795
Vivelle Transdermal System . . . 2288
Vivelle-Dot Transdermal System . . . 2293

DELIMON (Greece)
DICLOFENAC SODIUM
Voltaren Tablets . . . 2298
Voltaren-XR Tablets . . . 2301

DELIX (Germany)
RAMIPRIL
Altace Capsules . . . 1673

DELIXI (Germany)
PERMETHRIN
Acticin Cream . . . 2125

DELMUNO (Germany)
FELODIPINE
Plendil Extended-Release Tablets . . . 651

DELONAL (Germany, Switzerland)
ALCLOMETASONE DIPROPIONATE
Aclovate Cream . . . 1290
Aclovate Ointment . . . 1290

DELPHI (Belgium, The Netherlands)
TRIAMCINOLONE ACETONIDE
Azmacort Inhalation Aerosol . . . 1701
Nasacort AQ Nasal Spray . . . 2937

DELPHIMIX 1 (Germany)
DICLOFENAC SODIUM
Voltaren Tablets . . . 2298
Voltaren-XR Tablets . . . 2301

DELPHINAC (Germany)
DICLOFENAC SODIUM
Voltaren Tablets . . . 2298
Voltaren-XR Tablets . . . 2301

DELTA 80 (Italy)
BENZOYL PEROXIDE
Brevoxyl-4 Creamy Wash . . . 3212
Brevoxyl-4 Gel . . . 3211
Brevoxyl-8 Creamy Wash . . . 3212
Brevoxyl-8 Gel . . . 3211
Triaz Cleanser . . . 1864
Triaz Gel . . . 1864

DELTA T (Hong Kong)
CLINDAMYCIN PHOSPHATE
Clindets Pledgets . . . 3212

DELTACEF (Italy)
CEFUROXIME SODIUM
Zinacef Injection . . . 1604

DELTASORALEN (Irish Republic)
METHOXSALEN
Oxsoralen Lotion 1% . . . 3354
Oxsoralen-Ultra Capsules . . . 3354

DELTAZEN (France)
DILTIAZEM HYDROCHLORIDE
Cardizem LA Extended Release Tablets . . . 1699
Tiazac Capsules . . . 1204

DELVAS (United Kingdom)
AMILORIDE HYDROCHLORIDE/HYDROCHLOROTHIAZIDE
Moduretic Tablets . . . 2003

DENACLOF (Greece)
DICLOFENAC SODIUM
Voltaren Tablets . . . 2298
Voltaren-XR Tablets . . . 2301

DENAN (Germany)
SIMVASTATIN
Zocor Tablets . . . 2078

DENAPRIL (Portugal)
ENALAPRIL MALEATE
Vasotec I.V. Injection . . . 2076

DENAXPREN (Spain)
NAPROXEN
EC-Naprosyn Delayed-Release Tablets . . . 2769
Naprosyn Suspension . . . 2769
Naprosyn Tablets . . . 2769

DENAZOX (Thailand)
DILTIAZEM HYDROCHLORIDE
Cardizem LA Extended Release Tablets . . . 1699
Tiazac Capsules . . . 1204

DENCORUB ANTI-INFLAMMATORY (Australia)
DICLOFENAC SODIUM
Voltaren Tablets . . . 2298
Voltaren-XR Tablets . . . 2301

DENERVAL (Portugal)
PAROXETINE HYDROCHLORIDE
Paxil Oral Suspension . . . 1501
Paxil Tablets . . . 1501

DENIREN (Mexico)
AMOXICILLIN
Amoxil Pediatric Drops for Oral Suspension . . . 1315
Amoxil Tablets . . . 1315

DENKACORT (Hong Kong)
TRIAMCINOLONE ACETONIDE
Azmacort Inhalation Aerosol . . . 1701
Nasacort AQ Nasal Spray . . . 2937

DENTOMYCIN (Germany)
CLINDAMYCIN HYDROCHLORIDE
Cleocin Vaginal Ovules . . . 2613

DENULCER (Spain)
RANITIDINE HYDROCHLORIDE
Zantac 25 EFFERdose Tablets . . . 1597
Zantac 150 EFFERdose Tablets . . . 1597
Zantac 150 Tablets . . . 1597
Zantac 300 Tablets . . . 1597
Zantac Injection . . . 1593
Zantac Injection Premixed . . . 1593
Zantac Syrup . . . 1597

DENVAR (Mexico, Spain)
CEFIXIME
Suprax . . . 1811

DENZAPINE (United Kingdom)
CLOZAPINE
Clozapine Tablets . . . 2141
Clozaril Tablets . . . 2174

DEPAKENE (Argentina, Brazil, Canada, Chile)
VALPROIC ACID
Depakene Capsules . . . 417
Depakene Syrup . . . 417

DEPAKINE ZUUR (The Netherlands)
VALPROIC ACID
Depakene Capsules . . . 417
Depakene Syrup . . . 417

DEPEN (Canada)
PENICILLAMINE
Cuprimine Capsules . . . 1925

DEPICOR (India)
NIFEDIPINE
Adalat CC Tablets . . . 2978

DEPIN (India)
NIFEDIPINE
Adalat CC Tablets . . . 2978

DEPO MODERIN (Spain)
METHYLPREDNISOLONE ACETATE
Depo-Medrol Injectable Suspension . . . 2615

DEPO-CLINOVIR (Germany)
MEDROXYPROGESTERONE ACETATE
Depo-Medrol Single-Dose Vial 2617

DEPOCON (Austria)
MEDROXYPROGESTERONE ACETATE
Depo-Medrol Single-Dose Vial 2617

DEPO-GESTIN (Thailand)
MEDROXYPROGESTERONE ACETATE
Depo-Medrol Single-Dose Vial 2617

DEPO-MEDRATE (Germany)
METHYLPREDNISOLONE ACETATE
Depo-Medrol Injectable Suspension 2615

DEPO-MEDROL (Australia, Austria, Belgium, Brazil, Canada, Chile, Czech Republic, Denmark, Finland, France, Hong Kong, Hungary, India, Israel, Italy, Malaysia, Mexico, New Zealand, Norway, Portugal, South Africa, Sweden, Switzerland, Thailand, The Netherlands)
METHYLPREDNISOLONE ACETATE
Depo-Medrol Injectable Suspension 2615

DEPO-MEDRONE (Irish Republic, Sweden, United Kingdom)
METHYLPREDNISOLONE ACETATE
Depo-Medrol Injectable Suspension 2615

DEPO-NISOLONE (Australia)
METHYLPREDNISOLONE ACETATE
Depo-Medrol Injectable Suspension 2615

DEPO-PRODASONE (Chile, France)
MEDROXYPROGESTERONE ACETATE
Depo-Medrol Single-Dose Vial 2617

DEPO-PROGESNO (Thailand)
MEDROXYPROGESTERONE ACETATE
Depo-Medrol Single-Dose Vial 2617

DEPO-PROGESTA (Thailand)
MEDROXYPROGESTERONE ACETATE
Depo-Medrol Single-Dose Vial 2617

DEPO-PROGEVERA (Spain)
MEDROXYPROGESTERONE ACETATE
Depo-Medrol Single-Dose Vial 2617

DEPO-PROVERA (Argentina, Australia, Austria, Belgium, Brazil, Canada, Czech Republic, Denmark, Finland, France, Greece, Hong Kong, Hungary, India, Irish Republic, Israel, Italy, Malaysia, Mexico, New Zealand, Norway, Portugal, Singapore, South Africa, Sweden, Switzerland, Thailand, The Netherlands, United Kingdom)
MEDROXYPROGESTERONE ACETATE
Depo-Medrol Single-Dose Vial 2617

DEPO-RALOVERA (Australia)
MEDROXYPROGESTERONE ACETATE
Depo-Medrol Single-Dose Vial 2617

DEPRENYL (France, Germany)
SELEGILINE HYDROCHLORIDE
Eldepryl Capsules 3209

DEPRILAN (Brazil)
SELEGILINE HYDROCHLORIDE
Eldepryl Capsules 3209

DEPROCID (Chile)
METRONIDAZOLE
MetroGel-Vaginal Gel 1822
Noritate Cream, 1% 1051

DEPTEN (India)
ATENOLOL
Tenormin I.V. Injection 698

DEPUROL (Chile)
VENLAFAXINE HYDROCHLORIDE
Effexor Tablets 3405
Effexor XR Capsules 3411

DERALIN (Australia, Israel)
PROPRANOLOL HYDROCHLORIDE
Inderal LA Long-Acting Capsules 3421

DERCOME (Germany)
BENZOYL PEROXIDE
Brevoxyl-4 Creamy Wash 3212
Brevoxyl-4 Gel 3211
Brevoxyl-8 Creamy Wash 3212
Brevoxyl-8 Gel 3211
Triaz Cleanser 1864
Triaz Gel 1864

DERCUTANE (Spain)
ISOTRETINOIN
Accutane Capsules 2740

DERICIP (India)
THEOPHYLLINE
Uniphyl Tablets 2708

DERICIP PLUS (India)
THEOPHYLLINE
Uniphyl Tablets 2708

DERIPIL (Spain)
ERYTHROMYCIN
Ery-Tab Tablets 447
Erythromycin Base Filmtab Tablets 454
Erythromycin Delayed-Release Capsules, USP 456
PCE Dispertab Tablets 510

DERIVA (India)
ADAPALENE
Differin Gel 1211

DERIVA-C (India)
ADAPALENE
Differin Gel 1211

DERMABAZ (Hong Kong)
TRETINOIN
Avita Cream 2136
Avita Gel 2138
Renova 0.05% Cream 2387
Retin-A Micro 0.1%/0.04% 2388
Vesanoid Capsules 2823

DERMABEL (Chile)
CLINDAMYCIN PHOSPHATE
Clindets Pledgets 3212

DERMACARE (Brazil)
CLOBETASOL PROPIONATE
Temovate Cream 1549
Temovate E Emollient 1552
Temovate Gel 1550
Temovate Ointment 1549
Temovate Scalp Application 1551

DERMACNE (Canada)
BENZOYL PEROXIDE
Brevoxyl-4 Creamy Wash 3212
Brevoxyl-4 Gel 3211
Brevoxyl-8 Creamy Wash 3212
Brevoxyl-8 Gel 3211
Triaz Cleanser 1864
Triaz Gel 1864

DERMACORT (Finland, Hong Kong, Malaysia, Singapore, United Kingdom)
HYDROCORTISONE
Hydrocortone Tablets 1963

DERMADEX (Argentina)
CLOBETASOL PROPIONATE
Temovate Cream 1549
Temovate E Emollient 1552
Temovate Gel 1550
Temovate Ointment 1549
Temovate Scalp Application 1551

DERM-AID (Australia, Hong Kong, Malaysia, New Zealand, Singapore)
HYDROCORTISONE
Hydrocortone Tablets 1963

DERMAIROL (Sweden)
TRETINOIN
Avita Cream 2136
Avita Gel 2138
Renova 0.05% Cream 2387
Retin-A Micro 0.1%/0.04% 2388
Vesanoid Capsules 2823

DERMALLERG (Germany)
HYDROCORTISONE
Hydrocortone Tablets 1963

DERMANCE (Canada)
BENZOYL PEROXIDE
Brevoxyl-4 Creamy Wash 3212
Brevoxyl-4 Gel 3211
Brevoxyl-8 Creamy Wash 3212
Brevoxyl-8 Gel 3211
Triaz Cleanser 1864
Triaz Gel 1864

DERMAORAL (Denmark)
ISOTRETINOIN
Accutane Capsules 2740

DERMAREST DRICORT ANTI-ITCH (Canada)
HYDROCORTISONE
Hydrocortone Tablets 1963

DERMASIL (Thailand)
CLOBETASOL PROPIONATE
Temovate Cream 1549
Temovate E Emollient 1552
Temovate Gel 1550
Temovate Ointment 1549
Temovate Scalp Application 1551

DERMASONE (Canada, Hong Kong)
CLOBETASOL PROPIONATE
Temovate Cream 1549
Temovate E Emollient 1552
Temovate Gel 1550
Temovate Ointment 1549
Temovate Scalp Application 1551

DERMASPRAY DEMANGEAISON (France)
HYDROCORTISONE
Hydrocortone Tablets 1963

DERMASTEN (Mexico)
CLOTRIMAZOLE
Lotrimin Cream 3053
Lotrimin Lotion 1% 3053
Lotrimin Topical Solution 1% 3053

DERMATEN (Thailand)
CLOTRIMAZOLE
Lotrimin Cream 3053
Lotrimin Lotion 1% 3053
Lotrimin Topical Solution 1% 3053

DERMATOVATE (Mexico)
CLOBETASOL PROPIONATE
Temovate Cream 1549
Temovate E Emollient 1552
Temovate Gel 1550
Temovate Ointment 1549
Temovate Scalp Application 1551

DERMATRANS (Chile)
ESTRADIOL
Climara Transdermal System 795
Vivelle Transdermal System 2288
Vivelle-Dot Transdermal System 2293

DERMAZOL (Brazil, France, Italy)
ECONAZOLE NITRATE
Spectazole Cream 2390

DERMAZOLE (Australia, Hong Kong, New Zealand, Singapore)
ECONAZOLE NITRATE
Spectazole Cream 2390

DERMENET (Chile)
MOMETASONE FUROATE
Elocon Cream 0.1% 3019
Elocon Lotion 0.1% 3020
Elocon Ointment 0.1% 3021
Nasonex Nasal Spray 3058

DERMESTRIL (Australia, Austria, Belgium, Czech Republic, Finland, France, Germany, Greece, Hong Kong, Hungary, Irish Republic, Israel, Italy, Portugal, Spain, Switzerland, The Netherlands, United Kingdom)
ESTRADIOL
Climara Transdermal System 795
Vivelle Transdermal System 2288
Vivelle-Dot Transdermal System 2293

DERMEXANE (Argentina)
CLOBETASOL PROPIONATE
Temovate Cream 1549
Temovate E Emollient 1552
Temovate Gel 1550
Temovate Ointment 1549
Temovate Scalp Application 1551

DERMIL (Denmark)
HYDROCORTISONE
Hydrocortone Tablets 1963

DERMIMADE HIDROCORTISONA (Portugal)
HYDROCORTISONE
Hydrocortone Tablets 1963

DERMINOIN (Greece)
ISOTRETINOIN
Accutane Capsules 2740

DERMO (Hong Kong)
CLOBETASOL PROPIONATE
Temovate Cream 1549
Temovate E Emollient 1552
Temovate Gel 1550
Temovate Ointment 1549
Temovate Scalp Application 1551

DERMO POSTERISAN (Germany)
HYDROCORTISONE
Hydrocortone Tablets 1963

DERMOBENE (Brazil)
CLOTRIMAZOLE
Lotrimin Cream 3053
Lotrimin Lotion 1% 3053
Lotrimin Topical Solution 1% 3053

DERMOCORTAL (Italy)
HYDROCORTISONE
Hydrocortone Tablets 1963

DERMODAN (Chile)
TRETINOIN
Avita Cream 2136
Avita Gel 2138
Renova 0.05% Cream 2387
Retin-A Micro 0.1%/0.04% 2388
Vesanoid Capsules 2823

DERMOFENAC (France)
HYDROCORTISONE
Hydrocortone Tablets 1963

DERMOJUVENTUS (Spain)
TRETINOIN
Avita Cream 2136
Avita Gel 2138
Renova 0.05% Cream 2387
Retin-A Micro 0.1%/0.04% 2388
Vesanoid Capsules 2823

DERMOL (New Zealand)
CLOBETASOL PROPIONATE
Temovate Cream 1549
Temovate E Emollient 1552
Temovate Gel 1550
Temovate Ointment 1549
Temovate Scalp Application 1551

DERMOPER (Argentina)
PERMETHRIN
Acticin Cream 2125

DERMOPERATIVE (Argentina)
HYDROCORTISONE
Hydrocortone Tablets 1963

DERMORETIN (Brazil)
TRETINOIN
Avita Cream 2136
Avita Gel 2138
Renova 0.05% Cream 2387
Retin-A Micro 0.1%/0.04% 2388
Vesanoid Capsules 2823

DERMOSOL (Malaysia, Singapore)
CLOBETASOL PROPIONATE
Temovate Cream 1549
Temovate E Emollient 1552
Temovate Gel 1550
Temovate Ointment 1549
Temovate Scalp Application 1551

DERMOSONA (Chile)
MOMETASONE FUROATE
Elocon Cream 0.1% 3019
Elocon Lotion 0.1% 3020
Elocon Ointment 0.1% 3021
Nasonex Nasal Spray 3058

DERMOVAGISIL (Spain)
LIDOCAINE
Lidoderm Patch 1107

DERMOVAL (France)
CLOBETASOL PROPIONATE
Temovate Cream 1549
Temovate E Emollient 1552
Temovate Gel 1550
Temovate Ointment 1549
Temovate Scalp Application 1551

DERMOVAT (Denmark, Finland, Norway, Sweden)
CLOBETASOL PROPIONATE
Temovate Cream 1549
Temovate E Emollient 1552
Temovate Gel 1550
Temovate Ointment 1549
Temovate Scalp Application 1551

DERMOVATE (Austria, Belgium, Canada, Chile, Czech Republic, Hong Kong, Hungary, Irish Republic, Israel, Malaysia, New Zealand, Portugal, Singapore, South Africa, Switzerland, Thailand, The Netherlands, United Kingdom)
CLOBETASOL PROPIONATE
Temovate Cream 1549
Temovate E Emollient 1552
Temovate Gel 1550
Temovate Ointment 1549
Temovate Scalp Application 1551

DERMOX (Mexico)
METHOXSALEN
Oxsoralen Lotion 1% 3354
Oxsoralen-Ultra Capsules 3354

DERMOXIN (Germany)
CLOBETASOL PROPIONATE
Temovate Cream 1549
Temovate E Emollient 1552
Temovate Gel 1550
Temovate Ointment 1549
Temovate Scalp Application 1551

DERMOXINALE (Germany)
CLOBETASOL PROPIONATE
Temovate Cream 1549
Temovate E Emollient 1552
Temovate Gel 1550
Temovate Ointment 1549
Temovate Scalp Application 1551

DERMOXYL (Canada, Chile)
BENZOYL PEROXIDE
Brevoxyl-4 Creamy Wash 3212
Brevoxyl-4 Gel 3211
Brevoxyl-8 Creamy Wash 3212
Brevoxyl-8 Gel 3211
Triaz Cleanser 1864
Triaz Gel 1864

DERONGA HEILPASTE (Germany)
NATAMYCIN
Natacyn Antifungal Ophthalmic Suspension .... ⊙207

DERONIL (Canada)
DEXAMETHASONE
Decadron Tablets 1929

DEROXAT (France, Switzerland)
PAROXETINE HYDROCHLORIDE
Paxil Oral Suspension 1501
Paxil Tablets 1501

DESALARK (Italy)
DEXAMETHASONE
Decadron Tablets 1929
DEXAMETHASONE SODIUM PHOSPHATE
Decadron Phosphate Injection 1931

DESAMIN SAME (Italy)
NAPHAZOLINE HYDROCHLORIDE
Albalon Ophthalmic Solution .... ⊙216

DESANDEN (Switzerland)
BENZOYL PEROXIDE
Brevoxyl-4 Creamy Wash 3212
Brevoxyl-4 Gel 3211
Brevoxyl-8 Creamy Wash 3212
Brevoxyl-8 Gel 3211
Triaz Cleanser 1864
Triaz Gel 1864

DESERONIL (Italy)
DEXAMETHASONE
Decadron Tablets 1929

DESIKEN (Mexico)
RIBAVIRIN
Virazole for Inhalation Solution 3365

DESINFLAM (Argentina)
DICLOFENAC SODIUM
Voltaren Tablets 2298
Voltaren-XR Tablets 2301

DESINTAN P (Portugal)
PERMETHRIN
Acticin Cream 2125

DESITAL (Norway)
CITALOPRAM HYDROBROMIDE
Celexa Tablets 1177

DESITICLOPIDIN (Germany)
TICLOPIDINE HYDROCHLORIDE
Ticlid Tablets 2813

DESMOGALEN (Germany)
DESMOPRESSIN ACETATE
DDAVP Injection 4 mcg/mL 2893
DDAVP Nasal Spray 2894
DDAVP Tablets 2895
Desmopressin Acetate Injection 1143
Desmopressin Acetate Rhinal Tube 1144

DESMOSPRAY (Irish Republic, Portugal, United Kingdom)
DESMOPRESSIN ACETATE
DDAVP Injection 4 mcg/mL 2893
DDAVP Nasal Spray 2894
DDAVP Tablets 2895
Desmopressin Acetate Injection 1143
Desmopressin Acetate Rhinal Tube 1144

DESMOTABS (Irish Republic, United Kingdom)
DESMOPRESSIN ACETATE
DDAVP Injection 4 mcg/mL 2893
DDAVP Nasal Spray 2894
DDAVP Tablets 2895
Desmopressin Acetate Injection 1143
Desmopressin Acetate Rhinal Tube 1144

DESOCORT (France)
DEXAMETHASONE SODIUM PHOSPHATE
Decadron Phosphate Injection 1931

DESQUAM-X (Canada)
BENZOYL PEROXIDE
Brevoxyl-4 Creamy Wash 3212
Brevoxyl-4 Gel 3211
Brevoxyl-8 Creamy Wash 3212
Brevoxyl-8 Gel 3211
Triaz Cleanser 1864
Triaz Gel 1864

DETEBENCIL (Argentina)
PERMETHRIN
Acticin Cream 2125

DETENSOL (Canada)
PROPRANOLOL HYDROCHLORIDE
Inderal LA Long-Acting Capsules 3421

DETIDRON (Austria)
ETIDRONATE DISODIUM
Didronel Tablets 2693

DETROL (Canada)
TOLTERODINE TARTRATE
Detrol Tablets 2626

DETRUSITOL (Argentina, Austria, Belgium, Brazil, Chile, Czech Republic, Denmark, Finland, France, Germany, Greece, Hong Kong, India, Irish Republic, Israel, Italy, Malaysia, Mexico, New Zealand, Norway, Portugal, Russia, Singapore, South Africa, Spain, Sweden, Switzerland, Thailand, The Netherlands, United Kingdom)
TOLTERODINE TARTRATE
Detrol Tablets 2626

DETSEL (Austria, The Netherlands)
TOLTERODINE TARTRATE
Detrol Tablets 2626

DEUCOVAL (Chile)
NAPROXEN SODIUM
Anaprox DS Tablets 2769
Anaprox Tablets 2769

DEXA (Czech Republic, Germany, Hungary, Thailand)
DEXAMETHASONE SODIUM PHOSPHATE
Decadron Phosphate Injection 1931

DEXA ANB (Thailand)
DEXAMETHASONE SODIUM PHOSPHATE
Decadron Phosphate Injection 1931

DEXA IN DER OPHTIOLE (Germany)
DEXAMETHASONE SODIUM PHOSPHATE
Decadron Phosphate Injection 1931

DEXA TEOSONA (Argentina)
THEOPHYLLINE
Uniphyl Tablets 2708

DEXA-ALLVORAN (Germany)
DEXAMETHASONE SODIUM PHOSPHATE
Decadron Phosphate Injection 1931

DEXABENE (Austria, Germany)
DEXAMETHASONE SODIUM PHOSPHATE
Decadron Phosphate Injection 1931

DEXA-BRACHIALIN N (Germany)
DEXAMETHASONE SODIUM PHOSPHATE
Decadron Phosphate Injection 1931

DEXACAP (Hong Kong)
CAPTOPRIL
Captopril Tablets 2114

DEXACIP (India)
DEXAMETHASONE
Decadron Tablets 1929

DEXA-CLINIT (Germany)
DEXAMETHASONE SODIUM PHOSPHATE
Decadron Phosphate Injection 1931

DEXACLOR (Brazil)
DEXAMETHASONE
Decadron Tablets 1929

DEXACOLLYRE (Greece)
DEXAMETHASONE SODIUM PHOSPHATE
Decadron Phosphate Injection 1931

DEXACORT (Brazil, Israel)
DEXAMETHASONE
Decadron Tablets 1929

DEXACORTAL (Sweden)
DEXAMETHASONE
Decadron Tablets 1929

DEXACORTIN-K (Switzerland)
DEXAMETHASONE
Decadron Tablets 1929

DEXACORTISONE (Thailand)
DEXAMETHASONE SODIUM PHOSPHATE
Decadron Phosphate Injection 1931

DEXAEDO (Germany)
DEXAMETHASONE SODIUM PHOSPHATE
Decadron Phosphate Injection 1931

DEXA-EFFEKTON (Germany)
DEXAMETHASONE SODIUM PHOSPHATE
Decadron Phosphate Injection 1931

DEXAFARM (Argentina)
DEXAMETHASONE SODIUM PHOSPHATE
Decadron Phosphate Injection 1931

DEXAFLAM (Germany)
DEXAMETHASONE
Decadron Tablets 1929
DEXAMETHASONE SODIUM PHOSPHATE
Decadron Phosphate Injection 1931

DEXAFLAN (Brazil)
DEXAMETHASONE
Decadron Tablets 1929

DEXAGALEN (Germany)
DEXAMETHASONE
Decadron Tablets 1929

DEXAGEL (Germany)
DEXAMETHASONE SODIUM PHOSPHATE
Decadron Phosphate Injection 1931

DEXA-GENTAMICIN (Czech Republic)
DEXAMETHASONE
Decadron Tablets 1929

DEXA-HELVACORT (Switzerland)
DEXAMETHASONE SODIUM PHOSPHATE
Decadron Phosphate Injection 1931

DEXAHEXAL (Germany)
DEXAMETHASONE SODIUM PHOSPHATE
Decadron Phosphate Injection 1931

DEXA-INJEKT (Germany)
DEXAMETHASONE SODIUM PHOSPHATE
Decadron Phosphate Injection 1931

DEXALERGIN (Argentina)
DEXAMETHASONE SODIUM PHOSPHATE
Decadron Phosphate Injection 1931

DEXALOCAL (Hong Kong, Switzerland)
DEXAMETHASONE
Decadron Tablets 1929

DEXALTIN (Czech Republic, Malaysia, Singapore, Thailand)
DEXAMETHASONE
Decadron Tablets 1929

DEXAMED (Czech Republic, Germany, Hong Kong, Singapore)
DEXAMETHASONE SODIUM PHOSPHATE
Decadron Phosphate Injection 1931

DEXAMERAL (Argentina)
DEXAMETHASONE
Decadron Tablets 1929

DEXAMETAX (Brazil)
DEXAMETHASONE
Decadron Tablets 1929

DEXAMETONAL (Brazil)
DEXAMETHASONE
Decadron Tablets 1929

DEXAMINOR (Brazil)
DEXAMETHASONE
Decadron Tablets 1929

DEXAMISO (Spain)
DEXAMETHASONE
Decadron Tablets 1929

DEXAMONOZON (Germany)
DEXAMETHASONE
Decadron Tablets 1929

DEXAMONOZON N (Germany)
DEXAMETHASONE
Decadron Tablets 1929

DEXAMYTREX (Brazil)
GENTAMICIN SULFATE
Garamycin Injectable 3028
Genoptic Sterile Ophthalmic Solution .... ⊙227

DEXANO (Thailand)
DEXAMETHASONE
Decadron Tablets 1929

DEXAPLAST (Spain)
DEXAMETHASONE
Decadron Tablets 1929

DEXA-POS (The Netherlands)
DEXAMETHASONE SODIUM PHOSPHATE
Decadron Phosphate Injection 1931

DEXA-RATIOPHARM (Germany)
DEXAMETHASONE SODIUM PHOSPHATE
Decadron Phosphate Injection 1931

DEXA-SINE (Germany)
DEXAMETHASONE SODIUM PHOSPHATE
Decadron Phosphate Injection 1931

DEXASON (Czech Republic)
DEXAMETHASONE SODIUM PHOSPHATE
Decadron Phosphate Injection 1931

DEXASONE (Canada, Hong Kong, India, Malaysia)
DEXAMETHASONE
Decadron Tablets 1929

DEXATAM (Mexico)
DEXAMETHASONE
Decadron Tablets 1929

DEXATOTAL (Argentina)
DEXAMETHASONE
Decadron Tablets 1929

DEXICAR (Mexico)
DEXAMETHASONE
Decadron Tablets 1929

DEXIRON (Canada)
IRON DEXTRAN
Infed Injection 3381

DEXIVEN (Argentina)
CALCITRIOL
Calcijex Injection 411

DEXMETHSONE (Australia, Hong Kong)
DEXAMETHASONE
Decadron Tablets 1929

DEXNE (Mexico)
DEXAMETHASONE
Decadron Tablets 1929

DEXNON (Spain)
LEVOTHYROXINE SODIUM
Levothroid Tablets 1189

Levoxyl Tablets 1680
Synthroid Tablets 515

DEXOLAN (Switzerland)
DEXAMETHASONE
Decadron Tablets 1929

DEXOMON (United Kingdom)
DICLOFENAC SODIUM
Voltaren Tablets 2298
Voltaren-XR Tablets 2301

DEXON (Thailand)
DEXAMETHASONE SODIUM PHOSPHATE
Decadron Phosphate Injection 1931

DEXONA (Czech Republic, India, Mexico)
DEXAMETHASONE
Decadron Tablets 1929

DEXONA EYE/EAR (India)
DEXAMETHASONE SODIUM PHOSPHATE
Decadron Phosphate Injection 1931

DEXSOL (United Kingdom)
DEXAMETHASONE SODIUM PHOSPHATE
Decadron Phosphate Injection 1931

DEXTASONA (Brazil)
DEXAMETHASONE SODIUM PHOSPHATE
Decadron Phosphate Injection 1931

DEXTHASOL (Thailand)
DEXAMETHASONE SODIUM PHOSPHATE
Decadron Phosphate Injection 1931

DEXTON (Thailand)
DEXAMETHASONE SODIUM PHOSPHATE
Decadron Phosphate Injection 1931

DEXTRACIN (Malaysia)
DEXAMETHASONE SODIUM PHOSPHATE
Decadron Phosphate Injection 1931

DEZEPAN (Argentina)
DIAZEPAM
Diastat Rectal Delivery System 3344
Valium Tablets 2822

DEZOR (Malaysia, Singapore)
KETOCONAZOLE
Nizoral 2% Shampoo 1838

DEZORAL (Singapore)
KETOCONAZOLE
Nizoral 2% Shampoo 1838

DHABESOL (Hong Kong, Malaysia, Singapore)
CLOBETASOL PROPIONATE
Temovate Cream 1549
Temovate E Emollient 1552
Temovate Gel 1550
Temovate Ointment 1549
Temovate Scalp Application 1551

DHACTULOSE (Singapore)
LACTULOSE
Kristalose for Oral Solution 2149

DI RETARD (Spain)
DICLOFENAC SODIUM
Voltaren Tablets 2298
Voltaren-XR Tablets 2301

DIABEN (Argentina)
ROSIGLITAZONE MALEATE
Avandia Tablets 1348

DIABESTAT (Chile)
PIOGLITAZONE HYDROCHLORIDE
Actos Tablets 3224

DIACARDIN (Italy)
DILTIAZEM HYDROCHLORIDE
Cardizem LA Extended Release Tablets 1699
Tiazac Capsules 1204

DIACEPLEX (Spain)
DIAZEPAM
Diastat Rectal Delivery System 3344
Valium Tablets 2822

DIACEPLEX SIMPLE (Spain)
DIAZEPAM
Diastat Rectal Delivery System 3344
Valium Tablets 2822

DIA-COLON (Italy)
LACTULOSE
Kristalose for Oral Solution 2149

DIACOR (Chile, France)
MEBENDAZOLE
Vermox Chewable Tablets 1853

DIACORDIN (Czech Republic)
DILTIAZEM HYDROCHLORIDE
Cardizem LA Extended Release Tablets 1699
Tiazac Capsules 1204

DIACTAL (Argentina)
DIAZEPAM
Diastat Rectal Delivery System 3344
Valium Tablets 2822

DIACURE (The Netherlands)
LOPERAMIDE HYDROCHLORIDE
Imodium Capsules 1834

DIAFURAN (Brazil)
LOPERAMIDE HYDROCHLORIDE
Imodium Capsules 1834

DIAGLIM (India)
GLIMEPIRIDE
Amaryl Tablets 2864

DIAGLIT (India)
PIOGLITAZONE HYDROCHLORIDE
Actos Tablets 3224

DIAHALT (Canada)
LOPERAMIDE HYDROCHLORIDE
Imodium Capsules 1834

DIAH-LIMIT (United Kingdom)
LOPERAMIDE HYDROCHLORIDE
Imodium Capsules 1834

DIALAR (United Kingdom)
DIAZEPAM
Diastat Rectal Delivery System 3344
Valium Tablets 2822

DIANO (Thailand)
DIAZEPAM
Diastat Rectal Delivery System 3344
Valium Tablets 2822

DIAPAM (Finland, Thailand)
DIAZEPAM
Diastat Rectal Delivery System 3344
Valium Tablets 2822

DIAPANIL (Mexico)
DIAZEPAM
Diastat Rectal Delivery System 3344
Valium Tablets 2822

DIAPINE (Malaysia, Singapore, Thailand)
DIAZEPAM
Diastat Rectal Delivery System 3344
Valium Tablets 2822

DIAPIRIDE (Portugal)
GLIMEPIRIDE
Amaryl Tablets 2864

DIAPO (Malaysia)
DIAZEPAM
Diastat Rectal Delivery System 3344
Valium Tablets 2822

DIAPRIDE (Hong Kong, Singapore)
GLIMEPIRIDE
Amaryl Tablets 2864

DIAQUEL (South Africa)
DIAZEPAM
Diastat Rectal Delivery System 3344
Valium Tablets 2822

DIAQUITTE (United Kingdom)
LOPERAMIDE HYDROCHLORIDE
Imodium Capsules 1834

DIARENT (Thailand)
LOPERAMIDE HYDROCHLORIDE
Imodium Capsules 1834

DIARETYL (France)
LOPERAMIDE HYDROCHLORIDE
Imodium Capsules 1834

DIAREZE (United Kingdom)
LOPERAMIDE HYDROCHLORIDE
Imodium Capsules 1834

DIARLOP (India)
LOPERAMIDE HYDROCHLORIDE
Imodium Capsules 1834

DIARODIL (Thailand)
LOPERAMIDE HYDROCHLORIDE
Imodium Capsules 1834

DIARRESEC (Brazil)
LOPERAMIDE HYDROCHLORIDE
Imodium Capsules 1834

DIARR-EZE (Canada)
LOPERAMIDE HYDROCHLORIDE
Imodium Capsules 1834

DIARRHEA RELIEF (Canada)
LOPERAMIDE HYDROCHLORIDE
Imodium Capsules 1834

DIARSTOP (Italy)
LOPERAMIDE HYDROCHLORIDE
Imodium Capsules 1834

DIARSTOP L (Germany)
LOPERAMIDE HYDROCHLORIDE
Imodium Capsules 1834

DIARZERO (Italy)
LOPERAMIDE HYDROCHLORIDE
Imodium Capsules 1834

DIASEC (Brazil)
LOPERAMIDE HYDROCHLORIDE
Imodium Capsules 1834

DIASORB (United Kingdom)
LOPERAMIDE HYDROCHLORIDE
Imodium Capsules 1834

DIASTAT (Canada)
DIAZEPAM
Diastat Rectal Delivery System 3344
Valium Tablets 2822

DIASTONE (Argentina)
DICLOFENAC SODIUM
Voltaren Tablets 2298
Voltaren-XR Tablets 2301

DIATEX (Mexico)
DIAZEPAM
Diastat Rectal Delivery System 3344
Valium Tablets 2822

DIATIL (South Africa)
DILTIAZEM HYDROCHLORIDE
Cardizem LA Extended Release Tablets 1699
Tiazac Capsules 1204

DIATRACIN (Spain)
VANCOMYCIN HYDROCHLORIDE
Vancocin HCl Capsules, USP 3370

DIATROL (Malaysia)
LOPERAMIDE HYDROCHLORIDE
Imodium Capsules 1834

DIAZ (Israel)
DIAZEPAM
Diastat Rectal Delivery System 3344
Valium Tablets 2822

DIAZELONG (Brazil)
DIAZEPAM
Diastat Rectal Delivery System 3344
Valium Tablets 2822

DIAZEMULS (Australia, Canada, Germany, Hong Kong, Irish Republic, Italy, The Netherlands, United Kingdom)
DIAZEPAM
Diastat Rectal Delivery System 3344
Valium Tablets 2822

DIAZOLEN (Mexico)
MEBENDAZOLE
Vermox Chewable Tablets 1853

DIAZON (Hong Kong, Singapore, Thailand)
KETOCONAZOLE
Nizoral 2% Shampoo 1838

DIBASONA (Mexico)
DEXAMETHASONE SODIUM PHOSPHATE
Decadron Phosphate Injection 1931

DICAP (New Zealand)
LOPERAMIDE HYDROCHLORIDE
Imodium Capsules 1834

DICEPIN B6 (Spain)
DIAZEPAM
Diastat Rectal Delivery System 3344
Valium Tablets 2822

DICLAC (Australia, Austria, Brazil, Germany, Hungary, Irish Republic, Switzerland)
DICLOFENAC SODIUM
Voltaren Tablets 2298
Voltaren-XR Tablets 2301

DICLAX (New Zealand)
DICLOFENAC SODIUM
Voltaren Tablets 2298
Voltaren-XR Tablets 2301

DICLAXOL (Austria)
DICLOFENAC SODIUM
Voltaren Tablets 2298
Voltaren-XR Tablets 2301

DICLO (Irish Republic, Switzerland)
DICLOFENAC SODIUM
Voltaren Tablets 2298
Voltaren-XR Tablets 2301

DICLO P (Brazil)
DICLOFENAC POTASSIUM
Cataflam Tablets 2173

DICLO-ATTRITIN (Germany)
DICLOFENAC SODIUM
Voltaren Tablets 2298
Voltaren-XR Tablets 2301

DICLO-BASAN (Switzerland)
DICLOFENAC SODIUM
Voltaren Tablets 2298
Voltaren-XR Tablets 2301

DICLOBENE (Austria)
DICLOFENAC POTASSIUM
Cataflam Tablets 2173

DICLOBERL (Germany)
DICLOFENAC SODIUM
Voltaren Tablets 2298
Voltaren-XR Tablets 2301

DICLOCULAR (Italy)
DICLOFENAC SODIUM
Voltaren Tablets 2298
Voltaren-XR Tablets 2301

DICLO-DENK (Hong Kong, Singapore)
DICLOFENAC SODIUM
Voltaren Tablets 2298
Voltaren-XR Tablets 2301

DICLO-DIVIDO (Germany)
DICLOFENAC SODIUM
Voltaren Tablets 2298
Voltaren-XR Tablets 2301

DICLODOC (Germany)
DICLOFENAC SODIUM
Voltaren Tablets 2298
Voltaren-XR Tablets 2301

DICLODOL (Italy)
DICLOFENAC SODIUM
Voltaren Tablets 2298
Voltaren-XR Tablets 2301

DICLOFAN (Italy)
DICLOFENAC SODIUM
Voltaren Tablets 2298
Voltaren-XR Tablets 2301

DICLOFEN (Brazil, Czech Republic, Thailand)
DICLOFENAC POTASSIUM
Cataflam Tablets 2173

DICLOFENAX (Brazil)
DICLOFENAC POTASSIUM
Cataflam Tablets 2173

DICLOFENBETA (Germany)
DICLOFENAC SODIUM
Voltaren Tablets 2298
Voltaren-XR Tablets 2301

DICLOFLAM (South Africa)
DICLOFENAC SODIUM
Voltaren Tablets 2298
Voltaren-XR Tablets 2301

DICLOFLEX (United Kingdom)
DICLOFENAC SODIUM
Voltaren Tablets 2298
Voltaren-XR Tablets 2301

DICLOFTAL (Portugal)
DICLOFENAC SODIUM
Voltaren Tablets 2298
Voltaren-XR Tablets 2301

DICLOFTIL (Italy)
DICLOFENAC SODIUM
Voltaren Tablets 2298
Voltaren-XR Tablets 2301

DICLOGEA (Denmark)
DICLOFENAC SODIUM
Voltaren Tablets 2298
Voltaren-XR Tablets 2301

DICLO-GEL (Germany)
DICLOFENAC SODIUM
Voltaren Tablets 2298
Voltaren-XR Tablets 2301

DICLOGENOM (Brazil)
DICLOFENAC SODIUM
Voltaren Tablets 2298
Voltaren-XR Tablets 2301

DICLOGENTA (India)
DICLOFENAC SODIUM
Voltaren Tablets 2298
Voltaren-XR Tablets 2301

DICLOGESIC (Hong Kong)
DICLOFENAC SODIUM
Voltaren Tablets 2298
Voltaren-XR Tablets 2301

DICLOGESIC RELAX (Argentina)
DICLOFENAC SODIUM
Voltaren Tablets 2298
Voltaren-XR Tablets 2301

DICLOGRUN (Germany)
DICLOFENAC SODIUM
Voltaren Tablets 2298
Voltaren-XR Tablets 2301

DICLOHEXAL (Australia)
DICLOFENAC SODIUM
Voltaren Tablets 2298
Voltaren-XR Tablets 2301

DICLOLAN (Thailand)
DICLOFENAC SODIUM
Voltaren Tablets 2298
Voltaren-XR Tablets 2301

DICLOMAX (Irish Republic, United Kingdom)
DICLOFENAC SODIUM
Voltaren Tablets 2298
Voltaren-XR Tablets 2301

DICLOMEL (Hungary, Irish Republic)
DICLOFENAC SODIUM
Voltaren Tablets 2298
Voltaren-XR Tablets 2301

DICLOMELAN (Austria)
DICLOFENAC SODIUM
Voltaren Tablets 2298
Voltaren-XR Tablets 2301

DICLOMERCK (Germany)
DICLOFENAC SODIUM
Voltaren Tablets 2298
Voltaren-XR Tablets 2301

DICLOMETIN (Finland)
DICLOFENAC SODIUM
Voltaren Tablets 2298
Voltaren-XR Tablets 2301

DICLOMEX (Finland)
DICLOFENAC POTASSIUM
Cataflam Tablets 2173

DICLOMOL (India)
DICLOFENAC SODIUM
Voltaren Tablets 2298
Voltaren-XR Tablets 2301

DICLON (Denmark)
DICLOFENAC SODIUM
Voltaren Tablets 2298
Voltaren-XR Tablets 2301

DICLONAC (India)
DICLOFENAC SODIUM
Voltaren Tablets 2298
Voltaren-XR Tablets 2301

DICLO-OPT (Germany)
DICLOFENAC SODIUM
Voltaren Tablets 2298
Voltaren-XR Tablets 2301

DICLOPHLOGONT (Germany, Greece)
DICLOFENAC SODIUM
Voltaren Tablets 2298
Voltaren-XR Tablets 2301

DICLO-PUREN (Germany)
DICLOFENAC SODIUM
Voltaren Tablets 2298
Voltaren-XR Tablets 2301

DICLORAN (Mexico)
DICLOFENAC SODIUM
Voltaren Tablets 2298
Voltaren-XR Tablets 2301

DICLORAN-A (India)
DICLOFENAC SODIUM
Voltaren Tablets 2298
Voltaren-XR Tablets 2301

DICLOREKTAL (Germany)
DICLOFENAC SODIUM
Voltaren Tablets 2298
Voltaren-XR Tablets 2301

DICLORENGEL (Israel)
DICLOFENAC SODIUM
Voltaren Tablets 2298
Voltaren-XR Tablets 2301

DICLOREUM (Czech Republic)
DICLOFENAC SODIUM
Voltaren Tablets 2298
Voltaren-XR Tablets 2301

DICLO-SAAR (Germany)
DICLOFENAC SODIUM
Voltaren Tablets 2298
Voltaren-XR Tablets 2301

DICLOSIAN (Thailand)
DICLOFENAC SODIUM
Voltaren Tablets 2298
Voltaren-XR Tablets 2301

DICLOSIFAR (Switzerland)
DICLOFENAC SODIUM
Voltaren Tablets 2298
Voltaren-XR Tablets 2301

DICLO-SPONDYRIL (Germany)
DICLOFENAC SODIUM
Voltaren Tablets 2298
Voltaren-XR Tablets 2301

DICLOSTAD (Austria)
DICLOFENAC SODIUM
Voltaren Tablets 2298
Voltaren-XR Tablets 2301

DICLOSYL (Austria)
DICLOFENAC SODIUM
Voltaren Tablets 2298
Voltaren-XR Tablets 2301

DICLO-TABLINEN (Germany)
DICLOFENAC SODIUM
Voltaren Tablets 2298
Voltaren-XR Tablets 2301

DICLOTARD (United Kingdom)
DICLOFENAC SODIUM
Voltaren Tablets 2298
Voltaren-XR Tablets 2301

DICLOTEARS (Italy)
DICLOFENAC SODIUM
Voltaren Tablets 2298
Voltaren-XR Tablets 2301

DICLOTEC (Canada, Portugal)
DICLOFENAC SODIUM
Voltaren Tablets 2298
Voltaren-XR Tablets 2301

DICLOVIT (Russia)
DICLOFENAC SODIUM
Voltaren Tablets 2298
Voltaren-XR Tablets 2301

DICLOVOL (United Kingdom)
DICLOFENAC SODIUM
Voltaren Tablets 2298
Voltaren-XR Tablets 2301

DICLOWAL (Hong Kong, Singapore)
DICLOFENAC SODIUM
Voltaren Tablets 2298
Voltaren-XR Tablets 2301

DICLOZIP (United Kingdom)
DICLOFENAC SODIUM
Voltaren Tablets 2298
Voltaren-XR Tablets 2301

DIDAMOL (Belgium)
DIPYRIDAMOLE
Persantine Tablets 898

DIDRONATE (Denmark, Finland, Norway, Sweden)
ETIDRONATE DISODIUM
Didronel Tablets 2693

DIDRONEL (Austria, Belgium, Canada, France, Germany, Hong Kong, Irish Republic, Israel, Italy, Japan, New Zealand, Portugal, South Africa, Switzerland, The Netherlands, United Kingdom)
ETIDRONATE DISODIUM
Didronel Tablets 2693

DIENPAX (Brazil)
DIAZEPAM
Diastat Rectal Delivery System 3344
Valium Tablets 2822

DIFEN (Thailand)
DICLOFENAC SODIUM
Voltaren Tablets 2298
Voltaren-XR Tablets 2301

DIFENA (Hong Kong)
DICLOFENAC SODIUM
Voltaren Tablets 2298
Voltaren-XR Tablets 2301

DIFENAC (Argentina, Hong Kong, Singapore, South Africa, Thailand)
DICLOFENAC SODIUM
Voltaren Tablets 2298
Voltaren-XR Tablets 2301

DIFENAN (Brazil)
DICLOFENAC SODIUM
Voltaren Tablets 2298
Voltaren-XR Tablets 2301

DIFEND (Greece)
DICLOFENAC SODIUM
Voltaren Tablets 2298
Voltaren-XR Tablets 2301

DIFENE (Austria, Irish Republic)
DICLOFENAC SODIUM
Voltaren Tablets 2298
Voltaren-XR Tablets 2301

DIFENET (Denmark)
DICLOFENAC SODIUM
Voltaren Tablets 2298
Voltaren-XR Tablets 2301

DIFENO (Thailand)
DICLOFENAC SODIUM
Voltaren Tablets 2298
Voltaren-XR Tablets 2301

DIFENOL (Hong Kong)
DICLOFENAC SODIUM
Voltaren Tablets 2298
Voltaren-XR Tablets 2301

DIFERBEST (Mexico)
NAPROXEN SODIUM
Anaprox DS Tablets 2769
Anaprox Tablets 2769

DIFFERIN (Argentina, Australia, Austria, Belgium, Brazil, Canada, Chile, Finland, Germany, Hong Kong, Hungary, Irish Republic, Italy, Malaysia, New Zealand, Norway, Portugal, Russia, Singapore, South Africa, Sweden, Switzerland, Thailand, United Kingdom)
ADAPALENE
Differin Gel 1211

DIFFERINE (Czech Republic, France, Spain)
ADAPALENE
Differin Gel 1211

DIFFU-K (France)
POTASSIUM CHLORIDE
K-Dur Extended-Relase Tablets 3047
K-Lor Powder Packets 472
K-Tab Filmtab Tablets 473

DIFFUMAL (Italy)
THEOPHYLLINE
Uniphyl Tablets 2708

DIFIX (Italy)
CALCITRIOL
Calcijex Injection 411

DIFLERIX (Hong Kong, Malaysia)
INDAPAMIDE
Indapamide Tablets 2119

DIFLONID (Denmark, Norway, Sweden)
DIFLUNISAL
Dolobid Tablets 1937

DIFLUDOL (Italy)
DIFLUNISAL
Dolobid Tablets 1937

DIFLUNIL (Italy)
DIFLUNISAL
Dolobid Tablets 1937

DIFLUSAL (Belgium)
DIFLUNISAL
Dolobid Tablets 1937

DIFLUSAN (Italy)
DIFLUNISAL
Dolobid Tablets 1937

DIFNAL (Malaysia, Singapore)
DICLOFENAC POTASSIUM
Cataflam Tablets 2173

DIFOSFEN (Argentina, Singapore, Spain)
ETIDRONATE DISODIUM
Didronel Tablets 2693

DIFOXACIL (Mexico)
NORFLOXACIN
Noroxin Tablets 2009

DIGACIN (Germany)
DIGOXIN
Lanoxicaps Capsules 1458
Lanoxin Injection 1462
Lanoxin Injection Pediatric 1465
Lanoxin Tablets 1468

DIGAOL (France)
TIMOLOL MALEATE
Blocadren Tablets 1891
Timoptic Sterile Ophthalmic Solution 2058
Timoptic in Ocudose 2061
Timoptic-XE Sterile Ophthalmic Gel Forming Solution 2062

DIGARIL (Spain)
FLUVASTATIN SODIUM
Lescol Capsules 2227

DIGENAC (United Kingdom)
DICLOFENAC SODIUM
Voltaren Tablets 2298
Voltaren-XR Tablets 2301

DIGERVIN (Spain)
FAMOTIDINE
Pepcid Injection 2017
Pepcid Injection Premixed 2017
Pepcid Tablets 2014
Pepcid for Oral Suspension 2014

DIGESS (Canada)
PANCRELIPASE
Ultrase Capsules 735
Ultrase MT Capsules 736

DIGESTOSAN (Austria)
RANITIDINE HYDROCHLORIDE
Zantac 25 EFFERdose Tablets 1597
Zantac 150 EFFERdose Tablets 1597
Zantac 150 Tablets 1597
Zantac 300 Tablets 1597
Zantac Injection 1593
Zantac Injection Premixed 1593
Zantac Syrup 1597

DIGEZANOL (Mexico)
ALBENDAZOLE
Albenza Tablets 1310

DIGNOBETA (Germany)
ATENOLOL
Tenormin I.V. Injection 698

DIGNOFENAC (Chile, Germany)
DICLOFENAC SODIUM
Voltaren Tablets 2298
Voltaren-XR Tablets 2301

DIGNOKONSTANT (Germany)
NIFEDIPINE
Adalat CC Tablets 2978

DIGNORETIK (Germany)
AMILORIDE HYDROCHLORIDE/HYDROCHLOROTHIAZIDE
Moduretic Tablets 2003

DIGNOTRIMAZOL (Germany)
CLOTRIMAZOLE
Lotrimin Cream 3053

Lotrimin Lotion 1%. **3053**
Lotrimin Topical Solution 1% **3053**

DIGNOVER (Germany)
VERAPAMIL HYDROCHLORIDE
Covera-HS Tablets **3135**
Verelan PM Capsules **3120**

DIGOCARD-G (Argentina)
DIGOXIN
Lanoxicaps Capsules **1458**
Lanoxin Injection **1462**
Lanoxin Injection Pediatric **1465**
Lanoxin Tablets. **1468**

DIGOMAL (Italy)
DIGOXIN
Lanoxicaps Capsules **1458**
Lanoxin Injection **1462**
Lanoxin Injection Pediatric **1465**
Lanoxin Tablets. **1468**

DIGOREGEN (Germany)
DIGOXIN
Lanoxicaps Capsules **1458**
Lanoxin Injection **1462**
Lanoxin Injection Pediatric **1465**
Lanoxin Tablets. **1468**

DIGOSIN (Japan)
DIGOXIN
Lanoxicaps Capsules **1458**
Lanoxin Injection **1462**
Lanoxin Injection Pediatric **1465**
Lanoxin Tablets. **1468**

DIGOXIL (Brazil)
DIGOXIN
Lanoxicaps Capsules **1458**
Lanoxin Injection **1462**
Lanoxin Injection Pediatric **1465**
Lanoxin Tablets. **1468**

DILABAR (Spain)
CAPTOPRIL
Captopril Tablets **2114**

DILACARD (Brazil)
VERAPAMIL HYDROCHLORIDE
Covera-HS Tablets **3135**
Verelan PM Capsules **3120**

DILACLAN (Spain)
DILTIAZEM HYDROCHLORIDE
Cardizem LA Extended Release Tablets. . . **1699**
Tiazac Capsules **1204**

DILACOR (Brazil)
VERAPAMIL HYDROCHLORIDE
Covera-HS Tablets **3135**
Verelan PM Capsules **3120**

DILACORAN (Mexico)
VERAPAMIL HYDROCHLORIDE
Covera-HS Tablets **3135**
Verelan PM Capsules **3120**

DILACORON (Brazil)
VERAPAMIL HYDROCHLORIDE
Covera-HS Tablets **3135**
Verelan PM Capsules **3120**

DILADEL (Italy)
DILTIAZEM HYDROCHLORIDE
Cardizem LA Extended Release Tablets. . . **1699**
Tiazac Capsules **1204**

DILAFLUX (Brazil)
NIFEDIPINE
Adalat CC Tablets **2978**

DILAHIM (Argentina)
DILTIAZEM HYDROCHLORIDE
Cardizem LA Extended Release Tablets. . . **1699**
Tiazac Capsules **1204**

DILAMAX (Portugal)
SALMETEROL XINAFOATE
Serevent Diskus **1540**

DILANACIN (Germany)
DIGOXIN
Lanoxicaps Capsules **1458**
Lanoxin Injection **1462**
Lanoxin Injection Pediatric **1465**
Lanoxin Tablets. **1468**

DILAPLUS (Austria)
CARVEDILOL
Coreg Tablets. **1376**

DILATAM (Israel, South Africa, Thailand)
DILTIAZEM HYDROCHLORIDE
Cardizem LA Extended Release Tablets. . . **1699**
Tiazac Capsules **1204**

DILATAME (Austria)
DILTIAZEM HYDROCHLORIDE
Cardizem LA Extended Release Tablets. . . **1699**
Tiazac Capsules **1204**

DILATOL (Portugal)
ISRADIPINE
DynaCirc CR Tablets. **2726**

DILATREND (Argentina, Australia, Austria, Brazil, Chile, Czech Republic, Germany, Greece, Hong Kong, Hungary, Italy, Mexico, New Zealand, Norway, Singapore, South Africa, Switzerland, Thailand)
CARVEDILOL
Coreg Tablets. **1376**

DILAUDID (Australia, Austria, Canada, Germany, Irish Republic)
HYDROMORPHONE HYDROCHLORIDE
Dilaudid Ampules. **439**
Dilaudid Multiple Dose Vials **439**
Dilaudid Non-Sterile Powder **439**
Dilaudid Oral Liquid **443**
Dilaudid Rectal Suppositories **439**
Dilaudid Tablets. **439**
Dilaudid Tablets - 8 mg **443**
Dilaudid-HP Injection. **441**
Dilaudid-HP Lyophilized Powder 250 mg . . . **441**

DILBLOC (Portugal)
CARVEDILOL
Coreg Tablets. **1376**

DILCARD (Malaysia, New Zealand)
DILTIAZEM HYDROCHLORIDE
Cardizem LA Extended Release Tablets. . . **1699**
Tiazac Capsules **1204**

DILCARDIA (India, United Kingdom)
DILTIAZEM HYDROCHLORIDE
Cardizem LA Extended Release Tablets. . . **1699**
Tiazac Capsules **1204**

DILCEREN (Czech Republic)
NIMODIPINE
Nimotop Capsules **774**

DILCONTIN (India)
DILTIAZEM HYDROCHLORIDE
Cardizem LA Extended Release Tablets. . . **1699**
Tiazac Capsules **1204**

DILCOR (Denmark, Spain)
DILTIAZEM HYDROCHLORIDE
Cardizem LA Extended Release Tablets. . . **1699**
Tiazac Capsules **1204**

DILEM (Hong Kong, Italy, Malaysia, Thailand)
DILTIAZEM HYDROCHLORIDE
Cardizem LA Extended Release Tablets. . . **1699**
Tiazac Capsules **1204**

DILETAN (Portugal)
SUMATRIPTAN SUCCINATE
Imitrex Injection **1431**
Imitrex Tablets **1440**

DILFAR (Portugal)
DILTIAZEM HYDROCHLORIDE
Cardizem LA Extended Release Tablets. . . **1699**
Tiazac Capsules **1204**

DILGARD (India)
DILTIAZEM HYDROCHLORIDE
Cardizem LA Extended Release Tablets. . . **1699**
Tiazac Capsules **1204**

DILITER (Italy)
DILTIAZEM HYDROCHLORIDE
Cardizem LA Extended Release Tablets. . . **1699**
Tiazac Capsules **1204**

DILIZEM (Singapore, Thailand)
DILTIAZEM HYDROCHLORIDE
Cardizem LA Extended Release Tablets. . . **1699**
Tiazac Capsules **1204**

DILMIN (Finland)
DILTIAZEM HYDROCHLORIDE
Cardizem LA Extended Release Tablets. . . **1699**
Tiazac Capsules **1204**

DILOC (The Netherlands)
DILTIAZEM HYDROCHLORIDE
Cardizem LA Extended Release Tablets. . . **1699**
Tiazac Capsules **1204**

DILONGO (Portugal)
DILTIAZEM HYDROCHLORIDE
Cardizem LA Extended Release Tablets. . . **1699**
Tiazac Capsules **1204**

DILPRAL (Finland)
DILTIAZEM HYDROCHLORIDE
Cardizem LA Extended Release Tablets. . . **1699**
Tiazac Capsules **1204**

DILRENE (France, Hungary)
DILTIAZEM HYDROCHLORIDE
Cardizem LA Extended Release Tablets. . . **1699**
Tiazac Capsules **1204**

DILSAL (Germany)
DILTIAZEM HYDROCHLORIDE
Cardizem LA Extended Release Tablets. . . **1699**
Tiazac Capsules **1204**

DIL-SANORANIA (Germany)
DILTIAZEM HYDROCHLORIDE
Cardizem LA Extended Release Tablets. . . **1699**
Tiazac Capsules **1204**

DILTABETA (Germany)
DILTIAZEM HYDROCHLORIDE
Cardizem LA Extended Release Tablets. . . **1699**
Tiazac Capsules **1204**

DILTAHEXAL (Australia, Austria, Germany)
DILTIAZEM HYDROCHLORIDE
Cardizem LA Extended Release Tablets. . . **1699**
Tiazac Capsules **1204**

DILTAM (Irish Republic)
DILTIAZEM HYDROCHLORIDE
Cardizem LA Extended Release Tablets. . . **1699**
Tiazac Capsules **1204**

DILTAN (Hong Kong, Hungary, Thailand)
DILTIAZEM HYDROCHLORIDE
Cardizem LA Extended Release Tablets. . . **1699**
Tiazac Capsules **1204**

DILTAPHAM (Germany)
DILTIAZEM HYDROCHLORIDE
Cardizem LA Extended Release Tablets. . . **1699**
Tiazac Capsules **1204**

DILTARETARD (Germany)
DILTIAZEM HYDROCHLORIDE
Cardizem LA Extended Release Tablets. . . **1699**
Tiazac Capsules **1204**

DILTEC (Thailand)
DILTIAZEM HYDROCHLORIDE
Cardizem LA Extended Release Tablets. . . **1699**
Tiazac Capsules **1204**

DILTEM (Greece)
DILTIAZEM HYDROCHLORIDE
Cardizem LA Extended Release Tablets. . . **1699**
Tiazac Capsules **1204**

DILTI (Germany)
DILTIAZEM HYDROCHLORIDE
Cardizem LA Extended Release Tablets. . . **1699**
Tiazac Capsules **1204**

DILTIACOR (Argentina, Brazil)
DILTIAZEM HYDROCHLORIDE
Cardizem LA Extended Release Tablets. . . **1699**
Tiazac Capsules **1204**

DILTIAGAMMA (Germany)
DILTIAZEM HYDROCHLORIDE
Cardizem LA Extended Release Tablets. . . **1699**
Tiazac Capsules **1204**

DILTIAMAX (Australia)
DILTIAZEM HYDROCHLORIDE
Cardizem LA Extended Release Tablets. . . **1699**
Tiazac Capsules **1204**

DILTIAMERCK (Germany)
DILTIAZEM HYDROCHLORIDE
Cardizem LA Extended Release Tablets. . . **1699**
Tiazac Capsules **1204**

DILTIANGINA (Portugal)
DILTIAZEM HYDROCHLORIDE
Cardizem LA Extended Release Tablets. . . **1699**
Tiazac Capsules **1204**

DILTIASTAD (Austria)
DILTIAZEM HYDROCHLORIDE
Cardizem LA Extended Release Tablets. . . **1699**
Tiazac Capsules **1204**

DILTIEM (Portugal)
DILTIAZEM HYDROCHLORIDE
Cardizem LA Extended Release Tablets. . . **1699**
Tiazac Capsules **1204**

DILTI-ESSEX (Germany)
DILTIAZEM HYDROCHLORIDE
Cardizem LA Extended Release Tablets. . . **1699**
Tiazac Capsules **1204**

DILTIKARD (Norway)
DILTIAZEM HYDROCHLORIDE
Cardizem LA Extended Release Tablets. . . **1699**
Tiazac Capsules **1204**

DILTIPRESS (Brazil)
DILTIAZEM HYDROCHLORIDE
Cardizem LA Extended Release Tablets. . . **1699**
Tiazac Capsules **1204**

DILTIUC (Germany)
DILTIAZEM HYDROCHLORIDE
Cardizem LA Extended Release Tablets. . . **1699**
Tiazac Capsules **1204**

DILTIWAS (Spain)
DILTIAZEM HYDROCHLORIDE
Cardizem LA Extended Release Tablets. . . **1699**
Tiazac Capsules **1204**

DILTIZEM (Brazil)
DILTIAZEM HYDROCHLORIDE
Cardizem LA Extended Release Tablets. . . **1699**
Tiazac Capsules **1204**

DILUCID (Mexico)
LOVASTATIN
Mevacor Tablets **1996**

DILUTOL (Argentina)
ENOXAPARIN SODIUM
Lovenox Injection **2931**

DILVAS (India)
ENALAPRIL MALEATE
Vasotec I.V. Injection **2076**

DILVAS AM (India)
ENALAPRIL MALEATE
Vasotec I.V. Injection **2076**

DILZATYROL (Austria)
DILTIAZEM HYDROCHLORIDE
Cardizem LA Extended Release Tablets. . . **1699**
Tiazac Capsules **1204**

DILZEM (Australia, Austria, Czech Republic, Finland, Germany, Hong Kong, Hungary, India, Irish Republic, New Zealand, Switzerland, Thailand, United Kingdom)
DILTIAZEM HYDROCHLORIDE
Cardizem LA Extended Release Tablets. . . **1699**
Tiazac Capsules **1204**

DILZENE (Italy)
DILTIAZEM HYDROCHLORIDE
Cardizem LA Extended Release Tablets. . . **1699**
Tiazac Capsules **1204**

DILZEREAL (Germany)
DILTIAZEM HYDROCHLORIDE
Cardizem LA Extended Release Tablets. . . **1699**
Tiazac Capsules **1204**

DILZICARDIN (Germany)
DILTIAZEM HYDROCHLORIDE
Cardizem LA Extended Release Tablets. . . **1699**
Tiazac Capsules **1204**

DIMALAN (Argentina)
BICALUTAMIDE
Casodex Tablets **670**

DIMALOSIO (Italy)
LACTULOSE
Kristalose for Oral Solution **2149**

DIMENFORMON (The Netherlands)
ESTRADIOL
Climara Transdermal System **795**
Vivelle Transdermal System **2288**
Vivelle-Dot Transdermal System **2293**

DIMETIGAL (Mexico)
CIMETIDINE
Tagamet Tablets **1547**

DIMIREL (Australia)
GLIMEPIRIDE
Amaryl Tablets **2864**

DIMITONE (Belgium, Denmark, Israel)
CARVEDILOL
Coreg Tablets. **1376**

DIMOR (Sweden)
LOPERAMIDE HYDROCHLORIDE
Imodium Capsules **1834**

DIMORF (Brazil)
MORPHINE SULFATE
Kadian Capsules **572**
MS Contin Tablets **2703**

DINA (Italy)
CIMETIDINE
Tagamet Tablets **1547**

DINAC (Australia, Thailand)
DICLOFENAC SODIUM
Voltaren Tablets **2298**
Voltaren-XR Tablets **2301**

DINACLON (Greece)
DICLOFENAC SODIUM
Voltaren Tablets **2298**
Voltaren-XR Tablets **2301**

DINAVIR (Brazil)
INDINAVIR SULFATE
Crixivan Capsules **1918**

DINAZIDE (Thailand)
HYDROCHLOROTHIAZIDE/TRIAMTERENE
Dyazide Capsules **1389**
Maxzide Tablets **2150**
Maxzide-25 mg Tablets **2150**

DINEURIN (Chile)
GABAPENTIN
Neurontin Capsules **2498**

DINISOR (Spain)
DILTIAZEM HYDROCHLORIDE
Cardizem LA Extended Release Tablets . . . **1699**
Tiazac Capsules **1204**

DINUL (Portugal)
FAMOTIDINE
Pepcid Injection **2017**
Pepcid Injection Premixed **2017**
Pepcid Tablets **2014**
Pepcid for Oral Suspension **2014**

DIOCALM ULTRA (United Kingdom)
LOPERAMIDE HYDROCHLORIDE
Imodium Capsules **1834**

DIOCAM (Argentina)
CLONAZEPAM
Klonopin Tablets **2782**

DIOCAPS (United Kingdom)
LOPERAMIDE HYDROCHLORIDE
Imodium Capsules **1834**

DIODARONE (Brazil)
AMIODARONE HYDROCHLORIDE
Pacerone Tablets **3337**

DIODERM (Irish Republic, United Kingdom)
HYDROCORTISONE
Hydrocortone Tablets **1963**

DIODEX (Canada)
DEXAMETHASONE SODIUM PHOSPHATE
Decadron Phosphate Injection **1931**

DIOFLUOR (Canada)
FLUORESCEIN SODIUM
Fluorescite Injection . . . . ⊙**207**

DIOGENT (Canada)
GENTAMICIN SULFATE
Garamycin Injectable **3028**
Genoptic Sterile Ophthalmic Solution . . . . ⊙**227**

DIOMICETE (Portugal)
CLOTRIMAZOLE
Lotrimin Cream **3053**
Lotrimin Lotion 1% **3053**
Lotrimin Topical Solution 1% **3053**

DIOMYCIN (Canada)
ERYTHROMYCIN
Ery-Tab Tablets **447**
Erythromycin Base Filmtab Tablets **454**
Erythromycin Delayed-Release Capsules, USP **456**
PCE Dispertab Tablets **510**

DIOPTICON (Canada)
NAPHAZOLINE HYDROCHLORIDE
Albalon Ophthalmic Solution . . . . ⊙**216**

DIOSULF (Canada)
SULFACETAMIDE SODIUM
Klaron Lotion 10% **1050**

DIOVAN (Argentina, Austria, Brazil, Canada, Czech Republic, Denmark, Finland, Germany, Greece, Hong Kong, Hungary, India, Irish Republic, Israel, Malaysia, Mexico, New Zealand, Norway, Portugal, Russia, Singapore, South Africa, Spain, Sweden, Switzerland, Thailand, The Netherlands, United Kingdom)
VALSARTAN
Diovan Tablets **2191**

DIOVAN COMP (Denmark, Finland, Norway, Sweden)
HYDROCHLOROTHIAZIDE/VALSARTAN
Diovan HCT Tablets **2195**

DIOVAN D (Argentina)
VALSARTAN
Diovan Tablets **2191**

DIOVAN HCT (Brazil, Canada, Hungary, Mexico)
VALSARTAN
Diovan Tablets **2191**

DIOVANE (Belgium)
VALSARTAN
Diovan Tablets **2191**

DIOXAFLEX FORTE (Argentina)
DICLOFENAC SODIUM
Voltaren Tablets **2298**
Voltaren-XR Tablets **2301**

DIOXAFLEX GESIC (Argentina)
DICLOFENAC POTASSIUM
Cataflam Tablets **2173**

DIOXAFLEX PLUS (Argentina)
DICLOFENAC SODIUM
Voltaren Tablets **2298**
Voltaren-XR Tablets **2301**

DIPARENE (Belgium)
NAPROXEN
EC-Naprosyn Delayed-Release Tablets **2769**
Naprosyn Suspension **2769**
Naprosyn Tablets **2769**

DIPEDYNE (Mexico)
ZIDOVUDINE
Retrovir Capsules **1533**
Retrovir IV Infusion **1537**
Retrovir Syrup **1533**
Retrovir Tablets **1533**

DIPEZONA (Argentina)
DIAZEPAM
Diastat Rectal Delivery System **3344**
Valium Tablets **2822**

DIPHAR (France)
DIPYRIDAMOLE
Persantine Tablets **898**

DIPHOS (Germany)
ETIDRONATE DISODIUM
Didronel Tablets **2693**

DIPNI (Argentina)
NYSTATIN
Nystop Topical Powder USP **2490**

DIPRES (Mexico)
DIPYRIDAMOLE
Persantine Tablets **898**

DIPRIVAN (Argentina, Australia, Austria, Belgium, Brazil, Canada, Chile, Czech Republic, Denmark, Finland, France, Greece, Hong Kong, Hungary, Irish Republic, Israel, Italy, Malaysia, Mexico, New Zealand, Norway, Portugal, Russia, Singapore, South Africa, Spain, Sweden, Thailand, The Netherlands, United Kingdom)
PROPOFOL
Diprivan Injectable Emulsion **676**

DIPROFOL (Israel)
PROPOFOL
Diprivan Injectable Emulsion **676**

DI-PROMAL (Austria)
IPRATROPIUM BROMIDE
Atrovent Inhalation Solution **868**
Atrovent Nasal Spray 0.03% **869**
Atrovent Nasal Spray 0.06% **870**

DIPROX (Brazil)
LANSOPRAZOLE
Prevacid Delayed-Release Capsules **3268**

DIPSIN (Portugal)
FAMOTIDINE
Pepcid Injection **2017**
Pepcid Injection Premixed **2017**
Pepcid Tablets **2014**
Pepcid for Oral Suspension **2014**

DIPYRIDAN (Belgium)
DIPYRIDAMOLE
Persantine Tablets **898**

DIPYRIN (Finland)
DIPYRIDAMOLE
Persantine Tablets **898**

DIPYROL (South Africa)
DIPYRIDAMOLE
Persantine Tablets **898**

DIRINE (Malaysia, Singapore, Thailand)
FUROSEMIDE
Furosemide Tablets **2117**

DIRINOL (Mexico)
DIPYRIDAMOLE
Persantine Tablets **898**

DIROTON (Czech Republic, Russia)
LISINOPRIL
Prinivil Tablets **2029**
Zestril Tablets **704**

DIRRET (Mexico)
DICLOFENAC SODIUM
Voltaren Tablets **2298**
Voltaren-XR Tablets **2301**

DIRUNEZ (Greece)
NORFLOXACIN
Noroxin Tablets **2009**

DISCOID (Germany)
FUROSEMIDE
Furosemide Tablets **2117**

DISEL (Argentina)
NAPHAZOLINE HYDROCHLORIDE
Albalon Ophthalmic Solution . . . . ⊙**216**

DISEL HIDROCORTISONA (Argentina)
NAPHAZOLINE HYDROCHLORIDE
Albalon Ophthalmic Solution . . . . ⊙**216**

DISEQUENS (Argentina)
ESTRADIOL
Climara Transdermal System **795**
Vivelle Transdermal System **2288**
Vivelle-Dot Transdermal System **2293**

DISIPAN (Argentina)
DICLOFENAC SODIUM
Voltaren Tablets **2298**
Voltaren-XR Tablets **2301**

DISLIPINA (Portugal)
SIMVASTATIN
Zocor Tablets **2078**

DISLIPOR (Chile)
ATORVASTATIN CALCIUM
Lipitor Tablets **2495**

DISMAN SOBRES (Chile)
LACTULOSE
Kristalose for Oral Solution **2149**

DISMOLAN (Argentina)
ONDANSETRON HYDROCHLORIDE
Zofran Injection **1607**
Zofran Injection Premixed **1607**
Zofran Oral Solution **1613**
Zofran Tablets **1613**

DISNE ASMOL (Spain)
IPRATROPIUM BROMIDE
Atrovent Inhalation Solution **868**
Atrovent Nasal Spray 0.03% **869**
Atrovent Nasal Spray 0.06% **870**

DISOGRAM (United Kingdom)
DILTIAZEM HYDROCHLORIDE
Cardizem LA Extended Release Tablets . . . **1699**
Tiazac Capsules **1204**

DISOPAM (Israel)
DIAZEPAM
Diastat Rectal Delivery System **3344**
Valium Tablets **2822**

DISOPRIVAN (Germany, Switzerland)
PROPOFOL
Diprivan Injectable Emulsion **676**

DISPACLONIDIN (Germany)
CLONIDINE HYDROCHLORIDE
Catapres Tablets **874**

DISPAGENT (Germany)
GENTAMICIN SULFATE
Garamycin Injectable **3028**
Genoptic Sterile Ophthalmic Solution . . . . ⊙**227**

DISPASAN (Germany)
SODIUM HYALURONATE
Hyalgan Solution **2917**

DISPATIM (Austria, Germany)
TIMOLOL MALEATE
Blocadren Tablets **1891**
Timoptic Sterile Ophthalmic Solution **2058**
Timoptic in Ocudose **2061**
Timoptic-XE Sterile Ophthalmic Gel Forming Solution **2062**

DISPROMIL (Spain)
FAMOTIDINE
Pepcid Injection **2017**
Pepcid Injection Premixed **2017**
Pepcid Tablets **2014**
Pepcid for Oral Suspension **2014**

DISSENTEN (Czech Republic, Italy)
LOPERAMIDE HYDROCHLORIDE
Imodium Capsules **1834**

DISTALENE (Argentina)
ANASTROZOLE
Arimidex Tablets **665**

DISTAMINE (Austria, Irish Republic, New Zealand, The Netherlands, United Kingdom)
PENICILLAMINE
Cuprimine Capsules **1925**

DISTOBRAM (Portugal)
TOBRAMYCIN
TOBI Solution for Inhalation **1015**

DITENATE N (Germany)
THEOPHYLLINE
Uniphyl Tablets **2708**

DITENSIDE (Spain)
ENALAPRIL MALEATE/HYDROCHLOROTHIAZIDE
Vaseretic Tablets **2073**

DITENSOR (Spain)
ENALAPRIL MALEATE
Vasotec I.V. Injection **2076**

DITIZEM (Thailand)
DILTIAZEM HYDROCHLORIDE
Cardizem LA Extended Release Tablets . . . **1699**
Tiazac Capsules **1204**

DIU-ATENOLOL (Germany)
ATENOLOL
Tenormin I.V. Injection **698**

DIUBE (Italy)
ATENOLOL
Tenormin I.V. Injection **698**

DIUMIDE-K CONTINUS (United Kingdom)
FUROSEMIDE
Furosemide Tablets **2117**

DIURAL (Denmark, Norway, Sweden)
FUROSEMIDE
Furosemide Tablets **2117**

DIURAMIN (Finland)
AMILORIDE HYDROCHLORIDE/HYDROCHLOROTHIAZIDE
Moduretic Tablets **2003**

DIURAPID (Germany)
FUROSEMIDE
Furosemide Tablets **2117**

DIURENE (Portugal)
AMILORIDE HYDROCHLORIDE/HYDROCHLOROTHIAZIDE
Moduretic Tablets **2003**

DIURESAL (Switzerland)
FUROSEMIDE
Furosemide Tablets **2117**

DIURET (Brazil)
FUROSEMIDE
Furosemide Tablets **2117**

DIURETIKUM VERLA (Germany)
HYDROCHLOROTHIAZIDE/TRIAMTERENE
Dyazide Capsules **1389**

Maxzide Tablets 2150
Maxzide-25 mg Tablets 2150

DIUREX (Brazil, Finland)
AMILORIDE HYDROCHLORIDE/HYDROCHLOROTHIAZIDE
Moduretic Tablets 2003

DIUREX A (Argentina)
AMILORIDE HYDROCHLORIDE
Midamor Tablets 2000

DIURID (Austria)
HYDROCHLOROTHIAZIDE/TRIAMTERENE
Dyazide Capsules 1389
Maxzide Tablets 2150
Maxzide-25 mg Tablets 2150

DIURIN (New Zealand)
FUROSEMIDE
Furosemide Tablets 2117

DIURIT (Brazil)
FUROSEMIDE
Furosemide Tablets 2117

DIURIX (Brazil, Switzerland)
FUROSEMIDE
Furosemide Tablets 2117

DIUROLAN (Mexico)
FUROSEMIDE
Furosemide Tablets 2117

DIUROLASA (Spain)
FUROSEMIDE
Furosemide Tablets 2117

DIURSAN (Germany)
AMILORIDE HYDROCHLORIDE/HYDROCHLOROTHIAZIDE
Moduretic Tablets 2003

DIUTEC (South Africa)
AMILORIDE HYDROCHLORIDE/HYDROCHLOROTHIAZIDE
Moduretic Tablets 2003

DIUTENSAT (Germany)
HYDROCHLOROTHIAZIDE/TRIAMTERENE
Dyazide Capsules 1389
Maxzide Tablets 2150
Maxzide-25 mg Tablets 2150

DIU-TONOLYTRIL (Germany)
HYDROCHLOROTHIAZIDE/TRIAMTERENE
Dyazide Capsules 1389
Maxzide Tablets 2150
Maxzide-25 mg Tablets 2150

DIUZINE (Spain)
AMILORIDE HYDROCHLORIDE/HYDROCHLOROTHIAZIDE
Moduretic Tablets 2003

DIVANON (Chile)
CLINDAMYCIN PHOSPHATE
Clindets Pledgets 3212

DIVELOL (Brazil)
CARVEDILOL
Coreg Tablets 1376

DIVERMIL (Brazil)
MEBENDAZOLE
Vermox Chewable Tablets 1853

DIVIGEL (Czech Republic, Denmark, Finland, Hungary, Irish Republic, Malaysia, Singapore, Sweden, Switzerland, Thailand)
ESTRADIOL
Climara Transdermal System 795
Vivelle Transdermal System 2288
Vivelle-Dot Transdermal System .. 2293

DIXAMID (Greece)
INDAPAMIDE
Indapamide Tablets 2119

DIXARIT (Australia, Belgium, Canada, Germany, Hong Kong, Irish Republic, Malaysia, New Zealand, Singapore, South Africa, The Netherlands, United Kingdom)
CLONIDINE HYDROCHLORIDE
Catapres Tablets 874

DIZAN (Thailand)
DIAZEPAM
Diastat Rectal Delivery System .. 3344
Valium Tablets 2822

DIZEPAM (Thailand)
DIAZEPAM
Diastat Rectal Delivery System .. 3344
Valium Tablets 2822

DNAREN (Brazil)
DICLOFENAC SODIUM
Voltaren Tablets 2298
Voltaren-XR Tablets 2301

DOBUPAL (Spain)
VENLAFAXINE HYDROCHLORIDE
Effexor Tablets 3405
Effexor XR Capsules 3411

DOCEKEBIR (Argentina)
DOCETAXEL
Taxotere Injection Concentrate .. 2947

DOCETAX (India)
DOCETAXEL
Taxotere Injection Concentrate .. 2947

DOCITON (Germany)
PROPRANOLOL HYDROCHLORIDE
Inderal LA Long-Acting Capsules . 3421

DOCLIS (Spain)
DILTIAZEM HYDROCHLORIDE
Cardizem LA Extended Release Tablets ... 1699
Tiazac Capsules 1204

DOFEN (Mexico)
DICLOFENAC SODIUM
Voltaren Tablets 2298
Voltaren-XR Tablets 2301

DOFLEX (India)
DICLOFENAC SODIUM
Voltaren Tablets 2298
Voltaren-XR Tablets 2301

DOGOXINE (Mexico)
DIGOXIN
Lanoxicaps Capsules 1458
Lanoxin Injection 1462
Lanoxin Injection Pediatric 1465
Lanoxin Tablets 1468

DOLAK (Spain)
ISOSORBIDE MONONITRATE
Imdur Tablets 3032

DOLAUT (Italy)
DICLOFENAC SODIUM
Voltaren Tablets 2298
Voltaren-XR Tablets 2301

DOLCONTIN (Finland, Norway, Sweden)
MORPHINE SULFATE
Kadian Capsules 572
MS Contin Tablets 2703

DOLECTRAN (Argentina)
DOCETAXEL
Taxotere Injection Concentrate .. 2947

DOLFLAM (Mexico)
DICLOFENAC SODIUM
Voltaren Tablets 2298
Voltaren-XR Tablets 2301

DOLGIT-DICLO (Germany)
DICLOFENAC SODIUM
Voltaren Tablets 2298
Voltaren-XR Tablets 2301

DOLILUX (Italy)
RANITIDINE HYDROCHLORIDE
Zantac 25 EFFERdose Tablets 1597
Zantac 150 EFFERdose Tablets 1597
Zantac 150 Tablets 1597
Zantac 300 Tablets 1597
Zantac Injection 1593
Zantac Injection Premixed 1593
Zantac Syrup 1597

DOLISAL (Italy)
DIFLUNISAL
Dolobid Tablets 1937

DOLMIGRAL (Spain)
SUMATRIPTAN SUCCINATE
Imitrex Injection 1431
Imitrex Tablets 1440

DOLMINA (Czech Republic)
DICLOFENAC SODIUM
Voltaren Tablets 2298
Voltaren-XR Tablets 2301

DOLNAXEN (Mexico)
NAPROXEN
EC-Naprosyn Delayed-Release Tablets .. 2769
Naprosyn Suspension 2769
Naprosyn Tablets 2769

DOLO NERVOBION (Spain)
DICLOFENAC SODIUM
Voltaren Tablets 2298
Voltaren-XR Tablets 2301

DOLOATRIXEN (Mexico)
NAPROXEN
EC-Naprosyn Delayed-Release Tablets 2769
Naprosyn Suspension 2769
Naprosyn Tablets 2769

DOLOBASAN (Germany)
DICLOFENAC SODIUM
Voltaren Tablets 2298
Voltaren-XR Tablets 2301

DOLOBID (Australia, Canada, Hong Kong, Irish Republic, Israel, Italy, Mexico, Portugal, South Africa, Spain, Thailand, United Kingdom)
DIFLUNISAL
Dolobid Tablets 1937

DOLOBIS (France)
DIFLUNISAL
Dolobid Tablets 1937

DOLOCID (The Netherlands)
DIFLUNISAL
Dolobid Tablets 1937

DOLOCIDE K (India)
DICLOFENAC POTASSIUM
Cataflam Tablets 2173

DOLOCIDE KP (India)
DICLOFENAC POTASSIUM
Cataflam Tablets 2173

DOLONOVAG (Argentina)
HYDROMORPHONE HYDROCHLORIDE
Dilaudid Ampules 439
Dilaudid Multiple Dose Vials 439
Dilaudid Non-Sterile Powder 439
Dilaudid Oral Liquid 443
Dilaudid Rectal Suppositories 439
Dilaudid Tablets 439
Dilaudid Tablets - 8 mg 443
Dilaudid-HP Injection 441
Dilaudid-HP Lyophilized Powder 250 mg 441

DOLORMIN MIT NAPROXEN (Germany)
NAPROXEN
EC-Naprosyn Delayed-Release Tablets 2769
Naprosyn Suspension 2769
Naprosyn Tablets 2769

DOLOTANDAX (Mexico)
NAPROXEN SODIUM
Anaprox DS Tablets 2769
Anaprox Tablets 2769

DOLOVISANO DICLO (Germany)
DICLOFENAC SODIUM
Voltaren Tablets 2298
Voltaren-XR Tablets 2301

DOLO-VOLTAREN (Spain)
DICLOFENAC SODIUM
Voltaren Tablets 2298
Voltaren-XR Tablets 2301

DOLPASSE (Austria)
DICLOFENAC SODIUM
Voltaren Tablets 2298
Voltaren-XR Tablets 2301

DOLSINAL (Spain)
NABUMETONE
Relafen Tablets 1523

DOLTARD (Czech Republic, Denmark)
MORPHINE SULFATE
Kadian Capsules 572
MS Contin Tablets 2703

DOLVAN (Argentina)
DICLOFENAC SODIUM
Voltaren Tablets 2298
Voltaren-XR Tablets 2301

DOLXEN (Mexico)
NAPROXEN
EC-Naprosyn Delayed-Release Tablets 2769
Naprosyn Suspension 2769
Naprosyn Tablets 2769

DOMNAMID (Denmark)
ESTAZOLAM
ProSom Tablets 512

DONAPROX (Mexico)
NAPROXEN
EC-Naprosyn Delayed-Release Tablets .. 2769
Naprosyn Suspension 2769
Naprosyn Tablets 2769

DONATAXEL (Argentina)
DOCETAXEL
Taxotere Injection Concentrate .. 2947

DONAZ (India)
DONEPEZIL HYDROCHLORIDE
Aricept Tablets 1086

DONECEPT (India)
DONEPEZIL HYDROCHLORIDE
Aricept Tablets 1086

DONEKA (Spain)
LISINOPRIL
Prinivil Tablets 2029
Zestril Tablets 704

DONEKA PLUS (Spain)
HYDROCHLOROTHIAZIDE/LISINOPRIL
Prinzide Tablets 2033
Zestoretic Tablets 701

DONICER (Spain)
AMILORIDE HYDROCHLORIDE/HYDROCHLOROTHIAZIDE
Moduretic Tablets 2003

DONOBID (Denmark, Finland, Norway, Sweden)
DIFLUNISAL
Dolobid Tablets 1937

DOPSAN (Thailand)
DAPSONE
Dapsone Tablets USP 1656

DORANOL (Spain)
ERYTHROMYCIN STEARATE
Erythrocin Stearate Filmtab Tablets 452

DORBID (Brazil)
DIFLUNISAL
Dolobid Tablets 1937

DORCALOR (Portugal)
DICLOFENAC SODIUM
Voltaren Tablets 2298
Voltaren-XR Tablets 2301

DORGEN (Brazil)
DICLOFENAC SODIUM
Voltaren Tablets 2298
Voltaren-XR Tablets 2301

DORICOFLU (Italy)
FLUNISOLIDE
Aerobid Inhaler System 1172
Aerobid-M Inhaler System 1172
Nasarel Nasal Spray 1652

DORIMAN (Spain)
CIPROFLOXACIN HYDROCHLORIDE
Ciloxan Ophthalmic Ointment 554
Ciloxan Ophthalmic Solution ...... ⊙205
Cipro Tablets 2991

DORLAMIDA (Argentina)
DORZOLAMIDE HYDROCHLORIDE
Trusopt Sterile Ophthalmic Solution .. 2065

DORLAMIDA T (Argentina)
DORZOLAMIDE HYDROCHLORIDE
Trusopt Sterile Ophthalmic Solution .. 2065

DORMODOR (Spain)
FLURAZEPAM HYDROCHLORIDE
Dalmane Capsules 3343

DOROXAN (Italy)
DICLOFENAC SODIUM
Voltaren Tablets 2298
Voltaren-XR Tablets 2301

DORPANE (Thailand)
ORPHENADRINE CITRATE
Norflex Injection 1824

DORPIEL (Argentina)
TRETINOIN
Avita Cream 2136
Avita Gel 2138
Renova 0.05% Cream 2387
Retin-A Micro 0.1%/0.04% 2388
Vesanoid Capsules 2823

DORPIREN (Brazil)
DICLOFENAC POTASSIUM
Cataflam Tablets 2173

DORSOF T (Chile)
DORZOLAMIDE HYDROCHLORIDE/TIMOLOL MALEATE
Cosopt Sterile Ophthalmic Solution 1910

DORZOFLAX (Argentina)
DORZOLAMIDE HYDROCHLORIDE
Trusopt Sterile Ophthalmic Solution 2065

DORZONE (Brazil)
ORPHENADRINE CITRATE
Norflex Injection 1824

DORZOX (India)
DORZOLAMIDE HYDROCHLORIDE
Trusopt Sterile Ophthalmic Solution 2065

DOSIER (Argentina, Chile)
TICLOPIDINE HYDROCHLORIDE
Ticlid Tablets 2813

DOSTINEX (Argentina, Australia, Austria, Belgium, Brazil, Canada, Chile, Czech Republic, Denmark, Finland, France, Germany, Greece, Hong Kong, Irish Republic, Israel, Italy, Malaysia, Mexico, New Zealand, Norway, Portugal, Singapore, South Africa, Spain, Sweden, Switzerland, The Netherlands, United Kingdom)
CABERGOLINE
Dostinex Tablets 2631

DOTALSEC (Argentina)
LOPERAMIDE HYDROCHLORIDE
Imodium Capsules 1834

DOVAL (South Africa)
DIAZEPAM
Diastat Rectal Delivery System 3344
Valium Tablets 2822

DOVATE (South Africa)
CLOBETASOL PROPIONATE
Temovate Cream 1549
Temovate E Emollient 1552
Temovate Gel 1550
Temovate Ointment 1549
Temovate Scalp Application 1551

DOXAPRIL (Argentina)
LISINOPRIL
Prinivil Tablets 2029
Zestril Tablets 704

DOXETAL (Argentina)
DOCETAXEL
Taxotere Injection Concentrate 2947

DOXMIL (Argentina)
DOCETAXEL
Taxotere Injection Concentrate 2947

DOXTRAN FLEX (Argentina)
DICLOFENAC SODIUM
Voltaren Tablets 2298
Voltaren-XR Tablets 2301

DOZIC (Argentina)
RISPERIDONE
Risperdal Oral Solution 1658
Risperdal Tablets 1658

DP GESIC (India)
DICLOFENAC SODIUM
Voltaren Tablets 2298
Voltaren-XR Tablets 2301

DP HYDROCORTISONE (New Zealand)
HYDROCORTISONE
Hydrocortone Tablets 1963

D-PAM (New Zealand)
DIAZEPAM
Diastat Rectal Delivery System 3344
Valium Tablets 2822

D-PENAMINE (Australia, New Zealand)
PENICILLAMINE
Cuprimine Capsules 1925

DRAXON (Portugal)
FLUTAMIDE
Eulexin Capsules 3023

DRENIAN (Spain)
DIAZEPAM
Diastat Rectal Delivery System 3344
Valium Tablets 2822

DRIKEN (Mexico)
IRON DEXTRAN
Infed Injection 3381

DRILYNA (Argentina)
THEOPHYLLINE
Uniphyl Tablets 2708

DRIVERMIDE (Thailand)
MEBENDAZOLE
Vermox Chewable Tablets 1853

DROGENIL (Chile, Irish Republic, Italy, The Netherlands, United Kingdom)
FLUTAMIDE
Eulexin Capsules 3023

DROLASONA (Spain)
FLUTICASONE PROPIONATE
Cutivate Cream 1381
Cutivate Ointment 1384
Flonase Nasal Spray 1412

DRONAL (Italy)
ALENDRONATE SODIUM
Fosamax Tablets 1949

DRONATE-OS (India)
ETIDRONATE DISODIUM
Didronel Tablets 2693

DROPICINE (Argentina)
RISPERIDONE
Risperdal Oral Solution 1658
Risperdal Tablets 1658

DROPSTAR (Argentina, Italy)
SODIUM HYALURONATE
Hyalgan Solution 2917

DROPTIMOL (Italy)
TIMOLOL MALEATE
Blocadren Tablets 1891
Timoptic Sterile Ophthalmic Solution 2058
Timoptic in Ocudose 2061
Timoptic-XE Sterile Ophthalmic Gel Forming Solution 2062

DROSTEAKARD (Germany)
VERAPAMIL HYDROCHLORIDE
Covera-HS Tablets 3135
Verelan PM Capsules 3120

DRY & CLEAR (South Africa)
BENZOYL PEROXIDE
Brevoxyl-4 Creamy Wash 3212
Brevoxyl-4 Gel 3211
Brevoxyl-8 Creamy Wash 3212
Brevoxyl-8 Gel 3211
Triaz Cleanser 1864
Triaz Gel 1864

DRYPTAL (Czech Republic, Hong Kong, Irish Republic, United Kingdom)
FUROSEMIDE
Furosemide Tablets 2117

D-STOP (Germany)
LOPERAMIDE HYDROCHLORIDE
Imodium Capsules 1834

D-TATO (Mexico)
BENZONATATE
Tessalon Perles 1202

D-TRIOL (Greece)
CALCITRIOL
Calcijex Injection 411

DUAC ONCE DAILY (United Kingdom)
BENZOYL PEROXIDE
Brevoxyl-4 Creamy Wash 3212
Brevoxyl-4 Gel 3211
Brevoxyl-8 Creamy Wash 3212
Brevoxyl-8 Gel 3211
Triaz Cleanser 1864
Triaz Gel 1864

DUALIZOL (Mexico)
METRONIDAZOLE
MetroGel-Vaginal Gel 1822
Noritate Cream, 1% 1051

DUALTEN (Chile)
CARVEDILOL
Coreg Tablets 1376

DUBAGEST (India)
PROGESTERONE
Prometrium Capsules (100 mg, 200 mg) 3205

DUBE (Singapore)
LIDOCAINE
Lidoderm Patch 1107

DUCENE (Australia)
DIAZEPAM
Diastat Rectal Delivery System 3344
Valium Tablets 2822

DUCTELMIN (Brazil)
MEBENDAZOLE
Vermox Chewable Tablets 1853

DUCTONAR (Argentina)
RISEDRONATE SODIUM
Actonel Tablets 2679

DUCTOPRIL (Brazil)
CAPTOPRIL
Captopril Tablets 2114

DULAX (Irish Republic)
LACTULOSE
Kristalose for Oral Solution 2149

DUMOZOL (Portugal)
METRONIDAZOLE
MetroGel-Vaginal Gel 1822
Noritate Cream, 1% 1051

DUNCANKIL (Argentina)
PERMETHRIN
Acticin Cream 2125

DUNOX (Argentina)
AMOXICILLIN
Amoxil Pediatric Drops for Oral Suspension 1315
Amoxil Tablets 1315

DUO MINOXI (Argentina)
KETOCONAZOLE
Nizoral 2% Shampoo 1838

DUOBLOC (Argentina)
CARVEDILOL
Coreg Tablets 1376

DUOFLEX (Mexico)
DICLOFENAC SODIUM
Voltaren Tablets 2298
Voltaren-XR Tablets 2301

DUOGASTRIL (Spain)
CIMETIDINE
Tagamet Tablets 1547

DUOKLIMAN (Austria)
ESTRADIOL
Climara Transdermal System 795
Vivelle Transdermal System 2288
Vivelle-Dot Transdermal System 2293

DUOLAX (Spain)
LACTULOSE
Kristalose for Oral Solution 2149

DUOLIN (New Zealand)
IPRATROPIUM BROMIDE
Atrovent Inhalation Solution 868
Atrovent Nasal Spray 0.03% 869
Atrovent Nasal Spray 0.06% 870

DUOMET (Brazil, New Zealand, South Africa)
CIMETIDINE
Tagamet Tablets 1547

DUONASE (India)
AZELASTINE HYDROCHLORIDE
Astelin Nasal Spray 1876

DUORAN (Italy)
RANITIDINE HYDROCHLORIDE
Zantac 25 EFFERdose Tablets 1597
Zantac 150 EFFERdose Tablets 1597
Zantac 150 Tablets 1597
Zantac 300 Tablets 1597
Zantac Injection 1593
Zantac Injection Premixed 1593
Zantac Syrup 1597

DUOTRIC (Thailand)
CIMETIDINE
Tagamet Tablets 1547

DUOVIR (Brazil, India, South Africa)
LAMIVUDINE
Epivir Oral Solution 1394
Epivir Tablets 1394
Epivir-HBV Oral Solution 1398
Epivir-HBV Tablets 1398

DUOVIR N (India)
LAMIVUDINE
Epivir Oral Solution 1394
Epivir Tablets 1394
Epivir-HBV Oral Solution 1398
Epivir-HBV Tablets 1398

DUPHALAC (Australia, Austria, Belgium, Canada, Chile, Czech Republic, Finland, France, Greece, Hong Kong, Hungary, India, Irish Republic, Italy, Malaysia, New Zealand, Norway, Portugal, Russia, Singapore, South Africa, Spain, Sweden, Switzerland, Thailand, The Netherlands, United Kingdom)
LACTULOSE
Kristalose for Oral Solution 2149

DUPLAMIN (Italy)
PROMETHAZINE HYDROCHLORIDE
Phenergan Suppositories 3438
Phenergan Tablets 3438

DURACRALFAT (Germany)
SUCRALFATE
Carafate Suspension 727
Carafate Tablets 728

DURACTIN (Australia)
CIMETIDINE
Tagamet Tablets 1547

DURADIAZEPAM (Germany)
DIAZEPAM
Diastat Rectal Delivery System 3344
Valium Tablets 2822

DURADIURET (Germany)
HYDROCHLOROTHIAZIDE/TRIAMTERENE
Dyazide Capsules 1389
Maxzide Tablets 2150
Maxzide-25 mg Tablets 2150

DURAERYTHROMYCIN (Germany)
ERYTHROMYCIN STEARATE
Erythrocin Stearate Filmtab Tablets 452

DURAFENAT (Germany)
FENOFIBRATE
Tricor Tablets 523

DURAFUNGOL (Germany)
CLOTRIMAZOLE
Lotrimin Cream 3053
Lotrimin Lotion 1% 3053
Lotrimin Topical Solution 1% 3053

DURAFURID (Germany)
FUROSEMIDE
Furosemide Tablets 2117

DURAGENTAM (Germany)
GENTAMICIN SULFATE
Garamycin Injectable 3028
Genoptic Sterile Ophthalmic Solution ..... ⊙227

DURAGENTAMICIN (Germany)
GENTAMICIN SULFATE
Garamycin Injectable 3028
Genoptic Sterile Ophthalmic Solution ..... ⊙227

DURAGESIC (Canada)
FENTANYL
Duragesic Transdermal System 2448

DURAH2 (Germany)
CIMETIDINE
Tagamet Tablets 1547

DURALGIN (Denmark)
MORPHINE SULFATE
Kadian Capsules 572
MS Contin Tablets 2703

DURALITH (Canada)
LITHIUM CARBONATE
Eskalith CR Controlled-Release Tablets 1406
Eskalith Capsules 1406

DURALMOR (Mexico)
MORPHINE SULFATE
Kadian Capsules 572
MS Contin Tablets 2703

DURALOPID (Germany)
LOPERAMIDE HYDROCHLORIDE
Imodium Capsules 1834

DURAMONITAT (Germany)
ISOSORBIDE MONONITRATE
Imdur Tablets 3032

DURAMORPH (Argentina)
MORPHINE SULFATE
Kadian Capsules 572
MS Contin Tablets 2703

DURANIFIN (Germany)
NIFEDIPINE
Adalat CC Tablets 2978

(⊙ Described in PDR For Ophthalmic Medicines™)

DURANIFIN SALI (Germany)
NIFEDIPINE
Adalat CC Tablets 2978

DURANOL (Irish Republic)
PROPRANOLOL HYDROCHLORIDE
Inderal LA Long-Acting Capsules 3421

DURAPHYLLIN (Germany)
THEOPHYLLINE
Uniphyl Tablets 2708

DURARESE (Germany)
AMILORIDE HYDROCHLORIDE/HYDROCHLOROTHIAZIDE
Moduretic Tablets 2003

DURASOPTIN (Germany)
VERAPAMIL HYDROCHLORIDE
Covera-HS Tablets 3135
Verelan PM Capsules 3120

DURATENOL (Germany)
ATENOLOL
Tenormin I.V. Injection 698

DURATENOL COMP (Germany)
ATENOLOL
Tenormin I.V. Injection 698

DURATER (Mexico)
FAMOTIDINE
Pepcid Injection 2017
Pepcid Injection Premixed 2017
Pepcid Tablets 2014
Pepcid for Oral Suspension 2014

DURATIMOL (Germany)
TIMOLOL MALEATE
Blocadren Tablets 1891
Timoptic Sterile Ophthalmic Solution 2058
Timoptic in Ocudose 2061
Timoptic-XE Sterile Ophthalmic Gel Forming Solution 2062

DURAVOLTEN (Germany)
DICLOFENAC SODIUM
Voltaren Tablets 2298
Voltaren-XR Tablets 2301

DURA-ZOK (Denmark)
METOPROLOL SUCCINATE
Toprol-XL Tablets 660

DUREKAL (Finland)
POTASSIUM CHLORIDE
K-Dur Extended-Relase Tablets 3047
K-Lor Powder Packets 472
K-Tab Filmtab Tablets 473

DUREMID (Argentina)
INDAPAMIDE
Indapamide Tablets 2119

DURIDE (Australia, New Zealand)
ISOSORBIDE MONONITRATE
Imdur Tablets 3032

DUROGESIC (Argentina, Australia, Austria, Belgium, Brazil, Chile, Czech Republic, Denmark, Finland, France, Germany, Greece, Hong Kong, Hungary, India, Irish Republic, Israel, Italy, Malaysia, Mexico, New Zealand, Norway, Portugal, Russia, Singapore, South Africa, Spain, Sweden, Switzerland, Thailand, The Netherlands, United Kingdom)
FENTANYL
Duragesic Transdermal System 2448

DURO-K (Australia)
POTASSIUM CHLORIDE
K-Dur Extended-Relase Tablets 3047
K-Lor Powder Packets 472
K-Tab Filmtab Tablets 473

DURONITRIN (Italy)
ISOSORBIDE MONONITRATE
Imdur Tablets 3032

DUXIMA (Italy)
CEFUROXIME SODIUM
Zinacef Injection 1604

D-VOID (India)
DESMOPRESSIN ACETATE
DDAVP Injection 4 mcg/mL 2893
DDAVP Nasal Spray 2894
DDAVP Tablets 2895
Desmopressin Acetate Injection 1143
Desmopressin Acetate Rhinal Tube 1144

D-WORM (South Africa)
MEBENDAZOLE
Vermox Chewable Tablets 1853

DYAZIDE (Canada, Hong Kong, Irish Republic, Mexico, New Zealand, Portugal, Singapore, South Africa, Switzerland)
HYDROCHLOROTHIAZIDE/TRIAMTERENE
Dyazide Capsules 1389
Maxzide Tablets 2150
Maxzide-25 mg Tablets 2150

DYNABLOK (South Africa)
PROPRANOLOL HYDROCHLORIDE
Inderal LA Long-Acting Capsules 3421

DYNACIRC (Argentina, Canada, Chile, Hong Kong, Malaysia, Mexico, New Zealand, Singapore, South Africa, Thailand)
ISRADIPINE
DynaCirc CR Tablets 2726

DYNAFLOC (South Africa)
CIPROFLOXACIN
Cipro Oral Suspension 2991

DYNAMETRON (South Africa)
METRONIDAZOLE
MetroGel-Vaginal Gel 1822
Noritate Cream, 1% 1051

DYNAMIN (United Kingdom)
ISOSORBIDE MONONITRATE
Imdur Tablets 3032

DYNAPAM (South Africa)
DIAZEPAM
Diastat Rectal Delivery System 3344
Valium Tablets 2822

DYNASPOR (South Africa)
CLOTRIMAZOLE
Lotrimin Cream 3053
Lotrimin Lotion 1% 3053
Lotrimin Topical Solution 1% 3053

DYRENIUM (Canada, Switzerland)
TRIAMTERENE
Dyrenium Capsules 3390

DYSALFA (France)
TERAZOSIN HYDROCHLORIDE
Hytrin Capsules 469

DYSMENALGIT (Germany)
NAPROXEN
EC-Naprosyn Delayed-Release Tablets 2769
Naprosyn Suspension 2769
Naprosyn Tablets 2769

DYSPAGON (France)
LOPERAMIDE HYDROCHLORIDE
Imodium Capsules 1834

DYSPAMET (Irish Republic, United Kingdom)
CIMETIDINE
Tagamet Tablets 1547

DYTAC (Australia, Belgium, Irish Republic, The Netherlands, United Kingdom)
TRIAMTERENE
Dyrenium Capsules 3390

DYTA-URESE (Belgium, The Netherlands)
TRIAMTERENE
Dyrenium Capsules 3390

DYTENZIDE (Belgium, The Netherlands)
TRIAMTERENE
Dyrenium Capsules 3390

DYTERENE (Thailand)
HYDROCHLOROTHIAZIDE/TRIAMTERENE
Dyazide Capsules 1389
Maxzide Tablets 2150
Maxzide-25 mg Tablets 2150

DYTIDE H (Austria, Germany)
HYDROCHLOROTHIAZIDE/TRIAMTERENE
Dyazide Capsules 1389
Maxzide Tablets 2150
Maxzide-25 mg Tablets 2150

EASY DAYZ (India)
NAPROXEN SODIUM
Anaprox DS Tablets 2769
Anaprox Tablets 2769

EBERSEPT (Greece)
KETOCONAZOLE
Nizoral 2% Shampoo 1838

EBOREN (The Netherlands)
ERYTHROMYCIN
Ery-Tab Tablets 447
Erythromycin Base Filmtab Tablets 454
Erythromycin Delayed-Release Capsules, USP 456
PCE Dispertab Tablets 510

ECALIN (Russia)
ECONAZOLE NITRATE
Spectazole Cream 2390

ECAMAIS (Portugal)
LISINOPRIL
Prinivil Tablets 2029
Zestril Tablets 704

ECANOL (India)
ECONAZOLE NITRATE
Spectazole Cream 2390

ECAPRESAN (Mexico)
CAPTOPRIL
Captopril Tablets 2114

ECAPRIL (Mexico, Portugal)
CAPTOPRIL
Captopril Tablets 2114

ECATEN (Mexico)
CAPTOPRIL
Captopril Tablets 2114

ECLARAN (Argentina, Czech Republic, France, Portugal)
BENZOYL PEROXIDE
Brevoxyl-4 Creamy Wash 3212
Brevoxyl-4 Gel 3211
Brevoxyl-8 Creamy Wash 3212
Brevoxyl-8 Gel 3211
Triaz Cleanser 1864
Triaz Gel 1864

ECNAGEL PB (Argentina)
BENZOYL PEROXIDE
Brevoxyl-4 Creamy Wash 3212
Brevoxyl-4 Gel 3211
Brevoxyl-8 Creamy Wash 3212
Brevoxyl-8 Gel 3211
Triaz Cleanser 1864
Triaz Gel 1864

ECO MI (Italy)
ECONAZOLE NITRATE
Spectazole Cream 2390

ECOCORT (Malaysia)
ECONAZOLE NITRATE
Spectazole Cream 2390

ECODERGIN (Italy)
ECONAZOLE NITRATE
Spectazole Cream 2390

ECODERM (Malaysia, Singapore, South Africa)
ECONAZOLE NITRATE
Spectazole Cream 2390

ECODIPINE (Switzerland)
NIFEDIPINE
Adalat CC Tablets 2978

ECODUREX (Switzerland)
AMILORIDE HYDROCHLORIDE/HYDROCHLOROTHIAZIDE
Moduretic Tablets 2003

ECOFENAC (Switzerland)
DICLOFENAC SODIUM
Voltaren Tablets 2298
Voltaren-XR Tablets 2301

ECOLINE (Greece)
CEFUROXIME AXETIL
Ceftin Tablets 1369
Ceftin for Oral Suspension 1369

ECON (Thailand)
ECONAZOLE NITRATE
Spectazole Cream 2390

ECONAC (United Kingdom)
DICLOFENAC SODIUM
Voltaren Tablets 2298
Voltaren-XR Tablets 2301

ECONACORT (United Kingdom)
ECONAZOLE NITRATE
Spectazole Cream 2390

ECONAL-C (South Africa)
ECONAZOLE NITRATE
Spectazole Cream 2390

ECONAZINE (Malaysia, Singapore)
ECONAZOLE NITRATE
Spectazole Cream 2390

ECONITE (Hong Kong)
ECONAZOLE NITRATE
Spectazole Cream 2390

ECOPACE (United Kingdom)
CAPTOPRIL
Captopril Tablets 2114

E-COR (Czech Republic)
ENALAPRIL MALEATE
Vasotec I.V. Injection 2076

ECOREX (Italy)
ECONAZOLE NITRATE
Spectazole Cream 2390

ECOSONE (Hong Kong)
ECONAZOLE NITRATE
Spectazole Cream 2390

ECOSTATIN (Australia, Canada, Irish Republic, New Zealand, United Kingdom)
ECONAZOLE NITRATE
Spectazole Cream 2390

ECOSTERIL (Italy)
ECONAZOLE NITRATE
Spectazole Cream 2390

ECOTAM (Spain)
ECONAZOLE NITRATE
Spectazole Cream 2390

ECREME (New Zealand)
ECONAZOLE NITRATE
Spectazole Cream 2390

ECRINAL (Spain)
FLECAINIDE ACETATE
Tambocor Tablets 1824

ECTIVA (Italy, Mexico)
SIBUTRAMINE HYDROCHLORIDE
Meridia Capsules 485

ECURAL (Germany)
MOMETASONE FUROATE
Elocon Cream 0.1% 3019
Elocon Lotion 0.1% 3020
Elocon Ointment 0.1% 3021
Nasonex Nasal Spray 3058

EDALEN (Argentina)
RISPERIDONE
Risperdal Oral Solution 1658
Risperdal Tablets 1658

EDASON (Greece)
CLINDAMYCIN PHOSPHATE
Clindets Pledgets 3212

EDENOL (Mexico)
FUROSEMIDE
Furosemide Tablets 2117

EDEX (France, Greece)
ALPROSTADIL
Edex Injection 3103

EDICIN (Czech Republic, Hungary, Thailand)
VANCOMYCIN HYDROCHLORIDE
Vancocin HCl Capsules, USP 3370

EDICTUM (Argentina)
CLONAZEPAM
Klonopin Tablets 2782

EDIP (India)
NIFEDIPINE
Adalat CC Tablets 2978

EDISTOL (Spain)
ISOSORBIDE MONONITRATE
Imdur Tablets 3032

EDNYT (Czech Republic, Hungary, Irish Republic, Russia, United Kingdom)
ENALAPRIL MALEATE
Vasotec I.V. Injection 2076

EDOLGLAU (Portugal)
CLONIDINE HYDROCHLORIDE
Catapres Tablets 874

EFAVILEA (Argentina)
EFAVIRENZ
Sustiva Capsules 957

EFAVIR (India)
EFAVIRENZ
Sustiva Capsules 957

EFCORLIN (India)
HYDROCORTISONE
Hydrocortone Tablets . . . 1963

EFCORTELAN (United Kingdom)
HYDROCORTISONE
Hydrocortone Tablets . . . 1963

EFECTIN (Austria, Czech Republic, Hungary)
VENLAFAXINE HYDROCHLORIDE
Effexor Tablets . . . 3405
Effexor XR Capsules . . . 3411

EFEKTOLOL (Germany)
PROPRANOLOL HYDROCHLORIDE
Inderal LA Long-Acting Capsules . . . 3421

EFEMOLINA (Argentina)
FLUOROMETHOLONE
FML Ophthalmic Ointment . . . ⊙225

EFEROX (Germany)
LEVOTHYROXINE SODIUM
Levothroid Tablets . . . 1189
Levoxyl Tablets . . . 1680
Synthroid Tablets . . . 515

EFEROX JOD (Germany)
LEVOTHYROXINE SODIUM
Levothroid Tablets . . . 1189
Levoxyl Tablets . . . 1680
Synthroid Tablets . . . 515

EFEXOR (Argentina, Australia, Austria, Belgium, Brazil, Chile, Denmark, Finland, Greece, Hong Kong, Irish Republic, Israel, Italy, Malaysia, Mexico, New Zealand, Norway, Portugal, Singapore, South Africa, Switzerland, Thailand, The Netherlands, United Kingdom)
VENLAFAXINE HYDROCHLORIDE
Effexor Tablets . . . 3405
Effexor XR Capsules . . . 3411

EFEXOR XR (Greece)
VENLAFAXINE HYDROCHLORIDE
Effexor Tablets . . . 3405
Effexor XR Capsules . . . 3411

EFFACNE (France, Switzerland)
BENZOYL PEROXIDE
Brevoxyl-4 Creamy Wash . . . 3212
Brevoxyl-4 Gel . . . 3211
Brevoxyl-8 Creamy Wash . . . 3212
Brevoxyl-8 Gel . . . 3211
Triaz Cleanser . . . 1864
Triaz Gel . . . 1864

EFFECTSAL (Singapore)
NORFLOXACIN
Noroxin Tablets . . . 2009

EFFEDERM (France)
TRETINOIN
Avita Cream . . . 2136
Avita Gel . . . 2138
Renova 0.05% Cream . . . 2387
Retin-A Micro 0.1%/0.04% . . . 2388
Vesanoid Capsules . . . 2823

EFFEKTON (Germany)
DICLOFENAC SODIUM
Voltaren Tablets . . . 2298
Voltaren-XR Tablets . . . 2301

EFFEXOR (Canada)
VENLAFAXINE HYDROCHLORIDE
Effexor Tablets . . . 3405
Effexor XR Capsules . . . 3411

EFFLUMIDEX (Czech Republic, Germany, Hungary)
FLUOROMETHOLONE
FML Ophthalmic Ointment . . . ⊙225

EFFOX (Czech Republic)
ISOSORBIDE MONONITRATE
Imdur Tablets . . . 3032

EFIXANO (Argentina)
IRINOTECAN HYDROCHLORIDE
Camptosar Injection . . . 2602

EFLORAN (Czech Republic)
METRONIDAZOLE
MetroGel-Vaginal Gel . . . 1822
Noritate Cream, 1% . . . 1051

EFUDEX (Canada)
FLUOROURACIL
Efudex Topical Cream . . . 3348
Efudex Topical Solutions . . . 3348

EFUDIX (Argentina, Australia, Belgium, France, Germany, Hong Kong, Hungary, Irish Republic, Israel, Italy, Mexico, Irish Republic, Singapore, South Africa, Spain, Switzerland, Thailand, The Netherlands, United Kingdom)
FLUOROURACIL
Efudex Topical Cream . . . 3348
Efudex Topical Solutions . . . 3348

EFURIX (Brazil)
FLUOROURACIL
Efudex Topical Cream . . . 3348
Efudex Topical Solutions . . . 3348

EGERY (France)
ERYTHROMYCIN
Ery-Tab Tablets . . . 447
Erythromycin Base Filmtab Tablets . . . 454
Erythromycin Delayed-Release Capsules, USP . . . 456
PCE Dispertab Tablets . . . 510

EGIBREN (Italy)
SELEGILINE HYDROCHLORIDE
Eldepryl Capsules . . . 3209

EGIFILIN (Hungary)
THEOPHYLLINE
Uniphyl Tablets . . . 2708

EGLANDIN (Singapore)
ALPROSTADIL
Edex Injection . . . 3103

EGLIDON (Argentina)
TERAZOSIN HYDROCHLORIDE
Hytrin Capsules . . . 469

EGOCORT (Australia, Hong Kong, Malaysia, New Zealand, Singapore)
HYDROCORTISONE
Hydrocortone Tablets . . . 1963

EHLIFUNG (Mexico)
KETOCONAZOLE
Nizoral 2% Shampoo . . . 1838

EHLITEN (Mexico)
PRAZIQUANTEL
Biltricide Tablets . . . 2990

EHLIXACIN (Mexico)
CIPROFLOXACIN
Cipro Oral Suspension . . . 2991

EIFEL (Greece)
BETAXOLOL HYDROCHLORIDE
Betoptic S Ophthalmic Suspension . . . 554

EINALAT (Austria)
NIFEDIPINE
Adalat CC Tablets . . . 2978

EISMYCIN (Germany)
MUPIROCIN
Bactroban Ointment . . . 1358

ELAFAX (Argentina)
VENLAFAXINE HYDROCHLORIDE
Effexor Tablets . . . 3405
Effexor XR Capsules . . . 3411

ELAN (Italy)
ISOSORBIDE MONONITRATE
Imdur Tablets . . . 3032

ELANDUR (Argentina)
ALENDRONATE SODIUM
Fosamax Tablets . . . 1949

ELANTAN (Austria, Germany, Hong Kong, Irish Republic, Malaysia, Mexico, Singapore, South Africa, Switzerland, Thailand, United Kingdom)
ISOSORBIDE MONONITRATE
Imdur Tablets . . . 3032

ELANVER (Greece)
VERAPAMIL HYDROCHLORIDE
Covera-HS Tablets . . . 3135
Verelan PM Capsules . . . 3120

ELBAT (Greece)
FLUTAMIDE
Eulexin Capsules . . . 3023

ELBROL (Germany)
PROPRANOLOL HYDROCHLORIDE
Inderal LA Long-Acting Capsules . . . 3421

ELCAR (Russia)
LEVOCARNITINE
Carnitor Injection . . . 3185
Carnitor Tablets and Oral Solution . . . 3187

ELCION (India)
DIAZEPAM
Diastat Rectal Delivery System . . . 3344
Valium Tablets . . . 2822

ELCOMAN (Argentina)
LOPERAMIDE HYDROCHLORIDE
Imodium Capsules . . . 1834

ELDEPRINE (France)
SELEGILINE HYDROCHLORIDE
Eldepryl Capsules . . . 3209

ELDEPRYL (Australia, Belgium, Canada, Denmark, Finland, Irish Republic, New Zealand, Norway, South Africa, Sweden, The Netherlands, United Kingdom)
SELEGILINE HYDROCHLORIDE
Eldepryl Capsules . . . 3209

ELDORAL (Germany)
TRIMIPRAMINE MALEATE
Surmontil Capsules . . . 2347

ELEGELIN (Singapore, Thailand)
SELEGILINE HYDROCHLORIDE
Eldepryl Capsules . . . 3209

ELEM (Chile)
METHYLPHENIDATE HYDROCHLORIDE
Ritalin Hydrochloride Tablets . . . 2254
Ritalin-SR Tablets . . . 2254

ELEQUINE (Mexico)
LEVOFLOXACIN
Levaquin Injection . . . 2453
Levaquin Tablets . . . 2453

ELEVAT (South Africa)
DRONABINOL
Marinol Capsules . . . 3334

ELFAXONE (The Netherlands)
CEFTRIAXONE SODIUM
Rocephin Injectable Vials, ADD-Vantage, Galaxy, Bulk . . . 2801

ELICA (Mexico, South Africa, Spain)
MOMETASONE FUROATE
Elocon Cream 0.1% . . . 3019
Elocon Lotion 0.1% . . . 3020
Elocon Ointment 0.1% . . . 3021
Nasonex Nasal Spray . . . 3058

ELISOR (France)
PRAVASTATIN SODIUM
Pravachol Tablets . . . 943

ELISSAN (Spain)
LOPERAMIDE HYDROCHLORIDE
Imodium Capsules . . . 1834

ELITAR (Portugal)
NABUMETONE
Relafen Tablets . . . 1523

ELIUR (Argentina)
FUROSEMIDE
Furosemide Tablets . . . 2117

ELIXIFILIN (Spain)
THEOPHYLLINE
Uniphyl Tablets . . . 2708

ELIXINE (Chile)
THEOPHYLLINE
Uniphyl Tablets . . . 2708

ELIXOFILINA (Mexico)
THEOPHYLLINE
Uniphyl Tablets . . . 2708

ELIXOPHYLLIN (Australia, Canada)
THEOPHYLLINE
Uniphyl Tablets . . . 2708

ELLANCO (Hong Kong)
LOVASTATIN
Mevacor Tablets . . . 1996

ELLECI (Italy)
LEVOCARNITINE
Carnitor Injection . . . 3185
Carnitor Tablets and Oral Solution . . . 3187

ELLESTE (Czech Republic)
ESTRADIOL
Climara Transdermal System . . . 795
Vivelle Transdermal System . . . 2288
Vivelle-Dot Transdermal System . . . 2293

ELLESTE-SOLO (United Kingdom)
ESTRADIOL
Climara Transdermal System . . . 795
Vivelle Transdermal System . . . 2288
Vivelle-Dot Transdermal System . . . 2293

ELMENDOS (Australia, Germany)
LAMOTRIGINE
Lamictal Chewable Dispersible Tablets . . . 1449
Lamictal Tablets . . . 1449

ELMETIN (Hong Kong, Thailand)
MEBENDAZOLE
Vermox Chewable Tablets . . . 1853

ELMIRON (Argentina, Australia, Canada, Hong Kong)
PENTOSAN POLYSULFATE SODIUM
Elmiron Capsules . . . 2393

ELOBACT (Germany)
CEFUROXIME AXETIL
Ceftin Tablets . . . 1369
Ceftin for Oral Suspension . . . 1369

ELOCIN (Thailand)
ERYTHROMYCIN STEARATE
Erythrocin Stearate Filmtab Tablets . . . 452

ELOCOM (Belgium, Brazil, Canada, Chile, Czech Republic, Hungary, Israel, Portugal, Spain, Switzerland)
MOMETASONE FUROATE
Elocon Cream 0.1% . . . 3019
Elocon Lotion 0.1% . . . 3020
Elocon Ointment 0.1% . . . 3021
Nasonex Nasal Spray . . . 3058

ELOCON (Argentina, Australia, Austria, Denmark, Finland, Greece, India, Irish Republic, Italy, New Zealand, Norway, South Africa, Sweden, The Netherlands, United Kingdom)
MOMETASONE FUROATE
Elocon Cream 0.1% . . . 3019
Elocon Lotion 0.1% . . . 3020
Elocon Ointment 0.1% . . . 3021
Nasonex Nasal Spray . . . 3058

ELOCOR (Mexico)
NIFEDIPINE
Adalat CC Tablets . . . 2978

ELOCORT (Brazil)
HYDROCORTISONE
Hydrocortone Tablets . . . 1963

ELOMET (Hong Kong, Malaysia, Mexico, Singapore, Thailand)
MOMETASONE FUROATE
Elocon Cream 0.1% . . . 3019
Elocon Lotion 0.1% . . . 3020
Elocon Ointment 0.1% . . . 3021
Nasonex Nasal Spray . . . 3058

ELONGAL (Chile)
DIAZEPAM
Diastat Rectal Delivery System . . . 3344
Valium Tablets . . . 2822

ELOSALIC (Argentina, Austria, Brazil, Hong Kong, South Africa, Sweden, Thailand)
MOMETASONE FUROATE
Elocon Cream 0.1% . . . 3019
Elocon Lotion 0.1% . . . 3020
Elocon Ointment 0.1% . . . 3021
Nasonex Nasal Spray . . . 3058

ELOVENT (Austria, The Netherlands)
MOMETASONE FUROATE
Elocon Cream 0.1% . . . 3019
Elocon Lotion 0.1% . . . 3020
Elocon Ointment 0.1% . . . 3021
Nasonex Nasal Spray . . . 3058

ELPRADIL (Switzerland)
ENALAPRIL MALEATE
Vasotec I.V. Injection . . . 2076

ELPRADIL HCT (Switzerland)
ENALAPRIL MALEATE
Vasotec I.V. Injection . . . 2076

ELSPAR (Brazil, Hong Kong)
ASPARAGINASE
Elspar for Injection . . . 1943

ELSTATIN (Singapore)
LOVASTATIN
Mevacor Tablets . . . 1996

ELTHYRONE (Belgium)
LEVOTHYROXINE SODIUM
Levothroid Tablets . . . 1189

(⊙ Described in PDR For Ophthalmic Medicines™)

Levoxyl Tablets . . . 1680
Synthroid Tablets . . . 515

ELTOCIN (India)
ERYTHROMYCIN
Ery-Tab Tablets . . . 447
Erythromycin Base Filmtab Tablets . . . 454
Erythromycin Delayed-Release Capsules, USP . . . 456
PCE Dispertab Tablets . . . 510

ELTROXIN (Canada, Czech Republic, Denmark, Hong Kong, India, Irish Republic, Israel, New Zealand, Singapore, South Africa, Thailand, The Netherlands, United Kingdom)
LEVOTHYROXINE SODIUM
Levothroid Tablets . . . 1189
Levoxyl Tablets . . . 1680
Synthroid Tablets . . . 515

ELTROXINE (Switzerland)
LEVOTHYROXINE SODIUM
Levothroid Tablets . . . 1189
Levoxyl Tablets . . . 1680
Synthroid Tablets . . . 515

ELVENAVIR (Argentina)
INDINAVIR SULFATE
Crixivan Capsules . . . 1918

ELYZOL (Finland, Hong Kong, Mexico, Singapore, Thailand, The Netherlands)
METRONIDAZOLE
MetroGel-Vaginal Gel . . . 1822
Noritate Cream, 1% . . . 1051

ELZOGRAM (Germany)
CEFAZOLIN SODIUM
Ancef for Injection . . . 1318

EMANTHAL (India)
ALBENDAZOLE
Albenza Tablets . . . 1310

EMEDAL (Greece)
METRONIDAZOLE
MetroGel-Vaginal Gel . . . 1822
Noritate Cream, 1% . . . 1051

EMESET (Czech Republic, India, Thailand)
ONDANSETRON HYDROCHLORIDE
Zofran Injection . . . 1607
Zofran Injection Premixed . . . 1607
Zofran Oral Solution . . . 1613
Zofran Tablets . . . 1613

EMESTID (France)
ERYTHROMYCIN STEARATE
Erythrocin Stearate Filmtab Tablets . . . 452

EMETRON (Czech Republic, Hungary)
ONDANSETRON HYDROCHLORIDE
Zofran Injection . . . 1607
Zofran Injection Premixed . . . 1607
Zofran Oral Solution . . . 1613
Zofran Tablets . . . 1613

EMFORAL (Thailand)
PROPRANOLOL HYDROCHLORIDE
Inderal LA Long-Acting Capsules . . . 3421

EMIVOX (Argentina)
ONDANSETRON
Zofran ODT Orally Disintegrating Tablets . . . 1613

EMLA (Czech Republic, Finland, United Kingdom)
LIDOCAINE
Lidoderm Patch . . . 1107

EMOCAL (Finland)
CITALOPRAM HYDROBROMIDE
Celexa Tablets . . . 1177

EMO-CORT (Canada)
HYDROCORTISONE
Hydrocortone Tablets . . . 1963

EMOSINT (Argentina, Italy)
DESMOPRESSIN ACETATE
DDAVP Injection 4 mcg/mL . . . 2893
DDAVP Nasal Spray . . . 2894
DDAVP Tablets . . . 2895
Desmopressin Acetate Injection . . . 1143
Desmopressin Acetate Rhinal Tube . . . 1144

EMPECID (Argentina)
CLOTRIMAZOLE
Lotrimin Cream . . . 3053
Lotrimin Lotion 1% . . . 3053
Lotrimin Topical Solution 1% . . . 3053

EMPECID CORT (Argentina)
CLOTRIMAZOLE
Lotrimin Cream . . . 3053
Lotrimin Lotion 1% . . . 3053
Lotrimin Topical Solution 1% . . . 3053

EMPURINE (Thailand)
MERCAPTOPURINE
Purinethol Tablets . . . 1222

EMU-V (Australia, Czech Republic, South Africa)
ERYTHROMYCIN
Ery-Tab Tablets . . . 447
Erythromycin Base Filmtab Tablets . . . 454
Erythromycin Delayed-Release Capsules, USP . . . 456
PCE Dispertab Tablets . . . 510

EMUVIN (Austria)
ERYTHROMYCIN
Ery-Tab Tablets . . . 447
Erythromycin Base Filmtab Tablets . . . 454
Erythromycin Delayed-Release Capsules, USP . . . 456
PCE Dispertab Tablets . . . 510

E-MYCIN (Canada, Hong Kong, Israel, Singapore)
ERYTHROMYCIN
Ery-Tab Tablets . . . 447
Erythromycin Base Filmtab Tablets . . . 454
Erythromycin Delayed-Release Capsules, USP . . . 456
PCE Dispertab Tablets . . . 510

ENA-BASAN (Switzerland)
ENALAPRIL MALEATE
Vasotec I.V. Injection . . . 2076

ENABETA (Germany)
ENALAPRIL MALEATE
Vasotec I.V. Injection . . . 2076

ENABETA COMP (Germany)
ENALAPRIL MALEATE
Vasotec I.V. Injection . . . 2076

ENAC (Austria)
ENALAPRIL MALEATE
Vasotec I.V. Injection . . . 2076

ENACARD (United Kingdom)
ENALAPRIL MALEATE
Vasotec I.V. Injection . . . 2076

ENACE (India)
ENALAPRIL MALEATE
Vasotec I.V. Injection . . . 2076

ENACE-D (India)
ENALAPRIL MALEATE
Vasotec I.V. Injection . . . 2076

ENACODAN (Denmark)
ENALAPRIL MALEATE
Vasotec I.V. Injection . . . 2076

ENACOSTAD (Austria, The Netherlands)
ENALAPRIL MALEATE
Vasotec I.V. Injection . . . 2076

ENACOZID (Denmark)
ENALAPRIL MALEATE
Vasotec I.V. Injection . . . 2076

ENADIL (Denmark)
ENALAPRIL MALEATE
Vasotec I.V. Injection . . . 2076

ENADURA (Germany)
ENALAPRIL MALEATE
Vasotec I.V. Injection . . . 2076

ENAHEXAL (Australia, Germany, New Zealand)
ENALAPRIL MALEATE
Vasotec I.V. Injection . . . 2076

ENAHEXAL COMP (Germany)
ENALAPRIL MALEATE
Vasotec I.V. Injection . . . 2076

ENAL (Germany)
ENALAPRIL MALEATE
Vasotec I.V. Injection . . . 2076

ENALABAL (Brazil)
ENALAPRIL MALEATE
Vasotec I.V. Injection . . . 2076

ENALABENE (Austria)
ENALAPRIL MALEATE
Vasotec I.V. Injection . . . 2076

ENALADEX (Israel)
ENALAPRIL MALEATE
Vasotec I.V. Injection . . . 2076

ENALADIL (Mexico)
ENALAPRIL MALEATE
Vasotec I.V. Injection . . . 2076

ENALAFEL (Argentina)
ENALAPRIL MALEATE
Vasotec I.V. Injection . . . 2076

ENALAGAMMA (Germany)
ENALAPRIL MALEATE
Vasotec I.V. Injection . . . 2076

ENALAPRIL PLUS (Germany)
ENALAPRIL MALEATE
Vasotec I.V. Injection . . . 2076

ENALAPRIL/HCT (Austria)
ENALAPRIL MALEATE
Vasotec I.V. Injection . . . 2076

ENALDUN (Hong Kong)
ENALAPRIL MALEATE
Vasotec I.V. Injection . . . 2076

ENALICH (Germany)
ENALAPRIL MALEATE
Vasotec I.V. Injection . . . 2076

ENALIND (Germany)
ENALAPRIL MALEATE
Vasotec I.V. Injection . . . 2076

ENALOC (Finland)
ENALAPRIL MALEATE
Vasotec I.V. Injection . . . 2076

ENALOC COMP (Finland)
ENALAPRIL MALEATE/HYDROCHLOROTHIAZIDE
Vaseretic Tablets . . . 2073

ENALPRIN (Brazil)
ENALAPRIL MALEATE
Vasotec I.V. Injection . . . 2076

ENALTEN (Chile)
ENALAPRIL MALEATE
Vasotec I.V. Injection . . . 2076

ENALTEN D (Chile)
ENALAPRIL MALEATE/HYDROCHLOROTHIAZIDE
Vaseretic Tablets . . . 2073

ENALTEN DN (Chile)
ENALAPRIL MALEATE/HYDROCHLOROTHIAZIDE
Vaseretic Tablets . . . 2073

ENAM (Thailand)
ENALAPRIL MALEATE
Vasotec I.V. Injection . . . 2076

ENAP (Czech Republic, Hungary, Irish Republic, Russia, Singapore, South Africa)
ENALAPRIL MALEATE
Vasotec I.V. Injection . . . 2076

ENAP HL (Singapore)
ENALAPRIL MALEATE
Vasotec I.V. Injection . . . 2076

ENAP-CO (South Africa)
ENALAPRIL MALEATE
Vasotec I.V. Injection . . . 2076

ENAP-H (Czech Republic)
ENALAPRIL MALEATE
Vasotec I.V. Injection . . . 2076

ENAP-HL (Czech Republic, Hungary)
ENALAPRIL MALEATE
Vasotec I.V. Injection . . . 2076

ENAPIREX (Czech Republic)
ENALAPRIL MALEATE
Vasotec I.V. Injection . . . 2076

ENAPREN (Italy)
ENALAPRIL MALEATE
Vasotec I.V. Injection . . . 2076

ENAPRESS (Finland)
ENALAPRIL MALEATE
Vasotec I.V. Injection . . . 2076

ENAPRIL (Austria, Brazil, Czech Republic, Hungary, Thailand)
ENALAPRIL MALEATE
Vasotec I.V. Injection . . . 2076

ENAPROTEC (Brazil)
ENALAPRIL MALEATE
Vasotec I.V. Injection . . . 2076

ENA-PUREN (Germany)
ENALAPRIL MALEATE
Vasotec I.V. Injection . . . 2076

ENARAN (Austria)
ENALAPRIL MALEATE
Vasotec I.V. Injection . . . 2076

ENARENAL (Russia)
ENALAPRIL MALEATE
Vasotec I.V. Injection . . . 2076

ENARIL (Singapore, Thailand)
ENALAPRIL MALEATE
Vasotec I.V. Injection . . . 2076

ENASIFAR (Switzerland)
ENALAPRIL MALEATE
Vasotec I.V. Injection . . . 2076

ENATEC (Brazil, Switzerland)
ENALAPRIL MALEATE
Vasotec I.V. Injection . . . 2076

ENATEC F (Brazil)
ENALAPRIL MALEATE
Vasotec I.V. Injection . . . 2076

ENATIA (Portugal)
ENALAPRIL MALEATE/HYDROCHLOROTHIAZIDE
Vaseretic Tablets . . . 2073

ENATRIAL (Argentina)
ENALAPRIL MALEATE
Vasotec I.V. Injection . . . 2076

ENATYROL (Austria)
ENALAPRIL MALEATE
Vasotec I.V. Injection . . . 2076

ENBREL (Argentina, Australia, Belgium, Canada, Chile, Czech Republic, Denmark, Finland, France, Germany, Greece, Hong Kong, Hungary, Irish Republic, Israel, Italy, Mexico, New Zealand, Norway, Portugal, Spain, Sweden, Switzerland, Thailand, United Kingdom)
ETANERCEPT
Enbrel for Injection . . . 580

ENDANTADINE (Canada)
AMANTADINE HYDROCHLORIDE
Symmetrel Syrup . . . 1115
Symmetrel Tablets . . . 1115

ENDIAL (Argentina)
GLIMEPIRIDE
Amaryl Tablets . . . 2864

ENDIARON (Germany)
LOPERAMIDE HYDROCHLORIDE
Imodium Capsules . . . 1834

ENDOCLAR (Argentina)
DONEPEZIL HYDROCHLORIDE
Aricept Tablets . . . 1086

ENDOERITRIN (Spain)
ERYTHROMYCIN
Ery-Tab Tablets . . . 447
Erythromycin Base Filmtab Tablets . . . 454
Erythromycin Delayed-Release Capsules, USP . . . 456
PCE Dispertab Tablets . . . 510

ENDOMETRIN (Hong Kong, Israel)
PROGESTERONE
Prometrium Capsules (100 mg, 200 mg) . . . 3205

ENDOMINA (Spain)
ESTRADIOL
Climara Transdermal System . . . 795
Vivelle Transdermal System . . . 2288
Vivelle-Dot Transdermal System . . . 2293

ENDONE (Australia)
OXYCODONE HYDROCHLORIDE
OxyContin Tablets . . . 2699
OxyFast Oral Concentrate Solution . . . 2704
OxyIR Capsules . . . 2704

ENDRONAX (Brazil)
ALENDRONATE SODIUM
Fosamax Tablets . . . 1949

ENEAS (Germany, Spain)
ENALAPRIL MALEATE
Vasotec I.V. Injection . . . 2076

ENI (Mexico)
CIPROFLOXACIN HYDROCHLORIDE
Ciloxan Ophthalmic Ointment ... 554
Ciloxan Ophthalmic Solution ... ⊙205
Cipro Tablets ... 2991

ENIT (Spain)
ENALAPRIL MALEATE
Vasotec I.V. Injection ... 2076

ENOXIN (Malaysia)
CIPROFLOXACIN HYDROCHLORIDE
Ciloxan Ophthalmic Ointment ... 554
Ciloxan Ophthalmic Solution ... ⊙205
Cipro Tablets ... 2991

ENPER (Argentina)
ZIDOVUDINE
Retrovir Capsules ... 1533
Retrovir IV Infusion ... 1537
Retrovir Syrup ... 1533
Retrovir Tablets ... 1533

ENPOTT (Thailand)
POTASSIUM CHLORIDE
K-Dur Extended-Relase Tablets ... 3047
K-Lor Powder Packets ... 472
K-Tab Filmtab Tablets ... 473

ENROMIC (Argentina)
LOSARTAN POTASSIUM
Cozaar Tablets ... 1913

ENSIAL (Greece)
LEVOCARNITINE
Carnitor Injection ... 3185
Carnitor Tablets and Oral Solution ... 3187

ENTERMID (Thailand)
LOPERAMIDE HYDROCHLORIDE
Imodium Capsules ... 1834

ENTEROBENE (Austria, Hungary)
LOPERAMIDE HYDROCHLORIDE
Imodium Capsules ... 1834

ENTERONORM (Brazil)
LOPERAMIDE HYDROCHLORIDE
Imodium Capsules ... 1834

ENTIZOL (Czech Republic)
METRONIDAZOLE
MetroGel-Vaginal Gel ... 1822
Noritate Cream, 1% ... 1051

ENTOPLUS (Mexico)
ALBENDAZOLE
Albenza Tablets ... 1310

ENTROCALM (United Kingdom)
LOPERAMIDE HYDROCHLORIDE
Imodium Capsules ... 1834

ENTRYDIL (Irish Republic)
DILTIAZEM HYDROCHLORIDE
Cardizem LA Extended Release Tablets ... 1699
Tiazac Capsules ... 1204

ENULID (Italy)
MOEXIPRIL HYDROCHLORIDE
Univasc Tablets ... 3118

ENVAS (India, Thailand)
ENALAPRIL MALEATE
Vasotec I.V. Injection ... 2076

ENZACE (Australia)
CAPTOPRIL
Captopril Tablets ... 2114

ENZIPAN (Italy)
PANCRELIPASE
Ultrase Capsules ... 735
Ultrase MT Capsules ... 736

EPADOREN (Greece)
RANITIDINE HYDROCHLORIDE
Zantac 25 EFFERdose Tablets ... 1597
Zantac 150 EFFERdose Tablets ... 1597
Zantac 150 Tablets ... 1597
Zantac 300 Tablets ... 1597
Zantac Injection ... 1593
Zantac Injection Premixed ... 1593
Zantac Syrup ... 1597

EPALAT EPS (Italy)
LACTULOSE
Kristalose for Oral Solution ... 2149

EPALFEN (Italy)
LACTULOSE
Kristalose for Oral Solution ... 2149

EPAQ (Argentina, Mexico)
METRONIDAZOLE
MetroGel-Vaginal Gel ... 1822
Noritate Cream, 1% ... 1051

EPHELIA (Germany, Italy)
ESTRADIOL
Climara Transdermal System ... 795
Vivelle Transdermal System ... 2288
Vivelle-Dot Transdermal System ... 2293

EPI-ABEREL (Germany)
TRETINOIN
Avita Cream ... 2136
Avita Gel ... 2138
Renova 0.05% Cream ... 2387
Retin-A Micro 0.1%/0.04% ... 2388
Vesanoid Capsules ... 2823

EPICLODINA (Mexico)
CLONIDINE
Catapres-TTS ... 875

EPICORDIN (Austria, Germany)
ISOSORBIDE MONONITRATE
Imdur Tablets ... 3032

EPIESTROL (Chile, Irish Republic, Italy, Switzerland)
ESTRADIOL
Climara Transdermal System ... 795
Vivelle Transdermal System ... 2288
Vivelle-Dot Transdermal System ... 2293

EPILENIL (Brazil)
VALPROIC ACID
Depakene Capsules ... 417
Depakene Syrup ... 417

EPILEPAX (Argentina)
LAMOTRIGINE
Lamictal Chewable Dispersible Tablets ... 1449
Lamictal Tablets ... 1449

EPIMAZ (United Kingdom)
CARBAMAZEPINE
Carbatrol Capsules ... 3174
Tegretol Chewable Tablets ... 2278
Tegretol Suspension ... 2278
Tegretol Tablets ... 2278
Tegretol-XR Tablets ... 2278

EPIMORPH (Canada)
MORPHINE SULFATE
Kadian Capsules ... 572
MS Contin Tablets ... 2703

EPI-PEVARYL (Germany)
ECONAZOLE NITRATE
Spectazole Cream ... 2390

EPITOMAX (France)
TOPIRAMATE
Topamax Sprinkle Capsules ... 2438
Topamax Tablets ... 2438

EPITRIAM (The Netherlands)
TRIAMTERENE
Dyrenium Capsules ... 3390

EPITRIL (India)
CLONAZEPAM
Klonopin Tablets ... 2782

EPIVIR (Austria, Belgium, Brazil, Czech Republic, Denmark, Finland, France, Germany, Greece, Irish Republic, Israel, Italy, Japan, Norway, Portugal, Singapore, Spain, Sweden, Thailand, The Netherlands, United Kingdom)
LAMIVUDINE
Epivir Oral Solution ... 1394
Epivir Tablets ... 1394
Epivir-HBV Oral Solution ... 1398
Epivir-HBV Tablets ... 1398

EPIZAM (India)
CLONAZEPAM
Klonopin Tablets ... 2782

EPOGEN (Argentina)
EPOETIN ALFA
Epogen for Injection ... 586
Procrit for Injection ... 2374

EPOPEN (Spain)
EPOETIN ALFA
Epogen for Injection ... 586
Procrit for Injection ... 2374

EPOSAL (Chile)
CARBAMAZEPINE
Carbatrol Capsules ... 3174
Tegretol Chewable Tablets ... 2278
Tegretol Suspension ... 2278
Tegretol Tablets ... 2278
Tegretol-XR Tablets ... 2278

EPOXIDE (Thailand)
CHLORDIAZEPOXIDE HYDROCHLORIDE
Librium Capsules ... 3349

EPOXITIN (Italy)
EPOETIN ALFA
Epogen for Injection ... 586
Procrit for Injection ... 2374

EPREX (Argentina, Australia, Belgium, Brazil, Canada, Chile, Czech Republic, Denmark, Finland, France, Germany, Greece, Hong Kong, Hungary, Irish Republic, Israel, Italy, Malaysia, Mexico, New Zealand, Norway, Russia, Singapore, South Africa, Spain, Sweden, Switzerland, Thailand, The Netherlands, United Kingdom)
EPOETIN ALFA
Epogen for Injection ... 586
Procrit for Injection ... 2374

EPRIL (Switzerland)
ENALAPRIL MALEATE
Vasotec I.V. Injection ... 2076

EPROFIL (Chile)
KETOCONAZOLE
Nizoral 2% Shampoo ... 1838

EPSITRON (Hong Kong, Thailand)
CAPTOPRIL
Captopril Tablets ... 2114

EQUASYM (Denmark, Germany, Irish Republic, The Netherlands, United Kingdom)
METHYLPHENIDATE HYDROCHLORIDE
Ritalin Hydrochloride Tablets ... 2254
Ritalin-SR Tablets ... 2254

EQUIPAX (Spain)
GABAPENTIN
Neurontin Capsules ... 2498

ERADIX (Austria)
FAMOTIDINE
Pepcid Injection ... 2017
Pepcid Injection Premixed ... 2017
Pepcid Tablets ... 2014
Pepcid for Oral Suspension ... 2014

ERANZ (Argentina, Chile, Mexico)
DONEPEZIL HYDROCHLORIDE
Aricept Tablets ... 1086

ERAVERM (Brazil)
MEBENDAZOLE
Vermox Chewable Tablets ... 1853

ERCESTOP (France)
LOPERAMIDE HYDROCHLORIDE
Imodium Capsules ... 1834

ERCESTOPYL (Belgium)
LOPERAMIDE HYDROCHLORIDE
Imodium Capsules ... 1834

ERGOMICON (Mexico)
KETOCONAZOLE
Nizoral 2% Shampoo ... 1838

ERI (Argentina)
ERYTHROMYCIN
Ery-Tab Tablets ... 447
Erythromycin Base Filmtab Tablets ... 454
Erythromycin Delayed-Release Capsules, USP ... 456
PCE Dispertab Tablets ... 510

ERIBEC (Mexico)
ERYTHROMYCIN
Ery-Tab Tablets ... 447
Erythromycin Base Filmtab Tablets ... 454
Erythromycin Delayed-Release Capsules, USP ... 456
PCE Dispertab Tablets ... 510

ERIBER (Mexico)
ERYTHROMYCIN
Ery-Tab Tablets ... 447
Erythromycin Base Filmtab Tablets ... 454
Erythromycin Delayed-Release Capsules, USP ... 456
PCE Dispertab Tablets ... 510

ERIBUS (Mexico)
ERYTHROMYCIN
Ery-Tab Tablets ... 447
Erythromycin Base Filmtab Tablets ... 454
Erythromycin Delayed-Release Capsules, USP ... 456
PCE Dispertab Tablets ... 510

ERICIN (Thailand)
ERYTHROMYCIN STEARATE
Erythrocin Stearate Filmtab Tablets ... 452

ERICOSOL (Switzerland)
ERYTHROMYCIN STEARATE
Erythrocin Stearate Filmtab Tablets ... 452

ERIDAN (Italy)
DIAZEPAM
Diastat Rectal Delivery System ... 3344
Valium Tablets ... 2822

ERIDOSIS (Spain)
ERYTHROMYCIN
Ery-Tab Tablets ... 447
Erythromycin Base Filmtab Tablets ... 454
Erythromycin Delayed-Release Capsules, USP ... 456
PCE Dispertab Tablets ... 510

ERIFOSTINE (Argentina)
AMIFOSTINE
Ethyol for Injection ... 1869

ERIGRAND (Argentina)
ERYTHROMYCIN
Ery-Tab Tablets ... 447
Erythromycin Base Filmtab Tablets ... 454
Erythromycin Delayed-Release Capsules, USP ... 456
PCE Dispertab Tablets ... 510

ERIMICIN (Argentina)
BENZOYL PEROXIDE
Brevoxyl-4 Creamy Wash ... 3212
Brevoxyl-4 Gel ... 3211
Brevoxyl-8 Creamy Wash ... 3212
Brevoxyl-8 Gel ... 3211
Triaz Cleanser ... 1864
Triaz Gel ... 1864

ERIMICINA (Mexico)
ERYTHROMYCIN
Ery-Tab Tablets ... 447
Erythromycin Base Filmtab Tablets ... 454
Erythromycin Delayed-Release Capsules, USP ... 456
PCE Dispertab Tablets ... 510

ERIPRODIN (Spain)
ERYTHROMYCIN
Ery-Tab Tablets ... 447
Erythromycin Base Filmtab Tablets ... 454
Erythromycin Delayed-Release Capsules, USP ... 456
PCE Dispertab Tablets ... 510

ERISOL (Argentina)
ERYTHROMYCIN
Ery-Tab Tablets ... 447
Erythromycin Base Filmtab Tablets ... 454
Erythromycin Delayed-Release Capsules, USP ... 456
PCE Dispertab Tablets ... 510

ERISUSPEN (Mexico)
ERYTHROMYCIN
Ery-Tab Tablets ... 447
Erythromycin Base Filmtab Tablets ... 454
Erythromycin Delayed-Release Capsules, USP ... 456
PCE Dispertab Tablets ... 510

ERIT (Argentina)
ERYTHROMYCIN
Ery-Tab Tablets ... 447
Erythromycin Base Filmtab Tablets ... 454
Erythromycin Delayed-Release Capsules, USP ... 456
PCE Dispertab Tablets ... 510

ERITOLAT (Mexico)
ERYTHROMYCIN
Ery-Tab Tablets ... 447
Erythromycin Base Filmtab Tablets ... 454
Erythromycin Delayed-Release Capsules, USP ... 456
PCE Dispertab Tablets ... 510

ERITRERBA (Mexico)
ERYTHROMYCIN
Ery-Tab Tablets ... 447
Erythromycin Base Filmtab Tablets ... 454
Erythromycin Delayed-Release Capsules, USP ... 456
PCE Dispertab Tablets ... 510

ERITREX A (Brazil)
ERYTHROMYCIN
Ery-Tab Tablets ... 447

Erythromycin Base Filmtab Tablets 454
Erythromycin Delayed-Release Capsules, USP 456
PCE Dispertab Tablets 510

ERITRIL (Brazil)
ERYTHROMYCIN
Ery-Tab Tablets 447
Erythromycin Base Filmtab Tablets 454
Erythromycin Delayed-Release Capsules, USP 456
PCE Dispertab Tablets 510

ERITRODERM (Argentina)
ERYTHROMYCIN
Ery-Tab Tablets 447
Erythromycin Base Filmtab Tablets 454
Erythromycin Delayed-Release Capsules, USP 456
PCE Dispertab Tablets 510

ERITROFARMIN (Mexico)
ERYTHROMYCIN
Ery-Tab Tablets 447
Erythromycin Base Filmtab Tablets 454
Erythromycin Delayed-Release Capsules, USP 456
PCE Dispertab Tablets 510

ERITROLAT (Mexico)
ERYTHROMYCIN
Ery-Tab Tablets 447
Erythromycin Base Filmtab Tablets 454
Erythromycin Delayed-Release Capsules, USP 456
PCE Dispertab Tablets 510

ERITROMED (Argentina)
ERYTHROMYCIN
Ery-Tab Tablets 447
Erythromycin Base Filmtab Tablets 454
Erythromycin Delayed-Release Capsules, USP 456
PCE Dispertab Tablets 510

ERITROQUIM (Mexico)
ERYTHROMYCIN
Ery-Tab Tablets 447
Erythromycin Base Filmtab Tablets 454
Erythromycin Delayed-Release Capsules, USP 456
PCE Dispertab Tablets 510

ERITROSOL (Mexico)
ERYTHROMYCIN
Ery-Tab Tablets 447
Erythromycin Base Filmtab Tablets 454
Erythromycin Delayed-Release Capsules, USP 456
PCE Dispertab Tablets 510

ERITROWEL (Mexico)
ERYTHROMYCIN
Ery-Tab Tablets 447
Erythromycin Base Filmtab Tablets 454
Erythromycin Delayed-Release Capsules, USP 456
PCE Dispertab Tablets 510

ERLADEXONE (Singapore)
DEXAMETHASONE
Decadron Tablets 1929

ERLMETIN (Singapore)
CIMETIDINE
Tagamet Tablets 1547

ERMOFAN (Greece)
OFLOXACIN
Floxin Otic Solution 1043

ERMYCIN (Singapore)
ERYTHROMYCIN STEARATE
Erythrocin Stearate Filmtab Tablets 452

EROMEL (South Africa)
ERYTHROMYCIN STEARATE
Erythrocin Stearate Filmtab Tablets 452

EROTAB (Malaysia, Singapore)
ERYTHROMYCIN STEARATE
Erythrocin Stearate Filmtab Tablets 452

ERROLON (Argentina)
FUROSEMIDE
Furosemide Tablets 2117

ERWINASE (Greece)
ASPARAGINASE
Elspar for Injection 1943

ERXETILAN (Greece)
ENALAPRIL MALEATE
Vasotec I.V. Injection 2076

ERY (Germany)
ERYTHROMYCIN STEARATE
Erythrocin Stearate Filmtab Tablets 452

ERYACNE (Argentina, Australia, France, Greece, Hong Kong, Italy, New Zealand, Singapore, Thailand, The Netherlands, United Kingdom)
ERYTHROMYCIN
Ery-Tab Tablets 447
Erythromycin Base Filmtab Tablets 454
Erythromycin Delayed-Release Capsules, USP 456
PCE Dispertab Tablets 510

ERYACNEN (Brazil, Chile, Mexico)
ERYTHROMYCIN
Ery-Tab Tablets 447
Erythromycin Base Filmtab Tablets 454
Erythromycin Delayed-Release Capsules, USP 456
PCE Dispertab Tablets 510

ERYAKNEN (Austria, Germany, Switzerland)
ERYTHROMYCIN
Ery-Tab Tablets 447
Erythromycin Base Filmtab Tablets 454
Erythromycin Delayed-Release Capsules, USP 456
PCE Dispertab Tablets 510

ERYBID (Canada)
ERYTHROMYCIN
Ery-Tab Tablets 447
Erythromycin Base Filmtab Tablets 454
Erythromycin Delayed-Release Capsules, USP 456
PCE Dispertab Tablets 510

ERYC (Australia, Canada, Hong Kong, Hungary, Israel, New Zealand, The Netherlands)
ERYTHROMYCIN
Ery-Tab Tablets 447
Erythromycin Base Filmtab Tablets 454
Erythromycin Delayed-Release Capsules, USP 456
PCE Dispertab Tablets 510

ERYCEN (United Kingdom)
ERYTHROMYCIN
Ery-Tab Tablets 447
Erythromycin Base Filmtab Tablets 454
Erythromycin Delayed-Release Capsules, USP 456
PCE Dispertab Tablets 510

ERYCETTE (South Africa)
ERYTHROMYCIN
Ery-Tab Tablets 447
Erythromycin Base Filmtab Tablets 454
Erythromycin Delayed-Release Capsules, USP 456
PCE Dispertab Tablets 510

ERYCIN (India, Thailand)
ERYTHROMYCIN
Ery-Tab Tablets 447
Erythromycin Base Filmtab Tablets 454
Erythromycin Delayed-Release Capsules, USP 456
PCE Dispertab Tablets 510

ERYCINUM (Austria)
ERYTHROMYCIN
Ery-Tab Tablets 447
Erythromycin Base Filmtab Tablets 454
Erythromycin Delayed-Release Capsules, USP 456
PCE Dispertab Tablets 510

ERYCIP (India)
ERYTHROMYCIN STEARATE
Erythrocin Stearate Filmtab Tablets 452

ERYDERM (Belgium, Israel, Malaysia, Mexico, Singapore, South Africa, Switzerland, The Netherlands)
ERYTHROMYCIN
Ery-Tab Tablets 447
Erythromycin Base Filmtab Tablets 454
Erythromycin Delayed-Release Capsules, USP 456
PCE Dispertab Tablets 510

ERYDERMEC (Germany)
ERYTHROMYCIN
Ery-Tab Tablets 447
Erythromycin Base Filmtab Tablets 454
Erythromycin Delayed-Release Capsules, USP 456
PCE Dispertab Tablets 510

ERYFLUID (Argentina, Czech Republic, France, Portugal)
ERYTHROMYCIN
Ery-Tab Tablets 447
Erythromycin Base Filmtab Tablets 454
Erythromycin Delayed-Release Capsules, USP 456
PCE Dispertab Tablets 510

ERYLAR (Mexico)
ERYTHROMYCIN
Ery-Tab Tablets 447
Erythromycin Base Filmtab Tablets 454
Erythromycin Delayed-Release Capsules, USP 456
PCE Dispertab Tablets 510

ERYLIK (France, Hong Kong)
ERYTHROMYCIN
Ery-Tab Tablets 447
Erythromycin Base Filmtab Tablets 454
Erythromycin Delayed-Release Capsules, USP 456
PCE Dispertab Tablets 510

ERYMAX (Irish Republic, South Africa, Switzerland, United Kingdom)
ERYTHROMYCIN
Ery-Tab Tablets 447
Erythromycin Base Filmtab Tablets 454
Erythromycin Delayed-Release Capsules, USP 456
PCE Dispertab Tablets 510

ERY-MAX (Spain)
ERYTHROMYCIN
Ery-Tab Tablets 447
Erythromycin Base Filmtab Tablets 454
Erythromycin Delayed-Release Capsules, USP 456
PCE Dispertab Tablets 510

ERYPO (Austria, Germany)
EPOETIN ALFA
Epogen for Injection 586
Procrit for Injection 2374

ERYSAFE (India)
ERYTHROMYCIN
Ery-Tab Tablets 447
Erythromycin Base Filmtab Tablets 454
Erythromycin Delayed-Release Capsules, USP 456
PCE Dispertab Tablets 510

ERYSOL (Canada)
ERYTHROMYCIN
Ery-Tab Tablets 447
Erythromycin Base Filmtab Tablets 454
Erythromycin Delayed-Release Capsules, USP 456
PCE Dispertab Tablets 510

ERYSTAD (Austria)
ERYTHROMYCIN STEARATE
Erythrocin Stearate Filmtab Tablets 452

ERYTAB (Israel)
ERYTHROMYCIN
Ery-Tab Tablets 447
Erythromycin Base Filmtab Tablets 454
Erythromycin Delayed-Release Capsules, USP 456
PCE Dispertab Tablets 510

ERY-TAB (Thailand)
ERYTHROMYCIN
Ery-Tab Tablets 447
Erythromycin Base Filmtab Tablets 454
Erythromycin Delayed-Release Capsules, USP 456
PCE Dispertab Tablets 510

ERYTAB-S (Singapore)
ERYTHROMYCIN STEARATE
Erythrocin Stearate Filmtab Tablets 452

ERYTHROCIN (India, United Kingdom)
ERYTHROMYCIN
Ery-Tab Tablets 447
Erythromycin Base Filmtab Tablets 454
Erythromycin Delayed-Release Capsules, USP 456
PCE Dispertab Tablets 510

ERYTHRODERM (Israel)
ERYTHROMYCIN
Ery-Tab Tablets 447
Erythromycin Base Filmtab Tablets 454
Erythromycin Delayed-Release Capsules, USP 456
PCE Dispertab Tablets 510

ERYTHROGEL (France, Greece)
ERYTHROMYCIN
Ery-Tab Tablets 447
Erythromycin Base Filmtab Tablets 454
Erythromycin Delayed-Release Capsules, USP 456
PCE Dispertab Tablets 510

ERYTHRO-HEFA (Germany)
ERYTHROMYCIN STEARATE
Erythrocin Stearate Filmtab Tablets 452

ERYTHROMID (Canada, Irish Republic, South Africa, United Kingdom)
ERYTHROMYCIN
Ery-Tab Tablets 447
Erythromycin Base Filmtab Tablets 454
Erythromycin Delayed-Release Capsules, USP 456
PCE Dispertab Tablets 510

ERYTHROSKID (Czech Republic)
ERYTHROMYCIN
Ery-Tab Tablets 447
Erythromycin Base Filmtab Tablets 454
Erythromycin Delayed-Release Capsules, USP 456
PCE Dispertab Tablets 510

ERYTOP (Germany)
ERYTHROMYCIN
Ery-Tab Tablets 447
Erythromycin Base Filmtab Tablets 454
Erythromycin Delayed-Release Capsules, USP 456
PCE Dispertab Tablets 510

ERYTRAN (Switzerland)
ERYTHROMYCIN STEARATE
Erythrocin Stearate Filmtab Tablets 452

ERYTROCICLIN (Italy)
ERYTHROMYCIN STEARATE
Erythrocin Stearate Filmtab Tablets 452

ESALFON (Chile)
ENALAPRIL MALEATE
Vasotec I.V. Injection 2076

ESALFON-D (Chile)
ENALAPRIL MALEATE/HYDROCHLOROTHIAZIDE
Vaseretic Tablets 2073

ESCLEBIN (Spain)
NORFLOXACIN
Noroxin Tablets 2009

ESCLIMA (Italy)
ESTRADIOL
Climara Transdermal System 795
Vivelle Transdermal System 2288
Vivelle-Dot Transdermal System 2293

ESCODARONE (Switzerland)
AMIODARONE HYDROCHLORIDE
Pacerone Tablets 3337

ESCORETIC (Switzerland)
AMILORIDE HYDROCHLORIDE/HYDROCHLOROTHIAZIDE
Moduretic Tablets 2003

ESCOZEM (Switzerland)
DILTIAZEM HYDROCHLORIDE
Cardizem LA Extended Release Tablets 1699
Tiazac Capsules 1204

ESCUDO (Italy)
SUCRALFATE
Carafate Suspension 727
Carafate Tablets 728

ESGIPYRIN (India)
DICLOFENAC SODIUM
Voltaren Tablets 2298
Voltaren-XR Tablets 2301

ESGIPYRIN DS (India)
DICLOFENAC SODIUM
Voltaren Tablets 2298
Voltaren-XR Tablets 2301

ESILGAN (Italy)
ESTAZOLAM
ProSom Tablets 512

ESITEREN (Germany)
HYDROCHLOROTHIAZIDE/TRIAMTERENE
Dyazide Capsules 1389
Maxzide Tablets 2150
Maxzide-25 mg Tablets 2150

ESKAZOLE (Australia, Austria, France, Germany, Israel, Mexico, Spain, The Netherlands, United Kingdom)
ALBENDAZOLE
Albenza Tablets 1310

ESMERON (Australia, Austria, Belgium, Brazil, Chile, Czech Republic, Denmark, Finland, France, Germany, Greece, Hong Kong, Hungary, Irish Republic, Israel, Italy, Malaysia, New Zealand, Norway, Portugal, Russia, Singapore, South Africa, Spain, Sweden, Switzerland, Thailand, The Netherlands, United Kingdom)
ROCURONIUM BROMIDE
Zemuron Injection 2363

ESOFEX (Finland)
RANITIDINE HYDROCHLORIDE
Zantac 25 EFFERdose Tablets 1597
Zantac 150 EFFERdose Tablets. . . . 1597
Zantac 150 Tablets 1597
Zantac 300 Tablets 1597
Zantac Injection 1593
Zantac Injection Premixed 1593
Zantac Syrup 1597

ESOLUT (Italy)
PROGESTERONE
Prometrium Capsules (100 mg, 200 mg) . 3205

ESOTRAN (Spain)
ESTRADIOL
Climara Transdermal System 795
Vivelle Transdermal System 2288
Vivelle-Dot Transdermal System 2293

ESPA-LEPSIN (Germany)
CARBAMAZEPINE
Carbatrol Capsules 3174
Tegretol Chewable Tablets 2278
Tegretol Suspension. . . . 2278
Tegretol Tablets 2278
Tegretol-XR Tablets 2278

ESPARIL (Germany)
CAPTOPRIL
Captopril Tablets. . . . 2114

ESPASEVIT (Argentina)
ONDANSETRON
Zofran ODT Orally Disintegrating Tablets . . 1613

ESPEDEN (Spain)
NORFLOXACIN
Noroxin Tablets. . . . 2009

ESPO (Japan)
EPOETIN ALFA
Epogen for Injection. . . . 586
Procrit for Injection 2374

ESPONTAL (Argentina)
TAMSULOSIN HYDROCHLORIDE
Flomax Capsules. . . . 881

ESRADIN (Italy)
ISRADIPINE
DynaCirc CR Tablets. . . . 2726

ESSELDON (Greece)
FAMOTIDINE
Pepcid Injection 2017
Pepcid Injection Premixed 2017
Pepcid Tablets 2014
Pepcid for Oral Suspension 2014

ESTALIS (Argentina, Austria, Brazil, Canada, Czech Republic, Irish Republic, Norway, Portugal, Spain, Switzerland)
ESTRADIOL
Climara Transdermal System 795
Vivelle Transdermal System 2288
Vivelle-Dot Transdermal System 2293

ESTALIS CONTINUOUS (Australia)
ESTRADIOL
Climara Transdermal System 795
Vivelle Transdermal System 2288
Vivelle-Dot Transdermal System 2293

ESTEROMICIN (Mexico)
ERYTHROMYCIN
Ery-Tab Tablets 447
Erythromycin Base Filmtab Tablets. . . . 454
Erythromycin Delayed-Release Capsules, USP 456
PCE Dispertab Tablets 510

ESTILOMICIN (Argentina)
METRONIDAZOLE
MetroGel-Vaginal Gel 1822
Noritate Cream, 1% 1051

ESTIMA (France)
PROGESTERONE
Prometrium Capsules (100 mg, 200 mg) . 3205

ESTOMIL (Spain)
LANSOPRAZOLE
Prevacid Delayed-Release Capsules 3268

ESTRABETA (Germany)
ESTRADIOL
Climara Transdermal System 795
Vivelle Transdermal System 2288
Vivelle-Dot Transdermal System 2293

ESTRACE (Canada, Czech Republic)
ESTRADIOL
Climara Transdermal System 795
Vivelle Transdermal System 2288
Vivelle-Dot Transdermal System 2293

ESTRACE-C (Czech Republic)
ESTRADIOL
Climara Transdermal System 795
Vivelle Transdermal System 2288
Vivelle-Dot Transdermal System 2293

ESTRACUTAN (Austria)
ESTRADIOL
Climara Transdermal System 795
Vivelle Transdermal System 2288
Vivelle-Dot Transdermal System 2293

ESTRADELLE (Brazil)
ESTRADIOL
Climara Transdermal System 795
Vivelle Transdermal System 2288
Vivelle-Dot Transdermal System 2293

ESTRADERM (Argentina, Australia, Austria, Belgium, Brazil, Canada, Czech Republic, Denmark, Finland, France, Germany, Hong Kong, Hungary, India, Irish Republic, Israel, Italy, Mexico, New Zealand, Norway, Portugal, Singapore, South Africa, Spain, Sweden, Switzerland, The Netherlands, United Kingdom)
ESTRADIOL
Climara Transdermal System 795
Vivelle Transdermal System 2288
Vivelle-Dot Transdermal System 2293

ESTRADERM TTS (Greece)
ESTRADIOL
Climara Transdermal System 795
Vivelle Transdermal System 2288
Vivelle-Dot Transdermal System 2293

ESTRADOT (Argentina, Australia, Austria, Canada, Finland, Germany, Hungary, Irish Republic, Norway, Portugal, Spain, Sweden, Switzerland, The Netherlands, United Kingdom)
ESTRADIOL
Climara Transdermal System 795
Vivelle Transdermal System 2288
Vivelle-Dot Transdermal System 2293

ESTRAGEST (Argentina, Brazil, Czech Republic, Hungary)
ESTRADIOL
Climara Transdermal System 795
Vivelle Transdermal System 2288
Vivelle-Dot Transdermal System 2293

ESTRAHEXAL (Czech Republic)
ESTRADIOL
Climara Transdermal System 795
Vivelle Transdermal System 2288
Vivelle-Dot Transdermal System 2293

ESTRAMON (Austria, Germany, Greece, Hungary, Irish Republic, Switzerland)
ESTRADIOL
Climara Transdermal System 795
Vivelle Transdermal System 2288
Vivelle-Dot Transdermal System 2293

ESTRAPATCH (France)
ESTRADIOL
Climara Transdermal System 795
Vivelle Transdermal System 2288
Vivelle-Dot Transdermal System 2293

ESTRENA (Finland)
ESTRADIOL
Climara Transdermal System 795
Vivelle Transdermal System 2288
Vivelle-Dot Transdermal System 2293

ESTREVA (Argentina, Belgium, Brazil, Chile, Czech Republic, Germany, Hong Kong, Monaco, Singapore, Switzerland)
ESTRADIOL
Climara Transdermal System 795
Vivelle Transdermal System 2288
Vivelle-Dot Transdermal System 2293

ESTRIFAM (Germany)
ESTRADIOL
Climara Transdermal System 795
Vivelle Transdermal System 2288
Vivelle-Dot Transdermal System 2293

ESTRIMAX (Czech Republic, Hungary, Russia)
ESTRADIOL
Climara Transdermal System 795
Vivelle Transdermal System 2288
Vivelle-Dot Transdermal System 2293

ESTRING (Argentina, Australia, Austria, Canada, Czech Republic, Denmark, Finland, Germany, Greece, New Zealand, Norway, South Africa, Switzerland, The Netherlands, United Kingdom)
ESTRADIOL
Climara Transdermal System 795
Vivelle Transdermal System 2288
Vivelle-Dot Transdermal System 2293

ESTROACT (India)
RALOXIFENE HYDROCHLORIDE
Evista Tablets. . . . 1735

ESTROCLIM (Italy)
ESTRADIOL
Climara Transdermal System 795
Vivelle Transdermal System 2288
Vivelle-Dot Transdermal System 2293

ESTRODOSE (Italy)
ESTRADIOL
Climara Transdermal System 795
Vivelle Transdermal System 2288
Vivelle-Dot Transdermal System 2293

ESTROFEM (Argentina, Australia, Austria, Belgium, Brazil, Czech Republic, Denmark, Finland, France, Hong Kong, Hungary, Irish Republic, Israel, Italy, Malaysia, New Zealand, Portugal, Singapore, South Africa, Thailand, The Netherlands)
ESTRADIOL
Climara Transdermal System 795
Vivelle Transdermal System 2288
Vivelle-Dot Transdermal System 2293

ESTROFEM N (Switzerland)
ESTRADIOL
Climara Transdermal System 795
Vivelle Transdermal System 2288
Vivelle-Dot Transdermal System 2293

ESTROFFIK (Spain)
ESTRADIOL
Climara Transdermal System 795
Vivelle Transdermal System 2288
Vivelle-Dot Transdermal System 2293

ESTROGEL (Austria, Canada, Denmark, Finland)
ESTRADIOL
Climara Transdermal System 795
Vivelle Transdermal System 2288
Vivelle-Dot Transdermal System 2293

ESTRONAR (Portugal)
ESTRADIOL
Climara Transdermal System 795
Vivelle Transdermal System 2288
Vivelle-Dot Transdermal System 2293

ESTRONORM (Germany)
ESTRADIOL
Climara Transdermal System 795
Vivelle Transdermal System 2288
Vivelle-Dot Transdermal System 2293

ETACONIL (Chile)
FLUTAMIDE
Eulexin Capsules 3023

ETACORTILEN (Italy)
DEXAMETHASONE SODIUM PHOSPHATE
Decadron Phosphate Injection. . . . 1931

ETAMUCIN (Austria)
SODIUM HYALURONATE
Hyalgan Solution 2917

ETHEOPHYL (Germany)
THEOPHYLLINE
Uniphyl Tablets 2708

ETHIMIL (United Kingdom)
VERAPAMIL HYDROCHLORIDE
Covera-HS Tablets 3135
Verelan PM Capsules 3120

ETHIMYCIN (South Africa)
ERYTHROMYCIN STEARATE
Erythrocin Stearate Filmtab Tablets 452

ETHIPAM (South Africa)
DIAZEPAM
Diastat Rectal Delivery System 3344
Valium Tablets 2822

ETHYFEN (Greece)
NABUMETONE
Relafen Tablets 1523

ETHYOL (Argentina, Australia, Belgium, Brazil, Canada, Chile, Czech Republic, Denmark, Finland, France, Germany, Greece, Hong Kong, Hungary, Israel, Italy, Malaysia, Mexico, New Zealand, Portugal, Singapore, South Africa, Spain, Sweden, Switzerland, Thailand, The Netherlands, United Kingdom)
AMIFOSTINE
Ethyol for Injection. . . . 1869

ETIDRATE (New Zealand)
ETIDRONATE DISODIUM
Didronel Tablets 2693

ETIDRON (Greece, Italy)
ETIDRONATE DISODIUM
Didronel Tablets 2693

ETIMONIS (Switzerland)
ISOSORBIDE MONONITRATE
Imdur Tablets 3032

ETIPLUS (Greece)
ETIDRONATE DISODIUM
Didronel Tablets 2693

ETISUX (Argentina)
ERYTHROMYCIN
Ery-Tab Tablets 447
Erythromycin Base Filmtab Tablets. . . . 454
Erythromycin Delayed-Release Capsules, USP 456
PCE Dispertab Tablets 510

ETIZEM (Czech Republic, Portugal)
DILTIAZEM HYDROCHLORIDE
Cardizem LA Extended Release Tablets. . . 1699
Tiazac Capsules 1204

ETRAMON (Spain)
ECONAZOLE NITRATE
Spectazole Cream. . . . 2390

E-TROCIMA-P (Mexico)
ERYTHROMYCIN
Ery-Tab Tablets 447
Erythromycin Base Filmtab Tablets. . . . 454
Erythromycin Delayed-Release Capsules, USP 456
PCE Dispertab Tablets 510

ETRONIL (Argentina)
METRONIDAZOLE
MetroGel-Vaginal Gel 1822
Noritate Cream, 1% 1051

ETYOFIL (India)
THEOPHYLLINE
Uniphyl Tablets 2708

ETYZEM (Italy)
DILTIAZEM HYDROCHLORIDE
Cardizem LA Extended Release Tablets. . . 1699
Tiazac Capsules 1204

EUBINE (France)
OXYCODONE HYDROCHLORIDE
OxyContin Tablets 2699
OxyFast Oral Concentrate Solution. . . . 2704
OxyIR Capsules. . . . 2704

EUCARDIC (Irish Republic, Sweden, The Netherlands, United Kingdom)
CARVEDILOL
Coreg Tablets. . . . 1376

EUCARNIL (Italy)
LEVOCARNITINE
Carnitor Injection. . . . 3185
Carnitor Tablets and Oral Solution 3187

EUCOPROST (Spain)
FINASTERIDE
Propecia Tablets 2036
Proscar Tablets. . . . 2040

EUCOR (Thailand)
SIMVASTATIN
Zocor Tablets 2078

EUDEMINE (Irish Republic, United Kingdom)
DIAZOXIDE
Hyperstat I.V. Injection 3031

EUDIGOX (Italy)
DIGOXIN
Lanoxicaps Capsules 1458
Lanoxin Injection 1462
Lanoxin Injection Pediatric 1465
Lanoxin Tablets 1468

EUDYNA (Austria, Germany, Hong Kong, India, Mexico, Singapore)
TRETINOIN
Avita Cream 2136
Avita Gel 2138
Renova 0.05% Cream 2387
Retin-A Micro 0.1%/0.04% 2388
Vesanoid Capsules 2823

EUFILINA (Portugal, Spain)
THEOPHYLLINE
Uniphyl Tablets 2708

EUFLEX (Canada)
FLUTAMIDE
Eulexin Capsules 3023

EUGALAC (Austria, Germany)
LACTULOSE
Kristalose for Oral Solution 2149

EUGERIAL (Argentina, Brazil)
NIMODIPINE
Nimotop Capsules 774

EUGLIM (India)
GLIMEPIRIDE
Amaryl Tablets 2864

EUKODAL (Germany)
OXYCODONE HYDROCHLORIDE
OxyContin Tablets 2699
OxyFast Oral Concentrate Solution 2704
OxyIR Capsules 2704

EULEXIN (Argentina, Australia, Belgium, Brazil, Denmark, Finland, Israel, Italy, Mexico, New Zealand, Norway, Portugal, South Africa, Spain, Sweden, The Netherlands)
FLUTAMIDE
Eulexin Capsules 3023

EULEXINE (France)
FLUTAMIDE
Eulexin Capsules 3023

EUMICEL (Argentina)
KETOCONAZOLE
Nizoral 2% Shampoo 1838

EUPHYLLIN (Belgium, Czech Republic, Finland, Germany, Norway, South Africa)
THEOPHYLLINE
Uniphyl Tablets 2708

EUPHYLLIN 200 (Germany)
THEOPHYLLINE
Uniphyl Tablets 2708

EUPHYLLINA (Italy)
THEOPHYLLINE
Uniphyl Tablets 2708

EUPHYLLINE (France)
THEOPHYLLINE
Uniphyl Tablets 2708

EUPHYLONG (Czech Republic, Germany, Hong Kong, Hungary, Sweden, Switzerland, The Netherlands)
THEOPHYLLINE
Uniphyl Tablets 2708

EUPRESSIN (Brazil)
ENALAPRIL MALEATE
Vasotec I.V. Injection 2076

EUPRESSIN H (Brazil)
ENALAPRIL MALEATE/HYDROCHLOROTHIAZIDE
Vaseretic Tablets 2073

EURALBEN (Mexico)
ALBENDAZOLE
Albenza Tablets 1310

EURECEPTOR (Italy)
CIMETIDINE
Tagamet Tablets 1547

EURITSIN (Argentina)
ADENOSINE
Adenocard Injection 612
Adenoscan 613

EURODIN (Japan)
ESTAZOLAM
ProSom Tablets 512

EUROFLU (Italy)
FLUNISOLIDE
Aerobid Inhaler System 1172
Aerobid-M Inhaler System 1172
Nasarel Nasal Spray 1652

EUROGESIC GEL (Chile)
NAPROXEN
EC-Naprosyn Delayed-Release Tablets 2769
Naprosyn Suspension 2769
Naprosyn Tablets 2769

EUROLAT (Mexico)
KETOCONAZOLE
Nizoral 2% Shampoo 1838

EUROMICINA (Chile)
CLARITHROMYCIN
Biaxin Filmtab Tablets 402
Biaxin Granules 402

EUROSAN (Switzerland)
CLOTRIMAZOLE
Lotrimin Cream 3053
Lotrimin Lotion 1% 3053
Lotrimin Topical Solution 1% 3053

EUROTRETIN (Argentina)
TRETINOIN
Avita Cream 2136
Avita Gel 2138
Renova 0.05% Cream 2387
Retin-A Micro 0.1%/0.04% 2388
Vesanoid Capsules 2823

EURYTHMIC (India)
AMIODARONE HYDROCHLORIDE
Pacerone Tablets 3337

EUSEDON MONO (Germany)
PROMETHAZINE HYDROCHLORIDE
Phenergan Suppositories 3438
Phenergan Tablets 3438

EUSKIN (Spain)
ERYTHROMYCIN
Ery-Tab Tablets 447
Erythromycin Base Filmtab Tablets 454
Erythromycin Delayed-Release Capsules, USP 456
PCE Dispertab Tablets 510

EUSTIDIL (Portugal)
FLUTICASONE PROPIONATE
Cutivate Cream 1381
Cutivate Ointment 1384
Flonase Nasal Spray 1412

EUTHYROX (Argentina, Belgium, Brazil, Czech Republic, Germany, Hungary, Russia, Singapore, Sweden, Switzerland, The Netherlands)
LEVOTHYROXINE SODIUM
Levothroid Tablets 1189
Levoxyl Tablets 1680
Synthroid Tablets 515

EUTIMIL (Italy)
PAROXETINE HYDROCHLORIDE
Paxil Oral Suspension 1501
Paxil Tablets 1501

EUTIROX (Italy, Mexico, Spain)
LEVOTHYROXINE SODIUM
Levothroid Tablets 1189
Levoxyl Tablets 1680
Synthroid Tablets 515

EUTIZ (Argentina)
FINASTERIDE
Propecia Tablets 2036
Proscar Tablets 2040

EUTROXSIG (Australia)
LEVOTHYROXINE SODIUM
Levothroid Tablets 1189
Levoxyl Tablets 1680
Synthroid Tablets 515

EUXAT (Italy)
NIFEDIPINE
Adalat CC Tablets 2978

EVACALM (United Kingdom)
DIAZEPAM
Diastat Rectal Delivery System 3344
Valium Tablets 2822

EVADOL (Mexico)
DICLOFENAC SODIUM
Voltaren Tablets 2298
Voltaren-XR Tablets 2301

EVAFILM (France)
ESTRADIOL
Climara Transdermal System 795
Vivelle Transdermal System 2288
Vivelle-Dot Transdermal System 2293

EVAPAUSE (France)
PROGESTERONE
Prometrium Capsules (100 mg, 200 mg) . 3205

EVIANTRINA (Spain)
FAMOTIDINE
Pepcid Injection 2017
Pepcid Injection Premixed 2017
Pepcid Tablets 2014
Pepcid for Oral Suspension 2014

EVICER (Portugal)
CIMETIDINE
Tagamet Tablets 1547

EVIMAL (Chile)
DONEPEZIL HYDROCHLORIDE
Aricept Tablets 1086

EVINOPON (Greece)
DICLOFENAC SODIUM
Voltaren Tablets 2298
Voltaren-XR Tablets 2301

EVISTA (Argentina, Australia, Austria, Belgium, Brazil, Canada, Chile, Czech Republic, Denmark, Finland, France, Germany, Hong Kong, Hungary, Irish Republic, Israel, Italy, Malaysia, Mexico, New Zealand, Norway, Portugal, Singapore, South Africa, Spain, Sweden, Switzerland, The Netherlands, United Kingdom)
RALOXIFENE HYDROCHLORIDE
Evista Tablets 1735

EVITOCOR (Germany)
ATENOLOL
Tenormin I.V. Injection 698

EVITOCOR PLUS (Germany)
ATENOLOL
Tenormin I.V. Injection 698

EVOPAD (Spain)
ESTRADIOL
Climara Transdermal System 795
Vivelle Transdermal System 2288
Vivelle-Dot Transdermal System 2293

EVOREL (Argentina, Denmark, Finland, Germany, Irish Republic, Israel, Mexico, Norway, South Africa, Sweden, United Kingdom)
ESTRADIOL
Climara Transdermal System 795
Vivelle Transdermal System 2288
Vivelle-Dot Transdermal System 2293

EVOREL CONTI (Argentina, Irish Republic, Israel, United Kingdom)
ESTRADIOL
Climara Transdermal System 795
Vivelle Transdermal System 2288
Vivelle-Dot Transdermal System 2293

EVORELCONTI (Mexico)
ESTRADIOL
Climara Transdermal System 795
Vivelle Transdermal System 2288
Vivelle-Dot Transdermal System 2293

EXAFENIL (Mexico)
DEXAMETHASONE
Decadron Tablets 1929

EXAMICYN (Mexico)
ERYTHROMYCIN
Ery-Tab Tablets 447
Erythromycin Base Filmtab Tablets 454
Erythromycin Delayed-Release Capsules, USP 456
PCE Dispertab Tablets 510

EXAMIDA (Mexico)
SULFACETAMIDE SODIUM
Klaron Lotion 10% 1050

EXAVERM (Mexico)
MEBENDAZOLE
Vermox Chewable Tablets 1853

EXBENZOL (Mexico)
MEBENDAZOLE
Vermox Chewable Tablets 1853

EXE-CORT (United Kingdom)
HYDROCORTISONE
Hydrocortone Tablets 1963

EXERMET GM (India)
GLIMEPIRIDE
Amaryl Tablets 2864

EXERTIAL (Argentina)
CIPROFLOXACIN
Cipro Oral Suspension 2991

EXFLAM (Chile)
DICLOFENAC POTASSIUM
Cataflam Tablets 2173

EXFOLIUM (Argentina)
TRIAMCINOLONE ACETONIDE
Azmacort Inhalation Aerosol 1701
Nasacort AQ Nasal Spray 2937

EXIBRAL (Argentina)
VALPROIC ACID
Depakene Capsules 417
Depakene Syrup 417

EXIFINE (Malaysia)
TERBINAFINE HYDROCHLORIDE
Lamisil Tablets 2226

EXIMIUS (Argentina)
CLOTRIMAZOLE
Lotrimin Cream 3053
Lotrimin Lotion 1% 3053
Lotrimin Topical Solution 1% 3053

EXIREL (Austria)
PIRBUTEROL ACETATE
Maxair Autohaler 1820

EXOCIN (Denmark, Finland, Greece, Irish Republic, Italy, Portugal, South Africa, Spain, United Kingdom)
OFLOXACIN
Floxin Otic Solution 1043

EXOCINE (France)
OFLOXACIN
Floxin Otic Solution 1043

EXODERIL (Austria, Czech Republic, Germany, Hong Kong, Hungary, Israel, Malaysia, Singapore, Switzerland)
NAFTIFINE HYDROCHLORIDE
Naftin Cream 2097
Naftin Gel 2097

EXOGRAN (The Netherlands)
CEFTRIAXONE SODIUM
Rocephin Injectable Vials, ADD-Vantage, Galaxy, Bulk 2801

EXOVIR (Argentina)
ZIDOVUDINE
Retrovir Capsules 1533
Retrovir IV Infusion 1537
Retrovir Syrup 1533
Retrovir Tablets 1533

EXPIT (Argentina)
SILDENAFIL CITRATE
Viagra Tablets 2552

EXPLANER (Argentina)
NIMODIPINE
Nimotop Capsules 774

EXPROS (Finland)
TAMSULOSIN HYDROCHLORIDE
Flomax Capsules 881

EXTENY (Mexico)
MEBENDAZOLE
Vermox Chewable Tablets 1853

EXTISER Q (Mexico)
PRAZIQUANTEL
Biltricide Tablets 2990

EXTRACORT (Germany)
TRIAMCINOLONE ACETONIDE
Azmacort Inhalation Aerosol 1701
Nasacort AQ Nasal Spray 2937

EXTUR (Spain)
INDAPAMIDE
Indapamide Tablets 2119

EYEBREX (Greece)
TOBRAMYCIN
TOBI Solution for Inhalation 1015

EYEBREX-DEXA (Greece)
DEXAMETHASONE/TOBRAMYCIN
TobraDex Ophthalmic Ointment 558
TobraDex Ophthalmic Suspension 558

EYECLOF (Greece)
DICLOFENAC SODIUM
Voltaren Tablets 2298
Voltaren-XR Tablets 2301

EYECON (Israel)
SODIUM HYALURONATE
Hyalgan Solution 2917

EYESTIL (Canada)
SODIUM HYALURONATE
Hyalgan Solution 2917

EYETOBRIN (Greece)
TOBRAMYCIN
TOBI Solution for Inhalation 1015

EZOPTA (Greece)
RANITIDINE HYDROCHLORIDE
Zantac 25 EFFERdose Tablets 1597
Zantac 150 EFFERdose Tablets........ 1597
Zantac 150 Tablets 1597
Zantac 300 Tablets 1597
Zantac Injection 1593
Zantac Injection Premixed 1593
Zantac Syrup 1597

EZOSINA (Italy)
TERAZOSIN HYDROCHLORIDE
Hytrin Capsules................... 469

FABAMOX (Argentina)
AMOXICILLIN
Amoxil Pediatric Drops for Oral Suspension.................. 1315
Amoxil Tablets 1315

FABOFUROX (Argentina)
FUROSEMIDE
Furosemide Tablets 2117

FABOTENOL (Argentina)
ATENOLOL
Tenormin I.V. Injection.............. 698

FABOTRANIL (Argentina)
DIAZEPAM
Diastat Rectal Delivery System 3344
Valium Tablets 2822

FABRALGINA (Argentina)
NAPROXEN
EC-Naprosyn Delayed-Release Tablets.... 2769
Naprosyn Suspension.............. 2769
Naprosyn Tablets 2769

FABUTIN (Mexico)
FAMOTIDINE
Pepcid Injection 2017
Pepcid Injection Premixed 2017
Pepcid Tablets 2014
Pepcid for Oral Suspension 2014

FACORT (Thailand)
TRIAMCINOLONE ACETONIDE
Azmacort Inhalation Aerosol.......... 1701
Nasacort AQ Nasal Spray 2937

FACTION (Argentina)
KETOCONAZOLE
Nizoral 2% Shampoo 1838

FACTODIN (Greece)
CLOTRIMAZOLE
Lotrimin Cream................... 3053
Lotrimin Lotion 1%............... 3053
Lotrimin Topical Solution 1% 3053

FADALIVIO (Argentina)
NAPROXEN
EC-Naprosyn Delayed-Release Tablets.... 2769
Naprosyn Suspension.............. 2769
Naprosyn Tablets 2769

FADAMETASONA (Argentina)
DEXAMETHASONE
Decadron Tablets 1929

FADINE (Hong Kong, India, Malaysia, Thailand)
FAMOTIDINE
Pepcid Injection 2017
Pepcid Injection Premixed 2017
Pepcid Tablets 2014
Pepcid for Oral Suspension 2014

FADOL (Mexico)
HYDROCORTISONE
Hydrocortone Tablets 1963

FADUL (Germany)
FAMOTIDINE
Pepcid Injection 2017
Pepcid Injection Premixed 2017
Pepcid Tablets 2014
Pepcid for Oral Suspension 2014

FAGASTRIL (Spain)
FAMOTIDINE
Pepcid Injection 2017
Pepcid Injection Premixed 2017
Pepcid Tablets 2014
Pepcid for Oral Suspension 2014

FAGATRIM (Mexico)
FAMOTIDINE
Pepcid Injection 2017
Pepcid Injection Premixed 2017
Pepcid Tablets 2014
Pepcid for Oral Suspension 2014

FAGIZOL (Mexico)
METRONIDAZOLE
MetroGel-Vaginal Gel 1822
Noritate Cream, 1%................ 1051

FAGUS (Spain)
RANITIDINE HYDROCHLORIDE
Zantac 25 EFFERdose Tablets 1597
Zantac 150 EFFERdose Tablets........ 1597
Zantac 150 Tablets 1597
Zantac 300 Tablets 1597
Zantac Injection 1593
Zantac Injection Premixed 1593
Zantac Syrup 1597

FALICARD (Germany)
VERAPAMIL HYDROCHLORIDE
Covera-HS Tablets................ 3135
Verelan PM Capsules 3120

FALITONSIN (Germany)
ATENOLOL
Tenormin I.V. Injection.............. 698

FAMILY MEDICATED SUNBURN RELIEF (Canada)
LIDOCAINE
Lidoderm Patch 1107

FAMINE (Hong Kong)
FAMOTIDINE
Pepcid Injection 2017
Pepcid Injection Premixed 2017
Pepcid Tablets 2014
Pepcid for Oral Suspension 2014

FAMO (Israel)
FAMOTIDINE
Pepcid Injection 2017
Pepcid Injection Premixed 2017
Pepcid Tablets 2014
Pepcid for Oral Suspension 2014

FAMOBETA (Germany)
FAMOTIDINE
Pepcid Injection 2017
Pepcid Injection Premixed 2017
Pepcid Tablets 2014
Pepcid for Oral Suspension 2014

FAMOC (Singapore, Thailand)
FAMOTIDINE
Pepcid Injection 2017
Pepcid Injection Premixed 2017
Pepcid Tablets 2014
Pepcid for Oral Suspension 2014

FAMOCID (Singapore, Thailand)
FAMOTIDINE
Pepcid Injection 2017
Pepcid Injection Premixed 2017
Pepcid Tablets 2014
Pepcid for Oral Suspension 2014

FAMODIL (Italy)
FAMOTIDINE
Pepcid Injection 2017
Pepcid Injection Premixed 2017
Pepcid Tablets 2014
Pepcid for Oral Suspension 2014

FAMODIN (India)
FAMOTIDINE
Pepcid Injection 2017
Pepcid Injection Premixed 2017
Pepcid Tablets 2014
Pepcid for Oral Suspension 2014

FAMODINE (Brazil, Hong Kong)
FAMOTIDINE
Pepcid Injection 2017
Pepcid Injection Premixed 2017
Pepcid Tablets 2014
Pepcid for Oral Suspension 2014

FAMOHEXAL (Australia)
FAMOTIDINE
Pepcid Injection 2017
Pepcid Injection Premixed 2017
Pepcid Tablets 2014
Pepcid for Oral Suspension 2014

FAMOKEY (Spain)
FAMOTIDINE
Pepcid Injection 2017
Pepcid Injection Premixed 2017
Pepcid Tablets 2014
Pepcid for Oral Suspension 2014

FAMOLTA (Hong Kong)
FAMOTIDINE
Pepcid Injection 2017
Pepcid Injection Premixed 2017
Pepcid Tablets 2014
Pepcid for Oral Suspension 2014

FAMONERTON (Germany)
FAMOTIDINE
Pepcid Injection 2017
Pepcid Injection Premixed 2017
Pepcid Tablets 2014
Pepcid for Oral Suspension 2014

FAMONOX (Thailand)
FAMOTIDINE
Pepcid Injection 2017
Pepcid Injection Premixed 2017
Pepcid Tablets 2014
Pepcid for Oral Suspension 2014

FAMOPRIL (Singapore)
FAMOTIDINE
Pepcid Injection 2017
Pepcid Injection Premixed 2017
Pepcid Tablets 2014
Pepcid for Oral Suspension 2014

FAMOPSIN (Hong Kong, Malaysia, Singapore, Thailand)
FAMOTIDINE
Pepcid Injection 2017
Pepcid Injection Premixed 2017
Pepcid Tablets 2014
Pepcid for Oral Suspension 2014

FAMOSAN (Czech Republic)
FAMOTIDINE
Pepcid Injection 2017
Pepcid Injection Premixed 2017
Pepcid Tablets 2014
Pepcid for Oral Suspension 2014

FAMOSET (Brazil)
FAMOTIDINE
Pepcid Injection 2017
Pepcid Injection Premixed 2017
Pepcid Tablets 2014
Pepcid for Oral Suspension 2014

FAMOSIA (Thailand)
FAMOTIDINE
Pepcid Injection 2017
Pepcid Injection Premixed 2017
Pepcid Tablets 2014
Pepcid for Oral Suspension 2014

FAMOSIN (Austria)
FAMOTIDINE
Pepcid Injection 2017
Pepcid Injection Premixed 2017
Pepcid Tablets 2014
Pepcid for Oral Suspension 2014

FAMOTAB (Thailand)
FAMOTIDINE
Pepcid Injection 2017
Pepcid Injection Premixed 2017
Pepcid Tablets 2014
Pepcid for Oral Suspension 2014

FAMOTAL (Norway)
FAMOTIDINE
Pepcid Injection 2017
Pepcid Injection Premixed 2017
Pepcid Tablets 2014
Pepcid for Oral Suspension 2014

FAMOTEC (United Arab Emirates)
FAMOTIDINE
Pepcid Injection 2017
Pepcid Injection Premixed 2017
Pepcid Tablets 2014
Pepcid for Oral Suspension 2014

FAMOTID (Brazil)
FAMOTIDINE
Pepcid Injection 2017
Pepcid Injection Premixed 2017
Pepcid Tablets 2014
Pepcid for Oral Suspension 2014

FAMOTIL (Brazil)
FAMOTIDINE
Pepcid Injection 2017
Pepcid Injection Premixed 2017
Pepcid Tablets 2014
Pepcid for Oral Suspension 2014

FAMOTIN (Hong Kong, Singapore, Thailand)
FAMOTIDINE
Pepcid Injection 2017
Pepcid Injection Premixed 2017
Pepcid Tablets 2014
Pepcid for Oral Suspension 2014

FAMOWAL (India)
FAMOTIDINE
Pepcid Injection 2017
Pepcid Injection Premixed 2017
Pepcid Tablets 2014
Pepcid for Oral Suspension 2014

FAMOX (Brazil, Hong Kong, New Zealand)
FAMOTIDINE
Pepcid Injection 2017
Pepcid Injection Premixed 2017
Pepcid Tablets 2014
Pepcid for Oral Suspension 2014

FAMOXAL (Mexico)
FAMOTIDINE
Pepcid Injection 2017
Pepcid Injection Premixed 2017
Pepcid Tablets 2014
Pepcid for Oral Suspension 2014

FAMOXIL (Brazil)
FAMOTIDINE
Pepcid Injection 2017
Pepcid Injection Premixed 2017
Pepcid Tablets 2014
Pepcid for Oral Suspension 2014

FAMTAC (India)
FAMOTIDINE
Pepcid Injection 2017
Pepcid Injection Premixed 2017
Pepcid Tablets 2014
Pepcid for Oral Suspension 2014

FAMULCER (Spain)
FAMOTIDINE
Pepcid Injection 2017
Pepcid Injection Premixed 2017
Pepcid Tablets 2014
Pepcid for Oral Suspension 2014

FANCIADAZOL (Mexico)
MEBENDAZOLE
Vermox Chewable Tablets 1853

FANGAN (Argentina)
KETOCONAZOLE
Nizoral 2% Shampoo 1838

FANOSIN (Spain)
FAMOTIDINE
Pepcid Injection 2017
Pepcid Injection Premixed 2017
Pepcid Tablets 2014
Pepcid for Oral Suspension 2014

FANOX (Spain)
FAMOTIDINE
Pepcid Injection 2017
Pepcid Injection Premixed 2017
Pepcid Tablets 2014
Pepcid for Oral Suspension 2014

FARAXEN (Mexico)
NAPROXEN
EC-Naprosyn Delayed-Release Tablets.... 2769
Naprosyn Suspension.............. 2769
Naprosyn Tablets 2769

FARCEF (Greece)
CEFTRIAXONE SODIUM
Rocephin Injectable Vials, ADD-Vantage, Galaxy, Bulk 2801

FARGANESSE (Italy)
PROMETHAZINE HYDROCHLORIDE
Phenergan Suppositories............ 3438
Phenergan Tablets................ 3438

FARGO (Australia)
LIDOCAINE
Lidoderm Patch 1107

FARLAC (Brazil)
LACTULOSE
Kristalose for Oral Solution 2149

FARLUTAL (Australia, Austria, Belgium, Brazil, Chile, Finland, France, Germany, Hong Kong, Italy, Malaysia, Mexico, New Zealand, Norway, Singapore, South Africa, Spain, Sweden, Switzerland, Thailand, The Netherlands, United Kingdom)
MEDROXYPROGESTERONE ACETATE
Depo-Medrol Single-Dose Vial 2617

FARLUTALE (Argentina)
MEDROXYPROGESTERONE ACETATE
Depo-Medrol Single-Dose Vial 2617

FARMACICLIN (Italy)
VANCOMYCIN HYDROCHLORIDE
Vancocin HCl Capsules, USP 3370

FARMIN (Mexico)
DIAZEPAM
Diastat Rectal Delivery System 3344
Valium Tablets 2822

FARMOTEX (Mexico)
FAMOTIDINE
Pepcid Injection 2017
Pepcid Injection Premixed 2017
Pepcid Tablets 2014
Pepcid for Oral Suspension 2014

FARM-X DUO (Argentina)
METRONIDAZOLE
MetroGel-Vaginal Gel 1822
Noritate Cream, 1% 1051

FARM-X GINECOLOGICO (Argentina)
METRONIDAZOLE
MetroGel-Vaginal Gel 1822
Noritate Cream, 1% 1051

FARNITIN (Italy)
LEVOCARNITINE
Carnitor Injection 3185
Carnitor Tablets and Oral Solution 3187

FARPRESSE (Portugal)
LISINOPRIL
Prinivil Tablets 2029
Zestril Tablets 704

FARXEN (Mexico)
NAPROXEN
EC-Naprosyn Delayed-Release Tablets 2769
Naprosyn Suspension 2769
Naprosyn Tablets 2769

FASE (Italy)
APROTININ
Trasylol Injection 779

FASELUT (Argentina)
PROGESTERONE
Prometrium Capsules (100 mg, 200 mg) . 3205

FASIDINE (Thailand)
FAMOTIDINE
Pepcid Injection 2017
Pepcid Injection Premixed 2017
Pepcid Tablets 2014
Pepcid for Oral Suspension 2014

FASTIN (Canada)
PHENTERMINE HYDROCHLORIDE
Adipex-P Capsules 1216
Adipex-P Tablets 1216

FATEC (Thailand)
CETIRIZINE HYDROCHLORIDE
Zyrtec Syrup 2589
Zyrtec Tablets 2589

FATIDIN (Portugal)
FAMOTIDINE
Pepcid Injection 2017
Pepcid Injection Premixed 2017
Pepcid Tablets 2014
Pepcid for Oral Suspension 2014

FATORIL (Mexico)
FAMOTIDINE
Pepcid Injection 2017
Pepcid Injection Premixed 2017
Pepcid Tablets 2014
Pepcid for Oral Suspension 2014

FAULTENOCAN (Portugal)
IRINOTECAN HYDROCHLORIDE
Camptosar Injection 2602

FAUSTAN (Germany)
DIAZEPAM
Diastat Rectal Delivery System 3344
Valium Tablets 2822

FAWODIN (Mexico)
FAMOTIDINE
Pepcid Injection 2017
Pepcid Injection Premixed 2017
Pepcid Tablets 2014
Pepcid for Oral Suspension 2014

FAXINE (Italy)
VENLAFAXINE HYDROCHLORIDE
Effexor Tablets 3405
Effexor XR Capsules 3411

FAZOPLEX (Spain)
CEFAZOLIN SODIUM
Ancef for Injection 1318

FEACEF (Greece)
CEFUROXIME AXETIL
Ceftin Tablets 1369
Ceftin for Oral Suspension 1369

FEALIN (Greece)
ATENOLOL
Tenormin I.V. Injection 698

FEBRAX (Mexico)
NAPROXEN SODIUM
Anaprox DS Tablets 2769
Anaprox Tablets 2769

FEDIP (Austria, Switzerland)
NIFEDIPINE
Adalat CC Tablets 2978

FEGENOR (France)
FENOFIBRATE
Tricor Tablets 523

FELANOR (Argentina)
CLONAZEPAM
Klonopin Tablets 2782

FELIBERAL (Mexico)
ENALAPRIL MALEATE
Vasotec I.V. Injection 2076

FELISELIN (Greece)
SELEGILINE HYDROCHLORIDE
Eldepryl Capsules 3209

FELIXENE (Spain)
CIPROFLOXACIN HYDROCHLORIDE
Ciloxan Ophthalmic Ointment 554
Ciloxan Ophthalmic Solution . . . . ⊙205
Cipro Tablets 2991

FELLER (Brazil)
MEBENDAZOLE
Vermox Chewable Tablets 1853

FELO (New Zealand)
FELODIPINE
Plendil Extended-Release Tablets 651

FELOBETA (Germany)
FELODIPINE
Plendil Extended-Release Tablets 651

FELOBITS (Argentina)
ATENOLOL
Tenormin I.V. Injection 698

FELOCOR (Germany)
FELODIPINE
Plendil Extended-Release Tablets 651

FELODAY (Italy)
FELODIPINE
Plendil Extended-Release Tablets 651

FELODIL (Switzerland)
FELODIPINE
Plendil Extended-Release Tablets 651

FELODIN (Denmark)
FELODIPINE
Plendil Extended-Release Tablets 651

FELODIP (Russia)
FELODIPINE
Plendil Extended-Release Tablets 651

FELODUR (Australia)
FELODIPINE
Plendil Extended-Release Tablets 651

FELOGAMMA (Germany)
FELODIPINE
Plendil Extended-Release Tablets 651

FELOGARD (India)
FELODIPINE
Plendil Extended-Release Tablets 651

FELO-PUREN (Germany)
FELODIPINE
Plendil Extended-Release Tablets 651

FELORAN (Czech Republic)
DICLOFENAC SODIUM
Voltaren Tablets 2298
Voltaren-XR Tablets 2301

FELOTENS (United Kingdom)
FELODIPINE
Plendil Extended-Release Tablets 651

FEM 7 (Argentina, Brazil, Chile, Czech Republic, Germany, Hong Kong, Mexico, Singapore, Switzerland, The Netherlands)
ESTRADIOL
Climara Transdermal System 795
Vivelle Transdermal System 2288
Vivelle-Dot Transdermal System 2293

FEMALON (Chile)
ESTRADIOL
Climara Transdermal System 795
Vivelle Transdermal System 2288
Vivelle-Dot Transdermal System 2293

FEMANEST (Denmark, Sweden)
ESTRADIOL
Climara Transdermal System 795
Vivelle Transdermal System 2288
Vivelle-Dot Transdermal System 2293

FEMATAB (Irish Republic)
ESTRADIOL
Climara Transdermal System 795
Vivelle Transdermal System 2288
Vivelle-Dot Transdermal System 2293

FEMATRIX (Irish Republic, United Kingdom)
ESTRADIOL
Climara Transdermal System 795
Vivelle Transdermal System 2288
Vivelle-Dot Transdermal System 2293

FEMEX (The Netherlands)
NAPROXEN SODIUM
Anaprox DS Tablets 2769
Anaprox Tablets 2769

FEMIDERM (Chile)
ESTRADIOL
Climara Transdermal System 795
Vivelle Transdermal System 2288
Vivelle-Dot Transdermal System 2293

FEMIGEL (South Africa)
ESTRADIOL
Climara Transdermal System 795
Vivelle Transdermal System 2288
Vivelle-Dot Transdermal System 2293

FEMINOFLEX (Greece)
ETIDRONATE DISODIUM
Didronel Tablets 2693

FEMINOVA (Belgium)
ESTRADIOL
Climara Transdermal System 795
Vivelle Transdermal System 2288
Vivelle-Dot Transdermal System 2293

FEMIPRES (Italy)
MOEXIPRIL HYDROCHLORIDE
Univasc Tablets 3118

FEMIPRES PLUS (Italy)
HYDROCHLOROTHIAZIDE/MOEXIPRIL HYDROCHLORIDE
Uniretic Tablets 3114

FEMISAN (Mexico)
KETOCONAZOLE
Nizoral 2% Shampoo 1838

FEMIZOL (Australia)
CLOTRIMAZOLE
Lotrimin Cream 3053
Lotrimin Lotion 1% 3053
Lotrimin Topical Solution 1% 3053

FEMME FREE (Australia)
NAPROXEN
EC-Naprosyn Delayed-Release Tablets 2769
Naprosyn Suspension 2769
Naprosyn Tablets 2769

FEM-MONO (Denmark, Sweden)
ISOSORBIDE MONONITRATE
Imdur Tablets 3032

FEMOSTON 1/5 (Portugal)
ESTRADIOL
Climara Transdermal System 795
Vivelle Transdermal System 2288
Vivelle-Dot Transdermal System 2293

FEMOSTON CONTI (Austria, Belgium, Finland, Germany, Italy, Switzerland, United Kingdom)
ESTRADIOL
Climara Transdermal System 795
Vivelle Transdermal System 2288
Vivelle-Dot Transdermal System 2293

FEMOSTON MONO (Germany)
ESTRADIOL
Climara Transdermal System 795
Vivelle Transdermal System 2288
Vivelle-Dot Transdermal System 2293

FEMPHASCYL CONTI (Austria)
ESTRADIOL
Climara Transdermal System 795
Vivelle Transdermal System 2288
Vivelle-Dot Transdermal System 2293

FEMPRESS (Austria, Germany, Switzerland)
MOEXIPRIL HYDROCHLORIDE
Univasc Tablets 3118

FEMPRESS PLUS (Austria, Germany)
HYDROCHLOROTHIAZIDE/MOEXIPRIL HYDROCHLORIDE
Uniretic Tablets 3114

FEMSEPT (France)
ESTRADIOL
Climara Transdermal System 795
Vivelle Transdermal System 2288
Vivelle-Dot Transdermal System 2293

FEMSEVEN (Austria, Denmark, Finland, Italy, Sweden, Switzerland, United Kingdom)
ESTRADIOL
Climara Transdermal System 795
Vivelle Transdermal System 2288
Vivelle-Dot Transdermal System 2293

FEMSEVEN CONTI (United Kingdom)
ESTRADIOL
Climara Transdermal System 795
Vivelle Transdermal System 2288
Vivelle-Dot Transdermal System 2293

FEMSIEBEN (Austria)
ESTRADIOL
Climara Transdermal System 795
Vivelle Transdermal System 2288
Vivelle-Dot Transdermal System 2293

FEMTAB CONTINUOUS (United Kingdom)
ESTRADIOL
Climara Transdermal System 795
Vivelle Transdermal System 2288
Vivelle-Dot Transdermal System 2293

FEMTRAN (Australia, New Zealand)
ESTRADIOL
Climara Transdermal System 795
Vivelle Transdermal System 2288
Vivelle-Dot Transdermal System 2293

FENAC (Australia)
DICLOFENAC SODIUM
Voltaren Tablets 2298
Voltaren-XR Tablets 2301

FENACTOL (United Kingdom)
DICLOFENAC SODIUM
Voltaren Tablets 2298
Voltaren-XR Tablets 2301

FENADIUM (Malaysia)
DICLOFENAC SODIUM
Voltaren Tablets 2298
Voltaren-XR Tablets 2301

FENADOL (Italy)
DICLOFENAC SODIUM
Voltaren Tablets 2298
Voltaren-XR Tablets 2301

FENAFLAN (Brazil)
DICLOFENAC POTASSIUM
Cataflam Tablets 2173

FENAMON (Hong Kong, Malaysia, Singapore, Thailand)
NIFEDIPINE
Adalat CC Tablets 2978

FENAPLUS (India)
DICLOFENAC SODIUM
Voltaren Tablets 2298
Voltaren-XR Tablets 2301

(⊙ Described in PDR For Ophthalmic Medicines™)

FENAREN (Austria)
DICLOFENAC SODIUM
Voltaren Tablets 2298
Voltaren-XR Tablets 2301

FENAX (Chile)
FEXOFENADINE HYDROCHLORIDE
Allegra Capsules 2857

FENAZIL (Italy)
PROMETHAZINE HYDROCHLORIDE
Phenergan Suppositories 3438
Phenergan Tablets 3438

FENBURIL (Brazil)
DICLOFENAC SODIUM
Voltaren Tablets 2298
Voltaren-XR Tablets 2301

FENDER (Italy)
DICLOFENAC SODIUM
Voltaren Tablets 2298
Voltaren-XR Tablets 2301

FENERGAN (Argentina, Portugal)
PROMETHAZINE HYDROCHLORIDE
Phenergan Suppositories 3438
Phenergan Tablets 3438

FENIDINA (Italy)
NIFEDIPINE
Adalat CC Tablets 2978

FENIKEN (Mexico)
NIFEDIPINE
Adalat CC Tablets 2978

FENIL-V (Portugal)
DICLOFENAC SODIUM
Voltaren Tablets 2298
Voltaren-XR Tablets 2301

FENOBETA (Germany)
FENOFIBRATE
Tricor Tablets 523

FENOBRAT (Hungary)
FENOFIBRATE
Tricor Tablets 523

FENOBRATE (Argentina)
FENOFIBRATE
Tricor Tablets 523

FENOCLOF (Greece)
DICLOFENAC SODIUM
Voltaren Tablets 2298
Voltaren-XR Tablets 2301

FENODID (Mexico)
FENTANYL CITRATE
Actiq 993

FENOGAL (Belgium, United Kingdom)
FENOFIBRATE
Tricor Tablets 523

FENOGAL LIDOSE (Singapore)
FENOFIBRATE
Tricor Tablets 523

FENOLIP (Argentina, Austria, India)
FENOFIBRATE
Tricor Tablets 523

FENORIT (Italy)
PROPAFENONE HYDROCHLORIDE
Rythmol SR Capsules 2736

FENSAIDE (India)
DICLOFENAC SODIUM
Voltaren Tablets 2298
Voltaren-XR Tablets 2301

FENSAIDE-P (India)
DICLOFENAC SODIUM
Voltaren Tablets 2298
Voltaren-XR Tablets 2301

FENSARTAN (Argentina)
LOSARTAN POTASSIUM
Cozaar Tablets 1913

FENSARTAN D (Argentina)
LOSARTAN POTASSIUM
Cozaar Tablets 1913

FENSEL (Spain)
FELODIPINE
Plendil Extended-Release Tablets 651

FENTABBOTT (Brazil)
FENTANYL CITRATE
Actiq 993

FENTANEST (Brazil, Italy, Mexico, Spain)
FENTANYL CITRATE
Actiq 993

FENTAX (Argentina)
FENTANYL CITRATE
Actiq 993

FERCAYL (Belgium)
IRON DEXTRAN
Infed Injection 3381

FERMATHRON (Australia, Germany, United Kingdom)
SODIUM HYALURONATE
Hyalgan Solution 2917

FERMAVISC (Switzerland)
SODIUM HYALURONATE
Hyalgan Solution 2917

FERMENTMYCIN (South Africa)
GENTAMICIN SULFATE
Garamycin Injectable 3028
Genoptic Sterile Ophthalmic Solution . . . . ⊙227

FERROCEL (Mexico)
IRON DEXTRAN
Infed Injection 3381

FERROIN (Mexico)
IRON DEXTRAN
Infed Injection 3381

FEXIGRA (India)
FEXOFENADINE HYDROCHLORIDE
Allegra Capsules 2857

FEXIRON (Argentina)
IRON DEXTRAN
Infed Injection 3381

FEXOFEN (Argentina, India)
FEXOFENADINE HYDROCHLORIDE
Allegra Capsules 2857

FEXOTABS (Australia)
FEXOFENADINE HYDROCHLORIDE
Allegra Capsules 2857

FEXOVA (India)
FEXOFENADINE HYDROCHLORIDE
Allegra Capsules 2857

FIAGRA (India)
SILDENAFIL CITRATE
Viagra Tablets 2552

FIBONEL (Chile, Spain)
FAMOTIDINE
Pepcid Injection 2017
Pepcid Injection Premixed 2017
Pepcid Tablets 2014
Pepcid for Oral Suspension 2014

FIBRASE (Italy)
PENTOSAN POLYSULFATE SODIUM
Elmiron Capsules 2393

FIBREZYM (Germany)
PENTOSAN POLYSULFATE SODIUM
Elmiron Capsules 2393

FIBRIN GLUE (Thailand)
THROMBIN
Thrombin-JMI 1693

FIBROCARD (Belgium)
VERAPAMIL HYDROCHLORIDE
Covera-HS Tablets 3135
Verelan PM Capsules 3120

FIBROCID (Spain)
PENTOSAN POLYSULFATE SODIUM
Elmiron Capsules 2393

FIBROCIDE (Portugal)
PENTOSAN POLYSULFATE SODIUM
Elmiron Capsules 2393

FIBROXYN (South Africa)
NAPROXEN
EC-Naprosyn Delayed-Release Tablets 2769
Naprosyn Suspension 2769
Naprosyn Tablets 2769

FIBSOL (Australia)
LISINOPRIL
Prinivil Tablets 2029
Zestril Tablets 704

FIDECAINA (Argentina)
LIDOCAINE
Lidoderm Patch 1107

FIGOZANT (Greece)
NIMODIPINE
Nimotop Capsules 774

FIGREL (Greece)
DICLOFENAC SODIUM
Voltaren Tablets 2298
Voltaren-XR Tablets 2301

FILARTROS (Argentina)
LEFLUNOMIDE
Arava Tablets 2881

FILE (Argentina)
SILDENAFIL CITRATE
Viagra Tablets 2552

FILGINASE (Argentina)
EFAVIRENZ
Sustiva Capsules 957

FILNARINE (United Kingdom)
MORPHINE SULFATE
Kadian Capsules 572
MS Contin Tablets 2703

FILOKLIN (Spain)
CEFAZOLIN SODIUM
Ancef for Injection 1318

FILTEN (Argentina)
CARVEDILOL
Coreg Tablets 1376

FINABAND (Argentina)
BICALUTAMIDE
Casodex Tablets 670

FINABER (Argentina)
ONDANSETRON
Zofran ODT Orally Disintegrating Tablets . . 1613

FINACILEN (Argentina)
NIMODIPINE
Nimotop Capsules 774

FINALOP (Brazil)
FINASTERIDE
Propecia Tablets 2036
Proscar Tablets 2040

FINASEPT (Argentina)
CLARITHROMYCIN
Biaxin Filmtab Tablets 402
Biaxin Granules 402

FINASTERIN (Argentina)
FINASTERIDE
Propecia Tablets 2036
Proscar Tablets 2040

FINASTID (Italy)
FINASTERIDE
Propecia Tablets 2036
Proscar Tablets 2040

FINASTIL (Brazil)
FINASTERIDE
Propecia Tablets 2036
Proscar Tablets 2040

FINCAR (India)
FINASTERIDE
Propecia Tablets 2036
Proscar Tablets 2040

FINDALER (Chile)
CETIRIZINE HYDROCHLORIDE
Zyrtec Syrup 2589
Zyrtec Tablets 2589

FINDECLIN (Argentina)
ALENDRONATE SODIUM
Fosamax Tablets 1949

FINEX (Brazil, Czech Republic)
TERBINAFINE HYDROCHLORIDE
Lamisil Tablets 2226

FINIBRON (Italy)
BUPRENORPHINE HYDROCHLORIDE
Buprenex Injectable 2718

FINLEPSIN (Germany, Hungary)
CARBAMAZEPINE
Carbatrol Capsules 3174
Tegretol Chewable Tablets 2278
Tegretol Suspension 2278
Tegretol Tablets 2278
Tegretol-XR Tablets 2278

FINOXI (Argentina)
ONDANSETRON
Zofran ODT Orally Disintegrating Tablets . . 1613

FINPECIA (India)
FINASTERIDE
Propecia Tablets 2036
Proscar Tablets 2040

FINPROSTAT (Argentina)
FINASTERIDE
Propecia Tablets 2036
Proscar Tablets 2040

FINTOP (India)
BUTENAFINE HYDROCHLORIDE
Mentax Cream 2152

FIRIN (Germany)
NORFLOXACIN
Noroxin Tablets 2009

FIRMACEF (Italy)
CEFAZOLIN SODIUM
Ancef for Injection 1318

FIRMALONE (Italy)
DEXAMETHASONE
Decadron Tablets 1929

FISOPRED (Mexico)
PREDNISOLONE SODIUM PHOSPHATE
Pediapred Oral Solution 3319

FITAXAL (France)
LACTULOSE
Kristalose for Oral Solution 2149

FITONAL (Argentina)
KETOCONAZOLE
Nizoral 2% Shampoo 1838

FITZECALM (United Arab Emirates)
CARBAMAZEPINE
Carbatrol Capsules 3174
Tegretol Chewable Tablets 2278
Tegretol Suspension 2278
Tegretol Tablets 2278
Tegretol-XR Tablets 2278

FIVEFLURO (India)
FLUOROURACIL
Efudex Topical Cream 3348
Efudex Topical Solutions 3348

FIVEROCIL (Mexico)
FLUOROURACIL
Efudex Topical Cream 3348
Efudex Topical Solutions 3348

FIVOFLU (Thailand)
FLUOROURACIL
Efudex Topical Cream 3348
Efudex Topical Solutions 3348

FIXCA (Spain)
ONDANSETRON HYDROCHLORIDE
Zofran Injection 1607
Zofran Injection Premixed 1607
Zofran Oral Solution 1613
Zofran Tablets 1613

FIXIM (The Netherlands)
CEFIXIME
Suprax 1811

FIXIME (South Africa)
CEFIXIME
Suprax 1811

FIXX (India)
CEFIXIME
Suprax 1811

FLADEX (Singapore)
METRONIDAZOLE
MetroGel-Vaginal Gel 1822
Noritate Cream, 1% 1051

FLAGINAZOL (Mexico)
METRONIDAZOLE
MetroGel-Vaginal Gel 1822
Noritate Cream, 1% 1051

FLAGYL (Argentina, Australia, Austria, Belgium, Brazil, Canada, Finland, Germany, Greece, Hong Kong, India, Israel, Italy, Malaysia, Mexico, Portugal, Singapore, South Africa, Switzerland)
METRONIDAZOLE
MetroGel-Vaginal Gel 1822
Noritate Cream, 1% 1051

FLAGYL COMP (Finland)
METRONIDAZOLE
MetroGel-Vaginal Gel 1822
Noritate Cream, 1% 1051

FLAGYL NISTATINA (Brazil)
METRONIDAZOLE
MetroGel-Vaginal Gel 1822
Noritate Cream, 1% 1051

FLAGYSTATIN (Argentina)
METRONIDAZOLE
MetroGel-Vaginal Gel ... 1822
Noritate Cream, 1% ... 1051

FLAGYSTATIN V (Mexico)
METRONIDAZOLE
MetroGel-Vaginal Gel ... 1822
Noritate Cream, 1% ... 1051

FLAMATAK (United Kingdom)
DICLOFENAC SODIUM
Voltaren Tablets ... 2298
Voltaren-XR Tablets ... 2301

FLAMIN (Mexico)
METRONIDAZOLE
MetroGel-Vaginal Gel ... 1822
Noritate Cream, 1% ... 1051

FLAMIN 400 (Mexico)
METRONIDAZOLE
MetroGel-Vaginal Gel ... 1822
Noritate Cream, 1% ... 1051

FLAMON (Switzerland)
VERAPAMIL HYDROCHLORIDE
Covera-HS Tablets ... 3135
Verelan PM Capsules ... 3120

FLAMRASE (United Kingdom)
DICLOFENAC SODIUM
Voltaren Tablets ... 2298
Voltaren-XR Tablets ... 2301

FLANAKIN (Brazil)
DICLOFENAC POTASSIUM
Cataflam Tablets ... 2173

FLANAREN (Brazil)
DICLOFENAC SODIUM
Voltaren Tablets ... 2298
Voltaren-XR Tablets ... 2301

FLANAX (Brazil, Mexico)
NAPROXEN SODIUM
Anaprox DS Tablets ... 2769
Anaprox Tablets ... 2769

FLANIZOL (Brazil)
METRONIDAZOLE
MetroGel-Vaginal Gel ... 1822
Noritate Cream, 1% ... 1051

FLANKOL (Mexico)
DICLOFENAC SODIUM
Voltaren Tablets ... 2298
Voltaren-XR Tablets ... 2301

FLAVIX (India)
VENLAFAXINE HYDROCHLORIDE
Effexor Tablets ... 3405
Effexor XR Capsules ... 3411

FLAXIN (Brazil)
FINASTERIDE
Propecia Tablets ... 2036
Proscar Tablets ... 2040

FLAXVAN (Argentina)
NAPROXEN
EC-Naprosyn Delayed-Release Tablets ... 2769
Naprosyn Suspension ... 2769
Naprosyn Tablets ... 2769

FLECADURA (Germany)
FLECAINIDE ACETATE
Tambocor Tablets ... 1824

FLECAINE (France)
FLECAINIDE ACETATE
Tambocor Tablets ... 1824

FLECATAB (Australia)
FLECAINIDE ACETATE
Tambocor Tablets ... 1824

FLECOR-N (Greece)
NIFEDIPINE
Adalat CC Tablets ... 2978

FLEMEX (Mexico)
HYDROCORTISONE
Hydrocortone Tablets ... 1963

FLEMINOSAN (Hong Kong)
CLINDAMYCIN PHOSPHATE
Clindets Pledgets ... 3212

FLEMOXIN (Russia, Switzerland)
AMOXICILLIN
Amoxil Pediatric Drops for Oral Suspension ... 1315
Amoxil Tablets ... 1315

FLENVERME (Brazil)
MEBENDAZOLE
Vermox Chewable Tablets ... 1853

FLEXAGEN (South Africa)
DICLOFENAC SODIUM
Voltaren Tablets ... 2298
Voltaren-XR Tablets ... 2301

FLEXAMINA (Brazil)
DICLOFENAC SODIUM
Voltaren Tablets ... 2298
Voltaren-XR Tablets ... 2301

FLEXEN (Mexico)
NAPROXEN
EC-Naprosyn Delayed-Release Tablets ... 2769
Naprosyn Suspension ... 2769
Naprosyn Tablets ... 2769

FLEXIN (Israel)
ORPHENADRINE CITRATE
Norflex Injection ... 1824

FLEXOTARD (United Kingdom)
DICLOFENAC SODIUM
Voltaren Tablets ... 2298
Voltaren-XR Tablets ... 2301

FLIXODERM (Italy)
FLUTICASONE PROPIONATE
Cutivate Cream ... 1381
Cutivate Ointment ... 1384
Flonase Nasal Spray ... 1412

FLIXONASE (Argentina, Australia, Austria, Belgium, Brazil, Chile, Czech Republic, Denmark, Finland, France, Hong Kong, Hungary, Irish Republic, Israel, Italy, Malaysia, Mexico, New Zealand, Russia, Singapore, South Africa, Spain, Thailand, The Netherlands, United Kingdom)
FLUTICASONE PROPIONATE
Cutivate Cream ... 1381
Cutivate Ointment ... 1384
Flonase Nasal Spray ... 1412

FLIXOTAIDE (Portugal)
FLUTICASONE PROPIONATE
Cutivate Cream ... 1381
Cutivate Ointment ... 1384
Flonase Nasal Spray ... 1412

FLIXOTIDE (Argentina, Australia, Austria, Belgium, Brazil, Chile, Czech Republic, Denmark, Finland, France, Greece, Hong Kong, Hungary, Irish Republic, Israel, Italy, Malaysia, Mexico, New Zealand, Russia, Singapore, South Africa, Spain, Thailand, The Netherlands, United Kingdom)
FLUTICASONE PROPIONATE
Cutivate Cream ... 1381
Cutivate Ointment ... 1384
Flonase Nasal Spray ... 1412

FLIXOVATE (France)
FLUTICASONE PROPIONATE
Cutivate Cream ... 1381
Cutivate Ointment ... 1384
Flonase Nasal Spray ... 1412

FLOBAC (Brazil)
CIPROFLOXACIN
Cipro Oral Suspension ... 2991

FLOBACIN (Italy)
OFLOXACIN
Floxin Otic Solution ... 1043

FLOCOFIL (Mexico)
MERCAPTOPURINE
Purinethol Tablets ... 1222

FLODIL (France)
FELODIPINE
Plendil Extended-Release Tablets ... 651

FLOGEN (Mexico)
NAPROXEN SODIUM
Anaprox DS Tablets ... 2769
Anaprox Tablets ... 2769

FLOGENAC (Argentina)
DICLOFENAC SODIUM
Voltaren Tablets ... 2298
Voltaren-XR Tablets ... 2301

FLOGESIC (Brazil)
DICLOFENAC SODIUM
Voltaren Tablets ... 2298
Voltaren-XR Tablets ... 2301

FLOGINAX (Italy)
NAPROXEN
EC-Naprosyn Delayed-Release Tablets ... 2769
Naprosyn Suspension ... 2769
Naprosyn Tablets ... 2769

FLOGOCEFAL (Argentina)
NAPROXEN
EC-Naprosyn Delayed-Release Tablets ... 2769
Naprosyn Suspension ... 2769
Naprosyn Tablets ... 2769

FLOGOCORT (Chile)
MOMETASONE FUROATE
Elocon Cream 0.1% ... 3019
Elocon Lotion 0.1% ... 3020
Elocon Ointment 0.1% ... 3021
Nasonex Nasal Spray ... 3058

FLOGOGIN (Italy)
NAPROXEN SODIUM
Anaprox DS Tablets ... 2769
Anaprox Tablets ... 2769

FLOGOLISIN (Argentina)
DICLOFENAC SODIUM
Voltaren Tablets ... 2298
Voltaren-XR Tablets ... 2301

FLOGONAC (Brazil)
DICLOFENAC POTASSIUM
Cataflam Tablets ... 2173

FLOHALE (India)
FLUTICASONE PROPIONATE
Cutivate Cream ... 1381
Cutivate Ointment ... 1384
Flonase Nasal Spray ... 1412

FLOLAN (Australia, Austria, Belgium, Canada, Czech Republic, Denmark, France, Irish Republic, Israel, Italy, Norway, Singapore, Spain, Switzerland, The Netherlands, United Kingdom)
EPOPROSTENOL SODIUM
Flolan for Injection ... 1408

FLOMAX (Australia, Canada, New Zealand, South Africa, United Kingdom)
TAMSULOSIN HYDROCHLORIDE
Flomax Capsules ... 881

FLOMAXTRA (United Kingdom)
TAMSULOSIN HYDROCHLORIDE
Flomax Capsules ... 881

FLOMEX (India)
FLUOROMETHOLONE
FML Ophthalmic Ointment ... ⊙225

FLOMEX N (India)
FLUOROMETHOLONE
FML Ophthalmic Ointment ... ⊙225

FLOMIST (India)
FLUTICASONE PROPIONATE
Cutivate Cream ... 1381
Cutivate Ointment ... 1384
Flonase Nasal Spray ... 1412

FLONASE (Canada)
FLUTICASONE PROPIONATE
Cutivate Cream ... 1381
Cutivate Ointment ... 1384
Flonase Nasal Spray ... 1412

FLORAC (India)
FLUOROURACIL
Efudex Topical Cream ... 3348
Efudex Topical Solutions ... 3348

FLORALAC (Austria)
LACTULOSE
Kristalose for Oral Solution ... 2149

FLORAXINA (Argentina)
CIPROFLOXACIN HYDROCHLORIDE
Ciloxan Ophthalmic Ointment ... 554
Ciloxan Ophthalmic Solution ... ⊙205
Cipro Tablets ... 2991

FLORAZOLE (Canada)
METRONIDAZOLE
MetroGel-Vaginal Gel ... 1822
Noritate Cream, 1% ... 1051

FLOSEF (India)
FLUOROMETHOLONE
FML Ophthalmic Ointment ... ⊙225

FLOSSAC (Italy)
NORFLOXACIN
Noroxin Tablets ... 2009

FLOTRIN (Germany)
TERAZOSIN HYDROCHLORIDE
Hytrin Capsules ... 469

FLOVENT (Canada)
FLUTICASONE PROPIONATE
Cutivate Cream ... 1381
Cutivate Ointment ... 1384
Flonase Nasal Spray ... 1412

FLOVID (Hong Kong, Malaysia)
OFLOXACIN
Floxin Otic Solution ... 1043

FLOX (Brazil)
NORFLOXACIN
Noroxin Tablets ... 2009

FLOXACIN (Austria, Brazil, Mexico)
NORFLOXACIN
Noroxin Tablets ... 2009

FLOXACIPRON (Portugal)
CIPROFLOXACIN
Cipro Oral Suspension ... 2991

FLOXAGER (Mexico)
CIPROFLOXACIN HYDROCHLORIDE
Ciloxan Ophthalmic Ointment ... 554
Ciloxan Ophthalmic Solution ... ⊙205
Cipro Tablets ... 2991

FLOXAKIN (Mexico)
CIPROFLOXACIN
Cipro Oral Suspension ... 2991

FLOXAL (Austria, Czech Republic, Germany, Hungary, Switzerland)
OFLOXACIN
Floxin Otic Solution ... 1043

FLOXALIN (Italy)
NAPROXEN SODIUM
Anaprox DS Tablets ... 2769
Anaprox Tablets ... 2769

FLOXAMICIN (Argentina)
NORFLOXACIN
Noroxin Tablets ... 2009

FLOXAN (Brazil)
CIPROFLOXACIN
Cipro Oral Suspension ... 2991

FLOXANOR (Brazil)
NORFLOXACIN
Noroxin Tablets ... 2009

FLOXANTINA (Mexico)
CIPROFLOXACIN HYDROCHLORIDE
Ciloxan Ophthalmic Ointment ... 554
Ciloxan Ophthalmic Solution ... ⊙205
Cipro Tablets ... 2991

FLOXATRAL (Argentina)
NORFLOXACIN
Noroxin Tablets ... 2009

FLOXATRAT (Brazil)
NORFLOXACIN
Noroxin Tablets ... 2009

FLOXEDOL (Portugal)
OFLOXACIN
Floxin Otic Solution ... 1043

FLOXELENA (Mexico)
CIPROFLOXACIN
Cipro Oral Suspension ... 2991

FLOXEN (Hong Kong)
NORFLOXACIN
Noroxin Tablets ... 2009

FLOXENOR (Thailand)
NORFLOXACIN
Noroxin Tablets ... 2009

FLOXIL (Argentina, Mexico)
OFLOXACIN
Floxin Otic Solution ... 1043

FLOXIN (Canada, South Africa)
OFLOXACIN
Floxin Otic Solution ... 1043

FLOXINOL (Brazil)
NORFLOXACIN
Noroxin Tablets ... 2009

FLOXLEVO (Argentina)
LEVOFLOXACIN
Levaquin Injection ... 2453
Levaquin Tablets ... 2453

FLOXSTAT (Brazil, Mexico)
OFLOXACIN
Floxin Otic Solution ... 1043

FLOXUR (India)
OFLOXACIN
Floxin Otic Solution 1043

FLOXY (Thailand)
OFLOXACIN
Floxin Otic Solution 1043

FLU OPH (Thailand)
FLUOROMETHOLONE
FML Ophthalmic Ointment ⊙225

FLUATON (Italy)
FLUOROMETHOLONE
FML Ophthalmic Ointment ⊙225

FLUCINOM (Czech Republic, Greece)
FLUTAMIDE
Eulexin Capsules 3023

FLUCINOME (Switzerland)
FLUTAMIDE
Eulexin Capsules 3023

FLUCON (Australia, Belgium, Czech Republic, France, Greece, Hong Kong, Hungary, New Zealand, South Africa, Switzerland, Thailand, The Netherlands)
FLUOROMETHOLONE
FML Ophthalmic Ointment ⊙225

FLUDAPAMIDE (Switzerland)
INDAPAMIDE
Indapamide Tablets 2119

FLUDEX (Austria, Belgium, Denmark, France, Greece, Portugal, Switzerland, The Netherlands)
INDAPAMIDE
Indapamide Tablets 2119

FLUFORTE (Chile, Mexico)
FLUOROMETHOLONE
FML Ophthalmic Ointment ⊙225

FLUFORTE N (Mexico)
FLUOROMETHOLONE
FML Ophthalmic Ointment ⊙225

FLUGEN (Spain)
FLUOROMETHOLONE
FML Ophthalmic Ointment ⊙225

FLUIDEMA (Portugal)
INDAPAMIDE
Indapamide Tablets 2119

FLUILAST (Italy)
TICLOPIDINE HYDROCHLORIDE
Ticlid Tablets 2813

FLUINOL (Spain)
FLUTICASONE PROPIONATE
Cutivate Cream 1381
Cutivate Ointment 1384
Flonase Nasal Spray 1412

FLUI-THEOPHYLLINE (Germany)
THEOPHYLLINE
Uniphyl Tablets 2708

FLUKEN (Mexico)
FLUTAMIDE
Eulexin Capsules 3023

FLULEM (Chile, Mexico)
FLUTAMIDE
Eulexin Capsules 3023

FLUMADINE (Israel)
RIMANTADINE HYDROCHLORIDE
Flumadine Syrup 1186
Flumadine Tablets 1186

FLUMARC (Argentina)
TERAZOSIN HYDROCHLORIDE
Hytrin Capsules 469

FLUMETHOLON (Hong Kong)
FLUOROMETHOLONE
FML Ophthalmic Ointment ⊙225

FLUMETOL (Greece)
TIMOLOL MALEATE
Blocadren Tablets 1891
Timoptic Sterile Ophthalmic Solution 2058
Timoptic in Ocudose 2061
Timoptic-XE Sterile Ophthalmic Gel Forming Solution 2062

FLUMETOL S (Czech Republic)
FLUOROMETHOLONE
FML Ophthalmic Ointment ⊙225

FLUMETOL SEMPLICE (Italy)
FLUOROMETHOLONE
FML Ophthalmic Ointment ⊙225

FLUMEX (Brazil)
FLUOROMETHOLONE
FML Ophthalmic Ointment ⊙225

FLUMID (Germany)
FLUTAMIDE
Eulexin Capsules 3023

FLUMINEX (Italy)
FLUNISOLIDE
Aerobid Inhaler System 1172
Aerobid-M Inhaler System 1172
Nasarel Nasal Spray 1652

FLUMOX (South Africa)
AMOXICILLIN
Amoxil Pediatric Drops for Oral Suspension 1315
Amoxil Tablets 1315

FLUNASE (Israel)
FLUNISOLIDE
Aerobid Inhaler System 1172
Aerobid-M Inhaler System 1172
Nasarel Nasal Spray 1652

FLUNIDOR (Portugal)
DIFLUNISAL
Dolobid Tablets 1937

FLUNIGAR (Italy)
FLUNISOLIDE
Aerobid Inhaler System 1172
Aerobid-M Inhaler System 1172
Nasarel Nasal Spray 1652

FLUNIGET (Austria, Germany)
DIFLUNISAL
Dolobid Tablets 1937

FLUNITEC (Argentina, Brazil, Denmark, Norway)
FLUNISOLIDE
Aerobid Inhaler System 1172
Aerobid-M Inhaler System 1172
Nasarel Nasal Spray 1652

FLUNITOP (Italy)
FLUNISOLIDE
Aerobid Inhaler System 1172
Aerobid-M Inhaler System 1172
Nasarel Nasal Spray 1652

FLUODONIL (Italy)
DIFLUNISAL
Dolobid Tablets 1937

FLUOFTAL (Austria)
FLUORESCEIN SODIUM
Fluorescite Injection ⊙207

FLUORALFA (Italy)
FLUORESCEIN SODIUM
Fluorescite Injection ⊙207

FLUOR-AMPS (United Kingdom)
FLUORESCEIN SODIUM
Fluorescite Injection ⊙207

FLUORE STAIN STRIPS (India)
FLUORESCEIN SODIUM
Fluorescite Injection ⊙207

FLUORES (South Africa)
FLUORESCEIN SODIUM
Fluorescite Injection ⊙207

FLUORESCITE (Argentina, Australia, Canada, Hong Kong, Malaysia, New Zealand, Singapore, South Africa, Thailand)
FLUORESCEIN SODIUM
Fluorescite Injection ⊙207

FLUORETS (Australia, Canada, Hong Kong, Irish Republic, New Zealand, Singapore, South Africa)
FLUORESCEIN SODIUM
Fluorescite Injection ⊙207

FLUOR-I-STRIP AT (Canada)
FLUORESCEIN SODIUM
Fluorescite Injection ⊙207

FLUORO-OPHTAL (Germany)
FLUOROMETHOLONE
FML Ophthalmic Ointment ⊙225

FLUOROPLEX (Australia, Canada)
FLUOROURACIL
Efudex Topical Cream 3348
Efudex Topical Solutions 3348

FLUOROPOS (Czech Republic, Germany)
FLUOROMETHOLONE
FML Ophthalmic Ointment ⊙225

FLUPID (Italy)
TICLOPIDINE HYDROCHLORIDE
Ticlid Tablets 2813

FLUPROSIN (Denmark)
FLUTAMIDE
Eulexin Capsules 3023

FLUPROST (Italy)
FLUTAMIDE
Eulexin Capsules 3023

FLURABLASTIN (Denmark, Finland, Norway)
FLUOROURACIL
Efudex Topical Cream 3348
Efudex Topical Solutions 3348

FLURACEDYL (Israel, Malaysia, Norway)
FLUOROURACIL
Efudex Topical Cream 3348
Efudex Topical Solutions 3348

FLURACIL (India)
FLUOROURACIL
Efudex Topical Cream 3348
Efudex Topical Solutions 3348

FLURESS (Australia)
FLUORESCEIN SODIUM
Fluorescite Injection ⊙207

FLUROBLASTIN (Australia, Germany, South Africa)
FLUOROURACIL
Efudex Topical Cream 3348
Efudex Topical Solutions 3348

FLUROBLASTINE (Switzerland)
FLUOROURACIL
Efudex Topical Cream 3348
Efudex Topical Solutions 3348

FLUROLON (Denmark)
FLUOROMETHOLONE
FML Ophthalmic Ointment ⊙225

FLUROP (Portugal)
FLUOROMETHOLONE
FML Ophthalmic Ointment ⊙225

FLUROX (Mexico, Thailand)
FLUOROURACIL
Efudex Topical Cream 3348
Efudex Topical Solutions 3348

FLUSEMINAL (Greece)
NORFLOXACIN
Noroxin Tablets 2009

FLUSONAL (Spain)
FLUTICASONE PROPIONATE
Cutivate Cream 1381
Cutivate Ointment 1384
Flonase Nasal Spray 1412

FLUSPIRAL (Italy)
FLUTICASONE PROPIONATE
Cutivate Cream 1381
Cutivate Ointment 1384
Flonase Nasal Spray 1412

FLUSTAR (Italy)
DIFLUNISAL
Dolobid Tablets 1937

FLUTABENE (Austria)
FLUTAMIDE
Eulexin Capsules 3023

FLUTACAN (Czech Republic, Denmark, Sweden)
FLUTAMIDE
Eulexin Capsules 3023

FLUTAHEXAL (Austria, South Africa)
FLUTAMIDE
Eulexin Capsules 3023

FLUTAIDE (Portugal)
FLUTICASONE PROPIONATE
Cutivate Cream 1381
Cutivate Ointment 1384
Flonase Nasal Spray 1412

FLUTAM (Hungary)
FLUTAMIDE
Eulexin Capsules 3023

FLUTAMEX (Germany)
FLUTAMIDE
Eulexin Capsules 3023

FLUTAMID (Russia)
FLUTAMIDE
Eulexin Capsules 3023

FLUTAMIN (Australia, New Zealand)
FLUTAMIDE
Eulexin Capsules 3023

FLUTAN (Hong Kong, Malaysia, Thailand)
FLUTAMIDE
Eulexin Capsules 3023

FLUTANDRONA (Spain)
FLUTAMIDE
Eulexin Capsules 3023

FLUTAPLEX (Argentina, Belgium, Denmark, Malaysia, South Africa, Spain)
FLUTAMIDE
Eulexin Capsules 3023

FLUTASTAD (Austria)
FLUTAMIDE
Eulexin Capsules 3023

FLUTAX (Argentina)
FLUTAMIDE
Eulexin Capsules 3023

FLUTEPAN (Argentina)
FLUTAMIDE
Eulexin Capsules 3023

FLUTIAMIK (Argentina)
FINASTERIDE
Propecia Tablets 2036
Proscar Tablets 2040

FLUTICORT (Argentina)
FLUTICASONE PROPIONATE
Cutivate Cream 1381
Cutivate Ointment 1384
Flonase Nasal Spray 1412

FLUTIDE (Norway, Sweden)
FLUTICASONE PROPIONATE
Cutivate Cream 1381
Cutivate Ointment 1384
Flonase Nasal Spray 1412

FLUTI-K (Argentina)
FLUTICASONE PROPIONATE
Cutivate Cream 1381
Cutivate Ointment 1384
Flonase Nasal Spray 1412

FLUTINASE (Switzerland)
FLUTICASONE PROPIONATE
Cutivate Cream 1381
Cutivate Ointment 1384
Flonase Nasal Spray 1412

FLUTIVATE (Brazil, Chile, Germany, Norway, Sweden)
FLUTICASONE PROPIONATE
Cutivate Cream 1381
Cutivate Ointment 1384
Flonase Nasal Spray 1412

FLUTOL (New Zealand)
FLUTAMIDE
Eulexin Capsules 3023

FLUTRAX (Argentina)
FLUTAMIDE
Eulexin Capsules 3023

FLUXIDIN (Italy)
TICLOPIDINE HYDROCHLORIDE
Ticlid Tablets 2813

FLUXIL (Brazil)
FUROSEMIDE
Furosemide Tablets 2117

FLUXINAM (Greece)
FLUOROMETHOLONE
FML Ophthalmic Ointment ⊙225

FLUXOCOR (Brazil)
DIPYRIDAMOLE
Persantine Tablets 898

FLUXPIREN (Argentina)
DICLOFENAC SODIUM
Voltaren Tablets 2298
Voltaren-XR Tablets 2301

FLUZORAL (Hong Kong)
KETOCONAZOLE
Nizoral 2% Shampoo 1838

(⊙ Described in PDR For Ophthalmic Medicines™)

FML (Argentina, Australia, Belgium, Canada, Finland, Greece, Hong Kong, Irish Republic, Israel, Malaysia, Mexico, New Zealand, Portugal, Singapore, South Africa, Spain, Switzerland, Thailand, The Netherlands, United Kingdom)
FLUOROMETHOLONE
FML Ophthalmic Ointment .... ⊙225

FML NEO (Argentina)
FLUOROMETHOLONE
FML Ophthalmic Ointment .... ⊙225

FOILLE INSETTI (Italy)
HYDROCORTISONE
Hydrocortone Tablets 1963

FOKALEPSIN (Germany)
CARBAMAZEPINE
Carbatrol Capsules 3174
Tegretol Chewable Tablets 2278
Tegretol Suspension 2278
Tegretol Tablets 2278
Tegretol-XR Tablets 2278

FOLCRES (Argentina)
FINASTERIDE
Propecia Tablets 2036
Proscar Tablets 2040

FOLITABS (Spain)
FINASTERIDE
Propecia Tablets 2036
Proscar Tablets 2040

FONGERYL (France)
ECONAZOLE NITRATE
Spectazole Cream 2390

FONX (France)
OXICONAZOLE NITRATE
Oxistat Cream 1498
Oxistat Lotion 1498

FORDRIM (Argentina)
FLURAZEPAM HYDROCHLORIDE
Dalmane Capsules 3343

FOREXIN (Thailand)
CIPROFLOXACIN
Cipro Oral Suspension 2991

FORKEN (Mexico)
AMIODARONE HYDROCHLORIDE
Pacerone Tablets 3337

FORMAT (Argentina)
METRONIDAZOLE
MetroGel-Vaginal Gel 1822
Noritate Cream, 1% 1051

FORMISTIN (Italy)
CETIRIZINE HYDROCHLORIDE
Zyrtec Syrup 2589
Zyrtec Tablets 2589

FORPAR (India)
CEFEPIME HYDROCHLORIDE
Maxipime for Injection 1093

FORTAM (Spain, Switzerland)
CEFTAZIDIME
Fortaz for Injection 1422

FORTASEC (Spain)
LOPERAMIDE HYDROCHLORIDE
Imodium Capsules 1834

FORTAZ (Brazil, Canada)
CEFTAZIDIME
Fortaz for Injection 1422

FORTECORTIN (Czech Republic, Spain)
DEXAMETHASONE
Decadron Tablets 1929

FORTEDOL (Hungary)
DICLOFENAC POTASSIUM
Cataflam Tablets 2173

FORTENAC (Switzerland)
DICLOFENAC SODIUM
Voltaren Tablets 2298
Voltaren-XR Tablets 2301

FORTERRA (Greece)
CIPROFLOXACIN HYDROCHLORIDE
Ciloxan Ophthalmic Ointment 554
Ciloxan Ophthalmic Solution .... ⊙205
Cipro Tablets 2991

FORTFEN (South Africa)
DICLOFENAC SODIUM
Voltaren Tablets 2298
Voltaren-XR Tablets 2301

FORTIMAX (Spain)
NORFLOXACIN
Noroxin Tablets 2009

FORTIPINE (United Kingdom)
NIFEDIPINE
Adalat CC Tablets 2978

FORTUM (Argentina, Australia, Austria, Chile, Czech Republic, Denmark, France, Germany, Hong Kong, Hungary, India, Irish Republic, Israel, Malaysia, Mexico, New Zealand, Norway, Singapore, South Africa, Sweden, Thailand, The Netherlands, United Kingdom)
CEFTAZIDIME
Fortaz for Injection 1422

FORTUMSET (France)
CEFTAZIDIME
Fortaz for Injection 1422

FORTZAAR (Denmark, France, Malaysia, Portugal, South Africa, Spain, Thailand, The Netherlands)
LOSARTAN POTASSIUM
Cozaar Tablets 1913

FORVERM (Brazil)
MEBENDAZOLE
Vermox Chewable Tablets 1853

FORZAAR (Italy)
LOSARTAN POTASSIUM
Cozaar Tablets 1913

FORZID (Thailand)
CEFTAZIDIME
Fortaz for Injection 1422

FOSALAN (Israel)
ALENDRONATE SODIUM
Fosamax Tablets 1949

FOSAMAX (Argentina, Australia, Austria, Belgium, Brazil, Canada, Chile, Czech Republic, Denmark, Finland, France, Germany, Greece, Hong Kong, Hungary, Irish Republic, Italy, Malaysia, Mexico, New Zealand, Norway, Portugal, Russia, Singapore, South Africa, Spain, Sweden, Switzerland, Thailand, The Netherlands, United Kingdom)
ALENDRONATE SODIUM
Fosamax Tablets 1949

FOSSYOL (Germany)
METRONIDAZOLE
MetroGel-Vaginal Gel 1822
Noritate Cream, 1% 1051

FOSVAL (Chile)
ALENDRONATE SODIUM
Fosamax Tablets 1949

FOTADEX (Argentina)
TOBRAMYCIN
TOBI Solution for Inhalation 1015

FOTEX (Argentina)
TOBRAMYCIN
TOBI Solution for Inhalation 1015

FOUCACILLIN (Greece)
CEFUROXIME AXETIL
Ceftin Tablets 1369
Ceftin for Oral Suspension 1369

FOURNOX (Thailand)
CEFTAZIDIME
Fortaz for Injection 1422

FOXIN (Thailand)
NORFLOXACIN
Noroxin Tablets 2009

FOXINON (Thailand)
NORFLOXACIN
Noroxin Tablets 2009

FOXTIL (Brazil)
CEFOXITIN SODIUM
Mefoxin Premixed Intravenous Solution 1990
Mefoxin for Injection 1987

FP TAB (Japan)
SELEGILINE HYDROCHLORIDE
Eldepryl Capsules 3209

FRACTAL (France)
FLUVASTATIN SODIUM
Lescol Capsules 2227

FRAGMIN (Australia, Austria, Belgium, Brazil, Canada, Chile, Czech Republic, Denmark, Finland, Germany, Hong Kong, Hungary, Israel, Italy, New Zealand, Norway, Portugal, Russia, Singapore, South Africa, Spain, Sweden, Switzerland, The Netherlands, United Kingdom)
DALTEPARIN SODIUM
Fragmin Injection 2638

FRAGMINE (France)
DALTEPARIN SODIUM
Fragmin Injection 2638

FRANOL (Thailand)
THEOPHYLLINE
Uniphyl Tablets 2708

FRECUENTAL (Argentina)
FUROSEMIDE
Furosemide Tablets 2117

FREDYR (Greece)
CEFUROXIME SODIUM
Zinacef Injection 1604

FREMET (Spain)
CIMETIDINE
Tagamet Tablets 1547

FRESENIZOL (Mexico)
METRONIDAZOLE
MetroGel-Vaginal Gel 1822
Noritate Cream, 1% 1051

FRESOFOL (Argentina, Mexico, Thailand)
PROPOFOL
Diprivan Injectable Emulsion 676

FREUDAL (Mexico)
DIAZEPAM
Diastat Rectal Delivery System 3344
Valium Tablets 2822

FRIDALIT (Argentina)
HYDROCORTISONE
Hydrocortone Tablets 1963

FRINOVA (Spain)
PROMETHAZINE HYDROCHLORIDE
Phenergan Suppositories 3438
Phenergan Tablets 3438

FRIPI (Argentina)
PERMETHRIN
Acticin Cream 2125

FRISOL (Portugal)
KETOCONAZOLE
Nizoral 2% Shampoo 1838

FRISOLAC (Portugal)
KETOCONAZOLE
Nizoral 2% Shampoo 1838

FRIVENT (Italy)
THEOPHYLLINE
Uniphyl Tablets 2708

FROIDIR (Finland)
CLOZAPINE
Clozapine Tablets 2141
Clozaril Tablets 2174

FROMILID (Czech Republic, Hungary, Russia)
CLARITHROMYCIN
Biaxin Filmtab Tablets 402
Biaxin Granules 402

FROOP (United Kingdom)
FUROSEMIDE
Furosemide Tablets 2117

FROSINOR (Spain)
PAROXETINE HYDROCHLORIDE
Paxil Oral Suspension 1501
Paxil Tablets 1501

FROTIN (Malaysia)
METRONIDAZOLE
MetroGel-Vaginal Gel 1822
Noritate Cream, 1% 1051

FROXAL (Mexico)
CEFUROXIME SODIUM
Zinacef Injection 1604

FRUDEMISAN (Mexico)
FUROSEMIDE
Furosemide Tablets 2117

FRUMAX (United Kingdom)
FUROSEMIDE
Furosemide Tablets 2117

FRUMERON (Hong Kong, Thailand)
INDAPAMIDE
Indapamide Tablets 2119

FRUSEHEXAL (Australia)
FUROSEMIDE
Furosemide Tablets 2117

FRUSEMIX (India)
FUROSEMIDE
Furosemide Tablets 2117

FRUSENE (Irish Republic, United Kingdom)
FUROSEMIDE
Furosemide Tablets 2117

FRUSENEX (India)
FUROSEMIDE
Furosemide Tablets 2117

FRUSETIC (United Kingdom)
FUROSEMIDE
Furosemide Tablets 2117

FRUSID (Australia, Hong Kong, New Zealand, Singapore, United Kingdom)
FUROSEMIDE
Furosemide Tablets 2117

FRUSIDE (Irish Republic)
FUROSEMIDE
Furosemide Tablets 2117

FRUSIX (India)
FUROSEMIDE
Furosemide Tablets 2117

FRUSOL (United Kingdom)
FUROSEMIDE
Furosemide Tablets 2117

FTDA (Argentina)
FLUTAMIDE
Eulexin Capsules 3023

FTONAVIL (Greece)
CAPTOPRIL
Captopril Tablets 2114

FTOROCORT (Hungary, Russia, Thailand)
TRIAMCINOLONE ACETONIDE
Azmacort Inhalation Aerosol 1701
Nasacort AQ Nasal Spray 2937

FUCEROX (Mexico)
CEFUROXIME SODIUM
Zinacef Injection 1604

FUDERMEX (Chile)
LANSOPRAZOLE
Prevacid Delayed-Release Capsules 3268

FUDIRINE (Thailand)
FUROSEMIDE
Furosemide Tablets 2117

FUDONE (India)
FAMOTIDINE
Pepcid Injection 2017
Pepcid Injection Premixed 2017
Pepcid Tablets 2014
Pepcid for Oral Suspension 2014

FUGACAR (Thailand)
MEBENDAZOLE
Vermox Chewable Tablets 1853

FUGEREL (Australia, Austria, Germany, Hong Kong, Hungary, Malaysia, Singapore, Thailand)
FLUTAMIDE
Eulexin Capsules 3023

FULCRO (Italy)
FENOFIBRATE
Tricor Tablets 523

FUL-GLO (Australia, New Zealand)
FLUORESCEIN SODIUM
Fluorescite Injection .... ⊙207

FULGRAM (Italy)
NORFLOXACIN
Noroxin Tablets 2009

FULGRAM 400 (Chile)
NORFLOXACIN
Noroxin Tablets 2009

(⊙ Described in PDR For Ophthalmic Medicines™)

FUMARENID (Germany)
FUROSEMIDE
Furosemide Tablets **2117**

FUNAZOLE (India)
KETOCONAZOLE
Nizoral 2% Shampoo **1838**

FUNDAN (Sweden)
KETOCONAZOLE
Nizoral 2% Shampoo **1838**

FUNDUSCEIN (Canada)
FLUORESCEIN SODIUM
Fluorescite Injection . . . . **⊙207**

FUNGAMIZOL (Mexico)
KETOCONAZOLE
Nizoral 2% Shampoo **1838**

FUNGAREST (Chile, Spain)
KETOCONAZOLE
Nizoral 2% Shampoo **1838**

FUNGAZOL (Hong Kong, Malaysia, Mexico, Thailand)
KETOCONAZOLE
Nizoral 2% Shampoo **1838**

FUNGEDERM (United Kingdom)
CLOTRIMAZOLE
Lotrimin Cream **3053**
Lotrimin Lotion 1% **3053**
Lotrimin Topical Solution 1% **3053**

FUNGICIDE (India, Thailand)
KETOCONAZOLE
Nizoral 2% Shampoo **1838**

FUNGICIDIN (Czech Republic)
NYSTATIN
Nystop Topical Powder USP **2490**

FUNGICIL (Argentina)
KETOCONAZOLE
Nizoral 2% Shampoo **1838**

FUNGICON (Thailand)
CLOTRIMAZOLE
Lotrimin Cream **3053**
Lotrimin Lotion 1% **3053**
Lotrimin Topical Solution 1% **3053**

FUNGIDERM (Germany, Thailand)
CLOTRIMAZOLE
Lotrimin Cream **3053**
Lotrimin Lotion 1% **3053**
Lotrimin Topical Solution 1% **3053**

FUNGIDERM-K (Thailand)
KETOCONAZOLE
Nizoral 2% Shampoo **1838**

FUNGIDERMO (Spain)
CLOTRIMAZOLE
Lotrimin Cream **3053**
Lotrimin Lotion 1% **3053**
Lotrimin Topical Solution 1% **3053**

FUNGIMAX (Brazil)
METRONIDAZOLE
MetroGel-Vaginal Gel **1822**
Noritate Cream, 1% **1051**

FUNGINOX (Malaysia, Thailand)
KETOCONAZOLE
Nizoral 2% Shampoo **1838**

FUNGIREDUCT (Germany)
NYSTATIN
Nystop Topical Powder USP **2490**

FUNGISPOR (South Africa)
CLOTRIMAZOLE
Lotrimin Cream **3053**
Lotrimin Lotion 1% **3053**
Lotrimin Topical Solution 1% **3053**

FUNGISTEN (Norway)
CLOTRIMAZOLE
Lotrimin Cream **3053**
Lotrimin Lotion 1% **3053**
Lotrimin Topical Solution 1% **3053**

FUNGIUM (Chile)
KETOCONAZOLE
Nizoral 2% Shampoo **1838**

FUNGIZID (Germany, Hong Kong, New Zealand)
CLOTRIMAZOLE
Lotrimin Cream **3053**
Lotrimin Lotion 1% **3053**
Lotrimin Topical Solution 1% **3053**

FUNGO FARMASIERRA (Spain)
KETOCONAZOLE
Nizoral 2% Shampoo **1838**

FUNGORAL (Austria, Brazil, Greece, Mexico, Norway, Sweden)
KETOCONAZOLE
Nizoral 2% Shampoo **1838**

FUNGOTERBINE (Russia)
TERBINAFINE HYDROCHLORIDE
Lamisil Tablets **2226**

FUNGOTOX (Switzerland)
CLOTRIMAZOLE
Lotrimin Cream **3053**
Lotrimin Lotion 1% **3053**
Lotrimin Topical Solution 1% **3053**

FUNZAL (Chile)
CLOTRIMAZOLE
Lotrimin Cream **3053**
Lotrimin Lotion 1% **3053**
Lotrimin Topical Solution 1% **3053**

FURAGRAND (Argentina)
FUROSEMIDE
Furosemide Tablets **2117**

FURANTHRIL (Czech Republic, Germany)
FUROSEMIDE
Furosemide Tablets **2117**

FURAXIL (Greece)
CEFUROXIME AXETIL
Ceftin Tablets **1369**
Ceftin for Oral Suspension **1369**

FURAZOLON (Brazil)
HYDROCORTISONE
Hydrocortone Tablets **1963**

FURESE (Denmark)
FUROSEMIDE
Furosemide Tablets **2117**

FURESIN (Brazil)
FUROSEMIDE
Furosemide Tablets **2117**

FURESIS (Finland)
FUROSEMIDE
Furosemide Tablets **2117**

FURESIS COMP (Finland)
FUROSEMIDE
Furosemide Tablets **2117**

FURETIC (Thailand)
FUROSEMIDE
Furosemide Tablets **2117**

FURIDE (Thailand)
FUROSEMIDE
Furosemide Tablets **2117**

FURINE (Thailand)
FUROSEMIDE
Furosemide Tablets **2117**

FURITAL (Argentina)
FUROSEMIDE
Furosemide Tablets **2117**

FURIX (Argentina, Denmark, Norway, Sweden)
FUROSEMIDE
Furosemide Tablets **2117**

FURMIDAL (Mexico)
FUROSEMIDE
Furosemide Tablets **2117**

FURMIDE (Malaysia)
FUROSEMIDE
Furosemide Tablets **2117**

FURO-BASAN (Switzerland)
FUROSEMIDE
Furosemide Tablets **2117**

FURO-BASF (Germany)
FUROSEMIDE
Furosemide Tablets **2117**

FUROBETA (Germany)
FUROSEMIDE
Furosemide Tablets **2117**

FUROGAMMA (Germany)
FUROSEMIDE
Furosemide Tablets **2117**

FUROMED (Germany)
FUROSEMIDE
Furosemide Tablets **2117**

FUROMIL (Mexico)
FUROSEMIDE
Furosemide Tablets **2117**

FUROMIN (Finland)
FUROSEMIDE
Furosemide Tablets **2117**

FURON (Czech Republic, Hungary)
FUROSEMIDE
Furosemide Tablets **2117**

FURONET (Denmark)
FUROSEMIDE
Furosemide Tablets **2117**

FURONEX (Mexico)
FUROSEMIDE
Furosemide Tablets **2117**

FURO-PUREN (Germany)
FUROSEMIDE
Furosemide Tablets **2117**

FURORESE (Czech Republic)
FUROSEMIDE
Furosemide Tablets **2117**

FUROSAL (Germany)
FUROSEMIDE
Furosemide Tablets **2117**

FUROSAN (Brazil, Mexico)
FUROSEMIDE
Furosemide Tablets **2117**

FUROSCAND (Sweden)
FUROSEMIDE
Furosemide Tablets **2117**

FUROSEM (Brazil)
FUROSEMIDE
Furosemide Tablets **2117**

FUROSEMIX (France)
FUROSEMIDE
Furosemide Tablets **2117**

FUROSETRON (Brazil)
FUROSEMIDE
Furosemide Tablets **2117**

FUROSIFAR (Switzerland)
FUROSEMIDE
Furosemide Tablets **2117**

FUROSIX (Brazil)
FUROSEMIDE
Furosemide Tablets **2117**

FUROTER (Mexico)
FUROSEMIDE
Furosemide Tablets **2117**

FUROVITE (Israel)
FUROSEMIDE
Furosemide Tablets **2117**

FUROXIM (Austria)
CEFUROXIME AXETIL
Ceftin Tablets **1369**
Ceftin for Oral Suspension **1369**

FUROZIX (Brazil)
FUROSEMIDE
Furosemide Tablets **2117**

FURSEMIDA (Brazil)
FUROSEMIDE
Furosemide Tablets **2117**

FURSOL (Switzerland)
FUROSEMIDE
Furosemide Tablets **2117**

FURTENK (Argentina)
FUROSEMIDE
Furosemide Tablets **2117**

FUSANIDAZOL (Mexico)
METRONIDAZOLE
MetroGel-Vaginal Gel **1822**
Noritate Cream, 1% **1051**

FUSEPINA (Mexico)
NIFEDIPINE
Adalat CC Tablets **2978**

FUSERIDE (Thailand)
FUROSEMIDE
Furosemide Tablets **2117**

FUSID (Israel, The Netherlands)
FUROSEMIDE
Furosemide Tablets **2117**

FUSTAREN (Mexico)
DICLOFENAC SODIUM
Voltaren Tablets **2298**
Voltaren-XR Tablets **2301**

FUXEN (Mexico)
NAPROXEN
EC-Naprosyn Delayed-Release Tablets **2769**
Naprosyn Suspension **2769**
Naprosyn Tablets **2769**

G-80 (India)
GENTAMICIN SULFATE
Garamycin Injectable **3028**
Genoptic Sterile Ophthalmic Solution . . . . **⊙227**

GABAMOX (Portugal)
GABAPENTIN
Neurontin Capsules **2498**

GABATAL (Austria)
GABAPENTIN
Neurontin Capsules **2498**

GABATRIL (Mexico)
TIAGABINE HYDROCHLORIDE
Gabitril Tablets **998**

GABATUR (Spain)
GABAPENTIN
Neurontin Capsules **2498**

GABITRIL (Australia, Austria, Belgium, Brazil, Czech Republic, Denmark, Finland, France, Germany, Greece, Hungary, Irish Republic, Italy, Portugal, Spain, Switzerland, United Kingdom)
TIAGABINE HYDROCHLORIDE
Gabitril Tablets **998**

GADOPRIL (Argentina)
ENALAPRIL MALEATE
Vasotec I.V. Injection **2076**

GADOPRIL D (Argentina)
ENALAPRIL MALEATE
Vasotec I.V. Injection **2076**

GALEBIRON (Greece)
RANITIDINE HYDROCHLORIDE
Zantac 25 EFFERdose Tablets **1597**
Zantac 150 EFFERdose Tablets **1597**
Zantac 150 Tablets **1597**
Zantac 300 Tablets **1597**
Zantac Injection **1593**
Zantac Injection Premixed **1593**
Zantac Syrup **1597**

GALECIN (Mexico)
CLINDAMYCIN PHOSPHATE
Clindets Pledgets **3212**

GALEDOL (Mexico)
DICLOFENAC SODIUM
Voltaren Tablets **2298**
Voltaren-XR Tablets **2301**

GALEMIN (Greece)
CEFUROXIME SODIUM
Zinacef Injection **1604**

GALENAMET (Irish Republic, United Kingdom)
CIMETIDINE
Tagamet Tablets **1547**

GALENTROMICINA (Mexico)
ERYTHROMYCIN
Ery-Tab Tablets **447**
Erythromycin Base Filmtab Tablets **454**
Erythromycin Delayed-Release Capsules, USP **456**
PCE Dispertab Tablets **510**

GALIDRIN (Mexico)
RANITIDINE HYDROCHLORIDE
Zantac 25 EFFERdose Tablets **1597**
Zantac 150 EFFERdose Tablets **1597**
Zantac 150 Tablets **1597**
Zantac 300 Tablets **1597**
Zantac Injection **1593**
Zantac Injection Premixed **1593**
Zantac Syrup **1597**

GALOL (Greece)
ATENOLOL
Tenormin I.V. Injection **698**

GAMAVATE (United Arab Emirates)
CLOBETASOL PROPIONATE
Temovate Cream **1549**
Temovate E Emollient **1552**
Temovate Gel **1550**
Temovate Ointment **1549**
Temovate Scalp Application **1551**

GAMMAKINE (Italy)
INTERFERON GAMMA-1B
Actimmune **1646**

GANAVAX (Argentina)
VENLAFAXINE HYDROCHLORIDE
Effexor Tablets **3405**
Effexor XR Capsules **3411**

GANCIVIR (Brazil)
GANCICLOVIR SODIUM
Cytovene-IV **2763**

GANOR (Germany)
FAMOTIDINE
Pepcid Injection **2017**
Pepcid Injection Premixed **2017**
Pepcid Tablets **2014**
Pepcid for Oral Suspension **2014**

GANTIN (Australia)
GABAPENTIN
Neurontin Capsules **2498**

GANVIRAX (Brazil)
GANCICLOVIR SODIUM
Cytovene-IV **2763**

GANVIREL (Argentina)
LAMIVUDINE
Epivir Oral Solution **1394**
Epivir Tablets **1394**
Epivir-HBV Oral Solution **1398**
Epivir-HBV Tablets **1398**

GANVIREL DUO (Argentina)
LAMIVUDINE
Epivir Oral Solution **1394**
Epivir Tablets **1394**
Epivir-HBV Oral Solution **1398**
Epivir-HBV Tablets **1398**

GAOPTOL (Monaco)
TIMOLOL MALEATE
Blocadren Tablets **1891**
Timoptic Sterile Ophthalmic Solution **2058**
Timoptic in Ocudose **2061**
Timoptic-XE Sterile Ophthalmic Gel Forming Solution **2062**

GAPROXEN (Greece)
RANITIDINE HYDROCHLORIDE
Zantac 25 EFFERdose Tablets **1597**
Zantac 150 EFFERdose Tablets. **1597**
Zantac 150 Tablets **1597**
Zantac 300 Tablets **1597**
Zantac Injection **1593**
Zantac Injection Premixed **1593**
Zantac Syrup **1597**

GARACIN (Brazil)
GENTAMICIN SULFATE
Garamycin Injectable **3028**
Genoptic Sterile Ophthalmic Solution . . . . **⊙227**

GARACOL (The Netherlands)
GENTAMICIN SULFATE
Garamycin Injectable **3028**
Genoptic Sterile Ophthalmic Solution . . . . **⊙227**

GARACOLL (Mexico, South Africa)
GENTAMICIN SULFATE
Garamycin Injectable **3028**
Genoptic Sterile Ophthalmic Solution . . . . **⊙227**

GARALEN (Mexico)
GENTAMICIN SULFATE
Garamycin Injectable **3028**
Genoptic Sterile Ophthalmic Solution . . . . **⊙227**

GARALONE (Portugal)
GENTAMICIN SULFATE
Garamycin Injectable **3028**
Genoptic Sterile Ophthalmic Solution . . . . **⊙227**

GARAMYCIN (Australia, Austria, Canada, Czech Republic, Denmark, Greece, Hong Kong, Hungary, Israel, Malaysia, Norway, Singapore, South Africa, Sweden, Switzerland, Thailand, The Netherlands, United Kingdom)
GENTAMICIN SULFATE
Garamycin Injectable **3028**
Genoptic Sterile Ophthalmic Solution . . . . **⊙227**

GARANIL (Spain)
CAPTOPRIL
Captopril Tablets **2114**

GARASONE (Czech Republic, Hungary)
GENTAMICIN SULFATE
Garamycin Injectable **3028**
Genoptic Sterile Ophthalmic Solution . . . . **⊙227**

GARATEC (Canada)
GENTAMICIN SULFATE
Garamycin Injectable **3028**
Genoptic Sterile Ophthalmic Solution . . . . **⊙227**

GARDEX (Denmark, Finland)
CETIRIZINE HYDROCHLORIDE
Zyrtec Syrup **2589**
Zyrtec Tablets **2589**

GARDOTON (Chile)
ONDANSETRON
Zofran ODT Orally Disintegrating Tablets . . **1613**

GARIA (Spain)
CEFPODOXIME PROXETIL
Vantin Tablets and Oral Suspension **2650**

GARRANIL (Spain)
CAPTOPRIL
Captopril Tablets **2114**

GASCOP (Mexico)
ALBENDAZOLE
Albenza Tablets. **1310**

GASMILEN (Argentina)
GANCICLOVIR
Cytovene Capsules **2763**

GASTAB (Hong Kong)
CIMETIDINE
Tagamet Tablets **1547**

GASTENIN (Spain)
FAMOTIDINE
Pepcid Injection **2017**
Pepcid Injection Premixed **2017**
Pepcid Tablets **2014**
Pepcid for Oral Suspension **2014**

GASTER (Japan)
FAMOTIDINE
Pepcid Injection **2017**
Pepcid Injection Premixed **2017**
Pepcid Tablets **2014**
Pepcid for Oral Suspension **2014**

GASTEROGEN (Greece)
FAMOTIDINE
Pepcid Injection **2017**
Pepcid Injection Premixed **2017**
Pepcid Tablets **2014**
Pepcid for Oral Suspension **2014**

GASTIDIN (Brazil)
CIMETIDINE
Tagamet Tablets **1547**

GASTIDINE (Hong Kong)
CIMETIDINE
Tagamet Tablets **1547**

GASTOPRIDE (Portugal)
FAMOTIDINE
Pepcid Injection **2017**
Pepcid Injection Premixed **2017**
Pepcid Tablets **2014**
Pepcid for Oral Suspension **2014**

GASTRAL (Spain)
SUCRALFATE
Carafate Suspension **727**
Carafate Tablets **728**

GASTREX (Portugal)
LANSOPRAZOLE
Prevacid Delayed-Release Capsules **3268**

GASTRIDE (Chile)
LANSOPRAZOLE
Prevacid Delayed-Release Capsules **3268**

GASTRIDIN (Italy)
FAMOTIDINE
Pepcid Injection **2017**
Pepcid Injection Premixed **2017**
Pepcid Tablets **2014**
Pepcid for Oral Suspension **2014**

GASTRIDINA (Portugal)
RANITIDINE HYDROCHLORIDE
Zantac 25 EFFERdose Tablets **1597**
Zantac 150 EFFERdose Tablets. **1597**
Zantac 150 Tablets **1597**
Zantac 300 Tablets **1597**
Zantac Injection **1593**
Zantac Injection Premixed **1593**
Zantac Syrup **1597**

GASTRIFAM (Portugal)
FAMOTIDINE
Pepcid Injection **2017**
Pepcid Injection Premixed **2017**
Pepcid Tablets **2014**
Pepcid for Oral Suspension **2014**

GASTRIL (Hong Kong)
RANITIDINE HYDROCHLORIDE
Zantac 25 EFFERdose Tablets **1597**
Zantac 150 EFFERdose Tablets. **1597**
Zantac 150 Tablets **1597**
Zantac 300 Tablets **1597**
Zantac Injection **1593**
Zantac Injection Premixed **1593**
Zantac Syrup **1597**

GASTRION (Spain)
FAMOTIDINE
Pepcid Injection **2017**
Pepcid Injection Premixed **2017**
Pepcid Tablets **2014**
Pepcid for Oral Suspension **2014**

GASTRIUM (Chile)
FAMOTIDINE
Pepcid Injection **2017**
Pepcid Injection Premixed **2017**
Pepcid Tablets **2014**
Pepcid for Oral Suspension **2014**

GASTRO (Israel)
FAMOTIDINE
Pepcid Injection **2017**
Pepcid Injection Premixed **2017**
Pepcid Tablets **2014**
Pepcid for Oral Suspension **2014**

GASTRO H2 (Spain)
CIMETIDINE
Tagamet Tablets **1547**

GASTROBITAN (Norway)
CIMETIDINE
Tagamet Tablets **1547**

GASTROCOL (Chile)
SUCRALFATE
Carafate Suspension **727**
Carafate Tablets **728**

GASTRODIN (Thailand)
CIMETIDINE
Tagamet Tablets **1547**

GASTRODINA (Mexico)
CIMETIDINE
Tagamet Tablets **1547**

GASTRODINE (Brazil)
CIMETIDINE
Tagamet Tablets **1547**

GASTRODOMINA (Hong Kong, Spain)
FAMOTIDINE
Pepcid Injection **2017**
Pepcid Injection Premixed **2017**
Pepcid Tablets **2014**
Pepcid for Oral Suspension **2014**

GASTROGEL (Italy, Switzerland)
SUCRALFATE
Carafate Suspension **727**
Carafate Tablets **728**

GASTROLAV (Portugal)
RANITIDINE HYDROCHLORIDE
Zantac 150 EFFERdose Tablets. **1597**
Zantac 150 Tablets **1597**
Zantac 25 EFFERdose Tablets **1597**
Zantac 300 Tablets **1597**
Zantac Injection **1593**
Zantac Injection Premixed **1593**
Zantac Syrup **1597**

GASTROLEM (Mexico)
CIMETIDINE
Tagamet Tablets **1547**

GASTROLENE (Greece)
CIMETIDINE
Tagamet Tablets **1547**

GASTROLETS (Argentina)
RANITIDINE HYDROCHLORIDE
Zantac 25 EFFERdose Tablets **1597**
Zantac 150 EFFERdose Tablets. **1597**
Zantac 150 Tablets **1597**
Zantac 300 Tablets **1597**
Zantac Injection **1593**
Zantac Injection Premixed **1593**
Zantac Syrup **1597**

GASTROLIBER (Portugal)
LANSOPRAZOLE
Prevacid Delayed-Release Capsules **3268**

GASTROMET (Singapore)
CIMETIDINE
Tagamet Tablets **1547**

GASTRON (South Africa)
LOPERAMIDE HYDROCHLORIDE
Imodium Capsules **1834**

GASTROPEN (Spain)
FAMOTIDINE
Pepcid Injection **2017**
Pepcid Injection Premixed **2017**
Pepcid Tablets **2014**
Pepcid for Oral Suspension **2014**

GASTROPROTECT (Germany)
CIMETIDINE
Tagamet Tablets **1547**

GASTROSEDOL (Argentina)
RANITIDINE HYDROCHLORIDE
Zantac 25 EFFERdose Tablets **1597**
Zantac 150 EFFERdose Tablets. **1597**
Zantac 150 Tablets **1597**
Zantac 300 Tablets **1597**
Zantac Injection **1593**
Zantac Injection Premixed **1593**
Zantac Syrup **1597**

GASTRO-STOP (Australia)
LOPERAMIDE HYDROCHLORIDE
Imodium Capsules **1834**

GASTRULCER (Portugal)
RANITIDINE HYDROCHLORIDE
Zantac 25 EFFERdose Tablets **1597**
Zantac 150 EFFERdose Tablets. **1597**
Zantac 150 Tablets **1597**
Zantac 300 Tablets **1597**
Zantac Injection **1593**
Zantac Injection Premixed **1593**
Zantac Syrup **1597**

GATINAR (Spain, Switzerland)
LACTULOSE
Kristalose for Oral Solution **2149**

GAVILAST (United Kingdom)
RANITIDINE HYDROCHLORIDE
Zantac 25 EFFERdose Tablets **1597**
Zantac 150 EFFERdose Tablets. **1597**
Zantac 150 Tablets **1597**
Zantac 300 Tablets **1597**
Zantac Injection **1593**
Zantac Injection Premixed **1593**
Zantac Syrup **1597**

GAVISCON PREVENT (Canada)
CIMETIDINE
Tagamet Tablets **1547**

G-DIL (Greece)
ISOSORBIDE MONONITRATE
Imdur Tablets **3032**

GEABATAN (Finland)
GABAPENTIN
Neurontin Capsules **2498**

GEANGIN (Denmark, Norway, The Netherlands, United Kingdom)
VERAPAMIL HYDROCHLORIDE
Covera-HS Tablets **3135**
Verelan PM Capsules **3120**

GEFINA (Finland)
FINASTERIDE
Propecia Tablets **2036**
Proscar Tablets. **2040**

GELCAIN (Chile)
LIDOCAINE
Lidoderm Patch **1107**

GELERIT (Chile)
ERYTHROMYCIN
Ery-Tab Tablets **447**
Erythromycin Base Filmtab Tablets. **454**
Erythromycin Delayed-Release Capsules, USP **456**
PCE Dispertab Tablets **510**

GELESTRA (Italy)
ESTRADIOL
Climara Transdermal System **795**
Vivelle Transdermal System **2288**
Vivelle-Dot Transdermal System **2293**

GELMICIN (Mexico)
CLOTRIMAZOLE
Lotrimin Cream. **3053**
Lotrimin Lotion 1%. **3053**
Lotrimin Topical Solution 1% **3053**

GELODERM (Chile)
METRONIDAZOLE
MetroGel-Vaginal Gel **1822**
Noritate Cream, 1% **1051**

GEL-OSE (Canada)
LACTULOSE
Kristalose for Oral Solution **2149**

(⊙ Described in PDR For Ophthalmic Medicines™)

GEMCITE (India)
GEMCITABINE HYDROCHLORIDE
Gemzar for Injection 1743

GEMISTATIN (Argentina)
SIMVASTATIN
Zocor Tablets 2078

GEMTRO (Argentina)
GEMCITABINE HYDROCHLORIDE
Gemzar for Injection 1743

GEMZAR (Australia, Austria, Belgium, Brazil, Canada, Chile, Czech Republic, Denmark, Finland, France, Germany, Hong Kong, Hungary, Irish Republic, Israel, Italy, Malaysia, Mexico, New Zealand, Norway, Portugal, Russia, Singapore, South Africa, Spain, Sweden, Switzerland, Thailand, The Netherlands, United Kingdom)
GEMCITABINE HYDROCHLORIDE
Gemzar for Injection 1743

GEMZIL (Thailand)
CAPTOPRIL
Captopril Tablets 2114

GENALEN (Italy)
ALENDRONATE SODIUM
Fosamax Tablets 1949

GENALGEN (Mexico)
NAPROXEN
EC-Naprosyn Delayed-Release Tablets 2769
Naprosyn Suspension 2769
Naprosyn Tablets 2769

GENAPROST (Italy)
FINASTERIDE
Propecia Tablets 2036
Proscar Tablets 2040

GENCEFAL (Spain)
CEFAZOLIN SODIUM
Ancef for Injection 1318

GENCIN (Germany, South Africa)
GENTAMICIN SULFATE
Garamycin Injectable 3028
Genoptic Sterile Ophthalmic Solution . . . . ⊙227

GENDAZEL (Thailand)
ALBENDAZOLE
Albenza Tablets 1310

GENEPHOXAL (Greece)
CEFUROXIME AXETIL
Ceftin Tablets 1369
Ceftin for Oral Suspension 1369

GENERLOG (Thailand)
TRIAMCINOLONE ACETONIDE
Azmacort Inhalation Aerosol 1701
Nasacort AQ Nasal Spray 2937

GENFLOX (India)
OFLOXACIN
Floxin Otic Solution 1043

GENFLOX TZ (India)
OFLOXACIN
Floxin Otic Solution 1043

GENGIGEL (Portugal)
SODIUM HYALURONATE
Hyalgan Solution 2917

GENITOFLOX (Brazil)
NORFLOXACIN
Noroxin Tablets 2009

GENKOVA (Mexico)
GENTAMICIN SULFATE
Garamycin Injectable 3028
Genoptic Sterile Ophthalmic Solution . . . . ⊙227

GENLAC (Australia)
LACTULOSE
Kristalose for Oral Solution 2149

GEN-LAC (Canada)
LACTULOSE
Kristalose for Oral Solution 2149

GEN-MEDROXY (Canada)
MEDROXYPROGESTERONE ACETATE
Depo-Medrol Single-Dose Vial 2617

GENMOX (India)
AMOXICILLIN
Amoxil Pediatric Drops for Oral Suspension 1315
Amoxil Tablets 1315

GENOCOLAN (Argentina)
LACTULOSE
Kristalose for Oral Solution 2149

GENOPTIC (Australia, Belgium, Hong Kong, New Zealand, Singapore, South Africa, Spain)
GENTAMICIN SULFATE
Garamycin Injectable 3028
Genoptic Sterile Ophthalmic Solution . . . . ⊙227

GENOVOX (Greece)
NIMODIPINE
Nimotop Capsules 774

GENOXEN (Hong Kong, Irish Republic)
NAPROXEN
EC-Naprosyn Delayed-Release Tablets 2769
Naprosyn Suspension 2769
Naprosyn Tablets 2769

GENPROL (Spain)
CITALOPRAM HYDROBROMIDE
Celexa Tablets 1177

GENREX (Mexico)
GENTAMICIN SULFATE
Garamycin Injectable 3028
Genoptic Sterile Ophthalmic Solution . . . . ⊙227

GENSUMYCIN (Denmark, Finland, Norway, Sweden)
GENTAMICIN SULFATE
Garamycin Injectable 3028
Genoptic Sterile Ophthalmic Solution . . . . ⊙227

GENTA (Germany, Mexico, Thailand)
GENTAMICIN SULFATE
Garamycin Injectable 3028
Genoptic Sterile Ophthalmic Solution . . . . ⊙227

GENTA GOBENS (Portugal, Spain)
GENTAMICIN SULFATE
Garamycin Injectable 3028
Genoptic Sterile Ophthalmic Solution . . . . ⊙227

GENTABILLES (France)
GENTAMICIN SULFATE
Garamycin Injectable 3028
Genoptic Sterile Ophthalmic Solution . . . . ⊙227

GENTAC (Brazil, Thailand)
GENTAMICIN SULFATE
Garamycin Injectable 3028
Genoptic Sterile Ophthalmic Solution . . . . ⊙227

GENTACIDIN (Canada)
GENTAMICIN SULFATE
Garamycin Injectable 3028
Genoptic Sterile Ophthalmic Solution . . . . ⊙227

GENTACIN (Mexico, Thailand)
GENTAMICIN SULFATE
Garamycin Injectable 3028
Genoptic Sterile Ophthalmic Solution . . . . ⊙227

GENTACOLL (Denmark, Finland)
GENTAMICIN SULFATE
Garamycin Injectable 3028
Genoptic Sterile Ophthalmic Solution . . . . ⊙227

GENTACORT (Italy)
GENTAMICIN SULFATE
Garamycin Injectable 3028
Genoptic Sterile Ophthalmic Solution . . . . ⊙227

GENTADERM (Argentina)
GENTAMICIN SULFATE
Garamycin Injectable 3028
Genoptic Sterile Ophthalmic Solution . . . . ⊙227

GENTAGRAN (Brazil)
GENTAMICIN SULFATE
Garamycin Injectable 3028
Genoptic Sterile Ophthalmic Solution . . . . ⊙227

GENTAL (Thailand, United Arab Emirates)
GENTAMICIN SULFATE
Garamycin Injectable 3028
Genoptic Sterile Ophthalmic Solution . . . . ⊙227

GENTALLINE (France)
GENTAMICIN SULFATE
Garamycin Injectable 3028
Genoptic Sterile Ophthalmic Solution . . . . ⊙227

GENTALLORENS (Spain)
GENTAMICIN SULFATE
Garamycin Injectable 3028
Genoptic Sterile Ophthalmic Solution . . . . ⊙227

GENTALODINA (Spain)
GENTAMICIN SULFATE
Garamycin Injectable 3028
Genoptic Sterile Ophthalmic Solution . . . . ⊙227

GENTALYN (Chile, Italy)
GENTAMICIN SULFATE
Garamycin Injectable 3028
Genoptic Sterile Ophthalmic Solution . . . . ⊙227

GENTAMEDICAL (Spain)
GENTAMICIN SULFATE
Garamycin Injectable 3028
Genoptic Sterile Ophthalmic Solution . . . . ⊙227

GENTAMEN (Italy)
GENTAMICIN SULFATE
Garamycin Injectable 3028
Genoptic Sterile Ophthalmic Solution . . . . ⊙227

GENTAMIL (Brazil)
GENTAMICIN SULFATE
Garamycin Injectable 3028
Genoptic Sterile Ophthalmic Solution . . . . ⊙227

GENTAMIN (Spain)
GENTAMICIN SULFATE
Garamycin Injectable 3028
Genoptic Sterile Ophthalmic Solution . . . . ⊙227

GENTAMINA (Argentina)
GENTAMICIN SULFATE
Garamycin Injectable 3028
Genoptic Sterile Ophthalmic Solution . . . . ⊙227

GENTAMIVAL (Spain)
GENTAMICIN SULFATE
Garamycin Injectable 3028
Genoptic Sterile Ophthalmic Solution . . . . ⊙227

GENTAMIX (Germany)
GENTAMICIN SULFATE
Garamycin Injectable 3028
Genoptic Sterile Ophthalmic Solution . . . . ⊙227

GENTAMORGENS (Spain)
GENTAMICIN SULFATE
Garamycin Injectable 3028
Genoptic Sterile Ophthalmic Solution . . . . ⊙227

GENTAMYTREX (Belgium, Germany, Malaysia, Singapore, The Netherlands)
GENTAMICIN SULFATE
Garamycin Injectable 3028
Genoptic Sterile Ophthalmic Solution . . . . ⊙227

GENTA-OPH (Thailand)
GENTAMICIN SULFATE
Garamycin Injectable 3028
Genoptic Sterile Ophthalmic Solution . . . . ⊙227

GENTAPLUS (Brazil)
GENTAMICIN SULFATE
Garamycin Injectable 3028
Genoptic Sterile Ophthalmic Solution . . . . ⊙227

GENTAREN (Argentina)
GENTAMICIN SULFATE
Garamycin Injectable 3028
Genoptic Sterile Ophthalmic Solution . . . . ⊙227

GENTARIM (Mexico)
GENTAMICIN SULFATE
Garamycin Injectable 3028
Genoptic Sterile Ophthalmic Solution . . . . ⊙227

GENTASPORIN (India)
GENTAMICIN SULFATE
Garamycin Injectable 3028
Genoptic Sterile Ophthalmic Solution . . . . ⊙227

GENTATENK (Argentina)
GENTAMICIN SULFATE
Garamycin Injectable 3028
Genoptic Sterile Ophthalmic Solution . . . . ⊙227

GENTATRIM (Israel)
GENTAMICIN SULFATE
Garamycin Injectable 3028
Genoptic Sterile Ophthalmic Solution . . . . ⊙227

GENTAX (Austria, Brazil)
GENTAMICIN SULFATE
Garamycin Injectable 3028
Genoptic Sterile Ophthalmic Solution . . . . ⊙227

GENTAZAF Z (Mexico)
GENTAMICIN SULFATE
Garamycin Injectable 3028
Genoptic Sterile Ophthalmic Solution . . . . ⊙227

GENTIBIOPTAL (Italy)
GENTAMICIN SULFATE
Garamycin Injectable 3028
Genoptic Sterile Ophthalmic Solution . . . . ⊙227

GENTICIN (Irish Republic, United Kingdom)
GENTAMICIN SULFATE
Garamycin Injectable 3028
Genoptic Sterile Ophthalmic Solution . . . . ⊙227

GENTICINA (Spain)
GENTAMICIN SULFATE
Garamycin Injectable 3028
Genoptic Sterile Ophthalmic Solution . . . . ⊙227

GENTICOL (Argentina, Italy)
GENTAMICIN SULFATE
Garamycin Injectable 3028
Genoptic Sterile Ophthalmic Solution . . . . ⊙227

GENTICYN (India)
GENTAMICIN SULFATE
Garamycin Injectable 3028
Genoptic Sterile Ophthalmic Solution . . . . ⊙227

GENTICYN EYE/EAR (India)
GENTAMICIN SULFATE
Garamycin Injectable 3028
Genoptic Sterile Ophthalmic Solution . . . . ⊙227

GENTICYN HC (India)
GENTAMICIN SULFATE
Garamycin Injectable 3028
Genoptic Sterile Ophthalmic Solution . . . . ⊙227

GENTIPRESS (Italy)
ENALAPRIL MALEATE/HYDROCHLOROTHIAZIDE
Vaseretic Tablets 2073

GENTIRAN (Greece)
CETIRIZINE HYDROCHLORIDE
Zyrtec Syrup 2589
Zyrtec Tablets 2589

GENTISUM (Spain)
GENTAMICIN SULFATE
Garamycin Injectable 3028
Genoptic Sterile Ophthalmic Solution . . . . ⊙227

GENTOCIL (Portugal)
GENTAMICIN SULFATE
Garamycin Injectable 3028
Genoptic Sterile Ophthalmic Solution . . . . ⊙227

GENTOGRAM (France, The Netherlands)
GENTAMICIN SULFATE
Garamycin Injectable 3028
Genoptic Sterile Ophthalmic Solution . . . . ⊙227

GENTOLER (Argentina)
GENTAMICIN SULFATE
Garamycin Injectable 3028
Genoptic Sterile Ophthalmic Solution . . . . ⊙227

GENTOMIL (Italy)
GENTAMICIN SULFATE
Garamycin Injectable 3028
Genoptic Sterile Ophthalmic Solution . . . . ⊙227

GENT-OPHTAL (Germany)
GENTAMICIN SULFATE
Garamycin Injectable 3028
Genoptic Sterile Ophthalmic Solution . . . . ⊙227

GENTOPTINE (Monaco)
GENTAMICIN SULFATE
Garamycin Injectable 3028
Genoptic Sterile Ophthalmic Solution . . . . ⊙227

GENTRALAY (Spain)
GENTAMICIN SULFATE
Garamycin Injectable 3028
Genoptic Sterile Ophthalmic Solution . . . . ⊙227

GENTRASUL (Canada)
GENTAMICIN SULFATE
Garamycin Injectable 3028
Genoptic Sterile Ophthalmic Solution . . . . ⊙227

GEOMYCINE (Belgium)
GENTAMICIN SULFATE
Garamycin Injectable 3028
Genoptic Sterile Ophthalmic Solution . . . . ⊙227

GEOPHAGOL (Brazil)
MEBENDAZOLE
Vermox Chewable Tablets 1853

GEPEPROSTIN (Argentina)
BICALUTAMIDE
Casodex Tablets 670

GEPROMI (Mexico)
PROGESTERONE
Prometrium Capsules (100 mg, 200 mg) . 3205

GERAMET (Irish Republic)
CIMETIDINE
Tagamet Tablets 1547

GERELAX (Irish Republic, Israel)
LACTULOSE
Kristalose for Oral Solution 2149

GERICARB (Irish Republic)
CARBAMAZEPINE
Carbatrol Capsules 3174
Tegretol Chewable Tablets 2278
Tegretol Suspension 2278
Tegretol Tablets 2278
Tegretol-XR Tablets 2278

GERINAP (Irish Republic)
NAPROXEN
EC-Naprosyn Delayed-Release Tablets 2769
Naprosyn Suspension 2769
Naprosyn Tablets 2769

GERIPROST (Argentina)
TERAZOSIN HYDROCHLORIDE
Hytrin Capsules 469

GERODYL (The Netherlands)
PENICILLAMINE
Cuprimine Capsules 1925

GEROTEN (Irish Republic)
CAPTOPRIL
Captopril Tablets 2114

GEROXALEN (Denmark, Hungary, Norway, The Netherlands)
METHOXSALEN
Oxsoralen Lotion 1% 3354
Oxsoralen-Ultra Capsules 3354

GERTAC (Irish Republic)
RANITIDINE HYDROCHLORIDE
Zantac 25 EFFERdose Tablets 1597
Zantac 150 EFFERdose Tablets 1597
Zantac 150 Tablets 1597
Zantac 300 Tablets 1597
Zantac Injection 1593
Zantac Injection Premixed 1593
Zantac Syrup 1597

GERTOCALM (Greece)
RANITIDINE HYDROCHLORIDE
Zantac 25 EFFERdose Tablets 1597
Zantac 150 EFFERdose Tablets 1597
Zantac 150 Tablets 1597
Zantac 300 Tablets 1597
Zantac Injection 1593
Zantac Injection Premixed 1593
Zantac Syrup 1597

GERVAKEN (Mexico)
CLARITHROMYCIN
Biaxin Filmtab Tablets 402
Biaxin Granules 402

GESICAIN (India)
LIDOCAINE
Lidoderm Patch 1107

GESIPROX (Singapore)
NAPROXEN SODIUM
Anaprox DS Tablets 2769
Anaprox Tablets 2769

GESLUTIN (Mexico)
PROGESTERONE
Prometrium Capsules (100 mg, 200 mg) 3205

GESTAPOLAR (Germany)
MEDROXYPROGESTERONE ACETATE
Depo-Medrol Single-Dose Vial 2617

GESTAPURAN (Finland, Sweden)
MEDROXYPROGESTERONE ACETATE
Depo-Medrol Single-Dose Vial 2617

GESTER (Argentina)
PROGESTERONE
Prometrium Capsules (100 mg, 200 mg) 3205

GESTEROL (Canada)
PROGESTERONE
Prometrium Capsules (100 mg, 200 mg) 3205

GESTONE (Israel, New Zealand, Thailand, United Kingdom)
PROGESTERONE
Prometrium Capsules (100 mg, 200 mg) 3205

GESTORAL (France, Greece)
MEDROXYPROGESTERONE ACETATE
Depo-Medrol Single-Dose Vial 2617

GEVRAMYCIN (Spain)
GENTAMICIN SULFATE
Garamycin Injectable 3028
Genoptic Sterile Ophthalmic Solution ⊙227

GEVRAMYCIN TOPICA (Spain)
GENTAMICIN SULFATE
Garamycin Injectable 3028
Genoptic Sterile Ophthalmic Solution ⊙227

GEWACALM (Austria)
DIAZEPAM
Diastat Rectal Delivery System 3344
Valium Tablets 2822

GEWADILAT (Austria)
NIFEDIPINE
Adalat CC Tablets 2978

GEWAZEM (Austria)
DILTIAZEM HYDROCHLORIDE
Cardizem LA Extended Release Tablets 1699
Tiazac Capsules 1204

GEZON (Brazil)
DICLOFENAC POTASSIUM
Cataflam Tablets 2173

GEZT (Argentina)
GEMCITABINE HYDROCHLORIDE
Gemzar for Injection 1743

G-FARLUTAL (Germany)
MEDROXYPROGESTERONE ACETATE
Depo-Medrol Single-Dose Vial 2617

GI (Mexico)
GENTAMICIN SULFATE
Garamycin Injectable 3028
Genoptic Sterile Ophthalmic Solution ⊙227

GIARDYL (India)
METRONIDAZOLE
MetroGel-Vaginal Gel 1822
Noritate Cream, 1% 1051

GIBICEF (Italy)
CEFUROXIME SODIUM
Zinacef Injection 1604

GIBIFLU (Italy)
FLUNISOLIDE
Aerobid Inhaler System 1172
Aerobid-M Inhaler System 1172
Nasarel Nasal Spray 1652

GIBINAP (Italy)
NAPROXEN SODIUM
Anaprox DS Tablets 2769
Anaprox Tablets 2769

GIBIXEN (Italy)
NAPROXEN
EC-Naprosyn Delayed-Release Tablets 2769
Naprosyn Suspension 2769
Naprosyn Tablets 2769

GILT (Germany)
CLOTRIMAZOLE
Lotrimin Cream 3053
Lotrimin Lotion 1% 3053
Lotrimin Topical Solution 1% 3053

GIMABROL (Mexico)
AMOXICILLIN
Amoxil Pediatric Drops for Oral Suspension 1315
Amoxil Tablets 1315

GINAIKOS (Italy)
ESTRADIOL
Climara Transdermal System 795
Vivelle Transdermal System 2288
Vivelle-Dot Transdermal System 2293

GINATEX (Argentina)
ESTRADIOL
Climara Transdermal System 795
Vivelle Transdermal System 2288
Vivelle-Dot Transdermal System 2293

GINE CANESTEN (Spain)
CLOTRIMAZOLE
Lotrimin Cream 3053
Lotrimin Lotion 1% 3053
Lotrimin Topical Solution 1% 3053

GINECOSIDE (Brazil)
PROGESTERONE
Prometrium Capsules (100 mg, 200 mg) 3205

GINEDISC (Brazil, Mexico)
ESTRADIOL
Climara Transdermal System 795
Vivelle Transdermal System 2288
Vivelle-Dot Transdermal System 2293

GINEFLAVIR (Italy)
METRONIDAZOLE
MetroGel-Vaginal Gel 1822
Noritate Cream, 1% 1051

GINKAN (Argentina)
METRONIDAZOLE
MetroGel-Vaginal Gel 1822
Noritate Cream, 1% 1051

GINO CIRIAX (Argentina)
CIPROFLOXACIN HYDROCHLORIDE
Ciloxan Ophthalmic Ointment 554
Ciloxan Ophthalmic Solution ⊙205
Cipro Tablets 2991

GINO CLOTRIMIX (Brazil)
CLOTRIMAZOLE
Lotrimin Cream 3053
Lotrimin Lotion 1% 3053
Lotrimin Topical Solution 1% 3053

GINO-CANESTEN (Brazil, Portugal)
CLOTRIMAZOLE
Lotrimin Cream 3053
Lotrimin Lotion 1% 3053
Lotrimin Topical Solution 1% 3053

GINODERM (Chile)
ESTRADIOL
Climara Transdermal System 795
Vivelle Transdermal System 2288
Vivelle-Dot Transdermal System 2293

GINO-LOTREMINE (Portugal)
CLOTRIMAZOLE
Lotrimin Cream 3053
Lotrimin Lotion 1% 3053
Lotrimin Topical Solution 1% 3053

GINORECTOL (Greece, Singapore)
CIPROFLOXACIN HYDROCHLORIDE
Ciloxan Ophthalmic Ointment 554
Ciloxan Ophthalmic Solution ⊙205
Cipro Tablets 2991

GINOVAGIN (Brazil)
METRONIDAZOLE
MetroGel-Vaginal Gel 1822
Noritate Cream, 1% 1051

GIROFLOX (Portugal)
CIPROFLOXACIN
Cipro Oral Suspension 2991

GI-TAK (South Africa)
RANITIDINE HYDROCHLORIDE
Zantac 25 EFFERdose Tablets 1597
Zantac 150 EFFERdose Tablets 1597
Zantac 150 Tablets 1597
Zantac 300 Tablets 1597
Zantac Injection 1593
Zantac Injection Premixed 1593
Zantac Syrup 1597

GIVAIR (Italy)
FLUNISOLIDE
Aerobid Inhaler System 1172
Aerobid-M Inhaler System 1172
Nasarel Nasal Spray 1652

GLADEM (Austria, Germany, Switzerland)
SERTRALINE HYDROCHLORIDE
Zoloft Tablets 2581

GLADIUS (Greece)
CEFTRIAXONE SODIUM
Rocephin Injectable Vials, ADD-Vantage, Galaxy, Bulk 2801

GLAFEMAK (Greece)
TIMOLOL MALEATE
Blocadren Tablets 1891
Timoptic Sterile Ophthalmic Solution 2058
Timoptic in Ocudose 2061
Timoptic-XE Sterile Ophthalmic Gel Forming Solution 2062

GLATIM (Argentina)
TIMOLOL MALEATE
Blocadren Tablets 1891
Timoptic Sterile Ophthalmic Solution 2058
Timoptic in Ocudose 2061
Timoptic-XE Sterile Ophthalmic Gel Forming Solution 2062

GLAUCOL (United Kingdom)
TIMOLOL MALEATE
Blocadren Tablets 1891
Timoptic Sterile Ophthalmic Solution 2058
Timoptic in Ocudose 2061
Timoptic-XE Sterile Ophthalmic Gel Forming Solution 2062

GLAUCO-OPH (Hong Kong, Thailand)
TIMOLOL MALEATE
Blocadren Tablets 1891
Timoptic Sterile Ophthalmic Solution 2058
Timoptic in Ocudose 2061
Timoptic-XE Sterile Ophthalmic Gel Forming Solution 2062

GLAUCOSAN (South Africa)
TIMOLOL MALEATE
Blocadren Tablets 1891
Timoptic Sterile Ophthalmic Solution 2058
Timoptic in Ocudose 2061
Timoptic-XE Sterile Ophthalmic Gel Forming Solution 2062

GLAUCOSTAT (Argentina)
LATANOPROST
Xalatan Ophthalmic Solution ⊙280

GLAUCOTENSIL (Chile)
DORZOLAMIDE HYDROCHLORIDE
Trusopt Sterile Ophthalmic Solution 2065

GLAUCOTENSIL T (Chile)
DORZOLAMIDE HYDROCHLORIDE/TIMOLOL MALEATE
Cosopt Sterile Ophthalmic Solution 1910

GLAUSINE (Austria)
CLONIDINE HYDROCHLORIDE
Catapres Tablets 874

GLAUSOLETS (Chile)
TIMOLOL MALEATE
Blocadren Tablets 1891
Timoptic Sterile Ophthalmic Solution 2058
Timoptic in Ocudose 2061
Timoptic-XE Sterile Ophthalmic Gel Forming Solution 2062

GLAUTIMOL (Brazil)
TIMOLOL MALEATE
Blocadren Tablets 1891
Timoptic Sterile Ophthalmic Solution 2058
Timoptic in Ocudose 2061
Timoptic-XE Sterile Ophthalmic Gel Forming Solution 2062

GLAZIDIM (Belgium, Finland, Italy)
CEFTAZIDIME
Fortaz for Injection 1422

GLEMAZ (Argentina)
GLIMEPIRIDE
Amaryl Tablets 2864

GLEVO (India)
LEVOFLOXACIN
Levaquin Injection 2453
Levaquin Tablets 2453

GLEVOMICINA (Argentina)
GENTAMICIN SULFATE
Garamycin Injectable 3028
Genoptic Sterile Ophthalmic Solution ⊙227

GLICEMIN (Brazil)
DIAZOXIDE
Hyperstat I.V. Injection 3031

GLICOBASE (Italy)
ACARBOSE
Precose Tablets 776

GLIFAPEN (Argentina)
AMOXICILLIN
Amoxil Pediatric Drops for Oral Suspension 1315
Amoxil Tablets 1315

GLIMCIP (India)
GLIMEPIRIDE
Amaryl Tablets 2864

GLIMEPIL (Brazil)
GLIMEPIRIDE
Amaryl Tablets 2864

GLIMESEC (Brazil)
GLIMEPIRIDE
Amaryl Tablets 2864

GLIMIAL (Portugal)
GLIMEPIRIDE
Amaryl Tablets 2864

GLIMIDE (Argentina)
ROSIGLITAZONE MALEATE
Avandia Tablets 1348

GLIMIPREX (India)
GLIMEPIRIDE
Amaryl Tablets 2864

GLIMIPREX MF (India)
GLIMEPIRIDE
Amaryl Tablets 2864

GLIMITAB (India)
GLIMEPIRIDE
Amaryl Tablets 2864

GLIMULIN (India)
GLIMEPIRIDE
Amaryl Tablets 2864

GLIMULIN-MF (India)
GLIMEPIRIDE
Amaryl Tablets 2864

GLIOSARTAN (Argentina)
TELMISARTAN
Micardis Tablets 884

GLIOSARTAN PLUS (Argentina)
TELMISARTAN
Micardis Tablets 884

GLIOTEN (Argentina, Brazil, Chile, Mexico)
ENALAPRIL MALEATE
Vasotec I.V. Injection 2076

GLIOTENZIDE (Argentina, Brazil)
ENALAPRIL MALEATE
Vasotec I.V. Injection 2076

GLITA (India)
PIOGLITAZONE HYDROCHLORIDE
Actos Tablets 3224

GLOBUCE (Spain)
CIPROFLOXACIN HYDROCHLORIDE
Ciloxan Ophthalmic Ointment 554
Ciloxan Ophthalmic Solution . . . . ⊙205
Cipro Tablets 2991

GLOBUREN (Italy)
EPOETIN ALFA
Epogen for Injection 586
Procrit for Injection 2374

GLOPIR (Greece)
NIFEDIPINE
Adalat CC Tablets 2978

GLORIXONE (Greece)
CEFTRIAXONE SODIUM
Rocephin Injectable Vials, ADD-Vantage, Galaxy, Bulk 2801

GLOSSYFIN (Greece)
CIPROFLOXACIN HYDROCHLORIDE
Ciloxan Ophthalmic Ointment 554
Ciloxan Ophthalmic Solution . . . . ⊙205
Cipro Tablets 2991

GLUBOSE (India)
ACARBOSE
Precose Tablets 776

GLUCAGEN (Argentina, Australia, Austria, Belgium, Czech Republic, Denmark, Finland, France, Germany, Greece, Hong Kong, Hungary, India, Irish Republic, Israel, Italy, Malaysia, New Zealand, Portugal, Russia, Singapore, South Africa, Switzerland, Thailand, United Kingdom)
GLUCAGON HYDROCHLORIDE
Glucagon for Injection Vials and Emergency Kit 1749

GLUCAR (India)
ACARBOSE
Precose Tablets 776

GLUCERIDE (Argentina)
GLIMEPIRIDE
Amaryl Tablets 2864

GLUCOBAY (Argentina, Australia, Austria, Belgium, Brazil, Chile, Czech Republic, Denmark, Finland, Germany, Greece, Hong Kong, Hungary, India, Irish Republic, Italy, Malaysia, Mexico, New Zealand, Norway, Portugal, Singapore, South Africa, Spain, Sweden, Switzerland, Thailand, The Netherlands, United Kingdom)
ACARBOSE
Precose Tablets 776

GLUCOMOL (India)
TIMOLOL MALEATE
Blocadren Tablets 1891
Timoptic Sterile Ophthalmic Solution 2058
Timoptic in Ocudose 2061
Timoptic-XE Sterile Ophthalmic Gel Forming Solution 2062

GLUCONORM (Brazil, Canada)
REPAGLINIDE
Prandin Tablets (0.5, 1, and 2 mg) 2337

GLUCOPIRIDA (Argentina)
GLIMEPIRIDE
Amaryl Tablets 2864

GLUCOR (France)
ACARBOSE
Precose Tablets 776

GLUCOSULMID (Germany)
SULFACETAMIDE SODIUM
Klaron Lotion 10% 1050

GLUCOTIM (India)
TIMOLOL MALEATE
Blocadren Tablets 1891
Timoptic Sterile Ophthalmic Solution 2058
Timoptic in Ocudose 2061
Timoptic-XE Sterile Ophthalmic Gel Forming Solution 2062

GLUDEX (Argentina)
ROSIGLITAZONE MALEATE
Avandia Tablets 1348

GLUMIDA (Spain)
ACARBOSE
Precose Tablets 776

GLUTASEDAN (Argentina)
DIAZEPAM
Diastat Rectal Delivery System 3344
Valium Tablets 2822

GLUTASEY (Spain)
SIMVASTATIN
Zocor Tablets 2078

GLYREE (India)
GLIMEPIRIDE
Amaryl Tablets 2864

GLYREE M (India)
GLIMEPIRIDE
Amaryl Tablets 2864

GLYTOP (Argentina)
TRIAMCINOLONE ACETONIDE
Azmacort Inhalation Aerosol 1701
Nasacort AQ Nasal Spray 2937

GNOSTOCARDIN (Greece)
ENALAPRIL MALEATE
Vasotec I.V. Injection 2076

GNOSTOL (Greece)
METRONIDAZOLE
MetroGel-Vaginal Gel 1822
Noritate Cream, 1% 1051

GNOSTOVAL (Greece)
LISINOPRIL
Prinivil Tablets 2029
Zestril Tablets 704

GOBANAL (Spain)
DIAZEPAM
Diastat Rectal Delivery System 3344
Valium Tablets 2822

GOBBICAINA (Argentina)
LIDOCAINE
Lidoderm Patch 1107

GOBBIFOL (Argentina)
PROPOFOL
Diprivan Injectable Emulsion 676

GODAFILIN (Spain)
THEOPHYLLINE
Uniphyl Tablets 2708

GOLAN (Mexico)
FUROSEMIDE
Furosemide Tablets 2117

GOLD CROSS ANTIHISTAMINE ELIXIR (Australia)
PROMETHAZINE HYDROCHLORIDE
Phenergan Suppositories 3438
Phenergan Tablets 3438

GONDONAR (Argentina)
ANASTROZOLE
Arimidex Tablets 665

GONIF (Greece)
CEFUROXIME SODIUM
Zinacef Injection 1604

GONNING (Hong Kong)
CIPROFLOXACIN
Cipro Oral Suspension 2991

GONORCIN (Thailand)
NORFLOXACIN
Noroxin Tablets 2009

GOODNIGHT (New Zealand)
PROMETHAZINE HYDROCHLORIDE
Phenergan Suppositories 3438
Phenergan Tablets 3438

GO-ON (Germany, Hong Kong, Italy, Malaysia)
SODIUM HYALURONATE
Hyalgan Solution 2917

GOPTEN (Australia, Austria, Brazil, Denmark, Finland, France, Germany, Hungary, Irish Republic, Italy, Mexico, New Zealand, Norway, Portugal, South Africa, Spain, Sweden, Switzerland, The Netherlands, United Kingdom)
TRANDOLAPRIL
Mavik Tablets 482

GORDOX (Czech Republic, Hungary, Russia)
APROTININ
Trasylol Injection 779

GOTABIOTIC (Argentina)
TOBRAMYCIN
TOBI Solution for Inhalation 1015

GOTABIOTIC F (Argentina)
TOBRAMYCIN
TOBI Solution for Inhalation 1015

GOTADEX (Mexico)
DEXAMETHASONE
Decadron Tablets 1929

GOTINAL (Argentina)
NAPHAZOLINE HYDROCHLORIDE
Albalon Ophthalmic Solution . . . . ⊙216

GOVAL (Chile)
RISPERIDONE
Risperdal Oral Solution 1658
Risperdal Tablets 1658

GRAMAXIN (Austria, Germany)
CEFAZOLIN SODIUM
Ancef for Injection 1318

GRAMMICIN (Thailand)
GENTAMICIN SULFATE
Garamycin Injectable 3028
Genoptic Sterile Ophthalmic Solution . . . . ⊙227

GRAMMIXIN (Thailand)
GENTAMICIN SULFATE
Garamycin Injectable 3028
Genoptic Sterile Ophthalmic Solution . . . . ⊙227

GRAN-VERM (Brazil)
MEBENDAZOLE
Vermox Chewable Tablets 1853

GRATEN (Mexico)
MORPHINE SULFATE
Kadian Capsules 572
MS Contin Tablets 2703

GRAVIDEX (Spain)
DINOPROSTONE
Cervidil Vaginal Insert 1182

GRAY-F (Argentina)
FENTANYL CITRATE
Actiq 993

GRENFUNG (Argentina)
KETOCONAZOLE
Nizoral 2% Shampoo 1838

GRENIS (Greece)
NORFLOXACIN
Noroxin Tablets 2009

GRENIS-CIPRO (Greece)
CIPROFLOXACIN HYDROCHLORIDE
Ciloxan Ophthalmic Ointment 554
Ciloxan Ophthalmic Solution . . . . ⊙205
Cipro Tablets 2991

GRENIS-OFLO (Greece)
OFLOXACIN
Floxin Otic Solution 1043

GREPIFLOX (Argentina)
LEVOFLOXACIN
Levaquin Injection 2453
Levaquin Tablets 2453

GREXIN (Thailand)
DIGOXIN
Lanoxicaps Capsules 1458
Lanoxin Injection 1462
Lanoxin Injection Pediatric 1465
Lanoxin Tablets 1468

GRIFOCIPROX (Chile)
CIPROFLOXACIN
Cipro Oral Suspension 2991

GRIFODILZEM (Chile)
DILTIAZEM HYDROCHLORIDE
Cardizem LA Extended Release Tablets . . . 1699
Tiazac Capsules 1204

GRIFONIMOD (Chile)
NIMODIPINE
Nimotop Capsules 774

GRIFOPRIL (Chile)
ENALAPRIL MALEATE
Vasotec I.V. Injection 2076

GRIFOPRIL-D (Chile)
ENALAPRIL MALEATE/HYDROCHLOROTHIAZIDE
Vaseretic Tablets 2073

GRIFOTENOL (Chile)
ATENOLOL
Tenormin I.V. Injection 698

GRIFOTRIAXONA (Chile)
CEFTRIAXONE SODIUM
Rocephin Injectable Vials, ADD-Vantage, Galaxy, Bulk 2801

GRINEVEL (Argentina)
GANCICLOVIR SODIUM
Cytovene-IV 2763

GRISETIN (Spain)
FLUTAMIDE
Eulexin Capsules 3023

GROFENAC (Hong Kong, Switzerland)
DICLOFENAC SODIUM
Voltaren Tablets 2298
Voltaren-XR Tablets 2301

GROFIBRAT (Czech Republic)
FENOFIBRATE
Tricor Tablets 523

GROMAZOL (Switzerland)
CLOTRIMAZOLE
Lotrimin Cream 3053
Lotrimin Lotion 1% 3053
Lotrimin Topical Solution 1% 3053

GROWART (Greece)
LEVOCARNITINE
Carnitor Injection 3185
Carnitor Tablets and Oral Solution 3187

GUTRON (Austria, Chile, Czech Republic, France, Germany, Hong Kong, Hungary, Israel, Italy, Mexico, New Zealand, Portugal, Singapore, Switzerland, Thailand)
MIDODRINE HYDROCHLORIDE
ProAmatine Tablets 3183

GYNEBO (Thailand)
CLOTRIMAZOLE
Lotrimin Cream 3053
Lotrimin Lotion 1% 3053
Lotrimin Topical Solution 1% 3053

GYNE-LOTREMIN (Hong Kong, Malaysia, Singapore)
CLOTRIMAZOLE
Lotrimin Cream 3053
Lotrimin Lotion 1% 3053
Lotrimin Topical Solution 1% 3053

GYNE-LOTRIMIN (Australia)
CLOTRIMAZOLE
Lotrimin Cream 3053
Lotrimin Lotion 1% 3053
Lotrimin Topical Solution 1% 3053

GYNERIUM (Argentina)
KETOCONAZOLE
Nizoral 2% Shampoo 1838

GYNESTEN-B (Thailand)
CLOTRIMAZOLE
Lotrimin Cream 3053
Lotrimin Lotion 1% 3053
Lotrimin Topical Solution 1% 3053

GYNESTREL (Italy)
NAPROXEN SODIUM
Anaprox DS Tablets 2769
Anaprox Tablets 2769

GYNEZOL (South Africa)
CLOTRIMAZOLE
Lotrimin Cream 3053

Lotrimin Lotion 1%. **3053**
Lotrimin Topical Solution 1% **3053**

GYNO OCERAL (Austria)
OXICONAZOLE NITRATE
Oxistat Cream **1498**
Oxistat Lotion. **1498**

GYNOCANESTEN (Chile)
CLOTRIMAZOLE
Lotrimin Cream. **3053**
Lotrimin Lotion 1%. **3053**
Lotrimin Topical Solution 1% **3053**

GYNO-CANESTEN (Germany, Italy)
CLOTRIMAZOLE
Lotrimin Cream. **3053**
Lotrimin Lotion 1%. **3053**
Lotrimin Topical Solution 1% **3053**

GYNO-CANESTENE (Belgium, Switzerland)
CLOTRIMAZOLE
Lotrimin Cream. **3053**
Lotrimin Lotion 1%. **3053**
Lotrimin Topical Solution 1% **3053**

GYNO-LIDERMAN (Austria)
OXICONAZOLE NITRATE
Oxistat Cream **1498**
Oxistat Lotion. **1498**

GYNO-MYFUNGAR (Czech Republic, Mexico, Switzerland)
OXICONAZOLE NITRATE
Oxistat Cream **1498**
Oxistat Lotion. **1498**

GYNO-PEVARYL (Austria, Belgium, Czech Republic, France, Germany, Hong Kong, Hungary, Irish Republic, Israel, Malaysia, New Zealand, Portugal, Russia, Singapore, South Africa, Spain, Switzerland, The Netherlands, United Kingdom)
ECONAZOLE NITRATE
Spectazole Cream. **2390**

GYNOPLIX (Hong Kong)
METRONIDAZOLE
MetroGel-Vaginal Gel **1822**
Noritate Cream, 1%. **1051**

GYNOSTATUM (Malaysia)
CLOTRIMAZOLE
Lotrimin Cream. **3053**
Lotrimin Lotion 1%. **3053**
Lotrimin Topical Solution 1% **3053**

GYNO-TRIMAZE (South Africa)
CLOTRIMAZOLE
Lotrimin Cream. **3053**
Lotrimin Lotion 1%. **3053**
Lotrimin Topical Solution 1% **3053**

GYNPOLAR (Germany)
ESTRADIOL
Climara Transdermal System **795**
Vivelle Transdermal System **2288**
Vivelle-Dot Transdermal System **2293**

GYRABLOCK (Czech Republic, Singapore, Thailand)
NORFLOXACIN
Noroxin Tablets. **2009**

GYROFLOX (Germany)
OFLOXACIN
Floxin Otic Solution **1043**

GY-SOL (Mexico)
GENTAMICIN SULFATE
Garamycin Injectable **3028**
Genoptic Sterile Ophthalmic Solution . . . . ⊙**227**

H2 OXYL (Germany)
BENZOYL PEROXIDE
Brevoxyl-4 Creamy Wash. **3212**
Brevoxyl-4 Gel **3211**
Brevoxyl-8 Creamy Wash. **3212**
Brevoxyl-8 Gel **3211**
Triaz Cleanser **1864**
Triaz Gel. **1864**

H2OXYL (Canada, Switzerland)
BENZOYL PEROXIDE
Brevoxyl-4 Creamy Wash. **3212**
Brevoxyl-4 Gel **3211**
Brevoxyl-8 Creamy Wash. **3212**
Brevoxyl-8 Gel **3211**
Triaz Cleanser **1864**
Triaz Gel. **1864**

HABITROL (Canada)
NICOTINE
Nicotrol Inhaler. **2594**
Nicotrol NS **2596**

HAEMITON (Germany)
CLONIDINE HYDROCHLORIDE
Catapres Tablets **874**

HAEMITON-AUGENTROPFEN (Germany)
CLONIDINE HYDROCHLORIDE
Catapres Tablets **874**

HAIMASERUM (Italy)
PLASMA PROTEIN FRACTION
Plasmanate **3252**

HAIRCLIN (Argentina)
PERMETHRIN
Acticin Cream. **2125**

HALDID (Denmark)
FENTANYL CITRATE
Actiq **993**

HALF BETADUR CR (United Kingdom)
PROPRANOLOL HYDROCHLORIDE
Inderal LA Long-Acting Capsules **3421**

HALF BETA-PROGRANE (United Kingdom)
PROPRANOLOL HYDROCHLORIDE
Inderal LA Long-Acting Capsules **3421**

HALF CAPOZIDE (Irish Republic)
CAPTOPRIL
Captopril Tablets **2114**

HALF INDERAL (Irish Republic, United Kingdom)
PROPRANOLOL HYDROCHLORIDE
Inderal LA Long-Acting Capsules **3421**

HALF SECURON (United Kingdom)
VERAPAMIL HYDROCHLORIDE
Covera-HS Tablets **3135**
Verelan PM Capsules **3120**

HALONIX (India)
SODIUM HYALURONATE
Hyalgan Solution **2917**

HAMOXILLIN (Hong Kong)
AMOXICILLIN
Amoxil Pediatric Drops for Oral Suspension. **1315**
Amoxil Tablets **1315**

HARMONISE (Australia)
LOPERAMIDE HYDROCHLORIDE
Imodium Capsules **1834**

HARNAL (Hong Kong, Japan, Thailand)
TAMSULOSIN HYDROCHLORIDE
Flomax Capsules **881**

HART (Argentina)
DILTIAZEM HYDROCHLORIDE
Cardizem LA Extended Release Tablets. . . **1699**
Tiazac Capsules **1204**

HAWKMIDE (Thailand)
FUROSEMIDE
Furosemide Tablets **2117**

HAYFEVER & ALLERGY RELIEF (United Kingdom)
CETIRIZINE HYDROCHLORIDE
Zyrtec Syrup **2589**
Zyrtec Tablets **2589**

HAYFEVER RELIEF (United Kingdom)
CETIRIZINE HYDROCHLORIDE
Zyrtec Syrup **2589**
Zyrtec Tablets **2589**

HEADS SHAMPOO (Hong Kong)
ECONAZOLE NITRATE
Spectazole Cream. **2390**

HEALON (Australia, Belgium, Brazil, Canada, Chile, Czech Republic, Finland, France, Germany, Hong Kong, Hungary, Israel, Italy, Malaysia, New Zealand, Norway, Singapore, South Africa, Sweden, Switzerland, Thailand, The Netherlands)
SODIUM HYALURONATE
Hyalgan Solution **2917**

HEALONID (Austria, France, Irish Republic, United Kingdom)
SODIUM HYALURONATE
Hyalgan Solution **2917**

HEARTBURN RELIEF (Australia)
RANITIDINE HYDROCHLORIDE
Zantac 25 EFFERdose Tablets **1597**
Zantac 150 EFFERdose Tablets. **1597**
Zantac 150 Tablets **1597**
Zantac 300 Tablets **1597**
Zantac Injection **1593**
Zantac Injection Premixed **1593**
Zantac Syrup **1597**

HEDAZOL (Mexico)
MEBENDAZOLE
Vermox Chewable Tablets **1853**

HEINIX (Finland)
CETIRIZINE HYDROCHLORIDE
Zyrtec Syrup **2589**
Zyrtec Tablets **2589**

HEITRIN (Germany)
TERAZOSIN HYDROCHLORIDE
Hytrin Capsules. **469**

HEKTULOSE (Germany)
LACTULOSE
Kristalose for Oral Solution **2149**

HELICLAR (Belgium)
CLARITHROMYCIN
Biaxin Filmtab Tablets. **402**
Biaxin Granules **402**

HELICODID (Brazil)
CLARITHROMYCIN
Biaxin Filmtab Tablets. **402**
Biaxin Granules **402**

HELIMOX (Italy)
AMOXICILLIN
Amoxil Pediatric Drops for Oral Suspension. **1315**
Amoxil Tablets **1315**

HELIPAC (India)
AMOXICILLIN
Amoxil Pediatric Drops for Oral Suspension. **1315**
Amoxil Tablets **1315**

HELMIB (Brazil)
MEBENDAZOLE
Vermox Chewable Tablets **1853**

HELMIBEN (Brazil)
MEBENDAZOLE
Vermox Chewable Tablets **1853**

HELMIDRAX (Brazil)
MEBENDAZOLE
Vermox Chewable Tablets **1853**

HELMINE (Spain)
ONDANSETRON HYDROCHLORIDE
Zofran Injection. **1607**
Zofran Injection Premixed **1607**
Zofran Oral Solution. **1613**
Zofran Tablets **1613**

HELMINT (Argentina)
MEBENDAZOLE
Vermox Chewable Tablets **1853**

HELMINTAL (Brazil)
ALBENDAZOLE
Albenza Tablets. **1310**

HELMINZOLE (Mexico)
MEBENDAZOLE
Vermox Chewable Tablets **1853**

HELMI-PED (Brazil)
MEBENDAZOLE
Vermox Chewable Tablets **1853**

HELMISONS (Mexico)
ALBENDAZOLE
Albenza Tablets. **1310**

HELMIZIL (Brazil)
MEBENDAZOLE
Vermox Chewable Tablets **1853**

HELMIZOL (Brazil)
METRONIDAZOLE
MetroGel-Vaginal Gel **1822**
Noritate Cream, 1%. **1051**

HELPP (Argentina)
PERMETHRIN
Acticin Cream. **2125**

HEMAX (Thailand)
EPOETIN ALFA
Epogen for Injection. **586**
Procrit for Injection **2374**

HEMIGOXINE NATIVELLE (France)
DIGOXIN
Lanoxicaps Capsules **1458**
Lanoxin Injection **1462**
Lanoxin Injection Pediatric **1465**
Lanoxin Tablets. **1468**

HEMIPRALON (France)
PROPRANOLOL HYDROCHLORIDE
Inderal LA Long-Acting Capsules **3421**

HEMOGENIN (Brazil)
OXYMETHOLONE
Anadrol-50 Tablets. **3329**

HEMON (Greece)
ATENOLOL
Tenormin I.V. Injection. **698**

HENEXAL (Mexico)
FUROSEMIDE
Furosemide Tablets **2117**

HEPALAC (Thailand)
LACTULOSE
Kristalose for Oral Solution **2149**

HEPA-MERZ LACT (Germany)
LACTULOSE
Kristalose for Oral Solution **2149**

HEPATICUM-LAC-MEDICE (Germany)
LACTULOSE
Kristalose for Oral Solution **2149**

HEPRONE (Spain)
SUCRALFATE
Carafate Suspension **727**
Carafate Tablets **728**

HEPTODINE (Argentina)
LAMIVUDINE
Epivir Oral Solution **1394**
Epivir Tablets **1394**
Epivir-HBV Oral Solution **1398**
Epivir-HBV Tablets **1398**

HEPTOVIR (Canada)
LAMIVUDINE
Epivir Oral Solution **1394**
Epivir Tablets **1394**
Epivir-HBV Oral Solution **1398**
Epivir-HBV Tablets **1398**

HERBESSER (Hong Kong, Japan, Malaysia, Portugal, Singapore, Thailand)
DILTIAZEM HYDROCHLORIDE
Cardizem LA Extended Release Tablets. . . **1699**
Tiazac Capsules **1204**

HERCEPTIN (Argentina, Australia, Belgium, Brazil, Canada, Chile, Czech Republic, Denmark, Finland, France, Germany, Greece, Hong Kong, Hungary, Irish Republic, Israel, Italy, Mexico, New Zealand, Norway, Portugal, Singapore, South Africa, Spain, Sweden, Switzerland, Thailand, United Kingdom)
TRASTUZUMAB
Herceptin I.V. **1234**

HERMOLEPSIN (Sweden)
CARBAMAZEPINE
Carbatrol Capsules **3174**
Tegretol Chewable Tablets **2278**
Tegretol Suspension. **2278**
Tegretol Tablets **2278**
Tegretol-XR Tablets **2278**

HERPHONAL (Germany)
TRIMIPRAMINE MALEATE
Surmontil Capsules **2347**

HERTEN (Spain)
ENALAPRIL MALEATE
Vasotec I.V. Injection **2076**

HETACLOXACIN (Greece)
OFLOXACIN
Floxin Otic Solution **1043**

HEVRONAZ (Greece)
MUPIROCIN
Bactroban Ointment. **1358**

HEXA-BLOK (South Africa)
ATENOLOL
Tenormin I.V. Injection. **698**

HEXABOTIN (Denmark)
ERYTHROMYCIN STEARATE
Erythrocin Stearate Filmtab Tablets **452**

HEXADILAT (Denmark)
NIFEDIPINE
Adalat CC Tablets 2978

HEXADROL (Canada)
DEXAMETHASONE
Decadron Tablets 1929
DEXAMETHASONE SODIUM PHOSPHATE
Decadron Phosphate Injection. . . . 1931

HEXAGASTRON (Denmark)
SUCRALFATE
Carafate Suspension 727
Carafate Tablets 728

HEXAL KONAZOL SHAMPOO (Australia)
KETOCONAZOLE
Nizoral 2% Shampoo 1838

HEXALEN (Australia, Canada, Israel, Norway, Russia, Sweden, Thailand, United Kingdom)
ALTRETAMINE
Hexalen Capsules 2101

HEXALID (Denmark)
DIAZEPAM
Diastat Rectal Delivery System 3344
Valium Tablets 2822

HEXAMET (South Africa)
CIMETIDINE
Tagamet Tablets 1547

HEXAMYCIN (Denmark)
GENTAMICIN SULFATE
Garamycin Injectable 3028
Genoptic Sterile Ophthalmic Solution . . . . ⊙227

HEXARONE (South Africa)
AMIODARONE HYDROCHLORIDE
Pacerone Tablets 3337

HEXASOPTIN (Denmark)
VERAPAMIL HYDROCHLORIDE
Covera-HS Tablets 3135
Verelan PM Capsules 3120

HEXASTAT (Canada, France, Hong Kong, Italy, Norway, The Netherlands)
ALTRETAMINE
Hexalen Capsules 2101

HEXINAWAS (Spain)
ALTRETAMINE
Hexalen Capsules 2101

HIALID (Hong Kong, Singapore, Thailand)
SODIUM HYALURONATE
Hyalgan Solution 2917

HIALUDORF (Argentina)
SODIUM HYALURONATE
Hyalgan Solution 2917

HICONCIL (The Netherlands)
AMOXICILLIN
Amoxil Pediatric Drops for Oral Suspension. . . . 1315
Amoxil Tablets 1315

HIDALONE (Portugal)
HYDROCORTISONE
Hydrocortone Tablets 1963

HIDERM (Australia)
CLOTRIMAZOLE
Lotrimin Cream. . . . 3053
Lotrimin Lotion 1%. . . . 3053
Lotrimin Topical Solution 1% 3053

HIDRASAL (Mexico)
FUROSEMIDE
Furosemide Tablets 2117

HIDROALTESONA (Spain)
HYDROCORTISONE
Hydrocortone Tablets 1963

HIDROCOL (Brazil)
HYDROCORTISONE
Hydrocortone Tablets 1963

HIDROCORTIN (Argentina)
HYDROCORTISONE
Hydrocortone Tablets 1963

HIDROFENIL (Mexico)
HYDROCORTISONE
Hydrocortone Tablets 1963

HIDROPRIL (Brazil)
CAPTOPRIL
Captopril Tablets 2114

HIDRORONOL T (Chile)
HYDROCHLOROTHIAZIDE/TRIAMTERENE
Dyazide Capsules 1389
Maxzide Tablets 2150
Maxzide-25 mg Tablets 2150

HIDROTISONA (Argentina)
HYDROCORTISONE
Hydrocortone Tablets 1963

HINCOMOX (Brazil)
AMOXICILLIN
Amoxil Pediatric Drops for Oral Suspension. . . . 1315
Amoxil Tablets 1315

HIPEN (India)
AMOXICILLIN
Amoxil Pediatric Drops for Oral Suspension. . . . 1315
Amoxil Tablets 1315

HIPERSON (Chile)
ENALAPRIL MALEATE
Vasotec I.V. Injection 2076

HIPERSON-D (Chile)
ENALAPRIL MALEATE/HYDROCHLOROTHIAZIDE
Vaseretic Tablets. . . . 2073

HIPERTAN (Argentina)
ENALAPRIL MALEATE
Vasotec I.V. Injection 2076

HIPERTEX (Mexico)
CAPTOPRIL
Captopril Tablets. . . . 2114

HIPERTIL (Portugal)
CAPTOPRIL
Captopril Tablets. . . . 2114

HIPERTIN (Brazil)
ENALAPRIL MALEATE
Vasotec I.V. Injection 2076

HIPOARTEL (Chile, Spain)
ENALAPRIL MALEATE
Vasotec I.V. Injection 2076

HIPOARTEL H (Chile)
ENALAPRIL MALEATE/HYDROCHLOROTHIAZIDE
Vaseretic Tablets. . . . 2073

HIPOARTEL PLUS (Spain)
ENALAPRIL MALEATE/HYDROCHLOROTHIAZIDE
Vaseretic Tablets. . . . 2073

HIPOCATRIL (Brazil)
CAPTOPRIL
Captopril Tablets. . . . 2114

HIPOSTEROL (Chile)
LOVASTATIN
Mevacor Tablets 1996

HIPOTEN (Brazil)
CAPTOPRIL
Captopril Tablets. . . . 2114

HIPOTENSIL (Portugal)
CAPTOPRIL
Captopril Tablets. . . . 2114

HIPOVASTIN (Argentina)
LOVASTATIN
Mevacor Tablets 1996

HIPRANOL (South Africa)
PROPRANOLOL HYDROCHLORIDE
Inderal LA Long-Acting Capsules 3421

HIPRES (India)
ATENOLOL
Tenormin I.V. Injection. . . . 698

HIPRESS (Brazil)
LOSARTAN POTASSIUM
Cozaar Tablets 1913

HIPTEN (Portugal)
ENALAPRIL MALEATE
Vasotec I.V. Injection 2076

HISTAC (Czech Republic, Hungary, India, Malaysia, Singapore, Thailand)
RANITIDINE HYDROCHLORIDE
Zantac 25 EFFERdose Tablets 1597
Zantac 150 EFFERdose Tablets. . . . 1597
Zantac 150 Tablets 1597
Zantac 300 Tablets 1597
Zantac Injection 1593
Zantac Injection Premixed 1593
Zantac Syrup 1597

HISTAFILIN (Spain)
THEOPHYLLINE
Uniphyl Tablets 2708

HISTAFREN (Greece)
CETIRIZINE HYDROCHLORIDE
Zyrtec Syrup 2589
Zyrtec Tablets 2589

HISTAK (South Africa)
RANITIDINE HYDROCHLORIDE
Zantac 25 EFFERdose Tablets 1597
Zantac 150 EFFERdose Tablets. . . . 1597
Zantac 150 Tablets 1597
Zantac 300 Tablets 1597
Zantac Injection 1593
Zantac Injection Premixed 1593
Zantac Syrup 1597

HISTALOC (United Arab Emirates)
PROMETHAZINE HYDROCHLORIDE
Phenergan Suppositories. . . . 3438
Phenergan Tablets 3438

HISTANTIL (Canada)
PROMETHAZINE HYDROCHLORIDE
Phenergan Suppositories. . . . 3438
Phenergan Tablets 3438

HISTATEC (Switzerland)
CETIRIZINE HYDROCHLORIDE
Zyrtec Syrup 2589
Zyrtec Tablets 2589

HISTAX (Chile)
CETIRIZINE HYDROCHLORIDE
Zyrtec Syrup 2589
Zyrtec Tablets 2589

HISTAZINE (Hong Kong)
CETIRIZINE HYDROCHLORIDE
Zyrtec Syrup 2589
Zyrtec Tablets 2589

HISTEC (Finland)
CETIRIZINE HYDROCHLORIDE
Zyrtec Syrup 2589
Zyrtec Tablets 2589

HISTEK (Irish Republic)
CETIRIZINE HYDROCHLORIDE
Zyrtec Syrup 2589
Zyrtec Tablets 2589

HISTICA (Thailand)
CETIRIZINE HYDROCHLORIDE
Zyrtec Syrup 2589
Zyrtec Tablets 2589

HISTODIL (Hungary, Russia)
CIMETIDINE
Tagamet Tablets 1547

HISTOP (Spain)
SIMVASTATIN
Zocor Tablets. . . . 2078

HIVIRUX (Argentina)
LAMIVUDINE
Epivir Oral Solution 1394
Epivir Tablets 1394
Epivir-HBV Oral Solution 1398
Epivir-HBV Tablets 1398

HIVIRUX COMPLEX (Argentina)
LAMIVUDINE
Epivir Oral Solution 1394
Epivir Tablets 1394
Epivir-HBV Oral Solution 1398
Epivir-HBV Tablets 1398

HIZAAR (Italy)
HYDROCHLOROTHIAZIDE/LOSARTAN POTASSIUM
Hyzaar 50-12.5 Tablets. . . . 1964

H-MIDE (Thailand)
FUROSEMIDE
Furosemide Tablets 2117

HOCIMIN (Denmark)
CIMETIDINE
Tagamet Tablets 1547

HOFCOMANT (Greece)
AMANTADINE HYDROCHLORIDE
Symmetrel Syrup 1115
Symmetrel Tablets. . . . 1115

HOLADREN (Chile)
ALENDRONATE SODIUM
Fosamax Tablets 1949

HOLETAR (Czech Republic)
LOVASTATIN
Mevacor Tablets 1996

HOLFUNGIN (Germany)
CLOTRIMAZOLE
Lotrimin Cream. . . . 3053
Lotrimin Lotion 1%. . . . 3053
Lotrimin Topical Solution 1% 3053

HONZIL (Mexico)
KETOCONAZOLE
Nizoral 2% Shampoo 1838

HOPECARD (India)
RAMIPRIL
Altace Capsules 1673

HOPRANOLOL (Hong Kong)
PROPRANOLOL HYDROCHLORIDE
Inderal LA Long-Acting Capsules 3421

HOREX (Mexico)
TIMOLOL MALEATE
Blocadren Tablets 1891
Timoptic Sterile Ophthalmic Solution 2058
Timoptic in Ocudose 2061
Timoptic-XE Sterile Ophthalmic Gel Forming Solution 2062

HORIZEM (United Kingdom)
DILTIAZEM HYDROCHLORIDE
Cardizem LA Extended Release Tablets. . . 1699
Tiazac Capsules 1204

HORMODIOL (Argentina)
ESTRADIOL
Climara Transdermal System 795
Vivelle Transdermal System 2288
Vivelle-Dot Transdermal System 2293

HORMODOSE (Brazil)
ESTRADIOL
Climara Transdermal System 795
Vivelle Transdermal System 2288
Vivelle-Dot Transdermal System 2293

HOSBOCIN (Spain)
CEFTRIAXONE SODIUM
Rocephin Injectable Vials, ADD-Vantage, Galaxy, Bulk 2801

HOSBOGEN (Spain)
GENTAMICIN SULFATE
Garamycin Injectable 3028
Genoptic Sterile Ophthalmic Solution . . . . ⊙227

HPB (Argentina)
FINASTERIDE
Propecia Tablets 2036
Proscar Tablets. . . . 2040

HUBERDINA (Spain)
FAMOTIDINE
Pepcid Injection 2017
Pepcid Injection Premixed 2017
Pepcid Tablets 2014
Pepcid for Oral Suspension 2014

HUBERPLEX (Spain)
CHLORDIAZEPOXIDE HYDROCHLORIDE
Librium Capsules. . . . 3349

HUMA-ATENOL (Hungary)
ATENOLOL
Tenormin I.V. Injection. . . . 698

HUMA-CAPTORIL (Hungary)
CAPTOPRIL
Captopril Tablets. . . . 2114

HUMA-DIFENAC (Hungary)
DICLOFENAC SODIUM
Voltaren Tablets 2298
Voltaren-XR Tablets 2301

HUMA-PRONOL (Hungary)
PROPRANOLOL HYDROCHLORIDE
Inderal LA Long-Acting Capsules 3421

HUMA-RANIDINE (Hungary)
RANITIDINE HYDROCHLORIDE
Zantac 25 EFFERdose Tablets 1597
Zantac 150 EFFERdose Tablets. . . . 1597
Zantac 150 Tablets 1597
Zantac 300 Tablets 1597
Zantac Injection 1593
Zantac Injection Premixed 1593
Zantac Syrup 1597

HUMA-SEMIDE (Hungary)
FUROSEMIDE
Furosemide Tablets 2117

HUMORAP (Argentina)
CITALOPRAM HYDROBROMIDE
Celexa Tablets 1177

HYABAK (Italy)
SODIUM HYALURONATE
Hyalgan Solution . . . 2917

HYA-JECT (Germany)
SODIUM HYALURONATE
Hyalgan Solution . . . 2917

HYAL (Malaysia)
SODIUM HYALURONATE
Hyalgan Solution . . . 2917

HYALART (Argentina, Germany, Greece, Italy, Portugal)
SODIUM HYALURONATE
Hyalgan Solution . . . 2917

HYAL-DROP (France, Switzerland)
SODIUM HYALURONATE
Hyalgan Solution . . . 2917

HYALEIN (Japan)
SODIUM HYALURONATE
Hyalgan Solution . . . 2917

HYALGAN (Austria, Canada, Chile, Czech Republic, Denmark, Finland, France, Hong Kong, Hungary, Irish Republic, Italy, Malaysia, Singapore, Spain, Sweden, Thailand, United Kingdom)
SODIUM HYALURONATE
Hyalgan Solution . . . 2917

HYALISTIL (Italy)
SODIUM HYALURONATE
Hyalgan Solution . . . 2917

HYAL-SYSTEM (Germany)
SODIUM HYALURONATE
Hyalgan Solution . . . 2917

HYALUBRIX (Germany)
SODIUM HYALURONATE
Hyalgan Solution . . . 2917

HYALUDERMIN (Brazil)
SODIUM HYALURONATE
Hyalgan Solution . . . 2917

HYANAC (Argentina)
DICLOFENAC SODIUM
Voltaren Tablets . . . 2298
Voltaren-XR Tablets . . . 2301

HYA-OPHTAL (Germany)
SODIUM HYALURONATE
Hyalgan Solution . . . 2917

HYASOL (Argentina)
SODIUM HYALURONATE
Hyalgan Solution . . . 2917

HYBRIDIL (Austria)
CARVEDILOL
Coreg Tablets . . . 1376

HYCAMTIN (Argentina, Australia, Austria, Belgium, Brazil, Canada, Chile, Denmark, Finland, France, Germany, Greece, Hong Kong, Hungary, Irish Republic, Israel, Italy, Norway, Portugal, Singapore, South Africa, Spain, Sweden, Switzerland, Thailand, The Netherlands, United Kingdom)
TOPOTECAN HYDROCHLORIDE
Hycamtin for Injection . . . 1427

HYCOR (Australia)
HYDROCORTISONE
Hydrocortone Tablets . . . 1963

HYCORT (Canada)
HYDROCORTISONE
Hydrocortone Tablets . . . 1963

HYCORTIN (Hong Kong)
HYDROCORTISONE
Hydrocortone Tablets . . . 1963

HYDAC (Denmark, Finland, Sweden)
FELODIPINE
Plendil Extended-Release Tablets . . . 651

HYDAL (Austria)
HYDROMORPHONE HYDROCHLORIDE
Dilaudid Ampules . . . 439
Dilaudid Multiple Dose Vials . . . 439
Dilaudid Non-Sterile Powder . . . 439
Dilaudid Oral Liquid . . . 443
Dilaudid Rectal Suppositories . . . 439
Dilaudid Tablets . . . 439
Dilaudid Tablets - 8 mg . . . 443
Dilaudid-HP Injection . . . 441
Dilaudid-HP Lyophilized Powder 250 mg . . . 441

HYDOFTAL SINE NEOMYCINO (Austria)
HYDROCORTISONE
Hydrocortone Tablets . . . 1963

HYDRACORT (France)
HYDROCORTISONE
Hydrocortone Tablets . . . 1963

HYDRENE (Australia)
TRIAMTERENE
Dyrenium Capsules . . . 3390

HYDREX (South Africa)
FUROSEMIDE
Furosemide Tablets . . . 2117

HYDROCOMP (Germany)
AMILORIDE HYDROCHLORIDE/HYDROCHLOROTHIAZIDE
Moduretic Tablets . . . 2003

HYDROCORT MILD (Germany)
HYDROCORTISONE
Hydrocortone Tablets . . . 1963

HYDROCORTISON MED TERRAMYCIN (Denmark)
HYDROCORTISONE
Hydrocortone Tablets . . . 1963

HYDROCORTISYL (Irish Republic, United Kingdom)
HYDROCORTISONE
Hydrocortone Tablets . . . 1963

HYDROCORTONE (Austria, Irish Republic, Switzerland, United Kingdom)
HYDROCORTISONE
Hydrocortone Tablets . . . 1963

HYDROCUTAN MILD (Germany)
HYDROCORTISONE
Hydrocortone Tablets . . . 1963

HYDRODERM (Austria)
HYDROCORTISONE
Hydrocortone Tablets . . . 1963

HYDRODERM HC (Germany)
HYDROCORTISONE
Hydrocortone Tablets . . . 1963

HYDRODERMED (Germany)
ERYTHROMYCIN
Ery-Tab Tablets . . . 447
Erythromycin Base Filmtab Tablets . . . 454
Erythromycin Delayed-Release Capsules, USP . . . 456
PCE Dispertab Tablets . . . 510

HYDROFLUX (Greece)
FUROSEMIDE
Furosemide Tablets . . . 2117

HYDROFORM (Australia)
HYDROCORTISONE
Hydrocortone Tablets . . . 1963

HYDROGALEN (Germany)
HYDROCORTISONE
Hydrocortone Tablets . . . 1963

HYDRO-LESS (South Africa)
INDAPAMIDE
Indapamide Tablets . . . 2119

HYDROLID (Switzerland)
AMILORIDE HYDROCHLORIDE/HYDROCHLOROTHIAZIDE
Moduretic Tablets . . . 2003

HYDROMET (Irish Republic)
HYDROCHLOROTHIAZIDE/METHYLDOPA
Aldoril Tablets . . . 1884

HYDROMORPH (Canada)
HYDROMORPHONE HYDROCHLORIDE
Dilaudid Ampules . . . 439
Dilaudid Multiple Dose Vials . . . 439
Dilaudid Non-Sterile Powder . . . 439
Dilaudid Oral Liquid . . . 443
Dilaudid Rectal Suppositories . . . 439
Dilaudid Tablets . . . 439
Dilaudid Tablets - 8 mg . . . 443
Dilaudid-HP Injection . . . 441
Dilaudid-HP Lyophilized Powder 250 mg . . . 441

HYDRONET (Denmark)
AMILORIDE HYDROCHLORIDE/HYDROCHLOROTHIAZIDE
Moduretic Tablets . . . 2003

HY-DROP (Italy)
SODIUM HYALURONATE
Hyalgan Solution . . . 2917

HYDRO-RAPID (Germany)
FUROSEMIDE
Furosemide Tablets . . . 2117

HYDRO-RAPID-TABLINEN (Switzerland)
FUROSEMIDE
Furosemide Tablets . . . 2117

HYDROSONE (Canada)
HYDROCORTISONE
Hydrocortone Tablets . . . 1963

HYDRO-WOLFF (Germany)
HYDROCORTISONE
Hydrocortone Tablets . . . 1963

HYDROZIDE (Hong Kong)
AMILORIDE HYDROCHLORIDE/HYDROCHLOROTHIAZIDE
Moduretic Tablets . . . 2003

HYDROZIDE PLUS (Thailand)
AMILORIDE HYDROCHLORIDE/HYDROCHLOROTHIAZIDE
Moduretic Tablets . . . 2003

HYDROZOLE (Australia)
HYDROCORTISONE
Hydrocortone Tablets . . . 1963

HYFLOX (Thailand)
OFLOXACIN
Floxin Otic Solution . . . 1043

HY-GAG (Germany)
SODIUM HYALURONATE
Hyalgan Solution . . . 2917

HYLAN (Germany)
SODIUM HYALURONATE
Hyalgan Solution . . . 2917

HYLO-COMOD (France, Germany, Israel, Italy, Portugal, Switzerland)
SODIUM HYALURONATE
Hyalgan Solution . . . 2917

HYLUPROTECT (Italy)
SODIUM HYALURONATE
Hyalgan Solution . . . 2917

HYLUPROTECT UD (France)
SODIUM HYALURONATE
Hyalgan Solution . . . 2917

HYPACE (South Africa)
ENALAPRIL MALEATE
Vasotec I.V. Injection . . . 2076

HYPAN (Belgium)
NIFEDIPINE
Adalat CC Tablets . . . 2978

HYPERMOL (New Zealand)
TIMOLOL MALEATE
Blocadren Tablets . . . 1891
Timoptic Sterile Ophthalmic Solution . . . 2058
Timoptic in Ocudose . . . 2061
Timoptic-XE Sterile Ophthalmic Gel Forming Solution . . . 2062

HYPERNOL (Hong Kong, Singapore)
ATENOLOL
Tenormin I.V. Injection . . . 698

HYPERRETIC (Thailand)
AMILORIDE HYDROCHLORIDE/HYDROCHLOROTHIAZIDE
Moduretic Tablets . . . 2003

HYPERSTAT (Australia, Belgium, Canada, France, Greece, Italy, Mexico, South Africa, Spain, Sweden, Switzerland, The Netherlands)
DIAZOXIDE
Hyperstat I.V. Injection . . . 3031

HYPERTANE (United Kingdom)
AMILORIDE HYDROCHLORIDE/HYDROCHLOROTHIAZIDE
Moduretic Tablets . . . 2003

HYPERTONALUM (Germany)
DIAZOXIDE
Hyperstat I.V. Injection . . . 3031

HYPERTORR (Germany)
HYDROCHLOROTHIAZIDE/TRIAMTERENE
Dyazide Capsules . . . 1389
Maxzide Tablets . . . 2150
Maxzide-25 mg Tablets . . . 2150

HYPHORAL (India)
KETOCONAZOLE
Nizoral 2% Shampoo . . . 1838

HYPNOREX (Germany, Switzerland)
LITHIUM CARBONATE
Eskalith CR Controlled-Release Tablets . . . 1406
Eskalith Capsules . . . 1406

HYPODINE (Thailand)
CLONIDINE HYDROCHLORIDE
Catapres Tablets . . . 874

HYPOLAR RETARD (United Kingdom)
NIFEDIPINE
Adalat CC Tablets . . . 2978

HYPOLIP (Czech Republic)
FENOFIBRATE
Tricor Tablets . . . 523

HYPOMED (Austria)
LISINOPRIL
Prinivil Tablets . . . 2029
Zestril Tablets . . . 704

HYPOTENSOR (Greece)
CAPTOPRIL
Captopril Tablets . . . 2114

HYPREN (Austria)
RAMIPRIL
Altace Capsules . . . 1673

HYRON (Hungary)
TERAZOSIN HYDROCHLORIDE
Hytrin Capsules . . . 469

HYRUAN (Hong Kong)
SODIUM HYALURONATE
Hyalgan Solution . . . 2917

HYSAN (Germany)
SODIUM HYALURONATE
Hyalgan Solution . . . 2917

HYSONE (Australia)
HYDROCORTISONE
Hydrocortone Tablets . . . 1963

HYTACAND (Portugal)
CANDESARTAN CILEXETIL
Atacand Tablets . . . 634

HYTENEZE (United Kingdom)
CAPTOPRIL
Captopril Tablets . . . 2114

HYTISONE (Hong Kong)
HYDROCORTISONE
Hydrocortone Tablets . . . 1963

HYTRIN (Australia, Belgium, Brazil, Canada, Chile, Czech Republic, Greece, Hong Kong, Hungary, India, Irish Republic, Israel, Malaysia, Mexico, New Zealand, Portugal, Singapore, South Africa, Thailand, The Netherlands, United Kingdom)
TERAZOSIN HYDROCHLORIDE
Hytrin Capsules . . . 469

HYTRIN BPH (Switzerland)
TERAZOSIN HYDROCHLORIDE
Hytrin Capsules . . . 469

HYTRINE (France)
TERAZOSIN HYDROCHLORIDE
Hytrin Capsules . . . 469

HYTRINEX (Sweden)
TERAZOSIN HYDROCHLORIDE
Hytrin Capsules . . . 469

HYZAAR (Brazil, Canada, Chile, Czech Republic, France, Greece, Hong Kong, Hungary, Malaysia, Mexico, Singapore, Thailand, The Netherlands)
LOSARTAN POTASSIUM
Cozaar Tablets . . . 1913

HYZAN (Hong Kong, Malaysia, Singapore)
RANITIDINE HYDROCHLORIDE
Zantac 25 EFFERdose Tablets . . . 1597
Zantac 150 EFFERdose Tablets . . . 1597
Zantac 150 Tablets . . . 1597
Zantac 300 Tablets . . . 1597
Zantac Injection . . . 1593
Zantac Injection Premixed . . . 1593
Zantac Syrup . . . 1597

IAL (Hong Kong, Hungary, Italy, Switzerland, Thailand)
SODIUM HYALURONATE
Hyalgan Solution 2917

IALECT (Italy)
SODIUM HYALURONATE
Hyalgan Solution 2917

IALUGEN (Switzerland)
SODIUM HYALURONATE
Hyalgan Solution 2917

IALUGEN PLUS (Czech Republic, Hungary)
SODIUM HYALURONATE
Hyalgan Solution 2917

IALUM (Italy)
SODIUM HYALURONATE
Hyalgan Solution 2917

IALUREX (Italy)
SODIUM HYALURONATE
Hyalgan Solution 2917

IALUSET (France)
SODIUM HYALURONATE
Hyalgan Solution 2917

IBAMOXIL (Brazil)
AMOXICILLIN
Amoxil Pediatric Drops for Oral Suspension 1315
Amoxil Tablets 1315

IBDAZOL (Brazil)
MEBENDAZOLE
Vermox Chewable Tablets 1853

IBIAMOX (Thailand)
AMOXICILLIN
Amoxil Pediatric Drops for Oral Suspension 1315
Amoxil Tablets 1315

IBIPROVIR (Italy)
TERAZOSIN HYDROCHLORIDE
Hytrin Capsules 469

ICAZ (France)
ISRADIPINE
DynaCirc CR Tablets 2726

ICHTHOCORTIN (Germany)
HYDROCORTISONE
Hydrocortone Tablets 1963

ICORAN (Greece)
LISINOPRIL
Prinivil Tablets 2029
Zestril Tablets 704

ICTAN (Spain)
CLOTRIMAZOLE
Lotrimin Cream 3053
Lotrimin Lotion 1% 3053
Lotrimin Topical Solution 1% 3053

IDAMYCIN (Canada, Mexico)
IDARUBICIN HYDROCHLORIDE
Idamycin PFS Injection 2645

IDARALEM (Mexico)
IDARUBICIN HYDROCHLORIDE
Idamycin PFS Injection 2645

IDENONA (Argentina)
HYDROCORTISONE
Hydrocortone Tablets 1963

IDRIL N SINE (Germany)
NAPHAZOLINE HYDROCHLORIDE
Albalon Ophthalmic Solution . . . . ⊙216

IDROLAC (Italy)
LACTULOSE
Kristalose for Oral Solution 2149

IDUVO (Argentina)
ZIDOVUDINE
Retrovir Capsules 1533
Retrovir IV Infusion 1537
Retrovir Syrup 1533
Retrovir Tablets 1533

IECATEC (Spain, Thailand)
ENALAPRIL MALEATE
Vasotec I.V. Injection 2076

IFA REDUCCING S (Mexico)
PHENTERMINE HYDROCHLORIDE
Adipex-P Capsules 1216
Adipex-P Tablets 1216

IFACIL (Mexico)
FLUOROURACIL
Efudex Topical Cream 3348
Efudex Topical Solutions 3348

IFADA (Spain)
FAMOTIDINE
Pepcid Injection 2017
Pepcid Injection Premixed 2017
Pepcid Tablets 2014
Pepcid for Oral Suspension 2014

IFAVAC (Mexico)
VANCOMYCIN HYDROCHLORIDE
Vancocin HCl Capsules, USP 3370

IFISTATIN (Singapore)
SIMVASTATIN
Zocor Tablets 2078

IFOCID (Argentina)
FLUOROURACIL
Efudex Topical Cream 3348
Efudex Topical Solutions 3348

IFOS (Chile)
OFLOXACIN
Floxin Otic Solution 1043

I-GESIC (India)
DICLOFENAC SODIUM
Voltaren Tablets 2298
Voltaren-XR Tablets 2301

IGUASSINA (Brazil)
HYDROCHLOROTHIAZIDE/TRIAMTERENE
Dyazide Capsules 1389
Maxzide Tablets 2150
Maxzide-25 mg Tablets 2150

IHD (India)
ISOSORBIDE MONONITRATE
Imdur Tablets 3032

IKACOR (Israel)
VERAPAMIL HYDROCHLORIDE
Covera-HS Tablets 3135
Verelan PM Capsules 3120

IKAPRESS (Israel)
VERAPAMIL HYDROCHLORIDE
Covera-HS Tablets 3135
Verelan PM Capsules 3120

IKATIN (Mexico)
GENTAMICIN SULFATE
Garamycin Injectable 3028
Genoptic Sterile Ophthalmic Solution . . . . ⊙227

IKOBEL (Greece)
TOBRAMYCIN
TOBI Solution for Inhalation 1015

IKOLAN (Argentina)
CLOTRIMAZOLE
Lotrimin Cream 3053
Lotrimin Lotion 1% 3053
Lotrimin Topical Solution 1% 3053

IKTORIVIL (Sweden)
CLONAZEPAM
Klonopin Tablets 2782

ILACEN (Spain)
DIFLUNISAL
Dolobid Tablets 1937

ILAGANE (Spain)
NAPROXEN
EC-Naprosyn Delayed-Release Tablets 2769
Naprosyn Suspension 2769
Naprosyn Tablets 2769

ILGEM (Greece)
KETOCONAZOLE
Nizoral 2% Shampoo 1838

ILOCAP (Australia)
ERYTHROMYCIN
Ery-Tab Tablets 447
Erythromycin Base Filmtab Tablets 454
Erythromycin Delayed-Release Capsules, USP 456
PCE Dispertab Tablets 510

ILOPAR (Greece)
LOVASTATIN
Mevacor Tablets 1996

ILOSIN (Mexico)
ERYTHROMYCIN
Ery-Tab Tablets 447
Erythromycin Base Filmtab Tablets 454
Erythromycin Delayed-Release Capsules, USP 456
PCE Dispertab Tablets 510

ILOTICINA (Argentina, Spain)
ERYTHROMYCIN
Ery-Tab Tablets 447
Erythromycin Base Filmtab Tablets 454
Erythromycin Delayed-Release Capsules, USP 456
PCE Dispertab Tablets 510

ILOTICINA ANTI ACNE (Spain)
ERYTHROMYCIN
Ery-Tab Tablets 447
Erythromycin Base Filmtab Tablets 454
Erythromycin Delayed-Release Capsules, USP 456
PCE Dispertab Tablets 510

ILOTREX (Brazil)
ERYTHROMYCIN STEARATE
Erythrocin Stearate Filmtab Tablets 452

ILOTYCIN TS (South Africa)
ERYTHROMYCIN
Ery-Tab Tablets 447
Erythromycin Base Filmtab Tablets 454
Erythromycin Delayed-Release Capsules, USP 456
PCE Dispertab Tablets 510

ILOTYCIN-A (South Africa)
TRETINOIN
Avita Cream 2136
Avita Gel 2138
Renova 0.05% Cream 2387
Retin-A Micro 0.1%/0.04% 2388
Vesanoid Capsules 2823

ILSATEC (Argentina, Brazil, Mexico)
LANSOPRAZOLE
Prevacid Delayed-Release Capsules 3268

IMACILLIN (Denmark)
AMOXICILLIN
Amoxil Pediatric Drops for Oral Suspension 1315
Amoxil Tablets 1315

IMAVERMIL (Brazil)
ALBENDAZOLE
Albenza Tablets 1310

IMAZOL (Czech Republic, Germany, Switzerland)
CLOTRIMAZOLE
Lotrimin Cream 3053
Lotrimin Lotion 1% 3053
Lotrimin Topical Solution 1% 3053

IMAZOL PLUS (Czech Republic)
CLOTRIMAZOLE
Lotrimin Cream 3053
Lotrimin Lotion 1% 3053
Lotrimin Topical Solution 1% 3053

IMD (Singapore)
LOPERAMIDE HYDROCHLORIDE
Imodium Capsules 1834

IMDA (Argentina)
BICALUTAMIDE
Casodex Tablets 670

IMDEX (Malaysia, Singapore)
ISOSORBIDE MONONITRATE
Imdur Tablets 3032

IMDUR (Australia, Austria, Canada, Czech Republic, Denmark, Finland, Greece, Hong Kong, Irish Republic, Malaysia, Mexico, New Zealand, Norway, Portugal, Singapore, South Africa, Spain, Sweden, Switzerland, Thailand, United Kingdom)
ISOSORBIDE MONONITRATE
Imdur Tablets 3032

IMEPAS (Mexico)
DIAZEPAM
Diastat Rectal Delivery System 3344
Valium Tablets 2822

IMFERDEX (Switzerland)
IRON DEXTRAN
Infed Injection 3381

IMFERON (Australia, Belgium, Canada, India, Mexico, South Africa, Spain, The Netherlands, United Kingdom)
IRON DEXTRAN
Infed Injection 3381

IMFLAC (Australia)
DICLOFENAC SODIUM
Voltaren Tablets 2298
Voltaren-XR Tablets 2301

IMIDIL (India)
CLOTRIMAZOLE
Lotrimin Cream 3053
Lotrimin Lotion 1% 3053
Lotrimin Topical Solution 1% 3053

IMIGRAN (Argentina, Australia, Brazil, Chile, Czech Republic, Germany, Greece, Hong Kong, Hungary, Irish Republic, Malaysia, New Zealand, Norway, Portugal, Russia, Singapore, South Africa, Spain, Thailand, United Kingdom)
SUMATRIPTAN SUCCINATE
Imitrex Injection 1431
Imitrex Tablets 1440

IMIJECT (France)
SUMATRIPTAN SUCCINATE
Imitrex Injection 1431
Imitrex Tablets 1440

IMIMORE (Argentina)
IMIQUIMOD
Aldara Cream, 5% 1814

IMIPEM (Italy)
CILASTATIN SODIUM/IMIPENEM
Primaxin I.M. 2022
Primaxin I.V. 2024

IMITREX (Argentina, Israel)
SUMATRIPTAN
Imitrex Nasal Spray 1435

IMMUKIN (Hong Kong, Irish Republic)
INTERFERON GAMMA-1B
Actimmune 1646

IMMUKINE (The Netherlands)
INTERFERON GAMMA-1B
Actimmune 1646

IMOCUR (Finland)
LOPERAMIDE HYDROCHLORIDE
Imodium Capsules 1834

IMODIUM (Australia, Austria, Belgium, Canada, Czech Republic, Denmark, Finland, France, Germany, Greece, Hong Kong, Hungary, Irish Republic, Israel, Italy, Malaysia, Mexico, New Zealand, Norway, Portugal, Russia, Singapore, South Africa, Spain, Sweden, Switzerland, Thailand, The Netherlands)
LOPERAMIDE HYDROCHLORIDE
Imodium Capsules 1834

IMODIUM ADVANCED (Australia)
LOPERAMIDE HYDROCHLORIDE
Imodium Capsules 1834

IMODIUM KOMPLETT (Hungary)
LOPERAMIDE HYDROCHLORIDE
Imodium Capsules 1834

IMODIUM MED SIMETHICON (Denmark)
LOPERAMIDE HYDROCHLORIDE
Imodium Capsules 1834

IMODIUM PLUS (Austria, Brazil, Hong Kong)
LOPERAMIDE HYDROCHLORIDE
Imodium Capsules 1834

IMODONL (Hong Kong)
LOPERAMIDE HYDROCHLORIDE
Imodium Capsules 1834

IMOSEC (Brazil, Spain)
LOPERAMIDE HYDROCHLORIDE
Imodium Capsules 1834

IMOSSEL (France)
LOPERAMIDE HYDROCHLORIDE
Imodium Capsules 1834

IMOSSELLINGUAL (France)
LOPERAMIDE HYDROCHLORIDE
Imodium Capsules 1834

IMPELIUM (Thailand)
LOPERAMIDE HYDROCHLORIDE
Imodium Capsules 1834

IMPORE (Thailand)
LOPERAMIDE HYDROCHLORIDE
Imodium Capsules 1834

IMPOSERGON (Greece)
FAMOTIDINE
Pepcid Injection 2017
Pepcid Injection Premixed 2017
Pepcid Tablets 2014
Pepcid for Oral Suspension 2014

IMPUGAN (Denmark, Sweden, Switzerland, Thailand)
FUROSEMIDE
Furosemide Tablets 2117

IMTRATE (Australia, New Zealand)
ISOSORBIDE MONONITRATE
Imdur Tablets 3032

IMUFOR (Argentina, Austria)
INTERFERON GAMMA-1B
Actimmune 1646

IMUKIN (Austria, Denmark, Finland, France, Germany, Italy, Norway, Portugal, Spain, Sweden)
INTERFERON GAMMA-1B
Actimmune 1646

IMUNOXA (Argentina)
LAMIVUDINE
Epivir Oral Solution 1394
Epivir Tablets 1394
Epivir-HBV Oral Solution 1398
Epivir-HBV Tablets 1398

IMUNOXA COMPLEX (Argentina)
LAMIVUDINE
Epivir Oral Solution 1394
Epivir Tablets 1394
Epivir-HBV Oral Solution 1398
Epivir-HBV Tablets 1398

IMUXGEN (Argentina)
MYCOPHENOLATE MOFETIL
CellCept Capsules 2751
CellCept Oral Suspension 2751
CellCept Tablets 2751

INAC (Singapore)
DICLOFENAC SODIUM
Voltaren Tablets 2298
Voltaren-XR Tablets 2301

INALACOR (Spain)
FLUTICASONE PROPIONATE
Cutivate Cream 1381
Cutivate Ointment 1384
Flonase Nasal Spray 1412

INALCORT (Italy)
FLUNISOLIDE
Aerobid Inhaler System 1172
Aerobid-M Inhaler System 1172
Nasarel Nasal Spray 1652

INAMIDE (Irish Republic)
INDAPAMIDE
Indapamide Tablets 2119

INASPIR (Spain)
SALMETEROL XINAFOATE
Serevent Diskus 1540

INASTMOL (Argentina)
THEOPHYLLINE
Uniphyl Tablets 2708

INCIDAL-OD (Thailand)
CETIRIZINE HYDROCHLORIDE
Zyrtec Syrup 2589
Zyrtec Tablets 2589

INCORIL (Argentina, Brazil, Chile)
DILTIAZEM HYDROCHLORIDE
Cardizem LA Extended Release Tablets 1699
Tiazac Capsules 1204

INDACAR (Denmark)
INDAPAMIDE
Indapamide Tablets 2119

INDAFLEX (Italy)
INDAPAMIDE
Indapamide Tablets 2119

INDAHEXAL (Australia)
INDAPAMIDE
Indapamide Tablets 2119

INDALIX (Hong Kong, South Africa)
INDAPAMIDE
Indapamide Tablets 2119

INDAMOL (Italy)
INDAPAMIDE
Indapamide Tablets 2119

INDANORM (United Arab Emirates)
INDAPAMIDE
Indapamide Tablets 2119

INDAP (Czech Republic, Russia)
INDAPAMIDE
Indapamide Tablets 2119

INDAPRESS (Chile)
INDAPAMIDE
Indapamide Tablets 2119

INDA-PUREN (Germany)
INDAPAMIDE
Indapamide Tablets 2119

INDARZONA-N (Mexico)
DEXAMETHASONE
Decadron Tablets 1929

INDERAL (Argentina, Australia, Austria, Belgium, Brazil, Canada, Denmark, Finland, Hong Kong, India, Irish Republic, Israel, Italy, Malaysia, Norway, Portugal, Singapore, South Africa, Sweden, Switzerland, Thailand, The Netherlands, United Kingdom)
PROPRANOLOL HYDROCHLORIDE
Inderal LA Long-Acting Capsules 3421

INDERALICI (Mexico)
PROPRANOLOL HYDROCHLORIDE
Inderal LA Long-Acting Capsules 3421

INDERM (Belgium, Germany, Switzerland, The Netherlands)
ERYTHROMYCIN
Ery-Tab Tablets 447
Erythromycin Base Filmtab Tablets 454
Erythromycin Delayed-Release Capsules, USP 456
PCE Dispertab Tablets 510

INDIARAL (France)
LOPERAMIDE HYDROCHLORIDE
Imodium Capsules 1834

INDICONTIN (India)
INDAPAMIDE
Indapamide Tablets 2119

INDITOR (India)
INDAPAMIDE
Indapamide Tablets 2119

INDIVAN (India)
INDINAVIR SULFATE
Crixivan Capsules 1918

INDOBLOC (Germany)
PROPRANOLOL HYDROCHLORIDE
Inderal LA Long-Acting Capsules 3421

INDOBLOK (South Africa)
PROPRANOLOL HYDROCHLORIDE
Inderal LA Long-Acting Capsules 3421

INDOLIN (Italy)
INDAPAMIDE
Indapamide Tablets 2119

INDUZEPAM (Argentina)
CLONAZEPAM
Klonopin Tablets 2782

INESFAY (Mexico)
CIMETIDINE
Tagamet Tablets 1547

INESTOM (Greece)
LEVOCARNITINE
Carnitor Injection 3185
Carnitor Tablets and Oral Solution 3187

INF (Argentina)
INTERFERON ALFA-2B
Intron A for Injection 3038

INFASURF (Israel)
CALFACTANT
Infasurf Intratracheal Suspension 1188

INFECTOCIN (South Africa)
ERYTHROMYCIN STEARATE
Erythrocin Stearate Filmtab Tablets 452

INFECTOCLONT (Germany)
METRONIDAZOLE
MetroGel-Vaginal Gel 1822
Noritate Cream, 1% 1051

INFECTOFLAM (Brazil, Czech Republic, Malaysia)
FLUOROMETHOLONE
FML Ophthalmic Ointment ⊙225

INFECTOFLU (Germany)
AMANTADINE HYDROCHLORIDE
Symmetrel Syrup 1115
Symmetrel Tablets 1115

INFECTOMOX (Germany)
AMOXICILLIN
Amoxil Pediatric Drops for Oral Suspension 1315
Amoxil Tablets 1315

INFECTOPEDICUL (Germany)
PERMETHRIN
Acticin Cream 2125

INFECTOPYODERM (Germany)
MUPIROCIN
Bactroban Ointment 1358

INFECTOSS (Brazil)
ERYTHROMYCIN
Ery-Tab Tablets 447
Erythromycin Base Filmtab Tablets 454
Erythromycin Delayed-Release Capsules, USP 456
PCE Dispertab Tablets 510

INFERAX (Germany)
INTERFERON ALFACON-1
Infergen 1647

INFERGEN (Belgium, Canada, Czech Republic, France, Greece, Hungary, Italy, The Netherlands)
INTERFERON ALFACON-1
Infergen 1647

INFESTAT (United Kingdom)
NYSTATIN
Nystop Topical Powder USP 2490

INFEX (Chile)
CLARITHROMYCIN
Biaxin Filmtab Tablets 402
Biaxin Granules 402

INFLA-BAN (South Africa)
DICLOFENAC SODIUM
Voltaren Tablets 2298
Voltaren-XR Tablets 2301

INFLAMAC (Switzerland)
DICLOFENAC SODIUM
Voltaren Tablets 2298
Voltaren-XR Tablets 2301

INFLAMASE (Canada)
PREDNISOLONE SODIUM PHOSPHATE
Pediapred Oral Solution 3319

INFLAMAX (Brazil)
DICLOFENAC SODIUM
Voltaren Tablets 2298
Voltaren-XR Tablets 2301

INFLANAC (Hong Kong, Singapore, Thailand)
DICLOFENAC SODIUM
Voltaren Tablets 2298
Voltaren-XR Tablets 2301

INFLOXA (Mexico)
CIPROFLOXACIN
Cipro Oral Suspension 2991

INFLU-A (Israel)
AMANTADINE HYDROCHLORIDE
Symmetrel Syrup 1115
Symmetrel Tablets 1115

INFOSTAT (Argentina)
INTERFERON ALFA-2A
Roferon-A Injection 2805

INFUFER (Canada)
IRON DEXTRAN
Infed Injection 3381

INGASTRI (Spain)
FAMOTIDINE
Pepcid Injection 2017
Pepcid Injection Premixed 2017
Pepcid Tablets 2014
Pepcid for Oral Suspension 2014

INHACORT (Germany)
FLUNISOLIDE
Aerobid Inhaler System 1172
Aerobid-M Inhaler System 1172
Nasarel Nasal Spray 1652

INHALEX (Thailand)
IPRATROPIUM BROMIDE
Atrovent Inhalation Solution 868
Atrovent Nasal Spray 0.03% 869
Atrovent Nasal Spray 0.06% 870

INHIBACE (Israel)
CAPTOPRIL
Captopril Tablets 2114

INIBIL (Italy)
APROTININ
Trasylol Injection 779

INIPROL (Belgium, France, Italy)
APROTININ
Trasylol Injection 779

INKAMIL (Spain)
CIPROFLOXACIN HYDROCHLORIDE
Ciloxan Ophthalmic Ointment 554
Ciloxan Ophthalmic Solution ⊙205
Cipro Tablets 2991

INMUNOARTRO (Argentina)
LEFLUNOMIDE
Arava Tablets 2881

INNOMEL (Irish Republic)
ENALAPRIL MALEATE
Vasotec I.V. Injection 2076

INNOVACE (Irish Republic, United Kingdom)
ENALAPRIL MALEATE
Vasotec I.V. Injection 2076

INNOZIDE (Irish Republic, United Kingdom)
ENALAPRIL MALEATE/HYDROCHLOROTHIAZIDE
Vaseretic Tablets 2073

INOFLOX (Malaysia, Singapore)
OFLOXACIN
Floxin Otic Solution 1043

INOSERT (India)
SERTRALINE HYDROCHLORIDE
Zoloft Tablets 2581

INOTRIN (Greece)
ISOTRETINOIN
Accutane Capsules 2740

INOVAL (Brazil)
FENTANYL CITRATE
Actiq 993

INPAMIDE (Thailand)
INDAPAMIDE
Indapamide Tablets 2119

INPANOL (Hong Kong, Singapore)
PROPRANOLOL HYDROCHLORIDE
Inderal LA Long-Acting Capsules 3421

INSECT ECRAN (France)
PERMETHRIN
Acticin Cream 2125

INSENSYE (Australia)
NORFLOXACIN
Noroxin Tablets 2009

INSERTEC (Argentina)
SERTRALINE HYDROCHLORIDE
Zoloft Tablets 2581

INSIDE (Sweden)
RANITIDINE HYDROCHLORIDE
Zantac 25 EFFERdose Tablets 1597
Zantac 150 EFFERdose Tablets 1597
Zantac 150 Tablets 1597
Zantac 300 Tablets 1597
Zantac Injection 1593
Zantac Injection Premixed 1593
Zantac Syrup 1597

INSIDE BRUS (Finland, Norway)
RANITIDINE HYDROCHLORIDE
Zantac 25 EFFERdose Tablets 1597
Zantac 150 EFFERdose Tablets 1597
Zantac 150 Tablets 1597
Zantac 300 Tablets 1597
Zantac Injection 1593
Zantac Injection Premixed 1593
Zantac Syrup 1597

INSIG (Australia)
INDAPAMIDE
Indapamide Tablets 2119

INSOMN-EZE (Australia)
PROMETHAZINE HYDROCHLORIDE
Phenergan Suppositories 3438
Phenergan Tablets 3438

INSTANA (Spain)
CEFPODOXIME PROXETİL
Vantin Tablets and Oral Suspension 2650

INSUP (Spain)
ENALAPRIL MALEATE
Vasotec I.V. Injection 2076

INTAPAN (Hong Kong)
NALBUPHINE HYDROCHLORIDE
Nubain Injection 1111

INTEGRILIN (Australia, Belgium, Brazil, Canada, Chile, Czech Republic, Denmark, Finland, France, Germany, Greece, Hong Kong, Hungary, Irish Republic, Israel, Italy, Malaysia, New Zealand, Norway, Portugal, Russia, Singapore, South Africa, Spain, Sweden, Switzerland, Thailand, The Netherlands, United Kingdom)
EPTIFIBATIDE
Integrilin Injection 3034

INTELECTA (Greece)
LEVOCARNITINE
Carnitor Injection. 3185
Carnitor Tablets and Oral Solution 3187

INTER 2-B (Argentina)
INTERFERON ALFA-2B
Intron A for Injection. 3038

INTERBERIN (Austria)
SARGRAMOSTIM
Leukine. 829

INTERBION (Greece)
CEFUROXIME AXETIL
Ceftin Tablets 1369
Ceftin for Oral Suspension. 1369

INTERCEFAL (Spain)
CEFAZOLIN SODIUM
Ancef for Injection 1318

INTERMIGRAN (Germany)
PROPRANOLOL HYDROCHLORIDE
Inderal LA Long-Acting Capsules 3421

INTOCEL (Argentina)
CLADRIBINE
Leustatin Injection 2368

INTRACEF (South Africa)
CEFUROXIME SODIUM
Zinacef Injection 1604

INTRAZOLINA (Spain)
CEFAZOLIN SODIUM
Ancef for Injection 1318

INTRON A (Canada, Czech Republic, Hong Kong, Hungary, Israel, Malaysia, Mexico, Portugal, Singapore, South Africa, Spain, Switzerland, The Netherlands)
INTERFERON ALFA-2B
Intron A for Injection. 3038

INTRONA (Austria, Denmark, Finland, France, Irish Republic, Norway, Sweden, Thailand)
INTERFERON ALFA-2B
Intron A for Injection. 3038

INVEOXEL (Chile)
NAPROXEN
EC-Naprosyn Delayed-Release Tablets. . . . 2769
Naprosyn Suspension. 2769
Naprosyn Tablets 2769

INVIGAN (Spain)
FAMOTIDINE
Pepcid Injection 2017
Pepcid Injection Premixed 2017
Pepcid Tablets 2014
Pepcid for Oral Suspension 2014

INVORIL (Czech Republic, Hungary, Malaysia, Singapore, Thailand)
ENALAPRIL MALEATE
Vasotec I.V. Injection 2076

INVOZIDE (India)
ENALAPRIL MALEATE
Vasotec I.V. Injection 2076

INZA (Australia, Hong Kong, Malaysia)
NAPROXEN
EC-Naprosyn Delayed-Release Tablets. . . . 2769
Naprosyn Suspension. 2769
Naprosyn Tablets 2769

IOR T3 (Chile, Mexico)
MUROMONAB-CD3
Orthoclone OKT3 Sterile Solution 2370

IPACEF (Italy)
CEFUROXIME SODIUM
Zinacef Injection 1604

IPAGASTRIL (Italy)
SUCRALFATE
Carafate Suspension 727
Carafate Tablets 728

IPAMIX (Italy)
INDAPAMIDE
Indapamide Tablets 2119

IPATON (Czech Republic, Hungary)
TICLOPIDINE HYDROCHLORIDE
Ticlid Tablets 2813

IPOMEX (Argentina)
SIBUTRAMINE HYDROCHLORIDE
Meridia Capsules. 485

IPOTENSIUM (Italy)
CLONIDINE HYDROCHLORIDE
Catapres Tablets 874

IPRA (New Zealand)
IPRATROPIUM BROMIDE
Atrovent Inhalation Solution 868
Atrovent Nasal Spray 0.03%. 869
Atrovent Nasal Spray 0.06%. 870

IPRABON (Brazil)
IPRATROPIUM BROMIDE
Atrovent Inhalation Solution 868
Atrovent Nasal Spray 0.03%. 869
Atrovent Nasal Spray 0.06%. 870

IPRABRON (Argentina)
IPRATROPIUM BROMIDE
Atrovent Inhalation Solution 868
Atrovent Nasal Spray 0.03%. 869
Atrovent Nasal Spray 0.06%. 870

IPRADUAL (Argentina)
IPRATROPIUM BROMIDE
Atrovent Inhalation Solution 868
Atrovent Nasal Spray 0.03%. 869
Atrovent Nasal Spray 0.06%. 870

IPRAMID (Greece)
SIMVASTATIN
Zocor Tablets. 2078

IPRANASE (India)
IPRATROPIUM BROMIDE
Atrovent Inhalation Solution 868
Atrovent Nasal Spray 0.03%. 869
Atrovent Nasal Spray 0.06%. 870

IPRANEO (Brazil)
IPRATROPIUM BROMIDE
Atrovent Inhalation Solution 868
Atrovent Nasal Spray 0.03%. 869
Atrovent Nasal Spray 0.06%. 870

IPRASALB (Argentina)
IPRATROPIUM BROMIDE
Atrovent Inhalation Solution 868
Atrovent Nasal Spray 0.03%. 869
Atrovent Nasal Spray 0.06%. 870

IPRATRIN (Australia)
IPRATROPIUM BROMIDE
Atrovent Inhalation Solution 868
Atrovent Nasal Spray 0.03%. 869
Atrovent Nasal Spray 0.06%. 870

IPRAVENT (Australia, Hong Kong, India)
IPRATROPIUM BROMIDE
Atrovent Inhalation Solution 868
Atrovent Nasal Spray 0.03%. 869
Atrovent Nasal Spray 0.06%. 870

IPVENT (South Africa)
IPRATROPIUM BROMIDE
Atrovent Inhalation Solution 868
Atrovent Nasal Spray 0.03%. 869
Atrovent Nasal Spray 0.06%. 870

IQFADINA (Mexico)
RANITIDINE HYDROCHLORIDE
Zantac 25 EFFERdose Tablets 1597
Zantac 150 EFFERdose Tablets. 1597
Zantac 150 Tablets 1597
Zantac 300 Tablets 1597
Zantac Injection 1593
Zantac Injection Premixed 1593
Zantac Syrup 1597

IQFAMICINA (Mexico)
ERYTHROMYCIN
Ery-Tab Tablets 447
Erythromycin Base Filmtab Tablets 454
Erythromycin Delayed-Release Capsules, USP 456
PCE Dispertab Tablets 510

IQFASOL (Mexico)
NAPROXEN
EC-Naprosyn Delayed-Release Tablets. . . . 2769
Naprosyn Suspension. 2769
Naprosyn Tablets 2769

IRBAN (Israel)
IRBESARTAN
Avapro Tablets 925

IRBAN PLUS (Israel)
IRBESARTAN
Avapro Tablets 925

IRENAX (Argentina)
IRINOTECAN HYDROCHLORIDE
Camptosar Injection 2602

IRICIL (Spain)
LISINOPRIL
Prinivil Tablets 2029
Zestril Tablets. 704

IRICIL PLUS (Spain)
LISINOPRIL
Prinivil Tablets 2029
Zestril Tablets. 704

IRIDINA DUE (Italy)
NAPHAZOLINE HYDROCHLORIDE
Albalon Ophthalmic Solution . . . . ⊙216

IRILENS (Italy)
SODIUM HYALURONATE
Hyalgan Solution 2917

IRINOGEN (Argentina)
IRINOTECAN HYDROCHLORIDE
Camptosar Injection 2602

IRINOTEL (Thailand)
IRINOTECAN HYDROCHLORIDE
Camptosar Injection 2602

IROVEL (India)
IRBESARTAN
Avapro Tablets 925

IRRADIAL (Argentina)
SERTRALINE HYDROCHLORIDE
Zoloft Tablets 2581

IRUMED (Czech Republic)
LISINOPRIL
Prinivil Tablets 2029
Zestril Tablets. 704

IS 5 MONO (Germany)
ISOSORBIDE MONONITRATE
Imdur Tablets 3032

ISADOL (Mexico)
ZIDOVUDINE
Retrovir Capsules 1533
Retrovir IV Infusion. 1537
Retrovir Syrup 1533
Retrovir Tablets. 1533

ISANGINA (Finland)
ISOSORBIDE MONONITRATE
Imdur Tablets 3032

ISAXION (Portugal)
TICLOPIDINE HYDROCHLORIDE
Ticlid Tablets 2813

ISCLOFEN (United Kingdom)
DICLOFENAC SODIUM
Voltaren Tablets 2298
Voltaren-XR Tablets 2301

ISCOVER (Argentina, Australia, Brazil, Germany, Greece, Italy, Mexico, Portugal, Spain, Switzerland)
CLOPIDOGREL BISULFATE
Plavix Tablets 940, 2942

ISDINIUM (Spain)
HYDROCORTISONE
Hydrocortone Tablets 1963

ISET (Argentina)
CLARITHROMYCIN
Biaxin Filmtab Tablets 402
Biaxin Granules 402

ISIB (United Kingdom)
ISOSORBIDE MONONITRATE
Imdur Tablets 3032

ISIMOXIN (Italy)
AMOXICILLIN
Amoxil Pediatric Drops for Oral Suspension. 1315
Amoxil Tablets 1315

ISLOPIR (Argentina)
GLIMEPIRIDE
Amaryl Tablets 2864

ISMEXIN (Finland)
ISOSORBIDE MONONITRATE
Imdur Tablets 3032

ISMIPUR (Italy)
MERCAPTOPURINE
Purinethol Tablets 1222

ISMO (Canada, Chile, Denmark, Germany, Hong Kong, India, Israel, Italy, New Zealand, Norway, Portugal, Singapore, South Africa, Spain, Sweden, Switzerland, Thailand, The Netherlands, United Kingdom)
ISOSORBIDE MONONITRATE
Imdur Tablets 3032

ISMOX (Finland)
ISOSORBIDE MONONITRATE
Imdur Tablets 3032

ISOACNE (Brazil)
ISOTRETINOIN
Accutane Capsules 2740

ISOBLOC (Argentina)
CARVEDILOL
Coreg Tablets. 1376

ISO-CARD (South Africa)
VERAPAMIL HYDROCHLORIDE
Covera-HS Tablets 3135
Verelan PM Capsules 3120

ISOCUTAN (Austria)
ISOTRETINOIN
Accutane Capsules 2740

ISODERM (Germany)
ISOTRETINOIN
Accutane Capsules 2740

ISODERMAL (Greece)
ISOTRETINOIN
Accutane Capsules 2740

ISODUR (Denmark, Sweden, United Kingdom)
ISOSORBIDE MONONITRATE
Imdur Tablets 3032

ISOFTAL (Austria)
NAPHAZOLINE HYDROCHLORIDE
Albalon Ophthalmic Solution . . . . ⊙216

ISOGLAUCON (Austria, Germany, Italy, Spain)
CLONIDINE HYDROCHLORIDE
Catapres Tablets 874

ISOHEXAL (Australia)
ISOTRETINOIN
Accutane Capsules 2740

ISOLAN (Argentina)
ISOSORBIDE MONONITRATE
Imdur Tablets 3032

ISOMEL (Irish Republic)
ISOSORBIDE MONONITRATE
Imdur Tablets 3032

ISOMIN (India)
ISOSORBIDE MONONITRATE
Imdur Tablets 3032

ISOMON (Greece)
ISOSORBIDE MONONITRATE
Imdur Tablets 3032

ISOMONAT (Austria)
ISOSORBIDE MONONITRATE
Imdur Tablets 3032

ISOMONIT (Australia, Denmark, Germany, Irish Republic)
ISOSORBIDE MONONITRATE
Imdur Tablets 3032

ISOMONOREAL (Germany)
ISOSORBIDE MONONITRATE
Imdur Tablets 3032

ISONITRIL (Spain)
ISOSORBIDE MONONITRATE
Imdur Tablets . . . 3032

ISONTYN (Argentina)
TERAZOSIN HYDROCHLORIDE
Hytrin Capsules . . . 469

ISOPAMIL (Thailand)
VERAPAMIL HYDROCHLORIDE
Covera-HS Tablets . . . 3135
Verelan PM Capsules . . . 3120

ISOPEN (Thailand)
ISOSORBIDE MONONITRATE
Imdur Tablets . . . 3032

ISOPTIN (Australia, Austria, Canada, Czech Republic, Denmark, Finland, Germany, Greece, Hong Kong, Hungary, Irish Republic, Italy, Malaysia, New Zealand, Norway, Portugal, Singapore, South Africa, Sweden, Switzerland, Thailand, The Netherlands)
VERAPAMIL HYDROCHLORIDE
Covera-HS Tablets . . . 3135
Verelan PM Capsules . . . 3120

ISOPTINE (Belgium, France)
VERAPAMIL HYDROCHLORIDE
Covera-HS Tablets . . . 3135
Verelan PM Capsules . . . 3120

ISOPTO CETAMIDE (Belgium, Canada)
SULFACETAMIDE SODIUM
Klaron Lotion 10% . . . 1050

ISOPTO CETAPRED (Belgium, Canada)
PREDNISOLONE ACETATE/SULFACETAMIDE SODIUM
Blephamide Ophthalmic Ointment . . . 563
Blephamide Ophthalmic Suspension . . . 564

ISOPTO DEX (Germany)
DEXAMETHASONE
Decadron Tablets . . . 1929

ISOPTO FLUCON (Germany, Spain)
FLUOROMETHOLONE
FML Ophthalmic Ointment . . . ⊙225

ISOPTO MAXIDEX (Argentina, Norway, Sweden)
DEXAMETHASONE
Decadron Tablets . . . 1929

ISOSOL (Austria)
ISOTRETINOIN
Accutane Capsules . . . 2740

ISOSPAN (Hungary)
ISOSORBIDE MONONITRATE
Imdur Tablets . . . 3032

ISOTANE (Thailand)
ISOTRETINOIN
Accutane Capsules . . . 2740

ISOTARD (United Kingdom)
ISOSORBIDE MONONITRATE
Imdur Tablets . . . 3032

ISOTRATE (Hong Kong, Singapore, United Kingdom)
ISOSORBIDE MONONITRATE
Imdur Tablets . . . 3032

ISOTRET (Germany)
ISOTRETINOIN
Accutane Capsules . . . 2740

ISOTREX (Argentina, Australia, Austria, Brazil, Canada, Czech Republic, Denmark, France, Germany, Hong Kong, Hungary, Irish Republic, Israel, Italy, Malaysia, Mexico, New Zealand, Portugal, Singapore, South Africa, Spain, Thailand, United Kingdom)
ISOTRETINOIN
Accutane Capsules . . . 2740

ISOTREX ERITROMICINA (Spain)
ISOTRETINOIN
Accutane Capsules . . . 2740

ISOTREX GEL (Chile)
ISOTRETINOIN
Accutane Capsules . . . 2740

ISOTREXIN (Austria, Brazil, Germany, Irish Republic, Italy, Portugal, Singapore, Thailand, United Kingdom)
ISOTRETINOIN
Accutane Capsules . . . 2740

ISOTROIN (Greece, India)
ISOTRETINOIN
Accutane Capsules . . . 2740

ISTOPRIL (Thailand)
ENALAPRIL MALEATE
Vasotec I.V. Injection . . . 2076

ITALNIK (Mexico)
CIPROFLOXACIN
Cipro Oral Suspension . . . 2991

ITOREX (Italy)
CEFUROXIME SODIUM
Zinacef Injection . . . 1604

ITRIN (Italy)
TERAZOSIN HYDROCHLORIDE
Hytrin Capsules . . . 469

ITROP (Austria, Czech Republic, Germany, Switzerland)
IPRATROPIUM BROMIDE
Atrovent Inhalation Solution . . . 868
Atrovent Nasal Spray 0.03% . . . 869
Atrovent Nasal Spray 0.06% . . . 870

IVIDOL (Greece)
AMILORIDE HYDROCHLORIDE/HYDROCHLOROTHIAZIDE
Moduretic Tablets . . . 2003

IVOFOL (Spain)
PROPOFOL
Diprivan Injectable Emulsion . . . 676

IWAMET (Thailand)
CIMETIDINE
Tagamet Tablets . . . 1547

IZACEF (South Africa)
CEFAZOLIN SODIUM
Ancef for Injection . . . 1318

IZADIMA (Mexico)
CEFTAZIDIME
Fortaz for Injection . . . 1422

JABASTATINA (Portugal)
SIMVASTATIN
Zocor Tablets . . . 2078

JANACIN (Hong Kong, Malaysia, Thailand)
NORFLOXACIN
Noroxin Tablets . . . 2009

JATROPUR (Germany)
TRIAMTERENE
Dyrenium Capsules . . . 3390

JATROSOM N (Germany)
TRANYLCYPROMINE SULFATE
Parnate Tablets . . . 1499

JEDIPIN (Germany, Thailand)
NIFEDIPINE
Adalat CC Tablets . . . 2978

JENAFENAC (Germany)
DICLOFENAC SODIUM
Voltaren Tablets . . . 2298
Voltaren-XR Tablets . . . 2301

JENAMAZOL (Czech Republic, Germany)
CLOTRIMAZOLE
Lotrimin Cream . . . 3053
Lotrimin Lotion 1% . . . 3053
Lotrimin Topical Solution 1% . . . 3053

JENAMETIDIN (Germany)
CIMETIDINE
Tagamet Tablets . . . 1547

JENAPAMIL (Germany)
VERAPAMIL HYDROCHLORIDE
Covera-HS Tablets . . . 3135
Verelan PM Capsules . . . 3120

JENATENOL (Germany)
ATENOLOL
Tenormin I.V. Injection . . . 698

JENATEREN COMP (Germany)
HYDROCHLOROTHIAZIDE/TRIAMTERENE
Dyazide Capsules . . . 1389
Maxzide Tablets . . . 2150
Maxzide-25 mg Tablets . . . 2150

JENOQUINE (United Arab Emirates)
LEVOFLOXACIN
Levaquin Injection . . . 2453
Levaquin Tablets . . . 2453

JODTHYROX (Czech Republic)
LEVOTHYROXINE SODIUM
Levothroid Tablets . . . 1189
Levoxyl Tablets . . . 1680
Synthroid Tablets . . . 515

JOHNSONS CLEAN & CLEAR PERSA GEL (Canada)
BENZOYL PEROXIDE
Brevoxyl-4 Creamy Wash . . . 3212
Brevoxyl-4 Gel . . . 3211
Brevoxyl-8 Creamy Wash . . . 3212
Brevoxyl-8 Gel . . . 3211
Triaz Cleanser . . . 1864
Triaz Gel . . . 1864

JOSIR (France)
TAMSULOSIN HYDROCHLORIDE
Flomax Capsules . . . 881

JOSSALIND (Germany)
SODIUM HYALURONATE
Hyalgan Solution . . . 2917

JOYZOL (India)
OLANZAPINE
Zyprexa Tablets . . . 1798

JUAN (India)
SILDENAFIL CITRATE
Viagra Tablets . . . 2552

JULAB (Hong Kong, Thailand)
SELEGILINE HYDROCHLORIDE
Eldepryl Capsules . . . 3209

JUMEX (Argentina, Austria, Czech Republic, Hong Kong, Hungary, Israel, Italy, Malaysia, Portugal, Singapore, Thailand)
SELEGILINE HYDROCHLORIDE
Eldepryl Capsules . . . 3209

JUMEXAL (Switzerland)
SELEGILINE HYDROCHLORIDE
Eldepryl Capsules . . . 3209

JUMEXIL (Brazil)
SELEGILINE HYDROCHLORIDE
Eldepryl Capsules . . . 3209

JUNGLE FORMULA STING RELIEF CREAM (United Kingdom)
HYDROCORTISONE
Hydrocortone Tablets . . . 1963

JUNO (Argentina)
LEVOTHYROXINE SODIUM
Levothroid Tablets . . . 1189
Levoxyl Tablets . . . 1680
Synthroid Tablets . . . 515

JUVENTAL (Germany)
ATENOLOL
Tenormin I.V. Injection . . . 698

K-10 (Canada)
POTASSIUM CHLORIDE
K-Dur Extended-Relase Tablets . . . 3047
K-Lor Powder Packets . . . 472
K-Tab Filmtab Tablets . . . 473

KAARMEPAKKAUS (Finland)
DEXAMETHASONE
Decadron Tablets . . . 1929

KADALEX (Italy)
POTASSIUM CHLORIDE
K-Dur Extended-Relase Tablets . . . 3047
K-Lor Powder Packets . . . 472
K-Tab Filmtab Tablets . . . 473

KADEFUNGIN (Germany)
CLOTRIMAZOLE
Lotrimin Cream . . . 3053
Lotrimin Lotion 1% . . . 3053
Lotrimin Topical Solution 1% . . . 3053

KADIAN (Canada)
MORPHINE SULFATE
Kadian Capsules . . . 572
MS Contin Tablets . . . 2703

KAILASA (Argentina)
CLARITHROMYCIN
Biaxin Filmtab Tablets . . . 402
Biaxin Granules . . . 402

KAINEVER (Portugal)
ESTAZOLAM
ProSom Tablets . . . 512

KAION RETARD (Chile)
POTASSIUM CHLORIDE
K-Dur Extended-Relase Tablets . . . 3047
K-Lor Powder Packets . . . 472
K-Tab Filmtab Tablets . . . 473

KAIZEM (India)
DILTIAZEM HYDROCHLORIDE
Cardizem LA Extended Release Tablets . . . 1699
Tiazac Capsules . . . 1204

KAJOS (Norway, Sweden)
POTASSIUM CITRATE
Urocit-K Tablets . . . 2109

KALDYUM (Czech Republic, Hungary)
POTASSIUM CHLORIDE
K-Dur Extended-Relase Tablets . . . 3047
K-Lor Powder Packets . . . 472
K-Tab Filmtab Tablets . . . 473

KALEORID (Denmark, France, Norway, Sweden)
POTASSIUM CHLORIDE
K-Dur Extended-Relase Tablets . . . 3047
K-Lor Powder Packets . . . 472
K-Tab Filmtab Tablets . . . 473

KALICET (Italy)
FEXOFENADINE HYDROCHLORIDE
Allegra Capsules . . . 2857

KALIGLUTOL (Switzerland)
POTASSIUM CHLORIDE
K-Dur Extended-Relase Tablets . . . 3047
K-Lor Powder Packets . . . 472
K-Tab Filmtab Tablets . . . 473

KALIJECT (Thailand)
POTASSIUM CHLORIDE
K-Dur Extended-Relase Tablets . . . 3047
K-Lor Powder Packets . . . 472
K-Tab Filmtab Tablets . . . 473

KALILENTE (Norway, Sweden)
POTASSIUM CHLORIDE
K-Dur Extended-Relase Tablets . . . 3047
K-Lor Powder Packets . . . 472
K-Tab Filmtab Tablets . . . 473

KALINORM (Denmark, Finland, Norway)
POTASSIUM CHLORIDE
K-Dur Extended-Relase Tablets . . . 3047
K-Lor Powder Packets . . . 472
K-Tab Filmtab Tablets . . . 473

KALINOR-RETARD P (Germany)
POTASSIUM CHLORIDE
K-Dur Extended-Relase Tablets . . . 3047
K-Lor Powder Packets . . . 472
K-Tab Filmtab Tablets . . . 473

KALIOLITE (Mexico)
POTASSIUM CHLORIDE
K-Dur Extended-Relase Tablets . . . 3047
K-Lor Powder Packets . . . 472
K-Tab Filmtab Tablets . . . 473

KALIPOR (Sweden)
POTASSIUM CHLORIDE
K-Dur Extended-Relase Tablets . . . 3047
K-Lor Powder Packets . . . 472
K-Tab Filmtab Tablets . . . 473

KALISOL (Finland)
POTASSIUM CHLORIDE
K-Dur Extended-Relase Tablets . . . 3047
K-Lor Powder Packets . . . 472
K-Tab Filmtab Tablets . . . 473

KALISTERIL (Finland)
POTASSIUM CHLORIDE
K-Dur Extended-Relase Tablets . . . 3047
K-Lor Powder Packets . . . 472
K-Tab Filmtab Tablets . . . 473

KALI-STEROP (Belgium)
POTASSIUM CHLORIDE
K-Dur Extended-Relase Tablets . . . 3047
K-Lor Powder Packets . . . 472
K-Tab Filmtab Tablets . . . 473

KALITABS (Sweden)
POTASSIUM CHLORIDE
K-Dur Extended-Relase Tablets . . . 3047
K-Lor Powder Packets . . . 472
K-Tab Filmtab Tablets . . . 473

KALITRANS RETARD (Germany)
POTASSIUM CHLORIDE
K-Dur Extended-Relase Tablets . . . 3047

(⊙ Described in PDR For Ophthalmic Medicines™)

K-Lor Powder Packets 472
K-Tab Filmtab Tablets 473

KALIUM (Germany, Hong Kong)
POTASSIUM CITRATE
Urocit-K Tablets. . . . 2109

KALIUM DURETTER (Finland, Sweden)
POTASSIUM CHLORIDE
K-Dur Extended-Relase Tablets 3047
K-Lor Powder Packets 472
K-Tab Filmtab Tablets 473

KALIUM DURETTES (Belgium, The Netherlands)
POTASSIUM CHLORIDE
K-Dur Extended-Relase Tablets 3047
K-Lor Powder Packets 472
K-Tab Filmtab Tablets 473

KALIUM DURULES (Canada, Hungary, Singapore)
POTASSIUM CHLORIDE
K-Dur Extended-Relase Tablets 3047
K-Lor Powder Packets 472
K-Tab Filmtab Tablets 473

KALIUM RETARD (Sweden)
POTASSIUM CHLORIDE
K-Dur Extended-Relase Tablets 3047
K-Lor Powder Packets 472
K-Tab Filmtab Tablets 473

KALIUM-DURILES (Germany)
POTASSIUM CHLORIDE
K-Dur Extended-Relase Tablets 3047
K-Lor Powder Packets 472
K-Tab Filmtab Tablets 473

KALIUM-R (Hungary)
POTASSIUM CHLORIDE
K-Dur Extended-Relase Tablets 3047
K-Lor Powder Packets 472
K-Tab Filmtab Tablets 473

KALIXOCIN (Australia)
CLARITHROMYCIN
Biaxin Filmtab Tablets 402
Biaxin Granules 402

KALNORMIN (Czech Republic)
POTASSIUM CHLORIDE
K-Dur Extended-Relase Tablets 3047
K-Lor Powder Packets 472
K-Tab Filmtab Tablets 473

KALPRESS (Spain)
VALSARTAN
Diovan Tablets 2191

KALPRESS PLUS (Spain)
VALSARTAN
Diovan Tablets 2191

KALTIN MF (India)
METRONIDAZOLE
MetroGel-Vaginal Gel 1822
Noritate Cream, 1% 1051

KALURIL (Australia, Israel)
AMILORIDE HYDROCHLORIDE
Midamor Tablets 2000

KAMICIN (Hong Kong)
CLOTRIMAZOLE
Lotrimin Cream. . . . 3053
Lotrimin Lotion 1%. . . . 3053
Lotrimin Topical Solution 1% 3053

KAMIDEX (Israel)
LOPERAMIDE HYDROCHLORIDE
Imodium Capsules 1834

KANDISTAT (Brazil)
NYSTATIN
Nystop Topical Powder USP. . . . 2490

KANEZIN (Thailand)
CLOTRIMAZOLE
Lotrimin Cream. . . . 3053
Lotrimin Lotion 1%. . . . 3053
Lotrimin Topical Solution 1% 3053

KANOLONE (Thailand)
TRIAMCINOLONE ACETONIDE
Azmacort Inhalation Aerosol. . . . 1701
Nasacort AQ Nasal Spray 2937

KAOCHLOR (Canada)
POTASSIUM CHLORIDE
K-Dur Extended-Relase Tablets 3047
K-Lor Powder Packets 472
K-Tab Filmtab Tablets 473

KAPABLOC (Austria)
MORPHINE SULFATE
Kadian Capsules 572
MS Contin Tablets 2703

KAPANOL (Australia, Austria, Belgium, Denmark, France, Germany, Israel, Mexico, New Zealand, Norway, Switzerland, The Netherlands)
MORPHINE SULFATE
Kadian Capsules 572
MS Contin Tablets 2703

KAPARLON-S (Greece)
ENALAPRIL MALEATE
Vasotec I.V. Injection 2076

KAPLON (United Kingdom)
CAPTOPRIL
Captopril Tablets. . . . 2114

KARA (Thailand)
KETOCONAZOLE
Nizoral 2% Shampoo 1838

KARBAC (Brazil)
CARBAMAZEPINE
Carbatrol Capsules 3174
Tegretol Chewable Tablets. . . . 2278
Tegretol Suspension. . . . 2278
Tegretol Tablets 2278
Tegretol-XR Tablets 2278

KARDIL (Norway)
DILTIAZEM HYDROCHLORIDE
Cardizem LA Extended Release Tablets. . . 1699
Tiazac Capsules 1204

KARIDINA (Spain)
CEFAZOLIN SODIUM
Ancef for Injection 1318

KARIN (Israel)
CLARITHROMYCIN
Biaxin Filmtab Tablets. . . . 402
Biaxin Granules. . . . 402

KARISON (Germany)
CLOBETASOL PROPIONATE
Temovate Cream. . . . 1549
Temovate E Emollient. . . . 1552
Temovate Gel. . . . 1550
Temovate Ointment 1549
Temovate Scalp Application 1551

KARLIT (Argentina)
LITHIUM CARBONATE
Eskalith CR Controlled-Release Tablets . . . 1406
Eskalith Capsules 1406

KARMELITUS (India)
GLIMEPIRIDE
Amaryl Tablets 2864

KARON (Czech Republic)
ALPROSTADIL
Edex Injection. . . . 3103

KARRER (Italy)
LEVOCARNITINE
Carnitor Injection. . . . 3185
Carnitor Tablets and Oral Solution 3187

KARVEA (Australia, Germany, Greece, Italy, Spain)
IRBESARTAN
Avapro Tablets 925

KARVEZIDE (Australia, Germany, Italy, Spain)
IRBESARTAN
Avapro Tablets 925

KASELE (Mexico)
POTASSIUM CHLORIDE
K-Dur Extended-Relase Tablets 3047
K-Lor Powder Packets 472
K-Tab Filmtab Tablets 473

KATA (Italy)
VERAPAMIL HYDROCHLORIDE
Covera-HS Tablets 3135
Verelan PM Capsules 3120

KATION (Italy)
POTASSIUM CITRATE
Urocit-K Tablets. . . . 2109

KATOPIL (Czech Republic)
CAPTOPRIL
Captopril Tablets. . . . 2114

KATOPRIL (Singapore)
CAPTOPRIL
Captopril Tablets. . . . 2114

KATSIN (Thailand)
KETOCONAZOLE
Nizoral 2% Shampoo 1838

KATTWILACT (Germany)
LACTULOSE
Kristalose for Oral Solution 2149

KAY CIEL (Australia, Canada)
POTASSIUM CHLORIDE
K-Dur Extended-Relase Tablets 3047
K-Lor Powder Packets 472
K-Tab Filmtab Tablets 473

KAY-CEE-L (Irish Republic, United Kingdom)
POTASSIUM CHLORIDE
K-Dur Extended-Relase Tablets 3047
K-Lor Powder Packets 472
K-Tab Filmtab Tablets 473

KAZINAL (Thailand)
KETOCONAZOLE
Nizoral 2% Shampoo 1838

K-CITRA (Canada)
POTASSIUM CITRATE
Urocit-K Tablets. . . . 2109

KCL-RETARD (Austria, Germany)
POTASSIUM CHLORIDE
K-Dur Extended-Relase Tablets 3047
K-Lor Powder Packets 472
K-Tab Filmtab Tablets 473

K-DUR (Canada, Mexico)
POTASSIUM CHLORIDE
K-Dur Extended-Relase Tablets 3047
K-Lor Powder Packets 472
K-Tab Filmtab Tablets 473

KEAL (France)
SUCRALFATE
Carafate Suspension 727
Carafate Tablets 728

KEBIRTECAN (Argentina)
IRINOTECAN HYDROCHLORIDE
Camptosar Injection. . . . 2602

KECIFLOX (Germany)
CIPROFLOXACIN
Cipro Oral Suspension 2991

KEDUO (Argentina)
KETOCONAZOLE
Nizoral 2% Shampoo 1838

KEEFLOXIN (Portugal)
CIPROFLOXACIN HYDROCHLORIDE
Ciloxan Ophthalmic Ointment 554
Ciloxan Ophthalmic Solution . . . . ⊙205
Cipro Tablets 2991

KEFADIM (Belgium, Brazil, Czech Republic, Thailand, United Kingdom)
CEFTAZIDIME
Fortaz for Injection 1422

KEFAMIN (Spain)
CEFTAZIDIME
Fortaz for Injection 1422

KEFAZIM (Austria)
CEFTAZIDIME
Fortaz for Injection 1422

KEFAZIN (Israel)
CEFAZOLIN SODIUM
Ancef for Injection 1318

KEFAZOL (Brazil)
CEFAZOLIN SODIUM
Ancef for Injection 1318

KEFNIR (India)
CEFDINIR
Omnicef Capsules 506
Omnicef for Oral Suspension 506

KEFOL (Spain)
CEFAZOLIN SODIUM
Ancef for Injection 1318

KEFOX (Italy)
CEFUROXIME SODIUM
Zinacef Injection 1604

KEFPOD (India)
CEFPODOXIME PROXETIL
Vantin Tablets and Oral Suspension 2650

KEFTRAGARD (India)
CEFTRIAXONE SODIUM
Rocephin Injectable Vials, ADD-Vantage, Galaxy, Bulk 2801

KEFTRIAXON (Israel)
CEFTRIAXONE SODIUM
Rocephin Injectable Vials, ADD-Vantage, Galaxy, Bulk 2801

KEFURIM (Israel)
CEFUROXIME SODIUM
Zinacef Injection 1604

KEFURION (Finland)
CEFUROXIME SODIUM
Zinacef Injection 1604

KEFUROX (Belgium, Canada)
CEFUROXIME SODIUM
Zinacef Injection 1604

KEFZIM (Chile, South Africa)
CEFTAZIDIME
Fortaz for Injection 1422

KEFZOL (Australia, Austria, Belgium, Canada, Chile, Czech Republic, France, Irish Republic, Israel, New Zealand, South Africa, Switzerland, Thailand, The Netherlands, United Kingdom)
CEFAZOLIN SODIUM
Ancef for Injection 1318

KELA (Thailand)
TRIAMCINOLONE ACETONIDE
Azmacort Inhalation Aerosol. . . . 1701
Nasacort AQ Nasal Spray 2937

KELATIN (Belgium, The Netherlands)
PENICILLAMINE
Cuprimine Capsules 1925

KELATINE (Portugal)
PENICILLAMINE
Cuprimine Capsules 1925

KELBIUM (Spain)
CEFPODOXIME PROXETIL
Vantin Tablets and Oral Suspension 2650

KELEFUSIN (Mexico)
POTASSIUM CHLORIDE
K-Dur Extended-Relase Tablets 3047
K-Lor Powder Packets 472
K-Tab Filmtab Tablets 473

KELOC (United Kingdom)
FELODIPINE
Plendil Extended-Release Tablets 651

KEMZID (Hong Kong, Singapore, Thailand)
TRIAMCINOLONE ACETONIDE
Azmacort Inhalation Aerosol. . . . 1701
Nasacort AQ Nasal Spray 2937

KENACORT (Belgium, France, Italy, Thailand)
TRIAMCINOLONE ACETONIDE
Azmacort Inhalation Aerosol. . . . 1701
Nasacort AQ Nasal Spray 2937

KENACORT-A (Argentina, Australia, Belgium, Chile, Greece, Hong Kong, Irish Republic, Malaysia, New Zealand, Singapore, Switzerland, The Netherlands)
TRIAMCINOLONE ACETONIDE
Azmacort Inhalation Aerosol. . . . 1701
Nasacort AQ Nasal Spray 2937

KENACORT-T (Finland, Norway, Sweden)
TRIAMCINOLONE ACETONIDE
Azmacort Inhalation Aerosol. . . . 1701
Nasacort AQ Nasal Spray 2937

KENALIN (Mexico)
SULINDAC
Clinoril Tablets 1899

KENALOG (Canada, Czech Republic, Denmark, Germany, Hungary, Irish Republic, Israel, United Kingdom)
TRIAMCINOLONE ACETONIDE
Azmacort Inhalation Aerosol. . . . 1701
Nasacort AQ Nasal Spray 2937

KENALOG IN ORABASE (Australia, Canada, Hong Kong, Israel, Malaysia, New Zealand, Singapore, South Africa, Spain, Thailand)
TRIAMCINOLONE ACETONIDE
Azmacort Inhalation Aerosol. . . . 1701
Nasacort AQ Nasal Spray 2937

(⊙ Described in PDR For Ophthalmic Medicines™)

KENALONE (Australia)
TRIAMCINOLONE ACETONIDE
Azmacort Inhalation Aerosol 1701
Nasacort AQ Nasal Spray 2937

KENALYN (Thailand)
KETOCONAZOLE
Nizoral 2% Shampoo 1838

KENAPRIL (Mexico)
CAPTOPRIL
Captopril Tablets 2114

KENAPROX (Mexico)
NAPROXEN
EC-Naprosyn Delayed-Release Tablets 2769
Naprosyn Suspension 2769
Naprosyn Tablets 2769

KENAZOL (Thailand)
KETOCONAZOLE
Nizoral 2% Shampoo 1838

KENAZOLE (Thailand)
KETOCONAZOLE
Nizoral 2% Shampoo 1838

KENERGON (Switzerland)
LIDOCAINE
Lidoderm Patch 1107

KENESIL (Spain)
NIMODIPINE
Nimotop Capsules 774

KENO (Thailand)
TRIAMCINOLONE ACETONIDE
Azmacort Inhalation Aerosol 1701
Nasacort AQ Nasal Spray 2937

KENOIDAL (Belgium)
TRIAMCINOLONE ACETONIDE
Azmacort Inhalation Aerosol 1701
Nasacort AQ Nasal Spray 2937

KENOKET (Mexico)
CLONAZEPAM
Klonopin Tablets 2782

KENOLAN (Mexico)
CAPTOPRIL
Captopril Tablets 2114

KENOPRIL (Mexico)
ENALAPRIL MALEATE
Vasotec I.V. Injection 2076

KENORAL (Thailand)
KETOCONAZOLE
Nizoral 2% Shampoo 1838

KENSTATIN (Mexico)
PRAVASTATIN SODIUM
Pravachol Tablets 943

KENZEN (France)
CANDESARTAN CILEXETIL
Atacand Tablets 634

KENZOFLEX (Mexico)
CIPROFLOXACIN HYDROCHLORIDE
Ciloxan Ophthalmic Ointment 554
Ciloxan Ophthalmic Solution . . . . ⊙205
Cipro Tablets 2991

KENZOLOL (Mexico)
NIMODIPINE
Nimotop Capsules 774

KEPROBIOZOL (Mexico)
KETOCONAZOLE
Nizoral 2% Shampoo 1838

KERLOCAL (France)
TRETINOIN
Avita Cream 2136
Avita Gel 2138
Renova 0.05% Cream 2387
Retin-A Micro 0.1%/0.04% 2388
Vesanoid Capsules 2823

KERLON (Denmark, Finland, Italy, Sweden, Switzerland, The Netherlands)
BETAXOLOL HYDROCHLORIDE
Betoptic S Ophthalmic Suspension 554

KERLONE (Austria, Belgium, France, Germany, Greece, Hong Kong, Israel, Malaysia, Singapore, Spain, Thailand, United Kingdom)
BETAXOLOL HYDROCHLORIDE
Betoptic S Ophthalmic Suspension 554

KERLONG (Japan)
BETAXOLOL HYDROCHLORIDE
Betoptic S Ophthalmic Suspension 554

KERNIT (Italy)
LEVOCARNITINE
Carnitor Injection 3185
Carnitor Tablets and Oral Solution 3187

KESINT (Italy)
CEFUROXIME SODIUM
Zinacef Injection 1604

KESS (Argentina)
LAMIVUDINE
Epivir Oral Solution 1394
Epivir Tablets 1394
Epivir-HBV Oral Solution 1398
Epivir-HBV Tablets 1398

KESS COMPLEX (Argentina)
LAMIVUDINE
Epivir Oral Solution 1394
Epivir Tablets 1394
Epivir-HBV Oral Solution 1398
Epivir-HBV Tablets 1398

KESTOMICOL (Mexico)
KETOCONAZOLE
Nizoral 2% Shampoo 1838

KETANINE (Singapore)
CAPTOPRIL
Captopril Tablets 2114

KETAZOL (South Africa, Thailand)
KETOCONAZOLE
Nizoral 2% Shampoo 1838

KETAZON (Thailand)
KETOCONAZOLE
Nizoral 2% Shampoo 1838

KETIDIN (Argentina)
RALOXIFENE HYDROCHLORIDE
Evista Tablets 1735

KETO (India)
KETOCONAZOLE
Nizoral 2% Shampoo 1838

KETOCINE (Thailand)
KETOCONAZOLE
Nizoral 2% Shampoo 1838

KETOCON (Brazil)
KETOCONAZOLE
Nizoral 2% Shampoo 1838

KETODERM (Canada, France)
KETOCONAZOLE
Nizoral 2% Shampoo 1838

KETOFAR (Mexico)
KETOCONAZOLE
Nizoral 2% Shampoo 1838

KETOGEL (Argentina)
KETOCONAZOLE
Nizoral 2% Shampoo 1838

KETOISDIN (Spain)
KETOCONAZOLE
Nizoral 2% Shampoo 1838

KETOLAN (Thailand)
KETOCONAZOLE
Nizoral 2% Shampoo 1838

KETOMED (Thailand)
KETOCONAZOLE
Nizoral 2% Shampoo 1838

KETOMICOL (Brazil)
KETOCONAZOLE
Nizoral 2% Shampoo 1838

KETOMIZOL (Mexico)
KETOCONAZOLE
Nizoral 2% Shampoo 1838

KETONAN (Brazil)
KETOCONAZOLE
Nizoral 2% Shampoo 1838

KETONAZOL (Argentina, Brazil)
KETOCONAZOLE
Nizoral 2% Shampoo 1838

KETONAZOLE (Thailand)
KETOCONAZOLE
Nizoral 2% Shampoo 1838

KETONE (Mexico)
KETOCONAZOLE
Nizoral 2% Shampoo 1838

KETONIL (Chile)
KETOCONAZOLE
Nizoral 2% Shampoo 1838

KETOPLUS (Malaysia)
KETOCONAZOLE
Nizoral 2% Shampoo 1838

KETORAL (Thailand)
KETOCONAZOLE
Nizoral 2% Shampoo 1838

KETOSIL (Thailand)
KETOCONAZOLE
Nizoral 2% Shampoo 1838

KETOSON (Sweden)
KETOCONAZOLE
Nizoral 2% Shampoo 1838

KETOZAL (Thailand)
KETOCONAZOLE
Nizoral 2% Shampoo 1838

KETOZOL (Argentina, Hong Kong, Switzerland)
KETOCONAZOLE
Nizoral 2% Shampoo 1838

KETOZOLE (Hong Kong, Malaysia, Singapore)
KETOCONAZOLE
Nizoral 2% Shampoo 1838

KETREL (France, Portugal)
TRETINOIN
Avita Cream 2136
Avita Gel 2138
Renova 0.05% Cream 2387
Retin-A Micro 0.1%/0.04% 2388
Vesanoid Capsules 2823

KEVAL (Mexico)
LANSOPRAZOLE
Prevacid Delayed-Release Capsules 3268

KEYERPRIL (Mexico)
CAPTOPRIL
Captopril Tablets 2114

KEYLYTE (India)
POTASSIUM CHLORIDE
K-Dur Extended-Relase Tablets 3047
K-Lor Powder Packets 472
K-Tab Filmtab Tablets 473

KEZ (South Africa)
KETOCONAZOLE
Nizoral 2% Shampoo 1838

KEZEPIN (Mexico)
CARBAMAZEPINE
Carbatrol Capsules 3174
Tegretol Chewable Tablets 2278
Tegretol Suspension 2278
Tegretol Tablets 2278
Tegretol-XR Tablets 2278

KEZON (Thailand)
KETOCONAZOLE
Nizoral 2% Shampoo 1838

KEZORAL (Denmark, Malaysia)
KETOCONAZOLE
Nizoral 2% Shampoo 1838

K-FENAC (India)
DICLOFENAC POTASSIUM
Cataflam Tablets 2173

KIATRIUM (Brazil)
DIAZEPAM
Diastat Rectal Delivery System 3344
Valium Tablets 2822

KIDROLASE (Argentina, Canada, Czech Republic, France, Israel)
ASPARAGINASE
Elspar for Injection 1943

KILLIT (Brazil)
FLUOROURACIL
Efudex Topical Cream 3348
Efudex Topical Solutions 3348

KILNITS (Chile)
PERMETHRIN
Acticin Cream 2125

KIMAFAN (Hong Kong)
CAPTOPRIL
Captopril Tablets 2114

KINABIDE (Argentina)
SELEGILINE HYDROCHLORIDE
Eldepryl Capsules 3209

KINASTEN (Brazil)
CLOTRIMAZOLE
Lotrimin Cream 3053
Lotrimin Lotion 1% 3053
Lotrimin Topical Solution 1% 3053

KINDAREN (Brazil)
DICLOFENAC SODIUM
Voltaren Tablets 2298
Voltaren-XR Tablets 2301

KINDELMIN (Brazil)
MEBENDAZOLE
Vermox Chewable Tablets 1853

KINDERVAL (Argentina)
PERMETHRIN
Acticin Cream 2125

KINFIL D (Argentina)
ENALAPRIL MALEATE
Vasotec I.V. Injection 2076

KINLINE (Thailand)
SELEGILINE HYDROCHLORIDE
Eldepryl Capsules 3209

KINZAL (Switzerland)
TELMISARTAN
Micardis Tablets 884

KINZALKOMB (Belgium, Denmark, Finland, Germany, Sweden)
TELMISARTAN
Micardis Tablets 884

KINZALMONO (Belgium, Denmark, Finland, Germany, Sweden)
TELMISARTAN
Micardis Tablets 884

KINZALPLUS (Switzerland)
TELMISARTAN
Micardis Tablets 884

KIPRES (Japan)
MONTELUKAST SODIUM
Singulair Chewable Tablets 2047
Singulair Tablets 2047

KIR RICHTER (Italy)
APROTININ
Trasylol Injection 779

KITACNE (Argentina)
ERYTHROMYCIN
Ery-Tab Tablets 447
Erythromycin Base Filmtab Tablets 454
Erythromycin Delayed-Release Capsules, USP 456
PCE Dispertab Tablets 510

KITACNE AR (Argentina)
ERYTHROMYCIN
Ery-Tab Tablets 447
Erythromycin Base Filmtab Tablets 454
Erythromycin Delayed-Release Capsules, USP 456
PCE Dispertab Tablets 510

KITACNE PB (Argentina)
ERYTHROMYCIN
Ery-Tab Tablets 447
Erythromycin Base Filmtab Tablets 454
Erythromycin Delayed-Release Capsules, USP 456
PCE Dispertab Tablets 510

KITON (Italy)
ISOSORBIDE MONONITRATE
Imdur Tablets 3032

KLACID (Australia, Czech Republic, Denmark, Finland, Germany, Hungary, Irish Republic, Israel, Italy, Malaysia, New Zealand, Norway, Portugal, Russia, Singapore, South Africa, Spain, Sweden, Thailand, The Netherlands)
CLARITHROMYCIN
Biaxin Filmtab Tablets 402
Biaxin Granules 402

KLACIPED (Switzerland)
CLARITHROMYCIN
Biaxin Filmtab Tablets 402
Biaxin Granules 402

KLAMACIN (Thailand)
CLOTRIMAZOLE
Lotrimin Cream 3053
Lotrimin Lotion 1% 3053
Lotrimin Topical Solution 1% 3053

KLAMIRAN (Hungary)
CLARITHROMYCIN
Biaxin Filmtab Tablets 402
Biaxin Granules 402

KLARI (Hungary)
CLARITHROMYCIN
Biaxin Filmtab Tablets . . . 402
Biaxin Granules . . . 402

KLARICID (Argentina, Brazil, Chile, Greece, The Netherlands, United Kingdom)
CLARITHROMYCIN
Biaxin Filmtab Tablets . . . 402
Biaxin Granules . . . 402

KLARIDEX (Israel)
CLARITHROMYCIN
Biaxin Filmtab Tablets . . . 402
Biaxin Granules . . . 402

KLARON (Israel)
SULFACETAMIDE SODIUM
Klaron Lotion 10% . . . 1050

KLERIMED (Hong Kong, Russia, Singapore)
CLARITHROMYCIN
Biaxin Filmtab Tablets . . . 402
Biaxin Granules . . . 402

KLEXANE (Denmark, Finland, Norway, Sweden)
ENOXAPARIN SODIUM
Lovenox Injection . . . 2931

KLIANE (Czech Republic)
ESTRADIOL
Climara Transdermal System . . . 795
Vivelle Transdermal System . . . 2288
Vivelle-Dot Transdermal System . . . 2293

KLIMAPUR (Austria)
ESTRADIOL
Climara Transdermal System . . . 795
Vivelle Transdermal System . . . 2288
Vivelle-Dot Transdermal System . . . 2293

KLIMAREDUCT (Austria)
ESTRADIOL
Climara Transdermal System . . . 795
Vivelle Transdermal System . . . 2288
Vivelle-Dot Transdermal System . . . 2293

KLIMICIN (Czech Republic, Hungary)
CLINDAMYCIN HYDROCHLORIDE
Cleocin Vaginal Ovules . . . 2613

KLIMOFOL (Germany)
PROPOFOL
Diprivan Injectable Emulsion . . . 676

KLINNA (Thailand)
CLINDAMYCIN PHOSPHATE
Clindets Pledgets . . . 3212

KLINOXID (Germany)
BENZOYL PEROXIDE
Brevoxyl-4 Creamy Wash . . . 3212
Brevoxyl-4 Gel . . . 3211
Brevoxyl-8 Creamy Wash . . . 3212
Brevoxyl-8 Gel . . . 3211
Triaz Cleanser . . . 1864
Triaz Gel . . . 1864

KLIOFEM (United Kingdom)
ESTRADIOL
Climara Transdermal System . . . 795
Vivelle Transdermal System . . . 2288
Vivelle-Dot Transdermal System . . . 2293

KLIOGEST (Argentina, Australia, Belgium, Brazil, Czech Republic, Hungary, Malaysia, New Zealand)
ESTRADIOL
Climara Transdermal System . . . 795
Vivelle Transdermal System . . . 2288
Vivelle-Dot Transdermal System . . . 2293

KLION (Czech Republic, Hungary, Russia, Thailand)
METRONIDAZOLE
MetroGel-Vaginal Gel . . . 1822
Noritate Cream, 1% . . . 1051

KLION-D (Czech Republic, Hungary)
METRONIDAZOLE
MetroGel-Vaginal Gel . . . 1822
Noritate Cream, 1% . . . 1051

KLIOVANCE (Australia, New Zealand)
ESTRADIOL
Climara Transdermal System . . . 795
Vivelle Transdermal System . . . 2288
Vivelle-Dot Transdermal System . . . 2293

KLODIN (Italy)
TICLOPIDINE HYDROCHLORIDE
Ticlid Tablets . . . 2813

KLODIPIN (Portugal)
TICLOPIDINE HYDROCHLORIDE
Ticlid Tablets . . . 2813

KLOMAZOLE (Argentina)
CLOTRIMAZOLE
Lotrimin Cream . . . 3053
Lotrimin Lotion 1% . . . 3053
Lotrimin Topical Solution 1% . . . 3053

KLONACID (Argentina)
CLARITHROMYCIN
Biaxin Filmtab Tablets . . . 402
Biaxin Granules . . . 402

KLONALFLOX (Argentina)
OFLOXACIN
Floxin Otic Solution . . . 1043

KLONALMOX (Argentina)
AMOXICILLIN
Amoxil Pediatric Drops for Oral Suspension . . . 1315
Amoxil Tablets . . . 1315

KLONAMICIN (Argentina)
TOBRAMYCIN
TOBI Solution for Inhalation . . . 1015

KLONAMICIN COMPUESTO (Argentina)
TOBRAMYCIN
TOBI Solution for Inhalation . . . 1015

KLONAPROST (Argentina)
LATANOPROST
Xalatan Ophthalmic Solution . . . ⊙280

KLONASTIN (Argentina)
SIMVASTATIN
Zocor Tablets . . . 2078

K-LONG (Canada)
POTASSIUM CHLORIDE
K-Dur Extended-Relase Tablets . . . 3047
K-Lor Powder Packets . . . 472
K-Tab Filmtab Tablets . . . 473

KLONT (Thailand)
METRONIDAZOLE
MetroGel-Vaginal Gel . . . 1822
Noritate Cream, 1% . . . 1051

K-LOR (Canada)
POTASSIUM CHLORIDE
K-Dur Extended-Relase Tablets . . . 3047
K-Lor Powder Packets . . . 472
K-Tab Filmtab Tablets . . . 473

KLOREN (Brazil)
POTASSIUM CHLORIDE
K-Dur Extended-Relase Tablets . . . 3047
K-Lor Powder Packets . . . 472
K-Tab Filmtab Tablets . . . 473

KLORPO (Singapore)
CHLORDIAZEPOXIDE HYDROCHLORIDE
Librium Capsules . . . 3349

KLOSARTAN D (Argentina)
LOSARTAN POTASSIUM
Cozaar Tablets . . . 1913

KLOTRICID (Finland)
CLOTRIMAZOLE
Lotrimin Cream . . . 3053
Lotrimin Lotion 1% . . . 3053
Lotrimin Topical Solution 1% . . . 3053

KLYNDAKEN (Mexico)
CLINDAMYCIN PHOSPHATE
Clindets Pledgets . . . 3212

K-LYTE (Canada)
POTASSIUM CITRATE
Urocit-K Tablets . . . 2109

K-LYTE/CL (Canada)
POTASSIUM CHLORIDE
K-Dur Extended-Relase Tablets . . . 3047
K-Lor Powder Packets . . . 472
K-Tab Filmtab Tablets . . . 473

K-MED 900 (Canada)
POTASSIUM CHLORIDE
K-Dur Extended-Relase Tablets . . . 3047
K-Lor Powder Packets . . . 472
K-Tab Filmtab Tablets . . . 473

K-MIC (Sweden)
POTASSIUM CHLORIDE
K-Dur Extended-Relase Tablets . . . 3047
K-Lor Powder Packets . . . 472
K-Tab Filmtab Tablets . . . 473

KODAKON (Mexico)
DEXAMETHASONE
Decadron Tablets . . . 1929

KOFRON (Spain)
CLARITHROMYCIN
Biaxin Filmtab Tablets . . . 402
Biaxin Granules . . . 402

KOLKIN (Argentina)
FUROSEMIDE
Furosemide Tablets . . . 2117

KOLPOVENT (Chile)
SALMETEROL XINAFOATE
Serevent Diskus . . . 1540

KONADERM (Mexico)
KETOCONAZOLE
Nizoral 2% Shampoo . . . 1838

KONATURIL (Mexico)
KETOCONAZOLE
Nizoral 2% Shampoo . . . 1838

KONAZIL (Brazil)
KETOCONAZOLE
Nizoral 2% Shampoo . . . 1838

KONAZOL (Thailand)
KETOCONAZOLE
Nizoral 2% Shampoo . . . 1838

KONIFUNGIL (Chile)
CLOTRIMAZOLE
Lotrimin Cream . . . 3053
Lotrimin Lotion 1% . . . 3053
Lotrimin Topical Solution 1% . . . 3053

KONOVID (Thailand)
OFLOXACIN
Floxin Otic Solution . . . 1043

KONTIC (Greece)
ENALAPRIL MALEATE
Vasotec I.V. Injection . . . 2076

KORANDIL (Singapore, Thailand)
ENALAPRIL MALEATE
Vasotec I.V. Injection . . . 2076

KORNAM (Czech Republic, Hungary, Russia)
TERAZOSIN HYDROCHLORIDE
Hytrin Capsules . . . 469

KORTIKOID-RATIOPHARM (Germany)
TRIAMCINOLONE ACETONIDE
Azmacort Inhalation Aerosol . . . 1701
Nasacort AQ Nasal Spray . . . 2937

KOSTEO (Australia)
CALCITRIOL
Calcijex Injection . . . 411

KRATIUM (Hong Kong)
DIAZEPAM
Diastat Rectal Delivery System . . . 3344
Valium Tablets . . . 2822

KREBSILASI (Italy)
PANCRELIPASE
Ultrase Capsules . . . 735
Ultrase MT Capsules . . . 736

KREDEX (Australia, Belgium, France, Italy, Norway, Portugal, Spain, Sweden)
CARVEDILOL
Coreg Tablets . . . 1376

KRENOSIN (France, Italy, Mexico)
ADENOSINE
Adenocard Injection . . . 612
Adenoscan . . . 613

KRENOSINE (Switzerland)
ADENOSINE
Adenocard Injection . . . 612
Adenoscan . . . 613

KRIADEX (Mexico)
CLONAZEPAM
Klonopin Tablets . . . 2782

KROL (Argentina)
KETOCONAZOLE
Nizoral 2% Shampoo . . . 1838

K-SAN (Australia)
POTASSIUM CHLORIDE
K-Dur Extended-Relase Tablets . . . 3047
K-Lor Powder Packets . . . 472
K-Tab Filmtab Tablets . . . 473

KSR (Australia, Hong Kong)
POTASSIUM CHLORIDE
K-Dur Extended-Relase Tablets . . . 3047
K-Lor Powder Packets . . . 472
K-Tab Filmtab Tablets . . . 473

K-SR (New Zealand)
POTASSIUM CHLORIDE
K-Dur Extended-Relase Tablets . . . 3047
K-Lor Powder Packets . . . 472
K-Tab Filmtab Tablets . . . 473

KURACID (Denmark)
RANITIDINE HYDROCHLORIDE
Zantac 25 EFFERdose Tablets . . . 1597
Zantac 150 EFFERdose Tablets . . . 1597
Zantac 150 Tablets . . . 1597
Zantac 300 Tablets . . . 1597
Zantac Injection . . . 1593
Zantac Injection Premixed . . . 1593
Zantac Syrup . . . 1597

KURGAN (Portugal, Spain)
CEFAZOLIN SODIUM
Ancef for Injection . . . 1318

KWELL (Argentina, Brazil)
PERMETHRIN
Acticin Cream . . . 2125

KWELLADA-P (Canada)
PERMETHRIN
Acticin Cream . . . 2125

KYMAZOL (Greece)
SIMVASTATIN
Zocor Tablets . . . 2078

KYYPAKKAUS (Finland)
HYDROCORTISONE
Hydrocortone Tablets . . . 1963

LA MORPH (New Zealand)
MORPHINE SULFATE
Kadian Capsules . . . 572
MS Contin Tablets . . . 2703

LABEL (Brazil)
RANITIDINE HYDROCHLORIDE
Zantac 25 EFFERdose Tablets . . . 1597
Zantac 150 EFFERdose Tablets . . . 1597
Zantac 150 Tablets . . . 1597
Zantac 300 Tablets . . . 1597
Zantac Injection . . . 1593
Zantac Injection Premixed . . . 1593
Zantac Syrup . . . 1597

LABENDA (Thailand)
ALBENDAZOLE
Albenza Tablets . . . 1310

LABENTROL (Greece)
CIPROFLOXACIN HYDROCHLORIDE
Ciloxan Ophthalmic Ointment . . . 554
Ciloxan Ophthalmic Solution . . . ⊙205
Cipro Tablets . . . 2991

LABILENO (Spain)
LAMOTRIGINE
Lamictal Chewable Dispersible Tablets . . . 1449
Lamictal Tablets . . . 1449

LABISTATIN (Argentina)
SIMVASTATIN
Zocor Tablets . . . 2078

LABITRIX (Mexico)
METRONIDAZOLE
MetroGel-Vaginal Gel . . . 1822
Noritate Cream, 1% . . . 1051

LABOCNE (Chile)
ERYTHROMYCIN
Ery-Tab Tablets . . . 447
Erythromycin Base Filmtab Tablets . . . 454
Erythromycin Delayed-Release Capsules, USP . . . 456
PCE Dispertab Tablets . . . 510

LABOPAL (Spain)
BENAZEPRIL HYDROCHLORIDE
Lotensin Tablets . . . 2232

LABOTENSIL (Chile)
ATENOLOL
Tenormin I.V. Injection . . . 698

LABOTEROL (Chile)
CLOTRIMAZOLE
Lotrimin Cream . . . 3053
Lotrimin Lotion 1% . . . 3053
Lotrimin Topical Solution 1% . . . 3053

LAC STOP (Argentina)
CABERGOLINE
Dostinex Tablets . . . 2631

LAC-DOL (Australia)
LACTULOSE
Kristalose for Oral Solution . . . 2149

(⊙ Described in PDR For Ophthalmic Medicines™)

LACEROL (Spain)
DILTIAZEM HYDROCHLORIDE
Cardizem LA Extended Release Tablets . . . 1699
Tiazac Capsules . . . 1204

LACIN (Thailand)
CLINDAMYCIN HYDROCHLORIDE
Cleocin Vaginal Ovules . . . 2613

LACRIPHARMA (Argentina)
SODIUM HYALURONATE
Hyalgan Solution . . . 2917

LACROMYCIN (Israel)
GENTAMICIN SULFATE
Garamycin Injectable . . . 3028
Genoptic Sterile Ophthalmic Solution . . . ⊙227

LACSON (South Africa)
LACTULOSE
Kristalose for Oral Solution . . . 2149

LACTAMAX (Argentina)
CABERGOLINE
Dostinex Tablets . . . 2631

LACTICARE-HC (Chile, Hong Kong, Mexico)
HYDROCORTISONE
Hydrocortone Tablets . . . 1963

LACTID HC (Argentina)
HYDROCORTISONE
Hydrocortone Tablets . . . 1963

LACTISONA (Portugal, Spain)
HYDROCORTISONE
Hydrocortone Tablets . . . 1963

LACTOCUR (Australia, Germany)
LACTULOSE
Kristalose for Oral Solution . . . 2149

LACTOFALK (Germany)
LACTULOSE
Kristalose for Oral Solution . . . 2149

LACTOGER (Italy)
LACTULOSE
Kristalose for Oral Solution . . . 2149

LACTUFLOR (Germany)
LACTULOSE
Kristalose for Oral Solution . . . 2149

LACTUGAL (United Kingdom)
LACTULOSE
Kristalose for Oral Solution . . . 2149

LACTUL (Malaysia)
LACTULOSE
Kristalose for Oral Solution . . . 2149

LACTULAX (Canada, Israel, Mexico)
LACTULOSE
Kristalose for Oral Solution . . . 2149

LACTULON (Argentina)
LACTULOSE
Kristalose for Oral Solution . . . 2149

LACTULONA (Brazil)
LACTULOSE
Kristalose for Oral Solution . . . 2149

LACTUMED (Malaysia)
LACTULOSE
Kristalose for Oral Solution . . . 2149

LACTUS (Singapore)
LACTULOSE
Kristalose for Oral Solution . . . 2149

LACTUVERLAN (Germany)
LACTULOSE
Kristalose for Oral Solution . . . 2149

LACTYL (Italy)
LACTULOSE
Kristalose for Oral Solution . . . 2149

LADIWIN (India)
LAMIVUDINE
Epivir Oral Solution . . . 1394
Epivir Tablets . . . 1394
Epivir-HBV Oral Solution . . . 1398
Epivir-HBV Tablets . . . 1398

LAEVILAC S (Germany)
LACTULOSE
Kristalose for Oral Solution . . . 2149

LAEVOLAC (Austria, Czech Republic, Hong Kong, Hungary, Israel, Italy, New Zealand, Portugal, South Africa, Switzerland, Thailand)
LACTULOSE
Kristalose for Oral Solution . . . 2149

LAFEDAM (Argentina)
ALENDRONATE SODIUM
Fosamax Tablets . . . 1949

LAFELAX (Argentina)
LACTULOSE
Kristalose for Oral Solution . . . 2149

LAFIGIN (Chile)
LAMOTRIGINE
Lamictal Chewable Dispersible Tablets . . . 1449
Lamictal Tablets . . . 1449

LA-FU (Czech Republic)
FLUOROURACIL
Efudex Topical Cream . . . 3348
Efudex Topical Solutions . . . 3348

LAFUREX (Italy)
CEFUROXIME SODIUM
Zinacef Injection . . . 1604

LAGARMICIN (Spain)
ERYTHROMYCIN STEARATE
Erythrocin Stearate Filmtab Tablets . . . 452

LAGOTRAN (Argentina)
LAMOTRIGINE
Lamictal Chewable Dispersible Tablets . . . 1449
Lamictal Tablets . . . 1449

LAGRICEL (Mexico)
SODIUM HYALURONATE
Hyalgan Solution . . . 2917

LAGRICEL OFTENO (Chile)
SODIUM HYALURONATE
Hyalgan Solution . . . 2917

LAGUR (Brazil)
CLARITHROMYCIN
Biaxin Filmtab Tablets . . . 402
Biaxin Granules . . . 402

LAGYLAN (Mexico)
METRONIDAZOLE
MetroGel-Vaginal Gel . . . 1822
Noritate Cream, 1% . . . 1051

LAKE (Spain)
RANITIDINE HYDROCHLORIDE
Zantac 25 EFFERdose Tablets . . . 1597
Zantac 150 EFFERdose Tablets . . . 1597
Zantac 150 Tablets . . . 1597
Zantac 300 Tablets . . . 1597
Zantac Injection . . . 1593
Zantac Injection Premixed . . . 1593
Zantac Syrup . . . 1597

LAKTIPEX (Sweden)
LACTULOSE
Kristalose for Oral Solution . . . 2149

LAKTULAX (Austria)
LACTULOSE
Kristalose for Oral Solution . . . 2149

LAMA (Thailand)
KETOCONAZOLE
Nizoral 2% Shampoo . . . 1838

LAMBLIT (Mexico)
METRONIDAZOLE
MetroGel-Vaginal Gel . . . 1822
Noritate Cream, 1% . . . 1051

LAMDA (India)
LAMIVUDINE
Epivir Oral Solution . . . 1394
Epivir Tablets . . . 1394
Epivir-HBV Oral Solution . . . 1398
Epivir-HBV Tablets . . . 1398

LAMDA-Z (India)
LAMIVUDINE
Epivir Oral Solution . . . 1394
Epivir Tablets . . . 1394
Epivir-HBV Oral Solution . . . 1398
Epivir-HBV Tablets . . . 1398

LAMEPIL (India)
LAMOTRIGINE
Lamictal Chewable Dispersible Tablets . . . 1449
Lamictal Tablets . . . 1449

LAMETEC (India)
LAMOTRIGINE
Lamictal Chewable Dispersible Tablets . . . 1449
Lamictal Tablets . . . 1449

LAMIBERGEN (Argentina)
LAMIVUDINE
Epivir Oral Solution . . . 1394
Epivir Tablets . . . 1394
Epivir-HBV Oral Solution . . . 1398
Epivir-HBV Tablets . . . 1398

LAMICTAL (Argentina, Australia, Austria, Belgium, Brazil, Canada, Chile, Czech Republic, Denmark, Finland, France, Germany, Greece, Hong Kong, Hungary, Irish Republic, Israel, Italy, Malaysia, Mexico, New Zealand, Norway, Portugal, Singapore, Spain, Sweden, Switzerland, Thailand, The Netherlands, United Kingdom)
LAMOTRIGINE
Lamictal Chewable Dispersible Tablets . . . 1449
Lamictal Tablets . . . 1449

LAMICTIN (South Africa)
LAMOTRIGINE
Lamictal Chewable Dispersible Tablets . . . 1449
Lamictal Tablets . . . 1449

LAMIDAC (India)
LAMIVUDINE
Epivir Oral Solution . . . 1394
Epivir Tablets . . . 1394
Epivir-HBV Oral Solution . . . 1398
Epivir-HBV Tablets . . . 1398

LAMIDEN (Brazil)
LAMIVUDINE
Epivir Oral Solution . . . 1394
Epivir Tablets . . . 1394
Epivir-HBV Oral Solution . . . 1398
Epivir-HBV Tablets . . . 1398

LAMILEA (Argentina)
LAMIVUDINE
Epivir Oral Solution . . . 1394
Epivir Tablets . . . 1394
Epivir-HBV Oral Solution . . . 1398
Epivir-HBV Tablets . . . 1398

LAMIRAX (Argentina)
LAMOTRIGINE
Lamictal Chewable Dispersible Tablets . . . 1449
Lamictal Tablets . . . 1449

LAMIREX (India)
LAMIVUDINE
Epivir Oral Solution . . . 1394
Epivir Tablets . . . 1394
Epivir-HBV Oral Solution . . . 1398
Epivir-HBV Tablets . . . 1398

LAMISIL (Argentina, Australia, Belgium, Canada, Czech Republic, Denmark, Finland, France, Germany, Hong Kong, India, Irish Republic, Israel, Italy, Malaysia, Mexico, New Zealand, Portugal, Singapore, South Africa, Spain, Thailand, The Netherlands, United Kingdom)
TERBINAFINE HYDROCHLORIDE
Lamisil Tablets . . . 2226

LAMITOR (The Netherlands)
LAMOTRIGINE
Lamictal Chewable Dispersible Tablets . . . 1449
Lamictal Tablets . . . 1449

LAMITRIN (Australia)
LAMOTRIGINE
Lamictal Chewable Dispersible Tablets . . . 1449
Lamictal Tablets . . . 1449

LAMIVIR (India)
LAMIVUDINE
Epivir Oral Solution . . . 1394
Epivir Tablets . . . 1394
Epivir-HBV Oral Solution . . . 1398
Epivir-HBV Tablets . . . 1398

LAMIVIR S (India)
LAMIVUDINE
Epivir Oral Solution . . . 1394
Epivir Tablets . . . 1394
Epivir-HBV Oral Solution . . . 1398
Epivir-HBV Tablets . . . 1398

LAMODEX (Israel)
LAMOTRIGINE
Lamictal Chewable Dispersible Tablets . . . 1449
Lamictal Tablets . . . 1449

LAMOGINE (Israel)
LAMOTRIGINE
Lamictal Chewable Dispersible Tablets . . . 1449
Lamictal Tablets . . . 1449

LAMPOCEF (Italy)
CEFAZOLIN SODIUM
Ancef for Injection . . . 1318

LAMPOSPORIN (Italy)
CEFUROXIME SODIUM
Zinacef Injection . . . 1604

LAMRA (Germany)
DIAZEPAM
Diastat Rectal Delivery System . . . 3344
Valium Tablets . . . 2822

LAMUZID (India)
LAMIVUDINE
Epivir Oral Solution . . . 1394
Epivir Tablets . . . 1394
Epivir-HBV Oral Solution . . . 1398
Epivir-HBV Tablets . . . 1398

LANACARD (Germany)
DIGOXIN
Lanoxicaps Capsules . . . 1458
Lanoxin Injection . . . 1462
Lanoxin Injection Pediatric . . . 1465
Lanoxin Tablets . . . 1468

LANACORDIN (Spain)
DIGOXIN
Lanoxicaps Capsules . . . 1458
Lanoxin Injection . . . 1462
Lanoxin Injection Pediatric . . . 1465
Lanoxin Tablets . . . 1468

LANACRIST (Sweden)
DIGOXIN
Lanoxicaps Capsules . . . 1458
Lanoxin Injection . . . 1462
Lanoxin Injection Pediatric . . . 1465
Lanoxin Tablets . . . 1468

LANATIN (Denmark)
LISINOPRIL
Prinivil Tablets . . . 2029
Zestril Tablets . . . 704

LANCUS (India)
LANSOPRAZOLE
Prevacid Delayed-Release Capsules . . . 3268

LANDOLAXIN (Greece)
LISINOPRIL
Prinivil Tablets . . . 2029
Zestril Tablets . . . 704

LANFAST (United Arab Emirates)
LANSOPRAZOLE
Prevacid Delayed-Release Capsules . . . 3268

LANICOR (Argentina, Austria, Germany, Italy, The Netherlands)
DIGOXIN
Lanoxicaps Capsules . . . 1458
Lanoxin Injection . . . 1462
Lanoxin Injection Pediatric . . . 1465
Lanoxin Tablets . . . 1468

LANOGASTRO (Brazil)
LANSOPRAZOLE
Prevacid Delayed-Release Capsules . . . 3268

LANOLEPT (Austria)
CLOZAPINE
Clozapine Tablets . . . 2141
Clozaril Tablets . . . 2174

LANOXICAPS (The Netherlands)
DIGOXIN
Lanoxicaps Capsules . . . 1458
Lanoxin Injection . . . 1462
Lanoxin Injection Pediatric . . . 1465
Lanoxin Tablets . . . 1468

LANOXIN (Argentina, Australia, Belgium, Brazil, Canada, Hong Kong, India, Irish Republic, Israel, Italy, Malaysia, Mexico, New Zealand, Norway, Portugal, Singapore, South Africa, Sweden, Switzerland, Thailand, The Netherlands, United Kingdom)
DIGOXIN
Lanoxicaps Capsules . . . 1458
Lanoxin Injection . . . 1462
Lanoxin Injection Pediatric . . . 1465
Lanoxin Tablets . . . 1468

LANSEK A (Argentina)
LOPERAMIDE HYDROCHLORIDE
Imodium Capsules . . . 1834

LANSONE (Czech Republic, Hungary)
LANSOPRAZOLE
Prevacid Delayed-Release Capsules . . . 3268

LANSOX (Italy, Portugal)
LANSOPRAZOLE
Prevacid Delayed-Release Capsules . . . 3268

LANTOGENT (Spain)
GENTAMICIN SULFATE
Garamycin Injectable . . . 3028
Genoptic Sterile Ophthalmic Solution . . . ⊙227

(⊙ Described in PDR For Ophthalmic Medicines™)

LANTON (Israel)
LANSOPRAZOLE
Prevacid Delayed-Release Capsules **3268**

LANURETIC (Austria)
AMILORIDE HYDROCHLORIDE/HYDROCHLOROTHIAZIDE
Moduretic Tablets **2003**

LANZ (Brazil)
LANSOPRAZOLE
Prevacid Delayed-Release Capsules **3268**

LANZO (Denmark, Norway, Sweden)
LANSOPRAZOLE
Prevacid Delayed-Release Capsules **3268**

LANZOGASTRO (Portugal)
LANSOPRAZOLE
Prevacid Delayed-Release Capsules **3268**

LANZOL (Brazil, India)
LANSOPRAZOLE
Prevacid Delayed-Release Capsules **3268**

LANZOPRAL (Argentina, Chile)
LANSOPRAZOLE
Prevacid Delayed-Release Capsules **3268**

LANZOR (France, Germany, South Africa)
LANSOPRAZOLE
Prevacid Delayed-Release Capsules **3268**

LANZUL (Czech Republic)
LANSOPRAZOLE
Prevacid Delayed-Release Capsules **3268**

LAPENAX (Argentina)
CLOZAPINE
Clozapine Tablets **2141**
Clozaril Tablets **2174**

LAPOL (Portugal)
LANSOPRAZOLE
Prevacid Delayed-Release Capsules **3268**

LAPRAZOL (Greece)
LANSOPRAZOLE
Prevacid Delayed-Release Capsules **3268**

LAPRIL (Hong Kong, Thailand)
ENALAPRIL MALEATE
Vasotec I.V. Injection **2076**

LAPRILEN (Portugal)
ENALAPRIL MALEATE/HYDROCHLOROTHIAZIDE
Vaseretic Tablets. **2073**

LARA (India)
LEFLUNOMIDE
Arava Tablets **2881**

LARAFLEX (United Kingdom)
NAPROXEN
EC-Naprosyn Delayed-Release Tablets. . . . **2769**
Naprosyn Suspension. **2769**
Naprosyn Tablets **2769**

LARIAM (Australia, Austria, Belgium, Canada, Chile, Czech Republic, Denmark, Finland, France, Germany, Greece, Hong Kong, Hungary, Irish Republic, Israel, Italy, New Zealand, Norway, Singapore, South Africa, Sweden, Switzerland, The Netherlands, United Kingdom)
MEFLOQUINE HYDROCHLORIDE
Lariam Tablets **2790**

LARIMEF (India)
MEFLOQUINE HYDROCHLORIDE
Lariam Tablets **2790**

LARJANCAINA (Argentina)
LIDOCAINE
Lidoderm Patch **1107**

LARMADEX (Argentina)
GOSERELIN ACETATE
Zoladex. **709**
Zoladex 3-month **712**

LAROFERON (France)
INTERFERON ALFA-2A
Roferon-A Injection. **2805**

LARRY (Hong Kong, Thailand)
KETOCONAZOLE
Nizoral 2% Shampoo **1838**

LARSEN (Argentina)
TOBRAMYCIN
TOBI Solution for Inhalation **1015**

LARSIMAL (Argentina)
FLUOROMETHOLONE
FML Ophthalmic Ointment. . . . . ⊙**225**

LASER (Italy)
NAPROXEN
EC-Naprosyn Delayed-Release Tablets. . . . **2769**
Naprosyn Suspension. **2769**
Naprosyn Tablets **2769**

LASERVIS (Germany, Malaysia, Switzerland)
SODIUM HYALURONATE
Hyalgan Solution **2917**

LASIKAL (United Kingdom)
FUROSEMIDE
Furosemide Tablets **2117**

LASILACTON (Mexico)
FUROSEMIDE
Furosemide Tablets **2117**

LASILACTONE (United Kingdom)
FUROSEMIDE
Furosemide Tablets **2117**

LASILETTEN (The Netherlands)
FUROSEMIDE
Furosemide Tablets **2117**

LASILIX (France)
FUROSEMIDE
Furosemide Tablets **2117**

LASIPRESSIN (United Kingdom)
FUROSEMIDE
Furosemide Tablets **2117**

LASIX (Argentina, Australia, Belgium, Brazil, Canada, Czech Republic, Denmark, Finland, Hong Kong, India, Irish Republic, Israel, Malaysia, Mexico, New Zealand, Norway, Portugal, Singapore, South Africa, Sweden, Thailand, The Netherlands, United Kingdom)
FUROSEMIDE
Furosemide Tablets **2117**

LASMA (Irish Republic, United Kingdom)
THEOPHYLLINE
Uniphyl Tablets **2708**

LASORIDE (United Kingdom)
FUROSEMIDE
Furosemide Tablets **2117**

L-ASP (Argentina)
ASPARAGINASE
Elspar for Injection **1943**

LASPAR (South Africa)
ASPARAGINASE
Elspar for Injection **1943**

LASSIFAR (Italy)
LACTULOSE
Kristalose for Oral Solution **2149**

LASTICOM (Austria, Italy)
AZELASTINE HYDROCHLORIDE
Astelin Nasal Spray **1876**

LASTIN (Finland, Norway, Sweden)
AZELASTINE HYDROCHLORIDE
Astelin Nasal Spray **1876**

LATICORT (Czech Republic, Germany, Hungary)
HYDROCORTISONE BUTYRATE
Locoid Cream **1138**
Locoid Lipocream Cream **1138**
Locoid Ointment **1138**
Locoid Topical Solution. **1138**

LATOF (Chile)
LATANOPROST
Xalatan Ophthalmic Solution . . . . ⊙**280**

LATOTRYD (Mexico)
ERYTHROMYCIN
Ery-Tab Tablets **447**
Erythromycin Base Filmtab Tablets. **454**
Erythromycin Delayed-Release Capsules, USP **456**
PCE Dispertab Tablets **510**

LATTUBIO (Italy)
LACTULOSE
Kristalose for Oral Solution **2149**

LATTULAC (Italy)
LACTULOSE
Kristalose for Oral Solution **2149**

LAURIMICINA (Mexico)
ERYTHROMYCIN
Ery-Tab Tablets **447**
Erythromycin Base Filmtab Tablets. **454**
Erythromycin Delayed-Release Capsules, USP **456**
PCE Dispertab Tablets **510**

LAVER (Thailand)
TRIAMCINOLONE ACETONIDE
Azmacort Inhalation Aerosol. **1701**
Nasacort AQ Nasal Spray **2937**

LAVERAN (Brazil)
CIMETIDINE
Tagamet Tablets **1547**

LAXARON (France)
LACTULOSE
Kristalose for Oral Solution **2149**

LAXEERSIROOP (The Netherlands)
LACTULOSE
Kristalose for Oral Solution **2149**

LAXETTE (South Africa)
LACTULOSE
Kristalose for Oral Solution **2149**

LAXILOSE (Canada)
LACTULOSE
Kristalose for Oral Solution **2149**

LAXOMUNDIN (Germany)
LACTULOSE
Kristalose for Oral Solution **2149**

LAXOSE (Irish Republic, United Kingdom)
LACTULOSE
Kristalose for Oral Solution **2149**

LAXULAC (Italy)
LACTULOSE
Kristalose for Oral Solution **2149**

LAXYL (Mexico)
DIAZEPAM
Diastat Rectal Delivery System **3344**
Valium Tablets **2822**

L-CARN (Germany)
LEVOCARNITINE
Carnitor Injection. **3185**
Carnitor Tablets and Oral Solution **3187**

LEDERCORT (Argentina, Sweden)
TRIAMCINOLONE ACETONIDE
Azmacort Inhalation Aerosol. **1701**
Nasacort AQ Nasal Spray **2937**

LEDERCORT CON NEOMICINA (Argentina)
TRIAMCINOLONE ACETONIDE
Azmacort Inhalation Aerosol. **1701**
Nasacort AQ Nasal Spray **2937**

LEDERCORT-N (India)
TRIAMCINOLONE ACETONIDE
Azmacort Inhalation Aerosol. **1701**
Nasacort AQ Nasal Spray **2937**

LEDERLIND (Germany)
NYSTATIN
Nystop Topical Powder USP. **2490**

LEDERPAX (Argentina, Mexico, Spain)
ERYTHROMYCIN
Ery-Tab Tablets **447**
Erythromycin Base Filmtab Tablets. **454**
Erythromycin Delayed-Release Capsules, USP **456**
PCE Dispertab Tablets **510**

LEDOX (Norway)
NAPROXEN
EC-Naprosyn Delayed-Release Tablets. . . . **2769**
Naprosyn Suspension. **2769**
Naprosyn Tablets **2769**

LEDOXID ACNE (Switzerland)
BENZOYL PEROXIDE
Brevoxyl-4 Creamy Wash. **3212**
Brevoxyl-4 Gel **3211**
Brevoxyl-8 Creamy Wash. **3212**
Brevoxyl-8 Gel **3211**
Triaz Cleanser **1864**
Triaz Gel. **1864**

LEFCAR (Italy)
LEVOCARNITINE
Carnitor Injection. **3185**
Carnitor Tablets and Oral Solution **3187**

LEFLUAR (Argentina)
LEFLUNOMIDE
Arava Tablets **2881**

LEGEDERM (Denmark, Finland, Italy, Sweden)
ALCLOMETASONE DIPROPIONATE
Aclovate Cream **1290**
Aclovate Ointment **1290**

LEGENDAL (Switzerland, The Netherlands)
LACTULOSE
Kristalose for Oral Solution **2149**

LEICESTER (Italy)
ISOSORBIDE MONONITRATE
Imdur Tablets **3032**

LEKOKLAR (Czech Republic)
CLARITHROMYCIN
Biaxin Filmtab Tablets **402**
Biaxin Granules **402**

LEKOPTIN (Czech Republic)
VERAPAMIL HYDROCHLORIDE
Covera-HS Tablets **3135**
Verelan PM Capsules **3120**

LELONG CONTUSIONS (France)
PENTOSAN POLYSULFATE SODIUM
Elmiron Capsules **2393**

LEMBROL (Argentina)
DIAZEPAM
Diastat Rectal Delivery System **3344**
Valium Tablets **2822**

LEMERON (Mexico)
INTERFERON ALFA-2B
Intron A for Injection. **3038**

LEMLAX (United Kingdom)
LACTULOSE
Kristalose for Oral Solution **2149**

LEMNIS FATTY CREAM HC (New Zealand)
HYDROCORTISONE
Hydrocortone Tablets **1963**

LEMORCAN (Greece)
NORFLOXACIN
Noroxin Tablets. **2009**

LEMOXOL (Greece)
CEFTAZIDIME
Fortaz for Injection **1422**

LEMTOSID (Mexico)
BENZONATATE
Tessalon Perles **1202**

LEMYFLOX (Mexico)
CIPROFLOXACIN HYDROCHLORIDE
Ciloxan Ophthalmic Ointment **554**
Ciloxan Ophthalmic Solution . . . . ⊙**205**
Cipro Tablets **2991**

LEMYTRIOL (Mexico)
CALCITRIOL
Calcijex Injection **411**

LENAMET (South Africa)
CIMETIDINE
Tagamet Tablets **1547**

LENAZINE (South Africa)
PROMETHAZINE HYDROCHLORIDE
Phenergan Suppositories. **3438**
Phenergan Tablets **3438**

LENDACIN (Czech Republic, Hungary, Russia)
CEFTRIAXONE SODIUM
Rocephin Injectable Vials, ADD-Vantage, Galaxy, Bulk **2801**

LENDREX (Brazil)
PERMETHRIN
Acticin Cream. **2125**

LENDRONAL (Argentina)
ALENDRONATE SODIUM
Fosamax Tablets **1949**

LENIARTRIL (Italy)
NAPROXEN
EC-Naprosyn Delayed-Release Tablets. . . . **2769**
Naprosyn Suspension. **2769**
Naprosyn Tablets **2769**

LENIDE-T (South Africa)
LOPERAMIDE HYDROCHLORIDE
Imodium Capsules **1834**

(⊙ Described in PDR For Ophthalmic Medicines™)

LENITIL (Argentina)
DICLOFENAC SODIUM
Voltaren Tablets . . . 2298
Voltaren-XR Tablets . . . 2301

LENOXICAPS (Germany)
DIGOXIN
Lanoxicaps Capsules . . . 1458
Lanoxin Injection . . . 1462
Lanoxin Injection Pediatric . . . 1465
Lanoxin Tablets . . . 1468

LENOXIN (Germany)
DIGOXIN
Lanoxicaps Capsules . . . 1458
Lanoxin Injection . . . 1462
Lanoxin Injection Pediatric . . . 1465
Lanoxin Tablets . . . 1468

LENPRYL (Mexico)
CAPTOPRIL
Captopril Tablets . . . 2114

LENTO-KALIUM (Italy)
POTASSIUM CHLORIDE
K-Dur Extended-Relase Tablets . . . 3047
K-Lor Powder Packets . . . 472
K-Tab Filmtab Tablets . . . 473

LENTOLITH (South Africa)
LITHIUM CARBONATE
Eskalith CR Controlled-Release Tablets . . . 1406
Eskalith Capsules . . . 1406

LEO K (Irish Republic, United Kingdom)
POTASSIUM CHLORIDE
K-Dur Extended-Relase Tablets . . . 3047
K-Lor Powder Packets . . . 472
K-Tab Filmtab Tablets . . . 473

LEO-400 (Thailand)
ALBENDAZOLE
Albenza Tablets . . . 1310

LEODRIN (Chile)
ALENDRONATE SODIUM
Fosamax Tablets . . . 1949

LEPHIN (Thailand)
CEFTRIAXONE SODIUM
Rocephin Injectable Vials, ADD-Vantage, Galaxy, Bulk . . . 2801

LEPOBRON (Portugal)
THEOPHYLLINE
Uniphyl Tablets . . . 2708

LEPONEX (Austria, Belgium, Brazil, Chile, Czech Republic, Denmark, Finland, France, Germany, Greece, Hungary, Israel, Italy, Mexico, Norway, Portugal, South Africa, Spain, Sweden, Switzerland, The Netherlands)
CLOZAPINE
Clozapine Tablets . . . 2141
Clozaril Tablets . . . 2174

LEPROFEN (Argentina)
ANASTROZOLE
Arimidex Tablets . . . 665

LEPTANAL (Norway, Sweden)
FENTANYL CITRATE
Actiq . . . 993

LEPTANAL COMP (Sweden)
FENTANYL CITRATE
Actiq . . . 993

LEPTIC (Argentina)
CLONAZEPAM
Klonopin Tablets . . . 2782

LEPUR (Greece)
SIMVASTATIN
Zocor Tablets . . . 2078

LERGIGAN (Sweden)
PROMETHAZINE HYDROCHLORIDE
Phenergan Suppositories . . . 3438
Phenergan Tablets . . . 3438

LERSA (Spain)
SULFACETAMIDE SODIUM
Klaron Lotion 10% . . . 1050

LERUZE (Greece)
LISINOPRIL
Prinivil Tablets . . . 2029
Zestril Tablets . . . 704

LESCOL (Argentina, Australia, Austria, Belgium, Brazil, Canada, Czech Republic, Denmark, Finland, France, Greece, Hong Kong, Hungary, Irish Republic, Israel, Italy, Malaysia, Mexico, New Zealand, Norway, Portugal, Russia, Singapore, South Africa, Spain, Sweden, Switzerland, Thailand, The Netherlands, United Kingdom)
FLUVASTATIN SODIUM
Lescol Capsules . . . 2227

LESFLAM (Singapore)
DICLOFENAC POTASSIUM
Cataflam Tablets . . . 2173

LESTRIC (Malaysia)
LOVASTATIN
Mevacor Tablets . . . 1996

LETANSIL (Brazil)
DIAZEPAM
Diastat Rectal Delivery System . . . 3344
Valium Tablets . . . 2822

LETEQUATRO (Portugal)
LEVOTHYROXINE SODIUM
Levothroid Tablets . . . 1189
Levoxyl Tablets . . . 1680
Synthroid Tablets . . . 515

LETIZEN (Czech Republic, Russia)
CETIRIZINE HYDROCHLORIDE
Zyrtec Syrup . . . 2589
Zyrtec Tablets . . . 2589

LETROX (Czech Republic, Hungary)
LEVOTHYROXINE SODIUM
Levothroid Tablets . . . 1189
Levoxyl Tablets . . . 1680
Synthroid Tablets . . . 515

LETTER (Portugal)
LEVOTHYROXINE SODIUM
Levothroid Tablets . . . 1189
Levoxyl Tablets . . . 1680
Synthroid Tablets . . . 515

LEUCOGEN (Spain)
ASPARAGINASE
Elspar for Injection . . . 1943

LEUKERAN (Argentina, Australia, Austria, Belgium, Brazil, Canada, Chile, Czech Republic, Denmark, Finland, Germany, Hong Kong, India, Irish Republic, Israel, Italy, Malaysia, Mexico, New Zealand, Norway, Portugal, Singapore, South Africa, Spain, Sweden, Switzerland, Thailand, The Netherlands, United Kingdom)
CHLORAMBUCIL
Leukeran Tablets . . . 1472

LEUKOMINERASE (Germany)
LITHIUM CARBONATE
Eskalith CR Controlled-Release Tablets . . . 1406
Eskalith Capsules . . . 1406

LEUNASE (Hong Kong, India, Japan, Malaysia, Mexico, Singapore, Thailand)
ASPARAGINASE
Elspar for Injection . . . 1943

LEUSTAT (Argentina, United Kingdom)
CLADRIBINE
Leustatin Injection . . . 2368

LEUSTATIN (Australia, Austria, Belgium, Brazil, Canada, Czech Republic, Denmark, Finland, Germany, Greece, Hong Kong, Israel, Italy, New Zealand, Norway, South Africa, Spain, Sweden, Switzerland, Thailand, The Netherlands)
CLADRIBINE
Leustatin Injection . . . 2368

LEUSTATINE (France)
CLADRIBINE
Leustatin Injection . . . 2368

LEVAMIN (Greece)
LEVOCARNITINE
Carnitor Injection . . . 3185
Carnitor Tablets and Oral Solution . . . 3187

LEVAQUIN (Argentina, Brazil, Canada)
LEVOFLOXACIN
Levaquin Injection . . . 2453
Levaquin Tablets . . . 2453

LEVAXIN (Norway, Sweden)
LEVOTHYROXINE SODIUM
Levothroid Tablets . . . 1189
Levoxyl Tablets . . . 1680
Synthroid Tablets . . . 515

LEVEDAD (Argentina)
DICLOFENAC SODIUM
Voltaren Tablets . . . 2298
Voltaren-XR Tablets . . . 2301

LEVIOGEL (Italy)
DICLOFENAC SODIUM
Voltaren Tablets . . . 2298
Voltaren-XR Tablets . . . 2301

LEVO (Israel)
LEVOFLOXACIN
Levaquin Injection . . . 2453
Levaquin Tablets . . . 2453

LEVOCARNIL (Greece)
LEVOCARNITINE
Carnitor Injection . . . 3185
Carnitor Tablets and Oral Solution . . . 3187

LEVOCARVIT (Italy)
LEVOCARNITINE
Carnitor Injection . . . 3185
Carnitor Tablets and Oral Solution . . . 3187

LEVOCIDE (India)
LEVOFLOXACIN
Levaquin Injection . . . 2453
Levaquin Tablets . . . 2453

LEVODEX (Israel)
DILTIAZEM HYDROCHLORIDE
Cardizem LA Extended Release Tablets . . . 1699
Tiazac Capsules . . . 1204

LEVOFF (India)
LEVOFLOXACIN
Levaquin Injection . . . 2453
Levaquin Tablets . . . 2453

LEVOFLOX (India)
LEVOFLOXACIN
Levaquin Injection . . . 2453
Levaquin Tablets . . . 2453

LEVOFLOX OZ KIT (India)
LEVOFLOXACIN
Levaquin Injection . . . 2453
Levaquin Tablets . . . 2453

LEVOLAC (Finland, Norway)
LACTULOSE
Kristalose for Oral Solution . . . 2149

LEVONIS (Italy)
FLUNISOLIDE
Aerobid Inhaler System . . . 1172
Aerobid-M Inhaler System . . . 1172
Nasarel Nasal Spray . . . 1652

LEVO-T (Canada)
LEVOTHYROXINE SODIUM
Levothroid Tablets . . . 1189
Levoxyl Tablets . . . 1680
Synthroid Tablets . . . 515

LEVOTEC (Canada)
LEVOTHYROXINE SODIUM
Levothroid Tablets . . . 1189
Levoxyl Tablets . . . 1680
Synthroid Tablets . . . 515

LEVOTHROID (Spain)
LEVOTHYROXINE SODIUM
Levothroid Tablets . . . 1189
Levoxyl Tablets . . . 1680
Synthroid Tablets . . . 515

LEVOTHYROX (France)
LEVOTHYROXINE SODIUM
Levothroid Tablets . . . 1189
Levoxyl Tablets . . . 1680
Synthroid Tablets . . . 515

LEVOTIROX (Italy)
LEVOTHYROXINE SODIUM
Levothroid Tablets . . . 1189
Levoxyl Tablets . . . 1680
Synthroid Tablets . . . 515

LEVOTRIN (Argentina)
LIOTHYRONINE SODIUM
Cytomel Tablets . . . 1678

LEVOVANOX (Italy)
VANCOMYCIN HYDROCHLORIDE
Vancocin HCl Capsules, USP . . . 3370

LEVOXACIN (Italy)
LEVOFLOXACIN
Levaquin Injection . . . 2453
Levaquin Tablets . . . 2453

LEXEMIN (Hong Kong, Singapore, Thailand)
FENOFIBRATE
Tricor Tablets . . . 523

LEXFOR (Thailand)
NORFLOXACIN
Noroxin Tablets . . . 2009

LEXIFLOX (Hong Kong)
NORFLOXACIN
Noroxin Tablets . . . 2009

LEXINOR (Finland, Hong Kong, Malaysia, Singapore, Sweden, Thailand)
NORFLOXACIN
Noroxin Tablets . . . 2009

LEXIS (Chile)
CLINDAMYCIN PHOSPHATE
Clindets Pledgets . . . 3212

LEXOBENE (Germany)
DICLOFENAC SODIUM
Voltaren Tablets . . . 2298
Voltaren-XR Tablets . . . 2301

LEZIDIM (Mexico)
CEFTAZIDIME
Fortaz for Injection . . . 1422

LEZOLE (Argentina)
ANASTROZOLE
Arimidex Tablets . . . 665

LGHYAL (India)
SODIUM HYALURONATE
Hyalgan Solution . . . 2917

LI 450 (Germany)
LITHIUM CARBONATE
Eskalith CR Controlled-Release Tablets . . . 1406
Eskalith Capsules . . . 1406

LIBERALGIUM (Spain)
DICLOFENAC SODIUM
Voltaren Tablets . . . 2298
Voltaren-XR Tablets . . . 2301

LIBERPROST (Argentina)
BICALUTAMIDE
Casodex Tablets . . . 670

LIBRIUM (Canada, Italy, United Kingdom)
CHLORDIAZEPOXIDE HYDROCHLORIDE
Librium Capsules . . . 3349

LICAB (India, Thailand)
LITHIUM CARBONATE
Eskalith CR Controlled-Release Tablets . . . 1406
Eskalith Capsules . . . 1406

LICARB (Thailand)
LITHIUM CARBONATE
Eskalith CR Controlled-Release Tablets . . . 1406
Eskalith Capsules . . . 1406

LICARBIUM (Israel)
LITHIUM CARBONATE
Eskalith CR Controlled-Release Tablets . . . 1406
Eskalith Capsules . . . 1406

LICUAGEN (Argentina)
CILOSTAZOL
Pletal Tablets . . . 2478

LIDERMA (Switzerland)
ISOTRETINOIN
Accutane Capsules . . . 2740

LIDERMAN (Austria)
OXICONAZOLE NITRATE
Oxistat Cream . . . 1498
Oxistat Lotion . . . 1498

LIDIAL (Brazil)
LIDOCAINE
Lidoderm Patch . . . 1107

LIDOCAINA SPRAY (Italy)
LIDOCAINE
Lidoderm Patch . . . 1107

LIDONOSTRUM (Portugal)
LIDOCAINE
Lidoderm Patch . . . 1107

LIDOPOSTERINE (Germany)
LIDOCAINE
Lidoderm Patch . . . 1107

LIDOSPRAY (Brazil)
LIDOCAINE
Lidoderm Patch **1107**

LIDOSTON (Brazil)
LIDOCAINE
Lidoderm Patch **1107**

LIFENAC (Mexico)
DICLOFENAC SODIUM
Voltaren Tablets **2298**
Voltaren-XR Tablets **2301**

LIFERXINA (Mexico)
CIPROFLOXACIN
Cipro Oral Suspension **2991**

LIFERZIT (Greece)
LOVASTATIN
Mevacor Tablets **1996**

LIFUROM (South Africa)
CEFUROXIME SODIUM
Zinacef Injection **1604**

LIFUROX (Czech Republic, Denmark, Finland, Norway, Spain, Sweden)
CEFUROXIME SODIUM
Zinacef Injection **1604**

LIGNOSPAN SPECIAL (South Africa)
LIDOCAINE
Lidoderm Patch **1107**

LIGOFRAGMIN (Argentina)
DALTEPARIN SODIUM
Fragmin Injection. **2638**

LIKENIL (Spain)
LISINOPRIL
Prinivil Tablets **2029**
Zestril Tablets. **704**

LIMAS (Japan)
LITHIUM CARBONATE
Eskalith CR Controlled-Release Tablets . . . **1406**
Eskalith Capsules **1406**

LIMED (Thailand)
LITHIUM CARBONATE
Eskalith CR Controlled-Release Tablets . . . **1406**
Eskalith Capsules **1406**

LIMOX (Greece)
CIPROFLOXACIN
Cipro Oral Suspension **2991**

LIMOXIN (Mexico)
AMOXICILLIN
Amoxil Pediatric Drops for Oral Suspension. **1315**
Amoxil Tablets **1315**

LIMPELE (Brazil)
ECONAZOLE NITRATE
Spectazole Cream. **2390**

LIMPIDEX (Italy)
LANSOPRAZOLE
Prevacid Delayed-Release Capsules **3268**

LINATIL (Finland, Norway, Sweden)
ENALAPRIL MALEATE
Vasotec I.V. Injection **2076**

LINATIL COMP (Finland)
ENALAPRIL MALEATE/HYDROCHLOROTHIAZIDE
Vaseretic Tablets. **2073**

LINDASOL (Greece)
CLINDAMYCIN PHOSPHATE
Clindets Pledgets **3212**

LINDISC (Argentina, Brazil)
ESTRADIOL
Climara Transdermal System **795**
Vivelle Transdermal System **2288**
Vivelle-Dot Transdermal System **2293**

LINFOL (Argentina)
METRONIDAZOLE
MetroGel-Vaginal Gel **1822**
Noritate Cream, 1% **1051**

LINFOLYSIN (Italy)
CHLORAMBUCIL
Leukeran Tablets. **1472**

LINOLADIOL (Austria)
ESTRADIOL
Climara Transdermal System **795**
Vivelle Transdermal System **2288**
Vivelle-Dot Transdermal System **2293**

LINOLADIOL N (Czech Republic, Germany, Hungary)
ESTRADIOL
Climara Transdermal System **795**
Vivelle Transdermal System **2288**
Vivelle-Dot Transdermal System **2293**

LINOLADIOL-H N (Czech Republic, Germany, Hungary)
ESTRADIOL
Climara Transdermal System **795**
Vivelle Transdermal System **2288**
Vivelle-Dot Transdermal System **2293**

LINOPRIL (Brazil)
LISINOPRIL
Prinivil Tablets **2029**
Zestril Tablets. **704**

LINORIL (India)
LISINOPRIL
Prinivil Tablets **2029**
Zestril Tablets. **704**

LINOTEN (Spain)
PAMIDRONATE DISODIUM
Aredia for Injection **2168**

LINVAS (India)
LISINOPRIL
Prinivil Tablets **2029**
Zestril Tablets. **704**

LION (Argentina)
STAVUDINE
Zerit Capsules **971**
Zerit for Oral Solution. **971**

LIOTREX (Chile)
SUMATRIPTAN SUCCINATE
Imitrex Injection **1431**
Imitrex Tablets **1440**

LIPANON (Brazil)
FENOFIBRATE
Tricor Tablets **523**

LIPANTHYL (Belgium, Finland, France, Germany, Greece, Hong Kong, Hungary, Italy, Malaysia, Portugal, Russia, Singapore, Sweden, Switzerland, Thailand)
FENOFIBRATE
Tricor Tablets **523**

LIPANTIL (Irish Republic, United Kingdom)
FENOFIBRATE
Tricor Tablets **523**

LIPAREX (Argentina)
ATORVASTATIN CALCIUM
Lipitor Tablets **2495**

LIPARISON (Spain)
FENOFIBRATE
Tricor Tablets **523**

LIPAXAN (Italy)
FLUVASTATIN SODIUM
Lescol Capsules **2227**

LIPAZ (Portugal)
SIMVASTATIN
Zocor Tablets. **2078**

LIPCOR (Austria)
FENOFIBRATE
Tricor Tablets **523**

LIPCUT (Finland)
SIMVASTATIN
Zocor Tablets. **2078**

LIPDAUNE (Portugal)
LOVASTATIN
Mevacor Tablets **1996**

LIPEMOL (Spain)
PRAVASTATIN SODIUM
Pravachol Tablets **943**

LIPEX (Australia, New Zealand)
SIMVASTATIN
Zocor Tablets. **2078**

LIPIBEC (Argentina)
ATORVASTATIN CALCIUM
Lipitor Tablets **2495**

LIPICARD (India)
FENOFIBRATE
Tricor Tablets **523**

LIPIDAL (Israel)
PRAVASTATIN SODIUM
Pravachol Tablets **943**

LIPIDAX (Italy)
FENOFIBRATE
Tricor Tablets **523**

LIPIDIL (Argentina, Australia, Brazil, Canada, Chile, Germany, Greece, Hungary, Mexico)
FENOFIBRATE
Tricor Tablets **523**

LIPIDLESS (Greece)
LOVASTATIN
Mevacor Tablets **1996**

LIPIL (Italy)
FENOFIBRATE
Tricor Tablets **523**

LIPIREX (Czech Republic, France)
FENOFIBRATE
Tricor Tablets **523**

LIPITIFI (The Netherlands)
PRAVASTATIN SODIUM
Pravachol Tablets **943**

LIPITOR (Argentina, Australia, Belgium, Brazil, Canada, Chile, Finland, Greece, Hong Kong, Irish Republic, Israel, Italy, Japan, Malaysia, Mexico, New Zealand, Norway, Singapore, South Africa, Sweden, Thailand, The Netherlands, United Kingdom)
ATORVASTATIN CALCIUM
Lipitor Tablets **2495**

LIPIVAS (Denmark)
LOVASTATIN
Mevacor Tablets **1996**

LIPLAT (Spain)
PRAVASTATIN SODIUM
Pravachol Tablets **943**

LIPLE (Japan)
ALPROSTADIL
Edex Injection. **3103**

LIPO RED (Spain)
FENOFIBRATE
Tricor Tablets **523**

LIPOCAMBI (Argentina)
ATORVASTATIN CALCIUM
Lipitor Tablets **2495**

LIPOCIDEN (Spain)
SIMVASTATIN
Zocor Tablets. **2078**

LIPOCLAR (Italy)
FENOFIBRATE
Tricor Tablets **523**

LIPOFEN (Portugal)
FENOFIBRATE
Tricor Tablets **523**

LIPOFENE (Italy)
FENOFIBRATE
Tricor Tablets **523**

LIPOFIN (Argentina)
ATORVASTATIN CALCIUM
Lipitor Tablets **2495**

LIPOFREN (Spain)
LOVASTATIN
Mevacor Tablets **1996**

LIPONORM (Argentina, Italy)
ATORVASTATIN CALCIUM
Lipitor Tablets **2495**

LIPOPLASMIN (Argentina)
FENOFIBRATE
Tricor Tablets **523**

LIPOREST (India)
ATORVASTATIN CALCIUM
Lipitor Tablets **2495**

LIPOREX (Greece)
SIMVASTATIN
Zocor Tablets. **2078**

LIPOSCLER (Spain)
LOVASTATIN
Mevacor Tablets **1996**

LIPOSIT (Italy)
FENOFIBRATE
Tricor Tablets **523**

LIPOSTAT (Czech Republic, Irish Republic, Israel, New Zealand, United Kingdom)
PRAVASTATIN SODIUM
Pravachol Tablets **943**

LIPOVAS (Spain)
FENOFIBRATE
Tricor Tablets **523**

LIPRACE (Australia)
LISINOPRIL
Prinivil Tablets **2029**
Zestril Tablets. **704**

LIPREREN (Chile)
LISINOPRIL
Prinivil Tablets **2029**
Zestril Tablets. **704**

LIPRIL (India, Portugal)
LISINOPRIL
Prinivil Tablets **2029**
Zestril Tablets. **704**

LIPRIMAR (Hungary, Russia)
ATORVASTATIN CALCIUM
Lipitor Tablets **2495**

LIPSIN (Austria, France, Italy, South Africa)
FENOFIBRATE
Tricor Tablets **523**

LIPUS (Portugal)
LOVASTATIN
Mevacor Tablets **1996**

LIROKEN (Mexico)
DICLOFENAC SODIUM
Voltaren Tablets **2298**
Voltaren-XR Tablets **2301**

LIS (Italy)
LACTULOSE
Kristalose for Oral Solution **2149**

LISAC (Argentina)
SIMVASTATIN
Zocor Tablets. **2078**

LISACNE (Chile)
ISOTRETINOIN
Accutane Capsules **2740**

LISDENE (Singapore)
LISINOPRIL
Prinivil Tablets **2029**
Zestril Tablets. **704**

LISI LICH (Germany)
LISINOPRIL
Prinivil Tablets **2029**
Zestril Tablets. **704**

LISIBETA (Germany)
LISINOPRIL
Prinivil Tablets **2029**
Zestril Tablets. **704**

LISICOSTAD (United Kingdom)
LISINOPRIL
Prinivil Tablets **2029**
Zestril Tablets. **704**

LISIFLEN (Italy)
DICLOFENAC SODIUM
Voltaren Tablets **2298**
Voltaren-XR Tablets **2301**

LISIGAMMA (Germany)
LISINOPRIL
Prinivil Tablets **2029**
Zestril Tablets. **704**

LISIHEXAL (Austria, Germany)
LISINOPRIL
Prinivil Tablets **2029**
Zestril Tablets. **704**

LISIKEN (Mexico)
CLINDAMYCIN HYDROCHLORIDE
Cleocin Vaginal Ovules **2613**

LISINAL (Argentina)
LISINOPRIL
Prinivil Tablets **2029**
Zestril Tablets. **704**

LISINOBELL (Australia)
LISINOPRIL
Prinivil Tablets **2029**
Zestril Tablets. **704**

LISINOGEN (Denmark)
LISINOPRIL
Prinivil Tablets **2029**
Zestril Tablets. **704**

LISINOSPES (Greece)
LISINOPRIL
Prinivil Tablets **2029**
Zestril Tablets. **704**

LISINOSTAD (Austria)
LISINOPRIL
Prinivil Tablets 2029
Zestril Tablets 704

LISINOTYROL (Austria)
LISINOPRIL
Prinivil Tablets 2029
Zestril Tablets 704

LISIPRIL (Finland)
LISINOPRIL
Prinivil Tablets 2029
Zestril Tablets 704

LISIPRIL COMP (Finland)
HYDROCHLOROTHIAZIDE/LISINOPRIL
Prinzide Tablets 2033
Zestoretic Tablets 701

LISI-PUREN (Germany)
LISINOPRIL
Prinivil Tablets 2029
Zestril Tablets 704

LISITRIL (Switzerland)
LISINOPRIL
Prinivil Tablets 2029
Zestril Tablets 704

LISKONUM (United Kingdom)
LITHIUM CARBONATE
Eskalith CR Controlled-Release Tablets 1406
Eskalith Capsules 1406

LISODER (Chile)
MOMETASONE FUROATE
Elocon Cream 0.1% 3019
Elocon Lotion 0.1% 3020
Elocon Ointment 0.1% 3021
Nasonex Nasal Spray 3058

LISODUR (Australia)
LISINOPRIL
Prinivil Tablets 2029
Zestril Tablets 704

LISODURA (Germany)
LISINOPRIL
Prinivil Tablets 2029
Zestril Tablets 704

LISONOTEC (Brazil)
LISINOPRIL
Prinivil Tablets 2029
Zestril Tablets 704

LISOPRESS (Hungary, Irish Republic)
LISINOPRIL
Prinivil Tablets 2029
Zestril Tablets 704

LISOPRIL (Switzerland)
LISINOPRIL
Prinivil Tablets 2029
Zestril Tablets 704

LISORIL (India, Singapore)
LISINOPRIL
Prinivil Tablets 2029
Zestril Tablets 704

LISORIL-5HT (India)
LISINOPRIL
Prinivil Tablets 2029
Zestril Tablets 704

LISOTRAN (Brazil)
ERYTHROMYCIN
Ery-Tab Tablets 447
Erythromycin Base Filmtab Tablets 454
Erythromycin Delayed-Release Capsules, USP 456
PCE Dispertab Tablets 510

LISOTREX (Brazil)
ERYTHROMYCIN
Ery-Tab Tablets 447
Erythromycin Base Filmtab Tablets 454
Erythromycin Delayed-Release Capsules, USP 456
PCE Dispertab Tablets 510

LISPOR (Chile)
LOVASTATIN
Mevacor Tablets 1996

LISPRIL (Irish Republic, Thailand)
LISINOPRIL
Prinivil Tablets 2029
Zestril Tablets 704

LISPRIL-HYDROCHLOROTHIAZIDE (Irish Republic)
LISINOPRIL
Prinivil Tablets 2029
Zestril Tablets 704

LISTRAN (Spain)
NABUMETONE
Relafen Tablets 1523

LISTRIL (Czech Republic)
LISINOPRIL
Prinivil Tablets 2029
Zestril Tablets 704

LIT-300 (Thailand)
LITHIUM CARBONATE
Eskalith CR Controlled-Release Tablets 1406
Eskalith Capsules 1406

LITAK (Australia, Israel, Switzerland)
CLADRIBINE
Leustatin Injection 2368

LITHANE (Canada)
LITHIUM CARBONATE
Eskalith CR Controlled-Release Tablets 1406
Eskalith Capsules 1406

LITHEUM (Mexico)
LITHIUM CARBONATE
Eskalith CR Controlled-Release Tablets 1406
Eskalith Capsules 1406

LITHICARB (Australia, Hong Kong, New Zealand)
LITHIUM CARBONATE
Eskalith CR Controlled-Release Tablets 1406
Eskalith Capsules 1406

LITHIMOLE (Greece)
TIMOLOL MALEATE
Blocadren Tablets 1891
Timoptic Sterile Ophthalmic Solution 2058
Timoptic in Ocudose 2061
Timoptic-XE Sterile Ophthalmic Gel Forming Solution 2062

LITHIUN (Argentina)
LITHIUM CARBONATE
Eskalith CR Controlled-Release Tablets 1406
Eskalith Capsules 1406

LITHIZINE (Canada)
LITHIUM CARBONATE
Eskalith CR Controlled-Release Tablets 1406
Eskalith Capsules 1406

LITHONATE (United Kingdom)
LITHIUM CARBONATE
Eskalith CR Controlled-Release Tablets 1406
Eskalith Capsules 1406

LITHOSUN (Singapore)
LITHIUM CARBONATE
Eskalith CR Controlled-Release Tablets 1406
Eskalith Capsules 1406

LITICARB (Hungary)
LITHIUM CARBONATE
Eskalith CR Controlled-Release Tablets 1406
Eskalith Capsules 1406

LITIOCAR (Brazil)
LITHIUM CARBONATE
Eskalith CR Controlled-Release Tablets 1406
Eskalith Capsules 1406

LITO (Finland)
LITHIUM CARBONATE
Eskalith CR Controlled-Release Tablets 1406
Eskalith Capsules 1406

LITOCIT (Brazil)
POTASSIUM CITRATE
Urocit-K Tablets 2109

LIVAROLE (Russia)
KETOCONAZOLE
Nizoral 2% Shampoo 1838

LIVESAN (France)
FENOFIBRATE
Tricor Tablets 523

LIVO LUK (India)
LACTULOSE
Kristalose for Oral Solution 2149

LIVOMONIL (Argentina)
CLOTRIMAZOLE
Lotrimin Cream 3053
Lotrimin Lotion 1% 3053
Lotrimin Topical Solution 1% 3053

LIXAMIDE (South Africa)
INDAPAMIDE
Indapamide Tablets 2119

LIXOGAN (Mexico)
NAPROXEN
EC-Naprosyn Delayed-Release Tablets 2769
Naprosyn Suspension 2769
Naprosyn Tablets 2769

LIZOVAG (Mexico)
KETOCONAZOLE
Nizoral 2% Shampoo 1838

LIZUL (Portugal)
LANSOPRAZOLE
Prevacid Delayed-Release Capsules 3268

LOBATE (India)
CLOBETASOL PROPIONATE
Temovate Cream 1549
Temovate E Emollient 1552
Temovate Gel 1550
Temovate Ointment 1549
Temovate Scalp Application 1551

LOBATE-G (India)
CLOBETASOL PROPIONATE
Temovate Cream 1549
Temovate E Emollient 1552
Temovate Gel 1550
Temovate Ointment 1549
Temovate Scalp Application 1551

LOBATE-M (India)
CLOBETASOL PROPIONATE
Temovate Cream 1549
Temovate E Emollient 1552
Temovate Gel 1550
Temovate Ointment 1549
Temovate Scalp Application 1551

LOBESOL (Malaysia)
CLOBETASOL PROPIONATE
Temovate Cream 1549
Temovate E Emollient 1552
Temovate Gel 1550
Temovate Ointment 1549
Temovate Scalp Application 1551

LOBEVAT (Chile, Mexico)
CLOBETASOL PROPIONATE
Temovate Cream 1549
Temovate E Emollient 1552
Temovate Gel 1550
Temovate Ointment 1549
Temovate Scalp Application 1551

LOCACID (Argentina, Czech Republic, France, Hong Kong, Israel, Portugal)
TRETINOIN
Avita Cream 2136
Avita Gel 2138
Renova 0.05% Cream 2387
Retin-A Micro 0.1%/0.04% 2388
Vesanoid Capsules 2823

LOCASYN (Denmark)
FLUNISOLIDE
Aerobid Inhaler System 1172
Aerobid-M Inhaler System 1172
Nasarel Nasal Spray 1652

LOCEPTIN (Sweden)
MORPHINE SULFATE
Kadian Capsules 572
MS Contin Tablets 2703

LOCHOL (Hungary, Japan, Thailand)
FLUVASTATIN SODIUM
Lescol Capsules 2227

LOCK-2 (Czech Republic)
CIMETIDINE
Tagamet Tablets 1547

LOCOID (Belgium, Brazil, Chile, Czech Republic, Denmark, Finland, France, Hungary, Irish Republic, Mexico, Norway, Portugal, Russia, South Africa, Sweden, Switzerland, The Netherlands, United Kingdom)
HYDROCORTISONE BUTYRATE
Locoid Cream 1138
Locoid Lipocream Cream 1138
Locoid Ointment 1138
Locoid Topical Solution 1138

LOCOID CRELO (Sweden)
HYDROCORTISONE BUTYRATE
Locoid Cream 1138
Locoid Lipocream Cream 1138
Locoid Ointment 1138
Locoid Topical Solution 1138

LOCOIDON (Austria, Italy)
HYDROCORTISONE BUTYRATE
Locoid Cream 1138
Locoid Lipocream Cream 1138
Locoid Ointment 1138
Locoid Topical Solution 1138

LOCOL (Germany)
FLUVASTATIN SODIUM
Lescol Capsules 2227

LOCTENK (Argentina)
LOSARTAN POTASSIUM
Cozaar Tablets 1913

LOCULA (India)
SULFACETAMIDE SODIUM
Klaron Lotion 10% 1050

LODALES (France)
SIMVASTATIN
Zocor Tablets 2078

LODIAR (United Kingdom)
LOPERAMIDE HYDROCHLORIDE
Imodium Capsules 1834

LODIARID (France)
LOPERAMIDE HYDROCHLORIDE
Imodium Capsules 1834

LODIMOL (Mexico)
DIPYRIDAMOLE
Persantine Tablets 898

LODIPRES (Chile)
CARVEDILOL
Coreg Tablets 1376

LODIS (Italy)
LOPERAMIDE HYDROCHLORIDE
Imodium Capsules 1834

LODIXAL (Belgium)
VERAPAMIL HYDROCHLORIDE
Covera-HS Tablets 3135
Verelan PM Capsules 3120

LODYFEN (Mexico)
DICLOFENAC SODIUM
Voltaren Tablets 2298
Voltaren-XR Tablets 2301

LOFACOL (Hong Kong)
LOVASTATIN
Mevacor Tablets 1996

LOFENSAID (United Kingdom)
DICLOFENAC SODIUM
Voltaren Tablets 2298
Voltaren-XR Tablets 2301

LOFOSTIN (Greece)
LEVOCARNITINE
Carnitor Injection 3185
Carnitor Tablets and Oral Solution 3187

LOFOTO (Greece)
DEXAMETHASONE/TOBRAMYCIN
TobraDex Ophthalmic Ointment 558
TobraDex Ophthalmic Suspension 558

LOGAT (Brazil)
RANITIDINE HYDROCHLORIDE
Zantac 25 EFFERdose Tablets 1597
Zantac 150 EFFERdose Tablets 1597
Zantac 150 Tablets 1597
Zantac 300 Tablets 1597
Zantac Injection 1593
Zantac Injection Premixed 1593
Zantac Syrup 1597

LOGECINE (France)
ERYTHROMYCIN
Ery-Tab Tablets 447
Erythromycin Base Filmtab Tablets 454
Erythromycin Delayed-Release Capsules, USP 456
PCE Dispertab Tablets 510

LOGESIC (Mexico)
DICLOFENAC SODIUM
Voltaren Tablets 2298
Voltaren-XR Tablets 2301

LOGIMAX (Czech Republic, Hungary, Israel, The Netherlands)
FELODIPINE
Plendil Extended-Release Tablets 651

LOGISTIC (Argentina)
GABAPENTIN
Neurontin Capsules 2498

LOGODERM (Australia, Chile, Mexico, New Zealand)
ALCLOMETASONE DIPROPIONATE
Aclovate Cream 1290
Aclovate Ointment 1290

LOGOMED AKNE-GEL (Germany)
BENZOYL PEROXIDE
Brevoxyl-4 Creamy Wash 3212
Brevoxyl-4 Gel 3211
Brevoxyl-8 Creamy Wash 3212
Brevoxyl-8 Gel 3211
Triaz Cleanser 1864
Triaz Gel 1864

LOGOMED DURCHFALL-KAPSELN (Germany)
LOPERAMIDE HYDROCHLORIDE
Imodium Capsules 1834

LOGOMED HAUTPILZ-SALBE (Germany)
CLOTRIMAZOLE
Lotrimin Cream 3053
Lotrimin Lotion 1% 3053
Lotrimin Topical Solution 1% 3053

LOKALICID (Germany)
CLOTRIMAZOLE
Lotrimin Cream 3053
Lotrimin Lotion 1% 3053
Lotrimin Topical Solution 1% 3053

LOKALISON-F (Germany)
DEXAMETHASONE
Decadron Tablets 1929

LOKALISON-UNIVERSALE (Germany)
DEXAMETHASONE
Decadron Tablets 1929

LOKILAN (Norway)
FLUNISOLIDE
Aerobid Inhaler System 1172
Aerobid-M Inhaler System 1172
Nasarel Nasal Spray 1652

LOKILAN NASAL (Sweden)
FLUNISOLIDE
Aerobid Inhaler System 1172
Aerobid-M Inhaler System 1172
Nasarel Nasal Spray 1652

LOKREN (Czech Republic, Hungary)
BETAXOLOL HYDROCHLORIDE
Betoptic S Ophthalmic Suspension 554

LOMADRYL (Greece)
RANITIDINE HYDROCHLORIDE
Zantac 25 EFFERdose Tablets 1597
Zantac 150 EFFERdose Tablets 1597
Zantac 150 Tablets 1597
Zantac 300 Tablets 1597
Zantac Injection 1593
Zantac Injection Premixed 1593
Zantac Syrup 1597

LOMAR (Hong Kong)
LOVASTATIN
Mevacor Tablets 1996

LOMESONE (Greece)
ALCLOMETASONE DIPROPIONATE
Aclovate Cream 1290
Aclovate Ointment 1290

LOMET (Argentina)
GLIMEPIRIDE
Amaryl Tablets 2864

LOMIDE (Thailand)
LOPERAMIDE HYDROCHLORIDE
Imodium Capsules 1834

LOMIR (Austria, Belgium, Brazil, Czech Republic, Denmark, Finland, Germany, Greece, Hungary, Italy, Norway, Portugal, Spain, Sweden, Switzerland, The Netherlands)
ISRADIPINE
DynaCirc CR Tablets 2726

LOMOTIL (Mexico)
LOPERAMIDE HYDROCHLORIDE
Imodium Capsules 1834

LOMPER (Spain)
MEBENDAZOLE
Vermox Chewable Tablets 1853

LOMY (Thailand)
LOPERAMIDE HYDROCHLORIDE
Imodium Capsules 1834

LONAVAR (Australia, Israel)
OXANDROLONE
Oxandrin Tablets 2977

LONCORD (Brazil)
NIFEDIPINE
Adalat CC Tablets 2978

LONESTIN (Mexico)
CLOTRIMAZOLE
Lotrimin Cream 3053
Lotrimin Lotion 1% 3053
Lotrimin Topical Solution 1% 3053

LONGACEPH (Czech Republic)
CEFTRIAXONE SODIUM
Rocephin Injectable Vials, ADD-Vantage, Galaxy, Bulk 2801

LONGAZEM (Italy)
DILTIAZEM HYDROCHLORIDE
Cardizem LA Extended Release Tablets 1699
Tiazac Capsules 1204

LONOL (India)
ATENOLOL
Tenormin I.V. Injection 698

LONTAX (The Netherlands)
CITALOPRAM HYDROBROMIDE
Celexa Tablets 1177

LOORTAN (Belgium)
LOSARTAN POTASSIUM
Cozaar Tablets 1913

LOORTAN PLUS (Belgium)
HYDROCHLOROTHIAZIDE/LOSARTAN POTASSIUM
Hyzaar 50-12.5 Tablets 1964

LOPALIND (Germany)
LOPERAMIDE HYDROCHLORIDE
Imodium Capsules 1834

LOPAMIDE (India)
LOPERAMIDE HYDROCHLORIDE
Imodium Capsules 1834

LOPAMINE (Thailand)
LOPERAMIDE HYDROCHLORIDE
Imodium Capsules 1834

LO-P-CAPS (Thailand)
CALCIUM ACETATE
PhosLo GelCaps 2158

LOP-DIA (Germany)
LOPERAMIDE HYDROCHLORIDE
Imodium Capsules 1834

LOPEDIAR (Chile)
LOPERAMIDE HYDROCHLORIDE
Imodium Capsules 1834

LOPEDIUM (Austria, Germany, Hungary, South Africa)
LOPERAMIDE HYDROCHLORIDE
Imodium Capsules 1834

LOPELA (Thailand)
LOPERAMIDE HYDROCHLORIDE
Imodium Capsules 1834

LOPELIN (France)
LOPERAMIDE HYDROCHLORIDE
Imodium Capsules 1834

LOPEMID (Italy)
LOPERAMIDE HYDROCHLORIDE
Imodium Capsules 1834

LOPEPHAM (Germany)
LOPERAMIDE HYDROCHLORIDE
Imodium Capsules 1834

LOPERA AKUT (Germany)
LOPERAMIDE HYDROCHLORIDE
Imodium Capsules 1834

LOPERACAP (Canada, Hungary)
LOPERAMIDE HYDROCHLORIDE
Imodium Capsules 1834

LOPERAGEN (United Kingdom)
LOPERAMIDE HYDROCHLORIDE
Imodium Capsules 1834

LOPERAMERCK (Germany)
LOPERAMIDE HYDROCHLORIDE
Imodium Capsules 1834

LOPERAMIL (Singapore)
LOPERAMIDE HYDROCHLORIDE
Imodium Capsules 1834

LOPERAN (Spain)
LOPERAMIDE HYDROCHLORIDE
Imodium Capsules 1834

LOPERASTAT (South Africa)
LOPERAMIDE HYDROCHLORIDE
Imodium Capsules 1834

LOPERAX (Hong Kong, Malaysia)
LOPERAMIDE HYDROCHLORIDE
Imodium Capsules 1834

LOPERCIN (Thailand)
LOPERAMIDE HYDROCHLORIDE
Imodium Capsules 1834

LOPERDIUM (Thailand)
LOPERAMIDE HYDROCHLORIDE
Imodium Capsules 1834

LOPERHOE (Germany)
LOPERAMIDE HYDROCHLORIDE
Imodium Capsules 1834

LOPERIA (Thailand)
LOPERAMIDE HYDROCHLORIDE
Imodium Capsules 1834

LOPERID (Israel)
LOPERAMIDE HYDROCHLORIDE
Imodium Capsules 1834

LOPERIUM (Hong Kong, Israel, Malaysia)
LOPERAMIDE HYDROCHLORIDE
Imodium Capsules 1834

LOPERKEY (Spain)
LOPERAMIDE HYDROCHLORIDE
Imodium Capsules 1834

LOPERMIDE (Hong Kong, Malaysia, Singapore, Thailand)
LOPERAMIDE HYDROCHLORIDE
Imodium Capsules 1834

LOPEROL (South Africa)
LOPERAMIDE HYDROCHLORIDE
Imodium Capsules 1834

LOPERON (Czech Republic)
LOPERAMIDE HYDROCHLORIDE
Imodium Capsules 1834

LOPERYL (Italy)
LOPERAMIDE HYDROCHLORIDE
Imodium Capsules 1834

LOPETRANS (Germany)
LOPERAMIDE HYDROCHLORIDE
Imodium Capsules 1834

LOPEX (Finland)
LOPERAMIDE HYDROCHLORIDE
Imodium Capsules 1834

LOPIMED (Switzerland)
LOPERAMIDE HYDROCHLORIDE
Imodium Capsules 1834

LOPIRETIC (Portugal)
CAPTOPRIL
Captopril Tablets 2114

LOPIRIN (Austria, Germany, Switzerland)
CAPTOPRIL
Captopril Tablets 2114

LOPLAC (Argentina)
LOSARTAN POTASSIUM
Cozaar Tablets 1913

LOPLAC-D (Argentina)
LOSARTAN POTASSIUM
Cozaar Tablets 1913

LOPRANOL LA (United Kingdom)
PROPRANOLOL HYDROCHLORIDE
Inderal LA Long-Acting Capsules 3421

LOPRATIN (The Netherlands)
CEFTRIAXONE SODIUM
Rocephin Injectable Vials, ADD-Vantage, Galaxy, Bulk 2801

LOPRIL (Brazil, Finland, France)
CAPTOPRIL
Captopril Tablets 2114

LOPTOMIT (The Netherlands)
TIMOLOL MALEATE
Blocadren Tablets 1891
Timoptic Sterile Ophthalmic Solution 2058
Timoptic in Ocudose 2061
Timoptic-XE Sterile Ophthalmic Gel Forming Solution 2062

LORADUR (Austria, Czech Republic)
AMILORIDE HYDROCHLORIDE/HYDROCHLOROTHIAZIDE
Moduretic Tablets 2003

LORAGA (Finland, Sweden)
LACTULOSE
Kristalose for Oral Solution 2149

LORAMIDE (Malaysia, Singapore)
LOPERAMIDE HYDROCHLORIDE
Imodium Capsules 1834

LORBIFLOXACINA (Argentina)
CIPROFLOXACIN
Cipro Oral Suspension 2991

LORBINAFIL (Argentina)
SILDENAFIL CITRATE
Viagra Tablets 2552

LORCAMIN (Greece)
NORFLOXACIN
Noroxin Tablets 2009

LORENTIN (Australia)
METHYLPHENIDATE HYDROCHLORIDE
Ritalin Hydrochloride Tablets 2254
Ritalin-SR Tablets 2254

LORETIC (South Africa)
HYDROCHLOROTHIAZIDE/TRIAMTERENE
Dyazide Capsules 1389
Maxzide Tablets 2150
Maxzide-25 mg Tablets 2150

LOREXEN (Mexico)
NAPROXEN
EC-Naprosyn Delayed-Release Tablets 2769
Naprosyn Suspension 2769
Naprosyn Tablets 2769

LORIDE (Portugal)
LOPERAMIDE HYDROCHLORIDE
Imodium Capsules 1834

LORISTA (Czech Republic)
LOSARTAN POTASSIUM
Cozaar Tablets 1913

LORITER (Argentina)
LOVASTATIN
Mevacor Tablets 1996

LORMINE (Argentina)
DEXAMETHASONE SODIUM PHOSPHATE
Decadron Phosphate Injection 1931

LORNAZOL (Mexico)
KETOCONAZOLE
Nizoral 2% Shampoo 1838

LOROXIDE (Canada)
BENZOYL PEROXIDE
Brevoxyl-4 Creamy Wash 3212
Brevoxyl-4 Gel 3211
Brevoxyl-8 Creamy Wash 3212
Brevoxyl-8 Gel 3211
Triaz Cleanser 1864
Triaz Gel 1864

LORSACOR (Brazil)
LOSARTAN POTASSIUM
Cozaar Tablets 1913

LORTAAN (Italy, Portugal)
LOSARTAN POTASSIUM
Cozaar Tablets 1913

LORTAAN PLUS (Portugal)
HYDROCHLOROTHIAZIDE/LOSARTAN POTASSIUM
Hyzaar 50-12.5 Tablets 1964

LORVAS (India, Thailand)
INDAPAMIDE
Indapamide Tablets 2119

LORZAAR (Germany)
LOSARTAN POTASSIUM
Cozaar Tablets 1913

LORZAAR PLUS (Germany)
HYDROCHLOROTHIAZIDE/LOSARTAN POTASSIUM
Hyzaar 50-12.5 Tablets 1964

LOSACAR (India)
LOSARTAN POTASSIUM
Cozaar Tablets 1913

LOSACAR-H (India)
LOSARTAN POTASSIUM
Cozaar Tablets 1913

LOSACOR (Argentina)
LOSARTAN POTASSIUM
Cozaar Tablets 1913

LOSACOR D (Argentina)
LOSARTAN POTASSIUM
Cozaar Tablets 1913

LOSANORM (India)
LOSARTAN POTASSIUM
Cozaar Tablets 1913

LOSAPRES (Chile)
LOSARTAN POTASSIUM
Cozaar Tablets 1913

LOSAPRES-D (Chile)
HYDROCHLOROTHIAZIDE/LOSARTAN POTASSIUM
Hyzaar 50-12.5 Tablets. . . . 1964

LOSAPREX (Italy)
LOSARTAN POTASSIUM
Cozaar Tablets 1913

LOSARTEC (Brazil)
LOSARTAN POTASSIUM
Cozaar Tablets 1913

LOSATAL (Brazil)
LOSARTAN POTASSIUM
Cozaar Tablets 1913

LOSAZID (Italy)
HYDROCHLOROTHIAZIDE/LOSARTAN POTASSIUM
Hyzaar 50-12.5 Tablets. . . . 1964

LOSE.LAX (Austria)
LACTULOSE
Kristalose for Oral Solution 2149

LOSIUM (India)
LOSARTAN POTASSIUM
Cozaar Tablets 1913

LOSTAPRES (Argentina)
RAMIPRIL
Altace Capsules 1673

LOSTATIN (Malaysia, Singapore)
LOVASTATIN
Mevacor Tablets 1996

LOTEN (Malaysia)
ATENOLOL
Tenormin I.V. Injection. . . . 698

LO-TEN (Hong Kong, New Zealand)
ATENOLOL
Tenormin I.V. Injection. . . . 698

LOTENSIN (Brazil, Canada, Hungary, Mexico)
BENAZEPRIL HYDROCHLORIDE
Lotensin Tablets 2232

LOTENSIN H (Brazil)
BENAZEPRIL HYDROCHLORIDE/HYDROCHLOROTHIAZIDE
Lotensin HCT Tablets 2235

LOTENSIN HCT (Hungary)
BENAZEPRIL HYDROCHLORIDE
Lotensin Tablets 2232

LOTIOBLANC (Argentina)
TRETINOIN
Avita Cream. . . . 2136
Avita Gel 2138
Renova 0.05% Cream. . . . 2387
Retin-A Micro 0.1%/0.04%. . . . 2388
Vesanoid Capsules. . . . 2823

LOTREMIN (Australia, Hong Kong, Malaysia, Singapore)
CLOTRIMAZOLE
Lotrimin Cream. . . . 3053
Lotrimin Lotion 1%. . . . 3053
Lotrimin Topical Solution 1% 3053

LOTREMINE (Portugal)
CLOTRIMAZOLE
Lotrimin Cream. . . . 3053
Lotrimin Lotion 1%. . . . 3053
Lotrimin Topical Solution 1% 3053

LOTRIAL (Chile)
ENALAPRIL MALEATE
Vasotec I.V. Injection 2076

LOTRIAL D (Argentina, Chile)
ENALAPRIL MALEATE
Vasotec I.V. Injection 2076

LOTRIMIN (Mexico)
CLOTRIMAZOLE
Lotrimin Cream. . . . 3053
Lotrimin Lotion 1%. . . . 3053
Lotrimin Topical Solution 1% 3053

LOTRIX (Argentina)
ENALAPRIL MALEATE
Vasotec I.V. Injection 2076

LOUTEN (Argentina, Chile)
LATANOPROST
Xalatan Ophthalmic Solution . . . . ⊙280

LOUTEN T (Argentina)
LATANOPROST
Xalatan Ophthalmic Solution . . . . ⊙280

LOVA (Germany)
LOVASTATIN
Mevacor Tablets 1996

LOVABETA (Germany)
LOVASTATIN
Mevacor Tablets 1996

LOVACARD (Czech Republic, India)
LOVASTATIN
Mevacor Tablets 1996

LOVACODAN (Denmark)
LOVASTATIN
Mevacor Tablets 1996

LOVACOL (Chile, Finland)
LOVASTATIN
Mevacor Tablets 1996

LOVACOR (Brazil)
SIMVASTATIN
Zocor Tablets 2078

LOVADRUG (Greece)
LOVASTATIN
Mevacor Tablets 1996

LOVADURA (Germany)
LOVASTATIN
Mevacor Tablets 1996

LOVAGAMMA (Germany)
LOVASTATIN
Mevacor Tablets 1996

LOVAHEXAL (Germany)
LOVASTATIN
Mevacor Tablets 1996

LOVALIP (Israel)
LOVASTATIN
Mevacor Tablets 1996

LOVAPEN (Greece)
LOVASTATIN
Mevacor Tablets 1996

LOVASC (Brazil)
LOVASTATIN
Mevacor Tablets 1996

LOVAST (Brazil)
LOVASTATIN
Mevacor Tablets 1996

LOVASTIN (Malaysia)
LOVASTATIN
Mevacor Tablets 1996

LOVATEX (Greece)
LOVASTATIN
Mevacor Tablets 1996

LOVATON (Brazil)
LOVASTATIN
Mevacor Tablets 1996

LOVENOX (Austria, Canada, France, Portugal, Switzerland)
ENOXAPARIN SODIUM
Lovenox Injection 2931

LOVERAL (Mexico)
ALBENDAZOLE
Albenza Tablets. . . . 1310

LOW LIQUEMINE (Switzerland)
DALTEPARIN SODIUM
Fragmin Injection. . . . 2638

LOWCHOLID (Greece)
SIMVASTATIN
Zocor Tablets 2078

LOWFIN (Chile)
SERTRALINE HYDROCHLORIDE
Zoloft Tablets 2581

LOWLIPID (Greece)
LOVASTATIN
Mevacor Tablets 1996

LOWPRE (Mexico)
CAPTOPRIL
Captopril Tablets. . . . 2114

LOWPRESS (Brazil)
ENALAPRIL MALEATE
Vasotec I.V. Injection 2076

LOXAZOL (Switzerland, The Netherlands)
PERMETHRIN
Acticin Cream. . . . 2125

LOXIFEN (Argentina)
RALOXIFENE HYDROCHLORIDE
Evista Tablets. . . . 1735

LOXIN (Germany)
AZELASTINE HYDROCHLORIDE
Astelin Nasal Spray 1876

LOZAN (Brazil)
KETOCONAZOLE
Nizoral 2% Shampoo 1838

LOZAP (Czech Republic)
LOSARTAN POTASSIUM
Cozaar Tablets 1913

LOZAPIN (India)
CLOZAPINE
Clozapine Tablets 2141
Clozaril Tablets 2174

LOZAPINE (Israel)
CLOZAPINE
Clozapine Tablets 2141
Clozaril Tablets 2174

LOZIDE (Canada)
INDAPAMIDE
Indapamide Tablets 2119

LOZITAN (India)
LOSARTAN POTASSIUM
Cozaar Tablets 1913

L-THYROX (Germany)
LEVOTHYROXINE SODIUM
Levothroid Tablets 1189
Levoxyl Tablets. . . . 1680
Synthroid Tablets. . . . 515

L-TINE (India)
LEVOCARNITINE
Carnitor Injection. . . . 3185
Carnitor Tablets and Oral Solution 3187

LTK250 (Argentina)
POTASSIUM CITRATE
Urocit-K Tablets. . . . 2109

LUASE (Spain)
DICLOFENAC SODIUM
Voltaren Tablets 2298
Voltaren-XR Tablets 2301

LUBEXYL (Hungary, Switzerland)
BENZOYL PEROXIDE
Brevoxyl-4 Creamy Wash. . . . 3212
Brevoxyl-4 Gel 3211
Brevoxyl-8 Creamy Wash. . . . 3212
Brevoxyl-8 Gel 3211
Triaz Cleanser 1864
Triaz Gel. . . . 1864

LUFI (India)
LEVOFLOXACIN
Levaquin Injection 2453
Levaquin Tablets 2453

LUGACIN (United Kingdom)
GENTAMICIN SULFATE
Garamycin Injectable 3028
Genoptic Sterile Ophthalmic Solution . . . . ⊙227

LUGESTERON (Finland)
PROGESTERONE
Prometrium Capsules (100 mg, 200 mg) . 3205

LUITASE (Italy)
PANCRELIPASE
Ultrase Capsules. . . . 735
Ultrase MT Capsules 736

LUKAIR (Argentina)
MONTELUKAST SODIUM
Singulair Chewable Tablets 2047
Singulair Tablets 2047

LUKASM (Italy)
MONTELUKAST SODIUM
Singulair Chewable Tablets 2047
Singulair Tablets 2047

LUMAREN (Greece, Singapore)
RANITIDINE HYDROCHLORIDE
Zantac 25 EFFERdose Tablets 1597
Zantac 150 EFFERdose Tablets. . . . 1597
Zantac 150 Tablets 1597
Zantac 300 Tablets 1597
Zantac Injection 1593
Zantac Injection Premixed 1593
Zantac Syrup 1597

LUMAT (Argentina)
PERMETHRIN
Acticin Cream. . . . 2125

LUMBICID (Mexico)
MEBENDAZOLE
Vermox Chewable Tablets 1853

LUMIX (Argentina)
SILDENAFIL CITRATE
Viagra Tablets 2552

LUMOX (Mexico)
AMOXICILLIN
Amoxil Pediatric Drops for Oral Suspension. . . . 1315
Amoxil Tablets 1315

LUNDIRAN (Spain)
NAPROXEN
EC-Naprosyn Delayed-Release Tablets. . . . 2769
Naprosyn Suspension. . . . 2769
Naprosyn Tablets 2769

LUNIBRON (Italy)
FLUNISOLIDE
Aerobid Inhaler System. . . . 1172
Aerobid-M Inhaler System 1172
Nasarel Nasal Spray 1652

LUNIS (Italy)
FLUNISOLIDE
Aerobid Inhaler System. . . . 1172
Aerobid-M Inhaler System 1172
Nasarel Nasal Spray 1652

LUPAREN (Brazil)
DICLOFENAC SODIUM
Voltaren Tablets 2298
Voltaren-XR Tablets 2301

LUPERZOL (Mexico)
KETOCONAZOLE
Nizoral 2% Shampoo 1838

LURDEX (Mexico)
ALBENDAZOLE
Albenza Tablets. . . . 1310

LUSTRAL (Irish Republic, Israel, United Kingdom)
SERTRALINE HYDROCHLORIDE
Zoloft Tablets 2581

LUTAMIDAL (Chile)
BICALUTAMIDE
Casodex Tablets 670

LUTOGIN (Italy)
PROGESTERONE
Prometrium Capsules (100 mg, 200 mg) . 3205

LUTOPOLAR (Finland)
MEDROXYPROGESTERONE ACETATE
Depo-Medrol Single-Dose Vial 2617

LUTORAL (Italy)
MEDROXYPROGESTERONE ACETATE
Depo-Medrol Single-Dose Vial 2617

LUXAZONE (Italy)
DEXAMETHASONE
Decadron Tablets 1929

LYCEFT (India)
CEFTRIAXONE SODIUM
Rocephin Injectable Vials, ADD-Vantage, Galaxy, Bulk 2801

LYCLEAR (Australia, Irish Republic, Israel, New Zealand, South Africa, United Kingdom)
PERMETHRIN
Acticin Cream. . . . 2125

LYDERM (New Zealand)
PERMETHRIN
Acticin Cream. . . . 2125

LYMETEL (Spain)
FLUVASTATIN SODIUM
Lescol Capsules 2227

LYNDAK (Italy)
SULINDAC
Clinoril Tablets 1899

LYOTRET (Greece)
ISOTRETINOIN
Accutane Capsules 2740

LYOVAC COSMEGEN (Belgium, Germany, The Netherlands)
DACTINOMYCIN
Cosmegen for Injection. . . . 1907

LYPHOCIN (Hong Kong)
VANCOMYCIN HYDROCHLORIDE
Vancocin HCl Capsules, USP 3370

LYSOVIR (United Kingdom)
AMANTADINE HYDROCHLORIDE
Symmetrel Syrup 1115
Symmetrel Tablets 1115

LYSTIN (Hong Kong, Thailand)
NYSTATIN
Nystop Topical Powder USP 2490

MAALOX H2 ACID CONTROLLER (Canada)
FAMOTIDINE
Pepcid Injection 2017
Pepcid Injection Premixed 2017
Pepcid Tablets 2014
Pepcid for Oral Suspension 2014

MABICROL (Mexico)
CLARITHROMYCIN
Biaxin Filmtab Tablets 402
Biaxin Granules 402

MABTHERA (Argentina, Australia, Austria, Belgium, Brazil, Chile, Czech Republic, Denmark, Finland, France, Germany, Greece, Hong Kong, Hungary, Irish Republic, Israel, Italy, Mexico, New Zealand, Norway, Portugal, Singapore, South Africa, Spain, Sweden, Switzerland, Thailand, The Netherlands, United Kingdom)
RITUXIMAB
Rituxan I.V. 1251
Rituxan for Infusion 845

MACLADIN (Italy)
CLARITHROMYCIN
Biaxin Filmtab Tablets 402
Biaxin Granules 402

MACLAR (Austria, Belgium, India, Portugal)
CLARITHROMYCIN
Biaxin Filmtab Tablets 402
Biaxin Granules 402

MACOBAL (Argentina)
NIMODIPINE
Nimotop Capsules 774

MACOREL (Greece)
NIFEDIPINE
Adalat CC Tablets 2978

MACROLIN (France)
ALDESLEUKIN
Proleukin for Injection 1007

MACROMICINA (Argentina)
CLARITHROMYCIN
Biaxin Filmtab Tablets 402
Biaxin Granules 402

MACSORALEN (India)
METHOXSALEN
Oxsoralen Lotion 1% 3354
Oxsoralen-Ultra Capsules 3354

MADAPROX (Spain)
NAPROXEN
EC-Naprosyn Delayed-Release Tablets 2769
Naprosyn Suspension 2769
Naprosyn Tablets 2769

MADICURE (The Netherlands)
MEBENDAZOLE
Vermox Chewable Tablets 1853

MAFEL (Argentina)
PROGESTERONE
Prometrium Capsules (100 mg, 200 mg) . 3205

MAFENA (Mexico)
DICLOFENAC SODIUM
Voltaren Tablets 2298
Voltaren-XR Tablets 2301

MAFORAN (Thailand)
WARFARIN SODIUM
Coumadin Tablets 932
Coumadin for Injection 932

MAGICUL (Australia)
CIMETIDINE
Tagamet Tablets 1547

MAGLUPHEN (Austria)
DICLOFENAC SODIUM
Voltaren Tablets 2298
Voltaren-XR Tablets 2301

MAGNASPOR (Thailand)
CEFUROXIME AXETIL
Ceftin Tablets 1369
Ceftin for Oral Suspension 1369

MAGNITON-R (Greece)
INDAPAMIDE
Indapamide Tablets 2119

MAGNOGEN (Argentina)
BUPRENORPHINE HYDROCHLORIDE
Buprenex Injectable 2718

MAGNUROL (Spain)
TERAZOSIN HYDROCHLORIDE
Hytrin Capsules 469

MAGNUS (Argentina)
SILDENAFIL CITRATE
Viagra Tablets 2552

MAJOLAT (Austria)
NIFEDIPINE
Adalat CC Tablets 2978

MALANIL (South Africa)
ATOVAQUONE
Mepron Suspension 1487

MALARONE (Australia, Brazil, Israel, Italy, New Zealand, Norway, Spain, The Netherlands, United Kingdom)
ATOVAQUONE
Mepron Suspension 1487

MALASTOP (Belgium)
PYRIMETHAMINE
Daraprim Tablets 1385

MALEAPRIL (Brazil)
ENALAPRIL MALEATE
Vasotec I.V. Injection 2076

MALEDROL (Greece)
LEVOCARNITINE
Carnitor Injection 3185
Carnitor Tablets and Oral Solution 3187

MALEN (Portugal)
ENALAPRIL MALEATE
Vasotec I.V. Injection 2076

MALEXIN (Germany)
NAPROXEN
EC-Naprosyn Delayed-Release Tablets 2769
Naprosyn Suspension 2769
Naprosyn Tablets 2769

MALFIN (Denmark)
MORPHINE SULFATE
Kadian Capsules 572
MS Contin Tablets 2703

MALIMED (Switzerland)
CIMETIDINE
Tagamet Tablets 1547

MALOCEF (Greece)
CEFTAZIDIME
Fortaz for Injection 1422

MALOCIDE (France)
PYRIMETHAMINE
Daraprim Tablets 1385

MALOCIN (Thailand)
ERYTHROMYCIN STEARATE
Erythrocin Stearate Filmtab Tablets 452

MALOPRIM (Belgium, Irish Republic)
PYRIMETHAMINE
Daraprim Tablets 1385

MANDROLAX LACTU (Germany)
LACTULOSE
Kristalose for Oral Solution 2149

MANDROS DIARSTOP (Germany)
LOPERAMIDE HYDROCHLORIDE
Imodium Capsules 1834

MANDRO-ZEP (Germany)
DIAZEPAM
Diastat Rectal Delivery System 3344
Valium Tablets 2822

MANIALIT (Italy)
LITHIUM CARBONATE
Eskalith CR Controlled-Release Tablets . . . 1406
Eskalith Capsules 1406

MANIDON (Spain)
VERAPAMIL HYDROCHLORIDE
Covera-HS Tablets 3135
Verelan PM Capsules 3120

MANIPREX (Belgium)
LITHIUM CARBONATE
Eskalith CR Controlled-Release Tablets . . . 1406
Eskalith Capsules 1406

MANODEPO (Thailand)
MEDROXYPROGESTERONE ACETATE
Depo-Medrol Single-Dose Vial 2617

MANOFLOX (Thailand)
NORFLOXACIN
Noroxin Tablets 2009

MANOKETO (Thailand)
KETOCONAZOLE
Nizoral 2% Shampoo 1838

MANOLONE (Thailand)
TRIAMCINOLONE ACETONIDE
Azmacort Inhalation Aerosol 1701
Nasacort AQ Nasal Spray 2937

MANOMAZOLE (Thailand)
CLOTRIMAZOLE
Lotrimin Cream 3053
Lotrimin Lotion 1% 3053
Lotrimin Topical Solution 1% 3053

MANOMET (Thailand)
CIMETIDINE
Tagamet Tablets 1547

MANSAL (Spain)
CIMETIDINE
Tagamet Tablets 1547

MANTADAN (Italy)
AMANTADINE HYDROCHLORIDE
Symmetrel Syrup 1115
Symmetrel Tablets 1115

MANTADINE (United Kingdom)
AMANTADINE HYDROCHLORIDE
Symmetrel Syrup 1115
Symmetrel Tablets 1115

MANTADIX (Belgium, France)
AMANTADINE HYDROCHLORIDE
Symmetrel Syrup 1115
Symmetrel Tablets 1115

MANTIDAN (Brazil)
AMANTADINE HYDROCHLORIDE
Symmetrel Syrup 1115
Symmetrel Tablets 1115

MAOTIL (Germany)
SELEGILINE HYDROCHLORIDE
Eldepryl Capsules 3209

MAP AN (Argentina)
MEDROXYPROGESTERONE ACETATE
Depo-Medrol Single-Dose Vial 2617

MAPELOR (The Netherlands)
TAMSULOSIN HYDROCHLORIDE
Flomax Capsules 881

MAPEZINE (Thailand)
CARBAMAZEPINE
Carbatrol Capsules 3174
Tegretol Chewable Tablets 2278
Tegretol Suspension 2278
Tegretol Tablets 2278
Tegretol-XR Tablets 2278

MAPIN (Hong Kong, Malaysia)
NALOXONE HYDROCHLORIDE
Narcan Injection 1109

MAPLUXIN (Mexico)
DIGOXIN
Lanoxicaps Capsules 1458
Lanoxin Injection 1462
Lanoxin Injection Pediatric 1465
Lanoxin Tablets 1468

MARBEN (Mexico)
MEBENDAZOLE
Vermox Chewable Tablets 1853

MARDUK (Germany)
BENZOYL PEROXIDE
Brevoxyl-4 Creamy Wash 3212
Brevoxyl-4 Gel 3211
Brevoxyl-8 Creamy Wash 3212
Brevoxyl-8 Gel 3211
Triaz Cleanser 1864
Triaz Gel 1864

MAREVAN (Australia, Belgium, Brazil, Denmark, Finland, Greece, New Zealand, Norway, Singapore, United Kingdom)
WARFARIN SODIUM
Coumadin Tablets 932
Coumadin for Injection 932

MARFLOXACIN (Hong Kong)
OFLOXACIN
Floxin Otic Solution 1043

MARINOL (Canada)
DRONABINOL
Marinol Capsules 3334

MARITIDINE (Hong Kong)
CIMETIDINE
Tagamet Tablets 1547

MARMODINE (Hong Kong)
FAMOTIDINE
Pepcid Injection 2017
Pepcid Injection Premixed 2017
Pepcid Tablets 2014
Pepcid for Oral Suspension 2014

MARPHAZOLE (Hong Kong)
METRONIDAZOLE
MetroGel-Vaginal Gel 1822
Noritate Cream, 1% 1051

MARTENOL (Hong Kong)
ATENOLOL
Tenormin I.V. Injection 698

MARTIGENTA (France)
GENTAMICIN SULFATE
Garamycin Injectable 3028
Genoptic Sterile Ophthalmic Solution . . . . ⊙227

MARTULOSE (Hong Kong)
LACTULOSE
Kristalose for Oral Solution 2149

MARVIL (Argentina)
ALENDRONATE SODIUM
Fosamax Tablets 1949

MASAROL (Thailand)
KETOCONAZOLE
Nizoral 2% Shampoo 1838

MASAWORM (Thailand)
ALBENDAZOLE
Albenza Tablets 1310

MASAWORM-1 (Thailand)
MEBENDAZOLE
Vermox Chewable Tablets 1853

MASDIL (Spain)
DILTIAZEM HYDROCHLORIDE
Cardizem LA Extended Release Tablets . . . 1699
Tiazac Capsules 1204

MASNODERM (United Kingdom)
CLOTRIMAZOLE
Lotrimin Cream 3053
Lotrimin Lotion 1% 3053
Lotrimin Topical Solution 1% 3053

MATULANE (Canada)
PROCARBAZINE HYDROCHLORIDE
Matulane Capsules 3188

MAURAN (Italy)
RANITIDINE HYDROCHLORIDE
Zantac 25 EFFERdose Tablets 1597
Zantac 150 EFFERdose Tablets 1597
Zantac 150 Tablets 1597
Zantac 300 Tablets 1597
Zantac Injection 1593
Zantac Injection Premixed 1593
Zantac Syrup 1597

MAVID (Germany)
CLARITHROMYCIN
Biaxin Filmtab Tablets 402
Biaxin Granules 402

MAVIK (Canada, South Africa)
TRANDOLAPRIL
Mavik Tablets 482

MAXAIR (Canada, France, Switzerland)
PIRBUTEROL ACETATE
Maxair Autohaler 1820

MAXALT (Argentina, Austria, Belgium, Brazil, Canada, Chile, Czech Republic, Denmark, Finland, Germany, Greece, Hungary, Italy, Mexico, New Zealand, Norway, Portugal, South Africa, Spain, Sweden, Switzerland, The Netherlands, United Kingdom)
RIZATRIPTAN BENZOATE
Maxalt Tablets 1983
Maxalt-MLT Orally Disintegrating Tablets . . 1983

MAXCEF (Argentina, Brazil, Israel)
CEFEPIME HYDROCHLORIDE
Maxipime for Injection 1093

MAXDOSA (Argentina)
SILDENAFIL CITRATE
Viagra Tablets 2552

(⊙ Described in PDR For Ophthalmic Medicines™)

MAXIBONE (Israel)
ALENDRONATE SODIUM
Fosamax Tablets 1949

MAXIBRAL (Greece)
ETIDRONATE DISODIUM
Didronel Tablets 2693

MAXICARDIL (Argentina)
DIPYRIDAMOLE
Persantine Tablets 898

MAXIDEX (Australia, Belgium, Brazil, Canada, Chile, Denmark, France, Greece, Hong Kong, Hungary, Irish Republic, Israel, Malaysia, New Zealand, Singapore, South Africa, Spain, Switzerland, The Netherlands, United Kingdom)
DEXAMETHASONE
Decadron Tablets 1929

MAXIDON (Sweden)
MORPHINE SULFATE
Kadian Capsules 572
MS Contin Tablets 2703

MAXIMO (Argentina)
SILDENAFIL CITRATE
Viagra Tablets 2552

MAXIOSTENIL (Argentina)
SODIUM HYALURONATE
Hyalgan Solution 2917

MAXIPIME (Australia, Austria, Belgium, Canada, Chile, Czech Republic, Denmark, Finland, Germany, Greece, Hong Kong, Hungary, Irish Republic, Italy, Malaysia, Mexico, New Zealand, Portugal, Russia, Singapore, South Africa, Spain, Sweden, Switzerland, Thailand, The Netherlands)
CEFEPIME HYDROCHLORIDE
Maxipime for Injection 1093

MAXIPRIL (Italy)
CAPTOPRIL
Captopril Tablets 2114

MAXIVANIL (Italy)
VANCOMYCIN HYDROCHLORIDE
Vancocin HCl Capsules, USP 3370

MAXTRAL (Argentina)
ALENDRONATE SODIUM
Fosamax Tablets 1949

MAXUDIN (Greece)
PRAVASTATIN SODIUM
Pravachol Tablets 943

MAXZIDE (Belgium)
TRIAMTERENE
Dyrenium Capsules 3390

MAZEPINE (Canada)
CARBAMAZEPINE
Carbatrol Capsules 3174
Tegretol Chewable Tablets 2278
Tegretol Suspension 2278
Tegretol Tablets 2278
Tegretol-XR Tablets 2278

MAZETOL (India)
CARBAMAZEPINE
Carbatrol Capsules 3174
Tegretol Chewable Tablets 2278
Tegretol Suspension 2278
Tegretol Tablets 2278
Tegretol-XR Tablets 2278

M-BENTABS (Mexico)
MEBENDAZOLE
Vermox Chewable Tablets 1853

M-BETA (Germany)
MORPHINE SULFATE
Kadian Capsules 572
MS Contin Tablets 2703

MCR (Israel)
MORPHINE SULFATE
Kadian Capsules 572
MS Contin Tablets 2703

MCR-50 (United Kingdom)
ISOSORBIDE MONONITRATE
Imdur Tablets 3032

MDILTIWAS (Spain)
DILTIAZEM HYDROCHLORIDE
Cardizem LA Extended Release Tablets 1699
Tiazac Capsules 1204

M-DOLOR (Austria, Germany)
MORPHINE SULFATE
Kadian Capsules 572
MS Contin Tablets 2703

MEBA (Thailand)
MEBENDAZOLE
Vermox Chewable Tablets 1853

MEBAN (Mexico)
MEBENDAZOLE
Vermox Chewable Tablets 1853

MEBANDOZER (Mexico)
MEBENDAZOLE
Vermox Chewable Tablets 1853

MEBECICLOL (Mexico)
MEBENDAZOLE
Vermox Chewable Tablets 1853

MEBELMIN (Mexico)
MEBENDAZOLE
Vermox Chewable Tablets 1853

MEBEN (Brazil, Thailand)
MEBENDAZOLE
Vermox Chewable Tablets 1853

MEBENDAN (Spain)
MEBENDAZOLE
Vermox Chewable Tablets 1853

MEBENDA-P (Thailand)
MEBENDAZOLE
Vermox Chewable Tablets 1853

MEBENDAZOTIL (Brazil)
MEBENDAZOLE
Vermox Chewable Tablets 1853

MEBENDIL (Brazil)
MEBENDAZOLE
Vermox Chewable Tablets 1853

MEBENIX (Brazil)
ALBENDAZOLE
Albenza Tablets 1310

MEBENLAX (Thailand)
MEBENDAZOLE
Vermox Chewable Tablets 1853

MEBENSOLE (Mexico)
MEBENDAZOLE
Vermox Chewable Tablets 1853

MEBENTAL (Brazil)
MEBENDAZOLE
Vermox Chewable Tablets 1853

MEBENTIASIS (Mexico)
MEBENDAZOLE
Vermox Chewable Tablets 1853

MEBENTINE (Mexico)
MEBENDAZOLE
Vermox Chewable Tablets 1853

MEBENTRAL (Mexico)
MEBENDAZOLE
Vermox Chewable Tablets 1853

MEBEX (India)
MEBENDAZOLE
Vermox Chewable Tablets 1853

MEBEX PLUS (India)
MEBENDAZOLE
Vermox Chewable Tablets 1853

MEB-OVEROID (Mexico)
MEBENDAZOLE
Vermox Chewable Tablets 1853

MEBUTAN (The Netherlands)
NABUMETONE
Relafen Tablets 1523

MEBUTAR (Argentina)
MEBENDAZOLE
Vermox Chewable Tablets 1853

MEBUTAR COMPUESTO (Argentina)
MEBENDAZOLE
Vermox Chewable Tablets 1853

MEBZOL (United Arab Emirates)
MEBENDAZOLE
Vermox Chewable Tablets 1853

MECTIZAN (France)
IVERMECTIN
Stromectol Tablets 2053

MEDAMET (South Africa)
METRONIDAZOLE
MetroGel-Vaginal Gel 1822
Noritate Cream, 1% 1051

MEDAMOR (Finland)
AMILORIDE HYDROCHLORIDE
Midamor Tablets 2000

MEDAREN (Thailand)
DICLOFENAC SODIUM
Voltaren Tablets 2298
Voltaren-XR Tablets 2301

MEDASPOR (South Africa)
CLOTRIMAZOLE
Lotrimin Cream 3053
Lotrimin Lotion 1% 3053
Lotrimin Topical Solution 1% 3053

MEDAZOL (Czech Republic, Mexico)
METRONIDAZOLE
MetroGel-Vaginal Gel 1822
Noritate Cream, 1% 1051

MEDAZOL GEL (Chile)
METRONIDAZOLE
MetroGel-Vaginal Gel 1822
Noritate Cream, 1% 1051

MEDAZOLE (Thailand)
MEBENDAZOLE
Vermox Chewable Tablets 1853

MEDAZYL (Thailand)
METRONIDAZOLE
MetroGel-Vaginal Gel 1822
Noritate Cream, 1% 1051

MEDETON (Thailand)
MEDROXYPROGESTERONE ACETATE
Depo-Medrol Single-Dose Vial 2617

MED-GASTRAMET (Thailand)
CIMETIDINE
Tagamet Tablets 1547

MEDGESIC (Thailand)
ORPHENADRINE CITRATE
Norflex Injection 1824

MEDICLEAR (United Kingdom)
BENZOYL PEROXIDE
Brevoxyl-4 Creamy Wash 3212
Brevoxyl-4 Gel 3211
Brevoxyl-8 Creamy Wash 3212
Brevoxyl-8 Gel 3211
Triaz Cleanser 1864
Triaz Gel 1864

MEDIFUNGOL (Argentina)
CLOTRIMAZOLE
Lotrimin Cream 3053
Lotrimin Lotion 1% 3053
Lotrimin Topical Solution 1% 3053

MEDIKINET (Germany)
METHYLPHENIDATE HYDROCHLORIDE
Ritalin Hydrochloride Tablets 2254
Ritalin-SR Tablets 2254

MEDILAX (Denmark)
LACTULOSE
Kristalose for Oral Solution 2149

MEDILET (Austria, Germany)
LACTULOSE
Kristalose for Oral Solution 2149

MEDILIUM (Canada)
CHLORDIAZEPOXIDE HYDROCHLORIDE
Librium Capsules 3349

MEDINOX MONO (Germany)
PENTOBARBITAL SODIUM
Nembutal Sodium Solution, USP 2484

MEDIPAM (Finland)
DIAZEPAM
Diastat Rectal Delivery System 3344
Valium Tablets 2822

MEDIPHYLLIN CHRONO (Greece)
THEOPHYLLINE
Uniphyl Tablets 2708

MEDIPINA (Portugal)
NIFEDIPINE
Adalat CC Tablets 2978

MEDIPO (Italy)
SIMVASTATIN
Zocor Tablets 2078

MEDISPORT ATHLETE'S FOOT (United Kingdom)
CLOTRIMAZOLE
Lotrimin Cream 3053
Lotrimin Lotion 1% 3053
Lotrimin Topical Solution 1% 3053

MEDIURESIX (Thailand)
FUROSEMIDE
Furosemide Tablets 2117

MEDIXIL (Chile)
SIBUTRAMINE HYDROCHLORIDE
Meridia Capsules 485

MEDIXIN (Argentina)
LACTULOSE
Kristalose for Oral Solution 2149

MEDIZOL (Mexico)
METRONIDAZOLE
MetroGel-Vaginal Gel 1822
Noritate Cream, 1% 1051

MEDOCARNITIN (Italy)
LEVOCARNITINE
Carnitor Injection 3185
Carnitor Tablets and Oral Solution 3187

MEDOCIPRIN (Hong Kong, Thailand)
CIPROFLOXACIN HYDROCHLORIDE
Ciloxan Ophthalmic Ointment 554
Ciloxan Ophthalmic Solution . . . . ⊙205
Cipro Tablets 2991

MEDOCOR (Argentina)
ISOSORBIDE MONONITRATE
Imdur Tablets 3032

MEDODERMONE (Hong Kong, Singapore, Thailand)
CLOBETASOL PROPIONATE
Temovate Cream 1549
Temovate E Emollient 1552
Temovate Gel 1550
Temovate Ointment 1549
Temovate Scalp Application 1551

MEDOFLOXINE (Malaysia)
OFLOXACIN
Floxin Otic Solution 1043

MEDOSTATIN (Czech Republic, Hong Kong, Malaysia, Russia, Singapore)
LOVASTATIN
Mevacor Tablets 1996

MEDOVASCIN (Greece)
LOVASTATIN
Mevacor Tablets 1996

MEDOXEM (Greece)
CEFUROXIME SODIUM
Zinacef Injection 1604

MEDOXIM (Italy)
CEFUROXIME SODIUM
Zinacef Injection 1604

MEDOXONUM (Hong Kong)
CEFTRIAXONE SODIUM
Rocephin Injectable Vials, ADD-Vantage, Galaxy, Bulk 2801

MEDOZEM (Thailand)
DILTIAZEM HYDROCHLORIDE
Cardizem LA Extended Release Tablets 1699
Tiazac Capsules 1204

MEDOZIDE (Italy)
HYDROCHLOROTHIAZIDE/METHYLDOPA
Aldoril Tablets 1884

MED-PHYLLINE (Thailand)
THEOPHYLLINE
Uniphyl Tablets 2708

MEDROCIL (Argentina)
HYDROCORTISONE
Hydrocortone Tablets 1963

MEDROL VERIDERM (Canada, Italy)
METHYLPREDNISOLONE ACETATE
Depo-Medrol Injectable Suspension 2615

MEDROSTERONA (Argentina)
MEDROXYPROGESTERONE ACETATE
Depo-Medrol Single-Dose Vial 2617

MEDROXITEST (Brazil)
MEDROXYPROGESTERONE ACETATE
Depo-Medrol Single-Dose Vial 2617

MEDROXYHEXAL (Australia)
MEDROXYPROGESTERONE ACETATE
Depo-Medrol Single-Dose Vial 2617

(⊙ Described in PDR For Ophthalmic Medicines™)

MED-TRICOCIDE (Thailand)
METRONIDAZOLE
MetroGel-Vaginal Gel . . . 1822
Noritate Cream, 1% . . . 1051

MEFIRON (Thailand)
METRONIDAZOLE
MetroGel-Vaginal Gel . . . 1822
Noritate Cream, 1% . . . 1051

MEFLIAM (India, South Africa)
MEFLOQUINE HYDROCHLORIDE
Lariam Tablets . . . 2790

MEFLOC (India)
MEFLOQUINE HYDROCHLORIDE
Lariam Tablets . . . 2790

MEFOXIL (Greece)
CEFOXITIN SODIUM
Mefoxin Premixed Intravenous Solution . . . 1990
Mefoxin for Injection . . . 1987

MEFOXIN (Argentina, Australia, Belgium, Brazil, Canada, Czech Republic, Finland, France, Hong Kong, Irish Republic, Italy, New Zealand, Portugal, South Africa, The Netherlands, United Kingdom)
CEFOXITIN SODIUM
Mefoxin Premixed Intravenous Solution . . . 1990
Mefoxin for Injection . . . 1987

MEFOXITIN (Austria, Germany, Norway, Spain, Sweden, Switzerland)
CEFOXITIN SODIUM
Mefoxin Premixed Intravenous Solution . . . 1990
Mefoxin for Injection . . . 1987

MEGACINA (Portugal)
OFLOXACIN
Floxin Otic Solution . . . 1043

MEGACORT (Italy)
DEXAMETHASONE SODIUM PHOSPHATE
Decadron Phosphate Injection . . . 1931

MEGADIN (Hong Kong)
CIMETIDINE
Tagamet Tablets . . . 1547

MEGAFLOX (Portugal)
CIPROFLOXACIN HYDROCHLORIDE
Ciloxan Ophthalmic Ointment . . . 554
Ciloxan Ophthalmic Solution . . . ⊙205
Cipro Tablets . . . 2991

MEGALAT (Israel)
NIFEDIPINE
Adalat CC Tablets . . . 2978

MEGALEX (Argentina)
RANITIDINE HYDROCHLORIDE
Zantac 25 EFFERdose Tablets . . . 1597
Zantac 150 EFFERdose Tablets . . . 1597
Zantac 150 Tablets . . . 1597
Zantac 300 Tablets . . . 1597
Zantac Injection . . . 1593
Zantac Injection Premixed . . . 1593
Zantac Syrup . . . 1597

MEGAPRESS (Greece)
ENALAPRIL MALEATE
Vasotec I.V. Injection . . . 2076

MEGASIN (Portugal)
OFLOXACIN
Floxin Otic Solution . . . 1043

MEGAVIS (Italy)
LEVOCARNITINE
Carnitor Injection . . . 3185
Carnitor Tablets and Oral Solution . . . 3187

MEGENTAL (Czech Republic)
GENTAMICIN SULFATE
Garamycin Injectable . . . 3028
Genoptic Sterile Ophthalmic Solution . . . ⊙227

MEGENTAL PEDIATRICO (Italy)
GENTAMICIN SULFATE
Garamycin Injectable . . . 3028
Genoptic Sterile Ophthalmic Solution . . . ⊙227

MEGION (Hungary)
CEFTRIAXONE SODIUM
Rocephin Injectable Vials, ADD-Vantage, Galaxy, Bulk . . . 2801

MELADININA (Mexico)
METHOXSALEN
Oxsoralen Lotion 1% . . . 3354
Oxsoralen-Ultra Capsules . . . 3354

MELADININE (France, Germany, Malaysia, Switzerland, Thailand, The Netherlands)
METHOXSALEN
Oxsoralen Lotion 1% . . . 3354
Oxsoralen-Ultra Capsules . . . 3354

MELANOCYL (India)
METHOXSALEN
Oxsoralen Lotion 1% . . . 3354
Oxsoralen-Ultra Capsules . . . 3354

MELAOLINE (Greece)
METHOXSALEN
Oxsoralen Lotion 1% . . . 3354
Oxsoralen-Ultra Capsules . . . 3354

MELAXOSE (France)
LACTULOSE
Kristalose for Oral Solution . . . 2149

MELERIL (Spain)
THIORIDAZINE HYDROCHLORIDE
Thioridazine Hydrochloride Tablets . . . 2122

MELGAR (Argentina)
NAPROXEN
EC-Naprosyn Delayed-Release Tablets . . . 2769
Naprosyn Suspension . . . 2769
Naprosyn Tablets . . . 2769

MELLERETTEN (Germany, The Netherlands)
THIORIDAZINE HYDROCHLORIDE
Thioridazine Hydrochloride Tablets . . . 2122

MELLERETTES (Switzerland)
THIORIDAZINE HYDROCHLORIDE
Thioridazine Hydrochloride Tablets . . . 2122

MELLERIL (Austria, Belgium, Brazil, Denmark, Finland, Greece, Hong Kong, Hungary, Irish Republic, Israel, Italy, Malaysia, New Zealand, Norway, Portugal, South Africa, Switzerland, The Netherlands)
THIORIDAZINE HYDROCHLORIDE
Thioridazine Hydrochloride Tablets . . . 2122

MELZINE (Irish Republic)
THIORIDAZINE HYDROCHLORIDE
Thioridazine Hydrochloride Tablets . . . 2122

MEMAC (Italy)
DONEPEZIL HYDROCHLORIDE
Aricept Tablets . . . 1086

MEMENTO NF (Argentina)
NORFLOXACIN
Noroxin Tablets . . . 2009

MENAELLE (Monaco)
PROGESTERONE
Prometrium Capsules (100 mg, 200 mg) . 3205

MENISOLE (Thailand)
METRONIDAZOLE
MetroGel-Vaginal Gel . . . 1822
Noritate Cream, 1% . . . 1051

MENOGRAINE (South Africa)
CLONIDINE HYDROCHLORIDE
Catapres Tablets . . . 874

MENO-IMPLANT (Belgium, The Netherlands)
ESTRADIOL
Climara Transdermal System . . . 795
Vivelle Transdermal System . . . 2288
Vivelle-Dot Transdermal System . . . 2293

MENO-PATCH (Israel)
ESTRADIOL
Climara Transdermal System . . . 795
Vivelle Transdermal System . . . 2288
Vivelle-Dot Transdermal System . . . 2293

MENOREST (Australia, Austria, Brazil, Czech Republic, Denmark, Finland, France, Germany, Greece, Irish Republic, Italy, Norway, Portugal, South Africa, Spain, Sweden, Switzerland, The Netherlands, United Kingdom)
ESTRADIOL
Climara Transdermal System . . . 795
Vivelle Transdermal System . . . 2288
Vivelle-Dot Transdermal System . . . 2293

MENSOMA (Portugal)
FAMOTIDINE
Pepcid Injection . . . 2017
Pepcid Injection Premixed . . . 2017
Pepcid Tablets . . . 2014
Pepcid for Oral Suspension . . . 2014

MENTAX (Brazil, Israel, Japan)
BUTENAFINE HYDROCHLORIDE
Mentax Cream . . . 2152

MEPAGYL (Thailand)
METRONIDAZOLE
MetroGel-Vaginal Gel . . . 1822
Noritate Cream, 1% . . . 1051

MEPASTAT (Finland)
MEDROXYPROGESTERONE ACETATE
Depo-Medrol Single-Dose Vial . . . 2617

MEPHAMESONE (Switzerland)
DEXAMETHASONE SODIUM PHOSPHATE
Decadron Phosphate Injection . . . 1931

MEPHAQUIN (Brazil, Czech Republic, Hong Kong, Israel, Malaysia, Portugal, Singapore, Thailand)
MEFLOQUINE HYDROCHLORIDE
Lariam Tablets . . . 2790

MEPHAQUINE (Switzerland)
MEFLOQUINE HYDROCHLORIDE
Lariam Tablets . . . 2790

MEPLAR (Argentina)
PAROXETINE HYDROCHLORIDE
Paxil Oral Suspension . . . 1501
Paxil Tablets . . . 1501

MEPRATE (India)
MEDROXYPROGESTERONE ACETATE
Depo-Medrol Single-Dose Vial . . . 2617

MEPRIL (Austria)
ENALAPRIL MALEATE
Vasotec I.V. Injection . . . 2076

MEPRON (Canada)
ATOVAQUONE
Mepron Suspension . . . 1487

MEQUIN (Thailand)
MEFLOQUINE HYDROCHLORIDE
Lariam Tablets . . . 2790

MERAPRIL (Italy)
CAPTOPRIL
Captopril Tablets . . . 2114

MERCAP (Germany)
MERCAPTOPURINE
Purinethol Tablets . . . 1222

MERCAPTINA (Brazil)
MERCAPTOPURINE
Purinethol Tablets . . . 1222

MERCAPTYL (Switzerland)
PENICILLAMINE
Cuprimine Capsules . . . 1925

MEREDAZOL (Mexico)
METRONIDAZOLE
MetroGel-Vaginal Gel . . . 1822
Noritate Cream, 1% . . . 1051

MEREPRINE (Portugal)
CAPTOPRIL
Captopril Tablets . . . 2114

MERIDIA (Austria, Canada)
SIBUTRAMINE HYDROCHLORIDE
Meridia Capsules . . . 485

MERLIT (Greece)
LEVOCARNITINE
Carnitor Injection . . . 3185
Carnitor Tablets and Oral Solution . . . 3187

MERONEM (Belgium, Brazil, Chile, Czech Republic, Denmark, Finland, Germany, Greece, Hong Kong, Hungary, Irish Republic, Israel, Malaysia, Norway, Portugal, Russia, Singapore, South Africa, Spain, Sweden, Switzerland, Thailand, The Netherlands, United Kingdom)
MEROPENEM
Merrem I.V. . . . 687

MEROPEN (Japan)
MEROPENEM
Merrem I.V. . . . 687

MEROZEN (Argentina)
MEROPENEM
Merrem I.V. . . . 687

MERREM (Australia, Canada, Italy, Mexico, New Zealand)
MEROPENEM
Merrem I.V. . . . 687

MERTAN (Austria)
NAPHAZOLINE HYDROCHLORIDE
Albalon Ophthalmic Solution . . . ⊙216

MERXIL (Mexico)
DICLOFENAC SODIUM
Voltaren Tablets . . . 2298
Voltaren-XR Tablets . . . 2301

MESACTOL (Argentina)
LANSOPRAZOLE
Prevacid Delayed-Release Capsules . . . 3268

MESIN (Thailand)
ALBENDAZOLE
Albenza Tablets . . . 1310

M-ESLON (Canada, Chile, Czech Republic, Hong Kong, Hungary)
MORPHINE SULFATE
Kadian Capsules . . . 572
MS Contin Tablets . . . 2703

MESOLEX (Thailand)
METRONIDAZOLE
MetroGel-Vaginal Gel . . . 1822
Noritate Cream, 1% . . . 1051

MESONEX (Greece)
ATENOLOL
Tenormin I.V. Injection . . . 698

MESPORIN (Hong Kong, Malaysia, Portugal)
CEFTRIAXONE SODIUM
Rocephin Injectable Vials, ADD-Vantage, Galaxy, Bulk . . . 2801

META (Thailand)
PROMETHAZINE HYDROCHLORIDE
Phenergan Suppositories . . . 3438
Phenergan Tablets . . . 3438

METADATE (Israel)
METHYLPHENIDATE HYDROCHLORIDE
Ritalin Hydrochloride Tablets . . . 2254
Ritalin-SR Tablets . . . 2254

METAFLEX NF (Argentina)
DICLOFENAC POTASSIUM
Cataflam Tablets . . . 2173

METAFLEX PLUS NF (Argentina)
DICLOFENAC SODIUM
Voltaren Tablets . . . 2298
Voltaren-XR Tablets . . . 2301

METAGYL (South Africa)
METRONIDAZOLE
MetroGel-Vaginal Gel . . . 1822
Noritate Cream, 1% . . . 1051

METALCAPTASE (Czech Republic, Germany, Japan, South Africa)
PENICILLAMINE
Cuprimine Capsules . . . 1925

METAMIDOL (Portugal)
DIAZEPAM
Diastat Rectal Delivery System . . . 3344
Valium Tablets . . . 2822

METAPTYL (Greece)
CEFOXITIN SODIUM
Mefoxin Premixed Intravenous Solution . . . 1990
Mefoxin for Injection . . . 1987

METASON (Argentina)
MOMETASONE FUROATE
Elocon Cream 0.1% . . . 3019
Elocon Lotion 0.1% . . . 3020
Elocon Ointment 0.1% . . . 3021
Nasonex Nasal Spray . . . 3058

METASPRAY (India)
MOMETASONE FUROATE
Elocon Cream 0.1% . . . 3019
Elocon Lotion 0.1% . . . 3020
Elocon Ointment 0.1% . . . 3021
Nasonex Nasal Spray . . . 3058

METAZEM (Hong Kong, Singapore, Thailand, United Kingdom)
DILTIAZEM HYDROCHLORIDE
Cardizem LA Extended Release Tablets . . . 1699
Tiazac Capsules . . . 1204

METAZOL (South Africa)
METRONIDAZOLE
MetroGel-Vaginal Gel . . . 1822
Noritate Cream, 1% . . . 1051

METHYLIN (Argentina)
METHYLPHENIDATE HYDROCHLORIDE
Ritalin Hydrochloride Tablets 2254
Ritalin-SR Tablets 2254

METICEL (Spain)
RANITIDINE HYDROCHLORIDE
Zantac 25 EFFERdose Tablets 1597
Zantac 150 EFFERdose Tablets 1597
Zantac 150 Tablets 1597
Zantac 300 Tablets 1597
Zantac Injection 1593
Zantac Injection Premixed 1593
Zantac Syrup 1597

METIFEX-L (Germany)
LOPERAMIDE HYDROCHLORIDE
Imodium Capsules 1834

METILBETASONE SOLUBILE (Italy)
METHYLPREDNISOLONE ACETATE
Depo-Medrol Injectable Suspension 2615

METIMYD (Canada, Sweden)
PREDNISOLONE ACETATE/SULFACETAMIDE SODIUM
Blephamide Ophthalmic Ointment 563
Blephamide Ophthalmic Suspension 564

METINET (Denmark)
CIMETIDINE
Tagamet Tablets 1547

METLIGINE (Japan)
MIDODRINE HYDROCHLORIDE
ProAmatine Tablets 3183

METOLE (Hong Kong)
METRONIDAZOLE
MetroGel-Vaginal Gel 1822
Noritate Cream, 1% 1051

METORAL (Thailand)
TRIAMCINOLONE ACETONIDE
Azmacort Inhalation Aerosol 1701
Nasacort AQ Nasal Spray 2937

METRAL (Argentina)
METRONIDAZOLE
MetroGel-Vaginal Gel 1822
Noritate Cream, 1% 1051

METRAZOLE (South Africa, Thailand)
METRONIDAZOLE
MetroGel-Vaginal Gel 1822
Noritate Cream, 1% 1051

METRICOM (Mexico)
METRONIDAZOLE
MetroGel-Vaginal Gel 1822
Noritate Cream, 1% 1051

METRIZOL (Mexico, Switzerland)
METRONIDAZOLE
MetroGel-Vaginal Gel 1822
Noritate Cream, 1% 1051

METROCEV (Argentina)
METRONIDAZOLE
MetroGel-Vaginal Gel 1822
Noritate Cream, 1% 1051

METROCIDE (Thailand)
METRONIDAZOLE
MetroGel-Vaginal Gel 1822
Noritate Cream, 1% 1051

METROCREAM (Canada. Chile, Mexico)
METRONIDAZOLE
MetroGel-Vaginal Gel 1822
Noritate Cream, 1% 1051

METROCREME (Germany)
METRONIDAZOLE
MetroGel-Vaginal Gel 1822
Noritate Cream, 1% 1051

METRODAX (Brazil)
METRONIDAZOLE
MetroGel-Vaginal Gel 1822
Noritate Cream, 1% 1051

METRODERME (Portugal)
METRONIDAZOLE
MetroGel-Vaginal Gel 1822
Noritate Cream, 1% 1051

METROFUR (Mexico)
METRONIDAZOLE
MetroGel-Vaginal Gel 1822
Noritate Cream, 1% 1051

METROGEL (Canada, Chile, Denmark, Germany, Irish Republic, Mexico, The Netherlands, United Kingdom)
METRONIDAZOLE
MetroGel-Vaginal Gel 1822
Noritate Cream, 1% 1051

METROGYL (Australia, Greece, Hong Kong, India, Israel)
METRONIDAZOLE
MetroGel-Vaginal Gel 1822
Noritate Cream, 1% 1051

METROLEX (Thailand)
METRONIDAZOLE
MetroGel-Vaginal Gel 1822
Noritate Cream, 1% 1051

METROLYL (United Kingdom)
METRONIDAZOLE
MetroGel-Vaginal Gel 1822
Noritate Cream, 1% 1051

METRONIB (Brazil)
METRONIDAZOLE
MetroGel-Vaginal Gel 1822
Noritate Cream, 1% 1051

METRONIDE (Australia, Brazil, Irish Republic)
METRONIDAZOLE
MetroGel-Vaginal Gel 1822
Noritate Cream, 1% 1051

METRONID-PUREN (Germany)
METRONIDAZOLE
MetroGel-Vaginal Gel 1822
Noritate Cream, 1% 1051

METRONIMERCK (Germany)
METRONIDAZOLE
MetroGel-Vaginal Gel 1822
Noritate Cream, 1% 1051

METRONIX (Brazil)
METRONIDAZOLE
MetroGel-Vaginal Gel 1822
Noritate Cream, 1% 1051

METRONOM (Austria)
PROPAFENONE HYDROCHLORIDE
Rythmol SR Capsules 2736

METRONOUR (Germany)
METRONIDAZOLE
MetroGel-Vaginal Gel 1822
Noritate Cream, 1% 1051

METRONT (Germany)
METRONIDAZOLE
MetroGel-Vaginal Gel 1822
Noritate Cream, 1% 1051

METROPAST (Chile)
METRONIDAZOLE
MetroGel-Vaginal Gel 1822
Noritate Cream, 1% 1051

METROSA (United Kingdom)
METRONIDAZOLE
MetroGel-Vaginal Gel 1822
Noritate Cream, 1% 1051

METROSON (Mexico)
METRONIDAZOLE
MetroGel-Vaginal Gel 1822
Noritate Cream, 1% 1051

METROSTAT (South Africa)
METRONIDAZOLE
MetroGel-Vaginal Gel 1822
Noritate Cream, 1% 1051

METROTOP (Irish Republic, United Kingdom)
METRONIDAZOLE
MetroGel-Vaginal Gel 1822
Noritate Cream, 1% 1051

METROVAL (Brazil)
METRONIDAZOLE
MetroGel-Vaginal Gel 1822
Noritate Cream, 1% 1051

METROZINE (Australia, Hong Kong)
METRONIDAZOLE
MetroGel-Vaginal Gel 1822
Noritate Cream, 1% 1051

METROZOL (Brazil, United Kingdom)
METRONIDAZOLE
MetroGel-Vaginal Gel 1822
Noritate Cream, 1% 1051

METROZOLE (Singapore)
METRONIDAZOLE
MetroGel-Vaginal Gel 1822
Noritate Cream, 1% 1051

METRYL (South Africa)
METRONIDAZOLE
MetroGel-Vaginal Gel 1822
Noritate Cream, 1% 1051

MEVACOR (Austria, Brazil, Canada, Czech Republic, Denmark, Finland, Greece, Hong Kong, Hungary, Malaysia, Mexico, Norway, Spain)
LOVASTATIN
Mevacor Tablets 1996

MEVAL (Canada)
DIAZEPAM
Diastat Rectal Delivery System 3344
Valium Tablets 2822

MEVALOTIN (Brazil, Germany, Japan, Switzerland, Thailand)
PRAVASTATIN SODIUM
Pravachol Tablets 943

MEVAMYST (Greece)
LEVOCARNITINE
Carnitor Injection 3185
Carnitor Tablets and Oral Solution 3187

MEVASTEROL (Spain)
LOVASTATIN
Mevacor Tablets 1996

MEVASTIN (Greece)
LOVASTATIN
Mevacor Tablets 1996

MEVECAN (Greece)
CEFUROXIME AXETIL
Ceftin Tablets 1369
Ceftin for Oral Suspension 1369

MEVEDAL (Greece)
NABUMETONE
Relafen Tablets 1523

MEVINACOR (Germany, Portugal)
LOVASTATIN
Mevacor Tablets 1996

MEVINOL (Greece)
LOVASTATIN
Mevacor Tablets 1996

MEVLOR (Argentina, Portugal)
LOVASTATIN
Mevacor Tablets 1996

MEXASONE (Singapore)
DEXAMETHASONE
Decadron Tablets 1929

MEXCYN (Mexico)
ERYTHROMYCIN
Ery-Tab Tablets 447
Erythromycin Base Filmtab Tablets 454
Erythromycin Delayed-Release Capsules, USP 456
PCE Dispertab Tablets 510

MEXONA (Mexico)
DEXAMETHASONE
Decadron Tablets 1929

MEZARID (Greece)
ATENOLOL
Tenormin I.V. Injection 698

M-FLOX (Thailand)
NORFLOXACIN
Noroxin Tablets 2009

MIBAZOL (Mexico)
METRONIDAZOLE
MetroGel-Vaginal Gel 1822
Noritate Cream, 1% 1051

MICARDIS (Argentina, Australia, Austria, Belgium, Brazil, Canada, Chile, Czech Republic, Denmark, Finland, France, Germany, Greece, Hong Kong, Hungary, Irish Republic, Italy, Japan, Malaysia, Mexico, Norway, Portugal, Russia, Singapore, South Africa, Spain, Sweden, Switzerland, Thailand, The Netherlands, United Kingdom)
TELMISARTAN
Micardis Tablets 884

MICARDIS PLUS (Australia, Canada, Hong Kong, Italy, Malaysia, Portugal, Singapore, Spain, Sweden, The Netherlands)
TELMISARTAN
Micardis Tablets 884

MICARDISPLUS (Austria, Belgium, Denmark, Finland, France, Germany, Irish Republic, Norway, Switzerland, United Kingdom)
TELMISARTAN
Micardis Tablets 884

MICLONAZOL (Brazil)
CLOTRIMAZOLE
Lotrimin Cream 3053
Lotrimin Lotion 1% 3053
Lotrimin Topical Solution 1% 3053

MICOBAN (Greece)
MUPIROCIN
Bactroban Ointment 1358

MICOCIDE (Argentina)
ECONAZOLE NITRATE
Spectazole Cream 2390

MICOCLIN (Argentina)
CLOTRIMAZOLE
Lotrimin Cream 3053
Lotrimin Lotion 1% 3053
Lotrimin Topical Solution 1% 3053

MICOESPEC (Spain)
ECONAZOLE NITRATE
Spectazole Cream 2390

MICOESPEC K (Argentina)
KETOCONAZOLE
Nizoral 2% Shampoo 1838

MICOFITEX (Argentina)
ECONAZOLE NITRATE
Spectazole Cream 2390

MICOGAL (Mexico)
KETOCONAZOLE
Nizoral 2% Shampoo 1838

MICOGIN (Italy)
ECONAZOLE NITRATE
Spectazole Cream 2390

MICOLIS (Argentina, Chile)
ECONAZOLE NITRATE
Spectazole Cream 2390

MICOMAX (Argentina)
CLOTRIMAZOLE
Lotrimin Cream 3053
Lotrimin Lotion 1% 3053
Lotrimin Topical Solution 1% 3053

MICOMAZOL (Argentina)
CLOTRIMAZOLE
Lotrimin Cream 3053
Lotrimin Lotion 1% 3053
Lotrimin Topical Solution 1% 3053

MICOMAZOL B (Argentina)
CLOTRIMAZOLE
Lotrimin Cream 3053
Lotrimin Lotion 1% 3053
Lotrimin Topical Solution 1% 3053

MICOMAZOL DEO (Argentina)
CLOTRIMAZOLE
Lotrimin Cream 3053
Lotrimin Lotion 1% 3053
Lotrimin Topical Solution 1% 3053

MICOMISAN (South Africa, Spain)
CLOTRIMAZOLE
Lotrimin Cream 3053
Lotrimin Lotion 1% 3053
Lotrimin Topical Solution 1% 3053

MICONACINA (Mexico)
NATAMYCIN
Natacyn Antifungal Ophthalmic Suspension . . . . ⊙207

MICONAN (Brazil)
KETOCONAZOLE
Nizoral 2% Shampoo 1838

MICORAL (Argentina, Brazil)
KETOCONAZOLE
Nizoral 2% Shampoo 1838

MICOSEP (Argentina)
CLOTRIMAZOLE
Lotrimin Cream 3053

(⊙ Described in PDR For Ophthalmic Medicines™)

Lotrimin Lotion 1% 3053
Lotrimin Topical Solution 1% 3053

MICOSEP B (Argentina)
CLOTRIMAZOLE
Lotrimin Cream 3053
Lotrimin Lotion 1% 3053
Lotrimin Topical Solution 1% 3053

MICOSEPTIL (Spain)
ECONAZOLE NITRATE
Spectazole Cream 2390

MICOSER (Mexico)
KETOCONAZOLE
Nizoral 2% Shampoo 1838

MICOSET (Chile)
TERBINAFINE HYDROCHLORIDE
Lamisil Tablets 2226

MICOSIL (Brazil)
TERBINAFINE HYDROCHLORIDE
Lamisil Tablets 2226

MICOSONA (Spain)
NAFTIFINE HYDROCHLORIDE
Naftin Cream 2097
Naftin Gel 2097

MICOSTATIN (Argentina, Brazil, Chile, Mexico)
NYSTATIN
Nystop Topical Powder USP 2490

MICOSTEN (Brazil, Italy)
CLOTRIMAZOLE
Lotrimin Cream 3053
Lotrimin Lotion 1% 3053
Lotrimin Topical Solution 1% 3053

MICOSTOP (Chile)
TERBINAFINE HYDROCHLORIDE
Lamisil Tablets 2226

MICOSTYL (Brazil, Mexico)
ECONAZOLE NITRATE
Spectazole Cream 2390

MICOTER (Malaysia, Spain)
CLOTRIMAZOLE
Lotrimin Cream 3053
Lotrimin Lotion 1% 3053
Lotrimin Topical Solution 1% 3053

MICOTICUM (Spain)
KETOCONAZOLE
Nizoral 2% Shampoo 1838

MICOTRAT (Brazil)
CLOTRIMAZOLE
Lotrimin Cream 3053
Lotrimin Lotion 1% 3053
Lotrimin Topical Solution 1% 3053

MICOTRIM (Argentina)
CLOTRIMAZOLE
Lotrimin Cream 3053
Lotrimin Lotion 1% 3053
Lotrimin Topical Solution 1% 3053

MICOTRIZOL (Brazil)
CLOTRIMAZOLE
Lotrimin Cream 3053
Lotrimin Lotion 1% 3053
Lotrimin Topical Solution 1% 3053

MICRANIL (Argentina)
SUMATRIPTAN SUCCINATE
Imitrex Injection 1431
Imitrex Tablets 1440

MICRO-K (Canada, South Africa)
POTASSIUM CHLORIDE
K-Dur Extended-Relase Tablets 3047
K-Lor Powder Packets 472
K-Tab Filmtab Tablets 473

MICROKALEORID (France)
POTASSIUM CHLORIDE
K-Dur Extended-Relase Tablets 3047
K-Lor Powder Packets 472
K-Tab Filmtab Tablets 473

MICRO-KALIUM (Austria)
POTASSIUM CHLORIDE
K-Dur Extended-Relase Tablets 3047
K-Lor Powder Packets 472
K-Tab Filmtab Tablets 473

MICRONOAN (Italy)
DIAZEPAM
Diastat Rectal Delivery System 3344
Valium Tablets 2822

MICROPHYLLIN (South Africa)
THEOPHYLLINE
Uniphyl Tablets 2708

MICRORGAN (Mexico)
CIPROFLOXACIN HYDROCHLORIDE
Ciloxan Ophthalmic Ointment 554
Ciloxan Ophthalmic Solution . . . . ⊙205
Cipro Tablets 2991

MICROSONA (Argentina)
HYDROCORTISONE
Hydrocortone Tablets 1963

MICROSONA OTICA (Argentina)
HYDROCORTISONE
Hydrocortone Tablets 1963

MICROSULF (Argentina)
CIPROFLOXACIN HYDROCHLORIDE
Ciloxan Ophthalmic Ointment 554
Ciloxan Ophthalmic Solution . . . . ⊙205
Cipro Tablets 2991

MICROXIN (Mexico)
NORFLOXACIN
Noroxin Tablets 2009

MIDAMOR (Australia, Austria, Canada, Hong Kong, New Zealand, Norway, Sweden, Switzerland, The Netherlands, United Kingdom)
AMILORIDE HYDROCHLORIDE
Midamor Tablets 2000

MIDAX (Argentina)
OLANZAPINE
Zyprexa Tablets 1798

MIDON (Irish Republic)
MIDODRINE HYDROCHLORIDE
ProAmatine Tablets 3183

MIDORIDE (Australia)
AMILORIDE HYDROCHLORIDE
Midamor Tablets 2000

MIDRAN (Italy, South Africa)
APROTININ
Trasylol Injection 779

MIDRAT (Mexico)
CAPTOPRIL
Captopril Tablets 2114

MIDURET (Thailand)
AMILORIDE HYDROCHLORIDE/HYDROCHLOROTHIAZIDE
Moduretic Tablets 2003

MIELUCIN (Brazil)
BUSULFAN
Myleran Tablets 1492

MIGRIL (Brazil)
SUMATRIPTAN SUCCINATE
Imitrex Injection 1431
Imitrex Tablets 1440

MI-KE-SONS (Mexico)
KETOCONAZOLE
Nizoral 2% Shampoo 1838

MIKETOS (Mexico)
KETOCONAZOLE
Nizoral 2% Shampoo 1838

MIKOSTAT (United Arab Emirates)
NYSTATIN
Nystop Topical Powder USP 2490

MIKOSTAT BABY OINTMENT (United Arab Emirates)
NYSTATIN
Nystop Topical Powder USP 2490

MILAMET (Thailand)
CIMETIDINE
Tagamet Tablets 1547

MILANIDAZOLE (Thailand)
METRONIDAZOLE
MetroGel-Vaginal Gel 1822
Noritate Cream, 1% 1051

MILANOLONE (Thailand)
TRIAMCINOLONE ACETONIDE
Azmacort Inhalation Aerosol 1701
Nasacort AQ Nasal Spray 2937

MILDISON (Denmark, Finland, Irish Republic, Norway, Sweden, The Netherlands, United Kingdom)
HYDROCORTISONE
Hydrocortone Tablets 1963

MILICAL (Chile)
SIBUTRAMINE HYDROCHLORIDE
Meridia Capsules 485

MILITHIN (Greece)
LITHIUM CARBONATE
Eskalith CR Controlled-Release Tablets 1406
Eskalith Capsules 1406

MILLIBAR (Hong Kong, Italy, Singapore)
INDAPAMIDE
Indapamide Tablets 2119

MILLICORTENE (Switzerland)
DEXAMETHASONE
Decadron Tablets 1929

MILLICORTENOL (India)
DEXAMETHASONE
Decadron Tablets 1929

MILODERME (Portugal)
ALCLOMETASONE DIPROPIONATE
Aclovate Cream 1290
Aclovate Ointment 1290

MILOREX (Thailand)
AMILORIDE HYDROCHLORIDE/HYDROCHLOROTHIAZIDE
Moduretic Tablets 2003

MILORIDE (Finland)
AMILORIDE HYDROCHLORIDE/HYDROCHLOROTHIAZIDE
Moduretic Tablets 2003

MINARTINE (Greece)
LEVOCARNITINE
Carnitor Injection 3185
Carnitor Tablets and Oral Solution 3187

MINDOL (New Zealand)
MEBENDAZOLE
Vermox Chewable Tablets 1853

MINEGYL (Brazil)
METRONIDAZOLE
MetroGel-Vaginal Gel 1822
Noritate Cream, 1% 1051

MINEGYL C/NISTATINA (Brazil)
METRONIDAZOLE
MetroGel-Vaginal Gel 1822
Noritate Cream, 1% 1051

MINIBLOCK (India)
ESMOLOL HYDROCHLORIDE
Brevibloc Injection 766

MINICAM (Argentina)
LOPERAMIDE HYDROCHLORIDE
Imodium Capsules 1834

MINIDEX (Brazil)
DEXAMETHASONE
Decadron Tablets 1929

MINIOSTENIL (Argentina)
SODIUM HYALURONATE
Hyalgan Solution 2917

MINIRIN (Australia, Austria, Belgium, Canada, Czech Republic, Denmark, Finland, France, Germany, Greece, Hong Kong, Hungary, Israel, Malaysia, Mexico, Norway, Portugal, Russia, Singapore, Sweden, Switzerland, Thailand)
DESMOPRESSIN ACETATE
DDAVP Injection 4 mcg/mL 2893
DDAVP Nasal Spray 2894
DDAVP Tablets 2895
Desmopressin Acetate Injection 1143
Desmopressin Acetate Rhinal Tube 1144

MINIRIN/DDAVP (Italy)
DESMOPRESSIN ACETATE
DDAVP Injection 4 mcg/mL 2893
DDAVP Nasal Spray 2894
DDAVP Tablets 2895
Desmopressin Acetate Injection 1143
Desmopressin Acetate Rhinal Tube 1144

MINOBESE (South Africa)
PHENTERMINE HYDROCHLORIDE
Adipex-P Capsules 1216
Adipex-P Tablets 1216

MINOR (Brazil)
LOVASTATIN
Mevacor Tablets 1996

MINOREMED (Germany)
AMILORIDE HYDROCHLORIDE/HYDROCHLOROTHIAZIDE
Moduretic Tablets 2003

MINPROG (Austria, Germany)
ALPROSTADIL
Edex Injection 3103

MINPROSTIN (Denmark, Finland, Norway, Sweden)
DINOPROSTONE
Cervidil Vaginal Insert 1182

MINPROSTIN E2 (Germany)
DINOPROSTONE
Cervidil Vaginal Insert 1182

MINRIN (The Netherlands)
DESMOPRESSIN ACETATE
DDAVP Injection 4 mcg/mL 2893
DDAVP Nasal Spray 2894
DDAVP Tablets 2895
Desmopressin Acetate Injection 1143
Desmopressin Acetate Rhinal Tube 1144

MINUSLIP (Argentina)
FENOFIBRATE
Tricor Tablets 523

MINUSORB (Brazil)
ALENDRONATE SODIUM
Fosamax Tablets 1949

MIOCALM (Argentina)
DICLOFENAC SODIUM
Voltaren Tablets 2298
Voltaren-XR Tablets 2301

MIOCARDIN (Italy)
LEVOCARNITINE
Carnitor Injection 3185
Carnitor Tablets and Oral Solution 3187

MIOCOR (Italy)
LEVOCARNITINE
Carnitor Injection 3185
Carnitor Tablets and Oral Solution 3187

MIOCORON (Brazil)
AMIODARONE HYDROCHLORIDE
Pacerone Tablets 3337

MIODARID (Brazil)
AMIODARONE HYDROCHLORIDE
Pacerone Tablets 3337

MIODARON (Brazil)
AMIODARONE HYDROCHLORIDE
Pacerone Tablets 3337

MIODRONE (Portugal)
AMIODARONE HYDROCHLORIDE
Pacerone Tablets 3337

MIOPOTASIO (Spain)
POTASSIUM CHLORIDE
K-Dur Extended-Relase Tablets 3047
K-Lor Powder Packets 472
K-Tab Filmtab Tablets 473

MIOSEN (Spain)
DIPYRIDAMOLE
Persantine Tablets 898

MIOTENK (Argentina)
AMIODARONE HYDROCHLORIDE
Pacerone Tablets 3337

MIOTONAL (Italy)
LEVOCARNITINE
Carnitor Injection 3185
Carnitor Tablets and Oral Solution 3187

MIO-VIROBRON NF (Argentina)
DICLOFENAC SODIUM
Voltaren Tablets 2298
Voltaren-XR Tablets 2301

MIPHAR (Israel)
FUROSEMIDE
Furosemide Tablets 2117

MIQUIMOD (Argentina)
IMIQUIMOD
Aldara Cream, 5% 1814

MIR (Israel)
MORPHINE SULFATE
Kadian Capsules 572
MS Contin Tablets 2703

MIRACLAR (Spain)
NAPHAZOLINE HYDROCHLORIDE
Albalon Ophthalmic Solution . . . . ⊙216

MIRAMYCIN (Hong Kong, Malaysia, Singapore, Thailand)
GENTAMICIN SULFATE
Garamycin Injectable 3028
Genoptic Sterile Ophthalmic Solution . . . . ⊙227

MIRANAX (Austria, Denmark, Finland, Sweden)
NAPROXEN SODIUM
Anaprox DS Tablets 2769
Anaprox Tablets 2769

MIRASAN (Argentina)
NAPHAZOLINE HYDROCHLORIDE
Albalon Ophthalmic Solution . . . . . ⊙216

MIRATON (Malaysia)
LOPERAMIDE HYDROCHLORIDE
Imodium Capsules 1834

MIRETIC (Thailand)
AMILORIDE HYDROCHLORIDE/HYDROCHLOROTHIAZIDE
Moduretic Tablets 2003

MIRFAT (Germany)
CLONIDINE HYDROCHLORIDE
Catapres Tablets 874

MIRUS-S (Argentina)
NAPHAZOLINE HYDROCHLORIDE
Albalon Ophthalmic Solution . . . . . ⊙216

MISODOMIN (Greece)
LOVASTATIN
Mevacor Tablets 1996

MISOFENAC (Italy)
DICLOFENAC SODIUM
Voltaren Tablets 2298
Voltaren-XR Tablets 2301

MISORDIL (Argentina)
ISOSORBIDE MONONITRATE
Imdur Tablets 3032

MISULBAN (Italy, Monaco)
BUSULFAN
Myleran Tablets 1492

MITEN (Spain)
VALSARTAN
Diovan Tablets 2191

MITEN PLUS (Spain)
VALSARTAN
Diovan Tablets 2191

MITE-X (Israel)
PERMETHRIN
Acticin Cream 2125

MITOCORTYL (France)
HYDROCORTISONE
Hydrocortone Tablets 1963

MITROKEN (Mexico)
CIPROFLOXACIN HYDROCHLORIDE
Ciloxan Ophthalmic Ointment 554
Ciloxan Ophthalmic Solution . . . . . ⊙205
Cipro Tablets 2991

MIVACRON (Argentina, Australia, Austria, Belgium, Brazil, Canada, Chile, Czech Republic, Denmark, Finland, France, Germany, Greece, Hong Kong, Hungary, Irish Republic, Israel, Italy, Malaysia, Mexico, New Zealand, Norway, Portugal, Singapore, South Africa, Spain, Sweden, Switzerland, Thailand, The Netherlands, United Kingdom)
MIVACURIUM CHLORIDE
Mivacron Injection 489

MIVALEN (Brazil)
SIMVASTATIN
Zocor Tablets 2078

MIXCILIN (Argentina)
AMOXICILLIN
Amoxil Pediatric Drops for Oral Suspension 1315
Amoxil Tablets 1315

MIXER (Italy)
ATENOLOL
Tenormin I.V. Injection 698

MIZOLMEX (Mexico)
MEBENDAZOLE
Vermox Chewable Tablets 1853

MIZORON (Thailand)
KETOCONAZOLE
Nizoral 2% Shampoo 1838

M-LONG (Austria, Germany)
MORPHINE SULFATE
Kadian Capsules 572
MS Contin Tablets 2703

MND (Singapore)
METRONIDAZOLE
MetroGel-Vaginal Gel 1822
Noritate Cream, 1% 1051

MOBAN (Hong Kong)
MOLINDONE HYDROCHLORIDE
Moban Tablets 1108

MOBEN (Brazil)
MEBENDAZOLE
Vermox Chewable Tablets 1853

MODAMIDE (France)
AMILORIDE HYDROCHLORIDE
Midamor Tablets 2000

MODAPLATE (United Kingdom)
DIPYRIDAMOLE
Persantine Tablets 898

MODASOMIL (Austria, Switzerland)
MODAFINIL
Provigil Tablets 1002

MODAVIGIL (Australia, New Zealand)
MODAFINIL
Provigil Tablets 1002

MODIFENAC (Denmark, Norway, Sweden)
DICLOFENAC SODIUM
Voltaren Tablets 2298
Voltaren-XR Tablets 2301

MODIFICAL (Brazil)
ONDANSETRON HYDROCHLORIDE
Zofran Injection 1607
Zofran Injection Premixed 1607
Zofran Oral Solution 1613
Zofran Tablets 1613

MODINA (Portugal)
NIMODIPINE
Nimotop Capsules 774

MODINOL (Greece)
RIZATRIPTAN BENZOATE
Maxalt Tablets 1983
Maxalt-MLT Orally Disintegrating Tablets . . 1983

MODIODAL (Denmark, France, Greece, Norway, Portugal, Spain, Sweden, The Netherlands)
MODAFINIL
Provigil Tablets 1002

MODIP (Germany)
FELODIPINE
Plendil Extended-Release Tablets 651

MODISAL (Switzerland, United Kingdom)
ISOSORBIDE MONONITRATE
Imdur Tablets 3032

MODIZIDE (Australia)
AMILORIDE HYDROCHLORIDE/HYDROCHLOROTHIAZIDE
Moduretic Tablets 2003

MODRADERM (Belgium)
ALCLOMETASONE DIPROPIONATE
Aclovate Cream 1290
Aclovate Ointment 1290

MODRASONE (Irish Republic, United Kingdom)
ALCLOMETASONE DIPROPIONATE
Aclovate Cream 1290
Aclovate Ointment 1290

MODUCREN (United Kingdom)
AMILORIDE HYDROCHLORIDE/HYDROCHLOROTHIAZIDE
Moduretic Tablets 2003

MODUL'AID (France)
PERMETHRIN
Acticin Cream 2125

MODULAN (Thailand)
AMILORIDE HYDROCHLORIDE
Midamor Tablets 2000

MODU-PUREN (Germany)
AMILORIDE HYDROCHLORIDE/HYDROCHLOROTHIAZIDE
Moduretic Tablets 2003

MODURET (Canada, Irish Republic, United Kingdom)
AMILORIDE HYDROCHLORIDE/HYDROCHLOROTHIAZIDE
Moduretic Tablets 2003

MODURETIC (Argentina, Australia, Austria, Belgium, Brazil, Czech Republic, Denmark, Finland, France, Greece, Hong Kong, Irish Republic, Italy, Malaysia, Mexico, New Zealand, Norway, Portugal, South Africa, Sweden, Switzerland, Thailand, The Netherlands, United Kingdom)
AMILORIDE HYDROCHLORIDE
Midamor Tablets 2000

MODURETIK (Germany)
AMILORIDE HYDROCHLORIDE/HYDROCHLOROTHIAZIDE
Moduretic Tablets 2003

MODUS (Spain)
NIMODIPINE
Nimotop Capsules 774

MOEX (Czech Republic, Denmark, France, Hong Kong)
MOEXIPRIL HYDROCHLORIDE
Univasc Tablets 3118

MOGETIC (Germany)
MORPHINE SULFATE
Kadian Capsules 572
MS Contin Tablets 2703

MOKCAN (India)
AMOXICILLIN
Amoxil Pediatric Drops for Oral Suspension 1315
Amoxil Tablets 1315

MOLAGAR (Argentina)
LEFLUNOMIDE
Arava Tablets 2881

MOMATE (India)
MOMETASONE FUROATE
Elocon Cream 0.1% 3019
Elocon Lotion 0.1% 3020
Elocon Ointment 0.1% 3021
Nasonex Nasal Spray 3058

MOMATE-S (India)
MOMETASONE FUROATE
Elocon Cream 0.1% 3019
Elocon Lotion 0.1% 3020
Elocon Ointment 0.1% 3021
Nasonex Nasal Spray 3058

MOMEN (Spain)
NAPROXEN
EC-Naprosyn Delayed-Release Tablets 2769
Naprosyn Suspension 2769
Naprosyn Tablets 2769

MOMENDOL (Italy, Portugal)
NAPROXEN SODIUM
Anaprox DS Tablets 2769
Anaprox Tablets 2769

MONARIT (Argentina)
NAPROXEN SODIUM
Anaprox DS Tablets 2769
Anaprox Tablets 2769

MONASIN (Switzerland)
METRONIDAZOLE
MetroGel-Vaginal Gel 1822
Noritate Cream, 1% 1051

MONAXIN (Belgium)
CLARITHROMYCIN
Biaxin Filmtab Tablets 402
Biaxin Granules 402

MONDRIAN (Chile)
BUPROPION HYDROCHLORIDE
Wellbutrin SR Sustained-Release Tablets . . . 1583
Wellbutrin Tablets 1579
Zyban Sustained-Release Tablets 1620

MONICOR (France, India)
ISOSORBIDE MONONITRATE
Imdur Tablets 3032

MONIGEN (United Kingdom)
ISOSORBIDE MONONITRATE
Imdur Tablets 3032

MONILAC (Japan)
LACTULOSE
Kristalose for Oral Solution 2149

MONI-SANORANIA (Germany)
ISOSORBIDE MONONITRATE
Imdur Tablets 3032

MONISOL (Russia)
ISOSORBIDE MONONITRATE
Imdur Tablets 3032

MONIT (United Kingdom)
ISOSORBIDE MONONITRATE
Imdur Tablets 3032

MONIT-PUREN (Germany)
ISOSORBIDE MONONITRATE
Imdur Tablets 3032

MONIZOLE (India)
METRONIDAZOLE
MetroGel-Vaginal Gel 1822
Noritate Cream, 1% 1051

MONO ACIS (Germany)
ISOSORBIDE MONONITRATE
Imdur Tablets 3032

MONO BAYCUTEN (Germany)
CLOTRIMAZOLE
Lotrimin Cream 3053
Lotrimin Lotion 1% 3053
Lotrimin Topical Solution 1% 3053

MONO CORAX (Germany)
ISOSORBIDE MONONITRATE
Imdur Tablets 3032

MONO MACK (Austria, Chile, Czech Republic, Germany, Hong Kong, Hungary, Mexico, Singapore, South Africa, Thailand, The Netherlands)
ISOSORBIDE MONONITRATE
Imdur Tablets 3032

MONO WOLFF (Germany)
ISOSORBIDE MONONITRATE
Imdur Tablets 3032

MONO-A (India)
ISOSORBIDE MONONITRATE
Imdur Tablets 3032

MONOBETA (Germany)
ISOSORBIDE MONONITRATE
Imdur Tablets 3032

MONOBRACIN (Greece)
TOBRAMYCIN
TOBI Solution for Inhalation 1015

MONO-CEDOCARD (The Netherlands, United Kingdom)
ISOSORBIDE MONONITRATE
Imdur Tablets 3032

MONOCEF (India)
CEFTRIAXONE SODIUM
Rocephin Injectable Vials, ADD-Vantage, Galaxy, Bulk 2801

MONOCEF-O (India)
CEFPODOXIME PROXETIL
Vantin Tablets and Oral Suspension 2650

MONOCID (Austria)
CLARITHROMYCIN
Biaxin Filmtab Tablets 402
Biaxin Granules 402

MONOCINQUE (Hong Kong, Italy)
ISOSORBIDE MONONITRATE
Imdur Tablets 3032

MONOCLAIR (Germany)
ISOSORBIDE MONONITRATE
Imdur Tablets 3032

MONOCONTIN (India)
ISOSORBIDE MONONITRATE
Imdur Tablets 3032

MONOCORD (Israel)
ISOSORBIDE MONONITRATE
Imdur Tablets 3032

MONOCORDIL (Brazil)
ISOSORBIDE MONONITRATE
Imdur Tablets 3032

MONODUR (Australia)
ISOSORBIDE MONONITRATE
Imdur Tablets 3032

MONOFLAM (Germany)
DICLOFENAC SODIUM
Voltaren Tablets 2298
Voltaren-XR Tablets 2301

MONOFLOCET (France)
OFLOXACIN
Floxin Otic Solution 1043

MONOGINAL (Greece)
ISOSORBIDE MONONITRATE
Imdur Tablets 3032

MONOKET (Argentina, Austria, Greece, Italy, Norway, Portugal, Sweden)
ISOSORBIDE MONONITRATE
Imdur Tablets 3032

MONOLIN (Thailand)
ISOSORBIDE MONONITRATE
Imdur Tablets 3032

MONOLITUM (Portugal, Spain)
LANSOPRAZOLE
Prevacid Delayed-Release Capsules 3268

MONOLONG (Germany, Israel)
ISOSORBIDE MONONITRATE
Imdur Tablets 3032

MONOMAX (United Kingdom)
ISOSORBIDE MONONITRATE
Imdur Tablets 3032

MONONIT (Israel)
ISOSORBIDE MONONITRATE
Imdur Tablets 3032

MONONITRAT (Germany)
ISOSORBIDE MONONITRATE
Imdur Tablets 3032

MONONITRIL (Portugal)
ISOSORBIDE MONONITRATE
Imdur Tablets 3032

MONOPRONT (Portugal)
ISOSORBIDE MONONITRATE
Imdur Tablets 3032

MONOPUR (Germany)
ISOSORBIDE MONONITRATE
Imdur Tablets 3032

MONOSAN (Czech Republic)
ISOSORBIDE MONONITRATE
Imdur Tablets 3032

MONOSORB (France, United Kingdom)
ISOSORBIDE MONONITRATE
Imdur Tablets 3032

MONOSORBITRATE (India)
ISOSORBIDE MONONITRATE
Imdur Tablets 3032

MONOSORDIL (Greece)
ISOSORBIDE MONONITRATE
Imdur Tablets 3032

MONOSTENASE (Germany)
ISOSORBIDE MONONITRATE
Imdur Tablets 3032

MONOTAX (India)
CEFTRIAXONE SODIUM
Rocephin Injectable Vials, ADD-Vantage, Galaxy, Bulk 2801

MONOTAX-O (India)
CEFPODOXIME PROXETIL
Vantin Tablets and Oral Suspension 2650

MONO-TILDIEM (France, Malaysia, Singapore, Thailand)
DILTIAZEM HYDROCHLORIDE
Cardizem LA Extended Release Tablets. . . 1699
Tiazac Capsules 1204

MONOTOBRIN (Greece)
TOBRAMYCIN
TOBI Solution for Inhalation 1015

MONOTRATE (India, Singapore, Thailand)
ISOSORBIDE MONONITRATE
Imdur Tablets 3032

MONOTRIN (Argentina)
ISOSORBIDE MONONITRATE
Imdur Tablets 3032

MONOZOL (Brazil)
ALBENDAZOLE
Albenza Tablets. 1310

MONSALIC (Czech Republic)
MOMETASONE FUROATE
Elocon Cream 0.1% 3019
Elocon Lotion 0.1% 3020
Elocon Ointment 0.1% 3021
Nasonex Nasal Spray 3058

MONTAIR (India)
MONTELUKAST SODIUM
Singulair Chewable Tablets 2047
Singulair Tablets 2047

MONTAIR PLUS (India)
MONTELUKAST SODIUM
Singulair Chewable Tablets 2047
Singulair Tablets 2047

MONTEGEN (Italy)
MONTELUKAST SODIUM
Singulair Chewable Tablets 2047
Singulair Tablets 2047

MOPSORALEN (Belgium)
METHOXSALEN
Oxsoralen Lotion 1% 3354
Oxsoralen-Ultra Capsules. 3354

MORAPID (Austria)
MORPHINE SULFATE
Kadian Capsules 572
MS Contin Tablets 2703

MORAXEN (United Kingdom)
MORPHINE SULFATE
Kadian Capsules 572
MS Contin Tablets 2703

MORCAP (United Kingdom)
MORPHINE SULFATE
Kadian Capsules 572
MS Contin Tablets 2703

MORCONTIN (India)
MORPHINE SULFATE
Kadian Capsules 572
MS Contin Tablets 2703

MORETAL (Hungary)
MORPHINE SULFATE
Kadian Capsules 572
MS Contin Tablets 2703

MORFEX (Portugal)
FLURAZEPAM HYDROCHLORIDE
Dalmane Capsules. 3343

MORONAL (Germany)
NYSTATIN
Nystop Topical Powder USP. 2490

MORPH (Germany)
MORPHINE SULFATE
Kadian Capsules 572
MS Contin Tablets 2703

MORPHGESIC (United Kingdom)
MORPHINE SULFATE
Kadian Capsules 572
MS Contin Tablets 2703

MORSTEL (Irish Republic)
MORPHINE SULFATE
Kadian Capsules 572
MS Contin Tablets 2703

MOSALAN (Greece)
CEFUROXIME SODIUM
Zinacef Injection 1604

MOSALAN-ORAL (Greece)
CEFUROXIME AXETIL
Ceftin Tablets 1369
Ceftin for Oral Suspension. 1369

MOSCONTIN (France)
MORPHINE SULFATE
Kadian Capsules 572
MS Contin Tablets 2703

MOSKIZOL (France)
PERMETHRIN
Acticin Cream. 2125

MOSTRELAN (Greece)
FAMOTIDINE
Pepcid Injection 2017
Pepcid Injection Premixed 2017
Pepcid Tablets 2014
Pepcid for Oral Suspension 2014

MOTIAX (Italy)
FAMOTIDINE
Pepcid Injection 2017
Pepcid Injection Premixed 2017
Pepcid Tablets 2014
Pepcid for Oral Suspension 2014

MOTIDIN (Hungary)
FAMOTIDINE
Pepcid Injection 2017
Pepcid Injection Premixed 2017
Pepcid Tablets 2014
Pepcid for Oral Suspension 2014

MOTIDINE (Hong Kong, Singapore, Thailand)
FAMOTIDINE
Pepcid Injection 2017
Pepcid Injection Premixed 2017
Pepcid Tablets 2014
Pepcid for Oral Suspension 2014

MOTIFENE (Belgium, Finland, United Kingdom)
DICLOFENAC SODIUM
Voltaren Tablets 2298
Voltaren-XR Tablets 2301

MOTIRON (Denmark)
METHYLPHENIDATE HYDROCHLORIDE
Ritalin Hydrochloride Tablets. 2254
Ritalin-SR Tablets. 2254

MOTIVAN (Spain)
PAROXETINE HYDROCHLORIDE
Paxil Oral Suspension. 1501
Paxil Tablets. 1501

MOUSTICOLOGNE (France)
PERMETHRIN
Acticin Cream. 2125

MOUSTIDOSE (France)
PERMETHRIN
Acticin Cream. 2125

MOVERGAN (Germany)
SELEGILINE HYDROCHLORIDE
Eldepryl Capsules 3209

MOVIN (Portugal)
TICLOPIDINE HYDROCHLORIDE
Ticlid Tablets 2813

MOX (India)
AMOXICILLIN
Amoxil Pediatric Drops for Oral Suspension. 1315
Amoxil Tablets 1315

MOXADENT (Portugal)
AMOXICILLIN
Amoxil Pediatric Drops for Oral Suspension. 1315
Amoxil Tablets 1315

MOXAN (South Africa)
AMOXICILLIN
Amoxil Pediatric Drops for Oral Suspension. 1315
Amoxil Tablets 1315

MOXICEL (Mexico)
AMOXICILLIN
Amoxil Pediatric Drops for Oral Suspension. 1315
Amoxil Tablets 1315

MOXIPEN (Portugal, Singapore)
AMOXICILLIN
Amoxil Pediatric Drops for Oral Suspension. 1315
Amoxil Tablets 1315

MOXIPLUS (Brazil)
AMOXICILLIN
Amoxil Pediatric Drops for Oral Suspension. 1315
Amoxil Tablets 1315

MOXITRAL (Argentina)
AMOXICILLIN
Amoxil Pediatric Drops for Oral Suspension. 1315
Amoxil Tablets 1315

MOXYCARB (India)
AMOXICILLIN
Amoxil Pediatric Drops for Oral Suspension. 1315
Amoxil Tablets 1315

MOXYCLAV (South Africa)
AMOXICILLIN
Amoxil Pediatric Drops for Oral Suspension. 1315
Amoxil Tablets 1315

MOXYMAX (South Africa)
AMOXICILLIN
Amoxil Pediatric Drops for Oral Suspension. 1315
Amoxil Tablets 1315

MPA (Germany)
MEDROXYPROGESTERONE ACETATE
Depo-Medrol Single-Dose Vial 2617

MPA GYN (Germany)
MEDROXYPROGESTERONE ACETATE
Depo-Medrol Single-Dose Vial 2617

MPA-BETA (Germany)
MEDROXYPROGESTERONE ACETATE
Depo-Medrol Single-Dose Vial 2617

MPA-NOURY (Germany)
MEDROXYPROGESTERONE ACETATE
Depo-Medrol Single-Dose Vial 2617

MS CONTIN (Australia, Belgium, Canada, Italy, The Netherlands)
MORPHINE SULFATE
Kadian Capsules 572
MS Contin Tablets 2703

MS DIRECT (Belgium)
MORPHINE SULFATE
Kadian Capsules 572
MS Contin Tablets 2703

MS MONO (Australia)
MORPHINE SULFATE
Kadian Capsules 572
MS Contin Tablets 2703

MSI (Germany)
MORPHINE SULFATE
Kadian Capsules 572
MS Contin Tablets 2703

MSIR (Canada)
MORPHINE SULFATE
Kadian Capsules 572
MS Contin Tablets 2703

MS-LONG (Brazil)
MORPHINE SULFATE
Kadian Capsules 572
MS Contin Tablets 2703

MSP (Israel)
MORPHINE SULFATE
Kadian Capsules 572
MS Contin Tablets 2703

MSR (Germany)
MORPHINE SULFATE
Kadian Capsules 572
MS Contin Tablets 2703

MST (Portugal)
MORPHINE SULFATE
Kadian Capsules 572
MS Contin Tablets 2703

MST CONTINUS (Argentina, Brazil, Hong Kong, Irish Republic, Mexico, New Zealand, Singapore, South Africa, Spain, Switzerland, United Kingdom)
MORPHINE SULFATE
Kadian Capsules 572
MS Contin Tablets 2703

MST UNICONTINUS (Spain)
MORPHINE SULFATE
Kadian Capsules 572
MS Contin Tablets 2703

MST UNO (Czech Republic)
MORPHINE SULFATE
Kadian Capsules 572
MS Contin Tablets 2703

MUCLOX (Spain)
FAMOTIDINE
Pepcid Injection 2017
Pepcid Injection Premixed 2017
Pepcid Tablets 2014
Pepcid for Oral Suspension 2014

MULCATEL (Chile)
SUCRALFATE
Carafate Suspension 727
Carafate Tablets 728

MULTIELMIN (Brazil)
MEBENDAZOLE
Vermox Chewable Tablets 1853

MULTILIND (Germany, United Kingdom)
NYSTATIN
Nystop Topical Powder USP. 2490

MUNDIDOL (Austria)
MORPHINE SULFATE
Kadian Capsules 572
MS Contin Tablets 2703

MUNDIL (Germany)
CAPTOPRIL
Captopril Tablets 2114

MUNITREN H (Germany)
HYDROCORTISONE
Hydrocortone Tablets. 1963

MUNOBAL (Argentina, Austria, Germany, Mexico, Switzerland)
FELODIPINE
Plendil Extended-Release Tablets 651

MUNOTRAS (Argentina)
MYCOPHENOLATE MOFETIL
CellCept Capsules 2751
CellCept Oral Suspension 2751
CellCept Tablets 2751

MUPAX (Argentina)
MUPIROCIN
Bactroban Ointment 1358

MUPIDERM (France)
MUPIROCIN
Bactroban Ointment 1358

MUPIROX (Argentina)
MUPIROCIN
Bactroban Ointment 1358

MUPORIN (Thailand)
MUPIROCIN
Bactroban Ointment 1358

MURINE (Portugal, United Kingdom)
NAPHAZOLINE HYDROCHLORIDE
Albalon Ophthalmic Solution . . . . . ⊙216

MURINE CLEAR EYES (South Africa)
NAPHAZOLINE HYDROCHLORIDE
Albalon Ophthalmic Solution . . . . . ⊙216

MUS (Chile)
CLARITHROMYCIN
Biaxin Filmtab Tablets 402
Biaxin Granules 402

MUSE (Australia, Austria, Brazil, Canada, Czech Republic, Denmark, Finland, France, Germany, Hong Kong, Irish Republic, Israel, Mexico, New Zealand, Singapore, South Africa, Spain, Switzerland, Thailand, United Kingdom)
ALPROSTADIL
Edex Injection 3103

MUSTOPIC (India)
TACROLIMUS
Prograf Capsules and Injection 624

MUVIDINA (Argentina)
ZIDOVUDINE
Retrovir Capsules 1533
Retrovir IV Infusion 1537
Retrovir Syrup 1533
Retrovir Tablets 1533

MXL (Irish Republic, Portugal, United Kingdom)
MORPHINE SULFATE
Kadian Capsules 572
MS Contin Tablets 2703

MYCANDEN (Argentina)
CLOTRIMAZOLE
Lotrimin Cream 3053
Lotrimin Lotion 1% 3053
Lotrimin Topical Solution 1% 3053

MYCARZEM (Greece)
DILTIAZEM HYDROCHLORIDE
Cardizem LA Extended Release Tablets . . . 1699
Tiazac Capsules 1204

MYCELLA (Thailand)
KETOCONAZOLE
Nizoral 2% Shampoo 1838

MYCEPT (India)
MYCOPHENOLATE MOFETIL
CellCept Capsules 2751
CellCept Oral Suspension 2751
CellCept Tablets 2751

MYCIL GOLD (United Kingdom)
CLOTRIMAZOLE
Lotrimin Cream 3053
Lotrimin Lotion 1% 3053
Lotrimin Topical Solution 1% 3053

MYCINOPRED (Switzerland)
NEOMYCIN SULFATE/POLYMYXIN B SULFATE/PREDNISOLONE ACETATE
Poly-Pred Liquifilm Ophthalmic Suspension . . . . . ⊙231

MYCLO-DERM (Canada)
CLOTRIMAZOLE
Lotrimin Cream 3053
Lotrimin Lotion 1% 3053
Lotrimin Topical Solution 1% 3053

MYCLO-GYNE (Canada)
CLOTRIMAZOLE
Lotrimin Cream 3053
Lotrimin Lotion 1% 3053
Lotrimin Topical Solution 1% 3053

MYCOAPAISYL (France)
ECONAZOLE NITRATE
Spectazole Cream 2390

MYCOBACTER (Greece)
ECONAZOLE NITRATE
Spectazole Cream 2390

MYCOBAN (South Africa)
CLOTRIMAZOLE
Lotrimin Cream 3053
Lotrimin Lotion 1% 3053
Lotrimin Topical Solution 1% 3053

MYCOCID (India)
CLOTRIMAZOLE
Lotrimin Cream 3053
Lotrimin Lotion 1% 3053
Lotrimin Topical Solution 1% 3053

MYCODERM-C (India)
CLOTRIMAZOLE
Lotrimin Cream 3053
Lotrimin Lotion 1% 3053
Lotrimin Topical Solution 1% 3053

MYCODIB (Mexico)
KETOCONAZOLE
Nizoral 2% Shampoo 1838

MYCOFEBRIN (Greece)
KETOCONAZOLE
Nizoral 2% Shampoo 1838

MYCOFUG (Austria, Germany)
CLOTRIMAZOLE
Lotrimin Cream 3053
Lotrimin Lotion 1% 3053
Lotrimin Topical Solution 1% 3053

MYCOHAUG C (Germany)
CLOTRIMAZOLE
Lotrimin Cream 3053
Lotrimin Lotion 1% 3053
Lotrimin Topical Solution 1% 3053

MYCO-HERMAL (Israel, Singapore)
CLOTRIMAZOLE
Lotrimin Cream 3053
Lotrimin Lotion 1% 3053
Lotrimin Topical Solution 1% 3053

MYCOHEXAL (South Africa)
CLOTRIMAZOLE
Lotrimin Cream 3053
Lotrimin Lotion 1% 3053
Lotrimin Topical Solution 1% 3053

MYCO-INTRADERMI (Germany)
NYSTATIN
Nystop Topical Powder USP 2490

MYCORAL (Singapore, Thailand)
KETOCONAZOLE
Nizoral 2% Shampoo 1838

MYCORIL (Hong Kong, Singapore)
CLOTRIMAZOLE
Lotrimin Cream 3053
Lotrimin Lotion 1% 3053
Lotrimin Topical Solution 1% 3053

MYCOSORAL (Russia)
KETOCONAZOLE
Nizoral 2% Shampoo 1838

MYCOSTATIN (Australia, Austria, Denmark, Finland, Greece, Hong Kong, India, Irish Republic, Italy, Malaysia, New Zealand, Norway, Portugal, Singapore, South Africa, Spain, Sweden, Thailand)
NYSTATIN
Nystop Topical Powder USP 2490

MYCOSTATINE (France, Switzerland)
NYSTATIN
Nystop Topical Powder USP 2490

MYCOTEL (Thailand)
ALBENDAZOLE
Albenza Tablets 1310

MYCOTRICIDE (Thailand)
PRAZIQUANTEL
Biltricide Tablets 2990

MYCOZOLE (Thailand)
CLOTRIMAZOLE
Lotrimin Cream 3053
Lotrimin Lotion 1% 3053
Lotrimin Topical Solution 1% 3053

MYDA-B (Thailand)
CLOTRIMAZOLE
Lotrimin Cream 3053
Lotrimin Lotion 1% 3053
Lotrimin Topical Solution 1% 3053

MYFLOXIN (Thailand)
NORFLOXACIN
Noroxin Tablets 2009

MYFUNGAR (Czech Republic, Germany, Mexico, Switzerland)
OXICONAZOLE NITRATE
Oxistat Cream 1498
Oxistat Lotion 1498

MYKO CORDES (Austria, Germany)
CLOTRIMAZOLE
Lotrimin Cream 3053
Lotrimin Lotion 1% 3053
Lotrimin Topical Solution 1% 3053

MYKODERM HEILSALBE (Germany)
NYSTATIN
Nystop Topical Powder USP 2490

MYKOFUNGIN (Germany)
CLOTRIMAZOLE
Lotrimin Cream 3053
Lotrimin Lotion 1% 3053
Lotrimin Topical Solution 1% 3053

MYKOHAUG (Germany)
CLOTRIMAZOLE
Lotrimin Cream 3053
Lotrimin Lotion 1% 3053
Lotrimin Topical Solution 1% 3053

MYKOPOSTERINE N (Germany)
NYSTATIN
Nystop Topical Powder USP 2490

MYKUNDEX (Germany)
NYSTATIN
Nystop Topical Powder USP 2490

MYKUNDEX HEILSALBE (Germany)
NYSTATIN
Nystop Topical Powder USP 2490

MYKUNDEX MONO (Germany)
NYSTATIN
Nystop Topical Powder USP 2490

MYKUNDEX OVULA (Germany)
NYSTATIN
Nystop Topical Powder USP 2490

MYLERAN (Argentina, Australia, Austria, Belgium, Brazil, Canada, Chile, Czech Republic, France, Germany, Greece, Hong Kong, India, Irish Republic, Israel, Italy, Malaysia, Mexico, New Zealand, Norway, Portugal, Singapore, South Africa, Sweden, Switzerland, Thailand, The Netherlands, United Kingdom)
BUSULFAN
Myleran Tablets 1492

MYLPROIN (Germany)
VALPROIC ACID
Depakene Capsules 417
Depakene Syrup 417

MYOCARDON MONO (Austria)
ISOSORBIDE MONONITRATE
Imdur Tablets 3032

MYOCARDON N (Germany)
THEOPHYLLINE
Uniphyl Tablets 2708

MYOCORD (Argentina)
ATENOLOL
Tenormin I.V. Injection 698

MYODIPINE (Greece)
NIMODIPINE
Nimotop Capsules 774

MYOGARD (India)
NIFEDIPINE
Adalat CC Tablets 2978

MYOGIT (Czech Republic, Germany)
DICLOFENAC SODIUM
Voltaren Tablets 2298
Voltaren-XR Tablets 2301

MYONIL (Denmark)
DILTIAZEM HYDROCHLORIDE
Cardizem LA Extended Release Tablets . . . 1699
Tiazac Capsules 1204

MYOPAX (Denmark)
ATENOLOL
Tenormin I.V. Injection 698

MYOSPA (Thailand)
ORPHENADRINE CITRATE
Norflex Injection 1824

MYTOLAC (Sweden)
BENZOYL PEROXIDE
Brevoxyl-4 Creamy Wash 3212
Brevoxyl-4 Gel 3211
Brevoxyl-8 Creamy Wash 3212
Brevoxyl-8 Gel 3211
Triaz Cleanser 1864
Triaz Gel 1864

NABACT (South Africa)
METRONIDAZOLE
MetroGel-Vaginal Gel 1822
Noritate Cream, 1% 1051

NABESAC (Thailand)
ORPHENADRINE CITRATE
Norflex Injection 1824

NABICORTIN (Greece)
LOVASTATIN
Mevacor Tablets 1996

NABONE (Thailand)
NABUMETONE
Relafen Tablets 1523

NABONET (Thailand)
NABUMETONE
Relafen Tablets 1523

NABOREL (Greece)
NIMODIPINE
Nimotop Capsules 774

NABRATIN (Argentina)
CLOPIDOGREL BISULFATE
Plavix Tablets 940, 2942

NABUCO (Israel)
NABUMETONE
Relafen Tablets 1523

NABUCOX (France)
NABUMETONE
Relafen Tablets 1523

NABUFLAM (India)
NABUMETONE
Relafen Tablets 1523

NABUSER (Italy)
NABUMETONE
Relafen Tablets 1523

NABUTIL (France)
LOPERAMIDE HYDROCHLORIDE
Imodium Capsules 1834

NABUTON (Greece)
NABUMETONE
Relafen Tablets 1523

NAC (India)
DICLOFENAC SODIUM
Voltaren Tablets 2298
Voltaren-XR Tablets 2301

NACLOF (Austria, Czech Republic, Norway, South Africa, Sweden, Thailand, The Netherlands)
DICLOFENAC SODIUM
Voltaren Tablets 2298
Voltaren-XR Tablets 2301

NACOR (Spain)
ENALAPRIL MALEATE
Vasotec I.V. Injection 2076

NACTOL (Mexico)
BENZONATATE
Tessalon Perles 1202

NADIPINIA (Hong Kong)
NIFEDIPINE
Adalat CC Tablets 2978

NADITONE (Greece)
NABUMETONE
Relafen Tablets 1523

NADOSTINE (Canada, Hong Kong)
NYSTATIN
Nystop Topical Powder USP 2490

(⊙ Described in PDR For Ophthalmic Medicines™)

NAFASOL (South Africa)
NAPROXEN
EC-Naprosyn Delayed-Release Tablets.... 2769
Naprosyn Suspension.............. 2769
Naprosyn Tablets................ 2769

NAFLAPEN (Mexico)
NAPROXEN
EC-Naprosyn Delayed-Release Tablets.... 2769
Naprosyn Suspension.............. 2769
Naprosyn Tablets................ 2769

NAFLEX (Thailand)
NABUMETONE
Relafen Tablets.................. 1523

NAFLUVENT (Argentina)
FENTANYL
Duragesic Transdermal System........ 2448

NAFORDYL (Greece)
LISINOPRIL
Prinivil Tablets.................. 2029
Zestril Tablets.................... 704

NAFTAZOLINA (Italy)
NAPHAZOLINE HYDROCHLORIDE
Albalon Ophthalmic Solution .... ⊙216

NAFTIN (Canada)
NAFTIFINE HYDROCHLORIDE
Naftin Cream.................... 2097
Naftin Gel...................... 2097

NAKLOFEN (Czech Republic)
DICLOFENAC SODIUM
Voltaren Tablets................. 2298
Voltaren-XR Tablets.............. 2301

NALAPRES (Italy)
HYDROCHLOROTHIAZIDE/LISINOPRIL
Prinzide Tablets.................. 2033
Zestoretic Tablets................. 701

NALAPRIX (Brazil)
ENALAPRIL MALEATE
Vasotec I.V. Injection.............. 2076

NALGESIN (Czech Republic)
NAPROXEN SODIUM
Anaprox DS Tablets............... 2769
Anaprox Tablets................. 2769

NALGISA (Italy)
DIFLUNISAL
Dolobid Tablets.................. 1937

NALION (Spain)
NORFLOXACIN
Noroxin Tablets.................. 2009

NALONE (France)
NALOXONE HYDROCHLORIDE
Narcan Injection.................. 1109

NALOPRIL (Thailand)
ENALAPRIL MALEATE
Vasotec I.V. Injection.............. 2076

NALOSELECT (Germany)
NALOXONE HYDROCHLORIDE
Narcan Injection.................. 1109

NALOX (Argentina)
METRONIDAZOLE
MetroGel-Vaginal Gel.............. 1822
Noritate Cream, 1%............... 1051

NALOXON (Russia)
NALOXONE HYDROCHLORIDE
Narcan Injection.................. 1109

NAMETONE (Thailand)
NABUMETONE
Relafen Tablets.................. 1523

NAPAMIDE (Australia, Hong Kong, Malaysia, New Zealand, Singapore, Thailand)
INDAPAMIDE
Indapamide Tablets............... 2119

NAPFLAM (South Africa)
NAPROXEN
EC-Naprosyn Delayed-Release Tablets.... 2769
Naprosyn Suspension.............. 2769
Naprosyn Tablets................ 2769

NAPHACEL (Mexico)
NAPHAZOLINE HYDROCHLORIDE
Albalon Ophthalmic Solution .... ⊙216

NAPHASAL (Israel)
NAPHAZOLINE HYDROCHLORIDE
Albalon Ophthalmic Solution .... ⊙216

NAPHCON (Australia, Belgium, Hungary, New Zealand, Thailand)
NAPHAZOLINE HYDROCHLORIDE
Albalon Ophthalmic Solution .... ⊙216

NAPHCON FORTE (Canada, Israel)
NAPHAZOLINE HYDROCHLORIDE
Albalon Ophthalmic Solution .... ⊙216

NAPHCON-A (Australia, Malaysia)
NAPHAZOLINE HYDROCHLORIDE
Albalon Ophthalmic Solution .... ⊙216

NAPLIN (New Zealand)
INDAPAMIDE
Indapamide Tablets............... 2119

NAPMEL (Hungary, Irish Republic)
NAPROXEN
EC-Naprosyn Delayed-Release Tablets.... 2769
Naprosyn Suspension.............. 2769
Naprosyn Tablets................ 2769

NAPRATEC (United Kingdom)
NAPROXEN
EC-Naprosyn Delayed-Release Tablets.... 2769
Naprosyn Suspension.............. 2769
Naprosyn Tablets................ 2769

NAPREL (South Africa)
NAPROXEN
EC-Naprosyn Delayed-Release Tablets.... 2769
Naprosyn Suspension.............. 2769
Naprosyn Tablets................ 2769

NAPRELAN (Sweden)
NAPROXEN SODIUM
Anaprox DS Tablets............... 2769
Anaprox Tablets................. 2769

NAPREN (Norway)
NAPROXEN
EC-Naprosyn Delayed-Release Tablets.... 2769
Naprosyn Suspension.............. 2769
Naprosyn Tablets................ 2769

NAPREX (Irish Republic, Israel)
NAPROXEN SODIUM
Anaprox DS Tablets............... 2769
Anaprox Tablets................. 2769

NAPRILENE (Italy, Spain)
ENALAPRIL MALEATE
Vasotec I.V. Injection.............. 2076

NAPRIUM (Italy)
NAPROXEN
EC-Naprosyn Delayed-Release Tablets.... 2769
Naprosyn Suspension.............. 2769
Naprosyn Tablets................ 2769

NAPRIUS (Italy)
NAPROXEN
EC-Naprosyn Delayed-Release Tablets.... 2769
Naprosyn Suspension.............. 2769
Naprosyn Tablets................ 2769

NAPRIX (Brazil)
RAMIPRIL
Altace Capsules.................. 1673

NAPRIX D (Brazil)
RAMIPRIL
Altace Capsules.................. 1673

NAPRIZIDE (Israel)
ENALAPRIL MALEATE
Vasotec I.V. Injection.............. 2076

NAPROBENE (Austria, Czech Republic)
NAPROXEN
EC-Naprosyn Delayed-Release Tablets.... 2769
Naprosyn Suspension.............. 2769
Naprosyn Tablets................ 2769

NAPROCOAT (The Netherlands)
NAPROXEN
EC-Naprosyn Delayed-Release Tablets.... 2769
Naprosyn Suspension.............. 2769
Naprosyn Tablets................ 2769

NAPRODIL (Mexico)
NAPROXEN
EC-Naprosyn Delayed-Release Tablets.... 2769
Naprosyn Suspension.............. 2769
Naprosyn Tablets................ 2769

NAPRODOL (Italy)
NAPROXEN SODIUM
Anaprox DS Tablets............... 2769
Anaprox Tablets................. 2769

NAPRO-DORSCH (Germany)
NAPROXEN
EC-Naprosyn Delayed-Release Tablets.... 2769
Naprosyn Suspension.............. 2769
Naprosyn Tablets................ 2769

NAPROFIDEX (Argentina)
NAPROXEN
EC-Naprosyn Delayed-Release Tablets.... 2769
Naprosyn Suspension.............. 2769
Naprosyn Tablets................ 2769

NAPROGEN (Argentina)
NAPROXEN
EC-Naprosyn Delayed-Release Tablets.... 2769
Naprosyn Suspension.............. 2769
Naprosyn Tablets................ 2769

NAPROGESIC (Australia, Chile, New Zealand)
NAPROXEN SODIUM
Anaprox DS Tablets............... 2769
Anaprox Tablets................. 2769

NAPROKES (Spain)
NAPROXEN
EC-Naprosyn Delayed-Release Tablets.... 2769
Naprosyn Suspension.............. 2769
Naprosyn Tablets................ 2769

NAPROLAG (Switzerland)
NAPROXEN
EC-Naprosyn Delayed-Release Tablets.... 2769
Naprosyn Suspension.............. 2769
Naprosyn Tablets................ 2769

NAPROMETIN (Finland)
NAPROXEN
EC-Naprosyn Delayed-Release Tablets.... 2769
Naprosyn Suspension.............. 2769
Naprosyn Tablets................ 2769

NAPROMEX (Finland)
NAPROXEN
EC-Naprosyn Delayed-Release Tablets.... 2769
Naprosyn Suspension.............. 2769
Naprosyn Tablets................ 2769

NAPRONET (Denmark)
NAPROXEN
EC-Naprosyn Delayed-Release Tablets.... 2769
Naprosyn Suspension.............. 2769
Naprosyn Tablets................ 2769

NAPRONTAG (Argentina)
NAPROXEN
EC-Naprosyn Delayed-Release Tablets.... 2769
Naprosyn Suspension.............. 2769
Naprosyn Tablets................ 2769

NAPRONTAG FLEX (Argentina)
NAPROXEN
EC-Naprosyn Delayed-Release Tablets.... 2769
Naprosyn Suspension.............. 2769
Naprosyn Tablets................ 2769

NAPROREX (Hong Kong, Italy)
NAPROXEN
EC-Naprosyn Delayed-Release Tablets.... 2769
Naprosyn Suspension.............. 2769
Naprosyn Tablets................ 2769

NAPROSCRIPT (South Africa)
NAPROXEN
EC-Naprosyn Delayed-Release Tablets.... 2769
Naprosyn Suspension.............. 2769
Naprosyn Tablets................ 2769

NAPROSIAN (Thailand)
NAPROXEN
EC-Naprosyn Delayed-Release Tablets.... 2769
Naprosyn Suspension.............. 2769
Naprosyn Tablets................ 2769

NAPROSO (Thailand)
NAPROXEN SODIUM
Anaprox DS Tablets............... 2769
Anaprox Tablets................. 2769

NAPROSYN (Australia, Brazil, Canada, Czech Republic, Denmark, Finland, Greece, Hong Kong, Hungary, India, Irish Republic, Italy, New Zealand, Norway, Portugal, Singapore, South Africa, Spain, Sweden, Switzerland, Thailand, United Kingdom)
NAPROXEN
EC-Naprosyn Delayed-Release Tablets.... 2769
Naprosyn Suspension.............. 2769
Naprosyn Tablets................ 2769

NAPROSYNE (Belgium, France, The Netherlands)
NAPROXEN
EC-Naprosyn Delayed-Release Tablets.... 2769
Naprosyn Suspension.............. 2769
Naprosyn Tablets................ 2769

NAPROVAL (Spain)
NAPROXEN
EC-Naprosyn Delayed-Release Tablets.... 2769
Naprosyn Suspension.............. 2769
Naprosyn Tablets................ 2769

NAPROVITE (The Netherlands)
NAPROXEN SODIUM
Anaprox DS Tablets............... 2769
Anaprox Tablets................. 2769

NAPROX (Brazil)
NAPROXEN
EC-Naprosyn Delayed-Release Tablets.... 2769
Naprosyn Suspension.............. 2769
Naprosyn Tablets................ 2769

NAPROXI (Israel)
NAPROXEN
EC-Naprosyn Delayed-Release Tablets.... 2769
Naprosyn Suspension.............. 2769
Naprosyn Tablets................ 2769

NAPRUX (Argentina)
NAPROXEN
EC-Naprosyn Delayed-Release Tablets.... 2769
Naprosyn Suspension.............. 2769
Naprosyn Tablets................ 2769

NAPSEN (Thailand)
NAPROXEN
EC-Naprosyn Delayed-Release Tablets.... 2769
Naprosyn Suspension.............. 2769
Naprosyn Tablets................ 2769

NAPSYN (Czech Republic)
NAPROXEN
EC-Naprosyn Delayed-Release Tablets.... 2769
Naprosyn Suspension.............. 2769
Naprosyn Tablets................ 2769

NAPXEN (Hong Kong, Thailand)
NAPROXEN
EC-Naprosyn Delayed-Release Tablets.... 2769
Naprosyn Suspension.............. 2769
Naprosyn Tablets................ 2769

NAQUA (Portugal)
FUROSEMIDE
Furosemide Tablets............... 2117

NARAGRAN (Denmark)
NARATRIPTAN HYDROCHLORIDE
Amerge Tablets.................. 1312

NARAMIG (Argentina, Australia, Austria, Belgium, Brazil, Chile, Czech Republic, Finland, France, Greece, Hungary, Israel, Mexico, Norway, Portugal, Singapore, South Africa, Spain, Sweden, Switzerland, Thailand, The Netherlands, United Kingdom)
NARATRIPTAN HYDROCHLORIDE
Amerge Tablets.................. 1312

NARAPRIL (United Arab Emirates)
ENALAPRIL MALEATE
Vasotec I.V. Injection.............. 2076

NARCAN (Australia, Belgium, Brazil, Canada, France, Greece, Irish Republic, Israel, Italy, Malaysia, New Zealand, Portugal, Singapore, South Africa, Switzerland, Thailand, United Kingdom)
NALOXONE HYDROCHLORIDE
Narcan Injection.................. 1109

NARCANTI (Argentina, Austria, Denmark, Finland, Germany, Hungary, Mexico, Norway, Sweden)
NALOXONE HYDROCHLORIDE
Narcan Injection.................. 1109

NARCOTAN (India)
NALOXONE HYDROCHLORIDE
Narcan Injection.................. 1109

NARIAL (Brazil)
NAPHAZOLINE HYDROCHLORIDE
Albalon Ophthalmic Solution .... ⊙216

NARIDE (Australia)
INDAPAMIDE
Indapamide Tablets............... 2119

NARIDEX (Brazil)
NAPHAZOLINE HYDROCHLORIDE
Albalon Ophthalmic Solution .... ⊙216

NARIGEN (Greece)
RANITIDINE HYDROCHLORIDE
Zantac 25 EFFERdose Tablets........ 1597
Zantac 150 EFFERdose Tablets........ 1597

(⊙ Described in PDR For Ophthalmic Medicines™)

Zantac 150 Tablets **1597**
Zantac 300 Tablets **1597**
Zantac Injection **1593**
Zantac Injection Premixed **1593**
Zantac Syrup **1597**

NARILET (Spain)
IPRATROPIUM BROMIDE
Atrovent Inhalation Solution **868**
Atrovent Nasal Spray 0.03%. **869**
Atrovent Nasal Spray 0.06%. **870**

NARITEC (Thailand)
ENALAPRIL MALEATE
Vasotec I.V. Injection **2076**

NAROBIC (South Africa)
METRONIDAZOLE
MetroGel-Vaginal Gel **1822**
Noritate Cream, 1% **1051**

NAROCIN (Israel)
NAPROXEN SODIUM
Anaprox DS Tablets **2769**
Anaprox Tablets **2769**

NAROP (Israel, Sweden)
ROPIVACAINE HYDROCHLORIDE
Naropin Injection **640**

NAROPEINE (France, Greece, Portugal)
ROPIVACAINE HYDROCHLORIDE
Naropin Injection **640**

NAROPIN (Argentina, Australia, Austria, Belgium, Brazil, Canada, Chile, Denmark, Finland, Germany, Hong Kong, Hungary, Irish Republic, Malaysia, Mexico, New Zealand, Norway, Singapore, South Africa, Spain, Switzerland, Thailand, The Netherlands, United Kingdom)
ROPIVACAINE HYDROCHLORIDE
Naropin Injection **640**

NAROPIN WITH FENTANYL (Australia, New Zealand)
ROPIVACAINE HYDROCHLORIDE
Naropin Injection **640**

NAROPINA (Italy)
ROPIVACAINE HYDROCHLORIDE
Naropin Injection **640**

NARZEN (Thailand)
NAPROXEN
EC-Naprosyn Delayed-Release Tablets **2769**
Naprosyn Suspension **2769**
Naprosyn Tablets **2769**

NASACOR (South Africa)
TRIAMCINOLONE ACETONIDE
Azmacort Inhalation Aerosol **1701**
Nasacort AQ Nasal Spray **2937**

NASACORT (Argentina, Austria, Brazil, Canada, Chile, Czech Republic, Denmark, Finland, France, Germany, Greece, Hong Kong, Irish Republic, Italy, Mexico, New Zealand, Norway, Singapore, Spain, Sweden, Switzerland, Thailand, The Netherlands, United Kingdom)
TRIAMCINOLONE ACETONIDE
Azmacort Inhalation Aerosol **1701**
Nasacort AQ Nasal Spray **2937**

NASACORT AQ (Australia, Malaysia)
TRIAMCINOLONE ACETONIDE
Azmacort Inhalation Aerosol **1701**
Nasacort AQ Nasal Spray **2937**

NASALIDE (France)
FLUNISOLIDE
Aerobid Inhaler System **1172**
Aerobid-M Inhaler System **1172**
Nasarel Nasal Spray **1652**

NASOCAN (Mexico)
NAPROXEN SODIUM
Anaprox DS Tablets **2769**
Anaprox Tablets **2769**

NASOFAN (United Kingdom)
FLUTICASONE PROPIONATE
Cutivate Cream **1381**
Cutivate Ointment **1384**
Flonase Nasal Spray **1412**

NASOMET (Portugal)
MOMETASONE FUROATE
Elocon Cream 0.1% **3019**
Elocon Lotion 0.1% **3020**
Elocon Ointment 0.1% **3021**
Nasonex Nasal Spray **3058**

NASONEX (Argentina, Australia, Austria, Belgium, Brazil, Canada, Chile, Czech Republic, Denmark, Finland, France, Germany, Greece, Hong Kong, Hungary, Irish Republic, Israel, Italy, Malaysia, Norway, Russia, Singapore, South Africa, Spain, Sweden, Switzerland, Thailand, The Netherlands, United Kingdom)
MOMETASONE FUROATE
Elocon Cream 0.1% **3019**
Elocon Lotion 0.1% **3020**
Elocon Ointment 0.1% **3021**
Nasonex Nasal Spray **3058**

NASTERID (Brazil)
FINASTERIDE
Propecia Tablets **2036**
Proscar Tablets **2040**

NASTERIL (Argentina)
FINASTERIDE
Propecia Tablets **2036**
Proscar Tablets **2040**

NASTIL (Mexico)
KETOCONAZOLE
Nizoral 2% Shampoo **1838**

NATACYN (Argentina, Singapore, South Africa, Thailand)
NATAMYCIN
Natacyn Antifungal Ophthalmic Suspension . . . . **⊙207**

NATADROPS (India)
NATAMYCIN
Natacyn Antifungal Ophthalmic Suspension . . . . **⊙207**

NATAFUCIN (Italy)
NATAMYCIN
Natacyn Antifungal Ophthalmic Suspension . . . . **⊙207**

NATRAMID (United Kingdom)
INDAPAMIDE
Indapamide Tablets **2119**

NATRILIX (Argentina, Australia, Brazil, Denmark, Finland, Germany, Hong Kong, India, Irish Republic, Italy, Malaysia, New Zealand, Singapore, South Africa, Thailand, United Kingdom)
INDAPAMIDE
Indapamide Tablets **2119**

NATRIOXEN (Italy)
NAPROXEN SODIUM
Anaprox DS Tablets **2769**
Anaprox Tablets **2769**

NATULAN (Australia, Austria, Belgium, Canada, France, Germany, Greece, Hungary, Israel, Italy, Mexico, New Zealand, Norway, South Africa, Spain, Switzerland, The Netherlands, United Kingdom)
PROCARBAZINE HYDROCHLORIDE
Matulane Capsules **3188**

NATULANAR (Brazil, Sweden)
PROCARBAZINE HYDROCHLORIDE
Matulane Capsules **3188**

NATULAX (Germany)
LACTULOSE
Kristalose for Oral Solution **2149**

NATURA FENAC (Argentina)
DICLOFENAC SODIUM
Voltaren Tablets **2298**
Voltaren-XR Tablets **2301**

NATUROGEST (India)
PROGESTERONE
Prometrium Capsules (100 mg, 200 mg) . **3205**

NATYL (Switzerland)
DIPYRIDAMOLE
Persantine Tablets **898**

NAUSEDRON (Brazil)
ONDANSETRON HYDROCHLORIDE
Zofran Injection **1607**
Zofran Injection Premixed **1607**
Zofran Oral Solution **1613**
Zofran Tablets **1613**

NAVELBIN (Hungary)
VINORELBINE TARTRATE
Navelbine Injection **1494**

NAVELBINE (Argentina, Australia, Austria, Belgium, Brazil, Canada, Chile, Czech Republic, Denmark, Finland, France, Germany, Greece, Israel, Italy, Malaysia, Mexico, Norway, Portugal, Russia, Singapore, South Africa, Spain, Sweden, Switzerland, Thailand, United Kingdom)
VINORELBINE TARTRATE
Navelbine Injection **1494**

NAVIXEN (Mexico)
NAPROXEN
EC-Naprosyn Delayed-Release Tablets **2769**
Naprosyn Suspension **2769**
Naprosyn Tablets **2769**

NAXAN (Portugal)
NALOXONE HYDROCHLORIDE
Narcan Injection **1109**

NAXEN (Australia, Canada, Mexico, New Zealand, South Africa)
NAPROXEN
EC-Naprosyn Delayed-Release Tablets **2769**
Naprosyn Suspension **2769**
Naprosyn Tablets **2769**

NAXIL (Mexico)
NAPROXEN
EC-Naprosyn Delayed-Release Tablets **2769**
Naprosyn Suspension **2769**
Naprosyn Tablets **2769**

NAXOCLINDA (Argentina)
CLINDAMYCIN PHOSPHATE
Clindets Pledgets **3212**

NAXODOL (Mexico)
NAPROXEN
EC-Naprosyn Delayed-Release Tablets **2769**
Naprosyn Suspension **2769**
Naprosyn Tablets **2769**

NAXOLAN (Portugal)
NALOXONE HYDROCHLORIDE
Narcan Injection **1109**

NAXOPREN (Finland)
NAPROXEN
EC-Naprosyn Delayed-Release Tablets **2769**
Naprosyn Suspension **2769**
Naprosyn Tablets **2769**

NAXY (France)
CLARITHROMYCIN
Biaxin Filmtab Tablets **402**
Biaxin Granules **402**

NAXYN (Israel)
NAPROXEN
EC-Naprosyn Delayed-Release Tablets **2769**
Naprosyn Suspension **2769**
Naprosyn Tablets **2769**

NAZICOL (Brazil)
NAPHAZOLINE HYDROCHLORIDE
Albalon Ophthalmic Solution . . . . **⊙216**

NAZOBIO (Brazil)
NAPHAZOLINE HYDROCHLORIDE
Albalon Ophthalmic Solution . . . . **⊙216**

NAZOLFARM (Mexico)
KETOCONAZOLE
Nizoral 2% Shampoo **1838**

NEATENOL (Spain)
ATENOLOL
Tenormin I.V. Injection **698**

NEBAPUL (Chile)
METHYLPHENIDATE HYDROCHLORIDE
Ritalin Hydrochloride Tablets **2254**
Ritalin-SR Tablets **2254**

NEBULCORT (Italy)
FLUNISOLIDE
Aerobid Inhaler System **1172**
Aerobid-M Inhaler System **1172**
Nasarel Nasal Spray **1652**

NECAMIN (Brazil)
MEBENDAZOLE
Vermox Chewable Tablets **1853**

NECOPEN (Spain)
CEFIXIME
Suprax **1811**

NEDAX (Brazil)
PERMETHRIN
Acticin Cream **2125**

NEDAX PLUS (Brazil)
PERMETHRIN
Acticin Cream **2125**

NEFAZAN (Argentina)
CLOPIDOGREL BISULFATE
Plavix Tablets **940, 2942**

NEFAZOL (Italy)
CEFAZOLIN SODIUM
Ancef for Injection **1318**

NEFELID (Greece)
NIFEDIPINE
Adalat CC Tablets **2978**

NEFOBEN (Argentina)
THEOPHYLLINE
Uniphyl Tablets **2708**

NEFROCARNIT (Germany)
LEVOCARNITINE
Carnitor Injection **3185**
Carnitor Tablets and Oral Solution **3187**

NEGACEF (United Arab Emirates)
CEFTAZIDIME
Fortaz for Injection **1422**

NELABOCIN (Greece)
CEFUROXIME AXETIL
Ceftin Tablets **1369**
Ceftin for Oral Suspension **1369**

NELAPINE (Thailand)
NIFEDIPINE
Adalat CC Tablets **2978**

NELBINEX (Greece)
NIMODIPINE
Nimotop Capsules **774**

NEMAPRES (Mexico)
MEBENDAZOLE
Vermox Chewable Tablets **1853**

NEMASOLE (Argentina)
MEBENDAZOLE
Vermox Chewable Tablets **1853**

NEMBUTAL (Australia, Canada, Hong Kong, Thailand)
PENTOBARBITAL SODIUM
Nembutal Sodium Solution, USP **2484**

NEMOZOLE (India)
ALBENDAZOLE
Albenza Tablets **1310**

NEO BENDAZOL (Brazil)
ALBENDAZOLE
Albenza Tablets **1310**

NEO CARDIOL (Italy)
LEVOCARNITINE
Carnitor Injection **3185**
Carnitor Tablets and Oral Solution **3187**

NEO CEFIX (Brazil)
CEFIXIME
Suprax **1811**

NEO CLODIL (Brazil)
CLONIDINE HYDROCHLORIDE
Catapres Tablets **874**

NEO CLOTRIMAZYL (Brazil)
CLOTRIMAZOLE
Lotrimin Cream **3053**
Lotrimin Lotion 1% **3053**
Lotrimin Topical Solution 1% **3053**

NEO EBLIMON (Italy)
NAPROXEN
EC-Naprosyn Delayed-Release Tablets **2769**
Naprosyn Suspension **2769**
Naprosyn Tablets **2769**

NEO ELIXIFILIN (Spain)
THEOPHYLLINE
Uniphyl Tablets **2708**

NEO FEDIPINA (Brazil)
NIFEDIPINE
Adalat CC Tablets **2978**

NEO GASTRAUSIL (Italy)
CIMETIDINE
Tagamet Tablets **1547**

NEO KEF (Argentina)
LOPERAMIDE HYDROCHLORIDE
Imodium Capsules **1834**

NEO MEBEND (Brazil)
MEBENDAZOLE
Vermox Chewable Tablets **1853**

NEO METRODAZOL (Brazil)
METRONIDAZOLE
MetroGel-Vaginal Gel **1822**
Noritate Cream, 1% **1051**

NEO MISTATIN (Brazil)
NYSTATIN
Nystop Topical Powder USP **2490**

NEO PROPRANOL (Brazil)
PROPRANOLOL HYDROCHLORIDE
Inderal LA Long-Acting Capsules **3421**

NEO STRATA ASTRINGENT ACNE TREATMENT (Canada)
BENZOYL PEROXIDE
Brevoxyl-4 Creamy Wash **3212**
Brevoxyl-4 Gel **3211**
Brevoxyl-8 Creamy Wash **3212**
Brevoxyl-8 Gel **3211**
Triaz Cleanser **1864**
Triaz Gel **1864**

NEO STRATA BLEMISH SPOT (Canada)
BENZOYL PEROXIDE
Brevoxyl-4 Creamy Wash **3212**
Brevoxyl-4 Gel **3211**
Brevoxyl-8 Creamy Wash **3212**
Brevoxyl-8 Gel **3211**
Triaz Cleanser **1864**
Triaz Gel **1864**

NEO VERPAMIL (Brazil)
VERAPAMIL HYDROCHLORIDE
Covera-HS Tablets **3135**
Verelan PM Capsules **3120**

NEOCARDON (Greece)
ATENOLOL
Tenormin I.V. Injection **698**

NEOCEF (Portugal)
CEFIXIME
Suprax **1811**

NEOCEFTRIONA (Brazil)
CEFTRIAXONE SODIUM
Rocephin Injectable Vials, ADD-Vantage, Galaxy, Bulk **2801**

NEOCEL (Argentina)
DOCETAXEL
Taxotere Injection Concentrate **2947**

NEOCIP (India)
CIPROFLOXACIN
Cipro Oral Suspension **2991**

NEOCIP M (India)
CIPROFLOXACIN
Cipro Oral Suspension **2991**

NEOCITEC (Argentina)
VINORELBINE TARTRATE
Navelbine Injection **1494**

NEOCOLPOBEN (Argentina)
METRONIDAZOLE
MetroGel-Vaginal Gel **1822**
Noritate Cream, 1% **1051**

NEOCORTIGAMMA (Italy)
HYDROCORTISONE
Hydrocortone Tablets **1963**

NEO-CURRINO (Argentina)
NAPHAZOLINE HYDROCHLORIDE
Albalon Ophthalmic Solution . . . . **⊙216**

NEO-DECA (Malaysia)
DEXAMETHASONE SODIUM PHOSPHATE
Decadron Phosphate Injection **1931**

NEODEX (Thailand)
DEXAMETHASONE
Decadron Tablets **1929**

NEO-DEX (IMPROVED) (Hong Kong)
DEXAMETHASONE SODIUM PHOSPHATE
Decadron Phosphate Injection **1931**

NEO-DISTERIN (Greece)
FENOFIBRATE
Tricor Tablets **523**

NEODOLPASSE (Czech Republic, Hungary)
DICLOFENAC SODIUM
Voltaren Tablets **2298**
Voltaren-XR Tablets **2301**

NEO-EGMOL (Greece)
KETOCONAZOLE
Nizoral 2% Shampoo **1838**

NEOFAZOL (Spain)
CEFAZOLIN SODIUM
Ancef for Injection **1318**

NEOFEL (United Kingdom)
FELODIPINE
Plendil Extended-Release Tablets **651**

NEOFLOXIN (Brazil, Singapore)
NORFLOXACIN
Noroxin Tablets **2009**

NEOFLUOR (Germany)
FLUOROURACIL
Efudex Topical Cream **3348**
Efudex Topical Solutions **3348**

NEOGASTRO (Australia)
LOPERAMIDE HYDROCHLORIDE
Imodium Capsules **1834**

NEO-IPERTAS (Greece)
CAPTOPRIL
Captopril Tablets **2114**

NEOLAPRIL (Brazil)
ENALAPRIL MALEATE
Vasotec I.V. Injection **2076**

NEOLIPID (Brazil)
LOVASTATIN
Mevacor Tablets **1996**

NEO-LOTAN (Italy)
LOSARTAN POTASSIUM
Cozaar Tablets **1913**

NEO-LOTAN PLUS (Italy)
HYDROCHLOROTHIAZIDE/LOSARTAN POTASSIUM
Hyzaar 50-12.5 Tablets **1964**

NEO-METRIC (Canada)
METRONIDAZOLE
MetroGel-Vaginal Gel **1822**
Noritate Cream, 1% **1051**

NEONAXIL (Mexico)
NAPROXEN
EC-Naprosyn Delayed-Release Tablets **2769**
Naprosyn Suspension **2769**
Naprosyn Tablets **2769**

NEO-PENOTRAN (Malaysia, Singapore)
METRONIDAZOLE
MetroGel-Vaginal Gel **1822**
Noritate Cream, 1% **1051**

NEO-PREOCIL (Portugal)
FLUOROMETHOLONE
FML Ophthalmic Ointment . . . . **⊙225**

NEOPRESS (Brazil)
LOSARTAN POTASSIUM
Cozaar Tablets **1913**

NEOPREX (Italy)
ENALAPRIL MALEATE/HYDROCHLOROTHIAZIDE
Vaseretic Tablets **2073**

NEO-PYRAZON (Malaysia, Singapore)
DICLOFENAC SODIUM
Voltaren Tablets **2298**
Voltaren-XR Tablets **2301**

NEORINOL (Chile)
IPRATROPIUM BROMIDE
Atrovent Inhalation Solution **868**
Atrovent Nasal Spray 0.03% **869**
Atrovent Nasal Spray 0.06% **870**

NEOSAC (Brazil)
RANITIDINE HYDROCHLORIDE
Zantac 25 EFFERdose Tablets **1597**
Zantac 150 EFFERdose Tablets **1597**
Zantac 150 Tablets **1597**
Zantac 300 Tablets **1597**
Zantac Injection **1593**
Zantac Injection Premixed **1593**
Zantac Syrup **1597**

NEOSEMID (Brazil)
FUROSEMIDE
Furosemide Tablets **2117**

NEOSORO (Brazil)
NAPHAZOLINE HYDROCHLORIDE
Albalon Ophthalmic Solution . . . . **⊙216**

NEOSTATIN (Brazil)
NYSTATIN
Nystop Topical Powder USP **2490**

NEOTAREN (Brazil)
DICLOFENAC SODIUM
Voltaren Tablets **2298**
Voltaren-XR Tablets **2301**

NEOTENOL (Brazil)
ATENOLOL
Tenormin I.V. Injection **698**

NEOTENSIN (Spain)
ENALAPRIL MALEATE
Vasotec I.V. Injection **2076**

NEOTENSIN DIU (Spain)
ENALAPRIL MALEATE/HYDROCHLOROTHIAZIDE
Vaseretic Tablets **2073**

NEOTIGASON (Argentina, Australia, Austria, Belgium, Brazil, Chile, Czech Republic, Denmark, Finland, Germany, Greece, Hong Kong, Irish Republic, Israel, Italy, Mexico, New Zealand, Norway, Portugal, Singapore, South Africa, Spain, Sweden, Switzerland, Thailand, The Netherlands, United Kingdom)
ACITRETIN
Soriatane Capsules **1028**

NEO-TIROIMADE (Portugal)
LIOTHYRONINE SODIUM
Cytomel Tablets **1678**

NEOTRETIN (Argentina)
TRETINOIN
Avita Cream **2136**
Avita Gel **2138**
Renova 0.05% Cream **2387**
Retin-A Micro 0.1%/0.04% **2388**
Vesanoid Capsules **2823**

NEOTUL (Spain)
FAMOTIDINE
Pepcid Injection **2017**
Pepcid Injection Premixed **2017**
Pepcid Tablets **2014**
Pepcid for Oral Suspension **2014**

NEOVERMIN (Brazil)
MEBENDAZOLE
Vermox Chewable Tablets **1853**

NEOVISC (Canada)
SODIUM HYALURONATE
Hyalgan Solution **2917**

NEO-ZOL (Canada)
CLOTRIMAZOLE
Lotrimin Cream **3053**
Lotrimin Lotion 1% **3053**
Lotrimin Topical Solution 1% **3053**

NEPHRAL (Germany)
HYDROCHLOROTHIAZIDE/TRIAMTERENE
Dyazide Capsules **1389**
Maxzide Tablets **2150**
Maxzide-25 mg Tablets **2150**

NEPHREX (Australia, Hong Kong)
CALCIUM ACETATE
PhosLo GelCaps **2158**

NEREFLUN (Italy)
FLUNISOLIDE
Aerobid Inhaler System **1172**
Aerobid-M Inhaler System **1172**
Nasarel Nasal Spray **1652**

NERGADAN (Spain)
LOVASTATIN
Mevacor Tablets **1996**

NERICUR (United Kingdom)
BENZOYL PEROXIDE
Brevoxyl-4 Creamy Wash **3212**
Brevoxyl-4 Gel **3211**
Brevoxyl-8 Creamy Wash **3212**
Brevoxyl-8 Gel **3211**
Triaz Cleanser **1864**
Triaz Gel **1864**

NEROLID (Mexico)
DIAZEPAM
Diastat Rectal Delivery System **3344**
Valium Tablets **2822**

NESBILER (Argentina)
FLUOROMETHOLONE
FML Ophthalmic Ointment . . . . **⊙225**

NESTIC (Thailand)
CLOTRIMAZOLE
Lotrimin Cream **3053**
Lotrimin Lotion 1% **3053**
Lotrimin Topical Solution 1% **3053**

NETUNAL (Argentina)
SUCRALFATE
Carafate Suspension **727**
Carafate Tablets **728**

NEUGAL (Mexico)
RANITIDINE HYDROCHLORIDE
Zantac 25 EFFERdose Tablets **1597**
Zantac 150 EFFERdose Tablets **1597**
Zantac 150 Tablets **1597**
Zantac 300 Tablets **1597**
Zantac Injection **1593**
Zantac Injection Premixed **1593**
Zantac Syrup **1597**

NEUGERON (Mexico)
CARBAMAZEPINE
Carbatrol Capsules **3174**
Tegretol Chewable Tablets **2278**
Tegretol Suspension **2278**
Tegretol Tablets **2278**
Tegretol-XR Tablets **2278**

NEUMEGA (Argentina, Brazil, Chile, Mexico)
OPRELVEKIN
Neumega for Injection **3433**

NEURALPRONA (Argentina)
NAPROXEN
EC-Naprosyn Delayed-Release Tablets **2769**
Naprosyn Suspension **2769**
Naprosyn Tablets **2769**

NEURIL (Denmark, Finland)
GABAPENTIN
Neurontin Capsules **2498**

NEURIUM (Brazil)
LAMOTRIGINE
Lamictal Chewable Dispersible Tablets . . . **1449**
Lamictal Tablets **1449**

NEUROCEFAL TRANQUI (Spain)
DIAZEPAM
Diastat Rectal Delivery System **3344**
Valium Tablets **2822**

NEURODOL TISSUGEL (Switzerland)
LIDOCAINE
Lidoderm Patch **1107**

NEUROGERON (Chile)
NIMODIPINE
Nimotop Capsules **774**

NEUROLEP (Mexico)
CARBAMAZEPINE
Carbatrol Capsules **3174**
Tegretol Chewable Tablets **2278**
Tegretol Suspension **2278**
Tegretol Tablets **2278**
Tegretol-XR Tablets **2278**

NEUROLEPSIN (Austria)
LITHIUM CARBONATE
Eskalith CR Controlled-Release Tablets . . . **1406**
Eskalith Capsules **1406**

NEUROLITHIUM (Brazil)
LITHIUM CARBONATE
Eskalith CR Controlled-Release Tablets . . . **1406**
Eskalith Capsules **1406**

NEUROLYTRIL (Germany)
DIAZEPAM
Diastat Rectal Delivery System **3344**
Valium Tablets **2822**

NEURONTIN (Argentina, Australia, Austria, Belgium, Brazil, Canada, Czech Republic, Finland, France, Greece, Hong Kong, Hungary, India, Irish Republic, Israel, Italy, Malaysia, Mexico, New Zealand, Norway, Portugal, Singapore, South Africa, Spain, Sweden, Switzerland, Thailand, The Netherlands, United Kingdom)
GABAPENTIN
Neurontin Capsules **2498**

NEUROSTIL (Irish Republic)
GABAPENTIN
Neurontin Capsules **2498**

NEUROTOL (Finland)
CARBAMAZEPINE
Carbatrol Capsules **3174**

Tegretol Chewable Tablets 2278
Tegretol Suspension. 2278
Tegretol Tablets 2278
Tegretol-XR Tablets 2278

NEUROTOP (Austria, Czech Republic, Hungary, Singapore, Switzerland)
CARBAMAZEPINE
Carbatrol Capsules 3174
Tegretol Chewable Tablets 2278
Tegretol Suspension. 2278
Tegretol Tablets 2278
Tegretol-XR Tablets 2278

NEURYL (Argentina, Chile)
CLONAZEPAM
Klonopin Tablets 2782

NEUTOP (Argentina)
TOPIRAMATE
Topamax Sprinkle Capsules 2438
Topamax Tablets 2438

NEUTROGENA ACNE MASK (Australia, Canada)
BENZOYL PEROXIDE
Brevoxyl-4 Creamy Wash. 3212
Brevoxyl-4 Gel 3211
Brevoxyl-8 Creamy Wash. 3212
Brevoxyl-8 Gel 3211
Triaz Cleanser 1864
Triaz Gel. 1864

NEUTROGENA LONG LASTING DANDRUFF CONTROL (United Kingdom)
KETOCONAZOLE
Nizoral 2% Shampoo 1838

NEUTROGENA ON THE SPOT ACNE TREATMENT (Canada)
BENZOYL PEROXIDE
Brevoxyl-4 Creamy Wash. 3212
Brevoxyl-4 Gel 3211
Brevoxyl-8 Creamy Wash. 3212
Brevoxyl-8 Gel 3211
Triaz Cleanser 1864
Triaz Gel. 1864

NEUTROMED (Austria)
CIMETIDINE
Tagamet Tablets 1547

NEUTRONORM (Austria, Hong Kong)
CIMETIDINE
Tagamet Tablets 1547

NEWFLOX (Argentina)
OFLOXACIN
Floxin Otic Solution 1043

NEW-NOK (Israel)
PERMETHRIN
Acticin Cream. 2125

NEXADRON (Argentina)
DEXAMETHASONE
Decadron Tablets 1929

NEXADRON COMPUESTO (Argentina)
DEXAMETHASONE
Decadron Tablets 1929

NIACEL (Mexico)
METRONIDAZOLE
MetroGel-Vaginal Gel 1822
Noritate Cream, 1%. 1051

NIAR (Brazil, Mexico)
SELEGILINE HYDROCHLORIDE
Eldepryl Capsules 3209

NICABATE (Australia, New Zealand, United Kingdom)
NICOTINE
Nicotrol Inhaler 2594
Nicotrol NS 2596

NICARDIA (India)
NIFEDIPINE
Adalat CC Tablets 2978

NICHOGENCIN (Germany)
GENTAMICIN SULFATE
Garamycin Injectable 3028
Genoptic Sterile Ophthalmic Solution . . . . ⊙227

NICODERM (Canada)
NICOTINE
Nicotrol Inhaler 2594
Nicotrol NS 2596

NICODISC (Spain)
NICOTINE
Nicotrol Inhaler 2594
Nicotrol NS 2596

NICOGUM (France)
NICOTINE
Nicotrol Inhaler 2594
Nicotrol NS 2596

NICOLAN (Austria, Brazil, Sweden)
NICOTINE
Nicotrol Inhaler 2594
Nicotrol NS 2596

NICONIL (Irish Republic, United Kingdom)
NICOTINE
Nicotrol Inhaler 2594
Nicotrol NS 2596

NICOPASS (France)
NICOTINE
Nicotrol Inhaler 2594
Nicotrol NS 2596

NICOPATCH (France)
NICOTINE
Nicotrol Inhaler 2594
Nicotrol NS 2596

NICORETTE (Australia, Brazil, Canada, Chile, Czech Republic, Germany, Greece, Irish Republic, Israel, Malaysia, Mexico, New Zealand, Portugal, Singapore)
NICOTINE
Nicotrol Inhaler 2594
Nicotrol NS 2596

NICOSTOP TTS (Switzerland)
NICOTINE
Nicotrol Inhaler 2594
Nicotrol NS 2596

NICOTEX (India)
BUPROPION HYDROCHLORIDE
Wellbutrin SR Sustained-Release Tablets . . 1583
Wellbutrin Tablets 1579
Zyban Sustained-Release Tablets. 1620

NICOTINELL (Australia, Austria, Belgium, Chile, Czech Republic, Denmark, France, Germany, Greece, Hungary, Irish Republic, Israel, Malaysia, New Zealand, Norway, Singapore, Spain, Thailand)
NICOTINE
Nicotrol Inhaler 2594
Nicotrol NS 2596

NICOTINELL TTS (Argentina, Brazil, India, Italy, Mexico, Portugal, South Africa)
NICOTINE
Nicotrol Inhaler 2594
Nicotrol NS 2596

NICOTRANS (Italy, Spain)
NICOTINE
Nicotrol Inhaler 2594
Nicotrol NS 2596

NICOTROL (Austria, Canada, New Zealand, Spain)
NICOTINE
Nicotrol Inhaler 2594
Nicotrol NS 2596

NIDAGEL (Canada)
METRONIDAZOLE
MetroGel-Vaginal Gel 1822
Noritate Cream, 1%. 1051

NIDATRON (South Africa)
METRONIDAZOLE
MetroGel-Vaginal Gel 1822
Noritate Cream, 1%. 1051

NIDAZOL (United Kingdom)
METRONIDAZOLE
MetroGel-Vaginal Gel 1822
Noritate Cream, 1%. 1051

NIDAZOLEM (Mexico)
METRONIDAZOLE
MetroGel-Vaginal Gel 1822
Noritate Cream, 1%. 1051

NIDAZOLIN (Brazil)
NYSTATIN
Nystop Topical Powder USP. 2490

NIDRALON (Mexico)
METRONIDAZOLE
MetroGel-Vaginal Gel 1822
Noritate Cream, 1%. 1051

NIFADIL (Brazil)
NIFEDIPINE
Adalat CC Tablets 2978

NIFAL (Austria)
NIFEDIPINE
Adalat CC Tablets 2978

NIFANGIN (Finland)
NIFEDIPINE
Adalat CC Tablets 2978

NIFATENOL (Germany)
ATENOLOL
Tenormin I.V. Injection. 698

NIFDEMIN (Finland)
NIFEDIPINE
Adalat CC Tablets 2978

NIFE (Germany)
NIFEDIPINE
Adalat CC Tablets 2978

NIFE UNO (Germany)
NIFEDIPINE
Adalat CC Tablets 2978

NIFE-BASAN (Switzerland)
NIFEDIPINE
Adalat CC Tablets 2978

NIFEBENE (Austria)
NIFEDIPINE
Adalat CC Tablets 2978

NIFECARD (Australia, Austria, Czech Republic, Hong Kong, Hungary, Singapore, Thailand)
NIFEDIPINE
Adalat CC Tablets 2978

NIFECARD XL (Russia)
NIFEDIPINE
Adalat CC Tablets 2978

NIFECLAIR (Germany)
NIFEDIPINE
Adalat CC Tablets 2978

NIFECODAN (Denmark)
NIFEDIPINE
Adalat CC Tablets 2978

NIFECOR (Argentina, Finland, Germany)
NIFEDIPINE
Adalat CC Tablets 2978

NIFED (Irish Republic)
NIFEDIPINE
Adalat CC Tablets 2978

NIFED SOL (Argentina)
NIFEDIPINE
Adalat CC Tablets 2978

NIFEDALAT (South Africa)
NIFEDIPINE
Adalat CC Tablets 2978

NIFEDAX (Brazil)
NIFEDIPINE
Adalat CC Tablets 2978

NIFEDEL (Argentina)
NIFEDIPINE
Adalat CC Tablets 2978

NIFEDICOR (Italy, Switzerland)
NIFEDIPINE
Adalat CC Tablets 2978

NIFEDICRON (Italy)
NIFEDIPINE
Adalat CC Tablets 2978

NIFEDI-DENK (Singapore)
NIFEDIPINE
Adalat CC Tablets 2978

NIFEDIGEL (Mexico)
NIFEDIPINE
Adalat CC Tablets 2978

NIFEDIN (Brazil, Italy)
NIFEDIPINE
Adalat CC Tablets 2978

NIFEDINE (India)
NIFEDIPINE
Adalat CC Tablets 2978

NIFEDIPAT (Germany, Greece)
NIFEDIPINE
Adalat CC Tablets 2978

NIFEDIPRES (Mexico)
NIFEDIPINE
Adalat CC Tablets 2978

NIFEDIPRESS (United Kingdom)
NIFEDIPINE
Adalat CC Tablets 2978

NIFEDOTARD (United Kingdom)
NIFEDIPINE
Adalat CC Tablets 2978

NIFEHEXAL (Australia, Austria, Brazil, Czech Republic, Germany)
NIFEDIPINE
Adalat CC Tablets 2978

NIFEHEXAL SALI (Germany)
NIFEDIPINE
Adalat CC Tablets 2978

NIFELAT (Argentina, Brazil, Germany, India, Singapore, Thailand)
NIFEDIPINE
Adalat CC Tablets 2978

NIFELATE (France)
NIFEDIPINE
Adalat CC Tablets 2978

NIFELEASE (Irish Republic, United Kingdom)
NIFEDIPINE
Adalat CC Tablets 2978

NIFENSAR (Irish Republic)
NIFEDIPINE
Adalat CC Tablets 2978

NIFENSAR XL (United Kingdom)
NIFEDIPINE
Adalat CC Tablets 2978

NIFESAL (Italy)
NIFEDIPINE
Adalat CC Tablets 2978

NIFETOLOL (India)
ATENOLOL
Tenormin I.V. Injection. 698

NIFEZZARD (Mexico)
NIFEDIPINE
Adalat CC Tablets 2978

NIFICAL (Germany)
NIFEDIPINE
Adalat CC Tablets 2978

NIFICARD (Thailand)
NIFEDIPINE
Adalat CC Tablets 2978

NIFIDINE (South Africa)
NIFEDIPINE
Adalat CC Tablets 2978

NIFIRAN (Thailand)
NIFEDIPINE
Adalat CC Tablets 2978

NIFLAM (Argentina)
CELECOXIB
Celebrex Capsules. 3130

NIFOPRESS (United Kingdom)
NIFEDIPINE
Adalat CC Tablets 2978

NIFREAL (Germany)
NIFEDIPINE
Adalat CC Tablets 2978

NIF-TEN (Finland, Germany, Hong Kong, Italy)
ATENOLOL
Tenormin I.V. Injection. 698

NIJ-TEROL (Chile)
LOVASTATIN
Mevacor Tablets 1996

NIKION (Argentina)
ENALAPRIL MALEATE
Vasotec I.V. Injection 2076

NIKOFRENON (Germany)
NICOTINE
Nicotrol Inhaler 2594
Nicotrol NS 2596

NIKORAZOL (Mexico)
KETOCONAZOLE
Nizoral 2% Shampoo 1838

NILPERIDOL (Brazil)
FENTANYL CITRATE
Actiq . . . 993

NILSTAT (Australia, Belgium, Canada, New Zealand)
NYSTATIN
Nystop Topical Powder USP . . . 2490

NIM (Germany)
NIMODIPINE
Nimotop Capsules . . . 774

NIMAZ (France)
LOPERAMIDE HYDROCHLORIDE
Imodium Capsules . . . 1834

NIMEGEN (Singapore)
ISOTRETINOIN
Accutane Capsules . . . 2740

NIMICOR (Chile)
SIMVASTATIN
Zocor Tablets . . . 2078

NIMODIL (Greece)
NIMODIPINE
Nimotop Capsules . . . 774

NIMODILAT (Argentina)
NIMODIPINE
Nimotop Capsules . . . 774

NIMODILAT PLUS (Argentina)
NIMODIPINE
Nimotop Capsules . . . 774

NIMODREL (United Kingdom)
NIFEDIPINE
Adalat CC Tablets . . . 2978

NIMOREAGIN (Argentina)
NIMODIPINE
Nimotop Capsules . . . 774

NIMOTOP (Argentina, Australia, Austria, Belgium, Brazil, Canada, Chile, Czech Republic, Denmark, Finland, France, Germany, Greece, Hong Kong, Hungary, Irish Republic, Israel, Italy, Malaysia, Mexico, New Zealand, Norway, Portugal, Singapore, South Africa, Spain, Sweden, Switzerland, Thailand, The Netherlands, United Kingdom)
NIMODIPINE
Nimotop Capsules . . . 774

NIMOVAS (Brazil)
NIMODIPINE
Nimotop Capsules . . . 774

NINAZOL (Thailand)
KETOCONAZOLE
Nizoral 2% Shampoo . . . 1838

NINDAXA (United Kingdom)
INDAPAMIDE
Indapamide Tablets . . . 2119

NIPENT (Belgium, Canada, France, Germany, Greece, Italy, Portugal, Spain, United Kingdom)
PENTOSTATIN
Nipent for Injection . . . 3216

NIPIN (Italy, Singapore)
NIFEDIPINE
Adalat CC Tablets . . . 2978

NIPODUR (Greece)
RANITIDINE HYDROCHLORIDE
Zantac 25 EFFERdose Tablets . . . 1597
Zantac 150 EFFERdose Tablets. . . . 1597
Zantac 150 Tablets . . . 1597
Zantac 300 Tablets . . . 1597
Zantac Injection . . . 1593
Zantac Injection Premixed . . . 1593
Zantac Syrup . . . 1597

NIPOGALIN (Greece)
CEFUROXIME SODIUM
Zinacef Injection . . . 1604

NIPRESS (Chile)
NIFEDIPINE
Adalat CC Tablets . . . 2978

NIQUITIN (Belgium, Brazil, Czech Republic, Denmark, France, Germany, Hungary, Irish Republic, Israel, Mexico, Sweden, The Netherlands, United Kingdom)
NICOTINE
Nicotrol Inhaler . . . 2594
Nicotrol NS . . . 2596

NIRULID (Denmark)
AMILORIDE HYDROCHLORIDE
Midamor Tablets . . . 2000

NISIS (France)
VALSARTAN
Diovan Tablets . . . 2191

NISISCO (France)
HYDROCHLOROTHIAZIDE/VALSARTAN
Diovan HCT Tablets . . . 2195

NISODIPEN (Argentina)
NISOLDIPINE
Sular Tablets . . . 1163

NISOLID (Italy)
FLUNISOLIDE
Aerobid Inhaler System. . . . 1172
Aerobid-M Inhaler System . . . 1172
Nasarel Nasal Spray . . . 1652

NISTAGRAND (Argentina)
NYSTATIN
Nystop Topical Powder USP . . . 2490

NISTAGYN (Brazil)
NYSTATIN
Nystop Topical Powder USP . . . 2490

NISTAKEN (Mexico)
PROPAFENONE HYDROCHLORIDE
Rythmol SR Capsules . . . 2736

NISTAN (Mexico)
NYSTATIN
Nystop Topical Powder USP . . . 2490

NISTANIL (Brazil)
NYSTATIN
Nystop Topical Powder USP . . . 2490

NISTAQUIM (Mexico)
NYSTATIN
Nystop Topical Powder USP . . . 2490

NISTAT (Argentina)
NYSTATIN
Nystop Topical Powder USP . . . 2490

NISTAVAL (Brazil)
NYSTATIN
Nystop Topical Powder USP . . . 2490

NISTAX (Brazil)
NYSTATIN
Nystop Topical Powder USP . . . 2490

NISTINOL (Argentina)
NYSTATIN
Nystop Topical Powder USP . . . 2490

NISTORAL (Chile)
NYSTATIN
Nystop Topical Powder USP . . . 2490

NITAGON (South Africa)
PERMETHRIN
Acticin Cream . . . 2125

NITASTIN (Greece)
SIMVASTATIN
Zocor Tablets . . . 2078

NITEN (Argentina)
LOSARTAN POTASSIUM
Cozaar Tablets . . . 1913

NITEN D (Argentina)
LOSARTAN POTASSIUM
Cozaar Tablets . . . 1913

NITEREY (Argentina)
TRETINOIN
Avita Cream . . . 2136
Avita Gel . . . 2138
Renova 0.05% Cream . . . 2387
Retin-A Micro 0.1%/0.04% . . . 2388
Vesanoid Capsules . . . 2823

NITRAMIN (Greece)
ISOSORBIDE MONONITRATE
Imdur Tablets . . . 3032

NITREX (Italy)
ISOSORBIDE MONONITRATE
Imdur Tablets . . . 3032

NITRILAN (Greece)
ISOSORBIDE MONONITRATE
Imdur Tablets . . . 3032

NITROCIT (South Africa)
POTASSIUM CITRATE
Urocit-K Tablets . . . 2109

NITROLERG (Brazil)
HYDROCORTISONE
Hydrocortone Tablets . . . 1963

NITROMIDAGER (Mexico)
METRONIDAZOLE
MetroGel-Vaginal Gel . . . 1822
Noritate Cream, 1% . . . 1051

NIVADOR (Spain)
CEFUROXIME AXETIL
Ceftin Tablets . . . 1369
Ceftin for Oral Suspension . . . 1369

NIVAS (Argentina, Chile)
NIMODIPINE
Nimotop Capsules . . . 774

NIVAS PLUS (Argentina)
NIMODIPINE
Nimotop Capsules . . . 774

NIVATEN (United Kingdom)
NIFEDIPINE
Adalat CC Tablets . . . 2978

NIVELIPOL (Argentina)
SIMVASTATIN
Zocor Tablets . . . 2078

NIVOFLOX (Mexico)
CIPROFLOXACIN HYDROCHLORIDE
Ciloxan Ophthalmic Ointment . . . 554
Ciloxan Ophthalmic Solution . . . ⊙205
Cipro Tablets . . . 2991

NIX (Australia, Belgium, Canada, Denmark, Finland, France, Greece, Italy, Norway, Portugal, Sweden)
PERMETHRIN
Acticin Cream . . . 2125

NIXAL (Mexico)
NAPROXEN SODIUM
Anaprox DS Tablets . . . 2769
Anaprox Tablets . . . 2769

NIXIN (Brazil, Portugal)
CIPROFLOXACIN HYDROCHLORIDE
Ciloxan Ophthalmic Ointment . . . 554
Ciloxan Ophthalmic Solution . . . ⊙205
Cipro Tablets . . . 2991

NIZALE (Portugal)
KETOCONAZOLE
Nizoral 2% Shampoo . . . 1838

NIZCREME (South Africa)
KETOCONAZOLE
Nizoral 2% Shampoo . . . 1838

NIZOLE (Singapore)
METRONIDAZOLE
MetroGel-Vaginal Gel . . . 1822
Noritate Cream, 1% . . . 1051

NIZORAL (Australia, Austria, Belgium, Brazil, Canada, Czech Republic, Denmark, France, Germany, Hong Kong, Hungary, Irish Republic, Israel, Italy, Malaysia, Mexico, New Zealand, Portugal, Singapore, South Africa, Switzerland, Thailand, The Netherlands)
KETOCONAZOLE
Nizoral 2% Shampoo . . . 1838

NIZORELLE (South Africa)
KETOCONAZOLE
Nizoral 2% Shampoo . . . 1838

NIZORETIC (Brazil)
KETOCONAZOLE
Nizoral 2% Shampoo . . . 1838

NIZOVULES (South Africa)
KETOCONAZOLE
Nizoral 2% Shampoo . . . 1838

NIZSHAMPOO (South Africa)
KETOCONAZOLE
Nizoral 2% Shampoo . . . 1838

NM POWDER (India)
NORFLOXACIN
Noroxin Tablets . . . 2009

NOALDOL (Italy)
DIFLUNISAL
Dolobid Tablets . . . 1937

NOAN (Brazil, Italy)
DIAZEPAM
Diastat Rectal Delivery System . . . 3344
Valium Tablets . . . 2822

NOCEPTIN (The Netherlands)
MORPHINE SULFATE
Kadian Capsules . . . 572
MS Contin Tablets . . . 2703

NOCTAL (Brazil)
ESTAZOLAM
ProSom Tablets . . . 512

NOCUTIL (Austria, Czech Republic, Germany, Hungary, Switzerland, United Kingdom)
DESMOPRESSIN ACETATE
DDAVP Injection 4 mcg/mL . . . 2893
DDAVP Nasal Spray . . . 2894
DDAVP Tablets . . . 2895
Desmopressin Acetate Injection . . . 1143
Desmopressin Acetate Rhinal Tube . . . 1144

NODOL (Italy)
RANITIDINE HYDROCHLORIDE
Zantac 25 EFFERdose Tablets . . . 1597
Zantac 150 EFFERdose Tablets. . . . 1597
Zantac 150 Tablets . . . 1597
Zantac 300 Tablets . . . 1597
Zantac Injection . . . 1593
Zantac Injection Premixed . . . 1593
Zantac Syrup . . . 1597

NOFLAM (New Zealand)
NAPROXEN
EC-Naprosyn Delayed-Release Tablets. . . . 2769
Naprosyn Suspension . . . 2769
Naprosyn Tablets . . . 2769

NOFLAM-N (Hong Kong)
NAPROXEN SODIUM
Anaprox DS Tablets . . . 2769
Anaprox Tablets . . . 2769

NOITRON (Greece)
ISOTRETINOIN
Accutane Capsules . . . 2740

NOK (Israel)
PERMETHRIN
Acticin Cream . . . 2125

NOKLOT (India)
CLOPIDOGREL BISULFATE
Plavix Tablets . . . 940, 2942

NOKTONE (Norway)
RANITIDINE HYDROCHLORIDE
Zantac 25 EFFERdose Tablets . . . 1597
Zantac 150 EFFERdose Tablets. . . . 1597
Zantac 150 Tablets . . . 1597
Zantac 300 Tablets . . . 1597
Zantac Injection . . . 1593
Zantac Injection Premixed . . . 1593
Zantac Syrup . . . 1597

NOLICIN (Czech Republic, Hungary, Russia)
NORFLOXACIN
Noroxin Tablets . . . 2009

NOLIPAX (Italy)
FENOFIBRATE
Tricor Tablets . . . 523

NOLIPREL (Czech Republic, Hungary)
PERINDOPRIL ERBUMINE
Aceon Tablets (2 mg, 4 mg, 8 mg) . . . 3191

NOLOL (South Africa, Thailand)
PROPRANOLOL HYDROCHLORIDE
Inderal LA Long-Acting Capsules . . . 3421

NOODIPINA (Brazil)
NIMODIPINE
Nimotop Capsules . . . 774

NOPUCID (Argentina)
PERMETHRIN
Acticin Cream . . . 2125

NOR 2 (Argentina)
NORFLOXACIN
Noroxin Tablets . . . 2009

NOR T (India)
NORFLOXACIN
Noroxin Tablets . . . 2009

NORA (Thailand)
KETOCONAZOLE
Nizoral 2% Shampoo . . . 1838

NORACIN (Brazil, Thailand)
NORFLOXACIN
Noroxin Tablets . . . 2009

NORANAT (Argentina)
INDAPAMIDE
Indapamide Tablets **2119**

NORAXIN (Thailand)
NORFLOXACIN
Noroxin Tablets. **2009**

NORBACTIN (India, Malaysia, Singapore, Thailand)
NORFLOXACIN
Noroxin Tablets. **2009**

NORCIN (Thailand)
NORFLOXACIN
Noroxin Tablets. **2009**

NORDOTOL (Denmark)
CARBAMAZEPINE
Carbatrol Capsules **3174**
Tegretol Chewable Tablets **2278**
Tegretol Suspension. **2278**
Tegretol Tablets **2278**
Tegretol-XR Tablets **2278**

NORDURINE (Irish Republic)
DESMOPRESSIN ACETATE
DDAVP Injection 4 mcg/mL **2893**
DDAVP Nasal Spray **2894**
DDAVP Tablets **2895**
Desmopressin Acetate Injection **1143**
Desmopressin Acetate Rhinal Tube **1144**

NORELBIN (Brazil)
VINORELBINE TARTRATE
Navelbine Injection. **1494**

NORFCIN (Thailand)
NORFLOXACIN
Noroxin Tablets. **2009**

NORFENON (Mexico)
PROPAFENONE HYDROCHLORIDE
Rythmol SR Capsules **2736**

NORFLAMIN (Brazil)
NORFLOXACIN
Noroxin Tablets. **2009**

NORFLEX (Australia, Austria, Belgium, Canada, Denmark, Finland, Germany, Greece, Malaysia, Mexico, New Zealand, Portugal, Singapore, South Africa, Sweden, Switzerland, Thailand, United Kingdom)
ORPHENADRINE CITRATE
Norflex Injection **1824**

NORFLO (Thailand)
NORFLOXACIN
Noroxin Tablets. **2009**

NORFLOCIN (Thailand)
NORFLOXACIN
Noroxin Tablets. **2009**

NORFLOCINE (Switzerland)
NORFLOXACIN
Noroxin Tablets. **2009**

NORFLOHEXAL (Australia, Germany)
NORFLOXACIN
Noroxin Tablets. **2009**

NORFLOK (Spain)
NORFLOXACIN
Noroxin Tablets. **2009**

NORFLOL (Argentina)
NORFLOXACIN
Noroxin Tablets. **2009**

NORFLOSAL (Germany)
NORFLOXACIN
Noroxin Tablets. **2009**

NORFLOSTAD (Austria)
NORFLOXACIN
Noroxin Tablets. **2009**

NORFLOX (India)
NORFLOXACIN
Noroxin Tablets. **2009**

NORFLOX TZ (India)
NORFLOXACIN
Noroxin Tablets. **2009**

NORFLOXASAN (Brazil)
NORFLOXACIN
Noroxin Tablets. **2009**

NORFLOX-AZU (Germany)
NORFLOXACIN
Noroxin Tablets. **2009**

NORFLOXBETA (Germany)
NORFLOXACIN
Noroxin Tablets. **2009**

NORFLOXIN (Thailand)
NORFLOXACIN
Noroxin Tablets. **2009**

NORFLOXINOR (Malaysia)
NORFLOXACIN
Noroxin Tablets. **2009**

NORFLOX-PUREN (Germany)
NORFLOXACIN
Noroxin Tablets. **2009**

NORGESIC (Australia, Malaysia)
ORPHENADRINE CITRATE
Norflex Injection **1824**

NORIDERM (Brazil)
KETOCONAZOLE
Nizoral 2% Shampoo **1838**

NORIMODE (South Africa, United Kingdom)
LOPERAMIDE HYDROCHLORIDE
Imodium Capsules **1834**

NORIMOX (South Africa)
AMOXICILLIN
Amoxil Pediatric Drops for Oral Suspension. **1315**
Amoxil Tablets **1315**

NORIPLEX (Hungary)
INDAPAMIDE
Indapamide Tablets **2119**

NORITATE (Argentina, Canada, Chile, Hong Kong, Israel, United Kingdom)
METRONIDAZOLE
MetroGel-Vaginal Gel **1822**
Noritate Cream, 1% **1051**

NORIZAL (Brazil)
KETOCONAZOLE
Nizoral 2% Shampoo **1838**

NORMAFENAC (Greece)
CEFUROXIME SODIUM
Zinacef Injection **1604**

NORMALIP PRO (Germany)
FENOFIBRATE
Tricor Tablets **523**

NORMALOE (United Kingdom)
LOPERAMIDE HYDROCHLORIDE
Imodium Capsules **1834**

NORMALOL (Israel)
ATENOLOL
Tenormin I.V. Injection. **698**

NORMAPRIL (Brazil)
CAPTOPRIL
Captopril Tablets **2114**

NORMASE (Italy)
LACTULOSE
Kristalose for Oral Solution **2149**

NORMATEN (Chile, Hong Kong, Malaysia, Singapore)
ENALAPRIL MALEATE/HYDROCHLOROTHIAZIDE
Vaseretic Tablets **2073**

NORMATEN PLUS (Chile)
ENALAPRIL MALEATE/HYDROCHLOROTHIAZIDE
Vaseretic Tablets **2073**

NORMATENSIL (Argentina)
HYDROCHLOROTHIAZIDE/METHYLDOPA
Aldoril Tablets. **1884**

NORMATOL (Chile)
GABAPENTIN
Neurontin Capsules **2498**

NORMAX (India, Russia)
NORFLOXACIN
Noroxin Tablets. **2009**

NORMAX TZ (India)
NORFLOXACIN
Noroxin Tablets. **2009**

NORMETIC (United Kingdom)
AMILORIDE HYDROCHLORIDE/HYDROCHLOROTHIAZIDE
Moduretic Tablets **2003**

NORMITEN (Israel)
ATENOLOL
Tenormin I.V. Injection. **698**

NORMOLOSE (Greece)
CAPTOPRIL
Captopril Tablets **2114**

NORMOMENSIL (Brazil)
PROGESTERONE
Prometrium Capsules (100 mg, 200 mg) . **3205**

NORMOPRES (Brazil)
NIFEDIPINE
Adalat CC Tablets **2978**

NORMOPRESAN (Israel)
CLONIDINE HYDROCHLORIDE
Catapres Tablets **874**

NORMOPRESS (Italy)
ATENOLOL
Tenormin I.V. Injection. **698**

NORMOPRIL (India)
LISINOPRIL
Prinivil Tablets **2029**
Zestril Tablets. **704**

NORMORIX (Norway, Sweden)
AMILORIDE HYDROCHLORIDE/HYDROCHLOROTHIAZIDE
Moduretic Tablets **2003**

NORMORYTMIN (Argentina, Irish Republic)
PROPAFENONE HYDROCHLORIDE
Rythmol SR Capsules **2736**

NORMOSPOR (South Africa)
CLOTRIMAZOLE
Lotrimin Cream. **3053**
Lotrimin Lotion 1%. **3053**
Lotrimin Topical Solution 1% **3053**

NORMOTENSOR (Brazil)
FUROSEMIDE
Furosemide Tablets **2117**

NORMOTHERIN (Greece)
SIMVASTATIN
Zocor Tablets. **2078**

NORMOTIL (Portugal)
CAPTOPRIL
Captopril Tablets **2114**

NORMPRESS (Thailand)
PROPRANOLOL HYDROCHLORIDE
Inderal LA Long-Acting Capsules **3421**

NORMULEN (Spain)
DICLOFENAC SODIUM
Voltaren Tablets **2298**
Voltaren-XR Tablets **2301**

NOROCIN (Greece)
NORFLOXACIN
Noroxin Tablets. **2009**

NORONAL (Brazil)
KETOCONAZOLE
Nizoral 2% Shampoo **1838**

NOROXIN (Argentina, Australia, Canada, Chile, Finland, Italy, Mexico, New Zealand, Portugal, South Africa, Spain, Switzerland, The Netherlands, United Kingdom)
NORFLOXACIN
Noroxin Tablets. **2009**

NOROXINE (France)
NORFLOXACIN
Noroxin Tablets. **2009**

NORPHIN (India)
BUPRENORPHINE HYDROCHLORIDE
Buprenex Injectable **2718**

NORPRIL (Mexico)
ENALAPRIL MALEATE
Vasotec I.V. Injection **2076**

NORPRO (South Africa)
PROPRANOLOL HYDROCHLORIDE
Inderal LA Long-Acting Capsules **3421**

NORSA (Thailand)
NORFLOXACIN
Noroxin Tablets. **2009**

NORSOL (Argentina, Switzerland)
NORFLOXACIN
Noroxin Tablets. **2009**

NORTELOL (Thailand)
ATENOLOL
Tenormin I.V. Injection. **698**

NORTENSIN (Argentina)
TRANDOLAPRIL
Mavik Tablets **482**

NORTOLAN (Greece)
NIMODIPINE
Nimotop Capsules **774**

NORTON (Brazil)
NIMODIPINE
Nimotop Capsules **774**

NORVIR (Australia, Belgium, Canada, Chile, Czech Republic, Denmark, Finland, France, Germany, Greece, Hong Kong, Hungary, Irish Republic, Israel, Italy, Japan, Malaysia, Mexico, New Zealand, Norway, Portugal, South Africa, Spain, Sweden, Switzerland, Thailand, The Netherlands, United Kingdom)
RITONAVIR
Norvir Oral Solution **499**
Norvir Soft Gelatin Capsules. **499**

NORXACIN (Thailand)
NORFLOXACIN
Noroxin Tablets. **2009**

NORXIA (Thailand)
NORFLOXACIN
Noroxin Tablets. **2009**

NORXIN (Brazil)
NORFLOXACIN
Noroxin Tablets. **2009**

NOS (Spain)
FAMOTIDINE
Pepcid Injection **2017**
Pepcid Injection Premixed **2017**
Pepcid Tablets **2014**
Pepcid for Oral Suspension **2014**

NOSTEROL (Argentina)
SIMVASTATIN
Zocor Tablets. **2078**

NOTEN (Australia, Malaysia, Singapore, Thailand)
ATENOLOL
Tenormin I.V. Injection. **698**

NO-TON (Thailand)
NABUMETONE
Relafen Tablets **1523**

NOVA (Canada)
PENTOBARBITAL SODIUM
Nembutal Sodium Solution, USP **2484**

NOVA RECTAL (Canada)
PENTOBARBITAL SODIUM
Nembutal Sodium Solution, USP **2484**

NOVACEF (Argentina, Mexico)
CEFIXIME
Suprax **1811**

NOVACETOL (Chile)
CLOTRIMAZOLE
Lotrimin Cream. **3053**
Lotrimin Lotion 1%. **3053**
Lotrimin Topical Solution 1% **3053**

NOVACIL (Brazil)
AMOXICILLIN
Amoxil Pediatric Drops for Oral Suspension. **1315**
Amoxil Tablets **1315**

NOVACILINA (Chile)
LEVOFLOXACIN
Levaquin Injection **2453**
Levaquin Tablets **2453**

NOVACLAV (India)
AMOXICILLIN
Amoxil Pediatric Drops for Oral Suspension. **1315**
Amoxil Tablets **1315**

NOVACLOX LB (India)
AMOXICILLIN
Amoxil Pediatric Drops for Oral Suspension. **1315**
Amoxil Tablets **1315**

NOVACRIUM (Austria)
MIVACURIUM CHLORIDE
Mivacron Injection **489**

NOVADEX (Mexico)
NAPROXEN
EC-Naprosyn Delayed-Release Tablets 2769
Naprosyn Suspension 2769
Naprosyn Tablets 2769

NOVAL (Greece)
TIMOLOL MALEATE
Blocadren Tablets 1891
Timoptic Sterile Ophthalmic Solution 2058
Timoptic in Ocudose 2061
Timoptic-XE Sterile Ophthalmic Gel Forming Solution 2062

NOVAMET (Denmark, Mexico)
CIMETIDINE
Tagamet Tablets 1547

NOVAMILOR (Canada)
AMILORIDE HYDROCHLORIDE/HYDROCHLOROTHIAZIDE
Moduretic Tablets 2003

NOVAMOX (India)
AMOXICILLIN
Amoxil Pediatric Drops for Oral Suspension 1315
Amoxil Tablets 1315

NOVAMOX AX (India)
AMOXICILLIN
Amoxil Pediatric Drops for Oral Suspension 1315
Amoxil Tablets 1315

NOVAMOX LB (India)
AMOXICILLIN
Amoxil Pediatric Drops for Oral Suspension 1315
Amoxil Tablets 1315

NOVAPAM (New Zealand)
CHLORDIAZEPOXIDE HYDROCHLORIDE
Librium Capsules 3349

NOVAPAMYL (France)
VERAPAMIL HYDROCHLORIDE
Covera-HS Tablets 3135
Verelan PM Capsules 3120

NOVAPHYLLINE (Greece)
THEOPHYLLINE
Uniphyl Tablets 2708

NOVAPIRINA (Italy)
DICLOFENAC SODIUM
Voltaren Tablets 2298
Voltaren-XR Tablets 2301

NOVAPRES (Mexico)
CAPTOPRIL
Captopril Tablets 2114

NOVAPSYL (Mexico)
BENZONATATE
Tessalon Perles 1202

NOVASONE (Argentina, Australia)
MOMETASONE FUROATE
Elocon Cream 0.1% 3019
Elocon Lotion 0.1% 3020
Elocon Ointment 0.1% 3021
Nasonex Nasal Spray 3058

NOVASULFON (Mexico)
DAPSONE
Dapsone Tablets USP 1656

NOVATEC (Belgium, The Netherlands)
LISINOPRIL
Prinivil Tablets 2029
Zestril Tablets 704

NOVATIV (Brazil)
SERTRALINE HYDROCHLORIDE
Zoloft Tablets 2581

NOVAVIR (Mexico)
ZIDOVUDINE
Retrovir Capsules 1533
Retrovir IV Infusion 1537
Retrovir Syrup 1533
Retrovir Tablets 1533

NOVAXEN (Mexico)
NAPROXEN
EC-Naprosyn Delayed-Release Tablets 2769
Naprosyn Suspension 2769
Naprosyn Tablets 2769

NOVAZAM (France)
DIAZEPAM
Diastat Rectal Delivery System 3344
Valium Tablets 2822

NOVAZYD (Belgium, The Netherlands)
LISINOPRIL
Prinivil Tablets 2029
Zestril Tablets 704

NOVELIAN (Spain)
SUMATRIPTAN SUCCINATE
Imitrex Injection 1431
Imitrex Tablets 1440

NOVELMIN (Brazil)
MEBENDAZOLE
Vermox Chewable Tablets 1853

NOVIDAT (Argentina)
CIPROFLOXACIN HYDROCHLORIDE
Ciloxan Ophthalmic Ointment 554
Ciloxan Ophthalmic Solution . . . . ⊙205
Cipro Tablets 2991

NOVO RINO (Brazil)
NAPHAZOLINE HYDROCHLORIDE
Albalon Ophthalmic Solution . . . . ⊙216

NOVO-ATENOL (Canada)
ATENOLOL
Tenormin I.V. Injection 698

NOVO-AZT (Canada)
ZIDOVUDINE
Retrovir Capsules 1533
Retrovir IV Infusion 1537
Retrovir Syrup 1533
Retrovir Tablets 1533

NOVO-CAPTORIL (Canada, Hong Kong)
CAPTOPRIL
Captopril Tablets 2114

NOVO-CARBAMAZ (Canada)
CARBAMAZEPINE
Carbatrol Capsules 3174
Tegretol Chewable Tablets 2278
Tegretol Suspension 2278
Tegretol Tablets 2278
Tegretol-XR Tablets 2278

NOVO-CIMETINE (Canada)
CIMETIDINE
Tagamet Tablets 1547

NOVOCRAL (Greece)
CEFTAZIDIME
Fortaz for Injection 1422

NOVO-DIFENAC (Hong Kong)
DICLOFENAC SODIUM
Voltaren Tablets 2298
Voltaren-XR Tablets 2301

NOVODIL (Italy)
DIPYRIDAMOLE
Persantine Tablets 898

NOVO-DILTAZEM (Canada)
DILTIAZEM HYDROCHLORIDE
Cardizem LA Extended Release Tablets . . . 1699
Tiazac Capsules 1204

NOVO-DIPAM (Canada)
DIAZEPAM
Diastat Rectal Delivery System 3344
Valium Tablets 2822

NOVO-DIPIRADOL (Canada)
DIPYRIDAMOLE
Persantine Tablets 898

NOVO-FLUPAM (Canada)
FLURAZEPAM HYDROCHLORIDE
Dalmane Capsules 3343

NOVO-HERKLIN 2000 (Mexico)
PERMETHRIN
Acticin Cream 2125

NOVO-HYDROCORT (Canada)
HYDROCORTISONE
Hydrocortone Tablets 1963

NOVO-IPRAMIDE (Canada)
IPRATROPIUM BROMIDE
Atrovent Inhalation Solution 868
Atrovent Nasal Spray 0.03% 869
Atrovent Nasal Spray 0.06% 870

NOVOLENTE-K (Canada)
POTASSIUM CHLORIDE
K-Dur Extended-Relase Tablets 3047
K-Lor Powder Packets 472
K-Tab Filmtab Tablets 473

NOVO-MEDRONE (Canada)
MEDROXYPROGESTERONE ACETATE
Depo-Medrol Single-Dose Vial 2617

NOVO-NAPROX (Canada)
NAPROXEN
EC-Naprosyn Delayed-Release Tablets 2769
Naprosyn Suspension 2769
Naprosyn Tablets 2769

NOVO-NIDAZOL (Canada)
METRONIDAZOLE
MetroGel-Vaginal Gel 1822
Noritate Cream, 1% 1051

NOVO-NIFEDIN (Canada)
NIFEDIPINE
Adalat CC Tablets 2978

NOVONORM (Argentina, Australia, Austria, Belgium, Brazil, Chile, Czech Republic, Denmark, Finland, France, Germany, Greece, Hong Kong, Hungary, Irish Republic, Israel, Italy, Malaysia, New Zealand, Norway, Russia, Singapore, South Africa, Spain, Sweden, Switzerland, Thailand, The Netherlands, United Kingdom)
REPAGLINIDE
Prandin Tablets (0.5, 1, and 2 mg) 2337

NOVO-POXIDE (Canada)
CHLORDIAZEPOXIDE HYDROCHLORIDE
Librium Capsules 3349

NOVO-PRANOL (Canada)
PROPRANOLOL HYDROCHLORIDE
Inderal LA Long-Acting Capsules 3421

NOVOQUIN (Mexico)
CIPROFLOXACIN HYDROCHLORIDE
Ciloxan Ophthalmic Ointment 554
Ciloxan Ophthalmic Solution . . . . ⊙205
Cipro Tablets 2991

NOVO-RANIDINE (Canada, Hong Kong)
RANITIDINE HYDROCHLORIDE
Zantac 25 EFFERdose Tablets 1597
Zantac 150 EFFERdose Tablets 1597
Zantac 150 Tablets 1597
Zantac 300 Tablets 1597
Zantac Injection 1593
Zantac Injection Premixed 1593
Zantac Syrup 1597

NOVO-RIDAZINE (Canada)
THIORIDAZINE HYDROCHLORIDE
Thioridazine Hydrochloride Tablets 2122

NOVO-RYTHRO (Canada)
ERYTHROMYCIN
Ery-Tab Tablets 447
Erythromycin Base Filmtab Tablets 454
Erythromycin Delayed-Release Capsules, USP 456
PCE Dispertab Tablets 510

NOVOSEF (Czech Republic)
CEFTRIAXONE SODIUM
Rocephin Injectable Vials, ADD-Vantage, Galaxy, Bulk 2801

NOVO-SEMIDE (Canada)
FUROSEMIDE
Furosemide Tablets 2117

NOVO-SUCRALATE (Canada)
SUCRALFATE
Carafate Suspension 727
Carafate Tablets 728

NOVO-SUNDAC (Canada)
SULINDAC
Clinoril Tablets 1899

NOVO-THEOPHYL (Canada, Hong Kong)
THEOPHYLLINE
Uniphyl Tablets 2708

NOVO-TIMOL (Canada)
TIMOLOL MALEATE
Blocadren Tablets 1891
Timoptic Sterile Ophthalmic Solution 2058
Timoptic in Ocudose 2061
Timoptic-XE Sterile Ophthalmic Gel Forming Solution 2062

NOVO-TRIAMZIDE (Canada)
HYDROCHLOROTHIAZIDE/TRIAMTERENE
Dyazide Capsules 1389
Maxzide Tablets 2150
Maxzide-25 mg Tablets 2150

NOVO-TRIPRAMINE (Canada)
TRIMIPRAMINE MALEATE
Surmontil Capsules 2347

NOVO-VERAMIL (Canada)
VERAPAMIL HYDROCHLORIDE
Covera-HS Tablets 3135
Verelan PM Capsules 3120

NOVOXIL (Brazil)
AMOXICILLIN
Amoxil Pediatric Drops for Oral Suspension 1315
Amoxil Tablets 1315

NOVRAL (Brazil)
LISINOPRIL
Prinivil Tablets 2029
Zestril Tablets 704

NOXINE (Thailand)
NORFLOXACIN
Noroxin Tablets 2009

NOXINOR (Thailand)
NORFLOXACIN
Noroxin Tablets 2009

NOXUFEN (Switzerland)
NORFLOXACIN
Noroxin Tablets 2009

NOXWORM (Thailand)
MEBENDAZOLE
Vermox Chewable Tablets 1853

N-STATIN (Australia)
NYSTATIN
Nystop Topical Powder USP 2490

NUARDIN (Belgium)
CIMETIDINE
Tagamet Tablets 1547

NU-ATENOL (Canada)
ATENOLOL
Tenormin I.V. Injection 698

NUBAIN (Austria, Brazil, Canada, France, Germany, Greece, Hungary, Israel, Malaysia, Mexico, New Zealand, Singapore, South Africa, Switzerland, Thailand, United Kingdom)
NALBUPHINE HYDROCHLORIDE
Nubain Injection 1111

NUBAINA (Argentina)
NALBUPHINE HYDROCHLORIDE
Nubain Injection 1111

NU-CAPTO (Canada)
CAPTOPRIL
Captopril Tablets 2114

NU-CIMET (Canada)
CIMETIDINE
Tagamet Tablets 1547

NUCLOGEN (Spain)
GENTAMICIN SULFATE
Garamycin Injectable 3028
Genoptic Sterile Ophthalmic Solution . . . . ⊙227

NUCTALON (France)
ESTAZOLAM
ProSom Tablets 512

NU-DICLO (Canada)
DICLOFENAC SODIUM
Voltaren Tablets 2298
Voltaren-XR Tablets 2301

NU-DILTIAZ (Canada)
DILTIAZEM HYDROCHLORIDE
Cardizem LA Extended Release Tablets . . . 1699
Tiazac Capsules 1204

NUELIN (Australia, Denmark, Finland, Hong Kong, Malaysia, New Zealand, Norway, Singapore, South Africa, Thailand, United Kingdom)
THEOPHYLLINE
Uniphyl Tablets 2708

NUFLOXIB (Australia)
NORFLOXACIN
Noroxin Tablets 2009

NU-K (United Kingdom)
POTASSIUM CHLORIDE
K-Dur Extended-Relase Tablets 3047
K-Lor Powder Packets 472
K-Tab Filmtab Tablets 473

NULCERAN (Portugal)
FAMOTIDINE
Pepcid Injection . . . 2017
Pepcid Injection Premixed . . . 2017
Pepcid Tablets . . . 2014
Pepcid for Oral Suspension . . . 2014

NULCERIN (Spain)
FAMOTIDINE
Pepcid Injection . . . 2017
Pepcid Injection Premixed . . . 2017
Pepcid Tablets . . . 2014
Pepcid for Oral Suspension . . . 2014

NU-LOTAN (Japan)
LOSARTAN POTASSIUM
Cozaar Tablets . . . 1913

NUMORPHAN (Canada)
OXYMORPHONE HYDROCHLORIDE
Numorphan Injection . . . 1112
Numorphan Suppositories . . . 1112

NU-NAPROX (Canada)
NAPROXEN
EC-Naprosyn Delayed-Release Tablets . . . 2769
Naprosyn Suspension . . . 2769
Naprosyn Tablets . . . 2769

NU-NIFED (Canada)
NIFEDIPINE
Adalat CC Tablets . . . 2978

NUPENTIN (Australia)
GABAPENTIN
Neurontin Capsules . . . 2498

NUPRAFEN (Singapore)
NAPROXEN
EC-Naprosyn Delayed-Release Tablets . . . 2769
Naprosyn Suspension . . . 2769
Naprosyn Tablets . . . 2769

NU-RANIT (Canada)
RANITIDINE HYDROCHLORIDE
Zantac 25 EFFERdose Tablets . . . 1597
Zantac 150 EFFERdose Tablets . . . 1597
Zantac 150 Tablets . . . 1597
Zantac 300 Tablets . . . 1597
Zantac Injection . . . 1593
Zantac Injection Premixed . . . 1593
Zantac Syrup . . . 1597

NURIL (India)
ENALAPRIL MALEATE
Vasotec I.V. Injection . . . 2076

NUROCAIN (New Zealand)
LIDOCAINE
Lidoderm Patch . . . 1107

NUROLASTS (Australia)
NAPROXEN SODIUM
Anaprox DS Tablets . . . 2769
Anaprox Tablets . . . 2769

NUTRACORT (Brazil, Greece, Mexico)
HYDROCORTISONE
Hydrocortone Tablets . . . 1963

NUTRALONA (Chile)
HYDROCORTISONE
Hydrocortone Tablets . . . 1963

NU-TRIAZIDE (Canada)
HYDROCHLOROTHIAZIDE/TRIAMTERENE
Dyazide Capsules . . . 1389
Maxzide Tablets . . . 2150
Maxzide-25 mg Tablets . . . 2150

NU-VERAP (Canada)
VERAPAMIL HYDROCHLORIDE
Covera-HS Tablets . . . 3135
Verelan PM Capsules . . . 3120

NYADERM (Canada)
NYSTATIN
Nystop Topical Powder USP . . . 2490

NYAL PLUS+ ALLERGY RELIEF (Australia)
PROMETHAZINE HYDROCHLORIDE
Phenergan Suppositories . . . 3438
Phenergan Tablets . . . 3438

NYCOPIN (Denmark, Norway)
NIFEDIPINE
Adalat CC Tablets . . . 2978

NYCOPREN (Austria, Belgium, Denmark, Finland, Greece, Switzerland, The Netherlands, United Kingdom)
NAPROXEN
EC-Naprosyn Delayed-Release Tablets . . . 2769
Naprosyn Suspension . . . 2769
Naprosyn Tablets . . . 2769

NYEFAX (Australia, New Zealand, Thailand)
NIFEDIPINE
Adalat CC Tablets . . . 2978

NYOGEL (Australia, France, Germany, Greece, Irish Republic, Italy, Portugal, South Africa, United Kingdom)
TIMOLOL MALEATE
Blocadren Tablets . . . 1891
Timoptic Sterile Ophthalmic Solution . . . 2058
Timoptic in Ocudose . . . 2061
Timoptic-XE Sterile Ophthalmic Gel Forming Solution . . . 2062

NYOLOL (Brazil, Chile, France, Greece, Hong Kong, Israel, Malaysia, Mexico, Portugal, Singapore, Spain, Switzerland, Thailand)
TIMOLOL MALEATE
Blocadren Tablets . . . 1891
Timoptic Sterile Ophthalmic Solution . . . 2058
Timoptic in Ocudose . . . 2061
Timoptic-XE Sterile Ophthalmic Gel Forming Solution . . . 2062

NYPINE (Australia)
NIFEDIPINE
Adalat CC Tablets . . . 2978

NYSPES (United Kingdom)
NYSTATIN
Nystop Topical Powder USP . . . 2490

NYSTACID (South Africa)
NYSTATIN
Nystop Topical Powder USP . . . 2490

NYSTADERM (Austria, Germany)
NYSTATIN
Nystop Topical Powder USP . . . 2490

NYSTADERMAL (United Kingdom)
NYSTATIN
Nystop Topical Powder USP . . . 2490

NYSTAFORM (United Kingdom)
NYSTATIN
Nystop Topical Powder USP . . . 2490

NYSTAMONT (Greece, United Kingdom)
NYSTATIN
Nystop Topical Powder USP . . . 2490

NYSTAN (United Kingdom)
NYSTATIN
Nystop Topical Powder USP . . . 2490

NYSTASAN (Mexico)
NYSTATIN
Nystop Topical Powder USP . . . 2490

NYSTATIN-DOME (United Kingdom)
NYSTATIN
Nystop Topical Powder USP . . . 2490

NYSTAVESCENT (United Kingdom)
NYSTATIN
Nystop Topical Powder USP . . . 2490

NYZOC (Austria)
SIMVASTATIN
Zocor Tablets . . . 2078

OASIL (Greece)
CHLORDIAZEPOXIDE HYDROCHLORIDE
Librium Capsules . . . 3349

OBESTAT (India)
SIBUTRAMINE HYDROCHLORIDE
Meridia Capsules . . . 485

OBLIOSER (Italy, Spain)
MORPHINE SULFATE
Kadian Capsules . . . 572
MS Contin Tablets . . . 2703

OBRY (Mexico)
TOBRAMYCIN
TOBI Solution for Inhalation . . . 1015

OBRYPRE (Mexico)
TOBRAMYCIN
TOBI Solution for Inhalation . . . 1015

OBSIDAN (Germany)
PROPRANOLOL HYDROCHLORIDE
Inderal LA Long-Acting Capsules . . . 3421

OBSTAR (Brazil)
LOPERAMIDE HYDROCHLORIDE
Imodium Capsules . . . 1834

OCCIDAL (Thailand)
OFLOXACIN
Floxin Otic Solution . . . 1043

OCEFAX (Argentina)
CIPROFLOXACIN
Cipro Oral Suspension . . . 2991

OCERAL (Austria, Brazil, Switzerland)
OXICONAZOLE NITRATE
Oxistat Cream . . . 1498
Oxistat Lotion . . . 1498

OCERAL GB (Germany)
OXICONAZOLE NITRATE
Oxistat Cream . . . 1498
Oxistat Lotion . . . 1498

OCLOVIR (Argentina)
RIMANTADINE HYDROCHLORIDE
Flumadine Syrup . . . 1186
Flumadine Tablets . . . 1186

OCM (Argentina)
CHLORDIAZEPOXIDE HYDROCHLORIDE
Librium Capsules . . . 3349

OCSAAR (Israel)
LOSARTAN POTASSIUM
Cozaar Tablets . . . 1913

OCSAAR PLUS (Israel)
HYDROCHLOROTHIAZIDE/LOSARTAN POTASSIUM
Hyzaar 50-12.5 Tablets . . . 1964

OCTELMIN (Brazil)
MEBENDAZOLE
Vermox Chewable Tablets . . . 1853

OCTIL (Israel)
TIMOLOL MALEATE
Blocadren Tablets . . . 1891
Timoptic Sterile Ophthalmic Solution . . . 2058
Timoptic in Ocudose . . . 2061
Timoptic-XE Sterile Ophthalmic Gel Forming Solution . . . 2062

OCTIM (France, United Kingdom)
DESMOPRESSIN ACETATE
DDAVP Injection 4 mcg/mL . . . 2893
DDAVP Nasal Spray . . . 2894
DDAVP Tablets . . . 2895
Desmopressin Acetate Injection . . . 1143
Desmopressin Acetate Rhinal Tube . . . 1144

OCTIN (South Africa)
OFLOXACIN
Floxin Otic Solution . . . 1043

OCTOCAINE (Spain)
LIDOCAINE
Lidoderm Patch . . . 1107

OCTODIOL (Czech Republic)
ESTRADIOL
Climara Transdermal System . . . 795
Vivelle Transdermal System . . . 2288
Vivelle-Dot Transdermal System . . . 2293

OCTORAX (Greece)
ENALAPRIL MALEATE
Vasotec I.V. Injection . . . 2076

OCTOSTIM (Argentina, Australia, Austria, Brazil, Canada, Chile, Denmark, Finland, Germany, Hong Kong, Hungary, Israel, Norway, Singapore, Sweden, Switzerland, The Netherlands)
DESMOPRESSIN ACETATE
DDAVP Injection 4 mcg/mL . . . 2893
DDAVP Nasal Spray . . . 2894
DDAVP Tablets . . . 2895
Desmopressin Acetate Injection . . . 1143
Desmopressin Acetate Rhinal Tube . . . 1144

OCUBRAX (Belgium, Hungary, Spain)
DICLOFENAC SODIUM
Voltaren Tablets . . . 2298
Voltaren-XR Tablets . . . 2301

OCUDEX (Canada)
DEXAMETHASONE SODIUM PHOSPHATE
Decadron Phosphate Injection . . . 1931

OCUFLOX (Australia, Canada, Mexico)
OFLOXACIN
Floxin Otic Solution . . . 1043

OCUGRAM (Canada)
GENTAMICIN SULFATE
Garamycin Injectable . . . 3028
Genoptic Sterile Ophthalmic Solution . . . ⊙227

OCULASTIN (Austria, Switzerland)
AZELASTINE HYDROCHLORIDE
Astelin Nasal Spray . . . 1876

OCUPROST (Argentina)
LATANOPROST
Xalatan Ophthalmic Solution . . . ⊙280

OCUSOL (United Kingdom)
SULFACETAMIDE SODIUM
Klaron Lotion 10% . . . 1050

OCUSTIL (Italy)
SODIUM HYALURONATE
Hyalgan Solution . . . 2917

OCUSTRESS (India)
NAPHAZOLINE HYDROCHLORIDE
Albalon Ophthalmic Solution . . . ⊙216

OCU-SULF (India)
SULFACETAMIDE SODIUM
Klaron Lotion 10% . . . 1050

OCUTIM (India)
TIMOLOL MALEATE
Blocadren Tablets . . . 1891
Timoptic Sterile Ophthalmic Solution . . . 2058
Timoptic in Ocudose . . . 2061
Timoptic-XE Sterile Ophthalmic Gel Forming Solution . . . 2062

OCUTOB (India)
TOBRAMYCIN
TOBI Solution for Inhalation . . . 1015

OCUTOB-D (India)
TOBRAMYCIN
TOBI Solution for Inhalation . . . 1015

ODANET (Greece)
RANITIDINE HYDROCHLORIDE
Zantac 25 EFFERdose Tablets . . . 1597
Zantac 150 EFFERdose Tablets . . . 1597
Zantac 150 Tablets . . . 1597
Zantac 300 Tablets . . . 1597
Zantac Injection . . . 1593
Zantac Injection Premixed . . . 1593
Zantac Syrup . . . 1597

ODANEX (Chile)
ONDANSETRON
Zofran ODT Orally Disintegrating Tablets . . . 1613

ODEMASE (Germany)
FUROSEMIDE
Furosemide Tablets . . . 2117

ODIFEX (India)
FEXOFENADINE HYDROCHLORIDE
Allegra Capsules . . . 2857

ODIVIR KIT (India)
EFAVIRENZ
Sustiva Capsules . . . 957

ODRIC (Japan)
TRANDOLAPRIL
Mavik Tablets . . . 482

ODRIK (Australia, Brazil, Denmark, France, Greece, Irish Republic, New Zealand, Portugal, Spain, United Kingdom)
TRANDOLAPRIL
Mavik Tablets . . . 482

ODUPRIL (Greece)
CAPTOPRIL
Captopril Tablets . . . 2114

OECOZOL (Austria)
METRONIDAZOLE
MetroGel-Vaginal Gel . . . 1822
Noritate Cream, 1% . . . 1051

OEDEMEX (Switzerland)
FUROSEMIDE
Furosemide Tablets . . . 2117

OESCLIM (Austria, Brazil, Canada, Chile, Czech Republic, France, Greece, Hungary, Sweden)
ESTRADIOL
Climara Transdermal System . . . 795
Vivelle Transdermal System . . . 2288
Vivelle-Dot Transdermal System . . . 2293

OESTRACLIN (Spain)
ESTRADIOL
Climara Transdermal System . . . 795

Vivelle Transdermal System 2288
Vivelle-Dot Transdermal System 2293

OESTRING (Sweden)
ESTRADIOL
Climara Transdermal System 795
Vivelle Transdermal System 2288
Vivelle-Dot Transdermal System 2293

OESTRO GEL (Argentina)
ESTRADIOL
Climara Transdermal System 795
Vivelle Transdermal System 2288
Vivelle-Dot Transdermal System 2293

OESTRODOSE (France, Israel, Spain)
ESTRADIOL
Climara Transdermal System 795
Vivelle Transdermal System 2288
Vivelle-Dot Transdermal System 2293

OESTROGEL (Belgium, Brazil, Czech Republic, France, Hong Kong, Hungary, Irish Republic, Israel, Malaysia, Mexico, Russia, Singapore, Switzerland, Thailand, United Kingdom)
ESTRADIOL
Climara Transdermal System 795
Vivelle Transdermal System 2288
Vivelle-Dot Transdermal System 2293

OFAL (Argentina)
TIMOLOL MALEATE
Blocadren Tablets 1891
Timoptic Sterile Ophthalmic Solution 2058
Timoptic in Ocudose 2061
Timoptic-XE Sterile Ophthalmic Gel Forming Solution 2062

OFAL P (Argentina)
TIMOLOL MALEATE
Blocadren Tablets 1891
Timoptic Sterile Ophthalmic Solution 2058
Timoptic in Ocudose 2061
Timoptic-XE Sterile Ophthalmic Gel Forming Solution 2062

OFCIN (Malaysia, Singapore)
OFLOXACIN
Floxin Otic Solution 1043

OFLER (India)
OFLOXACIN
Floxin Otic Solution 1043

OFLER-TZ (India)
OFLOXACIN
Floxin Otic Solution 1043

OFLIN (India)
OFLOXACIN
Floxin Otic Solution 1043

OFLO (Germany)
OFLOXACIN
Floxin Otic Solution 1043

OFLOCEE (Thailand)
OFLOXACIN
Floxin Otic Solution 1043

OFLOCET (Australia, France, New Zealand)
OFLOXACIN
Floxin Otic Solution 1043

OFLOCIN (Italy)
OFLOXACIN
Floxin Otic Solution 1043

OFLODEX (Israel)
OFLOXACIN
Floxin Otic Solution 1043

OFLODURA (Germany)
OFLOXACIN
Floxin Otic Solution 1043

OFLOHEXAL (Germany)
OFLOXACIN
Floxin Otic Solution 1043

OFLONO (Chile)
CIPROFLOXACIN HYDROCHLORIDE
Ciloxan Ophthalmic Ointment 554
Ciloxan Ophthalmic Solution ⊙205
Cipro Tablets 2991

OFLOVIR (Spain)
OFLOXACIN
Floxin Otic Solution 1043

OFLOX (Argentina, Austria, Brazil, Chile, India, Israel)
OFLOXACIN
Floxin Otic Solution 1043

O-FLOX (Thailand)
OFLOXACIN
Floxin Otic Solution 1043

OFLOX D (India)
OFLOXACIN
Floxin Otic Solution 1043

OFLOX TZ (India)
OFLOXACIN
Floxin Otic Solution 1043

OFLOXA (Thailand)
OFLOXACIN
Floxin Otic Solution 1043

OFLOXAN (Brazil)
OFLOXACIN
Floxin Otic Solution 1043

OFLOXBETA (Germany)
OFLOXACIN
Floxin Otic Solution 1043

OFLOXCIN (Thailand)
OFLOXACIN
Floxin Otic Solution 1043

OFLOXIN (Brazil, Czech Republic)
OFLOXACIN
Floxin Otic Solution 1043

O-FLUOR (Germany)
FLUOROURACIL
Efudex Topical Cream 3348
Efudex Topical Solutions 3348

OFNIFENIL (Greece)
ENALAPRIL MALEATE
Vasotec I.V. Injection 2076

OFOXIN (Brazil)
CIPROFLOXACIN HYDROCHLORIDE
Ciloxan Ophthalmic Ointment 554
Ciloxan Ophthalmic Solution ⊙205
Cipro Tablets 2991

OFRAMAX (Czech Republic, India, Singapore, South Africa, Thailand)
CEFTRIAXONE SODIUM
Rocephin Injectable Vials, ADD-Vantage, Galaxy, Bulk 2801

OFTACILOX (Italy, Portugal, Spain)
CIPROFLOXACIN HYDROCHLORIDE
Ciloxan Ophthalmic Ointment 554
Ciloxan Ophthalmic Solution ⊙205
Cipro Tablets 2991

OFTACIPROX (Chile)
CIPROFLOXACIN HYDROCHLORIDE
Ciloxan Ophthalmic Ointment 554
Ciloxan Ophthalmic Solution ⊙205
Cipro Tablets 2991

OFTAGEN (Chile)
GENTAMICIN SULFATE
Garamycin Injectable 3028
Genoptic Sterile Ophthalmic Solution ⊙227

OFTALBRAX (Argentina)
TOBRAMYCIN
TOBI Solution for Inhalation 1015

OFTALMOLOSA CUSI (Malaysia)
ERYTHROMYCIN
Ery-Tab Tablets 447
Erythromycin Base Filmtab Tablets 454
Erythromycin Delayed-Release Capsules, USP 456
PCE Dispertab Tablets 510

OFTAMOLOL (Denmark, Norway)
TIMOLOL MALEATE
Blocadren Tablets 1891
Timoptic Sterile Ophthalmic Solution 2058
Timoptic in Ocudose 2061
Timoptic-XE Sterile Ophthalmic Gel Forming Solution 2062

OFTAN (Hong Kong, Israel, Norway, Switzerland, Thailand)
TIMOLOL MALEATE
Blocadren Tablets 1891
Timoptic Sterile Ophthalmic Solution 2058
Timoptic in Ocudose 2061
Timoptic-XE Sterile Ophthalmic Gel Forming Solution 2062

OFTAQUIN (Mexico)
CIPROFLOXACIN
Cipro Oral Suspension 2991

OFTAQUIX (Denmark, Finland, Germany, Sweden, The Netherlands)
LEVOFLOXACIN
Levaquin Injection 2453
Levaquin Tablets 2453

OFTENSIN (Czech Republic)
TIMOLOL MALEATE
Blocadren Tablets 1891
Timoptic Sterile Ophthalmic Solution 2058
Timoptic in Ocudose 2061
Timoptic-XE Sterile Ophthalmic Gel Forming Solution 2062

OFTIC (Chile)
DICLOFENAC SODIUM
Voltaren Tablets 2298
Voltaren-XR Tablets 2301

OFTIMOLO (Italy)
TIMOLOL MALEATE
Blocadren Tablets 1891
Timoptic Sterile Ophthalmic Solution 2058
Timoptic in Ocudose 2061
Timoptic-XE Sterile Ophthalmic Gel Forming Solution 2062

OFUS (Hong Kong)
OFLOXACIN
Floxin Otic Solution 1043

OGAST (France)
LANSOPRAZOLE
Prevacid Delayed-Release Capsules 3268

OGASTO (Argentina, Chile, Portugal)
LANSOPRAZOLE
Prevacid Delayed-Release Capsules 3268

OGASTRO (Brazil, Mexico)
LANSOPRAZOLE
Prevacid Delayed-Release Capsules 3268

OKAFLOX M (India)
OFLOXACIN
Floxin Otic Solution 1043

OKALAN D (India)
LANSOPRAZOLE
Prevacid Delayed-Release Capsules 3268

OKAMYCIN (India)
ERYTHROMYCIN
Ery-Tab Tablets 447
Erythromycin Base Filmtab Tablets 454
Erythromycin Delayed-Release Capsules, USP 456
PCE Dispertab Tablets 510

OKLARICID (Greece)
CLARITHROMYCIN
Biaxin Filmtab Tablets 402
Biaxin Granules 402

OLDINOT (Argentina)
DONEPEZIL HYDROCHLORIDE
Aricept Tablets 1086

OLEO-LAX (Argentina)
PROPOFOL
Diprivan Injectable Emulsion 676

OLEXAR (India)
OLANZAPINE
Zyprexa Tablets 1798

OLFEN (Brazil, Czech Republic, Hong Kong, Hungary, Israel, Malaysia, Portugal, Singapore, Thailand)
DICLOFENAC SODIUM
Voltaren Tablets 2298
Voltaren-XR Tablets 2301

OLFI (India)
OFLOXACIN
Floxin Otic Solution 1043

OLFI TZ (India)
OFLOXACIN
Floxin Otic Solution 1043

OLICARD (Czech Republic, Germany, Hungary, Spain, Switzerland)
ISOSORBIDE MONONITRATE
Imdur Tablets 3032

OLICARD RETARD (Russia)
ISOSORBIDE MONONITRATE
Imdur Tablets 3032

OLICARDIN (Austria)
ISOSORBIDE MONONITRATE
Imdur Tablets 3032

OLIMER (Argentina)
CLONAZEPAM
Klonopin Tablets 2782

OLMORAN (Spain)
ZAFIRLUKAST
Accolate Tablets 663

OLTENS (France)
CAPTOPRIL
Captopril Tablets 2114

OLTER (Argentina)
FLUTAMIDE
Eulexin Capsules 3023

OLUX (The Netherlands)
CLOBETASOL PROPIONATE
Temovate Cream 1549
Temovate E Emollient 1552
Temovate Gel 1550
Temovate Ointment 1549
Temovate Scalp Application 1551

OLWORM (India)
ALBENDAZOLE
Albenza Tablets 1310

OLYSTER (India)
TERAZOSIN HYDROCHLORIDE
Hytrin Capsules 469

OMAFLAXINA (Argentina)
CIPROFLOXACIN
Cipro Oral Suspension 2991

OMCILON A ORABASE (Brazil)
TRIAMCINOLONE ACETONIDE
Azmacort Inhalation Aerosol 1701
Nasacort AQ Nasal Spray 2937

OMIC (Belgium)
TAMSULOSIN HYDROCHLORIDE
Flomax Capsules 881

OMINOL (Mexico)
PROGESTERONE
Prometrium Capsules (100 mg, 200 mg) 3205

OMIX (Austria, France)
TAMSULOSIN HYDROCHLORIDE
Flomax Capsules 881

OMNALIO (Spain)
CHLORDIAZEPOXIDE HYDROCHLORIDE
Librium Capsules 3349

OMNIC (Argentina, Brazil, Chile, Denmark, Finland, Germany, Hungary, Irish Republic, Israel, Italy, Norway, Portugal, Russia, Spain, The Netherlands)
TAMSULOSIN HYDROCHLORIDE
Flomax Capsules 881

OMNICEF (Austria, Thailand)
CEFDINIR
Omnicef Capsules 506
Omnicef for Oral Suspension 506

ONAPAN (Mexico)
DIAZEPAM
Diastat Rectal Delivery System 3344
Valium Tablets 2822

ONCASPAR (Argentina, Canada, Germany)
PEGASPARGASE
Oncaspar 1123

ONCLAST (Japan)
ALENDRONATE SODIUM
Fosamax Tablets 1949

ONCOFU (Argentina)
FLUOROURACIL
Efudex Topical Cream 3348
Efudex Topical Solutions 3348

ONCOGEM (India)
GEMCITABINE HYDROCHLORIDE
Gemzar for Injection 1743

ONCOSAL (Spain)
FLUTAMIDE
Eulexin Capsules 3023

ONDEMET (Czech Republic)
ONDANSETRON HYDROCHLORIDE
Zofran Injection 1607
Zofran Injection Premixed 1607
Zofran Oral Solution 1613
Zofran Tablets 1613

ONKOFLUOR (Germany)
FLUOROURACIL
Efudex Topical Cream 3348
Efudex Topical Solutions 3348

ONKOMORPHIN (Germany)
MORPHINE SULFATE
Kadian Capsules 572
MS Contin Tablets 2703

ONOFIN-K (Mexico)
KETOCONAZOLE
Nizoral 2% Shampoo 1838

ONSIA (Thailand)
ONDANSETRON HYDROCHLORIDE
Zofran Injection 1607
Zofran Injection Premixed 1607
Zofran Oral Solution 1613
Zofran Tablets 1613

ONTRAX (Brazil)
ONDANSETRON HYDROCHLORIDE
Zofran Injection 1607
Zofran Injection Premixed 1607
Zofran Oral Solution 1613
Zofran Tablets 1613

ONYCHON (Czech Republic)
TERBINAFINE HYDROCHLORIDE
Lamisil Tablets 2226

ONYMYKEN (Germany)
CLOTRIMAZOLE
Lotrimin Cream 3053
Lotrimin Lotion 1% 3053
Lotrimin Topical Solution 1% 3053

OPATANOL (Belgium, Denmark, Finland, France, Germany, Irish Republic, Italy, Norway, Portugal, Spain, Sweden, Switzerland, United Kingdom)
OLOPATADINE HYDROCHLORIDE
Patanol Ophthalmic Solution 557

OPCON (Canada)
NAPHAZOLINE HYDROCHLORIDE
Albalon Ophthalmic Solution ⊙216

OPERIUM (Thailand)
LOPERAMIDE HYDROCHLORIDE
Imodium Capsules 1834

OPHTAGRAM (Czech Republic, France, Germany, Portugal, Singapore, Switzerland)
GENTAMICIN SULFATE
Garamycin Injectable 3028
Genoptic Sterile Ophthalmic Solution ⊙227

OPHTALIN (Italy)
SODIUM HYALURONATE
Hyalgan Solution 2917

OPHTHALIN (Australia, Hong Kong, Irish Republic, Israel, New Zealand, Singapore, Thailand, United Kingdom)
SODIUM HYALURONATE
Hyalgan Solution 2917

OPHTHO-SULF (Canada)
SULFACETAMIDE SODIUM
Klaron Lotion 10% 1050

OPHTILAN (Austria)
TIMOLOL MALEATE
Blocadren Tablets 1891
Timoptic Sterile Ophthalmic Solution 2058
Timoptic in Ocudose 2061
Timoptic-XE Sterile Ophthalmic Gel Forming Solution 2062

OPHTIM (France)
TIMOLOL MALEATE
Blocadren Tablets 1891
Timoptic Sterile Ophthalmic Solution 2058
Timoptic in Ocudose 2061
Timoptic-XE Sterile Ophthalmic Gel Forming Solution 2062

OPIDOL (Denmark, Finland, Sweden)
HYDROMORPHONE HYDROCHLORIDE
Dilaudid Ampules 439
Dilaudid Multiple Dose Vials 439
Dilaudid Non-Sterile Powder 439
Dilaudid Oral Liquid 443
Dilaudid Rectal Suppositories 439
Dilaudid Tablets 439
Dilaudid Tablets - 8 mg 443
Dilaudid-HP Injection 441
Dilaudid-HP Lyophilized Powder 250 mg 441

OPIRAN (France)
PIMOZIDE
Orap Tablets 1220

OPIREN (Spain)
LANSOPRAZOLE
Prevacid Delayed-Release Capsules 3268

OPNOL (Sweden)
DEXAMETHASONE SODIUM PHOSPHATE
Decadron Phosphate Injection 1931

OPRIDAN (Greece)
ISOTRETINOIN
Accutane Capsules 2740

OPSAR (Thailand)
SULFACETAMIDE SODIUM
Klaron Lotion 10% 1050

OPTAL (Thailand)
SULFACETAMIDE SODIUM
Klaron Lotion 10% 1050

OPTAMID (Italy)
SULFACETAMIDE SODIUM
Klaron Lotion 10% 1050

OPTAMIDE (Australia)
SULFACETAMIDE SODIUM
Klaron Lotion 10% 1050

OPTAZINE (Australia)
NAPHAZOLINE HYDROCHLORIDE
Albalon Ophthalmic Solution ⊙216

OPTERON (Italy)
TICLOPIDINE HYDROCHLORIDE
Ticlid Tablets 2813

OPTHAFLOX (Mexico)
CIPROFLOXACIN HYDROCHLORIDE
Ciloxan Ophthalmic Ointment 554
Ciloxan Ophthalmic Solution ⊙205
Cipro Tablets 2991

OPTICET (South Africa)
SULFACETAMIDE SODIUM
Klaron Lotion 10% 1050

OPTICIDE (Thailand)
PRAZIQUANTEL
Biltricide Tablets 2990

OPTIFLUOR (Mexico)
FLUORESCEIN SODIUM
Fluorescite Injection ⊙207

OPTIGEN (Hong Kong)
GENTAMICIN SULFATE
Garamycin Injectable 3028
Genoptic Sterile Ophthalmic Solution ⊙227

OPTI-GENTA (Israel)
GENTAMICIN SULFATE
Garamycin Injectable 3028
Genoptic Sterile Ophthalmic Solution ⊙227

OPTIL (United Kingdom)
DILTIAZEM HYDROCHLORIDE
Cardizem LA Extended Release Tablets 1699
Tiazac Capsules 1204

OPTILAST (Israel, United Kingdom)
AZELASTINE HYDROCHLORIDE
Astelin Nasal Spray 1876

OPTIMOL (Australia, Denmark, Hong Kong, Sweden)
TIMOLOL MALEATE
Blocadren Tablets 1891
Timoptic Sterile Ophthalmic Solution 2058
Timoptic in Ocudose 2061
Timoptic-XE Sterile Ophthalmic Gel Forming Solution 2062

OPTINATE (Finland, Italy, Norway, Sweden)
RISEDRONATE SODIUM
Actonel Tablets 2679

OPTINEM (Austria)
MEROPENEM
Merrem I.V. 687

OPTIPAR (Finland)
PAROXETINE HYDROCHLORIDE
Paxil Oral Suspension 1501
Paxil Tablets 1501

OPTIPRES (India)
BETAXOLOL HYDROCHLORIDE
Betoptic S Ophthalmic Suspension 554

OPTISOL (Israel)
SULFACETAMIDE SODIUM
Klaron Lotion 10% 1050

OPTOBET (Greece)
DICLOFENAC SODIUM
Voltaren Tablets 2298
Voltaren-XR Tablets 2301

OPTOMICIN (Mexico)
ERYTHROMYCIN STEARATE
Erythrocin Stearate Filmtab Tablets 452

OPTROL (Australia)
SALMETEROL XINAFOATE
Serevent Diskus 1540

OPTRUMA (Austria, Finland, France, Germany, Italy, Portugal, Spain)
RALOXIFENE HYDROCHLORIDE
Evista Tablets 1735

OPUMIDE (United Kingdom)
INDAPAMIDE
Indapamide Tablets 2119

ORABIOT UD (Argentina)
CLARITHROMYCIN
Biaxin Filmtab Tablets 402
Biaxin Granules 402

ORACORT (Canada, Israel, New Zealand, Thailand)
TRIAMCINOLONE ACETONIDE
Azmacort Inhalation Aerosol 1701
Nasacort AQ Nasal Spray 2937

ORADAY (Malaysia, Thailand)
ATENOLOL
Tenormin I.V. Injection 698

ORADEXON (Belgium, Chile, Greece, Hungary, Portugal, South Africa, Switzerland, Thailand, United Kingdom)
DEXAMETHASONE
Decadron Tablets 1929

ORAKIT (Argentina)
POTASSIUM CHLORIDE
K-Dur Extended-Relase Tablets 3047
K-Lor Powder Packets 472
K-Tab Filmtab Tablets 473

ORALMUV (Argentina)
LAMIVUDINE
Epivir Oral Solution 1394
Epivir Tablets 1394
Epivir-HBV Oral Solution 1398
Epivir-HBV Tablets 1398

ORAL-T (Thailand)
TRIAMCINOLONE ACETONIDE
Azmacort Inhalation Aerosol 1701
Nasacort AQ Nasal Spray 2937

ORALTEN TROCHE (Israel)
CLOTRIMAZOLE
Lotrimin Cream 3053
Lotrimin Lotion 1% 3053
Lotrimin Topical Solution 1% 3053

ORAMEDY (Singapore)
TRIAMCINOLONE ACETONIDE
Azmacort Inhalation Aerosol 1701
Nasacort AQ Nasal Spray 2937

ORAMINAX (Portugal)
AMOXICILLIN
Amoxil Pediatric Drops for Oral Suspension 1315
Amoxil Tablets 1315

ORAMORPH (Austria, Canada, Czech Republic, Irish Republic, Italy, Sweden, The Netherlands, United Kingdom)
MORPHINE SULFATE
Kadian Capsules 572
MS Contin Tablets 2703

ORANOR (Mexico)
NORFLOXACIN
Noroxin Tablets 2009

ORAP (Argentina, Australia, Austria, Belgium, Brazil, Canada, Chile, Czech Republic, Denmark, France, Germany, Hong Kong, India, Irish Republic, Israel, Italy, Japan, New Zealand, Norway, Singapore, South Africa, Spain, Sweden, Switzerland, Thailand, The Netherlands, United Kingdom)
PIMOZIDE
Orap Tablets 1220

ORAQIX (Sweden)
LIDOCAINE
Lidoderm Patch 1107

ORA-SED LOTION (Australia)
LIDOCAINE
Lidoderm Patch 1107

ORASORBIL (Germany, Italy, Portugal)
ISOSORBIDE MONONITRATE
Imdur Tablets 3032

ORATANE (Australia, Hong Kong, Malaysia, New Zealand, Singapore, South Africa)
ISOTRETINOIN
Accutane Capsules 2740

ORAXIM (Italy)
CEFUROXIME AXETIL
Ceftin Tablets 1369
Ceftin for Oral Suspension 1369

ORCILONE (Thailand)
TRIAMCINOLONE ACETONIDE
Azmacort Inhalation Aerosol 1701
Nasacort AQ Nasal Spray 2937

ORELOX (Australia, Brazil, Czech Republic, Denmark, France, Germany, Italy, Mexico, South Africa, Spain, Sweden, Switzerland, The Netherlands, United Kingdom)
CEFPODOXIME PROXETIL
Vantin Tablets and Oral Suspension 2650

ORFARIN (Malaysia, Singapore, Thailand)
WARFARIN SODIUM
Coumadin Tablets 932
Coumadin for Injection 932

ORFENACE (Canada)
ORPHENADRINE CITRATE
Norflex Injection 1824

ORIFUNGAL (Argentina)
KETOCONAZOLE
Nizoral 2% Shampoo 1838

ORIVAN (Finland)
VANCOMYCIN HYDROCHLORIDE
Vancocin HCl Capsules, USP 3370

ORIZOLIN (Czech Republic)
CEFAZOLIN SODIUM
Ancef for Injection 1318

ORLAMIX (Brazil)
DEXAMETHASONE
Decadron Tablets 1929

ORMOX (Finland)
ISOSORBIDE MONONITRATE
Imdur Tablets 3032

OROKEN (France)
CEFIXIME
Suprax 1811

OROMONE (France)
ESTRADIOL
Climara Transdermal System 795
Vivelle Transdermal System 2288
Vivelle-Dot Transdermal System 2293

OROTREX (Portugal)
ISOTRETINOIN
Accutane Capsules 2740

OROXINE (Australia, Malaysia, Singapore)
LEVOTHYROXINE SODIUM
Levothroid Tablets 1189
Levoxyl Tablets 1680
Synthroid Tablets 515

OROZANOL (Czech Republic)
KETOCONAZOLE
Nizoral 2% Shampoo 1838

ORPHENADOL (Malaysia, Singapore)
ORPHENADRINE CITRATE
Norflex Injection 1824

ORPHENGESIC (Thailand)
ORPHENADRINE CITRATE
Norflex Injection 1824

ORPIC (South Africa)
CIPROFLOXACIN HYDROCHLORIDE
Ciloxan Ophthalmic Ointment 554
Ciloxan Ophthalmic Solution ⊙205
Cipro Tablets 2991

ORREPASTE (Malaysia, Singapore)
TRIAMCINOLONE ACETONIDE
Azmacort Inhalation Aerosol 1701
Nasacort AQ Nasal Spray 2937

ORTACRONE (Spain)
AMIODARONE HYDROCHLORIDE
Pacerone Tablets 3337

ORTHOCEL (India)
CELECOXIB
Celebrex Capsules 3130

ORTHOCLONE (Greece, South Africa)
MUROMONAB-CD3
Orthoclone OKT3 Sterile Solution 2370

ORTHOCLONE OKT3 (Australia, Belgium, Brazil, Canada, Czech Republic, Finland, France, Germany, Hong Kong, Israel, Italy, Malaysia, Mexico, New Zealand, Norway, Sweden, Switzerland, Thailand, The Netherlands)
MUROMONAB-CD3
Orthoclone OKT3 Sterile Solution 2370

ORTHOVISC (Canada, Germany, Israel, United Kingdom)
SODIUM HYALURONATE
Hyalgan Solution 2917

ORTOCICLINA (Brazil)
ERYTHROMYCIN
Ery-Tab Tablets 447
Erythromycin Base Filmtab Tablets 454
Erythromycin Delayed-Release Capsules, USP 456
PCE Dispertab Tablets 510

ORTOFLAN (Brazil)
DICLOFENAC SODIUM
Voltaren Tablets 2298
Voltaren-XR Tablets 2301

ORTOPSIQUE (Mexico)
DIAZEPAM
Diastat Rectal Delivery System 3344
Valium Tablets 2822

ORTRIZOL (Mexico)
METRONIDAZOLE
MetroGel-Vaginal Gel 1822
Noritate Cream, 1% 1051

ORULOP (Spain)
LOPERAMIDE HYDROCHLORIDE
Imodium Capsules 1834

OSDRON (Brazil)
ALENDRONATE SODIUM
Fosamax Tablets 1949

OSEMIN (Mexico)
FUROSEMIDE
Furosemide Tablets 2117

OSEOTENK (Argentina)
ALENDRONATE SODIUM
Fosamax Tablets 1949

OSFO (Greece)
ETIDRONATE DISODIUM
Didronel Tablets 2693

OSKANA (Greece)
LEVOCARNITINE
Carnitor Injection 3185
Carnitor Tablets and Oral Solution 3187

OSMO-ADALAT (Israel)
NIFEDIPINE
Adalat CC Tablets 2978

OSMOLAC (Italy)
LACTULOSE
Kristalose for Oral Solution 2149

OSPAMOX (Greece, Hungary, Portugal)
AMOXICILLIN
Amoxil Pediatric Drops for Oral Suspension 1315
Amoxil Tablets 1315

OSPOCARD (Austria)
NIFEDIPINE
Adalat CC Tablets 2978

OSSOMAX (Brazil)
ALENDRONATE SODIUM
Fosamax Tablets 1949

OSTAREN (Thailand)
DICLOFENAC SODIUM
Voltaren Tablets 2298
Voltaren-XR Tablets 2301

OSTEDRON (Greece)
ETIDRONATE DISODIUM
Didronel Tablets 2693

OSTENAN (Brazil)
ALENDRONATE SODIUM
Fosamax Tablets 1949

OSTENIL (France, Germany, Switzerland, United Kingdom)
SODIUM HYALURONATE
Hyalgan Solution 2917

OSTEO D (Israel)
CALCITRIOL
Calcijex Injection 411

OSTEODIDRONEL (Belgium)
ETIDRONATE DISODIUM
Didronel Tablets 2693

OSTEODRUG (Greece)
ETIDRONATE DISODIUM
Didronel Tablets 2693

OSTEOFEM (Chile)
ALENDRONATE SODIUM
Fosamax Tablets 1949

OSTEOFENE (Argentina)
ALENDRONATE SODIUM
Fosamax Tablets 1949

OSTEOFORM (Brazil)
ALENDRONATE SODIUM
Fosamax Tablets 1949

OSTEOFOS (India)
ALENDRONATE SODIUM
Fosamax Tablets 1949

OSTEONATE (Argentina)
ALENDRONATE SODIUM
Fosamax Tablets 1949

OSTEORAL (Brazil)
ALENDRONATE SODIUM
Fosamax Tablets 1949

OSTEOSAN (Chile)
ALENDRONATE SODIUM
Fosamax Tablets 1949

OSTEOTOP (Chile)
ETIDRONATE DISODIUM
Didronel Tablets 2693

OSTEOTRAT (Brazil)
ALENDRONATE SODIUM
Fosamax Tablets 1949

OSTEOTRIOL (Germany, Russia)
CALCITRIOL
Calcijex Injection 411

OSTEPAM (France)
PAMIDRONATE DISODIUM
Aredia for Injection 2168

OSTEUM (Spain)
ETIDRONATE DISODIUM
Didronel Tablets 2693

OSTOGENE (Greece)
ETIDRONATE DISODIUM
Didronel Tablets 2693

OSTOPOR (Greece)
ETIDRONATE DISODIUM
Didronel Tablets 2693

OTEX HC (Argentina)
CIPROFLOXACIN HYDROCHLORIDE
Ciloxan Ophthalmic Ointment 554
Ciloxan Ophthalmic Solution ⊙205
Cipro Tablets 2991

OTO BIOTAER (Argentina)
CIPROFLOXACIN
Cipro Oral Suspension 2991

OTOBACID N (Czech Republic)
DEXAMETHASONE
Decadron Tablets 1929

OTOCIPRO (Argentina)
HYDROCORTISONE
Hydrocortone Tablets 1963

OTOFLOX (Argentina)
OFLOXACIN
Floxin Otic Solution 1043

OTOIAL (Italy)
SODIUM HYALURONATE
Hyalgan Solution 2917

OTOSPORIN C CIPROFLOXACINA (Argentina)
CIPROFLOXACIN HYDROCHLORIDE
Ciloxan Ophthalmic Ointment 554
Ciloxan Ophthalmic Solution ⊙205
Cipro Tablets 2991

OTRASEL (France)
SELEGILINE HYDROCHLORIDE
Eldepryl Capsules 3209

OTREON (Austria, Italy, Spain)
CEFPODOXIME PROXETIL
Vantin Tablets and Oral Suspension 2650

OTRIFLU (Norway, The Netherlands)
DICLOFENAC POTASSIUM
Cataflam Tablets 2173

OTRIVIN NEUSALLERGIE AZELASTINE (The Netherlands)
AZELASTINE HYDROCHLORIDE
Astelin Nasal Spray 1876

OTRIVIN RHUME DES FOINS (Switzerland)
AZELASTINE HYDROCHLORIDE
Astelin Nasal Spray 1876

OTRIVINE ANTI-ALLERGIE (Belgium)
AZELASTINE HYDROCHLORIDE
Astelin Nasal Spray 1876

OTROZOL (Mexico)
METRONIDAZOLE
MetroGel-Vaginal Gel 1822
Noritate Cream, 1% 1051

OTSUKA CEZ (Japan)
CEFAZOLIN SODIUM
Ancef for Injection 1318

OVEX (United Kingdom)
MEBENDAZOLE
Vermox Chewable Tablets 1853

OVINOL (Greece)
NORFLOXACIN
Noroxin Tablets 2009

OVIS NEU (Germany)
CLOTRIMAZOLE
Lotrimin Cream 3053
Lotrimin Lotion 1% 3053
Lotrimin Topical Solution 1% 3053

OXA FORTE (Argentina)
DICLOFENAC SODIUM
Voltaren Tablets 2298
Voltaren-XR Tablets 2301

OXAFEM (Argentina)
DICLOFENAC POTASSIUM
Cataflam Tablets 2173

OXAGESIC (Argentina)
DICLOFENAC POTASSIUM
Cataflam Tablets 2173

OXALGIN (India)
DICLOFENAC SODIUM
Voltaren Tablets 2298
Voltaren-XR Tablets 2301

OXALGIN-DP (India)
DICLOFENAC SODIUM
Voltaren Tablets 2298
Voltaren-XR Tablets 2301

OXANDRIN (Australia)
OXANDROLONE
Oxandrin Tablets 2977

OXANEST (Finland)
OXYCODONE HYDROCHLORIDE
OxyContin Tablets 2699
OxyFast Oral Concentrate Solution 2704
OxyIR Capsules 2704

OXAPROST (Argentina)
DICLOFENAC SODIUM
Voltaren Tablets 2298
Voltaren-XR Tablets 2301

OXCORD (Brazil)
NIFEDIPINE
Adalat CC Tablets 2978

OXEPAR (Portugal)
PAROXETINE HYDROCHLORIDE
Paxil Oral Suspension 1501
Paxil Tablets 1501

OXET (Germany)
PAROXETINE HYDROCHLORIDE
Paxil Oral Suspension 1501
Paxil Tablets 1501

OXETINE (Australia, Denmark)
PAROXETINE HYDROCHLORIDE
Paxil Oral Suspension 1501
Paxil Tablets 1501

OXIDERMA (Spain)
BENZOYL PEROXIDE
Brevoxyl-4 Creamy Wash 3212
Brevoxyl-4 Gel 3211
Brevoxyl-8 Creamy Wash 3212
Brevoxyl-8 Gel 3211
Triaz Cleanser 1864
Triaz Gel 1864

OXIGEN (Brazil)
NIMODIPINE
Nimotop Capsules 774

OXINOVAG (Argentina)
OXYCODONE HYDROCHLORIDE
OxyContin Tablets 2699
OxyFast Oral Concentrate Solution 2704
OxyIR Capsules 2704

OXINOVAG COMPLEX (Argentina)
OXYCODONE HYDROCHLORIDE
OxyContin Tablets 2699
OxyFast Oral Concentrate Solution 2704
OxyIR Capsules 2704

OXISTAT (Argentina, Mexico)
OXICONAZOLE NITRATE
Oxistat Cream 1498
Oxistat Lotion 1498

OXITOSONA (Spain)
OXYMETHOLONE
Anadrol-50 Tablets 3329

OXITOVER (Spain)
MEBENDAZOLE
Vermox Chewable Tablets 1853

OXITRAT (Brazil)
OXICONAZOLE NITRATE
Oxistat Cream 1498
Oxistat Lotion 1498

OXIZOLE (Canada, Mexico)
MEBENDAZOLE
Vermox Chewable Tablets 1853

OXODAL (Spain)
BETAXOLOL HYDROCHLORIDE
Betoptic S Ophthalmic Suspension 554

OXSORALEN (Australia, Austria, Canada, Czech Republic, Hong Kong, Israel, Italy, Japan, Malaysia, Mexico, New Zealand, Singapore, South Africa, Spain, The Netherlands)
METHOXSALEN
Oxsoralen Lotion 1% 3354
Oxsoralen-Ultra Capsules 3354

OXSORALON (Belgium)
METHOXSALEN
Oxsoralen Lotion 1% 3354
Oxsoralen-Ultra Capsules 3354

OXY (Australia, Canada, Czech Republic, Germany, Hong Kong, Israel, Mexico, United Kingdom)
BENZOYL PEROXIDE
Brevoxyl-4 Creamy Wash 3212
Brevoxyl-4 Gel 3211
Brevoxyl-8 Creamy Wash 3212
Brevoxyl-8 Gel 3211
Triaz Cleanser 1864
Triaz Gel 1864

OXY IR (Canada)
OXYCODONE HYDROCHLORIDE
OxyContin Tablets 2699
OxyFast Oral Concentrate Solution 2704
OxyIR Capsules 2704

OXY SENSITIVE (Israel)
BENZOYL PEROXIDE
Brevoxyl-4 Creamy Wash 3212
Brevoxyl-4 Gel 3211
Brevoxyl-8 Creamy Wash 3212
Brevoxyl-8 Gel 3211
Triaz Cleanser 1864
Triaz Gel 1864

OXYCARDIN (France)
ISOSORBIDE MONONITRATE
Imdur Tablets 3032

OXYCOD (Israel)
OXYCODONE HYDROCHLORIDE
OxyContin Tablets 2699
OxyFast Oral Concentrate Solution 2704
OxyIR Capsules 2704

OXYCONTIN (Argentina, Australia, Brazil, Canada, Chile, Czech Republic, Denmark, Finland, France, Irish Republic, Israel, Mexico, Norway, Sweden, Switzerland, The Netherlands, United Kingdom)
OXYCODONE HYDROCHLORIDE
OxyContin Tablets . . . 2699
OxyFast Oral Concentrate Solution . . . 2704
OxyIR Capsules . . . 2704

OXYDERM (Canada)
BENZOYL PEROXIDE
Brevoxyl-4 Creamy Wash . . . 3212
Brevoxyl-4 Gel . . . 3211
Brevoxyl-8 Creamy Wash . . . 3212
Brevoxyl-8 Gel . . . 3211
Triaz Cleanser . . . 1864
Triaz Gel . . . 1864

OXYGESIC (Germany)
OXYCODONE HYDROCHLORIDE
OxyContin Tablets . . . 2699
OxyFast Oral Concentrate Solution . . . 2704
OxyIR Capsules . . . 2704

OXYNORM (Australia, Denmark, Finland, France, Irish Republic, Norway, Sweden, Switzerland, The Netherlands, United Kingdom)
OXYCODONE HYDROCHLORIDE
OxyContin Tablets . . . 2699
OxyFast Oral Concentrate Solution . . . 2704
OxyIR Capsules . . . 2704

OXYTOKO (Spain)
BENZOYL PEROXIDE
Brevoxyl-4 Creamy Wash . . . 3212
Brevoxyl-4 Gel . . . 3211
Brevoxyl-8 Creamy Wash . . . 3212
Brevoxyl-8 Gel . . . 3211
Triaz Cleanser . . . 1864
Triaz Gel . . . 1864

OZAPIN (India)
OLANZAPINE
Zyprexa Tablets . . . 1798

OZEPAM (India)
CLONAZEPAM
Klonopin Tablets . . . 2782

PABALAT (Chile)
NIFEDIPINE
Adalat CC Tablets . . . 2978

PACEUM (Switzerland)
DIAZEPAM
Diastat Rectal Delivery System . . . 3344
Valium Tablets . . . 2822

PACINAX (Chile)
DIAZEPAM
Diastat Rectal Delivery System . . . 3344
Valium Tablets . . . 2822

PACIUM (Spain)
DIAZEPAM
Diastat Rectal Delivery System . . . 3344
Valium Tablets . . . 2822

PACTENS (Mexico)
NAPROXEN SODIUM
Anaprox DS Tablets . . . 2769
Anaprox Tablets . . . 2769

PADET (Argentina)
METRONIDAZOLE
MetroGel-Vaginal Gel . . . 1822
Noritate Cream, 1% . . . 1051

PADIKEN (Mexico)
AMANTADINE HYDROCHLORIDE
Symmetrel Syrup . . . 1115
Symmetrel Tablets . . . 1115

PAFTEC (Portugal)
FLUNISOLIDE
Aerobid Inhaler System . . . 1172
Aerobid-M Inhaler System . . . 1172
Nasarel Nasal Spray . . . 1652

PAHTLISAN (Mexico)
CHLOROTHIAZIDE
Diuril Oral Suspension . . . 1936
Diuril Tablets . . . 1936

PAINEX (Portugal)
DICLOFENAC SODIUM
Voltaren Tablets . . . 2298
Voltaren-XR Tablets . . . 2301

PALANE (Mexico)
ENALAPRIL MALEATE
Vasotec I.V. Injection . . . 2076

PALDAR (Argentina)
MUPIROCIN
Bactroban Ointment . . . 1358

PALIATIN (Spain)
CHLORDIAZEPOXIDE HYDROCHLORIDE
Librium Capsules . . . 3349

PALISTOP (Greece)
FLUTAMIDE
Eulexin Capsules . . . 3023

PALLADON (Germany, Switzerland, The Netherlands)
HYDROMORPHONE HYDROCHLORIDE
Dilaudid Ampules . . . 439
Dilaudid Multiple Dose Vials . . . 439
Dilaudid Non-Sterile Powder . . . 439
Dilaudid Oral Liquid . . . 443
Dilaudid Rectal Suppositories . . . 439
Dilaudid Tablets . . . 439
Dilaudid Tablets - 8 mg . . . 443
Dilaudid-HP Injection . . . 441
Dilaudid-HP Lyophilized Powder 250 mg . . . 441

PALLADONE (Irish Republic, Israel, United Kingdom)
HYDROMORPHONE HYDROCHLORIDE
Dilaudid Ampules . . . 439
Dilaudid Multiple Dose Vials . . . 439
Dilaudid Non-Sterile Powder . . . 439
Dilaudid Oral Liquid . . . 443
Dilaudid Rectal Suppositories . . . 439
Dilaudid Tablets . . . 439
Dilaudid Tablets - 8 mg . . . 443
Dilaudid-HP Injection . . . 441
Dilaudid-HP Lyophilized Powder 250 mg . . . 441

PALLIA (Hong Kong)
CIMETIDINE
Tagamet Tablets . . . 1547

PALON (Hong Kong, Thailand)
PROPRANOLOL HYDROCHLORIDE
Inderal LA Long-Acting Capsules . . . 3421

PALUX (Japan)
ALPROSTADIL
Edex Injection . . . 3103

PALUXETIL (Austria)
PAROXETINE HYDROCHLORIDE
Paxil Oral Suspension . . . 1501
Paxil Tablets . . . 1501

PAMDOSA (Argentina)
PAMIDRONATE DISODIUM
Aredia for Injection . . . 2168

PAMERGAN (Brazil)
PROMETHAZINE HYDROCHLORIDE
Phenergan Suppositories . . . 3438
Phenergan Tablets . . . 3438

PAMID (Israel)
INDAPAMIDE
Indapamide Tablets . . . 2119

PAMIDRIA (India)
PAMIDRONATE DISODIUM
Aredia for Injection . . . 2168

PAMIFOS (India)
PAMIDRONATE DISODIUM
Aredia for Injection . . . 2168

PAMISOL (Australia, Hong Kong, Malaysia, Singapore, Thailand)
PAMIDRONATE DISODIUM
Aredia for Injection . . . 2168

PAMITOR (Austria, Hungary)
PAMIDRONATE DISODIUM
Aredia for Injection . . . 2168

PAMPE (Portugal)
LANSOPRAZOLE
Prevacid Delayed-Release Capsules . . . 3268

PANALBA (Greece)
FAMOTIDINE
Pepcid Injection . . . 2017
Pepcid Injection Premixed . . . 2017
Pepcid Tablets . . . 2014
Pepcid for Oral Suspension . . . 2014

PANALDINE (Japan)
TICLOPIDINE HYDROCHLORIDE
Ticlid Tablets . . . 2813

PANALENE (Argentina)
ADAPALENE
Differin Gel . . . 1211

PANBESY (Belgium, Hong Kong, Singapore, Thailand)
PHENTERMINE HYDROCHLORIDE
Adipex-P Capsules . . . 1216
Adipex-P Tablets . . . 1216

PANCARDIOL (Spain)
ISOSORBIDE MONONITRATE
Imdur Tablets . . . 3032

PANCLOFLEX (Argentina)
DICLOFENAC SODIUM
Voltaren Tablets . . . 2298
Voltaren-XR Tablets . . . 2301

PANCREASE (Australia, Belgium, Brazil, Canada, Denmark, Finland, Israel, Italy, Mexico, New Zealand, Norway, Spain, Sweden, The Netherlands)
PANCRELIPASE
Ultrase Capsules . . . 735
Ultrase MT Capsules . . . 736

PANDERMIL (Portugal)
HYDROCORTISONE
Hydrocortone Tablets . . . 1963

PANDERMIN CICATRIZANTE (Spain)
SODIUM HYALURONATE
Hyalgan Solution . . . 2917

PANDRAT (Argentina)
PAMIDRONATE DISODIUM
Aredia for Injection . . . 2168

PANFUGAN (Brazil)
MEBENDAZOLE
Vermox Chewable Tablets . . . 1853

PAN-FUNGEX (Portugal)
CLOTRIMAZOLE
Lotrimin Cream . . . 3053
Lotrimin Lotion 1% . . . 3053
Lotrimin Topical Solution 1% . . . 3053

PANFUNGOL (Spain)
KETOCONAZOLE
Nizoral 2% Shampoo . . . 1838

PANGEL (Belgium)
BENZOYL PEROXIDE
Brevoxyl-4 Creamy Wash . . . 3212
Brevoxyl-4 Gel . . . 3211
Brevoxyl-8 Creamy Wash . . . 3212
Brevoxyl-8 Gel . . . 3211
Triaz Cleanser . . . 1864
Triaz Gel . . . 1864

PANGRAF (India)
TACROLIMUS
Prograf Capsules and Injection . . . 624

PANITOL (Thailand)
CARBAMAZEPINE
Carbatrol Capsules . . . 3174
Tegretol Chewable Tablets . . . 2278
Tegretol Suspension . . . 2278
Tegretol Tablets . . . 2278
Tegretol-XR Tablets . . . 2278

PANKREADEN (Italy)
PANCRELIPASE
Ultrase Capsules . . . 735
Ultrase MT Capsules . . . 736

PANKREASE (South Africa)
PANCRELIPASE
Ultrase Capsules . . . 735
Ultrase MT Capsules . . . 736

PANMICOL (Argentina)
CLOTRIMAZOLE
Lotrimin Cream . . . 3053
Lotrimin Lotion 1% . . . 3053
Lotrimin Topical Solution 1% . . . 3053

PANNOGEL (France)
BENZOYL PEROXIDE
Brevoxyl-4 Creamy Wash . . . 3212
Brevoxyl-4 Gel . . . 3211
Brevoxyl-8 Creamy Wash . . . 3212
Brevoxyl-8 Gel . . . 3211
Triaz Cleanser . . . 1864
Triaz Gel . . . 1864

PANOTILE CIPRO (Germany)
CIPROFLOXACIN HYDROCHLORIDE
Ciloxan Ophthalmic Ointment . . . 554
Ciloxan Ophthalmic Solution . . . ⊙205
Cipro Tablets . . . 2991

PANOXYL (Australia, Austria, Brazil, Canada, Finland, France, Germany, Hong Kong, Irish Republic, Israel, Italy, Malaysia, Mexico, New Zealand, Norway, Portugal, Singapore, South Africa, Spain, Switzerland, Thailand, United Kingdom)
BENZOYL PEROXIDE
Brevoxyl-4 Creamy Wash . . . 3212
Brevoxyl-4 Gel . . . 3211
Brevoxyl-8 Creamy Wash . . . 3212
Brevoxyl-8 Gel . . . 3211
Triaz Cleanser . . . 1864
Triaz Gel . . . 1864

PANQUIL (Australia)
PROMETHAZINE HYDROCHLORIDE
Phenergan Suppositories . . . 3438
Phenergan Tablets . . . 3438

PANSULFOX (Chile)
BENZOYL PEROXIDE
Brevoxyl-4 Creamy Wash . . . 3212
Brevoxyl-4 Gel . . . 3211
Brevoxyl-8 Creamy Wash . . . 3212
Brevoxyl-8 Gel . . . 3211
Triaz Cleanser . . . 1864
Triaz Gel . . . 1864

PANTASOL (Italy)
FLUNISOLIDE
Aerobid Inhaler System . . . 1172
Aerobid-M Inhaler System . . . 1172
Nasarel Nasal Spray . . . 1652

PANTELMIN (Austria, Brazil, Portugal)
MEBENDAZOLE
Vermox Chewable Tablets . . . 1853

PANTESTONE (Argentina)
ANASTROZOLE
Arimidex Tablets . . . 665

PANTINOL (Austria)
APROTININ
Trasylol Injection . . . 779

PANTODRIN (Spain)
ERYTHROMYCIN
Ery-Tab Tablets . . . 447
Erythromycin Base Filmtab Tablets . . . 454
Erythromycin Delayed-Release Capsules, USP . . . 456
PCE Dispertab Tablets . . . 510

PANTOK (Spain)
SIMVASTATIN
Zocor Tablets . . . 2078

PANTOMICINA (Argentina, Brazil)
ERYTHROMYCIN
Ery-Tab Tablets . . . 447
Erythromycin Base Filmtab Tablets . . . 454
Erythromycin Delayed-Release Capsules, USP . . . 456
PCE Dispertab Tablets . . . 510

PANTOSTIN (Germany)
ESTRADIOL
Climara Transdermal System . . . 795
Vivelle Transdermal System . . . 2288
Vivelle-Dot Transdermal System . . . 2293

PANTYSON (Finland)
HYDROCORTISONE
Hydrocortone Tablets . . . 1963

PANVERM (Brazil)
MEBENDAZOLE
Vermox Chewable Tablets . . . 1853

PANVERMIN (Mexico)
MEBENDAZOLE
Vermox Chewable Tablets . . . 1853

PANWARFIN (Greece)
WARFARIN SODIUM
Coumadin Tablets . . . 932
Coumadin for Injection . . . 932

PANZID (Italy)
CEFTAZIDIME
Fortaz for Injection . . . 1422

PANZYTRAT (Australia, New Zealand)
PANCRELIPASE
Ultrase Capsules . . . 735
Ultrase MT Capsules . . . 736

PAPASINE (Argentina)
NAPROXEN
EC-Naprosyn Delayed-Release Tablets . . . 2769

(⊙ Described in PDR For Ophthalmic Medicines™)

Naprosyn Suspension 2769
Naprosyn Tablets 2769

PARABACT (India)
NORFLOXACIN
Noroxin Tablets 2009

PARACEFAN (Belgium)
CLONIDINE HYDROCHLORIDE
Catapres Tablets 874

PARACNE (Argentina)
BENZOYL PEROXIDE
Brevoxyl-4 Creamy Wash 3212
Brevoxyl-4 Gel 3211
Brevoxyl-8 Creamy Wash 3212
Brevoxyl-8 Gel 3211
Triaz Cleanser 1864
Triaz Gel 1864

PARANTHIL (South Africa)
ALBENDAZOLE
Albenza Tablets 1310

PARANZOL (Mexico)
MEBENDAZOLE
Vermox Chewable Tablets 1853

PARAPRES (Spain)
CANDESARTAN CILEXETIL
Atacand Tablets 634

PARAPRES PLUS (Spain)
CANDESARTAN CILEXETIL
Atacand Tablets 634

PARAQUEIMOL (Brazil)
SULFACETAMIDE SODIUM
Klaron Lotion 10% 1050

PARASIN (Brazil)
ALBENDAZOLE
Albenza Tablets 1310

PARASTHMAN (Germany)
THEOPHYLLINE
Uniphyl Tablets 2708

PARAVERM (Brazil)
MEBENDAZOLE
Vermox Chewable Tablets 1853

PARCETIN (Argentina)
NORFLOXACIN
Noroxin Tablets 2009

PARELMIN (Brazil)
MEBENDAZOLE
Vermox Chewable Tablets 1853

PAREXAT (Switzerland)
PAROXETINE HYDROCHLORIDE
Paxil Oral Suspension 1501
Paxil Tablets 1501

PARGIN (Italy)
ECONAZOLE NITRATE
Spectazole Cream 2390

PARI (India)
PAROXETINE HYDROCHLORIDE
Paxil Oral Suspension 1501
Paxil Tablets 1501

PARITREL (Israel)
AMANTADINE HYDROCHLORIDE
Symmetrel Syrup 1115
Symmetrel Tablets 1115

PARKADINA (Portugal)
AMANTADINE HYDROCHLORIDE
Symmetrel Syrup 1115
Symmetrel Tablets 1115

PARKEXIN (Brazil)
SELEGILINE HYDROCHLORIDE
Eldepryl Capsules 3209

PARLAZIN (Hungary)
CETIRIZINE HYDROCHLORIDE
Zyrtec Syrup 2589
Zyrtec Tablets 2589

PARNATE (Argentina, Australia, Brazil, Canada, Czech Republic, Germany, Irish Republic, New Zealand, South Africa, Spain)
TRANYLCYPROMINE SULFATE
Parnate Tablets 1499

PAROCETAN (Austria)
PAROXETINE HYDROCHLORIDE
Paxil Oral Suspension 1501
Paxil Tablets 1501

PAROLICH (Germany)
PAROXETINE HYDROCHLORIDE
Paxil Oral Suspension 1501
Paxil Tablets 1501

PARONAL (Belgium)
ASPARAGINASE
Elspar for Injection 1943

PAROSER (Irish Republic)
PAROXETINE HYDROCHLORIDE
Paxil Oral Suspension 1501
Paxil Tablets 1501

PAROTIN (India)
PAROXETINE HYDROCHLORIDE
Paxil Oral Suspension 1501
Paxil Tablets 1501

PAROX (Irish Republic)
PAROXETINE HYDROCHLORIDE
Paxil Oral Suspension 1501
Paxil Tablets 1501

PAROXAT (Austria, Germany, Hungary)
PAROXETINE HYDROCHLORIDE
Paxil Oral Suspension 1501
Paxil Tablets 1501

PAROXEDURA (Germany)
PAROXETINE HYDROCHLORIDE
Paxil Oral Suspension 1501
Paxil Tablets 1501

PAROXIFLEX (Sweden)
PAROXETINE HYDROCHLORIDE
Paxil Oral Suspension 1501
Paxil Tablets 1501

PARSILID (Italy)
TICLOPIDINE HYDROCHLORIDE
Ticlid Tablets 2813

PARVEMAXOL (The Netherlands)
CLOTRIMAZOLE
Lotrimin Cream 3053
Lotrimin Lotion 1% 3053
Lotrimin Topical Solution 1% 3053

PASALEN (Thailand)
KETOCONAZOLE
Nizoral 2% Shampoo 1838

PATANOL (Argentina, Australia, Brazil, Canada, Chile, Hong Kong, Malaysia, Mexico, Singapore, South Africa, Thailand)
OLOPATADINE HYDROCHLORIDE
Patanol Ophthalmic Solution 557

PATXEN (Mexico)
NAPROXEN
EC-Naprosyn Delayed-Release Tablets 2769
Naprosyn Suspension 2769
Naprosyn Tablets 2769

PAUSOGEST (Czech Republic, Hungary)
ESTRADIOL
Climara Transdermal System 795
Vivelle Transdermal System 2288
Vivelle-Dot Transdermal System 2293

PAX (South Africa)
DIAZEPAM
Diastat Rectal Delivery System 3344
Valium Tablets 2822

PAXAM (Australia)
CLONAZEPAM
Klonopin Tablets 2782

PAXATE (Mexico)
DIAZEPAM
Diastat Rectal Delivery System 3344
Valium Tablets 2822

PAXETIL (Portugal)
PAROXETINE HYDROCHLORIDE
Paxil Oral Suspension 1501
Paxil Tablets 1501

PAXIL (Argentina, Canada, Mexico, Russia)
PAROXETINE HYDROCHLORIDE
Paxil Oral Suspension 1501
Paxil Tablets 1501

PAXON (Argentina)
LOSARTAN POTASSIUM
Cozaar Tablets 1913

PAXON-D (Argentina)
LOSARTAN POTASSIUM
Cozaar Tablets 1913

PAXTINE (Australia)
PAROXETINE HYDROCHLORIDE
Paxil Oral Suspension 1501
Paxil Tablets 1501

PAXUM (India)
DIAZEPAM
Diastat Rectal Delivery System 3344
Valium Tablets 2822

PAXXET (Israel)
PAROXETINE HYDROCHLORIDE
Paxil Oral Suspension 1501
Paxil Tablets 1501

PAZOLINI (Brazil)
DIAZEPAM
Diastat Rectal Delivery System 3344
Valium Tablets 2822

PB GEL (Argentina)
BENZOYL PEROXIDE
Brevoxyl-4 Creamy Wash 3212
Brevoxyl-4 Gel 3211
Brevoxyl-8 Creamy Wash 3212
Brevoxyl-8 Gel 3211
Triaz Cleanser 1864
Triaz Gel 1864

PCE (Canada, Hong Kong)
ERYTHROMYCIN
Ery-Tab Tablets 447
Erythromycin Base Filmtab Tablets 454
Erythromycin Delayed-Release Capsules, USP 456
PCE Dispertab Tablets 510

PEAULINE (The Netherlands)
BENZOYL PEROXIDE
Brevoxyl-4 Creamy Wash 3212
Brevoxyl-4 Gel 3211
Brevoxyl-8 Creamy Wash 3212
Brevoxyl-8 Gel 3211
Triaz Cleanser 1864
Triaz Gel 1864

PEBEGAL (Mexico)
BENZONATATE
Tessalon Perles 1202

PEDIAPHYLLIN PL (The Netherlands)
THEOPHYLLINE
Uniphyl Tablets 2708

PEDIAPRED (Canada)
PREDNISOLONE SODIUM PHOSPHATE
Pediapred Oral Solution 3319

PEDIKUROL (Austria)
CLOTRIMAZOLE
Lotrimin Cream 3053
Lotrimin Lotion 1% 3053
Lotrimin Topical Solution 1% 3053

PEDISAFE (Germany)
CLOTRIMAZOLE
Lotrimin Cream 3053
Lotrimin Lotion 1% 3053
Lotrimin Topical Solution 1% 3053

PEKTROL (Russia)
ISOSORBIDE MONONITRATE
Imdur Tablets 3032

PELICREP (Argentina)
FINASTERIDE
Propecia Tablets 2036
Proscar Tablets 2040

PELO LIBRE (Argentina)
PERMETHRIN
Acticin Cream 2125

PELVICILLIN NF (Argentina)
METRONIDAZOLE
MetroGel-Vaginal Gel 1822
Noritate Cream, 1% 1051

PENDINE (Australia)
GABAPENTIN
Neurontin Capsules 2498

PENDRAMINE (United Kingdom)
PENICILLAMINE
Cuprimine Capsules 1925

PENEDIL (Israel)
FELODIPINE
Plendil Extended-Release Tablets 651

PENEGRA (India)
SILDENAFIL CITRATE
Viagra Tablets 2552

PENESTER (Czech Republic)
FINASTERIDE
Propecia Tablets 2036
Proscar Tablets 2040

PENGON (Greece)
DICLOFENAC SODIUM
Voltaren Tablets 2298
Voltaren-XR Tablets 2301

PENLES (Japan)
LIDOCAINE
Lidoderm Patch 1107

PENMOX (South Africa)
AMOXICILLIN
Amoxil Pediatric Drops for Oral Suspension 1315
Amoxil Tablets 1315

PENNSAID (Canada, Italy, Portugal, United Kingdom)
DICLOFENAC SODIUM
Voltaren Tablets 2298
Voltaren-XR Tablets 2301

PENTACARD (Belgium, Thailand)
ISOSORBIDE MONONITRATE
Imdur Tablets 3032

PENTAZOLE (Brazil)
MEBENDAZOLE
Vermox Chewable Tablets 1853

PENTICLOX (Mexico)
AMOXICILLIN
Amoxil Pediatric Drops for Oral Suspension 1315
Amoxil Tablets 1315

PENTILZENO (Portugal)
DILTIAZEM HYDROCHLORIDE
Cardizem LA Extended Release Tablets 1699
Tiazac Capsules 1204

PENTOCLAVE (Argentina)
ERYTHROMYCIN
Ery-Tab Tablets 447
Erythromycin Base Filmtab Tablets 454
Erythromycin Delayed-Release Capsules, USP 456
PCE Dispertab Tablets 510

PENTOREL (India)
BUPRENORPHINE HYDROCHLORIDE
Buprenex Injectable 2718

PENVICILIN (Brazil)
AMOXICILLIN
Amoxil Pediatric Drops for Oral Suspension 1315
Amoxil Tablets 1315

PEPAR (India)
PIOGLITAZONE HYDROCHLORIDE
Actos Tablets 3224

PEPCID (Australia, Austria, Canada, Finland, Germany, Hong Kong, Irish Republic, New Zealand, Norway, South Africa, Spain, Sweden, Switzerland, The Netherlands)
FAMOTIDINE
Pepcid Injection 2017
Pepcid Injection Premixed 2017
Pepcid Tablets 2014
Pepcid for Oral Suspension 2014

PEPCIDAC (France)
FAMOTIDINE
Pepcid Injection 2017
Pepcid Injection Premixed 2017
Pepcid Tablets 2014
Pepcid for Oral Suspension 2014

PEPCIDIN (Denmark, Finland, Norway, Sweden, The Netherlands)
FAMOTIDINE
Pepcid Injection 2017
Pepcid Injection Premixed 2017
Pepcid Tablets 2014
Pepcid for Oral Suspension 2014

PEPCIDINA (Portugal)
FAMOTIDINE
Pepcid Injection 2017
Pepcid Injection Premixed 2017
Pepcid Tablets 2014
Pepcid for Oral Suspension 2014

PEPCIDINE (Australia, Austria, Belgium, Hong Kong, Malaysia, Mexico, New Zealand, Singapore, Switzerland, Thailand)
FAMOTIDINE
Pepcid Injection 2017

Pepcid Injection Premixed . . . 2017
Pepcid Tablets . . . 2014
Pepcid for Oral Suspension . . . 2014

PEPCINE (Thailand)
FAMOTIDINE
Pepcid Injection . . . 2017
Pepcid Injection Premixed . . . 2017
Pepcid Tablets . . . 2014
Pepcid for Oral Suspension . . . 2014

PEPDENAL (Thailand)
FAMOTIDINE
Pepcid Injection . . . 2017
Pepcid Injection Premixed . . . 2017
Pepcid Tablets . . . 2014
Pepcid for Oral Suspension . . . 2014

PEPDINE (France)
FAMOTIDINE
Pepcid Injection . . . 2017
Pepcid Injection Premixed . . . 2017
Pepcid Tablets . . . 2014
Pepcid for Oral Suspension . . . 2014

PEPDUL (Germany)
FAMOTIDINE
Pepcid Injection . . . 2017
Pepcid Injection Premixed . . . 2017
Pepcid Tablets . . . 2014
Pepcid for Oral Suspension . . . 2014

PEPFAMIN (Thailand)
FAMOTIDINE
Pepcid Injection . . . 2017
Pepcid Injection Premixed . . . 2017
Pepcid Tablets . . . 2014
Pepcid for Oral Suspension . . . 2014

PEP-RANI (Portugal)
RANITIDINE HYDROCHLORIDE
Zantac 25 EFFERdose Tablets . . . 1597
Zantac 150 EFFERdose Tablets . . . 1597
Zantac 150 Tablets . . . 1597
Zantac 300 Tablets . . . 1597
Zantac Injection . . . 1593
Zantac Injection Premixed . . . 1593
Zantac Syrup . . . 1597

PEPTAB (Portugal)
RANITIDINE HYDROCHLORIDE
Zantac 25 EFFERdose Tablets . . . 1597
Zantac 150 EFFERdose Tablets . . . 1597
Zantac 150 Tablets . . . 1597
Zantac 300 Tablets . . . 1597
Zantac Injection . . . 1593
Zantac Injection Premixed . . . 1593
Zantac Syrup . . . 1597

PEPTAN (Greece)
FAMOTIDINE
Pepcid Injection . . . 2017
Pepcid Injection Premixed . . . 2017
Pepcid Tablets . . . 2014
Pepcid for Oral Suspension . . . 2014

PEPTIC GUARD (Canada)
FAMOTIDINE
Pepcid Injection . . . 2017
Pepcid Injection Premixed . . . 2017
Pepcid Tablets . . . 2014
Pepcid for Oral Suspension . . . 2014

PEPTIC RELIEF (Canada)
RANITIDINE HYDROCHLORIDE
Zantac 25 EFFERdose Tablets . . . 1597
Zantac 150 EFFERdose Tablets . . . 1597
Zantac 150 Tablets . . . 1597
Zantac 300 Tablets . . . 1597
Zantac Injection . . . 1593
Zantac Injection Premixed . . . 1593
Zantac Syrup . . . 1597

PEPTICA (Thailand)
CIMETIDINE
Tagamet Tablets . . . 1547

PEPTIFAR (Portugal)
RANITIDINE HYDROCHLORIDE
Zantac 25 EFFERdose Tablets . . . 1597
Zantac 150 EFFERdose Tablets . . . 1597
Zantac 150 Tablets . . . 1597
Zantac 300 Tablets . . . 1597
Zantac Injection . . . 1593
Zantac Injection Premixed . . . 1593
Zantac Syrup . . . 1597

PEPTIGAL (Hungary)
FAMOTIDINE
Pepcid Injection . . . 2017
Pepcid Injection Premixed . . . 2017
Pepcid Tablets . . . 2014
Pepcid for Oral Suspension . . . 2014

PEPTIMAX (United Kingdom)
CIMETIDINE
Tagamet Tablets . . . 1547

PEPTOCI (Thailand)
FAMOTIDINE
Pepcid Injection . . . 2017
Pepcid Injection Premixed . . . 2017
Pepcid Tablets . . . 2014
Pepcid for Oral Suspension . . . 2014

PEPTOL (Canada)
CIMETIDINE
Tagamet Tablets . . . 1547

PEPTONORM (Greece)
SUCRALFATE
Carafate Suspension . . . 727
Carafate Tablets . . . 728

PEPZAN (Australia, Hong Kong, Malaysia, New Zealand, Singapore)
FAMOTIDINE
Pepcid Injection . . . 2017
Pepcid Injection Premixed . . . 2017
Pepcid Tablets . . . 2014
Pepcid for Oral Suspension . . . 2014

PEPZOL (Portugal)
LANSOPRAZOLE
Prevacid Delayed-Release Capsules . . . 3268

PERACEL (France)
LOPERAMIDE HYDROCHLORIDE
Imodium Capsules . . . 1834

PERASIAN (Thailand)
LOPERAMIDE HYDROCHLORIDE
Imodium Capsules . . . 1834

PERASTHMAN N (Germany)
THEOPHYLLINE
Uniphyl Tablets . . . 2708

PERATIVE (Argentina)
KETOCONAZOLE
Nizoral 2% Shampoo . . . 1838

PERCAPYL (Argentina)
PERMETHRIN
Acticin Cream . . . 2125

PERCLODIN (Irish Republic)
DIPYRIDAMOLE
Persantine Tablets . . . 898

PERCORINA (Spain)
ISOSORBIDE MONONITRATE
Imdur Tablets . . . 3032

PERDERM (Hong Kong, Hungary, Malaysia, Singapore)
ALCLOMETASONE DIPROPIONATE
Aclovate Cream . . . 1290
Aclovate Ointment . . . 1290

PERDIX (Denmark, Finland, Irish Republic, Israel, South Africa, Sweden, United Kingdom)
MOEXIPRIL HYDROCHLORIDE
Univasc Tablets . . . 3118

PERENAL (Greece)
LISINOPRIL
Prinivil Tablets . . . 2029
Zestril Tablets . . . 704

PERFUDAL (Spain)
FELODIPINE
Plendil Extended-Release Tablets . . . 651

PERICHOL (Denmark)
SIMVASTATIN
Zocor Tablets . . . 2078

PERILOX (Switzerland)
METRONIDAZOLE
MetroGel-Vaginal Gel . . . 1822
Noritate Cream, 1% . . . 1051

PERINAL (United Kingdom)
HYDROCORTISONE
Hydrocortone Tablets . . . 1963

PERIPLUM (Italy)
NIMODIPINE
Nimotop Capsules . . . 774

PERISET (India)
ONDANSETRON HYDROCHLORIDE
Zofran Injection . . . 1607
Zofran Injection Premixed . . . 1607
Zofran Oral Solution . . . 1613
Zofran Tablets . . . 1613

PERKOD (France)
DIPYRIDAMOLE
Persantine Tablets . . . 898

PERLICE (India)
PERMETHRIN
Acticin Cream . . . 2125

PERLOL (Thailand)
PROPRANOLOL HYDROCHLORIDE
Inderal LA Long-Acting Capsules . . . 3421

PERLUTEX (Denmark, Norway)
MEDROXYPROGESTERONE ACETATE
Depo-Medrol Single-Dose Vial . . . 2617

PERMETEL (Brazil)
PERMETHRIN
Acticin Cream . . . 2125

PERMETRIX (Brazil)
PERMETHRIN
Acticin Cream . . . 2125

PERMITE (India)
PERMETHRIN
Acticin Cream . . . 2125

PEROXACNE (Spain)
BENZOYL PEROXIDE
Brevoxyl-4 Creamy Wash . . . 3212
Brevoxyl-4 Gel . . . 3211
Brevoxyl-8 Creamy Wash . . . 3212
Brevoxyl-8 Gel . . . 3211
Triaz Cleanser . . . 1864
Triaz Gel . . . 1864

PEROXIBEN (Spain)
BENZOYL PEROXIDE
Brevoxyl-4 Creamy Wash . . . 3212
Brevoxyl-4 Gel . . . 3211
Brevoxyl-8 Creamy Wash . . . 3212
Brevoxyl-8 Gel . . . 3211
Triaz Cleanser . . . 1864
Triaz Gel . . . 1864

PEROXIBEN PLUS (Chile)
BENZOYL PEROXIDE
Brevoxyl-4 Creamy Wash . . . 3212
Brevoxyl-4 Gel . . . 3211
Brevoxyl-8 Creamy Wash . . . 3212
Brevoxyl-8 Gel . . . 3211
Triaz Cleanser . . . 1864
Triaz Gel . . . 1864

PEROXIMICINA (Argentina)
BENZOYL PEROXIDE
Brevoxyl-4 Creamy Wash . . . 3212
Brevoxyl-4 Gel . . . 3211
Brevoxyl-8 Creamy Wash . . . 3212
Brevoxyl-8 Gel . . . 3211
Triaz Cleanser . . . 1864
Triaz Gel . . . 1864

PERSA-GEL W (Australia)
BENZOYL PEROXIDE
Brevoxyl-4 Creamy Wash . . . 3212
Brevoxyl-4 Gel . . . 3211
Brevoxyl-8 Creamy Wash . . . 3212
Brevoxyl-8 Gel . . . 3211
Triaz Cleanser . . . 1864
Triaz Gel . . . 1864

PERSANTIN (Argentina, Australia, Austria, Brazil, Chile, Czech Republic, Denmark, Finland, Germany, Hong Kong, India, Irish Republic, Italy, Japan, Malaysia, Mexico, New Zealand, Norway, Portugal, Singapore, South Africa, Sweden, Thailand, The Netherlands, United Kingdom)
DIPYRIDAMOLE
Persantine Tablets . . . 898

PERSANTIN PLUS (Hong Kong)
DIPYRIDAMOLE
Persantine Tablets . . . 898

PERSANTIN S (Brazil)
DIPYRIDAMOLE
Persantine Tablets . . . 898

PERSANTINE (Belgium, Canada, France, Switzerland)
DIPYRIDAMOLE
Persantine Tablets . . . 898

PERSOL (India)
BENZOYL PEROXIDE
Brevoxyl-4 Creamy Wash . . . 3212
Brevoxyl-4 Gel . . . 3211
Brevoxyl-8 Creamy Wash . . . 3212
Brevoxyl-8 Gel . . . 3211
Triaz Cleanser . . . 1864
Triaz Gel . . . 1864

PERSOL FORTE (India)
BENZOYL PEROXIDE
Brevoxyl-4 Creamy Wash . . . 3212
Brevoxyl-4 Gel . . . 3211
Brevoxyl-8 Creamy Wash . . . 3212
Brevoxyl-8 Gel . . . 3211
Triaz Cleanser . . . 1864
Triaz Gel . . . 1864

PERTACILON (Greece, Singapore)
CAPTOPRIL
Captopril Tablets . . . 2114

PERTAXOL (Greece)
BETAXOLOL HYDROCHLORIDE
Betoptic S Ophthalmic Suspension . . . 554

PERTENSAL (Spain)
NIFEDIPINE
Adalat CC Tablets . . . 2978

PERTENSO (Argentina)
CLONIDINE
Catapres-TTS . . . 875

PERTIL (Spain)
ISOSORBIDE MONONITRATE
Imdur Tablets . . . 3032

PETOGEN (South Africa)
MEDROXYPROGESTERONE ACETATE
Depo-Medrol Single-Dose Vial . . . 2617

PETSIX (India)
FUROSEMIDE
Furosemide Tablets . . . 2117

PEVARYL (Australia, Denmark, Greece, Hong Kong, Hungary, Irish Republic, Israel, Malaysia, New Zealand, Portugal, Singapore, Spain, Switzerland, The Netherlands, United Kingdom)
ECONAZOLE NITRATE
Spectazole Cream . . . 2390

PEVISONE (Malaysia)
ECONAZOLE NITRATE
Spectazole Cream . . . 2390

P-GLITZ (India)
PIOGLITAZONE HYDROCHLORIDE
Actos Tablets . . . 3224

PHACOVIT (Greece)
LEVOCARNITINE
Carnitor Injection . . . 3185
Carnitor Tablets and Oral Solution . . . 3187

PHAMOPRIL (Germany)
CAPTOPRIL
Captopril Tablets . . . 2114

PHAMORANIT (Germany)
RANITIDINE HYDROCHLORIDE
Zantac 25 EFFERdose Tablets . . . 1597
Zantac 150 EFFERdose Tablets . . . 1597
Zantac 150 Tablets . . . 1597
Zantac 300 Tablets . . . 1597
Zantac Injection . . . 1593
Zantac Injection Premixed . . . 1593
Zantac Syrup . . . 1597

PHANATE (Thailand)
LITHIUM CARBONATE
Eskalith CR Controlled-Release Tablets . . . 1406
Eskalith Capsules . . . 1406

PHARCINA (Mexico)
CIPROFLOXACIN HYDROCHLORIDE
Ciloxan Ophthalmic Ointment . . . 554
Ciloxan Ophthalmic Solution . . . ⊙205
Cipro Tablets . . . 2991

PHARMAFLAM (South Africa)
DICLOFENAC SODIUM
Voltaren Tablets . . . 2298
Voltaren-XR Tablets . . . 2301

PHARMAFLEX (Belgium)
METRONIDAZOLE
MetroGel-Vaginal Gel . . . 1822
Noritate Cream, 1% . . . 1051

PHARMALOSE (Canada)
LACTULOSE
Kristalose for Oral Solution . . . 2149

PHARMAMOX (Switzerland)
AMOXICILLIN
Amoxil Pediatric Drops for Oral Suspension . . . 1315
Amoxil Tablets . . . 1315

PHARMAPRESS (South Africa)
ENALAPRIL MALEATE
Vasotec I.V. Injection . . . 2076

PHARMAPRESS CO (South Africa)
ENALAPRIL MALEATE
Vasotec I.V. Injection **2076**

PHARMOTIDINE (Thailand)
FAMOTIDINE
Pepcid Injection **2017**
Pepcid Injection Premixed **2017**
Pepcid Tablets **2014**
Pepcid for Oral Suspension **2014**

PHARPHYLLINE (The Netherlands)
THEOPHYLLINE
Uniphyl Tablets **2708**

PHARYNGOCIN (Germany)
ERYTHROMYCIN
Ery-Tab Tablets **447**
Erythromycin Base Filmtab Tablets **454**
Erythromycin Delayed-Release Capsules, USP **456**
PCE Dispertab Tablets **510**

PHASAL (United Kingdom)
LITHIUM CARBONATE
Eskalith CR Controlled-Release Tablets ... **1406**
Eskalith Capsules **1406**

PHENEDRINE (Hong Kong)
THEOPHYLLINE
Uniphyl Tablets **2708**

PHENERGAN (Australia, Belgium, Canada, Denmark, Hong Kong, India, Irish Republic, New Zealand, Norway, Singapore, South Africa, Thailand, The Netherlands, United Kingdom)
PROMETHAZINE HYDROCHLORIDE
Phenergan Suppositories **3438**
Phenergan Tablets **3438**

PHENHALAL (United Kingdom)
PROMETHAZINE HYDROCHLORIDE
Phenergan Suppositories **3438**
Phenergan Tablets **3438**

PHENSEDYL (Malaysia)
PROMETHAZINE HYDROCHLORIDE
Phenergan Suppositories **3438**
Phenergan Tablets **3438**

PHIMETIN (United Kingdom)
CIMETIDINE
Tagamet Tablets **1547**

PHOS-EX (Austria, Denmark, Finland, Germany, Norway, Sweden, United Kingdom)
CALCIUM ACETATE
PhosLo GelCaps **2158**

PHOSFORID (India)
CALCIUM ACETATE
PhosLo GelCaps **2158**

PHOSLO (Chile)
CALCIUM ACETATE
PhosLo GelCaps **2158**

PHOSTARAC (Argentina)
ALENDRONATE SODIUM
Fosamax Tablets **1949**

PHYLOBID (India)
THEOPHYLLINE
Uniphyl Tablets **2708**

PHYLODAY (India)
THEOPHYLLINE
Uniphyl Tablets **2708**

PHYZIDINE (Hong Kong)
FAMOTIDINE
Pepcid Injection **2017**
Pepcid Injection Premixed **2017**
Pepcid Tablets **2014**
Pepcid for Oral Suspension **2014**

PIAMFUCIN (Russia)
NATAMYCIN
Natacyn Antifungal Ophthalmic Suspension .... ⊙**207**

PIDILAT (Germany)
NIFEDIPINE
Adalat CC Tablets **2978**

PILOTIM (Argentina)
TIMOLOL MALEATE
Blocadren Tablets **1891**
Timoptic Sterile Ophthalmic Solution **2058**
Timoptic in Ocudose **2061**
Timoptic-XE Sterile Ophthalmic Gel Forming Solution **2062**

PIMA BICIRON N (Germany)
NATAMYCIN
Natacyn Antifungal Ophthalmic Suspension .... ⊙**207**

PIMAFUCIN (Belgium, Czech Republic, Finland, Germany, Hungary, United Kingdom)
NATAMYCIN
Natacyn Antifungal Ophthalmic Suspension .... ⊙**207**

PIMAFUCORT (Hungary)
HYDROCORTISONE
Hydrocortone Tablets **1963**

PINAMET (Irish Republic)
CIMETIDINE
Tagamet Tablets **1547**

PINAMOX (Irish Republic)
AMOXICILLIN
Amoxil Pediatric Drops for Oral Suspension **1315**
Amoxil Tablets **1315**

PINIFED (Irish Republic)
NIFEDIPINE
Adalat CC Tablets **2978**

PINIOL (Germany)
NAPHAZOLINE HYDROCHLORIDE
Albalon Ophthalmic Solution .... ⊙**216**

PINIOL NASENSPRAY (Germany)
NAPHAZOLINE HYDROCHLORIDE
Albalon Ophthalmic Solution .... ⊙**216**

PIOGLIT (Argentina)
PIOGLITAZONE HYDROCHLORIDE
Actos Tablets **3224**

PIOLHOL (Brazil)
PERMETHRIN
Acticin Cream **2125**

PIOLHOL PLUS (Brazil)
PERMETHRIN
Acticin Cream **2125**

PIOMED (India)
PIOGLITAZONE HYDROCHLORIDE
Actos Tablets **3224**

PIOSAFE (India)
PIOGLITAZONE HYDROCHLORIDE
Actos Tablets **3224**

PIOSAN (Brazil)
PERMETHRIN
Acticin Cream **2125**

PIOSOL (Brazil)
PERMETHRIN
Acticin Cream **2125**

PIOSTOP (Brazil)
PERMETHRIN
Acticin Cream **2125**

PIOZULIN (India)
PIOGLITAZONE HYDROCHLORIDE
Actos Tablets **3224**

PIPOLPHEN (Hungary, Russia)
PROMETHAZINE HYDROCHLORIDE
Phenergan Suppositories **3438**
Phenergan Tablets **3438**

PIPROL (Spain)
CIPROFLOXACIN HYDROCHLORIDE
Ciloxan Ophthalmic Ointment **554**
Ciloxan Ophthalmic Solution .... ⊙**205**
Cipro Tablets **2991**

PIREXYL (Chile)
DICLOFENAC SODIUM
Voltaren Tablets **2298**
Voltaren-XR Tablets **2301**

PIRIDASMIN (Spain)
THEOPHYLLINE
Uniphyl Tablets **2708**

PIRIMECIDAN (Spain)
PYRIMETHAMINE
Daraprim Tablets **1385**

PIRITEZE (United Kingdom)
CETIRIZINE HYDROCHLORIDE
Zyrtec Syrup **2589**
Zyrtec Tablets **2589**

PIRIUM (Greece)
PIMOZIDE
Orap Tablets **1220**

PIROBAC (Chile)
BENZOYL PEROXIDE
Brevoxyl-4 Creamy Wash **3212**
Brevoxyl-4 Gel **3211**
Brevoxyl-8 Creamy Wash **3212**
Brevoxyl-8 Gel **3211**
Triaz Cleanser **1864**
Triaz Gel **1864**

PISTOFIL (Greece)
NORFLOXACIN
Noroxin Tablets **2009**

PIZIDE (Thailand)
PIMOZIDE
Orap Tablets **1220**

PLACIDOX (India)
DIAZEPAM
Diastat Rectal Delivery System **3344**
Valium Tablets **2822**

PLAKET (Brazil)
TICLOPIDINE HYDROCHLORIDE
Ticlid Tablets **2813**

PLAN (Argentina)
ATORVASTATIN CALCIUM
Lipitor Tablets **2495**

PLANITRIX (Greece)
FENOFIBRATE
Tricor Tablets **523**

PLANIZOL (Mexico)
METRONIDAZOLE
MetroGel-Vaginal Gel **1822**
Noritate Cream, 1% **1051**

PLAQUETAL (Portugal)
TICLOPIDINE HYDROCHLORIDE
Ticlid Tablets **2813**

PLAQUETIL (Chile)
TICLOPIDINE HYDROCHLORIDE
Ticlid Tablets **2813**

PLASIMINE (Spain)
MUPIROCIN
Bactroban Ointment **1358**

PLASMANATE (Brazil, Malaysia)
PLASMA PROTEIN FRACTION
Plasmanate **3252**

PLASMATEIN (United Kingdom)
PLASMA PROTEIN FRACTION
Plasmanate **3252**

PLASMAVIRAL (Italy)
PLASMA PROTEIN FRACTION
Plasmanate **3252**

PLATELET (Italy)
DIPYRIDAMOLE
Persantine Tablets **898**

PLATIGREN (Czech Republic)
TICLOPIDINE HYDROCHLORIDE
Ticlid Tablets **2813**

PLATO (South Africa)
DIPYRIDAMOLE
Persantine Tablets **898**

PLAUCINA (Spain)
ENOXAPARIN SODIUM
Lovenox Injection **2931**

PLAVIX (Argentina, Australia, Austria, Belgium, Brazil, Canada, Chile, Czech Republic, Denmark, France, Germany, Greece, Hungary, Irish Republic, Israel, Italy, Malaysia, Mexico, New Zealand, Norway, Portugal, Singapore, South Africa, Spain, Sweden, Switzerland, Thailand, The Netherlands, United Kingdom)
CLOPIDOGREL BISULFATE
Plavix Tablets **940, 2942**

PLENACOR (Argentina, Brazil, Mexico)
ATENOLOL
Tenormin I.V. Injection **698**

PLENACTOL (Chile)
ORPHENADRINE CITRATE
Norflex Injection **1824**

PLENASTRIL (Germany)
OXYMETHOLONE
Anadrol-50 Tablets **3329**

PLENAX (Brazil)
CEFIXIME
Suprax **1811**

PLENDIL (Argentina, Australia, Austria, Belgium, Canada, Czech Republic, Denmark, Finland, Greece, Hong Kong, Irish Republic, Italy, Malaysia, Mexico, New Zealand, Norway, Singapore, South Africa, Spain, Sweden, Switzerland, Thailand, The Netherlands, United Kingdom)
FELODIPINE
Plendil Extended-Release Tablets **651**

PLENDUR (Denmark)
FELODIPINE
Plendil Extended-Release Tablets **651**

PLENISH-K (South Africa)
POTASSIUM CHLORIDE
K-Dur Extended-Relase Tablets **3047**
K-Lor Powder Packets **472**
K-Tab Filmtab Tablets **473**

PLENOLYT (Spain)
CIPROFLOXACIN HYDROCHLORIDE
Ciloxan Ophthalmic Ointment **554**
Ciloxan Ophthalmic Solution .... ⊙**205**
Cipro Tablets **2991**

PLENOMICINA (Brazil)
ERYTHROMYCIN STEARATE
Erythrocin Stearate Filmtab Tablets **452**

PLENTY (Brazil)
SIBUTRAMINE HYDROCHLORIDE
Meridia Capsules **485**

PLENUR (Spain)
LITHIUM CARBONATE
Eskalith CR Controlled-Release Tablets ... **1406**
Eskalith Capsules **1406**

PLETAAL (Argentina, Hong Kong, Japan, Thailand)
CILOSTAZOL
Pletal Tablets **2478**

PLETAL (United Kingdom)
CILOSTAZOL
Pletal Tablets **2478**

PLETOZ (India)
CILOSTAZOL
Pletal Tablets **2478**

PLEXOL (Argentina)
LOPERAMIDE HYDROCHLORIDE
Imodium Capsules **1834**

PLEXXO (The Netherlands)
LAMOTRIGINE
Lamictal Chewable Dispersible Tablets ... **1449**
Lamictal Tablets **1449**

PLEYAR (Argentina)
CLOPIDOGREL BISULFATE
Plavix Tablets **940, 2942**

PLIDAN (Argentina)
DIAZEPAM
Diastat Rectal Delivery System **3344**
Valium Tablets **2822**

PLIDEX (Argentina)
DIAZEPAM
Diastat Rectal Delivery System **3344**
Valium Tablets **2822**

PLIMYCOL (Czech Republic)
CLOTRIMAZOLE
Lotrimin Cream **3053**
Lotrimin Lotion 1% **3053**
Lotrimin Topical Solution 1% **3053**

PLOSTIM (Argentina)
TIMOLOL MALEATE
Blocadren Tablets **1891**
Timoptic Sterile Ophthalmic Solution **2058**
Timoptic in Ocudose **2061**
Timoptic-XE Sterile Ophthalmic Gel Forming Solution **2062**

PLURICEFO (Argentina)
CEFOXITIN SODIUM
Mefoxin Premixed Intravenous Solution ... **1990**
Mefoxin for Injection **1987**

PLURIMEN (Spain)
SELEGILINE HYDROCHLORIDE
Eldepryl Capsules **3209**

PLURIVERM (Brazil)
MEBENDAZOLE
Vermox Chewable Tablets **1853**

PLURIVERMIL (Brazil)
MEBENDAZOLE
Vermox Chewable Tablets **1853**

PLUS KALIUM RETARD (Switzerland)
POTASSIUM CHLORIDE
K-Dur Extended-Relase Tablets ... 3047
K-Lor Powder Packets ... 472
K-Tab Filmtab Tablets ... 473

PLUSGIN (Argentina)
CIPROFLOXACIN
Cipro Oral Suspension ... 2991

PLUSTAXANO (Argentina)
DOCETAXEL
Taxotere Injection Concentrate ... 2947

PMS-DOPAZIDE (Canada)
HYDROCHLOROTHIAZIDE/METHYLDOPA
Aldoril Tablets ... 1884

POCIN (Thailand)
ERYTHROMYCIN STEARATE
Erythrocin Stearate Filmtab Tablets ... 452

PODIUM (Spain)
DIAZEPAM
Diastat Rectal Delivery System ... 3344
Valium Tablets ... 2822

PODOMEXEF (Germany, Switzerland)
CEFPODOXIME PROXETIL
Vantin Tablets and Oral Suspension ... 2650

POENFLOX (Chile)
OFLOXACIN
Floxin Otic Solution ... 1043

POENTIMOL (Argentina)
TIMOLOL MALEATE
Blocadren Tablets ... 1891
Timoptic Sterile Ophthalmic Solution ... 2058
Timoptic in Ocudose ... 2061
Timoptic-XE Sterile Ophthalmic Gel Forming Solution ... 2062

POENTOBRAL PLUS (Chile)
DEXAMETHASONE/TOBRAMYCIN
TobraDex Ophthalmic Ointment ... 558
TobraDex Ophthalmic Suspension ... 558

POFOL (Singapore, Thailand)
PROPOFOL
Diprivan Injectable Emulsion ... 676

POINT (Israel)
NAPROXEN SODIUM
Anaprox DS Tablets ... 2769
Anaprox Tablets ... 2769

POLIBAC (Brazil)
AMOXICILLIN
Amoxil Pediatric Drops for Oral Suspension ... 1315
Amoxil Tablets ... 1315

POLIBEN (Brazil)
MEBENDAZOLE
Vermox Chewable Tablets ... 1853

POLICANO (Greece)
ISOTRETINOIN
Accutane Capsules ... 2740

POLI-CIFLOXIN (Thailand)
CIPROFLOXACIN
Cipro Oral Suspension ... 2991

POLICOR (Argentina)
CILOSTAZOL
Pletal Tablets ... 2478

POLIDELTAXIN (Mexico)
DEXAMETHASONE
Decadron Tablets ... 1929

POLIMOXIL (Brazil)
AMOXICILLIN
Amoxil Pediatric Drops for Oral Suspension ... 1315
Amoxil Tablets ... 1315

POLINAZOLO (Italy)
ECONAZOLE NITRATE
Spectazole Cream ... 2390

POLIOFTAL (Argentina)
TOBRAMYCIN
TOBI Solution for Inhalation ... 1015

POLIREUMIN (Brazil)
SODIUM HYALURONATE
Hyalgan Solution ... 2917

POLITELMIN (Brazil)
MEBENDAZOLE
Vermox Chewable Tablets ... 1853

POLI-URETIC (Thailand)
AMILORIDE HYDROCHLORIDE/HYDROCHLOROTHIAZIDE
Moduretic Tablets ... 2003

POLIXIMA (Italy)
CEFUROXIME SODIUM
Zinacef Injection ... 1604

POLY PRED (Spain)
NEOMYCIN SULFATE/POLYMYXIN B SULFATE/PREDNISOLONE ACETATE
Poly-Pred Liquifilm Ophthalmic Suspension ... ⊙231

POLYANION (Austria)
PENTOSAN POLYSULFATE SODIUM
Elmiron Capsules ... 2393

POLYCITRA-K (Canada)
POTASSIUM CITRATE
Urocit-K Tablets ... 2109

POLY-COF (Thailand)
PROMETHAZINE HYDROCHLORIDE
Phenergan Suppositories ... 3438
Phenergan Tablets ... 3438

POLYFLAM (Belgium)
DICLOFENAC SODIUM
Voltaren Tablets ... 2298
Voltaren-XR Tablets ... 2301

POLYTRIM (Canada)
POLYMYXIN B SULFATE/TRIMETHOPRIM SULFATE
Polytrim Ophthalmic Solution ... 570

POLYXEN (Thailand)
NAPROXEN
EC-Naprosyn Delayed-Release Tablets ... 2769
Naprosyn Suspension ... 2769
Naprosyn Tablets ... 2769

PONDARMETT (Thailand)
CIMETIDINE
Tagamet Tablets ... 1547

PONDERA (Brazil)
PAROXETINE HYDROCHLORIDE
Paxil Oral Suspension ... 1501
Paxil Tablets ... 1501

PONDTROXIN (Thailand)
LEVOTHYROXINE SODIUM
Levothroid Tablets ... 1189
Levoxyl Tablets ... 1680
Synthroid Tablets ... 515

PORPHYROCIN (Hong Kong)
ERYTHROMYCIN STEARATE
Erythrocin Stearate Filmtab Tablets ... 452

PORUXIN (Greece)
FINASTERIDE
Propecia Tablets ... 2036
Proscar Tablets ... 2040

POSANIN (Thailand)
DIPYRIDAMOLE
Persantine Tablets ... 898

POSE-CM (Thailand)
CIMETIDINE
Tagamet Tablets ... 1547

POSIVYL (Chile)
PAROXETINE HYDROCHLORIDE
Paxil Oral Suspension ... 1501
Paxil Tablets ... 1501

POSNAC (Thailand)
DICLOFENAC SODIUM
Voltaren Tablets ... 2298
Voltaren-XR Tablets ... 2301

POTASIO C (Argentina)
POTASSIUM CHLORIDE
K-Dur Extended-Relase Tablets ... 3047
K-Lor Powder Packets ... 472
K-Tab Filmtab Tablets ... 473

POTASION (Spain)
POTASSIUM CHLORIDE
K-Dur Extended-Relase Tablets ... 3047
K-Lor Powder Packets ... 472
K-Tab Filmtab Tablets ... 473

POTASSRIDE (Thailand)
POTASSIUM CHLORIDE
K-Dur Extended-Relase Tablets ... 3047
K-Lor Powder Packets ... 472
K-Tab Filmtab Tablets ... 473

POTCIT (Malaysia)
POTASSIUM CITRATE
Urocit-K Tablets ... 2109

POTENCORT (United Arab Emirates)
FLUTICASONE PROPIONATE
Cutivate Cream ... 1381
Cutivate Ointment ... 1384
Flonase Nasal Spray ... 1412

POTENDAL (Spain)
CEFTAZIDIME
Fortaz for Injection ... 1422

POTKLOR (India)
POTASSIUM CHLORIDE
K-Dur Extended-Relase Tablets ... 3047
K-Lor Powder Packets ... 472
K-Tab Filmtab Tablets ... 473

POWERCEF (India)
CEFTRIAXONE SODIUM
Rocephin Injectable Vials, ADD-Vantage, Galaxy, Bulk ... 2801

POWERGYL (India)
NORFLOXACIN
Noroxin Tablets ... 2009

PPS (Italy)
PLASMA PROTEIN FRACTION
Plasmanate ... 3252

PRACAP (Brazil)
FINASTERIDE
Propecia Tablets ... 2036
Proscar Tablets ... 2040

PRACEM (Mexico)
DIPYRIDAMOLE
Persantine Tablets ... 898

PRADIF (Greece, Italy, Portugal, Switzerland)
TAMSULOSIN HYDROCHLORIDE
Flomax Capsules ... 881

PRADINOLOL (Brazil)
PROPRANOLOL HYDROCHLORIDE
Inderal LA Long-Acting Capsules ... 3421

PRAECICOR (Germany)
VERAPAMIL HYDROCHLORIDE
Covera-HS Tablets ... 3135
Verelan PM Capsules ... 3120

PRALENAL (United Kingdom)
ENALAPRIL MALEATE
Vasotec I.V. Injection ... 2076

PRALOL (Thailand)
PROPRANOLOL HYDROCHLORIDE
Inderal LA Long-Acting Capsules ... 3421

PRAM (Austria)
CITALOPRAM HYDROBROMIDE
Celexa Tablets ... 1177

PRAMACE (Irish Republic, Sweden)
RAMIPRIL
Altace Capsules ... 1673

PRAMIDAL (Mexico)
LOPERAMIDE HYDROCHLORIDE
Imodium Capsules ... 1834

PRANADOX (Mexico)
ZIDOVUDINE
Retrovir Capsules ... 1533
Retrovir IV Infusion ... 1537
Retrovir Syrup ... 1533
Retrovir Tablets ... 1533

PRANDASE (Canada, Israel)
ACARBOSE
Precose Tablets ... 776

PRANDIN (Brazil, Spain)
REPAGLINIDE
Prandin Tablets (0.5, 1, and 2 mg) ... 2337

PRANDIN E2 (South Africa)
DINOPROSTONE
Cervidil Vaginal Insert ... 1182

PRANDIOL (France)
DIPYRIDAMOLE
Persantine Tablets ... 898

PRANOLOL (Norway)
PROPRANOLOL HYDROCHLORIDE
Inderal LA Long-Acting Capsules ... 3421

PRANOXEN (South Africa)
NAPROXEN
EC-Naprosyn Delayed-Release Tablets ... 2769
Naprosyn Suspension ... 2769
Naprosyn Tablets ... 2769

PRANOXEN CONTINUS (United Kingdom)
NAPROXEN
EC-Naprosyn Delayed-Release Tablets ... 2769
Naprosyn Suspension ... 2769
Naprosyn Tablets ... 2769

PRAQUANTEL (Thailand)
PRAZIQUANTEL
Biltricide Tablets ... 2990

PRAREDUCT (Belgium, Spain)
PRAVASTATIN SODIUM
Pravachol Tablets ... 943

PRASCOLEND (Mexico)
PRAVASTATIN SODIUM
Pravachol Tablets ... 943

PRASIKON (Thailand)
PRAZIQUANTEL
Biltricide Tablets ... 2990

PRASTEROL (Italy)
PRAVASTATIN SODIUM
Pravachol Tablets ... 943

PRAVA (South Africa)
PRAVASTATIN SODIUM
Pravachol Tablets ... 943

PRAVACHOL (Australia, Austria, Canada, Denmark, Finland, Greece, Hong Kong, Malaysia, Norway, Singapore, Sweden)
PRAVASTATIN SODIUM
Pravachol Tablets ... 943

PRAVACOL (Argentina, Brazil, Chile, Mexico, Portugal)
PRAVASTATIN SODIUM
Pravachol Tablets ... 943

PRAVAMEL (Irish Republic)
PRAVASTATIN SODIUM
Pravachol Tablets ... 943

PRAVASELECT (Italy)
PRAVASTATIN SODIUM
Pravachol Tablets ... 943

PRAVASIN (Germany)
PRAVASTATIN SODIUM
Pravachol Tablets ... 943

PRAVASINE (Belgium)
PRAVASTATIN SODIUM
Pravachol Tablets ... 943

PRAVITIN (Irish Republic)
PRAVASTATIN SODIUM
Pravachol Tablets ... 943

PRAYANOL (Chile)
AMANTADINE HYDROCHLORIDE
Symmetrel Syrup ... 1115
Symmetrel Tablets ... 1115

PRAZITE (Thailand)
PRAZIQUANTEL
Biltricide Tablets ... 2990

PRAZITRAL (Argentina)
PRAZIQUANTEL
Biltricide Tablets ... 2990

PRAZOL (Brazil)
LANSOPRAZOLE
Prevacid Delayed-Release Capsules ... 3268

PRE CLEAN MOM (Italy)
PERMETHRIN
Acticin Cream ... 2125

PRE-CLAR (Chile)
CLARITHROMYCIN
Biaxin Filmtab Tablets ... 402
Biaxin Granules ... 402

PRED-CLYSMA (Denmark, Norway, Sweden)
PREDNISOLONE SODIUM PHOSPHATE
Pediapred Oral Solution ... 3319

PREDMIX (Australia)
PREDNISOLONE SODIUM PHOSPHATE
Pediapred Oral Solution ... 3319

PREDMYCIN (Thailand)
NEOMYCIN SULFATE/POLYMYXIN B SULFATE/PREDNISOLONE ACETATE
Poly-Pred Liquifilm Ophthalmic Suspension ... ⊙231

PREDMYCIN P (Belgium)
NEOMYCIN SULFATE/POLYMYXIN B SULFATE/PREDNISOLONE ACETATE
Poly-Pred Liquifilm Ophthalmic Suspension ⊙231

PREDMYCIN-P (Singapore)
NEOMYCIN SULFATE/POLYMYXIN B SULFATE/PREDNISOLONE ACETATE
Poly-Pred Liquifilm Ophthalmic Suspension ⊙231

PREDMYCIN-P LIQUIFILM (The Netherlands)
NEOMYCIN SULFATE/POLYMYXIN B SULFATE/PREDNISOLONE ACETATE
Poly-Pred Liquifilm Ophthalmic Suspension ⊙231

PREDNABENE (Germany)
PREDNISOLONE SODIUM PHOSPHATE
Pediapred Oral Solution 3319

PREDNESOL (Irish Republic, United Kingdom)
PREDNISOLONE SODIUM PHOSPHATE
Pediapred Oral Solution 3319

PREDNI-F-TABLINEN (Germany)
DEXAMETHASONE
Decadron Tablets 1929

PREDNIMENT (Denmark, Finland)
PREDNISOLONE SODIUM PHOSPHATE
Pediapred Oral Solution 3319

PREDONIUM (Austria, Portugal, The Netherlands)
PERINDOPRIL ERBUMINE
Aceon Tablets (2 mg, 4 mg, 8 mg) 3191

PREDSOL (Australia, Irish Republic, New Zealand, South Africa, United Kingdom)
PREDNISOLONE SODIUM PHOSPHATE
Pediapred Oral Solution 3319

PREFACE (India)
RAMIPRIL
Altace Capsules 1673

PREFEST (Brazil)
ESTRADIOL
Climara Transdermal System 795
Vivelle Transdermal System 2288
Vivelle-Dot Transdermal System 2293

PREFIN (Spain)
BUPRENORPHINE HYDROCHLORIDE
Buprenex Injectable 2718

PRELECTAL (Italy)
PERINDOPRIL ERBUMINE
Aceon Tablets (2 mg, 4 mg, 8 mg) 3191

PREMJACT (United Kingdom)
LIDOCAINE
Lidoderm Patch 1107

PRENALON (Mexico)
KETOCONAZOLE
Nizoral 2% Shampoo 1838

PRENOLOL (Singapore, Thailand)
ATENOLOL
Tenormin I.V. Injection 698

PRENORETIC (Argentina)
ATENOLOL
Tenormin I.V. Injection 698

PRENORMINE (Argentina)
ATENOLOL
Tenormin I.V. Injection 698

PREPIDIL (Austria, Belgium, Canada, Czech Republic, France, Germany, Hong Kong, Hungary, Irish Republic, Israel, Italy, Mexico, New Zealand, South Africa, Spain, Switzerland, The Netherlands, United Kingdom)
DINOPROSTONE
Cervidil Vaginal Insert 1182

PRERAN (Japan)
TRANDOLAPRIL
Mavik Tablets 482

PRES (Germany)
ENALAPRIL MALEATE
Vasotec I.V. Injection 2076

PRES PLUS (Germany)
ENALAPRIL MALEATE/HYDROCHLOROTHIAZIDE
Vaseretic Tablets 2073

PRESCAL (Irish Republic, United Kingdom)
ISRADIPINE
DynaCirc CR Tablets 2726

PRESI REGUL (Argentina)
ENALAPRIL MALEATE
Vasotec I.V. Injection 2076

PRESI REGUL D (Argentina)
ENALAPRIL MALEATE
Vasotec I.V. Injection 2076

PRESID (Czech Republic, Hungary)
FELODIPINE
Plendil Extended-Release Tablets 651

PRESINEX (United Kingdom)
DESMOPRESSIN ACETATE
DDAVP Injection 4 mcg/mL 2893
DDAVP Nasal Spray 2894
DDAVP Tablets 2895
Desmopressin Acetate Injection 1143
Desmopressin Acetate Rhinal Tube 1144

PRESINOR (Argentina)
LOSARTAN POTASSIUM
Cozaar Tablets 1913

PRESINOR D (Argentina)
LOSARTAN POTASSIUM
Cozaar Tablets 1913

PRESLOW (Portugal, Spain)
FELODIPINE
Plendil Extended-Release Tablets 651

PRESOCOR (Chile)
VERAPAMIL HYDROCHLORIDE
Covera-HS Tablets 3135
Verelan PM Capsules 3120

PRESOKIN (Chile)
LISINOPRIL
Prinivil Tablets 2029
Zestril Tablets 704

PRESOLAR (India)
ATENOLOL
Tenormin I.V. Injection 698

PRESS-12 (Greece)
LISINOPRIL
Prinivil Tablets 2029
Zestril Tablets 704

PRESSANOL (South Africa)
PROPRANOLOL HYDROCHLORIDE
Inderal LA Long-Acting Capsules 3421

PRESSEL (Brazil)
ENALAPRIL MALEATE
Vasotec I.V. Injection 2076

PRESSITAN (Spain)
ENALAPRIL MALEATE
Vasotec I.V. Injection 2076

PRESSITAN PLUS (Spain)
ENALAPRIL MALEATE/HYDROCHLOROTHIAZIDE
Vaseretic Tablets 2073

PRESSOLAT (Israel)
NIFEDIPINE
Adalat CC Tablets 2978

PRESSOMAX (Brazil)
CAPTOPRIL
Captopril Tablets 2114

PRESSOTEC (Brazil)
ENALAPRIL MALEATE
Vasotec I.V. Injection 2076

PRESSURAL (Italy)
INDAPAMIDE
Indapamide Tablets 2119

PRESTARIUM (Czech Republic)
PERINDOPRIL ERBUMINE
Aceon Tablets (2 mg, 4 mg, 8 mg) 3191

PRESTOLE (France)
HYDROCHLOROTHIAZIDE/TRIAMTERENE
Dyazide Capsules 1389
Maxzide Tablets 2150
Maxzide-25 mg Tablets 2150

PRESYNDRAL (Spain)
ENALAPRIL MALEATE
Vasotec I.V. Injection 2076

PRETANIX (Hungary)
INDAPAMIDE
Indapamide Tablets 2119

PRETERAX (Argentina, Austria, Belgium, Brazil, Canada, Germany, Irish Republic, Italy, Portugal, Singapore, South Africa, Spain, The Netherlands)
PERINDOPRIL ERBUMINE
Aceon Tablets (2 mg, 4 mg, 8 mg) 3191

PREVACID (Canada, Japan, Malaysia, Singapore, Thailand)
LANSOPRAZOLE
Prevacid Delayed-Release Capsules 3268

PREVENCOR (Spain)
ATORVASTATIN CALCIUM
Lipitor Tablets 2495

PREVEX (Italy)
FELODIPINE
Plendil Extended-Release Tablets 651

PREVEX HC (Canada, Thailand)
HYDROCORTISONE
Hydrocortone Tablets 1963

PREXAN (Italy)
NAPROXEN
EC-Naprosyn Delayed-Release Tablets 2769
Naprosyn Suspension 2769
Naprosyn Tablets 2769

PREXUM (South Africa)
PERINDOPRIL ERBUMINE
Aceon Tablets (2 mg, 4 mg, 8 mg) 3191

PREZAL (The Netherlands)
LANSOPRAZOLE
Prevacid Delayed-Release Capsules 3268

PRIADEL (Australia, Belgium, Malaysia, New Zealand, Portugal, Singapore, South Africa, Switzerland, The Netherlands, United Kingdom)
LITHIUM CARBONATE
Eskalith CR Controlled-Release Tablets 1406
Eskalith Capsules 1406

PRILACE (Italy)
RAMIPRIL
Altace Capsules 1673

PRILAN (Portugal)
ENALAPRIL MALEATE
Vasotec I.V. Injection 2076

PRILOSIN (South Africa)
LISINOPRIL
Prinivil Tablets 2029
Zestril Tablets 704

PRILOVASE (Portugal)
CAPTOPRIL
Captopril Tablets 2114

PRILTENK (Argentina)
ENALAPRIL MALEATE
Vasotec I.V. Injection 2076

PRIMAMET (Czech Republic)
CIMETIDINE
Tagamet Tablets 1547

PRIMAQUIN (Chile)
ESTRADIOL
Climara Transdermal System 795
Vivelle Transdermal System 2288
Vivelle-Dot Transdermal System 2293

PRIMATENOL (Switzerland)
ATENOLOL
Tenormin I.V. Injection 698

PRIMATENOL PLUS (Switzerland)
ATENOLOL
Tenormin I.V. Injection 698

PRIMAXIN (Canada, Greece, United Kingdom)
CILASTATIN SODIUM/IMIPENEM
Primaxin I.M. 2022
Primaxin I.V. 2024

PRIMERAL (Italy)
NAPROXEN SODIUM
Anaprox DS Tablets 2769
Anaprox Tablets 2769

PRIMESIN (Italy)
FLUVASTATIN SODIUM
Lescol Capsules 2227

PRIMIPROST (India)
DINOPROSTONE
Cervidil Vaginal Insert 1182

PRIMOFENAC (Switzerland)
DICLOFENAC SODIUM
Voltaren Tablets 2298
Voltaren-XR Tablets 2301

PRIMOXIL (Italy)
MOEXIPRIL HYDROCHLORIDE
Univasc Tablets 3118

PRIMULEX (Hungary)
SELEGILINE HYDROCHLORIDE
Eldepryl Capsules 3209

PRINCESS PROLIB (Spain)
FLUVASTATIN SODIUM
Lescol Capsules 2227

PRINCIPROX (Switzerland)
CIPROFLOXACIN HYDROCHLORIDE
Ciloxan Ophthalmic Ointment 554
Ciloxan Ophthalmic Solution ⊙205
Cipro Tablets 2991

PRINDERIN (Spain)
CEFAZOLIN SODIUM
Ancef for Injection 1318

PRINIL (Switzerland)
LISINOPRIL
Prinivil Tablets 2029
Zestril Tablets 704

PRINIVIL (Australia, Austria, Brazil, Canada, Czech Republic, France, Greece, Hong Kong, Italy, Malaysia, Mexico, New Zealand, Portugal, Singapore, South Africa, Spain)
LISINOPRIL
Prinivil Tablets 2029
Zestril Tablets 704

PRINIVIL PLUS (Spain)
HYDROCHLOROTHIAZIDE/LISINOPRIL
Prinzide Tablets 2033
Zestoretic Tablets 701

PRINORM (Hungary)
ATENOLOL
Tenormin I.V. Injection 698

PRINZIDE (Austria, Brazil, Canada, France, Italy, Mexico, New Zealand, Portugal, Switzerland)
HYDROCHLOROTHIAZIDE/LISINOPRIL
Prinzide Tablets 2033
Zestoretic Tablets 701

PRIPSEN (United Kingdom)
MEBENDAZOLE
Vermox Chewable Tablets 1853

PRISDAL (Spain)
CITALOPRAM HYDROBROMIDE
Celexa Tablets 1177

PRISTINE (Hong Kong, Malaysia, Singapore)
KETOCONAZOLE
Nizoral 2% Shampoo 1838

PRISTINEX (Hong Kong, Malaysia, Singapore)
KETOCONAZOLE
Nizoral 2% Shampoo 1838

PRITANOL (Portugal)
PRAVASTATIN SODIUM
Pravachol Tablets 943

PRITOR (Argentina, Australia, Brazil, Czech Republic, France, Greece, Hungary, Italy, Portugal, Spain)
TELMISARTAN
Micardis Tablets 884

PRITOR PLUS (Portugal, Spain)
TELMISARTAN
Micardis Tablets 884

PRITORAL (Chile)
TELMISARTAN
Micardis Tablets 884

PRITORPLUS (France)
TELMISARTAN
Micardis Tablets 884

PRITORPLUS (Hungary)
TELMISARTAN
Micardis Tablets 884

PRITORPLUS (Italy)
TELMISARTAN
Micardis Tablets 884

PRIVACOM (United Kingdom)
CLOTRIMAZOLE
Lotrimin Cream 3053
Lotrimin Lotion 1% 3053
Lotrimin Topical Solution 1% 3053

PRIVINE (Canada)
NAPHAZOLINE HYDROCHLORIDE
Albalon Ophthalmic Solution . . . . ⊙216

PRIXAR (Italy)
LEVOFLOXACIN
Levaquin Injection 2453
Levaquin Tablets 2453

PRIZEM (Mexico)
DIAZEPAM
Diastat Rectal Delivery System 3344
Valium Tablets 2822

PRO ULCO (Spain)
LANSOPRAZOLE
Prevacid Delayed-Release Capsules 3268

PROAIR (Argentina)
FLUTICASONE PROPIONATE
Cutivate Cream 1381
Cutivate Ointment 1384
Flonase Nasal Spray 1412

PROBENXIL (Brazil)
DICLOFENAC POTASSIUM
Cataflam Tablets 2173

PROBETA LA (United Kingdom)
PROPRANOLOL HYDROCHLORIDE
Inderal LA Long-Acting Capsules 3421

PROCAPTAN (Italy)
PERINDOPRIL ERBUMINE
Aceon Tablets (2 mg, 4 mg, 8 mg) 3191

PROCARDIN (Singapore)
DIPYRIDAMOLE
Persantine Tablets 898

PROCARDOL (Greece)
ISOSORBIDE MONONITRATE
Imdur Tablets 3032

PROCETOKEN (Argentina)
FENOFIBRATE
Tricor Tablets 523

PROCIMETI (Mexico)
CIMETIDINE
Tagamet Tablets 1547

PROCIN (Brazil)
CIPROFLOXACIN
Cipro Oral Suspension 2991

PROCIP (India)
CIPROFLOXACIN
Cipro Oral Suspension 2991

PROCLIM (Canada)
MEDROXYPROGESTERONE ACETATE
Depo-Medrol Single-Dose Vial 2617

PROCOR (Brazil, Israel)
DIPYRIDAMOLE
Persantine Tablets 898

PROCOR S (Brazil)
DIPYRIDAMOLE
Persantine Tablets 898

PROCTOCREM (Argentina)
LIDOCAINE
Lidoderm Patch 1107

PROCULIN (Czech Republic, Germany, Hungary)
NAPHAZOLINE HYDROCHLORIDE
Albalon Ophthalmic Solution . . . . ⊙216

PRO-CURE (Israel)
FINASTERIDE
Propecia Tablets 2036
Proscar Tablets 2040

PROCUTA (France)
ISOTRETINOIN
Accutane Capsules 2740

PROCUTAN (South Africa)
HYDROCORTISONE
Hydrocortone Tablets 1963

PROCYTHOL (Greece)
SELEGILINE HYDROCHLORIDE
Eldepryl Capsules 3209

PRODAFEM (Austria, Switzerland)
MEDROXYPROGESTERONE ACETATE
Depo-Medrol Single-Dose Vial 2617

PRODASONE (Chile, France)
MEDROXYPROGESTERONE ACETATE
Depo-Medrol Single-Dose Vial 2617

PRODAZOL (Mexico)
MEBENDAZOLE
Vermox Chewable Tablets 1853

PRODIUM (South Africa)
LOPERAMIDE HYDROCHLORIDE
Imodium Capsules 1834

PRODOLOR (Germany)
NAPROXEN
EC-Naprosyn Delayed-Release Tablets 2769
Naprosyn Suspension 2769
Naprosyn Tablets 2769

PRODOROL (South Africa)
PROPRANOLOL HYDROCHLORIDE
Inderal LA Long-Acting Capsules 3421

PRODOXIN (Brazil)
CEFTRIAXONE SODIUM
Rocephin Injectable Vials, ADD-Vantage, Galaxy, Bulk 2801

PRODUVIR (Brazil)
ZIDOVUDINE
Retrovir Capsules 1533
Retrovir IV Infusion 1537
Retrovir Syrup 1533
Retrovir Tablets 1533

PROFAMID (Denmark, Finland)
FLUTAMIDE
Eulexin Capsules 3023

PROFENAC (India)
DICLOFENAC SODIUM
Voltaren Tablets 2298
Voltaren-XR Tablets 2301

PROFENZOL (Mexico)
MEBENDAZOLE
Vermox Chewable Tablets 1853

PROFERGAN (Brazil)
PROMETHAZINE HYDROCHLORIDE
Phenergan Suppositories 3438
Phenergan Tablets 3438

PROFEX (Israel)
PROPAFENONE HYDROCHLORIDE
Rythmol SR Capsules 2736

PROFINE (India)
PROGESTERONE
Prometrium Capsules (100 mg, 200 mg) . 3205

PROFIUM (Brazil)
MEBENDAZOLE
Vermox Chewable Tablets 1853

PROFLAG (Mexico)
METRONIDAZOLE
MetroGel-Vaginal Gel 1822
Noritate Cream, 1% 1051

PROFLAX (Argentina)
TIMOLOL MALEATE
Blocadren Tablets 1891
Timoptic Sterile Ophthalmic Solution 2058
Timoptic in Ocudose 2061
Timoptic-XE Sterile Ophthalmic Gel Forming Solution 2062

PROFLOX (Brazil, Thailand)
CIPROFLOXACIN
Cipro Oral Suspension 2991

PROFLOXIN (Australia)
CIPROFLOXACIN HYDROCHLORIDE
Ciloxan Ophthalmic Ointment 554
Ciloxan Ophthalmic Solution . . . . ⊙205
Cipro Tablets 2991

PROFOLEN (Brazil)
PROPOFOL
Diprivan Injectable Emulsion 676

PROFUNGAL (Singapore)
KETOCONAZOLE
Nizoral 2% Shampoo 1838

PROGAN (Australia)
PROMETHAZINE HYDROCHLORIDE
Phenergan Suppositories 3438
Phenergan Tablets 3438

PROGEFFIK (Italy, Spain)
PROGESTERONE
Prometrium Capsules (100 mg, 200 mg) . 3205

PROGENAR (Portugal)
PROGESTERONE
Prometrium Capsules (100 mg, 200 mg) . 3205

PROGENDO (Chile)
PROGESTERONE
Prometrium Capsules (100 mg, 200 mg) . 3205

PROGEST (Argentina, India)
PROGESTERONE
Prometrium Capsules (100 mg, 200 mg) . 3205

PROGESTAN (The Netherlands)
PROGESTERONE
Prometrium Capsules (100 mg, 200 mg) . 3205

PROGESTASERT (Canada, France)
PROGESTERONE
Prometrium Capsules (100 mg, 200 mg) . 3205

PROGESTERONE IMPLANTS (United Kingdom)
PROGESTERONE
Prometrium Capsules (100 mg, 200 mg) . 3205

PROGESTOGEL (Belgium, France, Germany, Hong Kong, Italy, Portugal, Russia, Spain, Switzerland, Thailand)
PROGESTERONE
Prometrium Capsules (100 mg, 200 mg) . 3205

PROGESTOL (Italy)
PROGESTERONE
Prometrium Capsules (100 mg, 200 mg) . 3205

PROGESTOSOL (France, Spain, Switzerland)
PROGESTERONE
Prometrium Capsules (100 mg, 200 mg) . 3205

PROGEVERA (Greece, Spain)
MEDROXYPROGESTERONE ACETATE
Depo-Medrol Single-Dose Vial 2617

PROGEVERA 250 (Spain)
MEDROXYPROGESTERONE ACETATE
Depo-Medrol Single-Dose Vial 2617

PROGLICEM (Argentina, France, Germany, Italy, Switzerland, The Netherlands)
DIAZOXIDE
Hyperstat I.V. Injection 3031

PROGLYCEM (Canada, Greece)
DIAZOXIDE
Hyperstat I.V. Injection 3031

PROGOR (Belgium)
DILTIAZEM HYDROCHLORIDE
Cardizem LA Extended Release Tablets . 1699
Tiazac Capsules 1204

PROGRAF (Argentina, Australia, Austria, Brazil, Canada, Chile, Czech Republic, Denmark, Finland, France, Germany, Greece, Hong Kong, Hungary, Irish Republic, Israel, Italy, Japan, Malaysia, Mexico, New Zealand, Norway, Portugal, Singapore, South Africa, Spain, Sweden, Switzerland, Thailand, United Kingdom)
TACROLIMUS
Prograf Capsules and Injection 624

PROGRAFT (Belgium, The Netherlands)
TACROLIMUS
Prograf Capsules and Injection 624

PROGRESSE (Brazil)
GABAPENTIN
Neurontin Capsules 2498

PROGYNOVA (United Kingdom)
ESTRADIOL
Climara Transdermal System 795
Vivelle Transdermal System 2288
Vivelle-Dot Transdermal System 2293

PROHAIR (Brazil, Chile)
FINASTERIDE
Propecia Tablets 2036
Proscar Tablets 2040

PRO-HDL (India)
LOVASTATIN
Mevacor Tablets 1996

PROHELMIN (Brazil)
MEBENDAZOLE
Vermox Chewable Tablets 1853

PROHIST (South Africa)
PROMETHAZINE HYDROCHLORIDE
Phenergan Suppositories 3438
Phenergan Tablets 3438

PROLEKOFEN (Czech Republic)
PROPAFENONE HYDROCHLORIDE
Rythmol SR Capsules 2736

PROLEUKIN (Argentina, Australia, Austria, Belgium, Brazil, Canada, Czech Republic, Denmark, France, Germany, Greece, Hong Kong, Hungary, Israel, Italy, Mexico, New Zealand, Portugal, Singapore, Spain, Switzerland, The Netherlands, United Kingdom)
ALDESLEUKIN
Proleukin for Injection 1007

PROLIDON (Mexico)
PROGESTERONE
Prometrium Capsules (100 mg, 200 mg) . 3205

PROLIPASE (Argentina, Austria, Switzerland)
PANCRELIPASE
Ultrase Capsules 735
Ultrase MT Capsules 736

PROLISINA E2 (Argentina)
DINOPROSTONE
Cervidil Vaginal Insert 1182

PROLISINA VR (Argentina)
ALPROSTADIL
Edex Injection 3103

PROLOL (Hong Kong, Israel, Thailand)
PROPRANOLOL HYDROCHLORIDE
Inderal LA Long-Acting Capsules 3421

PROLONG (Chile)
LIDOCAINE
Lidoderm Patch 1107

PROLUTON (Argentina, Australia, Italy, Thailand)
PROGESTERONE
Prometrium Capsules (100 mg, 200 mg) . 3205

PROMAHIST (South Africa)
PROMETHAZINE HYDROCHLORIDE
Phenergan Suppositories 3438
Phenergan Tablets 3438

PROMAL (Austria)
ATOVAQUONE
Mepron Suspension 1487

PROMET (Thailand)
CIMETIDINE
Tagamet Tablets 1547

PROMETIDINE (Brazil)
CIMETIDINE
Tagamet Tablets 1547

PROMETRIUM (Canada, Italy)
PROGESTERONE
Prometrium Capsules (100 mg, 200 mg) . 3205

PROMIBASOL (Mexico)
METRONIDAZOLE
MetroGel-Vaginal Gel 1822
Noritate Cream, 1% 1051

PROMKIDDI (Germany)
PROMETHAZINE HYDROCHLORIDE
Phenergan Suppositories 3438
Phenergan Tablets 3438

PROMOCARD (Belgium, The Netherlands)
ISOSORBIDE MONONITRATE
Imdur Tablets 3032

PRONASTERON (Brazil)
FINASTERIDE
Propecia Tablets 2036
Proscar Tablets 2040

PRONAT (Mexico)
NAPROXEN
EC-Naprosyn Delayed-Release Tablets 2769
Naprosyn Suspension 2769
Naprosyn Tablets 2769

PRONAXEN (Finland, Sweden)
NAPROXEN
EC-Naprosyn Delayed-Release Tablets 2769
Naprosyn Suspension 2769
Naprosyn Tablets 2769

PRONAXIL (Mexico)
NAPROXEN
EC-Naprosyn Delayed-Release Tablets 2769

(⊙ Described in PDR For Ophthalmic Medicines™)

Naprosyn Suspension . . . 2769
Naprosyn Tablets . . . 2769

PRONAX-P (Mexico)
NAPROXEN SODIUM
Anaprox DS Tablets . . . 2769
Anaprox Tablets . . . 2769

PRONEST (Brazil)
PROPOFOL
Diprivan Injectable Emulsion . . . 676

PRONEURIN (Germany)
PROMETHAZINE HYDROCHLORIDE
Phenergan Suppositories . . . 3438
Phenergan Tablets . . . 3438

PRONOSIL (Thailand)
PROPRANOLOL HYDROCHLORIDE
Inderal LA Long-Acting Capsules . . . 3421

PRONOVAN (Norway)
PROPRANOLOL HYDROCHLORIDE
Inderal LA Long-Acting Capsules . . . 3421

PRONOXEN (Mexico)
NAPROXEN
EC-Naprosyn Delayed-Release Tablets . . . 2769
Naprosyn Suspension . . . 2769
Naprosyn Tablets . . . 2769

PRONTAMID (Italy)
SULFACETAMIDE SODIUM
Klaron Lotion 10% . . . 1050

PRONTOGEST (Italy)
PROGESTERONE
Prometrium Capsules (100 mg, 200 mg) . 3205

PROPABLOC (Germany)
PROPRANOLOL HYDROCHLORIDE
Inderal LA Long-Acting Capsules . . . 3421

PROPACOR (Brazil)
PROPRANOLOL HYDROCHLORIDE
Inderal LA Long-Acting Capsules . . . 3421

PROPAFEN (Germany)
PROPAFENONE HYDROCHLORIDE
Rythmol SR Capsules . . . 2736

PROPAL (Denmark)
PROPRANOLOL HYDROCHLORIDE
Inderal LA Long-Acting Capsules . . . 3421

PROPALEM (Mexico)
PROPRANOLOL HYDROCHLORIDE
Inderal LA Long-Acting Capsules . . . 3421

PROPALONG (Argentina)
PROPRANOLOL HYDROCHLORIDE
Inderal LA Long-Acting Capsules . . . 3421

PROPAM (New Zealand)
DIAZEPAM
Diastat Rectal Delivery System . . . 3344
Valium Tablets . . . 2822

PRO-PAM (Australia)
DIAZEPAM
Diastat Rectal Delivery System . . . 3344
Valium Tablets . . . 2822

PROPAMERCK (Germany)
PROPAFENONE HYDROCHLORIDE
Rythmol SR Capsules . . . 2736

PROPANIX (United Kingdom)
PROPRANOLOL HYDROCHLORIDE
Inderal LA Long-Acting Capsules . . . 3421

PROPANOL (Malaysia)
PROPRANOLOL HYDROCHLORIDE
Inderal LA Long-Acting Capsules . . . 3421

PROPANORM (Czech Republic, Russia)
PROPAFENONE HYDROCHLORIDE
Rythmol SR Capsules . . . 2736

PROPA-ORAMON (Germany)
PROPAFENONE HYDROCHLORIDE
Rythmol SR Capsules . . . 2736

PROPASTAD (Germany)
PROPAFENONE HYDROCHLORIDE
Rythmol SR Capsules . . . 2736

PROPA-TABLETTEN (Czech Republic)
PROPAFENONE HYDROCHLORIDE
Rythmol SR Capsules . . . 2736

PROPAYERST (Argentina)
PROPRANOLOL HYDROCHLORIDE
Inderal LA Long-Acting Capsules . . . 3421

PROPAYERST PLUS (Argentina)
PROPRANOLOL HYDROCHLORIDE
Inderal LA Long-Acting Capsules . . . 3421

PROPECIA (Argentina, Australia, Austria, Brazil, Canada, Czech Republic, Denmark, Finland, France, Germany, Hong Kong, Israel, Italy, Malaysia, New Zealand, Portugal, Singapore, South Africa, Spain, Sweden, Switzerland, Thailand, The Netherlands, United Kingdom)
FINASTERIDE
Propecia Tablets . . . 2036
Proscar Tablets . . . 2040

PROPERIL (Chile)
CAPTOPRIL
Captopril Tablets . . . 2114

PROPESHIA (Mexico)
FINASTERIDE
Propecia Tablets . . . 2036
Proscar Tablets . . . 2040

PROPESS (Argentina, Austria, Czech Republic, Denmark, Finland, France, Germany, Greece, Hong Kong, Hungary, Irish Republic, Israel, Italy, Mexico, Portugal, South Africa, Spain, Sweden, Switzerland, The Netherlands, United Kingdom)
DINOPROSTONE
Cervidil Vaginal Insert . . . 1182

PROPHYLUX (Germany)
PROPRANOLOL HYDROCHLORIDE
Inderal LA Long-Acting Capsules . . . 3421

PROPIDEN (Denmark)
LOPERAMIDE HYDROCHLORIDE
Imodium Capsules . . . 1834

PROPIOSOL (Brazil)
CLOBETASOL PROPIONATE
Temovate Cream . . . 1549
Temovate E Emollient . . . 1552
Temovate Gel . . . 1550
Temovate Ointment . . . 1549
Temovate Scalp Application . . . 1551

PROPOABBOTT (Brazil)
PROPOFOL
Diprivan Injectable Emulsion . . . 676

PROPOCAM (Mexico)
PROPOFOL
Diprivan Injectable Emulsion . . . 676

PROPOTEN (Brazil)
CEFOXITIN SODIUM
Mefoxin Premixed Intravenous Solution . . . 1990
Mefoxin for Injection . . . 1987

PROPOVAN (Brazil)
PROPOFOL
Diprivan Injectable Emulsion . . . 676

PROPRA (Germany)
PROPRANOLOL HYDROCHLORIDE
Inderal LA Long-Acting Capsules . . . 3421

PROPRAHEXAL (Austria)
PROPRANOLOL HYDROCHLORIDE
Inderal LA Long-Acting Capsules . . . 3421

PROPRAL (Finland)
PROPRANOLOL HYDROCHLORIDE
Inderal LA Long-Acting Capsules . . . 3421

PROPRANET (Denmark)
PROPRANOLOL HYDROCHLORIDE
Inderal LA Long-Acting Capsules . . . 3421

PROPRANUR (Germany)
PROPRANOLOL HYDROCHLORIDE
Inderal LA Long-Acting Capsules . . . 3421

PROQUIN (Australia)
CIPROFLOXACIN HYDROCHLORIDE
Ciloxan Ophthalmic Ointment . . . 554
Ciloxan Ophthalmic Solution . . . ⊙205
Cipro Tablets . . . 2991

PRORYNORM (Germany)
PROPAFENONE HYDROCHLORIDE
Rythmol SR Capsules . . . 2736

PROSAID (United Kingdom)
NAPROXEN
EC-Naprosyn Delayed-Release Tablets . . . 2769
Naprosyn Suspension . . . 2769
Naprosyn Tablets . . . 2769

PROSCAR (Argentina, Australia, Austria, Belgium, Brazil, Canada, Chile, Czech Republic, Denmark, Finland, Germany, Greece, Hong Kong, Hungary, Irish Republic, Italy, Malaysia, Mexico, New Zealand, Norway, Portugal, Russia, Singapore, South Africa, Spain, Sweden, Switzerland, Thailand, The Netherlands, United Kingdom)
FINASTERIDE
Propecia Tablets . . . 2036
Proscar Tablets . . . 2040

PROSERINE (Thailand)
CYCLOSERINE
Seromycin Capsules . . . 1783

PROSMIN (Argentina)
FINASTERIDE
Propecia Tablets . . . 2036
Proscar Tablets . . . 2040

PROSOM (Canada)
ESTAZOLAM
ProSom Tablets . . . 512

PROSTACUR (Spain)
FLUTAMIDE
Eulexin Capsules . . . 3023

PROSTADIREX (France)
FLUTAMIDE
Eulexin Capsules . . . 3023

PROSTALL (Chile)
TAMSULOSIN HYDROCHLORIDE
Flomax Capsules . . . 881

PROSTAMID (India)
FLUTAMIDE
Eulexin Capsules . . . 3023

PROSTANDRIL (Czech Republic)
FLUTAMIDE
Eulexin Capsules . . . 3023

PROSTANIL (Argentina)
FINASTERIDE
Propecia Tablets . . . 2036
Proscar Tablets . . . 2040

PROSTANOVAG (Argentina)
FINASTERIDE
Propecia Tablets . . . 2036
Proscar Tablets . . . 2040

PROSTATIL (Italy)
TERAZOSIN HYDROCHLORIDE
Hytrin Capsules . . . 469

PROSTENE (Argentina)
FINASTERIDE
Propecia Tablets . . . 2036
Proscar Tablets . . . 2040

PROSTEP (Australia, Canada)
NICOTINE
Nicotrol Inhaler . . . 2594
Nicotrol NS . . . 2596

PROSTERID (Hungary)
FINASTERIDE
Propecia Tablets . . . 2036
Proscar Tablets . . . 2040

PROSTICA (Germany)
FLUTAMIDE
Eulexin Capsules . . . 3023

PROSTIDE (Brazil, Italy)
FINASTERIDE
Propecia Tablets . . . 2036
Proscar Tablets . . . 2040

PROSTIN E2 (Australia, Austria, Belgium, Canada, Czech Republic, Greece, Hong Kong, Hungary, Irish Republic, Israel, Italy, Malaysia, New Zealand, Portugal, Singapore, South Africa, Switzerland, Thailand, The Netherlands, United Kingdom)
DINOPROSTONE
Cervidil Vaginal Insert . . . 1182

PROSTIN PEDIATRICO (Chile)
ALPROSTADIL
Edex Injection . . . 3103

PROSTIN VR (Australia, Belgium, Canada, Czech Republic, Greece, Hong Kong, Hungary, India, Israel, Italy, Malaysia, New Zealand, Portugal, South Africa, Switzerland, Thailand, The Netherlands, United Kingdom)
ALPROSTADIL
Edex Injection . . . 3103

PROSTINE E (France)
DINOPROSTONE
Cervidil Vaginal Insert . . . 1182

PROSTINE VR (France)
ALPROSTADIL
Edex Injection . . . 3103

PROSTIVAS (Denmark, Finland, Norway, Sweden)
ALPROSTADIL
Edex Injection . . . 3103

PROSTOGENAT (Germany)
FLUTAMIDE
Eulexin Capsules . . . 3023

PROTANGIX (France)
DIPYRIDAMOLE
Persantine Tablets . . . 898

PROTENATE (Hong Kong)
PLASMA PROTEIN FRACTION
Plasmanate . . . 3252

PROTEVAL (Mexico)
VALPROIC ACID
Depakene Capsules . . . 417
Depakene Syrup . . . 417

PROTEVIS (Argentina)
TIMOLOL MALEATE
Blocadren Tablets . . . 1891
Timoptic Sterile Ophthalmic Solution . . . 2058
Timoptic in Ocudose . . . 2061
Timoptic-XE Sterile Ophthalmic Gel Forming Solution . . . 2062

PROTEXIN (Spain)
AMANTADINE HYDROCHLORIDE
Symmetrel Syrup . . . 1115
Symmetrel Tablets . . . 1115

PROTHAZIN (Germany)
PROMETHAZINE HYDROCHLORIDE
Phenergan Suppositories . . . 3438
Phenergan Tablets . . . 3438

PROTHAZINE (Australia, Malaysia)
PROMETHAZINE HYDROCHLORIDE
Phenergan Suppositories . . . 3438
Phenergan Tablets . . . 3438

PROTHIAZINE (Israel)
PROMETHAZINE HYDROCHLORIDE
Phenergan Suppositories . . . 3438
Phenergan Tablets . . . 3438

PROTININ (Mexico)
APROTININ
Trasylol Injection . . . 779

PROTOGYL (Hong Kong, Malaysia, Singapore)
METRONIDAZOLE
MetroGel-Vaginal Gel . . . 1822
Noritate Cream, 1% . . . 1051

PROTOPIC (Argentina, Austria, Belgium, Canada, Denmark, Finland, France, Germany, Hong Kong, Irish Republic, Israel, Italy, Japan, Norway, Portugal, Spain, Sweden, Switzerland, United Kingdom)
TACROLIMUS
Prograf Capsules and Injection . . . 624

PROTOSOL (Israel)
APROTININ
Trasylol Injection . . . 779

PROTOSTAT (Australia)
METRONIDAZOLE
MetroGel-Vaginal Gel . . . 1822
Noritate Cream, 1% . . . 1051

PROVAMES (France)
ESTRADIOL
Climara Transdermal System . . . 795
Vivelle Transdermal System . . . 2288
Vivelle-Dot Transdermal System . . . 2293

PRO-VENT (Irish Republic, United Kingdom)
THEOPHYLLINE
Uniphyl Tablets . . . 2708

(⊙ Described in PDR For Ophthalmic Medicines™)

PROVERA (Australia, Austria, Belgium, Brazil, Canada, Chile, Czech Republic, Denmark, Finland, Greece, Hong Kong, Hungary, Irish Republic, Israel, Italy, Malaysia, Mexico, New Zealand, Norway, Portugal, Singapore, South Africa, Sweden, Switzerland, Thailand, The Netherlands, United Kingdom)
MEDROXYPROGESTERONE ACETATE
Depo-Medrol Single-Dose Vial **2617**

PROVETAL (Mexico)
VALPROIC ACID
Depakene Capsules **417**
Depakene Syrup **417**

PROVIGIL (Belgium, Irish Republic, Israel, Italy, South Africa, United Kingdom)
MODAFINIL
Provigil Tablets **1002**

PROVISC (Argentina, Australia, Austria, Belgium, France, Germany, Hong Kong, Hungary, Irish Republic, Italy, Malaysia, New Zealand, Norway, Singapore, South Africa, Thailand, United Kingdom)
SODIUM HYALURONATE
Hyalgan Solution **2917**

PROVISUAL (Argentina)
GENTAMICIN SULFATE
Garamycin Injectable **3028**
Genoptic Sterile Ophthalmic Solution . . . . ⊙**227**

PROVIVE (Brazil)
PROPOFOL
Diprivan Injectable Emulsion **676**

PROXACIN (Brazil)
CIPROFLOXACIN HYDROCHLORIDE
Ciloxan Ophthalmic Ointment **554**
Ciloxan Ophthalmic Solution . . . . ⊙**205**
Cipro Tablets **2991**

PROXALIN (Mexico)
NAPROXEN
EC-Naprosyn Delayed-Release Tablets **2769**
Naprosyn Suspension **2769**
Naprosyn Tablets **2769**

PROXALIN-PLUS (Mexico)
NAPROXEN
EC-Naprosyn Delayed-Release Tablets **2769**
Naprosyn Suspension **2769**
Naprosyn Tablets **2769**

PROXATAN (Argentina)
TERAZOSIN HYDROCHLORIDE
Hytrin Capsules **469**

PROXEN (Australia, Austria, Germany, Hong Kong, South Africa, Switzerland, Thailand)
NAPROXEN
EC-Naprosyn Delayed-Release Tablets **2769**
Naprosyn Suspension **2769**
Naprosyn Tablets **2769**

PROXINE (Italy)
NAPROXEN
EC-Naprosyn Delayed-Release Tablets **2769**
Naprosyn Suspension **2769**
Naprosyn Tablets **2769**

PROXINOR (Thailand)
NORFLOXACIN
Noroxin Tablets **2009**

PROXITEC (Mexico)
CIPROFLOXACIN
Cipro Oral Suspension **2991**

PROZINE (South Africa)
CARBAMAZEPINE
Carbatrol Capsules **3174**
Tegretol Chewable Tablets **2278**
Tegretol Suspension **2278**
Tegretol Tablets **2278**
Tegretol-XR Tablets **2278**

PROZITEL (Mexico)
PRAZIQUANTEL
Biltricide Tablets **2990**

PRUDENCIAL (Argentina)
NIFEDIPINE
Adalat CC Tablets **2978**

PSICOASTEN (Argentina)
PAROXETINE HYDROCHLORIDE
Paxil Oral Suspension **1501**
Paxil Tablets **1501**

PSICOFAR (Italy)
CHLORDIAZEPOXIDE HYDROCHLORIDE
Librium Capsules **3349**

PSICONOR (Argentina)
CITALOPRAM HYDROBROMIDE
Celexa Tablets **1177**

PSICOTERINA (Italy)
CHLORDIAZEPOXIDE HYDROCHLORIDE
Librium Capsules **3349**

PSOREX (Brazil)
CLOBETASOL PROPIONATE
Temovate Cream **1549**
Temovate E Emollient **1552**
Temovate Gel **1550**
Temovate Ointment **1549**
Temovate Scalp Application **1551**

PSORIN (Brazil)
CLOBETASOL PROPIONATE
Temovate Cream **1549**
Temovate E Emollient **1552**
Temovate Gel **1550**
Temovate Ointment **1549**
Temovate Scalp Application **1551**

PSYCHOLANZ (India)
OLANZAPINE
Zyprexa Tablets **1798**

PSYCHOPAX (Austria, Switzerland)
DIAZEPAM
Diastat Rectal Delivery System **3344**
Valium Tablets **2822**

PTINOLIN (Greece)
RANITIDINE HYDROCHLORIDE
Zantac 25 EFFERdose Tablets **1597**
Zantac 150 EFFERdose Tablets **1597**
Zantac 150 Tablets **1597**
Zantac 300 Tablets **1597**
Zantac Injection **1593**
Zantac Injection Premixed **1593**
Zantac Syrup **1597**

PUIRITOL (Hong Kong)
OFLOXACIN
Floxin Otic Solution **1043**

PULMENO (Spain)
THEOPHYLLINE
Uniphyl Tablets **2708**

PULMIDUR (Austria, Germany)
THEOPHYLLINE
Uniphyl Tablets **2708**

PULMILIDE (Austria)
FLUNISOLIDE
Aerobid Inhaler System **1172**
Aerobid-M Inhaler System **1172**
Nasarel Nasal Spray **1652**

PULMIST (Italy)
FLUNISOLIDE
Aerobid Inhaler System **1172**
Aerobid-M Inhaler System **1172**
Nasarel Nasal Spray **1652**

PULMOPHYLLIN (South Africa)
THEOPHYLLINE
Uniphyl Tablets **2708**

PULMOPHYLLINE (Canada)
THEOPHYLLINE
Uniphyl Tablets **2708**

PULMO-TIMELETS (Denmark, Germany)
THEOPHYLLINE
Uniphyl Tablets **2708**

PULSOL (Mexico)
ENALAPRIL MALEATE
Vasotec I.V. Injection **2076**

PURAN T4 (Brazil)
LEVOTHYROXINE SODIUM
Levothroid Tablets **1189**
Levoxyl Tablets **1680**
Synthroid Tablets **515**

PUR-BLOKA (South Africa)
PROPRANOLOL HYDROCHLORIDE
Inderal LA Long-Acting Capsules **3421**

PURESIS (South Africa)
FUROSEMIDE
Furosemide Tablets **2117**

PURGOLAC (Greece)
LACTULOSE
Kristalose for Oral Solution **2149**

PURGOXIN (South Africa)
DIGOXIN
Lanoxicaps Capsules **1458**
Lanoxin Injection **1462**
Lanoxin Injection Pediatric **1465**
Lanoxin Tablets **1468**

PURI-NETHOL (Argentina, Australia, Austria, Belgium, Brazil, Canada, Chile, Czech Republic, France, Germany, Hong Kong, India, Irish Republic, Israel, Italy, Mexico, New Zealand, Norway, Singapore, South Africa, Sweden, Switzerland, Thailand, The Netherlands, United Kingdom)
MERCAPTOPURINE
Purinethol Tablets **1222**

PUTAREN (Thailand)
DICLOFENAC SODIUM
Voltaren Tablets **2298**
Voltaren-XR Tablets **2301**

PUVASORALEN (United Kingdom)
METHOXSALEN
Oxsoralen Lotion 1% **3354**
Oxsoralen-Ultra Capsules **3354**

P-VATE (Thailand)
CLOBETASOL PROPIONATE
Temovate Cream **1549**
Temovate E Emollient **1552**
Temovate Gel **1550**
Temovate Ointment **1549**
Temovate Scalp Application **1551**

PYLOKIT (India)
LANSOPRAZOLE
Prevacid Delayed-Release Capsules **3268**

PYRALFIN (India)
PYRIMETHAMINE
Daraprim Tablets **1385**

PYRAMET (India)
PYRIMETHAMINE
Daraprim Tablets **1385**

PYRIDAMEL (Irish Republic)
DIPYRIDAMOLE
Persantine Tablets **898**

PYRIFOAM (Australia, New Zealand)
PERMETHRIN
Acticin Cream **2125**

PYRIMON (India)
DEXAMETHASONE
Decadron Tablets **1929**

PYTAZEN (New Zealand)
DIPYRIDAMOLE
Persantine Tablets **898**

QINOLON (Thailand)
OFLOXACIN
Floxin Otic Solution **1043**

Q-MAZINE (United Kingdom)
PROMETHAZINE HYDROCHLORIDE
Phenergan Suppositories **3438**
Phenergan Tablets **3438**

QUADION (Argentina)
KETOCONAZOLE
Nizoral 2% Shampoo **1838**

QUAGU-TEST (Argentina)
APROTININ
Trasylol Injection **779**

QUALECON (Argentina)
FENOFIBRATE
Tricor Tablets **523**

QUAMATEL (Czech Republic, Hong Kong, Hungary, Russia)
FAMOTIDINE
Pepcid Injection **2017**
Pepcid Injection Premixed **2017**
Pepcid Tablets **2014**
Pepcid for Oral Suspension **2014**

QUANTOR (Spain)
RANITIDINE HYDROCHLORIDE
Zantac 25 EFFERdose Tablets **1597**
Zantac 150 EFFERdose Tablets **1597**
Zantac 150 Tablets **1597**
Zantac 300 Tablets **1597**
Zantac Injection **1593**
Zantac Injection Premixed **1593**
Zantac Syrup **1597**

QUARDIN (Portugal)
RANITIDINE HYDROCHLORIDE
Zantac 25 EFFERdose Tablets **1597**
Zantac 150 EFFERdose Tablets **1597**
Zantac 150 Tablets **1597**
Zantac 300 Tablets **1597**
Zantac Injection **1593**
Zantac Injection Premixed **1593**
Zantac Syrup **1597**

QUARK (Italy)
RAMIPRIL
Altace Capsules **1673**

QUASAR (Italy)
VERAPAMIL HYDROCHLORIDE
Covera-HS Tablets **3135**
Verelan PM Capsules **3120**

QUEL (India)
QUETIAPINE FUMARATE
Seroquel Tablets **691**

QUELLADA (Australia, Hong Kong)
PERMETHRIN
Acticin Cream **2125**

QUELLADA P (New Zealand)
PERMETHRIN
Acticin Cream **2125**

QUEMOX (Malaysia)
MEBENDAZOLE
Vermox Chewable Tablets **1853**

QUERTO (Germany)
CARVEDILOL
Coreg Tablets **1376**

QUIBRON (Thailand)
THEOPHYLLINE
Uniphyl Tablets **2708**

QUIBRON-T (Canada)
THEOPHYLLINE
Uniphyl Tablets **2708**

QUIDEX (Argentina)
CIPROFLOXACIN
Cipro Oral Suspension **2991**

QUIFLOX (Brazil)
CIPROFLOXACIN HYDROCHLORIDE
Ciloxan Ophthalmic Ointment **554**
Ciloxan Ophthalmic Solution . . . . ⊙**205**
Cipro Tablets **2991**

QUIFLOXONA (Mexico)
CIPROFLOXACIN
Cipro Oral Suspension **2991**

QUILONUM (Australia, South Africa)
LITHIUM CARBONATE
Eskalith CR Controlled-Release Tablets . . . **1406**
Eskalith Capsules **1406**

QUIMALAN (Mexico)
ENALAPRIL MALEATE
Vasotec I.V. Injection **2076**

QUIMOBROM (Mexico)
ERYTHROMYCIN
Ery-Tab Tablets **447**
Erythromycin Base Filmtab Tablets **454**
Erythromycin Delayed-Release Capsules, USP **456**
PCE Dispertab Tablets **510**

QUIMOLAURIL (Mexico)
ERYTHROMYCIN
Ery-Tab Tablets **447**
Erythromycin Base Filmtab Tablets **454**
Erythromycin Delayed-Release Capsules, USP **456**
PCE Dispertab Tablets **510**

QUINOBACT (India)
CIPROFLOXACIN
Cipro Oral Suspension **2991**

QUINOBIOT (Chile)
LEVOFLOXACIN
Levaquin Injection **2453**
Levaquin Tablets **2453**

QUINOFLEX (Portugal)
NORFLOXACIN
Noroxin Tablets **2009**

QUINOFORM (Brazil)
NORFLOXACIN
Noroxin Tablets **2009**

QUINOMED (Argentina)
OFLOXACIN
Floxin Otic Solution **1043**

QUINOX (Portugal)
CIPROFLOXACIN
Cipro Oral Suspension **2991**

(⊙ Described in PDR For Ophthalmic Medicines™)

QUINOXAN (Brazil)
OFLOXACIN
- Floxin Otic Solution 1043

QUINTAMICINA (Spain)
GENTAMICIN SULFATE
- Garamycin Injectable 3028
- Genoptic Sterile Ophthalmic Solution ⊙227

QUINTELMIN (Brazil)
MEBENDAZOLE
- Vermox Chewable Tablets 1853

QUINTOR (Czech Republic)
CIPROFLOXACIN HYDROCHLORIDE
- Ciloxan Ophthalmic Ointment 554
- Ciloxan Ophthalmic Solution ⊙205
- Cipro Tablets 2991

QUIPRO (Czech Republic, Spain)
CIPROFLOXACIN HYDROCHLORIDE
- Ciloxan Ophthalmic Ointment 554
- Ciloxan Ophthalmic Solution ⊙205
- Cipro Tablets 2991

QUISEGEN (Argentina)
CIPROFLOXACIN HYDROCHLORIDE
- Ciloxan Ophthalmic Ointment 554
- Ciloxan Ophthalmic Solution ⊙205
- Cipro Tablets 2991

QUIT (South Africa)
NICOTINE
- Nicotrol Inhaler 2594
- Nicotrol NS 2596

QUITOSO NF (Argentina)
PERMETHRIN
- Acticin Cream 2125

QUITX (Australia)
NICOTINE
- Nicotrol Inhaler 2594
- Nicotrol NS 2596

QUOMEM (Austria, Italy, Spain, Thailand)
BUPROPION HYDROCHLORIDE
- Wellbutrin SR Sustained-Release Tablets 1583
- Wellbutrin Tablets 1579
- Zyban Sustained-Release Tablets 1620

RABLAS (Greece)
ENALAPRIL MALEATE
- Vasotec I.V. Injection 2076

RADAN (Brazil)
RANITIDINE HYDROCHLORIDE
- Zantac 25 EFFERdose Tablets 1597
- Zantac 150 EFFERdose Tablets 1597
- Zantac 150 Tablets 1597
- Zantac 300 Tablets 1597
- Zantac Injection 1593
- Zantac Injection Premixed 1593
- Zantac Syrup 1597

RADICACINE (Argentina)
CELECOXIB
- Celebrex Capsules 3130

RADIGEN (Chile)
RISPERIDONE
- Risperdal Oral Solution 1658
- Risperdal Tablets 1658

RADIKAL (Germany)
CLOTRIMAZOLE
- Lotrimin Cream 3053
- Lotrimin Lotion 1% 3053
- Lotrimin Topical Solution 1% 3053

RADILEM (Mexico)
METHYLPREDNISOLONE ACETATE
- Depo-Medrol Injectable Suspension 2615

RADIN (Hong Kong)
RANITIDINE HYDROCHLORIDE
- Zantac 25 EFFERdose Tablets 1597
- Zantac 150 EFFERdose Tablets 1597
- Zantac 150 Tablets 1597
- Zantac 300 Tablets 1597
- Zantac Injection 1593
- Zantac Injection Premixed 1593
- Zantac Syrup 1597

RADINA (Argentina)
TOBRAMYCIN
- TOBI Solution for Inhalation 1015

RADINA DEX (Argentina)
TOBRAMYCIN
- TOBI Solution for Inhalation 1015

RADINE (Thailand)
RANITIDINE HYDROCHLORIDE
- Zantac 25 EFFERdose Tablets 1597
- Zantac 150 EFFERdose Tablets 1597
- Zantac 150 Tablets 1597
- Zantac 300 Tablets 1597
- Zantac Injection 1593
- Zantac Injection Premixed 1593
- Zantac Syrup 1597

RADUCTIL (Argentina, Mexico)
SIBUTRAMINE HYDROCHLORIDE
- Meridia Capsules 485

RAFFOLUTIL (Argentina)
BICALUTAMIDE
- Casodex Tablets 670

RAFFONIN (Chile)
FLUTICASONE PROPIONATE
- Cutivate Cream 1381
- Cutivate Ointment 1384
- Flonase Nasal Spray 1412

RAFOCILINA (Argentina)
OFLOXACIN
- Floxin Otic Solution 1043

RALISTA (India)
RALOXIFENE HYDROCHLORIDE
- Evista Tablets 1735

RALOVERA (Australia)
MEDROXYPROGESTERONE ACETATE
- Depo-Medrol Single-Dose Vial 2617

RAMACE (Australia, Belgium, Denmark, Finland, Mexico, South Africa)
RAMIPRIL
- Altace Capsules 1673

RAMCOR (India)
RAMIPRIL
- Altace Capsules 1673

RAMCOR H (India)
RAMIPRIL
- Altace Capsules 1673

RAMIPRES (Chile, India)
RAMIPRIL
- Altace Capsules 1673

RAMIPRES H (India)
RAMIPRIL
- Altace Capsules 1673

RAN (Italy, Portugal)
RANITIDINE HYDROCHLORIDE
- Zantac 25 EFFERdose Tablets 1597
- Zantac 150 EFFERdose Tablets 1597
- Zantac 150 Tablets 1597
- Zantac 300 Tablets 1597
- Zantac Injection 1593
- Zantac Injection Premixed 1593
- Zantac Syrup 1597

RAN H2 (Spain)
RANITIDINE HYDROCHLORIDE
- Zantac 25 EFFERdose Tablets 1597
- Zantac 150 EFFERdose Tablets 1597
- Zantac 150 Tablets 1597
- Zantac 300 Tablets 1597
- Zantac Injection 1593
- Zantac Injection Premixed 1593
- Zantac Syrup 1597

RAN LICH (Germany)
RANITIDINE HYDROCHLORIDE
- Zantac 25 EFFERdose Tablets 1597
- Zantac 150 EFFERdose Tablets 1597
- Zantac 150 Tablets 1597
- Zantac 300 Tablets 1597
- Zantac Injection 1593
- Zantac Injection Premixed 1593
- Zantac Syrup 1597

RANACID (Norway)
RANITIDINE HYDROCHLORIDE
- Zantac 25 EFFERdose Tablets 1597
- Zantac 150 EFFERdose Tablets 1597
- Zantac 150 Tablets 1597
- Zantac 300 Tablets 1597
- Zantac Injection 1593
- Zantac Injection Premixed 1593
- Zantac Syrup 1597

RANAPS (United Kingdom)
RANITIDINE HYDROCHLORIDE
- Zantac 25 EFFERdose Tablets 1597
- Zantac 150 EFFERdose Tablets 1597
- Zantac 150 Tablets 1597
- Zantac 300 Tablets 1597
- Zantac Injection 1593
- Zantac Injection Premixed 1593
- Zantac Syrup 1597

RANGIN (Hungary)
ISOSORBIDE MONONITRATE
- Imdur Tablets 3032

RANI (Germany, Singapore)
RANITIDINE HYDROCHLORIDE
- Zantac 25 EFFERdose Tablets 1597
- Zantac 150 EFFERdose Tablets 1597
- Zantac 150 Tablets 1597
- Zantac 300 Tablets 1597
- Zantac Injection 1593
- Zantac Injection Premixed 1593
- Zantac Syrup 1597

RANI 2 (Australia)
RANITIDINE HYDROCHLORIDE
- Zantac 25 EFFERdose Tablets 1597
- Zantac 150 EFFERdose Tablets 1597
- Zantac 150 Tablets 1597
- Zantac 300 Tablets 1597
- Zantac Injection 1593
- Zantac Injection Premixed 1593
- Zantac Syrup 1597

RANIBEN (Italy)
RANITIDINE HYDROCHLORIDE
- Zantac 25 EFFERdose Tablets 1597
- Zantac 150 EFFERdose Tablets 1597
- Zantac 150 Tablets 1597
- Zantac 300 Tablets 1597
- Zantac Injection 1593
- Zantac Injection Premixed 1593
- Zantac Syrup 1597

RANIBERL (Czech Republic, Germany)
RANITIDINE HYDROCHLORIDE
- Zantac 25 EFFERdose Tablets 1597
- Zantac 150 EFFERdose Tablets 1597
- Zantac 150 Tablets 1597
- Zantac 300 Tablets 1597
- Zantac Injection 1593
- Zantac Injection Premixed 1593
- Zantac Syrup 1597

RANIBETA (Germany)
RANITIDINE HYDROCHLORIDE
- Zantac 25 EFFERdose Tablets 1597
- Zantac 150 EFFERdose Tablets 1597
- Zantac 150 Tablets 1597
- Zantac 300 Tablets 1597
- Zantac Injection 1593
- Zantac Injection Premixed 1593
- Zantac Syrup 1597

RANIBLOC (Germany, Italy)
RANITIDINE HYDROCHLORIDE
- Zantac 25 EFFERdose Tablets 1597
- Zantac 150 EFFERdose Tablets 1597
- Zantac 150 Tablets 1597
- Zantac 300 Tablets 1597
- Zantac Injection 1593
- Zantac Injection Premixed 1593
- Zantac Syrup 1597

RANIC (Austria, Belgium)
RANITIDINE HYDROCHLORIDE
- Zantac 25 EFFERdose Tablets 1597
- Zantac 150 EFFERdose Tablets 1597
- Zantac 150 Tablets 1597
- Zantac 300 Tablets 1597
- Zantac Injection 1593
- Zantac Injection Premixed 1593
- Zantac Syrup 1597

RANICEL (Chile)
RANITIDINE HYDROCHLORIDE
- Zantac 25 EFFERdose Tablets 1597
- Zantac 150 EFFERdose Tablets 1597
- Zantac 150 Tablets 1597
- Zantac 300 Tablets 1597
- Zantac Injection 1593
- Zantac Injection Premixed 1593
- Zantac Syrup 1597

RANICID (Thailand)
RANITIDINE HYDROCHLORIDE
- Zantac 25 EFFERdose Tablets 1597
- Zantac 150 EFFERdose Tablets 1597
- Zantac 150 Tablets 1597
- Zantac 300 Tablets 1597
- Zantac Injection 1593
- Zantac Injection Premixed 1593
- Zantac Syrup 1597

RANICLON (Greece)
RANITIDINE HYDROCHLORIDE
- Zantac 25 EFFERdose Tablets 1597
- Zantac 150 EFFERdose Tablets 1597
- Zantac 150 Tablets 1597
- Zantac 300 Tablets 1597
- Zantac Injection 1593
- Zantac Injection Premixed 1593
- Zantac Syrup 1597

RANICODAN (Denmark)
RANITIDINE HYDROCHLORIDE
- Zantac 25 EFFERdose Tablets 1597
- Zantac 150 EFFERdose Tablets 1597
- Zantac 150 Tablets 1597
- Zantac 300 Tablets 1597
- Zantac Injection 1593
- Zantac Injection Premixed 1593
- Zantac Syrup 1597

RANICUR (Finland)
RANITIDINE HYDROCHLORIDE
- Zantac 25 EFFERdose Tablets 1597
- Zantac 150 EFFERdose Tablets 1597
- Zantac 150 Tablets 1597
- Zantac 300 Tablets 1597
- Zantac Injection 1593
- Zantac Injection Premixed 1593
- Zantac Syrup 1597

RANICUX (Germany)
RANITIDINE HYDROCHLORIDE
- Zantac 25 EFFERdose Tablets 1597
- Zantac 150 EFFERdose Tablets 1597
- Zantac 150 Tablets 1597
- Zantac 300 Tablets 1597
- Zantac Injection 1593
- Zantac Injection Premixed 1593
- Zantac Syrup 1597

RANIDIL (Italy)
RANITIDINE HYDROCHLORIDE
- Zantac 25 EFFERdose Tablets 1597
- Zantac 150 EFFERdose Tablets 1597
- Zantac 150 Tablets 1597
- Zantac 300 Tablets 1597
- Zantac Injection 1593
- Zantac Injection Premixed 1593
- Zantac Syrup 1597

RANIDIN (Brazil, Spain)
RANITIDINE HYDROCHLORIDE
- Zantac 25 EFFERdose Tablets 1597
- Zantac 150 EFFERdose Tablets 1597
- Zantac 150 Tablets 1597
- Zantac 300 Tablets 1597
- Zantac Injection 1593
- Zantac Injection Premixed 1593
- Zantac Syrup 1597

RANIDINA (Brazil)
RANITIDINE HYDROCHLORIDE
- Zantac 25 EFFERdose Tablets 1597
- Zantac 150 EFFERdose Tablets 1597
- Zantac 150 Tablets 1597
- Zantac 300 Tablets 1597
- Zantac Injection 1593
- Zantac Injection Premixed 1593
- Zantac Syrup 1597

RANIDURA T (Germany)
RANITIDINE HYDROCHLORIDE
- Zantac 25 EFFERdose Tablets 1597
- Zantac 150 EFFERdose Tablets 1597
- Zantac 150 Tablets 1597
- Zantac 300 Tablets 1597
- Zantac Injection 1593
- Zantac Injection Premixed 1593
- Zantac Syrup 1597

RANIFLEX (Brazil)
RANITIDINE HYDROCHLORIDE
- Zantac 25 EFFERdose Tablets 1597
- Zantac 150 EFFERdose Tablets 1597
- Zantac 150 Tablets 1597
- Zantac 300 Tablets 1597
- Zantac Injection 1593
- Zantac Injection Premixed 1593
- Zantac Syrup 1597

RANIHEXAL (Australia, South Africa)
RANITIDINE HYDROCHLORIDE
- Zantac 25 EFFERdose Tablets 1597
- Zantac 150 EFFERdose Tablets 1597
- Zantac 150 Tablets 1597
- Zantac 300 Tablets 1597
- Zantac Injection 1593
- Zantac Injection Premixed 1593
- Zantac Syrup 1597

RANIL (Finland)
RANITIDINE HYDROCHLORIDE
- Zantac 25 EFFERdose Tablets 1597
- Zantac 150 EFFERdose Tablets 1597
- Zantac 150 Tablets 1597
- Zantac 300 Tablets 1597
- Zantac Injection 1593
- Zantac Injection Premixed 1593
- Zantac Syrup 1597

RANILONGA (Spain)
RANITIDINE HYDROCHLORIDE
- Zantac 25 EFFERdose Tablets 1597
- Zantac 150 EFFERdose Tablets 1597

Zantac 150 Tablets 1597
Zantac 300 Tablets 1597
Zantac Injection 1593
Zantac Injection Premixed 1593
Zantac Syrup 1597

RANIMED (Argentina, Switzerland)
RANITIDINE HYDROCHLORIDE
Zantac 25 EFFERdose Tablets 1597
Zantac 150 EFFERdose Tablets 1597
Zantac 150 Tablets 1597
Zantac 300 Tablets 1597
Zantac Injection 1593
Zantac Injection Premixed 1593
Zantac Syrup 1597

RANIMERCK (Germany)
RANITIDINE HYDROCHLORIDE
Zantac 25 EFFERdose Tablets 1597
Zantac 150 EFFERdose Tablets 1597
Zantac 150 Tablets 1597
Zantac 300 Tablets 1597
Zantac Injection 1593
Zantac Injection Premixed 1593
Zantac Syrup 1597

RANIMEX (Finland)
RANITIDINE HYDROCHLORIDE
Zantac 25 EFFERdose Tablets 1597
Zantac 150 EFFERdose Tablets 1597
Zantac 150 Tablets 1597
Zantac 300 Tablets 1597
Zantac Injection 1593
Zantac Injection Premixed 1593
Zantac Syrup 1597

RANI-NERTON (Germany)
RANITIDINE HYDROCHLORIDE
Zantac 25 EFFERdose Tablets 1597
Zantac 150 EFFERdose Tablets 1597
Zantac 150 Tablets 1597
Zantac 300 Tablets 1597
Zantac Injection 1593
Zantac Injection Premixed 1593
Zantac Syrup 1597

RANINORM (Austria)
RANITIDINE HYDROCHLORIDE
Zantac 25 EFFERdose Tablets 1597
Zantac 150 EFFERdose Tablets 1597
Zantac 150 Tablets 1597
Zantac 300 Tablets 1597
Zantac Injection 1593
Zantac Injection Premixed 1593
Zantac Syrup 1597

RANIPLEX (France)
RANITIDINE HYDROCHLORIDE
Zantac 25 EFFERdose Tablets 1597
Zantac 150 EFFERdose Tablets 1597
Zantac 150 Tablets 1597
Zantac 300 Tablets 1597
Zantac Injection 1593
Zantac Injection Premixed 1593
Zantac Syrup 1597

RANIPROTECT (Germany)
RANITIDINE HYDROCHLORIDE
Zantac 25 EFFERdose Tablets 1597
Zantac 150 EFFERdose Tablets 1597
Zantac 150 Tablets 1597
Zantac 300 Tablets 1597
Zantac Injection 1593
Zantac Injection Premixed 1593
Zantac Syrup 1597

RANI-Q (Sweden)
RANITIDINE HYDROCHLORIDE
Zantac 25 EFFERdose Tablets 1597
Zantac 150 EFFERdose Tablets 1597
Zantac 150 Tablets 1597
Zantac 300 Tablets 1597
Zantac Injection 1593
Zantac Injection Premixed 1593
Zantac Syrup 1597

RANISAN (Czech Republic)
RANITIDINE HYDROCHLORIDE
Zantac 25 EFFERdose Tablets 1597
Zantac 150 EFFERdose Tablets 1597
Zantac 150 Tablets 1597
Zantac 300 Tablets 1597
Zantac Injection 1593
Zantac Injection Premixed 1593
Zantac Syrup 1597

RANISEN (Mexico)
RANITIDINE HYDROCHLORIDE
Zantac 25 EFFERdose Tablets 1597
Zantac 150 EFFERdose Tablets 1597
Zantac 150 Tablets 1597
Zantac 300 Tablets 1597
Zantac Injection 1593
Zantac Injection Premixed 1593
Zantac Syrup 1597

RANISIFAR (Switzerland)
RANITIDINE HYDROCHLORIDE
Zantac 25 EFFERdose Tablets 1597
Zantac 150 EFFERdose Tablets 1597
Zantac 150 Tablets 1597
Zantac 300 Tablets 1597
Zantac Injection 1593
Zantac Injection Premixed 1593
Zantac Syrup 1597

RANITAB (Germany)
RANITIDINE HYDROCHLORIDE
Zantac 25 EFFERdose Tablets 1597
Zantac 150 EFFERdose Tablets 1597
Zantac 150 Tablets 1597
Zantac 300 Tablets 1597
Zantac Injection 1593
Zantac Injection Premixed 1593
Zantac Syrup 1597

RANITAK (Brazil)
RANITIDINE HYDROCHLORIDE
Zantac 25 EFFERdose Tablets 1597
Zantac 150 EFFERdose Tablets 1597
Zantac 150 Tablets 1597
Zantac 300 Tablets 1597
Zantac Injection 1593
Zantac Injection Premixed 1593
Zantac Syrup 1597

RANITAL (Czech Republic)
RANITIDINE HYDROCHLORIDE
Zantac 25 EFFERdose Tablets 1597
Zantac 150 EFFERdose Tablets 1597
Zantac 150 Tablets 1597
Zantac 300 Tablets 1597
Zantac Injection 1593
Zantac Injection Premixed 1593
Zantac Syrup 1597

RANITIC (Argentina, Australia, Germany, Hungary, Irish Republic, United Kingdom)
RANITIDINE HYDROCHLORIDE
Zantac 25 EFFERdose Tablets 1597
Zantac 150 EFFERdose Tablets 1597
Zantac 150 Tablets 1597
Zantac 300 Tablets 1597
Zantac Injection 1593
Zantac Injection Premixed 1593
Zantac Syrup 1597

RANITIDOC (Germany)
RANITIDINE HYDROCHLORIDE
Zantac 25 EFFERdose Tablets 1597
Zantac 150 EFFERdose Tablets 1597
Zantac 150 Tablets 1597
Zantac 300 Tablets 1597
Zantac Injection 1593
Zantac Injection Premixed 1593
Zantac Syrup 1597

RANITIL (Brazil, United Kingdom)
RANITIDINE HYDROCHLORIDE
Zantac 25 EFFERdose Tablets 1597
Zantac 150 EFFERdose Tablets 1597
Zantac 150 Tablets 1597
Zantac 300 Tablets 1597
Zantac Injection 1593
Zantac Injection Premixed 1593
Zantac Syrup 1597

RANITIN (Czech Republic)
RANITIDINE HYDROCHLORIDE
Zantac 25 EFFERdose Tablets 1597
Zantac 150 EFFERdose Tablets 1597
Zantac 150 Tablets 1597
Zantac 300 Tablets 1597
Zantac Injection 1593
Zantac Injection Premixed 1593
Zantac Syrup 1597

RANITINE (Portugal)
RANITIDINE HYDROCHLORIDE
Zantac 25 EFFERdose Tablets 1597
Zantac 150 EFFERdose Tablets 1597
Zantac 150 Tablets 1597
Zantac 300 Tablets 1597
Zantac Injection 1593
Zantac Injection Premixed 1593
Zantac Syrup 1597

RANITINOL (Brazil)
RANITIDINE HYDROCHLORIDE
Zantac 25 EFFERdose Tablets 1597
Zantac 150 EFFERdose Tablets 1597
Zantac 150 Tablets 1597
Zantac 300 Tablets 1597
Zantac Injection 1593
Zantac Injection Premixed 1593
Zantac Syrup 1597

RANITION (Brazil)
RANITIDINE HYDROCHLORIDE
Zantac 25 EFFERdose Tablets 1597
Zantac 150 EFFERdose Tablets 1597
Zantac 150 Tablets 1597
Zantac 300 Tablets 1597
Zantac Injection 1593
Zantac Injection Premixed 1593
Zantac Syrup 1597

RANITRAL (Argentina)
RANITIDINE HYDROCHLORIDE
Zantac 25 EFFERdose Tablets 1597
Zantac 150 EFFERdose Tablets 1597
Zantac 150 Tablets 1597
Zantac 300 Tablets 1597
Zantac Injection 1593
Zantac Injection Premixed 1593
Zantac Syrup 1597

RANITRAT (Brazil)
RANITIDINE HYDROCHLORIDE
Zantac 25 EFFERdose Tablets 1597
Zantac 150 EFFERdose Tablets 1597
Zantac 150 Tablets 1597
Zantac 300 Tablets 1597
Zantac Injection 1593
Zantac Injection Premixed 1593
Zantac Syrup 1597

RANITYROL (Austria)
RANITIDINE HYDROCHLORIDE
Zantac 25 EFFERdose Tablets 1597
Zantac 150 EFFERdose Tablets 1597
Zantac 150 Tablets 1597
Zantac 300 Tablets 1597
Zantac Injection 1593
Zantac Injection Premixed 1593
Zantac Syrup 1597

RANIVEL (Spain)
RANITIDINE HYDROCHLORIDE
Zantac 25 EFFERdose Tablets 1597
Zantac 150 EFFERdose Tablets 1597
Zantac 150 Tablets 1597
Zantac 300 Tablets 1597
Zantac Injection 1593
Zantac Injection Premixed 1593
Zantac Syrup 1597

RANIX (Spain)
RANITIDINE HYDROCHLORIDE
Zantac 25 EFFERdose Tablets 1597
Zantac 150 EFFERdose Tablets 1597
Zantac 150 Tablets 1597
Zantac 25
Zantac 300 Tablets 1597
Zantac Injection 1593
Zantac Injection Premixed 1593
Zantac Syrup 1597

RANIXAL (Finland)
RANITIDINE HYDROCHLORIDE
Zantac 25 EFFERdose Tablets 1597
Zantac 150 EFFERdose Tablets 1597
Zantac 150 Tablets 1597
Zantac 300 Tablets 1597
Zantac Injection 1593
Zantac Injection Premixed 1593
Zantac Syrup 1597

RANIZAC (Greece)
RANITIDINE HYDROCHLORIDE
Zantac 25 EFFERdose Tablets 1597
Zantac 150 EFFERdose Tablets 1597
Zantac 150 Tablets 1597
Zantac 300 Tablets 1597
Zantac Injection 1593
Zantac Injection Premixed 1593
Zantac Syrup 1597

RANLOL (Malaysia)
ATENOLOL
Tenormin I.V. Injection 698

RANOLTA (Hong Kong)
RANITIDINE HYDROCHLORIDE
Zantac 25 EFFERdose Tablets 1597
Zantac 150 EFFERdose Tablets 1597
Zantac 150 Tablets 1597
Zantac 300 Tablets 1597
Zantac Injection 1593
Zantac Injection Premixed 1593
Zantac Syrup 1597

RANOPINE (Irish Republic)
RANITIDINE HYDROCHLORIDE
Zantac 25 EFFERdose Tablets 1597
Zantac 150 EFFERdose Tablets 1597
Zantac 150 Tablets 1597
Zantac 300 Tablets 1597
Zantac Injection 1593
Zantac Injection Premixed 1593
Zantac Syrup 1597

RANOPRIL (Malaysia)
LISINOPRIL
Prinivil Tablets 2029
Zestril Tablets 704

RANOPRIN (Finland)
PROPRANOLOL HYDROCHLORIDE
Inderal LA Long-Acting Capsules 3421

RANOXYL (Australia)
RANITIDINE HYDROCHLORIDE
Zantac 25 EFFERdose Tablets 1597
Zantac 150 EFFERdose Tablets 1597
Zantac 150 Tablets 1597
Zantac 300 Tablets 1597
Zantac Injection 1593
Zantac Injection Premixed 1593
Zantac Syrup 1597

RANTAC (India)
RANITIDINE HYDROCHLORIDE
Zantac 25 EFFERdose Tablets 1597
Zantac 150 EFFERdose Tablets 1597
Zantac 150 Tablets 1597
Zantac 300 Tablets 1597
Zantac Injection 1593
Zantac Injection Premixed 1593
Zantac Syrup 1597

RANTAG (United Arab Emirates)
RANITIDINE HYDROCHLORIDE
Zantac 25 EFFERdose Tablets 1597
Zantac 150 EFFERdose Tablets 1597
Zantac 150 Tablets 1597
Zantac 300 Tablets 1597
Zantac Injection 1593
Zantac Injection Premixed 1593
Zantac Syrup 1597

RANTEC (United Kingdom)
RANITIDINE HYDROCHLORIDE
Zantac 25 EFFERdose Tablets 1597
Zantac 150 EFFERdose Tablets 1597
Zantac 150 Tablets 1597
Zantac 300 Tablets 1597
Zantac Injection 1593
Zantac Injection Premixed 1593
Zantac Syrup 1597

RANTEEN (South Africa)
RANITIDINE HYDROCHLORIDE
Zantac 25 EFFERdose Tablets 1597
Zantac 150 EFFERdose Tablets 1597
Zantac 150 Tablets 1597
Zantac 300 Tablets 1597
Zantac Injection 1593
Zantac Injection Premixed 1593
Zantac Syrup 1597

RANUBER (Spain)
RANITIDINE HYDROCHLORIDE
Zantac 25 EFFERdose Tablets 1597
Zantac 150 EFFERdose Tablets 1597
Zantac 150 Tablets 1597
Zantac 300 Tablets 1597
Zantac Injection 1593
Zantac Injection Premixed 1593
Zantac Syrup 1597

RANZAC (United Kingdom)
RANITIDINE HYDROCHLORIDE
Zantac 25 EFFERdose Tablets 1597
Zantac 150 EFFERdose Tablets 1597
Zantac 150 Tablets 1597
Zantac 300 Tablets 1597
Zantac Injection 1593
Zantac Injection Premixed 1593
Zantac Syrup 1597

RANZOL (South Africa)
CEFAZOLIN SODIUM
Ancef for Injection 1318

RAPAMIC (Portugal)
KETOCONAZOLE
Nizoral 2% Shampoo 1838

RAPICLAV (India)
AMOXICILLIN
Amoxil Pediatric Drops for Oral Suspension 1315
Amoxil Tablets 1315

RAPILIN (India)
REPAGLINIDE
Prandin Tablets (0.5, 1, and 2 mg) 2337

RAPTEN RAPID (Russia)
DICLOFENAC POTASSIUM
Cataflam Tablets 2173

RASITOL (Malaysia)
FUROSEMIDE
Furosemide Tablets 2117

RATACAND (Italy)
CANDESARTAN CILEXETIL
Atacand Tablets **634**

RATACAND PLUS (Italy)
CANDESARTAN CILEXETIL
Atacand Tablets **634**

RATHIMED (Germany)
METRONIDAZOLE
MetroGel-Vaginal Gel **1822**
Noritate Cream, 1% **1051**

RATHIMED N (Germany)
METRONIDAZOLE
MetroGel-Vaginal Gel **1822**
Noritate Cream, 1% **1051**

RATIC (Singapore)
RANITIDINE HYDROCHLORIDE
Zantac 25 EFFERdose Tablets **1597**
Zantac 150 EFFERdose Tablets........ **1597**
Zantac 150 Tablets **1597**
Zantac 300 Tablets **1597**
Zantac Injection **1593**
Zantac Injection Premixed **1593**
Zantac Syrup **1597**

RATICINA (Argentina)
RANITIDINE HYDROCHLORIDE
Zantac 25 EFFERdose Tablets **1597**
Zantac 150 EFFERdose Tablets........ **1597**
Zantac 150 Tablets **1597**
Zantac 300 Tablets **1597**
Zantac Injection **1593**
Zantac Injection Premixed **1593**
Zantac Syrup **1597**

RATIOALLERG (Austria, Germany)
HYDROCORTISONE
Hydrocortone Tablets **1963**

RATIO-IPRA SAL UDV (Canada)
IPRATROPIUM BROMIDE
Atrovent Inhalation Solution **868**
Atrovent Nasal Spray 0.03%........... **869**
Atrovent Nasal Spray 0.06%........... **870**

RATIO-MPA (Canada)
MEDROXYPROGESTERONE ACETATE
Depo-Medrol Single-Dose Vial **2617**

RAVALTON (Greece)
CIPROFLOXACIN HYDROCHLORIDE
Ciloxan Ophthalmic Ointment **554**
Ciloxan Ophthalmic Solution .... ⊙**205**
Cipro Tablets **2991**

RAVAMIL (South Africa)
VERAPAMIL HYDROCHLORIDE
Covera-HS Tablets **3135**
Verelan PM Capsules **3120**

RAVOTRIL (Chile)
CLONAZEPAM
Klonopin Tablets **2782**

RAYNE (Mexico)
DIAZEPAM
Diastat Rectal Delivery System **3344**
Valium Tablets **2822**

RAZENE (New Zealand)
CETIRIZINE HYDROCHLORIDE
Zyrtec Syrup **2589**
Zyrtec Tablets **2589**

REACEL-A (Mexico)
TRETINOIN
Avita Cream.................... **2136**
Avita Gel...................... **2138**
Renova 0.05% Cream.............. **2387**
Retin-A Micro 0.1%/0.04%........... **2388**
Vesanoid Capsules................ **2823**

REACTINE (Belgium, Canada, France, Germany, Norway, Spain, Sweden, The Netherlands)
CETIRIZINE HYDROCHLORIDE
Zyrtec Syrup **2589**
Zyrtec Tablets **2589**

REACUR (Argentina)
HYDROCORTISONE
Hydrocortone Tablets **1963**

REALDIRON (Russia)
INTERFERON ALFA-2B
Intron A for Injection.............. **3038**

REBATEN (Brazil)
PROPRANOLOL HYDROCHLORIDE
Inderal LA Long-Acting Capsules **3421**

REBETOL (Austria, Belgium, Brazil, Chile, Czech Republic, Denmark, Finland, France, Germany, Greece, Hong Kong, Hungary, Irish Republic, Israel, Italy, Malaysia, Norway, Portugal, Singapore, Spain, Sweden, Switzerland, Thailand, The Netherlands, United Kingdom)
RIBAVIRIN
Virazole for Inhalation Solution **3365**

REBETRON (South Africa)
INTERFERON ALFA-2B
Intron A for Injection.............. **3038**

REBIF (Argentina, Australia, Austria, Belgium, Brazil, Canada, Czech Republic, Denmark, Finland, France, Germany, Greece, Hong Kong, Hungary, India, Irish Republic, Israel, Italy, Malaysia, Mexico, Norway, Portugal, Russia, South Africa, Spain, Sweden, Switzerland, Thailand, The Netherlands, United Kingdom)
INTERFERON BETA-1A
Avonex **839**

RECA (Spain)
ENALAPRIL MALEATE
Vasotec I.V. Injection **2076**

RECAMICINA (Chile)
LEVOFLOXACIN
Levaquin Injection **2453**
Levaquin Tablets **2453**

REC-DZ (India)
DIAZEPAM
Diastat Rectal Delivery System **3344**
Valium Tablets **2822**

RECEANT (Greece)
CEFUROXIME SODIUM
Zinacef Injection **1604**

RECEF (Italy)
CEFAZOLIN SODIUM
Ancef for Injection **1318**

RECEPTOZINE (South Africa)
PROMETHAZINE HYDROCHLORIDE
Phenergan Suppositories............ **3438**
Phenergan Tablets **3438**

RECITAL (Israel)
CITALOPRAM HYDROBROMIDE
Celexa Tablets **1177**

RECO (Argentina)
RANITIDINE HYDROCHLORIDE
Zantac 25 EFFERdose Tablets **1597**
Zantac 150 EFFERdose Tablets........ **1597**
Zantac 150 Tablets **1597**
Zantac 300 Tablets **1597**
Zantac Injection **1593**
Zantac Injection Premixed **1593**
Zantac Syrup **1597**

RECOFOL (Argentina, Australia, Czech Republic, Denmark, Finland, Germany, Hungary, Israel, Mexico, New Zealand, Norway, Portugal, Russia, Singapore, South Africa, Spain, Sweden, Switzerland, Thailand, The Netherlands)
PROPOFOL
Diprivan Injectable Emulsion **676**

RECTOPRED (Austria)
PREDNISOLONE SODIUM PHOSPHATE
Pediapred Oral Solution **3319**

RED AWAY (Canada)
NAPHAZOLINE HYDROCHLORIDE
Albalon Ophthalmic Solution .... ⊙**216**

REDAP (Denmark)
ADAPALENE
Differin Gel **1211**

REDIPRED (Australia, Hong Kong, New Zealand)
PREDNISOLONE SODIUM PHOSPHATE
Pediapred Oral Solution **3319**

REDUCOL (Brazil)
LOVASTATIN
Mevacor Tablets **1996**

REDUCTEL (Mexico)
CAPTOPRIL
Captopril Tablets................. **2114**

REDUCTIL (Australia, Austria, Belgium, Brazil, Chile, Denmark, Finland, Germany, Greece, Hong Kong, Hungary, Irish Republic, Israel, Italy, New Zealand, Norway, Portugal, Singapore, South Africa, Spain, Sweden, Switzerland, Thailand, The Netherlands, United Kingdom)
SIBUTRAMINE HYDROCHLORIDE
Meridia Capsules................. **485**

REDUPRES (Spain)
VERAPAMIL HYDROCHLORIDE
Covera-HS Tablets **3135**
Verelan PM Capsules **3120**

REDUPRESS (Brazil)
LOSARTAN POTASSIUM
Cozaar Tablets **1913**

REDUSA (Hong Kong)
PHENTERMINE HYDROCHLORIDE
Adipex-P Capsules................ **1216**
Adipex-P Tablets **1216**

REDUSCAR (Brazil)
FINASTERIDE
Propecia Tablets **2036**
Proscar Tablets.................. **2040**

REDUSTEROL (Argentina)
SIMVASTATIN
Zocor Tablets................... **2078**

REDUTEN (Chile)
SIBUTRAMINE HYDROCHLORIDE
Meridia Capsules................. **485**

REDUTENSIL (Argentina)
VALSARTAN
Diovan Tablets **2191**

REDUXADE (Italy)
SIBUTRAMINE HYDROCHLORIDE
Meridia Capsules................. **485**

REFENAX COLIRIO (Argentina)
NAPHAZOLINE HYDROCHLORIDE
Albalon Ophthalmic Solution .... ⊙**216**

REFLIN (India)
CEFAZOLIN SODIUM
Ancef for Injection **1318**

REFOBACIN (Austria)
GENTAMICIN SULFATE
Garamycin Injectable **3028**
Genoptic Sterile Ophthalmic Solution .... ⊙**227**

REGENESIS (Argentina)
ALENDRONATE SODIUM
Fosamax Tablets................. **1949**

REGENTAL (Chile)
NIMODIPINE
Nimotop Capsules **774**

REGEPAR (Austria, Switzerland)
SELEGILINE HYDROCHLORIDE
Eldepryl Capsules **3209**

REGIOCAINA (Argentina)
LIDOCAINE
Lidoderm Patch **1107**

REGOMED (Austria)
ENALAPRIL MALEATE
Vasotec I.V. Injection **2076**

REGULACT (Mexico)
LACTULOSE
Kristalose for Oral Solution **2149**

REGULANE (Argentina)
LOPERAMIDE HYDROCHLORIDE
Imodium Capsules................ **1834**

REGULANE AF (Argentina)
LOPERAMIDE HYDROCHLORIDE
Imodium Capsules................ **1834**

REGULOSE (United Kingdom)
LACTULOSE
Kristalose for Oral Solution **2149**

REJUVA-A (Canada)
TRETINOIN
Avita Cream.................... **2136**
Avita Gel...................... **2138**
Renova 0.05% Cream.............. **2387**
Retin-A Micro 0.1%/0.04%........... **2388**
Vesanoid Capsules................ **2823**

REKAMIDE (Israel)
LOPERAMIDE HYDROCHLORIDE
Imodium Capsules................ **1834**

REKAWAN (Austria, Germany)
POTASSIUM CHLORIDE
K-Dur Extended-Relase Tablets **3047**
K-Lor Powder Packets **472**
K-Tab Filmtab Tablets **473**

RELAFEN (Canada)
NABUMETONE
Relafen Tablets.................. **1523**

RELANIUM (Russia)
DIAZEPAM
Diastat Rectal Delivery System **3344**
Valium Tablets **2822**

RELASAN (Mexico)
DIAZEPAM
Diastat Rectal Delivery System **3344**
Valium Tablets **2822**

RELASTEF (Italy)
TRETINOIN
Avita Cream.................... **2136**
Avita Gel...................... **2138**
Renova 0.05% Cream.............. **2387**
Retin-A Micro 0.1%/0.04%........... **2388**
Vesanoid Capsules................ **2823**

RELAXYL (India)
DICLOFENAC SODIUM
Voltaren Tablets **2298**
Voltaren-XR Tablets **2301**

RELAXYL PLUS (India)
DICLOFENAC SODIUM
Voltaren Tablets **2298**
Voltaren-XR Tablets **2301**

RELAZEPAM (Mexico)
DIAZEPAM
Diastat Rectal Delivery System **3344**
Valium Tablets **2822**

RELIBERAN (Italy)
CHLORDIAZEPOXIDE HYDROCHLORIDE
Librium Capsules................. **3349**

RELIF (Spain)
NABUMETONE
Relafen Tablets.................. **1523**

RELIFEN (Japan, South Africa)
NABUMETONE
Relafen Tablets.................. **1523**

RELIFEX (Belgium, Brazil, Czech Republic, Denmark, Finland, Greece, Hong Kong, Hungary, Irish Republic, Israel, Italy, Mexico, Norway, Singapore, Sweden, Thailand, United Kingdom)
NABUMETONE
Relafen Tablets.................. **1523**

RELIGER (Irish Republic)
NABUMETONE
Relafen Tablets.................. **1523**

RELIPAIN (Italy)
MORPHINE SULFATE
Kadian Capsules **572**
MS Contin Tablets **2703**

RELISAN (South Africa)
NABUMETONE
Relafen Tablets.................. **1523**

RELITONE (South Africa)
NABUMETONE
Relafen Tablets.................. **1523**

RELOXYL (Italy)
BENZOYL PEROXIDE
Brevoxyl-4 Creamy Wash............ **3212**
Brevoxyl-4 Gel **3211**
Brevoxyl-8 Creamy Wash............ **3212**
Brevoxyl-8 Gel **3211**
Triaz Cleanser **1864**
Triaz Gel..................... **1864**

REMAFEN (Hong Kong, Malaysia, Singapore)
DICLOFENAC SODIUM
Voltaren Tablets **2298**
Voltaren-XR Tablets **2301**

REMEDERM HC (Germany)
HYDROCORTISONE
Hydrocortone Tablets.............. **1963**

REMENA (Greece)
CIPROFLOXACIN HYDROCHLORIDE
Ciloxan Ophthalmic Ointment **554**
Ciloxan Ophthalmic Solution .... ⊙**205**
Cipro Tablets **2991**

REMETHAN (Hong Kong, Malaysia)
DICLOFENAC SODIUM
Voltaren Tablets . . . 2298
Voltaren-XR Tablets . . . 2301

REMICADE (Argentina, Australia, Belgium, Brazil, Canada, Chile, Czech Republic, Denmark, Finland, France, Germany, Greece, Hong Kong, Hungary, Irish Republic, Israel, Italy, Japan, Mexico, New Zealand, Norway, Portugal, Singapore, Spain, Sweden, Switzerland, The Netherlands, United Kingdom)
INFLIXIMAB
Remicade for IV Injection . . . 987

REMIK (The Netherlands)
RAMIPRIL
Altace Capsules . . . 1673

REMITEX (Chile)
CETIRIZINE HYDROCHLORIDE
Zyrtec Syrup . . . 2589
Zyrtec Tablets . . . 2589

REMONTAL (Spain)
NIMODIPINE
Nimotop Capsules . . . 774

RENACIDIN (Argentina)
FINASTERIDE
Propecia Tablets . . . 2036
Proscar Tablets . . . 2040

RENACOR (Germany)
ENALAPRIL MALEATE/HYDROCHLOROTHIAZIDE
Vaseretic Tablets . . . 2073

RENALAPRIL (Brazil)
ENALAPRIL MALEATE
Vasotec I.V. Injection . . . 2076

RENASE (Thailand)
AMILORIDE HYDROCHLORIDE/HYDROCHLOROTHIAZIDE
Moduretic Tablets . . . 2003

RENATON (Singapore)
ENALAPRIL MALEATE
Vasotec I.V. Injection . . . 2076

RENCEF (Chile)
LACTULOSE
Kristalose for Oral Solution . . . 2149

RENEDIL (Belgium, Canada, The Netherlands)
FELODIPINE
Plendil Extended-Release Tablets . . . 651

RENEZIDE (South Africa)
HYDROCHLOROTHIAZIDE/TRIAMTERENE
Dyazide Capsules . . . 1389
Maxzide Tablets . . . 2150
Maxzide-25 mg Tablets . . . 2150

RENIDUR (Portugal)
ENALAPRIL MALEATE/HYDROCHLOROTHIAZIDE
Vaseretic Tablets . . . 2073

RENIPRESS (Brazil)
ENALAPRIL MALEATE
Vasotec I.V. Injection . . . 2076

RENIPRIL (Portugal)
ENALAPRIL MALEATE
Vasotec I.V. Injection . . . 2076

RENIPRIL PLUS (Portugal)
ENALAPRIL MALEATE
Vasotec I.V. Injection . . . 2076

RENISTAD (Austria)
ENALAPRIL MALEATE
Vasotec I.V. Injection . . . 2076

RENITEC (Argentina, Australia, Belgium, Czech Republic, Denmark, France, Greece, Hong Kong, Hungary, Malaysia, Mexico, New Zealand, Portugal, Russia, Singapore, South Africa, Thailand, The Netherlands)
ENALAPRIL MALEATE
Vasotec I.V. Injection . . . 2076

RENITEC COMP (Finland, Norway, Sweden)
ENALAPRIL MALEATE/HYDROCHLOROTHIAZIDE
Vaseretic Tablets . . . 2073

RENITEC PLUS (Australia, Austria, Finland, Hungary, The Netherlands)
ENALAPRIL MALEATE
Vasotec I.V. Injection . . . 2076

RENITECMAX (Spain)
ENALAPRIL MALEATE/HYDROCHLOROTHIAZIDE
Vaseretic Tablets . . . 2073

RENITEN PLUS (Switzerland)
ENALAPRIL MALEATE/HYDROCHLOROTHIAZIDE
Vaseretic Tablets . . . 2073

RENOTENS (South Africa)
LISINOPRIL
Prinivil Tablets . . . 2029
Zestril Tablets . . . 704

RENOVA (Canada, Malaysia, South Africa, Thailand)
TRETINOIN
Avita Cream . . . 2136
Avita Gel . . . 2138
Renova 0.05% Cream . . . 2387
Retin-A Micro 0.1%/0.04% . . . 2388
Vesanoid Capsules . . . 2823

RENOXACIN (Italy)
NORFLOXACIN
Noroxin Tablets . . . 2009

REOPRO (Argentina, Australia, Austria, Belgium, Brazil, Canada, Chile, Czech Republic, Denmark, Finland, France, Germany, Hong Kong, India, Irish Republic, Israel, Italy, Malaysia, Mexico, New Zealand, Norway, Singapore, South Africa, Spain, Sweden, Switzerland, Thailand, The Netherlands, United Kingdom)
ABCIXIMAB
ReoPro Vials . . . 1779

REPLASYN (Argentina)
ESTRADIOL
Climara Transdermal System . . . 795
Vivelle Transdermal System . . . 2288
Vivelle-Dot Transdermal System . . . 2293

REPLIGEN (Argentina)
METRONIDAZOLE
MetroGel-Vaginal Gel . . . 1822
Noritate Cream, 1% . . . 1051

REPRIADOL (Denmark)
MORPHINE SULFATE
Kadian Capsules . . . 572
MS Contin Tablets . . . 2703

REPROST (Chile)
NAPROXEN
EC-Naprosyn Delayed-Release Tablets . . . 2769
Naprosyn Suspension . . . 2769
Naprosyn Tablets . . . 2769

REQUIP (Argentina, Austria, Belgium, Canada, Chile, Czech Republic, Denmark, Finland, France, Germany, Greece, Hong Kong, Irish Republic, Israel, Italy, Malaysia, Norway, Portugal, Singapore, South Africa, Spain, Sweden, Switzerland, The Netherlands, United Kingdom)
ROPINIROLE HYDROCHLORIDE
Requip Tablets . . . 1528

RESIDEX P55 (United Kingdom)
PERMETHRIN
Acticin Cream . . . 2125

RESMA (Belgium)
ZAFIRLUKAST
Accolate Tablets . . . 663

RESPEXIL (Brazil)
NORFLOXACIN
Noroxin Tablets . . . 2009

RESPICORT (Switzerland)
TRIAMCINOLONE ACETONIDE
Azmacort Inhalation Aerosol . . . 1701
Nasacort AQ Nasal Spray . . . 2937

RESPICUR (Austria, Italy)
THEOPHYLLINE
Uniphyl Tablets . . . 2708

RESPONTIN (Norway, United Kingdom)
IPRATROPIUM BROMIDE
Atrovent Inhalation Solution . . . 868
Atrovent Nasal Spray 0.03% . . . 869
Atrovent Nasal Spray 0.06% . . . 870

RESTELEA (Argentina)
RISPERIDONE
Risperdal Oral Solution . . . 1658
Risperdal Tablets . . . 1658

RESTOPON (Greece)
RANITIDINE HYDROCHLORIDE
Zantac 25 EFFERdose Tablets . . . 1597
Zantac 150 EFFERdose Tablets . . . 1597
Zantac 150 Tablets . . . 1597
Zantac 300 Tablets . . . 1597
Zantac Injection . . . 1593
Zantac Injection Premixed . . . 1593
Zantac Syrup . . . 1597

RETACNYL (Argentina, Brazil, Chile, France, Hong Kong, Malaysia, Mexico, Singapore, South Africa, Thailand)
TRETINOIN
Avita Cream . . . 2136
Avita Gel . . . 2138
Renova 0.05% Cream . . . 2387
Retin-A Micro 0.1%/0.04% . . . 2388
Vesanoid Capsules . . . 2823

RETAFYLLIN (Finland, Hungary, Malaysia, Singapore, Thailand)
THEOPHYLLINE
Uniphyl Tablets . . . 2708

RETALZEM (Hong Kong)
DILTIAZEM HYDROCHLORIDE
Cardizem LA Extended Release Tablets . . . 1699
Tiazac Capsules . . . 1204

RET-A-PRES (Mexico)
TRETINOIN
Avita Cream . . . 2136
Avita Gel . . . 2138
Renova 0.05% Cream . . . 2387
Retin-A Micro 0.1%/0.04% . . . 2388
Vesanoid Capsules . . . 2823

RETAVIT (Israel)
TRETINOIN
Avita Cream . . . 2136
Avita Gel . . . 2138
Renova 0.05% Cream . . . 2387
Retin-A Micro 0.1%/0.04% . . . 2388
Vesanoid Capsules . . . 2823

RETCIN (United Kingdom)
ERYTHROMYCIN
Ery-Tab Tablets . . . 447
Erythromycin Base Filmtab Tablets . . . 454
Erythromycin Delayed-Release Capsules, USP . . . 456
PCE Dispertab Tablets . . . 510

RETEP (Argentina)
FUROSEMIDE
Furosemide Tablets . . . 2117

RETICNE (Argentina)
TRETINOIN
Avita Cream . . . 2136
Avita Gel . . . 2138
Renova 0.05% Cream . . . 2387
Retin-A Micro 0.1%/0.04% . . . 2388
Vesanoid Capsules . . . 2823

RETIN-A (Argentina, Australia, Austria, Brazil, Canada, Chile, Czech Republic, France, Hong Kong, Irish Republic, Israel, Italy, Malaysia, Mexico, New Zealand, Portugal, Singapore, South Africa, Switzerland, Thailand, United Kingdom)
TRETINOIN
Avita Cream . . . 2136
Avita Gel . . . 2138
Renova 0.05% Cream . . . 2387
Retin-A Micro 0.1%/0.04% . . . 2388
Vesanoid Capsules . . . 2823

RETINIDE (Argentina)
ISOTRETINOIN
Accutane Capsules . . . 2740

RETINOVA (Belgium, Brazil, Denmark, France, New Zealand, Singapore, Spain, Sweden, United Kingdom)
TRETINOIN
Avita Cream . . . 2136
Avita Gel . . . 2138
Renova 0.05% Cream . . . 2387
Retin-A Micro 0.1%/0.04% . . . 2388
Vesanoid Capsules . . . 2823

RETIRIDES (Spain)
TRETINOIN
Avita Cream . . . 2136
Avita Gel . . . 2138
Renova 0.05% Cream . . . 2387
Retin-A Micro 0.1%/0.04% . . . 2388
Vesanoid Capsules . . . 2823

RETISOL-A (Canada)
TRETINOIN
Avita Cream . . . 2136
Avita Gel . . . 2138
Renova 0.05% Cream . . . 2387
Retin-A Micro 0.1%/0.04% . . . 2388
Vesanoid Capsules . . . 2823

RETITOP (France)
TRETINOIN
Avita Cream . . . 2136
Avita Gel . . . 2138
Renova 0.05% Cream . . . 2387
Retin-A Micro 0.1%/0.04% . . . 2388
Vesanoid Capsules . . . 2823

RETOFAR (Mexico)
METRONIDAZOLE
MetroGel-Vaginal Gel . . . 1822
Noritate Cream, 1% . . . 1051

RETRIEVE (Australia, Hong Kong)
TRETINOIN
Avita Cream . . . 2136
Avita Gel . . . 2138
Renova 0.05% Cream . . . 2387
Retin-A Micro 0.1%/0.04% . . . 2388
Vesanoid Capsules . . . 2823

RETROVIR (Argentina, Australia, Austria, Belgium, Brazil, Canada, Chile, Czech Republic, Denmark, Finland, France, Germany, Greece, Hong Kong, India, Irish Republic, Israel, Italy, Malaysia, Mexico, New Zealand, Norway, Portugal, Singapore, South Africa, Spain, Sweden, Switzerland, Thailand, The Netherlands, United Kingdom)
ZIDOVUDINE
Retrovir Capsules . . . 1533
Retrovir IV Infusion . . . 1537
Retrovir Syrup . . . 1533
Retrovir Tablets . . . 1533

REUFLOS (Italy)
DIFLUNISAL
Dolobid Tablets . . . 1937

REUMAREN (Brazil)
DICLOFENAC SODIUM
Voltaren Tablets . . . 2298
Voltaren-XR Tablets . . . 2301

REUMYL (Italy)
SULINDAC
Clinoril Tablets . . . 1899

REUSAN (Mexico)
DEXAMETHASONE
Decadron Tablets . . . 1929

REUTAREN (Brazil)
DICLOFENAC POTASSIUM
Cataflam Tablets . . . 2173

REUXEN (Portugal)
NAPROXEN
EC-Naprosyn Delayed-Release Tablets . . . 2769
Naprosyn Suspension . . . 2769
Naprosyn Tablets . . . 2769

REVALINTABS (The Netherlands)
CETIRIZINE HYDROCHLORIDE
Zyrtec Syrup . . . 2589
Zyrtec Tablets . . . 2589

REVANGE (Brazil)
ISOSORBIDE MONONITRATE
Imdur Tablets . . . 3032

REVAPOL (Mexico)
MEBENDAZOLE
Vermox Chewable Tablets . . . 1853

REVASTIN (Brazil)
SIMVASTATIN
Zocor Tablets . . . 2078

REVECTINA (Brazil)
IVERMECTIN
Stromectol Tablets . . . 2053

REVELLEX (Argentina, South Africa)
INFLIXIMAB
Remicade for IV Injection . . . 987

REVELOL (India)
METOPROLOL SUCCINATE
Toprol-XL Tablets 660

REVION (Greece)
CIPROFLOXACIN HYDROCHLORIDE
Ciloxan Ophthalmic Ointment 554
Ciloxan Ophthalmic Solution . . . . ⊙205
Cipro Tablets 2991

REVIRAX (Brazil)
ZIDOVUDINE
Retrovir Capsules 1533
Retrovir IV Infusion 1537
Retrovir Syrup 1533
Retrovir Tablets 1533

REVIXIL (Argentina)
STAVUDINE
Zerit Capsules 971
Zerit for Oral Solution 971

REWODINA (Czech Republic, Germany)
DICLOFENAC SODIUM
Voltaren Tablets 2298
Voltaren-XR Tablets 2301

REXACIN (Hong Kong, Thailand)
NORFLOXACIN
Noroxin Tablets 2009

REXAMAT (Argentina)
CALCITRIOL
Calcijex Injection 411

REXETIN (Russia)
PAROXETINE HYDROCHLORIDE
Paxil Oral Suspension 1501
Paxil Tablets 1501

REXGENTA (Spain)
GENTAMICIN SULFATE
Garamycin Injectable 3028
Genoptic Sterile Ophthalmic Solution . . . . ⊙227

REXIGEN (South Africa)
PROPRANOLOL HYDROCHLORIDE
Inderal LA Long-Acting Capsules 3421

REXIMIDE (Hong Kong)
LOPERAMIDE HYDROCHLORIDE
Imodium Capsules 1834

REXNER (Argentina)
CIPROFLOXACIN HYDROCHLORIDE
Ciloxan Ophthalmic Ointment 554
Ciloxan Ophthalmic Solution . . . . ⊙205
Cipro Tablets 2991

REZAMID (Argentina)
TRIAMCINOLONE ACETONIDE
Azmacort Inhalation Aerosol 1701
Nasacort AQ Nasal Spray 2937

REZAMID D, REZAMID F, REZAMID M (Argentina)
TRIAMCINOLONE ACETONIDE
Azmacort Inhalation Aerosol 1701
Nasacort AQ Nasal Spray 2937

REZULT (India)
ROSIGLITAZONE MALEATE
Avandia Tablets 1348

RFG-KIT (Argentina)
FLUORESCEIN SODIUM
Fluorescite Injection . . . . ⊙207

R-FLEX (South Africa)
SULINDAC
Clinoril Tablets 1899

RHEFLUIN (Czech Republic, Germany, Switzerland)
AMILORIDE HYDROCHLORIDE
Midamor Tablets 2000

RHEMOFENAX (Hong Kong)
DICLOFENAC SODIUM
Voltaren Tablets 2298
Voltaren-XR Tablets 2301

RHEUFENAC (Switzerland)
DICLOFENAC SODIUM
Voltaren Tablets 2298
Voltaren-XR Tablets 2301

RHEUFLEX (United Kingdom)
NAPROXEN
EC-Naprosyn Delayed-Release Tablets 2769
Naprosyn Suspension 2769
Naprosyn Tablets 2769

RHEUMABENE (Austria)
DICLOFENAC SODIUM
Voltaren Tablets 2298
Voltaren-XR Tablets 2301

RHEUMASAN D (Germany)
DICLOFENAC SODIUM
Voltaren Tablets 2298
Voltaren-XR Tablets 2301

RHEUMATAC (United Kingdom)
DICLOFENAC SODIUM
Voltaren Tablets 2298
Voltaren-XR Tablets 2301

RHEUMAVEK (Greece)
DICLOFENAC SODIUM
Voltaren Tablets 2298
Voltaren-XR Tablets 2301

RHEWLIN (Malaysia)
DICLOFENAC SODIUM
Voltaren Tablets 2298
Voltaren-XR Tablets 2301

RHINALAR (Australia, Canada, Hong Kong)
FLUNISOLIDE
Aerobid Inhaler System 1172
Aerobid-M Inhaler System 1172
Nasarel Nasal Spray 1652

RHINARIS-F (Canada)
FLUNISOLIDE
Aerobid Inhaler System 1172
Aerobid-M Inhaler System 1172
Nasarel Nasal Spray 1652

RHINEX (Germany)
NAPHAZOLINE HYDROCHLORIDE
Albalon Ophthalmic Solution . . . . ⊙216

RHINISAN (Germany)
TRIAMCINOLONE ACETONIDE
Azmacort Inhalation Aerosol 1701
Nasacort AQ Nasal Spray 2937

RHINOGEN (Switzerland)
SODIUM HYALURONATE
Hyalgan Solution 2917

RHINOLAST (Irish Republic, Israel, New Zealand, South Africa, United Kingdom)
AZELASTINE HYDROCHLORIDE
Astelin Nasal Spray 1876

RHINO-MEX-N (Canada)
NAPHAZOLINE HYDROCHLORIDE
Albalon Ophthalmic Solution . . . . ⊙216

RHINON (Austria)
NAPHAZOLINE HYDROCHLORIDE
Albalon Ophthalmic Solution . . . . ⊙216

RHINOPERD (Austria)
NAPHAZOLINE HYDROCHLORIDE
Albalon Ophthalmic Solution . . . . ⊙216

RHINOVENT (Switzerland)
IPRATROPIUM BROMIDE
Atrovent Inhalation Solution 868
Atrovent Nasal Spray 0.03% 869
Atrovent Nasal Spray 0.06% 870

RHIZIN (Singapore)
CETIRIZINE HYDROCHLORIDE
Zyrtec Syrup 2589
Zyrtec Tablets 2589

RHODIALAX (Canada)
LACTULOSE
Kristalose for Oral Solution 2149

RHODIALOSE (Canada)
LACTULOSE
Kristalose for Oral Solution 2149

RHODIAPROX (Canada)
NAPROXEN
EC-Naprosyn Delayed-Release Tablets 2769
Naprosyn Suspension 2769
Naprosyn Tablets 2769

RHONURACIL (Mexico)
FLUOROURACIL
Efudex Topical Cream 3348
Efudex Topical Solutions 3348

RHOTARD (United Kingdom)
MORPHINE SULFATE
Kadian Capsules 572
MS Contin Tablets 2703

RHOTRIMINE (Canada)
TRIMIPRAMINE MALEATE
Surmontil Capsules 2347

RHUMALGAN (Switzerland, United Kingdom)
DICLOFENAC SODIUM
Voltaren Tablets 2298
Voltaren-XR Tablets 2301

RHUMANTIN (Denmark)
PENICILLAMINE
Cuprimine Capsules 1925

RHYTHMOCOR (Austria)
PROPAFENONE HYDROCHLORIDE
Rythmol SR Capsules 2736

RIATUL (Argentina)
RISPERIDONE
Risperdal Oral Solution 1658
Risperdal Tablets 1658

RIBASTAMIN (Argentina)
RISEDRONATE SODIUM
Actonel Tablets 2679

RIBATRA (Argentina)
CLOBETASOL PROPIONATE
Temovate Cream 1549
Temovate E Emollient 1552
Temovate Gel 1550
Temovate Ointment 1549
Temovate Scalp Application 1551

RIBAV (Brazil)
RIBAVIRIN
Virazole for Inhalation Solution 3365

RIBAVIN (India)
RIBAVIRIN
Virazole for Inhalation Solution 3365

RIBAVIRON C (Brazil)
RIBAVIRIN
Virazole for Inhalation Solution 3365

RIBEX FLU (Italy)
DICLOFENAC SODIUM
Voltaren Tablets 2298
Voltaren-XR Tablets 2301

RIBOFLUOR (Germany)
FLUOROURACIL
Efudex Topical Cream 3348
Efudex Topical Solutions 3348

RIBOLIN (Greece)
RANITIDINE HYDROCHLORIDE
Zantac 25 EFFERdose Tablets 1597
Zantac 150 EFFERdose Tablets 1597
Zantac 150 Tablets 1597
Zantac 300 Tablets 1597
Zantac Injection 1593
Zantac Injection Premixed 1593
Zantac Syrup 1597

RIBOMICIN (Italy)
GENTAMICIN SULFATE
Garamycin Injectable 3028
Genoptic Sterile Ophthalmic Solution . . . . ⊙227

RIDAZIN (Israel)
THIORIDAZINE HYDROCHLORIDE
Thioridazine Hydrochloride Tablets 2122

RIDAZINE (South Africa, Thailand)
THIORIDAZINE HYDROCHLORIDE
Thioridazine Hydrochloride Tablets 2122

RIDRON (Argentina)
RISEDRONATE SODIUM
Actonel Tablets 2679

RIDRON PACK (Argentina)
RISEDRONATE SODIUM
Actonel Tablets 2679

RIFAXI (Argentina)
RITONAVIR
Norvir Oral Solution 499
Norvir Soft Gelatin Capsules 499

RIGIX (Austria)
CETIRIZINE HYDROCHLORIDE
Zyrtec Syrup 2589
Zyrtec Tablets 2589

RILATINE (Belgium)
METHYLPHENIDATE HYDROCHLORIDE
Ritalin Hydrochloride Tablets 2254
Ritalin-SR Tablets 2254

RILCAPTON (Hong Kong, Singapore)
CAPTOPRIL
Captopril Tablets 2114

RILUTEK (Argentina, Australia, Austria, Belgium, Brazil, Canada, Czech Republic, Denmark, Finland, France, Germany, Greece, Hong Kong, Hungary, Irish Republic, Israel, Italy, Japan, Mexico, Norway, Portugal, Singapore, South Africa, Spain, Sweden, Switzerland, Thailand, The Netherlands, United Kingdom)
RILUZOLE
Rilutek Tablets 2945

RIMAPAM (United Kingdom)
DIAZEPAM
Diastat Rectal Delivery System 3344
Valium Tablets 2822

RIMIDOL (Sweden)
NAPHAZOLINE HYDROCHLORIDE
Albalon Ophthalmic Solution . . . . ⊙216

RIMOXYN (United Kingdom)
NAPROXEN
EC-Naprosyn Delayed-Release Tablets 2769
Naprosyn Suspension 2769
Naprosyn Tablets 2769

RINADINE (Thailand)
CIMETIDINE
Tagamet Tablets 1547

RINALIX (Malaysia, Singapore)
INDAPAMIDE
Indapamide Tablets 2119

RINATEC (Irish Republic, United Kingdom)
IPRATROPIUM BROMIDE
Atrovent Inhalation Solution 868
Atrovent Nasal Spray 0.03% 869
Atrovent Nasal Spray 0.06% 870

RINELON (Italy, Mexico, South Africa, Spain, Thailand)
MOMETASONE FUROATE
Elocon Cream 0.1% 3019
Elocon Lotion 0.1% 3020
Elocon Ointment 0.1% 3021
Nasonex Nasal Spray 3058

RINISONA (Argentina)
FLUTICASONE PROPIONATE
Cutivate Cream 1381
Cutivate Ointment 1384
Flonase Nasal Spray 1412

RINO NAFTAZOLINA (Italy)
NAPHAZOLINE HYDROCHLORIDE
Albalon Ophthalmic Solution . . . . ⊙216

RINO-AZETIN (Brazil)
AZELASTINE HYDROCHLORIDE
Astelin Nasal Spray 1876

RINOBEREN (Spain)
IPRATROPIUM BROMIDE
Atrovent Inhalation Solution 868
Atrovent Nasal Spray 0.03% 869
Atrovent Nasal Spray 0.06% 870

RINO-LASTIN (Brazil)
AZELASTINE HYDROCHLORIDE
Astelin Nasal Spray 1876

RINOS-A (Brazil)
NAPHAZOLINE HYDROCHLORIDE
Albalon Ophthalmic Solution . . . . ⊙216

RINOSONE (Spain)
FLUTICASONE PROPIONATE
Cutivate Cream 1381
Cutivate Ointment 1384
Flonase Nasal Spray 1412

RINOVAGOS (Italy)
IPRATROPIUM BROMIDE
Atrovent Inhalation Solution 868
Atrovent Nasal Spray 0.03% 869
Atrovent Nasal Spray 0.06% 870

RINOVAL (Chile)
MOMETASONE FUROATE
Elocon Cream 0.1% 3019
Elocon Lotion 0.1% 3020
Elocon Ointment 0.1% 3021
Nasonex Nasal Spray 3058

RINSTEAD TEETHING GEL (United Kingdom)
LIDOCAINE
Lidoderm Patch 1107

RIOWORM (South Africa)
MEBENDAZOLE
Vermox Chewable Tablets 1853

RIPHENIDATE (Canada)
METHYLPHENIDATE HYDROCHLORIDE
Ritalin Hydrochloride Tablets. 2254
Ritalin-SR Tablets. 2254

RISEDON (Argentina)
RISEDRONATE SODIUM
Actonel Tablets. 2679

RISELLE (Brazil, Czech Republic)
ESTRADIOL
Climara Transdermal System 795
Vivelle Transdermal System 2288
Vivelle-Dot Transdermal System 2293

RISNIA (India)
RISPERIDONE
Risperdal Oral Solution 1658
Risperdal Tablets. 1658

RISOFOS (India)
RISEDRONATE SODIUM
Actonel Tablets. 2679

RISPEN (Czech Republic)
RISPERIDONE
Risperdal Oral Solution 1658
Risperdal Tablets. 1658

RISPER (Argentina)
RISPERIDONE
Risperdal Oral Solution 1658
Risperdal Tablets. 1658

RISPERDAL (Argentina, Australia, Austria, Belgium, Brazil, Chile, Czech Republic, Denmark, Finland, Germany, Greece, Hong Kong, Hungary, India, Irish Republic, Israel, Italy, Japan, Malaysia, Mexico, New Zealand, Norway, Portugal, Singapore, South Africa, Spain, Sweden, Switzerland, Thailand, The Netherlands, United Kingdom)
RISPERIDONE
Risperdal Oral Solution 1658
Risperdal Tablets 1658

RISPERIN (Argentina)
RISPERIDONE
Risperdal Oral Solution 1658
Risperdal Tablets. 1658

RISPEX (Argentina)
RISPERIDONE
Risperdal Oral Solution 1658
Risperdal Tablets. 1658

RISPID (India)
RISPERIDONE
Risperdal Oral Solution 1658
Risperdal Tablets. 1658

RISPOLIN (Austria)
RISPERIDONE
Risperdal Oral Solution 1658
Risperdal Tablets. 1658

RISTALEN (Spain)
ENALAPRIL MALEATE
Vasotec I.V. Injection 2076

RISTO (Thailand)
TRIAMCINOLONE ACETONIDE
Azmacort Inhalation Aerosol. 1701
Nasacort AQ Nasal Spray 2937

RITALIN (Australia, Austria, Canada, Chile, Czech Republic, Denmark, Germany, Hong Kong, Hungary, Irish Republic, Israel, Malaysia, Mexico, New Zealand, Norway, Singapore, South Africa, The Netherlands, United Kingdom)
METHYLPHENIDATE HYDROCHLORIDE
Ritalin Hydrochloride Tablets. 2254
Ritalin-SR Tablets. 2254

RITALINA (Argentina, Brazil, Portugal)
METHYLPHENIDATE HYDROCHLORIDE
Ritalin Hydrochloride Tablets. 2254
Ritalin-SR Tablets. 2254

RITALINE (France, Switzerland)
METHYLPHENIDATE HYDROCHLORIDE
Ritalin Hydrochloride Tablets. 2254
Ritalin-SR Tablets. 2254

RITAPHEN (South Africa)
METHYLPHENIDATE HYDROCHLORIDE
Ritalin Hydrochloride Tablets. 2254
Ritalin-SR Tablets. 2254

RITECHOL (Irish Republic)
SIMVASTATIN
Zocor Tablets 2078

RITHMIK (Australia)
AMIODARONE HYDROCHLORIDE
Pacerone Tablets 3337

RITMOCARDYL (Chile)
AMIODARONE HYDROCHLORIDE
Pacerone Tablets 3337

RITMOCOR (Chile)
PROPAFENONE HYDROCHLORIDE
Rythmol SR Capsules 2736

RITMONORM (Brazil)
PROPAFENONE HYDROCHLORIDE
Rythmol SR Capsules 2736

RITOMUNE (India)
RITONAVIR
Norvir Oral Solution 499
Norvir Soft Gelatin Capsules. 499

RITROCEL (Chile)
METHYLPHENIDATE HYDROCHLORIDE
Ritalin Hydrochloride Tablets. 2254
Ritalin-SR Tablets. 2254

RITROMINE (Argentina)
NORFLOXACIN
Noroxin Tablets. 2009

RITUXAN (Canada, Japan)
RITUXIMAB
Rituxan I.V. 1251
Rituxan for Infusion 845

RIUCLONAZ (Argentina)
CLONAZEPAM
Klonopin Tablets 2782

RIVATRIL (Finland)
CLONAZEPAM
Klonopin Tablets 2782

RIVERVAN (Argentina)
VANCOMYCIN HYDROCHLORIDE
Vancocin HCl Capsules, USP 3370

RIVILINA (Argentina)
APROTININ
Trasylol Injection 779

RIVODARONE (Switzerland)
AMIODARONE HYDROCHLORIDE
Pacerone Tablets 3337

RIVOSTATIN (Switzerland)
NYSTATIN
Nystop Topical Powder USP. 2490

RIVOTRIL (Argentina, Australia, Austria, Belgium, Brazil, Canada, Czech Republic, Denmark, France, Germany, Hong Kong, Hungary, Irish Republic, Israel, Italy, Mexico, New Zealand, Norway, Portugal, Singapore, South Africa, Spain, Switzerland, Thailand, The Netherlands, United Kingdom)
CLONAZEPAM
Klonopin Tablets 2782

RIVOXICILLIN (Switzerland)
AMOXICILLIN
Amoxil Pediatric Drops for Oral Suspension. 1315
Amoxil Tablets 1315

RIZACT (India)
RIZATRIPTAN BENZOATE
Maxalt Tablets 1983
Maxalt-MLT Orally Disintegrating Tablets . . 1983

RIZALIEF (Austria)
RIZATRIPTAN BENZOATE
Maxalt Tablets 1983
Maxalt-MLT Orally Disintegrating Tablets . . 1983

RIZALIV (Italy)
RIZATRIPTAN BENZOATE
Maxalt Tablets 1983
Maxalt-MLT Orally Disintegrating Tablets . . 1983

R-LOC (India)
RANITIDINE HYDROCHLORIDE
Zantac 25 EFFERdose Tablets 1597
Zantac 150 EFFERdose Tablets. 1597
Zantac 150 Tablets 1597
Zantac 300 Tablets 1597
Zantac Injection 1593
Zantac Injection Premixed 1593
Zantac Syrup 1597

RMS (New Zealand)
MORPHINE SULFATE
Kadian Capsules 572
MS Contin Tablets 2703

ROACCUTAN (Argentina, Austria, Denmark, Finland, Germany, Greece, Hungary, Italy, Mexico, Portugal)
ISOTRETINOIN
Accutane Capsules 2740

ROACCUTANE (Australia, Belgium, Czech Republic, France, Hong Kong, Irish Republic, Israel, New Zealand, Singapore, South Africa, Switzerland, Thailand, The Netherlands, United Kingdom)
ISOTRETINOIN
Accutane Capsules 2740

ROACNETAN (Chile)
ISOTRETINOIN
Accutane Capsules 2740

ROACUTAN (Brazil, Spain)
ISOTRETINOIN
Accutane Capsules 2740

ROBAZ (Greece, Thailand)
METRONIDAZOLE
MetroGel-Vaginal Gel 1822
Noritate Cream, 1% 1051

ROCALTROL (Australia, Austria, Belgium, Brazil, Canada, Chile, Czech Republic, Denmark, France, Germany, Hong Kong, Hungary, Irish Republic, Italy, Japan, Mexico, New Zealand, Norway, Portugal, Singapore, South Africa, Spain, Sweden, Switzerland, Thailand, The Netherlands, United Kingdom)
CALCITRIOL
Calcijex Injection 411

ROCEFALIN (Spain)
CEFTRIAXONE SODIUM
Rocephin Injectable Vials, ADD-Vantage, Galaxy, Bulk 2801

ROCEFIN (Brazil, Italy)
CEFTRIAXONE SODIUM
Rocephin Injectable Vials, ADD-Vantage, Galaxy, Bulk 2801

ROCEPHALIN (Denmark, Finland, Norway, Sweden)
CEFTRIAXONE SODIUM
Rocephin Injectable Vials, ADD-Vantage, Galaxy, Bulk 2801

ROCEPHIN (Australia, Austria, Canada, Czech Republic, Germany, Greece, Hong Kong, Hungary, Irish Republic, Israel, Japan, Mexico, New Zealand, Portugal, Singapore, South Africa, Thailand, The Netherlands, United Kingdom)
CEFTRIAXONE SODIUM
Rocephin Injectable Vials, ADD-Vantage, Galaxy, Bulk 2801

ROCEPHINE (Belgium, France, Switzerland)
CEFTRIAXONE SODIUM
Rocephin Injectable Vials, ADD-Vantage, Galaxy, Bulk 2801

ROCERON (Norway)
INTERFERON ALFA-2A
Roferon-A Injection. 2805

ROCERON-A (Denmark)
INTERFERON ALFA-2A
Roferon-A Injection. 2805

ROCHE (Canada)
NAPROXEN SODIUM
Anaprox DS Tablets 2769
Anaprox Tablets 2769

RODANOL S (Czech Republic, Hungary)
NABUMETONE
Relafen Tablets. 1523

RODERMIL (Portugal)
METRONIDAZOLE
MetroGel-Vaginal Gel 1822
Noritate Cream, 1% 1051

RO-DEXSONE (Canada)
DEXAMETHASONE SODIUM PHOSPHATE
Decadron Phosphate Injection. 1931

RODINAC BIOTIC (Argentina)
AMOXICILLIN
Amoxil Pediatric Drops for Oral Suspension. 1315
Amoxil Tablets 1315

ROFANTEN (Spain)
NAPROXEN
EC-Naprosyn Delayed-Release Tablets. . . . 2769
Naprosyn Suspension. 2769
Naprosyn Tablets 2769

ROFERON-A (Argentina, Austria, Belgium, Brazil, Czech Republic, Finland, Germany, Hong Kong, Hungary, India, Israel, Italy, Japan, Mexico, New Zealand, Portugal, Singapore, South Africa, Spain, Sweden, Switzerland, Thailand, The Netherlands)
INTERFERON ALFA-2A
Roferon-A Injection. 2805

ROFLUAL (France)
RIMANTADINE HYDROCHLORIDE
Flumadine Syrup 1186
Flumadine Tablets 1186

ROFOXIN (Brazil)
CEFTRIAXONE SODIUM
Rocephin Injectable Vials, ADD-Vantage, Galaxy, Bulk 2801

ROGASTI (Israel)
FAMOTIDINE
Pepcid Injection 2017
Pepcid Injection Premixed 2017
Pepcid Tablets 2014
Pepcid for Oral Suspension 2014

RO-GENTYCIN (Canada)
GENTAMICIN SULFATE
Garamycin Injectable 3028
Genoptic Sterile Ophthalmic Solution . . . . ⊙227

ROGLIN (India)
ROSIGLITAZONE MALEATE
Avandia Tablets. 1348

ROGLIN-M (India)
ROSIGLITAZONE MALEATE
Avandia Tablets. 1348

ROICAL (Malaysia, Singapore)
CALCITRIOL
Calcijex Injection 411

ROKO (India)
LOPERAMIDE HYDROCHLORIDE
Imodium Capsules 1834

ROLAB-AMOCLAV (South Africa)
AMOXICILLIN
Amoxil Pediatric Drops for Oral Suspension. 1315
Amoxil Tablets 1315

ROLSICAL (India)
CALCITRIOL
Calcijex Injection 411

ROMESA (Mexico)
WARFARIN SODIUM
Coumadin Tablets 932
Coumadin for Injection 932

ROMIR (Mexico)
CAPTOPRIL
Captopril Tablets. 2114

ROMMIX (United Kingdom)
ERYTHROMYCIN
Ery-Tab Tablets 447
Erythromycin Base Filmtab Tablets. 454
Erythromycin Delayed-Release Capsules, USP 456
PCE Dispertab Tablets 510

RONABIN (Israel)
DRONABINOL
Marinol Capsules. 3334

RONAME (Spain)
GLIMEPIRIDE
Amaryl Tablets 2864

RO-NAPHZ (Canada)
NAPHAZOLINE HYDROCHLORIDE
Albalon Ophthalmic Solution . . . . ⊙216

RONIC (Portugal)
DEXAMETHASONE
Decadron Tablets 1929

RONMIX (United Kingdom)
ERYTHROMYCIN
Ery-Tab Tablets 447
Erythromycin Base Filmtab Tablets 454
Erythromycin Delayed-Release Capsules, USP 456
PCE Dispertab Tablets 510

RONTAGEL (Argentina)
ESTRADIOL
Climara Transdermal System 795
Vivelle Transdermal System 2288
Vivelle-Dot Transdermal System 2293

RONTILONA (Portugal, Spain)
FLUTICASONE PROPIONATE
Cutivate Cream 1381
Cutivate Ointment 1384
Flonase Nasal Spray 1412

RO-PREDPHATE (Canada)
PREDNISOLONE SODIUM PHOSPHATE
Pediapred Oral Solution 3319

ROPRIL (Hong Kong)
CAPTOPRIL
Captopril Tablets 2114

ROSAGENUS (Greece)
FAMOTIDINE
Pepcid Injection 2017
Pepcid Injection Premixed 2017
Pepcid Tablets 2014
Pepcid for Oral Suspension 2014

ROSALOX (Czech Republic, Switzerland)
METRONIDAZOLE
MetroGel-Vaginal Gel 1822
Noritate Cream, 1% 1051

ROSASED (Italy)
METRONIDAZOLE
MetroGel-Vaginal Gel 1822
Noritate Cream, 1% 1051

ROSASOL (Canada)
METRONIDAZOLE
MetroGel-Vaginal Gel 1822
Noritate Cream, 1% 1051

ROSAZOL (Finland)
METRONIDAZOLE
MetroGel-Vaginal Gel 1822
Noritate Cream, 1% 1051

ROSICED (France, The Netherlands)
METRONIDAZOLE
MetroGel-Vaginal Gel 1822
Noritate Cream, 1% 1051

ROSICON (India)
ROSIGLITAZONE MALEATE
Avandia Tablets 1348

ROSICON MF (India)
ROSIGLITAZONE MALEATE
Avandia Tablets 1348

ROSIL (Thailand)
CLINDAMYCIN HYDROCHLORIDE
Cleocin Vaginal Ovules 2613

ROSITAL (Greece)
NIMODIPINE
Nimotop Capsules 774

ROTHONAL (Greece)
RANITIDINE HYDROCHLORIDE
Zantac 25 EFFERdose Tablets 1597
Zantac 150 EFFERdose Tablets 1597
Zantac 150 Tablets 1597
Zantac 300 Tablets 1597
Zantac Injection 1593
Zantac Injection Premixed 1593
Zantac Syrup 1597

ROTIAZ (Argentina)
TERAZOSIN HYDROCHLORIDE
Hytrin Capsules 469

ROUG-MYCIN (Greece)
ERYTHROMYCIN
Ery-Tab Tablets 447
Erythromycin Base Filmtab Tablets 454
Erythromycin Delayed-Release Capsules, USP 456
PCE Dispertab Tablets 510

ROVACOR (India, Singapore)
LOVASTATIN
Mevacor Tablets 1996

ROXATINE (Australia)
PAROXETINE HYDROCHLORIDE
Paxil Oral Suspension 1501
Paxil Tablets 1501

ROXEN (Thailand)
NAPROXEN
EC-Naprosyn Delayed-Release Tablets 2769
Naprosyn Suspension 2769
Naprosyn Tablets 2769

ROXIN (Australia)
NORFLOXACIN
Noroxin Tablets 2009

ROYCEFAX (Brazil)
CEFTAZIDIME
Fortaz for Injection 1422

ROYCHLOR (Canada)
POTASSIUM CHLORIDE
K-Dur Extended-Relase Tablets 3047
K-Lor Powder Packets 472
K-Tab Filmtab Tablets 473

ROYEN (Argentina, Spain)
CALCIUM ACETATE
PhosLo GelCaps 2158

ROZACREME (France)
METRONIDAZOLE
MetroGel-Vaginal Gel 1822
Noritate Cream, 1% 1051

ROZAGEL (France)
METRONIDAZOLE
MetroGel-Vaginal Gel 1822
Noritate Cream, 1% 1051

ROZEX (Argentina, Australia, Austria, Belgium, Brazil, Czech Republic, Denmark, Finland, France, Hong Kong, Irish Republic, Israel, Italy, Malaysia, New Zealand, Norway, Singapore, South Africa, Spain, Sweden, Switzerland, The Netherlands, United Kingdom)
METRONIDAZOLE
MetroGel-Vaginal Gel 1822
Noritate Cream, 1% 1051

R-PRIL (India)
RAMIPRIL
Altace Capsules 1673

RUBACINA (Spain)
FAMOTIDINE
Pepcid Injection 2017
Pepcid Injection Premixed 2017
Pepcid Tablets 2014
Pepcid for Oral Suspension 2014

RUBIFEN (Argentina, New Zealand, Singapore, Spain, The Netherlands)
METHYLPHENIDATE HYDROCHLORIDE
Ritalin Hydrochloride Tablets 2254
Ritalin-SR Tablets 2254

RUBILEM (Mexico)
DAUNORUBICIN HYDROCHLORIDE
Cerubidine for Injection 788

RUBIMYCIN (South Africa)
ERYTHROMYCIN STEARATE
Erythrocin Stearate Filmtab Tablets 452

RUBIULCER (Spain)
RANITIDINE HYDROCHLORIDE
Zantac 25 EFFERdose Tablets 1597
Zantac 150 EFFERdose Tablets 1597
Zantac 150 Tablets 1597
Zantac 300 Tablets 1597
Zantac Injection 1593
Zantac Injection Premixed 1593
Zantac Syrup 1597

RUBOCORD (Greece)
CLOBETASOL PROPIONATE
Temovate Cream 1549
Temovate E Emollient 1552
Temovate Gel 1550
Temovate Ointment 1549
Temovate Scalp Application 1551

RUCAINA (Mexico)
LIDOCAINE
Lidoderm Patch 1107

RUDOLAC (Switzerland)
LACTULOSE
Kristalose for Oral Solution 2149

RUMATAB (Thailand)
DICLOFENAC SODIUM
Voltaren Tablets 2298
Voltaren-XR Tablets 2301

RUPEDEX (Argentina)
DEXAMETHASONE
Decadron Tablets 1929

RUPEDIZ (Argentina)
DIAZEPAM
Diastat Rectal Delivery System 3344
Valium Tablets 2822

RUSSEDYL (Malaysia)
PROMETHAZINE HYDROCHLORIDE
Phenergan Suppositories 3438
Phenergan Tablets 3438

RUSYDE (United Kingdom)
FUROSEMIDE
Furosemide Tablets 2117

RUVOMINOX (Greece)
DICLOFENAC SODIUM
Voltaren Tablets 2298
Voltaren-XR Tablets 2301

RYTHMARONE (France)
AMIODARONE HYDROCHLORIDE
Pacerone Tablets 3337

RYTHMEX (Israel)
PROPAFENONE HYDROCHLORIDE
Rythmol SR Capsules 2736

RYTHMOL (Canada, France, South Africa)
PROPAFENONE HYDROCHLORIDE
Rythmol SR Capsules 2736

RYTHMONOPM (Greece)
PROPAFENONE HYDROCHLORIDE
Rythmol SR Capsules 2736

RYTHOCIN (Thailand)
ERYTHROMYCIN
Ery-Tab Tablets 447
Erythromycin Base Filmtab Tablets 454
Erythromycin Delayed-Release Capsules, USP 456
PCE Dispertab Tablets 510

RYTMOGENAT (Germany)
PROPAFENONE HYDROCHLORIDE
Rythmol SR Capsules 2736

RYTMONORM (Belgium, Chile, Denmark, Finland, Germany, Hong Kong, Hungary, Italy, Malaysia, New Zealand, Portugal, Singapore, Spain, Sweden, Switzerland, Thailand, The Netherlands)
PROPAFENONE HYDROCHLORIDE
Rythmol SR Capsules 2736

RYTMONORMA (Austria)
PROPAFENONE HYDROCHLORIDE
Rythmol SR Capsules 2736

RYTMO-PUREN (Germany)
PROPAFENONE HYDROCHLORIDE
Rythmol SR Capsules 2736

RYVEL (Hong Kong)
CETIRIZINE HYDROCHLORIDE
Zyrtec Syrup 2589
Zyrtec Tablets 2589

SABAX GENTAMIX (South Africa)
GENTAMICIN SULFATE
Garamycin Injectable 3028
Genoptic Sterile Ophthalmic Solution . . . . ⊙227

SABIDAL RECTIOL (Italy)
THEOPHYLLINE
Uniphyl Tablets 2708

SAB-PENTASONE (Canada)
GENTAMICIN SULFATE
Garamycin Injectable 3028
Genoptic Sterile Ophthalmic Solution . . . . ⊙227

SAB-PREDNASE (Canada)
PREDNISOLONE SODIUM PHOSPHATE
Pediapred Oral Solution 3319

SAGITTOL (Germany)
PROPRANOLOL HYDROCHLORIDE
Inderal LA Long-Acting Capsules 3421

SAL DIETETICA (Chile)
POTASSIUM CHLORIDE
K-Dur Extended-Relase Tablets 3047
K-Lor Powder Packets 472
K-Tab Filmtab Tablets 473

SALAC (Argentina)
CLOBETASOL PROPIONATE
Temovate Cream 1549
Temovate E Emollient 1552
Temovate Gel 1550
Temovate Ointment 1549
Temovate Scalp Application 1551

SALDAC (Australia, New Zealand)
SULINDAC
Clinoril Tablets 1899

SALI-ADALAT (Germany)
NIFEDIPINE
Adalat CC Tablets 2978

SALICORT (Argentina)
TRIAMCINOLONE ACETONIDE
Azmacort Inhalation Aerosol 1701
Nasacort AQ Nasal Spray 2937

SALI-PUREN (Germany)
HYDROCHLOROTHIAZIDE/TRIAMTERENE
Dyazide Capsules 1389
Maxzide Tablets 2150
Maxzide-25 mg Tablets 2150

SALMETEDUR (Italy)
SALMETEROL XINAFOATE
Serevent Diskus 1540

SALODIUR (Austria)
HYDROCHLOROTHIAZIDE/TRIAMTERENE
Dyazide Capsules 1389
Maxzide Tablets 2150
Maxzide-25 mg Tablets 2150

SALONGO (Spain)
OXICONAZOLE NITRATE
Oxistat Cream 1498
Oxistat Lotion 1498

SALTERMOX (South Africa)
AMOXICILLIN
Amoxil Pediatric Drops for Oral Suspension 1315
Amoxil Tablets 1315

SALURIC (Irish Republic, United Kingdom)
CHLOROTHIAZIDE
Diuril Oral Suspension 1936
Diuril Tablets 1936

SALURIN (United Arab Emirates)
FUROSEMIDE
Furosemide Tablets 2117

SALVACOLINA NF (Spain)
LOPERAMIDE HYDROCHLORIDE
Imodium Capsules 1834

SALVALERG (Argentina)
CETIRIZINE HYDROCHLORIDE
Zyrtec Syrup 2589
Zyrtec Tablets 2589

SAMERTAN (Chile)
TELMISARTAN
Micardis Tablets 884

SAMIL-02 (Italy)
BENZOYL PEROXIDE
Brevoxyl-4 Creamy Wash 3212
Brevoxyl-4 Gel 3211
Brevoxyl-8 Creamy Wash 3212
Brevoxyl-8 Gel 3211
Triaz Cleanser 1864
Triaz Gel 1864

SAMONIL (Mexico)
METRONIDAZOLE
MetroGel-Vaginal Gel 1822
Noritate Cream, 1% 1051

SAMOX (Thailand)
AMOXICILLIN
Amoxil Pediatric Drops for Oral Suspension 1315
Amoxil Tablets 1315

SAMOXIN (Thailand)
AMOXICILLIN
Amoxil Pediatric Drops for Oral Suspension 1315
Amoxil Tablets 1315

SANALER (Chile)
CETIRIZINE HYDROCHLORIDE
Zyrtec Syrup 2589
Zyrtec Tablets 2589

SANAPRAV (Austria, Italy, Portugal)
PRAVASTATIN SODIUM
Pravachol Tablets 943

SANATISON MONO (Germany)
HYDROCORTISONE
Hydrocortone Tablets 1963

(⊙ Described in PDR For Ophthalmic Medicines™)

SANCAP (Greece)
CAPTOPRIL
Captopril Tablets . . . 2114

SANCIPRO (Denmark)
CIPROFLOXACIN HYDROCHLORIDE
Ciloxan Ophthalmic Ointment . . . 554
Ciloxan Ophthalmic Solution . . . ⊙205
Cipro Tablets . . . 2991

SANDOSTATIN (Canada, Finland, Germany, Irish Republic, Singapore, United Kingdom)
OCTREOTIDE ACETATE
Sandostatin LAR Depot . . . 2264

SANDOSTATINE (France, Switzerland, The Netherlands)
OCTREOTIDE ACETATE
Sandostatin LAR Depot . . . 2264

SANDOZ K (South Africa)
POTASSIUM CHLORIDE
K-Dur Extended-Relase Tablets . . . 3047
K-Lor Powder Packets . . . 472
K-Tab Filmtab Tablets . . . 473

SANDRENA (Australia, Austria, Brazil, Chile, Denmark, Germany, Italy, Mexico, New Zealand, Switzerland, The Netherlands, United Kingdom)
ESTRADIOL
Climara Transdermal System . . . 795
Vivelle Transdermal System . . . 2288
Vivelle-Dot Transdermal System . . . 2293

SANELOR (Chile)
LOVASTATIN
Mevacor Tablets . . . 1996

SANIFUG (Germany)
LOPERAMIDE HYDROCHLORIDE
Imodium Capsules . . . 1834

SANIPRESIN (Chile)
LOSARTAN POTASSIUM
Cozaar Tablets . . . 1913

SANIPRESIN-D (Chile)
HYDROCHLOROTHIAZIDE/LOSARTAN POTASSIUM
Hyzaar 50-12.5 Tablets . . . 1964

SANIPROSTOL (Chile)
FINASTERIDE
Propecia Tablets . . . 2036
Proscar Tablets . . . 2040

SANOXIT (Germany)
BENZOYL PEROXIDE
Brevoxyl-4 Creamy Wash . . . 3212
Brevoxyl-4 Gel . . . 3211
Brevoxyl-8 Creamy Wash . . . 3212
Brevoxyl-8 Gel . . . 3211
Triaz Cleanser . . . 1864
Triaz Gel . . . 1864

SANPRONOL (Brazil)
PROPRANOLOL HYDROCHLORIDE
Inderal LA Long-Acting Capsules . . . 3421

SANSACNE (Mexico)
ERYTHROMYCIN
Ery-Tab Tablets . . . 447
Erythromycin Base Filmtab Tablets . . . 454
Erythromycin Delayed-Release Capsules, USP . . . 456
PCE Dispertab Tablets . . . 510

SANSANAL (Germany)
CAPTOPRIL
Captopril Tablets . . . 2114

SANVAPRESS (Brazil)
ENALAPRIL MALEATE
Vasotec I.V. Injection . . . 2076

SAPUCAI (Argentina)
PERMETHRIN
Acticin Cream . . . 2125

SARCOP (Spain)
PERMETHRIN
Acticin Cream . . . 2125

SARF (United Arab Emirates)
CIPROFLOXACIN HYDROCHLORIDE
Ciloxan Ophthalmic Ointment . . . 554
Ciloxan Ophthalmic Solution . . . ⊙205
Cipro Tablets . . . 2991

SARNA HC (Canada)
HYDROCORTISONE
Hydrocortone Tablets . . . 1963

SAROMET (Argentina)
DIAZEPAM
Diastat Rectal Delivery System . . . 3344
Valium Tablets . . . 2822

SARTON (Czech Republic)
VALSARTAN
Diovan Tablets . . . 2191

SASTID ANTI-FUNGAL (Singapore)
CLOTRIMAZOLE
Lotrimin Cream . . . 3053
Lotrimin Lotion 1% . . . 3053
Lotrimin Topical Solution 1% . . . 3053

SATIGENE (Argentina)
IRINOTECAN HYDROCHLORIDE
Camptosar Injection . . . 2602

SAYOMOL (Spain)
PROMETHAZINE HYDROCHLORIDE
Phenergan Suppositories . . . 3438
Phenergan Tablets . . . 3438

SBOB (Thailand)
LOPERAMIDE HYDROCHLORIDE
Imodium Capsules . . . 1834

SCALPE (India)
KETOCONAZOLE
Nizoral 2% Shampoo . . . 1838

SCALPICIN (Italy)
HYDROCORTISONE
Hydrocortone Tablets . . . 1963

SCALPICIN CAPILAR (Spain)
HYDROCORTISONE
Hydrocortone Tablets . . . 1963

SCALPIN (Greece)
KETOCONAZOLE
Nizoral 2% Shampoo . . . 1838

SCF (Australia)
SUCRALFATE
Carafate Suspension . . . 727
Carafate Tablets . . . 728

SCHEINPHARM TRIAMCINE-A (Canada)
TRIAMCINOLONE ACETONIDE
Azmacort Inhalation Aerosol . . . 1701
Nasacort AQ Nasal Spray . . . 2937

SCHERICUR (Argentina, Austria, Germany, Spain)
HYDROCORTISONE
Hydrocortone Tablets . . . 1963

SCHERITONIN (Argentina)
ISOTRETINOIN
Accutane Capsules . . . 2740

SCHEROGEL (Austria, Belgium, Germany, Italy, Spain)
BENZOYL PEROXIDE
Brevoxyl-4 Creamy Wash . . . 3212
Brevoxyl-4 Gel . . . 3211
Brevoxyl-8 Creamy Wash . . . 3212
Brevoxyl-8 Gel . . . 3211
Triaz Cleanser . . . 1864
Triaz Gel . . . 1864

SCHOLL ATHLETE'S FOOT (Canada)
BUTENAFINE HYDROCHLORIDE
Mentax Cream . . . 2152

SCLERIL (Italy)
FENOFIBRATE
Tricor Tablets . . . 523

SCLEROFIN (Argentina)
FENOFIBRATE
Tricor Tablets . . . 523

SCRIPTOPAM (South Africa)
DIAZEPAM
Diastat Rectal Delivery System . . . 3344
Valium Tablets . . . 2822

SD-HERMAL (Germany)
CLOTRIMAZOLE
Lotrimin Cream . . . 3053
Lotrimin Lotion 1% . . . 3053
Lotrimin Topical Solution 1% . . . 3053

SEALDIN (Spain)
SERTRALINE HYDROCHLORIDE
Zoloft Tablets . . . 2581

SEBERCIM (Italy)
NORFLOXACIN
Noroxin Tablets . . . 2009

SEBIZOLE (Australia, Hong Kong, Malaysia, New Zealand, Singapore)
KETOCONAZOLE
Nizoral 2% Shampoo . . . 1838

SECADINE (South Africa)
CIMETIDINE
Tagamet Tablets . . . 1547

SECALIP (France, Spain)
FENOFIBRATE
Tricor Tablets . . . 523

SECOTEX (Argentina, Brazil, Chile, Mexico)
TAMSULOSIN HYDROCHLORIDE
Flomax Capsules . . . 881

SECUBAR (Spain)
LISINOPRIL
Prinivil Tablets . . . 2029
Zestril Tablets . . . 704

SECUBAR DIU (Spain)
HYDROCHLOROTHIAZIDE/LISINOPRIL
Prinzide Tablets . . . 2033
Zestoretic Tablets . . . 701

SECURO (Argentina)
IVERMECTIN
Stromectol Tablets . . . 2053

SECURON (United Kingdom)
VERAPAMIL HYDROCHLORIDE
Covera-HS Tablets . . . 3135
Verelan PM Capsules . . . 3120

SEDACORON (Austria, Czech Republic, Hong Kong)
AMIODARONE HYDROCHLORIDE
Pacerone Tablets . . . 3337

SEDACRIS (Argentina)
THEOPHYLLINE
Uniphyl Tablets . . . 2708

SEDALIN (Thailand)
CEFTRIAXONE SODIUM
Rocephin Injectable Vials, ADD-Vantage, Galaxy, Bulk . . . 2801

SEDANIUM-R (Greece)
FAMOTIDINE
Pepcid Injection . . . 2017
Pepcid Injection Premixed . . . 2017
Pepcid Tablets . . . 2014
Pepcid for Oral Suspension . . . 2014

SEDESTEROL (Argentina)
DEXAMETHASONE
Decadron Tablets . . . 1929

SEDILIX (Malaysia)
PROMETHAZINE HYDROCHLORIDE
Phenergan Suppositories . . . 3438
Phenergan Tablets . . . 3438

SEDIVER (Mexico)
DIAZEPAM
Diastat Rectal Delivery System . . . 3344
Valium Tablets . . . 2822

SEDONERVIL COMPLEX (Spain)
DIAZEPAM
Diastat Rectal Delivery System . . . 3344
Valium Tablets . . . 2822

SEDOPAN (Greece)
CEFUROXIME AXETIL
Ceftin Tablets . . . 1369
Ceftin for Oral Suspension . . . 1369

SEDOTENSIL (Argentina)
LISINOPRIL
Prinivil Tablets . . . 2029
Zestril Tablets . . . 704

SEDOVANON (Argentina)
CLONAZEPAM
Klonopin Tablets . . . 2782

SEDUXEN (Czech Republic, Hungary, Russia)
DIAZEPAM
Diastat Rectal Delivery System . . . 3344
Valium Tablets . . . 2822

SEDUXEN RG (Czech Republic)
DIAZEPAM
Diastat Rectal Delivery System . . . 3344
Valium Tablets . . . 2822

SEFARETIC (Hong Kong, Thailand)
AMILORIDE HYDROCHLORIDE
Midamor Tablets . . . 2000

SEFDIN (India)
CEFDINIR
Omnicef Capsules . . . 506
Omnicef for Oral Suspension . . . 506

SEFMEX (Hong Kong, Thailand)
SELEGILINE HYDROCHLORIDE
Eldepryl Capsules . . . 3209

SEFNOR (Singapore)
NORFLOXACIN
Noroxin Tablets . . . 2009

SEFULKEN (Mexico)
DIAZOXIDE
Hyperstat I.V. Injection . . . 3031

SEGALIN (Czech Republic)
SELEGILINE HYDROCHLORIDE
Eldepryl Capsules . . . 3209

SEGUREX (Argentina)
SILDENAFIL CITRATE
Viagra Tablets . . . 2552

SEGURIL (Spain)
FUROSEMIDE
Furosemide Tablets . . . 2117

SELADIN (Malaysia, Singapore)
NAPROXEN
EC-Naprosyn Delayed-Release Tablets . . . 2769
Naprosyn Suspension . . . 2769
Naprosyn Tablets . . . 2769

SELAN (Spain)
CEFUROXIME AXETIL
Ceftin Tablets . . . 1369
Ceftin for Oral Suspension . . . 1369

SELECIM (Switzerland)
SELEGILINE HYDROCHLORIDE
Eldepryl Capsules . . . 3209

SELECOM (Italy)
SELEGILINE HYDROCHLORIDE
Eldepryl Capsules . . . 3209

SELECTIN (Italy)
PRAVASTATIN SODIUM
Pravachol Tablets . . . 943

SELECTOFEN (Mexico)
DICLOFENAC SODIUM
Voltaren Tablets . . . 2298
Voltaren-XR Tablets . . . 2301

SELECTOFUR (Mexico)
FUROSEMIDE
Furosemide Tablets . . . 2117

SELEDAT (Italy)
SELEGILINE HYDROCHLORIDE
Eldepryl Capsules . . . 3209

SELEGAM (Germany)
SELEGILINE HYDROCHLORIDE
Eldepryl Capsules . . . 3209

SELEGOS (Hong Kong, Malaysia, Singapore)
SELEGILINE HYDROCHLORIDE
Eldepryl Capsules . . . 3209

SELEKTINE (The Netherlands)
PRAVASTATIN SODIUM
Pravachol Tablets . . . 943

SELEMERCK (Germany)
SELEGILINE HYDROCHLORIDE
Eldepryl Capsules . . . 3209

SELEPARK (Germany)
SELEGILINE HYDROCHLORIDE
Eldepryl Capsules . . . 3209

SELER (Chile)
SILDENAFIL CITRATE
Viagra Tablets . . . 2552

SELERIN (India)
SELEGILINE HYDROCHLORIDE
Eldepryl Capsules . . . 3209

SELES BETA (Italy)
ATENOLOL
Tenormin I.V. Injection . . . 698

SELGENE (Australia, New Zealand, Thailand)
SELEGILINE HYDROCHLORIDE
Eldepryl Capsules . . . 3209

SELGIMED (Germany)
SELEGILINE HYDROCHLORIDE
Eldepryl Capsules . . . 3209

SELGIN (India)
SELEGILINE HYDROCHLORIDE
Eldepryl Capsules **3209**

SELGINA (Chile)
SELEGILINE HYDROCHLORIDE
Eldepryl Capsules **3209**

SELINE (Thailand)
SELEGILINE HYDROCHLORIDE
Eldepryl Capsules **3209**

SELINOL (Sweden)
ATENOLOL
Tenormin I.V. Injection **698**

SELIPRAN (Austria, Switzerland)
PRAVASTATIN SODIUM
Pravachol Tablets **943**

SELOBLOC (Switzerland)
ATENOLOL
Tenormin I.V. Injection **698**

SELOKEN (Austria, Mexico, Spain)
METOPROLOL SUCCINATE
Toprol-XL Tablets **660**

SELOKEN ZOC (Finland, Sweden)
METOPROLOL SUCCINATE
Toprol-XL Tablets **660**

SELOZOK (France)
METOPROLOL SUCCINATE
Toprol-XL Tablets **660**

SELO-ZOK (Belgium, Brazil, Denmark, Norway)
METOPROLOL SUCCINATE
Toprol-XL Tablets **660**

SELPAR (Italy)
SELEGILINE HYDROCHLORIDE
Eldepryl Capsules **3209**

SEMUELE (Greece)
RANITIDINE HYDROCHLORIDE
Zantac 25 EFFERdose Tablets **1597**
Zantac 150 EFFERdose Tablets **1597**
Zantac 150 Tablets **1597**
Zantac 300 Tablets **1597**
Zantac Injection **1593**
Zantac Injection Premixed **1593**
Zantac Syrup **1597**

SENRO (Spain)
NORFLOXACIN
Noroxin Tablets **2009**

SENSATON (Argentina)
CLONAZEPAM
Klonopin Tablets **2782**

SENSIGARD (Italy)
RANITIDINE HYDROCHLORIDE
Zantac 25 EFFERdose Tablets **1597**
Zantac 150 EFFERdose Tablets **1597**
Zantac 150 Tablets **1597**
Zantac 300 Tablets **1597**
Zantac Injection **1593**
Zantac Injection Premixed **1593**
Zantac Syrup **1597**

SENTIAL HYDROCORTISONE (Belgium)
HYDROCORTISONE
Hydrocortone Tablets **1963**

SEPATREM (Czech Republic)
SELEGILINE HYDROCHLORIDE
Eldepryl Capsules **3209**

SEPCEN (Spain)
CIPROFLOXACIN HYDROCHLORIDE
Ciloxan Ophthalmic Ointment **554**
Ciloxan Ophthalmic Solution . . . . . **⊙205**
Cipro Tablets **2991**

SEPRAFILM (United Kingdom)
SODIUM HYALURONATE
Hyalgan Solution **2917**

SEPRAM (Finland, Germany)
CITALOPRAM HYDROBROMIDE
Celexa Tablets **1177**

SEPTICIDE (Argentina)
CIPROFLOXACIN HYDROCHLORIDE
Ciloxan Ophthalmic Ointment **554**
Ciloxan Ophthalmic Solution . . . . . **⊙205**
Cipro Tablets **2991**

SEPTOPAL (Australia, Malaysia)
GENTAMICIN SULFATE
Garamycin Injectable **3028**
Genoptic Sterile Ophthalmic Solution . . . . . **⊙227**

SEQUAX (Argentina)
CLOZAPINE
Clozapine Tablets **2141**
Clozaril Tablets **2174**

SEQUINAN (Argentina)
RISPERIDONE
Risperdal Oral Solution **1658**
Risperdal Tablets **1658**

SERACIN (Thailand)
OFLOXACIN
Floxin Otic Solution **1043**

SERAD (Italy)
SERTRALINE HYDROCHLORIDE
Zoloft Tablets **2581**

SERALGAN (Austria)
CITALOPRAM HYDROBROMIDE
Celexa Tablets **1177**

SERASA (Mexico)
ASPARAGINASE
Elspar for Injection **1943**

SERCERIN (Brazil)
SERTRALINE HYDROCHLORIDE
Zoloft Tablets **2581**

SERCIM (Mexico)
CIMETIDINE
Tagamet Tablets **1547**

SERDEP (India)
SERTRALINE HYDROCHLORIDE
Zoloft Tablets **2581**

SEREDYN (Mexico)
DIAZEPAM
Diastat Rectal Delivery System **3344**
Valium Tablets **2822**

SEREN (Italy)
CHLORDIAZEPOXIDE HYDROCHLORIDE
Librium Capsules **3349**

SEREN VITA (Italy)
CHLORDIAZEPOXIDE HYDROCHLORIDE
Librium Capsules **3349**

SERETIDE (Argentina, Australia, Belgium, Czech Republic, Hong Kong, Hungary, India, Malaysia)
SALMETEROL XINAFOATE
Serevent Diskus **1540**

SERETRAN (Chile)
PAROXETINE HYDROCHLORIDE
Paxil Oral Suspension **1501**
Paxil Tablets **1501**

SEREUPIN (Italy)
PAROXETINE HYDROCHLORIDE
Paxil Oral Suspension **1501**
Paxil Tablets **1501**

SEREVENT (Argentina, Australia, Austria, Belgium, Brazil, Canada, Chile, Czech Republic, Denmark, Finland, France, Germany, Greece, Hong Kong, Hungary, Irish Republic, Israel, Italy, Malaysia, Mexico, New Zealand, Norway, Portugal, Russia, Singapore, South Africa, Spain, Sweden, Switzerland, Thailand, The Netherlands, United Kingdom)
SALMETEROL XINAFOATE
Serevent Diskus **1540**

SERITAL (Germany)
CITALOPRAM HYDROBROMIDE
Celexa Tablets **1177**

SERIVO (Chile)
SERTRALINE HYDROCHLORIDE
Zoloft Tablets **2581**

SERLAIN (Belgium)
SERTRALINE HYDROCHLORIDE
Zoloft Tablets **2581**

SERLIFE (South Africa)
SERTRALINE HYDROCHLORIDE
Zoloft Tablets **2581**

SERLIFT (Czech Republic, Malaysia)
SERTRALINE HYDROCHLORIDE
Zoloft Tablets **2581**

SERLINA (Argentina)
SERTRALINE HYDROCHLORIDE
Zoloft Tablets **2581**

SEROBID (India)
SALMETEROL XINAFOATE
Serevent Diskus **1540**

SERODUR (Denmark)
PAROXETINE HYDROCHLORIDE
Paxil Oral Suspension **1501**
Paxil Tablets **1501**

SEROMYCIN (Canada, Hong Kong)
CYCLOSERINE
Seromycin Capsules **1783**

SEROPRAM (Argentina, Hungary, Spain)
CITALOPRAM HYDROBROMIDE
Celexa Tablets **1177**

SEROQUEL (Argentina, Australia, Austria, Belgium, Brazil, Canada, Chile, Czech Republic, Denmark, Finland, Germany, Greece, Hong Kong, Hungary, Irish Republic, Israel, Italy, Japan, Malaysia, Mexico, New Zealand, Norway, Portugal, Russia, Singapore, South Africa, Spain, Sweden, Switzerland, Thailand, The Netherlands, United Kingdom)
QUETIAPINE FUMARATE
Seroquel Tablets **691**

SEROQUIN (India)
QUETIAPINE FUMARATE
Seroquel Tablets **691**

SEROVIDINA (Mexico)
ZIDOVUDINE
Retrovir Capsules **1533**
Retrovir IV Infusion **1537**
Retrovir Syrup **1533**
Retrovir Tablets **1533**

SEROXAT (Austria, Belgium, Czech Republic, Denmark, Finland, Germany, Greece, Hong Kong, Hungary, Irish Republic, Israel, Italy, Malaysia, Norway, Portugal, Singapore, Spain, Sweden, Thailand, The Netherlands, United Kingdom)
PAROXETINE HYDROCHLORIDE
Paxil Oral Suspension **1501**
Paxil Tablets **1501**

SERTA (India)
SERTRALINE HYDROCHLORIDE
Zoloft Tablets **2581**

SERTIDINE (Mexico)
FAMOTIDINE
Pepcid Injection **2017**
Pepcid Injection Premixed **2017**
Pepcid Tablets **2014**
Pepcid for Oral Suspension **2014**

SERTINAL (Argentina)
SIBUTRAMINE HYDROCHLORIDE
Meridia Capsules **485**

SERTRIXEN (Mexico)
NAPROXEN
EC-Naprosyn Delayed-Release Tablets **2769**
Naprosyn Suspension **2769**
Naprosyn Tablets **2769**

SERVANOLOL (Switzerland)
PROPRANOLOL HYDROCHLORIDE
Inderal LA Long-Acting Capsules **3421**

SERVAZOLIN (Austria)
CEFAZOLIN SODIUM
Ancef for Injection **1318**

SERVICEF (Switzerland)
CEFAZOLIN SODIUM
Ancef for Injection **1318**

SERVIDIPINE (Switzerland)
NIFEDIPINE
Adalat CC Tablets **2978**

SERVIFLOX (Singapore, Thailand)
CIPROFLOXACIN HYDROCHLORIDE
Ciloxan Ophthalmic Ointment **554**
Ciloxan Ophthalmic Solution . . . . . **⊙205**
Cipro Tablets **2991**

SERVIGENTA (Mexico, Switzerland)
GENTAMICIN SULFATE
Garamycin Injectable **3028**
Genoptic Sterile Ophthalmic Solution . . . . . **⊙227**

SERVINAPROX (Switzerland)
NAPROXEN
EC-Naprosyn Delayed-Release Tablets **2769**
Naprosyn Suspension **2769**
Naprosyn Tablets **2769**

SERVIPEP (Hong Kong, Hungary, Singapore)
FAMOTIDINE
Pepcid Injection **2017**
Pepcid Injection Premixed **2017**
Pepcid Tablets **2014**
Pepcid for Oral Suspension **2014**

SERVIRADINE (Mexico)
RANITIDINE HYDROCHLORIDE
Zantac 25 EFFERdose Tablets **1597**
Zantac 150 EFFERdose Tablets **1597**
Zantac 150 Tablets **1597**
Zantac 300 Tablets **1597**
Zantac Injection **1593**
Zantac Injection Premixed **1593**
Zantac Syrup **1597**

SERVITENOL (Switzerland)
ATENOLOL
Tenormin I.V. Injection **698**

SERVIZOL (Singapore)
METRONIDAZOLE
MetroGel-Vaginal Gel **1822**
Noritate Cream, 1% **1051**

SESAREN (Argentina)
VENLAFAXINE HYDROCHLORIDE
Effexor Tablets **3405**
Effexor XR Capsules **3411**

SESTRINE (Argentina)
REPAGLINIDE
Prandin Tablets (0.5, 1, and 2 mg) **2337**

SETANOL (Greece)
NORFLOXACIN
Noroxin Tablets **2009**

SETEGIS (Hungary)
TERAZOSIN HYDROCHLORIDE
Hytrin Capsules **469**

SETIN (Thailand)
CETIRIZINE HYDROCHLORIDE
Zyrtec Syrup **2589**
Zyrtec Tablets **2589**

SETRON (Czech Republic)
ONDANSETRON HYDROCHLORIDE
Zofran Injection **1607**
Zofran Injection Premixed **1607**
Zofran Oral Solution **1613**
Zofran Tablets **1613**

SETRONIL (Chile)
CITALOPRAM HYDROBROMIDE
Celexa Tablets **1177**

SETROZOLE (Malaysia)
METRONIDAZOLE
MetroGel-Vaginal Gel **1822**
Noritate Cream, 1% **1051**

SEVACOL (Argentina)
SIMVASTATIN
Zocor Tablets **2078**

SEVREDOL (Czech Republic, France, Germany, Irish Republic, New Zealand, Portugal, Spain, Switzerland, The Netherlands, United Kingdom)
MORPHINE SULFATE
Kadian Capsules **572**
MS Contin Tablets **2703**

SEVRE-LONG (Switzerland)
MORPHINE SULFATE
Kadian Capsules **572**
MS Contin Tablets **2703**

SFINAC (Greece)
DICLOFENAC SODIUM
Voltaren Tablets **2298**
Voltaren-XR Tablets **2301**

SHAMPOUX (Belgium)
PERMETHRIN
Acticin Cream **2125**

SHEMOL (Mexico)
TIMOLOL MALEATE
Blocadren Tablets **1891**
Timoptic Sterile Ophthalmic Solution **2058**
Timoptic in Ocudose **2061**
Timoptic-XE Sterile Ophthalmic Gel Forming Solution **2062**

SHINCEF (Singapore)
CEFUROXIME SODIUM
Zinacef Injection **1604**

SHINCORT (Malaysia, Singapore, Thailand)
TRIAMCINOLONE ACETONIDE
Azmacort Inhalation Aerosol 1701
Nasacort AQ Nasal Spray 2937

SHINTAMET (Malaysia, Singapore)
CIMETIDINE
Tagamet Tablets 1547

SIAMIDINE (Thailand)
CIMETIDINE
Tagamet Tablets 1547

SIBUNAR (Denmark)
CIPROFLOXACIN HYDROCHLORIDE
Ciloxan Ophthalmic Ointment 554
Ciloxan Ophthalmic Solution .... ⊙205
Cipro Tablets 2991

SIBUTRAL (France)
SIBUTRAMINE HYDROCHLORIDE
Meridia Capsules 485

SIBU-TRATOBES (Argentina)
SIBUTRAMINE HYDROCHLORIDE
Meridia Capsules 485

SICADENTOL PLUS (Argentina)
NAPROXEN
EC-Naprosyn Delayed-Release Tablets 2769
Naprosyn Suspension 2769
Naprosyn Tablets 2769

SICCO (Germany)
INDAPAMIDE
Indapamide Tablets 2119

SICEF (Italy)
CEFAZOLIN SODIUM
Ancef for Injection 1318

SICLOT (Thailand)
TICLOPIDINE HYDROCHLORIDE
Ticlid Tablets 2813

SICO RELAX (Spain)
DIAZEPAM
Diastat Rectal Delivery System 3344
Valium Tablets 2822

SICOR (Hungary)
SIMVASTATIN
Zocor Tablets 2078

SICRIT (Chile)
MEDROXYPROGESTERONE ACETATE
Depo-Medrol Single-Dose Vial 2617

SIGABLOC (Germany)
ATENOLOL
Tenormin I.V. Injection 698

SIGACAP COR (Germany)
CAPTOPRIL
Captopril Tablets 2114

SIGACIMET (Germany)
CIMETIDINE
Tagamet Tablets 1547

SIGACORA (Germany)
ISOSORBIDE MONONITRATE
Imdur Tablets 3032

SIGAFAM (Mexico)
FAMOTIDINE
Pepcid Injection 2017
Pepcid Injection Premixed 2017
Pepcid Tablets 2014
Pepcid for Oral Suspension 2014

SIGAFENAC (Germany)
DICLOFENAC SODIUM
Voltaren Tablets 2298
Voltaren-XR Tablets 2301

SIGAMOPEN (Switzerland)
AMOXICILLIN
Amoxil Pediatric Drops for Oral Suspension 1315
Amoxil Tablets 1315

SIGAPAEDIL (Germany)
ERYTHROMYCIN
Ery-Tab Tablets 447
Erythromycin Base Filmtab Tablets 454
Erythromycin Delayed-Release Capsules, USP 456
PCE Dispertab Tablets 510

SIGASALUR (Germany)
FUROSEMIDE
Furosemide Tablets 2117

SIGMATRIOL (Brazil)
CALCITRIOL
Calcijex Injection 411

SIGMAXIN (Australia)
DIGOXIN
Lanoxicaps Capsules 1458
Lanoxin Injection 1462
Lanoxin Injection Pediatric 1465
Lanoxin Tablets 1468

SIGMETADINE (Australia)
CIMETIDINE
Tagamet Tablets 1547

SILAGRA (India)
SILDENAFIL CITRATE
Viagra Tablets 2552

SILCOR (Argentina)
CALCITRIOL
Calcijex Injection 411

SILDEFIL (Argentina)
SILDENAFIL CITRATE
Viagra Tablets 2552

SILDER (Greece)
ATENOLOL
Tenormin I.V. Injection 698

SILFOX (Argentina)
DICLOFENAC SODIUM
Voltaren Tablets 2298
Voltaren-XR Tablets 2301

SILFOX FLEX (Argentina)
DICLOFENAC SODIUM
Voltaren Tablets 2298
Voltaren-XR Tablets 2301

SILIDRAL (Argentina)
ALENDRONATE SODIUM
Fosamax Tablets 1949

SILINO (Germany)
DICLOFENAC SODIUM
Voltaren Tablets 2298
Voltaren-XR Tablets 2301

SILKIS (Austria, Belgium, Brazil, Finland, France, Germany, Irish Republic, Norway, Portugal, Singapore, Switzerland, The Netherlands, United Kingdom)
CALCITRIOL
Calcijex Injection 411

SILZOLIN (Italy)
CEFAZOLIN SODIUM
Ancef for Injection 1318

SIMAGLEN (Hong Kong, Thailand)
CIMETIDINE
Tagamet Tablets 1547

SIMATOR (Irish Republic)
SIMVASTATIN
Zocor Tablets 2078

SIMCARD (India)
SIMVASTATIN
Zocor Tablets 2078

SIMCHOL (India)
SIMVASTATIN
Zocor Tablets 2078

SIMCORA (Switzerland)
SIMVASTATIN
Zocor Tablets 2078

SIMCORHEXAL (Austria)
SIMVASTATIN
Zocor Tablets 2078

SIMETAC (Hong Kong)
RANITIDINE HYDROCHLORIDE
Zantac 25 EFFERdose Tablets 1597
Zantac 150 EFFERdose Tablets 1597
Zantac 150 Tablets 1597
Zantac 300 Tablets 1597
Zantac Injection 1593
Zantac Injection Premixed 1593
Zantac Syrup 1597

SIMEX (Thailand)
CIMETIDINE
Tagamet Tablets 1547

SIMGAL (Russia)
SIMVASTATIN
Zocor Tablets 2078

SIMIREX (Czech Republic)
SIMVASTATIN
Zocor Tablets 2078

SIMLO (India, Russia)
SIMVASTATIN
Zocor Tablets 2078

SIMOVIL (Israel)
SIMVASTATIN
Zocor Tablets 2078

SIMPERTEN (Chile)
LOSARTAN POTASSIUM
Cozaar Tablets 1913

SIMPERTEN-D (Chile)
HYDROCHLOROTHIAZIDE/LOSARTAN POTASSIUM
Hyzaar 50-12.5 Tablets 1964

SIMSTIN (Austria)
SIMVASTATIN
Zocor Tablets 2078

SIMTAN (Irish Republic)
SIMVASTATIN
Zocor Tablets 2078

SIMTEC (Malaysia)
CETIRIZINE HYDROCHLORIDE
Zyrtec Syrup 2589
Zyrtec Tablets 2589

SIMTIN (Hong Kong, Singapore)
SIMVASTATIN
Zocor Tablets 2078

SIMULECT (Argentina, Australia, Belgium, Brazil, Canada, Chile, Czech Republic, Denmark, Finland, France, Germany, Greece, Hong Kong, Irish Republic, Israel, Italy, Malaysia, Mexico, New Zealand, Norway, Portugal, Russia, Singapore, South Africa, Spain, Sweden, Switzerland, Thailand, The Netherlands, United Kingdom)
BASILIXIMAB
Simulect for Injection 2268

SIMULTAN (Argentina, Chile)
VALSARTAN
Diovan Tablets 2191

SIMULTAN D (Argentina)
VALSARTAN
Diovan Tablets 2191

SIMVAAPS (Germany)
SIMVASTATIN
Zocor Tablets 2078

SIMVABETA (Germany)
SIMVASTATIN
Zocor Tablets 2078

SIMVACARD (Czech Republic, Germany)
SIMVASTATIN
Zocor Tablets 2078

SIMVACHOL (Greece)
SIMVASTATIN
Zocor Tablets 2078

SIMVACOL (Hungary, Portugal)
SIMVASTATIN
Zocor Tablets 2078

SIMVACOR (Germany, Greece, Israel, Malaysia, Singapore, South Africa)
SIMVASTATIN
Zocor Tablets 2078

SIMVADOR (United Kingdom)
SIMVASTATIN
Zocor Tablets 2078

SIMVADURA (Germany)
SIMVASTATIN
Zocor Tablets 2078

SIMVAGAMMA (Germany)
SIMVASTATIN
Zocor Tablets 2078

SIMVAHEXAL (Australia)
SIMVASTATIN
Zocor Tablets 2078

SIMVAR (Australia)
SIMVASTATIN
Zocor Tablets 2078

SIMVASINE (Switzerland)
SIMVASTATIN
Zocor Tablets 2078

SIMVAST (Switzerland)
SIMVASTATIN
Zocor Tablets 2078

SIMVASTAD (Austria)
SIMVASTATIN
Zocor Tablets 2078

SIMVASTEN (Spain)
SIMVASTATIN
Zocor Tablets 2078

SIMVASTIN (Switzerland)
SIMVASTATIN
Zocor Tablets 2078

SIMVASTOL (Russia)
SIMVASTATIN
Zocor Tablets 2078

SIMVASTUR (Spain)
SIMVASTATIN
Zocor Tablets 2078

SIMVATIN (Austria)
SIMVASTATIN
Zocor Tablets 2078

SIMVAX (Czech Republic)
SIMVASTATIN
Zocor Tablets 2078

SIMVOR (Czech Republic, Hungary, Malaysia, Singapore, Thailand)
SIMVASTATIN
Zocor Tablets 2078

SIMVOTIN (India, South Africa)
SIMVASTATIN
Zocor Tablets 2078

SIMZOR (Irish Republic)
SIMVASTATIN
Zocor Tablets 2078

SINALFA (Denmark, Norway, Sweden)
TERAZOSIN HYDROCHLORIDE
Hytrin Capsules 469

SINAMIDA ECONAZOL (Argentina)
ECONAZOLE NITRATE
Spectazole Cream 2390

SINARONA (Mexico)
AMIODARONE HYDROCHLORIDE
Pacerone Tablets 3337

SINCERCK (Mexico)
PRAZIQUANTEL
Biltricide Tablets 2990

SINEGASTRIN (Mexico)
CIMETIDINE
Tagamet Tablets 1547

SINERTEC (Italy)
ENALAPRIL MALEATE/HYDROCHLOROTHIAZIDE
Vaseretic Tablets 2073

SINGULAIR (Argentina, Australia, Austria, Belgium, Brazil, Canada, Chile, Czech Republic, Denmark, Finland, France, Germany, Greece, Hong Kong, Hungary, Irish Republic, Israel, Italy, Malaysia, Mexico, New Zealand, Norway, Portugal, Singapore, South Africa, Spain, Sweden, Switzerland, Thailand, The Netherlands, United Kingdom)
MONTELUKAST SODIUM
Singulair Chewable Tablets 2047
Singulair Tablets 2047

SINOBID (Greece)
NORFLOXACIN
Noroxin Tablets 2009

SINOPREN (South Africa)
LISINOPRIL
Prinivil Tablets 2029
Zestril Tablets 704

SINOPRIL (Russia)
LISINOPRIL
Prinivil Tablets 2029
Zestril Tablets 704

SINOVIAL (France)
SODIUM HYALURONATE
Hyalgan Solution 2917

SINPET (Mexico)
PHENTERMINE HYDROCHLORIDE
Adipex-P Capsules 1216
Adipex-P Tablets 1216

(⊙ Described in PDR For Ophthalmic Medicines™)

SINPOR (Portugal)
SIMVASTATIN
Zocor Tablets . . . 2078

SINTENYL (Switzerland)
FENTANYL CITRATE
Actiq . . . 993

SINTOFENAC (Brazil)
DICLOFENAC SODIUM
Voltaren Tablets . . . 2298
Voltaren-XR Tablets . . . 2301

SINTOLATT (Italy)
LACTULOSE
Kristalose for Oral Solution . . . 2149

SINVACOR (Italy)
SIMVASTATIN
Zocor Tablets . . . 2078

SINVASCOR (Brazil)
SIMVASTATIN
Zocor Tablets . . . 2078

SINVASTACOR (Brazil)
SIMVASTATIN
Zocor Tablets . . . 2078

SINVASTIL (Portugal)
SIMVASTATIN
Zocor Tablets . . . 2078

SINVATROX (Brazil)
SIMVASTATIN
Zocor Tablets . . . 2078

SIPAM (Thailand)
DIAZEPAM
Diastat Rectal Delivery System . . . 3344
Valium Tablets . . . 2822

SIPRION (Finland)
CIPROFLOXACIN HYDROCHLORIDE
Ciloxan Ophthalmic Ointment . . . 554
Ciloxan Ophthalmic Solution . . . ⊙205
Cipro Tablets . . . 2991

SIRBEN (Brazil)
MEBENDAZOLE
Vermox Chewable Tablets . . . 1853

SIROLAX (Israel)
LACTULOSE
Kristalose for Oral Solution . . . 2149

SIROTAMICIN HC (Argentina)
HYDROCORTISONE
Hydrocortone Tablets . . . 1963

SIRTAL (Austria, Germany)
CARBAMAZEPINE
Carbatrol Capsules . . . 3174
Tegretol Chewable Tablets . . . 2278
Tegretol Suspension . . . 2278
Tegretol Tablets . . . 2278
Tegretol-XR Tablets . . . 2278

SISARE MONO (Germany)
ESTRADIOL
Climara Transdermal System . . . 795
Vivelle Transdermal System . . . 2288
Vivelle-Dot Transdermal System . . . 2293

SITERIN (Finland)
CETIRIZINE HYDROCHLORIDE
Zyrtec Syrup . . . 2589
Zyrtec Tablets . . . 2589

SITRIOL (Australia)
CALCITRIOL
Calcijex Injection . . . 411

SIVASTIN (Italy)
SIMVASTATIN
Zocor Tablets . . . 2078

SIVATIN (Irish Republic)
SIMVASTATIN
Zocor Tablets . . . 2078

SIVLOR (Argentina)
LOVASTATIN
Mevacor Tablets . . . 1996

SIZOPIN (India)
CLOZAPINE
Clozapine Tablets . . . 2141
Clozaril Tablets . . . 2174

SIZORISP (India)
RISPERIDONE
Risperdal Oral Solution . . . 1658
Risperdal Tablets . . . 1658

SKENAN (Belgium, Czech Republic, France, Italy, Portugal, Spain, The Netherlands)
MORPHINE SULFATE
Kadian Capsules . . . 572
MS Contin Tablets . . . 2703

SKEZIDE (Thailand)
HYDROCHLOROTHIAZIDE/TRIAMTERENE
Dyazide Capsules . . . 1389
Maxzide Tablets . . . 2150
Maxzide-25 mg Tablets . . . 2150

SKID E (Germany)
ERYTHROMYCIN
Ery-Tab Tablets . . . 447
Erythromycin Base Filmtab Tablets . . . 454
Erythromycin Delayed-Release Capsules, USP . . . 456
PCE Dispertab Tablets . . . 510

SKILAR (Italy)
ECONAZOLE NITRATE
Spectazole Cream . . . 2390

SKINCALM (South Africa)
HYDROCORTISONE
Hydrocortone Tablets . . . 1963

SKINFECT (Thailand)
GENTAMICIN SULFATE
Garamycin Injectable . . . 3028
Genoptic Sterile Ophthalmic Solution . . . ⊙227

SKITZ (Australia)
BENZOYL PEROXIDE
Brevoxyl-4 Creamy Wash . . . 3212
Brevoxyl-4 Gel . . . 3211
Brevoxyl-8 Creamy Wash . . . 3212
Brevoxyl-8 Gel . . . 3211
Triaz Cleanser . . . 1864
Triaz Gel . . . 1864

SLIMIN (Germany)
HYDROCHLOROTHIAZIDE/TRIAMTERENE
Dyazide Capsules . . . 1389
Maxzide Tablets . . . 2150
Maxzide-25 mg Tablets . . . 2150

SLO-BID (Australia, Canada, Hong Kong, Mexico)
THEOPHYLLINE
Uniphyl Tablets . . . 2708

SLOFEDIPINE (United Kingdom)
NIFEDIPINE
Adalat CC Tablets . . . 2978

SLOFENAC (United Kingdom)
DICLOFENAC SODIUM
Voltaren Tablets . . . 2298
Voltaren-XR Tablets . . . 2301

SLO-MORPH (Irish Republic)
MORPHINE SULFATE
Kadian Capsules . . . 572
MS Contin Tablets . . . 2703

SLO-PHYLLIN (Irish Republic, Italy, United Kingdom)
THEOPHYLLINE
Uniphyl Tablets . . . 2708

SLO-PRO (United Kingdom)
PROPRANOLOL HYDROCHLORIDE
Inderal LA Long-Acting Capsules . . . 3421

SLOPROLOL (United Kingdom)
PROPRANOLOL HYDROCHLORIDE
Inderal LA Long-Acting Capsules . . . 3421

SLO-THEO (Hong Kong)
THEOPHYLLINE
Uniphyl Tablets . . . 2708

SLOVALGIN (Czech Republic)
MORPHINE SULFATE
Kadian Capsules . . . 572
MS Contin Tablets . . . 2703

SLOW DERALIN (Israel)
PROPRANOLOL HYDROCHLORIDE
Inderal LA Long-Acting Capsules . . . 3421

SLOW K (Chile)
POTASSIUM CHLORIDE
K-Dur Extended-Relase Tablets . . . 3047
K-Lor Powder Packets . . . 472
K-Tab Filmtab Tablets . . . 473

SLOW-K (Australia, Brazil, Canada, Hong Kong, Irish Republic, Israel, Malaysia, New Zealand, South Africa, The Netherlands)
POTASSIUM CHLORIDE
K-Dur Extended-Relase Tablets . . . 3047
K-Lor Powder Packets . . . 472
K-Tab Filmtab Tablets . . . 473

SLOZEM (United Kingdom)
DILTIAZEM HYDROCHLORIDE
Cardizem LA Extended Release Tablets . . . 1699
Tiazac Capsules . . . 1204

SMARIL (Greece)
RANITIDINE HYDROCHLORIDE
Zantac 25 EFFERdose Tablets . . . 1597
Zantac 150 EFFERdose Tablets . . . 1597
Zantac 150 Tablets . . . 1597
Zantac 300 Tablets . . . 1597
Zantac Injection . . . 1593
Zantac Injection Premixed . . . 1593
Zantac Syrup . . . 1597

SNOFFOCIN (Thailand)
NORFLOXACIN
Noroxin Tablets . . . 2009

SOBREPINA (Portugal)
NIMODIPINE
Nimotop Capsules . . . 774

SOBRONIL (Spain)
NAPROXEN
EC-Naprosyn Delayed-Release Tablets . . . 2769
Naprosyn Suspension . . . 2769
Naprosyn Tablets . . . 2769

SOCALM (India)
QUETIAPINE FUMARATE
Seroquel Tablets . . . 691

SOCOSEP (Argentina)
KETOCONAZOLE
Nizoral 2% Shampoo . . . 1838

SODEN (Hong Kong, Singapore)
NAPROXEN SODIUM
Anaprox DS Tablets . . . 2769
Anaprox Tablets . . . 2769

SODEXX CIMETIDINE (Austria)
CIMETIDINE
Tagamet Tablets . . . 1547

SODEXX FAMOTIDINE (Austria)
FAMOTIDINE
Pepcid Injection . . . 2017
Pepcid Injection Premixed . . . 2017
Pepcid Tablets . . . 2014
Pepcid for Oral Suspension . . . 2014

SODICLO (South Africa)
DICLOFENAC SODIUM
Voltaren Tablets . . . 2298
Voltaren-XR Tablets . . . 2301

SODIP-PHYLLINE (Switzerland)
THEOPHYLLINE
Uniphyl Tablets . . . 2708

SODIUM SULAMYD (Canada)
SULFACETAMIDE SODIUM
Klaron Lotion 10% . . . 1050

SODIXEN (Mexico)
NAPROXEN SODIUM
Anaprox DS Tablets . . . 2769
Anaprox Tablets . . . 2769

SOFASIN (Greece)
NORFLOXACIN
Noroxin Tablets . . . 2009

SOFLAX (United Arab Emirates)
LACTULOSE
Kristalose for Oral Solution . . . 2149

SOGILEN (Spain)
CABERGOLINE
Dostinex Tablets . . . 2631

SOKARAL (Germany)
DEXAMETHASONE
Decadron Tablets . . . 1929

SOLARAZE (Denmark, Finland, France, Germany, Irish Republic, Italy, Sweden, United Kingdom)
DICLOFENAC SODIUM
Voltaren Tablets . . . 2298
Voltaren-XR Tablets . . . 2301

SOLARCAINE (Switzerland)
LIDOCAINE
Lidoderm Patch . . . 1107

SOLDESAM (Italy)
DEXAMETHASONE SODIUM PHOSPHATE
Decadron Phosphate Injection . . . 1931

SOLDESANIL (Greece)
DEXAMETHASONE SODIUM PHOSPHATE
Decadron Phosphate Injection . . . 1931

SOLEXA (Austria, Italy, Portugal, The Netherlands)
CELECOXIB
Celebrex Capsules . . . 3130

SOLFIDIN (Argentina)
CLONAZEPAM
Klonopin Tablets . . . 2782

SOLGERETIK (Germany)
NADOLOL
Nadolol Tablets . . . 2121

SOLGOL (Austria, Germany, Spain)
NADOLOL
Nadolol Tablets . . . 2121

SOLIS (United Kingdom)
DIAZEPAM
Diastat Rectal Delivery System . . . 3344
Valium Tablets . . . 2822

SOLIUM (Canada)
CHLORDIAZEPOXIDE HYDROCHLORIDE
Librium Capsules . . . 3349

SOLONE (Spain)
DEXAMETHASONE SODIUM PHOSPHATE
Decadron Phosphate Injection . . . 1931

SOLOSA (Greece, Italy)
GLIMEPIRIDE
Amaryl Tablets . . . 2864

SOLOSIN (Germany)
THEOPHYLLINE
Uniphyl Tablets . . . 2708

SOLOSPRIN (India)
ISOSORBIDE MONONITRATE
Imdur Tablets . . . 3032

SOLSOLONA (Mexico)
METHYLPREDNISOLONE ACETATE
Depo-Medrol Injectable Suspension . . . 2615

SOLTRIC (Mexico)
MEBENDAZOLE
Vermox Chewable Tablets . . . 1853

SOLUCEL (Spain)
BENZOYL PEROXIDE
Brevoxyl-4 Creamy Wash . . . 3212
Brevoxyl-4 Gel . . . 3211
Brevoxyl-8 Creamy Wash . . . 3212
Brevoxyl-8 Gel . . . 3211
Triaz Cleanser . . . 1864
Triaz Gel . . . 1864

SOLUCORT (France)
PREDNISOLONE SODIUM PHOSPHATE
Pediapred Oral Solution . . . 3319

SOLUDAMIN (Greece)
LEVOCARNITINE
Carnitor Injection . . . 3185
Carnitor Tablets and Oral Solution . . . 3187

SOLUDECADRON (France)
DEXAMETHASONE SODIUM PHOSPHATE
Decadron Phosphate Injection . . . 1931

SOLUGEL (Argentina, Brazil, Canada, Chile, Mexico)
BENZOYL PEROXIDE
Brevoxyl-4 Creamy Wash . . . 3212
Brevoxyl-4 Gel . . . 3211
Brevoxyl-8 Creamy Wash . . . 3212
Brevoxyl-8 Gel . . . 3211
Triaz Cleanser . . . 1864
Triaz Gel . . . 1864

SOLUMIDAZOL (Mexico)
METRONIDAZOLE
MetroGel-Vaginal Gel . . . 1822
Noritate Cream, 1% . . . 1051

SOLUPEN N (Germany)
DEXAMETHASONE SODIUM PHOSPHATE
Decadron Phosphate Injection . . . 1931

SOLUTIO CORDES DEXA N (Germany)
DEXAMETHASONE
Decadron Tablets . . . 1929

SOLVENTE INDOLORO (Argentina)
LIDOCAINE
Lidoderm Patch . . . 1107

SOLVETAN (Greece)
CEFTAZIDIME
Fortaz for Injection . . . 1422

SOMAFLEX (Greece)
ETIDRONATE DISODIUM
Didronel Tablets . . . 2693

SOMALGESIC (Mexico)
NAPROXEN
EC-Naprosyn Delayed-Release Tablets 2769
Naprosyn Suspension 2769
Naprosyn Tablets 2769

SOMAPLUS (Brazil)
DIAZEPAM
Diastat Rectal Delivery System 3344
Valium Tablets 2822

SOMATRAN (Chile)
SUMATRIPTAN
Imitrex Nasal Spray 1435

SOMINEX (United Kingdom)
PROMETHAZINE HYDROCHLORIDE
Phenergan Suppositories 3438
Phenergan Tablets 3438

SOMNATROL (Argentina)
ESTAZOLAM
ProSom Tablets 512

SOMOFILLINA (Italy)
THEOPHYLLINE
Uniphyl Tablets 2708

SOMOPHYLLIN (Canada, South Africa)
THEOPHYLLINE
Uniphyl Tablets 2708

SONAP (Thailand)
NAPROXEN SODIUM
Anaprox DS Tablets 2769
Anaprox Tablets 2769

SONSUUR (South Africa)
CIMETIDINE
Tagamet Tablets 1547

SOPENTAL (South Africa)
PENTOBARBITAL SODIUM
Nembutal Sodium Solution, USP 2484

SOPHIDONE (France)
HYDROMORPHONE HYDROCHLORIDE
Dilaudid Ampules 439
Dilaudid Multiple Dose Vials 439
Dilaudid Non-Sterile Powder 439
Dilaudid Oral Liquid 443
Dilaudid Rectal Suppositories 439
Dilaudid Tablets 439
Dilaudid Tablets - 8 mg 443
Dilaudid-HP Injection 441
Dilaudid-HP Lyophilized Powder 250 mg 441

SOPHIXIN (Mexico)
CIPROFLOXACIN HYDROCHLORIDE
Ciloxan Ophthalmic Ointment 554
Ciloxan Ophthalmic Solution .... ⊙205
Cipro Tablets 2991

SOPORIL (Germany)
PROMETHAZINE HYDROCHLORIDE
Phenergan Suppositories 3438
Phenergan Tablets 3438

SOPROXEN (Singapore, Thailand)
NAPROXEN SODIUM
Anaprox DS Tablets 2769
Anaprox Tablets 2769

SORBIMON (Austria, Czech Republic, Hungary)
ISOSORBIDE MONONITRATE
Imdur Tablets 3032

SOREDINE (Greece)
RANITIDINE HYDROCHLORIDE
Zantac 25 EFFERdose Tablets 1597
Zantac 150 EFFERdose Tablets 1597
Zantac 150 Tablets 1597
Zantac 300 Tablets 1597
Zantac Injection 1593
Zantac Injection Premixed 1593
Zantac Syrup 1597

SOREN (Hong Kong)
NAPROXEN SODIUM
Anaprox DS Tablets 2769
Anaprox Tablets 2769

SORIATANE (Canada, France)
ACITRETIN
Soriatane Capsules 1028

SORIDERMAL (Chile)
KETOCONAZOLE
Nizoral 2% Shampoo 1838

SORMON (Irish Republic)
ISOSORBIDE MONONITRATE
Imdur Tablets 3032

SORTIS (Austria, Czech Republic, Hungary, Switzerland)
ATORVASTATIN CALCIUM
Lipitor Tablets 2495

SOSTATIN (Greece)
KETOCONAZOLE
Nizoral 2% Shampoo 1838

SOSTILAR (Belgium)
CABERGOLINE
Dostinex Tablets 2631

SOSTRIL (Germany)
RANITIDINE HYDROCHLORIDE
Zantac 25 EFFERdose Tablets 1597
Zantac 150 EFFERdose Tablets 1597
Zantac 150 Tablets 1597
Zantac 300 Tablets 1597
Zantac Injection 1593
Zantac Injection Premixed 1593
Zantac Syrup 1597

SOTAZIDEN N (Germany)
NADOLOL
Nadolol Tablets 2121

SOTOMYCIN (Greece)
CLINDAMYCIN PHOSPHATE
Clindets Pledgets 3212

SOTOVASTIN (Greece)
SIMVASTATIN
Zocor Tablets 2078

SP 54 (Hungary)
PENTOSAN POLYSULFATE SODIUM
Elmiron Capsules 2393

SP54 (Hong Kong)
PENTOSAN POLYSULFATE SODIUM
Elmiron Capsules 2393

SPAN-K (Australia, Hong Kong, New Zealand)
POTASSIUM CHLORIDE
K-Dur Extended-Relase Tablets 3047
K-Lor Powder Packets 472
K-Tab Filmtab Tablets 473

SPARKAL (Denmark, Finland, Sweden)
AMILORIDE HYDROCHLORIDE/HYDROCHLOROTHIAZIDE
Moduretic Tablets 2003

SPECTROBAK (Spain)
GENTAMICIN SULFATE
Garamycin Injectable 3028
Genoptic Sterile Ophthalmic Solution .... ⊙227

SPECTROXYL (Switzerland)
AMOXICILLIN
Amoxil Pediatric Drops for Oral Suspension 1315
Amoxil Tablets 1315

SPECTRUM (Italy)
CEFTAZIDIME
Fortaz for Injection 1422

SPERSACET (Hong Kong, Switzerland)
SULFACETAMIDE SODIUM
Klaron Lotion 10% 1050

SPERSADEX (Canada, Germany, Hong Kong, Norway, South Africa, Switzerland)
DEXAMETHASONE SODIUM PHOSPHATE
Decadron Phosphate Injection 1931

SPERSADEX COMP (Hungary, Malaysia)
DEXAMETHASONE SODIUM PHOSPHATE
Decadron Phosphate Injection 1931

SPERSADEX COMPOSITUM (Czech Republic)
DEXAMETHASONE SODIUM PHOSPHATE
Decadron Phosphate Injection 1931

SPERSAMIDE (South Africa)
SULFACETAMIDE SODIUM
Klaron Lotion 10% 1050

SPIROLAIR (Belgium)
PIRBUTEROL ACETATE
Maxair Autohaler 1820

SPIRON (Chile)
RISPERIDONE
Risperdal Oral Solution 1658
Risperdal Tablets 1658

SPLENDIL (Brazil, Chile, Japan)
FELODIPINE
Plendil Extended-Release Tablets 651

SPOFALYT-KALIUM (Czech Republic)
POTASSIUM CHLORIDE
K-Dur Extended-Relase Tablets 3047
K-Lor Powder Packets 472
K-Tab Filmtab Tablets 473

SPONDY-DEXA (Germany)
DEXAMETHASONE SODIUM PHOSPHATE
Decadron Phosphate Injection 1931

SPONIF (Czech Republic)
NIFEDIPINE
Adalat CC Tablets 2978

SPOPHYLLIN (Czech Republic)
THEOPHYLLINE
Uniphyl Tablets 2708

SPOROXYL (Thailand)
KETOCONAZOLE
Nizoral 2% Shampoo 1838

SPOZAL (Singapore)
KETOCONAZOLE
Nizoral 2% Shampoo 1838

SPREDIOL (Italy)
ESTRADIOL
Climara Transdermal System 795
Vivelle Transdermal System 2288
Vivelle-Dot Transdermal System 2293

SQWORM (Australia)
MEBENDAZOLE
Vermox Chewable Tablets 1853

SRM-RHOTARD (Singapore, South Africa)
MORPHINE SULFATE
Kadian Capsules 572
MS Contin Tablets 2703

STACER (Portugal)
RANITIDINE HYDROCHLORIDE
Zantac 25 EFFERdose Tablets 1597
Zantac 150 EFFERdose Tablets 1597
Zantac 150 Tablets 1597
Zantac 300 Tablets 1597
Zantac Injection 1593
Zantac Injection Premixed 1593
Zantac Syrup 1597

STACIN (Thailand)
ERYTHROMYCIN
Ery-Tab Tablets 447
Erythromycin Base Filmtab Tablets 454
Erythromycin Delayed-Release Capsules, USP 456
PCE Dispertab Tablets 510

STACORT-A (Hong Kong)
TRIAMCINOLONE ACETONIDE
Azmacort Inhalation Aerosol 1701
Nasacort AQ Nasal Spray 2937

STADA K (Hong Kong)
KETOCONAZOLE
Nizoral 2% Shampoo 1838

STADELANT (Greece)
ENALAPRIL MALEATE
Vasotec I.V. Injection 2076

STAMAR (Argentina)
STAVUDINE
Zerit Capsules 971
Zerit for Oral Solution 971

STARCEF (Italy)
CEFTAZIDIME
Fortaz for Injection 1422

STARVAL (India)
VALSARTAN
Diovan Tablets 2191

STATEX (Canada, Singapore)
MORPHINE SULFATE
Kadian Capsules 572
MS Contin Tablets 2703

STATICIN (Canada)
ERYTHROMYCIN
Ery-Tab Tablets 447
Erythromycin Base Filmtab Tablets 454
Erythromycin Delayed-Release Capsules, USP 456
PCE Dispertab Tablets 510

STATICINE (Switzerland)
ERYTHROMYCIN
Ery-Tab Tablets 447
Erythromycin Base Filmtab Tablets 454
Erythromycin Delayed-Release Capsules, USP 456
PCE Dispertab Tablets 510

STATINAL (Greece)
SIMVASTATIN
Zocor Tablets 2078

STAURODORM (Austria)
FLURAZEPAM HYDROCHLORIDE
Dalmane Capsules 3343

STAVIR (India, South Africa)
STAVUDINE
Zerit Capsules 971
Zerit for Oral Solution 971

STAVUBERGEN (Argentina)
STAVUDINE
Zerit Capsules 971
Zerit for Oral Solution 971

STAZEPINE (Hungary)
CARBAMAZEPINE
Carbatrol Capsules 3174
Tegretol Chewable Tablets 2278
Tegretol Suspension 2278
Tegretol Tablets 2278
Tegretol-XR Tablets 2278

STEDON (Greece)
DIAZEPAM
Diastat Rectal Delivery System 3344
Valium Tablets 2822

STEINACLOX (Greece)
NORFLOXACIN
Noroxin Tablets 2009

STELEA (Argentina)
STAVUDINE
Zerit Capsules 971
Zerit for Oral Solution 971

STENOCOR (Italy)
DIPYRIDAMOLE
Persantine Tablets 898

STERICEF (India)
CEFTRIAXONE SODIUM
Rocephin Injectable Vials, ADD-Vantage, Galaxy, Bulk 2801

STERIGIN (Austria)
ESTRADIOL
Climara Transdermal System 795
Vivelle Transdermal System 2288
Vivelle-Dot Transdermal System 2293

STERODEX (Israel)
DEXAMETHASONE SODIUM PHOSPHATE
Decadron Phosphate Injection 1931

STERODOME (Greece)
ETIDRONATE DISODIUM
Didronel Tablets 2693

STERONASE AQ (Israel)
TRIAMCINOLONE ACETONIDE
Azmacort Inhalation Aerosol 1701
Nasacort AQ Nasal Spray 2937

STEROPOTASSIUM (Belgium)
POTASSIUM CHLORIDE
K-Dur Extended-Relase Tablets 3047
K-Lor Powder Packets 472
K-Tab Filmtab Tablets 473

STEROSTATINE (Belgium)
NYSTATIN
Nystop Topical Powder USP 2490

STESOLID (Austria, Czech Republic, Denmark, Finland, Germany, Greece, Hong Kong, Hungary, Irish Republic, Israel, Norway, Portugal, Singapore, Spain, Sweden, Switzerland, Thailand, The Netherlands, United Kingdom)
DIAZEPAM
Diastat Rectal Delivery System 3344
Valium Tablets 2822

STEVENCILLIN (Greece)
AMOXICILLIN
Amoxil Pediatric Drops for Oral Suspension 1315
Amoxil Tablets 1315

(⊙ Described in PDR For Ophthalmic Medicines™)

STIEBENYL (Greece)
RAMIPRIL
Altace Capsules 1673

STIEFCORTIL (Argentina, Brazil)
HYDROCORTISONE
Hydrocortone Tablets 1963

STIEFOTREX (Greece)
ISOTRETINOIN
Accutane Capsules 2740

STIEMAZOL (Germany, South Africa)
CLOTRIMAZOLE
Lotrimin Cream 3053
Lotrimin Lotion 1% 3053
Lotrimin Topical Solution 1% 3053

STIEMYCIN (Argentina, Brazil, Hong Kong, Irish Republic, Malaysia, Mexico, New Zealand, Singapore, South Africa, Thailand, The Netherlands, United Kingdom)
ERYTHROMYCIN
Ery-Tab Tablets 447
Erythromycin Base Filmtab Tablets 454
Erythromycin Delayed-Release Capsules, USP 456
PCE Dispertab Tablets 510

STIEMYCINE (Austria, Germany, Switzerland)
ERYTHROMYCIN
Ery-Tab Tablets 447
Erythromycin Base Filmtab Tablets 454
Erythromycin Delayed-Release Capsules, USP 456
PCE Dispertab Tablets 510

STIEVA-A (Australia, Canada, Chile, Hong Kong, Malaysia, Mexico, Singapore, Thailand)
TRETINOIN
Avita Cream 2136
Avita Gel 2138
Renova 0.05% Cream 2387
Retin-A Micro 0.1%/0.04% 2388
Vesanoid Capsules 2823

STIEVAMYCIN (Argentina, Canada, Mexico)
TRETINOIN
Avita Cream 2136
Avita Gel 2138
Renova 0.05% Cream 2387
Retin-A Micro 0.1%/0.04% 2388
Vesanoid Capsules 2823

STIGMICARPIN (Greece)
NIMODIPINE
Nimotop Capsules 774

STILL (Brazil)
DICLOFENAC SODIUM
Voltaren Tablets 2298
Voltaren-XR Tablets 2301

STILLINE (United Kingdom)
SELEGILINE HYDROCHLORIDE
Eldepryl Capsules 3209

STILOZ (India)
CILOSTAZOL
Pletal Tablets 2478

STIMOLCARDIO (Italy)
DIPYRIDAMOLE
Persantine Tablets 898

STIMULOTON (Hungary, Russia)
SERTRALINE HYDROCHLORIDE
Zoloft Tablets 2581

STIMYCINE (France)
ERYTHROMYCIN
Ery-Tab Tablets 447
Erythromycin Base Filmtab Tablets 454
Erythromycin Delayed-Release Capsules, USP 456
PCE Dispertab Tablets 510

STIOXYL (Sweden)
BENZOYL PEROXIDE
Brevoxyl-4 Creamy Wash 3212
Brevoxyl-4 Gel 3211
Brevoxyl-8 Creamy Wash 3212
Brevoxyl-8 Gel 3211
Triaz Cleanser 1864
Triaz Gel 1864

STIVATE (Thailand)
CLOBETASOL PROPIONATE
Temovate Cream 1549
Temovate E Emollient 1552
Temovate Gel 1550
Temovate Ointment 1549
Temovate Scalp Application 1551

STOCRIN (Argentina, Australia, Austria, Belgium, Brazil, Chile, Czech Republic, Denmark, Finland, Greece, Hong Kong, Israel, Malaysia, Mexico, New Zealand, Norway, Portugal, Russia, Singapore, South Africa, Sweden, Switzerland, Thailand, The Netherlands)
EFAVIRENZ
Sustiva Capsules 957

STOMAKON (Brazil)
CIMETIDINE
Tagamet Tablets 1547

STOMEDINE (France)
CIMETIDINE
Tagamet Tablets 1547

STOMET (Brazil, Italy)
CIMETIDINE
Tagamet Tablets 1547

STOP ESPINILLA NORMADERM (Spain)
BENZOYL PEROXIDE
Brevoxyl-4 Creamy Wash 3212
Brevoxyl-4 Gel 3211
Brevoxyl-8 Creamy Wash 3212
Brevoxyl-8 Gel 3211
Triaz Cleanser 1864
Triaz Gel 1864

STOPIT (Israel)
LOPERAMIDE HYDROCHLORIDE
Imodium Capsules 1834

STOPPERS (United Kingdom)
NICOTINE
Nicotrol Inhaler 2594
Nicotrol NS 2596

STOVAREN (Italy)
CEFOXITIN SODIUM
Mefoxin Premixed Intravenous Solution 1990
Mefoxin for Injection 1987

STROMECTOL (Australia, France, Japan, The Netherlands)
IVERMECTIN
Stromectol Tablets 2053

STROX (India)
CIPROFLOXACIN HYDROCHLORIDE
Ciloxan Ophthalmic Ointment 554
Ciloxan Ophthalmic Solution . . . . ⊙205
Cipro Tablets 2991

STUBIT (United Kingdom)
NICOTINE
Nicotrol Inhaler 2594
Nicotrol NS 2596

STUD (United Kingdom)
LIDOCAINE
Lidoderm Patch 1107

STUD 100 (Australia, Israel)
LIDOCAINE
Lidoderm Patch 1107

STV (Argentina)
STAVUDINE
Zerit Capsules 971
Zerit for Oral Solution 971

SUADIAN (Italy)
NAFTIFINE HYDROCHLORIDE
Naftin Cream 2097
Naftin Gel 2097

SUBLIMAZE (Argentina, Australia, Canada, Irish Republic, New Zealand, South Africa, United Kingdom)
FENTANYL CITRATE
Actiq 993

SUBSTITOL (Austria)
ESTRADIOL
Climara Transdermal System 795
Vivelle Transdermal System 2288
Vivelle-Dot Transdermal System 2293
MORPHINE SULFATE
Kadian Capsules 572
MS Contin Tablets 2703

SUBSYDE (Thailand)
DICLOFENAC SODIUM
Voltaren Tablets 2298
Voltaren-XR Tablets 2301

SUBUTEX (Australia, Austria, Belgium, Czech Republic, Denmark, Finland, France, Germany, Greece, Hong Kong, Israel, Italy, Malaysia, Norway, Portugal, Singapore, South Africa, Spain, Sweden, Switzerland, United Kingdom)
BUPRENORPHINE HYDROCHLORIDE
Buprenex Injectable 2718

SUCARI (Hong Kong)
SUCRALFATE
Carafate Suspension 727
Carafate Tablets 728

SUCCOSA (Sweden)
SUCRALFATE
Carafate Suspension 727
Carafate Tablets 728

SUCRABEST (Germany)
SUCRALFATE
Carafate Suspension 727
Carafate Tablets 728

SUCRAFEN (Thailand)
SUCRALFATE
Carafate Suspension 727
Carafate Tablets 728

SUCRAFILM (Brazil)
SUCRALFATE
Carafate Suspension 727
Carafate Tablets 728

SUCRAGER (Italy)
SUCRALFATE
Carafate Suspension 727
Carafate Tablets 728

SUCRAL (Italy, Thailand)
SUCRALFATE
Carafate Suspension 727
Carafate Tablets 728

SUCRALAN (Austria, Czech Republic)
SUCRALFATE
Carafate Suspension 727
Carafate Tablets 728

SUCRALBENE (Austria)
SUCRALFATE
Carafate Suspension 727
Carafate Tablets 728

SUCRALFIN (Italy)
SUCRALFATE
Carafate Suspension 727
Carafate Tablets 728

SUCRALMAX (Argentina)
SUCRALFATE
Carafate Suspension 727
Carafate Tablets 728

SUCRALOSE (PREPARATION) (United Arab Emirates)
SUCRALFATE
Carafate Suspension 727
Carafate Tablets 728

SUCRALSTAD (Austria)
SUCRALFATE
Carafate Suspension 727
Carafate Tablets 728

SUCRALUM (Portugal)
SUCRALFATE
Carafate Suspension 727
Carafate Tablets 728

SUCRAMAL (Italy)
SUCRALFATE
Carafate Suspension 727
Carafate Tablets 728

SUCRAMED (Austria)
SUCRALFATE
Carafate Suspension 727
Carafate Tablets 728

SUCRAPHIL (Germany)
SUCRALFATE
Carafate Suspension 727
Carafate Tablets 728

SUCRASE (India)
SUCRALFATE
Carafate Suspension 727
Carafate Tablets 728

SUCRATE (Greece, Italy, Thailand)
SUCRALFATE
Carafate Suspension 727
Carafate Tablets 728

SUCRATYROL (Austria)
SUCRALFATE
Carafate Suspension 727
Carafate Tablets 728

SUCRORIL (Italy)
SUCRALFATE
Carafate Suspension 727
Carafate Tablets 728

SUDAC (Italy)
SULINDAC
Clinoril Tablets 1899

SUFIL (Spain)
MEBENDAZOLE
Vermox Chewable Tablets 1853

SUFORTAN (Italy, Mexico)
PENICILLAMINE
Cuprimine Capsules 1925

SUFORTANON (Spain)
PENICILLAMINE
Cuprimine Capsules 1925

SUGAR (Italy)
SUCRALFATE
Carafate Suspension 727
Carafate Tablets 728

SUGAST (Italy)
SUCRALFATE
Carafate Suspension 727
Carafate Tablets 728

SUIFLOX (Mexico)
CIPROFLOXACIN HYDROCHLORIDE
Ciloxan Ophthalmic Ointment 554
Ciloxan Ophthalmic Solution . . . . ⊙205
Cipro Tablets 2991

SUL 10 (Mexico)
SULFACETAMIDE SODIUM
Klaron Lotion 10% 1050

SULAR (Belgium, Mexico, Spain, The Netherlands)
NISOLDIPINE
Sular Tablets 1163

SULARTRENE (Italy)
SULINDAC
Clinoril Tablets 1899

SULCRAN (Chile)
SUCRALFATE
Carafate Suspension 727
Carafate Tablets 728

SULCRATE (Canada)
SUCRALFATE
Carafate Suspension 727
Carafate Tablets 728

SULEN (Italy)
SULINDAC
Clinoril Tablets 1899

SULFA 10 (Belgium)
SULFACETAMIDE SODIUM
Klaron Lotion 10% 1050

SULFABLEPH N LIQUIFILM (Germany)
SULFACETAMIDE SODIUM
Klaron Lotion 10% 1050

SULFACET (Spain)
SULFACETAMIDE SODIUM
Klaron Lotion 10% 1050

SULFACETA (Spain)
SULFACETAMIDE SODIUM
Klaron Lotion 10% 1050

SULFACETAM (Spain)
SULFACETAMIDE SODIUM
Klaron Lotion 10% 1050

SULFACID (Israel)
SULFACETAMIDE SODIUM
Klaron Lotion 10% 1050

SULFACOLLYRE (Belgium)
SULFACETAMIDE SODIUM
Klaron Lotion 10% 1050

SULFAMYLON (Canada, United Kingdom)
MAFENIDE ACETATE
Sulfamylon Cream 2154
Sulfamylon for 5% Topical Solution 2155

(⊙ Described in PDR For Ophthalmic Medicines™)

SULFEX (Canada, Hong Kong)
SULFACETAMIDE SODIUM
Klaron Lotion 10% . . . 1050

SULFIL (Spain)
MEBENDAZOLE
Vermox Chewable Tablets . . . 1853

SULFINAV (Argentina)
EFAVIRENZ
Sustiva Capsules . . . 957

SULFONA (Portugal, Spain)
DAPSONE
Dapsone Tablets USP . . . 1656

SULFO-SELENIUM (Belgium)
HYDROCORTISONE
Hydrocortone Tablets . . . 1963

SULFOXYL (Canada)
BENZOYL PEROXIDE
Brevoxyl-4 Creamy Wash . . . 3212
Brevoxyl-4 Gel . . . 3211
Brevoxyl-8 Creamy Wash . . . 3212
Brevoxyl-8 Gel . . . 3211
Triaz Cleanser . . . 1864
Triaz Gel . . . 1864

SULINDAL (Spain)
SULINDAC
Clinoril Tablets . . . 1899

SULINOL (Italy)
SULINDAC
Clinoril Tablets . . . 1899

SULMYCIN (Austria, Germany)
GENTAMICIN SULFATE
Garamycin Injectable . . . 3028
Genoptic Sterile Ophthalmic Solution . . . ⊙227

SULOCTEN (Argentina)
ENALAPRIL MALEATE
Vasotec I.V. Injection . . . 2076

SULORANE (Israel)
DESFLURANE
Suprane Liquid for Inhalation . . . 770

SULOTIL (Chile)
NIFEDIPINE
Adalat CC Tablets . . . 2978

SULPHAMIDE (Israel)
SULFACETAMIDE SODIUM
Klaron Lotion 10% . . . 1050

SULREUMA (Italy)
SULINDAC
Clinoril Tablets . . . 1899

SUMACLINA (Portugal)
SIMVASTATIN
Zocor Tablets . . . 2078

SUMADOL (Italy)
SUMATRIPTAN SUCCINATE
Imitrex Injection . . . 1431
Imitrex Tablets . . . 1440

SUMAX (Brazil)
SUMATRIPTAN SUCCINATE
Imitrex Injection . . . 1431
Imitrex Tablets . . . 1440

SUMIAL (Spain)
PROPRANOLOL HYDROCHLORIDE
Inderal LA Long-Acting Capsules . . . 3421

SUMIGRENE (Italy)
SUMATRIPTAN SUCCINATE
Imitrex Injection . . . 1431
Imitrex Tablets . . . 1440

SUMINAT (India)
SUMATRIPTAN SUCCINATE
Imitrex Injection . . . 1431
Imitrex Tablets . . . 1440

SUNAZOL (Malaysia)
KETOCONAZOLE
Nizoral 2% Shampoo . . . 1838

SUNITON (Malaysia)
ORPHENADRINE CITRATE
Norflex Injection . . . 1824

SUNPROX (Malaysia, Singapore)
NAPROXEN SODIUM
Anaprox DS Tablets . . . 2769
Anaprox Tablets . . . 2769

SUPARTZ (United Kingdom)
SODIUM HYALURONATE
Hyalgan Solution . . . 2917

SUPERAMIN (Greece)
LEVOCARNITINE
Carnitor Injection . . . 3185
Carnitor Tablets and Oral Solution . . . 3187

SUPERO (Italy)
CEFUROXIME SODIUM
Zinacef Injection . . . 1604

SUPEUDOL (Canada)
OXYCODONE HYDROCHLORIDE
OxyContin Tablets . . . 2699
OxyFast Oral Concentrate Solution . . . 2704
OxyIR Capsules . . . 2704

SUPIROCIN (India)
MUPIROCIN
Bactroban Ointment . . . 1358

SUPIROCIN-B (India)
MUPIROCIN
Bactroban Ointment . . . 1358

SUPLASYN (Canada, France, Germany, United Kingdom)
SODIUM HYALURONATE
Hyalgan Solution . . . 2917

SUPOTRON (Greece)
ENALAPRIL MALEATE
Vasotec I.V. Injection . . . 2076

SUPPLIN (Hungary)
METRONIDAZOLE
MetroGel-Vaginal Gel . . . 1822
Noritate Cream, 1% . . . 1051

SUPRACEF (Finland)
CEFIXIME
Suprax . . . 1811

SUPRACORDIN (Czech Republic)
NIFEDIPINE
Adalat CC Tablets . . . 2978

SUPRAGENTA (Spain)
GENTAMICIN SULFATE
Garamycin Injectable . . . 3028
Genoptic Sterile Ophthalmic Solution . . . ⊙227

SUPRALIP (Thailand, United Kingdom)
FENOFIBRATE
Tricor Tablets . . . 523

SUPRAMOX (Switzerland)
AMOXICILLIN
Amoxil Pediatric Drops for Oral Suspension . . . 1315
Amoxil Tablets . . . 1315

SUPRAN (Israel)
CEFIXIME
Suprax . . . 1811

SUPRANE (Argentina, Australia, Austria, Belgium, Brazil, Canada, Denmark, Finland, Germany, Greece, Hungary, Irish Republic, Italy, Mexico, New Zealand, Norway, Singapore, South Africa, Spain, Sweden, Switzerland, Thailand, The Netherlands, United Kingdom)
DESFLURANE
Suprane Liquid for Inhalation . . . 770

SUPRAX (Canada, Czech Republic, Germany, Hungary, Irish Republic, Italy, Russia, United Kingdom)
CEFIXIME
Suprax . . . 1811

SUPRES (Canada)
CHLOROTHIAZIDE/METHYLDOPA
Aldoclor Tablets . . . 1881

SUPRIMOX (India)
AMOXICILLIN
Amoxil Pediatric Drops for Oral Suspension . . . 1315
Amoxil Tablets . . . 1315

SURAZEM (The Netherlands)
DILTIAZEM HYDROCHLORIDE
Cardizem LA Extended Release Tablets . . . 1699
Tiazac Capsules . . . 1204

SURFAZ (India)
CLOTRIMAZOLE
Lotrimin Cream . . . 3053
Lotrimin Lotion 1% . . . 3053
Lotrimin Topical Solution 1% . . . 3053

SURFONT (Germany)
MEBENDAZOLE
Vermox Chewable Tablets . . . 1853

SURIL (Italy)
SUCRALFATE
Carafate Suspension . . . 727
Carafate Tablets . . . 728

SURMONTIL (Canada, Denmark, Finland, Hong Kong, Irish Republic, New Zealand, Norway, Portugal, Sweden, The Netherlands, United Kingdom)
TRIMIPRAMINE MALEATE
Surmontil Capsules . . . 2347

SUSTAC (Argentina)
RANITIDINE HYDROCHLORIDE
Zantac 25 EFFERdose Tablets . . . 1597
Zantac 150 EFFERdose Tablets . . . 1597
Zantac 150 Tablets . . . 1597
Zantac 300 Tablets . . . 1597
Zantac Injection . . . 1593
Zantac Injection Premixed . . . 1593
Zantac Syrup . . . 1597

SUSTIVA (Canada, France, Germany, Irish Republic, Italy, Spain, United Kingdom)
EFAVIRENZ
Sustiva Capsules . . . 957

SUTAC (Thailand)
CETIRIZINE HYDROCHLORIDE
Zyrtec Syrup . . . 2589
Zyrtec Tablets . . . 2589

SUTIF (Spain)
TERAZOSIN HYDROCHLORIDE
Hytrin Capsules . . . 469

SUTRICO (Argentina)
FINASTERIDE
Propecia Tablets . . . 2036
Proscar Tablets . . . 2040

SUVALAN (Australia)
SUMATRIPTAN SUCCINATE
Imitrex Injection . . . 1431
Imitrex Tablets . . . 1440

SVELTANET (Greece)
RANITIDINE HYDROCHLORIDE
Zantac 25 EFFERdose Tablets . . . 1597
Zantac 150 EFFERdose Tablets . . . 1597
Zantac 150 Tablets . . . 1597
Zantac 300 Tablets . . . 1597
Zantac Injection . . . 1593
Zantac Injection Premixed . . . 1593
Zantac Syrup . . . 1597

SVIROXIT (Greece)
ETIDRONATE DISODIUM
Didronel Tablets . . . 2693

SWISS-KAL SR (South Africa)
POTASSIUM CHLORIDE
K-Dur Extended-Release Tablets . . . 3047
K-Lor Powder Packets . . . 472
K-Tab Filmtab Tablets . . . 473

SYMBYAX (Argentina)
OLANZAPINE
Zyprexa Tablets . . . 1798

SYMMETREL (Australia, Austria, Canada, Germany, Greece, Hong Kong, Irish Republic, Israel, New Zealand, Norway, Singapore, South Africa, Sweden, Switzerland, The Netherlands, United Kingdom)
AMANTADINE HYDROCHLORIDE
Symmetrel Syrup . . . 1115
Symmetrel Tablets . . . 1115

SYMOXYL (India)
AMOXICILLIN
Amoxil Pediatric Drops for Oral Suspension . . . 1315
Amoxil Tablets . . . 1315

SYNAGIS (Argentina, Australia, Belgium, Brazil, Canada, Czech Republic, Denmark, Finland, France, Germany, Greece, Hong Kong, Hungary, Irish Republic, Italy, Malaysia, Mexico, New Zealand, Norway, Singapore, South Africa, Spain, Sweden, Switzerland, The Netherlands, United Kingdom)
PALIVIZUMAB
Synagis Intramuscular Powder . . . 1868

SYNAROME (Greece)
ATENOLOL
Tenormin I.V. Injection . . . 698

SYNASTERON (Belgium)
OXYMETHOLONE
Anadrol-50 Tablets . . . 3329

SYNCLAR (India)
CLARITHROMYCIN
Biaxin Filmtab Tablets . . . 402
Biaxin Granules . . . 402

SYNCOMET (Hong Kong)
CIMETIDINE
Tagamet Tablets . . . 1547

SYNERPRIL (Austria, Denmark, Sweden)
ENALAPRIL MALEATE
Vasotec I.V. Injection . . . 2076

SYNFLEX (Australia, Canada, Hong Kong, Irish Republic, Italy, New Zealand, Singapore, South Africa, Thailand, United Kingdom)
NAPROXEN SODIUM
Anaprox DS Tablets . . . 2769
Anaprox Tablets . . . 2769

SYNITIDINE (Hong Kong)
RANITIDINE HYDROCHLORIDE
Zantac 25 EFFERdose Tablets . . . 1597
Zantac 150 EFFERdose Tablets . . . 1597
Zantac 150 Tablets . . . 1597
Zantac 300 Tablets . . . 1597
Zantac Injection . . . 1593
Zantac Injection Premixed . . . 1593
Zantac Syrup . . . 1597

SYNIZORAL (Hong Kong)
KETOCONAZOLE
Nizoral 2% Shampoo . . . 1838

SYNOGIL (Germany)
NATAMYCIN
Natacyn Antifungal Ophthalmic Suspension . . . ⊙207

SYNOGIN (Thailand)
NAPROXEN
EC-Naprosyn Delayed-Release Tablets . . . 2769
Naprosyn Suspension . . . 2769
Naprosyn Tablets . . . 2769

SYNTARIS (Austria, Belgium, Czech Republic, Germany, Irish Republic, Italy, South Africa, Switzerland, The Netherlands, United Kingdom)
FLUNISOLIDE
Aerobid Inhaler System . . . 1172
Aerobid-M Inhaler System . . . 1172
Nasarel Nasal Spray . . . 1652

SYNTHOMANET (Greece)
RANITIDINE HYDROCHLORIDE
Zantac 25 EFFERdose Tablets . . . 1597
Zantac 150 EFFERdose Tablets . . . 1597
Zantac 150 Tablets . . . 1597
Zantac 300 Tablets . . . 1597
Zantac Injection . . . 1593
Zantac Injection Premixed . . . 1593
Zantac Syrup . . . 1597

SYNTHROID (Brazil, Canada)
LEVOTHYROXINE SODIUM
Levothroid Tablets . . . 1189
Levoxyl Tablets . . . 1680
Synthroid Tablets . . . 515

SYNTONOL (Thailand)
PROPRANOLOL HYDROCHLORIDE
Inderal LA Long-Acting Capsules . . . 3421

SYNURETIC (United Kingdom)
AMILORIDE HYDROCHLORIDE/HYDROCHLOROTHIAZIDE
Moduretic Tablets . . . 2003

SYPROL (United Kingdom)
PROPRANOLOL HYDROCHLORIDE
Inderal LA Long-Acting Capsules . . . 3421

SYSCOR (Austria, Belgium, Brazil, Czech Republic, Finland, Greece, Italy, Mexico, South Africa, Spain, Sweden, Switzerland, The Netherlands, United Kingdom)
NISOLDIPINE
Sular Tablets . . . 1163

SYSTEN (Austria, Belgium, Brazil, Czech Republic, France, Hungary, Italy, Mexico, Switzerland, The Netherlands)
ESTRADIOL
Climara Transdermal System . . . 795

(⊙ Described in PDR For Ophthalmic Medicines™)

Vivelle Transdermal System 2288
Vivelle-Dot Transdermal System 2293

SYSTEN CONTI (Czech Republic)
ESTRADIOL
Climara Transdermal System 795
Vivelle Transdermal System 2288
Vivelle-Dot Transdermal System 2293

SYSTEPIN (Irish Republic)
NIFEDIPINE
Adalat CC Tablets 2978

SYSTRAL HYDROCORT (Germany)
HYDROCORTISONE
Hydrocortone Tablets 1963

T.O.VIR (Thailand)
ZIDOVUDINE
Retrovir Capsules 1533
Retrovir IV Infusion. 1537
Retrovir Syrup 1533
Retrovir Tablets. 1533

T/H-BASAN (Switzerland)
HYDROCHLOROTHIAZIDE/TRIAMTERENE
Dyazide Capsules 1389
Maxzide Tablets 2150
Maxzide-25 mg Tablets 2150

T3 (Greece)
LIOTHYRONINE SODIUM
Cytomel Tablets 1678

T4 (Argentina, Greece)
LEVOTHYROXINE SODIUM
Levothroid Tablets 1189
Levoxyl Tablets 1680
Synthroid Tablets. 515

TA OSOTH (Thailand)
TRIAMCINOLONE ACETONIDE
Azmacort Inhalation Aerosol 1701
Nasacort AQ Nasal Spray 2937

TABAZUR (France)
NICOTINE
Nicotrol Inhaler 2594
Nicotrol NS 2596

TACEX (Mexico)
CEFTRIAXONE SODIUM
Rocephin Injectable Vials, ADD-Vantage, Galaxy, Bulk 2801

TACHYDARON (Germany)
AMIODARONE HYDROCHLORIDE
Pacerone Tablets 3337

TACHYFENON (Germany)
PROPAFENONE HYDROCHLORIDE
Rythmol SR Capsules 2736

TACICUL (Argentina)
LOSARTAN POTASSIUM
Cozaar Tablets 1913

TACINOL (Thailand)
TRIAMCINOLONE ACETONIDE
Azmacort Inhalation Aerosol 1701
Nasacort AQ Nasal Spray 2937

TACRAF (Argentina)
TACROLIMUS
Prograf Capsules and Injection 624

TACRON (Singapore, Spain)
TICLOPIDINE HYDROCHLORIDE
Ticlid Tablets 2813

TACRO-TIC (Argentina)
TACROLIMUS
Prograf Capsules and Injection 624

TACROZ (India)
TACROLIMUS
Prograf Capsules and Injection 624

TAFENIL (Mexico)
FLUTAMIDE
Eulexin Capsules 3023

TAFLOC (South Africa)
OFLOXACIN
Floxin Otic Solution 1043

TAFLOX (Portugal)
NORFLOXACIN
Noroxin Tablets. 2009

TAGADINE (Hong Kong)
CIMETIDINE
Tagamet Tablets 1547

TAGAGEL (Germany)
CIMETIDINE
Tagamet Tablets 1547

TAGAL (Mexico)
CEFTAZIDIME
Fortaz for Injection 1422

TAGALIV (Brazil)
CIMETIDINE
Tagamet Tablets 1547

TAGAMET (Argentina, Australia, Denmark, Greece, Hong Kong, Irish Republic, Israel, Italy, Malaysia, Mexico, New Zealand, Norway, Portugal, Singapore, South Africa, Spain, Switzerland, Thailand, The Netherlands, United Kingdom)
CIMETIDINE
Tagamet Tablets 1547

TAGAMET DUAL ACTION (United Kingdom)
CIMETIDINE
Tagamet Tablets 1547

TAGONIS (Germany)
PAROXETINE HYDROCHLORIDE
Paxil Oral Suspension 1501
Paxil Tablets. 1501

TAGREN (Czech Republic)
TICLOPIDINE HYDROCHLORIDE
Ticlid Tablets 2813

TAGUINOL (Spain)
LOPERAMIDE HYDROCHLORIDE
Imodium Capsules 1834

TAHOR (France)
ATORVASTATIN CALCIUM
Lipitor Tablets 2495

TAIRAL (Spain)
FAMOTIDINE
Pepcid Injection 2017
Pepcid Injection Premixed 2017
Pepcid Tablets 2014
Pepcid for Oral Suspension 2014

TAKEPRON (Hong Kong, Japan)
LANSOPRAZOLE
Prevacid Delayed-Release Capsules 3268

TAKS (Malaysia, Thailand)
DICLOFENAC SODIUM
Voltaren Tablets 2298
Voltaren-XR Tablets 2301

TALAM (Australia)
CITALOPRAM HYDROBROMIDE
Celexa Tablets 1177

TALGESIL (Malaysia)
FENTANYL
Duragesic Transdermal System. 2448

TALICIX (Spain)
CLARITHROMYCIN
Biaxin Filmtab Tablets 402
Biaxin Granules 402

TALIRAX (Greece)
FLUOROMETHOLONE
FML Ophthalmic Ointment . . . . ⊙225

TALLITON (Hungary)
CARVEDILOL
Coreg Tablets. 1376

TALNUR (Argentina)
FENTANYL
Duragesic Transdermal System. 2448

TALOFILINA (Brazil)
THEOPHYLLINE
Uniphyl Tablets 2708

TALOHEXAL (Australia)
CITALOPRAM HYDROBROMIDE
Celexa Tablets 1177

TALOKEN (Mexico)
CEFTAZIDIME
Fortaz for Injection 1422

TALOMIL (South Africa)
CITALOPRAM HYDROBROMIDE
Celexa Tablets 1177

TAM (Spain)
CIPROFLOXACIN HYDROCHLORIDE
Ciloxan Ophthalmic Ointment 554
Ciloxan Ophthalmic Solution . . . . ⊙205
Cipro Tablets 2991

TAMBAC (India)
CEFPODOXIME PROXETIL
Vantin Tablets and Oral Suspension 2650

TAMBOCOR (Argentina, Australia, Belgium, Canada, Chile, Czech Republic, Denmark, Finland, Germany, Hong Kong, Irish Republic, Israel, Malaysia, Mexico, New Zealand, Norway, Singapore, South Africa, Sweden, Switzerland, Thailand, The Netherlands, United Kingdom)
FLECAINIDE ACETATE
Tambocor Tablets 1824

TAMERAN (Spain)
FAMOTIDINE
Pepcid Injection 2017
Pepcid Injection Premixed 2017
Pepcid Tablets 2014
Pepcid for Oral Suspension 2014

TAMETIN (Italy)
CIMETIDINE
Tagamet Tablets 1547

TAMIN (Spain)
FAMOTIDINE
Pepcid Injection 2017
Pepcid Injection Premixed 2017
Pepcid Tablets 2014
Pepcid for Oral Suspension 2014

TAMPER (Greece)
CIMETIDINE
Tagamet Tablets 1547

TAMSUNA (Argentina)
TAMSULOSIN HYDROCHLORIDE
Flomax Capsules 881

TANAVAT (Argentina)
SIMVASTATIN
Zocor Tablets. 2078

TANDAX (Mexico)
NAPROXEN SODIUM
Anaprox DS Tablets 2769
Anaprox Tablets 2769

TANDIAL (Mexico)
DIAZEPAM
Diastat Rectal Delivery System 3344
Valium Tablets 2822

TANDIX (Portugal)
INDAPAMIDE
Indapamide Tablets 2119

TANIDINA (Spain)
RANITIDINE HYDROCHLORIDE
Zantac 25 EFFERdose Tablets 1597
Zantac 150 EFFERdose Tablets. 1597
Zantac 150 Tablets 1597
Zantac 300 Tablets 1597
Zantac Injection 1593
Zantac Injection Premixed 1593
Zantac Syrup 1597

TANIZONA (Mexico)
NAPROXEN
EC-Naprosyn Delayed-Release Tablets. . . . 2769
Naprosyn Suspension 2769
Naprosyn Tablets 2769

TANSER (Spain)
ATENOLOL
Tenormin I.V. Injection. 698

TANYL (Israel, South Africa)
FENTANYL CITRATE
Actiq 993

TAPRODEX (Mexico)
DEXAMETHASONE
Decadron Tablets 1929

TARASKON (Germany)
ATENOLOL
Tenormin I.V. Injection. 698

TARATEN (Thailand)
CLOTRIMAZOLE
Lotrimin Cream. 3053
Lotrimin Lotion 1%. 3053
Lotrimin Topical Solution 1% 3053

TARDOTOL (Denmark)
CARBAMAZEPINE
Carbatrol Capsules 3174
Tegretol Chewable Tablets. 2278
Tegretol Suspension. 2278
Tegretol Tablets 2278
Tegretol-XR Tablets 2278

TAREG (Brazil, Chile, France, Italy, Portugal)
VALSARTAN
Diovan Tablets 2191

TAREG-D (Chile)
HYDROCHLOROTHIAZIDE/VALSARTAN
Diovan HCT Tablets 2195

TAREMIS (Argentina)
METRONIDAZOLE
MetroGel-Vaginal Gel 1822
Noritate Cream, 1%. 1051

TARGET (Hong Kong)
ATENOLOL
Tenormin I.V. Injection. 698

TARIFLOX (India)
OFLOXACIN
Floxin Otic Solution 1043

TARIFLOX PLUS (India)
OFLOXACIN
Floxin Otic Solution 1043

TARIVID (Czech Republic, Denmark, Finland, Hungary, India, Israel, Malaysia, Singapore, South Africa, Sweden, Switzerland, Thailand)
OFLOXACIN
Floxin Otic Solution 1043

TARJEN (Thailand)
DICLOFENAC SODIUM
Voltaren Tablets 2298
Voltaren-XR Tablets 2301

TARJENA (Thailand)
DICLOFENAC SODIUM
Voltaren Tablets 2298
Voltaren-XR Tablets 2301

TARKA (Argentina, Austria, Brazil, Canada, Czech Republic, Denmark, Finland, France, Germany, Greece, Hungary, Italy, Mexico, Russia, South Africa, Spain, Sweden, Switzerland, The Netherlands, United Kingdom)
VERAPAMIL HYDROCHLORIDE
Covera-HS Tablets 3135
Verelan PM Capsules 3120

TAROFLOX (Czech Republic)
OFLOXACIN
Floxin Otic Solution 1043

TASEDAN (Mexico)
ESTAZOLAM
ProSom Tablets 512

TASEP (Spain)
CEFAZOLIN SODIUM
Ancef for Injection 1318

TASMAR (Argentina, Austria, Brazil, Chile, Denmark, Greece, Hong Kong, Irish Republic, Mexico, New Zealand, Norway, Singapore, South Africa, Sweden, Switzerland, Thailand, United Kingdom)
TOLCAPONE
Tasmar Tablets. 3360

TATIG (Italy)
SERTRALINE HYDROCHLORIDE
Zoloft Tablets 2581

TAUCOR (Spain)
LOVASTATIN
Mevacor Tablets 1996

TAVANIC (Argentina, Austria, Belgium, Brazil, Chile, Czech Republic, Finland, France, Germany, Greece, Hungary, India, Irish Republic, Israel, Italy, Mexico, Portugal, Russia, South Africa, Spain, Sweden, Switzerland, The Netherlands, United Kingdom)
LEVOFLOXACIN
Levaquin Injection 2453
Levaquin Tablets 2453

TAVAN-SP 54 (South Africa)
PENTOSAN POLYSULFATE SODIUM
Elmiron Capsules 2393

TAVER (Malaysia, Thailand)
CARBAMAZEPINE
Carbatrol Capsules 3174
Tegretol Chewable Tablets. 2278
Tegretol Suspension. 2278
Tegretol Tablets 2278
Tegretol-XR Tablets 2278

TAVOR (Mexico)
OXYBUTYNIN CHLORIDE
Ditropan XL Extended Release Tablets . . . 2391

TAXIFUR (Mexico)
CEFTAZIDIME
Fortaz for Injection 1422

TAXOTERE (Argentina, Australia, Austria, Belgium, Brazil, Canada, Czech Republic, Denmark, Finland, France, Germany, Greece, Hong Kong, Hungary, Irish Republic, Israel, Italy, Japan, Malaysia, Mexico, New Zealand, Norway, Portugal, Russia, Singapore, South Africa, Spain, Sweden, Switzerland, Thailand, The Netherlands, United Kingdom)
DOCETAXEL
Taxotere Injection Concentrate. . . . 2947

TAXYL (Mexico)
DEXAMETHASONE
Decadron Tablets 1929

TAZEPIN (Brazil)
RANITIDINE HYDROCHLORIDE
Zantac 25 EFFERdose Tablets 1597
Zantac 150 EFFERdose Tablets. . . . 1597
Zantac 150 Tablets 1597
Zantac 300 Tablets 1597
Zantac Injection 1593
Zantac Injection Premixed 1593
Zantac Syrup 1597

TAZIDEM (Brazil)
CEFTAZIDIME
Fortaz for Injection 1422

TAZIDIME (Canada)
CEFTAZIDIME
Fortaz for Injection 1422

TAZOBAC (Germany, Italy, Portugal, Switzerland)
PIPERACILLIN SODIUM/TAZOBACTAM SODIUM
Zosyn. . . . 3492
Zosyn in Galaxy Containers 3492

TAZOCILLINE (France)
PIPERACILLIN SODIUM/TAZOBACTAM SODIUM
Zosyn. . . . 3492
Zosyn in Galaxy Containers 3492

TAZOCIN (Belgium, Denmark, Finland, Greece, Hong Kong, Irish Republic, Israel, Italy, Mexico, New Zealand, Singapore, South Africa, Sweden, Thailand, The Netherlands)
PIPERACILLIN SODIUM/TAZOBACTAM SODIUM
Zosyn. . . . 3492
Zosyn in Galaxy Containers 3492

TAZONAM (Austria, Chile)
PIPERACILLIN SODIUM/TAZOBACTAM SODIUM
Zosyn. . . . 3492
Zosyn in Galaxy Containers 3492

TAZUSIN (Spain)
TERAZOSIN HYDROCHLORIDE
Hytrin Capsules. . . . 469

TEALEP (Argentina)
FINASTERIDE
Propecia Tablets 2036
Proscar Tablets. . . . 2040

TEBLOC (Italy)
LOPERAMIDE HYDROCHLORIDE
Imodium Capsules. . . . 1834

TECFAZOLINA (Spain)
CEFAZOLIN SODIUM
Ancef for Injection. . . . 1318

TECHNIPHYLLINE (Monaco)
THEOPHYLLINE
Uniphyl Tablets 2708

TECNOFLUT (Brazil)
FLUTAMIDE
Eulexin Capsules. . . . 3023

TECNOLIP (Portugal)
LOVASTATIN
Mevacor Tablets 1996

TECNOMAX (Argentina)
SILDENAFIL CITRATE
Viagra Tablets 2552

TECNOTECAN (Brazil)
IRINOTECAN HYDROCHLORIDE
Camptosar Injection. . . . 2602

TEDICUMAR (Spain)
WARFARIN SODIUM
Coumadin Tablets 932
Coumadin for Injection 932

TEDOL (Portugal)
KETOCONAZOLE
Nizoral 2% Shampoo 1838

TEDRAL (United Kingdom)
THEOPHYLLINE
Uniphyl Tablets 2708

TEDRALAN (Monaco)
THEOPHYLLINE
Uniphyl Tablets 2708

TEGRETAL (Chile, Germany)
CARBAMAZEPINE
Carbatrol Capsules 3174
Tegretol Chewable Tablets 2278
Tegretol Suspension. . . . 2278
Tegretol Tablets 2278
Tegretol-XR Tablets 2278

TEGRETARD (Brazil)
CARBAMAZEPINE
Carbatrol Capsules 3174
Tegretol Chewable Tablets 2278
Tegretol Suspension. . . . 2278
Tegretol Tablets 2278
Tegretol-XR Tablets 2278

TEGRETOL (Argentina, Australia, Austria, Belgium, Brazil, Canada, Czech Republic, Denmark, Finland, France, Greece, Hong Kong, Hungary, Irish Republic, Israel, Italy, Malaysia, Mexico, New Zealand, Norway, Portugal, Russia, Singapore, South Africa, Spain, Sweden, Switzerland, Thailand, The Netherlands, United Kingdom)
CARBAMAZEPINE
Carbatrol Capsules. . . . 3174
Tegretol Chewable Tablets 2278
Tegretol Suspension 2278
Tegretol Tablets. . . . 2278
Tegretol-XR Tablets. . . . 2278

TEGREX (Brazil)
CARBAMAZEPINE
Carbatrol Capsules 3174
Tegretol Chewable Tablets. . . . 2278
Tegretol Suspension. . . . 2278
Tegretol Tablets 2278
Tegretol-XR Tablets 2278

TEGREZIN (Brazil)
CARBAMAZEPINE
Carbatrol Capsules 3174
Tegretol Chewable Tablets 2278
Tegretol Suspension. . . . 2278
Tegretol Tablets 2278
Tegretol-XR Tablets 2278

TEGRITAL (India)
CARBAMAZEPINE
Carbatrol Capsules 3174
Tegretol Chewable Tablets. . . . 2278
Tegretol Suspension. . . . 2278
Tegretol Tablets 2278
Tegretol-XR Tablets 2278

TELARIX (Greece)
CETIRIZINE HYDROCHLORIDE
Zyrtec Syrup 2589
Zyrtec Tablets 2589

TELFAST (Australia, Austria, Belgium, Czech Republic, Denmark, Finland, France, Hong Kong, Hungary, Irish Republic, Israel, Italy, Malaysia, New Zealand, Norway, Portugal, Russia, Singapore, South Africa, Spain, Sweden, Switzerland, Thailand, The Netherlands, United Kingdom)
FEXOFENADINE HYDROCHLORIDE
Allegra Capsules. . . . 2857

TELFAST D (Malaysia)
FEXOFENADINE HYDROCHLORIDE/PSEUDOEPHEDRINE HYDROCHLORIDE
Allegra-D 12 Hour Extended-Release Tablets 2860

TELFAST DECONGESTANT (New Zealand)
FEXOFENADINE HYDROCHLORIDE/PSEUDOEPHEDRINE HYDROCHLORIDE
Allegra-D 12 Hour Extended-Release Tablets 2860

TELFAST-D (Singapore)
FEXOFENADINE HYDROCHLORIDE/PSEUDOEPHEDRINE HYDROCHLORIDE
Allegra-D 12 Hour Extended-Release Tablets 2860

TELMA (India)
TELMISARTAN
Micardis Tablets 884

TELMA-H (India)
TELMISARTAN
Micardis Tablets 884

TELNASE (Australia)
TRIAMCINOLONE ACETONIDE
Azmacort Inhalation Aerosol. . . . 1701
Nasacort AQ Nasal Spray 2937

TELUGREN (Chile)
CLOTRIMAZOLE
Lotrimin Cream. . . . 3053
Lotrimin Lotion 1%. . . . 3053
Lotrimin Topical Solution 1% 3053

TELVODIN (Argentina)
ATENOLOL
Tenormin I.V. Injection. . . . 698

TEMACO (Thailand)
THEOPHYLLINE
Uniphyl Tablets 2708

TEMGESIC (Argentina, Australia, Austria, Belgium, Czech Republic, Denmark, Finland, France, Germany, Hong Kong, Irish Republic, Italy, Malaysia, Mexico, New Zealand, Norway, Singapore, South Africa, Sweden, Switzerland, Thailand, The Netherlands, United Kingdom)
BUPRENORPHINE HYDROCHLORIDE
Buprenex Injectable 2718

TEMGESIC-NX (New Zealand)
BUPRENORPHINE HYDROCHLORIDE
Buprenex Injectable 2718

TEMIC (Italy)
CIMETIDINE
Tagamet Tablets 1547

TEMISARTAN (Argentina)
LOSARTAN POTASSIUM
Cozaar Tablets 1913

TEMPERAX (Chile)
CITALOPRAM HYDROBROMIDE
Celexa Tablets 1177

TEMPOROL (Irish Republic, South Africa)
CARBAMAZEPINE
Carbatrol Capsules 3174
Tegretol Chewable Tablets. . . . 2278
Tegretol Suspension. . . . 2278
Tegretol Tablets 2278
Tegretol-XR Tablets 2278

TEMSERIN (Germany, Greece)
TIMOLOL MALEATE
Blocadren Tablets 1891
Timoptic Sterile Ophthalmic Solution 2058
Timoptic in Ocudose 2061
Timoptic-XE Sterile Ophthalmic Gel Forming Solution 2062

TENACID (Italy)
CILASTATIN SODIUM/IMIPENEM
Primaxin I.M. 2022
Primaxin I.V. 2024

TENAT (Switzerland)
ATENOLOL
Tenormin I.V. Injection. . . . 698

TENBEN (United Kingdom)
ATENOLOL
Tenormin I.V. Injection. . . . 698

TEN-BLOKA (South Africa)
ATENOLOL
Tenormin I.V. Injection. . . . 698

TENCAS (Argentina)
ENALAPRIL MALEATE
Vasotec I.V. Injection 2076

TENCHLOR (Irish Republic, United Kingdom)
ATENOLOL
Tenormin I.V. Injection. . . . 698

TENERETIC (Germany)
ATENOLOL
Tenormin I.V. Injection. . . . 698

TENIBEX (Mexico)
ALBENDAZOLE
Albenza Tablets. . . . 1310

TENIDON (Denmark)
ATENOLOL
Tenormin I.V. Injection. . . . 698

TENIF (Belgium, United Kingdom)
ATENOLOL
Tenormin I.V. Injection. . . . 698

TENIKEN (Mexico)
PRAZIQUANTEL
Biltricide Tablets 2990

TENKAFRUSE (United Kingdom)
FUROSEMIDE
Furosemide Tablets 2117

TENLOL (Australia)
ATENOLOL
Tenormin I.V. Injection. . . . 698

TENO (Germany, India)
ATENOLOL
Tenormin I.V. Injection. . . . 698

TENO-BASAN (Germany)
ATENOLOL
Tenormin I.V. Injection. . . . 698

TENOBLOCK (Finland)
ATENOLOL
Tenormin I.V. Injection. . . . 698

TENOCARD (Argentina)
NIMODIPINE
Nimotop Capsules 774

TENOCHEK (India)
ATENOLOL
Tenormin I.V. Injection. . . . 698

TENOCLOR (India)
ATENOLOL
Tenormin I.V. Injection. . . . 698

TENOCOR (Thailand)
ATENOLOL
Tenormin I.V. Injection. . . . 698

TENOFED (India)
ATENOLOL
Tenormin I.V. Injection. . . . 698

TENOL (Thailand)
ATENOLOL
Tenormin I.V. Injection. . . . 698

TENOLIN (Canada)
ATENOLOL
Tenormin I.V. Injection. . . . 698

TENOLOL (India, Singapore, Thailand)
ATENOLOL
Tenormin I.V. Injection. . . . 698

TENOLOL-AM (India)
ATENOLOL
Tenormin I.V. Injection. . . . 698

TENOLOL-D (India)
ATENOLOL
Tenormin I.V. Injection. . . . 698

TENOMAX (Italy)
ATENOLOL
Tenormin I.V. Injection. . . . 698

TENOPRES (Argentina)
LOSARTAN POTASSIUM
Cozaar Tablets 1913

TENOPRES D (Argentina)
LOSARTAN POTASSIUM
Cozaar Tablets 1913

TENOPRIN (Finland)
ATENOLOL
Tenormin I.V. Injection. . . . 698

TENOPT (Australia)
TIMOLOL MALEATE
Blocadren Tablets 1891

Timoptic Sterile Ophthalmic Solution 2058
Timoptic in Ocudose 2061
Timoptic-XE Sterile Ophthalmic Gel Forming Solution 2062

TENORET (Hong Kong, Malaysia, New Zealand, Thailand, United Kingdom)
ATENOLOL
Tenormin I.V. Injection 698

TENORETIC (Belgium, Brazil, Czech Republic, Denmark, France, Hong Kong, Malaysia, Mexico, New Zealand, Portugal, United Kingdom)
ATENOLOL
Tenormin I.V. Injection 698

TENORIC (India)
ATENOLOL
Tenormin I.V. Injection 698

TENORMIN (Australia, Austria, Belgium, Chile, Czech Republic, Denmark, Germany, Greece, Hong Kong, India, Irish Republic, Italy, Malaysia, Mexico, New Zealand, Norway, Portugal, Singapore, South Africa, Spain, Sweden, Switzerland, Thailand, The Netherlands, United Kingdom)
ATENOLOL
Tenormin I.V. Injection 698

TENORMINE (France)
ATENOLOL
Tenormin I.V. Injection 698

TENOVATE (India)
CLOBETASOL PROPIONATE
Temovate Cream 1549
Temovate E Emollient 1552
Temovate Gel 1550
Temovate Ointment 1549
Temovate Scalp Application 1551

TENOVATE G (India)
CLOBETASOL PROPIONATE
Temovate Cream 1549
Temovate E Emollient 1552
Temovate Gel 1550
Temovate Ointment 1549
Temovate Scalp Application 1551

TENOVATE M (India)
CLOBETASOL PROPIONATE
Temovate Cream 1549
Temovate E Emollient 1552
Temovate Gel 1550
Temovate Ointment 1549
Temovate Scalp Application 1551

TENPRIL (Italy)
CAPTOPRIL
Captopril Tablets 2114

TENSADIUR (Italy)
BENAZEPRIL HYDROCHLORIDE/HYDROCHLOROTHIAZIDE
Lotensin HCT Tablets 2235

TENSANIL (Italy)
BENAZEPRIL HYDROCHLORIDE
Lotensin Tablets 2232

TENSAZOL (Portugal)
ENALAPRIL MALEATE
Vasotec I.V. Injection 2076

TENSIG (Australia)
ATENOLOL
Tenormin I.V. Injection 698

TENSIKEY (Spain)
LISINOPRIL
Prinivil Tablets 2029
Zestril Tablets 704

TENSIKEY COMPLEX (Spain)
LISINOPRIL
Prinivil Tablets 2029
Zestril Tablets 704

TENSIMIN (India)
ATENOLOL
Tenormin I.V. Injection 698

TENSIOMIN (Czech Republic, Germany, Hong Kong, Hungary, Thailand)
CAPTOPRIL
Captopril Tablets 2114

TENSIOMIN-COR (Germany)
CAPTOPRIL
Captopril Tablets 2114

TENSIPINE (United Kingdom)
NIFEDIPINE
Adalat CC Tablets 2978

TENSIUM (United Kingdom)
DIAZEPAM
Diastat Rectal Delivery System 3344
Valium Tablets 2822

TENSOBON (Germany, Switzerland)
CAPTOPRIL
Captopril Tablets 2114

TENSOBON COMP (Germany)
CAPTOPRIL
Captopril Tablets 2114

TENSOPREL (Singapore, Spain)
CAPTOPRIL
Captopril Tablets 2114

TENSOPRIL (Argentina, Irish Republic, Israel, Portugal, United Kingdom)
CAPTOPRIL
Captopril Tablets 2114

TENSOPRIL D (Argentina)
LISINOPRIL
Prinivil Tablets 2029
Zestril Tablets 704

TENSOSTAD (Germany)
CAPTOPRIL
Captopril Tablets 2114

TENSOTEC (Malaysia)
MOEXIPRIL HYDROCHLORIDE
Univasc Tablets 3118

TENSO-TIMELETS (Germany)
CLONIDINE HYDROCHLORIDE
Catapres Tablets 874

TENSOTIN (United Arab Emirates)
ATENOLOL
Tenormin I.V. Injection 698

TENSURIL (Brazil)
DIAZOXIDE
Hyperstat I.V. Injection 3031

TENUALAX (Argentina)
LACTULOSE
Kristalose for Oral Solution 2149

TEOBID (Italy)
THEOPHYLLINE
Uniphyl Tablets 2708

TEODELIN (Spain)
THEOPHYLLINE
Uniphyl Tablets 2708

TEODOSIS (Argentina)
THEOPHYLLINE
Uniphyl Tablets 2708

TEOGEL (Spain)
THEOPHYLLINE
Uniphyl Tablets 2708

TEOLIXIR (Spain)
THEOPHYLLINE
Uniphyl Tablets 2708

TEOLONG (Brazil, Mexico)
THEOPHYLLINE
Uniphyl Tablets 2708

TEONIBSA (Portugal)
THEOPHYLLINE
Uniphyl Tablets 2708

TEONOVA (Italy)
THEOPHYLLINE
Uniphyl Tablets 2708

TEOPHYL (Brazil)
THEOPHYLLINE
Uniphyl Tablets 2708

TEOPLUS (Italy)
THEOPHYLLINE
Uniphyl Tablets 2708

TEOSONA (Argentina)
THEOPHYLLINE
Uniphyl Tablets 2708

TEOSONA SOL (Argentina)
THEOPHYLLINE
Uniphyl Tablets 2708

TEOSTON (Brazil)
THEOPHYLLINE
Uniphyl Tablets 2708

TEOTARD (Czech Republic)
THEOPHYLLINE
Uniphyl Tablets 2708

TEOVAL/R (Italy)
THEOPHYLLINE
Uniphyl Tablets 2708

TEOVENT (Portugal)
THEOPHYLLINE
Uniphyl Tablets 2708

TERA (Germany)
TERAZOSIN HYDROCHLORIDE
Hytrin Capsules 469

TERAFLUSS (Italy)
TERAZOSIN HYDROCHLORIDE
Hytrin Capsules 469

TERALITHE (France)
LITHIUM CARBONATE
Eskalith CR Controlled-Release Tablets 1406
Eskalith Capsules 1406

TERANAR (Germany)
TERAZOSIN HYDROCHLORIDE
Hytrin Capsules 469

TERAPROST (Italy)
TERAZOSIN HYDROCHLORIDE
Hytrin Capsules 469

TERAUMON (Spain)
TERAZOSIN HYDROCHLORIDE
Hytrin Capsules 469

TERAZID (Germany)
TERAZOSIN HYDROCHLORIDE
Hytrin Capsules 469

TERAZOFLO (Germany)
TERAZOSIN HYDROCHLORIDE
Hytrin Capsules 469

TERBAC (Mexico)
CEFTRIAXONE SODIUM
Rocephin Injectable Vials, ADD-Vantage, Galaxy, Bulk 2801

TERBIDERM (The Netherlands)
TERBINAFINE HYDROCHLORIDE
Lamisil Tablets 2226

TERBIFIN (India)
TERBINAFINE HYDROCHLORIDE
Lamisil Tablets 2226

TERBISIL (Czech Republic, Hungary)
TERBINAFINE HYDROCHLORIDE
Lamisil Tablets 2226

TEREKOL (Argentina)
TERBINAFINE HYDROCHLORIDE
Lamisil Tablets 2226

TERFEX (Chile)
TERBINAFINE HYDROCHLORIDE
Lamisil Tablets 2226

TERFIN (Argentina)
TERBINAFINE HYDROCHLORIDE
Lamisil Tablets 2226

TERIAM (France)
TRIAMTERENE
Dyrenium Capsules 3390

TERIL (Australia, Hong Kong, Israel, New Zealand, United Kingdom)
CARBAMAZEPINE
Carbatrol Capsules 3174
Tegretol Chewable Tablets 2278
Tegretol Suspension 2278
Tegretol Tablets 2278
Tegretol-XR Tablets 2278

TERMIZOL (Mexico)
KETOCONAZOLE
Nizoral 2% Shampoo 1838

TERNOLOL (Hong Kong, Malaysia, Singapore)
ATENOLOL
Tenormin I.V. Injection 698

TERODUL (Mexico)
RANITIDINE HYDROCHLORIDE
Zantac 25 EFFERdose Tablets 1597
Zantac 150 EFFERdose Tablets 1597
Zantac 150 Tablets 1597
Zantac 300 Tablets 1597
Zantac Injection 1593
Zantac Injection Premixed 1593
Zantac Syrup 1597

TEROL (India)
TOLTERODINE TARTRATE
Detrol Tablets 2626

TEROLINAL (Greece)
LISINOPRIL
Prinivil Tablets 2029
Zestril Tablets 704

TEROMOL (Spain)
THEOPHYLLINE
Uniphyl Tablets 2708

TEROST (Brazil)
ALENDRONATE SODIUM
Fosamax Tablets 1949

TERPOSEN (Spain)
RANITIDINE HYDROCHLORIDE
Zantac 25 EFFERdose Tablets 1597
Zantac 150 EFFERdose Tablets 1597
Zantac 150 Tablets 1597
Zantac 300 Tablets 1597
Zantac Injection 1593
Zantac Injection Premixed 1593
Zantac Syrup 1597

TERRAMYCIN N (Germany)
GENTAMICIN SULFATE
Garamycin Injectable 3028
Genoptic Sterile Ophthalmic Solution .... ⊙227

TERSIF (Argentina)
LISINOPRIL
Prinivil Tablets 2029
Zestril Tablets 704

TERSODERM PLUS (Argentina)
KETOCONAZOLE
Nizoral 2% Shampoo 1838

TERTENSIF (Czech Republic, Spain)
INDAPAMIDE
Indapamide Tablets 2119

TERTROXIN (Australia, Czech Republic, Irish Republic, New Zealand, South Africa, Thailand, United Kingdom)
LIOTHYRONINE SODIUM
Cytomel Tablets 1678

TERVESON (Greece)
LOVASTATIN
Mevacor Tablets 1996

TERZINE (Thailand)
CETIRIZINE HYDROCHLORIDE
Zyrtec Syrup 2589
Zyrtec Tablets 2589

TERZOLIN (Germany, Switzerland)
KETOCONAZOLE
Nizoral 2% Shampoo 1838

TESALON (Mexico)
BENZONATATE
Tessalon Perles 1202

TESICAL (Argentina)
MEBENDAZOLE
Vermox Chewable Tablets 1853

TESOPEN (Mexico)
BENZONATATE
Tessalon Perles 1202

TESS (India)
TRIAMCINOLONE ACETONIDE
Azmacort Inhalation Aerosol 1701
Nasacort AQ Nasal Spray 2937

TESSALON (Canada)
BENZONATATE
Tessalon Perles 1202

TESSIFOL (Portugal)
ATENOLOL
Tenormin I.V. Injection 698

TESTAC (Germany)
FLUTAMIDE
Eulexin Capsules 3023

TESTOTARD (Germany)
FLUTAMIDE
Eulexin Capsules 3023

TETACID (Austria)
FAMOTIDINE
Pepcid Injection 2017

Pepcid Injection Premixed 2017
Pepcid Tablets 2014
Pepcid for Oral Suspension 2014

TETRAHELMIN (Brazil)
MEBENDAZOLE
Vermox Chewable Tablets 1853

TETROID (Brazil)
LEVOTHYROXINE SODIUM
Levothroid Tablets 1189
Levoxyl Tablets 1680
Synthroid Tablets 515

TEXA (South Africa)
CETIRIZINE HYDROCHLORIDE
Zyrtec Syrup 2589
Zyrtec Tablets 2589

TEXACORT (Canada)
HYDROCORTISONE
Hydrocortone Tablets 1963

TEXOT (Argentina)
DOCETAXEL
Taxotere Injection Concentrate 2947

TEXOVEN (Mexico)
BENZONATATE
Tessalon Perles 1202

TEYLOR (Spain)
SIMVASTATIN
Zocor Tablets 2078

THAIS (France)
ESTRADIOL
Climara Transdermal System 795
Vivelle Transdermal System 2288
Vivelle-Dot Transdermal System 2293

THALIX (India)
THALIDOMIDE
Thalomid Capsules 979

THELBAN (Malaysia)
ALBENDAZOLE
Albenza Tablets 1310

THELMOX (Malaysia)
MEBENDAZOLE
Vermox Chewable Tablets 1853

THEO (Germany)
THEOPHYLLINE
Uniphyl Tablets 2708

THEO MAX (Spain)
THEOPHYLLINE
Uniphyl Tablets 2708

THEO PA (India)
THEOPHYLLINE
Uniphyl Tablets 2708

THEO2 (The Netherlands)
THEOPHYLLINE
Uniphyl Tablets 2708

THEO-24 (Italy)
THEOPHYLLINE
Uniphyl Tablets 2708

THEOBID (India)
THEOPHYLLINE
Uniphyl Tablets 2708

THEO-BROS (Greece)
THEOPHYLLINE
Uniphyl Tablets 2708

THEOCHRON (Canada)
THEOPHYLLINE
Uniphyl Tablets 2708

THEODAY (India)
THEOPHYLLINE
Uniphyl Tablets 2708

THEODUR (Japan)
THEOPHYLLINE
Uniphyl Tablets 2708

THEO-DUR (Argentina, Australia, Belgium, Canada, Czech Republic, Denmark, Finland, Greece, Hong Kong, Irish Republic, Italy, New Zealand, Norway, Singapore, South Africa, Spain, Sweden, Thailand, United Kingdom)
THEOPHYLLINE
Uniphyl Tablets 2708

THEOFOL (Finland)
THEOPHYLLINE
Uniphyl Tablets 2708

THEOFOL COMP (Finland)
THEOPHYLLINE
Uniphyl Tablets 2708

THEOHEXAL (Austria)
THEOPHYLLINE
Uniphyl Tablets 2708

THEOLAIR (Belgium, Canada, France, Germany, Italy, Spain, Switzerland, The Netherlands)
THEOPHYLLINE
Uniphyl Tablets 2708

THEOLAN (Irish Republic)
THEOPHYLLINE
Uniphyl Tablets 2708

THEOLIN (Malaysia, Singapore, The Netherlands)
THEOPHYLLINE
Uniphyl Tablets 2708

THEOLONG (Japan)
THEOPHYLLINE
Uniphyl Tablets 2708

THEON (Switzerland)
THEOPHYLLINE
Uniphyl Tablets 2708

THEOPED (India)
THEOPHYLLINE
Uniphyl Tablets 2708

THEOPEXINE (France)
THEOPHYLLINE
Uniphyl Tablets 2708

THEOPHAR (United Arab Emirates)
THEOPHYLLINE
Uniphyl Tablets 2708

THEOPHTARD (Hungary)
THEOPHYLLINE
Uniphyl Tablets 2708

THEOPHYLLARD (Belgium, Czech Republic, Germany)
THEOPHYLLINE
Uniphyl Tablets 2708

THEOPHYLLINE SEDATIVE BRUNEAU (Belgium)
THEOPHYLLINE
Uniphyl Tablets 2708

THEOPLUS (Czech Republic, South Africa, Spain)
THEOPHYLLINE
Uniphyl Tablets 2708

THEOSPIREX (Hungary)
THEOPHYLLINE
Uniphyl Tablets 2708

THEO-SR (Canada)
THEOPHYLLINE
Uniphyl Tablets 2708

THEOTARD (Israel)
THEOPHYLLINE
Uniphyl Tablets 2708

THEOTRIM (Hong Kong, Israel, Thailand)
THEOPHYLLINE
Uniphyl Tablets 2708

THEOVENT (Hong Kong)
THEOPHYLLINE
Uniphyl Tablets 2708

THERACORT (Brazil)
TRIAMCINOLONE ACETONIDE
Azmacort Inhalation Aerosol 1701
Nasacort AQ Nasal Spray 2937

THERADERM (United Kingdom)
BENZOYL PEROXIDE
Brevoxyl-4 Creamy Wash 3212
Brevoxyl-4 Gel 3211
Brevoxyl-8 Creamy Wash 3212
Brevoxyl-8 Gel 3211
Triaz Cleanser 1864
Triaz Gel 1864

THERAPAS (United Kingdom)
AMINOSALICYLIC ACID
Paser Granules 1657

THERAPSOR (Brazil)
CLOBETASOL PROPIONATE
Temovate Cream 1549
Temovate E Emollient 1552
Temovate Gel 1550
Temovate Ointment 1549
Temovate Scalp Application 1551

THERASONA (Brazil)
HYDROCORTISONE
Hydrocortone Tablets 1963

THEVIER (Germany)
LEVOTHYROXINE SODIUM
Levothroid Tablets 1189
Levoxyl Tablets 1680
Synthroid Tablets 515

THIAZID-COMP (Germany)
HYDROCHLOROTHIAZIDE/TRIAMTERENE
Dyazide Capsules 1389
Maxzide Tablets 2150
Maxzide-25 mg Tablets 2150

THILO-MICINE (Greece)
TOBRAMYCIN
TOBI Solution for Inhalation 1015

THILOTIM (Greece)
TIMOLOL MALEATE
Blocadren Tablets 1891
Timoptic Sterile Ophthalmic Solution 2058
Timoptic in Ocudose 2061
Timoptic-XE Sterile Ophthalmic Gel Forming Solution 2062

THILOXEDINE (Greece)
DEXAMETHASONE
Decadron Tablets 1929

THIOMED (Thailand)
THIORIDAZINE HYDROCHLORIDE
Thioridazine Hydrochloride Tablets 2122

THIORIL (India)
THIORIDAZINE HYDROCHLORIDE
Thioridazine Hydrochloride Tablets 2122

THIOSIA (Thailand)
THIORIDAZINE HYDROCHLORIDE
Thioridazine Hydrochloride Tablets 2122

THIOZINE (Irish Republic)
THIORIDAZINE HYDROCHLORIDE
Thioridazine Hydrochloride Tablets 2122

THRIONIREN (Greece)
NIMODIPINE
Nimotop Capsules 774

THRIUSEDON (Greece)
LISINOPRIL
Prinivil Tablets 2029
Zestril Tablets 704

THROMBINAR (Australia, Canada)
THROMBIN
Thrombin-JMI 1693

THROMBOCID (Germany, Spain)
PENTOSAN POLYSULFATE SODIUM
Elmiron Capsules 2393

THROMBOCOLL (Germany)
THROMBIN
Thrombin-JMI 1693

THROMBODINE (Austria)
TICLOPIDINE HYDROCHLORIDE
Ticlid Tablets 2813

THROMBOHEXAL (Austria)
DIPYRIDAMOLE
Persantine Tablets 898

THROMBOREDUCTIN (Austria)
ANAGRELIDE HYDROCHLORIDE
Agrylin Capsules 3172

THROMBOSTAT (Australia, Canada, New Zealand, Singapore)
THROMBIN
Thrombin-JMI 1693

THYRADIN-S (Japan)
LEVOTHYROXINE SODIUM
Levothroid Tablets 1189
Levoxyl Tablets 1680
Synthroid Tablets 515

THYRAX (Belgium, Czech Republic, Portugal, Spain, The Netherlands)
LEVOTHYROXINE SODIUM
Levothroid Tablets 1189
Levoxyl Tablets 1680
Synthroid Tablets 515

THYRO-4 (Greece)
LEVOTHYROXINE SODIUM
Levothroid Tablets 1189
Levoxyl Tablets 1680
Synthroid Tablets 515

THYROGEN (Austria, Brazil, Canada, Denmark, Germany, Israel, Italy, Norway, Spain, Sweden, United Kingdom)
THYROTROPIN ALFA
Thyrogen for Injection 1270

THYROHORMONE (Greece)
LEVOTHYROXINE SODIUM
Levothroid Tablets 1189
Levoxyl Tablets 1680
Synthroid Tablets 515

THYROSIT (Thailand)
LEVOTHYROXINE SODIUM
Levothroid Tablets 1189
Levoxyl Tablets 1680
Synthroid Tablets 515

TIADEN (Greece)
AMILORIDE HYDROCHLORIDE/HYDROCHLOROTHIAZIDE
Moduretic Tablets 2003

TIADIL (Portugal, The Netherlands)
DILTIAZEM HYDROCHLORIDE
Cardizem LA Extended Release Tablets . . . 1699
Tiazac Capsules 1204

TIADYL (Argentina)
CANDESARTAN CILEXETIL
Atacand Tablets 634

TIADYL PLUS (Argentina)
CANDESARTAN CILEXETIL
Atacand Tablets 634

TIAKEM (Czech Republic, Italy)
DILTIAZEM HYDROCHLORIDE
Cardizem LA Extended Release Tablets . . . 1699
Tiazac Capsules 1204

TIARIX (Argentina)
PAROXETINE HYDROCHLORIDE
Paxil Oral Suspension 1501
Paxil Tablets 1501

TIAZAC (Canada)
DILTIAZEM HYDROCHLORIDE
Cardizem LA Extended Release Tablets . . . 1699
Tiazac Capsules 1204

TIAZEN (Italy)
DILTIAZEM HYDROCHLORIDE
Cardizem LA Extended Release Tablets . . . 1699
Tiazac Capsules 1204

TIBLEX (Spain)
SUCRALFATE
Carafate Suspension 727
Carafate Tablets 728

TICAVENT (Italy)
FLUTICASONE PROPIONATE
Cutivate Cream 1381
Cutivate Ointment 1384
Flonase Nasal Spray 1412

TICDINE (Thailand)
TICLOPIDINE HYDROCHLORIDE
Ticlid Tablets 2813

TICLID (Argentina, Australia, Belgium, Brazil, Canada, Chile, Czech Republic, France, Greece, Hong Kong, Hungary, Malaysia, Mexico, New Zealand, Norway, Singapore, South Africa, Sweden, Switzerland, Thailand, United Kingdom)
TICLOPIDINE HYDROCHLORIDE
Ticlid Tablets 2813

TICLIDIL (Israel)
TICLOPIDINE HYDROCHLORIDE
Ticlid Tablets 2813

TICLO (Thailand)
TICLOPIDINE HYDROCHLORIDE
Ticlid Tablets 2813

TICLOBAL (Brazil)
TICLOPIDINE HYDROCHLORIDE
Ticlid Tablets 2813

TICLOBEST (India)
TICLOPIDINE HYDROCHLORIDE
Ticlid Tablets 2813

TICLODIX (Portugal)
TICLOPIDINE HYDROCHLORIDE
Ticlid Tablets 2813

TICLODONE (Austria, Italy, Spain)
TICLOPIDINE HYDROCHLORIDE
Ticlid Tablets **2813**

TICLOGI (Italy)
TICLOPIDINE HYDROCHLORIDE
Ticlid Tablets **2813**

TICLOMED (France)
TICLOPIDINE HYDROCHLORIDE
Ticlid Tablets **2813**

TICLOP (India)
TICLOPIDINE HYDROCHLORIDE
Ticlid Tablets **2813**

TICLOPAT (Portugal)
TICLOPIDINE HYDROCHLORIDE
Ticlid Tablets **2813**

TICLOPID (India)
TICLOPIDINE HYDROCHLORIDE
Ticlid Tablets **2813**

TICLOPROGE (Italy)
TICLOPIDINE HYDROCHLORIDE
Ticlid Tablets **2813**

TICLOSAN (Italy)
TICLOPIDINE HYDROCHLORIDE
Ticlid Tablets **2813**

TIDACT (Malaysia, Singapore)
CLINDAMYCIN HYDROCHLORIDE
Cleocin Vaginal Ovules **2613**

TIENAM (Chile, France, Italy, Norway, Russia, Singapore, South Africa, Spain, Sweden, Switzerland, Thailand, The Netherlands)
CILASTATIN SODIUM/IMIPENEM
Primaxin I.M. **2022**
Primaxin I.V. **2024**

TIFINIDAT (The Netherlands)
METHYLPHENIDATE HYDROCHLORIDE
Ritalin Hydrochloride Tablets. **2254**
Ritalin-SR Tablets **2254**

TIFISTAT (The Netherlands)
PRAVASTATIN SODIUM
Pravachol Tablets **943**

TIFOX (Italy)
CEFOXITIN SODIUM
Mefoxin Premixed Intravenous Solution . . . **1990**
Mefoxin for Injection. **1987**

TIKALAC (Sweden)
LACTULOSE
Kristalose for Oral Solution **2149**

TIKL (Argentina)
KETOCONAZOLE
Nizoral 2% Shampoo **1838**

TIKLEEN (India)
TICLOPIDINE HYDROCHLORIDE
Ticlid Tablets **2813**

TIKLID (Austria, Italy, Spain)
TICLOPIDINE HYDROCHLORIDE
Ticlid Tablets **2813**

TIKLYD (Germany, Portugal)
TICLOPIDINE HYDROCHLORIDE
Ticlid Tablets **2813**

TIKOL (Thailand)
TICLOPIDINE HYDROCHLORIDE
Ticlid Tablets **2813**

TILAZEM (Argentina, Chile, Mexico, South Africa)
DILTIAZEM HYDROCHLORIDE
Cardizem LA Extended Release Tablets. . . **1699**
Tiazac Capsules **1204**

TILDIEM (Belgium, Chile, France, Greece, Hong Kong, Irish Republic, Italy, Singapore, Switzerland, Thailand, The Netherlands, United Kingdom)
DILTIAZEM HYDROCHLORIDE
Cardizem LA Extended Release Tablets. . . **1699**
Tiazac Capsules **1204**

TILENE (Italy)
FENOFIBRATE
Tricor Tablets **523**

TILEXIM (Italy)
CEFUROXIME AXETIL
Ceftin Tablets **1369**
Ceftin for Oral Suspension **1369**

TILFERAN (Greece)
ETIDRONATE DISODIUM
Didronel Tablets **2693**

TILIOS (Argentina)
ALENDRONATE SODIUM
Fosamax Tablets **1949**

TILKER (Denmark, Norway, Spain)
DILTIAZEM HYDROCHLORIDE
Cardizem LA Extended Release Tablets. . . **1699**
Tiazac Capsules **1204**

TILODENE (Australia)
TICLOPIDINE HYDROCHLORIDE
Ticlid Tablets **2813**

TILOETCA COMBI (United Kingdom)
ETIDRONATE DISODIUM
Didronel Tablets **2693**

TILOPIN (Thailand)
TICLOPIDINE HYDROCHLORIDE
Ticlid Tablets **2813**

TILOPTIC (Israel)
TIMOLOL MALEATE
Blocadren Tablets **1891**
Timoptic Sterile Ophthalmic Solution **2058**
Timoptic in Ocudose **2061**
Timoptic-XE Sterile Ophthalmic Gel Forming Solution **2062**

TILORYTH (United Kingdom)
ERYTHROMYCIN
Ery-Tab Tablets **447**
Erythromycin Base Filmtab Tablets. **454**
Erythromycin Delayed-Release Capsules, USP **456**
PCE Dispertab Tablets **510**

TILTAB (Brazil)
ROSIGLITAZONE MALEATE
Avandia Tablets. **1348**

TILTIS (Argentina)
BENZOYL PEROXIDE
Brevoxyl-4 Creamy Wash. **3212**
Brevoxyl-4 Gel **3211**
Brevoxyl-8 Creamy Wash. **3212**
Brevoxyl-8 Gel **3211**
Triaz Cleanser **1864**
Triaz Gel. **1864**

TIMAB (Argentina)
DIAZEPAM
Diastat Rectal Delivery System **3344**
Valium Tablets **2822**

TIMABAK (Austria, Brazil, Chile, France, Greece, Hong Kong, Singapore, Spain)
TIMOLOL MALEATE
Blocadren Tablets **1891**
Timoptic Sterile Ophthalmic Solution **2058**
Timoptic in Ocudose **2061**
Timoptic-XE Sterile Ophthalmic Gel Forming Solution **2062**

TIMACAR (Denmark)
TIMOLOL MALEATE
Blocadren Tablets **1891**
Timoptic Sterile Ophthalmic Solution **2058**
Timoptic in Ocudose **2061**
Timoptic-XE Sterile Ophthalmic Gel Forming Solution **2062**

TIMACOR (France)
TIMOLOL MALEATE
Blocadren Tablets **1891**
Timoptic Sterile Ophthalmic Solution **2058**
Timoptic in Ocudose **2061**
Timoptic-XE Sterile Ophthalmic Gel Forming Solution **2062**

TIM-AK (Canada)
TIMOLOL MALEATE
Blocadren Tablets **1891**
Timoptic Sterile Ophthalmic Solution **2058**
Timoptic in Ocudose **2061**
Timoptic-XE Sterile Ophthalmic Gel Forming Solution **2062**

TIMAX (Austria)
TIMOLOL MALEATE
Blocadren Tablets **1891**
Timoptic Sterile Ophthalmic Solution **2058**
Timoptic in Ocudose **2061**
Timoptic-XE Sterile Ophthalmic Gel Forming Solution **2062**

TIMED (Argentina)
TIMOLOL MALEATE
Blocadren Tablets **1891**
Timoptic Sterile Ophthalmic Solution **2058**
Timoptic in Ocudose **2061**
Timoptic-XE Sterile Ophthalmic Gel Forming Solution **2062**

TIMED D (Argentina)
TIMOLOL MALEATE
Blocadren Tablets **1891**
Timoptic Sterile Ophthalmic Solution **2058**
Timoptic in Ocudose **2061**
Timoptic-XE Sterile Ophthalmic Gel Forming Solution **2062**

TIMISOL (Switzerland)
TIMOLOL MALEATE
Blocadren Tablets **1891**
Timoptic Sterile Ophthalmic Solution **2058**
Timoptic in Ocudose **2061**
Timoptic-XE Sterile Ophthalmic Gel Forming Solution **2062**

TIMOCOMOD (France)
TIMOLOL MALEATE
Blocadren Tablets **1891**
Timoptic Sterile Ophthalmic Solution **2058**
Timoptic in Ocudose **2061**
Timoptic-XE Sterile Ophthalmic Gel Forming Solution **2062**

TIMO-COMOD (Czech Republic, Germany, Malaysia, The Netherlands)
TIMOLOL MALEATE
Blocadren Tablets **1891**
Timoptic Sterile Ophthalmic Solution **2058**
Timoptic in Ocudose **2061**
Timoptic-XE Sterile Ophthalmic Gel Forming Solution **2062**

TIMOCORT (United Kingdom)
HYDROCORTISONE
Hydrocortone Tablets **1963**

TIMODINE (United Kingdom)
NYSTATIN
Nystop Topical Powder USP **2490**

TIMODOSE (Greece)
TIMOLOL MALEATE
Blocadren Tablets **1891**
Timoptic Sterile Ophthalmic Solution **2058**
Timoptic in Ocudose **2061**
Timoptic-XE Sterile Ophthalmic Gel Forming Solution **2062**

TIMODROP (Thailand)
TIMOLOL MALEATE
Blocadren Tablets **1891**
Timoptic Sterile Ophthalmic Solution **2058**
Timoptic in Ocudose **2061**
Timoptic-XE Sterile Ophthalmic Gel Forming Solution **2062**

TIMOEDO (Germany)
TIMOLOL MALEATE
Blocadren Tablets **1891**
Timoptic Sterile Ophthalmic Solution **2058**
Timoptic in Ocudose **2061**
Timoptic-XE Sterile Ophthalmic Gel Forming Solution **2062**

TIMOFTAL (Austria)
TIMOLOL MALEATE
Blocadren Tablets **1891**
Timoptic Sterile Ophthalmic Solution **2058**
Timoptic in Ocudose **2061**
Timoptic-XE Sterile Ophthalmic Gel Forming Solution **2062**

TIMOFTOL (Spain)
TIMOLOL MALEATE
Blocadren Tablets **1891**
Timoptic Sterile Ophthalmic Solution **2058**
Timoptic in Ocudose **2061**
Timoptic-XE Sterile Ophthalmic Gel Forming Solution **2062**

TIMOGAL (Czech Republic)
TIMOLOL MALEATE
Blocadren Tablets **1891**
Timoptic Sterile Ophthalmic Solution **2058**
Timoptic in Ocudose **2061**
Timoptic-XE Sterile Ophthalmic Gel Forming Solution **2062**

TIMOGEL (Spain)
TIMOLOL MALEATE
Blocadren Tablets **1891**
Timoptic Sterile Ophthalmic Solution **2058**
Timoptic in Ocudose **2061**
Timoptic-XE Sterile Ophthalmic Gel Forming Solution **2062**

TIMOGLAU (Portugal)
TIMOLOL MALEATE
Blocadren Tablets **1891**
Timoptic Sterile Ophthalmic Solution **2058**
Timoptic in Ocudose **2061**
Timoptic-XE Sterile Ophthalmic Gel Forming Solution **2062**

TIMOHEXAL (Austria, Czech Republic, Germany)
TIMOLOL MALEATE
Blocadren Tablets **1891**
Timoptic Sterile Ophthalmic Solution **2058**
Timoptic in Ocudose **2061**
Timoptic-XE Sterile Ophthalmic Gel Forming Solution **2062**

TIMOLABAK (Italy)
TIMOLOL MALEATE
Blocadren Tablets **1891**
Timoptic Sterile Ophthalmic Solution **2058**
Timoptic in Ocudose **2061**
Timoptic-XE Sterile Ophthalmic Gel Forming Solution **2062**

TIMOLEN (Portugal)
TIMOLOL MALEATE
Blocadren Tablets **1891**
Timoptic Sterile Ophthalmic Solution **2058**
Timoptic in Ocudose **2061**
Timoptic-XE Sterile Ophthalmic Gel Forming Solution **2062**

TIMOLER (Argentina)
TIMOLOL MALEATE
Blocadren Tablets **1891**
Timoptic Sterile Ophthalmic Solution **2058**
Timoptic in Ocudose **2061**
Timoptic-XE Sterile Ophthalmic Gel Forming Solution **2062**

TIMOLIDE (Canada)
HYDROCHLOROTHIAZIDE/TIMOLOL MALEATE
Timolide Tablets **2056**

TIMOLO (India)
TIMOLOL MALEATE
Blocadren Tablets **1891**
Timoptic Sterile Ophthalmic Solution **2058**
Timoptic in Ocudose **2061**
Timoptic-XE Sterile Ophthalmic Gel Forming Solution **2062**

TIMOLUX (Italy)
TIMOLOL MALEATE
Blocadren Tablets **1891**
Timoptic Sterile Ophthalmic Solution **2058**
Timoptic in Ocudose **2061**
Timoptic-XE Sterile Ophthalmic Gel Forming Solution **2062**

TIMOMANN (Germany)
TIMOLOL MALEATE
Blocadren Tablets **1891**
Timoptic Sterile Ophthalmic Solution **2058**
Timoptic in Ocudose **2061**
Timoptic-XE Sterile Ophthalmic Gel Forming Solution **2062**

TIMONIL (Czech Republic, Germany, Hong Kong, Hungary, Israel, Switzerland, United Kingdom)
CARBAMAZEPINE
Carbatrol Capsules **3174**
Tegretol Chewable Tablets **2278**
Tegretol Suspension. **2278**
Tegretol Tablets **2278**
Tegretol-XR Tablets **2278**

TIMO-OPTAL (Thailand)
TIMOLOL MALEATE
Blocadren Tablets **1891**
Timoptic Sterile Ophthalmic Solution **2058**
Timoptic in Ocudose **2061**
Timoptic-XE Sterile Ophthalmic Gel Forming Solution **2062**

TIMOP (Chile)
TIMOLOL MALEATE
Blocadren Tablets **1891**
Timoptic Sterile Ophthalmic Solution **2058**
Timoptic in Ocudose **2061**
Timoptic-XE Sterile Ophthalmic Gel Forming Solution **2062**

TIM-OPHTAL (Austria, Germany)
TIMOLOL MALEATE
Blocadren Tablets **1891**
Timoptic Sterile Ophthalmic Solution **2058**
Timoptic in Ocudose **2061**
Timoptic-XE Sterile Ophthalmic Gel Forming Solution **2062**

TIMOPOS COMOD (Germany)
TIMOLOL MALEATE
Blocadren Tablets **1891**

Timoptic Sterile Ophthalmic Solution 2058
Timoptic in Ocudose 2061
Timoptic-XE Sterile Ophthalmic Gel Forming Solution 2062

TIMOPTIC (Argentina, Austria, Canada, Switzerland)
TIMOLOL MALEATE
Blocadren Tablets 1891
Timoptic Sterile Ophthalmic Solution 2058
Timoptic in Ocudose 2061
Timoptic-XE Sterile Ophthalmic Gel Forming Solution 2062

TIMOPTOL (Australia, Belgium, Brazil, Czech Republic, France, Hong Kong, Irish Republic, Italy, Japan, Malaysia, Mexico, New Zealand, Portugal, Singapore, South Africa, Thailand, The Netherlands, United Kingdom)
TIMOLOL MALEATE
Blocadren Tablets 1891
Timoptic Sterile Ophthalmic Solution 2058
Timoptic in Ocudose 2061
Timoptic-XE Sterile Ophthalmic Gel Forming Solution 2062

TIMOPTOL-XE (Australia, Chile)
TIMOLOL MALEATE
Blocadren Tablets 1891
Timoptic Sterile Ophthalmic Solution 2058
Timoptic in Ocudose 2061
Timoptic-XE Sterile Ophthalmic Gel Forming Solution 2062

TIMOSAN (Denmark, Finland, Norway, Sweden)
TIMOLOL MALEATE
Blocadren Tablets 1891
Timoptic Sterile Ophthalmic Solution 2058
Timoptic in Ocudose 2061
Timoptic-XE Sterile Ophthalmic Gel Forming Solution 2062

TIMOSIL (Thailand)
TIMOLOL MALEATE
Blocadren Tablets 1891
Timoptic Sterile Ophthalmic Solution 2058
Timoptic in Ocudose 2061
Timoptic-XE Sterile Ophthalmic Gel Forming Solution 2062

TIMOSINE (Germany)
TIMOLOL MALEATE
Blocadren Tablets 1891
Timoptic Sterile Ophthalmic Solution 2058
Timoptic in Ocudose 2061
Timoptic-XE Sterile Ophthalmic Gel Forming Solution 2062

TIMOSOFT (Italy)
TIMOLOL MALEATE
Blocadren Tablets 1891
Timoptic Sterile Ophthalmic Solution 2058
Timoptic in Ocudose 2061
Timoptic-XE Sterile Ophthalmic Gel Forming Solution 2062

TIMO-STULLN (Germany)
TIMOLOL MALEATE
Blocadren Tablets 1891
Timoptic Sterile Ophthalmic Solution 2058
Timoptic in Ocudose 2061
Timoptic-XE Sterile Ophthalmic Gel Forming Solution 2062

TIMOZZARD (Mexico)
TIMOLOL MALEATE
Blocadren Tablets 1891
Timoptic Sterile Ophthalmic Solution 2058
Timoptic in Ocudose 2061
Timoptic-XE Sterile Ophthalmic Gel Forming Solution 2062

TIMPILO (Argentina, Australia, Czech Republic, Malaysia)
TIMOLOL MALEATE
Blocadren Tablets 1891
Timoptic Sterile Ophthalmic Solution 2058
Timoptic in Ocudose 2061
Timoptic-XE Sterile Ophthalmic Gel Forming Solution 2062

TIMPRON (United Kingdom)
NAPROXEN
EC-Naprosyn Delayed-Release Tablets 2769
Naprosyn Suspension 2769
Naprosyn Tablets 2769

TIMSOPT (Austria)
DORZOLAMIDE HYDROCHLORIDE/TIMOLOL MALEATE
Cosopt Sterile Ophthalmic Solution 1910

TINACEF (Argentina)
CEFTAZIDIME
Fortaz for Injection 1422

TINADERM EXTRA (Australia)
CLOTRIMAZOLE
Lotrimin Cream 3053
Lotrimin Lotion 1% 3053
Lotrimin Topical Solution 1% 3053

TINAGEL (Belgium, The Netherlands)
BENZOYL PEROXIDE
Brevoxyl-4 Creamy Wash 3212
Brevoxyl-4 Gel 3211
Brevoxyl-8 Creamy Wash 3212
Brevoxyl-8 Gel 3211
Triaz Cleanser 1864
Triaz Gel 1864

TINIAZOL (Mexico)
KETOCONAZOLE
Nizoral 2% Shampoo 1838

TIOF (Chile, Mexico)
TIMOLOL MALEATE
Blocadren Tablets 1891
Timoptic Sterile Ophthalmic Solution 2058
Timoptic in Ocudose 2061
Timoptic-XE Sterile Ophthalmic Gel Forming Solution 2062

TIOSALIS (Argentina)
ONDANSETRON
Zofran ODT Orally Disintegrating Tablets 1613

TIPAC (Chile)
RANITIDINE HYDROCHLORIDE
Zantac 25 EFFERdose Tablets 1597
Zantac 150 EFFERdose Tablets 1597
Zantac 150 Tablets 1597
Zantac 300 Tablets 1597
Zantac Injection 1593
Zantac Injection Premixed 1593
Zantac Syrup 1597

TIPERAL (Irish Republic)
PROPRANOLOL HYDROCHLORIDE
Inderal LA Long-Acting Capsules 3421

TIPIDIN (Hong Kong, Malaysia, Singapore)
TICLOPIDINE HYDROCHLORIDE
Ticlid Tablets 2813

TIPIDINE (Thailand)
TICLOPIDINE HYDROCHLORIDE
Ticlid Tablets 2813

TIPODEX (Spain)
FAMOTIDINE
Pepcid Injection 2017
Pepcid Injection Premixed 2017
Pepcid Tablets 2014
Pepcid for Oral Suspension 2014

TIRACRIN (Italy)
LEVOTHYROXINE SODIUM
Levothroid Tablets 1189
Levoxyl Tablets 1680
Synthroid Tablets 515

TIRIZIN (Austria)
CETIRIZINE HYDROCHLORIDE
Zyrtec Syrup 2589
Zyrtec Tablets 2589

TIROCAL (Mexico)
CALCITRIOL
Calcijex Injection 411

TIROIDINE (Mexico)
LEVOTHYROXINE SODIUM
Levothroid Tablets 1189
Levoxyl Tablets 1680
Synthroid Tablets 515

TIROSINT (Italy)
LEVOTHYROXINE SODIUM
Levothroid Tablets 1189
Levoxyl Tablets 1680
Synthroid Tablets 515

TISOGEN (Argentina)
TOPOTECAN HYDROCHLORIDE
Hycamtin for Injection 1427

TISOREK (Argentina)
CELECOXIB
Celebrex Capsules 3130

TITANOX (Greece, Thailand)
PROMETHAZINE HYDROCHLORIDE
Phenergan Suppositories 3438
Phenergan Tablets 3438

TITRANE (Spain)
ISOSORBIDE MONONITRATE
Imdur Tablets 3032

TI-TRE (Italy)
LIOTHYRONINE SODIUM
Cytomel Tablets 1678

TI-U-LAC HC (Canada)
HYDROCORTISONE
Hydrocortone Tablets 1963

TIVIRLON (Greece)
LISINOPRIL
Prinivil Tablets 2029
Zestril Tablets 704

TIXYLIX (Malaysia)
PROMETHAZINE HYDROCHLORIDE
Phenergan Suppositories 3438
Phenergan Tablets 3438

TIXYLIX NIGHTIME (Australia)
PROMETHAZINE HYDROCHLORIDE
Phenergan Suppositories 3438
Phenergan Tablets 3438

TKC (Chile)
KETOCONAZOLE
Nizoral 2% Shampoo 1838

TOBACIN (India)
TOBRAMYCIN
TOBI Solution for Inhalation 1015

TOBAZON (India)
TOBRAMYCIN
TOBI Solution for Inhalation 1015

TOBI (Argentina, Australia, Austria, Belgium, Canada, Denmark, Finland, France, Germany, Greece, Irish Republic, Israel, Italy, Norway, Spain, Sweden, Switzerland, United Kingdom)
TOBRAMYCIN
TOBI Solution for Inhalation 1015

TOBIN (Switzerland)
CETIRIZINE HYDROCHLORIDE
Zyrtec Syrup 2589
Zyrtec Tablets 2589

TOBRABACT (Italy, Spain)
TOBRAMYCIN
TOBI Solution for Inhalation 1015

TOBRABIOTIC (Argentina)
TOBRAMYCIN
TOBI Solution for Inhalation 1015

TOBRABIOTIC D (Argentina)
TOBRAMYCIN
TOBI Solution for Inhalation 1015

TOBRACORT (Argentina, Brazil)
TOBRAMYCIN
TOBI Solution for Inhalation 1015

TOBRADEX (Argentina, Austria, Belgium, Brazil, Canada, Chile, Czech Republic, France, Greece, Hong Kong, Hungary, Italy, Malaysia, Mexico, New Zealand, Singapore, South Africa, Spain, Switzerland, Thailand, The Netherlands, United Kingdom)
TOBRAMYCIN
TOBI Solution for Inhalation 1015

TOBRADICLO (Argentina)
TOBRAMYCIN
TOBI Solution for Inhalation 1015

TOBRAFEN (Switzerland)
DICLOFENAC SODIUM
Voltaren Tablets 2298
Voltaren-XR Tablets 2301

TOBRAGAN (Argentina, Brazil, Chile)
TOBRAMYCIN
TOBI Solution for Inhalation 1015

TOBRAGAN D (Argentina)
TOBRAMYCIN
TOBI Solution for Inhalation 1015

TOBRAL (Italy)
TOBRAMYCIN
TOBI Solution for Inhalation 1015

TOBRALEX (Irish Republic, United Kingdom)
TOBRAMYCIN
TOBI Solution for Inhalation 1015

TOBRA-M (Brazil)
TOBRAMYCIN
TOBI Solution for Inhalation 1015

TOBRAMAXIN (Germany)
TOBRAMYCIN
TOBI Solution for Inhalation 1015

TOBRANOM (Brazil)
TOBRAMYCIN
TOBI Solution for Inhalation 1015

TOBRASTILL (Italy)
TOBRAMYCIN
TOBI Solution for Inhalation 1015

TOBRATLAS (Argentina)
DICLOFENAC SODIUM
Voltaren Tablets 2298
Voltaren-XR Tablets 2301

TOBREX (Argentina, Australia, Austria, Belgium, Brazil, Canada, Chile, Czech Republic, Denmark, Finland, France, Greece, Hong Kong, Hungary, Israel, Malaysia, Mexico, New Zealand, Norway, Portugal, Singapore, South Africa, Spain, Sweden, Switzerland, Thailand, The Netherlands)
TOBRAMYCIN
TOBI Solution for Inhalation 1015

TOBRIDAVI (Portugal)
TOBRAMYCIN
TOBI Solution for Inhalation 1015

TOBRIN (Chile)
TOBRAMYCIN
TOBI Solution for Inhalation 1015

TOBRIN-D (Chile)
DEXAMETHASONE/TOBRAMYCIN
TobraDex Ophthalmic Ointment 558
TobraDex Ophthalmic Suspension 558

TOCOMIZOL (Mexico)
KETOCONAZOLE
Nizoral 2% Shampoo 1838

TOCONAL (Mexico)
KETOCONAZOLE
Nizoral 2% Shampoo 1838

TODEXONA (Chile)
DEXAMETHASONE/TOBRAMYCIN
TobraDex Ophthalmic Ointment 558
TobraDex Ophthalmic Suspension 558

TOFLAMIXINA (Argentina, Brazil)
TOBRAMYCIN
TOBI Solution for Inhalation 1015

TOFLAMIXINA PLUS (Argentina)
TOBRAMYCIN
TOBI Solution for Inhalation 1015

TOLBIN (Argentina)
METRONIDAZOLE
MetroGel-Vaginal Gel 1822
Noritate Cream, 1% 1051

TOLERABIOTICO (Spain)
ERYTHROMYCIN STEARATE
Erythrocin Stearate Filmtab Tablets 452

TOLOXIM (Portugal)
MEBENDAZOLE
Vermox Chewable Tablets 1853

TOLOXIN (Thailand)
DIGOXIN
Lanoxicaps Capsules 1458
Lanoxin Injection 1462
Lanoxin Injection Pediatric 1465
Lanoxin Tablets 1468

TOLREST (Brazil)
SERTRALINE HYDROCHLORIDE
Zoloft Tablets 2581

TOLTEM (Argentina)
TOLTERODINE TARTRATE
Detrol Tablets 2626

TOMAG (Argentina)
RANITIDINE HYDROCHLORIDE
Zantac 25 EFFERdose Tablets 1597
Zantac 150 EFFERdose Tablets 1597
Zantac 150 Tablets 1597

Zantac 300 Tablets 1597
Zantac Injection 1593
Zantac Injection Premixed 1593
Zantac Syrup 1597

TOMYCINE (Canada)
TOBRAMYCIN
TOBI Solution for Inhalation 1015

TONAVIR (Argentina)
STAVUDINE
Zerit Capsules 971
Zerit for Oral Solution 971

TONDEX (Mexico)
GENTAMICIN SULFATE
Garamycin Injectable 3028
Genoptic Sterile Ophthalmic Solution . . . . ⊙227

TONOBEXOL (Argentina)
BETAXOLOL HYDROCHLORIDE
Betoptic S Ophthalmic Suspension 554

TONOFTAL-N (Germany)
NYSTATIN
Nystop Topical Powder USP 2490

TONOPROTECT (Germany)
ATENOLOL
Tenormin I.V. Injection 698

TONOTENSIL (Chile)
LISINOPRIL
Prinivil Tablets 2029
Zestril Tablets 704

TONOTENSIL D (Chile)
HYDROCHLOROTHIAZIDE/LISINOPRIL
Prinzide Tablets 2033
Zestoretic Tablets 701

TONOVIT (Greece)
LEVOCARNITINE
Carnitor Injection 3185
Carnitor Tablets and Oral Solution 3187

TOPACE (Australia)
CAPTOPRIL
Captopril Tablets 2114

TOPAMAC (Argentina, Greece, India)
TOPIRAMATE
Topamax Sprinkle Capsules 2438
Topamax Tablets 2438

TOPAMATE (India)
TOPIRAMATE
Topamax Sprinkle Capsules 2438
Topamax Tablets 2438

TOPAMAX (Australia, Austria, Belgium, Brazil, Canada, Chile, Czech Republic, Germany, Hong Kong, Hungary, Irish Republic, Israel, Italy, Malaysia, Mexico, New Zealand, Portugal, Singapore, South Africa, Spain, Switzerland, Thailand, The Netherlands, United Kingdom)
TOPIRAMATE
Topamax Sprinkle Capsules 2438
Topamax Tablets 2438

TOPCORT (India)
MOMETASONE FUROATE
Elocon Cream 0.1% 3019
Elocon Lotion 0.1% 3020
Elocon Ointment 0.1% 3021
Nasonex Nasal Spray 3058

TOP-DAL (Mexico)
LOPERAMIDE HYDROCHLORIDE
Imodium Capsules 1834

TOPERIT (Argentina)
ERYTHROMYCIN
Ery-Tab Tablets 447
Erythromycin Base Filmtab Tablets 454
Erythromycin Delayed-Release Capsules, USP 456
PCE Dispertab Tablets 510

TOPESTIN (Argentina)
TOPOTECAN HYDROCHLORIDE
Hycamtin for Injection 1427

TOPEX (Australia)
BENZOYL PEROXIDE
Brevoxyl-4 Creamy Wash 3212
Brevoxyl-4 Gel 3211
Brevoxyl-8 Creamy Wash 3212
Brevoxyl-8 Gel 3211
Triaz Cleanser 1864
Triaz Gel 1864

TOPFANS (Italy)
DICLOFENAC SODIUM
Voltaren Tablets 2298
Voltaren-XR Tablets 2301

TOPICIL (Hong Kong, Malaysia, New Zealand, Singapore)
CLINDAMYCIN PHOSPHATE
Clindets Pledgets 3212

TOPICTAL (Argentina)
TOPIRAMATE
Topamax Sprinkle Capsules 2438
Topamax Tablets 2438

TOPIFORT (India)
CLOBETASOL PROPIONATE
Temovate Cream 1549
Temovate E Emollient 1552
Temovate Gel 1550
Temovate Ointment 1549
Temovate Scalp Application 1551

TOPILONE (Thailand)
TRIAMCINOLONE ACETONIDE
Azmacort Inhalation Aerosol 1701
Nasacort AQ Nasal Spray 2937

TOPIMAX (Denmark, Finland, Norway, Sweden)
TOPIRAMATE
Topamax Sprinkle Capsules 2438
Topamax Tablets 2438

TOPISTIN (Greece)
CIPROFLOXACIN
Cipro Oral Suspension 2991

TOPIZOL (Australia)
CLOTRIMAZOLE
Lotrimin Cream 3053
Lotrimin Lotion 1% 3053
Lotrimin Topical Solution 1% 3053

TOPLA (South Africa)
LIDOCAINE
Lidoderm Patch 1107

TOPOKEBIR (Argentina)
TOPOTECAN HYDROCHLORIDE
Hycamtin for Injection 1427

TOPOSTASIN (Germany, Italy, The Netherlands)
THROMBIN
Thrombin-JMI 1693

TOPOTAG (Argentina)
TOPOTECAN HYDROCHLORIDE
Hycamtin for Injection 1427

TOPOTEL (India)
TOPOTECAN HYDROCHLORIDE
Hycamtin for Injection 1427

TOPPYC (Brazil)
PERMETHRIN
Acticin Cream 2125

TOPREL (Chile)
TOPIRAMATE
Topamax Sprinkle Capsules 2438
Topamax Tablets 2438

TOPRILEM (Mexico)
CAPTOPRIL
Captopril Tablets 2114

TOPROL (Australia)
METOPROLOL SUCCINATE
Toprol-XL Tablets 660

TORACIN (Hong Kong)
TOBRAMYCIN
TOBI Solution for Inhalation 1015

TORIAC (Belgium)
LOPERAMIDE HYDROCHLORIDE
Imodium Capsules 1834

TORIO (Thailand)
SIMVASTATIN
Zocor Tablets 2078

TORIOL (Spain)
RANITIDINE HYDROCHLORIDE
Zantac 25 EFFERdose Tablets 1597
Zantac 150 EFFERdose Tablets 1597
Zantac 150 Tablets 1597
Zantac 300 Tablets 1597
Zantac Injection 1593
Zantac Injection Premixed 1593
Zantac Syrup 1597

TORIVAS (Argentina)
ATORVASTATIN CALCIUM
Lipitor Tablets 2495

TORVAST (Italy)
ATORVASTATIN CALCIUM
Lipitor Tablets 2495

TORYXIL (Germany)
DICLOFENAC SODIUM
Voltaren Tablets 2298
Voltaren-XR Tablets 2301

TOTACEF (Hungary, Israel, Italy)
CEFAZOLIN SODIUM
Ancef for Injection 1318

TOTALIP (Italy)
ATORVASTATIN CALCIUM
Lipitor Tablets 2495

TOTAMOL (United Kingdom)
ATENOLOL
Tenormin I.V. Injection 698

TOTARETIC (United Kingdom)
ATENOLOL
Tenormin I.V. Injection 698

TOTATROM (Mexico)
ERYTHROMYCIN
Ery-Tab Tablets 447
Erythromycin Base Filmtab Tablets 454
Erythromycin Delayed-Release Capsules, USP 456
PCE Dispertab Tablets 510

TOTELLE (Sweden)
ESTRADIOL
Climara Transdermal System 795
Vivelle Transdermal System 2288
Vivelle-Dot Transdermal System 2293

TOTELLE CONTINUO (Argentina)
ESTRADIOL
Climara Transdermal System 795
Vivelle Transdermal System 2288
Vivelle-Dot Transdermal System 2293

TOTELMIN (Brazil)
ALBENDAZOLE
Albenza Tablets 1310

TOTOCORTIN (Germany)
DEXAMETHASONE SODIUM PHOSPHATE
Decadron Phosphate Injection 1931

TOZOLDEN (Argentina)
ATENOLOL
Tenormin I.V. Injection 698

TRACIX (Spain)
CILASTATIN SODIUM/IMIPENEM
Primaxin I.M. 2022
Primaxin I.V. 2024

TRADELIA (Germany)
ESTRADIOL
Climara Transdermal System 795
Vivelle Transdermal System 2288
Vivelle-Dot Transdermal System 2293

TRADIVER (Greece)
ATENOLOL
Tenormin I.V. Injection 698

TRADOX (Chile)
LAMOTRIGINE
Lamictal Chewable Dispersible Tablets . . . 1449
Lamictal Tablets 1449

TRAFLOXAL (Belgium, The Netherlands)
OFLOXACIN
Floxin Otic Solution 1043

TRAMSILIONE (Thailand)
TRIAMCINOLONE ACETONIDE
Azmacort Inhalation Aerosol 1701
Nasacort AQ Nasal Spray 2937

TRANCOCARD (Italy)
DIPYRIDAMOLE
Persantine Tablets 898

TRANGINA (United Kingdom)
ISOSORBIDE MONONITRATE
Imdur Tablets 3032

TRANGOREX (Spain)
AMIODARONE HYDROCHLORIDE
Pacerone Tablets 3337

TRANIMET (Brazil)
CIMETIDINE
Tagamet Tablets 1547

TRANQUASE (Germany)
DIAZEPAM
Diastat Rectal Delivery System 3344
Valium Tablets 2822

TRANQUILYN (United Kingdom)
METHYLPHENIDATE HYDROCHLORIDE
Ritalin Hydrochloride Tablets 2254
Ritalin-SR Tablets 2254

TRANQUIRIT (Italy)
DIAZEPAM
Diastat Rectal Delivery System 3344
Valium Tablets 2822

TRANQUO (Germany)
DIAZEPAM
Diastat Rectal Delivery System 3344
Valium Tablets 2822

TRANSDERMA H (Argentina)
HYDROCORTISONE
Hydrocortone Tablets 1963

TRANSDIOL (Argentina)
ESTRADIOL
Climara Transdermal System 795
Vivelle Transdermal System 2288
Vivelle-Dot Transdermal System 2293

TRANSIPEN (Greece)
INDAPAMIDE
Indapamide Tablets 2119

TRANSPULMINA RINO (Italy)
NAPHAZOLINE HYDROCHLORIDE
Albalon Ophthalmic Solution . . . . . ⊙216

TRANSVITAL (Chile)
ESTRADIOL
Climara Transdermal System 795
Vivelle Transdermal System 2288
Vivelle-Dot Transdermal System 2293

TRANTALOL (Irish Republic)
ATENOLOL
Tenormin I.V. Injection 698

TRANTIL (Mexico)
CARBAMAZEPINE
Carbatrol Capsules 3174
Tegretol Chewable Tablets 2278
Tegretol Suspension 2278
Tegretol Tablets 2278
Tegretol-XR Tablets 2278

TRASTOCIR (Argentina)
CILOSTAZOL
Pletal Tablets 2478

TRASYLOL (Australia, Austria, Belgium, Brazil, Canada, Chile, Czech Republic, Denmark, Finland, France, Germany, Greece, Hong Kong, Hungary, Irish Republic, Italy, Malaysia, Mexico, New Zealand, Singapore, South Africa, Spain, Sweden, Switzerland, Thailand, The Netherlands, United Kingdom)
APROTININ
Trasylol Injection 779

TRATACNE (Argentina)
TRETINOIN
Avita Cream 2136
Avita Gel 2138
Renova 0.05% Cream 2387
Retin-A Micro 0.1%/0.04% 2388
Vesanoid Capsules 2823

TRAUMOX (South Africa)
NAPROXEN
EC-Naprosyn Delayed-Release Tablets 2769
Naprosyn Suspension 2769
Naprosyn Tablets 2769

TRAVELLO (Denmark, Norway, Sweden)
LOPERAMIDE HYDROCHLORIDE
Imodium Capsules 1834

TRAVIATA (Chile)
PAROXETINE HYDROCHLORIDE
Paxil Oral Suspension 1501
Paxil Tablets 1501

TRAVILAN (Greece)
CEFTRIAXONE SODIUM
Rocephin Injectable Vials, ADD-Vantage, Galaxy, Bulk 2801

TRAZOTEVA (Argentina)
DOCETAXEL
Taxotere Injection Concentrate 2947

TREDOL (Hong Kong)
ATENOLOL
Tenormin I.V. Injection 698

TREMEXAL (Greece)
FLUTAMIDE
Eulexin Capsules 3023

TREMOREX (Denmark)
SELEGILINE HYDROCHLORIDE
Eldepryl Capsules 3209

TREPOL (Mexico)
DIPYRIDAMOLE
Persantine Tablets 898

TRESLEEN (Austria)
SERTRALINE HYDROCHLORIDE
Zoloft Tablets 2581

TRETAX (Czech Republic)
ALTRETAMINE
Hexalen Capsules 2101

TRETIN (Greece)
ISOTRETINOIN
Accutane Capsules 2740

TRETINODERM (Argentina)
TRETINOIN
Avita Cream 2136
Avita Gel 2138
Renova 0.05% Cream 2387
Retin-A Micro 0.1%/0.04% 2388
Vesanoid Capsules 2823

TRETINOINE KEFRANE (France)
TRETINOIN
Avita Cream 2136
Avita Gel 2138
Renova 0.05% Cream 2387
Retin-A Micro 0.1%/0.04% 2388
Vesanoid Capsules 2823

TRETINON (Malaysia, Mexico)
TRETINOIN
Avita Cream 2136
Avita Gel 2138
Renova 0.05% Cream 2387
Retin-A Micro 0.1%/0.04% 2388
Vesanoid Capsules 2823

TREVILOR (Germany)
VENLAFAXINE HYDROCHLORIDE
Effexor Tablets 3405
Effexor XR Capsules 3411

TREWILOR (Austria)
VENLAFAXINE HYDROCHLORIDE
Effexor Tablets 3405
Effexor XR Capsules 3411

TREXEN (Mexico)
CLINDAMYCIN PHOSPHATE
Clindets Pledgets 3212

TREXOFIN (Singapore)
CEFTRIAXONE SODIUM
Rocephin Injectable Vials, ADD-Vantage, Galaxy, Bulk 2801

TRIACORT (Italy)
TRIAMCINOLONE ACETONIDE
Azmacort Inhalation Aerosol 1701
Nasacort AQ Nasal Spray 2937

TRIADERM (Canada)
TRIAMCINOLONE ACETONIDE
Azmacort Inhalation Aerosol 1701
Nasacort AQ Nasal Spray 2937

TRIAKEN (Mexico)
CEFTRIAXONE SODIUM
Rocephin Injectable Vials, ADD-Vantage, Galaxy, Bulk 2801

TRIAKLIM (Hungary)
ESTRADIOL
Climara Transdermal System 795
Vivelle Transdermal System 2288
Vivelle-Dot Transdermal System 2293

TRIAL GEL (Argentina)
ESTRADIOL
Climara Transdermal System 795
Vivelle Transdermal System 2288
Vivelle-Dot Transdermal System 2293

TRIAL GEST (Argentina)
ESTRADIOL
Climara Transdermal System 795
Vivelle Transdermal System 2288
Vivelle-Dot Transdermal System 2293

TRIAL SAT (Argentina)
ESTRADIOL
Climara Transdermal System 795
Vivelle Transdermal System 2288
Vivelle-Dot Transdermal System 2293

TRIALIX (Austria, Irish Republic)
RAMIPRIL
Altace Capsules 1673

TRIALONA (Spain)
FLUTICASONE PROPIONATE
Cutivate Cream 1381
Cutivate Ointment 1384
Flonase Nasal Spray 1412

TRIAM (Hong Kong, Singapore)
TRIAMCINOLONE ACETONIDE
Azmacort Inhalation Aerosol 1701
Nasacort AQ Nasal Spray 2937

TRIAMA (Thailand)
TRIAMCINOLONE ACETONIDE
Azmacort Inhalation Aerosol 1701
Nasacort AQ Nasal Spray 2937

TRIAMAXCO (United Kingdom)
HYDROCHLOROTHIAZIDE/TRIAMTERENE
Dyazide Capsules 1389
Maxzide Tablets 2150
Maxzide-25 mg Tablets 2150

TRIAMCINOLON COMPOSITUM (Czech Republic)
TRIAMCINOLONE ACETONIDE
Azmacort Inhalation Aerosol 1701
Nasacort AQ Nasal Spray 2937

TRIAMCINOLON E (Czech Republic)
TRIAMCINOLONE ACETONIDE
Azmacort Inhalation Aerosol 1701
Nasacort AQ Nasal Spray 2937

TRIAMCINOLON S (Czech Republic)
TRIAMCINOLONE ACETONIDE
Azmacort Inhalation Aerosol 1701
Nasacort AQ Nasal Spray 2937

TRIAMCO (United Kingdom)
HYDROCHLOROTHIAZIDE/TRIAMTERENE
Dyazide Capsules 1389
Maxzide Tablets 2150
Maxzide-25 mg Tablets 2150

TRIAM-CO (Hong Kong)
HYDROCHLOROTHIAZIDE/TRIAMTERENE
Dyazide Capsules 1389
Maxzide Tablets 2150
Maxzide-25 mg Tablets 2150

TRIAMCORT (Switzerland)
TRIAMCINOLONE ACETONIDE
Azmacort Inhalation Aerosol 1701
Nasacort AQ Nasal Spray 2937

TRIAMCREME (Germany)
TRIAMCINOLONE ACETONIDE
Azmacort Inhalation Aerosol 1701
Nasacort AQ Nasal Spray 2937

TRIAMGALEN (Germany)
TRIAMCINOLONE ACETONIDE
Azmacort Inhalation Aerosol 1701
Nasacort AQ Nasal Spray 2937

TRIAMHEXAL (Germany)
TRIAMCINOLONE ACETONIDE
Azmacort Inhalation Aerosol 1701
Nasacort AQ Nasal Spray 2937

TRIAMIZIDE (New Zealand)
HYDROCHLOROTHIAZIDE/TRIAMTERENE
Dyazide Capsules 1389
Maxzide Tablets 2150
Maxzide-25 mg Tablets 2150

TRIAMPUR COMPOSITUM (Germany)
HYDROCHLOROTHIAZIDE/TRIAMTERENE
Dyazide Capsules 1389
Maxzide Tablets 2150
Maxzide-25 mg Tablets 2150

TRIAMSALBE (Germany)
TRIAMCINOLONE ACETONIDE
Azmacort Inhalation Aerosol 1701
Nasacort AQ Nasal Spray 2937

TRIAMTEREN COMP (Austria, Germany)
HYDROCHLOROTHIAZIDE/TRIAMTERENE
Dyazide Capsules 1389
Maxzide Tablets 2150
Maxzide-25 mg Tablets 2150

TRIAMTEREN/HCT (Austria, Germany)
TRIAMTERENE
Dyrenium Capsules 3390

TRIAMTEREN-H (Germany)
HYDROCHLOROTHIAZIDE/TRIAMTERENE
Dyazide Capsules 1389
Maxzide Tablets 2150
Maxzide-25 mg Tablets 2150

TRIAMTERIL COMPLEX (Italy)
HYDROCHLOROTHIAZIDE/TRIAMTERENE
Dyazide Capsules 1389
Maxzide Tablets 2150
Maxzide-25 mg Tablets 2150

TRIAMTHIAZID (Germany)
HYDROCHLOROTHIAZIDE/TRIAMTERENE
Dyazide Capsules 1389
Maxzide Tablets 2150
Maxzide-25 mg Tablets 2150

TRIAM-TIAZIDA R (Portugal)
HYDROCHLOROTHIAZIDE/TRIAMTERENE
Dyazide Capsules 1389
Maxzide Tablets 2150
Maxzide-25 mg Tablets 2150

TRIAMVIRGI (Italy)
TRIAMCINOLONE ACETONIDE
Azmacort Inhalation Aerosol 1701
Nasacort AQ Nasal Spray 2937

TRIAN (Greece)
LEVOCARNITINE
Carnitor Injection 3185
Carnitor Tablets and Oral Solution 3187

TRIANCIL (Brazil)
TRIAMCINOLONE ACETONIDE
Azmacort Inhalation Aerosol 1701
Nasacort AQ Nasal Spray 2937

TRI-ANEMUL (Germany)
TRIAMCINOLONE ACETONIDE
Azmacort Inhalation Aerosol 1701
Nasacort AQ Nasal Spray 2937

TRIAPIN (Austria, The Netherlands, United Kingdom)
FELODIPINE
Plendil Extended-Release Tablets 651

TRIARESE (Germany)
HYDROCHLOROTHIAZIDE/TRIAMTERENE
Dyazide Capsules 1389
Maxzide Tablets 2150
Maxzide-25 mg Tablets 2150

TRIASPAR (Argentina)
CABERGOLINE
Dostinex Tablets 2631

TRIASTAD HCT (Austria)
HYDROCHLOROTHIAZIDE/TRIAMTERENE
Dyazide Capsules 1389
Maxzide Tablets 2150
Maxzide-25 mg Tablets 2150

TRIASYN (Czech Republic, Hungary)
FELODIPINE
Plendil Extended-Release Tablets 651

TRIATEC (Brazil, Chile, Denmark, France, Greece, Italy, Norway, Portugal, Sweden, Switzerland)
RAMIPRIL
Altace Capsules 1673

TRIATEC COMP (Denmark)
RAMIPRIL
Altace Capsules 1673

TRIATEC COMPOSTO (Portugal)
RAMIPRIL
Altace Capsules 1673

TRIATEC D (Brazil)
RAMIPRIL
Altace Capsules 1673

TRIATEC HCT (Italy)
RAMIPRIL
Altace Capsules 1673

TRIATOP (Argentina, Austria, Italy, Thailand)
KETOCONAZOLE
Nizoral 2% Shampoo 1838

TRIAX (Israel)
CEFTRIAXONE SODIUM
Rocephin Injectable Vials, ADD-Vantage, Galaxy, Bulk 2801

TRIAXONE (United Arab Emirates)
CEFTRIAXONE SODIUM
Rocephin Injectable Vials, ADD-Vantage, Galaxy, Bulk 2801

TRIAZID (Germany)
HYDROCHLOROTHIAZIDE/TRIAMTERENE
Dyazide Capsules 1389
Maxzide Tablets 2150
Maxzide-25 mg Tablets 2150

TRIAZOL (France)
CLOTRIMAZOLE
Lotrimin Cream 3053
Lotrimin Lotion 1% 3053
Lotrimin Topical Solution 1% 3053

TRICEF (Austria, Chile, Portugal, Sweden)
CEFIXIME
Suprax 1811

TRICEFIN (Singapore)
CEFTRIAXONE SODIUM
Rocephin Injectable Vials, ADD-Vantage, Galaxy, Bulk 2801

TRICEN (Spain)
TRANDOLAPRIL/VERAPAMIL HYDROCHLORIDE
Tarka Tablets 519

TRICEPHIN (Thailand)
CEFTRIAXONE SODIUM
Rocephin Injectable Vials, ADD-Vantage, Galaxy, Bulk 2801

TRICHAZOLE (South Africa)
METRONIDAZOLE
MetroGel-Vaginal Gel 1822
Noritate Cream, 1% 1051

TRICHEX (Austria)
METRONIDAZOLE
MetroGel-Vaginal Gel 1822
Noritate Cream, 1% 1051

TRICHO CORDES (Germany)
METRONIDAZOLE
MetroGel-Vaginal Gel 1822
Noritate Cream, 1% 1051

TRICHOPOL (Russia)
METRONIDAZOLE
MetroGel-Vaginal Gel 1822
Noritate Cream, 1% 1051

TRICHOZOLE (Australia, New Zealand)
METRONIDAZOLE
MetroGel-Vaginal Gel 1822
Noritate Cream, 1% 1051

TRICIN (Brazil)
DICLOFENAC POTASSIUM
Cataflam Tablets 2173

TRICLODERM (Hong Kong)
CLOTRIMAZOLE
Lotrimin Cream 3053
Lotrimin Lotion 1% 3053
Lotrimin Topical Solution 1% 3053

TRICOCET (Brazil)
NYSTATIN
Nystop Topical Powder USP 2490

TRICOFARMA (Argentina)
FINASTERIDE
Propecia Tablets 2036
Proscar Tablets 2040

TRICOFIN (Argentina)
METRONIDAZOLE
MetroGel-Vaginal Gel 1822
Noritate Cream, 1% 1051

TRICOMED (Thailand)
METRONIDAZOLE
MetroGel-Vaginal Gel 1822
Noritate Cream, 1% 1051

TRICORTONE (Australia)
TRIAMCINOLONE ACETONIDE
Azmacort Inhalation Aerosol 1701
Nasacort AQ Nasal Spray 2937

TRICOSTEN (Brazil)
CLOTRIMAZOLE
Lotrimin Cream 3053
Lotrimin Lotion 1% 3053
Lotrimin Topical Solution 1% 3053

TRICOWAS B (Spain)
METRONIDAZOLE
MetroGel-Vaginal Gel 1822
Noritate Cream, 1% 1051

TRIFAMOX (Argentina)
AMOXICILLIN
Amoxil Pediatric Drops for Oral Suspension 1315
Amoxil Tablets 1315

TRIGEN (Mexico)
CIPROFLOXACIN HYDROCHLORIDE
Ciloxan Ophthalmic Ointment . . . 554
Ciloxan Ophthalmic Solution . . . ⊙205
Cipro Tablets . . . 2991

TRIGGER (Italy)
RANITIDINE HYDROCHLORIDE
Zantac 25 EFFERdose Tablets . . . 1597
Zantac 150 EFFERdose Tablets. . . 1597
Zantac 150 Tablets . . . 1597
Zantac 300 Tablets . . . 1597
Zantac Injection . . . 1593
Zantac Injection Premixed . . . 1593
Zantac Syrup . . . 1597

TRIGON DEPOT (Spain)
TRIAMCINOLONE ACETONIDE
Azmacort Inhalation Aerosol. . . 1701
Nasacort AQ Nasal Spray . . . 2937

TRIIODOTHYRONINE INJECTION (United Kingdom)
LIOTHYRONINE SODIUM
Cytomel Tablets . . . 1678

TRIKACIDE (Canada)
METRONIDAZOLE
MetroGel-Vaginal Gel . . . 1822
Noritate Cream, 1% . . . 1051

TRIKOZOL (Finland)
METRONIDAZOLE
MetroGel-Vaginal Gel . . . 1822
Noritate Cream, 1% . . . 1051

TRILOSIL (Thailand)
TRIAMCINOLONE ACETONIDE
Azmacort Inhalation Aerosol. . . 1701
Nasacort AQ Nasal Spray . . . 2937

TRIM (Malaysia, Thailand)
TRIAMCINOLONE ACETONIDE
Azmacort Inhalation Aerosol. . . 1701
Nasacort AQ Nasal Spray . . . 2937

TRIMASONE (Thailand)
TRIAMCINOLONE ACETONIDE
Azmacort Inhalation Aerosol. . . 1701
Nasacort AQ Nasal Spray . . . 2937

TRIMAZE (South Africa)
CLOTRIMAZOLE
Lotrimin Cream. . . 3053
Lotrimin Lotion 1%. . . 3053
Lotrimin Topical Solution 1% . . . 3053

TRIMAZOL (Argentina, Malaysia)
CLOTRIMAZOLE
Lotrimin Cream. . . 3053
Lotrimin Lotion 1%. . . 3053
Lotrimin Topical Solution 1% . . . 3053

TRIMIDURA (Germany)
TRIMIPRAMINE MALEATE
Surmontil Capsules . . . 2347

TRIMINE (Switzerland)
TRIMIPRAMINE MALEATE
Surmontil Capsules . . . 2347

TRIMINEURIN (Germany)
TRIMIPRAMINE MALEATE
Surmontil Capsules . . . 2347

TRIMOLEX (South Africa)
AMILORIDE HYDROCHLORIDE/HYDROCHLOROTHIAZIDE
Moduretic Tablets . . . 2003

TRIMONIL (Denmark, Finland, Norway, Sweden)
CARBAMAZEPINE
Carbatrol Capsules . . . 3174
Tegretol Chewable Tablets . . . 2278
Tegretol Suspension. . . 2278
Tegretol Tablets . . . 2278
Tegretol-XR Tablets . . . 2278

TRIMOX (Brazil)
AMOXICILLIN
Amoxil Pediatric Drops for Oral Suspension. . . 1315
Amoxil Tablets . . . 1315

TRIMSTAT (Argentina)
METRONIDAZOLE
MetroGel-Vaginal Gel . . . 1822
Noritate Cream, 1% . . . 1051

TRIMYSTEN (France)
CLOTRIMAZOLE
Lotrimin Cream. . . 3053
Lotrimin Lotion 1%. . . 3053
Lotrimin Topical Solution 1% . . . 3053

TRINALIN (Greece)
LEVOCARNITINE
Carnitor Injection. . . 3185
Carnitor Tablets and Oral Solution . . . 3187

TRINALION (Portugal)
NIMODIPINE
Nimotop Capsules . . . 774

TRINOLONE (Singapore)
TRIAMCINOLONE ACETONIDE
Azmacort Inhalation Aerosol. . . 1701
Nasacort AQ Nasal Spray . . . 2937

TRINOTECAN (Argentina)
IRINOTECAN HYDROCHLORIDE
Camptosar Injection. . . 2602

TRIOMUNE (India)
LAMIVUDINE
Epivir Oral Solution . . . 1394
Epivir Tablets . . . 1394
Epivir-HBV Oral Solution . . . 1398
Epivir-HBV Tablets . . . 1398

TRIORAL/HCT (Austria)
TRIAMTERENE
Dyrenium Capsules . . . 3390

TRIOSULES (Argentina)
FLUOROURACIL
Efudex Topical Cream. . . 3348
Efudex Topical Solutions . . . 3348

TRIOX NF (Chile)
NAPROXEN SODIUM
Anaprox DS Tablets . . . 2769
Anaprox Tablets . . . 2769

TRI-PLEN (South Africa)
RAMIPRIL
Altace Capsules . . . 1673

TRIPRESS (New Zealand)
TRIMIPRAMINE MALEATE
Surmontil Capsules . . . 2347

TRISORCIN (Germany)
PENICILLAMINE
Cuprimine Capsules . . . 1925

TRITACE (Argentina, Australia, Austria, Belgium, Hong Kong, Hungary, Irish Republic, Israel, Malaysia, Mexico, Singapore, South Africa, Thailand, The Netherlands, United Kingdom)
RAMIPRIL
Altace Capsules . . . 1673

TRITACE COMP (Israel)
RAMIPRIL
Altace Capsules . . . 1673

TRITACE-HCT (Argentina)
RAMIPRIL
Altace Capsules . . . 1673

TRITAZIDE (Belgium, Czech Republic, Mexico, The Netherlands)
RAMIPRIL
Altace Capsules . . . 1673

TRI-THIAZID (Germany)
HYDROCHLOROTHIAZIDE/TRIAMTERENE
Dyazide Capsules . . . 1389
Maxzide Tablets . . . 2150
Maxzide-25 mg Tablets. . . 2150

TRI-THIAZID RESERPIN (Germany)
HYDROCHLOROTHIAZIDE/TRIAMTERENE
Dyazide Capsules . . . 1389
Maxzide Tablets . . . 2150
Maxzide-25 mg Tablets. . . 2150

TRIVUDIN (Argentina)
LAMIVUDINE
Epivir Oral Solution . . . 1394
Epivir Tablets . . . 1394
Epivir-HBV Oral Solution . . . 1398
Epivir-HBV Tablets . . . 1398

TRIXNE (Argentina)
ERYTHROMYCIN
Ery-Tab Tablets . . . 447
Erythromycin Base Filmtab Tablets. . . 454
Erythromycin Delayed-Release Capsules, USP . . . 456
PCE Dispertab Tablets . . . 510

TRIXONE (Thailand)
CEFTRIAXONE SODIUM
Rocephin Injectable Vials, ADD-Vantage, Galaxy, Bulk . . . 2801

TRIXOTENE (Argentina)
DOCETAXEL
Taxotere Injection Concentrate . . . 2947

TRIYOTEX (Mexico)
LIOTHYRONINE SODIUM
Cytomel Tablets . . . 1678

TRIZ (Thailand)
CETIRIZINE HYDROCHLORIDE
Zyrtec Syrup . . . 2589
Zyrtec Tablets . . . 2589

TRIZELE (Hong Kong)
METRONIDAZOLE
MetroGel-Vaginal Gel . . . 1822
Noritate Cream, 1% . . . 1051

TRIZID (Hong Kong, New Zealand)
HYDROCHLOROTHIAZIDE/TRIAMTERENE
Dyazide Capsules . . . 1389
Maxzide Tablets . . . 2150
Maxzide-25 mg Tablets. . . 2150

TRIZOLIN (Malaysia, Singapore, Thailand)
NORFLOXACIN
Noroxin Tablets. . . 2009

TROFENTYL (India)
FENTANYL CITRATE
Actiq . . . 993

TROKEN (Argentina)
CLOPIDOGREL BISULFATE
Plavix Tablets . . . 940, 2942

TROLIP (Hong Kong)
FENOFIBRATE
Tricor Tablets . . . 523

TROLOVOL (Czech Republic, France, Germany)
PENICILLAMINE
Cuprimine Capsules . . . 1925

TROMAGESIC (India)
DICLOFENAC SODIUM
Voltaren Tablets . . . 2298
Voltaren-XR Tablets . . . 2301

TROMAX (India)
DICLOFENAC SODIUM
Voltaren Tablets . . . 2298
Voltaren-XR Tablets . . . 2301

TROMBENAL (Argentina)
TICLOPIDINE HYDROCHLORIDE
Ticlid Tablets . . . 2813

TROMBENOX (Italy)
ENOXAPARIN SODIUM
Lovenox Injection . . . 2931

TROMBISTAT (The Netherlands)
THROMBIN
Thrombin-JMI . . . 1693

TROMBONOT (Argentina)
CILOSTAZOL
Pletal Tablets . . . 2478

TROMBOPAT (Portugal)
TICLOPIDINE HYDROCHLORIDE
Ticlid Tablets . . . 2813

TROMBOXANIL (Brazil)
DIPYRIDAMOLE
Persantine Tablets . . . 898

TROMIGAL (Mexico)
ERYTHROMYCIN
Ery-Tab Tablets . . . 447
Erythromycin Base Filmtab Tablets. . . 454
Erythromycin Delayed-Release Capsules, USP . . . 456
PCE Dispertab Tablets . . . 510

TROMPERSANTIN (Mexico)
DIPYRIDAMOLE
Persantine Tablets . . . 898

TROMPHYLLIN (Germany)
THEOPHYLLINE
Uniphyl Tablets . . . 2708

TROPICUR (Argentina)
MEFLOQUINE HYDROCHLORIDE
Lariam Tablets . . . 2790

TROPIOVENT (United Kingdom)
IPRATROPIUM BROMIDE
Atrovent Inhalation Solution . . . 868
Atrovent Nasal Spray 0.03%. . . 869
Atrovent Nasal Spray 0.06%. . . 870

TROPISOL (Mexico)
CAPTOPRIL
Captopril Tablets . . . 2114

TROPIUM (United Kingdom)
CHLORDIAZEPOXIDE HYDROCHLORIDE
Librium Capsules. . . 3349

TRORIX (Chile)
ONDANSETRON
Zofran ODT Orally Disintegrating Tablets . . 1613

TROZOLET (Chile)
ANASTROZOLE
Arimidex Tablets . . . 665

TROZOLITE (Argentina)
ANASTROZOLE
Arimidex Tablets . . . 665

TRU COMPUESTO (Argentina)
MEBENDAZOLE
Vermox Chewable Tablets . . . 1853

TRUMSAL (Spain)
DILTIAZEM HYDROCHLORIDE
Cardizem LA Extended Release Tablets. . . 1699
Tiazac Capsules . . . 1204

TRUOXIN (Irish Republic)
CIPROFLOXACIN
Cipro Oral Suspension . . . 2991

TRUSOPT (Argentina, Australia, Austria, Belgium, Brazil, Canada, Chile, Czech Republic, Denmark, Finland, France, Germany, Greece, Hong Kong, Hungary, Irish Republic, Israel, Italy, Malaysia, Mexico, New Zealand, Norway, Portugal, Singapore, South Africa, Spain, Sweden, Switzerland, Thailand, The Netherlands, United Kingdom)
DORZOLAMIDE HYDROCHLORIDE
Trusopt Sterile Ophthalmic Solution. . . . 2065

T-STAT (Canada, Mexico, Singapore)
ERYTHROMYCIN
Ery-Tab Tablets . . . 447
Erythromycin Base Filmtab Tablets. . . 454
Erythromycin Delayed-Release Capsules, USP . . . 456
PCE Dispertab Tablets . . . 510

TUBERBUT (Argentina)
TOBRAMYCIN
TOBI Solution for Inhalation . . . 1015

TULOTRACT (Germany)
LACTULOSE
Kristalose for Oral Solution . . . 2149

TUNDRA (Argentina)
NAPROXEN
EC-Naprosyn Delayed-Release Tablets. . . . 2769
Naprosyn Suspension. . . 2769
Naprosyn Tablets . . . 2769

TUPAST (Greece)
RANITIDINE HYDROCHLORIDE
Zantac 25 EFFERdose Tablets . . . 1597
Zantac 150 EFFERdose Tablets. . . 1597
Zantac 150 Tablets . . . 1597
Zantac 300 Tablets . . . 1597
Zantac Injection . . . 1593
Zantac Injection Premixed . . . 1593
Zantac Syrup . . . 1597

TURFA (Germany)
HYDROCHLOROTHIAZIDE/TRIAMTERENE
Dyazide Capsules . . . 1389
Maxzide Tablets . . . 2150
Maxzide-25 mg Tablets. . . 2150

TURIMONIT (Germany)
ISOSORBIDE MONONITRATE
Imdur Tablets . . . 3032

TURIMYCIN (Germany)
CLINDAMYCIN HYDROCHLORIDE
Cleocin Vaginal Ovules . . . 2613

TURIXIN (Germany)
MUPIROCIN CALCIUM
Bactroban Cream . . . 1356
Bactroban Nasal . . . 1357

TUSEHLI (Mexico)
BENZONATATE
Tessalon Perles . . . 1202

TUSICAL (Mexico)
BENZONATATE
Tessalon Perles . . . 1202

TUSITATO (Mexico)
BENZONATATE
Tessalon Perles 1202

TUZZIL (Mexico)
BENZONATATE
Tessalon Perles 1202

TWICE (Italy)
MORPHINE SULFATE
Kadian Capsules 572
MS Contin Tablets 2703

TWINA (Thailand)
CLOTRIMAZOLE
Lotrimin Cream 3053
Lotrimin Lotion 1% 3053
Lotrimin Topical Solution 1% 3053

TYKLID (India)
TICLOPIDINE HYDROCHLORIDE
Ticlid Tablets 2813

TYMASIL (United Kingdom)
NATAMYCIN
Natacyn Antifungal Ophthalmic Suspension . . . . ⊙207

T-ZA (Thailand)
ZIDOVUDINE
Retrovir Capsules 1533
Retrovir IV Infusion 1537
Retrovir Syrup 1533
Retrovir Tablets 1533

UBICOR (Switzerland)
DILTIAZEM HYDROCHLORIDE
Cardizem LA Extended Release Tablets . . . 1699
Tiazac Capsules 1204

UBIZOL (Portugal)
FLUTICASONE PROPIONATE
Cutivate Cream 1381
Cutivate Ointment 1384
Flonase Nasal Spray 1412

UDIMA ERY (Germany)
ERYTHROMYCIN
Ery-Tab Tablets 447
Erythromycin Base Filmtab Tablets 454
Erythromycin Delayed-Release Capsules, USP 456
PCE Dispertab Tablets 510

UDRAMIL (Germany)
TRANDOLAPRIL/VERAPAMIL HYDROCHLORIDE
Tarka Tablets 519

UDRIK (Germany)
TRANDOLAPRIL
Mavik Tablets 482

ULCAID (South Africa)
RANITIDINE HYDROCHLORIDE
Zantac 25 EFFERdose Tablets 1597
Zantac 150 EFFERdose Tablets 1597
Zantac 150 Tablets 1597
Zantac 300 Tablets 1597
Zantac Injection 1593
Zantac Injection Premixed 1593
Zantac Syrup 1597

ULCAR (France)
SUCRALFATE
Carafate Suspension 727
Carafate Tablets 728

ULCECUR (Portugal)
RANITIDINE HYDROCHLORIDE
Zantac 25 EFFERdose Tablets 1597
Zantac 150 EFFERdose Tablets 1597
Zantac 150 Tablets 1597
Zantac 300 Tablets 1597
Zantac Injection 1593
Zantac Injection Premixed 1593
Zantac Syrup 1597

ULCEDIN (Italy, Mexico)
CIMETIDINE
Tagamet Tablets 1547

ULCEDINE (Brazil)
CIMETIDINE
Tagamet Tablets 1547

ULCEDOR (Brazil)
CIMETIDINE
Tagamet Tablets 1547

ULCEFATE (South Africa, Thailand)
SUCRALFATE
Carafate Suspension 727
Carafate Tablets 728

ULCEKON (India)
SUCRALFATE
Carafate Suspension 727
Carafate Tablets 728

ULCELAC (Argentina)
FAMOTIDINE
Pepcid Injection 2017
Pepcid Injection Premixed 2017
Pepcid Tablets 2014
Pepcid for Oral Suspension 2014

ULCEMET (Thailand)
CIMETIDINE
Tagamet Tablets 1547

ULCENON (Brazil)
CIMETIDINE
Tagamet Tablets 1547

ULCERAC (Brazil)
CIMETIDINE
Tagamet Tablets 1547

ULCERACID (Brazil)
CIMETIDINE
Tagamet Tablets 1547

ULCERAL (Austria)
SUCRALFATE
Carafate Suspension 727
Carafate Tablets 728

ULCERAN (Czech Republic, Hong Kong, Hungary, Malaysia, Singapore, Thailand)
FAMOTIDINE
Pepcid Injection 2017
Pepcid Injection Premixed 2017
Pepcid Tablets 2014
Pepcid for Oral Suspension 2014

ULCERASE (Brazil)
CIMETIDINE
Tagamet Tablets 1547

ULCERFEN (Argentina)
CIMETIDINE
Tagamet Tablets 1547

ULCERIDINE (Portugal)
CIMETIDINE
Tagamet Tablets 1547

ULCERIM (Mexico)
CIMETIDINE
Tagamet Tablets 1547

ULCERIT (Brazil)
RANITIDINE HYDROCHLORIDE
Zantac 25 EFFERdose Tablets 1597
Zantac 150 EFFERdose Tablets 1597
Zantac 150 Tablets 1597
Zantac 300 Tablets 1597
Zantac Injection 1593
Zantac Injection Premixed 1593
Zantac Syrup 1597

ULCERLMIN (Japan)
SUCRALFATE
Carafate Suspension 727
Carafate Tablets 728

ULCERMIN (Portugal, Spain)
SUCRALFATE
Carafate Suspension 727
Carafate Tablets 728

ULCEROL (Portugal)
RANITIDINE HYDROCHLORIDE
Zantac 25 EFFERdose Tablets 1597
Zantac 150 EFFERdose Tablets 1597
Zantac 150 Tablets 1597
Zantac 300 Tablets 1597
Zantac Injection 1593
Zantac Injection Premixed 1593
Zantac Syrup 1597

ULCERTEC (Malaysia, Portugal, Singapore)
SUCRALFATE
Carafate Suspension 727
Carafate Tablets 728

ULCETAB (South Africa)
SUCRALFATE
Carafate Suspension 727
Carafate Tablets 728

ULCETIC (South Africa)
SUCRALFATE
Carafate Suspension 727
Carafate Tablets 728

ULCETRAX (Spain)
FAMOTIDINE
Pepcid Injection 2017
Pepcid Injection Premixed 2017
Pepcid Tablets 2014
Pepcid for Oral Suspension 2014

ULCEX (Italy)
RANITIDINE HYDROCHLORIDE
Zantac 25 EFFERdose Tablets 1597
Zantac 150 EFFERdose Tablets 1597
Zantac 150 Tablets 1597
Zantac 300 Tablets 1597
Zantac Injection 1593
Zantac Injection Premixed 1593
Zantac Syrup 1597

ULCIDINE (Canada, Switzerland)
FAMOTIDINE
Pepcid Injection 2017
Pepcid Injection Premixed 2017
Pepcid Tablets 2014
Pepcid for Oral Suspension 2014

ULCIMAX (India)
FAMOTIDINE
Pepcid Injection 2017
Pepcid Injection Premixed 2017
Pepcid Tablets 2014
Pepcid for Oral Suspension 2014

ULCIMET (Brazil, Thailand)
CIMETIDINE
Tagamet Tablets 1547

ULCINAX (Brazil)
CIMETIDINE
Tagamet Tablets 1547

ULCIREX (France)
RANITIDINE HYDROCHLORIDE
Zantac 25 EFFERdose Tablets 1597
Zantac 150 EFFERdose Tablets 1597
Zantac 150 Tablets 1597
Zantac 300 Tablets 1597
Zantac Injection 1593
Zantac Injection Premixed 1593
Zantac Syrup 1597

ULCITAG (Brazil)
CIMETIDINE
Tagamet Tablets 1547

ULCITRAT (Brazil)
CIMETIDINE
Tagamet Tablets 1547

ULCODINA (Italy)
CIMETIDINE
Tagamet Tablets 1547

ULCOFALK (Italy)
CIMETIDINE
Tagamet Tablets 1547

ULCOFAM (Thailand)
FAMOTIDINE
Pepcid Injection 2017
Pepcid Injection Premixed 2017
Pepcid Tablets 2014
Pepcid for Oral Suspension 2014

ULCOGANT (Austria, Belgium, Czech Republic, Germany, Hungary, Switzerland, The Netherlands)
SUCRALFATE
Carafate Suspension 727
Carafate Tablets 728

ULCOLIND H2 (Germany)
CIMETIDINE
Tagamet Tablets 1547

ULCOLIND METRO (Germany)
METRONIDAZOLE
MetroGel-Vaginal Gel 1822
Noritate Cream, 1% 1051

ULCOLIND RANI (Germany)
RANITIDINE HYDROCHLORIDE
Zantac 25 EFFERdose Tablets 1597
Zantac 150 EFFERdose Tablets 1597
Zantac 150 Tablets 1597
Zantac 300 Tablets 1597
Zantac Injection 1593
Zantac Injection Premixed 1593
Zantac Syrup 1597

ULCOMEDINA (Italy)
CIMETIDINE
Tagamet Tablets 1547

ULCOMET (Hong Kong)
CIMETIDINE
Tagamet Tablets 1547

ULCONA (Spain)
SUCRALFATE
Carafate Suspension 727
Carafate Tablets 728

ULCOREN (Brazil)
RANITIDINE HYDROCHLORIDE
Zantac 25 EFFERdose Tablets 1597
Zantac 150 EFFERdose Tablets 1597
Zantac 150 Tablets 1597
Zantac 300 Tablets 1597
Zantac Injection 1593
Zantac Injection Premixed 1593
Zantac Syrup 1597

ULCOSIN (Hungary)
RANITIDINE HYDROCHLORIDE
Zantac 25 EFFERdose Tablets 1597
Zantac 150 EFFERdose Tablets 1597
Zantac 150 Tablets 1597
Zantac 300 Tablets 1597
Zantac Injection 1593
Zantac Injection Premixed 1593
Zantac Syrup 1597

ULCOTENK (Argentina)
RANITIDINE HYDROCHLORIDE
Zantac 25 EFFERdose Tablets 1597
Zantac 150 EFFERdose Tablets 1597
Zantac 150 Tablets 1597
Zantac 300 Tablets 1597
Zantac Injection 1593
Zantac Injection Premixed 1593
Zantac Syrup 1597

ULCRAFATE (Thailand)
SUCRALFATE
Carafate Suspension 727
Carafate Tablets 728

ULCRAST (Italy)
SUCRALFATE
Carafate Suspension 727
Carafate Tablets 728

ULCUBLOC (Germany)
CIMETIDINE
Tagamet Tablets 1547

ULCUFATO (Spain)
SUCRALFATE
Carafate Suspension 727
Carafate Tablets 728

ULCUSAN (Austria)
FAMOTIDINE
Pepcid Injection 2017
Pepcid Injection Premixed 2017
Pepcid Tablets 2014
Pepcid for Oral Suspension 2014

ULCYTE (Australia)
SUCRALFATE
Carafate Suspension 727
Carafate Tablets 728

ULDAPRIL (Mexico)
LANSOPRAZOLE
Prevacid Delayed-Release Capsules 3268

ULFAMET (Thailand)
FAMOTIDINE
Pepcid Injection 2017
Pepcid Injection Premixed 2017
Pepcid Tablets 2014
Pepcid for Oral Suspension 2014

ULFAMID (Czech Republic)
FAMOTIDINE
Pepcid Injection 2017
Pepcid Injection Premixed 2017
Pepcid Tablets 2014
Pepcid for Oral Suspension 2014

ULGARINE (Spain)
FAMOTIDINE
Pepcid Injection 2017
Pepcid Injection Premixed 2017
Pepcid Tablets 2014
Pepcid for Oral Suspension 2014

ULGASTRIN (Brazil)
CIMETIDINE
Tagamet Tablets 1547

ULIS (Italy)
CIMETIDINE
Tagamet Tablets 1547

ULKOBRIN (Italy)
RANITIDINE HYDROCHLORIDE
Zantac 25 EFFERdose Tablets 1597
Zantac 150 EFFERdose Tablets 1597
Zantac 150 Tablets 1597
Zantac 300 Tablets 1597
Zantac Injection 1593
Zantac Injection Premixed 1593
Zantac Syrup 1597

(⊙ Described in PDR For Ophthalmic Medicines™)

ULKUSAL (Germany)
CIMETIDINE
Tagamet Tablets . . . 1547

ULMET (South Africa)
CIMETIDINE
Tagamet Tablets . . . 1547

ULOGEN (Mexico)
CIMETIDINE
Tagamet Tablets . . . 1547

ULPAX (Mexico)
LANSOPRAZOLE
Prevacid Delayed-Release Capsules . . . 3268

ULRAN (Czech Republic)
RANITIDINE HYDROCHLORIDE
Zantac 25 EFFERdose Tablets . . . 1597
Zantac 150 EFFERdose Tablets . . . 1597
Zantac 150 Tablets . . . 1597
Zantac 300 Tablets . . . 1597
Zantac Injection . . . 1593
Zantac Injection Premixed . . . 1593
Zantac Syrup . . . 1597

ULSAL (Austria)
RANITIDINE HYDROCHLORIDE
Zantac 25 EFFERdose Tablets . . . 1597
Zantac 150 EFFERdose Tablets . . . 1597
Zantac 150 Tablets . . . 1597
Zantac 300 Tablets . . . 1597
Zantac Injection . . . 1593
Zantac Injection Premixed . . . 1593
Zantac Syrup . . . 1597

ULSANIC (Hong Kong, Israel, South Africa, Thailand)
SUCRALFATE
Carafate Suspension . . . 727
Carafate Tablets . . . 728

ULSAVEN (Mexico)
RANITIDINE HYDROCHLORIDE
Zantac 25 EFFERdose Tablets . . . 1597
Zantac 150 EFFERdose Tablets . . . 1597
Zantac 150 Tablets . . . 1597
Zantac 300 Tablets . . . 1597
Zantac Injection . . . 1593
Zantac Injection Premixed . . . 1593
Zantac Syrup . . . 1597

ULSERRAL (Mexico)
CIMETIDINE
Tagamet Tablets . . . 1547

ULTAK (South Africa)
RANITIDINE HYDROCHLORIDE
Zantac 25 EFFERdose Tablets . . . 1597
Zantac 150 EFFERdose Tablets . . . 1597
Zantac 150 Tablets . . . 1597
Zantac 300 Tablets . . . 1597
Zantac Injection . . . 1593
Zantac Injection Premixed . . . 1593
Zantac Syrup . . . 1597

ULTEC (Hong Kong, United Kingdom)
CIMETIDINE
Tagamet Tablets . . . 1547

ULTICADEX (Greece)
ENALAPRIL MALEATE
Vasotec I.V. Injection . . . 2076

ULTIDIN (Mexico)
FAMOTIDINE
Pepcid Injection . . . 2017
Pepcid Injection Premixed . . . 2017
Pepcid Tablets . . . 2014
Pepcid for Oral Suspension . . . 2014

ULTRA (Belgium)
SULFACETAMIDE SODIUM
Klaron Lotion 10% . . . 1050

ULTRA CLEARASIL (United Kingdom)
BENZOYL PEROXIDE
Brevoxyl-4 Creamy Wash . . . 3212
Brevoxyl-4 Gel . . . 3211
Brevoxyl-8 Creamy Wash . . . 3212
Brevoxyl-8 Gel . . . 3211
Triaz Cleanser . . . 1864
Triaz Gel . . . 1864

ULTRA HEARTBURN RELIEF (United Kingdom)
FAMOTIDINE
Pepcid Injection . . . 2017
Pepcid Injection Premixed . . . 2017
Pepcid Tablets . . . 2014
Pepcid for Oral Suspension . . . 2014

ULTRABETA (Portugal)
SALMETEROL XINAFOATE
Serevent Diskus . . . 1540

ULTRABIOTIC (Chile)
MUPIROCIN
Bactroban Ointment . . . 1358

ULTRACELE (India)
CELECOXIB
Celebrex Capsules . . . 3130

ULTRA-CLEAR-A-MED (Austria)
BENZOYL PEROXIDE
Brevoxyl-4 Creamy Wash . . . 3212
Brevoxyl-4 Gel . . . 3211
Brevoxyl-8 Creamy Wash . . . 3212
Brevoxyl-8 Gel . . . 3211
Triaz Cleanser . . . 1864
Triaz Gel . . . 1864

ULTRADERMIS (Argentina)
GENTAMICIN SULFATE
Garamycin Injectable . . . 3028
Genoptic Sterile Ophthalmic Solution . . . ⊙227

ULTRAFINA (India)
FINASTERIDE
Propecia Tablets . . . 2036
Proscar Tablets . . . 2040

ULTRAMICINA (Spain)
CIPROFLOXACIN HYDROCHLORIDE
Ciloxan Ophthalmic Ointment . . . 554
Ciloxan Ophthalmic Solution . . . ⊙205
Cipro Tablets . . . 2991

ULTRAMICINA PLUS (Spain)
CIPROFLOXACIN
Cipro Oral Suspension . . . 2991

ULTRAMOP (Canada)
METHOXSALEN
Oxsoralen Lotion 1% . . . 3354
Oxsoralen-Ultra Capsules . . . 3354

ULTRAMOX (Brazil)
AMOXICILLIN
Amoxil Pediatric Drops for Oral Suspension . . . 1315
Amoxil Tablets . . . 1315

ULTRANEURAL (Argentina)
GABAPENTIN
Neurontin Capsules . . . 2498

ULTRASE (Brazil, Canada)
PANCRELIPASE
Ultrase Capsules . . . 735
Ultrase MT Capsules . . . 736

ULTRAVIRAL (Argentina)
LAMIVUDINE
Epivir Oral Solution . . . 1394
Epivir Tablets . . . 1394
Epivir-HBV Oral Solution . . . 1398
Epivir-HBV Tablets . . . 1398

ULTRAVIRAL DUO (Argentina)
LAMIVUDINE
Epivir Oral Solution . . . 1394
Epivir Tablets . . . 1394
Epivir-HBV Oral Solution . . . 1398
Epivir-HBV Tablets . . . 1398

ULTROXIM (Italy)
CEFUROXIME SODIUM
Zinacef Injection . . . 1604

UMAN-SERUM (Italy)
PLASMA PROTEIN FRACTION
Plasmanate . . . 3252

UMAREN (Hungary)
RANITIDINE HYDROCHLORIDE
Zantac 25 EFFERdose Tablets . . . 1597
Zantac 150 EFFERdose Tablets . . . 1597
Zantac 150 Tablets . . . 1597
Zantac 300 Tablets . . . 1597
Zantac Injection . . . 1593
Zantac Injection Premixed . . . 1593
Zantac Syrup . . . 1597

UMBRIUM (Austria)
DIAZEPAM
Diastat Rectal Delivery System . . . 3344
Valium Tablets . . . 2822

UMINE (New Zealand, Singapore)
PHENTERMINE HYDROCHLORIDE
Adipex-P Capsules . . . 1216
Adipex-P Tablets . . . 1216

UMODER (Greece)
ATENOLOL
Tenormin I.V. Injection . . . 698

UNDERACID (Spain)
RANITIDINE HYDROCHLORIDE
Zantac 25 EFFERdose Tablets . . . 1597
Zantac 150 EFFERdose Tablets . . . 1597
Zantac 150 Tablets . . . 1597
Zantac 300 Tablets . . . 1597
Zantac Injection . . . 1593
Zantac Injection Premixed . . . 1593
Zantac Syrup . . . 1597

UNDERAN (Chile)
MUPIROCIN
Bactroban Ointment . . . 1358

UNDEX (Switzerland)
CLOTRIMAZOLE
Lotrimin Cream . . . 3053
Lotrimin Lotion 1% . . . 3053
Lotrimin Topical Solution 1% . . . 3053

UNI CARBAMAZ (Brazil)
CARBAMAZEPINE
Carbatrol Capsules . . . 3174
Tegretol Chewable Tablets . . . 2278
Tegretol Suspension . . . 2278
Tegretol Tablets . . . 2278
Tegretol-XR Tablets . . . 2278

UNI DIAZEPAX (Brazil)
DIAZEPAM
Diastat Rectal Delivery System . . . 3344
Valium Tablets . . . 2822

UNI MASDIL (Spain)
DILTIAZEM HYDROCHLORIDE
Cardizem LA Extended Release Tablets . . . 1699
Tiazac Capsules . . . 1204

UNI MIST (Spain)
MORPHINE SULFATE
Kadian Capsules . . . 572
MS Contin Tablets . . . 2703

UNI PROPRALOL (Brazil)
PROPRANOLOL HYDROCHLORIDE
Inderal LA Long-Acting Capsules . . . 3421

UNIBLOC (Germany, The Netherlands)
ATENOLOL
Tenormin I.V. Injection . . . 698

UNICLAR (Argentina, Chile, Italy, Mexico)
MOMETASONE FUROATE
Elocon Cream 0.1% . . . 3019
Elocon Lotion 0.1% . . . 3020
Elocon Ointment 0.1% . . . 3021
Nasonex Nasal Spray . . . 3058

UNICLOPHEN (Czech Republic)
DICLOFENAC SODIUM
Voltaren Tablets . . . 2298
Voltaren-XR Tablets . . . 2301

UNICONTIN (India, Portugal)
THEOPHYLLINE
Uniphyl Tablets . . . 2708

UNICORT (Canada)
HYDROCORTISONE
Hydrocortone Tablets . . . 1963

UNIDERM (Denmark, Finland, Hong Kong, Singapore, Sweden)
HYDROCORTISONE
Hydrocortone Tablets . . . 1963

UNIDET (Canada)
TOLTERODINE TARTRATE
Detrol Tablets . . . 2626

UNIDIPIN (Austria)
NIFEDIPINE
Adalat CC Tablets . . . 2978

UNIDIPINE (Switzerland)
NIFEDIPINE
Adalat CC Tablets . . . 2978

UNIDROL (India)
METHYLPREDNISOLONE ACETATE
Depo-Medrol Injectable Suspension . . . 2615

UNI-DUR (Italy, Mexico, South Africa)
THEOPHYLLINE
Uniphyl Tablets . . . 2708

UNIF (Thailand)
TRIAMCINOLONE ACETONIDE
Azmacort Inhalation Aerosol . . . 1701
Nasacort AQ Nasal Spray . . . 2937

UNIFLOX (Argentina, France)
LEVOFLOXACIN
Levaquin Injection . . . 2453
Levaquin Tablets . . . 2453

UNIFYL (Austria, Switzerland)
THEOPHYLLINE
Uniphyl Tablets . . . 2708

UNIGET (Germany)
TIMOLOL MALEATE
Blocadren Tablets . . . 1891
Timoptic Sterile Ophthalmic Solution . . . 2058
Timoptic in Ocudose . . . 2061
Timoptic-XE Sterile Ophthalmic Gel Forming Solution . . . 2062

UNIGO (Hong Kong)
METRONIDAZOLE
MetroGel-Vaginal Gel . . . 1822
Noritate Cream, 1% . . . 1051

UNIKET (Spain)
ISOSORBIDE MONONITRATE
Imdur Tablets . . . 3032

UNILAIR (Czech Republic, Germany)
THEOPHYLLINE
Uniphyl Tablets . . . 2708

UNILOC (Denmark, Finland, Norway, Sweden)
ATENOLOL
Tenormin I.V. Injection . . . 698

UNILONG (Spain)
THEOPHYLLINE
Uniphyl Tablets . . . 2708

UNIMAX (Austria, Czech Republic, Finland, Switzerland, The Netherlands)
FELODIPINE
Plendil Extended-Release Tablets . . . 651

UNIMEST (Spain)
FELODIPINE
Plendil Extended-Release Tablets . . . 651

UNIMEZOL (India, Thailand)
METRONIDAZOLE
MetroGel-Vaginal Gel . . . 1822
Noritate Cream, 1% . . . 1051

UNIMOX (South Africa)
AMOXICILLIN
Amoxil Pediatric Drops for Oral Suspension . . . 1315
Amoxil Tablets . . . 1315

UNIPHYL (Canada, Hong Kong, South Africa)
THEOPHYLLINE
Uniphyl Tablets . . . 2708

UNIPHYLLIN (Germany, Greece)
THEOPHYLLINE
Uniphyl Tablets . . . 2708

UNIPHYLLIN CONTINUS (Irish Republic, United Kingdom)
THEOPHYLLINE
Uniphyl Tablets . . . 2708

UNIPINE XL (United Kingdom)
NIFEDIPINE
Adalat CC Tablets . . . 2978

UNIPRIL (Italy)
RAMIPRIL
Altace Capsules . . . 1673

UNIPRILDIUR (Italy)
RAMIPRIL
Altace Capsules . . . 1673

UNIREN (Hong Kong)
DICLOFENAC SODIUM
Voltaren Tablets . . . 2298
Voltaren-XR Tablets . . . 2301

UNISAL (Switzerland)
DIFLUNISAL
Dolobid Tablets . . . 1937

UNISEDIL (Portugal)
DIAZEPAM
Diastat Rectal Delivery System . . . 3344
Valium Tablets . . . 2822

UNITIMOFTOL (Spain)
TIMOLOL MALEATE
Blocadren Tablets . . . 1891
Timoptic Sterile Ophthalmic Solution . . . 2058
Timoptic in Ocudose . . . 2061
Timoptic-XE Sterile Ophthalmic Gel Forming Solution . . . 2062

UNIVAL (Chile, Mexico)
LANSOPRAZOLE
Prevacid Delayed-Release Capsules . . . 3268

UNIVATE (Malaysia, Singapore)
CLOBETASOL PROPIONATE
Temovate Cream . . . 1549
Temovate E Emollient . . . 1552
Temovate Gel . . . 1550
Temovate Ointment . . . 1549
Temovate Scalp Application . . . 1551

UNIVER (Spain, United Kingdom)
VERAPAMIL HYDROCHLORIDE
Covera-HS Tablets . . . 3135
Verelan PM Capsules . . . 3120

UNIWARFIN (India)
WARFARIN SODIUM
Coumadin Tablets . . . 932
Coumadin for Injection . . . 932

UNIXAN (Denmark)
THEOPHYLLINE
Uniphyl Tablets . . . 2708

UNIXIME (Italy)
CEFIXIME
Suprax . . . 1811

UNOCARDIL (Denmark)
DILTIAZEM HYDROCHLORIDE
Cardizem LA Extended Release Tablets . . . 1699
Tiazac Capsules . . . 1204

UNOPROST (Italy)
TERAZOSIN HYDROCHLORIDE
Hytrin Capsules . . . 469

UP MEP (Brazil)
CIMETIDINE
Tagamet Tablets . . . 1547

UPDERM (Greece)
CLINDAMYCIN PHOSPHATE
Clindets Pledgets . . . 3212

UPHANORMIN (Malaysia)
ATENOLOL
Tenormin I.V. Injection . . . 698

UPHASTATIN (Malaysia)
NYSTATIN
Nystop Topical Powder USP . . . 2490

U-PROXYN (Thailand)
NAPROXEN
EC-Naprosyn Delayed-Release Tablets . . . 2769
Naprosyn Suspension . . . 2769
Naprosyn Tablets . . . 2769

URASIN (Thailand)
FUROSEMIDE
Furosemide Tablets . . . 2117

URBAL (Spain)
SUCRALFATE
Carafate Suspension . . . 727
Carafate Tablets . . . 728

UREKOLIN (Chile)
NORFLOXACIN
Noroxin Tablets . . . 2009

UREMIDE (Australia, South Africa)
FUROSEMIDE
Furosemide Tablets . . . 2117

UREN (Chile)
HYDROCHLOROTHIAZIDE/TRIAMTERENE
Dyazide Capsules . . . 1389
Maxzide Tablets . . . 2150
Maxzide-25 mg Tablets . . . 2150

URETIC (South Africa)
FUROSEMIDE
Furosemide Tablets . . . 2117

UREX (Australia, Hong Kong)
FUROSEMIDE
Furosemide Tablets . . . 2117

URGINOL (Argentina)
TOLTERODINE TARTRATE
Detrol Tablets . . . 2626

URIFRON (Mexico)
INTERFERON ALFA-2B
Intron A for Injection . . . 3038

URIGON (Greece)
DICLOFENAC SODIUM
Voltaren Tablets . . . 2298
Voltaren-XR Tablets . . . 2301

URIMAX (Greece, India)
OFLOXACIN
Floxin Otic Solution . . . 1043

URIMAX F (India)
TAMSULOSIN HYDROCHLORIDE
Flomax Capsules . . . 881

URINOX (Malaysia, Thailand)
NORFLOXACIN
Noroxin Tablets . . . 2009

URITOL (Canada)
FUROSEMIDE
Furosemide Tablets . . . 2117

URITRAT (Brazil)
NORFLOXACIN
Noroxin Tablets . . . 2009

URIZIDE (South Africa)
HYDROCHLOROTHIAZIDE/TRIAMTERENE
Dyazide Capsules . . . 1389
Maxzide Tablets . . . 2150
Maxzide-25 mg Tablets . . . 2150

UROBACID (Austria, Malaysia, Singapore)
NORFLOXACIN
Noroxin Tablets . . . 2009

UROCAUDAL (Spain)
TRIAMTERENE
Dyrenium Capsules . . . 3390

UROCAUDAL TIAZIDA (Spain)
HYDROCHLOROTHIAZIDE/TRIAMTERENE
Dyazide Capsules . . . 1389
Maxzide Tablets . . . 2150
Maxzide-25 mg Tablets . . . 2150

URO-CEPHORAL (Germany)
CEFIXIME
Suprax . . . 1811

UROCIT-K (Australia, Hong Kong, Malaysia, Singapore)
POTASSIUM CITRATE
Urocit-K Tablets . . . 2109

UROCTAL (Hong Kong, Spain)
NORFLOXACIN
Noroxin Tablets . . . 2009

URODIE (Italy)
TERAZOSIN HYDROCHLORIDE
Hytrin Capsules . . . 469

UROFIN (Argentina)
FINASTERIDE
Propecia Tablets . . . 2036
Proscar Tablets . . . 2040

UROFLO (Austria)
TERAZOSIN HYDROCHLORIDE
Hytrin Capsules . . . 469

UROFLOX (Brazil, Portugal)
NORFLOXACIN
Noroxin Tablets . . . 2009

UROFOS (Argentina)
NORFLOXACIN
Noroxin Tablets . . . 2009

UROKIT (Argentina)
POTASSIUM CITRATE
Urocit-K Tablets . . . 2109

URO-LINFOL (Argentina)
NORFLOXACIN
Noroxin Tablets . . . 2009

UROLOSIN (Spain)
TAMSULOSIN HYDROCHLORIDE
Flomax Capsules . . . 881

UROMETRON (South Africa)
METRONIDAZOLE
MetroGel-Vaginal Gel . . . 1822
Noritate Cream, 1% . . . 1051

UROMYKOL (Germany)
CLOTRIMAZOLE
Lotrimin Cream . . . 3053
Lotrimin Lotion 1% . . . 3053
Lotrimin Topical Solution 1% . . . 3053

URONOVAG (Argentina)
NORFLOXACIN
Noroxin Tablets . . . 2009

UROPLEX (Brazil)
NORFLOXACIN
Noroxin Tablets . . . 2009

UROSEPTAL (Argentina, Brazil)
NORFLOXACIN
Noroxin Tablets . . . 2009

UROSIN (Malaysia)
ATENOLOL
Tenormin I.V. Injection . . . 698

UROSPES-N (Greece)
NORFLOXACIN
Noroxin Tablets . . . 2009

URO-TARIVID (Germany, Israel)
OFLOXACIN
Floxin Otic Solution . . . 1043

UROTEM (Argentina)
NORFLOXACIN
Noroxin Tablets . . . 2009

UROTRICEF (Chile)
CEFIXIME
Suprax . . . 1811

UROTROL (Spain)
TOLTERODINE TARTRATE
Detrol Tablets . . . 2626

UROXACIN (Argentina)
NORFLOXACIN
Noroxin Tablets . . . 2009

UROXAZOL-N (Brazil)
NORFLOXACIN
Noroxin Tablets . . . 2009

UROXIN (Hong Kong, Singapore, Thailand, United Arab Emirates)
CIPROFLOXACIN HYDROCHLORIDE
Ciloxan Ophthalmic Ointment . . . 554
Ciloxan Ophthalmic Solution . . . ⊙205
Cipro Tablets . . . 2991

URPROSAN (Spain)
FINASTERIDE
Propecia Tablets . . . 2036
Proscar Tablets . . . 2040

UTAC (Thailand)
RANITIDINE HYDROCHLORIDE
Zantac 25 EFFERdose Tablets . . . 1597
Zantac 150 EFFERdose Tablets . . . 1597
Zantac 150 Tablets . . . 1597
Zantac 300 Tablets . . . 1597
Zantac Injection . . . 1593
Zantac Injection Premixed . . . 1593
Zantac Syrup . . . 1597

UTAHZONE (Hong Kong)
CIPROFLOXACIN HYDROCHLORIDE
Ciloxan Ophthalmic Ointment . . . 554
Ciloxan Ophthalmic Solution . . . ⊙205
Cipro Tablets . . . 2991

UTICINA (Italy)
NORFLOXACIN
Noroxin Tablets . . . 2009

UTIN (South Africa)
NORFLOXACIN
Noroxin Tablets . . . 2009

UTINOR (Italy, United Kingdom)
NORFLOXACIN
Noroxin Tablets . . . 2009

UTORAL (Brazil)
FLUOROURACIL
Efudex Topical Cream . . . 3348
Efudex Topical Solutions . . . 3348

UTROGESTAN (Argentina, Austria, Belgium, Brazil, Czech Republic, France, Greece, Hong Kong, Hungary, Irish Republic, Israel, Malaysia, Mexico, Portugal, Russia, Singapore, South Africa, Spain, Switzerland, Thailand)
PROGESTERONE
Prometrium Capsules (100 mg, 200 mg) . 3205

V DAY ZEPAM (Thailand)
DIAZEPAM
Diastat Rectal Delivery System . . . 3344
Valium Tablets . . . 2822

VACINOLONE (Thailand)
TRIAMCINOLONE ACETONIDE
Azmacort Inhalation Aerosol . . . 1701
Nasacort AQ Nasal Spray . . . 2937

VACONTIL (Hong Kong, Malaysia, Singapore, Thailand)
LOPERAMIDE HYDROCHLORIDE
Imodium Capsules . . . 1834

VACROMIL (Chile)
GOSERELIN ACETATE
Zoladex . . . 709
Zoladex 3-month . . . 712

VADINAR (Mexico)
DIPYRIDAMOLE
Persantine Tablets . . . 898

VADITON (Spain)
FLUVASTATIN SODIUM
Lescol Capsules . . . 2227

VAFLUSON (Greece)
KETOCONAZOLE
Nizoral 2% Shampoo . . . 1838

VAGAKA (Thailand)
MEBENDAZOLE
Vermox Chewable Tablets . . . 1853

VAGIFEM (Australia, Austria, Belgium, Canada, Czech Republic, Denmark, Finland, Germany, Greece, Hungary, Irish Republic, Israel, Italy, New Zealand, Norway, Portugal, Singapore, South Africa, Spain, Sweden, Switzerland, Thailand, The Netherlands, United Kingdom)
ESTRADIOL
Climara Transdermal System . . . 795
Vivelle Transdermal System . . . 2288
Vivelle-Dot Transdermal System . . . 2293

VAGIL (Thailand)
METRONIDAZOLE
MetroGel-Vaginal Gel . . . 1822
Noritate Cream, 1% . . . 1051

VAGILEN (Italy)
METRONIDAZOLE
MetroGel-Vaginal Gel . . . 1822
Noritate Cream, 1% . . . 1051

VAGIMAX (Brazil)
METRONIDAZOLE
MetroGel-Vaginal Gel . . . 1822
Noritate Cream, 1% . . . 1051

VAGIMID (Germany)
METRONIDAZOLE
MetroGel-Vaginal Gel . . . 1822
Noritate Cream, 1% . . . 1051

VAGINYL (United Kingdom)
METRONIDAZOLE
MetroGel-Vaginal Gel . . . 1822
Noritate Cream, 1% . . . 1051

VAGISIL (United Kingdom)
LIDOCAINE
Lidoderm Patch . . . 1107

VAGMICOR (Mexico)
KETOCONAZOLE
Nizoral 2% Shampoo . . . 1838

VAGOLISAL (Italy)
CIMETIDINE
Tagamet Tablets . . . 1547

VAGOSTAL (Spain)
FAMOTIDINE
Pepcid Injection . . . 2017
Pepcid Injection Premixed . . . 2017
Pepcid Tablets . . . 2014
Pepcid for Oral Suspension . . . 2014

VAGYL (Thailand)
METRONIDAZOLE
MetroGel-Vaginal Gel . . . 1822
Noritate Cream, 1% . . . 1051

VALAXONA (Denmark, Germany)
DIAZEPAM
Diastat Rectal Delivery System . . . 3344
Valium Tablets . . . 2822

VALCAPS (Mexico)
VALPROIC ACID
Depakene Capsules . . . 417
Depakene Syrup . . . 417

VALCLAIR (United Kingdom)
DIAZEPAM
Diastat Rectal Delivery System . . . 3344
Valium Tablets . . . 2822

VALCOTE (Argentina)
VALPROIC ACID
Depakene Capsules . . . 417
Depakene Syrup . . . 417

VALDERMA ACTIVE (United Kingdom)
BENZOYL PEROXIDE
Brevoxyl-4 Creamy Wash . . . 3212
Brevoxyl-4 Gel . . . 3211
Brevoxyl-8 Creamy Wash . . . 3212
Brevoxyl-8 Gel . . . 3211
Triaz Cleanser . . . 1864
Triaz Gel . . . 1864

VALENAC (United Kingdom)
DICLOFENAC SODIUM
Voltaren Tablets 2298
Voltaren-XR Tablets 2301

VALENIUM (Thailand)
DIAZEPAM
Diastat Rectal Delivery System 3344
Valium Tablets 2822

VALIQUID (Germany)
DIAZEPAM
Diastat Rectal Delivery System 3344
Valium Tablets 2822

VALITRAN (Italy)
DIAZEPAM
Diastat Rectal Delivery System 3344
Valium Tablets 2822

VALIUM (Argentina, Australia, Austria, Belgium, Brazil, Canada, Denmark, France, Germany, India, Irish Republic, Israel, Italy, Mexico, Norway, Portugal, Singapore, South Africa, Spain, Sweden, Switzerland, Thailand, The Netherlands, United Kingdom)
DIAZEPAM
Diastat Rectal Delivery System 3344
Valium Tablets 2822

VALIX (Brazil)
DIAZEPAM
Diastat Rectal Delivery System 3344
Valium Tablets 2822

VALKEN (Mexico)
VALPROIC ACID
Depakene Capsules 417
Depakene Syrup 417

VALMAGEN (Italy)
CIMETIDINE
Tagamet Tablets 1547

VALOCORDIN-DIAZEPAM (Germany)
DIAZEPAM
Diastat Rectal Delivery System 3344
Valium Tablets 2822

VALPAM (Australia)
DIAZEPAM
Diastat Rectal Delivery System 3344
Valium Tablets 2822

VALPAX (Chile)
CLONAZEPAM
Klonopin Tablets 2782

VALPEX (Argentina)
DONEPEZIL HYDROCHLORIDE
Aricept Tablets 1086

VALPRESSION (Italy)
VALSARTAN
Diovan Tablets 2191

VALPROLIM (Portugal)
VALPROIC ACID
Depakene Capsules 417
Depakene Syrup 417

VALROX (United Kingdom)
NAPROXEN
EC-Naprosyn Delayed-Release Tablets 2769
Naprosyn Suspension 2769
Naprosyn Tablets 2769

VALS (Spain)
VALSARTAN
Diovan Tablets 2191

VALSARTAN/HCTZ (Austria)
VALSARTAN
Diovan Tablets 2191

VAMAZOLE (Thailand)
CLOTRIMAZOLE
Lotrimin Cream 3053
Lotrimin Lotion 1% 3053
Lotrimin Topical Solution 1% 3053

VAMISTOL (Greece)
VANCOMYCIN HYDROCHLORIDE
Vancocin HCl Capsules, USP 3370

VANAURUS (Mexico)
VANCOMYCIN HYDROCHLORIDE
Vancocin HCl Capsules, USP 3370

VANCAM (Mexico)
VANCOMYCIN HYDROCHLORIDE
Vancocin HCl Capsules, USP 3370

VANCLOMIN (Brazil)
VANCOMYCIN HYDROCHLORIDE
Vancocin HCl Capsules, USP 3370

VANCO (Germany, Italy)
VANCOMYCIN HYDROCHLORIDE
Vancocin HCl Capsules, USP 3370

VANCOABBOTT (Brazil)
VANCOMYCIN HYDROCHLORIDE
Vancocin HCl Capsules, USP 3370

VANCOCIN (Argentina, Australia, Belgium, Canada, Czech Republic, Denmark, Finland, Hong Kong, Hungary, India, Irish Republic, Israel, Malaysia, Mexico, New Zealand, Norway, South Africa, Sweden, Switzerland, Thailand, The Netherlands, United Kingdom)
VANCOMYCIN HYDROCHLORIDE
Vancocin HCl Capsules, USP 3370

VANCOCINA (Brazil, Chile, Italy, Portugal)
VANCOMYCIN HYDROCHLORIDE
Vancocin HCl Capsules, USP 3370

VANCOCINE (France)
VANCOMYCIN HYDROCHLORIDE
Vancocin HCl Capsules, USP 3370

VANCOLAN (United Arab Emirates)
VANCOMYCIN HYDROCHLORIDE
Vancocin HCl Capsules, USP 3370

VANCOLED (Australia, Czech Republic, Israel, Sweden, Switzerland)
VANCOMYCIN HYDROCHLORIDE
Vancocin HCl Capsules, USP 3370

VANCOPLUS (Brazil)
VANCOMYCIN HYDROCHLORIDE
Vancocin HCl Capsules, USP 3370

VANCO-SAAR (Germany)
VANCOMYCIN HYDROCHLORIDE
Vancocin HCl Capsules, USP 3370

VANCOSCAND (Sweden)
VANCOMYCIN HYDROCHLORIDE
Vancocin HCl Capsules, USP 3370

VANCOTENK (Argentina)
VANCOMYCIN HYDROCHLORIDE
Vancocin HCl Capsules, USP 3370

VANCO-TEVA (Hong Kong, Israel)
VANCOMYCIN HYDROCHLORIDE
Vancocin HCl Capsules, USP 3370

VANCOTEX (Italy)
VANCOMYCIN HYDROCHLORIDE
Vancocin HCl Capsules, USP 3370

VANCOX (Mexico)
VANCOMYCIN HYDROCHLORIDE
Vancocin HCl Capsules, USP 3370

VANDRAL (Spain)
VENLAFAXINE HYDROCHLORIDE
Effexor Tablets 3405
Effexor XR Capsules 3411

VANESTEN (Singapore, Thailand)
CLOTRIMAZOLE
Lotrimin Cream 3053
Lotrimin Lotion 1% 3053
Lotrimin Topical Solution 1% 3053

VANMICINA (Mexico)
VANCOMYCIN HYDROCHLORIDE
Vancocin HCl Capsules, USP 3370

VANTICON (Argentina)
ZAFIRLUKAST
Accolate Tablets 663

VANZOR (Mexico)
DIAZEPAM
Diastat Rectal Delivery System 3344
Valium Tablets 2822

VAPRESAN (Argentina)
ENALAPRIL MALEATE
Vasotec I.V. Injection 2076

VAPRESAN DIUR (Argentina)
ENALAPRIL MALEATE/HYDROCHLOROTHIAZIDE
Vaseretic Tablets 2073

VARFINE (Portugal)
WARFARIN SODIUM
Coumadin Tablets 932
Coumadin for Injection 932

VARIMER (Argentina)
MERCAPTOPURINE
Purinethol Tablets 1222

VARTALAN (Chile)
VALSARTAN
Diovan Tablets 2191

VARTALAN D (Chile)
HYDROCHLOROTHIAZIDE/VALSARTAN
Diovan HCT Tablets 2195

VARTELON (Hong Kong)
DICLOFENAC SODIUM
Voltaren Tablets 2298
Voltaren-XR Tablets 2301

VASAD (United Kingdom)
NIFEDIPINE
Adalat CC Tablets 2978

VASATEN (United Kingdom)
ATENOLOL
Tenormin I.V. Injection 698

VASCAL (Germany)
ISRADIPINE
DynaCirc CR Tablets 2726

VASCALPHA (United Kingdom)
FELODIPINE
Plendil Extended-Release Tablets 651

VASCARD (South Africa)
NIFEDIPINE
Adalat CC Tablets 2978

VASCOR (Malaysia, Singapore, Thailand)
SIMVASTATIN
Zocor Tablets 2078

VASCORIM (Portugal)
SIMVASTATIN
Zocor Tablets 2078

VASCOTEN (Hong Kong, Malaysia, Singapore, Thailand)
ATENOLOL
Tenormin I.V. Injection 698

VASDALAT (Singapore)
NIFEDIPINE
Adalat CC Tablets 2978

VASDILAT (Italy)
ISOSORBIDE MONONITRATE
Imdur Tablets 3032

VASERETIC (Canada)
ENALAPRIL MALEATE/HYDROCHLOROTHIAZIDE
Vaseretic Tablets 2073

VASETIC (United Kingdom)
AMILORIDE HYDROCHLORIDE/HYDROCHLOROTHIAZIDE
Moduretic Tablets 2003

VASILIP (Czech Republic, Russia)
SIMVASTATIN
Zocor Tablets 2078

VASLAN (Spain)
ISRADIPINE
DynaCirc CR Tablets 2726

VASLIP (Brazil)
SIMVASTATIN
Zocor Tablets 2078

VASOCARDOL (Australia)
DILTIAZEM HYDROCHLORIDE
Cardizem LA Extended Release Tablets . . . 1699
Tiazac Capsules 1204

VASOCON (Canada)
NAPHAZOLINE HYDROCHLORIDE
Albalon Ophthalmic Solution . . . . . ⊙216

VASOCONSTRICTOR PENSA (Spain)
NAPHAZOLINE HYDROCHLORIDE
Albalon Ophthalmic Solution . . . . . ⊙216

VASOCOR (Switzerland)
ENALAPRIL MALEATE
Vasotec I.V. Injection 2076

VASODIPINA (Brazil)
NIMODIPINE
Nimotop Capsules 774

VASOFED (Irish Republic, South Africa)
NIFEDIPINE
Adalat CC Tablets 2978

VASOFLEX (Chile)
NIMODIPINE
Nimotop Capsules 774

VASOJET (Brazil)
LISINOPRIL
Prinivil Tablets 2029
Zestril Tablets 704

VASOLAN (Japan)
VERAPAMIL HYDROCHLORIDE
Covera-HS Tablets 3135
Verelan PM Capsules 3120

VASOLAT (Chile)
ENALAPRIL MALEATE
Vasotec I.V. Injection 2076

VASOMED (Chile)
SIMVASTATIN
Zocor Tablets 2078

VASOMIL (South Africa)
VERAPAMIL HYDROCHLORIDE
Covera-HS Tablets 3135
Verelan PM Capsules 3120

VASOPRIL (Brazil)
ENALAPRIL MALEATE
Vasotec I.V. Injection 2076

VASOPRIL PLUS (Brazil)
ENALAPRIL MALEATE
Vasotec I.V. Injection 2076

VASOPTEN (Thailand)
VERAPAMIL HYDROCHLORIDE
Covera-HS Tablets 3135
Verelan PM Capsules 3120

VASORETIC (Italy)
ENALAPRIL MALEATE/HYDROCHLOROTHIAZIDE
Vaseretic Tablets 2073

VASOTENAL (Argentina, Chile)
SIMVASTATIN
Zocor Tablets 2078

VASOTOP (India)
NIMODIPINE
Nimotop Capsules 774

VASTATIFIX (The Netherlands)
PRAVASTATIN SODIUM
Pravachol Tablets 943

VASTEN (France)
PRAVASTATIN SODIUM
Pravachol Tablets 943

VASTIN (Australia, New Zealand)
FLUVASTATIN SODIUM
Lescol Capsules 2227

VASTRIPINE (Greece)
NIMODIPINE
Nimotop Capsules 774

VASTUS (Argentina, Chile)
ALBENDAZOLE
Albenza Tablets 1310

VASYROL (United Kingdom)
DIPYRIDAMOLE
Persantine Tablets 898

VATRAN (Italy)
DIAZEPAM
Diastat Rectal Delivery System 3344
Valium Tablets 2822

VATRIX-S (Mexico)
METRONIDAZOLE
MetroGel-Vaginal Gel 1822
Noritate Cream, 1% 1051

VECLAM (Italy)
CLARITHROMYCIN
Biaxin Filmtab Tablets 402
Biaxin Granules 402

VEENAC (Thailand)
DICLOFENAC SODIUM
Voltaren Tablets 2298
Voltaren-XR Tablets 2301

VEKFAZOLIN (Greece)
CEFUROXIME SODIUM
Zinacef Injection 1604

VELAMOX (Brazil)
AMOXICILLIN
Amoxil Pediatric Drops for Oral Suspension 1315
Amoxil Tablets 1315

(⊙ Described in PDR For Ophthalmic Medicines™)

VELMONIT (Spain)
CIPROFLOXACIN HYDROCHLORIDE
Ciloxan Ophthalmic Ointment 554
Ciloxan Ophthalmic Solution . . . . ⊙205
Cipro Tablets 2991

VELORIN (Hong Kong, Singapore, Thailand)
ATENOLOL
Tenormin I.V. Injection 698

VELPRO (Mexico)
BENZONATATE
Tessalon Perles 1202

VELSAY (Mexico)
NAPROXEN
EC-Naprosyn Delayed-Release Tablets 2769
Naprosyn Suspension 2769
Naprosyn Tablets 2769

VELTEX (South Africa)
DICLOFENAC SODIUM
Voltaren Tablets 2298
Voltaren-XR Tablets 2301

VELTION (Greece)
MUPIROCIN
Bactroban Ointment 1358

VEMIZOL (Malaysia)
ALBENDAZOLE
Albenza Tablets 1310

VENACHLOR (South Africa)
ATENOLOL
Tenormin I.V. Injection 698

VENAPULSE (South Africa)
ATENOLOL
Tenormin I.V. Injection 698

VENDREX (Brazil)
DICLOFENAC SODIUM
Voltaren Tablets 2298
Voltaren-XR Tablets 2301

VENLA (Israel)
VENLAFAXINE HYDROCHLORIDE
Effexor Tablets 3405
Effexor XR Capsules 3411

VENLOR (India)
VENLAFAXINE HYDROCHLORIDE
Effexor Tablets 3405
Effexor XR Capsules 3411

VENOGYL (Israel)
METRONIDAZOLE
MetroGel-Vaginal Gel 1822
Noritate Cream, 1% 1051

VENOPRIL (Brazil)
CAPTOPRIL
Captopril Tablets 2114

VENT RETARD (Spain)
THEOPHYLLINE
Uniphyl Tablets 2708

VENTER (Czech Republic, Hungary)
SUCRALFATE
Carafate Suspension 727
Carafate Tablets 728

VENTOFLU (Italy)
FLUNISOLIDE
Aerobid Inhaler System 1172
Aerobid-M Inhaler System 1172
Nasarel Nasal Spray 1652

VERABETA (Germany)
VERAPAMIL HYDROCHLORIDE
Covera-HS Tablets 3135
Verelan PM Capsules 3120

VERACAPS (Australia)
VERAPAMIL HYDROCHLORIDE
Covera-HS Tablets 3135
Verelan PM Capsules 3120

VERACIM (Switzerland)
VERAPAMIL HYDROCHLORIDE
Covera-HS Tablets 3135
Verelan PM Capsules 3120

VERACOL (Greece)
CEFTRIAXONE SODIUM
Rocephin Injectable Vials, ADD-Vantage, Galaxy, Bulk 2801

VERACOR (Israel)
VERAPAMIL HYDROCHLORIDE
Covera-HS Tablets 3135
Verelan PM Capsules 3120

VERACORON (Brazil)
VERAPAMIL HYDROCHLORIDE
Covera-HS Tablets 3135
Verelan PM Capsules 3120

VERADAY (Austria)
VERAPAMIL HYDROCHLORIDE
Covera-HS Tablets 3135
Verelan PM Capsules 3120

VERADIL (Australia)
VERAPAMIL HYDROCHLORIDE
Covera-HS Tablets 3135
Verelan PM Capsules 3120

VERADOL (Argentina)
NAPROXEN
EC-Naprosyn Delayed-Release Tablets 2769
Naprosyn Suspension 2769
Naprosyn Tablets 2769

VERADURAT (Germany)
VERAPAMIL HYDROCHLORIDE
Covera-HS Tablets 3135
Verelan PM Capsules 3120

VERAGAMMA (Germany)
VERAPAMIL HYDROCHLORIDE
Covera-HS Tablets 3135
Verelan PM Capsules 3120

VERAHEXAL (Australia, Czech Republic, Germany, South Africa)
VERAPAMIL HYDROCHLORIDE
Covera-HS Tablets 3135
Verelan PM Capsules 3120

VERAKARD (Norway)
VERAPAMIL HYDROCHLORIDE
Covera-HS Tablets 3135
Verelan PM Capsules 3120

VERAL (Argentina, Czech Republic, Hungary)
VERAPAMIL HYDROCHLORIDE
Covera-HS Tablets 3135
Verelan PM Capsules 3120

VERALAN (Mexico)
VERAPAMIL HYDROCHLORIDE
Covera-HS Tablets 3135
Verelan PM Capsules 3120

VERA-LICH (Germany)
VERAPAMIL HYDROCHLORIDE
Covera-HS Tablets 3135
Verelan PM Capsules 3120

VERALOC (Denmark, Sweden)
VERAPAMIL HYDROCHLORIDE
Covera-HS Tablets 3135
Verelan PM Capsules 3120

VERAMEX (Germany)
VERAPAMIL HYDROCHLORIDE
Covera-HS Tablets 3135
Verelan PM Capsules 3120

VERAMIL (Brazil, Irish Republic)
VERAPAMIL HYDROCHLORIDE
Covera-HS Tablets 3135
Verelan PM Capsules 3120

VERANORM (Germany)
VERAPAMIL HYDROCHLORIDE
Covera-HS Tablets 3135
Verelan PM Capsules 3120

VERANZOL (Mexico)
ALBENDAZOLE
Albenza Tablets 1310

VERAP (Irish Republic)
VERAPAMIL HYDROCHLORIDE
Covera-HS Tablets 3135
Verelan PM Capsules 3120

VERAPABENE (Austria)
VERAPAMIL HYDROCHLORIDE
Covera-HS Tablets 3135
Verelan PM Capsules 3120

VERAPAL (Argentina)
VERAPAMIL HYDROCHLORIDE
Covera-HS Tablets 3135
Verelan PM Capsules 3120

VERAPAM (Switzerland)
VERAPAMIL HYDROCHLORIDE
Covera-HS Tablets 3135
Verelan PM Capsules 3120

VERAPIN (Thailand)
VERAPAMIL HYDROCHLORIDE
Covera-HS Tablets 3135
Verelan PM Capsules 3120

VERAPLEX (Argentina, Malaysia)
MEDROXYPROGESTERONE ACETATE
Depo-Medrol Single-Dose Vial 2617

VERAPRESS (Israel, United Kingdom)
VERAPAMIL HYDROCHLORIDE
Covera-HS Tablets 3135
Verelan PM Capsules 3120

VERAPTIN (Italy, Switzerland)
VERAPAMIL HYDROCHLORIDE
Covera-HS Tablets 3135
Verelan PM Capsules 3120

VERASAL (Germany)
VERAPAMIL HYDROCHLORIDE
Covera-HS Tablets 3135
Verelan PM Capsules 3120

VERASIFAR (Switzerland)
VERAPAMIL HYDROCHLORIDE
Covera-HS Tablets 3135
Verelan PM Capsules 3120

VERASPIR (Portugal)
SALMETEROL XINAFOATE
Serevent Diskus 1540

VERASTAD (Austria)
VERAPAMIL HYDROCHLORIDE
Covera-HS Tablets 3135
Verelan PM Capsules 3120

VERATEN (Argentina)
CARVEDILOL
Coreg Tablets 1376

VERATENSIN (Spain)
VERAPAMIL HYDROCHLORIDE
Covera-HS Tablets 3135
Verelan PM Capsules 3120

VERATYROL (Austria)
VERAPAMIL HYDROCHLORIDE
Covera-HS Tablets 3135
Verelan PM Capsules 3120

VERAVAL (Brazil)
VERAPAMIL HYDROCHLORIDE
Covera-HS Tablets 3135
Verelan PM Capsules 3120

VERCOL (Greece)
LISINOPRIL
Prinivil Tablets 2029
Zestril Tablets 704

VERELAIT (Italy)
LACTULOSE
Kristalose for Oral Solution 2149

VERELAN (Canada, Irish Republic)
VERAPAMIL HYDROCHLORIDE
Covera-HS Tablets 3135
Verelan PM Capsules 3120

VEREXAMIL (Austria)
VERAPAMIL HYDROCHLORIDE
Covera-HS Tablets 3135
Verelan PM Capsules 3120

VERICORDIN (Argentina)
ATENOLOL
Tenormin I.V. Injection 698

VERIDERM MEDROL (France)
METHYLPREDNISOLONE ACETATE
Depo-Medrol Injectable Suspension 2615

VERISOP (Irish Republic)
VERAPAMIL HYDROCHLORIDE
Covera-HS Tablets 3135
Verelan PM Capsules 3120

VERLOST (Greece)
RANITIDINE HYDROCHLORIDE
Zantac 25 EFFERdose Tablets 1597
Zantac 150 EFFERdose Tablets 1597
Zantac 150 Tablets 1597
Zantac 300 Tablets 1597
Zantac Injection 1593
Zantac Injection Premixed 1593
Zantac Syrup 1597

VERMEPEN (Brazil)
MEBENDAZOLE
Vermox Chewable Tablets 1853

VERMICIDIN (Switzerland)
MEBENDAZOLE
Vermox Chewable Tablets 1853

VERMICLASE (Brazil)
ALBENDAZOLE
Albenza Tablets 1310

VERMICOL (Mexico)
MEBENDAZOLE
Vermox Chewable Tablets 1853

VERMIDIL (Mexico)
MEBENDAZOLE
Vermox Chewable Tablets 1853

VERMILAN (Mexico)
ALBENDAZOLE
Albenza Tablets 1310

VERMIN (Finland)
VERAPAMIL HYDROCHLORIDE
Covera-HS Tablets 3135
Verelan PM Capsules 3120

VERMIN-DAZOL (Mexico)
MEBENDAZOLE
Vermox Chewable Tablets 1853

VERMINE (Thailand)
VERAPAMIL HYDROCHLORIDE
Covera-HS Tablets 3135
Verelan PM Capsules 3120

VERMINON (Brazil)
MEBENDAZOLE
Vermox Chewable Tablets 1853

VERMIN-PLUS (Mexico)
ALBENDAZOLE
Albenza Tablets 1310

VERMIRAX (Brazil)
MEBENDAZOLE
Vermox Chewable Tablets 1853

VERMISEN (Mexico)
ALBENDAZOLE
Albenza Tablets 1310

VERMITAL (Brazil)
ALBENDAZOLE
Albenza Tablets 1310

VERMIXIDE (Thailand)
ALBENDAZOLE
Albenza Tablets 1310

VERMOL (Brazil)
MEBENDAZOLE
Vermox Chewable Tablets 1853

VERMONON (Brazil)
MEBENDAZOLE
Vermox Chewable Tablets 1853

VERMOPLEX (Brazil)
MEBENDAZOLE
Vermox Chewable Tablets 1853

VERMORAL (Brazil)
MEBENDAZOLE
Vermox Chewable Tablets 1853

VERMOX (Australia, Belgium, Canada, Czech Republic, Denmark, Germany, Greece, Hong Kong, Hungary, Irish Republic, Israel, Italy, Malaysia, Mexico, New Zealand, Norway, South Africa, Sweden, Switzerland, The Netherlands, United Kingdom)
MEBENDAZOLE
Vermox Chewable Tablets 1853

VERNTHOL (South Africa)
THEOPHYLLINE
Uniphyl Tablets 2708

VEROGALID (Hungary)
VERAPAMIL HYDROCHLORIDE
Covera-HS Tablets 3135
Verelan PM Capsules 3120

VEROPTINSTADA (Germany)
VERAPAMIL HYDROCHLORIDE
Covera-HS Tablets 3135
Verelan PM Capsules 3120

VERORAB (South Africa)
RABIES VACCINE
Rabies Vaccine RabAvert 1011

VEROXIL (Greece, Italy)
LISINOPRIL
Prinivil Tablets 2029
Zestril Tablets 704

VERPACOR (Finland)
VERAPAMIL HYDROCHLORIDE
Covera-HS Tablets 3135
Verelan PM Capsules 3120

VERPAMIL (Finland, Malaysia, New Zealand, Singapore, South Africa)
VERAPAMIL HYDROCHLORIDE
Covera-HS Tablets . . . 3135
Verelan PM Capsules . . . 3120

VERRUMAL (Portugal)
FLUOROURACIL
Efudex Topical Cream. . . 3348
Efudex Topical Solutions . . . 3348

VERTAB (United Kingdom)
VERAPAMIL HYDROCHLORIDE
Covera-HS Tablets . . . 3135
Verelan PM Capsules . . . 3120

VERTEX (Mexico)
MEBENDAZOLE
Vermox Chewable Tablets . . . 1853

VERTIZOLE (Mexico)
MEBENDAZOLE
Vermox Chewable Tablets . . . 1853

VERYTRACIN (Mexico)
ERYTHROMYCIN
Ery-Tab Tablets . . . 447
Erythromycin Base Filmtab Tablets. . . 454
Erythromycin Delayed-Release Capsules, USP . . . 456
PCE Dispertab Tablets . . . 510

VERZOL (Brazil)
MEBENDAZOLE
Vermox Chewable Tablets . . . 1853

VESALION FLEX (Argentina)
DICLOFENAC SODIUM
Voltaren Tablets . . . 2298
Voltaren-XR Tablets . . . 2301

VESALION GESIC (Argentina)
DICLOFENAC POTASSIUM
Cataflam Tablets . . . 2173

VESANOID (Argentina, Australia, Austria, Belgium, Brazil, Canada, Chile, Czech Republic, Finland, France, Germany, Greece, Hong Kong, Hungary, Irish Republic, Israel, Italy, Mexico, New Zealand, Norway, Portugal, Singapore, South Africa, Sweden, Switzerland, Thailand, The Netherlands, United Kingdom)
TRETINOIN
Avita Cream. . . 2136
Avita Gel. . . 2138
Renova 0.05% Cream. . . 2387
Retin-A Micro 0.1%/0.04%. . . 2388
Vesanoid Capsules. . . 2823

VESDIL (Germany, Switzerland)
RAMIPRIL
Altace Capsules . . . 1673

VESIX (Finland, The Netherlands)
FUROSEMIDE
Furosemide Tablets . . . 2117

VESTACLAV (Malaysia)
AMOXICILLIN
Amoxil Pediatric Drops for Oral Suspension. . . 1315
Amoxil Tablets . . . 1315

VETAMOL (Greece)
NORFLOXACIN
Noroxin Tablets. . . 2009

VETIPROST (Argentina)
FINASTERIDE
Propecia Tablets . . . 2036
Proscar Tablets. . . 2040

VIAFUROX (Argentina)
FUROSEMIDE
Furosemide Tablets . . . 2117

VIAGRA (Argentina, Australia, Austria, Belgium, Brazil, Canada, Chile, Czech Republic, Denmark, Finland, France, Germany, Greece, Hong Kong, Hungary, Irish Republic, Israel, Italy, Japan, Malaysia, Mexico, New Zealand, Norway, Portugal, Russia, Singapore, South Africa, Spain, Sweden, Switzerland, Thailand, United Kingdom)
SILDENAFIL CITRATE
Viagra Tablets . . . 2552

VIARTRIL NF (Argentina)
DICLOFENAC SODIUM
Voltaren Tablets . . . 2298
Voltaren-XR Tablets . . . 2301

VIATOPIN (Hungary)
TOPOTECAN HYDROCHLORIDE
Hycamtin for Injection. . . 1427

VIAZEM (Denmark, Sweden, United Kingdom)
DILTIAZEM HYDROCHLORIDE
Cardizem LA Extended Release Tablets. . . 1699
Tiazac Capsules . . . 1204

VIBUZOL (Argentina)
RIBAVIRIN
Virazole for Inhalation Solution . . . 3365

VICARD (Austria, Switzerland)
TERAZOSIN HYDROCHLORIDE
Hytrin Capsules. . . 469

VICK-ZYRT (Hong Kong)
CETIRIZINE HYDROCHLORIDE
Zyrtec Syrup . . . 2589
Zyrtec Tablets . . . 2589

VI-CLARO (Chile)
NAPHAZOLINE HYDROCHLORIDE
Albalon Ophthalmic Solution . . . ⊙216

VICMAFEN (Mexico)
DICLOFENAC SODIUM
Voltaren Tablets . . . 2298
Voltaren-XR Tablets . . . 2301

VICNAS (Spain)
NORFLOXACIN
Noroxin Tablets. . . 2009

VICORTIN (Mexico)
HYDROCORTISONE
Hydrocortone Tablets . . . 1963

VIDA FAMODINE (Hong Kong)
FAMOTIDINE
Pepcid Injection . . . 2017
Pepcid Injection Premixed . . . 2017
Pepcid Tablets . . . 2014
Pepcid for Oral Suspension . . . 2014

VIDALAT (Hong Kong)
NIFEDIPINE
Adalat CC Tablets . . . 2978

VIDAPERAMIDE (Hong Kong)
LOPERAMIDE HYDROCHLORIDE
Imodium Capsules . . . 1834

VIDAPRIL (Portugal)
CAPTOPRIL
Captopril Tablets. . . 2114

VIDOX (Argentina)
MUPIROCIN
Bactroban Ointment . . . 1358

VIEPAX (Israel)
VENLAFAXINE HYDROCHLORIDE
Effexor Tablets . . . 3405
Effexor XR Capsules . . . 3411

VIFAZOLIN (Greece)
CEFAZOLIN SODIUM
Ancef for Injection . . . 1318

VIGICER (Argentina)
MODAFINIL
Provigil Tablets . . . 1002

VIGIL (Czech Republic, Germany)
MODAFINIL
Provigil Tablets . . . 1002

VIKING (Greece)
LOVASTATIN
Mevacor Tablets . . . 1996

VILACRIL (Greece)
DICLOFENAC SODIUM
Voltaren Tablets . . . 2298
Voltaren-XR Tablets . . . 2301

VILADIL (Thailand)
TICLOPIDINE HYDROCHLORIDE
Ticlid Tablets . . . 2813

VILONA (Mexico)
RIBAVIRIN
Virazole for Inhalation Solution . . . 3365

VILONIT (Greece)
DICLOFENAC SODIUM
Voltaren Tablets . . . 2298
Voltaren-XR Tablets . . . 2301

VIMAX (Argentina)
SILDENAFIL CITRATE
Viagra Tablets . . . 2552

VIMULTISA (Argentina)
DICLOFENAC POTASSIUM
Cataflam Tablets . . . 2173

VINCOSEDAN (Spain)
DIAZEPAM
Diastat Rectal Delivery System . . . 3344
Valium Tablets . . . 2822

VINGIONAL (Argentina)
RANITIDINE HYDROCHLORIDE
Zantac 25 EFFERdose Tablets . . . 1597
Zantac 150 EFFERdose Tablets. . . 1597
Zantac 150 Tablets . . . 1597
Zantac 300 Tablets . . . 1597
Zantac Injection . . . 1593
Zantac Injection Premixed . . . 1593
Zantac Syrup . . . 1597

VINORGEN (Argentina)
VINORELBINE TARTRATE
Navelbine Injection. . . 1494

VINSEN (Thailand)
NAPROXEN
EC-Naprosyn Delayed-Release Tablets. . . 2769
Naprosyn Suspension . . . 2769
Naprosyn Tablets . . . 2769

VIOKASE (Belgium, Canada)
PANCRELIPASE
Ultrase Capsules . . . 735
Ultrase MT Capsules . . . 736

VIOTISONE (Hong Kong, Thailand)
OFLOXACIN
Floxin Otic Solution . . . 1043

VIPLUS (Mexico)
NAPROXEN SODIUM
Anaprox DS Tablets . . . 2769
Anaprox Tablets . . . 2769

VIPRES (Spain)
ENALAPRIL MALEATE
Vasotec I.V. Injection . . . 2076

VIRACEPT (Sweden)
NELFINAVIR MESYLATE
Viracept Oral Powder . . . 2556
Viracept Tablets . . . 2556

VIRAFERON (France, Mexico, Spain)
INTERFERON ALFA-2B
Intron A for Injection. . . 3038

VIRAMID (Brazil, Italy)
RIBAVIRIN
Virazole for Inhalation Solution . . . 3365

VIRAZID (Spain)
RIBAVIRIN
Virazole for Inhalation Solution . . . 3365

VIRAZIDE (Australia, Italy, Mexico)
RIBAVIRIN
Virazole for Inhalation Solution . . . 3365

VIRAZOLE (Belgium, Brazil, Canada, Germany, Hong Kong, Hungary, Irish Republic, Italy, Singapore, Spain, Sweden, Switzerland, The Netherlands, United Kingdom)
RIBAVIRIN
Virazole for Inhalation Solution . . . 3365

VIRDOX (Spain)
CETIRIZINE HYDROCHLORIDE
Zyrtec Syrup . . . 2589
Zyrtec Tablets . . . 2589

VIREGYT (Germany, Hungary)
AMANTADINE HYDROCHLORIDE
Symmetrel Syrup . . . 1115
Symmetrel Tablets. . . 1115

VIREGYT-K (Czech Republic)
AMANTADINE HYDROCHLORIDE
Symmetrel Syrup . . . 1115
Symmetrel Tablets. . . 1115

VIRFEN (Greece)
ENALAPRIL MALEATE
Vasotec I.V. Injection . . . 2076

VIRFLUTAM (Italy)
FLUTAMIDE
Eulexin Capsules. . . 3023

VIRGAN (Argentina, France, United Kingdom)
GANCICLOVIR
Cytovene Capsules . . . 2763

VIRILON (Argentina)
SILDENAFIL CITRATE
Viagra Tablets . . . 2552

VIRIPOTENS (Argentina)
SILDENAFIL CITRATE
Viagra Tablets . . . 2552

VIRLIX (Austria, Czech Republic, Denmark, France, Italy, Mexico, Norway, Portugal, Spain)
CETIRIZINE HYDROCHLORIDE
Zyrtec Syrup . . . 2589
Zyrtec Tablets . . . 2589

VIROBRON NF (Argentina)
DICLOFENAC SODIUM
Voltaren Tablets . . . 2298
Voltaren-XR Tablets . . . 2301

VIROFRAL (Denmark, Sweden)
AMANTADINE HYDROCHLORIDE
Symmetrel Syrup . . . 1115
Symmetrel Tablets. . . 1115

VIRORREVER (Argentina)
EFAVIRENZ
Sustiva Capsules. . . 957

VIROSOL (Argentina)
AMANTADINE HYDROCHLORIDE
Symmetrel Syrup . . . 1115
Symmetrel Tablets. . . 1115

VIROSTAV (Malaysia)
STAVUDINE
Zerit Capsules . . . 971
Zerit for Oral Solution. . . 971

VIROZID (Brazil)
ZIDOVUDINE
Retrovir Capsules . . . 1533
Retrovir IV Infusion. . . 1537
Retrovir Syrup . . . 1533
Retrovir Tablets. . . 1533

VIRUCID (Austria)
AMANTADINE HYDROCHLORIDE
Symmetrel Syrup . . . 1115
Symmetrel Tablets. . . 1115

VIRUSTAT (Brazil)
ZIDOVUDINE
Retrovir Capsules . . . 1533
Retrovir IV Infusion. . . 1537
Retrovir Syrup . . . 1533
Retrovir Tablets. . . 1533

VISCARD (Greece)
NIFEDIPINE
Adalat CC Tablets . . . 2978

VISCOR (Italy)
DIPYRIDAMOLE
Persantine Tablets . . . 898

VISCOSEAL (Germany, Malaysia, Switzerland, United Kingdom)
SODIUM HYALURONATE
Hyalgan Solution . . . 2917

VISIAL (India)
SODIUM HYALURONATE
Hyalgan Solution . . . 2917

VISINE ALLERGY WITH ANTIHISTAMINE (Australia, New Zealand)
NAPHAZOLINE HYDROCHLORIDE
Albalon Ophthalmic Solution . . . ⊙216

VISIOL (Germany, Malaysia)
SODIUM HYALURONATE
Hyalgan Solution . . . 2917

VISLUBE (Germany, Malaysia, Switzerland)
SODIUM HYALURONATE
Hyalgan Solution . . . 2917

VISMED (Australia, France, Germany, Hong Kong, Italy, Switzerland)
SODIUM HYALURONATE
Hyalgan Solution . . . 2917

VISTALBALON (Germany)
NAPHAZOLINE HYDROCHLORIDE
Albalon Ophthalmic Solution . . . ⊙216

VISTHESIA (Germany)
SODIUM HYALURONATE
Hyalgan Solution . . . 2917

VISUMETAZONE (Italy)
DEXAMETHASONE
Decadron Tablets . . . 1929

VITACID (Portugal)
TRETINOIN
Avita Cream. . . 2136

(⊙ Described in PDR For Ophthalmic Medicines™)

Avita Gel . . . 2138
Renova 0.05% Cream . . . 2387
Retin-A Micro 0.1%/0.04% . . . 2388
Vesanoid Capsules . . . 2823

VITAMIN A ACID (Hong Kong)
TRETINOIN
Avita Cream . . . 2136
Avita Gel . . . 2138
Renova 0.05% Cream . . . 2387
Retin-A Micro 0.1%/0.04% . . . 2388
Vesanoid Capsules . . . 2823

VITANOL (Spain)
TRETINOIN
Avita Cream . . . 2136
Avita Gel . . . 2138
Renova 0.05% Cream . . . 2387
Retin-A Micro 0.1%/0.04% . . . 2388
Vesanoid Capsules . . . 2823

VITANOL-A (Argentina, Brazil)
TRETINOIN
Avita Cream . . . 2136
Avita Gel . . . 2138
Renova 0.05% Cream . . . 2387
Retin-A Micro 0.1%/0.04% . . . 2388
Vesanoid Capsules . . . 2823

VITASEPTINE (France)
SULFACETAMIDE SODIUM
Klaron Lotion 10% . . . 1050

VITINOIN (Canada)
TRETINOIN
Avita Cream . . . 2136
Avita Gel . . . 2138
Renova 0.05% Cream . . . 2387
Retin-A Micro 0.1%/0.04% . . . 2388
Vesanoid Capsules . . . 2823

VITOBEL (Greece)
ENALAPRIL MALEATE
Vasotec I.V. Injection . . . 2076

VITRASERT (Australia, Spain, United Kingdom)
GANCICLOVIR
Cytovene Capsules . . . 2763

VITRAX (France)
SODIUM HYALURONATE
Hyalgan Solution . . . 2917

VITULPAS (Chile)
HYDROCORTISONE
Hydrocortone Tablets . . . 1963

VIVAL (Norway)
DIAZEPAM
Diastat Rectal Delivery System . . . 3344
Valium Tablets . . . 2822

VIVAPRYL (United Kingdom)
SELEGILINE HYDROCHLORIDE
Eldepryl Capsules . . . 3209

VIVATEC (Denmark, Finland, Norway, Sweden)
LISINOPRIL
Prinivil Tablets . . . 2029
Zestril Tablets . . . 704

VIVATEC COMP (Finland, Norway)
HYDROCHLOROTHIAZIDE/LISINOPRIL
Prinzide Tablets . . . 2033
Zestoretic Tablets . . . 701

VIVAZID (Denmark)
HYDROCHLOROTHIAZIDE/LISINOPRIL
Prinzide Tablets . . . 2033
Zestoretic Tablets . . . 701

VIVELLE (Belgium, Canada)
ESTRADIOL
Climara Transdermal System . . . 795
Vivelle Transdermal System . . . 2288
Vivelle-Dot Transdermal System . . . 2293

VIVELLE DOT (Denmark)
ESTRADIOL
Climara Transdermal System . . . 795
Vivelle Transdermal System . . . 2288
Vivelle-Dot Transdermal System . . . 2293

VIVELLEDOT (France)
ESTRADIOL
Climara Transdermal System . . . 795
Vivelle Transdermal System . . . 2288
Vivelle-Dot Transdermal System . . . 2293

VIVERDAL (Brazil)
RISPERIDONE
Risperdal Oral Solution . . . 1658
Risperdal Tablets . . . 1658

VIVIDRIN AKUT AZELASTIN (Germany)
AZELASTINE HYDROCHLORIDE
Astelin Nasal Spray . . . 1876

VIVOL (Canada)
DIAZEPAM
Diastat Rectal Delivery System . . . 3344
Valium Tablets . . . 2822

VIXCEF (Argentina)
CEFIXIME
Suprax . . . 1811

VIXIDERM E (Argentina)
BENZOYL PEROXIDE
Brevoxyl-4 Creamy Wash . . . 3212
Brevoxyl-4 Gel . . . 3211
Brevoxyl-8 Creamy Wash . . . 3212
Brevoxyl-8 Gel . . . 3211
Triaz Cleanser . . . 1864
Triaz Gel . . . 1864

VIXIDONE (Argentina)
DEXAMETHASONE
Decadron Tablets . . . 1929

VIXIDONE T (Argentina)
DEXAMETHASONE
Decadron Tablets . . . 1929

VIZERUL (Argentina)
RANITIDINE HYDROCHLORIDE
Zantac 25 EFFERdose Tablets . . . 1597
Zantac 150 EFFERdose Tablets . . . 1597
Zantac 150 Tablets . . . 1597
Zantac 300 Tablets . . . 1597
Zantac Injection . . . 1593
Zantac Injection Premixed . . . 1593
Zantac Syrup . . . 1597

VOFENAL (Canada)
DICLOFENAC SODIUM
Voltaren Tablets . . . 2298
Voltaren-XR Tablets . . . 2301

VOKER (Malaysia)
FAMOTIDINE
Pepcid Injection . . . 2017
Pepcid Injection Premixed . . . 2017
Pepcid Tablets . . . 2014
Pepcid for Oral Suspension . . . 2014

VOLDAL (France)
DICLOFENAC SODIUM
Voltaren Tablets . . . 2298
Voltaren-XR Tablets . . . 2301

VOLFENAC (Thailand)
DICLOFENAC SODIUM
Voltaren Tablets . . . 2298
Voltaren-XR Tablets . . . 2301

VOLNAC (Thailand)
DICLOFENAC SODIUM
Voltaren Tablets . . . 2298
Voltaren-XR Tablets . . . 2301

VOLOGEN (Irish Republic)
DICLOFENAC SODIUM
Voltaren Tablets . . . 2298
Voltaren-XR Tablets . . . 2301

VOLON A (Austria, Germany)
TRIAMCINOLONE ACETONIDE
Azmacort Inhalation Aerosol . . . 1701
Nasacort AQ Nasal Spray . . . 2937

VOLONIMAT (Germany)
TRIAMCINOLONE ACETONIDE
Azmacort Inhalation Aerosol . . . 1701
Nasacort AQ Nasal Spray . . . 2937

VOLONIMAT N (Germany)
TRIAMCINOLONE ACETONIDE
Azmacort Inhalation Aerosol . . . 1701
Nasacort AQ Nasal Spray . . . 2937

VOLRAMAN (United Kingdom)
DICLOFENAC SODIUM
Voltaren Tablets . . . 2298
Voltaren-XR Tablets . . . 2301

VOLSAID (United Kingdom)
DICLOFENAC SODIUM
Voltaren Tablets . . . 2298
Voltaren-XR Tablets . . . 2301

VOLTA (Thailand)
DICLOFENAC SODIUM
Voltaren Tablets . . . 2298
Voltaren-XR Tablets . . . 2301

VOLTAFLEX (Brazil)
DICLOFENAC SODIUM
Voltaren Tablets . . . 2298
Voltaren-XR Tablets . . . 2301

VOLTAMICIN (Austria, Brazil, Czech Republic, Hungary, Singapore)
DICLOFENAC SODIUM
Voltaren Tablets . . . 2298
Voltaren-XR Tablets . . . 2301

VOLTAREN (Brazil, Greece, Norway, Spain, Sweden)
DICLOFENAC SODIUM
Voltaren Tablets . . . 2298
Voltaren-XR Tablets . . . 2301

VOLTAREN COLIRIO (Argentina, Brazil)
DICLOFENAC SODIUM
Voltaren Tablets . . . 2298
Voltaren-XR Tablets . . . 2301

VOLTAREN FLEX (Argentina)
DICLOFENAC SODIUM
Voltaren Tablets . . . 2298
Voltaren-XR Tablets . . . 2301

VOLTAREN FORTE (Argentina)
DICLOFENAC SODIUM
Voltaren Tablets . . . 2298
Voltaren-XR Tablets . . . 2301

VOLTAREN OPHTA (Hungary, Switzerland)
DICLOFENAC SODIUM
Voltaren Tablets . . . 2298
Voltaren-XR Tablets . . . 2301

VOLTAREN OPHTHA (Australia, Canada, Germany, Hong Kong, Israel, New Zealand, Norway, Singapore, South Africa, Sweden)
DICLOFENAC SODIUM
Voltaren Tablets . . . 2298
Voltaren-XR Tablets . . . 2301

VOLTAREN PLUS (Germany)
DICLOFENAC SODIUM
Voltaren Tablets . . . 2298
Voltaren-XR Tablets . . . 2301

VOLTAREN T (Sweden)
DICLOFENAC POTASSIUM
Cataflam Tablets . . . 2173

VOLTARENE (France)
DICLOFENAC SODIUM
Voltaren Tablets . . . 2298
Voltaren-XR Tablets . . . 2301

VOLTAROL OPHTHA (Irish Republic, United Kingdom)
DICLOFENAC SODIUM
Voltaren Tablets . . . 2298
Voltaren-XR Tablets . . . 2301

VOLTFAST (Italy)
DICLOFENAC POTASSIUM
Cataflam Tablets . . . 2173

VOLTRIC (Spain)
CETIRIZINE HYDROCHLORIDE
Zyrtec Syrup . . . 2589
Zyrtec Tablets . . . 2589

VOLUTINE (Italy)
FENOFIBRATE
Tricor Tablets . . . 523

VOLUTOL (Mexico)
CARBAMAZEPINE
Carbatrol Capsules . . . 3174
Tegretol Chewable Tablets . . . 2278
Tegretol Suspension . . . 2278
Tegretol Tablets . . . 2278
Tegretol-XR Tablets . . . 2278

VOLVERAC (Thailand)
DICLOFENAC SODIUM
Voltaren Tablets . . . 2298
Voltaren-XR Tablets . . . 2301

VOMITRON (Thailand)
ONDANSETRON HYDROCHLORIDE
Zofran Injection . . . 1607
Zofran Injection Premixed . . . 1607
Zofran Oral Solution . . . 1613
Zofran Tablets . . . 1613

V-OPTIC (Israel)
TIMOLOL MALEATE
Blocadren Tablets . . . 1891
Timoptic Sterile Ophthalmic Solution . . . 2058
Timoptic in Ocudose . . . 2061
Timoptic-XE Sterile Ophthalmic Gel Forming Solution . . . 2062

VOREN (Malaysia, Thailand)
DICLOFENAC SODIUM
Voltaren Tablets . . . 2298
Voltaren-XR Tablets . . . 2301

VOREN PLUS (Malaysia)
DICLOFENAC SODIUM
Voltaren Tablets . . . 2298
Voltaren-XR Tablets . . . 2301

VORST (Argentina)
SILDENAFIL CITRATE
Viagra Tablets . . . 2552

VOSTAR (Denmark)
DICLOFENAC SODIUM
Voltaren Tablets . . . 2298
Voltaren-XR Tablets . . . 2301

VOTAMED (Thailand)
DICLOFENAC SODIUM
Voltaren Tablets . . . 2298
Voltaren-XR Tablets . . . 2301

VOXIN (Greece)
VANCOMYCIN HYDROCHLORIDE
Vancocin HCl Capsules, USP . . . 3370

VUCLODIR (Argentina)
LAMIVUDINE
Epivir Oral Solution . . . 1394
Epivir Tablets . . . 1394
Epivir-HBV Oral Solution . . . 1398
Epivir-HBV Tablets . . . 1398

VUDIRAX (Brazil)
LAMIVUDINE
Epivir Oral Solution . . . 1394
Epivir Tablets . . . 1394
Epivir-HBV Oral Solution . . . 1398
Epivir-HBV Tablets . . . 1398

VULMIZOLIN (Czech Republic)
CEFAZOLIN SODIUM
Ancef for Injection . . . 1318

VURDON (Greece)
DICLOFENAC SODIUM
Voltaren Tablets . . . 2298
Voltaren-XR Tablets . . . 2301

WARAN (Sweden)
WARFARIN SODIUM
Coumadin Tablets . . . 932
Coumadin for Injection . . . 932

WARCA (Thailand)
MEBENDAZOLE
Vermox Chewable Tablets . . . 1853

WARF (India)
WARFARIN SODIUM
Coumadin Tablets . . . 932
Coumadin for Injection . . . 932

WARFILONE (Canada)
WARFARIN SODIUM
Coumadin Tablets . . . 932
Coumadin for Injection . . . 932

WARI-DICLOWAL (Malaysia)
DICLOFENAC SODIUM
Voltaren Tablets . . . 2298
Voltaren-XR Tablets . . . 2301

WARIDIPIN (Hong Kong)
NIFEDIPINE
Adalat CC Tablets . . . 2978

WARIMAZOL (Hong Kong)
CLOTRIMAZOLE
Lotrimin Cream . . . 3053
Lotrimin Lotion 1% . . . 3053
Lotrimin Topical Solution 1% . . . 3053

WASPEZE HYDROCORTISONE (United Kingdom)
HYDROCORTISONE
Hydrocortone Tablets . . . 1963

WAUCOSIN (Greece)
TIMOLOL MALEATE
Blocadren Tablets . . . 1891
Timoptic Sterile Ophthalmic Solution . . . 2058
Timoptic in Ocudose . . . 2061
Timoptic-XE Sterile Ophthalmic Gel Forming Solution . . . 2062

WAYCITAL (Mexico)
PRAZIQUANTEL
Biltricide Tablets . . . 2990

WAYTRAX (Mexico)
CEFTAZIDIME
Fortaz for Injection . . . 1422

WELLBUTRIN (Argentina, Brazil, Canada, Chile, Czech Republic, Hungary, Mexico)
BUPROPION HYDROCHLORIDE
Wellbutrin SR Sustained-Release Tablets . . 1583
Wellbutrin Tablets 1579
Zyban Sustained-Release Tablets 1620

WELLCID (Brazil)
PERMETHRIN
Acticin Cream. 2125

WELLVONE (Australia, Austria, Belgium, Denmark, France, Germany, Greece, Italy, South Africa, Spain, Sweden, Switzerland, The Netherlands, United Kingdom)
ATOVAQUONE
Mepron Suspension 1487

WENFLOX (Argentina)
NORFLOXACIN
Noroxin Tablets. 2009

WEPOX (India)
EPOETIN ALFA
Epogen for Injection. 586
Procrit for Injection 2374

WINOL (Argentina)
IRINOTECAN HYDROCHLORIDE
Camptosar Injection. 2602

WITROMIN (Mexico)
ERYTHROMYCIN
Ery-Tab Tablets 447
Erythromycin Base Filmtab Tablets. 454
Erythromycin Delayed-Release Capsules, USP 456
PCE Dispertab Tablets 510

WITTY (Argentina)
PERMETHRIN
Acticin Cream. 2125

WONTIZEM (Hong Kong)
DILTIAZEM HYDROCHLORIDE
Cardizem LA Extended Release Tablets. . . 1699
Tiazac Capsules 1204

WORMGO (South Africa)
MEBENDAZOLE
Vermox Chewable Tablets 1853

WORMICIDE (Thailand)
PRAZIQUANTEL
Biltricide Tablets 2990

WORMIN (India)
MEBENDAZOLE
Vermox Chewable Tablets 1853

WORMSTOP (South Africa)
MEBENDAZOLE
Vermox Chewable Tablets 1853

WYMESONE (India)
DEXAMETHASONE
Decadron Tablets 1929

XACIN (Thailand)
NORFLOXACIN
Noroxin Tablets. 2009

XADAREN (Czech Republic)
FLUTAMIDE
Eulexin Capsules. 3023

XAGRID (Switzerland, United Kingdom)
ANAGRELIDE HYDROCHLORIDE
Agrylin Capsules 3172

XALACOM (Argentina, Australia, Austria, Belgium, Canada, Czech Republic, France, Germany, Hong Kong, Hungary, Irish Republic, Israel, Italy, Malaysia, Portugal, Singapore, South Africa, Spain, Switzerland, Thailand, The Netherlands, United Kingdom)
LATANOPROST
Xalatan Ophthalmic Solution . . . . ⊙280

XALATAN (Argentina, Australia, Austria, Belgium, Brazil, Canada, Chile, Denmark, Finland, France, Germany, Greece, Hong Kong, Hungary, Irish Republic, Israel, Italy, Malaysia, Mexico, New Zealand, Norway, Portugal, Russia, Singapore, South Africa, Spain, Sweden, Switzerland, Thailand, The Netherlands, United Kingdom)
LATANOPROST
Xalatan Ophthalmic Solution 280

XALCOM (Denmark, Finland, Norway, Sweden)
LATANOPROST
Xalatan Ophthalmic Solution . . . . ⊙280

XALOTINA (Argentina)
AMOXICILLIN
Amoxil Pediatric Drops for Oral Suspension. 1315
Amoxil Tablets 1315

XANAES (Argentina)
AZELASTINE HYDROCHLORIDE
Astelin Nasal Spray 1876

XANIDINE (Thailand)
RANITIDINE HYDROCHLORIDE
Zantac 25 EFFERdose Tablets 1597
Zantac 150 EFFERdose Tablets. 1597
Zantac 150 Tablets 1597
Zantac 300 Tablets 1597
Zantac Injection 1593
Zantac Injection Premixed 1593
Zantac Syrup 1597

XANOMEL (Hungary, Irish Republic)
RANITIDINE HYDROCHLORIDE
Zantac 25 EFFERdose Tablets 1597
Zantac 150 EFFERdose Tablets. 1597
Zantac 150 Tablets 1597
Zantac 300 Tablets 1597
Zantac Injection 1593
Zantac Injection Premixed 1593
Zantac Syrup 1597

XANTHIUM (France, Thailand)
THEOPHYLLINE
Uniphyl Tablets 2708

XANTIVENT (Switzerland)
THEOPHYLLINE
Uniphyl Tablets 2708

XAO T (Argentina)
TOBRAMYCIN
TOBI Solution for Inhalation 1015

XAO-DEX (Argentina)
TOBRAMYCIN
TOBI Solution for Inhalation 1015

XARATOR (Italy)
ATORVASTATIN CALCIUM
Lipitor Tablets 2495

XASMUN (Spain)
NORFLOXACIN
Noroxin Tablets. 2009

XATEN (France)
ATENOLOL
Tenormin I.V. Injection. 698

XEDENOL (Argentina)
DICLOFENAC SODIUM
Voltaren Tablets 2298
Voltaren-XR Tablets 2301

XEDENOL FLEX (Argentina)
DICLOFENAC SODIUM
Voltaren Tablets 2298
Voltaren-XR Tablets 2301

XEDENOL GESIC (Argentina)
DICLOFENAC POTASSIUM
Cataflam Tablets 2173

XELODA (Argentina, Australia, Austria, Belgium, Brazil, Canada, Chile, Czech Republic, Denmark, Finland, France, Germany, Greece, Hong Kong, Hungary, Irish Republic, Israel, Italy, Mexico, New Zealand, Norway, Portugal, Singapore, South Africa, Spain, Sweden, Switzerland, Thailand, United Kingdom)
CAPECITABINE
Xeloda Tablets 2825

XENAR (Italy)
NAPROXEN
EC-Naprosyn Delayed-Release Tablets. . . . 2769
Naprosyn Suspension. 2769
Naprosyn Tablets 2769

XENICAL (Argentina, Australia, Austria, Belgium, Brazil, Canada, Chile, Czech Republic, Denmark, Finland, France, Germany, Greece, Hong Kong, Hungary, Irish Republic, Israel, Italy, Mexico, New Zealand, Norway, Portugal, Singapore, South Africa, Spain, Sweden, Switzerland, Thailand, The Netherlands, United Kingdom)
ORLISTAT
Xenical Capsules 2834

XENOBID (India)
NAPROXEN
EC-Naprosyn Delayed-Release Tablets. . . . 2769
Naprosyn Suspension. 2769
Naprosyn Tablets 2769

XENOPAN (Austria)
NAPROXEN
EC-Naprosyn Delayed-Release Tablets. . . . 2769
Naprosyn Suspension. 2769
Naprosyn Tablets 2769

XENOVATE (South Africa)
CLOBETASOL PROPIONATE
Temovate Cream. 1549
Temovate E Emollient. 1552
Temovate Gel 1550
Temovate Ointment 1549
Temovate Scalp Application 1551

XEPAGAN (Singapore)
PROMETHAZINE HYDROCHLORIDE
Phenergan Suppositories. 3438
Phenergan Tablets 3438

XEPAMET (Malaysia, Singapore)
CIMETIDINE
Tagamet Tablets 1547

XERASPOR (South Africa)
CLOTRIMAZOLE
Lotrimin Cream. 3053
Lotrimin Lotion 1%. 3053
Lotrimin Topical Solution 1% 3053

XERGIC (Australia)
FEXOFENADINE HYDROCHLORIDE
Allegra Capsules 2857

XETIN (Spain)
PAROXETINE HYDROCHLORIDE
Paxil Oral Suspension. 1501
Paxil Tablets. 1501

XICANE (Argentina)
NAPROXEN
EC-Naprosyn Delayed-Release Tablets. . . . 2769
Naprosyn Suspension. 2769
Naprosyn Tablets 2769

XILANIC (Argentina)
PAROXETINE HYDROCHLORIDE
Paxil Oral Suspension. 1501
Paxil Tablets. 1501

XILOCLER (Argentina)
LIDOCAINE
Lidoderm Patch 1107

XILONIBSA (Portugal)
LIDOCAINE
Lidoderm Patch 1107

XILOPAR (Austria, Germany, Italy, Portugal)
SELEGILINE HYDROCHLORIDE
Eldepryl Capsules 3209

XIM (India)
CEFIXIME
Suprax 1811

XIMAKEN (Mexico)
CEFUROXIME SODIUM
Zinacef Injection 1604

XINA (Argentina)
DICLOFENAC SODIUM
Voltaren Tablets 2298
Voltaren-XR Tablets 2301

XIPRAL (Mexico)
PRAVASTATIN SODIUM
Pravachol Tablets 943

XIPROCAN (Mexico)
AMOXICILLIN
Amoxil Pediatric Drops for Oral Suspension. 1315
Amoxil Tablets 1315

XISMOX (United Kingdom)
ISOSORBIDE MONONITRATE
Imdur Tablets 3032

XOLOF (Chile)
TOBRAMYCIN
TOBI Solution for Inhalation 1015

XOLOF D (Chile)
DEXAMETHASONE/TOBRAMYCIN
TobraDex Ophthalmic Ointment 558
TobraDex Ophthalmic Suspension 558

XORIM (Hungary)
CEFUROXIME SODIUM
Zinacef Injection 1604

XSERT (India)
SERTRALINE HYDROCHLORIDE
Zoloft Tablets 2581

X'TAC (Malaysia)
RANITIDINE HYDROCHLORIDE
Zantac 25 EFFERdose Tablets 1597
Zantac 150 EFFERdose Tablets. 1597
Zantac 150 Tablets 1597
Zantac 300 Tablets 1597
Zantac Injection 1593
Zantac Injection Premixed 1593
Zantac Syrup 1597

X'TOR (India)
ATORVASTATIN CALCIUM
Lipitor Tablets 2495

XYDEP (Australia)
SERTRALINE HYDROCHLORIDE
Zoloft Tablets 2581

XYLESTESIN (Czech Republic)
LIDOCAINE
Lidoderm Patch 1107

XYLOCAINA 2% (Chile)
LIDOCAINE
Lidoderm Patch 1107

XYLOCAINE (Czech Republic, India, Israel, Malaysia, South Africa, United Kingdom)
LIDOCAINE
Lidoderm Patch 1107

XYLODASE (United Kingdom)
LIDOCAINE
Lidoderm Patch 1107

XYLOPROCT (Hong Kong)
LIDOCAINE
Lidoderm Patch 1107

YANURAX (Argentina)
NORFLOXACIN
Noroxin Tablets. 2009

YARA (Greece)
RANITIDINE HYDROCHLORIDE
Zantac 25 EFFERdose Tablets 1597
Zantac 150 EFFERdose Tablets. 1597
Zantac 150 Tablets 1597
Zantac 300 Tablets 1597
Zantac Injection 1593
Zantac Injection Premixed 1593
Zantac Syrup 1597

YATROX (Spain)
ONDANSETRON HYDROCHLORIDE
Zofran Injection. 1607
Zofran Injection Premixed 1607
Zofran Oral Solution. 1613
Zofran Tablets 1613

YECTAMICINA (Mexico)
GENTAMICIN SULFATE
Garamycin Injectable 3028
Genoptic Sterile Ophthalmic Solution . . . . ⊙227

YEDOC (Switzerland)
GENTAMICIN SULFATE
Garamycin Injectable 3028
Genoptic Sterile Ophthalmic Solution . . . . ⊙227

YESAN (Greece)
TIMOLOL MALEATE
Blocadren Tablets 1891
Timoptic Sterile Ophthalmic Solution 2058
Timoptic in Ocudose 2061
Timoptic-XE Sterile Ophthalmic Gel Forming Solution 2062

YOKEL (Greece)
CEFUROXIME SODIUM
Zinacef Injection 1604

YRELAN (Brazil)
ENALAPRIL MALEATE
Vasotec I.V. Injection 2076

YUCOMY (Malaysia, Singapore)
KETOCONAZOLE
Nizoral 2% Shampoo 1838

YUREMID (Mexico)
FUROSEMIDE
Furosemide Tablets 2117

ZAART-H (India)
LOSARTAN POTASSIUM
Cozaar Tablets 1913

ZACTOS (Mexico)
PIOGLITAZONE HYDROCHLORIDE
Actos Tablets 3224

ZADINE (Brazil)
RANITIDINE HYDROCHLORIDE
Zantac 25 EFFERdose Tablets 1597
Zantac 150 EFFERdose Tablets 1597
Zantac 150 Tablets 1597
Zantac 300 Tablets 1597
Zantac Injection 1593
Zantac Injection Premixed 1593
Zantac Syrup 1597

ZADIPINA (Italy)
NISOLDIPINE
Sular Tablets 1163

ZADOLINA (Mexico)
CEFTAZIDIME
Fortaz for Injection 1422

ZADSTAT (Israel, United Kingdom)
METRONIDAZOLE
MetroGel-Vaginal Gel 1822
Noritate Cream, 1% 1051

ZAEDOC (United Kingdom)
RANITIDINE HYDROCHLORIDE
Zantac 25 EFFERdose Tablets 1597
Zantac 150 EFFERdose Tablets 1597
Zantac 150 Tablets 1597
Zantac 300 Tablets 1597
Zantac Injection 1593
Zantac Injection Premixed 1593
Zantac Syrup 1597

ZAFIMIDA (Mexico)
FUROSEMIDE
Furosemide Tablets 2117

ZAFIRASMAL (Argentina)
ZAFIRLUKAST
Accolate Tablets 663

ZAFIRST (Italy)
ZAFIRLUKAST
Accolate Tablets 663

ZAGASTROL (Brazil)
CIMETIDINE
Tagamet Tablets 1547

ZAGYL (South Africa)
METRONIDAZOLE
MetroGel-Vaginal Gel 1822
Noritate Cream, 1% 1051

ZALVOR (Belgium)
PERMETHRIN
Acticin Cream 2125

ZAMACORT (Mexico)
TRIAMCINOLONE ACETONIDE
Azmacort Inhalation Aerosol 1701
Nasacort AQ Nasal Spray 2937

ZAMOCILLINE (France)
AMOXICILLIN
Amoxil Pediatric Drops for Oral Suspension 1315
Amoxil Tablets 1315

ZANDINE (Irish Republic)
RANITIDINE HYDROCHLORIDE
Zantac 25 EFFERdose Tablets 1597
Zantac 150 EFFERdose Tablets 1597
Zantac 150 Tablets 1597
Zantac 300 Tablets 1597
Zantac Injection 1593
Zantac Injection Premixed 1593
Zantac Syrup 1597

ZANIDEX (Israel)
RANITIDINE HYDROCHLORIDE
Zantac 25 EFFERdose Tablets 1597
Zantac 150 EFFERdose Tablets 1597
Zantac 150 Tablets 1597
Zantac 300 Tablets 1597
Zantac Injection 1593
Zantac Injection Premixed 1593
Zantac Syrup 1597

ZANIDIN (New Zealand)
RANITIDINE HYDROCHLORIDE
Zantac 25 EFFERdose Tablets 1597
Zantac 150 EFFERdose Tablets 1597
Zantac 150 Tablets 1597
Zantac 300 Tablets 1597
Zantac Injection 1593
Zantac Injection Premixed 1593
Zantac Syrup 1597

ZANOC (Brazil)
KETOCONAZOLE
Nizoral 2% Shampoo 1838

ZANOCIN (Czech Republic, Hungary, India, Malaysia, South Africa)
OFLOXACIN
Floxin Otic Solution 1043

ZANTAB (Israel)
RANITIDINE HYDROCHLORIDE
Zantac 25 EFFERdose Tablets 1597
Zantac 150 EFFERdose Tablets 1597
Zantac 150 Tablets 1597
Zantac 300 Tablets 1597
Zantac Injection 1593
Zantac Injection Premixed 1593
Zantac Syrup 1597

ZANTAC (Australia, Austria, Belgium, Canada, Chile, Czech Republic, Denmark, Finland, Greece, Hong Kong, Hungary, Irish Republic, Israel, Italy, Malaysia, New Zealand, Norway, Portugal, Singapore, South Africa, Spain, Sweden, Thailand, The Netherlands, United Kingdom)
RANITIDINE HYDROCHLORIDE
Zantac 25 EFFERdose Tablets 1597
Zantac 150 EFFERdose Tablets 1597
Zantac 150 Tablets 1597
Zantac 300 Tablets 1597
Zantac Injection 1593
Zantac Injection Premixed 1593
Zantac Syrup 1597

ZANTARAC (Austria)
RANITIDINE HYDROCHLORIDE
Zantac 25 EFFERdose Tablets 1597
Zantac 150 EFFERdose Tablets 1597
Zantac 150 Tablets 1597
Zantac 300 Tablets 1597
Zantac Injection 1593
Zantac Injection Premixed 1593
Zantac Syrup 1597

ZANTIC (Germany, Switzerland)
RANITIDINE HYDROCHLORIDE
Zantac 25 EFFERdose Tablets 1597
Zantac 150 EFFERdose Tablets 1597
Zantac 150 Tablets 1597
Zantac 300 Tablets 1597
Zantac Injection 1593
Zantac Injection Premixed 1593
Zantac Syrup 1597

ZAPONEX (United Kingdom)
CLOZAPINE
Clozapine Tablets 2141
Clozaril Tablets 2174

ZAPTO (South Africa)
CAPTOPRIL
Captopril Tablets 2114

ZAPTO CO (South Africa)
CAPTOPRIL
Captopril Tablets 2114

ZARATOR (Argentina, Chile, Denmark, Greece, Portugal, Spain)
ATORVASTATIN CALCIUM
Lipitor Tablets 2495

ZAREX (Israel)
FAMOTIDINE
Pepcid Injection 2017
Pepcid Injection Premixed 2017
Pepcid Tablets 2014
Pepcid for Oral Suspension 2014

ZARGUS (Brazil)
RISPERIDONE
Risperdal Oral Solution 1658
Risperdal Tablets 1658

ZART (India)
LOSARTAN POTASSIUM
Cozaar Tablets 1913

ZAVEDOS (Argentina, Australia, Austria, Belgium, Brazil, Chile, Czech Republic, Denmark, Finland, France, Germany, Greece, Hong Kong, Hungary, Irish Republic, Israel, Italy, Malaysia, New Zealand, Norway, Portugal, Singapore, South Africa, Spain, Sweden, Switzerland, Thailand, The Netherlands, United Kingdom)
IDARUBICIN HYDROCHLORIDE
Idamycin PFS Injection 2645

ZAXEM (Austria)
BUTENAFINE HYDROCHLORIDE
Mentax Cream 2152

ZAYASEL (Spain)
TERAZOSIN HYDROCHLORIDE
Hytrin Capsules 469

Z-BEC (Greece)
LISINOPRIL
Prinivil Tablets 2029
Zestril Tablets 704

ZEBEN (Thailand)
ALBENDAZOLE
Albenza Tablets 1310

ZECLAR (Czech Republic, Finland, France)
CLARITHROMYCIN
Biaxin Filmtab Tablets 402
Biaxin Granules 402

ZECLAREN OD (Greece)
CLARITHROMYCIN
Biaxin Filmtab Tablets 402
Biaxin Granules 402

ZEDDAN (Italy)
TRANDOLAPRIL
Mavik Tablets 482

ZEFA (Thailand)
CEFAZOLIN SODIUM
Ancef for Injection 1318

ZEFAXONE (Thailand)
CEFTRIAXONE SODIUM
Rocephin Injectable Vials, ADD-Vantage, Galaxy, Bulk 2801

ZEFFIX (Argentina, Australia, Austria, Belgium, Brazil, Czech Republic, Denmark, Finland, France, Germany, Greece, Hong Kong, Hungary, Irish Republic, Israel, Italy, Malaysia, New Zealand, Portugal, Singapore, Spain, Sweden, Switzerland, Thailand, United Kingdom)
LAMIVUDINE
Epivir Oral Solution 1394
Epivir Tablets 1394
Epivir-HBV Oral Solution 1398
Epivir-HBV Tablets 1398

ZEFTAM (Thailand)
CEFTAZIDIME
Fortaz for Injection 1422

ZEHU-ZE (Israel)
PERMETHRIN
Acticin Cream 2125

ZEISIN (Germany)
PIRBUTEROL ACETATE
Maxair Autohaler 1820

ZELAPAR (United Kingdom)
SELEGILINE HYDROCHLORIDE
Eldepryl Capsules 3209

ZELFIN (Mexico)
ALBENDAZOLE
Albenza Tablets 1310

ZEM (Greece)
DILTIAZEM HYDROCHLORIDE
Cardizem LA Extended Release Tablets . . . 1699
Tiazac Capsules 1204

ZEMON (United Kingdom)
ISOSORBIDE MONONITRATE
Imdur Tablets 3032

ZEMOX (Germany)
SIMVASTATIN
Zocor Tablets 2078

ZEMPLAR (Austria, Portugal, Spain, United Kingdom)
PARICALCITOL
Zemplar Injection 538

ZEMTARD (United Kingdom)
DILTIAZEM HYDROCHLORIDE
Cardizem LA Extended Release Tablets . . . 1699
Tiazac Capsules 1204

ZEMURON (Argentina, Canada)
ROCURONIUM BROMIDE
Zemuron Injection 2363

ZENAPAX (Argentina, Australia, Austria, Belgium, Brazil, Canada, Chile, Czech Republic, Denmark, Finland, France, Germany, Greece, Hong Kong, Hungary, Irish Republic, Israel, Italy, Mexico, New Zealand, Portugal, Singapore, South Africa, Spain, Sweden, Switzerland, Thailand, The Netherlands, United Kingdom)
DACLIZUMAB
Zenapax for Injection 2838

ZENAXIN (Mexico)
ALBENDAZOLE
Albenza Tablets 1310

ZENDHIN (Hong Kong, Malaysia, Singapore)
RANITIDINE HYDROCHLORIDE
Zantac 25 EFFERdose Tablets 1597
Zantac 150 EFFERdose Tablets 1597
Zantac 150 Tablets 1597
Zantac 300 Tablets 1597
Zantac Injection 1593
Zantac Injection Premixed 1593
Zantac Syrup 1597

ZENGAC (Italy)
VANCOMYCIN HYDROCHLORIDE
Vancocin HCl Capsules, USP 3370

ZENODIAN (Italy)
SUCRALFATE
Carafate Suspension 727
Carafate Tablets 728

ZENOXONE (United Kingdom)
HYDROCORTISONE
Hydrocortone Tablets 1963

ZENSIL (Thailand)
CETIRIZINE HYDROCHLORIDE
Zyrtec Syrup 2589
Zyrtec Tablets 2589

ZENTEL (Australia, Brazil, Chile, Czech Republic, France, Greece, India, Italy, Malaysia, Mexico, Portugal, Singapore, South Africa, Switzerland, Thailand)
ALBENDAZOLE
Albenza Tablets 1310

ZENTIUS (Argentina, Chile)
CITALOPRAM HYDROBROMIDE
Celexa Tablets 1177

ZENUSIN (Portugal, Thailand)
NIFEDIPINE
Adalat CC Tablets 2978

ZENZERA (Thailand)
ALBENDAZOLE
Albenza Tablets 1310

ZEPAN (Mexico)
DIAZEPAM
Diastat Rectal Delivery System 3344
Valium Tablets 2822

ZEPHOLIN (Greece, Irish Republic)
CETIRIZINE HYDROCHLORIDE
Zyrtec Syrup 2589
Zyrtec Tablets 2589

ZEPIKEN (Mexico)
CARBAMAZEPINE
Carbatrol Capsules 3174
Tegretol Chewable Tablets 2278
Tegretol Suspension 2278
Tegretol Tablets 2278
Tegretol-XR Tablets 2278

ZEPILEN (Thailand)
CEFAZOLIN SODIUM
Ancef for Injection 1318

ZEPOSE (India)
DIAZEPAM
Diastat Rectal Delivery System 3344
Valium Tablets 2822

ZEPRAT (Mexico)
DIAZEPAM
Diastat Rectal Delivery System 3344
Valium Tablets 2822

ZEPTOL (Russia, Thailand)
CARBAMAZEPINE
Carbatrol Capsules 3174
Tegretol Chewable Tablets 2278
Tegretol Suspension 2278
Tegretol Tablets 2278
Tegretol-XR Tablets 2278

ZERA (Portugal)
SIMVASTATIN
Zocor Tablets 2078

ZERELLA (Austria, Italy)
ESTRADIOL
Climara Transdermal System 795
Vivelle Transdermal System 2288
Vivelle-Dot Transdermal System 2293

ZERIT (Argentina, Australia, Austria, Belgium, Canada, Chile, Czech Republic, Denmark, Finland, France, Germany, Greece, Hong Kong, Hungary, Irish Republic, Israel, Italy, Japan, Malaysia, Mexico, New Zealand, Norway, Portugal, Singapore, South Africa, Spain, Sweden, Switzerland, Thailand, The Netherlands, United Kingdom)
STAVUDINE
Zerit Capsules 971
Zerit for Oral Solution 971

ZERITAVIR (Brazil)
STAVUDINE
Zerit Capsules 971
Zerit for Oral Solution 971

ZERLUBRON (Greece)
FENOFIBRATE
Tricor Tablets 523

ZERMED (Thailand)
CETIRIZINE HYDROCHLORIDE
Zyrtec Syrup 2589
Zyrtec Tablets 2589

ZEROPENEM (Argentina)
MEROPENEM
Merrem I.V. 687

ZERTINE (Hong Kong, Thailand)
CETIRIZINE HYDROCHLORIDE
Zyrtec Syrup 2589
Zyrtec Tablets 2589

ZESGER (Irish Republic)
LISINOPRIL
Prinivil Tablets 2029
Zestril Tablets 704

ZESTAN (Irish Republic)
LISINOPRIL
Prinivil Tablets 2029
Zestril Tablets 704

ZESTOMAX (South Africa)
LISINOPRIL
Prinivil Tablets 2029
Zestril Tablets 704

ZESTORETIC (Argentina, Austria, Belgium, Brazil, Canada, Chile, Denmark, France, Hong Kong, Irish Republic, Italy, Mexico, New Zealand, Norway, Portugal, South Africa, Spain, Sweden, Switzerland, The Netherlands, United Kingdom)
LISINOPRIL
Prinivil Tablets 2029
Zestril Tablets 704

ZESTRIL (Argentina, Australia, Belgium, Brazil, Canada, Chile, Denmark, Finland, France, Greece, Hong Kong, Irish Republic, Italy, Malaysia, Mexico, New Zealand, Norway, Portugal, Singapore, South Africa, Spain, Sweden, Switzerland, Thailand, The Netherlands, United Kingdom)
LISINOPRIL
Prinivil Tablets 2029
Zestril Tablets 704

ZETAGAL (Greece)
CEFUROXIME SODIUM
Zinacef Injection 1604

ZETALERG (Brazil)
CETIRIZINE HYDROCHLORIDE
Zyrtec Syrup 2589
Zyrtec Tablets 2589

ZETAVUDIN (Argentina)
ZIDOVUDINE
Retrovir Capsules 1533
Retrovir IV Infusion 1537
Retrovir Syrup 1533
Retrovir Tablets 1533

ZETIR (Brazil, Germany)
CETIRIZINE HYDROCHLORIDE
Zyrtec Syrup 2589
Zyrtec Tablets 2589

ZETOMAX (South Africa)
LISINOPRIL
Prinivil Tablets 2029
Zestril Tablets 704

ZETOP (South Africa)
CETIRIZINE HYDROCHLORIDE
Zyrtec Syrup 2589
Zyrtec Tablets 2589

ZETRON (Thailand)
ONDANSETRON HYDROCHLORIDE
Zofran Injection 1607
Zofran Injection Premixed 1607
Zofran Oral Solution 1613
Zofran Tablets 1613

ZETROTAX (Argentina)
ZIDOVUDINE
Retrovir Capsules 1533
Retrovir IV Infusion 1537
Retrovir Syrup 1533
Retrovir Tablets 1533

ZIAGEN (Australia, Austria, Belgium, Canada, Chile, Czech Republic, Denmark, Finland, France, Germany, Greece, Hong Kong, Irish Republic, Israel, Italy, New Zealand, Norway, Portugal, Singapore, South Africa, Spain, Sweden, Switzerland, United Kingdom)
ABACAVIR SULFATE
Ziagen Oral Solution 1600
Ziagen Tablets 1600

ZIAGENAVIR (Argentina, Brazil, Mexico, Thailand)
ABACAVIR SULFATE
Ziagen Oral Solution 1600
Ziagen Tablets 1600

ZIAXEL (Greece)
TRANDOLAPRIL/VERAPAMIL HYDROCHLORIDE
Tarka Tablets 519

ZICET (Hong Kong)
CETIRIZINE HYDROCHLORIDE
Zyrtec Syrup 2589
Zyrtec Tablets 2589

ZIDAC (France)
RANITIDINE HYDROCHLORIDE
Zantac 25 EFFERdose Tablets 1597
Zantac 150 EFFERdose Tablets 1597
Zantac 150 Tablets 1597
Zantac 300 Tablets 1597
Zantac Injection 1593
Zantac Injection Premixed 1593
Zantac Syrup 1597

ZIDA-CO (United Kingdom)
AMILORIDE HYDROCHLORIDE/HYDROCHLOROTHIAZIDE
Moduretic Tablets 2003

ZIDICEF (Mexico)
CEFTAZIDIME
Fortaz for Injection 1422

ZIDIMA (Argentina)
CEFTAZIDIME
Fortaz for Injection 1422

ZIDIS (Thailand)
ZIDOVUDINE
Retrovir Capsules 1533
Retrovir IV Infusion 1537
Retrovir Syrup 1533
Retrovir Tablets 1533

ZIDIX (Brazil)
ZIDOVUDINE
Retrovir Capsules 1533
Retrovir IV Infusion 1537
Retrovir Syrup 1533
Retrovir Tablets 1533

ZIDOLAM (Brazil)
LAMIVUDINE
Epivir Oral Solution 1394
Epivir Tablets 1394
Epivir-HBV Oral Solution 1398
Epivir-HBV Tablets 1398

ZIDOREX (India)
ZIDOVUDINE
Retrovir Capsules 1533
Retrovir IV Infusion 1537
Retrovir Syrup 1533
Retrovir Tablets 1533

ZIDOVAL (Denmark, Finland, Israel, Italy, Norway, Sweden, United Kingdom)
METRONIDAZOLE
MetroGel-Vaginal Gel 1822
Noritate Cream, 1% 1051

ZIDOVIR (Brazil, India, Mexico)
ZIDOVUDINE
Retrovir Capsules 1533
Retrovir IV Infusion 1537
Retrovir Syrup 1533
Retrovir Tablets 1533

ZIDOVUSAN (Brazil)
ZIDOVUDINE
Retrovir Capsules 1533
Retrovir IV Infusion 1537
Retrovir Syrup 1533
Retrovir Tablets 1533

ZIENAM (Austria)
CILASTATIN SODIUM/IMIPENEM
Primaxin I.M. 2022
Primaxin I.V. 2024

ZIFARTEL (Mexico)
PRAZIQUANTEL
Biltricide Tablets 2990

ZILACTIN-L (Canada)
LIDOCAINE
Lidoderm Patch 1107

ZILAK (Brazil)
RANITIDINE HYDROCHLORIDE
Zantac 25 EFFERdose Tablets 1597
Zantac 150 EFFERdose Tablets 1597
Zantac 150 Tablets 1597
Zantac 300 Tablets 1597
Zantac Injection 1593
Zantac Injection Premixed 1593
Zantac Syrup 1597

ZILAST (India)
CILOSTAZOL
Pletal Tablets 2478

ZILDEM (South Africa)
DILTIAZEM HYDROCHLORIDE
Cardizem LA Extended Release Tablets . . . 1699
Tiazac Capsules 1204

ZILDEN (Greece, Italy)
DILTIAZEM HYDROCHLORIDE
Cardizem LA Extended Release Tablets . . . 1699
Tiazac Capsules 1204

ZILION (India)
ZIDOVUDINE
Retrovir Capsules 1533
Retrovir IV Infusion 1537
Retrovir Syrup 1533
Retrovir Tablets 1533

ZILISTEN (Greece)
CEFUROXIME SODIUM
Zinacef Injection 1604

ZIMEROL (Mexico)
CIMETIDINE
Tagamet Tablets 1547

ZIMETIN (Switzerland)
CIMETIDINE
Tagamet Tablets 1547

ZIMMEX (Thailand)
SIMVASTATIN
Zocor Tablets 2078

ZIMSTAT (Australia)
SIMVASTATIN
Zocor Tablets 2078

ZINACEF (Belgium, Brazil, Canada, Czech Republic, Denmark, Finland, Germany, Greece, Hong Kong, Hungary, Irish Republic, Israel, Malaysia, New Zealand, Norway, Singapore, South Africa, Sweden, Switzerland, Thailand, The Netherlands, United Kingdom)
CEFUROXIME SODIUM
Zinacef Injection 1604

ZINADIUR (Italy)
BENAZEPRIL HYDROCHLORIDE/HYDROCHLOROTHIAZIDE
Lotensin HCT Tablets 2235

ZINADOL (Greece)
CEFUROXIME AXETIL
Ceftin Tablets 1369
Ceftin for Oral Suspension 1369

ZINADRIL (Italy)
BENAZEPRIL HYDROCHLORIDE
Lotensin Tablets 2232

ZINAT (Switzerland)
CEFUROXIME AXETIL
Ceftin Tablets 1369
Ceftin for Oral Suspension 1369

ZINCO SULPHA (India)
SULFACETAMIDE SODIUM
Klaron Lotion 10% 1050

ZINDACLIN (Germany, Israel, United Kingdom)
CLINDAMYCIN PHOSPHATE
Clindets Pledgets 3212

ZINDACLINE (France)
CLINDAMYCIN PHOSPHATE
Clindets Pledgets 3212

ZINECARD (Canada)
DEXRAZOXANE
Zinecard for Injection 2659

ZINERYT (Belgium, Czech Republic, Hungary, Irish Republic, Portugal, South Africa, Spain)
ERYTHROMYCIN
Ery-Tab Tablets 447
Erythromycin Base Filmtab Tablets 454
Erythromycin Delayed-Release Capsules, USP 456
PCE Dispertab Tablets 510

ZINETAC (India)
RANITIDINE HYDROCHLORIDE
Zantac 25 EFFERdose Tablets 1597
Zantac 150 EFFERdose Tablets 1597
Zantac 150 Tablets 1597
Zantac 300 Tablets 1597
Zantac Injection 1593
Zantac Injection Premixed 1593
Zantac Syrup 1597

ZINNAT (Australia, Austria, Belgium, Brazil, Chile, Czech Republic, Denmark, Finland, Germany, Hong Kong, Hungary, Irish Republic, Israel, Italy, Malaysia, New Zealand, Singapore, South Africa, Spain, Sweden, Thailand, The Netherlands, United Kingdom)
CEFUROXIME AXETIL
Ceftin Tablets 1369
Ceftin for Oral Suspension 1369

ZINOCEP (Italy)
CEFUROXIME SODIUM
Zinacef Injection 1604

ZINOPRIL (Brazil)
LISINOPRIL
Prinivil Tablets 2029
Zestril Tablets 704

ZIPOS (Portugal)
CEFUROXIME AXETIL
Ceftin Tablets 1369
Ceftin for Oral Suspension 1369

ZIPRA (Mexico)
CIPROFLOXACIN HYDROCHLORIDE
Ciloxan Ophthalmic Ointment 554
Ciloxan Ophthalmic Solution . . . . . ⊙205
Cipro Tablets 2991

ZIPRAX (India)
CEFIXIME
Suprax 1811

ZIREMEX (Greece)
NIMODIPINE
Nimotop Capsules 774

ZIRPINE (Irish Republic)
CETIRIZINE HYDROCHLORIDE
Zyrtec Syrup 2589
Zyrtec Tablets 2589

ZIRTEC (Italy)
CETIRIZINE HYDROCHLORIDE
Zyrtec Syrup 2589
Zyrtec Tablets 2589

ZIRTEK (Austria, Greece, Irish Republic, United Kingdom)
CETIRIZINE HYDROCHLORIDE
Zyrtec Syrup **2589**
Zyrtec Tablets **2589**

ZITA (United Kingdom)
CIMETIDINE
Tagamet Tablets **1547**

ZIZ (United Kingdom)
PROMETHAZINE HYDROCHLORIDE
Phenergan Suppositories. **3438**
Phenergan Tablets **3438**

ZNUPRIL (Greece)
CETIRIZINE HYDROCHLORIDE
Zyrtec Syrup **2589**
Zyrtec Tablets **2589**

ZOBACIDE (South Africa)
METRONIDAZOLE
MetroGel-Vaginal Gel **1822**
Noritate Cream, 1% **1051**

ZOBEN (Malaysia)
ALBENDAZOLE
Albenza Tablets. **1310**

ZOCOLIP (Denmark)
SIMVASTATIN
Zocor Tablets **2078**

ZOCOR (Argentina, Australia, Belgium, Brazil, Canada, Chile, Czech Republic, Denmark, Finland, France, Germany, Greece, Hong Kong, Hungary, Irish Republic, Italy, Malaysia, Mexico, New Zealand, Norway, Portugal, Russia, Singapore, South Africa, Spain, Switzerland, Thailand, The Netherlands, United Kingdom)
SIMVASTATIN
Zocor Tablets **2078**

ZOCORD (Austria, Sweden)
SIMVASTATIN
Zocor Tablets **2078**

ZODAC (Czech Republic)
CETIRIZINE HYDROCHLORIDE
Zyrtec Syrup **2589**
Zyrtec Tablets **2589**

ZODERM (India)
OXICONAZOLE NITRATE
Oxistat Cream **1498**
Oxistat Lotion. **1498**

ZOFLUT (India)
FLUTICASONE PROPIONATE
Cutivate Cream. **1381**
Cutivate Ointment **1384**
Flonase Nasal Spray **1412**

ZOFRAN (Argentina, Australia, Belgium, Brazil, Czech Republic, Germany, Hong Kong, Hungary, Irish Republic, Israel, Italy, Malaysia, Mexico, New Zealand, Norway, Portugal, Singapore, South Africa, Spain, Sweden, Switzerland, The Netherlands, United Kingdom)
ONDANSETRON HYDROCHLORIDE
Zofran Injection. **1607**
Zofran Injection Premixed **1607**
Zofran Oral Solution. **1613**
Zofran Tablets **1613**

ZOFRON (Greece)
ONDANSETRON HYDROCHLORIDE
Zofran Injection. **1607**
Zofran Injection Premixed **1607**
Zofran Oral Solution. **1613**
Zofran Tablets **1613**

ZOLADEX (Argentina, Australia, Austria, Belgium, Brazil, Canada, Chile, Czech Republic, Denmark, Finland, France, Germany, Greece, Hong Kong, Hungary, Irish Republic, Israel, Italy, Malaysia, Mexico, New Zealand, Norway, Portugal, Russia, Singapore, South Africa, Spain, Sweden, Switzerland, Thailand, The Netherlands, United Kingdom)
GOSERELIN ACETATE
Zoladex **709**
Zoladex 3-month **712**

ZOLAPIN (Brazil)
CLOZAPINE
Clozapine Tablets **2141**
Clozaril Tablets **2174**

ZOLBEN (Brazil)
ALBENDAZOLE
Albenza Tablets. **1310**

ZOLEROL (South Africa)
METRONIDAZOLE
MetroGel-Vaginal Gel **1822**
Noritate Cream, 1% **1051**

ZOLES (Brazil)
MEBENDAZOLE
Vermox Chewable Tablets **1853**

ZOLICEF (Austria)
CEFAZOLIN SODIUM
Ancef for Injection **1318**

ZOLIDEN (Greece)
RANITIDINE HYDROCHLORIDE
Zantac 25 EFFERdose Tablets **1597**
Zantac 150 EFFERdose Tablets. **1597**
Zantac 150 Tablets **1597**
Zantac 300 Tablets **1597**
Zantac Injection **1593**
Zantac Injection Premixed **1593**
Zantac Syrup **1597**

ZOLIN (Italy)
CEFAZOLIN SODIUM
Ancef for Injection **1318**

ZOLISINT (Italy)
CEFAZOLIN SODIUM
Ancef for Injection **1318**

ZOLIVAL (Spain)
CEFAZOLIN SODIUM
Ancef for Injection **1318**

ZOLOFT (Argentina, Australia, Austria, Brazil, Canada, Czech Republic, Denmark, Finland, France, Greece, Hong Kong, Hungary, Italy, Malaysia, New Zealand, Portugal, Russia, Singapore, South Africa, Sweden, Switzerland, Thailand, The Netherlands)
SERTRALINE HYDROCHLORIDE
Zoloft Tablets **2581**

ZOLT (Finland)
LANSOPRAZOLE
Prevacid Delayed-Release Capsules **3268**

ZOLTEROL (Malaysia, Singapore)
DICLOFENAC SODIUM
Voltaren Tablets **2298**
Voltaren-XR Tablets **2301**

ZOL-TRIQ (Brazil)
MEBENDAZOLE
Vermox Chewable Tablets **1853**

ZOLVERA (United Kingdom)
VERAPAMIL HYDROCHLORIDE
Covera-HS Tablets **3135**
Verelan PM Capsules **3120**

ZOMORPH (United Kingdom)
MORPHINE SULFATE
Kadian Capsules **572**
MS Contin Tablets **2703**

ZONATIAN (Argentina)
ISOTRETINOIN
Accutane Capsules **2740**

ZOPAM (Thailand)
DIAZEPAM
Diastat Rectal Delivery System **3344**
Valium Tablets **2822**

ZOPIROL (Argentina)
TIMOLOL MALEATE
Blocadren Tablets **1891**
Timoptic Sterile Ophthalmic Solution **2058**
Timoptic in Ocudose **2061**
Timoptic-XE Sterile Ophthalmic Gel Forming Solution **2062**

ZORAIL (Spain)
ENALAPRIL MALEATE
Vasotec I.V. Injection **2076**

ZORAN (Singapore)
RANITIDINE HYDROCHLORIDE
Zantac 25 EFFERdose Tablets **1597**
Zantac 150 EFFERdose Tablets. **1597**
Zantac 150 Tablets **1597**
Zantac 300 Tablets **1597**
Zantac Injection **1593**
Zantac Injection Premixed **1593**
Zantac Syrup **1597**

ZOREF (Italy, Portugal)
CEFUROXIME AXETIL
Ceftin Tablets **1369**
Ceftin for Oral Suspension. **1369**

ZORINAX (Singapore)
KETOCONAZOLE
Nizoral 2% Shampoo **1838**

ZOROTOP (Switzerland)
LOPERAMIDE HYDROCHLORIDE
Imodium Capsules **1834**

ZOROXIN (Austria, Belgium, Denmark)
NORFLOXACIN
Noroxin Tablets. **2009**

ZOTON (Australia, Irish Republic, Israel, Italy, New Zealand, United Kingdom)
LANSOPRAZOLE
Prevacid Delayed-Release Capsules **3268**

ZUMENON (Australia, Austria, Belgium, Finland, Portugal, Switzerland, The Netherlands, United Kingdom)
ESTRADIOL
Climara Transdermal System **795**
Vivelle Transdermal System **2288**
Vivelle-Dot Transdermal System **2293**

ZUVAIR (India)
ZAFIRLUKAST
Accolate Tablets **663**

ZYBAN (Australia, Austria, Belgium, Brazil, Canada, Czech Republic, Denmark, Finland, France, Germany, Greece, Hong Kong, Hungary, India, Irish Republic, Israel, Italy, New Zealand, Norway, Portugal, Singapore, South Africa, Sweden, Switzerland, United Kingdom)
BUPROPION HYDROCHLORIDE
Wellbutrin SR Sustained-Release Tablets . . **1583**
Wellbutrin Tablets **1579**
Zyban Sustained-Release Tablets **1620**

ZYCEL (India)
CELECOXIB
Celebrex Capsules. **3130**

ZYDOWIN (India)
ZIDOVUDINE
Retrovir Capsules **1533**
Retrovir IV Infusion. **1537**
Retrovir Syrup **1533**
Retrovir Tablets. **1533**

ZYLIUM (Brazil)
RANITIDINE HYDROCHLORIDE
Zantac 25 EFFERdose Tablets **1597**
Zantac 150 EFFERdose Tablets. **1597**
Zantac 150 Tablets **1597**
Zantac 300 Tablets **1597**
Zantac Injection **1593**
Zantac Injection Premixed **1593**
Zantac Syrup **1597**

ZYLLERGY (Israel)
CETIRIZINE HYDROCHLORIDE
Zyrtec Syrup **2589**
Zyrtec Tablets **2589**

ZYMAMED (Austria)
DICLOFENAC POTASSIUM
Cataflam Tablets **2173**

ZYMED (Thailand)
CETIRIZINE HYDROCHLORIDE
Zyrtec Syrup **2589**
Zyrtec Tablets **2589**

ZYMEROL (Mexico)
CIMETIDINE
Tagamet Tablets **1547**

ZYNACE (Malaysia)
ENALAPRIL MALEATE
Vasotec I.V. Injection **2076**

ZYNAL (Singapore)
NAPROXEN SODIUM
Anaprox DS Tablets **2769**
Anaprox Tablets **2769**

ZYNOR (Irish Republic)
CETIRIZINE HYDROCHLORIDE
Zyrtec Syrup **2589**
Zyrtec Tablets **2589**

ZYNOX (South Africa)
NALOXONE HYDROCHLORIDE
Narcan Injection **1109**

ZYNTABAC (Spain, The Netherlands)
BUPROPION HYDROCHLORIDE
Wellbutrin SR Sustained-Release Tablets . . **1583**
Wellbutrin Tablets **1579**
Zyban Sustained-Release Tablets **1620**

ZYOMET (United Kingdom)
METRONIDAZOLE
MetroGel-Vaginal Gel **1822**
Noritate Cream, 1% **1051**

ZYPREXA (Argentina, Australia, Austria, Belgium, Brazil, Canada, Chile, Czech Republic, Denmark, Finland, France, Germany, Hong Kong, Hungary, Irish Republic, Israel, Italy, Malaysia, México, New Zealand, Norway, Portugal, Russia, Singapore, South Africa, Spain, Sweden, Switzerland, Thailand, The Netherlands, United Kingdom)
OLANZAPINE
Zyprexa Tablets **1798**

ZYRAC (Thailand)
CETIRIZINE HYDROCHLORIDE
Zyrtec Syrup **2589**
Zyrtec Tablets **2589**

ZYRAZINE (Thailand)
CETIRIZINE HYDROCHLORIDE
Zyrtec Syrup **2589**
Zyrtec Tablets **2589**

ZYRCON (Thailand)
CETIRIZINE HYDROCHLORIDE
Zyrtec Syrup **2589**
Zyrtec Tablets **2589**

ZYREX (Thailand)
CETIRIZINE HYDROCHLORIDE
Zyrtec Syrup **2589**
Zyrtec Tablets **2589**

ZYRLEX (Sweden)
CETIRIZINE HYDROCHLORIDE
Zyrtec Syrup **2589**
Zyrtec Tablets **2589**

ZYRTEC (Argentina, Australia, Austria, Belgium, Brazil, Canada, Chile, Czech Republic, Denmark, Finland, France, Germany, Hong Kong, Hungary, India, Israel, Japan, Malaysia, Mexico, New Zealand, Norway, Portugal, Russia, Singapore, South Africa, Spain, Switzerland, Thailand, The Netherlands)
CETIRIZINE HYDROCHLORIDE
Zyrtec Syrup **2589**
Zyrtec Tablets **2589**

ZYRZINE (Thailand)
CETIRIZINE HYDROCHLORIDE
Zyrtec Syrup **2589**
Zyrtec Tablets **2589**

ZYTAZ (India)
CEFTAZIDIME
Fortaz for Injection **1422**

ZYTINE (Thailand)
CETIRIZINE HYDROCHLORIDE
Zyrtec Syrup **2589**
Zyrtec Tablets **2589**

SECTION 7

GENERIC AVAILABILITY GUIDE

This section allows you to quickly determine which forms and strengths of a brand-name drug are also available generically. The entries are organized alphabetically by brand name and dosage form, with strengths in ascending order. Generic availability is indicated by a mark in the "Yes" column. Included are all prescription products described in *PDR*® and *PDR for Ophthalmic Medicines™*. Generic availability information is drawn from the *Red Book*® *Drug Database* maintained by *PDR*'s parent organization, Thomson Healthcare.

STRENGTH	GENERIC YES	GENERIC NO
Abelcet Injection		
5 mg/ml	■	
Abilify Tablets		
5 mg		■
10 mg		■
15 mg		■
20 mg		■
30 mg		■
Accolate Tablets		
10 mg		■
20 mg		■
AccuNeb Inhalation Solution		
0.021%		■
0.042%	■	
Accutane Capsules		
10 mg	■	
20 mg	■	
40 mg	■	
Accuzyme Debriding Ointment		
1.1 million u/gm-100 mg/	■	
Aceon Tablets		
2 mg		■
4 mg		■
8 mg		■
Acthrel for Injection		
0.1 mg		■
Acticin Cream		
5%	■	
Actimmune		
2 million iu/0.5 ml		■
Actiq		
0.2 mg		■
0.4 mg		■
0.6 mg		■
0.8 mg		■
1.2 mg		■
1.6 mg		■
Activase I.V.		
20 mg		■
50 mg		■
100 mg		■
Activella Tablets		
1 mg-0.5 mg	■	
Actonel Tablets		
5 mg		■
30 mg		■
35 mg		■
Actos Tablets		
15 mg		■
30 mg		■
45 mg		■
Acular Ophthalmic Solution		
0.5%		■
Acular LS Ophthalmic Solution		
0.4%		■
Adacel Vaccine		■
Adalat CC Tablets		
30 mg	■	
60 mg	■	
90 mg	■	
Adderall Tablets		
5 mg	■	
7.5 mg	■	
10 mg	■	
12.5 mg	■	
15 mg	■	
20 mg	■	
30 mg	■	
Adderall XR Capsules		
5 mg		■
10 mg		■
15 mg		■
20 mg		■
25 mg		■
30 mg		■
Adenocard Injection		
3 mg/ml	■	
Adenoscan		
3 mg/ml	■	
Adipex-P Capsules		
37.5 mg	■	
Adipex-P Tablets		
37.5 mg	■	
Adriamycin for Injection, USP		
10 mg	■	
20 mg	■	
50 mg	■	
150 mg		■
Adriamycin Injection, USP		
2 mg/ml	■	
Advair Diskus 100/50		
0.1 mg/actuation-0.05 mg		■
Advair Diskus 250/50		
0.25 mg/actuation-0.05 mg		■
Advair Diskus 500/50		
0.5 mg/actuation-0.05 mg		■
Advate Injection		
1 iu		■
Advicor Tablets		
20 mg-1000 mg		■
20 mg-500 mg		■
20 mg-750 mg		■
Aerobid Inhaler System		
0.25 mg/actuation		■
Aerobid-M Inhaler System		
0.25 mg/actuation		■
Agenerase Capsules		
50 mg		■
150 mg		■
Agenerase Oral Solution		
15 mg/ml		■
Aggrastat Injection		
0.05 mg/ml		■
0.25 mg/ml		■
Aggrastat Injection Premixed		
0.05 mg/ml		■
Aggrenox Capsules		
25 mg-200 mg		■
Agrylin Capsules		
0.5 mg	■	
1 mg	■	
Alacol DM Syrup		
2 mg/5 ml-10 mg/5 ml-5 mg/5ml	■	
Alamast Ophthalmic Solution		
0.1%		■
Albalon Ophthalmic Solution		
0.1%	■	
Albenza Tablets		
200 mg		■
Aldara Cream		
5%		■

Strength	Generic Yes	Generic No
Aldoclor Tablets		
150 mg-250 mg	■	
250 mg-250 mg	■	
Aldoril Tablets		
15 mg-250 mg	■	
25 mg-250 mg	■	
Aldurazyme for Intravenous Infusion		
0.58 mg/ml		■
Alesse-28 Tablets		
0.02 mg-0.1 mg	■	
Alferon N Injection		
5 million iu/ml		■
Alimta for Injection		
500 mg		■
Alinia for Oral Suspension		
100 mg/5 ml		■
Alinia Tablets		
500 mg		■
Allegra Capsules		
60 mg		■
Allegra Tablets		
30 mg		■
60 mg		■
180 mg		■
Allegra-D Extended Release Tablets		
60 mg-120 mg		■
Allegra-D 24 Hour Extended-Release Tablets		
180 mg-240 mg		■
Aloprim for Injection		
500 mg	■	
Aloxi Injection		
0.05 mg/ml		■
Alphagan P Ophthalmic Solution		
0.15%		■
Alrex Ophthalmic Suspension		
0.2%		■
Altace Capsules		
1.25 mg		■
2.5 mg		■
5 mg		■
10 mg		■
Altoprev Extended-Release Tablets		
10 mg		■
20 mg		■
40 mg		■
60 mg		■
Alupent Inhalation Aerosol		
0.65 mg/actuation	■	
Amaryl Tablets		
1 mg		■
2 mg		■
4 mg		■
Ambien Tablets		
5 mg		■
10 mg		■
AmBisome for Injection		
50 mg		■
Amerge Tablets		
1 mg		■
2.5 mg		■
Aminohippurate Sodium "PAH" Injection		
20%		■
Amnesteem Capsules		
10 mg	■	
20 mg	■	
40 mg	■	
Amoxil Capsules		
250 mg	■	
500 mg	■	
Amoxil Chewable Tablets		
125 mg	■	
200 mg	■	
250 mg	■	
400 mg	■	
Amoxil Pediatric Drops for Oral Suspension		
50 mg/ml	■	
125 mg/5 ml	■	
200 mg/5 ml	■	
250 mg/5 ml	■	
400 mg/5 ml	■	
Amoxil Powder for Oral Suspension		
125 mg/5 ml	■	
200 mg/5 ml	■	
250 mg/5 ml	■	
400 mg/5 ml	■	
Amoxil Tablets		
500 mg	■	
875 mg	■	
Anadrol-50 Tablets		
50 mg	■	
Analpram HC Cream		
1%-1%	■	
2.5%-1%		■
Analpram HC Lotion		
2.5%-1%	■	
Anaprox Tablets		
275 mg	■	
Anaprox DS Tablets		
550 mg	■	
Ancef for Injection		
1 gm	■	
10 gm	■	
500 mg	■	
AndroGel		
1%	■	
Angiomax for Injection		
250 mg		■
Antara Capsules		
43 mg		■
130 mg		■
Antivenin (Black Widow Spider Antivenin)		
6000 u		■
Anzemet Injection		
20 mg/ml	■	
Anzemet Tablets		
50 mg		■
100 mg		■
Apokyn Injection		
10 mg/ml		■
Appearex Tablets		
2.5 mg	■	
Aptivus Capsules		
250 mg		■
AquaMEPHYTON Injection		
1 mg/0.5 ml	■	
10 mg/ml	■	
Aralast		
1 mg	■	
Aramine Injection		
10 mg/ml		■
Aranesp for Injection		
0.025 mg/ml		■
0.04 mg/ml		■
0.06 mg/0.3 ml		■
0.06 mg/ml		■
0.1 mg/ml		■
0.15 mg/0.75 ml		■
0.2 mg/ml		■
0.3 mg/ml		■
Arava Tablets		
10 mg		■
20 mg		■
Aredia for Injection		
30 mg	■	
90 mg	■	
Argatroban Injection		
100 mg/ml		■
Arimidex Tablets		
1 mg		■
Aromasin Tablets		
25 mg		■
Arthrotec Tablets		
50 mg-0.2 mg		■
75 mg-0.2 mg		■
Asacol Delayed-Release Tablets		
400 mg		■
Astelin Nasal Spray		
137 mcg/actuation		■
Atacand Tablets		
4 mg		■
8 mg		■
16 mg		■
32 mg		■
Atacand HCT Tablets		
32 mg-12.5 mg		■
Atrovent HFA Inhalation Aerosol		
0.017 mg/actuation		■
Atrovent Inhalation Solution		
0.02%	■	
Atrovent Nasal Spray		
0.03%	■	
0.06%	■	
Attenuvax		
1000 tcid50		■
Augmentin Chewable Tablets		
125 mg-31.25 mg		■
200 mg-28.5 mg	■	
250 mg-62.5 mg		■
400 mg-57 mg	■	
Augmentin Powder for Oral Suspension		
125 mg/5 ml-31.25 mg/5 ml		■
200 mg/5 ml-28.5 mg/5 ml	■	
250 mg/5 ml-62.5 mg/5 ml		■
400 mg/5 ml-57 mg/5 ml	■	
Augmentin Tablets		
250 mg-125 mg		■
500 mg-125 mg	■	
875 mg-125 mg	■	
Augmentin XR Tablets		
1000 mg-62.5 mg		■
Augmentin ES-600 Powder for Oral Suspension		
600 mg/5 ml-42.9 mg/5 ml	■	
Avalide Tablets		
12.5 mg-150 mg		■
12.5 mg-300 mg		■
Avandamet Tablets		
500 mg-1 mg		■
500 mg-2 mg		■
500 mg-4 mg		■
1000 mg-2 mg		■
1000 mg-4 mg		■
Avandia Tablets		
2 mg		■
4 mg		■
8 mg		■
Avapro Tablets		
75 mg		■
150 mg		■
300 mg		■
Avar Cleanser		
10%-5%	■	
Avar Gel		
10%-5%	■	
Avar Green		
10%-5%	■	
Avastin IV		
25 mg/ml		■
Avelox Tablets		
400 mg		■
Avinza Capsules		
30 mg		■
60 mg		■
90 mg		■
120 mg		■
Avita Cream		
0.025%	■	
Avita Gel		
0.025%	■	
Avodart Soft Gelatin Capsules		
0.5 mg		■
Axert Tablets		
6.25 mg		■
12.5 mg		■
Axid Oral Solution		
150 mg	■	
300 mg	■	
Aygestin Tablets		
5 mg	■	
Azopt Ophthalmic Suspension		
1%		■
Bactroban Cream		
2%		■
Bactroban Nasal		
2%		■
Bactroban Ointment		
2%	■	
Balamine DM Oral Drops		
2 mg/ml-3.5 mg/ml-25 mg/ml	■	
Balamine DM Syrup		
4 mg/5 ml-12.5 mg/5 ml-60mg/5ml	■	
Baraclude Tablets		
0.5 mg		■
Beconase AQ Nasal Spray		
0.042 mg/actuation		■
BeneFix for Injection		
1 iu		■
Benicar Tablets		
5 mg		■
20 mg		■
40 mg		■
Benicar HCT Tablets		
12.5 mg-20 mg		■
12.5 mg-40 mg		■
25 mg-40 mg		■
Benzaclin Topical Gel		
5%-1%	■	
Betadine 5% Ophthalmic Solution		
5%	■	
Betagan Ophthalmic Solution, USP		
0.25%	■	
0.5%	■	
Betaseron for SC Injection		
0.3 mg		■
Betimol Ophthalmic Solution		
0.25%		■
0.5%		■
Betoptic S Ophthalmic Suspension		
0.25%		■
Biaxin Filmtab Tablets		
250 mg		■
500 mg		■

STRENGTH	GENERIC YES	GENERIC NO
Biaxin Granules		
125 mg/5 ml		■
187.5 mg/5 ml		■
250 mg/5 ml		■
Biaxin XL Filmtab Tablets		
500 mg		■
BiDil Tablets		
37.5 mg-20 mg		■
Biltricide Tablets		
600 mg		■
Bleph-10 Ophthalmic Solution		
10%	■	
Blephamide Ophthalmic Ointment		
0.2%-10%		■
Blephamide Ophthalmic Suspension		
0.2%-10%		■
Blocadren Tablets		
5 mg	■	
10 mg	■	
20 mg	■	
Boniva Tablets		
2.5 mg		■
150 mg		■
Boostrix		■
Botox Purified Neurotoxin Complex		
100 u		■
Bravelle for Intramuscular or Subcutaneous Injection		
75 iu		■
Brevibloc Concentrate		
250 mg/ml	■	
Brevibloc Injection		
10 mg/ml	■	
Brevibloc Double Strength Injection		
20 mg/ml		■
Brevibloc Premixed Injection		
10 mg/ml	■	
Brevibloc Double Strength Premixed Injection		
20 mg/ml		■
Brevoxyl-4 Creamy Wash		
4%		■
Brevoxyl-4 Gel		
4%		■
Brevoxyl-8 Creamy Wash		
8%		■
Brevoxyl-8 Gel		
8%		■
Brimonidine Tartrate Ophthalmic Solution 0.2%		
0.2%	■	
Buminate 5% Solution, USP		
5%	■	
Buminate 25% Solution, USP		
25%	■	
Buphenyl Powder		
3 gm/tsp		■
Buphenyl Tablets		
500 mg	■	
Buprenex Injectable		
0.3 mg/ml	■	
Byetta Injection		
250 mcg/ml		■
Caduet Tablets		
5 mg-10 mg		■
5 mg-20 mg		■
5 mg-40 mg		■
5 mg-80 mg		■
10 mg-10 mg		■
10 mg-20 mg		■
10 mg-40 mg		■
10 mg-80 mg		■
Calcijex Injection		
1 mcg/ml	■	
Calcium Disodium Versenate Injection		
200 mg/ml		■
Campath Ampules		
10 mg/ml		■
Camptosar Injection		
20 mg/ml		■
Canasa Rectal Suppositories		
500 mg	■	
Cancidas for Injection		
50 mg		■
70 mg		■
Captopril Tablets		
12.5 mg	■	
25 mg	■	
50 mg	■	
100 mg	■	
Carac Cream		
0.5%		■
Carafate Suspension		
1 gm/10 ml	■	
Carafate Tablets		
1 gm	■	
Carbatrol Capsules		
100 mg		■
200 mg		■
300 mg		■
Cardene I.V.		
2.5 mg/ml		■
Cardizem LA Extended Release Tablets		
120 mg		■
180 mg		■
240 mg		■
300 mg		■
360 mg		■
420 mg		■
Carnitor Injection		
100 mg/ml		■
200 mg/ml	■	
330 mg	■	
Carnitor Tablets and Oral Solution		
100 mg/ml		■
330 mg	■	
Carteolol Hydrochloride Ophthalmic Solution USP		
1%	■	
Casodex Tablets		
50 mg		■
Cataflam Tablets		
50 mg	■	
Catapres Tablets		
0.1 mg	■	
0.2 mg	■	
0.3 mg	■	
Catapres-TTS		
0.1 mg/24 hr		■
0.2 mg/24 hr		■
0.3 mg/24 hr		■
Cathflo Activase		
2 mg		■
Caverject Impulse Injection		
10 mcg	■	
20 mcg	■	
Ceftin for Oral Suspension		
125 mg/5 ml		■
250 mg/5 ml		■
Ceftin Tablets		
250 mg	■	
500 mg	■	
Celebrex Capsules		
100 mg		■
200 mg		■
400 mg		■
Celexa Oral Solution		
10 mg/5 ml	■	
Celexa Tablets		
10 mg	■	
20 mg	■	
40 mg	■	
CellCept Capsules		
250 mg		■
CellCept Intravenous		
500 mg		■
CellCept Oral Suspension		
200 mg/ml		■
CellCept Tablets		
500 mg		■
Cenestin Tablets		
0.3 mg		■
0.45 mg		■
0.625 mg		■
0.9 mg		■
1.25 mg		■
Centany Ointment		
2%	■	
Cerezyme for Injection		
200 u		■
400 u		■
Cerubidine for Injection		
20 mg	■	
Cervidil Vaginal Insert		
0.3 mg/hr		■
Cetacaine Topical Anesthetic		
14%-2%-2%		■
Chemet Capsules		
100 mg		■
Chromagen Soft Gelatin Capsules		
150 mg-0.01 mg-70 mg-100 mg	■	
Chromagen FA Soft Gelatin Capsules		
150 mg-0.1 mg-1 mg-70 mg		■
Chromagen Forte Soft Gelatin Capsules		
60 mg-0.01 mg-70 mg-81 mg		■
Cialis Tablets		
5 mg		■
10 mg		■
20 mg		■
Ciloxan Ophthalmic Ointment		
0.3%	■	
Ciloxan Ophthalmic Solution		
0.3%	■	
Cipro Oral Suspension		
250 mg/5 ml		■
500 mg/5 ml		■
Cipro Tablets		
100 mg		■
250 mg	■	
500 mg	■	
750 mg	■	
Cipro XR Tablets		
500 mg		■
1000 mg		■
Citracal Prenatal Rx Tablets		
120 mg-125 mg-2 mg-50 mg	■	
Clarinex Syrup		
0.5 mg/ml		■
Clarinex Tablets RediTabs		
5 mg		■
Clarinex-D 24-Hour Extended-Release Tablets		
5 mg-240 mg		■
Claripel Cream		
4%	■	
Cleocin Capsules		
75 mg	■	
150 mg	■	
300 mg	■	
Climara Transdermal System		
0.025 mg/24 hr	■	
0.0375 mg/24 hr	■	
0.05 mg/24 hr	■	
0.06 mg/24 hr		■
0.075 mg/24 hr	■	
0.1 mg/24 hr	■	
Clinac BPO 7 Gel USP		
7%		■
Clindagel		
1%	■	
Clindesse Vaginal Cream		
2%	■	
Clindets Pledgets		
1%	■	
Clinoril Tablets		
150 mg	■	
200 mg	■	
Clobevate Gel		
0.05%	■	
Clolar for Intravenous Infusion		
1 mg/ml		■
Clorpres Tablets		
15 mg-0.1 mg	■	
15 mg-0.2 mg	■	
15 mg-0.3 mg	■	
Clozapine Tablets		
25 mg	■	
100 mg	■	
Clozaril Tablets		
25 mg	■	
100 mg	■	
Cogentin Injection		
1 mg/ml		■
Colazal Capsules		
750 mg		■
Colyte with Flavor Packs for Oral Solution	■	
CombiPatch Transdermal System		
0.05 mg/24 hr-0.14 mg/24 hr		■
0.05 mg/24 hr-0.25 mg/24 hr		■
Combivent Inhalation Aerosol		
0.09 mg/actuation-0.018 mg		■
Combivir Tablets		
150 mg-300 mg	■	
Combunox Tablets		
400 mg-5 mg		■
Comtan Tablets		
200 mg		■
Comvax		
7.5 mcg/0.5 ml-5 mcg/0.5 ml		■
Concerta Extended-Release Tablets		
18 mg		■
27 mg		■
36 mg		■
54 mg		■
Copaxone for Injection		
20 mg/ml		■
Copegus Tablets		
200 mg		■

Strength	Generic Yes	Generic No
Coreg Tablets		
3.125 mg		■
6.25 mg		■
12.5 mg		■
25 mg		■
Cosmegen for Injection		
0.5 mg		■
Cosopt Sterile Ophthalmic Solution		
2%-0.5%		■
Coumadin for Injection		
5 mg		■
Coumadin Tablets		
1 mg	■	
2 mg	■	
2.5 mg	■	
3 mg	■	
4 mg	■	
5 mg	■	
6 mg	■	
7.5 mg	■	
10 mg	■	
Covera-HS Tablets		
180 mg		■
240 mg		■
Cozaar Tablets		
25 mg		■
50 mg		■
100 mg		■
Creon 5 Capsules		
16600 u-5000 u-18750 u	■	
Creon 10 Capsules		
33200 u-10000 u-37500 u	■	
Creon 20 Capsules		
66400 u-20000 u-75000 u	■	
Crixivan Capsules		
100 mg		■
200 mg		■
333 mg		■
400 mg		■
Crolom Cromolyn Sodium Sterile Ophthalmic Solution USP		
4%	■	
Cubicin for Injection		
500 mg		■
Cuprimine Capsules		
125 mg		■
250 mg		■
Curosurf Intratracheal Suspension		
80 mg/ml		■
Cytomel Tablets		
0.005 mg		■
0.025 mg		■
0.05 mg		■
Cytovene Capsules		
250 mg	■	
500 mg	■	
Cytovene-IV		
500 mg		■
Dalmane Capsules		
15 mg	■	
30 mg	■	
Dantrium Capsules		
25 mg	■	
50 mg	■	
100 mg	■	
Dapsone Tablets USP		
25 mg		■
100 mg		■
DAPTACEL		■
Daranide Tablets		
50 mg		■
Daraprim Tablets		
25 mg		■
DDAVP Injection		
4 mcg/ml	■	
DDAVP Nasal Spray		
0.01 mg/actuation	■	
DDAVP Tablets		
0.1 mg		■
0.2 mg		■
Decadron Phosphate Injection		
4 mg/ml	■	
24 mg/ml	■	
Decadron Tablets		
0.5 mg	■	
0.75 mg	■	
4 mg	■	
Delatestryl Injection		
200 mg/ml	■	
Demser Capsules		
250 mg		■
Denavir Cream		
1%		■
Depacon Injection		
100 mg/ml	■	
Depakene Capsules		
250 mg	■	
Depakene Syrup		
250 mg/5 ml	■	
Depakote Sprinkle Capsules		
125 mg		■
Depakote Tablets		
125 mg		■
250 mg		■
500 mg		■
Depakote ER Tablets		
250 mg		■
500 mg		■
DepoCyt Injection		
10 mg/ml		■
DepoDur Extended-Release Injection		
10 mg/ml		■
Depo-Medrol Injectable Suspension		
20 mg/ml	■	
40 mg/ml	■	
80 mg/ml	■	
Depo-Medrol Single-Dose Vial		
400 mg/ml		■
Desferal Vials		
2 gm	■	
500 mg	■	
Desmopressin Acetate Injection		
4 mcg/ml	■	
Desmopressin Acetate Rhinal Tube		
0.01%	■	
Desoxyn Tablets, USP		
15 mg		■
Detrol Tablets		
1 mg		■
2 mg		■
Detrol LA Capsules		
2 mg		■
4 mg		■
Dexedrine Spansule Capsules		
5 mg	■	
10 mg	■	
15 mg	■	
Dexedrine Tablets		
5 mg	■	
DextroStat Tablets		
5 mg	■	
10 mg	■	
Diastat Rectal Delivery System		
15 mg	■	
Dibenzyline Capsules		
10 mg		■
Didronel Tablets		
200 mg		■
400 mg		■
Differin Cream		
0.1%		■
Differin Gel		
0.1%		■
Digibind for Injection		
38 mg		■
Digitek Tablets		
0.125 mg	■	
0.25 mg	■	
Dilaudid Ampules		
1 mg/ml	■	
2 mg/ml	■	
4 mg/ml	■	
Dilaudid Multiple Dose Vials		
2 mg/ml	■	
Dilaudid Oral Liquid		
1 mg/ml	■	
Dilaudid Rectal Suppositories		
3 mg	■	
Dilaudid Tablets		
2 mg	■	
4 mg	■	
8 mg	■	
Dilaudid-HP Injection		
10 mg/ml	■	
Dilaudid-HP Lyophilized Powder		
250 mg		■
Diovan Tablets		
40 mg		■
80 mg		■
160 mg		■
320 mg		■
Diovan HCT Tablets		
12.5 mg-160 mg		■
12.5 mg-80 mg		■
25 mg-160 mg		■
Diprolene Gel		
0.05%	■	
Diprolene Lotion		
0.05%		■
Diprolene Ointment		
0.05%	■	
Diprolene AF Cream		
0.05%	■	
Diprosone Cream, USP		
0.05%	■	
Ditropan XL Tablets		
5 mg		■
10 mg		■
15 mg		■
Diuril Oral Suspension		
250 mg/5 ml		■
Diuril Tablets		
250 mg	■	
500 mg	■	
Diuril Sodium Intravenous		
0.5 gm		■
Dolobid Tablets		
250 mg	■	
500 mg	■	
Dostinex Tablets		
0.5 mg		■
Dovonex Cream		
0.005%		■
Dovonex Ointment		
0.005%		■
Dovonex Scalp Solution		
0.005%		■
Doxil Injection		
2 mg/ml		■
Drysol Solution		
20%	■	
Duac Topical Gel		
5%-1%	■	
DuoNeb Inhalation Solution		
3 mg/3 ml-0.5 mg/3 ml		■
Duragesic Transdermal System		
12.5 mcg/hr		■
25 mcg/hr	■	
50 mcg/hr	■	
75 mcg/hr	■	
100 mcg/hr	■	
Dyazide Capsules		
25 mg-37.5 mg	■	
25 mg-50 mg	■	
Dynacin Tablets		
50 mg	■	
75 mg	■	
100 mg	■	
DynaCirc Capsules		
2.5 mg		■
5 mg		■
DynaCirc CR Tablets		
5 mg		■
10 mg		■
Dyrenium Capsules		
50 mg	■	
100 mg	■	
EC-Naprosyn Delayed-Release Tablets		
500 mg	■	
Edecrin Tablets		
25 mg		■
50 mg		■
Edecrin Sodium Intravenous		
50 mg		■
Edex Injection		
10 mcg	■	
20 mcg	■	
40 mcg	■	
E.E.S. 200 Liquid		
200 mg/5 ml	■	
E.E.S. 400 Liquid		
400 mg/5 ml	■	
E.E.S. 400 Filmtab Tablets		
400 mg	■	
E.E.S. Granules		
200 mg/5 ml	■	
Effexor Tablets		
25 mg		■
37.5 mg		■
50 mg		■
75 mg		■
100 mg		■
Effexor XR Capsules		
37.5 mg		■
75 mg		■
150 mg		■
Efudex Topical Cream		
5%		■
Efudex Topical Solutions		
2%	■	
5%	■	
Eldepryl Capsules		
5 mg	■	
Elidel Cream		
1%		■
Eligard		
7.5 mg		■
22.5 mg		■
30 mg		■
45 mg		■
Elitek		
1.5 mg		■

STRENGTH	GENERIC YES	GENERIC NO
Ellence Injection		
2 mg/ml		■
Elmiron Capsules		
100 mg		■
Elocon Cream		
0.1%	■	
Elocon Lotion		
0.1%		■
Elocon Ointment		
0.1%	■	
Eloxatin for Injection		
50 mg		■
100 mg		■
Elspar for Injection		
10000 iu		■
Emcyt Capsules		
140 mg		■
Emend Capsules		
80 mg		■
125 mg		■
Emtriva Capsules		
200 mg		■
Enbrel for Injection		
25 mg		■
Engerix-B Vaccine		
20 mcg/ml		■
Entocort EC Capsules		
3 mg		■
EpiPen Auto-Injector		
1 mg/ml		■
EpiPen Jr. Auto-Injector		
0.5 mg/ml		■
Epivir Oral Solution		
10 mg/ml		■
Epivir Tablets		
300 mg		■
Epivir-HBV Oral Solution		
5 mg/ml		■
Epivir-HBV Tablets		
100 mg		■
Epogen for Injection		
2000 u/ml	■	
3000 u/ml	■	
4000 u/ml	■	
10000 u/ml	■	
20000 u/ml	■	
40000 u/ml	■	
Equetro Extended-Release Capsules		
100 mg		■
200 mg		■
300 mg		■
Erbitux		
2 mg/ml		■
Ertaczo Cream		
2%		■
Erygel Topical Gel		
2%	■	
EryPed		
200 mg/5 ml	■	
400 mg/5 ml		■
EryPed Drops		
100 mg/2.5 ml		■
EryPed Chewable Tablets		
200 mg		■
Ery-Tab Tablets		
250 mg	■	
333 mg	■	
500 mg	■	
Erythrocin Stearate Filmtab Tablets		
250 mg	■	
500 mg	■	
Erythromycin Base Filmtab Tablets		
250 mg	■	
500 mg	■	
Erythromycin Delayed-Release Capsules, USP		
250 mg	■	
Eskalith Capsules		
300 mg	■	
Eskalith CR Controlled-Release Tablets		
450 mg		■
Estratest Tablets		
1.25 mg-2.5 mg	■	
Estratest H.S. Tablets		
0.625 mg-1.25 mg	■	
Estrogel		
0.06%		■
Ethyol for Injection		
500 mg	■	
Eulexin Capsules		
125 mg	■	
Evista Tablets		
60 mg		■
Evoclin Foam		
1%		■
Evoxac Capsules		
30 mg		■
Exelon Capsules		
1.5 mg		■
3 mg		■
4.5 mg		■
6 mg		■
Fabrazyme for Intravenous Infusion		
35 mg		■
Factive Tablets		
320 mg		■
Famvir Tablets		
125 mg		■
250 mg		■
500 mg		■
Faslodex Injection		
50 mg/ml		■
Feiba VH		
1 iu	■	
Femara Tablets		
2.5 mg		■
Ferrlecit Injection		
62.5 mg/5 ml		■
Finacea Gel		
15%		■
Flexeril Tablets		
5 mg	■	
10 mg	■	
Flolan for Injection		
0.5 mg		■
1.5 mg		■
Flomax Capsules		
0.4 mg		■
Flonase Nasal Spray		
0.05 mg/actuation		■
Flovent HFA 44 mcg Inhalation Aerosol		
0.044 mg/actuation		■
Flovent HFA 110 mcg Inhalation Aerosol		
0.11 mg/actuation		■
Flovent HFA 220 mcg Inhalation Aerosol		
0.22 mg/actuation		■
Floxin Otic Singles		
0.3%		■
Floxin Otic Solution		
0.3%		■
Flumadine Syrup		
50 mg/5 ml		■
Flumadine Tablets		
100 mg	■	
Fluorescite Injection		
10%	■	
25%	■	
Fluor-I-Strip A.T. Ophthalmic Strips		
1 mg	■	
Fluor-I-Strip Ophthalmic Strips		
9 mg		■
FML Ophthalmic Ointment		
0.1%		■
FML Ophthalmic Suspension		
0.1%	■	
FML Forte Ophthalmic Suspension		
0.25%		■
FML-S Liquifilm Sterile Ophthalmic Suspension		
0.1%-10%		■
Follistim AQ Cartridge		
300 iu/0.36 ml		■
600 iu/0.72 ml		■
Foradil Aerolizer		
0.012 mg		■
Fortamet Extended-Release Tablets		
500 mg	■	
1000 mg	■	
Fortaz Injection		
1 gm	■	
2 gm	■	
6 gm	■	
500 mg	■	
Fortaz for Injection		
1 gm/50 ml-2.2 gm/50 ml		■
2 gm/50 ml-1.6 gm/50 ml		■
Forteo for Injection		
250 mcg/ml		■
Fosamax Oral Solution		
70 mg/75 ml		■
Fosamax Tablets		
5 mg		■
10 mg		■
35 mg		■
40 mg		■
70 mg		■
Fosamax Plus D Tablets		
70 mg-2800 iu		■
Fosrenol Chewable Tablets		
250 mg		■
500 mg		■
Fragmin Injection		
2500 iu/0.2 ml		■
5000 iu/0.2 ml		■
7500 iu/0.3 ml		■
10000 iu/ml		■
25000 iu/ml		■
Furosemide Tablets		
20 mg	■	
40 mg	■	
80 mg	■	
Fuzeon Injection		
90 mg		■
Gabitril Tablets		
2 mg		■
4 mg		■
12 mg		■
16 mg		■
20 mg		■
Gammagard Liquid		
100 mg/ml	■	
Gammagard S/D		
0.5 gm	■	
2.5 gm	■	
5 gm	■	
10 gm	■	
Garamycin Injectable		
40 mg/ml	■	
Gemzar for Injection		
1 gm		■
200 mg		■
Gengraf Capsules		
25 mg	■	
100 mg	■	
Genoptic Sterile Ophthalmic Solution		
3 mg/ml	■	
Genotropin Lyophilized Powder		
1.5 mg		■
5.8 mg		■
13.8 mg		■
Geodon Capsules		
20 mg		■
40 mg		■
60 mg		■
80 mg		■
Geodon for Injection		
20 mg		■
Gleevec Tablets		
100 mg		■
400 mg		■
GlucaGen for Injection		
1 mg	■	
Glucagon for Injection Vials and Emergency Kit		
1 mg	■	
Gonal-f RFF Pen for Injection		
300 iu/0.5 ml		■
450 iu/0.75 ml		■
900 iu/1.5 ml		■
Gordochom Solution		
3%-25%	■	
Grifulvin V Tablets Microsize and Oral Suspension Microsize		
125 mg/5 ml	■	
500 mg	■	
Gris-PEG Tablets		
125 mg	■	
250 mg	■	
Guanidine Hydrochloride Tablets		
125 mg		■
Gynazole-1 Vaginal Cream		
2%	■	
Havrix Vaccine		
1440 el u/ml		■
Hectorol Capsules		
2.5 mcg		■
Hectorol Injection		
2 mcg/ml		■
Hemofil M		
1 iu	■	
Hepsera Tablets		
10 mg		■
Herceptin I.V.		
440 mg		■
Hexalen Capsules		
50 mg		■
HibTITER		
10 mcg	■	
100 mcg		■
HMS Sterile Ophthalmic Suspension		
1%		■
Humalog-Pen		
100 u/ml		■
Humalog Mix 75/25-Pen		
75 u/ml-25 u/ml		■

STRENGTH	GENERIC YES	GENERIC NO
Humatrope Vials and Cartridges		
5 mg	■	
6 mg		■
12 mg		■
24 mg		■
Humira Injection		
40 mg/0.8 ml		■
Humulin 70/30 Pen		
70 u/ml-30 u/ml	■	
Humulin R (U-500)		
500 u/ml		■
Hyalgan Solution		
10 mg/ml	■	
Hycamtin for Injection		
4 mg		■
Hycodan Syrup		
1.5 mg/5 ml-5 mg/5 ml	■	
Hycodan Tablets		
1.5 mg-5 mg	■	
Hycomine Compound Tablets		
250 mg-30 mg-2 mg-5 mg-10 mg		■
Hycotuss Expectorant Syrup		
100 mg/5 ml-5 mg/5 ml	■	
Hydrocortone Tablets		
10 mg	■	
20 mg	■	
HyperRAB		
150 iu/ml	■	
Hyperstat I.V. Injection		
15 mg/ml		■
HyperTET		
250 u		■
Hytrin Capsules		
1 mg	■	
2 mg	■	
5 mg	■	
10 mg	■	
Hyzaar Tablets		
12.5 mg-50 mg		■
25 mg-100 mg		■
Idamycin PFS Injection		
1 mg/ml	■	
Imdur Tablets		
30 mg	■	
60 mg	■	
120 mg	■	
Imitrex Injection		
6 mg/0.5 ml		■
Imitrex Nasal Spray		
5 mg		■
20 mg		■
Imitrex Tablets		
25 mg		■
50 mg		■
100 mg		■
Indapamide Tablets		
1.25 mg	■	
2.5 mg	■	
Inderal LA Long-Acting Capsules		
60 mg	■	
80 mg	■	
120 mg	■	
160 mg	■	
Indocin Capsules		
25 mg	■	
50 mg	■	
Indocin I.V.		
1 mg		■
Indocin Oral Suspension		
25 mg/5 ml	■	
Indocin Suppositories		
50 mg	■	
Infanrix Vaccine		■
Infasurf Intratracheal Suspension		
35 mg/ml		■

STRENGTH	GENERIC YES	GENERIC NO
Infed Injection		
50 mg/ml	■	
Infergen		
30 mcg/ml		■
Inspra Tablets		
25 mg		■
50 mg		■
Integrilin Injection		
0.75 mg/ml		■
2 mg/ml		■
Intron A for Injection		
3 million iu		■
3 million iu/0.2 ml		■
3 million iu/0.5 ml		■
5 million iu		■
5 million iu/0.2 ml		■
5 million iu/0.5 ml		■
6 million iu/ml		■
10 million iu		■
10 million iu/0.2 ml		■
10 million iu/ml		■
18 million iu		■
25 million iu		■
50 million iu		■
Invanz for Injection		
1 gm		■
Iressa Tablets		
250 mg		■
Kaletra Capsules		
133.3 mg-33.3 mg		■
Kaletra Oral Solution		
80 mg/ml-20 mg/ml		■
K-Dur Extended-Release Tablets		
10 meq	■	
20 meq	■	
Kepivance		
6.25 mg		■
Keppra Tablets		
250 mg		■
500 mg		■
750 mg		■
Ketek Tablets		
400 mg		■
Kineret Injection		
100 mg/0.67 ml		■
Klaron Lotion		
10%	■	
Klonopin Tablets		
0.5 mg	■	
1 mg	■	
2 mg	■	
Klonopin Wafers		
0.125 mg		■
0.25 mg		■
0.5 mg		■
1 mg		■
2 mg		■
K-Lor Powder Packets		
15 meq	■	
20 meq	■	
Koate-DVI		
1 iu	■	
Kogenate FS		
1 iu	■	
K-Phos Neutral Tablets		
155 mg-852 mg-130 mg	■	
K-Phos Original (Sodium Free) Tablets		
500 mg		■
Kristalose for Oral Solution		
10 gm/packet		■
20 gm/packet		■
K-Tab Filmtab Tablets		
10 meq	■	
Kytril Injection		
1 mg/ml		■
Kytril Oral Solution		
2 mg/10 ml		■

STRENGTH	GENERIC YES	GENERIC NO
Lacrisert Sterile Ophthalmic Insert		
5 mg		■
Lamictal Tablets		
25 mg		■
100 mg		■
150 mg		■
200 mg		■
Lamictal Chewable Dispersible Tablets		
5 mg		■
25 mg		■
Lamisil Tablets		
250 mg		■
Lanoxicaps Capsules		
0.05 mg		■
0.1 mg		■
0.2 mg		■
Lanoxin Injection		
0.25 mg/ml	■	
Lanoxin Tablets		
0.125 mg	■	
0.25 mg	■	
0.5 mg	■	
Lanoxin Injection Pediatric		
0.1 mg/ml	■	
Lantus Injection		
100 u/ml		■
Lariam Tablets		
250 mg	■	
Lescol Capsules		
20 mg		■
40 mg		■
Lescol XL Tablets		
80 mg		■
Leukeran Tablets		
2 mg		■
Leukine		
250 mcg		■
500 mcg/ml		■
Leustatin Injection		
1 mg/ml	■	
Levaquin in 5% Dextrose Injection		
5 mg/ml		■
Levaquin Injection		
5 mg/ml		■
25 mg/ml		■
Levaquin Oral Solution		
25 mg/ml		■
Levaquin Tablets		
250 mg		■
500 mg		■
750 mg		■
Levitra Tablets		
2.5 mg		■
5 mg		■
10 mg		■
20 mg		■
Levothroid Tablets		
0.025 mg	■	
0.05 mg	■	
0.075 mg	■	
0.088 mg	■	
0.1 mg	■	
0.112 mg	■	
0.125 mg	■	
0.137 mg	■	
0.15 mg	■	
0.175 mg	■	
0.2 mg	■	
0.3 mg	■	
Levoxyl Tablets		
0.025 mg	■	
0.05 mg	■	
0.075 mg	■	
0.088 mg	■	
0.1 mg	■	
0.112 mg	■	
0.125 mg	■	
0.137 mg	■	
0.15 mg	■	

STRENGTH	GENERIC YES	GENERIC NO
0.175 mg	■	
0.2 mg	■	
0.3 mg	■	
Lexapro Oral Solution		
5 mg/5 ml		■
Lexapro Tablets		
5 mg		■
10 mg		■
20 mg		■
Lexiva Tablets		
700 mg		■
Librium Capsules		
5 mg	■	
10 mg	■	
25 mg	■	
Lidoderm Patch		
5%		■
Lipitor Tablets		
10 mg		■
20 mg		■
40 mg		■
80 mg		■
Lithobid Tablets		
300 mg	■	
Locoid Cream		
0.1%		■
Locoid Lipocream Cream		
0.1%		■
Locoid Ointment		
0.1%		■
Locoid Topical Solution		
0.1%	■	
Lofibra Capsules		
67 mg	■	
134 mg	■	
200 mg	■	
Lo/Ovral-28 Tablets		
30 mcg-0.3 mg	■	
Loprox Gel		
0.77%		■
Loprox Shampoo		
1%		■
Lortab Elixir		
500 mg/15 ml-7.5 mg/15 ml	■	
Lotemax Ophthalmic Suspension 0.5%		
0.5%		■
Lotensin Tablets		
5 mg	■	
10 mg	■	
20 mg	■	
40 mg	■	
Lotensin HCT Tablets		
5 mg-6.25 mg	■	
10 mg-12.5 mg	■	
20 mg-12.5 mg	■	
20 mg-25 mg	■	
Lotrel Capsules		
2.5 mg-10 mg		■
5 mg-10 mg		■
5 mg-20 mg		■
10 mg-20 mg		■
Lotrimin Cream		
1%	■	
Lotrimin Lotion		
1%	■	
Lotrimin Topical Solution		
1%	■	
Lotrisone Cream		
0.05%-1%	■	
Lotronex Tablets		
1 mg		■
Lovenox Injection		
30 mg/0.3 ml		■
40 mg/0.4 ml		■
60 mg/0.6 ml		■
80 mg/0.8 ml		■

STRENGTH	GENERIC YES	GENERIC NO
100 mg/ml		■
120 mg/0.8 ml		■
150 mg/ml		■
Lumigan Ophthalmic Solution		
0.03%		■
Lunesta Tablets		
1 mg		■
2 mg		■
3 mg		■
Lupron Depot 3.75 mg		
3.75 mg		■
Lupron Depot 7.5 mg		
7.5 mg		■
Lupron Depot--3 Month 11.25 mg		
11.25 mg		■
Lupron Depot-PED		
7.5 mg		■
11.25 mg		■
15 mg		■
Lustra Cream		
4%	■	
Lustra-AF Cream		
4%	■	
Luxiq Foam		
0.12%		■
Lyrica Capsules		
25 mg		■
50 mg		■
75 mg		■
100 mg		■
150 mg		■
200 mg		■
225 mg		■
300 mg		■
Malarone Tablets		
250 mg-100 mg		■
Malarone Pediatric Tablets		
62.5 mg-25 mg		■
Marinol Capsules		
2.5 mg		■
5 mg		■
10 mg		■
Matulane Capsules		
50 mg		■
Mavik Tablets		
1 mg		■
2 mg		■
4 mg		■
Maxair Autohaler		
0.2 mg/actuation		■
Maxalt Tablets		
5 mg		■
10 mg		■
Maxalt-MLT Orally Disintegrating Tablets		
5 mg		■
10 mg		■
Maxzide Tablets		
25 mg-37.5 mg	■	
50 mg-75 mg	■	
Mebaral Tablets, USP		
32 mg	■	
50 mg	■	
100 mg	■	
Mefoxin for Injection		
1 gm	■	
2 gm	■	
10 gm	■	
Mefoxin Premixed Intravenous Solution		
1 gm/50 ml		■
2 gm/50 ml		■
Menactra Vaccine		■
Menopur for Subcutaneous Injection		
75 iu-75 iu		■
Mentax Cream		
1%		■
Mephyton Tablets		
5 mg		■
Mepron Suspension		
750 mg/5 ml		■
Meridia Capsules		
5 mg		■
10 mg		■
15 mg		■
Merrem I.V.		
1 gm		■
500 mg		■
Meruvax II		■
Metadate CD Capsules		
10 mg	■	
20 mg	■	
30 mg	■	
Metrogel		
0.75%		■
1%		■
MetroGel-Vaginal		
0.75%		■
Mevacor Tablets		
10 mg	■	
20 mg	■	
40 mg	■	
Miacalcin Injection		
200 iu/ml	■	
Miacalcin Nasal Spray		
200 iu/actuation		■
Micardis Tablets		
20 mg		■
40 mg		■
80 mg		■
Micardis HCT Tablets		
12.5 mg-40 mg		■
12.5 mg-80 mg		■
Midamor Tablets		
5 mg	■	
Migranal Nasal Spray		
0.5 mg/actuation		■
Mintezol Suspension		
500 mg/5 ml		■
Mintezol Chewable Tablets		
500 mg		■
Mirapex Tablets		
0.125 mg		■
0.25 mg		■
0.5 mg		■
1 mg		■
1.5 mg		■
Mirena Intrauterine System		
52 mg		■
Mivacron Injection		
2 mg/ml	■	
Moban Tablets		
5 mg		■
10 mg		■
25 mg		■
50 mg		■
100 mg		■
Mobic Tablets		
7.5 mg		■
15 mg		■
Moduretic Tablets		
5 mg-50 mg	■	
MS Contin Tablets		
15 mg	■	
30 mg	■	
60 mg	■	
100 mg	■	
200 mg	■	
Mumpsvax		■
Mustargen for Injection		
10 mg		■
Mycamine for Injection		
50 mg		■
Myfortic Tablets		
180 mg		■
360 mg		■
Mylotarg for Injection		
5 mg		■
Nadolol Tablets		
20 mg	■	
40 mg	■	
80 mg	■	
Naftin Cream		
1%		■
Naftin Gel		
1%		■
Naprosyn Suspension		
25 mg/ml	■	
Naprosyn Tablets		
250 mg	■	
375 mg	■	
500 mg	■	
Narcan Injection		
0.02 mg/ml	■	
0.4 mg/ml	■	
1 mg/ml	■	
Naropin Injection		
2 mg/ml		■
5 mg/ml		■
7.5 mg/ml		■
10 mg/ml		■
Nasacort AQ Nasal Spray		
55 mcg/actuation		■
Nasarel Nasal Spray		
0.025 mg/actuation	■	
Nasonex Nasal Spray		
0.05 mg/actuation		■
Natacyn Antifungal Ophthalmic Suspension		
5%		■
Natrecor for Injection		
1.5 mg		■
Navelbine Injection		
10 mg/ml	■	
Nembutal Sodium Solution, USP		
50 mg/ml	■	
Neoral Soft Gelatin Capsules		
25 mg	■	
100 mg	■	
Neoral Oral Solution		
100 mg/ml	■	
Neulasta Injection		
6 mg/0.6 ml		■
Neumega for Injection		
5 mg		■
Neupogen for Injection		
300 mcg/0.5 ml		■
300 mcg/ml		■
480 mcg/0.8 ml		■
480 mcg/1.6 ml		■
Neurontin Capsules		
100 mg	■	
300 mg	■	
400 mg	■	
Neurontin Oral Solution		
250 mg/5 ml		■
Neurontin Tablets		
600 mg	■	
800 mg	■	
Nexium Delayed-Release Capsules		
20 mg		■
40 mg		■
Nexium I.V.		
20 mg		■
40 mg		■
Niaspan Extended-Release Tablets		
500 mg	■	
750 mg	■	
1000 mg	■	
Nicomide Tablets		
0.5 mg-750 mg-25 mg	■	
Nicotrol Inhaler		
4 mg/actuation		■
Nicotrol NS		
0.5 mg/actuation		■
Niferex-150 Forte Capsules		■
Nimotop Capsules		
30 mg		■
Nipent for Injection		
10 mg		■
Niravam Orally Disintegrating Tablets		
0.25 mg		■
0.5 mg		■
1 mg		■
2 mg		■
Nitro-Dur Transdermal Infusion System		
0.1 mg/hr	■	
0.2 mg/hr	■	
0.3 mg/hr	■	
0.4 mg/hr	■	
0.6 mg/hr	■	
0.8 mg/hr	■	
Nitrolingual Pumpspray		
0.4 mg/actuation		■
Nizoral Shampoo		
2%		■
Norditropin Cartridges		
5 mg/1.5 ml		■
15 mg/1.5 ml		■
Norflex Injection		
30 mg/ml	■	
Noritate Cream		
1%		■
Noroxin Tablets		
400 mg		■
Norvasc Tablets		
2.5 mg		■
5 mg		■
10 mg		■
Norvir Soft Gelatin Capsules		
100 mg		■
Norvir Oral Solution		
80 mg/ml		■
Novantrone for Injection Concentrate		
2 mg/ml		■
Novarel for Injection		
10000 u	■	
Novolin 70/30 Human Insulin 10 ml Vials		
70 u/ml-30 u/ml	■	
Novolin 70/30 InnoLet		
70 u/ml-30 u/ml	■	
Novolin 70/30 PenFill 3 ml Cartridges		
70 u/ml-30 u/ml	■	
Novolin N Human Insulin 10 ml Vials		
100 u/ml	■	
Novolin N PenFill 3 ml Cartridges		
100 u/ml	■	
Novolin R Human Insulin 10 ml Vials		
100 u/ml	■	
Novolin R PenFill 1.5 ml Cartridges		
100 u/ml	■	

STRENGTH	GENERIC YES	GENERIC NO
Novolin R PenFill 3 ml Cartridges		
100 u/ml	■	
NovoLog Injection		
100 u/ml		■
NovoLog Mix 70/30		
70 u/ml-30 u/ml		■
NovoSeven		
1 mcg		■
Nubain Injection		
10 mg/ml	■	
20 mg/ml	■	
Numorphan Injection		
1 mg/ml		■
1.5 mg/ml		■
Numorphan Suppositories		
5 mg		■
Nutropin for Injection		
5 mg	■	
10 mg		■
Nutropin AQ Injection		
5 mg/ml		■
Nutropin AQ Pen Cartridge		
5 mg/ml		■
NuvaRing		
0.015 mg/24 hr-0.12 mg/24 hr		■
Nystatin Vaginal Tablets, USP		
100000 u	■	
Nystop Topical Powder USP		
100000 u/gm	■	
Ocucoat		
0.1%-0.8%	■	
Ocufen Ophthalmic Solution		
0.03%	■	
Olux Foam		
0.05%		■
Omnicef Capsules		
300 mg		■
Omnicef for Oral Suspension		
125 mg/5 ml		■
250 mg/5 ml		■
Oncaspar		
750 iu/ml		■
Ontak Vials		
150 mcg/ml		■
Ophthetic Ophthalmic Solution		
0.5%	■	
OptiNate Omega-3 L-Vcaps		■
OptiPranolol Metipranolol Ophthalmic Solution		
0.3%	■	
Optivar Ophthalmic Solution		
0.05%		■
Orap Tablets		
1 mg		■
2 mg		■
Ortho-Cept Tablets		
0.15 mg-0.03 mg	■	
Ortho-Cyclen Tablets		
35 mcg-0.25 mg	■	
Ortho Evra Transdermal System		
0.02 mg/24 hr-0.15 mg/24 hr		■
Ortho Micronor Tablets		
0.35 mg	■	
Ortho Tri-Cyclen		
35 mcg-0.180 mg, 0.125 mg, 0.250 mg	■	
Ortho Tri-Cyclen Lo Tablets		
0.025 mg-0.18 mg		■
Orthoclone OKT3 Sterile Solution		
1 mg/ml		■
Orthovisc Injection		
15 mg/ml		■
Oxandrin Tablets		
2.5 mg		■
10 mg		■
Oxsoralen Lotion		
1%		■
Oxsoralen-Ultra Capsules		
10 mg		■
OxyContin Tablets		
10 mg	■	
20 mg	■	
40 mg	■	
80 mg	■	
160 mg		■
OxyFast Oral Concentrate Solution		
20 mg/ml	■	
OxyIR Capsules		
5 mg	■	
Oxytrol Transdermal System		
3.9 mg/24 hr		■
Pacerone Tablets		
200 mg	■	
400 mg		■
Panafil Ointment		
0.5%-10%-10%	■	
10%-10%		■
Parcopa Orally Disintegrating Tablets		
10 mg-100 mg		■
25 mg-100 mg		■
25 mg-250 mg		■
Parnate Tablets		
10 mg		■
Paser Granules		
4 gm/packet		■
Patanol Ophthalmic Solution		
0.1%		■
Paxil CR Controlled-Release Tablets		
12.5 mg		■
25 mg		■
37.5 mg		■
Paxil Oral Suspension		
10 mg/5 ml		■
40 mg	■	
Paxil Tablets		
10 mg	■	
20 mg	■	
30 mg	■	
40 mg	■	
PCE Dispertab Tablets		
333 mg		■
500 mg		■
Pediapred Oral Solution		
5 mg/5 ml	■	
PedvaxHIB Liquid		
7.5 mcg/0.5 ml		■
Peganone Tablets, USP		
250 mg		■
Pegasys		
180 mcg/0.5 ml		■
180 mcg/ml		■
Penlac Nail Lacquer, Topical Solution		
8%		■
Pentasa Capsules		
250 mg	■	
500 mg		■
Pepcid Injection		
0.4 mg/ml	■	
10 mg/ml	■	
Pepcid Injection Premixed		
0.4 mg/ml	■	
Pepcid for Oral Suspension		
0.4 mg/ml	■	
40 mg/5 ml		■
Pepcid Tablets		
20 mg	■	
40 mg	■	
Percocet Tablets		
325 mg-10 mg	■	
325 mg-2.5 mg		■
325 mg-5 mg	■	
325 mg-7.5 mg	■	
500 mg-7.5 mg	■	
650 mg-10 mg	■	
Percodan Tablets		
325 mg-4.5 mg-0.38 mg	■	
Permax Tablets		
0.05 mg	■	
0.25 mg	■	
Persantine Tablets		
25 mg	■	
50 mg	■	
75 mg	■	
Phenergan Suppositories		
12.5 mg	■	
25 mg	■	
50 mg	■	
Phenergan Tablets		
12.5 mg	■	
25 mg	■	
50 mg	■	
Phenytek Capsules		
200 mg		■
300 mg		■
PhosLo GelCaps		
667 mg		■
Photofrin for Injection		
75 mg		■
Plasbumin-5		
5%	■	
Plasbumin-20		
20%	■	
Plasbumin-25		
25%	■	
Plasmanate		
5%	■	
Plavix Tablets		
75 mg		■
Plendil Extended-Release Tablets		
2.5 mg	■	
5 mg	■	
10 mg	■	
Pletal Tablets		
50 mg	■	
Plexion Cleanser		
10%-5%	■	
Plexion Cleansing Cloths		
10%-5%		■
Plexion SCT		
10%-5%	■	
Plexion Topical Suspension		
10%-5%	■	
Pneumovax 23	■	
Poly-Pred Liquifilm Ophthalmic Suspension		
0.35%-10000 u/ml-0.5%		■
Polytrim Ophthalmic Solution		
10000 u/ml-1 mg/ml	■	
Potaba Envules		
2 gm/packet	■	
Potaba Tablets		
0.5 gm	■	
Pramosone Cream		
1%-1%	■	
2.5%-1%		■
Pramosone Lotion		
1%-1%	■	
2.5%-1%	■	
Pramosone Ointment		
1%-1%		■
2.5%-1%		■
Prandin Tablets		
0.5 mg		■
1 mg		■
2 mg		■
Pravachol Tablets		
10 mg		■
20 mg		■
40 mg		■
80 mg		■
PreCare Chewables Tablets	■	
PreCare Prenatal Caplets	■	
Precose Tablets		
25 mg		■
50 mg		■
100 mg		■
Pred Forte Ophthalmic Suspension		
1%	■	
Pred Mild Sterile Ophthalmic Suspension		
0.12%		■
Pred-G Ophthalmic Suspension		
0.3%-1%		■
Pred-G Sterile Ophthalmic Ointment		
0.12%	■	
Premarin Intravenous		
25 mg		■
Premarin Tablets		
0.3 mg		■
0.45 mg		■
0.625 mg		■
0.9 mg		■
1.25 mg		■
2.5 mg		■
Premarin Vaginal Cream		
0.625 mg/gm		■
PremesisRx Tablets	■	
Premphase Tablets		
0.625 mg-5 mg		■
Prempro Tablets		
0.625 mg-2.5 mg		■
0.625 mg-5 mg		■
Prenate Elite Tablets		
120 mg-0.03 mg-200 mg-6	■	
Prevacid for Delayed-Release Oral Suspension		
15 mg/packet		■
30 mg/packet		■
Prevacid Delayed-Release Capsules		
15 mg		■
30 mg		■
Prevacid I.V. for Injection		
30 mg		■
Prevacid NapraPAC 375		
15 mg-375 mg		■
Prevacid NapraPAC 500		
15 mg-500 mg		■
Prevacid SoluTab Delayed-Release Orally Disintegrating Tablets		
15 mg		■
30 mg		■

Strength	Generic Yes	Generic No
Prevnar for Injection		
16 mcg/0.5 ml		■
PREVPAC		
500 mg-500 mg-30 mg		■
PrimaCare AM Capsules	■	
PrimaCare PM Tablets	■	
Primaxin I.M.		
500 mg-500 mg		■
750 mg-750 mg		■
Primaxin I.V.		
250 mg-250 mg		■
500 mg-500 mg		■
Prinivil Tablets		
2.5 mg	■	
5 mg	■	
10 mg	■	
20 mg	■	
40 mg	■	
Prinzide Tablets		
12.5 mg-10 mg	■	
12.5 mg-20 mg	■	
25 mg-20 mg	■	
ProAmatine Tablets		
2.5 mg	■	
5 mg	■	
10 mg	■	
Prochieve Gel		
4%	■	
8%	■	
Procrit for Injection		
2000 u/ml	■	
3000 u/ml	■	
4000 u/ml	■	
10000 u/ml	■	
20000 u/ml	■	
40000 u/ml	■	
ProctoFoam-HC		
1%-1%	■	
Prograf Capsules and Injection		
0.5 mg		■
1 mg		■
5 mg		■
5 mg/ml		■
Prolastin		
1 mg	■	
Proleukin for Injection		
22 million iu		■
Prometrium Capsules		
100 mg		■
200 mg		■
Propecia Tablets		
1 mg		■
Propine Ophthalmic Solution		
0.1%	■	
Proscar Tablets		
5 mg		■
ProSom Tablets		
1 mg	■	
2 mg	■	
Protonix I.V.		
40 mg		■
Protonix Tablets		
20 mg		■
40 mg		■
Protopic Ointment		
0.03%		■
0.1%		■
Proventil Inhalation Aerosol		
0.09 mg/actuation	■	
Proventil HFA Inhalation Aerosol		
0.09 mg/actuation	■	
Provigil Tablets		
100 mg		■
200 mg		■
Prozac Pulvules and Liquid		
10 mg	■	
20 mg	■	
20 mg/5 ml	■	
40 mg	■	
Psoriatec Cream		
1%	■	
Pulmicort Respules		
0.25 mg/2 ml		■
0.5 mg/2 ml		■
Pulmozyme Inhalation Solution		
2.5 mg/2.5 ml		■
Purinethol Tablets		
50 mg	■	
Quixin Ophthalmic Solution		
0.5%		■
Qvar Inhalation Aerosol		
0.04 mg/actuation		■
0.08 mg/actuation		■
Rabies Vaccine RabAvert		
2.5 iu	■	
Rapamune Oral Solution and Tablets		
1 mg		■
1 mg/ml		■
2 mg		■
Raptiva for Injection		
125 mg	■	
Razadyne ER Capsules		
8 mg		■
16 mg		■
24 mg		■
Razadyne Tablets		
4 mg		■
8 mg		■
12 mg		■
Rebetol Capsules		
200 mg	■	
Rebetron Combination Therapy		
3 million iu/0.2 ml-200		■
3 million iu/0.5 ml-200		■
Rebif Prefilled Syringe for Injection		
22 mcg/0.5 ml		■
44 mcg/0.5 ml		■
Recombinate		
1 iu	■	
Recombivax HB		
10 mcg/ml		■
40 mcg/ml		■
ReFacto Vials		
1 iu	■	
Refludan for Injection		
50 mg		■
Relafen Tablets		
500 mg	■	
750 mg	■	
Relenza Rotadisk		
5 mg/actuation		■
Relpax Tablets		
20 mg		■
40 mg		■
Remicade for IV Injection		
100 mg		■
Renagel Tablets		
400 mg		■
800 mg		■
Renova Cream		
0.02%		■
0.05%	■	
ReoPro Vials		
2 mg/ml		■
Repronex for Intramuscular and Subcutaneous Injection		
75 iu-75 iu	■	
Requip Tablets		
0.25 mg		■
0.5 mg		■
1 mg		■
2 mg		■
3 mg		■
4 mg		■
5 mg		■
Rescriptor Tablets		
100 mg		■
200 mg		■
Restasis Ophthalmic Emulsion		
0.05%		■
Retisert Implant		
0.59 mg		■
Retrovir Capsules		
100 mg		■
Retrovir IV Infusion		
10 mg/ml		■
Retrovir Syrup		
50 mg/5 ml		■
Retrovir Tablets		
300 mg		■
Revatio Tablets		
20 mg		■
Rev-Eyes Ophthalmic Eyedrops		
0.5%		■
Reyataz Capsules		
100 mg		■
150 mg		■
200 mg		■
R-Gene 10 for Intravenous Use		
10%		■
Rhinocort Aqua Nasal Spray		
0.032 mg/actuation		■
Rilutek Tablets		
50 mg		■
Risperdal Consta Injection		
25 mg		■
37.5 mg		■
50 mg		■
Risperdal M-Tab Tablets		
0.5 mg		■
1 mg		■
2 mg		■
Risperdal Oral Solution		
1 mg/ml		■
Risperdal Tablets		
0.25 mg		■
0.5 mg		■
1 mg		■
2 mg		■
3 mg		■
4 mg		■
Ritalin Hydrochloride Tablets		
5 mg	■	
10 mg	■	
20 mg	■	
Ritalin LA Capsules		
20 mg	■	
30 mg	■	
40 mg		■
Ritalin-SR Tablets		
20 mg	■	
Rituxan for Infusion		
10 mg/ml		■
Rituxan I.V.		
10 mg/ml		■
Rocephin Injectable Vials, ADD-Vantage, Galaxy, Bulk		
1 gm		■
1 gm/50 ml		■
2 gm		■
2 gm/50 ml		■
10 gm		■
250 mg		■
500 mg		■
Roferon-A Injection		
3 million iu/0.5 ml	■	
3 million u/ml		■
6 million iu/0.5 ml	■	
6 million u/ml		■
9 million iu/0.5 ml	■	
9 million u/0.9 ml		■
36 million u/ml		■
Rozerem Tablets		
8 mg		■
Rythmol SR Capsules		
150 mg	■	
225 mg	■	
300 mg	■	
Sanctura Tablets		
20 mg		■
Sandimmune I.V. Ampuls for Infusion		
50 mg/ml	■	
Sandimmune Oral Solution		
100 mg/ml		■
Sandimmune Soft Gelatin Capsules		
25 mg		■
50 mg		■
100 mg		■
Sandostatin Injection		
50 mcg/ml		■
100 mcg/ml		■
200 mcg/ml		■
500 mcg/ml		■
1000 mcg/ml		■
Sandostatin LAR Depot		
10 mg		■
20 mg		■
30 mg		■
Seasonale Tablets		
30 mcg-0.15 mg	■	
Sedapap Tablets		
650 mg-50 mg	■	
Sensipar Tablets		
30 mg		■
60 mg		■
90 mg		■
Serevent Diskus		
0.046 mg/actuation		■
Seroquel Tablets		
25 mg		■
100 mg		■
200 mg		■
300 mg		■
Simulect for Injection		
10 mg		■
20 mg		■
Singulair Oral Granules		
4 mg/packet		■
Singulair Tablets		
10 mg		■
Singulair Chewable Tablets		
4 mg		■
5 mg		■
Skelaxin Tablets		
400 mg	■	
800 mg		■
Somavert Injection		
10 mg	■	
15 mg	■	
20 mg	■	
Sonata Capsules		
5 mg		■
Soriatane Capsules		
30 mg	■	
Spectracef Tablets		
200 mg	■	
Spiriva HandiHaler		
18 mcg		■
Stalevo Tablets		
12.5 mg-200 mg-50 mg		■

STRENGTH	GENERIC YES	GENERIC NO
Strattera Capsules		
10 mg		■
18 mg		■
25 mg		■
40 mg		■
60 mg		■
Striant Mucoadhesive		
30 mg		■
Stromectol Tablets		
3 mg		■
Suboxone Tablets		
2 mg-0.5 mg		■
8 mg-2 mg		■
Subutex Tablets		
2 mg	■	
8 mg	■	
Sular Tablets		
10 mg		■
20 mg		■
30 mg		■
40 mg		■
Sulfamylon Cream		
85 mg/gm		■
Sulfamylon Topical Solution		
50 gm/packet		■
Suprane Liquid for Inhalation		
99%		■
Suprax		
100 mg/5 ml		■
Surmontil Capsules		
25 mg		■
50 mg		■
100 mg		■
Sustiva Capsules		
50 mg		■
100 mg		■
200 mg		■
Symbyax Capsules		
25 mg-12 mg		■
25 mg-6 mg		■
50 mg-12 mg		■
50 mg-6 mg		■
Symlin Injection		
0.6 mg/ml		■
Symmetrel Syrup		
50 mg/5 ml	■	
Symmetrel Tablets		
100 mg	■	
Synagis Intramuscular Powder		
50 mg		■
100 mg		■
Synercid I.V.		
420 mg-180 mg		■
Synthroid Tablets		
0.025 mg	■	
0.05 mg	■	
0.075 mg	■	
0.088 mg	■	
0.1 mg	■	
0.112 mg	■	
0.125 mg	■	
0.137 mg	■	
0.15 mg	■	
0.175 mg	■	
0.2 mg	■	
0.3 mg	■	
Syprine Capsules		
250 mg		■
Tabloid Tablets		
40 mg		■
Tagamet Tablets		
200 mg	■	
300 mg	■	
400 mg	■	
800 mg	■	
Tambocor Tablets		
50 mg	■	
100 mg	■	
150 mg	■	
Tamiflu Capsules		
75 mg		■
Tamiflu Oral Suspension		
12 mg/ml		■
Tarceva Tablets		
25 mg		■
100 mg		■
150 mg		■
Targretin Capsules		
75 mg		■
Tarka Tablets		
1 mg-240 mg		■
2 mg-180 mg		■
2 mg-240 mg		■
4 mg-240 mg		■
Taxotere Injection Concentrate		
20 mg/0.5 ml		■
Tegretol Chewable Tablets		
100 mg	■	
Tegretol-XR Tablets		
100 mg		■
200 mg		■
400 mg		■
Temodar Capsules		
5 mg		■
20 mg		■
100 mg		■
250 mg		■
Tenormin I.V. Injection		
0.5 mg/ml		■
Tenormin Tablets		
25 mg	■	
50 mg	■	
100 mg	■	
Tequin Injection		
2 mg/ml		■
10 mg/ml		■
Tequin Tablets		
200 mg		■
400 mg		■
Tessalon Capsules		
100 mg	■	
Tessalon Perles		
100 mg	■	
200 mg	■	
Testim Gel		
1%	■	
Teveten Tablets		
400 mg		■
600 mg		■
Tev-Tropin for Injection		
5 mg	■	
Thalomid Capsules		
50 mg		■
100 mg		■
200 mg		■
Thioridazine Hydrochloride Tablets		
10 mg	■	
25 mg	■	
50 mg	■	
100 mg	■	
Thiothixene Capsules		
1 mg	■	
2 mg	■	
5 mg	■	
10 mg	■	
Thrombate III		
1 iu	■	
Thrombin-JMI		
1000 u	■	
5000 u	■	
10000 iu	■	
20000 iu	■	
50000 u	■	
Thymoglobulin for Injection		
25 mg		■
Thyrogen for Injection		
1.1 mg		■
Tiazac Capsules		
120 mg	■	
180 mg	■	
240 mg	■	
300 mg	■	
360 mg	■	
420 mg		■
Ticlid Tablets		
250 mg	■	
Timentin ADD-Vantage		
100 mg-3 gm		■
100 mg/100 ml-3 gm/100 m		■
Timentin IV Infusion		
100 mg-3 gm		■
Timentin Pharmacy Bulk Package		
1 gm-30 gm		■
Timolide Tablets		
25 mg-10 mg		■
Timoptic in Ocudose		
0.25%	■	
0.5%	■	
Timoptic Sterile Ophthalmic Solution		
0.25%	■	
0.5%	■	
Timoptic-XE Sterile Ophthalmic Gel Forming Solution		
0.25%	■	
0.5%	■	
0.25%	■	
0.5%	■	
Tindamax		
250 mg		■
500 mg		■
TNKase I.V.		
50 mg		■
TOBI Solution for Inhalation		
60 mg/ml		■
TobraDex Ophthalmic Ointment		
0.1%-0.3%		■
TobraDex Ophthalmic Suspension		
0.1%-0.3%		■
Topamax Sprinkle Capsules		
15 mg		■
25 mg		■
Topamax Tablets		
25 mg		■
100 mg		■
200 mg		■
Topicort Gel		
0.05%	■	
Topicort Cream		
0.25%	■	
Topicort Ointment		
0.25%	■	
Topicort LP Cream		
0.05%	■	
Toprol-XL Tablets		
25 mg		■
50 mg		■
100 mg		■
200 mg		■
Tracleer Tablets		
62.5 mg		■
125 mg		■
Transderm Scop Transdermal Therapeutic System		
0.33 mg/24 hr		■
Tranxene T-TAB Tablets		
3.75 mg	■	
7.5 mg	■	
15 mg	■	
Tranxene-SD Tablets		
22.5 mg		■
Trasylol Injection		
10000 kiu/ml		■
Travatan Ophthalmic Solution		
0.004%		■
Trecator Tablets		
250 mg		■
Trelstar Depot		
3.75 mg		■
Triaz Cleanser		
3%		■
6%	■	
10%	■	
Triaz Gel		
3%		■
6%	■	
10%	■	
Triaz Pads		
3%		■
6%		■
9%		■
Tricor Tablets		
48 mg		■
145 mg		■
Triglide Tablets		
50 mg		■
160 mg	■	
Trileptal Oral Suspension		
300 mg/5 ml		■
Trileptal Tablets		
150 mg		■
300 mg		■
600 mg		■
Tri-Luma Cream		
0.01%-4%-0.05%		■
TriLyte with Flavor Packs for Oral Solution		
420 gm-1.48 gm-5.72 gm-1		■
Trisenox Injection		
1 mg/ml		■
Trizivir Tablets		
300 mg-150 mg-300 mg		■
Trusopt Sterile Ophthalmic Solution		
2%		■
Truvada Tablets		
200 mg-300 mg		■
Tussionex Pennkinetic Extended-Release Suspension		
8 mg/5 ml-10 mg/5 ml		■
Twinrix Vaccine		
720 el u/ml-20 mcg/ml		■
Tylenol with Codeine Elixir		
120 mg/5 ml-12 mg/5 ml	■	
Tylenol with Codeine Tablets		
300 mg-7.5 mg	■	
300 mg-15 mg	■	
300 mg-30 mg	■	
300 mg-60 mg	■	
Ultane Liquid for Inhalation		
100%		■
Ultracet Tablets		
325 mg-37.5 mg	■	
Ultrase Capsules		
20000 u-4500 u-25000 u	■	
Ultrase MT Capsules		
39000 u-12000 u-39000 u	■	
58500 u-18000 u-58500 u	■	
65000 u-20000 u-65000 u	■	
Uniphyl Tablets		
400 mg	■	
600 mg	■	
Uniretic Tablets		
12.5 mg-7.5 mg		■
12.5 mg-15 mg		■
25 mg-15 mg		■

STRENGTH	GENERIC YES	GENERIC NO
Univasc Tablets		
7.5 mg	■	
15 mg	■	
Urecholine Tablets		
5 mg	■	
10 mg	■	
25 mg	■	
50 mg	■	
Urocit-K Tablets		
5 meq		■
10 meq		■
Uroqid-Acid No. 2 Tablets		
500 mg-500 mg		■
Uroxatral Tablets		
10 mg		■
Vagifem Tablets		
25 mcg	■	
Valcyte Tablets		
450 mg		■
Valium Tablets		
2 mg	■	
5 mg	■	
10 mg	■	
Valtrex Caplets		
1 gm		■
500 mg		■
Vancocin HCl Capsules, USP		
125 mg		■
250 mg		■
Vanos Cream		
0.1%		■
Vantas		
50 mg		■
Vantin Tablets and Oral Suspension		
50 mg/5 ml		■
100 mg	■	
100 mg/5 ml		■
200 mg	■	
Vaqta		
50 u/ml		■
Varivax		
1350 pfu		■
Vaseretic Tablets		
5 mg-12.5 mg	■	
10 mg-25 mg	■	
Velcade for Injection		
3.5 mg		■
Ventavis Inhalation Solution		
10 mcg/ml		■
Ventolin HFA Inhalation Aerosol		
0.09 mg/actuation	■	
Verelan PM Capsules		
100 mg		■
200 mg		■
300 mg		■
Vermox Chewable Tablets		
100 mg	■	
Vesanoid Capsules		
10 mg		■
VFEND I.V.		
200 mg		■
VFEND Oral Suspension		
40 mg/ml		■
VFEND Tablets		
50 mg		■
200 mg		■
Viadur Implant		
65 mg		■
Viagra Tablets		
25 mg		■
50 mg		■
100 mg		■
Vicodin Tablets		
500 mg-5 mg	■	
Vicodin ES Tablets		
750 mg-7.5 mg	■	
Vicodin HP Tablets		
660 mg-10 mg	■	
Vicoprofen Tablets		
7.5 mg-200 mg	■	
Vigamox Ophthalmic Solution		
0.5%		■
Viokase Powder		■
Viokase Tablets	■	
Viracept Oral Powder		
50 mg/gm		■
Viracept Tablets		
250 mg		■
Viramune Oral Suspension		
50 mg/5 ml		■
Viramune Tablets		
200 mg		■
Virazole for Inhalation Solution		
6 gm		■
Viread Tablets		
300 mg		■
Visudyne for Injection		
15 mg		■
Vivactil Tablets		
5 mg	■	
10 mg	■	
Vivelle Transdermal System		
0.025 mg/24 hr	■	
0.0375 mg/24 hr	■	
0.05 mg/24 hr	■	
0.075 mg/24 hr	■	
0.1 mg/24 hr	■	
Vivelle-Dot Transdermal System		
0.025 mg/24 hr	■	
0.0375 mg/24 hr	■	
0.05 mg/24 hr	■	
0.075 mg/24 hr	■	
0.1 mg/24 hr	■	
Voltaren Ophthalmic Solution		
0.1%	■	
Voltaren Tablets		
25 mg	■	
50 mg	■	
75 mg	■	
Voltaren-XR Tablets		
100 mg	■	
VoSpire Extended-Release Tablets		
4 mg	■	
8 mg	■	
WelChol Tablets		
625 mg		■
Wellbutrin Tablets		
75 mg	■	
100 mg	■	
Wellbutrin SR Sustained-Release Tablets		
100 mg	■	
150 mg	■	
200 mg	■	
Wellbutrin XL Extended-Release Tablets		
150 mg		■
300 mg		■
WinRho SDF		
600 iu		■
1500 iu		■
5000 iu		■
Xalatan Sterile Ophthalmic Solution		
0.005%		■
Xanax XR Tablets		
0.5 mg		■
1 mg		■
2 mg		■
3 mg		■
Xeloda Tablets		
150 mg		■
500 mg		■
Xenaderm Ointment		■
Xenical Capsules		
120 mg		■
Xerac AC Solution		
6.25%		■
Xifaxan Tablets		
200 mg		■
Xigris Powder for Intravenous Infusion		
5 mg		■
20 mg		■
Xolair		
150 mg		■
Xopenex Inhalation Solution		
1.25 mg/3 ml		■
Xopenex Inhalation Solution Concentrate		
1.25 mg/0.5 ml		■
Yasmin 28 Tablets		
3 mg-0.03 mg		■
Zaditor Ophthalmic Solution		
0.025%		■
Zantac 150 Tablets		
150 mg	■	
Zantac 300 Tablets		
300 mg	■	
Zantac 25 EFFERdose Tablets		
150 mg		■
150 mg/packet		■
Zantac 150 EFFERdose Tablets		
150 mg		■
Zantac Injection		
25 mg/ml	■	
Zantac Injection Premixed		
1 mg/ml		■
Zantac Syrup		
15 mg/ml	■	
Zavesca Capsules		
100 mg		■
Zegerid Powder for Oral Solution		
20 mg/packet		■
Zelnorm Tablets		
2 mg		■
6 mg		■
Zemaira		
1 mg	■	
Zemplar Injection		
0.002 mg/ml		■
0.005 mg/ml		■
Zemuron Injection		
10 mg/ml		■
Zenapax for Injection		
5 mg/ml		■
Zerit Capsules		
15 mg		■
20 mg		■
30 mg		■
40 mg		■
Zerit for Oral Solution		
1 mg/ml		■
Zestoretic Tablets		
12.5 mg-10 mg	■	
12.5 mg-20 mg	■	
25 mg-20 mg	■	
Zestril Tablets		
2.5 mg	■	
5 mg	■	
10 mg	■	
20 mg	■	
30 mg	■	
40 mg	■	
Ziagen Oral Solution		
20 mg/ml		■
Ziagen Tablets		
300 mg		■
Zinacef Injection		
1.5 gm	■	
1.5 gm/50 ml	■	
7.5 gm	■	
750 mg	■	
750 mg/50 ml	■	
Zinecard for Injection		
250 mg		■
500 mg		■
Zithromax for IV Infusion		
500 mg		■
Zithromax for Oral Suspension		
1 gm/packet		■
Zithromax for Oral Suspension		
100 mg/5 ml		■
200 mg/5 ml		■
Zithromax Tablets		
250 mg		■
500 mg		■
600 mg		■
Zocor Tablets		
5 mg		■
10 mg		■
20 mg		■
40 mg		■
80 mg		■
Zofran Injection		
2 mg/ml		■
32 mg/50 ml		■
Zofran Injection Premixed		
32 mg/50 ml		■
Zofran Oral Solution		
4 mg/5 ml		■
Zofran Tablets		
4 mg		■
8 mg		■
24 mg		■
Zofran ODT Orally Disintegrating Tablets		
4 mg		■
8 mg		■
Zoladex		
3.6 mg		■
10.8 mg		■
Zoladex 3-month		
3.6 mg		■
10.8 mg		■
Zoloft Oral Concentrate		
20 mg/ml		■
Zoloft Tablets		
25 mg		■
50 mg		■
100 mg		■
Zometa for Intravenous Infusion		
4 mg		■
4 mg/5 ml		■
Zosyn		
2 gm-0.25 gm		■
3 gm-0.375 gm		■
4 gm-0.5 gm		■
4 gm/100 ml-0.5 gm/100 m		■
36 gm-4.5 gm		■
40 mg/ml-5 mg/ml		■
60 mg/ml-7.5 mg/ml		■

Zosyn in Galaxy Containers

STRENGTH	GENERIC YES	GENERIC NO
4 gm/100 ml-0.5 gm/100 ml		■
40 mg/ml-5 mg/ml		■
60 mg/ml-7.5 mg/ml		■

Zovirax Capsules

STRENGTH	GENERIC YES	GENERIC NO
200 mg	■	

Zovirax Cream

STRENGTH	GENERIC YES	GENERIC NO
5%		■

Zovirax for Injection

STRENGTH	GENERIC YES	GENERIC NO
500 mg	■	
1000 mg	■	

Zovirax Ointment

STRENGTH	GENERIC YES	GENERIC NO
5%		■

Zovirax Suspension

STRENGTH	GENERIC YES	GENERIC NO
200 mg/5 ml	■	

Zovirax Tablets

STRENGTH	GENERIC YES	GENERIC NO
400 mg	■	
800 mg	■	

Zyban Sustained-Release Tablets

STRENGTH	GENERIC YES	GENERIC NO
150 mg	■	

Zydone Tablets

STRENGTH	GENERIC YES	GENERIC NO
400 mg-5 mg		■
400 mg-7.5 mg		■
400 mg-10 mg		■

Zymar Ophthalmic Solution

STRENGTH	GENERIC YES	GENERIC NO
0.3%		■

Zyprexa Tablets

STRENGTH	GENERIC YES	GENERIC NO
2.5 mg		■
5 mg		■
7.5 mg		■
10 mg		■
15 mg		■
20 mg		■

Zyprexa IntraMuscular

STRENGTH	GENERIC YES	GENERIC NO
10 mg		■

Zyprexa ZYDIS Orally Disintegrating Tablets

STRENGTH	GENERIC YES	GENERIC NO
5 mg		■
10 mg		■
15 mg		■
20 mg		■

Zyrtec Syrup

STRENGTH	GENERIC YES	GENERIC NO
1 mg/ml		■

Zyrtec Tablets

STRENGTH	GENERIC YES	GENERIC NO
5 mg		■
10 mg		■

Zyrtec-D 12 Hour Extended Release Tablets

STRENGTH	GENERIC YES	GENERIC NO
5 mg-120 mg		■

Zyvox Injection

STRENGTH	GENERIC YES	GENERIC NO
2 mg/ml		■

Zyvox for Oral Suspension

STRENGTH	GENERIC YES	GENERIC NO
100 mg/5 ml		■

Zyvox Tablets

STRENGTH	GENERIC YES	GENERIC NO
600 mg		■

SECTION 10

IMPRINT IDENTIFICATION GUIDE

Too often, patients on multiple medications have no idea what they're taking; and a ''brown-bag inventory'' may not help if it confronts you with a collection of unfamiliar tablets and capsules. This section of the *PDR Companion Guide*™ provides you with a handy solution.

The convenient table below allows you to identify thousands of solid oral medications by imprint alone. Imprints beginning with a number are listed first, in ascending order. All numbers with leading zeros, as in ''053'', are listed before numbers without leading zeros. Imprints beginning with a letter follow in alphabetical order. Virtually all commonly prescribed drugs are represented.

Each entry includes the full imprint code, the product's brand or generic name, and, to confirm identification, its strength, color, form, and shape. The name of the product's manufacturer completes each listing. The information is extracted, with permission, from the Identidex System produced by Micromedex, Inc.

IMPRINT	BRAND/GENERIC NAME	STRENGTH	COLOR	FORM	SHAPE	MANUFACTURER
+	Max Alert Mini-Tabs	25 mg	White	Tablet	Circle, Quarter Sectioned	Pdk Labs
0.1; RPR;	Ddavp	0.1 mg	White	Tablet	Oval, Scored on 1 Side	Aventis Pharmaceuticals
0.1879	Codeine Sulfate	30 mg	White	Tablet	Flat	Halsey Drug
.5; 273	Clonazepam	0.5 mg	Yellow	Tablet	Circle, Scored	Caraco Pharmaceutical
0015; 4426	Reserpine	0.1 mg		Tablet		Richlyn Laboratories
0027; V	Acetaminophen	325 mg	White	Tablet	Circle	Vintage Pharmaceuticals
00-29; V	Acetaminophen	500 mg	White	Tablet	Bisected Scored	Vintage Pharmaceuticals
0032; 1204	Multivitamins	5000 IU; 400 IU; 2.5 mg; 2.5 mg; 50 mg; 20 mg; 0.5 mg; 5 mg; 2 mcg; 10 IU	Brown	Capsule	Oval	Solvay Pharmaceuticals
0037; 0681	Tussizone-12 Rf	60 mg; 5 mg	Mauve	Tablet	Capsule-Shape, Scored	Mallinckrodt
0038; G	Etodolac	200 mg	Light Gray	Capsule		Par Pharmaceutical
0039; G	Etodolac	300 mg	Gray	Capsule		Par Pharmaceutical
0040; G	Etodolac	400 mg	Orange	Tablet	Oval	Par Pharmaceutical
0048; V	Phenazopyridine	95 mg	Maroon	Tablet	Circle	Vintage Pharmaceuticals
0063; 1261	X-Otag S.R.	100 mg	Yellow	Tablet	Circle	Solvay Pharmaceuticals
0063; 1650	Sprx-1	35 mg	Peach	Tablet	Triangle	Solvay Pharmaceuticals
0063; 2660	Sprx-3	35 mg	Black	Capsule		Solvay Pharmaceuticals
0063; 3006	R-P Mycin	250 mg	Red	Tablet		Solvay Pharmaceuticals
0065; 4410	Hydralazine Hydrochloride and Hydrochlorothiazide	25 mg; 25 mg	Light Celery	Capsule		Solvay Pharmaceuticals
0065; 4420	Hydralazine Hydrochloride and Hydrochlorothiazide	50 mg; 50 mg	Light Celery and Dark Green	Capsule		Solvay Pharmaceuticals
0093; HY-PAM 25 MG	HY-Pam	25 mg	Black or Lavender	Capsule		Teva Pharmaceuticals
0093; HY-PAM 50 MG	HY-Pam 50	50 mg	Dark Green and White Opaque	Capsule		Teva Pharmaceuticals
01A; BOEHRINGER INGELHEIM LOGO	Aggrenox	200 mg; 25 mg	Red and Ivory with Yellow Pellets	Capsule		Boehringer Ingelheim
01, ADVANCE LOGO	Mytab Gas	80 mg	White	Tablet, Chewable		Qualitest Products
03; 0088;	Allegra	30 mg	Peach	Coated Tablet		Aventis Pharmaceuticals
04, ADVANCE LOGO	Mytab Gas Max Strength	125 mg	White	Tablet, Chewable		Qualitest Products
04, ADVANCE LOGO	Pink Bismuth	262 mg	Pink	Tablet, Chewable	Circle	Qualitest Products
06; 0088;	Allegra	60 mg	Peach	Coated Tablet	Oblong	Aventis Pharmaceuticals
011; OHM	Acetaminophen	500 mg	White	Tablet	Bisected Scored	Ohm Laboratories
015; OHM	Aspirin and Caffeine	400 mg; 32 mg	White	Tablet		Ohm Laboratories
018; 0088;	Allegra	180 mg	Peach	Coated Tablet		Aventis Pharmaceuticals
019; DMSP	Cimetidine	200 mg	White	Tablet	Oval	Bristol-Myers Squibb
025;	Calcium	648 mg	White	Tablet	Circle, Convex	Rugby Laboratories
026; G	Piroxicam	10 mg	Opaque Olive and Dark Green	Capsule		Par Pharmaceutical
027; G	Piroxicam	20 mg	Opaque Dark Green	Capsule		Par Pharmaceutical
028; ALPHA SYMBOL	Guaifenesin	1200 mg	White	Tablet		Alphagen Laboratories

IMPRINT	BRAND/GENERIC NAME	STRENGTH	COLOR	FORM	SHAPE	MANUFACTURER
045; OHM	Acetaminophen, Phenylephrine Hcl and Chlorpheniramine Maleate	325 mg; 5 mg; 2 mg	Yellow and White	Tablet		Ohm Laboratories
050; DMSP	Cimetidine	300 mg	White	Tablet	Oval	Bristol-Myers Squibb
055; OHM	Acetaminophen, Aspirin and Caffeine	250 mg; 250 mg; 65 mg	White	Tablet		Ohm Laboratories
057; DMSP	Cimetidine	400 mg	White	Tablet	Oval	Bristol-Myers Squibb
058; DMSP	Cimetidine	800 mg	White	Tablet	Oval	Bristol-Myers Squibb
060; OHM	Aluminum Hydroxide and Magnesium Carbonate	160 mg; 105 mg	White	Tablet, Chewable		Ohm Laboratories
078; OHM	Acetaminophen and Phenyltoloxamine Citrate	325 mg; 30 mg	Peach	Tablet	Bisected Scored	Ohm Laboratories
082; OHM	Pseudoephedrine Hcl and Chlorpheniramine Maleate	60 mg; 4 mg	White	Tablet	Bisected Scored	Ohm Laboratories
082; OHM	Sudal-12	30 mg/5 ml; 6 mg/5 ml	Red	Suspension		Atley Pharmaceuticals
091; BRECKENRIDGE	Guiadex D	600 mg; 20 mg	White	Extended-Release Tablet	Oval	Breckenridge Pharmaceutical
0115; 0100	Vitamin A	25000 U		Capsule		Global Pharmaceutical
0115; 0101	Vitamin A	25000 U		Capsule		Global Pharmaceutical
0115; 0102	Vitamin A Palmitate	50000 U		Capsule		Global Pharmaceutical
0115; 0104	Vitamin A	25000 U		Capsule		Global Pharmaceutical
0115; 0105	Vitamin A	50000 U		Capsule		Global Pharmaceutical
0115; 0109	Vitamin A	50000 U		Capsule		Global Pharmaceutical
0115; 0140	Vitamin D	50000 IU		Capsule		Global Pharmaceutical
0115; 812	Thyroglobulin	1 Gr		Tablet		Global Pharmaceutical
0115; 823	Thyroid	0.5 Gr		Enteric-Coated Tablet		Global Pharmaceutical
0115; 1110	Diphenhydramine Hydrochloride	25 mg	Transparent Pink	Capsule		Richlyn Laboratories
0115; 1111	Diphenhydramine Hydrochloride	50 mg	Pink	Capsule, Liquid Filled		Richlyn Laboratories
0115; 1140	Ephedrine Sulfate	25 mg	Pink	Capsule		Global Pharmaceutical
0115; 1142	Ephedrine Sulfate - No. 4	0.375 Gr	Pink	Capsule		Richlyn Laboratories
0115; 1142	Ephedrine Sulphate - No. 3	0.75 Gr	Pink	Capsule, Liquid Filled		Richlyn Laboratories
0115; 1300	Oxytetracycline Hydrochloride	250 mg		Capsule, Liquid Filled		Global Pharmaceutical
0115; 1301	Oxytetracycline Hydrochloride	250 mg		Capsule, Liquid Filled		Global Pharmaceutical
0115; 1374	Quinine Sulfate	325 mg		Tablet		Global Pharmaceutical
0115; 1399	Tetracycline Hydrochloride	100 mg	Orange and Yellow	Capsule		Global Pharmaceutical
0115; 1400	Tetracycline Hydrochloride	250 mg	Orange and Yellow	Capsule		Global Pharmaceutical
0115; 1402	Tetracycline Hydrochloride	500 mg	Black and Yellow	Capsule		Global Pharmaceutical
0115; 1405	Tetracycline Hydrochloride	250 mg	Blue and Yellow	Capsule		Global Pharmaceutical
0115; 2005	Chloral Hydrate	500 mg		Capsule		Richlyn Laboratories
0115; 2150	Aminophylline	100 mg	White	Tablet		Richlyn Laboratories
0115; 2151	Aminophylline	1.5 Gr		Enteric-Coated Tablet		Richlyn Laboratories
0115; 2158	Aminophylline	200 mg	White	Tablet		Richlyn Laboratories
0115; 2162	Aminophylline	3 Gr		Enteric-Coated Tablet		Richlyn Laboratories
0115; 2174	Aminosalicylic Acid	7.7 Gr		Tablet		Richlyn Laboratories
0115; 2176	Aminosalicylic Acid	7.7 Gr		Enteric-Coated Tablet		Richlyn Laboratories
0115; 2390	Azo-Sulfisoxazole	50 mg; 0.5 GM	Red	Tablet	Circle	Richlyn Laboratories
0115; 2400	Bellophen	0.25 Gr; 0.0065 mg; 0.1037 mg; 0.0194 mg		Tablet		Richlyn Laboratories
0115; 2758	Chlordiazepoxide	5 mg	Green and Yellow	Capsule, Liquid Filled		Richlyn Laboratories
0115; 2760	Chlordiazepoxide	10 mg	Black and Green	Capsule, Liquid Filled		Richlyn Laboratories
0115; 2762	Chlordiazepoxide	25 mg	Green and White	Capsule, Liquid Filled		Richlyn Laboratories
0115; 2790	Chloroquine Phosphate	250 mg	White	Tablet		Richlyn Laboratories
0115; 2800	Chlorothiazide	500 mg		Tablet		Richlyn Laboratories
0115; 2810	Chlorpheniramine Maleate	4 mg	Yellow	Tablet		Richlyn Laboratories
0115; 2900	Conjugated Estrogens	0.625 mg		Coated Tablet		Richlyn Laboratories
0115; 2902	Conjugated Estrogen	1.25 mg		Coated Tablet		Richlyn Laboratories
0115; 2904	Conjugated Estrogen	2.5 mg		Coated Tablet		Richlyn Laboratories
0115; 2920	Cortisone Acetate	25 mg	White	Tablet		Richlyn Laboratories
0115; 3030	Dehydrocholic Acid	250 mg	White	Tablet	Circle, Scored	Richlyn Laboratories
0115; 3100	Dexamethasone	0.75 mg	Blue	Tablet	Five-Sided, Scored	Richlyn Laboratories
0115; 3200	Dicyclomine Hydrochloride	10 mg		Capsule, Liquid Filled		Richlyn Laboratories
0115; 3210	Dicyclomine Hydrochloride with Phenobarbital	10 mg; 15 mg		Capsule		Richlyn Laboratories
0115; 3220	Dicyclomine Hydrochloride	20 mg		Tablet		Richlyn Laboratories
0115; 3225	Dicyclomine Hydrochloride with Phenobarbital	20 mg; 15 mg		Tablet		Richlyn Laboratories
0115; 3250	Digestozyme	250 mg; 300 mg; 25 mg	White	Tablet		Richlyn Laboratories
0115; 3585	Folic Acid	1 mg	Yellow	Tablet	Circle, Scored	Richlyn Laboratories
0115; 3660	Hydralazine Hydrochloride	25 mg	Blue	Tablet	Circle	Richlyn Laboratories
0115; 3662	Hydralazine Hydrochloride	50 mg	Blue	Tablet	Circle	Richlyn Laboratories
0115; 3670	Hydrochlorothiazide	25 mg	Peach	Tablet	Circle, Scored	Richlyn Laboratories
0115; 3675	Hydrochlorothiazide	50 mg	Peach	Tablet	Circle, Scored	Richlyn Laboratories
0115; 3677	Hydrochlorothiazide	100 mg	Peach	Tablet	Circle, Scored	Richlyn Laboratories
0115; 3685	Hydrocortisone	20 mg	White	Tablet	Oval, Scored	Richlyn Laboratories
0115; 3706	Isoniazid	100 mg	White	Tablet	Circle, Scored	Richlyn Laboratories
0115; 3840	Mannitol Hexanitrate	0.5 Gr		Tablet		Richlyn Laboratories
0115; 3875	Meclizine Hydrochloride	25 mg	Pink	Tablet, Chewable	Circle	Global Pharmaceutical
0115; 3888	Meprobamate	200 mg	White	Tablet	Circle	Global Pharmaceutical
0115; 3890	Meprobamate	400 mg	White	Tablet	Circle, Scored	Global Pharmaceutical
0115; 3900	Methocarbamol	500 mg	White	Tablet	Circle, Scored	Global Pharmaceutical
0115; 3902	Methocarbamol	750 mg	White	Tablet	Circle, Scored	Global Pharmaceutical
0115; 3975	Methenamine Mandelate	0.25 G		Enteric-Coated Tablet		Richlyn Laboratories
0115; 3976	Methenamine Mandelate	0.5 G	Brown	Enteric-Coated Tablet		Richlyn Laboratories
0115; 3977	Methenamine Mandelate	1 G	Lavender	Enteric-Coated Tablet	Oval	Richlyn Laboratories
0115; 3982	Methyltestosterone	10 mg		Tablet		Richlyn Laboratories
0115; 3984	Methyltestosterone	10 mg	White	Tablet	Circle, Scored, Compressed	Global Pharmaceutical

IMPRINT	BRAND/GENERIC NAME	STRENGTH	COLOR	FORM	SHAPE	MANUFACTURER
0115; 3986	Methyltestosterone	25 mg	Yellow	Tablet	Circle, Scored, Compressed	Global Pharmaceutical
0115; 4095	Nitrofurantoin	100 mg		Tablet		Global Pharmaceutical
0115; 4214	Phenobarbital White	16.2 mg	White	Tablet	Circle	Global Pharmaceutical
0115; 4233	Phenobarbital White	30 mg	White	Tablet		Global Pharmaceutical
0115; 4262	Potassium Chloride	5 Gr		Enteric-Coated Tablet		Global Pharmaceutical
0115; 4264	Potassium Chloride	7.5 Gr		Enteric-Coated Tablet		Global Pharmaceutical
0115; 4266	Potassium Chloride	10 Gr		Enteric-Coated Tablet		Global Pharmaceutical
0115; 4268	Potassium Chloride	15 Gr		Enteric-Coated Tablet		Global Pharmaceutical
0115; 4280	Prednisolone	5 mg	Orange	Tablet	Compressed, Scored	Global Pharmaceutical
0115; 4294	Prednisone	5 mg	White	Tablet	Circle, Scored	Global Pharmaceutical
0115; 4302	Probenecid and Colchicine	500 mg; 0.5 mg		Tablet		Global Pharmaceutical
0115; 4306	Promethazine Hydrochloride	25 mg	White	Tablet	Circle, Double Scored, Compressed	Global Pharmaceutical
0115; 4308	Propantheline Bromide	15 mg	Peach	Tablet		Global Pharmaceutical
0115; 4310	Propoxyphene Hydrochloride	65 mg		Capsule		Global Pharmaceutical
0115; 4314	Acetaminophen and Propoxyphene Hydrochloride	65 mg; 325 mg		Capsule		Global Pharmaceutical
0115; 4322	Propylthiouracil	50 mg	White	Tablet	Circle, Scored	Global Pharmaceutical
0115; 4332	Pseudoephedrine Hydrochloride	60 mg	White	Tablet	Circle, Scored	Global Pharmaceutical
0115; 4334	Pyridiate	100 mg	Dark Red	Tablet	Circle	Global Pharmaceutical
0115; 4336	Pyridiate	200 mg	Dark Red	Tablet	Circle	Global Pharmaceutical
0115; 4380	Quinidine Sulfate	200 mg	White	Tablet	Circle, Scored	Global Pharmaceutical
0115; 4400	Rauwolfia Serpentina	50 mg	Orange	Tablet	Circle	Global Pharmaceutical
0115; 4404	Rauwolfia Serpentina	100 mg	Orange	Tablet	Circle	Global Pharmaceutical
0115; 4428	Reserpine	0.25 mg	White	Tablet	Circle, Single-Scored	Richlyn Laboratories
0115; 4631	Sodium Fluoride	1 mg	Pink	Tablet, Chewable	Circle, Scored	Global Pharmaceutical
0115; 4652	Haponal	16.2 mg; 0.1037 mg; 0.0194 mg; 0.0065 mg	White	Tablet		Richlyn Laboratories
0115; 4652	Spasmolin	16.2 mg;	White	Tablet	Circle, Scored	Global Pharmaceutical
0115; 4711	Triple Sulfas	2.5 Gr; 2.5 Gr; 2.5 Gr		Tablet		Richlyn Laboratories
0115; 4714	Sulfadiazine	7.7 Gr		Tablet		Richlyn Laboratories
0115; 4714	Sulfadiazine	500 mg	White	Tablet	Circle, Scored	Global Pharmaceutical
0115; 4747	Sulfisoxazole	500 mg	White	Tablet	Circle, Scored	Global Pharmaceutical
0115; 4824	Thyroid	60 mg	Beige	Tablet	Circle	Global Pharmaceutical
0115; 4840	Triamcinolone	4 mg	White	Tablet		Global Pharmaceutical
0115; 4860	Trichlormethiazide	4 mg	Blue-Green	Tablet	Circle, Scored	Global Pharmaceutical
0115; 4871	Tripelennamine Hydrochloride	50 mg	Blue	Tablet	Circle, Scored	Global Pharmaceutical
0115; 7001	Pancrelipase	4500 units; 20,000 units; 25,000 units	White	Capsule		Global Pharmaceutical
0115; 7017	Minocycline Hydrochloride	50 mg	Olive/brown	Capsule		Global Pharmaceutical
0115; 7018	Minocycline Hydrochloride	100 mg	White/olive	Capsule		Global Pharmaceutical
0115; 7023	Lipram-Pn16	48000 U; 16000 U; 48000 U	Flesh	Capsule		Global Pharmaceutical
0115; 7024	Lipram-Cr20	66400 U; 20000 U; 75000 U	Brown/white	Capsule		Global Pharmaceutical
0115; 7035	Lipram 4500	20000 U; 4500 U; 25000 U	White	Capsule		Global Pharmaceutical
0115; 7036	Lipram-Cr10	33200 U; 10000 U; 37500 U	Brown/flesh	Capsule		Global Pharmaceutical
0115; 7040	Lipram-Pn10	30000 U; 10000 U; 30000 U	Natural/brown	Capsule		Global Pharmaceutical
0115; 7041	Lipram-Ul18	56500 U; 18000 U; 56500 U	Flesh/white	Capsule		Global Pharmaceutical
0115; 7042	Lipram-Ul12	39000 U; 12000 U; 39000 U	Natural/white	Capsule		Global Pharmaceutical
0115; 7043	Lipram-Ul20	65000 U; 20000 U; 65000 U	Brown	Capsule		Global Pharmaceutical
0115; 7054	Minocycline Hydrochloride	75 mg	Olive	Capsule		Global Pharmaceutical
0115; 7055	Lipram-Pn20	56000 U; 20000 U; 44000 U	Flesh/natural	Capsule		Global Pharmaceutical
0115; 7057	Lipram-Cr5	16600 U; 5000 U; 18750 U	Natural/white Opaque	Capsule		Global Pharmaceutical
0145; P200	Pacerone	400 mg	Light Yellow	Tablet	Oval, Scored	Upsher-Smith Laboratories
0282; V	Quinine Sulfate	325 mg	Natural	Capsule		Vintage Pharmaceuticals
0310; A	Mobidin	600 mg	Yellow	Tablet	Capsule-Shape, Compressed, Scored	Ascher
0321; US	Magsal	600 mg; 25 mg	Light Green	Tablet	Oval	U.S. Pharmaceutical
0364; NIFEDIPINE; 10;	Nifedipine	10 mg	Yellow	Capsule, Liquid Filled		Schein Pharmaceutical
0364; NIFEDIPINE; 20	Nifedipine	20 mg	Orange and Brown	Capsule, Liquid Filled		Schein Pharmaceutical
0430; WALLACE	Felbatol	400 mg	Yellow	Tablet	Capsule-Shape, Scored	Wallace Laboratories
0431; WALLACE	Felbatol	600 mg	Peach	Tablet	Capsule-Shape, Scored	Wallace Laboratories
0497; DYNACIN; 50 MG	Dynacin	50 mg	White	Capsule		Medicis Pharmaceutical
0498; DYNACIN; 100 MG	Dynacin	100 mg	Dark Gray and White	Capsule		Medicis Pharmaceutical
0499; DYNACIN; 75 MG	Dynacin	75 mg	Light Gray	Capsule		Medicis Pharmaceutical
0524; 0405;	Allopurinol	100 mg	White to Off-White	Tablet	Circle	Knoll Laboratories
0524; 0410	Allopurinol	300 mg	Orange; Peach	Tablet	Circle	Knoll Laboratories
0527; 0500	Aspirin Compound	3.5 Gr; 2.5 Gr; 0.5 Gr	Clear	Capsule		Lannett
0527; 0501	Aspirin Compound	3.5 Gr; 2.5 Gr; 0.5 Gr	Pink	Capsule		Lannett
0527; 0502	Acetaminophen	500 mg	Red and White	Capsule		Lannett
0527; 0504	B Complex Vitamin	1.5 mg; 2 mg; 0.1 mg; 1 mg; 10 mg	Red	Capsule		Lannett
0527; 0505	Disanthrol	100 mg; 30 mg	Red	Capsule		Lannett

IMPRINT	BRAND/GENERIC NAME	STRENGTH	COLOR	FORM	SHAPE	MANUFACTURER
0527; 0507	Ephedrine Sulfate	0.375 Gr	Pink	Capsule		Lannett
0527; 0508	Pentobarbital Sodium	100 mg	Yellow	Capsule		Lannett
0527; 0510	P-D-M	35 mg	Black	Capsule		Lannett
0527; 0511	Pentobarbital Sodium	3/4 grain	Yellow and Clear	Capsule		Lannett
0527; 0512	Ergocalciferol	50000 IU	Green	Capsule		Lannett
0527; 0512	Vitamin D	50000 IU	Green	Capsule		Lannett
0527; 0513	Sulfinpyrazone	200 mg	Orange	Capsule		Lannett
0527; 0514	Diphenhydramine Hydrochloride	50 mg	Pink	Capsule		Lannett
0527; 0515	Amobarbital Sodium	200 mg	Light Blue	Capsule		Lannett
0527; 0518	Lanabutazone Compound	100 mg; 100 mg; 150 mg		Capsule		Lannett
0527; 0519	Vitamin A	25000 IU		Capsule		Lannett
0527; 0520	Diphenylan Sodium	1.5 Gr		Capsule		Lannett
0527; 0521	A and D Vitamin	5000 IU; 400 IU		Capsule		Lannett
0527; 0524	Vitamin E	100 IU		Capsule		Lannett
0527; 0526	Abdcg Vitamin	5000 IU; 400 IU; 1 mg; 2 mg; 30 mg	Brown	Capsule		Lannett
0527; 0527	Vitamin A	50000 IU		Capsule		Lannett
0527; 0528	Diphenhydramine Hydrochloride	25 mg	Pink and Clear	Capsule		Lannett
0527; 0530	Vitamin E	200 IU		Capsule		Lannett
0527; 0531	Oxytetracycline Hydrochloride	250 mg	Clear Yellow	Capsule		Lannett
0527; 0534	Cyclandelate	200 mg	Orange	Capsule		Lannett
0527; 0535	Tribarb	0.5 Gr; 0.5 Gr; 0.5 Gr		Capsule		Lannett
0527; 0536	Vitamin E	400 IU		Capsule		Lannett
0527; 0537	Hydroxyzine Pamoate	100 mg	Dark Green and Gray	Capsule		Lannett
0527; 0538	Quinine Sulfate	5 Gr	White	Capsule		Lannett
0527; 0539	Rubraplex	2.5 mg; 2 mg; 0.5 mg; 1 mg; 20 mg; 5 mcg	Yellow and Pink	Capsule		Lannett
0527; 0540	Rufolex	200 mg; 0.25 mg; 5 mcg; 50 mg; 1 mg; 1.5 mg; 1.5 mg; 10 mg; 200 mg	Clear Pink	Capsule		Lannett
0527; 0541	Tetralan-500	500 mg	Black and Yellow	Capsule		Lannett
0527; 0542	Doxycycline Hyclate	50 mg		Capsule		Lannett
0527; 0543	Lanamins	5000 IU; 400 IU; 3 mg; 2.5 mg; 0.75 mg; 1.5 mcg; 50 mg; 20 mg; 80 mg; 61 mg; 13.4 mg; 0.05 mg; 1.5 mg; 1.4 mg; 1 mg; 7.5 mg; 5 mg; 3 IU	Maroon	Coated Tablet	Capsule-Shape	Lannett
0527; 0544	Secobarbital Sodium	100 mg	Reddish-Orange	Capsule		Lannett
0527; 0546	Secobarbital Sodium	0.75 Gr	Reddish-Orange	Capsule		Lannett
0527; 0547	Triasyn B	2 mg; 3 mg; 20 mg		Capsule		Lannett
0527; 0548	Lanabee-C	15 mg; 10 mg; 5 mg; 50 mg; 10 mg; 300 mg	Yellow and Green	Capsule		Lannett
0527; 0549	Phentermine Hydrochloride	30 mg	Yellow	Capsule		Lannett
0527; 0551	Zylan	5000 IU; 400 IU; 100 mg; 5 mg; 4 mcg; 5 mg; 2 mg; 10 mg; 30 mg	Red	Capsule	Oval	Lannett
0527; 0553	Doxycycline Hyclate	100 mg		Capsule		Lannett
0527; 0555	Multalan	5000 IU; 400 IU; 2.5 mg; 2.5 mg; 0.5 mg; 2 mcg; 50 mg; 20 mg; 5 mg	Yellow	Capsule		Lannett
0527; 0556	Disonate	100 mg	Amber	Capsule		Lannett
0527; 0557	Chloral Hydrate	500 mg	Green	Capsule	Oval	Lannett
0527; 0559	Lanophyllin GG	150 mg; 90 mg	Yellow and Clear	Capsule		Lannett
0527; 0559	Vitamin A	25000 IU		Capsule		Lannett
0527; 0560	Therapeutic Vitamin	10000 IU; 400 IU; 12.5 mg; 12.5 mg; 100 mg; 5 mg; 5 mcg; 25 mg; 200 mg	Red	Capsule		Lannett
0527; 0563	Cyclandelate	400 mg	Blue and White	Capsule		Lannett
0527; 0565	Penamp 250	250 mg		Capsule		Lannett
0527; 0566	Lanabarb	50 mg; 50 mg	Orange and Blue	Capsule		Lannett
0527; 0567	Lanabarb	100 mg; 100 mg	Orange and Blue	Capsule		Lannett
0527; 0569	Vitamin A	50,000 units		Capsule		Lannett
0527; 0572	Ferralyn Lanacaps	250 mg	Red and Clear	Timed-Release Capsule		Lannett
0527; 0575	Disonate	240 mg	Amber	Capsule		Lannett
0527; 0576	Tetralan-250	250 mg	White and Orange	Capsule		Lannett
0527; 0579	Hesperidin C	100 mg; 100 mg	Pink	Capsule		Lannett
0527; 0580	Procainamide Hydrochloride	250 mg	Yellow	Capsule		Lannett
0527; 0583	Penamp 500	500 mg		Capsule		Lannett
0527; 0586	Dicyclomine Hydrochloride	10 mg	Blue	Capsule		Lannett
0527; 0587	Procainamide Hydrochloride	500 mg	Yellow and Orange	Capsule		Lannett
0527; 0588	Vitamin A	10000 IU		Capsule		Lannett
0527; 0589	Dicyclomine Hydrochloride with Phenobarbital	10 mg; 15 mg	Blue and White	Capsule		Lannett
0527; 0591	Chlordiazepoxide Hydrochloride	5 mg	Green and Yellow	Capsule		Lannett

IMPRINT	BRAND/GENERIC NAME	STRENGTH	COLOR	FORM	SHAPE	MANUFACTURER
0527; 0592	Chlordiazepoxide Hydrochloride	10 mg	Green and Black	Capsule		Lannett
0527; 0593	Chlordiazepoxide Hydrochloride	25 mg	Green and White	Capsule		Lannett
0527; 0595	Propoxyphene Hydrochloride	65 mg	Pink	Capsule		Lannett
0527; 0597	Phentermine Hydrochloride	30 mg	Black	Capsule		Lannett
0527; 0618	Hydroxyzine Pamoate	25 mg	Dark Green and Light Green	Capsule		Lannett
0527; 0619	Hydroxyzine Pamoate	50 mg	Dark Green and White	Capsule		Lannett
0527; 0621	Phentermine Hydrochloride	30 mg	Green and Clear	Capsule		Lannett
0527; 0622	Phentermine Hydrochloride	30 mg	Brown and Clear	Capsule		Lannett
0527; 0623	Phentermine Hydrochloride	30 mg	Blue and Clear	Capsule		Lannett
0527; 0624	Phentermine Hydrochloride	30 mg	Red and Yellow	Capsule		Lannett
0527; 0625	P-D-M	35 mg	Yellow	Capsule		Lannett
0527; 0626	P-D-M	35 mg	Blue and Clear	Capsule		Lannett
0527; 0627	P-D-M	35 mg	Brown and Clear	Capsule		Lannett
0527; 0628	P-D-M	35 mg	Green and Clear	Capsule		Lannett
0527; 0631	Difuleron	150 mg; 100 mg	Light Green and Dark Green	Capsule		Lannett
0527; 0633	Triamazide	50 mg; 25 mg	Maroon and White	Capsule		Lannett
0527; 0637	Obalan	35 mg	Brown and Clear	Capsule		Lannett
0527; 0638	Obalan	35 mg	Red and Yellow	Capsule		Lannett
0527; 0639	Obalan	35 mg	Green and Clear	Capsule		Lannett
0527; 0900	Acetaminophen and Codeine No. 3	30 mg; 300 mg		Tablet		Lannett
0527; 0903	Codalan No. 1	8 mg; 150 mg; 230 mg; 30 mg	Orange	Tablet		Lannett
0527; 0904	Codalan No. 2	15 mg; 150 mg; 230 mg; 30 mg	White	Tablet		Lannett
0527; 0905	Codalan No. 3	30 mg; 150 mg; 230 mg; 30 mg	Green	Tablet		Lannett
0527; 0908	Papaverine Hydrochloride	60 mg		Tablet		Lannett
0527; 0909	Papaverine Hydrochloride	100 mg		Tablet		Lannett
0527; 0912	Papaverine Hydrochloride	200 mg		Tablet		Lannett
0527; 0914	Paverolan Lanacaps	150 mg	Brown and Clear	Timed-Release Capsule		Lannett
0527; 1000	Spironolactone	25 mg		Tablet		Lannett
0527; 1001	Dipyridamole	25 mg		Coated Tablet		Lannett
0527; 1003	Warfarin Sodium	5 mg	Peach	Tablet		Lannett
0527; 1004	Aminophylline	100 mg		Tablet		Lannett
0527; 1005	Furosemide	20 mg		Tablet		Lannett
0527; 1006	Aminophylline	200 mg		Tablet		Lannett
0527; 1008	Furosemide	40 mg		Tablet		Lannett
0527; 1009	Ascorbic Acid	250 mg		Tablet		Lannett
0527; 1010	Ascorbic Acid	500 mg		Tablet		Lannett
0527; 1011	Ammonium Chloride	7.5 Gr	Red	Enteric-Coated Tablet		Lannett
0527; 1012	Acetaminophen	5 Gr		Tablet		Lannett
0527; 1013	Veltane	4 mg		Tablet		Lannett
0527; 1015	Ascorbic Acid	25 mg		Tablet		Lannett
0527; 1016	Ascorbic Acid	50 mg		Tablet		Lannett
0527; 1017	Ascorbic Acid	100 mg		Tablet		Lannett
0527; 1018	Aspirin	5 Gr	White	Tablet		Lannett
0527; 1019	Aspirin	5 Gr	Pink	Tablet		Lannett
0527; 1020	Aspirin	5 Gr	Green	Tablet		Lannett
0527; 1021	Aspirin Children's	1 Gr		Tablet		Lannett
0527; 1022	Aspirin Compound	3.5 Gr; 2.5 Gr; 0.5 Gr	White	Tablet		Lannett
0527; 1023	Aspirin Compound	3.5 Gr; 2.5 Gr; 0.5 Gr	Pink	Tablet		Lannett
0527; 1024	Aspirin Compound	3.5 Gr; 2.5 Gr; 0.5 Gr	Green	Tablet		Lannett
0527; 1025	Atropine and Phenobarbital	0.33 Gr; 0.25 Gr	Pink	Tablet		Lannett
0527; 1026	Belladonna and Phenobarbital	0.25 Gr; 0.125 Gr		Tablet		Lannett
0527; 1027	B Complex Vitamin	1.5 mg; 2 mg; 0.2 mg; 1 mg; 10 mg		Tablet		Lannett
0527; 1028	Magnatril	260 mg; 130 mg; 455 mg		Tablet, Chewable		Lannett
0527; 1029	Laniazid	50 mg		Tablet		Lannett
0527; 1031	Daily Multiple Vitamin	5000 IU; 400 IU; 1 mcg; 2 mg; 2.5 mg; 1 mg; 50 mg; 1 mg; 20 mg	Red	Coated Tablet		Lannett
0527; 1032	Allopurinol	100 mg	White	Tablet		Lannett
0527; 1033	Dipyridamole	75 mg		Coated Tablet		Lannett
0527; 1034	Calcium Gluconate	10 Gr		Tablet		Lannett
0527; 1036	Allopurinol	300 mg	Peach	Tablet		Lannett
0527; 1037	Furalan	100 mg		Tablet		Lannett
0527; 1039	Ephedrine-Phenobarbital Compound	0.375 Gr; 0.25 Gr	Yellow	Tablet		Lannett
0527; 1040	Colchicine	0.1 Gr		Tablet		Lannett
0527; 1041	Daily Multiple Vitamin with Iron	15 mg; 5000 IU; 400 IU; 1 mcg; 2 mg; 2.5 mg; 1 mg; 50 mg; 1 mg; 20 mg	Yellow	Coated Tablet		Lannett
0527; 1042	Ferrous Sulfate	5 Gr	Green	Tablet		Lannett
0527; 1043	Lanorinal	50 mg; 325 mg; 40 mg	White	Tablet		Lannett
0527; 1045	Chlorpromazine Hydrochloride	50 mg		Coated Tablet		Lannett
0527; 1047	Hydroxyzine Hydrochloride	10 mg	Light Lavender	Coated Tablet		Lannett
0527; 1048	Chlorpromazine Hydrochloride	100 mg		Coated Tablet		Lannett

IMPRINT	BRAND/GENERIC NAME	STRENGTH	COLOR	FORM	SHAPE	MANUFACTURER
0527; 1049	Niacinamide	100 mg		Tablet		Lannett
0527; 1050	Acetazolamide	250 mg		Tablet	Double-Scored	Lannett
0527; 1056	Chlorpromazine Hydrochloride	10 mg		Coated Tablet		Lannett
0527; 1058	Seralazide	15 mg; 0.1 mg; 25 mg		Tablet		Lannett
0527; 1059	Chlorpromazine Hydrochloride	25 mg		Coated Tablet		Lannett
0527; 1061	Erythromycin Stearate	250 mg		Coated Tablet		Lannett
0527; 1062	Chlorpromazine Hydrochloride	200 mg		Coated Tablet		Lannett
0527; 1063	Hydroxyzine Hydrochloride	25 mg	Lavender	Coated Tablet		Lannett
0527; 1064	Warfarin Sodium	2 mg	Lavender	Tablet		Lannett
0527; 1065	Sulfinpyrazone	100 mg		Tablet		Lannett
0527; 1067	Sodium Bicarbonate	325 mg		Tablet		Lannett
0527; 1068	Sodium Bicarbonate	650 mg		Tablet		Lannett
0527; 1071	Sodium Salicylate	5 Gr	Red	Enteric-Coated Tablet		Lannett
0527; 1072	Warfarin Sodium	2.5 mg	Green	Tablet		Lannett
0527; 1074	Sulfadiazine	500 mg		Tablet		Lannett
0527; 1075	Hydroserpalan	50 mg; 0.125 mg		Tablet		Lannett
0527; 1078	Methyltestosterone	10 mg		Tablet		Lannett
0527; 1079	Thiamine Hydrochloride	5 mg		Tablet		Lannett
0527; 1080	Thiamine Hydrochloride	10 mg		Tablet		Lannett
0527; 1081	Thyroid	0.25 Gr		Tablet		Lannett
0527; 1082	Thyroid	0.5 Gr		Tablet		Lannett
0527; 1083	Thyroid	1 Gr		Tablet		Lannett
0527; 1084	Thyroid	2 Gr		Tablet		Lannett
0527; 1085	Thyroid	5 Gr		Tablet		Lannett
0527; 1086	Probalan	500 mg		Tablet		Lannett
0527; 1087	Promethazine Hydrochloride	25 mg	White	Tablet		Lannett
0527; 1089	Hydroxyzine Hydrochloride	50 mg	Purple	Coated Tablet		Lannett
0527; 1092	Laniazid	100 mg		Tablet		Lannett
0527; 1093	Methylprednisolone	4 mg		Tablet	Oval	Lannett
0527; 1097	Lanacillin VK	500 mg		Tablet		Lannett
0527; 1098	Folic Acid	1 mg		Tablet		Lannett
0527; 1099	Trichlorex	4 mg	Blue	Tablet		Lannett
0527; 1101	Trofedrin	2.5 mg; 60 mg		Tablet		Lannett
0527; 1102	Prelan F.A.	1 mg; 4000 IU; 0.5 mg; 2 mg; 10 mg; 3 mg; 2 mcg; 400 IU; 50 mg; 200 mg; 30 mg	Pink	Coated Tablet		Lannett
0527; 1104	Calcium Lactate	10 Gr		Tablet		Lannett
0527; 1105	Sufedrin	60 mg	White	Tablet		Lannett
0527; 1106	Spironolactone with Hydrochlorothiazide	25 mg; 25 mg		Tablet		Lannett
0527; 1107	Isoxsuprine Hydrochloride	20 mg		Tablet		Lannett
0527; 1108	Propylthiouracil	50 mg		Tablet		Lannett
0527; 1111	Meclizine Hydrochloride	12.5 mg	Blue and White	Tablet	Oval, Multi-Layered, Scored	Lannett
0527; 1112	Metronidazole	250 mg		Tablet		Lannett
0527; 1114	Hydrochlorulan	25 mg	Peach	Tablet		Lannett
0527; 1115	Promethazine Hydrochloride	12.5 mg	Orange	Tablet		Lannett
0527; 1116	Sodium Chloride	16.6 Gr		Tablet		Lannett
0527; 1117	Isoxsuprine Hydrochloride	10 mg		Tablet		Lannett
0527; 1119	Quinidine Sulfate	3 Gr		Tablet		Lannett
0527; 1121	Ferrous Sulfate	5 Gr	Red	Coated Tablet		Lannett
0527; 1122	Sodium Salicylate	10 Gr	Red	Enteric-Coated Tablet		Lannett
0527; 1123	Dextroamphetamine Sulfate	15 mg	Green	Tablet	Double-Scored	Lannett
0527; 1126	Calcium Lactate	5 Gr		Tablet		Lannett
0527; 1127	Bisacodyl	5 mg		Enteric-Coated Tablet		Lannett
0527; 1130	Apacomp	3.5 Gr; 2.5 Gr; 0.5 Gr	Green	Tablet		Lannett
0527; 1133	Therapeutic Vitamin	10000 IU; 400 IU; 12.5 mg; 12.5 mg; 100 mg; 5 mg; 5 mcg; 25 mg; 200 mg	Red	Coated Tablet	Capsule-Shape	Lannett
0527; 1134	Bellafedrol A-H	12.5 mg; 1 mg; 2.5 mg; 6 mg	Purple	Tablet		Lannett
0527; 1135	Thiamine Hydrochloride	25 mg		Tablet		Lannett
0527; 1136	Thiamine Hydrochloride	50 mg		Tablet		Lannett
0527; 1137	Thiamine Hydrochloride	100 mg		Tablet		Lannett
0527; 1138	Amphetamine Sulfate	5 mg		Tablet		Lannett
0527; 1139	Amphetamine Sulfate	10 mg		Tablet	Double-Scored	Lannett
0527; 1140	Methyltestosterone	25 mg		Tablet		Lannett
0527; 1141	Lanacillin VK	250 mg		Tablet		Lannett
0527; 1144	Promethazine Hydrochloride	50 mg	Pink	Tablet		Lannett
0527; 1146	Chlorzoxazone and Acetaminophen	250 mg; 300 mg		Tablet	Six-Sided	Lannett
0527; 1148	Gylanphen	0.125 Gr; 0.1 Gr; 2 Gr; 1 Gr; 1 Gr		Tablet		Lannett
0527; 1151	Acetaminophen with Phenobarbital	16 mg; 325 mg		Tablet		Lannett
0527; 1154	Niacinamide	500 mg		Tablet		Lannett
0527; 1156	Niacin	100 mg		Tablet		Lannett
0527; 1157	Hydralazine Hydrochloride	50 mg	Light Blue	Tablet		Lannett
0527; 1159	Dimenhydrinate	50 mg	Yellow	Tablet		Lannett
0527; 1160	Furalan	50 mg		Tablet		Lannett
0527; 1162	Tolbutamide	0.5 GM		Tablet		Lannett
0527; 1163	Phenazodine	200 mg	Maroon	Coated Tablet		Lannett

IMPRINT	BRAND/GENERIC NAME	STRENGTH	COLOR	FORM	SHAPE	MANUFACTURER
0527; 1167	Spasmophen	15 mg; 0.1037 mg; 0.0194 mg; 0.0065 mg		Tablet		Lannett
0527; 1169	Propantheline Bromide	15 mg		Coated Tablet		Lannett
0527; 1170	Lofene	2.5 mg; 25 mcg		Tablet		Lannett
0527; 1171	Papaverine Hydrochloride	30 mg		Tablet		Lannett
0527; 1172	Dipyridamole	50 mg		Coated Tablet		Lannett
0527; 1173	Cortisone Acetate	25 mg		Tablet		Lannett
0527; 1174	Aspirin	5 Gr	Orange	Enteric-Coated Tablet		Lannett
0527; 1175	Aspirin	10 Gr	Yellow	Enteric-Coated Tablet		Lannett
0527; 1176	Serpalan	0.1 mg		Tablet		Lannett
0527; 1177	Serpalan	0.25 mg		Tablet		Lannett
0527; 1179	Butabarbital Sodium	0.25 Gr	Lavender	Tablet		Lannett
0527; 1180	Butabarbital Sodium	30 mg	Green	Tablet		Lannett
0527; 1181	Meclizine Hydrochloride	25 mg	Yellow and White	Tablet	Oval, Multi-Layered, Scored	Lannett
0527; 1182	Niacin	25 mg		Tablet		Lannett
0527; 1183	Niacin	50 mg		Tablet		Lannett
0527; 1184	Butabarbital Sodium	100 mg	Pink	Tablet		Lannett
0527; 1185	Dicyclomine Hydrochloride	20 mg		Tablet		Lannett
0527; 1186	Hydrocortisone	20 mg		Tablet		Lannett
0527; 1187	Hydralazine Hydrochloride	25 mg	Dark Blue	Tablet		Lannett
0527; 1192	S-A-C	150 mg; 230 mg; 30 mg	Orange	Tablet	Capsule-Shape	Lannett
0527; 1193	Lanased	0.03 mg; 0.03 mg; 40.8 mg; 5.4 mg; 18.1 mg; 4.5 mg	Blue	Tablet		Lannett
0527; 1194	Pyridoxine Hydrochloride	10 mg		Tablet		Lannett
0527; 1195	Pyridoxine Hydrochloride	25 mg		Tablet		Lannett
0527; 1196	Pyridoxine Hydrochloride	50 mg		Tablet		Lannett
0527; 1198	P-I-N Forte	100 mg; 5 mg	Orange	Tablet		Lannett
0527; 1199	Salagen	500 mg	Green Speckled	Tablet	Capsule-Shape, Scored	Lannett
0527; 1200	Prednisone	5 mg		Tablet		Lannett
0527; 1201	Prednisolone	5 mg	Orange	Tablet		Lannett
0527; 1202	Pentylan	10 mg	Light Green	Tablet		Lannett
0527; 1204	Orphenadrine Citrate	100 mg		Tablet		Lannett
0527; 1205	Phenetron Lanatabs	8 mg	Yellow	Timed-Release Tablet		Lannett
0527; 1207	Phenetron	4 mg	Yellow	Tablet		Lannett
0527; 1208	Pentylan	20 mg	Green	Tablet		Lannett
0527; 1210	Neomycin Sulfate	0.5 GM		Tablet		Lannett
0527; 1211	Phenazodine	100 mg	Maroon	Coated Tablet		Lannett
0527; 1212	Methenamine Mandelate	0.5 G	Brown	Enteric-Coated Tablet	Capsule-Shape	Lannett
0527; 1216	Phenetron Lanatabs	12 mg	Orange	Timed-Release Tablet		Lannett
0527; 1217	Lanatrate	1 mg; 100 mg	Peach	Tablet		Lannett
0527; 1218	Aspirin Buffered	5 Gr		Tablet		Lannett
0527; 1220	Phenetron Compound	390 mg; 32.4 mg; 2 mg	Red	Tablet		Lannett
0527; 1221	Hydrochlorulan	50 mg	Peach	Tablet		Lannett
0527; 1223	Hydralazine Hydrochloride	10 mg	Yellow	Tablet		Lannett
0527; 1224	Meprobamate	400 mg		Tablet		Lannett
0527; 1225	Niacinamide	50 mg		Tablet		Lannett
0527; 1228	Digoxin	0.25 mg		Tablet		Lannett
0527; 1229	Chlorulan	250 mg		Tablet		Lannett
0527; 1230	Chlorulan	500 mg		Tablet		Lannett
0527; 1231	Primidone	250 mg		Tablet		Lannett
0527; 1235	Prelan	4000 IU; 0.5 mg; 2 mg; 10 mg; 3 mg; 2 mcg; 400 IU; 50 mg; 200 mg; 30 mg	Orange	Coated Tablet	Capsule-Shape	Lannett
0527; 1240	Tripelennamine Hydrochloride	50 mg	Blue-Green	Tablet		Lannett
0527; 1243	Neostigmine Bromide	15 mg		Tablet		Lannett
0527; 1244	Ferrous Gluconate	5 Gr	Green	Coated Tablet		Lannett
0527; 1245	Salicylamide	5 Gr	Pink	Tablet		Lannett
0527; 1248	Isosorbide Dinitrate	10 mg		Tablet		Lannett
0527; 1249	Nycralan	10 mg; 10 Gr		Tablet		Lannett
0527; 1250	Meprobamate	200 mg		Tablet		Lannett
0527; 1252	Obalan	35 mg	Green	Tablet		Lannett
0527; 1253	Isosorbide Dinitrate	5 mg		Tablet		Lannett
0527; 1254	Sulfisoxazole	0.5 GM		Tablet		Lannett
0527; 1256	Isosorbide Dinitrate	5 mg		Tablet		Lannett
0527; 1257	Arithmin	100 mg	Orange	Tablet		Lannett
0527; 1258	Arithmin	200 mg	White	Tablet		Lannett
0527; 1259	Bethanechol Chloride	5 mg		Tablet		Lannett
0527; 1260	Bethanechol Chloride	10 mg	Pink	Tablet		Lannett
0527; 1261	Bethanechol Chloride	25 mg	Yellow	Tablet		Lannett
0527; 1262	Prednisone	20 mg		Tablet		Lannett
0527; 1263	Niacin	500 mg		Tablet		Lannett
0527; 1264	Cebralan M.T.	15 mg; 10 mg; 2 mg; 10 mg; 100 mg; 7.5 mcg; 150 mg; 5 IU; 10000 IU; 400 IU; 1 mg; 15 mg; 0.15 mg; 1 mg; 5 mg; 1.5 mg	Orange	Coated Tablet		Lannett
0527; 1265	Methenamine Mandelate	1 G	Purple	Enteric-Coated Tablet	Oval	Lannett
0527; 1267	Isosorbide Dinitrate	2.5 mg		Tablet		Lannett
0527; 1268	Trihexyphenidyl Hydrochloride	5 mg		Tablet		Lannett
0527; 1269	P-D-M	35 mg	Speckled	Tablet	Oval	Lannett
0527; 1270	P-D-M	35 mg	Pink	Tablet		Lannett

IMPRINT	BRAND/GENERIC NAME	STRENGTH	COLOR	FORM	SHAPE	MANUFACTURER
0527; 1271	P-D-M	35 mg	Yellow	Tablet		Lannett
0527; 1272	P-D-M	35 mg	Gray	Tablet		Lannett
0527; 1273	P-D-M	35 mg	White	Tablet		Lannett
0527; 1274	P-D-M	35 mg	Green and White Speckled	Tablet		Lannett
0527; 1552	Lanorinal	50 mg; 325 mg; 40 mg	Light Green and Green	Capsule		Lannett
0527; 3006	Phenetron Lanacaps	8 mg	Blue-Green and Clear	Timed-Release Capsule		Lannett
0527; 3007	Phenetron Lanacaps	12 mg	Blue-Green and Clear	Timed-Release Capsule		Lannett
0527; 3010	Prochlorbid Lanacaps	10 mg; 5 mg		Timed-Release Capsule		Lannett
0554; M; 5 MG	Oxycodone Hydrochloride	5 mg	Opaque Brown and Light Brown	Capsule		Mallinckrodt
0665; 1393	Reserpine, Hydralazine and Hydrochlorothiazide	0.1 mg; 25 mg; 15 mg	White	Tablet	Circle, Scored	Solvay Pharmaceuticals
0665; 4001	Medroxyprogesterone	10 mg	White	Tablet	Circle, Scored	Novartis Generics
0665; 4001	Medroxyprogesterone	10 mg	White	Tablet	Circle, Scored, Compressed	Warner Chilcott
0665; 4120;	Valproic Acid	250 mg	Orange	Capsule, Liquid Filled	Oval	Novartis Generics
0665; 4120	Valproic Acid	250 mg	Orange	Capsule		Solvay Pharmaceuticals
0665; 4140	Hydralazine and Hydrochlorothiazide	25 mg; 25 mg	Light Green	Capsule		H.L. Moore
0665; 4160	Lithium Carbonate	300 mg	White	Capsule		Novartis Generics
0665; 4160	Lithium Carbonate	300 mg	White	Capsule		Solvay Pharmaceuticals
0822; 0150	Hydroserpine No. 2	50 mg; 0.125 mg		Tablet		Knoll Pharmaceutical
0822; 0430	Butalbital with Aspirin and Caffeine	50 mg; 325 mg; 40 mg	White	Tablet	Circle	Knoll Pharmaceutical
0822; 0432	Fortabs	325 mg; 40 mg; 50 mg	White	Tablet		Knoll Pharmaceutical
0822; 0545	Hydrochlorothiazide	25 mg	Peach	Tablet		Knoll Pharmaceutical
0822; 0550	Hydrochlorothiazide	50 mg	Peach	Tablet		Knoll Pharmaceutical
0822; 0576	Meclizine Hydrochloride	25 mg	Pink	Tablet, Chewable	Circle, Scored	Knoll Pharmaceutical
0822; 0735	Triprolidine Hydrochloride and Pseudoephedrine Hydrochloride	2.5 mg; 60 mg		Tablet		Cenci Labs
0822; 0841	Sodium Fluoride	2.2 mg		Tablet		Cenci Labs
0822; 1	Meprobamate	400 mg	White	Tablet		Knoll Pharmaceutical
0822; 6	Apc with Butalbital	200 mg; 130 mg; 40 mg; 50 mg		Capsule		Knoll Pharmaceutical
0822; 1259	L-Thyroxine Sodium	0.1 mg	Yellow	Tablet		Knoll Pharmaceutical
0822; 1530	L-Thyroxine Sodium	0.2 mg	Pink	Tablet		Knoll Pharmaceutical
0822; 1531	L-Thyroxine Sodium	0.3 mg	Green	Tablet		Knoll Pharmaceutical
0822; 2000	Dicyclomine Hydrochloride	10 mg		Capsule		Knoll Pharmaceutical
0822; 2005	Dicyclomine Hydrochloride	20 mg	Blue	Tablet		Knoll Pharmaceutical
0822; 4075	Uni Lom	2.5 mg; 0.025 mg	White	Tablet		Knoll Pharmaceutical
0822; 0735	Triprolidine Hydrochloride with Pseudoephedrine Hydrochloride	2.5 mg; 60 mg	White	Tablet		Knoll Pharmaceutical
0822; 0841	Sodium Fluoride	2.2 mg	Pink	Tablet, Chewable	Circle, Scored	Knoll Pharmaceutical
0832; 2C	Diazepam	2 mg	White	Tablet	Flat, Beveled Edge, Compressed, Scored	Rosemont Pharmaceutical
0832; 5C	Diazepam	5 mg	Yellow	Tablet	Flat, Beveled Edge, Compressed, Scored	Rosemont Pharmaceutical
0832; 10C	Diazepam	10 mg	Light Blue	Tablet	Flat, Beveled Edge, Compressed, Scored	Rosemont Pharmaceutical
0993;	Multiple Symptom Cough/cold	250 mg; 10 mg; 30 mg; 100 mg		Gel/jelly		Leiner Health Products
0993;	Multiple Symptom Cough/cold	250 mg; 10 mg; 30 mg; 100 mg		Gel/jelly		Scherer Laboratories
1	Amphedex TDC Paracotes	15 mg		Capsule		Paddock Labs
1	Lo-Ten	0.1 mg; 25 mg; 15 mg		Tablet		Teva Pharmaceuticals
1	Metoprolol Tartrate	25 mg	White	Tablet	Circle	Caraco Pharmaceutical
1	Nitrogard	1 mg	Off-White	Sustained-Release Tablet	Circle, Standard Convex	Forest Pharmaceuticals
1	Nitrotab	0.3 mg	White	Tablet	Circle	Able Laboratories
1/90; JC; E2/N; OM	Prefest Estradiol/norgestimate	1 mg; 0.09 mg	White	Tablet		Monarch Pharmaceuticals
1; 274	Clonazepam	1 mg	Blue	Tablet	Circle, Scored	Caraco Pharmaceutical
1; 4036;	Estazolam	1 mg	White	Tablet	Square, Flat-Faced, Beveled-Edge, Scored	Ivax Pharmaceuticals
1; JC; E2; OM	Prefest Estradiol	1 mg	Pink	Tablet		Monarch Pharmaceuticals
1; R	Terazosin Hydrochloride	1 mg	Beige	Capsule		Ranbaxy Pharmaceuticals
2	Amphedex TDC Paracotes	10 mg		Capsule		Paddock Labs
2	Detrol LA	2 mg	Blue-Green with White Ink	Extended-Release Capsule		Pharmacia & Upjohn
2	Nitrogard	2 mg	Off-White	Sustained-Release Tablet	Circle, Standard Convex	Forest Pharmaceuticals
2	Nitrotab	0.4 mg	White	Tablet	Circle	Able Laboratories
2; 93; 50	Acetaminophen and Codeine No. 2	300 mg; 15 mg	White	Tablet	Circle, Flat, Beveled Edge	Teva Pharmaceuticals
2; 275	Clonazepam	2 mg	White	Tablet	Circle, Scored	Caraco Pharmaceutical
2; 4037;	Estazolam	2 mg	Salmon	Tablet	Square, Flat-Faced, Beveled-Edge, Scored	Ivax Pharmaceuticals
2; OB; AC15	Acetaminophen and Codeine	300 mg; 15 mg	White	Tablet	Flat, Beveled	Medicopharma
2; R	Terazosin Hydrochloride	2 mg	Yellow	Capsule		Ranbaxy Pharmaceuticals
2; VALIUM; R; ROCHE	Valium	2 mg	White	Tablet	Circle, Scored	Roche Products
2 1/2; U; 121	Loniten	2.5 mg	White	Tablet	Circle, Scored	Pharmacia & Upjohn
3	Nitrogard	3 mg	Off-White	Sustained-Release Tablet	Circle, Standard Convex	Forest Pharmaceuticals
3	Nitroglycerin	0.3 mg	White	Tablet		Endo Laboratories
3	Nitrotab	0.6 mg	White	Tablet	Circle	Able Laboratories

IMPRINT	BRAND/GENERIC NAME	STRENGTH	COLOR	FORM	SHAPE	MANUFACTURER
3; 93; 150	Acetaminophen and Codeine No. 3	300 mg; 30 mg	White	Tablet	Circle, Flat Beveled Edge	Teva Pharmaceuticals
3; 93; 150	Acetaminophen and Codeine No. 3	300 mg; 30 mg	White	Tablet	Circle, Flat Beveled Edge	Udl Laboratories
3; OB; AC3	Acetaminophen and Codeine	300 mg; 30 mg	White	Tablet	Flat, Beveled	Medicopharma
3M; 107;	Alu-Tab	500 mg	Green	Tablet		3m Pharmaceuticals
3M; 221	Norflex	100 mg	White	Tablet	Circle	3m Pharmaceuticals
3M; 221	Orphenadrine Citrate ER	100 mg	White	Extended-Release Tablet	Circle	Mylan Pharmaceuticals
3M; 342	Theolair	125 mg	White	Tablet	Circle, Scored	3m Pharmaceuticals
3M; ALU-CAP;	Alu-Cap	400 mg	Red and Green	Capsule		3m Pharmaceuticals
3M; SR; 200	Theolair-SR	200 mg	White	Sustained-Release Tablet	Circle, Scored	3m Pharmaceuticals
3M; SR; 250;	Theolair-SR	250 mg	White	Sustained-Release Tablet	Circle, Scored	3m Pharmaceuticals
3M; SR; 300;	Theolair-SR	300 mg	White	Sustained-Release Tablet	Oval, Scored	3m Pharmaceuticals
3M; SR; 500;	Theolair-SR	500 mg	White	Sustained-Release Tablet	Capsule-Shape, Scored	3m Pharmaceuticals
3M; THEOLAIR; 250	Theolair	250 mg	White	Tablet	Capsule-Shape, Scored	3m Pharmaceuticals
3M; TITRALAC;	Titralac	420 mg	White	Tablet, Chewable	Circle	3m Pharmaceuticals
3M; TR; 50	Tambocor	50 mg	White	Tablet	Circle	3m Pharmaceuticals
3M; TR; 100	Tambocor	100 mg	White	Tablet	Circle, Scored	3m Pharmaceuticals
3M; TR; 150	Tambocor	150 mg	White	Tablet	Oval, Scored	3m Pharmaceuticals
3M; UREX	Urex	1 G	White	Tablet	Capsule-Shape, Scored	3m Pharmaceuticals
4	Bisacodyl	5 mg	Yellow and Orange	Enteric-Coated Tablet		Paddock Labs
4	Detrol LA	4 mg	Blue with White Ink	Extended-Release Capsule		Pharmacia & Upjohn
4	Ibuprofen	400 mg	White	Coated Tablet	Circle	Norton, H.N.
4	Ibuprofen	400 mg	White	Coated Tablet	Circle	Purepac Pharmaceutical
4	Nitroglycerin	0.4 mg	White	Tablet		Endo Laboratories
4; 93; 350	Acetaminophen and Codeine No. 4	300 mg; 60 mg	White	Tablet	Circle, Flat Beveled Edge	Teva Pharmaceuticals
4; 93; 350	Acetaminophen and Codeine No. 4	300 mg; 60 mg	White	Tablet	Circle, Flat Beveled Edge	Udl Laboratories
4; 717; COPLEY	Guanabenz Acetate	4 mg	Peach	Tablet	Square	Copley Pharmaceutical
4; OB; AC6	Acetaminophen and Codeine	300 mg; 60 mg	White	Tablet	Flat, Beveled	Medicopharma
5	Aspirin	325 mg	White	Enteric-Coated Tablet		Paddock Labs
5	Buspirone Hydrochloride	5 mg	White	Tablet	Circle	Amide Pharmaceuticals
5	Buspirone Hydrochloride	5 mg	White	Tablet	Round, Bisected Scored	Major Pharmaceutical
5	Citalopram Hydrobromide	10 mg	Peach	Tablet	Circle	Caraco Pharmaceutical
5	Rhinspec	300 mg; 100 mg; 5 mg	Pink	Tablet		Teva Pharmaceuticals
5	Zyprexa Zydis	5 mg	Yellow	Disintegrating Tablet	Circle	Eli Lilly
5; ARICEPT	Aricept Odt	5 mg	White	Disintegrating Tablet		Eisai
5; ARICEPT	Aricept Odt	5 mg	White	Disintegrating Tablet		Pfizer
5 MG; WATSON 369	Loxapine Succinate	5 mg	White	Capsule		Watson Laboratories
5; R	Sotret	10 mg	Light Pink	Capsule		Ranbaxy Pharmaceuticals
5; R	Terazosin Hydrochloride	5 mg	Red	Capsule		Ranbaxy Pharmaceuticals
5; VALIUM; R; ROCHE	Valium	5 mg	Yellow	Tablet	Circle, Scored	Roche Products
6	Bevitone	20 mg; 3 mcg; 150 mg; 5 mg; 20 mg	Pink	Tablet		Teva Pharmaceuticals
6	Ibuprofen	600 mg	White	Coated Tablet	Oval	Norton, H.N.
6	Ibuprofen	600 mg	White	Coated Tablet	Oval	Purepac Pharmaceutical
6	Nitroglycerin	0.6 mg	White	Tablet		Endo Laboratories
6; R	Sotret	20 mg	Maroon	Capsule		Ranbaxy Pharmaceuticals
7	Acetaminophen	325 mg	White	Tablet		Paddock Labs
7	Luride	1 mg		Tablet, Chewable		Colgate Oral Pharmaceuticals
7; R	Sotret	40 mg	Yellow	Capsule		Ranbaxy Pharmaceuticals
7.5; DF	Enablex	7.5 mg	White	Tablet, Extended Release	Circle	Novartis Pharmaceuticals
8	Aspirin, Enteric Coated	81 mg	Yellow	Enteric-Coated Tablet	Circle	Time Cap Labs
8	Ibuprofen	800 mg	White	Coated Tablet	Oblong	Norton, H.N.
8	Ibuprofen	800 mg	White	Coated Tablet	Oval	Purepac Pharmaceutical
8; 711; COPLEY	Guanabenz Acetate	8 mg	Peach	Tablet	Square	Copley Pharmaceutical
9; 3; 27	Torsemide	5 mg	White to Off-White	Tablet	Oval, Scored	Teva Pharmaceuticals
9; 3; 28	Torsemide	10 mg	White to Off-White	Tablet	Oval, Scored	Teva Pharmaceuticals
9; 3; 29	Torsemide	20 mg	White to Off-White	Tablet	Oval, Scored	Teva Pharmaceuticals
9; 3; 30	Torsemide	100 mg	White to Off-White	Tablet	Oval	Teva Pharmaceuticals
9; 3; 72; 22	Fosinopril Sodium	10 mg	White to Off-White	Tablet	Capsule-Shape	Teva Pharmaceuticals
9; 3; 7127	Torsemide	5 mg	White to Off-White	Tablet	Oval, Scored	Teva Pharmaceuticals
9; 3; 7128	Torsemide	10 mg	White to Off-White	Tablet	Oval, Scored	Teva Pharmaceuticals
9; 3; 7129	Torsemide	20 mg	White to Off-White	Tablet	Oval, Scored	Teva Pharmaceuticals
9; 3; 7130	Torsemide	100 mg	White to Off-White	Tablet	Oval, Scored	Teva Pharmaceuticals
9; 3; 7159	Pergolide Mesylate	0.25 mg	Mottled Green	Tablet	Capsule-Shape, Scored	Teva Pharmaceuticals
9; 3; 7160	Pergolide Mesylate	0.05 mg	Ivory	Tablet	Capsule-Shape, Scored	Teva Pharmaceuticals
9; 3; 7161	Pergolide Mesylate	1 mg	Mottled Pink	Tablet	Capsule-Shape, Scored	Teva Pharmaceuticals
10	Buspirone Hydrochloride	10 mg	White	Tablet	Circle	Amide Pharmaceuticals
10	Buspirone Hydrochloride	10 mg	White	Tablet	Round, Bisected Scored	Major Pharmaceutical
10	Zyprexa Zydis	10 mg	Yellow	Disintegrating Tablet	Circle	Eli Lilly
10;	Ceenu	10 mg	Two-Tone White	Capsule		Bristol-Myers Oncology
10/100; SP; 341	Parcopa	10 mg; 100 mg	Blue	Disintegrating Tablet	Circle, Flat-Faced, Scored	Schwarz Pharma
10 300; TP	Xodol	10 mg; 300 mg	White	Tablet	Capsule-Shape	Teamm Pharmaceuticals
10; 1362	Yellow Capsule	25 mg	Yellow	Capsule		Pdk Labs
ANDRX LOGO 10	Altoprev	10 mg	Dark Orange	Tablet, Extended Release	Circle	Andrx Pharmaceuticals
10; ARICEPT	Aricept Odt	10 mg	Yellow	Disintegrating Tablet		Eisai
10; ARICEPT	Aricept Odt	10 mg	Yellow	Disintegrating Tablet		Pfizer

IMPRINT	BRAND/GENERIC NAME	STRENGTH	COLOR	FORM	SHAPE	MANUFACTURER
10; GILEAD; LIVER SYMBOL	Hepsera	10 mg	White	Tablet		Gilead Sciences
10 MG; WATSON 370	Loxapine Succinate	10 mg	White and Yellow	Capsule		Watson Laboratories
10; R	Terazosin Hydrochloride	10 mg	Blue	Capsule		Ranbaxy Pharmaceuticals
10; VALIUM; R; ROCHE	Valium	10 mg	Blue	Tablet		Roche Products
11	Akineton	2 mg	White	Tablet	Circle	Par Pharmaceutical
14	Dexchlorpheniramine Maleate	4 mg	Yellow	Tablet	Oval	Qualitest Products
14	Quadrinal	24 mg; 24 mg; 130 mg; 320 mg	White	Tablet	Circle	Knoll Laboratories
15	Zyprexa Zydis	15 mg	Yellow	Disintegrating Tablet	Circle	Eli Lilly
15; M	Mobic	15 mg	Pastel Yellow	Tablet	Oblong	Abbott Laboratories
15; M	Mobic	15 mg	Pastel Yellow	Tablet	Oblong	Boehringer Ingelheim
17	Moexipril Hydrochloride	7.5 mg	Pink	Tablet	Oval, Scored	Teva Pharmaceuticals
18; 370	Adapin	150 mg	Brown and Beige	Capsule		Fisons Pharmaceuticals
18; 892	Tussionex	5 mg; 10 mg	Green and Ivory	Capsule		Fisons Pharmaceuticals
18; 894	Tussionex	5 mg; 10 mg	Light Tan	Tablet	Four-Sided, Scored	Fisons Pharmaceuticals
18; 899	Biphetamine-T 12 1/2	6.25 mg; 6.25 mg; 40 mg	Green and Black	Capsule		Fisons Pharmaceuticals
18; 900	Biphetamine-T 20	10 mg; 10 mg; 40 mg	Red and Black	Capsule		Fisons Pharmaceuticals
19	Simethicone	80 mg	White	Tablet, Chewable	Circle	Rugby Laboratories
19; N025	Perchloracap	200 mg	Opaque Gray	Capsule		Mallinckrodt
20	Neospect	100 mg; 25 mg; 15 mg; 100 mg	Green	Tablet		Teva Pharmaceuticals
20	Zyprexa Zydis	20 mg	Yellow	Disintegrating Tablet	Circle	Eli Lilly
20; 185	Yellow Capsule	175 mg	Yellow	Capsule		Pdk Labs
ANDRX LOGO 20	Altoprev	20 mg	Orange	Tablet, Extended Release	Circle	Andrx Pharmaceuticals
20 MG	Nexium	20 mg	Amethyst with Two Yellow Bars	Timed-Release Capsule		Astra Zeneca
20 MG; LILLY; 3235	Cymbalta	20 mg	Opaque Green	Delayed-Release Capsule		Eli Lilly
22	Rhinex	150 mg; 1.25 mg; 2.5 mg	Pink and White	Tablet		Teva Pharmaceuticals
25	Sonazine	25 mg	Butterscotch	Tablet	Circle	Solvay Pharmaceuticals
25/100; SP; 342	Parcopa	25 mg; 100 mg	Yellow	Disintegrating Tablet	Circle, Flat-Faced, Scored	Schwarz Pharma
25/250; SP; 343	Parcopa	25 mg; 250 mg	Blue	Disintegrating Tablet	Circle, Flat-Faced, Scored	Schwarz Pharma
25; LL; A; 13	Asendin	25 mg	Off-White	Tablet	Seven-Sided	Lederle Laboratories
25 MG; WATSON 371	Loxapine Succinate	25 mg	White and Green	Capsule		Watson Laboratories
25; T4	Levothroid	25 mcg	Orange	Tablet	Capsule-Shape	Forest Pharmaceuticals
25 W 701	Effexor	25 mg	Peach	Tablet	Shield-Shape	Wyeth Pharmaceuticals
26	Aceta-Gesic	325 mg; 30 mg	Orange	Tablet	Circle	Rugby Laboratories
27	Rulox No. 1	225 mg; 200 mg	Off-White	Tablet, Chewable	Circle	Rugby Laboratories
28	Atrohist Sprinkle	4 mg; 60 mg		Sustained-Release Capsule		Medeva Pharmaceuticals
30 30	Caffeine	325 mg	Blue with Red Speckles	Tablet	Oblong	Pdk Labs
30 MG; LILLY; 3240	Cymbalta	30 mg	Opaque White and Opaque Blue	Delayed-Release Capsule		Eli Lilly
31; 86; V;	Guaifenesin and Codeine	300 mg; 10 mg	Red	Tablet		Vintage Pharmaceuticals
31; 89; V;	Guaifenesin and Pseudoephedrine	600 mg; 120 mg	White	Sustained-Release Tablet	Oval	Vintage Pharmaceuticals
31; BONE IMAGE	Fosamax	70 mg	White	Tablet	Oval	Merck
35; 91; V	Hydrocodone Bitartrate and Acetaminophen	2.5 mg; 500 mg	White with Red Specks	Tablet		Vintage Pharmaceuticals
35; 94; V;	Acetaminophen and Hydrocodone Bitartrate	500 mg; 7.5 mg	White with Green Specks	Tablet		Vintage Pharmaceuticals
35; 94; V	Hydrocodone Bitartrate and Acetaminophen	7.5 mg; 500 mg	White with Green Specks	Tablet	Capsule-Shape	Vintage Pharmaceuticals
35; 96; V;	Acetaminophen and Hydrocodone Bitartrate	750 mg; 7.5 mg	White	Tablet		Vintage Pharmaceuticals
35; 96; V	Hydrocodone Bitartrate and Acetaminophen	7.5 mg; 750 mg	White	Tablet	Capsule-Shape	Vintage Pharmaceuticals
35; 97; V;	Acetaminophen and Hydrocodone Bitartrate	650 mg; 10 mg	Light Blue	Tablet		Vintage Pharmaceuticals
35; 97; V	Hydrocodone Bitartrate and Acetaminophen	10 mg; 650 mg	Light Blue	Tablet	Capsule-Shape	Vintage Pharmaceuticals
35; 98; V	Hydrocodone Bitartrate and Acetaminophen	10 mg; 660 mg	White	Tablet	Oval	Vintage Pharmaceuticals
36; 01; V	Hydrocodone Bitartrate and Acetaminophen	10 mg; 325 mg	Light Yellow	Tablet	Capsule-Shape	Vintage Pharmaceuticals
37; 4401	Depen	250 mg	White	Tablet		Wallace Laboratories
37-4101/300 WALLACE	Rondomycin	300 mg	Blue and White	Capsule		Wallace Laboratories
37; WALLACE; 4224	Organidin	30 mg	Rose	Tablet	Circle	Wallace Laboratories
37.5 W 781	Effexor	37.5 mg	Peach	Tablet	Shield-Shape	Wyeth Pharmaceuticals
40;	Ceenu	40 mg	White and Green	Capsule		Bristol-Myers Oncology
40	Isoptin	40 mg	Blue	Coated Tablet	Circle, Scored	Knoll Laboratories
40	Simethicone Gas Relief	125 mg	White	Tablet, Chewable	Circle	Rugby Laboratories
ANDRX LOGO 40	Altoprev	40 mg	Peach	Tablet, Extended Release	Circle	Andrx Pharmaceuticals
40 MG	Nexium	40 mg	Amethyst with Three Yellow Bars	Timed-Release Capsule		Astra Zeneca
42	Diphenhist	25 mg	Pink	Tablet	Oval	Rugby Laboratories
42	Neosorb Plus	300 mg; 150 mg	Green and White	Tablet		Teva Pharmaceuticals
42; 16; V	Methylprednisolone	4 mg	White	Tablet	Quadrisected, Oval Scored	Vintage Pharmaceuticals

IMPRINT	BRAND/GENERIC NAME	STRENGTH	COLOR	FORM	SHAPE	MANUFACTURER
43	Vitamin B1	100 mg	White	Tablet	Circle	Rugby Laboratories
43 060; 59743	Brompheniramine and Pseudoephedrine	12 mg; 120 mg	Green and Clear	Capsule		Qualitest Products
43 061; 59743	Brompheniramine and Pseudoephedrine PD	6 mg; 60 mg	Blue-Green and Clear	Capsule		Qualitest Products
43; RH405	Antara	43 mg	Light Green and White	Capsule	Capsule-Shape	Reliant Pharmaceuticals
44	Vicks 44 Cold, Flu & Cough	250 mg; 2 mg; 30 mg; 10 mg	Blue	Capsule		Procter & Gamble
44	Vicks 44 Liquicaps Cold, Flu & Cough	250 mg; 2 mg; 30 mg; 10 mg	Blue	Capsule		Procter & Gamble
44	Vicks 44 Liquicaps Non-Drowsy Cold & Cough	30 mg; 60 mg	Transparent Red	Capsule		Procter & Gamble
44	Vicks 44 Liquicaps Non-Drowsy Cough & Cold Relief	30 mg; 60 mg	Transparent Red	Gel/jelly		Procter & Gamble
44	Vicks 44 Liquidaps Cough, Cold & Flu Relief	250 mg; 2 mg; 30 mg; 10 mg	Transparent Blue	Gel/jelly		Procter & Gamble
44; 159	Acetaminophen, Aspirin and Caffeine	250 mg; 250 mg; 65 mg	White to Off-White	Tablet	Circle, Compressed, Convex	Leiner Health Products
44-164	Pain Reliever, Adult Strength	400 mg; 32 mg	White	Tablet	Circle, Convex, Compressed	Leiner Health Products
44-183	Buffered Aspirin	325 mg;	White	Coated Tablet	Circle, Double-Layer, Convex	Leiner Health Products
44; 191	Diphenhydramine Hydrochloride	25 mg	Pink	Coated Tablet	Oval	Udl Laboratories
44; 194	Chlorpheniramine Maleate	4 mg	Yellow	Tablet	Round, Bisected Scored	Udl Laboratories
44;198	Dimenhydrinate	50 mg	White	Tablet	Compressed, Convex, Bisected Scored	Leiner Health Products
44-199	Acetaminophen, Phenylephrine Hydrochloride & Chlorpheniramine Maleate	325 mg; 5 mg; 2 mg	Yellow and White	Coated Tablet	Circle, Flat Faced, Beveled Edge	Leiner Health Products
44; 205	Caffeine	100 mg	White	Tablet	Circle, Compressed, Convex	Leiner Health Products
44; 226	Stay Awake	200 mg	Yellow	Tablet	Compressed, Round, Convex, Bisected Scored	Leiner Health Products
44; 227	Aspirin	325 mg	Orange	Enteric-Coated Tablet	Circle, Convex	Leiner Health Products
44-247	Aspirin Maximum Strength	500 mg	Orange	Enteric-Coated Tablet	Circle, Convex	Leiner Health Products
44; 255	Aspirin	81 mg	Yellow	Tablet	Circle, Convex	Udl Laboratories
45	Peptic Relief	262.5 mg	Light Pink	Tablet, Chewable	Circle	Rugby Laboratories
50	Manoplax	50 mg	White	Coated Tablet	Six-Sided	Boots Pharmaceuticals
50	Sonazine	50 mg	Butterscotch	Tablet	Circle	Solvay Pharmaceuticals
50; LL; A; 15	Asendin	50 mg	Orange	Tablet	Seven-Sided	Lederle Laboratories
50 MG; WATSON 372	Loxapine Succinate	50 mg	White and Blue	Capsule		Watson Laboratories
50; T4	Levothroid	50 mcg	White	Tablet	Capsule-Shape	Forest Pharmaceuticals
50 W 703	Effexor	50 mg	Peach	Tablet	Shield-Shape	Wyeth Pharmaceuticals
51H; BOEHRINGER INGELHEIM LOGO	Micardis	40 mg	White	Tablet	Oblong, Scored	Boehringer Ingelheim
52H; BOEHRINGER INGELHEIM LOGO	Micardis	80 mg	White	Tablet	Oblong, Scored	Boehringer Ingelheim
54; 007	Mirtazapine	45 mg	White	Tablet	Circle	Roxane Laboratories
54; 009	Propranolol Hydrochloride	20 mg	White	Tablet	Circle	Roxane Laboratories
54; 010	Diflunisal	250 mg	Orange	Coated Tablet	Capsule-Shape, Biconvex	Roxane Laboratories
54; 012	Amitriptyline Hydrochloride	25 mg	White	Tablet		Roxane Laboratories
54; 013	Leucovorin Calcium	25 mg	Yellow	Tablet	Circle, Scored	Roxane Laboratories
54; 019	Chlorpheniramine Maleate	4 mg	Yellow	Tablet		Roxane Laboratories
54; 024	Flecainide Acetate	50 mg	White	Tablet	Circle	Roxane Laboratories
54; 039	Naproxen	500 mg	Beige	Tablet	Capsule-Shape	Roxane Laboratories
54; 042	Nefazodone Hydrochloride	100 mg	White	Tablet	Oval	Roxane Laboratories
54; 042	Nefazodone Hydrochloride	100 mg	White	Tablet	Oval, Scored	Roxane Laboratories
54; 043	Azathioprine	50 mg	Yellow	Tablet	Circle, Scored	Roxane Laboratories
54; 050	Haloperidol	1 mg		Tablet		Roxane Laboratories
54; 053	Quinidine Sulfate	300 mg	White	Tablet		Roxane Laboratories
54; 062	Propranolol Hydrochloride	60 mg	White	Tablet	Circle	Roxane Laboratories
54; 063	Acetaminophen	325 mg	White	Tablet		Roxane Laboratories
54; 070	Flecainide Acetate	100 mg	White	Tablet	Circle	Roxane Laboratories
54; 072	Hydroxyurea	500 mg	Dark Green and Light Pink	Capsule		Roxane Laboratories
54; 080	Prednisone	25 mg		Tablet		Roxane Laboratories
54; 090	Roxanol SR	30 mg	White	Sustained-Release Tablet		Roxane Laboratories
54; 092	Prednisone	1 mg	White	Tablet		Roxane Laboratories
54; 093	Diflunisal	500 mg	Orange	Coated Tablet	Capsule-Shape, Biconvex	Roxane Laboratories
54; 099	Amitriptyline Hydrochloride	50 mg	White	Tablet		Roxane Laboratories
54; 103	Bisacodyl	5 mg	Orange	Tablet		Roxane Laboratories
54; 133	Calcium Carbonate	1250 mg	Off-White	Tablet, Chewable	Circle	Roxane Laboratories
54; 142	Methadone Hydrochloride	10 mg	White	Tablet		Roxane Laboratories
54; 143	Amitriptyline Hydrochloride	100 mg	White	Tablet		Roxane Laboratories
54; 150	Flecainide Acetate	150 mg	White	Tablet	Capsule-Shape	Roxane Laboratories
54; 162	Dolophine Hydrochloride	5 mg	White	Tablet	Circle	Roxane Laboratories
54; 163	Meperidine Hydrochloride	100 mg	White	Tablet	Circle, Scored	Roxane Laboratories
54; 169	Haloperidol	0.5 mg		Tablet		Roxane Laboratories
54; 172	Isoxsuprine Hydrochloride	10 mg	White	Tablet		Roxane Laboratories
54; 179	Chloral Hydrate	500 mg	Red	Capsule		Roxane Laboratories
54; 180	Naproxen Sodium Film-Coated	275 mg	Light Blue	Tablet	Oval	Roxane Laboratories
54; 183	Prednisolone	5 mg	White	Tablet		Roxane Laboratories
54; 193	Viramune	200 mg	White	Tablet	Oval, Biconvex, Bisected Scored	Boehringer Ingelheim
54; 193	Viramune	200 mg	White	Tablet	Oval, Biconvex, Bisected Scored	Roxane Laboratories
54; 199	Roxicodone	30 mg	Blue	Tablet		Roxane Laboratories
54; 201	Mirtazapine	15 mg	Yellow	Tablet	Circle	Roxane Laboratories
54; 210	Methadone Hydrochloride	5 mg	White	Tablet		Roxane Laboratories
54; 212	Neomycin Sulfate	500 mg	Off-White	Tablet		Roxane Laboratories

IMPRINT	BRAND/GENERIC NAME	STRENGTH	COLOR	FORM	SHAPE	MANUFACTURER
54; 213	Lithium Carbonate	150 mg	Opaque, White	Capsule		Roxane Laboratories
54; 223	Diphenhydramine Hydrochloride	50 mg	Pink	Capsule		Roxane Laboratories
54; 249	Propranolol Hydrochloride	80 mg	White	Tablet	Circle	Roxane Laboratories
54; 252	Acetaminophen	500 mg		Tablet		Roxane Laboratories
54; 253	Sulfamethoxazole and Trimethoprim	400 mg; 80 mg	White	Tablet	Capsule-Shape, Scored	Roxane Laboratories
54; 259	Ferrous Sulfate	300 mg	Red	Tablet		Roxane Laboratories
54; 262	Morphine Sulfate	30 mg	White	Tablet		Roxane Laboratories
54; 263	Phenobarbital	100 mg	White	Tablet		Roxane Laboratories
54; 280	Dht	0.125 mg	White	Tablet		Roxane Laboratories
54; 293	Leucovorin Calcium	5 mg	Off-White	Tablet	Circle, Scored	Roxane Laboratories
54; 299	Dexamethasone	0.5 mg	Yellow	Tablet		Roxane Laboratories
54; 302	Calcium Carbonate	1250 mg	White	Tablet	Capsule-Shape	Roxane Laboratories
54; 303	Propantheline Bromide	15 mg	White	Tablet		Roxane Laboratories
54; 310	Nefazodone Hydrochloride	200 mg	Speckled Yellow	Tablet	Oval	Roxane Laboratories
54; 310	Nefazodone Hydrochloride	200 mg	Yellow	Tablet	Oval	Roxane Laboratories
54; 323	Methotrexate	2.5 mg	Yellow	Tablet	Circle, Scored	Roxane Laboratories
54; 329	Indomethacin	50 mg	Light Green	Capsule		Roxane Laboratories
54; 333	Propranolol Hydrochloride	40 mg	White	Tablet	Circle	Roxane Laboratories
54; 339	Prednisone	2.5 mg	White	Tablet		Roxane Laboratories
54; 343	Prednisone	50 mg	White	Tablet		Roxane Laboratories
54; 346	Lithium Carbonate	450 mg	Off-White to Yellow	Extended-Release Tablet		Roxane Laboratories
54; 352	Megestrol Acetate	40 mg	White	Tablet	Circle, Scored	Roxane Laboratories
54; 353	Mirtazapine	30 mg	Biege	Tablet	Circle	Roxane Laboratories
54; 360	Amitriptyline Hydrochloride	75 mg	White	Tablet		Roxane Laboratories
54; 363	Mirtazapine	30 mg	Beige	Tablet	Circle	Roxane Laboratories
54; 369	Loperamide Hydrochloride	2 mg	Light Green	Capsule		Roxane Laboratories
54; 372	Calcium Gluconate	500 mg	White	Tablet		Roxane Laboratories
54; 379	Docusate Sodium	50 mg	Red	Capsule		Roxane Laboratories
54; 382	Haloperidol	10 mg		Tablet		Roxane Laboratories
54; 383	Methyldopa	500 mg		Tablet		Roxane Laboratories
54; 392	Oxycodone and Acetaminophen	500 mg; 5 mg		Capsule		Roxane Laboratories
54; 392	Roxilox	5 mg; 500 mg		Capsule		Roxane Laboratories
54; 403	Hydromorphone Hydrochloride	8 mg	White	Tablet	Circle, Scored	Roxane Laboratories
54; 409; 30	Morphine Sulfate SR	30 mg	White	Sustained-Release Tablet	Circle, Scored	Roxane Laboratories
54; 409; 30	Oramorph SR	30 mg	White	Sustained-Release Tablet		Roxane Laboratories
54; 410	Levorphanol Tartrate	2 mg	White	Tablet	Circle, Scored	Roxane Laboratories
54; 412	Codeine Sulfate	60 mg	White	Tablet		Roxane Laboratories
54; 422	Indomethacin	25 mg	Light Green	Capsule		Roxane Laboratories
54; 452	Lithium Carbonate	300 mg	White	Tablet		Roxane Laboratories
54; 460	Cimetidine	800 mg		Tablet		Roxane Laboratories
54; 463	Lithium Carbonate	300 mg	Opaque Flesh	Capsule		Roxane Laboratories
54; 472	Piroxicam	10 mg		Capsule		Roxane Laboratories
54; 479	Piroxicam	20 mg	Dark Blue	Capsule		Roxane Laboratories
54; 482	Tamoxifen	20 mg	White	Tablet	Circle	Roxane Laboratories
54; 489	Dexamethasone	1 mg	Yellow	Tablet		Roxane Laboratories
54; 492	Amitriptyline Hydrochloride	150 mg	White	Tablet		Roxane Laboratories
54; 499	Hydrochlorothiazide	50 mg	Peach	Tablet		Roxane Laboratories
54; 503	Phenobarbital	15 mg	White	Tablet		Roxane Laboratories
54; 512	Alprazolam	0.25 mg	White	Tablet	Oval, Scored	Roxane Laboratories
54; 519	Triazolam	0.125 mg	White	Tablet	Oval	Roxane Laboratories
54; 523	Mexiletine Hydrochloride	150 mg		Capsule		Roxane Laboratories
54; 529	Torecan	10 mg	Yellow	Tablet		Roxane Laboratories
54; 532	Pseudoephedrine Hydrochloride	60 mg	White	Tablet		Roxane Laboratories
54; 533	Furosemide	80 mg	White	Tablet	Circle	Roxane Laboratories
54; 539	Ascorbic Acid	250 mg	White	Tablet		Roxane Laboratories
54; 543	Roxicet	5 mg; 325 mg	White	Tablet		Roxane Laboratories
54; 549	Dolophine Hydrochloride	10 mg	White	Tablet	Circle	Roxane Laboratories
54; 570	Haloperidol	2 mg		Tablet		Roxane Laboratories
54; 572	Phenobarbital	30 mg	White	Tablet		Roxane Laboratories
54; 579	Isoxsuprine Hydrochloride	20 mg	White	Tablet		Roxane Laboratories
54; 582	Roxicodone	5 mg	White	Tablet		Roxane Laboratories
54; 583	Furosemide	40 mg	White	Tablet		Roxane Laboratories
54; 592	Diclofenac Sodium	50 mg	White	Timed-Release Tablet	Circle	Roxane Laboratories
54; 599	Alprazolam	0.5 mg	White	Tablet	Oval, Scored	Roxane Laboratories
54; 603	Naproxen Sodium Film-Coated	550 mg	Dark Blue	Tablet	Capsule-Shape	Roxane Laboratories
54; 609	Hydromorphone Hydrochloride	4 mg	White	Tablet	Circle, Scored	Roxane Laboratories
54; 612	Prednisone	5 mg	White	Tablet		Roxane Laboratories
54; 613	Codeine Sulfate	15 mg		Tablet		Roxane Laboratories
54; 620	Triazolam	0.25 mg	Light Blue	Tablet	Oval, Scored	Roxane Laboratories
54; 622	Methyldopa	250 mg		Tablet		Roxane Laboratories
54; 623	Acetaminophen and Codeine Phosphate	300 mg; 30 mg	White	Tablet		Roxane Laboratories
54; 632	Mexiletine Hydrochloride	200 mg		Capsule		Roxane Laboratories
54; 639	Cyclophosphamide	25 mg	Light Blue	Tablet	Circle	Roxane Laboratories
54; 643	Naproxen	250 mg	Beige	Tablet	Circle	Roxane Laboratories
54; 650	Leucovorin Calcium	15 mg	Yellow	Tablet	Circle, Scored	Roxane Laboratories
54; 659	Pseudoephedrine Hydrochloride and Triprolidine Hydrochloride	60 mg; 2.5 mg	White	Tablet		Roxane Laboratories
54; 659	Triprolidine with Pseudoephedrine Hydrochloride	2.5 mg; 60 mg		Tablet		Roxane Laboratories
54; 662	Dexamethasone	2 mg	White	Tablet		Roxane Laboratories
54; 663	Docusate Sodium	100 mg	Red	Capsule		Roxane Laboratories
54; 680	Ascorbic Acid	500 mg	White	Tablet		Roxane Laboratories
54; 690	Haloperidol	20 mg		Tablet		Roxane Laboratories
54; 699	Niacin	50 mg	White	Tablet		Roxane Laboratories
54; 702	Lithium Carbonate	600 mg	Flesh and White	Capsule		Roxane Laboratories

IMPRINT	BRAND/GENERIC NAME	STRENGTH	COLOR	FORM	SHAPE	MANUFACTURER
54; 703	Imipramine Hydrochloride	50 mg	Coral	Tablet		Roxane Laboratories
54; 710	Roxicodone	15 mg	Green	Tablet		Roxane Laboratories
54; 713	Nefazodone Hydrochloride	50 mg	Peach	Tablet	Oval	Roxane Laboratories
54; 713	Nefazodone Hydrochloride	50 mg	Speckled Peach	Tablet	Oval	Roxane Laboratories
54; 720	Docusate Sodium with Casanthranol	100 mg; 30 mg	Dark Red	Capsule		Roxane Laboratories
54; 730	Roxicet	5 mg; 500 mg	White	Tablet	Capsule-Shape	Roxane Laboratories
54; 732	Diphenoxylate Hydrochloride and Atropine Sulfate	2.5 mg; 0.025 mg	White	Tablet		Roxane Laboratories
54; 733	Morphine Sulfate	15 mg	White	Tablet		Roxane Laboratories
54; 743	Hydromorphone Hydrochloride	2 mg	White	Tablet	Circle, Scored	Roxane Laboratories
54; 749	Nefazodone Hydrochloride	150 mg	Peach	Tablet	Oval	Roxane Laboratories
54; 749	Nefazodone Hydrochloride	150 mg	Speckled Peach	Tablet	Oval, Scored	Roxane Laboratories
54; 760	Prednisone	20 mg	White	Tablet		Roxane Laboratories
54; 763	Megestrol Acetate	20 mg	White	Tablet	Circle, Scored	Roxane Laboratories
54; 769	Dexamethasone	6 mg	Aqua	Tablet		Roxane Laboratories
54; 772	Dht	0.4 mg		Tablet		Roxane Laboratories
54; 773	Haloperidol	5 mg	White	Tablet	Six-Sided, Scored	Roxane Laboratories
54; 779	Phenobarbital	60 mg	White	Tablet		Roxane Laboratories
54; 780	Tamoxifen	10 mg	White	Tablet	Circle	Roxane Laboratories
54; 782; 15	Oramorph SR	15 mg	Off-White	Sustained-Release Tablet	Circle	Roxane Laboratories
54; 783	Codeine Sulfate	30 mg	White	Tablet		Roxane Laboratories
54; 799	Cimetidine	400 mg		Tablet		Roxane Laboratories
54; 810	Propranolol Hydrochloride	90 mg	White	Tablet	Circle	Roxane Laboratories
54; 812	Hydrochlorothiazide	25 mg	Peach	Tablet		Roxane Laboratories
54; 819	Acetaminophen	650 mg	White	Tablet		Roxane Laboratories
54; 820	Ranitidine Hydrochloride	300 mg	Yellow	Coated Tablet	Capsule-Shape	Eon Labs
54; 822	Sulfamethoxazole and Trimethoprim Double Strength	800 mg; 160 mg	White	Tablet	Capsule-Shape, Scored	Roxane Laboratories
54; 823	Pseudoephedrine Hydrochloride	30 mg	White	Tablet		Roxane Laboratories
54; 833	Nefazodone Hydrochloride	250 mg	White	Tablet	Oval	Roxane Laboratories
54; 839	Diclofenac Sodium	75 mg	White	Timed-Release Tablet	Circle	Roxane Laboratories
54 840	Furosemide	20 mg	White	Tablet		Roxane Laboratories
54; 843	Methadone Hydrochloride	40 mg	White	Tablet	Square with Rounded Corners; Cross-Scored	Roxane Laboratories
54; 853	Methyldopa	125 mg		Tablet		Roxane Laboratories
54; 859	Aminophylline	100 mg	White	Tablet		Roxane Laboratories
54; 860	Alprazolam	1 mg	White	Tablet	Oval, Scored	Roxane Laboratories
54; 862; 100	Oramorph SR	100 mg	White	Sustained-Release Tablet	Circle	Roxane Laboratories
54; 879	Meperidine Hydrochloride	50 mg	White	Tablet	Circle, Compressed, Scored	Roxane Laboratories
54; 880	Imipramine Hydrochloride	25 mg	Coral	Tablet		Roxane Laboratories
54; 883	Methadone Hydrochloride	40 mg	Peach	Tablet		Roxane Laboratories
54; 892	Dexamethasone	4 mg	Green	Tablet		Roxane Laboratories
54; 899	Prednisone	10 mg	White	Tablet		Roxane Laboratories
54; 902	Roxiprin	4.5 mg; 0.38 mg; 325 mg	White	Tablet	Circle	Roxane Laboratories
54; 903	Dht	0.2 mg	Pink	Tablet		Roxane Laboratories
54; 912	Cimetidine	300 mg		Tablet		Roxane Laboratories
54; 919	Ranitidine	150 mg	Orange	Coated Tablet	Circle, Convex	Eon Labs
54; 930	Aminophylline	200 mg	White	Tablet		Roxane Laboratories
54; 932	Acetaminophen and Codeine No. 4	300 mg; 60 mg	White	Tablet		Roxane Laboratories
54; 933; 60	Oramorph SR	60 mg	White	Sustained-Release Tablet		Roxane Laboratories
54; 939	Imipramine Hydrochloride	10 mg	Coral	Tablet		Roxane Laboratories
54; 942	Leucovorin Calcium	10 mg	Off-White	Tablet	Circle, Scored	Roxane Laboratories
54; 943	Dexamethasone	1.5 mg	Pink	Tablet		Roxane Laboratories
54; 959	Mexiletine Hydrochloride	250 mg		Tablet		Roxane Laboratories
54; 960	Dexamethasone	0.75 mg	Pale Blue	Tablet		Roxane Laboratories
54; 969	Diazepam	2 mg	Peach	Tablet	Circle, Scored	Roxane Laboratories
54; 970	Propranolol Hydrochloride	10 mg	White	Tablet	Circle	Roxane Laboratories
54; 972	Propoxyphene Hydrochloride	65 mg	Pink	Capsule		Roxane Laboratories
54; 973	Diazepam	5 mg	Peach	Tablet	Circle, Scored	Roxane Laboratories
54; 979	Quinidine Sulfate	200 mg	White	Tablet		Roxane Laboratories
54; 980	Cyclophosphamide	50 mg	Light Blue	Tablet	Circle	Roxane Laboratories
54; 982	Diazepam	10 mg	Peach	Tablet	Circle, Scored	Roxane Laboratories
54; 983	Amitriptyline Hydrochloride	10 mg	White	Tablet		Roxane Laboratories
54; 992	Naproxen	375 mg	Pink	Tablet	Capsule-Shape	Roxane Laboratories
54; 997	Mirtazapine	45 mg	White	Tablet	Circle	Roxane Laboratories
56; 105	Symmetrel	100 mg	Red	Capsule, Liquid Filled		Endo Laboratories
57	Docusate Sodium & Casanthranol	30 mg; 100 mg	Maroon	Capsule	Oval	Purepac Pharmaceutical
57	Docusate Sodium & Casanthranol	30 mg; 100 mg	Maroon	Capsule	Oval	Scherer Laboratories
57	Zorprin	800 mg	White	Timed-Release Tablet		Knoll Laboratories
57	Zorprin	800 mg	White	Extended-Release Tablet	Oblong	Par Pharmaceutical
59; 35; V;	Tricosal	500 mg	Orange	Capsule		Vintage Pharmaceuticals
59; 36; V;	Tricosal	750 mg	White	Capsule		Vintage Pharmaceuticals
59; 37; V;	Tricosal	1000 mg	Red	Capsule		Vintage Pharmaceuticals
60	Terazosin Hydrochloride	1 mg	Grey	Capsule		Teva Pharmaceuticals
ANDRX LOGO 60	Altoprev	60 mg	Light Peach	Tablet, Extended Release	Circle	Andrx Pharmaceuticals
60 MG; LILLY; 3237	Cymbalta	60 mg	Opaque Green and Opaque Blue	Delayed-Release Capsule		Eli Lilly
61	Terazosin Hydrochloride	2 mg	Yellow	Capsule		Teva Pharmaceuticals
62	Terazosin Hydrochloride	5 mg	Red	Capsule		Teva Pharmaceuticals
62.5	Tracleer	62.5 mg	Orange-White	Coated Tablet	Circle, Biconvex	Actelion Pharmaceuticals
62.5	Tracleer	62.5 mg	Orange-White	Coated Tablet	Circle, Biconvex	Genentech
63	Terazosin Hydrochloride	10 mg	Blue	Capsule		Teva Pharmaceuticals

IMPRINT	BRAND/GENERIC NAME	STRENGTH	COLOR	FORM	SHAPE	MANUFACTURER
68; 7	Norpramin	10 mg	Blue	Coated Tablet		Aventis Pharmaceuticals
70	Adipex 8	8 mg	Blue and White	Tablet		Teva Pharmaceuticals
74; XX	Potassium Chloride	750 mg	Light Brown	Tablet	Oval	Abbott Laboratories
75	Manoplax	75 mg	White	Coated Tablet	Six-Sided	Boots Pharmaceuticals
75	Ranitidine Hydrochloride	75 mg	Pink	Tablet	Shield-Shape	Apotex
75	Slo-Bid Gyrocaps	75 mg	White and Clear	Extended-Release Capsule		Aventis Pharmaceuticals
75; 1171	Plavix	75 mg	Pink	Coated Tablet	Circle, Biconvex	Bristol-Myers Squibb
75; 1171	Plavix	75 mg	Pink	Coated Tablet	Circle, Biconvex	Sanofi-Synthelabo
75; T4	Levothroid	75 mcg	Violet	Tablet	Capsule-Shape	Forest Pharmaceuticals
75 W 704	Effexor	75 mg	Peach	Tablet	Shield-Shape	Wyeth Pharmaceuticals
77; BONE IMAGE	Fosamax	35 mg	White	Tablet	Oval	Merck
78/27	Belladenal-S	0.25 mg; 50 mg	Multi-Colored	Tablet	Cross-Scored	Novartis Pharmaceuticals
78; 28;	Belladenal	0.25 mg; 50 mg	White	Tablet	Cross-Scored	Novartis Pharmaceuticals
78; 31	Bellergal-S	40 mg; 0.6 mg; 0.2 mg	Dark Green, Orange, Yellow	Tablet	Circle, Compressed	Novartis
78; 52; SANDOZ S;	Mesantoin	100 mg	Pink	Tablet		Novartis Pharmaceuticals
78/212; 10;	Metaprel	10 mg	White	Tablet	Circle, Compressed	Novartis Pharmaceuticals
78/213; 20	Metaprel	20 mg	White	Tablet	Circle, Compressed	Novartis Pharmaceuticals
80; RD201; R	Innopran XL	80 mg	Gray and White	Capsule		Reliant Pharmaceuticals
81	Bayer Enteric Aspirin	81 mg	Yellow	Enteric-Coated Tablet	Circle	Bayer Consumer Care
83	Ibuprofen Cold and Sinus	200 mg; 30 mg	Red-Brown	Tablet		Good Neighbor Pharmacy
83	Ibuprofen Cold and Sinus	200 mg; 30 mg	Red-Brown	Tablet		Good Sense
83	Ibuprofen Cold and Sinus	200 mg; 30 mg	Red-Brown	Tablet		Major
83	Ibuprofen Cold and Sinus	200 mg; 30 mg	Red-Brown	Tablet		Medic
83	Ibuprofen Cold and Sinus	200 mg; 30 mg	Red-Brown	Tablet		Perfect Choice
83	Ibuprofen Cold and Sinus	200 mg; 30 mg	Red-Brown	Tablet		Sunmark
83	Ibuprofen Cold and Sinus	200 mg; 30 mg	Red-Brown	Tablet		Top Care
83	Ibuprofen Cold and Sinus	200 mg; 30 mg	Red-Brown	Tablet		Valu Rite
85; 05; M	Flecainide Acetate	50 mg	Round	Tablet	Circle, White	Mylan Pharmaceuticals
85; 10; M	Flecainide Acetate	100 mg	White	Tablet	Circle	Mylan Pharmaceuticals
85; 15; M	Flecainide Acetate	150 mg	White	Tablet	Capsule-Shape	Mylan Pharmaceuticals
85; WMH; 231	Disophrol Chronotab	6 mg; 120 mg	Red	Extended-Release Tablet		Schering-Plough
86	Women's Laxative	5 mg	Brown-Orange	Enteric-Coated Tablet	Circle	Perrigo
86	Women's Laxative	5 mg	Brown-Orange	Enteric-Coated Tablet	Circle	Select Brand
86; 62; C;	Skelaxin	400 mg	Pale Rose	Tablet	Circle, Scored	King Pharmaceuticals
86; 67; S;	Skelaxin	800 mg	Pink	Tablet	Oval, Scored	King Pharmaceuticals
87	Terramycin with Polymyxin B Sulfate	100 mg; 100000 U	Yellow	Tablet		Pfizer
87; RH405	Antara	87 mg	Dark Green and Light Green	Capsule	Capsule-Shape	Reliant Pharmaceuticals
88; T4	Levothroid	88 mcg	Mint Green	Tablet	Capsule-Shape	Forest Pharmaceuticals
93	Actihist	2.5 mg; 60 mg	White	Tablet		Paddock Labs
93; 027	Dipyridamole	25 mg		Tablet		Teva Pharmaceuticals
93; 068	Meprobamate	200 mg		Tablet		Teva Pharmaceuticals
93; 069	Meprobamate	400 mg		Tablet		Teva Pharmaceuticals
93; 088	Sulfamethoxazole and Trimethoprim	400 mg; 80 mg	White	Tablet	Circle, Convex, Scored	Teva Pharmaceuticals
93; 089	Sulfamethoxazole and Trimethoprim Double Strength	800 mg; 160 mg	White	Tablet	Oval, Convex, Scored	Teva Pharmaceuticals
93; 0924	Oxaprozin	600 mg	White to Off-White	Tablet	Capsule-Shape	Teva Pharmaceuticals
93; 5	Naproxen Delayed-Release	375 mg	White	Enteric-Coated Tablet	Capsule-Shape	Teva Pharmaceuticals
93; 6	Naproxen Delayed-Release	500 mg	White	Enteric-Coated Tablet	Capsule-Shape	Teva Pharmaceuticals
93; 7	Chlorpropamide	250 mg	Blue	Tablet	Circle, Convex, Scored	Teva Pharmaceuticals
93; 8	Indapamide	2.5 mg	White	Coated Tablet	Circle	Teva Pharmaceuticals
93; 10	Chlorpropamide	100 mg	Blue	Tablet	Circle, Convex, Scored	Teva Pharmaceuticals
93 11; 2	Aspirin and Codeine No. 2	325 mg; 15 mg	White	Tablet	Circle, Convex	Teva Pharmaceuticals
93; 12; 3	Aspirin and Codeine No. 3	325 mg; 30 mg	White	Tablet	Circle, Convex	Teva Pharmaceuticals
93; 13; 4	Aspirin and Codeine No. 4	325 mg; 60 mg	White	Tablet	Circle, Convex	Teva Pharmaceuticals
93; 15	Nabumetone	500 mg	White	Tablet	Oval	Teva Pharmaceuticals
93; 16	Nabumetone	750 mg	Beige	Tablet	Oval	Teva Pharmaceuticals
93; 21	Diltiazem ER	60 mg	Pink and White	Extended-Release Capsule		Teva Pharmaceuticals
93; 22	Diltiazem ER	90 mg	Pink and Yellow	Extended-Release Capsule		Teva Pharmaceuticals
93; 23	Diltiazem ER	120 mg	Pink and Orange	Extended-Release Capsule		Teva Pharmaceuticals
93; 26	Enalapril Maleate	2.5 mg	Yellow	Tablet	Oval, Scored	Teva Pharmaceuticals
93; 27	Enalapril Maleate	5 mg	White	Tablet	Oval, Scored	Teva Pharmaceuticals
93; 28	Enalapril Maleate	10 mg		Tablet		Teva Pharmaceuticals
93; 29	Enalapril Maleate	20 mg	Orange	Tablet	Oblong	Teva Pharmaceuticals
93; 33	Oxycodone Hydrochloride Extended Release	80 mg	Green	Extended-Release Tablet	Oval, Convex	Teva Pharmaceuticals
93; 41	Clomiphene Citrate	50 mg	White	Tablet	Circle, Flat, Beveled Edge, Scored	Teva Pharmaceuticals
93; 42	Fluoxetine Hydrochloride	10 mg	Light Blue	Capsule		Teva Pharmaceuticals
93; 43	Fluoxetine Hydrochloride	20 mg	Blue and White	Capsule		Teva Pharmaceuticals
93; 48	Metformin Hydrochloride	500 mg	White to Off-White	Tablet	Oval	Teva Pharmaceuticals
93; 49	Metformin Hydrochloride	850 mg	White to Off-White	Tablet	Oval	Teva Pharmaceuticals
93; 50; 2	Acetaminophen and Codeine	300 mg; 15 mg	White	Tablet	Circle	H.L. Moore
93; 53	Buspirone Hydrochloride	5 mg		Tablet		Teva Pharmaceuticals
93; 54	Buspirone Hydrochloride	10 mg		Tablet		Teva Pharmaceuticals
93; 58	Tramadol Hydrochloride	50 mg	White	Tablet	Oval	Teva Pharmaceuticals
93; 61	Sotalol Hydrochloride	80 mg	Light Blue	Tablet	Oblong	Teva Pharmaceuticals
93; 62	Sotalol Hydrochloride	160 mg	Light Blue	Tablet	Oval, Scored	Teva Pharmaceuticals
93; 63	Sotalol Hydrochloride	240 mg	Light Blue	Tablet	Oval, Scored	Teva Pharmaceuticals
93; 72; 14	Metformin Hydrochloride	1000 mg	White to Off-White	Tablet	Oval	Teva Pharmaceuticals
93; 76	Isosorbide Mononitrate	20 mg	Yellow	Tablet	Circle, Scored	Teva Pharmaceuticals
93; 91	Captopril	12.5 mg	White	Tablet	Oval, Scored	Teva Pharmaceuticals
93; 92	Captopril	25 mg	White	Tablet	Round, Quadrisected Scored	Teva Pharmaceuticals

IMPRINT	BRAND/GENERIC NAME	STRENGTH	COLOR	FORM	SHAPE	MANUFACTURER
93; 93; 778	Carbamazepine	100 mg	Pink with Red Specks	Tablet, Chewable	Circle, Scored, Debossed	Teva Pharmaceuticals
93; 93; 778	Carbamazepine	100 mg	Pink with Red Specks	Tablet, Chewable	Circle, Scored, Debossed	Udl Laboratories
93-93; 852	Metronidazole	500 mg	White	Tablet	Oblong, Scored, Debossed	Teva Pharmaceuticals
93-93; 852	Metronidazole	500 mg	White	Tablet	Oblong, Scored, Debossed	Udl Laboratories
93; 97	Captopril	50 mg	White	Tablet	Circle, Scored	Teva Pharmaceuticals
93; 98	Captopril	100 mg	White	Tablet	Circle, Scored	Teva Pharmaceuticals
93; 100	Labetalol Hydrochloride	100 mg		Tablet		Teva Pharmaceuticals
93; 102	Labetalol Hydrochloride	200 mg		Tablet		Teva Pharmaceuticals
93; 106	Labetalol Hydrochloride	300 mg		Tablet		Teva Pharmaceuticals
93; 111	Cimetidine	200 mg	White	Coated Tablet	Circle	Teva Pharmaceuticals
93; 112	Cimetidine	300 mg	White	Coated Tablet	Circle	Teva Pharmaceuticals
93; 113	Cimetidine	400 mg	White	Coated Tablet	Oblong, Scored	Teva Pharmaceuticals
93; 115	Haloperidol	0.5 mg	White	Tablet	Circle	Teva Pharmaceuticals
93; 116	Haloperidol	1 mg	Yellow	Tablet	Circle	Teva Pharmaceuticals
93; 117	Haloperidol	2 mg	Pink	Tablet	Circle	Teva Pharmaceuticals
93; 118	Haloperidol	5 mg	Green	Tablet	Circle	Teva Pharmaceuticals
93; 122	Cimetidine	800 mg	White	Coated Tablet	Oblong, Scored	Teva Pharmaceuticals
93; 129	Estazolam	1 mg	White	Tablet	Oval	Teva Pharmaceuticals
93; 130	Estazolam	2 mg	Coral	Tablet	Oval, Scored	Teva Pharmaceuticals
93; 132	Acetaminophen and Codeine No. 2	300 mg; 15 mg	Carmel Opaque and White	Capsule		Teva Pharmaceuticals
93; 138	Diphenhydramine Hydrochloride	25 mg	Pink Transparent and Clear	Capsule		Teva Pharmaceuticals
93; 139	Diphenhydramine Hydrochloride	50 mg	Pink Transparent	Capsule		Teva Pharmaceuticals
93; 147	Naproxen	250 mg	Mottled Light Brick Red	Tablet	Circle, Biconvex	Teva Pharmaceuticals
93; 148	Naproxen	375 mg	Mottled Peach	Tablet	Oval	Teva Pharmaceuticals
93; 149	Naproxen	500 mg	Mottled Light Brick Red	Tablet	Oval	Teva Pharmaceuticals
93; 150; 3	Acetaminophen and Codeine	300 mg; 30 mg	White	Tablet	Circle	H.L. Moore
93; 152	Acetaminophen and Codeine No. 3	300 mg; 30 mg	Coral and Scarlet, Opaque	Capsule		Teva Pharmaceuticals
93; 153	Phendimetrazine Tartrate	35 mg	Pink	Tablet	Oblong	Teva Pharmaceuticals
93; 154	Ticlopidine Hydrochloride	250 mg	White	Coated Tablet	Oval	Teva Pharmaceuticals
93; 154	Ticlopidine Hydrochloride	250 mg	White	Coated Tablet	Oval	Udl Laboratories
93; 157	Diethylpropion Hydrochloride	25 mg	White	Tablet	Circle, Flat Beveled Edge	Teva Pharmaceuticals
93; 172	Acetaminophen and Codeine No. 4	300 mg; 60 mg	Brown and Iron Gray, Opaque	Capsule		Teva Pharmaceuticals
93; 176	Captopril and Hydrochlorothiazide	25 mg; 15 mg	White	Tablet	Round, Quadrisected Scored	Teva Pharmaceuticals
93; 177	Captopril and Hydrochlorothiazide	25 mg; 25 mg	Tan	Tablet	Round, Quadrisected Scored	Teva Pharmaceuticals
93; 181	Captopril and Hydrochlorothiazide	50 mg; 15 mg	White	Tablet	Oval, Scored	Teva Pharmaceuticals
93; 182	Captopril and Hydrochlorothiazide	50 mg; 25 mg	Tan	Tablet	Oval, Scored	Teva Pharmaceuticals
93; 205; LEMMON	Donphen	0.02 mg; 0.1 mg; 15 mg; 6 mcg	Pink	Tablet	Circle, Convex, Scored	Teva Pharmaceuticals
93; 208	Galzin	50 mg	Opaque Orange	Capsule, Liquid Filled		Gate Pharmaceuticals
93; 214	Tolmetin Sodium	600 mg	Orange	Tablet	Oblong	Teva Pharmaceuticals
93; 215	Galzin	25 mg	Opaque Aqua Blue	Capsule, Liquid Filled		Gate Pharmaceuticals
93; 280	Bupropion Hydrochloride	75 mg	Yellow	Coated Tablet	Circle	Teva Pharmaceuticals
93; 290	Bupropion Hydrochloride	100 mg		Coated Tablet		Teva Pharmaceuticals
93; 292	Carbidopa and Levodopa	10 mg; 100 mg	Mottled Blue	Tablet	Circle, Scored	Teva Pharmaceuticals
93; 292	Carbidopa and Levodopa	10 mg; 100 mg	Mottled Blue	Tablet	Circle, Scored	Udl Laboratories
93; 293	Carbidopa and Levodopa	25 mg; 100 mg	Mottled Yellow	Tablet	Circle, Scored	Teva Pharmaceuticals
93; 293	Carbidopa and Levodopa	25 mg; 100 mg	Mottled Yellow	Tablet	Circle, Scored	Udl Laboratories
93; 294	Carbidopa and Levodopa	25 mg; 250 mg	Mottled Blue	Tablet	Circle, Scored	Teva Pharmaceuticals
93; 294	Carbidopa and Levodopa	25 mg; 250 mg	Mottled Blue	Tablet	Circle, Scored	Udl Laboratories
93; 307	Antihistamine 12 Hour	1.34 mg		Tablet		Perrigo
93; 307	Clemastine Fumarate	1.34 mg	White	Tablet	Circle, Convex, Scored	Leiner Health Products
93; 307	Clemastine Fumarate	1.34 mg	White	Tablet	Circle, Convex, Scored	Teva Pharmaceuticals
93; 307	Dailyhist-1 Original Prescription Strength	1.34 mg		Tablet		Fleming
93; 307	Dailyhist-1 Original Prescription Strength	1.34 mg		Tablet		Glendale Foods
93; 307	Dailyhist-1 Original Prescription Strength	1.34 mg		Tablet		Good Neighbor Pharmacy
93; 307	Dailyhist-1 Original Prescription Strength	1.34 mg		Tablet		Good Sense
93; 307	Dailyhist-1 Original Prescription Strength	1.34 mg		Tablet		Harco Drug
93; 307	Dailyhist-1 Original Prescription Strength	1.34 mg		Tablet		Kerr Drug
93; 307	Dailyhist-1 Original Prescription Strength	1.34 mg		Tablet		Major
93; 307	Dailyhist-1 Original Prescription Strength	1.34 mg		Tablet		Major Quality
93; 307	Dailyhist-1 Original Prescription Strength	1.34 mg		Tablet		Medalist
93; 307	Dailyhist-1 Original Prescription Strength	1.34 mg		Tablet		Perrigo
93; 307	Dailyhist-1 Original Prescription Strength	1.34 mg		Tablet		Preferred Products
93; 307	Dailyhist-1 Original Prescription Strength	1.34 mg		Tablet		Rockbottom Stores

IMPRINT	BRAND/GENERIC NAME	STRENGTH	COLOR	FORM	SHAPE	MANUFACTURER
93; 307	Dailyhist-1 Original Prescription Strength	1.34 mg		Tablet		Sunfresh
93; 307	Dailyhist-1 Original Prescription Strength	1.34 mg		Tablet		Top Care
93; 307	Dailyhist-1 Original Prescription Strength	1.34 mg		Tablet		Valu Rite
93; 308	Clemastine Fumarate	2.68 mg	White	Tablet	Circle, Convex, Scored	Teva Pharmaceuticals
93; 311	Loperamide Hydrochloride	2 mg	Light Brown and Dark Brown	Capsule		Teva Pharmaceuticals
93; 318	Diltiazem Hydrochloride	30 mg	Faint Orange	Coated Tablet	Circle, Biconvex	Teva Pharmaceuticals
93; 319	Diltiazem Hydrochloride	60 mg	Orange	Coated Tablet	Circle, Biconvex, Scored	Teva Pharmaceuticals
93; 320	Diltiazem Hydrochloride	90 mg	Faint Orange	Coated Tablet	Oblong, Scored	Teva Pharmaceuticals
93; 321	Diltiazem Hydrochloride	120 mg	Orange	Coated Tablet	Oblong, Scored	Teva Pharmaceuticals
93; 350; 4	Acetaminophen and Codeine	300 mg; 60 mg	White	Tablet	Circle	H.L. Moore
93; 431	Chlorthalidone	50 mg	Blue	Tablet	Circle, Flat, Beveled Edge	Teva Pharmaceuticals
93; 433	Chlorthalidone	100 mg	White	Tablet	Circle, Flat Beveled Edge, Scored	Teva Pharmaceuticals
93; 490	Acetaminophen and Propoxyphene Napsylate	650 mg; 100 mg	White	Coated Tablet	Oblong, Convex	Teva Pharmaceuticals
93; 494	Clonidine Hydrochloride	0.1 mg	Green	Tablet	Circle	Teva Pharmaceuticals
93; 495	Clonidine Hydrochloride	0.2 mg	Yellow	Tablet		Teva Pharmaceuticals
93; 496	Clonidine Hydrochloride	0.3 mg	Peach	Tablet	Circle	Teva Pharmaceuticals
93; 525	Amitriptyline Hydrochloride	10 mg	Pink	Coated Tablet	Circle, Biconvex	Teva Pharmaceuticals
93; 527	Amitriptyline Hydrochloride	25 mg	Green	Coated Tablet	Circle, Biconvex	Teva Pharmaceuticals
93; 529	Amitriptyline Hydrochloride	50 mg	Brown	Coated Tablet	Circle, Biconvex	Teva Pharmaceuticals
93; 531	Amitriptyline Hydrochloride	75 mg	Purple	Coated Tablet	Circle, Biconvex	Teva Pharmaceuticals
93; 533	Amitriptyline Hydrochloride	100 mg	Orange	Coated Tablet	Circle, Biconvex	Teva Pharmaceuticals
93; 535	Amitriptyline Hydrochloride	150 mg	Peach	Coated Tablet	Circle, Biconvex	Teva Pharmaceuticals
93; 536	Naproxen Sodium	275 mg	White to Off-White	Coated Tablet	Oval	Teva Pharmaceuticals
93; 537	Naproxen Sodium	550 mg	White to Off-White	Coated Tablet	Oval	Teva Pharmaceuticals
93; 539	Mepro Compound	150 mg; 250 mg; 75 mg		Tablet	Three-Layered	Teva Pharmaceuticals
93; 542	Chlorzoxazone	500 mg	White	Tablet	Oblong, Scored	H.L. Moore
93; 542	Chlorzoxazone	500 mg	White	Tablet	Oblong, Scored, Convex	Teva Pharmaceuticals
93; 545	Chlorzoxazone and Acetaminophen	300 mg; 250 mg	Light Green	Tablet	Circle, Flat, Beveled Edge, Scored	Teva Pharmaceuticals
93; 576	Lovastatin	20 mg	Blue	Tablet	Circle	Teva Pharmaceuticals
93; 585	Indo-Lemmon	25 mg	Light Green Opaque	Capsule		Teva Pharmaceuticals
93; 587	Indo-Lemmon	50 mg	Light Green Opaque	Capsule		Teva Pharmaceuticals
93; 613	Amoxicillin	250 mg	Carmel and Ivory, Opaque	Capsule		Teva Pharmaceuticals
93; 615	Amoxicillin	500 mg	Ivory Opaque	Capsule		Teva Pharmaceuticals
93; 617	Chlordinum Sealets	5 mg; 2.5 mg	White Opaque	Capsule		Teva Pharmaceuticals
93; 620	Propranolol Hydrochloride	20 mg	Blue	Tablet	Circle, Scored	Teva Pharmaceuticals
93; 637	Trazodone Hydrochloride	50 mg	White to Off-White	Coated Tablet	Circle, Scored, Convex	Teva Pharmaceuticals
93; 638	Trazodone Hydrochloride	100 mg	White to Off-White	Coated Tablet	Circle, Scored	Teva Pharmaceuticals
93; 640	Propranolol Hydrochloride	40 mg	Green	Tablet	Circle, Scored	Teva Pharmaceuticals
93; 653	Doxycycline Hyclate	100 mg	Aqua Blue Opaque	Capsule		Teva Pharmaceuticals
93; 657	Calcitriol	0.25 mcg	Red-Brown, Yellow-Brown	Capsule, Liquid Filled	Oval	Teva Pharmaceuticals
93; 658	Calcitriol	0.5 mcg	Brown and Pink	Capsule, Liquid Filled	Oval	Teva Pharmaceuticals
93; 665	Albuterol Sulfate	2 mg	White	Tablet	Circle, Scored	Teva Pharmaceuticals
93; 666	Albuterol	4 mg	White	Tablet	Circle, Scored	Teva Pharmaceuticals
93; 670	Gemcor	600 mg	White to Off-White	Coated Tablet	Oval, Scored	Upsher-Smith Laboratories
93; 670	Gemfibrozil	600 mg	White	Coated Tablet	Oval, Scored	Teva Pharmaceuticals
93; 670	Gemfibrozil	600 mg	White	Coated Tablet	Oval, Scored	Udl Laboratories
93; 686	Propoxyphene Compound	389 mg; 32.4 mg; 65 mg	Gray and Red	Capsule		Teva Pharmaceuticals
93; 711	Flurbiprofen	100 mg	Deep Sky Blue	Coated Tablet	Circle, Convex	Teva Pharmaceuticals
93; 727	Papaverine Hydrochloride	150 mg	Brown and Clear	Timed-Release Capsule		Teva Pharmaceuticals
93; 728	Sulindac	150 mg	Yellow	Tablet	Circle, Convex	Teva Pharmaceuticals
93; 729	Sulindac	200 mg	Yellow	Tablet	Circle, Convex, Scored	Teva Pharmaceuticals
93; 733	Metoprolol Tartrate	50 mg	Mottled-Red	Coated Tablet	Circle, Biconvex, Scored	Teva Pharmaceuticals
93; 734	Metoprolol Tartrate	100 mg	Mottled-Blue	Coated Tablet	Circle, Biconvex, Scored	Teva Pharmaceuticals
93; 741; 93; 741	Propoxyphene Hydrochloride	65 mg	Opaque Pink	Capsule		Teva Pharmaceuticals
93; 742	Doxycycline Hyclate	50 mg	White and Aqua Blue, Opaque	Capsule		Teva Pharmaceuticals
93; 742	Doxy-Lemmon	50 mg	White and Aqua Blue, Opaque	Capsule		Teva Pharmaceuticals
93; 743	Doxy-Lemmon	50 mg	Aqua Blue Opaque	Capsule		Teva Pharmaceuticals
93; 752	Atenolol	50 mg	White	Tablet	Circle, Flat, Scored	Teva Pharmaceuticals
93; 753	Atenolol	100 mg	White	Tablet	Circle, Flat	Teva Pharmaceuticals
93; 754	Diflunisal	250 mg	Blue/lavender	Tablet	Capsule-Shape	Teva Pharmaceuticals
93; 755	Diflunisal	500 mg	Blue	Coated Tablet	Oblong	Teva Pharmaceuticals
93; 755	Diflunisal	500 mg	Blue	Coated Tablet	Oblong	Udl Laboratories
93; 756	Piroxicam	10 mg	Dark Green and Olive	Capsule		Teva Pharmaceuticals
93; 757	Piroxicam	20 mg	Dark Green	Capsule		Teva Pharmaceuticals
93; 777	Hydrochlorothiazide	25 mg	Peach	Tablet	Circle, Flat, Beveled Edge, Scored	Teva Pharmaceuticals
93; 779	Hydrochlorothiazide	50 mg	Peach	Tablet	Circle, Flat, Beveled Edge, Scored	Teva Pharmaceuticals
93; 782	Tamoxifen	20 mg	White to Off-White	Tablet	Circle	Teva Pharmaceuticals
93; 782	Tamoxifen Citrate	20 mg	White	Tablet	Circle	Teva Pharmaceuticals
93; 784	Tamoxifen	10 mg	White	Tablet	Circle	Teva Pharmaceuticals
93; 784	Tamoxifen Citrate	10 mg	White	Tablet	Circle	Teva Pharmaceuticals
93; 788	Selegiline Hydrochloride	5 mg	White to Off-White	Tablet	Circle, Flat, Beveled Edge	Teva Pharmaceuticals
93; 793	Nicardipine	20 mg	Opaque White and Aqua Blue	Capsule, Liquid Filled		Teva Pharmaceuticals
93; 794	Nicardipine	30 mg	Opaque White and Light Blue	Capsule, Liquid Filled		Teva Pharmaceuticals
93; 798	Indomethacin	25 mg	Light Green Opaque	Capsule		Teva Pharmaceuticals
93; 799	Indomethacin	50 mg	Light Green Opaque	Capsule		Teva Pharmaceuticals

IMPRINT	BRAND/GENERIC NAME	STRENGTH	COLOR	FORM	SHAPE	MANUFACTURER
93; 802	Antispasmodic	16.2 mg; 0.1037 mg; 0.0194 mg; 0.0065 mg	Transparent Green and Clear	Capsule		Teva Pharmaceuticals
93; 804	Phentermine Hydrochloride Black and Scarlet	30 mg	Black and Scarlet, Opaque	Capsule		Teva Pharmaceuticals
93; 808	Phentermine Hydrochloride	8 mg	Green	Tablet	Circle	Teva Pharmaceuticals
93; 809	Phentermine Hydrochloride	8 mg	Peach	Tablet	Circle	Teva Pharmaceuticals
93; 810	Nortriptyline Hydrochloride	10 mg	White and Orange	Capsule		Teva Pharmaceuticals
93; 811	Nortriptyline Hydrochloride	25 mg	White and Orange	Capsule		Teva Pharmaceuticals
93; 812	Nortriptyline	50 mg	White	Capsule		Teva Pharmaceuticals
93; 812	Nortriptyline Hydrochloride	50 mg	White	Capsule		Teva Pharmaceuticals
93; 813	Nortriptyline Hydrochloride	75 mg	Orange	Capsule		Teva Pharmaceuticals
93; 816	Belladonna Alkaloids with Phenobarbital	16.2 mg; 0.1037 mg; 0.0194 mg; 0.0065 mg	White	Tablet	Circle, Convex, Scored	Teva Pharmaceuticals
93; 820	Pseudoephedrine Hydrochloride	30 mg	Red	Coated Tablet		Rosemont Pharmaceutical
93; 821	Reserpine	0.25 mg	White	Tablet	Circle, Flat, Beveled Edge, Scored	Teva Pharmaceuticals
93; 823	Uridon	0.03 mg; 0.03 mg; 50 mg; 5.5 mg; 20 mg; 5 mg	Blue	Coated Tablet		Teva Pharmaceuticals
93; 824	Pseudoephedrine Hydrochloride	60 mg	White	Tablet	Circle	Rosemont Pharmaceutical
93; 824	Pseudoephedrine Hydrochloride	60 mg	White	Tablet	Circle, Convex	Teva Pharmaceuticals
93; 827	Reserpine	0.1 mg	White	Tablet	Circle, Flat, Beveled Edge, Scored	Teva Pharmaceuticals
93; 828	Urinary Anteseptic No. 3	0.06 mg; 0.03 mg; 120 mg; 6 mg; 30 mg; 7.5 mg	Blue	Coated Tablet	Circle	Teva Pharmaceuticals
93; 828	Uritin	0.06 mg; 0.03 mg; 120 mg; 30 mg; 6 mg; 7.5 mg		Tablet		Teva Pharmaceuticals
93; 832	Clonazepam	0.5 mg	Yellow	Tablet	Circle, Single-Scored	Teva Pharmaceuticals
93; 833	Clonazepam	1 mg	Mottled Green	Tablet	Circle, Single-Scored	Teva Pharmaceuticals
93; 834	Clonazepam	2 mg	White to Off-White	Tablet	Circle, Single-Scored	Teva Pharmaceuticals
93; 838	Dicyclomine Hydrochloride with Phenobarbital	10 mg; 15 mg	Blue and Clear	Capsule		Teva Pharmaceuticals
93; 841	Dicyclomine Hydrochloride	10 mg	Blue Transparent	Capsule		Teva Pharmaceuticals
93; 845	Atrosept	0.03 mg; 0.03 mg; 40.8 mg; 18.1 mg; 4.5 mg; 5.4 mg	Dark Blue	Coated Tablet	Circle	Teva Pharmaceuticals
93; 845	Urinary Antiseptic No. 2	0.03 mg; 0.03 mg; 40.8 mg; 5.4 mg; 18.1 mg; 4.5 mg	Purple	Coated Tablet	Circle	Major Pharmaceutical
93; 845	Urinary Antiseptic No. 2	0.03 mg; 0.03 mg; 40.8 mg; 5.4 mg; 18.1 mg; 4.5 mg	Purple	Coated Tablet	Circle	Teva Pharmaceuticals
93; 845	Urinary Antiseptic No. 2	0.03 mg; 0.03 mg; 40.8 mg; 18.1 mg; 4.5 mg	Purple	Tablet		West-Ward
93; 845	Urisep	40.8 mg; 0.03 mg; 18.1 mg; 4.5 mg; 5.4 mg	Purple	Tablet	Circle	Solvay Pharmaceuticals
93; 845	Uroblue	0.03 mg; 0.03 mg; 40.8 mg; 5.4 mg; 18.1 mg; 4.5 mg	Purple	Tablet		Teva Pharmaceuticals
93; 846	Belladonna Extract and Phenobarbital	0.167 Gr; 0.25 Gr	Green	Tablet	Circle	Teva Pharmaceuticals
93; 848	Triphed	2.5 mg; 60 mg	White	Tablet	Circle, Convex, Scored	Teva Pharmaceuticals
93; 851	Metronidazole	250 mg	White	Tablet	Circle, Convex	Teva Pharmaceuticals
93; 851	Metronidazole	250 mg	White	Tablet	Circle, Convex	Udl Laboratories
93; 853	Phentermine Hydrochloride	30 mg	Blue and Clear with Blue and White Pellets	Capsule		Teva Pharmaceuticals
93; 858	VI-Forte	12500 IU; 50 IU; 150 mg; 80 mg; 70 mg; 25 mg; 10 mg; 10 mg; 5 mg; 4 mg; 2 mg	Black and Orange	Capsule		Teva Pharmaceuticals
93; 859	Phentermine Hydrochloride	30 mg	Brown and Clear with Orange and White Pellets	Capsule		Teva Pharmaceuticals
93; 860	Phentermine Hydrochloride Yellow	30 mg	Yellow Opaque	Capsule		Teva Pharmaceuticals
93; 861	Phentermine Hydrochloride	8 mg	Yellow	Capsule		Teva Pharmaceuticals
93; 862	Phentermine Hydrochloride	8 mg	Black	Capsule		Teva Pharmaceuticals
93; 866	Phendimetrazine Tartrate	35 mg	Black	Capsule		Teva Pharmaceuticals
93; 867	Phendimetrazine Tartrate	35 mg	Brown and Clear	Capsule		Teva Pharmaceuticals
93; 868	Phendimetrazine Tartrate	30 mg	Red and Yellow	Capsule		Teva Pharmaceuticals
93; 869	Phendimetrazine Tartrate	35 mg	Green and Clear	Capsule		Teva Pharmaceuticals
93; 872	Butabarbital Sodium	15 mg	Purple	Tablet	Circle, Convex, Scored	Teva Pharmaceuticals
93; 873	Butabarbital Sodium	30 mg	Green	Tablet	Circle, Convex, Scored	Teva Pharmaceuticals
93; 882	Phentermine Hydrochloride	15 mg	Gray and Yellow	Capsule		Teva Pharmaceuticals
93; 886	Drummergal	20 mg; 0.3 mg; 0.1 mg	Tan	Coated Tablet	Circle	Teva Pharmaceuticals
93; 886	Ergobel	0.3 mg; 0.1 mg; 20 mg		Tablet		Teva Pharmaceuticals
93; 888	Phentermine Hydrochloride Black	30 mg	Black Opaque	Capsule		Teva Pharmaceuticals
93; 890	Acetaminophen and Propoxyphene Napsylate	650 mg; 100 mg	Pink	Coated Tablet	Oblong, Convex	Teva Pharmaceuticals
93; 891	Dicyclomine Hydrochloride	20 mg	Blue	Tablet	Circle, Flat Beveled Edge	Teva Pharmaceuticals
93; 892	Etodolac	400 mg	Pink	Tablet	Capsule-Shape	Teva Pharmaceuticals

IMPRINT	BRAND/GENERIC NAME	STRENGTH	COLOR	FORM	SHAPE	MANUFACTURER
93; 896	Famotidine	20 mg	Beige	Coated Tablet	Circle, Biconvex	Teva Pharmaceuticals
93; 897	Famotidine	40 mg	Tan	Tablet	Circle	Teva Pharmaceuticals
93; 899	Phentermine Hydrochloride	30 mg	Red and Yellow	Capsule		Teva Pharmaceuticals
93; 900	Ketoconazole	200 mg	White	Tablet	Circle	Teva Pharmaceuticals
93; 911; 10	Isoxsuprine Hydrochloride	10 mg	White	Tablet	Circle, Convex	Teva Pharmaceuticals
93; 913; 20	Isoxsuprine Hydrochloride	20 mg	White	Tablet	Circle, Convex, Scored	Teva Pharmaceuticals
93; 926	Lovastatin	10 mg		Tablet		Teva Pharmaceuticals
93; 928	Lovastatin	40 mg		Tablet		Teva Pharmaceuticals
93; 943	Nystatin	100,000 units	Light Yellow	Tablet	Diamond	Teva Pharmaceuticals
93; 948	Diclofenac Potassium	50 mg	Orange	Tablet	Circle	Teva Pharmaceuticals
93; 956	Clomipramine Hydrochloride	25 mg	White and Orange	Capsule		Teva Pharmaceuticals
93; 957	Chlordiazepoxide Hydrochloride	5 mg	Light Green and Yellow, Opaque	Capsule		Teva Pharmaceuticals
93; 958	Clomipramine Hydrochloride	50 mg	White and Light Blue	Capsule		Teva Pharmaceuticals
93; 959	Chlordiazepoxide Hydrochloride	10 mg	Black and Light Green, Opaque	Capsule		Teva Pharmaceuticals
93; 960	Clomipramine Hydrochloride	75 mg	White and Tan	Capsule		Teva Pharmaceuticals
93; 961	Chlordiazepoxide Hydrochloride	25 mg	Light Green and White, Opaque	Capsule		Teva Pharmaceuticals
93; 968	Famotidine	10 mg	Pink	Coated Tablet	Circle, Biconvex	Teva Pharmaceuticals
93; 983	Nystatin	500,000 units	Brown	Coated Tablet	Circle, Convex	Teva Pharmaceuticals
93; 1003; 5	Buspirone Hydrochloride	15 mg		Tablet		Teva Pharmaceuticals
93; 1024	Nefazodone Hydrochloride	100 mg	White	Tablet	Capsule-Shape, Scored	Teva Pharmaceuticals
93; 1025	Nefazodone Hydrochloride	200 mg	Yellow	Tablet	Capsule-Shape, Scored	Teva Pharmaceuticals
93; 1026	Nefazodone Hydrochloride	250 mg	White	Tablet	Capsule-Shape, Scored	Teva Pharmaceuticals
93; 1035	Hydrochlorothiazide and Lisinopril	12.5 mg; 10 mg	Peach	Tablet	Circle	Teva Pharmaceuticals
93; 1036	Hydrochlorothiazide and Lisinopril	12.5 mg; 20 mg	White	Tablet	Circle	Teva Pharmaceuticals
93; 1037	Hydrochlorothiazide and Lisinopril	25 mg; 20 mg	Peach	Tablet	Circle	Teva Pharmaceuticals
93; 1041	Diclofenac Sodium	100 mg	Pink	Extended-Release Tablet	Circle	Teva Pharmaceuticals
93; 1044	Enalapril and Hydrochlorothiazide	5 mg; 12.5 mg	White	Tablet	Capsule-Shape	Teva Pharmaceuticals
93; 1052	Enalapril and Hydrochlorothiazide	10 mg; 25 mg	Rust	Tablet	Capsule-Shape	Teva Pharmaceuticals
93; 1060	Sotalol Hydrochloride	120 mg	Light Blue	Tablet	Oval, Scored	Teva Pharmaceuticals
93; 1087	Cefaclor	500 mg	Blue	Tablet	Oval	Teva Pharmaceuticals
93; 1111	Lisinopril	2.5 mg	White	Tablet	Circle	Teva Pharmaceuticals
93; 1112	Lisinopril	5 mg	Red	Tablet	Circle, Scored	Teva Pharmaceuticals
93; 1113	Lisinopril	10 mg	Red	Tablet	Circle	Teva Pharmaceuticals
93; 1114	Lisinopril	20 mg	Red	Tablet	Capsule-Shape	Teva Pharmaceuticals
93; 1115	Lisinopril	40 mg	Yellow	Tablet	Capsule-Shape	Teva Pharmaceuticals
93; 1118	Etodolac	600 mg	Light Blue	Extended-Release Tablet	Oval	Teva Pharmaceuticals
93; 1122	Etodolac ER	400 mg	Orange	Extended-Release Tablet	Oval	Teva Pharmaceuticals
93; 1177	Neomycin Sulfate	500 mg	Off-White	Tablet	Circle	Novartis Generics
93; 1177	Neomycin Sulfate	500 mg	Off-White	Tablet	Circle	Teva Pharmaceuticals
93; 1177	Neomycin Sulfate	500 mg	Off-White	Tablet	Circle	Udl Laboratories
93; 1215	Cefaclor	375 mg	Blue	Tablet	Oval	Teva Pharmaceuticals
93; 1893	Etodolac	500 mg	Blue	Tablet	Oval	Teva Pharmaceuticals
93; 2264	Amoxicillin	875 mg	Off White	Tablet	Capsule-Shape, Scored	Teva Pharmaceuticals
93; 2268	Amoxicillin	250 mg	Off White	Tablet, Chewable	Capsule-Shape	Teva Pharmaceuticals
93; 2274	Amoxicillin and Clavulanate Potassium	500 mg; 125 mg	White	Tablet	Oblong	Teva Pharmaceuticals
93; 2275	Amoxicillin and Clavulanate Potassium	875 mg; 125 mg	White	Tablet	Oblong	Teva Pharmaceuticals
93; 3107	Amoxicillin	250 mg	Caramel and Buff	Capsule		Teva Pharmaceuticals
93; 3109	Amoxicillin	500 mg	Buff	Capsule		Teva Pharmaceuticals
93; 3111	Ampicillin	250 mg	Scarlet and Grey	Capsule		Teva Pharmaceuticals
93; 3113	Ampicillin	500 mg	Scarlet and Gray	Capsule		Teva Pharmaceuticals
93; 3115	Oxacillin Sodium	250 mg	Blue Opaque	Capsule		Teva Pharmaceuticals
93; 3115	Oxacillin Sodium	250 mg	Blue Opaque	Capsule		Zenith Goldline Pharmaceuticals
93; 3117	Oxacillin Sodium	500 mg	Blue Opaque	Capsule		Novartis Generics
93; 3117	Oxacillin Sodium	500 mg	Blue Opaque	Capsule		Teva Pharmaceuticals
93; 3119	Cloxacillin	250 mg	Dark Green and Scarlet	Capsule		Teva Pharmaceuticals
93; 3119	Cloxacillin	250 mg	Dark Green and Scarlet	Capsule		Zenith Goldline Pharmaceuticals
93; 3121	Cloxacillin	500 mg	Dark Green and Scarlet	Capsule		Teva Pharmaceuticals
93; 3121	Cloxacillin	500 mg	Dark Green and Scarlet	Capsule		Zenith Goldline Pharmaceuticals
93; 3123	Dicloxacillin Sodium	250 mg	Green and Light Green	Capsule		Novartis Generics
93; 3123	Dicloxacillin Sodium	250 mg	Green and Light Green	Capsule		Teva Pharmaceuticals
93; 3125	Dicloxacillin Sodium	500 mg	Green and Light Green	Capsule		Novartis Generics
93; 3125	Dicloxacillin Sodium	500 mg	Green and Light Green	Capsule		Teva Pharmaceuticals
93; 3127	Disopyramide Phosphate	100 mg	Blue and Scarlet	Capsule		Teva Pharmaceuticals
93; 3129	Disopyramide Phosphate	150 mg	Buff and Scarlet	Capsule		Teva Pharmaceuticals
93; 3145	Cephalexin	250 mg	Gray and Dark Orange	Capsule	Oblong	Teva Pharmaceuticals
93; 3145	Cephalexin	250 mg	Gray and Swedish Orange	Capsule		Teva Pharmaceuticals
93; 3147	Cephalexin	500 mg	Dark Orange	Capsule	Oblong	Teva Pharmaceuticals
93; 3147	Cephalexin	500 mg	Swedish Orange	Capsule		Teva Pharmaceuticals
93; 3153	Cephradine	250 mg	Light Green and Pink	Capsule		Novartis
93; 3153	Cephradine	250 mg	Light Green and Pink	Capsule		Teva Pharmaceuticals
93; 3155	Cephradine	500 mg	Light Green	Capsule		Teva Pharmaceuticals
93; 3165	Minocycline Hydrochloride	50 mg	Pink	Capsule		Teva Pharmaceuticals
93; 3167	Minocycline Hydrochloride	100 mg	Pink and Maroon	Capsule		Teva Pharmaceuticals

IMPRINT	BRAND/GENERIC NAME	STRENGTH	COLOR	FORM	SHAPE	MANUFACTURER
93; 3171	Clindamycin Hydrochloride	150 mg	Red and Blue	Capsule		Teva Pharmaceuticals
93; 3171	Clindamycin Hydrochloride	150 mg	Red and Blue	Capsule		Udl Laboratories
93; 3193	Ketoprofen	50 mg	Blue and Light Blue	Capsule		Teva Pharmaceuticals
93; 3195	Ketoprofen	75 mg	Blue and White	Capsule		Teva Pharmaceuticals
93; 5124	Benazepril Hydrochloride	5 mg	Light Yellow	Tablet	Triangle	Teva Pharmaceuticals
93; 5125	Benazepril Hydrochloride	10 mg	Mustard Yellow	Tablet	Triangle	Teva Pharmaceuticals
93; 5126	Benazepril Hydrochloride	20 mg	Pink	Tablet	Triangle	Teva Pharmaceuticals
93; 5127	Benazepril Hydrochloride	40 mg	Pink	Tablet	Triangle	Teva Pharmaceuticals
93; 5150	Moexipril Hydrochloride	15 mg	Pink	Tablet	Oval, Scored	Teva Pharmaceuticals
93; 5157	Lisinopril	30 mg	White	Tablet	Circle	Teva Pharmaceuticals
93 5160	Tizanidine Hydrochloride	4 mg	White to Off-White	Tablet		Teva Pharmaceuticals
93 5163	Tizanidine Hydrochloride	2 mg		Tablet		Teva Pharmaceuticals
93; 5194	Penicillin V Potassium	250 mg	White	Tablet	Oval	Teva Pharmaceuticals
93; 5195	Penicillin V Potassium	500 mg	White	Tablet	Oval	Teva Pharmaceuticals
93; 7113	Nefazodone Hydrochloride	150 mg	Peach	Tablet	Capsule-Shape, Scored	Teva Pharmaceuticals
93; 7120	Flutamide	125 mg	Beige	Capsule		Teva Pharmaceuticals
93; 7172	Etodolac	500 mg	Gray	Extended-Release Tablet	Oval	Teva Pharmaceuticals
93; 7178	Nefazodone Hydrochloride	50 mg	Light Pink	Tablet	Capsule-Shape, Scored	Teva Pharmaceuticals
93; 7180	Ofloxacin	200 mg	Light Yellow	Tablet	Oval	Teva Pharmaceuticals
93; 7181	Ofloxacin	300 mg	White to Off-White	Tablet	Oval	Teva Pharmaceuticals
93; 7182	Ofloxacin	400 mg	Pale Gold	Tablet	Oval	Teva Pharmaceuticals
93; 7188	Fluoxetine Hydrochloride	10 mg	Blue	Tablet	Oval, Scored	Teva Pharmaceuticals
93; 7198	Fluoxetine Hyrochloride	40 mg	Blue and Orange	Capsule		Teva Pharmaceuticals
93; 7206	Mirtazapine	15 mg	Yellow	Tablet	Circle	Teva Pharmaceuticals
93; 7207	Mirtazapine	30 mg	Reddish Brown	Tablet	Circle	Teva Pharmaceuticals
93; 7208	Mirtazapine	45 mg	White to Off-White	Tablet	Circle	Teva Pharmaceuticals
93; 7223	Fosinopril Sodium	20 mg	White to Off-White	Tablet	Rectangle	Teva Pharmaceuticals
93; 7224	Fosinopril Sodium	40 mg	White to Off-White	Tablet	Circle	Teva Pharmaceuticals
93; 7267	Metformin Hydrochloride	500 mg	White to Off-White	Extended-Release Tablet	Oval	Teva Pharmaceuticals
93; 9111	Prenatal Plus Vitamins	200 mg; 2 mg; 12 mcg; 1 mg; 20 mg; 10 mg; 3 mg; 1.5 mg; 4000 IU; 120 mg; 400 IU; 22 mg; 25 mg; 65 mg	Mustard Yellow	Coated Tablet	Oval	Teva Pharmaceuticals
93; 9133	Amiodarone Hydrochloride	200 mg	Pink	Tablet	Circle, Scored	Teva Pharmaceuticals
93; 9158	Multivitamins with Fluoride	2500 IU; 60 mg; 400 IU; 15 IU; 1.05 mg; 1.2 mg; 13.5 mg; 1.05 mg; 0.3 mg; 4.5 mcg; 0.5 mg	Pink, Purple, Orange	Tablet, Chewable	Square	Teva Pharmaceuticals
93; 9159	Multivitamins with Fluoride and Iron	2500 IU; 60 mg; 400 IU; 15 IU; 1.05 mg; 1.2 mg; 13.5 mg; 1.05 mg; 0.3 mg; 4.5 mcg; 12 mg; 10 mg; 1 mg; 1 mg	Purple	Tablet, Chewable	Square	Teva Pharmaceuticals
93; 9166	Multivitamins with Fluoride	2500 IU; 60 mg; 400 IU; 15 IU; 1.05 mg; 1.2 mg; 13.5 mg; 1.05 mg; 0.3 mg; 4.5 mcg; 1 mg	Pink, Purple, Orange	Tablet, Chewable	Square	Teva Pharmaceuticals
93; 9197	Multivitamins with Fluoride and Iron	2500 IU; 60 mg; 400 IU; 15 IU; 1.05 mg; 1.2 mg; 13.5 mg; 1.05 mg; 0.3 mg; 4.5 mcg; 12 mg; 10 mg; 1 mg; 0.5 mg	Pink	Tablet, Chewable	Square	Teva Pharmaceuticals
93; 9411	Methazolamide	25 mg	White	Tablet	Square	Teva Pharmaceuticals
93; 9643	Prochlorperazine Maleate	5 mg	Yellow	Tablet	Circle	Teva Pharmaceuticals
93; 9652	Prochlorperazine Maleate	10 mg	Yellow	Tablet	Circle	Teva Pharmaceuticals
93; 9774	Hydroxychloroquine	200 mg	White	Tablet	Capsule-Shape	Akyma Pharmaceuticals
93; DOXY	Doxycycline Hyclate	100 mg	Orange	Coated Tablet	Circle	Teva Pharmaceuticals
93; DOXY	Doxy-Lemmon	100 mg	Orange	Coated Tablet	Circle	Teva Pharmaceuticals
93; SOFARIN; 2	Sofarin	2 mg	Lavender	Tablet	Circle, Scored	Teva Pharmaceuticals
93; SOFARIN; 2 1/2	Sofarin	2.5 mg	Orange	Tablet	Circle, Scored	Teva Pharmaceuticals
93; SOFARIN; 5	Sofarin	5 mg	Pink	Tablet	Circle, Scored	Teva Pharmaceuticals
99	Adipex 8	8 mg	Blue and White	Capsule		Teva Pharmaceuticals
99	Vibra-Tabs	100 mg	Peach	Coated Tablet	Circle	Pfizer Laboratories
100	Ceenu	100 mg	Two-Tone Green	Capsule		Bristol-Myers Oncology
100	Dicumarol	100 mg		Tablet		Abbott Laboratories
100	Manoplax	100 mg	White	Coated Tablet	Six-Sided	Boots Pharmaceuticals
100; LARODOPA; ROCHE	Larodopa	100 mg	Pink	Tablet	Oval, Scored	Roche Pharmaceuticals
100; LL; A; 17	Asendin	100 mg	Blue	Tablet	Seven-Sided	Lederle Laboratories
100; T4	Levothroid	100 mcg	Yellow	Tablet	Capsule-Shape	Forest Pharmaceuticals
100; W; 705	Effexor	100 mg	Peach	Tablet	Shield-Shape	Wyeth Pharmaceuticals
101	Azulfidine	500 mg	Yellow	Tablet	Circle	Pharmacia & Upjohn
101	Docusate Sodium	100 mg	Red-Orange	Capsule		Paddock Labs
102	Docusate Sodium	250 mg	Red-Orange	Capsule		Paddock Labs
102; 5; BOEHRINGER MANNHEIM LOGO	Demadex	5 mg	White	Tablet	Oval, Scored	Roche Laboratories

IMPRINT	BRAND/GENERIC NAME	STRENGTH	COLOR	FORM	SHAPE	MANUFACTURER
103	Docusate Sodium with Casanthranol	100 mg; 30 mg	Maroon	Capsule		Paddock Labs
103	Oxoids	20 mg; 0.3 mg; 8 mg	Blue	Tablet		Teva Pharmaceuticals
103; 10; BOEHRINGER MANNHEIM LOGO	Demadex	10 mg	White	Tablet	Oval, Scored	Boehringer Mannheim
103; 10; BOEHRINGER MANNHEIM LOGO	Demadex	10 mg	White	Tablet	Oval, Scored	Roche Laboratories
104; 20; BOEHRINGER MANNHEIM LOGO	Demadex	20 mg	White	Tablet	Oval, Scored	Boehringer Mannheim
104; 20; BOEHRINGER MANNHEIM LOGO	Demadex	20 mg	White	Tablet	Oval, Scored	Roche Laboratories
105; 100; BOEHRINGER MANNHEIM LOGO	Demadex	100 mg	White	Tablet	Capsule-Shape, Scored	Boehringer Mannheim
105; 100; BOEHRINGER MANNHEIM LOGO	Demadex	100 mg	White	Tablet	Capsule-Shape, Scored	Roche Laboratories
107	Nu'leven	100 mg; 10 mg; 150 mg	Aqua	Tablet	Circle, Concave	Teva Pharmaceuticals
108	Lemidyne with Codeine	30 mg; 230 mg; 150 mg; 30 mg	White	Tablet		Teva Pharmaceuticals
110	Amnesteem	10 mg	Reddish Brown	Capsule		Bertek Pharmaceuticals
110	Rhinex DM	2 mg; 10 mg; 5 mg	White	Tablet		Teva Pharmaceuticals
112; T4	Levothroid	112 mcg	Rose	Tablet	Capsule-Shape	Forest Pharmaceuticals
115	Feogen FA	200 mg; 250 mg; 1 mg; 10 mcg	Maroon and Black	Capsule, Liquid Filled	Oval	Rising Pharmaceuticals
117; C	Dezone	0.75 mg	Light Blue	Tablet	Five-Sided	Solvay Pharmaceuticals
120	Amnesteem	20 mg	Reddish Brown and Cream	Capsule		Bertek Pharmaceuticals
120	Diltiazem Hydrochloride	120 mg	Light Purple	Extended-Release Capsule		Biovail Pharmaceuticals
120; RD201; R	Innopran XL	120 mg	Gray and Off-White	Extended-Release Capsule		Reliant Pharmaceuticals
122	K-Pek II	2 mg	Light Green	Tablet	Capsule-Shape	Rugby Laboratories
122	Loperamide	2 mg	Green	Tablet	Oblong	Qualitest Products
122	Loperamide Hydrochloride	2 mg	Green	Tablet	Bisected Scored	Ohm Laboratories
125	Slo-Bid Gyrocaps	125 mg	White	Extended-Release Capsule		Aventis Pharmaceuticals
125	Tracleer	125 mg	Orange-White	Coated Tablet	Oval, Biconvex	Actelion Pharmaceuticals
125	Tracleer	125 mg	Orange-White	Coated Tablet	Oval, Biconvex	Genentech
125; T4	Levothroid	125 mcg	Brown	Tablet	Capsule-Shape	Forest Pharmaceuticals
126; OHM	Pseudoephedrine Hcl and Acetaminophen	30 mg; 500 mg	Peach	Tablet		Ohm Laboratories
130; RH405	Antara	130 mg	Dark Green and White	Capsule	Capsule-Shape	Reliant Pharmaceuticals
131; 07	Prednicen-M	5 mg	Red	Coated Tablet	Capsule-Shaped, Bisected Scored	Century Pharmaceuticals
131; 07	Prednicen-M Tablet 5 mg	5 mg	Red	Coated Tablet	Capsule-Shape	Schwarz Pharma
133	Extendryl Chewable	10 mg; 2 mg; 1.25 mg	Tan	Tablet		Fleming
135; OHM	Acetaminophen, Pseudoephedrine Hcl, Dextromethorphan Hbr and Chlorpheniramine Maleate	325 mg; 2 mg; 30 mg; 10 mg	Yellow	Tablet		Ohm Laboratories
140	Amnesteem	40 mg	Orange and Brown	Capsule		Bertek Pharmaceuticals
141	Trilafon Repetab	8 mg	Gray	Timed-Release Tablet		Schering
150	Acetaminophen and Codeine	325 mg; 30 mg	White	Tablet		Paddock Labs
150; LL; A; 18	Asendin	150 mg	Peach	Tablet	Seven-Sided	Lederle Laboratories
150; T4	Levothroid	150 mcg	Blue	Tablet	Capsule-Shape	Forest Pharmaceuticals
152	Guaifenesin LA	600 mg	Green	Extended-Release Tablet	Capsule-Shape, Scored	Caraco Pharmaceutical
153	Aquatensen	5 mg	Pink	Tablet		Wallace Laboratories
155	Lemidyne with Codeine	15 mg; 230 mg; 150 mg; 30 mg	White	Tablet		Teva Pharmaceuticals
160	Triprolidine Hydrochloride and Pseudoephedrine Hydrochloride	2.5 mg; 60 mg	White	Tablet	Circle, Scored	Ohm Laboratories
160	Triprolidine Hydrochloride and Pseudoephedrine Hydrochloride	2.5 mg; 60 mg	White	Tablet	Circle, Scored	Udl Laboratories
160; OHM	Pseudoephedrine Hcl and Triprolidine Hcl	60 mg; 2.5 mg	White	Tablet	Bisected Scored	Ohm Laboratories
166	Mandelamine	500 mg	Brown	Coated Tablet	Capsule-Shape	Warner Chilcott
166	Metoprolol	50 mg	White	Tablet		Qualitest Products
166	Metoprolol Tartrate	50 mg	White	Tablet	Capsule-Shape	Caraco Pharmaceutical
167	Mandelamine	1000 mg	Purple	Coated Tablet		Warner Chilcott
167	Metoprolol	100 mg	White	Tablet		Qualitest Products
167	Metoprolol Tartrate	100 mg	White	Tablet	Capsule-Shape, Scored	Caraco Pharmaceutical
170	Sulindac	150 mg	Yellow	Tablet	Six-Sided	Endo Laboratories
172	Meticorten	5 mg	White	Tablet		Schering
172	Tora I	30 mg	Black	Capsule		Solvay Pharmaceuticals
174	Women's Laxative	5 mg	Pink	Enteric-Coated Tablet	Circle	Good Neighbor Pharmacy

IMPRINT	BRAND/GENERIC NAME	STRENGTH	COLOR	FORM	SHAPE	MANUFACTURER
174	Women's Laxative	5 mg	Pink	Enteric-Coated Tablet	Circle	Good Sense
174	Women's Laxative	5 mg	Pink	Enteric-Coated Tablet	Circle	Kerr Drug
174	Women's Laxative	5 mg	Pink	Enteric-Coated Tablet	Circle	Nex
174	Women's Laxative	5 mg	Pink	Enteric-Coated Tablet	Circle	Perfect Choice
174	Women's Laxative	5 mg	Pink	Enteric-Coated Tablet	Circle	Perrigo
174	Women's Laxative	5 mg	Pink	Enteric-Coated Tablet	Circle	Quality Care
174	Women's Laxative	5 mg	Pink	Enteric-Coated Tablet	Circle	Sunmark
174	Women's Laxative	5 mg	Pink	Enteric-Coated Tablet	Circle	Top Care
174	Women's Laxative	5 mg	Pink	Enteric-Coated Tablet	Circle	Valu Rite
175	Synthroid	175 mcg	Lilac	Tablet		Abbott Laboratories
175 175	Paromomycin Sulfate	250 mg	Yellow-Green	Capsule		Caraco Pharmaceutical
175; T4	Levothroid	175 mcg	Lilac	Tablet	Capsule-Shape	Forest Pharmaceuticals
177; KU; 15	Moexipril Hydrochloride	15 mg	Salmon	Tablet	Circle, Biconvex, Scored	Kremers Urban
180	Diltiazem Hydrochloride	180 mg	White and Blue-Green	Extended-Release Capsule		Biovail Pharmaceuticals
200	Breonesin	200 mg	Red	Capsule		Winthrop Pharmaceuticals
200	Hydrochlorothiazide	50 mg	Peach	Tablet		Paddock Labs
200	Hytuss	200 mg	Red	Capsule		Hyrex Pharmaceuticals
200; T4	Levothroid	200 mcg	Pink	Tablet	Capsule-Shape	Forest Pharmaceuticals
201	Berovite Plus	5000 IU; 30 IU; 500 mg; 20 mg; 20 mg; 100 mg; 25 mg; 0.15 mg; 25 mg; 0.8 mg; 50 mcg; 27 mg; 0.1 mg; 50 mg; 5 mg; 3 mg; 22.5 mg	Clear	Tablet		Everett Laboratories
204	Amobarbital D-Lay	60 mg	Orange and White	Tablet		Teva Pharmaceuticals
207	Corgard	40 mg		Tablet		Monarch Pharmaceuticals
207; LEMMON; 207	Mepriam	400 mg	Yellow	Tablet	Oblong, Scored	Teva Pharmaceuticals
208	Corgard	120 mg		Tablet		Monarch Pharmaceuticals
215; ALRA	Ibu-Tab	200 mg	Orange	Coated Tablet	Circle	Alra Laboratories
215; Q	Meclodium	50 mg	Ivory	Capsule, Liquid Filled		Quantum Pharmics
216; Q	Meclodium	100 mg	Yellow	Capsule, Liquid Filled		Quantum Pharmics
219	Choline Magnesium Trisalicylate 500 mg	293 mg; 362 mg	Yellow	Tablet	Capsule-Shape, Scored	Caraco Pharmaceutical
220	Choline Magnesium Trisalicylate 750 mg	440 mg; 544 mg	Blue	Tablet	Capsule-Shape, Scored	Caraco Pharmaceutical
221	Choline Magnesium Trisalicylate 1000 mg	587 mg; 725 mg	Pink	Tablet	Capsule-Shape	Caraco Pharmaceutical
221	Glipizide	5 mg	White	Tablet	Circle, Scored	Schein Pharmaceutical
225; 105	Tolfrinic	600 mg; 25 mcg; 100 mg	Brown	Coated Tablet		Ascher
225; 295; A	Anaspaz	0.125 mg	Light Yellow	Tablet	Compressed, Scored	Ascher
225; 300; A	Anaspaz PB	0.125 mg; 15 mg	Pink	Tablet		Ascher
225; 356; A	Mobigesic	325 mg; 30 mg	White	Tablet	Circle, Scored	Ascher
225; 410; A	Metronid	250 mg	White	Tablet	Circle, Scored	Ascher
225; 425; A	Furose	40 mg	White	Tablet	Circle, Scored	Ascher
225; 450; A	HY-Phen	5 mg; 500 mg	White	Tablet	Capsule-Shape, Compressed, Scored	Ascher
225; 470	Adipost	105 mg	Clear and White with White Beads	Capsule		Ascher
225; 480; A	Allent	12 mg; 120 mg	Clear with White Beads	Extended-Release Capsule		Ascher
225; 490	Unilax	230 mg; 130 mg	Gold Tan	Capsule, Liquid Filled	Oval	Ascher
227; 555	Erythromycin Estolate	250 mg	Orange	Capsule		Teva Pharmaceuticals
230	Bisacodyl	5 mg	Yellow	Enteric-Coated Tablet	Circle, Convex	Leiner Health Products
230	Bisacodyl	5 mg	Yellow	Enteric-Coated Tablet	Circle	Ohm Laboratories
230	Bisacodyl	5 mg	Yellow	Enteric-Coated Tablet	Circle	Udl Laboratories
231	Ferrocol	150 mg	Blue	Capsule		Teva Pharmaceuticals
232	Corgard	20 mg		Tablet		Monarch Pharmaceuticals
235	Thyrocrine	2.5 Gr	Tan	Tablet		Teva Pharmaceuticals
235	Thyroid	2.5 Gr	Tan	Tablet		Teva Pharmaceuticals
240	Diltiazem Hydrochloride	240 mg	Blue-Green and Light Purple	Extended-Release Capsule		Biovail Pharmaceuticals
241	Clorazepate Dipotassium	3.75 mg	Blue	Tablet	T-Shaped, Scored	Purepac Pharmaceutical
241	Corgard	80 mg		Tablet		Monarch Pharmaceuticals
242	Clorazepate Dipotassium	7.5 mg	Peach	Tablet	T-Shaped, Scored	Purepac Pharmaceutical
243	Clorazepate Dipotassium	15 mg	Lavender	Tablet	T-Shaped, Scored	Purepac Pharmaceutical
246	Corgard	160 mg	Blue	Tablet	Oblong, Scored	Monarch Pharmaceuticals
250	Bendopa	0.25 GM	Clear	Capsule		Icn Pharmaceuticals
250	Cefaclor	250 mg	Blue and White	Capsule		Stada
250	Slo-Niacin	250 mg	Pink	Extended-Release Tablet	Capsule-Shape, Scored	Upsher-Smith Laboratories
250; LARODOPA; ROCHE	Larodopa	250 mg	Pink	Tablet	Circle, Scored	Roche Pharmaceuticals
251; DMSP	Carbidopa and Levodopa	25 mg; 250 mg	Light Dapple-Blue	Tablet	Oval, Scored	Bristol-Myers Squibb
252; 0220	Thyroid	129.6 mg		Tablet		Bowman Pharmaceuticals
252; 0494	Thyroid	32.4 mg		Tablet		Bowman Pharmaceuticals
252; 0495	Thyroid	64.8 mg	Tan	Tablet	Circle	Bowman Pharmaceuticals
255	Chlorpheniramine Maleate	4 mg	Yellow	Tablet	Compressed, Round, Convex, Bisected Scored	Leiner Health Products
258	Histex Ct	8 mg	Blue Film-Coated	Extended-Release Tablet	Circle, Scored	Teamm Pharmaceuticals
261	Codone	5 mg	White	Tablet		Teva Pharmaceuticals
271; DMSP	Carbidopa and Levodopa	10 mg; 100 mg	Dark Dapple-Blue	Tablet	Oval, Scored	Bristol-Myers Squibb
272; DMSP	Carbidopa and Levodopa	25 mg; 100 mg	Yellow	Tablet	Oval, Scored	Bristol-Myers Squibb
274; HEXAGON	Diutensen-R	2.5 mg; 0.1 mg	Red and White Mottled	Tablet		Mallinckrodt
283; 200 MCG	Baycol	0.2 mg	Light Yellow	Tablet		Bayer Pharmaceutical
284; 300 MCG	Baycol	0.3 mg	Yellow-Brown	Tablet		Bayer Pharmaceutical
285; 400 MCG	Baycol	0.4 mg	Ocher	Tablet		Bayer Pharmaceutical

IMPRINT	BRAND/GENERIC NAME	STRENGTH	COLOR	FORM	SHAPE	MANUFACTURER
286; 800 MCG	Baycol	0.8 mg	Brown-Orange	Tablet		Bayer Pharmaceutical
296	Phyldrox	100 mg; 25 mg; 15 mg	White	Tablet		Teva Pharmaceuticals
300	Diltiazem Hydrochloride	300 mg	White and Light Purple	Extended-Release Capsule		Biovail Pharmaceuticals
300; M30; MOVA	Cimetidine	300 mg	White	Coated Tablet	Round, Bisected Scored	Par Pharmaceutical
300; T4	Levothroid	300 mcg	Green	Tablet	Capsule-Shape	Forest Pharmaceuticals
301	Barbidonna	16 mg; 0.13 mg; 0.025 mg; 0.007 mg	White	Tablet	Oblong	Wallace Laboratories
301; VIRILON 10 MG	Virilon	10 mg	Black and Clear	Capsule		Star Pharmaceuticals
304	Pyradyne	210 mg; 30 mg; 150 mg; 15 mg	Red	Tablet		Teva Pharmaceuticals
305; MARLOP	Martinic	110 mg; 240 mg; 15 mcg; 75 mg; 0.5 mg	Light Blue	Capsule		Marlop Pharmaceuticals
306	Pyradyne Compound	15 mg; 120 mg; 100 mg; 8 mg; 10 mg; 0.12 mg; 8 mg;	Yellow	Tablet		Teva Pharmaceuticals
308AV	Allegra-D 24 Hour	180 mg; 240 mg	White	Extended-Release Tablet	Circle	Aventis Pharmaceuticals
311	Barbidonna No. 2	32 mg; 0.13 mg; 0.025 mg; 0.007 mg		Tablet		Wallace Laboratories
311	Vytorin 10/10	10 mg; 10 mg	White to Off-White	Tablet	Capsule-Shape	Merck
311; OHM	Acetaminophen	500 mg	White	Tablet		Ohm Laboratories
312	Vytorin 10/20	10 mg; 20 mg	White to Off-White	Tablet	Capsule-Shape	Merck
313	Vytorin 10/40	10 mg; 40 mg	White to Off-White	Tablet	Capsule-Shape	Merck
315	Vytorin 10/80	10 mg; 80 mg	White to Off-White	Tablet	Capsule-Shape	Merck
315; MARLOP	Promar	115 mcg; 15 mcg; 75 mg; 150 mg; 1 mg	Red	Capsule		Marlop Pharmaceuticals
320	Phenolphthalein	90 mg	Off-White	Coated Tablet	Circle, Convex	Leiner Health Products
320; OHM	Yellow Phenolphthalein	90 mg	White	Coated Tablet		Ohm Laboratories
321; ALRA	PP-Cap	65 mg	Grey and White	Capsule		Alra Laboratories
322	Lemivite	16 mg; 71 mg; 1.6 mg; 1 mcg; 3.33 mg; 0.33 mg; 55 mg; 0.166 mg; 1 mg; 1 mg; 0.4 mg; 0.4 IU; 1666 IU; 1.7 mg; 8 mg; 1 mg; 66 IU; 0.33 mg	Red	Tablet		Teva Pharmaceuticals
323; ALRA	Pc-Cap	65 mg; 389 mg; 32.4 mg	Grey and Orange	Capsule		Alra Laboratories
325; ALRA	Mb-Tab	200 mg	White	Tablet	Circle	Alra Laboratories
327	Ticlopidine Hydrochloride	250 mg	Peach	Tablet	Oval	Caraco Pharmaceutical
327; ALRA	Mb-Tab	400 mg	White	Tablet	Circle	Alra Laboratories
331	Regular Strength Laxative Pills	15 mg	Beige	Tablet	Circle	Good Neighbor Pharmacy
331	Regular Strength Laxative Pills	15 mg	Beige	Tablet	Circle	Kerr Drug
331	Regular Strength Laxative Pills	15 mg	Beige	Tablet	Circle	Major
331	Regular Strength Laxative Pills	15 mg	Beige	Tablet	Circle	Top Care
331	Regular Strength Laxative Pills	15 mg	Beige	Tablet	Circle	Valu Rite
333	Campral	333 mg	White	Enteric-Coated Tablet	Circle	Forest Pharmaceuticals
336	Diagnex Blue Test Sodium Benzoate and Caffeine	250 mg;		Tablet		Bristol-Myers Squibb
345	Clozapine	25 mg		Tablet	Circle, Scored on Blank Side	Caraco Pharmaceutical
347	Clozapine	100 mg		Tablet	Circle, Scored on Blank Side	Caraco Pharmaceutical
348	Glucoron with B12	250 mg; 1 mg; 0.5 mg; 1 mg; 2 mg; 3 mcg	Pink	Tablet		Teva Pharmaceuticals
351; RPR	Slo-Phyllin	100 mg	White	Tablet	Circle	Aventis Pharmaceuticals
355	Aluprin	300 mg;	Green and White	Tablet		Teva Pharmaceuticals
360	Diltiazem Hydrochloride	360 mg	Blue-Green	Extended-Release Capsule		Biovail Pharmaceuticals
375 MG; PILFA	Metronidazole	375 mg	Light Green	Capsule		Pliva
377	Tramadol Hydrochloride	50 mg	White	Tablet	Capsule-Shape	Caraco Pharmaceutical
386; ORGANON	Cotazym	8000 U; 30000 U; 30000 U; 25 mg	Red	Capsule		Organon
389	Axocet	50 mg; 650 mg	Blue	Tablet	Capsule-Shape	Savage Laboratories
391	Oxaprozin	600 mg	White to Off-White	Tablet	Capsule-Shape	Caraco Pharmaceutical
393	Diabinese	100 mg	Blue	Tablet	D-Shape, Scored	Pfizer Laboratories
394	Diabinese	250 mg	Blue	Tablet	D-Shape, Scored	Pfizer Laboratories
400	Ibuprofen	400 mg	White	Tablet	Circle	Winsor Pharmaceuticals
400; M40; MOVA	Cimetidine	400 mg	White	Coated Tablet	Capsule-Shaped, Bisected Scored	Par Pharmaceutical
403	Pseudoephedrine Hydrochloride	30 mg	Red	Coated Tablet	Circle	Ohm Laboratories
404	Acetaminophen	648 mg	White	Tablet	Oval	Jb Laboratories
405; HD	Amitriptyline Hydrochloride	10 mg	Pink	Coated Tablet		Halsey Drug
406; HD	Amitriptyline Hydrochloride	25 mg	Green	Coated Tablet		Halsey Drug
407; HD	Amitriptyline Hydrochloride	50 mg	Brown	Coated Tablet		Halsey Drug
408; HD	Amitriptyline Hydrochloride	75 mg	Purple	Coated Tablet		Halsey Drug
409; HD	Amitriptyline Hydrochloride	100 mg	Orange	Coated Tablet		Halsey Drug
414	Zetia	10 mg	Off-White	Tablet	Capsule-Shape	Schering
415; A	Niloric	1 mg	White	Tablet	Oval	Ascher
420	Ibuprofen	200 mg	White	Coated Tablet	Circle	Ohm Laboratories
420	Ibuprofen	200 mg	White	Coated Tablet	Circle	Udl Laboratories
420	Ibutab	200 mg	White	Tablet	Circle, Convex	Zee Medical
424; OHM	Ibuprofen	200 mg	White	Tablet		Ohm Laboratories

IMPRINT	BRAND/GENERIC NAME	STRENGTH	COLOR	FORM	SHAPE	MANUFACTURER
426; 27	Acetaminophen	325 mg	White	Tablet	Circle, Scored	Oakmont Pharmaceutical
426; 29	Acetaminophen	500 mg		Tablet	Circle	Oakmont Pharmaceutical
437	Digoxin	125 mcg	Yellow	Tablet	Circle	Caraco Pharmaceutical
437; PM	Extra Strength Mapap Pm/sleep Aid	500 mg; 25 mg	Blue	Tablet		Major Pharmaceutical
437; PM	Extra Strength Mapap Pm/sleep Aid	500 mg; 25 mg	Blue	Tablet		Major Quality
437; PM	Pain-A-Lieve Pm, Extra Strength	500 mg; 25 mg	Blue	Tablet		True Quality
437; PM	Pain-A-Lieve Pm, Extra Strength	500 mg; 25 mg	Blue	Tablet		True Quality Products
440; OHM	Ibuprofen	400 mg	Red	Coated Tablet		Ohm Laboratories
441	Digoxin	0.25 mg	White	Tablet	Circle	Caraco Pharmaceutical
446; OHM	Ibuprofen	400 mg	White	Coated Tablet		Ohm Laboratories
457	Laxative Pills Maximum Strength	25 mg	Blue	Tablet	Circle	Good Neighbor Pharmacy
457	Laxative Pills Maximum Strength	25 mg	Blue	Tablet	Circle	Kerr Drug
457	Senna Laxative Maximum Strength	25 mg	Blue	Tablet	Circle	Sunmark
457	Laxative Pills Maximum Strength	25 mg	Blue	Tablet	Circle	Top Care
457	Laxative Pills Maximum Strength	25 mg	Blue	Tablet	Circle	Valu Rite
461; 80 MG	Emend	80 mg	White	Capsule		Merck
462; 125 MG	Emend	125 mg	White and Pink	Capsule		Merck
465; 3	Acetaminophen and Codeine	300 mg; 30 mg	White	Tablet	Compressed	Rosemont Pharmaceutical
466; 4	Acetaminophen and Codeine	300 mg; 60 mg	White	Tablet	Compressed	Rosemont Pharmaceutical
477	Metoprolol Tartrate	50 mg	White	Tablet	Circle, Scored	Caraco Pharmaceutical
496	Adphen-G	35 mg	Green Speckled	Tablet	Oblong, Scored	Ferndale Laboratories
499; SCHERING	Oreton Methyl	25 mg	Peach	Tablet		Schering
500	Anacin Maximum Strength	500 mg; 32 mg	White	Coated Tablet	Circle	Whitehall Laboratories
500	Cefaclor	500 mg	Blue and Grey	Capsule		Stada
500	Niacor B3	500 mg	White	Tablet	Oblong, Scored	Upsher-Smith Laboratories
500	Slo-Niacin	500 mg	Pink	Extended-Release Tablet	Capsule-Shape, Scored	Upsher-Smith Laboratories
500; BAYER	Bayer Maximum	500 mg		Tablet		Bayer Consumer Care
500; LARODOPA; ROCHE	Larodopa	500 mg	Pink	Tablet	Oblong, Scored	Roche Pharmaceuticals
500; M50; MOVA	Naproxen	500 mg	Peach	Tablet	Oval	Mova Pharmaceutical
500; MG	Mono-Gesic	500 mg	Pink	Coated Tablet	Circle	Schwarz Pharma
500 MG; A5; LEDERLE	Achromycin V	500 mg	Yellow and Blue	Capsule		Lederle Laboratories
502	Advicor	500 mg; 20 mg	Light Yellow	Coated Tablet	Capsule-Shape	Kos Pharmaceuticals
502	Azene	6.5 mg	Orange	Tablet	Oblong	Endo Laboratories
502	Tizanidine Hydrochloride	2 mg	White to Off-White	Tablet	Circle	Caraco Pharmaceutical
503	Tizanidine Hydrochloride	4 mg	White to Off-White	Tablet		Caraco Pharmaceutical
508	Citalopram Hydrobromide	20 mg	Pink	Tablet	Oval	Caraco Pharmaceutical
508	Ferrous Gluconate	324 mg	Green	Capsule		Paddock Labs
509	Citalopram Hydrobromide	40 mg	White	Tablet	Oval	Caraco Pharmaceutical
511	Selegiline Hydrochloride	5 mg	White	Capsule		Stada
511; 0.5	Lorazepam	0.5 mg	White	Tablet	Five-Sided, Small	Esi Lederle
511; 1	Lorazepam	1 mg	White	Tablet	Five-Sided, Scored	Esi Lederle
511; 1 MG	Lorazepam	1 mg	White	Tablet	Five-Sided	Wyeth Pharmaceuticals
511; 2	Lorazepam	2 mg	White	Tablet	Five-Sided, Scored	Esi Lederle
511; 2 MG	Lorazepam	2 mg	White	Tablet	Five-Sided	Wyeth Pharmaceuticals
511; 3620; 400	Etodolac	400 mg	Light Orange	Extended-Release Tablet	Oval	Esi Lederle
511; 3621; 500	Etodolac	500 mg	Light Green	Extended-Release Tablet	Oval	Esi Lederle
511; 3622; 600	Etodolac	600 mg	White	Extended-Release Tablet	Oval	Esi Lederle
511; 7065	Bisoprolol and Hydrochlorothiazide	2.5 mg; 6.25 mg	Off-White to Yellow	Tablet	Circle	Esi Lederle
511; M; X	Methotrexate Sodium	2.5 mg	Yellow	Tablet	Circle	Esi Lederle
511; P77	Pentoxifylline	400 mg	White	Sustained-Release Tablet	Oval	Esi Lederle
512	Acetaminophen and Oxycodone	325 mg; 5 mg	White	Tablet	Circle, Scored	Mallinckrodt
512	Oxycodone and Acetaminophen	5 mg; 325 mg	White	Tablet	Circle	Mallinckrodt
521; SINEMET CR	Sinemet Cr 50-200	50 mg; 200 mg	Peach	Sustained-Release Tablet	Oval, Scored, Biconvex, Compressed	Bristol-Myers Squibb
538	Amitriptyline Hydrochloride	10 mg		Tablet		Circa Pharmaceuticals
539	Amitriptyline Hydrochloride	25 mg		Tablet		Circa Pharmaceuticals
541	Amitriptyline Hydrochloride	75 mg		Tablet		Circa Pharmaceuticals
543; 80	Zocor	80 mg	Brick Red	Coated Tablet	Capsule-Shape	Merck & Company
547	Wigrettes	2 mg	White	Tablet		Organon
555; 030	Colchicine	0.65 mg	White	Tablet		Barr Laboratories
555; 19	Hydrochlorothiazide Hydrochloride	25 mg	Peach	Tablet	Circle, Scored	Barr Laboratories
555; 20	Hydrochlorothiazide Hydrochloride	50 mg	Peach	Tablet	Circle, Scored	Barr Laboratories
555; 126	Dicyclomine Hydrochloride	20 mg	Blue	Tablet	Circle	Barr Laboratories
555; 279	Isosorbide Dinitrate	30 mg	Blue	Tablet	Circle, Scored	H.L. Moore
555; 429	Trimethoprim	100 mg	White	Tablet	Circle, Scored	Barr Laboratories
555; 430	Trimethoprim	200 mg		Tablet		Barr Laboratories
561; MD	Metadate ER	10 mg	White	Extended-Release Tablet	Oval	Medeva Pharmaceuticals
562; HD	Brotane	4 mg	Peach	Tablet		Halsey Drug
562; MD	Metadate ER	20 mg	White	Extended-Release Tablet	Circle	Medeva Pharmaceuticals
562; W615	Westhroid	129.6 mg	Various Colors	Tablet	Circle	Western Research Laboratories
591; A	Meprobamate	400 mg	White	Tablet	Circle, Scored	Watson Laboratories
591; B	Meprobamate	200 mg	White	Tablet	Scored, Circle	Watson Laboratories
592; ATHENA LOGO	Zanaflex	2 mg	White	Tablet	Circle	Athena Neurosciences
592; ATHENA LOGO	Zanaflex	2 mg	White	Tablet	Circle	Elan Pharma
594; ATHENA LOGO	Zanaflex	4 mg	White	Tablet	Circle, Cross-Scored	Athena Neurosciences
594; ATHENA LOGO	Zanaflex	4 mg	White	Tablet	Circle, Cross-Scored	Elan Pharma
600	Ibuprofen	600 mg	White	Tablet	Oval	Winsor Pharmaceuticals
600; 4141	Fenoprofen Calcium	600 mg	Peach	Coated Tablet	Oval, Bisected Scored	Ivax Pharmaceuticals
600; OHM	Acetaminophen	500 mg	Red and White	Capsule		Ohm Laboratories

IMPRINT	BRAND/GENERIC NAME	STRENGTH	COLOR	FORM	SHAPE	MANUFACTURER
601; SINEMET CR	Sinemet Cr 25-100	25 mg; 100 mg	Pink	Sustained-Release Tablet	Oval, Biconvex, Compressed	Bristol-Myers Squibb
603	Sumycin	500 mg	Pink	Tablet	Capsule-Shape	Par Pharmaceutical
603	Sumycin 500	500 mg	Pink	Tablet	Capsule-Shape	Par Pharmaceutical
607; 0.5 MG	Prograf	0.5 mg	Light Yellow	Capsule		Fujisawa
608	Ferrous Sulfate	324 mg	Red	Enteric-Coated Tablet		Paddock Labs
610; HD	Acetaminophen and Propoxyphene Napsylate	50 mg; 325 mg	Orange	Coated Tablet	Capsule-Shape	Halsey Drug
617; 1 MG	Prograf	1 mg	White	Capsule		Fujisawa
620; OHM	Acetaminophen, Pseudoephedrine Hcl, Dextromethorphan Hbr and Chlorpheniramine Maleate	325 mg; 2 mg; 30 mg; 10 mg	Orange and Yellow	Capsule		Ohm Laboratories
627	Belap Se	10.8 mg	Green	Tablet		Teva Pharmaceuticals
643; 2 1/2	Metolazone	2.5 mg	Pink	Tablet	Circle	Celltech
644	Prednisolone	5 mg	Orange	Tablet		Teva Pharmaceuticals
644; 5	Metolazone	5 mg	Blue	Tablet	Circle	Celltech
645	Prednisone	5 mg	White	Tablet		Teva Pharmaceuticals
645; 10	Metolazone	10 mg	Yellow	Tablet	Circle	Celltech
647 SINEMET	Sinemet 10-100	10 mg; 100 mg	Dark Dapple-Blue	Tablet	Oval, Scored	Bristol-Myers Squibb
650; SINEMET	Sinemet 25-100	25 mg; 100 mg	Yellow	Tablet	Oval, Scored	Bristol-Myers Squibb
654; SINEMET	Sinemet 25-250	25 mg; 250 mg	Light Dapple-Blue	Tablet	Oval, Scored	Bristol-Myers Squibb
657; 5 MG	Prograf	5 mg	Gray and Red	Capsule		Fujisawa
663	Sumycin	250 mg	Pink	Tablet	Capsule-Shape	Par Pharmaceutical
663	Sumycin 250	250 mg	Light Pink	Tablet	Capsule-Shape	Par Pharmaceutical
665	Lithium Carbonate	300 mg	Opaque White	Capsule		Solvay Pharmaceuticals
672	Pentoxifylline	400 mg	White	Extended-Release Tablet	Oblong	Copley Pharmaceutical
707	Rynatan	9 mg; 25 mg	Buff	Tablet	Capsule-Shape	Wallace Laboratories
707; SP; 7.5	Univasc	7.5 mg	Pink	Coated Tablet	Circle, Biconvex, Scored	Schwarz Pharma
710; LOGO	Fosamax Plus D	70 mg; 2800 IU	White to Off White	Tablet	Capsule-Shape	Merck & Company
715; SP; 15	Univasc	15 mg	Salmon	Coated Tablet	Circle, Biconvex, Scored	Schwarz Pharma
717; KU; 7.5	Moexipril Hydrochloride	7.5 mg	Pink	Tablet	Circle, Biconvex, Scored	Kremers Urban
730	Tamoxifen	10 mg	White	Tablet	Circle, Biconvex	Astra Zeneca
731	Tamoxifen	20 mg	White	Tablet	Circle, Biconvex	Astra Zeneca
733; 54	Morphine Sulfate	15 mg	White	Tablet		Roxane Laboratories
750	Slo-Niacin	750 mg	Pink	Extended-Release Tablet	Capsule-Shape, Scored	Upsher-Smith Laboratories
752	Advicor	750 mg; 20 mg	Light Orange	Coated Tablet	Capsule-Shape	Kos Pharmaceuticals
752; 2	Hydromorphone Hydrochloride	2 mg	White	Tablet	Circle	Endo Laboratories
753; TRIANGLE	Mirtazapine	15 mg	Yellow	Tablet	Circle, Scored	Andrx Pharmaceuticals
754; TRIANGLE	Mirtazapine	30 mg	Beige	Tablet	Circle, Scored	Andrx Pharmaceuticals
755; TRIANGLE	Mirtazapine	45 mg	White	Tablet	Circle, Scored	Andrx Pharmaceuticals
757; 4	Hydromorphone Hydrochloride	4 mg	Light Yellow	Tablet	Circle	Endo Laboratories
770	Acetaminophen	500 mg	White	Tablet	Oblong	Jb Laboratories
771	Acetaminophen	325 mg	White	Tablet	Circle	Jb Laboratories
773	Spasdel	0.125 mg	Yellow	Tablet		Marlop Pharmaceuticals
800	Ibuprofen	800 mg	White	Tablet	Capsule-Shape	Winsor Pharmaceuticals
800; M80; MOVA	Cimetidine	800 mg	White	Coated Tablet	Capsule-Shaped, Bisected Scored	Par Pharmaceutical
804	Tora 30	30 mg	Black and Scarlet	Capsule		Solvay Pharmaceuticals
810	Thyroid Green	5 Gr	Green	Tablet		Teva Pharmaceuticals
811	Dolmar	50 mg; 325 mg; 40 mg	White	Tablet		Marlop Pharmaceuticals
812	Thyroid	3 Gr	Blue	Tablet		Teva Pharmaceuticals
816	Chlorpheniramine Maleate	4 mg	Yellow	Tablet	Compressed	Rosemont Pharmaceutical
822; 6	Butalbital with Apc	50 mg; 200 mg; 130 mg; 40 mg	White	Tablet		Knoll Pharmaceutical
830	Proglycem	100 mg	Orange	Capsule		Schering
831; 10	Chlorpromazine Hydrochloride	10 mg	Tan	Coated Tablet	Circle	H.L. Moore
832; 05	Oxybutynin Chloride	5 mg	Pink	Tablet	Compressed, Scored	Rosemont Pharmaceutical
832; 10	Chlorpromazine	10 mg	Tan	Tablet	Circle, Scored	Qualitest Products
832; 10	Chlorpromazine Hydrochloride	10 mg	Butterscotch	Coated Tablet	Circle	Rosemont Pharmaceutical
832; 10	Chlorpromazine Hydrochloride	10 mg	Butterscotch	Coated Tablet	Circle	Udl Laboratories
832; 25	Chlorpromazine Hydrchoride	25 mg	Butterscotch	Coated Tablet	Circle	H.L. Moore
832; 25	Chlorpromazine	25 mg	Tan	Tablet	Circle, Scored	Qualitest Products
832; 25	Chlorpromazine Hydrochloride	25 mg	Butterscotch	Coated Tablet	Circle	Rosemont Pharmaceutical
832; 25	Chlorpromazine Hydrochloride	25 mg	Butterscotch	Coated Tablet	Circle	Udl Laboratories
832; 38;	Oxybutynin Chloride	5 mg	White	Tablet	Circle, Scored	Udl Laboratories
832; 50	Chlorpromazine Hydrochloride	50 mg	Tan	Coated Tablet	Circle	H.L. Moore
832; 50	Chlorpromazine	50 mg	Tan	Tablet	Circle, Scored	Qualitest Products
832; 50	Chlorpromazine Hydrochloride	50 mg	Butterscotch	Coated Tablet	Circle	Rosemont Pharmaceutical
832; 50	Chlorpromazine Hydrochloride	50 mg	Butterscotch	Coated Tablet	Circle	Udl Laboratories
832 86	Androxy	10 mg	Green	Tablet	Circle	Upsher-Smith Laboratories
832; 86	Fluoxymesterone	10 mg	Green	Tablet	Circle	Qualitest Products
832; 100	Chlorpromazine Hydrochloride	100 mg	Tan	Coated Tablet	Circle	H.L. Moore
832; 100	Chlorpromazine	100 mg	Tan	Tablet	Circle, Scored	Qualitest Products
832; 100	Chlorpromazine Hydrochloride	100 mg	Butterscotch	Coated Tablet	Circle	Rosemont Pharmaceutical
832; 100	Chlorpromazine Hydrochloride	100 mg	Butterscotch	Coated Tablet	Circle	Udl Laboratories
832; 200	Chlorpromazine Hydrochloride	200 mg	Tan	Coated Tablet	Circle	H.L. Moore
832; 200	Chlorpromazine	200 mg	Tan	Tablet	Circle, Scored	Qualitest Products
832; 200	Chlorpromazine Hydrochloride	200 mg	Butterscotch	Coated Tablet	Circle	Rosemont Pharmaceutical
832; 200	Chlorpromazine Hydrochloride	200 mg	Butterscotch	Coated Tablet	Circle	Udl Laboratories
832; BC10	Antispastic	10 mg	White	Tablet	Circle, Scored	Rosemont Pharmaceutical
832; BC20	Antispastic	20 mg	White	Tablet	Circle, Scored	Rosemont Pharmaceutical
832; BM05	Benztropine Mesylate	0.5 mg	White	Tablet	Circle, Scored	Rosemont Pharmaceutical
832; BM05	Benztropine Mesylate	0.5 mg	White	Tablet	Circle, Scored	Udl Laboratories
832; BM1	Benztropine Mesylate	1 mg	White	Tablet	Oval, Scored	Rosemont Pharmaceutical
832; BM1	Benztropine Mesylate	1 mg	White	Tablet	Oval, Scored	Udl Laboratories
832; BM2	Benztropine Mesylate	2 mg	White	Tablet	Circle, Scored	Rosemont Pharmaceutical
832; BM2	Benztropine Mesylate	2 mg	White	Tablet	Circle, Scored	Udl Laboratories
832; C; 614	Thyroid	1 Gr	Beige	Tablet	Circle	Solvay Pharmaceuticals
832C; TEM15	Temazepam	15 mg	White and Green	Capsule		Rosemont Pharmaceutical

IMPRINT	BRAND/GENERIC NAME	STRENGTH	COLOR	FORM	SHAPE	MANUFACTURER
832C; TEM30	Temazepam	30 mg	White	Capsule		Rosemont Pharmaceutical
832; C5C	Clinibrax	5 mg; 2.5 mg	Green and Blue	Capsule		Rosemont Pharmaceutical
832; D25	Dipyridamole	25 mg	Orange or White	Coated Tablet		Rosemont Pharmaceutical
832; D50	Dipyridamole	50 mg	White	Coated Tablet		Rosemont Pharmaceutical
832; D75	Dipyridamole	75 mg	White	Coated Tablet		Rosemont Pharmaceutical
832; G; 19C; 2;	Prazepam	5 mg	White and Ivory	Capsule		Rosemont Pharmaceutical
832; G31	Acetohexamide	250 mg	White	Tablet	Capsule-Shape, Compressed, Scored	Rosemont Pharmaceutical
832; G32	Acetohexamide	500 mg	White	Tablet	Capsule-Shape, Compressed, Scored	Rosemont Pharmaceutical
832; G55C	Amitriptyline Hydrochloride and Chlordiazepoxide	12.5 mg; 5 mg	Green	Coated Tablet		Pharmaceutical Basics
832; G55C	Chlordiazepoxide and Amitriptyline Hydrochloride	5 mg; 12.5 mg	Green	Coated Tablet	Circle	Pharmaceutical Basics
832; G56C	Amitriptyline Hydrochloride and Chlordiazepoxide	25 mg; 10 mg	White	Coated Tablet		Pharmaceutical Basics
832; G56C	Chlordiazepoxide and Amitriptyline Hydrochloride	10 mg; 25 mg	White	Coated Tablet	Circle	Pharmaceutical Basics
832; G; 133	Carbamazepine	200 mg	White	Tablet	Circle, Single-Scored	Pharmaceutical Basics
832; G; 197	Chlorpropamide	250 mg	Blue	Tablet	Circle, Compressed, Scored	Rosemont Pharmaceutical
832; G; 198	Chlorpropamide	100 mg	Blue	Tablet	Circle, Compressed, Scored	Rosemont Pharmaceutical
832; G; 203	Chlorthalidone	25 mg	Orange	Tablet	Flat, Beveled Edge, Compressed, Scored	Rosemont Pharmaceutical
832; G; 204	Chlorthalidone	50 mg	Blue	Tablet	Flat, Beveled Edge, Compressed, Scored	Rosemont Pharmaceutical
832; G; 220C	Clorazepate Dipotassium	3.75 mg	White	Capsule		Rosemont Pharmaceutical
832; G; 221C	Clorazepate Dipotassium	7.5 mg	White	Capsule		Rosemont Pharmaceutical
832; G; 222C	Clorazepate Dipotassium	15 mg	White	Capsule		Rosemont Pharmaceutical
832; G254	Desipramine Hydrochloride	25 mg	Lavender	Coated Tablet	Circle	H.L. Moore
832; G; 254	Desipramine Hydrochloride	25 mg	Lavender	Coated Tablet		Pharmaceutical Basics
832; G255	Desipramine Hydrochloride	50 mg	Blue	Coated Tablet	Circle	H.L. Moore
832; G; 255	Desipramine Hydrochloride	50 mg	Blue	Coated Tablet		Pharmaceutical Basics
832; G256	Desipramine Hydrochloride	75 mg	White	Coated Tablet	Circle	H.L. Moore
832; G; 256	Desipramine Hydrochloride	75 mg	White	Coated Tablet		Pharmaceutical Basics
832; G257	Desipramine Hydrochloride	100 mg	Butterscotch	Coated Tablet	Circle	H.L. Moore
832; G; 257	Desipramine Hydrochloride	100 mg	Butterscotch	Coated Tablet		Pharmaceutical Basics
832; G; 359	Fluoxymesterone	10 mg	Green	Tablet	Circle, Scored	Rosemont Pharmaceutical
832; G; 366C	Flurazepam Hydrochloride	15 mg	White and Light Blue	Capsule		Rosemont Pharmaceutical
832; G; 367C	Flurazepam Hydrochloride	30 mg	Light Blue and Dark Blue	Capsule		Rosemont Pharmaceutical
832; G; 420	Hydroflumethiazide and Reserpine	50 mg; 0.125 mg	Green	Tablet	Circle	Pharmaceutical Basics
832; G; 423	Hydroxyzine Hydrochloride	10 mg	Light Purple	Coated Tablet		Rosemont Pharmaceutical
832; G; 424	Hydroxyzine Hydrochloride	25 mg	Purple	Coated Tablet		Rosemont Pharmaceutical
832; G; 425	Hydroxyzine Hydrochloride	50 mg	Lavender	Coated Tablet		Rosemont Pharmaceutical
832; G; 463	Medroxyprogesterone Acetate	10 mg	White	Tablet	Circle, Scored	Qualitest Products
832; G; 465	Megestrol Acetate	20 mg	White	Tablet	Flat, Beveled Edge, Compressed, Scored	Rosemont Pharmaceutical
832; G; 466	Megestrol Acetate	40 mg	White	Tablet	Compressed, Scored	Rosemont Pharmaceutical
832; G; 506	Nystatin	500,000 units	Brown	Coated Tablet	Circle	Rosemont Pharmaceutical
832; G; 528C	Phendimetrazine Tartrate	35 mg	Yellow, Orange or Green	Tablet	Circle	Rosemont Pharmaceutical
832; G; 536C	Phentermine Hydrochloride	30 mg	Yellow, Black or Blue	Capsule		Pharmaceutical Basics
832; G; 563C	Phentermine Hydrochloride	30 mg	Blue and Clear with Blue and White Beads	Capsule		Rosemont Pharmaceutical
832; G; 602	Sulfamethoxazole and Trimethoprim	400 mg; 80 mg	White	Tablet	Compressed, Scored	Rosemont Pharmaceutical
832; G; 603	Sulfamethoxazole and Trimethoprim	800 mg; 160 mg		Tablet	Capsule-Shape, Compressed, Scored	Rosemont Pharmaceutical
832; G; 613;	Thyroid	0.5 G	Tan	Tablet	Circle	Rosemont Pharmaceutical
832; G; 614	Thyroid	1 G	Tan, Red, Blue, Yellow or Pink	Tablet	Circle	Rosemont Pharmaceutical
832; G; 615	Thyroid	2 G	Tan, Red, Blue, Yellow, Pink or Orange	Tablet		Rosemont Pharmaceutical
832; G; 616	Thyroid	3 G	Green, Tan or Blue	Tablet	Circle	Rosemont Pharmaceutical
832; G; 618	Tolazamide	100 mg	White	Tablet	Circle	Rosemont Pharmaceutical
832; G; 621	Tolazamide	500 mg	White	Tablet	Circle	Rosemont Pharmaceutical
832; G; 622	Tolazamide	250 mg	White	Tablet	Circle	Rosemont Pharmaceutical
832; GC; 100	Chlorthalidone	100 mg	White	Tablet	Compressed, Scored	Rosemont Pharmaceutical
832; LR1C	Lorazepam	1 mg	White	Tablet	Circle, Scored	Rosemont Pharmaceutical
832; LR2C	Lorazepam	2 mg	White	Tablet	Circle, Scored	Rosemont Pharmaceutical
832; M5	Methyclothiazide	5 mg	Orange	Tablet	Compressed, Scored	Rosemont Pharmaceutical
832; M; 400	Meprobase	25 mg; 400 mg	Yellow	Coated Tablet		Rosemont Pharmaceutical
832; MC50	Meclofenamate Sodium	50 mg	Maroon and Pink	Capsule		Rosemont Pharmaceutical
832; MC100	Meclofenamate Sodium	100 mg	Maroon and White	Capsule		Rosemont Pharmaceutical
832; MS10	Metaproterenol Sulfate	10 mg	White	Tablet	Circle, Scored	Rosemont Pharmaceutical
832; MS20	Metaproterenol Sulfate	20 mg	White	Tablet	Circle	Rosemont Pharmaceutical
832; P; 10C	Prazepam	10 mg	Green and White	Capsule		Rosemont Pharmaceutical
832; P19C	Hydrocodone Bitartrate and Acetaminophen	5 mg; 500 mg	White	Tablet	Rectangle, Flat, Beveled Edge, Compressed, Scored	Rosemont Pharmaceutical
832; P; 375C	Phentermine Hydrochloride	37.5 mg	Yellow	Capsule	Rectangle	Rosemont Pharmaceutical
832; S; 500	Salsalate	500 mg	Yellow or Blue	Coated Tablet		Rosemont Pharmaceutical
832; S; 750	Salsalate	750 mg	Yellow or Blue	Coated Tablet	Rectangle	Rosemont Pharmaceutical
832; TM25	Trimipramine Maleate	25 mg	Purple and Orange	Capsule		Pharmaceutical Basics
832; TM50	Trimipramine Maleate	50 mg	Pink and White	Capsule		Pharmaceutical Basics
832; TM100	Trimipramine Maleate	100 mg	Dark Green and Brown	Capsule		Pharmaceutical Basics
832; TZD50	Trazodone Hydrochloride	50 mg	White	Coated Tablet		Pharmaceutical Basics
832; TZD100	Trazodone Hydrochloride	100 mg	White	Coated Tablet		Pharmaceutical Basics

IMPRINT	BRAND/GENERIC NAME	STRENGTH	COLOR	FORM	SHAPE	MANUFACTURER
832; WARFARIN; 2	Warfarin Sodium	2 mg	Lavender	Tablet	Compressed, Scored	Rosemont Pharmaceutical
832; WARFARIN; 2.1/2	Warfarin Sodium	2.5 mg	Green	Tablet	Compressed, Scored	Rosemont Pharmaceutical
832; WARFARIN; 5	Warfarin Sodium	5 mg	Pink	Tablet	Compressed, Scored	Rosemont Pharmaceutical
844	Thyroid	2 Gr	Red	Tablet		Teva Pharmaceuticals
854	Thyroid Tan	5 Gr	Tan	Tablet		Teva Pharmaceuticals
861; SCHERING	Chlor-Trimeton Non-Drowsy Decongestant 4 Hour	60 mg	Light Tan	Tablet	Circle, Scored	Schering-Plough Healthcare Products
866	Disophrol	2 mg; 120 mg	Blue and White Mottled	Tablet	Circle	Schering-Plough
866	Docusate Calcium	240 mg	Red	Capsule	Oblong	Scherer Laboratories
872; CARACO LOGO	Nifedipine	10 mg	Yellow	Capsule, Liquid Filled		Caraco Pharmaceutical
872; CARACO LOGO	Nifedipine	10 mg	Yellow	Capsule, Liquid Filled		Geneva Generics
873; CARACO LOGO	Nifedipine	20 mg	Brown-Orange	Capsule, Liquid Filled		Caraco Pharmaceutical
873; CARACO LOGO	Nifedipine	20 mg	Orange and Brown	Capsule, Liquid Filled		Geneva Generics
879	Meperidine Hydrochloride	10 mg		Tablet		Halsey Drug
879; 0155	Propoxyphene Hydrochloride	65 mg	Pink	Capsule		Halsey Drug
879; 0158	Tetracycline Hydrochloride	250 mg	Opaque Yellow and Orange	Capsule		Halsey Drug
879; 027	Pentobarbital Sodium	100 mg	Yellow	Capsule		Halsey Drug
879; 113	Isoniazid	100 mg	White	Tablet	Circle, Scored	Halsey Drug
879; 129	Prednisone	5 mg	White	Tablet	Circle, Scored	Halsey Drug
879; 130	Propylthiouracil	50 mg	White	Tablet	Circle, Scored	Halsey Drug
879; 159	Tetracycline Hydrochloride	500 mg	Opaque Yellow and Black	Capsule		Halsey Drug
879; 317;	Dextroamphetamine Sulfate	10 mg	Yellow	Tablet	Double-Scored	Halsey Drug
879; 341	Isoniazid	300 mg	White	Tablet	Circle	Halsey Drug
879; 360	Triprolidine and Pseudoephedrine Hydrochloride	2.5 mg; 60 mg	White	Tablet		Halsey Drug
879; 364;	Chlordiazepoxide Hydrochloride	5 mg	Green and Yellow	Capsule		Halsey Drug
879; 365	Chlordiazepoxide Hydrochloride	10 mg	Green and Black	Capsule		Halsey Drug
879; 366	Chlordiazepoxide Hydrochloride	25 mg	Green and White	Capsule		Halsey Drug
879; 525	Doxycycline Hyclate	50 mg	Blue and White	Capsule		Novartis Generics
879; 526	Doxycycline Hyclate	100 mg	Blue	Capsule		Novartis Generics
879; G20C	Oxycodone Hydrochloride and Acetaminophen	5 mg; 325 mg	White	Tablet	Circle	Halsey Drug
879; G41	Aminophylline	100 mg	White	Tablet		Halsey Drug
879; G85C; 2	Aspirin with Codeine Phosphate	325 mg; 15 mg	White	Tablet	Circle	Halsey Drug
879; G86C; 3	Aspirin with Codeine Phosphate	325 mg; 30 mg	White	Tablet	Circle	Halsey Drug
879; G87C; 4	Aspirin with Codeine Phosphate	325 mg; 60 mg	White	Tablet	Circle	Halsey Drug
879; G88C	Diphenoxylate Hydrochloride and Atropine Sulfate	2.5 mg; 0.025 mg	White	Tablet	Circle	Halsey Drug
879; G88C	Diphenoxylate Hcl and Atropine Sulfate	2.5 mg; 0.025 mg	White	Tablet	Circle	Purepac Pharmaceutical
879; G122C	Butabarbital Sodium	30 mg	Green	Tablet		Halsey Drug
879; G302	Diphenhydramine Hydrochloride	25 mg	Pink and Clear	Capsule		Halsey Drug
879; G303	Diphenhydramine Hydrochloride	50 mg	Pink	Capsule		Halsey Drug
879; G368	Folic Acid	1 mg	Yellow	Tablet	Circle, Scored	Halsey Drug
879; G406	Hydro-D	25 mg	Peach	Tablet		Halsey Drug
879; G407	Hydro-D	50 mg	Peach	Tablet		Halsey Drug
879; G468;C;	Meperidine Hydrochloride	50 mg	White	Tablet	Circle	Halsey Drug
879; G469; C;	Meperidine Hydrochloride	100 mg	White	Tablet	Circle, Scored	Halsey Drug
879 G545	Prednisolone	5 mg	Light Orange	Tablet		Halsey Drug
879; G549	Prednisone	20 mg	Salmon	Tablet	Circle, Scored	Halsey Drug
879; G594C	Secobarbital Sodium	100 mg	Red-Orange	Capsule		Halsey Drug
879; G594C	Sodium Secobarbital	100 mg		Capsule		Halsey Drug
879; G650C	Oxycodone and Aspirin	4.5 mg; 0.38 mg; 325 mg	Yellow	Tablet	Circle, Scored	Halsey Drug
891	Docusate Potassium and Casanthranol	100 mg; 30 mg	Yellow	Capsule	Oblong	Scherer Laboratories
891	Docusate Potassium and Casanthranol	100 mg; 30 mg	Yellow	Capsule	Oblong	Udl Laboratories
895	Docusate Calcium and Yellow Phenolphthalein	60 mg; 65 mg	Red	Capsule	Oblong	Scherer Laboratories
895	Docusate Calcium and Yellow Phenolphthalein	60 mg; 65 mg	Red	Capsule	Oblong	Udl Laboratories
897	Docusate Sodium	100 mg	Orange	Capsule	Oval	Purepac Pharmaceutical
897	Docusate Sodium	100 mg	Orange	Capsule	Oval	Scherer Laboratories
897	Docusate Sodium	100 mg	Orange	Capsule	Oval	Udl Laboratories
898	Docusate Sodium	250 mg	Orange	Capsule	Oblong	Purepac Pharmaceutical
898	Docusate Sodium	250 mg	Orange	Capsule	Oblong	Scherer Laboratories
898	Docusate Sodium	250 mg	Orange	Capsule	Oblong	Udl Laboratories
901	Chlor-Trimeton Allergy Decongestant 4 Hour	4 mg; 60 mg	Light Blue	Tablet		Schering-Plough Healthcare Products
955	Famotidine	20 mg	White	Tablet	Circle	Andrx Pharmaceuticals
968;	Tindal	20 mg	Salmon	Tablet		Schering
989	Femcare	100 mg	White	Tablet	Torpedo-Shaped	Schering-Plough Healthcare Products
1002	Advicor	1000 mg; 20 mg	Light Purple/dark Pink	Coated Tablet	Capsule-Shape	Kos Pharmaceuticals
1024	Christodyne-Dhc	150 mg; 230 mg; 30 mg; 5 mg	Green and White Speckled	Tablet		Paddock Labs
1050	Formula Cold, Flu, & Cough	250 mg; 2 mg; 30 mg; 10 mg	Clear Blue	Gel/jelly		Leiner Health Products
1050	Formula Cold, Flu, & Cough	250 mg; 2 mg; 30 mg; 10 mg	Clear Blue	Gel/jelly		Scherer Laboratories
1051	Formula Cold & Cough	30 mg; 60 mg	Clear Red	Gel/jelly		Leiner Health Products
1051	Formula Cold & Cough	30 mg; 60 mg	Clear Red	Gel/jelly		Scherer Laboratories
1052	Diphenhydramine Hydrochloride	50 mg	Clear Blue	Gel/jelly		Leiner Health Products

IMPRINT	BRAND/GENERIC NAME	STRENGTH	COLOR	FORM	SHAPE	MANUFACTURER
1052	Diphenhydramine Hydrochloride	50 mg	Clear Blue	Gel/jelly		Scherer Laboratories
1101	Stool Softener	100 mg	Orange and White	Tablet	Oval	Scherer Laboratories
1105	Docusate Sodium	50 mg	Red	Capsule	Oval	Scherer Laboratories
1125	Prenatal-Z Advanced Formula	200 mg; 1 mg; 65 mg; 17 mg; 4000 IU; 2.2 mcg; 1.6 mg; 400 IU; 70 mg; 15 mg; 10 IU; 2.2 mg; 1.5 mg; 65 mcg; 100 mg; 175 mcg	White	Coated Tablet	Oval	Pecos Pharmaceutical
1190	Pain Reliever	500 mg	White	Tablet		Good Sense
1311	Dexchlorpheniramine Maleate	6 mg	Red	Tablet		Qualitest Products
1481	Carenate	250 mg; 2 mg; 40 mg; 2 mg; 6 mcg; 15 mg; 3.5 mg; 50 mg; 50 mg; 0.5 mg	Peach	Tablet	Oval	Pecos Pharmaceutical
1492	Monopril HCT	10 mg; 12.5 mg	Peach	Tablet	Circle	Bristol-Myers Squibb
1493	Monopril HCT	20 mg; 12.5 mg	Peach	Tablet	Circle, Scored	Bristol-Myers Squibb
2011; G	Orphenadrine Citrate	100 mg	White	Extended-Release Tablet	Circle	Global Pharmaceutical
2013	Chlorpheniramine Maleate	4 mg	Yellow	Tablet	Circle, Scored	Circa Pharmaceuticals
2013	Genericare Allergy Relief	4 mg	Yellow	Tablet	Circle, Scored	Circa Pharmaceuticals
2063; V; 2	Acetaminophen and Codeine Phosphate	300 mg; 15 mg	White	Tablet	Circle	Vintage Pharmaceuticals
2064; V; 3	Acetaminophen and Codeine Phosphate	300 mg; 30 mg	White	Tablet	Circle	Vintage Pharmaceuticals
2065; V; 4	Acetaminophen and Codeine Phosphate	300 mg; 60 mg	White	Tablet	Circle	Vintage Pharmaceuticals
2080	Axert	6.25 mg	White with Red Ink	Tablet	Circle, Compressed, Biconvex	Pharmacia & Upjohn
2083; V	Allopurinol	100 mg	White	Tablet	Circle	Vintage Pharmaceuticals
2084; V	Allopurinol	300 mg	Orange	Tablet	Circle	Vintage Pharmaceuticals
2112	Pentetra-TDC	80 mg	Clear and Green	Capsule		Paddock Labs
2120; V; 3	Aspirin and Codeine	325 mg; 30 mg	White	Tablet	Circle	Vintage Pharmaceuticals
2121; V; 3	Aspirin and Codeine	325 mg; 60 mg	White	Tablet	Circle	Vintage Pharmaceuticals
2205	Ferrous Sulfate	324 mg	Green	Tablet	Circle	Time Cap Labs
2320; V	Phenobarbital and Belladonna Alkaloids	16.2 mg; 0.1296 mg	White	Tablet	Circle	Vintage Pharmaceuticals
2323; V	Bellaspas	0.2 mg; 0.6 mg; 40 mg	Green	Tablet	Round, Quadrisected Scored	Qualitest Products
2500; V	Chlorpheniramine Maleate	8 mg	Natural and Green	Sustained-Release Capsule		Vintage Pharmaceuticals
2501; V	Chlorpheniramine Maleate	12 mg	Natural and Green	Sustained-Release Capsule		Vintage Pharmaceuticals
2611; G	Terbutaline Sulfate	2.5 mg	White	Tablet	Oval	Global Pharmaceutical
2622; G	Terbutaline Sulfate	5 mg	White	Tablet	Circle	Global Pharmaceutical
2711; G	Sotalol Hydrochloride	80 mg	Light Blue	Tablet	Capsule-Shape	Global Pharmaceutical
2722; G	Sotalol Hydrochloride	120 mg	Light Blue	Tablet	Capsule-Shape	Global Pharmaceutical
2729; 20	Fosinopril Sodium	20 mg	White to Off-White	Tablet	Oval	Sandoz
2732; 40	Fosinopril Sodium	40 mg	White to Off-White	Tablet	Six-Sided	Sandoz
2733; G	Sotalol Hydrochloride	160 mg	Light Blue	Tablet	Capsule-Shape	Global Pharmaceutical
2737; 10	Fosinopril Sodium	10 mg	White to Off-White	Tablet	Diamond	Sandoz
2744; G	Sotalol Hydrochloride	240 mg	Light Blue	Tablet	Capsule-Shape	Global Pharmaceutical
2771; HEART SHAPE	Avapro	75 mg	White	Tablet	Oval, Biconvex	Bristol-Myers Squibb
2771; HEART SHAPE	Avapro	75 mg	White	Tablet	Oval, Biconvex	Sanofi Pharmaceuticals
2772; HEART SHAPE	Avapro	150 mg	White	Tablet	Oval, Biconvex	Bristol-Myers Squibb
2772; HEART SHAPE	Avapro	150 mg	White	Tablet	Oval, Biconvex	Sanofi Pharmaceuticals
2773; HEART SHAPE	Avapro	300 mg	White	Tablet	Oval, Biconvex	Bristol-Myers Squibb
2773; HEART SHAPE	Avapro	300 mg	White	Tablet	Oval, Biconvex	Sanofi Pharmaceuticals
2775; HEART	Avalide	150 mg; 12.5 mg	Peach	Tablet	Oval, Biconvex	Bristol-Myers Squibb
2776; HEART	Avalide	300 mg; 12.5 mg	Peach	Tablet	Oval, Biconvex	Bristol-Myers Squibb
3000	Quinidine Gluconate	324 mg		Sustained-Release Tablet		Roxane Laboratories
3125; VANCOCIN HCL; 125 MG	Vancocin	125 mg	Blue and Brown	Capsule		Eli Lilly
3126; VANCOCIN HCL; 250 MG	Vancocin	250 mg	Blue and Lavender	Capsule		Eli Lilly
3344; SB; 10 MG	Compazine Spansule	10 mg	Black and Natural	Sustained-Release Capsule		Glaxosmithkline
3346; SB; 15 MG	Compazine Spansule	15 mg	Black and Natural	Sustained-Release Capsule		Glaxosmithkline
3438; APOTEX LOGO	Selegiline Hydrochloride	5 mg	White Slightly Mottled	Tablet		Apotex
3591; V	Hydrocodone Bitartrate and Acetaminophen	2.5 mg; 500 mg	White with Red Specks	Tablet	Capsule-Shape, Scored	Vintage Pharmaceuticals
3592; V	Hydrocodone Bitartrate and Acetaminophen	5 mg; 500 mg	White	Tablet	Capsule-Shape	Vintage Pharmaceuticals
3594; V	Hydrocodone Bitartrate and Acetaminophen	7.5 mg; 500 mg	White with Green Specks	Tablet	Capsule-Shape, Scored	Vintage Pharmaceuticals
3595; V	Hydrocodone Bitartrate and Acetaminophen	7.5 mg; 650 mg	White	Tablet	Capsule-Shape, Scored	Vintage Pharmaceuticals
3596; V	Hydrocodone Bitartrate and Acetaminophen	7.5 mg; 750 mg	White	Tablet	Capsule-Shape, Scored	Vintage Pharmaceuticals
3597; V	Hydrocodone Bitartrate and Acetaminophen	10 mg; 650 mg	Light Blue	Tablet	Capsule-Shape, Scored	Vintage Pharmaceuticals
3598; V	Hydrocodone Bitartrate and Acetaminophen	10 mg; 660 mg	White	Tablet	Oval, Scored	Vintage Pharmaceuticals
3600; V	Hydrocodone Bitartrate and Acetaminophen	10 mg; 500 mg	Pink	Tablet	Capsule-Shape, Scored	Vintage Pharmaceuticals

IMPRINT	BRAND/GENERIC NAME	STRENGTH	COLOR	FORM	SHAPE	MANUFACTURER
3601; V	Hydrocodone Bitartrate and Acetaminophen	10 mg; 325 mg	Light Yellow	Tablet	Capsule-Shape, Scored	Vintage Pharmaceuticals
3611; V	Hydromorphone	2 mg	Pink	Tablet	Circle	Vintage Pharmaceuticals
3612; V	Hydromorphone	4 mg	White	Tablet	Circle	Vintage Pharmaceuticals
3618; TSH	Fiber-Lax	500 mg	Cream Colored	Tablet	Capsule-Shape	Rugby Laboratories
3911; V	Levothyroxine	25 mcg	Peach	Tablet	Circle	Vintage Pharmaceuticals
3912; V	Levothyroxine	50 mcg	White	Tablet	Circle	Vintage Pharmaceuticals
3913; V	Levothyroxine	75 mcg	Purple	Tablet	Circle	Vintage Pharmaceuticals
3914; V	Levothyroxine	100 mcg	Yellow	Tablet	Circle	Vintage Pharmaceuticals
3915; V	Levothyroxine	150 mcg	Blue	Tablet	Circle	Vintage Pharmaceuticals
3916; V	Levothyroxine	200 mcg	Pink	Tablet	Circle	Vintage Pharmaceuticals
3917; V	Levothyroxine	300 mcg	Green	Tablet	Circle	Vintage Pharmaceuticals
3966	Atropine Sulfate and Diphenoxylate Hydrochloride	0.025 mg; 2.5 mg	White	Tablet	Circle	Mallinckrodt
3984; 3;	Aspirin and Codeine Phosphate	325 mg; 30 mg	White	Tablet	Circle	Ivax Pharmaceuticals
3985; 4;	Aspirin and Codeine Phosphate	325 mg; 60 mg	White	Tablet	Circle	Ivax Pharmaceuticals
4206; V	Meperidine Hydrochloride and Promethazine Hydrochloride	50 mg; 25 mg	Red	Capsule		Vintage Pharmaceuticals
4266; 200	Acyclovir	200 mg	White	Capsule		Watson Laboratories
4364; 100	Labetalol	100 mg	Yellow	Tablet	Circle, Bisected	Goldline Laboratories
4364; 100	Labetalol	100 mg	Yellow	Tablet	Circle, Bisected	Ivax Pharmaceuticals
4365; 200	Labetalol	200 mg	White	Tablet	Circle, Bisected	Goldline Laboratories
4365; 200	Labetalol	200 mg	White	Tablet	Circle, Bisected	Ivax Pharmaceuticals
4366; 300	Labetalol	300 mg	Green	Tablet	Circle	Ivax Pharmaceuticals
LOGO 4440; 100	Gabapentin	100 mg	White	Tablet	Circle	Ivax Pharmaceuticals
LOGO 4441; 300	Gabapentin	300 mg	White	Tablet	Circle	Ivax Pharmaceuticals
LOGO 4442; 400	Gabapentin	400 mg	White	Tablet	Oval	Ivax Pharmaceuticals
4832; V	Acetaminophen and Oxycodone	500 mg; 5 mg	Red	Capsule		Vintage Pharmaceuticals
4839; V	Acetaminophen and Oxycodone	325 mg; 5 mg	White	Tablet	Circle	Vintage Pharmaceuticals
4971; V	Phenazopyridine	100 mg	Maroon	Tablet	Circle	Vintage Pharmaceuticals
4972; V	Phenazopyridine	200 mg	Maroon	Tablet	Circle	Vintage Pharmaceuticals
5011; G	Spironolactone	25 mg	Light Yellow/off White	Tablet	Circle	Greenstone
5011; V	Phenobarbital	15 mg	White	Tablet	Circle	Vintage Pharmaceuticals
5012; G	Spironolactone	50 mg		Tablet		Greenstone
5012; V	Phenobarbital	30 mg	White	Tablet	Circle	Vintage Pharmaceuticals
5013; G	Spironolactone	100 mg		Tablet		Greenstone
5013; V	Phenobarbital	60 mg	White	Tablet	Circle	Vintage Pharmaceuticals
5014; G	Hydrochlorothiazide and Spironolactone	25 mg; 25 mg		Tablet		Greenstone
5014; V	Phenobarbital	100 mg	White	Tablet	Circle	Vintage Pharmaceuticals
5040; BMS	Atenolol	50 mg	White to Off-White, Slightly Mottled	Tablet	Circle, Biconvex	Apothecon
5044	Teveten	400 mg	Pink	Coated Tablet	Oval, Scored	Unimed
5124; V	Propafenone Hydrochloride	150 mg	White	Tablet	Circle, Scored	Qualitest Products
5125; V	Propafenone Hydrochloride	225 mg	White	Tablet	Circle, Scored	Qualitest Products
5126; V	Propafenone Hydrochloride	300 mg	White	Tablet	Circle, Scored	Qualitest Products
5161	Hydrocodone Bitartrate and Ibuprofen	7.5 mg; 200 mg	White	Tablet	Circle	Teva Pharmaceuticals
5240; BMS	Atenolol	100 mg	White to Off-White, Slightly Mottled	Tablet	Circle, Biconvex	Apothecon
5511	Chlorpheniramine Maleate	8 mg	Grey and Clear	Capsule		West-Ward
5512	Chlorpheniramine Maleate	12 mg	Grey and Clear	Timed-Release Capsule		West-Ward
5623; 150 MG;	Nizatidine	150 mg	Yellow and White	Capsule		Ivax Pharmaceuticals
5636; DAN	Meclofenamate Sodium	50 mg	Pink	Capsule		Watson Laboratories
5656; 10; HOURGLASS	Tamoxifen	10 mg	White	Tablet	Circle	Ivax Pharmaceuticals
5657; 20; HOURGLASS	Tamoxifen	20 mg	White	Tablet	Circle	Ivax Pharmaceuticals
LOGO 5710; 1.25/250	Glyburide (Micronized) and Metformin Hydrochloride	1.25 mg; 250 mg	Light Yellow	Tablet	Oval	Ivax Pharmaceuticals
LOGO 5711; 2.5/500	Glyburide (Micronized) and Metformin Hydrochloride	2.5 mg; 500 mg	Light Yellow	Tablet	Oval	Ivax Pharmaceuticals
LOGO 5712; 5/500	Glyburide (Micronized) and Metformin Hydrochloride	5 mg; 500 mg	Yellow	Tablet	Oval	Ivax Pharmaceuticals
5752; SCS	Piroxicam	10 mg	Opaque Light Blue and Orange	Capsule		Schiapparelli Searle
5752; SCS	Piroxicam	10 mg	Opaque Light Blue and Orange	Capsule		Scs Pharmaceuticals
5777; DAN; 50	Atenolol	50 mg	White	Tablet	Circle, Scored	Watson Laboratories
5778; DAN; 100	Atenolol	100 mg	White	Tablet	Circle	Watson Laboratories
5811; V	Salsalate	500 mg	Light Torquoise	Coated Tablet	Circle	Vintage Pharmaceuticals
5812	Salsalate	750 mg	Light Torquoise	Coated Tablet	Capsule-Shape	Vintage Pharmaceuticals
6057	Glyburide and Metformin Hydrochloride	1.25 mg; 250 mg	Pale Yellow	Coated Tablet	Capsule-Shape	Par Pharmaceutical
6058	Glyburide and Metformin Hydrochloride	2.5 mg; 500 mg	Pale Orange	Coated Tablet	Capsule-Shape	Par Pharmaceutical
6059	Glyburide and Metformin Hydrochloride	5 mg; 500 mg	Yellow	Coated Tablet	Capsule-Shape	Par Pharmaceutical
6211; V	Guaifenesin and Pseudoephedrine	600 mg; 120 mg	Yellow	Sustained-Release Tablet	Oval	Vintage Pharmaceuticals
6460	Rauwolfia Serpentina	50 mg	Red	Tablet		Bowman Pharmaceuticals
6462	Rauwolfia Serpentina	100 mg	Red	Tablet		Bowman Pharmaceuticals
6855	Cold Medicine Plus	325 mg; 2 mg; 30 mg	Blue	Capsule, Liquid Filled	Oblong	Ivax Pharmaceuticals
6857	Cold & Cough Medicine Plus	325 mg; 2 mg; 10 mg; 30 mg	Purple	Capsule, Liquid Filled	Oblong	Ivax Pharmaceuticals
7005	Mephobarbital	32 mg	White	Tablet	Circle, Scored	Global Pharmaceutical
7006	Mephobarbital	50 mg	White	Tablet	Circle	Global Pharmaceutical
7007	Mephobarbital	100 mg	White	Tablet	Circle	Global Pharmaceutical

IMPRINT	BRAND/GENERIC NAME	STRENGTH	COLOR	FORM	SHAPE	MANUFACTURER
7013	Guaifenesin and Pseudoephedrine ER	600 mg; 120 mg	Orange	Extended-Release Tablet	Oval, Scored	Global Pharmaceutical
7030;	Pancrelipase	60000 U; 16000 U; 60000 U	Buff Flecked and Tan	Tablet	Oval	Global Pharmaceutical
7030	Pancrelipase	60000 U; 16000 U; 60000 U	Buff-Flecked Tan	Tablet	Oval	Major Pharmaceutical
7033	Fludrocortisone Acetate	0.1 mg	White/off White	Tablet	Circle	Global Pharmaceutical
7066; 511	Bisoprolol and Hydrochlorothiazide	5 mg; 6.25 mg		Tablet		Esi Lederle
7067; 511	Bisoprolol and Hydrochlorothiazide	10 mg; 6.25 mg	White	Tablet	Circle, Scored	Esi Lederle
7112	Docusate Sodium	100 mg	Red	Capsule	Oval	Rugby Laboratories
7113	Docusate Sodium	250 mg	Red	Capsule	Oval	Rugby Laboratories
7115	Docusate Calcium	240 mg	Red	Capsule, Liquid Filled	Oblong	Rugby Laboratories
7117; 300;	Cimetidine	300 mg	White	Coated Tablet	Circle	Ivax Pharmaceuticals
7171; 400;	Cimetidine	400 mg	White	Tablet	Capsule-Shape, Scored	Ivax Pharmaceuticals
7489	Ampicillin	250 mg	Brown and White	Capsule		Bristol-Myers Squibb
7499	Ampicillin	500 mg	Brown and White	Capsule		Bristol-Myers Squibb
7663	Aromasin	25 mg	Light Grey	Tablet	Circle, Biconvex	Pharmacia & Upjohn
7711; 800;	Cimetidine	800 mg	White to Off White	Tablet	Oval, Scored	Ivax Pharmaceuticals
7711; 800;	Cimetidine	800 mg	White to Off White	Tablet	Oval, Scored	Lek Pharmaceuticals
7720; 250;	Cefzil	250 mg	Light Orange	Coated Tablet		Bristol-Myers Squibb
7721; 500;	Cefzil	500 mg	White	Coated Tablet		Bristol-Myers Squibb
7767; 100	Celebrex	100 mg	White with Blue Band	Capsule		Searle
7767; 200	Celebrex	200 mg	White with Gold Band	Capsule		Searle
7767; 400	Celebrex	400 mg	White with Green Band	Capsule		Searle
8225	Diphenoxylate Hydrochloride with Atropine Sulfate	2.5 mg; 0.025 mg		Tablet		Cenci Labs
8643	Minotal	325 mg; 15 mg	Yellow	Tablet		Carnrick Laboratories
8645	Capital	325 mg	White	Tablet		Carnrick Laboratories
9200; TRIANGLE TRIANGLE	Glipizide	10 mg	White	Tablet	Circle, Scored	Baker Norton
9515	Bensulfoid	130 mg		Tablet		Poythress Laboratories
9531	Uro-Phosphate	300 mg; 500 mg	White	Coated Tablet		Poythress Laboratories
9540	Antrocol	0.195 mg; 16 mg	Green	Tablet	Circle	Poythress Laboratories
9550	Mudrane	111 mg; 16 mg; 195 mg; 8 mg	Yellow	Tablet		Ecr Pharmaceuticals
51479; 007	Dura-Tap/PD	4 mg; 60 mg	Opaque Blue and Clear with White Beads	Capsule		Dura Pharmaceuticals
52273; 111	Nystatin	100000 U	White or Pale-Yellow	Tablet	Diamond	Quantum Pharmics
59010; 240	Bupap	50 mg; 650 mg	Light Blue	Tablet		Ecr Pharmaceuticals
59743; 002	Guaifenesine-P	120 mg; 250 mg	Natural and White	Capsule		Qualitest Products
59743; 003	Guaifenesin-P-PD	60 mg; 300 mg	Blue and Natural	Capsule		Qualitest Products
59911; 60	Propranolol Hydrochloride, Long-Acting	60 mg	White	Capsule		Esi Lederle
59911; 80	Propranolol Hydrochloride, Long-Acting	80 mg	White and Light Blue	Capsule		Esi Lederle
59911; 120	Propranolol Hydrochloride, Long-Acting	120 mg	White and Dark Blue	Capsule		Esi Lederle
59911; 160	Propranolol Hydrochloride, Long-Acting	160 mg	White/dark-Blue	Capsule		Esi Lederle
59911; 3606; 200	Etodolac	200 mg	White with Red Ink	Capsule		Esi Lederle
59911; 3607; 300	Etodolac	300 mg	White with Red Ink	Capsule		Esi Lederle
59911; 3608	Etodolac	400 mg	White	Tablet	Oblong	Esi Lederle
59911; 5806	Griseofulvin Ultra	330 mg	White	Tablet	Oblong, Scored	Esi Lederle
59911; 5808	Griseofulvin	500 mg	White	Tablet	Circle	Esi Lederle
59911; 5815	Metoclopramide	10 mg	White	Tablet	Oval, Scored	Esi Lederle
59911; 5869	Minocycline Hydrochloride	50 mg	Yellow and Clear Yellow	Capsule		Esi Lederle
59911; 5870	Minocycline Hydrochloride	100 mg	Green and Yellow	Capsule		Esi Lederle
59911; 5871	Promethazine Hydrochloride	12.5 mg	White	Tablet		Esi Lederle
59911; 5872	Promethazine Hydrochloride	25 mg	White	Tablet		Esi Lederle
59911; 5873	Promethazine Hydrochloride	50 mg	White	Tablet		Esi Lederle
59911; 5876	Oxazepam	10 mg	Pink and White	Capsule		Esi Lederle
59911; 5877	Oxazepam	15 mg	Orange and White	Capsule		Esi Lederle
59911; 5878	Oxazepam	30 mg	Blue and White	Capsule		Esi Lederle
59911; 5885	Potassium Chloride	8 meq	White	Extended-Release Capsule		Esi Lederle
59911; 5899	Potassium Chloride	10 meq	White	Extended-Release Capsule		Esi Lederle
59911; PLUS	Prenatal Plus	65 mg; 4000 IU; 400 IU; 11 mg; 120 mg; 1 mg; 1.5 mg; 3 mg; 20 mg; 10 mg; 12 mcg; 200 mg; 2 mg; 25 mg		Tablet		Esi Lederle
60274; 120MG	Verapamil Hydrochloride	120 mg	Yellow Opaque	Capsule		Watson Laboratories
60274; 180MG	Verapamil Hydrochloride	180 mg	Light Gray Yellow Opaque	Capsule		Watson Laboratories
60274; 240MG	Verapamil Hydrochloride	240 mg	Dark Blue and Yellow Opaque	Capsule		Watson Laboratories
60274; 360MG	Verapamil Hydrochloride	360 mg	Lavender and Yellow Opaque	Capsule		Watson Laboratories
A	Axert	12.5 mg	White with Blue Ink	Tablet	Circle, Compressed, Biconvex	Ortho-Mcneil Pharmaceutical

IMPRINT	BRAND/GENERIC NAME	STRENGTH	COLOR	FORM	SHAPE	MANUFACTURER
A	Cefol	750 mg; 100 mg; 20 mg; 15 mg; 10 mg; 5 mg; 0.5 mg; 6 mcg; 30 IU	Green	Coated Tablet	Oval	Abbott Laboratories
A	Children's Aspirin	75 mg	Bright Pink	Tablet, Chewable		Abbott Laboratories
A	Cough-X	5 mg; 2 mg	Cream, Pearlescent	Lozenge/troche	Square	Ascher
A	Ephedrine and Nembutal 25	25 mg; 25 mg	Black	Capsule		Abbott Laboratories
A	Fero-Gradumet	525 mg	Red	Tablet		Abbott Laboratories
A	Gerilets	27 mg; 5000 IU; 400 IU; 45 IU; 90 mg; 0.4 mg; 2.25 mg; 2.6 mg; 30 mg; 3 mg; 9 mcg; 0.45 mg; 15 mg	Green	Tablet		Abbott Laboratories
A	Iberet-500	525 mg; 500 mg; 25 mcg; 6 mg; 6 mg; 30 mg; 5 mg; 10 mg	Red	Coated Tablet	Oblong	Abbott Laboratories
A	Lidone	5 mg	Cream and Blue	Capsule		Abbott Laboratories
A	Lidone	10 mg	Cream and Red	Capsule		Abbott Laboratories
A	Lidone	25 mg	Cream and Brown	Capsule		Abbott Laboratories
A	Optilets 500	500 mg; 100 mg; 20 mg; 15 mg; 10000 U; 10 mg; 5 mg; 400 U; 12 mcg; 30 IU	Yellow	Tablet	Oblong	Abbott Laboratories
A	Phenazopyridine Hydrochloride	95 mg	Dark Maroon	Tablet	Circle	Able Laboratories
A	Surbex T	15 mg; 10 mg; 100 mg; 5 mg; 10 mcg; 20 mg; 500 mg	Orange	Tablet	Oblong	Abbott Laboratories
A	Tral with Phenobarbital Gradumet	50 mg; 30 mg	Blue	Tablet		Abbott Laboratories
A; 002	Aquatab DM	1200 mg; 60 mg	Light Blue	Coated Tablet	Circle, Scored	Adams Laboratories
A; 002	Tri-Vit with Fluoride	3000 IU; 400 IU; 60 mg; 0.5 mg	Assorted	Tablet, Chewable	Square	Qualitest Products
A; 003;	Phenazopyridine Hydrochloride	100 mg	Maroon	Tablet	Circle, Scored	Amide Pharmaceuticals
A; 003;	Phenazopyridine Hydrochloride	100 mg	Maroon	Tablet	Circle, Scored	Geneva Generics
A; 004;	Phenazopyridine Hydrochloride	200 mg	Maroon	Tablet	Circle, Scored	Amide Pharmaceuticals
A; 004;	Phenazopyridine Hydrochloride	200 mg	Maroon	Tablet	Circle, Scored	Geneva Generics
A; 008; 10	Abilify	10 mg	Pink	Tablet	Rectangle	Bristol-Myers Squibb
A; 009; 15	Abilify	15 mg	Yellow	Tablet	Circle	Bristol-Myers Squibb
A; 0010; 20	Abilify	20 mg	White	Tablet	Circle	Bristol-Myers Squibb
A; 0011; 30	Abilify	30 mg	Pink	Tablet	Circle	Bristol-Myers Squibb
A; 02; 400	Acyclovir	400 mg	White	Tablet		Stada
A; 03; 800	Acyclovir	800 mg	White	Capsule	Oval	Stada
A04; 400	Etodolac	400 mg	White	Tablet	Oval	Stada
A; 05; 200	Acyclovir	200 mg	Blue	Capsule		Stada
A; 07	Ketoconazole	200 mg	White	Tablet	Circle	Stada
A07; OB	Hycotab	500 mg; 5 mg		Tablet	Capsule-Shaped, Bisected Scored	Medicopharma
A; 018	Chlordiazepoxide Hydrochloride with Clidinium Bromide	5 mg; 2.5 mg	Green	Capsule		Watson Laboratories
A; 019;	Amigesic	500 mg	Yellow	Coated Tablet	Circle	Amide Pharmaceuticals
A; 020;	Amigesic	750 mg	Yellow	Tablet		Amide Pharmaceuticals
A; 024	Permax	0.05 mg	Ivory	Tablet		Eli Lilly
A; 025	Permax	0.25 mg	Green	Tablet		Eli Lilly
A; 026	Hyoscyamine	0.125 mg	White	Tablet		Qualitest Products
A; 026	Permax	1 mg	Pink	Tablet		Eli Lilly
A; 027	Amilac	420 mg	White	Tablet	Circle	Amide Pharmaceuticals
A; 031	Multivitamin with Fluoride	0.5 mg; 2500 IU; 400 IU; 15 IU; 60 mg; 0.3 mg; 1.05 mg; 1.2 mg; 13.5 mg; 1.05 mg; 4.5 mcg	Assorted	Tablet, Chewable	Circle	Qualitest Products
A; 031;	Multivita-Bets with Fluoride	2500 IU; 400 IU; 15 IU; 60 mg; 0.3 mg; 1.05 mg; 1.2 mg; 13.5 mg; 1.05 mg; 4.5 mcg; 0.5 mg	Orange, Pink or Purple	Tablet, Chewable		Amide Pharmaceuticals
A; 039;	Amidrine	325 mg; 65 mg; 100 mg	Maroon or Red and White	Capsule		Amide Pharmaceuticals
A; 041	Acetaminophen and Oxycodone	500 mg; 5 mg	White	Capsule		Amide Pharmaceuticals
A; 047	Bontril Slow-Release	105 mg	Green and Yellow	Extended-Release Capsule		Amarin Pharmaceuticals
A; 056	Chlorpheniramine Maleate	4 mg	Yellow	Tablet	Circle, Scored	Amide Pharmaceuticals
A; 056	Chlorpheniramine Maleate	4 mg	Yellow	Tablet	Circle, Scored	Geneva Generics
A; 060	Ursodiol	300 mg	Pink and White	Capsule		Amide Pharmaceuticals
A; 076;	Vitaplex	500 mg; 0.5 mg; 18 mg; 5 mcg; 15 mg; 4 mg; 15 mg; 100 mg	Green	Tablet	Capsule-Shape	Amide Pharmaceuticals
A; 085	Tricosal	750 mg	White	Tablet	Capsule-Shape	Qualitest Products
A; 1	Guanfacine	1 mg	White	Tablet	Circle	Qualitest Products
A2C	Lanoxicaps	0.05 mg	Red	Capsule, Liquid Filled	Oblong, Small	Glaxosmithkline
A; 2	Dilaudid	2 mg	Orange	Tablet	Circle	Abbott Laboratories
A; 2	Guanfacine	2 mg	Yellow	Tablet	Circle	Qualitest Products
A2; WYETH; 65	Ativan	2 mg	White	Tablet	Five-Sided	Wyeth Pharmaceuticals
A; 3	Indapamide	2.5 mg	White to Off-White	Coated Tablet		Rhone-Poulenc Rorer

IMPRINT	BRAND/GENERIC NAME	STRENGTH	COLOR	FORM	SHAPE	MANUFACTURER
A; 4	Dilaudid	4 mg	Yellow	Tablet	Circle	Abbott Laboratories
A; 5	Oxycodone Hydrochloride	5 mg	White	Tablet	Circle, Scored	Amide Pharmaceuticals
A9L; RD	Artane Sequels	5 mg	Clear Blue	Sustained-Release Capsule	Oval	Lederle Laboratories
A-10; 31;	Dermrax	10 mg	Light Tan	Tablet	Circle	Medeva Pharmaceuticals
A; 15	Buspirone Hydrochloride	15 mg	White	Tablet	Rectangle	Amide Pharmaceuticals
A; 15	Buspirone Hydrochloride	15 mg	White	Tablet	Rectangle, with Two Scores on Both Sides	Major Pharmaceutical
A; 21	Acetaminophen	325 mg	White	Tablet		Lederle Laboratories
A-25; 32;	Dermrax	25 mg	Light Green	Tablet	Circle	Medeva Pharmaceuticals
A; 40	Dimenhydrinate	50 mg	White	Tablet	Circle, Scored	Novartis Generics
A; 50; G	Atenolol	50 mg	White	Tablet	Circle, Flat; Bevelled Edge; Scored	Par Pharmaceutical
A75; 511	Acyclovir	400 mg	White	Tablet	Circle	Esi Lederle
A; 75	Acetaminophen and Oxycodone	325 mg; 5 mg	White	Tablet	Circle	Amide Pharmaceuticals
A77; 511	Acyclovir	800 mg		Tablet		Esi Lederle
A; 100; G	Atenolol	100 mg	White	Tablet	Circle, Flat; Bevelled Edge	Par Pharmaceutical
A; 105	Naltrexone Hydrochloride	50 mg	Yellow	Tablet	Capsule-Shape	Amide Pharmaceuticals
A; 105	Naltrexone Hydrochloride	50 mg	Yellow	Tablet	Capsule-Shape	Mallinckrodt
A; 106	Amibid LA	600 mg	Green	Extended-Release Tablet	Capsule-Shape	Amide Pharmaceuticals
A; 106	Ami-Tex LA	600 mg; 30 mg	Green	Extended-Release Tablet		Amide Pharmaceuticals
A; 111	Methenamine Mandelate	0.5 G	Brown	Tablet	Oval	Amide Pharmaceuticals
A; 115	Bellamine S	0.2 mg; 0.6 mg; 40 mg	Green	Tablet	Round, Quadrisected Scored	Amide Pharmaceuticals
A; 117	Meclizine Hydrochloride	25 mg	Pink	Tablet, Chewable	Circle	Amide Pharmaceuticals
A; 126	Hyoscyamine	0.125 mg	Blue	Tablet		Qualitest Products
A; 127	Sodium Fluoride	1.1 mg	Purple	Tablet	Circle	Amide Pharmaceuticals
A; 128	Sodium Fluoride	1 mg	Assorted	Tablet	Circle	Amide Pharmaceuticals
A; 133	Glyburide	1.5 mg	White	Tablet	Oval, Scored	Amide Pharmaceuticals
A; 134	Glyburide	3 mg	Blue	Tablet	Oval, Scored	Amide Pharmaceuticals
A; 135	Glyburide	6 mg	Yellow	Tablet	Oval, Scored	Amide Pharmaceuticals
A; 136	Carisoprodol	350 mg	White	Tablet	Circle, Scored	Amide Pharmaceuticals
A; 137	Aspirin and Carisoprodol	325 mg; 200 mg	Red/white	Tablet	Circle	Amide Pharmaceuticals
A; 137	Carisoprodol and Aspirin	200 mg; 325 mg	Red and White	Tablet	Circle	Amide Pharmaceuticals
A; 137	Carisoprodol and Aspirin	200 mg; 325 mg	Red and White	Tablet	Circle	Qualitest Products
A; 138	Aspirin, Carisoprodol and Codeine	325 mg; 200 mg; 16 mg	Yellow/white	Tablet	Circle	Amide Pharmaceuticals
A; 138	Carisoprodol, Aspirin and Codeine Phosphate	200 mg; 325 mg; 16 mg	White and Yellow	Tablet	Circle	Amide Pharmaceuticals
A; 139	Amibid DM	30 mg; 600 mg	Green	Extended-Release Tablet	Capsule-Shape	Amide Pharmaceuticals
A; 140	Homatropine and Hydrocodone	1.5 mg; 5 mg	White	Tablet	Circle, Scored	Amide Pharmaceuticals
A; 143	Hyoscyamine Sulfate	0.125 mg	White	Tablet	Circle	Amide Pharmaceuticals
A; 145	Digoxin	0.125 mg	Yellow	Tablet	Circle, Flat; Double-Scored	Amide Pharmaceuticals
A; 146	Digoxin	0.25 mg	White	Tablet	Circle	Amide Pharmaceuticals
A; 147	Digoxin	0.5 mg	Green	Tablet	Circle	Amide Pharmaceuticals
A; 150	Multivitamin with Fluoride	0.25 mg; 2500 IU; 400 IU; 15 IU; 60 mg; 0.3 mg; 1.05 mg; 1.2 mg; 13.5 mg; 1.05 mg; 4.5 mcg	Assorted	Tablet, Chewable	Circle	Qualitest Products
A; 155	Hyoscyamine Sulfate SL	0.125 mg	Blue	Tablet	Circle	Amide Pharmaceuticals
A; 156	Hyoscyamine Sulfate	0.375 mg	Orange	Extended-Release Tablet	Capsule-Shape	Amide Pharmaceuticals
A; 157	Meperidine Hydrochloride	100 mg	White	Tablet	Circle	Amide Pharmaceuticals
A; 158	Meperidine Hydrochloride	50 mg	White	Tablet	Circle	Amide Pharmaceuticals
A; 159	Phentermine Hydrochloride	37.5 mg	White with Blue Speckles	Tablet	Capsule-Shape	Amide Pharmaceuticals
A; 160	Phentermine Hydrochloride	30 mg	Yellow	Capsule		Amide Pharmaceuticals
A; 161	Pemoline	37.5 mg	Peach	Tablet	Circle	Amide Pharmaceuticals
A; 161	Pemoline	37.5 mg	Peach	Tablet	Circle, Scored	Mallinckrodt
A; 162	Pemoline	75 mg	Peach	Tablet	Circle	Amide Pharmaceuticals
A; 162	Pemoline	75 mg	Peach	Tablet	Circle, Scored	Mallinckrodt
A; 163	Hyoscyamine Sulfate ER	0.375 mg	Clear with White and Orange Beads	Extended-Release Capsule	Small	Amide Pharmaceuticals
A; 166	Pemoline	37.5 mg	Peach	Tablet, Chewable	Square, Scored	Mallinckrodt
A; 166	Trimethobenzamide Hydrochloride	250 mg	Aqua and Light Blue	Capsule		Amide Pharmaceuticals
A; 167	Phentermine Hydrochloride	37.5 mg	White and Blue	Capsule		Amide Pharmaceuticals
A; 170	Phentermine	15 mg	Gray, Orange, Yellow	Capsule		Amide Pharmaceuticals
A; 171	Prenatal RX	0.03 mg; 200 mg; 1 mg; 100 mg; 7 mg; 1.5 mg; 2.5 mcg; 80 mg; 4 mg; 25 mg; 15 IU; 400 IU; 4000 IU; 1.6 mg; 17 mg; 60 mg; 3 mg	White	Tablet	Oblong	Amide Pharmaceuticals
A; 172	Codeine Phosphate and Guaifenesin	10 mg; 300 mg	Red	Tablet		Amide Pharmaceuticals
A; 173	Phentermine	30 mg	Clear and Blue	Capsule		Amide Pharmaceuticals
A; 178	Prenatal Plus Iron	200 mg; 2 mg; 12 mcg; 1 mg; 20 mg; 10 mg; 3 mg; 1.5 mg; 4000 IU; 120 mg; 400 IU; 22 mg; 25 mg; 27 mg;	Yellow	Tablet	Oval	Qualitest Products
A; 179	Betaxolol Hydrochloride	10 mg	White	Tablet	Circle	Amide Pharmaceuticals
A; 180	Betaxolol Hydrochloride	20 mg	White	Tablet	Circle	Amide Pharmaceuticals
A; 185	Trimethobenzamide Hydrochloride	300 mg	Lavender	Capsule		Amide Pharmaceuticals
A; 186	Pemoline	37.5 mg	Peach	Tablet	Square	Amide Pharmaceuticals

IMPRINT	BRAND/GENERIC NAME	STRENGTH	COLOR	FORM	SHAPE	MANUFACTURER
A; 187	Oxycodone Hydrochloride	5 mg	Peach and Brown	Capsule		Amide Pharmaceuticals
A; 190	Meperidine and Promethazine	50 mg; 25 mg	Red	Capsule		Amide Pharmaceuticals
A; 197	Pemoline	18.75 mg	White	Tablet	Circle	Amide Pharmaceuticals
A; 197	Pemoline	18.75 mg	White	Tablet	Circle, Scored	Mallinckrodt
A; 211	Naloxone and Pentazocine	0.5 mg; 50 mg	Yellow	Tablet	Oblong, Scored	Amide Pharmaceuticals
A; 213	Acetaminophen and Pentazocine Hydrochloride	650 mg; 25 mg	Light Blue	Tablet	Capsule-Shape	Amide Pharmaceuticals
A; 213	Pentazocine Hydrochloride and Acetaminophen	25 mg; 650 mg	Light Blue	Tablet	Capsule-Shape	Amide Pharmaceuticals
A; 214	Oxycodone Hydrochloride	15 mg	Green	Tablet	Circle	Amide Pharmaceuticals
A; 215	Oxycodone Hydrochloride	30 mg	Blue	Tablet	Circle	Amide Pharmaceuticals
A; 216	Carbetapentane Tannate and Chlorpheniramine Tannate	60 mg; 5 mg	Dark Purple	Tablet	Circle	Amide Pharmaceuticals
A; 225	Rythmol SR	225 mg	White	Capsule		Abbott Laboratories
A; 226	Mirtazapine	15 mg	Yellow	Tablet	Oval	Amide Pharmaceuticals
A; 227	Mirtazapine	30 mg	Tan	Tablet	Oval	Amide Pharmaceuticals
A; 228	Mirtazapine	45 mg	White	Tablet	Oval	Amide Pharmaceuticals
A 234	Tizanidine Hydrochloride	4 mg	White	Tablet		Amide Pharmaceuticals
A; 235	Acetaminophen, Butalbital and Caffeine	500 mg; 50 mg; 40 mg		Tablet		Able Laboratories
A 236	Tizanidine Hydrochloride	2 mg	White	Tablet	Circle	Amide Pharmaceuticals
A; 236	Butalbital, Acetaminophen and Caffeine	50 mg; 325 mg; 40 mg	White	Tablet	Oblong	Able Laboratories
A; 237	Atropine Sulfate and Diphenoxylate Hydrochloride	0.025 mg; 2.5 mg	White to Off-White	Tablet	Circle	Able Laboratories
A; 237	Diphenoxylate Hydrochloride and Atropine Sulfate	2.5 mg; 0.025 mg	White	Tablet	Circle	Qualitest Products
A; 240	Butalbital, Acetaminophen, Caffeine, Codeine Phosphate	50 mg; 325 mg; 40 mg; 30 mg	Light Blue	Capsule		Able Laboratories
A; 245	Guaifenesin ER	1200 mg	White	Extended-Release Tablet	Capsule-Shape	Amide Pharmaceuticals
A; 246	Dextromethorphan and Guaifenesin	60 mg; 1200 mg	Blue	Extended-Release Tablet	Capsule-Shape	Amide Pharmaceuticals
A; 247	Guaifenesin and Pseudoephedrine	1200 mg; 120 mg	White	Extended-Release Tablet	Capsule-Shape	Amide Pharmaceuticals
A; 253	Ami-Tex LA	600 mg; 30 mg	White	Extended-Release Tablet	Capsule-Shape	Amide Pharmaceuticals
A; 253	Methylphenidate Hydrochloride	5 mg		Tablet		Able Laboratories
A; 254	Methylphenidate Hydrochloride	10 mg	White to Off-White	Tablet	Circle	Able Laboratories
A; 255	Methylphenidate Hydrochloride	20 mg	Orange Mottled	Tablet	Circle	Able Laboratories
A; 256	Acetaminophen, Propoxyphene Napsylate	650 mg; 100 mg	Pink	Tablet	Capsule-Shape	Able Laboratories
A; 257	Phentermine Hydrochloride	37.5 mg	Blue and White Mottled	Tablet	Oval	Able Laboratories
A; 258	Phentermine Hydrochloride	30 mg	Yellow	Capsule		Able Laboratories
A; 259	Phentermine Hydrochloride	30 mg	Dark Blue and Clear	Capsule		Able Laboratories
A; 261	Acetaminophen and Propoxyphene Napsylate	650 mg; 100 mg	White to Off-White	Tablet	Capsule-Shape	Able Laboratories
A; 262	Methylphenidate Hydrochloride	20 mg	White to Off-White	Extended-Release Tablet	Circle	Able Laboratories
A; 264	Methocarbamol	750 mg	White to- Off-White	Tablet	Capsule-Shape	Able Laboratories
A; 265	Methocarbamol	500 mg	White to- Off-White	Tablet	Capsule-Shape	Able Laboratories
A; 266	Carisoprodol	350 mg	White to Off-White	Tablet	Circle	Able Laboratories
A; 267	Indomethacin	25 mg	White and Green	Capsule		Able Laboratories
A; 268	Indomethacin	50 mg	White and Green	Capsule		Able Laboratories
A; 269	Indomethacin	75 mg	Green and Clear	Extended-Release Capsule		Able Laboratories
A; 270	Lithium Carbonate	300 mg	Pink	Capsule		Able Laboratories
A; 273	Tramadol Hydrochloride	50 mg	White to Off-White	Tablet	Circle	Able Laboratories
A; 273	Tramadol Hydrochloride	50 mg	White to Off-White	Tablet	Circle	Ivax Pharmaceuticals
A; 283	Lithium Carbonate	300 mg	White	Extended-Release Tablet	Circle	Able Laboratories
A; 283	Lithium Carbonate Extended Release	300 mg	White to Off-White	Extended-Release Tablet	Circle	Udl Laboratories
A; 285; 3	Acetaminophen and Codeine	300 mg; 30 mg	White to Off-White	Tablet	Circle, Flat Faced, Beveled Edges	Able Laboratories
A; 286; 4	Acetaminophen and Codeine	300 mg; 60 mg	White to Off-White	Tablet	Circle, Flat Faced, Beveled Edges	Able Laboratories
A; 325	Rythmol SR	325 mg	White	Capsule		Abbott Laboratories
A; 328	Hydrocodone Bitartrate and Acetaminophen	10 mg; 325 mg	White to Off-White	Tablet	Capsule-Shape	Able Laboratories
A; 329	Hydrocodone Bitartrate and Acetaminophen	5 mg; 500 mg	White to Off-White	Tablet	Capsule-Shape	Able Laboratories
A; 330	Hydrocodone Bitartrate and Acetaminophen	7.5 mg; 500 mg	Blue and White Mottled	Tablet	Capsule-Shape, Scored	Able Laboratories
A; 331	Hydrocodone Bitartrate and Acetaminophen	10 mg; 500 mg	Blue Mottled	Tablet	Oval	Able Laboratories
A; 332	Hydrocodone Bitartrate and Acetaminophen	7.5 mg; 650 mg	White to Off-White	Tablet	Capsule-Shape	Able Laboratories
A; 333	Hydrocodone Bitartrate and Acetaminophen	10 mg; 650 mg	Green Mottled	Tablet	Capsule-Shape	Able Laboratories
A; 334	Hydrocodone Bitartrate and Acetaminophen	7.5 mg; 750 mg	White to Off-White	Tablet	Capsule-Shape	Able Laboratories
A; 335	Hydrocodone Bitartrate and Acetaminophen	7.5 mg; 325 mg	Yellow Mottled	Tablet	Capsule-Shape	Able Laboratories
A; 338	Bethanechol Chloride	25 mg;	Light Peach	Tablet	Circle, Bisected	Able Laboratories
A; 339	Bethanechol Chloride	5 mg;	White to Off White	Tablet	Circle, Bisected	Able Laboratories
A; 340	Bethanechol Chloride	10 mg;	White to Off White	Tablet	Circle, Bisected	Able Laboratories
A; 341	Bethanechol Chloride	50 mg;	Light Peach	Tablet	Circle, Bisected	Able Laboratories
A; 345	Hydrocodone Bitartrate and Acetaminophen	5 mg; 325 mg	Blue and White Mottled	Tablet	Capsule-Shape	Able Laboratories
A; 352	Metronidazole	750 mg	Yellow	Extended-Release Tablet	Oval	Able Laboratories
A; 363	Naproxen	275 mg	White	Tablet	Oval	Able Laboratories
A; 364	Naproxen	550 mg	White	Tablet	Oval	Able Laboratories
A; 374	Metronidazole	250 mg	White to Off-White	Tablet	Circle	Able Laboratories

IMPRINT	BRAND/GENERIC NAME	STRENGTH	COLOR	FORM	SHAPE	MANUFACTURER
A; 375	Metronidazole	500 mg	White to Off-White	Tablet	Oval	Able Laboratories
A; 412	Atenolol	25 mg	White to Off White	Tablet	Circle	Able Laboratories
A; 413	Atenolol	50 mg	White to Off White	Tablet	Circle, Bisected	Able Laboratories
A; 414	Atenolol	100 mg	White to Off White	Tablet	Circle	Able Laboratories
A; 425	Rythmol SR	425 mg	White	Capsule		Abbott Laboratories
A; 500	Salsalate	500 mg	Light Turquoise	Coated Tablet	Circle	Novartis Generics
A; 554	Carbamazepine	200 mg	White	Tablet	Circle, Flat, Scored	Teva Pharmaceuticals
A; 585	Atamet	25 mg; 100 mg	Mottled Yellow	Tablet	Circle, Scored	Athena Neurosciences
A; 585	Atamet	25 mg; 100 mg	Mottled Yellow	Tablet	Circle, Scored	Elan Pharma
A; 585	Carbidopa and Levodopa	25 mg; 100 mg	Mottled Yellow	Tablet	Circle, Scored	Teva Pharmaceuticals
A; 585	Carbidopa and Levodopa	25 mg; 100 mg	Mottled Yellow	Tablet	Circle, Scored	Udl Laboratories
A; 587	Atamet	25 mg; 250 mg	Mottled Blue	Tablet	Circle, Scored	Athena Neurosciences
A; 587	Atamet	25 mg; 250 mg	Mottled Blue	Tablet	Circle, Scored	Elan Pharma
A; 587	Carbidopa and Levodopa	25 mg; 250 mg	Mottled Blue	Tablet	Circle, Scored	Teva Pharmaceuticals
A; 600; CAL	Uni-Rex 600 Calcium Chewable Tablet	600 mg		Tablet, Chewable		Nutritional Laboratories
A; 615	Permax	0.05 mg	Ivory	Tablet	Rectangle, Modified	Elan Pharma
A; 625	Permax	0.25 mg	Green	Tablet	Rectangle, Modified	Elan Pharma
A; 630	Permax	1 mg	Pink	Tablet	Rectangle, Modified	Elan Pharma
A; 633	Guaifenesin, Pseudoephedrine Hydrochloride, Dextromethorphan Hydrobromide	30 mg; 600 mg; 60 mg	White	Extended-Release Tablet	Capsule-Shape	United Research Laboratories
A; 750	Salsalate	750 mg	Light Turquoise	Coated Tablet	Capsule-Shape	Able Laboratories
A; 750	Salsalate	750 mg	Blue or Yellow	Tablet		Novartis Generics
A; 750	Salsalate	750 mg	Light Turquoise	Coated Tablet	Capsule-Shape	Novartis Generics
A; 1847	Phenylephrine Hydrochloride, Chlorpheniramine Maleate, and Methscopolamine Nitrate	20 mg; 8 mg; 2.5 mg		Tablet		Url
A; 1848	Pseudoephedrine Hydrochloride, Chlorpheniramine Maleate, and Methscopolamine Nitrate	90 mg; 8 mg; 2.5 mg	Whtie	Tablet		Url
A; 1861	Pseudoephedrine Hydrochloride, Guaifenesin, and Dextromethorphan Hydrobromide	60 mg; 1200 mg; 120 mg	White	Extended-Release Tablet	Capsule-Shape	Pharmafab
A; 1891	Pseudoephedrine Hydrochloride and Guaifenesin	595 mg; 48 mg	White	Extended-Release Tablet	Capsule-Shape	Url
A; A; 8	Dilaudid	8 mg	White	Tablet	Triangle	Abbott Laboratories
A; AA	Chlorthalidone	25 mg		Tablet		Abbott Laboratories
A; AB	Chlorthalidone	50 mg		Tablet		Abbott Laboratories
A; AD;	Peganone	250 mg	White	Tablet	Circle, Scored	Abbott Laboratories
A; AE;	Peganone	500 mg	White	Tablet	Circle, Scored	Abbott Laboratories
A; AF	Colchicine	0.6 mg		Tablet		Abbott Laboratories
A; AF; 500	Anacin Maximum Strength, Aspirin Free	500 mg	White	Coated Tablet		Whitehall Laboratories
A; AM	Tridione	300 mg		Capsule		Abbott Laboratories
A; AN	Dicumarol	25 mg		Tablet		Abbott Laboratories
A; ANTABUSE; 250	Antabuse	250 mg	White to Off-White	Tablet	Eight-Sided, Scored, Compressed	Wyeth Pharmaceuticals
A; ANTABUSE; 500	Antabuse	500 mg	White to Off-White	Tablet	Eight-Sided, Scored, Compressed	Wyeth Pharmaceuticals
A; AO	Dicumarol	50 mg		Tablet		Abbott Laboratories
A; B	Toprol Xl	25 mg		Extended-Release Tablet		Astra Zeneca
A; CE	Nembutal Sodium	30 mg	Yellow	Capsule		Abbott Laboratories
A; CP	A-Poxide	5 mg	Yellow and Green	Capsule		Abbott Laboratories
A; CS	A-Poxide	10 mg	Green and Evergreen	Capsule		Abbott Laboratories
A; CT	A-Poxide	25 mg		Capsule		Abbott Laboratories
A; EC	Ery-Tab	250 mg	White	Enteric-Coated Tablet	Oval	Abbott Laboratories
A; EE	E.E.S.-400 Filmtab	400 mg	Pink	Coated Tablet	Oblong	Abbott Laboratories
A; EH	Ery-Tab	333 mg	White	Enteric-Coated Tablet		Abbott Laboratories
A; FI	Tricor	48 mg	Yellow	Tablet		Abbott Laboratories
A; FO	Tricor	145 mg	White	Tablet		Abbott Laboratories
A; FT;	Mavik	1 mg	Salmon	Tablet	Circle, Scored	Abbott Laboratories
A; FX;	Mavik	2 mg	Yellow	Tablet	Circle, Compressed	Abbott Laboratories
A; FZ;	Mavik	4 mg	Rose	Tablet	Circle, Compressed	Abbott Laboratories
A; IA	Cartrol	2.5 mg	Gray	Tablet	Oval	Abbott Laboratories
A; ID	Isosorbide Mononitrate	60 mg	Yellow	Extended-Release Tablet	Circle, Scored	Warrick Pharmaceuticals
A; II	Phenurone	500 mg	White	Tablet		Abbott Laboratories
A; JC;	Rythmol	150 mg	White	Coated Tablet	Circle, Scored	Abbott Laboratories
A; JI;	Rythmol	225 mg	White	Coated Tablet	Circle, Scored	Abbott Laboratories
A; JN;	Rythmol	300 mg	White	Coated Tablet	Circle, Scored	Abbott Laboratories
A; KJ	Biaxin Xl	500 mg	Yellow	Extended-Release Tablet	Capsule-Shape	Abbott Laboratories
A; KL	Biaxin	500 mg	Yellow	Coated Tablet	Oval	Abbott Laboratories
A; KT	Biaxin	250 mg	Yellow	Coated Tablet	Oval	Abbott Laboratories
A; LE	Tridione Dulcet	150 mg		Tablet, Chewable		Abbott Laboratories
A; LF;	Panwarfin	10 mg	White	Tablet		Abbott Laboratories
A; LJ;	Harmonyl	0.1 mg	Light Yellow	Tablet		Abbott Laboratories
A; LK;	Harmonyl	0.25 mg	Salmon	Tablet		Abbott Laboratories
A; LM;	Panwarfin	2 mg	Purple	Tablet		Abbott Laboratories
A; LN;	Panwarfin	2.5 mg	Orange	Tablet		Abbott Laboratories
A; LO;	Panwarfin	5 mg	Salmon	Tablet		Abbott Laboratories
A; LR;	Panwarfin	7.5 mg	Yellow	Tablet		Abbott Laboratories
A; MC	Desoxyn Gradumet	5 mg	White	Tablet		Abbott Laboratories
A; ME	Desoxyn Gradumet	10 mg	Light Orange	Tablet		Abbott Laboratories
A; MF	Desoxyn Gradumet	15 mg	Yellow	Tablet		Abbott Laboratories
A; MO	Toprol Xl	50 mg	White	Sustained-Release Tablet	Circle, Biconvex, Scored	Astra Zeneca
A; MS	Toprol Xl	100 mg	White	Sustained-Release Tablet	Circle, Biconvex, Scored	Astra Zeneca
A; MY	Toprol Xl	200 mg	White	Sustained-Release Tablet	Oval, Biconvex, Scored	Astra Zeneca
A; NC	Nicobid	125 mg	Black and Clear	Capsule		Aventis Behring

IMPRINT	BRAND/GENERIC NAME	STRENGTH	COLOR	FORM	SHAPE	MANUFACTURER
A; ND	Nicobid	250 mg	Green and Clear	Capsule		Aventis Behring
A; NE	Nicolar	500 mg	Yellow	Tablet		Aventis Behring
A; NJ	Cefol	750 mg; 100 mg; 20 mg; 15 mg; 10 mg; 5 mg; 50 mcg; 6 mcg; 30 IU	Green	Coated Tablet	Oval	Abbott Laboratories
A; NR	Depakote	250 mg	Peach	Enteric-Coated Tablet		Abbott Laboratories
A; NS;	Depakote	500 mg	Lavender	Enteric-Coated Tablet		Abbott Laboratories
A; NT;	Depakote	125 mg	Salmon Pink	Enteric-Coated Tablet		Abbott Laboratories
A; P; ALOR; 5	Alor 5/500	5 mg; 500 mg	Pink	Tablet	Round with Rectangular Side, Bisected Scored	Atley Pharmaceuticals
A; PNV	Uni-Rex 600 Prenatal Vitamins	60 mg; 90 mg; 400 IU; 30 IU; 2 mg; 3 mg; 1 mg; 25 mg; 20 mg; 3500 IU; 12 mcg; 2 mg; 50 mg	Light Blue	Tablet	Capsule-Shape	Nutritional Laboratories
A; TC	Armour Thyroid 1/4 grain	15 mg	Light Tan	Tablet	Circle, Convex	Forest Pharmaceuticals
A; TC	Desoxyn	2.5 mg	White	Tablet		Abbott Laboratories
A; TD	Armour Thyroid 1/2 grain	30 mg	Light Tan	Tablet	Circle, Convex	Forest Pharmaceuticals
A; TE	Armour Thyroid 1 grain	60 mg	Light Tan	Tablet	Circle, Convex	Forest Pharmaceuticals
A; TE	Desoxyn	5 mg	White	Tablet		Abbott Laboratories
A; TF	Armour Thyroid 2 grains	120 mg	Light Tan	Tablet	Circle, Convex	Forest Pharmaceuticals
A; TG	Armour Thyroid 3 grains	180 mg	Light Tan	Tablet	Round, Bisected Scored	Forest Pharmaceuticals
A; TH	Armour Thyroid 4 grains	240 mg	Light Tan	Tablet	Circle, Convex	Forest Pharmaceuticals
A; TI	Armour Thyroid 5 grains	300 mg	Light Tan	Tablet	Round, Bisected Scored	Forest Pharmaceuticals
A; TJ	Armour Thyroid 1-1/2 grains	90 mg	Light Tan	Tablet	Circle, Convex	Forest Pharmaceuticals
A; TL	Tranxene T-Tab	3.75 mg	Blue	Tablet	T-Shaped, Scored	Abbott Laboratories
A; TM	Tranxene T-Tab	7.5 mg	Peach	Tablet	T-Shaped, Scored	Abbott Laboratories
A; TN	Tranxene T-Tab	15 mg	Lavender	Tablet	T-Shaped, Scored	Abbott Laboratories
A; TX	Tranxene-SD Half Strength	11.25 mg	Blue	Tablet	Circle	Abbott Laboratories
A; WYETH; 64	Ativan	1 mg	White	Tablet	Five-Sided	Wyeth Pharmaceuticals
A; WYETH; 81	Ativan	0.5 mg	White	Tablet	Circle, Pentagonal	Wyeth Pharmaceuticals
A; YC	Thyrolar-1/4	3.1 mcg; 12.5 mcg	Violet and White	Tablet		Forest Pharmaceuticals
A; YD	Thyrolar-1/2	6.25 mcg; 25 mcg	Peach and White	Tablet		Forest Pharmaceuticals
A; YE	Thyrolar-1	12.5 mcg; 50 mcg	Pink and White	Tablet		Forest Pharmaceuticals
A; YF	Thyrolar-2	25 mcg; 100 mcg	Green and White	Tablet		Forest Pharmaceuticals
A; YH	Thyrolar-3	37.5 mcg; 150 mcg	Yellow and White	Tablet		Forest Pharmaceuticals
A; Z	Azathioprine	50 mg	Yellow	Tablet	Circle, Scored	Mylan Pharmaceuticals
A; Z	Azathioprine	50 mg	Yellow	Tablet	Circle	Sandoz
AARP; 201	Chewable Antacid #201	200 mg; 200 mg	White	Tablet, Chewable	Round, Bisected Scored	Pharmaceutical Formulations
AARP; 242	Ganalac	420 mg	White	Tablet, Chewable	Circle	Pharmaceutical Formulations
AARP; 247	Chewable Antacid No. 247	80 mg; 80 mg; 200 mg	Off-White	Tablet, Chewable	Circle	Pharmaceutical Formulations
AARP; 263	Magnesia	311 mg	White	Tablet, Chewable	Circle	Pharmaceutical Formulations
AARP; 400	Laxative	100 mg; 65 mg	Beige	Tablet	Circle	Pharmaceutical Formulations
AARP; 428	Advanced Decongestant	325 mg; 5 mg; 2 mg	Yellow and White	Tablet	Circle	Pharmaceutical Formulations
AARP; 556	Backache Relief	325 mg	Dark Green	Tablet	Oval	Pharmaceutical Formulations
ABANA; 217	Obenix	37.5 mg	Green and Clear with Green Beads	Capsule, Liquid Filled	Capsule-Shape	Abana Pharmaceuticals
ABANA; 250	Nasabid	250 mg; 90 mg	Yellow with Black Imprint	Capsule, Liquid Filled		Abana Pharmaceuticals
ABBOTT LOGO; 25 MG; OR	Gengraf	25 mg	White with Blue Ink	Capsule		Abbott Laboratories
ABBOTT LOGO; 25 MG; OR	Gengraf	25 mg	White with Blue Ink	Capsule		Sangstat
ABBOTT LOGO; 100; DS	Norvir	100 mg	White	Capsule, Liquid Filled		Abbott Laboratories
ABBOTT LOGO; 100 MG; OT	Gengraf	100 mg	White, 2 Blue Stripes, Blue Ink	Capsule		Abbott Laboratories
ABBOTT LOGO; 100 MG; OT	Gengraf	100 mg	White, 2 Blue Stripes, Blue Ink	Capsule		Sangstat
ABBOTT LOGO; AR	Tricor, Micronized	134 mg	White	Capsule		Abbott Laboratories
ABBOTT LOGO; EB	Erythromycin	250 mg	Pink	Coated Tablet	Capsule-Shape	Abbott Laboratories
AC; 200; G	Acebutolol Hydrochloride	200 mg	Orange and Purple	Capsule		Alpharma
AC; 200; G	Acebutolol Hydrochloride	200 mg	Lavender and Orange	Capsule		Par Pharmaceutical
AC; 400; G	Acebutolol Hydrochloride	400 mg	Lavender and Orange	Capsule		Par Pharmaceutical
AC; 1000; 62.5	Augmentin Xr	1000 mg; 62.5 mg	White	Extended-Release Tablet	Oval	Glaxosmithkline
A-C	Maalox Antacid	100 mg;		Tablet		Novartis Consumer
ACCU; HIST; 010	Accuhist LA	20 mg; 8 mg; 0.19 mg; 0.04 mg; 0.01 mg	White	Extended-Release Tablet	Capsule-Shape, Scored	Pediamed Pharmaceuticals
ACCUTANE; 10; ROCHE	Accutane	10 mg	Light Pink	Capsule	Oval	Roche Laboratories
ACCUTANE; 20; ROCHE	Accutane	20 mg	Maroon	Capsule	Oval	Roche Laboratories
ACCUTANE; 40; ROCHE	Accutane	40 mg	Yellow	Capsule	Oval	Roche Laboratories
ACF; 004	Atacand	4 mg	White	Tablet	Circle, Biconvex	Astra Zeneca
ACG; 008	Atacand	8 mg	Pink	Tablet	Circle, Biconvex	Astra Zeneca
ACH; 016	Atacand	16 mg	Pink	Tablet	Circle, Biconvex	Astra Zeneca
ACIPHEX; 20;	Aciphex	20 mg	Light Yellow	Delayed-Release Tablet		Eisai
ACJ; 322	Atacand HCT	32 mg; 12.5 mg	Yellow	Tablet	Oval, Biconvex	Astra Zeneca
ACL; 032	Atacand	32 mg	Pink	Tablet	Circle, Biconvex	Astra Zeneca
ACS; 162	Atacand HCT	16 mg; 12.5 mg	Peach	Tablet	Oval, Biconvex	Astra Zeneca

IMPRINT	BRAND/GENERIC NAME	STRENGTH	COLOR	FORM	SHAPE	MANUFACTURER
ACTIFED; 12-HOUR	Actifed 12 Hour	120 mg; 5 mg	Yellow and Clear	Controlled-Release Capsule		Pfizer Consumer Health Care
ACTIFED C-S	Actifed Cold and Sinus Maximum Strength	500 mg; 30 mg; 2 mg		Tablet		Pfizer Consumer Health Care
ACTIFED DAY	Actifed Sinus Daytime/nighttime Daytime Tablet	30 mg; 325 mg	White	Tablet	Circle	Pfizer Consumer Health Care
ACTIFED; M2A	Actifed Tablet	2.5 mg; 60 mg	White	Tablet	Biconvex, Scored	Pfizer Consumer Health Care
ACTIFED NIGHT	Actifed Sinus Daytime/nighttime Nighttime Tablet	30 mg; 500 mg; 25 mg	Blue	Tablet	Circle	Pfizer Consumer Health Care
ACTIFED PLUS	Actifed Plus	500 mg; 30 mg; 1.25 mg	Aqua	Tablet		Warner Wellcome
ACTIFED; WELLCOME	Actifed Capsule	60 mg; 2.5 mg	Yellow and Orange	Capsule		Pfizer Consumer Health Care
ACTIGALL; 300 MG;	Actigall	300 mg	Pink and White	Capsule		Watson Laboratories
ACTOS; 15	Actos	15 mg	White to Off White	Tablet	Circle, Convex	Eli Lilly
ACTOS; 15	Actos	15 mg	White to Off White	Tablet	Circle, Convex	Takeda Pharmaceuticals
ACTOS; 30	Actos	30 mg	White to Off White	Tablet	Circle, Flat	Eli Lilly
ACTOS; 30	Actos	30 mg	White to Off White	Tablet	Circle, Flat	Takeda Pharmaceuticals
ACTOS; 45	Actos	45 mg	White to Off White	Tablet	Circle, Flat	Eli Lilly
ACTOS; 45	Actos	45 mg	White to Off White	Tablet	Circle, Flat	Takeda Pharmaceuticals
ACY; 200	Acyclovir	200 mg		Tablet		Mylan Pharmaceuticals
ACY; 400	Acyclovir	400 mg	White	Tablet	Oval	Mylan Pharmaceuticals
ACY; 800	Acyclovir	800 mg		Tablet		Mylan Pharmaceuticals
AD; 5	Adderall 5 mg Tablet	1.25 mg; 1.25 mg; 1.25 mg; 1.25 mg	Blue	Tablet	Double-Scored	Shire Pharmaceuticals
AD; 7.5	Adderall 7.5 mg Tablet	1.875 mg; 1.875 mg; 1.875 mg; 1.875 mg	Blue	Tablet	Circle, Double-Scored	Shire Pharmaceuticals
AD; 10	Adderall 10 mg Tablet	2.5 mg; 2.5 mg; 2.5 mg; 2.5 mg	Blue	Tablet	Double-Scored	Shire Pharmaceuticals
AD; 12.5	Adderall 12.5 mg Tablet	3.125 mg; 3.125 mg; 3.125 mg; 3.125 mg	Orange	Tablet	Circle, Double-Scored	Shire Pharmaceuticals
AD; 15	Adderall 15 mg Tablet	3.75 mg; 3.75 mg; 3.75 mg; 3.75 mg	Orange	Tablet	Oval, Double-Scored	Shire Pharmaceuticals
AD; 20	Adderall 20 mg Tablet	5 mg; 5 mg; 5 mg; 5 mg	Orange	Tablet	Double-Scored	Shire Pharmaceuticals
AD; 30	Adderall 30 mg Tablet	7.5 mg; 7.5 mg; 7.5 mg; 7.5 mg	Orange	Tablet	Double-Scored	Shire Pharmaceuticals
AD; RPR	Maalox Anti-Diarrheal	2 mg	Light Green	Tablet	Oblong	Novartis Consumer
ADALAT; 10	Adalat	20 mg	Orange and Light Brown	Capsule, Liquid Filled		Bayer Pharmaceutical
ADALAT; 20	Adalat	10 mg	Orange	Capsule, Liquid Filled		Bayer Pharmaceutical
ADALAT CC; 30	Adalat CC	30 mg	Pink	Sustained-Release Tablet	Circle	Bayer Pharmaceutical
ADALAT CC; 60	Adalat CC	60 mg	Salmon	Sustained-Release Tablet	Circle	Bayer Pharmaceutical
ADALAT CC; 90	Adalat CC	90 mg	Dark Red	Sustained-Release Tablet	Circle	Bayer Pharmaceutical
ADAMS; 006	Allerx Day/night Pack A.M. Tablet - Yellow	120 mg; 2.5 mg	Yellow	Controlled-Release Tablet	Elongated, Scored	Adams Laboratories
ADAMS; 006	Allerx Dose Pack AM Dose	2.5 mg; 120 mg	Yellow	Extended-Release Tablet	Elongated, Scored	Adams Laboratories
ADAMS; 007	Allerx Day/night Pack P.M. Tablet - Blue	8 mg; 2.5 mg	Blue	Controlled-Release Tablet	Elongated, Scored	Adams Laboratories
ADAMS; 012	Syn-RX Pm Treatment Phase	600 mg	Light Green	Tablet		Medeva Pharmaceuticals
ADAMS; 014;	Deconsal	60 mg; 200 mg	Blue and White	Capsule		Medeva Pharmaceuticals
ADAMS; 015;	Deconsal LA	400 mg; 120 mg	Light Blue	Tablet		Medeva Pharmaceuticals
ADAMS; 017	Deconsal II	600 mg; 60 mg	Dark Blue	Sustained-Release Tablet		Medeva Pharmaceuticals
ADAMS; 017	Syn-RX AM Treatment Phase	600 mg; 60 mg	Dark Blue	Extended-Release Tablet	Elongated, Scored	Medeva Pharmaceuticals
ADAMS; 018;	Humibid Sprinkle	300 mg	Light Green and White	Capsule		Medeva Pharmaceuticals
ADAMS; 019	Deconsal Sprinkle	10 mg; 200 mg	Blue and Clear	Capsule		Medeva Pharmaceuticals
ADAMS; 021;	Atrohist LA	4 mg; 50 mg; 120 mg; 0.0242 mg	Yellow	Tablet		Medeva Pharmaceuticals
ADAMS; 034	Humibid DM Sprinkle	15 mg; 300 mg	Green and Clear with White Beads	Capsule		Medeva Pharmaceuticals
ADAMS; 063	Aquatab C	60 mg; 1200 mg; 120 mg	Light Yellow	Extended-Release Tablet	Oval, Scored	Adams Laboratories
ADAMS; 068	Aquatab D	1200 mg; 75 mg	Light Green	Extended-Release Tablet	Oval, Scored	Adams Laboratories
ADAMS; 309	Syn-RX DM Pm Treatment Phase	30 mg; 600 mg	Yellow	Tablet	Elongated, Scored	Medeva Pharmaceuticals
ADAMS; 310	Syn-RX DM AM Treatment Phase	600 mg; 60 mg; 30 mg	Light Blue	Extended-Release Tablet	Elongated, Scored	Medeva Pharmaceuticals
ADAPIN; 10	Adapin	10 mg	Yellow-Orange	Capsule		Fisons Pharmaceuticals
ADAPIN; 25	Adapin	25 mg	Orange-Green	Capsule		Fisons Pharmaceuticals
ADAPIN; 50	Adapin	50 mg	Green	Capsule		Fisons Pharmaceuticals
ADAPIN; 75	Adapin	75 mg	White-Orange	Capsule		Fisons Pharmaceuticals
ADAPIN; 100	Adapin	100 mg	Green and White	Capsule		Fisons Pharmaceuticals
ADDERALL XR; 5 MG	Adderall Xr 5 mg Capsule	1.25 mg; 1.25 mg; 1.25 mg; 1.25 mg	Clear and Blue	Extended-Release Capsule		Shire Pharmaceuticals
ADDERALL XR; 15 MG	Adderall Xr 15 mg Capsule	3.75 mg; 3.75 mg; 3.75 mg; 3.75 mg	White and Blue	Extended-Release Capsule		Shire Pharmaceuticals
ADDERALL XR; 25 MG	Adderall Xr 25 mg Capsule	6.25 mg; 6.25 mg; 6.25 mg; 6.25 mg	Orange and White	Extended-Release Capsule		Shire Pharmaceuticals
ADEFLOR; CHEWABLE; 0.5	Adeflor	5 mg; 2 mcg; 18 mg; 2 mg; 0.5 mg; 4000 IU; 400 IU; 2 mg; 75 mg; 1 mg	Light Brown	Tablet, Chewable	Circle	Pharmacia & Upjohn

IMPRINT	BRAND/GENERIC NAME	STRENGTH	COLOR	FORM	SHAPE	MANUFACTURER
ADEFLOR; CHEWABLE; 1.0	Adeflor	5 mg; 2 mcg; 18 mg; 2 mg; 1 mg; 4000 IU; 400 IU; 2 mg; 75 mg; 1 mg	Brown	Tablet, Chewable	Circle	Pharmacia & Upjohn
ADEFLOR; M	Adeflor M	250 mg; 10 mg; 2 mcg; 20 mg; 1 mg; 100 mg; 2.5 mg; 400 IU; 6000 IU; 1.5 mg; 10 mg; 30 mg; 0.1 mg;	Pink	Tablet	Oval	Pharmacia & Upjohn
ADIPEX-P; 37.5	Adipex-P	37.5 mg	White and Blue	Capsule		Gate Pharmaceuticals
ADIPEX-P; 9-9	Adipex-P	37.5 mg	Blue and White	Tablet	Oblong, Scored	Gate Pharmaceuticals
ADRIA; 230	Octamide	10 mg	Yellow	Tablet	Eight-Sided, Scored	Adria Laboratories
ADRIA; 304	Kaon-CL	750 mg	Green	Sustained-Release Tablet		Savage Laboratories
ADRIA; 307	Kaon-CL	500 mg	Yellow	Sustained-Release Tablet		Savage Laboratories
ADRIA; 312	Kaon	5 meq	Purple	Tablet, Chewable		Savage Laboratories
ADVIL	Advil	200 mg	Light Brown	Coated Tablet	Circle	Wyeth Consumer Healthcare
ADVIL	Advil Liqui-Gels	200 mg	Green	Capsule, Liquid Filled	Oblong	Wyeth Consumer Healthcare
ADVIL; 50	Children's Advil Fruit Flavored Chewables	50 mg	Red	Tablet, Chewable	Circle	Wyeth Consumer Healthcare
ADVIL; 50	Children's Advil Grape Flavored Chewables	50 mg	Purple	Tablet, Chewable	Circle	Wyeth Consumer Healthcare
ADVIL; 100	Junior Strength Advil	100 mg	Orange-Brown	Coated Tablet	Circle	Wyeth Consumer Healthcare
ADVIL; 100	Junior Strength Advil Fruit Flavor	100 mg	Red	Tablet, Chewable	Circle	Wyeth Consumer Healthcare
ADVIL; 100	Junior Strength Advil Grape Flavor	100 mg	Purple	Tablet, Chewable	Circle	Wyeth Consumer Healthcare
ADVIL C&S	Advil Cold & Sinus Tablet	200 mg; 30 mg	Buff	Coated Tablet	Circle	Wyeth Consumer Healthcare
ADVIL COLD & SINUS	Advil Cold & Sinus Caplet	200 mg; 30 mg	Brown	Tablet	Oblong, Coated	Wyeth Consumer Healthcare
ADVIL FLU	Advil Flu & Body Ache	200 mg; 30 mg	White	Tablet	Oval, Film-Coated	Wyeth Consumer Healthcare
ADX; 1; A	Arimidex	1 mg	White	Coated Tablet	Biconvex	Astra Zeneca
AERO	Aerohist	8 mg; 2.5 mg	Blue	Tablet	Capsule-Shape, Scored	Aero Pharmaceuticals
AERO; 2376	Aerohist Plus	8 mg; 20 mg; 2.5 mg	White	Tablet	Capsule-Shape, Scored	Aero Pharmaceuticals
AEY; 420	Deronil	0.75 mg	Amber-Yellow	Tablet		Schering
AF; 1	Decongestant D	325 mg; 2 mg; 5 mg	Yellow and White	Coated Tablet	Circle, Convex, Two Layered	Genco Distributors
AF; 1	Decongestant D	325 mg; 2 mg; 5 mg	Yellow and White	Coated Tablet	Circle, Convex, Two Layered	Glendale Foods
AF; 1	Decongestant D	325 mg; 2 mg; 5 mg	Yellow and White	Coated Tablet	Circle, Convex, Two Layered	Good Sense
AF; 1	Decongestant D	325 mg; 2 mg; 5 mg	Yellow and White	Coated Tablet	Circle, Convex, Two Layered	Major Pharmaceutical
AF; 1	Decongestant D	325 mg; 2 mg; 5 mg	Yellow and White	Coated Tablet	Circle, Convex, Two Layered	Major Quality
AF; 1	Decongestant D	325 mg; 2 mg; 5 mg	Yellow and White	Coated Tablet	Circle, Convex, Two Layered	Nex
AF; 1	Decongestant D	325 mg; 2 mg; 5 mg	Yellow and White	Coated Tablet	Circle, Convex, Two Layered	Perrigo
AF; 1	Decongestant D	325 mg; 2 mg; 5 mg	Yellow and White	Coated Tablet	Circle, Convex, Two Layered	Regal Distributing
AF; 1	Decongestant D	325 mg; 2 mg; 5 mg	Yellow and White	Coated Tablet	Circle, Convex, Two Layered	Revco
AF; 1	Decongestant D	325 mg; 2 mg; 5 mg	Yellow and White	Coated Tablet	Circle, Convex, Two Layered	Sears
AF; 1	Decongestant D	325 mg; 2 mg; 5 mg	Yellow and White	Coated Tablet	Circle, Convex, Two Layered	Seaway
AF; 1	Decongestant D	325 mg; 2 mg; 5 mg	Yellow and White	Coated Tablet	Circle, Convex, Two Layered	Sunfresh
AF; 1	Decongestant D	325 mg; 2 mg; 5 mg	Yellow and White	Coated Tablet	Circle, Convex, Two Layered	Top Care
AF; 1	Decongestant D	325 mg; 2 mg; 5 mg	Yellow and White	Coated Tablet	Circle, Convex, Two Layered	United Drugs
AF; 1	Multi-Symptom Cold	5 mg; 2 mg; 325 mg		Tablet		Perrigo
AF ANACIN	Anacin Maximum Strength, Aspirin Free	500 mg	Blue or White	Capsule, Liquid Filled	Capsule-Shape	A.H. Robins
AF ANACIN	Anacin Aspirin Free Maximum Strength	500 mg	White	Tablet	Oblong	Whitehall Laboratories
AFRINOL; 258;	Afrinol	120 mg	Blue	Tablet		Schering-Plough Healthcare Products
AHR	Cough Calmers	52.5 mg; 7.5 mg	Red	Lozenge/troche	Square	Wyeth Consumer Healthcare
AHR	Dimacol	10 mg; 100 mg; 30 mg	Orange	Tablet	Oval	Wyeth Consumer Healthcare
AHR	Robalate	500 mg	White	Tablet, Chewable		Wyeth Pharmaceuticals
AHR;	Z-Bec	45 IU; 600 mg; 15 mg; 10.2 mg; 100 mg; 10 mg; 6 mcg; 25 mg; 22.5 mg	Green	Coated Tablet	Capsule-Shape	Wyeth Consumer Healthcare
AHR; 0677	Allbee C-800	45 IU; 800 mg; 15 mg; 17 mg; 100 mg; 25 mg; 12 mcg; 25 mg	Orange	Coated Tablet	Oblong	A.H. Robins

IMPRINT	BRAND/GENERIC NAME	STRENGTH	COLOR	FORM	SHAPE	MANUFACTURER
AHR; 0678	Allbee C-800 Plus Iron	27 mg; 45 IU; 800 mg; 0.4 mg; 15 mg; 17 mg; 100 mg; 25 mg; 12 mcg; 25 mg	Dark Red	Coated Tablet	Oblong	A.H. Robins
AHR; 160;	Rela	350 mg	Pink	Coated Tablet	Circle	Schering-Plough
AHR; 1535	Mitrolan	500 mg	Pale Yellow	Tablet, Chewable	Circle	Wyeth Pharmaceuticals
AHR; 1650	Dimacol	100 mg; 30 mg; 15 mg	Orange and Green	Capsule		Wyeth Consumer Healthcare
AHR; 1843;	Dimetane Extentabs	12 mg	Peach-Colored	Timed-Release Tablet		A.H. Robins
AHR; 1857;	Dimetane	4 mg	Peach-Colored	Tablet	Compressed, Scored	A.H. Robins
AHR; 1868;	Dimetane Extentabs	8 mg	Persian Rose-Colored	Timed-Release Tablet		A.H. Robins
AHR; 2117	Dimetane Decongestant	10 mg; 4 mg	Light Blue	Tablet		A.H. Robins
AHR; 2245	Dimetapp Decongestant Non-Drowsy Liqui-Gels	30 mg	Dark Blue	Capsule, Liquid Filled	Oval	Wyeth Consumer Healthcare
AHR; 2248	Dimetapp Allergy	4 mg	Peach	Tablet	Circle	A.H. Robins
AHR; 2250	Dimetapp Allergy Liqui-Gels	4 mg	Green	Capsule, Liquid Filled	Oval	Wyeth Consumer Healthcare
AHR; 5049	Entozyme	300 mg; 250 mg; 150 mg	White	Coated Tablet	Circle	A.H. Robins
AHR; 5449	Exna	50 mg	Yellow	Tablet	Circle, Scored	Wyeth Pharmaceuticals
AHR; 5650	Imavate	50 mg	Pink	Tablet	Circle	Wyeth Consumer Healthcare
AHR; 6207	Phenaphen	325 mg	Dark Brown, Black and Clear	Capsule		A.H. Robins
AHR; 6209	Phenaphen	325 mg	White	Coated Tablet	Capsule-Shape	A.H. Robins
AHR; 6242	Phenaphen with Codeine No. 2	15 mg; 325 mg	Black and Yellow	Capsule		A.H. Robins
AHR; 6251	Phenaphen-650 with Codeine	30 mg; 650 mg	White	Tablet	Capsule-Shape	A.H. Robins
AHR; 6257	Phenaphen with Codeine No. 3	30 mg; 325 mg	Black and Green	Capsule		A.H. Robins
AHR; 6274	Phenaphen with Codeine No. 4	60 mg; 325 mg	Green and White	Capsule		A.H. Robins
AHR; 6447	Pondimin	20 mg	Orange	Tablet	Scored, Compressed	Whitehall-Robins Healthcare
AHR; 8501	Robitussin Cold Severe Congestion Liquigels	200 mg; 30 mg	Aqua	Capsule, Liquid Filled	Oval	Wyeth Consumer Healthcare
AHR; 8600	Robitussin Cold & Cough Liquigels	10 mg; 200 mg; 30 mg	Red	Capsule, Liquid Filled	Oval	Wyeth Consumer Healthcare
AHR; 8601	Robitussin Severe Congestion Non-Drowsy Formula	200 mg; 30 mg	Aqua	Capsule, Liquid Filled	Oval	Wyeth Consumer Healthcare
AHR; 8831	Silain	50 mg		Tablet		Wyeth Pharmaceuticals
AHR; AHR	Robitussin Cough Calmers Cherry Flavor	5 mg	Red	Lozenge/troche	Square	Wyeth Consumer Healthcare
AHR; ROBAXISAL	Robaxisal	325 mg; 400 mg	Pink and White Layered	Tablet		A.H. Robins
AHR; ROBICAP; 8417	Robitet-250 Robicaps	250 mg	Pink and Brown	Capsule		Wyeth Pharmaceuticals
AHR; ROBICAP; 8427	Robitet-500 Robicaps	500 mg	Cream and Brown	Capsule		Wyeth Pharmaceuticals
AKH; 892;	Tremin	2 mg	White	Tablet		Schering
AKJ; 596;	Tremin	5 mg	Gray	Tablet		Schering
AL	Clorazepate Dipotassium	3.75 mg	Blue	Tablet	Circle	Able Laboratories
AL	Clorazepate Dipotassium	3.75 mg	Blue	Tablet	Circle, Scored, Compressed	Novartis Generics
AL	Clorazepate Dipotassium	3.75 mg	Blue	Tablet	Circle	Qualitest Products
AL 0.5; G	Alprazolam	0.5 mg	Dark Yellow	Tablet	Oval, Scored	Par Pharmaceutical
AL; 1.0; G;	Alprazolam	1 mg	White	Tablet	Oval, Scored	Par Pharmaceutical
ALBAMYCIN	Albamycin	250 mg	White and Maroon	Capsule		Pharmacia & Upjohn
ALEVE	Aleve	220 mg	Light Blue	Tablet	Oblong	Bayer Consumer Care
ALEVE COLD & SINUS	Aleve Cold and Sinus	220 mg; 120 mg	White with Blue Ink	Effervescent Tablet		Bayer Consumer Care
ALKA SELTZER	Alka-Seltzer	325 mg; 1916 mg; 1000 mg	White	Effervescent Tablet	Circle, Bevel-Edged, Embossed	Bayer Consumer Care
ALKA SELTZER; AF	Alka-Seltzer Advanced Formula	325 mg; 280 mg; 900 mg; 300 mg; 465 mg	White	Effervescent Tablet		Bayer Consumer Care
ALKA SELTZER; PM	Alka-Seltzer Pm	325 mg; 38 mg	White	Effervescent Tablet	Circle	Bayer Consumer Care
ALKA-MINTS	Alka-Mints	850 mg	White	Tablet, Chewable	Circle	Bayer Consumer Care
ALKA-SELTZER ANTACID	Alka-Seltzer	958 mg; 832 mg; 312 mg	White	Effervescent Tablet	Circle	Bayer Consumer Care
ALKA-SELTZER HR	Alka-Seltzer Heartburn Relief	1000 mg; 1940 mg	White	Effervescent Tablet	Circle, Large	Bayer Consumer Care
ALKA-SELTZER MR	Alka-Seltzer Morning Relief	500 mg; 65 mg	White	Effervescent Tablet	Circle, Large	Bayer Consumer Care
ALLBEE C; AHR	Allbee with C	300 mg; 15 mg; 10.2 mg; 50 mg; 5 mg; 10 mg	Yellow	Tablet	Capsule-Shape	A.H. Robins
ALLEGRA; 60 MG	Allegra	60 mg	White and Pink	Capsule		Aventis Pharmaceuticals
ALLEGRA-D	Allegra-D	60 mg; 120 mg	White and Tan	Extended-Release Tablet	Oblong	Aventis Pharmaceuticals
ALPHA; 028	Guaifenesin	1200 mg	White	Tablet	Oblong, Scored	Eli Lilly
ALPHAGEN	Drituss Gp	1200 mg; 120 mg	White	Extended-Release Tablet		Qualitest Products
ALRA; GX	Gen-Xene	3.75 mg	Gray	Tablet	Capsule-Shape	Alra Laboratories
ALRA; GN	Gen-Xene	15 mg	Light Green	Tablet	Capsule-Shape	Alra Laboratories
ALRA; GT	Gen-Xene	7.5 mg	Peach	Tablet	Capsule-Shape	Alra Laboratories
ALTACE; 1.25; HOECHST	Altace	1.25 mg	Yellow	Capsule		Monarch Pharmaceuticals
ALTACE; 2.5 MG; HOECHST	Altace	2.5 mg	Orange	Capsule		Monarch Pharmaceuticals
ALTACE; 5 MG; HOECHST	Altace	5 mg	Red	Capsule		Monarch Pharmaceuticals
ALTACE; 10 MG; HOECHST	Altace	10 mg	Blue	Capsule		Monarch Pharmaceuticals
ALTO; 401	Zinc-220	220 mg		Capsule		Alto Pharmaceuticals
ALZA; 5	Ditropan Xl	5 mg	Yellow	Extended-Release Tablet		Alza
ALZA; 10	Ditropan Xl	10 mg	Pink	Extended-Release Tablet		Alza
ALZA; 15	Ditropan Xl	15 mg	Gray	Extended-Release Tablet		Alza

IMPRINT	BRAND/GENERIC NAME	STRENGTH	COLOR	FORM	SHAPE	MANUFACTURER
ALZA; 18	Concerta	18 mg	Yellow	Extended-Release Tablet		Alza
ALZA; 27	Concerta	27 mg		Extended-Release Tablet		Alza
ALZA; 36	Concerta	36 mg	White	Extended-Release Tablet		Alza
ALZA; 54	Concerta	54 mg	Brown-Red	Extended-Release Tablet		Alza
AM	Clorazepate Dipotassium	7.5 mg	Peach	Tablet	Circle, Scored, Compressed	Able Laboratories
AM	Clorazepate Dipotassium	7.5 mg	Peach	Tablet		Qualitest Products
AM	Tridione	300 mg	White	Capsule		Abbott Laboratories
AM; 1	Methenamine Mandelate	1.0 G	Purple	Tablet	Oval	Amide Pharmaceuticals
AM; 200; G	Amiodarone Hydrochloride	200 mg	White	Tablet	Circle, Scored	Par Pharmaceutical
AM; PM	V-Dec-M	120 mg; 500 mg	White	Sustained-Release Tablet		Seatrace
AMARYL	Amaryl	1 mg	Pink	Tablet	Oblong, Flat-Faced, with Notched Sides at Double Bisect	Aventis Pharmaceuticals
AMARYL	Amaryl	2 mg	Green	Tablet	Oblong, Flat-Faced, with Notched Sides at Double Bisect	Aventis Pharmaceuticals
AMARYL	Amaryl	4 mg	Blue	Tablet	Oblong, Flat-Faced, with Notched Sides at Double Bisect	Aventis Pharmaceuticals
AMB 5; 5401	Ambien	5 mg	Pink	Tablet	Capsule-Shape	Sanofi-Synthelabo
AMB 10; 5421	Ambien	10 mg	White	Tablet	Capsule-Shape	Sanofi-Synthelabo
AMBI; G; AMBIFED; G	Ambifed-G	60 mg; 1000 mg	White	Tablet	Capsule-Shape, Score	Mcr/american Pharmaceuticals
AMBI; G; DM; AMBIFED; G	Ambifed-G DM	60 mg; 1000 mg; 30 mg	White	Tablet	Capsule-Shape	Mcr/american Pharmaceuticals
AMC; 500; 125;	Amoxicillin and Clavulanate Potassium	500 mg; 125 mg	White to Off White	Tablet	Oblong	Lek Pharmaceuticals
AMC; 875; 125;	Amoxicillin and Clavulanate Potassium	875 mg; 125 mg	White to Off White	Tablet	Oblong	Lek Pharmaceuticals
AMGEN; 30	Sensipar	30 mg	Light Green	Tablet	Oval	Amgen
AMGEN; 60	Sensipar	60 mg	Light Green	Tablet	Oval	Amgen
AMGEN; 90	Sensipar	90 mg	Light Green	Tablet	Oval	Amgen
AMIDE; 001	Multivita-Bets with Fluoride	2500 IU; 400 IU; 15 IU; 0.3 mg; 1.2 mg; 13.5 mg; 1 mg; 60 mg; 1.05 mg; 1.05 mg; 4.5 mcg	Orange, Pink and Purple	Tablet, Chewable	Circle	Novartis Generics
AMIDE; 005	Pseudoephedrine Hydrochloride	60 mg		Tablet		Amide Pharmaceuticals
AMIDE; 009; 10	Isoxsuprine Hydrochloride	10 mg	White	Tablet	Circle	Amide Pharmaceuticals
AMIDE; 0046	Tri-Tannate	25 mg; 8 mg; 25 mg	Buff	Tablet	Capsule-Shape	Amide Pharmaceuticals
AMIDE; 010; 20	Isoxsuprine Hydrochloride	20 mg	White	Tablet	Circle	Amide Pharmaceuticals
AMIDE; 012	Chlorzoxazone and Acetaminophen	250 mg; 300 mg		Tablet		Amide Pharmaceuticals
AMIDE; 013	Ami-Rax	130 mg; 25 mg; 10 mg	White	Tablet	Circle	Amide Pharmaceuticals
AMIDE; 014	Dexchlorpheniramine Maleate	4 mg	Yellow	Tablet	Oval	Watson Laboratories
AMIDE; 015	Dexchlorpheniramine Maleate	6 mg	White	Tablet	Oval	Watson Laboratories
AMIDE; 016	Ami-Natal Plus One	8000 IU; 400 IU; 30 IU; 90 mg; 1 mg; 2.55 mg; 3 mg; 20 mg; 10 mg; 12 mcg; 200 mg; 150 mcg; 65 mg; 100 mg		Tablet		Amide Pharmaceuticals
AMIDE; 024	Amidal	300 mg; 20 mg	White	Tablet	Capsule-Shape	Amide Pharmaceuticals
AMIDE; 025	Chlorzoxazone	500 mg	Green	Tablet	Capsule-Shape	Amide Pharmaceuticals
AMIDE; 028	Hydralazine Hydrochloride	25 mg		Tablet		Amide Pharmaceuticals
AMIDE; 029	Hydralazine Hydrochloride	50 mg		Tablet		Amide Pharmaceuticals
AMIDE; 041	Hydralazine Hydrochloride	10 mg		Tablet		Amide Pharmaceuticals
AMIDE; 043	Aminatal Plus One	200 mg; 2 mg; 12 mcg; 1 mg; 20 mg; 10 mg; 3 mg; 1.5 mg; 4000 IU; 120 mg; 400 IU; 22 mg; 25 mg; 65 mg	Yellow	Coated Tablet	Oval	Amide Pharmaceuticals
AMIDE; 046	Hexavitamin	5000 IU; 400 IU; 75 mg; 2 mg; 3 mg; 20 mg		Tablet		Amide Pharmaceuticals
AMIDE; 053;	Chlorzoxazone	250 mg	Peach	Tablet	Circle	Amide Pharmaceuticals
AMIDE; 055	Ami-Drix	6 mg; 120 mg		Sustained-Release Tablet		Amide Pharmaceuticals
AMIDE; 077	B-C with Folic Acid Plus	27 mg; 5000 IU; 30 IU; 100 mg; 0.15 mg; 25 mg; 0.8 mg; 0.1 mg; 50 mg; 5 mg; 3 mg; 22.5 mg; 500 mg; 20 mg; 20 mg; 25 mg; 50 mcg	Mustard Yellow	Coated Tablet	Oval	Amide Pharmaceuticals
AMIDE; 077	Vitaplex Plus	5000 IU; 30 IU; 500 mg; 20 mg; 20 mg; 100 mg; 25 mg; 0.15 mg; 25 mg; 0.8 mg; 50 mcg; 27 mg; 0.1 mg; 5 mg; 5 mg; 3 mg; 22.5 mg	Yellow	Coated Tablet	Oval	Amide Pharmaceuticals

IMPRINT	BRAND/GENERIC NAME	STRENGTH	COLOR	FORM	SHAPE	MANUFACTURER
AMIDE; 078	Vitacon Forte	8000 IU; 50 IU; 150 mg; 80 mg; 70 mg; 25 mg; 10 mg; 10 mg; 5 mg; 4 mg; 1 mg; 10 mcg; 2 mg	Orange and Black	Capsule		Amide Pharmaceuticals
AMIDE; 082	Cyclandelate	200 mg	Blue	Capsule		Amide Pharmaceuticals
AMIDE; 083	Cyclandelate	400 mg	Red and Blue	Capsule		Amide Pharmaceuticals
AMIDE; 084	Choline Magnesium Trisalicylate	500 mg	Peach	Tablet	Capsule-Shape	Amide Pharmaceuticals
AMIDE; 084	Tricosal	500 mg	Peach	Tablet	Capsule-Shape	Qualitest Products
AMIDE; 085	Choline Magnesium Trisalicylate	750 mg	White	Tablet	Capsule-Shape	Amide Pharmaceuticals
AMIDE; 512	Unipara Plus	250 mg; 300 mg	Green	Tablet		Amide Pharmaceuticals
AMITONE	Amitone	350 mg	White	Tablet, Chewable	Circle	Glaxosmithkline Consumer
AMITONE	Amitone Calcium Antacid	350 mg	White	Tablet	Circle	Perrigo
AMOXIL; 125	Amoxil	125 mg	Pink	Tablet, Chewable	Oval	Glaxosmithkline
AMOXIL; 200	Amoxil	200 mg	Pale Pink	Tablet, Chewable	Circle	Glaxosmithkline
AMOXIL; 250	Amoxil	250 mg	Pink	Tablet, Chewable	Oval	Glaxosmithkline
AMOXIL; 250	Amoxil	250 mg	Royal Blue and Pink	Capsule		Glaxosmithkline
AMOXIL; 400	Amoxil	400 mg	Pale Pink	Tablet, Chewable	Circle	Glaxosmithkline
AMOXIL; 500	Amoxil	500 mg	Pink	Coated Tablet	Capsule-Shape	Glaxosmithkline
AMOXIL; 500	Amoxil	500 mg	Royal Blue and Pink	Capsule		Glaxosmithkline
AMOXIL; 875	Amoxil	875 mg	Pink	Coated Tablet	Capsule-Shape, Scored	Glaxosmithkline
AMP; 500	Ampicillin	500 mg	Blue and White	Capsule		Teva Pharmaceuticals
AMT; 832	Amantadine Hydrochloride	100 mg	Peach	Tablet	Circle	Upsher-Smith Laboratories
AMX; 500	Amoxicillin	500 mg	Orange and White	Capsule		Par Pharmaceutical
AN	Clorazepate Dipotassium	15 mg	White	Tablet	Circle, Scored, Compressed	Able Laboratories
AN	Clorazepate Dipotassium	15 mg	White	Tablet		Qualitest Products
ANACIN	Anacin	400 mg; 32 mg	White	Tablet	Capsule-Shape	Whitehall Laboratories
ANAFRANIL; 25 MG	Anafranil	25 mg	Ivory and Melon Yellow	Capsule		Mallinckrodt
ANAFRANIL; 50 MG	Anafranil	50 mg	Ivory and Aqua Blue	Capsule		Mallinckrodt
ANAFRANIL; 75 MG	Anafranil	75 mg	Ivory and Yellow	Capsule		Mallinckrodt
ANAPROX DS; ROCHE;	Anaprox DS	550 mg	Dark Blue	Coated Tablet	Oblong	Roche Laboratories
ANCOBON; 250 ROCHE	Ancobon	250 mg	Green and Gray	Capsule		Icn Pharmaceuticals
ANCOBON; 500 ROCHE	Ancobon	500 mg	Gray and White	Capsule		Icn Pharmaceuticals
ANDRX; 333;	Entex LA	400 mg; 30 mg	Yellow and Blue	Capsule		Andrx Pharmaceuticals
ANDRX; 510; 100 MG	Ketoprofen	100 mg	White	Extended-Release Capsule		Andrx Pharmaceuticals
ANDRX; 515; 150 MG	Ketoprofen	150 mg	Light Turquoise Blue and White	Extended-Release Capsule		Andrx Pharmaceuticals
ANDRX; 520; 200 MG	Ketoprofen	200 mg	Light Turquoise Blue	Extended-Release Capsule		Andrx Pharmaceuticals
ANDRX; 548	Diltia Xt	120 mg	White	Extended-Release Capsule		Andrx Pharmaceuticals
ANDRX; 549	Diltia Xt	180 mg	Gray and White	Extended-Release Capsule		Andrx Pharmaceuticals
ANDRX; 550	Diltia Xt	240 mg	Gray	Extended-Release Capsule		Andrx Pharmaceuticals
ANDRX; 597	Cartia Xt	120 mg	Orange and White	Extended-Release Capsule		Andrx Pharmaceuticals
ANDRX; 598	Cartia Xt	180 mg	Orange and Yellow	Extended-Release Capsule		Andrx Pharmaceuticals
ANDRX; 599	Cartia Xt	240 mg	Orange and Brown	Extended-Release Capsule		Andrx Pharmaceuticals
ANDRX; 600	Cartia Xt	300 mg	Orange	Extended-Release Capsule		Andrx Pharmaceuticals
ANDRX; 605	Allergy and Congestion Relief	5 mg; 120 mg	White	Extended-Release Tablet		Andrx Pharmaceuticals
ANDRX; 605	Allergy and Congestion Relief	5 mg; 120 mg	White	Extended-Release Tablet		Good Sense
ANDRX; 605	Allergy and Congestion Relief Non-Drowsy	10 mg; 240 mg	White to Off-White	Extended-Release Tablet	Oval	Good Sense
ANDRX; 605	Allergy Relief D Non-Drowsy	10 mg; 240 mg	White to Off-White	Extended-Release Tablet	Oval	Sunmark
ANDRX; 605	Allergy Relief D24 Non-Drowsy	10 mg; 240 mg	White to Off-White	Extended-Release Tablet	Oval	Top Care
ANDRX; 605	Lorata-Dine D	10 mg; 240 mg	White to Off White	Extended-Release Tablet	Oval	Berkley & Jensen
ANDRX; 674; 500	Metformin Hydrochloride	500 mg	White	Tablet	Circle	Andrx Pharmaceuticals
ANDRX; 675; 850	Metformin Hydrochloride	850 mg	White	Tablet	Circle	Andrx Pharmaceuticals
ANDRX; 676; 1000	Metformin Hydrochloride	1000 mg	White	Tablet	Circle	Andrx Pharmaceuticals
ANDRX; 696; 120 MG	Taztia Xt	120 mg	Pink	Capsule		Andrx Pharmaceuticals
ANDRX; 697; 180 MG	Taztia Xt	180 mg	Blue and Cream	Capsule		Andrx Pharmaceuticals
ANDRX; 698; 240 MG	Taztia Xt	240 mg	Pink and Blue	Capsule		Andrx Pharmaceuticals
ANDRX; 699; 300 MG	Taztia Xt	300 mg	Pink and Cream	Capsule		Andrx Pharmaceuticals
ANDRX; 700; 360 MG	Taztia Xt	360 mg	Light Blue	Capsule		Andrx Pharmaceuticals
ANDRX; 827	Generic Entex LA	30 mg; 400 mg	Opaque Orange	Extended-Release Capsule		Andrx Pharmaceuticals
ANEXSIA; 5361	Anexsia	500 mg; 5 mg	White	Tablet	Capsule-Shaped, Bisected Scored	Mallinckrodt
ANEXSIA; 5362	Anexsia	650 mg; 7.5 mg	White	Tablet	Capsule-Shaped, Bisected Scored	Mallinckrodt
ANEXSIA; 5363;	Anexsia	10 mg; 660 mg	White	Tablet	Capsule-Shaped, Bisected Scored	Mallinckrodt
ANK; SP;	Miradon	50 mg	Pink	Tablet	Oval, Scored	Schering
ANOLOR; 300; 51674; 0009	Anolor 300	325 mg; 50 mg; 40 mg	White	Capsule		Blansett Pharmacal
ANSAID; 50 MG	Ansaid	50 mg	White	Coated Tablet	Oval	Pharmacia & Upjohn
ANSAID; 100 MG	Ansaid	100 mg	Blue	Coated Tablet	Oval	Pharmacia & Upjohn

IMPRINT	BRAND/GENERIC NAME	STRENGTH	COLOR	FORM	SHAPE	MANUFACTURER
ANSPOR; 250; SKF	Anspor	250 mg	Red and White	Capsule		Glaxosmithkline
ANSPOR; 500; SKF	Anspor	500 mg	Red	Capsule		Glaxosmithkline
ANTIVERT; 210;	Antivert	12.5 mg	White and Blue	Tablet	Oval	Roerig
ANTIVERT; 211;	Antivert	25 mg	Yellow and White	Tablet		Roerig
ANTIVERT; 212;	Antivert	25 mg	Pink	Tablet, Chewable		Roerig
ANTIVERT; 214	Antivert	50 mg	Blue and Yellow	Tablet	Oval	Roerig
ANTURANE; 200; CIBA; 168	Anturane	200 mg	Green	Capsule		Ciba-Geigy
ANX	Anx	25 mg	Light Green	Tablet		Economed Pharmaceuticals
ANZEMET; 50	Anzemet	50 mg	Light Pink	Coated Tablet	Circle	Aventis Pharmaceuticals
ANZEMET; 100	Anzemet	100 mg	Pink	Coated Tablet	Oval, Elongated	Aventis Pharmaceuticals
AO3; 800	Acyclovir	800 mg	White	Tablet	Oval	Mova Pharmaceutical
AP; 009	Children's Aspirin	81 mg	Orange	Tablet, Chewable	Circle, Convex	Rugby Laboratories
AP; 012	Apap	325 mg	White	Tablet	Circle	Advance Pharmaceutical
AP; 012	Pain & Fever Regular Strength	325 mg	White	Tablet	Circle, Flat, Bevel Edges	Rugby Laboratories
AP; 013	Pain & Fever Extra Strength	500 mg	White	Tablet	Circle, Flat, Bevel Edges	Rugby Laboratories
AP; 015;	Allerfrim	2.5 mg; 60 mg	White	Tablet	Circle, Scored	Rugby Laboratories
AP; 015	Pseudoephedrine Hcl and Triprolidine Hcl	60 mg; 2.5 mg	White	Tablet	Circle, Scored	Advance Pharmaceutical
AP; 016;	Aller-Chlor	4 mg	Yellow	Tablet	Circle, Scored	Rugby Laboratories
AP; 017	Nasal Decongestant	30 mg	Red	Coated Tablet	Circle, Convex	Rugby Laboratories
AP; 017	Pseudoephedrine Hydrochloride	30 mg	Red	Tablet	Circle	Advance Pharmaceutical
AP; 018	Nasal Decongestant Adult Strength	60 mg	White	Coated Tablet	Circle, Convex	Rugby Laboratories
AP; 019	Gas Relief	80 mg	White	Tablet, Chewable	Circle, Flat, Bevel Edges	Rugby Laboratories
AP; 025	Calcium Carbonate	650 mg	White	Tablet	Circle, Convex	Advance Pharmaceutical
AP; 025	Estradiol	0.5 mg	White	Tablet		Apothecon
AP; 026	Acetaminophen and Phenyltoloxamine	325 mg; 30 mg	Peach	Tablet	Circle	Advance Pharmaceutical
AP; 026	Estradiol	1 mg	Lavender	Tablet	Circle	Bristol-Myers Squibb
AP; 027	Estradiol	2 mg	Green	Tablet	Circle	Bristol-Myers Squibb
AP; 040	Maximum Strength Gas Relief	125 mg	White	Tablet, Chewable	Circle, Flat, Bevel Edges	Rugby Laboratories
AP; 043	Cal-Gest Assorted Flavors	500 mg	Yellow, Green, Peach and Pink	Tablet, Chewable		Rugby Laboratories
AP; 045	Peptic Relief	262 mg	Light Pink	Tablet, Chewable	Circle, Flat, Bevel Edged	Rugby Laboratories
AP; 051	Apap 80 mg Pain/fever Childs	80 mg	Light Pink	Tablet, Chewable	Circle	Rugby Laboratories
AP; 0812;	Doxycycline	100 mg		Coated Tablet		Apothecon
AP; 0814;	Doxycycline	100 mg	White	Capsule		Apothecon
AP; 0837;	Doxycycline	50 mg	White	Capsule		Apothecon
AP; 1	Phenazopyridine Hydrochloride	100 mg	Dark Maroon	Coated Tablet	Circle, Scored	Able Laboratories
AP; 1	Phenazopyridine Hydrochloride	100 mg	Dark Maroon	Coated Tablet	Circle, Scored	Novartis Generics
AP; 2	Phenazopyridine Hydrochloride	200 mg	Dark Maroon	Coated Tablet	Circle, Scored	Able Laboratories
AP; 2	Phenazopyridine Hydrochloride	200 mg	Dark Maroon	Coated Tablet	Circle, Scored	Novartis Generics
AP; 20	Diphenhist	25 mg	Natural and Pink	Capsule		Rugby Laboratories
AP; 20	Diphenhydramine	25 mg	Pink and White	Capsule		Qualitest Products
AP; 20	Diphenhydramine Hydrochloride	25 mg	Pink and White	Capsule		Advance Pharmaceutical
AP; 21	Diphenhydramine	50 mg	Pink	Capsule		Qualitest Products
AP; 21	Diphenhydramine Hydrochloride	50 mg	Bright Pink	Capsule	Small	Advance Pharmaceutical
AP; 35	Docusate Sodium	250 mg	Red and Yellow	Capsule		Advance Pharmaceutical
AP; 37	Acetaminophen	500 mg	Red and Clear with White Powder	Capsule		Advance Pharmaceutical
AP; 2461	Nadolol	20 mg	White	Tablet	Circle	Apothecon
AP; 2462	Nadolol	40 mg	White	Tablet	Circle	Apothecon
AP; 2463	Nadolol	80 mg	White	Tablet	Circle	Apothecon
AP; 2464	Nadolol	120 mg	White	Tablet	Capsule-Shape	Apothecon
AP; 2465	Nadolol	160 mg	White	Tablet	Capsule-Shape	Apothecon
AP; 2472	Nadolol and Bendroflumethiazide	5 mg; 40 mg	White	Tablet	Circle	Apothecon
AP; 2473	Nadolol and Bendroflumethiazide	5 mg; 80 mg	White	Tablet	Circle, Biconvex	Apothecon
AP; 3171; 50 50 50	Trazodone	150 mg		Tablet		Apothecon
AP; 4165	Acyclovir	400 mg	White	Tablet	Circle	Apothecon
AP; 5160	Captopril and Hydrochlorothiazide	25 mg; 15 mg	White and Orange Mottled	Tablet	Rounded Square, Quadrisected Scored	Bristol-Myers Squibb
AP; 5161	Captopril and Hydrochlorothiazide	25 mg; 25 mg	Peach	Tablet	Rounded Square, Quadrisected Scored	Bristol-Myers Squibb
AP; 5162	Captopril and Hydrochlorothiazide	50 mg; 15 mg	White and Orange Mottled	Tablet	Oval, Scored	Bristol-Myers Squibb
AP; 5163	Captopril and Hydrochlorothiazide	50 mg; 25 mg	Peach	Tablet	Oval, Scored	Bristol-Myers Squibb
AP; 5541	Enalapril Maleate	2.5 mg		Tablet		Apothecon
AP; 5542	Enalapril Maleate	5 mg		Tablet		Apothecon
AP; 5543	Enalapril Maleate	10 mg		Tablet		Apothecon
AP; 5544	Enalapril Maleate	20 mg		Tablet		Apothecon
AP; 6910; 10 MEQ	Potassium Chloride	10 meq	Orange	Sustained-Release Tablet	Circle	Apothecon
AP; 7045	Captopril	12.5 mg		Tablet		Apothecon
AP; 7045;	Captopril	12.5 mg	White	Tablet	Circle, Scored	Sandoz
AP; 7046	Captopril	25 mg		Tablet		Apothecon
AP; 7046	Captopril	25 mg	White	Tablet	Circle, Scored	Sandoz
AP; 7047	Captopril	50 mg		Tablet		Apothecon
AP; 7047	Captopril	50 mg	White	Tablet	Circle, Scored	Sandoz
AP; 7048	Captopril	100 mg		Tablet		Apothecon
AP; 7048	Captopril	100 mg	White	Tablet	Circle, Scored	Sandoz
AP; 7491; 250;	Cefaclor	250 mg	Light Yellow and Blue	Capsule		Apothecon
AP; 7494; 500;	Cefaclor	500 mg	Orange and Blue	Capsule		Apothecon
APO; 010	Omeprazole	10 mg	Pink and Reddish Brown	Delayed-Release Capsule		Apotex
APO; 014	Dilt-Xr	120 mg	Orange and White	Capsule, Extended Release		Apotex

IMPRINT	BRAND/GENERIC NAME	STRENGTH	COLOR	FORM	SHAPE	MANUFACTURER
APO; 015	Dilt-Xr	180 mg	Orange and White	Capsule, Extended Release	Capsule-Shape	Apotex
APO; 016	Dilt-Xr	240 mg	White and Brown	Capsule, Extended Release		Apotex
APO; 018	Cimetidine	200 mg	Green	Tablet	Circle	Apotex
APO; 019	Cimetidine	300 mg	Green	Tablet	Circle	Apotex
APO; 020	Cimetidine	400 mg	Green	Tablet	Oblong	Apotex
APO; 020	Omeprazole	20 mg;	Pink and Reddish Brown	Delayed-Release Capsule		Apotex
APO; 021	Cimetidine	800 mg	Green	Tablet	Circle	Apotex
APO; 025	Ranitidine Hydrochloride	150 mg	White	Tablet	Circle	Apotex
APO; 026;	Ranitidine Hydrochloride	300 mg	White	Tablet	Oblong	Apotex
APO; 027	Ticlopidine Hydrochloride	250 mg	White	Tablet	Oblong	Apotex
APO; 033	Pentoxifylline	400 mg	White	Extended-Release Tablet	Oblong	Apotex
APO; 033	Pentoxifylline Extended-Release	400 mg	White	Extended-Release Tablet	Oval	Akyma Pharmaceuticals
APO; 034; 600	Gemfibrozil	600 mg	White	Tablet	Oval, Scored	Apotex
APO; 039	Etodolac	200 mg	White and Gray	Capsule		Apotex
APO; 040	Etodolac	300 mg	White and Gray	Capsule		Apotex
APO; 040	Omeprazole	40 mg	Pink and Reddish Brown	Delayed-Release Capsule		Apotex
APO; 055	Selegiline Hydrochloride	5 mg	White and Aqua	Capsule		Apotex
APO; 078	Buspirone Hydrochloride	5 mg	Light Blue	Tablet	Barrel, Scored	Apotex
APO; 079	Buspirone Hydrochloride	10 mg	Light Blue	Tablet	Barrel, Scored	Apotex
APO; 083	Paroxetine Hydrochloride	20 mg	Off White	Tablet	Oval, Scored	Apotex
APO; 084	Paroxetine Hydrochloride	30 mg	Off White	Tablet	Oval	Apotex
APO; 093	Doxazosin Mesylate	1 mg	White to Off-White	Tablet	Circle, Scored with Partial Score on Other Side	Apotex
APO; 094	Doxazosin Mesylate	2 mg	White to Off-White	Tablet	Capsule-Shape, Scored with Partial Scored with Partial	Apotex
APO; 095	Doxazosin Mesylate	4 mg	White to Off-White	Tablet	Capsule-Shape, Scored with Partial Scored with Partial	Apotex
APO; 096	Doxazosin Mesylate	8 mg	White to Off-White	Tablet	Capsule-Shape, Scored with Partial Score on the Other Side	Apotex
APO; 097	Paroxetine Hydrochloride	10 mg	Off White	Tablet	Oval, Scored	Apotex
APO; 2.5	Lisinopril	2.5 mg	White	Tablet	Circle	Apotex
APO; 101	Paroxetine Hydrochloride	40 mg	Off White	Tablet	Oval	Apotex
APO; 103	Buspirone Hydrochloride	15 mg	Light Blue	Tablet	Rectangle, Tri-Sect on Both Sides	Apotex
APO; 115	Terazosin Hydrochloride	1 mg	Beige	Capsule		Apotex
APO; 116	Terazosin Hydrochloride	2 mg	Yellow	Capsule		Apotex
APO; 117	Terazosin Hydrochloride	5 mg	Red	Capsule		Apotex
APO; 118	Terazosin Hydrochloride	10 mg	Blue	Capsule		Apotex
APO; 133; 25	Cyclosporine	25 mg	Reddish-Brown	Capsule, Liquid Filled		Apotex
APO; 134; 100	Cyclosporine	100 mg	Reddish-Brown	Capsule, Liquid Filled		Apotex
APO; 150	Nizatidine	150 mg	White and Yellow	Capsule		Apotex
APO; 200	Carbamazepine	200 mg	White to Off-White	Tablet	Circle, Scored	Apotex
APO; 300	Nizatidine	300 mg	White and Light Brown	Capsule		Apotex
APO; 500; MET	Metformin Hydrochloride	500 mg	White to Off White	Tablet	Capsule-Shape	Apotex
APO; 850	Metformin Hydrochloride	850 mg	White to Off White	Tablet	Oval	Apotex
APO; 1000	Metformin Hydrochloride	1000 mg	White to Off White	Tablet	Scored, Capsule-Shape	Apotex
APO; AF; 80	Sotalol Hydrochloride Af	80 mg	White to Off-White	Tablet	Capsule-Shape, Scored	Apotex
APO; AF; 120	Sotalol Hydrochloride Af	120 mg	White to Off-White	Tablet	Capsule-Shape, Scored	Apotex
APO; AF; 160	Sotalol Hydrochloride Af	160 mg	White to Off-White	Tablet	Capsule-Shape, Scored	Apotex
APO; C-0.5	Clonazepam	0.5 mg	Orange	Tablet	Circle, Scored	Apotex
APO; C-1	Clonazepam	1 mg	Blue	Tablet	Circle	Apotex
APO; C-2	Clonazepam	2 mg	White to Off-White	Tablet	Circle	Apotex
APO; C250	Cefuroxime Axetil	250 mg	White	Tablet	Capsule-Shape	Apotex
APO; C500	Cefuroxime Axetil	500 mg	White	Tablet	Capsule-Shape	Apotex
APO; F25	Fluvoxamine Maleate	25 mg	White	Tablet	Circle	Apotex
APO; F50	Fluvoxamine Maleate	50 mg	Golden	Tablet	Circle, Scored	Apotex
APO; FCN; 50	Fluconazole	50 mg	Pink	Tablet	Circle	Apotex
APO; FCN; 100	Fluconazole	100 mg	Pink	Tablet	Circle	Apotex
APO; FCN; 150	Fluconazole	150 mg	Pink	Tablet	Circle	Apotex
APO; FCN; 200	Fluconazole	200 mg	Pink	Tablet	Circle	Apotex
APO; FLU100	Fluvoxamine Maleate	100 mg	Reddish Brown	Tablet	Ovoid-Rectangular, Scored	Apotex
APO; GLP; 5	Glipizide	5 mg	White to Off-White	Tablet	Circle, Scored	Apotex
APO; GLP; 10	Glipizide	10 mg	White to Off White	Tablet	Circle, Scored	Apotex
APO; KET; 200	Ketoconazole	200 mg	White to Off-White	Tablet	Circle, Scored	Apotex
APO; L; 5	Lisinopril	5 mg	Reddish-Brown	Tablet	Oval, Scored	Apotex
APO; L10	Lisinopril	10 mg	Reddish-Brown	Tablet	Oval	Apotex
APO; L20	Lisinopril	20 mg	Reddish-Brown	Tablet	Oval	Apotex
APO; L30	Lisinopril	30 mg	Reddish-Brown	Tablet	Oval	Apotex
APO; L40	Lisinopril	40 mg	Yellow	Tablet	Oval	Apotex
APO; OXA; 600	Oxaprozin	600 mg;	White to Off White	Tablet	Capsule-Shape, Scored	Apotex
APO; SO; 80	Sotalol Hydrochloride	80 mg	White to Off-White	Tablet	Capsule-Shape, Scored	Apotex
APO; SOT; 120	Sotalol Hydrochloride	120 mg	White to Off-White	Tablet	Capsule-Shape, Scored	Apotex
APO; SOT; 160	Sotalol Hydrochloride	160 mg	White to Off-White	Tablet	Capsule-Shape, Scored	Apotex
APO; SOT; 240	Sotalol Hydrochloride	240 mg	White to Off-White	Tablet	Capsule-Shape, Scored	Apotex
APO; TR; 50	Tramadol Hydrochloride	50 mg	White to Off White	Tablet	Capsule-Shape	Apotex
APO; TR50	Tramadol Hydrochloride	50 mg	White to Off-White	Tablet	Capsule-Shape	Major Pharmaceutical
APO; CI 10	Citalopram Hydrobromide	10 mg	Beige-Pink	Tablet	Oval	Apotex
APO; CI 20	Citalopram Hydrobromide	20 mg	Pink	Tablet	Oval	Apotex
APO; CI 40	Citalopram Hydrobromide	40 mg	White	Tablet	Oval	Apotex
APO 041; 400	Etodolac	400 mg	White to Off White	Tablet	Oval	Apotex
APO 102; 500	Etodolac	500 mg	White to Off White	Tablet	Oval	Apotex
APO 131	Carbidopa and Levodopa	25 mg; 100 mg	Reddish Brown	Tablet	Circle	Apotex
APO 132	Carbidopa and Levodopa	50 mg; 200 mg	Buff to Light Brown	Tablet	Circle	Apotex
APO TI-2	Tizanidine Hydrochloride	2 mg	White to Off-White	Tablet	Circle	Apotex
APO TI-4	Tizanidine Hydrochloride	4 mg	White to Off-White	Tablet	Circle	Apotex

IMPRINT	BRAND/GENERIC NAME	STRENGTH	COLOR	FORM	SHAPE	MANUFACTURER
APSE	Ami-Tex Pse	600 mg; 120 mg	Yellow	Tablet	Capsule-Shape	Amide Pharmaceuticals
APSE	Pseudoephedrine Hydrochloride and Guaifenesin	120 mg; 600 mg	Yellow	Tablet	Oval	Duramed Pharmaceuticals
ARE	Mol-Iron Panhemic	500 mg; 7.5 mcg; 75 mg; 2 mg; 2 mg; 10 mg	Orange and Black	Capsule		Schering-Plough Healthcare Products
ARROW; LIFT CAP UP	Feverall Sprinkle Caps	80 mg	White and Clear	Capsule		Upsher-Smith Laboratories
ARROW; LIFT CAP UP	Feverall Sprinkle Caps Powder, Junior Strength	160 mg	Red and Clear	Capsule		Upsher-Smith Laboratories
ARROW;	Anacin	400 mg; 32 mg	White	Coated Tablet	Circle	Whitehall Laboratories
ARTHA-G	Artha-G	750 mg	Lavender	Tablet		T.E. Williams Pharmaceuticals
AS	Comtrex Allergy/sinus Formula	500 mg; 30 mg; 2 mg	Green	Tablet		Bristol-Myers Squibb
AS	Isoclor	4 mg; 60 mg	White	Tablet	Circle	Novartis Consumer
AS+ C & C	Alka-Seltzer Plus Cold & Cough Medicine Liqui-Gels	10 mg; 2 mg; 30 mg; 325 mg	Purple	Capsule, Liquid Filled	Oblong	Bayer Consumer Care
AS+ C&F	Alka-Seltzer Plus Cold & Flu Medicine Liqui-Gels Non-Drowsy	325 mg; 30 mg; 10 mg	Orange	Capsule, Liquid Filled	Oblong	Bayer Consumer Care
AS+ C&S	Alka-Seltzer Plus Cold & Sinus Non-Drowsy	325 mg; 30 mg	Red	Capsule, Liquid Filled	Oblong	Bayer Consumer Care
AS+ COLD	Alka-Seltzer Plus Cold Medicine Liqui-Gels	2 mg; 30 mg; 325 mg	Clear Blue	Capsule, Liquid Filled	Oblong	Bayer Consumer Care
AS+ NT	Alka-Seltzer Plus Night-Time Cold Medicine Liqui-Gels	10 mg; 6.25 mg; 30 mg; 325 mg	Clear Green	Capsule, Liquid Filled	Oblong	Bayer Consumer Care
ASACOL; NE	Asacol	400 mg	Red-Brown	Timed-Release Tablet	Capsule-Shape	Procter & Gamble Pharmaceuticals
ASB	Bufferin Arthritis Strength	500 mg;	White	Tablet		Bristol-Myers Squibb
ASB	Bufferin Tri-Buffered Arthritis Strength	500 mg; 222.3 mg; 88.9 mg; 55.6 mg		Tablet		Bristol-Myers Squibb
ASBRON; G; 78/202;	Asbron G	100 mg; 300 mg	Green with White Inlay	Tablet		Novartis Pharmaceuticals
ASPIRIN	Aspirin	325 mg	White	Tablet	Circle	Baxter Healthcare
ASPIRIN	Aspirin	325 mg	White	Tablet	Circle	J.J. Balan
ASPIRIN	Aspirin	325 mg	White	Coated Tablet	Circle	Pfeiffer Pharmaceuticals
ASPIRIN	Aspirin	325 mg	White	Tablet	Circle	Republic Drug
ASPIRIN	Aspirin	325 mg	White	Tablet	Circle	Zee Medical
ASPIRIN	Aspercin	325 mg	White	Tablet	Circle	Otis Clapp
ASPIRIN; 44; 157	Aspirin	325 mg	White	Coated Tablet	Circle, Convex	Udl Laboratories
ASPIRIN; 44-250	Aspirin	325 mg	White to Off-White	Coated Tablet	Circle, Convex, Embossed	Leiner Health Products
ASPIRIN; 500	Aspirin Extra Strength	500 mg	White	Coated Tablet	Circle	Good Neighbor Pharmacy
ASPIRIN; 500	Aspirin Extra Strength	500 mg	White	Coated Tablet	Circle	Valu Rite
ASPIRIN; A2	Aspirin Lightly Coated Caffeine and Sodium Free	325 mg	White	Coated Tablet	Biconvex, Double	Top Care
ASPIRIN; L012;	Aspirin	325 mg	White to Off-White	Coated Tablet	Circle, Convex, Embossed	Leiner Health Products
ASPIRIN; L019;	Aspirin	325 mg	White to Off-White	Tablet	Circle, Convex, Embossed	Leiner Health Products
ASPIRIN; L	Aspirin	325 mg	White	Coated Tablet	Biconcave, Compressed, Punch	Good Neighbor Pharmacy
ASPIRIN; L	Aspirin	325 mg	White	Coated Tablet	Biconcave, Compressed, Punch	Perfect Choice
ASPIRIN; L	Aspirin	325 mg		Tablet		Perrigo
ASPIRIN; L	Aspirin	325 mg	White	Coated Tablet	Biconcave, Compressed, Punch	Valu Rite
ASPIRIN; L	Aspirin Regular Strength	325 mg	White	Tablet	Circle, Compressed, Concave	Good Neighbor Pharmacy
ASPIRIN; L	Aspirin Regular Strength	325 mg	White	Tablet	Circle, Compressed, Concave	Good Sense
ASPIRIN; L	Aspirin Regular Strength	325 mg	White	Tablet	Circle, Compressed, Concave	Harco Drug
ASPIRIN; L	Aspirin Regular Strength	325 mg	White	Tablet	Circle, Compressed, Concave	Inter-American Foods
ASPIRIN; L	Aspirin Regular Strength	325 mg	White	Tablet	Circle, Compressed, Concave	North Laboratories
ASPIRIN; L	Aspirin Regular Strength	325 mg	White	Tablet	Circle, Compressed, Concave	Perfect Choice
ASPIRIN; L	Aspirin Regular Strength	325 mg	White	Tablet	Circle, Compressed, Concave	Perrigo
ASPIRIN; L	Aspirin Regular Strength	325 mg	White	Tablet	Circle, Compressed, Concave	Regal Distributing
ASPIRIN; L	Aspirin Regular Strength	325 mg	White	Coated Tablet	Biconcave, Compressed, Punch	Sunmark
ASPIRIN; L	Aspirin Regular Strength	325 mg	White	Tablet	Circle, Compressed, Concave	Swan
ASPIRIN; L	Aspirin Regular Strength	325 mg	White	Tablet	Circle, Compressed, Concave	True Quality
ASPIRIN; L	Coated Aspirin	325 mg	White	Coated Tablet	Biconcave, Compressed, Punch	First Choice
ASPIRIN; L	Coated Aspirin	325 mg	White	Coated Tablet	Biconcave, Compressed, Punch	Fleming
ASPIRIN; L	Coated Aspirin	325 mg	White	Coated Tablet	Biconcave, Compressed, Punch	Good Sense
ASPIRIN; L	Coated Aspirin	325 mg	White	Coated Tablet	Biconcave, Compressed, Punch	Medalist
ASPIRIN; L	Coated Aspirin	325 mg	White	Coated Tablet	Biconcave, Compressed, Punch	Perrigo
ASPIRIN; L	Coated Aspirin	325 mg	White	Coated Tablet	Biconcave, Compressed, Punch	Sunfresh
ASPIRIN; L	Coated Aspirin	325 mg	White	Coated Tablet	Biconcave, Compressed, Punch	Top Care
ASPIRIN; L	Coated Aspirin	325 mg	White	Coated Tablet	Biconcave, Compressed, Punch	True Quality
ASPIRIN; L	Coated Aspirin	325 mg	White	Coated Tablet	Biconcave, Compressed, Punch	True Quality Pharmacies
ASPIRIN; L	Coated Aspirin Micro-Thin Coating	325 mg	White	Coated Tablet	Circle	Fleming
ASPIRIN; L	Coated Aspirin Micro-Thin Coating	325 mg	White	Coated Tablet	Circle	Glendale Foods
ASPIRIN; L	Coated Aspirin Micro-Thin Coating	325 mg	White	Coated Tablet	Circle	Good Neighbor Pharmacy
ASPIRIN; L	Coated Aspirin Micro-Thin Coating	325 mg	White	Coated Tablet	Circle	Good Sense
ASPIRIN; L	Coated Aspirin Micro-Thin Coating	325 mg	White	Coated Tablet	Circle	Hytop
ASPIRIN; L	Coated Aspirin Micro-Thin Coating	325 mg	White	Coated Tablet	Circle	Major
ASPIRIN; L	Coated Aspirin Micro-Thin Coating	325 mg	White	Coated Tablet	Circle	Medalist
ASPIRIN; L	Coated Aspirin Micro-Thin Coating	325 mg	White	Coated Tablet	Circle	Nex
ASPIRIN; L	Coated Aspirin Micro-Thin Coating	325 mg	White	Coated Tablet	Circle	Perfect Choice

IMPRINT	BRAND/GENERIC NAME	STRENGTH	COLOR	FORM	SHAPE	MANUFACTURER
ASPIRIN; L	Coated Aspirin Micro-Thin Coating	325 mg	White	Coated Tablet	Circle	Perrigo
ASPIRIN; L	Coated Aspirin Micro-Thin Coating	325 mg	White	Coated Tablet	Circle	Quality Care
ASPIRIN; L	Coated Aspirin Micro-Thin Coating	325 mg	White	Coated Tablet	Circle	Regal Distributing
ASPIRIN; L	Coated Aspirin Micro-Thin Coating	325 mg	White	Coated Tablet	Circle	Rexall
ASPIRIN; L	Coated Aspirin Micro-Thin Coating	325 mg	White	Coated Tablet	Circle	Swan
ASPIRIN; L	Coated Aspirin Micro-Thin Coating	325 mg	White	Coated Tablet	Circle	Top Care
ASPIRIN; L	Coated Aspirin Micro-Thin Coating	325 mg	White	Coated Tablet	Circle	True Quality
ASPIRIN; L	Coated Aspirin Micro-Thin Coating	325 mg	White	Coated Tablet	Circle	United Drugs
ASPIRIN; L	Coated Aspirin Micro-Thin Coating	325 mg	White	Coated Tablet	Circle	Valu Buy
ASPIRIN; L	Coated Aspirin Micro-Thin Coating	325 mg	White	Coated Tablet	Circle	Valu Rite
AT; 0.5; 56	Alzapam	0.5 mg	White	Tablet	Circle	Major Pharmaceutical
AT; 1.0; 58	Alzapam	1 mg	White	Tablet	Circle	Major Pharmaceutical
AT; 2.0; 60	Alzapam	2 mg	White	Tablet	Circle	Major Pharmaceutical
ATARAX; 10	Atarax	10 mg	Orange	Tablet	Triangle	Pfizer
ATARAX; 25	Atarax	25 mg	Green	Tablet	Triangle	Pfizer Laboratories
ATARAX; 50	Atarax	50 mg	Yellow	Tablet	Triangle	Pfizer Laboratories
ATARAX; 100	Atarax	100 mg	Red	Tablet	Triangle	Pfizer Laboratories
ATHENA LOGO	Carbatrol	200 mg	Light Gray and Blue-Green	Extended-Release Capsule		Shire Pharmaceuticals
ATHENA LOGO	Carbatrol	300 mg	Black and Blue-Green	Extended-Release Capsule		Shire Pharmaceuticals
ATRAL; 250	Cephalexin	250 mg	Opaque Scarlet and Grey	Capsule		Duramed Pharmaceuticals
ATRAL; 250	Tetracycline Hydrochloride	250 mg	Opaque Yellow and Orange	Capsule		Duramed Pharmaceuticals
ATRAL; 500	Tetracycline Hydrochloride	500 mg	Opaque Black and Yellow	Capsule		Duramed Pharmaceuticals
ATROMID-S; 500	Atromid-S	500 mg	Orange	Capsule, Liquid Filled	Oblong	Wyeth Pharmaceuticals
AUGMENTIN; 200	Augmentin	200 mg; 28.5 mg	Mottled Pink	Tablet, Chewable	Circle, Biconvex	Glaxosmithkline
AUGMENTIN; 250/ 125	Augmentin	250 mg; 125 mg	White	Coated Tablet	Oval	Glaxosmithkline
AUGMENTIN; 400	Augmentin	400 mg; 57 mg	Mottled Pink	Tablet, Chewable	Circle, Biconvex	Glaxosmithkline
AUGMENTIN; 500/ 125	Augmentin	500 mg; 125 mg	White	Coated Tablet	Oval	Glaxosmithkline
AUGMENTIN; 875;	Augmentin	875 mg; 125 mg	White	Coated Tablet	Capsule-Shape, Scored	Glaxosmithkline
AUGMENTIN XR	Augmentin Xr	1000 mg; 62.5 mg	White	Extended-Release Tablet	Oval, BI-Layered	Glaxosmithkline
AXID; 150; RELIANT;	Axid	150 mg	Opaque Dark Yellow and Opaque Pale Yellow	Capsule		Eli Lilly
AXID; 300; RELIANT;	Axid	300 mg	Opaque Brown and Opaque Pale Yellow	Capsule		Eli Lilly
AXID; AR	Axid AR	75 mg	Yellow	Tablet		Wyeth Consumer Healthcare
AYERST; 878	Premarin with Methyltestosterone	0.625 mg; 5 mg	White	Tablet	Circle	Wyeth Pharmaceuticals
AYERST; 879	Premarin with Methyltestosterone	1.25 mg; 10 mg	Yellow	Tablet	Circle	Wyeth Pharmaceuticals
AYERST; 880	Pmb-200	0.45 mg; 200 mg	Green	Tablet	Oblong	Wyeth Pharmaceuticals
AYERST; 881	Pmb-400	0.45 mg; 400 mg	Pink	Tablet	Oblong	Wyeth Pharmaceuticals
AYGESTIN; 5	Aygestin	5 mg	White	Tablet	Oval, Scored	Barr Laboratories
AYGESTIN; 5	Aygestin	5 mg	White	Tablet	Oval, Scored	Duramed Pharmaceuticals
B	Anolor Dh	5 mg; 325 mg; 50 mg; 40 mg	Orange	Capsule		Blansett Pharmacal
B	Bufferin	325 mg	White, Opaque	Tablet	Capsule-Shape	Bristol-Myers Squibb
B	Bufferin Tri-Buffered	325 mg; 158 mg; 63 mg; 34 mg	White	Coated Tablet	Circle, Scored	Bristol-Myers Squibb
B; 097	Guai-D	1000 mg; 60 mg	White, Scored	Tablet		Breckenridge Pharmaceutical
B2C	Lanoxicaps	0.1 mg	Yellow	Capsule, Liquid Filled	Oval, Small	Glaxosmithkline
B3; LL	Zebeta	10 mg	White	Coated Tablet	Heart-Shape, Biconvex	Lederle Laboratories
B; 11;	Zagam	200 mg	White	Coated Tablet	Circle, Biconvex	Bertek Pharmaceuticals
B; 21	Levlen 21	0.15 mg; 30 mcg	Orange	21-Day Tablet Pack	Circle	Berlex Laboratories
B; 21	Levlen 28 Orange Tablet	0.15 mg; 30 mcg	Orange	28-Day Tablet Pack	Circle	Berlex Laboratories
B; 25	Benadryl Allergy Tablet	25 mg	Bright Pink	Tablet	Capsule-Shape, Small	Pfizer Consumer Health Care
B; 30	Nifediac CC Extended Release	30 mg	Mustard Yellow	Tablet	Circle	Teva Pharmaceuticals
B; 30	Nifedical Xl	30 mg	Reddish Brown	Extended-Release Tablet	Circle	Teva Pharmaceuticals
B; 50; 902	Naltrexone Hydrochloride	50 mg	Beige	Tablet	Circle, Scored	Barr Laboratories
B; 60	Nifediac CC Extended Release	60 mg	Mustard Yellow	Tablet	Circle	Teva Pharmaceuticals
B; 60	Nifedical Xl	60 mg	Reddish Brown	Extended-Release Tablet	Circle	Teva Pharmaceuticals
B; 60	Nifedipine	60 mg	Yellow	Extended-Release Tablet	Circle	Teva Pharmaceuticals
B; 066; 100	Isoniazid	100 mg	White	Tablet	Circle, Scored, Flat-Faced	Barr Laboratories
B; 071; 300	Isoniazid	300 mg	White	Tablet	Circle, Scored, Flat-Faced	Barr Laboratories
B; 95	Tri-Levlen 21 Brown Tablet	0.05 mg; 0.03 mg	Brown	21-Day Tablet Pack	Circle	Berlex Laboratories
B; 95	Tri-Levlen 28 Brown Tablet	0.05 mg; 0.03 mg	Brown	28-Day Tablet Pack	Circle	Berlex Laboratories
B; 96	Tri-Levlen 21 White Tablet	0.075 mg; 0.04 mg	White	21-Day Tablet Pack	Circle	Berlex Laboratories
B; 96	Tri-Levlen 28 White Tablet	0.075 mg; 0.04 mg	White	28-Day Tablet Pack	Circle	Berlex Laboratories
B; 97	Tri-Levlen 21 Light Yellow Tablet	0.125 mg; 0.03 mg	Light Yellow	21-Day Tablet Pack	Circle	Berlex Laboratories
B; 97	Tri-Levlen 28 Light Yellow Tablet	0.125 mg; 0.03 mg	Light Yellow	28-Day Tablet Pack	Circle	Berlex Laboratories
B; 120 MG	Cardizem LA	120 mg	White	Extended-Release Tablet	Capsule-Shape	Biovail Pharmaceuticals

IMPRINT	BRAND/GENERIC NAME	STRENGTH	COLOR	FORM	SHAPE	MANUFACTURER
B; 133	Pyridostigmine Bromide	60 mg	White	Tablet	Round, Quadrisected Scored	Barr Laboratories
B; 145	Digitek	0.125 mg	Yellow	Tablet	Circle, Scored in Imprinted Side	Bertek Pharmaceuticals
B; 145	Digitek	0.125 mg	Yellow	Tablet	Circle, Scored in Imprinted Side	Udl Laboratories
B; 146	Digitek	0.25 mg	White	Tablet	Circle, Scored on Imprinted Side	Bertek Pharmaceuticals
B; 146	Digitek	0.25 mg	White	Tablet	Circle, Scored on Imprinted Side	Udl Laboratories
B; 151	Vinate Good Start	200 mg; 100 mg; 29 mg; 30 IU; 20 mg; 20 mg; 15 mg; 7 mg; 3 mg; 3 mg; 1 mg; 12 mcg; 1000 IU; 400 IU	Off White	Tablet, Chewable	Circle	Breckenridge Pharmaceutical
B; 171	Mefloquine Hydrochloride	250 mg	White	Tablet	Oval	Barr Laboratories
B; 180 MG	Cardizem LA	180 mg	White	Extended-Release Tablet	Capsule-Shape	Biovail Pharmaceuticals
B; 201; 10	Fluoxetine Hydrochloride	10 mg	Beige	Tablet	Scored, Oval	Barr Laboratories
B; 211; 5	Norethindrone Acetate	5 mg	White	Tablet	Oval	Barr Laboratories
B; 236	Crantex LA	600 mg; 30 mg	White	Tablet	Oval	Breckenridge Pharmaceutical
B237	Mindal	60 mg; 500 mg	White	Extended-Release Tablet	Capsule-Shape	Duramed Pharmaceuticals
B; 240 MG	Cardizem LA	240 mg	White	Extended-Release Tablet	Capsule-Shape	Biovail Pharmaceuticals
B; 241	Mirtazapine	15 mg	White	Disintegrating Tablet	Circle	Barr Laboratories
B; 242	Mirtazapine	30 mg	White to Off White	Disintegrating Tablet	Circle	Barr Laboratories
B; 247	Junel Fe 28 Day Brown Tablet	75 mg	Brown	Tablet	Circle	Barr Laboratories
B; 252	Dipyridamole	25 mg	White	Coated Tablet	Circle, Biconvex	Barr Laboratories
B; 252	Dipyridamole	25 mg	White	Coated Tablet	Circle, Biconvex	Udl Laboratories
B; 275; REVIA	Revia	50 mg	Beige	Tablet	Circle, Scored	Barr Laboratories
B; 285	Dipyridamole	50 mg	White	Coated Tablet	Circle, Biconvex	Barr Laboratories
B; 285	Dipyridamole	50 mg	White	Coated Tablet	Circle, Biconvex	Udl Laboratories
B; 298	Hydroxyzine Hydrochloride	25 mg	Orange	Tablet	Circle	Barr Laboratories
B; 300 MG	Cardizem LA	300 mg	White	Extended-Release Tablet	Capsule-Shape	Biovail Pharmaceuticals
B; 301	Hydroxyzine Hydrochloride	10 mg	Yellow	Tablet	Circle	Barr Laboratories
B; 302; 2;	Acetaminophen and Codeine	300 mg; 15 mg	White	Tablet	Circle, Scored	Barr Laboratories
B; 303; 3;	Acetaminophen and Codeine	300 mg; 30 mg	White	Tablet	Circle, Scored	Barr Laboratories
B; 304; 4;	Acetaminophen and Codeine	300 mg; 60 mg	White	Tablet	Circle, Scored	Barr Laboratories
B; 344	Errin	0.35 mg	Yellow	Tablet	Circle	Barr Laboratories
B; 345	Lithium Carbonate	300 mg	Off-White	Extended-Release Tablet	Circle	Barr Laboratories
B; 357	Methyldopa	125 mg	White	Coated Tablet	Circle	Barr Laboratories
B; 360 MG	Cardizem LA	360 mg	White	Extended-Release Tablet	Capsule-Shape	Biovail Pharmaceuticals
B; 381;	Meperidine Hydrochloride	50 mg	White	Tablet	Circle	Barr Laboratories
B; 385; 500	Metformin Hydrochloride	500 mg	White	Tablet	Oval	Barr Laboratories
B; 386; 850	Metformin Hydrochloride	850 mg	White	Tablet	Oval	Barr Laboratories
B; 387; 10; 00	Metformin Hydrochloride	1000 mg	White	Tablet	Oval	Barr Laboratories
B; 420 MG	Cardizem LA	420 mg	White	Extended-Release Tablet	Capsule-Shape	Biovail Pharmaceuticals
B; 484	Leucovorin Calcium	5 mg	White	Tablet	Circle	Barr Laboratories
B; 484	Leucovorin Calcium	5 mg	White	Tablet	Circle	Supergen
B; 485	Leucovorin Calcium	25 mg	Green	Tablet	Circle	Barr Laboratories
B; 485	Leucovorin Calcium	25 mg	Light Green	Tablet	Circle	Supergen
B; 555; 424	Metoclopramide	10 mg	White	Tablet	Circle, Scored, Convex	Barr Laboratories
B; 555; 606	Megestrol Acetate	20 mg	White	Tablet	Round, Flat-Faced, Beveled-Edge, Scored	Barr Laboratories
B; 555; 606	Megestrol Acetate	20 mg	White	Tablet	Round, Flat-Faced, Beveled-Edge, Scored	Supergen
B; 555; 606	Megestrol Acetate	20 mg	White	Tablet	Round, Flat-Faced, Beveled-Edge, Scored	Udl Laboratories
B; 555; 779	Medroxyprogesterone Acetate	10 mg	White	Tablet	Circle, Biconvex, Scored	Barr Laboratories
B; 555; 872	Medroxyprogesterone Acetate	2.5 mg	White	Tablet	Circle, Biconvex, Scored	Barr Laboratories
B; 555; 873	Medroxyprogesterone Acetate	5 mg	White	Tablet	Circle, Biconvex, Scored	Barr Laboratories
B; 572	Methotrexate	2.5 mg	Yellow	Tablet	Oval, Scored	Barr Laboratories
B; 572	Methotrexate	2.5 mg		Tablet		Supergen
B; 695	Hyoscyamine TR	0.375 mg	Light Orange	Tablet	Capsule-Shape, Scored	Breckenridge Pharmaceutical
B; 715	Camila	0.35 mg	Light Pink	Tablet	Circle	Barr Laboratories
B; 728	Doxycycline	50 mg	Yellow	Tablet	Circle	Bioglan Pharma
B; 729	Doxycycline	100 mg	Yellow	Tablet	Circle	Bioglan Pharma
B; 730	Doxycycline	75 mg	Light Orange	Tablet	Circle	Bioglan Pharma
B; 775; 7; 1/2	Dextroamphetamine Saccharate, Amphetamine Aspartate, Dextroamphetamine Sulfate, Amphetamine Sulfate 7.5 mg Tablet	1.875 mg; 1.875 mg; 1.875 mg; 1.875 mg	Blue	Tablet	Oval	Barr Laboratories
B; 776; 12; 1/2	Dextroamphetamine Saccharate, Amphetamine Aspartate, Dextroamphetamine Sulfate, Amphetamine Sulfate 12.5 mg Tablet	3.125 mg; 3.125 mg; 3.125 mg; 3.125 mg	Peach	Tablet	Oval	Barr Laboratories
B; 777; 1; 5	Dextroamphetamine Saccharate, Amphetamine Aspartate, Dextroamphetamine Sulfate, Amphetamine Sulfate 15 mg Tablet	3.75 mg; 3.75 mg; 3.75 mg; 3.75 mg	Peach	Tablet	Circle	Barr Laboratories
B; 814; 250	Ciprofloxacin	250 mg	Yellow	Tablet	Circle	Barr Laboratories
B; 815; 500	Ciprofloxacin	500 mg	Yellow	Tablet	Capsule-Shape	Barr Laboratories
B; 816; 750	Ciprofloxacin	750 mg	Yellow	Tablet	Capsule-Shape	Barr Laboratories
B; 859	Flecainide Acetate	50 mg	White to Off White	Tablet	Circle	Barr Laboratories
B; 860; 100	Flecainide Acetate	100 mg	White to Off White	Tablet	Oval, Scored	Barr Laboratories
B; 861; 150	Flecainide Acetate	150 mg	White to Off White	Tablet	Oval, Scored	Barr Laboratories
B; 886; 1	Estradiol	1 mg		Tablet		Barr Laboratories
B; 887; 2	Estradiol	2 mg	Green	Tablet	Oval	Barr Laboratories
B; 899; 1/2	Estradiol	0.5 mg		Tablet		Barr Laboratories
B; 917; 200	Amiodarone Hydrochloride	200 mg	White	Tablet	Circle, Scored	Barr Laboratories
B; 923; 400	Ethambutol Hydrochloride	400 mg	White	Tablet	Oval, Scored	Barr Laboratories

IMPRINT	BRAND/GENERIC NAME	STRENGTH	COLOR	FORM	SHAPE	MANUFACTURER
B; 927; 5	Trexall	5 mg	Green	Tablet	Oval	Barr Laboratories
B; 928; 7 1/2	Trexall	7.5 mg	Blue	Tablet	Oval, Scored	Barr Laboratories
B; 929; 10	Trexall	10 mg	Pink	Tablet	Oval, Scored	Barr Laboratories
B; 941	Nortrel .5/35	35 mcg; 0.5 mg	Light Yellow	Tablet	Circle	Barr Laboratories
B; 942	Nortrel 7/7/7 Blue Tablet	0.75 mg; 0.035 mg	Blue	28-Day Tablet Pack	Circle	Barr Laboratories
B; 943	Nortrel 7/7/7 Peach Tablet	1 mg; 0.035 mg	Peach	28-Day Tablet Pack	Circle	Barr Laboratories
B; 945; 15	Trexall	15 mg	Purple	Tablet	Oval	Barr Laboratories
B; 949	Nortrel 1/35	35 mcg; 1 mg	Yellow	Tablet	Circle	Barr Laboratories
B; 951	Nortrel 7/7/7 Light Yellow Tablet	0.5 mg; 0.035 mg	Light Yellow	28-Day Tablet Pack	Circle	Barr Laboratories
B; 952; 5	Dextroamphetamine Sulfate	5 mg	Peach	Tablet	Circle	Barr Laboratories
B; 953; 10	Dextroamphetamine Sulfate	10 mg	Pink	Tablet	Circle, Scored	Barr Laboratories
B; 965	Lessina 28 Pink Tablet	0.1 mg; 0.02 mg	Pink	Tablet	Circle	Barr Laboratories
B; 967	Fluvoxamine Maleate	25 mg	Off-White	Tablet	Oval	Barr Laboratories
B; 968; 50	Fluvoxamine Maleate	50 mg	Yellow	Tablet	Oval, Scored	Barr Laboratories
B; 969; 100	Fluvoxamine Maleate	100 mg	Brown	Tablet	Oval, Scored	Barr Laboratories
B; 971; 5	Dextroamphetamine Saccharate, Amphetamine Aspartate, Dextroamphetamine Sulfate, Amphetamine Sulfate 5 mg Tablet	1.25 mg; 1.25 mg; 1.25 mg; 1.25 mg	Blue	Tablet	Oval	Barr Laboratories
B; 972; 1; 0	Dextroamphetamine Saccharate, Amphetamine Aspartate, Dextroamphetamine Sulfate, Amphetamine Sulfate 10 mg Tablet	2.5 mg; 2.5 mg; 2.5 mg; 2.5 mg	Blue	Tablet	Oval, Scored, with Partial Bisects	Barr Laboratories
B; 973; 2; 0	Dextroamphetamine Saccharate, Amphetamine Aspartate, Dextroamphetamine Sulfate, Amphetamine Sulfate 20 mg Tablet	5 mg; 5 mg; 5 mg; 5 mg	Peach	Tablet	Oval	Barr Laboratories
B; 974; 3; 0	Dextroamphetamine Saccharate, Amphetamine Aspartate, Dextroamphetamine Sulfate, Amphetamine Sulfate 30 mg Tablet	7.5 mg; 7.5 mg; 7.5 mg; 7.5 mg	Peach	Tablet	Oval	Barr Laboratories
B; 977	Junel 21 Day Yellow Tablet	1 mg; 20 mcg	Light Yellow	Tablet	Circle	Barr Laboratories
B; 977	Junel Fe 28 Day Yellow Tablet	1 mg; 20 mcg	Light Yellow	Tablet		Barr Laboratories
B; 978	Junel 21 Day Pink Tablet	1.5 mg; 30 mcg	Pink	Tablet	Circle	Barr Laboratories
B; 978	Junel Fe 28 Day Pink Tablet	1.5 mg; 30 mcg	Light Yellow	Tablet		Barr Laboratories
B; 987	Sprintec	35 mcg; 0.25 mg	Blue	Tablet	Circle	Barr Laboratories
B; 992	Portia 28 Pink Tablet	0.15 mg; 30 mcg	Pink	28-Day Tablet Pack	Circle	Barr Laboratories
B; 997; 1/10	Fludrocortisone Acetate	0.1 mg	Yellow	Tablet	Oval	Barr Laboratories
B/B	Anolor Dh5	5 mg; 500 mg	Opaque White	Capsule		Blansett Pharmacal
B; WL; 28	Benadryl Severe Allergy and Sinus Headache	500 mg; 25 mg; 30 mg		Tablet		Warner Lambert Consumer Health Products
BAC; 10; 832	Baclofen	10 mg	White	Tablet	Circle, Scored	Rosemont Pharmaceutical
BACTRIM; ROCHE	Bactrim	80 mg; 400 mg	Light Green	Tablet	Capsule-Shape, Scored	Roche Laboratories
BACTRIM-DS; ROCHE	Bactrim DS	160 mg; 800 mg	White	Tablet	Capsule-Shape	Roche Laboratories
BARR; 010	Tetracycline Hydrochloride	500 mg	Black and Yellow	Capsule		Barr Laboratories
BARR; 011	Tetracycline Hydrochloride	250 mg	Orange and Yellow	Capsule		Barr Laboratories
BARR; 033	Chlordiazepoxide	10 mg	Green and Black	Capsule		Qualitest Products
BARR; 033	Chlordiazepoxide Hydrochloride	10 mg	Black and Green	Capsule		Barr Laboratories
BARR; 059;	Diphenhydramine Hydrochloride	50 mg	Pink	Capsule		Barr Laboratories
BARR; 059;	Diphenhydramine Hydrochloride	50 mg	Pink	Capsule		Udl Laboratories
BARR; 10 MG; 876	Fluoxetine Hydrochloride	10 mg	Blue and Yellow	Capsule		Barr Laboratories
BARR; 20 MG; 877	Fluoxetine Hydrochloride	20 mg	Blue and White	Capsule		Barr Laboratories
BARR; 128	Dicyclomine Hydrochloride	10 mg	Blue	Capsule		Barr Laboratories
BARR; 158	Chlordiazepoxide Hydrochloride	5 mg	Green and Yellow	Capsule		Barr Laboratories
BARR; 159	Chlordiazepoxide Hydrochloride	25 mg	Green and White	Capsule		Barr Laboratories
BARR; 281	Aminophylline	200 mg	White	Tablet	Circle	Barr Laboratories
BARR; 282	Aminophylline	100 mg	White	Tablet	Circle	Barr Laboratories
BARR; 286;	Dipyridamole	75 mg	White	Coated Tablet	Circle, Biconvex	Barr Laboratories
BARR; 286;	Dipyridamole	75 mg	White	Coated Tablet	Circle, Biconvex	Udl Laboratories
BARR; 299	Hydroxyzine Hydrochloride	50 mg	Orange	Tablet	Circle	Barr Laboratories
BARR; 300	Hydroxyzine Hydrochloride	100 mg	Orange	Tablet	Circle	Barr Laboratories
BARR; 302; 50	Hydroxyzine Pamoate	50 mg	Opaque Yellow and Opaque Maroon with Yellow Powder	Capsule, Liquid Filled		Barr Laboratories
BARR; 323; 25	Hydroxyzine Pamoate	25 mg	Opaque Yellow and Opaque Pink with Yellow Powder	Capsule, Liquid Filled		Barr Laboratories
BARR; 324; 100	Hydroxyzine Pamoate	100 mg	Opaque Yellow and Opaque Pink Filled with Yellow Powder	Capsule, Liquid Filled		Barr Laboratories
BARR; 325	Hydrocodone Bitartrate and Acetaminophen	5 mg; 500 mg	White	Tablet	Capsule-Shape, Scored	Barr Laboratories
BARR; 382;	Meperidine Hydrochloride	100 mg	White	Tablet	Circle, Biconvex	Barr Laboratories
BARR; 407	Doxepin Hydrochloride	100 mg	White and Green	Capsule		Barr Laboratories
BARR; 442	Acetohexamide	250 mg	White	Tablet	Oval, Biconvex, Scored	Barr Laboratories
BARR; 443	Acetohexamide	500 mg	White	Tablet	Capsule-Shape, Biconvex, Scored	Barr Laboratories
BARR; 446	Tamoxifen Citrate	10 mg	White	Tablet	Circle, Biconvex	Barr Laboratories
BARR; 555; 163	Diazepam	2 mg	White	Tablet	Round, Flat-Faced, Beveled-Edge, Scored	Barr Laboratories
BARR; 555; 164	Diazepam	10 mg	Blue	Tablet	Round, Flat-Faced, Beveled-Edge, Scored	Barr Laboratories
BARR; 555; 192	Hydrochlorothiazide Hydrochloride	100 mg	Peach	Tablet	Circle, Scored	Barr Laboratories

IMPRINT	BRAND/GENERIC NAME	STRENGTH	COLOR	FORM	SHAPE	MANUFACTURER
BARR; 555; 271	Sulfinpyrazone	100 mg	White	Tablet	Round, Flat-Faced, Beveled-Edge, Scored	Barr Laboratories
BARR; 555; 293	Oxycodone with Aspirin	4.5 mg; 0.38 mg; 325 mg	Yellow	Tablet	Circle, Scored	Barr Laboratories
BARR; 555; 363	Diazepam	5 mg	Yellow	Tablet	Round, Flat-Faced, Beveled-Edge, Scored	Barr Laboratories
BARR; 555; 444	Hydrochlorothiazide and Triamterene	50 mg; 75 mg	Yellow	Tablet	Oval	Barr Laboratories
BARR; 555; 444	Triamterene and Hydrochlorothiazide	75 mg; 50 mg	Yellow	Tablet	Oval, Biconvex, Scored	Barr Laboratories
BARR; 555; 483;	Amiloride Hydrochloride and Hydrochlorothiazide	5 mg; 50 mg	Light Yellow	Tablet	Circle, Biconvex, Scored	Barr Laboratories
BARR; 555; 489	Trazodone Hydrochloride	50 mg	White	Tablet	Circle, Biconvex, Scored	Barr Laboratories
BARR; 555; 489	Trazodone Hydrochloride	50 mg	White	Tablet	Circle, Biconvex, Scored	Udl Laboratories
BARR; 555; 490	Trazodone Hydrochloride	100 mg	White	Tablet	Circle, Biconvex, Scored	Barr Laboratories
BARR; 555; 490	Trazodone Hydrochloride	100 mg	White	Tablet	Circle, Biconvex, Scored	Udl Laboratories
BARR; 555; 585	Chlorzoxazone	500 mg	Light Green	Tablet	Circle, Scored	Barr Laboratories
BARR; 555; 585	Chlorzoxazone	500 mg	Light Green	Tablet	Circle, Scored	Udl Laboratories
BARR; 555; 607;	Megestrol Acetate	40 mg	White	Tablet	Round, Flat-Faced, Beveled-Edge, Scored	Barr Laboratories
BARR; 555; 607;	Megestrol Acetate	40 mg	White	Tablet	Round, Flat-Faced, Beveled-Edge, Scored	Supergen
BARR; 555; 607;	Megestrol Acetate	40 mg	White	Tablet	Round, Flat-Faced, Beveled-Edge, Scored	Udl Laboratories
BARR; 555; 643	Hydrochlorothiazide and Triamterene	25 mg; 37.5 mg	Green	Tablet	Oval	Barr Laboratories
BARR; 555; 643	Triamterene and Hydrochlorothiazide	37.5 mg; 25 mg	Green	Tablet	Oval, Scored	Barr Laboratories
BARR; 555; 727	Estropipate	0.75 mg	Yellow	Tablet	Circle, Scored	Barr Laboratories
BARR; 555; 728	Estropipate	1.5 mg	Peach	Tablet	Circle	Barr Laboratories
BARR; 555; 729	Estropipate	3 mg	Blue	Tablet	Circle, Scored	Barr Laboratories
BARR; 633	Danazol	50 mg	Yellow and White	Capsule		Barr Laboratories
BARR; 634	Danazol	100 mg	Yellow	Capsule		Barr Laboratories
BARR; 635	Danazol	200 mg	Opaque Orange and Transparent Orange	Capsule, Liquid Filled		Barr Laboratories
BARR; 658	Oxycodone and Acetaminophen	5 mg; 500 mg	Red and White	Capsule		Barr Laboratories
BARR; 732; 50 50 50	Trazodone Hydrochloride	150 mg	White	Tablet	Oblong	Barr Laboratories
BARR; 733; 100 100 100	Trazodone Hydrochloride	300 mg	White	Tablet	Oval	Barr Laboratories
BARR; 831; 1;	Warfarin Sodium	1 mg	Pink	Tablet	Oval, Flat-Faced, Beveled-Edge, Scored	Barr Laboratories
BARR; 832; 2 1/2;	Warfarin Sodium	2.5 mg	Green	Tablet	Oval, Flat-Faced, Beveled-Edge, Scored	Barr Laboratories
BARR; 833; 5	Warfarin Sodium	5 mg	Peach	Tablet	Oval, Flat-Faced, Beveled-Edge, Scored	Barr Laboratories
BARR; 834; 7 1/2;	Warfarin Sodium	7.5 mg	Yellow	Tablet	Oval, Flat-Faced, Beveled-Edge, Scored	Barr Laboratories
BARR; 835; 10;	Warfarin Sodium	10 mg	White	Tablet	Oval, Flat-Faced, Beveled-Edge, Scored	Barr Laboratories
BARR; 869; 2;	Warfarin Sodium	2 mg	Lavender	Tablet	Oval, Flat-Faced, Beveled-Edge, Scored	Barr Laboratories
BARR; 870	Flutamide	125 mg	Brown and White	Capsule		Barr Laboratories
BARR; 874; 4;	Warfarin Sodium	4 mg	Blue	Tablet	Oval, Flat-Faced, Beveled-Edge, Scored	Barr Laboratories
BARR; 882	Hydroxyurea	500 mg	Pink and Purple	Capsule		Barr Laboratories
BARR; 904	Tamoxifen Citrate	20 mg	White	Tablet	Circle, Biconvex	Barr Laboratories
BARR; 925; 3	Warfarin Sodium	3 mg	Tan	Tablet	Oval	Barr Laboratories
BARR; 926; 6	Warfarin Sodium	6 mg	Teal	Tablet	Oval	Barr Laboratories
BARR; 934	Claravis	10 mg	Light Gray	Capsule		Barr Laboratories
BARR; 935	Claravis	20 mg	Brown Orange and Brown	Capsule		Barr Laboratories
BARR; 936	Claravis	40 mg	Light Orange	Capsule		Barr Laboratories
BARR; 954	Dextroamphetamine Sulfate	5 mg	Beige	Extended-Release Capsule		Barr Laboratories
BARR; 955	Dextroamphetamine Sulfate	10 mg	Brown and Clear	Extended-Release Capsule		Barr Laboratories
BARR; 956	Dextroamphetamine Sulfate	15 mg	Brown and Clear	Extended-Release Capsule		Barr Laboratories
BAYER	Bayer 8-Hour Extended Release	650 mg	White	Sustained-Release Tablet	Oblong, Scored	Bayer Consumer Care
BAYER	Bayer Aspirin Children's Cherry Flavored	81 mg	Pink	Tablet, Chewable	Circle	Bayer Consumer Care
BAYER	Bayer Aspirin Children's Orange Flavored	81 mg	Orange	Tablet, Chewable	Circle	Bayer Consumer Care
BAYER	Bayer Genuine Aspirin	325 mg	White	Tablet		Bayer Consumer Care
BAYER; 2.5	Levitra	2.5 mg	Orange	Tablet	Circle	Bayer Pharmaceutical
BAYER; 5	Levitra	5 mg	Orange	Tablet	Circle	Bayer Pharmaceutical
BAYER; 10	Levitra	10 mg	Orange	Tablet	Circle	Bayer Pharmaceutical
BAYER; 20	Levitra	20 mg	Orange	Tablet	Circle	Bayer Pharmaceutical
BAYER; 325	Bayer Enteric Aspirin	325 mg	Yellow	Tablet		Bayer Consumer Care
BAYER; 500	Bayer Enteric 500	500 mg	Yellow	Delayed-Release Tablet		Bayer Consumer Care
BAYER; C500; QD	Cipro Xr	500 mg	White to Light Yellow	Extended-Release Tablet	Oblong	Bayer Pharmaceutical
BAYER; C1000; QD	Cipro Xr	1000 mg	White to Light Yellow	Extended-Release Tablet	Oblong	Bayer Pharmaceutical
BAYER; LG;	Biltricide	600 mg	White to Orange Tinged	Coated Tablet	Oblong, Triscored	Bayer Pharmaceutical
BAYER; M400	Avelox	400 mg	Red	Coated Tablet	Oblong	Bayer
BAYER; PM	Extra Strength Bayer Pm	500 mg; 25 mg	Light Blue	Tablet	Capsule-Shape	Bayer Consumer Care
BAYER BUFFERED	Bayer Buffered	325 mg;	White	Coated Tablet	Circle	Bayer Consumer Care
BAYER PLUS	Aspirin Plus	325 mg; 160 mg; 63 mg; 34		Tablet		Bayer Consumer Care
BAYER PLUS; 500	Bayer Plus	500 mg;	White	Tablet		Bayer Consumer Care
BAYER SELECT	Bayer Select Pain Relief Formula	200 mg	White	Tablet		Bayer Consumer Care
BAYER SELECT; ALLERGY SINUS	Bayer Select Allergy Sinus	500 mg; 30 mg; 2 mg		Tablet	Oval	Bayer Consumer Care
BAYER SELECT; BACKACHE	Bayer Select Backache	580 mg	Yellow	Tablet		Bayer Consumer Care

IMPRINT	BRAND/GENERIC NAME	STRENGTH	COLOR	FORM	SHAPE	MANUFACTURER
BAYER SELECT; CHEST COLD	Bayer Select Chest Cold	500 mg; 15 mg	Light Purple	Tablet		Bayer Consumer Care
BAYER SELECT; FLU RELIEF	Bayer Select Flu Relief	500 mg; 2 mg; 30 mg; 15 mg	Red	Tablet		Bayer Consumer Care
BAYER SELECT; HEAD COLD	Bayer Select Head Cold	500 mg; 30 mg	Light Green	Tablet		Bayer Consumer Care
BAYER SELECT; HEAD/CHEST COLD	Bayer Select Head & Chest Cold	325 mg; 10 mg; 100 mg; 30 mg	Light Orange	Tablet		Bayer Consumer Care
BAYER SELECT HEADACHE	Bayer Select	500 mg; 65 mg	White	Tablet	Capsule-Shape	Bayer Consumer Care
BAYER SELECT MENSTRUAL	Bayer Select Menstrual Maximum Strength Multi-Symptom	500 mg; 25 mg	Pink	Tablet	Capsule-Shape	Bayer Consumer Care
BAYER SELECT NIGHT TIME	Bayer Select Night Time Pain Relief	500 mg; 25 mg	Light Blue	Tablet		Bayer Consumer Care
BAYER SELECT; NIGHT TIME COLD	Bayer Select Night Time Cold	500 mg; 15 mg; 1.25 mg; 30 mg	Light Blue	Tablet	Oblong	Bayer Consumer Care
BAYER SELECT SINUS	Bayer Select Sinus Pain Relief Formula	500 mg; 30 mg	Green	Tablet		Bayer Consumer Care
BB	Bufferin Tri-Buffered	325 mg		Tablet		Bristol-Myers Squibb
BB; 2092	Trichlortension	4 mg; 0.1 mg		Tablet		Circa Pharmaceuticals
BC	Bc Fast Pain Relief	325 mg; 95 mg; 16 mg	White	Tablet	Circle	Block Drug
BC; 20; 832	Baclofen	20 mg	White	Tablet	Circle, Scored	Rosemont Pharmaceutical
BCD; AMIDE; 0	Multivitamin with Fluoride	1 mg; 2500 IU; 400 IU; 15 IU; 60 mg; 0.3 mg; 1.05 mg; 1.2 mg; 13.5 mg; 1.05 mg; 4.5 mcg	Assorted	Tablet, Chewable	Circle	Qualitest Products
BCI	Hectorol	2.5 mcg	Yellow	Capsule, Liquid Filled	Oval	Bone Care International
BCP; 7400	Tolmetin Sodium	492 mg	Orange and Orange	Capsule		Norton, H.N.
BCT; 2 1/2	Bromocriptine Mesylate	2.5 mg	White	Tablet	Circle	Rosemont Pharmaceutical
BCT; 5	Bromocriptine Mesylate	5 mg	Pink	Capsule		Rosemont Pharmaceutical
BEACH; 1111	K-Phos	500 mg	White	Tablet	Circle	Beach Pharmaceuticals
BEACH; 1112	Uroqid-Acid	350 mg; 200 mg	Yellow	Tablet	Circle	Beach Pharmaceuticals
BEACH; 1114	Uroqid-Acid No. 2	500 mg; 500 mg	Yellow	Coated Tablet	Capsule-Shape	Beach Pharmaceuticals
BEACH; 1115	Thiacide	500 mg; 250 mg;	Green	Tablet	Capsule-Shape	Beach Pharmaceuticals
BEACH; 1125	K-Phos Neutral	155 mg; 852 mg; 130 mg	White	Tablet	Capsule-Shape	Beach Pharmaceuticals
BEACH; 1134	K-Phos No. 2	305 mg; 700 mg; 250 mg	Brown	Tablet	Capsule-Shape	Beach Pharmaceuticals
BEACH; 1135	K-Phos M.F.	155 mg; 250 mg	White	Tablet	Circle	Beach Pharmaceuticals
BEACH; 1136	Citrolith	50 mg; 950 mg		Tablet		Beach Pharmaceuticals
BEECHAM; 185	Beepen - VK	250 mg	White	Tablet	Oval	Glaxosmithkline
BEECHAM; 186	Beepen - VK	500 mg	White	Tablet	Oval	Glaxosmithkline
BENADRYL; 12.5	Benadryl Allergy Chewable Tablet	12.5 mg	Purple	Tablet, Chewable	Circle, Scored	Pfizer Consumer Health Care
BENADRYL; ALLERGY SINUS HEADACHE	Benadryl Allergy Sinus Headache	500 mg; 12.5 mg; 30 mg	Light Green	Tablet	Oblong	Pfizer Consumer Health Care
BENADRYL; COLD	Benadryl Cold & Flu	12.5 mg; 30 mg; 500 mg	White	Tablet	Oval	Warner Wellcome
BENADRYL; D	Benadryl Allergy Sinus	25 mg; 60 mg	Blue	Tablet	Capsule-Shape	Pfizer Consumer Health Care
BENTYL; 10;	Bentyl	10 mg	Blue	Capsule		Aventis Pharmaceuticals
BENTYL; 20;	Bentyl	20 mg	Blue	Tablet	Circle	Aventis Pharmaceuticals
BERLEX	Elixophyllin SR	250 mg	Clear	Extended-Release Capsule		Forest Pharmaceuticals
BERLEX; 80 MG	Betapace Af	80 mg	White	Tablet	Capsule-Shape, Scored	Berlex Laboratories
BERLEX; 100	Elixophyllin	100 mg	White	Capsule		Forest Pharmaceuticals
BERLEX; 120 MG	Betapace Af	120 mg	White	Tablet	Capsule-Shape, Scored	Berlex Laboratories
BERLEX; 129	Elixophyllin SR	125 mg	White	Extended-Release Capsule		Forest Pharmaceuticals
BERLEX; 131	Aminodur Dura-Tabs	300 mg	White to Off-White	Tablet		Berlex Laboratories
BERLEX; 160 MG	Betapace Af	160 mg	White	Tablet	Capsule-Shape, Scored	Berlex Laboratories
BERLEX; 162	Bilivist	500 mg	Yellow-Tan	Capsule, Liquid Filled		Berlex Laboratories
BERLEX; 181	Deconamine SR	120 mg; 8 mg	Blue and Yellow	Sustained-Release Tablet		Kenwood Laboratories
BERLEX; 200	Elixophyllin	200 mg	White	Capsule		Forest Pharmaceuticals
BEROCCA; PLUS; ROCHE	Berocca Plus	5000 IU; 30 IU; 100 mg; 0.15 mg; 25 mg; 0.8 mg; 27 mg; 0.1 mg; 50 mg; 5 mg; 3 mg; 22.5 mg; 500 mg; 20; 20 mg; 25 mg; 50 mg	Yellow-Gold	Tablet	Oblong	Roche Pharmaceuticals
BEROCCA; ROCHE	Berocca	100 mg; 18 mg; 0.5 mg; 500 mg; 15 mg; 15 mg; 4 mg; 5 mcg	Light Green	Tablet	Capsule-Shape	Roche Pharmaceuticals
BERTEK; 560	Phenytoin	100 mg		Capsule		Bertek Pharmaceuticals
BERTEK; 670	Phenytek	200 mg	Dark Blue Cap, Blue Body	Extended-Release Capsule		Bertek Pharmaceuticals
BERTEK; 750	Phenytek	300 mg	Blue Cap and Body	Extended-Release Capsule		Bertek Pharmaceuticals
BETAPACE; 80 MG	Betapace	80 mg	Light Blue	Tablet	Capsule-Shape, Scored	Berlex Laboratories
BETAPACE; 120 MG	Betapace	120 mg	Light Blue	Tablet	Capsule-Shape, Scored	Berlex Laboratories
BETAPACE; 160 MG	Betapace	160 mg	Light Blue	Tablet	Capsule-Shape, Scored	Berlex Laboratories

IMPRINT	BRAND/GENERIC NAME	STRENGTH	COLOR	FORM	SHAPE	MANUFACTURER
BETAPACE; 240 MG	Betapace	240 mg	Light Blue	Tablet	Capsule-Shape, Scored	Berlex Laboratories
BI; 6	Catapres	0.1 mg	Tan	Tablet	Oval, Scored	Boehringer Ingelheim
BI; 7	Catapres	0.2 mg	Orange	Tablet	Oval, Scored	Boehringer Ingelheim
BI; 8	Combipres	0.1 mg; 15 mg	Pink	Tablet	Oval, Scored	Boehringer Ingelheim
BI; 9	Combipres	0.2 mg; 15 mg	Blue	Tablet	Oval, Scored	Boehringer Ingelheim
BI; 10	Combipres	0.3 mg; 15 mg	White	Tablet	Oval, Scored	Boehringer Ingelheim
BI; 11	Catapres	0.3 mg	Orange	Tablet	Oval, Scored	Boehringer Ingelheim
BI; 12	Dulcolax	5 mg	Tan	Enteric-Coated Tablet	Circle	Boehringer Ingelheim
BI; 12	Dulcolax Bowel Prep Kit Tablet	5 mg	Tan	Enteric-Coated Tablet	Circle	Novartis Consumer
BI; 17	Persantine	25 mg	Orange	Coated Tablet	Circle	Boehringer Ingelheim
BI; 18	Persantine	50 mg	Orange	Tablet	Circle	Boehringer Ingelheim
BI; 19	Persantine	75 mg	Orange	Coated Tablet	Circle	Boehringer Ingelheim
BI; 20	Serentil	10 mg	Red	Coated Tablet		Boehringer Ingelheim
BI; 28	Torecan	10 mg	Yellow	Tablet	Circle	Boehringer Ingelheim
BI; 48	Respbid	250 mg	White	Extended-Release Tablet		Boehringer Ingelheim
BI; 49	Respbid	500 mg	White	Extended-Release Tablet		Boehringer Ingelheim
BI; 49	Respid	500 mg	White	Tablet	Capsule-Shape	3m Pharmaceuticals
BI; 62	Preludin	75 mg	Pink	Tablet		Boehringer Ingelheim
BI; 64	Prelu-2	105 mg	Light and Dark Green	Extended-Release Capsule		Boehringer Ingelheim
BI; 66	Mexitil	150 mg	Red and Tan	Capsule		Boehringer Ingelheim
BI; 67	Mexitil	200 mg	Red	Capsule		Boehringer Ingelheim
BI; 68	Mexitil	250 mg	Red and Aqua Green	Capsule		Boehringer Ingelheim
BI; 79	Preludin	50 mg	White	Tablet	Circle	Boehringer Ingelheim
BI; 100	Serentil	100 mg	Red	Coated Tablet		Boehringer Ingelheim
BIOCAL	Biocal Calcium Supplement	625 mg	White	Tablet, Chewable		Bayer Consumer Care
BIOCAL	Biocal Calcium Supplement	1250 mg	White	Tablet		Bayer Consumer Care
BIOCRAFT; 16	Penicillin VK	250 mg	White	Tablet	Oval	Teva Pharmaceuticals
BIOCRAFT; 32	Sulfamethoxazole and Trimethoprim Single Strength	400 mg; 80 mg	White	Tablet	Circle, Scored	H.L. Moore
BIOCRAFT; 32	Sulfamethoxazole and Trimethoprim Single Strength	400 mg; 80 mg	White	Tablet	Circle, Scored	Teva Pharmaceuticals
BIOCRAFT; 33	Smz-Tmp DS	800 mg; 160 mg	White	Tablet	Oval, Scored	Teva Pharmaceuticals
BIOCRAFT; 34	Trimethoprim	100 mg	White	Tablet	Circle	Teva Pharmaceuticals
BIOCRAFT; 49	Penicillin-VK	500 mg	White	Tablet	Oval, Scored	Teva Pharmaceuticals
BIOCRAFT; 94	Cyclacillin	250 mg	White	Tablet	Capsule-Shape	Teva Pharmaceuticals
BIOCRAFT; 95	Cyclacillin	500 mg	White	Tablet	Capsule-Shape	Teva Pharmaceuticals
BIOCRAFT; 105 105	Sucralfate	1 G	White	Tablet	Capsule-Shape, Scored	Teva Pharmaceuticals
BIOCRAFT; 117	Cephalexin	500 mg	Orange	Capsule		Teva Pharmaceuticals
BIOCRAFT; 148	Clindamycin Hydrochloride	75 mg	Red	Capsule		Teva Pharmaceuticals
BIOCRAFT; 163	Cinoxacin	250 mg	Blue and Yellow	Capsule		Teva Pharmaceuticals
BIOCRAFT; 164	Cinoxacin	500 mg	Blue and Yellow	Capsule		Teva Pharmaceuticals
BIOCRAFT; 177	Potassium Chloride	600 mg	Opaque Blue and White	Extended-Release Capsule		Teva Pharmaceuticals
BIOCRAFT; 178	Potassium Chloride	750 mg	Opaque Blue	Extended-Release Capsule		Teva Pharmaceuticals
BIOCRAFT; 185	Ketoprofen	25 mg	White	Capsule		Teva Pharmaceuticals
BIOCRAFT; 223	Cefaclor	250 mg	Opaque White and Gray	Capsule		Teva Pharmaceuticals
BIOCRAFT; 224	Cefaclor	500 mg	Opaque Red and White	Capsule		Teva Pharmaceuticals
BIPHET; 12 1/2	Biphetamine	6.25 mg; 6.25 mg	Black and White	Capsule		Fisons Pharmaceuticals
BIPHET; 20	Biphetamine	10 mg; 10 mg	Black	Capsule		Fisons Pharmaceuticals
BJ; 675;	Oreton Propionate	10 mg	Pink	Tablet		Schering
BL; 07	Penicillin G Potassium	200,000 units	White	Tablet	Circle	Teva Pharmaceuticals
BL; 09	Penicillin G Potassium	250,000 units	White	Tablet	Circle	Teva Pharmaceuticals
BL; 10	Penicillin G Potassium	400,000 units	White	Tablet	Circle	Teva Pharmaceuticals
BL; 15	Penicillin-VK	250 mg	White	Tablet	Circle, Scored	Teva Pharmaceuticals
BL; 15	Penicillin-VK	250 mg	White	Tablet	Circle, Scored	Udl Laboratories
BL; 17	Penicillin-VK	500 mg	White	Tablet	Circle, Scored	Novartis Generics
BL; 17	Penicillin-VK	500 mg	White	Tablet	Circle, Scored	Teva Pharmaceuticals
BL; 17	Penicillin-VK	500 mg	White	Tablet	Circle, Scored	Udl Laboratories
BL; 19	Imipramine	10 mg	Yellow	Coated Tablet	Circle	H.L. Moore
BL; 19	Imipramine Hydrochloride	10 mg	Yellow	Tablet	Circle	Teva Pharmaceuticals
BL; 20	Imipramine	25 mg	Rust	Coated Tablet	Circle	H.L. Moore
BL; 20	Imipramine Hydrochloride	25 mg	Salmon	Tablet	Circle	Teva Pharmaceuticals
BL; 21	Imipramine	50 mg	Green	Coated Tablet	Circle	H.L. Moore
BL; 21	Imipramine Hydrochloride	50 mg	Green	Tablet	Circle	Teva Pharmaceuticals
BL; 22	Amitriptyline Hydrochloride	10 mg	Pink	Tablet	Circle	Teva Pharmaceuticals
BL; 23	Amitriptyline Hydrochloride	25 mg	Light Green	Tablet	Circle	Teva Pharmaceuticals
BL; 24	Amitriptyline Hydrochloride	50 mg	Brown	Tablet	Circle	Teva Pharmaceuticals
BL; 25	Amitriptyline Hydrochloride	75 mg	Lavender	Tablet	Circle	Teva Pharmaceuticals
BL; 26	Amitriptyline Hydrochloride	100 mg	Orange	Tablet	Circle	Teva Pharmaceuticals
BL; 32	Smz-Tmp	400 mg; 80 mg	White	Tablet	Circle	Teva Pharmaceuticals
BL; 35	Trimethoprim	200 mg	White	Tablet	Circle	Teva Pharmaceuticals
BL; 42	Thioridazine Hydrochloride	10 mg	Green	Tablet	Oval	Teva Pharmaceuticals
BL; 46	Thioridazine Hydrochloride	100 mg	Light-Green	Tablet	Oval	Teva Pharmaceuticals
BL; 52	Amiloride Hydrochloride and Hydrochlorothiazide	5 mg; 50 mg	Yellow	Tablet	Circle, Scored	Teva Pharmaceuticals
BL; 52	Amiloride Hydrochloride and Hydrochlorothiazide	5 mg; 50 mg	Yellow	Tablet	Circle, Scored	Warner Chilcott
BL; 82;	Saluron	50 mg	White	Tablet	Circle, Scored	Bristol-Myers Squibb
BL; 92	Metoclopramide	5 mg	White	Tablet	Circle	Teva Pharmaceuticals
BL; 92	Metoclopramide	5 mg	White	Tablet	Circle	Udl Laboratories
BL; 93	Metoclopramide	10 mg	White	Tablet	Circle, Scored	Duramed Pharmaceuticals
BL; 93	Metoclopramide	10 mg	White	Tablet	Circle, Scored	Teva Pharmaceuticals
BL; 130	Albuterol Sulfate	2 mg	White	Tablet	Circle	Teva Pharmaceuticals
BL; 131	Albuterol	4 mg	White	Tablet	Round, Bisected Scored	Teva Pharmaceuticals
BL; 131	Albuterol	4 mg	White	Tablet	Round, Bisected Scored	Udl Laboratories

IMPRINT	BRAND/GENERIC NAME	STRENGTH	COLOR	FORM	SHAPE	MANUFACTURER
BL; 132	Metaproterenol	10 mg	White	Tablet	Circle, Scored	Teva Pharmaceuticals
BL; 133	Metaproterenol	20 mg	White	Tablet	Circle	Teva Pharmaceuticals
BL; 136	Cephalexin	250 mg	White	Tablet	Capsule-Shape, Scored	Teva Pharmaceuticals
BL; 137	Cephalexin	500 mg	White	Tablet	Capsule-Shape	Teva Pharmaceuticals
BL; 141	Baclofen	10 mg	White	Tablet	Circle, Scored	Teva Pharmaceuticals
BL; 142	Baclofen	20 mg	White	Tablet	Circle, Scored	Teva Pharmaceuticals
BL; 207;	Corgard	40 mg	Blue	Tablet	Circle, Scored	Bristol Laboratories
BL; 208;	Corgard	120 mg	Blue	Tablet	Oblong, Scored	Bristol-Myers Squibb
BL; 221	Amoxicillin	125 mg	White to Off-White	Tablet, Chewable	Capsule-Shape	Teva Pharmaceuticals
BL; 222	Amoxicillin	250 mg	White	Tablet, Chewable	Capsule-Shape	Teva Pharmaceuticals
BL; 232;	Corgard	20 mg	Blue	Tablet	Circle, Scored	Bristol-Myers Squibb
BL; 241;	Corgard	80 mg	Blue	Tablet	Circle, Scored	Bristol-Myers Squibb
BL; C1	Ultracef	1 GM	White or Yellow	Tablet	Capsule-Shape	Bristol-Myers Squibb
BL; E1;	Bristamycin	250 mg	Orange	Tablet	Circle	Bristol-Myers Squibb
BL; L1	Lysodren	500 mg	White	Tablet	Scored, Circle	Bristol-Myers Squibb
BL; N2	Naldagesic	325 mg; 15 mg	Blue	Tablet	Capsule-Shape	Bristol-Myers Squibb
BL; S1	Salutensin	50 mg; 0.125 mg	Light Green	Tablet	Circle	Apothecon
BL; S3	Salutensin Demi	25 mg; 0.125 mg	Pale Yellow	Tablet	Circle	Apothecon
BL; V1;	Betapen-VK	250 mg	White	Coated Tablet		Bristol-Myers Squibb
BL; V2	Betapen-VK	500 mg	White	Coated Tablet	Circle	Apothecon
BLAINE	Mag-Ox 400	400 mg	White	Tablet	Circle, Scored	Blaine
BLAINE; 0054	Uro-Mag	140 mg	White	Capsule		Blaine
BLANSETT; 3; 08	Nalex-A	4 mg; 40 mg; 20 mg	Light Tan	Extended-Release Tablet	Capsule-Shape, Scored	Blansett Pharmacal
BLANSETT; 30	Nalex	120 mg; 250 mg	Clear and White	Extended-Release Capsule		Blansett Pharmacal
BMP; 108	Cotrol-D	60 mg; 4 mg	Green	Tablet		Glaxosmithkline
BMP; 109	Dasikon	2 mg; 32 mg; 195 mg; 130 mg; 0.065 mg	Natural and Blue	Capsule		Glaxosmithkline
BMP; 119	Hybephen	15 mg; 0.1277 mg; 0.0233 mg; 0.0094 mg	Green	Tablet		Glaxosmithkline
BMP; 121	Livitamin	100 mg; 3 mg; 3 mg; 10 mg; 100 mg; 3 mg; 5 mcg; 0.66 mg; 2 mg; 150 mg	Pink	Capsule		Glaxosmithkline
BMP; 122	Livitamin-If	100 mg; 3 mg; 3 mg; 10 mg; 100 mg; 3 mg; 5 mcg; 0.66 mg; 2 mg; 150 mg; 0.33 Nf U	Green	Capsule		Glaxosmithkline
BMP; 123	Livitamin	100 mg; 2 mg; 0.33 mg; 50 mg; 3 mg; 3 mg; 3 mg; 10 mg; 5 mcg	Orange	Tablet, Chewable		Glaxosmithkline
BMP; 124	Livitamin Prenatal	6000 U.S.P. units; 400 U.S.P. units; 100 mg; 20 mg; 10 mg; 5 mg; 3 Mgg; 3 mg; 0.5 mg; 5 mcg; 350 mg; 50 mg	Yellow	Tablet		Glaxosmithkline
BMP; 135	Semets	3 mg	Red	Troche		Glaxosmithkline
BMP; 139	Thalfed	8 mg; 0.12 G; 25 mg	White	Tablet		Glaxosmithkline
BMP; 140	Totacillin	250 mg	Brown and Orange	Capsule		Glaxosmithkline
BMP; 141	Totacillin	500 mg	Brown and Orange	Capsule		Glaxosmithkline
BMP; 143	Bactocill	250 mg	Brown and Yellow	Capsule		Glaxosmithkline
BMP; 144	Bactocill	500 mg	Brown and Yellow	Capsule		Glaxosmithkline
BMP; 145	Daricon	10 mg	White	Tablet	Circle, Grooved	Glaxosmithkline
BMP; 146	Daricon PB	5 mg; 15 mg	Pink	Tablet		Glaxosmithkline
BMP; 150	Obedrin-LA	10 mg		Tablet		Glaxosmithkline
BMP; 165	Dycill	250 mg	Light Blue and Creme	Capsule		Glaxosmithkline
BMP; 166	Dycill	500 mg	Light Blue and Creme	Capsule		Glaxosmithkline
BMP; 167	Actol Expectorant Tablet	30 mg; 200 mg	Red	Coated Tablet		Glaxosmithkline
BMP; 169	Cloxapen	250 mg	Lime and Beige	Capsule		Glaxosmithkline
BMP; 170	Cloxapen	500 mg	Lime and Beige	Capsule		Glaxosmithkline
BMP; 189	Augmentin	125 mg; 31.25 mg	Mottled Yellow	Tablet, Chewable	Circle	Glaxosmithkline
BMP; 190	Augmentin	250 mg; 62.5 mg	Mottled Yellow	Tablet, Chewable	Circle	Glaxosmithkline
BMP; 192	Maxolon	10 mg	Blue	Tablet	Circle, Scored	Glaxosmithkline
BMP; 194	Enarax White	5 mg; 25 mg	White	Tablet		Glaxosmithkline
BMP; 195	Enarax Black and White	10 mg; 25 mg	Black and White	Tablet		Glaxosmithkline
BMP; 211	Larotid	250 mg	Caramel and Buff	Capsule		Glaxosmithkline
BMS; 37	Amoxicillin	125 mg	Pink	Tablet, Chewable	Circle, Flat-Faced	Apothecon
BMS; 37.5 MG; 1555	Zerit Xr	37.5 mg	Red and Yellow	Extended-Release Capsule		Bristol-Myers Squibb
BMS; 38	Amoxicillin	250 mg	Pink	Tablet, Chewable	Circle, Flat-Faced	Apothecon
BMS; 50; 31	Serzone	50 mg	Light Pink	Tablet	Six-Sided	Bristol-Myers Squibb
BMS; 50 MG; 1656	Zerit Xr	50 mg	Orange	Extended-Release Capsule		Bristol-Myers Squibb
BMS; 52; 50	Diltiazem	30 mg	Green, Slightly Mottled	Coated Tablet	Circle, Biconvex	Apothecon
BMS; 55; 50	Diltiazem	60 mg	Yellow, Slightly Mottled	Coated Tablet	Circle, Biconvex	Apothecon
BMS; 57; 70	Diltiazem	90 mg	Green, Slightly Mottled	Coated Tablet	Capsule-Shape	Apothecon

IMPRINT	BRAND/GENERIC NAME	STRENGTH	COLOR	FORM	SHAPE	MANUFACTURER
BMS; 58; 50	Diltiazem	120 mg	Yellow, Slightly Mottled	Coated Tablet	Capsule-Shape	Apothecon
BMS; 75 MG; 1557	Zerit Xr	75 mg	Red	Extended-Release Capsule		Bristol-Myers Squibb
BMS; 80	Pravachol	80 mg	Yellow	Tablet	Oval	Bristol-Myers Squibb
BMS; 80;	Pravigard Pac	325 mg; 80 mg	Yellow Oval Tablet and White Tablet	Tablet		Bristol-Myers Squibb
BMS; 80;	Pravigard Pac	81 mg; 80 mg	Yellow Oval Tablet and White Tablet	Tablet		Bristol-Myers Squibb
BMS; 100; 32	Serzone	100 mg	White	Tablet	Hexagonal, Bisected, Scored Scored	Bristol-Myers Squibb
BMS; 100 MG; 1558	Zerit Xr	100 mg	Yellow	Extended-Release Capsule		Bristol-Myers Squibb
BMS; 100 MG; 3623	Reyataz	100 mg	Blue and White	Capsule		Bristol-Myers Squibb
BMS; 125 MG; 6671	Videx Ec	125 mg	White with Tan Ink	Extended-Release Capsule		Bristol-Myers Squibb
BMS; 150; 39	Serzone	150 mg	Peach	Tablet	Six-Sided, Bisect Scored	Bristol-Myers Squibb
BMS; 150 MG; 3624	Reyataz	150 mg	Blue and Light Blue	Capsule		Bristol-Myers Squibb
BMS; 200; 33	Serzone	200 mg	Light Yellow	Tablet	Six-Sided	Bristol-Myers Squibb
BMS; 200 MG; 3631	Reyataz	200 mg	Blue	Capsule		Bristol-Myers Squibb
BMS; 200 MG; 6672	Videx Ec	200 mg	White with Green Ink	Extended-Release Capsule		Bristol-Myers Squibb
BMS; 250; 41	Serzone	250 mg	White	Tablet	Six-Sided	Bristol-Myers Squibb
BMS; 250 MG; 6673	Videx Ec	250 mg	White with Blue Ink	Extended-Release Capsule		Bristol-Myers Squibb
BMS; 400 MG; 6674	Videx Ec	400 mg	White with Red Ink	Extended-Release Capsule		Bristol-Myers Squibb
BMS; 5040	Atenolol	50 mg	White	Tablet		Apothecon
BMS; 5240	Atenolol	100 mg	White	Tablet		Apothecon
BMS; 5250	Diltiazem Hydrochloride	30 mg	Green	Tablet	Circle, Biconvex	Apothecon
BMS; 5550	Diltiazem Hydrochloride	60 mg	Yellow	Tablet	Circle, Biconvex	Apothecon
BMS; 5770	Diltiazem Hydrochloride	90 mg	Green	Tablet	Capsule-Shape	Apothecon
BMS; 5850	Diltiazem Hydrochloride	120 mg	Yellow	Tablet	Capsule-Shape, Biconvex	Apothecon
BMS; 6060; 500	Glucophage	500 mg	White	Coated Tablet		Bristol-Myers Squibb
BMS; 6063; 500	Glucophage Xr	500 mg	White	Extended-Release Tablet	Capsule-Shape, Biconvex	Bristol-Myers Squibb
BMS; 6070; 850	Glucophage	850 mg	White	Coated Tablet		Bristol-Myers Squibb
BMS; 6071; 1000	Glucophage	1000 mg	White	Tablet	Oblong, Scored	Bristol-Myers Squibb
BMS; 6072	Glucovance	1.25 mg; 250 mg	Pale Yellow	Coated Tablet	Capsule-Shape, Bevel-Edged, Biconvex	Bristol-Myers Squibb
BMS; 6073	Glucovance	2.5 mg; 500 mg	Pale Orange	Coated Tablet	Capsule-Shape, Bevel-Edged, Biconvex	Bristol-Myers Squibb
BMS; 6074	Glucovance	5 mg; 500 mg	Yellow	Coated Tablet	Capsule-Shape, Bevel-Edged, Biconvex	Bristol-Myers Squibb
BMS; 6077	Metaglip	2.5 mg; 500 mg	White	Tablet	Oval	Bristol-Myers Squibb
BMS; 6078	Metaglip	5 mg; 500 mg	Pink	Tablet	Oval	Bristol-Myers Squibb
BMS; 6081	Metaglip	2.5 mg; 250 mg	Pink	Tablet	Oval	Bristol-Myers Squibb
BMS; MONOPRIL; 10;	Monopril	10 mg	White to Off-White	Tablet	Diamond, Biconvex Flat-End, Compressed, Partially Scored	Bristol-Myers Squibb
BMS; MONOPRIL; 20;	Monopril	20 mg	White to Off-White	Tablet	Oval, Compressed	Bristol-Myers Squibb
BMS; MONOPRIL; 40;	Monopril	40 mg	White to Off-White	Tablet	Six-Sided, Biconvex Hexagonal Shaped, Compressed	Bristol-Myers Squibb
BMS; TEQUIN; 200	Tequin	200 mg	White	Coated Tablet	Oval, Biconvex	Bristol-Myers Squibb
BMS; TEQUIN; 400	Tequin	400 mg	White	Coated Tablet	Oval, Biconvex	Bristol-Myers Squibb
BMS; W921	Metoprolol	50 mg	Pink	Coated Tablet	Capsule-Shape	Apothecon
BMS; W921	Metoprolol Tartrate	50 mg	Pink	Coated Tablet	Capsule-Shape	Apothecon
BMS; W933	Metoprolol Tartrate	100 mg	Blue	Coated Tablet	Capsule-Shape	Apothecon
BMS; W933	Metoprolol Tartrate	100 mg	Blue	Coated Tablet	Capsule-Shape	Apothecon
BMS; 1611	Baraclude	0.5 mg	White to Off White	Tablet	Triangle	Bristol-Myers Squibb
BMS; 1612	Baraclude	1 mg	Pink	Tablet	Triangle	Bristol-Myers Squibb
BMS 1964; 15	Zerit	15 mg	Light Yellow and Dark Red	Capsule		Bristol-Myers Squibb
BMS 1965; 20	Zerit	20 mg	Light Brown	Capsule		Bristol-Myers Squibb
BMS 1966; 30	Zerit	30 mg	Light Orange and Dark Orange	Capsule		Bristol-Myers Squibb
BMS 1967; 40	Zerit	40 mg	Dark Orange	Capsule		Bristol-Myers Squibb
BN 37; BN 37	Acetaminophen	500 mg	White	Tablet	Oblong	Neil Laboratories
BN; 51	Ephedrine and Guaifenesin	25 mg; 200 mg	White	Tablet	Circle, Scored	Neil Laboratories
BNP; 7600	Elmiron	100 mg	White	Capsule		Alza
BNVA; 150	Boniva	150 mg	White	Tablet	Oblong	Glaxosmithkline
BNVA; 150	Boniva	150 mg	White	Tablet	Oblong	Roche Laboratories
BOCA; 124	Pseudo GG TR	595 mg; 48 mg	White	Extended-Release Tablet	Capsule-Shape, Scored	Boca Pharmacal
BOCA; 125	Pcm Allergy Tab	20 mg; 12 mg; 2.5 mg	White	Tablet		Boca Pharmacal
BOCA; 131	Pcm	10 mg; 2 mg; 1.25 mg	Purple	Tablet, Chewable	Capsule-Shape	Boca Pharmacal
BOCK; 460	Zephrex	400 mg; 60 mg	White	Coated Tablet	Oval; Bisected Scored	Sanofi Pharmaceuticals
BOCK; HS 33	Hemaspan	110 mg; 20 mg; 200 mg	Tan	Tablet	Oblong	Sanofi Pharmaceuticals
BOCK; P; N	Prenate Ultra Prenatal Vitamins	90 mg; 1 mg; 2700 I.U.; 400 I.U.; 30 I.U.	White	Tablet	Oval, Scored	Sanofi Pharmaceuticals
BOLAR; 0084	Phenytoin	100 mg		Capsule		Bolar Pharmaceutical
BOLAR KV; 12/100	Disopyramide Phosphate	100 mg	Purple and Yellow	Controlled-Release Capsule		Bolar Pharmaceutical
BOLAR KV; 12/150	Disopyramide Phosphate	150 mg	Purple and Orange	Controlled-Release Capsule		Bolar Pharmaceutical
BOOTS; 0051	Lopurin	100 mg	White	Tablet	Circle	Boots Pharmaceuticals
BOOTS; 0052	Lopurin	300 mg	Orange	Tablet	Circle	Boots Pharmaceuticals
BP; 0002	Dicyclomine Hydrochloride with Phenobarbital	10 mg; 15 mg	Blue and Clear	Capsule		Bolar Pharmaceutical
BP; 0004	Primidone	250 mg		Tablet		Circa Pharmaceuticals
BP; 0005	Methocarbamol	500 mg	White	Tablet	Circle	Bolar Pharmaceutical

IMPRINT	BRAND/GENERIC NAME	STRENGTH	COLOR	FORM	SHAPE	MANUFACTURER
BP; 0006	Methocarbamol	750 mg	White	Tablet	Capsule-Shape	Bolar Pharmaceutical
BP; 0007	Trihexyphenidyl Hydrochloride	2 mg	White	Tablet		Bolar Pharmaceutical
BP; 0012	Furosemide	50 mg	Yellow	Tablet	Capsule-Shape	Bolar Pharmaceutical
BP; 0013;	Chlorothiazide	500 mg	White	Tablet	Circle	Bolar Pharmaceutical
BP; 0014	Oxtriphylline with Guaifenesin	200 mg; 100 mg		Tablet		Bolar Pharmaceutical
BP; 0017	Pentaerythritol Tetranitrate	80 mg	Light Green and Dark Green	Tablet		Bolar Pharmaceutical
BP; 0024;	Trihexane	5 mg		Tablet		Circa Pharmaceuticals
BP; 0026	Isosorbide Dinitrate	40 mg	Green	Timed-Release Tablet	Circle	Bolar Pharmaceutical
BP; 0029	Triprolidine Hydrochloride and Pseudoephedrine	2.5 mg; 60 mg		Tablet		Bolar Pharmaceutical
BP; 0035	Chlorthalidone	100 mg	White	Tablet	Circle	Bolar Pharmaceutical
BP; 0036;	Chlorothiazide	250 mg	White	Tablet	Circle	Bolar Pharmaceutical
BP; 0044	Warfarin Sodium	2.5 mg	Green	Tablet	Circle	Bolar Pharmaceutical
BP; 0045	Warfarin Sodium	5 mg	Pink	Tablet	Circle	Bolar Pharmaceutical
BP; 0046	Warfarin Sodium	7.5 mg	Yellow	Tablet	Circle	Bolar Pharmaceutical
BP; 0047	Warfarin Sodium	10 mg	White	Tablet	Circle	Bolar Pharmaceutical
BP; 0049	Isosorbide Dinitrate	20 mg	Green	Tablet	Circle	Bolar Pharmaceutical
BP; 0050	Warfarin Sodium	2 mg	Lavender	Tablet	Circle	Bolar Pharmaceutical
BP; 0052	Ergoloid Mesylates	0.167 mg; 0.167 mg; 0.167 mg	White	Tablet		Bolar Pharmaceutical
BP; 0058	Hydrochlorothiazide	100 mg	Orange	Tablet	Circle	Bolar Pharmaceutical
BP; 0059	Sulfasalazine	500 mg	Brown	Tablet		Bolar Pharmaceutical
BP; 0062	Methyclothiazide	2.5 mg	Red-Orange	Tablet	Circle	Bolar Pharmaceutical
BP; 0063	Methyclothiazide	5 mg	Red-Orange	Tablet	Circle	Bolar Pharmaceutical
BP; 0064;	Hydralazine Hydrochloride and Hydrochlorothiazide	100 mg; 50 mg	Blue	Capsule		Bolar Pharmaceutical
BP; 0065;	Hydralazine Hydrochloride and Hydrochlorothiazide	25 mg; 25 mg	White	Capsule		Bolar Pharmaceutical
BP; 0066;	Hydralazine Hydrochloride and Hydrochlorothiazide	50 mg; 50 mg	White and Black	Capsule		Bolar Pharmaceutical
BP; 0069	Ergoloid Mesylates	0.333 mg; 0.333 mg; 0.333 mg	White	Tablet		Bolar Pharmaceutical
BP; 0072	Hydroflumethiazide	50 mg	White	Tablet	Circle	Bolar Pharmaceutical
BP; 0073	Bethanechol Chloride	5 mg	White	Tablet	Circle	Bolar Pharmaceutical
BP; 0076	Oxtriphylline	100 mg	Red-Orange	Coated Tablet	Circle	Bolar Pharmaceutical
BP; 0077	Oxtriphylline	200 mg	Yellow	Coated Tablet	Circle	Bolar Pharmaceutical
BP; 0079;	Clonidine Hydrochloride	0.1 mg	White	Tablet	Circle	Circa Pharmaceuticals
BP; 0080	Clonidine Hydrochloride	0.2 mg	Orange	Tablet	Circle	Bolar Pharmaceutical
BP; 0081	Clonidine Hydrochloride	0.3 mg	Peach	Tablet	Circle	Bolar Pharmaceutical
BP; 0084	Phenytoin Sodium	100 mg	White	Extended-Release Capsule		Bolar Pharmaceutical
BP; 0087	Sulfamethoxazole	500 mg	Green	Tablet	Circle	Bolar Pharmaceutical
BP; 0088	Primidone	250 mg		Tablet		Circa Pharmaceuticals
BP; 0089	Hydroxyzine, Theophylline and Ephedrine Sulfate	10 mg; 130 mg; 25 mg		Tablet		Bolar Pharmaceutical
BP; 0091	Chlorzoxazone with Apap	250 mg; 300 mg	Green	Tablet		Bolar Pharmaceutical
BP; 0092	Prochlorperazine with Isopropamide	10 mg; 5 mg	Yellow and Clear	Timed-Release Capsule		Bolar Pharmaceutical
BP; 0094;	Carisoprodol	350 mg		Tablet		Bolar Pharmaceutical
BP; 0094;	Carisoprodol	350 mg		Tablet		Regal Labs
BP; 0123	Propranolol Hydrochloride	10 mg	Peach	Tablet	Circle	Bolar Pharmaceutical
BP; 0124	Propranolol Hydrochloride	20 mg	Light Blue	Tablet	Circle	Bolar Pharmaceutical
BP; 0125	Propranolol Hydrochloride	40 mg	Green	Tablet	Circle	Bolar Pharmaceutical
BP; 0126	Propranolol Hydrochloride	80 mg	Yellow	Tablet	Circle	Bolar Pharmaceutical
BP; 0127;	Hydroflumethiazide with Reserpine	25 mg; 0.125 mg	Yellow	Tablet	Circle	Bolar Pharmaceutical
BP; 0128;	Hydroflumethiazide with Reserpine	50 mg; 0.125 mg	Green	Tablet	Circle	Bolar Pharmaceutical
BP; 0129	Spironolactone with Hydrochlorothiazide	25 mg; 25 mg		Tablet		Bolar Pharmaceutical
BP; 0131	Sulfasalazine	500 mg	Brown	Enteric-Coated Tablet	Circle	Bolar Pharmaceutical
BP; 0132;	Chlorothiazide with Reserpine	500 mg; 0.125 mg	Pink	Tablet	Circle	Bolar Pharmaceutical
BP; 0133	Allopurinol	100 mg	White	Tablet	Circle	Bolar Pharmaceutical
BP; 0134	Allopurinol	300 mg	Peach	Tablet	Circle	Bolar Pharmaceutical
BP; 0135	Guanethidine Monosulfate	10 mg	Orange	Tablet	Circle	Bolar Pharmaceutical
BP; 0136	Guanethidine Monosulfate	25 mg	White	Tablet	Circle	Bolar Pharmaceutical
BP; 0137	Fluoxymesterone	2 mg	Peach	Tablet	Circle	Bolar Pharmaceutical
BP; 0138	Fluoxymesterone	5 mg	Green	Tablet	Circle	Bolar Pharmaceutical
BP; 0139	Fluoxymesterone	10 mg	Green	Tablet	Circle	Bolar Pharmaceutical
BP; 0145	Indomethacin	25 mg	Light Green and Dark Green	Capsule		Bolar Pharmaceutical
BP; 0146	Indomethacin	50 mg	Light Green	Capsule		Bolar Pharmaceutical
BP; 0157	Methyclothiazide with Deserpidine	5 mg; 0.5 mg	Grey	Tablet	Circle	Bolar Pharmaceutical
BP; 0158	Methyclothiazide with Deserpidine	5 mg; 0.25 mg	Yellow	Tablet	Circle	Bolar Pharmaceutical
BP; 0163	Fluphenazine Hydrochloride	1 mg	White	Coated Tablet	Circle	Bolar Pharmaceutical
BP; 0164	Fluphenazine Hydrochloride	2.5 mg	Beige	Coated Tablet	Circle	Bolar Pharmaceutical
BP; 0165	Fluphenazine Hydrochloride	5 mg	Blue	Coated Tablet	Circle	Bolar Pharmaceutical
BP; 0166	Fluphenazine Hydrochloride	10 mg	Red	Coated Tablet	Circle	Bolar Pharmaceutical
BP; 0167	Chlorpropamide	100 mg	Blue	Tablet	Circle	Bolar Pharmaceutical
BP; 0168	Chlorpropamide	250 mg	Blue	Tablet	Circle	Bolar Pharmaceutical
BP; 0181	Lorazepam	1 mg	White	Tablet	Circle	Bolar Pharmaceutical
BP; 0182	Lorazepam	2 mg	White	Tablet	Circle	Bolar Pharmaceutical
BP; 0187	Procainamide Hydrochloride SR	1000 mg	Pink	Sustained-Release Tablet	Capsule-Shape	Bolar Pharmaceutical
BP; 1	Thioridazine Hydrochloride	10 mg	Green	Tablet	Capsule-Shape	Bolar Pharmaceutical
BP; 10	Dipyridamole	25 mg		Tablet		Bolar Pharmaceutical

IMPRINT	BRAND/GENERIC NAME	STRENGTH	COLOR	FORM	SHAPE	MANUFACTURER
BP; 28;	Imipramine Hydrochloride	25 mg	Brown	Coated Tablet	Circle	Circa Pharmaceuticals
BP; 31	Thioridazine Hydrochloride	15 mg	Purple	Tablet	Capsule-Shape	Bolar Pharmaceutical
BP; 32	Dexamethasone	0.75 mg	Light Blue	Tablet		Bolar Pharmaceutical
BP; 33	Chlorthalidone	25 mg	Peach	Tablet	Circle	Bolar Pharmaceutical
BP; 34	Chlorthalidone	50 mg	Blue	Tablet	Circle	Bolar Pharmaceutical
BP; 39;	Imipramine Hydrochloride	10 mg	Yellow	Coated Tablet	Triangle	Circa Pharmaceuticals
BP; 40;	Imipramine Hydrochloride	50 mg	Green	Coated Tablet	Circle	Circa Pharmaceuticals
BP; 41	Ergoloid Mesylates	0.333 mg; 0.333 mg; 0.333 mg	White	Tablet		Bolar Pharmaceutical
BP; 60	Liothyronine Sodium	25 mcg	White	Tablet	Circle	Bolar Pharmaceutical
BP; 61	Liothyronine Sodium	50 mcg	White	Tablet	Circle	Bolar Pharmaceutical
BP; 78	Cyproheptadine Hydrochloride	4 mg	White	Tablet	Circle	Bolar Pharmaceutical
BP; 100	Hydroxyzine Pamoate	25 mg	Dark Green and Light Green	Capsule		Bolar Pharmaceutical
BP; 101	Hydroxyzine Pamoate	50 mg	White and Green	Capsule		Bolar Pharmaceutical
BP; 102	Hydroxyzine Pamoate	100 mg	Grey and Green	Capsule		Bolar Pharmaceutical
BP; 118	Thioridazine Hydrochloride	25 mg	Brown	Tablet	Capsule-Shape	Bolar Pharmaceutical
BP; 119	Thioridazine Hydrochloride	50 mg	White	Tablet		Bolar Pharmaceutical
BP; 120	Thioridazine Hydrochloride	100 mg	Yellow-Green	Tablet	Capsule-Shape	Bolar Pharmaceutical
BP; 121	Thioridazine Hydrochloride	150 mg	Yellow	Tablet	Capsule-Shape	Bolar Pharmaceutical
BP; 122	Thioridazine Hydrochloride	200 mg	Purple	Tablet	Capsule-Shape	Bolar Pharmaceutical
BP; 132	Beelith	600 mg; 25 mg	Golden Yellow	Coated Tablet		Beach Pharmaceuticals
BP; 143	Trimethobenzamide	250 mg	Blue	Capsule		Bolar Pharmaceutical
BP; 151	Trifluoperazine Hydrochloride	10 mg	Red	Tablet		Bolar Pharmaceutical
BP; 152	Procainamide SR	250 mg	White	Sustained-Release Tablet	Oval	Bolar Pharmaceutical
BP; 153	Procainamide SR	500 mg	Pink	Sustained-Release Tablet	Oval	Bolar Pharmaceutical
BP; 154	Procainamide SR	750 mg	Tan	Sustained-Release Tablet	Oval	Bolar Pharmaceutical
BP; 157	Methyclothiazide with Deserpidine	5 mg; 0.5 mg	Grey	Tablet	Biconcave	Bolar Pharmaceutical
BP; 158	Methyclothiazide with Deserpidine	5 mg; 0.25 mg	Yellow	Tablet	Biconcave	Bolar Pharmaceutical
BP; 171	Trifluoperazine Hydrochloride	1 mg	Red	Tablet		Bolar Pharmaceutical
BP; 172	Trifluoperazine Hydrochloride	2 mg	Red	Tablet		Bolar Pharmaceutical
BP; 195	Timolol Maleate	5 mg	White	Tablet	Circle	Bolar Pharmaceutical
BP; 196	Timolol Maleate	10 mg	White	Tablet	Circle, Scored	Bolar Pharmaceutical
BP; 197	Timolol Maleate	20 mg	White	Tablet	Capsule-Shape, Scored	Bolar Pharmaceutical
BP; 209	Amitriptyline	10 mg		Tablet	Circle	Circa Pharmaceuticals
BP; 211	Maprotiline Hydrochloride	25 mg	Blue	Tablet		Bolar Pharmaceutical
BP; 212	Maprotiline Hydrochloride	50 mg	Yellow	Tablet		Bolar Pharmaceutical
BP; 213	Maprotiline Hydrochloride	75 mg	White	Tablet		Bolar Pharmaceutical
BP; 1004	Dicyclomine Hydrochloride with Phenobarbital	20 mg; 15 mg	White	Tablet		Bolar Pharmaceutical
BP; 1007;	Trazodone Hydrochloride	50 mg	White	Tablet	Circle	Circa Pharmaceuticals
BP; 1008;	Trazodone Hydrochloride	100 mg	White	Tablet	Circle	Circa Pharmaceuticals
BP; 1015	Nitrofurantoin	100 mg	Yellow	Capsule		Bolar Pharmaceutical
BP; 1027;	Amantadine Hydrochloride	100 mg	Pink	Capsule, Liquid Filled	Oblong	Bolar Pharmaceutical
BP; 1045	Theophylline, Ephedrine and Phenobarbital	130 mg; 24 mg; 8 mg		Tablet		Bolar Pharmaceutical
BP; 2005	Disopyramide Phosphate	100 mg	White and Orange	Capsule		Bolar Pharmaceutical
BP; 2006	Disopyramide Phosphate	150 mg	Orange and Brown	Capsule		Bolar Pharmaceutical
BP; 2013	Chlorpheniramine Maleate	4 mg		Tablet		Bolar Pharmaceutical
BP; 2014	Methyldopa	125 mg	White	Coated Tablet	Circle	Bolar Pharmaceutical
BP; 2015	Methyldopa	250 mg	White	Coated Tablet	Circle	Bolar Pharmaceutical
BP; 2016	Methyldopa	500 mg	White	Coated Tablet	Circle	Bolar Pharmaceutical
BP; 2016	Nitrofurantoin	50 mg	Yellow	Capsule		Bolar Pharmaceutical
BP; 2017	Brompheniramine Maleate	4 mg		Tablet		Bolar Pharmaceutical
BP; 2023	Dicyclomine Hydrochloride	10 mg	Blue	Capsule		Bolar Pharmaceutical
BP; 2024	Meclofenamate Sodium	50 mg	Maroon and Pink	Capsule		Bolar Pharmaceutical
BP; 2025	Meclofenamate Sodium	100 mg	Maroon and White	Capsule		Bolar Pharmaceutical
BP; 2026	Dicyclomine Hydrochloride	20 mg	Blue	Tablet		Bolar Pharmaceutical
BP; 2027	Metoclopramide Hydrochloride	10 mg	White	Tablet	Circle	Bolar Pharmaceutical
BP; 2028	Dimenhydrinate	50 mg		Tablet		Bolar Pharmaceutical
BP; 2036	Methyldopa with Hydrochlorothiazide	250 mg; 15 mg	Chartreuse	Coated Tablet	Circle	Bolar Pharmaceutical
BP; 2037	Methyldopa with Hydrochlorothiazide	250 mg; 25 mg	Pink	Coated Tablet	Circle	Bolar Pharmaceutical
BP; 2038	Methyldopa with Hydrochlorothiazide	500 mg; 30 mg	Chartreuse	Coated Tablet	Oval	Bolar Pharmaceutical
BP; 2039	Methyldopa with Hydrochlorothiazide	500 mg; 50 mg	Pink	Coated Tablet	Oval	Bolar Pharmaceutical
BP; 2042	Verapamil Hydrochloride	80 mg	White	Tablet	Circle	Bolar Pharmaceutical
BP; 2043	Verapamil Hydrochloride	120 mg	White	Tablet	Circle	Bolar Pharmaceutical
BP; 2047	Hydrochlorothiazide with Reserpine	25 mg; 0.125 mg	Green	Tablet	Circle	Bolar Pharmaceutical
BP; 2048	Hydrochlorothiazide with Reserpine	50 mg; 0.125 mg	Green	Tablet	Circle	Bolar Pharmaceutical
BP; 2049	H.H.R.	25 mg; 15 mg; 0.1 mg		Tablet		Bolar Pharmaceutical
BP; 2049;	Hydrochlorothiazide with Reserpine and Hydralazine	15 mg; 25 mg; 0.1 mg	White or Pink	Tablet	Circle	Bolar Pharmaceutical
BP; 2051	Isosorbide Dinitrate	5 mg		Tablet		Bolar Pharmaceutical
BP; 2052	Isosorbide Dinitrate	10 mg		Tablet		Bolar Pharmaceutical
BP; 2053;	Perphenazine and Amitriptyline	2 mg; 25 mg	Orange	Coated Tablet	Circle	Circa Pharmaceuticals
BP; 2054;	Perphenazine and Amitriptyline	4 mg; 25 mg	Yellow	Coated Tablet	Circle	Circa Pharmaceuticals
BP; 2055;	Perphenazine and Amitriptyline	4 mg; 50 mg	Orange	Coated Tablet	Circle	Circa Pharmaceuticals
BP; 2056;	Perphenazine and Amitriptyline	2 mg; 10 mg	Blue	Coated Tablet	Circle	Circa Pharmaceuticals

IMPRINT	BRAND/GENERIC NAME	STRENGTH	COLOR	FORM	SHAPE	MANUFACTURER
BP; 2057;	Perphenazine and Amitriptyline	4 mg; 10 mg	Salmon	Coated Tablet	Circle	Circa Pharmaceuticals
BP; 2060	Propranolol Hydrochloride	60 mg	Yellow	Tablet	Circle	Bolar Pharmaceutical
BP; 2062	Tolbutamide	250 mg	White	Tablet	Circle	Bolar Pharmaceutical
BP; 2063	Tolbutamide	500 mg	White	Tablet	Circle	Bolar Pharmaceutical
BP; 2064	Pentaerythritol Tetranitrate	10 mg	Green	Tablet	Circle	Bolar Pharmaceutical
BP; 2066;	Lithium Carbonate	300 mg	White and Pink	Capsule		Circa Pharmaceuticals
BP; 2067	Pentaerythritol Tetranitrate	20 mg	Green	Tablet	Circle	Bolar Pharmaceutical
BP; 2068	Tolazamide	100 mg	White	Tablet	Circle	Bolar Pharmaceutical
BP; 2069	Tolazamide	250 mg	White	Tablet	Circle	Bolar Pharmaceutical
BP; 2070	Tolazamide	500 mg	White	Tablet	Circle	Bolar Pharmaceutical
BP; 2074	Probenecid with Colchicine	500 mg; 0.5 mg	White	Tablet	Capsule-Shape	Bolar Pharmaceutical
BP; 2075	Nitrofurantoin	50 mg	Yellow	Tablet	Circle	Bolar Pharmaceutical
BP; 2076	Procainamide Hydrochloride	250 mg	Yellow	Capsule		Bolar Pharmaceutical
BP; 2078	Procainamide Hydrochloride	500 mg	Yellow and Orange	Capsule		Bolar Pharmaceutical
BP; 2079	Propantheline Bromide	15 mg	Peach	Tablet	Circle	Bolar Pharmaceutical
BP; 2080	Nitrofurantoin	100 mg	Yellow	Tablet	Circle	Bolar Pharmaceutical
BP; 2081;	Flurazepam Hydrochloride	15 mg	White and Light Green	Capsule		Bolar Pharmaceutical
BP; 2082;	Flurazepam Hydrochloride	30 mg	White and Dark Green	Capsule		Bolar Pharmaceutical
BP; 2087	Temazepam	15 mg	Pink	Capsule		Bolar Pharmaceutical
BP; 2088	Temazepam	30 mg	Yellow and Pink	Capsule		Bolar Pharmaceutical
BP; 2092	Trichlormethiazide with Reserpine	4 mg; 0.1 mg	Lavender	Tablet	Circle	Bolar Pharmaceutical
BP; 2092	Trichlortension	4 mg; 0.1 mg		Tablet		Bolar Pharmaceutical
BP; 2093	Hydrochlorothiazide	25 mg	Orange	Tablet	Circle	Bolar Pharmaceutical
BP; 2094	Hydrochlorothiazide	50 mg	Orange	Tablet	Circle	Bolar Pharmaceutical
BP; 2126	Potassium Chloride	750 mg	White	Capsule		Bolar Pharmaceutical
BP; 2130	Tripelennamine Hydrochloride	50 mg	Blue	Tablet		Bolar Pharmaceutical
BP; 2147	Potassium Chloride ER	600 mg		Extended-Release Tablet		Bolar Pharmaceutical
BP; 2150	Isoniazid	100 mg	White	Tablet	Circle	Circa Pharmaceuticals
BP; 2155	Isoniazid	300 mg	White	Tablet	Circle	Circa Pharmaceuticals
BP; 2200	Folic Acid	1 mg		Tablet		Bolar Pharmaceutical
BP; 3000	Quinidine Gluconate	324 mg	White	Tablet		Bolar Pharmaceutical
BP; 3020	Trichlormethiazide	4 mg	Blue	Tablet	Circle	Bolar Pharmaceutical
BP; 5000	Spironolactone	25 mg	White	Tablet	Circle	Bolar Pharmaceutical
BP; 5010	Bethanechol Chloride	50 mg	Yellow	Tablet	Circle	Bolar Pharmaceutical
BP; 8037	Orphenadrine Citrate	100 mg	White	Tablet	Circle	Bolar Pharmaceutical
BP; 9000	Quinine Sulfate	260 mg	White	Tablet	Circle	Bolar Pharmaceutical
BRA; 200	Phoslo	667 mg	White	Tablet	Circle	Braintree Laboratories
BREON	Trancopal	100 mg	Peach	Tablet		Winthrop Pharmaceuticals
BREON; 100	Bronkodyl	100 mg	Brown and White	Capsule		Sanofi Winthrop Pharmaceuticals
BREON; 200	Bronkodyl	200 mg	Green and White	Capsule		Sanofi Winthrop Pharmaceuticals
BREON; SR300	Bronkodyl SR	300 mg	Blue and White	Sustained-Release Capsule		Sanofi Winthrop Pharmaceuticals
BREON; T 200	Trancopal	200 mg	Green	Tablet		Winthrop Pharmaceuticals
BRICANYL; 2 1/2;	Bricanyl	2.5 mg	White	Tablet	Circle	Aventis Pharmaceuticals
BRICANYL; 5;	Bricanyl	5 mg	White	Tablet	Square, Scored	Aventis Pharmaceuticals
BRISTOL	Bristacycline	250 mg	Green and Yellow	Capsule		Bristol-Myers Squibb
BRISTOL	Polycillin	125 mg	White	Tablet, Chewable		Apothecon
BRISTOL	Tetrex	100 mg	Yellow and Orange	Capsule		Bristol-Myers Squibb
BRISTOL	Tetrex-F	250 mg; 250000 U		Capsule		Bristol-Myers Squibb
BRISTOL; 500	Bristacycline	500 mg	Green and Yellow	Capsule		Bristol-Myers Squibb
BRISTOL; 518;	Quibron Plus	150 mg; 100 mg; 25 mg; 20 mg		Capsule		Bristol-Myers Squibb
BRISTOL; 732	Enkaid	25 mg	Green and Yellow	Capsule		Bristol-Myers Squibb
BRISTOL; 734	Enkaid	35 mg	Green and Orange	Capsule		Bristol-Myers Squibb
BRISTOL; 735	Enkaid	50 mg	Green and Brown	Capsule		Bristol-Myers Squibb
BRISTOL; 3091	Vepesid	50 mg	Pink	Capsule, Liquid Filled		Bristol-Myers Squibb
BRISTOL; 3506	Kantrex	500 mg	Opaque White	Capsule		Apothecon
BRISTOL; 7178	Polymox	250 mg		Capsule		Apothecon
BRISTOL; 7271	Cefadroxil	500 mg	Blue and Black	Capsule		Apothecon
BRISTOL; 7271	Cefadroxil	500 mg	Blue and Black	Capsule		Sandoz
BRISTOL; 7278	Trimox	250 mg	Maroon and Pink	Capsule		Bristol-Myers Squibb
BRISTOL; 7279	Trimox	500 mg	Maroon and Pink	Capsule		Bristol-Myers Squibb
BRISTOL; 7375	Cefanex	250 mg	Blue and Purple	Capsule		Apothecon
BRISTOL; 7376	Cefanex	500 mg	Blue	Capsule		Apothecon
BRISTOL; 7496	Tegopen	500 mg	Black and Orange	Capsule		Apothecon
BRISTOL; 7658	Dynapen	500 mg	Blue and White	Capsule		Apothecon
BRISTOL; 7892;	Dynapen	125 mg	Blue and White	Capsule		Apothecon
BRISTOL; 7893	Dynepen	250 mg	Blue and White	Capsule		Apothecon
BRISTOL; 7935;	Tegopen	250 mg	Black and Orange	Capsule		Apothecon
BRISTOL; 7977	Oxacillin Sodium	250 mg	Opaque Flesh	Capsule		Apothecon
BRISTOL; 7977	Prostaphlin	250 mg	Light Pink	Capsule		Apothecon
BRISTOL; 7982	Oxacillin Sodium	500 mg	Opaque Flesh	Capsule		Apothecon
BRISTOL; 7982	Prostaphlin	500 mg	Pink	Capsule		Apothecon
BRISTOL; 7992;	Polycillin	250 mg	Scarlet and Gray	Capsule		Apothecon
BRISTOL; 7993;	Polycillin	500 mg	Red and Gray	Capsule		Apothecon
BRISTOL-MYERS; COMTREX	Comtrex Multi-Symptom Cold Reliever	500 mg; 30 mg; 2 mg; 15 mg	Orange and Yellow	Capsule, Liquid Filled		Bristol-Myers Squibb
BRISTOL-MYERS; DATRIL; 500MG	Datril Extra Strength	500 mg	Green and White	Capsule		Bristol-Myers Squibb
BRONKAID	Bronkaid Dual Action Formula	25 mg; 400 mg	White	Tablet		Bayer Consumer Care
BUCET; UAD; 307	Bucet	650 mg; 50 mg	White	Capsule		Uad Laboratories
BUTIBEL; 37; 046	Butibel	15 mg; 15 mg	Red	Tablet	Circle	Wallace Laboratories
BUTISOL; 37-112	Butisol Sodium	15 mg	Lavender	Tablet	Circle	Wallace Laboratories
BUTISOL; 37-113	Butisol Sodium	30 mg		Tablet		Wallace Laboratories
BUTISOL; 37-114	Butisol Sodium	50 mg		Tablet		Wallace Laboratories

IMPRINT	BRAND/GENERIC NAME	STRENGTH	COLOR	FORM	SHAPE	MANUFACTURER
BUTISOL; 37-115	Butisol Sodium	100 mg		Tablet		Wallace Laboratories
BVF; 0117	Pentoxifylline	400 mg		Extended-Release Tablet	Oblong, Compressed	Teva Pharmaceuticals
BVF; 120	Diltiazem Hydrochloride	120 mg	Clear Light Green	Extended-Release Capsule		Teva Pharmaceuticals
BVF; 180	Diltiazem Hydrochloride	180 mg	Dark Green and Light Green	Extended-Release Capsule		Teva Pharmaceuticals
BVF; 240	Diltiazem Hydrochloride	240 mg	Clear Dark Green	Extended-Release Capsule		Teva Pharmaceuticals
BVF; 300	Diltiazem Hydrochloride	300 mg	Ivory and Dark Green	Extended-Release Capsule		Teva Pharmaceuticals
C	Calcitrel	585 mg; 120 mg;	White	Tablet	Circle	Sterling Health
C	Clarinex Reditabs	5 mg	Pink	Disintegrating Tablet	Circle	Schering-Plough
C	Comtrex Maximum Strength	500 mg; 2 mg; 30 mg; 15 mg	Yellow	Tablet		Bristol-Myers Squibb
C	Comtrex Maximum Strength Day/night - Tablet & Capsule	500 mg; 15 mg; 30 mg	Blue	Tablet	Circle	Bristol-Myers Squibb
C	Comtrex Maximum Strength Day/night - Tablet & Capsule	500 mg; 2 mg; 30 mg; 15 mg	Orange	Tablet	Capsule-Shape	Bristol-Myers Squibb
C	Comtrex Maximum Strength Non-Drowsy	500 mg; 15 mg; 30 mg	Orange	Tablet	Capsule-Shape	Bristol-Myers Squibb
C	Comtrex Multi-Symptom Cold Reliever	30 mg; 2 mg; 10 mg; 325 mg	Yellow	Tablet		Bristol-Myers Squibb
C	Congespirin Children	1.25 mg; 81 mg	Orange	Tablet, Chewable		Bristol-Myers Squibb
C	Congestac	60 mg; 400 mg	White	Tablet		Ascher
C	Humibid Plus	400 mg; 60 mg		Tablet		Menley & James
C	Myfortic	180 mg;	Lime Green	Enteric-Coated Tablet	Circle	Novartis
C	Prempro White Tablet	2.5 mg	White	Tablet	Oval, Scored	Wyeth-Ayerst Laboratories
C; 01; 70	Oxaprozin	600 mg	Yellow	Tablet	Oval	DR Reddy's Laboratories
C; 0170	Oxaprozin	600 mg	Yellow	Tablet		Warrick Pharmaceuticals
C; 1	Choline Magnesium Trisalicylate	1000 mg	Pink	Tablet	Capsule-Shape	Amide Pharmaceuticals
C; 1	Tricosal	1000 mg	Pink	Tablet	Capsule-Shape	Qualitest Products
C; 1	Triprolidine & Pseudoephedrine Hydrochloride	60 mg; 2.5 mg	White	Coated Tablet	Round, Convex, Bisected Scored	KV Pharmaceutical
C; 1	Triprolidine & Pseudoephedrine Hydrochloride	60 mg; 2.5 mg	White	Coated Tablet	Round, Convex, Bisected Scored	Leiner Health Products
C2C	Lanoxicaps	0.2 mg	Green	Capsule, Liquid Filled	Oblong	Glaxosmithkline
C; 5	Cialis	5 mg	Yellow	Tablet	Teardrop-Shape	Eli Lilly
C5	Clarinex	5 mg	Light Blue	Coated Tablet	Circle	Schering
C; 10	Cialis	10 mg	Yellow	Tablet	Teardrop-Shape	Eli Lilly
C; 20	Cialis	20 mg	Yellow	Tablet	Teardrop-Shape	Eli Lilly
C35	Docusate Calcium & Yellow Phenolphthalein	65 mg; 60 mg	Reddish Brown	Gel/jelly		Leiner Health Products
C; 39	Peri-Dos	30 mg; 100 mg	Maroon	Capsule, Liquid Filled	Oval	Zenith Goldline Pharmaceuticals
C; 83; LL	Centrum Singles	500 mg	White	Coated Tablet	Oval, Convex	Wyeth Consumer Healthcare
C; 86; 72	Salflex	750 mg	White	Coated Tablet	Oblong, Scored	Amarin Pharmaceuticals
C; 101; 400	Ibuprofen	400 mg	White	Tablet	Circle	DR Reddy's Laboratories
C; 102; 600	Ibuprofen	600 mg	White	Tablet	Capsule-Shape	DR Reddy's Laboratories
C; 103; 800	Ibuprofen	800 mg	White	Tablet	Capsule-Shape	DR Reddy's Laboratories
C; 119	Famotidine	20 mg	Pale Yellow	Tablet	Circle	Par Pharmaceutical
C; 120	Famotidine	40 mg	Yellow	Tablet	Circle	Par Pharmaceutical
C; 122	Amantadine Hydrochloride	100 mg	Yellow	Capsule, Liquid Filled	Oblong	Rosemont Pharmaceutical
C; 133	Valproic Acid	250 mg	Yellow	Capsule, Liquid Filled		Qualitest Products
C; 133	Valproic Acid	250 mg	Yellow	Capsule, Liquid Filled	Oblong	Udl Laboratories
C; 135	Doxylamine Succinate	25 mg	White	Tablet	Oval, Bisected Scored	Copley Pharmaceutical
C; 135	Doxylamine Succinate	25 mg	White	Tablet	Oval, Bisected Scored	Leiner Health Products
C; 135	Sleep Aid	25 mg	White	Tablet	Circle	Good Neighbor Pharmacy
C; 135	Sleep Aid	25 mg	White	Tablet	Circle	Good Sense
C; 135	Sleep Aid	25 mg	White	Tablet	Circle	Major
C; 135	Sleep Aid	25 mg	White	Tablet	Circle	Medalist
C; 135	Sleep Aid	25 mg	White	Tablet	Circle	Nex
C; 135	Sleep Aid	25 mg	White	Tablet	Circle	Perrigo
C; 135	Sleep Aid	25 mg	White	Tablet	Circle	Preferred Products
C; 135	Sleep Aid	25 mg	White	Tablet	Circle	Top Care
C; 135	Sleep Aid	25 mg	White	Tablet	Circle	Valu Rite
C; 151	Buspirone Hydrochloride	5 mg	White	Tablet	Circle	Ranbaxy Pharmaceuticals
C; 152	Buspirone Hydrochloride	10 mg	White	Tablet	Circle	Ranbaxy Pharmaceuticals
C; 229	Brompheril	120 mg; 6 mg	Dark Green	Sustained-Release Tablet	Circle, Convex	Copley Pharmaceutical
C; 229	Brompheril	120 mg; 6 mg	Dark Green	Sustained-Release Tablet	Circle, Convex	Leiner Health Products
C; 229	Dexaphen	6 mg; 120 mg		Sustained-Release Tablet		Major Pharmaceutical
C; 229	Dexaphen	6 mg; 120 mg		Sustained-Release Tablet		Major Quality
C; 229	Dexaphen	6 mg; 120 mg		Sustained-Release Tablet		Perrigo
C; 229	Dixaphed	6 mg; 120 mg		Sustained-Release Tablet		Preferred Products
C; 229	Dixaphedrine	6 mg; 120 mg	Green	Sustained-Release Tablet	Biconvex	Good Neighbor Pharmacy
C; 229	Dixaphedrine	6 mg; 120 mg	Green	Sustained-Release Tablet	Biconvex	Harco Drug
C; 229	Dixaphedrine	6 mg; 120 mg	Green	Sustained-Release Tablet	Biconvex	Nex
C; 229	Dixaphedrine	6 mg; 120 mg	Green	Sustained-Release Tablet	Biconvex	Park Lane
C; 229	Dixaphedrine	6 mg; 120 mg	Green	Sustained-Release Tablet	Biconvex	Perrigo

IMPRINT	BRAND/GENERIC NAME	STRENGTH	COLOR	FORM	SHAPE	MANUFACTURER
C; 229	Dixaphedrine	6 mg; 120 mg	Green	Sustained-Release Tablet	Biconvex	Regal Distributing
C; 229	Dixaphedrine	6 mg; 120 mg	Green	Sustained-Release Tablet	Biconvex	Stay-Well
C; 229	Dixaphedrine	6 mg; 120 mg	Green	Sustained-Release Tablet	Biconvex	Sunfresh
C; 229	Dixaphedrine	6 mg; 120 mg	Green	Sustained-Release Tablet	Biconvex	Swan
C; 229	Ephedrix	6 mg; 120 mg		Sustained-Release Tablet		True Quality
C229	12-Hour Antihistamine Nasal Decongestant	6 mg; 120 mg		Sustained-Release Tablet		Good Sense
C229	12-Hour Antihistamine Nasal Decongestant	6 mg; 120 mg		Sustained-Release Tablet		Legend Pharmaceuticals
C229	12-Hour Antihistamine Nasal Decongestant	6 mg; 120 mg		Sustained-Release Tablet		Medalist
C229	12-Hour Antihistamine Nasal Decongestant	6 mg; 120 mg		Sustained-Release Tablet		Perrigo
C229	12-Hour Antihistamine Nasal Decongestant	6 mg; 120 mg		Sustained-Release Tablet		Revco
C229	12-Hour Antihistamine Nasal Decongestant	6 mg; 120 mg		Sustained-Release Tablet		Select Brand
C229	12-Hour Antihistamine Nasal Decongestant	6 mg; 120 mg		Sustained-Release Tablet		Top Care
C229	12-Hour Antihistamine Nasal Decongestant	6 mg; 120 mg		Sustained-Release Tablet		Valu Rite
C; 333	Butinal with Codeine	325 mg; 50 mg; 30 mg; 40 mg	Blue and White	Capsule		Econolab
C; 402	Gabitril	2 mg	Orange-Peach	Tablet	Circle	Cephalon
C; 404;	Gabitril	4 mg	Yellow	Tablet	Circle	Cephalon
C; 412;	Gabitril	12 mg	Green	Tablet	Oval	Cephalon
C; 416;	Gabitril	16 mg	Blue	Tablet	Oval	Cephalon
C; 420;	Gabitril	20 mg	Pink	Tablet	Oval	Cephalon
C; 425	Ascomp with Codeine	325 mg; 50 mg; 30 mg; 40 mg	Blue and Yellow	Capsule		Econolab
C; 582	Cefadroxil	500 mg	Brown and White	Capsule		Ranbaxy Pharmaceuticals
C; 600; LL	Caltrate 600	600 mg	White	Coated Tablet	Oblong	Wyeth Consumer Healthcare
C; 3227	Nifedipine	10 mg	Tan	Capsule		Warner Chilcott
C; 3453	Nifedipine	20 mg	White	Capsule	Oval	Warner Chilcott
C; 8643	Minotal	325 mg; 15 mg	Tan	Tablet		Carnrick Laboratories
C; 8644	Capital with Codeine	325 mg; 30 mg	Pale Blue	Tablet		Carnrick Laboratories
C; 8648	Bontril Pdm	35 mg	Green and Yellow	Tablet	Circle, BI-Layered, Scored	Amarin Pharmaceuticals
C; 8650	Phrenilin	325 mg; 50 mg		Tablet		Amarin Pharmaceuticals
C; 8655	Phrenilin with Codeine No. 3	325 mg; 50 mg; 30 mg	Purple and White	Capsule		Carnrick Laboratories
C; 8656	Phrenilin Forte	50 mg; 650 mg	Amethyst	Capsule		Amarin Pharmaceuticals
C; 8657	Hydrocet	500 mg; 5 mg	Blue and White	Capsule		Amarin Pharmaceuticals
C; 8671	Salflex	500 mg	White	Coated Tablet	Circle	Amarin Pharmaceuticals
C; 8674	Motofen	0.025 mg; 1 mg	White	Tablet	Five-Sided, Scored	Amarin Pharmaceuticals
C; 86120	Midrin	65 mg; 100 mg; 325 mg	Red with Pink Band	Capsule		Carnrick Laboratories
C; AMEN	Amen	10 mg	Peach and White	Tablet	Circle, BI-Layered,scored	Carnrick Laboratories
C C	Robitussin Cold Cold & Congestion	200 mg; 30 mg; 10 mg	Red	Tablet	Film-Coated	Wyeth Consumer Healthcare
C; C+C	Coricidin Hbp Cough & Cold	4 mg; 30 mg	Red	Tablet	Circle	Schering-Plough Healthcare Products
C; CLOCK DESIGN	Quinaglute Dura-Tabs	324 mg	White	Extended-Release Tablet	Circle	Berlex Laboratories
C; DAY	Contac Day & Night Cold & Flu	650 mg; 30 mg; 60 mg	Yellow	Tablet		Glaxosmithkline
C F	Robitussin Cold Multi-Symptom Cold & Flu	325 mg; 200 mg; 30 mg; 10 mg	Yellow	Tablet	Film-Coated	Wyeth Consumer Healthcare
C S	Robitussin Cold Sinus & Congestion	325 mg; 200 mg; 30 mg	Light Blue	Tablet		Wyeth Consumer Healthcare
CAFFEDRINE	Caffedrine Maximum Strength Time-Released	200 mg	Yellow	Timed-Release Capsule	Oval	Thompson Medical
CALAN; 40	Calan	40 mg	Pink	Coated Tablet	Circle	Searle
CALAN; 80	Calan	80 mg	Peach	Coated Tablet	Oval, Scored	Searle
CALAN; 120	Calan	120 mg	Brown	Coated Tablet	Oval, Scored	Searle
CALAN; SR; 120	Calan SR	120 mg	Light Violet	Sustained-Release Tablet	Oval	Searle
CALAN; SR; 180	Calan SR	180 mg	Light Pink	Sustained-Release Tablet	Oval, Scored	Searle
CALAN; SR; 240	Calan SR	240 mg	Light Green	Sustained-Release Tablet	Capsule-Shape, Scored	Searle
CALTRATE	Caltrate 600 Plus D	200 IU; 600 mg	Light Pink	Tablet	Oval	Wyeth Consumer Healthcare
CALTRATE; M; 600	Caltrate Plus Calcium	600 mg; 200 IU; 40 mg; 7.5 mg; 1 mg; 1.8 mg;	Dusty Rose	Coated Tablet	Oval, Scored	Wyeth Consumer Healthcare
CAMA 500; DORSEY	Cama Arthritis Pain Reliever	150 mg; 500 mg; 150 mg	White with Salmon Inlay	Tablet	Oblong	Novartis Consumer
CAMA 500; DORSEY	Cama Arthritis Pain Reliever	150 mg; 500 mg; 150 mg	White with Salmon Inlay	Tablet	Oblong	Sandoz Consumer Pharmaceuticals
CAP; STAR	Certuss-D	600 mg; 40 mg; 60 mg	Red	Tablet	Eight-Sided	Capellon Pharmaceuticals
CAPOTEN; 12.5 MG;	Capoten	12.5 mg	White	Tablet	Oval, Biconvex, Partially Bisected Scored	Bristol-Myers Squibb
CAPOTEN; 25 MG;	Capoten	25 mg	White	Tablet	Oval, Biconvex with a Quadrisect Bar Scored	Bristol-Myers Squibb
CAPOTEN; 50 MG;	Capoten	50 mg	White	Tablet	Oval, Biconvex, Scored	Bristol-Myers Squibb

IMPRINT	BRAND/GENERIC NAME	STRENGTH	COLOR	FORM	SHAPE	MANUFACTURER
CAPOTEN; 100 MG;	Capoten	100 mg	White	Tablet	Oval, Biconvex, Scored	Bristol-Myers Squibb
CAPOZIDE; 25; 15;	Capozide 25/15	25 mg; 15 mg	White and Orange Speckled	Tablet	Square, Rounded, Double Scored	Bristol-Myers Squibb
CAPOZIDE; 25; 25;	Capozide 25/25	25 mg; 25 mg	Peach, Slightly Speckled	Tablet	Square, Rounded, Double Scored	Bristol-Myers Squibb
CAPOZIDE; 50; 15;	Capozide 50/15	50 mg; 15 mg	White and Orange Speckled	Tablet	Oval, Scored	Bristol-Myers Squibb
CAPOZIDE; 50; 25;	Capozide 50/25	50 mg; 25 mg	Peach, Slightly Speckled	Tablet	Oval, Scored	Bristol-Myers Squibb
CARACO; 105 105	Salsalate	750 mg	Blue	Tablet	Oval	Caraco Pharmaceutical
CARACO; 222	Miraphen Pse	600 mg; 120 mg	Yellow	Sustained-Release Tablet	Capsule-Shape, Scored	Caraco Pharmaceutical
CARACO LOGO; 103 103	Salsalate	500 mg	Blue	Tablet	Circle	Caraco Pharmaceutical
CARAFATE; 1712;	Carafate	1 G	Light Pink	Tablet	Capsule-Shape, Scored, Embossed	Aventis Pharmaceuticals
CARBEX	Carbex	5 mg	White	Tablet	Oval	Endo Laboratories
CARDENE; 20 MG; ROCHE	Cardene	20 mg	White with Blue Band	Capsule		Roche Laboratories
CARDENE; 30 MG; ROCHE	Cardene	30 mg	Light Blue with Blue Band	Capsule		Roche Laboratories
CARDENE SR; 30 MG; SYNTEX; 2440	Cardene SR	30 mg	Pink	Sustained-Release Capsule		Roche Laboratories
CARDENE SR; 45 MG; SYNTEX; 2441	Cardene SR	45 mg	Powder Blue	Sustained-Release Capsule		Roche Laboratories
CARDENE SR; 60 MG; SYNTEX; 2442	Cardene SR	60 mg	Light Blue and White	Sustained-Release Capsule		Roche Laboratories
CARDILATE; X7A	Cardilate	10 mg	White	Tablet, Chewable	Circle	Burroughs Wellcome
CARDILATE; X7A	Cardilate	10 mg	White	Tablet	Square	Glaxosmithkline
CARDILATE; X7A;	Cardilate	10 mg	White	Tablet	Square	Burroughs Wellcome
CARDIZEM; 90 MG	Cardizem	90 mg	Green	Tablet	Oblong, Scored	Biovail Pharmaceuticals
CARDIZEM; 120 MG	Cardizem	120 mg	Yellow	Tablet	Oblong, Scored	Biovail Pharmaceuticals
CARDIZEM CD; 120 MG	Cardizem Cd	120 mg	Light Turquoise	Extended-Release Capsule		Biovail Pharmaceuticals
CARDIZEM CD; 180 MG	Cardizem Cd	180 mg	Light Turquoise and Blue	Extended-Release Capsule		Biovail Pharmaceuticals
CARDIZEM CD; 240 MG	Cardizem Cd	240 mg	Blue	Extended-Release Capsule		Biovail Pharmaceuticals
CARDIZEM CD; 300 MG	Cardizem Cd	300 mg	Light Gray and Blue	Extended-Release Capsule		Biovail Pharmaceuticals
CARDIZEM CD; 360 MG	Cardizem Cd	360 mg	Light Blue and White	Extended-Release Capsule		Biovail Pharmaceuticals
CARDIZEM; SR; 60 MG	Cardizem SR	60 mg	Ivory and Brown	Sustained-Release Capsule		Biovail Pharmaceuticals
CARDIZEM; SR; 90 MG	Cardizem SR	90 mg	Gold and Brown	Sustained-Release Capsule		Biovail Pharmaceuticals
CARDIZEM SR; 120 MG	Cardizem SR	120 mg	Caramel and Brown	Sustained-Release Capsule		Biovail Pharmaceuticals
CARDURA; 1 MG	Cardura	1 mg	White	Tablet	Oblong, Scored	Pfizer Laboratories
CARDURA; 2 MG	Cardura	2 mg	Light Orange	Tablet	Oblong, Scored	Pfizer Laboratories
CARDURA; 4 MG	Cardura	4 mg	Orange	Tablet	Oblong, Scored	Pfizer Laboratories
CARDURA; 8 MG	Cardura	8 mg	Green	Tablet	Oblong, Scored	Pfizer Laboratories
CARNITOR ST	Carnitor	330 mg		Tablet		Sigma-Tau Pharmaceuticals
CATAFLAM; 25	Cataflam	25 mg	Light Pink	Tablet	Circle, Biconvex	Novartis Pharmaceuticals
CATAFLAM; 50;	Cataflam	50 mg	Light Brown	Tablet	Circle, Biconvex	Ciba-Geigy
CB; 300	Cimetidine	300 mg	Light Yellow	Coated Tablet	Circle	Lederle Laboratories
CB; 400	Cimetidine	400 mg	Light Yellow	Coated Tablet	Oval	Lederle Laboratories
CB; 800	Cimetidine	800 mg	Light Yellow	Coated Tablet	Oval	Lederle Laboratories
CBF	Nestabs Cbf	4000 IU; 400 IU; 30 IU; 120 mg; 1 mg; 3 mg; 3 mg; 20 mg; 3 mg; 8 mcg; 500 mg; 150 mcg; 15 mg; 50 mg	White	Coated Tablet	Circle, Scored	Fielding
CC	Cycrin	2.5 mg	White	Tablet	Oval, Scored	Esi Pharma
CC; 0147	Phentermine Hydrochloride	30 mg	Various	Capsule		Camall
CC; 37.5	Phentermine	37.5 mg	Black and Red	Capsule		Camall
CC; 101	Meclizine Hydrochloride	25 mg	Yellow	Tablet	Oval	Camall
CC; 105	Cam-Metrazine	35 mg	Pink	Tablet	Circle	Camall
CC; 108	Hydrochlorothiazide	50 mg	Peach	Tablet	Circle	Novartis Generics
CC; 116	Hydrochlorothiazide	25 mg	Peach	Tablet	Circle	Novartis Generics
CC; 123	Hydrochlorothiazide	50 mg	Yellow	Tablet	Circle	Camall
CC; 124	Cam-AP-Es	15 mg; 25 mg; 0.1 mg	Salmon	Tablet	Circle, Scored	Camall
CC; 125	Hydro-Reserp	50 mg; 0.125 mg	Green	Tablet	Circle, Scored	Camall
CC; 137	Meclizine Hydrochloride	12.5 mg	Blue	Tablet	Oval, Scored	Camall
CC; 255	Hydralazine Hydrochloride	10 mg	Orange	Tablet		Camall
CC; 256	Hydralazine Hydrochloride	25 mg	Orange	Tablet		Camall
CC; 257	Hydralazine Hydrochloride	50 mg	Orange	Tablet		Camall
CC; 258	Hydralazine Hydrochloride	100 mg	Orange	Tablet		Camall
CC; CYCRIN	Cycrin	5 mg	Light Purple	Tablet	Oval, Scored	Esi Lederle
CC; CYCRIN	Cycrin	10 mg	Peach	Tablet	Oval, Scored	Esi Pharma
CC-136	Phentermine Hydrochloride	8 mg	Orange	Tablet	Circle	Camall
CC-227	Thyroid	3 Gr	Tan	Tablet		Camall
CC-236	Cyproheptadine Hydrochloride	4 mg	White	Tablet	Circle	Camall
CC-238	Potassium Gluconate	500 mg	White	Tablet	Circle, Scored	Camall

IMPRINT	BRAND/GENERIC NAME	STRENGTH	COLOR	FORM	SHAPE	MANUFACTURER
CC-242	Thyroid	0.5 Gr	Tan	Tablet		Camall
CC-243	Thyroid	1 Gr	Tan	Tablet		Camall
CC-244	Thyroid	2 Gr	Tan	Tablet		Camall
CC-424	Super Ditex Blue/white	3 mg	Blue/white	Capsule		Camall
CC-425	Super Ditex Red/red	3 mg	Red/red	Capsule		Camall
CD; 129	Ranitidine Hydrochloride	150 mg	Tan	Capsule, Liquid Filled		Par Pharmaceutical
CDX50	Casodex	50 mg	White	Coated Tablet		Astra Zeneca
CECLOR CD; 375 MG	Ceclor Cd	375 mg	Blue	Extended-Release Tablet	Oblong	Dura Pharmaceuticals
CECLOR CD; 500	Ceclor Cd	500 mg	Blue	Extended-Release Tablet	Oblong	Dura Pharmaceuticals
CEDAX; 400 MG	Cedax	400 mg	White	Capsule		Biovail Pharmaceuticals
CEG	Correctol Extra Gentle Stool Softener	100 mg	Red	Capsule, Liquid Filled	Oval	Schering-Plough Healthcare Products
CELGENE; 50 MG; DO NOT GET PREGNANT LOGO	Thalomid	50 mg	White	Capsule		Celgene
CELGENE;100 MG; DO NOT GET PREGNANT LOGO	Thalomid	100 mg	Tan	Capsule		Celgene
CELGENE; 200 MG; DO NOT GET PREGNANT LOGO	Thalomid	200 mg	Blue	Capsule		Celgene
CELGENE; DO NOT GET PREGNANT LOGO	Thalomid	50 mg	White	Capsule		Celgene
CELLCEPT; 250; ROCHE	Cellcept	250 mg	Blue and Brown	Capsule, Liquid Filled		Roche
CELLCEPT; 500; ROCHE	Cellcept	500 mg	Lavender	Coated Tablet	Capsule-Shape	Roche Laboratories
CELLTECH; 575; 20 MG	Metadate Cd	20 mg	Blue and White	Extended-Release Capsule		Celltech
CELLTECH; 576; 30 MG	Metadate Cd	30 mg	Reddish Brown and White	Extended-Release Capsule		Celltech
CENTRAL	Niferex with Vitamin C	250 mg; 50 mg; 168.75 mg	Brown	Tablet, Chewable	Circle	Ther-RX
CENTRAL; 20	Niferex Daily	60 mg; 0.3 mg; 259 mg; 6 mcg; 150 mcg; 100 mg; 20 mg; 5.4 mg; 1.7 mg; 2 mg; 15 mg; 30 IU; 400 IU; 5000 IU; 1.5 mg; 10 mg; 5 mg; 18 mg; 0.4 mg; 2 mg	Lavender	Tablet	Capsule-Shape	Ther-RX
CENTRAL; 40	Codimal-L.A.	8 mg; 120 mg	Clear and Red with Blue Beads	Extended-Release Capsule		Schwarz Pharma
CENTRAL; 130 MG	Theoclear LA	130 mg	Clear	Timed-Release Capsule		Schwarz Pharma
CENTRAL; 260 MG	Theoclear LA	260 mg	Clear	Timed-Release Capsule		Schwarz Pharma
CENTRUM; C;1	Centrum Advanced Formula	18 mg; 5000 IU; 30 IU; 400 mcg; 20 mg; 400 IU; 30 mcg; 10 mg; 162 mg; 125 mg; 150 mcg; 100 mg; 2 mg; 15 mg; 2.5 mg; 40 mg; 25 mcg; 25 mcg; 25 mcg; 5 mcg; 10 mcg; 60 mg; 1.5 mg; 1.7 mg; 2 mg; 6 mcg; 25 mcg	Peach	Coated Tablet	Oblong, Scored	Wyeth Consumer Healthcare
CETAZONE	Cetazone	250 mg; 300 mg	Green	Capsule		Marnel Pharmaceuticals
CF; 512	Cefadroxil	500 mg	White	Coated Tablet	Oblong, Biconvex, Scored	Ranbaxy Pharmaceuticals
CF; A	Nembutal Sodium	50 mg	Orange and White	Capsule		Abbott Laboratories
CFL	Chocolate Laxative	90 mg	Dark Brown	Chewable Piece		H.L. Moore
CG; FXF	Foradil Aerolizer	12 mcg	Clear	Capsule		Novartis
CG; HGH	Diovan HCT	12.5 mg; 80 mg	Light Orange	Tablet	Oval	Novartis
CG; HHH	Diovan HCT	12.5 mg; 160 mg	Dark Red	Tablet	Oval	Novartis
CH; A	Nembutal Sodium	100 mg	Yellow	Capsule		Abbott Laboratories
CHARACTER IMPRINT	Sesame Street Complete Vitamins and Minerals	10 mg; 2250 IU; 500 IU; 200 IU; 10 mg; 5 mg; 10 IU; 200 mcg; 15 mcg; 75 mcg; 8 mg; 1 mg; 80 mg; 20 mg; 0.75 mg; 0.85 mg; 0.7 mg; 3 mcg; 40 mg		Tablet	Character-Shape	Johnson & Johnson
CHARACTER IMPRINT	Sesame Street Extra C Vitamins	2250 IU; 500 IU; 200 IU; 0.75 mg; 0.85 mg; 10 mg; 5 mg; 0.7 mg; 3 mcg; 80 mg; 10 IU; 200 mcg		Tablet	Character-Shape	Johnson & Johnson

IMPRINT	BRAND/GENERIC NAME	STRENGTH	COLOR	FORM	SHAPE	MANUFACTURER
CHEMET; 100	Chemet	100 mg	Opague White with Medicated Beads	Capsule		Sanofi Winthrop Pharmaceuticals
CHEW; EZ	Eryped	200 mg	White	Tablet, Chewable	Circle, Scored	Abbott Laboratories
CHILDREN; A; 3	Anacin-3 Children's	80 mg	Pink	Tablet, Chewable	Circle, Scored	Wyeth Consumer Healthcare
CHOLOXIN; 1	Choloxin	1 mg	Orange	Tablet	Circle, Convex, Scored	Knoll Pharmaceutical
CHOLOXIN; 2	Choloxin	2 mg	Yellow	Tablet	Circle, Convex, Scored	Knoll Pharmaceutical
CHOLOXIN; 4	Choloxin	4 mg	White	Tablet	Circle, Scored	Knoll Pharmaceutical
CHOLOXIN; 6	Choloxin	6 mg		Tablet		Knoll Pharmaceutical
CIBA	Pyribenzamine Lontabs	50 mg	Light Green	Tablet		Novartis
CIBA; 3	Ritalin	10 mg	Pale Green	Tablet	Circle, Scored	Novartis Pharmaceuticals
CIBA; 7	Ritalin	5 mg	Yellow	Tablet	Circle	Novartis Pharmaceuticals
CIBA; 13	Serpasil-Esidrix No. 1	25 mg; 0.1 mg	Light Orange	Tablet	Circle	Novartis
CIBA; 16	Ritalin SR	20 mg	White	Sustained-Release Tablet	Circle, Coated	Novartis Pharmaceuticals
CIBA; 22	Esidrix	25 mg	Pink	Tablet	Circle, Scored	Novartis
CIBA; 24	Cytadren	250 mg	White	Tablet	Circle, Cross-Scored	Novartis
CIBA; 26	Ludiomil	50 mg	Dark Orange	Tablet	Circle, Scored	Novartis
CIBA; 32	Metandren	25 mg	Yellow	Tablet	Circle, Scored	Novartis
CIBA; 33;	Pyribenzamine	50 mg	Light Blue	Tablet		Novartis
CIBA; 34	Ritalin	20 mg	Pale Yellow	Tablet	Circle, Scored	Novartis Pharmaceuticals
CIBA; 35	Serpasil	0.1 mg	White	Tablet	Circle	Novartis
CIBA; 36	Serpasil	0.25 mg	White	Tablet	Circle, Scored	Novartis
CIBA; 37	Apresoline Hydrochloride	10 mg	Yellow	Tablet	Circle	Ciba-Geigy
CIBA; 39	Apresoline Hydrochloride	25 mg	Blue	Tablet	Circle	Ciba-Geigy
CIBA; 40	Serpasil-Apresoline No. 1	25 mg; 0.1 mg	Yellow	Tablet	Circle	Novartis
CIBA; 41;	Anturane	100 mg	White	Tablet	Circle, Scored	Ciba-Geigy
CIBA; 45	Forhistal Lontabs	2.5 mg	Orange	Tablet	Oblong	Novartis
CIBA; 46	Esidrex	50 mg	Yellow	Tablet	Circle, Scored	Ciba-Geigy
CIBA; 47	Esimil	10 mg; 25 mg	White	Tablet	Circle, Scored	Novartis
CIBA; 49	Ismelin	10 mg	Yellow	Tablet	Circle, Scored	Novartis
CIBA; 64	Metandren Linguets	10 mg	Yellow	Tablet	Capsule-Shape	Novartis
CIBA; 65	Lithobid	300 mg	Peach	Sustained-Release Tablet		Novartis
CIBA; 71	Ser-AP-Es	25 mg; 15 mg; 0.1 mg	Pink	Tablet	Circle	Novartis
CIBA; 73	Apresoline Hydrochloride	50 mg	Light Blue	Tablet	Circle	Ciba-Geigy
CIBA; 92	Gammacorten	0.75 mg		Tablet		Novartis
CIBA; 95	Pyribenzamine	25 mg	Green	Tablet		Novartis
CIBA; 96	Ultandren	5 mg	Lavender	Tablet		Novartis
CIBA; 101	Apresoline Hydrochloride	100 mg	Peach	Tablet	Circle	Ciba-Geigy
CIBA; 103	Ismelin	25 mg	White	Tablet	Circle, Scored	Novartis
CIBA; 104	Serpasil-Apresoline No. 2	50 mg; 0.2 mg	Yellow	Tablet	Circle	Novartis
CIBA; 105	Dialog	300 mg; 15 mg	White	Tablet	Circle, Scored	Novartis
CIBA; 110	Ludiomil	25 mg	Orange	Tablet	Oval, Scored	Novartis
CIBA; 130	Metopirone	250 mg	White	Tablet	Circle, Scored	Novartis
CIBA; 134	Pyribenzamine with Ephedrine	12 mg; 25 mg	White	Tablet		Novartis
CIBA; 135	Ludiomil	75 mg	White	Coated Tablet	Oval	Novartis
CIBA; 135	Ludiomil	75 mg	White	Tablet	Oval, Scored	Novartis
CIBA; 139; APRESAZIDE; 25/25	Apresazide 25/25	25 mg; 25 mg	Light Blue and White	Capsule		Ciba-Geigy
CIBA; 149; APRESAZIDE; 50/50	Apresazide 50/50	50 mg; 50 mg	Pink and White	Capsule		Ciba-Geigy
CIBA; 152	Regitine	50 mg	White	Tablet		Novartis
CIBA; 154	Rimactane	300 mg	Scarlet and Caramel	Capsule		Geneva Generics
CIBA; 159; APRESAZIDE; 100/50	Apresazide 100/50	100 mg; 50 mg	White and Flesh Pink	Capsule		Ciba-Geigy
CIBA; 192	Esidrex	100 mg	Blue	Tablet	Circle, Scored	Novartis
CIBA; 192	Esidrix	100 mg	Blue	Tablet	Circle, Scored	Novartis
CIBA; 31 (ORANGE);	Forhistal	1 mg	Orange or Green	Tablet		Novartis
CIBA; NR	Slow Fe	160 mg	Yellowish-White	Extended-Release Tablet	Circle, Biconvex	Novartis Consumer
CIPRO; 100	Cipro Cystitis Pack	100 mg	Slightly Yellow	Tablet	Circle	Bayer Pharmaceutical
CIPRO; 250	Cipro	250 mg	Yellow	Coated Tablet	Circle	Bayer Pharmaceutical
CIPRO; 500	Cipro	500 mg	Yellow	Coated Tablet	Capsule-Shape	Bayer Pharmaceutical
CIPRO; 750	Cipro	750 mg	Yellow	Coated Tablet	Capsule-Shape	Bayer Pharmaceutical
CIR; 3 MG	Entocort Ec	3 mg	Light Grey and Pink	Capsule		Astra Zeneca
CL; 21	Furosemide	20 mg	White	Tablet		West-Ward
CL; 40	Amitriptyline Hydrochloride	10 mg	Pink	Tablet		West-Ward
CL; 44	Amitriptyline Hydrochloride	25 mg	Green	Tablet		West-Ward
CL; 53	Trifluoperazine Hydrochloride	2 mg	Lavender	Tablet	Circle	Rosemont Pharmaceutical
CL; 101	Methocarbamol	750 mg		Tablet		Roxane Laboratories
CL; 110	Acetachlor	250 mg; 300 mg	Light Green	Tablet		West-Ward
CL; 127	Regal-AM	260 mg	White	Tablet	Circle	Geneva Generics
CL; 141	Meclizine Hydrochloride	12.5 mg	Blue and White	Tablet		West-Ward
CL; 190	Methocarbamol	500 mg		Tablet		Roxane Laboratories
CL; 201	Furosemide	40 mg	White	Tablet		West-Ward
CL; 205	Sodium Bicarbonate	5 Gr	White	Tablet	Circle	Rugby Laboratories
CL; 206	Sodium Bicarbonate	10 Gr	White	Tablet	Circle	Rugby Laboratories
CL; 215	Senexon	8.6 mg	Brown	Tablet	Circle	Rugby Laboratories
CL; 229	Isosorbide Dinitrate	40 mg	Green	Timed-Release Tablet		West-Ward
CL; 261	Meclizine Hydrochloride	25 mg	Yellow and White	Tablet		West-Ward
CL; 400	Ercaf	100 mg; 1 mg	Beige	Coated Tablet	Circle, Scored	Novartis Generics
CL; 407	Chlorpromazine Hydrochloride	50 mg	Tan	Tablet		West-Ward
CL; 418	Phenylbutazone	100 mg	Red	Coated Tablet		Novartis Generics
CL; 431	Amitriptyline Hydrochloride	50 mg	Brown	Tablet		West-Ward
CL; 437	Chlorpromazine Hydrochloride	100 mg	Tan	Coated Tablet		West-Ward
CL; 455	Chlorpromazine Hydrochloride	10 mg	Tan	Coated Tablet		West-Ward

IMPRINT	BRAND/GENERIC NAME	STRENGTH	COLOR	FORM	SHAPE	MANUFACTURER
CL; 457	Chlorpromazine Hydrochloride	200 mg	Tan	Coated Tablet		West-Ward
CL; 476	Chlorpromazine Hydrochloride	25 mg	Tan	Coated Tablet		West-Ward
CL; 476	Chlorpromazine Hydrochloride	50 mg	Tan	Coated Tablet		West-Ward
CL; 501	Nitroglycerin	6.5 mg	Blue and Yellow	Sustained-Release Capsule		West-Ward
CL; 501	Trates	6.5 mg	Black Opaque and Clear Yellow	Capsule		Solvay Pharmaceuticals
CL; 503	Papaverine Hydrochloride	150 mg	Brown and Clear	Extended-Release Capsule		Roxane Laboratories
CL; 511	Nitroglycerin	2.5 mg	Purple and Clear	Sustained-Release Capsule		West-Ward
CL; 511	Trates S.R.	6.5 mg	Clear and Purple with White Beads	Capsule		Solvay Pharmaceuticals
CL; 581; 10;	Trifluoperazine Hydrochloride	10 mg	Lavender	Coated Tablet	Circle	Rosemont Pharmaceutical
CL; 751	Methyldopa	250 mg		Tablet		Novartis Generics
CL; 752	Methyldopa	500 mg		Tablet		Novartis Generics
CL; 753	Methyldopa and Hydrochlorothiazide	250 mg; 15 mg		Tablet		Novartis Generics
CL; 754	Methyldopa and Hydrochlorothiazide	250 mg; 25 mg		Tablet		Novartis Generics
CLARITIN 10; 458	Claritin	10 mg	White to Off-White	Tablet	Circle, Compressed	Schering
CLARITIN-D	Claritin-D 12 Hour	5 mg; 120 mg	White	Extended-Release Tablet		Schering
CLARITIN-D; 24 HOUR	Claritin-D 24 Hour	10 mg; 240 mg	White to Off-White	Extended-Release Tablet		Schering
CLEOCIN; 75 MG	Cleocin	75 mg	Green	Capsule		Pharmacia & Upjohn
CLEOCIN; 150 MG	Cleocin	150 mg	Blue and Green	Capsule		Pharmacia & Upjohn
CLEOCIN; 300 MG	Cleocin	300 mg	Blue	Capsule		Pharmacia & Upjohn
CLISTIN; MCNEIL	Clistin	4 mg	Pink	Tablet	Circle, Scored	Mcneil Pharmaceutical
CLOMID; 50;	Clomid	50 mg	White to Pale Yellow	Tablet	Circle, Scored	Aventis Pharmaceuticals
CLORFED	Clorfed	4 mg; 60 mg	White and Yellow	Extended-Release Tablet		Stewart-Jackson Pharmacal
CLOZARIL; 25	Clozaril	25 mg	Pale Yellow	Tablet	Circle, Compressed, Embossed	Novartis Pharmaceuticals
CLOZARIL; 100	Clozaril	100 mg	Pale Yellow	Tablet	Circle, Compressed	Novartis Pharmaceuticals
CM	Children's Mylanta	400 mg	Pink	Tablet, Chewable	Circle, Scored	Johnson & Johnson Merck
CN; 0.5; G	Clonazepam	0.5 mg	Light Yellow	Tablet	Circle, Scored	Par Pharmaceutical
CN; 1; G	Clonazepam	1 mg	Dark Yellow	Tablet	Circle, Scored	Par Pharmaceutical
CN; 2; G	Clonazepam	2 mg	White	Tablet	Circle, Scored	Par Pharmaceutical
C-NIGHT	Contac Day & Night Cold & Flu	650 mg; 60 mg; 50 mg; 30 mg	Blue	Tablet		Glaxosmithkline Consumer
COADVIL	CO-Advil	200 mg; 30 mg	Tan	Tablet		Whitehall
COGNEX; 10	Cognex	10 mg	Yellow and Dark Green	Capsule		First Horizon Pharmaceutical
COGNEX; 20	Cognex	20 mg	Yellow and Light Blue	Capsule		First Horizon Pharmaceutical
COGNEX; 30	Cognex	30 mg	Yellow and Orange	Capsule		First Horizon Pharmaceutical
COGNEX; 40	Cognex	40 mg	Yellow and Lavender	Capsule		First Horizon Pharmaceutical
COMBID; SKF	Combid	5 mg; 10 mg	Yellow and Clear	Capsule		Glaxosmithkline
COMHIST; 0149 044	Comhist	2 mg; 25 mg; 10 mg	Yellow	Tablet		Lee Pharmaceuticals
COMHIST LA; 01490466	Comhist LA	4 mg; 50 mg; 20 mg	Yellow and Clear	Capsule		Procter & Gamble Pharmaceuticals
COMPOZ	Compoz Maximum Strength Nighttime Sleep Aid	50 mg	Blue	Capsule, Liquid Filled	Circle	Medtech
COMPOZ	Compoz Maximum Strength Nighttime Sleep Aid	50 mg	White	Tablet	Oblong	Medtech
COMTAN	Comtan	200 mg	Brown-Orange	Coated Tablet	Oval	Novartis
COMTREX	Comtrex Maximum Strength	500 mg; 2 mg; 30 mg; 15 mg	Yellow	Tablet		Bristol-Myers Squibb
COMTREX; A S	Comtrex Allergy and Sinus	500 mg; 30 mg; 2 mg	Green	Tablet		Bristol-Myers Squibb
CONTAC; S	Contac Sinus	500 mg; 30 mg	Pink	Tablet	Capsule-Shape	Glaxosmithkline Consumer
COP; 014	Luride	0.5 mg		Tablet, Chewable		Colgate Oral Pharmaceuticals
COP; 186	Luride	0.25 mg		Tablet, Chewable		Colgate Oral Pharmaceuticals
COPE	Cope Extra Strength Formula	421 mg; 32 mg	White	Tablet	Oval	Lee Pharmaceuticals
COPLEY; 0519	Vitamins with Fluoride	2500 IU; 400 IU; 15 IU; 0.3 mg; 13.5 mg; 1 mg; 60 mg; 1.05 mg; 1.2 mg; 1.05 mg; 4.5 mcg	Multi-Colored	Tablet, Chewable	Square	Copley Pharmaceutical
COPLEY; 0519	Vitamins with Fluoride	2500 IU; 400 IU; 15 IU; 0.3 mg; 13.5 mg; 1 mg; 60 mg; 1.05 mg; 1.2 mg; 1.05 mg; 4.5 mcg	Multi-Colored	Tablet, Chewable	Square	Novartis Generics
COPLEY; 107	Mebendazole	100 mg	Light Peach	Tablet, Chewable	Circle	Teva Pharmaceuticals
COPLEY; 111	Prenatal 1+1	65 mg; 4000 IU; 400 IU; 11 mg; 1 mg; 1.5 mg; 3 mg; 20 mg; 200 mg; 2 mg; 25 mg; 120 mg; 10 mg; 12 mcg	Yellow	Coated Tablet	Capsule-Shape	Copley Pharmaceutical
COPLEY; 111	Prenatal 1+1	65 mg; 4000 IU; 400 IU; 11 mg; 1 mg; 1.5 mg; 3 mg; 20 mg; 200 mg; 2 mg; 25 mg; 120 mg; 10 mg; 12 mcg	Yellow	Coated Tablet	Capsule-Shape	Novartis Generics

IMPRINT	BRAND/GENERIC NAME	STRENGTH	COLOR	FORM	SHAPE	MANUFACTURER
COPLEY; 113	R-Tannate	25 mg; 8 mg; 25 mg	Beige	Tablet	Capsule-Shape, Compressed	Copley Pharmaceutical
COPLEY; 114	Procainamide Hydrochloride	750 mg	Tan	Sustained-Release Tablet	Capsule-Shape, Scored	Copley Pharmaceutical
COPLEY; 123	Sodium Fluoride	1.1 mg	Purple-Blue	Tablet, Chewable		Copley Pharmaceutical
COPLEY; 126	Multibret-Folic-500	525 mg; 30 mg; 10 mg; 800 mcg; 500 mg; 6 mg; 6 mg; 5 mg; 25 mcg	Fuchsia	Extended-Release Tablet	Oval	Copley Pharmaceutical
COPLEY; 126	Multibret-Folic-500	525 mg; 30 mg; 10 mg; 800 mcg; 500 mg; 6 mg; 6 mg; 5 mg; 25 mcg	Fuchsia	Extended-Release Tablet	Oval	Qualitest Products
COPLEY; 131	Sodium Fluoride	2.2 mg	Pink	Tablet, Chewable	Circle	Copley Pharmaceutical
COPLEY; 131	Sodium Fluoride	2.2 mg	Pink	Tablet, Chewable	Circle	Novartis Generics
COPLEY; 132	Albuterol Sulfate	2 mg	White	Tablet	Round; Flat; Bisected Scored	Copley Pharmaceutical
COPLEY; 133	Amiodarone Hydrochloride	200 mg	Pink	Tablet		Copley Pharmaceutical
COPLEY; 133	Amiodarone Hydrochloride	200 mg	Pink	Tablet		Udl Laboratories
COPLEY; 134	Albuterol Sulfate	4 mg	White	Tablet	Round; Flat; Bisected Scored	Copley Pharmaceutical
COPLEY; 136	Metoprolol Tartrate	50 mg	Pink	Tablet	Capsule-Shape	Copley Pharmaceutical
COPLEY; 143	Salsalate	500 mg	Aqua Blue	Tablet	Circle	Copley Pharmaceutical
COPLEY; 144	Salsalate	750 mg	Aqua Blue	Tablet	Capsule-Shape	Copley Pharmaceutical
COPLEY; 146	Naproxen	250 mg	Light Yellow	Tablet	Circle	Copley Pharmaceutical
COPLEY; 150	Naproxen	500 mg	Off-White	Tablet	Capsule-Shape	Copley Pharmaceutical
COPLEY; 151	B-Complex Vitamins	100 mg; 18 mg; 0.5 mg; 500 mg; 15 mg; 15 mg; 4 mg; 5 mcg	Chartreuse	Tablet	Oval	Copley Pharmaceutical
COPLEY; 152	B-Complex Vitamins Plus	500 mg; 0.15 mg; 3 mg; 0.8 mg; 5 mg; 25 mg; 5000 IU; 25 mg; 50 mcg; 22.5 mg; 30 IU; 100 mg; 20 mg; 100 mg; 50 mg; 27 mg; 0.1 mg	Light Yellow to Tan	Tablet	Capsule-Shape	Copley Pharmaceutical
COPLEY; 157	Prenatal 1/60	60 mg; 8000 IU; 400 IU; 30 IU; 1 mg; 3 mg; 3.4 mg; 20 mg; 250 mg; 0.3 mg; 25 mg; 2 mg; 25 mg; 50 mg; 100 mg; 4 mg; 12 mcg	Pink	Tablet	Capsule-Shape	Copley Pharmaceutical
COPLEY 158;	Multivitamins with Fluoride	2500 IU; 400 IU; 15 IU; 0.3 mg; 1.05 mg; 1.2 mg; 13.5 mg; 0.5 mg; 60 mg; 1.05 mg; 4.5 mcg	Multi-Colored	Tablet, Chewable	Square	Copley Pharmaceutical
COPLEY 158;	Multivitamins with Fluoride	2500 IU; 400 IU; 15 IU; 0.3 mg; 1.05 mg; 1.2 mg; 13.5 mg; 0.5 mg; 60 mg; 1.05 mg; 4.5 mcg	Multi-Colored	Tablet, Chewable	Square	Novartis Generics
COPLEY; 159	Chewable Multivitamins with Fluoride and Iron 1 mg Fluoride	1 mg; 0.3 mg; 13.5 mg; 1 mg; 2500 IU; 1.05 mg; 400 IU; 10 mg; 15 IU; 60 mg; 4.5 mcg; 1.05 mg; 1.2 mg; 12 mg	Purple	Tablet, Chewable	Square	Copley Pharmaceutical
COPLEY 159	Multivitamins with Fluoride and Iron	12 mg; 2500 IU; 400 IU; 15 IU; 0.3 mg; 1.05 mg; 1.2 mg; 13.5 mg; 1 mg; 1 mg; 10 mg; 60 mg; 1.05 mg; 4.5 mcg	Purple	Tablet, Chewable	Square	Copley Pharmaceutical
COPLEY; 165	Prenatal Vitamins	30 mg; 2000 IU; 200 IU; 7.5 IU; 40 mg; 0.5 mg; 0.75 mg; 0.8 mg; 8.5 mg; 2 mg; 1.25 mcg; 0.015 mg; 3.5 mg; 100 mg; 50 mg; 1.5 mg; 12.5 mg	White	Tablet	Oval	Copley Pharmaceutical

IMPRINT	BRAND/GENERIC NAME	STRENGTH	COLOR	FORM	SHAPE	MANUFACTURER
COPLEY; 166	Multivitamins with Fluoride	2.21 mg; 3.46 mg; 3.78 mg; 3.31 mg; Less Than 5.5 mg; Less Than 5.5 mg; 0.194 mg; 0.35 mg; 0.49 mg; 31.5 mg; 38.3 mg; 32.2 mg; 42.52 mg	Orange, Pink or Purple	Tablet, Chewable	Square	Copley Pharmaceutical
COPLEY 169	Prenatal RX with Beta-Carotene	60 mg; 4000 IU; 400 IU; 15 IU; 1 mg; 1.5 mg; 1.6 mg; 17 mg; 0.03 mg; 7 mg; 200 mg; 100 mg; 3 mg; 25 mg; 80 mg; 4 mg; 2.5 mcg	White	Tablet	Oval	Copley Pharmaceutical
COPLEY; 170	Prenatal FA	60 mg; 4000 IU; 400 IU; 100 mg; 1 mg; 3 mg; 2 mg; 10 mg; 5 mg; 3 mcg; 0.92 mg; 250 mg; 100 mcg; 0.15 mg	Blue	Tablet	Oval	Copley Pharmaceutical
COPLEY; 171	Azo Sulfamethoxazole	500 mg; 100 mg		Tablet		Copley Pharmaceutical
COPLEY; 175	Quinidine Sulfate	300 mg		Sustained-Release Tablet		Copley Pharmaceutical
COPLEY; 176	Triple Multivitamins with Fluoride	2800 IU; 400 IU; 1 mg; 60 mg		Tablet		Copley Pharmaceutical
COPLEY; 182; PIROXICAM 10	Piroxicam	10 mg		Capsule		Copley Pharmaceutical
COPLEY; 188	Procainamide Hydrochloride	500 mg	Pink	Sustained-Release Tablet	Capsule-Shape, Scored	Copley Pharmaceutical
COPLEY; 192	Chewable Multivitamins with Fluoride and Iron 0.5 mg Fluoride	1 mg; 0.3 mg; 13.5 mg; 0.5 mg; 2500 IU; 1.05 mg; 400 IU; 10 mg; 15 IU; 60 mg; 4.5 mcg; 1.05 mg; 1.2 mg; 12 mg	Pink	Tablet, Chewable	Square	Copley Pharmaceutical
COPLEY; 192	Prenatal Z	1 mg; 3.56 mg; 3.15 mg; 1.32 mg; 0.229 mg; 24.9 mg; 10.5 mg; 63 mg; 10.2 mg; 234 mg; 28.6 mg; 82 mg; 197.75 mg; 0.5 mg; 165.8 mg	Blue	Tablet	Capsule-Shape	Copley Pharmaceutical
COPLEY; 195; PIROXICAM 20	Piroxicam	20 mg		Capsule		Copley Pharmaceutical
COPLEY; 197	Multivitamins with Fluoride and Iron	2500 IU; 400 IU; 15 IU; 60 mg; 0.3 mg; 1.05 mg; 1.2 mg; 13.5 mg; 1.05 mg; 4.5 mcg; 12 mg; 1 mg; 10 mg; 0.5 mg	Pink	Tablet, Chewable	Square	Copley Pharmaceutical
COPLEY; 203	Phenazopyridine Hydrochloride	100 mg	Purple	Coated Tablet	Circle	Copley Pharmaceutical
COPLEY; 204	Phenazopyridine Hydrochloride	200 mg	Purple	Coated Tablet	Circle	Copley Pharmaceutical
COPLEY; 205	Potassium Chloride	25 meq		Effervescent Tablet		Copley Pharmaceutical
COPLEY; 206	Amitriptyline Hydrochloride	10 mg	Blue	Tablet	Circle	Copley Pharmaceutical
COPLEY; 207	Amitriptyline Hydrochloride	25 mg	Yellow	Tablet	Circle	Copley Pharmaceutical
COPLEY; 208	Amitriptyline Hydrochloride	50 mg	Beige	Tablet	Circle	Copley Pharmaceutical
COPLEY; 209	Amitriptyline Hydrochloride	75 mg	Orange	Tablet	Circle	Copley Pharmaceutical
COPLEY; 210	Amitriptyline Hydrochloride	100 mg	Mauve	Tablet	Circle	Copley Pharmaceutical
COPLEY; 211	Amitriptyline Hydrochloride	150 mg	Blue	Tablet	Capsule-Shape	Copley Pharmaceutical
COPLEY; 225	Potassium Chloride	600 mg	Peach	Extended-Release Tablet	Circle	Copley Pharmaceutical
COPLEY; 225	Potassium Chloride	8 meq	Orange	Extended-Release Tablet	Circle	Copley Pharmaceutical
COPLEY; 225	Potassium Chloride	8 meq	Orange	Extended-Release Tablet	Circle	Teva Pharmaceuticals
COPLEY; 225	Potassium Chloride	600 mg	Peach	Extended-Release Tablet	Circle	Teva Pharmaceuticals
COPLEY; 225	Potassium Chloride Extended Release	8 meq	Orange	Extended-Release Tablet	Circle	Akyma Pharmaceuticals
COPLEY; 381; 381	Micronized Glyburide	3 mg	Light Green	Tablet	Six-Sided, Rounded, Scored	Copley Pharmaceutical
COPLEY; 411	Methazolamide	25 mg		Tablet		Copley Pharmaceutical
COPLEY; 417	Metoprolol Tartrate	100 mg	Blue	Tablet	Capsule-Shape	Copley Pharmaceutical
COPLEY; 424	Methazolamide	50 mg		Tablet		Copley Pharmaceutical
COPLEY; 427	Diclofenac Sodium	75 mg	Pink	Timed-Release Tablet	Circle, Biconvex, Beveled Edge	Copley Pharmaceutical
COPLEY; 431	Diclofenac Sodium	25 mg	Pink	Timed-Release Tablet	Circle, Biconvex, Beveled Edge	Copley Pharmaceutical
COPLEY; 443	Naproxen	375 mg	Light Yellow	Tablet	Capsule-Shape	Copley Pharmaceutical
COPLEY; 447	Iodinated Glycerol	30 mg	Red-Orange	Tablet	Circle, Flat	Copley Pharmaceutical
COPLEY; 474	Diclofenac Sodium	50 mg	Pink	Timed-Release Tablet	Circle, Biconvex, Beveled Edge	Copley Pharmaceutical
COPLEY; 631	Diltiazem Hydrochloride	30 mg	Blue	Tablet	Circle	Copley Pharmaceutical
COPLEY; 643	Prochlorperazine Maleate	5 mg	Yellow	Coated Tablet	Circle	Copley Pharmaceutical
COPLEY; 652	Prochlorperazine Maleate	10 mg	Yellow	Coated Tablet	Circle	Copley Pharmaceutical
COPLEY; 652	Prochlorperazine Maleate	10 mg	Yellow	Coated Tablet	Circle	Copley Pharmaceutical
COPLEY; 662	Diltiazem Hydrochloride	60 mg	White	Tablet	Circle, Scored	Copley Pharmaceutical
COPLEY; 691	Diltiazem Hydrochloride	90 mg	Blue	Tablet	Oblong	Copley Pharmaceutical
COPLEY; 712	Atenolol	50 mg		Tablet		Copley Pharmaceutical
COPLEY; 713	Atenolol	100 mg		Tablet		Copley Pharmaceutical

IMPRINT	BRAND/GENERIC NAME	STRENGTH	COLOR	FORM	SHAPE	MANUFACTURER
COPLEY; 720	Diltiazem Hydrochloride	120 mg	White	Tablet	Oblong	Copley Pharmaceutical
COPLEY; 724	Nadolol	80 mg		Tablet		Copley Pharmaceutical
COPLEY; 725; 725	Micronized Glyburide	1.5 mg	Pink	Tablet	Six-Sided, Rounded, Scored	Copley Pharmaceutical
COPLEY; 727	Nadolol	120 mg		Tablet		Copley Pharmaceutical
COPLEY; 731	Nadolol	160 mg		Tablet		Copley Pharmaceutical
COPLEY; 741	Naproxen Sodium	275 mg		Tablet		Copley Pharmaceutical
COPLEY; 744	Naproxen Sodium	550 mg		Tablet		Copley Pharmaceutical
COPLEY; 774	Hydroxychloroquine Sulfate	200 mg	White	Coated Tablet	Capsule-Shape, Scored	Copley Pharmaceutical
COR; 103	Carisoprodol	350 mg	White	Tablet	Circle	Geneva Generics
COR; 103	Carisoprodol	350 mg	White	Tablet	Circle	Ohm Laboratories
COR; 103	Carisoprodol	350 mg	White	Tablet	Circle	Ranbaxy Pharmaceuticals
COR; 103;	Carisoprodol	350 mg	White	Tablet	Circle	Sandoz
COR; 108	Salsalate	500 mg	Yellow	Tablet	Circle, Scored	Richmond Pharmaceuticals
COR; 109	Salsalate	750 mg	Yellow	Tablet	Circle, Scored	Richmond Pharmaceuticals
COR; 111	Rimantadine Hydrochloride	100 mg	Orange	Tablet	Circle	Geneva Generics
COR; 118	Phenobarbital	15 mg	White	Tablet	Circle	Ohm Laboratories
COR; 119	Phenobarbital	30 mg	White	Tablet	Circle	Ohm Laboratories
COR; 120	Phenobarbital	60 mg	White	Tablet	Circle	Ohm Laboratories
COR; 121	Phenobarbital	100 mg	White	Tablet	Circle, Scored	Ohm Laboratories
COR; 123	Glyburide	1.25 mg	White	Tablet	Circle, Scored	Sandoz
COR; 124	Glyburide	2.5 mg	Yellow	Tablet	Circle, Scored	Sandoz
COR; 125	Glyburide	5 mg	Green	Tablet	Circle, Scored	Sandoz
COR; 127	Tramadol Hydrochloride	50 mg	White	Tablet	Circle	Akyma Pharmaceuticals
COR; 128	Pyridostigmine Bromide	60 mg	White	Tablet	Round, Quadrisected Scored	Geneva Generics
COR; 130	Dextroamphetamine Saccharate, Amphetamine Aspartate, Dextroamphetamine Sulfate, and Amphetamine Sulfate	1.25 mg; 1.25 mg; 1.25 mg; 1.25 mg	Blue	Tablet	Circle, Quadrisected	Ranbaxy Pharmaceuticals
COR; 132	Dextroamphetamine Saccharate, Amphetamine Aspartate, Dextroamphetamine Sulfate, and Amphetamine Sulfate	2.5 mg; 2.5 mg; 2.5 mg	Blue	Tablet	Quadrisected, Round Scored	Ranbaxy Pharmaceuticals
COR; 135	Dextroamphetamine Saccharate, Amphetamine Aspartate, Dextroamphetamine Sulfate, and Amphetamine Sulfate	5 mg; 5 mg; 5 mg; 5 mg	Pink	Tablet	Quadrisected, Round Scored	Ranbaxy Pharmaceuticals
COR; 136	Dextroamphetamine Saccharate, Amphetamine Aspartate, Dextroamphetamine Sulfate, and Amphetamine Sulfate	7.5 mg; 7.5 mg; 7.5 mg	Pink	Tablet	Quadrisected, Round Scored	Ranbaxy Pharmaceuticals
COR; 143	Benztropine Mesylate	0.5 mg	White	Tablet	Circle, Scored	Major Pharmaceutical
COR; 143	Benztropine Mesylate	0.5 mg	White	Tablet	Circle, Scored	Rising Pharmaceuticals
COR; 144	Benztropine Mesylate	1 mg	White	Tablet	Oval, Scored	Major Pharmaceutical
COR; 144	Benztropine Mesylate	1 mg	White	Tablet	Oval, Scored	Rising Pharmaceuticals
COR; 145	Benztropine Mesylate	2 mg	White	Tablet	Circle, Scored	Major Pharmaceutical
COR; 145	Benztropine Mesylate	2 mg	White	Tablet	Circle, Scored	Rising Pharmaceuticals
COR; 150	Cyproheptadine Hydrochloride	4 mg	White	Tablet	Circle, Scored	Rising Pharmaceuticals
COR; 153	Clindamycin Hydrochloride	150 mg		Capsule		Sandoz
COR; 154	Clindamycin Hydrochloride	300 mg		Capsule		Sandoz
COR 106	Tizanidine Hydrochloride	2 mg	White	Tablet	Circle	Akyma Pharmaceuticals
COR 138	Tizanidine Hydrochloride	4 mg	White	Tablet		Akyma Pharmaceuticals
CORRECTOL	Correctol	5 mg	Bright Pink	Tablet	Oblong	Schering-Plough Healthcare Products
CORRECTOL IN A HALF MOON	Correctol	5 mg	Bright Pink	Tablet	Circle	Schering-Plough Healthcare Products
CORTEF; 5	Cortef	5 mg	White	Tablet	Circle, Scored	Pharmacia & Upjohn
CORTEF; 10	Cortef	10 mg	White	Tablet	Circle, Scored	Pharmacia & Upjohn
CORTEF; 20	Cortef	20 mg	White	Tablet	Circle, Scored	Pharmacia & Upjohn
CORZIDE; 40/5; 283;	Corzide 40/5	5 mg; 40 mg	White to Bluish White with Dark Blue Specks	Tablet	Circle, Biconvex	Monarch Pharmaceuticals
CORZIDE; 80/5; 284;	Corzide 80/5	5 mg; 80 mg	White to Bluish White with Dark Blue Specks	Tablet	Circle, Biconvex	Monarch Pharmaceuticals
COSAMIN DS	Cosamin DS	500 mg; 400 mg;	Blue and White	Capsule		Nutramax Laboratories
COTRIM; 93 93	Cotrim	400 mg; 80 mg	White	Tablet	Circle, Convex, Scored	Teva Pharmaceuticals
COTRIM DS; 93 93	Cotrim DS	800 mg; 160 mg	White	Tablet	Oval, Convex, Scored	Teva Pharmaceuticals
COTYLENOL	Cotylenol Cold Medication	2 mg; 30 mg; 15 mg; 325 mg	Yellow	Tablet	Oblong	Mcneil Consumer Products
COUMADIN; 1;	Coumadin	1 mg	Pink	Tablet	Circle, Scored	Bristol-Myers Squibb
COUMADIN; 2;	Coumadin	2 mg	Lavender	Tablet	Circle, Scored	Bristol-Myers Squibb
COUMADIN; 2 1/2;	Coumadin	2.5 mg	Green	Tablet	Circle, Scored	Bristol-Myers Squibb
COUMADIN; 3;	Coumadin	3 mg	Tan	Tablet	Circle, Scored	Bristol-Myers Squibb
COUMADIN; 4;	Coumadin	4 mg	Blue	Tablet	Circle, Scored	Bristol-Myers Squibb
COUMADIN; 5;	Coumadin	5 mg	Peach	Tablet	Circle, Scored	Bristol-Myers Squibb
COUMADIN; 6;	Coumadin	6 mg	Teal	Tablet	Circle, Scored	Bristol-Myers Squibb
COUMADIN; 7 1/2;	Coumadin	7.5 mg	Yellow	Tablet	Circle, Scored	Bristol-Myers Squibb
COUMADIN; 10;	Coumadin	10 mg	White	Tablet	Circle, Scored	Bristol-Myers Squibb
COVERA-HS; 2011	Covera-Hs	180 mg	Lavender	Sustained-Release Tablet	Circle	Searle
COVERA-HS; 2021	Covera-Hs	240 mg	Pale Yellow	Sustained-Release Tablet	Circle	Searle
CP; 200	Humibid L.A.	600 mg; 200 mg	Light Green	Tablet	Capsule-Shape, Scored	Vintage Pharmaceuticals
CP; 253; NOTRIPTYLINE; 75 MG	Nortriptyline Hydrochloride	75 mg	Green	Capsule		Creighton Labs
CP; 253; NOTRIPTYLINE; 75 MG	Nortriptyline Hydrochloride	75 mg	Green	Capsule		Geneva Generics

IMPRINT	BRAND/GENERIC NAME	STRENGTH	COLOR	FORM	SHAPE	MANUFACTURER
CP; 264	Thioridazine Hcl	10 mg	Light Yellow-Green	Coated Tablet		Creighton Products
CP; 266	Thioridazine Hcl	25 mg	Butterscotch	Coated Tablet		Creighton Products
CP; 267	Thioridazine Hcl	50 mg	White	Coated Tablet		Creighton Products
CP; 268	Thioridazine Hcl	100 mg	Pale Lime Green	Coated Tablet		Creighton Products
CP; 269	Thioridazine Hcl	150 mg	Lemon Yellow	Coated Tablet		Creighton Products
CP; 270	Thioridazine Hcl	200 mg	White	Coated Tablet		Creighton Pharmaceutical
CP; 273; TEMAZEPAM; 30 MG	Temazepam	30 mg	Aqua	Capsule		Creighton Products
CP; 820	Amoxicillin	250 mg	Tan and Beige	Capsule		Consolidated Pharmaceutical
CP; 825	Amoxicillin	500 mg	Light Yellow	Capsule		Consolidated Midland
CP; 845	Penicillin V Potassium	500 mg	White	Tablet	Oval, Scored	Consolidated Midland
CPC; 737	Vica-Forte	8000 IU; 50 IU; 150 mg; 80 mg; 70 mg; 25 mg; 10 mg; 10 mg; 5 mg; 4 mg; 2 mg; 1 mg; 10 mcg	Orange and Black	Capsule		Qualitest Products
CPC; 1025	Therobec	500 mg; 15 mg; 15 mg; 100 mg; 4 mg; 18 mg; 0.5 mg; 5 mcg	Olive	Tablet		Qualitest Products
CPC; 1027	Therobec Plus	5000 IU; 30 IU; 500 mg; 20 mg; 20 mg; 100 mg; 25 mg; 0.15 mg; 25 mg; 0.8 mg; 50 mg; 27 mg; 0.1 mg; 50 mg; 5 mg; 3 mg; 22.5 mg	Yellow	Tablet		Qualitest Products
CPC; 1132	Q-Fed	30 mg	Red	Coated Tablet		Qualitest Products
CPC; 1327	Ferrocite F	324 mg; 1 mg	Light Blue	Tablet	Capsule-Shape	Breckenridge Pharmaceutical
CPI; AO2	Caffeine	200 mg	Pink	Tablet	Biconcave	Medicopharma
CPI; FO1	Folic Acid	1 mg	Yellow	Tablet	Concave, Bisected Scored	Medicopharma
CPM; PSE	Chlorpheniramine Maleate and Pseudoephedrine Hydrochloride	120 mg; 8 mg	Blue and Clear	Extended-Release Capsule		Pharmafab
CPM; PSE	De-Congestine	8 mg; 120 mg	Blue and Clear with White Beads	Extended-Release Capsule		Qualitest Products
CPM 8; CPM 8	Chlorpheniramine TR	8 mg	Green and Clear	Capsule		Qualitest Products
CRIXIVAN; 100 MG	Crixivan	100 mg	White Semi-Translucent	Capsule		Merck
CRIXIVAN; 200 MG	Crixivan	200 mg	White Semi-Translucent	Capsule		Merck & Company
CRIXIVAN; 333 MG	Crixivan	333 mg	White with a Red Band	Capsule		Merck & Company
CRIXIVAN; 400 MG	Crixivan	400 mg	White Semi-Translucent	Capsule		Merck
CS; 11; SILVER	Centrum Silver	9 mg; 6000 IU; 1.5 mg; 1.7 mg; 3 mg; 25 mcg; 30 mcg; 200 mcg; 20 mg; 10 mg; 60 mg; 400 IU; 45 IU; 10 mcg; 200 mg; 2 mg; 150 mcg; 100 mg; 48 mg; 15 mg; 72 mg; 100 mcg; 2.5 mg; 25 mcg; 5 mcg; 80 mg; 25 mcg; 10 mcg	Light Grey	Geltab		Wyeth Consumer Healthcare
CT	Myfortic	360 mg	Pale Orange-Red	Enteric-Coated Tablet	Oval	Novartis
CTA	Children's Tylenol Allergy-D	80 mg; 6.25 mg; 7.5 mg	Pink	Tablet, Chewable	Circle	Mcneil Consumer Products
CTS	Children's Tylenol Sinus	80 mg; 7.5 mg	Pink	Tablet, Chewable	Circle	Mcneil Consumer Products
CY	Cyklokapron	500 mg	White	Tablet	Circle, Flat, with Beveled Edges	Pharmacia & Upjohn
CYCRIN; C	Premphase Medroxyprogesterone	5 mg	Light Purple	Tablet	Oval, Scored	Wyeth Pharmaceuticals
CYP; 106	Mst 600	600 mg	Yellow	Tablet	Circle	Cypress Pharmaceutical
CYP; 179	Prenatal U	106.5 mg; 10 mg; 5 mg; 1 mg; 10 mg; 0.8 mg; 200 mg; 6 mg; 15 mcg; 30 mg; 1.3 mg	Blue	Capsule		Cypress Pharmaceutical
CYP; 227	G/p 1200/75	1200 mg; 75 mg	White	Extended-Release Tablet	Capsule-Shape, Scored	Cypress Pharmaceutical
CYP 241	Anextuss	600 mg; 40 mg; 60 mg	White	Tablet		Cypress Pharmaceutical
CYP; 242	Pendex	600 mg; 10 mg	White	Tablet	Capsule-Shape	Cypress Pharmaceutical
CYP; 250	Cpm 8/pe 20/msc 1.25	20 mg; 8 mg; 1.25 mg	White	Tablet	Capsule-Shape, Scored	Cypress Pharmaceutical
CYP; 253	Gfn 795/pse 85	795 mg; 85 mg		Extended-Release Tablet		Cypress Pharmaceutical
CYP; 254	Gfn 800 and Pse 60	800 mg; 60 mg	White	Extended-Release Tablet	Capsule-Shape	Cypress Pharmaceutical
CYP; 255	Gfn 1200/pse 50	1200 mg; 50 mg	White	Extended-Release Tablet	Capsule-Shape	Cypress Pharmaceutical
CYP; 268	Gfn 1200/DM 60/pse 60	60 mg; 1200 mg; 60 mg	White	Extended-Release Tablet	Capsule-Shape, Scored	Cypress Pharmaceutical
CYP; 276	Gfn 595/pse 48/DM 32	32 mg; 595 mg; 48 mg		Extended-Release Tablet		Cypress Pharmaceutical
CYP; 279	Gfn 550/pse 60	550 mg; 60 mg	White	Extended-Release Tablet	Capsule-Shape	Cypress Pharmaceutical

IMPRINT	BRAND/GENERIC NAME	STRENGTH	COLOR	FORM	SHAPE	MANUFACTURER
CYP; 280	Pcm LA	90 mg; 8 mg; 2.5 mg	Whtie	Tablet	Capsule-Shape, Scored	Cypress Pharmaceutical
CYP; 282	Pannaz	8 mg; 2.5 mg; 90 mg	White	Extended-Release Tablet	Capsule-Shape	Pamlab
CYP; 284	Gfn 1200 and Phenylephrine 40	1200 mg; 40 mg	White	Extended-Release Tablet	Oval	Cypress Pharmaceutical
CYP; 285	Gfn 595/pse 48	595 mg; 48 mg		Extended-Release Tablet		Cypress Pharmaceutical
CYP; 286	Gfn 500/DM 30	30 mg; 500 mg	White	Extended-Release Tablet	Capsule-Shape, Scored	Cypress Pharmaceutical
CYP; 287	Gfn 550/pse 60/DM 30	30 mg; 550 mg; 60 mg		Extended-Release Tablet		Cypress Pharmaceutical
CYP; 288	Gfn 1000/DM 50	50 mg; 1000 mg	White	Extended-Release Tablet	Capsule-Shape, Scored	Cypress Pharmaceutical
CYP; 292	Gfn 1200 and DM 60	30 mg; 800 mg	White to Off-White	Extended-Release Tablet	Capsule-Shape	Cypress Pharmaceutical
CYP; 294	Gfn 800/pe 25	800 mg; 25 mg	White	Extended-Release Tablet	Capsule-Shape	Cypress Pharmaceutical
CYP; 295	Pse 15/cpm 2	15 mg; 2 mg	Red	Tablet, Chewable	Circle	Cypress Pharmaceutical
CYP; 471	Bidhist	6 mg	White	Extended-Release Tablet	Oval	Cypress Pharmaceutical
CYP; 512	Msp-Blu	0.12 mg; 81.6 mg; 36.2 mg; 40.8 mg; 10.8 mg	Blue	Tablet	Circle	Cypress Pharmaceutical
CYP; 512	Utira	0.12 mg; 81.6 mg; 36.2 mg; 40.8 mg; 10.8 mg	Blue	Tablet	Circle	Cypress Pharmaceutical
CYP; 515	Mhp-A	0.03 mg; 0.03 mg; 40.8 mg; 5.4 mg; 18.1 mg; 4.5 mg	Green	Tablet	Circle	Cypress Pharmaceutical
CYP 810	Lapase	1200 U; 15000 U; 15000 U	Green, Yellow	Capsule		Cypress Pharmaceutical
CYSTA; 50; MYLAN	Cystagon	50 mg	White, Opaque	Capsule		Mylan Pharmaceuticals
CYSTAGON; 150; MYLAN	Cystagon	150 mg	White, Opaque	Capsule		Mylan Pharmaceuticals
CZ;	Colazal	750 mg	Beige with Black Ink	Capsule		Salix Pharmaceuticals
D	Bronkaid	24 mg; 400 mg; 100 mg	White	Coated Tablet	Circle, Scored	Bayer Consumer Care
D	Doan's Ibuprofen Backache Pills	200 mg	White	Tablet		Novartis Consumer
D	Dristan Cold Multi-Symptom	325 mg; 2 mg; 5 mg		Tablet		Wyeth Consumer Healthcare
D0	Yasmin Light Yellow Tablet	3 mg; 0.03 mg	Light Yellow	Coated Tablet	Circle	Berlex Laboratories
D; 2.5 MG	Focalin	2.5 mg	Blue	Tablet	D-Shape	Novartis
D; 5 MG	Focalin	5 mg	Yellow	Tablet	D-Shape	Novartis
D; 10 MG	Focalin	10 mg	White	Tablet	D-Shape	Novartis
D; 24	Clarinex-D 24 Hour	5 mg; 240 mg	Light Blue	Tablet, Extended Release	Oval	Schering
D; 31	Demerol Apap	50 mg; 300 mg	Red	Tablet	Circle	Sanofi Winthrop Pharmaceuticals
D; 92	Drisdol	50000 IU	Green	Capsule, Liquid Filled		Sanofi Winthrop Pharmaceuticals
D35; W	Demerol Hydrochloride	50 mg	White	Tablet	Circle, Scored	Sanofi Winthrop Pharmaceuticals
D37; W	Demerol Hydrochloride	100 mg	White	Tablet	Circle	Sanofi Winthrop Pharmaceuticals
DALLERGY; H12;	Dallergy	8 mg; 20 mg; 2.5 mg	White	Extended-Release Tablet	Capsule-Shape	Laser
DALLERGY JR; LASER; 176	Dallergy-JR.	60 mg; 6 mg	Yellow and Clear	Extended-Release Capsule		Laser
DALMANE; 15; ICN;	Dalmane	15 mg	Orange and Ivory	Capsule		Icn Pharmaceuticals
DALMANE; 30; ICN;	Dalmane	30 mg	Red and Ivory	Capsule		Icn Pharmaceuticals
DAN; 2; 5621	Diazepam	2 mg	White	Tablet	Circle, Scored	Watson Laboratories
DAN; 5; 5619	Diazepam	5 mg	Yellow	Tablet	Circle, Scored	Watson Laboratories
DAN; 5; 5882	Methylphenidate Hydrochloride	5 mg	Purple	Tablet	Circle	Watson Laboratories
DAN; 10; 5554	Propranolol Hydrochloride	10 mg	Orange	Tablet	Circle, Scored	Watson Laboratories
DAN; 10; 5620	Diazepam	10 mg	Light Blue	Tablet	Circle, Scored	Watson Laboratories
DAN; 10; 5883	Methylphenidate Hydrochloride	10 mg	Green	Tablet	Circle	Watson Laboratories
DAN; 20; 5884	Methylphenidate Hydrochloride	20 mg	Peach	Tablet	Circle	Watson Laboratories
DAN; 50; 5777	Atenolol	50 mg	White	Tablet	Circle	Watson Laboratories
DAN; 59; 12	Captopril and Hydrochlorothiazide	50 mg; 25 mg	Blue	Tablet	Oval, Scored	Danbury Pharmacal
DAN; 944	Colchicine	0.6 mg	White	Tablet	Circle	Watson Laboratories
DAN; 3120	Clindamycin Hydrochloride	300 mg	Pink	Capsule		Watson Laboratories
DAN; 5017	Chlorpheniramine Maleate	12 mg	Green and Clear	Timed-Release Capsule		West-Ward
DAN; 5050	Hydralazine Hydrochloride	25 mg	Blue	Tablet		West-Ward
DAN; 5052;	Prednisone	5 mg	White	Tablet	Circle, Scored	Watson Laboratories
DAN; 5055	Hydralazine Hydrochloride	50 mg	Light Blue	Tablet		West-Ward
DAN; 5059 DAN	Prednisolone	5 mg	Peach	Tablet	Circle, Scored	Watson Laboratories
DAN; 5196	Papaverine Hydrochloride	150 mg	Brown and Clear	Timed-Release Capsule		West-Ward
DAN; 5216; DAN	Folic Acid	1 mg	Yellow	Tablet	Circle, Scored	Danbury Pharmacal
DAN; 5216; DAN	Folic Acid	1 mg	Yellow	Tablet	Circle, Scored	Watson Laboratories
DAN; 5257	Propantheline Bromide	15 mg		Tablet		West-Ward
DAN; 5307; DAN	Promethazine Hydrochloride	25 mg	White	Tablet	Circle, Scored	Watson Laboratories
DAN; 5319	Promethazine Hydrochloride	50 mg	White	Tablet	Circle	Watson Laboratories
DAN; 5321; DAN	Primidone	250 mg	White	Tablet	Circle, Scored	Watson Laboratories
DAN; 5325	Probenecid with Colchicine	500 mg; 0.5 mg	White	Tablet		West-Ward
DAN; 5325; DAN	Probenecid and Colchicine	0.5 mg; 500 mg	White	Tablet	Capsule-Shape, Scored	Watson Laboratories
DAN; 5333	Procainamide Hydrochloride	500 mg	Yellow and Orange	Capsule		West-Ward
DAN; 5335	Trihexane	2 mg		Tablet		Dan Pharmacal
DAN; 5335; DAN	Trihexyphenidyl Hydrochloride	2 mg	White	Tablet	Circle, Scored	Watson Laboratories
DAN; 5337; DAN	Trihexyphenidyl Hydrochloride	5 mg	White	Tablet	Circle, Scored	Watson Laboratories
DAN; 5347	Probenecid	0.5 G	Yellow	Tablet		West-Ward
DAN; 5347; DAN	Probenecid	500 mg	Yellow	Coated Tablet	Capsule-Shape, Scored	Watson Laboratories
DAN; 5368; DAN	Disulfiram	500 mg	Off-White	Tablet	Circle, Scored	Danbury Pharmacal
DAN; 5368; DAN	Disulfiram	500 mg	Off-White	Tablet	Circle, Scored	Schein Pharmaceutical
DAN; 5376; DAN	Disulfiram	250 mg	Off-White	Tablet	Circle, Scored	Danbury Pharmacal

IMPRINT	BRAND/GENERIC NAME	STRENGTH	COLOR	FORM	SHAPE	MANUFACTURER
DAN; 5376; DAN	Disulfiram	250 mg	Off-White	Tablet	Circle, Scored	Schein Pharmaceutical
DAN; 5379	Erythromycin Estolate	250 mg	Orange and White	Capsule		Danbury Pharmacal
DAN; 5381; DAN	Methocarbamol	500 mg	White	Tablet	Circle, Scored	Danbury Pharmacal
DAN; 5381; DAN	Methocarbamol	500 mg	White	Tablet	Circle, Scored	Schein Pharmaceutical
DAN; DAN; 5382	Methocarbamol	750 mg	White	Tablet	Oval, Scored	Watson Laboratories
DAN; DAN; 5406	Hydroserpine	25 mg	Green	Tablet	Circle, Scored	H.L. Moore
DAN; DAN; 5407	Hydroserpine	50 mg	Green	Tablet	Circle, Scored	H.L. Moore
DAN; 5428	Hydralazine Complex	15 mg; 25 mg; 0.1 mg	Pink	Tablet		Danbury Pharmacal
DAN; 5428	Hydralazine Complex	15 mg; 25 mg; 0.1 mg	Pink	Tablet		West-Ward
DAN; 5428	Reserpine, Hydralazine Hydrochloride and Hydrochlorothiazide	25 mg; 15 mg; 0.1 mg	Yellow	Tablet	Circle	Danbury Pharmacal
DAN; 5428	Reserpine, Hydralazine Hydrochloride and Hydrochlorothiazide	25 mg; 15 mg; 0.1 mg	Yellow	Tablet	Circle	Schein Pharmaceutical
DAN; 5430; DAN	Acetazolamide	250 mg	White	Tablet	Circle, Scored	Watson Laboratories
DAN; 5438 DAN	Quinidine Sulfate	200 mg	White	Tablet	Scored, Circle	Watson Laboratories
DAN; 5440	Doxycycline Hyclate	100 mg	Light Blue	Capsule		Watson Laboratories
DAN; 5442 DAN	Prednisone	10 mg	White	Tablet	Circle, Scored	Watson Laboratories
DAN; 5443 DAN	Prednisone	20 mg	Peach	Tablet	Circle, Scored	Watson Laboratories
DAN; 5453	Quinidine Sulfate	100 mg		Tablet		Danbury Pharmacal
DAN; 5454; DAN	Quinidine Sulfate	300 mg	White	Tablet	Circle, Scored	Watson Laboratories
DAN; 5455; DAN	Chlorpropamide	250 mg	Blue	Tablet	Circle, Scored	Danbury Pharmacal
DAN; 5455; DAN	Chlorpropamide	250 mg	Blue	Tablet	Circle, Scored	Schein Pharmaceutical
DAN; 5507	Chlorthalidone	25 mg	Yellow or Orange	Tablet	Circle	Danbury Pharmacal
DAN; 5507	Chlorthalidone	25 mg	Yellow or Orange	Tablet	Circle	Schein Pharmaceutical
DAN; 5513	Carisoprodol	350 mg	White	Tablet	Circle	H.L. Moore
DAN; 5513	Carisoprodol	350 mg	White	Tablet	Circle	Watson Laboratories
DAN; 5518	Chlorthalidone	50 mg	Light Green or Light Blue	Tablet	Circle	Danbury Pharmacal
DAN; 5518	Chlorthalidone	50 mg	Light Green or Light Blue	Tablet	Circle	Schein Pharmaceutical
DAN; 5522;	Hydroxyzine Hydrochloride	10 mg	Orange	Coated Tablet	Circle	Watson Laboratories
DAN; 5523	Hydroxyzine Hydrochloride	25 mg	Green	Coated Tablet	Circle	Watson Laboratories
DAN; 5535;	Doxycycline Hyclate	50 mg	LT. Blue and White	Capsule		Watson Laboratories
DAN; 5540	Metronidazole	250 mg	White to Off-White	Tablet	Circle	Watson Laboratories
DAN; 5543; DAN	Allopurinol	100 mg	White	Tablet	Circle, Scored	Watson Laboratories
DAN; DAN; 5543	Allopurinol	100 mg	White	Tablet	Circle, Scored	Watson Laboratories
DAN; 5544; DAN	Allopurinol	300 mg	Orange	Tablet	Circle, Scored	Watson Laboratories
DAN; DAN; 5544	Allopurinol	300 mg	Orange	Tablet	Circle, Scored	Watson Laboratories
DAN; 5552; DAN	Metronidazole	500 mg	White to Off-White	Tablet	Circle, Scored	Watson Laboratories
DAN; 5553	Doxycycline Hyclate	100 mg	Orange	Coated Tablet	Circle	Watson Laboratories
DAN; 5555; 20	Propranolol Hydrochloride	20 mg	Light Blue	Tablet	Circle, Scored	Watson Laboratories
DAN; 5556; 40	Propranolol Hydrochloride	40 mg	Light Green	Tablet	Circle, Scored	Watson Laboratories
DAN; 5557; 80	Propranolol Hydrochloride	80 mg	Yellow	Tablet	Circle, Scored	Watson Laboratories
DAN; 5560	Disopyramide Phosphate	100 mg	Opaque Orange	Capsule		Watson Laboratories
DAN; 5561	Disopyramide Phosphate	150 mg	Opaque Brown	Capsule		Watson Laboratories
DAN; 5579; DAN	Chlorpropamide	100 mg	Blue	Tablet	Circle, Scored	Danbury Pharmacal
DAN; 5579; DAN	Chlorpropamide	100 mg	Blue	Tablet	Circle, Scored	Schein Pharmaceutical
DAN; 5582; DAN	Tolazamide	250 mg	White	Tablet	Circle, Scored	Danbury Pharmacal
DAN; 5582; DAN	Tolazamide	250 mg	White	Tablet	Circle, Scored	Schein Pharmaceutical
DAN; 5584	Ibuprofen	400 mg	White	Coated Tablet	Circle	Danbury Pharmacal
DAN; 5586	Ibuprofen	600 mg	White	Coated Tablet	Oval	Danbury Pharmacal
DAN; 5590; DAN	Tolazamide	500 mg	White	Tablet	Circle, Scored	Danbury Pharmacal
DAN; 5590; DAN	Tolazamide	500 mg	White	Tablet	Circle, Scored	Schein Pharmaceutical
DAN; 5591; DAN	Tolazamide	100 mg	White	Tablet	Circle, Scored	Danbury Pharmacal
DAN; 5591; DAN	Tolazamide	100 mg	White	Tablet	Circle, Scored	Schein Pharmaceutical
DAN; 5593	Thiothixene	1 mg	Yellow	Capsule		H.L. Moore
DAN; 5599; DAN	Trazodone Hcl	100 mg	White	Coated Tablet	Circle, Scored	Watson Laboratories
DAN DAN; 5600;	Trazodone Hydrochloride	50 mg	White	Coated Tablet	Circle, Scored	Watson Laboratories
DAN; 5629	Doxepin Hydrochloride	10 mg	Buff	Capsule		Watson Laboratories
DAN; 5630	Doxepin Hydrochloride	25 mg	White and Ivory	Capsule		Watson Laboratories
DAN; 5631	Doxepin Hydrochloride	50 mg	Ivory	Capsule		Watson Laboratories
DAN; 5632	Doxepin Hydrochloride	75 mg	Light Green	Capsule		Watson Laboratories
DAN; 5633	Doxepin Hydrochloride	100 mg	Green and White	Capsule		Watson Laboratories
DAN; 5642; 2.5	Minoxidil	2.5 mg	White	Tablet	Circle, Scored	Watson Laboratories
DAN; 5643; 10	Minoxidil	10 mg	White	Tablet	Circle, Scored	Watson Laboratories
DAN; 5644	Ibuprofen	800 mg	White	Coated Tablet	Oval	Danbury Pharmacal
DAN; 5658	Cyclobenzaprine Hydrochloride	10 mg	White	Tablet	Circle	Vangard Labs
DAN; 5658	Cyclobenzaprine Hydrochloride	10 mg	White	Coated Tablet	Circle	Watson Laboratories
DAN; 5660; DAN	Sulindac	200 mg	Yellow	Tablet	Circle, Scored	Watson Laboratories
DAN; 5661	Sulindac	150 mg	Yellow	Tablet	Circle	Watson Laboratories
DAN; 5682	Triamterene and Hydrochlorothiazide	75 mg; 50 mg	Yellow	Tablet	Circle, Scored	Danbury Pharmacal
DAN; 5694; MINOCYCLINE; 50	Minocycline Hydrochloride	50 mg	Yellow	Capsule		Watson Laboratories
DAN; 5695; MINOCYCLINE; 100	Minocycline Hydrochloride	100 mg	Gray and Yellow	Capsule		Watson Laboratories
DAN; 5708	Clindamycin Hydrochloride	150 mg	Gray and Pink	Capsule		Danbury Pharmacal
DAN; 5708	Clindamycin Hydrochloride	150 mg	Gray and Pink	Capsule		Schein Pharmaceutical
DAN; 5726	Hydroxyzine Pamoate	25 mg	Dark Green and Light Green	Capsule		Watson Laboratories
DAN; 5730; 10	Baclofen	10 mg	White	Tablet	Circle, Scored	Watson Laboratories
DAN; 5731; 20	Baclofen	20 mg	White	Tablet	Circle, Scored	Watson Laboratories
DAN; 5778; 100	Atenolol	100 mg	White	Tablet	Circle	Watson Laboratories

IMPRINT	BRAND/GENERIC NAME	STRENGTH	COLOR	FORM	SHAPE	MANUFACTURER
DAN; 5782	Atenolol and Chlorthalidone	50 mg; 25 mg	White	Tablet	Circle, Scored	Watson Laboratories
DAN; 5783	Atenolol and Chlorthalidone	100 mg; 25 mg	White	Tablet	Circle	Watson Laboratories
DANOCRINE; WINTHROP; D05; 200 MG;	Danocrine	200 mg	Orange	Capsule		Winthrop Pharmaceuticals
DANTRIUM 25 MG; 0149 0030	Dantrium	25 mg	Opaque, Orange and Tan	Capsule		Procter & Gamble Pharmaceuticals
DANTRIUM 50 MG; 0149 0031	Dantrium	50 mg	Opaque, Orange and Tan	Capsule		Procter & Gamble Pharmaceuticals
DANTRIUM 100 MG; 0149 0033	Dantrium	100 mg	Opaque, Orange and Tan	Capsule		Procter & Gamble Pharmaceuticals
DARAPRIM; A3A	Daraprim	25 mg	White	Tablet		Glaxosmithkline
DARVON COMP	Darvon Compound	32 mg; 389 mg; 32.4 mg	Pink	Capsule		Eli Lilly
DAY	Day Time Cold Medicine Liquid Caps	250 mg; 10 mg; 30 mg; 100 mg	Dark Orange	Capsule, Liquid Filled		Leiner Health Products
DAY	Day Time Cold Medicine Liquid Caps	250 mg; 10 mg; 30 mg; 100 mg	Dark Orange	Capsule, Liquid Filled		Scherer Laboratories
DAYPRO; 1381	Daypro	600 mg	White	Coated Tablet	Capsule-Shape, Scored	Searle
DAYQUIL; SINUS PAIN	Dayquil Sinus Pressure and Pain Relief with Ibuprofen	30 mg; 200 mg	White	Tablet		Procter & Gamble
DCI; PANCRECARB MS-4	Pancrecarb Ms-4	4000 U; 25000 U; 25000 U	Clear with Blue Ink	Extended-Release Capsule		Digestive Care
DCI; PANCRECARB MS-8	Pancrecarb Ms-8	8000 U; 40000 U; 45000 U	Clear with Blue Ink	Extended-Release Capsule		Digestive Care
DDAVP; 0.2; RPR;	Ddavp	0.2 mg	White	Tablet	Circle, Scored on 1 Side	Aventis Pharmaceuticals
DECONGEST; 12 HOUR	Decongest 12 Hour Maximum Strength	120 mg; 12 mg	Red and White	Tablet	Oval	Thompson Medical
DEFEN	Defen-LA	60 mg; 600 mg	White	Sustained-Release Tablet		First Horizon Pharmaceutical
DELTASONE; 2.5	Deltasone	2.5 mg	Pink	Tablet	Circle, Scored	Pharmacia & Upjohn
DELTASONE; 5	Deltasone	5 mg	White	Tablet	Circle, Scored	Pharmacia & Upjohn
DELTASONE; 10	Deltasone	10 mg	White	Tablet	Circle, Scored	Pharmacia & Upjohn
DELTASONE; 20	Deltasone	20 mg	Peach	Tablet	Circle, Scored	Pharmacia & Upjohn
DELTASONE; 50;	Deltasone	50 mg	White	Tablet	Circle, Scored	Pharmacia & Upjohn
DEPADE; 50	Depade	50 mg	Pastel Orange	Tablet	Circle, Scored	Mallinckrodt
DEPAKENE	Depakene	250 mg	Orange	Capsule, Liquid Filled		Abbott Laboratories
DEPAKOTE SPRINKLE 125 MG; THIS END UP	Depakote Sprinkle	125 mg	White Opaque/blue	Capsule		Abbott Laboratories
DERMIK; 044	Durrax	10 mg	Lavender	Tablet	Circle	Dermik Laboratories
DERMIK; 045	Durrax	25 mg	Lavender	Tablet	Circle	Dermik Laboratories
DF; 15	Enablex	15 mg	Light Peach	Tablet, Extended Release	Circle	Novartis Pharmaceuticals
DIA; B;	Diabeta	1.25 mg	Peach	Tablet	Oblong, Scored	Aventis Pharmaceuticals
DIA; B;	Diabeta	2.5 mg	Peach	Tablet	Oblong, Scored	Aventis Pharmaceuticals
DIA; B;	Diabeta	5 mg	Light Green	Tablet	Oblong, Scored	Aventis Pharmaceuticals
DIAMOX; D3	Diamox Sequels	500 mg	Orange	Extended-Release Capsule		Lederle Laboratories
DIAMOX; D3	Diamox Sequels	500 mg	Orange	Extended-Release Capsule		Wyeth Pharmaceuticals
DIAMOX; D3	Diamox Sequels	500 mg	Orange	Extended-Release Capsule		Wyeth-Ayerst Laboratories
DIASORB	Diasorb	750 mg	Pink	Tablet	Circle	Columbia Laboratories
DIFIL-G; MD; 305	Difil-G	200 mg; 200 mg	White	Coated Tablet	Circle	Med-Derm Pharmaceuticals
DIFLUCAN; 50; ROERIG	Diflucan	50 mg	Pink	Tablet	Four-Sided	Pfizer Roerig
DIFLUCAN; 100; ROERIG	Diflucan	100 mg	Pink	Tablet	Four-Sided	Pfizer Roerig
DIFLUCAN; 150; ROERIG	Diflucan	150 mg	Pink	Tablet	Oval	Pfizer Roerig
DIFLUCAN; 200; ROERIG	Diflucan	200 mg	Pink	Tablet	Four-Sided	Pfizer Roerig
DI-GEL	Di-Gel	25 mg; 280 mg; 128 mg	Yellow and White	Tablet		Schering-Plough
DIGOXIN; 233; ALRA	Digoxin	0.125 mg	Light Yellow	Tablet	Round, Bisected Scored	Alra Laboratories
DIGOXIN; 234; ALRA	Digoxin	0.25 mg	White	Tablet	Round, Bisected Scored	Alra Laboratories
DIGOXIN; 235; ALRA	Digoxin	0.5 mg	White	Tablet	Round, Bisected Scored	Alra Laboratories
DILANTIN; 100 MG	Dilantin Kapseals	100 mg	White with Orange Band	Extended-Release Capsule		Parke-Davis
DIPENTUM; 250 MG	Dipentum	250 mg	Beige	Capsule		Pharmacia & Upjohn
DISALCID; 750; 3M	Disalcid	750 mg	Aqua	Coated Tablet	Capsule-Shaped, Bisected Scored	3m Pharmaceuticals
DISALCID; 3M	Disalcid	500 mg	Aqua	Coated Tablet	Round, Bisected Scored	3m Pharmaceuticals
DISALCID; 3M	Disalcid	500 mg	Aqua and White	Capsule		3m Pharmaceuticals
DISTA; 3055; CINOBAC 250 MG	Cinobac	250 mg	Orange and Green	Capsule		Dista Products
DISTA; 3056; CINOBAC 500 MG	Cinobac	500 mg	Orange and Green	Capsule		Dista Products
DISTA; 3104; PROZAC; 10 MG	Prozac	10 mg	Green and Gray	Capsule		Dista Products
DISTA; 3105; PROZAC; 20 MG	Prozac	20 mg	Green and Off-White	Capsule		Dista Products
DISTA; 3107; PROZAC 40 MG	Prozac	40 mg	Green and Orange	Capsule		Dista Products
DISTA; 3122	CO-Pyronil 2	2 mg; 30 mg	Red	Capsule		Dista Products
DISTA; 3123	CO-Pyronil 2	4 mg; 60 mg	Yellow and Green	Capsule		Dista Products

IMPRINT	BRAND/GENERIC NAME	STRENGTH	COLOR	FORM	SHAPE	MANUFACTURER
DISTA; 4142	Keftab	250 mg	Light Green	Tablet	Circle	Dista Products
DISTA; C19	MI-Cebrin	10 mg; 5 mg; 1.7 mg; 10 mg; 30 mg; 3 mcg; 100 mg; 5.5 mg; 10000 IU; 400 IU	Yellow	Tablet		Dista Products
DISTA; C20	MI-Cebrin T	15 mg; 10 mg; 2 mg; 10 mg; 100 mg; 7.5 mcg; 150 mg; 10000 IU; 400 IU	Orange	Coated Tablet		Dista Products
DISTA; C22	Becotin-T	15 mg; 10 mg; 5 mg; 100 mg; 20 mg; 4 mcg; 300 mg	Orange	Coated Tablet	Oval	Dista Products
DISTA; F62	Becotin	10 mg; 10 mg; 4.1 mg; 50 mg; 25 mg; 1 mcg		Tablet		Dista Products
DISTA; F77	Becotin with Vitamin C	10 mg; 10 mg; 4.1 mg; 50 mg; 25 mg; 1 mcg; 150 mg	Green and Black	Tablet		Dista Products
DISTA; H09	Ilosone	250 mg	Ivory and Red	Capsule		Dista Products
DISTA; H69; KEFLEX; 250 MG	Keflex	250 mg	White and Dark Green	Capsule		Dista Products
DISTA; H71; KEFLEX; 500 MG	Keflex	500 mg	Light Green and Dark Green	Capsule		Dista Products
DISTA; H76; NALFON 200	Nalfon	200 mg	Ocher and White	Capsule		Dista Products
DISTA; U26	Ilosone	500 mg	Pink or White	Coated Tablet	Capsule-Shape, Scored	Dista Products
DISTA; U60	Keflex	1 G	Green	Tablet	Capsule-Shape	Dista Products
DITROPAN; 92; 00;	Ditropan	5 mg	Blue	Tablet	Biconvex, Scored	Alza
DIUCARDIN; 50	Diucardin	50 mg	White	Tablet	Oval, Scored	Wyeth Pharmaceuticals
DO; NVR	Diovan	40 mg	Yellow	Tablet	Circle, Bevel-Edged	Novartis
DOAN'S	Doan's, Extra Strength	467.2 mg	White	Tablet	Capsule-Shape	Novartis Consumer
DOAN'S PM	Extra Strength Doan's Pm	580 mg; 25 mg	Light Blue	Tablet	Capsule-Shape	Novartis Consumer
DORAL; 7.5	Doral	7.5 mg	Light Orange with White Speckles	Tablet	Capsule-Shape	Wallace Laboratories
DORAL; 15	Doral	15 mg	Light Orange with White Speckles	Tablet	Capsule-Shape	Wallace Laboratories
DORMALIN; 722	Dormalin	15 mg	Light Orange	Tablet	Capsule-Shape	Schering
DORMIN; 25	Dormin	25 mg	Pink	Capsule		West-Ward
DORSEY	Kanulase	9 mg; 500 mg; 200 mg; 100 mg; 150 mg	Pink	Tablet		Novartis Consumer
DORSEY	Kanulase	9 mg; 500 mg; 200 mg; 100 mg; 150 mg	Pink	Tablet		Sandoz Consumer Pharmaceuticals
DORSEY	Rautensin	2 mg	Orange	Tablet	Circle, Scored	Novartis Pharmaceuticals
DORSEY	Wilpo	8 mg	Green	Tablet		Novartis Pharmaceuticals
DOW; 11	Novahistine Fortis	10 mg; 2 mg	Green and White	Capsule		Glaxosmithkline Consumer
DOW; 71	Novahistine Sinus	325 mg; 30 mg; 2 mg	White	Tablet	Circle	Glaxosmithkline Consumer
DOW; 603	Phenoxene	50 mg	Beige	Tablet	Circle	Aventis Pharmaceuticals
DOXIDAN	Doxidan	30 mg; 100 mg	Dark Red	Capsule		Pharmacia & Upjohn
DOXYCHEL; 50 MG	Doxychel Hyclate	50 mg	Blue and White	Capsule		Rachelle Laboratories
DOXYCHEL; 100 MG	Doxychel Hyclate	100 mg	Blue	Capsule		Rachelle Laboratories
DOXY-TAB; 100; 581; RACHELLE	Doxy-Tabs	100 mg	Beige	Tablet		Rachelle Laboratories
DP; 01	Clonidine Hydrochloride	0.1 mg	Tan	Tablet	Hexagonal on Back and Round on Front, Scored	Duramed Pharmaceuticals
DP; 02	Clonidine Hydrochloride	0.2 mg	Orange	Tablet	Hexagonal on Back and Round on Front, Scored	Duramed Pharmaceuticals
DP; 03	Clonidine Hydrochloride	0.3 mg	Peach	Tablet	Hexagonal on Front and Round on Back, Scored	Duramed Pharmaceuticals
DP; 016	Aviane 28 Orange Tablet	0.02 mg; 0.1 mg	Orange	28-Day Tablet Pack	Circle	Barr Laboratories
DP; 021	Kariva White	0.15 mg; 0.02 mg	White	Tablet	Circle	Barr Laboratories
DP; 022	Kariva Light Blue	0.01 mg	Light Blue	Tablet	Circle	Barr Laboratories
DP; 042	V-Throid	300 mcg	Green	Tablet	Circle	Daniels Pharmaceuticals
DP; 048	V-Throid	500 mcg	White	Tablet	Circle	Daniels Pharmaceuticals
DP; 068	V-Throid	100 mcg	Yellow	Tablet	Circle	Daniels Pharmaceuticals
DP; 069	V-Throid	200 mcg	Pink	Tablet	Circle	Daniels Pharmaceuticals
DP; 099; DIAMYCIN	Diamycin	50 mg; 0.5 mg	Off-White	Tablet	Circle	Daniels Pharmaceuticals
DP; 10	Propranolol Hydrochloride	10 mg	Orange	Tablet	Circle, Scored	Duramed Pharmaceuticals
DP; 11	Trifluoperazine Hydrochloride	1 mg	Lavender	Coated Tablet		Duramed Pharmaceuticals
DP; 12	Trifluoperazine Hydrochloride	2 mg	Lavender	Coated Tablet		Duramed Pharmaceuticals
DP; 13	Trifluoperazine Hydrochloride	5 mg	Lavender	Coated Tablet		Duramed Pharmaceuticals
DP; 14	Trifluoperazine Hydrochloride	10 mg	Lavender	Coated Tablet		Duramed Pharmaceuticals
DP; 15	Diazepam	2 mg	White	Tablet	Circle, Scored	Duramed Pharmaceuticals
DP; 20	Propranolol Hydrochloride	20 mg	Blue	Tablet	Circle, Scored	Duramed Pharmaceuticals
DP; 25	Dipyridamole	25 mg	White	Tablet	Circle	Duramed Pharmaceuticals
DP; 25	Levoxyl	25 mcg	Orange	Tablet	Oval, Notched	Monarch Pharmaceuticals
DP; 30	Conjugated Estrogens	0.3 mg		Tablet		Duramed Pharmaceuticals
DP; 31	Conjugated Estrogens	0.625 mg		Tablet		Duramed Pharmaceuticals
DP; 32	Conjugated Estrogens	1.25 mg		Tablet		Duramed Pharmaceuticals
DP; 33	Conjugated Estrogen	2.5 mg		Tablet		Duramed Pharmaceuticals
DP; 34	Conjugated Estrogens	2.5 mg		Tablet		Duramed Pharmaceuticals
DP; 40	Propranolol Hydrochloride	40 mg	Green	Tablet	Circle, Scored	Duramed Pharmaceuticals

IMPRINT	BRAND/GENERIC NAME	STRENGTH	COLOR	FORM	SHAPE	MANUFACTURER
DP; 41	Cenestin	0.3 mg	Green	Tablet	Circle	Barr Laboratories
DP; 41	Cenestin	0.3 mg	Green	Tablet	Circle	Duramed Pharmaceuticals
DP; 42	Cenestin	0.625 mg	Red	Tablet	Circle	Barr Laboratories
DP; 42	Cenestin	0.625 mg	Red	Coated Tablet	Circle	Duramed Pharmaceuticals
DP; 42	Cenestin	0.625 mg	Red	Tablet	Circle	Duramed Pharmaceuticals
DP; 43	Cenestin	0.9 mg	White	Tablet	Circle	Barr Laboratories
DP; 43	Cenestin	0.9 mg	White	Coated Tablet	Circle	Duramed Pharmaceuticals
DP; 43	Cenestin	0.9 mg	White	Tablet	Circle	Duramed Pharmaceuticals
DP; 44	Cenestin	1.25 mg	Blue	Tablet	Circle	Barr Laboratories
DP; 44	Cenestin	1.25 mg	Blue	Tablet	Circle	Duramed Pharmaceuticals
DP; 50	Dipyridamole	50 mg	White	Tablet	Circle	Duramed Pharmaceuticals
DP; 50;	Levoxyl	50 mcg	White	Tablet	Oval, Notched	Monarch Pharmaceuticals
DP; 60	Propranolol Hydrochloride	60 mg	Pink	Tablet	Circle, Scored	Duramed Pharmaceuticals
DP; 75	Dipyridamole	75 mg	White	Tablet	Circle	Duramed Pharmaceuticals
DP; 75	Levoxyl	75 mcg	Purple	Tablet	Oval, Notched	Monarch Pharmaceuticals
DP; 80	Propranolol Hydrochloride	80 mg	Yellow	Tablet	Circle, Scored	Duramed Pharmaceuticals
DP; 88	Levoxyl	88 mcg	Olive	Tablet	Oval, Notched	Monarch Pharmaceuticals
DP; 90	Propranolol Hydrochloride	90 mg	Lavender	Tablet	Circle, Scored	Duramed Pharmaceuticals
DP; 100	Levoxyl	100 mcg	Yellow	Tablet	Oval, Notched	Monarch Pharmaceuticals
DP; 112	Levoxyl	112 mcg	Rose	Tablet	Oval, Notched	Monarch Pharmaceuticals
DP; 125	Levoxyl	125 mcg	Brown	Tablet	Oval, Notched	Monarch Pharmaceuticals
DP; 137	Levoxyl	137 mcg	Dark Blue	Tablet	Oval, Notched	Monarch Pharmaceuticals
DP; 150	Levoxyl	150 mcg	Blue	Tablet	Oval, Notched	Monarch Pharmaceuticals
DP; 175	Levoxyl	175 mcg	Turquoise	Tablet	Oval, Notched	Monarch Pharmaceuticals
DP; 200	Levoxyl	200 mcg	Pink	Tablet	Oval, Notched	Monarch Pharmaceuticals
DP; 215	Chlorzoxazone and Acetaminophen	250 mg; 300 mg		Tablet		Duramed Pharmaceuticals
DP; 223	Aminophylline	100 mg	White	Tablet	Circle, Scored	Duramed Pharmaceuticals
DP; 224	Aminophylline	200 mg	White	Tablet	Circle, Scored	Duramed Pharmaceuticals
DP; 225	Haloperidol	0.5 mg	White	Tablet	Circle, Scored	Duramed Pharmaceuticals
DP; 226	Haloperidol	1 mg	Yellow	Tablet	Circle, Scored	Duramed Pharmaceuticals
DP; 227	Haloperidol	2 mg	Lavender	Tablet	Circle, Scored	Duramed Pharmaceuticals
DP; 228	Haloperidol	5 mg	Green	Tablet	Circle, Scored	Duramed Pharmaceuticals
DP; 246	Cyproheptadine Hydrochloride	4 mg	White	Tablet	Circle	Duramed Pharmaceuticals
DP; 249	Iodoquinol	650 mg		Tablet		Duramed Pharmaceuticals
DP; 251	Chlorpropamide	250 mg	Blue	Tablet	Circle, Scored	Duramed Pharmaceuticals
DP; 252	Chlorpropamide	100 mg	Blue	Tablet	Circle, Scored	Duramed Pharmaceuticals
DP; 265	Hydroxyzine Pamoate	25 mg	Green	Capsule		Duramed Pharmaceuticals
DP; 266	Hydroxyzine Pamoate	50 mg	White and Green	Capsule		Duramed Pharmaceuticals
DP; 267	Hydroxyzine Pamoate	100 mg	Gray and Green	Capsule		Duramed Pharmaceuticals
DP; 274	Isoniazid	100 mg	White	Tablet	Circle, Scored	Duramed Pharmaceuticals
DP; 275	Indomethacin	25 mg		Capsule		Duramed Pharmaceuticals
DP; 276	Indomethacin	50 mg		Capsule		Duramed Pharmaceuticals
DP; 277	Isoniazid	300 mg	White	Tablet	Circle, Scored	Duramed Pharmaceuticals
DP; 296	Salsalate	500 mg	Blue or Yellow	Tablet	Circle	Duramed Pharmaceuticals
DP; 297	Salsalate	750 mg	Blue or Yellow	Tablet	Capsule-Shape, Scored	Duramed Pharmaceuticals
DP; 300	Levoxyl	300 mcg	Green	Tablet	Oval, Notched	Monarch Pharmaceuticals
DP; 301	Methylprednisolone	4 mg	White	Tablet	Oval, Scored	Barr Laboratories
DP; 305	Papaverine Hydrochloride	150 mg		Timed-Release Capsule		Duramed Pharmaceuticals
DP; 311	Prednisone	5 mg	White	Tablet	Circle, Scored	Duramed Pharmaceuticals
DP; 312	Prednisone	10 mg	White	Tablet	Circle, Scored	Duramed Pharmaceuticals
DP; 313	Prednisone	20 mg	Orange	Tablet	Circle, Scored	Duramed Pharmaceuticals
DP; 314	Prochlorperazine	5 mg	Yellow	Coated Tablet	Circle	H.L. Moore
DP; 314	Prochlorperazine Maleate	5 mg	Yellow	Tablet	Circle	Duramed Pharmaceuticals
DP; 315	Prochlorperazine Maleate	10 mg	Yellow	Tablet	Circle	Duramed Pharmaceuticals
DP; 316	Prochlorperazine Maleate	25 mg		Tablet		Duramed Pharmaceuticals
DP; 325	Tolazamide	100 mg	White	Tablet	Circle, Scored	Duramed Pharmaceuticals
DP; 326	Tolazamide	250 mg	White	Tablet	Circle, Scored	Duramed Pharmaceuticals
DP; 327	Tolazamide	500 mg	White	Tablet	Circle, Scored	Duramed Pharmaceuticals
DP; 332	Propranolol Hydrochloride and Hydrochlorothiazide	40 mg; 25 mg	Pale Yellow	Tablet	Circle, Scored	Duramed Pharmaceuticals
DP; 333	Propranolol Hydrochloride and Hydrochlorothiazide	80 mg; 25 mg		Tablet		Duramed Pharmaceuticals
DP; 371	Methyldopa	250 mg	White	Tablet	Circle	Duramed Pharmaceuticals
DP; 372	Methyldopa	500 mg	White	Tablet	Circle	Duramed Pharmaceuticals
DP; 401	Guaifenesin and Pseudoephedrine Hydrochloride	600 mg; 120 mg	Yellow	Extended-Release Tablet	Capsule-Shape, Scored	Duramed Pharmaceuticals
DP; 417	Guaifenesin	600 mg	Green	Extended-Release Tablet	Capsule-Shape, Scored	Duramed Pharmaceuticals
DP; 417	S-Pack P.M. Treatment Phase	600 mg	Green	Controlled-Release Tablet	Capsule-Shape, Scored	Duramed Pharmaceuticals
DP; 420	Guaifenesin DM	600 mg; 30 mg	White	Tablet	Capsule-Shape, Scored	Duramed Pharmaceuticals
DP; 420	S-Pack-DM P.M. Treatment Phase	600 mg; 30 mg	White	Controlled-Release Tablet	Capsule-Shape, Scored	Duramed Pharmaceuticals
DP; 480	Verapamil Hydrochloride SR	120 mg	Light Pink	Sustained-Release Tablet	Capsule-Shape	Duramed Pharmaceuticals
DP; 482	Verapamil Hydrochloride SR	240 mg	Light Tan	Sustained-Release Tablet	Capsule-Shape	Duramed Pharmaceuticals
DP; 501	Estradiol	0.5 mg	Lavender	Tablet	Round, Bisected Scored	Duramed Pharmaceuticals
DP; 502	Estradiol	1 mg	Rose	Tablet	Round, Bisected Scored	Duramed Pharmaceuticals
DP; 504	Estradiol	2 mg	Blue	Tablet	Round, Bisected Scored	Duramed Pharmaceuticals
DP; 509	Methotrexate Sodium	2.5 mg	Yellow	Tablet	Oval, Scored	Duramed Pharmaceuticals
DP; 510	Enpresse 28 Pink Tablets	0.03 mg; 0.05 mg	Pink	Tablet	Circle	Barr Laboratories
DP; 511	Enpresse 28 White Tablets	0.04 mg; 0.075 mg	White	28-Day Tablet Pack	Circle	Barr Laboratories
DP; 512	Enpresse 28 Orange Tablets	0.03 mg; 0.125 mg	Orange	28-Day Tablet Pack	Circle	Barr Laboratories
DP; 521	Prochlorperazine Maleate	5 mg	Orange	Tablet	Circle	Barr Laboratories
DP; 521	Prochlorperazine Maleate	5 mg	Orange	Tablet	Circle	Duramed Pharmaceuticals
DP; 522	Prochlorperazine Maleate	10 mg	Yellow	Tablet	Circle	Barr Laboratories
DP; 541	Medroxyprogesterone Acetate	5 mg	Yellow	Tablet	Circle, Scored	Duramed Pharmaceuticals

IMPRINT	BRAND/GENERIC NAME	STRENGTH	COLOR	FORM	SHAPE	MANUFACTURER
DP; 543	Cryselle 28 White Tablet	0.3 mg; 0.03 mg	White	Tablet	Circle	Barr Laboratories
DP; 548	Hydroxyurea	500 mg	Buff and Dark Green	Capsule		Duramed Pharmaceuticals
DP; 575	Apri 28 Pink Tablets	0.15 mg; 0.03 mg	Pink	Tablet		Barr Laboratories
DP; 610	Acetaminophen and Oxycodone	325 mg; 5 mg	White to Off-White	Tablet	Round, Bisected Scored	Duramed Pharmaceuticals
DP; 622	Diazepam	5 mg	Yellow	Tablet	Circle, Scored	Duramed Pharmaceuticals
DP; 623	Diazepam	10 mg	Blue	Tablet	Circle, Scored	Duramed Pharmaceuticals
DP; 651	Phentermine Hydrochloride	30 mg	Blue and Clear	Capsule		Duramed Pharmaceuticals
DP; 660	Temazepam	15 mg	Green and White	Capsule		Duramed Pharmaceuticals
DP; 661	Temazepam	30 mg	White	Capsule		Duramed Pharmaceuticals
DP; 825	Triotann	25 mg; 8 mg; 25 mg	Beige	Tablet	Capsule-Shape, Scored	Duramed Pharmaceuticals
DP; 832	Choline Magnesium Trisalicylate	500 mg	Pale Pink	Tablet	Capsule-Shape	Duramed Pharmaceuticals
DP; 833	Choline Magnesium Trisalicylate	750 mg	White	Tablet	Capsule-Shape	Duramed Pharmaceuticals
DP; 840;	Amoxicillin	250 mg	Ivory or Buff Opaque and Brown	Capsule		Duramed Pharmaceuticals
DP; 841;	Amoxicillin	500 mg	Ivory or Buff Opaque	Capsule		Duramed Pharmaceuticals
DP; 842	Cephalexin	250 mg	Opaque Scarlet and Gray	Capsule		Duramed Pharmaceuticals
DP; 843;	Cephalexin	500 mg	Opaque Scarlet	Capsule		Duramed Pharmaceuticals
DP; 844	Tetracycline Hydrochloride	250 mg	Yellow and Orange Opaque	Capsule		Duramed Pharmaceuticals
DP; 845	Tetracycline Hydrochloride	500 mg	Black and Yellow Opaque	Capsule		Duramed Pharmaceuticals
DP; 857	Guaifenesin	1200 mg		Extended-Release Tablet		Duramed Pharmaceuticals
DP; 896	Durasal II	600 mg; 60 mg	Blue	Extended-Release Tablet	Capsule-Shape	Duramed Pharmaceuticals
DP; 896	S-Pack A.M. Treatment Phase	600 mg; 60 mg	Blue	Controlled-Release Tablet	Capsule-Shape, Scored	Duramed Pharmaceuticals
DP; 896	S-Pack-DM A.M. Treatment Phase	600 mg; 60 mg	Blue	Controlled-Release Tablet	Capsule-Shape, Scored	Duramed Pharmaceuticals
DP; 907	Duragal-S	0.2 mg; 0.6 mg; 40 mg	Green	Tablet	Round, Quadrisected Scored	Duramed Pharmaceuticals
DP; 932	Hyoscyamine Sulfate	0.125 mg	White	Tablet	Circle	Duramed Pharmaceuticals
DP; 933	Hyoscyamine Sulfate	0.375 mg	Orange	Extended-Release Tablet	Capsule-Shape	Duramed Pharmaceuticals
DP; 933	Hyoscyamine Sulfate	0.375 mg	White	Extended-Release Tablet	Capsule-Shape, Scored	Duramed Pharmaceuticals
DP; 935	Hyocyamine Sulfate SL	0.125 mg	Blue	Tablet	Circle	Duramed Pharmaceuticals
DP; 970	Digoxin	0.125 mg	Yellow	Tablet	Circle, Scored	Duramed Pharmaceuticals
DP; 971	Digoxin	0.25 mg	White	Tablet	Circle, Scored	Duramed Pharmaceuticals
DP; 972	Digoxin	0.5 mg	Green	Tablet	Circle, Scored	Duramed Pharmaceuticals
DPI; 2	Acetaminophen and Codeine Phosphate	300 mg; 15 mg	White	Tablet	Circle	Duramed Pharmaceuticals
DPI; 3	Acetaminophen and Codeine Phosphate	300 mg; 30 mg	White	Tablet	Circle	Duramed Pharmaceuticals
DPI; 4	Acetaminophen and Codeine Phosphate	300 mg; 60 mg	White	Tablet	Circle	Duramed Pharmaceuticals
DPI; 125	Estropipate	1.5 mg	White	Tablet	Diamond, Scored	Duramed Pharmaceuticals
DPI; 288	Triamterene and Hydrochlorothiazide	37.5 mg; 25 mg	White	Capsule		Barr Laboratories
DPI; 364	Duradrin	325 mg; 65 mg; 100 mg	White and Scarlet	Capsule		Barr Laboratories
DPI; 488	Hydrochlorothiazide and Triamterene	25 mg; 37.5 mg	White	Capsule		Barr Laboratories
DPI; 488	Triamterene and Hydrochlorothiazide	37.5 mg; 25 mg	White and Clear	Capsule		Duramed Pharmaceuticals
DPI; 625	Estropipate	0.75 mg	Light Orange	Tablet	Diamond, Scored	Duramed Pharmaceuticals
DPI; 644	Acetaminophen and Oxycodone	5 mg; 500 mg	Red and White	Capsule		Duramed Pharmaceuticals
DPI; 658	Acetaminophen and Oxycodone	5 mg; 500 mg	Red and White	Capsule		Duramed Pharmaceuticals
DPI; 855	Pseudoephderine and Guaifenesin	120 mg; 250 mg	White and Clear	Timed-Release Capsule		Duramed Pharmaceuticals
DPI; 856	Pseudoephedrine and Guaifenesin	60 mg; 300 mg	Blue and Clear	Timed-Release Capsule		Duramed Pharmaceuticals
DQSP	Vicks Dayquil Sinus Pressure & Pain Relief	500 mg; 30 mg	Red	Tablet		Procter & Gamble
DRISTAN ALLERGY	Dristan Allergy	60 mg; 4 mg	Green	Tablet		Whitehall Laboratories
DRISTAN COLD	Dristan Cold Multi-Symptom	500 mg; 30 mg; 2 mg	White and Red	Capsule, Liquid Filled	Oblong	Whitehall Laboratories
DRISTAN COLD ND	Dristan Cold NO-Drowsiness	500 mg; 30 mg	Yellow	Tablet	Oblong	Whitehall Laboratories
DRISTAN; COLD; ND	Dristan Cold NO Drowsiness Formula	500 mg; 30 mg	Brick Red and Yellow	Capsule, Liquid Filled		Wyeth Consumer Healthcare
DRISTAN SINUS	Dristan Sinus	200 mg; 30 mg	White	Tablet	Oval	Whitehall Laboratories
DRISTAN; ULTRA	Dristan Ultra Colds Formula	500 mg; 30 mg; 15 mg; 2 mg	Orange and White	Capsule		Whitehall-Robins Healthcare
DRIXORAL	Drixoral Cold & Allergy	120 mg; 6 mg	Polished Dark Green	Extended-Release Tablet	Circle	Schering-Plough Healthcare Products
DRIXORAL; C&C	Drixoral Cough & Congestion	30 mg; 60 mg	Red	Capsule	Oval	Schering-Plough Healthcare Products
DRIXORAL; C&ST	Drixoral Cough & Sore Throat	325 mg; 15 mg	Blue	Capsule	Oval	Schering-Plough Healthcare Products
DRIXORAL; NDF	Drixoral Non-Drowsy	120 mg	Polished Blue	Sustained-Release Tablet	Circle	Schering-Plough Healthcare Products
DRIXORAL; PLUS	Drixoral Plus	500 mg; 3 mg; 60 mg	Green	Sustained-Release Tablet		Schering-Plough Healthcare Products
DRIXORAL;	Drixoral	6 mg; 120 mg	Green	Coated Tablet		Schering-Plough Healthcare Products
DRIXORAL A/S	Drixoral Allergy Sinus	500 mg; 3 mg; 60 mg	Bright Yellow	Sustained-Release Tablet	Oblong	Schering-Plough Healthcare Products
DRIXORAL C+F	Drixoral Cold & Flu	60 mg; 3 mg; 500 mg	Green	Sustained-Release Tablet	Oval	Schering-Plough Healthcare Products
DRIXORAL COUGH	Drixoral Cough	30 mg	Purple	Capsule	Oval	Schering-Plough Healthcare Products

IMPRINT	BRAND/GENERIC NAME	STRENGTH	COLOR	FORM	SHAPE	MANUFACTURER
DRL; 50; 1	Nefazodone Hydrochloride	50 mg	White	Tablet	Oval	Par Pharmaceutical
DRL; 100; 2	Nefazodone Hydrochloride	100 mg	White	Tablet	Oval	Par Pharmaceutical
DRL; 150; 3	Nefazodone Hydrochloride	150 mg	White	Tablet	Oval	Par Pharmaceutical
DRL; 200; 4	Nefazodone Hydrochloride	200 mg	White	Tablet	Oval	Par Pharmaceutical
DRL; 250; 5	Nefazodone Hydrochloride	250 mg	White	Tablet	Oval	Par Pharmaceutical
DROXIA; 6335	Droxia	200 mg	Blue-Green	Capsule		Bristol-Myers Squibb
DROXIA; 6336	Droxia	300 mg	Purple	Capsule		Bristol-Myers Squibb
DROXIA; 6337	Droxia	400 mg	Red-Orange	Capsule		Bristol-Myers Squibb
DT	Detrol	2 mg	White	Coated Tablet	Circle, Biconvex	Pharmacia & Upjohn
DT; I	Pec-Dec	60 mg	Light Brown	Tablet	Circle	Glaxosmithkline
DUOCET	Duocet	5 mg; 500 mg	White	Tablet		Mason Pharmaceuticals
DUPONT; 1 1;	Revia	50 mg	Pale Yellow	Coated Tablet	Capsule-Shape, Scored	Bristol-Myers Squibb
DUPONT; TREXAN	Trexan	50 mg	White	Tablet	Circle, Scored	Bristol-Myers Squibb
DUPONT; VALPIN	Valpin 50	50 mg	Beige	Tablet		Bristol-Myers Squibb
DURA; 009	Fenesin	600 mg	Light Blue	Tablet		Biovail Pharmaceuticals
DURA; 015	Guai-Vent/pse	600 mg; 120 mg	White	Sustained-Release Tablet		Biovail Pharmaceuticals
DURA; CHEW	D.A. Chewable	2 mg; 1.25 mg; 10 mg	Orange	Tablet, Chewable		Biovail Pharmaceuticals
DURA; DA	Dura-Vent/da	8 mg; 2.5 mg; 20 mg	Light Brown	Tablet		Biovail Pharmaceuticals
DURA; DA II	D.A. II	4 mg; 10 mg; 1.25 mg	White	Extended-Release Tablet	Capsule-Shape	Biovail Pharmaceuticals
DURA; FDM; 014	Fenesin DM	600 mg; 30 mg	Dark Blue	Tablet		Biovail Pharmaceuticals
DURACT	Duract	25 mg	Opaque Light Yellow Body and Opaque Red Cap with 2 Blue Bands	Capsule		Wyeth-Ayerst Laboratories
DURATION	Duration 12-Hour	120 mg	Blue	Tablet	Circle	Schering-Plough Healthcare Products
DV; NVR	Diovan	80 mg	Pale Red	Tablet	Teardrop-Shape, Bevel-Edged	Novartis
DX; 2; G	Doxazosin Mesylate	2 mg	White	Tablet	Capsule-Shape, Scored	Par Pharmaceutical
DX; 4; G	Doxazosin Mesylate	4 mg	White	Tablet	Capsule-Shape, Scored	Par Pharmaceutical
DX; 8; G	Doxazosin Mesylate	8 mg	White	Tablet	Capsule-Shape, Scored	Par Pharmaceutical
DX; 41	Diclofenac Sodium	100 mg	Pink	Extended-Release Tablet	Circle	Watson Laboratories
DX; NVR	Diovan	160 mg	Grey-Orange	Tablet	Teardrop-Shape, Bevel-Edged	Novartis
DX1; G	Doxazosin Mesylate	1 mg	White	Tablet	Circle	Par Pharmaceutical
DXL; NVR	Diovan	320 mg	Dark Grey-Violet	Tablet	Teardrop-Shape, Bevel-Edged	Novartis
DYAZIDE; SB	Dyazide	25 mg; 37.5 mg	Red and White	Capsule		Glaxosmithkline
DYFLEX; 400	Dyflex	400 mg	White	Tablet	Circle, Concave, Scored	Teva Pharmaceuticals
DYFLEX-G	Dyflex-G	200 mg; 200 mg	White	Tablet		Economed Pharmaceuticals
DYN-50; 747	Dynacin	50 mg	White	Tablet	Capsule-Shape	Medicis Pharmaceutical
DYN-75; 748	Dynacin	75 mg	Gray	Tablet	Capsule-Shape	Medicis Pharmaceutical
DYN-100; 749	Dynacin	100 mg	Dark Gray	Tablet	Capsule-Shape	Medicis Pharmaceutical
DYNABAC; UC; 5364	Dynabac	250 mg	White	Enteric-Coated Tablet	Circle	Muro Pharmaceutical
DYNACIRC; 2.5; S	Dynacirc	2.5 mg	White	Capsule		Novartis Pharmaceuticals
DYNACIRC; 5; S	Dynacirc	5 mg	Light Pink	Capsule		Novartis Pharmaceuticals
DYNACIRC CR; 5	Dynacirc Cr	5 mg	Light Pink	Timed-Release Tablet	Circle, Biconvex	Sandoz
DYNACIRC CR; 10	Dynacirc Cr	10 mg	Beige	Timed-Release Tablet	Circle, Biconvex	Sandoz
DYRENIUM; SKF; 50	Dyrenium	50 mg	Opaque Red	Capsule		Glaxosmithkline
DYRENIUM; SKF; 100	Dyrenium	100 mg	Opaque Red	Capsule		Glaxosmithkline
E	Equalactin	500 mg		Tablet, Chewable		Numark
E	Excedrin Extra Strength	250 mg; 250 mg; 65 mg	White	Tablet		Bristol-Myers Squibb
E	Excedrin Migraine	250 mg; 250 mg; 65 mg	White	Coated Tablet		Bristol-Myers Products
E; 0932	Cyclosporine	25 mg	Clear	Capsule, Liquid Filled		Eon Labs
E; 0933	Cyclosporine	100 mg	Clear	Capsule, Liquid Filled	Oblong	Eon Labs
E; 2	Hydromorphone Hydrochloride	2 mg	Blue	Tablet	Circle	Ethex
E; 3	Enjuvia	0.625 mg	Pink	Tablet	Oval	Duramed Pharmaceuticals
E; 4	Enjuvia	1.25 mg	Yellow	Tablet	Oval	Duramed Pharmaceuticals
E; 4	Hydromorphone Hydrochloride	4 mg	Tan	Tablet	Circle	Ethex
E; 5	Benazepril Hydrochloride	5 mg	Yellow-Orange	Tablet	Circle	Eon Labs
E; 5	Zydone 5/400	5 mg; 400 mg	Yellow	Tablet	Eight-Sided, Elongated, Convex	Endo Laboratories
E; 7.5	Zydone 7.5/400	7.5 mg; 400 mg	Blue	Tablet	Eight-Sided, Elongated, Convex	Endo Laboratories
E; 10	Labetalol Hydrochloride	100 mg	White	Tablet		Eon Labs
E; 10	Labetalol Hydrochloride	100 mg	White	Tablet		Udl Laboratories
E; 10	Zydone 10/400	10 mg; 400 mg	Red	Tablet	Eight-Sided, Elongated, Convex	Endo Laboratories
E; 14;	Chlorpheniramine Maleate	4 mg	Yellow	Tablet	Circle, Scored, Compressed	Eon Labs
E; 16	Nefazodone Hydrochloride	100 mg	White	Tablet	Capsule-Shape	Eon Labs
E; 17	Fluvoxamine Maleate	25 mg	White	Tablet	Circle	Eon Labs
E; 19;	Desipramine Hydrochloride	25 mg	Light Blue	Coated Tablet	Circle	Eon Labs
E; 20	Mirtazapine	15 mg	Yellow	Tablet	Round, Bisected Scored	Eon Labs
E; 22	Orphenadrine Citrate	100 mg	White	Extended-Release Tablet	Circle	Eon Labs
E; 24	Diphenoxylate Hydrochloride with Atropine Sulfate	2.5 mg; 0.025 mg	White	Tablet	Compressed	Eon Labs
E; 25	Lisinopril	2.5 mg	White	Tablet	Oval	Eon Labs
E; 27	Fluvoxamine Maleate	50 mg	Yellow	Tablet	Circle	Eon Labs
E; 29;	Desipramine Hydrochloride	10 mg	White	Coated Tablet	Circle	Eon Labs
E; 30	Isosorbide Mononitrate	30 mg	Red-Pink	Extended-Release Tablet	Oval	Ethex
E; 30 MG; 505	Avinza	30 mg	Yellow and White	Extended-Release Capsule		Ligand Pharmaceuticals
E; 31	Captopril	12.5 mg	White	Tablet	Circle	Eon Labs
E; 32;	Reserpine	0.1 mg	White	Tablet	Circle, Scored, Compressed	Eon Labs
E; 32;	Reserpine	0.1 mg	White	Tablet	Circle, Scored, Compressed	Novartis Generics
E 34	Tizanidine Hydrochloride	2 mg	White	Tablet	Circle	Eon Labs
E; 38	Nefazodone Hydrochloride	50 mg	Light Pink	Tablet	Capsule-Shape	Eon Labs
E; 39	Naltrexone Hydrochloride	50 mg	White	Tablet	Oblong	Eon Labs

IMPRINT	BRAND/GENERIC NAME	STRENGTH	COLOR	FORM	SHAPE	MANUFACTURER
E; 40	Midodrine Hydrochloride	2.5 mg	White	Tablet	Circle	Eon Labs
E; 43	Midodrine Hydrochloride	5 mg	Reddish Orange	Tablet	Circle	Eon Labs
E 44	Tizanidine Hydrochloride	4 mg	White	Tablet	Circle	Eon Labs
E; 48	Benazepril Hydrochloride	40 mg	Red	Tablet	Circle	Eon Labs
E; 53	Benazepril Hydrochloride	10 mg	Orange	Tablet	Circle	Eon Labs
E; 54	Lisinopril	5 mg	Pink	Tablet	Oval	Eon Labs
E; 60	Isosorbide Mononitrate	60 mg	Yellow	Extended-Release Tablet		Ethex
E; 60 MG; 506	Avinza	60 mg	Blue-Green and White	Extended-Release Capsule		Ligand Pharmaceuticals
E; 61	Captopril	25 mg	White	Tablet	Circle, Scored	Eon Labs
E; 63	Clonazepam	0.5 mg	Light Yellow	Tablet	Circle, Biconvex, Scored	Eon Labs
E; 64	Clonazepam	1 mg	Light Blue	Tablet	Circle, Biconvex, Scored	Eon Labs
E; 65	Clonazepam	2 mg	White	Tablet	Circle, Biconvex, Scored	Eon Labs
E; 70	Lovastatin	10 mg	Peach	Tablet	Circle	Eon Labs
E; 71	Hydrochlorothiazide and Lisinopril	12.5 mg; 10 mg	Light Pink	Tablet	Circle	Eon Labs
E; 72	Lovastatin	20 mg	Light Blue	Tablet	Circle	Eon Labs
E; 74	Lovastatin	40 mg	Light Green	Tablet	Circle	Eon Labs
E; 75;	Phendimetrazine Tartrate	35 mg	Pink, White and Blue	Tablet		Eon Labs
E; 76;	Phendimetrazine Tartrate	35 mg	Yellow	Tablet	Circle, Scored	Eon Labs
E; 77	Frova	2.5 mg	White	Coated Tablet	Circle	Elan Pharma
E; 77;	Phendimetrazine Tartrate	35 mg	Pink	Tablet		Eon Labs
E; 80	Fluoxetine Hydrochloride	10 mg	Light Green	Capsule		Eon Labs
E; 81	Nefazodone Hydrochloride	150 mg	Peach	Tablet	Capsule-Shape	Eon Labs
E; 82	Benazepril Hydrochloride	20 mg	Pink	Tablet	Circle	Eon Labs
E; 84	Dextroamphetamine Saccharate, Amphetamine Aspartate, Dextroamphetamine Sulfate, Amphetamine Sulfate 5 mg Tablet	1.25 mg; 1.25 mg; 1.25 mg; 1.25 mg	Blue	Tablet	Double-Scored	Eon Labs
E; 84	Iodinated Glycerol	30 mg	Orange	Tablet	Round, Bisected Scored	Eon Labs
E; 85	Fluoxetine Hydrochloride	20 mg	White and Green	Capsule		Eon Labs
E; 90 MG; 507	Avinza	90 mg	Red and White	Extended-Release Capsule		Ligand Pharmaceuticals
E; 101	Lisinopril	10 mg	Pink	Tablet	Oval	Eon Labs
E; 102	Lisinopril	20 mg	Peach	Tablet	Oval	Eon Labs
E; 103	Lisinopril	30 mg	Red	Tablet	Oval	Eon Labs
E; 104	Lisinopril	40 mg	Yellow	Tablet	Oval	Eon Labs
E; 111	Dextroamphetamine Saccharate, Amphetamine Aspartate, Dextroamphetamine Sulfate, Amphetamine Sulfate 10 mg Tablet	2.5 mg; 2.5 mg; 2.5 mg; 2.5 mg	Blue	Tablet	Double-Scored	Eon Labs
E; 112;	Sulfamethoxazole and Trimethoprim Double Strength	800 mg; 160 mg	White	Tablet	Oval, Scored, Compressed	Eon Labs
E; 114	Enalapril Maleate	2.5 mg	Yellow	Tablet	Circle, Scored	Eon Labs
E; 117	Labetalol Hydrochloride	200 mg	White	Tablet		Eon Labs
E; 117	Labetalol Hydrochloride	200 mg	White	Tablet		Udl Laboratories
E; 118	Labetalol Hydrochloride	300 mg		Tablet		Eon Labs
E; 120	Isosorbide Mononitrate	120 mg	White	Extended-Release Tablet		Ethex
E; 120 MG; 508	Avinza	120 mg	Blue-Violet and White	Extended-Release Capsule		Ligand Pharmaceuticals
E; 121	Captopril	12.5 mg	White	Tablet	Circle, Scored	Par Pharmaceutical
E; 122	Captopril	25 mg	White	Tablet	Round, Quadrisected Scored	Par Pharmaceutical
E; 123	Captopril	50 mg	White	Tablet	Circle, Scored	Par Pharmaceutical
E; 124	Benazepril Hydrochloride and Hydrochlorothiazide	5 mg; 6.25 mg	White to Off-White	Tablet	Oblong, Scored	Eon Labs
E; 124	Captopril	100 mg	White	Tablet	Circle, Scored	Par Pharmaceutical
E; 126	Nefazodone Hydrochloride	200 mg	Light Yellow	Tablet	Capsule-Shape	Eon Labs
E; 127	Enalapril Maleate	5 mg	White	Tablet	Circle, Scored	Eon Labs
E; 128	Bumetanide	0.5 mg	Green	Tablet	Bisected, Round Scored	Eon Labs
E; 128	Bumetanide	0.5 mg	Green	Tablet	Bisected, Round Scored	Udl Laboratories
E; 129	Bumetanide	1 mg	Yellow	Tablet	Round, Bisected Scored	Eon Labs
E; 129	Bumetanide	1 mg	Yellow	Tablet	Round, Bisected Scored	Udl Laboratories
E; 130	Bumetanide	2 mg	Beige to Light Brown	Tablet	Round, Bisected Scored	Eon Labs
E; 130	Bumetanide	2 mg	Beige to Light Brown	Tablet	Round, Bisected Scored	Udl Laboratories
E; 132	Methadone Hydrochloride	40 mg	White	Tablet	Circle	Eon Labs
E; 134;	Reserpine	0.25 mg	White	Tablet	Scored, Compressed, Circle	Eon Labs
E; 134;	Reserpine	0.25 mg	White	Tablet	Scored, Compressed, Circle	Novartis Generics
E; 139	Etodolac	500 mg	White	Tablet	Oblong	Eon Labs
E; 140	Etodolac	400 mg	White	Coated Tablet	Oval	Eon Labs
E; 141	Oxaprozin	600 mg	White	Tablet		Eon Labs
E; 144	Amiodarone Hydrochloride	200 mg	Yellow	Tablet		Eon Labs
E; 145	Nabumetone	500 mg	White	Tablet	Oblong	Eon Labs
E; 146	Nabumetone	750 mg	White	Tablet	Oblong	Eon Labs
E; 147	Enalapril Maleate	10 mg	Salmon	Tablet	Circle	Eon Labs
E; 148	Nefazodone Hydrochloride	250 mg	White	Tablet	Capsule-Shape	Eon Labs
E; 150	Nizatidine	150 mg	Yellow and White	Capsule		Eon Labs
E; 152	Hydrochlorothiazide and Lisinopril	12.5 mg; 20 mg	White	Tablet	Circle	Eon Labs
E; 157	Fluvoxamine Maleate	100 mg	Tan	Tablet	Circle	Eon Labs
E; 170	Sotalol Hydrochloride	120 mg	Blue	Tablet	Capsule-Shape	Eon Labs
E; 171	Sotalol Hydrochloride	80 mg		Tablet		Eon Labs
E; 173	Hydrochlorothiazide and Lisinopril	25 mg; 20 mg	Light Pink	Tablet	Circle	Eon Labs
E; 174	Sotalol Hydrochloride	240 mg	Blue	Tablet	Capsule-Shape	Eon Labs
E; 177	Sotalol Hydrochloride	160 mg	Blue	Tablet	Capsule-Shape	Eon Labs
E; 204	Benazepril Hydrochloride and Hydrochlorothiazide	10 mg; 12.5 mg	Pink	Tablet	Oblong, Scored	Eon Labs
E; 205	Methimazole	5 mg		Tablet		Eon Labs
E; 210	Methimazole	10 mg		Tablet		Eon Labs

IMPRINT	BRAND/GENERIC NAME	STRENGTH	COLOR	FORM	SHAPE	MANUFACTURER
E; 211	Benazepril Hydrochloride and Hydrochlorothiazide	20 mg; 12.5 mg	Lavendar	Tablet	Oblong, Scored	Eon Labs
E; 212	Mirtazapine	30 mg	Red Brown	Tablet	Round, Bisected Scored	Eon Labs
E; 213	Metformin Hydrochloride	500 mg	White	Tablet	Circle	Eon Labs
E; 214	Enalapril Maleate	20 mg	Peach	Tablet	Circle	Eon Labs
E; 215	Metformin Hydrochloride	850 mg	White	Tablet	Circle	Eon Labs
E; 220;	Urinary Antiseptic No. 2	0.03 mg; 4.5 mg; 40.8 mg; 18.1 mg; 5.4 mg; 0.03 mg	Dark Blue	Coated Tablet	Circle	Geneva Generics
E; 221	Metformin Hydrochloride	1000 mg	White	Tablet	Oval	Eon Labs
E; 222	Mirtazapine	45 mg	White	Tablet	Circle	Eon Labs
E; 245; 5	Aricept	5 mg	White	Coated Tablet	Circle	Eisai
E; 245; 5	Aricept	5 mg	White	Coated Tablet	Circle	Pfizer
E; 246; 10	Aricept	10 mg	Yellow	Coated Tablet	Circle	Eisai
E; 246; 10	Aricept	10 mg	Yellow	Coated Tablet	Circle	Pfizer
E; 277	Benazepril Hydrochloride and Hydrochlorothiazide	20 mg; 25 mg	Maroon	Tablet	Oblong, Scored	Eon Labs
E; 300	Nizatidine	300 mg	White and Orange	Capsule		Eon Labs
E; 311	Tramadol Hydrochloride	50 mg	White to Off-White	Tablet	Circle	Eon Labs
E 371	Citalopram Hydrobromide	10 mg	Orange	Tablet	Capsule-Shape	Eon Labs
E 372	Citalopram Hydrobromide	20 mg	Dark Pink	Tablet	Capsule-Shape	Eon Labs
E 373	Citalopram Hydrobromide	40 mg	White to Off White	Tablet	Capsule-Shape	Eon Labs
E; 401	Dextroamphetamine Saccharate, Amphetamine Aspartate, Dextroamphetamine Sulfate, Amphetamine Sulfate 20 mg Tablet	5 mg; 5 mg; 5 mg; 5 mg	Dark Orange	Tablet	Double-Scored	Eon Labs
E; 404	Dextroamphetamine Saccharate, Amphetamine Aspartate, Dextroamphetamine Sulfate, Amphetamine Sulfate 30 mg Tablet	7.5 mg; 7.5 mg; 7.5 mg; 7.5 mg	Dark Orange	Tablet	Double-Scored	Eon Labs
E; 410	Bupropion Hydrochloride Extended Release	100 mg	Aquamarine	Extended-Release Tablet	Circle	Eon Labs
E; 471	Captopril	50 mg	White	Tablet	Circle, Scored	Eon Labs
E; 511;	Quinidine Sulfate	200 mg	White	Tablet	Scored, Compressed	Eon Labs
E; 512;	Quinidine Sulfate	300 mg	White	Tablet	Scored, Compressed	Eon Labs
E; 530; 10	Isoxsuprine Hydrochloride	10 mg	White	Tablet	Circle, Scored, Compressed	Eon Labs
E; 531; 20	Isoxsuprine Hydrochloride	20 mg	White	Tablet	Circle, Scored, Compressed	Eon Labs
E; 591	Captopril	100 mg	White	Tablet	Circle, Scored	Eon Labs
E; 613;	Hydroxyzine Pamoate	25 mg	Light Green and Dark Green	Capsule		Eon Labs
E; 613;	Hydroxyzine Pamoate	25 mg	Light Green and Dark Green	Capsule		Novartis Generics
E; 615;	Hydroxyzine Pamoate	50 mg	Dark Green and White	Capsule		Eon Labs
E; 615;	Hydroxyzine Pamoate	50 mg	Dark Green and White	Capsule		Novartis Generics
E; 616	Dicyclomine	20 mg	Blue	Tablet		Chelsea Laboratories
E; 617;	Chlordiazepoxide Hydrochloride and Clidinium Bromide	5 mg; 2.5 mg	White	Capsule		Eon Labs
E; 647;	Phentermine Hydrochloride Yellow	30 mg	Yellow	Capsule		Eon Labs
E; 648;	Diphenhydramine Hydrochloride	25 mg	Pink and Clear	Capsule		Eon Labs
E; 649;	Diphenhydramine Hydrochloride	50 mg	Pink	Capsule		Eon Labs
E; 652; 15	Morphine Sulfate ER	15 mg	Blue	Extended-Release Tablet	Circle	Endo Laboratories
E; 653; 30	Morphine Sulfate ER	30 mg	Green	Extended-Release Tablet	Circle	Endo Laboratories
E; 655; 60	Morphine Sulfate ER	60 mg	Orange	Extended-Release Tablet	Capsule-Shape	Endo Laboratories
E; 658; 100	Morphine Sulfate ER	100 mg	Blue	Extended-Release Tablet	Capsule-Shape	Endo Laboratories
E; 659; 200	Morphine Sulfate ER	200 mg	Green	Extended-Release Tablet	Oval	Endo Laboratories
E; 660	Oxycodone and Acetaminophen	5 mg; 500 mg	Red-Orange	Capsule		Endo Laboratories
E; 675	Aspirin, Butalbital, Caffeine and Codeine	325 mg; 50 mg; 40 mg; 30 mg	Yellow and Blue	Capsule		Endo Laboratories
E; 700; 7.5/325	Endocet	325 mg; 7.5 mg	Peach	Tablet	Capsule-Shape	Endo Laboratories
E; 701	Bisoprolol and Hydrochlorothiazide	2.5 mg; 6.25 mg	Orange	Tablet		Eon Labs
E; 704	Bisoprolol and Hydrochlorothiazide	5 mg; 6.25 mg	Red	Tablet	Circle	Eon Labs
E; 707	Bisoprolol and Hydrochlorothiazide	10 mg; 6.25 mg	White	Tablet	Circle	Eon Labs
E; 712; 10/325	Endocet	325 mg; 10 mg	Yellow	Tablet	Oval	Endo Laboratories
E; 713;	Orphenadrine Compound Ss	25 mg; 385 mg; 60 mg	Green, White and Green	Tablet	Three-Layered, Scored	Eon Labs
E; 714;	Orphenadrine Compound DS	50 mg; 770 mg; 60 mg	Green, White and Green	Tablet	Three-Layered, Scored	Eon Labs
E; 716;	Meprobamate	200 mg	White	Tablet	Circle	Eon Labs
E; 717;	Meprobamate	400 mg	White	Tablet	Round, Bisected Scored	Eon Labs
E; 720;	Indomethacin ER	75 mg	Green and Clear	Sustained-Release Capsule		Eon Labs
E; 721;	Desipramine Hydrochloride	50 mg	Blue	Tablet	Circle	Eon Labs
E; 722;	Desipramine Hydrochloride	75 mg	Light Blue	Coated Tablet	Circle	Eon Labs
E; 724	Carisoprodol and Aspirin	200 mg; 325 mg	White and Lavender	Tablet	Circle, Bilayered	Eon Labs
E; 736;	Desipramine Hydrochloride	100 mg	Medium Blue	Tablet		Eon Labs
E; 749	Carisoprodol, Aspirin and Codeine Phosphate	200 mg; 325 mg; 16 mg	Yellow and White	Tablet	Circle	Eon Labs
E; 757	Sulfadiazine	500 mg	White	Tablet	Capsule-Shape, Biconvex	Eon Labs
E; 757	Sulfadiazine	500 mg	White	Tablet	Capsule-Shape, Biconvex	Udl Laboratories
E; 760;	Desipramine Hydrochloride	150 mg	White	Coated Tablet	Circle	Eon Labs
E; 771	Bisoprolol Fumarate	5 mg	Pink	Tablet	Circle	Eon Labs

IMPRINT	BRAND/GENERIC NAME	STRENGTH	COLOR	FORM	SHAPE	MANUFACTURER
E; 774	Bisoprolol Fumarate	10 mg		Tablet		Eon Labs
E; 784	Guiapax Pse	600 mg; 120 mg	White	Tablet	Oval, Bisected Scored	Eon Labs
E; 796; 7.5	Endocet	500 mg; 7.5 mg	Peach	Tablet	Capsule-Shape	Endo Laboratories
E; 797; 10	Endocet	650 mg; 10 mg	Yellow	Tablet	Oval, Large	Endo Laboratories
E; 799	Rifampin	300 mg	Red	Capsule		Eon Labs
E; 799	Rifampin	300 mg	Red	Capsule		Udl Laboratories
E; 801	Rifampin	150 mg	Orange	Capsule		Eon Labs
E; 805	Doxycycline Monohydrate	50 mg	Yellow	Capsule		Eon Labs
E; 810	Doxycycline Monohydrate	100 mg	Brown	Capsule		Eon Labs
E; 882;	Phentermine Hydrochloride	15 mg	Grey and Yellow	Capsule		Eon Labs
E; 968	Chlordiazepoxide Hydrochloride with Clidinium Bromide	5 mg; 2.5 mg	Light Green	Capsule		Eon Labs
E; 1125	Flutamide	125 mg	Brown and White	Capsule		Eon Labs
E; 1217;	Nitroglycerin	9 mg	Green and Yellow	Sustained-Release Capsule		Eon Labs
E; 1235;	Nitroglycerin	6.5 mg	Dark Blue and Dark Yellow	Sustained-Release Capsule		Eon Labs
E; 1304	Chlorpheniramine Maleate and Pseudoephedrine Hydrochloride	8 mg; 120 mg	Dark Blue and Clear	Extended-Release Capsule		Eon Labs
E; 4350	Isoniazid	300 mg	White	Tablet	Circle, Scored, Compressed	Eon Labs
E; 4354	Isoniazid	100 mg	White	Tablet	Circle, Scored, Compressed	Eon Labs
E; 5000;	Phentermine Hydrochloride Blue/ clear	30 mg	Blue and Clear	Capsule		Novartis Generics
E; 5156	Papaverine Hydrochloride	150 mg	Brown and Clear	Sustained-Release Capsule		Eon Labs
E; 5174; E; 5174;	Nitroglycerin	2.5 mg	Amethyst and Clear	Sustained-Release Capsule		Eon Labs
E; 5254	Phendimetrazine Tartrate	105 mg	Brown and Clear	Extended-Release Capsule		Eon Labs
E; 5380;	Contrin	0.5 mg; 110 mg; 240 mg; 15 mcg; 75 mg	Maroon and Red	Capsule		Novartis Generics
E; 5380;	Foltrin	240 mg; 110 mg; 75 mg; 0.5 mg; 15 mcg	Red and Scarlet	Capsule		Eon Labs
E; T; 7	Tritan	25 mg; 8 mg; 25 mg	Tan	Tablet	Oblong, Bisected Scored	Eon Labs
E50	Etoposide	50 mg	Dark Pink with Black Ink	Capsule	Oblong	Mylan Pharmaceuticals
EA	Erythromycin	500 mg	Pink	Coated Tablet	Capsule-Shape	Abbott Laboratories
EATON; 007	Macrodantin	25 mg	White	Capsule		Norwich Eaton
EATON; 008	Macrodantin	50 mg	White and Yellow	Capsule		Norwich Eaton
EATON; 009;	Macrodantin	100 mg	Yellow	Capsule		Norwich Eaton
EATON; 013	Dopar	100 mg	Opaque, Green	Capsule		Norwich Eaton
EATON; 014	Dopar	250 mg	Opaque Green and White	Capsule		Norwich Eaton
EATON; 015	Dopar	500 mg	Opaque Green	Capsule		Norwich Eaton
EATON; 030	Dantrium	25 mg	Brown and Orange	Capsule		Norwich Eaton
EATON; 031	Dantrium	50 mg	Orange and Brown	Capsule		Norwich Eaton
EATON; 033	Dantrium	100 mg	Orange and Brown	Capsule		Norwich Eaton
EATON; 036	Furadantin	50 mg	Yellow	Tablet		Procter & Gamble Pharmaceuticals
EATON; 072	Furoxone	100 mg	Brown	Tablet		Norwich Eaton
EC-NAPROSYN; 375	Ec-Naprosyn	375 mg	White	Delayed-Release Tablet	Capsule-Shape	Roche Laboratories
EC-NAPROSYN; 500	Ec-Naprosyn	500 mg	White	Delayed-Release Tablet	Capsule-Shape	Roche Laboratories
ECOTRIN; LOW	Ecotrin Adult Low Strength	81 mg	Orange	Enteric-Coated Tablet		Glaxosmithkline Consumer
ECOTRIN; REG	Ecotrin	325 mg	Orange	Tablet	Circle	Glaxosmithkline Consumer
ECOTRIN MAX	Ecotrin	500 mg	Orange	Enteric-Coated Tablet	Circle	Glaxosmithkline Consumer
ECOTRIN REG	Ecotrin	325 mg	Orange	Tablet		Glaxosmithkline Consumer
ECR; 6006	Lodrane Ld	60 mg; 6 mg	Clear	Capsule		Ecr Pharmaceuticals
ED; A	Ery-Tab	500 mg	Pink	Enteric-Coated Tablet		Abbott Laboratories
ED-F	Ed Cyte F	324 mg; 1 mg; 50 mg	Green	Tablet		Edwards
E-DUAL	Excedrin Dual Aspirin Free	500 mg	Pink	Tablet		Bristol-Myers Squibb
EEF; 20	Methazolamide	50 mg	White	Tablet	Circle	Qualitest Products
EEF; 21	Methazolamide	25 mg	White	Tablet	Circle	Qualitest Products
EF	E.E.S.	200 mg	White	Tablet, Chewable	Circle, Scored	Abbott Laboratories
EFF; 12	Pyrazinamide	500 mg	White	Tablet		Mikart
EFF; 20	Methazolamide	50 mg	White	Tablet	Circle, Scored	Effcon Laboratories
EFF; 21	Methazolamide	25 mg	White	Tablet	Circle	Effcon Laboratories
EFF; 26	Isoniazid	100 mg	White	Tablet	Circle, Debossed	Mikart
EFF; 27	Isoniazid	300 mg	White	Tablet	Circle, Debossed	Mikart
EK; ABBOTT LOGO	Pce Dispertab	500 mg	White	Tablet	Oval	Abbott Laboratories
EL; 040	Mucobid LA	600 mg	Green	Tablet	Capsule-Shape, Single Scored	Econolab
EL; 069	Flumezide	4 mg; 50 mg	Light Blue	Tablet	Circle	Econolab
EL; 077	Andec TR	4 mg; 120 mg	Violet	Tablet	Oval	Econolab
EL; 082	Andec	4 mg; 60 mg	White	Tablet	Oval	Econolab
EL; 090	Mucobid DM	60 mg; 600 mg	Light Green	Tablet		Econolab
EL; 111	Hyospaz	0.15 mg	Light Blue	Tablet		Econolab
EL; 122	Tuss Tan	60 mg; 5 mg; 10 mg; 10 mg	Light Pink	Tablet	Oval, Single Scored	Econolab
EL; 124	Spastrin	0.2 mg; 0.6 mg; 40 mg	Turquoise	Tablet	Circle, Single Scored	Econolab
EL; 125	Nalfed	12 mg; 120 mg	Blue and Clear	Capsule		Econolab
EL; 125	Nalfed PD	6 mg; 60 mg	Dark Blue and Clear	Capsule		Econolab
EL; 130	Hyoscyamine Sulfate	0.125 mg	White	Tablet	Circle, Scored	Econolab
EL; 140	Demibid II	60 mg; 600 mg	Blue	Tablet		Econolab
EL; 145	Spastrin	0.2 mg; 0.6 mg; 40 mg	Turquoise	Tablet	Circle, Scored	Breckenridge Pharmaceutical

IMPRINT	BRAND/GENERIC NAME	STRENGTH	COLOR	FORM	SHAPE	MANUFACTURER
EL; 158	Polycarb	625 mg	Beige	Tablet	Single Scored	Econolab
EL; 175	Rexin	1 mg; 400 mg	Pink	Tablet		Econolab
EL; 191	Tanoral	8 mg; 25 mg; 25 mg	Beige	Tablet	Oval, Single Scored	Econolab
EL; 250	Iodrol	30 mg	Pink	Tablet	Circle, Scored	Econolab
EL; 320	Panokase	30000 U; 8000 U; 30000 U	Off-White	Tablet	Circle, Scored	Econolab
EL; 444	Trimethobenzamide Hydrochloride	250 mg	Light Blue and Blue	Capsule		Econolab
EL; 514	Sloprin	800 mg	White	Tablet	Oval, Single Scored	Econolab
EL; 518	Drinex	650 mg; 4 mg; 60 mg	Pink	Tablet	Oval	Econolab
EL; 522	Dyphylline with Guaifenesin	200 mg; 200 mg	White	Tablet	Circle, Scored	Econolab
EL; 524	Linhist LA	4 mg; 20 mg; 50 mg	Yellow and Clear	Capsule		Econolab
EL; 525	Micomp-PB	0.125 mg; 100 mg; 1 mg; 30 mg	Green	Tablet	Circle	Econolab
EL; 717	Hyosol/SL	0.125 mg	Blue	Tablet	Circle, Scored	Econolab
EL; 740	Colfed-A	8 mg; 120 mg	Blue and Clear	Sustained-Release Capsule		Breckenridge Pharmaceutical
EL; 840	Obnate-90	250 mg; 2 mg; 1 mg; 90 mg; 4000 IU; 12 mcg; 3.4 mg; 400 IU; 120 mg; 25 mg; 30 IU; 20 mg; 3 mg; 20 mg; 0.15 mg; 50 mg	White	Coated Tablet	Oblong, Single Scored	Econolab
EL; 860	Guaibid D	250 mg; 120 mg	Light Gray and Clear	Timed-Release Capsule		Econolab
EL; 870	Guaibid D Pediatric	300 mg; 60 mg	Light Blue and Clear	Timed-Release Capsule		Econolab
EL; 880	Encron-10	30000 U; 8000 U; 13000 U	White and Clear	Capsule	Capsule-Shape	Econolab
EL; 890	Preterna	30 mcg; 250 mg; 2 mg; 1 mg; 20 mg; 5000 IU; 12 mcg; 3.4 mg; 10 mg; 25 mg; 30 IU; 400 IU; 100 mg; 3 mg; 150 mcg; 25 mg; 60 mg; 10 mg	White	Coated Tablet	Oblong, Single Scored	Econolab
EL; 950	Zitamin	200 mg; 65 mg; 100 mg; 175 mcg; 4000 IU; 2.2 mcg; 1.6 mg; 400 IU; 70 mg; 15 mg; 10 IU; 2.2 mg; 1.5 mg; 65 mcg; 17 mg; 1 mg	White	Coated Tablet	Oblong, Single Scored	Econolab
ELAVIL; 40	Elavil	10 mg	Blue	Coated Tablet	Circle	Astra Zeneca
ELAVIL; 41	Elavil	50 mg	Beige	Coated Tablet	Circle	Astra Zeneca
ELAVIL; 42	Elavil	75 mg	Orange	Coated Tablet	Circle	Astra Zeneca
ELAVIL; 43	Elavil	100 mg	Mauve	Coated Tablet	Circle	Astra Zeneca
ELAVIL; 45	Elavil	25 mg	Yellow	Coated Tablet	Circle	Astra Zeneca
ELAVIL; 47	Elavil	150 mg	Blue	Coated Tablet	Capsule-Shape	Astra Zeneca
ELDEPRYL; 5 MG; SOMERSET LOGO	Eldepryl	5 mg	Aqua Blue	Capsule		Somerset Pharmaceuticals
ELDEPRYL; 5 MG; SOMERSET LOGO	Eldepryl	5 mg	Aqua Blue	Capsule		Udl Laboratories
ELN; 30	Afeditab Cr	30 mg	Brick Red	Extended-Release Tablet	Circle	Watson Laboratories
ELN; 30	Nifedipine	30 mg	Red-Brown	Extended-Release Tablet	Circle	Teva Pharmaceuticals
ELN; 30	Nifedipine	30 mg	Red-Brown	Extended-Release Tablet	Circle	Watson Laboratories
ELN; 60	Afeditab Cr	60 mg	Brick Red	Extended-Release Tablet	Circle	Watson Laboratories
ELN; 60	Nifedipine ER	60 mg	Red-Brown	Extended-Release Tablet	Circle	Watson Laboratories
ELP; 5	Enalapril Maleate	5 mg	Pink	Tablet	Circle	Lek Pharmaceuticals
ELP; 10	Enalapril Maleate	10 mg	Pink	Tablet	Circle	Lek Pharmaceuticals
ELP; 20	Enalapril Maleate	20 mg	Gray	Tablet	Circle	Lek Pharmaceuticals
ELP; 212	Enalapril Maleate	2.5 mg	Light Yellow	Tablet	Circle	Lek Pharmaceuticals
EM	Dyflex 200	200 mg	White	Tablet	Circle, Concave, Scored	Teva Pharmaceuticals
EM; SP	Estinyl	0.05 mg	Pink	Coated Tablet		Schering
EMCYT; PHARMACIA; 132	Emcyt	140 mg	White	Capsule		Pharmacia & Upjohn
EMPIRIN; 3	Empirin with Codeine No. 3	30 mg; 325 mg	White	Tablet		Glaxosmithkline
EMPIRIN; 4	Empirin with Codeine No. 4	60 mg; 325 mg	White	Tablet		Glaxosmithkline
E-MYCIN; 250 MG	E-Mycin	250 mg	Orange	Timed-Release Tablet	Circle	Knoll Pharmaceutical
E-MYCIN; 250 MG	E-Mycin	250 mg	Orange	Timed-Release Tablet	Circle	Pharmacia & Upjohn
E-MYCIN; 333 MG	E-Mycin	333 mg	White	Timed-Release Tablet	Circle	Knoll Pharmaceutical
E-MYCIN; 333 MG	E-Mycin	333 mg	White	Timed-Release Tablet	Circle	Pharmacia & Upjohn
EN; 2.5; G	Enalapril Maleate	2.5 mg	White	Tablet	Circle	Par Pharmaceutical
EN; 5; G; G	Enalapril Maleate	5 mg	White	Tablet	Oval	Par Pharmaceutical
EN; 10; G	Enalapril Maleate	10 mg	Rusty Red	Tablet	Oval	Par Pharmaceutical
EN; 20; G	Enalapril Maleate	20 mg	Peach	Tablet	Oval	Par Pharmaceutical
ENDEP; 10; ROCHE	Endep	10 mg	Orange	Coated Tablet	Circle, Scored	Hoffmann-LA Roche
ENDEP; 25; ROCHE	Endep	25 mg	Orange	Coated Tablet	Circle, Scored	Hoffmann-LA Roche
ENDEP; 50; ROCHE	Endep	50 mg	Orange	Coated Tablet	Circle, Scored	Roche Laboratories
ENDEP; 75; ROCHE	Endep	75 mg	Yellow	Coated Tablet	Circle, Scored	Roche Laboratories
ENDEP; 100; ROCHE	Endep	100 mg	Peach	Coated Tablet	Circle, Scored	Hoffmann-LA Roche
ENDEP; 150; ROCHE	Endep	150 mg	Salmon	Coated Tablet	Circle, Scored	Hoffmann-LA Roche

IMPRINT	BRAND/GENERIC NAME	STRENGTH	COLOR	FORM	SHAPE	MANUFACTURER
ENDO	Selegiline	5 mg	White	Tablet	Oblong	Endo Laboratories
ENDO; 048	Hycomine Compound	250 mg; 30 mg; 2 mg; 10 mg; 5 mg	Pink	Tablet	Circle, Scored	Endo Laboratories
ENDO; 051	Remsed	50 mg	Light Blue	Tablet		Dupont Merck
ENDO; 501	Azene	3.25 mg	Tan	Capsule		Endo Laboratories
ENDO; 502	Clorazepate	6.5 mg	Orange	Capsule		Endo Laboratories
ENDO; 503	Azene	13 mg	Blue	Capsule		Endo Laboratories
ENDO; 570	Percobarb	4.5 mg; 0.38 mg; 100 mg; 224 mg; 160 mg; 32 mg	Blue and Yellow	Capsule		Endo Laboratories
ENDO; 602	Oxycodone and Acetaminophen	5 mg; 325 mg	White	Tablet		Endo Laboratories
ENDO; 603	Carbidopa and Levodopa	10 mg; 100 mg	Dark Dapple-Blue	Tablet	Oval, Scored	Endo Laboratories
ENDO; 605	Carbidopa and Levodopa	25 mg; 100 mg	Yellow	Tablet	Oval, Scored	Endo Laboratories
ENDO; 607	Carbidopa and Levodopa	25 mg; 250 mg	Light Dapple-Blue	Tablet	Oval, Scored	Endo Laboratories
ENDO; 610	Endodan	4.5 mg; 0.38 mg; 325 mg	Yellow	Tablet		Endo Laboratories
ENDO; 630	Cimetidine	200 mg	White	Coated Tablet	Oval	Endo Laboratories
ENDO; 631	Cimetidine	300 mg	White	Coated Tablet	Oval	Endo Laboratories
ENDO; 633	Cimetidine	800 mg	White	Coated Tablet	Oval	Endo Laboratories
ENDO; 714	Glipizide	10 mg	White	Tablet	Circle, Scored	Endo Laboratories
ENDO; 731	Captopril and Hydrochlorothiazide	50 mg; 25 mg	Peach	Tablet	Round, Bisected on One Side Scored	Endo Laboratories
ENDO; 733	Captopril and Hydrochlorothiazide	25 mg; 15 mg	White	Tablet	Round, Quadrisected on One Side Scored	Endo Laboratories
ENDO; 739	Captopril and Hydrochlorothiazide	50 mg; 15 mg	White	Tablet	Round, Bisected on One Side Scored	Endo Laboratories
ENDO; 741	Captopril and Hydrochlorothiazide	25 mg; 25 mg	Peach	Tablet	Round, Quadrisected on One Side Scored	Endo Laboratories
ENDO; 744	Etodolac	400 mg	Pale Yellow	Tablet	Oval	Bristol-Myers Squibb
ENDURON	Enduron	2.5 mg	Orange	Tablet	Square, Scored	Abbott Laboratories
ENDURON	Enduron	5 mg	Salmon	Tablet	Square, Scored	Abbott Laboratories
ENTAB; DM	Entab-DM	60 mg; 1200 mg	White	Extended-Release Tablet	Oval	Rising Pharmaceuticals
ENTEX; ER; 334	Entex ER	300 mg; 10 mg		Extended-Release Tablet		Andrx Pharmaceuticals
ENTEX PSE; 032 032	Entex Pse	600 mg; 120 mg	Yellow	Sustained-Release Tablet	Oval, Elongated, Scored	Andrx Pharmaceuticals
ENTOLASE; AHR	Entolase	25,000 USP units; 20,000 USP units; 4000 USP units		Capsule		Wyeth Pharmaceuticals
ENTOLASE-HP; AHR	Entolase-Hp	40,000 USP units; 8000 USP units; 50,000 USP units		Capsule		Wyeth Pharmaceuticals
EP; 102	Eperbel-S	40 mg; 0.6 mg; 0.2 mg	Green	Tablet		Excellium Pharmaceuticals
EP; 103	Pseudoephedrine Hydrochloride	60 mg	White	Tablet	Circle, Scored	Excellium Pharmaceuticals
EP; 104	Colchicine	0.6 mg	White	Tablet	Circle	Excellium Pharmaceuticals
EP-105	Aspirin	800 mg	White	Tablet	Capsule-Shape	Cypress Pharmaceutical
EP; 106	Aspirin	800 mg	White	Tablet	Capsule-Shape	Excellium Pharmaceuticals
EP; 107	Acetaminophen	500 mg	White	Tablet	Circle, Scored	Excellium Pharmaceuticals
EP; 110	Hyoscyamine	0.375 mg	Orange	Extended-Release Tablet	Capsule-Shape	Qualitest Products
EP; 121	Quinine Sulfate	260 mg	White	Tablet	Circle	Excellium Pharmaceuticals
EPI; 101	Migratine	65 mg; 100 mg; 325 mg	Red and White	Capsule		Excellium Pharmaceuticals
EPI; 132	Percolone	5 mg	White	Tablet	Round, Biconvex, Bisected, Debossed Scored	Endo Laboratories
EPITOL; 93; 93	Epitol	200 mg	White	Tablet	Circle, Scored, Flat	Teva Pharmaceuticals
EPITOL; 93; 758	Epitol	100 mg	Pink with Red Speckles	Tablet, Chewable	Circle, Flat, Beveled Edge, Scored	Teva Pharmaceuticals
ER; ABBOTT LOGO	Erythromycin Delayed-Release	250 mg	Clear and Maroon with Pink and Yellow Particles	Capsule		Abbott Laboratories
ER; SP	Estinyl	0.02 mg	Beige	Coated Tablet		Schering
ES	Erythrocin Stearate Filmtab	250 mg	Pink	Coated Tablet	Circle	Abbott Laboratories
ES;	Excedrin Sinus	500 mg; 30 mg	Orange	Tablet	Capsule-Shape	Bristol-Myers Squibb
ESB	Bufferin Extra Strength	500 mg; 222.3 mg; 88.9 mg; 55.6 mg	White	Coated Tablet	Oval	Bristol-Myers Squibb
ESKALITH; SB	Eskalith	300 mg	Gray and Yellow	Capsule		Glaxosmithkline
ESP 4177; SECTRAL; 200	Sectral	200 mg	Purple and Orange	Capsule		Esp Pharma
ESP; 4179; SECTRAL; 400	Sectral	400 mg	Brown and Orange	Capsule		Esp Pharma
ESR; 1174; MARION	Gaviscon	160 mg; 105 mg	White	Tablet, Chewable	Circle	Glaxosmithkline Consumer
ET	Erythrocin Stearate Filmtab	500 mg	Pink	Coated Tablet	Oblong	Abbott Laboratories
ETH; 042	Anemagen	200 mg; 250 mg; 10 mcg; 100 mg	Maroon	Capsule, Liquid Filled		Ethex
ETH; 043	Anemagen FA	200 mg; 10 mcg; 250 mg	Brown and Green	Capsule, Liquid Filled		Ethex
ETH; 052	Anemagen Ob	60 mg; 200 mg; 28 mg; 400 IU; 30 IU; 1.6 mg; 1.8 mg; 20 mg; 12 mcg; 25 mg; 1 mg	Green with White Ink	Capsule, Liquid Filled		Ethex
ETH; 4;	Nitroquick	0.4 mg	White	Tablet	Oval	Ethex
ETH; 15	Morphine Sulfate	15 mg	Brown	Tablet	Round, Partially Bisected Scored	Ethex
ETH; 227	Ed A-Hist	8 mg; 20 mg	Brown	Tablet	Capsule-Shape, Scored	Edwards
ETH; 227	Hista-Vent Da	8 mg; 20 mg; 2.5 mg	Brown	Extended-Release Tablet	Capsule-Shape	Ethex
ETH; 255	Hyoscyamine Sulfate	0.125 mg	White	Tablet		Ethex

IMPRINT	BRAND/GENERIC NAME	STRENGTH	COLOR	FORM	SHAPE	MANUFACTURER
ETH; 266; 1 MG	Doxazosin Mesylate	1 mg	Gray	Tablet		Ethex
ETH; 266; 1 MG	Doxazosin Mesylate	1 mg	Gray	Tablet		Stada
ETH; 267; 2 MG	Doxazosin Mesylate	2 mg	Yellow	Tablet		Ethex
ETH; 267; 2 MG	Doxazosin Mesylate	2 mg	Yellow	Tablet		Stada
ETH; 268; 4 MG	Doxazosin Mesylate	4 mg	Pink	Tablet		Ethex
ETH; 268; 4 MG	Doxazosin Mesylate	4 mg	Pink	Tablet		Stada
ETH; 269; 8 MG	Doxazosin Mesylate	8 mg	Blue	Tablet		Ethex
ETH; 269; 8 MG	Doxazosin Mesylate	8 mg	Blue	Tablet		Stada
ETH; 274	Hyoscyamine Sulfate	0.125 mg	White	Tablet	Oval	Ethex
ETH; 309; 5 5 5	Buspirone Hydrochloride	15 mg	Yellow	Tablet	Capsule-Shape, Trisected	Ethex
ETH; 315	Oxycodone Hydrochloride	5 mg	Orange	Tablet	Round, Flat-Faced, Beveled-Edge, Partially Bisected Scored	Ethex
ETH;331	Propafenone Hydrochloride	150 mg	White	Tablet	Circle	Ethex
ETH; 341	Benazepril Hydrochloride	5 mg	White	Tablet		Ethex
ETH; 342	Benazepril Hydrochloride	10 mg	Red	Tablet		Ethex
ETH; 343	Benazepril Hydrochloride	20 mg	Gray	Tablet		Ethex
ETH; 344	Benazepril Hydrochloride	40 mg	Blue	Tablet		Ethex
ETH; 416	Plaretase 8000	8000 U; 30000 U; 30000 U	Tan	Tablet	Circle	Ethex
ETH; 423	Hyoscyamine Sulfate	0.125 mg	White	Disintegrating Tablet	Circle	Ethex
ETHEX; 001	Potassium Chloride	750 mg	Clear	Extended-Release Capsule		Ethex
ETHEX; 002	Disopyramide Phosphate	150 mg	Purple and Orange	Extended-Release Capsule		Ethex
ETHEX; 003	Disopyramide Phosphate	100 mg	Purple and Yellow	Extended-Release Capsule		Ethex
ETHEX; 004	Nitroglycerin	2.5 mg	Lavender and Clear with White Beads	Extended-Release Capsule		Ethex
ETHEX; 005	Nitroglycerin	6.5 mg	Dark Blue and Yellow	Extended-Release Capsule		Ethex
ETHEX; 006	Nitroglycerin	9 mg	Clear	Extended-Release Capsule		Ethex
ETHEX; 015	Guaivent PD	300 mg; 60 mg	Opaque Black and Clear	Capsule		Ethex
ETHEX; 015	Pseudovent Ped	300 mg; 60 mg	Blue and Clear with White Beads	Extended-Release Capsule		Ethex
ETHEX; 016	Guaivent	250 mg; 120 mg	Opaque White and Clear	Capsule		Ethex
ETHEX; 016	Pseudovent	250 mg; 60 mg	White and Clear with White Beads	Extended-Release Capsule		Ethex
ETHEX; 017	Hyoscyamine Sulfate	0.375 mg	Clear	Extended-Release Capsule		Ethex
ETHEX; 019	Bromfenex	12 mg; 120 mg	Green and Clear	Extended-Release Capsule		Ethex
ETHEX; 020	Bromfenex PD Pediatric	6 mg; 60 mg	Green and Clear	Extended-Release Capsule		Ethex
ETHEX; 024	Fe-Tinic 150	150 mg	Orange	Capsule		Ethex
ETHEX; 025	Fe-Tinic 150 Forte	150 mg; 1 mg; 25 mcg	Maroon	Capsule		Ethex
ETHEX; 027	Meperidine Hcl and Promethazine Hcl	50 mg; 25 mg	Maroon	Capsule		Ethex
ETHEX; 028	Pangestyme Mt16	48000 U; 16000 U; 48000 U	Red	Capsule	Capsule-Shape	Ethex
ETHEX; 029	Pangestyme Cn-10	33200 U; 10000 U; 37500 U	Pink and Clear	Capsule	Capsule-Shape	Ethex
ETHEX; 030	Pangestyme Cn-20	75000 U; 20000 U; 66400 U	Red and Clear	Capsule	Capsule-Shape	Ethex
ETHEX; 031	Pangestyme Ec	20000 U; 4500 U; 25000 U	White	Capsule	Capsule-Shape	Ethex
ETHEX; 037	Trimethobenzamide Hydrochloride	250 mg	Green	Capsule		Ethex
ETHEX; 041	Oxycodone Hydrochloride	5 mg	Buff and White	Capsule		Ethex
ETHEX; 044	Conison	240 mg; 15 mcg; 110 mg; 75 mg; 0.5 mg	Maroon	Capsule		Ethex
ETHEX; 048	Pangestyme Ul12	39000 U; 12000 U; 39000 U	Blue and Clear	Capsule	Capsule-Shape	Ethex
ETHEX; 049	Pangestyme Ul18	58500 U; 18000 U; 58500 U	Blue	Capsule	Capsule-Shape	Ethex
ETHEX; 050	Pangestyme Ul20	65000 U; 20000 U; 65000 U	Green and Clear	Capsule	Capsule-Shape	Ethex
ETHEX; 076	Bromfenex Pe Pediatric	7.5 mg; 6 mg	Green and Clear	Capsule		Ethex
ETHEX; 077	Bromfenex Pe	15 mg; 12 mg	Light Green and Clear	Capsule		Ethex
ETHEX; 3	Nitroquick	0.3 mg	White	Tablet	Oval	Ethex
ETHEX; 6	Nitroquick	0.6 mg	White	Tablet	Oval	Ethex
ETHEX; 30	Morphine Sulfate	30 mg	Brown	Tablet	Capsule-Shaped, Partially Bisected Scored	Ethex
ETHEX; 205	Guaifenex LA	600 mg	White	Sustained-Release Tablet	Capsule-Shape	Ethex
ETHEX; 208	Guaifenex Pse 120	600 mg; 120 mg	White	Extended-Release Tablet	Capsule-Shape	Ethex
ETHEX; 212	Prenatal MR 90	250 mg; 2 mg; 1 mg; 90 mg; 4,000 I.U.; 12 mcg; 3.4 mg; 400 I.U.; 120 mg; 25 mg; 30 I.U.; 20 mg; 3 mg; 20 mg; 0.15 mg; 50 mg	Pink or White	Coated Tablet	Oval	Ethex
ETHEX; 213	Guaifenex DM	30 mg; 600 mg	Green	Extended-Release Tablet	Capsule-Shape	Ethex

IMPRINT	BRAND/GENERIC NAME	STRENGTH	COLOR	FORM	SHAPE	MANUFACTURER
ETHEX; 214	Guaifenex Pse 60	600 mg; 60 mg	Blue	Extended-Release Tablet	Capsule-Shaped; Bisected Scored	Ethex
ETHEX; 216	Prenatal RX 1	4000 IU; 15 IU; 80 mg; 1 mg; 1.5 mg; 1.6 mg; 17 mg; 4 mg; 2.5 mcg; 0.03 mg; 7 mg; 200 mg; 60 mg; 100 mg; 3 mg; 25 mg; 400 IU	White	Tablet	Oval	Ethex
ETHEX; 217	Prenatal Mtr Multivitamin and Mineral	5000 IU; 30 IU; 100 mg; 1 mg; 3 mg; 3.4 mg; 20 mg; 10 mg; 12 mcg; 30 mcg; 10 mg; 250 mg; 150 mcg; 60 mg; 25 mg; 2 mg; 25 mg; 25 mcg; 25 mcg; 5 mg; 400 IU	Tan	Tablet	Capsule-Shape	Ethex
ETHEX; 223	Codeine Phosphate and Guaifenesin	300 mg; 10 mg	Red	Tablet	Oval	Ethex
ETHEX; 232	Natal Care Multivitamin	250 mg; 2 mg; 1 mg; 50 mg; 50 mg; 15 mg; 3.6 mg; 2 mg; 40 mg; 250 IU		Tablet	Capsule-Shape	Ethex
ETHEX; 234	R-Tannate	25 mg; 8 mg; 25 mg	Off-White	Tablet	Capsule-Shape	Ethex
ETHEX; 236	Carisoprodol with Aspirin	200 mg; 325 mg	White and Orange	Tablet	Biconvex, Two Layered	Ethex
ETHEX; 237	Hyoscyamine Sulfate	0.375 mg		Sustained-Release Tablet		Ethex
ETHEX; 264; 5 MG	Buspirone Hydrochloride	5 mg	Yellow	Tablet	Oval	Ethex
ETHEX; 265; 10 MG	Buspirone Hydrochloride	10 mg	Yellow	Tablet	Oval	Ethex
ETHEX; 276	Guaifenex-RX AM Treatment Phase	600 mg; 60 mg	Blue	Extended-Release Tablet		Ethex
ETHEX; 276	Guaifenex-RX Pm Treatment Phase	600 mg	White	Extended-Release Tablet		Ethex
ETHEX; 277	Guaifenex-RX DM AM Treatment Phase	600 mg; 60 mg	Blue	Extended-Release Tablet		Ethex
ETHEX; 277	Guaifenex-RX DM Pm Treatment Phase	600 mg	White	Extended-Release Tablet		Ethex
ETHEX; 292	Ultra Natalcare	2700 IU; 120 mg; 200 mg; 90 mg; 400 IU; 30 IU; 3 mg; 3.4 mg; 20 mg; 20 mg; 1 mg; 12 mcg; 150 mcg; 25 mg; 2 mg; 50 mg	Beige	Tablet	Oval, Bisected Scored	Ethex
ETHEX; 301	Ketorolac Tromethamine	10 mg	White	Coated Tablet	Circle	Ethex
ETHEX; 302	Enteric Coated Naproxen	375 mg	White	Delayed-Release Tablet	Capsule-Shape	Ethex
ETHEX; 302	Enteric Coated Naproxen	375 mg	White	Enteric-Coated Tablet	Capsule-Shape	Ethex
ETHEX; 303	Enteric Coated Naproxen	500 mg	White	Delayed-Release Tablet	Capsule-Shape	Ethex
ETHEX; 303	Enteric Coated Naproxen	500 mg	White	Enteric-Coated Tablet	Capsule-Shape	Ethex
ETHEX; 308	Guaifenex G	1200 mg	White	Extended-Release Tablet	Capsule-Shape, or Round, Scored	Ethex
ETHEX; 311	Dextroamphetamine Sulfate	5 mg	Orange	Tablet	Circle, Scored	Ethex
ETHEX; 316	Prenatal Mtr with Selenium	5000 IU; 120 mg; 200 mg; 27 mg; 400 IU; 30 IU; 3 mg; 3.4 mg; 20 mg; 10 mg; 1 mg; 12 mcg; 30 mcg; 10 mg; 150 mcg; 25 mg; 25 mg; 20 mcg; 2 mg; 5 mg; 25 mcg; 25 mcg	Tan	Coated Tablet	Modified Capsule-Shaped, Partially Bisected Scored	Ethex
ETHEX; 322	Natalcare Cfe 60	1000 IU; 120 mg; 60 mg; 400 IU; 11 IU; 2 mg; 3 mg; 20 mg; 10 mg; 1 mg	Orange	Tablet	Oval	Ethex
ETHEX; 350	Advanced Natalcare	2700 IU; 120 mg; 200 mg; 90 mg; 400 IU; 30 IU; 3 mg; 3.4 mg; 20 mg; 20 mg; 1 mg; 12 mcg; 25 mg; 2 mg; 30 mg; 50 mg	White	Tablet	Oval, Bisected Scored	Ethex
ETHEX; 418	Natalcare Glosstabs	2700 IU; 120 mg; 200 mg; 90 mg; 400 IU; 10 IU; 3 mg; 3.4 mg; 20 mg; 20 mg; 1 mg; 12 mcg; 15 mg; 2 mg; 30 mg; 0.03 mg; 50 mg; 6 mg	Pink	Tablet		Ethex
ETHEX; 426	Hista-Vent Pse	120 mg; 8 mg; 2.5	White	Tablet		Ethex

IMPRINT	BRAND/GENERIC NAME	STRENGTH	COLOR	FORM	SHAPE	MANUFACTURER
ETHEX; 427	Histaclear-D	2.5 mg; 120 mg	Yellow	Tablet	Capsule-Shape	Ethex
ETHEX; 435	Carenate 600	600 mg; 2 mg; 90 mg; 3 mg; 400 IU; 20 mg; 30 IU; 60 mg; 25 mg; 1 mg; 2 mg; 3 mg; 3500 IU; 12 mcg; 50 mg	Yellow	Tablet	Oval	Ethex
ETHEX; 436	Carenate 600	600 mg; 2 mg; 90 mg; 3 mg; 400 IU; 20 mg; 30 IU; 60 mg; 25 mg; 1 mg; 2 mg; 3 mg; 3500 IU; 12 mcg; 50 mg	Yellow	Tablet, Chewable	Circle	Ethex
ETHEX; 439	Cal-Nate	2700 IU; 120 mg; 125 mg; 27 mg; 400 IU; 30 IU; 3 mg; 3.4 mg; 20 mg; 20 mg; 1 mg; 150 mcg; 25 mg; 2 mg; 50 mg	White	Tablet	Oval	Ethex
ETHEX; 458	Advanced-Rf Natalcare	120 mg; 200 mg; 90 mg; 30 IU; 3 mg; 3.4 mg; 20 mg; 20 mg; 1 mg; 12 mcg; 25 mg; 2 mg; 30 mg; 50 mg	White	Tablet		Ethex
ETHEX; KCL; 10	Potassium Chloride	750 mg	Clear	Extended-Release Capsule		KV Pharmaceutical
ETO; 200	Etodolac	200 mg	Dark Pink and Black	Capsule		Taro Pharmaceuticals
ETO; 300	Etodolac	300 mg	Pink and Black	Capsule		Taro Pharmaceuticals
EV; 0471	Tussall ER	20 mg; 30 mg; 6 mg	White	Tablet	Capsule-Shape	Everett Laboratories
EV; 0661	Trituss-ER	600 mg; 30 mg; 10 mg	White	Extended-Release Tablet	Capsule-Shape	Everett Laboratories
EVERETT	Anafed	8 mg; 120 mg	Yellow and Clear	Capsule		Everett Laboratories
EVERETT	Pavatym	150 mg	Blue and Brown	Capsule		Everett Laboratories
EVERETT; 0072	Vitafol	6000 IU; 400 IU; 30 IU; 1 mg; 60 mg; 1.1 mg; 1.8 mg; 2.5 mg; 5 mcg; 15 mg; 125 mg; 65 mg	Pink	Coated Tablet	Capsule-Shape	Everett Laboratories
EVERETT; 0201	Strovite Plus	27 mg; 500 I.U.; 30 I.U.; 500 mg; 20 mg; 20 mg; 100 mg; 25 mg; 0.15 mg; 25 mg; 0.8 mg; 50 mcg; 0.1 mg; 5 mg; 3 mg; 22.5 mg	Deep Red	Tablet	Oval	Everett Laboratories
EVERETT; 162	Repan	50 mg; 325 mg; 40 mg	White	Tablet	Circle	Everett Laboratories
EVOXAC; 30 MG	Evoxac	30 mg	White	Capsule		Daiichi Pharmaceutical
EXCEDRIN	Excedrin Tri-Buffered Arthritis Strength	500 mg	White	Tablet		Bristol-Myers Squibb
EXCEDRIN; AF	Aspirin Free Excedrin Extra Strength Geltab	500 mg; 65 mg	Red	Geltab	Capsule-Shape	Bristol-Myers Squibb
EXCEDRIN IB	Excedrin Ib Tablet	200 mg	White	Tablet	Circle	Bristol-Myers Squibb
EXCEDRIN PM	Excedrin Pm Aspirin Free Tablet	500 mg; 38 mg	Light Blue	Tablet	Circle	Bristol-Myers Products
EXELON; 1.5 MG	Exelon	1.5 mg	Yellow with Red Ink	Capsule		Novartis
EXELON; 3 MG	Exelon	3 mg	Orange with Red Ink	Capsule		Novartis
EXELON; 4.5 MG	Exelon	4.5 mg	Red with White Ink	Capsule		Novartis
EXELON; 6 MG	Exelon	6 mg	Orange and Red with Red Ink	Capsule		Novartis
EX-LAX	Ex-Lax	100 mg	Green	Tablet	Oblong	Sandoz Consumer
EZOL	Ezol	50 mg; 325 mg; 40 mg		Capsule		Stewart-Jackson Pharmacal
F; 1	Sodium Fluoride	2.2 mg	Pink	Tablet	Circular, Flat-Faced, Bevel-Edged, Bisected, Compressed Scored	Trinity Technologies
F2F	Actifed Plus Extra Strength	500 mg; 60 mg; 2.5 mg	White	Tablet		Pfizer Consumer Health Care
F; 16;	Principen with Probenecid	389 mg; 111 mg	Orange and Red	Capsule		Apothecon
F; 66; LL	Fibercon	500 mg	Clear	Coated Tablet		Lederle Laboratories
F; III	Aerolate Iii	65 mg	Red and Clear	Timed-Release Capsule		Fleming
F; JR	Aerolate JR.	130 mg	Red and Clear	Timed-Release Capsule		Fleming
F; JR; F; JR	Extendryl JR.	10 mg; 4 mg; 1.25 mg	Green and Red	Sustained-Release Capsule		Fleming
F; L; 10	Lexapro	10 mg	White to Off White	Coated Tablet	Circle, Scored	Forest Pharmaceuticals
F; L; 20	Lexapro	20 mg	White to Off White	Coated Tablet	Circle	Forest Pharmaceuticals
F; SR	Aerolate SR.	260 mg	Red and Clear	Timed-Release Capsule		Fleming
F; SR; SR	Extendryl SR.	20 mg; 8 mg; 2.5 mg	Green and Red	Sustained-Release Capsule		Fleming
F P; 5400	Combunox	5 mg; 400 mg	Off White, White	Tablet	Capsule-Shape	Forest Pharmaceuticals
FAMVIR; 125	Famvir	125 mg	White	Coated Tablet	Circle	Novartis
FAMVIR; 250	Famvir	250 mg	White	Coated Tablet	Circle	Novartis
FAMVIR; 500	Famvir	500 mg	White	Coated Tablet	Oval	Novartis

IMPRINT	BRAND/GENERIC NAME	STRENGTH	COLOR	FORM	SHAPE	MANUFACTURER
FANSIDAR; ROCHE	Fansidar	25 mg; 500 mg	White	Tablet	Circle, Scored	Roche Laboratories
FASTIN; BEECHAM	Fastin	30 mg	Blue and Clear with Blue and White Beads	Capsule		Glaxosmithkline
FC; 50; G	Flecainide Acetate	50 mg	White	Tablet	Circle	Par Pharmaceutical
FC; 100	Somophyllin-T	100 mg	White	Capsule		Fisons Pharmaceuticals
FC; 100; G	Flecainide Acetate	100 mg	White	Tablet	Circle, Scored	Par Pharmaceutical
FC; 150; G	Flecainide Acetate	150 mg	White	Tablet	Oval, Scored	Par Pharmaceutical
FC; 200	Somophyllin-T	200 mg	White	Capsule		Fisons Pharmaceuticals
FC; 250	Somophyllin-T	250 mg	White	Capsule		Fisons Pharmaceuticals
FE	Feratab	300 mg	Red	Tablet	Circle	Upsher-Smith Laboratories
FE	Ferrous Gluconate	300 mg	Green	Coated Tablet	Circle	Upsher-Smith Laboratories
FEEN-A-MINT	Feen-A-Mint	5 mg	White	Enteric-Coated Tablet	Circle	Schering-Plough Healthcare Products
FELDENE; PFIZER 322	Feldene	10 mg	Maroon and Blue	Capsule		Pfizer Laboratories
FELDENE; PFIZER 323	Feldene	20 mg	Maroon	Capsule		Pfizer Laboratories
FEOSOL	Feosol	159 mg		Extended-Release Capsule		Glaxosmithkline Consumer
FERGON	Fergon	320 mg		Tablet		Bayer Consumer Care
FHF	Pentone	100 mg	White	Capsule		Faulding Laboratories
FIORICET; CODEINE; FOUR-HEAD PROFILE	Fioricet with Codeine	30 mg; 50 mg; 40 mg; 325 mg	Dark Blue and Gray	Capsule		Watson Laboratories
FIORICET; S	Fioricet	50 mg; 40 mg; 325 mg	Blue	Tablet	Circle	Watson Laboratories
FIORINAL; 78; 103	Fiorinal	325 mg; 50 mg; 40 mg	Kelly Green and Lime Green	Capsule		Watson Laboratories
FISONS; 101	Gastrocrom	100 mg	Clear	Capsule		Fisons Pharmaceuticals
FL	Adphen	35 mg	Peach	Tablet	Circle, Scored	Ferndale Laboratories
FL	Chlorzoxazone	500 mg	Light Green	Tablet	Oblong	Econolab
FL	Migrex	325 mg; 100 mg; 65 mg	Red and White	Capsule		Econolab
FL	Phendimetrazine Tartrate	35 mg	Yellow or Pink	Tablet	Circle	Ferndale Laboratories
FL	Strifon Forte Dsc	500 mg	Light Green	Tablet	Circle, Scored	Ferndale Laboratories
FL; 5	Lexapro	5 mg	White to Off White	Coated Tablet	Circle	Forest Pharmaceuticals
FL; 5	Namenda	5 mg	Tan	Tablet	Capsule-Shape	Forest Pharmaceuticals
FL; 10	Namenda	10 mg	Gray	Tablet	Capsule-Shape	Forest Pharmaceuticals
FL; 10; G	Fluoxetine Hydrochloride	10 mg	White	Tablet	Oval	Par Pharmaceutical
FL; 20; G	Fluoxetine Hydrochloride	20 mg	White	Tablet	Oval	Par Pharmaceutical
FL; 1033	Spastrin	40 mg; 0.6 mg; 0.2 mg	Blue	Tablet	Circle, Scored	Novartis Generics
FL; DOUBLE HEART	Dapex	37.5 mg	Opaque Blue and Clear	Capsule		Ferndale Laboratories
FL; DOUBLE HEART	Kronofed-A	120 mg; 8 mg	White, Clear	Sustained-Release Capsule		Ferndale Laboratories
FL; DOUBLE HEART	Kronofed-A JR	60 mg; 4 mg	White and Clear	Sustained-Release Capsule		Ferndale Laboratories
FL; DOUBLE HEART	Obestin	30 mg	Blue and Clear with Blue and White Beads	Capsule		Ferndale Laboratories
FLAGYL; 375	Flagyl	375 mg	Grey and Green	Capsule	Oblong	Searle
FLAGYL; 500	Flagyl	500 mg	Blue	Coated Tablet	Oblong	Searle
FLEXERIL	Flexeril	5 mg	Yellow-Orange	Coated Tablet	D-Shape	Alza
FLOMAX 0.4 MG; BI; 58	Flomax	0.4 mg	Green Opaque Cap and Orange Opaque Body	Capsule		Boehringer Ingelheim
FLOXIN; 200 MG	Floxin	200 mg	Pale Yellow	Coated Tablet		Ortho-Mcneil Pharmaceutical
FLOXIN; 300 MG	Floxin	300 mg	White	Coated Tablet		Ortho-Mcneil Pharmaceutical
FLOXIN; 400 MG	Floxin	400 mg	Pale Gold	Coated Tablet		Ortho-Mcneil Pharmaceutical
FLUMADINE 100; FOREST	Flumadine	100 mg	Orange	Coated Tablet	Oval	Forest Pharmaceuticals
FLUOXETINE; R; 149	Fluoxetine Hydrochloride	40 mg	White	Capsule		Par Pharmaceutical
FLZ; 50	Fluconazole	50 mg	Pink	Tablet	Four-Sided	Greenstone
FLZ; 100	Fluconazole	100 mg	Pink	Tablet	Four-Sided	Greenstone
FLZ; 150	Fluconazole	150 mg	Pink	Tablet	Oval	Greenstone
FLZ; 200	Fluconazole	200 mg	Pink	Tablet	Four-Sided	Greenstone
FOREST; 372;	Feostat	100 mg	Brown	Tablet, Chewable	Circle	Forest Pharmaceuticals
FOREST; 0372; ESGIC PLUS	Esgic-Plus	500 mg; 50 mg; 40 mg	Red	Capsule		Forest Pharmaceuticals
FOREST; 642	Elixophyllin Df 100	100 mg	White	Gel/jelly		Forest Pharmaceuticals
FOREST; 643	Elixophyllin Df 200	200 mg	White	Capsule, Liquid Filled		Forest Pharmaceuticals
FOREST; 677	Esgic with Codeine	50 mg; 325 mg; 40 mg; 30 mg	Black and Opaque Blue	Capsule		Forest Pharmaceuticals
FOREST; 678	Esgic-Plus	50 mg; 500 mg; 40 mg	White	Tablet	Capsule-Shape, Scored	Forest Pharmaceuticals
FOREST; 610A	Bancap Hc	500 mg; 5 mg	Yellow and Orange	Capsule		Forest Pharmaceuticals
FOREST; 610A	Hydrocodone Bitartrate and Acetaminophen	5 mg; 500 mg	Orange and Yellow	Capsule		Forest Pharmaceuticals
FP; 10 MG	Celexa	10 mg	Beige	Coated Tablet	Oval	Forest Pharmaceuticals
FP; 20 MG	Celexa	20 mg	Pink	Coated Tablet	Oval, Scored	Forest Pharmaceuticals
FP; 40 MG	Celexa	40 mg	White	Coated Tablet	Oval, Scored	Forest Pharmaceuticals
FR; ABBOTT LOGO	Tricor, Micronized	67 mg	Yellow	Capsule		Abbott Laboratories
FULVICIN; P/G; 352	Fulvicin P/g	330 mg	White	Tablet	Oval, Compressed, Scored	Schering
FULVICIN; P/G; 654	Fulvicin P/g	165 mg	White	Tablet	Oval, Compressed, Scored	Schering
FV; CG	Femara	2.5 mg	Dark Yellow	Coated Tablet	Circle	Novartis
G	Gelpirin	125 mg; 240 mg; 32 mg	Orange	Tablet	Circle	Alra Laboratories

IMPRINT	BRAND/GENERIC NAME	STRENGTH	COLOR	FORM	SHAPE	MANUFACTURER
G	Geritol Extend	1250 IU; 130 mg; 150 mcg; 35 mg; 100 mg; 3333 IU; 15 mg; 15 IU; 200 IU; 70 mcg; 15 mg; 10 mg; 0.2 mg; 2 mcg; 1.4 mg; 2 mg; 80 mcg; 60 mg; 1.2 mg	Maroon	Tablet	Oblong	Glaxosmithkline Consumer
G; 00	Laxative for Women	65 mg; 100 mg	Pink	Coated Tablet	Circle	G & W Laboratories
G; 00; 30	Ranitidine Hydrochloride	150 mg	White	Tablet	Circle	Mylan Pharmaceuticals
G; 00; 53	Oxaprozin	600 mg	White	Tablet	Oval	Par Pharmaceutical
G; 0031	Ranitidine Hydrochloride	300 mg	White	Tablet	Capsule-Shape	Mylan Pharmaceuticals
G; 0034	Acyclovir	200 mg	Blue, Opaque	Capsule		Par Pharmaceutical
G; 0036	Acyclovir	400 mg	White	Tablet	Five-Sided	Par Pharmaceutical
G; 0037	Acyclovir	800 mg	Blue	Tablet	Oval	Par Pharmaceutical
G; 0041	Nicardipine Hydrochloride	20 mg	White and Blue	Capsule		Par Pharmaceutical
G; 0042	Nicardipine Hydrochloride	30 mg	Light Blue	Capsule		Par Pharmaceutical
G; 0506	Ser-A-Gen	15 mg; 25 mg; 0.1 mg	Salmon	Tablet	Circle	Zenith Goldline Pharmaceuticals
G; 1	Glyburide	1.5 mg	White	Tablet	Capsule-Shape	West-Ward
G; 2	Benzocaine	15 mg	Yellow	Lozenge/troche	Circle, Flat	Gemini Pharmaceuticals
G; 2	Genac	2.5 mg; 60 mg	White	Tablet	Circle	Ivax Pharmaceuticals
G; 2	Glyburide	3 mg	Blue	Tablet	Capsule-Shape, Scored	West-Ward
G; 25	Atenolol	25 mg	White	Tablet	Circle, Flat; Bevelled Edge; Scored	Par Pharmaceutical
G; 50; BAYER LOGO	Glucobay	50 mg	White to Brown Tinged	Tablet	Circle, Convex	Bayer Pharmaceutical
G; 100; BAYER LOGO	Glucobay	100 mg	White to Brown Tinged	Tablet	Circle, Convex, Scored	Bayer Pharmaceutical
G; 150 MG; 3328	Clindamycin Hydrochloride	150 mg	Blue-Green	Capsule		Greenstone
G; 181	Flavoxate Hydrochloride	100 mg	Off-White	Tablet	Circle	Global Pharmaceutical
G; 300 MG; 5010	Clindamycin Hydrochloride	300 mg	Light Blue	Capsule		Greenstone
G; 400	Ibuprofen	400 mg	White	Tablet	Circle	Greenstone
G; 800	Ibuprofen	800 mg	White	Tablet	Capsule-Shape	Greenstone
G; 891	Preven	0.25 mg; 0.05 mg	Blue	Tablet		Gynetics
G; 1911	Rimantadine Hydrochloride	100 mg	Orange	Tablet	Oval	Global Pharmaceutical
G; 2442	Budeprion SR	100 mg	Yellow	Extended-Release Tablet	Circle	Teva Pharmaceuticals
G; 2444	Budeprion SR	150 mg	Light Yellow	Extended-Release Tablet	Circle	Teva Pharmaceuticals
G; 3327; 4	Methylprednisolone Acetate	4 mg	White	Tablet	Oval	Pharmacia & Upjohn
G; 3717	Triazolam	0.125 mg	White	Tablet	Flat Beveled Edge	Greenstone
G; 3718	Triazolam	0.25 mg	Light Blue	Tablet	Oval, Scored	Greenstone
G; 3719	Alprazolam	0.25 mg	White	Tablet	Oval, Scored	Greenstone
G; 3720	Alprazolam	0.5 mg	Peach	Tablet	Oval, Scored	Greenstone
G; 3721	Alprazolam	1 mg	Blue	Tablet	Oval, Scored	Greenstone
G; 3722	Alprazolam	2 mg	White	Tablet	Oblong, Quadrisected Scored	Greenstone
G; 3723	Flurbiprofen	50 mg	White	Tablet	Oval	Greenstone
G; 3724	Flurbiprofen	100 mg	Blue	Tablet	Oval	Greenstone
G; 3725	Glyburide	1.25 mg	White	Tablet	Circle, Scored	Greenstone
G; 3726	Glyburide	2.5 mg	Dark Pink	Tablet	Circle, Scored	Greenstone
G; 3727	Glyburide	5 mg	Blue	Tablet	Circle, Scored	Greenstone
G; 3740	Medroxyprogesterone Acetate	2.5 mg	Orange	Tablet	Circle, Scored	Greenstone
G; 3741	Medroxyprogesterone Acetate	5 mg	White	Tablet	Six-Sided, Scored	Greenstone
G; 3742	Medroxyprogesterone Acetate	10 mg	White	Tablet	Circle, Scored	Greenstone
G; 3781	Glyburide, Micronized	1.5 mg	White	Tablet	Egg-Shape, Contour, Scored	Greenstone
G; 3782	Glyburide, Micronized	3 mg	Blue	Tablet	Egg-Shape, Contour, Scored	Greenstone
G; 3783	Glyburide, Micronized	6 mg	Yellow	Tablet	Egg-Shape, Contour, Scored	Greenstone
G; ANTACID	Antacid	311 mg; 232 mg	Clear and Aqua	Capsule, Liquid Filled		Leiner Health Products
G; ET; 500	Etodolac	500 mg	Light Blue	Tablet	Oval	Par Pharmaceutical
G; FL; 10	Fluoxetine Hydrochloride	10 mg	Purple and Green	Capsule		Par Pharmaceutical
G; FL; 20	Fluoxetine Hydrochloride	20 mg	Purple and Green	Capsule		Par Pharmaceutical
G; GU; 1	Guanfacine Hydrochloride	1 mg	White	Tablet	Oval	Par Pharmaceutical
G; GU; 2	Guanfacine Hydrochloride	2 mg	White	Tablet	Oval	Par Pharmaceutical
G; S; 80	Sotalol Hydrochloride	80 mg	White	Tablet	Capsule-Shape	Par Pharmaceutical
G; S; 120	Sotalol Hydrochloride	120 mg	White	Tablet	Capsule-Shape	Par Pharmaceutical
G; S; 160	Sotalol Hydrochloride	160 mg	White	Tablet	Capsule-Shape	Par Pharmaceutical
G; S; 240	Sotalol Hydrochloride	240 mg	White	Tablet	Capsule-Shape	Par Pharmaceutical
G; SE; 5	Selegiline Hydrochloride	5 mg	White	Tablet	Circle	Par Pharmaceutical
G; T250	Ticlopidine Hydrochloride	250 mg	White to Off-White	Tablet	Oval	Par Pharmaceutical
G; FL 50	Fluconazole	50 mg	Pink	Tablet	Rectangle	Par Pharmaceutical
G; FL 100	Fluconazole	100 mg	Pink	Tablet	Rectangle	Par Pharmaceutical
G; FL 150	Fluconazole	150 mg	Pink	Tablet	Oval	Par Pharmaceutical
G; FL 200	Fluconazole	200 mg	Pink	Tablet	Rectangle	Par Pharmaceutical
G3511	Pyridostigmine Bromide	60 mg	White	Tablet	Round, Quadrisected Scored	Global Pharmaceutical
G4; 832; 63	Medroxyprogesterone Acetate	10 mg	White	Tablet	Circle	Rosemont Pharmaceutical
GANTANOL; ROCHE	Gantanol	0.5 G	Pale Green	Tablet	Circle, Scored	Roche Laboratories
GANTANOL-DS; ROCHE	Gantanol-DS	1 G	Light Orange	Tablet	Capsule-Shape, Scored	Roche Laboratories
GAS-X	Gas-X	80 mg	White	Tablet, Chewable		Novartis Consumer
GAS-X	Gas-X Extra Strength	125 mg		Tablet, Chewable		Novartis Consumer
GDC; 113	Calcium Antacid	500 mg	White	Tablet, Chewable	Circle	Qualitest Products
GDC; 119	Alenic Alka	80 mg; 20 mg	White	Tablet, Chewable	Circle	Rugby Laboratories
GDC; 119	Foaming Antacid	80 mg; 20 mg		Tablet, Chewable		Qualitest Products
GDC; 127	Antacid Extra Strength	750 mg	Multi	Tablet, Chewable		Ivax Pharmaceuticals
GDC; 127	Calcium Antacid Extra Strength	750 mg	Assorted	Tablet	Circle	Qualitest Products
GDC; 128	Foaming Antacid Es	160 mg; 105 mg	White	Tablet, Chewable	Circle	Qualitest Products
GDC; 143	Corrective Laxative	5 mg	Pink	Enteric-Coated Tablet	Circle	Qualitest Products
GDC; 144	Calcium Antacid Extra Strength	750 mg	White	Tablet	Circle	Qualitest Products

IMPRINT	BRAND/GENERIC NAME	STRENGTH	COLOR	FORM	SHAPE	MANUFACTURER
GE; 320	Factive	320 mg	White to Off-White	Tablet	Oval	Lg Life Science
GE; 320	Factive	320 mg	White to Off-White	Tablet	Oval	Oscient Pharmaceuticals
GEIGY; 14	Butazolidin	100 mg	Red	Coated Tablet	Circle	Novartis
GEIGY; 20	Tofranil-Pm	75 mg	Coral	Capsule		Mallinckrodt
GEIGY; 22	Tofranil-Pm	150 mg	Coral	Capsule		Mallinckrodt
GEIGY; 32	Tofranil	10 mg	Coral	Tablet	Triangle	Mallinckrodt
GEIGY; 35 35	Lopressor HCT	25 mg; 50 mg	White and Blue	Tablet		Novartis
GEIGY; 35 35	Lopressor HCT 50/25	50 mg; 25 mg	Light Blue	Tablet	Capsule-Shape, Scored	Ciba-Geigy
GEIGY; 40	Tofranil-Pm	100 mg	Dark Yellow and Coral	Capsule		Mallinckrodt
GEIGY; 42	Constant-T	200 mg	Pink	Timed-Release Tablet	Oval, Scored	Geigy
GEIGY; 44; BUTAZOLIDIN; 100 MG	Butazolidin	100 mg	Orange and White	Capsule		Novartis
GEIGY; 45	Tofranil-Pm	125 mg	Light Yellow and Coral	Capsule		Mallinckrodt
GEIGY; 48	Pbz-SR	100 mg	Lavender	Extended-Release Tablet	Circle	Novartis
GEIGY; 51	Lopressor	50 mg	Pink	Tablet	Capsule-Shape, Scored	Ciba-Geigy
GEIGY; 53 53	Lopressor HCT 100/25	100 mg; 25 mg	Pink	Tablet	Capsule-Shape, Scored	Ciba-Geigy
GEIGY; 57	Constant-T	300 mg	Blue	Timed-Release Tablet	Oval, Scored	Geigy
GEIGY; 71; 71	Lopressor	100 mg	Light Blue	Tablet	Capsule-Shape, Scored	Ciba-Geigy
GEIGY; 72	Brethine	2.5 mg	White	Tablet	Oval	Ciba-Geigy
GEIGY; 73 73	Lopressor HCT 100/50	100 mg; 50 mg	Yellow	Tablet	Capsule-Shape, Scored	Ciba-Geigy
GEIGY; 105	Brethine	5 mg	White	Tablet	Circle, Scored	Ciba-Geigy
GEIGY; 111	Pbz	25 mg	White	Tablet	Circle, Scored	Novartis
GEIGY; 117	Pbz	50 mg	White	Tablet	Circle, Scored	Novartis
GEIGY; 136	Tofranil	50 mg	Coral	Coated Tablet	Circle	Mallinckrodt
GEIGY; 140	Tofranil	25 mg	Coral	Coated Tablet	Circle	Mallinckrodt
GEIGY GM	Lamprene	50 mg	Brown	Capsule	Oblong	Novartis
GEIGY; GM	Lamprene	100 mg	Brown	Capsule	Oblong	Novartis
GERITOL	Geritol Complete	45 mcg; 162 mg; 2 mg; 150 mcg; 100 mg; 15 mcg; 10 mg; 25 mcg; 125 mg; 400 IU; 60 mg; 1.7 mg; 2 mg; 6 mcg; 1.5 mg; 6000 IU; 15 mcg; 15 mg; 30 IU; 37.5 mg; 20 mg; 2.5 mg; 18 mg; 400 mcg; 15 mcg	Red	Coated Tablet	Oblong	Glaxosmithkline Consumer
GF; DM	Q-Bid DM	30 mg; 600 mg	Green	Tablet	Oval	Qualitest Products
GG; 3	Phenobarbital	15 mg	White	Tablet	Circle	Geneva Generics
GG; 4;	Lonox	0.025 mg; 2.5 mg	White	Tablet	Circle	Sandoz
GG; 9;	Dexamethasone	0.75 mg	Blue	Tablet	Five-Sided	Novartis Generics
GG; 11;	Chlorthalidone	25 mg	Yellow	Tablet	Circle	Novartis Generics
GG; 12	Medroxyprogesterone	10 mg	White	Tablet	Circle, Scored	Novartis Generics
GG; 13;	Chlorthalidone	50 mg	Green	Tablet	Circle, Scored	Novartis Generics
GG; 14;	Prednisolone	5 mg	Peach	Tablet	Circle, Scored	Novartis Generics
GG; 15	Nylidrin Hydrochloride	12 mg	White	Tablet	Circle	Geneva Generics
GG; 17	Chlorthalidone and Reserpine	50 mg; 0.25 mg		Tablet		Novartis Generics
GG; 18	Perphenazine	2 mg	White	Coated Tablet	Circle, Debossed	Geneva Generics
GG; 21;	Furosemide	20 mg	White	Tablet	Circle, Scored	Sandoz
GG; 22;	Pseudoephedrine Hydrochloride	60 mg	White	Tablet	Circle, Scored	Geneva Generics
GG; 23	T.E.P.	130 mg; 24.3 mg; 8.1 mg	White	Tablet	Circle	Novartis Generics
GG; 24;	T.E.H.	25 mg; 10 mg; 130 mg	White	Tablet	Circle, Scored; Compressed	Novartis Generics
GG; 26	Isdn	10 mg	White	Tablet	Circle, Scored, Debossed	Sandoz
GG; 27;	Hydrochlorothiazide	50 mg	Peach	Tablet	Circle, Scored	Novartis Generics
GG; 28;	Hydrochlorothiazide	25 mg	Peach	Tablet	Circle, Scored	Novartis Generics
GG; 29;	Triamcinolone	4 mg	White	Tablet	Capsule-Shape	Novartis Generics
GG; 30	Thioridazine Hydrochloride	10 mg	Orange	Coated Tablet	Circle	Geneva Generics
GG; 31; 15	Thioridazine Hydrochloride	15 mg	Orange	Coated Tablet	Circle	Geneva Generics
GG; 32; 25	Thioridazine Hydrochloride	25 mg	Orange	Coated Tablet	Circle	Geneva Generics
GG; 33; 50	Thioridazine Hydrochloride	50 mg	Orange	Coated Tablet	Circle	Geneva Generics
GG; 34; 100	Thioridazine Hydrochloride	100 mg	Orange	Coated Tablet	Circle	Geneva Generics
GG; 35	Thioridazine Hydrochloride	150 mg	Orange	Coated Tablet	Circle	Geneva Generics
GG; 36	Thioridazine Hydrochloride	200 mg	Orange	Coated Tablet	Circle	Geneva Generics
GG; 37	Hydroxyzine Hydrochloride	10 mg	Lavender	Coated Tablet		Novartis Generics
GG; 38	Hydroxyzine Hydrochloride	25 mg	Lavender	Coated Tablet	Circle	Novartis Generics
GG; 39	Hydroxyzine Hydrochloride	50 mg	Purple	Coated Tablet		Novartis Generics
GG; 40;	Amitriptyline Hydrochloride	10 mg	Pink with White Core	Coated Tablet	Circle	Sandoz
GG; 41	Imipramine Hydrochloride	10 mg	Yellow	Coated Tablet	Circle, Debossed	Sandoz
GG; 42	Imipramine Hydrochloride	50 mg	Green	Coated Tablet	Circle, Debossed	Sandoz
GG; 45;	Dipyridamole	50 mg	White	Coated Tablet	Circle	Novartis Generics
GG; 47	Imipramine Hydrochloride	25 mg	Beige	Coated Tablet	Circle, Debossed	Sandoz
GG; 48;	Pseudoephedrine Hydrochloride	30 mg	Red	Coated Tablet	Circle	Geneva Generics
GG; 49;	Dipyridamole	25 mg	White	Coated Tablet	Circle	Novartis Generics
GG; 51; 1	Trifluoperazine Hydrochloride	1 mg	Lavender	Coated Tablet	Circle	Geneva Generics
GG; 52;	Levothyroxine Sodium	0.1 mg	Yellow	Tablet	Circle, Scored	Novartis Generics
GG; 53; 2	Trifluoperazine Hydrochloride	2 mg	Lavender	Coated Tablet	Circle	Geneva Generics
GG; 54;	Levothyroxine Sodium	0.2 mg	White	Tablet	Circle, Scored	Novartis Generics
GG; 55; 5	Trifluoperazine Hydrochloride	5 mg	Lavender	Coated Tablet	Circle	Geneva Generics
GG; 56	Disopyramide Phosphate	100 mg	Opaque Orange	Capsule		Novartis Generics
GG; 57	Disopyramide Phosphate	150 mg		Capsule		Novartis Generics
GG; 58; 10	Trifluoperazine Hydrochloride	10 mg	Lavender	Coated Tablet	Circle	Geneva Generics

IMPRINT	BRAND/GENERIC NAME	STRENGTH	COLOR	FORM	SHAPE	MANUFACTURER
GG; 61	Chlorpropamide	100 mg	White	Tablet	Circle, Scored	Novartis Generics
GG; 62	Sodium Fluoride	2.2 mg	Pink	Tablet	Circle	Novartis Generics
GG; 63	Desipramine Hydrochloride	10 mg	White	Coated Tablet	Circle, Debossed	Sandoz
GG; 64	Desipramine Hydrochloride	25 mg	White	Coated Tablet	Circle, Debossed	Sandoz
GG; 65	Desipramine Hydrochloride	50 mg	White	Coated Tablet	Circle, Debossed	Sandoz
GG; 66	Diazepam	2 mg	White	Tablet	Circle, Scored	Novartis Generics
GG; 67	Diazepam	5 mg	Orange	Tablet	Circle, Scored	Novartis Generics
GG; 68	Diazepam	10 mg	Green	Tablet	Circle, Scored	Novartis Generics
GG; 70	Propranolol Hydrochloride	90 mg		Tablet		Novartis Generics
GG; 71	Propranolol Hydrochloride	10 mg	Peach Colored	Tablet	Circle, Scored	Novartis Generics
GG; 72	Propranolol Hydrochloride	20 mg	Blue	Tablet	Circle, Scored	Novartis Generics
GG; 73	Propranolol Hydrochloride	40 mg	Green	Tablet	Circle, Scored	Novartis Generics
GG; 74	Propranolol Hydrochloride	60 mg	Salmon Colored	Tablet	Circle, Scored	Novartis Generics
GG; 75	Propranolol Hydrochloride	80 mg	Yellow	Tablet	Circle, Scored	Novartis Generics
GG; 76	Levothyroxine Sodium	0.3 mg	Green	Tablet	Circle, Scored	Novartis Generics
GG; 77	Levothyroxine Sodium	0.15 mg	Blue	Tablet	Circle, Scored	Novartis Generics
GG; 78	Methazolamide	25 mg	White	Tablet	Circle, Scored, Debossed	Sandoz
GG; 79	Prednisone	5 mg	White	Tablet	Circle, Scored	Novartis Generics
GG; 80	Furosemide	80 mg	White	Tablet	Circle, Scored, Beveled-Edge	Sandoz
GG; 81	Clonidine Hydrochloride	0.1 mg	Light Green	Tablet	Circle, Scored	Novartis Generics
GG; 82	Clonidine Hydrochloride	0.2 mg	Yellow	Tablet	Circle, Scored	Novartis Generics
GG; 83	Clonidine Hydrochloride	0.3 mg	Blue	Tablet	Circle, Scored	Novartis Generics
GG; 84	Timolol Maleate	5 mg	White	Tablet	Circle	Novartis Generics
GG; 85	Spironolactone	25 mg	White	Tablet	Circle, Scored, Debossed	Geneva Generics
GG; 86	Clonidine Hydrochloride and Chlorthalidone	15 mg; 0.1 mg		Tablet		Novartis Generics
GG; 87	Clonidine Hydrochloride and Chlorthalidone	15 mg; 0.2 mg		Tablet		Novartis Generics
GG; 88	Clonidine Hydrochloride and Chlorthalidone	15 mg; 0.3 mg		Tablet		Novartis Generics
GG; 91	Lorazepam	0.5 mg	White	Tablet	Circle	Sandoz
GG; 92	Lorazepam	1 mg	White	Tablet	Circle, Scored	Sandoz
GG; 93	Lorazepam	2 mg	White	Tablet	Circle, Scored	Sandoz
GG; 95	Spironolactone and Hydrochlorothiazide	25 mg; 25 mg	White	Coated Tablet	Circle, Scored	Geneva Generics
GG; 96	Clorazepate Dipotassium	3.75 mg	Blue	Tablet	Circle, Scored, Compressed	Novartis Generics
GG; 97	Fluphenazine Hydrochloride	1 mg	Rust	Coated Tablet	Circle	Sandoz
GG; 98	Clorazepate Dipotassium	7.5 mg	Peach	Tablet	Circle, Scored, Compressed	Novartis Generics
GG; 99	Clorazepate Dipotassium	15 mg	White	Tablet	Circle, Scored, Compressed	Novartis Generics
GG; 101;	Methocarbamol	750 mg	White	Tablet	Oblong	Novartis Generics
GG; 103;	Metronidazole	250 mg	White	Coated Tablet	Circle, Scored	Novartis Generics
GG; 104	Methyldopa	125 mg	White	Coated Tablet	Circle	Novartis Generics
GG; 105	Haloperidol	0.5 mg	White	Tablet	Circle, Partially Scored	Sandoz
GG; 107	Perphenazine	4 mg	White	Coated Tablet	Circle, Debossed	Geneva Generics
GG; 108	Perphenazine	8 mg	White	Coated Tablet	Circle, Debossed	Geneva Generics
GG; 109	Perphenazine	16 mg	White	Coated Tablet	Circle, Debossed	Geneva Generics
GG; 111	Methyldopa	250 mg	White	Coated Tablet	Circle	Novartis Generics
GG; 113	Metoclopramide Hydrochloride	10 mg	White	Tablet	Circle, Scored	Novartis Generics
GG; 119;	Butal Compound	50 mg; 325 mg; 40 mg	White	Tablet	Circle	Novartis Generics
GG; 122	Sulfasalazine	500 mg	Butterscotch	Tablet	Circle	Novartis Generics
GG; 123	Haloperidol	1 mg	Yellow	Tablet	Circle, Partially Scored	Sandoz
GG; 124	Haloperidol	2 mg	Pink	Tablet	Circle, Scored	Sandoz
GG; 125	Haloperidol	5 mg	Green	Tablet	Circle, Partially Scored	Sandoz
GG; 126	Haloperidol	10 mg	Light Green	Tablet	Circle, Scored	Sandoz
GG; 127	Quiphile	260 mg	White	Tablet	Circle	Novartis Generics
GG; 128	Oxazepam	10 mg		Tablet		Geneva Generics
GG; 129	Oxazepam	30 mg		Tablet		Geneva Generics
GG; 131	Oxazepam	15 mg		Tablet		Geneva Generics
GG; 132	Verapamil Hydrochloride	80 mg	White	Coated Tablet	Circle, Scored	Geneva Generics
GG; 133	Verapamil Hydrochloride	120 mg	White	Coated Tablet	Circle, Scored	Geneva Generics
GG; 134	Haloperidol	20 mg	Coral	Tablet	Circle, Scored	Sandoz
GG; 135	Clorazepate Dipotassium	11.25 mg		Sustained-Release Tablet		Novartis Generics
GG; 136	Clorazepate Dipotassium	22.5 mg		Sustained-Release Tablet		Novartis Generics
GG; 138;	Sulfamethoxazole	500 mg	Green	Tablet	Circle, Scored	Novartis Generics
GG; 139	Buspirone Hydrochloride	5 mg		Tablet		Novartis Generics
GG; 140	Buspirone Hydrochloride	10 mg		Tablet		Novartis Generics
GG; 141	Meclizine Hydrochloride Otc	12.5 mg	Blue	Tablet	Oval, Scored	Sandoz
GG; 141	Meclizine Hydrochloride RX	12.5 mg	Blue	Tablet	Oval, Scored	Sandoz
GG; 144	Chlorpropamide	250 mg	White	Tablet	Circle, Scored	Novartis Generics
GG; 145;	Dimenhydrinate	50 mg	Yellow	Tablet	Circle, Scored	Novartis Generics
GG; 146	Hydrochlorothiazide and Reserpine	50 mg; 0.125 mg		Tablet		Novartis Generics
GG; 150;	Meprobamate	400 mg	White	Tablet	Circle, Scored	Novartis Generics
GG; 153	Propranolol Hydrochloride and Hydrochlorothiazide	25 mg; 40 mg	White	Tablet	Circle, Scored	Novartis Generics
GG; 154	Propranolol Hydrochloride and Hydrochlorothiazide	80 mg; 25 mg	White	Tablet	Circle, Scored	Novartis Generics
GG; 155;	Prednisone	20 mg	Peach-Colored	Tablet	Circle, Scored	Novartis Generics
GG; 156	Prednisone	10 mg	White	Tablet	Circle	Novartis Generics
GG; 157	Prednisone	50 mg	White	Tablet	Circle, Scored	Novartis Generics
GG; 158;	Sulfisoxazole	500 mg	White	Tablet	Circle	Novartis Generics
GG; 159	Clemastine Fumarate	1.34 mg	White	Tablet	Capsule-Shape, Scored, Debossed	Sandoz
GG; 160	Clemastine Fumarate	2.68 mg	White	Tablet	Circle, Scored, Debossed	Sandoz
GG; 162	Triazolam	0.125 mg	White	Tablet		Geneva Generics
GG; 163	Triazolam	0.25 mg	Blue	Tablet		Geneva Generics
GG; 164	Triazolam	0.5 mg		Tablet		Geneva Generics

IMPRINT	BRAND/GENERIC NAME	STRENGTH	COLOR	FORM	SHAPE	MANUFACTURER
GG; 165	Triamterene and Hydrochlorothiazide	25 mg; 37.5 mg	Green	Tablet	Circle, Scored	Geneva Generics
GG; 166	Desipramine Hydrochloride	75 mg	White	Coated Tablet	Circle, Debossed	Sandoz
GG; 167	Desipramine Hydrochloride	100 mg	White	Coated Tablet	Circle, Debossed	Sandoz
GG; 168	Desipramine Hydrochloride	150 mg	White	Coated Tablet	Circle, Debossed	Sandoz
GG; 169	Verapamil Hydrochloride	40 mg	White	Coated Tablet	Circle	Geneva Generics
GG; 172	Triamterene and Hydrochlorothiazide	50 mg; 75 mg	Yellow	Tablet	Circle, Scored	Geneva Generics
GG; 173	Methotrexate	2.5 mg		Tablet		Novartis Generics
GG; 174	Sulfamethoxazole and Trimethoprim	400 mg; 80 mg	White	Tablet	Circle, Scored	Geneva Generics
GG; 175	Sulfamethoxazole and Trimethoprim	800 mg; 160 mg	White	Tablet	Oval	Geneva Generics
GG; 177	Captopril	25 mg		Tablet		Novartis Generics
GG; 178	Captopril	50 mg		Tablet		Novartis Generics
GG; 179	Captopril	100 mg		Tablet		Novartis Generics
GG; 181	Methazolamide	50 mg	White	Tablet	Circle, Scored, Debossed	Sandoz
GG; 182	Timolol Maleate	10 mg	White	Tablet	Circle, Scored	Novartis Generics
GG; 183	Timolol Maleate	20 mg	Blue	Tablet	Circle, Scored	Novartis Generics
GG; 184	Oxybutynin Chloride	5 mg	Light Blue	Tablet	Round, Convex, Bisected Scored	Novartis Generics
GG; 186	Metaproterenol Sulfate	10 mg		Tablet		Novartis Generics
GG; 187	Metaproterenol Sulfate	20 mg		Tablet		Novartis Generics
GG; 188	Guanabenz Acetate	4 mg		Tablet		Novartis Generics
GG; 189	Guanabenz Acetate	8 mg		Tablet		Novartis Generics
GG; 190;	Methocarbamol	500 mg	White	Tablet	Circle, Scored	Novartis Generics
GG; 193	Naloxone and Pentazocine	0.5 mg; 50 mg		Tablet		Novartis Generics
GG; 194	Indapamide	2.5 mg		Tablet		Novartis Generics
GG; 195;	Metronidazole	500 mg	White	Coated Tablet	Oblong	Novartis Generics
GG; 201	Furosemide	40 mg	White	Tablet	Circle, Scored	Sandoz
GG; 204	Tolmetin Sodium	200 mg		Tablet		Novartis Generics
GG; 206	Captopril and Hydrochlorothiazide	25 mg; 15 mg		Tablet		Novartis Generics
GG; 207	Captopril and Hydrochlorothiazide	25 mg; 25 mg		Tablet		Novartis Generics
GG; 208	Captopril and Hydrochlorothiazide	50 mg; 15 mg		Tablet		Novartis Generics
GG; 209	Captopril and Hydrochlorothiazide	50 mg; 25 mg		Tablet		Novartis Generics
GG; 211	Bromocriptine Mesylate	2.5 mg	White	Tablet	Scored, Circle	Sandoz
GG; 213	Perphenazine and Amitriptyline Hydrochloride	10 mg; 2 mg	Blue	Coated Tablet	Circle, Debossed	Geneva Generics
GG; 214	Perphenazine and Amitriptyline Hydrochloride	25 mg; 2 mg	Orange	Coated Tablet	Circle, Debossed	Geneva Generics
GG; 215	Perphenazine and Amitriptyline Hydrochloride	10 mg; 4 mg	Salmon	Coated Tablet	Circle, Debossed	Geneva Generics
GG; 216	Perphenazine and Amitriptyline Hydrochloride	4 mg; 25 mg	Yellow	Coated Tablet	Circle	Geneva Generics
GG; 217	Perphenazine and Amitriptyline Hydrochloride	50 mg; 4 mg	Orange	Coated Tablet	Circle	Geneva Generics
GG; 219	Methyldopa and Hydrochlorothiazide	15 mg; 250 mg	Light Green	Coated Tablet	Circle	Novartis Generics
GG; 221	Theophylline	100 mg		Tablet		Novartis Generics
GG; 222	Theophylline	200 mg		Tablet		Novartis Generics
GG; 223	Theophylline	300 mg		Tablet		Novartis Generics
GG; 225	Promethazine Hydrochloride	25 mg	White	Tablet	Circle, Scored, Debossed	Geneva Generics
GG; 226	Lovastatin	20 mg	Blue	Tablet	Oval	Sandoz
GG; 227	Isdn	20 mg	Green	Tablet	Circle, Scored, Debossed	Sandoz
GG; 227	Isoxsuprine Hydrochloride	10 mg	Green	Tablet	Circle, Scored	Sandoz
GG; 234	Methylprednisolone	4 mg	White	Tablet	Oval, Scored	Novartis Generics
GG; 235	Promethazine Hydrochloride	50 mg	Pink	Tablet	Circle	Geneva Generics
GG; 236	Sulindac	150 mg	Yellow	Tablet	Circle, Scored, Debossed	Geneva Generics
GG; 237	Sulindac	200 mg	Yellow	Tablet	Circle, Scored, Debossed	Geneva Generics
GG; 238	Glyburide	1.25 mg	White	Tablet	Circle, Scored	Novartis Generics
GG; 239	Glyburide	2.5 mg	Dark Pink	Tablet	Circle, Scored	Novartis Generics
GG; 240	Glyburide	5 mg	Blue	Tablet	Circle, Scored	Novartis Generics
GG; 242	Methyclothiazide	5 mg	Salmon-Colored	Tablet	Circle, Scored	Novartis Generics
GG; 243	Methyldopa and Hydrochlorothiazide	30 mg; 500 mg	Light Green	Coated Tablet	Circle	Novartis Generics
GG; 244	Methyclothiazide	2.5 mg	Orange	Tablet	Circle, Scored	Novartis Generics
GG; 246	Bumetanide	0.5 mg		Tablet		Novartis Generics
GG; 247	Bumetanide	1 mg		Tablet		Novartis Generics
GG; 248	Bumetanide	2 mg		Tablet		Novartis Generics
GG; 249	Alprazolam	2 mg	White	Tablet	Rectangle, Tri-Scored	Sandoz
GG; 250	Quinidine Gluconate	324 mg	White	Sustained-Release Tablet	Circle	Novartis Generics
GG; 251	Carbidopa and Levodopa	10 mg; 100 mg	Blue	Tablet	Circle, Scored	Novartis Generics
GG; 252	Carbidopa and Levodopa	25 mg; 100 mg	Yellow	Tablet	Circle, Scored	Novartis Generics
GG; 253	Carbidopa and Levodopa	25 mg; 250 mg	Light Blue	Tablet	Circle, Scored	Novartis Generics
GG; 254	Fenoprofen Calcium	600 mg	White	Coated Tablet	Oval, Scored, Embossed	Novartis Generics
GG; 255	Disobrom	6 mg; 120 mg	White	Timed-Release Tablet	Circle	Novartis Generics
GG; 256	Alprazolam	0.25 mg	White	Tablet	Oval, Scored	Sandoz
GG; 257	Alprazolam	0.5 mg	Peach	Tablet	Oval, Scored	Sandoz
GG; 258	Alprazolam	1 mg	Blue	Tablet	Oval, Scored	Sandoz
GG; 259	Isdn	5 mg	Pink	Tablet	Circle, Scored, Debossed	Sandoz
GG; 260	Hydroxychloroquine Sulfate	200 mg	White	Coated Tablet	Circle, Scored	Sandoz
GG; 261	Meclizine Hydrochloride Otc	25 mg	Yellow	Tablet	Oval, Scored	Sandoz
GG; 261	Meclizine Hydrochloride RX	25 mg	Yellow	Tablet	Oval, Scored	Sandoz
GG; 263	Atenolol	50 mg	White	Tablet	Circle, Scored	Sandoz
GG; 264	Atenolol	100 mg	White	Tablet	Circle	Sandoz

IMPRINT	BRAND/GENERIC NAME	STRENGTH	COLOR	FORM	SHAPE	MANUFACTURER
GG; 265	Methyldopa and Hydrochlorothiazide	25 mg; 250 mg	White	Coated Tablet	Circle	Novartis Generics
GG; 268	Oxaprozin	600 mg		Tablet		Geneva Generics
GG; 270	Tolazamide	100 mg	White	Tablet	Circle, Scored	Novartis Generics
GG; 271	Tolazamide	250 mg	White	Tablet	Circle, Scored	Novartis Generics
GG; 272	Tolazamide	500 mg	White	Tablet	Circle, Scored	Novartis Generics
GG; 273	Quinidine Sulfate	300 mg		Sustained-Release Tablet		Novartis Generics
GG; 277	Sucralfate	1 GM		Tablet		Novartis Generics
GG; 280	Minocycline	50 mg		Tablet		Novartis Generics
GG; 281	Minocycline	100 mg		Tablet		Novartis Generics
GG; 284	Isoxsuprine Hydrochloride	20 mg	White	Tablet	Circle, Scored	Sandoz
GG; 285;	Quinidine Sulfate	200 mg	White	Tablet	Circle, Scored	Novartis Generics
GG; 286	Quinidine Sulfate	300 mg	White	Tablet	Circle, Scored	Novartis Generics
GG; 289	Methyldopa and Hydrochlorothiazide	50 mg; 500 mg	White	Coated Tablet	Circle	Novartis Generics
GG; 296	Loratadine	10 mg	White	Tablet	Circle	Sandoz
GG; 297	Doxycycline Hyclate	100 mg		Tablet		Novartis Generics
GG; 364	Benazepril and Hydrochlorothiazide	5 mg; 6.25 mg	White	Tablet	Oval	Sandoz
GG; 365	Benazepril and Hydrochlorothiazide	10 mg; 12.5 mg	Light Pink	Tablet	Oval	Sandoz
GG; 366	Benazepril and Hydrochlorothiazide	20 mg; 12.5 mg	Grayish Violet	Tablet	Oval	Sandoz
GG; 367	Benazepril and Hydrochlorothiazide	20 mg; 25 mg	Red	Tablet	Oval	Sandoz
GG; 406	Probucol	250 mg		Tablet		Novartis Generics
GG; 407;	Chlorpromazine Hydrochloride	50 mg	Off-White	Coated Tablet	Circle	Novartis Generics
GG; 407; 50	Chlorpromazine Hydrochloride	50 mg	Butterscotch	Coated Tablet	Circle	Sandoz
GG; 409	Leucovorin Calcium	5 mg		Tablet		Novartis Generics
GG; 410	Leucovorin Calcium	25 mg		Tablet		Novartis Generics
GG; 412	Carisoprodol Compound	325 mg; 200 mg		Tablet		Novartis Generics
GG; 414	Metoprolol Tartrate	50 mg	White	Coated Tablet	Circle, Scored	Geneva Generics
GG; 414	Probenecid	500 mg	Yellow	Coated Tablet	Capsule-Shape	Novartis Generics
GG; 415	Metoprolol Tartrate	100 mg	White	Coated Tablet	Circle, Scored	Geneva Generics
GG; 417	Naproxen Sodium	275 mg	Yellow	Tablet	Oval, Debossed	Geneva Generics
GG; 418	Naproxen Sodium	550 mg	White	Coated Tablet	Oval, Debossed	Geneva Generics
GG; 419	Trazodone Hydrochloride	50 mg	White	Coated Tablet	Circle, Scored	Geneva Generics
GG; 420	Trazodone Hydrochloride	100 mg	White	Coated Tablet	Circle, Scored	Geneva Generics
GG; 421	Chlorzoxazone	250 mg	Orange	Tablet	Circle, Scored	Novartis Generics
GG; 422	Chlorzoxazone	500 mg	Orange	Tablet	Circle, Scored	Novartis Generics
GG; 424	Tamoxifen Citrate	10 mg		Tablet		Cibageneva Pharmaceuticals
GG; 425	Erythromycin Ethylsuccinate	400 mg		Coated Tablet		Novartis Generics
GG; 431;	Amitriptyline Hydrochloride	50 mg	Brown with White Core	Coated Tablet	Circle	Sandoz
GG; 436	Nystatin	500,000 units	Brown	Coated Tablet	Circle	Novartis Generics
GG; 437;	Chlorpromazine Hydrochloride	100 mg	Off-White	Coated Tablet	Circle	Novartis Generics
GG; 437; 100	Chlorpromazine Hydrochloride	100 mg	Butterscotch	Coated Tablet	Circle	Sandoz
GG; 438	Pindolol	5 mg	White	Tablet	Circle, Scored, Debossed	Geneva Generics
GG; 439	Pindolol	10 mg	White	Tablet	Circle, Scored, Debossed	Geneva Generics
GG; 442	Ranitidine Hydrochloride	150 mg		Tablet		Geneva Generics
GG; 443	Ranitidine Hydrochloride	300 mg		Tablet		Geneva Generics
GG; 447	Pentoxifylline	400 mg		Sustained-Release Tablet		Novartis Generics
GG; 449	Verapamil Hydrochloride	240 mg		Sustained-Release Tablet		Geneva Generics
GG; 450;	Amitriptyline Hydrochloride	150 mg	Light Green	Coated Tablet	Circle	Sandoz
GG; 451;	Amitriptyline Hydrochloride	75 mg	Purple with White Core	Coated Tablet	Circle	Sandoz
GG; 452	Orphenadrine Citrate, Aspirin and Caffeine	385 mg; 30 mg; 25 mg		Tablet		Novartis Generics
GG; 453	Orphenadrine Citrate, Aspirin and Caffeine	770 mg; 60 mg; 50 mg		Tablet		Novartis Generics
GG; 454	Diflunisal	250 mg		Tablet		Novartis Generics
GG; 455;	Chlorpromazine Hydrochloride	10 mg	Off-White	Coated Tablet	Circle	Novartis Generics
GG; 455; 10	Chlorpromazine Hydrochloride	10 mg	Butterscotch	Coated Tablet	Circle	Sandoz
GG; 456	Diflunisal	500 mg		Tablet		Novartis Generics
GG; 457;	Chlorpromazine Hydrochloride	200 mg	Off-White	Coated Tablet	Circle	Novartis Generics
GG; 457; 200	Chlorpromazine Hydrochloride	200 mg	Butterscotch	Coated Tablet	Circle	Sandoz
GG; 461;	Amitriptyline Hydrochloride	100 mg	Orange with White Core	Coated Tablet	Circle	Sandoz
GG; 462	Tocainide	400 mg		Tablet		Novartis Generics
GG; 463	Tocainide	600 mg		Tablet		Novartis Generics
GG; 464;	Dipyridamole	75 mg	White	Coated Tablet	Circle	Novartis Generics
GG; 465	Nadolol	20 mg		Tablet		Novartis Generics
GG; 466	Nadolol	40 mg		Tablet		Novartis Generics
GG; 467	Nadolol	80 mg		Tablet		Novartis Generics
GG; 468	Nadolol	120 mg		Tablet		Novartis Generics
GG; 469	Nadolol	160 mg		Tablet		Novartis Generics
GG; 471	Methyldopa	500 mg	White	Coated Tablet	Circle	Novartis Generics
GG; 472	Procainamide Hydrochloride	250 mg	White	Sustained-Release Tablet	Oblong	Novartis Generics
GG; 473	Procainamide Hydrochloride	500 mg	White	Sustained-Release Tablet	Oblong, Scored	Novartis Generics
GG; 476;	Chlorpromazine Hydrochloride	25 mg	Off-White	Coated Tablet	Circle	Novartis Generics
GG; 476; 25	Chlorpromazine Hydrochloride	25 mg	Butterscotch	Coated Tablet	Circle	Sandoz
GG; 487	Probenecid and Colchicine	0.5 mg; 500 mg	White	Tablet	Oblong	Novartis Generics
GG; 488	Fluphenazine Hydrochloride	2.5 mg	Beige	Coated Tablet	Circle	Sandoz
GG; 489	Fluphenazine Hydrochloride	5 mg	Light Rust	Coated Tablet	Circle	Sandoz

IMPRINT	BRAND/GENERIC NAME	STRENGTH	COLOR	FORM	SHAPE	MANUFACTURER
GG; 490	Fluphenazine Hydrochloride	10 mg	Rust	Coated Tablet	Circle, Debossed	Sandoz
GG; 492	Divalproex Sodium	125 mg		Tablet		Novartis Generics
GG; 493	Divalproex Sodium	250 mg		Tablet		Novartis Generics
GG; 494	Divalproex Sodium	500 mg		Tablet		Novartis Generics
GG; 501;	Nitroglycerin	6.5 mg	Blue and Dark Yellow	Sustained-Release Capsule		Novartis Generics
GG; 503	Papaverine Hydrochloride	150 mg	Brown and Clear	Sustained-Release Capsule		Geneva Generics
GG; 504	Tolmetin Sodium	400 mg		Capsule		Novartis Generics
GG; 505	Oxazepam	10 mg	White with Pink and Black Bands	Capsule		Geneva Generics
GG; 506	Oxazepam	15 mg	White with Red and Black Bands	Capsule		Geneva Generics
GG; 507	Oxazepam	30 mg	Opaque White with Maroon and Black Bands	Capsule		Geneva Generics
GG; 508;	Pseudoephedrine Hydrochloride	120 mg	Brown and Orange	Sustained-Release Capsule		Geneva Generics
GG; 509;	Cyclandelate	400 mg	Blue and Red	Capsule		Novartis Generics
GG; 510	Sulfinpyrazone	200 mg		Capsule		Novartis Generics
GG; 511;	Nitroglycerin	2.5 mg	Lavender and Clear	Sustained-Release Capsule		Novartis Generics
GG; 512;	Nitroglycerin SR	9 mg	Clear Yellow and Green	Sustained-Release Capsule		Novartis Generics
GG; 513	Gemfibrozil	300 mg		Capsule		Novartis Generics
GG; 514;	Phenylbutazone	100 mg	Light Blue	Capsule		Novartis Generics
GG; 515	Quinidine Sulfate	325 mg		Tablet		Novartis Generics
GG; 516;	Phendimetrazine	105 mg	Blue and Clear with Blue Beads	Sustained-Release Capsule		Novartis Generics
GG; 517	Indomethacin	25 mg	Light Green	Capsule		Novartis Generics
GG; 518	Indomethacin	50 mg	Light Green	Capsule		Novartis Generics
GG; 519	Indomethacin	75 mg		Extended-Release Capsule		Novartis Generics
GG; 520;	Butal Compound	50 mg; 325 mg; 40 mg		Capsule		Novartis Generics
GG; 522	Flurazepam	15 mg	Powder Blue and White	Capsule		Novartis Generics
GG; 523	Flurazepam	30 mg	Powder Blue	Capsule		Novartis Generics
GG; 524	Meclofenamate Sodium	50 mg	Maroon and Pink	Capsule		Novartis Generics
GG; 525	Meclofenamate Sodium	100 mg	Maroon and White	Capsule		Novartis Generics
GG; 526	Clorazepate Dipotassium	3.75 mg	Opaque White with Bands	Capsule		Novartis Generics
GG; 527	Clorazepate	7.5 mg	Opaque White with Bands	Capsule		Novartis Generics
GG; 528	Clorazepate	15 mg	Opaque White with Bands	Capsule		Novartis Generics
GG; 529;	Cyclandelate	200 mg	Powder Blue	Capsule		Novartis Generics
GG; 531	Temazepam	15 mg	Dark Green and White	Capsule		Geneva Generics
GG; 532	Temazepam	30 mg	White	Capsule		Geneva Generics
GG; 533;	Diphenhydramine Hydrochloride	25 mg	Pink and Clear with White Powder	Capsule		Novartis Generics
GG; 534	Clofibrate	500 mg		Capsule		Novartis Generics
GG; 538	Nitrofurantoin Macrocrystals	25 mg	Opaque White	Capsule		Geneva Generics
GG; 540	Fluoxetine Hydrochloride	40 mg	White with a Single Orange Band	Capsule		Sandoz
GG; 541;	Diphenhydramine Hydrochloride	50 mg	Pink	Capsule		Novartis Generics
GG; 542	Prazepam	5 mg		Capsule		Novartis Generics
GG; 543	Prazepam	10 mg		Capsule		Novartis Generics
GG; 544	Prazepam	20 mg		Capsule		Novartis Generics
GG; 545	Cephalexin	250 mg	Opaque Orange and Gray	Capsule		Novartis Generics
GG; 546	Cephalexin	500 mg	Opaque Orange and Gray	Capsule		Novartis Generics
GG; 549	Ursodiol	300 mg		Capsule		Geneva Generics
GG; 550	Fluoxetine Hydrochloride	20 mg	White with a Single Black Band	Capsule		Sandoz
GG; 554;	Niacin	125 mg	Black and Clear	Sustained-Release Capsule		Novartis Generics
GG; 555	Cephalexin	500 mg	Swedish Orange	Capsule		Novartis Generics
GG; 556	Cephalexin	250 mg	Swedish Orange and Gray	Capsule		Novartis Generics
GG; 557	Nifedipine	10 mg		Capsule		Geneva Generics
GG; 558	Fenoprofen Calcium	200 mg	White with Gold and Black Bands	Capsule		Novartis Generics
GG; 559	Fenoprofen Calcium	300 mg	White with Gold Bands	Capsule		Novartis Generics
GG; 560	Ferrous Sulfate	250 mg		Sustained-Release Capsule		Novartis Generics
GG; 560;	Ferrous Sulfate	250 mg	Red and Clear with Brown and White Beads	Sustained-Release Capsule		Novartis Generics
GG; 561	Danazol	50 mg		Capsule		Novartis Generics
GG; 564;	Niacin	250 mg	Green and Clear	Sustained-Release Capsule		Novartis Generics
GG; 571	Clinoxide	5 mg; 2.5 mg	Opaque White	Capsule		Novartis Generics
GG; 572	Doxepin Hydrochloride	25 mg	Opaque White with Pink and Gold Bands	Capsule		Novartis Generics

IMPRINT	BRAND/GENERIC NAME	STRENGTH	COLOR	FORM	SHAPE	MANUFACTURER
GG; 573	Doxepin Hydrochloride	50 mg	Opaque White with Pink and Green Bands	Capsule		Novartis Generics
GG; 574	Doxepin Hydrochloride	75 mg	Opaque White with Black and Gold Bands	Capsule		Novartis Generics
GG; 575	Fluoxetine Hydrochloride	10 mg	White with Green Band	Capsule		Sandoz
GG; 576	Doxepin Hydrochloride	10 mg	White with Red and Gold Band	Capsule		Novartis Generics
GG; 577	Doxepin Hydrochloride	100 mg	White with Blue and Green Bands	Capsule		Novartis Generics
GG; 578	Doxepin Hydrochloride	150 mg		Capsule		Novartis Generics
GG; 580	Triamterene and Hydrochlorothiazide	25 mg; 50 mg	Red	Capsule		Geneva Generics
GG; 582	Hydroxyzine Pamoate	25 mg	Two-Toned Green	Capsule		Novartis Generics
GG; 583	Hydroxyzine Pamoate	50 mg	Opaque White and Green	Capsule		Novartis Generics
GG; 584	Hydroxyzine Pamoate	100 mg		Capsule		Novartis Generics
GG; 585	Loxapine Succinate	5 mg		Capsule		Novartis Generics
GG; 586	Loxapine Succinate	10 mg		Capsule		Novartis Generics
GG; 587	Loxapine Succinate	25 mg		Capsule		Novartis Generics
GG; 588	Loxapine Succinate	50 mg		Capsule		Novartis Generics
GG; 589	Thiothixene	1 mg	White, Orange and Gold	Capsule		Geneva Generics
GG; 591;	Propoxyphene Hydrochloride	65 mg	Opaque Pale Pink	Capsule		Novartis Generics
GG; 592	Prazosin Hydrochloride	1 mg	White with Black Ink Bands	Capsule		Novartis Generics
GG; 593	Prazosin Hydrochloride	2 mg	White with Pink and Black Ink Bands	Capsule		Novartis Generics
GG; 594	Prazosin Hydrochloride	5 mg	White with Blue and Black Ink Bands	Capsule		Novartis Generics
GG; 596	Thiothixene	2 mg	White, Blue and Gold	Capsule		Geneva Generics
GG; 597	Thiothixene	5 mg	Opaque White, Orange and Black	Capsule		Geneva Generics
GG; 598	Thiothixene	10 mg	Black and Blue	Capsule		Geneva Generics
GG; 599	Thiothixene	20 mg		Capsule		Geneva Generics
GG; 601	Isotretinoin	10 mg		Capsule		Novartis Generics
GG; 602	Isotretinoin	20 mg		Capsule		Novartis Generics
GG; 603	Isotretinoin	40 mg		Capsule		Novartis Generics
GG; 604	Cyclosporine	25 mg		Capsule		Novartis Generics
GG; 605	Cyclosporine	100 mg		Capsule		Novartis Generics
GG; 614	Ranitidine Hydrochloride	150 mg	Opaque Caramel	Capsule		Geneva Generics
GG; 615	Ranitidine Hydrochloride	300 mg	Opaque Caramel	Capsule		Geneva Generics
GG; 616	Ranitidine Hydrochloride	150 mg		Capsule		Geneva Generics
GG; 617	Ranitidine Hydrochloride	300 mg		Capsule		Geneva Generics
GG; 621	Terazosin Hydrochloride	1 mg		Capsule		Geneva Generics
GG; 622	Terazosin Hydrochloride	2 mg		Capsule		Geneva Generics
GG; 623	Terazosin Hydrochloride	5 mg		Capsule		Geneva Generics
GG; 624	Terazosin Hydrochloride	10 mg		Capsule		Geneva Generics
GG; 625	Flutamide	125 mg		Capsule		Novartis Generics
GG; 633;	Rifampin	300 mg	Scarlet, Caramel	Capsule		Geneva Generics
GG; 634	Amantadine Hydrochloride	100 mg	Red and White	Capsule		Sandoz
GG; 702	Isosorbide Mononitrate	20 mg		Tablet		Novartis Generics
GG; 704	Tolmetin Sodium	600 mg		Tablet		Novartis Generics
GG; 705	Ranitidine Hydrochloride	150 mg	Pink	Coated Tablet	Circle	Geneva Generics
GG; 706	Ranitidine Hydrochloride	300 mg	Orange	Coated Tablet	Circle	Geneva Generics
GG; 714	Erythromycin Stearate	250 mg		Tablet		Novartis Generics
GG; 715	Erythromycin Stearate	500 mg		Tablet		Novartis Generics
GG; 721	Terazosin Hydrochloride	1 mg		Tablet		Geneva Generics
GG; 722	Terazosin Hydrochloride	2 mg		Tablet		Geneva Generics
GG; 723	Terazosin Hydrochloride	5 mg		Tablet		Geneva Generics
GG; 724	Naproxen	250 mg	Yellow	Tablet	Circle	Geneva Generics
GG; 725	Naproxen	375 mg	Orange	Tablet	Capsule-Shape	Geneva Generics
GG; 726	Naproxen	500 mg	Yellow	Tablet	Capsule-Shape	Geneva Generics
GG; 730	Pseudoephedrine and Terfenadine	60 mg; 120 mg		Sustained-Release Tablet		Novartis Generics
GG; 731	Trazodone Hydrochloride	150 mg		Tablet		Geneva Generics
GG; 733	Salsalate	500 mg	Light Green	Coated Tablet	Circle	Novartis Generics
GG; 734	Salsalate	750 mg		Coated Tablet	Capsule-Shape, Scored	Novartis Generics
GG; 737	Diclofenac Sodium	25 mg	Yellow	Timed-Release Tablet	Circle	Sandoz
GG; 738	Diclofenac Sodium	50 mg	Light Brown	Timed-Release Tablet	Circle	Sandoz
GG; 739	Diclofenac Sodium	75 mg	Pink	Delayed-Release Tablet	Circle	Sandoz
GG; 741	Ciprofloxacin	250 mg	White	Tablet	Circle	Sandoz
GG; 742	Ciprofloxacin	500 mg	White	Tablet	Capsule-Shape	Sandoz
GG; 743	Ciprofloxacin	750 mg	White	Tablet	Capsule-Shape	Sandoz
GG; 744	Verapamil Hydrochloride	120 mg		Sustained-Release Tablet		Geneva Generics
GG; 745	Verapamil Hydrochloride	180 mg		Sustained-Release Tablet		Geneva Generics
GG; 746	Benazepril	5 mg	Yellow	Tablet	Circle	Sandoz
GG; 747	Benazepril	10 mg	Dark Yellow	Tablet	Circle	Sandoz
GG; 748	Benazepril	20 mg	Pink	Tablet	Circle	Sandoz
GG; 749	Benazepril	40 mg	Dark Rose	Tablet	Circle	Sandoz
GG; 755	Doxazosin	1 mg		Tablet		Novartis Generics
GG; 756	Doxazosin	2 mg		Tablet		Novartis Generics
GG; 757	Doxazosin	4 mg		Tablet		Novartis Generics
GG; 758	Doxazosin	8 mg		Tablet		Novartis Generics
GG; 770	Lovastatin	10 mg	White	Tablet	Circle	Sandoz

IMPRINT	BRAND/GENERIC NAME	STRENGTH	COLOR	FORM	SHAPE	MANUFACTURER
GG; 771	Glipizide	5 mg	White	Tablet	Circle, Scored, Debossed	Sandoz
GG; 772	Glipizide	10 mg	White	Tablet	Circle, Scored, Debossed	Sandoz
GG; 773	Lovastatin	40 mg	Green	Tablet	Oval	Sandoz
GG; 774	Etodolac	400 mg		Tablet		Novartis Generics
GG; 801	Ketoprofen	75 mg		Capsule		Novartis Generics
GG; 802	Ketoprofen	50 mg		Capsule		Novartis Generics
GG; 805	Piroxicam	10 mg		Capsule		Novartis Generics
GG; 806	Piroxicam	20 mg		Capsule		Novartis Generics
GG; 808	Tetracycline Hydrochloride	250 mg	Yellow and Orange	Capsule		Novartis Generics
GG; 809	Tetracycline Hydrochloride	500 mg	Yellow and Black	Capsule		Novartis Generics
GG; 810	Oxytetracycline	250 mg		Capsule		Novartis Generics
GG; 811	Erythromycin Estolate	250 mg	Orange and Buff	Capsule		Novartis Generics
GG; 812	Minocycline	50 mg		Capsule		Novartis Generics
GG; 813	Minocycline	100 mg		Capsule		Novartis Generics
GG; 814	Doxycycline	50 mg	Blue and White	Capsule		Novartis Generics
GG; 815	Doxycycline	100 mg	Blue	Capsule		Novartis Generics
GG; 816	Nizatidine	150 mg		Capsule		Novartis Generics
GG; 817	Nizatidine	300 mg		Capsule		Novartis Generics
GG; 818	Propranolol	60 mg		Sustained-Release Capsule		Novartis Generics
GG; 819	Propranolol	80 mg		Sustained-Release Capsule		Novartis Generics
GG; 820	Propranolol	120 mg		Sustained-Release Capsule		Novartis Generics
GG; 821	Propranolol	160 mg		Sustained-Release Capsule		Novartis Generics
GG; 822	Clomipramine Hydrochloride	25 mg	White and Orange with Yellow Band	Capsule		Sandoz
GG; 823	Clomipramine Hydrochloride	50 mg	Opaque White	Capsule		Sandoz
GG; 824	Clomipramine Hydrochloride	75 mg	Dark Yellow with Yellow Band	Capsule		Sandoz
GG; 828	Rifampin	150 mg		Capsule		Geneva Generics
GG; 832	Etodolac	200 mg		Capsule		Novartis Generics
GG; 833	Etodolac	300 mg		Capsule		Novartis Generics
GG; 835	Erythromycin	250 mg		Capsule		Novartis Generics
GG; 842	Nicardipine Hydrochloride	20 mg		Capsule		Novartis Generics
GG; 843	Nicardipine Hydrochloride	30 mg		Capsule		Novartis Generics
GG; 850	Ampicillin	250 mg	White	Capsule		Sandoz
GG; 851	Ampicillin	500 mg	White	Capsule		Sandoz
GG; 855	Dicloxacillin	500 mg	Blue	Capsule		Sandoz
GG; 904	Diclofenac Sodium	100 mg	Light Pink	Extended-Release Tablet	Circle	Sandoz
GG; 929	Bupropion Hydrochloride	75 mg	Lavender	Coated Tablet	Circle	Sandoz
GG; 930	Bupropion Hydrochloride	100 mg	Lavender	Coated Tablet	Circle	Sandoz
GG; 931	Orphenadrine Citrate	100 mg	White	Extended-Release Tablet	Circle	Geneva Generics
GG; 932	Pemoline	18.75 mg	White	Tablet	Circle, Scored	Geneva Generics
GG; 933	Pemoline	37.5 mg	White	Tablet	Circle, Scored	Geneva Generics
GG; 934	Pemoline	75 mg	White	Tablet	Circle, Scored	Geneva Generics
GG; 935	Naproxen Delayed-Release	375 mg	White	Delayed-Release Tablet	Capsule-Shape	Geneva Generics
GG; 936	Naproxen Delayed-Release	500 mg	White	Delayed-Release Tablet	Capsule-Shape	Geneva Generics
GG949; PVK250	Penicillin VK	250 mg	White	Tablet	Circle, Scored	Geneva Generics
GG950; PVK500	Penicillin VK Potassium	500 mg	Off White	Tablet	Oblong	Geneva Generics
GG; 952; 5	Prochlorperazine Maleate	5 mg	Light Yellow	Tablet	Circle	Geneva Generics
GG; 953; 10	Prochlorperazine Maleate	10 mg	Pale Yellow	Tablet	Circle	Geneva Generics
GG; 957	Methylprednisolone	4 mg	White	Tablet	Oval, Quadrisect Scored on Blank Side	Geneva Generics
GG; 958;	Metoclopramide	5 mg	White	Tablet	Circle	Novartis Generics
GG; 963; 250	Cefuroxime Axetil	250 mg	White to Off-White	Tablet	Oval	Sandoz
GG; 964; 500	Cefuroxime Axetil	500 mg	White to Off-White	Tablet	Oval	Sandoz
GG; 977	Diclofenac Potassium	50 mg	White	Coated Tablet	Circle	Sandoz
GG; 9533	Mudrane GG-2	111 mg; 100 mg	Green Mottled	Tablet		Ecr Pharmaceuticals
GG; 9551	Mudrane GG	111 mg; 16 mg; 100 mg; 8 mg	Yellow Mottled	Tablet		Ecr Pharmaceuticals
GG; C1	Terazosin Hydrochloride	10 mg		Tablet		Geneva Generics
GG; C7	Levothyroxine Sodium	0.025 mg		Tablet		Novartis Generics
GG; D5	Selegiline Hydrochloride	5 mg		Tablet		Novartis Generics
GG; L7	Atenolol	25 mg	White	Tablet	Circle	Sandoz
GG; M1	Metoclopramide Hydrochloride	1 mg		Tablet		Novartis Generics
GG; N2	Amoxicillin and Clavulanate Potassium	200 mg; 28.5 mg	Pink	Tablet, Chewable	Circle	Sandoz
GG; N4	Amoxicillin and Clavulanate Potassium	400 mg; 57 mg	Pink	Tablet, Chewable	Circle	Sandoz
GG; N6	Amoxicillin and Clavulanate Potassium	500 mg; 125 mg	White to Slight Yellow	Tablet	Oblong	Sandoz
GG; N7	Amoxicillin and Clavulanate Potassium	875 mg; 125 mg	White to Slight Yellow	Tablet	Oblong	Sandoz
GILEAD; 200 MG	Emtriva	200 mg	Blue and White	Capsule		Gilead Sciences
GILEAD; 701	Truvada	200 mg; 300 mg	Blue	Tablet	Capsule-Shape	Gilead Sciences
GILEAD; 4331; 300	Viread	300 mg	Light Blue	Coated Tablet	Teardrop-Shape	Gilead Sciences
GL; 81	Renoquid	250 mg	White	Tablet	Circle, Scored	Glenwood
GL; 535-11;	Esgic	325 mg; 40 mg; 50 mg	White	Tablet	Circle, Compressed	Gilbert Laboratories
GL; 535-12;	Esgic	325 mg; 40 mg; 50 mg	White	Capsule		Gilbert Laboratories
GLAXO	Vicon Plus	4000 IU; 50 IU; 150 mg; 80 mg; 70 mg; 25 mg; 10 mg; 10 mg; 5 mg; 4 mg; 2 mg	Red and Beige	Capsule		Glaxosmithkline

IMPRINT	BRAND/GENERIC NAME	STRENGTH	COLOR	FORM	SHAPE	MANUFACTURER
GLAXO	Vicon-C	100 mg; 80 mg; 70 mg; 20 mg; 20 mg; 10 mg; 5 mg; 300 mg	Orange and Yellow	Capsule		Glaxosmithkline
GLAXO	VI-Zac	5000 IU; 80 mg; 50 IU; 500 mg	Orange	Capsule		Glaxosmithkline
GLAXO; 268	Theobid Duracap	260 mg	Blue and Clear	Sustained-Release Capsule		Glaxosmithkline
GLAXO; 295	Theobid Duracap JR.	130 mg	Two-Tone Blue	Sustained-Release Capsule		Glaxosmithkline
GLAXO; 316	Vicon Forte	8000 IU; 50 IU; 150 mg; 80 mg; 70 mg; 25 mg; 10 mg; 10 mg; 5 mg; 4 mg; 2 mg; 1 mg; 10 mcg	Orange and Black	Capsule		Glaxosmithkline
GLAXO; 371	Trandate HCT	100 mg; 25 mg	Pale Peach	Coated Tablet	Oval	Glaxosmithkline
GLAXO; 372	Trandate HCT	200 mg; 25 mg	White	Coated Tablet	Oval	Glaxosmithkline
GLAXO; 373	Trandate HCT	300 mg; 25 mg	Medium Peach	Coated Tablet	Oval	Glaxosmithkline
GLAXO; AMESEC	Amesec	130 mg; 25 mg	Orange and Blue	Capsule		Glaxosmithkline
GLAXO; TRINSICON	Trinsicon	0.5 mg; 75 mg; 110 mg; 240 mg; 15 mcg	Dark Pink and Dark Red	Capsule		Glaxosmithkline
GLAXO; VENTOLIN; 2	Ventolin	2 mg	White	Tablet	Circle, Compressed	Glaxosmithkline
GLAXO; ZANTAC; 150	Zantac 150 Maximum Strength	150 mg	Peach	Coated Tablet	Five-Sided	Glaxosmithkline
GLAXO; ZANTAC; 300	Zantac 300	300 mg	Yellow	Coated Tablet	Capsule-Shape	Glaxosmithkline
GLUCOTROL XL; 2.5	Glucotrol Xl	2.5 mg	Blue	Extended-Release Tablet		Pfizer Laboratories
GLUCOTROL XL; 5	Glucotrol Xl	5 mg	White	Extended-Release Tablet	Circle, Biconvex	Pfizer Laboratories
GLUCOTROL XL; 10	Glucotrol Xl	10 mg	White	Extended-Release Tablet	Circle, Biconvex	Pfizer Laboratories
GLYBUR; 477; 477	Glyburide	1.25 mg	White	Tablet	Oblong, Scored	Copley Pharmaceutical
GLYBUR 364; 364	Glyburide	5 mg	Blue	Tablet	Oblong	Teva Pharmaceuticals
GLYBUR 433; 433	Glyburide	2.5 mg	Pink	Tablet	Oblong, Scored	Teva Pharmaceuticals
GLYNASE 1.5; PT; PT	Glynase Prestab	1.5 mg	White	Tablet	Egg-Shape, Contour, Scored	Pharmacia & Upjohn
GLYNASE 3; PT; PT	Glynase Prestab	3 mg	Blue	Tablet	Egg-Shape, Contour, Scored	Pharmacia & Upjohn
GLYNASE 6; PT; PT	Glynase Prestab	6 mg	Yellow	Tablet	Egg-Shape, Contour, Scored	Pharmacia & Upjohn
GLYSET; 25	Glyset	25 mg	White	Coated Tablet	Circle	Pharmacia & Upjohn
GLYSET; 50	Glyset	50 mg	White	Coated Tablet	Circle	Pharmacia & Upjohn
GLYSET; 100	Glyset	100 mg	White	Coated Tablet	Circle	Pharmacia & Upjohn
GOODY'S	Goody's Extra Strength Tablets	260 mg; 130 mg; 16.25 mg	White	Tablet	Circle	Block Drug
GOODY'S	Pain Relief	260 mg; 130 mg; 16.25 mg	White	Tablet	Circle	Goody's
GP; 0026	Cefaclor	250 mg	Blue and White	Capsule		World Gen
GP; 0027	Cefaclor	500 mg	Blue and Gray	Capsule		World Gen
GP; 3;	Cephalexin	250 mg	White and Light Green	Capsule		Stada
GP; 3; GP; 3	Cephalexin	250 mg	Dark Green and White	Capsule		World Gen
GP; 4;	Cephalexin	500 mg	White and Light Green	Capsule		Stada
GP; 4; GP; 4	Cephalexin	500 mg	Dark Green and Light Green	Capsule		World Gen
GP 5; G	Glipizide	5 mg	White	Tablet	Oval, Convex	Par Pharmaceutical
GP 10; G	Glipizide	10 mg	White	Tablet	Oval, Convex	Par Pharmaceutical
GP; 111	Lisinopril	2.5 mg	White	Coated Tablet	Circle	Sandoz
GP; 112	Lisinopril	5 mg	Pink	Coated Tablet	Circle	Sandoz
GP; 113	Lisinopril	10 mg	White	Coated Tablet	Circle	Sandoz
GP; 114	Lisinopril	20 mg	Peach	Coated Tablet	Circle	Sandoz
GP; 115	Lisinopril	40 mg	Rose	Coated Tablet	Circle	Sandoz
GP; 118	Mefloquine Hydrochloride	250 mg	White	Tablet	Circle, Scored	Sandoz
GP; 124	Metformin Hydrochloride	500 mg	White	Coated Tablet	Circle	Sandoz
GP; 127	Metformin Hydrochloride	850 mg	White	Coated Tablet	Circle	Sandoz
GP; 128	Metformin Hydrochloride	1000 mg	White	Tablet	Oval	Sandoz
GP; 142	Fluvoxamine Maleate	50 mg	White	Tablet	Circle	Sandoz
GP; 150	Lisinopril	30 mg	Peach	Coated Tablet	Circle	Sandoz
GPC	Cevi Fer	300 mg; 60 mg; 1 mg	Orange and Green	Sustained-Release Capsule		Geriatric Pharmaceutical
GPI; 20	Caffeine	200 mg	Pink with White Specks	Tablet	Heart-Shape	Gemini Pharmaceuticals
GPI; 35	Caffeine	150 mg		Tablet		Gemini Pharmaceuticals
GPI; 52	Calcium Carbonate	500 mg	White	Tablet	Circle	Gemini Pharmaceuticals
GPI; 325	Acetaminophen	325 mg	White	Tablet		Gemini Pharmaceuticals
GPI; 325	Diphenhydramine	25 mg	Orange	Tablet		Gemini Pharmaceuticals
GPI; A5	Acetaminophen	500 mg	White	Tablet	Circle, Flat, Scored	Gemini Pharmaceuticals
GPI; P60	Pseudoephedrine	60 mg	White	Tablet		Gemini Pharmaceuticals
GRISACTIN; 125	Grisactin	125 mg	Orange	Capsule, Liquid Filled		Wyeth Pharmaceuticals
GRISACTIN; 250	Grisactin	250 mg	Yellow	Capsule, Liquid Filled		Wyeth Pharmaceuticals
GRISACTIN; 500	Grisactin	500 mg	Pink	Tablet	Circle	Wyeth Pharmaceuticals
GRISACTIN ULTRA; 125	Grisactin Ultra	125 mg	White	Tablet		Wyeth Pharmaceuticals
GRISACTIN ULTRA; 250	Grisactin Ultra	250 mg	White	Tablet		Wyeth Pharmaceuticals
GRISACTIN ULTRA; 330	Grisactin Ultra	330 mg	White	Tablet		Wyeth Pharmaceuticals
GRIS-PEG; 125	Gris-Peg	125 mg	White	Coated Tablet	Circle, Scored	Pedinol

IMPRINT	BRAND/GENERIC NAME	STRENGTH	COLOR	FORM	SHAPE	MANUFACTURER
GRIS-PEG; 250	Gris-Peg	250 mg	White	Coated Tablet	Capsule-Shape, Scored	Pedinol
GS; 25C	Zantac 25 Efferdose	25 mg	White to Pale Yellow	Effervescent Tablet	Circle, Flat-Faced, Bevel-Edged	Glaxosmithkline
GS; FC2	Epzicom	600 mg; 300 mg	Orange	Tablet	Capsule-Shape, Modified	Glaxosmithkline
GSK; 1/500	Avandamet	1 mg; 500 mg	Yellow	Tablet	Oval	Glaxosmithkline
GSK; 2/500	Avandamet	2 mg; 500 mg	Light Pink	Tablet	Oval	Glaxosmithkline
GSK; 2/1000	Avandamet	2 mg; 1000 mg	Yellow	Tablet	Oval	Glaxosmithkline
GSK; 4/500	Avandamet	4 mg; 500 mg	Orange	Tablet	Oval	Glaxosmithkline
GSK; 4/1000	Avandamet	4 mg; 1000 mg	Pink	Tablet	Oval	Glaxosmithkline
GUAIFED; MURO 120-250	Guaifed	120 mg; 250 mg	White and Clear	Extended-Release Capsule		Muro Pharmaceutical
GUAIFED-PD	Guaifed-PD	60 mg; 300 mg	Blue and Clear	Extended-Release Capsule		Muro Pharmaceutical
GUAIMAX-D; SP; 2055	Guaimax-D	600 mg; 120 mg	White	Extended-Release Tablet	Capsule-Shape, Scored	Schwarz Pharma
GX; 623	Ziagen	300 mg	Yellow	Coated Tablet	Capsule-Shape, Biconvex	Glaxosmithkline
GX; CC1	Agenerase	50 mg	White	Capsule, Liquid Filled	Capsule-Shape	Glaxosmithkline
GX; CC2	Agenerase	150 mg	White	Capsule, Liquid Filled	Capsule-Shape	Glaxosmithkline
GX; CE2	Avodart	0.5 mg	Opaque Yellow with Red Ink	Capsule, Liquid Filled		Glaxosmithkline
GX; CE3	Amerge	1 mg	White	Coated Tablet	D-Shape	Glaxosmithkline
GX; CE5	Amerge	2.5 mg	Green	Coated Tablet	D-Shape	Glaxosmithkline
GX; CF7; 24	Zofran	24 mg	Pink	Coated Tablet	Oval	Glaxosmithkline
GX; CG5	Epivir-Hbv	100 mg	Butterscotch	Coated Tablet	Capsule-Shape, Biconvex	Glaxosmithkline
GX; CG7	Malarone Pediatric	62.5 mg; 25 mg	Pink	Coated Tablet	Circle, Biconvex	Glaxosmithkline
GX; CJ7; 150;	Epivir	150 mg	White	Coated Tablet	Diamond, Modified	Glaxosmithkline
GX; CK3	Raxar	200 mg	White to Pale Yellow	Coated Tablet	Circle, Biconvex, Bevel-Edged	Glaxosmithkline
GX; CL2	Lamictal	5 mg	White	Tablet, Chewable	Capsule-Shape	Glaxosmithkline
GX; CL5	Lamictal	25 mg	White	Tablet, Chewable	Circle	Glaxosmithkline
GX; CM3	Malarone	250 mg; 100 mg	Pink	Coated Tablet	Circle, Biconvex	Glaxosmithkline
GX; CT1	Lotronex	1 mg	Blue	Coated Tablet	Oval	Glaxosmithkline
GX; EF3; M;	Myleran	2 mg	White	Tablet	Circle	Glaxosmithkline
GX; EG2	Ceftin	500 mg	White	Tablet	Capsule-Shape	Glaxosmithkline
GX; EG2	Cefuroxime	500 mg	White	Tablet	Capsule-Shape	Ivax Pharmaceuticals
GX; EG2	Cefuroxime Axetil	500 mg	White	Tablet	Capsule-Shape	Stada
GX; EG3; L	Leukeran	2 mg	Brown	Tablet	Circle, Biconvex	Glaxosmithkline
GX; EH3; A	Alkeran	2 mg	White	Coated Tablet	Circle, Biconvex	Celgene
GX; EH3; A	Alkeran	2 mg	White	Coated Tablet	Circle, Biconvex	Glaxosmithkline
GX; EJ7	Epivir	300 mg	Gray	Coated Tablet	Diamond, Modified	Glaxosmithkline
GX; ES7	Ceftin	250 mg	White	Tablet	Capsule-Shape	Glaxosmithkline
GX; ES7	Cefuroxime	250 mg	White	Tablet	Capsule-Shape	Ivax Pharmaceuticals
GX; ES7	Cefuroxime Axetil	250 mg	White	Tablet	Capsule-Shape	Stada
GX; EX1	Lotronex	0.5 mg	White	Coated Tablet	Oval	Glaxosmithkline
GXFC3	Combivir	150 mg; 300 mg	White	Coated Tablet	Capsule-Shape	Glaxosmithkline
GX; LL1	Trizivir	300 mg; 150 mg; 300 mg	Blue-Green	Coated Tablet	Capsule-Shape	Glaxosmithkline
GX; LL7	Lexiva	700 mg	Pink	Tablet	Capsule-Shape	Glaxosmithkline
GX CW3; 300	Retrovir	300 mg	White	Coated Tablet	Circle, Biconvex	Glaxosmithkline
H; 1	Captopril	12.5 mg	White	Tablet	Circle, Scored	Duramed Pharmaceuticals
H; 1; LL	Hydromox	50 mg	White	Tablet	Circle, Flat, Scored, Beveled	Lederle Laboratories
H; 5	Glyburide	6 mg	Yellow	Tablet	Capsule-Shape, Scored	West-Ward
H; 11	Captopril	25 mg	White	Tablet	Round, Quadrisected Scored	Duramed Pharmaceuticals
H; 12	Captopril	100 mg	White	Tablet	Circle, Scored	Duramed Pharmaceuticals
H; 111	Captopril	50 mg	White	Tablet	Circle, Scored	Duramed Pharmaceuticals
H; 111	Hyospaz	0.15 mg	Light Blue	Tablet	Circle	Econolab
H; 114	Glipizide	5 mg	White	Tablet	Round, Bisected Scored	Duramed Pharmaceuticals
H; 115	Glipizide	10 mg	White	Tablet	Round, Bisected Scored	Duramed Pharmaceuticals
H; 214	Tetracycline Hydrochloride	250 mg	Yellow and Orange	Capsule		Solvay Pharmaceuticals
H; 302; 2	Acetaminophen and Codeine	300 mg; 15 mg	White	Tablet	Circle	Duramed Pharmaceuticals
H; 303	Acetaminophen and Codeine Phosphate	300 mg; 30 mg	White	Tablet	Circle	Duramed Pharmaceuticals
H; 304; 4	Acetaminophen and Codeine Phosphate	300 mg; 60 mg	White	Tablet	Circle	Duramed Pharmaceuticals
H3647; 400	Ketek	400 mg	Light Orange	Tablet	Oval	Aventis Pharmaceuticals
HALCION; 0.125	Halcion	0.125 mg	White	Tablet	Oval	Pharmacia & Upjohn
HALCION; 0.25;	Halcion	0.25 mg	Powder-Blue	Tablet	Oval, Scored	Pharmacia & Upjohn
HALCION; 0.5	Halcion	0.5 mg	White	Tablet	Oval, Scored	Pharmacia & Upjohn
HALDOL; 1; MCNEIL	Haldol	1 mg	Yellow	Tablet,u-Shape, with H Cut Out in Center, Scored,ortho-Mcneil Pharmaceutical		
HALDOL; 2; MCNEIL	Haldol	2 mg	Pink	Tablet	U-Shape, with H Cut Out in Center, Scored,ortho-Mcneil Pharmaceutical	
HALDOL; 5; MCNEIL	Haldol	5 mg	Green	Tablet	U-Shape, with H Cut Out in Center, Scored,ortho-Mcneil Pharmaceutical	
HALDOL; 10; MCNEIL	Haldol	10 mg	Aqua	Tablet	U-Shape, with H Cut Out in Center, Scored,ortho-Mcneil Pharmaceutical	
HALDOL; 20; MCNEIL	Haldol	20 mg	Salmon	Tablet,u-Shape, with H Cut Out in Center, Scored,ortho-Mcneil Pharmaceutical		
HALFAN	Halfan	250 mg	White	Tablet	Capsule-Shape,glaxosmithkline	
HALOTESTIN; 2;	Halotestin	2 mg	Peach	Tablet	Circle, Scored	Pharmacia & Upjohn
HALOTESTIN; 5;	Halotestin	5 mg	Light Green	Tablet	Circle, Scored	Pharmacia & Upjohn
HALOTESTIN; 10;	Halotestin	10 mg	Green	Tablet	Circle, Scored	Pharmacia & Upjohn
HALTRAN	Haltran	200 mg	White	Tablet	Oval	Lee Pharmaceuticals
HAW; 240	Xpect-AT	600 mg; 60 mg	White	Tablet	Capsule-Shape, Bisect	Hawthorn Pharmaceuticals
HAW; 251	Xpect	400 mg	White	Tablet		Hawthorn Pharmaceuticals
HAW; 571	Dytan	25 mg		Tablet, Chewable	Oval	Hawthorn Pharmaceuticals
HAW; 577	Dytan-D	25 mg; 10 mg	Blue	Tablet, Chewable	Triangle	Hawthorn Pharmaceuticals

IMPRINT	BRAND/GENERIC NAME	STRENGTH	COLOR	FORM	SHAPE	MANUFACTURER
HAW 581	Dytan-Cs	25 mg; 10 mg; 30 mg	Tan	Tablet	Triangle	Hawthorn Pharmaceuticals
HB; 93; 614	Belap	16.2 mg; 10.8 mg	Green	Tablet	Circle, Convex	Teva Pharmaceuticals
HC; ABBOTT LOGO	Depakote ER	500 mg	Gray	Extended-Release Tablet		Abbott Laboratories
HD; 125	Digoxin	0.125 mg	White	Tablet	Circle, Scored	Halsey Drug
HD; 157	Quinine Sulfate	325 mg	Clear	Capsule		Halsey Drug
HD; 250	Digoxin	0.25 mg	White	Tablet	Circle, Scored	Halsey Drug
HD; 467	Dipyridamole	75 mg	White	Coated Tablet		Halsey Drug
HD; 479	Dipyridamole	50 mg	White	Coated Tablet		Halsey Drug
HD; 494	Dipyridamole	25 mg	White	Coated Tablet		Halsey Drug
HD; 503	Chlorpropamide	250 mg	Blue	Tablet		Halsey Drug
HD; 506	Metronidazole	250 mg	White	Tablet	Circle	Halsey Drug
HD; 507	Indomethacin	25 mg	Green	Capsule		Halsey Drug
HD; 508	Indomethacin	50 mg	Green	Capsule		Halsey Drug
HD; 512	Oxycodone and Acetaminophen	5 mg; 325 mg	White	Tablet		Halsey Drug
HD; 522	Chlorpropamide	100 mg	Blue	Tablet	Circle, Scored	Halsey Drug
HD; 524	Cyproheptadine Hydrochloride	4 mg	White	Tablet	Circle	Halsey Drug
HD; 532	Oxycodone and Acetaminophen	5 mg; 500 mg	Red and Buff	Capsule		Halsey Drug
HD; 532	Oxycodone and Acetaminophen	500 mg; 5 mg	Red and Off-White	Capsule		Halsey Drug
HD; 532	Roxilox	5 mg; 500 mg	Scarlet Red and Buff White	Capsule		Halsey Drug
HD; 532	Roxilox	5 mg; 500 mg	Scarlet Red and Buff White	Capsule		Roxane Laboratories
HD; 533	Flurazepam Hydrochloride	30 mg	Blue	Capsule		Halsey Drug
HD; 534	Flurazepam Hydrochloride	15 mg	Blue and White	Capsule		Halsey Drug
HD; 535	Hydralazine Hydrochloride	10 mg	Pink or Pale Yellow	Tablet		Halsey Drug
HD; 536	Hydralazine Hydrochloride	25 mg	Peach	Tablet	Circle, Scored	Halsey Drug
HD; 537	Hydralazine Hydrochloride	50 mg	Orange	Tablet	Circle	Halsey Drug
HD; 538	Hydralazine Hydrochloride	100 mg	Orange	Tablet	Circle	Halsey Drug
HD; 540	Metronidazole	500 mg	White	Tablet	Circle, Scored	Halsey Drug
HD; 543	Butalbital and Acetaminophen	50 mg; 325 mg	White	Tablet		Halsey Drug
HD; 544	Diazepam	5 mg	Yellow	Tablet	Circle, Scored	Warner Chilcott
HD; 546	Diazepam	2 mg	White	Tablet	Circle, Scored	Warner Chilcott
HD; 549	Diazepam	10 mg	Blue	Tablet	Circle, Scored	Warner Chilcott
HD; 557	Ibuprofen	200 mg	White	Coated Tablet	Circle	Halsey Drug
HD; 559	Ibuprofen	400 mg	White	Coated Tablet	Circle	Halsey Drug
HD; 560	Ibuprofen	600 mg	White	Coated Tablet	Oval	Halsey Drug
HD; 561	Metoclopramide Hydrochloride	10 mg	White	Tablet	Capsule-Shape	Halsey Drug
HD; 565; 0.5	Lorazepam	0.5 mg	White	Tablet	Circle, Scored	Halsey Drug
HD; 566	Butalbital, Aspirin and Caffeine	50 mg; 325 mg; 40 mg	White	Tablet	Circle	Halsey Drug
HD; 567	Butalbital, Acetaminophen and Caffeine	50 mg; 325 mg; 40 mg	White	Tablet	Circle	Watson Laboratories
HD; 572; 1	Lorazepam	1 mg	White	Tablet	Circle, Scored	Halsey Drug
HD; 573; 2	Lorazepam	2 mg	White	Tablet	Circle, Scored	Halsey Drug
HD; 607	Methyldopa	250 mg	White	Coated Tablet	Circle	Halsey Drug
HD; 608	Methyldopa	500 mg	White	Coated Tablet	Circle	Halsey Drug
HD; 622	Ibuprofen	800 mg	White	Coated Tablet	Capsule-Shape, Scored	Halsey Drug
HD; 632	Fenoprofen Calcium	200 mg	Lavender and Light Pink	Capsule		Halsey Drug
HD; 633	Fenoprofen Calcium	300 mg	Orange and Light Pink	Capsule		Halsey Drug
HD; 634	Fenoprofen Calcium	600 mg	Peach	Coated Tablet	Capsule-Shape	Halsey Drug
HD; 647	Aspirin, Butalbital, Caffeine and Codeine No. 3	325 mg; 50 mg; 40 mg; 30 mg	Blue and White	Capsule		Halsey Drug
HD; 648	Aspirin, Butalbital, Caffeine and Codeine No. 2	325 mg; 50 mg; 40 mg; 15 mg	Gray and White	Capsule		Halsey Drug
HD; 714	Hydromorphone Hydrochloride	1 mg	White	Tablet	Circle	Halsey Drug
HD; 715; 2	Hydromorphone Hydrochloride	2 mg	White	Tablet	Circle	Halsey Drug
HD; 716	Hydromorphone Hydrochloride	3 mg	White	Tablet	Circle	Halsey Drug
HD; 717; 4	Hydromorphone Hydrochloride	4 mg	White	Tablet	Circle	Halsey Drug
HD; 725	Doxycycline Hyclate	100 mg	Beige	Coated Tablet	Circle	Novartis Generics
HD; 765	Hydrocodone Bitartrate and Acetaminophen	5 mg; 500 mg	White	Tablet	Capsule-Shape, Scored	Halsey Drug
HD; 765	Hydrocodone Bitartrate and Acetaminophen	500 mg; 5 mg	White	Tablet		Halsey Drug
HD; 778	Acetaminophen and Hydrocodone Bitartrate	650 mg; 10 mg	White	Tablet	Oblong	Halsey Drug
HD; 779	Acetaminophen and Hydrocodone Bitartrate	750 mg; 7.5 mg	White	Tablet	Oblong	Halsey Drug
HD; 780	Acetaminophen and Hydrocodone Bitartrate	650 mg; 7.5 mg		Tablet		Halsey Drug
HEART	Miniprin Analgesic	81 mg	Yellow	Tablet, Enteric Coated	Circle	Time Cap Labs
HEART SHAPE	Healthprin	81 mg	White	Tablet	Heart Shape; Bisected Scored	Smart Pharmaceuticals
HEART SHAPE	Healthprin	162.5 mg	Pink	Tablet	Heart Shape; Bisected Scored	Smart Pharmaceuticals
HEART SHAPE; SMART	Healthprin	325 mg		Tablet	Heart Shape; Bisected Scored	Smart Pharmaceuticals
HEMAX	Hemax	150 mg; 500 mg; 60 mcg; 75 mg; 1 mg; 30 IU; 50 mg; 3 mg; 5 mcg; 150 mcg; 150 mcg	Amber and Beige	Extended-Release Tablet	Capsule-Shape	Pronova
HF; ABBOTT LOGO	Depakote ER	250 mg	White	Extended-Release Tablet	Oval	Abbott Laboratories
HH; ABBOTT LOGO	Hytrin	1 mg	Grey	Capsule		Abbott Laboratories
HISTEX I/E; 050	Histex I/e	2 mg/8 mg	Green and White	Capsule		Teamm Pharmaceuticals
HIVID; 0.375; ROCHE	Hivid	0.375 mg	Beige	Coated Tablet	Oval	Roche Pharmaceuticals
HIVID; 0.750; ROCHE	Hivid	0.75 mg	Gray	Coated Tablet	Oval	Roche Pharmaceuticals
HK; ABBOTT LOGO	Hytrin	5 mg	Red	Capsule		Abbott Laboratories
HL; T41	Temaril	2.5 mg	Gray	Coated Tablet	Circle	Allergan Pharmaceuticals

IMPRINT	BRAND/GENERIC NAME	STRENGTH	COLOR	FORM	SHAPE	MANUFACTURER
HL; T50	Temaril	5 mg	Gray and Natural	Extended-Release Capsule		Allergan Pharmaceuticals
HN; ABBOTT LOGO	Hytrin	10 mg	Blue	Capsule		Abbott Laboratories
HOECHST; 73	Festalan	30,000 units; 1 mg; 6000 units; 20,000 units	Orange	Tablet	Circle	Aventis Pharmaceuticals
HOECHST; LASIX	Lasix	20 mg	White	Tablet	Oval	Aventis Pharmaceuticals
HOPE; 742	Sal-Tropine	0.4 mg		Tablet		Hope Pharmaceuticals
HORIZON; 205	Robinul Forte	2 mg	White	Tablet	Circle, Compressed, Scored	First Horizon Pharmaceutical
HOURGLASS; 56; 65; 5; 5; 5	Buspirone Hydrochloride	15 mg	White	Tablet	Capsule-Shape	Ivax Pharmaceuticals
HOURGLASS; 120	Verapamil Hydrochloride	120 mg	Ivory	Extended-Release Tablet	Circle	Ivax Pharmaceuticals
HOURGLASS; 200;	Cimetidine	200 mg	White	Tablet	Circle	Ivax Pharmaceuticals
HOURGLASS; 3667	Perphenazine	2 mg	White	Coated Tablet	Circle	Ivax Pharmaceuticals
HOURGLASS; 3668	Perphenazine	4 mg	White	Coated Tablet	Oval	Ivax Pharmaceuticals
HOURGLASS; 3669	Perphenazine	8 mg	White	Coated Tablet	Circle	Ivax Pharmaceuticals
HOURGLASS; 3670	Perphenazine	16 mg	White	Coated Tablet	Oval	Ivax Pharmaceuticals
HOURGLASS; 3685; 1	Doxazosin Mesylate	1 mg	White	Tablet	Circle	Ivax Pharmaceuticals
HOURGLASS; 3686; 2	Doxazosin Mesylate	2 mg	White	Tablet	Circle	Ivax Pharmaceuticals
HOURGLASS; 3687; 4	Doxazosin Mesylate	4 mg	Orange	Tablet	Circle	Ivax Pharmaceuticals
HOURGLASS; 3688; 8	Doxazosin Mesylate	8 mg	Green	Tablet	Circle	Ivax Pharmaceuticals
HOURGLASS; 3757	Lisinopril	2.5 mg	White	Tablet	Circle	Ivax Pharmaceuticals
HOURGLASS; 3758	Lisinopril	5 mg	White	Tablet	Square	Ivax Pharmaceuticals
HOURGLASS; 3759	Lisinopril	10 mg	White	Tablet	Oval	Ivax Pharmaceuticals
HOURGLASS; 3760	Lisinopril	20 mg	White	Tablet	Five-Sided	Ivax Pharmaceuticals
HOURGLASS; 3761	Lisinopril	40 mg	White	Tablet	Circle	Ivax Pharmaceuticals
HOURGLASS; 3762	Lisinopril	30 mg	White	Tablet	Oval	Ivax Pharmaceuticals
HOURGLASS; 3966	Diphenoxylate Hydrochloride and Atropine Sulfate	2.5 mg; 0.025 mg	White	Tablet	Circle	Ivax Pharmaceuticals
HOURGLASS; 4058	Cefadroxil	500 mg	Clear and White	Capsule		Ivax Pharmaceuticals
HOURGLASS; 4059;	Cefadroxil	1000 mg	White	Tablet	Oval, Bisected on One Side Scored	Ivax Pharmaceuticals
HOURGLASS; 4194; 500	Cefaclor Extended-Release	500 mg	Blue	Extended-Release Tablet	Oval	Ivax Pharmaceuticals
HOURGLASS; 4195; 2.5	Enalapril Maleate	2.5 mg	Yellow	Tablet	Circle, Scored	Ivax Pharmaceuticals
HOURGLASS; 4196; 5	Enalapril Maleate	5 mg	White	Tablet	Circle, Scored	Ivax Pharmaceuticals
HOURGLASS; 4197; 10	Enalapril Maleate	10 mg	Salmon	Tablet	Circle	Ivax Pharmaceuticals
HOURGLASS; 4198; 20	Enalapril Maleate	20 mg	Peach	Tablet	Circle	Ivax Pharmaceuticals
HOURGLASS; 4267; 400;	Acyclovir	400 mg	White	Tablet	Circle, Flat-Faced, Beveled-Edge	Ivax Pharmaceuticals
HOURGLASS; 4268; 800;	Acyclovir	800 mg	White	Tablet	Oval	Ivax Pharmaceuticals
HOURGLASS; 4303	Clozapine	12.5 mg	Pale Yellow	Tablet	Oval	Ivax Pharmaceuticals
HOURGLASS 4330; 850	Metformin Hydrochloride	850 mg	White	Tablet	Oval	Ivax Pharmaceuticals
HOURGLASS 4331; 500	Metformin Hydrochloride	500 mg	White	Tablet	Oval	Ivax Pharmaceuticals
HOURGLASS; 4332; 100	Nefazodone Hydrochloride	100 mg	Peach	Tablet	Oval	Ivax Pharmaceuticals
HOURGLASS; 4333; 150	Nefazodone Hydrochloride	150 mg	Peach	Tablet	Circle	Ivax Pharmaceuticals
HOURGLASS; 4334; 200	Nefazodone Hydrochloride	200 mg	Peach	Tablet	Oval	Ivax Pharmaceuticals
HOURGLASS; 4335; 250	Nefazodone Hydrochloride	250 mg	Peach	Tablet	Circle	Ivax Pharmaceuticals
HOURGLASS; 4343; 50	Nefazodone Hydrochloride	50 mg	Peach	Tablet	Oval	Ivax Pharmaceuticals
HOURGLASS; 4359; 25;	Clozapine	25 mg	Pale Yellow	Tablet	Circle	Ivax Pharmaceuticals
HOURGLASS; 4360; 100;	Clozapine	100 mg	Pale Yellow	Tablet	Circle	Ivax Pharmaceuticals
HOURGLASS; 4389	Fluvoxamine Maleate	25 mg	White	Tablet	Circle	Ivax Pharmaceuticals
HOURGLASS; 4391	Fluvoxamine Maleate	50 mg	Yellow	Tablet	Circle, Scored	Ivax Pharmaceuticals
HOURGLASS; 4392	Fluvoxamine Maleate	100 mg	Beige	Tablet	Circle	Ivax Pharmaceuticals
HOURGLASS; 4430; 100	Misoprostol	100 mcg		Tablet		Ivax Pharmaceuticals
HOURGLASS; 4431; 200	Misoprostol	200 mcg	White	Tablet	Circle, Scored	Ivax Pharmaceuticals
HOURGLASS 4432; 1000	Metformin Hydrochloride	1000 mg	White	Tablet	Oval	Ivax Pharmaceuticals
HOURGLASS; 4510	Fluoxetine Hydrochloride	10 mg	Light Green	Tablet	Oval, Scored	Ivax Pharmaceuticals
HOURGLASS 4740; 10	Citalopram Hydrobromide	10 mg	Light Beige	Tablet	Capsule-Shape	Ivax Pharmaceuticals
HOURGLASS 4741; 20	Citalopram Hydrobromide	20 mg	Light Pink	Tablet	Capsule-Shape	Ivax Pharmaceuticals
HOURGLASS 4742; 40	Citalopram Hydrobromide	40 mg	White	Tablet	Capsule-Shape	Ivax Pharmaceuticals
HOURGLASS; 4960	Flutamide	125 mg	Light Brown Opaque	Capsule		Ivax Pharmaceuticals
HOURGLASS; 4980	Propoxyphene Napsylate and Acetaminophen	100 mg; 650 mg	Pink	Coated Tablet	Capsule-Shape	Ivax Pharmaceuticals
HOURGLASS; 5032; 20/25	Lisinopril and Hydrochlorothiazide	20 mg; 25 mg	Peach	Tablet	Circle	Ivax Pharmaceuticals

IMPRINT	BRAND/GENERIC NAME	STRENGTH	COLOR	FORM	SHAPE	MANUFACTURER
HOURGLASS; 5033; 10/12.5	Lisinopril and Hydrochlorothiazide	10 mg; 12.5 mg	Blue	Tablet	Circle	Ivax Pharmaceuticals
HOURGLASS; 5034; 20/12.5	Lisinopril and Hydrochlorothiazide	20 mg; 12.5 mg	Yellow	Tablet	Circle	Ivax Pharmaceuticals
HOURGLASS; 5350; 5	Benazepril Hydrochloride	5 mg	Light Yellow	Tablet	Capsule-Shape	Ivax Pharmaceuticals
HOURGLASS; 5351; 10	Benazepril Hydrochloride	10 mg	Dark Yellow	Tablet	Capsule-Shape	Ivax Pharmaceuticals
HOURGLASS; 5352; 20	Benazepril Hydrochloride	20 mg	Pink	Tablet	Capsule-Shape	Ivax Pharmaceuticals
HOURGLASS; 5353; 40	Benazepril Hydrochloride	40 mg	Pink	Tablet	Capsule-Shape	Ivax Pharmaceuticals
HOURGLASS; 5663; 5	Buspirone Hydrochloride	5 mg	White	Tablet	Oval	Ivax Pharmaceuticals
HOURGLASS; 5664; 10	Buspirone Hydrochloride	10 mg	White	Tablet	Oval	Ivax Pharmaceuticals
HOURGLASS; 5675; 15	Mirtazapine	15 mg	Yellow	Tablet	Circle, Scored	Ivax Pharmaceuticals
HOURGLASS; 5676; 30	Mirtazapine	30 mg	Tan	Tablet	Circle, Scored	Ivax Pharmaceuticals
HOURGLASS; 5695; 45	Mirtazapine	45 mg	White	Tablet	Circle	Ivax Pharmaceuticals
HOURGLASS; 5728; 20;	Famotidine	20 mg	Off-White to Light Tan	Tablet	Circle	Ivax Pharmaceuticals
HOURGLASS; 5729; 40	Famotidine	40 mg	Tan	Tablet	Circle	Ivax Pharmaceuticals
HOURGLASS; 7300	Verapamil Hydrochloride	240 mg	Ivory	Sustained-Release Tablet	Oblong	Norton, H.N.
HOURGLASS; 7300;	Verapamil Hydrochloride	240 mg	Ivory	Extended-Release Tablet	Oblong	Ivax Pharmaceuticals
HOURGLASS; 7301;	Verapamil Hydrochloride	180 mg	Orange	Extended-Release Tablet	Oblong, Scored	Ivax Pharmaceuticals
HOURGLASS; 9200	Glipizide	10 mg	White	Tablet	Circle, Scored	Ivax Pharmaceuticals
HOURGLASS; 9201	Glipizide	5 mg	White	Tablet	Circle	Ivax Pharmaceuticals
HOYT; 052	Phos-Flur	2.2 mg		Tablet, Chewable		Colgate Hoyt
HP; 15	Mescolor	8 mg; 120 mg; 2.5 mg	White	Sustained-Release Tablet	Film-Coated, Scored	First Horizon Pharmaceutical
HP; 81	Aspirin	81 mg	Pink	Coated Tablet	Circle	Pdk Labs
HPC; 170; HORIZON LOGO	Zebutal	500 mg; 50 mg; 40 mg	Pink and Red	Capsule		First Horizon Pharmaceutical
HPC; 200	Robinul	1 mg	White	Tablet	Circle, Compressed, Scored	First Horizon Pharmaceutical
HSS; 375	Hyoscyamine	0.375 mg	Brown and Natural	Extended-Release Capsule		Qualitest Products
HSS; 375	Hyoscyamine TR	0.375 mg	Brown and White	Capsule		Breckenridge Pharmaceutical
HTI; 77;	Thalitone	15 mg	White	Tablet	Kidney-Shape, Compressed	Monarch Pharmaceuticals
HUMIBID DM; CAROLINA PHARMA	Humibid DM	50 mg; 400 mg; 200 mg	Blue and White	Extended-Release Capsule, 12 Hour		Pharmafab
HY	Hytuss	100 mg	White	Tablet		Hyrex Pharmaceuticals
HY; 310	Panzyme Tabs	0.0519 mg; 0.2885 mg; 0.0033 mg; 8.1 mg; 300 mg; 150 mg	Light Blue	Tablet		Hyrex Pharmaceuticals
HY; 408	Trac Tabs 2x	0.06 mg; 0.03 mg; 120 mg; 6 mg; 30 mg; 7.5 mg		Tablet		Hyrex Pharmaceuticals
HY; ABBOTT LOGO	Hytrin	2 mg	Yellow	Capsule		Abbott Laboratories
HYCODAN	Hycodan	5 mg; 1.5 mg	White	Tablet	Circle, Scored	Dupont Pharma
HYCODAN	Hycodan	5 mg; 1.5 mg	White	Tablet	Circle, Scored	Endo Laboratories
HYDERGINE; 0.5; S;	Hydergine	0.167 mg; 0.167 mg; 0.167 mg	White	Tablet	Circle	Novartis
HYDREA; 830	Hydrea	500 mg	Pink and Green	Capsule		Bristol-Myers Squibb
HYLOREL; 10	Hylorel	10 mg	Light Orange	Tablet	Circle, Scored	Medeva Pharmaceuticals
HYLOREL; 25	Hylorel	25 mg	White	Tablet	Circle, Scored	Medeva Pharmaceuticals
HZ	Halls Zinc Defense Cold Season Dietary Supplement	5 mg		Lozenge/troche		Pfizer Consumer Health Care
I	Visicol	1.102 GM; 0.398 GM	White to Off-White	Tablet	Oval	Inkine Pharmaceuticals
I; 2	Ibu-200	200 mg	White	Coated Tablet	Circle, Biconvex	Major
I; 2	Ibuprofen	200 mg	Brown	Coated Tablet	Circle, Biconvex	Fleming
I; 2	Ibuprofen	200 mg	Brown	Coated Tablet	Circle, Biconvex	Good Neighbor Pharmacy
I; 2	Ibuprofen	200 mg	Brown	Coated Tablet	Circle, Biconvex	Good Sense
I; 2	Ibuprofen	200 mg	Brown	Coated Tablet	Circle, Biconvex	Hytop
I; 2	Ibuprofen	200 mg	Brown	Coated Tablet	Circle, Biconvex	Kerr Drug
I; 2	Ibuprofen	200 mg	Brown	Coated Tablet	Circle, Biconvex	Major
I; 2	Ibuprofen	200 mg	Brown	Coated Tablet	Circle, Biconvex	Medic
I; 2	Ibuprofen	200 mg	Brown	Coated Tablet	Circle, Biconvex	Nex
I; 2	Ibuprofen	200 mg	Brown	Coated Tablet	Circle, Biconvex	Perfect Choice
I; 2	Ibuprofen	200 mg	Brown	Coated Tablet	Circle, Biconvex	Perrigo
I; 2	Ibuprofen	200 mg	Brown	Coated Tablet	Circle, Biconvex	Pharm X
I; 2	Ibuprofen	200 mg	Brown	Coated Tablet	Circle, Biconvex	Quality Care
I; 2	Ibuprofen	200 mg	Brown	Coated Tablet	Circle, Biconvex	Revco
I; 2	Ibuprofen	200 mg	Brown	Coated Tablet	Circle, Biconvex	Seaway
I; 2	Ibuprofen	200 mg	Brown	Coated Tablet	Circle, Biconvex	Sunmark
I; 2	Ibuprofen	200 mg	Brown	Coated Tablet	Circle, Biconvex	Swan
I; 2	Ibuprofen	200 mg	Brown	Coated Tablet	Circle, Biconvex	Top Care
I; 2	Ibuprofen	200 mg	Brown	Coated Tablet	Circle, Biconvex	Valu Rite
I; 2	Ibuprofen	200 mg	White	Coated Tablet	Circle, Biconvex	Kerr Drug
I; 2	Ibuprofen	200 mg	White	Coated Tablet	Circle, Biconvex	Major
I; 2	Ibuprofen	200 mg	White	Coated Tablet	Circle, Biconvex	Major Quality
I; 2	Ibuprofen	200 mg	White	Coated Tablet	Circle, Biconvex	North Laboratories

IMPRINT	BRAND/GENERIC NAME	STRENGTH	COLOR	FORM	SHAPE	MANUFACTURER
I; 2	Ibuprofen	200 mg	White	Tablet		Perfect Choice
I; 2	Ibuprofen	200 mg	White	Tablet		Perrigo
I; 2	Ibuprofen	200 mg	White	Tablet		Pharmx
I; 2	Ibuprofen	200 mg	White	Coated Tablet	Circle, Biconvex	Top Care
I; 2	Ibuprofen	200 mg	White	Coated Tablet	Circle, Biconvex	Valu Rite
I-2	Ibuprofen	200 mg	Brown	Tablet		Fleming
I-2	Ibuprofen	200 mg	Brown	Tablet		Glendale Foods
I-2	Ibuprofen	200 mg	Brown	Tablet	Oblong	Good Neighbor Pharmacy
I-2	Ibuprofen	200 mg	Brown	Tablet		Good Neighbor Pharmacy
I-2	Ibuprofen	200 mg	Brown	Tablet		Good Sense
I-2	Ibuprofen	200 mg	Brown	Tablet		Hytop
I-2	Ibuprofen	200 mg	Brown	Tablet		Kerr Drug
I-2	Ibuprofen	200 mg	Brown	Tablet		Major
I-2	Ibuprofen	200 mg	Brown	Tablet		Medalist
I-2	Ibuprofen	200 mg	Brown	Tablet		Medic
I-2	Ibuprofen	200 mg	Brown	Tablet		Moore Medical
I-2	Ibuprofen	200 mg	Brown	Tablet		Park Lane
I-2	Ibuprofen	200 mg	Brown	Coated Tablet	Circle	Perfect Choice
I-2	Ibuprofen	200 mg	Brown	Tablet		Perfect Choice
I-2	Ibuprofen	200 mg	Brown	Tablet		Perrigo
I-2	Ibuprofen	200 mg	Brown	Tablet		Pharm X
I-2	Ibuprofen	200 mg	Brown	Tablet		Preferred Products
I-2	Ibuprofen	200 mg	Brown	Tablet		Quality Care
I-2	Ibuprofen	200 mg	Brown	Tablet		Regal Distributing
I-2	Ibuprofen	200 mg	Brown	Tablet		Rexall
I-2	Ibuprofen	200 mg	Brown	Tablet		Sunfresh
I-2	Ibuprofen	200 mg	Brown	Tablet		Sunmark
I-2	Ibuprofen	200 mg	Brown	Tablet		Swan
I-2	Ibuprofen	200 mg	Brown	Tablet	Oblong	Top Care
I-2	Ibuprofen	200 mg	Brown	Tablet		Valu Buy
I-2	Ibuprofen	200 mg	Brown	Tablet		Valu Rite
I-2	Ibuprofen	200 mg	Brown	Tablet		Valumed
I-2	Ibuprofen Ib	200 mg	White	Coated Tablet	Circle	Perfect Choice
I-2	Ibuprofen Ib	200 mg	White	Coated Tablet	Circle	Valu Rite
I-2	Ibu-200	200 mg	White	Tablet		Major
I; 25	Imitrex	25 mg	White	Coated Tablet	Triangle	Glaxosmithkline
I L; 20 MG	Citalopram Hydrobromide	20 mg	Pink	Tablet	Oval	Inwood Laboratories
I L; 40 MG	Citalopram Hydrobromide	40 mg	White	Tablet	Oval	Inwood Laboratories
IB; 2;	Ibuprofen	200 mg	Brown or White	Tablet	Circle	Genco Distributors
IB; 2;	Ibuprofen	200 mg	Brown or White	Tablet	Circle	Harco Drug
IB; 2;	Ibuprofen	200 mg	Brown or White	Tablet	Circle	Perfect Choice
IB; 2;	Ibuprofen	200 mg	Brown or White	Tablet	Circle	Perrigo
IB; 2;	Ibuprofen	200 mg	Brown or White	Tablet	Circle	True Quality
IBU; 400	Ibuprofen	400 mg	White	Tablet	Oblong	Vangard Labs
IBU; 400	Ibuprofen	400 mg	White	Tablet		Warner Chilcott
IBU; 600	Ibuprofen	600 mg	White	Coated Tablet		Warner Chilcott
IBU; 800	Ibuprofen	800 mg	White	Tablet		Warner Chilcott
IC	Cartrol	5 mg	White	Tablet	Oval	Abbott Laboratories
ICN; 0901	Testred	10 mg	Red	Capsule		Icn Pharmaceuticals
ICN; 311	Android-10	10 mg	White	Capsule		Icn Pharmaceuticals
ICN; 600	8-Mop	10 mg	Pink	Capsule	Oblong	Icn Pharmaceuticals
ICN; 600;	Oxsoralen	10 mg		Capsule		Icn Pharmaceuticals
ICN; 650	Oxsoralen-Ultra	10 mg		Capsule		Icn Pharmaceuticals
ICN; M180;	Mestinon Timespan	180 mg		Sustained-Release Tablet	Capsule-Shape, Scored	Icn Pharmaceuticals
ID; 112	Iobid DM	30 mg; 600 mg	Light Green	Tablet	Oblong, Scored	Iopharm
ID; 121	Iotex Pse	600 mg; 120 mg	Yellow	Tablet	Oblong, Scored	Iopharm
ID; 122	Iosal II	600 mg; 60 mg	Light Blue	Tablet	Oblong, Scored	Iopharm
ID; 125	Guaifenesin	600 mg	White	Tablet	Oblong, Scored	Iopharm
ID; 152	Drixomed	6 mg; 120 mg	Green	Tablet	Circle	Iopharm
ID; 155	Hyoscyamine Sulfate	0.375 mg	White	Tablet	Oblong, Scored	Iopharm
ID; 156	Hyoscyamine Sulfate	0.125 mg	Blue	Tablet	Circle, Scored	Iopharm
ID; 172	Guaifenesin	1200 mg	White	Tablet	Oblong, Scored	Iopharm
IDMUR; 30 MG	Imdur	30 mg	Rose	Sustained-Release Tablet		Key Pharmaceuticals
IE; 1.25; G	Indapamide	1.25 mg	Orange	Tablet	Circle	Par Pharmaceutical
IE; 2.5; G	Indapamide	2.5 mg	White	Tablet	Circle	Par Pharmaceutical
IF; 400; ALRA	Ibu-Tab	400 mg	Orange	Coated Tablet	Circle	Alra Laboratories
IF; 600; ALRA	Ibu-Tab	600 mg	Light Orange	Coated Tablet	Capsule-Shape	Alra Laboratories
IF; 800; ALRA	Ibu-Tab	800 mg	Pale Orange	Coated Tablet	Oblong	Alra Laboratories
IKA	Serophene	50 mg	White	Tablet		Serono Labs
IL	Diphenoxylate Hydrochoride and Atropine Sulfate	2.5 mg; 0.025 mg	White	Tablet		Inwood Laboratories
IL; 10 MG	Citalopram Hydrobromide	10 mg	Beige	Tablet	Oval	Inwood Laboratories
IL; 360	Indomethacin E.R.	40 mg	Lavender and Clear	Extended-Release Capsule		Inwood Laboratories
IL; 3309	Betachron	60 mg	Brown and Clear	Extended-Release Capsule		Inwood Laboratories
IL; 3521	Nitrobon	2.5 mg		Timed-Release Capsule		Inwood Laboratories
IL; 3522	Nitrobon	6.5 mg		Timed-Release Capsule		Inwood Laboratories
IL; 3530	Cyclandelate	200 mg	Orange	Capsule		Inwood Laboratories
IL; 3535	Cyclandelate	400 mg	Green and White	Capsule		Inwood Laboratories
IL; 3549	Isosorbide Dinitrate	40 mg	Peach	Sustained-Release Tablet	Circle, Scored	Inwood Laboratories
IL; 3575	Isosorbide Dinitrate	40 mg	White and Clear	Capsule		H.L. Moore
IL; 3575	Isosorbide Dinitrate	40 mg	White and Clear	Extended-Release Tablet		Inwood Laboratories
IL; 3577	Pentaerythritol Tetranitrate	80 mg	White with White Pellets	Controlled-Release Capsule		Inwood Laboratories
IL; 3581	Theochron	300 mg	White	Extended-Release Tablet	Capsule-Shape, Scored	Forest Pharmaceuticals

IMPRINT	BRAND/GENERIC NAME	STRENGTH	COLOR	FORM	SHAPE	MANUFACTURER
IL; 3581	Theophylline Cr	300 mg	White	Tablet	Capsule-Shape	Qualitest Products
IL; 3581	Theophylline Extended Release	300 mg	White	Extended-Release Tablet	Capsule-Shape, Scored	Akyma Pharmaceuticals
IL; 3583	Theochron	200 mg	White	Extended-Release Tablet	Oval, Convex, Scored	Forest Pharmaceuticals
IL; 3583	Theophylline Cr	200 mg	White	Tablet	Oval	Qualitest Products
IL; 3583	Theophylline Extended Release	200 mg	White	Extended-Release Tablet	Oval, Convex, Scored	Akyma Pharmaceuticals
IL; 3584	Theochron	100 mg	White	Extended-Release Tablet	Circle, Convex, Scored	Forest Pharmaceuticals
IL; 3584	Theophylline Cr	100 mg	White	Tablet	Circle	Qualitest Products
IL; 3584	Theophylline Extended Release	100 mg	White	Extended-Release Tablet	Circle, Convex, Scored	Akyma Pharmaceuticals
IL; 3587	Carbamazepine	200 mg	White	Tablet	Round, Bisected, Scored Scored	Inwood Laboratories
IL; 3607	Indochron	75 mg	Lavender and Clear with White Beads	Extended-Release Capsule		Inwood Laboratories
IL; 3607	Indomethacin	75 mg	Clear and Lavender	Extended-Release Capsule		Inwood Laboratories
IL; 3609	Propranolol Hydrochloride	60 mg	Brown and Clear	Extended-Release Capsule		Novartis Generics
IL; 3610	Betachron	80 mg	Opaque Blue and Clear	Extended-Release Capsule		Inwood Laboratories
IL; 3610	Propranolol Hydrochloride	80 mg	Opaque Blue and Clear	Extended-Release Capsule		Novartis Generics
IL; 3611	Betachron	120 mg	Opaque Blue and Clear	Extended-Release Capsule		Inwood Laboratories
IL; 3611	Propranolol Hydrochloride	120 mg	Opaque Blue and Clear	Extended-Release Capsule		Novartis Generics
IL; 3612	Betachron	160 mg	Opaque Blue and Clear	Extended-Release Capsule		Inwood Laboratories
IL; 3612	Propranolol Hydrochloride	160 mg	Opaque Blue and Clear	Extended-Release Capsule		Novartis Generics
IL; 3613	Isochron	40 mg	Peach	Extended-Release Capsule	Circle, Scored	Forest Pharmaceuticals
IL; 3614; 450	Theophylline Extended Release	450 mg	Off White	Extended-Release Tablet	Capsule-Shape, Scored	Akyma Pharmaceuticals
IL; 3622	Hydrocodone Bitartrate and Acetaminophen	650 mg; 7.5 mg		Tablet		Inwood Laboratories
IL; 3625	Theocap	300 mg	Clear with Off-White Beads	Capsule		Forest Pharmaceuticals
IL; 3625	Theophylline	300 mg	White and Clear	Extended-Release Capsule		Inwood Laboratories
IL; 3625	Theophylline ER	300 mg	White and Clear	Extended-Release Capsule		Qualitest Products
IL; 3634	Theocap	200 mg	Clear and White with Off-White Beads	Capsule		Forest Pharmaceuticals
IL; 3634	Theophylline	200 mg	Clear and Opaque	Extended-Release Capsule		Inwood Laboratories
IL; 3634	Theophylline ER	200 mg	White and Clear	Extended-Release Capsule		Qualitest Products
IL; 3637	Theophylline	100 mg	White and Clear	Extended-Release Capsule		Inwood Laboratories
IL; 3638	Theocap	125 mg	Clear with Off-White Beads	Capsule		Forest Pharmaceuticals
IL; 3638	Theophylline	125 mg	Clear and Clear	Extended-Release Capsule		Inwood Laboratories
IL; 3638	Theophylline ER	125 mg	Clear	Extended-Release Capsule		Qualitest Products
IL; 3657	Acetaminophen, Butalbital and Caffeine	500 mg; 50 mg; 40 mg	White	Tablet	Capsule-Shape, Scored	Inwood Laboratories
IL; 3658	Hydrocodone Bitartrate and Acetaminophen	10 mg; 650 mg	Powder Blue	Tablet	Capsule-Shaped, Bisected Scored	Inwood Laboratories
IMDUR; 60 MG	Imdur	60 mg	Yellow	Sustained-Release Tablet		Key Pharmaceuticals
IMDUR; 120 MG	Imdur	120 mg	White	Sustained-Release Tablet		Key Pharmaceuticals
IMITREX; 50; CHEVRON SHAPE	Imitrex	50 mg	White	Coated Tablet	Triangle	Glaxosmithkline
IMITREX; 100; CHEVRON SHAPE	Imitrex	100 mg	Pink	Coated Tablet	Triangle	Glaxosmithkline
IMODIUM; 2/125	Imodium Advanced	2 mg; 125 mg	Light Green	Tablet, Chewable	Circle, Scored	Mcneil Consumer Products
IMODIUM AD; 2 MG	Imodium A-D Antidiarrheal	2 mg	Pale Green	Tablet		Mcneil Consumer Products
IMODIUM A-D	Imodium A-D	2 mg	Green	Tablet		Mcneil Consumer Products
IMURAN; 50	Imuran	50 mg	Yellow to White	Tablet	Oval, Overlapping, Scored	Faro Pharmaceuticals
INDERAL; 10;	Inderal	10 mg	Orange	Tablet	Six-Sided, Scored	Wyeth Pharmaceuticals
INDERAL; 20	Inderal	20 mg	Blue	Tablet	Six-Sided, Scored	Wyeth Pharmaceuticals
INDERAL; 40;	Inderal	40 mg	Green	Tablet	Six-Sided, Scored	Wyeth Pharmaceuticals
INDERAL; 60; I	Inderal	60 mg	Pink	Tablet	Six-Sided, Scored	Wyeth Pharmaceuticals
INDERAL; 80; I	Inderal	80 mg	Yellow	Tablet	Six-Sided, Scored	Wyeth Pharmaceuticals
INDERAL; 90; I	Inderal	90 mg	Lavender	Tablet	Six-Sided, Scored	Wyeth Pharmaceuticals
INDERAL; LA; 60	Inderal LA	60 mg	White and Light Blue	Capsule		Wyeth Pharmaceuticals
INDERAL; LA; 80	Inderal LA	80 mg	Light Blue	Capsule		Wyeth Pharmaceuticals
INDERAL; LA; 120	Inderal LA	120 mg	Light Blue and Dark Blue	Capsule		Wyeth Pharmaceuticals
INDERAL; LA; 160	Inderal LA	160 mg	Dark Blue	Capsule		Wyeth Pharmaceuticals
INDERIDE; 40/25; I	Inderide	25 mg; 40 mg	Off-White	Tablet	Six-Sided, Scored	Wyeth Pharmaceuticals
INDERIDE; 80/25; I	Inderide	80 mg; 25 mg	Off-White	Tablet	Six-Sided, Scored	Wyeth Pharmaceuticals
INDERIDE LA; 80/50	Inderide LA	80 mg; 50 mg	Beige with 4 Gold Bands	Extended-Release Capsule		Wyeth Pharmaceuticals
INDERIDE LA; 120/50	Inderide LA	120 mg; 50 mg	Beige and Brown with 4 Gold Bands	Extended-Release Capsule		Wyeth Pharmaceuticals
INDERIDE LA; 160/50	Inderide LA	160 mg; 50 mg	Brown with 4 Gold Bands	Extended-Release Capsule		Wyeth Pharmaceuticals
INOR	Plan B	0.75 mg	White	Tablet	Circle	Women's Capital

IMPRINT	BRAND/GENERIC NAME	STRENGTH	COLOR	FORM	SHAPE	MANUFACTURER
INV; 140	Asprimox E/p	325 mg; 75 mg; 75 mg	White	Coated Tablet	Capsule-Shape	Invamed
INV; 208	Benztropine Mesylate	0.5 mg	White	Tablet	Circle, Compressed, Scored	Apothecon
INV; 208	Benztropine Mesylate	0.5 mg	White	Tablet	Circle, Compressed, Scored	Invamed
INV; 258	Iodur	30 mg	White	Tablet	Circle, Scored	Duramed Pharmaceuticals
INV; 260	Methazolamide	50 mg	White	Tablet	Round, Compressed, Bisected Scored	Apothecon
INV; 260	Methazolamide	50 mg	White	Tablet	Round, Compressed, Bisected Scored	Invamed
INV; 261	Methazolamide	25 mg	White	Tablet	Circle, Compressed	Apothecon
INV; 261	Methazolamide	25 mg	White	Tablet	Circle, Compressed	Invamed
INV; 278	Trifluoperazine Hydrochloride	1 mg	Lavender	Coated Tablet	Circle	Apothecon
INV; 278	Trifluoperazine Hydrochloride	1 mg	Lavender	Coated Tablet	Circle	Invamed
INV; 279; 2	Trifluoperazine Hydrochloride	2 mg	Lavender	Coated Tablet	Circle	Apothecon
INV; 279; 2	Trifluoperazine Hydrochloride	2 mg	Lavender	Coated Tablet	Circle	Invamed
INV; 280; 5	Trifluoperazine Hydrochloride	5 mg	Lavender	Coated Tablet	Circle	Apothecon
INV; 280; 5	Trifluoperazine Hydrochloride	5 mg	Lavender	Coated Tablet	Circle	Invamed
INV; 281; 10	Trifluoperazine Hydrochloride	10 mg	Lavender	Coated Tablet	Circle	Apothecon
INV; 281; 10	Trifluoperazine Hydrochloride	10 mg	Lavender	Coated Tablet	Circle	Invamed
INV; 290	Naproxen DR	500 mg	White	21-Day Tablet Pack	Capsule-Shape	Geneva Generics
INV; 309	Warfarin Sodium	1 mg	Pink	Tablet	Square	Geneva Generics
INV; 310; 5	Warfarin Sodium	2 mg	Light Purple	Tablet	Square	Geneva Generics
INV; 311; 2.5	Warfarin Sodium	2.5 mg	Green	Tablet	Square	Geneva Generics
INV; 312; 4	Warfarin Sodium	4 mg	Blue	Tablet	Square	Geneva Generics
INV; 313; 5	Warfarin Sodium	5 mg	Peach	Tablet	Square	Geneva Generics
INV; 314; 7.5	Warfarin Sodium	7.5 mg	Yellow	Tablet	Square	Geneva Generics
INV; 315; 10	Warfarin Sodium	10 mg	White	Tablet	Square	Geneva Generics
INV; 351	Methylprednisolone	4 mg	White	Tablet	Oval,quadrisect Scored	Apothecon
INV; 353	Clonazepam	0.5 mg	Yellow	Tablet	Circle	Apothecon
INV; 354	Clonazepam	1 mg	Green	Tablet	Round, Bisected Scored	Apothecon
INV; 355	Clonazepam	2 mg	White	Tablet	Round, Bisected Scored	Apothecon
INV; 359	Etodolac	200 mg	Grey and White Opaque	Capsule		Apothecon
INV; 359	Etodolac	200 mg	Grey and White Opaque	Capsule		Invamed
INV; 360	Etodolac	300 mg	Grey Opaque	Capsule		Apothecon
INV; 360	Etodolac	300 mg	Grey Opaque	Capsule		Invamed
INV; 375	Ticlopidine Hcl	250 mg	Light Orange	Coated Tablet	Circle	Geneva Generics
INV; 423; 3	Warfarin Sodium	3 mg	Tan	Tablet	Square, Scored	Geneva Generics
INV; 424; 6	Warfarin Sodium	6 mg	Teal	Tablet	Square	Geneva Generics
IONAMIN; 15	Ionamin	15 mg	Yellow and Gray	Capsule		Medeva Pharmaceuticals
IONAMIN; 30	Ionamin	30 mg	Yellow	Capsule		Medeva Pharmaceuticals
IP; 001	Acetaminophen	500 mg	White	Tablet	Circle, Scored	Interpharm
IP; 050	Cold Tablets	325 mg; 30 mg	Pink	Tablet	Circle	Interpharm
IP; 059	Doxycycline Hyclate	58.14 mg	Blue and White	Capsule		Interpharm
IP; 060	Doxycycline Hyclate	116.28 mg	Blue	Capsule		Interpharm
IP; 061	Doxycycline Hyclate	100 mg	Tan	Coated Tablet	Circle	Interpharm
IP; 26	Acetaminophen and Diphenhydramine Hydrochloride	500 mg; 25 mg	Blue	Tablet	Capsule-Shape	Interpharm
IP; 45	Clonidine Hydrochloride	0.1 mg	Light Green	Tablet	Circle, Scored	Interpharm
IP; 46	Clonidine Hydrochloride	0.2 mg	Yellow	Tablet	Circle, Scored	Interpharm
IP; 47	Clonidine Hydrochloride	0.3 mg	Blue	Tablet	Circle, Scored	Interpharm
IP; 62	Disopyramide Phosphate	150 mg	Scarlet and Buff	Capsule		Interpharm
IP; 63	Disopyramide Phosphate	100 mg	Scarlet and Blue	Capsule		Interpharm
IP; 131; 400	Ibuprofen	400 mg	White	Tablet	Circle, Convex	Akyma Pharmaceuticals
IP; 131; 400	Ibuprofen	400 mg	White	Tablet	Circle, Debossed	Interpharm
IP131; 400	Ibuprofen	400 mg	White	Coated Tablet	Circle	Qualitest Products
IP; 132; 600	Ibuprofen	600 mg	White	Tablet	Oval	Akyma Pharmaceuticals
IP; 132; 600	Ibuprofen	600 mg	White	Tablet	Oval	Interpharm
IP132; 600	Ibuprofen	600 mg	White	Coated Tablet	Oval	Qualitest Products
IP; 135	Ibuprofen	200 mg	White	Tablet	Circle	Interpharm
IP; 136	Migrend	325 mg; 100 mg; 65 mg	Red and White	Capsule		Econolab
IP; 137; 800	Ibuprofen	800 mg	White	Tablet	Capsule-Shape	Akyma Pharmaceuticals
IP; 137; 800	Ibuprofen	800 mg	White	Tablet	Capsule-Shape	Interpharm
IP137; 800	Ibuprofen	800 mg	White	Coated Tablet	Oval	Qualitest Products
IP; 138	Ibuprofen	200 mg	White	Tablet		Interpharm
IP; 141	Migquin	65 mg; 100 mg; 325 mg	Red	Capsule		Qualitest Products
IP; 141	Migrazone	325 mg; 65 mg; 100 mg	Red or White and Red	Capsule		Interpharm
IP; 142	Ibuprofen	200 mg	Brown	Coated Tablet	Capsule-Shape	Interpharm
IP 146	Reprexain	5 mg; 200 mg	White	Tablet	Oval	Watson Laboratories
IP; 175	Metoclopramide Hydrochloride	10 mg	White	Tablet	Oblong, Notched	Interpharm
IP; 188; 250	Naproxen	250 mg	White	Tablet	Circle, Biconvex	Akyma Pharmaceuticals
IP; 188; 250	Naproxen	250 mg	White	Tablet	Circle	Interpharm
IP; 189; 375	Naproxen	375 mg	White	Tablet	Capsule-Shape, Biconvex	Akyma Pharmaceuticals
IP; 189; 375	Naproxen	375 mg	White	Tablet	Capsule-Shape	Interpharm
IP; 190; 500	Naproxen	500 mg	White	Tablet	Capsule-Shape, Biconvex	Akyma Pharmaceuticals
IP; 190; 500	Naproxen	500 mg	White	Tablet	Capsule-Shape	Interpharm
IP; 217	Propranolol Hydrochloride	20 mg	Blue	Tablet	Circle, Scored	Interpharm
IP; 218	Propranolol Hydrochloride	10 mg	Peach	Tablet	Circle, Scored	Interpharm
IP; 219	Propranolol Hydrochloride	40 mg	Green	Tablet	Circle, Scored	Interpharm
IP; 220	Propranolol Hydrochloride	80 mg	Yellow	Tablet	Circle, Scored	Interpharm
IP; 229	Prednisone	5 mg	White	Tablet	Circle, Scored	Interpharm
IP; 230	Prednisone	10 mg	White	Tablet	Circle, Scored	Interpharm
IP; 231	Prednisone	20 mg	Peach	Tablet	Circle, Scored	Interpharm
IP; 271	Sulfamethoxazole and Trimethoprim Single Strength	400 mg; 80 mg	White	Tablet	Circle, Compressed, Scored	Interpharm
IP; 272	Sulfamethoxazole and Trimethoprim Double Strength	800 mg; 160 mg	White	Tablet	Capsule-Shape, Scored	Interpharm

IMPRINT	BRAND/GENERIC NAME	STRENGTH	COLOR	FORM	SHAPE	MANUFACTURER
IP; 286	Tolazamide	250 mg	White	Tablet	Circle, Scored	Interpharm
IP; 287	Tolazamide	500 mg	White	Tablet	Circle, Scored	Interpharm
IRCON;	Ircon	200 mg		Tablet		Key Pharmaceuticals
ISMO; 20	Ismo	20 mg	Orange	Coated Tablet	Circle, Scored	Wyeth Pharmaceuticals
ISOPTIN SR; 180 MG	Isoptin SR	180 mg	Light Pink	Sustained-Release Tablet	Oval, Scored	Knoll Laboratories
ISOPTIN SR/TWO KNOLL TRIANGLES	Isoptin SR	240 mg	Light Green	Sustained-Release Tablet	Capsule-Shape, Scored	Knoll Laboratories
IT; L3	Boniva	2.5 mg	White	Tablet	Oblong	Glaxosmithkline
IT; L3	Boniva	2.5 mg	White	Tablet	Oblong	Roche Laboratories
J05	Caffeine, Citrated	65 mg		Tablet		Eli Lilly
J; 19	Potassium Permanganate	300 mg		Tablet		Eli Lilly
J; 37	Phenobarbital	60 mg	White	Tablet	Circle	Eli Lilly
J75;	Isuprel	10 mg	White	Tablet		Sanofi Winthrop Pharmaceuticals
J77;	Isuprel	15 mg	White	Tablet		Sanofi Winthrop Pharmaceuticals
J; 94	Tapazole	5 mg	White	Tablet	Circle, Scored	Jones Pharma
J; 95	Tapazole	10 mg	White	Tablet	Circle, Scored	Jones Pharma
JACOBUS; 101; 100	Dapsone	100 mg	White	Tablet		Jacobus Pharmaceutical
JACOBUS; 102; 25	Dapsone	25 mg	White	Tablet		Jacobus Pharmaceutical
JANSSEN; AST; 10	Hismanal	10 mg	White	Tablet		Janssen Pharmaceutica
JANSSEN; CIS; 10	Prepulsid	10 mg		Tablet		Janssen Pharmaceutica
JANSSEN; G; 4	Reminyl	4 mg	Off-White	Coated Tablet	Circle, Biconvex	Janssen Pharmaceutica
JANSSEN; G; 8	Reminyl	8 mg	Pink	Coated Tablet	Circle, Biconvex, Scored	Janssen Pharmaceutica
JANSSEN; G; 12	Reminyl	12 mg	Orange-Brown	Coated Tablet	Circle, Biconvex	Janssen Pharmaceutica
JANSSEN; IMODIUM	Imodium	2 mg	Light Green and Dark Green	Capsule		Mcneil Consumer Products
JANSSEN; L; 50	Ergamisol	50 mg	White	Coated Tablet		Janssen Pharmaceutica
JANSSEN; NIZORAL	Nizoral	200 mg	White	Tablet		Janssen Pharmaceutica
JANSSEN; P; 10	Propulsid	10 mg	White	Tablet	Circle, Small, Scored	Janssen Pharmaceutica
JANSSEN; P; 20	Propulsid	20 mg	Blue	Tablet	Oval	Janssen Pharmaceutica
JANSSEN; R; 1	Risperdal	1 mg	White	Tablet		Janssen Pharmaceutica
JANSSEN; R; 2	Risperdal	2 mg	Orange	Tablet		Janssen Pharmaceutica
JANSSEN; R; 3	Risperdal	3 mg	Yellow	Tablet		Janssen Pharmaceutica
JANSSEN; R; 4	Risperdal	4 mg	Green	Tablet		Janssen Pharmaceutica
JANSSEN RIS 0.25	Risperdal	0.25 mg	Dark Yellow	Tablet		Janssen Pharmaceutica
JANSSEN RIS 0.5	Risperdal	0.5 mg	Red-Brown	Tablet		Janssen Pharmaceutica
JANSSEN; SPORANOX; 100	Sporanox	100 mg	Blue and Pink	Capsule		Janssen Pharmaceutica
JANSSEN; VERMOX	Vermox	100 mg	Orange	Tablet, Chewable		Mcneil Consumer Products
JMI; 626	Thyroid Strong 0.5 grain	0.75 Gr	Orange or Reddish Brown	Coated Tablet		Western Research Laboratories
JMI; 627	Thyroid Strong 1 grain	1.5 Gr	Orange or Reddish Brown	Coated Tablet		Western Research Laboratories
JMI; 628	Thyroid Strong 2 grains	3 Gr	Red or Reddish Brown	Coated Tablet		Western Research Laboratories
JMI; 629	Thyroid Strong 3 grains	4.5 Gr	Red or Reddish Brown	Coated Tablet		Western Research Laboratories
JMI; 674	Thyroid Strong 1 grain Natural	1.5 Gr	Tan	Tablet	Compressed	Western Research Laboratories
JMI; 675	Thyroid Strong 2 grains Natural	3 Gr	Tan	Tablet	Compressed	Western Research Laboratories
JMI; 686	Thyroid Strong 0.5 grain Natural	0.75 Gr	Tan	Tablet	Compressed	Western Research Laboratories
JMI; APT	Thyroid with Pituitary	194.4 mg;	Lemon Yellow	Coated Tablet	Circle	Western Research Laboratories
JMI; D16	Cytomel	25 mcg	White	Tablet	Circle	Jones Pharma
JMI; D17	Cytomel	50 mcg		Tablet		Jones Medical
JPS; 515	Levotabs	75 mcg	Lavender	Tablet	Circle	Pecos Pharmaceutical
JSP; 490	Methocarbamol and Aspirin	400 mg; 325 mg	Pink and White	Tablet	Circle, Bilayered, Compressed	Jerome Stevens Pharmaceuticals
JSP; 507	Aspirin, Butalbital, Caffeine and Codeine	325 mg; 50 mg; 40 mg; 30 mg	Yellow and Blue	Capsule		Duramed Pharmaceuticals
JSP; 507	Aspirin, Butalbital, Caffeine and Codeine	325 mg; 50 mg; 40 mg; 30 mg	Yellow and Blue	Capsule		Jerome Stevens Pharmaceuticals
JSP; 508	Acetaminophen/isometheptene Mucate/dichloralphenazone	325 mg; 100 mg; 65 mg	Red and White	Capsule		Jerome Stevens Pharmaceuticals
JSP; 508	Migraine	65 mg; 100 mg; 325 mg	Red and White	Capsule		Jerome Stevens Pharmaceuticals
JSP; 510	Decongestant S.R.	8 mg; 120 mg	Blue and White	Sustained-Release Capsule		Pecos Pharmaceutical
JSP; 510	Decongestant SR	8 mg; 120 mg	Blue and Clear	Sustained-Release Capsule		Jerome Stevens Pharmaceuticals
JSP; 513	Levotabs	25 mcg	Peach	Tablet	Circle	Pecos Pharmaceutical
JSP; 513	Levothyroxine Sodium	25 mcg	Peach	Tablet	Circle	Jerome Stevens Pharmaceuticals
JSP; 513	Unithroid	25 mcg	Peach	Tablet	Round, Partially Bisected Scored	Jerome Stevens Pharmaceuticals
JSP; 513	Unithroid	25 mcg	Peach	Tablet	Round, Partially Bisected Scored	Watson Laboratories
JSP; 514	Levotabs	50 mcg	White	Tablet	Circle	Pecos Pharmaceutical
JSP; 514	Levothyroxine Sodium	50 mcg	White	Tablet	Circle	Jerome Stevens Pharmaceuticals
JSP; 514	Unithroid	50 mcg	White	Tablet	Round, Partially Bisected Scored	Jerome Stevens Pharmaceuticals
JSP; 514	Unithroid	50 mcg	White	Tablet	Round, Partially Bisected Scored	Watson Laboratories
JSP; 515	Levothyroxine Sodium	75 mcg	Light Purple	Tablet	Circle	Jerome Stevens Pharmaceuticals
JSP; 515	Unithroid	75 mcg	Purple	Tablet	Round, Partially Bisected Scored	Jerome Stevens Pharmaceuticals
JSP; 515	Unithroid	75 mcg	Purple	Tablet	Round, Partially Bisected Scored	Watson Laboratories
JSP; 516	Levotabs	100 mcg	Yellow	Tablet	Circle	Pecos Pharmaceutical

IMPRINT	BRAND/GENERIC NAME	STRENGTH	COLOR	FORM	SHAPE	MANUFACTURER
JSP; 516	Levothyroxine Sodium	0.1 mg	Yellow	Tablet	Round, Compressed, Bisected Scored	Jerome Stevens Pharmaceuticals
JSP; 516	Unithroid	100 mcg	Yellow	Tablet	Round, Partially Bisected Scored	Jerome Stevens Pharmaceuticals
JSP; 516	Unithroid	100 mcg	Yellow	Tablet	Round, Partially Bisected Scored	Watson Laboratories
JSP; 519	Levotabs	125 mcg	Tan	Tablet	Circle	Pecos Pharmaceutical
JSP; 519	Levothyroxine Sodium	125 mcg	Tan	Tablet	Circle	Jerome Stevens Pharmaceuticals
JSP; 519	Unithroid	125 mcg	Tan	Tablet	Round, Partially Bisected Scored	Jerome Stevens Pharmaceuticals
JSP; 519	Unithroid	125 mcg	Tan	Tablet	Round, Partially Bisected Scored	Watson Laboratories
JSP; 520	Levotabs	150 mcg	Light Blue	Tablet	Circle	Pecos Pharmaceutical
JSP; 520	Levothyroxine Sodium	0.15 mg	Blue	Tablet	Round, Compressed, Bisected Scored	Jerome Stevens Pharmaceuticals
JSP; 520	Unithroid	150 mcg	Blue	Tablet	Round, Partially Bisected Scored	Jerome Stevens Pharmaceuticals
JSP; 520	Unithroid	150 mcg	Blue	Tablet	Round, Partially Bisected Scored	Watson Laboratories
JSP; 522	Levotabs	200 mcg	Pink	Tablet	Circle	Pecos Pharmaceutical
JSP; 522	Levothyroxine Sodium	200 mcg	Pink	Tablet	Circle	Jerome Stevens Pharmaceuticals
JSP; 522	Unithroid	200 mcg	Pink	Tablet	Round, Partially Bisected Scored	Jerome Stevens Pharmaceuticals
JSP; 522	Unithroid	200 mcg	Pink	Tablet	Round, Partially Bisected Scored	Watson Laboratories
JSP; 523	Levotabs	300 mcg	Green	Tablet	Circle	Pecos Pharmaceutical
JSP; 523	Levothyroxine Sodium	300 mcg	Light Green	Tablet	Circle	Jerome Stevens Pharmaceuticals
JSP; 523	Unithroid	300 mcg	Green	Tablet	Round, Partially Bisected Scored	Jerome Stevens Pharmaceuticals
JSP; 523	Unithroid	300 mcg	Green	Tablet	Round, Partially Bisected Scored	Watson Laboratories
JSP; 526	B-Fedrine PD	6 mg; 60 mg	Green and White	Timed-Release Capsule		Pecos Pharmaceutical
JSP; 526	Nasal Decongestant PD	6 mg; 60 mg	Dark Green and Clear with White Beads	Timed-Release Capsule		Jerome Stevens Pharmaceuticals
JSP; 527	B-Fedrine	12 mg; 120 mg	Light Green and White	Timed-Release Capsule		Pecos Pharmaceutical
JSP; 527	Nasal Decongestant	12 mg; 120 mg	Light Green and Clear with White Beads	Timed-Release Capsule		Jerome Stevens Pharmaceuticals
JSP; 533	Isosorbide 40 mg S.R.	40 mg	Peach	Tablet	Circle	Pecos Pharmaceutical
JSP; 533	Isosorbide Dinitrate	40 mg	Peach	Tablet		Jerome Stevens Pharmaceuticals
JSP; 544	Digoxin	0.125 mg	White	Tablet	Circle	Jerome Stevens Pharmaceuticals
JSP; 545	Digoxin	0.25 mg	White	Tablet	Circle	Jerome Stevens Pharmaceuticals
JSP; 548	Guaifenesin L.A.	600 mg	Green	Sustained-Release Tablet	Capsule-Shaped, Bisected Scored	Rugby Laboratories
JSP; 553	Codeine Phosphate Guaifenesin	10 mg; 300 mg	Red	Tablet	Capsule-Shape	Pecos Pharmaceutical
JSP; 553	Codeine Phosphate Guaifenesin	10 mg; 300 mg	Red	Tablet	Capsule-Shape	Rugby Laboratories
JSP; 561	Levothyroxine Sodium	88 mcg	Olive Green	Tablet	Circle	Jerome Stevens Pharmaceuticals
JSP; 561	Unithroid	88 mcg	Olive	Tablet	Round, Partially Bisected Scored	Jerome Stevens Pharmaceuticals
JSP; 561	Unithroid	88 mcg	Olive	Tablet	Round, Partially Bisected Scored	Watson Laboratories
JSP; 562	Levothyroxine Sodium	112 mcg	Rose	Tablet	Circle	Jerome Stevens Pharmaceuticals
JSP; 562	Unithroid	112 mcg	Rose	Tablet	Round, Partially Bisected Scored	Jerome Stevens Pharmaceuticals
JSP; 562	Unithroid	112 mcg	Rose	Tablet	Round, Partially Bisected Scored	Watson Laboratories
JSP; 563	Levothyroxine Sodium	175 mcg	Lilac	Tablet	Circle	Jerome Stevens Pharmaceuticals
JSP; 563	Unithroid	175 mcg	Lilac	Tablet	Round, Partially Bisected Scored	Jerome Stevens Pharmaceuticals
JSP; 563	Unithroid	175 mcg	Lilac	Tablet	Round, Partially Bisected Scored	Watson Laboratories
JSP; 873	Thyrox	25 mcg	Peach	Tablet		Watson Laboratories
JSP; 874	Thyrox	50 mcg	White	Tablet		Watson Laboratories
JSP; 875	Thyrox	75 mcg	Purple	Tablet		Watson Laboratories
JSP; 876	Thyrox	88 mcg	Olive	Tablet		Watson Laboratories
JSP; 877	Thyrox	100 mcg	Yellow	Tablet		Watson Laboratories
JSP; 878	Thyrox	112 mcg	Rose	Tablet		Watson Laboratories
JSP; 879	Thyrox	125 mcg	Tan	Tablet		Watson Laboratories
JSP; 880	Thyrox	150 mcg	Blue	Tablet		Watson Laboratories
JSP; 881	Thyrox	175 mcg	Lilac	Tablet		Watson Laboratories
JSP; 882	Thyrox	200 mcg	Pink	Tablet		Watson Laboratories
JSP; 883	Thyrox	300 mcg	Green	Tablet		Watson Laboratories
K	Aspirin	81 mg	Yellow	Enteric-Coated Tablet	Circle, Convex	Pdk Labs
K	Aspirin	81 mg	Yellow	Tablet	Circle	Rugby Laboratories
K	Aspirin	325 mg	Orange	Enteric-Coated Tablet	Circle, Convex	Pdk Labs
K	Aspirin	325 mg	Orange	Tablet, Enteric Coated		Rugby Laboratories
K	Potassium Chloride	25 meq	Orange	Extended-Release Tablet	Circle	Qualitest Products
K+8; ALRA;	K+8	8 meq	Orange	Sustained-Release Tablet		Alra Laboratories
K+10; ALRA;	K+10	10 meq	Yellow	Sustained-Release Tablet	Capsule-Shape	Alra Laboratories
K; 0659	Ergoloid Mesylates	0.333 mg; 0.333 mg; 0.333 mg	White	Tablet	Oval	KV Pharmaceutical
K; 0675; 2	Acetaminophen and Codeine Phosphate	325 mg; 15 mg	White	Tablet		KV Pharmaceutical
K; 0678	Acetaminophen and Codeine Phosphate	325 mg; 45 mg	White	Tablet		KV Pharmaceutical

IMPRINT	BRAND/GENERIC NAME	STRENGTH	COLOR	FORM	SHAPE	MANUFACTURER
K; 0679; 4	Acetaminophen and Codeine Phosphate	300 mg; 60 mg	White	Tablet		KV Pharmaceutical
K; 0712	Ergoloid Mesylates	0.167 mg; 0.167 mg; 0.167 mg	White	Tablet	Circle	KV Pharmaceutical
K; 0;	Apap 325 mg Pain/fever	325 mg	White	Tablet	Circle	Rugby Laboratories
K; 0	Pain Reliever	325 mg	White	Tablet	Circle, Flat-Faced, Bevel-Edged	Pdk Labs
K1	Kytril	1 mg	White	Coated Tablet	Triangle, Biconvex	Roche Laboratories
K; 6	Diphenhydramine Hydrochloride	50 mg	Blue	Tablet	Circle, Biconvex, Scored	Pdk Labs
K; 6	Diphenhydramine Hydrochloride	50 mg	Blue	Tablet	Circle	Rugby Laboratories
K; 10;	Apap 500 mg Pain/fever X-Str	500 mg	White	Tablet	Capsule-Shape	Rugby Laboratories
K; 10;	Apap 500 mg Pain/fever X-Str	500 mg	White	Tablet	Circle	Rugby Laboratories
K; 10	Hydroxyzine Hydrochloride	10 mg	Beige	Tablet	Circle	KV Pharmaceutical
K; 10	Pain Reliever Extra Strength	500 mg	White	Tablet	Circle, Flat-Faced, Bevel-Edged	Pdk Labs
K; 17	Multi-Symptom Cold	325 mg; 30 mg; 10 mg	White	Tablet	Circle	Pdk Labs
K; 25	Hydroxyzine Hydrochloride	25 mg	Green	Tablet	Circle	KV Pharmaceutical
K; 27	Pseudoephedrine	60 mg	White	Tablet	Round, Quadrisected Scored	Pdk Labs
K; 28	Aspirin Children's	81 mg	Orange	Tablet, Chewable	Circle, Convex, Scored	Pdk Labs
K; 28	Aspirin Children's	81 mg	Orange	Tablet, Chewable		Rugby Laboratories
K; 30	Codeine Sulfate	30 mg	White	Tablet	Circle	Knoll Pharmaceutical
K; 30	Non-Aspirin Pain Reliever Children's Fruit Flavor	80 mg	Light Pink	Tablet, Chewable	Circle, Flat-Faced, Bevel-Edged, Scored	Pdk Labs
K; 30	Non-Aspirin Pain Reliever Children's Grape Flavor	80 mg	Purple	Tablet, Chewable	Circle, Flat-Faced, Bevel-Edged, Scored	Pdk Labs
K; 48	Aspirin Tri-Buffered	325 mg	White	Tablet	Circle, Convex	Pdk Labs
K48; ASPIRIN	Aspirin	325 mg	White	Tablet	Circle, Convex	Pdk Labs
K; 50	Hydroxyzine Hydrochloride	50 mg	Brown	Tablet	Circle	KV Pharmaceutical
K; 56	Acetaminophen, Aspirin, and Caffeine	250 mg; 250 mg; 65 mg	White	Tablet	Circle	Pdk Labs
K 60	Codeine Sulfate	60 mg	White	Tablet	Circle, Tablet	Knoll Laboratories
K; 100	Hydroxyzine Hydrochloride	100 mg	Pink	Tablet	Circle	KV Pharmaceutical
K; 102	Bisacodyl Laxative	5 mg	Orange	Enteric-Coated Tablet	Circle, Convex	Pdk Labs
K; 102	Laxative	5 mg	Orange	Tablet	Circle	Rugby Laboratories
K; 105	Senna Lax	8.6 mg	Brown	Tablet	Circle	Qualitest Products
K; 106	Docusate Sodium and Senna	50 mg; 8.6 mg	Red	Tablet	Circle	Rugby Laboratories
K; 115	Diphenhist	25 mg	Clear and Pink	Capsule		Rugby Laboratories
K; 115	Diphenhydramine	25 mg	Pink	Tablet	Oval	Pdk Labs
K; 117	Cold Relief Multi-Symptom	500 mg; 2 mg; 15 mg; 30 mg	Yellow	Tablet	Circle	Pdk Labs
K; 130	Pse and Cpm	60 mg; 4 mg	White	Tablet	Circle, Scored	Pdk Labs
K; 200	Dimenhydrinate	50 mg	White	Tablet	Circle	Qualitest Products
K; 398	Meclizine Hydrochloride	12.5 mg	White	Tablet	Capsule-Shape	Pdk Labs
K; 399	Meclizine Hydrochloride	25 mg	Light Maroon Red	Tablet, Chewable	Circle, Convex, Scored	Pdk Labs
K; 399	Meclizine Hydrochloride	25 mg	Yellow	Tablet	Circle, Flat-Faced, Bevel-Edged	Pdk Labs
K; 490	Chlorpromazine Hydrochloride	200 mg	Tan	Tablet	Circle	KV Pharmaceutical
K; 491	Chlorpromazine Hydrochloride	25 mg	Tan	Tablet	Circle	KV Pharmaceutical
K; 492	Chlorpromazine Hydrochloride	10 mg	Tan	Tablet	Circle	KV Pharmaceutical
K; 493	Chlorpromazine Hydrochloride	50 mg	Tan	Tablet	Circle	KV Pharmaceutical
K; 494	Chlorpromazine Hydrochloride	100 mg	Tan	Coated Tablet		KV Pharmaceutical
K; 634	Nitroglycerin	2.5 mg	Lavender	Extended-Release Capsule	Triangle	KV Pharmaceutical
K; 635	Nitroglycerin	6.5 mg	Blue	Extended-Release Capsule	Triangle	KV Pharmaceutical
K; 676; 3	Acetaminophen and Codeine Phosphate	300 mg; 30 mg	White	Tablet		KV Pharmaceutical
K; 698	Nitroglycerin	9 mg		Extended-Release Tablet	Triangle	KV Pharmaceutical
K; 699	Nitroglycerin	13 mg		Extended-Release Tablet	Triangle	KV Pharmaceutical
K; 789	Quinidine Sulfate	200 mg	White	Tablet	Circle	KV Pharmaceutical
K; 804	Chlorthalidone	25 mg	Orange	Tablet		KV Pharmaceutical
K; 805	Chlorthalidone	50 mg	Blue	Tablet		KV Pharmaceutical
K; 887	Meclizine Hydrochloride	12.5 mg	Blue	Tablet	Oval	KV Pharmaceutical
K; 888	Meclizine Hydrochloride	25 mg	Yellow	Tablet	Oval	KV Pharmaceutical
K; 896	Diphenoxylate Hydrochloride and Atropine Sulfate	2.5 mg; 0.025 mg	White	Tablet	Circle	KV Pharmaceutical
K; ARROW;	Aspirin	325 mg	Orange	Enteric-Coated Tablet	Circle, Scored	Watson Laboratories
K; U	Levsin Forte	0.25 mg	White	Tablet		Schwarz Pharma
KADIAN; 20 MG	Kadian	20 mg	Yellow	Sustained-Release Capsule		Purepac Pharmaceutical
KADIAN; 30 MG	Kadian	30 mg	Blue-Violet	Sustained-Release Capsule		Purepac Pharmaceutical
KADIAN; 50 MG	Kadian	50 mg	Blue	Sustained-Release Capsule		Purepac Pharmaceutical
KADIAN; 60 MG	Kadian	60 mg	Pink	Sustained-Release Capsule		Purepac Pharmaceutical
KADIAN; 100 MG	Kadian	100 mg	Green	Sustained-Release Capsule		Purepac Pharmaceutical
KALI; 280	Citalopram Hydrobromide	10 mg	Beige	Tablet	Circle	Perrigo
KALI; 281	Citalopram Hydrobromide	20 mg	Pink	Tablet	Circle	Perrigo
KALI; 282	Citalopram Hydrobromide	40 mg	White	Tablet	Circle	Perrigo
KC; M10	Klor-Con M10	10 meq	White	Extended-Release Tablet	Oblong	Upsher-Smith Laboratories
KC; M20	Klor-Con M20	20 meq	White	Extended-Release Tablet	Oblong, Scored	Upsher-Smith Laboratories
KC; M20	Klor-Con M20	1500 mg	White	Tablet	Oblong	Upsher-Smith Laboratories
K-DUR; 10;	K-Dur	750 mg	White	Sustained-Release Tablet	Oblong	Key Pharmaceuticals
K-DUR; 20;	K-Dur	1500 mg	White	Sustained-Release Tablet	Oblong, Scored	Key Pharmaceuticals
KEFLET; 250	Keflet	250 mg	Light Blue-Green	Tablet	Capsule-Shape	Dista Products
KEFLET; 500	Keflet	500 mg	Dark Green	Tablet	Capsule-Shape	Dista Products
KEFTAB; 500	Keftab	500 mg	Dark Green	Tablet	Circle	Biovail Pharmaceuticals

IMPRINT	BRAND/GENERIC NAME	STRENGTH	COLOR	FORM	SHAPE	MANUFACTURER
KEMADRIN; S3A	Kemadrin	5 mg	White	Tablet		Glaxosmithkline
KENWOOD; 181	Deconamine SR	8 mg; 120 mg	Blue and Yellow	Capsule		Kenwood Laboratories
KENWOOD; 184	Deconamine	60 mg; 4 mg	White	Tablet	Circle, Scored	Kenwood Laboratories
KERLONE; 10	Kerlone	10 mg	White	Coated Tablet	Circle, Scored	Searle
KERLONE; 20; B	Kerlone	20 mg	White	Coated Tablet	Circle	Searle
KG	Keep Going-Alertness Aid, Maximum Strength	200 mg	White	Tablet	Oval	Block Drug
KL; 142	R-Tanna	25 mg; 9 mg	Mottled Tan	Tablet	Capsule-Shape	Prasco Laboratories
KL; 161	K-Tan 4	25 mg; 60 mg	Tan	Tablet	Oval, Scored	Prasco Laboratories
KLOR-CON; 8	Klor-Con 8	600 mg	Blue	Coated Tablet	Circle, Bevel-Edged	Upsher-Smith Laboratories
KLOR-CON 10	Klor-Con 10	750 mg	Yellow	Coated Tablet	Circle, Bevel-Edged	Upsher-Smith Laboratories
KLOTRIX; BL; 10MEQ; 770	Klotrix	750 mg	Orange	Timed-Release Tablet	Circle	Bristol-Myers Squibb
KNOLL; 120SR	Isoptin SR	120 mg	Light Violet	Sustained-Release Tablet	Oval	Knoll Laboratories
KNOLL; ISOPTIN; 80	Isoptin	80 mg	Yellow	Coated Tablet	Circle, Scored	Knoll Laboratories
KNOLL; ISOPTIN; 120	Isoptin	120 mg	White	Coated Tablet		Knoll Laboratories
K-NORM; 10	K-Norm	10 meq	Clear with White Granules	Extended-Release Capsule		Medeva Pharmaceuticals
KO	Gentle Comfort	325 mg	White	Tablet	Circle	Pdk Labs
KOS; 500	Niaspan	500 mg	Off-White	Extended-Release Tablet	Capsule-Shape	Kos Pharmaceuticals
KOS; 750	Niaspan	750 mg	Off-White	Extended-Release Tablet	Capsule-Shape	Kos Pharmaceuticals
KOS; 1000	Niaspan	1000 mg	Off-White	Extended-Release Tablet	Capsule-Shape	Kos Pharmaceuticals
KPH; 102	Azulfidine En-Tabs	500 mg	Gold	Enteric-Coated Tablet	Oval	Pharmacia & Upjohn
KPI; 1	Acetaminophen and Hydrocodone Bitartrate	500 mg; 5 mg		Tablet		King Pharmaceuticals
KPI; 2	Acetaminophen and Hydrocodone Bitartrate	750 mg; 7.5 mg	Light Blue	Tablet	Circle	King Pharmaceuticals
KREM	Krem	400 mg; 200 mg		Tablet, Chewable		Wallace Laboratories
KREMERS URBAN; 320	Nitrocine Timecaps	2.5 mg	Violet and Clear	Sustained-Release Capsule		Schwarz Pharma
KREMERS URBAN; 330	Nitrocine Timecaps	6.5 mg	Blue and Orange	Sustained-Release Capsule		Schwarz Pharma
KREMERS URBAN; 340	Nitrocine Timecaps	9 mg	Clear	Sustained-Release Capsule		Schwarz Pharma
KU; 101	Hyoscyamine Sulfate	0.125 mg	White	Tablet	Circle, Scored	Kremers Urban
KU; 102	Hyoscyamine Sulfate	0.125 mg	White	Tablet	Circle, Flat, Bevel Edged, Scored	Kremers Urban
KU; 103	Hyoscyamine Sulfate	0.375 mg	Brown and White	Extended-Release Capsule		Kremers Urban
KU; 106; 10	Isosorbide Mononitrate	10 mg	White	Tablet	Circle, Scored	Kremers Urban
KU; 107; 20	Isosorbide Mononitrate	20 mg	White	Tablet	Circle, Scored	Kremers Urban
KU; 108	Hyoscyamine Sulfate	0.375 mg	Light Orange	Extended-Release Tablet	Capsule-Shape, Scored	Kremers Urban
KU; 114	Omeprazole	10 mg	White	Delayed-Release Capsule		Kremers Urban
KU; 114	Omeprazole	10 mg	White	Delayed-Release Capsule		Schwarz Pharma
KU; 118	Omeprazole	20 mg	White and Gold	Delayed-Release Capsule		Kremers Urban
KU; 118	Omeprazole	20 mg	White and Gold	Delayed-Release Capsule		Schwarz Pharma
KU; 119	Isosorbide Mononitrate	60 mg	White	Extended-Release Tablet	Capsule-Shape, Scored	Kremers Urban
KU; 128	Isosorbide Mononitrate	30 mg	White	Extended-Release Tablet	Capsule-Shape, Scored	Kremers Urban
KU; 129	Isosorbide Mononitrate	120 mg	White	Extended-Release Tablet	Capsule-Shape	Kremers Urban
KV; 680	Prednisone	5 mg	White	Tablet		KV Pharmaceutical
KV DISO; 12/100	Disopyramide Phosphate	100 mg	Purple and Yellow	Extended-Release Capsule		KV Pharmaceutical
KV DISO; 12/150	Disopyramide Phosphate	150 mg	Purple and Yellow	Extended-Release Capsule		KV Pharmaceutical
L	Oridol	30 mg	Orange	Tablet	Circle	Norton, H.N.
L; 010	Acetaminophen	325 mg	White to Off-White	Tablet	Compressed, Round, Flat-Flace, Beveled Edge, Bisected Scored	Leiner Health Products
L; 011	Ibuprofen Ib	100 mg	White	Tablet		Sunmark
L; 011	Junior Strength Ibuprofen Ages 6 to 11	100 mg	White	Tablet		Good Sense
L; 011	Junior Strength Ibuprofen Ages 6 to 11	100 mg	White	Tablet		Valu Rite
L011	Pain Reliever, Adult Strength	400 mg; 32 mg	White to Off-White	Coated Tablet	Circle, Convex	Leiner Health Products
L; 014;	Acetaminophen	500 mg	White to Off-White	Tablet		Leiner Health Products
L; 015	Multi-Symptom Pain Relief Cold Non-Drowsy	325 mg; 15 mg; 200 mg; 30 mg	Yellow	Tablet		Top Care
L; 015	Non-Aspirin Cold Multi-Symptom Severe Congestion	30 mg; 15 mg; 325 mg; 200 mg	Yellow	Tablet		Good Sense
L; 015	Non-Aspirin Cold Multi-Symptom Severe Congestion	30 mg; 15 mg; 325 mg; 200 mg	Yellow	Tablet		Valu Rite
L; 015	Pain Reliever Cold Multi-Symptom	325 mg; 15 mg; 200 mg; 30 mg	Yellow	Tablet		Sunmark
L; 015;	Triprolidine & Pseudoephedrine Hydrochloride	60 mg; 2.5 mg	White	Tablet	Round, Compressed, Convex, Bisected Scored	Leiner Health Products
L; 016;	Acetaminophen	500 mg	White to Off-White	Tablet	Circle, Compressed, Flat Face, Beveled Edge	Leiner Health Products
L; 017	Mapap Sinus Maximum Strength	30 mg; 500 mg	White and Green	Geltab		Major
L; 017	Maximum Strength Non-Aspirin Sinus	30 mg; 500 mg	White and Green	Geltab		Valu Rite
L; 017	Pain Reliever Sinus Maximum Strength	500 mg; 30 mg	White and Green	Geltab		Genovese
L; 017	Pain Reliever Sinus Maximum Strength	500 mg; 30 mg	White and Green	Geltab		Major

IMPRINT	BRAND/GENERIC NAME	STRENGTH	COLOR	FORM	SHAPE	MANUFACTURER
L; 017	Pain Reliever Sinus Maximum Strength	500 mg; 30 mg	White and Green	Geltab		Perfect Choice
L; 017	Pain Reliever Sinus Maximum Strength	500 mg; 30 mg	White and Green	Geltab		Pharm X
L; 017	Pain Reliever Sinus Maximum Strength	500 mg; 30 mg	White and Green	Geltab		Sunmark
L; 017	Pain Reliever Sinus Maximum Strength	500 mg; 30 mg	White and Green	Geltab		Top Care
L; 017;	Acetaminophen Fruit Flavor	80 mg	Mottled Pink	Tablet, Chewable	Round, Flat Face, Beveled Edge, Bisected Scored	Leiner Health Products
L;021	Chlorpheniramine Maleate	4 mg	Yellow	Tablet	Compressed, Round, Convex, Bisected Scored	Leiner Health Products
L; 021	Natural Senna Laxative	8.6 mg	Green-Brown	Tablet	Circle	Good Sense
L; 021	Natural Senna Laxative	8.6 mg	Green-Brown	Tablet	Circle	Perfect Choice
L; 021	Natural Senna Laxative	8.6 mg	Green-Brown	Tablet	Circle	Sunmark
L; 021	Natural Senna Laxative	8.6 mg	Green-Brown	Tablet	Circle	Valu Rite
L; 022	Acid Reducer	200 mg	White	Tablet	Oval	Sunmark
L; 022	Acid Reducer	200 mg	White	Tablet	Oval	Valu Rite
L; 022	Acid Reducer 200	200 mg	White	Tablet	Oval	Major
L; 022	Cimetidine	200 mg	White	Tablet	Oval	Good Neighbor Pharmacy
L; 022	Cimetidine	200 mg	White	Tablet	Oval	Good Sense
L; 022	Cimetidine	200 mg	White	Tablet	Oval	Major
L; 022	Cimetidine	200 mg	White	Tablet	Oval	Nex
L; 022	Cimetidine	200 mg	White	Tablet	Oval	Perfect Choice
L; 022	Cimetidine	200 mg	White	Tablet	Oval	Pharmx
L; 022	Cimetidine	200 mg	White	Tablet	Oval	Top Care
L; 022	Heartburn Relief 200	200 mg	White	Tablet	Oval	Good Neighbor Pharmacy
L; 022	Heartburn Relief 200	200 mg	White	Tablet	Oval	Pharm X
L; 022;	Acetaminophen	80 mg	Mottled Purple	Tablet, Chewable	Round, Compressed, Flat Faced, Beveled Edge, Bisected Scored	Leiner Health Products
L;023	Pseudoephedrine Hydrochloride	30 mg	Red	Coated Tablet	Circle	Leiner Health Products
L; 024	Maximum Strength Sleep Aid	50 mg	Aqua	Capsule, Liquid Filled	Oval	Kerr Drug
L; 024	Maximum Strength Sleep Aid	50 mg	Aqua	Capsule, Liquid Filled	Oval	Valu Rite
L; 024	Sleep Aid Liquid Gels Maximum Strength	50 mg	Aqua	Capsule, Liquid Filled	Oval	Good Sense
L; 024	Sleep Aid Liquid Gels Maximum Strength	50 mg	Aqua	Capsule, Liquid Filled	Oval	Kerr Drug
L; 024	Sleep Aid Liquid Gels Maximum Strength	50 mg	Aqua	Capsule, Liquid Filled	Oval	Valu Rite
L; 024	Sleep Aid Nighttime	50 mg	Aqua	Capsule, Liquid Filled	Oval	Sunmark
L; 025	Antacid Peppermint Flavor	750 mg	Off-White	Tablet, Chewable	Circle	Leiner Health Products
L; 025;	Calcium Carbonate Peppermint Flavor	500 mg	Off-White	Tablet	Circle, Compressed, Flat Face, Beveled Edge	Leiner Health Products
L; 026	Antacid Assorted Flavors	750 mg	Various	Tablet, Chewable	Circle	Leiner Health Products
L; 026;	Calcium Carbonate Assorted Flavors	500 mg	Various	Tablet	Circle, Compressed, Flat Face, Beveled Edge	Leiner Health Products
L; 027	Extra Strength Calcium Carbonate	750 mg	Various	Tablet	Circle, Compressed, Flat Face, Beveled Edge	Leiner Health Products
L; 027	Extra Strength Chewable Antacid Cherry Flavor	750 mg	Pink	Tablet, Chewable	Circle	Leiner Health Products
L; 030	Allergy/sinus Headache Medicine	500 mg; 12.5 mg; 30 mg	Light Green	Tablet		Sunmark
L; 030	Diphedryl Allergy/sinus/headache	500 mg; 12.5 mg; 30 mg	Light Green	Tablet	Oblong	Good Neighbor Pharmacy
L; 030	Diphedryl Allergy/sinus/headache	500 mg; 12.5 mg; 30 mg	Light Green	Tablet	Oblong	Good Sense
L; 030	Diphedryl Allergy/sinus/headache	500 mg; 12.5 mg; 30 mg	Light Green	Tablet	Oblong	Perfect Choice
L; 030	Diphedryl Allergy/sinus/headache	500 mg; 12.5 mg; 30 mg	Light Green	Tablet	Oblong	Swan
L; 030	Valu-Dryl Allergy/sinus/headache	500 mg; 12.5 mg; 30 mg	Light Green	Tablet		Valu Rite
L; 031;	Bismuth Subsalicylate Wintergreen	262 mg	Pink with Slight Mottling	Tablet	Circle, Compressed, Flat Face, Beveled Edge	Leiner Health Products
L031	Pept-Eez	262 mg	Pink	Tablet	Circle	Zee Medical
L; 034	Diphenhydramine	25 mg	Pink	Tablet	Oval	Leiner Health Products
L; 036;	Acetaminophen & Diphenhydramine Hydrochloride	500 mg; 25 mg	Light Blue	Tablet		Leiner Health Products
L; 037;	Acetaminophen & Diphenhydramine Hydrochloride	500 mg; 25 mg	Light Blue	Tablet	Circle, Compressed, Flat Face, Beveled Edge	Leiner Health Products
L; 039	Motion Sickness Relief II	25 mg	Yellow	Tablet	Circle, Flat-Faced, Bevel-Edged	Perrigo
L; 040;	Diphenhydramine Hydrochloride	25 mg	Light Blue	Tablet	Compressed, Round Convex	Leiner Health Products
L; 043;	Acetaminophen	500 mg	Opaque Red, Opaque Yellow and Blue	Capsule, Liquid Filled		Leiner Health Products
L;047;	Bismuth Subsalicylate Cherry	262 mg	Cherry Red with Slight Mottling	Tablet	Circle, Compressed, Flat Face, Beveled Edge	Leiner Health Products
L;052;	Calcium Polycarbophil	625 mg	Off-White with Brown Specks	Tablet	Oblong, Bowed	Leiner Health Products
L; 053;	Meclizine Hydrochloride	25 mg	Yellow	Tablet	Circle, Compressed, Flat Faced, Beveled Edge	Leiner Health Products
L; 054	Nasal Decongestant Maximum Strength Non-Drowsy	120 mg	White	Extended-Release Tablet	Capsule-Shape, Coated	Good Sense
L; 054	Nasal Decongestant Maximum Strength Non-Drowsy	120 mg	White	Extended-Release Tablet	Capsule-Shape, Coated	Top Care
L; 054	Sinus	325 mg; 30 mg; 4 mg	White	Tablet	Oblong	Leiner Health Products
L; 054	Sinus 12 Hour Maximum Strength	120 mg	White	Extended-Release Tablet	Capsule-Shape, Coated	Sunmark
L; 054	Suphedrin 12 Hour Non-Drowsy	120 mg	White	Extended-Release Tablet	Capsule-Shape, Coated	Good Neighbor Pharmacy
L; 054	Suphedrin 12 Hour Non-Drowsy	120 mg	White	Extended-Release Tablet	Capsule-Shape, Coated	Kerr Drug

IMPRINT	BRAND/GENERIC NAME	STRENGTH	COLOR	FORM	SHAPE	MANUFACTURER
L; 054	Suphedrin 12 Hour Non-Drowsy	120 mg	White	Extended-Release Tablet	Capsule-Shape, Coated	Perfect Choice
L; 054	Suphedrin 12 Hour Non-Drowsy	120 mg	White	Extended-Release Tablet	Capsule-Shape, Coated	Valu Rite
L; 055	Sinus	325 mg; 30 mg	Pink	Coated Tablet	Round, Convex, Bisected Scored	Leiner Health Products
L; 056;	Extra Strength Acetaminophen & Antacid	500 mg; 250 mg	White	Tablet		Leiner Health Products
L; 057;	Dihydroxyaluminum Sodium Carbonate	300 mg	White	Tablet	Circle, Compressed, Convex	Leiner Health Products
L; 059	Extra Strength Chewable Antacid Wintergreen	750 mg	Green	Tablet, Chewable	Circle	Leiner Health Products
L; 062;	Adult Micro-Coated Aspirin, Low Strength	81 mg	White	Tablet	Circle, Convex, Embossed	Leiner Health Products
L; 071	Super Strength Chewable Antacid Assorted Mint Flavors	1000 mg	Green or White	Tablet, Chewable	Circle	Leiner Health Products
L; 072	Super Strength Chewable Antacid Assorted Fruit Flavors	1000 mg	Various	Tablet, Chewable	Circle	Leiner Health Products
L; 074;	Multiple Symptom Cold	325 mg; 2 mg; 30 mg; 10 mg	Yellow	Tablet	Circle, Compressed, Convex	Leiner Health Products
L; 077;	Maximum Strength Non-Aspirin Sinus	500 mg; 30 mg	Light Orange	Tablet		Leiner Health Products
L; 077	Maximum Strength Sinus	500 mg; 30 mg	Orange	Tablet		Good Neighbor Pharmacy
L; 077	Sinus Maximum Strength without Drowsiness	500 mg; 30 mg	Orange	Tablet		Good Sense
L; 077	Sinus Maximum Strength without Drowsiness	500 mg; 30 mg	Orange	Tablet		Kerr Drug
L; 077	Sinus Maximum Strength without Drowsiness	500 mg; 30 mg	Orange	Tablet		Top Care
L; 077	Sinus Maximum Strength without Drowsiness	500 mg; 30 mg	Orange	Tablet		Valu Rite
L; 077	Sinus Relief Non-Drowsy	500 mg; 30 mg	Orange	Tablet		Sunmark
L; 079	Multi-Symptom Pain Relief Cold Non-Drowsy	30 mg; 15 mg; 325 mg	Orange/beige	Capsule, Liquid Filled		Good Sense
L; 079	Non-Aspirin Cold Multi-Symptom	325 mg; 15 mg; 30 mg	Orange/beige	Capsule, Liquid Filled		Kerr Drug
L; 079	Non-Aspirin Cold Multi-Symptom	325 mg; 15 mg; 30 mg	Orange/beige	Capsule, Liquid Filled		Top Care
L; 079;	Acetaminophen & Pseudoephedrine Hydrochloride	500 mg; 30 mg	Orange	Tablet	Circle, Compressed, Convex	Leiner Health Products
L; 089;	Phed Plus	60 mg; 4 mg	White	Tablet	Compressed, Round, Convex, Bisected Scored	Leiner Health Products
L; 091	Children's Chewable Non-Aspirin Acetaminophen	80 mg	Mottled Pink	Tablet, Chewable	Circle	Valu Rite
L; 091	Children's Pain Reliever Bubble Gum Flavored	80 mg	Mottled Pink	Tablet, Chewable	Circle	Good Neighbor Pharmacy
L; 091	Children's Pain Reliever Bubble Gum Flavored	80 mg	Mottled Pink	Tablet, Chewable	Circle	Good Sense
L; 091	Children's Pain Reliever Bubble Gum Flavored	80 mg	Mottled Pink	Tablet, Chewable	Circle	Kerr Drug
L; 091	Children's Pain Reliever Bubble Gum Flavored	80 mg	Mottled Pink	Tablet, Chewable	Circle	Major
L; 091	Children's Pain Reliever Bubble Gum Flavored	80 mg	Mottled Pink	Tablet, Chewable	Circle	Perfect Choice
L; 091	Children's Pain Reliever Bubble Gum Flavored	80 mg	Mottled Pink	Tablet, Chewable	Circle	Swan
L; 091	Children's Pain Reliever Bubble Gum Flavored	80 mg	Mottled Pink	Tablet, Chewable	Circle	Top Care
L1	Ferrous Sulfate	88 mg; 46 mg	Grey	Tablet	Circle	Nex
L1	Ferrous Sulfate	88 mg; 46 mg	Grey	Tablet	Circle	North Laboratories
L1	Ferrous Sulfate	88 mg; 46 mg	Grey	Tablet	Circle	Perrigo
L1	Ferrous Sulfate	88 mg; 46 mg	Grey	Tablet	Circle	Preferred Products
L1	Ferrous Sulfate	88 mg; 46 mg	Grey	Tablet	Circle	Valu Rite
L1	Ferrous Sulfate	88 mg; 46 mg	Grey	Tablet	Circle	Vita-Smart
L1	Iron	88 mg; 46 mg	Grey	Tablet	Circle	Sunmark
L1	Iron	88 mg; 46 mg	Grey	Tablet	Circle	Vita-Smart
L; 2	Antidiarrheal	2 mg	Green	Tablet	Bisected Scored	Fleming
L; 2	Antidiarrheal	2 mg	Green	Tablet	Bisected Scored	Glendale Foods
L; 2	Antidiarrheal	2 mg	Green	Tablet	Bisected Scored	Goldline Laboratories
L; 2	Antidiarrheal	2 mg	Green	Tablet	Bisected Scored	Harco Drug
L; 2	Antidiarrheal	2 mg	Green	Tablet	Bisected Scored	Kerr Drug
L; 2	Antidiarrheal	2 mg	Green	Tablet	Bisected Scored	Major
L; 2	Antidiarrheal	2 mg	Green	Tablet	Bisected Scored	Medalist
L; 2	Antidiarrheal	2 mg	Green	Tablet	Bisected Scored	Perfect Choice
L; 2	Antidiarrheal	2 mg	Green	Tablet	Bisected Scored	Perrigo
L; 2	Antidiarrheal	2 mg	Green	Tablet	Bisected Scored	Pharmacist Value
L; 2	Antidiarrheal	2 mg	Green	Tablet	Bisected Scored	Preferred Products
L; 2	Antidiarrheal	2 mg	Green	Tablet	Bisected Scored	Quality Care
L; 2	Antidiarrheal	2 mg	Green	Tablet	Bisected Scored	Regal Distributing
L; 2	Antidiarrheal	2 mg	Green	Tablet	Bisected Scored	Revco
L; 2	Antidiarrheal	2 mg	Green	Tablet	Bisected Scored	True Quality
L; 2	Antidiarrheal	2 mg	Green	Tablet	Bisected Scored	United Drugs
L; 2	Antidiarrheal	2 mg	Green	Tablet	Bisected Scored	Valu Rite
L; 2	Anti-Diarrheal	2 mg	Light Green	Tablet	Bisected Scored	Good Neighbor Pharmacy
L; 2	Anti-Diarrheal	2 mg	Light Green	Tablet	Bisected Scored	Hytop
L; 2	Anti-Diarrheal	2 mg	Light Green	Tablet	Bisected Scored	Legend Pharmaceuticals
L; 2	Anti-Diarrheal	2 mg	Light Green	Tablet	Bisected Scored	Major
L; 2	Anti-Diarrheal	2 mg	Light Green	Tablet	Bisected Scored	Medic
L; 2	Anti-Diarrheal	2 mg	Light Green	Tablet	Bisected Scored	Nex
L; 2	Anti-Diarrheal	2 mg	Light Green	Tablet	Bisected Scored	Perfect Choice
L; 2	Anti-Diarrheal	2 mg	Light Green	Tablet	Bisected Scored	Perrigo
L; 2	Anti-Diarrheal	2 mg	Light Green	Tablet	Bisected Scored	Sunfresh

IMPRINT	BRAND/GENERIC NAME	STRENGTH	COLOR	FORM	SHAPE	MANUFACTURER
L; 2	Anti-Diarrheal	2 mg	Light Green	Tablet	Bisected Scored	Swan
L; 2	Anti-Diarrheal	2 mg	Light Green	Tablet	Bisected Scored	Top Care
L; 2	Anti-Diarrheal	2 mg	Light Green	Tablet	Bisected Scored	United Drugs
L; 2	Anti-Diarrheal	2 mg	Light Green	Tablet	Bisected Scored	Valu Rite
L; 2	Ferrous Gluconate	240 mg	Green	Tablet	Circle, Convex	Perrigo
L; 2	Ferrous Gluconate	240 mg	Green	Tablet	Circle, Convex	True Quality
L; 2	Ferrous Gluconate	240 mg	Green	Tablet	Circle, Convex	Vita-Smart
L2	Anti Diarrheal	2 mg	Green	Tablet	Capsule, Bisected Scored	Berkley & Jensen
L2	Anti Diarrheal	2 mg	Green	Tablet	Capsule, Bisected Scored	Good Neighbor Pharmacy
L2	Anti Diarrheal	2 mg	Green	Tablet	Capsule, Bisected Scored	Good Sense
L2	Anti Diarrheal	2 mg	Green	Tablet	Capsule, Bisected Scored	Major
L2	Anti Diarrheal	2 mg	Green	Tablet	Capsule, Bisected Scored	Sunmark
L2	Anti Diarrheal	2 mg	Green	Tablet	Capsule, Bisected Scored	Swan
L2	Anti Diarrheal	2 mg	Green	Tablet	Capsule, Bisected Scored	Top Care
L2	Anti Diarrheal	2 mg	Green	Tablet	Capsule, Bisected Scored	Valu Rite
L-2	Anti-Diarrheal Original Strength	2 mg	Light Green	Tablet		Good Neighbor Pharmacy
L-2	Anti-Diarrheal Original Strength	2 mg	Light Green	Tablet		Perfect Choice
L; 4	Prenatal Vitamins	4000 IU; 100 mg; 400 IU; 11 IU; 1.84 mg; 1.7 mg; 18 mg; 2.6 mg; 800 mcg; 4 mcg; 200 mg; 27 mg; 25 mg	Pink	Tablet	Circle	Good Neighbor Pharmacy
L; 4	Prenatal Vitamins	4000 IU; 100 mg; 400 IU; 11 IU; 1.84 mg; 1.7 mg; 18 mg; 2.6 mg; 800 mcg; 4 mcg; 200 mg; 27 mg; 25 mg	Pink	Tablet	Circle	Good Sense
L; 4	Prenatal Vitamins	4000 IU; 100 mg; 400 IU; 11 IU; 1.84 mg; 1.7 mg; 18 mg; 2.6 mg; 800 mcg; 4 mcg; 200 mg; 27 mg; 25 mg	Pink	Tablet	Circle	Nex
L; 4	Prenatal Vitamins	4000 IU; 100 mg; 400 IU; 11 IU; 1.84 mg; 1.7 mg; 18 mg; 2.6 mg; 800 mcg; 4 mcg; 200 mg; 27 mg; 25 mg	Pink	Tablet	Circle	Perrigo
L; 4	Prenatal Vitamins	4000 IU; 100 mg; 400 IU; 11 IU; 1.84 mg; 1.7 mg; 18 mg; 2.6 mg; 800 mcg; 4 mcg; 200 mg; 27 mg; 25 mg	Pink	Tablet	Circle	Sunmark
L; 4	Prenatal Vitamins	4000 IU; 100 mg; 400 IU; 11 IU; 1.84 mg; 1.7 mg; 18 mg; 2.6 mg; 800 mcg; 4 mcg; 200 mg; 27 mg; 25 mg	Pink	Tablet	Circle	Top Care
L; 4	Prenatal Vitamins	4000 IU; 100 mg; 400 IU; 11 IU; 1.84 mg; 1.7 mg; 18 mg; 2.6 mg; 800 mcg; 4 mcg; 200 mg; 27 mg; 25 mg	Pink	Tablet	Circle	True Quality
L; 4	Prenatal Vitamins	4000 IU; 100 mg; 400 IU; 11 IU; 1.84 mg; 1.7 mg; 18 mg; 2.6 mg; 800 mcg; 4 mcg; 200 mg; 27 mg; 25 mg	Pink	Tablet	Circle	Valu Rite
L; 4	Prenatal Vitamins	4000 IU; 100 mg; 400 IU; 11 IU; 1.84 mg; 1.7 mg; 18 mg; 2.6 mg; 800 mcg; 4 mcg; 200 mg; 27 mg; 25 mg	Pink	Tablet	Circle	Vita-Smart
L4;	Prenatal Vitamins	60 mg	Beige	Tablet	Circle	Perrigo
L; 4; M	Levothyroxine Sodium	25 mcg	Orange	Tablet	Capsule-Shape, Scored	Mylan Pharmaceuticals
L; 5; M	Levothyroxine Sodium	50 mcg	White	Tablet	Capsule-Shape, Scored	Mylan Pharmaceuticals
L; 6; M	Levothyroxine Sodium	75 mcg	Purple	Tablet	Capsule-Shape, Scored	Mylan Pharmaceuticals
L; 7; M	Levothyroxine Sodium	88 mcg	Light Green	Tablet	Capsule-Shape, Scored	Mylan Pharmaceuticals
L; 8; M	Levothyroxine Sodium	100 mcg	Yellow	Tablet	Capsule-Shape, Scored	Mylan Pharmaceuticals
L; 9; LL	Ledercillin VK	500 mg	White	Tablet	Round, Convex, Bisected Scored	Lederle Laboratories
L; 9; M	Levothyroxine Sodium	112 mcg	Rose	Tablet	Capsule-Shape, Scored	Mylan Pharmaceuticals
L; 10; LL	Ledercillin VK	250 mg	White	Tablet	Round, Convex, Bisected Scored	Lederle Laboratories

IMPRINT	BRAND/GENERIC NAME	STRENGTH	COLOR	FORM	SHAPE	MANUFACTURER
L; 10; M	Levothyroxine Sodium	125 mcg	Gray	Tablet	Capsule-Shape, Scored	Mylan Pharmaceuticals
L11	Thyroid, Usp 3 grain	114 mcg; 18 mcg	Tan	Tablet	Circle	Norton, H.N.
L; 11; M	Levothyroxine Sodium	150 mcg	Blue	Tablet	Capsule-Shape, Scored	Mylan Pharmaceuticals
L; 12; M	Levothyroxine Sodium	175 mcg	Light Purple	Tablet	Capsule-Shape, Scored	Mylan Pharmaceuticals
L; 13; M	Levothyroxine Sodium	200 mcg	Pink	Tablet	Capsule-Shape, Scored	Mylan Pharmaceuticals
L; 14; M	Levothyroxine Sodium	300 mcg	Green	Tablet	Capsule-Shape, Scored	Mylan Pharmaceuticals
L; 100	Acetaminophen	160 mg	White	Tablet	Bisected Scored	Leiner Health Products
L; 101	Non-Aspirin Sinus	500 mg; 30 mg	Pale Yellow	Capsule, Liquid Filled	Capsule-Shape	Perrigo
L; 102	Maximum Strength Allergy Sinus	500 mg; 2 mg; 30 mg	Yellow	Tablet		Leiner Health Products
L; 105	Acetaminophen & Pseudoephedrine Hydrochloride	500 mg; 30 mg	Light Green	Tablet		Leiner Health Products
L110	Low Dose Adult Chewable Aspirin	81 mg	Light Yellow	Tablet	Capsule-Shape, Compressed	Leiner Health Products
L;111	Anti-Allergy	30 mg; 2 mg	Blue	Tablet	Circle, Compressed, Convex	Leiner Health Products
L; 124; 200	Acid Reducer 200	200 mg	White	Coated Tablet	Oval	Hytop
L; 124; 200	Acid Reducer 200	200 mg	White	Coated Tablet	Oval	Major
L; 124; 200	Acid Reducer Cimetidine	200 mg	White	Coated Tablet	Oval	Good Neighbor Pharmacy
L; 124; 200	Acid Reducer Cimetidine	200 mg	White	Coated Tablet	Oval	Nex
L; 126	Multi-Symptom Pain Relief Cold Non-Drowsy	30 mg; 15 mg; 325 mg	White	Tablet		Good Sense
L; 126	Pain Reliever Cold Multi-Symptom	325 mg; 15 mg; 30 mg	White	Tablet		Good Neighbor Pharmacy
L; 126	Pain Reliever Cold Multi-Symptom	325 mg; 15 mg; 30 mg	White	Tablet		Good Sense
L; 126	Pain Reliever Cold Multi-Symptom	325 mg; 15 mg; 30 mg	White	Tablet		Kerr Drug
L; 126	Pain Reliever Cold Multi-Symptom	325 mg; 15 mg; 30 mg	White	Tablet		Perrigo
L; 128	Antacid	311 mg; 232 mg	Blue and White with Blue Sealing Band	Capsule, Liquid Filled		Perrigo
L; 128	Antacid	311 mg; 232 mg	Blue and White with Blue Sealing Band	Capsule, Liquid Filled		Sunfresh
L; 128	Antacid	311 mg; 232 mg	Blue and White with Blue Sealing Band	Capsule, Liquid Filled		Top Care
L; 137	Junior Strength Non-Aspirin Fruit Splash Flavor - Ages 6-12	160 mg	Pink	Tablet, Chewable	Circle	Valu Rite
L; 137	Junior Strength Pain Reliever Fruit Splash Flavor - Ages 6-12	160 mg	Pink	Tablet, Chewable	Circle	Kerr Drug
L; 137	Junior Strength Pain Reliever Fruit Splash Flavor - Ages 6-12	160 mg	Pink	Tablet, Chewable	Circle	Top Care
L; 137	Junior's Chewable Acetaminophen	160 mg	Pink	Tablet, Chewable	Circle	Good Sense
L; 137	Pain Reliever Junior Strength Chewable	160 mg	Pink	Tablet, Chewable	Circle	Sunmark
L; 143	Children's Non Aspirin Fruit Splash Flavor	80 mg	Mottled Pink	Tablet, Chewable	Circle	Valu Rite
L; 143	Children's Pain Reliever without Aspirin Fruit Splash Flavor	80 mg	Mottled Pink	Tablet, Chewable	Circle	Good Neighbor Pharmacy
L; 143	Children's Pain Reliever without Aspirin Fruit Splash Flavor	80 mg	Mottled Pink	Tablet, Chewable	Circle	Major
L; 143	Children's Pain Reliever without Aspirin Fruit Splash Flavor	80 mg	Mottled Pink	Tablet, Chewable	Circle	Perfect Choice
L; 143	Children's Pain Reliever without Aspirin Fruit Splash Flavor	80 mg	Mottled Pink	Tablet, Chewable	Circle	Perrigo
L; 143	Children's Pain Reliever without Aspirin Fruit Splash Flavor	80 mg	Mottled Pink	Tablet, Chewable	Circle	United Drugs
L; 143	Pain Reliever	80 mg	Mottled Pink	Tablet, Chewable	Circle	Sunmark
L; 148	Children's Non-Aspirin Cold Plus Cough	80 mg; 0.5 mg; 7.5 mg; 2.5 mg	Pale Pink	Tablet, Chewable	Circle	Revco
L; 148	Children's Non-Aspirin Cold Plus Cough	80 mg; 0.5 mg; 7.5 mg; 2.5 mg	Pale Pink	Tablet, Chewable	Circle	Top Care
L; 148	Children's Non-Aspirin Cold Plus Cough	80 mg; 0.5 mg; 7.5 mg; 2.5 mg	Pale Pink	Tablet, Chewable	Circle	Valu Rite
L; 156	Acid Reducer	75 mg	Pink	Tablet	Six-Sided	Good Sense
L; 156	Heartburn Relief	75 mg	Pink	Tablet	Six-Sided	Pharmx
L; 156	Ranitidine 75	75 mg	Pink	Tablet	Six-Sided	Good Neighbor Pharmacy
L; 156	Ranitidine 75	75 mg	Pink	Tablet	Six-Sided	Top Care
L; 159	Antacid	311 mg; 232 mg	White and Aqua	Capsule, Liquid Filled	Capsule-Shape	Masanti
L; 159	Antacid	311 mg; 232 mg	White and Aqua	Capsule, Liquid Filled	Capsule-Shape	Nex
L; 159	Antacid	311 mg; 232 mg	White and Aqua	Capsule, Liquid Filled	Capsule-Shape	Perrigo
L; 171	Pain Reliever Pm, Extra Strength	500 mg; 25 mg	Pale Blue and White with Blue Band	Tablet		Good Sense
L; 171	Pain Reliever Pm, Extra Strength	500 mg; 25 mg	Pale Blue and White with Blue Band	Tablet		Perrigo
L; 172	Junior Strength Pain Reliever	160 mg	Mottled Pink	Tablet, Chewable	Flat-Face, Bevel-Edged, Bisected, Round Scored	Glendale Foods
L; 172	Junior Strength Pain Reliever	160 mg	Mottled Pink	Tablet, Chewable	Flat-Face, Bevel-Edged, Bisected, Round Scored	Good Neighbor Pharmacy
L; 172	Junior Strength Pain Reliever	160 mg	Mottled Pink	Tablet, Chewable	Flat-Face, Bevel-Edged, Bisected, Round Scored	Good Sense
L; 172	Junior Strength Pain Reliever	160 mg	Mottled Pink	Tablet, Chewable	Flat-Face, Bevel-Edged, Bisected, Round Scored	Major Pharmaceutical
L; 172	Junior Strength Pain Reliever	160 mg	Mottled Pink	Tablet, Chewable	Flat-Face, Bevel-Edged, Bisected, Round Scored	Major Quality
L; 172	Junior Strength Pain Reliever	160 mg	Mottled Pink	Tablet, Chewable	Flat-Face, Bevel-Edged, Bisected, Round Scored	Perrigo
L; 172	Junior Strength Pain Reliever	160 mg	Mottled Pink	Tablet, Chewable	Flat-Face, Bevel-Edged, Bisected, Round Scored	Regal Distributing

IMPRINT	BRAND/GENERIC NAME	STRENGTH	COLOR	FORM	SHAPE	MANUFACTURER
L; 172	Junior Strength Pain Reliever	160 mg	Mottled Pink	Tablet, Chewable	Flat-Face, Bevel-Edged, Bisected, Round Scored	Sunfresh
L; 172	Junior Strength Pain Reliever	160 mg	Mottled Pink	Tablet, Chewable	Flat-Face, Bevel-Edged, Bisected, Round Scored	Top Care
L; 172	Junior Strength Pain Reliever	160 mg	Mottled Pink	Tablet, Chewable	Flat-Face, Bevel-Edged, Bisected, Round Scored	Valu Rite
L; 173	Non-Aspirin Allergy Sinus	500 mg; 2 mg; 30 mg	Yellow and Pale Green with Dark Green Band	Capsule, Liquid Filled	Capsule-Shape	Good Neighbor Pharmacy
L; 173	Non-Aspirin Allergy Sinus	500 mg; 2 mg; 30 mg	Yellow and Pale Green with Dark Green Band	Capsule, Liquid Filled	Capsule-Shape	Perrigo
L; 179	Calcium Antacid Extra Strength Assorted Flavors	750 mg	Yellow, Red, Orange and Green	Tablet	Circle	Good Neighbor Pharmacy
L; 179	Calcium Antacid Extra Strength Assorted Flavors	750 mg	Yellow, Red, Orange and Green	Tablet	Circle	Kerr Drug
L; 179	Calcium Antacid Extra Strength Assorted Flavors	750 mg	Yellow, Red, Orange and Green	Tablet	Circle	Major
L; 179	Calcium Antacid Extra Strength Assorted Flavors	750 mg	Yellow, Red, Orange and Green	Tablet	Circle	Perrigo
L; 179	Calcium Antacid Extra Strength Assorted Flavors	750 mg	Yellow, Red, Orange and Green	Tablet	Circle	Revco
L; 179	Calcium Antacid Extra Strength Assorted Flavors	750 mg	Yellow, Red, Orange and Green	Tablet	Circle	Sunmark
L; 179	Calcium Antacid Extra Strength Assorted Flavors	750 mg	Yellow, Red, Orange and Green	Tablet	Circle	Top Care
L; 179	Calcium Antacid Extra Strength Assorted Flavors	750 mg	Yellow, Red, Orange and Green	Tablet	Circle	Valu Rite
L; 185	Acetaminophen Pm	500 mg; 25 mg	Blue and White	Capsule, Liquid Filled	Capsule-Shape	Genovese
L; 185	Acetaminophen Pm	500 mg; 25 mg	Blue and White	Capsule, Liquid Filled	Capsule-Shape	Good Sense
L; 185	Acetaminophen Pm	500 mg; 25 mg	Blue and White	Capsule, Liquid Filled	Capsule-Shape	Nex
L; 185	Acetaminophen Pm	500 mg; 25 mg	Blue and White	Capsule, Liquid Filled	Capsule-Shape	Perrigo
L; 185	Acetaminophen Pm	500 mg; 25 mg	Blue and White	Capsule, Liquid Filled	Capsule-Shape	Valu Rite
L; 187	Mapap Extra Strength	500 mg	Red-Orange and Yellow	Geltab	Circle	Major
L; 187	Non-Aspirin Extra Strength	500 mg	Red and Yellow	Geltab		Perfect Choice
L; 187	Non-Aspirin Pain Reliever Extra Strength	500 mg	Orange and Yellow	Geltab	Circle	Genovese
L; 187	Non-Aspirin Pain Reliever Extra Strength	500 mg	Orange and Yellow	Geltab	Circle	Good Sense
L; 187	Non-Aspirin Pain Reliever Extra Strength	500 mg	Orange and Yellow	Geltab	Circle	Harco Drug
L; 187	Non-Aspirin Pain Reliever Extra Strength	500 mg	Orange and Yellow	Geltab	Circle	Hytop
L; 187	Non-Aspirin Pain Reliever Extra Strength	500 mg	Orange and Yellow	Geltab	Circle	Medic
L; 187	Non-Aspirin Pain Reliever Extra Strength	500 mg	Orange and Yellow	Geltab	Circle	Perrigo
L; 187	Non-Aspirin Pain Reliever Extra Strength	500 mg	Orange and Yellow	Geltab	Circle	Pharmacist Value
L; 187	Non-Aspirin Pain Reliever Extra Strength	500 mg	Orange and Yellow	Geltab	Circle	Quality Care
L; 187	Non-Aspirin Pain Reliever Extra Strength	500 mg	Orange and Yellow	Geltab	Circle	Rockbottom Stores
L; 187	Non-Aspirin Pain Reliever Extra Strength	500 mg	Orange and Yellow	Geltab	Circle	Top Care
L; 187	Non-Aspirin Pain Reliever Extra Strength	500 mg	Orange and Yellow	Geltab	Circle	Valu Rite
L; 193	Night Time Liquid Caps	250 mg; 10 mg; 30 mg; 6.25 mg	Light Green	Capsule, Liquid Filled	Oblong	Fleming
L; 193	Night Time Liquid Caps	250 mg; 10 mg; 30 mg; 6.25 mg	Light Green	Capsule, Liquid Filled	Oblong	Glendale Foods
L; 193	Night Time Liquid Caps	250 mg; 10 mg; 30 mg; 6.25 mg	Light Green	Capsule, Liquid Filled	Oblong	Good Neighbor Pharmacy
L; 193	Night Time Liquid Caps	250 mg; 10 mg; 30 mg; 6.25 mg	Light Green	Capsule, Liquid Filled	Oblong	Good Sense
L; 193	Night Time Liquid Caps	250 mg; 10 mg; 30 mg; 6.25 mg	Light Green	Capsule, Liquid Filled	Oblong	Harco Drug
L; 193	Night Time Liquid Caps	250 mg; 10 mg; 30 mg; 6.25 mg	Light Green	Capsule, Liquid Filled	Oblong	Kerr Drug
L; 193	Night Time Liquid Caps	250 mg; 10 mg; 30 mg; 6.25 mg	Light Green	Capsule, Liquid Filled	Oblong	Medalist
L; 193	Night Time Liquid Caps	250 mg; 10 mg; 30 mg; 6.25 mg	Light Green	Capsule, Liquid Filled	Oblong	Park Lane
L; 193	Night Time Liquid Caps	250 mg; 10 mg; 30 mg; 6.25 mg	Light Green	Capsule, Liquid Filled	Oblong	Perrigo
L; 193	Night Time Liquid Caps	250 mg; 10 mg; 30 mg; 6.25 mg	Light Green	Capsule, Liquid Filled	Oblong	Pharm X
L; 193	Night Time Liquid Caps	250 mg; 10 mg; 30 mg; 6.25 mg	Light Green	Capsule, Liquid Filled	Oblong	Regal Distributing
L; 193	Night Time Liquid Caps	250 mg; 10 mg; 30 mg; 6.25 mg	Light Green	Capsule, Liquid Filled	Oblong	Revco
L; 193	Night Time Liquid Caps	250 mg; 10 mg; 30 mg; 6.25 mg	Light Green	Capsule, Liquid Filled	Oblong	Sunfresh
L; 193	Night Time Liquid Caps	250 mg; 10 mg; 30 mg; 6.25 mg	Light Green	Capsule, Liquid Filled	Oblong	Swan
L; 193	Night Time Liquid Caps	250 mg; 10 mg; 30 mg; 6.25 mg	Light Green	Capsule, Liquid Filled	Oblong	Valu Buy

IMPRINT	BRAND/GENERIC NAME	STRENGTH	COLOR	FORM	SHAPE	MANUFACTURER
L; 193	Night Time Liquid Caps	250 mg; 10 mg; 30 mg; 6.25 mg	Light Green	Capsule, Liquid Filled	Oblong	Valu Rite
L; 193	Nite Time Liquid Caps Cold and Flu Relief	250 mg; 10 mg; 30 mg; 6.25 mg	Clear Green	Capsule, Liquid Filled	Oblong	Good Sense
L; 193	Nite Time Liquid Caps Cold and Flu Relief	250 mg; 10 mg; 30 mg; 6.25 mg	Clear Green	Capsule, Liquid Filled	Oblong	Kerr Drug
L; 193	Nite Time Liquid Caps Cold and Flu Relief	250 mg; 10 mg; 30 mg; 6.25 mg	Clear Green	Capsule, Liquid Filled	Oblong	Medic
L; 193	Nite Time Liquid Caps Cold and Flu Relief	250 mg; 10 mg; 30 mg; 6.25 mg	Clear Green	Capsule, Liquid Filled	Oblong	Nex
L; 193	Nite Time Liquid Caps Cold and Flu Relief	250 mg; 10 mg; 30 mg; 6.25 mg	Clear Green	Capsule, Liquid Filled	Oblong	Perfect Choice
L; 193	Nite Time Liquid Caps Cold and Flu Relief	250 mg; 10 mg; 30 mg; 6.25 mg	Clear Green	Capsule, Liquid Filled	Oblong	Perrigo
L; 193	Nite Time Liquid Caps Cold and Flu Relief	250 mg; 10 mg; 30 mg; 6.25 mg	Clear Green	Capsule, Liquid Filled	Oblong	Preferred Products
L; 193	Nite Time Liquid Caps Cold and Flu Relief	250 mg; 10 mg; 30 mg; 6.25 mg	Clear Green	Capsule, Liquid Filled	Oblong	Quality Care
L; 193	Nite Time Liquid Caps Cold and Flu Relief	250 mg; 10 mg; 30 mg; 6.25 mg	Clear Green	Capsule, Liquid Filled	Oblong	Revco
L; 193	Nite Time Liquid Caps Cold and Flu Relief	250 mg; 10 mg; 30 mg; 6.25 mg	Clear Green	Capsule, Liquid Filled	Oblong	Sunmark
L; 193	Nite Time Liquid Caps Cold and Flu Relief	250 mg; 10 mg; 30 mg; 6.25 mg	Clear Green	Capsule, Liquid Filled	Oblong	Top Care
L; 198	Non-Aspirin Allergy Sinus Maximum Strength	500 mg; 2 mg; 30 mg	Green and Yellow	Capsule, Liquid Filled	Oblong	Swan
L; 198	Pain Relief Allergy Sinus Maximum Strength	500 mg; 2 mg; 30 mg	Green and Yellow	Capsule, Liquid Filled	Oblong	Good Sense
L; 198	Pain Relief Allergy Sinus Maximum Strength	500 mg; 2 mg; 30 mg	Green and Yellow	Capsule, Liquid Filled	Oblong	Kerr Drug
L; 198	Pain Relief Allergy Sinus Maximum Strength	500 mg; 2 mg; 30 mg	Green and Yellow	Capsule, Liquid Filled	Oblong	Perfect Choice
L; 198	Pain Relief Allergy Sinus Maximum Strength	500 mg; 2 mg; 30 mg	Green and Yellow	Capsule, Liquid Filled	Oblong	Perrigo
L; 198	Pain Relief Allergy Sinus Maximum Strength	500 mg; 2 mg; 30 mg	Green and Yellow	Capsule, Liquid Filled	Oblong	Pharmx
L; 198	Pain Relief Allergy Sinus Maximum Strength	500 mg; 2 mg; 30 mg	Green and Yellow	Capsule, Liquid Filled	Oblong	Top Care
L; 198	Pain Relief Allergy Sinus Maximum Strength	500 mg; 2 mg; 30 mg	Green and Yellow	Capsule, Liquid Filled	Oblong	Valu Rite
L; 198	Pain Reliever Allergy Sinus Maximum Strength	500 mg; 2 mg; 30 mg	Green and Yellow	Capsule, Liquid Filled	Oblong	Sunmark
L; 216	Children's Pain & Cold Relief	80 mg; 0.5 mg; 7.5 mg	Purple	Tablet, Chewable	Circle	Top Care
L; 216	Children's Pain Reliever Cold Multi-Symptom Relief	80 mg; 0.5 mg; 7.5 mg	Purple	Tablet, Chewable	Circle	Good Neighbor Pharmacy
L; 216	Children's Pain Reliever Cold Multi-Symptom Relief	80 mg; 0.5 mg; 7.5 mg	Purple	Tablet, Chewable	Circle	Good Sense
L; 216	Children's Pain Reliever Cold Multi-Symptom Relief	80 mg; 0.5 mg; 7.5 mg	Purple	Tablet, Chewable	Circle	Kerr Drug
L; 216	Children's Pain Reliever Cold Multi-Symptom Relief	80 mg; 0.5 mg; 7.5 mg	Purple	Tablet, Chewable	Circle	Perrigo
L; 216	Children's Pain Reliever Cold Multi-Symptom Relief	80 mg; 0.5 mg; 7.5 mg	Purple	Tablet, Chewable	Circle	Swan
L; 216	Children's Pain Reliever Cold Multi-Symptom Relief	80 mg; 0.5 mg; 7.5 mg	Purple	Tablet, Chewable	Circle	Valu Rite
L; 226	Tussin Cold and Cough	10 mg; 200 mg; 30 mg	Red	Capsule, Liquid Filled	Oblong	Good Neighbor Pharmacy
L; 226	Tussin Cold and Cough	10 mg; 200 mg; 30 mg	Red	Capsule, Liquid Filled	Oblong	Perfect Choice
L; 226	Tussin Cold and Cough	10 mg; 200 mg; 30 mg	Red	Capsule, Liquid Filled	Oblong	Sunmark
L; 226	Tussin Cold and Cough	10 mg; 200 mg; 30 mg	Red	Capsule, Liquid Filled	Oblong	Valu Rite
L; 228	Non-Aspirin Sinus Non-Drowsy	500 mg; 30 mg	Green and White	Capsule, Liquid Filled	Oblong	Valu Rite
L; 228	Pain Relief Sinus Maximum Strength	500 mg; 30 mg	Green and White	Capsule, Liquid Filled	Oblong	Good Neighbor Pharmacy
L; 228	Pain Relief Sinus Maximum Strength	500 mg; 30 mg	Green and White	Capsule, Liquid Filled	Oblong	Kerr Drug
L; 228	Pain Relief Sinus Maximum Strength	500 mg; 30 mg	Green and White	Capsule, Liquid Filled	Oblong	Perfect Choice
L; 228	Pain Relief Sinus Maximum Strength	500 mg; 30 mg	Green and White	Capsule, Liquid Filled	Oblong	Perrigo
L; 228	Pain Relief Sinus Maximum Strength	500 mg; 30 mg	Green and White	Capsule, Liquid Filled	Oblong	Pharmx
L; 228	Pain Relief Sinus Maximum Strength	500 mg; 30 mg	Green and White	Capsule, Liquid Filled	Oblong	Top Care
L; 228	Pain Relief Sinus Maximum Strength	500 mg; 30 mg	Green and White	Capsule, Liquid Filled	Oblong	Valu Rite
L; 228	Pain Reliever Sinus Maximum Strength	500 mg; 30 mg	Green and White	Capsule, Liquid Filled	Oblong	Sunmark
L; 235	Acid Relief Regular	300 mg	White	Tablet	Circle, Concave-Faced	Good Sense
L; 235	Acid Relief Regular	300 mg	White	Tablet	Circle, Concave-Faced	Perrigo
L; 235	Acid Relief Regular	300 mg	White	Tablet	Circle, Concave-Faced	Revco
L; 235	Acid Relief Regular	300 mg	White	Tablet	Circle, Concave-Faced	True Quality
L; 235	Acid Relief Regular	300 mg	White	Tablet	Circle, Concave-Faced	True Quality Products
L; 240	Laxative Pills Regular Strength	90 mg	Beige	Coated Tablet	Circle, Convex	Good Neighbor Pharmacy
L; 240	Laxative Pills Regular Strength	90 mg	Beige	Coated Tablet	Circle, Convex	Good Sense
L; 240	Laxative Pills Regular Strength	90 mg	Beige	Coated Tablet	Circle, Convex	Hytop

IMPRINT	BRAND/GENERIC NAME	STRENGTH	COLOR	FORM	SHAPE	MANUFACTURER
L; 240	Laxative Pills Regular Strength	90 mg	Beige	Coated Tablet	Circle, Convex	Park Lane
L; 240	Laxative Pills Regular Strength	90 mg	Beige	Coated Tablet	Circle, Convex	Perrigo
L; 240	Laxative Pills Regular Strength	90 mg	Beige	Coated Tablet	Circle, Convex	Preferred Products
L; 240	Laxative Pills Regular Strength	90 mg	Beige	Coated Tablet	Circle, Convex	Sunfresh
L; 240	Laxative Pills Regular Strength	90 mg	Beige	Coated Tablet	Circle, Convex	Top Care
L; 240	Laxative Pills Regular Strength	90 mg	Beige	Coated Tablet	Circle, Convex	Valu Buy
L; 259	Aspirin Adult Chewable Low Strength	81 mg	Light Orange	Tablet, Chewable	Circle	Good Neighbor Pharmacy
L; 259	Aspirin Adult Chewable Low Strength	81 mg	Light Orange	Tablet, Chewable	Circle	Good Sense
L; 259	Aspirin Adult Chewable Low Strength	81 mg	Light Orange	Tablet, Chewable	Circle	Perrigo
L; 259	Aspirin Adult Chewable Low Strength	81 mg	Light Orange	Tablet, Chewable	Circle	Rockbottom Stores
L; 259	Aspirin Adult Chewable Low Strength	81 mg	Light Orange	Tablet, Chewable	Circle	Sunmark
L; 259	Aspirin Adult Chewable Low Strength	81 mg	Light Orange	Tablet, Chewable	Circle	Swan
L; 259	Aspirin Adult Chewable Low Strength	81 mg	Light Orange	Tablet, Chewable	Circle	Valu Rite
L; 267	Pain Relief Flu Maximum Strength	500 mg; 30 mg; 15 mg	Red and White	Capsule, Liquid Filled	Capsule-Shape	Good Sense
L; 267	Pain Relief Flu Maximum Strength	500 mg; 30 mg; 15 mg	Red and White	Capsule, Liquid Filled	Capsule-Shape	Hytop
L; 267	Pain Relief Flu Maximum Strength	500 mg; 30 mg; 15 mg	Red and White	Capsule, Liquid Filled	Capsule-Shape	Kerr Drug
L; 267	Pain Relief Flu Maximum Strength	500 mg; 30 mg; 15 mg	Red and White	Capsule, Liquid Filled	Capsule-Shape	Nex
L; 267	Pain Relief Flu Maximum Strength	500 mg; 30 mg; 15 mg	Red and White	Capsule, Liquid Filled	Capsule-Shape	Perfect Choice
L; 267	Pain Relief Flu Maximum Strength	500 mg; 30 mg; 15 mg	Red and White	Capsule, Liquid Filled	Capsule-Shape	Perrigo
L; 267	Pain Relief Flu Maximum Strength	500 mg; 30 mg; 15 mg	Red and White	Capsule, Liquid Filled	Capsule-Shape	Pharmx
L; 267	Pain Relief Flu Maximum Strength	500 mg; 30 mg; 15 mg	Red and White	Capsule, Liquid Filled	Capsule-Shape	Sunmark
L; 267	Pain Relief Flu Maximum Strength	500 mg; 30 mg; 15 mg	Red and White	Capsule, Liquid Filled	Capsule-Shape	Top Care
L; 267	Pain Relief Flu Maximum Strength	500 mg; 30 mg; 15 mg	Red and White	Capsule, Liquid Filled	Capsule-Shape	Valu Rite
L; 274	Children's Chewable Aspirin	81 mg	Pink	Tablet, Chewable	Circle	Good Neighbor Pharmacy
L; 274	Children's Chewable Aspirin	81 mg	Pink	Tablet, Chewable	Circle	Perrigo
L; 274	Children's Chewable Aspirin	81 mg	Pink	Tablet, Chewable	Circle	Pharmx
L; 274	Children's Chewable Aspirin	81 mg	Pink	Tablet, Chewable	Circle	Sunmark
L; 274	Children's Chewable Aspirin	81 mg	Pink	Tablet, Chewable	Circle	Valu Rite
L; 282	Allergy Relief	1.34 mg	Off-White	Tablet		Sunmark
L; 282	Dayhist Allergy	1.34 mg	Off-White	Tablet		Valu Rite
L; 282	Dayhist-1	1.34 mg	Off-White	Tablet	Capsule-Shape	Kerr Drug
L; 282	Dayhist-1	1.34 mg	Off-White	Tablet	Capsule-Shape	Perrigo
L: 282	Dayhist-1 Original Prescription Strength	1.34 mg	Off-White	Tablet		Revco
L; 299	Non-Aspirin with Antacid, Extra Strength	500 mg; 250 mg	White	Tablet		Good Neighbor Pharmacy
L; 299	Non-Aspirin with Antacid, Extra Strength	500 mg; 250 mg	White	Tablet		Good Sense
L; 299	Non-Aspirin with Antacid, Extra Strength	500 mg; 250 mg	White	Tablet		Perrigo
L; 299	Non-Aspirin with Antacid, Extra Strength	500 mg; 250 mg	White	Tablet		Swan
L; 314	Pain Relief Severe Allergy Maximum Strength	500 mg; 12.5 mg	Yellow	Tablet		Perrigo
L; 314	Pain Relief Severe Allergy Maximum Strength	500 mg; 12.5 mg	Yellow	Tablet		Top Care
L; 325	Clotrimazole	100 mg	White	Tablet	Bullet-Shaped	Perrigo
L; 326	Non-Aspirin Allergy Sinus Maximum Strength	2 mg; 30 mg; 500 mg	Green and Yellow	Geltab	Circle	Valu Rite
L; 326	Pain Relief Allergy Sinus Maximum Strength	2 mg; 30 mg; 500 mg	Green and Yellow	Geltab	Circle	Genovese
L; 326	Pain Reliever Allergy Sinus Maximum Strength	2 mg; 30 mg; 500 mg	Green and Yellow	Geltab	Circle	Sunmark
L; 355; PM	Pain Relief Pm Non-Aspirin	500 mg; 25 mg	Light Blue	Tablet	Circle	Good Neighbor Pharmacy
L; 355; PM	Pain Relief Pm Non-Aspirin	500 mg; 25 mg	Light Blue	Tablet	Circle	Good Sense
L; 355; PM	Pain Relief Pm Non-Aspirin	500 mg; 25 mg	Light Blue	Tablet	Circle	Perrigo
L; 355; PM	Pain Relief Pm Non-Aspirin	500 mg; 25 mg	Light Blue	Tablet	Circle	Top Care
L355; PM	Aspirin Free Headache Pm	500 mg; 25 mg	Light Blue	Tablet	Circle	Good Neighbor Pharmacy
L355; PM	Aspirin Free Headache Pm	500 mg; 25 mg	Light Blue	Tablet	Circle	Good Sense
L355; PM	Aspirin Free Headache Pm	500 mg; 25 mg	Light Blue	Tablet	Circle	Perrigo
L355; PM	Aspirin Free Headache Pm	500 mg; 25 mg	Light Blue	Tablet	Circle	Top Care
L355; PM	Headache Pm Formula	500 mg; 25 mg	Light Blue	Tablet	Circle	Valu Rite
L355; PM	Headache Relief Pm	500 mg; 25 mg	Light Blue	Tablet	Circle	Sunmark
L; 368	Naproxen Sodium	220 mg	Light Blue	Tablet	Oval	Good Neighbor Pharmacy
L; 368	Naproxen Sodium	220 mg	Light Blue	Tablet	Oval	Major
L; 368	Naproxen Sodium	220 mg	Light Blue	Tablet	Oval	Medic
L; 368	Naproxen Sodium	220 mg	Light Blue	Tablet	Oval	Perfect Choice
L; 368	Naproxen Sodium	220 mg	Light Blue	Tablet	Oval	Perrigo
L; 368	Naproxen Sodium	220 mg	Light Blue	Tablet	Oval	Top Care
L; 368	Naproxen Sodium	220 mg	Light Blue	Tablet	Oval	Valu Rite
L; 381	Headache Formula Added Strength	250 mg; 65 mg; 250 mg	White	Tablet	Capsule-Shape	Good Sense

IMPRINT	BRAND/GENERIC NAME	STRENGTH	COLOR	FORM	SHAPE	MANUFACTURER
L; 381	Headache Formula Added Strength	250 mg; 65 mg; 250 mg	White	Tablet	Capsule-Shape	Perrigo
L; 381	Headache Formula Added Strength	250 mg; 65 mg; 250 mg	White	Tablet	Capsule-Shape	Top Care
L; 381	Headache Formula Added Strength	250 mg; 65 mg; 250 mg	White	Tablet	Capsule-Shape	Valu Rite
L; 389	Day Time Multi-Symptom	30 mg; 250 mg; 10 mg	Orange	Capsule, Liquid Filled	Oblong	Good Sense
L; 389	Day Time Multi-Symptom	30 mg; 250 mg; 10 mg	Orange	Capsule, Liquid Filled	Oblong	Sunmark
L; 389	Day Time Multi-Symptom	30 mg; 250 mg; 10 mg	Orange	Capsule, Liquid Filled	Oblong	Valu Rite
L; 389	Day Time Non-Drowsy Multi-Symptom Cold/flu	30 mg; 250 mg; 10 mg	Orange	Capsule, Liquid Filled	Oblong	Good Neighbor Pharmacy
L; 389	Day Time Non-Drowsy Multi-Symptom Cold/flu	30 mg; 250 mg; 10 mg	Orange	Capsule, Liquid Filled	Oblong	Good Sense
L; 389	Day Time Non-Drowsy Multi-Symptom Cold/flu	30 mg; 250 mg; 10 mg	Orange	Capsule, Liquid Filled	Oblong	Hytop
L; 389	Day Time Non-Drowsy Multi-Symptom Cold/flu	30 mg; 250 mg; 10 mg	Orange	Capsule, Liquid Filled	Oblong	Kerr Drug
L; 389	Day Time Non-Drowsy Multi-Symptom Cold/flu	30 mg; 250 mg; 10 mg	Orange	Capsule, Liquid Filled	Oblong	Pharm X
L; 389	Day Time Non-Drowsy Multi-Symptom Cold/flu	30 mg; 250 mg; 10 mg	Orange	Capsule, Liquid Filled	Oblong	Top Care
L; 389	Day Time Non-Drowsy Multi-Symptom Cold/flu	30 mg; 250 mg; 10 mg	Orange	Capsule, Liquid Filled	Oblong	Valu Rite
L; 403	Acetaminophen Regular Strength	325 mg	White	Tablet	Circle, Flat-Faced, Bevel-Edged	First Choice
L; 403	Acetaminophen Regular Strength	325 mg	White	Tablet	Circle, Flat-Faced, Bevel-Edged	Good Neighbor Pharmacy
L; 403	Acetaminophen Regular Strength	325 mg	White	Tablet	Circle, Flat-Faced, Bevel-Edged	Hytop
L; 403	Acetaminophen Regular Strength	325 mg	White	Tablet	Circle, Flat-Faced, Bevel-Edged	Major
L; 403	Acetaminophen Regular Strength	325 mg	White	Tablet	Circle, Flat-Faced, Bevel-Edged	Medic
L; 403	Acetaminophen Regular Strength	325 mg	White	Tablet	Circle, Flat-Faced, Bevel-Edged	Mediguard
L; 403	Acetaminophen Regular Strength	325 mg	White	Tablet	Circle, Flat-Faced, Bevel-Edged	Nex
L; 403	Acetaminophen Regular Strength	325 mg	White	Tablet	Circle, Flat-Faced, Bevel-Edged	Paddock Labs
L; 403	Acetaminophen Regular Strength	325 mg	White	Tablet	Circle, Flat-Faced, Bevel-Edged	Park Lane
L; 403	Acetaminophen Regular Strength	325 mg	White	Tablet	Circle, Flat-Faced, Bevel-Edged	Perrigo
L; 403	Acetaminophen Regular Strength	325 mg	White	Tablet	Circle, Flat-Faced, Bevel-Edged	Preferred Products
L; 403	Acetaminophen Regular Strength	325 mg	White	Tablet	Circle, Flat-Faced, Bevel-Edged	Quality Care
L; 403	Acetaminophen Regular Strength	325 mg	White	Tablet	Circle, Flat-Faced, Bevel-Edged	Rexall
L; 403	Acetaminophen Regular Strength	325 mg	White	Tablet	Circle, Flat-Faced, Bevel-Edged	Ribordy Drugs
L; 403	Acetaminophen Regular Strength	325 mg	White	Tablet	Circle, Flat-Faced, Bevel-Edged	Sunfresh
L; 403	Acetaminophen Regular Strength	325 mg	White	Tablet	Circle, Flat-Faced, Bevel-Edged	Swan
L; 403	Acetaminophen Regular Strength	325 mg	White	Tablet	Circle, Flat-Faced, Bevel-Edged	United Drugs
L; 403	Pain Reliever Regular Strength	325 mg	White	Tablet	Circle, Flat-Faced, Bevel-Edged	Sunmark
L; 403	Pain Reliever Regular Strength without Aspirin	325 mg	White	Tablet	Circle	Good Neighbor Pharmacy
L; 403	Regular Strength Non-Aspirin Acetaminophen	325 mg	White	Tablet	Circle, Flat-Faced, Bevel-Edged	Valu Rite
L; 405	Extra Strength Non-Aspirin	500 mg	White	Tablet	Circle	Medic
L; 405	Extra Strength Non-Aspirin	500 mg	White	Tablet	Circle	Valu Rite
L; 405	Extra Strength Pain Reliever	500 mg	White	Tablet	Circle	First Choice
L; 405	Extra Strength Pain Reliever	500 mg	White	Tablet	Circle	Fleming
L; 405	Extra Strength Pain Reliever	500 mg	White	Tablet	Circle	Good Neighbor Pharmacy
L; 405	Extra Strength Pain Reliever	500 mg	White	Tablet	Circle	Good Sense
L; 405	Extra Strength Pain Reliever	500 mg	White	Tablet	Circle	Hytop
L; 405	Extra Strength Pain Reliever	500 mg	White	Tablet	Circle	Major
L; 405	Extra Strength Pain Reliever	500 mg	White	Tablet	Circle	Major Quality
L; 405	Extra Strength Pain Reliever	500 mg	White	Tablet	Circle	Medic
L; 405	Extra Strength Pain Reliever	500 mg	White	Tablet	Circle	Ms Pharmaceutical
L; 405	Extra Strength Pain Reliever	500 mg	White	Tablet	Circle	Nex
L; 405	Extra Strength Pain Reliever	500 mg	White	Tablet	Circle	Perfect Choice
L; 405	Extra Strength Pain Reliever	500 mg	White	Tablet	Circle	Preferred Products
L; 405	Extra Strength Pain Reliever	500 mg	White	Tablet	Circle	Quality Care
L; 405	Extra Strength Pain Reliever	500 mg	White	Tablet	Circle	Regal Distributing
L; 405	Extra Strength Pain Reliever	500 mg	White	Tablet	Circle	Rexall
L; 405	Extra Strength Pain Reliever	500 mg	White	Tablet	Circle	Seaway
L; 405	Extra Strength Pain Reliever	500 mg	White	Tablet	Circle	Sunfresh
L; 405	Extra Strength Pain Reliever	500 mg	White	Tablet	Circle	Swan
L; 405	Extra Strength Pain Reliever	500 mg	White	Tablet	Circle	Top Care
L; 405	Extra Strength Pain Reliever	500 mg	White	Tablet	Circle	True Quality
L; 405	Extra Strength Pain Reliever	500 mg	White	Tablet	Circle	United Drugs
L; 405	Extra Strength Pain Reliever	500 mg	White	Tablet	Circle	Valu Buy
L; 405	Pain Relief, Extra Strength Aspirin Free	500 mg	White	Tablet	Circle	Top Care
L; 405	Pain Reliever Extra Strength	500 mg	White	Tablet	Circle	Sunmark
L; 406; 325 MG	Sleep	25 mg	Light Blue	Tablet	Circle, Concave	Kerr Drug
L; 406; 325 MG	Sleep	25 mg	Light Blue	Tablet	Circle, Concave	Nex
L; 406; 325 MG	Sleep	25 mg	Light Blue	Tablet	Circle, Concave	Perrigo
L; 406; 325 MG	Sleep	25 mg	Light Blue	Tablet	Circle, Concave	Swan
L; 406; 325 MG	Sleep	25 mg	Light Blue	Tablet	Circle, Concave	Valu Buy
L; 409	Stay Awake	200 mg	Yellow	Tablet	Circle	Good Neighbor Pharmacy
L; 409	Stay Awake	200 mg	Yellow	Tablet	Circle	Good Sense
L; 409	Stay Awake	200 mg	Yellow	Tablet	Circle	Hytop
L; 409	Stay Awake	200 mg	Yellow	Tablet	Circle	Major Pharmaceutical
L; 409	Stay Awake	200 mg	Yellow	Tablet	Circle	Major Quality
L; 409	Stay Awake	200 mg	Yellow	Tablet	Circle	Medic
L; 409	Stay Awake	200 mg	Yellow	Tablet	Circle	Perrigo
L; 409	Stay Awake	200 mg	Yellow	Tablet	Circle	Sunmark
L; 409	Stay Awake	200 mg	Yellow	Tablet	Circle	Swan

IMPRINT	BRAND/GENERIC NAME	STRENGTH	COLOR	FORM	SHAPE	MANUFACTURER
L; 409	Stay Awake	200 mg	Yellow	Tablet	Circle	Top Care
L; 409	Stay Awake	200 mg	Yellow	Tablet	Circle	Valu Buy
L; 409	Stay Awake	200 mg	Yellow	Tablet	Circle	Valu Rite
L; 410	Suphedrine Sinus Maximum Strength	500 mg; 30 mg	Orange	Tablet		Good Sense
L; 410	Suphedrine Sinus Maximum Strength	500 mg; 30 mg	Orange	Tablet		Kerr Drug
L; 410	Suphedrine Sinus Maximum Strength	500 mg; 30 mg	Orange	Tablet		Rexall
L; 410	Suphedrine Sinus Maximum Strength	500 mg; 30 mg	Orange	Tablet		Top Care
L; 415	Adult Strength Analgesic	400 mg; 32 mg	White	Coated Tablet	Circle, Concave	Fleming
L; 415	Adult Strength Analgesic	400 mg; 32 mg	White	Coated Tablet	Circle, Concave	Glendale Foods
L; 415	Adult Strength Analgesic	400 mg; 32 mg	White	Coated Tablet	Circle, Concave	Good Neighbor Pharmacy
L; 415	Adult Strength Analgesic	400 mg; 32 mg	White	Coated Tablet	Circle, Concave	Good Sense
L; 415	Adult Strength Analgesic	400 mg; 32 mg	White	Coated Tablet	Circle, Concave	Major
L; 415	Adult Strength Analgesic	400 mg; 32 mg	White	Coated Tablet	Circle, Concave	Medalist
L; 415	Adult Strength Analgesic	400 mg; 32 mg	White	Coated Tablet	Circle, Concave	Nex
L; 415	Adult Strength Analgesic	400 mg; 32 mg	White	Coated Tablet	Circle, Concave	Perrigo
L; 415	Adult Strength Analgesic	400 mg; 32 mg	White	Coated Tablet	Circle, Concave	Regal Distributing
L; 415	Adult Strength Analgesic	400 mg; 32 mg	White	Coated Tablet	Circle, Concave	Sunfresh
L; 415	Adult Strength Analgesic	400 mg; 32 mg	White	Coated Tablet	Circle, Concave	Swan
L; 415	Adult Strength Analgesic	400 mg; 32 mg	White	Coated Tablet	Circle, Concave	Top Care
L; 415	Adult Strength Analgesic	400 mg; 32 mg	White	Coated Tablet	Circle, Concave	True Quality
L; 415	Adult Strength Analgesic	400 mg; 32 mg	White	Coated Tablet	Circle, Concave	Valu Rite
L; 418	Nasal Decongestant	200 mg; 30 mg	Blue	Capsule, Liquid Filled		Good Sense
L; 418	Nasal Decongestant	200 mg; 30 mg	Blue	Capsule, Liquid Filled		Top Care
L; 418	Non-Drying Sinus Maximum Strength	200 mg; 30 mg	Blue	Capsule, Liquid Filled		Sunmark
L; 418	Sinus Liquid Caps Non-Drying Relief	200 mg; 30 mg	Light Blue	Capsule, Liquid Filled		Top Care
L; 418	Suphedrine Non-Drying Sinus Liquid Caps	200 mg; 30 mg	Blue	Capsule, Liquid Filled	Capsule-Shape	Top Care
L; 418	Suphedrine Non-Drying Sinus Liquid Caps	200 mg; 30 mg	Blue	Capsule, Liquid Filled	Capsule-Shape	Valu Rite
L; 420	Complete Cold	325 mg; 2 mg; 30 mg; 10 mg	Yellow	Tablet	Biconvex	Good Sense
L; 420	Complete Cold	325 mg; 2 mg; 30 mg; 10 mg	Yellow	Tablet	Biconvex	Harco Drug
L; 420	Complete Cold	325 mg; 2 mg; 30 mg; 10 mg	Yellow	Tablet	Biconvex	Legend Pharmaceuticals
L; 420	Complete Cold	325 mg; 2 mg; 30 mg; 10 mg	Yellow	Tablet	Biconvex	Major Pharmaceutical
L; 420	Complete Cold	325 mg; 2 mg; 30 mg; 10 mg	Yellow	Tablet	Biconvex	Major Quality
L; 420	Complete Cold	325 mg; 2 mg; 30 mg; 10 mg	Yellow	Tablet	Biconvex	Medalist
L; 420	Complete Cold	325 mg; 2 mg; 30 mg; 10 mg	Yellow	Tablet	Biconvex	Swan
L; 420	Complete Cold	325 mg; 2 mg; 30 mg; 10 mg	Yellow	Tablet	Biconvex	Top Care
L; 420	Complete Cold	325 mg; 2 mg; 30 mg; 10 mg	Yellow	Tablet	Biconvex	True Quality
L; 420	Complete Cold	325 mg; 2 mg; 30 mg; 10 mg	Yellow	Tablet	Biconvex	United Drugs
L; 420	Complete Cold	325 mg; 2 mg; 30 mg; 10 mg	Yellow	Tablet	Biconvex	Valu Rite
L; 421	Effervescent Pain Reliever Original Flavor	325 mg; 1000 mg; 1916 mg	White	Effervescent Tablet	Circle, Flat-Faced, Beveled Edge	Genovese
L; 421	Effervescent Pain Reliever Original Flavor	325 mg; 1000 mg; 1916 mg	White	Effervescent Tablet	Circle, Flat-Faced, Beveled Edge	Good Neighbor Pharmacy
L; 421	Effervescent Pain Reliever Original Flavor	325 mg; 1000 mg; 1916 mg	White	Effervescent Tablet	Circle, Flat-Faced, Beveled Edge	Kerr Drug
L; 421	Effervescent Pain Reliever Original Flavor	325 mg; 1000 mg; 1916 mg	White	Effervescent Tablet	Circle, Flat-Faced, Beveled Edge	Major
L; 421	Effervescent Pain Reliever Original Flavor	325 mg; 1000 mg; 1916 mg	White	Effervescent Tablet	Circle, Flat-Faced, Beveled Edge	Medic
L; 421	Effervescent Pain Reliever Original Flavor	325 mg; 1000 mg; 1916 mg	White	Effervescent Tablet	Circle, Flat-Faced, Beveled Edge	Navarro
L; 421	Effervescent Pain Reliever Original Flavor	325 mg; 1000 mg; 1916 mg	White	Effervescent Tablet	Circle, Flat-Faced, Beveled Edge	Nex
L; 421	Effervescent Pain Reliever Original Flavor	325 mg; 1000 mg; 1916 mg	White	Effervescent Tablet	Circle, Flat-Faced, Beveled Edge	Perrigo
L; 421	Effervescent Pain Reliever Original Flavor	325 mg; 1000 mg; 1916 mg	White	Effervescent Tablet	Circle, Flat-Faced, Beveled Edge	Pharmacist Value
L; 421	Effervescent Pain Reliever Original Flavor	325 mg; 1000 mg; 1916 mg	White	Effervescent Tablet	Circle, Flat-Faced, Beveled Edge	Sunfresh
L; 421	Effervescent Pain Reliever Original Flavor	325 mg; 1000 mg; 1916 mg	White	Effervescent Tablet	Circle, Flat-Faced, Beveled Edge	Sunmark
L; 421	Effervescent Pain Reliever Original Flavor	325 mg; 1000 mg; 1916 mg	White	Effervescent Tablet	Circle, Flat-Faced, Beveled Edge	Swan
L; 421	Effervescent Pain Reliever Original Flavor	325 mg; 1000 mg; 1916 mg	White	Effervescent Tablet	Circle, Flat-Faced, Beveled Edge	Top Care
L; 421	Effervescent Pain Reliever Original Flavor	325 mg; 1000 mg; 1916 mg	White	Effervescent Tablet	Circle, Flat-Faced, Beveled Edge	True Quality
L; 421	My-Luck	325 mg; 1916 mg; 1000 mg		Effervescent Tablet		Mypharm
L; 427	Pain Reliever Allergy Sinus Maximum Strength	500 mg; 2 mg; 30 mg	Yellow	Tablet		Fleming

IMPRINT	BRAND/GENERIC NAME	STRENGTH	COLOR	FORM	SHAPE	MANUFACTURER
L; 427	Pain Reliever Allergy Sinus Maximum Strength	500 mg; 2 mg; 30 mg	Yellow	Tablet		Glendale Foods
L; 427	Pain Reliever Allergy Sinus Maximum Strength	500 mg; 2 mg; 30 mg	Yellow	Tablet		Good Neighbor Pharmacy
L; 427	Pain Reliever Allergy Sinus Maximum Strength	500 mg; 2 mg; 30 mg	Yellow	Tablet		Good Sense
L; 427	Pain Reliever Allergy Sinus Maximum Strength	500 mg; 2 mg; 30 mg	Yellow	Tablet		Hytop
L; 427	Pain Reliever Allergy Sinus Maximum Strength	500 mg; 2 mg; 30 mg	Yellow	Tablet		Kerr Drug
L; 427	Pain Reliever Allergy Sinus Maximum Strength	500 mg; 2 mg; 30 mg	Yellow	Tablet		Nex
L; 427	Pain Reliever Allergy Sinus Maximum Strength	500 mg; 2 mg; 30 mg	Yellow	Tablet		Perfect Choice
L; 427	Pain Reliever Allergy Sinus Maximum Strength	500 mg; 2 mg; 30 mg	Yellow	Tablet		Perrigo
L; 427	Pain Reliever Allergy Sinus Maximum Strength	500 mg; 2 mg; 30 mg	Yellow	Tablet		Preferred Products
L; 427	Pain Reliever Allergy Sinus Maximum Strength	500 mg; 2 mg; 30 mg	Yellow	Tablet		Regal Distributing
L; 427	Pain Reliever Allergy Sinus Maximum Strength	500 mg; 2 mg; 30 mg	Yellow	Tablet		Sunmark
L; 427	Pain Reliever Allergy Sinus Maximum Strength	500 mg; 2 mg; 30 mg	Yellow	Tablet		Swan
L; 427	Pain Reliever Allergy Sinus Maximum Strength	500 mg; 2 mg; 30 mg	Yellow	Tablet		Top Care
L; 427	Pain Reliever Allergy Sinus Maximum Strength	500 mg; 2 mg; 30 mg	Yellow	Tablet		Valu Rite
L; 427	Sinus Allergy Maximum Strength	500 mg; 30 mg; 2 mg	Yellow	Tablet	Capsule-Shape	Good Sense
L; 427	Sinus Allergy Maximum Strength	500 mg; 30 mg; 2 mg	Yellow	Tablet	Capsule-Shape	Kerr Drug
L; 427	Sinus Allergy Maximum Strength	500 mg; 30 mg; 2 mg	Yellow	Tablet	Capsule-Shape	Nex
L; 428	Gas Relief Extra Strength	125 mg	Green	Capsule, Liquid Filled		Good Neighbor Pharmacy
L; 428	Gas Relief Extra Strength	125 mg	Green	Capsule, Liquid Filled		Medic
L; 428	Gas Relief Extra Strength	125 mg	Green	Capsule, Liquid Filled		Sunmark
L; 428	Gas Relief Extra Strength	125 mg	Green	Capsule, Liquid Filled		Top Care
L; 428	Gas Relief Extra Strength	125 mg	Green	Capsule, Liquid Filled		Valu Rite
L; 428	Simethicone	Approximately 130 mg	Green	Capsule, Liquid Filled	Oval	Scherer Laboratories
L; 429	Aspirin Regular Strength	325 mg	Orange	Enteric-Coated Tablet	Circle	Good Neighbor Pharmacy
L; 429	Enteric Coated Aspirin Regular Strength	325 mg	Orange	Enteric-Coated Tablet	Circle, Concave	Glendale Foods
L; 429	Enteric Coated Aspirin Regular Strength	325 mg	Orange	Enteric-Coated Tablet	Circle, Concave	Good Neighbor Pharmacy
L; 429	Enteric Coated Aspirin Regular Strength	325 mg	Orange	Enteric-Coated Tablet	Circle, Concave	Good Sense
L; 429	Enteric Coated Aspirin Regular Strength	325 mg	Orange	Enteric-Coated Tablet	Circle, Concave	Hytop
L; 429	Enteric Coated Aspirin Regular Strength	325 mg	Orange	Enteric-Coated Tablet	Circle, Concave	Kerr Drug
L; 429	Enteric Coated Aspirin Regular Strength	325 mg	Orange	Enteric-Coated Tablet	Circle, Concave	Major
L; 429	Enteric Coated Aspirin Regular Strength	325 mg	Orange	Enteric-Coated Tablet	Circle, Concave	Major Quality
L; 429	Enteric Coated Aspirin Regular Strength	325 mg	Orange	Enteric-Coated Tablet	Circle, Concave	Medalist
L; 429	Enteric Coated Aspirin Regular Strength	325 mg	Orange	Enteric-Coated Tablet	Circle, Concave	Perrigo
L; 429	Enteric Coated Aspirin Regular Strength	325 mg	Orange	Enteric-Coated Tablet	Circle, Concave	Preferred Products
L; 429	Enteric Coated Aspirin Regular Strength	325 mg	Orange	Enteric-Coated Tablet	Circle, Concave	Sunfresh
L; 429	Enteric Coated Aspirin Regular Strength	325 mg	Orange	Enteric-Coated Tablet	Circle, Concave	Swan
L; 429	Enteric Coated Aspirin Regular Strength	325 mg	Orange	Enteric-Coated Tablet	Circle, Concave	Top Care
L; 429	Enteric Coated Aspirin Regular Strength	325 mg	Orange	Enteric-Coated Tablet	Circle, Concave	United Drugs
L; 429	Enteric Coated Aspirin Regular Strength	325 mg	Orange	Enteric-Coated Tablet	Circle, Concave	Valu Rite
L; 430	Added Strength Pain Reliever Headache Formula	250 mg; 250 mg; 65 mg	White	Coated Tablet	Circle, Convex-Faced	Fleming
L; 430	Added Strength Pain Reliever Headache Formula	250 mg; 250 mg; 65 mg	White	Coated Tablet	Circle, Convex-Faced	Glendale Foods
L; 430	Added Strength Pain Reliever Headache Formula	250 mg; 250 mg; 65 mg	White	Coated Tablet	Circle, Convex-Faced	Good Neighbor Pharmacy
L; 430	Added Strength Pain Reliever Headache Formula	250 mg; 250 mg; 65 mg	White	Coated Tablet	Circle, Convex-Faced	Good Sense
L; 430	Added Strength Pain Reliever Headache Formula	250 mg; 250 mg; 65 mg	White	Coated Tablet	Circle, Convex-Faced	Major
L; 430	Added Strength Pain Reliever Headache Formula	250 mg; 250 mg; 65 mg	White	Coated Tablet	Circle, Convex-Faced	Medalist
L; 430	Added Strength Pain Reliever Headache Formula	250 mg; 250 mg; 65 mg	White	Coated Tablet	Circle, Convex-Faced	Moore Medical
L; 430	Added Strength Pain Reliever Headache Formula	250 mg; 250 mg; 65 mg	White	Coated Tablet	Circle, Convex-Faced	Ms Pharmaceutical

IMPRINT	BRAND/GENERIC NAME	STRENGTH	COLOR	FORM	SHAPE	MANUFACTURER
L; 430	Added Strength Pain Reliever Headache Formula	250 mg; 250 mg; 65 mg	White	Coated Tablet	Circle, Convex-Faced	Nex
L; 430	Added Strength Pain Reliever Headache Formula	250 mg; 250 mg; 65 mg	White	Coated Tablet	Circle, Convex-Faced	Park Lane
L; 430	Added Strength Pain Reliever Headache Formula	250 mg; 250 mg; 65 mg	White	Coated Tablet	Circle, Convex-Faced	Perfect Choice
L; 430	Added Strength Pain Reliever Headache Formula	250 mg; 250 mg; 65 mg	White	Coated Tablet	Circle, Convex-Faced	Perrigo
L; 430	Added Strength Pain Reliever Headache Formula	250 mg; 250 mg; 65 mg	White	Coated Tablet	Circle, Convex-Faced	Preferred Products
L; 430	Added Strength Pain Reliever Headache Formula	250 mg; 250 mg; 65 mg	White	Coated Tablet	Circle, Convex-Faced	Regal Distributing
L; 430	Added Strength Pain Reliever Headache Formula	250 mg; 250 mg; 65 mg	White	Coated Tablet	Circle, Convex-Faced	Rexall
L; 430	Added Strength Pain Reliever Headache Formula	250 mg; 250 mg; 65 mg	White	Coated Tablet	Circle, Convex-Faced	Sunfresh
L; 430	Added Strength Pain Reliever Headache Formula	250 mg; 250 mg; 65 mg	White	Coated Tablet	Circle, Convex-Faced	Swan
L; 430	Added Strength Pain Reliever Headache Formula	250 mg; 250 mg; 65 mg	White	Coated Tablet	Circle, Convex-Faced	Top Care
L; 430	Added Strength Pain Reliever Headache Formula	250 mg; 250 mg; 65 mg	White	Coated Tablet	Circle, Convex-Faced	Valu Rite
L; 430	Added Strength Pain Reliever Headache Formula	250 mg; 250 mg; 65 mg	White	Coated Tablet	Circle, Convex-Faced	Valumed
L; 430	Headache Formula Added Strength	250 mg; 250 mg; 65 mg	White	Coated Tablet	Circle, Convex-Faced	Good Neighbor Pharmacy
L; 430	Headache Formula Added Strength	250 mg; 250 mg; 65 mg	White	Coated Tablet	Circle, Convex-Faced	Good Sense
L; 430	Headache Formula Added Strength	250 mg; 250 mg; 65 mg	White	Coated Tablet	Circle, Convex-Faced	Major
L; 430	Headache Formula Added Strength	250 mg; 250 mg; 65 mg	White	Coated Tablet	Circle, Convex-Faced	Pharmx
L; 431	Easy Sleep	25 mg	Light Blue	Tablet	Small	Major
L; 431	Night Time Sleep Aid	25 mg	Light Blue	Tablet	Small	Good Neighbor Pharmacy
L; 431	Night Time Sleep Aid	25 mg	Light Blue	Tablet	Small	Good Sense
L; 431	Night Time Sleep Aid	25 mg	Light Blue	Tablet	Small	Pharmx
L; 431	Night Time Sleep Aid	25 mg	Light Blue	Tablet	Small	Sunmark
L; 431	Night Time Sleep Aid	25 mg	Light Blue	Tablet	Small	Top Care
L; 431	Night Time Sleep Aid	25 mg	Light Blue	Tablet	Small	Valu Rite
L; 431	Sleep Aid Nighttime Sleep Aid	25 mg	Light Blue	Tablet	Small	Perfect Choice
L; 432	Pseudo-Tabs	30 mg	Red	Coated Tablet	Circle	Major Pharmaceutical
L; 432	Suphedrine Nasal Decongestant	30 mg	Red	Coated Tablet	Circle	First Choice
L; 432	Suphedrine Nasal Decongestant	30 mg	Red	Coated Tablet	Circle	Fleming
L; 432	Suphedrine Nasal Decongestant	30 mg	Red	Coated Tablet	Circle	Genovese
L; 432	Suphedrine Nasal Decongestant	30 mg	Red	Coated Tablet	Circle	Good Neighbor Pharmacy
L; 432	Suphedrine Nasal Decongestant	30 mg	Red	Coated Tablet	Circle	Good Sense
L; 432	Suphedrine Nasal Decongestant	30 mg	Red	Coated Tablet	Circle	Hytop
L; 432	Suphedrine Nasal Decongestant	30 mg	Red	Coated Tablet	Circle	Kerr Drug
L; 432	Suphedrine Nasal Decongestant	30 mg	Red	Coated Tablet	Circle	Major
L; 432	Suphedrine Nasal Decongestant	30 mg	Red	Coated Tablet	Circle	Major Quality
L; 432	Suphedrine Nasal Decongestant	30 mg	Red	Coated Tablet	Circle	Medalist
L; 432	Suphedrine Nasal Decongestant	30 mg	Red	Coated Tablet	Circle	Medic
L; 432	Suphedrine Nasal Decongestant	30 mg	Red	Coated Tablet	Circle	Mediguard
L; 432	Suphedrine Nasal Decongestant	30 mg	Red	Coated Tablet	Circle	Ms Pharmaceutical
L; 432	Suphedrine Nasal Decongestant	30 mg	Red	Coated Tablet	Circle	Nex
L; 432	Suphedrine Nasal Decongestant	30 mg	Red	Coated Tablet	Circle	Perfect Choice
L; 432	Suphedrine Nasal Decongestant	30 mg	Red	Coated Tablet	Circle	Perrigo
L; 432	Suphedrine Nasal Decongestant	30 mg	Red	Coated Tablet	Circle	Quality Care
L; 432	Suphedrine Nasal Decongestant	30 mg	Red	Coated Tablet	Circle	Regal Distributing
L; 432	Suphedrine Nasal Decongestant	30 mg	Red	Coated Tablet	Circle	Rexall
L; 432	Suphedrine Nasal Decongestant	30 mg	Red	Coated Tablet	Circle	Ribordy Drugs
L; 432	Suphedrine Nasal Decongestant	30 mg	Red	Coated Tablet	Circle	Sears
L; 432	Suphedrine Nasal Decongestant	30 mg	Red	Coated Tablet	Circle	Sunfresh
L; 432	Suphedrine Nasal Decongestant	30 mg	Red	Coated Tablet	Circle	Swan
L; 432	Suphedrine Nasal Decongestant	30 mg	Red	Coated Tablet	Circle	Top Care
L; 432	Suphedrine Nasal Decongestant	30 mg	Red	Coated Tablet	Circle	True Quality
L; 432	Suphedrine Nasal Decongestant	30 mg	Red	Coated Tablet	Circle	United Drugs
L; 432	Suphedrine Nasal Decongestant	30 mg	Red	Coated Tablet	Circle	Valu Buy
L; 432	Suphedrine Nasal Decongestant	30 mg	Red	Coated Tablet	Circle	Valu Rite
L; 434	Aphedrid	60 mg; 2.5 mg	White	Coated Tablet	Circle	Genovese
L; 434	Aphedrid	60 mg; 2.5 mg	White	Coated Tablet	Circle	Good Neighbor Pharmacy
L; 434	Aphedrid	60 mg; 2.5 mg	White	Coated Tablet	Circle	Harco Drug
L; 434	Aphedrid	60 mg; 2.5 mg	White	Coated Tablet	Circle	Major
L; 434	Aphedrid	60 mg; 2.5 mg	White	Coated Tablet	Circle	Major Quality
L; 434	Aphedrid	60 mg; 2.5 mg	White	Coated Tablet	Circle	Perrigo
L; 434	Aphedrid	60 mg; 2.5 mg	White	Coated Tablet	Circle	Revco
L; 434	Aphedrid	60 mg; 2.5 mg	White	Coated Tablet	Circle	Ribordy Drugs
L; 434	Aphedrid	60 mg; 2.5 mg	White	Coated Tablet	Circle	Top Care
L; 434	Aphedrid	60 mg; 2.5 mg	White	Coated Tablet	Circle	True Quality
L; 434	Aphedrid Cold & Allergy	60 mg; 2.5 mg	White	Coated Tablet	Circle	First Choice
L; 434	Aphedrid Cold & Allergy	60 mg; 2.5 mg	White	Coated Tablet	Circle	Fleming
L; 434	Aphedrid Cold & Allergy	60 mg; 2.5 mg	White	Coated Tablet	Circle	Good Neighbor Pharmacy
L; 434	Aphedrid Cold & Allergy	60 mg; 2.5 mg	White	Coated Tablet	Circle	Good Sense
L; 434	Aphedrid Cold & Allergy	60 mg; 2.5 mg	White	Coated Tablet	Circle	Medic
L; 434	Aphedrid Cold & Allergy	60 mg; 2.5 mg	White	Coated Tablet	Circle	Park Lane
L; 434	Aphedrid Cold & Allergy	60 mg; 2.5 mg	White	Coated Tablet	Circle	Perrigo
L; 434	Aphedrid Cold & Allergy	60 mg; 2.5 mg	White	Coated Tablet	Circle	Pharm X
L; 434	Aphedrid Cold & Allergy	60 mg; 2.5 mg	White	Coated Tablet	Circle	Quality Care
L; 434	Aphedrid Cold & Allergy	60 mg; 2.5 mg	White	Coated Tablet	Circle	Sunfresh

IMPRINT	BRAND/GENERIC NAME	STRENGTH	COLOR	FORM	SHAPE	MANUFACTURER
L; 434	Aphedrid Cold & Allergy	60 mg; 2.5 mg	White	Coated Tablet	Circle	Swan
L; 434	Aphedrid Cold & Allergy	60 mg; 2.5 mg	White	Coated Tablet	Circle	Top Care
L; 434	Aphedrid Cold & Allergy	60 mg; 2.5 mg	White	Coated Tablet	Circle	Valu Buy
L; 434	Aphedrid Cold & Allergy	60 mg; 2.5 mg	White	Coated Tablet	Circle	Valu Rite
L; 434	Aprodine Antihistamine and Nasal Decongestant	60 mg; 2.5 mg		Tablet		Major Pharmaceutical
L; 434	Aprodine Antihistamine and Nasal Decongestant	60 mg; 2.5 mg		Tablet		Major Quality
L; 434	Histafed	60 mg; 2.5 mg	White	Coated Tablet	Circle	Good Neighbor Pharmacy
L; 434	Histafed Head Cold & Allergy Medicine	60 mg; 2.5 mg	White	Tablet	Circle, Scored	Good Neighbor Pharmacy
L; 434	Nasal Decongestant Antihistamine	60 mg; 2.5 mg	White	Coated Tablet	Circle, Scored	Good Sense
L; 435	Non-Aspirin Cold Medicine Multi-Symptom	30 mg; 2 mg; 15 mg; 325 mg	Yellow	Tablet		Valu Rite
L; 435	Pain Relief Cold Multi-Symptom	30 mg; 2 mg; 15 mg; 325 mg	Yellow	Tablet		Good Sense
L; 435	Pain Relief Cold Multi-Symptom	30 mg; 2 mg; 15 mg; 325 mg	Yellow	Tablet		Top Care
L; 435	Pain Reliever Cold Multi Symptom	30 mg; 2 mg; 15 mg; 325 mg	Yellow	Tablet		Sunmark
L; 437	Extra Strength Acetaminophen Pm	500 mg; 25 mg	Light Blue	Tablet		Perrigo
L; 437; PM	Mapap Pm	500 mg; 25 mg	Light Blue	Tablet		Major
L; 437; PM	Non-Aspirin Pm Extra Strength	500 mg; 25 mg	Light Blue	Tablet		Fleming
L; 437; PM	Non-Aspirin Pm Extra Strength	500 mg; 25 mg	Light Blue	Tablet		Sunmark
L; 437; PM	Non-Aspirin Pm Extra Strength	500 mg; 25 mg	Light Blue	Tablet		Swan
L; 437; PM	Non-Aspirin Pm Extra Strength	500 mg; 25 mg	Light Blue	Tablet		Valu Rite
L; 437; PM	Pain Reliever Pm Extra Strength	500 mg; 25 mg	Light Blue	Tablet		Good Neighbor Pharmacy
L; 437; PM	Pain Reliever Pm Extra Strength	500 mg; 25 mg	Light Blue	Tablet		Good Sense
L; 437; PM	Pain Reliever Pm Extra Strength	500 mg; 25 mg	Light Blue	Tablet		Hytop
L; 437; PM	Pain Reliever Pm Extra Strength	500 mg; 25 mg	Light Blue	Tablet		Perrigo
L; 437; PM	Pain Reliever Pm Extra Strength	500 mg; 25 mg	Light Blue	Tablet		Pharm X
L; 437; PM	Pain Reliever Pm Extra Strength	500 mg; 25 mg	Light Blue	Tablet		Quality Care
L; 437; PM	Pain Reliever Pm Extra Strength	500 mg; 25 mg	Light Blue	Tablet		Regal Distributing
L; 437; PM	Pain Reliever Pm Extra Strength	500 mg; 25 mg	Light Blue	Tablet		Top Care
L; 437; PM	Pain Reliever Pm Extra Strength	500 mg; 25 mg	Light Blue	Tablet		United Drugs
L; 438	Mapap Sinus Maximum Strength	500 mg; 30 mg	Light Green	Tablet		Major
L; 438	Pain Reliever Sinus Maximum Strength	500 mg; 30 mg	Light Green	Tablet		Fleming
L; 438	Pain Reliever Sinus Maximum Strength	500 mg; 30 mg	Light Green	Tablet		Glendale Foods
L; 438	Pain Reliever Sinus Maximum Strength	500 mg; 30 mg	Light Green	Tablet		Goldline Laboratories
L; 438	Pain Reliever Sinus Maximum Strength	500 mg; 30 mg	Light Green	Tablet		Good Neighbor Pharmacy
L; 438	Pain Reliever Sinus Maximum Strength	500 mg; 30 mg	Light Green	Tablet		Good Sense
L; 438	Pain Reliever Sinus Maximum Strength	500 mg; 30 mg	Light Green	Tablet		Kerr Drug
L; 438	Pain Reliever Sinus Maximum Strength	500 mg; 30 mg	Light Green	Tablet		Nex
L; 438	Pain Reliever Sinus Maximum Strength	500 mg; 30 mg	Light Green	Tablet		Perfect Choice
L; 438	Pain Reliever Sinus Maximum Strength	500 mg; 30 mg	Light Green	Tablet		Perrigo
L; 438	Pain Reliever Sinus Maximum Strength	500 mg; 30 mg	Light Green	Tablet		Pharm X
L; 438	Pain Reliever Sinus Maximum Strength	500 mg; 30 mg	Light Green	Tablet		Preferred Products
L; 438	Pain Reliever Sinus Maximum Strength	500 mg; 30 mg	Light Green	Tablet		Regal Distributing
L; 438	Pain Reliever Sinus Maximum Strength	500 mg; 30 mg	Light Green	Tablet		Rockbottom Stores
L; 438	Pain Reliever Sinus Maximum Strength	500 mg; 30 mg	Light Green	Tablet		Sunmark
L; 438	Pain Reliever Sinus Maximum Strength	500 mg; 30 mg	Light Green	Tablet		Swan
L; 438	Pain Reliever Sinus Maximum Strength	500 mg; 30 mg	Light Green	Tablet		Top Care
L; 438	Pain Reliever Sinus Maximum Strength	500 mg; 30 mg	Light Green	Tablet		Valu Rite
L; 441	Sleep Aid	25 mg	Blue	Tablet	Capsule-Shape, Scored	Good Neighbor Pharmacy
L; 441	Sleep Aid	25 mg	Blue	Tablet	Capsule-Shape, Scored	Good Sense
L; 441	Sleep Aid	25 mg	Blue	Tablet	Capsule-Shape, Scored	Kerr Drug
L; 441	Sleep Aid	25 mg	Blue	Tablet	Capsule-Shape, Scored	Major
L; 441	Sleep Aid	25 mg	Blue	Tablet	Capsule-Shape, Scored	Nex
L; 441	Sleep Aid	25 mg	Blue	Tablet	Capsule-Shape, Scored	Perrigo
L; 441	Sleep Aid	25 mg	Blue	Tablet	Capsule-Shape, Scored	Sunmark
L; 441	Sleep Aid	25 mg	Blue	Tablet	Capsule-Shape, Scored	Top Care
L; 441	Sleep Aid	25 mg	Blue	Tablet	Capsule-Shape, Scored	Valu Rite
L; 442	Laxative Woman's	100 mg; 65 mg	Pink	Tablet	Oval	Fleming
L; 442	Laxative Woman's	100 mg; 65 mg	Pink	Tablet	Oval	Genco Distributors
L; 442	Laxative Woman's	100 mg; 65 mg	Pink	Tablet	Oval	Good Neighbor Pharmacy
L; 442	Laxative Woman's	100 mg; 65 mg	Pink	Tablet	Oval	Harco Drug
L; 442	Laxative Woman's	100 mg; 65 mg	Pink	Tablet	Oval	Nex
L; 442	Laxative Woman's	100 mg; 65 mg	Pink	Tablet	Oval	Perrigo
L; 442	Laxative Woman's	100 mg; 65 mg	Pink	Tablet	Oval	Quality Care
L; 442	Laxative Woman's	100 mg; 65 mg	Pink	Tablet	Oval	Swan

IMPRINT	BRAND/GENERIC NAME	STRENGTH	COLOR	FORM	SHAPE	MANUFACTURER
L; 442	Laxative Woman's	100 mg; 65 mg	Pink	Tablet	Oval	True Quality
L; 447	Maximum Strength Sinus	500 mg; 30 mg	Orange	Tablet	Oval	Fleming
L; 447	Maximum Strength Sinus	500 mg; 30 mg	Orange	Tablet	Oval	Glendale Foods
L; 447	Maximum Strength Sinus	500 mg; 30 mg	Orange	Tablet	Oval	Good Sense
L; 447	Maximum Strength Sinus	500 mg; 30 mg	Orange	Tablet	Oval	Harco Drug
L; 447	Maximum Strength Sinus	500 mg; 30 mg	Orange	Tablet	Oval	Hytop
L; 447	Maximum Strength Sinus	500 mg; 30 mg	Orange	Tablet	Oval	Medalist
L; 447	Maximum Strength Sinus	500 mg; 30 mg	Orange	Tablet	Oval	Perfect Choice
L; 447	Maximum Strength Sinus	500 mg; 30 mg	Orange	Tablet	Oval	Perrigo
L; 447	Maximum Strength Sinus	500 mg; 30 mg	Orange	Tablet	Oval	Preferred Products
L; 447	Maximum Strength Sinus	500 mg; 30 mg	Orange	Tablet	Oval	Regal Distributing
L; 447	Maximum Strength Sinus	500 mg; 30 mg	Orange	Tablet	Oval	Top Care
L; 447	Maximum Strength Sinus	500 mg; 30 mg	Orange	Tablet	Oval	Valu Rite
L; 449	Junior Strength Fever & Pain Reliever	160 mg	Mottled Lavender	Tablet, Chewable	Circle	Good Neighbor Pharmacy
L; 449	Junior Strength Mapap Ages 6-12	160 mg	Mottled Lavender	Tablet, Chewable	Round, Bisected Scored	Major
L; 449	Junior Strength Non-Aspirin Ages 6-12	160 mg	Mottled Lavender	Tablet, Chewable	Round, Bisected Scored	Valu Rite
L; 449	Junior Strength Pain Reliever Ages 6-12	160 mg	Mottled Lavender	Tablet, Chewable	Round, Bisected Scored	Good Neighbor Pharmacy
L; 449	Junior Strength Pain Reliever Ages 6-12	160 mg	Mottled Lavender	Tablet, Chewable	Round, Bisected Scored	Good Sense
L; 449	Junior Strength Pain Reliever Ages 6-12	160 mg	Mottled Lavender	Tablet, Chewable	Round, Bisected Scored	Hytop
L; 449	Junior Strength Pain Reliever Ages 6-12	160 mg	Mottled Lavender	Tablet, Chewable	Round, Bisected Scored	Major
L; 449	Junior Strength Pain Reliever Ages 6-12	160 mg	Mottled Lavender	Tablet, Chewable	Round, Bisected Scored	Nex
L; 449	Junior Strength Pain Reliever Ages 6-12	160 mg	Mottled Lavender	Tablet, Chewable	Round, Bisected Scored	Perfect Choice
L; 449	Junior Strength Pain Reliever Ages 6-12	160 mg	Mottled Lavender	Tablet, Chewable	Round, Bisected Scored	Perrigo
L; 449	Junior Strength Pain Reliever Ages 6-12	160 mg	Mottled Lavender	Tablet, Chewable	Round, Bisected Scored	Preferred Products
L; 449	Junior Strength Pain Reliever Ages 6-12	160 mg	Mottled Lavender	Tablet, Chewable	Round, Bisected Scored	Regal Distributing
L; 449	Junior Strength Pain Reliever Ages 6-12	160 mg	Mottled Lavender	Tablet, Chewable	Round, Bisected Scored	Rockbottom Stores
L; 449	Junior Strength Pain Reliever Ages 6-12	160 mg	Mottled Lavender	Tablet, Chewable	Round, Bisected Scored	Seaway
L; 449	Junior Strength Pain Reliever Ages 6-12	160 mg	Mottled Lavender	Tablet, Chewable	Round, Bisected Scored	Sunfresh
L; 449	Junior Strength Pain Reliever Ages 6-12	160 mg	Mottled Lavender	Tablet, Chewable	Round, Bisected Scored	Top Care
L; 449	Junior Strength Pain Reliever Ages 6-12	160 mg	Mottled Lavender	Tablet, Chewable	Round, Bisected Scored	Valu Rite
L; 450	Sinus & Allergy Maximum Strength	4 mg; 60 mg	White	Tablet	Circle	Sunmark
L; 450	Sinus & Allergy Maximum Strength	60 mg; 4 mg	White	Tablet	Circle, Scored	Sunmark
L; 450	Suphedrine Cold and Allergy	4 mg; 60 mg	White	Tablet	Circle	Perrigo
L; 450	Suphedrine Cold and Allergy	4 mg; 60 mg	White	Tablet	Circle	Valu Rite
L; 450	Suphedrine Plus Maximum Strength Cold & Allergy	4 mg; 60 mg	White	Tablet	Circle	Good Neighbor Pharmacy
L; 450	Suphedrine Plus Maximum Strength Cold & Allergy	4 mg; 60 mg	White	Tablet	Circle	Good Sense
L; 450	Suphedrine Plus Maximum Strength Cold & Allergy	4 mg; 60 mg	White	Tablet	Circle	Major
L; 450	Suphedrine Plus Maximum Strength Cold & Allergy	4 mg; 60 mg	White	Tablet	Circle	Major Quality
L; 450	Suphedrine Plus Maximum Strength Cold & Allergy	4 mg; 60 mg	White	Tablet	Circle	Perrigo
L; 450	Suphedrine Plus Maximum Strength Cold & Allergy	4 mg; 60 mg	White	Tablet	Circle	Top Care
L; 450	Suphedrine Plus Maximum Strength Cold & Allergy	4 mg; 60 mg	White	Tablet	Circle	True Quality
L; 450	Suphedrine Plus Maximum Strength Cold & Allergy	4 mg; 60 mg	White	Tablet	Circle	United Drugs
L; 450	Suphedrine Plus Maximum Strength Cold & Allergy	4 mg; 60 mg	White	Tablet	Circle	Valu Rite
L; 452	A.S.A. Drox Analgesic	325 mg; 50 mg; 50 mg;		Coated Tablet		True Quality
L; 452	A.S.A. Drox Analgesic	325 mg; 50 mg; 50 mg;		Coated Tablet		True Quality Pharmacies
L; 452	Aspir-Mox	325 mg; 50 mg; 50 mg		Coated Tablet		Major
L; 452	Non Irritating Aspirin	50 mg; 325 mg; 50 mg;	White	Coated Tablet	Circle	Good Sense
L; 452	Non Irritating Aspirin	50 mg; 325 mg; 50 mg;	White	Coated Tablet	Circle	Perrigo
L; 453	Acetaminophen Regular Strength	325 mg	White	Tablet		Fleming
L; 453	Acetaminophen Regular Strength	325 mg	White	Tablet		Good Neighbor Pharmacy
L; 453	Acetaminophen Regular Strength	325 mg	White	Tablet		Good Sense
L; 453	Acetaminophen Regular Strength	325 mg	White	Tablet		North Laboratories
L; 453	Acetaminophen Regular Strength	325 mg	White	Tablet		Perrigo
L; 453	Acetaminophen Regular Strength	325 mg	White	Tablet		Rexall
L; 453	Acetaminophen Regular Strength	325 mg	White	Tablet		Sunfresh
L; 453	Acetaminophen Regular Strength	325 mg	White	Tablet		Top Care

IMPRINT	BRAND/GENERIC NAME	STRENGTH	COLOR	FORM	SHAPE	MANUFACTURER
L; 453	Acetaminophen Regular Strength	325 mg	White	Tablet		Valu Rite
L; 462	Allergy Medicine	25 mg	Clear and Pink with White Powder	Capsule		Top Care
L; 462	Diphedryl Allergy	25 mg	Clear and Pink with White Powder	Capsule		Fleming
L; 462	Diphedryl Allergy	25 mg	Clear and Pink with White Powder	Capsule		Genovese
L; 462	Diphedryl Allergy	25 mg	Clear and Pink with White Powder	Capsule		Glendale Foods
L; 462	Diphedryl Allergy	25 mg	Clear and Pink with White Powder	Capsule		Good Neighbor Pharmacy
L; 462	Diphedryl Allergy	25 mg	Clear and Pink with White Powder	Capsule		Good Sense
L; 462	Diphedryl Allergy	25 mg	Clear and Pink with White Powder	Capsule		Harco Drug
L; 462	Diphedryl Allergy	25 mg	Clear and Pink with White Powder	Capsule		Hytop
L; 462	Diphedryl Allergy	25 mg	Clear and Pink with White Powder	Capsule		Kerr Drug
L; 462	Diphedryl Allergy	25 mg	Clear and Pink with White Powder	Capsule		Major
L; 462	Diphedryl Allergy	25 mg	Clear and Pink with White Powder	Capsule		Major Quality
L; 462	Diphedryl Allergy	25 mg	Clear and Pink with White Powder	Capsule		Medalist
L; 462	Diphedryl Allergy	25 mg	Clear and Pink with White Powder	Capsule		Medic
L; 462	Diphedryl Allergy	25 mg	Clear and Pink with White Powder	Capsule		Nex
L; 462	Diphedryl Allergy	25 mg	Clear and Pink with White Powder	Capsule		Park Lane
L; 462	Diphedryl Allergy	25 mg	Clear and Pink with White Powder	Capsule		Perfect Choice
L; 462	Diphedryl Allergy	25 mg	Clear and Pink with White Powder	Capsule		Perrigo
L; 462	Diphedryl Allergy	25 mg	Clear and Pink with White Powder	Capsule		Pharm X
L; 462	Diphedryl Allergy	25 mg	Clear and Pink with White Powder	Capsule		Preferred Products
L; 462	Diphedryl Allergy	25 mg	Clear and Pink with White Powder	Capsule		Quality Care
L; 462	Diphedryl Allergy	25 mg	Clear and Pink with White Powder	Capsule		Regal Distributing
L; 462	Diphedryl Allergy	25 mg	Clear and Pink with White Powder	Capsule		Rockbottom Stores
L; 462	Diphedryl Allergy	25 mg	Clear and Pink with White Powder	Capsule		Sunfresh
L; 462	Diphedryl Allergy	25 mg	Clear and Pink with White Powder	Capsule		Swan
L; 462	Diphedryl Allergy	25 mg	Clear and Pink with White Powder	Capsule		Top Care
L; 462	Diphedryl Allergy	25 mg	Clear and Pink with White Powder	Capsule		True Quality
L; 462	Diphedryl Allergy	25 mg	Clear and Pink with White Powder	Capsule		Valu Buy
L; 462	Valu-Dryl Allergy	25 mg	Clear and Pink	Capsule		Valu Rite
L; 463	4 Hour Antihistamine	4 mg		Tablet		Good Neighbor Pharmacy
L; 463	4 Hour Antihistamine	4 mg		Tablet		Kerr Drug
L; 463	4 Hour Antihistamine	4 mg		Tablet		Nex
L; 463	4 Hour Antihistamine	4 mg		Tablet		Perfect Choice
L; 463	4 Hour Antihistamine	4 mg		Tablet		Valu Rite
L; 463	Allergy 4 Hour Relief	4 mg	Yellow	Tablet	Circle, Compressed, Scored	First National Supermarkets
L; 463	Allergy 4 Hour Relief	4 mg	Yellow	Tablet	Circle, Compressed, Scored	Fleming
L; 463	Allergy 4 Hour Relief	4 mg	Yellow	Tablet	Circle, Compressed, Scored	Genco Distributors
L; 463	Allergy 4 Hour Relief	4 mg	Yellow	Tablet	Circle, Compressed, Scored	Genovese
L; 463	Allergy 4 Hour Relief	4 mg	Yellow	Tablet	Circle, Compressed, Scored	Good Neighbor Pharmacy
L; 463	Allergy 4 Hour Relief	4 mg	Yellow	Tablet	Circle, Compressed, Scored	Good Sense
L; 463	Allergy 4 Hour Relief	4 mg	Yellow	Tablet	Circle, Compressed, Scored	Hytop
L; 463	Allergy 4 Hour Relief	4 mg	Yellow	Tablet	Circle, Compressed, Scored	Kerr Drug
L; 463	Allergy 4 Hour Relief	4 mg	Yellow	Tablet	Circle, Compressed, Scored	Major
L; 463	Allergy 4 Hour Relief	4 mg	Yellow	Tablet	Circle, Compressed, Scored	Major Quality
L; 463	Allergy 4 Hour Relief	4 mg	Yellow	Tablet	Circle, Compressed, Scored	Medalist
L; 463	Allergy 4 Hour Relief	4 mg	Yellow	Tablet	Circle, Compressed, Scored	Medic
L; 463	Allergy 4 Hour Relief	4 mg	Yellow	Tablet	Circle, Compressed, Scored	Nex
L; 463	Allergy 4 Hour Relief	4 mg	Yellow	Tablet	Circle, Compressed, Scored	Perrigo
L; 463	Allergy 4 Hour Relief	4 mg	Yellow	Tablet	Circle, Compressed, Scored	Regal Distributing
L; 463	Allergy 4 Hour Relief	4 mg	Yellow	Tablet	Circle, Compressed, Scored	Rexall Managed Care
L; 463	Allergy 4 Hour Relief	4 mg	Yellow	Tablet	Circle, Compressed, Scored	Top Care
L; 463	Allergy 4 Hour Relief	4 mg	Yellow	Tablet	Circle, Compressed, Scored	True Quality
L; 463	Allergy Antihistamine	4 mg	Yellow	Tablet	Circle, Compressed, Scored	Sunmark
L; 465; PM	Acetaminophen Pm Extra Strength	500 mg; 25 mg	Mottled Light Blue	Tablet	Circle, Compressed, Flat-Faced, Bevel-Edged	Glendale Foods
L; 465; PM	Acetaminophen Pm Extra Strength	500 mg; 25 mg	Mottled Light Blue	Tablet	Circle, Compressed, Flat-Faced, Bevel-Edged	Good Sense
L; 465; PM	Acetaminophen Pm Extra Strength	500 mg; 25 mg	Mottled Light Blue	Tablet	Circle, Compressed, Flat-Faced, Bevel-Edged	Perrigo
L; 465; PM	Acetaminophen Pm Extra Strength	500 mg; 25 mg	Mottled Light Blue	Tablet	Circle, Compressed, Flat-Faced, Bevel-Edged	Preferred Products

IMPRINT	BRAND/GENERIC NAME	STRENGTH	COLOR	FORM	SHAPE	MANUFACTURER
L; 465; PM	Acetaminophen Pm Extra Strength	500 mg; 25 mg	Mottled Light Blue	Tablet	Circle, Compressed, Flat-Faced, Bevel-Edged	Regal Distributing
L; 465; PM	Acetaminophen Pm Extra Strength	500 mg; 25 mg	Mottled Light Blue	Tablet	Circle, Compressed, Flat-Faced, Bevel-Edged	Sunfresh
L; 465; PM	Acetaminophen Pm Extra Strength	500 mg; 25 mg	Mottled Light Blue	Tablet	Circle, Compressed, Flat-Faced, Bevel-Edged	Swan
L; 465; PM	Acetaminophen Pm Extra Strength	500 mg; 25 mg	Mottled Light Blue	Tablet	Circle, Compressed, Flat-Faced, Bevel-Edged	Top Care
L; 466	Antacid Calcium Rich	350 mg; 150 mg	White	Tablet, Chewable	Circle	Perrigo
L; 466	Antacid Calcium Rich	350 mg; 150 mg	White	Tablet, Chewable	Circle	Swan
L; 467	Children's Aspirin	81 mg;	Orange	Tablet, Chewable	Circle, Compressed, Concave Punch	Fleming
L; 467	Children's Aspirin	81 mg;	Orange	Tablet, Chewable	Circle, Compressed, Concave Punch	Good Neighbor Pharmacy
L; 467	Children's Aspirin	81 mg;	Orange	Tablet, Chewable	Circle, Compressed, Concave Punch	Good Sense
L; 467	Children's Aspirin	81 mg;	Orange	Tablet, Chewable	Circle, Compressed, Concave Punch	Kerr Drug
L; 467	Children's Aspirin	81 mg;	Orange	Tablet, Chewable	Circle, Compressed, Concave Punch	Medic
L; 467	Children's Aspirin	81 mg;	Orange	Tablet, Chewable	Circle, Compressed, Concave Punch	Perrigo
L; 467	Children's Aspirin	81 mg;	Orange	Tablet, Chewable	Circle, Compressed, Concave Punch	Quality Care
L; 467	Children's Aspirin	81 mg;	Orange	Tablet, Chewable	Circle, Compressed, Concave Punch	Revco
L; 467	Children's Aspirin	81 mg;	Orange	Tablet, Chewable	Circle, Compressed, Concave Punch	Rexall
L; 467	Children's Aspirin	81 mg;	Orange	Tablet, Chewable	Circle, Compressed, Concave Punch	Rockbottom Stores
L; 467	Children's Aspirin	81 mg;	Orange	Tablet, Chewable	Circle, Compressed, Concave Punch	Sunfresh
L; 467	Children's Aspirin	81 mg;	Orange	Tablet, Chewable	Circle, Compressed, Concave Punch	Sunmark
L; 467	Children's Aspirin	81 mg;	Orange	Tablet, Chewable	Circle, Compressed, Concave Punch	Swan
L; 467	Children's Aspirin	81 mg;	Orange	Tablet, Chewable	Circle, Compressed, Concave Punch	Top Care
L; 467	Children's Aspirin	81 mg;	Orange	Tablet, Chewable	Circle, Compressed, Concave Punch	Valu Rite
L; 468	Calcium Antacid Extra Strength Tropical Flavors	750 mg	Red, Green, White and Orange	Tablet	Circle	Kerr Drug
L; 468	Calcium Antacid Extra Strength Tropical Flavors	750 mg	Red, Green, White and Orange	Tablet	Circle	Perrigo
L; 468	Calcium Antacid Extra Strength Tropical Flavors	750 mg	Red, Green, White and Orange	Tablet	Circle	Sunmark
L; 468	Calcium Antacid Extra Strength Tropical Flavors	750 mg	Red, Green, White and Orange	Tablet	Circle	Top Care
L; 468	Calcium Antacid Extra Strength Tropical Flavors	750 mg	Red, Green, White and Orange	Tablet	Circle	Valu Rite
L; 469	Pink Bismuth	262 mg	Pink	Tablet, Chewable	Circle, Flat-Faced, Bevel-Edged	Good Sense
L; 469	Pink Bismuth	262 mg	Pink	Tablet, Chewable	Circle, Flat-Faced, Bevel-Edged	Hytop
L; 469	Pink Bismuth	262 mg	Pink	Tablet, Chewable	Circle, Flat-Faced, Bevel-Edged	Major Pharmaceutical
L; 469	Pink Bismuth	262 mg	Pink	Tablet, Chewable	Circle, Flat-Faced, Bevel-Edged	Major Quality
L; 469	Pink Bismuth	262 mg	Pink	Tablet, Chewable	Circle, Flat-Faced, Bevel-Edged	Perrigo
L; 469	Pink Bismuth	262 mg	Pink	Tablet, Chewable	Circle, Flat-Faced, Bevel-Edged	Pharmx
L; 469	Pink Bismuth	262 mg	Pink	Tablet, Chewable	Circle, Flat-Faced, Bevel-Edged	Quality Care
L; 469	Pink Bismuth	262 mg	Pink	Tablet, Chewable	Circle, Flat-Faced, Bevel-Edged	Regal Distributing
L; 469	Pink Bismuth	262 mg	Pink	Tablet, Chewable	Circle, Flat-Faced, Bevel-Edged	Rexall Drug
L; 469	Pink Bismuth	262 mg	Pink	Tablet, Chewable	Circle, Flat-Faced, Bevel-Edged	Sunfresh
L; 469	Pink Bismuth	262 mg	Pink	Tablet, Chewable	Circle, Flat-Faced, Bevel-Edged	Top Care
L; 469	Pink Bismuth	262 mg	Pink	Tablet, Chewable	Circle, Flat-Faced, Bevel-Edged	Valu Rite
L; 469	Stomach Relief	262 mg	Pink	Tablet, Chewable	Circle	Sunmark
L; 469	Stress Tablets	262 mg	Pink	Tablet, Chewable	Circle	Swan
L; 470	Acetaminophen	500 mg	Yellow and White	Capsule, Liquid Filled		First Choice
L; 470	Acetaminophen	500 mg	Yellow and White	Capsule, Liquid Filled		Fleming
L; 470	Acetaminophen	500 mg	Yellow and White	Capsule, Liquid Filled		Glendale Foods
L; 470	Acetaminophen	500 mg	Yellow and White	Capsule, Liquid Filled		Good Sense
L; 470	Acetaminophen	500 mg	Yellow and White	Capsule, Liquid Filled		Great Atlantic & Pacific Tea
L; 470	Acetaminophen	500 mg	Yellow and White	Capsule, Liquid Filled		Legend Pharmaceuticals
L; 470	Acetaminophen	500 mg	Yellow and White	Capsule, Liquid Filled		Major Pharmaceutical
L; 470	Acetaminophen	500 mg	Yellow and White	Capsule, Liquid Filled		Medalist
L; 470	Acetaminophen	500 mg	Yellow and White	Capsule, Liquid Filled		Ms Pharmaceutical
L; 470	Acetaminophen	500 mg	Yellow and White	Capsule, Liquid Filled		Park Lane
L; 470	Acetaminophen	500 mg	Yellow and White	Capsule, Liquid Filled		Perrigo
L; 470	Acetaminophen	500 mg	Yellow and White	Capsule, Liquid Filled		Preferred Products
L; 470	Acetaminophen	500 mg	Yellow and White	Capsule, Liquid Filled		Regal Distributing
L; 470	Acetaminophen	500 mg	Yellow and White	Capsule, Liquid Filled		Seaway
L; 470	Acetaminophen	500 mg	Yellow and White	Capsule, Liquid Filled		Sunfresh
L; 470	Acetaminophen	500 mg	Yellow and White	Capsule, Liquid Filled		Swan
L; 470	Acetaminophen	500 mg	Yellow and White	Capsule, Liquid Filled		Top Care
L; 470	Acetaminophen	500 mg	Yellow and White	Capsule, Liquid Filled		Valu Rite
L; 477	Fiber Laxative	625 mg	Light Brown	Tablet		Perfect Choice
L; 477	Fiber Laxative	625 mg	Light Brown	Tablet		Perrigo
L; 477	Fiber Laxative	625 mg	Light Brown	Tablet		Pharmx
L; 477	Fiber Laxative	625 mg	Light Brown	Tablet		Sunmark
L; 477	Fiber Laxative	625 mg	Light Brown	Tablet		Top Care
L; 477	Fiber Laxative	625 mg	Light Brown	Tablet		Valu Rite
L; 478	Calcium Antacid Regular Strength	200 mg	Yellow, Orange, Red and Green	Tablet, Chewable	Circle, Flat-Faced, Bevel-Edged	Fleming
L; 478	Calcium Antacid Regular Strength	200 mg	Yellow, Orange, Red and Green	Tablet, Chewable	Circle, Flat-Faced, Bevel-Edged	Glendale Foods
L; 478	Calcium Antacid Regular Strength	200 mg	Yellow, Orange, Red and Green	Tablet, Chewable	Circle, Flat-Faced, Bevel-Edged	Good Neighbor Pharmacy
L; 478	Calcium Antacid Regular Strength	200 mg	Yellow, Orange, Red and Green	Tablet, Chewable	Circle, Flat-Faced, Bevel-Edged	Good Sense
L; 478	Calcium Antacid Regular Strength	200 mg	Yellow, Orange, Red and Green	Tablet, Chewable	Circle, Flat-Faced, Bevel-Edged	Hytop
L; 478	Calcium Antacid Regular Strength	200 mg	Yellow, Orange, Red and Green	Tablet, Chewable	Circle, Flat-Faced, Bevel-Edged	Kerr Drug
L; 478	Calcium Antacid Regular Strength	200 mg	Yellow, Orange, Red and Green	Tablet, Chewable	Circle, Flat-Faced, Bevel-Edged	Major Pharmaceutical
L; 478	Calcium Antacid Regular Strength	200 mg	Yellow, Orange, Red and Green	Tablet, Chewable	Circle, Flat-Faced, Bevel-Edged	Major Quality

IMPRINT	BRAND/GENERIC NAME	STRENGTH	COLOR	FORM	SHAPE	MANUFACTURER
L; 478	Calcium Antacid Regular Strength	200 mg	Yellow, Orange, Red and Green	Tablet, Chewable	Circle, Flat-Faced, Bevel-Edged	Medalist
L; 478	Calcium Antacid Regular Strength	200 mg	Yellow, Orange, Red and Green	Tablet, Chewable	Circle, Flat-Faced, Bevel-Edged	Nex
L; 478	Calcium Antacid Regular Strength	200 mg	Yellow, Orange, Red and Green	Tablet, Chewable	Circle, Flat-Faced, Bevel-Edged	Park Lane
L; 478	Calcium Antacid Regular Strength	200 mg	Yellow, Orange, Red and Green	Tablet, Chewable	Circle, Flat-Faced, Bevel-Edged	Perfect Choice
L; 478	Calcium Antacid Regular Strength	200 mg	Yellow, Orange, Red and Green	Tablet, Chewable	Circle, Flat-Faced, Bevel-Edged	Perrigo
L; 478	Calcium Antacid Regular Strength	200 mg	Yellow, Orange, Red and Green	Tablet, Chewable	Circle, Flat-Faced, Bevel-Edged	Preferred Products
L; 478	Calcium Antacid Regular Strength	200 mg	Yellow, Orange, Red and Green	Tablet, Chewable	Circle, Flat-Faced, Bevel-Edged	Quality Care
L; 478	Calcium Antacid Regular Strength	200 mg	Yellow, Orange, Red and Green	Tablet, Chewable	Circle, Flat-Faced, Bevel-Edged	Regal Distributing
L; 478	Calcium Antacid Regular Strength	200 mg	Yellow, Orange, Red and Green	Tablet, Chewable	Circle, Flat-Faced, Bevel-Edged	Revco
L; 478	Calcium Antacid Regular Strength	200 mg	Yellow, Orange, Red and Green	Tablet, Chewable	Circle, Flat-Faced, Bevel-Edged	Rexall Drug
L; 478	Calcium Antacid Regular Strength	200 mg	Yellow, Orange, Red and Green	Tablet, Chewable	Circle, Flat-Faced, Bevel-Edged	Sunfresh
L; 478	Calcium Antacid Regular Strength	200 mg	Yellow, Orange, Red and Green	Tablet, Chewable	Circle, Flat-Faced, Bevel-Edged	Sunmark
L; 478	Calcium Antacid Regular Strength	200 mg	Yellow, Orange, Red and Green	Tablet, Chewable	Circle, Flat-Faced, Bevel-Edged	Swan
L; 478	Calcium Antacid Regular Strength	200 mg	Yellow, Orange, Red and Green	Tablet, Chewable	Circle, Flat-Faced, Bevel-Edged	Top Care
L; 478	Calcium Antacid Regular Strength	200 mg	Yellow, Orange, Red and Green	Tablet, Chewable	Circle, Flat-Faced, Bevel-Edged	True Quality
L; 478	Calcium Antacid Regular Strength	200 mg	Yellow, Orange, Red and Green	Tablet, Chewable	Circle, Flat-Faced, Bevel-Edged	Unilab
L; 478	Calcium Antacid Regular Strength	200 mg	Yellow, Orange, Red and Green	Tablet, Chewable	Circle, Flat-Faced, Bevel-Edged	United Drugs
L; 478	Calcium Antacid Regular Strength	200 mg	Yellow, Orange, Red and Green	Tablet, Chewable	Circle, Flat-Faced, Bevel-Edged	Valu Buy
L; 478	Calcium Antacid Regular Strength	200 mg	Yellow, Orange, Red and Green	Tablet, Chewable	Circle, Flat-Faced, Bevel-Edged	Valu Rite
L; 479	Allergy Medicine	25 mg	Dark Pink	Tablet	Capsule-Shape	Top Care
L; 479	Antihistamine	25 mg		Tablet		Medalist
L; 479	Antihistamine	25 mg		Tablet		Perrigo
L; 479	Antihistamine Allergy Relief	25 mg		Tablet		Good Sense
L; 479	Antihistamine Allergy Relief	25 mg		Tablet		Perrigo
L; 479	Diphedryl Allergy	25 mg	Dark Pink	Tablet	Capsule-Shape	Good Neighbor Pharmacy
L; 479	Diphedryl Allergy	25 mg	Dark Pink	Tablet	Capsule-Shape	Good Sense
L; 479	Diphedryl Allergy	25 mg	Dark Pink	Tablet	Capsule-Shape	Harco Drug
L; 479	Diphedryl Allergy	25 mg	Dark Pink	Tablet	Capsule-Shape	Hytop
L; 479	Diphedryl Allergy	25 mg	Dark Pink	Tablet	Capsule-Shape	Major
L; 479	Diphedryl Allergy	25 mg	Dark Pink	Tablet	Capsule-Shape	Major Quality
L; 479	Diphedryl Allergy	25 mg	Dark Pink	Tablet	Capsule-Shape	Medic
L; 479	Diphedryl Allergy	25 mg	Dark Pink	Tablet	Capsule-Shape	Park Lane
L; 479	Diphedryl Allergy	25 mg	Dark Pink	Tablet	Capsule-Shape	Perrigo
L; 479	Diphedryl Allergy	25 mg	Dark Pink	Tablet	Capsule-Shape	Pharm X
L; 479	Diphedryl Allergy	25 mg	Dark Pink	Tablet	Capsule-Shape	Rexall
L; 479	Diphedryl Allergy	25 mg	Dark Pink	Tablet	Capsule-Shape	Sunfresh
L; 479	Diphedryl Allergy	25 mg	Dark Pink	Tablet	Capsule-Shape	Top Care
L; 479	Diphedryl Allergy	25 mg	Dark Pink	Tablet	Capsule-Shape	True Quality
L; 479	Valu-Dryl	25 mg	Dark Pink	Tablet	Oval, Small	Valu Rite
L; 480	Sinus Maximum Strength	500 mg; 2 mg; 30 mg	Yellow	Tablet	Oval	Good Neighbor Pharmacy
L; 480	Sinus Maximum Strength	500 mg; 2 mg; 30 mg	Yellow	Tablet	Oval	Good Sense
L; 480	Sinus Maximum Strength	500 mg; 2 mg; 30 mg	Yellow	Tablet	Oval	Nex
L; 480	Sinus Maximum Strength	500 mg; 2 mg; 30 mg	Yellow	Tablet	Oval	Park Lane
L; 480	Sinus Maximum Strength	500 mg; 2 mg; 30 mg	Yellow	Tablet	Oval	Perrigo
L; 480	Sinus Maximum Strength	500 mg; 2 mg; 30 mg	Yellow	Tablet	Oval	Regal Distributing
L; 481	Children's Pain Reliever Grape Flavor	80 mg	Mottled Lavender	Tablet, Chewable	Round, Flat-Faced, Bevel-Edged, Bisected Scored	Fleming
L; 481	Children's Pain Reliever Grape Flavor	80 mg	Mottled Lavender	Tablet, Chewable	Round, Flat-Faced, Bevel-Edged, Bisected Scored	Glendale Foods
L; 481	Children's Pain Reliever Grape Flavor	80 mg	Mottled Lavender	Tablet, Chewable	Round, Flat-Faced, Bevel-Edged, Bisected Scored	Good Neighbor Pharmacy
L; 481	Children's Pain Reliever Grape Flavor	80 mg	Mottled Lavender	Tablet, Chewable	Round, Flat-Faced, Bevel-Edged, Bisected Scored	Good Sense
L; 481	Children's Pain Reliever Grape Flavor	80 mg	Mottled Lavender	Tablet, Chewable	Round, Flat-Faced, Bevel-Edged, Bisected Scored	Harco Drug
L; 481	Children's Pain Reliever Grape Flavor	80 mg	Mottled Lavender	Tablet, Chewable	Round, Flat-Faced, Bevel-Edged, Bisected Scored	Hytop
L; 481	Children's Pain Reliever Grape Flavor	80 mg	Mottled Lavender	Tablet, Chewable	Round, Flat-Faced, Bevel-Edged, Bisected Scored	Major
L; 481	Children's Pain Reliever Grape Flavor	80 mg	Mottled Lavender	Tablet, Chewable	Round, Flat-Faced, Bevel-Edged, Bisected Scored	Medalist
L; 481	Children's Pain Reliever Grape Flavor	80 mg	Mottled Lavender	Tablet, Chewable	Round, Flat-Faced, Bevel-Edged, Bisected Scored	Medic

IMPRINT	BRAND/GENERIC NAME	STRENGTH	COLOR	FORM	SHAPE	MANUFACTURER
L; 481	Children's Pain Reliever Grape Flavor	80 mg	Mottled Lavender	Tablet, Chewable	Round, Flat-Faced, Bevel-Edged, Bisected Scored	Nex
L; 481	Children's Pain Reliever Grape Flavor	80 mg	Mottled Lavender	Tablet, Chewable	Round, Flat-Faced, Bevel-Edged, Bisected Scored	Park Lane
L; 481	Children's Pain Reliever Grape Flavor	80 mg	Mottled Lavender	Tablet, Chewable	Round, Flat-Faced, Bevel-Edged, Bisected Scored	Perfect Choice
L; 481	Children's Pain Reliever Grape Flavor	80 mg	Mottled Lavender	Tablet, Chewable	Round, Flat-Faced, Bevel-Edged, Bisected Scored	Perrigo
L; 481	Children's Pain Reliever Grape Flavor	80 mg	Mottled Lavender	Tablet, Chewable	Round, Flat-Faced, Bevel-Edged, Bisected Scored	Quality Care
L; 481	Children's Pain Reliever Grape Flavor	80 mg	Mottled Lavender	Tablet, Chewable	Round, Flat-Faced, Bevel-Edged, Bisected Scored	Regal Distributing
L; 481	Children's Pain Reliever Grape Flavor	80 mg	Mottled Lavender	Tablet, Chewable	Round, Flat-Faced, Bevel-Edged, Bisected Scored	Revco
L; 481	Children's Pain Reliever Grape Flavor	80 mg	Mottled Lavender	Tablet, Chewable	Round, Flat-Faced, Bevel-Edged, Bisected Scored	Rexall
L; 481	Children's Pain Reliever Grape Flavor	80 mg	Mottled Lavender	Tablet, Chewable	Round, Flat-Faced, Bevel-Edged, Bisected Scored	Rockbottom Stores
L; 481	Children's Pain Reliever Grape Flavor	80 mg	Mottled Lavender	Tablet, Chewable	Round, Flat-Faced, Bevel-Edged, Bisected Scored	Seaway
L; 481	Children's Pain Reliever Grape Flavor	80 mg	Mottled Lavender	Tablet, Chewable	Round, Flat-Faced, Bevel-Edged, Bisected Scored	Sunfresh
L; 481	Children's Pain Reliever Grape Flavor	80 mg	Mottled Lavender	Tablet, Chewable	Round, Flat-Faced, Bevel-Edged, Bisected Scored	Swan
L; 481	Children's Pain Reliever Grape Flavor	80 mg	Mottled Lavender	Tablet, Chewable	Round, Flat-Faced, Bevel-Edged, Bisected Scored	Top Care
L; 481	Children's Pain Reliever Grape Flavor	80 mg	Mottled Lavender	Tablet, Chewable	Round, Flat-Faced, Bevel-Edged, Bisected Scored	True Quality
L; 481	Children's Pain Reliever Grape Flavor	80 mg	Mottled Lavender	Tablet, Chewable	Round, Flat-Faced, Bevel-Edged, Bisected Scored	United Drugs
L; 481	Children's Pain Reliever Grape Flavor	80 mg	Mottled Lavender	Tablet, Chewable	Round, Flat-Faced, Bevel-Edged, Bisected Scored	Valu Rite
L; 481	Pain Reliever Children's	80 mg	Mottled Lavender	Tablet, Chewable	Round, Flat-Faced, Bevel-Edged, Bisected Scored	Sunmark
L; 484	Extra Strength Non-Aspirin Acetaminophen	500 mg	White	Tablet	Oblong	Valu Rite
L; 484	Extra Strength Pain Reliever	500 mg	White	Tablet	Oblong	First Choice
L; 484	Extra Strength Pain Reliever	500 mg	White	Tablet	Oblong	Genovese
L; 484	Extra Strength Pain Reliever	500 mg	White	Tablet	Oblong	Glendale Foods
L; 484	Extra Strength Pain Reliever	500 mg	White	Tablet	Oblong	Good Neighbor Pharmacy
L; 484	Extra Strength Pain Reliever	500 mg	White	Tablet	Oblong	Good Sense
L; 484	Extra Strength Pain Reliever	500 mg	White	Tablet	Oblong	Hytop
L; 484	Extra Strength Pain Reliever	500 mg	White	Tablet	Oblong	Major
L; 484	Extra Strength Pain Reliever	500 mg	White	Tablet	Oblong	Major Quality
L; 484	Extra Strength Pain Reliever	500 mg	White	Tablet	Oblong	Medic
L; 484	Extra Strength Pain Reliever	500 mg	White	Tablet	Oblong	Mediguard
L; 484	Extra Strength Pain Reliever	500 mg	White	Tablet	Oblong	Nex
L; 484	Extra Strength Pain Reliever	500 mg	White	Tablet	Oblong	Park Lane
L; 484	Extra Strength Pain Reliever	500 mg	White	Tablet	Oblong	Perfect Choice
L; 484	Extra Strength Pain Reliever	500 mg	White	Tablet	Oblong	Perrigo
L; 484	Extra Strength Pain Reliever	500 mg	White	Tablet	Oblong	Pharm X
L; 484	Extra Strength Pain Reliever	500 mg	White	Tablet	Oblong	Quality Care
L; 484	Extra Strength Pain Reliever	500 mg	White	Tablet	Oblong	Regal Distributing
L; 484	Extra Strength Pain Reliever	500 mg	White	Tablet	Oblong	Rexall
L; 484	Extra Strength Pain Reliever	500 mg	White	Tablet	Oblong	Seaway
L; 484	Extra Strength Pain Reliever	500 mg	White	Tablet	Oblong	Top Care
L; 484	Extra Strength Pain Reliever	500 mg	White	Tablet	Oblong	Valu Buy
L; 484	Pain Reliever Extra Strength	500 mg	White	Tablet	Oblong	Sunmark
L; 485	Calcium Antacid Regular Strength	200 mg	White	Tablet, Chewable	Circle	Glendale Foods
L; 485	Calcium Antacid Regular Strength	200 mg	White	Tablet, Chewable	Circle	Good Neighbor Pharmacy
L; 485	Calcium Antacid Regular Strength	200 mg	White	Tablet, Chewable	Circle	Good Sense
L; 485	Calcium Antacid Regular Strength	200 mg	White	Tablet, Chewable	Circle	Kerr Drug
L; 485	Calcium Antacid Regular Strength	200 mg	White	Tablet, Chewable	Circle	Major
L; 485	Calcium Antacid Regular Strength	200 mg	White	Tablet, Chewable	Circle	Major Pharmaceutical
L; 485	Calcium Antacid Regular Strength	200 mg	White	Tablet, Chewable	Circle	Major Quality
L; 485	Calcium Antacid Regular Strength	200 mg	White	Tablet, Chewable	Circle	Perrigo
L; 485	Calcium Antacid Regular Strength	200 mg	White	Tablet, Chewable	Circle	Preferred Products
L; 485	Calcium Antacid Regular Strength	200 mg	White	Tablet, Chewable	Circle	Regal Distributing
L; 485	Calcium Antacid Regular Strength	200 mg	White	Tablet, Chewable	Circle	Revco
L; 485	Calcium Antacid Regular Strength	200 mg	White	Tablet, Chewable	Circle	Sunmark
L; 485	Calcium Antacid Regular Strength	200 mg	White	Tablet, Chewable	Circle	Top Care
L; 485	Calcium Antacid Regular Strength	200 mg	White	Tablet, Chewable	Circle	Unilab
L; 485	Calcium Antacid Regular Strength	200 mg	White	Tablet, Chewable	Circle	Valu Rite
L; 486	Stool Softener	100 mg	Red and White	Capsule, Liquid Filled	Oval	Good Sense
L; 486	Stool Softener	100 mg	Red and White	Capsule, Liquid Filled	Oval	Kerr Drug
L; 486	Stool Softener	100 mg	Red and White	Capsule, Liquid Filled	Oval	Perrigo
L; 486	Stool Softener	100 mg	Red and White	Capsule, Liquid Filled	Oval	Top Care
L; 489	Calcium Antacid Extra Strength Assorted Berries	600 mg	Red and Purple	Tablet, Chewable	Circle	Good Sense
L; 489	Calcium Antacid Extra Strength Assorted Berries	600 mg	Red and Purple	Tablet, Chewable	Circle	Major
L; 489	Calcium Antacid Extra Strength Assorted Berries	600 mg	Red and Purple	Tablet, Chewable	Circle	Pharmx
L; 489	Calcium Antacid Extra Strength Assorted Berries	600 mg	Red and Purple	Tablet, Chewable	Circle	Sunmark
L; 489	Calcium Antacid Extra Strength Assorted Berries	600 mg	Red and Purple	Tablet, Chewable	Circle	Top Care
L; 489	Extra Strength Antacid Assorted Berries	600 mg	Red and Purple	Tablet, Chewable	Circle	Perfect Choice

IMPRINT	BRAND/GENERIC NAME	STRENGTH	COLOR	FORM	SHAPE	MANUFACTURER
L; 490	Naproxen Sodium	220 mg	Light Blue	Tablet	Circle	Good Neighbor Pharmacy
L; 490	Naproxen Sodium	220 mg	Light Blue	Tablet	Circle	Major
L; 490	Naproxen Sodium	220 mg	Light Blue	Tablet	Circle	Medic
L; 490	Naproxen Sodium	220 mg	Light Blue	Tablet	Circle	Perrigo
L; 490	Naproxen Sodium	220 mg	Light Blue	Tablet	Circle	Pharm X
L; 490	Naproxen Sodium	220 mg	Light Blue	Tablet	Circle	Top Care
L; 490	Naproxen Sodium	220 mg	Light Blue	Tablet	Circle	Valu Rite
L; 492	Children's Pain Reliever Mixed Fruit Flavored	80 mg	Mottled Pink	Tablet, Chewable	Circle, Scored	First Choice
L; 492	Children's Pain Reliever Mixed Fruit Flavored	80 mg	Mottled Pink	Tablet, Chewable	Circle, Scored	Fleming
L; 492	Children's Pain Reliever Mixed Fruit Flavored	80 mg	Mottled Pink	Tablet, Chewable	Circle, Scored	Glendale Foods
L; 492	Children's Pain Reliever Mixed Fruit Flavored	80 mg	Mottled Pink	Tablet, Chewable	Circle, Scored	Good Neighbor Pharmacy
L; 492	Children's Pain Reliever Mixed Fruit Flavored	80 mg	Mottled Pink	Tablet, Chewable	Circle, Scored	Good Sense
L; 492	Children's Pain Reliever Mixed Fruit Flavored	80 mg	Mottled Pink	Tablet, Chewable	Circle, Scored	Hytop
L; 492	Children's Pain Reliever Mixed Fruit Flavored	80 mg	Mottled Pink	Tablet, Chewable	Circle, Scored	Legend Pharmaceuticals
L; 492	Children's Pain Reliever Mixed Fruit Flavored	80 mg	Mottled Pink	Tablet, Chewable	Circle, Scored	Major
L; 492	Children's Pain Reliever Mixed Fruit Flavored	80 mg	Mottled Pink	Tablet, Chewable	Circle, Scored	Major Quality
L; 492	Children's Pain Reliever Mixed Fruit Flavored	80 mg	Mottled Pink	Tablet, Chewable	Circle, Scored	Medalist
L; 492	Children's Pain Reliever Mixed Fruit Flavored	80 mg	Mottled Pink	Tablet, Chewable	Circle, Scored	Medic
L; 492	Children's Pain Reliever Mixed Fruit Flavored	80 mg	Mottled Pink	Tablet, Chewable	Circle, Scored	Ms Pharmaceutical
L; 492	Children's Pain Reliever Mixed Fruit Flavored	80 mg	Mottled Pink	Tablet, Chewable	Circle, Scored	Nex
L; 492	Children's Pain Reliever Mixed Fruit Flavored	80 mg	Mottled Pink	Tablet, Chewable	Circle, Scored	Our Choice
L; 492	Children's Pain Reliever Mixed Fruit Flavored	80 mg	Mottled Pink	Tablet, Chewable	Circle, Scored	Park Lane
L; 492	Children's Pain Reliever Mixed Fruit Flavored	80 mg	Mottled Pink	Tablet, Chewable	Circle, Scored	Perfect Choice
L; 492	Children's Pain Reliever Mixed Fruit Flavored	80 mg	Mottled Pink	Tablet, Chewable	Circle, Scored	Perrigo
L; 492	Children's Pain Reliever Mixed Fruit Flavored	80 mg	Mottled Pink	Tablet, Chewable	Circle, Scored	Preferred Products
L; 492	Children's Pain Reliever Mixed Fruit Flavored	80 mg	Mottled Pink	Tablet, Chewable	Circle, Scored	Quality Care
L; 492	Children's Pain Reliever Mixed Fruit Flavored	80 mg	Mottled Pink	Tablet, Chewable	Circle, Scored	Regal Distributing
L; 492	Children's Pain Reliever Mixed Fruit Flavored	80 mg	Mottled Pink	Tablet, Chewable	Circle, Scored	Rexall
L; 492	Children's Pain Reliever Mixed Fruit Flavored	80 mg	Mottled Pink	Tablet, Chewable	Circle, Scored	Seaway
L; 492	Children's Pain Reliever Mixed Fruit Flavored	80 mg	Mottled Pink	Tablet, Chewable	Circle, Scored	Sunfresh
L; 492	Children's Pain Reliever Mixed Fruit Flavored	80 mg	Mottled Pink	Tablet, Chewable	Circle, Scored	Swan
L; 492	Children's Pain Reliever Mixed Fruit Flavored	80 mg	Mottled Pink	Tablet, Chewable	Circle, Scored	Top Care
L; 492	Children's Pain Reliever Mixed Fruit Flavored	80 mg	Mottled Pink	Tablet, Chewable	Circle, Scored	United Drugs
L; 492	Children's Pain Reliever Mixed Fruit Flavored	80 mg	Mottled Pink	Tablet, Chewable	Circle, Scored	Valu Buy
L; 492	Children's Pain Reliever Mixed Fruit Flavored	80 mg	Mottled Pink	Tablet, Chewable	Circle, Scored	Valu Rite
L; 495	Laxative and Stool Softener	30 mg; 100 mg	Dark Red	Capsule, Liquid Filled	Oval	Good Neighbor Pharmacy
L; 495	Laxative and Stool Softener	30 mg; 100 mg	Dark Red	Capsule, Liquid Filled	Oval	Good Sense
L; 495	Laxative and Stool Softener	30 mg; 100 mg	Dark Red	Capsule, Liquid Filled	Oval	Kerr Drug
L; 495	Laxative and Stool Softener	30 mg; 100 mg	Dark Red	Capsule, Liquid Filled	Oval	Perrigo
L; 503	Nite Time Cold Formula	250 mg; 15 mg; 30 mg; 25 mg		Capsule, Liquid Filled		Top Care
L; 524	Sinus without Drowsiness Regular Strength	325 mg; 30 mg	Pink and White	Tablet	Round, Concave Punch, Bisected Scored	Genovese
L; 524	Sinus without Drowsiness Regular Strength	325 mg; 30 mg	Pink and White	Tablet	Round, Concave Punch, Bisected Scored	Good Neighbor Pharmacy
L; 524	Sinus without Drowsiness Regular Strength	325 mg; 30 mg	Pink and White	Tablet	Round, Concave Punch, Bisected Scored	Good Sense
L; 524	Sinus without Drowsiness Regular Strength	325 mg; 30 mg	Pink and White	Tablet	Round, Concave Punch, Bisected Scored	Hytop
L; 524	Sinus without Drowsiness Regular Strength	325 mg; 30 mg	Pink and White	Tablet	Round, Concave Punch, Bisected Scored	Major
L; 524	Sinus without Drowsiness Regular Strength	325 mg; 30 mg	Pink and White	Tablet	Round, Concave Punch, Bisected Scored	Major Quality
L; 524	Sinus without Drowsiness Regular Strength	325 mg; 30 mg	Pink and White	Tablet	Round, Concave Punch, Bisected Scored	Perrigo
L; 524	Sinus without Drowsiness Regular Strength	325 mg; 30 mg	Pink and White	Tablet	Round, Concave Punch, Bisected Scored	Revco
L; 524	Sinus without Drowsiness Regular Strength	325 mg; 30 mg	Pink and White	Tablet	Round, Concave Punch, Bisected Scored	Rexall
L; 524	Sinus without Drowsiness Regular Strength	325 mg; 30 mg	Pink and White	Tablet	Round, Concave Punch, Bisected Scored	Seaway

IMPRINT	BRAND/GENERIC NAME	STRENGTH	COLOR	FORM	SHAPE	MANUFACTURER
L; 524	Sinus without Drowsiness Regular Strength	325 mg; 30 mg	Pink and White	Tablet	Round, Concave Punch, Bisected Scored	Top Care
L; 525	Cold and Cough Maximum Strength	500 mg; 15 mg; 2 mg; 30 mg	Yellow	Coated Tablet	Circle	Sunmark
L; 525	Complete Maximum Strength	500 mg; 15 mg; 2 mg; 30 mg	Yellow	Coated Tablet	Circle	Good Neighbor Pharmacy
L; 525	Complete Maximum Strength	500 mg; 15 mg; 2 mg; 30 mg	Yellow	Coated Tablet	Circle	Valu Rite
L; 525	Multi-Symptom Cold Relief Maximum Strength	500 mg; 15 mg; 2 mg; 30 mg	Yellow	Coated Tablet	Circle	Hytop
L; 525	Multi-Symptom Cold Relief Maximum Strength	500 mg; 15 mg; 2 mg; 30 mg	Yellow	Coated Tablet	Circle	Kerr Drug
L; 525	Multi-Symptom Cold Relief Maximum Strength	500 mg; 15 mg; 2 mg; 30 mg	Yellow	Coated Tablet	Circle	Major
L; 525	Multi-Symptom Cold Relief Maximum Strength	500 mg; 15 mg; 2 mg; 30 mg	Yellow	Coated Tablet	Circle	Nex
L; 525	Multi-Symptom Cold Relief Maximum Strength	500 mg; 15 mg; 2 mg; 30 mg	Yellow	Coated Tablet	Circle	Perrigo
L; 527	Acid Relief Original Flavor	550 mg; 110 mg		Tablet, Chewable		Hytop
L; 527	Acid Relief Original Flavor	550 mg; 110 mg		Tablet, Chewable		Kerr Drug
L; 528	Antacid Extra Strength Wintergreen	750 mg	Green	Tablet, Chewable	Circle	Good Sense
L; 528	Antacid Extra Strength Wintergreen	750 mg	Green	Tablet, Chewable	Circle	Kerr Drug
L; 528	Antacid Extra Strength Wintergreen	750 mg	Green	Tablet, Chewable	Circle	Life
L; 528	Antacid Extra Strength Wintergreen	750 mg	Green	Tablet, Chewable	Circle	Perrigo
L; 528	Antacid Extra Strength Wintergreen	750 mg	Green	Tablet, Chewable	Circle	Top Care
L; 530	All-Nite Cold Medicine	250 mg; 15 mg; 30 mg; 25 mg		Capsule, Liquid Filled		Major Pharmaceutical
L; 530	All-Nite Cold Medicine	250 mg; 15 mg; 30 mg; 25 mg		Capsule, Liquid Filled		Major Quality
L; 530	Cold Caps Severe Cold and Flu	500 mg; 2 mg; 15 mg; 30 mg	Light Blue	Tablet		Good Sense
L; 530	Cold Caps Severe Cold and Flu	500 mg; 2 mg; 15 mg; 30 mg	Light Blue	Tablet		Pharmx
L; 530	Cold Caps Severe Cold and Flu	500 mg; 2 mg; 15 mg; 30 mg	Light Blue	Tablet		Valu Rite
L; 530	Maximum Strength Cold Severe Cold and Flu	500 mg; 2 mg; 15 mg; 30 mg	Light Blue	Tablet		Perfect Choice
L; 530	Maximum Strength Cold Severe Cold and Flu	500 mg; 2 mg; 15 mg; 30 mg	Light Blue	Tablet		Top Care
L; 530	Nite Time	250 mg; 15 mg; 30 mg; 25 mg		Capsule		Glendale Foods
L; 530	Nite Time	250 mg; 15 mg; 30 mg; 25 mg		Capsule		Good Neighbor Pharmacy
L; 530	Nite Time	250 mg; 15 mg; 30 mg; 25 mg		Capsule		Good Sense
L; 530	Nite Time	250 mg; 15 mg; 30 mg; 25 mg		Capsule		Kerr Drug
L; 530	Nite Time	250 mg; 15 mg; 30 mg; 25 mg		Capsule		Park Lane
L; 530	Nite Time	250 mg; 15 mg; 30 mg; 25 mg		Capsule		Perrigo
L; 530	Nite Time	250 mg; 15 mg; 30 mg; 25 mg		Capsule		Preferred Products
L; 530	Nite Time	250 mg; 15 mg; 30 mg; 25 mg		Capsule		Regal Distributing
L; 530	Nite Time	250 mg; 15 mg; 30 mg; 25 mg		Capsule		Swan
L; 530	Nite Time	250 mg; 15 mg; 30 mg; 25 mg		Capsule		True Quality
L; 530	Nite Time	250 mg; 15 mg; 30 mg; 25 mg		Capsule		Valu Rite
L; 530	Severe Cold and Flu Maximum Strength	500 mg; 2 mg; 15 mg; 30 mg	Light Blue	Tablet		Good Neighbor Pharmacy
L; 530	Severe Cold and Flu Maximum Strength	500 mg; 2 mg; 15 mg; 30 mg	Light Blue	Tablet		Good Sense
L; 531	Calcium Antacid Ultra Strength Assorted Mint	1000 mg	White or Green	Tablet, Chewable	Circle	Major
L; 531	Calcium Antacid Ultra Strength Assorted Mint	1000 mg	White or Green	Tablet, Chewable	Circle	Swan
L; 531	Calcium Antacid Ultra Strength Assorted Mint	1000 mg	White or Green	Tablet, Chewable	Circle	Top Care
L; 535	Aspirin 81 mg	81 mg	Yellow	Enteric-Coated Tablet	Circle	Medic
L; 535	Aspirin Adult Low Strength	81 mg	Yellow	Enteric-Coated Tablet	Circle	Good Neighbor Pharmacy
L; 535	Aspirin Adult Low Strength	81 mg	Yellow	Enteric-Coated Tablet	Circle	Good Sense
L; 535	Aspirin Adult Low Strength	81 mg	Yellow	Enteric-Coated Tablet	Circle	Hytop
L; 535	Aspirin Adult Low Strength	81 mg	Yellow	Enteric-Coated Tablet	Circle	Perrigo
L; 535	Aspirin Adult Low Strength	81 mg	Yellow	Enteric-Coated Tablet	Circle	Valu Rite
L; 535;	Aspirin Adult Low Strength	81 mg	Yellow	Delayed-Release Tablet	Circle, Enteric-Coated	Good Neighbor Pharmacy
L; 535;	Aspirin Adult Low Strength	81 mg	Yellow	Delayed-Release Tablet	Circle, Enteric-Coated	Perfect Choice
L; 535;	Aspirin Adult Low Strength	81 mg	Yellow	Delayed-Release Tablet	Circle, Enteric-Coated	Sunmark
L; 535;	Aspirin Adult Low Strength	81 mg	Yellow	Delayed-Release Tablet	Circle, Enteric-Coated	Valu Rite
L; 544	Arthritis Pain Relief Temporary Minor	650 mg	White	Tablet		Good Sense

IMPRINT	BRAND/GENERIC NAME	STRENGTH	COLOR	FORM	SHAPE	MANUFACTURER
L; 544	Arthritis Pain Relief Temporary Minor	650 mg	White	Tablet		Perfect Choice
L; 562	Cough & Cold Multi-Symptom	250 mg; 10 mg; 30 mg; 100 mg	Orange	Capsule, Liquid Filled		Sunmark
L; 562	Multi-Symptom Pseudoephedrine Cold and Cough	250 mg; 10 mg; 30 mg; 100 mg	Orange	Capsule, Liquid Filled	Oval	Good Sense
L; 562	Multi-Symptom Pseudoephedrine Cold and Cough	250 mg; 10 mg; 30 mg; 100 mg	Orange	Capsule, Liquid Filled	Oval	Rockbottom Stores
L; 562;	Day Time Liquid Caps Multi-Symptom Cold & Flu Relief	250 mg; 10 mg; 30 mg; 100 mg	Orange	Capsule, Liquid Filled	Oblong	Fleming
L; 562;	Day Time Liquid Caps Multi-Symptom Cold & Flu Relief	250 mg; 10 mg; 30 mg; 100 mg	Orange	Capsule, Liquid Filled	Oblong	Glendale Foods
L; 562;	Day Time Liquid Caps Multi-Symptom Cold & Flu Relief	250 mg; 10 mg; 30 mg; 100 mg	Orange	Capsule, Liquid Filled	Oblong	Good Neighbor Pharmacy
L; 562;	Day Time Liquid Caps Multi-Symptom Cold & Flu Relief	250 mg; 10 mg; 30 mg; 100 mg	Orange	Capsule, Liquid Filled	Oblong	Good Sense
L; 562;	Day Time Liquid Caps Multi-Symptom Cold & Flu Relief	250 mg; 10 mg; 30 mg; 100 mg	Orange	Capsule, Liquid Filled	Oblong	Kerr Drug
L; 562;	Day Time Liquid Caps Multi-Symptom Cold & Flu Relief	250 mg; 10 mg; 30 mg; 100 mg	Orange	Capsule, Liquid Filled	Oblong	Major
L; 562;	Day Time Liquid Caps Multi-Symptom Cold & Flu Relief	250 mg; 10 mg; 30 mg; 100 mg	Orange	Capsule, Liquid Filled	Oblong	Nex
L; 562;	Day Time Liquid Caps Multi-Symptom Cold & Flu Relief	250 mg; 10 mg; 30 mg; 100 mg	Orange	Capsule, Liquid Filled	Oblong	Perrigo
L; 562;	Day Time Liquid Caps Multi-Symptom Cold & Flu Relief	250 mg; 10 mg; 30 mg; 100 mg	Orange	Capsule, Liquid Filled	Oblong	Preferred Products
L; 562;	Day Time Liquid Caps Multi-Symptom Cold & Flu Relief	250 mg; 10 mg; 30 mg; 100 mg	Orange	Capsule, Liquid Filled	Oblong	Quality Care
L; 562;	Day Time Liquid Caps Multi-Symptom Cold & Flu Relief	250 mg; 10 mg; 30 mg; 100 mg	Orange	Capsule, Liquid Filled	Oblong	Revco
L; 562;	Day Time Liquid Caps Multi-Symptom Cold & Flu Relief	250 mg; 10 mg; 30 mg; 100 mg	Orange	Capsule, Liquid Filled	Oblong	Top Care
L 562	Multi-Symptom Suphedrin	250 mg; 10 mg; 30 mg; 100 mg	Orange	Capsule, Liquid Filled	Oval	Good Neighbor Pharmacy
L; 576	Non-Aspirin Cold	325 mg; 15 mg; 30 mg	Light Pink	Tablet	Capsule-Shape	Genco Distributors
L; 576	Non-Aspirin Cold	325 mg; 15 mg; 30 mg	Light Pink	Tablet	Capsule-Shape	Perrigo
L; 582	Aspirin	325 mg	White	Tablet	Capsule-Shaped, Bisected Scored	Perrigo
L; 595	Calcium Antacid Ultra Strength Assorted Fruit	1000 mg	Assorted	Tablet, Chewable	Circle	Kerr Drug
L; 595	Calcium Antacid Ultra Strength Assorted Fruit	1000 mg	Assorted	Tablet, Chewable	Circle	Major
L; 595	Calcium Antacid Ultra Strength Assorted Fruit	1000 mg	Assorted	Tablet, Chewable	Circle	Perrigo
L; 595	Calcium Antacid Ultra Strength Assorted Fruit	1000 mg	Assorted	Tablet, Chewable	Circle	Sunmark
L; 595	Calcium Antacid Ultra Strength Assorted Fruit	1000 mg	Assorted	Tablet, Chewable	Circle	Top Care
L; 595	Calcium Antacid Ultra Strength Assorted Fruit	1000 mg	Assorted	Tablet, Chewable	Circle	Valu Rite
L; 596	Pseudoephedrine Severe Cold Formula	500 mg; 15 mg; 30 mg	White	Tablet	Circle	Good Neighbor Pharmacy
L; 596	Pseudoephedrine Severe Cold Formula	500 mg; 15 mg; 30 mg	White	Tablet	Circle	Perrigo
L; 596	Pseudoephedrine Severe Cold Formula	500 mg; 15 mg; 30 mg	White	Tablet	Circle	Valu Rite
L; 596	Suphedrine Severe Cold Formula Maximum Strength	500 mg; 15 mg; 30 mg	White	Tablet	Capsule-Shape	Perrigo
L; 596	Suphedrine Severe Cold Formula Maximum Strength	500 mg; 15 mg; 30 mg	White	Tablet	Capsule-Shape	Valu Rite
L; 615	Woman's Laxative Gentle	100 mg	Red	Capsule, Liquid Filled		Perrigo
L; 615	Woman's Laxative Gentle	100 mg	Red	Capsule, Liquid Filled		Top Care
L; 615	Woman's Laxative Gentle	100 mg	Red	Capsule, Liquid Filled		Valu Rite
L; 617; 75	Acid Reducer	75 mg	Pink	Tablet	Circle	Valu Rite
L; 617; 75	Heartburn Relief	75 mg	Pink	Tablet	Circle	Good Sense
L; 617; 75	Heartburn Relief	75 mg	Pink	Tablet	Circle	Perfect Choice
L; 617; 75	Ranitidine	75 mg	Pink	Tablet	Circle	Good Neighbor Pharmacy
L; 617; 75	Ranitidine	75 mg	Pink	Tablet	Circle	Good Sense
L; 617; 75	Ranitidine	75 mg	Pink	Tablet	Circle	Major
L; 617; 75	Ranitidine	75 mg	Pink	Tablet	Circle	Top Care
L; 617; 75	Ranitidine	75 mg	Pink	Tablet	Circle	Valu Rite
L; 642	Buffered Aspirin	325 mg;	White	Coated Tablet	Circle, Biconvex, Two-Layered	Exel
L; 642	Buffered Aspirin	325 mg;	White	Coated Tablet	Circle, Biconvex, Two-Layered	First Choice
L; 642	Buffered Aspirin	325 mg;	White	Coated Tablet	Circle, Biconvex, Two-Layered	Fleming
L; 642	Buffered Aspirin	325 mg;	White	Coated Tablet	Circle, Biconvex, Two-Layered	Genovese
L; 642	Buffered Aspirin	325 mg;	White	Coated Tablet	Circle, Biconvex, Two-Layered	Good Neighbor Pharmacy
L; 642	Buffered Aspirin	325 mg;	White	Coated Tablet	Circle, Biconvex, Two-Layered	Good Sense
L; 642	Buffered Aspirin	325 mg;	White	Coated Tablet	Circle, Biconvex, Two-Layered	Hytop
L; 642	Buffered Aspirin	325 mg;	White	Coated Tablet	Circle, Biconvex, Two-Layered	Kerr Drug
L; 642	Buffered Aspirin	325 mg;	White	Coated Tablet	Circle, Biconvex, Two-Layered	Major
L; 642	Buffered Aspirin	325 mg;	White	Coated Tablet	Circle, Biconvex, Two-Layered	Major Quality
L; 642	Buffered Aspirin	325 mg;	White	Coated Tablet	Circle, Biconvex, Two-Layered	Medic
L; 642	Buffered Aspirin	325 mg;	White	Coated Tablet	Circle, Biconvex, Two-Layered	Nex
L; 642	Buffered Aspirin	325 mg;	White	Coated Tablet	Circle, Biconvex, Two-Layered	Regal Distributing
L; 642	Buffered Aspirin	325 mg;	White	Coated Tablet	Circle, Biconvex, Two-Layered	Rexall
L; 642	Buffered Aspirin	325 mg;	White	Coated Tablet	Circle, Biconvex, Two-Layered	Seaway
L; 642	Buffered Aspirin	325 mg;	White	Coated Tablet	Circle, Biconvex, Two-Layered	Sunfresh
L; 642	Buffered Aspirin	325 mg;	White	Coated Tablet	Circle, Biconvex, Two-Layered	Sunmark

IMPRINT	BRAND/GENERIC NAME	STRENGTH	COLOR	FORM	SHAPE	MANUFACTURER
L; 642	Buffered Aspirin	325 mg;	White	Coated Tablet	Circle, Biconvex, Two-Layered	Swan
L; 642	Buffered Aspirin	325 mg;	White	Coated Tablet	Circle, Biconvex, Two-Layered	Top Care
L; 642	Buffered Aspirin	325 mg;	White	Coated Tablet	Circle, Biconvex, Two-Layered	United Drugs
L; 642	Buffered Aspirin	325 mg;	White	Coated Tablet	Circle, Biconvex, Two-Layered	Valu Rite
L; 643	Sudogest Sinus Maximum Strength	500 mg; 30 mg	White	Coated Tablet	Circle	Major
L; 643	Suphedrine Sinus Maximum Strength	500 mg; 30 mg	White	Coated Tablet	Circle, Compressed, Flat-Faced, Bevel-Edged	Good Neighbor Pharmacy
L; 643	Suphedrine Sinus Maximum Strength	500 mg; 30 mg	White	Coated Tablet	Circle, Compressed, Flat-Faced, Bevel-Edged	Kerr Drug
L; 643	Suphedrine Sinus Maximum Strength	500 mg; 30 mg	White	Coated Tablet	Circle, Compressed, Flat-Faced, Bevel-Edged	Perrigo
L; 643	Suphedrine Sinus Maximum Strength	500 mg; 30 mg	White	Coated Tablet	Circle, Compressed, Flat-Faced, Bevel-Edged	Regal Distributing
L; 643	Suphedrine Sinus Maximum Strength	500 mg; 30 mg	White	Coated Tablet	Circle, Compressed, Flat-Faced, Bevel-Edged	Rockbottom Stores
L; 643	Suphedrine Sinus Maximum Strength	500 mg; 30 mg	White	Coated Tablet	Circle, Compressed, Flat-Faced, Bevel-Edged	Swan
L; 643	Suphedrine Sinus Maximum Strength	500 mg; 30 mg	White	Coated Tablet	Circle, Compressed, Flat-Faced, Bevel-Edged	Top Care
L; 643	Suphedrine Sinus Maximum Strength	500 mg; 30 mg	White	Coated Tablet	Circle, Compressed, Flat-Faced, Bevel-Edged	Valu Rite
L; 670	Quinine Sulfate	260 mg	White	Tablet	Circle	Norton, H.N.
L685	Thyroid, Usp 1/2 grain	10 mcg; 4.5 mcg	Tan	Tablet	Circle	Norton, H.N.
L686	Thyroid, Usp 1 grain	38 mcg; 9 mcg	Tan	Tablet	Circle	Norton, H.N.
L687	Thyroid, Usp 2 grain	76 mcg; 18 mcg	Tan	Tablet	Circle	Norton, H.N.
L; 754	Chemdal	20 mg; 300 mg	Green Speckled	Sustained-Release Tablet	Oblong	Norton, H.N.
L; 814	Allergy Medicine Dye Free	25 mg	Clear	Capsule, Liquid Filled		Top Care
L; 814	Antihistamine Allergy Relief Dye-Free	25 mg	Clear	Capsule, Liquid Filled	Oblong	Good Sense
L; 814	Diphedryl Dye-Free Allergy	25 mg	Clear	Capsule, Liquid Filled	Oblong	Good Neighbor Pharmacy
L; 814	Diphedryl Dye-Free Allergy	25 mg	Clear	Capsule, Liquid Filled	Oblong	Perfect Choice
L; 814	Valu-Dryl Clear Dye-Free Allergy Medicine	25 mg	Clear	Capsule, Liquid Filled	Oblong	Valu Rite
L; 816	Chlorpheniramine Maleate and Pseudoephedrine Hydrochloride	8 mg; 120 mg	Clear with White Beads	Sustained-Release Capsule		Norton, H.N.
L; 821	Women's Menstrual Relief	500 mg; 25 mg	White	Tablet		Good Neighbor Pharmacy
L; 821	Women's Menstrual Relief	500 mg; 25 mg	White	Tablet		Good Sense
L; 821	Women's Menstrual Relief	500 mg; 25 mg	White	Tablet		Perfect Choice
L; 821	Women's Menstrual Relief	500 mg; 25 mg	White	Tablet		Swan
L; 821	Women's Menstrual Relief	500 mg; 25 mg	White	Tablet		Top Care
L; 821	Women's Menstrual Relief	500 mg; 25 mg	White	Tablet		Valu Rite
L; 835	Severe Cold and Flu Non-Drowsy	325 mg; 15 mg; 30 mg	White	Tablet		Good Sense
L; 837	Acetaminophen Pm	500 mg; 25 mg	White and Blue	Geltab	Circle	Perrigo
L; 837	Acetaminophen Pm	500 mg; 25 mg	White and Blue	Geltab	Circle	Top Care
L; 837	Non-Aspirin Pm Extra Strength	500 mg; 25 mg	White and Blue	Geltab		Valu Rite
L; 855	Gas Relief Maximum Strength	125 mg	Red	Capsule, Liquid Filled	Oblong	Genovese
L; 855	Gas Relief Maximum Strength	125 mg	Red	Capsule, Liquid Filled	Oblong	Good Sense
L; 866	Laxative Women's	100 mg; 65 mg	Pink	Tablet	Capsule-Shape	Perrigo
L; 866	Laxative Women's	100 mg; 65 mg	Pink	Tablet	Capsule-Shape	Top Care
L; 877	Extra Strength Pain Reliever without Aspirin	500 mg	Yellow and Red	Capsule, Liquid Filled	Oblong	Genovese
L; 877	Extra Strength Pain Reliever without Aspirin	500 mg	Yellow and Red	Capsule, Liquid Filled	Oblong	Medic
L; 877	Extra Strength Pain Reliever without Aspirin	500 mg	Yellow and Red	Capsule, Liquid Filled	Oblong	Nex
L; 877	Extra Strength Pain Reliever without Aspirin	500 mg	Yellow and Red	Capsule, Liquid Filled	Oblong	Perfect Choice
L; 877	Extra Strength Pain Reliever without Aspirin	500 mg	Yellow and Red	Capsule, Liquid Filled	Oblong	Perrigo
L; 877	Extra Strength Pain Reliever without Aspirin	500 mg	Yellow and Red	Capsule, Liquid Filled	Oblong	Quality Care
L; 877	Extra Strength Pain Reliever without Aspirin	500 mg	Yellow and Red	Capsule, Liquid Filled	Oblong	Select Brand
L; 877	Extra Strength Pain Reliever without Aspirin	500 mg	Yellow and Red	Capsule, Liquid Filled	Oblong	True Quality
L; 877	Mapap Extra Strength	500 mg	Red-Orange and Yellow	Capsule, Liquid Filled		Major
L; 877	Non-Aspirin Extra Strength	500 mg	Red-Orange and Yellow	Capsule, Liquid Filled		Good Neighbor Pharmacy
L; 877	Non-Aspirin Extra Strength	500 mg	Red-Orange and Yellow	Capsule, Liquid Filled		Valu Rite
L; 877	Pain Relief Extra Strength	500 mg	Red-Orange and Yellow	Capsule, Liquid Filled		Perfect Choice
L; 877	Pain Reliever Non-Aspirin, Extra Strength	500 mg	Reddish Orange and Yellow	Capsule, Liquid Filled		Top Care
L; 880	Antacid Extra Strength	160 mg; 105 mg	White	Tablet, Chewable	Circle	Good Sense
L; 880	Antacid Extra Strength	160 mg; 105 mg	White	Tablet, Chewable	Circle	Major
L; 880	Antacid Extra Strength	160 mg; 105 mg	White	Tablet, Chewable	Circle	Perfect Choice
L; 880	Antacid Extra Strength	160 mg; 105 mg	White	Tablet, Chewable	Circle	Perrigo
L; 880	Antacid Extra Strength	160 mg; 105 mg	White	Tablet, Chewable	Circle	Revco
L; 880	Antacid Extra Strength	160 mg; 105 mg	White	Tablet, Chewable	Circle	Sunmark
L; 880	Antacid Extra Strength	160 mg; 105 mg	White	Tablet, Chewable	Circle	Top Care
L; 880	Antacid Extra Strength	160 mg; 105 mg	White	Tablet, Chewable	Circle	Valu Rite
L; 890	Motion Sickness Relief	50 mg	White	Tablet	Round, Convex, Bisected Scored	Good Sense
L; 890	Motion Sickness Relief	50 mg	White	Tablet	Round, Convex, Bisected Scored	Perrigo
L; 890	Motion Sickness Relief	50 mg	White	Tablet	Round, Convex, Bisected Scored	Top Care

IMPRINT	BRAND/GENERIC NAME	STRENGTH	COLOR	FORM	SHAPE	MANUFACTURER
L; 890	Original Travel Ease	50 mg	White	Tablet	Round, Convex, Bisected Scored	Good Sense
L; 890	Original Travel Ease	50 mg	White	Tablet	Round, Convex, Bisected Scored	Perrigo
L; 890	Original Travel Ease	50 mg	White	Tablet	Round, Convex, Bisected Scored	Top Care
L; 965	Dixaphedrine 12 Hour Relief	6 mg; 120 mg	Green	Sustained-Release Tablet	Circle	Perrigo
L; 965	Dixaphedrine 12 Hour Relief	6 mg; 120 mg	Green	Sustained-Release Tablet	Circle	Pharmacist Value
L; 965	Dixaphedrine 12 Hour Relief	6 mg; 120 mg	Green	Sustained-Release Tablet	Circle	Quality Care
L; O49;	Acetaminophen	160 mg	Mottled Pink	Tablet, Chewable	Round, Flat Face, Beveled Edge, Bisected Scored	Leiner Health Products
L; O99;	Acetaminophen	160 mg	Mottled Purple	Tablet, Chewable	Round, Compressed, Flat Faced, Beveled Edge, Bisected Scored	Leiner Health Products
LA; 500	Gp-500	120 mg; 500 mg	White	Sustained-Release Tablet	Capsule-Shape	Marnel Pharmaceuticals
LA; 500	Tuss-LA	120 mg; 500 mg	White	Sustained-Release Tablet	Capsule-Shape, Scored	Hyrex Pharmaceuticals
LA; CTM; D	Chlor-Trimeton Allergy Decongestant 12 Hour	8 mg; 120 mg	Polished Medium Green	Tablet	Circle	Schering-Plough Healthcare Products
LA; CTM; D;	Chlor-Trimeton Long-Acting Decongestant Repetabs	120 mg; 8 mg	Green	Timed-Release Tablet		Schering-Plough Healthcare Products
LAMICTAL; 25	Lamictal	25 mg	White	Tablet	Shield-Shape, Scored	Glaxosmithkline
LAMICTAL; 100	Lamictal	100 mg	Peach	Tablet	Shield-Shape, Scored	Glaxosmithkline
LAMICTAL; 150	Lamictal	150 mg	Cream	Tablet	Shield-Shape, Scored	Glaxosmithkline
LAMICTAL; 200	Lamictal	200 mg	Blue	Tablet	Shield-Shape, Scored	Glaxosmithkline
LAMISIL; 250	Lamisil	250 mg	White to Yellow-Tinged	Tablet	Circle, BI-Convex, Bevelled	Novartis
LAN; 0586	Dicyclomine	10 mg	Blue	Capsule		Qualitest Products
LAN; 0586	Dicyclomine Hydrochloride	10 mg	Blue	Capsule		Duramed Pharmaceuticals
LAN; 0586	Dicyclomine Hydrochloride	10 mg	Blue	Capsule		Lannett
LAN; 1143;	Dextroamphetamine Sulfate	5 mg	Yellow	Tablet		Lannett
LAN; 1152;	Methocarbamol	750 mg	White	Tablet	Capsule-Shape	Lannett
LAN; 1219;	Dextroamphetamine Sulfate	10 mg	Orange	Tablet	Double-Scored	Lannett
LAN; 1231	Primidone	250 mg	White	Tablet	Round, Flat Faced, Bevelled Edge, Bisected	Akyma Pharmaceuticals
LAN; 1231	Primidone	250 mg	White	Tablet	Circle, Scored	Lannett
LAN; 1231	Primidone	250 mg	White	Tablet	Circle, Scored	Qualitest Products
LAN; 1282	Dicyclomine	20 mg	Blue	Tablet	Circle	Qualitest Products
LAN; 1290	Pseudoephedrine	60 mg	White	Tablet	Circle	Lannett
LAN; 1292	Guaifenesin and Ephedrine Hydrochloride	200 mg; 25 mg	White	Tablet	Circle, Flat	Lannett
LAN; 1301	Primidone	50 mg	White	Tablet	Round, Flat Faced, Bevelled Edge, Scored	Akyma Pharmaceuticals
LAN; 1301	Primidone	50 mg		Tablet		Lannett
LAN; 1301	Primidone	50 mg	White	Tablet	Circle, Scored	Qualitest Products
LAN; 1302	Methocarbamol	500 mg	White	Tablet	Circle	Lannett
LAN; 1305	Pseudoephedrine	30 mg	White	Tablet	Circle	Lannett
LANNETT; 0527; 1552	Butalbital Compound	325 mg; 50 mg; 40 mg	Green and Clear	Capsule		Qualitest Products
LANNETT; 0527; 1552	Butalbital with Aspirin and Caffeine	325 mg; 50 mg; 40 mg	Dark Green and Light Green	Capsule		Lannett
LANOXIN; T9A	Lanoxin	0.5 mg	Green	Tablet	Circle, Scored	Glaxosmithkline
LANOXIN; X3A	Lanoxin	0.25 mg	White	Tablet	Circle, Scored	Glaxosmithkline
LANOXIN; Y3B	Lanoxin	0.125 mg	Yellow	Tablet	Circle, Scored	Glaxosmithkline
LARIAM; 250; ROCHE	Lariam	250 mg	White	Tablet	Circle, Scored	Roche Pharmaceuticals
LAROBEC; ROCHE	Larobec	100 mg; 18 mg; 0.5 mg; 500 mg; 15 mg; 15 mg; 5 mcg	Orange	Coated Tablet	Oblong	Roche Pharmaceuticals
LARODOPA; ROCHE; 100	Larodopa	100 mg	Pink and Scarlet	Capsule		Roche Pharmaceuticals
LARODOPA; ROCHE; 250	Larodopa	250 mg	Pink and Beige	Capsule		Roche Pharmaceuticals
LARODOPA; ROCHE; 500	Larodopa	500 mg	Pink	Capsule		Roche Pharmaceuticals
LAROTID; 500; BMP; 212	Larotid	500 mg	Buff	Capsule		Glaxosmithkline
LASER; 0169	Respaire-120 SR	120 mg; 250 mg	Orange and Clear	Extended-Release Capsule		Laser
LASER; 0172	Fumatinic	275 mg; 100 mg; 15 mcg; 1 mg; 20 mg	Orange and Clear with White, Orange and Brown Pellets	Capsule		Laser
LASER; 0174	Respaire-60 SR	60 mg; 200 mg	Green and Clear	Extended-Release Capsule		Laser
LASIX; 40; HOECHST	Lasix	40 mg	White	Tablet	Circle, Scored	Aventis Pharmaceuticals
LASIX; 80; HOECHST	Lasix	80 mg	White	Tablet	Circle	Aventis Pharmaceuticals
LB; 2	Ergomar	2 mg	Green	Tablet	Circle	Lotus Biochemical
LCE; 50	Stalevo 50	12.5 mg; 50 mg; 200 mg	Brown or Grey	Tablet	Circle	Novartis
LCE; 100	Stalevo 100	25 mg; 100 mg; 200 mg	Brown or Grey	Tablet	Oval	Novartis
LCE; 150	Stalevo 150	37.5 mg; 150 mg; 200 mg	Brown or Grey	Tablet	Oblong	Novartis
LCH	Protegra	200 IU; 250 mg; 3 mg; 7.5 mg; 1 mg; 15 mcg; 1.5 mg	Orange	Capsule, Liquid Filled	Oval, Scored	Lederle Consumer Health

IMPRINT	BRAND/GENERIC NAME	STRENGTH	COLOR	FORM	SHAPE	MANUFACTURER
LCH	Protegra	200 IU; 250 mg; 3 mg; 7.5 mg; 1 mg; 15 mcg; 1.5 mg	Orange	Capsule, Liquid Filled	Oval, Scored	Lederle Laboratories
LE	Tridione	150 mg	White	Tablet, Chewable		Abbott Laboratories
LEDERLE; A3; 250 MG	Achromycin V	250 mg	Yellow and Blue	Capsule		Lederle Laboratories
LEDERLE; A; 20	Acetaminophen	500 mg	Blue	Capsule		Lederle Laboratories
LEDERLE; A31	Ampicillin Trihydrate	250 mg	Green and White	Capsule		Lederle Laboratories
LEDERLE; A32	Ampicillin Trihydrate	500 mg	Green and White	Capsule		Lederle Laboratories
LEDERLE; A33	Amoxicillin	250 mg	Grey and Green	Capsule		Lederle Laboratories
LEDERLE; A34	Amoxicillin	500 mg	Gray and Green	Capsule		Lederle Laboratories
LEDERLE;C2;CENTRUM JR	Centrum JR. Plus Iron	18 mg; 5000 IU; 400 IU; 30 IU; 60 mg; 400 mcg; 1.5 mg; 1.7 mg; 20 mg; 2 mg; 6 mcg; 40 mg; 2 mg; 15 mg; 1 mg; 45 mcg; 150 mg; 20 mcg; 20 mcg; 10 mg; 10 mcg; 50 mg; 108 mg	Various	Tablet, Chewable	Oval, Scored	Wyeth Consumer Healthcare
LEDERLE; C54; CEFACLOR; 250MG	Cefaclor	250 mg	Opaque Pink and Blue	Capsule		Lederle Laboratories
LEDERLE; C55	Clorazepate Dipotassium	3.75 mg	White and Lavender	Capsule		Lederle Laboratories
LEDERLE; C56	Clorazepate Dipotassium	7.5 mg	Lavender and Maroon	Capsule		Lederle Laboratories
LEDERLE; C57	Clorazepate Dipotassium	15 mg	Lavender	Capsule		Lederle Laboratories
LEDERLE; C58; CEFACLOR; 500MG	Cefaclor	500 mg	Opaque Lavender and Blue	Capsule		Lederle Laboratories
LEDERLE; C; 61	Cephradine	250 mg	Green and Light Pink	Capsule		Lederle Laboratories
LEDERLE; C; 62	Cephradine	500 mg	Light Green	Capsule		Lederle Laboratories
LEDERLE; C; 64	Cephalexin	250 mg	Grey and Red	Capsule		Esi Lederle
LEDERLE; C; 65	Cephalexin	500 mg	Red	Capsule		Esi Lederle
LEDERLE; D16	Dicloxacillin Sodium	250 mg	Green	Capsule		Lederle Laboratories
LEDERLE; D17	Dicloxacillin Sodium	500 mg	Light Green	Capsule		Lederle Laboratories
LEDERLE; D25	Doxycycline Hyclate	100 mg	Blue	Capsule		Lederle Laboratories
LEDERLE; D36	Dolene	65 mg	Pink	Capsule		Lederle Laboratories
LEDERLE; D47	Doxepin Hydrochloride	25 mg	Ivory and Yellow	Capsule		Lederle Laboratories
LEDERLE; D48	Doxepin Hydrochloride	50 mg	Lavendar and Dark Red	Capsule		Lederle Laboratories
LEDERLE; D49	Doxepin Hydrochloride	75 mg	Purple and Dark Pink	Capsule		Lederle Laboratories
LEDERLE; D50	Doxepin Hydrochloride	10 mg	Buff or Blue	Capsule		Lederle Laboratories
LEDERLE; D54	Doxepin Hydrochloride	100 mg	Green and White	Capsule		Lederle Laboratories
LEDERLE; D55	Doxepin Hydrochloride	150 mg	Gray and Orange	Capsule		Lederle Laboratories
LEDERLE; D62	Disopyramide	100 mg	Dark Red and Blue	Capsule		Lederle Laboratories
LEDERLE; I19;	Indomethacin	25 mg	Pink and White	Capsule		Lederle Laboratories
LEDERLE; I20;	Indomethacin	50 mg	Opaque Pink and Opaque White	Capsule		Lederle Laboratories
LEDERLE; K1	Ketoprofen	25 mg	Dark Green	Capsule		Lederle Laboratories
LEDERLE; K2	Ketoprofen	50 mg	Light Green	Capsule		Lederle Laboratories
LEDERLE; K3	Ketoprofen	75 mg	White	Capsule		Lederle Laboratories
LEDERLE; O; P69	Prazosin Hydrochloride	1 mg	Flesh	Capsule		Lederle Laboratories
LEDERLE; O; P70	Prazosin Hydrochloride	2 mg	Pink	Capsule		Lederle Laboratories
LEDERLE; O; P71	Prazosin Hydrochloride	5 mg	Blue	Capsule		Lederle Laboratories
LEK; CT3	Cimetidine	300 mg	Off White	Tablet	Circle, Biconvex	Akyma Pharmaceuticals
LEK; CT; 3;	Cimetidine	300 mg	Off White	Tablet	Circle, Scored	Stada
LEK; CT4	Cimetidine	400 mg	Off White	Tablet	Bar, Biconvex, Scored	Akyma Pharmaceuticals
LEK; CT; 4;	Cimetidine	400 mg	Off White	Tablet	Capsule-Shape, Scored	Stada
LEK; CT8	Cimetidine	800 mg	Off White	Tablet	Oval, Biconvex	Akyma Pharmaceuticals
LEK; CT; 8	Cimetidine	800 mg	Off White	Tablet	Oval, Scored	Lek Pharmaceuticals
LEK; CT; 8;	Cimetidine	800 mg	Off White	Tablet	Oval, Scored	Stada
LEKCT3	Cimetidine	300 mg	Off White	Tablet	Circle	Lek Pharmaceuticals
LEKCT4	Cimetidine	400 mg	Off White	Tablet	Oblong, Scored	Lek Pharmaceuticals
LEMMON	Dralserp	25 mg; 0.1 mg	Orange	Tablet		Teva Pharmaceuticals
LEMMON	Promethazine Hydrochloride	25 mg	Blue	Tablet	Circle, Convex, Scored	Teva Pharmaceuticals
LEMMON; 30	Neothylline	200 mg	White	Tablet	Circle, Convex, Scored	Teva Pharmaceuticals
LEMMON; 37	Neothylline	400 mg	White	Tablet	Oblong, Scored	Teva Pharmaceuticals
LEMMON; 52	Uristat	0.03 mg; 5 mg; 0.03 mg; 5.5 mg; 20 mg; 50 mg	Blue	Tablet		Teva Pharmaceuticals
LEMMON; 71; 71	Statobex	35 mg	Green and White	Tablet	Oblong, Convex; Scored	Teva Pharmaceuticals
LEMMON; 77	Statobex-G	35 mg	Green	Tablet	Oblong, Scored	Teva Pharmaceuticals
LEMMON; 86; 86	S.B.P.	30 mg; 15 mg; 50 mg	White	Tablet	Circle, Flat, Beveled Edge, Scored	Teva Pharmaceuticals
LEMMON; 93-7; GLUCAMIDE; 250	Glucamide	250 mg	Blue	Tablet	Circle, Convex, Scored	Teva Pharmaceuticals
LEMMON; 93-10; GLUCAMIDE; 100	Glucamide	100 mg	Blue	Tablet	Circle, Convex, Scored	Teva Pharmaceuticals
LEMMON; 105	Dralzine	25 mg	Yellow	Tablet	Oblong	Teva Pharmaceuticals
LEMMON; 123	Sed-Tens S.E.	10 mg	Red and White Speckled	Tablet	Oblong	Teva Pharmaceuticals
LEMMON; 128 128	Neothylline GG	200 mg; 200 mg	White	Tablet	Circle, Flat, Beveled Edge, Scored	Teva Pharmaceuticals
LEMMON; 133	Dexampex	15 mg	Green Transparent and Clear	Capsule		Teva Pharmaceuticals
LEMMON; 137	Dipav	150 mg	Brown and Clear	Capsule		Teva Pharmaceuticals

IMPRINT	BRAND/GENERIC NAME	STRENGTH	COLOR	FORM	SHAPE	MANUFACTURER
LEMMON; 169	B.P.P.	1.2 mg; 120 mg; 15 mg; 120 mg; 15 mg	Yellow	Tablet	Circle, Convex	Teva Pharmaceuticals
LEMMON; 178 178	Methampex	10 mg	Pink	Tablet	Oblong, Scored	Teva Pharmaceuticals
LEMMON; 179	Dexampex	15 mg	Blue	Tablet	Oblong	Teva Pharmaceuticals
LEMMON; 180	Dexampex	10 mg	Pink	Tablet	Oblong	Teva Pharmaceuticals
LEMMON; 211	Lexor	50 mg	Peach	Tablet		Teva Pharmaceuticals
LEMMON; 238	Diacin	200 mg	Red and Clear with Red and White Pellets Inside	Capsule		Teva Pharmaceuticals
LEMMON; 277	Statobex	35 mg	Green and White, Opaque	Capsule		Teva Pharmaceuticals
LEMMON; 341	Ruhexatal with Reserpine	30 mg; 10 mg; 0.1 mg; 20 mg		Tablet		Teva Pharmaceuticals
LEMMON; ORAP; 2	Orap	2 mg	White	Tablet	Oval, Scored	Teva Pharmaceuticals
LESCOL XL; 80	Lescol Xl	80 mg	Yellow	Extended-Release Tablet	Circle	Novartis
LEVACET	Levacet	250 mg; 150 mg; 500 mg; 32.5 mg	Yellow	Tablet	Capsule-Shape	Wraser Pharmaceuticals
LEVALL; G	Levall G	400 mg; 90 mg	Red	Capsule		Athlon Pharmaceuticals
LEVAQUIN; 250	Levaquin	250 mg	Terra Cotta Pink	Coated Tablet		Ortho-Mcneil Pharmaceutical
LEVAQUIN; 500	Levaquin	500 mg	Peach	Coated Tablet		Ortho-Mcneil Pharmaceutical
LEVAQUIN; 750	Levaquin	750 mg	White	Coated Tablet	Rectangle, Modified	Ortho-Mcneil Pharmaceutical
LEVO	Levofloxacin	500 mg		Tablet		Unipharm
LEVO-DROMORAN; ROCHE;	Levo-Dromoran	2 mg	White	Tablet	Circle, Scored, Beveled	Icn Pharmaceuticals
LEXXEL; 1; 5-5	Lexxel	5 mg; 5 mg	White	Extended-Release Tablet	Circle, Biconvex	Astra Zeneca
LEXXEL 2; 5-2.5	Lexxel	5 mg; 2.5 mg	White	Extended-Release Tablet	Circle, Biconvex, Film-Coated	Astra Zeneca
LH; 12	Lohist 12	6 mg	White	Tablet, Extended Release		Larken Laboratories
LH; 12D	Lohist 12d	6 mg; 45 mg	White	Tablet, Extended Release		Larken Laboratories
LIBRAX; ICN;	Librax	5 mg; 2.5 mg	Blue-Green	Capsule, Liquid Filled		Icn Pharmaceuticals
LIBRITABS; 5; ROCHE	Libritabs	5 mg	Green	Coated Tablet	Circle, Scored	Roche Products
LIBRITABS; 10; ROCHE	Libritabs	10 mg	Green	Coated Tablet	Circle, Scored	Roche Products
LIBRITABS; 25; ROCHE	Libritabs	25 mg	Green	Coated Tablet	Circle, Scored	Roche Products
LIBRIUM 5; ROCHE	Librium	5 mg	Green and Yellow	Capsule		Icn Pharmaceuticals
LIBRIUM 10; ROCHE	Librium	10 mg	Green and Black	Capsule		Icn Pharmaceuticals
LIBRIUM 25; ROCHE	Librium	25 mg	Green and White	Capsule		Icn Pharmaceuticals
LILLY; 3004; 90 MG	Prozac Weekly	90 mg	Green and Clear with White Enteric-Coated Pellets	Timed-Release Capsule		Eli Lilly
LILLY; 3061	Ceclor	250 mg	White and Purple	Capsule		Eli Lilly
LILLY; 3062	Ceclor	500 mg	Gray and Purple	Capsule		Eli Lilly
LILLY; 3075	Histadyl and A.S.A. Compound	4 mg; 325 mg	White and Red	Capsule		Eli Lilly
LILLY; 3110; DARVON COMP	Darvon Compound	32 mg; 389 mg; 32.4 mg	Pink and Gray	Capsule		Eli Lilly
LILLY; 3111; DARVON COMP 65	Darvon Compound 65	389 mg; 32.4 mg; 65 mg	Red and Grey	Capsule		Eli Lilly
LILLY; 3132; PINDAC; 12.5	Pindac	12.5 mg	Blue and Clear with Orange Beads	Capsule		Eli Lilly
LILLY; 3133; PINDAC; 25	Pindac	25 mg	Blue and Clear with White Beads	Capsule		Eli Lilly
LILLY; 3170	Lorabid Pulvules	200 mg	Blue and Gray	Capsule		Monarch Pharmaceuticals
LILLY; 3210; 10 MG	Sarafem	10 mg	Lavender	Capsule		Eli Lilly
LILLY; 3220; 20 MG	Sarafem	20 mg	Lavender and Pink	Capsule		Eli Lilly
LILLY; 3227; 10 MG	Strattera	10 mg	White	Capsule		Eli Lilly
LILLY; 3228; 25 MG	Strattera	25 mg	Blue and White	Capsule		Eli Lilly
LILLY; 3229; 40 MG	Strattera	40 mg	Blue and Blue	Capsule		Eli Lilly
LILLY; 3231; 6/25	Symbyax	6 mg; 25 mg	Mustard and Light Yellow	Capsule		Eli Lilly
LILLY; 3232; 12/25	Symbyax	12 mg; 25 mg	Red and Light Yellow	Capsule		Eli Lilly
LILLY; 3233; 6/50	Symbyax	6 mg; 50 mg	Mustard and Light Grey	Capsule		Eli Lilly
LILLY; 3234; 12/50	Symbyax	12 mg; 50 mg	Red and Light Grey	Capsule		Eli Lilly
LILLY; 3238; 18 MG	Strattera	18 mg	White and Gold	Capsule		Eli Lilly
LILLY; 3239; 60 MG	Strattera	60 mg	Blue and Gold	Capsule		Eli Lilly
LILLY; 4112	Zyprexa	2.5 mg	White	Coated Tablet	Circle	Eli Lilly
LILLY; 4115	Zyprexa	5 mg	White with Blue Ink	Coated Tablet	Circle	Eli Lilly
LILLY; 4116	Zyprexa	7.5 mg	White	Coated Tablet	Circle	Eli Lilly
LILLY; 4117	Zyprexa	10 mg	White with Blue Ink	Coated Tablet	Circle	Eli Lilly
LILLY; 4165	Evista	60 mg	White with Blue Ink	Coated Tablet	Circle	Eli Lilly
LILLY; 4415	Zyprexa	15 mg	Blue	Tablet	Egg-Shape, Debossed	Eli Lilly
LILLY; 4420	Zyprexa	20 mg		Tablet		Eli Lilly
LILLY; A01	Ammonium Chloride	500 mg		Sustained-Release Tablet		Eli Lilly
LILLY; A02	Ferrous Sulfate	325 mg	Red	Sustained-Release Tablet		Eli Lilly
LILLY; A04	Pancreatin, Triple Strength	1 G		Sustained-Release Tablet		Eli Lilly
LILLY; A05	Potassium Chloride	300 mg		Tablet		Eli Lilly
LILLY; A06	Potassium Iodide	300 mg		Enteric-Coated Tablet		Eli Lilly
LILLY; A09	Sodium Chloride	1 GM		Enteric-Coated Tablet		Eli Lilly
LILLY; A10	Sodium Salicylate	325 mg		Coated Tablet		Eli Lilly
LILLY; A11	Sodium Salicylate	650 mg		Enteric-Coated Tablet		Eli Lilly

IMPRINT	BRAND/GENERIC NAME	STRENGTH	COLOR	FORM	SHAPE	MANUFACTURER
LILLY; A12	Ammonium Chloride	15 Gr		Sustained-Release Tablet		Eli Lilly
LILLY; A14	Thyroid	30 mg		Enteric-Coated Tablet		Eli Lilly
LILLY; A15	Thyroid	60 mg		Enteric-Coated Tablet		Eli Lilly
LILLY; A16	Thyroid	120 mg		Enteric-Coated Tablet		Eli Lilly
LILLY; A17	Thyroid	200 mg		Enteric-Coated Tablet		Eli Lilly
LILLY; A25	A.S.A.	325 mg		Enteric-Coated Tablet		Eli Lilly
LILLY; A27	Amesec	130 mg; 25 mg; 25 mg		Sustained-Release Tablet		Eli Lilly
LILLY; A30	Aminosalicylic Acid	500 mg		Sustained-Release Tablet		Eli Lilly
LILLY; A31	Potassium Chloride	1 GM		Enteric-Coated Tablet		Eli Lilly
LILLY; A32	A.S.A.	650 mg		Enteric-Coated Tablet		Eli Lilly
LILLY; A36	Ferrous Sulfate	325 mg	Green	Sustained-Release Tablet		Eli Lilly
LILLY; A39	Quinidine Sulfate	200 mg		Enteric-Coated Tablet		Eli Lilly
LILLY; B51	Alphalin	7.5 mg		Capsule		Eli Lilly
LILLY; B52	Alphalin	15 mg		Capsule		Eli Lilly
LILLY; B60	Deltalin	1.25 mg		Capsule, Liquid Filled		Eli Lilly
LILLY; C06	Cascara	325 mg	Chocolate	Coated Tablet		Eli Lilly
LILLY; C07	Cascara Compound	16 mg; 16 mg; 10 mg; 8 mg; 4 mg	Pink	Coated Tablet		Eli Lilly
LILLY; C11	Rhinitis, Full Strength	32.5 mg; 32.5 mg; 5.8 mg	Chocolate	Coated Tablet		Eli Lilly
LILLY; C13	Ferrous Sulfate	325 mg	Chocolate	Coated Tablet		Eli Lilly
LILLY; C27	V-Cillin K	125 mg	White	Tablet		Eli Lilly
LILLY; C29	V-Cillin K	250 mg	White	Tablet		Eli Lilly
LILLY; C31	Anhydron K	2 mg; 500 mg		Coated Tablet		Eli Lilly
LILLY; C32	Anhydron Kr	2 mg; 500 mg; 0.25 mg		Coated Tablet		Eli Lilly
LILLY; C36	Quinine Sulfate	325 mg	Chocolate	Coated Tablet		Eli Lilly
LILLY; C46	V-Cillin K	500 mg	White	Tablet		Eli Lilly
LILLY; C47	Hepicebrin	1.5 mg; 10 mcg; 20 mg; 75 mg; 2 mg; 3 mg		Coated Tablet		Eli Lilly
LILLY; C71	Multi-Cebrin	5 mg; 25 mg; 6 mg; 3 mg; 25 mcg; 3 mg; 3 mg; 1.2 mg; 3 mcg; 75 mg	Dark Red	Tablet		Eli Lilly
LILLY; DARVOCET-N 50	Darvocet-N 50	325 mg; 50 mg	Dark Orange	Coated Tablet	Capsule-Shape	Eli Lilly
LILLY; DARVOCET-N 100	Darvocet-N 100	100 mg; 650 mg	Dark Orange	Coated Tablet	Capsule-Shape	Eli Lilly
LILLY; DARVON-N; 100;	Darvon-N	100 mg	Buff	Tablet	Oblong	Eli Lilly
LILLY; DARVON-N; ASA	Darvon-N with A.S.A.	100 mg; 325 mg	Orange	Tablet	Circle	Eli Lilly
LILLY; F09	Seromycin with Isoniazid	250 mg; 150 mg		Capsule		Eli Lilly
LILLY; F11;	A.S.A.	325 mg	Clear or Pink	Capsule		Eli Lilly
LILLY; F13	A.S.A. Compound	227 mg; 32.5 mg; 160 mg	White Opaque	Capsule		Eli Lilly
LILLY; F14	Ephedrine and Amytal	25 mg; 50 mg	Yellow	Capsule		Eli Lilly
LILLY; F20	Ephedrine and Seconal Sodium	25 mg; 50 mg	Scarlet	Capsule		Eli Lilly
LILLY; F23	Amytal Sodium No. 4	65 mg	Blue	Capsule		Eli Lilly
LILLY; F24	Ephedrine Sulfate	25 mg	Pink	Capsule		Eli Lilly
LILLY; F25	Ephedrine Sulfate	50 mg	Pink	Capsule		Eli Lilly
LILLY; F26	Quinine Sulfate	130 mg	White Opaque	Capsule		Eli Lilly
LILLY; F27	Quinine Sulfate	200 mg	White Opaque	Capsule		Eli Lilly
LILLY; F29	Quinine Sulfate	325 mg	White Opaque	Capsule		Eli Lilly
LILLY; F30	A.S.A. Compound	227 mg; 160 mg; 32.5 mg	Pink	Capsule		Eli Lilly
LILLY; F33	Amytal Sodium No. 2	200 mg	Blue	Capsule		Eli Lilly
LILLY; F36	Copavin	15 mg; 15 mg	Clear	Capsule		Eli Lilly
LILLY; F39	Quinidine Sulfate	200 mg		Capsule		Eli Lilly
LILLY; F41	Bilron	300 mg	Green	Capsule		Eli Lilly
LILLY; F42	Seconal Sodium	50 mg	Red	Capsule		Eli Lilly
LILLY; F43	Betalin Compound	3.333 mg; 10 mg; 1 mg; 2 mg; 0.4 mg; 1 mcg	Pink	Capsule		Eli Lilly
LILLY; F45	Epragen	22 mg; 130 mg; 227 mg; 50 mg	Yellow and Brown	Capsule		Eli Lilly
LILLY; F47	Amesec	130 mg; 25 mg; 25 mg	Blue and Orange	Capsule		Eli Lilly
LILLY; F50	A.S.A. and Codeine, No. 2	230 mg; 30 mg; 15 mg; 150 mg	White and Light Gray	Capsule		Eli Lilly
LILLY; F51	A.S.A. and Codeine, No. 3	230 mg; 30 mg; 30 mg; 150 mg	White and Dark Gray	Capsule		Eli Lilly
LILLY; F52	Dibasic Calcium Phosphate with Vitamin D	500 mg; 0.825 mg	Clear	Capsule		Eli Lilly
LILLY; F53	Trisogel	4 1/2 grains	Pink	Capsule		Eli Lilly
LILLY; F56	Calcium Gluconate with Vitamin D	325 mg; 0.825 mcg	Opaque White	Capsule		Eli Lilly
LILLY; F57	Dicalcium Phosphate and Calcium Gluconate with Vitamin D	290 mg; 200 mg; 8.25 mcg	White Opaque	Capsule		Eli Lilly
LILLY; F61	Bilron	150 mg	Green	Capsule		Eli Lilly

IMPRINT	BRAND/GENERIC NAME	STRENGTH	COLOR	FORM	SHAPE	MANUFACTURER
LILLY; F62	Becotin	10 mg; 10 mg; 4.1 mg; 50 mg; 25 mg; 1 mcg	Dark Blue	Capsule		Eli Lilly
LILLY; F63	Dicalcium Phosphate with Vitamin D and Iron	500 mg; 33 IU; 10 mg	Pink	Capsule		Eli Lilly
LILLY; F64	Tuinal	25 mg; 25 mg	Blue and Orange	Capsule		Eli Lilly
LILLY; F67	A.S.A. and Codeine, No. 4	230 mg; 30 mg; 60 mg; 150 mg	Dark Gray	Capsule		Eli Lilly
LILLY; F76	Prenalac	0.25 mg; 0.5 mg; 1.25 mcg; 16.6 mg; 2.5 mg; 0.3 mg; 1.7 mcg; 2.5 mg; 0.8 mg; 1 mg;	Pink and Light Blue	Capsule		Eli Lilly
LILLY; F77	Becotin with Vitamin C	10 mg; 10 mg; 4.1 mg; 50 mg; 25 mg; 1 mcg; 150 mg	Green and Blue	Capsule		Eli Lilly
LILLY; F97	CO-Elorine	8 mg	Yellow and Turquoise	Capsule		Eli Lilly
LILLY; G01	Alphalin	3 mg		Capsule		Eli Lilly
LILLY; H03; DARVON	Darvon	65 mg	Pink	Capsule	Capsule-Shape	Eli Lilly
LILLY; H04; DARVON; C; ASA	Darvon with Asa	65 mg; 325 mg	Red and Light Pink	Capsule		Eli Lilly
LILLY; H10	En-Cebrin F	1.2 mg; 3 mg; 2 mg; 10 mg; 2 mg; 1 mg; 5 mcg; 5 mg; 50 mg; 10 mcg; 250 mg; 30 mg; 0.15 mg; 1 mg; 5 mg; 1 mg; 1.5 mg	Pink and Blue	Capsule		Eli Lilly
LILLY; H12	En-Cebrin	1.2 mg; 10 mg; 5 mg; 10 mcg; 250 mg; 30 mg; 0.15 mg; 1 mg; 5 mg; 1 mg; 1.5 mg; 3 mg; 2 mg; 1.7 mg; 5 mcg; 50 mg	Pink and Blue	Capsule		Eli Lilly
LILLY; H13	Novrad	50 mg	Ivory and Light Brown	Capsule		Eli Lilly
LILLY; H14	Novrad	100 mg	Ivory and Light Brown	Capsule		Eli Lilly
LILLY; H15	Novrad with A.S.A.	50 mg; 300 mg	Ivory and Dark Brown	Capsule		Eli Lilly
LILLY; H17	Aventyl	10 mg	White and Yellow	Capsule		Eli Lilly
LILLY; H19	Aventyl	25 mg	White and Yellow	Capsule		Eli Lilly
LILLY; H72	Theracebrin	20 mg; 150 mg; 12.5 mg; 7.5 mg; 37.5 mcg; 15 mg; 10 mg; 2.5 mg; 10 mcg; 150 mg	Black	Capsule		Eli Lilly
LILLY; H91	Doloxene Compound	100 mg; 375 mg; 30 mg	Red and Gray	Capsule		Eli Lilly
LILLY; HO2	Darvon	32 mg	Light Pink	Capsule		Eli Lilly
LILLY; J01	Ammonium Chloride	325 mg		Tablet	Compressed	Eli Lilly
LILLY; J02	Atropine Sulfate	0.4 mg		Tablet		Eli Lilly
LILLY; J03	Belladonna Extract	15 mg		Tablet	Compressed	Eli Lilly
LILLY; J05	Caffeine, Citrated	65 mg		Tablet	Compressed	Eli Lilly
LILLY; J09	Codeine Sulfate	15 mg		Tablet		Eli Lilly
LILLY; J11	Codeine Sulfate	60 mg		Tablet		Eli Lilly
LILLY; J13	Colchicine	0.6 mg		Tablet	Compressed	Eli Lilly
LILLY; J20	Quinidine Sulfate	200 mg		Tablet	Compressed	Eli Lilly
LILLY; J23	Soda Mint	5 Gr		Tablet	Compressed	Eli Lilly
LILLY; J24	Sodium Bicarbonate	325 mg		Tablet		Eli Lilly
LILLY; J25	Thyroid	60 mg		Tablet	Compressed	Eli Lilly
LILLY; J26	Thyroid	120 mg		Tablet	Compressed	Eli Lilly
LILLY; J29	Thyroid	30 mg		Tablet	Compressed	Eli Lilly
LILLY; J30	Thyroid	15 mg		Tablet	Compressed	Eli Lilly
LILLY; J31	Phenobarbital	15 mg		Tablet		Eli Lilly
LILLY; J32	Phenobarbital	30 mg		Tablet		Eli Lilly
LILLY; J33	Phenobarbital	100 mg	White	Tablet	Circle, Scored	Eli Lilly
LILLY; J36	Ergotrate Maleate	0.2 mg		Tablet		Eli Lilly
LILLY; J41	Niacin	20 mg		Tablet	Compressed	Eli Lilly
LILLY; J43	Niacin	50 mg		Tablet	Compressed, Scored	Eli Lilly
LILLY; J45	Hexa-Betalin	25 mg; 0.5%		Tablet	Compressed	Eli Lilly
LILLY; J46	Niacinamide	50 mg		Tablet	Compressed	Eli Lilly
LILLY; J47	Riboflavin	5 mg		Tablet	Compressed	Eli Lilly
LILLY; J49	Diethylstilbestrol	0.1 mg		Tablet		Eli Lilly
LILLY; J53	Pantholin	10 mg		Tablet	Compressed	Eli Lilly
LILLY; J55	Phenobarbital and Belladonna, No. 1	30 mg; 8 mg		Tablet	Compressed, Scored	Eli Lilly
LILLY; J56	Hexa-Betalin	10 mg		Tablet	Compressed	Eli Lilly
LILLY; J57	Crystodigin	0.2 mg	White	Tablet		Eli Lilly
LILLY; J59	Phenobarbital and Belladonna, No. 2	15 mg; 4 mg		Tablet	Compressed	Eli Lilly
LILLY; J60	Crystodigin	0.1 mg	Pink	Tablet		Eli Lilly
LILLY; J61	Papaverine Hydrochloride	30 mg		Tablet	Compressed	Eli Lilly
LILLY; J62	Papaverine Hydrochloride	60 mg		Tablet		Eli Lilly
LILLY; J63	Riboflavin	10 mg		Tablet		Eli Lilly

IMPRINT	BRAND/GENERIC NAME	STRENGTH	COLOR	FORM	SHAPE	MANUFACTURER
LILLY; J66	Folic Acid	5 mg		Tablet	Compressed	Eli Lilly
LILLY; J69	Propylthiouracil	50 mg		Tablet	Compressed, Scored	Eli Lilly
LILLY; J70	Phenobarbital and Belladonna, No. 3	15 mg; 8 mg		Tablet	Compressed	Eli Lilly
LILLY; J73	Methyltestosterone	10 mg		Tablet	Compressed, Scored	Eli Lilly
LILLY; J74	Methyltestosterone	25 mg		Tablet		Eli Lilly
LILLY; J75	Crystodigin	0.05 mg	Orange	Tablet		Eli Lilly
LILLY; J76	Crystodigin	0.15 mg	Yellow	Tablet		Eli Lilly
LILLY; J99	Sandril	0.1 mg	Orange	Tablet	Compressed	Eli Lilly
LILLY; L01	Sandril	0.25 mg	Green	Tablet	Compressed, Scored	Eli Lilly
LILLY; L02	Tylandril	0.25 mg; 5 mg; 0.1 mg		Tablet	Compressed	Eli Lilly
LILLY; S04	Metycaine Hydrochloride and Zinc Oxide Compound	12.5 mg; 125 mg; 250 mg		Suppository		Eli Lilly
LILLY; S05	Seconal Sodium Suppositories	120 mg		Suppository		Eli Lilly
LILLY; S06	Amytal Sodium	200 mg		Suppository		Eli Lilly
LILLY; S11	Seconal Sodium Suppositories	200 mg		Suppository		Eli Lilly
LILLY; S14	Seconal Sodium Suppositories	60 mg		Suppository		Eli Lilly
LILLY; S17	Seconal Sodium Suppositories	30 mg		Suppository		Eli Lilly
LILLY; T02	Novacebrin	4000 IU; 400 IU; 60 mg; 1.5 mg; 2 mg; 0.8 mg; 3 mcg; 12 mg; 2.5 mg	Yellow	Tablet, Chewable	Compressed	Eli Lilly
LILLY; T03	Novacebrin with Fluoride	1 mg; 1.2 mg; 10 mcg; 60 mg; 1.5 mg; 2 mg; 1 mg; 3 mcg; 12 mg; 2.5 mg	Orange	Tablet, Chewable		Eli Lilly
LILLY; T05	A.S.A.	325 mg		Tablet	Compressed	Eli Lilly
LILLY; T06	A.S.A.	325 mg	Pink	Tablet	Compressed	Eli Lilly
LILLY; T07	A.S.A. Compound	227 mg; 160 mg; 32.5 mg	White	Tablet	Compressed	Eli Lilly
LILLY; T13	Calcium Lactate	325 mg		Tablet	Compressed	Eli Lilly
LILLY; T14	Calcium Lactate	650 mg		Tablet	Compressed	Eli Lilly
LILLY; T19	Methenamine	325 mg		Tablet	Compressed	Eli Lilly
LILLY; T20	Methenamine	500 mg		Tablet	Compressed	Eli Lilly
LILLY; T21	Methenamine and Sodium Biphosphate	325 mg; 325 mg		Tablet	Compressed	Eli Lilly
LILLY; T23	Sodium Chloride	2.25 GM		Tablet	Compressed	Eli Lilly
LILLY; T24	Sodium Chloride	1 GM		Tablet	Compressed	Eli Lilly
LILLY; T26	Pancreatin	325 mg		Tablet	Compressed	Eli Lilly
LILLY; T29	Sodium Bicarbonate	650 mg		Tablet	Compressed	Eli Lilly
LILLY; T32	Amytal	100 mg	Pink	Tablet		Eli Lilly
LILLY; T35	Calcium Carbonate, Aromatic	650 mg		Tablet	Compressed	Eli Lilly
LILLY; T36	Calcium Gluconate	1 GM		Tablet	Compressed	Eli Lilly
LILLY; T37	Amytal	50 mg	Orange	Tablet		Eli Lilly
LILLY; T39	Calcium Gluconate	500 mg		Tablet	Compressed	Eli Lilly
LILLY; T40	Amytal	15 mg	Green	Tablet	Capsule-Shape	Eli Lilly
LILLY; T42	A.S.A. and Codeine, N0. 2	230 mg; 30 mg; 15 mg; 150 mg		Tablet	Compressed	Eli Lilly
LILLY; T44	Calcium Gluconate with Vitamin D	1 GM; 1.65 mcg		Tablet	Compressed	Eli Lilly
LILLY; T46	Sulfapyridine	0.5 GM		Tablet	Compressed	Eli Lilly
LILLY; T49	A.S.A. and Codeine, No. 3	230 mg; 30 mg; 30 mg; 150 mg		Tablet	Compressed	Eli Lilly
LILLY; T50	A.S.A. Compound	227 mg; 160 mg; 32.5 mg	Pink	Tablet	Compressed	Eli Lilly
LILLY; T52	Betalin S	10 mg		Tablet	Compressed	Eli Lilly
LILLY; T55	Papaverine Hydrochloride	100 mg		Tablet	Compressed	Eli Lilly
LILLY; T56	Amytal	30 mg	Yellow	Tablet		Eli Lilly
LILLY; T59	Betalin S	25 mg		Tablet	Compressed	Eli Lilly
LILLY; T61	Dicalcium Phosphate	500 mg		Tablet	Compressed	Eli Lilly
LILLY; T62	Betalin S	50 mg		Tablet	Compressed	Eli Lilly
LILLY; T63	Betalin S	100 mg		Tablet	Compressed	Eli Lilly
LILLY; T71	Sulfonamides Triplex	0.167 GM; 0.167 GM; 0.167 GM		Tablet	Compressed	Eli Lilly
LILLY; T72	Hexa-Betalin	50 mg		Tablet	Compressed	Eli Lilly
LILLY; T73	Papaverine Hydrochloride	200 mg		Tablet	Compressed	Eli Lilly
LILLY; T75	Neotrizine	167 mg; 167 mg; 167 mg		Tablet	Compressed, Scored	Eli Lilly
LILLY; T77	Neopenzine 150	167 mg; 167 mg; 167 mg; 150,000 units		Tablet	Compressed	Eli Lilly
LILLY; T92	Neopenzine 300	167 mg; 167 mg; 167 mg; 300,000 units		Tablet		Eli Lilly
LILLY; T95	V-Cillin Sulfa	125 mg; 167 mg; 167 mg; 167 mg		Tablet		Eli Lilly
LILLY; T96	Neomycin Sulfate	500 mg		Tablet		Eli Lilly
LILLY; U02	Sandril	1 mg		Tablet		Eli Lilly
LILLY; U03	Dymelor	250 mg	White	Tablet	Capsule-Shape, Scored	Eli Lilly
LILLY; U04	V-Cillin K Sulfa	125 mg; 0.167 GM; 0.167 GM; 0.167 GM		Tablet		Eli Lilly
LILLY; U07	Dymelor	500 mg	Yellow	Tablet	Capsule-Shape, Scored	Eli Lilly
LILLY; U09	Anhydron	2 mg	Pink	Tablet		Eli Lilly
LILLY; U; 29	Sandril	0.25 mg		Tablet		Eli Lilly

IMPRINT	BRAND/GENERIC NAME	STRENGTH	COLOR	FORM	SHAPE	MANUFACTURER
LILLY; U30	Tylandril	0.25 mg; 5 mg; 0.1 mg	Green	Tablet		Eli Lilly
LILLY; U56	Folic Acid	1 mg		Tablet		Eli Lilly
LILLY; Y18	Penicillin G Potassium Solvets	100,000 units		Tablet		Eli Lilly
LILLY; Y23	Castor Oil	0.62 ml		Capsule		Eli Lilly
LILLY; Y40	Apomorphine Hydrochloride	6 mg		Tablet		Eli Lilly
LILLY; Y41	Atropine Sulfate Hypodermic Tablet	0.3 mg		Tablet		Eli Lilly
LILLY; Y42	Atropine Sulfate Hypodermic Tablet	0.4 mg		Tablet		Eli Lilly
LILLY; Y43	Atropine Sulfate Hypodermic Tablet	0.6 mg		Tablet		Eli Lilly
LILLY; Y52	Morphine and Atropine Hypodermic	15 mg; 0.4 mg		Tablet		Eli Lilly
LILLY; Y53	Scopolamine Hydrobromide Hypodermic	0.6 mg		Tablet		Eli Lilly
LILLY; Y54	Scopolamine Hydrobromide Hypodermic	0.4 mg		Tablet		Eli Lilly
LILLY; Y56	Codeine Phosphate Hypodermic Tablet	15 mg		Tablet		Eli Lilly
LILLY; Y57	Codeine Phosphate	30 mg		Tablet		Eli Lilly
LILLY F04; LILLY F04	Seromycin	250 mg	Opaque Gray, Opaque Red	Capsule		Eli Lilly
LILLY F40	Seconal	100 mg	Orange or Red	Capsule		Eli Lilly
LIMBITROL	Limbitrol	5 mg; 12.5 mg	Blue	Coated Tablet	Circle	Icn Pharmaceuticals
LIMBITROL DS	Limbitrol DS	10 mg; 25 mg	White	Coated Tablet		Icn Pharmaceuticals
LINCOCIN; 250 MG;	Lincocin Pediatric	250 mg	Light Blue	Capsule		Pharmacia & Upjohn
LINCOCIN; 500 MG;	Lincocin	500 mg	Light Blue and Dark Blue	Capsule		Pharmacia & Upjohn
LIORESAL; 10/10	Lioresal	10 mg	White	Tablet	Oval, Scored	Novartis
LIORESAL; 20/20	Lioresal	20 mg	White	Tablet	Capsule-Shape, Scored	Novartis
LIQUIBID-D	Liquibid-D	600 mg; 40 mg	White	Extended-Release Tablet	Elongated, Scored	Capellon Pharmaceuticals
LL; 5; C; 33	Leucovorin Calcium	5 mg	Yellow-White	Tablet	Circle, Convex, Scored	Xanodyne Pharmaceuticals
LL; 10; C; 12	Leucovorin Calcium	10 mg	Light Yellow	Tablet	Square with Rounded Corners, Convex, Bisected Scored	Lederle Laboratories
LL; 15; C; 35	Leucovorin Calcium	15 mg	Yellow-White	Tablet	Oval, Convex, Scored	Xanodyne Pharmaceuticals
LL; A1;	Aristocort	1 mg	Yellow	Tablet	Oblong, Flat; Scored	Lederle Laboratories
LL; A2;	Triamcinolone	2 mg	Pink	Tablet	Oblong, Flat, Scored	Lederle Laboratories
LL; A4;	Aristocort	4 mg	White	Tablet	Oblong, Flat, Scored	Lederle Laboratories
LL; A; 7	Atenolol	25 mg	White	Tablet	Circle	Lederle Laboratories
LL; A8;	Aristocort	8 mg	Yellow	Tablet	Oblong, Flat, Scored	Lederle Laboratories
LL; A11; ARTANE; 2	Artane	2 mg	White	Tablet	Circle, Flat, Scored	Lederle Laboratories
LL; A11; ARTANE; 2	Artane	2 mg	White	Tablet	Circle, Flat, Scored	Udl Laboratories
LL; A12; ARTANE; 5	Artane	5 mg	White	Tablet	Circle, Flat, Scored	Lederle Laboratories
LL; A12; ARTANE; 5	Artane	5 mg	White	Tablet	Circle, Flat, Scored	Udl Laboratories
LL; A 24	Amitriptyline Hydrochloride	10 mg	Pink	Coated Tablet	Circle	Lederle Laboratories
LL; A 25	Amitriptyline Hydrochloride	25 mg	Green	Coated Tablet	Circle	Lederle Laboratories
LL; A 26	Amitriptyline Hydrochloride	50 mg	Brown	Coated Tablet	Circle	Lederle Laboratories
LL; A; 27	Amitriptyline Hydrochloride	75 mg	Light Purple	Coated Tablet	Circle	Lederle Laboratories
LL; A; 28	Amitriptyline Hydrochloride	100 mg	Red-Orange	Coated Tablet	Circle	Lederle Laboratories
LL; A; 45	Albuterol Sulfate	2 mg	White	Tablet	Round, Flat, Bisected Scored	Lederle Laboratories
LL; A; 46	Albuterol Sulfate	4 mg	White	Tablet	Round, Flat, Bisected Scored	Lederle Laboratories
LL; A; 49	Atenolol	50 mg	White	Tablet	Circle, Scored	Lederle Laboratories
LL; A; 51	Alprazolam	0.25 mg	White	Tablet	Oval, Convex, Scored	Lederle Laboratories
LL; A; 52	Alprazolam	0.5 mg	Yellow	Tablet	Oval, Convex, Scored	Lederle Laboratories
LL; A; 53	Alprazolam	1 mg	Green	Tablet	Oval, Convex, Scored	Lederle Laboratories
LL; A; 54	Alprazolam	2 mg	Green	Tablet	Oblong, Convex	Lederle Laboratories
LL; A; 71	Atenolol	100 mg	White	Tablet	Circle	Esi Lederle
LL;A 14	Amiloride and Hydrochlorothiazide	5 mg; 50 mg	Yellow	Tablet	Circle	Lederle Laboratories
LL; B1	Zebeta	5 mg	Pink	Coated Tablet	Heart-Shape	Lederle Laboratories
LL; B; 10	Benztropine Mesylate	1 mg	White	Tablet	Oval, Scored	Lederle Laboratories
LL; B; 11	Benztropine Mesylate	2 mg	White	Tablet	Circle, Scored	Lederle Laboratories
LL; C;7	Chlorthalidone	25 mg	Dark Orange	Tablet	Circle, Scored	Lederle Laboratories
LL; C; 15	Chlorthalidone	50 mg	Dark Blue	Tablet	Circle, Scored	Lederle Laboratories
LL; C16	Chlorpheniramine Maleate	4 mg	Yellow	Tablet	Circle, Scored	KV Pharmaceutical
LL; C37	Chlorpropamide	100 mg	White	Tablet	Circle, Scored	Lederle Laboratories
LL; C38	Chlorpropamide	250 mg	White	Tablet	Circle, Scored	Lederle Laboratories
LL; C; 40	Caltrate 600 Plus Vitamin D	125 IU; 600 mg	Light Brown	Coated Tablet	Oblong, Scored	Wyeth Consumer Healthcare
LL; C; 42	Clonidine Hydrochloride	0.1 mg	Blue	Tablet	Circle, Convex	Lederle Laboratories
LL; C; 43	Clonidine Hydrochloride	0.2 mg	Light Yellow	Tablet	Circle, Convex	Lederle Laboratories
LL; C; 44	Clonidine Hydrochloride	0.3 mg	Light Green	Tablet	Circle, Convex	Lederle Laboratories
LL; C; 45	Caltrate 600 Plus Iron and Vitamin D	600 mg; 18 mg; 125 IU	Red	Tablet	Oblong, Scored	Wyeth Consumer Healthcare
LL; C60; CENTRUM JR	Centrum JR. with Extra Calcium	18 mg; 5000 IU; 400 IU; 30 IU; 400 mcg; 45 mcg; 1.5 mg; 10 mg; 1.7 mg; 20 mg; 40 mg; 150 mcg; 2 mg; 50 mg; 160 mg; 15 mg; 1 mg; 20 mcg; 20 mcg; 60 mg; 2 mg; 6 mcg; 10 mcg	Red	Tablet	Oblong, Scored	Wyeth Consumer Healthcare
LL; C; 67	Chlordiazepoxide and Amitriptyline Hydrochloride	5 mg; 12.5 mg	Green	Coated Tablet	Circle	Lederle Laboratories
LL; C; 68	Chlordiazepoxide and Amitriptyline Hydrochloride	10 mg; 25 mg	White	Coated Tablet	Circle	Lederle Laboratories

IMPRINT	BRAND/GENERIC NAME	STRENGTH	COLOR	FORM	SHAPE	MANUFACTURER
LL; C; 69	Clorazepate Dipotassium	3.75 mg	Blue	Tablet	Circle, Scored	Lederle Laboratories
LL; C; 70	Clorazepate Dipotassium	7.5 mg	Peach	Tablet	Circle, Scored	Lederle Laboratories
LL; C; 71	Clorazepate Dipotassium	15 mg	White	Tablet	Circle, Scored	Lederle Laboratories
LL; C; 81	Cephalexin	250 mg	White	Coated Tablet	Oblong	Lederle Laboratories
LL; C; 82	Cephalexin	500 mg	White	Coated Tablet	Oblong	Lederle Laboratories
LL;CA85	Calcium Centrum Singles	500 mg	White	Tablet	Oblong	Lederle Laboratories
LL; D1; DIAMOX; 125	Diamox	125 mg	White	Tablet	Circle, Flat, Scored	Wyeth Pharmaceuticals
LL; D2; DIAMOX; 250	Diamox	250 mg	White	Tablet	Four-Sided, Convex	Lederle Laboratories
LL; D2; DIAMOX; 250	Diamox	250 mg	White	Tablet	Four-Sided, Convex	Wyeth Pharmaceuticals
LL; D2; DIAMOX; 250	Diamox	250 mg	White	Tablet	Four-Sided, Convex	Wyeth-Ayerst Laboratories
LL; D11	Declomycin	150 mg	Red	Coated Tablet	Circle, Convex	Lederle Laboratories
LL; D12	Declomycin	300 mg	Red	Coated Tablet	Circle, Convex	Lederle Laboratories
LL; D; 31	Diphenoxylate Hydrochloride and Atropine Sulfate	2.5 mg; 0.025 mg	White	Tablet	Circle	Lederle Laboratories
LL; D32	Docusate Sodium	100 mg	Red and Orange-Red	Capsule		Lederle Laboratories
LL; D34	Docusate Sodium with Casanthranol	100 mg; 30 mg	Maroon	Capsule		Lederle Laboratories
LL; D; 41	Doxycycline Hyclate	100 mg	Green	Coated Tablet	Circle	Lederle Laboratories
LL; D; 44	Dipyridamole	25 mg	Purple or White	Coated Tablet	Circle	Lederle Laboratories
LL; D; 45	Dipyridamole	50 mg	Purple or White	Coated Tablet	Circle	Lederle Laboratories
LL; D; 46	Dipyridamole	75 mg	Purple or White	Coated Tablet	Circle	Lederle Laboratories
LL; D; 51	Diazepam	2 mg	White	Tablet	Circle, Scored	Lederle Laboratories
LL; D52	Diazepam	5 mg	Light Brown	Tablet	Circle, Scored	Lederle Laboratories
LL; D53	Diazepam	10 mg	Light Green	Tablet	Circle, Scored	Lederle Laboratories
LL; D71	Diltiazem	30 mg	Blue	Coated Tablet	Circle, Convex	Lederle Laboratories
LL; D; 72	Diltiazem	60 mg	Blue	Coated Tablet	Round, Convex, Bisected Scored	Lederle Laboratories
LL; D; 75	Diltiazem	90 mg	Blue	Coated Tablet	Oblong, Convex, Bisected Scored	Lederle Laboratories
LL; D; 77	Diltiazem	120 mg	Blue	Coated Tablet	Oblong, Convex, Bisected Scored	Lederle Laboratories
LL; E2	Erythromycin Stearate	250 mg	Yellow	Coated Tablet	Circle	Lederle Laboratories
LL; E5;	Erythromycin Stearate	500 mg	Yellow	Coated Tablet	Oval	Lederle Laboratories
LL; E10	Erythromycin Ethylsuccinate	400 mg	Beige	Tablet	Oval	Lederle Laboratories
LL; EXTRA C; C39; CENTRUM JR	Centrum JR. Plus Extra C, Advanced Formula	18 mg; 5000 IU; 400 IU; 30 IU; 400 mcg; 45 mcg; 1.5 mg; 10 mg; 1.7 mg; 20 mg; 40 mg; 150 mcg; 2 mg; 50 mg; 108 mg; 15 mg; 1 mg; 20 mcg; 20 mcg; 300 mg; 2 mg; 6 mcg; 10 mcg		Tablet, Chewable	Oblong, Scored	Wyeth Consumer Healthcare
LL; F2	Ferro-Sequels, Dual-Action	150 mg; 100 mg	Green	Timed-Release Tablet	Oblong	Lederle Laboratories
LL; F11	Furosemide	20 mg	White to Off-White	Tablet	Circle	Lederle Laboratories
LL; F; 12	Furosemide	40 mg	White to Off-White	Tablet	Circle, Scored	Lederle Laboratories
LL; F; 13	Furosemide	80 mg	White to Off-White	Tablet	Circle, Scored	Lederle Laboratories
LL; F21	Ferrous Gluconate	300 mg	Green	Coated Tablet	Circle	Lederle Laboratories
LL; F; 22	Fenoprofen Calcium	600 mg	White	Coated Tablet	Capsule-Shape, Scored	Lederle Laboratories
LL; G2	Gevral T	27 mg; 5000 IU; 400 IU; 45 IU; 90 mg; 0.4 mg; 2.25 mg; 2.6 mg; 30 mg; 3 mg; 9 mcg; 162 mg; 225 mcg; 100 mg; 1.5 mg; 22.5 mg	Maroon	Coated Tablet	Oblong	Lederle Laboratories
LL; G17	Gemfibrozil	600 mg	White to Off-White	Coated Tablet	Oval, Scored	Lederle Laboratories
LL; H; 2	Hydromox R	50 mg; 0.125 mg	Yellow	Tablet	Circle, Scored	Lederle Laboratories
LL; H11	Hydralazine Hydrochloride	25 mg	Red	Coated Tablet	Circle, Convex	Lederle Laboratories
LL; H12	Hydralazine Hydrochloride	50 mg	Red	Coated Tablet	Circle, Convex	Lederle Laboratories
LL; H; 14	Hydrochlorothiazide	25 mg	Peach	Tablet	Circle, Scored	Lederle Laboratories
LL; H; 14	Hydrochlorothiazide	25 mg	Peach	Tablet	Circle, Scored	Udl Laboratories
LL; H; 15	Hydrochlorothiazide	50 mg	Peach	Tablet	Circle, Scored	Udl Laboratories
LL; HEART; B; 12	Ziac	2.5 mg; 6.25 mg	Yellow	Coated Tablet	Circle, Convex	Wyeth Pharmaceuticals
LL; HEART; B; 13	Ziac	5 mg; 6.25 mg	Pink	Coated Tablet	Circle, Convex	Wyeth Pharmaceuticals
LL; HEART; B; 14	Ziac	10 mg; 6.25 mg	White	Coated Tablet	Circle, Convex	Wyeth Pharmaceuticals
LL; I11	Imipramine Hydrochloride	10 mg	Yellow	Tablet	Circle	Lederle Laboratories
LL; I12	Imipramine Hydrochloride	25 mg	Rust	Tablet	Circle	Lederle Laboratories
LL; I13	Imipramine Hydrochloride	50 mg	Green	Tablet	Circle	Lederle Laboratories
LL; I; 27	Aches-N-Pain 200	200 mg	Orange	Coated Tablet	Circle, Convex	Lederle Laboratories
LL; J1	Methazolamide	25 mg	White	Tablet	Square, Convex	Lederle Laboratories
LL; J2	Methazolamide	50 mg	White	Tablet	Circle, Convex	Lederle Laboratories
LL; M; 1	Methotrexate	2.5 mg	Yellow	Tablet	Round, Convex, Bisected Scored	Lederle Laboratories
LL; M1	Rheumatrex	2.5 mg	Yellow	Tablet	Circle, Convex, Scored	Lederle Laboratories
LL; M3	Minocin	50 mg	Orange	Coated Tablet	Circle, Convex	Lederle Laboratories
LL; M5	Minocin	100 mg	Orange	Coated Tablet	Circle, Convex, Scored	Lederle Laboratories
LL; M6	Myambutol	100 mg	White	Coated Tablet	Circle, Convex	Lederle Laboratories
LL; M; 7	Myambutol	400 mg	White	Coated Tablet	Circle, Convex, Scored	Lederle Laboratories
LL; M8; MAXZIDE	Maxzide	50 mg; 75 mg	Yellow	Tablet	Bowtie	Lederle Laboratories
LL; M; 19	Methocarbamol	500 mg	White	Tablet	Circle, Scored	Lederle Laboratories
LL; M; 19	Methocarbamol	500 mg	White	Tablet	Circle, Scored	Udl Laboratories
LL; M; 20	Methocarbamol	750 mg	White	Tablet	Capsule-Shape, Scored	Lederle Laboratories
LL; M; 20	Methocarbamol	750 mg	White	Tablet	Capsule-Shape, Scored	Udl Laboratories
LL; M22	Methyldopa	250 mg	Peach	Coated Tablet	Circle	Lederle Laboratories
LL; M23	Methyldopa	500 mg	Peach	Coated Tablet	Circle	Lederle Laboratories

IMPRINT	BRAND/GENERIC NAME	STRENGTH	COLOR	FORM	SHAPE	MANUFACTURER
LL; M28	Metoclopramide Hydrochloride	10 mg	White		Circle, Scored	Lederle Laboratories
LL; M; 36	Methyldopa and Hydrochlorothiazide	250 mg; 15 mg	Yellow	Coated Tablet	Circle	Lederle Laboratories
LL; M; 37	Methyldopa and Hydrochlorothiazide	250 mg; 25 mg	Pink	Coated Tablet	Circle	Lederle Laboratories
LL; N; 1	Neptazane	50 mg	White	Tablet	Circle, Scored, Convex	Wyeth Pharmaceuticals
LL; N6	Nilstat	100,000 units	Yellow	Tablet	Oval, Convex	Lederle Laboratories
LL; N; 11	Naproxen	250 mg	Light Green	Tablet	Circle	Lederle Laboratories
LL; N; 17	Naproxen	375 mg	White	Tablet	Capsule-Shape	Lederle Laboratories
LL; N; 77	Naproxen	500 mg	Light Green	Tablet	Capsule-Shape	Lederle Laboratories
LL; P9	Pronemia	75 mg; 115 mg; 150 mg; 1 mg; 15 mcg	Red	Capsule		Lederle Laboratories
LL; P; 33	Propylthiouracil	50 mg	White	Tablet	Circle, Scored	Lederle Laboratories
LL; P; 36	Pyrazinamide	500 mg	White	Tablet	Circle, Scored, Convex	Lederle Laboratories
LL; P; 36	Pyrazinamide	500 mg	White	Tablet	Circle, Scored, Convex	Udl Laboratories
LL; P; 44	Propranolol Hydrochloride	10 mg	Gray	Tablet	Circle, Scored	Lederle Laboratories
LL; P; 45	Propranolol Hydrochloride	20 mg	Purple	Tablet	Circle, Scored	Lederle Laboratories
LL; P; 46	Propranolol Hydrochloride	40 mg	Light Brown	Tablet	Circle	Lederle Laboratories
LL; P; 47	Propranolol Hydrochloride	80 mg	Light Blue	Tablet	Circle, Scored	Lederle Laboratories
LL; P; 48	Procainamide Hydrochloride SR	250 mg	Light Blue	Coated Tablet	Oval, Scored	Lederle Laboratories
LL; P; 65	Propranolol Hydrochloride	60 mg	White	Tablet	Circle	Lederle Laboratories
LL; P72	Perphenazine and Amitriptyline Hydrochloride	2 mg; 10 mg	Blue	Coated Tablet	Circle	Lederle Laboratories
LL; P73	Perphenazine with Amitriptyline Hydrochloride	2 mg; 25 mg	Orange	Coated Tablet	Circle	Lederle Laboratories
LL; P74	Perphenazine and Amitriptyline Hydrochloride	4 mg; 10 mg	Light Peach	Coated Tablet	Circle	Lederle Laboratories
LL; P75	Perphenazine and Amitriptyline Hydrochloride	4 mg; 25 mg	Yellow	Coated Tablet	Circle	Lederle Laboratories
LL; P; 76	Perphenazine and Amitriptyline Hydrochloride	4 mg; 50 mg	Orange	Coated Tablet	Circle	Lederle Laboratories
LL; Q; 11	Quinidine Sulfate	200 mg	White	Tablet	Circle, Convex, Scored	Lederle Laboratories
LL; S; 1	Advanced Formula Stresstabs 600	45 mcg; 400 mcg; 100 mg; 15 mg; 5 mg; 500 mg; 30 IU; 15 mg; 12 mcg; 20 mg	Orange	Tablet	Oblong	Lederle Laboratories
LL; S; 1	Stresstabs	45 mcg; 400 mcg; 20 mg; 12 mcg; 10 mg; 30 IU; 500 mg; 5 mg; 10 mg; 100 mg	Orange	Tablet	Oblong, Scored	Lederle Laboratories
LL; S; 3	Stresstabs 600 Plus Zinc	30 IU; 600 mg; 400 mcg; 20 IU; 10 mg; 100 mg; 5 mg; 12 mcg; 45 mcg; 25 mg; 3 mg; 23.9 mg	Peach	Tablet	Oblong, Scored	Lederle Laboratories
LL; S; 3	Stresstabs Plus Zinc	30 IU; 500 mg; 400 mcg; 10 mg; 10 mg; 100 mg; 5 mg; 12 mcg; 45 mcg; 20 mg; 3 mg; 23.9 mg	Peach	Tablet	Oblong, Scored	Lederle Laboratories
LL; S11	Selegiline Hydrochloride	5 mg	White	Tablet	Circle	Esi Lederle
LL; S; 14	Sulfasalazine	500 mg	Brown	Tablet	Circle, Scored	Lederle Laboratories
LL; S; 16	Sulindac	150 mg	Yellow	Tablet	Circle, Scored	Lederle Laboratories
LL; S; 17	Sulindac	200 mg	Yellow	Tablet	Circle, Scored	Lederle Laboratories
LL; T1	Tri-Hemic 600	30 IU; 75 mg; 1 mg; 115 mg; 50 mg; 600 mg; 25 mcg	Red	Coated Tablet	Oblong	Lederle Laboratories
LL; T13	Sulfamethoxazole and Trimethoprim	400 mg; 80 mg	White	Tablet	Circle, Scored	Lederle Laboratories
LL; T16	Sulfamethoxazole and Trimethoprim	800 mg; 160 mg	White	Tablet	Oblong	Lederle Laboratories
LL; T; 29	Trazodone Hydrochloride	50 mg	White	Tablet	Circle, Scored	Lederle Laboratories
LL; T; 30	Trazodone Hydrochloride	100 mg	White	Tablet	Circle, Scored	Lederle Laboratories
LL; T31; 50; 100	Trazodone Hydrochloride	150 mg	White	Tablet	Four-Sided, Scored	Lederle Laboratories
LL; T; 34	Theophylline C.R.	100 mg	White	Timed-Release Tablet	Circle, Convex	Lederle Laboratories
LL; V; 5	Verapamil Hydrochloride	120 mg	White	Coated Tablet	Circle, Scored	Lederle Laboratories
LNK; 25	Diphenhydramine	25 mg	Clear and Pink	Capsule		Pioneer Pharmaceuticals
LODINE; 200	Lodine	200 mg	Light Grey with a Wide Red Band	Capsule		Wyeth Pharmaceuticals
LODINE; 300	Lodine	300 mg	Light Gray with a Wide Red Band, Light Gray with 2 Narrow Red Bands	Capsule		Wyeth Pharmaceuticals
LODINE; 400	Lodine	400 mg	Yellow-Orange	Coated Tablet	Oval	Wyeth Pharmaceuticals
LODINE; 500	Lodine	500 mg	Blue	Coated Tablet	Oval	Wyeth Pharmaceuticals
LODINE XL; 400	Lodine Xl	400 mg	Orange-Red	Extended-Release Tablet	Capsule-Shape, Biconvex	Wyeth Pharmaceuticals
LODINE XL; 500	Lodine Xl	500 mg	Grey-Green	Extended-Release Tablet	Capsule-Shape, Biconvex	Wyeth Pharmaceuticals
LODINE XL; 600	Lodine Xl	600 mg	Light Grey	Extended-Release Tablet	Capsule-Shape, Biconvex	Wyeth Pharmaceuticals
LONITEN; 10;	Loniten	10 mg	White	Tablet	Circle, Scored	Pharmacia & Upjohn
LORELCO; 250	Lorelco	250 mg	White	Coated Tablet	Circle	Hoechst Marion Roussel
LORELCO; 500	Lorelco	500 mg	White	Coated Tablet	Capsule-Shape	Hoechst Marion Roussel
LOTENSIN; 5;	Lotensin	5 mg	Light Yellow	Tablet	Circle	Novartis Pharmaceuticals
LOTENSIN; 10;	Lotensin	10 mg	Dark Yellow	Tablet	Circle	Novartis Pharmaceuticals

IMPRINT	BRAND/GENERIC NAME	STRENGTH	COLOR	FORM	SHAPE	MANUFACTURER
LOTENSIN; 20;	Lotensin	20 mg	Tan	Tablet	Circle	Novartis Pharmaceuticals
LOTENSIN; 40;	Lotensin	40 mg	Dark Rose	Tablet	Circle	Novartis Pharmaceuticals
LOTENSIN HCT; 57;	Lotensin HCT	5 mg; 6.25 mg	White	Tablet	Oblong, Scored	Novartis Pharmaceuticals
LOTENSIN HCT; 72;	Lotensin HCT	10 mg; 12.5 mg	Light Pink	Tablet	Oblong, Scored	Novartis Pharmaceuticals
LOTENSIN HCT; 74;	Lotensin HCT	20 mg; 12.5 mg	Grayish-Violet	Tablet	Oblong, Scored	Novartis Pharmaceuticals
LOTENSIN HCT; 75;	Lotensin HCT	20 mg; 25 mg	Red	Tablet	Scored, Oblong	Novartis Pharmaceuticals
LOTREL; 2255	Lotrel 2.5/10	2.5 mg; 10 mg	White with 2 Gold Bands	Capsule		Novartis Pharmaceuticals
LOTREL; 2260	Lotrel 5/10	5 mg; 10 mg	Light Brown with 2 White Bands	Capsule		Novartis Pharmaceuticals
LOTREL; 2265	Lotrel 5/20	5 mg; 20 mg	Pink with 2 White Bands	Capsule		Novartis Pharmaceuticals
LSP; 2 1/2	Lisinopril	2.5 mg	Light Yellow Mottled	Tablet	Circle	Lek Pharmaceuticals
LSP; 5	Lisinopril	5 mg	Green, Mottled	Tablet	Circle	Lek Pharmaceuticals
LSP; 10	Lisinopril	10 mg	Yellow, Mottled	Tablet	Circle	Lek Pharmaceuticals
LSP; 20	Lisinopril	20 mg	Light Gray, Mottled	Tablet	Circle	Lek Pharmaceuticals
LSP; 30	Lisinopril	30 mg	Light Gray Mottled	Tablet	Circle	Lek Pharmaceuticals
LSP; 40	Lisinopril	40 mg	Light Gray, Mottled	Tablet	Circle	Lek Pharmaceuticals
LTG; 2	Lamictal	2 mg	White	Tablet, Chewable	Circle	Glaxosmithkline
LUCHEM; 5	Hydrocodone Bitartrate and Acetaminophen	5 mg; 500 mg	White	Tablet	Oblong	Norton, H.N.
LUCHEM; 649	Dexophed	6 mg; 120 mg	Green	Sustained-Release Tablet	Circle	Norton, H.N.
LUCHEM; 663	Allay	5 mg; 500 mg	Black and Red	Capsule		Norton, H.N.
LUCHEM; 663	Hydrocodone Bitartrate and Acetaminophen	5 mg; 500 mg	Red and Black	Capsule		Norton, H.N.
LUCHEM; 743	Histatan	25 mg; 8 mg; 25 mg	Beige	Sustained-Release Tablet	Oblong	Norton, H.N.
LUCHEM; 990	Quinine Sulfate 5 grain	325 mg	Clear with White Powder	Capsule		Norton, H.N.
LUCHEM; 992	Chlorpheniramine Maleate	12 mg	Green and Clear with Red and White Beads	Sustained-Release Capsule		Norton, H.N.
LUCHEM; 993	Chlorpheniramine Maleate	8 mg	Green and Clear with Red and White Beads	Sustained-Release Capsule		Norton, H.N.
LUPIN; 302	Cefuroxime Axetil	250 mg	White to Off-White	Tablet	Capsule-Shape	Watson Laboratories
LUPIN; 303	Cefuroxime Axetil	500 mg	White to Off-White	Tablet	Capsule-Shape	Watson Laboratories
LV; 10; G	Lovastatin	10 mg	Peach	Tablet	Circle	Par Pharmaceutical
LV; 20; G	Lovastatin	20 mg	Light Blue	Tablet	Circle	Par Pharmaceutical
LV; 40; G	Lovastatin	40 mg	Green	Tablet	Circle	Par Pharmaceutical
M	Cepacol Anesthetic Lozenges	10 mg; 1.4 mg	Green	Lozenge/troche	Circle	J.B. Williams
M	Daily Vite with Iron	5000 IU; 60 mg; 400 IU; 30 IU; 1.5 mg; 1.7 mg; 20 mg; 2 mg; 400 mcg; 6 mcg; 10 mg; 18 mg	Yellow	Tablet	Circle	Rugby Laboratories
M	Momentum	500 mg; 15 mg	White	Tablet	Oval	Whitehall Laboratories
M	Mylanta Soothing Antacid Cherry Creme	600 mg	Pink	Lozenge/troche		Johnson & Johnson Merck Consumer Pharmaceuticals
M	Mylanta Soothing Antacid Cool Mint Creme	600 mg		Lozenge/troche		Johnson & Johnson Merck Consumer Pharmaceuticals
M; 01	Captopril	12.5 mg	White	Tablet	Oval	Stada
M01; MOVA	Captopril	12.5 mg		Tablet		Mova Pharmaceutical
M03; 1.5	Glyburide	1.5 mg	White	Tablet	Oval	Stada
M03; 1.5; MOVA	Glyburide Micronized	1.5 mg	White	Tablet	Oval, Bisected Scored	Mova Pharmaceutical
M03; 1.5; MOVA	Glyburide Micronized	1.5 mg	White	Tablet	Oval, Bisected Scored	Watson Laboratories
M04; 3.0	Glyburide	3 mg	Blue	Tablet	Oval	Stada
M04; 3.0; MOVA	Glyburide Micronized	3 mg	Blue	Tablet	Oval, Bisected Scored	Mova Pharmaceutical
M04; 3.0; MOVA	Glyburide Micronized	3 mg	Blue	Tablet	Oval, Bisected Scored	Watson Laboratories
M05; 50	Captopril	50 mg	White	Tablet	Capsule-Shape	Stada
M05; MOVA; 50	Captopril	50 mg		Tablet		Mova Pharmaceutical
M06; 4.5; MOVA	Glyburide (Micronized)	4.5 mg	Light Green	Tablet	Oval, Bisected Scored	Mova Pharmaceutical
M07; 6.0; MOVA	Glyburide Micronized	6 mg	Light Yellow	Tablet	Oval, Bisected Scored	Mova Pharmaceutical
M07; 6.0; MOVA	Glyburide Micronized	6 mg	Light Yellow	Tablet	Oval, Bisected Scored	Watson Laboratories
M07; 6.5	Glyburide	6 mg	Light Yellow	Tablet	Oval	Stada
M; 018;	Nucofed	20 mg; 60 mg	Green and Clear	Capsule		Monarch Pharmaceuticals
M; 019;	Quibron-T/SR	300 mg	White	Sustained-Release Tablet	Accudose (Triple-Scored)	Monarch Pharmaceuticals
M; 020	Quibron-T	300 mg	Ivory	Tablet	Accudose (Triple-Scored)	Monarch Pharmaceuticals
M; 022;	Quibron	150 mg; 90 mg	Clear Yellow	Capsule, Liquid Filled		Monarch Pharmaceuticals
M; 052;	Septra	400 mg; 80 mg	Pink	Tablet	Circle, Scored	Monarch Pharmaceuticals
M; 053;	Septra DS	800 mg; 160 mg	Pink	Tablet	Oval, Scored	Monarch Pharmaceuticals
M; 057	Sucralfate	1 GM	White	Tablet	Oblong, Scored	Akyma Pharmaceuticals
M; 057	Sucralfate	1 G	White	Tablet	Oblong, Scored	Eon Labs
M; 057	Sucralfate	1 G	White	Tablet	Oblong, Scored	Martec Pharmaceuticals
M; 064	Fluphenazine Hydrochloride	10 mg	Orange	Coated Tablet	Circle	H.L. Moore
M; 0661	Fluoxetine Hydrochloride	10 mg	Light Green	Capsule		Mallinckrodt
M; 0663	Fluoxetine Hydrochloride	20 mg	Green and White	Capsule		Mallinckrodt
M; 1	Clonidine Hydrochloride and Chlorthalidone	0.1 mg; 15 mg	Yellow	Tablet	Circle, Scored, Biconvex	Mylan Pharmaceuticals
M; 1	Clorpres	15 mg; 0.1 mg	Yellow	Tablet	Circle, Scored	Bertek Pharmaceuticals
M; 1	Rheumatrex	2.5 mg	Yellow	Tablet		Stada
M; 2	Acetaminophen and Codeine	300 mg; 15 mg	White	Tablet	Circle	Mallinckrodt
M; 2	Furosemide	20 mg	White	Tablet	Circle, Bevel-Edged	Mylan Pharmaceuticals
M; 2	Furosemide	20 mg	White	Tablet	Circle, Bevel-Edged	Udl Laboratories
M; 2	Hydromorphone Hydrochloride	2 mg	White	Tablet	Circle	Mallinckrodt
M; 3	Acetaminophen and Codeine	300 mg; 30 mg		Tablet		Mallinckrodt
M4	Mesnex	400 mg	White	Coated Tablet	Oblong, Scored Biconvex	Bristol-Myers Squibb
M; 4	Acetaminophen and Codeine	300 mg; 60 mg	White	Tablet	Circle	Mallinckrodt

IMPRINT	BRAND/GENERIC NAME	STRENGTH	COLOR	FORM	SHAPE	MANUFACTURER
M; 4	Fluphenazine Hydrochloride	1 mg	White	Coated Tablet	Triangle	Mylan Pharmaceuticals
M; 4	Fluphenazine Hydrochloride	1 mg	White	Coated Tablet	Triangle	Udl Laboratories
M; 4	Hydromorphone Hydrochloride	4 mg	White	Tablet	Circle	Mallinckrodt
M; 5	Dextroamphetamine Sulfate	5 mg	White	Tablet	Triangle	Mallinckrodt
M; 5	Methimazole	5 mg	White	Tablet	Circle, Score	Daniels Pharmaceuticals
M; 5	Methylin	5 mg	White	Tablet	Circle	Mallinckrodt
M; 5	Oxycodone Hydrochloride	5 mg	White	Tablet	Circle, Scored	Mallinckrodt
M; 6	Erythromycin Stearate	250 mg	Pink	Tablet		West-Ward
M; 9	Fluphenazine Hydrochloride	2.5 mg	Yellow	Coated Tablet	Triangle	Mylan Pharmaceuticals
M; 9	Fluphenazine Hydrochloride	2.5 mg	Yellow	Coated Tablet	Triangle	Udl Laboratories
M; 10	Dextroamphetamine Sulfate	10 mg	White	Tablet	Diamond	Mallinckrodt
M; 10	Donnamar	0.125 mg	Pink	Tablet		Marnel Pharmaceuticals
M; 10	Methimazole	10 mg	White	Tablet	Circle, Score	Daniels Pharmaceuticals
M; 10	Methylin	10 mg	White	Tablet	Circle, Scored	Mallinckrodt
M10; 100	Captopril	100 mg	White	Tablet	Capsule-Shape	Stada
M10; MOVA; 100	Captopril	100 mg		Tablet		Mova Pharmaceutical
M; 11	Donnamar PB	0.13 mg; 16.2 mg	Blue	Tablet		Marnel Pharmaceuticals
M; 11	Penicillin V Potassium	250 mg	White	Tablet	Oval	Mylan Pharmaceuticals
M; 12	Penicillin V Potassium	500 mg	White	Tablet	Circle, Scored	Mylan Pharmaceuticals
M; 12	Penicillin VK	500 mg		Tablet		Teva Pharmaceuticals
M; 13	Tolbutamide	500 mg	White	Tablet	Circle, Scored	Mylan Pharmaceuticals
M; 13	Tolbutamide	500 mg	White	Tablet	Circle, Scored	Udl Laboratories
M; 13	Tolbutamide	0.5 G	White	Tablet		West-Ward
M; 14	Methotrexate Sodium	2.5 mg	Orange	Tablet	Circle, Scored	Mylan Pharmaceuticals
M; 14	Methotrexate Sodium	2.5 mg	Orange	Tablet	Circle, Scored	Udl Laboratories
M; 15	Atropine Sulfate and Diphenoxylate Hydrochloride	0.025 mg; 2.5 mg	White	Tablet	Circle	Mylan Pharmaceuticals
M; 15	Atropine Sulfate and Diphenoxylate Hydrochloride	0.025 mg; 2.5 mg	White	Tablet	Circle	Udl Laboratories
M; 15	Klor-Con M15	1125 mg	White	Tablet	Oblong	Upsher-Smith Laboratories
M; 15	Morphine Sulfate	15 mg	Blue	Extended-Release Tablet	Circle	Mallinckrodt
M; 15	Oxycodone Hydrochloride	15 mg	Light Green	Tablet	Circle	Mallinckrodt
M; 16	Marcillin	250 mg	Red	Capsule		Marnel Pharmaceuticals
M; 17	Marcillin	500 mg	Red	Capsule		Marnel Pharmaceuticals
M; 17; 378	Ampicillin Trihydrate	250 mg	Grey and Maroon	Capsule		West-Ward
M; 18	Marpres	0.1 mg; 25 mg; 15 mg		Tablet		Marnel Pharmaceuticals
M; 20	Methylin	20 mg	White	Tablet	Circle, Scored	Mallinckrodt
M; 23	Diltiazem Hydrochloride	30 mg	White	Coated Tablet	Circle	Mylan Pharmaceuticals
M; 23	Diltiazem Hydrochloride	30 mg	White	Coated Tablet	Circle	Udl Laboratories
M; 25	L-Thyroxine	0.025 mg	Blue	Tablet	Circle, Scored	Mova Pharmaceutical
M; 25	L-Thyroxine	0.025 mg	Blue	Tablet	Circle, Scored	Warner Chilcott
M25; 250	Naproxen	250 mg	Rose	Tablet	Circle	Stada
M; 27	Clonidine Hydrochloride and Chlorthalidone	0.2 mg; 15 mg	Yellow	Tablet	Circle, Scored, Biconvex	Mylan Pharmaceuticals
M; 27	Clorpres	15 mg; 0.2 mg	Yellow	Tablet	Circle, Scored	Bertek Pharmaceuticals
M; 28	Nadolol	20 mg	Yellow	Tablet	Circle, Scored	Mylan Pharmaceuticals
M; 28	Nadolol	20 mg	Yellow	Tablet	Circle, Scored	Udl Laboratories
M; 29	Methyclothiazide	5 mg	Blue	Tablet	Circle, Scored	Mylan Pharmaceuticals
M; 30	Clorazepate Dipotassium	3.75 mg	Blue	Tablet	Circle, Scored, Flat Beveled Edge	Mylan Pharmaceuticals
M; 30	Clorazepate Dipotassium	3.75 mg	Blue	Tablet	Circle, Scored, Flat Beveled Edge	Udl Laboratories
M; 30	Morphine Sulfate	30 mg	Purple	Extended-Release Tablet	Circle	Mallinckrodt
M; 30	Oxycodone Hydrochloride	30 mg	Light Blue	Tablet	Circle	Mallinckrodt
M; 31	Allopurinol	100 mg	White	Tablet	Circle, Scored	Mylan Pharmaceuticals
M; 31	Allopurinol	100 mg	White	Tablet	Circle, Scored	Udl Laboratories
M; 32	Metoprolol Tartrate	50 mg	Pink	Coated Tablet	Circle, Scored	Mylan Pharmaceuticals
M; 32	Metoprolol Tartrate	50 mg	Pink	Coated Tablet	Circle, Scored	Udl Laboratories
M; 33	Chlorothiazide and Reserpine	0.125 mg; 250 mg	Light Orange	Tablet	Circle, Scored, Flat Beveled Edge	Mylan Pharmaceuticals
M; 33; 56	Orphenadrine Citrate, Aspirin and Caffeine Double Strength	50 mg; 770 mg; 60 mg	White and Yellow Layered	Tablet	Capsule-Shape	Mylan Pharmaceuticals
M; 35	Chlorthalidone	25 mg	Yellow	Tablet	Circle	Mylan Pharmaceuticals
M; 35	Chlorthalidone	25 mg	Yellow	Tablet	Circle	Udl Laboratories
M; 36	Amitriptyline Hydrochloride	50 mg	Brown	Coated Tablet	Circle	Mylan Pharmaceuticals
M; 36	Amitriptyline Hydrochloride	50 mg	Brown	Coated Tablet	Circle	Udl Laboratories
M; 37	Amitriptyline Hydrochloride	75 mg	Blue	Coated Tablet	Circle	Mylan Pharmaceuticals
M; 37	Amitriptyline Hydrochloride	75 mg	Blue	Coated Tablet	Circle	Udl Laboratories
M37; 375	Naproxen	375 mg	White	Tablet	Capsule-Shape	Stada
M; 38	Amitriptyline Hydrochloride	100 mg	Orange	Coated Tablet	Circle	Mylan Pharmaceuticals
M; 38	Amitriptyline Hydrochloride	100 mg	Orange	Coated Tablet	Circle	Udl Laboratories
M; 39	Amitriptyline Hydrochloride	150 mg	Flesh	Coated Tablet	Capsule-Shape	Mylan Pharmaceuticals
M; 39	Amitriptyline Hydrochloride	150 mg	Flesh	Coated Tablet	Capsule-Shape	Udl Laboratories
M; 40	Clorazepate Dipotassium	7.5 mg	Peach	Tablet	Circle, Scored, Flat Beveled Edge	Mylan Pharmaceuticals
M; 40	Clorazepate Dipotassium	7.5 mg	Peach	Tablet	Circle, Scored, Flat Beveled Edge	Udl Laboratories
M; 40; MATERNA	Materna Prenatal Vitamin and Mineral	100 mg; 30 mcg; 25 mcg; 1 mg; 60 mg; 5 mg; 20 mg; 5000 IU; 10 mg; 25 mg; 30 IU; 400 IU; 3.4 mg; 10 mg; 12 mcg; 3 mg; 25 mcg; 25 mg; 150 mcg; 2 mg; 250 mg	Off-White	Coated Tablet	Oval, Scored	Lederle Laboratories

IMPRINT	BRAND/GENERIC NAME	STRENGTH	COLOR	FORM	SHAPE	MANUFACTURER
M; 40; MATERNA	Materna Prenatal Vitamin and Mineral	100 mg; 30 mcg; 25 mcg; 1 mg; 60 mg; 5 mg; 20 mg; 5000 IU; 10 mg; 25 mg; 30 IU; 400 IU; 3.4 mg; 10 mg; 12 mcg; 3 mg; 25 mcg; 25 mg; 150 mcg; 2 mg; 250 mg	Off-White	Coated Tablet	Oval, Scored	Wyeth Pharmaceuticals
M; 40; MATERNA	Materna Prenatal Vitamin and Mineral	100 mg; 30 mcg; 25 mcg; 1 mg; 60 mg; 5 mg; 20 mg; 5000 IU; 10 mg; 25 mg; 30 IU; 400 IU; 3.4 mg; 10 mg; 12 mcg; 3 mg; 25 mcg; 25 mg; 150 mcg; 2 mg; 250 mg	Off-White	Coated Tablet	Oval, Scored	Wyeth-Ayerst Laboratories
M; 41	Spironolactone and Hydrochlorothiazide	25 mg; 25 mg	Ivory	Tablet	Circle, Scored, Compressed	Mylan Pharmaceuticals
M; 41	Spironolactone and Hydrochlorothiazide	25 mg; 25 mg	Ivory	Tablet	Circle, Scored, Compressed	Udl Laboratories
M; 43	Chlorothiazide and Reserpine	0.125 mg; 500 mg	Light Orange	Tablet	Circle, Scored, Flat Beveled Edge	Mylan Pharmaceuticals
M; 44	Cyproheptadine Hydrochloride	4 mg	White	Tablet		West-Ward
M 44	Cyproheptadine Hydrochloride	4 mg	White	Tablet	Circle, Scored, Flat Beveled Edge	Mylan Pharmaceuticals
M; 45	Diltiazem Hydrochloride	60 mg	White	Coated Tablet	Circle, Scored	Mylan Pharmaceuticals
M; 45	Diltiazem Hydrochloride	60 mg	White	Coated Tablet	Circle, Scored	Udl Laboratories
M45; LEDERLE; 50 MG	Minocin Pellet-Filled	50 mg	Yellow and Green	Capsule		Lederle Laboratories
M; 46	Spironolactone	25 mg	Orange	Tablet		Mylan Pharmaceuticals
M46; LEDERLE; 100 MG	Minocin Pellet-Filled	100 mg	Light Green and Green	Capsule		Lederle Laboratories
M; 47	Metoprolol Tartrate	100 mg	Blue	Coated Tablet	Circle, Scored	Mylan Pharmaceuticals
M; 47	Metoprolol Tartrate	100 mg	Blue	Coated Tablet	Circle, Scored	Udl Laboratories
M; 50	Chlorothiazide	250 mg	White	Tablet	Circle, Scored	Mylan Pharmaceuticals
M; 50	Chlorothiazide	250 mg	White	Tablet	Circle, Scored	Udl Laboratories
M; 50	L-Thyroxine	0.05 mg	Blue	Tablet	Circle, Scored	Mova Pharmaceutical
M; 50	L-Thyroxine	0.05 mg	Blue	Tablet	Circle, Scored	Warner Chilcott
M50; 500	Naproxen	500 mg	Rose	Tablet	Capsule-Shape	Stada
M; 51	Amitriptyline Hydrochloride	25 mg	Light Green	Coated Tablet	Circle	Mylan Pharmaceuticals
M; 51	Amitriptyline Hydrochloride	25 mg	Light Green	Coated Tablet	Circle	Udl Laboratories
M; 52	Pindolol	5 mg	White	Tablet	Circle, Scored, Biconvex	Mylan Pharmaceuticals
M; 53	Cimetidine	200 mg	Green	Coated Tablet	Five-Sided, House Shaped, Biconvex, Beveled Edge	Mylan Pharmaceuticals
M 54; 10	Thioridazine Hydrochloride	10 mg		Tablet		Roxane Laboratories
M; 54; 10	Thioridazine	10 mg	Orange	Coated Tablet	Circle	H.L. Moore
M; 54; 10	Thioridazine Hydrochloride	10 mg	Orange	Coated Tablet	Circle	Mylan Pharmaceuticals
M; 54; 10	Thioridazine Hydrochloride	10 mg	Orange	Coated Tablet	Circle	Udl Laboratories
M; 55	Timolol Maleate	5 mg	Green	Tablet	Circle, Flat Beveled Edge	Mylan Pharmaceuticals
M; 58; 25	Thioridazine	25 mg	Orange	Coated Tablet	Circle	H.L. Moore
M; 58; 25	Thioridazine Hydrochloride	25 mg	Orange	Coated Tablet	Circle	Mylan Pharmaceuticals
M; 58; 25	Thioridazine Hydrochloride	25 mg		Tablet		Roxane Laboratories
M; 58; 25	Thioridazine Hydrochloride	25 mg	Orange	Coated Tablet	Circle	Udl Laboratories
M; 59; 50	Thioridazine	50 mg	Orange	Coated Tablet	Circle	H.L. Moore
M; 59; 50	Thioridazine Hydrochloride	50 mg	Orange	Coated Tablet	Circle	Mylan Pharmaceuticals
M; 59; 50	Thioridazine Hydrochloride	50 mg		Tablet		Roxane Laboratories
M; 59; 50	Thioridazine Hydrochloride	50 mg	Orange	Coated Tablet	Circle	Udl Laboratories
M; 60	Maprotiline Hydrochloride	25 mg	White	Coated Tablet	Circle, Scored, Biconvex, Beveled Edge	Mylan Pharmaceuticals
M; 60	Morphine Sulfate	60 mg	Orange	Extended-Release Tablet	Circle	Mallinckrodt
M; 61; 100	Thioridazine	100 mg	Orange	Coated Tablet	Circle	H.L. Moore
M; 61; 100	Thioridazine Hydrochloride	100 mg	Orange	Coated Tablet	Circle	Mylan Pharmaceuticals
M; 61; 100	Thioridazine Hydrochloride	100 mg		Tablet		Roxane Laboratories
M; 61; 100	Thioridazine Hydrochloride	100 mg	Orange	Coated Tablet	Circle	Udl Laboratories
M; 63	Atenolol and Chlorthalidone	50 mg; 25 mg	White	Tablet	Circle, Scored, Biconvex	Mylan Pharmaceuticals
M; 64	Atenolol and Chlorthalidone	100 mg; 25 mg	White	Tablet	Circle, Biconvex	Mylan Pharmaceuticals
M; 65	Acetaminophen and Propoxyphene Hydrochloride	65 mg; 650 mg	Orange	Capsule		Mylan Pharmaceuticals
M; 65	Pancet	650 mg; 65 mg	Red-Orange	Tablet		Pamlab
M; 69	Indapamide	1.25 mg		Tablet		Mylan Pharmaceuticals
M; 70	Clorazepate Dipotassium	15 mg	White	Tablet	Circle, Scored, Flat Beveled Edge	Mylan Pharmaceuticals
M; 70	Clorazepate Dipotassium	15 mg	White	Tablet	Circle, Scored, Flat Beveled Edge	Udl Laboratories
M; 71	Allopurinol	300 mg	White	Tablet	Circle, Scored	Mylan Pharmaceuticals
M; 71	Allopurinol	300 mg	White	Tablet	Circle, Scored	Udl Laboratories
M; 72	Clonidine Hydrochloride and Chlorthalidone	0.3 mg; 15 mg	Yellow	Tablet	Circle, Scored, Biconvex	Mylan Pharmaceuticals
M; 72	Clorpres	15 mg; 0.3 mg	Yellow	Tablet	Circle, Scored	Bertek Pharmaceuticals
M; 72	Menest	0.3 mg	Yellow	Coated Tablet	Oblong	Monarch Pharmaceuticals
M; 73	Menest	0.625 mg	Orange	Coated Tablet	Oblong	Monarch Pharmaceuticals
M; 74	Fluphenazine Hydrochloride	5 mg	Green	Coated Tablet	Triangle	Mylan Pharmaceuticals
M; 74	Fluphenazine Hydrochloride	5 mg	Green	Coated Tablet	Triangle	Udl Laboratories
M; 74	Menest	1.25 mg	Green	Coated Tablet	Oblong	Monarch Pharmaceuticals
M; 75	Chlorthalidone	50 mg	Green	Tablet	Circle, Scored	Mylan Pharmaceuticals
M; 75	Chlorthalidone	50 mg	Green	Tablet	Circle, Scored	Udl Laboratories
M; 75	L-Thyroxine	0.075 mg	Blue	Tablet	Circle, Scored	Mova Pharmaceutical
M; 75	L-Thyroxine	0.075 mg	Blue	Tablet	Circle, Scored	Warner Chilcott
M; 75	Menest	2.5 mg	Pink	Coated Tablet	Oblong	Monarch Pharmaceuticals
M; 76	Flurbiprofen	50 mg	Beige	Coated Tablet	Circle	Mylan Pharmaceuticals

IMPRINT	BRAND/GENERIC NAME	STRENGTH	COLOR	FORM	SHAPE	MANUFACTURER
M; 77	Amitriptyline Hydrochloride	10 mg	White	Coated Tablet	Circle, Biconvex	Mylan Pharmaceuticals
M; 77	Amitriptyline Hydrochloride	10 mg	White	Coated Tablet	Circle, Biconvex	Udl Laboratories
M; 80	Indapamide	2.5 mg	White	Coated Tablet	Circle, Biconvex, Beveled Edge	Mylan Pharmaceuticals
M; 80	Indapamide	2.5 mg	White	Coated Tablet	Circle, Biconvex, Beveled Edge	Udl Laboratories
M; 81	Captopril and Hydrochlorothiazide	25 mg; 15 mg	White	Tablet	Circle, Scored	Mylan Pharmaceuticals
M; 83	Captopril and Hydrochlorothiazide	25 mg; 25 mg	Peach	Tablet	Circle, Scored	Mylan Pharmaceuticals
M; 84	Captopril and Hydrochlorothiazide	50 mg; 15 mg	White	Tablet	Capsule-Shape, Scored	Mylan Pharmaceuticals
M; 86	Captopril and Hydrochlorothiazide	50 mg; 25 mg	Peach	Tablet	Capsule-Shape, Scored	Mylan Pharmaceuticals
M; 87	Maprotiline Hydrochloride	50 mg	Blue	Coated Tablet	Circle, Scored, Biconvex, Beveled Edge	Mylan Pharmaceuticals
M; 90; W; 60MG	Modrastane	60 mg	Pink and Black	Capsule		Winthrop Pharmaceuticals
M; 91; W; 30MG	Modrastane	30 mg	Pink	Capsule		Winthrop Pharmaceuticals
M; 92	Maprotiline Hydrochloride	75 mg	White	Coated Tablet	Circle, Scored, Biconvex, Beveled Edge	Mylan Pharmaceuticals
M; 93	Flurbiprofen	100 mg	Beige	Coated Tablet	Circle	Mylan Pharmaceuticals
M; 93	Flurbiprofen	100 mg	Beige	Coated Tablet	Circle	Udl Laboratories
M; 95	Penicillin V Potassium	250 mg	White	Tablet	Circle, Scored	Mylan Pharmaceuticals
M; 97	Fluphenazine Hydrochloride	10 mg	Orange	Coated Tablet	Triangle	Mylan Pharmaceuticals
M; 97	Fluphenazine Hydrochloride	10 mg	Orange	Coated Tablet	Triangle	Udl Laboratories
M; 98	Penicillin V Potassium	500 mg	White	Tablet	Oval	Mylan Pharmaceuticals
M; 100	L-Thyroxine	0.1 mg	Blue	Tablet	Circle, Scored	Mova Pharmaceutical
M; 100	L-Thyroxine	0.1 mg	Blue	Tablet	Circle, Scored	Warner Chilcott
M; 100	Morphine Sulfate	100 mg	Gray	Extended-Release Tablet	Circle	Mallinckrodt
M; 100	Motrin	100 mg	White	Tablet	Capsule-Shape, Scored	Mcneil Consumer Products
M; 100; LEVO; T	L-Thyroxine	0.1 mg	Yellow	Tablet	Circle, Scored	Novartis Generics
M; 113	Glyburide, Micronized	1.5 mg	White	Tablet	Oval, Scored	Mylan Pharmaceuticals
M118	Pentazocine and Naloxone Hydrochloride	50 mg; 0.5 mg	Light Yellow	Tablet	Capsule-Shape, Scored	Ranbaxy Pharmaceuticals
M; 125	Glyburide, Micronized	3 mg	Light Yellow	Tablet	Oval, Scored	Mylan Pharmaceuticals
M; 125	L-Thyroxine	0.125 mg	Blue	Tablet	Circle, Scored	Mova Pharmaceutical
M; 125	L-Thyroxine	0.125 mg	Blue	Tablet	Circle, Scored	Warner Chilcott
M; 127	Pindolol	10 mg	White	Tablet	Circle, Scored, Biconvex	Mylan Pharmaceuticals
M; 132	Nadolol	80 mg	Yellow	Tablet	Circle, Scored	Mylan Pharmaceuticals
M; 132	Nadolol	80 mg	Yellow	Tablet	Circle, Scored	Udl Laboratories
M; 134	Ketorolac Tromethamine	10 mg	White	Tablet	Circle	Mylan Pharmaceuticals
M; 135	Diltiazem Hydrochloride	90 mg	White	Coated Tablet	Capsule-Shape, Scored	Mylan Pharmaceuticals
M; 135	Diltiazem Hydrochloride	90 mg	White	Coated Tablet	Capsule-Shape, Scored	Udl Laboratories
M; 142	Glyburide	6 mg	Green	Tablet	Oval, Scored	Mylan Pharmaceuticals
M; 144	Tamoxifen Citrate	10 mg	White	Tablet	Circle	Mylan Pharmaceuticals
M; 146	Spironolactone	25 mg	White	Coated Tablet	Circle, Biconvex, Bevel-Edged	Mylan Pharmaceuticals
M; 146	Spironolactone	25 mg	White	Coated Tablet	Circle, Biconvex, Bevel-Edged	Udl Laboratories
M; 150	L-Thyroxine	0.15 mg	Blue	Tablet	Circle, Scored	Warner Chilcott
M; 150; LEVO; T	L-Thyroxine	0.15 mg	Blue	Tablet	Circle, Scored	Novartis Generics
M; 171	Nadolol	40 mg	Yellow	Tablet	Circle, Scored	Mylan Pharmaceuticals
M; 171	Nadolol	40 mg	Yellow	Tablet	Circle, Scored	Udl Laboratories
M; 172	Metolazone	2.5 mg	Peach	Tablet	Circle	Mylan Pharmaceuticals
M; 200	L-Thyroxine	0.2 mg	Blue	Tablet	Circle, Scored	Mova Pharmaceutical
M; 200	L-Thyroxine	0.2 mg	Blue	Tablet	Circle, Scored	Warner Chilcott
M; 200	Morphine Sulfate	200 mg	Green	Extended-Release Tablet	Capsule-Shape	Mallinckrodt
M; 200; LEVO; T	L-Thyroxine	0.2 mg	Pink	Tablet	Circle, Scored	Novartis Generics
M; 221	Timolol Maleate	10 mg	Green	Tablet	Circle, Scored, Flat Beveled Edge	Mylan Pharmaceuticals
M; 231	Atenolol	50 mg	White	Tablet	Circle, Scored	Mylan Pharmaceuticals
M; 231	Atenolol	50 mg	White	Tablet	Circle, Scored	Udl Laboratories
M; 234	Metformin Hydrochloride	500 mg	White	Coated Tablet	Circle, Biconvex, Bevel Edged	Mylan Pharmaceuticals
M; 240	Metformin Hydrochloride	850 mg	White	Coated Tablet	Circle, Biconvex, Bevel Edged	Mylan Pharmaceuticals
M; 243	Spironolactone	50 mg	White	Coated Tablet	Circle, Biconvex, Bevel-Edged, Scored	Mylan Pharmaceuticals
M; 244	Metformin Hydrochloride	1000 mg	White	Coated Tablet	Oval, Biconvex, Bevel Edged	Mylan Pharmaceuticals
M; 253	Acyclovir	400 mg	White	Tablet	Circle	Mylan Pharmaceuticals
M; 255	Albuterol	2 mg	White	Tablet	Circle, Scored	Mylan Pharmaceuticals
M; 255	Albuterol	2 mg	White	Tablet	Circle, Scored	Udl Laboratories
M; 261	Ketoconazole	200 mg	White	Tablet	Circle	Mylan Pharmaceuticals
M; 273	Penicillin V Potassium	250 mg	White	Coated Tablet	Circle, Biconvex, Scored	Mylan Pharmaceuticals
M; 274	Tamoxifen Citrate	20 mg	White to Off-White	Tablet	Circle	Mylan Pharmaceuticals
M; 275	Penicillin V Potassium	500 mg	White	Coated Tablet	Oblong, Biconvex, Scored on Both Sides	Mylan Pharmaceuticals
M; 300	L-Thyroxine	0.3 mg	Blue	Tablet	Circle, Scored	Mova Pharmaceutical
M; 300	L-Thyroxine	0.3 mg	Blue	Tablet	Circle, Scored	Warner Chilcott
M; 300; LEVO; T	L-Thyroxine	0.3 mg	Green	Tablet	Circle, Scored	Novartis Generics
M; 302	Acyclovir	800 mg	White	Tablet	Oval	Mylan Pharmaceuticals
M; 305	Sotalol Hydrochloride	80 mg	Orange	Tablet	Circle, Scored	Mylan Pharmaceuticals
M; 310	Sotalol Hydrochloride	120 mg	Orange	Tablet	Circle, Scored	Mylan Pharmaceuticals
M; 312	Verapamil Hydrochloride	180 mg	Blue	Extended-Release Tablet	Oval, Scored	Mylan Pharmaceuticals
M; 312	Verapamil Hydrochloride	180 mg	Blue	Extended-Release Tablet	Oval, Scored	Udl Laboratories
M; 313	Tolmetin Sodium	600 mg	Beige	Coated Tablet	Oval	Mylan Pharmaceuticals
M; 314	Sotalol Hydrochloride	160 mg	Orange	Tablet	Circle, Scored	Mylan Pharmaceuticals
M; 316	Sotalol Hydrochloride	240 mg	Orange	Tablet	Circle, Scored	Mylan Pharmaceuticals
M; 317	Cimetidine	300 mg	Green	Coated Tablet	Five-Sided	Mylan Pharmaceuticals
M; 317	Cimetidine	300 mg	Green	Coated Tablet	Five-Sided	Udl Laboratories
M; 321	Lorazepam	0.5 mg	White	Tablet	Circle	Mylan Pharmaceuticals
M; 321	Lorazepam	0.5 mg	White	Tablet	Circle	Udl Laboratories
M; 355	Diclofenac Sodium	100 mg	Yellow	Extended-Release Tablet	Circle, Biconvex, Bevel-Edged	Mylan Pharmaceuticals
M; 357	Acetaminophen and Hydrocodone Bitartrate	500 mg; 5 mg	White	Tablet	Capsule-Shape, Scored	Mallinckrodt
M; 358	Acetaminophen and Hydrocodone Bitartrate	7.5 mg; 500 mg	White	Tablet	Capsule-Shape, Scored	Mallinckrodt
M; 359	Acetaminophen and Hydrocodone Bitartrate	7.5 mg; 650 mg	White	Tablet	Capsule-Shape, Scored	Mallinckrodt

IMPRINT	BRAND/GENERIC NAME	STRENGTH	COLOR	FORM	SHAPE	MANUFACTURER
M; 360	Acetaminophen and Hydrocodone Bitartrate	750 mg; 7.5 mg	White	Tablet	Capsule-Shape, Scored	Mallinckrodt
M; 361	Acetaminophen and Hydrocodone Bitartrate	10 mg; 650 mg	Blue	Tablet	Capsule-Shape, Scored	Mallinckrodt
M; 362	Acetaminophen and Hydrocodone Bitartrate	660 mg; 10 mg	White	Tablet	Capsule-Shape, Scored	Mallinckrodt
M; 362	Hydrocodone Bitartrate and Acetaminophen	10 mg; 660 mg	White	Tablet	Capsule-Shape	Mallinckrodt
M; 363	Acetaminophen and Hydrocodone Bitartrate	10 mg; 500 mg	White	Tablet	Capsule-Shape, Scored	Mallinckrodt
M; 365	Hydrocodone Bitartrate and Acetaminophen	5 mg; 325 mg	White	Tablet	Capsule-Shape, Scored	Mallinckrodt
M; 365	Procet	5 mg; 325 mg	White	Tablet	Capsule-Shape, Scored	Andrx Pharmaceuticals
M; 366	Hydrocodone Bitartrate and Acetaminophen	7.5 mg; 325 mg	White	Tablet	Oval, Scored	Mallinckrodt
M; 366	Procet	7.5 mg; 325 mg	White	Tablet	Oval, Scored	Andrx Pharmaceuticals
M; 367	Acetaminophen and Hydrocodone Bitartrate	325 mg; 10 mg	White	Tablet	Oval, Scored	Mallinckrodt
M; 372	Cimetidine	400 mg	Green	Coated Tablet	Five-Sided, House Shaped	Mylan Pharmaceuticals
M; 372	Cimetidine	400 mg	Green	Coated Tablet	Five-Sided, House Shaped	Udl Laboratories
M; 373	Hydroxychloroquine Sulfate	200 mg	White	Tablet	Circle	Mylan Pharmaceuticals
M; 400	Erythromycin Ethylsuccinate	400 mg	Beige	Coated Tablet	Capsule-Shape, Biconvex, Beveled Edge	Mylan Pharmaceuticals
M; 407	Fluvoxamine Maleate	25 mg	Off-White to Yellow	Tablet	Oval	Mylan Pharmaceuticals
M; 407	Fluvoxamine Maleate	25 mg	Orange	Tablet	Oval	Mylan Pharmaceuticals
M; 411	Verapamil Hydrochloride	240 mg	Blue	Extended-Release Tablet	Capsule-Shape, Modified	Mylan Pharmaceuticals
M; 411	Verapamil Hydrochloride	240 mg	Blue	Extended-Release Tablet	Capsule-Shape, Modified	Udl Laboratories
M; 412	Fluvoxamine Maleate	50 mg	Off-White to Yellow	Tablet	Oval, Scored	Mylan Pharmaceuticals
M; 412	Fluvoxamine Maleate	50 mg	Orange	Tablet	Oval, Scored	Mylan Pharmaceuticals
M; 414	Fluvoxamine Maleate	100 mg	Off-White to Yellow	Tablet	Oval, Scored	Mylan Pharmaceuticals
M; 414	Fluvoxamine Maleate	100 mg	Orange	Tablet	Oval, Scored	Mylan Pharmaceuticals
M; 433	Bupropion Hydrochloride	75 mg	Peach	Tablet	Circle	Mylan Pharmaceuticals
M; 433	Bupropion Hydrochloride	75 mg	Peach	Tablet	Circle	Udl Laboratories
M; 435	Bupropion Hydrochloride	100 mg	Light Blue	Tablet	Circle	Mylan Pharmaceuticals
M; 435	Bupropion Hydrochloride	100 mg	Light Blue	Tablet	Circle	Udl Laboratories
M; 437	Spironolactone	100 mg	White	Coated Tablet	Circle, Biconvex, Bevel-Edged, Scored	Mylan Pharmaceuticals
M; 441	Benazepril Hydrochloride	5 mg	White	Tablet	Circle	Mylan Pharmaceuticals
M; 443	Benazepril Hydrochloride	10 mg	White	Tablet	Circle	Mylan Pharmaceuticals
M; 444	Benazepril Hydrochloride	20 mg	White	Tablet	Circle	Mylan Pharmaceuticals
M; 447	Benazepril Hydrochloride	40 mg	White	Tablet	Oval	Mylan Pharmaceuticals
M; 450	Atenolol and Chlorthalidone	50 mg; 25 mg	White	Coated Tablet	Round, Bisected Scored	Martec Pharmaceuticals
M; 451	Atenolol and Chlorthalidone	100 mg; 25 mg	White	Coated Tablet	Circle	Martec Pharmaceuticals
M; 471	Fenoprofen Calcium	600 mg	Orange	Coated Tablet	Capsule-Shape, Scored	Mylan Pharmaceuticals
M; 475	Nifedipine ER	30 mg	Rose-Pink	Extended-Release Tablet	Circle	Mylan Pharmaceuticals
M; 482	Nifedipine ER	60 mg	Rose-Pink	Extended-Release Tablet	Circle	Mylan Pharmaceuticals
M; 495	Nifedipine ER	90 mg	Rose-Pink	Extended-Release Tablet	Circle	Mylan Pharmaceuticals
M; 501	Bisoprolol and Hydrochlorothiazide	2.5 mg; 6.25 mg	Orange	Tablet	Circle	Mylan Pharmaceuticals
M; 501	Bisoprolol and Hydrochlorothiazide	2.5 mg; 6.25 mg	Orange	Tablet	Circle	Udl Laboratories
M; 503	Bisoprolol and Hydrochlorothiazide	5 mg; 6.25 mg	Blue	Tablet	Circle	Mylan Pharmaceuticals
M; 503	Bisoprolol and Hydrochlorothiazide	5 mg; 6.25 mg	Blue	Tablet	Circle	Udl Laboratories
M; 505	Bisoprolol and Hydrochlorothiazide	10 mg; 6.25 mg	White	Tablet	Circle	Mylan Pharmaceuticals
M; 505	Bisoprolol and Hydrochlorothiazide	10 mg; 6.25 mg	White	Tablet	Circle	Udl Laboratories
M; 515	Mirtazapine	15 mg	Beige	Tablet	Circle	Mylan Pharmaceuticals
M522; 7.5; 325	Oxycodone and Acetaminophen	7.5 mg; 325 mg	White to Off-White	Tablet	Capsule-Shape	Mallinckrodt
M523; 10; 325	Oxycodone and Acetaminophen	10 mg; 325 mg	White to Off-White	Tablet	Capsule-Shape	Mallinckrodt
M; 525	Diltiazem Hydrochloride	120 mg	White with Clear Film Coat	Coated Tablet	Capsule-Shape, Scored	Mylan Pharmaceuticals
M; 530	Mirtazapine	30 mg	Beige	Tablet	Circle	Mylan Pharmaceuticals
M; 532	Acetaminophen and Oxycodone	500 mg; 5 mg	Red and Beige	Capsule		Mallinckrodt
M 532; M 532	Oxycodone and Acetaminophen	5 mg; 500 mg	Beige, Red	Capsule		Mallinckrodt
M; 537	Naproxen Sodium	275 mg	Light Blue	Coated Tablet	Circle	Mylan Pharmaceuticals
M; 541	Cimetidine	800 mg	Green	Coated Tablet	Oval, Scored	Mylan Pharmaceuticals
M; 541	Cimetidine	800 mg	Green	Coated Tablet	Oval, Scored	Udl Laboratories
M; 545	Mirtazapine	45 mg	Beige	Tablet	Circle	Mylan Pharmaceuticals
M562	Oxycodone and Acetaminophen	10 mg; 650 mg	White to Off-White	Tablet	Capsule-Shape	Mallinckrodt
M; 572	Albuterol	4 mg	White	Tablet	Circle, Scored, Flat Beveled Edge	Mylan Pharmaceuticals
M; 572	Albuterol	4 mg	White	Tablet	Circle, Scored, Flat Beveled Edge	Udl Laboratories
M; 577	Amiloride Hydrochloride and Hydrochlorothiazide	5 mg; 50 mg	Orange	Tablet	Circle, Scored	Mylan Pharmaceuticals
M; 577	Amiloride Hydrochloride and Hydrochlorothiazide	5 mg; 50 mg	Orange	Tablet	Circle, Scored	Udl Laboratories
M582	Oxycodone and Acetaminophen	7.5 mg; 500 mg	White to Off-White	Tablet	Oval	Mallinckrodt
M; 633	Nifedipine	90 mg	Brown	Tablet, Extended Release	Circle	Andrx Pharmaceuticals
M; 712	Enalapril and Hydrochlorothiazide	5 mg; 12.5 mg	White	Tablet	Circle, Biconvex	Mylan Pharmaceuticals
M; 715	Timolol Maleate	20 mg	Green	Tablet	Capsule-Shape, Scored, Biconvex, Beveled Edge	Mylan Pharmaceuticals
M; 723	Enalapril and Hydrochlorothiazide	10 mg; 25 mg	White	Tablet	Circle, Biconvex	Mylan Pharmaceuticals
M 724	Tizanidine Hydrochloride	4 mg	White to Off-White	Tablet		Mylan Pharmaceuticals
M; 725	Benazepril Hydrochloride and Hydrochlorothiazide	5 mg; 6.25 mg	Beige	Tablet	Oval, Scored	Mylan Pharmaceuticals
M; 735	Benazepril Hydrochloride and Hydrochlorothiazide	10 mg; 12.5 mg	Beige	Tablet	Circle, Scored	Mylan Pharmaceuticals

IMPRINT	BRAND/GENERIC NAME	STRENGTH	COLOR	FORM	SHAPE	MANUFACTURER
M; 745	Benazepril Hydrochloride and Hydrochlorothiazide	20 mg; 12.5 mg	Beige	Tablet	Capsule-Shape, Scored	Mylan Pharmaceuticals
M; 751	Cyclobenzaprine Hydrochloride	10 mg	Butterscotch Yellow	Coated Tablet	Circle	Mylan Pharmaceuticals
M; 751	Cyclobenzaprine Hydrochloride	10 mg	Butterscotch Yellow	Coated Tablet	Circle	Udl Laboratories
M; 757	Atenolol	100 mg	White	Tablet	Circle	Mylan Pharmaceuticals
M; 757	Atenolol	100 mg	White	Tablet	Circle	Udl Laboratories
M; 775	Benazepril Hydrochloride and Hydrochlorothiazide	20 mg; 25 mg	Beige	Tablet	Oval, Scored	Mylan Pharmaceuticals
M; 970	Acetaminophen, Butalbital and Caffeine	325 mg; 50 mg; 40 mg	White	Tablet	Circle	Mallinckrodt
M; 1423	Methylin ER	10 mg	White	Extended-Release Tablet	Circle, Flat-Faced, Bevel-Edged	Mallinckrodt
M; 1451	Methylin ER	20 mg	White	Extended-Release Tablet	Circle, Convex	Mallinckrodt
M; 1721	Acetaminophen and Propoxyphene Napsylate	650 mg; 100 mg		Tablet		Mallinckrodt
M; 1771	Propoxyphene Napsylate and Acetaminophen	650 mg; 100 mg	White	Tablet	Capsule-Shape	Mallinckrodt
M; 1772	Propoxyphene Napsylate and Acetaminophen	650 mg; 100 mg	Pink	Tablet	Capsule-Shape	Mallinckrodt
M; 3354	Orphenadrine Citrate, Aspirin and Caffeine	25 mg; 385 mg; 30 mg	White and Yellow Layered	Tablet	Circle	Mylan Pharmaceuticals
M; 3358	Orphenadrine Citrate	100 mg	White	Extended-Release Tablet	Circle	Mylan Pharmaceuticals
M; 4357	Acetaminophen and Hydrocodone Bitartrate	500 mg; 5 mg	Maroon	Capsule		Mallinckrodt
M; 7113	Meperidine Hydrochloride	50 mg	White	Tablet	Circle	Mallinckrodt
M; 7115	Meperidine Hydrochloride	100 mg		Tablet		Mallinckrodt
M; 7171	Tramadol Hydrochloride	50 mg	White	Tablet	Capsule-Shape	Mallinckrodt
M; 8960	Dextroamphetamine Sulfate	5 mg	White	Extended-Release Capsule		Mallinckrodt
M; 8961	Dextroamphetamine Sulfate	10 mg	White	Extended-Release Capsule		Mallinckrodt
M; 8962	Dextroamphetamine Sulfate	15 mg	White	Extended-Release Capsule		Mallinckrodt
M; A2	Atenolol	25 mg	White	Tablet	Circle	Mylan Pharmaceuticals
M; A2	Atenolol	25 mg	White	Tablet	Circle	Udl Laboratories
M; B1	Buspirone Hydrochloride	5 mg	White	Tablet	Oval, Biconvex, Scored	Mylan Pharmaceuticals
M; B2	Buspirone Hydrochloride	10 mg	White	Tablet	Oval, Biconvex, Scored	Mylan Pharmaceuticals
M; B3; 5 5 5	Buspirone Hydrochloride	15 mg	White	Tablet	Capsule-Shape, Flat, Beveled Edge, Tri-Sected	Mylan Pharmaceuticals
M; B3; 5 5 5	Buspirone Hydrochloride	15 mg	White	Tablet	Capsule-Shape, Flat, Beveled Edge, Tri-Sected	Udl Laboratories
M; B4; 10 10 10	Buspirone Hydrochloride	30 mg	White	Tablet	Capsule-Shape, Bevel-Edged,trisected	Mylan Pharmaceuticals
M; BOEHRINGER INGELHEIM LOGO	Mobic	7.5 mg	Pastel Yellow	Tablet	Circle, Biconvex	Abbott Laboratories
M; BOEHRINGER INGELHEIM LOGO	Mobic	7.5 mg	Pastel Yellow	Tablet	Circle, Biconvex	Boehringer Ingelheim
M; C1	Captopril	12.5 mg	White	Tablet	Oval, Partially Scored	Mylan Pharmaceuticals
M; C1	Captopril	12.5 mg	White	Tablet	Oval, Partially Scored	Udl Laboratories
M; C2	Captopril	25 mg	White	Tablet	Circle, Scored	Mylan Pharmaceuticals
M; C2	Captopril	25 mg	White	Tablet	Circle, Scored	Udl Laboratories
M; C3	Captopril	50 mg	White	Tablet	Circle, Scored	Mylan Pharmaceuticals
M; C4	Captopril	100 mg	White	Tablet	Circle, Scored	Mylan Pharmaceuticals
M; C; 7	Clozapine	25 mg	Peach	Tablet	Circle, Scored	Mylan Pharmaceuticals
M; C; 7	Clozapine	25 mg	Peach	Tablet	Circle, Scored	Udl Laboratories
M; C; 11	Clozapine	100 mg	Green	Tablet	Circle, Scored	Mylan Pharmaceuticals
M; C; 11	Clozapine	100 mg	Green	Tablet	Circle, Scored	Udl Laboratories
M; C; 13	Clonazepam	0.5 mg	Yellow	Tablet	Circle, Scored	Mylan Pharmaceuticals
M; C; 13	Clonazepam	0.5 mg	Yellow	Tablet	Circle, Scored	Udl Laboratories
M; C; 14	Clonazepam	1 mg	Green	Tablet	Circle, Scored	Mylan Pharmaceuticals
M; C; 14	Clonazepam	1 mg	Green	Tablet	Circle, Scored	Udl Laboratories
M; C; 15	Clonazepam	2 mg	White	Tablet	Circle, Scored	Mylan Pharmaceuticals
M; C; 15	Clonazepam	2 mg	White	Tablet	Circle, Scored	Udl Laboratories
M; D5	Diclofenac Potassium	50 mg	White	Coated Tablet	Circle, Biconvex	Mylan Pharmaceuticals
M; D6	Dicyclomine Hydrochloride	20 mg	Blue	Tablet	Circle, Flat-Faced, Beveled Edge	Mylan Pharmaceuticals
M; D6	Dicyclomine Hydrochloride	20 mg	Blue	Tablet	Circle, Flat-Faced, Beveled Edge	Udl Laboratories
M; D9	Doxazosin Mesylate	1 mg	White	Tablet	Circle, Scored	Mylan Pharmaceuticals
M; D9	Doxazosin Mesylate	1 mg	White	Tablet	Circle, Scored	Udl Laboratories
M; D10	Doxazosin Mesylate	2 mg	Pink	Tablet	Circle, Scored	Mylan Pharmaceuticals
M; D10	Doxazosin Mesylate	2 mg	Pink	Tablet	Circle, Scored	Udl Laboratories
M; D11	Doxazosin Mesylate	4 mg	Blue	Tablet	Circle, Scored	Mylan Pharmaceuticals
M; D11	Doxazosin Mesylate	4 mg	Blue	Tablet	Circle, Scored	Udl Laboratories
M; D12	Doxazosin Mesylate	8 mg	Purple	Tablet	Circle, Scored	Mylan Pharmaceuticals
M; D-C	Damacet-P	5 mg; 500 mg	Light Blue	Tablet		Mason Pharmaceuticals
M; D-P	Damason-P	5 mg; 500 mg	Pink	Tablet		Mason Pharmaceuticals
M; E3	Estradiol	0.5 mg	White	Tablet	Circle	Mylan Pharmaceuticals
M; E4	Estradiol	1 mg	Pink	Tablet	Circle	Mylan Pharmaceuticals
M; E5	Estradiol	2 mg	Blue	Tablet	Circle	Mylan Pharmaceuticals
M; E7	Estropipate	0.75 mg	Yellow	Tablet	Circle	Mylan Pharmaceuticals
M; E8	Estropipate	1.5 mg	Peach	Tablet	Circle	Mylan Pharmaceuticals
M; E9	Estropipate	3 mg	Blue	Tablet	Circle	Mylan Pharmaceuticals
M; E15	Enalapril Maleate	2.5 mg	White	Tablet	Circle, Scored	Mylan Pharmaceuticals
M; E15	Enalapril Maleate	2.5 mg	White	Tablet	Circle, Scored	Udl Laboratories
M; E16	Enalapril Maleate	5 mg	White	Tablet	Circle, Scored	Mylan Pharmaceuticals
M; E16	Enalapril Maleate	5 mg	White	Tablet	Circle, Scored	Udl Laboratories
M; E17	Enalapril Maleate	10 mg	Light Blue	Tablet	Circle	Mylan Pharmaceuticals
M; E17	Enalapril Maleate	10 mg	Light Blue	Tablet	Circle	Udl Laboratories
M; E18	Enalapril Maleate	20 mg	Blue	Tablet	Circle	Mylan Pharmaceuticals
M; E18	Enalapril Maleate	20 mg	Blue	Tablet	Circle	Udl Laboratories

IMPRINT	BRAND/GENERIC NAME	STRENGTH	COLOR	FORM	SHAPE	MANUFACTURER
M; F1	Famotidine	20 mg	Yellow	Coated Tablet	Circle, Biconvex, Bevel-Edgied	Mylan Pharmaceuticals
M; F1	Famotidine	20 mg	Yellow	Coated Tablet	Circle, Biconvex, Bevel-Edgied	Udl Laboratories
M; F2	Famotidine	40 mg	Green	Coated Tablet	Circle, Biconvex, Bevel-Edged	Mylan Pharmaceuticals
M; G4	Guanfacine	1 mg	White	Tablet	Circle	Mylan Pharmaceuticals
M; G5	Guanfacine	2 mg	Blue	Tablet	Circle	Mylan Pharmaceuticals
M; IB;	Midol Ib	200 mg	White	Coated Tablet		Bayer Consumer Care
M; L19	Lovastatin	10 mg	White to Off-White	Tablet	Circle, Flat-Faced, Bevel-Edged	Mylan Pharmaceuticals
M; L20	Lovastatin	20 mg	Yellow	Tablet	Circle, Flat-Faced, Bevel-Edged	Mylan Pharmaceuticals
M; L21	Lovastatin	40 mg	Pink	Tablet	Circle, Flat-Faced, Bevel-Edged	Mylan Pharmaceuticals
M; L22	Lisinopril	2.5 mg	Light Blue	Tablet	Circle	Mylan Pharmaceuticals
M; L23	Lisinopril	5 mg	Peach	Tablet	Circle	Mylan Pharmaceuticals
M; L24	Lisinopril	10 mg	White	Tablet	Circle	Mylan Pharmaceuticals
M; L25	Lisinopril	20 mg	Light Yellow	Tablet	Circle	Mylan Pharmaceuticals
M; L26	Lisinopril	40 mg	Light Green	Tablet	Circle	Mylan Pharmaceuticals
M; L27	Lisinopril	30 mg	Light Blue	Tablet	Circle	Mylan Pharmaceuticals
M; LH1	Hydrochlorothiazide and Lisinopril	12.5 mg; 10 mg		Tablet		Mylan Pharmaceuticals
M; LH2	Hydrochlorothiazide and Lisinopril	12.5 mg; 20 mg		Tablet		Mylan Pharmaceuticals
M; LH3	Hydrochlorothiazide and Lisinopril	25 mg; 20 mg		Tablet		Mylan Pharmaceuticals
M; N; 52	Nefazodone Hydrochloride	100 mg	White	Tablet	Circle	Mylan Pharmaceuticals
M; N; 53	Nefazodone Hydrochloride	150 mg	White	Tablet	Circle	Mylan Pharmaceuticals
M; N; 54	Nefazodone Hydrochloride	200 mg	White	Tablet	Circle	Mylan Pharmaceuticals
M; N; 55	Nefazodone Hydrochloride	250 mg	White	Tablet	Circle	Mylan Pharmaceuticals
M; P1	Prochlorperazine Maleate	5 mg	Maroon	Tablet	Circle	Mylan Pharmaceuticals
M; P1	Prochlorperazine Maleate	5 mg	Maroon	Tablet	Circle	Udl Laboratories
M; P2	Prochlorperazine Maleate	10 mg	Maroon	Tablet	Circle	Mylan Pharmaceuticals
M; P2	Prochlorperazine Maleate	10 mg	Maroon	Tablet	Circle	Udl Laboratories
M/R; 0379	Anatuss	400 mg; 120 mg	Off-White	Tablet	Oval, Deep-Scored	Mayrand Pharmaceutical
M; R	Buff-A	5 Gr	Pink and White Mottled	Tablet	Square	Merz
M; R	Hydrotensin-50	50 mg; 0.125 mg	Light Green	Tablet	Circle, Scored	Mayrand Pharmaceutical
M; R	Nu-Iron 150	150 mg	Red and White	Capsule		Merz
M; R	Nu-Iron-V	60 mg; 1 mg; 50 mg; 3 mcg; 4000 IU; 400 IU; 3 mg; 3 mg; 2 mg; 10 mg; 312 mg	Red	Tablet	Oblong, Scored	Merz
M; R; 1278	Sedapap	650 mg; 50 mg	White	Tablet	Capsule-Shape, Scored	Mayrand Pharmaceutical
M; T3	Trifluoperazine Hydrochloride	1 mg	White	Coated Tablet	Circle	Mylan Pharmaceuticals
M; T3	Trifluoperazine Hydrochloride	1 mg	White	Coated Tablet	Circle	Udl Laboratories
M; T4	Trifluoperazine Hydrochloride	2 mg	White	Coated Tablet	Circle	Mylan Pharmaceuticals
M; T4	Trifluoperazine Hydrochloride	2 mg	White	Coated Tablet	Circle	Udl Laboratories
M; T5	Trifluoperazine Hydrochloride	5 mg	Lavender	Coated Tablet	Circle	Mylan Pharmaceuticals
M; T5	Trifluoperazine Hydrochloride	5 mg	Lavender	Coated Tablet	Circle	Udl Laboratories
M; T6	Trifluoperazine Hydrochloride	10 mg	Lavender	Coated Tablet	Circle	Mylan Pharmaceuticals
M; T6	Trifluoperazine Hydrochloride	10 mg	Lavender	Coated Tablet	Circle	Udl Laboratories
M; T7	Tramadol Hydrochloride	50 mg	White	Tablet	Circle	Mylan Pharmaceuticals
MAALOX; RPR	Maalox	200 mg; 200 mg	White	Tablet, Chewable	Circle	Novartis Consumer
MAALOX PLUS; RPR	Maalox Plus	200 mg; 200 mg; 25 mg		Tablet, Chewable		Novartis Consumer
MACROBID; NORWICH EATON	Macrobid	100 mg	Opaque, Black and Yellow	Capsule		Procter & Gamble Pharmaceuticals
MACRODANTIN; 25 MG; 0149; 0007	Macrodantin	25 mg	Opaque, White	Capsule		Procter & Gamble Pharmaceuticals
MACRODANTIN; 50 MG; 0149-0008	Macrodantin	50 mg	Opaque, Yellow and White	Capsule		Procter & Gamble Pharmaceuticals
MACRODANTIN; 100 MG; 0149; 0009	Macrodantin	100 mg	Opaque, Yellow	Capsule		Procter & Gamble Pharmaceuticals
MAG; 357	Max Alert Magnum	200 mg	White/pink with Blue Specks	Tablet	Bullet-Shaped, Double Layered	Pdk Labs
MAOLATE	Maolate	400 mg	Tan	Tablet	Circle, Scored	Upjohn
MAR; 750MG	Marthritic	750 mg	White	Tablet	Oval	Marnel Pharmaceuticals
MAR; NATAL; F	Mar Natal-F	8000 IU; 400 IU; 30 IU; 100 mg; 1 mg; 3 mg; 3.4 mg; 20 mg; 5 mg; 12 mcg; 250 mg; 0.2 mg; 60 mg; 25 mg; 2 mg; 25 mg	Pink	Tablet		Marnel Pharmaceuticals
MAREZINE; T4A	Marezine	50 mg	White	Tablet		Glaxosmithkline
MARGESIC	Margesic	325 mg; 50 mg; 40 mg	Blue and White	Capsule		Marnel Pharmaceuticals
MARGESIC; #3	Margesic No. 3	650 mg; 30 mg	White	Tablet	Capsule-Shape	Marnel Pharmaceuticals
MARGESIC; NO. 3	Margesic No. 3	325 mg; 50 mg; 40 mg; 30 mg	Blue and White Speckled	Tablet		Marnel Pharmaceuticals
MARGESIC-H	Margesic-H	500 mg; 5 mg	Grey and Lavender	Capsule		Marnel Pharmaceuticals
MARION; 1525	Duotrate	30 mg	Black and Clear with White Pellets	Capsule		Aventis Pharmaceuticals
MARION; 1530	Duotrate	45 mg	Black and Light Blue with White Pellets	Capsule		Aventis Pharmaceuticals
MARION; 1555	Pavabid	150 mg		Extended-Release Capsule		Aventis Pharmaceuticals
MARION; 1555	Pavabid Plateau	150 mg		Timed-Release Capsule		Aventis Pharmaceuticals
MARION; 1555; PAVABID	Pavabid	150 mg	Black and White	Capsule		Aventis Pharmaceuticals
MARION; 1656	Os-Cal-Gesic	400 mg; 100 mg; 50 U	Blue-Green	Tablet	Oblong	Aventis Pharmaceuticals
MARION; 1771	Cardizem	30 mg	Green	Tablet	Circle	Biovail Pharmaceuticals
MARION; 1772	Cardizem	60 mg	Yellow	Tablet	Circle, Scored	Biovail Pharmaceuticals

IMPRINT	BRAND/GENERIC NAME	STRENGTH	COLOR	FORM	SHAPE	MANUFACTURER
MARION; GAVISCON; 1175	Gaviscon	80 mg; 20 mg	White	Tablet, Chewable	Circle	Glaxosmithkline Consumer
MARION; OS-CAL; 1650	Os-Cal 250	625 mg; 250 mg; 125 units;	Light Green	Tablet	Circle	Aventis Pharmaceuticals
MARION; OS-CAL; 1650	Os-Cal 250 + D	625 mg; 125 units		Tablet		Aventis Pharmaceuticals
MARION; PAVABID; HP	Pavabid Hp	300 mg	Light Orange	Capsule		Aventis Pharmaceuticals
MARION; PAVABID HP	Pavabid Hp Capsulets	300 mg	Light Orange	Tablet		Aventis Pharmaceuticals
MARION; PRETTS; 1177	Pretts Diet Aid	200 mg; 100 mg; 70 mg	Yellow	Tablet	Circle	Aventis Pharmaceuticals
MARLOP	Broncomar	100 mg; 100 mg; 30 mg	Purple	Tablet		Marlop Pharmaceuticals
MARLOP	Calcio Del Mar	1250 mg; 500 mg	Light Green	Tablet		Marlop Pharmaceuticals
MARLOP	Hipotest	50 mg; 10000 IU; 400 IU; 25 mg; 25 mg; 50 mcg; 150 mg; 15 mg; 50 mg; 12.5 mg; 12.5 IU; 150 mg; 25 mg; 15 mg; 5 mg; 15 mg; 1 mcg; 50 mg; 162 mg; 0.25 mg; 7.2 mg; 6.15 mg; 2.2 mg; 76 mcg; 53.5 mg; 24.3 mg	Brown	Tablet		Marlop Pharmaceuticals
MARLOP	Ternamar	60 mg; 5000 IU; 400 IU; 30 IU; 100 mg; 1 mg; 3 mg; 3.4 mg; 10 mg; 20 mg; 12 mcg; 30 mcg; 10 mg; 250 mg; 150 mcg; 25 mg; 2 mg; 25 mg; 25 mcg; 25 mcg; 5 mg	Peach	Tablet		Marlop Pharmaceuticals
MARSAM; 0530	Cefaclor	250 mg	Purple	Capsule		Marsam Pharmaceuticals
MARTEC; 972	Piroxicam	10 mg	Opaque Ivory and Orange	Capsule, Liquid Filled		Pliva
MARTEC; 973	Piroxicam	20 mg	Swedish Orange	Capsule, Liquid Filled		Pliva
MARTET	Martet	250 mg	Purple	Capsule		Marnel Pharmaceuticals
MATULANE; O; SIGMA-TAU;	Matulane	50 mg	Ivory	Capsule		Sigma-Tau Pharmaceuticals
MAXALT; MRK; 267	Maxalt	10 mg	Pink	Tablet	Capsule-Shape	Merck
MAXAQUIN; 400	Maxaquin	400 mg	White	Coated Tablet	Oval, Scored	Searle
MAXIDONE; 634	Maxidone	750 mg; 10 mg	Yellow	Tablet	Capsule-Shape, Scored	Watson Laboratories
MAXZIDE; B; M8	Maxzide	75 mg; 50 mg	Yellow	Tablet	Bowtie	Bertek Pharmaceuticals
MAXZIDE; B; M9	Maxzide	37.5 mg; 25 mg	Green	Tablet	Bowtie	Bertek Pharmaceuticals
MAYRAND	Eldercaps	4000 IU; 400 IU; 25 IU; 200 mg; 10 mg; 5 mg; 2 mg; 25 mg; 10 mg; 110 mg; 70 mg; 5 mg; 1 mg	Opaque Red	Capsule		Merz
MAYRAND	Trimcaps	105 mg	Lavender and White	Sustained-Release Capsule		Merz
MAYRAND/ ANAMINE; 1234	Anamine T.D.	8 mg; 120 mg	White and Clear with Green and White Beads	Capsule		Mayrand Pharmaceutical
MC	Desoxyn	5 mg	White	Sustained-Release Tablet		Abbott Laboratories
MCNEIL; 1/2; HALDOL	Haldol	0.5 mg	White	Tablet,u-Shape, with °°h" Cut Out in Center, Scored	Ortho-Mcneil Pharmaceutical	
MCNEIL; 058;	Butibel-Zyme	15 mg; 15 mg	Pink	Tablet		Mcneil Pharmaceutical
MCNEIL; 151	Clistin-Ra	8 mg	Orange	Coated Tablet		Mcneil Pharmaceutical
MCNEIL; 153	Clistin-Ra	12 mg	Yellow	Coated Tablet		Mcneil Pharmaceutical
MCNEIL; 659;	Ultram	50 mg	White	Coated Tablet	Capsule-Shape, Scored	Ortho-Mcneil Pharmaceutical
MCNEIL; BUTIBEL;	Butibel	15 mg; 15 mg	Red	Tablet		Mcneil Pharmaceutical
MCNEIL; BUTICAPS;	Buticaps	15 mg	Lavender and White	Capsule		Mcneil Pharmaceutical
MCNEIL; BUTICAPS;	Buticaps	30 mg	Aqua-Green and White	Capsule		Mcneil Pharmaceutical
MCNEIL; BUTICAPS;	Buticaps	50 mg	Orange and White	Capsule		Mcneil Pharmaceutical
MCNEIL; BUTICAPS;	Buticaps	100 mg	Pink and White	Capsule		Mcneil Pharmaceutical
MCNEIL; BUTISOL SODIUM;	Butisol Sodium	30 mg	Green	Tablet	Circle, Scored	Mcneil Pharmaceutical
MCNEIL; BUTISOL SODIUM;	Butisol Sodium	50 mg	Orange	Tablet	Circle, Scored	Mcneil Pharmaceutical
MCNEIL; BUTISOL SODIUM;	Butisol Sodium	100 mg	Pink	Tablet		Mcneil Pharmaceutical
MCNEIL; PANCREASE	Pancrease	4500 U; 20000 U; 25000 U	White	Capsule		Ortho-Mcneil Pharmaceutical
MCNEIL; PANCREASE; MT 4	Pancrease Mt 4	4000 USP units; 12,000 USP units; 12,000 USP units	Yellow and Clear	Capsule		Mcneil Pharmaceutical

IMPRINT	BRAND/GENERIC NAME	STRENGTH	COLOR	FORM	SHAPE	MANUFACTURER
MCNEIL; PANCREASE; MT 10	Pancrease Mt 10	10,000 USP units; 30,000 USP units; 30,000 USP units	Pink and Clear	Capsule		Mcneil Pharmaceutical
MCNEIL; PANCREASE; MT 16	Pancrease Mt 16	16,000 USP units; 48,000 USP units; 48,000 USP units	Salmon and Clear	Capsule		Mcneil Pharmaceutical
MCNEIL; PANCREASE; MT 25	Pancrease Mt 25	25000 U; 75000 U; 75000 U	White	Capsule		Mcneil Pharmaceutical
MCNEIL; PANCREASE; MT 32	Pancrease Mt 32	32000 U; 90000 U; 70000 U	White	Capsule		Mcneil Pharmaceutical
MCNEIL; TYLENOL; CODEINE 1;	Tylenol with Codeine No. 1	7.5 mg; 300 mg	White	Tablet	Circle	Mcneil Pharmaceutical
MCNEIL; TYLENOL CODEINE 2;	Tylenol with Codeine No. 2	15 mg; 300 mg	White	Tablet		Mcneil Pharmaceutical
MD; 451	Guai-Sudo	120 mg; 600 mg	Dark Blue	Tablet	Capsule-Shape, Scored	MD Pharmaceutical
MD; 500	Degen II	60 mg; 600 mg	Blue	Tablet	Capsule-Shape, Scored	MD Pharmaceutical
MD; 501	Humigen L.A.	600 mg	White to Off-White	Tablet	Capsule-Shape, Scored	MD Pharmaceutical
MD; 502	Humigen DM	30 mg; 600 mg	White with Green Specks	Tablet	Capsule-Shape, Scored	MD Pharmaceutical
MD; 514	Tagafed	2.5 mg; 60 mg	White	Tablet	Circle	Solvay Pharmaceuticals
MD; 518	Depletite	25 mg	Light Blue	Tablet	Circle	Solvay Pharmaceuticals
MD; 518	Diethylpropion Hydrochloride	25 mg	Medium Blue		Circle	MD Pharmaceutical
MD; 518	Diethylpropion Hydrochloride	25 mg	Medium Blue		Circle	Novartis Generics
MD; 530	Methylphenidate Hydrochloride	10 mg	Pale Blue-Green	Tablet	Circle, Scored	Apothecon
MD; 530	Methylphenidate Hydrochloride	10 mg	Pale Blue-Green	Tablet	Circle, Scored	Medeva Pharmaceuticals
MD; 530	Methylphenidate Hydrochloride	10 mg	Pale Blue-Green	Tablet	Circle, Scored	Novopharm
MD; 530	Methylphenidate Hydrochloride	10 mg	Pale Blue-Green	Tablet	Circle, Scored	Purepac Pharmaceutical
MD; 531	Methylphenidate Hydrochloride	5 mg	Yellow	Tablet	Circle	Apothecon
MD; 531	Methylphenidate Hydrochloride	5 mg	Yellow	Tablet	Circle	Medeva Pharmaceuticals
MD; 531	Methylphenidate Hydrochloride	5 mg	Yellow	Tablet	Circle	Novopharm
MD; 531	Methylphenidate Hydrochloride	5 mg	Yellow	Tablet	Circle	Purepac Pharmaceutical
MD; 531	Methylphenidate Ir	5 mg	Yellow	Tablet	Circle, Scored	Sandoz
MD; 532	Methylphenidate Hydrochloride	20 mg	Orange	Tablet	Circle, Scored	Apothecon
MD; 532	Methylphenidate Hydrochloride	20 mg	Orange	Tablet	Circle, Scored	Medeva Pharmaceuticals
MD; 532	Methylphenidate Hydrochloride	20 mg	Orange	Tablet	Circle, Scored	Novopharm
MD; 535	Di-Atro	2.5 mg; 0.025 mg	White	Tablet		MD Pharmaceutical
MD; 543	Amitriptyline Hydrochloride	150 mg	Flesh	Coated Tablet		H.L. Moore
MD; 547	Cyproheptadine Hydrochloride	4 mg	White	Tablet	Circle	MD Pharmaceutical
MD; 562	Methylphenidate ER	20 mg	White	Tablet	Circle	Sandoz
MD; 562	Methylphenidate Hydrochloride	20 mg	White	Extended-Release Tablet	Circle	Apothecon
MD; 562	Methylphenidate Hydrochloride	20 mg	White	Extended-Release Tablet	Circle	Medeva Pharmaceuticals
MD; 562	Methylphenidate Hydrochloride	20 mg	White	Extended-Release Tablet	Circle	Purepac Pharmaceutical
MD; 711	Triprolidine with Pseudoephedrine	2.5 mg; 60 mg	White	Tablet	Circle, Curved	MD Pharmaceutical
ME	Desoxyn	10 mg	Orange	Sustained-Release Tablet		Abbott Laboratories
MEDACID	Medacid Antacid	223 mg; 127 mg; 59 mg	Blue	Tablet		Bristol-Myers Squibb
MEDEVA; 400;	Atrohist Pediatric	4 mg; 60 mg	White and Yellow	Extended-Release Capsule		Medeva Pharmaceuticals
MEDEVA; 402	Humibid Pediatric	300 mg	Light Green and Clear with White Beads	Sustained-Release Capsule		Medeva Pharmaceuticals
MEDICO; 350	Duospaz	5 mg; 1.5 mg	Opaque Green	Capsule		Medicopharma
MEDIPREN	Medipren	200 mg	White	Tablet		Mcneil Consumer Products
MEDROL; 2	Medrol	2 mg	Pink	Tablet	Oval, Scored	Pharmacia & Upjohn
MEDROL; 4;	Medrol	4 mg	White	Tablet	Oval, Scored	Pharmacia & Upjohn
MEDROL; 8;	Medrol	8 mg	Peach	Tablet	Oval, Scored	Pharmacia & Upjohn
MEDROL; 16;	Medrol	16 mg	White	Tablet	Oval, Scored	Pharmacia & Upjohn
MEDROL; 24;	Medrol	24 mg	Yellow	Tablet	Oval, Scored	Pharmacia & Upjohn
MEDROL; 32;	Medrol	32 mg	Peach	Tablet	Oval, Scored	Pharmacia & Upjohn
MED-TEK	Hycomed	500 mg; 5 mg	Black and Red	Capsule		Med-Tek Pharmaceuticals
MED-TEK	Medex-LA	75 mg; 400 mg		Extended-Release Tablet		Med-Tek Pharmaceuticals
MED-TEK	Medex-LA	120 mg; 400 mg	Blue	Tablet	Capsule-Shape	Med-Tek Pharmaceuticals
MED-TEK	Med-Hist	120 mg; 8 mg	Ivory with Green Speckles	Tablet	Oblong, Scored	Med-Tek Pharmaceuticals
MED-TEK	Medispaz	0.125 mg	Pink	Tablet	Circle, Scored	Med-Tek Pharmaceuticals
MED-TEK	Medivert	30 mg	Aqua Blue	Tablet	Circle, Scored	Med-Tek Pharmaceuticals
MED-TEK	Sinumed	2 mg; 30 mg; 500 mg	Orange	Tablet	Oblong, Scored	Med-Tek Pharmaceuticals
MED-TEK	Vitamed	65 mg; 6000 IU; 400 IU; 1 mg; 60 mg; 1.1 mg; 1.8 mg; 2.5 mg; 5 mcg; 15 mg; 125 mg	Peach	Tablet	Oblong	Med-Tek Pharmaceuticals
MERIDIA; 5	Meridia	5 mg	Blue and Yellow	Capsule		Abbott Laboratories
MERIDIA; 10	Meridia	10 mg	Blue and White	Capsule		Abbott Laboratories
MERIDIA; 15	Meridia	15 mg	Yellow and White	Capsule		Abbott Laboratories
MERRELL; 37	Cantil	25 mg	Yellow	Tablet		Aventis Pharmaceuticals
MERRELL; 56	Ircon-FA	250 mg; 1 mg	Red	Tablet		Key Pharmaceuticals
MERRELL; 62	Metahydrin	2 mg	Pink	Tablet	Circle, Debossed	Aventis Pharmaceuticals
MERRELL; 63	Metahydrin	4 mg	Aqua Blue	Tablet	Circle, Debossed	Aventis Pharmaceuticals
MERRELL; 64	Metatensin	2 mg; 0.1 mg	Yellow	Tablet		Aventis Pharmaceuticals
MERRELL; 65	Metatensin	4 mg; 0.1 mg	Lavender	Tablet		Aventis Pharmaceuticals
MERRELL; 277	Hiprex	1000 mg	Yellow	Tablet	Capsule-Shape	Aventis Pharmaceuticals
MESTINON; 60; ICN;	Mestinon	60 mg		Tablet		Icn Pharmaceuticals
MET; 10; 832	Metoclopramide Hydrochloride	10 mg	White	Tablet	Compressed, Scored	Rosemont Pharmaceutical

IMPRINT	BRAND/GENERIC NAME	STRENGTH	COLOR	FORM	SHAPE	MANUFACTURER
METHADOSE; 5	Methadose	5 mg	White	Tablet		Mallinckrodt
METHADOSE; 10	Methadose	10 mg	White	Tablet		Mallinckrodt
METHADOSE; 40	Methadose	40 mg	White	Tablet	Quadrisect Scored	Mallinckrodt
METRYL; 93	Metryl	250 mg	White	Tablet	Circle, Convex	Teva Pharmaceuticals
METRYL; 500; 93; 93	Metryl	500 mg	White	Tablet	Oblong, Scored	Teva Pharmaceuticals
MF	Desoxyn	15 mg	Yellow	Sustained-Release Tablet		Abbott Laboratories
MF	Mifeprex	200 mg	Light Yellow	Tablet	Biconvex, Cylindrical	Danco Laboratories
MF; 1; G	Metformin Hydrochloride	500 mg	White	Tablet	Circle	Par Pharmaceutical
MF; 2; G	Metformin Hydrochloride	850 mg	White	Tablet	Circle	Par Pharmaceutical
MF; 3; G	Metformin Hydrochloride	1000 mg	White	Tablet	Oblong	Par Pharmaceutical
MG	Magnesium Gluconate	500 mg	Buff	Tablet		Western Research
MH; 1; M	Midodrine Hydrochloride	2.5 mg	White to Off White	Tablet	Circle, Scored	Mylan Pharmaceuticals
MH; 2; M	Midodrine Hydrochloride	5 mg	White to Off White	Tablet	Circle, Scored	Mylan Pharmaceuticals
MH; 3; M	Midodrine Hydrochloride	10 mg	White to Off White	Tablet	Circle, Scored	Mylan Pharmaceuticals
MIA; 106	Acetaminophen and Butalbital	325 mg; 50 mg	White	Tablet	Oval, Scored	Mikart
MIA; 106	Butalbital and Acetaminophen	325 mg; 50 mg	White	Tablet	Capsule-Shape	Qualitest Products
MIA; 110	Butalbital, Acetaminophen and Caffeine	325 mg; 50 mg; 40 mg	White	Tablet	Capsule-Shape, Scored	Akyma Pharmaceuticals
MIA; 110	Butalbital, Acetaminophen and Caffeine	325 mg; 50 mg; 40 mg	White	Tablet	Capsule-Shape, Scored	Novartis Generics
MICRO-K 10; THER-RX 009	Micro-K 10	10 meq	Light Orange and White	Extended-Release Capsule		Ther-RX
MICRO-K; THER-RX 010	Micro-K	8 meq	Light Orange	Extended-Release Capsule		Ther-RX
MICRONASE; 1.25	Micronase	1.25 mg	White	Tablet	Circle, Scored	Pharmacia & Upjohn
MICRONASE; 2.5	Micronase	2.5 mg	Dark Pink	Tablet	Circle, Scored	Pharmacia & Upjohn
MICRONASE; 5	Micronase	5 mg	Blue	Tablet	Circle, Scored	Pharmacia & Upjohn
MICROZIDE; 12.5	Microzide	12.5 mg	Opaque Teal	Capsule, Liquid Filled		Watson Laboratories
MICTRIN; 38130	Mictrin	50 mg		Tablet		Economed Pharmaceuticals
MIDOL	Midol Maximum Strength Multi-Symptom	500 mg; 60 mg; 15 mg	Light Blue and Dark Blue	Capsule, Liquid Filled		Bayer Consumer Care
MIDOL	Midol Multi-Symptom Formula Regular Strength	325 mg; 12.5 mg	White	Tablet		Bayer Consumer Care
MIDOL MAXIMUM	Midol Multi-Symptom Formula Maximum Strength	500 mg; 15 mg; 60 mg	White	Tablet		Bayer Consumer Care
MIDOL; MENSTRUAL	Midol Maximum Strength Menstrual Formula	500 mg; 60 mg; 15 mg	White	Tablet	Oblong	Bayer Consumer Care
MIDOL PM	Midol Pm Night Time Formula	500 mg; 25 mg	Blue	Tablet	Capsule-Shape	Bayer Consumer Care
MIDOL; PMS	Midol Pms Multi-Symptom Formula	500 mg; 25 mg; 15 mg	White	Tablet		Bayer Consumer Care
MIDRIN	Midrin	65 mg; 100 mg; 325 mg	Red with Pink Band	Capsule		Women First Healthcare
MILES; 093	Mycelex-G	100 mg	White	Tablet		Bayer Consumer Care
MILES; 121	Decholin	250 mg	White	Tablet		Bayer Pharmaceutical
MILES; 721	Niclocide	500 mg		Tablet		Bayer Pharmaceutical
MILES; 951	Lithane	300 mg	Green	Tablet	Circle, Scocred(Scored)	Bayer Pharmaceutical
MJ	Fer-in-Sol Iron Supplement	190 mg	Red	Capsule		Mead Johnson
MJ	Natalins	200 mg; 1.5 mg; 30 mg; 17 mg; 1.5 mg; 2.5 mcg; 70 mg; 15 IU; 400 IU; 15 mg; 2.6 mg; 4000 IU; 1.6 mg; 100 mg; 0.5 mg	Yellow	Tablet	Oval	Mead Johnson
MJ; 021	Estrace	0.5 mg		Tablet		Warner Chilcott
MJ; 5 MG;	Buspar	5 mg	White	Tablet	Ovoid-Rectangular, Scored	Mead Johnson
MJ; 10 MG;	Buspar	10 mg	White	Tablet	Ovoid-Rectangular, Scored	Mead Johnson
MJ; 468	Poly-VI-Flor	0.5 mg; 2500 IU; 400 IU; 15 IU; 60 mg; 0.3 mg; 1.05 mg; 1.2 mg; 13.5 mg; 1.05 mg; 4.5 mcg	Purple, Orange, or Pink	Tablet, Chewable	Rectangle	Mead Johnson
MJ; 474	Poly-VI-Flor	1 mg; 2500 U; 1.05 mg; 1.2 mg; 13.5 mg; 1.05 mg; 4.5 mcg; 60 mg; 400 U; 15 IU; 0.3 mg	Pink, Purple, or Orange	Tablet, Chewable	Square	Mead Johnson
MJ; 487	Poly-VI-Flor	60 mg; 0.3 mg; 0.25 mg; 15 IU; 400 IU; 1.05 mg; 2500 IU; 13.5 mg; 1.2 mg; 1.05 mg; 45 mcg	Light Purple	Tablet, Chewable	Circle	Mead Johnson
MJ; 503; 50	Cytoxan	50 mg	White with Blue Speckles	Tablet		Bristol-Myers Squibb
MJ; 504; 25	Cytoxan	25 mg	White with Blue Speckles	Tablet		Bristol-Myers Squibb
MJ; 543	Vasodilan	10 mg	White	Tablet		Bristol-Myers Squibb
MJ; 544	Vasodilan	20 mg	White	Tablet		Apothecon
MJ; 555	Deapril-ST	1 mg		Tablet		Mead Johnson
MJ; 583	Ovcon-35-21	0.4 mg; 35 mcg	Peach	21-Day Tablet Pack	Circle	Warner Chilcott
MJ; 583	Ovcon-35-28 Peach Tablet	0.4 mg; 35 mcg	Peach	28-Day Tablet Pack	Circle	Warner Chilcott
MJ; 584	Ovcon-50 Yellow Tablet	1 mg; 50 mcg	Yellow	28-Day Tablet Pack	Circle	Warner Chilcott
MJ; 595	Megace	20 mg	Light Blue	Tablet		Mead Johnson Oncology
MJ; 596	Megace	40 mg	Light Blue	Tablet		Mead Johnson Oncology

IMPRINT	BRAND/GENERIC NAME	STRENGTH	COLOR	FORM	SHAPE	MANUFACTURER
MJ; 702	Enfamil Natalins RX	4000 IU; 80 mg; 400 IU; 15 IU; 1.5 mg; 1.6 mg; 17 mg; 4 mg; 1 mg; 2.5 mcg; 30 mcg; 7 mg; 200 mg; 54 mg; 100 mg; 25 mg; 3 mg	White Speckled	Tablet	Oval	Mead Johnson
MJ; 702	Natalins RX	0.03 mg; 200 mg; 1 mg; 100 mg; 7 mg; 1.5 mg; 2.5 mcg; 80 mg; 4 mg; 25 mg; 15 IU; 400 IU; 4000 IU; 1.6 mg; 17 mg; 60 mg; 3 mg	White	Tablet	Oval	Mead Johnson
MJ; 755	Estrace	1 mg	Lavender	Tablet		Warner Chilcott
MJ; 756	Estrace	2 mg	Turquoise	Tablet		Warner Chilcott
MJ; 775; DESYREL	Desyrel	50 mg	Orange	Tablet	Circle, Scored	Apothecon
MJ; 776; DESYREL	Desyrel	100 mg	White	Tablet	Circle, Scored	Apothecon
MJ; 778; 50	Desyrel	150 mg	Orange	Tablet	Triple-Scored	Apothecon
MJ; 784; DURICEF; 500MG;	Duricef	500 mg	Maroon and White	Capsule		Bristol-Myers Squibb
MJ; 785	Duricef	1 G	White	Tablet		Bristol-Myers Squibb
MJ; 796; 100	Desyrel	300 mg	Yellow	Tablet	Triple-Scored	Apothecon
MJ; 822; 5	Buspar Dividose	15 mg	White	Tablet		Bristol-Myers Squibb
ML; 629	Thyroid	3 G		Coated Tablet		Rosemont Pharmaceutical
ML; 674	Thyroid Strong	65 mg	Light Tan	Tablet		Western Research Laboratories
ML; 674;	Thyroid	1 G	Red	Coated Tablet		Rosemont Pharmaceutical
ML; 675;	Thyroid	2 G	Light Tan	Tablet		Rosemont Pharmaceutical
ML; 824; 10	Buspar Dividose	30 mg	Pink	Tablet	Trisected	Bristol-Myers Squibb
MM; L083;	Milk of Magnesia	311 mg	White	Tablet, Chewable	Circle, Compressed, Convex	Leiner Health Products
MOBAN; 5	Moban	5 mg	Orange	Tablet	Circle, Biconvex	Endo Laboratories
MOBAN; 10	Moban	10 mg	Lavender	Tablet	Circle, Biconvex	Endo Laboratories
MOBAN; 25	Moban	25 mg	Green	Tablet	Circle, Biconvex, Scored	Endo Laboratories
MOBAN; 50	Moban	50 mg	Blue	Tablet	Circle, Biconvex, Scored	Endo Laboratories
MOBAN; 100	Moban	100 mg	Tan	Tablet	Circle, Biconvex, Scored	Endo Laboratories
MOLE	Caffeine	325 mg	Blue	Capsule		Pdk Labs
MONODOX; 50; M260	Monodox	50 mg	Yellow and White	Capsule		Watson Laboratories
MONODOX; 100; M259	Monodox	100 mg	Brown and Yellow	Capsule		Watson Laboratories
MOTRIN; 50	Motrin	50 mg	Orange	Tablet, Chewable	Circle, Scored	Mcneil Consumer Products
MOTRIN; 100	Motrin	100 mg	Orange	Tablet, Chewable	Circle, Scored	Mcneil Consumer Products
MOTRIN; 300 MG	Motrin	300 mg	White	Coated Tablet	Circle	Pharmacia & Upjohn
MOTRIN; 400 MG	Motrin	400 mg	Orange	Coated Tablet	Circle	Pharmacia & Upjohn
MOTRIN; 600 MG	Motrin	600 mg	Peach	Coated Tablet	Oval	Pharmacia & Upjohn
MOTRIN; 800 MG	Motrin	800 mg	Apricot	Coated Tablet	Oblong	Pharmacia & Upjohn
MOTRIN; IB; SINUS	Motrin Ib Sinus	200 mg; 30 mg	White	Tablet	Circle	Mcneil Consumer Products
MOTRIN COLD & FLU	Motrin Cold & Flu Non-Drowsy Formula	200 mg; 30 mg	Yellow	Tablet	Film-Coated	Mcneil Consumer Products
MOVA; 25	Captopril	25 mg		Tablet		Mova Pharmaceutical
MOVA; 25	Captopril	25 mg	White	Tablet	Circle	Stada
MOVA; 375; M; 37	Naproxen	375 mg	White	Tablet		Mova Pharmaceutical
MP; 3	Hydroxyzine Hydrochloride	10 mg	Purple	Coated Tablet		Mutual Pharmaceutical
MP; 4	Imipramine	10 mg	Yellow	Coated Tablet		Mutual Pharmaceutical
MP; 4	Imipramine	10 mg	Yellow	Tablet		Qualitest Products
MP; 6	Lorazepam	0.5 mg	White	Tablet		Mutual Pharmaceutical
MP; 7	Hydroxyzine Hydrochloride	25 mg	Purple	Coated Tablet		Mutual Pharmaceutical
MP; 8	Imipramine	25 mg	Brown	Coated Tablet		Mutual Pharmaceutical
MP; 9	Atenolol	25 mg	White	Tablet	Circle	Mutual Pharmaceutical
MP; 10	Amitriptyline Hydrochloride	10 mg	Pink	Coated Tablet	Circle	H.L. Moore
MP; 10	Amitriptyline Hydrochloride	10 mg	Purple	Coated Tablet	Circle	Mutual Pharmaceutical
MP; 11	Dipyridamole	25 mg	White	Coated Tablet		Mutual Pharmaceutical
MP; 12	Thioridazine	10 mg	Yellow	Tablet		Qualitest Products
MP; 12	Thioridazine Hydrochloride	10 mg	Yellow	Coated Tablet		Mutual Pharmaceutical
MP; 13	Hydroxyzine Hydrochloride	50 mg	Purple	Coated Tablet		Mutual Pharmaceutical
MP; 14	Thioridazine	25 mg	Yellow	Tablet		Qualitest Products
MP; 14	Thioridazine Hcl	25 mg	Yellow	Coated Tablet		Mutual Pharmaceutical
MP; 15	Dipyridamole	50 mg	White	Coated Tablet		Mutual Pharmaceutical
MP; 17	Thioridazine	50 mg	Yellow	Tablet		Qualitest Products
MP; 17	Thioridazine Hydrochloride	50 mg	Yellow	Coated Tablet		Mutual Pharmaceutical
MP; 18	Dipyridamole	75 mg	White	Coated Tablet		Mutual Pharmaceutical
MP; 20	Ergoloid Mesylate	1 mg	White	Tablet	Circle	Qualitest Products
MP; 20	Ergoloid Mesylates	1 mg	White	Tablet	Circle	Mutual Pharmaceutical
MP; 22	Hydralazine Hydrochloride	10 mg	White	Tablet		Mutual Pharmaceutical
MP; 25	Amitriptyline Hydrochloride	25 mg	Green	Coated Tablet	Circle	H.L. Moore
MP; 25	Amitriptyline Hydrochloride	25 mg	Light Green	Coated Tablet	Circle	Mutual Pharmaceutical
MP; 26	Amitriptyline Hydrochloride	50 mg	Brown	Coated Tablet	Circle	H.L. Moore
MP; 26	Amitriptyline Hydrochloride	50 mg	Dark Orange	Coated Tablet	Circle	Mutual Pharmaceutical
MP; 27	Amitriptyline Hydrochloride	75 mg	Purple	Coated Tablet	Circle	H.L. Moore
MP; 27	Amitriptyline Hydrochloride	75 mg	Purple	Coated Tablet	Circle	Mutual Pharmaceutical
MP; 28	Amitriptyline Hydrochloride	100 mg	Orange	Coated Tablet	Circle	H.L. Moore
MP; 28	Amitriptyline Hydrochloride	100 mg	Orange	Coated Tablet	Circle	Mutual Pharmaceutical
MP; 29	Amitriptyline Hydrochloride	150 mg	Peach	Coated Tablet	Capsule-Shape	H.L. Moore
MP; 29	Amitriptyline Hydrochloride	150 mg	Light Pink	Coated Tablet	Capsule-Shape	Mutual Pharmaceutical
MP; 30	Chlorthalidone	25 mg	Pale Yellow	Tablet		Mutual Pharmaceutical
MP; 35	Spironolactone	25 mg	White	Tablet	Circle, Scored	H.L. Moore
MP; 35	Spironolactone	25 mg	White	Tablet	Circle	Mutual Pharmaceutical

IMPRINT	BRAND/GENERIC NAME	STRENGTH	COLOR	FORM	SHAPE	MANUFACTURER
MP; 35	Spironolactone	25 mg	White	Tablet		Qualitest Products
MP; 36	Metoclopramide	10 mg	White	Tablet	Circle, Scored	Mutual Pharmaceutical
MP; 37	Doxycycline	100 mg	Orange	Tablet		Qualitest Products
MP; 37	Doxycycline Hyclate	100 mg	Light Pink	Coated Tablet	Circle	Mutual Pharmaceutical
MP; 39	Lorazepam	1 mg	White	Tablet	Circle, Scored	Mutual Pharmaceutical
MP; 40	Spironolactone and Hydrochlorothiazide	25 mg; 25 mg	Buff	Tablet		Mutual Pharmaceutical
MP; 40	Spironolactone and Hydrochlorothiazide	25 mg; 25 mg	Buff	Tablet		Qualitest Products
MP; 43	Chlorthalidone	50 mg	Light Green	Tablet		Mutual Pharmaceutical
MP; 44	Benztropine Mesylate	1 mg		Tablet		Mutual Pharmaceutical
MP; 45	Metronidazole	250 mg	White	Tablet	Circle, Compressed	Martec Pharmaceuticals
MP; 45	Metronidazole	250 mg	White	Tablet	Circle, Compressed	Mutual Pharmaceutical
MP; 46	Metronidazole	500 mg	White	Tablet	Capsule-Shape, Compressed	Martec Pharmaceuticals
MP; 46	Metronidazole	500 mg	White	Tablet	Capsule-Shape, Compressed	Mutual Pharmaceutical
MP; 47	Albuterol Sulfate	2 mg		Tablet		Mutual Pharmaceutical
MP; 50	Tolmetin Sodium	200 mg		Tablet		Mutual Pharmaceutical
MP; 51	Prednisone	5 mg	White	Tablet	Circle, Scored	Mutual Pharmaceutical
MP; 52	Prednisone	10 mg	White	Tablet	Circle, Scored	Mutual Pharmaceutical
MP; 53	Prednisone	20 mg	Peach	Tablet	Circle, Scored	Mutual Pharmaceutical
MP; 55	Hydralazine Hydrochloride	50 mg	Orange	Tablet		Mutual Pharmaceutical
MP; 58	Carisoprodol	350 mg	White	Tablet	Circle	Mutual Pharmaceutical
MP; 58	Carisoprodol	350 mg	White	Tablet	Circle	Udl Laboratories
MP; 64	Hydralazine Hydrochloride	25 mg	Orange	Tablet		Mutual Pharmaceutical
MP; 65	Acetazolamide	125 mg	White	Tablet		Mutual Pharmaceutical
MP; 66	Quinidine Gluconate	324 mg	White	Sustained-Release Tablet	Circle	Mutual Pharmaceutical
MP; 68	Tolazamide	100 mg	White	Tablet		Mutual Pharmaceutical
MP; 69	Verapamil Hydrochloride	80 mg	White	Coated Tablet		Mutual Pharmaceutical
MP; 70	Tolazamide	250 mg	White	Tablet		Mutual Pharmaceutical
MP; 71	Allopurinol	100 mg	White	Tablet		Mutual Pharmaceutical
MP; 71	Allopurinol	100 mg	White	Tablet		Qualitest Products
MP; 72	Tolazamide	500 mg	White	Tablet		Mutual Pharmaceutical
MP; 74	Chlorzoxazone	500 mg	Light Green	Tablet		Mutual Pharmaceutical
MP; 76	Verapamil Hydrochloride	120 mg	White	Coated Tablet		Mutual Pharmaceutical
MP; 77	Ibuprofen	200 mg	White	Coated Tablet		Mutual Pharmaceutical
MP; 79	Imipramine	50 mg	Green	Coated Tablet		Mutual Pharmaceutical
MP; 79	Imipramine	50 mg	Green	Tablet		Qualitest Products
MP; 80	Allopurinol	300 mg	Orange	Tablet		Mutual Pharmaceutical
MP; 80	Allopurinol	300 mg	Orange	Tablet		Qualitest Products
MP; 80	Imipramine	25 mg	Brown	Tablet		Qualitest Products
MP; 81	Sulfamethoxazole and Trimethoprim	400 mg; 80 mg	White	Tablet	Circle, Scored	Akyma Pharmaceuticals
MP; 81	Sulfamethoxazole and Trimethoprim	400 mg; 80 mg	White	Tablet		Mutual Pharmaceutical
MP; 83	Nystatin	500000 U	Brown	Coated Tablet		Mutual Pharmaceutical
MP; 84	Minoxidil	2.5 mg		Tablet		Mutual Pharmaceutical
MP; 85	Sulfamethoxazole and Trimethoprim	800 mg; 160 mg	White	Tablet	Oval, Scored	Akyma Pharmaceuticals
MP; 85	Sulfamethoxazole and Trimethoprim	800 mg; 160 mg	White	Tablet	Oval, Scored	Mutual Pharmaceutical
MP; 88	Albuterol Sulfate	4 mg		Tablet		Mutual Pharmaceutical
MP; 89	Minoxidil	10 mg		Tablet		Mutual Pharmaceutical
MP; 91	Sulfasalazine	500 mg	Golden Yellow	Tablet	Circle, Scored	Mutual Pharmaceutical
MP; 91	Sulfasalazine	500 mg	Yellow	Tablet		Qualitest Products
MP; 94	Ibuprofen	300 mg	White	Coated Tablet		Mutual Pharmaceutical
MP; 95	Ibuprofen	400 mg	White	Coated Tablet		Mutual Pharmaceutical
MP; 96	Ibuprofen	600 mg	White	Coated Tablet	Capsule-Shape	Mutual Pharmaceutical
MP; 96	Lorazepam	2 mg	White	Tablet	Circle, Scored	Mutual Pharmaceutical
MP; 99; 800	Ibuprofen	800 mg	White	Coated Tablet	Capsule-Shape	Mutual Pharmaceutical
MP; 108	Quinidine Sulfate	200 mg		Tablet		Mutual Pharmaceutical
MP; 111; 2	Acetaminophen and Codeine	300 mg; 15 mg	White	Tablet		Mutual Pharmaceutical
MP; 112	Sulindac	150 mg	Yellow	Tablet	Circle, Scored	Mutual Pharmaceutical
MP; 112	Sulindac	150 mg	Yellow	Tablet		Qualitest Products
MP; 114	Trazodone Hydrochloride	100 mg	White	Coated Tablet	Circle, Scored	Mutual Pharmaceutical
MP; 116	Sulindac	200 mg	Yellow	Tablet	Circle, Scored	Mutual Pharmaceutical
MP; 116	Sulindac	200 mg	Yellow	Tablet		Qualitest Products
MP; 118	Trazodone Hydrochloride	50 mg	White	Coated Tablet	Circle, Scored	Mutual Pharmaceutical
MP; 122; 3	Acetaminophen and Codeine	300 mg; 30 mg	White	Tablet		Mutual Pharmaceutical
MP; 124	Quinidine Sulfate	300 mg		Tablet		Mutual Pharmaceutical
MP; 127; 4	Acetaminophen and Codeine	300 mg; 60 mg	White	Tablet		Mutual Pharmaceutical
MP; 135	Acetaminophen	325 mg	White	Tablet		Mutual Pharmaceutical
MP; 140	Acetaminophen	500 mg	White	Tablet		Mutual Pharmaceutical
MP; 141	Acetazolamide	250 mg	White	Tablet	Circle	H.L. Moore
MP; 141	Acetazolamide	250 mg	White	Tablet	Circle	Mutual Pharmaceutical
MP; 142	Benztropine Mesylate	2 mg	White	Tablet	Circle	Mutual Pharmaceutical
MP; 145	Acetaminophen	500 mg	White	Tablet		Mutual Pharmaceutical
MP; 146	Atenolol	50 mg	White	Tablet	Circle, Scored	Mutual Pharmaceutical
MP; 147	Atenolol	100 mg	White	Tablet	Circle	Mutual Pharmaceutical
MP; 148	Metoclopramide	5 mg		Tablet		Mutual Pharmaceutical
MP; 148	Metoclopramide	5 mg	White	Tablet		Qualitest Products
MP; 152	Atenolol and Chlorthalidone	100 mg; 25 mg	White	Tablet	Circle	Mutual Pharmaceutical
MP; 153	Atenolol and Chlorthalidone	50 mg; 25 mg	White	Tablet	Circle, Scored	Mutual Pharmaceutical
MP; 155	Quinine Sulfate	260 mg		Tablet		Mutual Pharmaceutical
MP; 160	Thioridazine	100 mg	Yellow	Coated Tablet		Mutual Pharmaceutical
MP; 160	Thioridazine	100 mg	Yellow	Tablet		Qualitest Products
MP; 167	Fenoprofen Calcium	600 mg	Yellow	Tablet		Mutual Pharmaceutical
MP; 168; 25 25; 50 50;	Trazodone Hydrochloride	150 mg	White	Tablet	Quadrisected; Round Scored	Watson Laboratories

IMPRINT	BRAND/GENERIC NAME	STRENGTH	COLOR	FORM	SHAPE	MANUFACTURER
MP; 174	Salsalate	500 mg	Yellow	Coated Tablet	Circle	Mutual Pharmaceutical
MP; 177	Salsalate	750 mg	Yellow	Coated Tablet	Capsule-Shape	Mutual Pharmaceutical
MP; 178	Pindolol	5 mg	White	Tablet		Mutual Pharmaceutical
MP; 183	Pindolol	10 mg	White	Tablet		Mutual Pharmaceutical
MP; 184	Metoprolol Tartrate	50 mg	Light Orange	Coated Tablet	Capsule-Shape, Scored	Mutual Pharmaceutical
MP; 185	Metoprolol Tartrate	100 mg	Yellow	Coated Tablet	Capsule-Shape, Scored	Mutual Pharmaceutical
MP; 271	Labetalol Hydrochloride	200 mg	White	Coated Tablet		Mutual Pharmaceutical
MP; 272	Labetalol Hydrochloride	300 mg	Blue	Coated Tablet		Mutual Pharmaceutical
MP; 277	Labetalol Hydrochloride	100 mg	Beige	Coated Tablet		Mutual Pharmaceutical
MP; 303	Spironolactone	100 mg	White	Coated Tablet	Oval	Mutual Pharmaceutical
MP; 392	Sedapap	50 mg; 650 mg	White	Tablet		Mikart
MP; 423	Guaifenesin LA	600 mg	Green	Extended-Release Tablet	Capsule-Shape	Mutual Pharmaceutical
MP; 424	Guaifenesin with Pseudoephedrine	600 mg; 120 mg		Tablet		Mutual Pharmaceutical
MP; 425	Guaifenesin with Pseudoephedrine	600 mg; 60 mg		Tablet		Mutual Pharmaceutical
MP; 500	Ketoconazole	200 mg	White to Off-White	Tablet		Mutual Pharmaceutical
MP; 511	Propafenone Hydrochloride	150 mg	White	Tablet	Circle	Mutual Pharmaceutical
MP; 512	Propafenone Hydrochloride	225 mg	White	Tablet	Circle	Mutual Pharmaceutical
MP; 513	Propafenone Hydrochloride	300 mg	White	Tablet		Mutual Pharmaceutical
MP; 542	Spironolactone	50 mg	White	Coated Tablet	Circle	Mutual Pharmaceutical
MP; 711	Bisoprolol	5 mg	Red	Coated Tablet	Circle	Mutual Pharmaceutical
MP; 712	Bisoprolol	10 mg	White	Coated Tablet	Circle	Mutual Pharmaceutical
MP; 717	Tramadol Hydrochloride	50 mg	White	Tablet	Circle	Mutual Pharmaceutical
MP; 751	Metformin Hydrochloride	500 mg	White	Coated Tablet	Circle, Concave	Major Pharmaceutical
MP; 751	Metformin Hydrochloride	500 mg	White	Tablet		Mutual Pharmaceutical
MP; 752	Metformin Hydrochloride	850 mg	White	Coated Tablet	Circle, Concave	Major Pharmaceutical
MP; 752	Metformin Hydrochloride	850 mg	White	Tablet		Mutual Pharmaceutical
MP; 753	Metformin Hydrochloride	1000 mg	White	Coated Tablet	Oval	Major Pharmaceutical
MP; 753	Metformin Hydrochloride	1000 mg	White	Tablet	Oblong	Mutual Pharmaceutical
MPC; 100	Tussend	5 mg; 60 mg; 4 mg	Yellow	Tablet	Capsule-Shape, Scored	Monarch Pharmaceuticals
MR	Glytuss	200 mg	White	Tablet	Oblong	Mayrand Pharmaceutical
MR	Hydro-Z-50	50 mg	Peach	Tablet	Circle, Scored	Merz
MR	Sterapred	5 mg	Blue	Tablet	Circle	Merz
MR	Trimtabs	35 mg	Lavender	Tablet		Merz
MR; 15; G	Mirtazapine	15 mg	Yellow	Tablet	Circle	Par Pharmaceutical
MR; 30; G	Mirtazapine	30 mg	Buff	Tablet	Circle	Par Pharmaceutical
MR; 45; G	Mirtazapine	45 mg	White	Tablet	Circle	Par Pharmaceutical
MRK; 117; SINGULAIR	Singulair	10 mg	Beige	Coated Tablet	Square, Rounded	Merck & Company
MRK; 212; FOSAMAX	Fosamax	40 mg	White	Tablet	Triangle	Merck & Company
MRK; 266	Maxalt	5 mg	Pink	Tablet	Capsule-Shape, Compressed	Merck
MRK; 275; SINGULAIR	Singulair	5 mg	Pink	Tablet, Chewable	Circle, Biconvex	Merck & Company
MRK; 711; SINGULAIR	Singulair	4 mg	Pink	Tablet, Chewable	Oval, Biconvex	Merck & Company
MRK; 717; HYZAAR	Hyzaar	12.5 mg; 50 mg	Yellow	Coated Tablet	Teardrop-Shape	Merck
MRK; 747; HYZAAR	Hyzaar	25 mg; 100 mg	Light Yellow	Coated Tablet	Teardrop-Shape	Merck
MRK; 925	Fosamax	5 mg	White	Tablet	Circle	Merck & Company
MRK; 936	Fosamax	10 mg	White	Tablet	Oval	Merck & Company
MRK; 951	Cozaar	25 mg	Light Green	Coated Tablet	Teardrop-Shape	Merck
MRK; 952; COZAAR	Cozaar	50 mg	Green	Coated Tablet	Teardrop-Shape	Merck
MRK; 960	Cozaar	100 mg	Dark Green	Coated Tablet	Teardrop-Shape	Merck
MSAP	Arthritis Pain Formula	500 mg; 27 mg; 100 mg	Light Brown or White	Tablet		Wyeth Consumer Healthcare
MSD; 14; VASOTEC	Vasotec	2.5 mg	Yellow	Tablet	Barrel, Biconvex, Scored, Compressed	Merck & Company
MSD; 15	Prinivil	2.5 mg	White	Tablet	Circle, Small	Merck Sharp & Dohme
MSD; 19; PRINIVIL	Prinivil	5 mg	White	Tablet	Shield-Shape, Compressed, Scored	Merck & Company
MSD; 20	Decadron	0.25 mg	Orange	Tablet	Five-Sided, Compressed, Scored	Merck & Company
MSD; 21	Cogentin	0.5 mg	White	Tablet	Circle, Scored	Merck & Company
MSD; 25	Indocin	25 mg	Opaque Blue and White	Capsule		Merck & Company
MSD; 41	Decadron	0.5 mg	Yellow	Tablet	Five-Sided, Compressed, Score	Merck & Company
MSD; 42	Hydrodiuril	25 mg	Peach	Tablet	Circle, Scored, Compressed	Merck & Company
MSD; 43	Mephyton	5 mg	Yellow	Tablet	Circle, Scored, Compressed	Merck & Company
MSD; 49	Daranide	50 mg	Yellow	Tablet	Circle, Compressed, Scored	Merck Sharp & Dohme
MSD; 50	Indocin	50 mg	Opaque Blue and White	Capsule		Merck & Company
MSD; 52	Inversine	2.5 mg	Yellow	Tablet	Circle, Scored, Compressed	Merck & Company
MSD; 53	Hydropres-25	25 mg; 0.125 mg	Green	Tablet	Circle, Scored	Merck & Company
MSD; 59; BLOCADREN	Blocadren	5 mg	Light Blue	Tablet	Circle, Compressed	Merck & Company
MSD; 60	Cogentin	2 mg	White	Tablet	Circle, Scored, Compressed	Merck & Company
MSD; 62	Periactin	4 mg	White	Tablet	Circle, Compressed, Scored	Merck & Company
MSD; 63	Decadron	0.75 mg	Bluish-Green	Tablet	Five-Sided, Compressed, Scored	Merck & Company
MSD; 65	Edecrin	25 mg	White	Tablet	Capsule-Shape, Scored	Merck & Company
MSD; 67	Timolide	10 mg; 25 mg	Light Blue	Tablet		Merck & Company
MSD; 72; PROSCAR	Proscar	5 mg	Blue	Coated Tablet	Character-Shape, Modified Apple	Merck & Company
MSD; 90	Edecrin	50 mg	Green	Tablet	Capsule-Shape, Scored	Merck & Company
MSD; 92	Midamor	5 mg	Yellow	Tablet	Diamond-Shaped, Compressed	Merck & Company
MSD; 95	Decadron	1.5 mg	Pink	Tablet	Five-Sided, Compressed, Scored	Merck & Company
MSD; 97	Decadron	4 mg	White	Tablet	Five-Sided, Compressed, Scored	Merck & Company
MSD; 105	Hydrodiuril	50 mg	Peach	Tablet	Circle, Scored, Compressed	Merck & Company
MSD; 106; PRINIVIL	Prinivil	10 mg	Light Yellow	Tablet	Shield-Shape, Compressed	Merck & Company
MSD; 120	Inversine	10 mg	Yellow	Tablet	Circle, Cross-Scored	Merck & Company
MSD; 127	Hydropres-50	50 mg; 0.125 mg	Green	Tablet	Circle, Scored	Merck & Company
MSD; 135	Aldomet	125 mg	Yellow	Coated Tablet	Circle	Merck & Company

IMPRINT	BRAND/GENERIC NAME	STRENGTH	COLOR	FORM	SHAPE	MANUFACTURER
MSD; 136; BLOCADREN	Blocadren	10 mg	Light Blue	Tablet	Circle, Scored, Compressed	Merck & Company
MSD; 139	Stromectol	6 mg	White	Tablet	Scored, Beveled-Edge	Merck & Company
MSD; 140; PRINZIDE	Prinzide	12.5 mg; 20 mg	Yellow	Tablet	Circle, Fluted-Edge	Merck & Company
MSD; 142; PRINZIDE	Prinzide	25 mg; 20 mg	Peach	Tablet	Circle, Fluted-Edge	Merck & Company
MSD; 145; PRINZIDE	Prinzide	12.5 mg; 10 mg	Blue	Tablet	Six-Sided	Merck & Company
MSD; 147	Decadron	6 mg	Green	Tablet	Five-Sided, Compressed, Scored	Merck & Company
MSD; 173	Vaseretic	5 mg; 12.5 mg	Green	Tablet	Capsule-Shape, Squared, Compressed	Merck & Company
MSD; 207; PRINIVIL	Prinivil	20 mg	Peach	Tablet	Shield-Shape, Compressed	Merck & Company
MSD; 214	Diuril	250 mg	White	Tablet	Circle, Scored, Compressed	Merck & Company
MSD; 219	Cortone Acetate	25 mg	White	Tablet	Circle, Scored, Compressed	Merck & Company
MSD; 230	Diupres-250	250 mg; 0.125 mg	Pink	Tablet	Circle, Scored	Merck & Company
MSD; 237; PRINIVIL	Prinivil	40 mg	Rose-Red	Tablet	Shield-Shape, Compressed	Merck & Company
MSD; 401	Aldomet	250 mg	Yellow	Coated Tablet	Circle	Merck & Company
MSD; 403	Urecholine	5 mg	White	Tablet	Circle, Scored, Compressed	Merck & Company
MSD; 405	Diupres-500	500 mg; 0.125 mg	Pink	Tablet	Circle, Scored	Merck & Company
MSD; 410	Hydrodiuril	100 mg	Peach	Tablet	Circle, Scored, Compressed	Merck & Company
MSD; 412	Urecholine	10 mg	Pink	Tablet	Circle, Compressed, Scored	Merck & Company
MSD; 423	Aldoril-15	250 mg; 15 mg	Salmon	Coated Tablet	Circle	Merck & Company
MSD; 432	Diuril	500 mg	White	Tablet	Circle, Scored, Compressed	Merck & Company
MSD; 437; BLOCADREN	Blocadren	20 mg	Light Blue	Tablet	Capsule-Shape, Scored, Compressed	Merck & Company
MSD; 456	Aldoril-25	250 mg; 25 mg	White	Coated Tablet	Circle	Merck & Company
MSD; 457	Urecholine	25 mg	Yellow	Tablet	Circle, Compressed, Scored	Merck & Company
MSD; 460	Urecholine	50 mg	Yellow	Tablet	Circle, Compressed, Scored	Merck & Company
MSD; 501	Benemid	500 mg	Yellow	Coated Tablet	Capsule-Shape, Scored	Merck & Company
MSD; 516	Aldomet	500 mg	Yellow	Coated Tablet	Circle	Merck & Company
MSD; 517	Triavil 4-50	4 mg; 50 mg	Orange	Coated Tablet	Diamond	Merck & Company
MSD; 602	Cuprimine	250 mg	Ivory	Capsule		Merck & Company
MSD; 612	Aldoclor 150	250 mg; 150 mg	Beige	Coated Tablet	Oval	Merck & Company
MSD; 614	Colbenemid	0.5 GM; 0.5 mg	White to Off-White	Tablet	Capsule-Shape, Scored	Merck & Company
MSD; 619	Hydrocortone	10 mg	White	Tablet	Oval, Compressed, Scored	Merck & Company
MSD; 634	Aldoclor 250	250 mg; 250 mg	Green	Coated Tablet	Oval	Merck & Company
MSD; 635	Cogentin	1 mg	White	Tablet	Oval, Scored, Compressed	Merck & Company
MSD; 661	Syprine	250 mg	Light Brown, Opaque	Capsule		Merck & Company
MSD; 672	Cuprimine	125 mg	Opaque Ivory and Grey	Capsule		Merck & Company
MSD; 675	Dolobid	250 mg	Peach	Coated Tablet	Capsule-Shape	Merck & Company
MSD; 690; DEMSER	Demser	250 mg	Opaque Two-Tone Blue	Capsule		Merck & Company
MSD; 693	Indocin SR	75 mg	Blue and Clear with White Pellets	Extended-Release Capsule		Merck & Company
MSD; 694	Aldoril D30	500 mg; 30 mg	Salmon	Coated Tablet	Oval	Merck & Company
MSD; 697	Dolobid	500 mg	Orange	Coated Tablet	Capsule-Shape	Merck & Company
MSD; 705; NOROXIN	Noroxin	400 mg	Dark Pink	Coated Tablet	Oval	Merck Sharp & Dohme
MSD; 705; NOROXIN	Noroxin	400 mg	Dark Pink	Coated Tablet	Oval	Roberts Pharmaceutical
MSD; 712; VASOTEC	Vasotec	5 mg	White	Tablet	Barrel, Scored, Compressed	Merck & Company
MSD; 713; VASOTEC	Vasotec	10 mg	Salmon	Tablet	Barrel, Compressed	Merck & Company
MSD; 714; VASOTEC	Vasotec	20 mg	Peach	Tablet	Barrel, Compressed	Merck & Company
MSD; 720; VASERETIC	Vaseretic	10 mg; 25 mg	Rust	Tablet	Capsule-Shape, Squared, Compressed	Merck & Company
MSD; 726; ZOCOR	Zocor	5 mg	Buff	Coated Tablet	Shield-Shape	Merck & Company
MSD; 730; MEVACOR	Mevacor	10 mg	Peach	Tablet	Eight-Sided	Merck & Company
MSD; 731; MEVACOR	Mevacor	20 mg	Light Blue	Tablet	Eight-Sided	Merck & Company
MSD; 732; MEVACOR	Mevacor	40 mg	Green	Tablet	Eight-Sided	Merck & Company
MSD; 735; ZOCOR	Zocor	10 mg	Peach	Coated Tablet	Shield-Shape	Merck & Company
MSD; 740; ZOCOR	Zocor	20 mg	Tan	Coated Tablet	Shield-Shape	Merck & Company
MSD; 749; ZOCOR	Zocor	40 mg	Brick Red	Coated Tablet	Shield-Shape	Merck & Company
MSD; 907	Mintezol	500 mg	White	Tablet, Chewable	Circle, Scored	Merck & Company
MSD; 914	Triavil 2-10	2 mg; 10 mg	Blue	Coated Tablet	Triangle	Merck & Company
MSD; 917	Moduretic	5 mg; 50 mg	Peach	Tablet	Diamond	Merck & Company
MSD; 921	Triavil 2-25	2 mg; 25 mg	Orange	Coated Tablet	Triangle	Merck & Company
MSD; 931; FLEXERIL	Flexeril	10 mg	Butterscotch Yellow	Coated Tablet	D-Shape	Alza
MSD; 934	Triavil 4-10	4 mg; 10 mg	Salmon	Coated Tablet	Triangle	Merck & Company
MSD; 935	Aldoril D50	500 mg; 50 mg	White	Coated Tablet	Oval	Merck & Company
MSD; 941	Clinoril	150 mg	Yellow	Tablet	Six-Sided, Compressed	Merck & Company
MSD; 942	Clinoril	200 mg	Yellow	Tablet	Six-Sided, Scored, Compressed	Merck & Company
MSD; 946	Triavil 4-25	4 mg; 25 mg	Yellow	Coated Tablet	Triangle	Merck & Company
MSD; 963	Pepcid	20 mg	Beige	Coated Tablet	U-Shape	Merck & Company
MSD; 964	Pepcid	40 mg	Light Brownish-Orange	Coated Tablet	U-Shape	Merck & Company
MSM	Momentum Extra Strength	580 mg	White	Tablet	Oblong	Medtech

IMPRINT	BRAND/GENERIC NAME	STRENGTH	COLOR	FORM	SHAPE	MANUFACTURER
MULTI-42	Multi 42	5000 IU; 200 IU; 250 mg; 12.5 mg; 12.5 mg; 12.5 mg; 50 mcg; 200 mcg; 12.5 mg; 12.5 mg; 50 mg; 50 mg; 150 mcg; 25 mcg; 9.5 mg; 4.5 mg; 75 mcg; 25 mg; 12.5 mg; 7.5 mg; 75 mg; 1.5 mg; 7.5 mg; 15 IU; 25 mg; 12.5 mcg; 12.5 mg; 5 mg; 12.5 mg; 1 mg;		Capsule, Liquid Filled		Sundown Vitamins
MURO; 6-60;	Bromfed-PD	6 mg; 60 mg	Dark-Green and Clear with White Beads	Timed-Release Capsule		Muro Pharmaceutical
MURO; 12-120;	Bromfed	12 mg; 120 mg	Light Green and Clear	Timed-Release Capsule		Muro Pharmaceutical
MURO; 60/40	Guaitab	60 mg; 400 mg	Purple	Tablet	Layered, Scored	Muro Pharmaceutical
MURO; 4060	Bromfed	4 mg; 60 mg	White	Tablet		Muro Pharmaceutical
MUTUAL; 100	Doxycycline Hyclate	50 mg	Blue and White	Capsule		Mutual Pharmaceutical
MUTUAL; 101	Indomethacin	25 mg	Light Green	Capsule		Mutual Pharmaceutical
MUTUAL; 102	Quinine Sulfate	325 mg	Clear with White Powder	Capsule		Mutual Pharmaceutical
MUTUAL; 103	Diphenhydramine Hydrochloride	25 mg	Pink and Clear	Capsule		Mutual Pharmaceutical
MUTUAL; 105	Doxycycline Hyclate	100 mg	Light Blue	Capsule		Mutual Pharmaceutical
MUTUAL; 106	Indomethacin	50 mg	Light Green	Capsule		Mutual Pharmaceutical
MUTUAL; 107	Diphenhydramine Hydrochloride	50 mg	Pink	Capsule		Mutual Pharmaceutical
MUTUAL; 110	Acetaminophen	500 mg	Red and White	Capsule		Mutual Pharmaceutical
MUTUAL; 115	Disopyramide Phosphate	100 mg	Scarlet and Buff	Capsule		Mutual Pharmaceutical
MUTUAL; 120	Disopyramide Phosphate	150 mg	Blue and Scarlet	Capsule		Mutual Pharmaceutical
MUTUAL; 165	Piroxicam	10 mg	Lavender and White	Capsule		Mutual Pharmaceutical
MUTUAL; 166	Piroxicam	20 mg	Lavender	Capsule		Mutual Pharmaceutical
MUTUAL; 179	Tolmetin Sodium	400 mg		Capsule		Mutual Pharmaceutical
MUTUAL; 400	Trimethobenzamide	250 mg	Light Blue	Capsule		Qualitest Products
MUTUAL; 400	Trimethobenzamide Hydrochloride	250 mg	Light Blue	Capsule		Mutual Pharmaceutical
MUTUAL; 401	Trimethobenzamide Hydrochloride	300 mg	Orange Opaque	Capsule		Mutual Pharmaceutical
MUTUAL; 688	Pancrelipase 4500	20000 U; 4500 U; 25000 U	White	Capsule		Mutual Pharmaceutical
MUTUAL; 689	Pancrelipase 10,000	20000 U; 10000 U; 25000 U	Natural and Light Brown	Capsule		Mutual Pharmaceutical
MUTUAL; 698	Fluoxetine Hydrochloride	10 mg	Light Green	Capsule		Mutual Pharmaceutical
MUTUAL; 699	Fluoxetine Hydrochloride	20 mg	White and Green	Capsule		Mutual Pharmaceutical
MX 225	Nasatab LA	400 mg; 120 mg	White	Extended-Release Tablet	Oval, Scored	Medi-Plex Pharmaceuticals
MX; 405	Medipain 5	5 mg; 500 mg	Opaque White	Capsule		Medi-Plex Pharmaceuticals
MYCELEX; 10	Mycelex	10 mg	White	Troche	Circle	Alza
MYCOBUTIN; PHARMACIA	Mycobutin	150 mg	Red-Brown	Capsule		Pharmacia & Upjohn
MYKROX; 1/2	Mykrox	0.5 mg	White	Tablet	Circle, Flat Faced	Medeva Pharmaceuticals
MYL; GAS; 80	Mylanta Gas	80 mg	White or Pink	Tablet, Chewable	Circle, Scored	Johnson & Johnson Merck Consumer Pharmaceuticals
MYL; GAS; 125	Mylanta Gas Maximum Strength	125 mg	White or Pink	Tablet, Chewable	Circle, Scored	Johnson & Johnson Merck Consumer Pharmaceuticals
MYLAN; 9; 4	Carbidopa and Levodopa	50 mg; 200 mg	Purple	Extended-Release Tablet	Oval, Scored, Biconvex	Mylan Pharmaceuticals
MYLAN; 9; 4	Carbidopa and Levodopa	50 mg; 200 mg	Purple	Extended-Release Tablet	Oval, Scored, Biconvex	Udl Laboratories
MYLAN; 11; 77	Oxaprozin	600 mg	White	Coated Tablet	Oval, Biconvex, Bevel-Edged, Scored	Mylan Pharmaceuticals
MYLAN; 43	Reserpine and Chlorothiazide	500 mg; 0.125 mg	Peach	Tablet	Circle, Scored	Mylan Pharmaceuticals
MYLAN; 73	Perphenazine and Amitriptyline Hydrochloride	50 mg; 4 mg	Purple	Coated Tablet	Circle, Biconvex, Beveled Edge	Mylan Pharmaceuticals
MYLAN; 88	Carbidopa and Levodopa	25 mg; 100 mg	Purple	Extended-Release Tablet	Oval	Mylan Pharmaceuticals
MYLAN; 101	Tetracycline Hydrochloride	250 mg	Orange and Yellow	Capsule		Mylan Pharmaceuticals
MYLAN; 102	Tetracycline Hydrochloride	500 mg	Black and Yellow	Capsule		Mylan Pharmaceuticals
MYLAN; 106; 250	Erythromycin Stearate	250 mg	Yellow	Coated Tablet	Circle, Biconvex	Mylan Pharmaceuticals
MYLAN; 107; 500	Erythromycin Stearate	500 mg	Yellow	Coated Tablet	Oval, Biconvex	Mylan Pharmaceuticals
MYLAN; 115	Ampicillin Trihydrate	250 mg	Scarlet and Light Gray	Capsule		Mylan Pharmaceuticals
MYLAN; 116	Ampicillin Trihydrate	500 mg	Scarlet and Light Gray	Capsule		Mylan Pharmaceuticals
MYLAN; 129	Propoxyphene Hydrochloride	65 mg	Pink	Capsule		Mylan Pharmaceuticals
MYLAN; 131	Propoxyphene Compound	389 mg; 32.4 mg; 65 mg	Red and Grey	Capsule		Mylan Pharmaceuticals
MYLAN; 143	Indomethacin	25 mg	Light Green	Capsule		Mylan Pharmaceuticals
MYLAN; 143	Indomethacin	25 mg	Light Green	Capsule		Udl Laboratories
MYLAN; 145	Doxycycline Hyclate	50 mg	Aqua Blue and White	Capsule		Mylan Pharmaceuticals
MYLAN; 147	Indomethacin	50 mg	Light Green	Capsule		Mylan Pharmaceuticals
MYLAN; 147	Indomethacin	50 mg	Light Green	Capsule		Udl Laboratories
MYLAN; 148	Doxycycline Hyclate	100 mg	Aqua Blue	Capsule		Mylan Pharmaceuticals
MYLAN; 148	Doxycycline Hyclate	100 mg	Aqua Blue	Capsule		Udl Laboratories
MYLAN; 152	Clonidine Hydrochloride	0.1 mg	White	Tablet	Circle, Scored	Mylan Pharmaceuticals
MYLAN; 152	Clonidine Hydrochloride	0.1 mg	White	Tablet	Circle, Scored	Udl Laboratories
MYLAN; 155	Acetaminophen and Propoxyphene Napsylate	650 mg; 100 mg	Pink	Coated Tablet	Capsule-Shape	Mylan Pharmaceuticals
MYLAN; 156; 500	Probenecid	500 mg	Yellow	Coated Tablet	Capsule-Shape	Mylan Pharmaceuticals
MYLAN; 162	Chlorothiazide	500 mg	White	Tablet	Circle, Scored, Flat Beveled Edge	Mylan Pharmaceuticals
MYLAN; 162	Chlorothiazide	500 mg	White	Tablet	Circle, Scored, Flat Beveled Edge	Udl Laboratories
MYLAN; 167; 100	Doxycycline Hyclate	100 mg	Beige	Coated Tablet	Circle, Biconvex, Beveled Edge	Mylan Pharmaceuticals
MYLAN; 167; 100	Doxycycline Hyclate	100 mg	Beige	Coated Tablet	Circle, Biconvex, Beveled Edge	Udl Laboratories
MYLAN; 182; 10	Propranolol Hydrochloride	10 mg	Orange	Tablet	Circle, Scored, Flat Beveled Edge	Mylan Pharmaceuticals

IMPRINT	BRAND/GENERIC NAME	STRENGTH	COLOR	FORM	SHAPE	MANUFACTURER
MYLAN; 182; 10	Propranolol Hydrochloride	10 mg	Orange	Tablet	Circle, Scored, Flat Beveled Edge	Udl Laboratories
MYLAN; 183; 20	Propranolol Hydrochloride	20 mg	Blue	Tablet	Circle, Scored, Flat Beveled Edge	Mylan Pharmaceuticals
MYLAN; 183; 20	Propranolol Hydrochloride	20 mg	Blue	Tablet	Circle, Scored, Flat Beveled Edge	Udl Laboratories
MYLAN; 184; 40	Propranolol Hydrochloride	40 mg	Green	Tablet	Circle, Scored, Flat, Beveled Edge	Mylan Pharmaceuticals
MYLAN; 184; 40	Propranolol Hydrochloride	40 mg	Green	Tablet	Circle, Scored, Flat, Beveled Edge	Udl Laboratories
MYLAN; 185; 80	Propranolol Hydrochloride	80 mg	Yellow	Tablet	Circle, Scored, Flat Beveled Edge	Mylan Pharmaceuticals
MYLAN; 185; 80	Propranolol Hydrochloride	80 mg	Yellow	Tablet	Circle, Scored, Flat Beveled Edge	Udl Laboratories
MYLAN; 186	Clonidine Hydrochloride	0.2 mg	White	Tablet	Circle, Scored	Mylan Pharmaceuticals
MYLAN; 186	Clonidine Hydrochloride	0.2 mg	White	Tablet	Circle, Scored	Udl Laboratories
MYLAN; 197; 100	Chlorpropamide	100 mg	Green	Tablet	Circle, Scored	Mylan Pharmaceuticals
MYLAN; 197; 100	Chlorpropamide	100 mg	Green	Tablet	Circle, Scored	Udl Laboratories
MYLAN; 199	Clonidine Hydrochloride	0.3 mg	White	Tablet	Circle, Scored	Mylan Pharmaceuticals
MYLAN; 199	Clonidine Hydrochloride	0.3 mg	White	Tablet	Circle, Scored	Udl Laboratories
MYLAN; 204	Amoxicillin Trihydrate	250 mg	Caramel and Buff	Capsule		Mylan Pharmaceuticals
MYLAN; 205	Amoxicillin Trihydrate	500 mg	Buff	Capsule		Mylan Pharmaceuticals
MYLAN; 210; 250	Chlorpropamide	250 mg	Green	Tablet	Circle, Scored	Mylan Pharmaceuticals
MYLAN; 210; 250	Chlorpropamide	250 mg	Green	Tablet	Circle, Scored	Udl Laboratories
MYLAN; 211	Chlordiazepoxide and Amitriptyline	5 mg; 12.5 mg	Green	Coated Tablet	Circle	H.L. Moore
MYLAN; 211	Chlordiazepoxide and Amitriptyline Hydrochloride	12.5 mg; 5 mg	Green	Coated Tablet	Circle, Biconvex	Mylan Pharmaceuticals
MYLAN; 214	Haloperidol	2 mg	Orange	Tablet	Circle, Scored	Mylan Pharmaceuticals
MYLAN; 216; 40	Furosemide	40 mg	White	Tablet	Circle, Scored, Flat Beveled Edge	Mylan Pharmaceuticals
MYLAN; 216; 40	Furosemide	40 mg	White	Tablet	Circle, Scored, Flat Beveled Edge	Udl Laboratories
MYLAN; 217; 250	Tolazamide	250 mg	White	Tablet	Circle, Scored, Biconvex	Mylan Pharmaceuticals
MYLAN; 232; 80	Furosemide	80 mg	White	Tablet	Circle, Scored, Flat Beveled Edge	Mylan Pharmaceuticals
MYLAN; 232; 80	Furosemide	80 mg	White	Tablet	Circle, Scored, Flat Beveled Edge	Udl Laboratories
MYLAN; 237	Etodolac	400 mg	White	Tablet	Oval	Mylan Pharmaceuticals
MYLAN; 242	Etodolac	500 mg	Pink	Coated Tablet	Oval, Biconvex	Mylan Pharmaceuticals
MYLAN; 244	Verapamil Hydrochloride	120 mg	Blue	Extended-Release Tablet	Oval	Mylan Pharmaceuticals
MYLAN; 244	Verapamil Hydrochloride	120 mg	Blue	Extended-Release Tablet	Oval	Udl Laboratories
MYLAN; 245	Bumetanide	0.5 mg	Light Green	Tablet	Oval, Scored	Mylan Pharmaceuticals
MYLAN; 251	Trazodone Hydrochloride	50 mg	Clear	Coated Tablet	Circle, Scored, Biconvex, Beveled Edge	Mylan Pharmaceuticals
MYLAN; 252	Trazodone Hydrochloride	100 mg	Clear	Coated Tablet	Circle, Scored, Biconvex, Beveled Edge	Mylan Pharmaceuticals
MYLAN; 257	Haloperidol	1 mg	Orange	Tablet	Circle, Scored	Mylan Pharmaceuticals
MYLAN; 271	Diazepam	2 mg	White	Tablet	Circle, Scored, Flat Beveled Edge	Mylan Pharmaceuticals
MYLAN; 271	Diazepam	2 mg	White	Tablet	Circle, Scored, Flat Beveled Edge	Udl Laboratories
MYLAN; 277	Chlordiazepoxide and Amitriptyline	10 mg; 25 mg	White	Coated Tablet	Circle	H.L. Moore
MYLAN; 277	Chlordiazepoxide and Amitriptyline Hydrochloride	25 mg; 10 mg	White	Coated Tablet	Circle, Biconvex	Mylan Pharmaceuticals
MYLAN; 327	Haloperidol	5 mg	Orange	Tablet	Circle, Scored	Mylan Pharmaceuticals
MYLAN; 330	Perphenazine and Amitriptyline Hydrochloride	2 mg; 10 mg	White	Coated Tablet	Circle, Biconvex, Beveled Edge	Mylan Pharmaceuticals
MYLAN; 345	Diazepam	5 mg	Orange	Tablet	Circle, Scored, Flat Beveled Edge	Mylan Pharmaceuticals
MYLAN; 345	Diazepam	5 mg	Orange	Tablet	Circle, Scored, Flat Beveled Edge	Udl Laboratories
MYLAN; 347	Propranolol Hydrochloride and Hydrochlorothiazide	80 mg; 25 mg	White	Tablet	Circle, Scored, Biconvex	Mylan Pharmaceuticals
MYLAN; 351	Haloperidol	0.5 mg	Orange	Tablet	Circle, Scored	Mylan Pharmaceuticals
MYLAN; 357	Pentoxifylline	400 mg	Lavender	Sustained-Release Tablet	Capsule-Shape	Mylan Pharmaceuticals
MYLAN; 357	Pentoxifylline	400 mg	Lavender	Sustained-Release Tablet	Capsule-Shape	Udl Laboratories
MYLAN; 370	Bumetanide	1 mg	Yellow	Tablet	Oval, Scored	Mylan Pharmaceuticals
MYLAN; 377	Naproxen	250 mg	White	Tablet	Circle	Mylan Pharmaceuticals
MYLAN; 377	Naproxen	250 mg	White	Tablet	Circle	Udl Laboratories
MYLAN; 417	Bumetanide	2 mg	Peach	Tablet	Oval, Scored	Mylan Pharmaceuticals
MYLAN; 421	Methyldopa	500 mg	Beige	Coated Tablet	Capsule-Shape, Biconvex, Beveled Edge	Mylan Pharmaceuticals
MYLAN; 421	Methyldopa	500 mg	Beige	Coated Tablet	Capsule-Shape, Biconvex, Beveled Edge	Udl Laboratories
MYLAN; 427	Sulindac	150 mg	Yellow-Orange	Tablet	Circle, Biconvex	Mylan Pharmaceuticals
MYLAN; 427	Sulindac	150 mg	Yellow-Orange	Tablet	Circle, Biconvex	Udl Laboratories
MYLAN; 442	Perphenazine and Amitriptyline Hydrochloride	2 mg; 25 mg	Purple	Coated Tablet	Circle, Biconvex, Beveled Edge	Mylan Pharmaceuticals
MYLAN; 451	Naproxen	500 mg	White	Tablet	Capsule-Shape	Mylan Pharmaceuticals
MYLAN; 451	Naproxen	500 mg	White	Tablet	Capsule-Shape	Udl Laboratories
MYLAN; 457	Lorazepam	1 mg	White	Tablet	Circle, Scored	Mylan Pharmaceuticals
MYLAN; 457	Lorazepam	1 mg	White	Tablet	Circle, Scored	Udl Laboratories
MYLAN; 477	Diazepam	10 mg	Green	Tablet	Circle, Scored	Mylan Pharmaceuticals
MYLAN; 507	Methyldopa and Hydrochlorothiazide	250 mg; 15 mg	Green	Coated Tablet	Circle, Biconvex, Beveled Edge	Mylan Pharmaceuticals
MYLAN; 512	Verapamil Hydrochloride	80 mg	White	Coated Tablet	Circle, Scored	Mylan Pharmaceuticals
MYLAN; 512	Verapamil Hydrochloride	80 mg	White	Coated Tablet	Circle, Scored	Udl Laboratories
MYLAN; 517	Gemfibrozil	600 mg	White	Coated Tablet	Oval, Partially Scored	Mylan Pharmaceuticals
MYLAN; 521	Acetaminophen and Propoxyphene Napsylate	650 mg; 100 mg	White	Coated Tablet	Capsule-Shape, Biconvex, Beveled Edge	Mylan Pharmaceuticals
MYLAN; 531	Sulindac	200 mg	Yellow-Orange	Tablet	Circle, Scored, Biconvex	Mylan Pharmaceuticals
MYLAN; 531	Sulindac	200 mg	Yellow-Orange	Tablet	Circle, Scored, Biconvex	Udl Laboratories
MYLAN; 551	Tolazamide	500 mg	White	Tablet	Circle, Scored, Biconvex	Mylan Pharmaceuticals
MYLAN; 555	Naproxen	375 mg	White	Tablet	Capsule-Shape	Mylan Pharmaceuticals
MYLAN; 555	Naproxen	375 mg	White	Tablet	Capsule-Shape	Udl Laboratories
MYLAN; 574	Perphenazine and Amitriptyline Hydrochloride	25 mg; 4 mg	Orange	Coated Tablet	Circle, Biconvex, Beveled Edge	Mylan Pharmaceuticals
MYLAN; 611	Methyldopa	250 mg	Beige	Coated Tablet	Circle, Biconvex, Beveled Edge	Mylan Pharmaceuticals
MYLAN; 611	Methyldopa	250 mg	Beige	Coated Tablet	Circle, Biconvex, Beveled Edge	Udl Laboratories
MYLAN; 711	Methyldopa and Hydrochlorothiazide	250 mg; 25 mg	Green	Coated Tablet	Capsule-Shape, Biconvex	Mylan Pharmaceuticals

IMPRINT	BRAND/GENERIC NAME	STRENGTH	COLOR	FORM	SHAPE	MANUFACTURER
MYLAN; 727	Perphenazine and Amitriptyline Hydrochloride	4 mg; 10 mg	Blue	Coated Tablet	Circle, Biconvex, Beveled Edge	Mylan Pharmaceuticals
MYLAN; 731	Propranolol Hydrochloride and Hydrochlorothiazide	40 mg; 25 mg	White	Tablet	Circle, Scored, Biconvex	Mylan Pharmaceuticals
MYLAN; 733	Naproxen Sodium	550 mg	Light Blue	Coated Tablet	Oval, Modified	Mylan Pharmaceuticals
MYLAN; 772	Verapamil Hydrochloride	120 mg	White	Coated Tablet	Circle, Scored	Mylan Pharmaceuticals
MYLAN; 772	Verapamil Hydrochloride	120 mg	White	Coated Tablet	Circle, Scored	Udl Laboratories
MYLAN; 777	Lorazepam	2 mg	White	Tablet	Circle, Scored	Mylan Pharmaceuticals
MYLAN; 777	Lorazepam	2 mg	White	Tablet	Circle, Scored	Udl Laboratories
MYLAN; 810	Hydrochlorothiazide	12.5 mg	White	Capsule		Mylan Pharmaceuticals
MYLAN; 1001	Thiothixene	1 mg	Tan and Blue	Capsule		Mylan Pharmaceuticals
MYLAN; 1001	Thiothixene	1 mg	Tan and Blue	Capsule		Udl Laboratories
MYLAN; 1010	Piroxicam	10 mg	Green and Olive	Capsule		Mylan Pharmaceuticals
MYLAN; 1010	Piroxicam	10 mg	Green and Olive	Capsule		Udl Laboratories
MYLAN; 1020	Nicardipine Hydrochloride	20 mg	Opaque Blue-Green and Yellow	Capsule		Mylan Pharmaceuticals
MYLAN; 1049	Doxepin	10 mg	Buff and Buff	Capsule		H.L. Moore
MYLAN; 1049	Doxepin Hydrochloride	10 mg	Buff	Capsule		Mylan Pharmaceuticals
MYLAN; 1049	Doxepin Hydrochloride	10 mg	Buff	Capsule		Udl Laboratories
MYLAN; 1101	Prazosin Hydrochloride	1 mg	Green and Brown	Capsule		Mylan Pharmaceuticals
MYLAN; 1101	Prazosin Hydrochloride	1 mg	Green and Brown	Capsule		Udl Laboratories
MYLAN; 1155	Acetaminophen and Propoxyphene Napsylate	100 mg; 650 mg	White	Tablet	Capsule-Shape	Mylan Pharmaceuticals
MYLAN; 1155	Acetaminophen and Propoxyphene Napsylate	650 mg; 100 mg	White	Tablet	Capsule-Shape, Biconvex, Beveled Edge	Mylan Pharmaceuticals
MYLAN; 1200	Acebutolol Hydrochloride	200 mg	Medium Orange Opaque	Capsule		Mylan Pharmaceuticals
MYLAN; 1204	Amoxicillin	250 mg	Yellow	Capsule		Mylan Pharmaceuticals
MYLAN; 1205	Amoxicillin	500 mg	Yellow	Capsule		Mylan Pharmaceuticals
MYLAN; 1400	Acebutolol Hydrochloride	400 mg	Medium Orange Opaque	Capsule		Mylan Pharmaceuticals
MYLAN; 1401	Ibuprofen	400 mg	White	Coated Tablet	Circle	Mylan Pharmaceuticals
MYLAN; 1401;	Ibuprofen	400 mg	White	Coated Tablet	Circle, Biconvex, Beveled Edge	Mylan Pharmaceuticals
MYLAN; 1410	Nortriptyline Hydrochloride	10 mg	Opaque Swedish Orange	Capsule		Mylan Pharmaceuticals
MYLAN; 1410	Nortriptyline Hydrochloride	10 mg	Opaque Swedish Orange	Capsule		Udl Laboratories
MYLAN; 1430	Nicardipine Hydrochloride	30 mg	Opaque Blue-Green and Yellow	Capsule		Mylan Pharmaceuticals
MYLAN; 1560;	Extended Phenytoin Sodium	100 mg	Lavender and White	Extended-Release Capsule		Mylan Pharmaceuticals
MYLAN; 1560;	Extended Phenytoin Sodium	100 mg	Lavender and White	Extended-Release Capsule		Udl Laboratories
MYLAN; 1570	Terazosin Hydrochloride	10 mg	Lavender	Capsule		Mylan Pharmaceuticals
MYLAN; 1570	Terazosin Hydrochloride	10 mg	Lavender	Capsule		Udl Laboratories
MYLAN; 1601	Ibuprofen	600 mg	White	Coated Tablet	Oval	Mylan Pharmaceuticals
MYLAN; 1601;	Ibuprofen	600 mg	White	Coated Tablet	Capsule-Shape, Biconvex, Beveled Edge	Mylan Pharmaceuticals
MYLAN; 1610	Dicyclomine Hydrochloride	10 mg	Light Turquoise Blue	Capsule		Mylan Pharmaceuticals
MYLAN; 1610	Dicyclomine Hydrochloride	10 mg	Light Turquoise Blue	Capsule		Udl Laboratories
MYLAN; 1650	Nitrofurantoin Macrocrystals	50 mg	Opaque Light Brown	Capsule		Mylan Pharmaceuticals
MYLAN; 1650	Nitrofurantoin Macrocrystals	50 mg	Opaque Light Brown	Capsule		Udl Laboratories
MYLAN; 1700	Nitrofurantoin Macrocrystals	100 mg	Opaque Grey	Capsule		Mylan Pharmaceuticals
MYLAN; 1700	Nitrofurantoin Macrocrystals	100 mg	Opaque Grey	Capsule		Udl Laboratories
MYLAN; 1801	Ibuprofen	800 mg	White	Coated Tablet	Capsule-Shape	Mylan Pharmaceuticals
MYLAN; 1801;	Ibuprofen	800 mg	White	Coated Tablet	Oval, Biconvex, Beveled Edge	Mylan Pharmaceuticals
MYLAN; 2002	Thiothixene	2 mg	Tan and Yellow	Capsule		Mylan Pharmaceuticals
MYLAN; 2002	Thiothixene	2 mg	Tan and Yellow	Capsule		Udl Laboratories
MYLAN; 2020	Piroxicam	20 mg	Green	Capsule		Mylan Pharmaceuticals
MYLAN; 2020	Piroxicam	20 mg	Green	Capsule		Udl Laboratories
MYLAN; 2100	Loperamide Hydrochloride	2 mg	Brown	Capsule		Mylan Pharmaceuticals
MYLAN; 2100	Loperamide Hydrochloride	2 mg	Brown	Capsule		Udl Laboratories
MYLAN; 2115	Ampicillin	250 mg	White Opaque	Capsule		Mylan Pharmaceuticals
MYLAN; 2116	Ampicillin	500 mg	White	Capsule		Mylan Pharmaceuticals
MYLAN; 2150	Meclofenamate Sodium	50 mg	Coral	Capsule		Mylan Pharmaceuticals
MYLAN; 2200	Acyclovir	200 mg	Purple	Capsule		Mylan Pharmaceuticals
MYLAN; 2252	Selegiline Hydrochloride	5 mg	Light Blue Opaque and Aqua Blue	Capsule		Mylan Pharmaceuticals
MYLAN; 2260	Terazosin Hydrochloride	1 mg	Rich Yellow and Light Lavender	Capsule		Mylan Pharmaceuticals
MYLAN; 2260	Terazosin Hydrochloride	1 mg	Rich Yellow and Light Lavender	Capsule		Udl Laboratories
MYLAN; 2264	Terazosin Hydrochloride	2 mg	Black and Light Lavender	Capsule		Mylan Pharmaceuticals
MYLAN; 2264	Terazosin Hydrochloride	2 mg	Black and Light Lavender	Capsule		Udl Laboratories
MYLAN; 2268	Terazosin Hydrochloride	5 mg	Gray and Lavender	Capsule		Mylan Pharmaceuticals
MYLAN; 2268	Terazosin Hydrochloride	5 mg	Gray and Lavender	Capsule		Udl Laboratories
MYLAN; 2302	Prazosin Hydrochloride	2 mg	Brown	Capsule		Mylan Pharmaceuticals
MYLAN; 2302	Prazosin Hydrochloride	2 mg	Brown	Capsule		Udl Laboratories
MYLAN; 2325	Nortriptyline Hydrochloride	25 mg	Opaque Orange and Opaque Swedish Orange	Capsule		Mylan Pharmaceuticals
MYLAN; 2325	Nortriptyline Hydrochloride	25 mg	Opaque Orange and Opaque Swedish Orange	Capsule		Udl Laboratories
MYLAN; 2537	Triamterene and Hydrochlorothiazide	25 mg; 37.5 mg	Olive and Yellow	Capsule		Mylan Pharmaceuticals

IMPRINT	BRAND/GENERIC NAME	STRENGTH	COLOR	FORM	SHAPE	MANUFACTURER
MYLAN; 2537	Triamterene and Hydrochlorothiazide	25 mg; 37.5 mg	Olive and Yellow	Capsule		Udl Laboratories
MYLAN; 3000	Meclofenamate Sodium	100 mg	Coral and White	Capsule		Mylan Pharmaceuticals
MYLAN; 3005	Thiothixene	5 mg	Tan and White	Capsule		Mylan Pharmaceuticals
MYLAN; 3005	Thiothixene	5 mg	Tan and White	Capsule		Udl Laboratories
MYLAN; 3025	Clomipramine Hydrochloride	25 mg	Orange and Flesh	Capsule		Mylan Pharmaceuticals
MYLAN; 3050	Clomipramine Hydrochloride	50 mg	Yellow and Flesh	Capsule		Mylan Pharmaceuticals
MYLAN; 3075	Clomipramine Hydrochloride	75 mg	Orange and Flesh	Capsule		Mylan Pharmaceuticals
MYLAN; 3125	Doxepin	25 mg	Ivory and White	Capsule		H.L. Moore
MYLAN; 3125	Doxepin Hydrochloride	25 mg	Ivory and White	Capsule		Mylan Pharmaceuticals
MYLAN; 3125	Doxepin Hydrochloride	25 mg	Ivory and White	Capsule		Udl Laboratories
MYLAN; 3205	Prazosin Hydrochloride	5 mg	Blue and Brown	Capsule		Mylan Pharmaceuticals
MYLAN; 3205	Prazosin Hydrochloride	5 mg	Blue and Brown	Capsule		Udl Laboratories
MYLAN; 3250	Nortriptyline Hydrochloride	50 mg	Opaque Yellow and Opaque Swedish Orange	Capsule		Mylan Pharmaceuticals
MYLAN; 3250	Nortriptyline Hydrochloride	50 mg	Opaque Yellow and Opaque Swedish Orange	Capsule		Udl Laboratories
MYLAN; 3422	Nitrofurantoin Monohydrate/ macrocrystals	25 mg; 75 mg	Light Gray and Light Brown	Capsule		Mylan Pharmaceuticals
MYLAN; 4010	Temazepam	15 mg	Peach	Capsule		Mylan Pharmaceuticals
MYLAN; 4010	Temazepam	15 mg	Peach	Capsule		Udl Laboratories
MYLAN; 4070	Ketoprofen	50 mg	Light Green	Capsule		Mylan Pharmaceuticals
MYLAN; 4175	Nortriptyline Hydrochloride	75 mg	Brown and Orange	Capsule		Mylan Pharmaceuticals
MYLAN; 4210	Fluoxetine Hydrochloride	10 mg	White and Flesh	Capsule		Mylan Pharmaceuticals
MYLAN; 4220	Fluoxetine Hydrochloride	20 mg	Turquoise and Flesh	Capsule		Mylan Pharmaceuticals
MYLAN; 4250	Doxepin	50 mg	Ivory and White	Capsule		H.L. Moore
MYLAN; 4250	Doxepin Hydrochloride	50 mg	Ivory	Capsule		Mylan Pharmaceuticals
MYLAN; 4250	Doxepin Hydrochloride	50 mg	Ivory	Capsule		Udl Laboratories
MYLAN; 4415	Flurazepam Hydrochloride	15 mg	White and Blue	Capsule		Mylan Pharmaceuticals
MYLAN; 4415	Flurazepam Hydrochloride	15 mg	White and Blue	Capsule		Udl Laboratories
MYLAN; 4430	Flurazepam Hydrochloride	30 mg	Blue	Capsule		Mylan Pharmaceuticals
MYLAN; 4430	Flurazepam Hydrochloride	30 mg	Blue	Capsule		Udl Laboratories
MYLAN; 4700	Gemfibrozil	300 mg	Swedish Orange and White	Capsule		Mylan Pharmaceuticals
MYLAN; 5010	Thiothixene	10 mg	Tan and Peach	Capsule		Mylan Pharmaceuticals
MYLAN; 5010	Thiothixene	10 mg	Tan and Peach	Capsule		Udl Laboratories
MYLAN; 5050	Temazepam	30 mg	Yellow	Capsule		Mylan Pharmaceuticals
MYLAN; 5050	Temazepam	30 mg	Yellow	Capsule		Udl Laboratories
MYLAN; 5200	Tolmetin Sodium	400 mg	Light Blue	Capsule		Mylan Pharmaceuticals
MYLAN; 5211	Omeprazole	10 mg	Dark Green	Delayed-Release Capsule		Mylan Pharmaceuticals
MYLAN; 5211	Omeprazole	10 mg	Green	Delayed-Release Capsule		Udl Laboratories
MYLAN; 5220	Diltiazem Hydrochloride	120 mg	Light Pink and Flesh	Extended-Release Capsule		Mylan Pharmaceuticals
MYLAN; 5220	Diltiazem Hydrochloride	120 mg	Light Pink and Flesh	Extended-Release Capsule		Udl Laboratories
MYLAN; 5280	Diltiazem Hydrochloride	180 mg	Lavender and Flesh	Extended-Release Capsule		Mylan Pharmaceuticals
MYLAN; 5280	Diltiazem Hydrochloride	180 mg	Lavender and Flesh	Extended-Release Capsule		Udl Laboratories
MYLAN; 5340	Diltiazem Hydrochloride	240 mg	Light Blue and Flesh	Extended-Release Capsule		Mylan Pharmaceuticals
MYLAN; 5340	Diltiazem Hydrochloride	240 mg	Light Blue and Flesh	Extended-Release Capsule		Udl Laboratories
MYLAN; 5375	Doxepin	75 mg	Green	Capsule		H.L. Moore
MYLAN; 5375	Doxepin Hydrochloride	75 mg	Brite Light Green	Capsule		Mylan Pharmaceuticals
MYLAN; 5375	Doxepin Hydrochloride	75 mg	Brite Light Green	Capsule		Udl Laboratories
MYLAN; 5750	Ketoprofen	75 mg		Capsule		Mylan Pharmaceuticals
MYLAN; 6025	Cephalexin	250 mg	Dark Blue and Opaque White	Capsule		Mylan Pharmaceuticals
MYLAN; 6050	Cephalexin	500 mg	Dark Blue and Light Blue	Capsule		Mylan Pharmaceuticals
MYLAN; 6060	Diltiazem Hydrochloride	60 mg	Coral and White	Extended-Release Capsule		Mylan Pharmaceuticals
MYLAN; 6060	Diltiazem Hydrochloride	60 mg	Coral and White	Extended-Release Capsule		Udl Laboratories
MYLAN; 6090	Diltiazem Hydrochloride	90 mg	Coral and Ivory	Extended-Release Capsule		Mylan Pharmaceuticals
MYLAN; 6090	Diltiazem Hydrochloride	90 mg	Coral and Ivory	Extended-Release Capsule		Udl Laboratories
MYLAN; 6120	Diltiazem Hydrochloride	120 mg	Coral	Extended-Release Capsule		Mylan Pharmaceuticals
MYLAN; 6120	Diltiazem Hydrochloride	120 mg	Coral	Extended-Release Capsule		Udl Laboratories
MYLAN; 6150	Omeprazole	20 mg	Dark Green and Blue Green	Delayed-Release Capsule		Mylan Pharmaceuticals
MYLAN; 6150	Omeprazole	20 mg	Dark Green and Blue Green	Delayed-Release Capsule		Udl Laboratories
MYLAN; 6320	Verapamil Hydrochloride	120 mg	Blue-Green and White	Extended-Release Capsule		Mylan Pharmaceuticals
MYLAN; 6320	Verapamil Hydrochloride	120 mg	Blue-Green and White	Extended-Release Capsule		Udl Laboratories
MYLAN; 6380	Verapamil Hydrochloride	180 mg	Blue-Green and Light Green	Extended-Release Capsule		Mylan Pharmaceuticals
MYLAN; 6380	Verapamil Hydrochloride	180 mg	Blue-Green and Light Green	Extended-Release Capsule		Udl Laboratories

IMPRINT	BRAND/GENERIC NAME	STRENGTH	COLOR	FORM	SHAPE	MANUFACTURER
MYLAN; 6410	Doxepin	100 mg	Green and White	Capsule		H.L. Moore
MYLAN; 6410	Doxepin Hydrochloride	100 mg	Bright Light Green and White	Capsule		Mylan Pharmaceuticals
MYLAN; 6410	Doxepin Hydrochloride	100 mg	Bright Light Green and White	Capsule		Udl Laboratories
MYLAN; 6440	Verapamil Hydrochloride	240 mg	Blue-Green	Extended-Release Capsule		Mylan Pharmaceuticals
MYLAN; 6440	Verapamil Hydrochloride	240 mg	Blue-Green	Extended-Release Capsule		Udl Laboratories
MYLAN; 7200	Etodolac	200 mg	Brown Opaque	Capsule		Mylan Pharmaceuticals
MYLAN; 7233	Etodolac	300 mg	Light Brown Opaque	Capsule		Mylan Pharmaceuticals
MYLAN; 7250	Cefaclor	250 mg	Pink and White	Capsule		Mylan Pharmaceuticals
MYLAN; 7500	Cefaclor	500 mg	Pink and Grey	Capsule		Mylan Pharmaceuticals
MYLAN; A	Alprazolam	0.25 mg	White	Tablet	Circle, Scored	Mylan Pharmaceuticals
MYLAN; A	Alprazolam	0.25 mg	White	Tablet	Circle, Scored	Udl Laboratories
MYLAN; A1	Alprazolam	1 mg	Blue	Tablet	Circle	Mylan Pharmaceuticals
MYLAN; A1	Alprazolam	1 mg	Blue	Tablet	Circle	Udl Laboratories
MYLAN; A3	Alprazolam	0.5 mg	Peach	Tablet	Circle	Mylan Pharmaceuticals
MYLAN; A3	Alprazolam	0.5 mg	Peach	Tablet	Circle	Udl Laboratories
MYLAN; A4	Alprazolam	2 mg	White	Tablet	Circle	Mylan Pharmaceuticals
MYLAN; G1	Glipizide	5 mg	White	Tablet	Circle, Scored, Biconvex	Mylan Pharmaceuticals
MYLAN; G1	Glipizide	5 mg	White	Tablet	Circle, Scored, Biconvex	Udl Laboratories
MYLAN; G2	Glipizide	10 mg	White	Tablet	Circle, Scored, Biconvex	Mylan Pharmaceuticals
MYLAN; G2	Glipizide	10 mg	White	Tablet	Circle, Scored, Biconvex	Udl Laboratories
MYLAN; TH; 2	Triamterene and Hydrochlorothiazide	50 mg; 75 mg	Yellow	Tablet	Circle, Scored	Mylan Pharmaceuticals
MYLAN; TH; 2	Triamterene and Hydrochlorothiazide	50 mg; 75 mg	Yellow	Tablet	Circle, Scored	Udl Laboratories
MYLANTA; GELCAP	Mylanta Gelcaps	550 mg; 125 mg	Light Blue and White	Capsule, Liquid Filled		Johnson & Johnson Merck Consumer Pharmaceuticals
MYLANTA DS	Mylanta Double Strength	700 mg; 300 mg	Red or Green	Tablet, Chewable		Johnson & Johnson Merck
MYLICON; 125	Mylicon 125	125 mg	Pink	Tablet, Chewable		Johnson & Johnson Merck
MYSOLINE; 50	Mysoline	50 mg	White	Tablet		Xcel Pharmaceuticals
MYSOLINE; 250	Mysoline	250 mg	White	Tablet		Xcel Pharmaceuticals
N	Nytol Quick Caps	25 mg	White to Off-White	Tablet	Oblong	Block Drug
N; 1.5; 034	Glyburide	1.5 mg		Tablet		Teva Pharmaceuticals
N; 3	Nitrostat	0.3 mg	White	Tablet	Circle, Flat-Faced	Parke-Davis
N; 3; 035	Glyburide	3 mg	Pale Blue	Tablet	Oval, Scored	Teva Pharmaceuticals
N; 4	Nitrostat	0.4 mg	White	Tablet	Circle, Flat-Faced	Parke-Davis
N; 6	Nitrostat	0.6 mg	White	Tablet	Circle, Flat-Faced	Parke-Davis
N; 126; 0.25	Alprazolam	0.25 mg	White	Tablet	Circle, Scored	Warner Chilcott
N; 127; 0.5	Alprazolam	0.5 mg	Orange	Tablet	Circle, Scored	Warner Chilcott
N; 131; 1.0	Alprazolam	1 mg	Blue	Tablet	Circle, Scored	Warner Chilcott
N; 132; 12.5	Captopril	12.5 mg	White	Tablet	Oval, Scored	Teva Pharmaceuticals
N; 133; 25	Captopril	25 mg	White	Tablet	Round, Quadrisect Scored	Novopharm
N; 134; 50	Captopril	50 mg	White	Tablet	Oval, Scored	Teva Pharmaceuticals
N; 135; 100	Captopril	100 mg	White	Tablet	Oval, Scored	Teva Pharmaceuticals
N; 171; 10	Nifedipine	10 mg	Brown	Capsule		Teva Pharmaceuticals
N; 181; 200	Cimetidine	200 mg	Green	Coated Tablet	Oval	Teva Pharmaceuticals
N; 192; 300	Cimetidine	300 mg	Green	Coated Tablet	Oval	Teva Pharmaceuticals
N; 204; 400	Cimetidine	400 mg	Green	Coated Tablet	Oval, Scored	Teva Pharmaceuticals
N; 235	Norwich Aspirin, Regular Strength	325 mg	White	Coated Tablet	Circle	Chattem Consumer Products
N; 235; 800	Cimetidine	800 mg	Green	Coated Tablet	Oval, Scored	Teva Pharmaceuticals
N; 240; 67	Fenofibrate	67 mg	Pink	Capsule		Teva Pharmaceuticals
N; 240; 67	Lofibra	67 mg	Pink	Capsule		Gate Pharmaceuticals
N; 325	Acetaminophen	325 mg	White	Tablet	Circle	Chattem Consumer Products
N; 342; 1.25	Glyburide	1.25 mg	White	Tablet	Circle, Scored	Teva Pharmaceuticals
N; 343; 2.5	Glyburide	2.5 mg	Peach	Tablet	Circle, Scored	Teva Pharmaceuticals
N; 344; 5	Glyburide	5 mg	Light Green	Tablet	Circle, Scored	Teva Pharmaceuticals
N; 397; 300	Etodolac	300 mg	Red	Capsule		Teva Pharmaceuticals
N; 411; 134	Fenofibrate	134 mg	Light Blue	Capsule		Teva Pharmaceuticals
N; 411; 134	Lofibra	134 mg	Light Blue	Capsule		Gate Pharmaceuticals
N; 412; 200	Fenofibrate	200 mg	Orange	Capsule		Teva Pharmaceuticals
N; 412; 200	Lofibra	200 mg	Orange	Capsule		Gate Pharmaceuticals
N; 544; 150	Ranitidine Hydrochloride	150 mg	White	Tablet	Circle	Teva Pharmaceuticals
N; 547; 300	Ranitidine Hydrochloride	300 mg	White	Tablet	Capsule-Shape	Teva Pharmaceuticals
N; 590; 1	Doxazosin Mesylate	1 mg	White to Off-White	Tablet	Circle, Scored	Teva Pharmaceuticals
N; 593; 2	Doxazosin Mesylate	2 mg	White to Off-White	Tablet	Capsule-Shape	Teva Pharmaceuticals
N; 596; 4	Doxazosin Mesylate	4 mg	White to Off-White	Tablet	Diamond, Scored	Teva Pharmaceuticals
N; 598; 8	Doxazosin Mesylate	8 mg	White to Off-White	Tablet	Circle	Teva Pharmaceuticals
N; 739; 150	Mexiletine Hydrochloride	150 mg	Light Orange and Tan	Capsule		Teva Pharmaceuticals
N; 740; 200	Mexiletine Hydrochloride	200 mg	Light Orange	Capsule		Teva Pharmaceuticals
N; 741; 250	Mexiletine Hydrochloride	250 mg	Light Orange and Dark Green	Capsule		Teva Pharmaceuticals
N; 815; 400	Tolmetin Sodium	400 mg	Red	Capsule		Teva Pharmaceuticals
N; 894; 150	Nizatidine	150 mg	Tan and White	Capsule		Teva Pharmaceuticals
N; 899; 300	Nizatidine	300 mg	Tan	Capsule		Teva Pharmaceuticals
N; 940; 200	Acyclovir	200 mg		Capsule		Teva Pharmaceuticals
N; 943; 400	Acyclovir	400 mg		Tablet		Teva Pharmaceuticals
N; 947; 800	Acyclovir	800 mg		Tablet		Teva Pharmaceuticals
N;	Nytol	50 mg	Blue	Tablet	Circle, Scored	Block Drug
N;	Nytol	25 mg		Tablet		Block Drug
N2; N	Neptazane	25 mg	White	Tablet	Square	Lederle Laboratories
N2; N	Neptazane	25 mg	White	Tablet	Square	Wyeth Pharmaceuticals
N2; SWORD LOGO	Suboxone	2 mg; 0.5 mg	Orange	Tablet	Six-Sided	Reckitt Benckiser
N5; LL	Nilstat	500,000 units	Pink	Coated Tablet	Circle, Convex	Lederle Laboratories
N8; SWORD LOGO	Suboxone	8 mg; 2 mg	Orange	Tablet	Six-Sided	Reckitt Benckiser
NALFON; DISTA	Nalfon	600 mg	Yellow	Tablet	Capsule-Shape, Paracapsule-Shaped, Scored	Dista Products

IMPRINT	BRAND/GENERIC NAME	STRENGTH	COLOR	FORM	SHAPE	MANUFACTURER
NALFON; DISTA; H77	Nalfon	300 mg	Yellow and Ocher	Capsule		Dista Products
NAP	Spancap No. 1	15 mg	Black and Yellow	Sustained-Release Capsule		Vortech Pharmaceuticals
NAPROSYN; 250; ROCHE;	Naprosyn	250 mg	Yellow	Tablet	Circle, Biconvex	Roche Laboratories
NAPROSYN; 375;	Naprosyn	375 mg	Peach	Tablet	Capsule-Shape	Roche Laboratories
NAPROSYN; 500;	Naprosyn	500 mg	Yellow	Tablet	Capsule-Shape	Roche Laboratories
NATAFORT	Natafort	1000 IU; 400 IU; 11 IU; 120 mg; 1 mg; 2 mg; 3 mg; 20 mg; 10 mg; 12 mcg; 60 mg	White	Coated Tablet		Warner Chilcott
NAVANE; ROERIG; 571;	Navane	1 mg	Orange and Yellow	Capsule		Roerig
NAVANE; ROERIG; 572;	Navane	2 mg	Blue and Yellow	Capsule		Roerig
NAVANE; ROERIG; 573;	Navane	5 mg	Orange and White	Capsule		Roerig
NAVANE; ROERIG; 574;	Navane	10 mg	Blue and White	Capsule		Roerig
NAVANE; ROERIG; 577;	Navane	20 mg	Blue and White	Capsule		Roerig
N-BACK	Nuprin Backache	500 mg	White	Tablet	Capsule-Shape	Bristol-Myers Squibb
ND; A;	Janimine	10 mg	Orange	Coated Tablet		Abbott Laboratories
ND; SCF	Contac Severe Cold & Flu Non-Drowsy Formula	325 mg; 30 mg; 15 mg	White	Tablet		Glaxosmithkline Consumer
NE; 406	Didronel	400 mg	White	Tablet	Capsule-Shape, Scored	Procter & Gamble Pharmaceuticals
NE; A;	Janimine	25 mg	Yellow	Coated Tablet		Abbott Laboratories
NEORAL; 25 MG	Neoral	25 mg	Blue-Gray	Capsule, Liquid Filled	Oval	Novartis
NEORAL; 100 MG	Neoral	100 mg	Blue-Gray	Capsule, Liquid Filled	Oblong	Novartis
NEO-SYNEPHRINOL	Neo-Synephrinol	120 mg	Clear with White Pellets	Capsule		Sanofi Winthrop
NICHE; 420	Mag-Tab SR	84 mg	Yellow	Sustained-Release Tablet	Capsule-Shape	Niche Pharmaceuticals
NICOTINE; 7 MG/ DAY	Nicotine Transdermal System	7 mg/24 Hours	Tan, Opaque	Patch	Square, Round Edges	Watson Laboratories
NICOTINE; 14 MG/ DAY	Nicotine Transdermal System	14 mg/24 Hours	Tan, Opaque	Patch	Square, Round Edges	Watson Laboratories
NICOTINE; 21 MG/ DAY	Nicotine Transdermal System	21 mg/24 Hours	Tan, Opaque	Patch	Square, Round Edges	Watson Laboratories
NIMOTOP	Nimotop	30 mg	Ivory	Capsule, Liquid Filled		Bayer Pharmaceutical
NITE;	Night Time Cold Medicine Liquid Caps	250 mg; 10 mg; 30 mg; 6.25 mg	Green	Capsule, Liquid Filled		Leiner Health Products
NITE;	Night Time Cold Medicine Liquid Caps	250 mg; 10 mg; 30 mg; 6.25 mg	Green	Capsule, Liquid Filled		Scherer Laboratories
NL; 18	Pseudoephedrine Hydrochloride and Guaifenesin	90 mg; 800 mg	White	Tablet	Capsule-Shape, Scored	Neil Laboratories
NL; 105	Acetaminophen	500 mg	White	Tablet	Oblong	Neil Laboratories
NL; 715	Pseudoephedrine 90/guaifenesin 1200	90 mg; 1200 mg		Extended-Release Tablet	Capsule-Shape, Scored	United Research Laboratories
NL; 718	Guaifenesin and Pseudoephedrine Hydrochloride	800 mg; 90 mg	White	Tablet	Capsule-Shape	Neil Laboratories
NL; 719	Dextromethorphan Hydrobromide, Pseudoephedrine Hydrochloride, and Guaifenesin	60 mg; 800 mg; 90 mg	White	Tablet	Capsule-Shape	Neil Laboratories
NL; 720	Guaifenesin and Phenylephrine Hydrochloride	1200 mg; 40 mg	Light Green	Extended-Release Tablet	Capsule-Shape	Neil Laboratories
NL; 732	Pseudoephedrine Hydrochloride, and Guaifenesin	50 mg; 1200 mg	White	Extended-Release Tablet	Capsule-Shape	Neil Laboratories
NL; 736	Dextromethorphan Hydrobromide and Guaifenesin	30 mg; 500 mg		Tablet		United Research Laboratories
NL; A;	Janimine	50 mg	Peach	Coated Tablet		Abbott Laboratories
NM	K-Tab	10 meq	Yellow	Extended-Release Tablet		Abbott Laboratories
NMI	Fe50	50 mg	Off White	Tablet		Ucb Pharma
NO DOZ	NO Doz	100 mg	White	Tablet	Circle	Bristol-Myers Squibb
NO DOZ	NO Doz Maximum Strength	200 mg	White	Tablet	Capsule-Shape	Bristol-Myers Squibb
NO DOZ; CHEW	NO Doz	100 mg	White	Tablet, Chewable		Bristol-Myers Squibb
NOLUDAR	Noludar	300 mg	Amethyst and White	Capsule		Roche Laboratories
NOLVADEX; 600; CAMEO	Nolvadex	10 mg	White	Tablet	Circle, Biconvex	Astra Zeneca
NOLVADEX; 604; CAMEO	Nolvadex	20 mg	White	Tablet	Circle, Biconvex	Astra Zeneca
NORCO; 539	Norco 10/325	10 mg; 325 mg	Yellow	Tablet	Capsule-Shape, Scored	Watson Laboratories
NORCO; 729	Norco 7.5/325	7.5 mg; 325 mg	Light Orange	Tablet	Capsule-Shape, Scored	Watson Laboratories
NORGESIC; 3M	Norgesic	25 mg; 385 mg; 30 mg	Light Green, White and Yellow	Tablet	Circle, Three-Layered	3m Pharmaceuticals
NORGESIC; FORTE; 3M	Norgesic Forte	770 mg; 60 mg; 50 mg	Light Green, White and Yellow	Tablet	Capsule-Shape, Three-Layered	3m Pharmaceuticals
NORMOZIDE; 227	Normozide	200 mg; 25 mg	White	Coated Tablet	Capsule-Shape, Scored	Schering
NORMOZIDE; 235	Normozide	100 mg; 25 mg	Light Brown	Coated Tablet	Capsule-Shape, Scored	Schering
NORMOZIDE; 391;	Normozide	300 mg; 25 mg	Blue	Coated Tablet	Capsule-Shape, Scored	Schering
NORPRAMIN; 25;	Norpramin	25 mg	Yellow	Coated Tablet		Aventis Pharmaceuticals
NORPRAMIN; 50;	Norpramin	50 mg	Green	Coated Tablet		Aventis Pharmaceuticals
NORPRAMIN; 75;	Norpramin	75 mg	Orange	Tablet		Aventis Pharmaceuticals
NORPRAMIN; 100;	Norpramin	100 mg	Peach	Tablet		Aventis Pharmaceuticals
NORPRAMIN; 150;	Norpramin	150 mg	White	Tablet		Aventis Pharmaceuticals

IMPRINT	BRAND/GENERIC NAME	STRENGTH	COLOR	FORM	SHAPE	MANUFACTURER
NORTRIPTYLINE; 10 MG; 250; CP	Nortripyline Hydrochloride	10 mg	Green and White	Capsule		Creighton Labs
NORTRIPTYLINE; 25 MG; 251; CP	Nortriptyline Hydrochloride	25 mg	Green and White	Capsule		Creighton Labs
NORTRIPTYLINE; DAN; 10 MG	Nortriptyline Hydrochloride	10 mg	Opaque Deep Green and Opaque White	Capsule		Watson Laboratories
NORTRIPTYLINE; DAN; 25 MG	Nortriptyline Hydrochloride	25 mg	Opaque Deep Green and Opaque White	Capsule		Watson Laboratories
NORTRIPTYLINE; DAN; 50 MG	Nortriptyline Hydrochloride	50 mg	Opaque White	Capsule		Watson Laboratories
NORTRIPTYLINE; DAN; 75 MG	Nortriptyline Hydrochloride	75 mg	Opaque Deep Green	Capsule		Watson Laboratories
NORTYRIPTYLINE; 50 MG; 252; CP	Nortriptyline Hydrochloride	50 mg	Green and Yellow	Capsule		Creighton Labs
NORVASC; 2.5;	Norvasc	2.5 mg	White	Tablet	Diamond-Shaped, Flat-Faced, Beveled Edge	Pfizer
NORVASC; 5;	Norvasc	5 mg	White	Tablet	Eight-Sided, Elongated, Flat-Aced, Beveled Edge	Pfizer
NORVASC; 10;	Norvasc	10 mg	White	Tablet	Circle, Flat-Faced, Beveled Edge	Pfizer
NORWICH	Norwich Aspirin, Extra Strength	500 mg	White	Coated Tablet	Capsule-Shape	Chattem Consumer Products
NORWICH; 325	Norwich Enteric Safety Coated Aspirin	325 mg	Orange	Coated Tablet	Circle, Convex	Chattem Consumer Products
NORWICH; 500	Norwich Enteric Safety Coated Maximum Strength Aspirin	500 mg	Orange	Coated Tablet	Circle, Convex	Chattem Consumer Products
NOVAFED; 104	Novafed	120 mg	Orange and Brown	Controlled-Release Capsule	Capsule-Shape	Aventis Pharmaceuticals
NOVAFED A;	Novafed A	120 mg; 8 mg	Red and Orange	Extended-Release Capsule	Capsule-Shape, Red Opaque with Orange Transparent Body	Aventis Pharmaceuticals
NOVO; 288; APIS BULL LOGO	Activella	1 mg; 0.5 mg	White	Coated Tablet	Circle, BI-Convex	Pharmacia & Upjohn
NOVO NORDISK LOGO (BULL)	Prandin	0.5 mg	White	Tablet	Biconvex	Novo Nordisk
NOVO NORDISK LOGO (BULL)	Prandin	1 mg	Yellow	Tablet	Biconvex	Novo Nordisk
NOVO NORDISK LOGO (BULL)	Prandin	2 mg	Peach	Tablet	Biconvex	Novo Nordisk
NPL 51081; 831	Aclophen	40 mg; 8 mg; 500 mg		Tablet	Capsule-Shape	Nutripharm Laboratories
NPR; LE; 375	Naprosyn	375 mg	Pink	Tablet	Oval	Roche Laboratories
NPR; LE; 375;	Prevacid Naprapac	15 mg; 375 mg	Pink	Tablet	Oval	Tap Pharmaceuticals
NR	Nature's Remedy	43 mg	Beige	Tablet	Circle	Block Drug
NRX	Nestabs RX	4000 IU; 400 IU; 30 IU; 120 mg; 1 mg; 3 mg; 3 mg; 20 mg; 3 mg; 8 mcg; 30 mcg; 7 mg; 200 mg; 150 mcg; 15 mg; 100 mg; 29 mg; 3 mg	Light Blue	Coated Tablet	Circle, Scored	Fielding
NT; 0; RJS	Nature-Throid	32.4 mg	Tan	Tablet	Round, Compressed, Bisected Scored	Western Research Laboratories
NT; 1; RJS;	Nature-Throid	64.8 mg	Tan	Tablet	Round, Compressed, Bisected Scored	Western Research Laboratories
NT; 2; RJS;	Nature-Throid	129.6 mg	Tan	Tablet	Round, Compressed, Bisected Scored	Western Research Laboratories
NT; 3; RJS;	Nature-Throid	194.4 mg	Tan	Tablet	Circle, Compressed	Western Research Laboratories
NT; 16;	Neurontin	600 mg	White	Coated Tablet	Circle	Parke-Davis
NT; 26;	Neurontin	800 mg	White	Coated Tablet	Circle	Parke-Davis
NTBC; 2 MG	Orfadin	2 mg	White	Capsule		Rare Disease Therapeutics
NTBC; 5 MG	Orfadin	5 mg	White	Capsule		Rare Disease Therapeutics
NTBC; 10 MG	Orfadin	10 mg	White	Capsule		Rare Disease Therapeutics
NUPRIN	Nuprin	200 mg	Yellow	Tablet	Capsule-Shape	Bristol-Myers Squibb
NUPRIN; 200	Nuprin	200 mg	Yellow	Tablet	Circle	Bristol-Myers Squibb
NVR; DL	Zelnorm	2 mg	White to Yellow Marbled	Tablet	Circle, Flat	Novartis
NVR; EH	Zelnorm	6 mg	White to Yellow Marbled	Tablet	Circle, Flat	Novartis
NVR; EH	Zelnorm	6 mg	White to Yellow Marbled	Tablet	Circle, Flat	Novartis Pharmaceuticals
NVR; R20	Ritalin LA	20 mg	White	Extended-Release Capsule	Capsule-Shape	Novartis Pharmaceuticals
NVR; R30	Ritalin LA	30 mg	Yellow	Extended-Release Capsule	Capsule-Shape	Novartis Pharmaceuticals
NVR; R40	Ritalin LA	40 mg	Light Brown	Extended-Release Capsule	Capsule-Shape	Novartis Pharmaceuticals
NVR; SA	Gleevec	100 mg	Dark Yellow to Brownish Orange	Tablet	Circle, Scored	Novartis
NVR; SL	Gleevec	400 mg	Dark Yellow to Brownish Orange	Tablet	Oval	Novartis
NVR SI	Gleevec	100 mg	Orange with Red Ink	Capsule		Novartis
NYQUIL	Vicks Nyquil Multi-Symptom Cold/flu Relief	250 mg; 10 mg; 30 mg; 6.25 mg	Transparent Green	Capsule, Liquid Filled		Procter & Gamble
NZ; 150; G	Nizatidine	150 mg	Light Yellow and Dark Yellow	Capsule		Par Pharmaceutical
NZ; 300; G	Nizatidine	300 mg	Light Brown	Capsule		Par Pharmaceutical
OC; 10	Oxycontin	10 mg	White	Controlled-Release Tablet	Circle, Convex	Purdue
OC; 20	Oxycontin	20 mg	Pink	Controlled-Release Tablet	Circle, Convex	Purdue
OC; 40	Oxycontin	40 mg	Yellow	Controlled-Release Tablet	Circle, Convex	Purdue

IMPRINT	BRAND/GENERIC NAME	STRENGTH	COLOR	FORM	SHAPE	MANUFACTURER
OC; 80	Oxycontin	80 mg	Green	Controlled-Release Tablet	Circle, Convex	Purdue
OC; 160	Oxycontin	160 mg	Blue	Controlled-Release Tablet	Capsule-Shape, Convex	Purdue
OCL; 55; CINOBAC 250 MG	Cinobac	250 mg	Orange and Green	Capsule		Oclassen
OCL; 56; CINOBAC 500 MG	Cinobac	500 mg	Orange and Green	Capsule		Oclassen
OGT; 918	Zavesca	100 mg;	White	Capsule		Actelion Pharmaceuticals
OHM; 010	Acetaminophen	325 mg	White	Tablet	Circle, Scored	Ohm Laboratories
OHM; 021	Buffered Aspirin	325 mg	White	Tablet	Circle, Convex	Udl Laboratories
OHM; 076	Pseudoephedrine Hydrochloride	60 mg	White	Tablet	Circle, Scored	Ohm Laboratories
OHM; 078	Uni Perr	325 mg; 30 mg	Light Orange	Tablet	Circle	Url
OHM; 117	Senna Concentrate	8.6 mg	Green-Brown	Tablet	Circle, Convex	Ohm Laboratories
O-IR; PF5MG	Oxyir	5 mg	Beige and Orange	Capsule		Purdue Pharmaceutical Products
OIXCAL	Oxical Antioxidant	2700 IU; 200 mg; 30 IU; 25 mg; 100 mcg; 3.5 mg; 20 mg; 250 mcg; 1 mg; 275 mcg; 50 mg; 5 mg; 20 mg; 20 mg; 225 mg	Blue	Tablet	Capsule-Shape	Delta Pharmaceuticals
OIXCAL CHEWABLE	Oxical Calcium	400 mg; 200 IU	Orange	Tablet, Chewable	Circle	Delta Pharmaceuticals
O-M; 180	Ortho Tri-Cyclen Lo White Tablet	0.18 mg; 0.025 mg	White	28-Day Tablet Pack	Circle	Ortho-Mcneil Pharmaceutical
O-M; 215	Ortho Tri-Cyclen Lo Light Blue Tablet	0.215 mg; 0.025 mg	Light Blue	28-Day Tablet Pack	Circle	Ortho-Mcneil Pharmaceutical
O-M; 250	Ortho Tri-Cyclen Lo Dark Blue Tablet	0.25 mg; 0.025 mg	Dark Blue	28-Day Tablet Pack	Circle	Ortho-Mcneil Pharmaceutical
O-M; 650	Ultracet	325 mg; 37.5 mg	Light Yellow	Coated Tablet	Capsule-Shape	Ortho-Mcneil Pharmaceutical
OME; 10	Omeprazole	10 mg	Light Brown Opaque	Delayed-Release Capsule		Lek Pharmaceuticals
OME; 20	Omeprazole	20 mg	White	Delayed-Release Capsule		Lek Pharmaceuticals
OMNICEF	Omnicef	300 mg	Lavender and Turquoise	Capsule		Abbott Laboratories
ONE A DAY	One-A-Day Plus Extra C Adult Formula	5000 IU; 500 mg; 1.5 mg; 1.7 mg; 20 mg; 400 IU; 15 IU; 2 mg; 0.4 mg; 6 mcg		Tablet		Bayer Consumer Care
ONE-A-DAY	One-A-Day Multivitamin Supplement	5,000 units; 400 units; 1.5 mg; 1.7 mg; 2 mg; 6 mcg; 60 mg; 20 mg; 15 units; 0.4 mg	Red	Coated Tablet	Circle	Bayer Consumer Care
OP; 32	Obetrol	2.5 mg; 2.5 mg; 2.5 mg; 2.5 mg	Blue	Tablet		Rexar Pharmacal
OP; 33	Obetrol	5 mg; 5 mg; 5 mg; 5 mg	Orange	Tablet		Rexar Pharmacal
OP; 701	Vivactil	5 mg	Orange	Coated Tablet	Oval	Odyssey Pharmaceuticals
OP; 702	Vivactil	10 mg	Yellow	Coated Tablet	Oval	Odyssey Pharmaceuticals
OP; 704	Urecholine	25 mg	Yellow	Tablet	Circle, Compressed, Scored	Odyssey Pharmaceuticals
OP; 706	Disulfiram	250 mg	White	Tablet	Circle	Odyssey Pharmaceuticals
OP; 718;	Surmontil	25 mg	Blue and Yellow	Capsule		Odyssey Pharmaceuticals
OP; 719;	Surmontil	50 mg	Blue and Orange	Capsule		Odyssey Pharmaceuticals
OP; 720;	Surmontil	100 mg	Blue and White	Capsule		Odyssey Pharmaceuticals
OR; 606	Ranitidine Hydrochloride	75 mg	Pink	Tablet	Circle	Ranbaxy Pharmaceuticals
ORAP; 1	Orap	1 mg	White	Tablet	Oval, Scored	Teva Pharmaceuticals
ORETIC	Oretic	25 mg	White	Tablet	Circle	Abbott Laboratories
ORETIC	Oretic	50 mg	White	Tablet	Circle, Scored	Abbott Laboratories
ORG; 07	Jenest 28 White Tablet	35 mcg; 0.5 mg	White	28-Day Tablet Pack	Circle	Organon Teknika
ORG; 14	Jenest 28 Peach Tablet	35 mcg; 1 mg	Peach	28-Day Tablet Pack	Circle	Organon Teknika
ORGANON; 388	Cotazyme-S	5,000 USP units; 20,000 USP units; 20,000 USP units		Capsule		Organon
ORGANON; 393	Zymase	12,000 USP units; 24,000 USP units; 24,000 USP units	White and Green	Capsule		Organon
ORGANON; 542	Wigraine	1 mg; 100 mg	White	Tablet	Circle	Organon
ORGANON; 790	Hexadrol	1.5 mg	Peach	Tablet		Organon
ORGANON; 791	Hexadrol	0.75 mg	White	Tablet		Organon
ORGANON; 792	Hexadrol	0.5 mg	Yellow	Tablet		Organon
ORGANON; 798	Hexadrol	4 mg	Green	Tablet		Organon
ORGANON; K2S	Mircette Yellow Tablet	0.01 mg	Yellow	Tablet	Circle	Organon
ORGANON; T4R;	Mircette White Tablet	0.15 mg; 0.02 mg	White	28-Day Tablet Pack	Circle	Organon
ORGANON; TR5	Desogen White Tablet	0.15 mg; 0.03 mg	White	28-Day Tablet Pack	Circle	Organon
ORGANON; TZ3;	Remeron	15 mg	Yellow	Coated Tablet	Oval, Scored	Organon
ORGANON; TZ5;	Remeron	30 mg	Red-Brown	Coated Tablet	Oval, Scored	Organon
ORGANON; TZ7	Remeron	45 mg	White	Coated Tablet	Oval	Organon
ORINASE; 250	Orinase	250 mg	White	Tablet	Circle, Scored	Upjohn
ORINASE; 500	Orinase	500 mg	White	Tablet	Circle, Scored	Pharmacia & Upjohn
ORNEX	Ornex	325 mg; 30 mg	Blue	Tablet		Ascher
ORNEX; MAX	Ornex Maximum Strength	500 mg; 30 mg	White	Tablet		Ascher
ORNEX; SC	Ornex Severe Cold Formula	30 mg; 500 mg; 15 mg	Yellow	Tablet		Menley & James
ORTHO; 0.35	Micronor	0.35 mg	Light Green	28-Day Tablet Pack	Circle	Ortho-Mcneil Pharmaceutical

IMPRINT	BRAND/GENERIC NAME	STRENGTH	COLOR	FORM	SHAPE	MANUFACTURER
ORTHO; 75	Ortho-Novum 7/7/7-21 Light Peach Tablet	35 mcg; 0.75 mg	Light Peach	21-Day Tablet Pack	Circle	Ortho-Mcneil Pharmaceutical
ORTHO; 75	Ortho-Novum 7/7/7-28 Light Peach Tablet	35 mcg; 0.75 mg	Light Peach	28-Day Tablet Pack	Circle	Ortho-Mcneil Pharmaceutical
ORTHO; 135	Ortho-Novum 1/35-21	1 mg; 35 mcg	Peach	21-Day Tablet Pack	Circle	Ortho-Mcneil Pharmaceutical
ORTHO; 135	Ortho-Novum 1/35-28 Peach Tablet	1 mg; 35 mcg	Peach	28-Day Tablet Pack	Circle	Ortho-Mcneil Pharmaceutical
ORTHO; 135	Ortho-Novum 10/11-21 Peach Tablet	1 mg; 35 mcg	Peach	21-Day Tablet Pack	Circle	Ortho-Mcneil Pharmaceutical
ORTHO; 135	Ortho-Novum 10/11-28 Peach Tablet	1 mg; 35 mcg	Peach	28-Day Tablet Pack	Circle	Ortho-Mcneil Pharmaceutical
ORTHO; 135	Ortho-Novum 7/7/7-21 Peach Tablet	1 mg; 35 mcg	Peach	21-Day Tablet Pack	Circle	Ortho-Mcneil Pharmaceutical
ORTHO; 135	Ortho-Novum 7/7/7-28 Peach Tablet	1 mg; 35 mcg	Peach	28-Day Tablet Pack	Circle	Ortho-Mcneil Pharmaceutical
ORTHO; 150	Ortho-Novum 1/50-21	1 mg; 50 mcg	Yellow	21-Day Tablet Pack	Circle	Ortho-Mcneil Pharmaceutical
ORTHO; 150	Ortho-Novum 1/50-28 Yellow Tablet	1 mg; 50 mcg	Yellow	28-Day Tablet Pack	Circle	Ortho-Mcneil Pharmaceutical
ORTHO; 180	Ortho Tri-Cyclen 21 White Tablet	0.18 mg; 0.035 mg	White	21-Day Tablet Pack	Circle	Ortho-Mcneil Pharmaceutical
ORTHO; 180	Ortho Tri-Cyclen 28 White Tablet	0.18 mg; 0.035 mg	White	28-Day Tablet Pack	Circle	Ortho-Mcneil Pharmaceutical
ORTHO; 211	Grifulvin V	250 mg	White	Tablet		Ortho-Mcneil Pharmaceutical
ORTHO; 0214	Grifulvin V	500 mg	White	Tablet		Ortho-Mcneil Pharmaceutical
ORTHO; 215	Ortho Tri-Cyclen 21 Light Blue Tablet	0.215 mg; 0.035 mg	Light Blue	21-Day Tablet Pack	Circle	Ortho-Mcneil Pharmaceutical
ORTHO; 215	Ortho Tri-Cyclen 28 Light Blue Tablet	0.215 mg; 0.035 mg	Light Blue	28-Day Tablet Pack	Circle	Ortho-Mcneil Pharmaceutical
ORTHO; 250	Ortho Tri-Cyclen 21 Blue Tablet	0.25 mg; 0.035 mg	Blue	21-Day Tablet Pack	Circle	Ortho-Mcneil Pharmaceutical
ORTHO; 250	Ortho Tri-Cyclen 28 Blue Tablet	0.25 mg; 0.035 mg	Blue	28-Day Tablet Pack	Circle	Ortho-Mcneil Pharmaceutical
ORTHO; 250	Ortho-Cyclen 21	0.25 mg; 0.035 mg	Blue	21-Day Tablet Pack	Circle	Ortho-Mcneil Pharmaceutical
ORTHO; 250	Ortho-Cyclen 28 Blue Tablet	0.25 mg; 0.035 mg	Blue	28-Day Tablet Pack	Circle	Ortho-Mcneil Pharmaceutical
ORTHO; 535	Modicon 21	0.5 mg; 35 mcg	White	21-Day Tablet Pack	Circle	Ortho-Mcneil Pharmaceutical
ORTHO; 535	Modicon 28 White Tablet	0.5 mg; 35 mcg	White	28-Day Tablet Pack	Circle	Ortho-Mcneil Pharmaceutical
ORTHO; 535	Ortho-Novum 10/11-21 White Tablet	0.5 mg; 35 mcg	White	21-Day Tablet Pack	Circle	Ortho-Mcneil Pharmaceutical
ORTHO; 535	Ortho-Novum 10/11-28 White Tablet	0.5 mg; 35 mcg	White	28-Day Tablet Pack	Circle	Ortho-Mcneil Pharmaceutical
ORTHO; 535	Ortho-Novum 7/7/7-21 White Tablet	0.5 mg; 35 mcg	White	21-Day Tablet Pack	Circle	Ortho-Mcneil Pharmaceutical
ORTHO; 535	Ortho-Novum 7/7/7-28 White Tablet	0.5 mg; 35 mcg	White	28-Day Tablet Pack	Circle	Ortho-Mcneil Pharmaceutical
ORTHO; 1570	Protostat	250 mg	White	Tablet	Capsule-Shape	Ortho-Mcneil Pharmaceutical
ORTHO; 1571	Protostat	500 mg	White	Tablet	Capsule-Shape	Ortho-Mcneil Pharmaceutical
ORTHO; 1800	Ortho-Est	1.5 mg	Lavender	Tablet	Diamond, Scored	Women First Healthcare
ORTHO; 1801	Ortho-Est	0.75 mg	White	Tablet	Diamond, Scored	Women First Healthcare
ORTHO; D; 150	Ortho-Cept 21	0.15 mg; 0.03 mg	Orange	21-Day Tablet Pack	Circle	Ortho-Mcneil Pharmaceutical
ORTHO; D; 150	Ortho-Cept 28 Orange Tablet	0.15 mg; 0.03 mg	Orange	28-Day Tablet Pack	Circle	Ortho-Mcneil Pharmaceutical
ORUDIS; KT	Orudis Kt	12.5 mg	Lime Green	Tablet		Wyeth Consumer Healthcare
ORUVAIL; 100	Oruvail	100 mg	Pink and Dark Green with Two Radial Bands	Capsule		Wyeth Pharmaceuticals
ORUVAIL; 150	Oruvail	150 mg	Pink and Light Green with Two Radial Bands	Capsule		Wyeth Pharmaceuticals
ORUVAIL; 200	Oruvail	200 mg	Pink and White with Two Radial Bands	Capsule		Wyeth Pharmaceuticals
OS CAL	Os-Cal 500	500 mg		Tablet, Chewable		Aventis Pharmaceuticals
OTIS CLAP & SON	Emagrin Forte	260.2 mg; 32.7 mg; 5.36 mg; 0.066 mg	Light Red	Tablet	Circle	Otis Clapp
OTIS CLAPP & SON	Diatrol	300 mg	White	Tablet	Circle	Otis Clapp
OTIS CLAPP & SON	Valorin	325 mg	Light Yellow	Tablet	Circle	Otis Clapp
OV; 12	Desoxyn	5 mg	White	Tablet		Ovation Pharmaceuticals
OV; 31; T	Tranxene T-Tab	3.75 mg	Blue	Tablet	T-Shaped, Scored	Ovation Pharmaceuticals
OV; 32; T	Tranxene T-Tab	7.5 mg	Peach	Tablet	T-Shaped, Scored	Ovation Pharmaceuticals
OV; 33; T	Tranxene T-Tab	15 mg	Lavender	Tablet	T-Shaped, Scored	Ovation Pharmaceuticals
OV; 44	Tranxene-SD Half Strength	11.25 mg	Blue	Tablet		Ovation Pharmaceuticals
OV; 45	Tranxene-SD	22.5 mg	Tan	Extended-Release Tablet		Ovation Pharmaceuticals
OXYROL; 3.9 MG/ DAY	Oxytrol	3.9 mg/24 Hours		Patch	Rectangle	Watson Laboratories
P	Panadol Junior	160 mg	White	Tablet	Oval	Bayer Consumer Care
P	Panadol, Children's Aspirin Free	80 mg	Pink	Tablet, Chewable		Bayer Consumer Care
P	Phillips Liqu-Gels	100 mg	Clear Blue	Capsule, Liquid Filled	Oval	Bayer Consumer Care
P	Primatene P	130 mg; 24 mg; 8 mg	Yellow	Tablet		Whitehall
P	Senokot-S	8.6 mg; 50 mg	Yellow-Orange	Coated Tablet	Circle	Purdue Pharmaceutical Products
P; 0031	Nystatin	10000 U		Tablet		Pharmaderm
P; 02	Mercaptopurine	50 mg	Light Yellow	Tablet	Diamond	Par Pharmaceutical
P; 054	Peri-Colace Stool Softener/ stimulant Laxative	50 mg; 8.6 mg	Dark Red	Tablet	Circle	Purdue
P; 087;	Diphenhydramine Hydrochloride	25 mg		Capsule		Leiner Health Products
P; 087;	Diphenhydramine Hydrochloride	25 mg		Capsule		Pharmaceutical Formulations
P; 1	Ibuprofen	200 mg	Reddish Brown	Coated Tablet	Circle, Convex	Leiner Health Products

IMPRINT	BRAND/GENERIC NAME	STRENGTH	COLOR	FORM	SHAPE	MANUFACTURER
P; 1	Ibuprofen	200 mg	Reddish Brown	Coated Tablet	Circle, Convex	Pharmaceutical Formulations
P; 1	Q-Profen	200 mg	Brown	Tablet	Circle	Qualitest Products
P1; G	Paroxetine Hydrochloride	10 mg	White	Tablet	Circle	Andrx Pharmaceuticals
P2	Ibuprofen White	200 mg	White	Coated Tablet	Circle	Pharmaceutical Formulations
P; 2	Ibuprofen	200 mg	White	Coated Tablet	Circle, Convex	Leiner Health Products
P2; G	Paroxetine Hydrochloride	20 mg	White	Tablet	Circle	Andrx Pharmaceuticals
P; 3	Revinol Junior	160 mg	White	Tablet	Capsule-Shaped, Bisected Scored	Pharmaceutical Formulations
P3; G	Paroxetine Hydrochloride	30 mg	White	Tablet	Circle	Andrx Pharmaceuticals
P; 4	Pseudoephedrine Plus	60 mg; 4 mg	White	Tablet	Round, Bisected Scored	Pharmaceutical Formulations
P4; G	Paroxetine Hydrochloride	40 mg	White	Tablet	Circle	Andrx Pharmaceuticals
P4; LL	Pathilon	25 mg	Pink	Coated Tablet	Circle, Convex	Lederle Laboratories
P5; G	Pindolol	5 mg	White	Tablet	Circle	Par Pharmaceutical
P; 7	Antihistamine	4 mg	Yellow	Tablet	Circle, Scored	Pharmaceutical Formulations
P; 8	Decongestant	60 mg; 2.5 mg	White	Tablet	Round, Bisected Scored	Pharmaceutical Formulations
P; 10	Travel Sickness II	25 mg	Yellow	Tablet	Circle	Pharmaceutical Formulations
P10; G	Pindolol	10 mg	White	Tablet	Circle	Par Pharmaceutical
P; 11	Pseudoephedrine	60 mg	White	Tablet	Circle	Pharmaceutical Formulations
P11; P11	Fluoride	1.1 mg	Purple	Tablet, Chewable		Qualitest Products
P; 12	Allergy	30 mg; 2 mg	Blue	Tablet	Circle	Pharmaceutical Formulations
P; 13	Enteric Coated Aspirin	500 mg	Orange	Enteric-Coated Tablet	Circle	Pharmaceutical Formulations
P; 19	Enteric Coated Aspirin	325 mg	Orange	Enteric-Coated Tablet	Circle	Pharmaceutical Formulations
P20	Protonix	20 mg	Yellow with Brown Ink	Delayed-Release Tablet	Oval, Biconvex	Wyeth Pharmaceuticals
P; 20	Genericare Nasal Decongestant	60 mg	White	Tablet	Circle	Circa Pharmaceuticals
P; 20	Pseudoephedrine Hydrochloride	60 mg	White	Coated Tablet	Circle, Scored	Circa Pharmaceuticals
P; 21	Aid to Sleep II	25 mg	Blue	Tablet	Circle	Pharmaceutical Formulations
P; 22	Revinol	325 mg	White	Tablet		Pharmaceutical Formulations
P22; P22	Fluoride	2.2 mg	Orange	Tablet, Chewable		Qualitest Products
P; 23	Adult Strength Pain Relief	400 mg; 32 mg	White	Tablet	Circle	Pharmaceutical Formulations
P; 25	Motion Sickness	50 mg	White	Tablet	Round, Bisected Scored	Pharmaceutical Formulations
P; 32	Chewable Aspirin	81 mg	Orange	Tablet, Chewable	Circle	Pharmaceutical Formulations
P; 32	Reserpine	0.1 mg	White	Tablet	Circle	H.L. Moore
P; 33	Sleep Aid	25 mg	White	Tablet	Circle	Pharmaceutical Formulations
P; 35	Children's Acetaminophen Fruit Burst Flavor	80 mg	Pink	Tablet, Chewable	Circle, Scored	Pharmaceutical Formulations
P; 35	Genericare Nasal Decongestant	30 mg	Red	Coated Tablet	Circle	Circa Pharmaceuticals
P; 35	Pseudoephedrine Hydrochloride	30 mg	Red	Coated Tablet	Circle	Circa Pharmaceuticals
P; 36	Pyrazinamide	500 mg	White	Tablet	Circle	Stada
P; 41	Pain Reliever	325 mg	White	Tablet	Round; Bisected Scored	Pharmaceutical Formulations
P; 42	Ibuprofen	200 mg	White	Tablet		Leiner Health Products
P; 42	Ibuprofen	200 mg	White	Tablet		Pharmaceutical Formulations
P; 42	Q-Profen	200 mg	White	Tablet	Oblong	Qualitest Products
P; 43	Ibuprofen	200 mg	Brown	Tablet		Pharmaceutical Formulations
P; 44	Aid to Sleep	50 mg	Blue	Tablet	Round, Bisected Scored	Pharmaceutical Formulations
P46;	Amytal Sodium	250 mg/ampule		Solution for Injection		Eli Lilly
P47	Acetaminophen, Children's	80 mg	Purple	Tablet, Chewable		Pharmaceutical Formulations
P; 53; LEDERLE	Ext Phenytoin Sodium	100 mg	Clear	Capsule		Lederle Laboratories
P; 60; GF	Decongest II	600 mg; 60 mg	Blue	Tablet		Qualitest Products
P; 67	Cimetidine	200 mg		Tablet		Pharmaceutical Formulations
P; 71	Tussin Severe Congestion	200 mg; 30 mg	Green	Gel/jelly		Leiner Health Products
P; 72	Tussin Cold & Cough	10 mg; 200 mg; 30 mg	Red Clear	Gel/jelly		Leiner Health Products
P; 73	Enteric Coated Aspirin	81 mg	Yellow	Tablet	Circle	Pharmaceutical Formulations
P; 74; TRIANGLE;	Liquid Capsules Adult Nighttime Multi-Symptom Cold/flu Medicine	6.25 mg; 10 mg; 250 mg; 30 mg	Green	Capsule, Liquid Filled		Perfect Choice
P; 75	Magnesium Salicylate	325 mg	White	Tablet		Pharmaceutical Formulations
P; 77	Buffered Aspirin	325 mg;	White	Coated Tablet	Circle, Double-Layer, Convex	Leiner Health Products
P; 77	Buffered Aspirin	325 mg;	White	Coated Tablet	Circle, Double-Layer, Convex	Pharmaceutical Formulations
P; 77	Tri-Buffered Aspirin	325 mg	White	Tablet	Circle	Pharmaceutical Formulations
P77; P77	Fluoride	0.25 mg	White	Tablet, Chewable		Qualitest Products
P; 111	X-Str Pain Relief	500 mg	White	Tablet	Capsule-Shape	Pharmaceutical Formulations
P; 114	Alertness Aid	200 mg	Yellow	Tablet	Circle	Pharmaceutical Formulations
P; 115	Multiple Symptom Cold Relief	325 mg; 2 mg; 15 mg; 30 mg	Yellow	Tablet	Circle	Pharmaceutical Formulations
P; 121	X-Strength Pain Reliever	500 mg	White	Tablet	Circle	Pharmaceutical Formulations
P; 122	Anti-Diarrheal	2 mg	Green	Tablet	Capsule-Shape	Pharmaceutical Formulations
P; 122	Non-Drowsy Multi-Symptom Cold	325 mg; 15 mg; 30 mg	White	Tablet		Pharmaceutical Formulations
P; 125	Allergy Sinus Headache Relief	500 mg; 30 mg; 12.5 mg	Green	Tablet		Pharmaceutical Formulations
P; 141	Multi-Symptom Allergy Sinus	500 mg; 30 mg; 2 mg	Yellow	Tablet		Pharmaceutical Formulations
P; 142	Sinus Tablet II	500 mg; 30 mg	Orange	Tablet	Circle	Pharmaceutical Formulations
P; 144	Chewable Junior Apap	160 mg	Purple	Tablet, Chewable	Round, Bisected Scored	Pharmaceutical Formulations
P; 147	Maximum Strength Sinus Relief	500 mg; 30 mg	Orange	Tablet		Pharmaceutical Formulations
P; 152	Non-Aspirin Extra Strength Pain Relief Plus Antacid	500 mg; 250 mg	White	Tablet	Capsule-Shape	Pharmaceutical Formulations
P; 171	Day Time Cold Relief	650 mg; 30 mg; 60 mg	Yellow	Tablet	Capsule-Shape	Pharmaceutical Formulations
P; 172	Night Time Cold Relief	650 mg; 60 mg; 50 mg	Blue	Tablet	Capsule-Shape	Pharmaceutical Formulations
P; 174	Multi-Symptom Cold	325 mg; 2 mg; 15 mg; 30 mg	Yellow	Tablet		Pharmaceutical Formulations
P; 177	Decongestant Allergy Medicine	25 mg; 60 mg	White	Tablet	Oval	Pharmaceutical Formulations
P; 207	Sucralfate	1000 mg	White	Tablet	Capsule-Shape	Pharmaceutical Formulations
P; 214	NO Drowsy Complete Cold Symptom Relief	325 mg; 10 mg; 30 mg	Orange	Tablet	Capsule-Shape	Pharmaceutical Formulations
P; 219	Allergy/decongestant	60 mg; 25 mg	Blue	Tablet	Capsule-Shape	Pharmaceutical Formulations
P; 221	Maximum Strength Sinus Relief	500 mg; 30 mg	Orange	Tablet	Circle	Pharmaceutical Formulations

IMPRINT	BRAND/GENERIC NAME	STRENGTH	COLOR	FORM	SHAPE	MANUFACTURER
P; 225	Back Ache Relief	580 mg	White	Tablet	Capsule-Shape	Pharmaceutical Formulations
P; 225	Magnesium Salicylate, Extra Strength	500 mg	White	Tablet		Pharmaceutical Formulations
P; 241	Maximum Strength Decongestant	500 mg; 30 mg	Yellow	Tablet	Capsule-Shape	Pharmaceutical Formulations
P; 252	Complete Symptom Cold Relief	325 mg; 2 mg; 10 mg; 30 mg	Yellow	Tablet	Circle	Pharmaceutical Formulations
P; 253	Complete Symptom Cold Relief	325 mg; 2 mg; 10 mg; 30 mg	Yellow	Tablet		Pharmaceutical Formulations
P; 254	Ibuprofen	200 mg	Brown and Tan	Capsule		Pharmaceutical Formulations
P; 255	Diphenhydramine Plus	500 mg; 30 mg; 12.5 mg	White	Tablet	Circle	Pharmaceutical Formulations
P; 300	Allergy Sinus Relief	500 mg; 30 mg; 2 mg	Green and Ivory	Capsule		Pharmaceutical Formulations
P; 301	NO Drowsy Allergy/sinus	500 mg; 30 mg	Green and White	Capsule		Pharmaceutical Formulations
P; 316	Extra Strength Pain Relief without Aspirin	500 mg	Red and White	Capsule		Pharmaceutical Formulations
P; 316	Extra Strength Pain Relief without Aspirin	500 mg	Red and White	Capsule		Revco
P; 325	Acetaminophen Pm	500 mg; 25 mg	Blue	Tablet		Pharmaceutical Formulations
P; 334	Night Time Pain Relief	500 mg; 25 mg	Blue	Tablet	Circle	Pharmaceutical Formulations
P; 337	Maximum Strength Severe Cold	500 mg; 15 mg; 30 mg	White	Tablet	Capsule-Shape	Pharmaceutical Formulations
P; 337	Severe Cold Suphedrine	500 mg; 15 mg; 30 mg	White	Tablet		Pharmaceutical Formulations
P; 345	Antacid	311 mg; 232 mg	Aqua and Ivory	Tablet	Capsule-Shape	Pharmaceutical Formulations
P; 346	NO Drowsy Cold	325 mg; 15 mg; 30 mg	Red and Orange	Tablet	Capsule-Shape	Pharmaceutical Formulations
P; 349	Extra Strength Non-Aspirin Pm	500 mg; 25 mg	Dark Blue Opaque, Light Blue Opaque and Clear	Capsule, Liquid Filled		Leiner Health Products
P; 349	Night Time Pain Reliever	500 mg; 25 mg	Light Blue	Tablet	Capsule-Shape	Pharmaceutical Formulations
P; 384	Children's Non-Aspirin Cold	80 mg; 7.5 mg; 0.5 mg	Purple	Tablet, Chewable	Round, Bisected Scored	Pharmaceutical Formulations
P; 411	Diphenhydramine Hydrochloride	25 mg		Coated Tablet		Pharmaceutical Formulations
P; 412	Pain Relief	250 mg; 250 mg; 65 mg	White	Tablet	Circle	Pharmaceutical Formulations
P; 416	Maximum Relief Laxative	135 mg	Blue	Tablet	Circle	Pharmaceutical Formulations
P; 419	Maximum Strength Non-Aspirin Flu	500 mg; 15 mg; 30 mg	Red and Clear	Capsule, Liquid Filled		Pharmaceutical Formulations
P; 420	Maximum Strength Non-Aspirin Nighttime Flu	500 mg; 30 mg; 25 mg	Blue and Beige	Capsule		Pharmaceutical Formulations
P; 422	Multi-Symptom Suphedrine Severe Cold	500 mg; 15 mg; 30 mg	White	Coated Tablet	Circle	Pharmaceutical Formulations
P; 431	Night Time Allergy Sinus	500 mg; 30 mg; 25 mg	Blue	Tablet	Capsule-Shape	Pharmaceutical Formulations
P; 440	Maximum Strength Pms Relief	500 mg; 25 mg; 15 mg	White	Tablet	Capsule-Shape	Pharmaceutical Formulations
P; 441	Maximum Strength Sinus II	500 mg; 30 mg	Orange	Tablet	Capsule-Shape	Pharmaceutical Formulations
P; 445	Naproxen Sodium	200 mg	Light Blue	Tablet	Oval	Pharmaceutical Formulations
P; 452	Non-Aspirin Cold and Cough	0.5 mg; 2.5 mg; 7.5 mg	Red	Tablet	Circle	Pharmaceutical Formulations
P; 458	Acetaminophen and Diphenhydramine	500 mg; 38 mg	Blue	Tablet	Circle	Pharmaceutical Formulations
P; 459	Complete Allergy Children's	12.5 mg	Lavender	Tablet, Chewable	Circle, Scored	Pharmaceutical Formulations
P; 484	Acetaminophen, Aspirin, and Caffeine	250 mg; 250 mg; 65 mg	White	Tablet	Circle	Pharmaceutical Formulations
P; 499	Bisacodyl	5 mg	Pink	Tablet	Circle	Pharmaceutical Formulations
P; 500	Panadol Maximum Strength	500 mg	White	Tablet		Bayer Consumer Care
P; 511	Advanced Formula Decongestant	325 mg; 2 mg; 5 mg	White and Yellow	Tablet	Circle	Pharmaceutical Formulations
P; 537	Acetaminophen, Extra Strength	500 mg	Red and Yellow with Blue-Green Band	Capsule		Pharmaceutical Formulations
P; 542	Naproxen Sodium	220 mg	Light Blue	Tablet	Circle	Par Pharmaceutical
P; 543	Naproxen Sodium	220 mg	Blue	Tablet	Oblong	Par Pharmaceutical
P; 771	Atropine and Diphenoxylate Hydrochloride	0.025 mg; 2.5 mg	White	Tablet	Circle	Par Pharmaceutical
P; 771	Diphenoxylate Hydrochloride and Atropine Sulfate	2.5 mg; 0.025 mg	White	Tablet	Circle, Convex	Purepac Pharmaceutical
P; 912	Correct Laxative	100 mg; 90 mg	Pink	Tablet	Circle	Pharmaceutical Formulations
P; 2120	Valproic Acid	250 mg	White	Capsule, Liquid Filled	Oblong	Aligen Independent Laboratories
P; 2120	Valproic Acid	250 mg	White	Capsule, Liquid Filled	Oblong	H.L. Moore
P; 2120	Valproic Acid	250 mg	White	Gel/jelly		Pharmacaps
P; 2120	Valproic Acid	250 mg	White	Capsule, Liquid Filled	Oblong	Qualitest Products
P; 3900	Glyceryl-T	150 mg; 90 mg	Yellow	Capsule		Pharmacaps
P; 4600	Benzonatate	100 mg	Yellow	Capsule, Liquid Filled	Oval	Warner Chilcott
P; 5124	Fluoxetine	10 mg	White and Blue	Capsule		Purepac Pharmaceutical
P; 5124	Fluoxetine	10 mg	White and Blue	Capsule		Siegfried
P; 5125	Fluoxetine	20 mg	White and Violet	Capsule		Purepac Pharmaceutical
P; 5125	Fluoxetine	20 mg	White and Violet	Capsule		Siegfried
P; 9523	Solfoton	16 mg		Coated Tablet		Poythress Laboratories
P; PRAVACOL 20;;	Pravigard Pac	81 mg; 20 mg	Yellow Tablet and White Tablet	Tablet		Bristol-Myers Squibb
P; PRAVACOL 20;;	Pravigard Pac	325 mg; 20 mg	Yellow Tablet and White Tablet	Tablet		Bristol-Myers Squibb
P; PRAVACOL 40;;	Pravigard Pac	81 mg; 40 mg	Green Tablet and White Tablet	Tablet		Bristol-Myers Squibb
P; PRAVACOL 40;;	Pravigard Pac	325 mg; 40 mg	Green Tablet and White Tablet	Tablet		Bristol-Myers Squibb

IMPRINT	BRAND/GENERIC NAME	STRENGTH	COLOR	FORM	SHAPE	MANUFACTURER
P; T222	Acetaminophen	500 mg	Opaque Red, Opaque Yellow and Blue	Capsule, Liquid Filled		Leiner Health Products
P; UNDERSCORED	Prilosec Otc	20 mg	Salmon/pink	Delayed-Release Tablet	Oval	Procter & Gamble
P; US; 144	Amiodarone Hydrochloride	100 mg	White	Tablet	Circle	Upsher-Smith Laboratories
P&G; 402	Didronel	200 mg	White	Tablet	Rectangle	Procter & Gamble Pharmaceuticals
PA; 07;	Hydroxyzine	10 mg	White	Tablet	Circle, Scored	Pliva
PA; 08;	Hydroxyzine	25 mg	White	Tablet	Circle	Pliva
PA; 09;	Cyclosporine	25 mg	Off-White	Capsule, Liquid Filled	Capsule-Shape	Pliva
PA; 20;	Cyclosporine	100 mg	White	Capsule		Pliva
PA; 46;	Benzonatate	100 mg	Yellow	Capsule	Oval	Pliva
PA; 140;	Vitamin D	1.25 mg	Green	Capsule, Liquid Filled	Oval	Pliva
PA; 307;	Hydroxyzine Hydrochloride	10 mg	Lavender	Coated Tablet	Circle	Pliva
PA; 308;	Hydroxyzine Hydrochloride	25 mg	White	Coated Tablet	Circle	Pliva
PA; 309;	Hydroxyzine	50 mg	White	Tablet	Circle	Pliva
PA; 309;	Hydroxyzine Hydrochloride	50 mg	White	Coated Tablet	Circle	Pliva
PA; 550;	Cimetidine	300 mg	White	Tablet	Circle	Pliva
PA; 551;	Cimetidine	400 mg	White	Coated Tablet	Capsule-Shape, Scored	Pliva
PA; 552;	Cimetidine	800 mg	White	Tablet	Capsule-Shape, Scored	Pliva
PA; 608;	Ketorolac Tromethamine	10 mg	White	Tablet	Circle	Pliva
PA; 1000;	Ethosuximide	250 mg	Orange	Capsule, Liquid Filled	Oval	Pliva
PA; 2120;	Valproic Acid	250 mg	White	Capsule		Pliva
PAL	Panritis Forte C.T.	600 mg; 250 mg	Yellow	Coated Tablet	Capsule-Shape, Scored	Pamlab
PAL; 0016	Panlor Dc	356.4 mg; 30 mg; 16 mg	Red with White Ink	Capsule		Pamlab
PAL; 07; 54	Panmist DM	30 mg; 600 mg; 45 mg	Green	Extended-Release Tablet	Capsule-Shape	Pamlab
PAL; 07; 75	Panmist LA	90 mg; 600 mg	White with Red Specks	Extended-Release Tablet	Capsule-Shape, Scored	Pamlab
PAL; 032	Panlor Ss	712.8 mg; 60 mg; 32 mg	Lavender	Tablet	Oval, Scored	Pamlab
PAL; 0305	Panfil-G	200 mg; 100 mg	Orange and Green	Capsule		Pamlab
PAL; 0762	Panmist JR	45 mg; 600 mg	White	Tablet	Capsule-Shape	Pamlab
PAL; 2	Foltx	2.5 mg; 1 mg; 25 mg	Peach	Tablet	Circle	Pamlab
PAL; 4	Palgic	4 mg	White	Tablet	Circle, Scored	Pamlab
PAL; 5	Diatx	5 mg; 20 mg; 1 mg; 10 mg; 50 mg; 300 mcg; 1.5 mg; 60 mg; 1.5 mg	Yellow	Tablet	Circle	Pamlab
PAL; 5FE	Diatx Fe	5 mg; 20 mg; 1 mg; 10 mg; 50 mg; 300 mcg; 1.5 mg; 60 mg; 1.5 mg; 217 mg	Brown	Tablet	Circle	Pamlab
PAL; 8; 8	Pannaz	8 mg; 2.5 mg; 90 mg	Light Green	Extended-Release Tablet	Oblong, Scored	Pamlab
PAL; 61/31	Palgic-D	8 mg; 80 mg	White	Tablet	Capsule-Shape	Pamlab
PAMPRIN	Pamprin Maximum Cramp Relief Formula	500 mg; 25 mg; 15 mg	White	Tablet	Circle	Chattem Consumer Products
PAMPRIN	Pamprin, Maximum Pain Relief	250 mg; 250 mg; 25 mg	White with Blue Ink	Tablet		Chattem
PAMPRIN	Pamprin Multi-Symptom	500 mg; 25 mg; 15 mg	White	Tablet	Circle	Chattem
PAMPRIN	Pamprin, Multi-Symptom Caplet	500 mg; 25 mg; 15 mg	White	Tablet	Capsule-Shape	Chattem Consumer Products
PAMPRIN	Pamprin, Multi-Symptom Gelcap	500 mg; 25 mg; 15 mg	Sky Blue and Aqua Blue	Capsule, Liquid Filled	Capsule-Shape	Chattem Consumer Products
PAMPRIN	Pamprin, Multi-Symptom Tablet	500 mg; 25 mg; 15 mg	White	Tablet	Circle	Chattem Consumer Products
PANADOL; 500;	Panadol Maximum Strength	500 mg	White	Coated Tablet	Circle	Bayer Consumer Care
PANADOL PLUS	Panadol Plus	500 mg; 65 mg	White	Tablet		Bayer Consumer Care
PANADOL-3; CODEINE; W	Panadol with Codeine No. 3	300 mg; 30 mg	White	Tablet	Circle	Winthrop Pharmaceuticals
PANMYCIN; 250 MG	Panmycin	250 mg	Yellow and Gray	Capsule		Upjohn
PAR	Berovite	500 mg; 15 mg; 15 mg; 100 mg; 4 mg; 18 mg; 0.5 mg; 5 mcg	Red	Tablet		Everett Laboratories
PAR; 009	Isosorbide Dinitrate	30 mg	Blue	Tablet	Circle, Scored	H.L. Moore
PAR; 009	Isosorbide Dinitrate	30 mg	Blue	Tablet	Circle	Par Pharmaceutical
PAR; 015	Meclizine Hydrochloride	50 mg	Yellow and Blue	Tablet	Oval, Scored; Multiple Layered	Par Pharmaceutical
PAR; 016	Chlorzoxazone	250 mg	Orange	Tablet	Circle, Scored	Par Pharmaceutical
PAR; 020	Isosorbide Dinitrate	5 mg	White	Tablet	Circle, Scored	Par Pharmaceutical
PAR; 021	Isosorbide Dinitrate	10 mg	White	Tablet	Circle, Scored	Par Pharmaceutical
PAR; 022	Isosorbide Dinitrate	20 mg	Green	Tablet	Circle, Scored	Par Pharmaceutical
PAR; 027	Hydralazine Hydrochloride	25 mg	Peach	Tablet	Circle, Convex	Par Pharmaceutical
PAR; 028	Hydralazine Hydrochloride	50 mg	Peach or Blue	Tablet	Round or Oval	Par Pharmaceutical
PAR; 029	Hydralazine Hydrochloride	10 mg	Pink	Tablet	Circle	Par Pharmaceutical
PAR; 034	Meclizine Hydrochloride	12.5 mg	Blue and White	Tablet	Oval	Par Pharmaceutical
PAR; 034	Meclizine Hydrochloride	12.5 mg	Blue and White	Tablet	Oval	Udl Laboratories
PAR; 035	Meclizine Hydrochloride	25 mg	Yellow and White	Tablet	Teardrop-Shape	Par Pharmaceutical
PAR; 035	Meclizine Hydrochloride	25 mg	Yellow and White	Tablet	Teardrop-Shape	Udl Laboratories
PAR; 043	Cyproheptadine Hydrochloride	4 mg	White	Tablet	Circle, Scored; Compressed	Par Pharmaceutical
PAR; 054	Imipramine Hydrochloride	10 mg	Yellow	Tablet	Triangle	Par Pharmaceutical
PAR; 055	Imipramine Hydrochloride	25 mg	Brown	Tablet	Circle	Par Pharmaceutical
PAR; 056	Imipramine Hydrochloride	50 mg	Green	Coated Tablet		Par Pharmaceutical
PAR; 056	Imipramine Hydrochloride	50 mg	Green	Coated Tablet		United Research Laboratories

IMPRINT	BRAND/GENERIC NAME	STRENGTH	COLOR	FORM	SHAPE	MANUFACTURER
PAR; 061	Fluphenazine Hydrochloride	1 mg	White	Coated Tablet	Circle	H.L. Moore
PAR; 061	Fluphenazine Hydrochloride	1 mg	White	Coated Tablet	Circle	Par Pharmaceutical
PAR; 062	Fluphenazine Hydrochloride	2.5 mg	Blue	Coated Tablet	Circle	H.L. Moore
PAR; 062	Fluphenazine Hydrochloride	2.5 mg	Blue	Coated Tablet	Circle	Par Pharmaceutical
PAR; 064	Fluphenazine Hydrochloride	10 mg	Orange	Coated Tablet	Circle	Par Pharmaceutical
PAR; 067	Indomethacin	25 mg	Light Green or White and Blue	Capsule		Par Pharmaceutical
PAR; 068	Indomethacin	50 mg	Light Green or White and Blue	Capsule		Par Pharmaceutical
PAR; 076	Fluphenazine Hydrochloride	5 mg	Pink	Coated Tablet	Circle	H.L. Moore
PAR; 076	Fluphenazine Hydrochloride	5 mg	Dark Pink	Coated Tablet	Circle	Par Pharmaceutical
PAR; 083	Dexamethasone	0.25 mg	Pale Orange	Tablet	Five-Sided, Scored	Par Pharmaceutical
PAR; 084	Dexamethasone	0.5 mg	Pale Yellow	Tablet	Five-Sided, Scored	Par Pharmaceutical
PAR; 085	Dexamethasone	0.75 mg	Pale Blue	Tablet	Five-Sided, Scored	Par Pharmaceutical
PAR; 085	Dexamethasone Dspk	0.75 mg	Blue	Tablet	Five-Sided	Qualitest Products
PAR; 086	Dexamethasone	1.5 mg	Pale Pink	Tablet	Five-Sided, Scored	Par Pharmaceutical
PAR; 087	Dexamethasone	4 mg	White	Tablet	Five-Sided, Scored	Par Pharmaceutical
PAR; 095	Metronidazole	250 mg	White	Coated Tablet	Circle	Par Pharmaceutical
PAR; 104	Allopurinol	100 mg	White	Tablet	Circle, Flat Bevel	Par Pharmaceutical
PAR; 105	Allopurinol	300 mg	Orange	Tablet	Circle	Par Pharmaceutical
PAR; 110	Clonidine Hydrochloride	0.1 mg	Green	Tablet	Round; Bisected Scored	Major Pharmaceutical
PAR; 110	Clonidine Hydrochloride	0.1 mg	Green	Tablet	Round; Bisected Scored	Par Pharmaceutical
PAR; 111	Clonidine Hydrochloride	0.2 mg	Yellow	Tablet	Round; Bisected Scored	Major Pharmaceutical
PAR; 111	Clonidine Hydrochloride	0.2 mg	Yellow	Tablet	Round; Bisected Scored	Par Pharmaceutical
PAR; 112	Clonidine Hydrochloride	0.3 mg	Blue	Tablet	Round; Bisected Scored	Major Pharmaceutical
PAR; 112	Clonidine Hydrochloride	0.3 mg	Blue	Tablet	Round; Bisected Scored	Par Pharmaceutical
PAR; 113	Clonidine Hydrochloride and Chlorthalidone	15 mg; 0.1 mg	White	Tablet	Round; Flat-Faced; Beveled Edge; Bisected Scored	Par Pharmaceutical
PAR; 114	Metronidazole	500 mg	White	Tablet	Capsule-Shape	Par Pharmaceutical
PAR; 115	Clonidine Hydrochloride and Chlorthalidone	15 mg; 0.2 mg	Blue	Tablet	Circle, Flat-Faced; Beveled Edge	Par Pharmaceutical
PAR; 116	Clonidine Hydrochloride and Chlorthalidone	15 mg; 0.3 mg	White	Tablet	Round; Concave; Bisected Scored	Par Pharmaceutical
PAR; 117	Amiloride Hydrochloride	5 mg	Yellow	Tablet	Circle, Compressed	Par Pharmaceutical
PAR; 118	Propantheline Bromide	15 mg	Light Peach	Tablet	Circle	Par Pharmaceutical
PAR; 119	Nystatin	500,000 units	Brown	Coated Tablet	Circle	Par Pharmaceutical
PAR; 121	Hydralazine Hydrochloride	100 mg	Peach	Tablet	Circle	Par Pharmaceutical
PAR; 129	Dexamethasone	6 mg	Pale Green	Tablet	Five-Sided, Scored	Par Pharmaceutical
PAR; 133	Amitriptyline Hydrochloride	10 mg	Pink	Tablet	Circle	Par Pharmaceutical
PAR; 134	Amitriptyline Hydrochloride	25 mg	Green	Tablet	Circle	Par Pharmaceutical
PAR; 135	Amitriptyline Hydrochloride	50 mg	Brown	Tablet	Circle	Par Pharmaceutical
PAR; 136	Amitriptyline Hydrochloride	75 mg	Purple	Tablet	Circle	Par Pharmaceutical
PAR; 137	Amitriptyline Hydrochloride	100 mg	Orange	Tablet	Circle	Par Pharmaceutical
PAR; 138	Amitriptyline Hydrochloride	150 mg	Peach	Tablet	Circle	Par Pharmaceutical
PAR; 139	Sulfamethoxazole and Trimethoprim	400 mg; 80 mg	White	Tablet		Par Pharmaceutical
PAR; 140	Sulfamethoxazole and Trimethoprim	800 mg; 160 mg	White	Tablet		Par Pharmaceutical
PAR; 143	Hydralazine Hydrochloride and Hydrochlorothiazide	25 mg; 25 mg	White	Capsule		Par Pharmaceutical
PAR; 143	Hydralazine with HCTz	25 mg; 25 mg	White	Capsule		H.L. Moore
PAR; 144	Hydralazine Hydrocloride and Hydrochlorothiazide	50 mg; 50 mg	White and Black	Capsule		Par Pharmaceutical
PAR; 144	Hydralazine with HCTz	50 mg; 50 mg	White and Black	Capsule		H.L. Moore
PAR; 145	Hydralazine Hydrochloride and Hydrochlorothiazide	100 mg; 50 mg	Powder Blue and Light Blue	Capsule		Par Pharmaceutical
PAR; 148	Hydroflumethiazide with Reserpine	50 mg; 0.125 mg	Green	Tablet	Circle, Scored	H.L. Moore
PAR; 162; 400	Ibuprofen	400 mg	White	Coated Tablet	Circle	Par Pharmaceutical
PAR; 162; 400	Ibuprofen	400 mg	White	Coated Tablet	Circle	Udl Laboratories
PAR; 163; 600	Ibuprofen	600 mg	White	Coated Tablet	Oval	Par Pharmaceutical
PAR; 163; 600	Ibuprofen	600 mg	White	Coated Tablet	Oval	Udl Laboratories
PAR; 164	Benztropine Mesylate	0.5 mg	White	Tablet	Circle, Scored	Par Pharmaceutical
PAR; 165	Benztropine Mesylate	1 mg	White	Tablet	Oval, Scored	Par Pharmaceutical
PAR; 166	Benztropine Mesylate	2 mg	White	Tablet	Circle, Scored	Par Pharmaceutical
PAR; 181	Perphenazine and Amitriptyline Hydrochloride	2 mg; 10 mg	Blue	Coated Tablet	Circle	Par Pharmaceutical
PAR; 182	Perphenazine and Amitriptyline Hydrochloride	2 mg; 25 mg	Orange	Coated Tablet	Circle	Par Pharmaceutical
PAR; 183	Perphenazine and Amitriptyline Hydrochloride	4 mg; 10 mg	Salmon	Coated Tablet	Circle	Par Pharmaceutical
PAR; 184	Perphenazine and Amitriptyline Hydrochloride	4 mg; 25 mg	Yellow	Coated Tablet	Circle	Par Pharmaceutical
PAR; 185	Perphenazine and Amitriptyline Hydrochloride	4 mg; 50 mg	Orange	Coated Tablet	Circle	Par Pharmaceutical
PAR; 186	Methyldopa and Hydrochlorothiazide	250 mg; 15 mg	Green	Coated Tablet	Circle	Par Pharmaceutical
PAR; 187	Methyldopa and Hydrochlorothiazide	250 mg; 25 mg	White	Coated Tablet	Capsule-Shape	Par Pharmaceutical
PAR; 188	Methyldopa and Hydrochlorothiazide	30 mg; 500 mg	Yellow	Coated Tablet	Oval	Par Pharmaceutical
PAR; 189	Methyldopa and Hydrochlorothiazide	50 mg; 500 mg	Pink	Coated Tablet	Oval	Par Pharmaceutical
PAR; 193	Flurazepam Hydrochloride	15 mg	White and Powder Blue	Capsule		Par Pharmaceutical
PAR; 194	Flurazepam Hydrochloride	30 mg	Powder Blue	Capsule		Par Pharmaceutical
PAR; 200; 682	Ofloxacin	200 mg	White	Tablet	Capsule-Shape	Par Pharmaceutical
PAR; 202	Methyldopa and Chlorothiazide	250 mg; 150 mg	Beige	Coated Tablet	Circle	Major Pharmaceutical
PAR; 202	Methyldopa and Chlorothiazide	250 mg; 150 mg	Beige	Coated Tablet	Circle	Par Pharmaceutical

IMPRINT	BRAND/GENERIC NAME	STRENGTH	COLOR	FORM	SHAPE	MANUFACTURER
PAR; 203	Methyldopa and Chlorothiazide	250 mg; 250 mg	Green	Coated Tablet	Circle	Major Pharmaceutical
PAR; 203	Methyldopa and Chlorothiazide	250 mg; 250 mg	Green	Coated Tablet	Circle	Par Pharmaceutical
PAR; 213	Orphengesic	25 mg; 30 mg; 385 mg	White and Green	Tablet	Circle, Flat; Double Layered	Par Pharmaceutical
PAR; 214	Orphengesic Forte	50 mg; 60 mg; 770 mg	White and Green	Tablet	Capsule-Shaped; Bisected; Double Layered Scored	Par Pharmaceutical
PAR; 216; 800	Ibuprofen	800 mg	White	Coated Tablet	Capsule-Shape	Par Pharmaceutical
PAR; 216; 800	Ibuprofen	800 mg	White	Coated Tablet	Capsule-Shape	Udl Laboratories
PAR; 217	Doxepin Hydrochloride	10 mg	Opaque Buff	Capsule		Par Pharmaceutical
PAR; 218	Doxepin Hydrochloride	25 mg	Opaque Ivory and White	Capsule		Par Pharmaceutical
PAR; 219	Doxepin Hydrochloride	50 mg	Opaque Ivory	Capsule		Par Pharmaceutical
PAR; 220	Doxepin Hydrochloride	75 mg	Bright Light Green	Capsule		Par Pharmaceutical
PAR; 221	Doxepin Hydrochloride	100 mg	White and Bright Light Green	Capsule		Par Pharmaceutical
PAR; 222	Doxepin Hydrochloride	150 mg	Opaque White and Blue	Capsule		Par Pharmaceutical
PAR; 223	Haloperidol	0.5 mg	White	Tablet		H.L. Moore
PAR; 223	Haloperidol	0.5 mg	White	Tablet	Circle, Scored; Flat; Compressed	Par Pharmaceutical
PAR; 224	Haloperidol	1 mg	Yellow	Tablet	Circle, Scored	H.L. Moore
PAR; 224	Haloperidol	1 mg	Yellow	Tablet	Circle, Scored; Flat; Compressed	Par Pharmaceutical
PAR; 225	Haloperidol	2 mg	Pink	Tablet	Circle, Scored	H.L. Moore
PAR; 225	Haloperidol	2 mg	Pink	Tablet	Circle, Scored; Flat; Compressed	Par Pharmaceutical
PAR; 226	Haloperidol	5 mg	Green	Tablet	Circle, Scored	H.L. Moore
PAR; 226	Haloperidol	5 mg	Green	Tablet	Circle, Scored; Flat; Compressed	Par Pharmaceutical
PAR; 227	Haloperidol	10 mg	Aqua	Tablet	Circle, Scored	H.L. Moore
PAR; 227	Haloperidol	10 mg	Aqua	Tablet	Circle, Scored; Flat; Compressed	Par Pharmaceutical
PAR; 240	Temazepam	15 mg	Opaque White and Dark Green	Capsule		Par Pharmaceutical
PAR; 241	Temazepam	30 mg	Opaque White	Capsule		Par Pharmaceutical
PAR; 246	Carisoprodol and Aspirin	325 mg; 200 mg	White and Light Lavender	Tablet	Circle, Double-Layered	Par Pharmaceutical
PAR; 249	Methocarbamol and Aspirin	325 mg; 400 mg	White and Pink	Tablet	Circle, Double Layered; Compressed	Par Pharmaceutical
PAR; 258	Metaproterenol Sulfate	10 mg	White	Tablet	Circle, Scored; Compressed	Par Pharmaceutical
PAR; 259	Metaproterenol Sulfate	20 mg	White	Tablet	Circle, Scored; Compressed	Par Pharmaceutical
PAR; 289	Megestrol Acetate	20 mg	White	Tablet	Circle, Scored	H.L. Moore
PAR; 289	Megestrol Acetate	20 mg	White	Tablet	Round, Bisected Scored	Par Pharmaceutical
PAR; 290	Megestrol Acetate	40 mg	White	Tablet	Circle, Scored	H.L. Moore
PAR; 290	Megestrol Acetate	40 mg	White	Tablet	Round, Bisected Scored	Par Pharmaceutical
PAR; 300; 683	Ofloxacin	300 mg	White	Tablet	Capsule-Shape	Par Pharmaceutical
PAR; 400; 684	Ofloxacin	400 mg	White	Tablet	Capsule-Shape	Par Pharmaceutical
PAR; 412	Metoprolol Tartrate	50 mg	Light Pink	Coated Tablet	Circle	Par Pharmaceutical
PAR; 413	Metoprolol Tartrate	100 mg	Light Blue	Coated Tablet	Circle	Par Pharmaceutical
PAR; 444	Captopril	12.5 mg	White	Tablet	Oval	Par Pharmaceutical
PAR; 445	Captopril	25 mg	White	Tablet	Circle	Par Pharmaceutical
PAR; 446	Captopril	50 mg	White	Tablet	Circle	Par Pharmaceutical
PAR; 447	Captopril	100 mg	White	Tablet	Circle	Par Pharmaceutical
PAR; 448;	Alprazolam	0.25 mg	Light Yellow	Tablet	Oval, Scored	Par Pharmaceutical
PAR; 449	Alprazolam	0.5 mg	Dark Yellow	Tablet	Oval	Par Pharmaceutical
PAR; 467	Ibuprofen	400 mg	White	Coated Tablet	Capsule-Shape	Par Pharmaceutical
PAR; 468	Ibuprofen	600 mg	White	Coated Tablet	Capsule-Shape	Par Pharmaceutical
PAR; 469	Ibuprofen	800 mg	White	Coated Tablet	Capsule-Shape	Knoll Pharmaceutical
PAR; 473	Orphengesic Forte	100 mg; 60 mg; 770 mg	Blue and White	Tablet	Capsule-Shape, BI-Layered, Scored	Par Pharmaceutical
PAR; 544	Ranitidine Hydrochloride	150 mg		Tablet		Par Pharmaceutical
PAR; 545	Ranitidine Hydrochloride	300 mg		Tablet		Par Pharmaceutical
PAR; 556	Lisinopril	2.5 mg	White	Tablet	Oval	Par Pharmaceutical
PAR; 557	Lisinopril	5 mg	White	Tablet	Capsule-Shape	Par Pharmaceutical
PAR; 558	Lisinopril	10 mg	White	Tablet	Circle	Par Pharmaceutical
PAR; 559	Lisinopril	20 mg	White	Tablet	Circle	Par Pharmaceutical
PAR; 560	Lisinopril	40 mg	White	Tablet	Circle	Par Pharmaceutical
PAR; 635	Lisinopril	30 mg	White	Tablet	Circle	Par Pharmaceutical
PAR; 651; 5	Torsemide	5 mg	White	Tablet	Circle, Scored	Par Pharmaceutical
PAR; 652; 10	Torsemide	10 mg	White	Tablet	Circle, Scored	Par Pharmaceutical
PAR; 653; 20	Torsemide	20 mg	White	Tablet	Circle, Scored	Par Pharmaceutical
PAR; 654; 100	Torsemide	100 mg	White	Tablet	Circle, Scored	Par Pharmaceutical
PAR; 701	Clomiphene Citrate	50 mg	White	Tablet	Circle, Scored	Par Pharmaceutical
PAR; 707; 5	Buspirone Hydrochloride	5 mg	Peach	Tablet	Oval	Par Pharmaceutical
PAR; 708; 10	Buspirone Hydrochloride	10 mg	Peach	Tablet	Oval	Par Pharmaceutical
PAR; 721; 555	Buspirone Hydrochloride	15 mg	Peach	Tablet	Rectangle, Scored	Par Pharmaceutical
PAR; 724	Hydroxyurea	500 mg		Capsule		Par Pharmaceutical
PAR; 725; 7.5	Buspirone Hydrochloride	7.5 mg	Peach	Tablet	Oval	Par Pharmaceutical
PAR; 726	Doxycycline Hyclate	50 mg	Buff and White	Capsule		Par Pharmaceutical
PAR; 727	Doxycycline Hyclate	100 mg	Brown and Cream	Capsule		Par Pharmaceutical
PAR; 876	Paroxetine Hydrochloride	10 mg	White	Tablet		Par
PAR; 877	Paroxetine Hydrochloride	20 mg	White	Tablet		Par
PAR; 878	Paroxetine Hydrochloride	30 mg	White	Tablet		Par
PAR; 879	Paroxetine Hydrochloride	40 mg	White	Tablet		Par
PAR; 962	Chlordiazepoxide and Amitriptyline Hydrochloride	10 mg; 25 mg	White	Coated Tablet		Par Pharmaceutical
PAR 256; MINOXIDIL; 2 1/2	Minoxidil	2.5 mg	White	Tablet	Round; Bisected Scored	Par Pharmaceutical
PAR 257; MINOXIDIL 10	Minoxidil	10 mg	White	Tablet	Round; Bisected Scored	Par Pharmaceutical
PARAFLEX; MCNEIL	Paraflex	250 mg	Orange or Peach	Tablet		Ortho-Mcneil Pharmaceutical
PARAFON FORTE DSC; MCNEIL	Parafon Forte Dsc	500 mg	Light Green	Tablet		Mcneil Pharmaceutical
PARLODEL; 2 1/2;	Parlodel	2.5 mg	White	Tablet	Square, Scored	Novartis

IMPRINT	BRAND/GENERIC NAME	STRENGTH	COLOR	FORM	SHAPE	MANUFACTURER
PARLODEL; 5 MG; TRIANGLE(S)	Parlodel	5 mg	Caramel and White	Capsule, Liquid Filled		Novartis
PARNATE; SKF	Parnate	10 mg	Rose-Red	Tablet	Circle	Glaxosmithkline
PAVAMAR	Pavamar	150 mg	Orange and White	Capsule		Marnel Pharmaceuticals
PAXIL; 10	Paxil	10 mg	Yellow	Coated Tablet	Oval	Glaxosmithkline
PAXIL; 20	Paxil	20 mg	Pink	Coated Tablet	Oval, Modified, Scored	Glaxosmithkline
PAXIL; 30	Paxil	30 mg	Blue	Coated Tablet	Oval, Modified	Glaxosmithkline
PAXIL; 40	Paxil	40 mg	Green	Coated Tablet	Oval	Glaxosmithkline
PAXIL CR; 12.5	Paxil Cr	12.5 mg	Yellow	Controlled-Release Tablet	Circle, Enteric Film-Coated	Glaxosmithkline
PAXIL CR; 25	Paxil Cr	25 mg	Pink	Controlled-Release Tablet	Circle, Enteric Film-Coated	Glaxosmithkline
PAXIL CR; 37.5	Paxil Cr	37.5 mg	Blue	Controlled-Release Tablet	Circle, Enteric Film-Coated	Glaxosmithkline
PBA;	Proglycem	50 mg	Orange and Clear	Capsule		Schering
PCE; ABBOTT LOGO	Pce Dispertab	333 mg	White with Pink Speckles	Tablet	Oval	Abbott Laboratories
PD; 144	Femhrt	1 mg; 5 mcg	White	Tablet	D-Shape	Parke-Davis
PD; 155; 10	Lipitor	10 mg	White	Coated Tablet	Circle	Parke-Davis
PD; 156; 20	Lipitor	20 mg	White	Coated Tablet	Circle	Parke-Davis
PD; 157; 40	Lipitor	40 mg	White	Coated Tablet	Circle	Parke-Davis
PD; 158; 80	Lipitor	80 mg	White	Coated Tablet	Circle	Parke-Davis
PD; 220	Accuretic	20 mg; 12.5 mg	Pink	Coated Tablet	Triangle, Scored	Parke-Davis
PD; 222	Accuretic	10 mg; 12.5 mg	Pink	Coated Tablet	Biconvex, Elliptical, Scored	Parke-Davis
PD; 223	Accuretic	20 mg; 25 mg	Pink	Coated Tablet	Circle, Biconvex	Parke-Davis
PD; 352; 200	Rezulin	200 mg	Yellow	Coated Tablet	Oval	Parke-Davis
PD; 353; 400	Rezulin	400 mg	Tan	Coated Tablet	Oval	Parke-Davis
PD; 357; 300	Rezulin	300 mg	White	Coated Tablet	Oval	Parke-Davis
PD; 527; 5	Accupril	5 mg	Brown	Coated Tablet	Circle, Scored	Parke-Davis
PD; 530; 10	Accupril	10 mg	Brown	Coated Tablet	Triangle	Parke-Davis
PD; 532; 20	Accupril	20 mg	Brown	Coated Tablet	Circle	Parke-Davis
PD; 535; 40	Accupril	40 mg	Brown	Coated Tablet	Circle	Parke-Davis
PD; BRECKENRIDGE	Guiadex PD	600 mg; 10 mg	White	Extended-Release Tablet	Oval	Breckenridge Pharmaceutical
PD; NEURONTIN 100 MG	Neurontin	100 mg	White	Capsule		Parke-Davis
PD; NEURONTIN 300 MG	Neurontin	300 mg	Yellow	Capsule		Parke-Davis
PD; NEURONTIN 400 MG	Neurontin	400 mg	Orange	Capsule		Parke-Davis
P-D; 007	Dilantin Infatabs	50 mg	Yellow	Tablet, Chewable	Triangle, Scored	Parke-Davis
P-D; 043	Gelusil-II Chewable Tablet	400 mg; 400 mg; 30 mg	White and Orange	Tablet, Chewable		Pfizer Consumer Health Care
P-D; 045	Gelusil-M Chewable Tablet	300 mg; 200 mg; 25 mg	White	Tablet, Chewable		Pfizer Consumer Health Care
P-D; 141; 2	Diazepam	2 mg	White	Tablet	Oval	Parke-Davis
P-D; 142; 5	Diazepam	5 mg		Tablet	Triangle	Parke-Davis
P-D; 143; 10	Diazepam	10 mg	White	Tablet	Circle	Parke-Davis
P-D; 160	Pyridium Plus	150 mg; 0.3 mg; 15 mg		Tablet		Warner Chilcott
P-D; 200	Brondecon	200 mg; 100 mg		Tablet		Parke-Davis
P-D; 201	Brondecon	200 mg; 100 mg	Pink	Tablet		Parke-Davis
P-D; 202	Procan SR	250 mg	Green	Sustained-Release Tablet	Circle	Parke-Davis
P-D; 207	Procan SR	1000 mg	Red	Sustained-Release Tablet	Circle, Scored	Parke-Davis
P-D; 214	Choledyl SA	400 mg	Pink	Extended-Release Tablet		Parke-Davis
P-D; 221	Choledyl SA	600 mg	Tan	Extended-Release Tablet		Parke-Davis
P-D; 237	Zarontin	250 mg	Orange	Capsule		Parke-Davis
P-D; 248	D-S-S Plus	30 mg; 100 mg		Capsule		Parke-Davis Consumer Health Products
P-D; 260	Euthroid-1/2	30 mcg; 7.5 mcg		Tablet		Parke-Davis
P-D; 261	Euthroid-1	60 mcg; 15 mcg		Tablet		Parke-Davis
P-D; 262	Euthroid-2	120 mcg; 30 mcg		Tablet		Parke-Davis
P-D; 263	Euthroid-3	180 mcg; 45 mcg		Tablet		Parke-Davis
P-D; 270	Nardil	15 mg	Orange	Coated Tablet	Circle, Biconvex	Parke-Davis
P-D; 271	Amitril	100 mg	Brown and Mustard	Coated Tablet		Parke-Davis
P-D; 272	Amitril	10 mg	Tan	Coated Tablet		Parke-Davis
P-D; 273	Amitril	25 mg	Coral	Coated Tablet		Parke-Davis
P-D; 274	Amitril	50 mg	Blue-Purple	Coated Tablet		Parke-Davis
P-D; 275	Amitril	75 mg	Green	Coated Tablet		Parke-Davis
P-D; 276	Centrax	10 mg	Blue	Tablet		Parke-Davis
P-D; 278	Amitril	150 mg	Orange	Coated Tablet		Parke-Davis
P-D; 365;	Dilantin Kapseals	30 mg	White with Pink Band	Extended-Release Capsule		Parke-Davis
P-D; 373	Benadryl Capsule	50 mg	Pink	Capsule		Pfizer Consumer Health Care
P-D; 382	Geriplex	30 mg; 1.5 mg; 20 mg; 15 mg; 5 IU; 4 mg; 4 mg; 2 mg; 200 mg; 2.5 Gr; 50 mg; 5 mg; 5 mg; 2 mcg		Capsule		Parke-Davis Consumer Health Products
P-D; 390	Natabec	30 mg; 4000 IU; 400 IU; 50 mg; 3 mg; 2 mg; 3 mg; 5 mcg; 10 mg; 600 mg	Pink and Blue	Capsule		Parke-Davis Consumer Health Products
P-D; 393	Milontin	500 mg		Capsule		Parke-Davis
P-D; 407	Cyclopar	250 mg	Scarlet and Flesh	Capsule		Parke-Davis
P-D; 471	Benadryl Capsule	25 mg	Pink and White	Capsule		Pfizer Consumer Health Care

IMPRINT	BRAND/GENERIC NAME	STRENGTH	COLOR	FORM	SHAPE	MANUFACTURER
P-D; 525	Celontin	300 mg	Yellow with Orange Band	Capsule		Parke-Davis
P-D; 529	Humatin	250 mg		Capsule		Monarch Pharmaceuticals
P-D; 531	Dilantin with Phenobarbital	100 mg; 32 mg	White and Purple with Black Band	Capsule		Parke-Davis
P-D; 537	Celontin	150 mg	Yellow with Brown Band	Capsule		Parke-Davis
P-D; 540	Ponstel	250 mg	Ivory with a Blue Band	Capsule		First Horizon Pharmaceutical
P-D; 541	Natabec-FA	30 mg; 4000 IU; 0.1 mg; 10 mg; 600 mg; 50 mg; 3 mg; 2 mg; 3 mg; 5 mcg; 400 IU		Capsule		Parke-Davis Consumer Health Products
P-D; 557	Verapamil Hydrochloride	80 mg		Tablet		Warner Chilcott
P-D; 573	Verapamil Hydrochloride	120 mg		Tablet		Warner Chilcott
P-D; 622	Loestrin Fe 1/20 Brown Tablet	75 mg	Brown	28-Day Tablet Pack	Circle	Pfizer Laboratories
P-D; 697	Cyclopar	500 mg	Orange and Flesh	Capsule		Warner Chilcott
P-D; 730	Utimox	250 mg		Capsule		Warner Chilcott
P-D; 731	Utimox	500 mg		Capsule		Warner Chilcott
P-D; 737; LOPID	Lopid	600 mg	White	Coated Tablet	Circle, Scored	Parke-Davis
P-D; 849	Quinidine Sulfate	200 mg		Tablet		Parke-Davis
P-D; 915	Loestrin Fe 1/20 White Tablet	20 mcg; 1 mg	White	28-Day Tablet Pack	Circle	Pfizer Laboratories
P-D; CENTRAX; 552	Centrax	5 mg	Celery	Capsule		Parke-Davis
P-D; CENTRAX; 553	Centrax	10 mg	Aqua	Capsule		Parke-Davis
P-D; CENTRAX; 554	Centrax	20 mg	Yellow	Capsule		Parke-Davis
PDK	Caffeine	200 mg	Pink	Tablet	Heart-Shape	Pdk Labs
PDK	Caffeine	200 mg	White and Pink with Blue Speckles	Tablet	Teardrop-Shape, Bilayered	Pdk Labs
PDK; 10-362	Caffeine	275 mg	Dark Blue	Capsule		Pdk Labs
PDK; 10-1362	Caffeine	200 mg	Blue	Capsule		Pdk Labs
PDK; 10-1362	Caffeine	275 mg	Green and Clear with Green and White Pellets	Capsule		Pdk Labs
PDK; 1362	Caffeine	200 mg	Blue and Clear with White Pellets	Capsule		Pdk Labs
PE; 614	Duraphen DM	1200 mg; 40 mg; 20 mg	White	Tablet		Proethic Laboratories
PE; 723	Duraflu	200 mg; 60 mg; 20 mg; 500 mg	Dye-Free	Tablet		Proethic Laboratories
PE; 822	Duraphen II	800 mg; 25 mg	White	Extended-Release Tablet	Capsule-Shape, Scored	Proethic Laboratories
PE; I; 425	Durahist Pe	20 mg; 8 mg; 1.25 mg	White	Tablet		Proethic Laboratories
PEC; 101	Maternal Vitamin and Mineral Formula	100 mg; 30 mcg; 25 mcg; 1 mg; 60 mg; 5 mg; 20 mg; 5000 IU; 10 mg; 25 mg; 30 IU; 400 IU; 3.4 mg; 10 mg; 12 mcg; 3 mg; 25 mcg; 25 mg; 150 mcg; 2 mg; 250 mg	Tan	Coated Tablet	Oval	Pecos Pharmaceutical
PEC; 102	Maternal 90	250 mg; 2 mg; 1 mg; 90 mg; 3.4 mg; 3 mg; 12 mcg; 400 IU; 120 mg; 25 mg; 30 IU; 20 mg; 4000 IU; 20 mg; 0.15 mg; 50 mg	White	Coated Tablet	Oval	Pecos Pharmaceutical
PEC; 103	Prenatal Plus New Formula	200 mg; 12 mcg; 20 mg; 3 mg; 4000 IU; 400 IU; 25 mg; 11 mg; 120 mg; 1.5 mg; 10 mg; 1 mg; 2 mg	Yellow	Coated Tablet	Oval	Pecos Pharmaceutical
PEC; 105	Polysaccharide Iron 150 Complex	150 mg	Brown and Orange	Capsule		Pecos Pharmaceutical
PEC; 110	Phenobel Extentabs	0.064 mg; 0.3422 mg; 0.0215 mg; 48.6 mg	Light Green	Sustained-Release Tablet	Circle	Pecos Pharmaceutical
PEC; 114	Hyoscyamine	0.375 mg	Light Orange	Extended-Release Tablet	Oblong	Mutual Pharmaceutical
PEC; 114	Hyoscyamine	0.375 mg	Light Orange	Extended-Release Tablet	Oblong	Pecos Pharmaceutical
PEC; 115	Trimethobenzamide	250 mg	Dark Blue and Light Blue	Capsule		Pecos Pharmaceutical
PEC; 118	Ferragen	250 mg; 10 mcg; 200 mg; 100 mg	Burgundy	Capsule, Liquid Filled		Pecos Pharmaceutical
PEC; 121	Bellaphen-S	0.2 mg; 0.6 mg; 40 mg	Aqua	Tablet	Circle	Mutual Pharmaceutical
PEC; 121	Bellaphen-S	0.2 mg; 0.6 mg; 40 mg	Aqua	Tablet	Circle	Pecos Pharmaceutical
PEC; 122	Pancrelipase Mt 16	48,000 USP units; 16,000 USP units; 48,000 USP units	Orange and Clear	Capsule		Pecos Pharmaceutical
PEC; 126	Pancron 20	20000 U	White	Extended-Release Capsule		Pecos Pharmaceutical
PEC; 301	Hyoscyamine	0.125 mg	Blue	Tablet	Circle	Mutual Pharmaceutical
PEC; 301	Hyoscyamine	0.125 mg	Blue	Tablet	Circle	Pecos Pharmaceutical

IMPRINT	BRAND/GENERIC NAME	STRENGTH	COLOR	FORM	SHAPE	MANUFACTURER
PEC; 505	Hyoscyamine	0.375 mg	Clear with Brown Beads	Capsule		Mutual Pharmaceutical
PEC; 505	Hyoscyamine	0.375 mg	Clear with Brown Beads	Capsule		Pecos Pharmaceutical
PEC; 505	Pancron 10	33,200 USP units; 10,000 USP units; 37,500 USP units	Brown and Clear	Capsule		Pecos Pharmaceutical
PEC; 512	Guaifenesin and Codeine	10 mg; 300 mg	Red	Tablet	Oblong	Pecos Pharmaceutical
PEDIACARE; 3	Pediacare Cough-Cold	0.5 mg; 2.5 mg; 7.5 mg	Pink	Tablet, Chewable		Pharmacia & Upjohn
PEDIACARE; CC	Pediacare for Ages 6-12 Cough-Cold	1 mg; 5 mg; 15 mg	Pink	Tablet, Chewable		Pharmacia & Upjohn
PENTOX; 672	Pentoxifylline	400 mg	White	Tablet	Oval	Merrell
PEPCID AC	Pepcid Ac	10 mg	Peach	Tablet	Square	Johnson & Johnson Merck
PEPTO-BISMOL	Pepto Bismol	262 mg	Pink	Tablet, Chewable	Oval	Procter & Gamble
PEPTO-BISMOL	Pepto-Bismol	262 mg	Pink	Tablet, Chewable	Circle	Procter & Gamble Pharmaceuticals
PERCOCET; 2.5	Percocet 2.5/325	325 mg; 2.5 mg	Pink	Tablet	Oval	Endo Laboratories
PERCOCET; 5	Percocet 5/325	325 mg; 5 mg	Blue	Tablet	Circle, Scored	Endo Laboratories
PERCOCET; 7.5	Percocet 7.5/500	500 mg; 7.5 mg	Peach	Tablet	Capsule-Shape	Endo Laboratories
PERCOCET; 7.5/325	Percocet 7.5/325	325 mg; 7.5 mg	Peach	Tablet	Oval	Endo Laboratories
PERCOCET; 10	Percocet 10/650	650 mg; 10 mg	Yellow	Tablet	Oval	Endo Laboratories
PERCOCET; 10/325	Percocet 10/325	325 mg; 10 mg	Yellow	Tablet	Capsule-Shape	Endo Laboratories
PERCODAN	Percodan	325 mg; 4.5 mg; 0.38 mg	Yellow	Tablet		Endo Laboratories
PERCOGESIC	Percogesic	325 mg; 30 mg	Light Orange	Coated Tablet		Medtech
PF; 100;	Ms Contin	100 mg	Gray	Timed-Release Tablet	Circle	Purdue Pharmaceutical Products
PF; C275	Cardioquin	275 mg	White	Tablet		Purdue Pharmaceutical Products
PF; M15	Ms Contin	15 mg	Blue	Timed-Release Tablet	Circle	Purdue Pharmaceutical Products
PF; M30	Ms Contin	30 mg	Lavender	Timed-Release Tablet	Circle	Purdue Pharmaceutical Products
PF; M60	Ms Contin	60 mg	Orange	Timed-Release Tablet	Circle	Purdue Pharmaceutical Products
PF; M200	Ms Contin	200 mg	Green	Timed-Release Tablet	Capsule-Shape	Purdue Pharmaceutical Products
PF; MI; 15	Msir	15 mg	White	Tablet	Circle, Scored	Purdue Pharmaceutical Products
PF; MI; 30	Msir	30 mg	White	Tablet	Capsule-Shape, Scored	Purdue Pharmaceutical Products
PF; MSIR; 15; THIS END UP	Msir	15 mg	White and Blue	Capsule		Purdue Pharmaceutical Products
PF; MSIR; 30; THIS END UP	Msir	30 mg	Gray and Lavender	Capsule		Purdue Pharmaceutical Products
PF; T; 500	Trilisate 500 mg	293 mg; 362 mg	Salmon	Coated Tablet		Purdue Pharmaceutical Products
PF; T; 750	Trilisate 750 mg	440 mg; 544 mg	White	Coated Tablet		Purdue Pharmaceutical Products
PF; T; 1000	Trilisate 1000 mg	587 mg; 725 mg	Red	Coated Tablet		Purdue Pharmaceutical Products
PF; U200	T-Phyl	200 mg	White	Extended-Release Tablet		Purdue Pharmaceutical Products
PF; U; 200	Uniphyl	200 mg	White	Controlled-Release Tablet	Circle	Purdue Pharmaceutical Products
PF; U; 400	Uniphyl	400 mg	White	Timed-Release Tablet		Purdue Pharmaceutical Products
PF; U; 600	Uniphyl	600 mg		Extended-Release Tablet		Purdue Pharmaceutical Products
PFEIFFER	Mycinettes	15 mg; 2.5 mg	Yellow	Lozenge/troche	Circle	Pfeiffer Pharmaceuticals
PFI; 048	Ibuprofen	400 mg		Tablet		Pharmaceutical Formulations
PFI; 049	Ibuprofen	600 mg		Tablet		Pharmaceutical Formulations
PFI; 22108	Doxycycline Hyclate	100 mg	Blue	Capsule		Pharmaceutical Formulations
PFIZER; 015	Tetracyn	250 mg	Black and White	Capsule		Pfizer
PFIZER; 016	Tetracyn	500 mg	Blue and White	Capsule		Pfizer
PFIZER; 072; TERRAMYCIN	Terramycin	125 mg		Capsule		Pfizer
PFIZER; 073	Terramycin	250 mg	Clear Yellow	Capsule		Pfizer
PFIZER; 073; TERRAMYCIN	Terramycin	250 mg	Yellow	Capsule		Pfizer
PFIZER; 084	Terramycin	250 mg	Yellow	Coated Tablet		Pfizer
PFIZER; 088	Terrastatin	250 mg; 250000 U	Pink and Yellow	Capsule		Pfizer
PFIZER; 092	Urobiotic	250 mg; 250 mg; 50 mg	Yellow and Green	Capsule		Roerig
PFIZER; 094	Vibramycin Hyclate	50 mg	Blue and White	Capsule		Pfizer
PFIZER; 094; VIBRA	Vibramycin	50 mg	Blue and White	Capsule		Pfizer Laboratories
PFIZER; 095	Vibramycin Hyclate	100 mg	Blue	Capsule		Pfizer
PFIZER; 095; VIBRA;	Vibramycin	100 mg	Blue	Capsule		Pfizer
PFIZER; 099; VIBRA-TABS;	Vibra-Tabs	100 mg		Coated Tablet	Circle	Pfizer
PFIZER; 105	Pfizerpen VK	250 mg	White	Tablet		Pfizer
PFIZER; 106	Pfizerpen VK	500 mg	White	Tablet		Pfizer
PFIZER; 180	Vistrax 5	5 mg; 25 mg	White	Tablet		Pfizer
PFIZER; 181	Vistrax 10	10 mg; 25 mg	Black and White	Tablet		Pfizer
PFIZER; 220; SUSTAIRE;	Sustaire	100 mg	White	Delayed-Release Tablet		Pfizer
PFIZER; 221; SUSTAIRE;	Sustaire	300 mg	White	Delayed-Release Tablet		Pfizer

IMPRINT	BRAND/GENERIC NAME	STRENGTH	COLOR	FORM	SHAPE	MANUFACTURER
PFIZER; 306	Zithromax	250 mg	Pink	Coated Tablet	Capsule-Shape	Pfizer Laboratories
PFIZER; 308	Zithromax	600 mg	White	Coated Tablet	Oval, Modified	Pfizer Laboratories
PFIZER; 335	Sterane	5 mg	White	Tablet	Oval	Pfizer Laboratories
PFIZER; 375	Renese	1 mg	White	Tablet	Circle, Scored	Pfizer
PFIZER; 376	Renese	2 mg	Yellow	Tablet	Circle, Scored	Pfizer
PFIZER; 377	Renese	4 mg	White	Tablet	Circle, Scored	Pfizer
PFIZER; 378	Trovan	100 mg	Blue	Coated Tablet	Circle	Pfizer
PFIZER; 378	Trovan/zithromax Compliance Pak Trovafloxacin	100 mg	Blue	Coated Tablet	Circle	Pfizer Laboratories
PFIZER; 379	Trovan	200 mg	Blue	Coated Tablet	Oval	Pfizer
PFIZER; 396	Geodon	20 mg	Blue and White	Capsule		Pfizer Laboratories
PFIZER; 397	Geodon	40 mg	Blue	Capsule		Pfizer Laboratories
PFIZER; 398	Geodon	60 mg	White	Capsule		Pfizer Laboratories
PFIZER; 399	Geodon	80 mg	Blue and White	Capsule		Pfizer Laboratories
PFIZER; 411	Glucotrol	5 mg	White	Tablet	Diamond Shaped, Scored	Pfizer Us Pharmaceuticals Group
PFIZER; 412	Glucotrol	10 mg	White	Tablet	Diamond Shaped, Scored	Pfizer Us Pharmaceuticals Group
PFIZER; 430; MINIZIDE	Minizide 1	1 mg; 0.5 mg	Blue-Green	Capsule		Pfizer
PFIZER; 431; MINIPRESS	Minipress	1 mg	White	Capsule		Pfizer
PFIZER 432; MINIZIDE	Minizide 2	2 mg; 0.5 mg	Blue-Green and Pink	Capsule		Pfizer
PFIZER; 436; MINIZIDE	Minizide 5	5 mg; 0.5 mg	Blue-Green and Blue	Capsule		Pfizer
PFIZER; 437; MINIPRESS	Minipress	2 mg	Pink and White	Capsule		Pfizer
PFIZER; 438; MINIPRESS	Minipress	5 mg	Blue and White	Capsule		Pfizer
PFIZER; 441	Moderil	0.25 mg	Yellow	Tablet	Oval, Scored	Pfizer
PFIZER; 442	Moderil	0.5 mg	Salmon; Orange	Tablet	Oval, Scored	Pfizer
PFIZER; 446	Renese-R	2 mg; 0.25 mg	White	Tablet		Pfizer
PFIZER; 541; VISTARIL;	Vistaril	25 mg	Dark Green and Light Green	Capsule		Pfizer
PFIZER; 542; VISTARIL;	Vistaril	50 mg	Dark Green and White	Capsule		Pfizer
PFIZER; 543; VISTARIL;	Vistaril	50 mg	Dark Green and Pink	Capsule		Pfizer
PFIZER; 550	Zyrtec	5 mg	White	Coated Tablet	Rectangle, Rounded-Off	Pfizer Laboratories
PFIZER; 551;	Zyrtec	10 mg	White	Coated Tablet	Rectangle, Rounded-Off	Pfizer Laboratories
PFIZER; CDT; 051	Caduet	5 mg; 10 mg	White	Tablet		Pfizer
PFIZER; CDT; 052	Caduet	5 mg; 20 mg	White	Tablet		Pfizer
PFIZER; CDT; 054	Caduet	5 mg; 40 mg	White	Tablet		Pfizer
PFIZER; CDT; 058	Caduet	5 mg; 80 mg	White	Tablet		Pfizer
PFIZER; CDT; 101	Caduet	10 mg; 10 mg	Blue	Tablet		Pfizer
PFIZER; CDT; 102	Caduet	10 mg; 20 mg	Blue	Tablet		Pfizer
PFIZER; CDT; 104	Caduet	10 mg; 40 mg	Blue	Tablet		Pfizer
PFIZER; CDT; 108	Caduet	10 mg; 80 mg	Blue	Tablet		Pfizer
PFIZER; CDT; 251	Caduet	2.5 mg; 10 mg	White	Tablet		Pfizer
PFIZER; CDT; 252	Caduet	2.5 mg; 20 mg	White	Tablet		Pfizer
PFIZER; CDT; 254	Caduet	2.5 mg; 40 mg	White	Tablet		Pfizer
PFIZER; NSR; 25;	Inspra	25 mg	Yellow	Tablet	Diamond	Pfizer
PFIZER; NSR; 25;	Inspra	25 mg	Yellow	Tablet	Diamond	Searle
PFIZER; NSR; 50;	Inspra	50 mg	Pink	Tablet	Diamond	Pfizer
PFIZER; NSR; 50;	Inspra	50 mg	Pink	Tablet	Diamond	Searle
PFIZER; TKN; 125	Tikosyn	125 mcg	Light Orange and White	Capsule		Pfizer Laboratories
PFIZER; TKN; 250	Tikosyn	250 mcg	Peach	Capsule		Pfizer Laboratories
PFIZER; TKN; 500	Tikosyn	500 mcg	Peach and White	Capsule		Pfizer Laboratories
PFIZER;VOR200	Vfend	200 mg	White	Coated Tablet	Capsule-Shape	Pfizer Laboratories
PFIZER;VOR50	Vfend	50 mg	White	Coated Tablet	Circle	Pfizer Laboratories
PG; 11	Helidac Therapy: Part I	262.4 mg	Pink	Tablet, Chewable	Circle	Procter & Gamble Pharmaceuticals
PG; 12	Helidac Therapy: Part Iii	500 mg	Pale Orange and White	Capsule		Procter & Gamble Pharmaceuticals
PHA; 1730	Inspra	100 mg	Red	Tablet	Diamond	Searle
PHAZYME	Phazyme	60 mg	Pink	Sustained-Release Tablet	Circle	Block Drug
PHAZYME	Phazyme	60 mg	Pink	Sustained-Release Tablet	Circle	Reed & Carnrick Pharmaceuticals
PHAZYME; 95	Phazyme 95 Sf	95 mg	Red	Coated Tablet	Circle	Block Drug
PHAZYME; 125	Phazyme Quick Dissolve	125 mg	White to Off-White	Tablet	Circle	Block Drug
PHAZYME; 125	Phazyme, Maximum Strength	125 mg	White with Green Nonpareils	Tablet, Chewable	Circle	Reed & Carnrick Pharmaceuticals
PHAZYME; 166	Phazyme Extra Strength	166 mg	White with Green Specks	Tablet, Chewable	Circle, Bevel-Edge	Block Drug
PHAZYME 95	Phazyme-95	95 mg	Red	Sustained-Release Tablet	Oblong	Block Drug
PHAZYME 95	Phazyme-95	95 mg	Red	Sustained-Release Tablet	Oblong	Reed & Carnrick Pharmaceuticals
PHILLIPS	Phillips' Gelcaps	90 mg; 83 mg	White	Capsule, Liquid Filled		Bayer Consumer Care
PHILLIPS'	Phillips' Fibercaps	625 mg	White	Tablet		Bayer Consumer Care
PIROXICAM; EGIS; 111	Piroxicam	10 mg	Blue and Red	Capsule		Ranbaxy Pharmaceuticals
PIROXICAM; EGIS; 112	Piroxicam	20 mg	Red	Capsule		Ranbaxy Pharmaceuticals
PK; ABBOTT LOGO	Kaletra	133.3 mg; 33.3 mg	Orange	Capsule		Abbott Laboratories

IMPRINT	BRAND/GENERIC NAME	STRENGTH	COLOR	FORM	SHAPE	MANUFACTURER
P L; 250	Tindamax	250 mg	Pink	Tablet	Circle, Scored	Presutti Laboratories
P L; 500	Tindamax	500 mg	Pink	Tablet	Capsule-Shape, Scored	Presutti Laboratories
PL; AT8	Amoxicillin	875 mg	Pink	Tablet	Capsule-Shape, Scored	Ivax Pharmaceuticals
PL; CT4	Amoxicillin	400 mg	Pale Pink	Tablet, Chewable	Circle	Ivax Pharmaceuticals
PLACIDYL; 500	Placidyl	500 mg	Red	Capsule, Liquid Filled		Abbott Laboratories
PLACIDYL; 750	Placidyl	750 mg	Green	Capsule, Liquid Filled		Abbott Laboratories
PLAQUENIL	Hydroxychloroquine Sulfate	200 mg	White with Black Ink	Tablet	Oval	Sanofi Winthrop Pharmaceuticals
PLAQUENIL; P62	Plaquenil	200 mg	White	Coated Tablet	Capsule-Shape	Sanofi Pharmaceuticals
PLEGINE; 35	Plegine	35 mg		Tablet		Wyeth Pharmaceuticals
PLENDIL; 450	Plendil	2.5 mg	Sage Green	Extended-Release Tablet	Circle, Convex	Astra Zeneca
PLENDIL; 451	Plendil	5 mg	Red-Brown	Extended-Release Tablet	Circle, Convex	Astra Zeneca
PLENDIL; 452	Plendil	10 mg	Red-Brown	Extended-Release Tablet	Circle, Convex	Astra Zeneca
PLETAL; 50	Pletal	50 mg	White	Tablet	Triangle	Otsuka America Pharmaceutical
PLETAL; 100	Pletal	100 mg	White	Tablet	Circle	Otsuka America Pharmaceutical
PLIVA; 314;	Cyproheptadine Hydrochloride	4 mg	White	Tablet	Round, Flat-Faced, Bisected Scored	Pliva
PLIVA; 323;	Bethanechol Chloride	5 mg	White	Tablet	Circle, Scored	Pliva
PLIVA; 324;	Bethanechol Chloride	10 mg	White	Tablet	Circle, Scored	Pliva
PLIVA; 325;	Bethanechol Chloride	25 mg	Yellow	Tablet	Circle, Scored	Pliva
PLIVA; 326	Bethanechol Chloride	50 mg	Yellow	Tablet	Circle, Scored	Pliva
PLIVA; 327;	Hydralazine Hydrochloride	25 mg		Tablet		Pliva
PLIVA; 328;	Hydralazine Hydrochloride	50 mg		Tablet		Pliva
PLIVA; 333	Metronidazole	250 mg	White	Tablet	Circle, Convex	Akyma Pharmaceuticals
PLIVA; 333;	Metronidazole	250 mg	White	Tablet	Circle, Convex	Pliva
PLIVA; 334	Metronidazole	500 mg	White	Tablet	Oblong, Convex	Akyma Pharmaceuticals
PLIVA; 334;	Metronidazole	500 mg	White	Tablet	Oblong, Convex	Martec Pharmaceuticals
PLIVA; 334;	Metronidazole	500 mg	White	Tablet	Oblong, Convex	Pliva
PLIVA; 362;	Chlorthalidone	25 mg	Orange	Tablet	Circle, Flat-Faced	Pliva
PLIVA; 363;	Chlorthalidone	50 mg	Blue	Tablet	Round, Flat-Faced, Bisected Scored	Pliva
PLIVA; 364;	Chlorthalidone	100 mg	White	Tablet	Round, Flat-Faced, Bisected Scored	Pliva
PLIVA; 372;	Chlorpropamide	100 mg	Blue	Tablet	Round, Flat-Faced, Bisected Scored	Pliva
PLIVA; 373;	Chlorpropamide	250 mg	Blue	Tablet	Round, Flat-Faced, Bisected Scored	Pliva
PLIVA; 390;	Salsalate	500 mg	Yellow	Coated Tablet	Circle, Convex	Pliva
PLIVA; 391;	Salsalate	750 mg	Yellow	Coated Tablet	Capsule-Shape	Pliva
PLIVA; 393;	Benztropine Mesylate	0.5 mg	White	Tablet	Round, Flat-Faced, Bisected Scored	Pliva
PLIVA; 394;	Benztropine Mesylate	1 mg	White	Tablet	Oval, Bisected Scored	Pliva
PLIVA; 395;	Benztropine Mesylate	2 mg	White	Tablet	Round, Flat-Faced, Bisected Scored	Pliva
PLIVA; 397;	Hydralazine Hydrochloride	100 mg	Orange	Tablet	Circle, Convex	Pliva
PLIVA; 398;	Hydralazine Hydrochloride	10 mg	Orange	Tablet	Circle, Convex	Pliva
PLIVA; 430;	Metoclopramide Hydrochloride	10 mg	White	Tablet	Round, Convex, Bisected Scored	Pliva
PLIVA; 433;	Trazodone Hydrochloride	50 mg	White	Tablet	Round, Convex, Bisected Scored	Pliva
PLIVA; 434;	Trazodone Hydrochloride	100 mg	White	Tablet	Round, Convex, Bisected Scored	Pliva
PLIVA; 441;	Trazodone Hydrochloride	150 mg	White	Tablet	Trapezoidal, Flat-Faced, Bisected Scored	Pliva
PLIVA; 456;	Oxybutynin Chloride	5 mg	Very Pale Blue	Tablet	Circle, Scored	Pliva
PLIVA; 459;	Theophylline	300 mg	White	Extended-Release Tablet	Oblong, Scored	Pliva
PLIVA; 467;	Propranolol Hydrochloride	10 mg	Orange	Tablet	Round, Convex, Bisected Scored	Pliva
PLIVA; 468;	Propanolol	20 mg	Blue	Tablet	Circle, Scored	Pliva
PLIVA; 468;	Propranolol Hydrochloride	20 mg	Blue	Tablet	Round, Convex, Bisected Scored	Pliva
PLIVA; 469;	Propranolol Hydrochloride	40 mg	Green	Tablet	Round, Convex, Bisected Scored	Pliva
PLIVA; 470;	Propranolol Hydrochloride	60 mg	Pink	Tablet	Round, Convex, Bisected Scored	Pliva
PLIVA; 471;	Propranolol Hydrochloride	80 mg	Yellow	Tablet	Round, Convex, Bisected Scored	Pliva
PLIVA; 473;	Propranolol Hydrochloride and Hydrochlorothiazide	40 mg; 25 mg	White	Tablet	Circle, Convex	Pliva
PLIVA; 474;	Propranolol Hydrochloride and Hydrochlorothiazide	80 mg; 25 mg	White	Tablet	Circle, Convex	Sidmak Laboratories
PLIVA; 482;	Theophylline	200 mg	White	Extended-Release Tablet	Oval, Convex, Bisected Scored	Pliva
PLIVA; 483;	Theophylline	100 mg	White	Extended-Release Tablet	Round, Convex, Bisected Scored	Pliva
PLIVA; 505;	Triamterene and Hydrochlorothiazide	75 mg; 50 mg	Yellow	Tablet	Rectangle	Pliva
PLIVA; 517;	Metoclopramide Hydrochloride	5 mg	Light Green	Tablet	Circle	Pliva
PLIVA; 518;	Theophylline	450 mg	White	Extended-Release Tablet	Capsule-Shaped, Bisected Scored	Pliva
PLIVA; 528;	Choline Magnesium Trisalicylate	500 mg	Yellow	Coated Tablet	Capsule-Shaped, Bisected Scored	Pliva
PLIVA; 529;	Choline Magnesium Trisalicylate	750 mg	Blue	Coated Tablet	Capsule-Shape, Scored	Pliva
PLIVA; 530;	Choline Magnesium Trisalicylate	1000 mg	Pink	Coated Tablet	Capsule-Shaped, Bisected Scored	Pliva
PLIVA; 534;	Triamterene and Hydrochlorothiazide	37.5 mg; 25 mg	Peach	Tablet	Rectangle, Scored	Pliva
PLIVA; 563;	Cyclobenzaprine Hydrochloride	10 mg	Yellow	Coated Tablet	Circle	Pliva
PLIVA; 609;	Pentoxifylline ER	400 mg	Yellow	Extended-Release Tablet	Capsule-Shape	Pliva
PLIVA; 616;	Tramadol Hydrochloride	50 mg	White	Tablet	Oval	Pliva
PLIVA; 621;	Ketoconazole	200 mg	White	Tablet	Circle	Pliva
PLIVA; 647	Fluoxetine Hydrochloride	10 mg	Opaque, White, Green Band	Capsule		Akyma Pharmaceuticals
PLIVA; 647;	Fluoxetine Hydrochloride	10 mg	White and Green	Capsule		Pliva
PLIVA; 648	Fluoxetine Hydrochloride	20 mg	Opaque, White	Capsule		Akyma Pharmaceuticals
PLIVA; 648;	Fluoxetine Hydrochloride	20 mg	White and Green	Capsule		Pliva
PLIVA; 651;	Doxazosin Mesylate	1 mg	White	Tablet	Circle, Scored	Pliva
PLIVA; 652;	Doxazosin Mesylate	2 mg	Yellow	Tablet	Circle, Scored	Pliva
PLIVA; 653;	Doxazosin Mesylate	4 mg	Orange	Tablet	Circle, Scored	Pliva
PLIVA; 654;	Doxazosin Mesylate	8 mg	Green	Tablet	Circle, Scored	Pliva
PLIVA 708	Propafenone Hydrochloride	150 mg	White	Tablet	Circle	Pliva
PLIVA 709	Propafenone Hydrochloride	225 mg	White	Tablet	Circle	Pliva
PLIVA 710	Propafenone Hydrochloride	300 mg	White	Tablet	Circle	Pliva
PM 12; CPM 1	Chlorpheniramine TR	12 mg	Green and Clear	Capsule		Qualitest Products

IMPRINT	BRAND/GENERIC NAME	STRENGTH	COLOR	FORM	SHAPE	MANUFACTURER
PN; SANOFI	Prenatal Vitamin Ultra	90 mg; 0.15 mg; 250 mg; 2 mg; 25 mg; 1 mg; 4000 IU; 400 IU; 30 IU; 120 mg; 3 mg; 3.4 mg; 20 mg; 12 mcg; 20 mg; 50 mg	Beige	Coated Tablet	Egg-Shape	Sanofi Pharmaceuticals
PO	Nasal Decongestant	30 mg	Red	Tablet	Circle	Pharmaceutical Formulations
POLY; 500	Polygesic	5 mg; 500 mg	Opaque White	Capsule		Poly Pharmaceuticals
POLY; 500; FLEXTRA	Flextra-DS	500 mg; 50 mg		Tablet		Poly Pharmaceuticals
POT; 10	Pexeva	10 mg	White	Tablet	Oval, Modified	Synthon Pharmaceuticals
POT; 20	Pexeva	20 mg	Dark Orange	Tablet	Oval, Modified	Synthon Pharmaceuticals
POT; 30	Pexeva	30 mg	Yellow	Tablet	Oval, Modified	Synthon Pharmaceuticals
POT; 40	Pexeva	40 mg	Rose	Tablet	Oval, Modified	Synthon Pharmaceuticals
PP; 134	Reserpine	0.25 mg	White	Tablet	Circle	H.L. Moore
PP; 551	Metizol	250 mg	White	Tablet	Circle	Glenwood
PP; 1217	Nitroglycerin	9 mg	Green and Yellow	Capsule		H.L. Moore
PP; 1235	Nitroglycerin	6.5 mg	Blue and Yellow	Capsule		H.L. Moore
PP; 1304	Pseudo-Chlor SR	8 mg; 120 mg	Blue and Clear	Sustained-Release Capsule		Novartis Generics
PP; 2007	Papaverine Hydrochloride	150 mg	Clear Brown and Natural with White Beads	Capsule		Pioneer Pharmaceuticals
PP; 4001	Cyclandelate	200 mg	Opaque Blue	Capsule		Pioneer Pharmaceuticals
PP; 4002	Cyclandelate	400 mg	Red and Blue	Capsule		Pioneer Pharmaceuticals
PP; 4005	Indomethacin	25 mg	Opaque Green	Capsule		Pioneer Pharmaceuticals
PP; 4006	Indomethacin	50 mg	Opaque Green	Capsule		Pioneer Pharmaceuticals
PP; 4008	Diphenhydramine	50 mg	Clear Pink	Capsule		Pioneer Pharmaceuticals
PP; 4009	Chlordiazepoxide Hydrochloride with Clidinium	5 mg; 2.5 mg	Opaque Green	Capsule		Pioneer Pharmaceuticals
PP; 4010	Chlordiazepoxide Hydrochloride	5 mg	Yellow and Green	Capsule		Pioneer Pharmaceuticals
PP; 4011	Chlordiazepoxide Hydrochloride	10 mg	Black and Green	Capsule		Pioneer Pharmaceuticals
PP; 4012	Chlordiazepoxide Hydrochloride	25 mg	Green and White	Capsule		Pioneer Pharmaceuticals
PP; 4013	Diphenhydramine	25 mg	Clear Pink and Natural	Capsule		Pioneer Pharmaceuticals
PP; 4017	Dicyclomine Hydrochloride	10 mg	Blue	Capsule		Pioneer Pharmaceuticals
PP; 5174	Nitroglycerin	2.5 mg	Lavender and Clear	Capsule		H.L. Moore
PP; 6001	Therax	25 mg; 10 mg; 130 mg	Light Blue	Tablet		Pioneer Pharmaceuticals
PP; 6004	Folic Acid	1 mg	Yellow	Tablet	Circle, Scored	Pioneer Pharmaceuticals
PP; 6007	Diazepam	2 mg	White	Tablet	Circle, Scored	Pioneer Pharmaceuticals
PP; 6008	Diazepam	5 mg	Yellow	Tablet	Circle, Scored	Pioneer Pharmaceuticals
PP; 6009	Diazepam	10 mg	Blue	Tablet	Circle, Scored	Pioneer Pharmaceuticals
PP; 6012	Chlorzoxazone	250 mg	Peach	Tablet	Circle	Pioneer Pharmaceuticals
PP; 6013	Dicyclomine Hydrochloride	20 mg	Light Blue	Tablet	Biconcave, Scored	Pioneer Pharmaceuticals
PP; 6015	Cyproheptadine	4 mg	White	Tablet	Circle, Scored	Pioneer Pharmaceuticals
PP; 6017	Chlorzoxazone with Acetaminophen	300 mg; 250 mg	Green	Tablet	Six-Sided	Pioneer Pharmaceuticals
PP; 6018	Carisoprodol	350 mg	White	Tablet	Circle	Pioneer Pharmaceuticals
PP; 6036	Methocarbamol	500 mg	White	Tablet	Circle, Scored	Pioneer Pharmaceuticals
PP; 6038	Methocarbamol	750 mg	White	Tablet	Oblong	Pioneer Pharmaceuticals
PP; 6048	Chlorzoxazone	500 mg	Green	Tablet	Capsule-Shape	Pioneer Pharmaceuticals
PP; 6062	Chlorthalidone	25 mg	Peach	Tablet	Circle	Pioneer Pharmaceuticals
PP; 6063	Chlorthalidone	50 mg	Light Blue	Tablet	Circle	Pioneer Pharmaceuticals
PP; N338	Methocarbamol	750 mg	White	Tablet	Oblong	Pioneer Pharmaceuticals
PPP; 431;	Pronestyl	250 mg		Tablet		Apothecon
PPP; 434;	Pronestyl	375 mg	Orange	Tablet	Capsule-Shape	Apothecon
PPP; 438;	Pronestyl	500 mg	Red to Orange	Tablet	Capsule-Shape	Apothecon
PPP; 618;	Naturetin	10 mg	Orange	Tablet	Circle, Biconvex, Scored	Apothecon
PPP; 713;	Raudixin	50 mg	Red	Tablet		Apothecon
PPP; 756;	Pronestyl	375 mg	Orange and White	Capsule		Apothecon
PPP; 757;	Pronestyl	500 mg	Yellow and Orange	Capsule		Apothecon
PPP; 758;	Pronestyl	250 mg	Yellow	Capsule		Apothecon
PPP; 769;	Rauzide	50 mg; 4 mg	Green	Tablet	Circle	Apothecon
PPP; 775;	Pronestyl-SR	500 mg	Greenish-Yellow	Sustained-Release Tablet	Oval, Biconvex, Elongated	Apothecon
PPP; 776;	Raudixin	100 mg	Red	Tablet		Apothecon
PPP; 784; DURICEF; 500 MG	Duricef	500 mg	Maroon and Whtie	Capsule		Bristol-Myers Squibb
PPP; 785	Duricef	1 GM	White to Off White	Tablet	Oval	Bristol-Myers Squibb
PPP; 863	Prolixin	1 mg	White	Coated Tablet	Circle, Biconvex	Apothecon
PPP; 864	Prolixin	2.5 mg	Blue	Coated Tablet	Circle, Biconvex	Apothecon
PPP; 877	Prolixin	5 mg	Green	Coated Tablet	Circle, Biconvex	Apothecon
PPP; 956	Prolixin	10 mg	Pink	Tablet	Circle, Biconvex	Apothecon
PPP 606; NATURETIN 5;	Naturetin	5 mg	Green	Tablet	Circle, Biconvex, Scored	Apothecon
PRASCO; 315	Wellbid-D	600 mg; 40 mg	White	Extended-Release Tablet	Oval	Prasco Laboratories
PRASCO; 316	Wellbid-D 1200	1200 mg; 40 mg	Light Green	Extended-Release Tablet	Capsule-Shape	Prasco Laboratories
PRASCO LOGO; 120	Amdry-D	2.5 mg; 120 mg	Yellow	Extended-Release Tablet	Capsule-Shape	Prasco Laboratories
PRASCO LOGO; 312	Guaifenesin DM	1000 mg; 60 mg	White	Tablet	Capsule-Shape	Prasco Laboratories
PRASCO LOGO; 322	Guaifenesin	1000 mg	White	Extended-Release Tablet	Capsule-Shape	Prasco Laboratories
PRASCO TRIANGLE; 100	Drihist SR	8 mg; 20 mg; 2.5 mg	White	Tablet	Capsule-Shape	Prasco Laboratories
PRASCO TRIANGLE; 120	Amdry-D	2.5 mg; 120 mg	Yellow	Tablet	Capsule-Shape, Scored	Prasco Laboratories
PRASCO TRIANGLE; 124	Amdry-C	8 mg; 2.5 mg; 120 mg	White	Tablet		Prasco Laboratories

IMPRINT	BRAND/GENERIC NAME	STRENGTH	COLOR	FORM	SHAPE	MANUFACTURER
PRASCO TRIANGLE; 300	Guaifenesin and Pseudoephedrine	60 mg; 600 mg	Mottled Blue	Tablet	Capsule-Shape, Scored	Prasco Laboratories
PRASCO TRIANGLE; 310	Guaifenesin DM	30 mg; 600 mg	Green	Tablet	Capsule-Shape, Scored	Prasco Laboratories
PRASCO TRIANGLE; 312	Guaifenesin DM	60 mg; 1000 mg	White	Extended-Release Tablet	Capsule-Shape, Scored	Prasco Laboratories
PRASCO TRIANGLE; 320	Guaifenesin	600 mg	White	Extended-Release Tablet	Capsule-Shape, Scored	Prasco Laboratories
PRASCO TRIANGLE; 322	Guaifenesin	1000 mg	White	Extended-Release Tablet	Capsule-Shape, Scored	Prasco Laboratories
PRASCO TRIANGLE; 324	Guaifenesin	1200 mg	White	Extended-Release Tablet	Capsule-Shape, Scored	Prasco Laboratories
PRASCO TRIANGLE; 330	Pse/guaifenesin ER	600 mg; 120 mg	Yellow	Sustained-Release Tablet	Capsule-Shape, Scored	Prasco Laboratories
PRASCO TRIANGLE; 332	Pse/guaifenesin ER	1200 mg; 120 mg	White	Extended-Release Tablet	Capsule-Shape, Scored	Prasco Laboratories
PRASCO TRIANGLE; 400	Hyoscyamine Sulfate	0.125 mg	Blue	Tablet	Circle, Scored	Prasco Laboratories
PRASCO TRIANGLE; 402	Hyoscyamine Sulfate	0.15 mg	White	Tablet	Circle	Prasco Laboratories
PRASCO TRIANGLE; 404	Hyoscyamine Sulfate ER	0.375 mg	White	Tablet	Capsule-Shape, Scored	Prasco Laboratories
PRASCO TRIANGLE; 514	P-Tuss DM	600 mg; 60 mg; 30 mg	White	Tablet	Capsule-Shape, Scored	Prasco Laboratories
PRAVACHOL; 10; P;	Pravachol	10 mg	Pale Pink or Peach	Tablet	Rectangle, Biconvex, Rounded	Bristol-Myers Squibb
PRAVACHOL; 20; P;	Pravachol	20 mg	Yellow	Tablet	Rectangle, Rounded, Biconvex	Bristol-Myers Squibb
PRAVACHOL; 40; P;	Pravachol	40 mg	Green	Tablet	Rectangle, Rounded, Biconvex	Bristol-Myers Squibb
PRECOSE; 25	Precose	25 mg	White	Tablet	Circle	Bayer Pharmaceutical
PRECOSE; 50	Precose	50 mg	White to Yellow	Tablet		Bayer Pharmaceutical
PRECOSE; 100	Precose	100 mg	White to Yellow	Tablet		Bayer Pharmaceutical
PREHIST	Prehist	8 mg; 20 mg	Pink and White	Capsule		Marnel Pharmaceuticals
PREHIST D	Prehist-D	8 mg; 20 mg; 2.5 mg	Red and White	Capsule		Marnel Pharmaceuticals
PREMARIN; 0.3	Premarin	0.3 mg	Green	Tablet	Oval	Wyeth Pharmaceuticals
PREMARIN; .45	Premarin	0.45 mg	Blue	Tablet	Oval	Wyeth Pharmaceuticals
PREMARIN; 0.625	Premarin	0.625 mg	Maroon	Tablet	Oval	Wyeth Pharmaceuticals
PREMARIN; 0.9	Premarin	0.9 mg	White	Tablet	Oval	Wyeth Pharmaceuticals
PREMARIN; 1.25	Premarin	1.25 mg	Yellow	Tablet	Oval	Wyeth Pharmaceuticals
PREMARIN; 2.5	Premarin	2.5 mg	Purple	Tablet	Oval	Wyeth Pharmaceuticals
PREMPRO	Premphase Conjugated Estrogens and Medroxyprogesterone	0.625 mg; 5 mg	Light-Blue	Coated Tablet	Oval	Wyeth Pharmaceuticals
PREMPRO	Prempro Single Tablet	0.625 mg; 2.5 mg	Peach	Coated Tablet	Oval	Wyeth Pharmaceuticals
PREMSYN; PMS	Premsyn Pms	500 mg; 25 mg; 15 mg	Dark Pink and Pink	Capsule		Chattem
PREMSYN; PMS	Premsyn Pms	500 mg; 25 mg; 15 mg	White	Tablet	Capsule-Shape	Chattem
PRENATE; ADVANCE	Prenate Advance	90 mg; 200 mg; 2 mg; 25 mg; 1 mg; 400 IU; 30 IU; 120 mg; 3 mg; 3.4 mg; 20 mg; 2 mcg; 20 mg; 30 mg; 50 mg	White	Tablet	Oval	First Horizon Pharmaceutical
PRIADEL	Priadel	400 mg	White	Timed-Release Tablet		Protea Pharmaceuticals
PRILOSEC; 10; 606	Prilosec	10 mg	Apricot and Amethyst	Enteric-Coated Tablet		Astra Zeneca
PRILOSEC; 20; 742	Prilosec	20 mg	Amethyst	Timed-Release Capsule		Astra Zeneca
PRO DM	Protuss DM	600 mg; 60 mg; 30 mg	White	Sustained-Release Tablet	Film-Coated, Scored	First Horizon Pharmaceutical
PROCANBID; 500	Procanbid	500 mg	White	Extended-Release Tablet	Circle	Monarch Pharmaceuticals
PROCANBID; 1000	Procanbid	1000 mg	Gray	Extended-Release Tablet	Circle	Monarch Pharmaceuticals
PROCARDIA; PFIZER 260	Procardia	10 mg	Orange	Capsule, Liquid Filled		Pfizer Laboratories
PROCARDIA 20; PFIZER 261	Procardia	20 mg	Orange and Light Brown	Capsule, Liquid Filled		Pfizer Laboratories
PROCARDIA XL; 30	Procardia Xl	30 mg	Rose Pink	Extended-Release Tablet	Circle, Biconvex	Pfizer Laboratories
PROCARDIA XL; 60	Procardia Xl	60 mg	Rose Pink	Extended-Release Tablet	Circle, Biconvex	Pfizer Laboratories
PROCARDIA XL; 90	Procardia Xl	90 mg	Rose Pink	Extended-Release Tablet	Circle, Biconvex	Pfizer Laboratories
PROLOPRIM; 09A	Proloprim	100 mg	White	Tablet	Circle, Scored	Monarch Pharmaceuticals
PROPACET	Propacet 100	650 mg; 100 mg	White	Coated Tablet	Oblong, Convex	Teva Pharmaceuticals
PROPACET; 100; LEMMON	Propacet	650 mg; 100 mg	White	Coated Tablet	Oblong	Teva Pharmaceuticals
PROPECIA; P	Propecia	1 mg	Tan	Coated Tablet	Eight-Sided, Convex	Merck & Company
PROSTIGMIN; 15; ICN	Prostigmin	15 mg	White	Tablet	Flat, Bevel-Edged	Icn Pharmaceuticals
PROTONIX	Protonix	40 mg	Yellow with Brown Ink	Enteric-Coated Tablet	Oval, Biconvex	Wyeth Pharmaceuticals
PROTOPAM; 500	Protopam	500 mg	White	Tablet	Circle	Wyeth Pharmaceuticals
PROVENTIL; 2; 252	Proventil	2 mg	White	Tablet	Circle	Schering
PROVENTIL; 4; 573	Proventil	4 mg	White	Tablet	Circle, Scored, Compressed	Schering
PROVERA; 2.5	Provera	2.5 mg	Orange	Tablet	Circle, Scored	Pharmacia & Upjohn
PROVERA; 5	Provera	5 mg	White	Tablet	Six-Sided, Scored	Pharmacia & Upjohn
PROVERA; 10	Provera	10 mg	White	Tablet	Circle, Scored	Pharmacia & Upjohn
PROVIGIL; 100 MG	Provigil	100 mg	White	Tablet	Capsule-Shape	Cephalon
PROVIGIL; 200 MG	Provigil	200 mg	White	Tablet	Capsule-Shape, Scored	Cephalon
PROZAC; 10	Prozac	10 mg	Green	Tablet	Elliptical-Shaped, Scored	Eli Lilly
PSL; 333	Metronidazole	250 mg	White	Tablet	Circle	Qualitest Products
PSL; 407	Indomethacin	50 mg	Green	Capsule		Qualitest Products
PSL; 470	Propranolol	60 mg	Pink	Tablet	Circle	Qualitest Products
PSL; 550	Cimetidine	300 mg	White	Tablet	Circle	Qualitest Products

IMPRINT	BRAND/GENERIC NAME	STRENGTH	COLOR	FORM	SHAPE	MANUFACTURER
PU; 700	Dostinex	0.5 mg	White	Tablet	Capsule-Shape, Scored	Pharmacia & Upjohn
PURDUE	Dhc Plus	16 mg; 256.4 mg; 30 mg	Light Aqua and Bluish-Green	Capsule		Purdue Pharmaceutical Products
PURDUE; 200 MG	Spectracef	200 mg	White with Blue Ink	Tablet	Circle	Purdue
PURINETHOL; 04A	Purinethol	50 mg	Light Yellow	Tablet		Glaxosmithkline
PVK; 250; GG; 949	Penicillin-VK	250 mg	White	Tablet	Circle	Geneva Generics
PVK; 500; GG; 950	Penicillin VK	500 mg	White	Tablet	Oblong	Geneva Generics
P-XL; 12 MG	Palladone	12 mg	Cinnamon	Extended-Release Capsule		Purdue Pharma
P-XL; 16 MG	Palladone	16 mg	Pink	Extended-Release Capsule		Purdue Pharma
P-XL; 24 MG	Palladone	24 mg	Blue	Extended-Release Capsule		Purdue Pharma
P-XL; 32 MG	Palladone	32 mg	White	Extended-Release Capsule		Purdue Pharma
PZ; 125	Phazyme Softgels 125 mg	125 mg	Blue with White Ink	Capsule, Liquid Filled		Block Drug
PZ; 166	Phazyme Maximum Strength	166 mg	Red	Capsule, Liquid Filled	Oval	Block Drug
PZ; 180	Phazyme Ultra Strength	180 mg	Orange with White Ink	Capsule, Liquid Filled	Circle	Block Drug
Q; 192	Razapam	15 mg	White and Green	Capsule		Quantum Pharmics
Q; 192;	Somaz	15 mg	Dark Green and White Opaque	Capsule		Quantum Pharmics
Q; 192	Temaz	15 mg	Dark Green and White Opaque	Capsule		Quantum Pharmics
Q; 193	Razapam	30 mg	White	Capsule		Quantum Pharmics
Q; 193	Somaz	30 mg	White Opaque	Capsule		Quantum Pharmics
Q; 193;	Temaz	30 mg	White Opaque	Capsule		Quantum Pharmics
Q; QPL; 238	Fenoprofen Calcium	600 mg	Peach	Coated Tablet	Capsule-Shape	Quantum Pharmics
Q; QPL; 245	Oxybutynin Chloride	5 mg	White	Tablet	Biconvex, Scored	Quantum Pharmics
QD; 112	Pseudoephedrine Hydrochloride and Chlorpheniramine Maleate	12 mg; 100 mg	Blue and Yellow with Off-White Beads	Extended-Release Capsule		Atley Pharmaceuticals
QPL; 114	Nystatin	500000 U	Brown	Coated Tablet	Circle	Quantum Pharmics
QPL; 115; Q;	Benztropine Mesylate	2 mg	White	Tablet	Circle	Quantum Pharmics
QPL; 116; Q;	Benztropine Mesylate	0.5 mg	White	Tablet	Circle, Scored	Quantum Pharmics
QPL; 117; Q;	Benztropine Mesylate	1 mg	White	Tablet	Oval	Quantum Pharmics
QPL; 154	Phenazopyridine Hydrochloride	100 mg	Maroon	Coated Tablet	Circle	Quantum Pharmics
QPL; 155	Phenazopyridine Hydrochloride	200 mg	Maroon	Coated Tablet	Circle	Quantum Pharmics
QPL; 156; Q;	Loraz	0.5 mg	White	Tablet	Circle	Quantum Pharmics
QPL; 157; Q;	Loraz	1 mg	White	Tablet	Circle	Quantum Pharmics
QPL; 158; Q;	Loraz	2 mg	White	Tablet	Circle	Quantum Pharmics
QPL; 171	Mepro Compound	150 mg; 250 mg; 75 mg		Tablet	Three Layered	Quantum Pharmics
QPL; 179	Phentermine Resin Complex	30 mg	Blue	Capsule		Quantum Pharmics
QPL; 184	Doxepin Hydrochloride	10 mg	Buff	Capsule		Quantum Pharmics
QPL; 185	Doxepin Hydrochloride	25 mg	Ivory and White	Capsule		Quantum Pharmics
QPL; 186	Doxepin Hydrochloride	50 mg	Ivory	Capsule		Quantum Pharmics
QPL; 187	Doxepin Hydrochloride	75 mg	Green	Capsule		Quantum Pharmics
QPL; 188	Doxepin Hydrochloride	100 mg	Green and White	Capsule		Quantum Pharmics
QPL; 189	Doxepin Hydrochloride	150 mg	White and Blue	Capsule		Quantum Pharmics
QPL; 192	Temazepam	15 mg	Dark Green and White Opaque	Capsule		Quantum Pharmics
QPL; 193	Temazepam	30 mg	White Opaque	Capsule		Quantum Pharmics
QPL; 194; Q	Halperon	0.5 mg	White	Tablet	Circle, Scored	Quantum Pharmics
QPL; 195; Q	Halperon	1 mg	Yellow	Tablet	Circle, Scored	Quantum Pharmics
QPL; 196; Q	Halperon	2 mg	Lavender	Tablet	Circle, Scored	Quantum Pharmics
QPL; 197; Q	Halperon	5 mg	Green	Tablet	Circle, Scored	Quantum Pharmics
QPL; 212; Q;	Meprogesic Q	200 mg; 325 mg	Green and Orange or Salmon and Blue-Green	Tablet	Circle, Scored	Quantum Pharmics
QPL; 213; Q	Trialodine	50 mg	White	Tablet	Circle	Quantum Pharmics
QPL; 214; Q	Trialodine	100 mg	White	Tablet	Circle	Quantum Pharmics
QPL; 217; Q	Clopra	10 mg	White	Tablet	Circle, Scored	Quantum Pharmics
QPL; 225; Q	Clorazepate Dipotassium	3.75 mg	Blue	Tablet	Circle	Quantum Pharmics
QPL; 226; Q	Clorazepate Dipotassium	7.5 mg	Peach	Tablet	Circle	Quantum Pharmics
QPL; 227; Q	Clorazepate Dipotassium	15 mg	Lavender	Tablet	Circle	Quantum Pharmics
QPL; 228; 10;	Minodyl	10 mg	White	Tablet	Circle	Quantum Pharmics
QPL; 236	Fenoprofen Calcium	200 mg	Lavender Opaque and Flesh	Capsule		Quantum Pharmics
QPL; 237	Fenoprofen Calcium	300 mg	Swedish Orange Opaque and Flesh	Capsule		Quantum Pharmics
QPL; 242; Q	Q-Gesic	200 mg; 325 mg	Green and Yellow	Tablet	Circle, Double-Layered	Quantum Pharmics
QPL; 243; 2.5;	Minodyl	2.5 mg	White	Tablet	Bisected, Round Scored	Quantum Pharmics
QUANTUM; 181; 2; Q	Q-Pam	2 mg	White	Tablet	Circle, Scored	Quantum Pharmics
QUANTUM; 182; 5; Q	Q-Pam	5 mg	Yellow	Tablet	Circle, Scored	Quantum Pharmics
QUANTUM; 183; 10; Q	Q-Pam	10 mg	Blue	Tablet	Circle, Scored	Quantum Pharmics
QUARZAN; 2.5; ROCHE	Quarzan	2.5 mg	Green and Red Opaque	Capsule		Roche Products
QUARZAN; 5; ROCHE	Quarzan	5 mg	Green and Grey Opaque	Capsule		Roche Products
QUINIDEX; AHR	Quinidex Extentabs	300 mg	White	Extended-Release Tablet		Wyeth Consumer Healthcare
QUINORA; 200	Quinora	200 mg	White	Tablet		Key Pharmaceuticals
QUINORA; 300	Quinora	300 mg	White	Tablet		Key Pharmaceuticals

IMPRINT	BRAND/GENERIC NAME	STRENGTH	COLOR	FORM	SHAPE	MANUFACTURER
R	VI-Daylin Multivitamin Plus Iron Chewable Tablet	12 mg; 2500 IU; 400 IU; 15 IU; 0.3 mg; 13.5 mg; 60 mg; 1.05 mg; 1.05 mg; 1.2 mg; 4.5 mcg		Tablet, Chewable		Ross Products
R; 001; 3;	Acetaminophen and Codeine No. 3	300 mg; 30 mg; 38 mg	White	Tablet	Circle, Scored	Purepac Pharmaceutical
R 003; 4;	Acetaminophen and Codeine Phosphate	60 mg; 300 mg	White	Tablet	Circle	Purepac Pharmaceutical
R; 003; 4;	Acetaminophen and Codeine No. 4	300 mg; 60 mg	White	Tablet	Circle, Scored	Purepac Pharmaceutical
R; 006	A.P.C. with Butalbital	50 mg; 200 mg; 130 mg; 40 mg	White	Tablet	Circle	Rondex Laboratories
R; 016	Meprobamate	200 mg	White	Tablet	Circle	Rondex Laboratories
R; 018	Meprobamate	400 mg	White	Tablet		Rondex Laboratories
R021	Flurazepam Hydrochloride	15 mg	Blue and White	Capsule		Purepac Pharmaceutical
R022	Flurazepam Hydrochloride	30 mg	Blue	Capsule		Purepac Pharmaceutical
R; 023	Butalbital, Aspirin and Caffeine	50 mg; 325 mg; 40 mg	White	Tablet	Circle, Convex	Purepac Pharmaceutical
R; 026	Phenobarbital	15 mg	White	Tablet	Circle	Purepac Pharmaceutical
R; 026	Phenobarbital	15 mg	White	Tablet	Circle	Udl Laboratories
R; 027	Alprazolam	0.25 mg	White	Tablet	Circle, Scored	Purepac Pharmaceutical
R; 028	Phenobarbital	30 mg	White	Tablet	Circle, Scored	Purepac Pharmaceutical
R; 028	Phenobarbital	30 mg	White	Tablet	Circle, Scored	Udl Laboratories
R; 029	Alprazolam	0.5 mg	Peach	Tablet	Circle, Scored	Purepac Pharmaceutical
R; 031	Alprazolam	1 mg	Blue	Tablet	Circle, Scored	Purepac Pharmaceutical
R; 039	Alprazolam	2 mg	Yellow	Tablet	Rectangle, Multi-Scored	Purepac Pharmaceutical
R; 049;	Diphenoxylate Hydrochloride and Atropine Sulfate	2.5 mg; 0.025 mg	White	Tablet	Circle, Convex	Purepac Pharmaceutical
R; 051	Diazepam	2 mg	White	Tablet	Round, Bisected, Flat Faced, Beveled Edge Scored	Purepac Pharmaceutical
R; 052	Diazepam	5 mg	Yellow	Tablet	Round, Bisected, Flat Faced, Beveled Edge Scored	Purepac Pharmaceutical
R; 053	Diazepam	10 mg	Blue	Tablet	Circle, Scored, Flat Faced, Beveled Edge	Purepac Pharmaceutical
R; 060	Chlordiazepoxide Hydrochloride	5 mg	Green and Yellow	Capsule		Rondex Laboratories
R; 061	Chlordiazepoxide Hydrochloride	10 mg	Black and Green	Capsule		Rondex Laboratories
R; 063	Lorazepam	2 mg	White	Tablet	Round; Bisected Scored	Purepac Pharmaceutical
R; 064	Chlordiazepoxide Hydrochloride	25 mg	White and Green	Capsule		Rondex Laboratories
R; 067	Oxazepam	10 mg	Pink	Capsule		Purepac Pharmaceutical
R; 069	Oxazepam	15 mg	Red	Capsule		Purepac Pharmaceutical
R; 073	Oxazepam	30 mg	Maroon	Capsule		Purepac Pharmaceutical
R; 076	Temazepam	15 mg	Green and White	Capsule		Purepac Pharmaceutical
R; 077	Temazepam	30 mg	White	Capsule		Purepac Pharmaceutical
R; 078;	Clorazepate Dipotassium	3.75 mg	Blue	Tablet	Round; Bisected Scored	Purepac Pharmaceutical
R; 080	Propoxyphene Compound	65 mg; 227 mg; 162 mg; 33.4 mg	Red and Gray	Capsule		Rondex Laboratories
R; 081;	Clorazepate Dipotassium	7.5 mg	Peach	Tablet	Round; Bisected Scored	Purepac Pharmaceutical
R; 082	Propoxyphene Hydrochloride	65 mg	Pink	Capsule		Rondex Laboratories
R; 082;	Propoxyphene Hydrochloride	65 mg	Opaque Pink	Capsule, Liquid Filled		Purepac Pharmaceutical
R; 083;	Clorazepate Dipotassium	15 mg	Pink	Tablet	Round; Bisected Scored	Purepac Pharmaceutical
R; 085	Acetaminophen and Propoxyphene Napsylate	650 mg; 100 mg	Pink	Coated Tablet	Capsule-Shape	Purepac Pharmaceutical
R; 085	Propoxyphene Napsylate and Acetaminophen	100 mg; 650 mg	Pink	Coated Tablet	Capsule-Shape	Purepac Pharmaceutical
R0.5	Risperdal M-Tab	0.5 mg	Light Coral	Disintegrating Tablet	Circle, Biconvex	Janssen Pharmaceutica
R1	Risperdal M-Tab	1 mg	Light Coral	Disintegrating Tablet	Square, Biconvex	Janssen Pharmaceutica
R2	Risperdal M-Tab	2 mg	Light Coral	Disintegrating Tablet	Circle, Biconvex	Janssen Pharmaceutica
R3	Risperdal M-Tab	3 mg	Coral	Disintegrating Tablet	Circle, Biconvex	Janssen Pharmaceutica
R; 4;	Ibuprofen	400 mg	White	Coated Tablet	Circle	Purepac Pharmaceutical
R4	Risperdal M-Tab	4 mg	Coral	Disintegrating Tablet	Circle, Biconvex	Janssen Pharmaceutica
R; 6;	Ibuprofen	600 mg	White	Coated Tablet	Oval	Purepac Pharmaceutical
R; 7	Lozol	1.25 mg	Orange	Coated Tablet	Eight-Sided	Aventis Pharmaceuticals
R; 8	Lozol	2.5 mg	White	Coated Tablet	Eight-Sided	Aventis Pharmaceuticals
R; 8;	Ibuprofen	800 mg		Tablet		Purepac Pharmaceutical
R; 10	Charco Caps	250 mg	Black	Tablet	Circle	Requa
R; 20; 3	Acetaminophen and Codeine Phosphate	300 mg; 30 mg	White	Tablet	Circle	Omj Pharmaceuticals
R; 20; 3	Acetaminophen and Codeine Phosphate	300 mg; 30 mg	White	Tablet	Circle	Purepac Pharmaceutical
R; 21; 4	Acetaminophen and Codeine Phosphate	300 mg; 60 mg	White	Tablet	Circle	Omj Pharmaceuticals
R; 21; 4	Acetaminophen and Codeine Phosphate	300 mg; 60 mg	White	Tablet	Circle	Purepac Pharmaceutical
R; 27	Propranolol Hydrochloride	10 mg	Orange	Tablet	Circle, Scored	Purepac Pharmaceutical
R; 29	Propranolol Hydrochloride	20 mg	Blue	Tablet	Circle, Scored	Purepac Pharmaceutical
R31;	Amitriptyline Hydrochloride	10 mg	Pink	Coated Tablet	Circle	Purepac Pharmaceutical
R; 32	Demi-Regroton	25 mg; 0.25 mg	White	Tablet		Usv Laboratories
R; 32;	Amitriptyline Hydrochloride	25 mg	Green	Coated Tablet	Circle, Convex	Purepac Pharmaceutical
R; 33	Clonazepam	0.5 mg	Pink	Tablet	Circle, Scored	Purepac Pharmaceutical
R; 34	Clonazepam	1 mg	Yellow	Tablet	Circle, Scored	Purepac Pharmaceutical
R; 35	Clonazepam	2 mg	White	Tablet	Circle, Scored	Purepac Pharmaceutical
R; 50	Doxy-Tabs	50 mg	Light Green	Tablet		Rachelle Laboratories
R50	Doxycycline Hyclate	50 mg	Beige	Coated Tablet	Circle	Halsey Drug
R; 56; 3	Acetaminophen and Codeine Phosphate	300 mg; 30 mg	White to Off White	Tablet	Circle	Mallinckrodt
R; 56; 3	Acetaminophen and Codeine Phosphate	300 mg; 30 mg	White to Off White	Tablet	Circle	Purepac Pharmaceutical

IMPRINT	BRAND/GENERIC NAME	STRENGTH	COLOR	FORM	SHAPE	MANUFACTURER
R; 57	Lorazepam	0.5 mg	White	Tablet	Circle, Scored	Purepac Pharmaceutical
R; 58; 4	Acetaminophen and Codeine Phosphate	300 mg; 30 mg	White to Off White	Tablet	Circle	Mallinckrodt
R; 58; 4	Acetaminophen and Codeine Phosphate	300 mg; 30 mg	White to Off White	Tablet	Circle	Purepac Pharmaceutical
R; 59	Lorazepam	1 mg	White	Tablet	Circle, Scored	Purepac Pharmaceutical
R; 101;	Acetazolamide	250 mg	White	Tablet	Circle, Scored	Purepac Pharmaceutical
R; 102;	Allopurinol	100 mg	White	Tablet	Circle, Scored	Purepac Pharmaceutical
R; 103;	Allopurinol	300 mg	Peach	Tablet	Circle, Scored	Purepac Pharmaceutical
R; 105	Aminophylline	100 mg	White	Tablet	Circle	Rondex Laboratories
R; 107	Aminophylline	200 mg	White	Tablet	Circle	Rondex Laboratories
R; 111	Ibuprofen	800 mg		Tablet		Purepac Pharmaceutical
R; 112	Ampicillin Trihydrate	250 mg	Gray-Maroon	Capsule		Rondex Laboratories
R; 114	Ampicillin Trihydrate	500 mg	Gray-Maroon	Capsule		Rondex Laboratories
R; 118	Belladonna Alkaloids with Phenobarbital	16.2 mg; 0.1037 mg; 0.0194 mg; 0.0065 mg	White	Tablet	Circle	Rondex Laboratories
R; 121	Pramilet FA	40 mg; 4000 IU; 400 IU; 1 mg; 10 mg; 1 mg; 250 mg; 100 mcg; 10 mg; 0.15 mg; 0.085 mg; 60 mg; 3; 2 mg; 3 mg; 3 mcg		Coated Tablet		Ross Products
R; 124;	Ibuprofen	400 mg	White	Coated Tablet	Circle	Purepac Pharmaceutical
R; 125;	Ibuprofen	600 mg	White	Coated Tablet	Oval	Purepac Pharmaceutical
R; 127	Clonidine Hydrochloride	0.1 mg	Orange	Tablet	Round, Bisected Scored	Purepac Pharmaceutical
R; 128	Clonidine Hydrochloride	0.2 mg	Orange	Tablet	Round, Bisected Scored	Purepac Pharmaceutical
R; 129	Clonidine Hydrochloride	0.3 mg	Orange	Tablet	Round, Bisected Scored	Purepac Pharmaceutical
R133;	Amitriptyline Hydrochloride	50 mg	Reddish-Brown or Tan	Coated Tablet	Circle, Convex	Purepac Pharmaceutical
R134;	Amitriptyline Hydrochloride	75 mg	Purple or Orange	Coated Tablet	Circle, Convex	Purepac Pharmaceutical
R135;	Amitriptyline Hydrochloride	100 mg	Orange or Lavender	Coated Tablet	Circle, Convex	Purepac Pharmaceutical
R; 143	Carbamazepine	200 mg	White	Tablet	Circle, Scored	Purepac Pharmaceutical
R; 147	Pramet FA	1 mg; 100 mg; 10 mg; 5 mg; 3 mg; 2 mg; 1.2 mg; 0.92 mg; 400 IU; 3 mcg; 60 mg; 0.1 mg; 250 mg; 0.15 mg	Blue	Coated Tablet	Capsule-Shape	Ross Laboratories
R; 154	Colchicine	0.6 mg	White	Tablet	Circle	Rondex Laboratories
R; 158	Cortisone Acetate	25 mg	White	Tablet	Circle	Rondex Laboratories
R; 161;	Chlorthalidone	25 mg	Yellow	Tablet	Circle, Scored	Purepac Pharmaceutical
R; 163;	Chlorthalidone	50 mg	Bluish-Green	Tablet	Circle, Scored	Purepac Pharmaceutical
R; 176	Digitoxin	0.1 mg	Pink	Tablet	Circle	Rondex Laboratories
R; 176	Digitoxin	0.2 mg	White	Tablet	Circle	Rondex Laboratories
R 179	Tizanidine	2 mg		Tablet		DR Reddy's Laboratories
R 179	Tizanidine Hydrochloride	2 mg	White to Off White	Tablet	Oval	Par Pharmaceutical
R 180	Tizanidine	4 mg	White	Tablet	Oval	DR Reddy's Laboratories
R 180	Tizanidine Hydrochloride	4 mg	White to Off White	Tablet		Par Pharmaceutical
R; 182	Digoxin	0.25 mg	White	Tablet	Circle	Rondex Laboratories
R; 183;	Dipyridamole	50 mg	White	Coated Tablet	Circle	Purepac Pharmaceutical
R185;	Dipyridamole	75 mg	White	Coated Tablet	Circle	Purepac Pharmaceutical
R; 191;	Diphenhydramine Hydrochloride	25 mg	Clear and Pink	Capsule, Liquid Filled		Purepac Pharmaceutical
R; 192;	Diphenhydramine Hydrochloride	50 mg	Pink	Capsule, Liquid Filled		Purepac Pharmaceutical
R; 193;	Dipyridamole	25 mg	White or Orange	Coated Tablet	Circle	Purepac Pharmaceutical
R; 194;	Doxycycline Hyclate	50 mg	Aqua and Cream	Capsule		Purepac Pharmaceutical
R; 201	Ergonovine Maleate	0.2 mg	White	Tablet	Circle	Rondex Laboratories
R; 204	Erythromycin Stearate	250 mg	Pink	Tablet	Circle, Convex	Purepac Pharmaceutical
R; 204	Erythromycin Steareate	250 mg	Pink	Tablet	Circle	Rondex Laboratories
R; 210	Folic Acid	1 mg	Yellow	Tablet	Circle	Rondex Laboratories
R; 212	Hydrocortisone	10 mg	White	Tablet	Circle	Rondex Laboratories
R; 214	Hydrocortisone	20 mg	White	Tablet	Circle	Rondex Laboratories
R; 221	Hydrochlorothiazide	25 mg	Peach	Tablet	Round; Partially Bisected Scored	Purepac Pharmaceutical
R; 222	Hydrochlorothiazide	50 mg	Peach	Tablet	Round; Bisected Scored	Purepac Pharmaceutical
R; 224; 2.5	Minoxidil	2.5 mg	White	Tablet	Circle, Scored	Watson Laboratories
R; 225	Hydrochlorothiazide with Reserpine	50 mg; 0.125 mg	Green	Tablet	Circle	Purepac Pharmaceutical
R; 225; 10	Minoxidal	10 mg	White	Tablet	Circle, Scored	Watson Laboratories
R; 227	Hydrochlorothiazide with Reserpine and Hydralazine	25 mg; 15 mg; 0.1 mg	Salmon	Tablet	Circle	Purepac Pharmaceutical
R; 229; 0.5	Haloperidol	0.5 mg	White	Tablet	Circle	Watson Laboratories
R; 230; 1	Haloperidol	1 mg	Yellow	Tablet	Circle	Watson Laboratories
R; 231	Chlorpheniramine Maleate	4 mg	Yellow	Tablet	Circle	Rondex Laboratories
R; 231;	Imipramine Hydrochloride	10 mg		Tablet		Purepac Pharmaceutical
R; 231; 2	Haloperidol	2 mg	Purple	Tablet	Circle	Watson Laboratories
R; 232;	Imipramine Hydrochloride	25 mg	Brown	Tablet	Circle	Purepac Pharmaceutical
R; 232; 5	Haloperidol	5 mg	Green	Tablet	Circle	Watson Laboratories
R; 233;	Imipramine Hydrochloride	50 mg	Rust	Tablet	Circle	Purepac Pharmaceutical
R; 233; 10	Haloperidol	10 mg	Green-Blue	Tablet	Circle	Watson Laboratories
R; 234; 20	Haloperidol	20 mg	Salmon	Tablet	Circle	Watson Laboratories
R; 236	Isoniazid	100 mg	White	Tablet		Rondex Laboratories
R; 237	Isosorbide Dinitrate	5 mg	Pink	Tablet		Rondex Laboratories
R; 238	Isosorbide Dinitrate	10 mg	White	Tablet		Rondex Laboratories
R; 247	Methocarbamol	500 mg	White	Tablet	Circle	Rondex Laboratories
R; 249	Methocarbamol	750 mg	White	Tablet	Oblong	Rondex Laboratories
R; 269	Metoclopramide	10 mg	White	Tablet	Circle, Scored	Purepac Pharmaceutical

IMPRINT	BRAND/GENERIC NAME	STRENGTH	COLOR	FORM	SHAPE	MANUFACTURER
R; 269	Metoclopramide	10 mg	White	Tablet	Circle, Scored	Udl Laboratories
R; 278	Oxytetracycline Hydrochloride	250 mg	Yellow Opaque	Capsule		Rondex Laboratories
R; 280;	Haloperidol	1 mg	Yellow	Tablet	Round, Bisected Scored	Purepac Pharmaceutical
R; 281;	Haloperidol	2 mg	Light Pink	Tablet	Round, Bisected Scored	Purepac Pharmaceutical
R; 282;	Haloperidol	5 mg	Green	Tablet	Round, Bisected Scored	Purepac Pharmaceutical
R; 286;	Haloperidol	10 mg	Aqua	Tablet	Round, Bisected Scored	Purepac Pharmaceutical
R; 287;	Haloperidol	20 mg	Salmon	Tablet	Round, Bisected Scored	Purepac Pharmaceutical
R; 289;	Haloperidol	0.5 mg	White	Tablet	Round, Bisected Scored	Purepac Pharmaceutical
R; 292	Papaverine Hydrochloride	150 mg	Brown and Clear	Capsule		Rondex Laboratories
R; 300	Penicillin G	250,000 units	White	Tablet		Rondex Laboratories
R; 304	Penicillin G	400,000 units	White	Tablet	Circle	Rondex Laboratories
R; 316	Phentermine Hydrochloride	37.5 mg	White	Tablet	Capsule-Shape, Scored	Purepac Pharmaceutical
R; 317	Fenoprofen Calcium	600 mg	Yellow	Tablet	Capsule-Shaped; Bisected Scored	Purepac Pharmaceutical
R; 321	Propranolol Hydrochloride	60 mg	Pink	Tablet	Circle, Scored	Purepac Pharmaceutical
R; 324	Penicillin V	400,000 units	White	Tablet		Rondex Laboratories
R; 331	Propranolol Hydrochloride	40 mg	Green	Tablet	Circle, Scored	Purepac Pharmaceutical
R; 332	Prednisolone	5 mg	Orange	Tablet	Circle	Rondex Laboratories
R; 333	Propranolol Hydrochloride	80 mg	Yellow	Tablet	Circle, Scored	Purepac Pharmaceutical
R; 336	Prednisone	5 mg	White	Tablet	Circle	Rondex Laboratories
R; 337	Prednisone	20 mg	Light Orange	Tablet	Circle	Rondex Laboratories
R; 338	Prednisone	10 mg	White	Tablet	Circle	Rondex Laboratories
R; 348	Propylthiouracil	50 mg	White	Tablet	Circle, Scored	Purepac Pharmaceutical
R; 356	Quinidine Sulfate	200 mg	White	Tablet	Circle	Rondex Laboratories
R; 356;	Quinidine Sulfate	200 mg	White	Tablet	Circle, Scored	Purepac Pharmaceutical
R; 358	Propranolol Hydrochloride and Hydrochlorothiazide	40 mg; 25 mg	White	Tablet	Circle, Scored	Purepac Pharmaceutical
R; 360	Propranolol Hydrochloride and Hydrochlorothiazide	80 mg; 25 mg	White	Tablet	Circle, Scored	Purepac Pharmaceutical
R; 370	Rauwolfia Serpentina	100 mg	Red	Coated Tablet		West-Ward
R; 404	Tetracycline Hydrochloride	250 mg	Yellow and Orange	Capsule		Rondex Laboratories
R; 404;	Tetracycline Hydrochloride	250 mg	Yellow and Orange	Capsule, Liquid Filled		Purepac Pharmaceutical
R; 406	Tetracycline Hydrochloride	500 mg	Yellow and Black	Capsule		Rondex Laboratories
R; 406;	Tetracycline Hydrochloride	500 mg	Yellow and Black	Capsule, Liquid Filled		Purepac Pharmaceutical
R; 418;	Cephalexin	500 mg	Red	Capsule		Purepac Pharmaceutical
R; 439	Trazodone Hydrochloride	50 mg	White	Coated Tablet	Circle	H.L. Moore
R; 439	Trazodone Hydrochloride	50 mg	White	Coated Tablet	Circle	Purepac Pharmaceutical
R; 441	Trazodone Hydrochloride	100 mg	White	Coated Tablet	Circle	H.L. Moore
R; 441	Trazodone Hydrochloride	100 mg	White	Coated Tablet	Circle	Purepac Pharmaceutical
R; 454	Triamcinolone	4 mg	White	Tablet	Circle	Rondex Laboratories
R; 473	Verapamil Hydrochloride	80 mg	White	Coated Tablet	Circle, Scored	Purepac Pharmaceutical
R; 475	Verapamil Hydrochloride	120 mg	White	Coated Tablet	Circle, Scored	Purepac Pharmaceutical
R; 480	Tolmetin Sodium	600 mg	White	Coated Tablet	Oval	Purepac Pharmaceutical
R; 497	Nifedipine	10 mg	Yellow	Capsule, Liquid Filled		H.L. Moore
R; 497	Nifedipine	10 mg	Yellow	Capsule, Liquid Filled		Purepac Pharmaceutical
R; 500	Prazosin Hydrochloride	1 mg	White	Capsule		Purepac Pharmaceutical
R; 500; 239	Chlorzoxazone	500 mg	Light Green	Tablet	Capsule-Shape, Scored	H.L. Moore
R; 501	Prazosin Hydrochloride	2 mg	Pink	Capsule		Purepac Pharmaceutical
R; 502	Prazosin Hydrochloride	5 mg	Blue	Capsule		Purepac Pharmaceutical
R; 507	Quinine Sulfate	325 mg	White	Tablet	Circle	Rondex Laboratories
R; 511	Quinine Sulfate	650 mg	Clear	Capsule		Rondex Laboratories
R; 520	Tolmetin Sodium	400 mg	Orange and White	Capsule		Purepac Pharmaceutical
R; 521	Naproxen	250 mg	White	Tablet	Circle	Purepac Pharmaceutical
R; 522	Naproxen	375 mg	White	Tablet	Capsule-Shape	Purepac Pharmaceutical
R; 523	Naproxen	500 mg	White	Tablet	Capsule-Shape	Purepac Pharmaceutical
R; 530	Nifedipine	20 mg	Yellow	Capsule		H.L. Moore
R; 530	Nifedipine	20 mg	Red-Brown	Capsule, Liquid Filled		Purepac Pharmaceutical
R; 534;	Pindolol	5 mg	White	Tablet	Circle	Purepac Pharmaceutical
R; 535;	Pindolol	10 mg	White	Tablet	Circle	Purepac Pharmaceutical
R; 538	Carbidopa and Levodopa	10 mg; 100 mg	Dark Blue Mottled	Tablet	Round, Bisected Scored	Purepac Pharmaceutical
R; 539	Carbidopa and Levodopa	25 mg; 100 mg	Mottled Yellow	Tablet	Round, Bisected Scored	Purepac Pharmaceutical
R; 540	Carbidopa and Levodopa	25 mg; 250 mg	Mottled Light Blue	Tablet	Round, Bisected Scored	Purepac Pharmaceutical
R; 545	Diflunisal	250 mg	Peach	Coated Tablet	Circle	Purepac Pharmaceutical
R; 546	Diflunisal	500 mg	Orange	Coated Tablet	Circle	Purepac Pharmaceutical
R; 547	Naproxen	275 mg	White	Coated Tablet	Oval	Purepac Pharmaceutical
R; 548	Naproxen	550 mg	White	Coated Tablet	Oval	Purepac Pharmaceutical
R; 550	Diclofenac Sodium	50 mg	White	Delayed-Release Tablet	Circle, Enteric-Coated	Purepac Pharmaceutical
R; 551	Diclofenac Sodium	75 mg	White	Delayed-Release Tablet	Circle, Enteric-Coated	Purepac Pharmaceutical
R; 552;	Gemfibrozil	600 mg	White	Coated Tablet	Capsule-Shape, Partially Scored	Purepac Pharmaceutical
R; 553	Doxycycline Hyclate	100 mg	Blue Opaque	Capsule		West-Ward
R; 553	Erythromycin	250 mg	Natural with White Enteric-Coated Pellets	Timed-Release Capsule		Purepac Pharmaceutical
R; 554;	Metoprolol Tartrate	50 mg	Pink	Coated Tablet	Round; Partially Bisected Scored	Purepac Pharmaceutical
R; 555;	Metoprolol Tartrate	100 mg	White	Coated Tablet	Round; Partially Bisected Scored	Purepac Pharmaceutical
R; 557	Doxycycline Hyclate	100 mg	Blue	Capsule		West-Ward
R; 571	Indapamide	2.5 mg	White	Coated Tablet	Circle	Purepac Pharmaceutical
R; 597	Indapamide	1.25 mg	Orange	Coated Tablet	Circle	Purepac Pharmaceutical
R; 599	Etodolac	400 mg	Light Gray	Coated Tablet	Egg-Shape	Purepac Pharmaceutical
R; 605	Acyclovir	200 mg	Green	Capsule		Purepac Pharmaceutical
R; 606	Acyclovir	400 mg	White	Tablet	Circle, Flat Faced, Beveled Edged	Purepac Pharmaceutical
R; 607	Acyclovir	800 mg	Pastel Green	Tablet	Oval	Purepac Pharmaceutical
R; 611	Pentoxifylline	400 mg	Yellow	Extended-Release Tablet	Oblong, Film-Coated	Purepac Pharmaceutical
R; 613	Ticlopidine Hydrochloride	250 mg	White	Coated Tablet	Oval	Purepac Pharmaceutical
R; 614	Oxaprozin	600 mg	Orange	Coated Tablet	Capsule-Shape	Purepac Pharmaceutical
R; 617	Naproxen Delayed-Release	375 mg	Yellow	Enteric-Coated Tablet	Capsule-Shape	Purepac Pharmaceutical
R; 618	Naproxen Delayed-Release	500 mg	Yellow	Enteric-Coated Tablet	Capsule-Shape	Purepac Pharmaceutical
R; 620	Isosorbide Mononitrate	20 mg	Blue	Tablet	Circle, Scored	Purepac Pharmaceutical
R; 631	Isosorbide Mononitrate	10 mg	Blue	Tablet	Circle, Scored	Purepac Pharmaceutical
R; 632	Etodolac	500 mg	White	Coated Tablet	Egg-Shape	Purepac Pharmaceutical

IMPRINT	BRAND/GENERIC NAME	STRENGTH	COLOR	FORM	SHAPE	MANUFACTURER
R; 633	Lovastatin	10 mg	White	Tablet	Circle, Flat Faced, Beveled Edge	Purepac Pharmaceutical
R; 634	Lovastatin	20 mg	Pink	Tablet	Circle, Flat Faced, Beveled Edge	Purepac Pharmaceutical
R; 635	Lovastatin	40 mg	Yellow	Tablet	Circle, Flat Faced, Beveled Edge	Purepac Pharmaceutical
R; 641	Famotidine	40 mg	Beige	Coated Tablet	Circle	Purepac Pharmaceutical
R; 642	Doxazosin Mesylate	1 mg	White	Tablet	Circle, Scored	Purepac Pharmaceutical
R; 643	Doxazosin Mesylate	2 mg	White	Tablet	Capsule-Shape, Scored	Purepac Pharmaceutical
R; 644	Doxazosin Mesylate	4 mg	White	Tablet	Capsule-Shape, Scored	Purepac Pharmaceutical
R; 645	Doxazosin Mesylate	8 mg	White	Tablet	Circle, Scored	Purepac Pharmaceutical
R; 650	Bisoprolol and Hydrochlorothiazide	2.5 mg; 6.25 mg	Yellow	Coated Tablet	Capsule-Shape	Purepac Pharmaceutical
R; 651	Bisoprolol and Hydrochlorothiazide	5 mg; 6.25 mg	Pink	Coated Tablet	Capsule-Shape	Purepac Pharmaceutical
R; 652	Bisoprolol and Hydrochlorothiazide	10 mg; 6.25 mg	White	Coated Tablet	Capsule-Shape	Purepac Pharmaceutical
R; 655	Fluvoxamine Maleate	50 mg	Blue	Coated Tablet	Capsule-Shape, Scored	Purepac Pharmaceutical
R; 656	Fluvoxamine Maleate	100 mg	White	Coated Tablet	Capsule-Shape, Scored	Purepac Pharmaceutical
R; 657	Metformin Hydrochloride	500 mg	White to Off-White	Coated Tablet	Oval	Purepac Pharmaceutical
R; 671	Etodolac	400 mg	Peach	Extended-Release Tablet	Oval, Film-Coated	Purepac Pharmaceutical
R; 672	Spironolactone	50 mg	White	Coated Tablet	Oval	Purepac Pharmaceutical
R; 673	Spironolactone	100 mg	White	Coated Tablet	Circle	Purepac Pharmaceutical
R; 679	Famotidine	20 mg	Yellow	Coated Tablet	Circle	Purepac Pharmaceutical
R; 704	Fluvoxamine Maleate	25 mg	Green	Coated Tablet	Capsule-Shape	Purepac Pharmaceutical
R; 706	Lisinopril and Hydrocholorthiazide	10 mg; 12.5 mg	White to Off White	Tablet	Circle	Purepac Pharmaceutical
R; 707	Lisinopril and Hydrochlorothiazide	20 mg; 12.5 mg	Yellow	Tablet	Circle	Purepac Pharmaceutical
R; 708	Lisinopril and Hydrochlorothiazide	20 mg; 25 mg	Pink, Mottled	Tablet	Circle	Purepac Pharmaceutical
R; 711	Isosorbide Mononitrate	60 mg	Tan	Extended-Release Tablet	Oval, Bisected, Film-Coated Scored	Purepac Pharmaceutical
R; 713	Isosorbide Mononitrate	30 mg	White	Extended-Release Tablet	Oval, Bisected, Film-Coated Scored	Purepac Pharmaceutical
R; 714	Tramadol Hydrochloride	50 mg	White	Coated Tablet	Oval	Purepac Pharmaceutical
R; 715	Metformin Hydrochloride	850 mg	White to Off-White	Coated Tablet	Oval	Purepac Pharmaceutical
R; 717	Diclofenac Sodium	100 mg	Yellow	Extended-Release Tablet	Circle, Coated, Beveled Edge	Purepac Pharmaceutical
R; 718	Metformin Hydrochloride	1000 mg	White to Off-White	Coated Tablet	Oval	Purepac Pharmaceutical
R 741	Tizanidine Hydrochloride	4 mg	Yellow	Tablet	Circle	Purepac Pharmaceutical
R 742	Tizanidine Hydrochloride	2 mg	Yellow	Tablet	Capsule-Shape	Purepac Pharmaceutical
R; 743	Diclofenac Sodium Delayed-Release	50 mg	White	Enteric-Coated Tablet	Circle	Purepac Pharmaceutical
R; 743	Diclofenac Sodium Delayed-Release	50 mg	White	Enteric-Coated Tablet	Circle	Sidmak Laboratories
R; 744	Diclofenac Sodium Delayed-Release	75 mg	White	Enteric-Coated Tablet	Circle	Purepac Pharmaceutical
R; 744	Diclofenac Sodium Delayed-Release	75 mg	White	Enteric-Coated Tablet	Circle	Sidmak Laboratories
R; 745	Naproxen Delayed-Release	375 mg	Yellow	Delayed-Release Tablet	Capsule-Shape	Pliva
R; 745	Naproxen Delayed-Release	375 mg	Yellow	Enteric-Coated Tablet	Capsule-Shape	Purepac Pharmaceutical
R; 745	Naproxen Delayed-Release	375 mg	Yellow	Enteric-Coated Tablet	Capsule-Shape	Sidmak Laboratories
R; 746	Naproxen Delayed-Release	500 mg	Green	Delayed-Release Tablet	Capsule-Shape	Pliva
R; 746	Naproxen Delayed-Release	500 mg	Green	Enteric-Coated Tablet	Capsule-Shape	Purepac Pharmaceutical
R; 746	Naproxen Delayed-Release	500 mg	Green	Enteric-Coated Tablet	Capsule-Shape	Sidmak Laboratories
R; 747	Pentoxifylline	400 mg	Yellow	Extended-Release Tablet	Capsule-Shape, Film-Coated	Purepac Pharmaceutical
R; 747	Pentoxifylline	400 mg	Yellow	Extended-Release Tablet	Capsule-Shape, Film-Coated	Sidmak Laboratories
R; 1103;	Acetaminophen	325 mg	White	Tablet	Circle, Scored	Purepac Pharmaceutical
R; 1511;	Quinine Sulfate	325 mg	Clear	Capsule		Purepac Pharmaceutical
R; 1840	Pramocon	18 mg; 5000 IU; 400 IU; 30 IU; 120 mg; 800 mcg; 1.5 mg; 1.7 mg; 20 mg; 4 mg; 12 mcg; 250 mg; 150 mcg; 100 mg		Coated Tablet		Ross Laboratories
R; 2577	Diltiazem Hydrochloride	180 mg	Dark Green and Aqua Blue	Extended-Release Capsule		Purepac Pharmaceutical
R; 2578	Diltiazem Hydrochloride	240 mg	Dark Green	Extended-Release Capsule		Purepac Pharmaceutical
R; 2579	Diltiazem Hydrochloride	300 mg	Dark Green and Light Gray	Extended-Release Capsule		Purepac Pharmaceutical
R; 2588	Diltiazem Hydrochloride	120 mg	Light Gray	Extended-Release Capsule		Purepac Pharmaceutical
R; 2598	Doxycycline Hyclate	100 mg	Dark Yellow, Clear Body and Cap with Yellow Pellets	Timed-Release Capsule		Purepac Pharmaceutical
R; 4374	Propoxyphene with Aspirin and Caffeine	389 mg; 32.4 mg; 65 mg		Capsule		Rugby Laboratories
R; 4374	Propoxyphene with Aspirin and Caffeine	389 mg; 32.4 mg; 65 mg		Capsule		Teva Pharmaceuticals
R; 4956	Triamterene and Hydrochlorothiazide	75 mg; 50 mg	Yellow	Tablet		Watson Laboratories
R; 5726	Rondec	4 mg; 60 mg	Orange	Coated Tablet		Biovail Pharmaceuticals
R; 6240	Rondec-TR	8 mg; 120 mg	Blue	Timed-Release Tablet		Biovail Pharmaceuticals
R; 7621	VI-Daylin/f Multivitamin Plus Iron Chewable Tablet	12 mg; 1 mg; 2500 IU; 400 IU; 15 IU; 60 mg; 0.3 mg; 1.05 mg; 1.2 mg; 1.05 mg; 4.5 mcg; 13.5 mg		Tablet, Chewable		Ross Products
R; 7626	VI-Daylin/f Multivitamin Chewable Tablet	1 mg; 2500 IU; 400 IU; 15 IU; 0.3 mg; 1.05 mg; 1.2 mg; 13.5 mg; 60 mg; 1.05 mg; 4.5 mg		Tablet, Chewable		Ross Products

IMPRINT	BRAND/GENERIC NAME	STRENGTH	COLOR	FORM	SHAPE	MANUFACTURER
R (PUREPAC LOGO); 334	Prednisone	2.5 mg	White	Tablet	Circle	Purepac Pharmaceutical
R (PUREPAC LOGO); 336	Prednisone	5 mg	White	Tablet	Circle, Flat Beveled; Scored	Purepac Pharmaceutical
R (PUREPAC LOGO); 337	Prednisone	20 mg	Peach	Tablet	Circle, Flat Beveled; Scored	Purepac Pharmaceutical
R (PUREPAC LOGO); 338	Prednisone	10 mg	White	Tablet	Circle, Flat Beveled; Scored	Purepac Pharmaceutical
R&C; 730	Syntrogel	120 mg; 220 mg		Tablet, Chewable		Reed & Carnrick Pharmaceuticals
RACHELLE; 202	Tetrachel	250 mg	Orange and Yellow	Capsule		Rachelle Laboratories
RACHELLE; 315	Chlordiazachel	5 mg	Green and Yellow	Capsule		Rachelle Laboratories
RACHELLE; 316	Chlordiazachel	10 mg	Black and Green	Capsule		Rachelle Laboratories
RACHELLE; 317	Chlordiazachel	25 mg	Green and Gray	Capsule		Rachelle Laboratories
RACHELLE; 556	Doxycycline	50 mg	Blue and White	Capsule		Rachelle Laboratories
RACHELLE; 557	Doxycycline	100 mg	Blue	Capsule		Rachelle Laboratories
RAPAMUNE; 1 MG	Rapamune	1 mg	White	Tablet	Triangle	Wyeth Pharmaceuticals
RC; 80	Panixine Disperdose	125 mg	Light Yellow	Tablet	Capsule-Shape, Scored	Ranbaxy Pharmaceuticals
RC; 81	Panixine Disperdose	250 mg	Light Yellow	Tablet	Capsule-Shape, Scored	Ranbaxy Pharmaceuticals
RD; 12	Nephro-Vite RX Vitamin B Complex and C Supplement	10 mg; 1.5 mg; 60 mcg; 1.7 mg; 60 mg; 1 mg; 300 mcg; 20 mg; 10 mg	Yellow	Tablet	Circle	Watson Laboratories
RD; 13	Nephro-Fer	350 mg	Brown	Capsule		Watson Laboratories
RDY; 342	Citalopram Hydrobromide	10 mg	Brown	Tablet	Circle	DR Reddy's Laboratories
RDY; 343	Citalopram Hydrobromide	20 mg	Pink	Tablet	Circle	DR Reddy's Laboratories
RDY 344	Citalopram Hydrobromide	40 mg	White	Tablet	Circle	DR Reddy's Laboratories
REBETOL; 200 MG; SCHERING LOGO	Rebetol	200 mg	White	Capsule		Schering
REDUX	Redux	15 mg	Opaque White	Capsule		Wyeth-Ayerst Laboratories
REGLAN; 5; SP;	Reglan	5 mg	Green	Tablet	Circle	Schwarz Pharma
REGLAN; SP; 10;	Reglan	10 mg	Pink	Tablet	Capsule-Shape	Schwarz Pharma
RELAFEN; 500	Relafen	500 mg	White	Coated Tablet	Oval	Glaxosmithkline
RELAFEN; 750	Relafen	750 mg	Beige	Tablet	Oblong	Glaxosmithkline
RENAGEL; 400	Renagel	400 mg	White	Coated Tablet	Oval	Genzyme
RENAGEL; 800	Renagel	800 mg	White	Coated Tablet	Oval	Genzyme
REP; 20; PFIZER	Relpax	20 mg	Orange	Tablet	Circle	Pfizer Laboratories
REP; 40; PFIZER	Relpax	40 mg	Orange	Tablet	Circle	Pfizer Laboratories
RESCON JR	Rescon JR	60 mg; 4 mg	White and Clear	Extended-Release Capsule		Capellon Pharmaceuticals
RESCON-ED	Rescon-Ed	120 mg; 8 mg	Green and Clear	Timed-Release Capsule		Capellon Pharmaceuticals
RESCRIPTOR; 200 MG	Rescriptor	200 mg	White	Tablet	Capsule-Shape	Agouron Pharmaceuticals
RESTORIL 7.5 MG; FOR SLEEP	Restoril	7.5 mg	Blue and Pink	Capsule		Mallinckrodt
RESTORIL 15 MG; FOR SLEEP	Restoril	15 mg	Maroon and Pink	Capsule		Mallinckrodt
RESTORIL 30 MG; FOR SLEEP	Restoril	30 mg	Maroon and Blue	Capsule		Mallinckrodt
RG; F50	Fluconazole	50 mg	White or Almost White	Tablet	Rounded Rectangle	Barr Laboratories
RG; F100	Fluconazole	100 mg	White or Almost White	Tablet	Rounded Rectangle	Barr Laboratories
RG; F150	Fluconazole	150 mg	White or Almost White	Tablet	Oblong, Convex	Barr Laboratories
RG; F200	Fluconazole	200 mg	White or Almost White	Tablet	Rounded Rectangle	Barr Laboratories
RHEABAN	Rheaban Maximum Strength	750 mg	White	Tablet		Pfizer Consumer Health Care
RIB; 200; ROCHE	Copegus	200 mg	Light Pink	Tablet	Oval	Roche Laboratories
RIFADIN; 150;	Rifadin	150 mg	Maroon and Scarlet	Capsule		Aventis Pharmaceuticals
RIFADIN; 300;	Rifadin	300 mg	Maroon and Scarlet	Capsule		Aventis Pharmaceuticals
RIFAMATE	Rifamate	300 mg; 150 mg	Red	Capsule		Aventis Pharmaceuticals
RIFATER	Rifater	120 mg; 50 mg; 300 mg	Light Beige	Coated Tablet	Circle	Aventis Pharmaceuticals
RIKER; 125; PLUS	Theolair-Plus	125 mg; 100 mg		Tablet	Circle	3m Pharmaceuticals
RIKER; 161	Disipal	50 mg	Green	Tablet	Circle	3m Pharmaceuticals
RIKER; 193	Estomul-M	500 mg; 45 mg	Pink	Tablet	Capsule-Shape	3m Pharmaceuticals
RIKER; 250; PLUS	Theolair-Plus	250 mg; 200 mg		Tablet		3m Pharmaceuticals
RIKER; 265	Rauwiloid	2 mg	Brown	Tablet	Circle	3m Pharmaceuticals
RIKER; TEPANIL	Tepanil	25 mg	White	Tablet		3m Pharmaceuticals
RIKER; TEPANIL; TEN-TAB	Tepanil Ten-Tab	75 mg	White	Timed-Release Tablet		3m Pharmaceuticals
RIOPAN	Riopan	480 mg		Tablet, Chewable		Wyeth Consumer Healthcare
RIOPAN;	Riopan	480 mg		Tablet		Wyeth Consumer Healthcare
RIOPAN PLUS	Riopan Plus	480 mg; 20 mg		Tablet, Chewable		Wyeth Consumer Healthcare
RIS; 120	Natafolic-Ob	2700 IU; 70 mg; 400 IU; 30 IU; 1.6 mg; 1.8 mg; 19 mg; 12 mcg; 100 mg; 65 mg; 25 mg; 25 mg; 2 mg	Light Blue	Tablet	Capsule-Shape	Rising Pharmaceuticals
RL	Antacid No. 2	356 mg; 162 mg	White	Tablet	Circle	Richlyn Laboratories
RL	Calcium Gluconate	650 mg	White	Tablet	Circle	Richlyn Laboratories
RL;	Marinol	2.5 mg	White	Capsule, Liquid Filled	Circle	Roxane Laboratories
RL;	Marinol	2.5 mg	White	Capsule, Liquid Filled	Circle	Unimed
RL;	Marinol	5 mg	Dark Brown	Capsule, Liquid Filled	Circle	Roxane Laboratories
RL;	Marinol	5 mg	Dark Brown	Capsule, Liquid Filled	Circle	Unimed
RL;	Marinol	10 mg	Orange	Capsule, Liquid Filled		Roxane Laboratories

IMPRINT	BRAND/GENERIC NAME	STRENGTH	COLOR	FORM	SHAPE	MANUFACTURER
RL;	Marinol	10 mg	Orange	Capsule, Liquid Filled		Unimed
RO; L3	Boniva	2.5 mg	White	Tablet	Oblong	Roche Laboratories
ROBAXIN; 500; SP	Robaxin	500 mg	Light Orange	Coated Tablet	Circle	Schwarz Pharma
ROBAXIN; 750; SP	Robaxin-750	750 mg	Orange	Coated Tablet	Capsule-Shape	Schwarz Pharma
ROBITAB; 8217	Robicillin VK	250 mg	White	Tablet	Circle, Scored	Wyeth Consumer Healthcare
ROBITAB; 8227	Robicillin VK	500 mg	White	Tablet	Circle, Scored	Wyeth Consumer Healthcare
ROBITAB; 8317	Robimycin	250 mg	Green	Enteric-Coated Tablet		Wyeth Consumer Healthcare
ROCALTROL; 0.25; ROCHE;	Rocaltrol	0.25 mcg	Light Orange	Capsule, Liquid Filled	Oval	Roche Laboratories
ROCALTROL; 0.5; ROCHE;	Rocaltrol	0.5 mcg	Dark Orange	Capsule, Liquid Filled	Oblong	Roche Laboratories
ROCHE; 0245	Invirase	200 mg	Opaque Light Brown and Green	Capsule, Liquid Filled		Roche Laboratories
ROCHE; 0246	Fortovase	200 mg	Opaque Beige	Capsule, Liquid Filled		Roche Laboratories
ROCHE; 05; KLONOPIN	Klonopin	0.5 mg	Orange	Tablet	Circle, K-Shaped Perforation	Roche Pharmaceuticals
ROCHE; 1; KLONOPIN	Klonopin	1 mg	Blue	Tablet	Circle, K-Shaped Perforation	Roche Pharmaceuticals
ROCHE; 2; KLONOPIN	Klonopin	2 mg	White	Tablet	Circle, K-Shaped Perforation	Roche Pharmaceuticals
ROCHE; 16	Noludar	50 mg	White	Tablet		Roche Laboratories
ROCHE; 17	Noludar	200 mg	White	Tablet		Roche Laboratories
ROCHE; 19	Noludar	50 mg	Purple and White	Capsule		Roche Laboratories
ROCHE; 75 MG	Tamiflu	75 mg	Grey and Light Yellow with Blue Ink	Capsule		Hoffmann-LA Roche
ROCHE; 136	Valcaps	2 mg	Blue and White	Capsule		Roche Pharmaceuticals
ROCHE; 137	Valcaps	5 mg	Blue and Yellow	Capsule		Roche Pharmaceuticals
ROCHE; 139	Valcaps	10 mg	Black and Blue	Capsule		Roche Pharmaceuticals
ROCHE; 274	Anaprox	275 mg	Blue	Tablet	Oval, Biconvex	Roche Laboratories
ROCHE; BUMEX 0.5	Bumex	0.5 mg	Light Green	Tablet	Oval	Roche Pharmaceuticals
ROCHE; BUMEX 1	Bumex	1 mg	Yellow	Tablet	Oval	Roche Pharmaceuticals
ROCHE; BUMEX 2	Bumex	2 mg	Peach	Tablet	Oval	Roche Pharmaceuticals
ROCHE; AZO; GANTANOL	Azo Gantanol	0.5 GM; 100 mg	Red	Coated Tablet		Roche Pharmaceuticals
ROCHE; AZO; GANTRISIN	Azo Gantrisin	500 mg; 50 mg	Red	Coated Tablet		Roche Pharmaceuticals
ROCHE; C; MOGADON; 5	Mogadon	5 mg	White	Tablet	Barrel, Biplane, Scored	Icn Pharmaceuticals
ROCHE; C; MOGADON; 10	Mogadon	10 mg	White	Tablet	Barrel, Biplane, Scored	Icn Pharmaceuticals
ROCHE; CYTOVENE; 250	Cytovene	250 mg	Opaque Green	Capsule		Roche Laboratories
ROCHE; GANTRISIN	Gantrisin	0.5 GM	White	Tablet	Circle, Scored	Roche Pharmaceuticals
ROCHE; MARPLAN	Marplan	10 mg	Peach	Tablet	Circle, Scored	Hoffmann-LA Roche
ROCHE; POSICOR; 50	Posicor	50 mg	Pale Yellow	Tablet	Biconvex, Hexagon	Roche Laboratories
ROCHE; POSICOR; 100	Posicor	100 mg	Light Orange	Tablet	Biconvex, Hexagon	Roche Laboratories
ROCHE; PROSTIGMIN	Prostigmin	15 mg	White	Tablet		Roche Laboratories
ROCHE; XENICAL; 120	Xenical	120 mg	Dark Blue	Capsule		Roche Laboratories
ROERIG; 038	Unasyn	375 mg		Tablet		Roerig
ROERIG; 143	Geocillin	382 mg	Yellow	Tablet		Roerig
ROERIG; 159; TAO;	Tao	250 mg	White	Capsule		Roerig
ROERIG; 201	Bonine	25 mg		Tablet, Chewable		Pfizer Consumer Health Care
ROERIG; 254; MARAX	Marax	10 mg; 25 mg; 130 mg	White	Tablet	Four-Sided	Roerig
ROERIG; 338	Diflucan	50 mg		Capsule		Roerig
ROERIG; 339	Diflucan	100 mg		Capsule		Roerig
ROERIG; 340	Diflucan	200 mg		Capsule		Roerig
ROERIG; 504; HEPTUNA PLUS;	Heptuna Plus	311 mg; 50 mg; 5 mcg; 25 mg; 3.1 mg; 2 mg; 1.6 mg; 150 mg; 15 mg; 0.9 mg; 1 mg; 0.2 mg; 37.4 mg; 0.05 mg; 0.033 mg; 2 mg; 29 mg; 1.7 mg	Red and White	Capsule	Oval	Roerig
ROERIG; 566	Lithane	300 mg	Green	Tablet		Roerig
ROERIG; 627	Vitamin E	200 IU	Clear Yellow	Capsule, Liquid Filled		Pfizer Roerig
ROERIG; 628	Vitamin E	400 IU	Light Yellow	Capsule, Liquid Filled		Pfizer Roerig
ROERIG; 991	Vitamin E	600 IU	Light Yellow	Capsule, Liquid Filled		Pfizer Roerig
RORER; 82	Lozol	2.5 mg	White	Tablet	Circle	Aventis Pharmaceuticals
ROWELL; 1224	Vio-Geric	18 mg; 5,000 units; 400 units; 30 units; 60 mg; 0.4 mg; 5 mg; 5 mg; 20 mg; 2.4 mg; 6 mcg; 0.22 GM; 0.125 GM; 150 mcg; 100 mg; 2 mg; 15 mg	Red	Tablet	Oval	Solvay Pharmaceuticals
ROWELL; 2406	C-Ron FA	200 mg; 600 mg	Red	Tablet	Circle	Reid-Rowell Pharmaceutical
ROWELL; 3604	Colrex	2 mg; 5 mg; 325 mg	Orange	Capsule		Solvay Pharmaceuticals
RP; 51	Dextroamphetamine Sulfate	5 mg	Yellow	Tablet		Rexar Pharmacal
RP; 51	Dextrostat	5 mg	Yellow	Tablet	Circle, Scored	Shire Pharmaceuticals

IMPRINT	BRAND/GENERIC NAME	STRENGTH	COLOR	FORM	SHAPE	MANUFACTURER
RP; 52	Dextroamphetamine Sulfate	10 mg	Yellow	Tablet	Circle, Scored	Rexar Pharmacal
RP; 52	Dextrostat	10 mg	Yellow	Tablet	Circle, Double-Scored	Shire Pharmaceuticals
RPC	Dextroamphetamine Sulfate	15 mg		Timed-Release Capsule		Rexar Pharmacal
RPC; 052	Colace	50 mg	Clear Dark Red with Clear Pink Fill	Capsule, Liquid Filled	Oval	Purdue
RPC; 053	Colace	100 mg	Pink-Red and Light Beige	Capsule, Liquid Filled	Oval	Purdue
RPL; 1011	Supen	250 mg		Capsule		Solvay Pharmaceuticals
RPL; 1080	G-Recillin-T	400,000 units		Tablet		Solvay Pharmaceuticals
RPL; 1101	Retet	250 mg		Capsule		Solvay Pharmaceuticals
RPL; 1108	Sumox	250 mg	Yellow and White	Capsule		Solvay Pharmaceuticals
RPL; 1109	Sumox	500 mg	Yellow and White	Capsule		Solvay Pharmaceuticals
RPL; 1222	Zide	50 mg	Peach	Tablet	Circle	Solvay Pharmaceuticals
RPL; 1234	Aquatag	50 mg	Aqua	Tablet	Circle, Scored	Solvay Pharmaceuticals
RPL; 1270	Vaso-80 Unicelles	80 mg	Grey and Clear	Capsule		Solvay Pharmaceuticals
RPL; 1340	Tora	8 mg	Orange	Tablet	Circle	Solvay Pharmaceuticals
RPL; 1501	Tuzon	250 mg; 300 mg	Purple	Tablet	Circle	Solvay Pharmaceuticals
RPL; 1654	Bacarate	35 mg	Pink	Tablet	Circle, Scored	Solvay Pharmaceuticals
RPL; 2580	Sprx-105	105 mg	Brown and Clear with White Beads	Capsule		Solvay Pharmaceuticals
RPR; 0514	Combipatch	0.05 mg/day; 0.14 mg/day		Patch	Square	Novartis
RPR; 0525	Combipatch	0.05 mg/day; 0.25 mg/day		Patch	Square	Novartis
RPR; 202	Rilutek	50 mg	White	Coated Tablet	Capsule-Shape	Aventis Pharmaceuticals
RPR; 352	Slo-Phyllin	200 mg	White	Tablet	Circle	Aventis Pharmaceuticals
RPR; 5100	Penetrex	200 mg	Light Blue	Coated Tablet	Circle	Aventis Pharmaceuticals
RPR; 5140	Penetrex	400 mg	Dark Blue	Coated Tablet	Circle	Aventis Pharmaceuticals
RPR; AD	Anti Diarrheal	2 mg	Green	Tablet		Perrigo
RR; 1	Orasone	1 mg	Pink	Tablet	Circle, Scored	Solvay Pharmaceuticals
RR; 5	Orasone 5	5 mg	White	Tablet	Circle, Scored	Solvay Pharmaceuticals
RR; 10	Orasone 10	10 mg	Blue	Tablet	Circle, Scored	Solvay Pharmaceuticals
RR; 20	Orasone 20	20 mg	Yellow	Tablet	Circle, Scored	Solvay Pharmaceuticals
RR; 50	Orasone 50	50 mg	White	Tablet	Circle, Scored	Solvay Pharmaceuticals
RR; 4140	Amantadine	100 mg	Red	Capsule		H.L. Moore
RR; 4140	Amantadine Hydrochloride	100 mg	Red	Capsule	Oval	Solvay Pharmaceuticals
RR; 7516	Lithotabs	300 mg	White	Coated Tablet		Solvay Pharmaceuticals
R-R; 4140	Amantadine Hydrochloride	100 mg	Red	Capsule	Oval	Solvay Pharmaceuticals
RS; 117	Ergoloid Mesylate	0.5 mg	White	Tablet	Oval	3m Pharmaceuticals
RS; 119	Ergoloid Mesylate	1 mg	White	Tablet	Oval	3m Pharmaceuticals
RS; 142;	Diethylpropion Hydrochloride	75 mg	White	Tablet	Oval	3m Pharmaceuticals
RSN; 5 MG	Actonel	5 mg	Yellow	Coated Tablet		Procter & Gamble
RSN; 30 MG	Actonel	30 mg	White	Coated Tablet	Oval	Procter & Gamble
RSN; 35 MG	Actonel	35 mg	Orange	Coated Tablet	Oval	Aventis Pharmaceuticals
RSN; 35 MG	Actonel	35 mg	Orange	Coated Tablet	Oval	Procter & Gamble Pharmaceuticals
RUFEN; 400	Rufen	400 mg	White	Coated Tablet	Circle	Boots Pharmaceuticals
RUFEN; 400 MG	Ibuprofen	400 mg	Pink	Tablet	Circle	Vangard Labs
RUFEN; 600	Rufen	600 mg	White	Coated Tablet	Capsule-Shape	Boots Pharmaceuticals
RUFEN; 800	Rufen	800 mg	White	Coated Tablet	Circle	Boots Pharmaceuticals
RUGBY; 3015	Aller-Chlor	4 mg; 60 mg	Light Blue	Tablet	Circle	Rugby Laboratories
RUGBY; 3406	Clorazepate Dipotassium	3.75 mg		Capsule		Rugby Laboratories
RUGBY; 3407	Clorazepate Dipotassium	7.5 mg		Capsule		Rugby Laboratories
RUGBY; 3408	Clorazepate Dipotassium	15 mg		Capsule		Rugby Laboratories
RUGBY; 3478	Aller-Chlor	12 mg	Orange	Timed-Release Tablet		Rugby Laboratories
RUGBY; 3479	Aller-Chlor	8 mg	Green and Clear	Capsule		Rugby Laboratories
RUGBY; 3730;	Doxepin Hydrochloride	100 mg	Opaque White and Yellow	Capsule		Rugby Laboratories
RUGBY; 3737	Doxepin Hydrochloride	75 mg		Capsule		Rugby Laboratories
RUGBY; 3738	Doxepin Hydrochloride	150 mg		Capsule		Rugby Laboratories
RUGBY; 3895	Hydroxyzine Pamoate	100 mg	Green and Gray	Capsule		Rugby Laboratories
RUGBY; 3899	Hydroxyzine Hydrochloride	100 mg	Fuschia	Coated Tablet	Circle	Rugby Laboratories
RUGBY; 3919	Hydrochlorothiazide	50 mg	Peach	Tablet		Rugby Laboratories
RUGBY; 3921	Hydrochlorothiazide	50 mg	Yellow	Tablet		Rugby Laboratories
RUGBY; 3922	Hydrochlorothiazide	25 mg	Peach	Tablet		Rugby Laboratories
RUGBY; 3923	Hydrochlorothiazide	100 mg	Peach	Tablet		Rugby Laboratories
RUGBY; 3990	Meclizine Hydrochloride	25 mg		Tablet, Chewable		Rugby Laboratories
RUGBY; 4028	Methocarbamol with Aspirin	400 mg; 325 mg	White and Pink	Tablet	Circle, Double-Layered	Rugby Laboratories
RUGBY; 4083	Nitroglycerin TD	2.5 mg	Amethyst and Natural	Timed-Release Capsule		Rugby Laboratories
RUGBY; 4084	Nitroglycerin TD	6.5 mg	Dark Blue and Amber	Timed-Release Capsule		Rugby Laboratories
RUGBY; 4090	Nitroglycerin TD	9 mg		Timed-Release Capsule		Rugby Laboratories
RUGBY; 4094	Nystatin	500,000 units	Brown	Coated Tablet	Circle, Convex	Rugby Laboratories
RUGBY; 4147	Perphenazine Fc	8 mg		Coated Tablet		Rugby Laboratories
RUGBY; 4339	Prenatal Plus Improved Vitamin Supplement	65 mg; 4000 IU; 400 IU; 11 mg; 1 mg; 1.5 mg; 3 mg; 20 mg; 200 mg; 2 mg; 25 mg; 120 mg; 10 mg; 12 mcg		Tablet		Rugby Laboratories
RUGBY; 4382	Propoxyphene Hydrochloride	65 mg	Pink Opaque	Capsule		Rugby Laboratories
RUGBY; 4402	Propranolol Hydrochloride and Hydrochlorothiazide	40 mg; 25 mg	White	Tablet	Circle, BI-Convex, Half-Scored	Rugby Laboratories
RUGBY; 4403	Propranolol Hydrochloride and Hydrochlorothiazide	80 mg; 25 mg	White	Tablet	Circle, BI-Convex, Half-Scored	Rugby Laboratories
RUGBY; 4427	Quinine Sulfate	325 mg		Tablet		Rugby Laboratories

IMPRINT	BRAND/GENERIC NAME	STRENGTH	COLOR	FORM	SHAPE	MANUFACTURER
RUGBY; 4579	Therapeutic Vitamin	500 mg; 15 mg; 15 mg; 100 mg; 4 mg; 18 mg; 0.5 mg; 5 mcg		Tablet		Amide Pharmaceuticals
RUGBY; 4738	Tolazamide	100 mg	White	Tablet	Circle, Biconvex, Half-Scored	Chelsea Laboratories
RUGBY; 4739	Tolazamide	250 mg	White	Tablet	Circle, Biconvex, Half-Scored	Chelsea Laboratories
RUGBY; 4744	Tolazamide	500 mg	White	Tablet	Circle, Biconvex, Half-Scored	Chelsea Laboratories
RUSS; 702	Femcet	50 mg; 325 mg; 40 mg	Lavender	Capsule		Ucb Pharma
RX; 5	Lisinopril	2.5 mg	Light Pink	Tablet		Ranbaxy Pharmaceuticals
RX; 7	Lorazepam	0.5 mg	White	Tablet	Circle	Ranbaxy Pharmaceuticals
RX; 504	Acyclovir	400 mg	White	Tablet	Oval	Akyma Pharmaceuticals
RX; 504	Acyclovir	400 mg	White	Tablet	Oval	Ranbaxy Pharmaceuticals
RX; 505	Acyclovir	800 mg	White	Tablet	Oval	Akyma Pharmaceuticals
RX; 505	Acyclovir	800 mg	White	Tablet	Oval	Ranbaxy Pharmaceuticals
RX; 509	Amoxicillin and Clavulanate Potassium	875 mg; 125 mg	White	Tablet	Oval, Scored	Ranbaxy Pharmaceuticals
RX; 514	Amoxicillin	125 mg	Pink Mottled	Tablet, Chewable	Oval, Biconvex	Purepac Pharmaceutical
RX; 514	Amoxicillin	125 mg	Pink	Tablet, Chewable	Oval	Ranbaxy Pharmaceuticals
RX; 514	Dispermox	125 mg	Pink	Tablet, Chewable	Circle	Ranbaxy Pharmaceuticals
RX; 515	Amoxicillin	250 mg	Pink Mottled	Tablet, Chewable	Circle, Flat-Faced, Bevel-Edged	Purepac Pharmaceutical
RX; 515	Amoxicillin	250 mg	Pink	Tablet, Chewable	Circle	Ranbaxy Pharmaceuticals
RX; 515	Dispermox	250 mg	Pink	Tablet, Chewable	Oval	Ranbaxy Pharmaceuticals
RX; 522	Enalapril Maleate	2.5 mg	Yellow	Tablet	Circle, Biconvex, Scored	Ohm Laboratories
RX; 522	Enalapril Maleate	2.5 mg	Yellow	Tablet	Circle, Biconvex, Scored	Purepac Pharmaceutical
RX; 522	Enalapril Maleate	2.5 mg	Yellow	Tablet	Circle, Biconvex, Scored	Ranbaxy Pharmaceuticals
RX; 523	Enalapril Maleate	5 mg	White	Tablet	Circle, Biconvex, Scored	Ohm Laboratories
RX; 523	Enalapril Maleate	5 mg	White	Tablet	Circle, Biconvex, Scored	Purepac Pharmaceutical
RX; 523	Enalapril Maleate	5 mg	White	Tablet	Circle, Biconvex, Scored	Ranbaxy Pharmaceuticals
RX; 524	Enalapril Maleate	10 mg	Red-Brown	Tablet	Circle, Biconvex	Ohm Laboratories
RX; 524	Enalapril Maleate	10 mg	Red-Brown	Tablet	Circle, Biconvex	Purepac Pharmaceutical
RX; 524	Enalapril Maleate	10 mg	Red-Brown	Tablet	Circle, Biconvex	Ranbaxy Pharmaceuticals
RX; 525	Enalapril Maleate	20 mg	Orange	Tablet	Circle, Biconvex	Ohm Laboratories
RX; 525	Enalapril Maleate	20 mg	Orange	Tablet	Circle, Biconvex	Purepac Pharmaceutical
RX; 525	Enalapril Maleate	20 mg	Orange	Tablet	Circle, Biconvex	Ranbaxy Pharmaceuticals
RX; 532	Lisinopril	5 mg	Light Pink	Tablet	Circle	Ranbaxy Pharmaceuticals
RX; 533	Lisinopril	10 mg	Light Pink	Tablet	Circle	Ranbaxy Pharmaceuticals
RX; 534	Lisinopril	20 mg		Tablet		Ranbaxy Pharmaceuticals
RX; 535	Lisinopril	40 mg		Tablet		Ranbaxy Pharmaceuticals
RX; 536	Hydrochlorothiazide and Lisinopril	12.5 mg; 10 mg	Pale Blue	Tablet	Circle	Ranbaxy Pharmaceuticals
RX; 537	Hydrochlorothiazide and Lisinopril	12.5 mg; 20 mg	Yellow	Tablet	Circle	Ranbaxy Pharmaceuticals
RX; 538	Hydrochlorothiazide and Lisinopril	25 mg; 20 mg	Peach	Tablet	Circle	Ranbaxy Pharmaceuticals
RX; 561; 4	Acetaminophen and Codeine	300 mg; 60 mg	White	Tablet	Circle	Ranbaxy Pharmaceuticals
RX; 562; 3	Acetaminophen and Codeine	300 mg; 30 mg	White	Tablet	Circle	Ranbaxy Pharmaceuticals
RX; 565	Dispermox	200 mg	Light Pink	Tablet for Suspension	Circle	Ranbaxy Pharmaceuticals
RX; 567	Dispermox	400 mg	Light Pink	Tablet for Suspension	Circle	Ranbaxy Pharmaceuticals
RX; 652	Acyclovir	200 mg	White	Capsule		Ranbaxy Pharmaceuticals
RX; 654	Amoxicillin	250 mg	Yellow	Capsule		Purepac Pharmaceutical
RX; 654	Amoxicillin	250 mg	Yellow	Capsule		Ranbaxy Pharmaceuticals
RX; 654	Dispermox	250 mg	Yellow	Capsule		Ranbaxy Pharmaceuticals
RX; 655	Amoxicillin	500 mg	Maroon and Yellow	Capsule		Purepac Pharmaceutical
RX; 655	Amoxicillin	500 mg	Maroon and Yellow	Capsule		Ranbaxy Pharmaceuticals
RX; 655	Dispermox	500 mg	Maroon	Capsule		Ranbaxy Pharmaceuticals
RX; 656	Cephalexin	250 mg	Dark Green and White	Capsule		Ranbaxy Pharmaceuticals
RX; 657	Cephalexin	500 mg	Dark Green and Light Green	Capsule		Ranbaxy Pharmaceuticals
RX; 658	Cefaclor	250 mg	Blue and Green	Capsule		Ranbaxy Pharmaceuticals
RX; 659	Cefaclor	500 mg	Blue and Green	Capsule		Ranbaxy Pharmaceuticals
RX; 675	Cephalexin	250 mg	Green and White	Capsule		Ranbaxy Pharmaceuticals
RX; 676	Cephalexin	500 mg	Dark Green and Light Green	Capsule		Ranbaxy Pharmaceuticals
RX; 677	Propoxyphene Hydrochloride	65 mg	Pink	Capsule		Ranbaxy Pharmaceuticals
RX; 678	Propoxyphene Hydrochloride Compound	389 mg; 32.4 mg; 65 mg	White and Red	Capsule		Ranbaxy Pharmaceuticals
RX; 679	Seconal Sodium	100 mg	Orange	Capsule		Ranbaxy Pharmaceuticals
RX; 680	Tuinal	50 mg; 50 mg	Blue and Orange	Capsule		Ranbaxy Pharmaceuticals
RX; 681	Nalfon 200	200 mg	White and Ocher	Capsule		Ranbaxy Pharmaceuticals
RX; 682	Nalfon	300 mg	Yellow and Ocher	Capsule		Ranbaxy Pharmaceuticals
RX; 692	Clindamycin Hydrochloride	150 mg	Blue and Light Green	Capsule		Ranbaxy Pharmaceuticals
RX; 693	Clindamycin Hydrochloride	300 mg		Capsule		Ranbaxy Pharmaceuticals
RX; 694	Minocycline Hydrochloride	50 mg	White Opaque	Capsule		Ranbaxy Pharmaceuticals
RX; 695	Minocycline Hydrochloride	75 mg	Gray Opaque	Capsule		Ranbaxy Pharmaceuticals
RX; 696	Minocycline Hydrochloride	100 mg	Opaque Gray and White	Capsule		Ranbaxy Pharmaceuticals
RX; 701	Etodolac	400 mg	Yellow	Coated Tablet	Oval	Ranbaxy Pharmaceuticals
RX; 713	Amoxicillin and Clavulanate Potassium	500 mg; 125 mg	White	Tablet	Oval, Scored	Ranbaxy Pharmaceuticals
RX; 714	Etodolac	500 mg	Blue	Coated Tablet	Oval	Ranbaxy Pharmaceuticals
RX; 715	Ofloxacin	300 mg	White	Tablet	Oblong	Ranbaxy Pharmaceuticals
RX; 716	Ofloxacin	200 mg	White	Tablet	Oblong	Ranbaxy Pharmaceuticals
RX; 717	Ofloxacin	400 mg	White	Tablet	Oblong	Ranbaxy Pharmaceuticals
RX; 736	Benazepril Hydrochloride	5 mg	Light Yellow	Tablet	Circle	Ranbaxy Pharmaceuticals
RX; 737	Benazepril Hydrochloride	10 mg	Dark Yellow	Tablet	Circle	Ranbaxy Pharmaceuticals
RX; 738	Benazepril Hydrochloride	20 mg	Light Pink	Tablet	Circle	Ranbaxy Pharmaceuticals
RX; 739	Benazepril Hydrochloride	40 mg	Dark Pink	Tablet	Circle	Ranbaxy Pharmaceuticals
RX; 741	Phenobarbital	15 mg	White	Tablet		Ranbaxy Pharmaceuticals
RX; 742	Phenobarbital	30 mg	White	Tablet		Ranbaxy Pharmaceuticals
RX; 743	Phenobarbital	60 mg	White	Tablet		Ranbaxy Pharmaceuticals

IMPRINT	BRAND/GENERIC NAME	STRENGTH	COLOR	FORM	SHAPE	MANUFACTURER
RX; 744	Phenobarbital	100 mg	White	Tablet		Ranbaxy Pharmaceuticals
RX; 745	Morphine Sulfate	10 mg	White	Tablet		Ranbaxy Pharmaceuticals
RX; 746	Morphine Sulfate	15 mg	White	Tablet		Ranbaxy Pharmaceuticals
RX; 747	Morphine Sulfate	30 mg	White	Tablet		Ranbaxy Pharmaceuticals
RX; 748	Codeine Phosphate	30 mg	White	Tablet		Ranbaxy Pharmaceuticals
RX; 749	Codeine Phosphate	60 mg	White	Tablet		Ranbaxy Pharmaceuticals
RX; 751	Cefuroxime Axetil	250 mg	Blue	Tablet	Capsule-Shape	Ranbaxy Pharmaceuticals
RX; 751	Cefuroxime Axetil	250 mg	Blue	Tablet	Capsule-Shape	Udl Laboratories
RX; 752	Cefuroxime	500 mg	Blue	Tablet	Oblong	Ranbaxy Pharmaceuticals
RX; 752	Cefuroxime Axetil	500 mg	Blue	Tablet		Ranbaxy Pharmaceuticals
RX; 752	Cefuroxime Axetil	500 mg	Blue	Tablet	Capsule-Shape	Udl Laboratories
RX; 753	Amoxicillin and Clavulanate Potassium Chewable	200 mg; 28.5 mg	Pink	Tablet	Circle	Ranbaxy Pharmaceuticals
RX; 754	Amoxicillin and Clavulanate Potassium Chewable	400 mg; 57 mg	Pink	Tablet	Circle	Ranbaxy Pharmaceuticals
RX; 760	Amoxicillin	200 mg	Pink	Tablet, Chewable		Ranbaxy Pharmaceuticals
RX; 760	Dispermox	200 mg	Pink	Tablet, Chewable	Circle	Ranbaxy Pharmaceuticals
RX; 761	Amoxicillin	400 mg	Pink	Tablet, Chewable		Ranbaxy Pharmaceuticals
RX; 761	Dispermox	400 mg	Pink	Tablet, Chewable	Circle	Ranbaxy Pharmaceuticals
RX; 762	Amoxicillin	500 mg	Pink	Tablet	Capsule-Shape	Ranbaxy Pharmaceuticals
RX; 762	Dispermox	500 mg	Pink	Tablet	Capsule-Shape	Ranbaxy Pharmaceuticals
RX; 763	Amoxicillin	875 mg	Pink	Tablet	Capsule-Shape	Ranbaxy Pharmaceuticals
RX; 763	Dispermox	875 mg	Pink	Tablet	Capsule-Shape	Ranbaxy Pharmaceuticals
RX; 773	Lorazepam	1 mg		Tablet		Ranbaxy Pharmaceuticals
RX; 774	Lorazepam	2 mg	White	Tablet	Circle	Ranbaxy Pharmaceuticals
RX860	Metformin Hydrochloride	500 mg	Off White	Tablet, Extended Release	Capsule-Shape	Ranbaxy Pharmaceuticals
RYMED	Rymed	30 mg; 250 mg	Maroon and Clear	Capsule		Edwards
RYNA; 1708	Ryna-12x	25 mg; 60 mg; 200 mg	Blue	Tablet	Oval, Scored	Medpointe
S	Brexin	60 mg; 30 mg; 100 mg	Maroon and Yellow	Capsule		Savage Laboratories
S	Sanctura	20 mg	Brownish Yellow	Tablet	Circle	Odyssey Pharmaceuticals
S	Senokot	8.6 mg	Brown	Tablet		Purdue Pharmaceutical Products
S	Sleep-Eze 3	25 mg	Yellow	Tablet		Whitehall Laboratories
S	Sominex Maximum Strength Formula	50 mg	Light Blue	Tablet	Oblong	Glaxosmithkline Consumer
S	Sominex Original Formula	25 mg	Light Blue	Tablet	Circle	Glaxosmithkline Consumer
S; 009;	Chlor-Trimeton Allergy 12 Hour	12 mg	Yellow-Orange	Sustained-Release Tablet	Circle	Schering-Plough Healthcare Products
S 063	Agrylin	0.5 mg	White	Capsule		Shire
S 064	Agrylin	1 mg	Gray	Capsule		Shire
S; 5	Selegiline Hydrochloride	5 mg	White	Tablet	Shield-Shape	Mylan Pharmaceuticals
S; 11	Selegiline Hydrochloride	5 mg	White	Tablet	Circle	Stada
S; 15; WYETH; 317	Serax	15 mg	Yellow	Tablet	Five-Sided	Faulding Laboratories
S; 19; STORZ	Storzolamide	250 mg	White	Tablet	Circle	Lederle Laboratories
S; 20	Penicillin V Potassium	250 mg	White	Tablet	Oval	Stada
S; 20; LESCOL	Lescol	20 mg	Brown and Light Brown	Capsule		Novartis Pharmaceuticals
S; 21	Penicillin V Potassium	500 mg	White	Tablet	Oval	Stada
S; 40; LESCOL	Lescol	40 mg	Brown and Gold	Capsule		Novartis Pharmaceuticals
S; 62	Seasonale	0.15 mg; 0.03 mg	Pink	Tablet	Circle	Barr Laboratories
S; 78-2	Mellaril	10 mg	Bright Chartreuse	Coated Tablet		Novartis
S; 78-8	Mellaril	15 mg	Pink	Coated Tablet		Novartis
S; 78/22;	Bellergal	20 mg; 0.3 mg; 0.1 mg	Pink	Coated Tablet	Circle	Novartis Pharmaceuticals
S; 78; 240	Sandimmune	25 mg	Pink	Capsule	Oval	Novartis Pharmaceuticals
S; 78; 241	Sandimmune	100 mg	Dusty Rose	Capsule	Oblong	Novartis Pharmaceuticals
S; 78; 242	Sandimmune	50 mg	Yellow	Capsule	Oblong	Novartis Pharmaceuticals
S190	Lunesta	1 mg	Light Blue	Tablet	Circle	Sepracor
S191	Lunesta	2 mg	White	Tablet	Circle	Sepracor
S193	Lunesta	3 mg	Dark Blue	Tablet	Circle	Sepracor
S; 374	Chlor-Trimeton Allergy	8 mg	Yellow	Sustained-Release Tablet		Schering-Plough Healthcare Products
S405; 250	Fosrenol	250 mg	White to Off White	Tablet, Chewable		Shire Pharmaceuticals
S405; 500	Fosrenol	500 mg	White to Off White	Tablet, Chewable		Shire Pharmaceuticals
S; 770	Sorbitrate	5 mg	Green	Tablet	Oval, Scored	Astra Zeneca
S; 780	Sorbitrate	10 mg	Yellow	Tablet	Oval, Scored	Astra Zeneca
S; 810	Sorbitrate	5 mg	Green	Tablet, Chewable	Circle, Scored	Astra Zeneca
S; 820	Sorbitrate	20 mg	Blue	Tablet	Oval, Scored	Astra Zeneca
S; 820	Sorbitrate	20 mg	Blue	Tablet	Oval, Scored	Professional Pharmaceutical
S; 3581	Satric	250 mg	White	Tablet	Circle	Savage Laboratories
S; 3681	Satric	250 mg	White	Tablet	Circle, Convex	Savage Laboratories
S; 3688	Satric	500 mg		Tablet		Savage Laboratories
S; 4140;	Symadine	100 mg	Red	Capsule, Liquid Filled		Solvay Pharmaceuticals
S; 5182	Estrocon	0.625 mg		Tablet		Savage Laboratories
S; 5185	Estrocon	1.25 mg		Tablet		Savage Laboratories
S; AHG;	Naqua	2 mg	Pink	Tablet	Character-Shape, Scored	Schering
S; AHH;	Naqua	4 mg	Aqua	Tablet	Character-Shape, Scored	Schering
S; ANB;	Etrafon-A	4 mg; 10 mg	Orange	Coated Tablet		Schering
S; ANE;	Etrafon-Forte	25 mg; 4 mg	Red	Coated Tablet		Schering-Plough
S; CAFERGOT	Cafergot	100 mg; 1 mg	Tan	Coated Tablet		Novartis Pharmaceuticals
S; HYDERGINE; LC; 1 MG	Hydergine Lc	1 mg	Off White	Capsule		Novartis
S; HYDERGINE 1;	Hydergine	1 mg	White	Tablet	Circle	Novartis
S; MELLARIL; 25	Mellaril	25 mg	Light Tan	Coated Tablet		Novartis
S; MELLARIL; 50	Mellaril	50 mg	White	Coated Tablet		Novartis
S; MELLARIL; 100	Mellaril	100 mg	Light Green	Coated Tablet		Novartis

IMPRINT	BRAND/GENERIC NAME	STRENGTH	COLOR	FORM	SHAPE	MANUFACTURER
S; MELLARIL; 150	Mellaril	150 mg	Yellow	Coated Tablet		Novartis
S; MELLARIL; 200	Mellaril	200 mg	Pink	Coated Tablet		Novartis
S CAFERGOT; P-B 78/35 SUPPOSITORY	Cafergot P-B	2 mg; 100 mg; 0.25 mg; 60 mg		Suppository		Novartis Pharmaceuticals
S F C; SANDOZ 78-107;	Fiorinal with Codeine	325 mg; 50 mg; 40 mg; 30 mg	Blue and Yellow	Capsule		Watson Laboratories
S/T; DS; 911	Sulfamethoxazole and Trimethoprim	800 mg; 160 mg	White	Tablet	Oval, Convex, Scored	Teva Pharmaceuticals
SAL; 5;	Salagen	5 mg	White	Coated Tablet	Circle	Mgi Pharma
SAL; 7.5	Salagen	7.5 mg	Blue	Tablet	Circle	Mgi Pharma
SANDOZ; 78; 36;	Cafergot P-B	0.125 mg; 100 mg; 1 mg; 30 mg	Green	Coated Tablet		Novartis Pharmaceuticals
SANDOZ; 78; 38	Cedilanid	0.5 mg	Salmon	Coated Tablet		Novartis Pharmaceuticals
SANDOZ; 78; 45;	Glysennid	12 mg	Rose	Coated Tablet		Novartis Consumer
SANDOZ; 78; 45;	Glysennid	12 mg	Rose	Coated Tablet		Sandoz Consumer Pharmaceuticals
SANDOZ; 78; 48	Gynergen	1 mg	Ivory Gray	Coated Tablet		Novartis
SANDOZ; 78; 54	Methergine	0.2 mg	Purple	Tablet		Novartis Pharmaceuticals
SANDOZ; 78; 58	Sansert	2 mg	Yellow	Coated Tablet	Circle	Novartis Pharmaceuticals
SANDOZ; 78; 64	Torecan	10 mg	Yellow	Tablet		Novartis Consumer
SANDOZ; 78; 64	Torecan	10 mg	Yellow	Tablet		Sandoz Consumer Pharmaceuticals
SANDOZ; 78; 66	Sanorex	2 mg	White	Tablet	Circle, Scored	Novartis Pharmaceuticals
SANDOZ; 78/71;	Sanorex	1 mg	White	Tablet	Elliptical; Scored	Novartis Pharmaceuticals
SANDOZ; PAMELOR 10 MG	Pamelor	10 mg	Orange and White	Capsule		Mallinckrodt
SANDOZ; PAMELOR 25 MG	Pamelor	25 mg	Orange and White	Capsule		Mallinckrodt
SANDOZ; PAMELOR 50 MG	Pamelor	50 mg	White	Capsule		Mallinckrodt
SANDOZ; PAMELOR 75 MG	Pamelor	75 mg	Orange	Capsule		Mallinckrodt
SANDOZ; S	Belladenal Spacetabs	0.25 mg; 50 mg	Multi-Colored	Tablet		Novartis Pharmaceuticals
SANDOZ-S; 78; 33	Caffergot	2 mg; 100 mg;		Suppository		Novartis Pharmaceuticals
SANDOZ-S;	Bellergal Spacetabs	0.2 mg; 0.6 mg; 40 mg	Multi-Colored	Tablet		Novartis
SANKYO; C; 12	Benicar	5 mg	Yellow	Coated Tablet	Circle	Sankyo
SANKYO; C; 14	Benicar	20 mg	White	Coated Tablet	Circle	Sankyo
SANKYO; C01	Welchol	625 mg	White	Coated Tablet		Sankyo
SANKYO; C22	Benicar HCT	20 mg; 12.5 mg	Reddish-Yellow	Tablet	Circle	Sankyo
SANKYO; C23	Benicar HCT	40 mg; 12.5 mg	Reddish-Yellow	Tablet	Oval	Sankyo
SANKYO; C25	Benicar HCT	40 mg; 25 mg	Pink	Tablet	Oval	Sankyo
SAVAGE LOGO; 0259	Chromagen FA	200 mg; 1 mg; 10 mcg; 250 mg	Maroon and Brown	Capsule, Liquid Filled		Savage Laboratories
SAVAGE LOGO; 0262	Chromagen Forte	460 mg; 1 mg; 10 mcg; 60 mg	Brown	Capsule, Liquid Filled		Savage Laboratories
SB; 2	Avandia	2 mg	Pink	Coated Tablet	Five-Sided	Glaxosmithkline
SB; 4	Avandia	4 mg	Orange	Coated Tablet	Five-Sided	Glaxosmithkline
SB; 8	Avandia	8 mg	Red-Brown	Coated Tablet	Five-Sided	Glaxosmithkline
SB; 39	Coreg	3.125 mg	White	Coated Tablet	Oval	Glaxosmithkline
SB; 3512; 5 MG	Dexedrine Spansule	5 mg	Brown and Clear	Extended-Release Capsule		Glaxosmithkline
SB; 3513; 10 MG	Dexedrine Spansule	10 mg	Brown and Clear	Extended-Release Capsule		Glaxosmithkline
SB; 3514; 15 MG	Dexedrine Spansule	15 mg	Brown and Clear	Extended-Release Capsule		Glaxosmithkline
SB; 4140	Coreg	6.25 mg	White	Coated Tablet	Oval	Glaxosmithkline
SB; 4141	Coreg	12.5 mg	White	Coated Tablet	Oval	Glaxosmithkline
SB; 4142	Coreg	25 mg	White	Coated Tablet	Oval	Glaxosmithkline
SB; 4890	Requip	0.25 mg	White	Coated Tablet	Five-Sided, Bevel Edged	Glaxosmithkline
SB; 4891	Requip	0.5 mg	Yellow	Coated Tablet	Five-Sided, Bevel Edged	Glaxosmithkline
SB; 4892	Requip	1 mg	Green	Coated Tablet	Five-Sided, Bevel Edged	Glaxosmithkline
SB; 4893	Requip	2 mg	Yellowish Pink	Coated Tablet	Five-Sided, Bevel Edged	Glaxosmithkline
SB; 4894	Requip	5 mg	Blue	Coated Tablet	Five-Sided, Bevel Edged	Glaxosmithkline
SB; 4895	Requip	3 mg	Red-Purple	Coated Tablet	Five-Sided, Bevel Edged	Glaxosmithkline
SB; 4896	Requip	4 mg	Pale Brown	Coated Tablet	Five-Sided, Bevel-Edged	Glaxosmithkline
SB; 5500	Albenza	200 mg	White to Off-White	Coated Tablet	Circle, Biconvex, Bevel-Edged	Glaxosmithkline
SCF	Contac Severe Cold and Flu	500 mg; 15 mg; 30 mg; 2 mg	Blue	Tablet		Glaxosmithkline Consumer
SCHEIN; 0765; 400	Ibuprofen	400 mg	White	Coated Tablet	Oblong	Schein Pharmaceutical
SCHEIN; 0766; 600	Ibuprofen	600 mg	White	Coated Tablet	Oval	Schein Pharmaceutical
SCHEIN; 2137; 800	Ibuprofen	800 mg	White	Coated Tablet	Oval	Schein Pharmaceutical
SCHERING; 011	Celestone	0.6 mg	Pink	Tablet	Circle, Compressed, Scored	Schering
SCHERING; 080	Chlor-Trimeton Allergy	4 mg		Tablet		Schering-Plough Healthcare Products
SCHERING; 095;	Polaramine Repetabs	4 mg	Light Red	Timed-Release Tablet	Oval	Schering
SCHERING; 148;	Polaramine Repetabs	6 mg	Bright Red	Timed-Release Tablet	Oval	Schering
SCHERING; 228	Fulvicin P/g	125 mg	White	Tablet	Scored, Compressed	Schering
SCHERING; 244; NORMODYNE; 100	Normodyne	100 mg	Light Brown	Coated Tablet	Circle, Scored	Key Pharmaceuticals
SCHERING; 251	Paxipam	20 mg	Orange	Tablet	Compressed, Scored	Schering
SCHERING; 311;	Oreton Methyl	10 mg	White	Tablet	Circle	Schering
SCHERING; 394;	Naquival	4 mg; 0.1 mg	Peach	Tablet		Schering-Plough Healthcare Products
SCHERING 402;	Theovent Long-Acting	125 mg	Dark Green and Yellow	Timed-Release Capsule		Schering

IMPRINT	BRAND/GENERIC NAME	STRENGTH	COLOR	FORM	SHAPE	MANUFACTURER
SCHERING; 432;	Coriforte	190 mg; 130 mg; 30 mg; 500 G; 4 mg	Red and Yellow	Capsule		Schering
SCHERING; 438; NORMODYNE; 300	Normodyne	300 mg	Blue	Coated Tablet	Circle	Key Pharmaceuticals
SCHERING; 507	Fulvicin P/g	250 mg	White	Tablet	Scored, Compressed	Schering
SCHERING; 522	Coricidin Hbp Cold & Flu	2 mg; 325 mg	Dark Pink	Tablet	Oblong	Schering-Plough Healthcare Products
SCHERING; 525	Eulexin	125 mg	Opaque, Two-Toned Brown	Capsule		Schering
SCHERING; 538	Paxipam	40 mg	White	Tablet	Compressed, Scored	Schering
SCHERING; 734	Gyne-Lotrimin	100 mg	White	Insert	Tombstone	Schering-Plough Healthcare Products
SCHERING; 752; NORMODYNE; 200	Normodyne	200 mg	White	Coated Tablet	Circle, Scored	Key Pharmaceuticals
SCHERING; 753;	Theovent Long-Acting	250 mg	Dark Green and Clear	Timed-Release Capsule		Schering
SCHERING; 820	Polaramine	2 mg	Red	Tablet	Oval, Compressed	Schering
SCHERING; 901	Chlor-Trimeton Decongestant	4 mg; 60 mg	Blue	Tablet		Schering-Plough
SCHERING; 970;	Oreton Methyl	10 mg	Pink to Lavender	Tablet	Oval	Schering
SCHERING; AGT;	Polaramine Repetabs	2 mg	Red	Tablet	Oval, Compressed	Schering
SCHERING; AUF;	Fulvicin-U/f	250 mg	White	Tablet	Compressed, Scored	Schering
SCHERING; AUG;	Fulvicin-U/f	500 mg	White	Tablet	Compressed, Scored	Schering
SCHERING; JE;	Oreton Methyl	25 mg	Peach	Tablet	Circle	Schering
SCHERING; KEM;	Meticorten	1 mg	White	Tablet	Compressed	Schering
SCHERING LOGO	Children's Coricidin Medilets	1 mg; 80 mg	Pink with Green Speckles	Tablet		Schering-Plough Healthcare Products
SCHWARZ; 053;	Fedahist Gyrocaps	10 mg; 65 mg	White and Yellow	Timed-Release Capsule		Schwarz Pharma
SCHWARZ; 055;	Fedahist Timecaps	8 mg; 120 mg	Clear	Timed-Release Capsule		Schwarz Pharma
SCHWARZ; 0920	Dilatrate-SR	40 mg	Pink and Clear with White Beads	Sustained-Release Capsule		Schwarz Pharma
SCHWARZ; 525	Ku-Zyme Hp	30000 U; 8000 U; 30000 U	White	Capsule		Schwarz Pharma
SCHWARZ; 531	Levsin	0.125 mg	White	Tablet	Circle, Scored	Schwarz Pharma
SCHWARZ; 532	Levsin SL	0.125 mg	White or Pale Blue-Green	Tablet	Eight-Sided, Scored	Schwarz Pharma
SCHWARZ; 534;	Levsin-PB	0.125 mg; 15 mg	Pink	Tablet	Circle, Scored	Schwarz Pharma
SCHWARZ; 537	Levsinex	0.375 mg	Brown and White	Extended-Release Capsule		Schwarz Pharma
SCHWARZ; 610; 10	Monoket	10 mg	White	Tablet	Circle, Scored	Schwarz Pharma
SCHWARZ 620; 20	Monoket	20 mg	White	Tablet	Circle, Scored	Schwarz Pharma
SCHWARZ; 2489; VERELAN; 180 MG	Verelan	180 mg	Yellow and Gray	Sustained-Release Capsule		Schwarz Pharma
SCHWARZ; 2490; VERELAN; 120 MG	Verelan	120 mg	Yellow	Sustained-Release Capsule		Schwarz Pharma
SCHWARZ; 2491; VERELAN; 240 MG	Verelan	240 mg	Blue and Yellow	Sustained-Release Capsule		Schwarz Pharma
SCHWARZ; 2495; VERELAN; 360 MG	Verelan	360 mg	Lavender and Yellow	Sustained-Release Capsule		Schwarz Pharma
SCHWARZ; 4085; 100 MG	Verelan Pm	100 mg	White and Amethyst	Extended-Release Capsule		Schwarz Pharma
SCHWARZ; 4086; 200 MG	Verelan Pm	200 mg	Amethyst	Extended-Release Capsule		Schwarz Pharma
SCHWARZ; 4087; 300 MG	Verelan Pm	300 mg	Lavender and Amethyst	Extended-Release Capsule		Schwarz Pharma
SCHWARZ; 4122	Ku-Zyme	1200 U; 15000 U; 15000 U	Yellow and White	Capsule		Schwarz Pharma
SCHWARZ; 4175	Kutrase	2400 U; 30000 U; 30000 U	Green and White	Capsule		Schwarz Pharma
S-CRT; 100	Somophyllin-Crt	100 mg	White and Clear	Timed-Release Capsule		Fisons Pharmaceuticals
S-CRT; 200	Somaphyllin-Crt	200 mg		Capsule, Liquid Filled		Fisons Pharmaceuticals
S-CRT; 200	Somophyllin-Crt	200 mg	White and Clear	Timed-Release Capsule		Fisons Pharmaceuticals
S-CRT; 250	Somophyllin-Crt	250 mg	White and Clear	Timed-Release Capsule		Fisons Pharmaceuticals
S-CRT; 300	Somophyllin-Crt	300 mg	White and Clear	Timed-Release Capsule		Fisons Pharmaceuticals
SCS; 3; 30	Low-Ogestrel White Tablet	0.3 mg; 0.03 mg	White	28-Day Tablet Pack	Circle	Watson Laboratories
SCS; 5658	Cyclobenzaprine Hydrochloride	10 mg	White	Coated Tablet	Circle	Schiapparelli Searle
SCS; 5762	Piroxicam	20 mg	Orange Opaque	Capsule		Schiapparelli Searle
SCS; 5762	Piroxicam	20 mg	Orange Opaque	Capsule		Scs Pharmaceuticals
SEARLE; 1/2	Haloperidol	0.5 mg	White	Tablet	Circle	Searle
SEARLE; 6	Tri-Norinyl 21-Day	0.5 mg; 35 mcg	Blue	21-Day Tablet Pack	Circle	Watson Laboratories
SEARLE; 7	Tri-Norinyl 21 Day Yellow-Green Tablet	1 mg; 35 mcg	Yellow-Green	21-Day Tablet Pack	Circle	Watson Laboratories
SEARLE; 51; 5	Enovid	5 mg; 75 mcg	Tan	Tablet	Circle	Searle
SEARLE; 61	Lomotil Tablet	2.5 mg; 0.025 mg	White	Tablet	Circle	Searle
SEARLE; 71	Demulen 1/50-21	1 mg; 50 mcg	White	21-Day Tablet Pack	Circle	Searle
SEARLE; 71	Demulen 1/50-28 White Tablet	1 mg; 50 mcg	White	28-Day Tablet Pack	Circle	Searle
SEARLE; 101; 10	Enovid	10 mg; 75 mcg	Brown	Tablet	Circle	Searle
SEARLE; 151	Demulen 1/35-21	1 mg; 0.035 mg	White	21-Day Tablet Pack	Circle	Searle
SEARLE; 151	Demulen 1/35-28 White Tablet	1 mg; 35 mcg	White	28-Day Tablet Pack	Circle	Searle
SEARLE; 501	Diulo	2.5 mg	Pink	Sustained-Release Tablet		Schiapparelli Searle
SEARLE; 511	Diulo	5 mg	Blue	Sustained-Release Tablet		Schiapparelli Searle

IMPRINT	BRAND/GENERIC NAME	STRENGTH	COLOR	FORM	SHAPE	MANUFACTURER
SEARLE; 521	Diulo	10 mg	Yellow	Sustained-Release Tablet		Schiapparelli Searle
SEARLE; 531	Chlorthalidone	25 mg	Yellow	Tablet	Circle, Scored	Searle
SEARLE; 541	Chlorthalidone	50 mg	Green	Tablet	Circle, Scored	Searle
SEARLE; 571	Furosemide	20 mg	White	Tablet	Circle, Scored	Searle
SEARLE; 581	Furosemide	40 mg	White	Tablet	Circle, Scored	Searle
SEARLE; 631	Pro-Banthine with Phenobarbital	15 mg; 15 mg	Ivory	Tablet		Searle
SEARLE; 651	Pro-Banthine P.A.	30 mg	Peach	Tablet	Capsule-Shape	Searle
SEARLE; 661	Probital	7.5 mg; 15 mg	Pink	Tablet		Searle
SEARLE; 841; 1	Haloperidol	1 mg	White	Tablet	Circle, Scored	Searle
SEARLE; 851; 2	Haloperidol	2 mg	White	Tablet	Circle, Scored	Schiapparelli Searle
SEARLE; 861; 1	Haloperidol	5 mg	White	Tablet	Circle, Scored	Schiapparelli Searle
SEARLE; 871; 10	Haloperidol	10 mg	White	Tablet	Circle, Scored	Searle
SEARLE; 881; 20	Haloperidol	20 mg	White	Tablet	Circle, Scored	Searle
SEARLE; 1001; ALDACTONE; 25	Aldactone	25 mg	Light Yellow	Coated Tablet	Circle	Searle
SEARLE; 1011; ALDACTAZIDE; 25	Aldactazide	25 mg; 25 mg	Tan	Coated Tablet	Circle	Searle
SEARLE; 1021; ALDACTAZIDE; 50	Aldactazide	50 mg; 50 mg	Tan	Coated Tablet	Circle, Scored	Searle
SEARLE; 1031; ALDACTONE; 100	Aldactone	100 mg	Peach	Coated Tablet	Circle, Scored	Searle
SEARLE; 1041; ALDACTONE; 50	Aldactone	50 mg	Light Orange	Coated Tablet	Oval, Scored	Searle
SEARLE; 1231	Aminophyllin	100 mg	White	Tablet	Circle, Scored	Searle
SEARLE; 1251	Aminophyllin	200 mg	White	Tablet	Oval, Scored	Searle
SEARLE; 1291	Amodrine	100 mg; 25 mg; 8 mg	Salmon	Tablet	Oval	Searle
SEARLE; 1301	Kiophyllin	150 mg; 15 mg; 125 mg	White	Tablet	Circle	Searle
SEARLE; 1401	Anavar	2.5 mg	White	Tablet	Oval, Scored	Searle
SEARLE; 1411; AAAA; 50	Arthrotec	50 mg; 200 mcg	White	Tablet	Circle	Searle
SEARLE; 1421; AAAA; 75	Arthrotec	75 mg; 200 mcg	White	Tablet	Circle	Searle
SEARLE; 1451	Cytotec	100 mcg	White	Tablet	Circle	Searle
SEARLE; 1461; STOMACH (2 STOMACHS LAYERED)	Cytotec	200 mcg	White	Tablet	Six-Sided, Scored	Searle
SEARLE; 1501;	Pro-Banthine	50 mg	Peach	Tablet	Circle, Scored	Searle
SEARLE; 1611	Floraquin	100 mg; 60 mg; 20 mg		Tablet		Searle
SEARLE; 1831; FLAGYL; 250	Flagyl	250 mg	Blue	Coated Tablet	Circle	Searle
SEARLE; 1961; FLAGYL ER	Flagyl ER	750 mg	Blue	Extended-Release Tablet	Oval	Searle
SEARLE; 2101	Ketochol	250 mg	Red	Tablet		Searle
SEARLE; 2732, NORPACE CR; 100 MG	Norpace Cr	100 mg	Green and White	Controlled-Release Capsule		Searle
SEARLE; 2742, NORPACE CR; 150 MG	Norpace Cr	150 mg	Green and Brown	Controlled-Release Capsule		Searle
SEARLE; 2752, NORPACE; 100 MG	Norpace	100 mg	White and Orange	Capsule		Searle
SEARLE; 2762, NORPACE; 150 MG	Norpace	150 mg	Brown and Orange	Capsule		Searle
SEARLE; E; 131	Enovid-E	2.5 mg; 0.1 mg	Pink	Tablet	Circle	Searle
SEMPREX-D; WELLCOME	Semprex-D	8 mg; 60 mg	Green and White with Yellow Band	Capsule		Medeva Pharmaceuticals
SERAX; 10; 51; WYETH	Serax	10 mg	Pink and White	Capsule		Faulding Laboratories
SERAX; 15; 6; WYETH	Serax	15 mg	Red and White	Capsule		Faulding Laboratories
SERAX; 30; 52; WYETH	Serax	30 mg	Maroon and White	Capsule		Faulding Laboratories
SEROQUEL; 25 MG	Seroquel	25 mg	Peach	Coated Tablet	Circle, Biconvex	Astra Zeneca
SEROQUEL; 100 MG	Seroquel	100 mg	Yellow	Coated Tablet	Circle, Biconvex	Astra Zeneca
SEROQUEL; 200 MG	Seroquel	200 mg	White	Coated Tablet	Circle, Biconvex	Astra Zeneca
SHIRE; 381; 10 MG	Adderall Xr 10 mg Capsule	2.5 mg; 2.5 mg; 2.5 mg; 2.5 mg	Blue	Extended-Release Capsule		Shire Pharmaceuticals
SHIRE; 381; 20 MG	Adderall Xr 20 mg Capsule	5 mg; 5 mg; 5 mg; 5 mg	Orange	Extended-Release Capsule		Shire Pharmaceuticals
SHIRE; 381; 30 MG	Adderall Xr 30 mg Capsule	7.5 mg; 7.5 mg; 7.5 mg; 7.5 mg	Natural and Orange	Extended-Release Capsule		Shire Pharmaceuticals
SHOALS	Agesic	600 mg	Peach	Tablet	Capsule-Shape	Shoals Pharmaceuticals
SHOALS	D-Vert 15	15 mg		Capsule		Shoals Pharmaceuticals
SHOALS	D-Vert 30	30 mg		Capsule		Shoals Pharmaceuticals
SHOALS	E-D	60 mg; 400 mg		Tablet		Shoals Pharmaceuticals
SHOALS	Histafed-LA	120 mg; 8 mg		Capsule		Shoals Pharmaceuticals
SHOALS	Histafed-S.R.	4 mg; 20 mg	Red	Extended-Release Tablet	Circle	Shoals Pharmaceuticals
SINA; 6301	Sina-12x	25 mg; 200 mg	Purple	Tablet	Capsule-Shape, Scored	Medpointe
SINAREST	Sinarest Sinus	325 mg; 30 mg; 2 mg	Yellow	Tablet	Circle	Novartis Consumer

IMPRINT	BRAND/GENERIC NAME	STRENGTH	COLOR	FORM	SHAPE	MANUFACTURER
SINE-AID; IB	Sine-Aid Ib, Ibuprofen Strength	200 mg; 30 mg	Light Yellow with Red Ink	Tablet		Mcneil Consumer Products
SINE-OFF	Sine-Off Allergy/sinus Maximum Strength	2 mg; 30 mg; 500 mg	Yellow	Tablet		Glaxosmithkline Consumer
SINE-OFF	Sine-Off Maximum Strength	30 mg; 500 mg		Tablet		Glaxosmithkline Consumer
SINEQUAN; ROERIG; 534	Sinequan	10 mg	Pink and Red	Capsule		Pfizer Roerig
SINEQUAN; ROERIG; 535	Sinequan	25 mg	Pink and Blue	Capsule		Pfizer Roerig
SINEQUAN; ROERIG; 536	Sinequan	50 mg	Pink and White	Capsule		Pfizer Roerig
SINEQUAN; ROERIG; 537	Sinequan	150 mg	Blue	Capsule		Pfizer Roerig
SINEQUAN; ROERIG; 538	Sinequan	100 mg	Blue and White	Capsule		Pfizer Roerig
SINEQUAN; ROERIG; 539	Sinequan	75 mg	White	Capsule		Pfizer Roerig
SINGLES; 1	Beta Carotene Centrum Singles	25000 IU	Brown	Gel/jelly	Oblong	Lederle Laboratories
SINGLES; 2	Vitamin E Centrum Singles	400 IU	Pale Clear Yellow	Capsule, Liquid Filled	Oblong	Lederle Laboratories
SINUS; EXCEDRIN	Excedrin Extra Strength Sinus	30 mg; 500 mg	Orange	Tablet	Circle	Bristol-Myers Squibb
SINUTAB	Sinutab Non-Drying Liquid-Capsule	30 mg; 200 mg	Blue	Capsule	Oval	Pfizer Consumer Health Care
SJ	Ezol No. 3	325 mg; 50 mg; 40 mg; 30 mg	Orange and White	Tablet		Stewart-Jackson Pharmacal
SJ; 631	Bidex	800 mg	Pink	Sustained-Release Tablet	Capsule-Shape, Scored	Stewart-Jackson Pharmacal
SJ; 638	Bidex-DM	800 mg; 30 mg	White	Extended-Release Tablet	Trisected	Stewart-Jackson Pharmacal
SJ; 641	Medent-DM	30 mg; 800 mg; 60 mg	White	Extended-Release Tablet	Oval, Scored, Trisected	Stewart-Jackson Pharmacal
SJ; 642	Medent Ld	800 mg; 60 mg	White	Extended-Release Tablet	Oval, Trisected	Stewart-Jackson Pharmacal
SJ; 647	Difil G	200 mg; 200 mg	White	Tablet	Capsule-Shape	Stewart-Jackson Pharmacal
SKF; 25	Vontrol	25 mg	Orange	Tablet	Circle	Glaxosmithkline
SKF; 101	SK-Ampicillin	250 mg	Yellow and White	Capsule		Glaxosmithkline
SKF; 102	SK-Ampicillin	500 mg	Yellow and White	Capsule		Glaxosmithkline
SKF; 107	SK-Ampicillin	125 mg	White, Scored	Tablet, Chewable		Glaxosmithkline
SKF; 111	SK-Penicillin G	400,000 units	White	Tablet		Glaxosmithkline
SKF; 112	SK-Penicillin G	800000 U	White	Tablet	Capsule-Shape	Glaxosmithkline
SKF; 116	SK-Penicillin VK	250 mg	White	Tablet		Glaxosmithkline
SKF; 117	SK-Penicillin VK	500 mg		Tablet		Glaxosmithkline
SKF; 120	SK-Amitriptyline	10 mg	White	Tablet		Glaxosmithkline
SKF; 121	SK-Amitriptyline	25 mg	Green	Tablet		Glaxosmithkline
SKF; 122	SK-Digoxin	0.25 mg	White	Tablet		Glaxosmithkline
SKF; 123	SK-Amitriptyline	50 mg	Yellow	Tablet		Glaxosmithkline
SKF; 124	SK-Amitriptyline	75 mg	Green	Tablet		Glaxosmithkline
SKF; 126	SK-Tetracycline	250 mg	Pink and White	Capsule		Glaxosmithkline
SKF; 126	SK-Tetracycline	250 mg	Pink and White	Capsule		Glaxosmithkline
SKF; 127	SK-Tetracycline	500 mg	Pink and White	Capsule		Glaxosmithkline
SKF; 129	SK-Niacin	50 mg	White	Tablet		Glaxosmithkline
SKF; 130	SK-Niacin	100 mg	White	Tablet		Glaxosmithkline
SKF; 131	SK-Amitriptyline	100 mg	Yellow	Tablet		Glaxosmithkline
SKF; 132	SK-Amitriptyline	150 mg	White	Tablet		Glaxosmithkline
SKF; 133	SK-Bamate	200 mg		Tablet		Glaxosmithkline
SKF; 134	SK-Bamate	400 mg	White	Tablet		Glaxosmithkline
SKF; 136	SK-Phenobarbital	15 mg	White	Tablet		Glaxosmithkline
SKF; 137	SK-Phenobarbital	30 mg	White	Tablet		Glaxosmithkline
SKF; 163	SK-Soxazole	500 mg	White	Tablet		Glaxosmithkline
SKF; 169	SK-Reserpine	0.25 mg	White	Tablet		Glaxosmithkline
SKF; 171	SK-Quinidine Sulfate	200 mg	White	Tablet		Glaxosmithkline
SKF; 173	SK-Apap	650 mg	White	Tablet	Capsule-Shape	Glaxosmithkline
SKF; 174	SK-Apap	325 mg	White	Tablet		Glaxosmithkline
SKF; 176	SK-Chloral Hydrate	500 mg	Green	Tablet		Glaxosmithkline
SKF; 303	SK-Diphenhydramine	25 mg	Green	Capsule		Glaxosmithkline
SKF; 304	SK-Diphenhydramine	50 mg	White and Green	Capsule		Glaxosmithkline
SKF; 310	SK-Propantheline	15 mg	White	Tablet	Circle	Glaxosmithkline
SKF; 316	SK-Petn	10 mg	White	Tablet		Glaxosmithkline
SKF; 317	SK-Petn	20 mg	White	Tablet		Glaxosmithkline
SKF; 319	SK-Oxycodone with Aspirin	325 mg; 4.5 mg; 0.38 mg	White	Tablet	Oval	Glaxosmithkline
SKF; 320	SK-Oxycodone with Acetaminophen	325 mg; 5 mg	White	Tablet	Circle	Glaxosmithkline
SKF; 321	SK-Pramine	10 mg	Blue	Tablet		Glaxosmithkline
SKF; 322	SK-Pramine	25 mg	Blue	Tablet		Glaxosmithkline
SKF; 323	SK-Pramine	50 mg	Blue	Tablet		Glaxosmithkline
SKF; 324	SK-Apap	325 mg; 15 mg	White	Tablet		Glaxosmithkline Consumer
SKF; 326	SK-Apap	325 mg; 30 mg	White	Tablet		Glaxosmithkline
SKF; 327	SK-Apap	325 mg; 60 mg	White	Tablet		Glaxosmithkline
SKF; 339	SK-Prednisone	5 mg	White	Tablet		Glaxosmithkline
SKF; 340	SK-Furosemide	20 mg		Tablet		Glaxosmithkline
SKF; 341	SK-Furosemide	40 mg		Tablet		Glaxosmithkline
SKF; 363	SK-Hydrochlorothiazide	25 mg		Tablet		Glaxosmithkline
SKF; 364	SK-Hydrochlorothiazide	50 mg		Tablet		Glaxosmithkline
SKF; 367	SK-Erythromycin	250 mg	Yellow	Tablet		Glaxosmithkline
SKF; 369	SK-Erythromycin	500 mg	Yellow	Coated Tablet	Capsule-Shape	Glaxosmithkline
SKF; 371	SK-Thioridazine Hydrochloride	10 mg		Tablet		Glaxosmithkline
SKF; 372	SK-Thioridazine	25 mg		Tablet		Glaxosmithkline
SKF; 373	SK-Thioridazine	50 mg		Tablet		Glaxosmithkline
SKF; 374	SK-Dexamethasone	0.5 mg	Light Yellow	Tablet		Glaxosmithkline
SKF; 375	SK-Thioridazine Hydrochloride	100 mg		Tablet		Glaxosmithkline
SKF; 376	SK-Dexamethasone	0.75 mg	Light Blue	Tablet		Glaxosmithkline

IMPRINT	BRAND/GENERIC NAME	STRENGTH	COLOR	FORM	SHAPE	MANUFACTURER
SKF; 377	SK-Dexamethasone	1.5 mg	Pink	Tablet		Glaxosmithkline
SKF; 379	SK-Dipyridamole	25 mg		Tablet		Glaxosmithkline
SKF; 380; 50MG	SK-Dipyridamole	50 mg		Tablet		Glaxosmithkline
SKF; 381; 75MG	SK-Dipyridamole	75 mg		Tablet		Glaxosmithkline
SKF; 403	SK-Triamcinolone	2 mg	Pink	Tablet		Glaxosmithkline
SKF; 404	SK-Triamcinolone	4 mg	White	Tablet		Glaxosmithkline
SKF; 406	SK-Triamcinolone	8 mg	Yellow	Tablet		Glaxosmithkline
SKF; 409	SK-Tolbutamide	500 mg	Peach-Orange	Tablet	Circle	Glaxosmithkline
SKF; 419	SK-Chlorothiazide	250 mg	White	Tablet	Circle	Glaxosmithkline
SKF; 420	SK-Chlorothiazide	500 mg	White	Tablet	Circle	Glaxosmithkline
SKF; 423	SK-Diphenoxylate	0.025 mg; 2.5 mg	White	Tablet		Glaxosmithkline
SKF; 426	SK Metronidazole	250 mg	Off-White	Tablet		Glaxosmithkline
SKF; 441	SK-Lygen	5 mg	Pink	Capsule		Glaxosmithkline
SKF; 442	SK-Lygen	10 mg	Pink and Orange	Capsule		Glaxosmithkline
SKF; 443	SK-Lygen	25 mg	Orange	Capsule		Glaxosmithkline
SKF; 463	SK-65	65 mg	Gray and White	Capsule		Glaxosmithkline
SKF; 468	SK-65 Compound	32.4 mg; 65 mg; 389 mg	Orange and Gray	Capsule		Glaxosmithkline
SKF; 470	SK-Methocarbamol	500 mg	White	Tablet	Oval	Glaxosmithkline
SKF; 471	SK-Methocarbamol	750 mg	White	Tablet	Oval	Glaxosmithkline
SKF; 474	SK-65	650 mg; 65 mg	Orange	Tablet	Capsule-Shape	Glaxosmithkline
SKF; 494	SK-Apap	300 mg; 15 mg	White	Tablet	Circle	Glaxosmithkline
SKF; 499	SK-Probenecid	500 mg	White	Coated Tablet		Glaxosmithkline
SKF; 499	SK-Probenecid	500 mg	White	Tablet	Capsule-Shape, Scored	Glaxosmithkline
SKF; A70	Anspor	250 mg	Orange and White	Capsule		Glaxosmithkline Consumer
SKF; A71	Anspor	500 mg	Orange	Capsule		Glaxosmithkline
SKF; A90	Benzedrine	15 mg	Purple and Clear	Capsule		Glaxosmithkline
SKF; A91	Benzedrine	5 mg		Tablet		Glaxosmithkline
SKF; A92	Benzedrine	10 mg	Peach	Tablet		Glaxosmithkline
SKF; C26	Combid	10 mg; 5 mg	Yellow & Clear	Capsule		Glaxosmithkline Consumer
SKF; C66	Compazine	5 mg	Yellow-Green	Coated Tablet	Circle	Glaxosmithkline
SKF; C67	Compazine	10 mg	Yellow-Green	Coated Tablet	Circle	Glaxosmithkline
SKF; D14	Cytomel	5 mcg	White	Tablet	Circle	Glaxosmithkline
SKF; D16	Cytomel	25 mcg	White	Tablet	Circle, Scored	Glaxosmithkline
SKF; D17	Cytomel	50 mcg	White	Tablet	Circle, Scored	Glaxosmithkline
SKF; D62	Darbid	5 mg	Pink	Tablet	Circle	Glaxosmithkline
SKF; E19	Dexedrine	5 mg	Orange	Tablet	Triangle	Glaxosmithkline
SKF; E33	Dibenzyline	10 mg	Red, Coral	Capsule		Glaxosmithkline Consumer
SKF; H06	Dyrenium	50 mg		Capsule		Glaxosmithkline Consumer
SKF; H07	Dyrenium	100 mg	Red	Capsule		Glaxosmithkline Consumer
SKF; H24	Ecotrin	325 mg	Orange	Enteric-Coated Tablet		Glaxosmithkline Consumer
SKF; H26	Ecotrin	10 Gr	Orange	Enteric-Coated Tablet		Glaxosmithkline
SKF; H74	Eskabarb	65 mg		Capsule		Glaxosmithkline Consumer
SKF; H76	Eskabarb	97 mg	Blue & Clear	Capsule		Glaxosmithkline Consumer
SKF; J10	Eskalith Cr	450 mg	Buff	Timed-Release Tablet	Circle, Scored	Glaxosmithkline
SKF; J20	Eskaphen B	0.25 Gr; 5 mg	Peach	Tablet		Glaxosmithkline
SKF; J66	Eskatrol	15 mg; 7.5 mg	White and Clear	Capsule		Glaxosmithkline
SKF; K32	Feosol	200 mg	Green	Tablet	Triangle	Glaxosmithkline Consumer
SKF; K33	Feosol Plus	200 mg; 0.4 mg; 50 mg; 2 mg; 2 mg; 1 mg; 325 mg; 10 mg; 2 mg; 1.7 mcg	Green and Red	Capsule		Glaxosmithkline
SKF; K60	Fortespan	6 mg; 6 mg; 6 mg; 15 mcg; 60 mg; 150 mg; 10,000 USP units; 400 USP units	Red and Clear	Capsule		Glaxosmithkline
SKF; P36	Prydon	0.4 mg; 0.305 mg; 0.06 mg; 0.035 mg; 1 Gr	Blue and Clear	Capsule		Glaxosmithkline
SKF; RIDAURA	Ridaura	3 mg	Opaque Brown and Opaque Tan	Capsule		Connetics
SKF; S03	Stelazine	1 mg	Blue	Coated Tablet	Circle	Glaxosmithkline
SKF; S04	Stelazine	2 mg	Blue	Coated Tablet	Circle	Glaxosmithkline
SKF; S06	Stelazine	5 mg	Blue	Coated Tablet	Circle	Glaxosmithkline
SKF; S07	Stelazine	10 mg	Blue	Coated Tablet	Circle	Glaxosmithkline
SKF; S72	Teldrin	8 mg	Green & Clear with Pink & White Pellets	Timed-Release Capsule		Glaxosmithkline Consumer
SKF; T01	Temaril	5 mg	Gray and Clear	Capsule		Glaxosmithkline
SKF; T03	Temaril	2.5 mg	Gray Blue	Tablet		Glaxosmithkline
SKF; T63	Thorazine	30 mg	Orange and Natural	Sustained-Release Capsule		Glaxosmithkline
SKF; T64	Thorazine	75 mg	Orange and Natural	Sustained-Release Capsule		Glaxosmithkline
SKF; T66	Thorazine	150 mg	Orange and Natural	Sustained-Release Capsule		Glaxosmithkline
SKF; T67	Thorazine	200 mg	Opaque Orange Cap and Natural Body	Sustained-Release Capsule		Glaxosmithkline
SKF; T69	Thorazine	300 mg	Opaque Orange Cap and Natural Body	Sustained-Release Capsule		Glaxosmithkline
SKF; T73	Thorazine	10 mg	Orange	Coated Tablet	Circle	Glaxosmithkline
SKF; T74	Thorazine	25 mg	Orange	Coated Tablet	Circle	Glaxosmithkline
SKF; T76	Thorazine	50 mg	Orange	Coated Tablet	Circle	Glaxosmithkline
SKF; T77	Thorazine	100 mg	Orange	Coated Tablet	Circle	Glaxosmithkline
SKF; T79	Thorazine	200 mg	Orange	Coated Tablet	Circle	Glaxosmithkline
SKF; V23	Trophite	10 mg; 25 mcg	Pink	Tablet		Glaxosmithkline
SKF; V24	Troph-Iron	10 mg; 25 mcg	Pink	Tablet		Glaxosmithkline

IMPRINT	BRAND/GENERIC NAME	STRENGTH	COLOR	FORM	SHAPE	MANUFACTURER
SKF S73	Teldrin	12 mg	Green & Clear with Pink & White Pellets	Timed-Release Capsule		Glaxosmithkline Consumer
SL	Simply Sleep	25 mg	Blue	Tablet		Mcneil Consumer Products
SL	Verapamil Hydrochloride	40 mg		Coated Tablet		Pliva
SL; 11	Dipyridamole	25 mg	White	Coated Tablet	Circle, Convex	Pliva
SL; 36	Desipramine	25 mg	Light Yellow	Coated Tablet	Circle	H.L. Moore
SL; 36	Desipramine Hydrochloride	25 mg	Light Yellow	Coated Tablet	Circle	Pliva
SL; 66	Amitriptyline Hydrochloride	10 mg	Pink	Coated Tablet	Circle, Convex	Pliva
SL; 67	Amitriptyline Hydrochloride	25 mg	Green	Coated Tablet	Circle, Convex	Pliva
SL; 301	Nitroglycerin	2.5 mg	Lavender and Clear	Capsule, Liquid Filled		Pliva
SL; 302	Nitroglycerin	6.5 mg	Dark Blue and Yellow	Capsule, Liquid Filled		Pliva
SL; 303	Nitroglycerin	9 mg	Green and Yellow	Capsule		Pliva
SL; 312	Dipyridamole	50 mg	White	Coated Tablet	Circle, Convex	Pliva
SL; 313	Dipyridamole	75 mg	White	Coated Tablet	Circle, Convex	Pliva
SL; 318	Papaverine Hydrochloride	150 mg	Brown and Clear with White Beads	Capsule		Pliva
SL; 320	Chewable Multivitamins with Fluoride	1 mg; 2500 units; 13.5 mg; 1.05 mg; 60 mg; 400 units; 15 IU; 0.3 mg; 1.05 mg; 1.2 mg; 4.5 mcg	Buff with Orange Flecks	Tablet, Chewable	Circle	Pliva
SL; 320	Florvite Chewable Tablet	2500 IU; 400 IU; 15 IU; 0.3 mg; 1.05 mg; 1.2 mg; 13.5 mg; 1 mg; 60 mg; 1.05 mg; 4.5 mcg	Red, Orange or Purple	Tablet, Chewable	Circle	Sidmak Laboratories
SL; 323	Bethanechol Chloride	5 mg	White	Tablet	Circle, Scored	Pliva
SL; 325	Bethanechol Chloride	25 mg	Yellow	Tablet	Circle, Scored	Pliva
SL; 326	Bethanechol Chloride	50 mg	Yellow	Tablet	Circle, Scored	Pliva
SL; 327	Hydralazine Hydrochloride	25 mg	Orange	Tablet	Circle	H.L. Moore
SL; 327	Hydralazine Hydrochloride	25 mg	Orange	Tablet	Circle, Convex	Sidmak Laboratories
SL; 328	Hydralazine Hydrochloride	50 mg	Orange	Tablet	Circle	H.L. Moore
SL; 328	Hydralazine Hydrochloride	50 mg	Orange	Tablet	Circle, Convex	Sidmak Laboratories
SL; 329	Cyclandelate	200 mg	Blue or Orange Opaque	Capsule		Pliva
SL; 330	Cyclandelate	400 mg	Blue and Red or Opaque Green and White	Capsule		Pliva
SL; 331	Disulfiram	250 mg	White to Off-White	Tablet	Circle, Convex	Pliva
SL; 332	Disulfiram	500 mg	White to Off-White	Tablet	Round, Convex, Bisected Scored	Pliva
SL; 337	Nylidrin Hydrochloride	6 mg	White	Tablet	Circle	Pliva
SL; 338	Nylidrin Hydrochloride	12 mg	White	Tablet		Pliva
SL; 339	Procainamide Hydrochloride	250 mg	Blue	Sustained-Release Tablet	Oval, Convex	Pliva
SL; 340	Procainamide Hydrochloride	500 mg	Pink	Sustained-Release Tablet	Oval, Convex, Bisected Scored	Pliva
SL; 341	Sulfamethoxazole and Trimethoprim	400 mg; 80 mg	White	Tablet	Round, Convex, Bisected Scored	Pliva
SL; 342	Sulfamethoxazole and Trimethoprim	800 mg; 160 mg	White	Tablet	Oval, Convex, Bisected Scored	Pliva
SL; 342	Sulfamethoxazole and Trimethoprim Double Strength	800 mg; 160 mg	White	Tablet	Oval, Scored	H.L. Moore
SL; 342	Sulfamethoxazole and Trimethoprim Double Strength	800 mg; 160 mg	White	Tablet	Oval, Scored	Pliva
SL; 343	Papaverine Hydrochloride	300 mg	Peach	Tablet	Oval	Pliva
SL; 355	Meclizine Hydrochloride	25 mg	Pink	Tablet, Chewable	Circle, Convex	Pliva
SL; 359	Dexchlorpheniramine Maleate	2 mg	Pink	Tablet	Oval	Pliva
SL; 368	Amitriptyline Hydrochloride	50 mg	Brown	Coated Tablet	Circle, Convex	Pliva
SL; 369	Amitriptyline Hydrochloride	75 mg	Lavender	Coated Tablet	Circle, Convex	Pliva
SL; 370	Amitriptyline Hydrochloride	100 mg	Orange	Coated Tablet	Circle, Convex	Pliva
SL; 371	Amitriptyline Hydrochloride	150 mg	Light Peach	Coated Tablet	Oval, Convex	Pliva
SL; 377	Doxycycline Hyclate	100 mg	Teal Blue and Clear Lemon Yellow with Yellow Beads	Capsule, Liquid Filled		Pliva
SL; 383	Sidcon TD	6 mg; 120 mg	White	Sustained-Release Tablet	Circle	Pliva
SL; 387	Ibuprofen	400 mg	White	Coated Tablet	Circle, Convex	Pliva
SL; 388	Ibuprofen	600 mg	White	Coated Tablet	Oval, Convex	Pliva
SL; 397	Hydralazine Hydrochloride	100 mg	Orange	Tablet	Circle	H.L. Moore
SL; 398	Hydralazine Hydrochloride	10 mg	Orange	Tablet	Circle	H.L. Moore
SL; 404	Phenytoin Sodium	100 mg	White	Extended-Release Capsule		Pliva
SL; 406	Indomethacin	25 mg	Green	Capsule		Pliva
SL; 410	Carbamazepine	200 mg	White	Tablet	Round, Flat-Faced, Bisected Scored	Pliva
SL; 415	Griseofulvin	165 mg	White	Tablet	Oval	Pliva
SL; 415	Ultramicrosize Griseofulvin	165 mg	White	Tablet	Oval, Bisected Scored	Pliva
SL; 416	Griseofulvin	330 mg	White	Tablet	Oval, Bisected Scored	Pliva
SL; 416	Ultramicrosize Griseofulvin	330 mg	White	Tablet	Oval, Bisected Scored	Pliva
SL; 425	Maxiprin-15	15 Gr	Salmon Pink	Enteric-Coated Tablet	Capsule-Shape	Pliva
SL; 433	Trazodone	50 mg	White	Tablet	Circle, Scored	Warner Chilcott
SL; 434	Trazodone	100 mg	White	Tablet	Circle, Scored	Warner Chilcott
SL; 437	Desipramine	50 mg	Light Green	Coated Tablet	Circle	H.L. Moore
SL; 437	Desipramine Hydrochloride	50 mg	Light Green	Coated Tablet	Circle, Convex	Pliva
SL; 438	Desipramine	75 mg	Light Orange	Coated Tablet	Circle	H.L. Moore
SL; 438	Desipramine Hydrochloride	75 mg	Light Orange	Coated Tablet	Circle, Convex	Pliva
SL; 439	Desipramine Hydrochloride	100 mg	Peach	Coated Tablet	Circle	Pliva
SL; 440	Desipramine Hydrochloride	150 mg	White	Coated Tablet	Circle	Pliva

IMPRINT	BRAND/GENERIC NAME	STRENGTH	COLOR	FORM	SHAPE	MANUFACTURER
SL; 451	Ibuprofen	800 mg	White	Coated Tablet	Capsule-Shape	Pliva
SL; 459	Theophylline	300 mg	White	Sustained-Release Tablet	Capsule-Shaped, Bisected Scored	Novartis Generics
SL; 460	Clonidine Hydrochloride	0.1 mg	Light Green	Tablet	Circle, Scored	Pliva
SL; 461	Clonidine Hydrochloride	0.2 mg	Light Yellow	Tablet	Circle, Scored	Pliva
SL; 462	Clonidine Hydrochloride	0.3 mg	Blue	Tablet	Circle, Scored	Pliva
SL; 463	Clonidine Hydrochloride with Chlorthalidone 0.1/15 mg Tablet	0.1 mg; 5 mg	Pink	Tablet	Circle, Scored	Pliva
SL; 464	Clonidine Hydrochloride with Chlorthalidone 0.2/15 mg Tablet	0.2 mg; 15 mg	Blue	Tablet	Circle, Scored	Pliva
SL; 465	Clonidine Hydrochloride with Chlorthalidone 0.3/15 mg Tablet	0.3 mg; 15 mg	White	Tablet	Circle, Scored	Pliva
SL; 472	Propranolol Hydrochloride	90 mg	Light Blue	Tablet	Round, Convex, Bisected Scored	Pliva
SL; 475	Methyldopa	125 mg	Beige	Coated Tablet	Circle, Convex	Pliva
SL; 476	Methyldopa	250 mg	Beige	Coated Tablet	Circle, Convex	Pliva
SL; 477	Methyldopa	500 mg	Beige	Coated Tablet	Circle, Convex	Pliva
SL; 484	Sulindac	150 mg	Yellow	Tablet	Circle	Pliva
SL; 485	Sulindac	200 mg	Yellow	Tablet	Round, Bisected Scored	Pliva
SL; 486	Verapamil Hydrochloride	80 mg	White	Coated Tablet	Round, Convex, Bisected Scored	Pliva
SL; 487	Verapamil Hydrochloride	120 mg	White	Coated Tablet	Round, Convex, Bisected Scored	Pliva
SL; 491	Albuterol	2 mg	White	Tablet	Round, Flat-Faced, Bisected Scored	Pliva
SL; 492	Albuterol	4 mg	White	Tablet	Round, Flat-Faced, Bisected Scored	Pliva
SL; 506	Atenolol	50 mg	White	Tablet	Round, Flat-Faced, Beveled Edge, Bisected Scored	Pliva
SL; 507	Atenolol	100 mg	White	Tablet	Circle, Flat-Faced, Beveled Edge	Pliva
SL; 516	Verapamil Hydrochloride	40 mg	White	Tablet	Circle, Scored	Pliva
SL; 521	Decotuss	60 mg; 10 mg; 10 mg; 5 mg	Pink	Tablet	Bisected, Capsule Shaped, Debossed Scored	Pliva
SL; 523	Protriptyline Hydrochloride	5 mg		Tablet		Pliva
SL; 524	Protriptyline Hydrochloride	10 mg	Yellow	Tablet		Pliva
SL; 534	Triamterene and Hydrochlorothiazide	37 mg; 25 mg	Orange	Tablet	Rectangle	Sidmak Laboratories
SL; 535	Guaifenesin LA	600 mg	White	Extended-Release Tablet	Capsule Shaped, Bisected Scored	Pliva
SL; 546	Diclofenac Sodium	50 mg	Peach	Enteric-Coated Tablet	Circle	Pliva
SL; 547	Diclofenac Sodium	75 mg	Beige	Enteric-Coated Tablet	Circle	Pliva
SL; 553	Atenolol	25 mg	White	Tablet	Circle, Flat-Faced, Beveled Edge	Pliva
SLEEPINAL	Sleepinal Night-Time Sleep Aid	50 mg	Navy and Turquoise	Capsule		Thompson Medical
SLO-BID; 50 MG; RPR	Slo-Bid Gyrocaps	50 mg	White and Clear with White Pellets	Capsule	Oblong	Aventis Pharmaceuticals
SLO-BID; 75 MG; RPR	Slo-Bid Gyrocaps	75 mg	White and Clear with White Pellets	Extended-Release Capsule	Oblong	Aventis Pharmaceuticals
SLO-BID; 100 MG; RPR	Slo-Bid Gyrocaps	100 mg	White and Clear with White Pellets	Capsule	Oblong	Aventis Pharmaceuticals
SLO-BID; 125 MG; RPR	Slo-Bid Gyrocaps	125 mg	White and Clear with White Pellets	Extended-Release Capsule	Oblong	Aventis Pharmaceuticals
SLO-BID; 200 MG; RPR	Slo-Bid Gyrocaps	200 mg	White and Clear with White Pellets	Capsule	Oblong	Aventis Pharmaceuticals
SLO-BID; 300 MG; RPR	Slo-Bid Gyrocaps	300 mg	White and Clear with White Pellets	Extended-Release Capsule	Oblong	Aventis Pharmaceuticals
SLOW-MAG	Slow-Mag	64 mg	White with Blue Ink	Enteric-Coated Tablet	Circle, Biconvex	Purdue
SLV; SLV; ACN 2;	Aceon	2 mg	White	Tablet	Oblong, Scored	Solvay Pharmaceuticals
SLV; SLV; ACN 4;	Aceon	4 mg	Pink	Tablet	Oblong, Scored	Solvay Pharmaceuticals
SLV; SLV; ACN 8;	Aceon	8 mg	Salmon	Tablet	Oblong, Scored	Solvay Pharmaceuticals
SMS	Sudafed Cold & Cough Liquid-Capsule	250 mg; 10 mg; 100 mg; 30 mg	Orange	Capsule	Oval	Pfizer Consumer Health Care
SOCCER BALL	Kids Complete	5000 IU; 80 mg; 400 IU; 30 IU; 5 mcg; 1.6 mg; 1.75 mg; 20 mg; 2.2 mg; 400 mcg; 7 mcg; 43 mcg; 10 mg; 105 mg; 18 mg; 50 mg; 150 mg; 20 mg; 15 mg; 2 mg; 5 mg		Tablet, Chewable		Good Neighbor Pharmacy
SOCCER BALL	Kids Complete	5000 IU; 80 mg; 400 IU; 30 IU; 5 mcg; 1.6 mg; 1.75 mg; 20 mg; 2.2 mg; 400 mcg; 7 mcg; 43 mcg; 10 mg; 105 mg; 18 mg; 50 mg; 150 mg; 20 mg; 15 mg; 2 mg; 5 mg		Tablet, Chewable		Millenium
SOLATENE; ROCHE	Solatene	30 mg	Blue and Green	Capsule		Roche Pharmaceuticals
SOLOXINE; DP; 0.1	Soloxine	0.1 mg	Yellow	Tablet	Oval	Daniels Pharmaceuticals
SOLOXINE; DP; 0.2	Soloxine	0.2 mg	Pink	Tablet	Oval, Scored	Daniels Pharmaceuticals
SOLOXINE; DP; 0.3	Soloxine	0.3 mg	Green	Tablet	Oval	Daniels Pharmaceuticals
SOLOXINE; DP; 0.4	Soloxine	0.4 mg	Maroon	Tablet	Oval	Daniels Pharmaceuticals
SOLOXINE; DP; 0.5	Soloxine	0.5 mg	White	Tablet	Oval, Scored	Daniels Pharmaceuticals
SOLOXINE; DP; 0.6	Soloxine	0.6 mg	Purple	Tablet	Oval	Daniels Pharmaceuticals
SOLOXINE; DP; 0.7	Soloxine	0.7 mg	Orange	Tablet	Oval	Daniels Pharmaceuticals
SOLOXINE; DP; 0.8	Soloxine	0.8 mg	Blue	Tablet	Oval	Daniels Pharmaceuticals
SOLVAY; 0147;	Unifast Unicelle	30 mg	Blue and Clear	Capsule		Solvay Pharmaceuticals
SOLVAY; 0840;	Colrex Compound	16 mg; 325 mg; 10 mg; 2 mg	Opaque Yellow	Capsule		Solvay Pharmaceuticals
SOLVAY; 1007;	Curretab	10 mg	White	Tablet	Circle, Scored	Solvay Pharmaceuticals
SOLVAY; 1010;	RP-Mycin	250 mg	Red	Coated Tablet		Solvay Pharmaceuticals

IMPRINT	BRAND/GENERIC NAME	STRENGTH	COLOR	FORM	SHAPE	MANUFACTURER
SOLVAY; 1014	Estratab	0.3 mg	Blue	Coated Tablet		Solvay Pharmaceuticals
SOLVAY; 1022	Estratab	0.625 mg	Yellow	Coated Tablet		Solvay Pharmaceuticals
SOLVAY; 1023	Estratest H.S.	0.625 mg; 1.25 mg	Light Green	Coated Tablet	Capsule-Shape	Solvay Pharmaceuticals
SOLVAY; 1026	Estratest	1.25 mg; 2.5 mg	Dark Green	Coated Tablet	Capsule-Shape	Solvay Pharmaceuticals
SOLVAY; 1030;	Fumatrin Forte	100 mg; 100 mg; 3 mg; 100 mg; 0.5 mg; 12 mcg	Orange	Coated Tablet	Oval	Solvay Pharmaceuticals
SOLVAY; 1040;	Proaqua	50 mg	Aqua	Tablet	Circle, Scored	Solvay Pharmaceuticals
SOLVAY; 1044;	Pavacap Unicelle	150 mg	Blue and Clear	Capsule		Solvay Pharmaceuticals
SOLVAY; 1050;	Histalet X	120 mg; 400 mg	White with Green Specks	Tablet	Circle, Scored	Solvay Pharmaceuticals
SOLVAY; 1054;	Tranmep	400 mg	White	Tablet	Circle, Scored	Solvay Pharmaceuticals
SOLVAY; 1075;	Proval No. 3	325 mg; 30 mg	Green	Capsule		Solvay Pharmaceuticals
SOLVAY; 1079;	Melfiat	35 mg	Peach	Tablet	Circle, Scored	Solvay Pharmaceuticals
SOLVAY; 1082;	Melfiat Unicelle	105 mg	Orange and Clear with White Beads	Capsule		Solvay Pharmaceuticals
SOLVAY; 1091	P-V-Tussin	5 mg; 60 mg	Orange	Tablet	Capsule-Shape	Solvay Pharmaceuticals
SOLVAY; 1132;	Unipres	25 mg; 0.1 mg; 15 mg	Yellow	Tablet	Scored, Circle	Solvay Pharmaceuticals
SOLVAY; 1139;	Calinate FA	60 mg; 0.2 mg; 0.2 mg; 0.1 mg; 0.02 mg; 250 mg; 4000 IU; 400 IU; 3 mg; 1 mg; 5 mg; 3 mg; 20 mg; 50 mg; 1 mg; 1 mcg	Yellow	Tablet	Oval	Solvay Pharmaceuticals
SOLVAY; 1200	Creon	8000 U; 30000 U; 13000 U	Brown and Clear Yellow	Capsule		Solvay Pharmaceuticals
SOLVAY; 1205	Creon 5	5,000 units; 18,750 units; 16,600 units	Orange Opaque and Blue Opaque	Sustained-Release Capsule		Solvay Pharmaceuticals
SOLVAY; 1210	Creon 10	10,000 units; 37,500 units; 33,200 units	Brown Opaque and Natural	Sustained-Release Capsule		Solvay Pharmaceuticals
SOLVAY; 1216;	Vio-Bec	25 mg; 26 mg; 25 mg; 500 mg; 40 mg; 100 mg	Brown	Capsule		Solvay Pharmaceuticals
SOLVAY; 1218;	Vio-Bec Forte	0.5 mg; 25 mg; 25 mg; 25 mg; 500 mg; 40 mg; 100 mg	Brown	Coated Tablet	Capsule-Shape	Solvay Pharmaceuticals
SOLVAY; 1220	Creon 20	20,000 units; 75,000 units; 66,400 units	Orange Opaque and Natural Transparent	Sustained-Release Capsule		Solvay Pharmaceuticals
SOLVAY; 1290;	Compal	16 mg; 356 mg; 30 mg	Blue-Green and Aqua	Capsule		Solvay Pharmaceuticals
SOLVAY; 1472	Advanced Formula Zenate	65 mg; 400 IU; 10 IU; 70 mg; 1 mg; 1.5 mg; 1.6 mg; 17 mg; 2.2 mg; 2.2 mcg; 200 mg; 175 mcg; 100 mg; 15 mg; 3000 IU	White	Coated Tablet	Capsule-Shape, Scored	Solvay Pharmaceuticals
SOLVAY; 1610;	Norlac	60 mg; 8000 IU; 400 IU; 30 IU; 90 mg; 0.4 mg; 2 mg; 2 mg; 20 mg; 4 mg; 8 mcg; 0.2 G; 150 mcg; 100 mg; 2 mg; 15 mg	Pink	Coated Tablet	Oval	Solvay Pharmaceuticals
SOLVAY; 1611;	Norlac RX	60 mg; 8000 IU; 400 IU; 30 IU; 90 mg; 1 mg; 2 mg; 2 mg; 20 mg; 4 mg; 8 mcg; 0.2 G; 150 mcg; 100 mg; 2 mg; 15 mg	Peach	Coated Tablet	Oval	Solvay Pharmaceuticals
SOLVAY; 2046;	C-Ron Forte	200 mg; 600 mg	Red	Coated Tablet	Circle	Solvay Pharmaceuticals
SOLVAY; 2080;	S.A.S.-500	500 mg	Dark Gold	Tablet	Circle	Solvay Pharmaceuticals
SOLVAY; 2404;	C-Ron	200 mg; 100 mg	Red	Coated Tablet	Circle	Solvay Pharmaceuticals
SOLVAY; 2805;	Uproco	200 mg; 30 mg	Orange	Capsule		Solvay Pharmaceuticals
SOLVAY; 2808	Orasone	1 mg	Pink	Tablet	Circle, Scored	Solvay Pharmaceuticals
SOLVAY; 2810	Orasone 5	5 mg	White	Tablet	Circle, Scored	Solvay Pharmaceuticals
SOLVAY; 2812	Orasone 10	10 mg	Blue	Tablet	Circle, Scored	Solvay Pharmaceuticals
SOLVAY; 2814	Orasone	20 mg	Yellow	Tablet	Circle, Scored	Solvay Pharmaceuticals
SOLVAY; 2816	Orasone 50	50 mg	White	Coated Tablet	Circle, Scored	Solvay Pharmaceuticals
SOLVAY; 3205;	Dexone	0.5 mg	Yellow	Tablet	Circle, Scored	Solvay Pharmaceuticals
SOLVAY; 3210;	Dexone	0.75 mg	Light Green	Tablet	Circle, Scored	Solvay Pharmaceuticals
SOLVAY; 3215;	Dexone	1.5 mg	Pink	Tablet	Circle, Scored	Solvay Pharmaceuticals
SOLVAY; 3220;	Dexone 4	4 mg	White	Tablet	Circle, Scored	Solvay Pharmaceuticals
SOLVAY; 4016;	Cin-Quin 200	200 mg	Clear	Capsule		Solvay Pharmaceuticals
SOLVAY; 4020;	Cin-Quin 300	300 mg	Clear	Capsule		Solvay Pharmaceuticals
SOLVAY; 4024;	Cin-Quin 100	100 mg	White	Tablet	Circle	Solvay Pharmaceuticals
SOLVAY; 4032;	Cin-Quin 300	300 mg	White	Tablet	Circle, Scored	Solvay Pharmaceuticals
SOLVAY; 4120;	Deproic	250 mg	Orange	Capsule		Solvay Pharmaceuticals
SOLVAY; 4202	Luvox	25 mg	White	Coated Tablet	Circle	Solvay Pharmaceuticals
SOLVAY; 4205	Luvox	50 mg	Yellow	Coated Tablet	Circle, Scored	Solvay Pharmaceuticals
SOLVAY; 4210	Luvox	100 mg	Beige	Coated Tablet	Circle, Scored	Solvay Pharmaceuticals

IMPRINT	BRAND/GENERIC NAME	STRENGTH	COLOR	FORM	SHAPE	MANUFACTURER
SOLVAY; 4412;	Quine 300	300 mg	Clear	Capsule		Solvay Pharmaceuticals
SOLVAY; 4492	Lithobid	300 mg	Peach	Timed-Release Tablet		Solvay Pharmaceuticals
SOLVAY; 4520;	Dihydrocodeine Compound	16 mg; 356 mg; 30 mg	Blue	Capsule		Solvay Pharmaceuticals
SOLVAY; 4710;	Ronase 100	100 mg	White	Tablet		Solvay Pharmaceuticals
SOLVAY; 4725;	Ronase 250	250 mg	White	Tablet		Solvay Pharmaceuticals
SOLVAY; 4750;	Ronase 500	500 mg	White	Tablet		Solvay Pharmaceuticals
SOLVAY; 4825;	Procamide SR 250	250 mg	Pastel Blue	Sustained-Release Tablet		Solvay Pharmaceuticals
SOLVAY; 4850;	Procamide SR 500	500 mg	Pastel Pink	Sustained-Release Tablet		Solvay Pharmaceuticals
SOLVAY; 4875;	Procamide SR 750	750 mg	Tan	Sustained-Release Tablet		Solvay Pharmaceuticals
SOLVAY; 5044	Teveten	400 mg	Pink	Coated Tablet	Oval	Biovail Pharmaceuticals
SOLVAY; 5046	Teveten	600 mg	White	Tablet	Capsule-Shape	Biovail Pharmaceuticals
SOLVAY; 5046	Teveten	600 mg	White	Coated Tablet	Capsule-Shape	Unimed
SOLVAY; 5147	Teveten HCT	600 mg; 12.5 mg	Butterscotch	Coated Tablet	Capsule-Shape	Solvay Pharmaceuticals
SOLVAY; 5150	Teveten HCT	600 mg; 25 mg	Brick Red	Coated Tablet	Capsule-Shape	Solvay Pharmaceuticals
SOLVAY; 7025;	Ruvert M	25 mg	Red	Coated Tablet	Circle	Solvay Pharmaceuticals
SOLVAY; 7415;	Lithobid	300 mg		Tablet		Solvay Pharmaceuticals
SOLVAY; 7512;	Lithonate	300 mg	Peach	Capsule		Solvay Pharmaceuticals
SOLVAY; 7516;	Lithotabs	300 mg	White	Coated Tablet	Circle, Scored	Solvay Pharmaceuticals
SOLVAY; CREON;	Creon	30,000 units; 8,000 units; 13,000 units	Opaque Brown and Clear Yellow with Buff Microspheres	Capsule		Solvay Pharmaceuticals
SOMA; 37; WALLACE; 2001	Soma	350 mg	White	Tablet	Circle, Convex	Wallace Laboratories
SONATA; 5 MG	Sonata	5 mg	Green and Light Green	Capsule		Wyeth Pharmaceuticals
SONATA; 10 MG	Sonata	10 mg	Green and Light Green	Capsule		Wyeth Pharmaceuticals
SORIATANE; 10; ROCHE	Soriatane	10 mg	Brown and White	Capsule		Roche Laboratories
SORIATANE; 25; ROCHE	Soriatane	25 mg	Brown and Yellow	Capsule		Roche Laboratories
SP22;	Levatol	20 mg	Yellow	Tablet	Capsule-Shape, Scored	Schwarz Pharma
SP; 111	Nulev	0.125 mg	White	Tablet	Circle	Schwarz Pharma
SP; 130	Hydrochlorothiazide	50 mg		Tablet		Superpharm
SP 321; 0.25	Niravam	0.25 mg	Yellow	Tablet, Disintegrating	Circle	Schwarz Pharma
SP 322; 0.5	Niravam	0.5 mg	Yellow	Tablet, Disintegrating	Circle	Schwarz Pharma
SP 323; 1	Niravam	1 mg	White	Tablet, Disintegrating	Circle	Schwarz Pharma
SP 324; 2	Niravam	2 mg	White	Tablet, Disintegrating	Circle	Schwarz Pharma
SP; 351	Kemstro	10 mg	White	Disintegrating Tablet	Circle	Schwarz Pharma
SP; 352	Kemstro	20 mg	White	Disintegrating Tablet	Circle	Schwarz Pharma
SP371; 20	Fluxid	20 mg	White	Disintegrating Tablet	Circle, Biconvex	Schwarz Pharma
SP372; 40	Fluxid	40 mg	White	Disintegrating Tablet	Circle, Biconvex	Schwarz Pharma
SP; 431;	Proventil Repetabs	4 mg	White	Timed-Release Tablet	Circle	Schering
SP; 538	Levbid	0.375 mg	Light Orange	Extended-Release Tablet	Capsule-Shape, Scored	Schwarz Pharma
SP; 712	Uniretic	12.5 mg; 7.5 mg	Yellow	Coated Tablet	Oval, Scored	Schwarz Pharma
SP; 720	Uniretic	12.5 mg; 15 mg	White	Coated Tablet	Oval, Scored	Schwarz Pharma
SP; 725	Uniretic	25 mg; 15 mg	Yellow	Coated Tablet	Oval, Scored	Schwarz Pharma
SP; 2104; 500; 5	CO-Gesic	5 mg; 500 mg	White	Tablet	Oval, Compressed, Scored	Schwarz Pharma
SP; 2164; 750 MG	Mono-Gesic	750 mg	Pink	Coated Tablet	Oval, Scored	Schwarz Pharma
SP; 2200	Niferex	50 mg	Brown	Coated Tablet	Circle	Ther-RX
SP; 2209; 131/05	Niferex-Pn	312 mg; 10 mg; 4000 IU; 400 IU; 80 mg; 60 mg; 50 mg; 3 mg; 3 mcg; 3 mg; 2 mg	Blue	Coated Tablet	Oval	Ther-RX
SP 2309 1 0	Niferex-Pn Forte	250 mg; 2 mg; 1 mg; 60 mg; 20 mg; 3 mg; 30 IU; 400 IU; 25 mg; 5000 IU; 3.4 mg; 10 mg; 0.2 mg; 12 mcg; 80 mg; 4 mg	White	Coated Tablet	Capsule-Shape	Ther-RX
SP; 4220	Niferex-150	150 mg	Orange and Clear with Brown Beads	Capsule		Ther-RX
SP; 4330	Niferex-150 Forte	1 mg; 150 mg; 25 mcg	Red and Clear with Brown Beads	Capsule		Ther-RX
SP; ADH;	Trilafon	2 mg	Gray	Coated Tablet		Schering
SP; ADJ;	Trilafon	8 mg	Gray	Coated Tablet		Schering
SP; ADK;	Trilafon	4 mg	Gray	Coated Tablet		Schering
SP; ADM;	Trilafon	16 mg	Gray	Coated Tablet		Schering
SP; ANA;	Etrafon 2-10	10 mg; 2 mg	Deep Yellow	Coated Tablet		Schering
SP; ANC;	Etrafon	25 mg; 2 mg	Pink	Coated Tablet		Schering
SP; WDR;	Permitil	2.5 mg	Light Orange	Tablet	Oval, Compressed, Scored	Schering
SP; WEG;	Permitil	10 mg	Light Red	Tablet	Oval, Compressed, Scored	Schering
SP; WFF;	Permitil	5 mg	Purple-Pink	Tablet	Oval, Compressed, Scored	Schering
LOGO; SPD417 100 MG	Equetro	100 mg	Bluish Green, Yellow	Capsule, Extended Release		Shire
LOGO; SPD417 200	Equetro	200 mg	Blue, Yellow	Capsule, Extended Release		Shire
LOGO; SPD417 300 MG	Equetro	300 mg	Blue, Yellow	Capsule, Extended Release		Shire
SPECTROBID; 035;	Spectrobid	400 mg	White	Coated Tablet		Roerig
SQUARE	Maxalt-Mlt	10 mg	White	Tablet	Circle	Merck
SQUIBB; 28	Imipramine Hydrochloride	25 mg		Tablet		Bristol-Myers Squibb

IMPRINT	BRAND/GENERIC NAME	STRENGTH	COLOR	FORM	SHAPE	MANUFACTURER
SQUIBB; 39	Imipramine Hydrochloride	10 mg		Tablet		Bristol-Myers Squibb
SQUIBB; 40	Imipramine Hydrochloride	50 mg		Tablet		Bristol-Myers Squibb
SQUIBB; 45	Desipramine Hydrochloride	25 mg		Tablet		Bristol-Myers Squibb
SQUIBB; 63	Ergoloid Mesylates	1 mg		Tablet		Bristol-Myers Squibb
SQUIBB; 105	Sulindac	150 mg		Tablet		Bristol-Myers Squibb
SQUIBB; 107	Sulindac	200 mg		Tablet		Bristol-Myers Squibb
SQUIBB; 109	Vitamin A	25000 IU		Capsule		Bristol-Myers Squibb
SQUIBB; 110	Vitamin A	50000 IU		Capsule		Bristol-Myers Squibb
SQUIBB; 111	Vitamin A	10000 IU		Capsule		Bristol-Myers Squibb
SQUIBB; 112	Vitamin C	250 mg		Tablet		Bristol-Myers Squibb
SQUIBB; 113	Velosef	250 mg	Blue and Orange	Capsule		Apothecon
SQUIBB; 114	Velosef	500 mg	Blue	Capsule		Apothecon
SQUIBB; 133	Clorazepate	3.75 mg		Tablet		Bristol-Myers Squibb
SQUIBB; 138	Smz-Tmp 400/80	400 mg; 80 mg	White	Tablet	Circle, Scored	Bristol-Myers Squibb
SQUIBB; 139	Chlorpropamide	100 mg	Blue	Tablet	Circle	Bristol-Myers Squibb
SQUIBB; 147	Velosef	1 G	Light Yellow	Tablet	Oblong	Apothecon
SQUIBB; 152	Chlorpropamide	250 mg	Blue	Tablet	Circle	Bristol-Myers Squibb
SQUIBB; 157	Clorazepate Dipotassium	7.5 mg	Peach	Tablet	Circle, Scored	Bristol-Myers Squibb
SQUIBB; 159	Oxazepam	30 mg		Capsule		Bristol-Myers Squibb
SQUIBB; 160	Ethril	250 mg	Pink	Tablet		Bristol-Myers Squibb
SQUIBB; 161	Ethril	500 mg	Pink	Tablet		Bristol-Myers Squibb
SQUIBB; 162	Chlorthalidone	25 mg	Yellow	Tablet	Circle	Bristol-Myers Squibb
SQUIBB; 163	Clorazepate	15 mg	Pink	Tablet	Circle, Scored	Bristol-Myers Squibb
SQUIBB; 164	Pentids	125 mg	White	Tablet	Oval	Apothecon
SQUIBB; 165	Pentids 400	250 mg	White	Tablet		Apothecon
SQUIBB; 167	Pentids 400	250 mg		Capsule		Apothecon
SQUIBB; 168	Pentids	500 mg	Yellow	Tablet		Apothecon
SQUIBB; 168	Pentids 800	500 mg	Yellow	Tablet	Oval	Apothecon
SQUIBB; 171	Smz-Tmp 800/160	800 mg; 160 mg	White	Tablet	Oval, Scored	Bristol-Myers Squibb
SQUIBB; 180	Chlorthalidone	50 mg		Tablet		Bristol-Myers Squibb
SQUIBB; 181	Cephalexin	250 mg	Opaque Orange Body with Gray Cap	Capsule		Apothecon
SQUIBB; 185	Diazepam	2 mg	White	Tablet	Bisected Scored	Bristol-Myers Squibb
SQUIBB; 187	Chlorthalidone	100 mg	White	Tablet	Circle	Bristol-Myers Squibb
SQUIBB; 192	Ascorbic Acid	50 mg		Tablet		Bristol-Myers Squibb
SQUIBB; 193	Perphenazine with Amitriptyline 2/10	2 mg; 10 mg	Blue	Coated Tablet	Circle	Bristol-Myers Squibb
SQUIBB; 195	Tolazamide	100 mg	White	Tablet	Circle	Bristol-Myers Squibb
SQUIBB; 196	Ascorbic Acid	250 mg		Tablet		Bristol-Myers Squibb
SQUIBB 196	Vitamin C Squibb 196	100 mg		Tablet		E.R. Squibb & Sons
SQUIBB; 197	Ascorbic Acid Squibb 197	500 mg		Tablet		E.R. Squibb & Sons
SQUIBB; 202	Dicloxacillin Sodium	250 mg	Blue and White or Green and Light Green	Capsule		Bristol-Myers Squibb
SQUIBB; 203	Dicloxacillin Sodium	500 mg	Blue and White or Green and Light Green	Capsule		Bristol-Myers Squibb
SQUIBB; 204	B Complex Vitamin	9 mg; 0.7 mg; 0.7 mg; 0.9 mg; 2 mcg		Tablet		Bristol-Myers Squibb
SQUIBB; 211	Cloxacillin Sodium	250 mg		Capsule		Bristol-Myers Squibb
SQUIBB; 212	Cloxacillin Sodium	500 mg		Capsule		Bristol-Myers Squibb
SQUIBB; 230	Trimox	250 mg	Green	Capsule		Bristol-Myers Squibb
SQUIBB; 238	Diazepam	5 mg	Yellow	Tablet	Bisected Scored	Bristol-Myers Squibb
SQUIBB; 243	Corgard	100 mg		Tablet		Bristol-Myers Squibb
SQUIBB; 245	Diazepam	10 mg	Light Blue	Tablet	Bisected Scored	Bristol-Myers Squibb
SQUIBB; 259	Perphenazine and Amitriptyline 2/25	2 mg; 25 mg	Orange	Coated Tablet	Circle	Bristol-Myers Squibb
SQUIBB; 267	Perphenazine and Amitriptyline 4/10	4 mg; 10 mg	Salmon	Coated Tablet	Circle	Bristol-Myers Squibb
SQUIBB; 271	Perphenazine and Amitriptyline 4/25	4 mg; 25 mg	Yellow	Coated Tablet	Circle	Bristol-Myers Squibb
SQUIBB; 274	Trazodone	50 mg	White	Tablet	Circle	Bristol-Myers Squibb
SQUIBB; 275	Triamterene and Hydrochlorothiazide	25 mg; 50 mg		Capsule		Bristol-Myers Squibb
SQUIBB; 277	Tolazamide	250 mg		Tablet		Bristol-Myers Squibb
SQUIBB; 279	Isosorbide Dinitrate	40 mg		Tablet		Bristol-Myers Squibb
SQUIBB; 280	Indomethacin	25 mg	Green	Capsule		Bristol-Myers Squibb
SQUIBB; 286	Quinidine Gluconate	324 mg	White	Sustained-Release Tablet	Circle	Bristol-Myers Squibb
SQUIBB; 288;	Allopurinol	300 mg	Peach	Tablet	Circle	Bristol-Myers Squibb
SQUIBB; 289	Clonidine	0.1 mg		Tablet		Bristol-Myers Squibb
SQUIBB; 295	Indomethacin	50 mg	Green	Capsule		Bristol-Myers Squibb
SQUIBB; 297	Engran	6000 U; 400 U; 3 mg; 3 mg; 2 mg; 2 mcg; 20 mg; 5 mg; 75 mg; 100 mg; 0.15 mg; 45 mg; 1 mg; 1 mg; 1.5 mg	Blue	Tablet		Bristol-Myers Squibb
SQUIBB; 298	Lorazepam	0.5 mg	White	Tablet	Circle	Bristol-Myers Squibb
SQUIBB; 300	Prazosin Hydrochloride	1 mg		Capsule		Bristol-Myers Squibb
SQUIBB; 325	Trifluoperazine	10 mg	Lavender	Coated Tablet	Circle	Bristol-Myers Squibb
SQUIBB; 327	Triamterene and Hydrochlorothiazide	25 mg; 50 mg		Tablet		Bristol-Myers Squibb

IMPRINT	BRAND/GENERIC NAME	STRENGTH	COLOR	FORM	SHAPE	MANUFACTURER
SQUIBB; 341	Theragran-Z	12 mg; 10000 IU; 400 IU; 15 mg; 100 mg; 20 mg; 150 mcg; 2 mg; 22.5 mg; 1 mg; 0.6 mg; 0.68 mg; 200 mg; 10 mg; 10 mg; 5 mg; 5 mcg	Brown	Tablet	Capsule-Shape	Bristol-Myers Squibb
SQUIBB; 348	Indomethacin SR	75 mg	Green and Clear	Capsule		Bristol-Myers Squibb
SQUIBB; 355	Valadol	325 mg	White	Tablet		Bristol-Myers Squibb
SQUIBB; 357	Valadol	120 mg	Yellow	Tablet, Chewable		Bristol-Myers Squibb
SQUIBB; 359	Furosemide	20 mg	White	Tablet	Oval	Bristol-Myers Squibb
SQUIBB; 360	Furosemide	40 mg	White	Tablet	Circle	Bristol-Myers Squibb
SQUIBB; 365	Trifluoperazine	1 mg	Lavender	Coated Tablet	Circle	Bristol-Myers Squibb
SQUIBB; 368	Trifluoperazine	2 mg	Lavender	Coated Tablet	Circle	Bristol-Myers Squibb
SQUIBB; 371	Digitoxin	0.1 mg		Tablet		Bristol-Myers Squibb
SQUIBB; 386	Carisoprodol	350 mg	White	Tablet	Circle	Bristol-Myers Squibb
SQUIBB; 399	Trifluoperazine	5 mg	Lavender	Coated Tablet	Circle	Bristol-Myers Squibb
SQUIBB; 400	Prazosin Hydrochloride	2 mg		Capsule		Bristol-Myers Squibb
SQUIBB; 408	Lorazepam	1 mg	White	Tablet	Circle	Bristol-Myers Squibb
SQUIBB; 429	Florinef Acetate	0.1 mg	Pink	Tablet	Circle, Biconvex, Scored	Apothecon
SQUIBB; 433	Methyldopa	500 mg	White	Coated Tablet	Circle	Bristol-Myers Squibb
SQUIBB; 447	Methyldopa	250 mg	White	Coated Tablet	Circle	Bristol-Myers Squibb
SQUIBB; 457	Mycostatin	100000 U	Ivory	Tablet		Bristol-Myers Squibb
SQUIBB; 476;	Engram-Hp	9 mg; 4000 IU; 200 IU; 10 mg; 0.4 mg; 325 mg; 75 mcg; 50 mg; 0.85 mg; 1.25 mg; 4 mcg; 30 mg		Tablet		Bristol-Myers Squibb
SQUIBB; 487	Lorazepam	2 mg	White	Tablet	Circle	Bristol-Myers Squibb
SQUIBB; 488	Metronidazole	250 mg	White	Tablet	Circle	Bristol-Myers Squibb
SQUIBB; 500	Prazosin Hydrochloride	5 mg		Capsule		Bristol-Myers Squibb
SQUIBB; 504	Kenacort	2 mg	White	Tablet		Bristol-Myers Squibb
SQUIBB; 511	Kenacort	1 mg	White	Tablet		Bristol-Myers Squibb
SQUIBB; 512	Kenacort	4 mg	White	Tablet		Bristol-Myers Squibb
SQUIBB; 518	Kenacort	8 mg	Yellow	Tablet		Bristol-Myers Squibb
SQUIBB; 520	B Complex with Vitamin C	10 mg; 10 mg; 2 mg; 4 mcg; 300 mg; 100 mg		Tablet		Bristol-Myers Squibb
SQUIBB; 534	Clonidine	0.3 mg		Tablet		Bristol-Myers Squibb
SQUIBB; 535	Theragran Hemantinic	66.7 mg; 2.5 mg; 3.3 mcg; 3.3 mg; 3.3 mg; 3.3 mg; 33.3 mg; 11.7 mg; 4.13 mg; 0.67 mg; 41.7 mg; 0.5 mg; 50 mcg; 100 mg	Pink	Tablet		Apothecon
SQUIBB; 537	Niacin	500 mg	White	Tablet	Circle, Biconvex	Apothecon
SQUIBB; 538	Rautrax-N Modified	50 mg; 2 mg; 400 mg		Tablet		Bristol-Myers Squibb
SQUIBB; 539	Rautrax-N	50 mg; 4 mg; 400 mg		Tablet		Bristol-Myers Squibb
SQUIBB; 549	Iron with Vitamin C	50 mg; 25 mg		Tablet		Bristol-Myers Squibb
SQUIBB; 560	Disopyramide	100 mg		Capsule		Bristol-Myers Squibb
SQUIBB; 567	Disopyramide	150 mg		Capsule		Bristol-Myers Squibb
SQUIBB; 572	Metronidazole	500 mg	White	Tablet	Oblong	Bristol-Myers Squibb
SQUIBB; 573	Ora-Testryl	5 mg		Tablet		Bristol-Myers Squibb
SQUIBB; 574	Oxazepam	10 mg		Capsule		Bristol-Myers Squibb
SQUIBB; 580	Mycostatin	500000 U	Light Yellow to Light Brown	Tablet	Circle, Biconvex	Apothecon
SQUIBB; 598	Neomycin Sulfate	350 mg		Tablet		Bristol-Myers Squibb
SQUIBB; 599	Oxazepam	15 mg		Capsule		Bristol-Myers Squibb
SQUIBB; 602	Naturetin with K	2.5 mg; 500 mg		Tablet		Bristol-Myers Squibb
SQUIBB; 603	Sumycin	500 mg	Pink	Tablet	Oblong	Apothecon
SQUIBB; 605	Naturetin	2.5 mg	Green	Tablet	Circle	Apothecon
SQUIBB; 608	Naturetin with K	5 mg; 500 mg		Tablet		Apothecon
SQUIBB; 610	Niacin	25 mg		Tablet		Apothecon
SQUIBB; 611	Niacin	50 mg	White	Tablet	Circle, Biconvex	Apothecon
SQUIBB; 612	Niacin	100 mg	White	Tablet	Circle, Biconvex	Apothecon
SQUIBB; 615	Propoxyphene Hydrochloride	65 mg	Green and Orange	Capsule		Bristol-Myers Squibb
SQUIBB; 619	Propoxyphene Hydrochloride and A.P.C.	65 mg; 227 mg; 162 mg; 32.4 mg	Green and Gray	Capsule		Bristol-Myers Squibb
SQUIBB; 622	Meclofenamate	50 mg	Maroon and Pink	Capsule		Bristol-Myers Squibb
SQUIBB; 623	Noctec	250 mg	Red	Capsule		Bristol-Myers Squibb
SQUIBB; 626	Noctec	500 mg	Red	Capsule		Bristol-Myers Squibb
SQUIBB; 629	Meclofenamate	100 mg	Maroon and White	Capsule		Bristol-Myers Squibb
SQUIBB; 630	Methyldopa and Hydrochlorothiazide	250 mg; 15 mg	Red	Coated Tablet	Circle	Bristol-Myers Squibb
SQUIBB; 637	Nydrazid	100 mg		Tablet		Bristol-Myers Squibb
SQUIBB; 645	Methyldopa and Hydrochlorothiazide	250 mg; 25 mg	Pink	Coated Tablet	Circle	Bristol-Myers Squibb
SQUIBB; 648	Veetids	500 mg	White	Coated Tablet		Apothecon
SQUIBB; 649	Trigot	0.5 mg	White	Tablet		Bristol-Myers Squibb
SQUIBB; 652	Methyldopa and Hydrochlorothiazide	500 mg; 30 mg	Red	Coated Tablet	Oval	Bristol-Myers Squibb
SQUIBB; 654	Trigot	1 mg	White	Tablet		Bristol-Myers Squibb
SQUIBB; 655	Sumycin	250 mg	Pink	Capsule		Apothecon

IMPRINT	BRAND/GENERIC NAME	STRENGTH	COLOR	FORM	SHAPE	MANUFACTURER
SQUIBB; 663	Sumycin	250 mg	Pink	Tablet		Apothecon
SQUIBB; 671	Methyldopa and Hydrochlorothiazide	500 mg; 50 mg	Pink	Coated Tablet	Oval	Bristol-Myers Squibb
SQUIBB; 684	Veetids	250 mg	Orange	Coated Tablet		Apothecon
SQUIBB; 685	Rautrax	50 mg; 400 mg; 400 mg		Tablet		Bristol-Myers Squibb
SQUIBB; 690	Teslac	50 mg	White	Tablet	Biconvex	Bristol-Myers Squibb
SQUIBB; 692	Tolbutamide	500 mg	White	Tablet		Bristol-Myers Squibb
SQUIBB; 693;	Hydrochlorothiazide	25 mg	White	Tablet		Bristol-Myers Squibb
SQUIBB; 694;	Hydrochlorothiazide	50 mg	White	Tablet		Bristol-Myers Squibb
SQUIBB; 718	Chlordiazepoxide Hydrochloride	5 mg	Carmel and Yellow	Capsule		Bristol-Myers Squibb
SQUIBB; 723	Phenytoin Sodium	100 mg	White	Extended-Release Capsule		Bristol-Myers Squibb
SQUIBB; 727	Chlordiazepoxide Hydrochloride	10 mg	Carmel and Black	Capsule		Bristol-Myers Squibb
SQUIBB; 736	Chlordiazepoxide Hydrochloride	25 mg	Carmel and White	Capsule		Bristol-Myers Squibb
SQUIBB; 738	Temazepam	15 mg	Pink	Capsule		Bristol-Myers Squibb
SQUIBB; 749;	Cephalexin	250 mg	Swedish Orange and Gray	Capsule		Bristol-Myers Squibb
SQUIBB; 763	Sumycin	500 mg	Pink and White	Capsule		Apothecon
SQUIBB; 780	Rau-Sed	0.25 mg		Tablet		Bristol-Myers Squibb
SQUIBB; 788	Vitamin B-12	25 mcg		Capsule		Bristol-Myers Squibb
SQUIBB; 802	Clorazepate Dipotassium	3.75 mg	White	Capsule		Bristol-Myers Squibb
SQUIBB; 829	Chlorothiazide	500 mg	White	Tablet	Compressed	Bristol-Myers Squibb
SQUIBB; 831	Vitamin E	200 mg		Tablet		Bristol-Myers Squibb
SQUIBB; 838	Clorazepate	7.5 mg		Capsule		Bristol-Myers Squibb
SQUIBB; 842	Theragran	5000 IU; 3 mg; 9 mcg; 90 mg; 400 IU; 30 IU; 30 mg; 0.4 mg; 10 mg; 30 mcg		Coated Tablet		Bristol-Myers Squibb
SQUIBB; 845	Allopurinol	100 mg	White	Tablet	Circle	Bristol-Myers Squibb
SQUIBB; 849	Multiple Vitamins and Minerals	5000 IU; 30 IU; 500 mg; 20 mg; 20 mg; 100 mg; 25 mg; 0.15 mg; 25 mg; 0.8 mg; 50 mcg; 27 mg; 0.1 mg; 50 mg; 5 mg; 3 mg; 22.5 mg		Tablet		Bristol-Myers Squibb
SQUIBB; 851	Triamterene and Hydrochlorothiazide	75 mg; 50 mg	Yellow	Tablet	Circle, Scored	Bristol-Myers Squibb
SQUIBB; 874	Cephalexin	500 mg	Opaque Orange and Orange	Capsule		Apothecon
SQUIBB; 876	Trigesic	125 mg; 230 mg; 30 mg		Tablet		Bristol-Myers Squibb
SQUIBB; 883	Doxycycline Hyclate	50 mg	White and Brown	Capsule, Liquid Filled		Bristol-Myers Squibb
SQUIBB; 884	Doxycycline Hyclate	100 mg	Brown	Capsule, Liquid Filled		Bristol-Myers Squibb
SQUIBB; 889	Vitamin E	74 mg		Capsule		Bristol-Myers Squibb
SQUIBB; 897	Doxycycline Hyclate	100 mg	Orange	Coated Tablet		Bristol-Myers Squibb
SQUIBB; 915	Vitamin B-1	50 mg		Tablet		Bristol-Myers Squibb
SQUIBB; 916	Vitamin B-1	100 mg		Tablet		Bristol-Myers Squibb
SQUIBB; 921	Vesprin	10 mg	Pink	Tablet		Bristol-Myers Squibb
SQUIBB; 922	Vesprin	25 mg	White and Orange	Tablet		Bristol-Myers Squibb
SQUIBB; 923	Vesprin	50 mg	Green	Tablet		Bristol-Myers Squibb
SQUIBB; 955	Amitid	100 mg	Purple-Red	Tablet		Squibb & Sons
SQUIBB; 963	Trazodone	100 mg		Tablet		Bristol-Myers Squibb
SQUIBB; 971;	Principen	250 mg	Gray	Capsule		Apothecon
SQUIBB; 974;	Principen	500 mg	Gray and Dark Gray	Capsule		Apothecon
SQUIBB; 1535	Loxapine Succinate	50 mg		Capsule		Bristol-Myers Squibb
SQUIBB; E.T.	E.T. the Extraterrestrial Children's Chewable Vitamins	5000 IU; 400 IU; 30 IU; 60 mg; 0.4 mg; 1.5 mg; 1.7 mg; 20 mg; 2 mg; 6 mcg	Purple, Orange and Pink	Tablet, Chewable		Bristol-Myers Squibb
SQUIBB; E.T.	E.T. the Extraterrestrial Children's Chewable Vitamins with Iron	5000 IU; 400 IU; 30 IU; 60 mg; 0.4 mg; 1.5 mg; 1.7 mg; 20 mg; 2 mg; 6 mcg; 18 mg	Purple, Orange and Pink	Tablet, Chewable		Bristol-Myers Squibb
SQUIBB; W028	Cloxacillin Sodium	250 mg	Opaque Orange	Capsule		Apothecon
SQUIBB; W028	Cloxacillin Sodium	250 mg	Orange	Capsule		Apothecon
SQUIBB; W038	Cloxacillin Sodium	500 mg	Opaque Orange	Capsule		Apothecon
SQUIBB; W048	Dicloxacillin	250 mg	Blue	Capsule		Sandoz
SQUIBB; W048	Dicloxacillin Sodium	250 mg		Capsule		Bristol-Myers Squibb
SQUIBB; W058	Dicloxacillin Sodium	500 mg		Capsule		Bristol-Myers Squibb
SQUIBB; W134	Lithium Carbonate	300 mg		Capsule		Bristol-Myers Squibb
SQUIBB; W460	Desipramine Hydrochloride	50 mg		Tablet		Bristol-Myers Squibb
SQUIBB; W470	Desipramine Hydrochloride	75 mg		Tablet		Bristol-Myers Squibb
SQUIBB; WO38	Cloxacillin Sodium	500 mg	Orange	Capsule		Apothecon
SR; 089	Histex SR	10 mg; 120 mg	Peach/clear Capsule	Extended-Release Capsule		Teamm Pharmaceuticals
SR; ABBOTT LOGO	Tricor, Micronized	200 mg	Orange	Capsule		Abbott Laboratories
STA; HIST	Stahist	25 mg; 40 mg; 8 mg; 0.19 mg; 0.04 mg; 0.01 mg	White	Tablet		Magna Pharmaceuticals
STA-D	Sta-D	25 mg; 40 mg; 0.19 mg; 0.04 mg; .01	Blue	Tablet		Magna Pharmaceuticals
STAFLEX	Staflex	500 mg; 60 mg	Orange	Tablet		Magna Pharmaceuticals

IMPRINT	BRAND/GENERIC NAME	STRENGTH	COLOR	FORM	SHAPE	MANUFACTURER
STAGESIC	Stagesic	5 mg; 500 mg	White	Capsule		Magna Pharmaceuticals
STAMOIST E;	Stamoist E	500 mg; 120 mg	White	Extended-Release Tablet		Magna Pharmaceuticals
STAR; 109	Uro-Kp-Neutral	250 mg; 250 mg; 49.25 mg	Peach	Tablet		Star Pharmaceuticals
STAR; 1200	Liquibid-D	1200 mg; 40 mg	Light Green	Extended-Release Tablet	Capsule-Shape	Capellon Pharmaceuticals
STAR; PHE	Rescon Mx	8 mg; 2.5 mg; 120 mg	Green and White	Extended-Release Tablet	Capsule-Shape	Capellon Pharmaceuticals
STAR; UROLENE BLUE	Urolene Blue	65 mg	Blue	Tablet	Circle	Star Pharmaceuticals
STAR SHAPE	Liquibid - PD	275 mg; 25 mg	White and Blue	Extended-Release Tablet	Triangle, Scored	Capellon Pharmaceuticals
STARLIX; 60	Starlix	60 mg	Pink	Tablet	Circle, Bevel Edged	Novartis
STARLIX; 120	Starlix	120 mg	Yellow	Tablet	Oval	Novartis
STASON; 10/11	Captopril	12.5 mg	White	Tablet	Diamond, Scored	Stason Pharmaceuticals
STASON; 10/12	Captopril	25 mg	White	Tablet	Diamond-Shaped, Quadrisected Scored	Stason Pharmaceuticals
STASON; 10/13	Captopril	50 mg	White	Tablet	Diamond, Scored	Stason Pharmaceuticals
STASON; 10/14	Captopril	100 mg	White	Tablet	Capsule-Shape, Scored	Stason Pharmaceuticals
STASON; 1020	Selegiline Hydrochloride	5 mg	White	Tablet	Circle	Stason Pharmaceuticals
STASON; 1020	Selegiline Hydrochloride	5 mg	White	Tablet	Circle	Duramed Pharmaceuticals
STUART	Orexin Softab	10 mg; 5 mg; 25 mcg	Pink	Tablet	Circle, Biconvex	Stason Pharmaceuticals
STUART; 380	Kasof	240 mg	Brown	Capsule		Johnson & Johnson Merck Consumer Pharmaceuticals
STUART; 450	Mylicon	40 mg	White	Tablet	Circle, Biconvex	Johnson & Johnson Merck Consumer Pharmaceuticals
STUART; 650	Ferancee	3.1 Gr; 150 mg	Brown and Gold	Tablet, Chewable		Johnson & Johnson Merck Consumer Pharmaceuticals
STUART; 851	Mylanta II	400 mg; 400 mg; 40 mg	Green and White	Tablet, Chewable		Johnson & Johnson Merck Consumer Pharmaceuticals
STUART; 858	Mylicon 80	80 mg	Pink	Tablet, Chewable	Circle, Beveled	Johnson & Johnson Merck Consumer Pharmaceuticals
SU	Sudafed	30 mg	Red	Coated Tablet		Johnson & Johnson Merck Consumer Pharmaceuticals
SU; 24	Sudafed 24 Hour	240 mg		Extended-Release Tablet	Oval	Pfizer Consumer Health Care
SUDAFED; 60	Sudafed	60 mg	Red	Tablet		Pfizer Consumer Health Care
SUDAFED; SCF	Maximum Strength Sudafed Severe Cold Formula Tablet	500 mg; 15 mg; 30 mg	White	Tablet	Circle	Pfizer Consumer Health Care
SUDAFED; SCF	Sudafed Severe Cold Formula	500 mg; 15 mg; 30 mg	White	Coated Tablet	Circle	Burroughs Wellcome
SUDAFED; SCF	Sudafed Severe Cold Formula	500 mg; 15 mg; 30 mg	White	Tablet	Circle	Pfizer Consumer Health Care
SUDAFED; SINUS	Sudafed Non-Drying Sinus Liquid Caps	200 mg; 30 mg	Clear Turquoise	Capsule		Pfizer Consumer Health Care
SUDAFED; SINUS	Sudafed Sinus Headache	500 mg; 30 mg	Peach	Tablet		Pfizer Consumer Health Care
SUDAFED 12 HOUR; H9B	Sudafed 12 Hour	120 mg	Red and Clear	Extended-Release Capsule		Pfizer Consumer Health Care
SUDAFED C&S	Sudafed Cold and Sinus Liquid Caps	325 mg; 30 mg	Blue	Capsule, Liquid Filled	Oval	Pfizer Consumer Health Care
SUDAFED PLUS;	Sudafed Plus Tablet	60 mg; 4 mg		Tablet		Pfizer Consumer Health Care
SUDAL; 60; A; P	Sudal 60/500	60 mg; 500 mg	White	Tablet	Capsule-Shape, Scored	Atley Pharmaceuticals
SUDAL; SR; A; P	Sudal SR	50 mg; 1200 mg	White	Extended-Release Tablet	Capsule-Shape	Atley Pharmaceuticals
SUMMIT; 165;	Slow-K	600 mg	Buff	Sustained-Release Tablet	Circle	Summit Pharmaceuticals
SUNKIST 60, SUNKIST LOGO, ORANGE SLICE	Sunkist Vitamin C	60 mg	White, Flat	Tablet, Chewable	Circle	Novartis Consumer
SUNKIST 250, SUNKIST LOGO, ORANGE SLICE	Sunkist Vitamin C	250 mg	White, Flat	Tablet, Chewable	Circle	Novartis Consumer
SUNKIST 500, SUNKIST LOGO, ORANGE SLICE	Sunkist Vitamin C	500 mg	White, Flat	Tablet, Chewable	Circle	Novartis Consumer
SUNKIST V	Sunkist Multivitamins, Children's Regular	2500 IU; 15 IU; 0.3 mg; 13.5 mg; 400 IU; 60 mg; 1.05 mg; 4.5 mcg; 1.05 mg; 1.2 mg; 5 mcg	Orange, Yellow and Pinkish-Rose	Tablet, Chewable	Circle, Flat	Novartis Consumer
SUNKIST; V+FE	Sunkist Multivitamins with Iron Children's	15 mg; 2500 IU; 15 IU; 0.3 mg; 13.5 mg; 400 IU; 60 mg; 1.05 mg; 4.5 mcg; 1.05 mg; 1.2 mg; 5 mcg	Orange, Yellow and Pinkish-Rose	Tablet, Chewable	Circle	Novartis Consumer
SUNKIST V+M	Sunkist Multivitamins Children's	10 mg; 5000 IU; 400 IU; 30 IU; 60 mg; 0.4 mg; 40 mcg; 10 mg; 20 mg; 2 mg; 6 mcg; 1.5 mg; 1.7 mg; 10 mcg; 20 mg; 150 mcg; 10 mg; 1 mg; 100 mg; 78 mg; 2 mg	Yellow, Orange and Pinkish-Rose	Tablet, Chewable	Circle	Novartis Consumer
SUNKIST XC	Sunkist Multivitamins Plus Extra C	2500 IU; 400 IU; 15 IU; 250 mg; 0.3 mg; 13.5 mg; 1.05 mg; 4.5 mcg; 1.05 mg; 1.2 mg; 5 mcg	Yellow, Orange and Pinkish-Rose	Tablet	Circle, Flat	Novartis Consumer
SUPRAX; LL; 200	Suprax	200 mg	White	Coated Tablet	Rectangle, Scored, Convex	Lederle Laboratories

IMPRINT	BRAND/GENERIC NAME	STRENGTH	COLOR	FORM	SHAPE	MANUFACTURER
SUPRAX; LL; 400	Suprax	400 mg	White	Coated Tablet	Rectangle, Scored, Convex	Lederle Laboratories
SURFAK	Surfak Liqui-Gels	240 mg	Dark Purple	Capsule, Liquid Filled	Oblong	Pharmacia & Upjohn
SUSTIVA; 50 MG	Sustiva	50 mg	Gold and White	Capsule		Bristol-Myers Squibb
SUSTIVA; 100 MG	Sustiva	100 mg	White	Capsule		Bristol-Myers Squibb
SUSTIVA; 200 MG	Sustiva	200 mg	Gold	Capsule		Bristol-Myers Squibb
SUSTIVA; SUSTIVA	Sustiva	600 mg	Yellow	Coated Tablet	Capsule-Shape	Bristol-Myers Squibb
SV	Prometrium	100 mg	Peach	Capsule	Circle	Solvay Pharmaceuticals
SV2	Prometrium	200 mg	Pale Yellow	Capsule	Oval	Solvay Pharmaceuticals
SW; 200	Skelid	200 mg	White to Off-White	Tablet	Circle, Biconvex	Sanofi Winthrop Pharmaceuticals
SX	Xifaxan	200 mg	Pink	Tablet	Circle	Salix Pharmaceuticals
SYMMETREL	Symmetrel	100 mg	Light Orange	Tablet	Triangle, Convex	Endo Laboratories
SYNTEX	Norminest Fe-28 Blue Tablet	0.5 mg; 0.035 mg	Blue	28-Day Tablet Pack		Roche Laboratories
SYNTEX; 2902	Anadrol	50 mg	White	Tablet		Roche Laboratories
SYNTEX; TORADOL; T	Toradol Oral	10 mg		Coated Tablet	Circle	Roche Laboratories
SYNTHROID; 25;	Synthroid	25 mcg	Orange	Tablet		Abbott Laboratories
SYNTHROID; 50;	Synthroid	50 mcg	White	Tablet		Abbott Laboratories
SYNTHROID; 75;	Synthroid	75 mcg	Violet	Tablet		Abbott Laboratories
SYNTHROID; 88;	Synthroid	88 mcg	Olive	Tablet	Circle, Scored	Abbott Laboratories
SYNTHROID; 100;	Synthroid	100 mcg	Yellow	Tablet		Abbott Laboratories
SYNTHROID; 112;	Synthroid	112 mcg	Rose	Tablet		Abbott Laboratories
SYNTHROID; 125;	Synthroid	125 mcg	Brown	Tablet		Abbott Laboratories
SYNTHROID; 137	Synthroid	137 mcg	Turquoise	Tablet		Abbott Laboratories
SYNTHROID; 150;	Synthroid	150 mcg	Blue	Tablet		Abbott Laboratories
SYNTHROID; 175	Synthroid	175 mcg	Lilac	Tablet		Abbott Laboratories
SYNTHROID; 200;	Synthroid	200 mcg	Pink	Tablet		Abbott Laboratories
SYNTHROID; 300;	Synthroid	300 mcg	Green	Tablet		Abbott Laboratories
T	Aspirin	325 mg	Red	Tablet	Circle, Scored	Rugby Laboratories
T	Aspirin Enteric Coated	325 mg	Orange	Delayed-Release Tablet	Circle, Biconvex, Enteric-Coated	Time Cap Labs
T	Aspirin Enteric Coated	325 mg	Orange	Delayed-Release Tablet	Circle, Biconvex, Enteric-Coated	Udl Laboratories
T	Benzonatate	100 mg	Light Gold	Capsule	Circle	Inwood Laboratories
T	K-Effervescent	25 Meg	Orange	Effervescent Tablet	Circle	Qualitest Products
T	Potassium Bicarbonate	25 meq	Orange	Effervescent Tablet	Circle	Watson Laboratories
T	Teldrin	4 mg	Green	Tablet	Circle	Glaxosmithkline Consumer
T	Tessalon Perles	100 mg	Yellow	Capsule		Forest Pharmaceuticals
T0R; ORGANON	Cyclessa Light Yellow Tablet	0.1 mg; 0.025 mg	Light Yellow	Coated Tablet	Circle	Organon
T1R; ORGANON	Cyclessa Red Tablet	0.15 mg; 0.025 mg	Red	Coated Tablet	Circle	Organon
T; 2	Enalapril Maleate	2.5 mg	Yellow	Tablet	Circle, Scored	Taro Pharmaceuticals
T3	Enalapril and Hydrochlorothiazide	10 mg; 25 mg	Peach	Tablet	Capsule-Shape	Taro Pharmaceuticals
T4	Enalapril and Hydrochlorothiazide	5 mg; 12.5 mg	Ivory	Tablet	Capsule-Shape	Taro Pharmaceuticals
T; 5	Enalapril Maleate	5 mg	Yellow	Tablet	Circle, Scored	Taro Pharmaceuticals
T6R; ORGANON	Cyclessa Orange Tablet	0.125 mg; 0.025 mg	Orange	Coated Tablet	Circle	Organon
T; 10	Enalapril Maleate	10 mg	Round	Tablet	Circle, Pink	Taro Pharmaceuticals
T; 12	Trinlet LA	500 mg; 40 mg; 8 mg	Pink	Tablet		Trinity Technologies
T; 20	Enalapril Maleate	20 mg	Orange	Tablet	Circle	Taro Pharmaceuticals
T 25	Tarceva	25 mg	White	Tablet	Circle	Genentech
T 25	Tarceva	25 mg	White	Tablet	Circle	Osi Pharmaceuticals
T31;	Telepaque	500 mg	Off-White or Light Buff	Tablet	Circle, Scored	Nycomed
T; 31	Warfarin Sodium	1 mg	Pink	Tablet	Capsule-Shape, Scored	Taro Pharmaceuticals
T; 32	Warfarin Sodium	2 mg	Lavender	Tablet	Capsule-Shape, Scored	Taro Pharmaceuticals
T; 33	Warfarin Sodium	2.5 mg	Green	Tablet	Capsule-Shape, Scored	Taro Pharmaceuticals
T; 34	Warfarin Sodium	4 mg	Blue	Tablet	Capsule-Shape, Scored	Taro Pharmaceuticals
T; 35	Warfarin Sodium	5 mg	Peach	Tablet	Capsule-Shape, Scored	Taro Pharmaceuticals
T36	Calcium Gluconate	1 GM		Tablet		Eli Lilly
T; 36	Warfarin Sodium	7.5 mg	Yellow	Tablet	Capsule-Shape, Scored	Taro Pharmaceuticals
T; 37	Warfarin Sodium	10 mg	White	Tablet	Capsule-Shape, Scored	Taro Pharmaceuticals
T; 38	Warfarin Sodium	3 mg	Tan	Tablet	Capsule-Shape, Scored	Taro Pharmaceuticals
T; 39	Warfarin Sodium	6 mg	Greenish-Yellow	Tablet	Capsule-Shape, Scored	Taro Pharmaceuticals
T; 41	Phenazopyridine Hydrochloride	100 mg	Maroon	Coated Tablet	Circle	Trinity Technologies
T; 45	Clorazepate Dipotassium	3.75 mg	Pale Violet	Tablet	Circle, Flat, Scored	Taro Pharmaceuticals
T; 46	Clorazepate Dipotassium	7.5 mg	Orange	Tablet	Circle, Flat, Scored	Taro Pharmaceuticals
T; 47	Clorazepate Dipotassium	15 mg	Pale Pink	Tablet	Circle, Flat, Scored	Taro Pharmaceuticals
T; 52	Acetazolamide	125 mg	White	Tablet	Circle, Scored	Taro Pharmaceuticals
T; 53	Acetazolamide	250 mg	White	Tablet	Round, Quadrisected Scored	Taro Pharmaceuticals
T; 57	Ketoconazole	200 mg	White to Off-White	Tablet	Flat, Scored	Taro Pharmaceuticals
T; 88	Etodolac	400 mg	Peach	Coated Tablet	Oval	Taro Pharmaceuticals
T; 93	Isoniazid	100 mg		Tablet		Eli Lilly
T 100	Tarceva	100 mg	White	Tablet	Circle	Genentech
T; 100 MG	Tegretol-Xr	100 mg	Yellow	Extended-Release Tablet	Circle	Novartis
T; 103	Hyoscyamine Sulfate	0.125 mg	White	Tablet	Standard Cup, Bisected Scored	Trinity Technologies
T; 107	Tenormin	25 mg	White	Tablet	Circle, Flat	Astra Zeneca
T; 109	Carbamazepine	200 mg	White	Tablet	Circle, Single Scored	Teva Pharmaceuticals
T; 109	Carbamazepine	200 mg	White	Tablet	Circle, Single Scored	Udl Laboratories
T; 121	Urinary Antiseptic	40.8 mg; 18.1 mg; 4.5 mg; 5.4 mg; 0.03 mg; 0.03 mg	Deep Blue	Coated Tablet	Circle	H.L. Moore
T; 121	Urinary Antiseptic	40.8 mg; 18.1 mg; 4.5 mg; 5.4 mg; 0.03 mg; 0.03 mg	Deep Blue	Coated Tablet	Circle	Trinity Technologies
T; 142	Phenazopyridine Hydrochloride	200 mg	Maroon	Coated Tablet	Circle	Trinity Technologies
T 150	Tarceva	150 mg	White	Tablet	Circle	Genentech
T; 177	Pseudoephedrine Hydrochloride Guaifenesin	120 mg; 600 mg	Yellow	Tablet	Capsule-Shape	Trinity Technologies
T; 200 MG	Tegretol-Xr	200 mg	Pink	Extended-Release Tablet	Circle	Novartis

IMPRINT	BRAND/GENERIC NAME	STRENGTH	COLOR	FORM	SHAPE	MANUFACTURER
T; 203	Colchicine	0.5 mg	White	Tablet	Circle, Standard Cup, Compressed	Trinity Technologies
T; 204	Colchicine	0.6 mg	White	Tablet	Circle, Standard Cup, Compressed	Trinity Technologies
T; 400	Etodolac	400 mg	Pink	Extended-Release Tablet	Circle	Taro Pharmaceuticals
T; 400 MG	Tegretol-Xr	400 mg	Brown	Extended-Release Tablet	Circle	Novartis
T; 500	Etodolac	500 mg	Green	Extended-Release Tablet	Oblong	Taro Pharmaceuticals
T; 600	Etodolac	600 mg	Grey	Extended-Release Tablet	Oval	Taro Pharmaceuticals
TAGAMET; 200; SKF	Tagamet	200 mg	Light-Green	Coated Tablet	Circle	Glaxosmithkline
TAGAMET; 300; SB	Tagamet	300 mg	Light-Green	Coated Tablet	Circle	Glaxosmithkline
TAGAMET; 400; SB	Tagamet	400 mg	Light-Green	Coated Tablet	Oval	Glaxosmithkline
TAGAMET; 800; SB	Tagamet	800 mg	Light-Green	Coated Tablet	Oval	Glaxosmithkline
TAGAMET; HB; SB	Tagamet Hb	100 mg	White	Coated Tablet	Circle	Glaxosmithkline
TAGAMET HB; 200	Tagamet Hb 200	200 mg	White	Tablet	Diamond	Glaxosmithkline Consumer
TAP; 200 MG	Spectracef	200 mg	White with Blue Ink	Coated Tablet	Circle	Tap Pharmaceuticals
TAP; PREVACID; 15	Prevacid	15 mg	Pink and Green	Delayed-Release Capsule		Tap Pharmaceuticals
TAP; PREVACID; 30	Prevacid	30 mg	Pink and Black	Delayed-Release Capsule		Tap Pharmaceuticals
TARACTAN; ROCHE 10	Taractan	10 mg	Light Coral	Coated Tablet		Roche Pharmaceuticals
TARACTAN; ROCHE 25	Taractan	25 mg	Coral	Coated Tablet		Roche Pharmaceuticals
TARACTAN; ROCHE 50	Taractan	50 mg	Pinkish Orange	Coated Tablet		Roche Pharmaceuticals
TARACTAN; ROCHE 100	Taractan	100 mg	Reddish Brown	Coated Tablet		Roche Pharmaceuticals
TARGRETIN	Targretin	75 mg	Off-White	Capsule	Oblong	Ligand Pharmaceuticals
TARKA; 182; KNOLL TRIANGLE;	Tarka 2/180 mg	2 mg; 180 mg	Pink	Sustained-Release Tablet	Oval	Abbott Laboratories
TARKA; 241; KNOLL TRIANGLE;	Tarka 1/240 mg	1 mg; 240 mg	White	Sustained-Release Tablet	Oval	Abbott Laboratories
TARKA; 242; KNOLL TRIANGLE;	Tarka 2/240 mg	2 mg; 240 mg	Gold	Sustained-Release Tablet	Oval	Abbott Laboratories
TARKA; 244; KNOLL TRIANGLE;	Tarka 4/240 mg	4 mg; 240 mg	Red-Brown	Sustained-Release Tablet	Oval	Abbott Laboratories
TARO; 11	Carbamazepine	200 mg	White	Tablet	Circle, Flat Beveled-Edge, Scored	Taro Pharmaceuticals
TARO; 11	Carbamazepine	200 mg	White	Tablet	Round, Scored, Flat Beveled-Edge	Akyma Pharmaceuticals
TARO; 16	Carbamazepine	100 mg	White, Pink	Tablet, Chewable	Circle, Scored	Taro Pharmaceuticals
TARO; 25	Clomipramine Hydrochloride	25 mg	Dark Blue and Light Blue	Capsule		Taro Pharmaceuticals
TARO; 50	Clomipramine Hydrochloride	50 mg	Yellow	Capsule		Taro Pharmaceuticals
TARO; 75	Clomipramine Hydrochloride	75 mg	White	Capsule		Taro Pharmaceuticals
TARO; 89	Etodolac	500 mg	Blue	Coated Tablet	Oval	Taro Pharmaceuticals
TASMAR; 100; ROCHE	Tasmar	100 mg	Beige	Coated Tablet	Six-Sided, Biconvex	Roche Pharmaceuticals
TASMAR; 200; ROCHE	Tasmar	200 mg	Red-Brown	Coated Tablet	Six-Sided, Biconvex	Roche Pharmaceuticals
TAVIST	Tavist Sinus	500 mg; 30 mg	Red and White	Capsule, Liquid Filled		Novartis Consumer
TAVIST; 78/72;	Tavist	2.68 mg	White	Tablet	Circle, Scored	Novartis Pharmaceuticals
TAVIST; ALLERGY	Tavist Allergy	1.34 mg	White	Tablet	Oblong, Scored	Novartis Consumer
TC; TYLENOL COLD	Children's Tylenol Cold	80 mg; 0.5 mg; 7.5 mg	Purple	Tablet, Chewable	Circle	Mcneil Consumer Products
TCL; 001	Aspirin	325 mg	Orange	Enteric-Coated Tablet	Circle, Biconvex	Time Cap Labs
TCL; 002	Aspirin	650 mg	Red	Tablet	Circle	Rugby Laboratories
TCL; 002	Aspirin, Enteric Coated	650 mg	Red	Coated Tablet	Circle	Time Cap Labs
TCL; 003	Bisacodyl	5 mg	Yellow	Coated Tablet	Circle	Able Laboratories
TCL; 003	Bisacodyl	5 mg	Yellow and Orange	Enteric-Coated Tablet	Circle	Time Cap Labs
TCL; 005	Aspirin, Enteric Coated Maximum Strength	500 mg	Orange	Enteric-Coated Tablet	Circle	Time Cap Labs
TCL; 005;	Maximum Strength Aspirin	500 mg	Orange	Enteric-Coated Tablet	Circle	Good Neighbor Pharmacy
TCL; 005;	Maximum Strength Aspirin	500 mg	Orange	Enteric-Coated Tablet	Circle	Good Sense
TCL; 005;	Maximum Strength Aspirin	500 mg	Orange	Enteric-Coated Tablet	Circle	Kerr Drug
TCL; 005;	Maximum Strength Aspirin	500 mg	Orange	Enteric-Coated Tablet	Circle	Perrigo
TCL; 005;	Maximum Strength Aspirin	500 mg	Orange	Enteric-Coated Tablet	Circle	Top Care
TCL; 005;	Maximum Strength Aspirin	500 mg	Orange	Enteric-Coated Tablet	Circle	Valu Rite
TCL; 006	Ferro-Time	250 mg	Red and Clear with Maroon and White Pellets	Extended-Release Capsule		Time Cap Labs
TCL; 011	Aspirin	325 mg	White	Tablet	Circle	Rugby Laboratories
TCL; 011	Aspirin, Film Coated	325 mg	Clear	Coated Tablet	Circle	Time Cap Labs
TCL; 016	Pseudoephedrine Hydrochloride	30 mg	Red	Tablet	Circle	Time Cap Labs
TCL; 019	Papaverine	150 mg	Brown and Clear	Capsule		Qualitest Products
TCL; 019	Para-Time	150 mg	Brown and Clear with Natural Pellets	Extended-Release Capsule		Time Cap Labs
TCL; 019	Para-Time	150 mg	Brown and Clear with Natural Pellets	Extended-Release Capsule		Udl Laboratories
TCL; 020	Correct	100 mg; 65 mg	Pink	Coated Tablet	Circle, Convex	Leiner Health Products
TCL; 020	Correct	100 mg; 65 mg	Pink	Coated Tablet	Circle, Convex	Time Cap Labs
TCL; 021	Thyroid	32.5 mg	Natural	Tablet	Circle, Compressed	Time Cap Labs
TCL; 021	Thyroid	0.5 Gr	Beige	Tablet	Circle	Qualitest Products
TCL; 022	Thyroid	65 mg	Natural	Tablet	Circle, Compressed	Time Cap Labs
TCL; 022	Thyroid	1 Gr	Beige	Tablet	Circle	Qualitest Products
TCL; 023	Thyroid	130 mg	Natural to Light Tan	Tablet	Circle, Compressed	Time Cap Labs
TCL; 023	Thyroid	2 Gr	Beige	Tablet	Circle	Qualitest Products
TCL; 025	Adults Low Strength Aspirin	81 mg	Yellow	Enteric-Coated Tablet	Circle, Convex	Leiner Health Products
TCL; 025	Adults Low Strength Aspirin	81 mg	Yellow	Enteric-Coated Tablet	Circle, Convex	Time Cap Labs
TCL; 027	Ferrous Sulfate	324 mg	Red	Coated Tablet	Circle	Time Cap Labs
TCL; 031	Ferro-Dss	150 mg; 100 mg	Light Green	Tablet		Time Cap Labs
TCL; 032	Aspirin, Enteric Coated	325 mg	Red	Enteric-Coated Tablet	Circle	Time Cap Labs
TCL; 033	Vitamin C	500 mg		Tablet		Time Cap Labs

IMPRINT	BRAND/GENERIC NAME	STRENGTH	COLOR	FORM	SHAPE	MANUFACTURER
TCL; 036	Com-Time	4 mg; 50 mg; 20 mg	Yellow and Clear with Natural and Yellow Pellets	Extended-Release Capsule		Time Cap Labs
TCL; 038	Thyroid	195 mg	Natural	Tablet	Circle, Compressed	Time Cap Labs
TCL; 038	Thyroid	3 Gr	Beige	Tablet	Circle	Qualitest Products
TCL; 041	Chlorpheniramine Maleate	8 mg	Blue Green and Clear with Pink and White Pellets	Extended-Release Capsule		Time Cap Labs
TCL; 043	Chlorpheniramine Maleate	12 mg	Blue Green and Clear with Pink and White Pellets	Extended-Release Capsule		Time Cap Labs
TCL; 057	Correct	5 mg	Pink	Coated Tablet	Circle	Time Cap Labs
TCL; 090	Allerfrim	2.5 mg; 60 mg	White	Tablet	Circle	Rugby Laboratories
TCL; 224	Megaprin	15 Gr	White	Tablet	Oval	Econolab
TCL; 1221	Nitroglycerin	2.5 mg	Pink and Clear	Capsule		Qualitest Products
TCL; 1221	Nitro-Time	2.5 mg	Lavender and Clear with Natural Pellets	Extended-Release Capsule		Time Cap Labs
TCL; 1222	Nitroglycerin	6.5 mg	Blue and Yellow	Capsule		Qualitest Products
TCL; 1222	Nitro-Time	6.5 mg	Blue and Yellow with Natural Pellets	Extended-Release Capsule		Time Cap Labs
TCL; 1223	Nitroglycerin	9 mg	Green and Yellow	Capsule		Qualitest Products
TCL; 1223	Nitro-Time	9 mg	Blue and Yellow with Natural Pellets	Extended-Release Capsule		Time Cap Labs
TD; CG	Trileptal	150 mg	Yellow	Coated Tablet	Oval, Biconvex, Scored Both Sides	Novartis
TE TE; CG CG	Trileptal	300 mg	Yellow	Coated Tablet	Oval, Biconvex, Scored Both Sides	Novartis
TEGISON; 10; ROCHE	Tegison	10 mg	Brown and Green	Capsule	Oval	Roche Pharmaceuticals
TEGISON; 25; ROCHE	Tegison	25 mg	Brown and Caramel	Capsule	Oval	Roche Pharmaceuticals
TEGRETOL; 27; 27;	Tegretol	200 mg	Pink	Tablet	Capsule-Shape, Single-Scored	Novartis
TEGRETOL; 52 52;	Tegretol	100 mg	Pink with Red Speckles	Tablet, Chewable	Circle, Scored	Novartis
TELDRIN; 12 MG	Teldrin	12 mg	Clear, Green	Timed-Release Capsule		Glaxosmithkline Consumer
TEMAZEPAM; 7.5 MG; 271; CP	Temazepam	7.5 mg	White and Pink	Capsule		Geneva Generics
TEMAZEPAM; 15 MG; 272; CP	Temazepam	15 mg	Aqua and White	Capsule		Creighton Products
TEMOZOLOMIDE; 5 MG; SP	Temodar	5 mg	Off-White with Green Ink	Capsule		Schering
TEMOZOLOMIDE; 20 MG; SP	Temodar	20 mg	Off-White with Brown Ink	Capsule		Schering
TEMOZOLOMIDE; 100 MG; SP	Temodar	100 mg	Off-White with Blue Ink	Capsule		Schering
TEMOZOLOMIDE; 250 MG; SP	Temodar	250 mg	Off-White with Black Ink	Capsule		Schering
TEN K	Ten-K	750 mg	White	Timed-Release Tablet	Capsule-Shape, Scored	Novartis
TENEX; 1; AHR	Tenex	1 mg	Light Pink	Tablet	Diamond	A.H. Robins
TENEX/2 AHR	Tenex	2 mg	Yellow	Tablet	Diamond	A.H. Robins
TENORETIC; 115	Tenoretic 50	25 mg; 50 mg	White	Tablet	Round, Biconvex, Bisected Scored	Astra Zeneca
TENORETIC; 117;	Tenoretic 100	25 mg; 100 mg	White	Tablet	Circle, Biconvex	Astra Zeneca
TENORMIN; 101	Tenormin	100 mg	White	Tablet	Circle, Flat	Astra Zeneca
TENORMIN; 105	Tenormin	50 mg	White	Tablet	Round, Flat, Bisected Scored	Astra Zeneca
TENUATE; 25	Tenuate	25 mg	White	Tablet	Circle	Aventis Pharmaceuticals
TENUATE; 75	Tenuate Dospan	75 mg	White	Timed-Release Tablet	Capsule-Shape	Aventis Pharmaceuticals
TEW; PRE-H-CAL	Pre-H-Cal	4000 IU; 400 IU; 50 mg; 3 mg; 3 mg; 5 mg; 2.5 mcg; 3 mg; 0.5 mg; 125 mg; 32.4 mg; 32.5 mg; 1 mg; 500 mg	Pink	Coated Tablet		T.E. Williams Pharmaceuticals
TEW; THEO-TUSS	Theo-Tuss	165 mg; 15 mg; 25 mg; 300 mg	Red	Coated Tablet		T.E. Williams Pharmaceuticals
TF TF; CG CG	Trileptal	600 mg	Yellow	Coated Tablet	Oval, Biconvex, Scored Both Sides	Novartis
T-GESIC; TEW	T-Gesic	5 mg; 500 mg	White	Capsule		T.E. Williams Pharmaceuticals
TH; 0; RJS;	Westhroid	32.4 mg	Tan	Tablet	Round, Compressed, Bisected Scored	Western Research Laboratories
TH; 1; RJS;	Westhroid	64.8 mg	Tan	Tablet	Round, Compressed, Bisected Scored	Western Research Laboratories
TH; 2; RJS;	Westhroid	130 mg	Tan	Tablet	Circle, Compressed	Western Research Laboratories
TH; A	Cylert	18.75 mg	White	Tablet	Monogrammed, Grooved	Abbott Laboratories
THEO; 250	Theo-250	250 mg	Clear	Sustained-Release Capsule		Shoals Pharmaceuticals
THEO-24; 100 MG; UCB; 2832;	Theo-24	100 mg	Yellow-Orange and Clear	Extended-Release Capsule		Ucb Pharma
THEO-24; 200 MG; UCB; 2842;	Theo-24	200 mg	Red-Orange and Clear	Extended-Release Capsule		Ucb Pharma
THEO-24; 300 MG; UCB; 2852;	Theo-24	300 mg	Red and Clear	Extended-Release Capsule		Ucb Pharma
THEO-24; 400 MG; UCB; 2902;	Theo-24	400 mg	Pink and Clear	Extended-Release Capsule		Ucb Pharma
THEOBID; 130;	Theobid Duracap JR.	130 mg	Clear with White Beads	Capsule		Ucb Pharma
THEOBID; 260;	Theobid Duracap	260 mg	Clear with White Beads	Capsule		Ucb Pharma
THEO-BID; 260	Theo-Bid Duracap	260 mg	Clear	Extended-Release Capsule		Ucb Pharma
THEO-DUR; 100	Theo-Dur	100 mg	White to Off-White	Sustained-Release Tablet	Circle, Scored	Key Pharmaceuticals
THEO-DUR; 200	Theo-Dur	200 mg	White to Off-White	Sustained-Release Tablet	Oval, Scored	Key Pharmaceuticals

IMPRINT	BRAND/GENERIC NAME	STRENGTH	COLOR	FORM	SHAPE	MANUFACTURER
THEO-DUR; 300	Theo-Dur	300 mg	White to Off-White	Sustained-Release Tablet	Capsule-Shape, Scored	Key Pharmaceuticals
THEO-DUR; 450	Theo-Dur	450 mg	White to Off-White	Sustained-Release Tablet	Capsule-Shape, Scored	Key Pharmaceuticals
THEOPHYL	Theophyl-SR	250 mg	Green and Clear	Timed-Release Capsule		Mcneil Pharmaceutical
THEOPHYL; 100	Theophyl Chewable	100 mg	White	Tablet, Chewable	Circle	Mcneil Pharmaceutical
THEOPHYL; 125	Theophyl-SR	125 mg	Yellow and Clear	Timed-Release Capsule		Mcneil Pharmaceutical
THEOPHYL; 225	Theophyl-225	225 mg	White	Tablet	Triangle, Scored	Mcneil Pharmaceutical
THERAFLU	Theraflu Maximum Strength Flu, Cold & Cough Non-Drowsy Formula	500 mg; 15 mg; 30 mg	Yellow	Tablet		Novartis Consumer
THERAFLU	Theraflu Maximum Strength Nighttime Flu, Cold & Cough	500 mg; 30 mg; 15 mg; 2 mg	Green	Tablet		Novartis Consumer
THERAFLU	Thera-Flu Maximum Strength Nighttime Formula	500 mg; 30 mg; 15 mg; 2 mg	Green	Tablet	Oblong	Sandoz Consumer
THER-RX; 014	Precare Conceive	60 mg; 200 mg; 30 mg; 30 IU; 3 mg; 3.4 mg; 20 mg; 50 mg; 1 mg; 100 mg; 12 mcg; 15 mg; 2 mg	Yellow	Coated Tablet	Diamond	Ther-RX
THER-RX; 019	Premesis RX	75 mg; 12 mcg; 1 mg; 200 mg;	Blue	Tablet	Oval	Ther-RX
THER-RX; 025	Precare	50 mg; 250 mg; 40 mg; 3.5 mg; 6 mcg; 3 mg; 3.4 mg; 20 mg; 20 mg; 1 mg; 12 mcg; 50 mg; 15 mg; 2 mg	Peach	Tablet	Coated, Partially Bisected Scored	Ther-RX
THER-RX; 128	Strongstart	225 mg; 50 mg; 40 mg; 30 IU; 50 mg; 15 mg; 20 mg; 7 mg; 3 mg; 3.4 mg; 1 mg; 12 mg; 400 IU; 90 mcg; 35 mg; 2 mg; 75 mcg; 45 mcg; 50 mcg; 30 mg; 25 mg	White	Tablet	Oval	Ther-RX
THER-RX; 137	Strongstart	250 mg; 50 mg; 35 mg; 3.5 mg; 15 mg; 50 mg; 1 mg; 6 mcg; 2 mg; 10 mg	Orange	Tablet, Chewable		Ther-RX
THIS END UP; THEO-DUR SPRINKLE 50 MG	Theo-Dur Sprinkle	50 mg	White and Clear	Timed-Release Capsule		Key Pharmaceuticals
THIS END UP; THEO-DUR SPRINKLE 75 MG	Theo-Dur Sprinkle	75 mg	White and Clear	Timed-Release Capsule		Key Pharmaceuticals
THIS END UP; THEO-DUR SPRINKLE 125 MG	Theo-Dur Sprinkle	125 mg	White and Clear	Timed-Release Capsule		Key Pharmaceuticals
THIS END UP; THEO-DUR SPRINKLE 200 MG	Theo-Dur Sprinkle	200 mg	White and Clear	Timed-Release Capsule		Key Pharmaceuticals
THX; 024	Precare	50 mg; 250 mg; 40 mg; 6 mcg; 3.5 mg; 2 mg; 1 mg; 50 mg; 15 mg; 2 mg	Orange Speckled	Tablet, Chewable	Circle	Ther-RX
THX; 0129	Chromagen	70 mg; 150 mg; 100 mg; 10 mcg	Red	Capsule, Liquid Filled	Capsule-Shape	Ther-RX
THX; 0130	Chromagen FA	70 mg; 1 mg; 10 mcg; 150 mg	Green and Brown	Capsule, Liquid Filled		Savage Laboratories
THX; 0130	Chromagen FA	70 mg; 150 mg; 1 mg; 10 mcg	Green and Brown	Capsule, Liquid Filled	Capsule-Shape	Ther-RX
THX; 0131	Chromagen Forte	70 mg; 81 mg; 60 mg; 1 mg; 10 mcg	Brown	Capsule, Liquid Filled	Capsule-Shape	Ther-RX
THX; 0134	Niferex	40 mg; 20 mg	Brown and Clear	Capsule		Ther-RX
THX; 0135	Niferex 150	80 mg; 70 mg; 50 mg	Orange and Clear	Capsule		Ther-RX
THX; 0136	Niferex 150 Forte	80 mg; 70 mg; 1 mg; 60 mg; 25 mcg	Red and Clear	Capsule		Ther-RX
TI; 01	Spiriva	18 mcg	Light Green	Capsule		Pfizer
TI; A	Cylert	37.5 mg	Orange	Tablet	Monogrammed, Grooved	Abbott Laboratories
TIAZAC; 120	Tiazac	120 mg	Lavender	Extended-Release Capsule		Forest Pharmaceuticals
TIAZAC; 180	Tiazac	180 mg	White and Blue-Green	Extended-Release Capsule		Forest Pharmaceuticals
TIAZAC; 240	Tiazac	240 mg	Blue-Green and Lavender	Extended-Release Capsule		Forest Pharmaceuticals
TIAZAC; 300	Tiazac	300 mg	White and Lavender	Extended-Release Capsule		Forest Pharmaceuticals

IMPRINT	BRAND/GENERIC NAME	STRENGTH	COLOR	FORM	SHAPE	MANUFACTURER
TIAZAC; 360	Tiazac	360 mg	Blue-Green	Extended-Release Capsule		Forest Pharmaceuticals
TIAZAC; 420	Tiazac	420 mg	White	Extended-Release Capsule		Forest Pharmaceuticals
TICLID; 250	Ticlid	250 mg	White	Coated Tablet	Oval	Syntex
TIGAN; M079	Tigan	300 mg	Purple	Capsule		Monarch Pharmaceuticals
TITRALAC; EXTRA	Titralac Extra Strength	750 mg	White	Tablet, Chewable	Circle	3m Pharmaceuticals
TITRALAC PLUS	Titralac Plus	420 mg; 21 mg		Tablet, Chewable		3m Pharmaceuticals
TJ; A	Cylert	75 mg	Tan	Tablet	Monogrammed, Grooved	Abbott Laboratories
TK; A	Cylert	37.5 mg	Orange	Tablet, Chewable	Monogrammed, Grooved	Abbott Laboratories
TL; 001	Methylprednisolone	4 mg	White	Tablet	Oval; Quadrisected Scored	Breckenridge Pharmaceutical
TL; 001	Methylprednisolone	4 mg	White	Tablet	Oval, Quadrisected Scored	Ranbaxy Pharmaceuticals
TL; 113	Prochlorperazine Maleate	5 mg	Yellow-Green	Tablet	Circle, Scored	Par Pharmaceutical
TL; 115	Prochlorperazine Maleate	10 mg	Light Green	Tablet	Circle, Scored	Par Pharmaceutical
TL; Q	Tramadol Hydrochloride	50 mg	White	Tablet		Par Pharmaceutical
TO	Detrol	1 mg	White	Coated Tablet	Circle, Biconvex	Pharmacia & Upjohn
TO; 60	Fareston	60 mg	White to Off-White	Tablet	Circle, Convex	Schering
TOLECTIN; 200; MCNEIL	Tolectin	200 mg	White	Tablet		Ortho-Mcneil Pharmaceutical
TOLECTIN; 600; MCNEIL	Tolectin 600	600 mg	Orange	Tablet	Oval	Ortho-Mcneil Pharmaceutical
TOLECTIN DS; MCNEIL	Tolectin DS	400 mg	Orange	Capsule		Ortho-Mcneil Pharmaceutical
TOLINASE; 100;	Tolinase	100 mg	White	Tablet	Circle, Scored	Pharmacia & Upjohn
TOLINASE; 250;	Tolinase	250 mg	White	Tablet	Circle, Scored	Pharmacia & Upjohn
TOLINASE; 500;	Tolinase	500 mg	White	Tablet	Circle, Scored	Pharmacia & Upjohn
TOLMETIN; 200	Tolmetin Sodium	200 mg	White	Tablet	Circle, Scored	Duramed Pharmaceuticals
TOLMETIN; 400	Tolmetin Sodium	400 mg	Orange	Capsule		Duramed Pharmaceuticals
TOLMETIN; 600	Tolmetin Sodium	600 mg	Orange	Tablet	Egg-Shape, Scored	Duramed Pharmaceuticals
TONOCARD; 707	Tonocard	400 mg	Yellow	Coated Tablet	Oval, Scored	Astra Zeneca
TONOCARD; 709	Tonocard	600 mg	Yellow	Coated Tablet	Oblong, Scored	Astra Zeneca
TOP; 15 MG	Topamax Sprinkle Capsule	15 mg	White and Clear with White Spheres	Capsule		Ortho-Mcneil Pharmaceutical
TOP; 25	Topamax	25 mg	White	Coated Tablet	Circle	Ortho-Mcneil Pharmaceutical
TOP; 25 MG	Topamax Sprinkle Capsule	25 mg	White and Clear with White Spheres	Capsule		Ortho-Mcneil Pharmaceutical
TOPAMAX; 100	Topamax	100 mg	Yellow	Coated Tablet	Circle	Ortho-Mcneil Pharmaceutical
TOPAMAX; 200	Topamax	200 mg	Salmon	Coated Tablet	Circle	Ortho-Mcneil Pharmaceutical
TORADOL; ROCHE	Toradol	10 mg	White	Tablet	Circle	Roche Laboratories
TP; 373	Folic Acid	1 mg	Pale Yellow	Tablet	Single Bisect, Compressed	Rosemont Pharmaceutical
TP; 404	Hydrochlorothiazide	25 mg	Peach	Tablet	Compressed	Rosemont Pharmaceutical
TP; 407	Hydrochlorothiazide with Reserpine	50 mg; 0.125 mg		Tablet		Bolar Pharmaceutical
TP; 758;	Acetaminophen	325 mg	White	Tablet		Rosemont Pharmaceutical
TR; 1; ORGANON	Cesia Red Tablet	0.15 mg; 0.025 mg	Red	28-Day Tablet Pack	Circle	Prasco Laboratories
TR; 6; ORGANON	Cesia Orange Tablet	0.125 mg; 0.025 mg	Orange	28-Day Tablet Pack	Circle	Prasco Laboratories
TR; 125; G	Triazolam	0.125 mg	White	Tablet	Oval	Par Pharmaceutical
TR; 250; G	Triazolam	0.25 mg	Pale Yellow	Tablet	Oval, Scored	Par Pharmaceutical
TR; O; ORGANON	Cesia Light Yellow Tablet	0.1 mg; 0.025 mg	Light Yellow	28-Day Tablet Pack	Circle	Prasco Laboratories
TRANDATE; 100	Trandate	100 mg	Orange	Coated Tablet	Circle, Scored	Glaxosmithkline
TRANDATE; 200	Trandate	200 mg	White	Coated Tablet	Circle, Scored	Glaxosmithkline
TRANDATE; 300	Trandate	300 mg	Peach	Coated Tablet	Circle, Scored	Glaxosmithkline
TRANSDERM-NITRO; 0.1 MG/HR	Transderm-Nitro	0.1 mg/hr	Tan	Patch	Circle	Novartis Generics
TRANSDERM-NITRO; 0.2 MG/HR	Transderm-Nitro	0.2 mg/hr	Tan	Patch	Oblong	Novartis Generics
TRANSDERM-NITRO; 0.4 MG/HR	Transderm-Nitro	0.4 mg/hr	Tan	Patch	Oblong	Novartis Generics
TRANSDERM-NITRO; 0.6 MG/HR	Transderm-Nitro	0.6 mg/hr	Tan	Patch	Oblong	Novartis Generics
TRANSDERM-NITRO; 0.8 MG/HR	Transderm-Nitro	0.8 mg/hr	Tan	Patch	Circle	Novartis Generics
TRAVIST; SINUS	Tavist Sinus	500 mg; 30 mg	White	Tablet		Novartis Consumer
TRENTAL	Trental	400 mg	Pink	Timed-Release Tablet	Oblong	Aventis Pharmaceuticals
TRIAD; UAD; 305	Triad	325 mg; 50 mg; 40 mg	White	Capsule		Uad Laboratories
TRIANGEL; 567	Hydrocodone Bitartrate and Acetaminophen	10 mg; 660 mg	White	Tablet	Capsule-Shape, Scored	Andrx Pharmaceuticals
TRIANGLE	Maxalt-Mlt	5 mg	White	Tablet	Circle	Merck
TRIANGLE	Phentermine Hydrochloride	8 mg	Red	Tablet	Circle	Rosemont Pharmaceutical
TRIANGLE; 516	Benazepril Hydrochloride	5 mg	Light Orange	Tablet	Circle	Andrx Pharmaceuticals
TRIANGLE; 517	Benazepril Hydrochloride	10 mg	Orange	Tablet	Circle	Andrx Pharmaceuticals
TRIANGLE; 518	Benazepril Hydrochloride	20 mg	Peach	Tablet	Circle	Andrx Pharmaceuticals
TRIANGLE; 519	Benazepril Hydrochloride	40 mg	Orange-Red	Tablet	Circle	Andrx Pharmaceuticals
TRIANGLE; 521; 3	Acetaminophen and Codeine Phosphate	300 mg; 15 mg	White	Tablet	Circle, Scored	Andrx Pharmaceuticals
TRIANGLE; 522; 3	Acetaminophen and Codeine Phosphate	300 mg; 30 mg	White	Tablet	Circle, Scored	Andrx Pharmaceuticals
TRIANGLE; 523; 4	Acetaminophen and Codeine Phosphate	300 mg; 60 mg	White	Tablet	Circle, Scored	Andrx Pharmaceuticals
TRIANGLE; 756	Benazepril Hydrochloride and Hydrochlorothiazide	5 mg; 6.25 mg	White	Tablet		Andrx Pharmaceuticals
TRIANGLE; 757	Benazepril Hydrochloride and Hydrochlorothiazide	10 mg; 12.5 mg	Purple	Tablet		Andrx Pharmaceuticals
TRIANGLE; 758	Benazepril Hydrochloride and Hydrochlorothiazide	20 mg; 12.5 mg	Pink	Tablet		Andrx Pharmaceuticals

IMPRINT	BRAND/GENERIC NAME	STRENGTH	COLOR	FORM	SHAPE	MANUFACTURER
TRIANGLE; 759	Benazepril Hydrochloride and Hydrochlorothiazide	20 mg; 25 mg	Red	Tablet		Andrx Pharmaceuticals
TRIANGLE; 791	Lovastatin	10 mg	White to Off-White	Tablet	Circle	Andrx Pharmaceuticals
TRIANGLE; 792	Lovastatin	20 mg	White to Off-White	Tablet	Circle	Andrx Pharmaceuticals
TRIANGLE; 793	Lovastatin	40 mg	White to Off-White	Tablet	Circle	Andrx Pharmaceuticals
TRIANGLE; 871	Glipizide Extended-Release	2.5 mg	Blue	Extended-Release Tablet	Circle	Andrx Pharmaceuticals
TRIANGLE; 872	Glipizide Extended-Release	5 mg	White	Extended-Release Tablet	Circle	Andrx Pharmaceuticals
TRIANGLE; 873	Glipizide Extended-Release	10 mg	White	Extended-Release Tablet	Circle	Andrx Pharmaceuticals
TRIANGLE; P; 71;	Tussin Severe Congestion Non-Drowsy Formula	200 mg; 30 mg	Green	Capsule, Liquid Filled		Good Neighbor Pharmacy
TRIANGLE; P; 71;	Tussin Severe Congestion Non-Drowsy Formula	200 mg; 30 mg	Green	Capsule, Liquid Filled		Good Sense
TRIANGLE; P; 71;	Tussin Severe Congestion Non-Drowsy Formula	200 mg; 30 mg	Green	Capsule, Liquid Filled		Hytop
TRIANGLE; P; 71;	Tussin Severe Congestion Non-Drowsy Formula	200 mg; 30 mg	Green	Capsule, Liquid Filled		Kerr Drug
TRIANGULAR LOGO; 168	Nilandron	50 mg	White	Tablet	Biconvex, Cylindrical	Hoechst-Roussel Pharmaceuticals
TRIMEN; TRIMEN	Dyrexan-OD	105 mg	Brown and Clear	Sustained-Release Capsule		Trimen Laboratories
TRIMPEX; 100; ROCHE	Trimpex	100 mg	White	Tablet	Circle, Scored	Roche Pharmaceuticals
TRIMPEX; 100; ROCHE	Trimpex	100 mg	White	Tablet	Oval, Scored	Roche Laboratories
TRINALIN; 703	Trinalin Repetabs	1 mg; 120 mg	Coral	Coated Tablet		Key Pharmaceuticals
TRINITY; G 600	Guaifenesin	600 mg	Light Green	Sustained-Release Tablet	Capsule, Bisected Scored	Trinity Technologies
TRINSICON-M; GLAXO	Trinsicon M	75 mg; 110 mg; 240 mg; 15 mcg	Dark Pink and Dark Red	Capsule		Glaxosmithkline
TRITEC; STOMACH-SHAPED LOGO	Tritec	400 mg	Blue	Coated Tablet	Eight-Sided, Elongated	Glaxosmithkline
TSH; 8441;	Almacone	200 mg; 200 mg; 25 mg	Yellow and White	Tablet, Chewable	Circle	Rugby Laboratories
TT	Trinprin	800 mg	White	Tablet		Trinity Technologies
TT; 500	Choline Magnesium Trisalicylate	500 mg	Orange	Tablet	Bisected Scored	Trinity Technologies
TT; 750	Choline Magnesium Trisalicylate	750 mg	Off-White	Tablet	Bisected Scored	Trinity Technologies
TT; 1000	Choline Magnesium Trisalicylate	1000 mg	Red	Coated Tablet	Bisected Scored	Trinity Technologies
TT; S500	Salsalate	500 mg	Blue or Yellow	Coated Tablet	Circle, Standard Cup, Compressed	Trinity Technologies
TT; S750	Salsalate	750 mg	Blue or Yellow	Tablet		Trinity Technologies
TTC; 091	Anaplex SR	8 mg; 120 mg	Blue and Clear	Sustained-Release Capsule		Ecr Pharmaceuticals
TTC; 091	Chlorpheniramine Maleate and D-Pseudoephedrine Hydrochloride SR	8 mg; 120 mg	Opaque Blue and Clear	Capsule		Trinity Technologies
TTC; 104	Brompheniramine and Pseudoephedrine	6 mg; 60 mg	Dark Green and Clear	Capsule		Trinity Technologies
TTC; 138	Pancrelipase	4000 U; 20000 U; 25000 U	White	Capsule		Trinity Technologies
TTC; 140	Comtrin LA	4 mg; 20 mg; 50 mg	Opaque Blue and Clear or Opaque Yellow and Clear	Capsule		Trinity Technologies
TUMS	Tums Anti-Gas/antacid	500 mg; 20 mg	Assorted	Tablet	Circle	Glaxosmithkline Consumer
TUMS	Tums Assorted Flavors	500 mg	Pink, Orange, Yellow or Green	Tablet, Chewable	Circle	Glaxosmithkline Consumer
TUSSIGON; DP; 082	Tussigon	5 mg; 1.5 mg	Blue	Tablet	Circle	Daniels Pharmaceuticals
TUTAG	Sprx-2	35 mg	Yellow and White Layered	Tablet		Solvay Pharmaceuticals
TUTAG	Unproco	200 mg; 30 mg	Orange	Capsule		Solvay Pharmaceuticals
TY; 80	Children's Tylenol Soft-Chews Bubblegum Flavor	80 mg	Pink	Tablet, Chewable	Oval	Mcneil Consumer Products
TY; 80	Children's Tylenol Soft-Chews Fruit Flavor	80 mg	Pink	Tablet, Chewable	Oval	Mcneil Consumer Products
TY; 80	Children's Tylenol Soft-Chews Grape Flavor	80 mg	Purple	Tablet, Chewable	Oval	Mcneil Consumer Products
TY; A	Tranxene-SD	22.5 mg	Peach	Extended-Release Tablet	Circle	Abbott Laboratories
TYLENOL	Children's Tylenol Bubblegum Flavor	80 mg	Pink	Tablet, Chewable	Circle, Scored	Mcneil Consumer Products
TYLENOL	Children's Tylenol Fruit-Flavored	80 mg	Pink	Tablet, Chewable		Mcneil Consumer Products
TYLENOL	Children's Tylenol Grape Flavored	80 mg	Purple	Tablet, Chewable		Mcneil Consumer Products
TYLENOL	Children's Tylenol Meltaways - Bubble Gum Burst	80 mg		Disintegrating Tablet	Circle	Mcneil Consumer Products
TYLENOL	Children's Tylenol Meltaways - Grape Punch	80 mg		Disintegrating Tablet	Circle	Mcneil Consumer Products
TYLENOL	Children's Tylenol Meltaways - Wacky Watermelon	80 mg		Disintegrating Tablet	Circle	Mcneil Consumer Products
TYLENOL	Junior Strength Tylenol Meltaways - Bubble Gum Burst	160 mg		Disintegrating Tablet	Circle	Mcneil Consumer Products
TYLENOL	Junior Strength Tylenol Meltaways - Grape Punch	160 mg		Disintegrating Tablet	Circle	Mcneil Consumer Products
TYLENOL	Tylenol Extra Strength	500 mg	White	Tablet	Circle	Mcneil Consumer Products
TYLENOL	Tylenol Regular Strength	325 mg	White	Tablet	Circle	Mcneil Consumer Products
TYLENOL; 160	Junior Strength Tylenol	160 mg	White	Tablet		Mcneil Consumer Products
TYLENOL; 160	Junior Strength Tylenol Fruit Flavor	160 mg	Pink	Tablet, Chewable	Circle	Mcneil Consumer Products
TYLENOL; 160	Junior Strength Tylenol Grape Flavor	160 mg	Purple	Tablet, Chewable	Circle	Mcneil Consumer Products
TYLENOL; 325	Tylenol Regular Strength	325 mg	White	Tablet		Mcneil Consumer Products
TYLENOL; 500	Tylenol Extra Strength Caplets	500 mg	White	Tablet		Mcneil Consumer Products
TYLENOL; 500	Tylenol Extra Strength Gelcaps	500 mg	Yellow and Red	Capsule, Liquid Filled		Mcneil Consumer Products

IMPRINT	BRAND/GENERIC NAME	STRENGTH	COLOR	FORM	SHAPE	MANUFACTURER
TYLENOL; 500	Tylenol Extra Strength Geltabs	500 mg	Yellow and Red	Geltab		Mcneil Consumer Products
TYLENOL; A/S	Tylenol Allergy Sinus Maximum Strength Gelcaps	2 mg; 30 mg; 500 mg	Green and Yellow	Capsule, Liquid Filled		Mcneil Consumer Products
TYLENOL; A/S	Tylenol Allergy Sinus Maximum Strength Geltabs	2 mg; 30 mg; 500 mg	Green and Yellow	Geltab	Circle	Mcneil Consumer Products
TYLENOL; A/S; NIGHT TIME	Tylenol Allergy Sinus Nighttime Maximum Strength	500 mg; 30 mg; 25 mg	Light Blue	Capsule, Liquid Filled		Mcneil Consumer Products
TYLENOL; ALLERGY SINUS	Tylenol Allergy Sinus Maximum Strength Caplets	2 mg; 30 mg; 500 mg	Dark Yellow	Tablet	Oblong	Mcneil Consumer Products
TYLENOL; C/C; TC/C	Children's Tylenol Cold Plus Cough	80 mg; 0.5 mg; 7.5 mg; 2.5 mg	Pink	Tablet, Chewable		Mcneil Consumer Products
TYLENOL; CODEINE; 2	Tylenol with Codeine No. 2	300 mg; 15 mg	White	Tablet	Circle	Mcneil Pharmaceutical
TYLENOL; CODEINE; 3;	Tylenol with Codeine No. 3	300 mg; 30 mg	White	Tablet	Circle	Mcneil Pharmaceutical
TYLENOL; CODEINE; 4;	Tylenol with Codeine No. 4	300 mg; 60 mg	White	Tablet	Circle	Mcneil Pharmaceutical
TYLENOL; COLD	Tylenol Cold Multi-Symptom	325 mg; 2 mg; 30 mg; 15 mg	Light Yellow	Tablet		Mcneil Consumer Products
TYLENOL; COLD; DM; 80	Children's Tylenol Cold DM	0.5 mg; 80 mg; 3.75 mg; 7.5 mg		Tablet, Chewable	Flat-Faced, Beveled	Mcneil Consumer Products
TYLENOL; COLD; SC	Tylenol Cold Severe Congestion Non-Drowsy	30 mg; 200 mg; 15 mg; 325 mg	Yellow	Tablet	Capsule-Shape	Mcneil Consumer Products
TYLENOL; ER	Tylenol Arthritis Extended Relief	650 mg	White	Extended-Release Capsule	Oblong	Mcneil Consumer Products
TYLENOL; HEADACHE PLUS	Tylenol Extra Strength Headache Plus Tablet	500 mg; 250 mg	White	Tablet		Mcneil Consumer Products
TYLENOL; SEVERE ALLERGY	Tylenol Severe Allergy Fast Relief	500 mg; 12.5 mg	Bright Yellow	Tablet	Oblong	Mcneil Consumer Products
TYLENOL; SINUS	Tylenol Sinus Maximum Strength Non-Drowsy	500 mg; 30 mg	Light Green	Tablet	Circle	Mcneil Consumer Products
TYLENOL; SINUS	Tylenol Sinus Maximum Strength Non-Drowsy Caplets	500 mg; 30 mg	Light Green	Tablet		Mcneil Consumer Products
TYLENOL; SINUS	Tylenol Sinus Maximum Strength Non-Drowsy Gelcaps	30 mg; 500 mg	Green and White	Capsule, Liquid Filled		Mcneil Consumer Products
TYLENOL COLD	Tylenol Cold Multi-Symptom Non-Drowsy Caplets	325 mg; 15 mg; 30 mg	White	Tablet	Oblong	Mcneil Consumer Products
TYLENOL COLD	Tylenol Cold Multi-Symptom Non-Drowsy Gelcaps	325 mg; 15 mg; 30 mg	Yellow and Orange	Capsule, Liquid Filled		Mcneil Consumer Products
TYLENOL FLU	Extra Strength Tylenol Flu Convenience Pack Daytime Relief	500 mg; 30 mg; 15 mg	Red and White	Capsule, Liquid Filled	Capsule-Shape	Mcneil Consumer Products
TYLENOL FLU	Extra Strength Tylenol Flu Daytime Relief	500 mg; 30 mg; 15 mg	Red and White	Capsule, Liquid Filled	Capsule-Shape	Mcneil Consumer Products
TYLENOL FLU	Tylenol Flu Maximum Strength	500 mg; 15 mg; 30 mg	Burgundy and White	Capsule, Liquid Filled		Mcneil Consumer Products
TYLENOL FLU; NT	Tylenol Flu Nighttime Maximum Strength	500 mg; 30 mg; 25 mg	White and Dark Blue	Capsule, Liquid Filled		Mcneil Consumer Products
TYLENOL PM	Tylenol Pm Extra Strength Caplets	500 mg; 25 mg	Light Blue	Tablet		Mcneil Consumer Products
TYLENOL PM	Tylenol Pm Extra Strength - Gelcaps	500 mg; 25 mg	Blue and White	Capsule, Liquid Filled		Mcneil Consumer Products
TYLENOL PM	Tylenol Pm Extra Strength Geltabs	500 mg; 25 mg	Blue and White	Geltab	Circle	Mcneil Consumer Products
TYLENOL SINUS	Tylenol Sinus Maximum Strength Non-Drowsy Geltabs	30 mg; 500 mg	Green and White	Geltab	Circle	Mcneil Consumer Products
TYLOX; MCNEIL	Tylox	5 mg; 500 mg	Red	Capsule		Ortho-Mcneil Pharmaceutical
TYME	Tylenol Women's Menstrual Relief	500 mg; 25 mg	White	Tablet		Mcneil Consumer Products
TZ; 1	Remeron Soltab	15 mg	White	Tablet	Circle	Organon
TZ; 2	Remeron Soltab	30 mg	White	Tablet	Circle	Organon
TZ; 4	Remeron Soltab	45 mg	White	Tablet	Circle	Organon
U	Colestid	1 GM	Yellow	Coated Tablet	Circle	Pharmacia & Upjohn
U	Unicap	5000 IU; 400 IU; 15 IU; 60 mg; 0.4 mg; 1.5 mg; 1.7 mg; 20 mg; 2 mg; 6 mcg	Yellow	Capsule		Upjohn
U	Unicap M	5000 IU; 400 IU; 15 IU; 60 mg; 0.4 mg; 1.5 mg; 1.7 mg; 20 mg; 2 mg; 6 mcg; 10 mg; 150 mcg; 18 mg; 2 mg; 15 mg; 1 mg; 5 mg	Tan	Coated Tablet		Upjohn
U	Unicap M Plus Iron	1.5 mg; 10 mcg; 2.5 mg; 2.5 mg; 50 mg; 20 mg; 0.5 mg; 5 mg; 2 mcg; 10 IU; 50 mg; 0.15 mg; 1 mg; 1 mg; 6 mg; 5 mg; 35 mg	Tan	Coated Tablet		Upjohn
U	Unicap Plus Iron	18 mg; 5000 IU; 400 IU; 15 IU; 0.4 mg; 1.5 mg; 1.7 mg; 20 mg; 10 mg; 60 mg; 2 mg; 6 mcg	Red	Coated Tablet		Upjohn

IMPRINT	BRAND/GENERIC NAME	STRENGTH	COLOR	FORM	SHAPE	MANUFACTURER
U	Unicap Senior	10 mg; 5000 IU; 15 IU; 0.4 mg; 1.2 mg; 1.7 mg; 14 mg; 10 mg; 150 mcg; 2 mg; 15 mg; 1 mg; 5 mg; 60 mg; 2 mg; 6 mcg	Blue	Coated Tablet		Upjohn
U	Uristat	95 mg	Red-Brown	Tablet	Circle	Ortho Advanced
U; 2	Mirapex	0.125 mg	White	Tablet	Circle	Boehringer Ingelheim
U; 4	Mirapex	0.25 mg	White	Tablet	Oval, Scored	Boehringer Ingelheim
U; 6	Mirapex	1 mg	White	Tablet	Circle, Scored	Boehringer Ingelheim
U; 8	Mirapex	0.5 mg	White	Tablet	Oval, Scored	Boehringer Ingelheim
U; 26;	Sandril	0.25 mg	Green	Tablet		Eli Lilly
U; 37	Mirapex	1.5 mg	White	Tablet	Circle, Scored	Boehringer Ingelheim
U; 60	Keflex	1 GM	Green	Tablet		Eli Lilly
U; 94;	Xanax	2 mg	White	Tablet	Oblong, Multi-Scored	Pharmacia & Upjohn
U; 201;	Lorcet Plus	650 mg; 7.5 mg	White	Tablet	Capsule-Shape, Scored	Uad Laboratories
U; 3617	Vantin	100 mg	Light Orange	Coated Tablet	Circle	Pharmacia & Upjohn
U; 3618	Vantin	200 mg	Coral Red	Coated Tablet	Circle	Pharmacia & Upjohn
U; 3761	Rescriptor	100 mg	White	Tablet	Capsule-Shape	Agouron Pharmaceuticals
UAA	Urinary Antiseptic Antispasmodic	0.03 mg; 0.03 mg; 40.8 mg; 5.4 mg; 18.1 mg; 4.5 mg		Coated Tablet	Compressed	Economed Pharmaceuticals
UAD; 111	E-Lor	650 mg; 65 mg	Orange	Tablet	Capsule-Shape, Film-Coated	Uad Laboratories
UAD; 400	Eudal-SR	120 mg; 400 mg	White	Sustained-Release Tablet	Capsule-Shape, Scored	Uad Laboratories
UAD; 1120	Lorcet-HD	5 mg; 500 mg	Maroon	Capsule		Uad Laboratories
UAD; 2304	Dital	105 mg	Lavender and Clear	Extended-Release Capsule		Uad Laboratories
UAD; 2404	Vertab	50 mg	Opaque Blue	Capsule		Uad Laboratories
UAD; 6350	Lorcet 10/650	10 mg; 650 mg	Light Blue	Tablet	Capsule-Shape, Scored	Uad Laboratories
UAD; CEZIN S; 811	Cezin-S	10000 IU; 50 IU; 50 IU; 200 mg; 50 mg; 10 mg; 10 mg; 5 mg; 4 mg; 2 mg; 80 mg; 0.5 mg; 70 mg	Yellow	Capsule		Uad Laboratories
UAD; ENDAFED; 206	Endafed	120 mg; 12 mg	Blue and Clear	Sustained-Release Capsule		Uad Laboratories
UC; ABBOTT LOGO	Prosom	1 mg	White	Tablet		Abbott Laboratories
UCB; 250	Keppra	250 mg	Blue	Coated Tablet	Oblong, Scored	Ucb Pharma
UCB; 316;	Vicon Forte	150 mg; 10 mg; 70 mg; 25 mg; 5 mg; 8000 IU; 50 IU; 80 mg; 10 mcg; 10 mg; 2 mg; 4 mg; 1 mg	Orange and Black	Capsule		Ucb Pharma
UCB; 364;	Trinsicon	0.5 mg; 240 mg; 15 mcg; 75 mg; 110 mg	Dark Pink and Dark Red	Capsule		Ucb Pharma
UCB; 500	Keppra	500 mg	Yellow	Coated Tablet	Oblong, Scored	Ucb Pharma
UCB; 500;	Lortab Asa	500 mg; 5 mg	Dark Pink	Tablet	Capsule-Shape	Ucb Pharma
UCB; 612;	Duratuss	600 mg; 120 mg	White	Extended-Release Tablet	Oval, Scored	Ucb Pharma
UCB; 620;	Duratuss G	1200 mg	White	Extended-Release Tablet	Capsule-Shape, Scored	Ucb Pharma
UCB; 640	Duratuss Gp	1200 mg; 120 mg	White	Extended-Release Tablet	Oval, Coated, Scored	Ucb Pharma
UCB; 750	Keppra	750 mg	Orange	Coated Tablet	Oblong, Scored	Ucb Pharma
UCB; 901;	Lortab 2.5/500	500 mg; 2.5 mg	White with Pink Specks	Tablet	Capsule-Shaped, Bisected Scored	Ucb Pharma
UCB; 902;	Lortab 5/500	500 mg; 5 mg	White with Blue Specks	Tablet	Capsule-Shaped, Bisected Scored	Ucb Pharma
UCB; 903;	Lortab 7.5/500	500 mg; 7.5 mg	White with Green Specks	Tablet	Capsule-Shaped; Bisected Scored	Ucb Pharma
UCB; 910;	Lortab 10/500	500 mg; 10 mg	Pink	Tablet	Capsule-Shape	Ucb Pharma
UCB; UCB;	Vicon Plus	150 mg; 10 mg; 4 mg; 2 mg; 10 mg; 50 IU; 80 mg; 4000 IU; 5 mg; 25 mg; 70 mg	Red and Light Yellow with Blue Band	Capsule		Ucb Pharma
UCB; UCB;	Vicon-C	300 mg; 7 mg; 18 mg; 10 mg; 18 mg; 20 mg; 4 mg; 99 mg	Orange and Yellow with Blue Band	Capsule		Ucb Pharma
UCB UCB;	VI-Zac	5000 IU; 18 mg; 50 IU; 500 mg	Orange with Blue Band	Capsule		Ucb Pharma
UCY; 500	Buphenyl	500 mg	Off-White	Tablet	Oval	Ucyclyd Pharma
UD; ABBOTT LOGO	Prosom	2 mg	Pink	Tablet		Abbott Laboratories
ULTRAGESIC	Ultragesic	5 mg; 500 mg	White	Capsule		Stewart-Jackson Pharmacal
ULTRASE; MT6	Ultrase Mt6	19500 U; 6000 U; 19500 U	Yellow	Extended-Release Capsule		Axcan Scandipharm
ULTRASE; MT12	Ultrase Mt12	39,000 units; 12,000 units; 39,000 units	White and Yellow	Capsule		Axcan Scandipharm
ULTRASE; MT18	Ultrase Mt18	58,500 units; 18,000 units; 58,500 units	Gray and White	Capsule		Axcan Scandipharm
ULTRASE; MT20	Ultrase Mt20	65,000 units; 20,000 units; 65,000 units	Light Gray and Yellow	Capsule		Axcan Scandipharm

IMPRINT	BRAND/GENERIC NAME	STRENGTH	COLOR	FORM	SHAPE	MANUFACTURER
ULTRASE; MT24	Ultrase Mt24	78,000 units; 24,000 units; 78,000 units	Gray and Orange	Capsule		Axcan Scandipharm
ULTRASE; MT30	Ultrase Mt30	97500 U; 30000 U; 97500 U	Gray	Extended-Release Capsule		Axcan Scandipharm
UNI-DUR; 400	Uni-Dur	400 mg	Mottled White	Timed-Release Tablet	Capsule-Shape, Scored	Dura Pharmaceuticals
UNI-DUR; 400	Uni-Dur	400 mg	Mottled White	Timed-Release Tablet	Capsule-Shape, Scored	Key Pharmaceuticals
UNI-DUR; 600	Uni-Dur	600 mg	Mottled White	Timed-Release Tablet	Capsule-Shape, Scored	Dura Pharmaceuticals
UNI-DUR; 600	Uni-Dur	600 mg	Mottled White	Timed-Release Tablet	Capsule-Shape, Scored	Key Pharmaceuticals
UNIMED; 8633	Anadrol-50	50 mg	White	Tablet		Unimed
UNISOM	Unisom	25 mg	Blue	Tablet	Oval, Bisected Scored	Pfizer Consumer Health Care
UNISOM	Unisom Sleepgels	50 mg	Clear Blue	Capsule	Oval	Pfizer Consumer Health Care
UPJOHN	Uticillin K	250 mg		Tablet		Upjohn
UPJOHN; 15	Cortisone Acetate	5 mg	White	Tablet	Circle, Scored	Pharmacia & Upjohn
UPJOHN; 23	Cortisone Acetate	10 mg	White	Tablet	Circle, Scored	Pharmacia & Upjohn
UPJOHN; 34	Cortisone Acetate	25 mg	White	Tablet	Circle, Scored	Pharmacia & Upjohn
UPJOHN; 243	Alkets	780 mg; 130 mg; 65 mg	Pink	Tablet, Chewable		Pharmacia & Upjohn
UPJOHN 949	Uracil Mustard	1 mg	Yellow and Dark Blue	Capsule		Upjohn
UPR	Unisom with Pain Relief	650 mg; 50 mg	Pale Blue	Coated Tablet	Capsule-Shape	Pfizer Consumer Health Care
URIMAR-T	Urimar-T	81.6 mg; 40.8 mg; 36.2 mg; 10.8 mg; 0.12 mg	Purple	Tablet		Marnel Pharmaceuticals
URISPAS; SKF	Urispas	100 mg	White	Coated Tablet	Circle	Alza
UROEZE; DP; 079	Uroeze	400 mg	Brown	Tablet, Chewable	Circle	Daniels Pharmaceuticals
UROEZE; DP; 103	Uroeze	400 mg	Light Brown	Tablet	Circle	Daniels Pharmaceuticals
URS; 785	Urso 250	250 mg	White	Tablet		Axcan Scandipharm
US	Hemocyte	324 mg	Maroon	Tablet	Circle	U.S. Pharmaceutical
US	Hemocyte-C	50 mg; 250 mg	Light Brown	Tablet, Chewable	Circle, Scored	U.S. Pharmaceutical
US	Hemocyte-F Film-Coated	324 mg; 1 mg	Maroon	Tablet	Circle	U.S. Pharmaceutical
US	Hemocyte Plus	324 mg; 10 mg; 6 mg; 5 mg; 15 mcg; 1 mg; 30 mg; 10 mg; 80 mg; 70 mg; 4 mg; 2 mg; 200 mg	Maroon	Capsule		Us Pharmaceutical Corporation
US; 016	Folgard RX 2.2	2.2 mg; 25 mg; 0.5 mg	Yellow	Tablet	Oval	Upsher-Smith Laboratories
US; 017	Folgard	0.8 mg; 10 mg; 0.115 mg	Green	Tablet	Circle	Upsher-Smith Laboratories
US; 027	Pentoxil	400 mg	Light Pink	Extended-Release Tablet	Capsule-Shape	Upsher-Smith Laboratories
US; 0147; P200	Pacerone	200 mg	Pink	Tablet	Circle, Score	Upsher-Smith Laboratories
US; 10	Potassium Chloride	10 meq	White	Extended-Release Tablet	Oblong	Qualitest Products
US; 12; 80	Sorine	80 mg	White	Tablet	Capsule-Shape	Upsher-Smith Laboratories
US; 13; 120	Sorine	120 mg	White	Tablet	Capsule-Shape	Upsher-Smith Laboratories
US; 14; 160	Sorine	160 mg	White	Tablet	Capsule-Shape	Upsher-Smith Laboratories
US; 15; 240	Sorine	240 mg	White	Tablet	Capsule-Shape	Upsher-Smith Laboratories
US; 20	Potassium Chloride	20 meq	White	Extended-Release Tablet	Oblong	Qualitest Products
US; 67; 500	Niacor	500 mg	White	Tablet	Oval, Scored	Upsher-Smith Laboratories
US; 200; A;	Amiodarone Hydrochloride	200 mg	White	Tablet	Circle, Scored	Sandoz
US; 500	Salsitab	500 mg	Blue	Tablet	Circle	Upsher-Smith Laboratories
US; 750	Salsitab	750 mg	Blue	Tablet	Capsule-Shape	Upsher-Smith Laboratories
US; CENOGEN ULTRA; 140	Cenogen Ultra	324 mg; 200 mg; 10 mg; 6 mg; 5 mg; 15 mcg; 1 mg; 30 mg; 10 mg; 1.3 mg; 0.8 mg	Blue and Pink	Capsule		Us Pharmaceutical Corporation
USB; 001	Hexalen	50 mg	Clear	Capsule		Medimmune
USB; 001	Hexalen	50 mg	Clear	Capsule		Mgi Pharma
USL; 8	Potassium Chloride	8 meq	Blue	Tablet	Circle	Qualitest Products
USL; 8	Potassium Chloride	600 mg	Blue	Sustained-Release Tablet	Circle	Geneva Generics
USL; 8	Potassium Chloride	600 mg	Blue	Sustained-Release Tablet	Circle	Upsher-Smith Laboratories
USL; 10	Potassium Chloride	10 meq	White	Extended-Release Tablet	Circle	Geneva Generics
USL; 10	Potassium Chloride	10 meq	White	Tablet	Circle	Qualitest Products
USL; 10	Potassium Chloride	750 mg	White	Sustained-Release Tablet	Circle	Geneva Generics
USL; 10	Potassium Chloride	750 mg	White	Sustained-Release Tablet	Circle	Upsher-Smith Laboratories
USL; 80	Zinc Sulfate	220 mg	Pink	Capsule		Upsher-Smith Laboratories
USV	Fedrine	30 mg	White	Tablet		Usv Laboratories
USV	Presamine	25 mg	Tan	Coated Tablet		Usv Laboratories
USV	Presamine	50 mg	Dark Blue	Coated Tablet		Usv Laboratories
USV; 31	Regroton	50 mg; 0.25 mg	Pink	Tablet		Usv Laboratories
USV; 32	Demi-Regroton	25 mg; 0.125 mg	White	Tablet		Usv Laboratories
USV; 45	Arlidin	6 mg	White	Tablet		Usv Laboratories
USV; 46	Arlidin	12 mg	White	Tablet		Usv Laboratories
USV; 82	Lozol	2.5 mg	White	Tablet	Circle	Aventis Pharmaceuticals
USV; 160;	Pertofrane	25 mg	Pink	Capsule		Usv Laboratories
USV; 161;	Pertofrane	50 mg	Maroon and Pink	Capsule		Usv Laboratories
V	Vivarin	200 mg	Yellow	Tablet		Glaxosmithkline Consumer
V; 0027	Q-Pap	325 mg	White	Tablet	Circle	Qualitest Products
V; 0029	Q-Pap ES	500 mg	White	Tablet	Circle	Qualitest Products
V; 0031	Acetaminophen	500 mg	White	Tablet	Circle, Scored	Vintage Pharmaceuticals
V; 0031	Q-Pap	500 mg	White	Tablet	Circle	Qualitest Products
V; 4	Vospire ER	4 mg	Green	Coated Tablet	Circle	Odyssey Pharmaceuticals
V; 8	Vospire ER	8 mg	White	Extended-Release Tablet	Circle	Odyssey Pharmaceuticals

IMPRINT	BRAND/GENERIC NAME	STRENGTH	COLOR	FORM	SHAPE	MANUFACTURER
V; 60	Bisacodyl	5 mg	Orange	Tablet	Circle	Qualitest Products
V60; FLT	Bisacodyl	5 mg	Orange	Tablet	Circle	Vintage Pharmaceuticals
V; 625	Viracept	625 mg	White	Coated Tablet	Oval	Agouron Pharmaceuticals
V; 2101	Amitriptyline	10 mg	Blue	Tablet	Circle	Qualitest Products
V; 2101	Amitriptyline Hydrochloride	10 mg	Blue	Tablet	Circle, Small	Vintage Pharmaceuticals
V; 2102	Amitriptyline	25 mg	Yellow	Tablet	Circle	Qualitest Products
V; 2102	Amitriptyline Hydrochloride	25 mg	Yellow	Tablet	Circle	Vintage Pharmaceuticals
V; 2103	Amitriptyline	50 mg	Beige	Tablet	Circle	Qualitest Products
V; 2103	Amitriptyline Hydrochloride	50 mg	Beige	Tablet	Circle	Vintage Pharmaceuticals
V; 2104	Amitriptyline	75 mg	Orange	Tablet	Circle	Qualitest Products
V; 2104	Amitriptyline Hydrochloride	75 mg	Orange	Tablet		Vintage Pharmaceuticals
V; 2105	Amitriptyline	100 mg	Mauve	Tablet	Circle	Qualitest Products
V; 2105	Amitriptyline Hydrochloride	100 mg		Tablet		Vintage Pharmaceuticals
V; 2106	Amitriptyline	150 mg	Blue	Tablet	Oval	Qualitest Products
V; 2106	Amitriptyline Hydrochloride	150 mg	Blue	Coated Tablet	Circle, Biconvex	Vintage Pharmaceuticals
V; 2410	Carisoprodol	350 mg	White	Tablet		Qualitest Products
V; 2410	Carisoprodol	350 mg	White	Tablet	Circle	Vintage Pharmaceuticals
V; 2520	Clomiphene Citrate	50 mg	White	Tablet	Circle, Scored	Qualitest Products
V; 2577	Colchicine	0.6 mg	Yellow	Tablet	Circle	Qualitest Products
V; 2577	Colchicine	0.6 mg	Yellow	Tablet	Circle	Vintage Pharmaceuticals
V; 2690	Diethylpropion Hydrochloride	75 mg	White	Tablet		Vintage Pharmaceuticals
V; 2732	Chlordiazepoxide and Clidinium	5 mg; 2.5 mg	Green	Capsule		Vintage Pharmaceuticals
V; 3169	Furosemide	20 mg	White	Tablet	Oval	Vintage Pharmaceuticals
V; 3170	Furosemide	40 mg	White	Tablet	Circle, Scored	Vintage Pharmaceuticals
V; 3171	Furosemide	80 mg	White	Tablet	Circle, Scored	Vintage Pharmaceuticals
V; 3186	Guaifenesin and Codeine	10 mg; 300 mg	Red	Tablet	Oblong	Qualitest Products
V; 3566	Hydrochlorothiazide	12.5 mg	Opaque Teal	Capsule		Qualitest Products
V; 3571	Hydrochlorothiazide	25 mg	Peach	Tablet	Circle	Qualitest Products
V; 3572	Hydrochlorothiazide	50 mg	Peach	Tablet	Circle	Qualitest Products
V; 3591	Acetaminophen and Hydrocodone	500 mg; 2.5 mg	White	Tablet	Oblong	Qualitest Products
V; 3592	Acetaminophen and Hydrocodone	500 mg; 5 mg	White	Tablet	Oblong	Qualitest Products
V; 3594	Acetaminophen and Hydrocodone	500 mg; 7.5 mg	White and Green Speckled	Tablet		Qualitest Products
V; 3595	Acetaminophen and Hydrocodone	650 mg; 7.5 mg	White	Tablet	Oblong	Qualitest Products
V; 3596	Acetaminophen and Hydrocodone	750 mg; 7.5 mg	White	Tablet	Oblong	Qualitest Products
V; 3597	Acetaminophen and Hydrocodone	650 mg; 10 mg	Light Blue	Tablet	Oblong	Qualitest Products
V; 3598	Acetaminophen and Hydrocodone	660 mg; 10 mg	White	Tablet	Oblong	Qualitest Products
V; 3598	Acetaminophen and Hydrocodone Bitartrate	660 mg; 10 mg	White	Tablet	Oblong	Vintage Pharmaceuticals
V; 3600	Acetaminophen and Hydrocodone	500 mg; 10 mg	Pink	Tablet	Oblong	Qualitest Products
V; 3600	Acetaminophen and Hydrocodone Bitartrate	500 mg; 10 mg	Pink	Tablet	Oval, Large	Vintage Pharmaceuticals
V; 3601	Acetaminophen and Hydrocodone	325 mg; 10 mg	Yellow	Tablet	Oblong	Qualitest Products
V; 3601	Acetaminophen and Hydrocodone Bitartrate	325 mg; 10 mg	Light Yellow	Tablet	Capsule-Shape	Vintage Pharmaceuticals
V; 3611	Hydromorphone	2 mg	White	Tablet	Circle	Qualitest Products
V; 3612	Hydromorphone	4 mg	White	Tablet	Circle	Qualitest Products
V; 3917	Levothyroxine Sodium	0.3 mg	Green	Tablet		Qualitest Products
V; 3918	Levothyroxine Sodium	0.112 mg	Rose	Tablet	Circle	Qualitest Products
V; 3920	Levothyroxine Sodium	0.175 mg	Turquoise	Tablet	Circle	Qualitest Products
V; 3921	Levothyroxine Sodium	0.088 mg	Olive	Tablet	Circle	Qualitest Products
V; 3922	Levothyroxine Sodium	0.137 mg	Blue	Tablet	Circle	Qualitest Products
V; 4171	Meperitab	50 mg	White	Tablet	Circle	Qualitest Products
V; 4172	Meperitab	100 mg	White	Tablet	Circle	Qualitest Products
V; 4206	Meprozine	50 mg; 25 mg	Red	Capsule		Qualitest Products
V; 4211	Methocarbamol	500 mg	White	Tablet	Circle, Scored	Vintage Pharmaceuticals
V; 4216	Methylprednisolone	4 mg	White	Tablet	Oval	Qualitest Products
V; 4740	Organ-I NR	200 mg	Salmon	Tablet	Circle	Qualitest Products
V; 4853	Oxybutynin Chloride	5 mg	Light Blue	Tablet		Qualitest Products
V; 4853	Oxybutynin Chloride	5 mg	Blue	Tablet	Circle, Scored	Vintage Pharmaceuticals
V; 4929	Pemoline	18.75 mg	White	Tablet	Round, Bisected Scored	Qualitest Products
V; 4930	Pemoline	37.5 mg	Orange	Tablet	Round, Bisected Scored	Qualitest Products
V; 4931	Pemoline	75 mg	Tan	Tablet	Round, Bisected Scored	Qualitest Products
V; 4940	Perphenazine	2 mg	Gray	Tablet		Qualitest Products
V; 4942	Perphenazine	8 mg	Gray	Tablet		Qualitest Products
V; 4943	Perphenazine	16 mg	Gray	Tablet		Qualitest Products
V; 4971	Phenazopyridine	100 mg	Maroon	Tablet	Circle	Qualitest Products
V; 4972	Phenazopyridine	200 mg	Maroon	Tablet	Circle	Qualitest Products
V; 4991	Perphenazine	4 mg	Gray	Tablet		Qualitest Products
V; 5011	Phenobarbital	0.25 Gr	White	Tablet	Circle	Qualitest Products
V; 5013	Phenobarbital	1 Gr	White	Tablet	Circle	Qualitest Products
V; 5014	Phenobarbital	1.5 Gr	White	Tablet	Circle	Qualitest Products
V; 5030	Phentermine Hydrochloride	37.5 mg	White and Black Speckled	Tablet	Oblong	Qualitest Products
V; 5093	Prednisone	10 mg	White	Tablet	Circle, Scored	Qualitest Products
V; 5094	Prednisone	5 mg	White	Tablet	Circle, Scored	Qualitest Products
V; 5111	Propoxyphene Napsylate and Acetaminophen	325 mg; 50 mg	Orange	Tablet	Oblong	Qualitest Products
V; 5112	Acetaminophen and Propoxyphene Napsylate	650 mg; 100 mg	Rust Orange to Brown	Tablet		Vintage Pharmaceuticals
V; 5112	Propoxyphene Napsylate and Acetaminophen	650 mg; 100 mg	Orange	Tablet	Oblong	Qualitest Products
V; 5113	Acetaminophen and Propoxyphene Napsylate	650 mg; 100 mg	White	Tablet		Vintage Pharmaceuticals
V; 5113	Propoxyphene Napsylate and Acetaminophen	650 mg; 100 mg	White	Tablet	Oblong	Qualitest Products
V; 5114	Acetaminophen and Propoxyphene Napsylate	650 mg; 100 mg	Pink	Tablet		Vintage Pharmaceuticals

IMPRINT	BRAND/GENERIC NAME	STRENGTH	COLOR	FORM	SHAPE	MANUFACTURER
V; 5114	Propoxyphene Napsylate and Acetaminophen	650 mg; 100 mg	Pink	Tablet	Oblong	Qualitest Products
V; 5311	Q-Bid DM	30 mg; 600 mg	Green	Tablet	Oblong	Qualitest Products
V; 5312	Q-Bid LA	600 mg	Light Green	Tablet	Capsule-Shape	Qualitest Products
V; 5401	Quinine Sulfate	260 mg	White	Tablet	Circle	Qualitest Products
V; 5811	Salsalate	500 mg	Aqua	Tablet	Circle	Qualitest Products
V; 5812	Salsalate	750 mg	Aqua	Tablet	Oblong	Qualitest Products
V; 5905	Sulfazine Ec	500 mg	Gold	Enteric-Coated Tablet	Oval	Qualitest Products
V; 5971	Trihexyphenidyl	2 mg	White	Tablet	Circle	Qualitest Products
V; 5972	Trihexyphenidyl	5 mg	White	Tablet	Circle	Qualitest Products
V; 5972	Trihexyphenidyl Hydrochloride	5 mg		Tablet		Vintage Pharmaceuticals
V; 6211	Guaifen-Pse	600 mg; 120 mg	Yellow	Tablet	Oblong	Qualitest Products
VALPROIC; 250; 0364	Valproic Acid	250 mg	Off-White	Capsule		Watson Laboratories
VALRELEASE 15; ROCHE	Valrelease	15 mg	Yellow and Blue	Sustained-Release Capsule		Roche Pharmaceuticals
VALTREX; 500 MG	Valtrex	500 mg	Blue	Tablet	Film-Coated	Glaxosmithkline
VALTREX; 1 GRAM	Valtrex	1 G	Blue	Tablet	Film-Coated	Glaxosmithkline
VANACHOL	Vanachol	10 mg; 200 mg; 200 mg; 12.5 mg; 200 mcg; 500 mcg	Dark Amber	Capsule, Liquid Filled	Oblong	GM Pharmaceuticals
VANQUISH	Vanquish	227 mg; 194 mg; 33 mg		Tablet		Bayer Consumer Care
VENTOLIN; 4; GLAXO	Ventolin	4 mg	White	Tablet	Circle, Compressed	Glaxosmithkline
VENTOLIN; 200; GLAXO	Ventolin Rotacaps	200 mcg	Light Blue and Clear	Capsule, Liquid Filled		Glaxosmithkline
VERGON	Vergon	25 mg; 50 mg	Blue and White	Capsule		Marnel Pharmaceuticals
VESANOID 10; ROCHE	Vesanoid	10 mg	Orange-Yellow and Red-Brown	Capsule		Roche Laboratories
VGC; 450	Valcyte	450 mg	Pink	Tablet	Oval, Convex	Roche Laboratories
VGR; 25; PFIZER	Viagra	25 mg	Blue	Coated Tablet	Diamond, Rounded	Pfizer Laboratories
VGR; 50; PFIZER	Viagra	50 mg	Blue	Coated Tablet	Diamond, Rounded	Pfizer Laboratories
VGR; 100; PFIZER	Viagra	100 mg	Blue	Coated Tablet	Diamond, Rounded	Pfizer Laboratories
VICODIN	Vicodin	5 mg; 500 mg	White	Tablet		Abbott Laboratories
VICODIN; ES	Vicodin Es	7.5 mg; 750 mg	White	Tablet	Oval, Scored	Abbott Laboratories
VICODIN HP	Vicodin Hp	10 mg; 660 mg	White	Tablet	Oval	Abbott Laboratories
VIDEX; 25 MG	Videx	25 mg	Light Orange-Yellow	Tablet, Chewable	Circle	Bristol-Myers Squibb
VIDEX; 50 MG	Videx	50 mg	Light Orange-Yellow	Tablet, Chewable	Circle	Bristol-Myers Squibb
VIDEX; 100 MG	Videx	100 mg	Light Orange-Yellow	Tablet, Chewable	Circle	Bristol-Myers Squibb
VIDEX; 150 MG	Videx	150 mg	Light Orange-Yellow	Tablet, Chewable	Circle	Bristol-Myers Squibb
VIDEX; 200 MG	Videx	200 mg	Light Orange-Yellow	Tablet, Chewable	Circle	Bristol-Myers Squibb
VIOKASE; 9111	Viokase 8	8000 U; 30000 U; 30000 U	Tan	Tablet	Circle, Compressed	Paddock Labs
VIRACEPT; 250	Viracept	250 mg	Light Blue	Coated Tablet	Capsule-Shape	Agouron Pharmaceuticals
VIRAVAN-DM	Viravan-DM	25 mg; 30 mg; 25 mg	Brown	Tablet, Chewable		Pediamed Pharmaceuticals
VISKEN; 5; 78/111	Visken	5 mg	White	Tablet	Circle, Scored	Novartis Pharmaceuticals
VISKEN; 10; 78/73	Visken	10 mg	White	Tablet	Circle, Scored	Novartis Pharmaceuticals
VITRON C+	Vitron-C Plus	400 mg; 250 mg; 25 mcg; 1 mg	Dark Brown	Coated Tablet	Circle	Heritage Consumer Products
VL; 3	Apc with Codeine	30 mg		Tablet		Vangard Labs
VL; 4	Apc with Codeine	60 mg		Tablet		Vangard Labs
VL; 406	Butabarbital	15 mg		Tablet		Vangard Labs
VL; 407	Butabarbital	30 mg		Tablet		Vangard Labs
VL; 413	Chloral Hydrate	500 mg		Capsule		Vangard Labs
VL; 414	Meprobamate	200 mg		Tablet		Vangard Labs
VL; 415	Meprobamate	400 mg		Tablet		Vangard Labs
VL; 420	Phenobarbital	15 mg		Tablet		Vangard Labs
VL; 421	Phenobarbital	30 mg		Tablet		Vangard Labs
VL; 430	Acetaminophen and Codeine	325 mg; 30 mg		Tablet		Vangard Labs
VL; 432	Acetaminophen and Codeine NO.4	325 mg; 60 mg		Tablet	Circle	Vangard Labs
VL; 435	Chlordiazepoxide	5 mg		Capsule		Vangard Labs
VL; 437	Chlordiazepoxide	25 mg		Capsule		Vangard Labs
VL; 439	Propoxyphene	65 mg		Capsule		Vangard Labs
VL; 440	Propoxyphene Compound 65	65 mg; 227 mg; 162 mg; 32.4 mg		Capsule		Vangard Labs
VL; 512	Reserpine	0.25 mg		Tablet		Vangard Labs
VL; 515	Quinidine Sulfate	200 mg		Tablet		Vangard Labs
VL; 536	Prednisone	5 mg		Tablet		Vangard Labs
VL; 591	Acetaminophen	325 mg		Tablet		Vangard Labs
VOLMAX; 4	Volmax	4 mg	Light Blue	Extended-Release Tablet	Six-Sided	Muro Pharmaceutical
VOLMAX; 4	Volmax	4 mg	Light Blue	Sustained-Release Tablet	Six-Sided	Muro Pharmaceutical
VOLMAX; 8	Volmax	8 mg	White	Extended-Release Tablet	Six-Sided	Muro Pharmaceutical
VOLMAX; 8	Volmax	8 mg	White	Sustained-Release Tablet	Six-Sided	Muro Pharmaceutical
VOLTAREN; 25	Voltaren	25 mg	Yellow	Timed-Release Tablet	Triangle, Biconvex	Ciba-Geigy
VOLTAREN; 50	Voltaren	50 mg	Light Brown	Timed-Release Tablet	Triangle, Biconvex	Ciba-Geigy
VOLTAREN; 75	Voltaren	75 mg	Light Pink	Timed-Release Tablet	Triangle, Biconvex	Ciba-Geigy
VOLTAREN; XR; 100	Voltaren Xr	100 mg	Light Pink	Sustained-Release Tablet	Circle, Biconvex	Ciba-Geigy
VP; A;	Vicoprofen	7.5 mg; 200 mg	White	Coated Tablet	Circle, Convex	Abbott Laboratories
W	Bronkotabs	100 mg; 100 mg; 24 mg; 8 mg	White	Tablet	Circle, Scored	Winthrop Pharmaceuticals
W	Hytakerol	0.125 mg	Brown	Capsule, Liquid Filled	Circle, Soft	Winthrop Pharmaceuticals
W	Mytelase Chloride	25 mg	Yellow	Tablet		Winthrop Pharmaceuticals

IMPRINT	BRAND/GENERIC NAME	STRENGTH	COLOR	FORM	SHAPE	MANUFACTURER
W	Pipanol	2 mg	White	Tablet		Winthrop Pharmaceuticals
W; 0.45/1.5	Prempro Single Tablet	0.45 mg; 1.5 mg	Gold	Tablet	Oval	Wyeth Pharmaceuticals
W; 0.625/5	Prempro Single Tablet	0.625 mg; 5 mg	Light Blue	Coated Tablet	Oval	Wyeth Pharmaceuticals
W; 2.5	Isordil	2.5 mg	Yellow	Tablet	Circle	Wyeth Pharmaceuticals
W3	Isosorbide Dinitrate	5 mg	Pink	Tablet		West-Ward
W; 5	Isordil	5 mg	Pink	Tablet	Circle	Wyeth Pharmaceuticals
W; 7	Captopril	12.5 mg	White	Tablet	Bisect Scored	West-Ward
W53	Winstrol	2 mg	Pink	Tablet	Circle, Scored	Sanofi Pharmaceuticals
W; 100	Theophylline	100 mg	Brown and Clear	Capsule		KV Pharmaceutical
W; 200	Theophylline	200 mg	Green and Clear	Capsule		KV Pharmaceutical
W; 332	Vitalize Plus	5000 I.U.; 30 I.U.; 500 mg; 20 mg; 20 mg; 100 mg; 25 mg; 0.15 mg; 25 mg; 0.8 mg; 50 mcg; 27 mg; 0.1 mg; 50 mg; 5 mg; 3 mg; 22.5 mg	Golden Yellow	Tablet	Capsule-Shape	West-Ward
W; 530	Reserpine	0.1 mg		Tablet		West-Ward
W; 641	Triphasil-21 Brown Tablet	0.03 mg; 0.05 mg	Brown	21-Day Tablet Pack	Circle	Wyeth Pharmaceuticals
W; 641	Triphasil-28 Brown Tablet	0.03 mg; 0.05 mg	Brown	28-Day Tablet Pack	Circle	Wyeth Pharmaceuticals
W; 642	Triphasil-21 White Tablet	0.04 mg; 75 mcg	White	21-Day Tablet Pack	Circle	Wyeth Pharmaceuticals
W; 642	Triphasil-28 White Tablet	0.04 mg; 75 mcg	White	28-Day Tablet Pack	Circle	Wyeth Pharmaceuticals
W; 643	Triphasil-21 Light Yellow Tablet	0.03 mg; 0.125 mg	Light Yellow	21-Day Tablet Pack	Circle	Wyeth Pharmaceuticals
W; 643	Triphasil-28 Light Yellow Tablet	0.03 mg; 0.125 mg	Light Yellow	28-Day Tablet Pack	Circle	Wyeth Pharmaceuticals
W; 718	Buspirone Hydrochloride	15 mg	White	Tablet	Oval, Scored	Watson Laboratories
W; 901	Naprelan	375 mg	White	Controlled-Release Tablet	Capsule-Shape	Carnrick Laboratories
W; 902	Naprelan	500 mg	White	Controlled-Release Tablet	Capsule-Shape	Carnrick Laboratories
W; 906;	Ranitidine Hydrochloride	150 mg	White	Tablet	Six-Sided	Ranbaxy Pharmaceuticals
W906	Ranitidine Hydrochloride	150 mg	White	Tablet	Six Sided	Akyma Pharmaceuticals
W; 907;	Ranitidine Hydrochloride	300 mg	White	Tablet	Capsule-Shape	Ranbaxy Pharmaceuticals
W907	Ranitidine	300 mg	White	Tablet	Capsule-Shape	Akyma Pharmaceuticals
W; 912	Alesse 21	20 mcg; 0.1 mg	Pink	21-Day Tablet Pack	Circle	Wyeth Pharmaceuticals
W; 912	Alesse 28 Pink Tablet	20 mcg; 0.1 mg	Pink	28-Day Tablet Pack	Circle	Wyeth Pharmaceuticals
W; 923	Enalapril Maleate	2.5 mg	White	Tablet	Circle, Flat Faced	Major Pharmaceutical
W; 924	Enalapril Maleate	5 mg	White	Tablet	Circle, Flat Faced	Major Pharmaceutical
W; 925	Enalapril Maleate	10 mg	Light Salmon	Tablet	Circle, Flat Faced	Major Pharmaceutical
W; 926	Enalapril Maleate	20 mg	Light Beige	Tablet	Circle, Flat Faced	Major Pharmaceutical
W; 965	Bethanechol Chloride	5 mg	White	Tablet	Oval	Ranbaxy Pharmaceuticals
W; 966	Bethanechol Chloride	10 mg	Pink	Tablet	Oval	Ranbaxy Pharmaceuticals
W; 967	Bethanechol Chloride	25 mg	Light Yellow	Tablet	Oval	Ranbaxy Pharmaceuticals
W; 968	Bethanechol Chloride	50 mg	Yellow	Tablet	Oval	Ranbaxy Pharmaceuticals
W; 1600	Perphenazine	2 mg		Tablet		Warrick Pharmaceuticals
W; 1603	Perphenazine	4 mg		Tablet		Warrick Pharmaceuticals
W; 1605	Perphenazine	8 mg		Tablet		Warrick Pharmaceuticals
W; 1610	Perphenazine	16 mg		Tablet		Warrick Pharmaceuticals
W; 1620	Griseofulvin	125 mg		Tablet		Warrick Pharmaceuticals
W; 1621	Griseofulvin	250 mg		Tablet		Warrick Pharmaceuticals
W; 1624	Griseofulvin	330 mg		Tablet		Warrick Pharmaceuticals
W; 1650	Theophylline	100 mg		Sustained-Release Tablet		Warrick Pharmaceuticals
W; 1670	Theophylline	300 mg		Sustained-Release Tablet		Warrick Pharmaceuticals
W; 1680	Theophylline	450 mg		Sustained-Release Tablet		Warrick Pharmaceuticals
W; 2183	Urised	0.03 mg; 0.03 mg; 40.8 mg; 5.4 mg; 18.1 mg; 4.5 mg	Purple	Coated Tablet	Circle	Polymedica Pharmaceuticals
W; 2183	Urised	0.03 mg; 0.03 mg; 40.8 mg; 5.4 mg; 18.1 mg; 4.5 mg	Purple	Coated Tablet	Circle	Polymedica Pharmaceuticals
W; 2183	Urised	0.03 mg; 0.03 mg; 40.8 mg; 5.4 mg; 18.1 mg; 4.5 mg	Purple	Coated Tablet	Circle	Webcon
W; 2225	Cystospaz	0.15 mg	Aqua	Tablet	Circle	Polymedica Pharmaceuticals
W; 2260	Cystospaz-M	0.375 mg	Light Blue	Timed-Release Capsule		Polymedica Pharmaceuticals
W; 7300	Tacaryl	4 mg	Pink	Tablet, Chewable		Westwood-Squibb Pharmaceuticals
W; 7400	Tacaryl	8 mg	Peach	Tablet		Westwood-Squibb Pharmaceuticals
W; A79	Aralen Phosphate and Primaquine Phosphate	500 mg; 79 mg	Orange	Coated Tablet	Circle	Sanofi Winthrop Pharmaceuticals
W; B; 34	Bilopaque	750 mg; 54.7%	Orange and Yellow	Capsule		Nycomed
W; C; 270	Nardil	15 mg	Orange	Tablet		Pfizer
W; DILACOR XR; 120 MG;	Dilacor Xr	120 mg	Pink and Flesh	Extended-Release Capsule		Watson Laboratories
W; DILACOR XR; 180 MG;	Dilacor Xr	180 mg	Lavender and Flesh	Extended-Release Capsule		Watson Laboratories
W; DILACOR XR; 240 MG;	Dilacor Xr	240 mg	Light Blue and Flesh	Extended-Release Capsule		Watson Laboratories
W; M; 31;	Mebaral	32 mg	White	Tablet		Ovation Pharmaceuticals
W; M; 31;	Mebaral	32 mg	White	Tablet		Sanofi Winthrop
W; M; 32;	Mebaral	50 mg	White	Tablet		Ovation Pharmaceuticals
W; M; 32;	Mebaral	50 mg	White	Tablet		Sanofi Winthrop
W; M; 33;	Mebaral	100 mg	White	Tablet		Ovation Pharmaceuticals

IMPRINT	BRAND/GENERIC NAME	STRENGTH	COLOR	FORM	SHAPE	MANUFACTURER
W; M; 33;	Mebaral	100 mg	White	Tablet		Sanofi Winthrop
W; M; 87;	Mytelase	10 mg	White	Tablet		Winthrop Pharmaceuticals
W; MERRELL; 547	Quinamm	260 mg	White	Tablet	Circle	Aventis Pharmaceuticals
W; T51	Talwin Nx	50 mg; 0.5 mg	Yellow	Tablet	Oblong, Scored	Sanofi Winthrop Pharmaceuticals
W; A77	Aralen	500 mg	White	Film-Coated, Discoid Tablet	Circle	Sanofi Winthrop Pharmaceuticals
W A; 82 (AFTER 1982);	Atabrine	100 mg	Yellow	Tablet		Winthrop Pharmaceuticals
W EFFEXOR XR 37.5	Effexor-Xr	37.5 mg	Gray and Peach	Extended-Release Capsule		Wyeth Pharmaceuticals
W EFFEXOR XR 75	Effexor-Xr	75 mg	Peach	Extended-Release Capsule		Wyeth Pharmaceuticals
W EFFEXOR XR 150	Effexor-Xr	150 mg	Orange	Extended-Release Capsule		Wyeth Pharmaceuticals
WAH S7C	Caniheptin	276 mg; 110 mg; 83 mg; 1 mcg;		Capsule		Wellcome Animal Health
WALLACE; 37; 4001; 150	Rondomycin	150 mg	Blue and White	Capsule		Wallace Laboratories
WALLACE; 153	Aquatensen	5 mg	Peach	Tablet	Rectangle, Scored	Wallace Laboratories
WALLACE; 272	Diutensen	2.5 mg; 2 mg	Blue and White Mottled	Tablet	Circle	Wallace Laboratories
WALLACE; 274	Diutensen-R	2.5 mg; 0.1 mg	Pink and White	Tablet	Circle, Mottled	Wallace Laboratories
WALLACE; 301	Barbidonna	16 mg; 0.1286 mg; 0.025 mg; 0.0074 mg	White	Tablet	Circle	Wallace Laboratories
WALLACE; 311	Barbidonna No. 2	32 mg; 0.1286 mg; 0.025 mg; 0.0074 mg	Light Brown	Tablet	Circle	Wallace Laboratories
WALLACE; 400; 37-1301	Meprospan 400	400 mg	Blue	Timed-Release Capsule		Wallace Laboratories
WALLACE; 431	Lufyllin-400	400 mg	White	Tablet	Capsule-Shape	Wallace Laboratories
WALLACE; 521	Lufyllin	200 mg	White	Tablet		Wallace Laboratories
WALLACE; 541	Lufyllin-GG	200 mg; 200 mg	Yellow	Tablet	Circle	Wallace Laboratories
WALLACE; 561	Lufyllin-Epg	200 mg; 100 mg; 16 mg; 16 mg	Pink	Tablet	Circle	Wallace Laboratories
WALLACE; 0640	Tussi-12	60 mg; 5 mg; 10 mg	Mauve	Tablet		Wallace Laboratories
WALLACE; 673	Ryna-12	25 mg; 60 mg	Buff	Tablet	Oblong	Wallace Laboratories
WALLACE; 713	Rynatan	25 mg; 25 mg; 8 mg	Buff	Tablet	Capsule-Shape, Scored	Wallace Laboratories
WALLACE; 717	Rynatuss	60 mg; 5 mg; 10 mg; 10 mg	Brown	Tablet	Capsule-Shape	Wallace Laboratories
WALLACE; 2103	Soma Compound	200 mg; 325 mg	White and Orange	Tablet		Wallace Laboratories
WALLACE; 2403	Soma Compound with Codeine	200 mg; 325 mg; 16 mg	White and Yellow	Tablet		Wallace Laboratories
WALLACE; 37-0120	Micrainin	325 mg; 200 mg	Orange and White	Coated Tablet		Wallace Laboratories
WALLACE; 37-0120	Micrainin	325 mg; 200 mg	Peach and White	Tablet	Oblong	Wallace Laboratories
WALLACE; 37-1001	Miltown	400 mg	White	Tablet		Wallace Laboratories
WALLACE; 37-1101	Miltown	200 mg	White	Coated Tablet		Wallace Laboratories
WALLACE; 37-1601	Miltown 600	600 mg	White	Tablet		Wallace Laboratories
WALLACE; 37-5301	Miltrate-20	200 mg; 20 mg	Oral	Tablet		Wallace Laboratories
WALLACE; 37-5401	Milprem-400	400 mg; 0.45 mg	Dark Pink	Tablet		Wallace Laboratories
WALLACE; 37-5501	Milprem-200	200 mg; 0.45 mg	Light Pink	Tablet		Wallace Laboratories
WALLACE; BUTICAPS; 0061; 30	Buticaps	30 mg		Capsule		Wallace Laboratories
WALLACE 200; 37-1401	Meprospan	200 mg	Yellow	Sustained-Release Capsule		Wallace Laboratories
WALLCE; BUTICAPS; 0060; 15	Buticaps	15 mg		Capsule		Wallace Laboratories
WARRICK; 1520	Albuterol Sulfate	2 mg		Tablet		Warrick Pharmaceuticals
WARRICK; 1530	Albuterol Sulfate	4 mg	White	Tablet	Circle, Compressed	Warrick Pharmaceuticals
WARRICK; 1602; 100	Labetalol Hydrochloride	100 mg	Brown	Tablet	Small	Warrick Pharmaceuticals
WARRICK; 1636; 200	Labetalol Hydrochloride	200 mg		Tablet		Warrick Pharmaceuticals
WARRICK; 1650	Theophylline	100 mg	White	Sustained-Release Tablet	Circle	Warrick Pharmaceuticals
WARRICK; 1653; 300	Labetalol Hydrochloride	300 mg		Tablet		Warrick Pharmaceuticals
WARRICK; 1660;	Theophylline	200 mg		Sustained-Release Tablet		Warrick Pharmaceuticals
WARRICK; 1670	Theophylline	300 mg	White to Off-White	Sustained-Release Tablet	Capsule-Shape	Warrick Pharmaceuticals
WARRICK; 1680	Theophylline	450 mg	White to Off-White	Extended-Release Tablet	Capsule-Shape	Warrick Pharmaceuticals
WATSON; 235;	Nor-Qd	0.35 mg	Yellow	Tablet	Circle	Watson Laboratories
WATSON; 240; 0.5;	Lorazepam	0.5 mg	White	Tablet	Circle	Watson Laboratories
WATSON; 241; 1;	Lorazepam	1 mg	White	Tablet	Circle	Watson Laboratories
WATSON; 242; 2;	Lorazepam	2 mg	White	Tablet	Circle, Scored	Watson Laboratories
WATSON; 254	Brevicon 28-Day Blue Tablet	0.5 mg; 0.035 mg	Blue	28-Day Tablet Pack	Circle	Watson Laboratories
WATSON; 254;	Tri-Norinyl 28 Day Blue Tablet	0.5 mg; 35 mcg	Blue	28-Day Tablet Pack	Circle	Watson Laboratories
WATSON; 259	Norinyl 1/35 Yellow-Green Tablet	1 mg; 35 mcg	Yellow-Green	28-Day Tablet Pack	Circle	Watson Laboratories
WATSON; 259;	Tri-Norinyl 28 Day Yellow-Green Tablet	1 mg; 35 mcg	Yellow-Green	28-Day Tablet Pack	Circle	Watson Laboratories
WATSON; 265	Norinyl 1/50 White Tablet	1 mg; 50 mcg	White	28-Day Tablet Pack	Circle	Watson Laboratories
WATSON; 300	Furosemide	20 mg	White	Tablet	Circle	Watson Laboratories
WATSON; 301;	Furosemide	40 mg	White	Tablet	Circle	Watson Laboratories
WATSON; 302;	Furosemide	80 mg	White	Tablet	Circle	Watson Laboratories
WATSON; 303	Indomethacin	25 mg	Green	Capsule		Watson Laboratories
WATSON; 304	Indomethacin	50 mg	Green	Capsule		Watson Laboratories
WATSON; 305;	Propranolol Hydrochloride	10 mg	Orange	Tablet	Circle	Watson Laboratories

IMPRINT	BRAND/GENERIC NAME	STRENGTH	COLOR	FORM	SHAPE	MANUFACTURER
WATSON; 306;	Propranolol Hydrochloride	20 mg	Blue	Tablet	Circle	Watson Laboratories
WATSON; 307;	Propranolol Hydrochloride	40 mg	Green	Tablet	Circle	Watson Laboratories
WATSON; 308;	Propranolol Hydrochloride	80 mg	Yellow	Tablet	Circle	Watson Laboratories
WATSON; 309; 50	Doxycycline	50 mg	Green and Yellow	Capsule		Watson Laboratories
WATSON; 310; 100	Doxycycline	100 mg	Green	Capsule		Watson Laboratories
WATSON; 311;	Furosemide	20 mg	White	Tablet	Oval	Watson Laboratories
WATSON; 312	Metoclopramide Hydrochloride	10 mg	White	Tablet	Round; Bisected Scored	Watson Laboratories
WATSON; 332	Lorazepam	0.5 mg	White	Tablet	Circle, Scored	Watson Laboratories
WATSON; 333	Lorazepam	1 mg	White	Tablet	Circle, Scored	Watson Laboratories
WATSON; 334;	Lorazepam	2 mg	White	Tablet	Circle, Scored	Watson Laboratories
WATSON; 335	Acyclovir	400 mg	White to Off-White	Tablet	Oval	Watson Laboratories
WATSON; 336	Acyclovir	800 mg	White to Off-White	Tablet	Oval	Watson Laboratories
WATSON; 338	Diclofenac Sodium	50 mg	White to Off-White	Delayed-Release Tablet	Circle, Biconvex, Enteric-Coated	Watson Laboratories
WATSON; 339	Diclofenac Sodium	75 mg	White to Off-White	Delayed-Release Tablet	Circle, Biconvex, Enteric-Coated	Watson Laboratories
WATSON; 343;	Verapamil Hydrochloride	80 mg	White	Tablet	Circle, Scored	Watson Laboratories
WATSON; 344;	Verapamil Hydrochloride	80 mg	Light Peach	Tablet	Circle, Scored	Watson Laboratories
WATSON; 345;	Verapamil Hydrochloride	120 mg	White	Tablet	Circle, Scored	Watson Laboratories
WATSON; 346;	Verapamil Hydrochloride	120 mg	Peach	Tablet	Circle, Scored	Watson Laboratories
WATSON; 347; 12.5;	Hydrochlorothiazide	12.5 mg	Teal and White	Capsule		Watson Laboratories
WATSON; 348;	Triamterene and Hydrochlorothiazide	75 mg; 50 mg	Yellow	Tablet	Circle, Scored	Watson Laboratories
WATSON; 349;	Hydrocodone Bitartrate and Acetaminophen	500 mg; 5 mg	White	Tablet	Capsule-Shape	Udl Laboratories
WATSON; 349;	Hydrocodone Bitartrate and Acetaminophen	500 mg; 5 mg	White	Tablet	Capsule-Shape	Watson Laboratories
WATSON; 352;	Propranolol Hydrochloride	60 mg	Pink	Tablet	Circle	Watson Laboratories
WATSON; 353	Propranolol Hydrochloride	90 mg	Lavender	Tablet	Circle	Watson Laboratories
WATSON; 357	Methyldopa and Hydrochlorothiazide	250 mg; 15 mg	Off-White	Coated Tablet	Circle	Watson Laboratories
WATSON; 358	Methyldopa and Hydrochlorothiazide	250 mg; 25 mg	White	Coated Tablet	Circle	Watson Laboratories
WATSON; 359	Methyldopa and Hydrochlorothiazide	500 mg; 30 mg	Off-White	Coated Tablet	Circle	Watson Laboratories
WATSON; 360	Methyldopa and Hydrochlorothiazide	500 mg; 50 mg	White	Coated Tablet	Circle	Watson Laboratories
WATSON 363	Clorazepate Dipotassium	3.75 mg	Light Blue	Tablet	Circle	Watson Laboratories
WATSON 364	Clorazepate Dipotassium	7.5 mg	Light Beige	Tablet	Circle	Watson Laboratories
WATSON 365	Clorazepate Dipotassium	15 mg	Pink	Tablet	Circle	Watson Laboratories
WATSON; 366	Fenoprofen Calcium	600 mg;	Peach	Coated Tablet	Oblong, Scored	Watson Laboratories
WATSON; 367	Fenoprofen Calcium	200 mg	White and Yellow	Capsule		Watson Laboratories
WATSON; 368	Fenoprofen Calcium	300 mg	Yellow	Capsule		Watson Laboratories
WATSON; 373	Maprotiline Hydrochloride	25 mg	Peach	Coated Tablet	Oval	Watson Laboratories
WATSON; 374	Maprotiline Hydrochloride	50 mg	Peach	Coated Tablet	Circle	Watson Laboratories
WATSON; 375	Maprotiline Hydrochloride	75 mg	White	Coated Tablet	Oval	Watson Laboratories
WATSON; 379;	Amoxapine	25 mg	White	Tablet	Circle, Scored	Watson Laboratories
WATSON; 380;	Amoxapine	50 mg	Orange	Tablet	Circle, Scored	Watson Laboratories
WATSON; 381;	Amoxapine	100 mg	Blue	Tablet	Circle, Scored	Watson Laboratories
WATSON; 382;	Amoxapine	150 mg	Orange	Tablet	Circle, Scored	Watson Laboratories
WATSON; 383	Zovia 1/35e-21	1 mg; 35 mcg	Light Pink	21-Day Tablet Pack	Circle	Watson Laboratories
WATSON; 383	Zovia 1/35e-28 Light Pink Tablet	1 mg; 35 mcg	Light Pink	28-Day Tablet Pack	Circle	Watson Laboratories
WATSON; 384	Zovia 1/50e-21	1 mg; 50 mcg	Pink	21-Day Tablet Pack	Circle	Watson Laboratories
WATSON; 384	Zovia 1/50e-28 Pink Tablet	1 mg; 50 mcg	Pink	28-Day Tablet Pack	Circle	Watson Laboratories
WATSON; 385;	Hydrocodone Bitartrate and Acetaminophen	500 mg; 7.5 mg	White	Tablet	Capsule-Shape	Udl Laboratories
WATSON; 385;	Hydrocodone Bitartrate and Acetaminophen	500 mg; 7.5 mg	White	Tablet	Capsule-Shape	Watson Laboratories
WATSON; 387;	Hydrocodone Bitartrate and Acetaminophen	750 mg; 7.5 mg	White	Tablet	Oblong	Udl Laboratories
WATSON; 387;	Hydrocodone Bitartrate and Acetaminophen	750 mg; 7.5 mg	White	Tablet	Oblong	Watson Laboratories
WATSON; 388;	Hydrocodone Bitartrate and Acetaminophen	2.5 mg; 500 mg	White	Tablet	Oblong	Watson Laboratories
WATSON; 395; 50; 0.5;	Pentazocine and Naloxone Hydrochloride	0.5 mg; 50 mg	Green	Tablet	Capsule-Shape, Scored	Watson Laboratories
WATSON; 396; 25; 650	Pentazocine and Acetaminophen	25 mg; 650 mg	Light Aqua	Tablet	Capsule-Shape	Watson Laboratories
WATSON; 401	Albuterol Sulfate	2 mg	White	Tablet	Circle	Watson Laboratories
WATSON; 402	Albuterol Sulfate	4 mg	White	Tablet	Circle	Watson Laboratories
WATSON; 403	Verapamil Hydrochloride	40 mg	White	Tablet	Circle, Scored	Watson Laboratories
WATSON; 404	Verapamil Hydrochloride	40 mg	Peach	Tablet	Circle	Watson Laboratories
WATSON; 405	Lisinopril	2.5 mg	White	Tablet	Circle	Watson Laboratories
WATSON; 406	Lisinopril	5 mg	White	Tablet	Capsule-Shape	Watson Laboratories
WATSON; 407	Lisinopril	10 mg	Light Blue	Tablet	Circle	Watson Laboratories
WATSON; 408	Lisinopril	20 mg	Yellow	Tablet	Circle	Watson Laboratories
WATSON; 409	Lisinopril	40 mg	Yellow	Tablet	Circle	Watson Laboratories
WATSON; 414	Estropipate	0.75 mg	Yellow	Tablet	Circle, Scored	Watson Laboratories
WATSON; 415	Estropipate	1.5 mg	Peach	Tablet	Circle, Scored	Watson Laboratories
WATSON; 416	Estropipate	3 mg	Blue	Tablet	Circle, Scored	Watson Laboratories
WATSON; 418;	Cyclobenzaprine Hydrochloride	10 mg	White	Coated Tablet	Circle	Watson Laboratories
WATSON; 424	Triamterene and Hydrochlorothiazide	37.5 mg; 25 mg	Light Green	Tablet	Circle, Scored	Watson Laboratories
WATSON; 425	Butalbital, Aspirin, Caffeine and Codeine Phosphate	50 mg; 325 mg; 40 mg; 30 mg	Blue and Yellow	Capsule		Watson Laboratories
WATSON; 430	Carbidopa and Levodopa	10 mg; 100 mg	Blue	Tablet	Circle, Scored	Watson Laboratories
WATSON; 431	Carbidopa and Levodopa	25 mg; 100 mg	Tan	Tablet	Circle, Scored	Watson Laboratories
WATSON; 432	Carbidopa and Levodopa	25 mg; 250 mg	Blue	Tablet	Circle, Scored	Watson Laboratories
WATSON; 437	Acebutolol Hydrochloride	200 mg	Red and Gray	Capsule		Watson Laboratories
WATSON; 438	Acebutolol Hydrochloride	400 mg	Maroon and Green	Capsule		Watson Laboratories
WATSON; 444	Guanfacine Hydrochloride	1 mg	Pink	Tablet	Circle	Watson Laboratories

IMPRINT	BRAND/GENERIC NAME	STRENGTH	COLOR	FORM	SHAPE	MANUFACTURER
WATSON; 451	Guanabenz Acetate	4 mg	Orange	Tablet	Circle	Watson Laboratories
WATSON; 452	Guanabenz Acetate	8 mg	Gray	Tablet	Circle	Watson Laboratories
WATSON; 453	Guanfacine Hydrochloride	2 mg	Peach	Tablet	Circle	Watson Laboratories
WATSON; 454	Gemfibrozil	600 mg	White	Coated Tablet	Oval, Scored	Watson Laboratories
WATSON; 460	Glipizide	5 mg	White	Tablet	Circle, Scored	Watson Laboratories
WATSON; 461	Glipizide	10 mg	White	Tablet	Circle, Scored	Watson Laboratories
WATSON; 462	Metoprolol Tartrate	50 mg	Pink	Tablet	Circle, Scored	Watson Laboratories
WATSON; 463	Metoprolol Tartrate	100 mg	Blue	Tablet	Circle, Scored	Watson Laboratories
WATSON; 466	Tramadol Hydrochloride	50 mg	White	Tablet	Circle	Watson Laboratories
WATSON; 485	Acetaminophen, Butalbital and Caffeine	325 mg; 50 mg; 40 mg	White	Tablet		Watson Laboratories
WATSON; 487	Estradiol	1 mg	Gray	Tablet	Scored, Circle	Watson Laboratories
WATSON; 488	Estradiol	2 mg	Light Green	Tablet	Circle, Scored	Watson Laboratories
WATSON; 491; 150MG	Mexiletine Hydrochloride	150 mg	Brown and Light Brown	Capsule		Watson Laboratories
WATSON; 492; 200MG;	Mexiletine Hydrochloride	200 mg	Brown	Capsule		Watson Laboratories
WATSON; 493; 250MG;	Mexiletine Hydrochloride	250 mg	Brown and Light Green	Capsule		Watson Laboratories
WATSON; 498	Doxycycline Hyclate	100 mg	Blue	Capsule		Watson Laboratories
WATSON; 499	Doxycycline Hyclate	100 mg	Beige	Coated Tablet	Circle	Watson Laboratories
WATSON; 500; 50MG;	Doxycycline Hyclate	50 mg	Blue and White	Capsule		Watson Laboratories
WATSON; 502;	Hydrocodone Bitartrate and Acetaminophen	650 mg; 7.5 mg	Pink	Tablet	Capsule-Shape	Watson Laboratories
WATSON; 503;	Hydrocodone Bitartrate and Acetaminophen	650 mg; 10 mg	Light Green	Tablet	Capsule-Shape	Watson Laboratories
WATSON; 504	Indapamide	2.5 mg	White	Coated Tablet	Circle	Watson Laboratories
WATSON; 507	Necon 0.5/35-21	0.5 mg; 35 mcg	Light Yellow	21-Day Tablet Pack	Circle	Watson Laboratories
WATSON; 507	Necon 0.5/35-28 Light Yellow Tablet	0.5 mg; 35 mcg	Light Yellow	28-Day Tablet Pack	Circle	Watson Laboratories
WATSON; 507	Necon 10/11-21 Light Yellow Tablet	0.5 mg; 35 mcg	Light Yellow	21-Day Tablet Pack	Circle	Watson Laboratories
WATSON; 507	Necon 10/11-28 Light Yellow Tablet	0.5 mg; 35 mcg	Light Yellow	28-Day Tablet Pack	Circle	Watson Laboratories
WATSON; 508	Necon 1/35-21	1 mg; 35 mcg	Yellow	21-Day Tablet Pack	Circle	Watson Laboratories
WATSON; 508	Necon 1/35-28 Yellow Tablet	1 mg; 35 mcg	Yellow	28-Day Tablet Pack	Circle	Watson Laboratories
WATSON; 508	Necon 10/11-21 Yellow Tablet	1 mg; 35 mcg	Yellow	21-Day Tablet Pack	Circle	Watson Laboratories
WATSON; 508	Necon 10/11-28 Yellow Tablet	1 mg; 35 mcg	Yellow	28-Day Tablet Pack	Circle	Watson Laboratories
WATSON; 510	Necon 1/50-21	1 mg; 50 mcg	Blue	21-Day Tablet Pack	Circle	Watson Laboratories
WATSON; 510	Necon 1/50-28 Blue Tablet	1 mg; 50 mcg	Blue	28-Day Tablet Pack	Circle	Watson Laboratories
WATSON; 517	Hydrocodone Bitartrate and Acetaminophen	10 mg; 660 mg	White	Tablet	Oval	Watson Laboratories
WATSON; 524	Trinessa White Tablet	0.18 mg; 0.035 mg	White	28-Day Tablet Pack	Circle	Watson Laboratories
WATSON; 525	Trinessa Light Blue Tablet	0.215 mg; 0.035 mg	Light Blue	28-Day Tablet Pack	Circle	Watson Laboratories
WATSON; 526	Mononessa	0.25 mg; 0.035 mg	Blue	Tablet	Circle	Watson Laboratories
WATSON; 526	Trinessa Blue Tablet	0.25 mg; 0.035 mg	Blue	28-Day Tablet Pack	Circle	Watson Laboratories
WATSON; 527	Indapamide	1.25 mg	Orange	Coated Tablet	Circle	Watson Laboratories
WATSON; 528	Estradiol	0.5 mg	White	Tablet	Circle, Scored	Watson Laboratories
WATSON; 540	Hydrocodone Bitartrate and Acetaminophen	10 mg; 500 mg	Blue	Tablet	Capsule-Shape	Watson Laboratories
WATSON; 544;	Desipramine Hydrochloride	75 mg	Orange	Coated Tablet	Circle	Watson Laboratories
WATSON; 545;	Desipramine Hydrochloride	100 mg	Peach	Coated Tablet	Circle	Watson Laboratories
WATSON; 575	Trihexyphenidyl Hydrochloride	2 mg	White	Tablet	Circle, Scored	Watson Laboratories
WATSON; 576	Trihexyphenidyl Hydrochloride	5 mg	White	Tablet	Circle, Scored	Watson Laboratories
WATSON; 582	Propafenone Hydrochloride	150 mg	White	Coated Tablet	Circle, Scored	Watson Laboratories
WATSON; 583	Propafenone Hydrochloride	225 mg	White	Coated Tablet	Circle, Scored	Watson Laboratories
WATSON; 585	Diclofenac Potassium	50 mg	Brown	Coated Tablet	Circle	Watson Laboratories
WATSON; 594; 25 MG	Clomipramine Hydrochloride	25 mg	Blue	Capsule		Watson Laboratories
WATSON; 595; 50 MG	Clomipramine Hydrochloride	50 mg	Yellow	Capsule		Watson Laboratories
WATSON; 596; 75 MG	Clomipramine Hydrochloride	75 mg	Green	Capsule		Watson Laboratories
WATSON; 605;	Labetalol Hydrochloride	100 mg	Beige	Coated Tablet	Circle, Scored	Watson Laboratories
WATSON; 606;	Labetalol Hydrochloride	200 mg	White	Coated Tablet	Circle, Scored	Watson Laboratories
WATSON; 607;	Labetalol Hydrochloride	300 mg	Blue	Coated Tablet	Circle, Scored	Watson Laboratories
WATSON; 613	Butalbital, Acetaminophen and Caffeine	50 mg; 500 mg; 40 mg	Light Blue	Tablet	Capsule-Shape, Scored	Watson Laboratories
WATSON; 617	Morphine Sulfate	100 mg	Gray	Extended-Release Tablet	Circle	Watson Laboratories
WATSON; 629	Nora-Be	0.35 mg	White	Tablet	Circle	Watson Laboratories
WATSON; 630	Microgestin Fe 1/20 White Tablet	20 mcg; 1 mg	White	28-Day Tablet Pack	Circle	Watson Laboratories
WATSON; 631	Microgestin Fe 1.5/30 Green Tablet	1.5 mg; 30 mcg	Green	28-Day Tablet Pack	Circle	Watson Laboratories
WATSON; 632	Microgestin Fe 1.5/30 Brown Tablet	75 mg	Brown	28-Day Tablet Pack	Circle	Watson Laboratories
WATSON; 632	Microgestin Fe 1/20 Brown Tablet	75 mg	Brown	28-Day Tablet Pack	Circle	Watson Laboratories
WATSON; 632	Microgestin Fe Brown Tablet	75 mg	Brown	Tablet	Circle	Watson Laboratories
WATSON; 637	Pentoxifylline	400 mg	Red	Extended-Release Tablet	Oblong	Andrx Pharmaceuticals
WATSON; 639	Doxazosin Mesylate	1 mg	White	Tablet	Circle, Biconvex, Scored	Watson Laboratories
WATSON; 640	Doxazosin Mesylate	2 mg	Light Orange	Tablet	Circle, Biconvex, Scored	Watson Laboratories
WATSON; 641	Doxazosin Mesylate	4 mg	Light Orange	Tablet	Circle, Biconvex, Scored	Watson Laboratories
WATSON; 642	Doxazosin Mesylate	8 mg	Green	Tablet	Circle, Biconvex, Scored	Watson Laboratories
WATSON; 654	Sotalol Hydrochloride	80 mg	Light Blue	Tablet	Oval, Scored	Watson Laboratories

IMPRINT	BRAND/GENERIC NAME	STRENGTH	COLOR	FORM	SHAPE	MANUFACTURER
WATSON; 655	Sotalol Hydrochloride	160 mg	Light Blue	Tablet	Oval, Scored	Watson Laboratories
WATSON; 656	Sotalol Hydrochloride	240 mg	Light Blue	Tablet	Oval, Scored	Watson Laboratories
WATSON; 657	Buspirone Hydrochloride	5 mg	White	Tablet	Oval, Biconvex, Scored	Watson Laboratories
WATSON; 658	Buspirone Hydrochloride	10 mg	White	Tablet	Oval, Biconvex, Scored	Watson Laboratories
WATSON; 662; 120	Diltiazem Hydrochloride	120 mg	Pink and White	Extended-Release Capsule		Watson Laboratories
WATSON; 663; 180	Diltiazem Hydrochloride	180 mg	Pink and White	Extended-Release Capsule		Watson Laboratories
WATSON; 664; 240	Diltiazem Hydrochloride	240 mg	Red and White	Extended-Release Capsule		Watson Laboratories
WATSON; 665	Sotalol Hydrochloride	120 mg	Light Blue	Tablet	Oval, Scored	Watson Laboratories
WATSON; 667; 400;	Etodolac	400 mg	Yellow	Coated Tablet	Capsule-Shape	Watson Laboratories
WATSON; 668	Enalapril Maleate	2.5 mg	White to Off-White	Tablet	Circle, Biconvex, Scored	Watson Laboratories
WATSON; 669	Enalapril Maleate	5 mg	White to Off-White	Tablet	Circle, Biconvex	Watson Laboratories
WATSON; 670	Enalapril Maleate	10 mg	Pink with White Speckles	Tablet	Circle, Biconvex	Watson Laboratories
WATSON; 671	Enalapril Maleate	20 mg	Peach with White Speckles	Tablet	Circle, Biconvex	Watson Laboratories
WATSON; 682; 0.25;	Alprazolam	0.25 mg	White	Tablet	Oval, BI-Convex	Watson Laboratories
WATSON; 683; 0.5;	Alprazolam	0.5 mg	Peach	Tablet	Oval, BI-Convex	Watson Laboratories
WATSON; 684; 1;	Alprazolam	1 mg	Blue	Tablet	Oval, BI-Convex	Watson Laboratories
WATSON 685; 5-50;	Amiloride Hydrochloride and Hydrochlorothiazide	5 mg; 50 mg	Peach	Tablet	Circle	Watson Laboratories
WATSON; 686; 10;	Baclofen	10 mg	White	Tablet	Oval	Watson Laboratories
WATSON; 687; 20;	Baclofen	20 mg	White	Tablet	Circle	Watson Laboratories
WATSON; 688; 12.5;	Captopril	12.5 mg	White	Tablet	Capsule-Shape, Scored	Watson Laboratories
WATSON; 689; 25;	Captopril	25 mg	White	Tablet	Circle, Quadrisect-Scored	Watson Laboratories
WATSON; 690; 50;	Captopril	50 mg	White	Tablet	Egg-Shape	Watson Laboratories
WATSON; 691; 100;	Captopril	100 mg	White	Tablet	Egg-Shape	Watson Laboratories
WATSON; 693; 500;	Chlorzoxazone	500 mg	Green	Tablet	Capsule-Shape, Partial-Scored	Watson Laboratories
WATSON; 695; 10;	Doxepin Hydrochloride	10 mg	Scarlet and Pink	Capsule		Watson Laboratories
WATSON; 696; 25;	Doxepin Hydrochloride	25 mg	Blue and Pink	Capsule		Watson Laboratories
WATSON; 697; 50;	Doxepin Hydrochloride	50 mg	Pink and Flesh	Capsule		Watson Laboratories
WATSON; 698; 200;	Hydroxychloroquine Sulfate	200 mg	White	Coated Tablet	Oval	Watson Laboratories
WATSON; 700; 25;	Hydroxyzine Hydrochloride	25 mg	Green	Coated Tablet	Circle	Watson Laboratories
WATSON; 704; 50;	Hydroxyzine Hydrochloride	50 mg	Yellow	Coated Tablet	Circle	Watson Laboratories
WATSON 706; 2-10;	Perphenazine and Amitriptyline Hydrochloride	10 mg; 2.04 mg	Blue	Coated Tablet	Circle	Watson Laboratories
WATSON 707; 2-25;	Perphenazine and Amitriptyline Hydrochloride	25 mg; 2 mg	Orange	Coated Tablet	Circle	Watson Laboratories
WATSON 708; 4-10;	Perphenazine and Amitriptyline Hydrochloride	10 mg; 4 mg	Salmon	Coated Tablet	Circle	Watson Laboratories
WATSON 709; 4-25;	Perphenazine and Amitriptyline Hydrochloride	25 mg; 4 mg	Yellow	Coated Tablet	Circle	Watson Laboratories
WATSON; 710; 5;	Pindolol	5 mg	White	Tablet	Circle, Scored	Watson Laboratories
WATSON; 711; 10;	Pindolol	10 mg	White	Tablet	Circle, Scored	Watson Laboratories
WATSON; 712; 10 MG;	Piroxicam	10 mg	Light Blue and White	Capsule		Watson Laboratories
WATSON; 713; 20 MG;	Piroxicam	20 mg	Light Blue	Capsule		Watson Laboratories
WATSON 714; 65-650;	Acetaminophen and Propoxyphene Hydrochloride	65 mg; 650 mg	Orange	Coated Tablet	Oblong	Watson Laboratories
WATSON; 715; 260;	Quinine Sulfate	260 mg	White	Tablet	Circle	Watson Laboratories
WATSON; 716; 325;	Quinine Sulfate	325 mg	White	Capsule		Watson Laboratories
WATSON; 726; 50	Meperidine Hydrochloride	50 mg	White	Tablet	Circle, Biconvex	Watson Laboratories
WATSON; 727; 100	Meperidine Hydrochloride	100 mg	White	Tablet	Circle, Biconvex	Watson Laboratories
WATSON; 728; 500	Etodolac	500 mg	Blue	Coated Tablet	Capsule-Shape	Watson Laboratories
WATSON; 735; 200	Etodolac	200 mg	Gray and Brown	Capsule		Watson Laboratories
WATSON; 736; 300	Etodolac	300 mg	Gray and Swedish Orange	Capsule		Watson Laboratories
WATSON; 737; 5; 500 MG	Oxycodone and Acetaminophen	5 mg; 500 mg	White and Red	Capsule		Watson Laboratories
WATSON; 744; 1	Estazolam	1 mg	White	Tablet	Diamond, Scored	Watson Laboratories
WATSON; 745; 2	Estazolam	2 mg	Pink	Tablet	Diamond, Scored	Watson Laboratories
WATSON; 746	Clonazepam	0.5 mg	Yellow	Tablet	Circle, Scored	Watson Laboratories
WATSON; 747	Clonazepam	1 mg	Aqua	Tablet	Circle, Scored	Watson Laboratories
WATSON; 748	Clonazepam	2 mg	White	Tablet	Circle, Scored	Watson Laboratories
WATSON; 749	Oxycodone and Acetaminophen	325 mg; 5 mg	White	Tablet	Circle, Scored	Watson Laboratories
WATSON; 760;	Ranitidine	150 mg	Beige	Coated Tablet	Circle	Watson Laboratories
WATSON; 761;	Ranitidine	300 mg	Beige	Coated Tablet	Capsule-Shape	Watson Laboratories
WATSON; 764;	Nefazodone	100 mg	White	Tablet	Capsule-Shape, Scored	Watson Laboratories
WATSON; 765;	Nefazodone	150 mg	Orange	Tablet	Capsule-Shape, Scored	Watson Laboratories
WATSON; 766;	Nefazodone	200 mg	Yellow	Tablet	Capsule-Shape, Scored	Watson Laboratories
WATSON; 767;	Nefazodone	250 mg	White	Tablet	Capsule-Shape	Watson Laboratories
WATSON; 771; 18.75	Pemoline	75 mg	White	Tablet	Circle, Scored	Watson Laboratories
WATSON; 772; 37.5	Pemoline	37.5 mg	Peach	Tablet	Circle, Scored	Watson Laboratories
WATSON; 773; 18.75	Pemoline	75 mg	Yellow	Tablet	Circle, Scored	Watson Laboratories
WATSON; 774	Oxycodone Hydrochloride	5 mg	White	Tablet	Circle, Scored	Watson Laboratories
WATSON; 775;	Diltiazem Hydrochloride	30 mg	Blue	Tablet	Circle, Scored	Watson Laboratories
WATSON; 776;	Diltiazem Hydrochloride	60 mg	White	Tablet	Circle	Watson Laboratories
WATSON; 777;	Diltiazem Hydrochloride	90 mg	Blue	Tablet	Oblong, Scored	Watson Laboratories
WATSON; 778;	Diltiazem Hydrochloride	120 mg	White	Tablet	Oblong, Scored	Watson Laboratories
WATSON; 779;	Oxybutynin Chloride	5 mg	Pale Blue	Tablet	Circle	Watson Laboratories
WATSON; 780;	Sucralfate	1 G	Light Blue	Tablet	Oblong	Watson Laboratories
WATSON; 781;	Clomiphene	50 mg	White	Tablet	Circle	Watson Laboratories
WATSON; 782;	Diethylpropion Hydrochloride	75 mg	White	Extended-Release Tablet	Capsule-Shape	Watson Laboratories
WATSON; 783;	Diethylpropion Hydrochloride	25 mg	White	Tablet	Circle	Watson Laboratories
WATSON; 784;	Carisoprodol	350 mg	White	Tablet	Circle	Watson Laboratories
WATSON; 785; 5MG;	Chlordiazepoxide Hydrochloride	5 mg	Green and Yellow	Capsule		Watson Laboratories

IMPRINT	BRAND/GENERIC NAME	STRENGTH	COLOR	FORM	SHAPE	MANUFACTURER
WATSON; 786; 10MG;	Chlordiazepoxide Hydrochloride	10 mg	Green and Black	Capsule		Watson Laboratories
WATSON; 787; 25MG;	Chlordiazepoxide Hydrochloride	25 mg	Green and White	Capsule		Watson Laboratories
WATSON; 790;	Methylprednisolone	4 mg	White	Tablet	Oval, Quadrisect Scored	Watson Laboratories
WATSON; 791;	Naproxen	500 mg	White	Tablet	Capsule-Shape	Watson Laboratories
WATSON; 792;	Naproxen Sodium	275 mg	White	Coated Tablet	Oval	Watson Laboratories
WATSON; 793;	Naproxen Sodium	550 mg	Green	Coated Tablet	Oval	Watson Laboratories
WATSON; 794; 10MG;	Dicyclomine	10 mg	Dark Blue	Capsule		Watson Laboratories
WATSON; 795;	Dicyclomine Hydrochloride	20 mg	Blue	Tablet	Circle	Watson Laboratories
WATSON; 796;	Sulfasalazine	500 mg	Mustard	Tablet	Round, Bisected Scored	Watson Laboratories
WATSON; 797;	Prednisone	50 mg	White	Tablet	Circle	Watson Laboratories
WATSON; 800; 25;	Hydroxyzine Pamoate	25 mg	Dark Green and Light Green	Capsule		Watson Laboratories
WATSON; 801; 50MG;	Hydroxyzine Pamoate	50 mg	Green and White	Capsule		Watson Laboratories
WATSON; 802;	Meclizine Hydrochloride	12.5 mg	Blue and White	Tablet	Oval	Watson Laboratories
WATSON; 803;	Meclizine Hydrochloride	25 mg	Yellow and White	Tablet	Oval	Watson Laboratories
WATSON; 804;	Meprobamate	200 mg	White	Tablet	Circle	Watson Laboratories
WATSON; 805;	Meprobamate	400 mg	White	Tablet	Circle, Convex	Watson Laboratories
WATSON; 806;	Methocarbamol	500 mg	White	Tablet	Circle	Watson Laboratories
WATSON; 807;	Methocarbamol	750 mg	White	Tablet	Capsule-Shape	Watson Laboratories
WATSON; 808;	Desipramine Hydrochloride	25 mg	Yellow	Coated Tablet	Circle	Watson Laboratories
WATSON; 809;	Desipramine Hydrochloride	50 mg	Green	Coated Tablet	Circle	Watson Laboratories
WATSON; 820	Oxycodone and Aspirin	4.5 mg; 0.38 mg; 325 mg	Yellow	Tablet	Circle, Scored	Watson Laboratories
WATSON; 821;	Naproxen	250 mg	White	Tablet	Circle	Watson Laboratories
WATSON; 822;	Naproxen	375 mg	Gray	Tablet	Capsule-Shape	Watson Laboratories
WATSON; 824	Oxycodone and Acetaminophen	500 mg; 7.5 mg	White	Tablet	Capsule-Shape, Scored	Watson Laboratories
WATSON; 825	Oxycodone and Acetaminophen	650 mg; 10 mg	White	Tablet	Capsule-Shape, Scored	Watson Laboratories
WATSON; 826; 20 MG	Fluoxetine Hydrochloride	10 mg	Light Green	Capsule		Watson Laboratories
WATSON; 827; 20 MG	Fluoxetine Hydrochloride	20 mg	Light Green and White	Capsule		Watson Laboratories
WATSON; 830;	Prednisone	5 mg	White	Tablet	Circle	Watson Laboratories
WATSON; 831;	Prednisone	10 mg	White	Tablet	Circle	Watson Laboratories
WATSON; 832;	Prednisone	20 mg	Peach	Tablet	Circle	Watson Laboratories
WATSON; 838	Ketorolac Tromethamine	10 mg	White	Coated Tablet	Circle, Convex	Watson Laboratories
WATSON; 841	Bisoprolol and Hydrochlorothiazide	2.5 mg; 6.25 mg	Yellow	Tablet	Circle, Biconvex	Watson Laboratories
WATSON; 842	Bisoprolol and Hydrochlorothiazide	5 mg; 6.25 mg	Pink	Tablet	Circle, Biconvex	Watson Laboratories
WATSON; 843	Bisoprolol and Hydrochlorothiazide	10 mg; 6.25 mg	White	Coated Tablet	Circle, Biconvex	Watson Laboratories
WATSON; 847	Ogestrel White Tablet	0.5 mg; 0.5 mg	White	28-Day Tablet Pack	Circle	Watson Laboratories
WATSON; 848;	Ogestrel White Tablet	0.5 mg; 0.05 mg	White	28-Day Tablet Pack	Circle	Watson Laboratories
WATSON; 850;	Acetaminophen and Codeine Phosphate	300 mg; 15 mg	White	Tablet	Circle, Flat-Faced, Beveled Edge	Watson Laboratories
WATSON; 851;	Acetaminophen and Codeine Phosphate	300 mg; 30 mg	White	Tablet	Circle, Scored	Watson Laboratories
WATSON; 852;	Acetaminophen and Codeine Phosphate	300 mg; 60 mg	White	Tablet	Circle, Scored	Watson Laboratories
WATSON; 853	Acetaminophen and Hydrocodone Bitartrate	325 mg; 10 mg	Yellow	Tablet	Capsule-Shape	Watson Laboratories
WATSON; 860	Lisinopril and Hydrochlorothiazide	10 mg; 12.5 mg	Pink	Tablet	Circle	Watson Laboratories
WATSON; 861	Lisinopril and Hydrochlorothiazide	20 mg; 12.5 mg	Light Blue	Tablet	Circle	Watson Laboratories
WATSON; 862	Lisinopril and Hydrochlorothiazide	20 mg; 25 mg	Pink	Tablet	Circle	Watson Laboratories
WATSON; 885	Lisinopril	30 mg	Yellow	Tablet	Circle	Watson Laboratories
WATSON; 892	Jolivette	0.35 mg	Green	Tablet		Watson Laboratories
WATSON; 913	Norco 5/325	5 mg; 325 mg	White with Orange Specks	Tablet	Capsule-Shape, Scored	Watson Laboratories
WATSON; 932	Oxycodone and Acetaminophen	325 mg; 10 mg	White	Tablet	Circle	Watson Laboratories
WATSON; 933	Oxycodone and Acetaminophen	325 mg; 7.5 mg	White	Tablet	Circle	Watson Laboratories
WATSON; 3159	Ursodiol	300 mg	White	Capsule		Watson Laboratories
WATSON; 3191	Pyridostigmine Bromide	60 mg	White	Tablet	Round, Quadrisected Scored	Watson Laboratories
WATSON; 3202	Hydrocodone Bitartrate and Acetaminophen	5 mg; 325 mg	White with Orange Specks	Tablet	Capsule-Shape	Watson Laboratories
WATSON; 3203	Hydrocodone Bitartrate and Acetaminophen	7.5 mg; 325 mg	Light Orange	Tablet	Capsule; Bisected Scored	Watson Laboratories
WATSON; 3219	Aspirin, Caffeine and Butalbital	325 mg; 50 mg; 40 mg	Yellow and Green	Capsule		Watson Laboratories
WATSON; 3220	Butalbital, Acetaminophen, Caffeine, and Codeine Phosphate	50 mg; 325 mg; 40 mg; 30 mg	Opaque Dark Blue, Opaque White	Capsule		Watson Laboratories
WATSON; 125/30	Trivora-21 Pink Tablet	30 mcg; 125 mcg	Pink	21-Day Tablet Pack	Circle	Watson Laboratories
WATSON; 125/30	Trivora-28 Pink Tablet	30 mcg; 125 mcg	Pink	28-Day Tablet Pack	Circle	Watson Laboratories
WATSON; 15/30	Levora 0.15/30-28 White Tablet	0.15 mg; 30 mcg	White	28-Day Tablet Pack	Circle	Watson Laboratories
WATSON; 15-30	Levora 0.15/30-21	0.15 mg; 30 mcg	White	21-Day Tablet Pack	Circle	Watson Laboratories
WATSON; 50/30	Trivora-21 Blue Tablet	30 mcg; 50 mcg	Blue	21-Day Tablet Pack	Circle	Watson Laboratories
WATSON; 50/30	Trivora-28 Blue Tablet	30 mcg; 50 mcg	Blue	28-Day Tablet Pack	Circle	Watson Laboratories
WATSON; 75/40	Trivora-21 White Tablet	40 mcg; 75 mcg	White	21-Day Tablet Pack	Circle	Watson Laboratories
WATSON; 75/40	Trivora-28 White Tablet	40 mcg; 75 mcg	White	28-Day Tablet Pack	Circle	Watson Laboratories
WATSON; LOXITANE; 5 MG;	Loxitane	5 mg	Opaque Green	Capsule		Watson Laboratories
WATSON; LOXITANE; 10 MG;	Loxitane	10 mg	Dark Green and Yellow	Capsule		Watson Laboratories

IMPRINT	BRAND/GENERIC NAME	STRENGTH	COLOR	FORM	SHAPE	MANUFACTURER
WATSON; LOXITANE; 25 MG;	Loxitane	25 mg	Dark Green and Light Green	Capsule		Watson Laboratories
WATSON; LOXITANE; 50 MG;	Loxitane	50 mg	Dark Green and Blue	Capsule		Watson Laboratories
WBA	Mol-Iron with Vitamin C	195 mg; 75 mg	Burgundy	Tablet		Schering-Plough Healthcare Products
WBB	Mol-Iron	195 mg	Brown	Tablet		Schering-Plough Healthcare Products
WC	Tedral Expectorant	130 mg; 24 mg; 8 mg	White	Tablet		Parke-Davis
WC; 010	Chlorpromazine Hydrochloride	10 mg		Tablet		Warner Chilcott
WC; 025	Chlorpromazine Hydrochloride	25 mg		Tablet		Warner Chilcott
WC; 030	Methyldopa and Hydrochlorothiazide	250 mg; 15 mg		Tablet		Warner Chilcott
WC; 031	Methyldopa and Hydrochlorothiazide	250 mg; 25 mg		Tablet		Warner Chilcott
WC; 032	Methyldopa and Hydrochlorothiazide	500 mg; 30 mg	Dark Red	Tablet	Circle	Warner Chilcott
WC; 033	Methyldopa and Hydrochlorothiazide	500 mg; 50 mg	Grey	Tablet	Circle	Warner Chilcott
WC; 050	Chlorpromazine Hydrochloride	50 mg		Tablet		Warner Chilcott
WC; 070;	Propranolol Hydrochloride	10 mg		Tablet		Warner Chilcott
WC; 071;	Propranolol Hydrochloride	20 mg		Tablet		Warner Chilcott
WC; 072;	Propranolol Hydrochloride	40 mg		Tablet		Warner Chilcott
WC; 073;	Propranolol Hydrochloride	60 mg		Tablet		Warner Chilcott
WC; 074;	Propranolol Hydrochloride	80 mg		Tablet		Warner Chilcott
WC; 084	Gemfibrozil	600 mg	White	Coated Tablet	Circle, Scored	Warner Chilcott
WC; 100	Chlorpromazine Hydrochloride	100 mg		Tablet		Warner Chilcott
WC; 117	Diphenoxylate Hydrochloride and Atropine	2.5 mg; 0.025 mg	White	Tablet	Circle	Warner Chilcott
WC; 121	Chlorthalidone	50 mg		Tablet		Warner Chilcott
WC; 123	Chlorthalidone	25 mg		Tablet		Warner Chilcott
WC; 141	Diazepam	2 mg		Tablet		Warner Chilcott
WC; 142	Diazepam	5 mg		Tablet		Warner Chilcott
WC; 176	Isotrate ER	60 mg	White	Extended-Release Tablet	Capsule-Shape, Scored(Both Sides)	Apothecon
WC; 201	Chlorpromazine Hydrochloride	200 mg		Tablet		Warner Chilcott
WC; 227	Natachew	1000 IU; 400 IU; 11 IU; 120 mg; 1 mg; 2 mg; 3 mg; 20 mg; 10 mg; 12 mcg; 29 mg	Tan Speckled	Tablet, Chewable	Circle, Scored	Warner Chilcott
WC; 230	Tedral	130 mg; 24 mg; 8 mg	White	Tablet		Parke-Davis
WC; 238	Tedral-25	130 mg; 24 mg; 25 mg	Salmon and Pink	Tablet		Parke-Davis
WC; 242	Carbamazepine	100 mg	Pink	Tablet, Chewable	Circle, Scored	H.L. Moore
WC; 242	Carbamazepine	100 mg	Pink Speckled	Tablet, Chewable	Circle, Scored	Warner Chilcott
WC; 243	Carbamazepine	200 mg		Tablet		Warner Chilcott
WC; 271	Amitriptyline	100 mg		Tablet		Warner Chilcott
WC; 272	Amitriptyline	10 mg		Tablet		Warner Chilcott
WC; 273	Amitriptyline	25 mg		Tablet		Warner Chilcott
WC; 274	Amitriptyline	50 mg		Tablet		Warner Chilcott
WC; 275	Amitriptyline	75 mg		Tablet		Warner Chilcott
WC; 278	Amitriptyline	150 mg		Tablet		Warner Chilcott
WC; 402	Amcill	250 mg		Capsule		Warner Chilcott
WC; 402	Ampicillin	250 mg	Grey and Blue	Capsule		Stada
WC; 404	Amcill	500 mg		Capsule		Warner Chilcott
WC; 404	Ampicillin	500 mg	Grey and Blue	Capsule		Stada
WC; 420;	Quinine Sulfate	5 Gr		Capsule		Warner Chilcott
WC; 440	Furosemide	20 mg	White	Tablet	Oval	Warner Chilcott
WC; 441;	Furosemide	40 mg	White	Tablet	Circle	Warner Chilcott
WC; 442;	Furosemide	80 mg	White	Tablet	Circle	Warner Chilcott
WC; 443	Clonidine Hydrochloride	0.1 mg		Tablet		Warner Chilcott
WC; 444	Clonidine Hydrochloride	0.2 mg		Tablet		Warner Chilcott
WC; 445	Clonidine Hydrochloride	0.3 mg		Tablet		Warner Chilcott
WC; 451	Clorazepate Dipotassium	3.75 mg		Tablet		Warner Chilcott
WC; 452	Clorazepate Dipotassium	7.5 mg		Tablet		Warner Chilcott
WC; 453	Clorazepate Dipotassium	15 mg		Tablet		Warner Chilcott
WC; 551	Oxazepam	15 mg	Yellow	Tablet	Circle, Biconvex	Warner Chilcott
WC; 557	Verapamil Hydrochloride	80 mg	White	Tablet		Warner Chilcott
WC; 573	Verapamil Hydrochloride	120 mg	White	Tablet		Warner Chilcott
WC; 606	Aspirin	5 Gr	White	Tablet		Warner Chilcott
WC; 615	Minocycline Hcl	50 mg	Olive and Brown	Capsule		Warner Chilcott
WC; 615	Minocycline Hydrochloride	50 mg	Green and Brown	Capsule		H.L. Moore
WC; 616	Minocycline Hcl	100 mg	White and Olive	Capsule		Warner Chilcott
WC; 616	Minocycline Hydrochloride	100 mg	Green and White	Capsule		H.L. Moore
WC; 634;	Acetaminophen and Codeine No. 2	300 mg; 15 mg		Tablet		Warner Chilcott
WC; 635;	Acetaminophen and Codeine No. 3	300 mg; 30 mg	White	Tablet	Circle	Warner Chilcott
WC; 637;	Acetaminophen and Codeine No. 4	300 mg; 60 mg	White	Tablet	Flat	Warner Chilcott
WC; 640	Acetaminophen	325 mg	White	Tablet	Circle	Warner Chilcott
WC; 648	Penapar VK	250 mg		Tablet		Warner Chilcott
WC; 672	Erythromycin Stearate	250 mg		Tablet		Warner Chilcott
WC; 673	Penapar VK	500 mg		Tablet		Warner Chilcott
WC; 702	Hydrochlorothiazide	25 mg		Tablet		Warner Chilcott

IMPRINT	BRAND/GENERIC NAME	STRENGTH	COLOR	FORM	SHAPE	MANUFACTURER
WC; 710	Hydrochlorothiazide	50 mg		Tablet		Warner Chilcott
WC; 712	Spironolactone with Hydrochlorothiazide	25 mg; 25 mg		Tablet		Warner Chilcott
WC; 713	Spironolactone	25 mg		Tablet		Warner Chilcott
WC; 725	Aspirin with Codeine Phosphate No. 2	15 mg; 325 mg		Tablet		Warner Chilcott
WC; 726	Aspirin with Codeine Phosphate No. 3	30 mg; 325 mg		Tablet		Warner Chilcott
WC; 727	Aspirin with Codeine Phosphate No. 4	60 mg; 325 mg		Tablet		Warner Chilcott
WC; 730	Amoxicillin	250 mg	Red and Pink	Capsule		Stada
WC; 730	Amoxicillin	250 mg		Capsule		Warner Chilcott
WC; 731	Amoxicillin	500 mg	Red and Pink	Capsule		Stada
WC; 731	Amoxicillin	500 mg	Red and Pink	Capsule		Warner Chilcott
WC; 784	Potassium Chloride	10 meq		Extended-Release Tablet		Warner Chilcott
WC; 800	Chlordiazepoxide Hydrochloride	5 mg		Capsule		Warner Chilcott
WC; 801	Chlordiazepoxide Hydrochloride	10 mg		Capsule		Warner Chilcott
WC; 802	Chlordiazepoxide Hydrochloride	25 mg		Capsule		Warner Chilcott
WC; 808	Cephradine	250 mg		Capsule		Warner Chilcott
WC; 809	Cephradine	500 mg		Capsule		Warner Chilcott
WC; 813;	Doxycycline Hyclate	100 mg		Tablet		Warner Chilcott
WC; 829;	Doxycycline Hyclate	50 mg		Capsule		Warner Chilcott
WC; 830;	Doxycycline Hyclate	100 mg		Capsule		Warner Chilcott
WC; 832	Amiloride Hydrochloride and Hydrochlorothiazide	5 mg; 50 mg	Yellow	Tablet	Circle	Warner Chilcott
WC; 833	Triamterene and Hydrochlorothiazide	50 mg; 75 mg	Yellow	Tablet	Round, Bisected Scored	Warner Chilcott
WC; 849	Quinidine Sulfate	200 mg		Tablet		Warner Chilcott
WC; 850	Duraquin	330 mg	White	Sustained-Release Tablet		Warner Chilcott
WC; 850	Quinidine Gluconate	330 mg		Tablet		Warner Chilcott
WC; 865;	Methyldopa	250 mg	Blue	Tablet	Circle	Warner Chilcott
WC; 866;	Methyldopa	500 mg	Blue	Tablet	Circle	Warner Chilcott
WC; 878	Metoclopramide Hydrochloride	10 mg		Tablet		Warner Chilcott
WC; 919	Erythromycin Stearate	500 mg		Tablet		Warner Chilcott
WC; 929	Nelova 0.5/35e-21	0.5 mg; 35 mcg	Light Yellow	21-Day Tablet Pack	Circle	Warner Chilcott
WC; 929	Nelova 0.5/35e-28 Light Yellow Tablet	0.5 mg; 35 mcg	Light Yellow	28-Day Tablet Pack	Circle	Warner Chilcott
WC; 929	Nelova 10/11-21 Light Yellow Tablet	0.5 mg; 35 mcg	Light Yellow	21-Day Tablet Pack	Circle	Warner Chilcott
WC; 929	Nelova 10/11-28 Light Yellow Tablet	0.5 mg; 35 mcg	Light Yellow	28-Day Tablet Pack	Circle	Warner Chilcott
WC; 930	Nelova 1/35e-21	1 mg; 35 mcg	Dark Yellow	21-Day Tablet Pack	Circle	Warner Chilcott
WC; 930	Nelova 1/35e-28 Dark Yellow Tablet	1 mg; 35 mcg	Dark Yellow	28-Day Tablet Pack	Circle	Warner Chilcott
WC; 930	Nelova 10/11-21 Dark Yellow Tablet	1 mg; 35 mcg	Dark Yellow	21-Day Tablet Pack	Circle	Warner Chilcott
WC; 930	Nelova 10/11-28 Dark Yellow Tablet	1 mg; 35 mcg	Dark Yellow	28-Day Tablet Pack	Circle	Warner Chilcott
WC; 940	R-Tannate	25 mg; 8 mg; 25 mg	Buff	Tablet	Capsule-Shape	Warner Chilcott
WC; 942	Nelova 1/50m-21	1 mg; 50 mcg	Light Blue	21-Day Tablet Pack	Circle	Warner Chilcott
WC; 942	Nelova 1/50m-28 Light Blue Tablet	1 mg; 50 mcg	Light Blue	28-Day Tablet Pack	Circle	Warner Chilcott
WC; 945	Dicloxacillin Sodium	250 mg		Capsule		Warner Chilcott
WC; 946	Dicloxacillin Sodium	500 mg		Capsule		Warner Chilcott
WC; 951	Potassium Chloride	8 meq		Extended-Release Capsule		Warner Chilcott
WC; 977	Temazepam	15 mg		Capsule		Warner Chilcott
WC; 978	Temazepam	30 mg		Capsule		Warner Chilcott
WC; 979	Acetaminophen and Propoxyphene Hydrochloride	65 mg; 650 mg		Tablet		Warner Chilcott
WC; 980	Acetaminophen and Propoxyphene Napsylate	100 mg; 650 mg		Tablet		Warner Chilcott
WC; 981	Haloperidol	0.5 mg		Tablet		Warner Chilcott
WC; 982	Haloperidol	1 mg		Tablet		Warner Chilcott
WC; 983	Haloperidol	2 mg		Tablet		Warner Chilcott
WC; 984	Haloperidol	5 mg		Tablet		Warner Chilcott
WC; 985	Clonidine Hydrochloride and Chlorthalidone	0.1 mg; 15 mg		Tablet		Warner Chilcott
WC; 986	Clonidine Hydrochloride and Chlorthalidone	0.2 mg; 15 mg		Tablet		Warner Chilcott
WC; 987	Clonidine Hydrochloride and Chlorthalidone	0.3 mg; 15 mg		Tablet		Warner Chilcott
WC; 988	Flurazepam Hydrochloride	15 mg	Peach and Orange	Capsule		Warner Chilcott
WC; 989	Flurazepam Hydrochloride	30 mg	Peach and Strawberry	Capsule		Warner Chilcott
WDF	Mol-Iron Chronosule	390 mg	Pink and Red, Clear	Capsule		Schering-Plough Healthcare Products
WE; 04	Ultrabrom PD	6 mg; 60 mg	Purple and Clear	Timed-Release Capsule		We Pharmaceuticals
WE; 05	D-Feda	600 mg; 60 mg	Blue	Tablet	Oblong	We Pharmaceuticals
WE; 65	We Mist II LA	800 mg; 80 mg	White	Extended-Release Tablet	Oval, Scored	We Pharmaceuticals
WE O2;	Omnihist L.A.	20 mg; 8 mg; 2.5 mg	White	Tablet	Oblong, Bisected, Scored Scored	We Pharmaceuticals
WE; O3	Ah-Chew	10 mg; 2 mg; 1.25 mg	Purple	Tablet, Chewable	Oblong, Scored	We Pharmaceuticals
WELLBUTRIN; 75	Wellbutrin	75 mg	Yellow-Gold	Coated Tablet	Circle, Biconvex	Glaxosmithkline
WELLBUTRIN; 100	Wellbutrin	100 mg	Red	Coated Tablet	Circle, Biconvex	Glaxosmithkline

IMPRINT	BRAND/GENERIC NAME	STRENGTH	COLOR	FORM	SHAPE	MANUFACTURER
WELLBUTRIN; SR; 200	Wellbutrin SR	200 mg	Light Pink	Sustained-Release Tablet	Circle, Biconvex	Glaxosmithkline
WELLBUTRIN; XL; 150	Wellbutrin Xl	150 mg	Creamy White to Pale Yellow	Extended-Release Tablet	Circle	Glaxosmithkline
WELLBUTRIN; XL; 300	Wellbutrin Xl	300 mg	Creamy White to Pale Yellow	Extended-Release Tablet	Circle	Glaxosmithkline
WELLBUTRIN SR; 100	Wellbutrin SR	100 mg	Blue	Sustained-Release Tablet	Circle, Biconvex	Glaxosmithkline
WELLBUTRIN SR; 150	Wellbutrin SR	150 mg	Purple	Sustained-Release Tablet	Circle, Biconvex	Glaxosmithkline
WELLBUTRIN XL; 150	Wellbutrin Xl	150 mg	White to Yellow	Tablet	Circle	Glaxosmithkline
WELLBUTRIN XL; 300	Wellbutrin Xl	300 mg	White to Yellow	Tablet	Circle	Glaxosmithkline
WELLCOME; U3B	Tabloid	40 mg	Green-Yellow	Tablet	Circle, Scored	Glaxosmithkline
WELLCOME; Y9C; 100; UNICORN LOGO	Retrovir	100 mg	White with Dark Blue Band	Capsule		Glaxosmithkline
WELLCOME; ZOVIRAX; 200	Zovirax	200 mg	Blue	Capsule		Glaxosmithkline
WER	Mol-Iron Panhemic Chronosule	390 mg; 25 mcg; 150 mg; 6 mg; 6 mg; 5 mg; 30 mg	Clear, Red and Yellow	Capsule		Schering-Plough Healthcare Products
WESTWARD; 445	Phenobarbital	15 mg	White	Tablet	Circle, Scored	West-Ward
WESTWARD; 765	Isosorbide Dinitrate Sublingual	2.5 mg	Yellow	Tablet	Circle	West-Ward
WESTWARD; 767	Isosorbide Dinitrate Sublingual	5 mg	White	Tablet	Circle	West-Ward
WESTWARD; 769	Isosorbide Dinitrate	5 mg	White	Tablet	Circle, Scored	West-Ward
WESTWARD; 771	Isosorbide Dinitrate	10 mg	White	Tablet	Circle, Scored	West-Ward
WESTWARD; 772	Isosorbide Dinitrate	20 mg	Green	Tablet	Circle, Scored	West-Ward
WESTWARD; 3142	Doxycycline	100 mg	Blue and Blue	Capsule		Qualitest Products
WESTWARD; FLURAZEPAM; 15	Flurazepam Hydrochloride	15 mg	Blue and White	Capsule		Novartis Generics
WESTWARD; FLURAZEPAM; 30	Flurazepam Hydrochloride	30 mg	Blue	Capsule	Oblong	Novartis Generics
WEST-WARD	Meclizine Hydrochloride	25 mg	Pink	Tablet, Chewable		West-Ward
WEST-WARD	Meclizine Hydrochloride	12.5 mg	White	Tablet	Capsule-Shape	West-Ward
WEST-WARD; 020	Aminophylline	100 mg	White	Tablet		West-Ward
WEST-WARD; 025	Aminophylline	200 mg	White	Tablet	Compressed	West-Ward
WEST-WARD; 090	Chlordiazepoxide Hydrochloride	5 mg	Green and Yellow	Capsule		West-Ward
WEST-WARD; 093	Chlordiazepoxide Hydrochloride	10 mg	Green and Black	Capsule		West-Ward
WEST-WARD; 095	Chlordiazepoxide Hydrochloride	25 mg	Green and White	Capsule		West-Ward
WEST-WARD; 110	Chloral Hydrate	500 mg	Green	Capsule	Oval	West-Ward
WEST-WARD; 137	Diphenhydramine Hydrochloride	50 mg	Pink	Capsule		West-Ward
WEST-WARD; 140	Belladonna Alkaloids with Phenobarbital	16.2 mg; 0.1037 mg; 0.0194 mg; 0.0065 mg	White	Tablet		West-Ward
WEST-WARD; 155	Butabarbital Sodium	15 mg	Lavender	Tablet		West-Ward
WEST-WARD; 157	Butabarbital Sodium	30 mg	Blue-Green	Tablet		West-Ward
WEST-WARD; 195	Chloroquine Phosphate	250 mg	White	Tablet		West-Ward
WEST-WARD; 195;	Chloroquine Phosphate	250 mg	White	Tablet	Circle, Scored, Compressed	Global Pharmaceutical
WEST-WARD; 201	Colchicine	0.6 mg		Tablet		West-Ward
WEST-WARD; 202	Cortisone Acetate	25 mg	White	Tablet	Circle, Scored	Qualitest Products
WEST-WARD; 202	Cortisone Acetate	25 mg	White	Tablet		West-Ward
WEST-WARD; 208	Nitroglycerin	2.5 mg	Purple and Clear	Capsule		West-Ward
WEST-WARD; 209	Chlorothiazide	250 mg	White	Tablet		West-Ward
WEST-WARD; 210	Chlorothiazide	500 mg	White	Tablet	Circle, Scored	Qualitest Products
WEST-WARD; 210	Chlorothiazide	500 mg	White	Tablet		West-Ward
WEST-WARD; 210	Oxytetracycline Hydrochloride	250 mg	Yellow	Capsule		West-Ward
WEST-WARD; 217	Chlorothiazide with Reserpine	0.125 mg; 250 mg	Pink	Tablet		West-Ward
WEST-WARD; 218	Chlorothiazide with Reserpine	0.125 mg; 500 mg	Pink	Tablet		West-Ward
WEST-WARD; 235	Propoxyphene	65 mg	Pink	Capsule		Qualitest Products
WEST-WARD; 235	Propoxyphene Hydrochloride	65 mg	Pink	Capsule		West-Ward
WEST-WARD; 245	Diphenoxylate with Atropine	2.5 mg; 0.025 mg	White	Tablet		West-Ward
WEST-WARD; 248	Folic Acid	1 mg	Yellow	Tablet	Circle	Qualitest Products
WEST-WARD; 248	Folic Acid	1 mg	Yellow	Tablet	Circle	Udl Laboratories
WEST-WARD; 248	Folic Acid	1 mg	Yellow	Tablet	Circle	West-Ward
WEST-WARD; 254	Hydrocortisone	20 mg	White	Tablet		West-Ward
WEST-WARD; 256	Hydrochlorothiazide	25 mg	Peach	Tablet		West-Ward
WEST-WARD; 257	Hydrochlorothiazide	50 mg	Peach	Tablet		West-Ward
WEST-WARD; 258	Isoxsuprine Hydrochloride	10 mg	White	Tablet		West-Ward
WEST-WARD; 259	Isoxsuprine Hydrochloride	20 mg	White	Tablet		West-Ward
WEST-WARD; 260	Isoniazid	100 mg	White	Tablet	Circle, Scored	Akyma Pharmaceuticals
WEST-WARD; 260	Isoniazid	100 mg		Tablet		West-Ward
WEST-WARD; 261	Isoniazid	300 mg	White	Tablet	Circle, Scored	Akyma Pharmaceuticals
WEST-WARD; 261	Isoniazid	300 mg	White	Tablet		West-Ward
WEST-WARD; 265	Hydrochlorothiazide and Reserpine	50 mg; 0.125 mg	Aqua	Tablet		West-Ward
WEST-WARD; 290	Methocarbamol	500 mg	White	Tablet	Circle, Scored	Qualitest Products
WEST-WARD; 290	Methocarbamol	500 mg	White	Tablet		West-Ward
WEST-WARD; 292	Methocarbamol	750 mg	White	Tablet	Oblong, Scored	Qualitest Products
WEST-WARD; 292	Methocarbamol	750 mg	White	Tablet		West-Ward
WEST-WARD; 295	Tetracycline Hydrochloride	250 mg	Orange and Yellow	Capsule		West-Ward
WEST-WARD; 330	Methyltestosterone	25 mg	Yellow	Tablet		West-Ward
WEST-WARD; 352	Niacin	500 mg	White	Tablet		West-Ward
WEST-WARD; 470	Prednisolone	5 mg	Yellow	Tablet		West-Ward
WEST-WARD; 473	Prednisone	10 mg	White	Tablet	Circle, Scored	Qualitest Products
WEST-WARD; 473	Prednisone	10 mg	White	Tablet	Circle, F-Faced, Beveled, Scored	West-Ward
WEST-WARD; 475	Prednisone	5 mg	White	Tablet		Novartis Generics
WEST-WARD; 475	Prednisone	5 mg	White	Tablet	Circle, Scored	Qualitest Products
WEST-WARD; 475	Prednisone	5 mg	White	Tablet	Circle, F-Faced, Beveled, Scored	West-Ward

IMPRINT	BRAND/GENERIC NAME	STRENGTH	COLOR	FORM	SHAPE	MANUFACTURER
WEST-WARD; 477	Prednisone	20 mg	Peach	Tablet	Circle, Scored	Novartis Generics
WEST-WARD; 477	Prednisone	20 mg	Peach	Tablet	Circle, Scored	Qualitest Products
WEST-WARD; 477	Prednisone	20 mg	Peach	Tablet	Circle, F-Faced, Beveled, Scored	West-Ward
WEST-WARD; 480	Propylthiouracil	50 mg	White	Tablet		West-Ward
WEST-WARD; 481	Prednisone	50 mg	White	Tablet	Circle, F-Faced, Beveled, Scored	West-Ward
WEST-WARD; 485	Pseudoephedrine Hydrochloride	60 mg	White	Tablet		West-Ward
WEST-WARD; 510	Quinidine Sulfate	200 mg	White	Tablet		West-Ward
WEST-WARD; 530	Reserpine	0.1 mg	White	Tablet		West-Ward
WEST-WARD; 535	Reserpine	0.25 mg	White	Tablet		West-Ward
WEST-WARD; 683	Sulfisoxazole	0.5 G	White	Tablet		West-Ward
WEST-WARD; 695	T-E-P	2 Gr; 0.375 Gr; 0.125 Gr		Tablet		West-Ward
WEST-WARD; 695	Theophylline, Ephedrine and Phenobarbital	118.2 mg; 24 mg; 8 mg	White	Tablet	Circle	West-Ward
WEST-WARD; 737	Butalbital, Acetaminophen, and Caffeine	50 mg; 325 mg; 40 mg	White	Tablet	Circle	West-Ward
WEST-WARD; 755	Triprolidine and Pseudoephedrine	2.5 mg; 60 mg		Tablet		West-Ward
WEST-WARD; 769	Isosorbide Dinitrate	5 mg	White	Tablet		West-Ward
WEST-WARD; 771	Isosorbide Dinitrate	10 mg	White	Tablet		West-Ward
WEST-WARD; 772	Isosorbide Dinitrate	20 mg	Green	Tablet	Circle, Scored	Qualitest Products
WEST-WARD; 785	Butalbital Compound	50 mg; 325 mg; 40 mg	White	Tablet	Circle	Qualitest Products
WEST-WARD; 785	Butalbital, Aspirin and Caffeine	50 mg; 325 mg; 40 mg	White	Tablet	Circle	West-Ward
WEST-WARD; 787	Butalbital, Acetaminophen and Caffeine	50 mg; 325 mg; 40 mg	Blue	Tablet	Circle	West-Ward
WEST-WARD; 3141	Doxycycline	50 mg	Blue and White	Capsule		Qualitest Products
WEST-WARD; 3141	Doxycycline Hyclate	50 mg	Opaque Blue and White	Capsule		Akyma Pharmaceuticals
WEST-WARD; 3141	Doxycycline Hyclate	50 mg	White and Blue	Capsule		West-Ward
WEST-WARD; 3142	Doxycycline Hyclate	100 mg	Blue	Capsule		West-Ward
WEST-WARD; 3142	Doxycycline Hyclate	100 mg	Opaque Blue	Capsule		Akyma Pharmaceuticals
WEST-WARD; 3145	Ephedrine Sulfate	25 mg	Pink	Capsule	Oblong	West-Ward
WEST-WARD; 3189	Lithium Carbonate	300 mg	Grey/yellow	Capsule		Ivax Pharmaceuticals
WEST-WARD; FLURAZEPAM; 15	Flurazepam	15 mg	Blue and White	Capsule		West-Ward
WEST-WARD; FLURAZEPAM; 30	Flurazepam	30 mg	Blue	Capsule		West-Ward
WFHC; 91	Equagesic	200 mg; 325 mg	Pink and Yellow	Tablet	Circle, Layered, Scored	Women First Healthcare
WFHC; 4191	Synalgos-Dc	16 mg; 356.4 mg; 30 mg	Blue and Gray	Capsule		Women First Healthcare
WH-SCS; 5752	Piroxicam	10 mg	Opaque Orange and Opaque Light Blue	Capsule		Lederle Laboratories
WH-SCS; 5762	Piroxicam	20 mg	Opaque Orange	Capsule		Lederle Laboratories
WI	Isosorbide Dinitrate	2.5 mg	Yellow	Tablet		West-Ward
WINTHROP; D03; 50 MG;	Danocrine	50 mg	Orange and White	Capsule		Winthrop Pharmaceuticals
WINTHROP; D04; 100 MG;	Danocrine	100 mg	Yellow	Capsule		Winthrop Pharmaceuticals
WINTHROP; T; 37	Talacen	25 mg; 650 mg	Pale Blue	Tablet		Sanofi Winthrop Pharmaceuticals
WKJ;	Permitil Chronotab	1 mg	Yellow	Tablet		Schering
WMM	Mol-Iron with Vitamin C Chronosule	390 mg; 150 mg	Clear, Red and Orange	Capsule		Schering-Plough Healthcare Products
WMP; 9525	Solfoton	16 mg	Brown and Yellow	Capsule		Poythress Laboratories
WMP; 9541	Antrocol	0.195 mg; 16 mg	Green	Capsule		Poythress Laboratories
WP; 97	Primaquine Phosphate	15 mg	White	Coated Tablet	Circle	Winthrop Pharmaceuticals
WPI; 839	Bupropion Hydrochloride	150 mg	White	Extended-Release Tablet	Circle, Biconvex	Watson Laboratories
WPI; 844	Glipizide Extended-Release	5 mg	Orange	Extended-Release Tablet	Circle	Watson Laboratories
WPI; 845	Glipizide Extended-Release	10 mg	White to Off-White	Extended-Release Tablet	Circle	Watson Laboratories
WPI; 858	Bupropion Hydrochloride	100 mg	White	Extended-Release Tablet	Circle, Biconvex	Watson Laboratories
WPI; 1117;	Mirtazapine	15 mg	White	Tablet	Oval, Scored	Watson Laboratories
WPI; 1118	Mirtazapine	30 mg	Yellow	Tablet	Oval, Scored	Watson Laboratories
WPI; 1119	Mirtazapine	45 mg	White	Tablet	Oval	Watson Laboratories
WPI; 2137	Ibuprofen	800 mg		Tablet		Watson Laboratories
WPI; 2455;	Metformin Hydrochloride	1000 mg	Light Peach	Coated Tablet	Capsule-Shaped; Bisected Scored	Watson Laboratories
WPI; 2713	Metformin Hydrochloride	500 mg	Light Peach	Coated Tablet	Capsule-Shape	Watson Laboratories
WPI; 2775	Metformin Hydrochloride	850 mg	Light Peach	Coated Tablet	Capsule-Shape	Watson Laboratories
WPI; 3111	Methylphenidate Hydrochloride	20 mg	White	Extended-Release Tablet	Oval	Watson Laboratories
WPI; 3137	Nizatidine	150 mg	Buff	Capsule		Watson Laboratories
WPI; 3138	Nizatidine	300 mg	Light Brown	Capsule		Watson Laboratories
WPI; 3176	Citalopram Hydrobromide	10 mg	White	Tablet	Circle	Watson Laboratories
WPI 3177	Citalopram Hydrobromide	20 mg	White	Tablet	Circle	Watson Laboratories
WPI 3177	Citalopram Hydrobromide	40 mg	White	Tablet	Circle	Watson Laboratories
WPI; 4010	Ibuprofen	400 mg	White	Tablet	Oblong	Watson Laboratories
WPI; 4011	Ibuprofen	600 mg	White	Tablet	Elongated	Watson Laboratories
WPI; MINOCYCLINE; 75	Minocycline Hydrochloride	75 mg	White and Yellow	Capsule		Watson Laboratories
WPPH	Diflunisal	250 mg	Peach	Tablet	Capsule-Shape	West Point Pharma
WPPH	Diflunisal	500 mg	Orange	Tablet	Capsule-Shape	West Point Pharma
WPPH; 153	Methyldopa and Hydrochlorothiazide	250 mg; 25 mg	White	Coated Tablet	Circle	Endo Laboratories
WPPH; 156	Cyclobenzaprine Hydrochloride	10 mg	Butterscotch Yellow	Coated Tablet	D-Shape	Endo Laboratories
WPPH; 162	Amiloride Hydrochloride and Hydrochlorothiazide	5 mg; 50 mg	Peach	Tablet	Diamond, Scored	Endo Laboratories
WPPH; 179	Methyldopa and Hydrochlorothiazide	250 mg; 15 mg	Salmon	Coated Tablet	Circle	Endo Laboratories
WPPH; 195	Diflunisal	250 mg	Peach	Coated Tablet	Capsule-Shape	Endo Laboratories
WPPH; 196	Diflunisal	500 mg	Orange	Coated Tablet	Capsule-Shape	Endo Laboratories

IMPRINT	BRAND/GENERIC NAME	STRENGTH	COLOR	FORM	SHAPE	MANUFACTURER
WW; 27	Dicyclomine Hydrochloride	20 mg	Light Blue	Tablet	Circle	West-Ward
WW; 33	Isosorbide Mononitrate	20 mg	White	Tablet	Circle, Scored	West-Ward
WW; 65	Lisinopril	2.5 mg	White	Tablet	Oblong	West-Ward
WW; 66	Lisinopril	5 mg	Red	Tablet	Oblong, Bisected Scored	West-Ward
WW; 112	Doxycycline Hyclate	100 mg	Orange	Tablet	Circle	West-Ward
WW; 115	Acetaminophen, Butalbital and Caffeine	500 mg; 50 mg; 40 mg	White	Tablet	Capsule-Shape, Scored	West-Ward
WW; 115	Butalbital, Acetaminophen, and Caffeine	50 mg; 40 mg; 500 mg	White	Tablet	Oblong	Qualitest Products
WW; 172	Captopril	25 mg	White	Tablet	Quadrisect Scored	West-Ward
WW; 173	Captopril	50 mg	White	Tablet	Bisect Scored	West-Ward
WW; 174	Captopril	100 mg	White	Tablet	Biconvex, Bisect Scored	West-Ward
WW; 174	Captopril	100 mg	White	Tablet	Oblong	Qualitest Products
WW; 176	Carisoprodol	350 mg	White	Tablet	Circle	West-Ward
WW; 267	Lisinopril	10 mg	Pink	Tablet	Circle	West-Ward
WW; 268	Lisinopril	20 mg	Red	Tablet	Circle	West-Ward
WW; 270	Lisinopril	40 mg	Yellow	Tablet	Circle	West-Ward
WW; 277	Lithium Carbonate Extended-Release	450 mg	Yellow	Extended-Release Tablet	Circle, Scored	West-Ward
WW; 450;	Phenobarbital	30 mg	White	Tablet	Circle, Scored	West-Ward
WW; 455	Phenobarbital	60 mg		Tablet		West-Ward
WW; 771	Isosorbide Dinitrate	10 mg		Tablet		West-Ward
WW; 772	Isosorbide Dinitrate	20 mg	Light Green	Tablet	Circle	Schein Pharmaceutical
WW; 772	Isosorbide Dinitrate	20 mg	Light Green	Tablet	Circle	West-Ward
WYETH; 1	Equanil	400 mg	White	Tablet		Wyeth Pharmaceuticals
WYETH; 2	Equanil	200 mg	White	Tablet		Wyeth Pharmaceuticals
WYETH; 10	Isordil	10 mg	White	Tablet	Circle	Wyeth Pharmaceuticals
WYETH; 13	Amphojel	600 mg	White	Tablet		Wyeth Pharmaceuticals
WYETH; 19	Phenergan	12.5 mg	Orange	Tablet		Wyeth Pharmaceuticals
WYETH; 22	Aludrox	233 mg; 83 mg		Tablet, Chewable		Wyeth Pharmaceuticals
WYETH; 27	Phenergan	25 mg	White	Tablet		Wyeth Pharmaceuticals
WYETH; 28	Sparine	50 mg	Orange	Coated Tablet	Circle	Wyeth Pharmaceuticals
WYETH; 29	Sparine	25 mg	Yellow	Coated Tablet	Circle	Wyeth Pharmaceuticals
WYETH; 33	Equanil Wyseals	400 mg	Yellow	Coated Tablet	Circle	Wyeth Pharmaceuticals
WYETH; 33	Wyseals	400 mg	Yellow	Coated Tablet		Wyeth Pharmaceuticals
WYETH; 53	Omnipen	250 mg	Violet and Pink	Capsule		Wyeth Pharmaceuticals
WYETH; 56	Ovral	0.5 mg; 50 mcg	White	21-Day Tablet Pack	Circle	Wyeth Pharmaceuticals
WYETH; 56	Ovral-28 White Tablet	0.5 mg; 50 mcg	White	28-Day Tablet Pack	Circle	Wyeth Pharmaceuticals
WYETH; 57	Unipen	250 mg	Green and Yellow	Capsule		Wyeth Pharmaceuticals
WYETH; 59	Pen-Vee K	250 mg	White	Tablet		Wyeth Pharmaceuticals
WYETH; 62	Ovrette	75 mcg	Yellow	28-Day Tablet Pack	Circle	Wyeth Pharmaceuticals
WYETH; 71	Mazanor	1 mg	White	Tablet	Circle, Scored	Wyeth Pharmaceuticals
WYETH; 73, W; 4	Wytensin	4 mg	Orange	Tablet	Five-Sided	Wyeth Pharmaceuticals
WYETH; 74; W; 8	Wytensin	8 mg	Grey	Tablet	Five-Sided	Wyeth Pharmaceuticals
WYETH; 75	Nordette-21	0.15 mg; 30 mcg	Light Orange	21-Day Tablet Pack	Circle	Wyeth Pharmaceuticals
WYETH; 75	Nordette-28 Light Orange Tablet	0.15 mg; 30 mcg	Light Orange	28-Day Tablet Pack	Circle	Wyeth Pharmaceuticals
WYETH; 78	Lo/ovral	0.3 mg; 30 mcg	White	21-Day Tablet Pack	Circle	Wyeth Pharmaceuticals
WYETH; 78	Lo/ovral-28 White Tablet	0.3 mg; 30 mcg	White	28-Day Tablet Pack	Circle	Wyeth Pharmaceuticals
WYETH; 91	Equagesic	200 mg; 325 mg	Orange and Pink	Tablet	Circle	Wyeth Pharmaceuticals
WYETH; 92; W; 16	Wytensin	16 mg	White	Tablet	Five-Sided	Wyeth Pharmaceuticals
WYETH; 119	Amphojel	300 mg	White	Tablet	Circle	Wyeth Pharmaceuticals
WYETH; 138	A-M-T	162 mg; 250 mg		Tablet		Wyeth Pharmaceuticals
WYETH; 200	Sparine	100 mg	Pink	Coated Tablet	Circle	Wyeth Pharmaceuticals
WYETH; 227	Phenergan	50 mg	Pink	Tablet		Wyeth Pharmaceuticals
WYETH; 261	Mepergan Fortis	50 mg; 25 mg	Maroon	Capsule		Wyeth Pharmaceuticals
WYETH; 308	Meperidine Hydrochloride	50 mg	Tablet	Tablet	Circle, Scored	Wyeth Pharmaceuticals
WYETH; 309	Omnipen	500 mg	Violet and Pink	Capsule		Wyeth Pharmaceuticals
WYETH; 313	Aspirin	300 mg		Tablet		Wyeth Pharmaceuticals
WYETH; 322	Chloral Hydrate	500 mg	Red	Capsule		Wyeth Pharmaceuticals
WYETH; 360	Pathocil	250 mg	Purple and White	Capsule		Wyeth Pharmaceuticals
WYETH; 389	Tetracycline Hydrochloride	250 mg	Blue and Yellow	Capsule		Wyeth Pharmaceuticals
WYETH; 390	Pen-Vee K	500 mg	White	Tablet		Wyeth Pharmaceuticals
WYETH; 434	Phenergan-D	6.25 mg; 60 mg	Orange and White	Tablet		Wyeth Pharmaceuticals
WYETH; 464	Unipen	500 mg	White	Coated Tablet		Wyeth Pharmaceuticals
WYETH; 471	Tetracycline Hydrochloride	500 mg	Blue and Yellow	Capsule		Wyeth Pharmaceuticals
WYETH; 472	Basaljel	608 mg		Capsule		Wyeth Pharmaceuticals
WYETH; 473	Basaljel	608 mg		Tablet		Wyeth Pharmaceuticals
WYETH; 559	Wymox	250 mg	Gray and Green	Capsule		Wyeth Pharmaceuticals
WYETH; 560	Wymox	500 mg	Gray and Green	Capsule		Wyeth Pharmaceuticals
WYETH; 576	Wyamycin S	250 mg	Yellow	Coated Tablet		Wyeth Pharmaceuticals
WYETH; 578	Wyamycin S	500 mg	Pink	Coated Tablet		Wyeth Pharmaceuticals
WYETH; 593	Pathocil	500 mg	Purple and White	Capsule		Wyeth Pharmaceuticals
WYETH; 614	Cyclapen W	250 mg	Yellow	Tablet	Capsule-Shape, Scored	Wyeth Pharmaceuticals
WYETH; 615	Cyclapen W	500 mg	Yellow	Tablet		Wyeth Pharmaceuticals
WYETH; 794	Stuart Prenatal Multivitamin/multimineral Supplement	4000 I.U.; 400 I.U.; 11 mg; 100 mg; 0.8 mg; 1.84 mg; 1.7 mg; 18 mg; 2.6 mg; 4 mcg; 200 mg; 60 mg; 25 mg	Pink	Tablet		Wyeth Pharmaceuticals
WYETH; 4120	Cyclospasmol	100 mg	Orange	Coated Tablet		Wyeth Pharmaceuticals
WYETH; 4124	Cyclospasmol	200 mg	Blue	Capsule		Wyeth Pharmaceuticals
WYETH; 4130	Trecator-Sc	250 mg	Orange	Coated Tablet		Wyeth Pharmaceuticals
WYETH; 4140	Isordil Tembids	40 mg	Clear Blue and Transparent	Capsule		Wyeth Pharmaceuticals
WYETH; 4148	Cyclospasmol	400 mg	Red and Blue	Capsule		Wyeth Pharmaceuticals
WYETH; 4152	Isordil Titradose	5 mg	Pink	Tablet		Wyeth Pharmaceuticals
WYETH; 4153	Isordil Titradose	10 mg	White	Tablet		Wyeth Pharmaceuticals

IMPRINT	BRAND/GENERIC NAME	STRENGTH	COLOR	FORM	SHAPE	MANUFACTURER
WYETH; 4154	Isordil Titradose	20 mg	Green	Tablet		Wyeth Pharmaceuticals
WYETH; 4159	Isordil Titradose	30 mg	Blue	Tablet		Wyeth Pharmaceuticals
WYETH; 4169	Synalgos	6.25 mg; 356.4 mg; 30 mg	Maroon and Gray	Capsule		Wyeth Pharmaceuticals
WYETH; 4175	Synalgos-Dc-A	16 mg; 356.4 mg; 30 mg	Green and Gray	Capsule		Wyeth Pharmaceuticals
WYETH; 4177; SECTRAL; 200	Sectral	200 mg	Purple and Orange	Capsule		Wyeth Pharmaceuticals
WYETH; 4179; SECTRAL; 400	Sectral	400 mg	Brown and Orange	Capsule		Wyeth Pharmaceuticals
WYETH; 4181; ORUDIS 50	Orudis	50 mg	Dark Green and Light Green	Capsule		Wyeth Pharmaceuticals
WYETH; 4186; ORUDIS 25	Orudis	25 mg	Dark Green and Red	Capsule		Wyeth Pharmaceuticals
WYETH; 4187; ORUDIS 75	Orudis	75 mg	Dark Green and White	Capsule		Wyeth Pharmaceuticals
WYETH; 4188; C	Cordarone	200 mg	Pink	Tablet	Circle, Convex-Faced	Wyeth Pharmaceuticals
WYETH; 4191	Synalgos-Dc	16 mg; 356.4 mg; 30 mg	Blue and Gray	Capsule		Women First Healthcare
WYETH; 4191	Synalgos-Dc	16 mg; 356.4 mg; 30 mg	Blue and Gray	Capsule		Wyeth-Ayerst Laboratories
WYETH; 4191	Synalgos-Dc	16 mg; 356.4 mg; 30 mg	Blue and Gray	Capsule		Wyeth Pharmaceuticals
WYETH; 4192	Isordil Titradose	40 mg	Green	Tablet		Wyeth Pharmaceuticals
X	Senokot Xtra	17 mg	Tan	Tablet	Circle	Purdue Pharmaceutical Products
X; 0.5	Alprazolam	0.5 mg	White	Extended-Release Tablet	Five-Sided	Pharmacia & Upjohn
X; 0.5	Xanax Xr	0.5 mg	White	Extended-Release Tablet	Five-Sided	Pharmacia & Upjohn
X; 1	Xanax Xr	1 mg	Yellow	Extended-Release Tablet	Square	Pharmacia & Upjohn
X; 2	Xanax Xr	2 mg	Blue	Extended-Release Tablet	Circle	Pharmacia & Upjohn
X; 3	Xanax Xr	3 mg	Green	Extended-Release Tablet	Triangle	Pharmacia & Upjohn
X; 10	Uroxatral	10 mg	White and Yellow	Extended-Release Tablet	Circle	Sanofi-Synthelabo
XANAX; 0.25	Xanax	0.25 mg	White	Tablet	Oval, Scored	Pharmacia & Upjohn
XANAX; 0.5	Xanax	0.5 mg	Peach	Tablet	Oval, Scored	Pharmacia & Upjohn
XANAX; 1.0	Xanax	1 mg	Blue	Tablet	Oval, Scored	Pharmacia & Upjohn
XELODA; 150	Xeloda	150 mg	Light Peach	Coated Tablet	Oblong	Roche Laboratories
XELODA; 500	Xeloda	500 mg	Peach	Coated Tablet	Oblong	Roche Laboratories
XP; A; 10	Amicar	500 mg	White	Tablet	Circle, Scored	Xanodyne Pharmaceuticals
XP; A; 20	Amicar	1000 mg	White	Tablet	Oblong, Scored	Xanodyne Pharmaceuticals
Z	Zomig-Zmt	2.5 mg	White	Disintegrating Tablet	Circle	Astra Zeneca
Z	Zomig-Zmt	2.5 mg	White	Disintegrating Tablet	Circle	Medpointe
Z; 4	Zofran Odt	4 mg	White	Disintegrating Tablet	Round, Plano-Convex	Glaxosmithkline
Z; 5	Zomig-Zmt	5 mg	White	Disintegrating Tablet	Circle, Flat Faced, Bevelled	Astra Zeneca
Z; 5	Zomig-Zmt	5 mg	White	Disintegrating Tablet	Circle, Flat Faced, Bevelled	Medpointe
Z; 8	Zofran Odt	8 mg	White	Disintegrating Tablet	Round, Plano-Convex	Glaxosmithkline
Z; 75	Zantac 75	75 mg	Pink	Tablet	Five-Sided	Pfizer Consumer Health Care
Z; 2057	Phenytoin Sodium	100 mg	Clear	Capsule		Ivax Pharmaceuticals
Z; 2058	Digoxin	0.25 mg	White	Tablet		Zenith Goldline Pharmaceuticals
Z; 2083	Hydrochlorothiazide	25 mg	Peach	Tablet	Circle	Ivax Pharmaceuticals
Z; 2089	Hydrochlorothiazide	50 mg	Peach	Tablet	Circle	Ivax Pharmaceuticals
Z; 2155	Prednisolone	5 mg	Orange	Tablet	Circle	Solvay Pharmaceuticals
Z; 2168	Hydroserpine No. 2	50 mg; 0.125 mg	Light Green	Tablet	Circle	Zenith Goldline Pharmaceuticals
Z; 2169	Hydroserpine No. 1	25 mg; 0.125 mg	Light Green	Tablet	Circle	Zenith Goldline Pharmaceuticals
Z; 2186	Propoxyphene Hydrochloride	65 mg	Pale Pink	Capsule		Ivax Pharmaceuticals
Z; 2190	Probenecid	500 mg	Yellow	Coated Tablet	Capsule-Shape	Novartis Generics
Z; 2193	Probenecid with Colchicine	0.5 mg; 500 mg	White	Tablet	Capsule-Shape	Novartis Generics
Z; 2198	Reserpine	0.1 mg	White	Tablet	Circle	Zenith Goldline Pharmaceuticals
Z; 2199	Reserpine	0.25 mg	White	Tablet	Circle	Zenith Goldline Pharmaceuticals
Z; 2218	Sulfisoxazole	500 mg	White	Tablet	Circle, Scored	Ivax Pharmaceuticals
Z; 2345	Procainamide Hydrochloride	250 mg	Yellow	Capsule		Ivax Pharmaceuticals
Z; 2345	Procainamide Hydrochloride	250 mg	Yellow	Capsule		West-Ward
Z; 2347	Procainamide Hydrochloride	500 mg	Yellow and Orange	Capsule		Ivax Pharmaceuticals
Z 2407;	Tetracycline Hydrochloride	500 mg	Black and Yellow	Capsule		Zenith Goldline Pharmaceuticals
Z 2416;	Tetracycline Hydrochloride	250 mg	Orange and Yellow	Capsule		Zenith Goldline Pharmaceuticals
Z; 2485	Hydrochlorothiazide	100 mg	Light Orange	Tablet	Circle	Ivax Pharmaceuticals
Z; 2662; 10	Famotidine	10 mg		Tablet		Ivax Pharmaceuticals
Z; 2907	Furosemide	40 mg	White	Tablet	Circle	Ivax Pharmaceuticals
Z; 2908	Furosemide	20 mg	White	Tablet	Oval	Ivax Pharmaceuticals
Z; 2909	Hydroxyzine Pamoate	50 mg	Green and White	Capsule		Ivax Pharmaceuticals
Z; 2911	Hydroxyzine Pamoate	25 mg	Dark Green and Light Green	Capsule		Ivax Pharmaceuticals
Z; 2929;	Cyproheptadine Hydrochloride	4 mg	White	Tablet	Round-Flat, Bisected Scored	Ivax Pharmaceuticals
Z; 2931	Methyldopa	250 mg	White	Coated Tablet	Circle	Ivax Pharmaceuticals
Z; 2932	Methyldopa	500 mg	White	Coated Tablet	Circle	Ivax Pharmaceuticals
Z; 2936	Amitriptyline Hydrochloride and Perphenazine	10 mg; 2 mg	Blue	Coated Tablet	Circle	H.L. Moore
Z; 2936	Perphenazine with Amitriptyline Hydrochloride	2 mg; 10 mg	Blue	Coated Tablet	Circle	Zenith Goldline Pharmaceuticals
Z; 2937	Amitriptyline Hydrochloride and Perphenazine	25 mg; 2 mg	Orange	Coated Tablet	Circle	H.L. Moore
Z; 2937	Perphenazine with Amitriptyline Hydrochloride	2 mg; 25 mg	Orange	Coated Tablet	Circle	Zenith Goldline Pharmaceuticals

IMPRINT	BRAND/GENERIC NAME	STRENGTH	COLOR	FORM	SHAPE	MANUFACTURER
Z; 2938	Amitriptyline Hydrochloride and Perphenazine	10 mg; 4 mg	Salmon	Coated Tablet	Circle	H.L. Moore
Z; 2938	Perphenazine with Amitriptyline Hydrochloride	4 mg; 10 mg	Salmon	Coated Tablet	Circle	Zenith Goldline Pharmaceuticals
Z; 2939	Amitriptyline Hydrochloride and Perphenazine	25 mg; 4 mg	Yellow	Coated Tablet	Circle	H.L. Moore
Z; 2939	Perphenazine with Amitriptyline Hydrochloride	4 mg; 25 mg	Yellow	Coated Tablet	Circle	Zenith Goldline Pharmaceuticals
Z; 2959	Ergoloid Mesylates SL	1 mg	White	Tablet	Oval	Ivax Pharmaceuticals
Z; 2971	Metronidazole	250 mg	White	Tablet	Circle, Convex	Ivax Pharmaceuticals
Z; 2971;	Helidac Therapy: Part II	250 mg	White	Tablet	Circle	Procter & Gamble Pharmaceuticals
Z; 2984	Doxycycline Hyclate	50 mg	Blue and White	Capsule		Ivax Pharmaceuticals
Z; 3001	Quinine Sulfate	260 mg	White	Tablet	Circle	Ivax Pharmaceuticals
Z; 3007	Metronidazole	500 mg	White	Tablet	Oblong, Convex	Ivax Pharmaceuticals
Z; 3626	Doxycycline Hyclate	100 mg	Orange	Coated Tablet	Circle	Ivax Pharmaceuticals
Z; 3667	Perphenazine	2 mg	Gray	Coated Tablet	Circle	H.L. Moore
Z; 3668	Perphenazine	4 mg	Gray	Coated Tablet	Circle	H.L. Moore
Z; 3669	Perphenazine	8 mg	Gray	Coated Tablet	Circle	H.L. Moore
Z; 3670	Perphenazine	16 mg	Gray	Coated Tablet	Circle	H.L. Moore
Z; 3671	Amitriptyline and Perphenazine	50 mg; 4 mg	Orange	Coated Tablet	Circle	H.L. Moore
Z; 3671	Perphenazine with Amitriptyline Hydrochloride	4 mg; 50 mg	Orange	Coated Tablet	Circle	Zenith Goldline Pharmaceuticals
Z; 3690; 5	Prochlorperazine Maleate	5 mg	Gold	Tablet	Circle	Ivax Pharmaceuticals
Z; 3691; 10	Prochlorperazine Maleate	10 mg	Gold	Tablet	Circle	Ivax Pharmaceuticals
Z; 3815	Dextroamphetamine Sulfate	10 mg	Brown and Clear	Capsule		Zenith Goldline Pharmaceuticals
Z; 3816	Dextroamphetamine Sulfate	15 mg	Brown and Clear	Capsule		Zenith Goldline Pharmaceuticals
Z; 3817	Dextroamphetamine Sulfate	15 mg	Red and Yellow	Capsule		Zenith Goldline Pharmaceuticals
Z; 3830	Dextroamphetamine Sulfate	5 mg	Yellow	Tablet		Zenith Goldline Pharmaceuticals
Z; 3921	Tora II	30 mg	Yellow Opaque	Capsule		Solvay Pharmaceuticals
Z; 3925; 2	Diazepam	2 mg	White	Tablet	Circle	Ivax Pharmaceuticals
Z; 3926; 5	Diazepam	5 mg	Yellow	Tablet	Circle	Ivax Pharmaceuticals
Z; 3927; 10	Diazepam	10 mg	Light Blue	Tablet	Circle	Ivax Pharmaceuticals
Z; 3984	Acetaminophen and Codeine	300 mg; 30 mg	White	Tablet	Circle, Scored	H.L. Moore
Z; 4029	Indomethacin	25 mg	Green	Capsule		Ivax Pharmaceuticals
Z; 4030	Indomethacin	50 mg	Green	Capsule		Ivax Pharmaceuticals
Z; 4067	Prazosin	1 mg	Ivory	Capsule		H.L. Moore
Z; 4067	Prazosin Hydrochloride	1 mg	Ivory	Capsule		Ivax Pharmaceuticals
Z; 4068	Prazosin	2 mg	Pink	Capsule		H.L. Moore
Z; 4068	Prazosin Hydrochloride	2 mg	Pink	Capsule		Ivax Pharmaceuticals
Z; 4069	Prazosin	5 mg	Blue	Capsule		H.L. Moore
Z; 4069	Prazosin Hydrochloride	5 mg	Blue	Capsule		Ivax Pharmaceuticals
Z; 4073	Cephalexin	250 mg	Grey and Red	Capsule		Ivax Pharmaceuticals
Z; 4074	Cephalexin	500 mg	Red	Capsule		Ivax Pharmaceuticals
Z; 4096; 10;	Baclofen	10 mg	White	Tablet	Circle, Flat, Scored	Ivax Pharmaceuticals
Z; 4097; 20;	Baclofen	20 mg	White	Tablet	Circle, Flat, Scored	Ivax Pharmaceuticals
Z; 4172	Quinine Sulfate	325 mg	White	Capsule		Ivax Pharmaceuticals
Z; 4217; 5	Pindolol	5 mg	White	Tablet	Circle	Ivax Pharmaceuticals
Z; 4218; 10	Pindolol	10 mg	White	Tablet	Circle	Ivax Pharmaceuticals
Z; 4226	Guanabenz Acetate	4 mg	Peach	Tablet	Circle, Compressed	Ivax Pharmaceuticals
Z; 4227	Guanabenz Acetate	8 mg	Grey	Tablet	Round, Compressed, Bisected Scored	Ivax Pharmaceuticals
Z; 4232; 0.5	Bumetanide	0.5 mg	Green	Tablet	Flat, Round, Bevel-Edged, Bisected Scored	Ivax Pharmaceuticals
Z; 4233; 1	Bumetanide	1 mg	Yellow	Tablet	Flat, Round, Bevel-Edged, Bisected Scored	Ivax Pharmaceuticals
Z; 4234; 2	Bumetanide	2 mg	Peach	Tablet	Flat, Round, Bevel-Edged, Bisected Scored	Ivax Pharmaceuticals
Z; 4235; 20	Nadolol	20 mg	White	Tablet	Circle	Ivax Pharmaceuticals
Z; 4236; 40	Nadolol	40 mg	White	Tablet	Circle	Ivax Pharmaceuticals
Z; 4237; 80	Nadolol	80 mg	White	Tablet	Circle	Ivax Pharmaceuticals
Z; 4238; 120	Nadolol	120 mg	White	Tablet	Oblong	Ivax Pharmaceuticals
Z; 4239; 160	Nadolol	160 mg	White	Tablet	Oblong	Ivax Pharmaceuticals
Z; 4259	Indapamide	2.5 mg	White	Coated Tablet	Circle	Ivax Pharmaceuticals
Z; 4262; 1.25	Indapamide	1.25 mg	Orange	Tablet	Circle	Ivax Pharmaceuticals
Z; 4288; 20 MG	Nicardipine Hydrochloride	20 mg	Opaque White	Capsule		Ivax Pharmaceuticals
Z; 4289; 30 MG	Nicardipine Hydrochloride	30 mg	Light Blue Opaque	Capsule		Ivax Pharmaceuticals
Z; 4338; 5 MG	Terazosin Hydrochloride	5 mg	Red and White	Capsule		Ivax Pharmaceuticals
Z; 4348; 600	Oxaprozin	600 mg	White	Tablet	Oval	Ivax Pharmaceuticals
Z; 4356; 20	Fluoxetine Hydrochloride	20 mg	Aqua Blue	Capsule	Oblong	Ivax Pharmaceuticals
Z; 4363; 10	Fluoxetine Hydrochloride	10 mg	Aqua Blue	Capsule	Oblong	Ivax Pharmaceuticals
Z; 4804	Oxazepam	10 mg	Blue and White	Capsule		Ivax Pharmaceuticals
Z; 4805	Oxazepam	15 mg	Clear	Capsule		Ivax Pharmaceuticals
Z; 4806	Oxazepam	30 mg	Orange and White	Capsule		Ivax Pharmaceuticals
Z; 5624; 300 MG	Nizatidine	300 mg	Light Brown and White	Capsule		Ivax Pharmaceuticals
Z; LA; BOCK	Zephrex-LA	120 mg; 600 mg	Orange	Timed-Release Tablet	Oval	Sanofi Pharmaceuticals
Z TUSS; MAGNA	Ztuss	300 mg; 5 mg; 30 mg	Red	Tablet	Triangle, Score	Magna Pharmaceuticals
ZANTAC; 150; 427	Zantac 150 Efferdose	150 mg	White to Pale Yellow	Effervescent Tablet	Circle, Flat-Faced, Bevel-Edged	Glaxosmithkline
ZANTAC; 150; GLAXO	Zantac 150 Geldose	150 mg	Beige	Gel/jelly		Glaxosmithkline
ZANTAC; 300; GLAXO	Zantac 300 Geldose	300 mg	Beige	Gel/jelly		Glaxosmithkline
ZAROXOLYN; 2 1/2	Zaroxolyn	2.5 mg	Pink	Sustained-Release Tablet		Medeva Pharmaceuticals

IMPRINT	BRAND/GENERIC NAME	STRENGTH	COLOR	FORM	SHAPE	MANUFACTURER
ZAROXOLYN; 5	Zaroxolyn	5 mg	Blue	Sustained-Release Tablet		Medeva Pharmaceuticals
ZAROXOLYN; 10	Zaroxolyn	10 mg	Yellow	Sustained-Release Tablet		Medeva Pharmaceuticals
ZAROXOLYN; 10;	Zaroxolyn	10 mg	Yellow	Tablet		Fisons Pharmaceuticals
ZBN	Arava	10 mg	White	Coated Tablet	Circle	Aventis Pharmaceuticals
ZBO	Arava	20 mg	Yellow	Coated Tablet	Triangle	Aventis Pharmaceuticals
ZBP	Arava	100 mg	White	Coated Tablet	Circle	Aventis Pharmaceuticals
ZD4522; 5	Crestor	5 mg	Yellow	Tablet	Circle	Astra Zeneca
ZD4522; 10	Crestor	10 mg	Pink	Tablet	Circle	Astra Zeneca
ZD4522; 20	Crestor	20 mg	Pink	Tablet	Circle	Astra Zeneca
ZD4522; 40	Crestor	40 mg	Pink	Tablet	Oval	Astra Zeneca
ZE; 74	Erythromycin Ethylsuccinate	400 mg	Mottled Pink	Tablet	Oval	Abbott Laboratories
ZEE; C; A	Congest-Aid	30 mg	Red	Tablet	Circle	Zee Medical
ZEE; ESP	Extra Strength Pain-Aid	250 mg; 250 mg; 65 mg	White	Coated Tablet		Zee Medical
ZEE; H/F	Histenol-Forte	325 mg; 10 mg; 30 mg	Bright Orange	Tablet		Zee Medical
ZEE; P/A	Pain-Aid	110 mg; 162 mg; 152 mg; 32.4 mg	Orange	Tablet	Circle	Zee Medical
ZEE; P/C	Precomp	226.8 mg; 194.4 mg; 32.4 mg	Yellow	Tablet	Circle	Zee Medical
ZEE; S/N	Sustain	220 mg; 15 mg; 18 mg	White	Tablet	Circle	Zee Medical
ZEE; T/B	Triple Buffered Aspirin	325 mg; 120 mg; 90 mg; 15 mg	White	Tablet	Circle	Zee Medical
ZEE; T/L	Trial Antacid	420 mg		Tablet	Circle	Zee Medical
ZEE; U/A	Un-Aspirin	325 mg	White	Tablet	Circle	Zee Medical
ZEE; X/U	Extra Strength Un-Aspirin	500 mg	White	Tablet	Circle	Zee Medical
ZENECA; 10; 891	Sular	10 mg	Oyster	Sustained-Release Tablet	Circle	Astra Zeneca
ZENECA; 20; 892	Sular	20 mg	Yellow Cream	Sustained-Release Tablet	Circle	Astra Zeneca
ZENECA; 30; 893	Sular	30 mg	Mustard	Sustained-Release Tablet	Circle	Astra Zeneca
ZENECA; 40; 894	Sular	40 mg	Burnt Orange	Sustained-Release Tablet	Circle	Astra Zeneca
ZENECA; ACCOLATE; 10	Accolate	10 mg	White	Coated Tablet	Circle, Biconvex, Mini	Astra Zeneca
ZENECA; ACCOLATE; 20	Accolate	20 mg	White	Coated Tablet	Circle, Biconvex	Astra Zeneca
ZENITH; 50 MG; 2130	Nitrofurantoin Macrocrystals	50 mg	Pink and White	Capsule		Ivax Pharmaceuticals
ZENITH; 100 MG; 2131	Nitrofurantoin Macrocrystals	100 mg	Pink	Capsule		Ivax Pharmaceuticals
ZENITH; 200 MG; 4171	Quinine Sulfate	200 mg	White	Capsule		Ivax Pharmaceuticals
ZENITH; 4266; 200	Acyclovir	200 mg	Opaque White	Capsule		Ivax Pharmaceuticals
ZESTORETIC; 141	Zestoretic	12.5 mg; 10 mg	Peach	Tablet	Circle, Biconvex	Astra Zeneca
ZESTORETIC; 142	Zestoretic	12.5 mg; 20 mg	White	Tablet	Circle, Biconvex	Astra Zeneca
ZESTORETIC; 145	Zestoretic	25 mg; 20 mg	Peach	Tablet	Circle, Biconvex	Astra Zeneca
ZESTRIL; 2 1/2; 135	Zestril	2.5 mg	White	Tablet	Circle, Biconvex	Astra Zeneca
ZESTRIL; 10; 131	Zestril	10 mg	Pink	Tablet	Circle, Biconvex	Astra Zeneca
ZESTRIL; 20; 132	Zestril	20 mg	Red	Tablet	Circle, Biconvex	Astra Zeneca
ZESTRIL; 30; 133	Zestril	30 mg	Red	Tablet	Circle, Biconvex	Astra Zeneca
ZESTRIL; 40; 134	Zestril	40 mg	Yellow	Tablet	Circle, Biconvex	Astra Zeneca
ZESTRIL; 130	Zestril	5 mg	Pink	Tablet	Capsule-Shape, Biconvex, Scored	Astra Zeneca
ZL; 600; ABBOTT LOGO	Zyflo	600 mg	White	Tablet	Oval, Single Bisect	Abbott Laboratories
ZOFRAN; 4	Zofran	4 mg	White	Coated Tablet	Oval	Glaxosmithkline
ZOFRAN; 8	Zofran	8 mg	Yellow	Coated Tablet	Oval	Glaxosmithkline
ZOLOFT; 25 MG	Zoloft	25 mg	Light Green	Coated Tablet	Capsule-Shape, Scored	Pfizer
ZOLOFT; 50 MG	Zoloft	50 mg	Light Blue	Coated Tablet	Capsule-Shape, Scored	Pfizer
ZOLOFT; 100 MG	Zoloft	100 mg	Light Yellow	Coated Tablet	Capsule-Shape, Scored	Pfizer
ZOMIG; 2.5	Zomig	2.5 mg	Yellow	Coated Tablet	Circle, Biconvex, Scored	Astra Zeneca
ZOMIG; 2.5	Zomig	2.5 mg	Yellow	Coated Tablet	Circle, Biconvex, Scored	Medpointe
ZOMIG; 5	Zomig	5 mg	Pink	Coated Tablet	Biconvex	Astra Zeneca
ZOMIG; 5	Zomig	5 mg	Pink	Coated Tablet	Biconvex	Medpointe
ZONEGRAN; 25	Zonegran	25 mg	White and White	Capsule		Elan Pharma
ZONEGRAN; 50	Zonegran	50 mg	White and Gray	Capsule		Elan Pharma
ZONEGRAN; 100	Zonegran	100 mg	White and Red	Capsule		Elan Pharma
ZONEGRAN; 100; ELAN LOGO	Zonegran	100 mg	White and Red	Capsule		Elan Pharma
ZOVIRAX; 800	Zovirax	800 mg	Light Blue	Tablet	Oval	Glaxosmithkline
ZOVIRAX; TRIANGLE	Zovirax	400 mg	White	Tablet	Shield-Shape	Glaxosmithkline
ZYBAN; 150	Zyban	150 mg	Purple	Sustained-Release Tablet	Circle, Biconvex	Glaxosmithkline
ZYBER; 105	Z-Cof LA	30 mg; 650 mg	White	Extended-Release Tablet		Zyber Pharmaceuticals
ZYBER; 650	Aldex	650 mg; 25 mg	White	Extended-Release Tablet	Oval, Scored	Zyber Pharmaceuticals
ZYLOPRIM; 100	Zyloprim	100 mg	White	Tablet	Circle, Flat, Scored with Raised Hexagon	Faro Pharmaceuticals
ZYLOPRIM; 300	Zyloprim	300 mg	Peach	Tablet	Circle, Flat, Scored with a Raised Hexagon	Faro Pharmaceuticals
ZYRTEC; C5	Zyrtec Chewable	5 mg	Purple	Tablet	Circle	Pfizer Laboratories
ZYRTEC; C10	Zyrtec Chewable	10 mg	Purple	Tablet	Circle	Pfizer Laboratories
ZYRTEC-D	Zyrtec-D 12 Hour	5 mg; 120 mg	White	Extended-Release Tablet	Circle, Biconvex, Bilayer	Pfizer Laboratories
ZYRTEC-D	Zyrtec-D 12 Hour	5 mg; 120 mg	White	Extended-Release Tablet	Circle, Biconvex, Bilayer	Ucb Pharma
ZYVOX; 400 MG	Zyvox	400 mg	White	Coated Tablet	Oblong, Compressed	Pharmacia & Upjohn
ZYVOX; 600 MG	Zyvox	600 mg	White	Coated Tablet	Capsule-Shape, Compressed	Pharmacia & Upjohn

Key to Controlled Substances Categories

Products listed with the symbols shown below are subject to the Controlled Substances Act of 1970. These drugs are categorized according to their potential for abuse. The greater the potential, the more severe the limitations on their prescription.

CATEGORY	INTERPRETATION
C-II	**HIGH POTENTIAL FOR ABUSE.** Use may lead to severe physical or psychological dependence. Prescriptions must be written in ink, or typewritten and signed by the practitioner. Verbal prescriptions must be confirmed in writing within 72 hours, and may be given only in a genuine emergency. No renewals are permitted.
C-III	**SOME POTENTIAL FOR ABUSE.** Use may lead to low-to-moderate physical dependence or high psychological dependence. Prescriptions may be oral or written. Up to 5 renewals are permitted within 6 months.
C-IV	**LOW POTENTIAL FOR ABUSE.** Use may lead to limited physical or psychological dependence. Prescriptions may be oral or written. Up to 5 renewals are permitted within 6 months.
C-V	**SUBJECT TO STATE AND LOCAL REGULATION.** Abuse potential is low; a prescription may not be required.

Key to FDA Use-in-Pregnancy Ratings

The U.S. Food and Drug Administration's use-in-pregnancy rating system weighs the degree to which available information has ruled out risk to the fetus against the drug's potential benefit to the patient. The ratings, and their interpretation, are as follows:

CATEGORY	INTERPRETATION
A	**CONTROLLED STUDIES SHOW NO RISK.** Adequate, well-controlled studies in pregnant women have failed to demonstrate a risk to the fetus in any trimester of pregnancy.
B	**NO EVIDENCE OF RISK IN HUMANS.** Adequate, well-controlled studies in pregnant women have not shown increased risk of fetal abnormalities despite adverse findings in animals, or, in the absence of adequate human studies, animal studies show no fetal risk. The chance of fetal harm is remote, but remains a possibility.
C	**RISK CANNOT BE RULED OUT.** Adequate, well-controlled human studies are lacking, and animal studies have shown a risk to the fetus or are lacking as well. There is a chance of fetal harm if the drug is administered during pregnancy; but the potential benefits may outweigh the potential risk.
D	**POSITIVE EVIDENCE OF RISK.** Studies in humans, or investigational or post-marketing data, have demonstrated fetal risk. Nevertheless, potential benefits from the use of the drug may outweigh the potential risk. For example, the drug may be acceptable if needed in a life-threatening situation or serious disease for which safer drugs cannot be used or are ineffective.
X	**CONTRAINDICATED IN PREGNANCY.** Studies in animals or humans, or investigational or post-marketing reports, have demonstrated positive evidence of fetal abnormalities or risk which clearly outweighs any possible benefit to the patient.

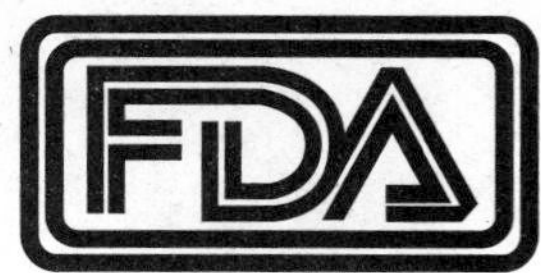

U.S. FOOD AND DRUG ADMINISTRATION

Medical Product Reporting Programs

MedWatch (24-hour service) **800-332-1088**
Reporting of problems with drugs, devices, biologics (except vaccines), medical foods, and dietary supplements.

Vaccine Adverse Event Reporting System (24-hour service) **800-822-7967**
Reporting of vaccine-related problems.

Mandatory Medical Device Reporting **301-827-0360**
Reporting required from user facilities regarding device-related deaths and serious injuries.

Veterinary Adverse Drug Reaction Program **888-332-8387**
Reporting of adverse drug events in animals.

Division of Drug Marketing, Advertising, and Communication (DDMAC) **301-827-2828**
Inquiries from health professionals regarding product promotion.

USP Medication Errors **800-233-7767**
Reporting of medication errors or near-errors to help avoid future problems through improvement in product names and packaging.

Information for Health Professionals

Center for Drug Evaluation and Research Drug Information Hotline **301-827-4573**
Information on human drugs including hormones.

Center for Biologics Office of Communications **301-827-2000**
Information on biological products including vaccines and blood.

Center for Devices and Radiological Health **301-443-4190**
Automated request for information on medical devices and radiation-emitting products.

Emergency Operations **301-443-1240**
Emergencies involving FDA-regulated products, tampering reports, and emergency Investigational New Drug requests.

Office of Orphan Products Development **301-827-3666**
Information on products for rare diseases.

General Information

General Consumer Inquiries **888-463-6332**
Consumer information on regulated products/issues.

Freedom of Information **301-827-6500**
Requests for publicly available FDA documents.

Office of Public Affairs **301-827-6250**
Interviews/press inquiries on FDA activities.

Center for Food Safety and Applied Nutrition **888-723-3366**
Information on food safety, seafood, dietary supplements, women's nutrition, and cosmetics.

Consumer Information Service, Center for Devices and Radiological Health **301-443-4190**
Information on medical devices, mammography facilities, and radiation-emitting products.

POISON CONTROL CENTERS

The American Association of Poison Control Centers (AAPCC) uses a single, nationwide emergency number to automatically link callers with their regional poison center. This toll-free number, **800-222-1222**, also works for **teletype lines (TTY)** for the hearing-impaired and **telecommunication devices (TTD)** for individuals who are deaf. However, a few local poison centers and the ASPCA/Animal Poison Control Center are not part of this nationwide system and continue to use separate numbers.

Most of the centers listed below are certified by the AAPCC. **Certified centers are marked by an asterisk after the name.** Each has to meet certain criteria. It must, for example, serve a large geographic area; it must be open 24 hours a day and provide direct-dial or toll-free access; it must be supervised by a medical director; and it must have registered pharmacists or nurses available to answer questions from the public.

Within each state, centers are listed alphabetically by city. Some state poison centers also list their original emergency numbers (including TTY/TDD) that only work within that state. For these listings, callers may use either the state number or the nationwide 800 number.

ALABAMA

BIRMINGHAM

Regional Poison Control Center, The Children's Hospital of Alabama (*)

1600 7th Ave. South
Birmingham, AL 35233-1711
Business: 205-939-9201
Emergency: 800-222-1222
800-292-6678 (AL)
www.chsys.org

TUSCALOOSA

Alabama Poison Center (*)

2503 Phoenix Dr.
Tuscaloosa, AL 35405
Business: 205-345-0600
Emergency: 800-222-1222
800-462-0800 (AL)
www.alapoisoncenter.org

ALASKA

JUNEAU

Alaska Poison Control System

Section of Community Health and EMS
410 Willoughby Ave., Room 109
Box 110616
Juneau, AK 99811-0616
Business: 907-465-3027
Emergency: 800-222-1222
www.chems.alaska.gov

(PORTLAND, OR)

**Oregon Poison Center (*)
Oregon Health Sciences University**

3181 SW Sam Jackson Park Rd.
CB550
Portland, OR 97239
Business: 503-494-8600
Emergency: 800-222-1222
www.oregonpoison.com

ARIZONA

PHOENIX

**Banner Poison Control Center (*)
Banner Good Samaritan Medical Center**

901 E. Willetta St.
Room 2701
Phoenix, AZ 85006
Business: 602-495-6360
Emergency: 800-222-1222
800-362-0101 (AZ)
602-253-3334 (AZ)
www.bannerpoisoncontrol.com

TUCSON

**Arizona Poison and Drug Information Center (*)
Arizona Health Sciences Center**

1501 N. Campbell Ave.
Room 1156
Tucson, AZ 85724
Business: 520-626-7899
Emergency: 800-222-1222

ARKANSAS

LITTLE ROCK

**Arkansas Poison and Drug Information Center
College of Pharmacy - UAMS**

4301 West Markham St.
Mail Slot 522-2
Little Rock, AR 72205-7122
Business: 501-686-5540
Emergency: 800-222-1222
800-376-4766 (AR)
TDD/TTY: 800-641-3805

ASPCA/ANIMAL POISON CONTROL CENTER

1717 South Philo Rd.
Suite 36
Urbana, IL 61802
Business: 217-337-5030
Emergency: 888-426-4435
800-548-2423
www.napcc.aspca.org

CALIFORNIA

FRESNO/MADERA

**California Poison Control System-Fresno/Madera Div.(*)
Children's Hospital of Central California**

9300 Valley Children's Place
MB 15
Madera, CA 93638-8762
Business: 559-622-2300
Emergency: 800-222-1222
800-876-4766 (CA)
TDD/TTY: 800-972-3323
www.calpoison.org

SACRAMENTO

**California Poison Control System-Sacramento Div.(*)
UC Davis Medical Center**

Room HSF 1024
2315 Stockton Blvd.
Sacramento, CA 95817
Business: 916-227-1400
Emergency: 800-222-1222
800-876-4766 (CA)
TDD/TTY: 800-972-3323
www.calpoison.org

SAN DIEGO

**California Poison Control System-San Diego Div. (*)
UC San Diego Medical Center**

200 West Arbor Dr.
San Diego, CA 92103-8925
Business: 858-715-6300
Emergency: 800-222-1222
800-876-4766 (CA)
TDD/TTY: 800-972-3323
www.calpoison.org

SAN FRANCISCO

**California Poison Control System-San Francisco Div.(*)
San Francisco General Hospital
University of California San Francisco**

Box 1369
San Francisco, CA 94143-1369
Business: 415-502-6000
Emergency: 800-222-1222
800-876-4766 (CA)
TDD/TTY: 800-972-3323
www.calpoison.org

COLORADO

DENVER

Rocky Mountain Poison and Drug Center (*)

777 Bannock St.
Mail Code 0180
Denver CO 80204-4507
Business: 303-739-1100
Emergency: 800-222-1222
TDD/TTY: 303-739-1127 (CO)
www.RMPDC.org

CONNECTICUT

FARMINGTON

Connecticut Regional Poison Control Center (*)
University of Connecticut Health Center

263 Farmington Ave.
Farmington, CT 06030-5365
Business: 860-679-4540
Emergency: 800-222-1222
TDD/TTY: 866-218-5372
http://poisoncontrol.uchc.edu

DELAWARE

(PHILADELPHIA, PA)

The Poison Control Center (*)
Children's Hospital of Philadelphia

34th St. & Civic Center Blvd.
Philadelphia, PA 19104-4303
Business: 215-590-2003
Emergency: 800-222-1222
800-722-7112 (DE)
TDD/TTY: 215-590-8789
www.poisoncontrol.chop.edu

DISTRICT OF COLUMBIA

WASHINGTON, DC

National Capital Poison Center (*)

3201 New Mexico Ave., NW
Suite 310
Washington, DC 20016
Business: 202-362-3867
Emergency: 800-222-1222
TDD/TTY: 202-362-8563
www.poison.org

FLORIDA

JACKSONVILLE

Florida Poison Information Center-Jacksonville (*)
SHANDS Hospital

655 West 8th St.
Jacksonville, FL 32209
Business: 904-244-4465
Emergency: 800-222-1222
http://fpicjax.org

MIAMI

Florida Poison Information Center-Miami (*)
University of Miami–Department of Pediatrics

P.O. Box 016960 (R-131)
Miami, FL 33101
Business: 305-585-5250
Emergency: 800-222-1222
www.miami.edu/poison-center

TAMPA

Florida Poison Information Center-Tampa (*)
Tampa General Hospital

P.O. Box 1289
Tampa, FL 33601-1289
Business: 813-844-7044
Emergency: 800-222-1222
www.poisoncentertampa.org

GEORGIA

ATLANTA

Georgia Poison Center (*)
Hughes Spalding Children's Hospital, Grady Health System

80 Jesse Hill Jr. Dr., SE
P.O. Box 26066
Atlanta, GA 30303-3050
Business: 404-616-9237
Emergency: 800-222-1222
404-616-9000 (Atlanta)
TDD: 404-616-9287
www.georgiapoisoncenter.org

HAWAII

(DENVER, CO)

Rocky Mountain Poison and Drug Center (*)

777 Bannock St.
Mail Code 0180
Denver CO 80204-4507
Business: 303-739-1100
Emergency: 800-222-1222
www.RMPDC.org

IDAHO

(DENVER, CO)

Rocky Mountain Poison and Drug Center (*)

777 Bannock St.
Mail Code 0180
Denver CO 80204-4507
Business: 303-739-1100
Emergency: 800-222-1222
www.RMPDC.org

ILLINOIS

CHICAGO

Illinois Poison Center (*)

222 South Riverside Plaza
Suite 1900
Chicago, IL 60606
Business: 312-906-6136
Emergency: 800-222-1222
TDD/TTY: 312-906-6185
www.illinoispoisoncenter.org

INDIANA

INDIANAPOLIS

Indiana Poison Control Center (*)
Clarian Health Partners Methodist Hospital

I-65 at 21st St.
Indianapolis, IN 46206-1367
Business: 317-962-2335
Emergency: 800-222-1222
800-382-9097
317-962-2323 (Indianapolis)
TTY: 317-962-2336
www.clarian.org/clinical/poisoncontrol

IOWA

SIOUX CITY

Iowa Statewide Poison Control Center
Iowa Health System and the University of Iowa Hospitals and Clinics

2910 Hamilton Blvd., Suite 101
Sioux City, IA 51104
Business: 712-279-3710
Emergency: 800-222-1222
712-277-2222 (IA)
www.iowapoison.org

KANSAS

KANSAS CITY

Mid-America Poison Control Center
University of Kansas Medical Center

3901 Rainbow Blvd.
Room B-400
Kansas City, KS 66160-7231
Business 913-588-6638
Emergency: 800-222-1222
800-332-6633 (KS)
TDD: 913-588-6639
www.kumc.edu/poison

KENTUCKY

LOUISVILLE

Kentucky Regional Poison Center (*)

PO Box 35070
Louisville, KY 40232-5070
Business: 502-629-7264
Emergency: 800-222-1222
502-589-8222 (Louisville)
www.krpc.com

LOUISIANA

MONROE

Louisiana Drug and Poison Information Center (*)
University of Louisiana at Monroe

700 University Ave.
Monroe, LA 71209-6430
Business: 318-342-3648
Emergency: 800-222-1222
www.lapcc.org

MAINE

PORTLAND

Northern New England Poison Center

Maine Medical Center
22 Bramhall St.
Portland, ME 04102
Business: 207-842-7220
Emergency: 800-222-1222
207-871-2879 (ME)
TDD/TTY: 877-299-4447 (ME)
207-871-2879 (ME)

MARYLAND

BALTIMORE

Maryland Poison Center (*)
University of Maryland at Baltimore
School of Pharmacy

20 North Pine St., PH 772
Baltimore, MD 21201
Business: 410-706-7604
Emergency: 800-222-1222
TDD: 410-706-1858
www.mdpoison.com

(WASHINGTON, DC)

National Capital Poison Center (*)

3201 New Mexico Ave., NW
Suite 310
Washington DC 20016
Business: 202-362-3867
Emergency: 800-222-1222
TDD/TTY: 202-362-8563 (MD)
www.poison.org

MASSACHUSETTS

BOSTON

Regional Center for Poison Control and Prevention (*)
(Serving Massachusetts and Rhode Island)

300 Longwood Ave.
Boston, MA 02115
Business: 617-355-6609
Emergency: 800-222-1222
TDD/TTY: 888-244-5313
www.maripoisoncenter.com

MICHIGAN

DETROIT

Regional Poison Control Center (*) Children's Hospital of Michigan

4160 John R. Harper
Professional Office Bldg.
Suite 616
Detroit, MI 48201
Business: 313-745-5335
Emergency: 800-222-1222
TDD/TTY: 800-356-3232
www.mitoxic.org/pcc

GRAND RAPIDS

DeVos Children's Hospital Regional Poison Center (*)

100 Michigan St., NE
Grand Rapids, MI 49503
Business: 616-391-3690
Emergency: 800-222-1222
http://poisoncenter.devoschildrens.org

MINNESOTA

MINNEAPOLIS

Minnesota Poison Control System (*) Hennepin County Medical Center

701 Park Ave.
Mail Code 820
Minneapolis, MN 55415
Business: 612-873-6000
Emergency: 800-222-1222
TTY: 612-904-4691
www.mnpoison.org

MISSISSIPPI

JACKSON

Mississippi Regional Poison Control Center, University of Mississippi Medical Center

2500 North State St.
Jackson, MS 39216
Business: 601-984-1675
Emergency: 800-222-1222

MISSOURI

ST. LOUIS

Missouri Regional Poison Center (*) Cardinal Glennon Children's Hospital

7980 Clayton Rd.
Suite 200
St. Louis, MO 63117
Business: 314-772-5200
Emergency: 800-222-1222
TDD/TTY: 314-612-5705
www.cardinalglennon.com

MONTANA

(DENVER, CO)

Rocky Mountain Poison and Drug Center (*)

777 Bannock St.
Mail Code 0180
Denver CO 80204-4507
Business: 303-739-1100
Emergency: 800-222-1222
TDD/TTY: 303-739-1127
www.RMPDC.org

NEBRASKA

OMAHA

The Poison Center (*) Children's Hospital

8200 Dodge St.
Omaha, NE 68114
Business: 402-955-5555
Emergency: 800-222-1222
www.poison-center.com

NEVADA

(DENVER, CO)

Rocky Mountain Poison and Drug Center (*)

777 Bannock St.
Mail Code 0180
Denver CO 80204-4507
Business: 303-739-1100
Emergency: 800-222-1222
www.RMPDC.org

(PORTLAND, OR)

Oregon Poison Center (*) Oregon Health Sciences University

3181 SW Sam Jackson Park Rd.
Portland, OR 97201
Business: 503-494-8600
Emergency: 800-222-1222
www.oregonpoison.com

NEW HAMPSHIRE

(PORTLAND, ME)

Northern New England Poison Center

Maine Medical Center
22 Bramhall St.
Portland, ME 04102
Business: 207-842-7220
Emergency: 800-222-1222

NEW JERSEY

NEWARK

New Jersey Poison Information and Education System (*) UMDNJ

65 Bergen St.
Newark, NJ 07101
Business: 973-972-9280
Emergency: 800-222-1222
TDD/TTY: 973-926-8008
www.njpies.org

NEW MEXICO

ALBUQUERQUE

New Mexico Poison and Drug Information Center (*)

MSC09-5080
1 University of New Mexico
Albuquerque, NM 87131-0001
Business: 505-272-4261
Emergency: 800-222-1222
http://HSC.UNM.edu/pharmacy/poison

NEW YORK

BUFFALO

Western New York Regional Poison Control Center (*) Children's Hospital of Buffalo

219 Bryant St.
Buffalo, NY 14222
Business: 716-878-7654
Emergency: 800-222-1222
www.fingerlakespoison.org

MINEOLA

Long Island Regional Poison and Drug Information Center (*) Winthrop University Hospital

259 First St.
Mineola, NY 11501
Business: 516-663-2650
Emergency: 800-222-1222
TDD: 516-747-3323 (Nassau)
516-924-8811 (Suffolk)
www.lirpdic.org

NEW YORK CITY

New York City Poison Control Center (*) NYC Dept. of Health

455 First Ave., Room 123
New York, NY 10016
Business: 212-447-8152
Emergency: 800-222-1222
(English) 212-340-4494
212-POISONS
(212-764-7667)

Emergency: 212-VENENOS
(Spanish) (212-836-3667)
TDD: 212-689-9014

ROCHESTER

Finger Lakes Regional Poison and Drug Information Center (*) University of Rochester Medical Center

601 Elmwood Ave.
Box 321
Rochester, NY 14642
Business: 585-273-4155
Emergency: 800-222-1222
TTY: 585-273-3854

SYRACUSE

Central New York Poison Center (*) SUNY Upstate Medical University

750 East Adams St.
Syracuse, NY 13210
Business: 315-464-7078
Emergency: 800-222-1222
www.cnypoison.org

NORTH CAROLINA

CHARLOTTE

Carolinas Poison Center (*) Carolinas Medical Center

PO Box 32861
Charlotte, NC 28232
Business: 704-395-3795
Emergency: 800-222-1222
TDD: 800-735-8262
TTY: 800-735-2962
www.ncpoisoncenter.org

NORTH DAKOTA

(MINNEAPOLIS, MN)

Minnesota Poison Control System (*) Hennepin County Medical Center

701 Park Ave.
Mail Code 820
Minneapolis, MN 55415
Business: 612-873-3144
Emergency: 800-222-1222
www.ndpoison.org

OHIO

CINCINNATI

Cincinnati Drug and Poison Information Center (*)
Regional Poison Control System

3333 Burnet Ave.
Vernon Place, 3rd Floor
Cincinnati, OH 45229
Business: 513-636-5111
Emergency: 800-222-1222
TDD/TTY: 800-253-7955
www.cincinnatichildrens.org/dpic

CLEVELAND

Greater Cleveland Poison Control Center

11100 Euclid Ave.
MP 6007
Cleveland, OH 44106-6007
Business: 216-844-1573
Emergency: 800-222-1222
216-231-4455 (OH)

COLUMBUS

Central Ohio Poison Center (*)

700 Children's Dr.
Room L032
Columbus, OH 43205-2696
Business: 614-722-2635
Emergency: 800-222-1222
614-228-1323
937-222-2227
(Dayton region)
TTY: 614-228-2272
www.bepoisonsmart.com

OKLAHOMA

OKLAHOMA CITY

Oklahoma Poison Control Center (*)
Children's Hospital at OU Medical Center

940 Northeast 13th St.
Room 3510
Oklahoma City, OK 73104
Business: 405-271-5062
Emergency: 800-222-1222
www.oklahomapoison.org

OREGON

PORTLAND

Oregon Poison Center (*)
Oregon Health Sciences University

3181 S.W. Sam Jackson Park Rd., CB550
Portland, OR 97239
Business: 503-494-8600
Emergency: 800-222-1222
www.oregonpoison.com

PENNSYLVANIA

PHILADELPHIA

The Poison Control Center (*)
Children's Hospital of Philadelphia

34th Street & Civic Center Blvd.
Philadelphia, PA 19104-4399
Business: 215-590-2003
Emergency: 800-222-1222
215-386-2100 (PA)
TDD/TTY: 215-590-8789
www.poisoncontrol.chop.edu

PITTSBURGH

Pittsburgh Poison Center (*)
Children's Hospital of Pittsburgh

3705 Fifth Ave.
Pittsburgh, PA 15213
Business: 412-390-3300
Emergency: 800-222-1222
412-681-6669
www.chp.edu/clinical/03a_poison.php

PUERTO RICO

SANTURCE

San Jorge Children's Hospital Poison Center

258 San Jorge St.
Santurce, PR 00912
Business: 787-726-5660
Emergency: 800-222-1222
TTY: 787-641-1934
www.poisoncenter.net

RHODE ISLAND

(BOSTON, MA)

Regional Center for Poison Control and Prevention (*)
(Serving Massachusetts and Rhode Island)

300 Longwood Ave.
Boston, MA 02115
Business: 617-355-6609
Emergency: 800-222-1222
TDD/TTY: 888-244-5313
www.maripoisoncenter.com

SOUTH CAROLINA

COLUMBIA

Palmetto Poison Center (*)
College of Pharmacy
University of South Carolina

Columbia, SC 29208
Business: 803-777-7909
Drug Info: 800-777-7804
Emergency: 800-222-1222
803-777-1117 (SC)
www.pharm.sc.edu/PPS/pps.htm

SOUTH DAKOTA

(MINNEAPOLIS, MN)

Hennepin Regional Poison Center (*) Hennepin County Medical Center

701 Park Ave.
Minneapolis, MN 55415
Business: 612-873-6000
Emergency: 800-222-1222
TTY: 612-904-4691
www.mnpoison.org

SIOUX FALLS

Provides education only—Does not manage exposure cases.

Sioux Valley Poison Control Center (*)

1305 W. 18th St.
Box 5039
Sioux Falls, SD 57117-5039
Business: 605-333-6638
www.sdpoison.org

TENNESSEE

NASHVILLE

Tennessee Poison Center (*)

1161 21st Ave. South
501 Oxford House
Nashville, TN 37232-4632
Business: 615-936-0760
Emergency: 800-222-1222
www.poisonlifeline.org

TEXAS

AMARILLO

Texas Panhandle Poison Center (*)
Northwest Texas Hospital

1501 S. Coulter Dr.
Amarillo, TX 79106
Business: 806-354-1630
Emergency: 800-222-1222
www.poisoncontrol.org

DALLAS

North Texas Poison Center (*)
Texas Poison Center Network
Parkland Health and Hospital System

5201 Harry Hines Blvd.
Dallas, TX 75235
Business: 214-589-0911
Emergency: 800-222-1222
www.poisoncontrol.org

EL PASO

West Texas Regional Poison Center (*)
Thomason Hospital

4815 Alameda Ave.
El Paso, TX 79905
Business 915-534-3800
Emergency: 800-222-1222
www.poisoncontrol.org

GALVESTON

Southeast Texas Poison Center (*)
The University of Texas Medical Branch

3.112 Trauma Bldg.
301 University Ave.
Galveston, TX 77555-1175
Business: 409-766-4403
Emergency: 800-222-1222
www.poisoncontrol.org

SAN ANTONIO

South Texas Poison Center (*)
The University of Texas Health Science Center–San Antonio

7703 Floyd Curl Dr., MC 7849
San Antonio, TX 78229-3900
Business: 210-567-5762
Emergency: 800-222-1222
www.poisoncontrol.org

TEMPLE

Central Texas Poison Center (*)
Scott & White Memorial Hospital

2401 South 31st St.
Temple, TX 76508
Business: 254-724-7401
Emergency: 800-222-1222
www.poisoncontrol.org

UTAH

SALT LAKE CITY

Utah Poison Control Center (*)

585 Komas Dr.
Suite 200
Salt Lake City, UT 84108
Business: 801-581-7504
Emergency: 800-222-1222
801-587-0600 (UT)
http://uuhsc.utah.edu/poison

VERMONT

(PORTLAND, ME)

Northern New England Poison Center

Maine Medical Center
22 Bramhall St.
Portland, ME 04102
Business: 207-842-7220
Emergency: 800-222-1222

VIRGINIA

CHARLOTTESVILLE

Blue Ridge Poison Center (*)
University of Virginia Health System

PO Box 800774
Charlottesville, VA 22908-0774
Business: 434-924-0347
Emergency: 800-222-1222
800-451-1428 (VA)
www.healthsystem.virginia.edu.brpc

RICHMOND

Virginia Poison Center (*)
Virginia Commonwealth University

P.O. Box 980522
Richmond, VA 23298-0522
Business: 804-828-4780
Emergency: 800-222-1222
804-828-9123
TDD/TTY: 804-828-9123

WASHINGTON

SEATTLE

Washington Poison Center (*)

155 NE 100th St.
Suite 400
Seattle, WA 98125-8011
Business: 206-517-2351
Emergency: 800-222-1222
206-526-2121 (WA)
TDD: 800-572-0638 (WA)
206-517-2394 (Seattle)
www.wapc.org

WEST VIRGINIA

CHARLESTON

West Virginia Poison Center (*)

3110 MacCorkle Ave. SE
Charleston, WV 25304
Business: 304-347-1212
Emergency: 800-222-1222
www.wvpoisoncontrol.org

WISCONSIN

MILWAUKEE

Children's Hospital of Wisconsin Statewide Poison Center

9000 W. Wisconsin Ave.
P.O. Box 1997, Mail Station 677A
Milwaukee, WI 53226
Business: 414-266-2000
Emergency: 800-222-1222
TDD/TTY: 414-964-3497
www.chw.org

WYOMING

(OMAHA, NE)

The Poison Center (*)
Children's Hospital

8200 Dodge St.
Omaha, NE 68114
Business: 402-955-5555
Emergency: 800-222-1222
www.poison-center.com

DRUG INFORMATION CENTERS

ALABAMA

BIRMINGHAM

Drug Information Service
University of Alabama
UAB Hospital Pharmacy
Drug Information-JT1720
619 S. 19th St.
Birmingham, AL 35249-6860
Mon.-Fri. 8 AM-5 PM
205-934-2162
www.health.uab.edu/pharmacy

Global Drug
Information Service
Samford University
McWhorter School
of Pharmacy
800 Lakeshore Dr.
Birmingham, AL 35229-7027
Mon.-Fri. 8 AM-4:30 PM
205-726-2659
www.samford.edu/schools/pharmacy/dic/index.html

HUNTSVILLE

Huntsville Hospital Drug Information Center
101 Sivley Rd.
Huntsville, AL 35801
Mon.-Fri. 7 AM-3:30 PM
256-265-8288

ARIZONA

TUCSON

Arizona Poison and Drug Information Center
Arizona Health Sciences Center
University Medical Center
1501 N. Campbell Ave.
Room 1156
Tucson, AZ 85724
7 days/week, 24 hours
520-626-6016
800-222-1222 (**Emergency**)
www.pharmacy.arizona.edu

ARKANSAS

LITTLE ROCK

Arkansas Poison and Drug Information Center
4301 W. Markham St.
Slot 522-2
Little Rock, AR 72205
Mon.-Fri. 8:30 AM-5 PM
501-686-5072
(Little Rock area only - **for healthcare professionals only**)
800-228-1233
(AR only - **for healthcare professionals only**)

CALIFORNIA

LOS ANGELES

Los Angeles Regional
Drug Information Center
LAC & USC Medical Center
1200 N. State St.
Trailer 25
Los Angeles, CA 90033
Mon.-Fri. 8:30 AM-4 PM
Closed 12 PM to 1 PM
323-226-7741

SAN DIEGO

Drug Information Service
University of California
San Diego Medical Center
200 West Arbor Dr.
MC 8925
San Diego, CA 92103-8925
Mon.-Fri. 9 AM-5 PM
900-226-7536
(**for healthcare professionals only**)

SAN FRANCISCO

Drug Information Analysis Service
University of California, San Francisco
Box 1262
521 Parnassus Ave.
Room C152
San Francisco, CA 94143-0622
Mon.-Fri. 8:30 AM-4:30 PM
415-502-9540
(**for healthcare professionals only**)

STANFORD

Drug Information Center
University of California
Stanford Hospital and Clinics
300 Pasteur Dr.
Room H-0301
Stanford, CA 94305
Mon.-Fri. 8 AM-4 PM
650-723-6422

COLORADO

DENVER

Rocky Mountain Poison and Drug Center
990 Bannock St.
(Physical address)
777 Bannock St.
(Mailing address)
Denver, CO 80264
303-739-1123
800-222-1222 (**Emergency**)
www.rmpdc.org

Drug Information Center
University of Colorado
Health Science Center
School of Pharmacy
4200 E. 9th Ave., Box C239
Denver, CO 80262
Mon.-Fri. 8 AM-5 PM
303-315-8489

CONNECTICUT

FARMINGTON

Drug Information Service
University of Connecticut Health Center
263 Farmington Ave.
Farmington, CT 06030
Mon.-Fri. 7:30 AM-4 PM
860-679-2783

HARTFORD

Drug Information Center Hartford Hospital
P.O. Box 5037
80 Seymour St.
Hartford, CT 06102
Mon.-Fri. 8:30 AM-5 PM
860-545-2221
860-545-2961(After 5 PM)
www.hartfordhospital.org

NEW HAVEN

Drug Information Center
Yale-New Haven Hospital
20 York St.
New Haven, CT 06540-3202
Mon.-Fri. 8:30 AM-5 PM
203-688-2248
www.ynhh.org

DISTRICT OF COLUMBIA

Drug Information Service
Howard University Hospital
Room BB06
2041 Georgia Ave. NW
Washington, DC 20060
Mon.-Fri. 8:30 AM-4:30 PM
202-865-1325
800-222-1222 (**Emergency**)

FLORIDA

FT. LAUDERDALE

Nova Southeastern University
College of Pharmacy
Drug Information Center
3200 S. University Dr.
Ft. Lauderdale, FL 33328
Mon.-Fri. 9 AM-5 PM
954-262-3103
http://pharmacy.nova.edu

GAINESVILLE

Drug Information &
Pharmacy Resource Center
Shands Hospital at
University of Florida
P.O. Box 100316
Gainesville, FL 32610-0316
Mon.-Fri. 9 AM-5 PM
352-265-0408
(**for healthcare professionals only**)
http://shands.org/professional/drugs

JACKSONVILLE

Drug Information Service
Shands Jacksonville
655 W. 8th St.
Jacksonville, FL 32209
Mon.-Fri. 9:30 AM-4 PM
904-244-4185
(**for healthcare professionals only**)
904-244-4700
(**for consumers, Mon.-Fri. 9 AM-4 PM**)

ORLANDO

Orlando Regional Drug Information Service
Orlando Regional Healthcare System
1414 Kuhl Ave., MP 192
Orlando, FL 32806
Mon.-Fri. 8 AM-4 PM
321-841-8717

TALLAHASSEE

Drug Information Education Center
Florida Agricultural and Mechanical University
College of Pharmacy and Pharmaceutical Sciences
Tallahassee, FL 32307
Mon.-Fri. 9 AM-5 PM
850-488-5239

WEST PALM BEACH

Drug Information Center
Nova Southeastern University, West Palm Beach
3970 RCA Blvd., Suite 7006A
Palm Beach Gardens, FL 33410
Mon.-Fri. 9 AM-5 PM
561-622-0658
(**for healthcare professionals only**)

GEORGIA

ATLANTA

Emory University Hospital
Dept. of Pharmaceutical Services-Drug Information
1364 Clifton Rd. NE
Atlanta, GA 30322
Mon.-Fri. 8:30 AM-5 PM
404-712-7150
(**for healthcare professionals only**)

Drug Information Service
Northside Hospital
1000 Johnson Ferry Rd. NE
Atlanta, GA 30342
Mon.-Fri. 9 AM-4 PM
404-851-8676 (GA only)

AUGUSTA
Drug Information Center
Medical College of Georgia
Hospital and Clinic
BI2101
1120 15th St.
Augusta, GA 30912
Mon.-Fri. 8:30 AM-5 PM
706-721-2887

COLUMBUS
Columbus Regional Drug
Information Center
710 Center St.
Columbus, GA 31902
Mon.-Fri. 8 AM-5 PM
706-571-1934
(for healthcare professionals only)

IDAHO

POCATELLO
Drug Information Center
Idaho State University
School of Pharmacy
970 S. 5th St.
Campus Box 8092
Pocatello, ID 83209
Mon.-Thur. 8:30 AM-5 PM
Fri. 8:30 AM-2:30 PM
Closed 12 PM to 1 PM
208-282-4689
800-334-7139 (ID only)
http://pharmacy.isu.edu

ILLINOIS

CHICAGO
Drug Information Center
Northwestern Memorial Hospital
Feinberg Pavilion, LC 700
251 E. Huron St.
Chicago, IL 60611
Mon.-Fri. 8:30 AM-5 PM
312-926-7573

Drug Information Services
University of Chicago Hospitals
5841 S. Maryland Ave.
MC 0010
Chicago, IL 60637-1470
Mon.-Fri. 9 AM-5 PM
773-702-1388

Drug Information Center
University of Illinois at Chicago
833 S. Wood St.
MC 886
Chicago, IL 60612-7231
Mon.-Fri. 8 AM-4 PM
312-996-3681
(for healthcare professionals only)
312-996-3682
(for consumers, Mon.-Fri. 9 AM-12 PM)
www.uic.edu/pharmacy/services/di/index.html

HARVEY
Drug Information Center
Ingalls Memorial Hospital
1 Ingalls Dr.
Harvey, IL 60426
Mon.-Fri. 8 AM-4:30 PM
708-333-2300

HINES
Drug Information Service
Hines Veterans Administration Hospital
2100 S. 5th Ave.
Pharmacy Services
MC119
P.O. Box 5000
Hines, IL 60141-5000
Mon.-Fri. 8 AM-4:30 PM
708-202-8387,
ext. 23780

PARK RIDGE
Drug Information Center
Advocate Lutheran General Hospital
1775 Dempster St.
Park Ridge, IL 60068
Mon.-Fri. 7:30 AM-4 PM
847-723-8128
(for healthcare professionals only)

INDIANA

INDIANAPOLIS
Drug Information Center
St. Vincent Hospital
and Health Services
2001 W. 86th St.
Indianapolis, IN 46260
Mon.-Fri. 8 AM-4 PM
317-338-3200
(for healthcare professionals only)

Drug Information Service
Clarian Health Partners
Pharmacy Department I-65
at 21st St.
Room CG04
Indianapolis, IN 46202
Mon.-Fri. 8 AM-4:30 PM
317-962-1750

MUNCIE
Drug Information Center
Ball Memorial Hospital
2401 University Ave.
Muncie, IN 47303
Mon.-Fri. 8 AM-4:30 PM
765-747-3035

IOWA

DES MOINES
Regional Drug
Information Center
Mercy Medical Center-Des Moines
1111 Sixth Ave.
Des Moines, IA 50314
Mon.-Fri. 8 AM-4:30 PM
(regional service; in-house service answered 7 days/week, 24 hours)
515-247-3286

IOWA CITY
Drug Information Center
University of Iowa
Hospitals and Clinics
200 Hawkins Dr.
Iowa City, IA 52242
Mon.-Fri. 8 AM-4:30 PM
319-356-2600
(for healthcare professionals only)

KANSAS

KANSAS CITY
Drug Information Center
University of Kansas
Medical Center
3901 Rainbow Blvd.
Kansas City, KS 66160
Mon.-Fri. 8:30 AM-4:30 PM
913-588-2328
(for healthcare professionals only)

KENTUCKY

LEXINGTON
University of Kentucky
Drug Information Center
Chandler Medical Center
800 Rose St., C-113
Lexington, KY 40536-0293
Mon.-Fri. 8 AM-5 PM
859-323-5320 or
859-323-5476

LOUISIANA

MONROE
Louisiana Drug and Poison
Information Center
University of Louisiana at Monroe
College of Pharmacy
Sugar Hall
Monroe, LA 71209-6430
Mon.-Fri. 8 AM-4:30 PM
318-342-1710

NEW ORLEANS
Xavier University Drug
Information Center
Tulane University
Hospital and Clinic
1440 Canal St.
Suite 808
New Orleans, LA 70112
Mon.-Fri. 9 AM-5 PM
504-588-5670

MARYLAND

ANDREWS AFB
Drug Information Services
89 MDTS/SGQP
1050 W. Perimeter Rd.
Suite D1-119
Andrews AFB, MD 20762-6660
Mon.-Fri. 7:30 AM-5 PM
240-857-4565

ANNAPOLIS
The Anne Arundel
Medical Center
Dept. of Pharmacy
2001 Medical Pkwy.
Annapolis, MD 21401
7 days/week, 24 hours
443-481-4155
www.aahs.org

BALTIMORE
Drug Information Service
Johns Hopkins Hospital
600 N. Wolfe St.
Carnegie 180
Baltimore, MD 21287-6180
Mon.-Fri. 8:30 AM-5 PM
410-955-6348

Drug Information Service
University of Maryland
School of Pharmacy Pharmacy Hall
Room 760
20 North Pine St.
Baltimore, MD 21201
Mon.-Fri. 8:30 AM-5 PM
410-706-7568
(consumers only)
410-706-0898
(for healthcare professionals only)
www.pharmacy.umaryland.edu/umdi

BETHESDA
Drug Information Service National Institutes of Health
Building 10, Room 1S-259
10 Center Dr. (MSC1196)
Bethesda, MD 20892-1196
Mon.-Fri. 8:30 AM-5 PM
301-496-2407
www.cc.nih.gov/phar

EASTON
Drug Information
Pharmacy Dept.
Memorial Hospital
219 S. Washington St.
Easton, MD 21601
7 days/week, 7 AM-5:30 PM
410-822-1000, ext. 5645

MASSACHUSETTS

BOSTON
Drug Information Services
Brigham and Women's Hospital
75 Francis St.
Boston, MA 02115
Mon.-Fri. 7 AM-3 PM
617-732-7166

WORCESTER
Drug Information Pharmacy
UMass Memorial
Medical Center
Healthcare Hospital
55 Lake Ave. North
Worcester, MA 01655
Mon.-Fri. 8:30 AM-5 PM
508-856-3456
508-856-2775 (24-hour)

MICHIGAN

ANN ARBOR

Drug Information Service Dept. of Pharmacy Services
University of Michigan Health System
1500 East Medical Center Dr.
UH B2D301
Box 0008
Ann Arbor, MI 48109-0008
Mon.-Fri. 8 AM-5 PM
734-936-8200

DETROIT

Drug Information Center
Department of Pharmacy Services
Detroit Receiving Hospital and University Health Center
4201 St. Antoine Blvd.
Detroit, MI 48201
Mon.-Fri. 9 AM-5 PM
313-745-4556
www.dmcpharmacy.org

LANSING

Drug Information Services
Sparrow Hospital
1215 East Michigan Ave.
Lansing, MI 48912
7 days/week, 24 hours
517-364-2444

PONTIAC

Drug Information Center
St. Joseph Mercy Oakland
44405 Woodward Ave.
Pontiac, MI 48341
Mon.-Fri. 8 AM-4:30 PM
248-858-3055

ROYAL OAK

Drug Information Services
William Beaumont Hospital
3601 West 13 Mile Rd.
Royal Oak, MI 48073-6769
Mon.-Fri. 8 AM-4:30 PM
248-898-4077

SOUTHFIELD

Drug Information Service
Providence Hospital
16001 West 9 Mile Rd.
Southfield, MI 48075
Mon.-Fri. 8 AM-4 PM
248-849-3125

MISSISSIPPI

JACKSON

Drug Information Center
University of Mississippi Medical Center
2500 N. State St.
Jackson, MS 39216
Mon.-Fri. 8 AM-4:30 PM
601-984-2060

MISSOURI

KANSAS CITY

University of Missouri-Kansas City
Drug Information Center
2411 Holmes St., MG-200
Kansas City, MO 64108
Mon.-Fri. 8 AM-5 PM
816-235-5490
http://druginfo.umkc.edu/

SPRINGFIELD

Drug Information Center
St. John's Hospital
1235 E. Cherokee St.
Springfield, MO 65804
Mon.-Fri. 7:30 AM-4:30 PM
417-820-3488

ST. JOSEPH

Regional Medical Center Pharmacy
5325 Faraon St.
St. Joseph, MO 64506
7 days/week, 24 hours
816-271-6141

MONTANA

MISSOULA

Drug Information Service
University of Montana School of Pharmacy and Allied Health Sciences
32 Campus Dr.
Skaggs Bldg. 217
Missoula, MT 59812-1522
Mon.-Fri. 8 AM-5 PM
406-243-5254
800-501-5491
www.umt.edu/druginfo

NEBRASKA

OMAHA

Drug Informatics Service
School of Pharmacy
Creighton University
2500 California Plaza
Omaha, NE 68178
Mon.-Fri. 8:30 AM-4:30 PM
402-280-5101
http://pharmacy.creighton.edu

NEW JERSEY

NEWARK

New Jersey Poison Information and Education System
65 Bergen St.
Newark, NJ 07107
Mon.-Fri. 8:30 AM- 5 PM
973-972-9280
800-222-1222 (**Emergency**)
www.njpies.org

NEW BRUNSWICK

Drug Information Service
Robert Wood Johnson University Hospital
Pharmacy Department
1 Robert Wood Johnson Pl.
New Brunswick, NJ 08901
Mon.-Fri. 8:30 AM-4:30 PM
732-937-8842

NEW MEXICO

ALBUQUERQUE

New Mexico Poison Center
University of New Mexico Health Sciences Center
MSC09 5080
1 University of New Mexico
Albuquerque, NM 87131
7 days/week, 24 hours
505-272-4261
800-222-1222 (**Emergency**)
http://hsc.unm.edu/pharmacy/poison

NEW YORK

BROOKLYN

International Drug Information Center
Long Island University
Arnold & Marie Schwartz College of Pharmacy & Health Sciences
1 University Plaza
RM-HS509
Brooklyn, NY 11201
Mon.-Fri. 9 AM-5 PM
718-780-4184
www.liu.edu

COOPERSTOWN

Drug Information Center
Bassett Healthcare
1 Atwell Rd.
Cooperstown, NY 13326
7 days/week, 24 hours
607-547-3686

NEW HYDE PARK

Drug Information Center
St. John's University at Long Island Jewish Medical Center
270-05 76th Ave.
New Hyde Park, NY 11040
Mon.-Fri. 8 AM-3 PM
718-470-DRUG (3784)

NEW YORK CITY

Drug Information Center
Memorial Sloan-Kettering Cancer Center
1275 York Ave.
RM S-712
New York, NY 10021
Mon.-Fri. 9 AM-5 PM
212-639-7552

Drug Information Center
Mount Sinai Medical Center
1 Gustave Levy Pl.
New York, NY 10029
Mon.-Fri. 9 AM-5 PM
212-241-6619

Drug Information Service
New York Presbyterian Hospital
Room K04
525 E. 68th St.
New York, NY 10021
Mon.-Fri. 9 AM-5 PM
212-746-0741

ROCHESTER

Finger Lakes Poison and Drug Information Center
University of Rochester
601 Elmwood Ave.
Rochester, NY 14642
Mon.-Fri. 8 AM-5 PM
585-275-3718

ROCKVILLE CENTER

Drug Information Center
Mercy Medical Center
1000 North Village Ave.
Rockville Center, NY 11571-9024
Mon.-Fri. 8 AM-4 PM
516-705-1053

NORTH CAROLINA

BUIES CREEK

Drug Information Center
School of Pharmacy
Campbell University
P.O. Box 1090
Buies Creek, NC 27506
Mon.-Fri. 8:30 AM-4:30 PM
910-893-1200
x2701
800-760-9697 (Toll free)
x2701
800-327-5467 (NC only)

CHAPEL HILL

University of North Carolina Hospitals
Drug Information Center
Dept. of Pharmacy
101 Manning Dr.
Chapel Hill, NC 27514
Mon.-Fri. 8 AM-4:30 PM
919-966-2373

DURHAM

Drug Information Center
Duke University Health Systems
DUMC Box 3089
Durham, NC 27710
Mon.-Fri. 8 AM-5 PM
919-684-5125

GREENVILLE

Eastern Carolina Drug Information Center
Pitt County Memorial Hospital
Dept. of Pharmacy Service
P.O. Box 6028
2100 Stantonsburg Rd.
Greenville, NC 27835
Mon.-Fri. 8 AM-5 PM
252-847-4257

WINSTON-SALEM

Drug Information Service Center
Wake-Forest University Baptist Medical Center
Medical Center Blvd.
Winston-Salem, NC 27157
Mon.-Fri. 8 AM-5 PM
336-716-2037
(**for healthcare professionals only**)

OHIO

ADA

Drug Information Center
Raabe College of Pharmacy
Ohio Northern University
Ada, OH 45810
Mon.-Thurs. 8:30 AM-5 PM,
7-10 PM
Fri. 8:30 AM- 5 PM;
Sun. 2 PM-10 PM
419-772-2307
www.onu.edu/pharmacy/druginfo

CINCINNATI

Drug and Poison Information Center
Children's Hospital Medical Center
3333 Burnet Ave. ML9004
Cincinnati, OH 45229
Mon.-Fri. 9 AM-5 PM
513-636-5054
(Administration)
513-636-5111
(7 days/week, 24 hours)

CLEVELAND

Drug Information Service
Cleveland Clinic Foundation
9500 Euclid Ave.
Cleveland, OH 44195
Mon.-Fri. 8:30 AM-4:30 PM
216-444-6456
(for healthcare professionals only)

COLUMBUS

Drug Information Center
Ohio State University Hospital
Dept. of Pharmacy
Doan Hall 368
410 W. 10th Ave.
Columbus, OH 43210-1228
7 days/week, 24 hours
614-293-8679

Drug Information Center
Riverside Methodist Hospital
3535 Olentangy River Road
Columbus, OH 43214
Mon.-Fri. 8:30 AM-4 PM
614-566-5425

TOLEDO

Drug Information Services
St. Vincent Mercy Medical Center
2213 Cherry St.
Toledo, Ohio 43608-2691
Mon.-Fri. 8 AM-4 PM
419-251-4227
www.rx.medctr.ohio-state.edu

OKLAHOMA

OKLAHOMA CITY

Drug Information Service
Integris Health
3300 Northwest Expressway
Oklahoma City, OK 73112
Mon.-Fri. 8 AM-4:30 PM
405-949-3660

Drug Information Center
OU Medical Center
Presbyterian Tower
700 NE 13th St.
Oklahoma City, OK 73104
Mon.-Fri. 8 AM-4:30 PM
405-271-6226
Fax: 405-271-6281

TULSA

Drug Information Center
Saint Francis Hospital
6161 S. Yale Ave.
Tulsa, OK 74136
Mon.-Fri. 8 AM-4:30 PM
918-494-6339
(for healthcare professionals only)

PENNSYLVANIA

PHILADELPHIA

Drug Information Center
Temple University Hospital
Dept. of Pharmacy
3401 N. Broad St.
Philadelphia, PA 19140
Mon.-Fri. 8 AM-4:30 PM
215-707-4644

Drug Information Service
Tenet Health System
Hahnemann University Hospital
Department of Pharmacy
MS 451
Broad and Vine Streets
Philadelphia, PA 19102
Mon.-Fri. 8 AM-4 PM
215-762-DRUG (3784)
(for healthcare professionals only)

Drug Information Service
Dept. of Pharmacy
Thomas Jefferson University Hospital
111 S. 11th St.
Philadelphia, PA 19107-5089
Mon.-Fri. 8 AM-5 PM
215-955-8877

University of Pennsylvania Health System Drug Information Service
Hospital of the University of Pennsylvania
Department of Pharmacy
3400 Spruce St.
Philadelphia, PA 19104
Mon.-Fri. 8:30 AM-4 PM
215-662-2903

PITTSBURGH

Pharmaceutical Information Center
Mylan School of Pharmacy
Duquesne University
431 Mellon Hall
Pittsburgh, PA 15282
Mon.-Fri. 8 AM-4 PM
412-396-4600

Drug Information Center
University of Pittsburgh
302 Scaife Hall
200 Lothrop St.
Pittsburgh, PA 15213
Mon.-Fri. 9 AM-3 PM
412-647-3784
(for healthcare professionals only)

UPLAND

Drug Information Center
Crozer-Chester Medical Center
Dept. of Pharmacy
1 Medical Center Blvd.
Upland, PA 19013
Mon.-Fri. 8 AM-4:30 PM
610-447-2851
(for in-house healthcare professionals only)

PUERTO RICO

PONCE

Centro Informacion Medicamentos
Escuela de Medicina de Ponce
P.O. Box 7004
Ponce, PR 00732-7004
Mon.-Fri. 8 AM-4:30 PM
787-840-2575

SAN JUAN

Centro de Informacion de Medicamentos-CIM
Escuela de Farmacia-RCM
P.O. Box 365067
San Juan, PR 00936-5067
Mon.-Fri. 8 AM-4:30 PM
787-758-2525, ext. 1516

SOUTH CAROLINA

CHARLESTON

Drug Information Service
Medical University of South Carolina
150 Ashley Ave.
Rutledge Tower Annex
Room 604
P.O. Box 250584
Charleston, SC 29425-0810
Mon.-Fri. 9 AM-5:30 PM
843-792-3896
800-922-5250

COLUMBIA

Drug Information Service
University of South Carolina
College of Pharmacy
Columbia, SC 29208
Mon.-Fri. 8 AM-Midnight
803-777-7804
www.pharm.sc.edu

SPARTANBURG

Drug Information Center
Spartanburg Regional Healthcare System
101 E. Wood St.
Spartanburg, SC 29303
Mon.-Fri. 8 AM-4:30 PM
864-560-6910

TENNESSEE

KNOXVILLE

Drug Information Center
University of Tennessee Medical Center at Knoxville
1924 Alcoa Highway
Knoxville, TN 37920-6999
Mon.-Fri. 8 AM-4:30 PM
865-544-9124

MEMPHIS

South East Regional Drug Information Center
VA Medical Center
1030 Jefferson Ave.
Memphis, TN 38104
Mon.-Fri. 6:30 AM-4 PM
901-523-8990, ext. 6720

Drug Information Center
University of Tennessee
875 Monroe Ave.
Suite 116
Memphis, TN 38163
Mon.-Fri. 8 AM-5 PM
901-448-5556

TEXAS

AMARILLO

Drug Information Center
Texas Tech Health Sciences Center
1300 Coulter Rd.
Amarillo, TX 79106
Mon.-Fri. 8 AM-5 PM
806-356-4008
(for healthcare professionals only)

GALVESTON

Drug Information Center
University of Texas Medical Branch
301 University Blvd.
Galveston, TX 77555-0701
Mon.-Fri. 8 AM-5 PM
409-772-2734

HOUSTON

Drug Information Center
Ben Taub General Hospital
Texas Southern University/HCHD
1504 Taub Loop
Houston, TX 77030
Mon.-Fri. 9 AM-5 PM
713-873-3710

LACKLAND A.F.B.

Drug Information Center
Dept. of Pharmacy
Wilford Hall Medical Center
2200 Bergquist Dr.
Suite 1
Lackland A.F.B., TX 78236
7 days/week, 24 hours
210-292-5414

LUBBOCK

Drug Information and Consultation Service
Covenant Medical Center
3615 19th St.
Lubbock, TX 79410
Mon.-Fri. 8 AM-5 PM
806-725-0408

SAN ANTONIO

Drug Information Service
University of Texas
Health Science Center
at San Antonio
Department of Pharmacology
7703 Floyd Curl Drive
San Antonio, TX 78229-3900
Mon.-Fri. 8 AM-4 PM
210-567-4280

TEMPLE

Drug Information Center
Scott and White
Memorial Hospital
2401 S. 31st St.
Temple, TX 76508
Mon.-Fri. 8 AM-6 PM
254-724-4636

UTAH

SALT LAKE CITY

Drug Information Service
University of Utah Hospital
421 Wakara Way
Suite 204
Salt Lake City, UT 84108
Mon.-Fri. 8:30 AM-4:30 PM
801-581-2073

VIRGINIA

HAMPTON

Drug Information Center
Hampton University School
of Pharmacy
Kittrell Hall Room 208
Hampton, VA 23668
Mon.-Fri. 9 AM-4 PM
757-728-6693

WEST VIRGINIA

MORGANTOWN

West Virginia Center for
Drug and Health Information
West Virginia University
Robert C. Byrd
Health Sciences Center
1124 HSN, P.O. Box 9550
Morgantown, WV 26506
Mon.-Fri. 8:30 AM-5 PM
304-293-6640
800-352-2501 (WV)
www.hsc.wvu.edu/SOP

WYOMING

LARAMIE

Drug Information Center
University of Wyoming
P.O. Box 3375
Laramie, WY 82071
Mon.-Fri. 8:30 AM-4:30 PM
307-766-6988

U.S. Department of Health and Human Services

Form Approved: OMB No. 0910-0291, Expires: 03/31/05
See OMB statement on reverse.

MEDWATCH

For VOLUNTARY reporting of adverse events and product problems

The FDA Safety Information and Adverse Event Reporting Program

Page ____ of ____

FDA USE ONLY

Triage unit sequence #

A. PATIENT INFORMATION

1. **Patient Identifier** — In confidence
2. **Age at Time of Event:** or ______ **Date of Birth:**
3. **Sex** — ☐ Female ☐ Male
4. **Weight** — ____ lbs or ____ kgs

B. ADVERSE EVENT OR PRODUCT PROBLEM

1. ☐ **Adverse Event** and/or ☐ **Product Problem** *(e.g., defects/malfunctions)*
2. **Outcomes Attributed to Adverse Event** *(Check all that apply)*
   - ☐ Death: ____________ *(mo/day/yr)*
   - ☐ Life-threatening
   - ☐ Hospitalization - initial or prolonged
   - ☐ Disability
   - ☐ Congenital Anomaly
   - ☐ Required Intervention to Prevent Permanent Impairment/Damage
   - ☐ Other: ____________
3. **Date of Event** *(mo/day/year)*
4. **Date of This Report** *(mo/day/year)*
5. **Describe Event or Problem**
6. **Relevant Tests/Laboratory Data, Including Dates**
7. **Other Relevant History, Including Preexisting Medical Conditions** *(e.g., allergies, race, pregnancy, smoking and alcohol use, hepatic/renal dysfunction, etc.)*

PLEASE TYPE OR USE BLACK INK

C. SUSPECT MEDICATION(S)

1. **Name** *(Give labeled strength & mfr/labeler, if known)*
   #1
   #2
2. **Dose, Frequency & Route Used**
   #1
   #2
3. **Therapy Dates** *(If unknown, give duration) from/to (or best estimate)*
   #1
   #2
4. **Diagnosis for Use** *(Indication)*
   #1
   #2
5. **Event Abated After Use Stopped or Dose Reduced?**
   #1 ☐ Yes ☐ No ☐ Doesn't Apply
   #2 ☐ Yes ☐ No ☐ Doesn't Apply
6. **Lot #** *(if known)*
   #1
   #2
7. **Exp. Date** *(if known)*
   #1
   #2
8. **Event Reappeared After Reintroduction?**
   #1 ☐ Yes ☐ No ☐ Doesn't Apply
   #2 ☐ Yes ☐ No ☐ Doesn't Apply
9. **NDC#** *(For product problems only)*
   – –
10. **Concomitant Medical Products and Therapy Dates** *(Exclude treatment of event)*

D. SUSPECT MEDICAL DEVICE

1. **Brand Name**
2. **Type of Device**
3. **Manufacturer Name, City and State**
4. **Model #** — **Lot #**
   Catalog # — **Expiration Date** *(mo/day/yr)*
   Serial # — **Other #**
5. **Operator of Device**
   ☐ Health Professional
   ☐ Lay User/Patient
   ☐ Other: ____________
6. **If Implanted, Give Date** *(mo/day/yr)*
7. **If Explanted, Give Date** *(mo/day/yr)*
8. **Is this a Single-use Device that was Reprocessed and Reused on a Patient?**
   ☐ Yes ☐ No
9. **If Yes to Item No. 8, Enter Name and Address of Reprocessor**
10. **Device Available for Evaluation?** *(Do not send to FDA)*
    ☐ Yes ☐ No ☐ Returned to Manufacturer on: ____________ *(mo/day/yr)*
11. **Concomitant Medical Products and Therapy Dates** *(Exclude treatment of event)*

E. REPORTER *(See confidentiality section on back)*

1. **Name and Address** — **Phone #**
2. **Health Professional?** ☐ Yes ☐ No
3. **Occupation**
4. **Also Reported to:**
   ☐ Manufacturer
   ☐ User Facility
   ☐ Distributor/Importer
5. **If you do NOT want your identity disclosed to the manufacturer, place an "X" in this box:** ☐

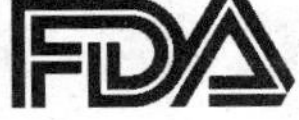

Mail to: **MEDWATCH**
5600 Fishers Lane
Rockville, MD 20852-9787

-or-

FAX to:
1-800-FDA-0178

FORM FDA 3500 (12/03) **Submission of a report does not constitute an admission that medical personnel or the product caused or contributed to the event.**

ADVICE ABOUT VOLUNTARY REPORTING

Report adverse experiences with:

- Medications *(drugs or biologics)*
- Medical devices *(including in-vitro diagnostics)*
- Special nutritional products *(dietary supplements, medical foods, infant formulas)*
- Cosmetics
- Medication errors

Report product problems - quality, performance or safety concerns such as:

- Suspected counterfeit product
- Suspected contamination
- Questionable stability
- Defective components
- Poor packaging or labeling
- Therapeutic failures

Report SERIOUS adverse events. An event is serious when the patient outcome is:

- Death
- Life-threatening *(real risk of dying)*
- Hospitalization *(initial or prolonged)*
- Disability *(significant, persistent or permanent)*
- Congenital anomaly
- Required intervention to prevent permanent impairment or damage

-Fold Here-

Report even if:

- You're not certain the product caused the event
- You don't have all the details

How to report:

- Just fill in the sections that apply to your report
- Use section C for all products except medical devices
- Attach additional blank pages if needed
- Use a separate form for each patient
- Report either to FDA or the manufacturer *(or both)*

Confidentiality: The patient's identity is held in strict confidence by FDA and protected to the fullest extent of the law. FDA will not disclose the reporter's identity in response to a request from the public, pursuant to the Freedom of Information Act. The reporter's identity, including the identity of a self-reporter, may be shared with the manufacturer unless requested otherwise.

If your report involves a serious adverse event with a device and it occurred in a facility outside a doctor's office, that facility may be legally required to report to FDA and/or the manufacturer. Please notify the person in that facility who would handle such reporting.

-Fold Here-

Important numbers:

- 1-800-FDA-0178 -- To FAX report
- 1-800-FDA-1088 -- To report by phone or for more information
- 1-800-822-7967 -- For a VAERS form for vaccines

To Report via the Internet:

http://www.fda.gov/medwatch/report.htm

The public reporting burden for this collection of information has been estimated to average 30 minutes per response, including the time for reviewing instructions, searching existing data sources, gathering and maintaining the data needed, and completing and reviewing the collection of information. Send comments regarding this burden estimate or any other aspect of this collection of information, including suggestions for reducing this burden to:

Department of Health and Human Services
Food and Drug Administration
MedWatch; HFD-410
5600 Fishers Lane
Rockville, MD 20857

Please DO NOT RETURN this form to this address.

OMB statement:
"An agency may not conduct or sponsor, and a person is not required to respond to, a collection of information unless it displays a currently valid OMB control number."

U.S. DEPARTMENT OF HEALTH AND HUMAN SERVICES
Food and Drug Administration

Please Use Address Provided Below -- Fold in Thirds, Tape and Mail